Fetal and Neonatal Physiology

Sixth Edition

Fetal and Neonatal Physiology

Richard A. Polin, MD
William T. Speck Professor of Pediatrics
College of Physicians and Surgeons
Columbia University
Executive Vice-Chair
Department of Pediatrics
Morgan Stanley Children's Hospital of New York–Presbyterian
Columbia University Irving Medical Center
New York, New York

Steven H. Abman, MD
Professor, Department of Pediatrics
Director, Pediatric Heart Lung Center
University of Colorado School of Medicine and Children's Hospital Colorado
Aurora, Colorado

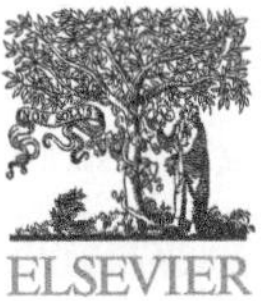

David H. Rowitch, MD ScD FMedSci FRS
Professor and Head
Department of Paediatrics
Wellcome Trust—Medical Research Council Stem Cell Institute
University of Cambridge
Cambridge, United Kingdom
Adjunct Professor
Department of Pediatrics
University of California, San Francisco
San Francisco, California

William E. Benitz, MD
Philip Sunshine Professor in Neonatology Emeritus
Division of Neonatal and Developmental Medicine
Stanford University School of Medicine
Stanford, California

William W. Fox, MD
Editor Emeritus
Perelman School of Medicine, The University of Pennsylvania

Elsevier
1600 John F. Kennedy Blvd.
Ste. 1800
Philadelphia, PA 19103-2899

FETAL AND NEONATAL PHYSIOLOGY: SIXTH EDITION

ISBN-13: 978-0-323-71284-2
Vol 1: 978-0-323-82555-9
Vol 2: 978-0-323-82556-6

Notice

Practitioners and researchers must always rely on their own experience and knowledge in evaluating and using any information, methods, compounds, or experiments described herein. Because of rapid advances in the medical sciences in particular, independent verification of diagnoses and drug dosages should be made. To the fullest extent of the law, no responsibility is assumed by Elsevier, authors, editors, or contributors for any injury and/or damage to persons or property as a matter of products liability, negligence or otherwise, or from any use or operation of any methods, products, instructions, or ideas contained in the material herein.

Library of Congress Control Number: 2021940940

Publisher: Sarah Barth
Senior Content Development Specialist: Mary Hegeler
Publishing Services Manager: Catherine Albright Jackson
Senior Project Manager: Doug Turner
Designer: Brian Salisbury

Printed in the United States of America

Last digit is the print number: 9 8 7 6 5 4 3 2

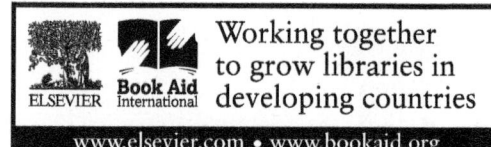

DEDICATED TO

Our spouses –
Helene Polin, Carolyn Abman, Risa Sorkin, and Andrea Benitz

Our children –
Allison Polin Steinbrenner, Mitchell Polin, Jessica Moseley, and Gregory Polin
Ryan Abman, Lauren Abman, Mark Abman, and Megan Abman
Sophie Rowitch
Lindsey Benitz, Maija Benitz, and Annika Benitz Chaloff

And our grandchildren –
Lindsey Steinbrenner, Eli Steinbrenner, Willa Polin, Jasper Polin, Elliot Polin, Lily Polin, Casey Moseley, Smith Moseley, Calla Moseley, Winslow Broderick, Mieke Broderick, Isla Abman, and Alina Abman

Contributors

Soraya Abbasi, MD
Professor
Department of Pediatrics
Perelman School of Medicine
University of Pennsylvania
Philadelphia, Pennsylvania
Evaluation of Pulmonary Function in the Neonate

Yalda Afshar, MD, PhD
Assistant Professor
Department of Obstetrics and Gynecology
Division of Maternal Fetal Medicine
David Geffen School of Medicine
University of California, Los Angeles
Los Angeles, California
Angiogenesis

Sun-Young Ahn, MD
Associate Professor
Pediatric Nephrology
Children's National Hospital
The George Washington University
Washington, District of Columbia
Organic Anion Transport in the Developing Kidney

Kurt H. Albertine, PhD
Professor
Edward B. Clark Endowed Chair IV in Pediatrics
Department of Pediatrics
University of Utah Health
Editor-in-Chief, *The Anatomical Record*
Salt Lake City, Utah
Impaired Lung Growth After Injury in Preterm Lung

Karel Allegaert, MD, PhD
Professor
Department of Development and Regeneration
Department of Pharmaceutical and Pharmacological Sciences
KU Leuven
Leuven, Belgium
Department of Clinical Pharmacy
Erasmus Medical Center
Rotterdam, The Netherlands
The Physiology of Placental Drug Disposition

Seth L. Alper, MD, PhD
Professor of Medicine
Harvard Medical School
Division of Nephrology and Vascular Biology Research Center
Beth Israel Deaconess Medical Center
Boston, Massachusetts
Urinary Acidification

Gabriel Altit, MDCM, MSc
Assistant Professor
Department of Pediatrics
McGill University
Neonatologist
Division of Neonatology
Montreal Children's Hospital
Montreal, Quebec, Canada
Basic Pharmacologic Principles

Ruben E. Alvaro, MD
Medical Director of Neonatology
St Boniface Hospital
Associate Professor
Department of Pediatrics
University of Manitoba
Winnipeg, Manitoba, Canada
Control of Breathing in Fetal Life and Onset and Control of Breathing in the Neonate

Cristina M. Alvira, MD
Associate Professor of Pediatrics
Division of Critical Care Medicine
Stanford University School of Medicine
Stanford, California
Developmental Biology of the Pulmonary Vasculature

Natália Carlos Maia Amorim, MS
Master in Nutrition
Postgraduate Program in Nutrition
Nutritionist of University Hospital Ana Bezerra-Federal University of Rio Grande do Norte
Santa Cruz, Brazil
Vitamin E Nutrition in Pregnancy and the Newborn Infant

Kelsey L. Anbuhl, PhD
Postdoctoral Fellow
Center for Neural Science
New York University
New York, New York
Early Development of the Human Auditory System

Claus Yding Andersen, MSc, DMSc
Professor
Laboratory of Reproductive Biology
University Hospital of Copenhagen
Copenhagen, Denmark
Differentiation of the Ovary

Richard A. Anderson, MD, PhD
Professor
MRC Centre for Reproductive Health
University of Edinburgh
Edinburgh, United Kingdom
Differentiation of the Ovary

Katrina A. Andrews, MB BChir
Department of Clinical Genetics
Cambridge University Hospitals NHS Foundation Trust
Department of Medical Genetics
University of Cambridge and NIHR Cambridge Biomedical Research Centre
Cancer Research UK Cambridge Centre
Cambridge Biomedical Campus
Cambridge, United Kingdom
Pathophysiology of Genetic Neonatal Disease

David J. Askenazi, MD, MSPH
Professor
Director, Pediatric and Infant Center for Acute Nephrology
Department of Pediatrics
Division of Nephrology
University of Alabama Birmingham
Birmingham, Alabama
Pathophysiology of Neonatal Acute Kidney Injury

Débora Gabriela Fernandes Assunção, MD
Nutritionist
Specialist in Neonate Intensive Care
Postgraduate Program in Nutrition
Federal University of Rio Grande do Norte
Natal, Brazil
Vitamin E Nutrition in Pregnancy and the Newborn Infant

Richard Lambert Auten Jr., MD
Professor
Department of Pediatrics (Neonatology)
Cone Health System
Greensboro, North Carolina
Mechanisms of Neonatal Lung Injury

Julie Autmizguine, MD, MHS
Associate Professor
Departments of Pharmacology and Pediatrics
University of Montreal
Infectious Disease Pediatrician
Department of Pediatrics
CHU Sainte-Justine
Montreal, Quebec, Canada
Basic Pharmacologic Principles

Timur Azhibekov, MD, MS CBTI
Assistant Professor
Department of Pediatrics
Case Western Reserve University School of Medicine
Department of Pediatrics
MetroHealth Medical Center
Cleveland, Ohio
Regulation of Acid-Base Balance in the Fetus and Neonate

Stephen A. Back, MD, PhD
Clyde and Elda Munson Professor of Pediatric Research
Department of Pediatrics
Oregon Health & Science University
Portland, Oregon
Pathophysiology of Neonatal White Matter Injury

Timothy M. Bahr, MD
Department of Pediatrics-Neonatology
University of Utah Health
Salt Lake City, Utah
Developmental Erythropoiesis

Peter Russell Baker II, MD
Associate Professor
Department of Pediatrics
Section of Clinical Genetics and Metabolism
University of Colorado School of Medicine
Aurora, Colorado
Fetal Origins of Adult Disease:A Classic Hypothesis With New Relevance

Eduardo H. Bancalari, MD
Professor
Department of Pediatrics—Neonatology
University of Miami Miller School of Medicine
Miami, Florida
Pathophysiology of Bronchopulmonary Dysplasia

Tatiana Barichello, PhD
Assistant Professor
Department of Psychiatric and Behavioral Sciences
The University of Texas Health Science Center at Houston
McGovern Medical School
Houston, Texas
Professor
Laboratory of Experimental Pathophysiology
Graduate Program in Health Sciences
University of Southern Santa Catarina
Criciúma, Brazil
Pathophysiology of Neonatal Acute Bacterial Meningitis

Frederick C. Battaglia, MD
Professor Emeritus
Department of Pediatrics
University of Colorado School of Medicine
Aurora, Colorado
Placental and Fetal Circulatory and Metabolic Changes Accompanying Fetal Growth Restriction

Andrew J. Bauer, MD
Director, The Thyroid Center
Division of Endocrinology and Diabetes
Children's Hospital of Philadelphia
Professor
Department of Pediatrics
Perelman School of Medicine
University of Pennsylvania
Philadelphia, Pennsylvania
Fetal and Neonatal Thyroid Physiology

Michel Baum, MD
Professor of Pediatrics and Internal Medicine
Sarah M. and Charles E. Seay Chair in Pediatric Research
UT Southwestern Medical Center
Dallas, Texas
Renal Transport of Sodium During Development

Ryan W. Bavis, PhD
Helen A. Papaioanou Professor of Biological Sciences
Department of Biology
Bates College
Lewiston, Maine
Pathophysiology of Apnea of Prematurity

Kathryn Beardsall, BSc, MBBS, MD
Lecturer
Department of Paediatrics
University of Cambridge
Physician
Department of Neonatology
Cambridge University Hospitals NHS Trust
Cambridge, United Kingdom
Role of Glucoregulatory Hormones in Hepatic Glucose Metabolism During the Perinatal Period

Simon Beggs, PhD
Associate Professor
UCL Great Ormond Street Institute of Child Health
London, United Kingdom
Developmental Aspects of Pain

Corinne Benchimol, DO
Assistant Professor
Department of Pediatrics
Mount Sinai Hospital
New York, New York
Potassium Homeostasis in the Fetus and Neonate

Manon J.N.L. Benders, MD, PhD
Professor
Department of Neonatology
University Medical Center Utrecht
Utrecht, The Netherlands
Cerebellar Development—The Impact of Preterm Birth and Comorbidities

Laura Bennet, PhD
Professor
Department of Physiology
The University of Auckland
Auckland, New Zealand
Neuroprotective Therapeutic Hypothermia

Phillip R. Bennett, MD, PhD
Clinical Professor
Faculty of Medicine
Department of Metabolism, Digestion, and Reproduction
Institute of Reproductive and Developmental Biology
Imperial College Parturition Research Group
Researcher
March of Dimes Prematurity Research Centre
Imperial College London
London, United Kingdom
Pathophysiology of Preterm Birth

Melvin Berger, MD, PhD
Adjunct Professor
Pediatrics and Pathology
Case Western Reserve University School of Medicine
Cleveland, Ohio
The Complement System of the Fetus and Newborn

Wolfgang Bernhard, MD
Professor
Department of Neonatology
Children's Hospital
Eberhard-Karls-University
Tübingen, Germany
Regulation of Surfactant-Associated Phospholipid Synthesis and Secretion

John F. Bertram, BSc, PhD, DSc
Head, Anatomy and Developmental Biology
Professor
Biomedicine Discovery Institute
Monash University
Melbourne, Victoria, Australia
Development of the Kidney: Morphology and Mechanisms

Shazia Bhombal, MD
Clinical Associate Professor of Pediatrics
Division of Neonatal and Developmental Medicine
Stanford University School of Medicine
Stanford, California
Developmental Biology of the Pulmonary Vasculature

Vinod K. Bhutani, MD
Professor
Department of Pediatrics
Lucile Packard Children's Hospital at Stanford
Stanford, California
Mechanistic Aspects of Phototherapy for Neonatal Hyperbilirubinemia

Mary Jane Black, BSc (Hons), PhD
Associate Professor
Deputy Head
Department of Anatomy and Developmental Biology
Biomedicine Discovery Institute
Monash University
Melbourne, Victoria, Australia
Development of the Kidney: Morphology and Mechanisms

Joseph M. Bliss, MD, PhD
Associate Professor
Department of Pediatrics
Women & Infants Hospital of Rhode Island
Warren Alpert Medical School of Brown University
Providence, Rhode Island
Normal and Abnormal Neutrophil Physiology in the Newborn

David L. Bolender, PhD
Professor
Cell Biology, Neurobiology, and Anatomy
Medical College of Wisconsin
Milwaukee, Wisconsin
Basic Embryology

Sarah C. Bowdin, MD
Department of Clinical Genetics
Cambridge University Hospitals NHS Foundation Trust
Cambridge, United Kingdom
Pathophysiology of Genetic Neonatal Disease

Scott D. Boyd, MD, PhD
Associate Professor
Department of Pathology
Stanford University School of Medicine
Stanford, California
B-Cell Development

Joline E. Brandenburg, MD
Assistant Professor
Physical Medicine and Rehabilitation
Pediatrics and Adolescent Medicine
Mayo Clinic
Rochester, Minnesota
Functional Development of Respiratory Muscles

Laura D. Brown, MD
Associate Professor
Department of Pediatrics
University of Colorado School of Medicine
Aurora, Colorado
Placental Transfer and Fetal Requirements of Amino Acids

Douglas G. Burrin, PhD
Research Physiologist and Professor
USDA-ARS Children's Nutrition Research Center
Department of Pediatrics
Baylor College of Medicine
Houston, Texas
Trophic Factors and Regulation of Gastrointestinal Tract and Liver Development

Barbara Cannon, BSc, PhD
Professor
Department of Molecular Biosciences
The Wenner-Gren Institute
Stockholm University
Stockholm, Sweden
Brown Adipose Tissue: Development and Function

Michael Caplan, MD
Chairman
Department of Pediatrics
NorthShore University HealthSystem
Evanston, Illinois
Clinical Professor
Department of Pediatrics
University of Chicago Pritzker School of Medicine
Chicago, Illinois
Pathophysiology and Prevention of Neonatal Necrotizing Enterocolitis

Susan E. Carlson, PhD
A. J. Rice Professor of Nutrition and University Distinguished Professor
Department of Dietetics and Nutrition
University of Kansas
Kansas City, Kansas
Long-Chain Polyunsaturated Fatty Acids in Neurodevelopment

David P. Carlton, MD
Marcus Professor and Chief
Division of Neonatology
Emory University
Atlanta, Georgia
Regulation of Liquid Secretion and Absorption by the Fetal and Neonatal Lung
Pathophysiology of Edema

Piya Chaemsaithong, MD, PhD
Division of Maternal Fetal Medicine
Department of Obstetrics and Gynecology
Faculty of Medicine
Ramathibodi Hospital
Mahidol University
Bangkok, Thailand
Intra-Amniotic Infection/Inflammation and the Fetal Inflammatory Response Syndrome

Jill Chang, MD
Assistant Professor
Department of Pediatrics
Division of Neonatology
Northwestern University Feinberg School of Medicine
Chicago, Illinois
Placental Function in Intrauterine Growth Restriction

Jennifer R. Charlton, MD
Associate Professor
Department of Pediatrics
Division of Nephrology
University of Virginia Children's Hospital
Charlottesville, Virginia
Response to Nephron Loss in Early Development
Pathophysiology of Neonatal Acute Kidney Injury

Sylvain Chemtob, MD, PhD
Professor
Departments of Pediatrics and Pharmacology
CHU Ste-Justine and University of Montreal
Professor
Department of Ophthalmology
Hospital Maisonneuve Rosemont and University of Montreal
Montreal, Quebec, Canada
Basic Pharmacologic Principles

Sadhana Chheda, MBBS, DTMH
Assistant Professor
Department of Pediatrics
Texas Tech University Health Sciences Center–El Paso
El Paso, Texas
Immunology of Human Milk

Andrew J. Childs, BSc (Hons), MSc, PhD
Lecturer
Institute of Reproductive and Developmental Biology
Imperial College London
London, United Kingdom
Differentiation of the Ovary

David H. Chu, MD, PhD
Staff Physician
Division of Dermatology and Cutaneous Surgery
Scripps Clinic Medical Group
La Jolla, California
Structure and Development of the Skin and Cutaneous Appendages

Wendy K. Chung, MD, PhD
Kennedy Family Professor of Pediatrics and Medicine
Department of Pediatrics
Division of Molecular Genetics
Columbia University Irving Medical Center
New York, New York
Basic Genetic Principles

Maria Roberta Cilio, MD, PhD
Professor
Department of Pediatrics
Saint-Luc University Hospital
Université Catholique de Louvain
Brussels, Belgium
Electroencephalography in the Preterm and Term Infant

David A. Clark, MD
Chairman and Professor
Department of Pediatrics
Albany Medical College
Albany, New York
Development of the Gastrointestinal Circulation in the Fetus and Newborn

Paul Clarke, MD, DCH DCCH
Professor
Neonatal Intensive Care Unit
Norfolk and Norwich University Hospitals NHS Foundation Trust
Professor
Norwich Medical School
University of East Anglia
Norwich, United Kingdom
Vitamin K Metabolism in the Fetus and Neonate

Jane K. Cleal, PhD
Lecturer in Epigenetics
School of Human Development and Health
Faculty of Medicine
University of Southampton
Southampton, United Kingdom
Mechanisms of Transfer Across the Human Placenta

Ethel G. Clemente, MD
Assistant Professor
Department of Pediatrics
Western Michigan University Homer Stryker MD School of Medicine
Kalamazoo, Michigan
Luteinizing Hormone and Follicle-Stimulating Hormone Secretion in the Fetus and Newborn Infant

John A. Clements, MD
Professor Emeritus
Department of Pediatrics
University of California, San Francisco
San Francisco, California
Historical Perspective

Ronald I. Clyman, MD
Professor Emeritus
Department of Pediatrics
University of California, San Francisco
San Francisco, California
Mechanisms Regulating Closure of the Ductus Arteriosus

Jennifer L. Cohen, MD
Assistant Professor
Department of Pediatrics
Division of Medical Genetics Pediatrics
Duke University School of Medicine
Durham, North Carolina
Genetic Variants and Neonatal Disease

Susan S. Cohen, MD
Associate Professor
Department of Pediatrics
Medical College of Wisconsin
Milwaukee, Wisconsin
Development of the Blood-Brain Barrier

Amélie Collins, MD, PhD
Assistant Professor
Department of Pediatrics
Columbia University Irving Medical Center
New York, New York
Developmental Biology of Hematopoietic Stem Cells

Allan Collodel, PhD
Laboratory of Experimental Pathophysiology
Graduate Program in Health Sciences
University of Southern Santa Catarina
Criciúma, Brazil
Pathophysiology of Neonatal Acute Bacterial Meningitis

John Colombo, PhD
Professor
Department of Psychology
University of Kansas
Lawrence, Kansas
Long-Chain Polyunsaturated Fatty Acids in Neurodevelopment

Alexander N. Combes, PhD
Senior Research Fellow
Monash Biomedicine Discovery Institute
Department of Anatomy and Developmental Biology
Biomedicine Discovery Institute
Monash University
Melbourne, Victoria, Australia
Development of the Kidney: Morphology and Mechanisms

Andrew J. Copp, MBBS, DPhil
Professor
GOS Institute of Child Health
University College London
London, United Kingdom
Pathophysiology of Neural Tube Defects

C. Michael Cotten, MD
Professor
Chief, Division of Pediatric Neonatology
Department of Pediatrics
Duke University School of Medicine
Durham, North Carolina
Genetic Variants and Neonatal Disease

Peter A. Crawford, MD, PhD
Professor
Vice Chair for Research
Department of Medicine
Director, Division of Molecular Medicine
University of Minnesota Medical School
Minneapolis, Minnesota
Ketone Body Metabolism in the Neonate

James E. Crowe, Jr., MD
Director
Vanderbilt Vaccine Center
Ann Scott Carell Chair
Pediatrics and Pathology, Microbiology and Immunology
Vanderbilt University Medical Center
Nashville, Tennessee
Host Defense Mechanisms Against Viruses

C.A. Crowther, MBChB, DCH, MD, CMFM
Professor
Liggins Institute
University of Auckland
Auckland, New Zealand
Antenatal Hormonal Therapy for Prevention of Respiratory Distress Syndrome

Luise A. Cullen-McEwen, BSc, PhD
Research Fellow
Department of Anatomy and Developmental Biology
Biomedicine Discovery Institute
Monash University
Melbourne, Victoria, Australia
Development of the Kidney: Morphology and Mechanisms

Wayne S. Cutfield, MD
Professor
Liggins Institute
University of Auckland
Auckland, New Zealand
Epigenetics

Chanèle Cyr-Depauw, MSc
PhD Candidate
Sinclair Centre for Regenerative Medicine
Ottawa Hospital Research Institute
Department of Cellular and Molecular Medicine
University of Ottawa
Ottawa, Ontario, Canada
Developmental Biology of Lung Stem Cells

Karla Danielly da S. Ribeiro, PhD
Nutritionist
Professor Adjunct
Department of Nutrition
Researcher
Postgraduate Program in Nutrition
Federal University of Rio Grande do Norte
Natal, Brazil
Vitamin E Nutrition in Pregnancy and the Newborn Infant

Nicolas Dauby, MD, PhD
Deputy Head of Clinic
Infectious Diseases
CHU Saint-Pierre
Post-Doctoral Researcher
Institute for Medical Immunology
Université Libre de Bruxelles
Brussels, Belgium
Host Defense Mechanisms Against Bacteria

Patricia Davenport, MD
Instructor of Pediatrics
Division of Newborn Medicine
Children's Hospital Boston and Harvard Medical School
Boston, Massachusetts
Developmental Megakaryopoiesis

Joanne O. Davidson, PhD
Senior Research Fellow
Department of Physiology
University of Auckland
Auckland, New Zealand
Neuroprotective Therapeutic Hypothermia

Diomel de la Cruz, MD
Assistant Professor
Department of Pediatrics
Division of Neonatology
University of Florida College of Medicine
Gainesville, Florida
Digestive-Absorptive Functions in Fetuses, Infants, and Children

Priscila Gomes de Oliveira, MD
Nutritionist
Specialist in Neonate Intensive Care
Postgraduate Program in Nutrition
Federal University of Rio Grande do Norte
Natal, Brazil
Vitamin E Nutrition in Pregnancy and the Newborn Infant

Barbra de Vrijer, MD
Associate Professor
Department of Obstetrics and Gynaecology
Western University
London, Ontario, Canada
Placental and Fetal Circulatory and Metabolic Changes Accompanying Fetal Growth Restriction

Andrew Del Colle, MS
Research Assistant
Department of Pediatrics
Columbia University Vagelos College of Physicians and Surgeons
New York, New York
Development of the Enteric Nervous System and Gastrointestinal Motility

Christophe Delacourt, MD, PhD
Physician
Department of Paediatric Pulmonology and Allergology
University Hospital Necker-Enfants Malades
Assistance Publique-Hôpitaux de Paris
Paris, France
Regulation of Alveolarization

Thomas G. Diacovo, MD
Professor
Department of Pediatrics
University of Pittsburgh School of Medicine
Chief, UMPC Division of Newborn Medicine
University of Pittsburgh Medical Center
Pittsburgh, Pennsylvania
Platelet–Vessel Wall Interactions

Clémence Disdier, PhD, PharmD
Postdoctoral Fellow
Department of Pediatrics
The Warren Alpert Medical School of Brown University
Providence, Rhode Island
Development of the Blood-Brain Barrier

John P. Dormans, MD
Chief, Pediatric Orthopedic Surgery
Riley Hospital for Children
Garceau Professor of Orthopedic Surgery
Indiana University School of Medicine
Indianapolis, Indiana
The Growth Plate: Embryologic Origin, Structure, and Function

François Duhamel, BPharm, MSc
PhD Candidate
Department of Pharmacology
University of Montreal
Montreal, Quebec, Canada
Basic Pharmacologic Principles

Minh Dien Duong, MD
Department of Pediatrics
Division of Nephrology
The Children's Hospital at Montefiore
Albert Einstein College of Medicine
Bronx, New York
Role of the Kidney in Calcium and Phosphorus Homeostasis

Kevin Dysart, MD
Associate Medical Director
Division of Neonatology
Children's Hospital of Philadelphia
Philadelphia, Pennsylvania
Evaluation of Pulmonary Function in the Neonate

Eric C. Eichenwald, MD
Professor of Pediatrics
Department of Pediatrics/Neonatology
Perelman School of Medicine
University of Pennsylvania
Chief, Division of Neonatology
Children's Hospital of Philadelphia
Philadelphia, Pennsylvania
Evaluation of Pulmonary Function in the Neonate

Afif F. El-Khuffash, MB, BCh, BAO, BA(Sci), MD, DCE
Consultant Neonatologist and Pediatrician
Department of Neonatology
The Rotunda Hospital
Clinical Professor
Department of Paediatrics
Royal College of Physicians in Ireland
Dublin, Ireland
Oxygen Transport and Delivery

Peter James Ivor Ellis, PhD
Senior Lecturer
School of Biosciences
University of Kent
Canterbury, United Kingdom
Genetics of Sex Determination and Differentiation

Kerry M. Empey, PharmD, PhD
Associate Professor
Department of Pharmacy and Therapeutics
Associate Professor (secondary appointment)
Clinical Translational Science Institute
Associate Professor (secondary appointment)
Department of Immunology
University of Pittsburgh
Pittsburgh, Pennsylvania
Neonatal Pulmonary Host Defense

Baris Ercal, MD, PhD
Instructor
Department of Psychiatry
Washington University School of Medicine
St. Louis, Missouri
Ketone Body Metabolism in the Neonate

Melinda Erdős, MD, PhD
Associate Professor
Primary Immunodeficiency Clinical Unit and Laboratory
Department of Dermatology, Venereology, and Dermatooncology
Faculty of Medicine
Semmelweis University
Budapest, Hungary
Host Defense Mechanisms Against Fungi
T-Cell Development

Mariella Errede, MD, PhD
Department of Basic Medical Sciences, Neurosciences, and Sensory Organs
Human Anatomy and Histology Unit
University of Bari School of Medicine
Bari, Italy
Development of the Blood-Brain Barrier

Brian J. Feldman, MD, PhD
Walter L. Miller Distinguished Professorship
Department of Pediatrics
University of California San Francisco
San Francisco, California
Development of the Hypothalamus-Pituitary-Adrenal Axis in the Fetus

Mario Fidanza, PhD
Postdoctoral Scientist
Systems Vaccinology
Telethon Kids Institute
Perth, Western Australia, Australia
Host Defense Mechanisms Against Bacteria

Matthew J. Fogarty, BVSc, PhD
Assistant Professor
Physiology and Biomedical Engineering
Mayo Clinic
Rochester, Minnesota
Functional Development of Respiratory Muscles

Philippe S. Friedlich, MD, MS Epi, MBA
Teresa and Byron Pollitt Family Chair in Fetal & Neonatal Medicine
Professor
Departments of Pediatrics and Surgery
Keck School of Medicine
University of Southern California
Co-Director, Fetal and Neonatal Institute
Children's Hospital Los Angeles
Chief, Division of Neonatology
Department of Pediatrics
Children's Hospital Los Angeles
Los Angeles, California
Regulation of Acid-Base Balance in the Fetus and Neonate
Pathophysiology of Shock in the Fetus and Neonate

Ryoichi Fujiwara, PhD
Assistant Professor
Department of Pharmaceutical Sciences
College of Pharmacy
University of Arkansas for Medical Sciences
Little Rock, Arkansas
Fetal and Neonatal Bilirubin Metabolism

Vittorio Gallo, PhD
Chief Research Officer
Center for Neuroscience Research
Children's National Research Institute and George Washington University School of Medicine and Health Sciences
Washington, District of Columbia
Cellular and Molecular Mechanisms of Neonatal Brain Injury and Neuroprotection

Abhrajit Ganguly, MD
Assistant Professor of Pediatrics
Section of Neonatal-Perinatal Medicine
Center for Pregnancy & Newborn Research
University of Oklahoma Health Science Center
Oklahoma City, Oklahoma
Regulation of Lower Airway Function

Yuansheng Gao, PhD
Professor
Department of Physiology and Pathophysiology
Peking University Health Science Center
Beijing, China
Regulation of Pulmonary Circulation

Marianne Garland, MB ChB
Associate Professor
Department of Pediatrics
Columbia University Vagelos College of Physicians and Surgeons
Attending Neonatologist
Department of Pediatrics
Children's Hospital of New York
New York, New York
Drug Distribution in Fetal Life

Donna Geddes, Post Grad Dip (Sci), PhD
Professor
School of Molecular Sciences
The University of Western Australia, Perth
Perth, Western Australia, Australia
Human Milk Composition and Function in the Infant

Michael K. Georgieff, MD
Professor
Department of Pediatrics
University of Minnesota Medical School
Minneapolis, Minnesota
Fetal and Neonatal Iron Metabolism

Jason Gien, MD
Associate Professor
Department of Pediatrics
Section of Neonatology
University of Colorado School of Medicine
Aurora, Colorado
Pathophysiology of Meconium Aspiration Syndrome

Dino A. Giussani, PhD, ScD
Professor
Department of Physiology Development and Neuroscience
Professorial Fellow
Gonville & Caius College
Cambridge, United Kingdom
Regulation of Cardiovascular Function During Fetal and Newborn Life

Armond S. Goldman, MD
Emeritus Professor
Department of Pediatrics
University of Texas Medical Branch
Galveston, Texas
Immunology of Human Milk

Nardhy Gomez-Lopez, PhD
Associate Professor
Division of Maternal-Fetal Medicine
Department of Obstetrics and Gynecology
Wayne State University School of Medicine
Detroit, Michigan
Intra-Amniotic Infection/Inflammation and the Fetal Inflammatory Response Syndrome

Misty Good, MD
Assistant Professor
Division of Newborn Medicine
Departments of Pediatrics, Pathology, and Immunology
Washington University School of Medicine
St. Louis, Missouri
Neonatal Pulmonary Host Defense
Pathophysiology and Prevention of Neonatal Necrotizing Enterocolitis

Pamela I. Good, MD
Instructor
Division of Neonatology-Perinatology
Department of Pediatrics
Columbia University Vagelos College of Physicians and Surgeons
New York, New York
Response to Nephron Loss in Early Development

Scott M. Gordon, MD, PhD
Attending Physician
Division of Neonatology
Children's Hospital of Philadelphia
Instructor
Perelman School of Medicine
University of Pennsylvania
Philadelphia, Pennsylvania
Cytokines and Inflammatory Response in the Fetus and Neonate

Lucy R. Green, BSc, PhD
Physician
Institute of Developmental Sciences
University of Southampton
Southampton, United Kingdom
Nutritional and Environmental Effects on the Fetal Circulation

Nicholas D.E. Greene, PhD
Professor
Great Ormond Street Institute of Child Health
University College London
London, United Kingdom
Pathophysiology of Neural Tube Defects

Zoya Gridneva, BSc, PhD
Research Associate
School of Molecular Sciences
The University of Western Australia, Crawley
Crawley, Western Australia, Australia
Human Milk Composition and Function in the Infant

Emmanouil Grigoriou, MD
Pediatric Orthopaedic Surgery
Texas Scottish Rite Hospital for Children
Dallas, Texas
The Growth Plate: Embryologic Origin, Structure, and Function

Adda Grimberg, MD
Professor
Department of Pediatrics
Perelman School of Medicine
University of Pennsylvania
Scientific Director
Diagnostic and Research Growth Center
Children's Hospital of Philadelphia
Philadelphia, Pennsylvania
Hypothalamus: Neuroendometabolic Center

Ruth E. Grunau, PhD
Professor
Department of Pediatrics
University of British Columbia
Vancouver, Canada
Developmental Aspects of Pain

Jean-Pierre Guignard, MD
Honorary Professor of Pediatric Nephrology
Lausanne University Medical School
Lausanne, Switzerland
Postnatal Development of Glomerular Filtration Rate in Neonates
Concentration and Dilution of Urine

Alistair J. Gunn, MBChB, PhD
Professor
Department of Physiology
University of Auckland
Auckland, New Zealand
Neuroprotective Therapeutic Hypothermia

Nursen Gurtunca, MD
Assistant Professor
Department of Pediatrics
Division of Endocrinology and Diabetes
Children's Hospital of Pittsburgh
Pittsburgh, Pennsylvania
Growth Hormone, Prolactin, and Placental Lactogen in the Fetus and Newborn

Kathleen M. Gustafson, PhD
Associate Professor
Department of Neurology
Hoglund Biomedical Imaging Center
University of Kansas Medical Center
Kansas City, Kansas
Long-Chain Polyunsaturated Fatty Acids in Neurodevelopment

Alice Hadchouel, MD, PhD
Physician
Department of Paediatric Pulmonology and Allergology
University Hospital Necker-Enfants Malades
Assistance Publique-Hôpitaux de Paris
Paris, France
Regulation of Alveolarization

Gabriel G. Haddad, MD
Professor
Department of Pediatrics
University of California, San Diego
La Jolla, California
Basic Mechanisms of Oxygen Sensing and Adaptation to Hypoxia

Thomas W. Hale, RPh, PhD
Professor
Associate Dean of Research
Texas Tech University Health Science Center
Department of Pediatrics
School of Medicine
Amarillo, Texas
Drug Transfer During Breastfeeding

K. Michael Hambidge, MD, ScD
Professor Emeritus
Department of Pediatrics
Section of Nutrition
University of Colorado School of Medicine
Aurora, Colorado
Zinc in the Fetus and Neonate

Cathy Hammerman, MD
Professor of Pediatrics
Faculty of Medicine
Hebrew University
Director, Newborn Nurseries Division
Neonatology
Shaare Zedek Medical Center
Jerusalem, Israel
Hereditary Contributions to Neonatal Hyperbilirubinemia

Thor Willy Ruud Hansen, MD, PhD, MHA
Professor Emeritus
Division of Pediatric and Adolescent Medicine
Oslo University Hospital and Institute of Clinical Medicine
Oslo, Norway
Pathophysiology of Kernicterus

Mark A. Hanson, MA, DPhil
Director
Institute of Developmental Sciences
University of Southampton
Southampton, United Kingdom
Nutritional and Environmental Effects on the Fetal Circulation

Danny Harbeson, PhD
Experimental Medicine
University of British Columbia
Vancouver, British Columbia, Canada
Host Defense Mechanisms Against Bacteria

J.E. Harding, MBChB, DPhil
Professor
Liggins Institute
University of Auckland
Auckland, New Zealand
Antenatal Hormonal Therapy for Prevention of Respiratory Distress Syndrome

Richard Harding, PhD, DSc
Emeritus Professor
Department of Anatomy and Developmental Biology
Monash University
Melbourne, Victoria, Australia
Physiologic Mechanisms of Normal and Altered Lung Growth Before and After Birth

Mary Catherine Harris, MD
Professor
Division of Neonatology
Department of Pediatrics
Children's Hospital of Philadelphia
Philadelphia, Pennsylvania
Cytokines and Inflammatory Response in the Fetus and Neonate

Peter Hartmann, BSc, PhD
Emeritus Professor
School of Molecular Sciences
The University of Western Australia, Perth
Perth, Western Australia, Australia
Human Milk Composition and Function in the Infant

M. Elizabeth Hartnett, MD
Distinguished Professor in Ophthalmology and Visual Sciences
Department of Ophthalmology
John A. Moran Eye Center
University of Utah Health
Salt Lake City, Utah
Pathophysiology of Retinopathy of Prematurity

Rodrigo Hasbun, MD, MPH
Professor
Division of Infectious Diseases
The University of Texas Health Science Center at Houston
McGovern Medical School
Houston, Texas
Pathophysiology of Neonatal Acute Bacterial Meningitis

Guttorm Haugen, MD
Consultant
Department of Fetal Medicine
Division of Obstetrics and Gynaecology
Oslo University Hospital
Professor
Institute of Clinical Medicine
Faculty of Medicine
University of Oslo
Oslo, Norway
Umbilical Circulation

Colin P. Hawkes, MD, PhD
Physician
Division of Endocrinology and Diabetes
Children's Hospital of Philadelphia
Adjunct Professor
Department of Pediatrics
Perelman School of Medicine
University of Pennsylvania
Philadelphia, Pennsylvania
Consultant Paediatric Endocrinologist
Department of Paediatrics and Child Health
University College Cork
Cork, Ireland
Growth Factor Regulation of Fetal Growth
Pathophysiology of Neonatal Hypoglycemia

William W. Hay, Jr., MD
Professor (Retired)
Department of Pediatrics
University of Colorado School of Medicine
Aurora, Colorado
Placental and Fetal Circulatory and Metabolic Changes Accompanying Fetal Growth Restriction
Placental Transfer and Fetal Requirements of Amino Acids

Vivi M. Heine, PhD
Assistant Professor
Pediatrics/Child Neurology
Vrije University Medical Center
Amsterdam, The Netherlands
Cerebellar Development—The Impact of Preterm Birth and Comorbidities

Michael A. Helmrath, MD
Professor
Division of Pediatric General and Thoracic Surgery
Cincinnati Children's Hospital Medical Center
Cincinnati, Ohio
Organogenesis of the Gastrointestinal Tract

Karen D. Hendricks-Muñoz, MD, MPH
William Tate Graham Professor
Chair, Neonatal Medicine
Department of Pediatrics
Virginia Commonwealth University School of Medicine
Richmond, Virginia
Structure and Development of Alveolar Epithelial Cells

Emilio Herrera, PhD
Emeritus Professor of Biochemistry and Molecular Biology
Department of Chemistry and Biochemistry
Faculties of Pharmacy and Medicine
University San Pablo-CEU
Madrid, Spain
Maternal-Fetal Transfer of Lipid Metabolites
Lipids as an Energy Source for the Premature and Term Neonate

Michael J. Hiatt, PhD
Senior Scientist Research and Development
Stemcell Technologies
Vancouver, British Columbia, Canada
Functional Development of the Kidney in Utero

Stuart B. Hooper, BSc (Hons), PhD
Professor
The Ritchie Centre
Hudson Institute for Medical Research
Professor
Department of Obstetrics and Gynaecology
Monash University
Melbourne, Victoria, Australia
Physiologic Mechanisms of Normal and Altered Lung Growth Before and After Birth
Physiology of Neonatal Resuscitation

Thomas A. Hooven, MD
Assistant Professor
Department of Pediatrics
University of Pittsburgh School of Medicine
Pittsburgh, Pennsylvania
Pathophysiology of Chorioamnionitis: Host Immunity and Microbial Virulence

Silvia Iacobelli, MD, PhD
Professor of Pediatrics
Réanimation Néonatale et Pédiatrique, Neonatologie
Centre Hospitalier Universitaire La Réunion
Saint Pierre, France
Centre d'Etudes Périnatales de l'Océan Indien
Université de la Réunion
Réunion, France
Postnatal Development of Glomerular Filtration Rate in Neonates
Concentration and Dilution of Urine

Terrie E. Inder, MBChB, MD
Chair
Pediatric Newborn Medicine
Brigham and Women's Hospital
Professor
Department of Pediatrics
Harvard Medical School
Boston, Massachusetts
Intraventricular Hemorrhage in the Neonate

M. Luisa Iruela-Arispe, PhD
Stephen Walter Ranson Professor and Chair
Department of Cell and Developmental Biology
Feinberg School of Medicine
Northwestern University
Chicago, Illinois
Angiogenesis

Sudarshan Rao Jadcherla, MD, DCH, AGAF
Professor
Department of Pediatrics
Sections of Neonatology and Pediatric Gastroenterology & Nutrition
The Ohio State University College of Medicine
Attending Neonatologist
Section of Neonatology
Director
Neonatal and Infant Feeding Disorders Program
Nationwide Children's Hospital
Principal Investigator
Center for Perinatal Research
Abigail Wexner Research Institute at Nationwide Children's Hospital
Columbus, Ohio
Pathophysiology of Gastroesophageal Reflux

Deepak Jain, MD
Associate Professor
Department of Pediatrics
Division of Neonatology
Rutgers Robert Wood Johnson Medical School
New Brunswick, New Jersey
Pathophysiology of Bronchopulmonary Dysplasia

Jennifer G. Jetton, MD
Medical Director, Pediatric Dialysis Unit
Clinical Associate Professor
Division of Nephrology
Stead Family Department of Pediatrics
University of Iowa Health Care
Iowa City, Iowa
Pathophysiology of Neonatal Acute Kidney Injury

Alan H. Jobe, MD, PhD
Professor
Department of Pediatrics
Director, Division of Perinatal Biology
Cincinnati Children's Hospital Medical Center
Cincinnati, Ohio
Antenatal Factors That Influence Postnatal Lung Development and Injury
Surfactant Treatment
Pathophysiology of Respiratory Distress Syndrome

Helen Jones, PhD
Associate Professor
Department of Physiology and Functional Genomics
Department of Obstetrics and Gynecology
University of Florida College of Medicine
Gainesville, Florida
Placental Development

Pedro A. Jose, MD, PhD
Professor
Departments of Medicine and Pharmacology-Physiology
The George Washington University School of Medicine & Health Sciences
Washington, District of Columbia
Development and Regulation of Renal Blood Flow in the Neonate

Eunjung Jung, MD
Assistant Professor
Division of Maternal-Fetal Medicine
Department of Obstetrics and Gynecology
Wayne State University School of Medicine
Detroit, Michigan
Intra-Amniotic Infection/Inflammation and the Fetal Inflammatory Response Syndrome

Suhas G. Kallapur, MD
Professor
Department of Pediatrics
Division of Neonatology
UCLA David Geffen School of Medicine
UCLA Mattel Children's Hospital
Los Angeles, California
Antenatal Factors That Influence Postnatal Lung Development and Injury
Surfactant Treatment

Michael Kaplan, MB ChB
Emeritus Director
Department of Neonatology
Shaare Zedek Medical Center
Professor of Pediatrics
Faculty of Medicine
Hebrew University
Jerusalem, Israel
Hereditary Contributions to Neonatal Hyperbilirubinemia

S. Ananth Karumanchi, MD
Professor
Department of Medicine
Harvard Medical School
Boston, Massachusetts
Staff Physician
Medallion Chair in Vascular Biology
Director, Nephrology
Cedars-Sinai Medical Center
Los Angeles, California
Pathophysiology of Preeclampsia

Frederick J. Kaskel, MD, PhD
Professor
Department of Pediatrics
Division of Nephrology
The Children's Hospital at Montefiore
Albert Einstein College of Medicine
Bronx, New York
Role of the Kidney in Calcium and Phosphorus Homeostasis

Lorraine E. Levitt Katz, MD
Physician
Division of Endocrinology and Diabetes
Children's Hospital of Philadelphia
Professor
Perelman School of Medicine
University of Pennsylvania
Philadelphia, Pennsylvania
Growth Factor Regulation of Fetal Growth

Haluk Kavus, MD
Medical Geneticist, Postdoctoral Research Scientist
Pediatrics, Division of Molecular Genetics
Columbia University Vagelos College of Physicians and Surgeons
New York, New York
Basic Genetic Principles

Susan E. Keeney, MD
Associate Professor
Department of Pediatrics
University of Texas Medical Branch
Galveston, Texas
Immunology of Human Milk

Steven E. Kern, PhD
Deputy Director, Quantitative Sciences
Global Health-Integrated Development
Bill & Melinda Gates Foundation
Seattle, Washington
Principles of Pharmacokinetics

Shirin Khanjani, MD, PhD
University College London Hospitals
London, United Kingdom
Pathophysiology of Preterm Birth

Julie Khlevner, MD
Associate Professor
Department of Pediatrics
Columbia University Vagelos College of Physicians and Surgeons
New York, New York
Development of the Enteric Nervous System and Gastrointestinal Motility

Laurie E. Kilpatrick, PhD
Professor
Department of Thoracic Medicine and Surgery
Lewis Katz School of Medicine
Temple University
Philadelphia, Pennsylvania
Cytokines and Inflammatory Response in the Fetus and Neonate

Chang-Ryul Kim, MD, PhD
Professor
Department of Pediatrics
Hanyang University College of Medicine
Seoul, South Korea
Director in NICU
Hanyang University Guri Hospital
Guri-si, South Korea
Fluid Distribution in the Fetus and Neonate

Paul S. Kingma, MD, PhD
Associate Professor of Pediatrics
Division of Neonatology
University of Cincinnati
Cincinnati Children's Hospital Medical Center
Cincinnati, Ohio
Surfactant Homeostasis: Composition and Function of Pulmonary Surfactant Lipids and Proteins

John P. Kinsella, MD
Professor
Department of Pediatrics
Section of Neonatology
University of Colorado School of Medicine
Aurora, Colorado
Pulmonary Gas Exchange in the Developing Lung
Pathophysiology of Meconium Aspiration Syndrome

Torvid Kiserud, MD, PhD
Professor
Department of Clinical Science
University of Bergen
Consultant
Fetal Medicine Unit
Department of Obstetrics and Gynecology
Haukeland University Hospital
Bergen, Norway
Umbilical Circulation

Joyce M. Koenig, MD
Professor
Division of Neonatal/Perinatal Medicine
Department of Pediatrics
Saint Louis University School of Medicine
St. Louis, Missouri
Normal and Abnormal Neutrophil Physiology in the Newborn

Rohit Kohli, MBBS, MS
Chief, Division of Gastroenterology
Children's Hospital Los Angeles
Professor of Pediatrics
Keck School of Medicine
University of Southern California
Los Angeles, California
Bile Acid Metabolism During Development

Tobias R. Kollmann, MD, PhD
Professor
Systems Biology and Pediatric Infectious Diseases
Telethon Kids Institute
Perth, Western Australia, Australia
Host Defense Mechanisms Against Bacteria

Jay K. Kolls, MD
Professor of Pediatrics
Medicine and Pediatrics
Tulane University School of Medicine
New Orleans, Louisiana
Neonatal Pulmonary Host Defense

Christina M. Konecny, MD
Postdoctoral Scholar
Department of Pediatrics
Stanford University School of Medicine
Stanford, California
Mechanistic Aspects of Phototherapy for Neonatal Hyperbilirubinemia

Panagiotis Kratimenos, MD, PhD
Assistant Professor
Center for Neuroscience Research
Children's National Research Institute and George Washington University School of Medicine and Health Sciences
Department of Pediatrics
Division of Neonatology
Children's National Hospital
Washington, District of Columbia
Cellular and Molecular Mechanisms of Neonatal Brain Injury and Neuroprotection

Nancy F. Krebs, MD
Professor
Department of Pediatrics
Section of Nutrition
University of Colorado School of Medicine
Aurora, Colorado
Zinc in the Fetus and Neonate

Kaytlin Krutsch, PharmD, MBA
Assistant Professor
Texas Tech University Health Sciences Center
Department of Obstetrics and Gynecology
School of Medicine
Amarillo, Texas
Drug Transfer During Breastfeeding

Kara Kuhn-Riordon, MD
Assistant Clinical Professor
Department of Pediatrics
Division of Neonatology
University of California Davis School of Medicine
Sacramento, California
Endocrine Factors Affecting Neonatal Growth

†Thomas J. Kulik, MD
Senior Associate in Cardiology
Department of Cardiology
Boston Children's Hospital
Associate Professor of Pediatrics
Harvard Medical School
Boston, Massachusetts
Physiology of Congenital Heart Disease in the Neonate

T. Rajendra Kumar, PhD
Professor and Edgar L. Patricia M. Makowski and Family Endowed Chair
Department of Obstetrics and Gynecology
University of Colorado School of Medicine
Aurora, Colorado
Luteinizing Hormone and Follicle-Stimulating Hormone Secretion in the Fetus and Newborn Infant

Jessica Katz Kutikov, MD
Pediatrics Specialist
Voorhees, New Jersey
Hypothalamus: Neuroendometabolic Center

Satyan Lakshminrusimha, MBBS, MD
Professor
Dennis and Nancy Marks Chair of Pediatrics
Pediatrician-in-Chief
UC Davis Children's Hospital
Sacramento, California
Pathophysiology of Persistent Pulmonary Hypertension of the Newborn

Miguel Angel Lasunción, PhD
Head, Servicio de Bioquímica-Investigación
Hospital Universitario Ramón y Cajal, IRyCIS, and CIBEROBN
Madrid, Spain
Maternal-Fetal Transfer of Lipid Metabolites

Pascal M. Lavoie, MDCM, PhD
Associate Professor
Department of Pediatrics
University of British Columbia
Clinician-Scientist
BC Children's Hospital Research Institute
Canada Staff Neonatologist
Children's & Women's Health Centre of British Columbia
Vancouver, British Columbia, Canada
Mononuclear Phagocyte System

Shelley M. Lawrence, MD
Associate Professor
Department of Pediatrics
Divisions of Neonatal-Perinatal Medicine and Host-Microbe Systems and Therapeutics
University of California, San Diego
La Jolla, California
Neutrophil Granulopoiesis and Homeostasis

Mark K. Lee, MD
Professor and Chief Physician
Nemours Children's Hospital
Wilmington, Delaware
Regulation of Embryogenesis

Mary M. Lee, MD
Professor
Department of Pediatrics
Sidney Kimmel Medical College
Jefferson University
Philadelphia, Pennsylvania
Physician-in-Chief
Nemours, AI duPont Hospital for Children
Chief Scientific Officer
Nemours Health Care System
Wilmington, Delaware
Testicular Development and Descent

†Deceased.

Yvonne K. Lee, MD
Pediatric Endocrinology
Department of Pediatrics
Kaiser Permanente
Oakland, California
Endocrine Factors Affecting Neonatal Growth

Sandra L. Leibel, MD
Assistant Professor
Department of Pediatrics
University of California, San Diego
La Jolla, California
The Extracellular Matrix in Development
Molecular Mechanisms of Lung Development and Lung Branching Morphogenesis

Ofer Levy, MD, PhD
Director, Precision Vaccines Program
Division of Infectious Diseases
Boston Children's Hospital
Professor
Department of Pediatrics
Harvard Medical School
Boston, Massachusetts
Associate Member
Broad Institute of MIT and Harvard
Cambridge, Massachusetts
Mononuclear Phagocyte System

Philip T. Levy, MD
Physician
Department of Neonatology
Division of Newborn Medicine
Boston Children's Hospital
Harvard Medical School
Boston, Massachusetts
Physiology of Congenital Heart Disease in the Neonate

Rohan M. Lewis, PhD
Professor
School of Human Development and Health
Faculty of Medicine
University of Southampton
Southampton, United Kingdom
Mechanisms of Transfer Across the Human Placenta
Placental Transfer and Fetal Requirements of Amino Acids

Changgong Li, PhD
Associate Professor
Department of Pediatrics
Keck School of Medicine
University of Southern California
Los Angeles County-University of Southern California Medical Center
Los Angeles, California
Regulation of Embryogenesis

Fangming Lin, MD, PhD
Director, Pediatric Nephrology
Department of Pediatrics
Columbia University Vagelos College of Physicians and Surgeons
New York, New York
Response to Nephron Loss in Early Development

Steven Lobritto, MD
Professor
Department of Pediatrics
NY Presbyterian-Columbia
New York, New York
Organogenesis and Histologic Development of the Liver

Cynthia A. Loomis, MD
Assistant Professor
Ronald O. Perelman Department of Dermatology
NYU Grossman School of Medicine
New York, New York
Structure and Development of the Skin and Cutaneous Appendages

Peter M. MacFarlane, PhD
Associate Professor
Department of Pediatrics
Division of Neonatology
Case Western Reserve University School of Medicine
Cleveland, Ohio
Regulation of Lower Airway Function
Pathophysiology of Apnea of Prematurity

David A. MacIntyre, PhD
Senior Lecturer
Faculty of Medicine
Department of Metabolism, Digestion, and Reproduction
Institute of Reproductive and Developmental Biology
Imperial College Parturition Research Group
Researcher
March of Dimes Prematurity Research Centre
Imperial College London
London, United Kingdom
Pathophysiology of Preterm Birth

Maxime M. Mahe, PhD
Assistant Professor
TENS, The Enteric Nervous System in Gut and Brain Diseases
INSERM
Université de Nantes
Nantes, France
Adjunct Assistant Professor
Department of Pediatric General and Thoracic Surgery
Cincinnati Children's Hospital Medical Center
Department of Pediatrics
University of Cincinnati
Cincinnati, Ohio
Organogenesis of the Gastrointestinal Tract

Linn Salto Mamsen, MSc, PhD
Researcher
Laboratory of Reproductive Biology
University Hospital of Copenhagen, Rigshospitalet
Copenhagen, Denmark
Differentiation of the Ovary

Anastasiya Mankouski, MD
Assistant Professor
Department of Pediatrics
Division of Neonatology
University of Utah Health
Salt Lake City, Utah
Mechanisms of Neonatal Lung Injury

Carlos B. Mantilla, MD, PhD
Professor and Chair
Anesthesiology and Perioperative Medicine
Professor
Physiology and Biomedical Engineering
Mayo Clinic
Rochester, Minnesota
Functional Development of Respiratory Muscles

Arnaud Marchant, MD, PhD
Director
Institute for Medical Immunology
Université Libre de Bruxelles
Brussels, Belgium
Host Defense Mechanisms Against Bacteria
Host Defense Mechanisms Against Viruses

Kara Gross Margolis, MD
Associate Professor
Department of Pediatrics
Columbia University Vagelos College of Physicians and Surgeons
New York, New York
Development of the Enteric Nervous System and Gastrointestinal Motility

László Maródi, MD, PhD
Professor
Primary Immunodeficiency Clinical Unit and Laboratory
Department of Dermatology, Venereology, and Dermatooncology
Faculty of Medicine
Semmelweis University
Budapest, Hungary
Host Defense Mechanisms Against Fungi
T-Cell Development

Karel Maršál, MD, PhD
Professor Emeritus
Department of Obstetrics and Gynecology
Lund University
Lund, Sweden
Fetal and Placental Circulation During Labor

Richard J. Martin, MBBS
Professor of Pediatrics, Reproductive Biology, and Physiology & Biophysics
Division of Neonatology
Case Western Reserve University School of Medicine
Drusinsky-Fanaroff Professor
Director, Neonatal Research
Department of Pediatrics/Neonatology
Rainbow Babies and Children's Hospital
Cleveland, Ohio
Regulation of Lower Airway Function

Jayne F. Martin Carli, PhD
Fellow
Department of Pediatrics
University of Colorado School of Medicine
Aurora, Colorado
Physiology of Lactation
Pathophysiology of Apnea of Prematurity

Hugo R. Martinez, MD
Assistant Professor
Department of Pediatrics
University of Tennessee Health Science Center
Cardiomyopathy and Transplant Cardiology
Cardio-Vascular Genetics Service
Le Bonheur Hospital
Cardio-Oncology Service
St. Jude Children's Research Hospital
Memphis, Tennessee
Pathophysiology of Cardiomyopathies

Douglas G. Matsell, MDCM
Head, Division of Nephrology
British Columbia Children's Hospital
University of British Columbia
Vancouver, British Columbia, Canada
Functional Development of the Kidney in Utero

Dwight E. Matthews, PhD
Professor Emeritus
Chemistry and Medicine
University of Vermont
Burlington, Vermont
General Concepts of Protein Metabolism

Harry J. McArdle, BSc (Hons), PhD
Professor
Rowett Institute of Nutrition and Health
University of Aberdeen
Aberdeen, United Kingdom
Fetal and Neonatal Iron Metabolism

C.J.D. McKinlay, MBChB, PhD
Senior Lecturer
Liggins Institute
University of Auckland
Auckland, New Zealand
Antenatal Hormonal Therapy for Prevention of Respiratory Distress Syndrome

James L. McManaman, PhD
Professor
Department of Obstetrics and Gynecology
University of Colorado School of Medicine
Aurora, Colorado
Physiology of Lactation

Patrick J. McNamara, MD, MRCPCH, MSc
Professor
Department of Pediatrics
Director, Division of Neonatology
University of Iowa Health Care
Iowa City, Iowa
Oxygen Transport and Delivery

Giacomo Meschia, MD
Emeritus Professor
Department of Physiology
University of Colorado School of Medicine
Aurora, Colorado
Placental and Fetal Circulatory and Metabolic Changes Accompanying Fetal Growth Restriction

Karen Mestan, MD
Associate Professor
Department of Pediatrics
Northwestern University Feinberg School of Medicine
Chicago, Illinois
Placental Function in Intrauterine Growth Restriction

Steven P. Miller, MDCM, MAS
Division Head, Neurology
Bloorview Children's Hospital
Chair, Paediatric Neuroscience
The Hospital for Sick Children
Professor
Department of Pediatrics
University of Toronto
Senior Scientist, Chair
Neuroscience and Mental Health
SickKids Research Institute
Toronto, Ontario, Canada
Pathophysiology of Neonatal White Matter Injury

Parviz Minoo, PhD
Professor
Department of Pediatrics
Keck School of Medicine
University of Southern California
Los Angeles County—University of Southern California Medical Center
Los Angeles, California
Regulation of Embryogenesis

Imran N. Mir, MD
Assistant Professor
Department of Pediatrics
University of Texas Southwestern Medical Center
Dallas, Texas
Regulation of the Placental Circulation

Lisa J. Mitchell, DO
Assistant Professor
Department of Pediatrics
F. Edward Hébert School of Medicine
Uniformed Services University of the Health Sciences
Bethesda, Maryland
Medical Director
Neonatal Intensive Care Unit
Carl R. Darnall Army Medical Center
Fort Hood, Texas
Pathophysiology of Apnea of Prematurity

Ivana Mižíková, PhD
Postdoctoral Fellow
Sinclair Centre for Regenerative Medicine
Ottawa Hospital Research Institute
Department of Cellular and Molecular Medicine
University of Ottawa
Ottawa, Ontario, Canada
Developmental Biology of Lung Stem Cells

Tomoyuki Mizuno, PhD
Assistant Professor
Division of Clinical Pharmacology
Cincinnati Children's Hospital Medical Center
Assistant Professor
Department of Pediatrics
University of Cincinnati College of Medicine
Cincinnati, Ohio
Pharmacogenomics

Jeremiah D. Momper, PharmD, PhD
Associate Professor
Skaggs School of Pharmacy and Pharmaceutical Sciences
University of California, San Diego
La Jolla, California
Organic Anion Transport in the Developing Kidney

Paul Monagle, MBBS, MD, MSC
Professor
Department Paediatrics
University of Melbourne
Haematologist
Department of Haematology
Royal Children's Hospital
Group Leader
Haematology Research
Murdoch Childrens Research Institute
Melbourne, Victoria, Australia
Staff Specialist
Kids Cancer Centre
Sydney Children's Hospital
Sydney, New South Wales, Australia
Developmental Hemostasis

Jenifer Monks, PhD
Assistant Professor
Department of Obstetrics and Gynecology
University of Colorado School of Medicine
Aurora, Colorado
Physiology of Lactation

Jacopo P. Mortola, MD
Professor
Department of Physiology
McGill University
Montreal, Quebec, Canada
Mechanics of Breathing

Louis J. Muglia, MD, PhD
Adjunct Professor
Department of Pediatrics
Cincinnati Children's Hospital Medical Center
Cincinnati, Ohio
President and CEO
Burroughs Wellcome Fund
Research Triangle Park, North Carolina
Fetal and Neonatal Adrenocortical Physiology

Upender K. Munshi, MBBS, MD
Associate Professor
Department of Pediatrics
Albany Medical Center
Albany, New York
Development of the Gastrointestinal Circulation in the Fetus and Newborn

Sumana Narasimhan, MD
Assistant Professor
Pediatric Endocrinology
Case Western Reserve University
Cleveland, Ohio
Luteinizing Hormone and Follicle-Stimulating Hormone Secretion in the Fetus and Newborn Infant

Vivek Narendran, MD, MRCP (UK), MBA
Professor of Pediatrics
Perinatal Institute
Cincinnati Children's Hospital and Medical Center
Director UCMC-NICU
University of Cincinnati Medical Center
Cincinnati Children's Hospital Medical Center
Cincinnati, Ohio
Physiologic Development of the Skin

Jan Nedergaard, PhD
Professor
Department of Molecular Biosciences
The Wenner-Gren Institute
Stockholm University
Stockholm, Sweden
Brown Adipose Tissue: Development and Function

Leif D. Nelin, MD
Dean W. Jeffers Chair in Neonatology
Nationwide Children's Hospital
Professor and Chief
Division of Neonatology
The Ohio State University
Columbus, Ohio
Pulmonary Gas Exchange in the Developing Lung

Josef Neu, MD
Professor
Department of Pediatrics
Division of Neonatology
University of Florida College of Medicine
Gainesville, Florida
Digestive-Absorptive Functions in Fetuses, Infants, and Children
The Developing Microbiome of the Fetus and Neonate: A Multiomic Approach

Sandra C.A. Nielsen, PhD
Scientist
Department of Pathology
Stanford University School of Medicine
Stanford, California
B-Cell Development

Sanjay K. Nigam, MD
Nancy Kaehr Chair in Research
Pediatrics and Medicine
University of California, San Diego
La Jolla, California
Organic Anion Transport in the Developing Kidney

Victor Nizet, MD
Distinguished Professor
Vice Chair for Basic Research
Department of Pediatrics
Distinguished Professor
Department of Pharmacy and Pharmaceutical Sciences
University of California, San Diego
La Jolla, California
Neutrophil Granulopoiesis and Homeostasis

Lawrence M. Nogee, MD
Professor
Eudowood Neonatal Pulmonary Division
Department of Pediatrics
Johns Hopkins University School of Medicine
Baltimore, Maryland
Genetics and Physiology of Surfactant Protein Deficiencies

Shahab Noori, MD, MS CBTI
Professor
Department of Pediatrics
Keck School of Medicine
University of Southern California
Administrative Director of Clinical Research
Division of Neonatology
Children's Hospital Los Angeles
Los Angeles, California
Pathophysiology of Shock in the Fetus and Neonate

Andrew W. Norris, MD, PhD
Professor
Department of Pediatrics
University of Iowa Health Care
Iowa City, Iowa
Glucose Metabolism in the Fetus and Newborn, and Methods for Its Investigation

Barbara M. O'Brien, MD
Beth Israel Deaconess Medical Center
Department of Obstetrics and Gynecology
Boston, Massachusetts
Prenatal Diagnosis

Lori L. O'Brien, PhD
Assistant Professor
Department of Cell Biology and Physiology
University of North Carolina at Chapel Hill
Chapel Hill, North Carolina
Development of the Kidney: Morphology and Mechanisms

Karen M. O'Callaghan, PhD
Research Fellow
Centre for Global Child Health
SickKids Research Institute
The Hospital for Sick Children
Toronto, Ontario, Canada
Fetal and Neonatal Calcium, Phosphorus, and Magnesium Homeostasis

Amanda Ogilvy-Stuart, BM, DM
Consultant Neonatologist
Department of Neonatology
Cambridge University Hospitals NHS Trust
Cambridge, United Kingdom
Role of Glucoregulatory Hormones in Hepatic Glucose Metabolism During the Perinatal Period

Robin K. Ohls, MD
Professor
Department of Pediatrics-Neonatology
University of Utah Health
Salt Lake City, Utah
Developmental Erythropoiesis

Henar Ortega-Senovilla, PhD
Adjunct Professor
Department of Chemistry and Biochemistry
Faculties of Pharmacy and Medicine
Universidad San Pablo-CEU
Madrid, Spain
Lipids as an Energy Source for the Premature and Term Neonate

Justin M. O'Sullivan, PhD
Professor
Deputy Director, Liggins Institute
University of Auckland
Auckland, New Zealand
Epigenetics

Howard B. Panitch, MD
Medical Director, Technology Dependence Program
Division of Pulmonary and Sleep Medicine
Children's Hospital of Philadelphia
Professor
Department of Pediatrics
Perelman School of Medicine
University of Pennsylvania
Philadelphia, Pennsylvania
Pathophysiology of Ventilator-Dependent Infants

Anna A. Penn, MD, PhD
Associate Professor
Department of Pediatrics
George Washington University School of Medicine
Attending Physician and Director
Translational Research for Hospital-Based Services
Co-Director, Cerebral Palsy Prevention Program
Fetal and Transitional Medicine, Neonatology
Investigator
Children's Research Institute Center for Neuroscience
Children's National Medical Center
Washington, District of Columbia
Endocrine and Paracrine Function of the Human Placenta

Raymond B. Penn, PhD
Robley Dunglison Professor of Pulmonary Research
Director, Center for Translational Medicine
Director, Pulmonary Research
Jefferson Jane and Leonard Korman Lung Institute
Vice Chair, Research
Department of Medicine
Division of Pulmonary, Allergy, and Critical Care Medicine
Thomas Jefferson University
Philadelphia, Pennsylvania
Upper Airway Structure: Function, Regulation, and Development

Margaret G. Petroff, PhD
Associate Professor
Pathobiology and Diagnostic Investigation
Michigan State University
East Lansing, Michigan
Placental Development

Anthony F. Philipps, AB, MD
Professor
Department of Pediatrics
University of California Davis School of Medicine
Sacramento, California
Oxygen Consumption and General Carbohydrate Metabolism of the Fetus

Francesco Pisani, MD, PhD
Professor
Child Neuropsychiatry Unit
Department of Medicine and Surgery
Neuroscience Section
University of Parma
Parma, Italy
Electroencephalography in the Preterm and Term Infant

David Pleasure, MD
Distinguished Professor
Department of Neurology and Pediatrics
University of California Davis School of Medicine
Sacramento, California
Trophic Factor, Nutritional, and Hormonal Regulation of Brain Development

Scott L. Pomeroy, MD, PhD
Bronson Crothers Professor
Department of Neurology
Harvard Medical School
Neurologist-in-Chief and Chairman
Department of Neurology
Boston Children's Hospital
Boston, Massachusetts
Development of the Nervous System

Martin Post, PhD
Senior Scientist
Translational Medicine
The Hospital for Sick Children
Professor
Department of Physiology
Laboratory Medicine and Pathobiology
University of Toronto
Toronto, Ontario, Canada
The Extracellular Matrix in Development
Molecular Mechanisms of Lung Development and Lung Branching Morphogenesis

Y.S. Prakash, MD, PhD
Professor
Anesthesiology and Physiology
Mayo Clinic
Rochester, Minnesota
Regulation of Lower Airway Function

Joshua D. Prozialeck, MD, MSA
Assistant Professor
Department of Pediatrics
Northwestern University Feinberg School of Medicine
Ann & Robert H. Lurie Children's Hospital of Chicago
Chicago, Illinois
Development of Gastric Secretory Function

Theodore J. Pysher, MD
Professor
Chief, Division of Pediatric Pathology
Department of Pathology
University of Utah Health
Salt Lake City, Utah
Impaired Lung Growth After Injury in Preterm Lung

Raymond Quigley, MD
Professor
Department of Pediatrics
UT Southwestern Medical Center
Dallas, Texas
Potassium Homeostasis in the Fetus and Neonate
Transport of Amino Acids in the Fetus and Neonate

Marlene Rabinovitch, MD
Professor of Pediatrics
Division of Cardiology
Stanford University School of Medicine
Stanford, California
Developmental Biology of the Pulmonary Vasculature

Thomas M. Raffay, MD
Assistant Professor of Pediatrics
Division of Neonatology
Case Western Reserve University
Rainbow Babies and Children's Hospital
Cleveland, Ohio
Regulation of Lower Airway Function

J. Usha Raj, MD, MHA
Anjuli S. Nayak Professor of Pediatrics
University of Illinois at Chicago
Chicago, Illinois
Regulation of Pulmonary Circulation

Laura B. Ramsey, PhD
Assistant Professor
Divisions of Clinical Pharmacology and Research in Patient Services
Cincinnati Children's Hospital Medical Center
Assistant Professor
Department of Pediatrics
University of Cincinnati College of Medicine
Co-Director, Genetic Pharmacology Service
Cincinnati Children's Hospital Medical Center
Cincinnati, Ohio
Pharmacogenomics

Sarosh Rana, MD, MPH
Professor
Division of Maternal Fetal Medicine
Department of Obstetrics and Gynecology
University of Chicago
Chicago, Illinois
Pathophysiology of Preeclampsia

Tara M. Randis, MD
Associate Professor
Department of Pediatrics and Molecular Medicine
USF Health Morsani College of Medicine
Tampa, Florida
Pathophysiology of Chorioamnionitis: Host Immunity and Microbial Virulence

Manon Ranger, PhD
Assistant Professor
School of Nursing
University of British Columbia
Vancouver, British Columbia, Canada
Developmental Aspects of Pain

Timothy R.H. Regnault, PhD
Associate Professor
Departments of Obstetrics/Gynaecology and Physiology/Pharmacology
Western University
London, Ontario, Canada
Placental and Fetal Circulatory and Metabolic Changes Accompanying Fetal Growth Restriction
Placental Transfer and Fetal Requirements of Amino Acids

Danielle R. Rios, MD
Associate Professor
Department of Pediatrics
Division of Neonatology
University of Iowa Health Care
Iowa City, Iowa
Oxygen Transport and Delivery

Roberto Romero, MD, DMedSci
Chief, Perinatology Research Branch
Eunice Kennedy Shriver National Institute for Child Health and Human Development
National Institutes of Health
U.S. Department of Health and Human Services
Detroit, Michigan
Intra-Amniotic Infection/Inflammation and the Fetal Inflammatory Response Syndrome

Charles R. Rosenfeld, MD
Professor Emeritus
Departments of Pediatrics, Obstetrics/Gynecology, Anesthesiology
University of Texas Southwestern Medical Center
Dallas, Texas
Regulation of the Placental Circulation

A. Catharine Ross, PhD
Professor of Nutrition and Physiology
Nutritional Sciences
Pennsylvania State University
University Park, Pennsylvania
Vitamin A Metabolism in the Fetus and Neonate

Daniel E. Roth, MD, PhD
Staff Pediatrician
Division of Pediatric Medicine
The Hospital for Sick Children
Associate Professor
Departments of Pediatrics and Nutritional Sciences
University of Toronto
Toronto, Ontario, Canada
Fetal and Neonatal Calcium, Phosphorus, and Magnesium Homeostasis

Henry J. Rozycki, MD
Professor and Vice Chair for Research
Department of Pediatrics
Children's Hospital of Richmond at VCU
Director, Children's Health Research Institute
Virginia Commonwealth University School of Medicine
Richmond, Virginia
Structure and Development of Alveolar Epithelial Cells

Thomas D. Ryan, MD, PhD
Associate Professor
Department of Pediatrics
University of Cincinnati College of Medicine
Director, Clinical Operations, Cardiomyopathy, and Heart Failure
Co-Director, Cardio-Oncology Program
The Heart Institute
Cincinnati Children's Hospital Medical Center
Cincinnati, Ohio
Pathophysiology of Cardiomyopathies

Rakesh Sahni, MBBS
Professor
Department of Pediatrics
Columbia University Vagelos College of Physicians and Surgeons
New York, New York
Temperature Control in Newborn Infants

Harvey B. Sarnat, MD
Professor
Departments of Paediatrics, Pathology (Neuropathology), and Clinical Neurosciences
University of Calgary Faculty of Medicine and Alberta Children's Hospital Research Institute
Calgary, Alberta, Canada
Development of Olfaction and Taste in the Human Fetus and Neonate
Ontogenesis of Striated Muscle

Lisa M. Satlin, MD
Professor and System Chair
Department of Pediatrics
Icahn School of Medicine at Mount Sinai
Pediatrician-in-Chief
Mount Sinai Kravis Children's Hospital
New York, New York
Potassium Homeostasis in the Fetus and Neonate

Joseph Scafidi, DO, MS
Associate Professor
Department of Neurology and Pediatrics
Kennedy Krieger Institute
Johns Hopkins School of Medicine
Baltimore, Maryland
Cellular and Molecular Mechanisms of Neonatal Brain Injury and Neuroprotection

Michael A. Schellpfeffer, MD
Professor
Departments of Cell Biology, Neurobiology, and Anatomy
Medical College of Wisconsin
Milwaukee, Wisconsin
Developmental Electrophysiology in the Fetus and Neonate

William Schierding, PhD
Senior Research Fellow
Liggins Institute
University of Auckland
Auckland, New Zealand
Epigenetics

George J. Schwartz, MD
Professor
Department of Pediatrics
Division of Nephrology
University of Rochester Medical Center and Golisano Children's Hospital
Rochester, New York
Urinary Acidification

Jeffrey L. Segar, MD
Physician
Department of Pediatrics
University of Iowa Children's Hospital
Iowa City, Iowa
Regulation of Cardiovascular Function During Fetal and Newborn Life

David T. Selewski, MD
Associate Professor
Department of Pediatrics
Division of Nephrology
Medical University of South Carolina
Charleston, South Carolina
Pathophysiology of Neonatal Acute Kidney Injury

Istvan Seri, MD, PhD, HonD
Professor
Pediatrics (Research)
First Department of Pediatrics
Semmelweis University
Budapest, Hungary, Professor of Pediatrics (Adjunct)
Pediatrics/Neonatology
Children's Hospital Los Angeles
Keck School of Medicine
University of Southern California
Los Angeles, California
Regulation of Acid-Base Balance in the Fetus and Neonate
Pathophysiology of Shock in the Fetus and Neonate

Thomas H. Shaffer, MSE, PhD
Professor Emeritus
Physiology, Pediatrics, and Medicine
Lewis Katz School of Medicine at Temple University
Professor of Pediatrics
Sidney Kimmel Medical College
Thomas Jefferson University
Philadelphia, Pennsylvania
Associate Director, Biomedical Research
Alfred I. duPont Hospital for Children
Wilmington, Delaware
Upper Airway Structure: Function, Regulation, and Development

Martin J. Shearer, BSc, PhD, FRCPath
Physician
Centre for Haemostasis and Thrombosis
St Thomas' Hospital
London, United Kingdom
Vitamin K Metabolism in the Fetus and Neonate

Noah F. Shroyer, PhD
Associate Professor
Department of Medicine
Section of Gastroenterology and Hepatology
Baylor College of Medicine
Houston, Texas
Organogenesis of the Gastrointestinal Tract

Gary C. Sieck, PhD
Professor
Physiology and Biomedical Engineering
Mayo Clinic
Rochester, Minnesota
Functional Development of Respiratory Muscles

Rebecca A. Simmons, MD
Hallam Hurt Professor Pediatrics
Department of Pediatrics
Children's Hospital of Philadelphia
Philadelphia, Pennsylvania
Cell Glucose Transport and Glucose Handling During Fetal and Neonatal Development

Neel Kamal Singh, MBBS, MD
NICU Fellow
Department of Pediatrics
Division of Neonatology
University of Florida College of Medicine
Gainesville, Florida
The Developing Microbiome of the Fetus and Neonate: A Multiomic Approach

Emidio Sivieri, MS, BE
Biomedical Engineer
Department of Neonatology
CHOP Newborn Care at Pennsylvania Hospital
Children's Hospital of Philadelphia
Philadelphia, Pennsylvania
Evaluation of Pulmonary Function in the Neonate

Laura Smith, MD
Beth Israel Deaconess Medical Center
Department of Obstetrics and Gynecology
Boston, Massachusetts
Prenatal Diagnosis

Ian M. Smyth, PhD
Group Leader
Department of Anatomy and Developmental Biology
Biomedicine Discovery Institute
Associate Professor of Pediatrics
Department of Biochemistry and Molecular Biology
Biomedicine Discovery Institute
Monash University
Melbourne, Victoria, Australia
Development of the Kidney: Morphology and Mechanisms

Martha C. Sola-Visner, MD
Associate Professor of Pediatrics
Department of Medicine
Division of Newborn Medicine
Children's Hospital Boston and Harvard Medical School
Boston, Massachusetts
Developmental Megakaryopoiesis

Michael J. Solhaug, MD
Professor of Pediatrics and Physiology
Physiological Sciences
Eastern Virginia Medical School
Norfolk, Virginia
Development and Regulation of Renal Blood Flow in the Neonate

Markus Sperandio, MD
Professor
Institute for Cardiovascular Physiology and Pathophysiology
Walter Brendel Center for Experimental Medicine
Ludwig-Maximilians-Universität
Munich, Germany
Normal and Abnormal Neutrophil Physiology in the Newborn

Mark A. Sperling, MBBS
Emeritus Professor and Chair
Department of Pediatrics
Children's Hospital University of Pittsburgh
Pittsburgh, Pennsylvania
Professorial Lecturer
Pediatric Endocrinology and Diabetes
Icahn School of Medicine at Mt. Sinai
New York, New York
Growth Hormone, Prolactin, and Placental Lactogen in the Fetus and Newborn

Lakshmi Srinivasan, MBBS
Assistant Professor
Department of Pediatrics
Children's Hospital of Philadelphia
Philadelphia, Pennsylvania
Cytokines and Inflammatory Response in the Fetus and Neonate

Diana E. Stanescu, MD
Assistant Professor
Department of Pediatrics
Perelman School of Medicine
University of Pennsylvania
Philadelphia, Pennsylvania
Pathophysiology of Neonatal Hypoglycemia

Charles A. Stanley, MD
Senior Endocrinologist
Division of Endocrinology and Diabetes
Children's Hospital of Philadelphia
Professor Emeritus
Department of Pediatrics
Perelman School of Medicine
University of Pennsylvania
Philadelphia, Pennsylvania
Pathophysiology of Neonatal Hypoglycemia

Robin H. Steinhorn, MD
Senior Vice President and Executive Director
Rady Children's Specialists of San Diego
Vice Dean, Children's Clinical Services
University of California, San Diego
La Jolla, California
Pathophysiology of Persistent Pulmonary Hypertension of the Newborn

Lisa Stinson, BSc, MMedSci, PhD
Research Fellow
School of Molecular Sciences
The University of Western Australia, Perth
Perth, Western Australia, Australia
Human Milk Composition and Function in the Infant

Barbara S. Stonestreet, MD
Professor
Department of Pediatrics
Women & Infants Hospital of Rhode Island
The Warren Alpert Medical School of Brown University
Providence, Rhode Island
Fluid Distribution in the Fetus and Neonate
Development of the Blood-Brain Barrier

Janette F. Strasburger, MD
Professor
Department of Pediatrics
Medical College of Wisconsin
Attending Cardiologist
Herma Heart Institute
Children's Hospital of Wisconsin
Milwaukee, Wisconsin
Developmental Electrophysiology in the Fetus and Neonate

Dennis M. Styne, MD
Yocha Dehe Chair of Pediatric Endocrinology
Professor
Department of Pediatrics
University of California Davis School of Medicine
Davis, California
Endocrine Factors Affecting Neonatal Growth

Xin Sun, PhD
Professor
Pediatrics and Biological Sciences
University of California, San Diego
La Jolla, California
Normal and Abnormal Structural Development of the Lung

Lori Sussel, PhD
Professor
Barbara Davis Center for Diabetes
University of Colorado School of Medicine
Aurora, Colorado
Development of the Endocrine and Exocrine Pancreas

Emily W.Y. Tam, MDCM, MAS
Associate Professor
Department of Paediatrics
University of Toronto
Toronto, Ontario, Canada
Cerebellar Development—The Impact of Preterm Birth and Comorbidities

Libo Tan, PhD
Assistant Professor
Human Nutrition and Hospitality Management
University of Alabama
Tuscaloosa, Alabama
Vitamin A Metabolism in the Fetus and Neonate

Arjan B. te Pas, MD, PhD
Professor
Department of Pediatrics
Leiden University Medical Center
Leiden, The Netherlands
Physiology of Neonatal Resuscitation

Vadim S. Ten, MD, PhD
Professor
Department of Pediatrics
Division of Neonatology
Columbia University Irving Medical Center
New York, New York
Pathophysiology of Neonatal Hypoxic-Ischemic Brain Injury

Bernard Thébaud, MD, PhD
Senior Scientist
Sinclair Centre for Regenerative Medicine
Ottawa Hospital Research Institute
Professor
Department of Pediatrics
Neonatologist
Children's Hospital of Eastern Ontario
University of Ottawa
Ottawa, Ontario, Canada
Developmental Biology of Lung Stem Cells

Claire Thornton, PhD
Senior Lecturer
Comparative Biomedical Sciences
Royal Veterinary College
London, United Kingdom
Mechanisms of Cell Death in the Developing Brain

Daniel J. Tollin, PhD
Professor
Department of Physiology and Biophysics
University of Colorado School of Medicine
Aurora, Colorado
Early Development of the Human Auditory System

Jeffrey A. Towbin, MD
Executive Co-Director
The Heart Institute
Le Bonheur Children's Hospital
Professor and Chief
Pediatric Cardiology
Medical Director, Cardiomyopathy, Heart Failure, and Transplant Services
University of Tennessee Health Science Center
Memphis, Tennessee
Pathophysiology of Cardiomyopathies

William E. Truog III, MD
Sosland Endowed Chair in Neonatal Research
Center for Infant Pulmonary Disorders
Children's Mercy Hospital
Professor
Department of Pediatrics
University of Missouri Kansas City School of Medicine
Kansas City, Missouri
Pulmonary Gas Exchange in the Developing Lung

Kristin M. Uhler, PhD
Audiologist/Associate Professor
Otolaryngology, Physical Medicine & Rehabilitation
University of Colorado School of Medicine
Chair
Audiology, Speech Pathology, and Learning
Children's Colorado Hospital
Aurora, Colorado
Early Development of the Human Auditory System

Chris H.P. van den Akker, MD, PhD
Pediatrician, Neonatologist
Amsterdam UMC—Emma Children's Hospital
Department of Pediatrics/Neonatology
University of Amsterdam and Vrije Universiteit Amsterdam
Amsterdam, The Netherlands
General Concepts of Protein Metabolism

John Nicolaas van den Anker, MD, PhD
Chief, Clinical Pharmacology
Department of Pediatrics
Children's National Health System
Washington, District of Columbia
Chair, Paediatric Pharmacology and Pharmacometrics
Department of Pediatrics
University Children's Hospital Basel
Basel, Switzerland
Faculty, Intensive Care
Pediatric Surgery
Erasmus Medical Center–Sophia Children's Hospital
Rotterdam, The Netherlands
The Physiology of Placental Drug Disposition

Maurice J.B. van den Hoff, PhD
Associate Professor
Department of Medical Biology
Amsterdam UMC
Amsterdam, The Netherlands
Cardiovascular Development

Johannes (Hans) B. van Goudoever, MD, PhD
Professor
Amsterdam UMC—Emma Children's Hospital
Department of Pediatrics
University of Amsterdam and Vrije Universiteit Amsterdam
Amsterdam, The Netherlands
General Concepts of Protein Metabolism

Mark H. Vickers, PhD
Professor
Liggins Institute
University of Auckland
Auckland, New Zealand
Epigenetics

Alexander A. Vinks, PhD, PharmD
Cincinnati Children's Research Foundation Endowed Chair
Professor of Pediatrics and Pharmacology
University of Cincinnati College of Medicine
Director, Division of Clinical Pharmacology
Director, Pediatric Clinical Pharmacology Fellowship Program
Scientific Director, Pharmacy Research in Patient Services
Cincinnati Children's Hospital Medical Center
Cincinnati, Ohio
Pharmacogenomics

Daniela Virgintino, MD
Professor
Department of Basic Medical Sciences, Neurosciences, and Sensory Organs
University of Bari School of Medicine
Bari, Italy
Development of the Blood-Brain Barrier

Marty O. Visscher, PhD
Professor
James L. Winkle College of Pharmacy
University of Cincinnati College of Medicine
Cincinnati, Ohio
Physiologic Development of the Skin

Caitlin E. Vonderohe, DVM, PhD
Postdoctoral Fellow
USDA-ARS Children's Nutrition Research Center
Department of Pediatrics
Baylor College of Medicine
Houston, Texas
Trophic Factors and Regulation of Gastrointestinal Tract and Liver Development

Neha V. Vyas, MD
Pediatric Endocrinology Fellow
Pediatric Endocrinology
Rainbow Babies and Children's Hospital
Cleveland, Ohio
Luteinizing Hormone and Follicle-Stimulating Hormone Secretion in the Fetus and Newborn Infant

Annette Wacker-Gussmann, MD
Department of Sport and Health Sciences
Institute of Preventive Pediatrics
Department of Pediatric Cardiology and Congenital Heart Defects
German Heart Center
Munich, Germany
Developmental Electrophysiology in the Fetus and Neonate

Abby Walch, MD
Clinical Fellow
Pediatric Endocrinology
University of California, San Francisco
San Francisco, California
Development of the Hypothalamus-Pituitary-Adrenal Axis in the Fetus

Megan J. Wallace, BSc, BSc (Hons), PhD
Associate Professor
Department of Obstetrics and Gynaecology
Director, Medical Student Research
School of Medicine
Monash University
Head, Lung Development Research Group
The Ritchie Centre
Hudson Institute of Medical Research
Clayton, Victoria, Australia
Physiologic Mechanisms of Normal and Altered Lung Growth Before and After Birth

Brian H. Walsh, MB, BCh, PhD
Physician
Department of Neonatology
Cork University Maternity Hospital
Cork, Ireland
Intraventricular Hemorrhage in the Neonate

Jennifer A. Wambach, MD
Associate Professor
Edward Mallinckrodt Department of Pediatrics
Washington University School of Medicine
St. Louis, Missouri
Genetics and Physiology of Surfactant Protein Deficiencies

Linda X. Wang, MD
Division of Gastroenterology
Children's Hospital Los Angeles
Clinical Instructor of Pediatrics
Keck School of Medicine
University of Southern California
Los Angeles, California
Bile Acid Metabolism During Development

David Warburton, DSc, MD
Professor
Developmental Biology and Regenerative Medicine Program
Saban Research Institute
Children's Hospital Los Angeles
Los Angeles, California
Regulation of Embryogenesis

Robert M. Ward, MD
Professor Emeritus
Department of Pediatrics
Division of Pediatric Clinical Pharmacology
Adjunct Professor
Department of Pharmacology/Toxicology
University of Utah Health
Salt Lake City, Utah
Principles of Pharmacokinetics

Kevin M. Watt, MD, PhD
Chief, Division of Clinical Pharmacology
Associate Professor
Department of Pediatrics
Division of Pediatric Critical Care Medicine
University of Utah Health
Salt Lake City, Utah
Principles of Pharmacokinetics

Kristi L. Watterberg, MD
Professor Emerita
Division of Neonatology
University of New Mexico
Albuquerque, New Mexico
Fetal and Neonatal Adrenocortical Physiology

Lynne A. Werner, PhD
Professor Emeritus
Department of Speech & Hearing Sciences
University of Washington
Seattle, Washington
Early Development of the Human Auditory System

Sarah A. Wernimont, MD, PhD
Assistant Professor
Department of Obstetrics, Gynecology, and Women's Health
University of Minnesota Medical School
Minneapolis, Minnesota
Glucose Metabolism in the Fetus and Newborn, and Methods for Its Investigation

Barry K. Wershil, MD
Professor
Department of Pediatrics
Feinberg School of Medicine at Northwestern
Chief, Division of Gastroenterology, Hepatology, and Nutrition
Department of Pediatrics
Ann & Robert H. Lurie Children's Hospital of Chicago
Chicago, Illinois
Development of Gastric Secretory Function

Andy Wessels, PhD
Professor
Regenerative Medicine and Cell Biology
Pediatric Cardiology
Medical University of South Carolina
Charleston, South Carolina
Cardiovascular Development

Jeffrey A. Whitsett, MD
Professor of Pediatrics
Divisions of Pulmonary Biology and Neonatology
Perinatal Institute
University of Cincinnati
Cincinnati Children's Hospital Medical Center
Cincinnati, Ohio
Surfactant Homeostasis: Composition and Function of Pulmonary Surfactant Lipids and Proteins

Fabienne Willems, PhD
Professor
Institute for Medical Immunology
Université Libre de Bruxelles
Brussels, Belgium
Host Defense Mechanisms Against Viruses

Myat Su Win, MBBS, MRCPCH
Physician
Department of Paediatrics
Cambridge University Hospitals NHS Trust
Cambridge, United Kingdom
Role of Glucoregulatory Hormones in Hepatic Glucose Metabolism During the Perinatal Period

Christoph Wohlmuth, MD, PhD
Department of Obstetrics and Gynecology
Paracelsus Medical University
Salzburg, Austria
The Pathophysiology of Twin-Twin Transfusion Syndrome, Twin-Anemia Polycythemia Sequence, and Twin-Reversed Arterial Perfusion

Matthias T. Wolf, MD
Associate Professor
Department of Pediatrics
UT Southwestern Medical Center
Dallas, Texas
Potassium Homeostasis in the Fetus and Neonate

Marla R. Wolfson, PhD
Professor
Departments of Physiology, Medicine, and Pediatrics
Center for Inflammation, Translational, and Clinical Lung Research
Associate Chair
Department of Physiology
Lead Researcher
CENTRe: Collaborative for Environmental and Neonatal Therapeutics Research
Lewis Katz School of Medicine
Temple University
Philadelphia, Pennsylvania
Upper Airway Structure: Function, Regulation, and Development

Ronald J. Wong, MD
Senior Research Scientist
Department of Pediatrics
Stanford University School of Medicine
Stanford, California
Mechanistic Aspects of Phototherapy for Neonatal Hyperbilirubinemia

James L. Wynn, MD
Professor
Departments of Pediatrics and Pathology, Immunology, and Laboratory Medicine
University of Florida College of Medicine
Gainesville, Florida
Pathophysiology of Neonatal Sepsis

Lami Yeo, MD
Professor
Division of Maternal-Fetal Medicine
Department of Obstetrics and Gynecology
Wayne State University School of Medicine
Director, Fetal Cardiology
Perinatology Research Branch, NICHD/NIH/DHHS
Detroit, Michigan
Intra-Amniotic Infection/Inflammation and the Fetal Inflammatory Response Syndrome

Bradley A. Yoder, MD
Professor
Department of Pediatrics
University of Utah Health
Salt Lake City, Utah
Impaired Lung Growth After Injury in Preterm Lung

Christopher J. Yuskaitis, MD, PhD
Assistant
Department of Neurology
Boston Children's Hospital
Instructor in Neurology
Harvard Medical School
Boston, Massachusetts
Development of the Nervous System

Jennifer Zabinsky, MD
Clinical Fellow
Pediatric Endocrinology
University of California, San Francisco
San Francisco, California
Development of the Hypothalamus-Pituitary-Adrenal Axis in the Fetus

Dan Zhou, PhD
Scientist
Department of Pediatrics
University of California San Diego
La Jolla, California
Basic Mechanisms of Oxygen Sensing and Adaptation to Hypoxia

Preface

The care of critically ill newborn infants has its foundations in neonatal physiology. Practitioners have traditionally used general physiologic principles in combination with clinical effectiveness studies to provide the most appropriate care. The sixth edition of *Fetal and Neonatal Physiology* marks the beginning of a new era in our specialty in which care providers will use genetic information, biomarkers, and big data to make clinical decisions. We are poised to rapidly diagnose and better understand the genetic basis of a variety of diseases affecting newborn infants, including chronic lung disease, necrotizing enterocolitis, retinopathy of prematurity, white matter injury, and sepsis. Whole genome sequencing (WGS) to identify the genetic basis for complex neonatal diseases (and to identify potentially treatable conditions) is becoming a bedside tool and will practically support pharmacogenomics to tailor treatments for neonatal conditions and limit side effects. Indeed, in the next 2 decades we expect WGS to augment newborn screening, providing information not only for NICU care but extending across the life span. In a critically ill infant, repeated RNA sequencing may be needed as a new parameter to monitor changes during the course of the illness. Well done randomized clinical trials will always be necessary to test the hypotheses that a new therapy is better or equivalent to a current therapy. However, success of any clinical trial begins with having a strong physiologic basis for any given intervention, and ensuring the enrollment of well-phenotyped and endotyped subjects will enhance the precision, success, and impact of such studies. Unfortunately, most randomized trials are based upon a best guess or power analysis of sample size and with limited insights into critical differences within the cohort that may affect outcomes. No matter how carefully patients are selected for a trial, underlying biases and physiologic differences will still exist and must be considered a priori. Data unable to demonstrate differences in two treatment arms does not mean an individual patient may not benefit. For precision medicine to be effective, genetic information must become available on a continuous and real-time basis and linked with ongoing assessment of organ function. This concept is not unique to neonatology and has been termed *personalized physiologic medicine* by Can Ince.[1] Dr. Ince has suggested four pillars of personalized physiology: fitness and frailty (to determine physiologic reserve), organ function response to therapy, hemodynamic coherence (assessment of the macro- and micro-circulations to determine appropriate resuscitation), and integration and feedback (which provides ongoing assessments and includes predictive models).

Our specialty is poised to apply these four pillars to neonatal intensive care, and we believe the sixth edition of *Fetal and Neonatal Physiology* will help support this. Most of the 174 chapters in the book have been extensively updated by nearly 400 authors. More than 1500 visual elements—photographs, illustrations, diagrams, charts, tables—are included, and we are pleased to offer over 100 brand new color illustrations and diagrams to illuminate the text. The genetics content has been expanded to include new chapters such as "Pathophysiology of Genetic Neonatal Disease" and "Genetic Variants and Neonatal Disease." Each of the chapters on disease pathophysiology has been extensively revised by leading experts in our specialty.

We want to thank many individuals who made this edition possible, including foremost the chapter authors who not only wrote superb chapters but who also adhered to the tight production schedule. We deeply appreciate the editorial help from two individuals at Elsevier. Mary Hegeler was our content development specialist, without whom we could never have done this revision. She was with us every step of the way and provided invaluable guidance as we moved through the stages of book development. We also wish to thank Sarah Barth at Elsevier who supported the decision to undertake the sixth edition.

Finally, we would like to thank the many readers of *Fetal and Neonatal Physiology*, who provided the stimulus and encouragement to revise the book.

RAP
SHA
WEB
DHR

[1]Ince C. Personalized physiological medicine. *Crit Care* 2017;21:308.

Contents

†Deceased.

SECTION XXIV ENDOCRINE FUNCTION

SECTION XXV OVARY AND TESTIS

SECTION XXVI PATHOPHYSIOLOGY OF NEONATAL DISEASES

Basic Genetic Principles

1

Haluk Kavus | Wendy K. Chung

INTRODUCTION

The human genome refers to the complete set of human DNA (with the suffix -ome arising from the Greek for "all" or "complete"). A copy of our genome comprises approximately 3 billion base pairs (bp) and about 20,000 protein-coding genes. The Human Genome Project was a significant contribution toward understanding the organization, structure, and sequence of the human genome.[1,2] With these developments, *genomic medicine* has emerged as a new discipline to analyze the genome and genetic information as a part of clinical care.

Having in-depth knowledge about the genome and the types and consequences of genomic variations is important for all medical professionals, especially neonatologists. Recognizing the most common chromosomal and monogenic disorders and genetic concepts such as inheritance, genomic imprinting, uniparental disomy (UPD), and X chromosome inactivation can help clinicians understand the origins of genetic conditions and risk of recurrence to patients and their families. Knowing the types of available clinical genomic tests, along with their utility and limitations, is critical for appropriate clinical use. In this chapter, we will also review prenatal diagnosis, clinical physical examination of the dysmorphic child, the future of newborn sequencing, and therapeutic approaches for monogenic diseases.

GENOMIC ORGANIZATION

DNA AND RNA

Deoxyribonucleic acid (DNA) and ribonucleic acid (RNA) are long polymers of nucleotides. Each nucleotide has three elements: (1) a nitrogenous base, (2) a sugar molecule, and (3) a phosphate molecule. The nitrogenous bases fall into two types: purines and pyrimidines. The purines include adenine and guanine; the pyrimidines include cytosine, thymine, and uracil. The primary difference between RNA and DNA is related to a base composition, such that RNA contains uracil, whereas DNA contains thymine. The other difference between RNA and DNA is in their sugar-phosphate backbones: RNA contains ribose, and DNA contains 2-deoxyribose. Deoxyribose confers resistance to hydrolysis, which gives DNA chemical stability, supporting the fidelity of the information as cells divide. While DNA is packaged in chromosomes in the nucleus, RNA carries that message from the nucleus to the cytoplasm, where it is made into proteins.

The double-helix structure of DNA was elucidated in 1953.[3] Hydrogen bonds zip up the complementary strands of DNA in which A pairs with T, and C pairs with G. Because of the complementary sequence of the two strands of DNA, there is redundancy in the information content, increasing the fidelity of the code. Replication of the double-stranded structure of DNA molecules requires a separation of the two strands followed by the synthesis of two new complementary strands. In contrast to DNA, RNA molecules are single-stranded and short-lived.

STRUCTURE OF CHROMOSOMES

Humans usually have 46 chromosomes in 23 pairs: 44 are autosomes, and 2 are the sex chromosomes (X and Y) involved in sex determination. The homologous pairs are numbered from 1 to 22 in order of decreasing size, with one member of each pair inherited from one parent.

Every chromosome consists of a long, single, and continuous DNA molecule located in the nucleus. DNA is packaged as chromatin complexed with histone proteins to condense the DNA into the nucleus. The five major types of histone proteins play a critical role in packaging of the chromatin. Two copies of the four core histones H2A, H2B, H3, and H4 constitute an octamer, around which a segment of DNA winds. A fifth histone, H1, binds to DNA at the tip of each nucleosome. Approximately 140 bp of DNA are linked with each histone core, making just under two turns around the octamer. After a short (20- to 60-bp) "spacer" segment of DNA, the pattern repeats, giving chromatin the look of beads on a string. Each complex of DNA with its core histones is called a *nucleosome*, which is the basic structural unit of chromatin.

Between cell divisions, the chromatin is unwound where genes are being expressed. With cell division, the chromosomes condense and become visible as the structures we observe in a karyotype. Noncoding RNA molecules play an essential role in gene regulation. For example, Xist, a noncoding RNA molecule, is a central regulator of X chromosome inactivation. It coats the inactivated X chromosome, which is structurally condensed, with most (but not all) genes being transcriptionally inactive.[4]

MITOCHONDRIAL GENOME

Mitochondria are organelles within cells that transform the energy from food into a form that cells can use. Each cell contains thousands of mitochondria, each containing several copies of a small circular mitochondrial chromosome. The mitochondrial DNA molecule is 16 kb in length and encodes 37 genes, all of which are fundamental for both normal mitochondrial function and also required for the function of ribosomal and transfer RNA molecules in the mitochondria. Mitochondrial genes are solely inherited from the mother.

STRUCTURE OF GENES

Genes in humans are composed of protein-coding sequences called *exons* and the intervening (noncoding) DNA sequences called *introns* (Fig. 1.1). Introns are initially transcribed into RNA in the nucleus and are spliced out to make the mature mRNA. Therefore, the information from the intronic sequences is not typically represented in the final protein product. Exonic sequences determine the amino acid sequence of the protein. Most genes contain at least one and usually numerous introns. The total length of the introns makes up a far greater proportion of a gene's total length for most genes. Genes are also flanked by additional sequences that are transcribed but untranslated, known as the 5′ and 3′ untranslated regions, which play a role in RNA stability and gene expression.

The human genome contains noncoding DNA sequences that act as *regulatory elements*. These sequences include promoters, enhancers, silencers, and locus control regions. They coordinate the regulation of genes in space and time. They include sequences for proteins called *transcription factors* to bind to and either increase or repress transcription. Promoter regions are responsible for the initiation of transcription and are typically found 5′ or upstream of a gene. Enhancers and silencers can be located either 5′ or 3′ of a gene, within the introns or sometimes farther away in neighboring genes. Promoters are binding sites for proteins that increase or repress transcription. Besides genes that are transcribed and made into proteins, there are genes known as non-coding RNAs (ncRNAs), whose functional product is RNA. Some ncRNAs can be quite long (long ncRNAs or lncRNAs) and play roles in gene regulation.[5] There are also small non-coding RNAs, known as *short interfering RNAs (siRNAs)* and *microRNAs (miRNAs)*, that control gene expression. MicroRNAs are short, non-coding RNAs, approximately 22 nucleotides in length, which post-transcriptionally regulate mRNA expression,[6] usually by decreasing expression. siRNAs are homologous to specific mRNAs and degrade the mRNA to decrease the expression of the target gene.

More than half of the human genome consists of various types of repeat sequences that are either clustered together or evenly distributed throughout the genome. These sequences can be short and consist of only a few nucleotides or can be as long as 5000 to 6000 nucleotides. The two best-studied dispersed repetitive elements are the Alu family and the long interspersed nuclear element (LINE) family. The Alu family makes up at least 10% of human DNA, and the LINE family accounts for nearly 20% of the genome. Segmental duplications are another repeat and are highly conserved and make up 5% of the human genome. When these duplicated sequences include genes, structural rearrangements can cause genetic diseases.

CELL DIVISION

Transmission of the genetic information from one generation to the next relies on accurate replication of DNA during reproduction. *Mitosis* is used during somatic cell division to support the development and cellular differentiation. In mitotic division, the usual complement of 46 chromosomes is maintained through a process of DNA replication and subsequent separation of the chromosomes. In contrast, *meiosis* occurs only in cells that become gametes, each of which has only 23 chromosomes (haploid genome). Thus errors in cell division in either somatic or germline cells can cause abnormalities of chromosome number or structure that can be clinically significant.

MOSAICISM

Mosaicism is the presence of at least two cell populations derived from the same zygote. Mitotic nondisjunction, trisomy rescue, or occurrence of a somatic new mutation can lead to the development of genetically different cell lines within the body. Mosaicism can affect any cells or tissue within a developing embryo at any point after conception to adulthood. If the mosaic cells are found only in the placenta and absent in the embryo, this known as *confined placental mosaicism (CPM)* (Fig. 1.2A).[7] CPM may be detectable on a chorionic villus sample and may be associated with intrauterine growth restriction but not with congenital anomalies or neurodevelopmental disorders if the genetic anomaly is not present in the fetus. Somatic mosaicism is the presence of two or more cell lineages in tissues that may have a clinically observable phenotype in the part of the body with the genetic aberration (see Fig. 1.2B). In gonadal mosaicism, the mosaic cells are restricted to the gametes and do not have a clinically observable phenotype but can be passed onto the next generation.

MEIOSIS

Meiosis is the process by which gametes are formed. In contrast with mitosis, in which a single cell division and an exact duplication of the genetic material occurs, meiosis involves two cell divisions, starting with a diploid parental cell and random reassortment and reduction of genetic material so that each of the four daughter cells has the haploid DNA content (i.e., 23 chromosomes). In this way, meiosis yields four haploid gametes (sperm or eggs). In female meiosis, the second meiotic division is completed only after fertilization, and advancing maternal age is associated with nondisjunction of the chromosomes. A polar body, containing a complete set of chromosomes, is extruded, leaving the egg with a single remaining haploid set of chromosomes. The second polar body is useful for preimplantation genetic diagnosis.

RECOMBINATION

During the prophase of the first meiotic division, homologous pairs of chromosomes are held together by the synaptonemal complex, which extends along the entire length of the paired chromosomes. Recombination between chromatids of the homologous chromosomes occurs at this stage, resulting in the exchange of DNA between the original parental chromosomes (Fig. 1.3). In males, the X and Y chromosomes are physically associated only at the tips of their short arms during meiotic prophase. This short region is called the *pseudoautosomal* region because recombination between the X and Y chromosomes occurs there (and thus it behaves as an autosome in terms of Mendelian inheritance). Recombination

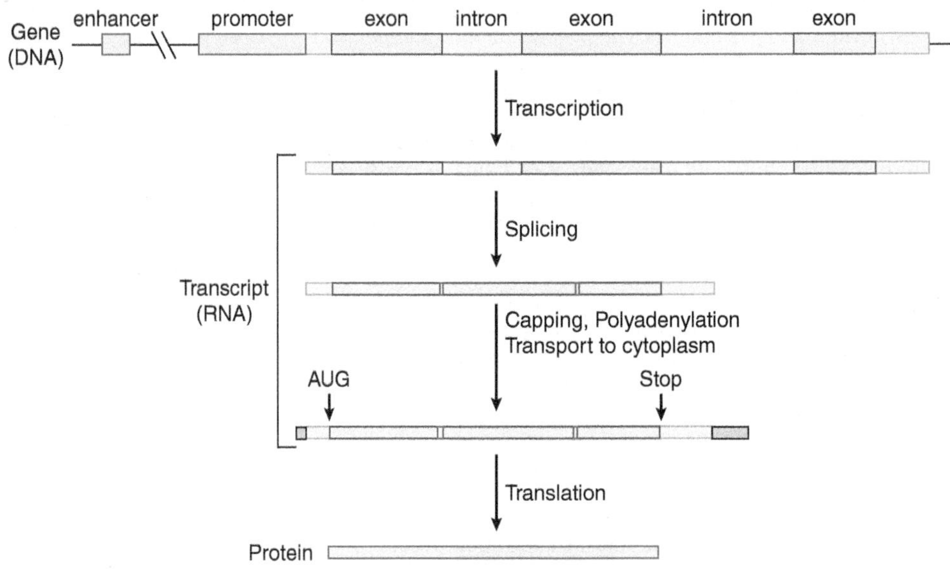

Fig. 1.1 Gene structure *(top)* and the flow of genetic information from DNA to protein. Tan boxes indicate the regions of exons that do not encode amino acid sequences; gray boxes indicate posttranscriptional modifications. AUG is a codon that specifies the amino acid methionine and is also used to specify the first amino acid of a protein.

involves the exchange of genetic material between the two homologs during meiosis I, and it is also critical for proper chromosome segregation during meiosis. Failure to recombine correctly can lead to nondisjunction of the chromosomes in meiosis I and is a frequent cause of aneuploidy (incorrect chromosome number) leading to pregnancy loss and congenital anomalies.

HOW GENES FUNCTION

FLOW OF GENETIC INFORMATION

TRANSCRIPTION

The first step in gene expression is the production of an RNA molecule from the DNA template. The RNA acts as a molecular messenger, carrying the genetic information out of the nucleus to the cytoplasm. The synthesis of mRNA is called *transcription* because the genetic information in DNA is transcribed. During transcription, the two DNA strands separate, and one functions as a template for the synthesis of single-stranded RNA molecules by RNA polymerases. The initial RNA transcripts are quite long because they include both introns and exons from the gene. The intronic sequences are cut out, and the remaining exons are spliced together. To form the mature mRNAs that leave the nucleus, a methylated guanine nucleotide called a *cap* is added to the 5′ end, and a string of 200 to 250 adenine (polyA tail) bases is added to the 3′ end. The cap is necessary for ribosomal binding to initiate protein synthesis, and the polyadenosine stretch at the 3′ end increases the stability of the mRNA.

Transcriptional control is central for the development and proper functioning of every organism. Transcriptional regulation is accomplished by modifying the DNA (e.g., cytosine methylation) or by protein binding to specific DNA sequences to activate or repress transcription of a gene. There are many sequence-specific transcription factors that are differentially active by cellular and tissue type and time in development. Several regulatory sequences have been identified in promoters that are important for transcriptional initiation by RNA polymerase II, including the TATA box, so-called because it consists of a run of T and A base pairs. The TATA box is located approximately 30 bases before the transcription start site and functions as the binding site for a large, multisubunit complex of transcription factors (including RNA polymerase). A second conserved region, the so-called *CAT box*, is a few dozen base pairs farther upstream. Specific sequence elements that form promoters and enhancers are required for binding the ~1400 sequence-specific proteins that bind to DNA and regulate transcription. Mutations in these regulatory sequence elements can lead to significant alterations in transcription and also can lead to genetic disorders.

The boundary between the introns and exons consists of a 5′ donor GT dinucleotide and a 3′ acceptor AG dinucleotide. Besides the canonical splice sequences, there are also splicing regulatory elements such as exonic splicing enhancers (ESEs) and exonic splicing silencers (ESSs). ESEs and ESSs correspond to six to eight nucleotides that serve as docking sites for splicing activator or splicing repressor proteins, thereby influencing the recruitment and activity of the splicing machinery.[8] Most human genes undergo alternative splicing and hence encode more than one protein for each gene. Alternative polyadenylation creates further diversity. Some genes have more than one promoter, and these alternative promoters may result in tissue-specific isoforms. Alternative splicing of exons is also seen with individual exons present in only some isoforms.

TRANSLATION

The production of protein from a mRNA template is called *translation* because the genetic information that is encoded in DNA is translated into a sequence of amino acids in the protein. The genetic information is stored in the genetic code. Each of the three adjacent nucleotides is a unit of information called a *codon* and specifies an amino acid or the start or stop of translation. The linear codons in the DNA sequence specify the sequence of amino acids in a protein. Because each of the three sites in a codon can be one of four possible nucleotides, a total of 4^3, or 64, different codons are possible. Three of these 64 possible codons, UAA, UAG, and UGA, are called *termination codons*. The remaining 61 codons specify one of the 20 amino acids, leading to some degeneracy in coding certain amino acids. A consequence of degeneracy is that some DNA variants do not result in a change in the amino acid sequence (synonymous variants).

EPIGENETICS

In addition to the classic transcription factors that bind to specific sequence elements in genes, gene expression is controlled by enzymes that modify DNA-bound proteins and DNA itself. The

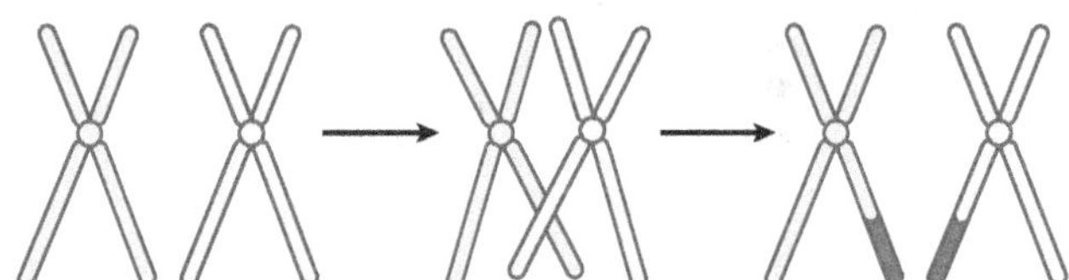

Fig. 1.3 Recombination. In this simplified view of recombination, the two members of a homologous pair of chromosomes line up during the first meiotic prophase. Segments of the two chromosomes "cross over," and breakage and rejoining of the DNA strands occur.

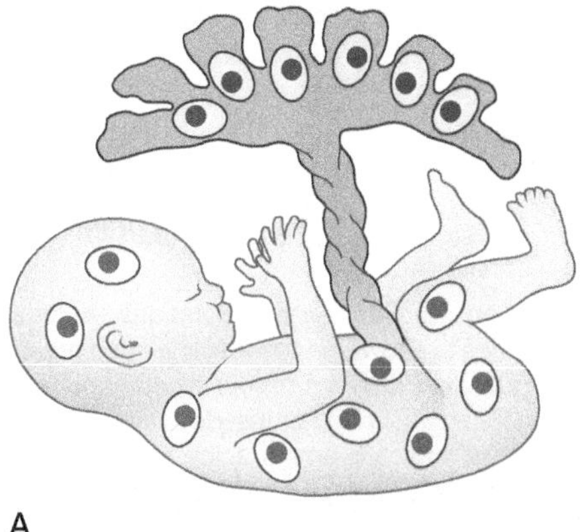

A

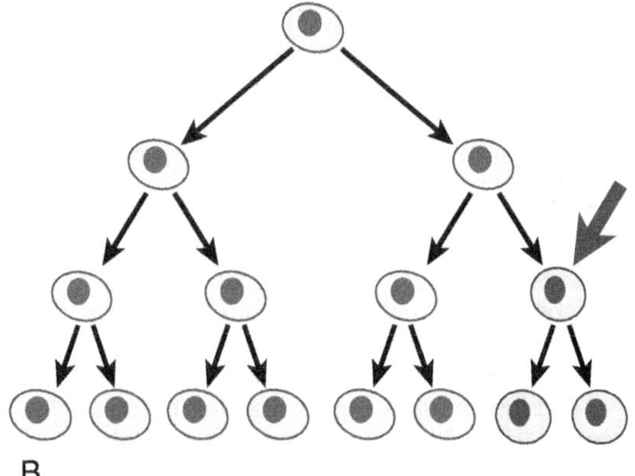

B

Fig. 1.2 Mosaicism. (A) Confined placental mosaicism. Presence of mutant cells only in the placental tissue, not in the fetus. (B) Somatic mosaicism. Presence of two or more mutant cell lineages in tissues and may have a clinically observable phenotype in the part of the body with the genetic aberration.

principal mechanism by which DNA is modified is by methylation of cytosine residues adjacent to guanosine. Methylation of these CpG dinucleotides by DNA methylases leads to transcriptional inactivation, while demethylation by demethylases alters the conformation of chromatin, leading to transcriptional activation. Histone proteins are extensively modified by many enzymes, including acetylases, kinases, and methylases. The pattern of histone modification, particularly on lysine residues, controls whether a particular region of chromatin will be transcriptionally active or inactive.

Modifications of chromatin proteins and DNA can be inherited through multiple cell divisions. Such alterations that do not change the DNA sequence itself and are called *epigenetic*. Genetic diseases that affect this process exemplify the importance of epigenetics. For example, mutations in MeCP2, a protein that binds to methylated DNA to repress the expression of associated genes, cause Rett syndrome, an X-linked neurodegenerative disease. Rubinstein-Taybi syndrome is caused by mutations in the CBP gene, encoding CREB-binding protein, which acts to acetylate the histone proteins that are major components of chromatin.

GENETIC VARIATION

A *locus* is a particular position on a chromosome for a specific gene and related DNA elements. *Alleles* refer to an alternative version of the DNA sequence at a locus. Generally, one of the alternative alleles is found in more than half of the population and is called is the *major allele*. The other versions of that gene refer to variants or minor alleles. Allele frequencies vary significantly in different populations. If an allele frequency is greater than 1%, it is said to be a *polymorphism* (multiple forms).

Mutation is generally meant to signify a DNA sequence that is deleterious and associated with a human disease. Mutations can be germline and inherited from one or both parents, or somatic and acquired over the life of an individual. Mutations can vary by the size of the altered DNA sequence. The size of mutations can range from a single nucleotide to the rearrangements of an entire chromosome. By convention, we have a reference genome that is used to compare genetic variants. This reference genome is updated as we understand the human genome better.

SINGLE NUCLEOTIDE VARIATIONS

When a "point mutation" of one or a small number of nucleotides occurs in a part of the gene that codes for a protein and alters the protein by changing the codon of which it is a part, it is called a ***nonsynonymous variant*** (Fig. 1.4A). Because the genetic code is degenerate, it is possible to have a point mutation that does not change the amino acid that is encoded. This is called a *synonymous variant*. Insertion or deletion of a nucleotide in the protein-coding portion of a gene is called a *frameshift mutation* because it changes the entire reading frame of the gene at every codon distal to the site of the mutation. *Nonsense mutations* are those point mutations that result in one of the three codons (UAA, UAG, UGA) that do not code for amino acids but rather truncate proteins, often producing proteins with little or no activity if they occur early enough in the protein. Point mutations occurring at the boundaries between introns and exons can cause improper splicing of RNA precursors, resulting in aberrant splicing or RNA instability.

Regulation of gene expression can be affected by mutations occurring in control elements, such as promoters and enhancers; the effect of such mutations is to quantitatively affect the amount of protein produced, such as occurs in some forms of thalassemia.

A different mutational mechanism involves the expansion of triplet repeat sequences *(dynamic mutations)*, caused by an increase in the number of copies of triplet repeats in the coding or noncoding region of a gene. These disorders include myotonic dystrophy, fragile X syndrome, and Huntington disease. The repeat size can increase with successive generations, and as the repeat number increases, the age of onset of the disease decreases, giving rise to the phenomenon of *anticipation*.

HOW MANY MENDELIAN CONDITIONS ARE THERE?

There are 8319 Mendelian phenotypes described. A total of 5489 of them (66%) have an associated known underlying gene. A total of 20% (3912/19,580) of human genes are known to underlie a Mendelian phenotype.[9] This information is curated in Online Mendelian Inheritance in Man (OMIM),[10] which is a continuation of Mendelian Inheritance in Man (MIM), published between 1966 and 1998.

CHROMOSOMAL MUTATIONS

Mutations in chromosome structure include deletions, duplications, inversions, and translocations. Because chromosomal alterations usually result in the disruption of multiple genes, they often have profound clinical consequences that include more than one organ system (see Fig. 1.4B).

If the total amount of genetic material is normal (just simply rearranged), then the karyotype is *balanced*. A *deletion* is the loss of a part of a chromosome and results in monosomy for that segment of the chromosome. An *insertion* is the addition of a segment of DNA into a chromosome. An insertion is often associated with an *unbalanced* chromosome complement. An *inversion* is a two-break rearrangement involving a single

A. Single-Gene Mutations

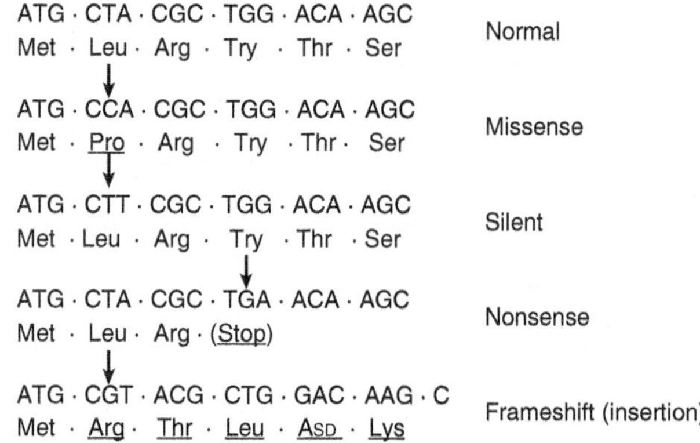

B. Chromosomal Mutations

Normal Deletions Duplication Inversions Translocation

Fig. 1.4 Mutation. (A) Single-gene mutations. A prototypical normal gene sequence is shown on the first line, with the corresponding amino acid sequence. Examples of four types of common mutations also are shown. The substituted or inserted nucleotides are indicated by arrows, and the affected amino acids are underlined. (B) Chromosomal mutations. A prototype normal chromosome is shown, with genes A through H. Examples of gross chromosomal mutations are shown to the right, and their effects on gene content and arrangement are indicated. In the translocation example, the two chromosomes are not members of a homologous pair.

chromosome in which a segment is flipped and reversed in position. If the inversion segment includes the centromere, it is termed a *pericentric inversion*. If it involves only one arm of the chromosome and does not involve the centromere, it is known as a *paracentric inversion*. A *translocation* refers to the transfer of genetic material from one chromosome to another. If two different chromosome breaks and the chromosome segments are exchanged, it is called a *reciprocal translocation*. If the translocation occurs between two acrocentric chromosomes or chromosomes with redundant genetic material on the p arm, it is called a *Robertsonian translocation*. Similar to inversions, translocations can be balanced or unbalanced. Individuals who carry translocations but who have a normal amount of genetic material are called *balanced translocation carriers*. Translocations can have severe effects on offspring if the progeny has an unbalanced complement. When counseling a carrier of a balanced reciprocal translocation or Robertsonian translocation, it is necessary to consider the particular rearrangement to determine what the probability is that it could result in the birth of an abnormal baby. Translocation carriers are at increased risk of miscarriage of unbalanced products of conception.

A *ring chromosome* is formed when a break occurs on each arm of a chromosome leaving two "sticky" ends on the central portion of the chromosome that reunite as a ring. The two distal chromosomal fragments are lost, so if the involved chromosome is an autosome, the effects are usually severe.

Structural variant (SV) refers to genomic rearrangements and includes deletions, insertions, inversions, duplications, and translocations. *Copy number variation* (CNV) describes a group of DNA sequence variants (including deletions and duplications) that result in an abnormal number of copies of segments of DNA.[11]

GENETIC DISORDERS

CHROMOSOMAL DISORDERS

Chromosome disorders compose an important category of genetic disease, occurring in approximately 1 out of every 150 live births.[12] They are a common cause of intellectual disability and pregnancy loss. Chromosomal disorders can be divided into two groups: numerical and structural abnormalities. Numerical abnormalities result from one or more chromosome gains or losses, referred to as an *aneuploidy* (e.g., trisomy, monosomy, tetrasomy) or the addition of one or more complete haploid genomes, referred to as *polyploidy* (e.g., triploidy, tetraploidy).

In addition to the loss or gain of whole chromosomes, parts of chromosomes can be lost or duplicated as gametes are formed, and the arrangement of portions of chromosomes can be altered. Structural chromosome abnormalities may be unbalanced (the rearrangement causes a gain or loss of chromosomal material) or balanced (the rearrangement does not produce a loss or gain of chromosome material). Molecular methods including chromosome microarrays are often helpful to sensitively detect gains, losses, and rearrangements that may be missed by standard karyotype alone. Unlike aneuploidy and polyploidy, balanced structural abnormalities less frequently produce serious health consequences, and many are compatible with normal health and behavior. However, unbalanced abnormalities of chromosome structure and even some that are balanced but that disrupt key genes can create severe disease in individuals or their offspring. The phenotype associated with the chromosome disorder tends to run true in the family when inherited, so testing the parents to determine if a chromosome disorder is inherited or de novo is often recommended by a geneticist. Some structural alterations can be caused by translocations (reciprocal or Robertsonian), insertion, deletion, or rearrangement of DNA sequences, so examination of the parents of a child with a complex rearrangement may be helpful in predicting recurrence risk for the parents. Some deletions and insertions involve only a few nucleotides and are generally most easily detected by sequencing the relevant part of the genome. In other cases, a large segment of a gene, an entire gene, or several adjacent genes are deleted, duplicated, inverted, or translocated and create a novel arrangement. Depending on the exact nature of the deletion, insertion, or rearrangement, a variety of different laboratory approaches can be used to detect the genomic alteration, including karyotype, fluorescent in situ hybridization (FISH), chromosome microarray, or sequencing methods.

ANEUPLOIDY

Aneuploidy refers to missing or additional individual chromosomes in the cell (a number other than 46 chromosomes). Aneuploidies of chromosomes 13, 18, and 21 are among the most clinically important of the chromosome abnormalities. They consist of monosomy (the presence of only one copy of a chromosome in an otherwise diploid cell) and trisomy (three copies of a chromosome). Nondisjunction causes errors in chromosome segregation and leads to aneuploidies. Multiple congenital anomalies, growth restriction, and intellectual disability are the most common phenotypes of these trisomies.

Nevertheless, each has a reasonably unique neonatal phenotype that is recognizable by an experienced clinician. Trisomy 13 and 18 are both less common than trisomy 21, and survival beyond the first year is rare for trisomy 13 and 18. In contrast, individuals with Down syndrome have a life expectancy of over 50 years. Most other autosomal trisomies result in early pregnancy loss, with trisomy 16 being a particularly common finding in first-trimester spontaneous miscarriages.

Trisomy 21, which causes Down syndrome, is the most common autosomal aneuploidy seen among live births. The most common features include intellectual disability, hypotonia, gastrointestinal obstruction, congenital heart defects, and dysmorphic facial features. In approximately 90% of cases, the third chromosome 21 is of maternal origin. About 95% of Down syndrome cases are caused by nondisjunction, and Robertsonian translocations cause most of the remaining cases. Mosaicism is seen in 2% to 4% of Down syndrome cases and is often associated with a milder phenotype. The most frequent cause of mosaicism in trisomies is a trisomic conception followed by loss of the extra chromosome during mitosis in some embryonic cells (trisomic rescue).

Trisomy 13 and 18 are sometimes compatible with survival to term, although 95% or more of affected fetuses are spontaneously aborted. These trisomies produce more severe disease than trisomy 21, with 90% to 95% mortality during the first year of life.

Turner syndrome is most commonly associated with 45, X. Although this disorder is common at conception, it is relatively rare among live births, reflecting a high rate of spontaneous abortion. Mosaicism, including confined placental mosaicism, appears to increase the probability of survival to term. Klinefelter syndrome occurs in men who receive two X chromosomes in addition to the Y chromosome. The presence of an extra sex chromosome (X or Y) has only mild phenotypic effects.

GENOMIC DISORDERS (MICRODELETION AND DUPLICATION SYNDROMES, STRUCTURAL VARIATIONS, COPY NUMBER VARIATIONS)

Chromosomal deletions and duplications are an important cause of human malformations and intellectual disability. Those caused by submicroscopic changes were not easily detectable with a standard karyotype (with a resolution of approximately 5 to 10 Mb). With the advent of high-resolution banding, it has become feasible to identify smaller deletions. Advances in molecular genetics, mainly the FISH and chromosome microarray techniques, have permitted the detection of deletions that are often too small to be observed microscopically (i.e., <5 Mb).

Because these syndromes generally involve the deletion or duplication of a series of adjacent genes, it is sometimes referred to as a *contiguous gene syndrome*. Recent studies show that this is caused by the presence of flanking repeat sequences, termed *low-copy repeats* (also termed *segmental duplications*), at the deletion borders. These repeat sequences favor unequal crossing-over, which then produces duplications and deletions of the region bounded by the repeat elements. These disorders are collectively called *genomic disorders*.[13]

Some of well-known genomic disorders and their associated clinical features are shown in Table 1.1.

GENOMIC IMPRINTING

There are regions of the genome with parent-of-origin effects as a result of genomic imprinting. *Genomic imprinting* is an epigenetic term describing monoallelic gene expression according to parental origin. This epigenetic "mark" or imprint affects the chromatin structures and silences expression of the gene/gene(s) that are imprinted. The imprint is maintained throughout the life of the organism, in virtually all tissues; however, germ cells erase and then reset imprints for transmission to the next generation. Imprinting disorders can be caused by:

(a) sequence mutation of the relevant gene (*UBE3A* for Angelman syndrome),
(b) deletion or duplication of imprinted genes,
(c) UPD, or
(d) epigenetic errors in imprinting centers causing faulty imprinting.

Prader-Willi syndrome, Angelman syndrome, and Beckwith-Wiedemann syndrome are the best-studied examples of the role of genomic imprinting in human disease.

Table 1.1 Examples of Microdeletion Syndromes.

Syndrome	Chromosomal Locus	Major Clinical Features
Deletion 1p36 Syndrome	1p36	Intellectual disability, seizures, hearing loss, heart defects, growth failure, behavioral symptoms
Wolf-Hirschhorn Syndrome	4p16.3	Pre- and postnatal growth failure, iris coloboma, seizure, microcephaly
Cri-du-chat Syndrome	5p	High-pitched cat-like cry, microcephaly, hypotonia, developmental delay, low-set ears
Williams-Beuren Syndrome	7q11.23	Supravalvular aortic stenosis, hypercalcemia, periorbital fullness, thick lips, friendly personality
WAGR Syndrome	11p13	Wilms tumor, aniridia, genitourinary abnormalities, intellectual disability, obesity
Prader-Willi Syndrome	15q11–q13	Intellectual disability, short stature, obesity, hypotonia, characteristic facies, small feet
Angelman Syndrome	15q11–q13	Intellectual disability, ataxia, behavioral abnormalities, seizures, hypotonia, wide-based gait
Rubinstein-Taybi Syndrome	16p13.3	Intellectual disability, broad thumbs and great toes, vertebral and sternal abnormalities, heart defects
Smith-Magenis Syndrome	17p11.2	Intellectual disability, hyperactivity, dysmorphic features, self-destructive behavior
Miller-Dieker Syndrome	17p13.3	Lissencephaly, microcephaly, seizures, growth retardation, facial dysmorphism, early death
DiGeorge/VCF Syndrome	22q11.2	Characteristic facies, cleft palate, heart defects, hypocalcemia, thymic hypoplasia

UNIPARENTAL DISOMY

Uniparental disomy (UPD) refers to the presence of a disomic cell line containing two chromosomes that are inherited from only one parent, rather than one chromosome being inherited from the mother and the other from the father. If the disomic chromosomes are received from identical sister chromatids, it is called *isodisomy* (the same copy of two chromosomes); if both homologs come from one parent, the situation is *heterodisomy*.

Trisomy rescue is the mechanism of loss of a chromosome that restores a disomic state and escape from trisomy. If it happens, the resulting cell might show UPD.

If UPD occurs and includes a chromosome with an imprinted region such as chromosome 15, this may cause disease. For example, Angelman syndrome is due to mutations/deletions in the maternally expressed gene *UBE3A* or paternal UPD 15, such that there is no functional UBE3A allele, as the maternal allele is missing. Angelman syndrome can also be due to epigenetic modifications of the imprinting center on chromosome 15q11, which results in the loss of expression of UBE3A.

SEX CHROMOSOME ABNORMALITIES

Sex chromosome aneuploidies are common and may not be diagnosed for decades, if ever. Males with Klinefelter syndrome (47, XXY) are taller than average, may have slightly reduced IQ, and are usually infertile. The 47, XXX and 47, XYY karyotypes are present in about 1/1000 female and male births, respectively. Each involves a slight reduction in IQ and potentially behavioral issues, including attention deficit hyperactivity disorder, but are associated with few physical or medical problems.

X INACTIVATION

The principle of *X inactivation* is that in somatic cells in normal females (but not in normal males), one X chromosome is inactivated early in development, thus equalizing the expression of X-linked genes in the two sexes. In normal female development, because the choice of which X chromosome is to be inactivated is random and then clonally maintained, females are mosaic with respect to X-linked gene expression. In patients with extra X chromosomes (whether male or female), additional X chromosomes are randomly inactivated, leaving only one active X per cell. Thus all diploid somatic cells in both males and females have a single active X chromosome, regardless of the total number of X or Y chromosomes present.

The X chromosome contains approximately 1000 genes, but not all of them are subject to inactivation. Notably, the genes that continue to be expressed from the inactive X are not distributed randomly along the X chromosome. Many of the genes that "escape" inactivation are on distal Xp (as many as 50%) rather than on Xq (just a few percent). This finding has important implications for genetic counseling in cases of a partial X chromosome aneuploidy, because imbalance for genes on Xp may have greater clinical significance than imbalance for genes on Xq, where the effect is mostly normalized by X inactivation.

SINGLE-GENE DISORDERS

A trait or disorder that is determined by a gene on an autosome is said to show *autosomal inheritance*, whereas a trait or disorder determined by a gene on one of the sex chromosomes is said to show *sex-linked inheritance*. For autosomal loci, the genotype of a person at a locus consists of both of the alleles occupying that locus on the two homologous chromosomes. If two alleles are the same for a particular locus, the genotype is *homozygous*. When the alleles are different, and one of the alleles is the reference allele (common variant in the population), it is called *heterozygous*. If the two alleles are different and neither is the reference allele, it is called *compound heterozygote*. The term *hemizygous* refers to one abnormal allele located on the X chromosome in a male. Mitochondrial loci are present in thousands of copies per cell; thus the terms mentioned herein are not used to describe mitochondrial genotypes.

There are two types of genetic heterogeneity. *Allelic heterogeneity* is when many different mutations in one gene cause similar phenotypes. *Locus heterogeneity* is when mutations in several different genes all cause a similar phenotype. *Phenotype* is the expression of genotype as a morphologic, clinical, cellular, or biochemical trait, which may be clinically observable or may only be detected by blood or tissue testing. The phenotype can be discrete or can be a measured quantity, such as body mass index or blood glucose levels.

AUTOSOMAL DOMINANT DISORDERS

Autosomal dominant (AD) disorders manifest in heterozygous individuals who have a single copy of the mutant allele. Many molecular mechanisms are associated with AD inheritance, including haploinsufficiency (loss of function of one amorphic allele), hypomorphic alleles with decreased function, hypermorphic alleles exhibiting gain of function (constitutive protein activity), neomorphic alleles that acquire a new function (such as altered substrate specificity), and toxic (antimorphic) effects of a protein, leading to dominant-negative (DN) mechanisms (Fig. 1.5A).

Principles of Autosomal Dominant Inheritance

- Males and females are affected equally.
- Males and females can both transmit the disorder.
- There is a 50% risk to offspring in any pregnancy in which one parent carries a mutation.
- The severity of the disorder in the offspring may vary, being similar, more severe, or less severe than in the parent.
- Many AD disorders are due to de novo mutations.

Dominant diseases show the same phenotype in either the heterozygous or homozygous state. The majority of AD disorders are incompletely dominant or semidominant, which means homozygous individuals have a more severe phenotype than heterozygous individuals. In codominant inheritance, both alleles are phenotypically expressed (e.g., ABO blood group).

Penetrance is the percentage of individuals who carry the relevant genotype and have signs or symptoms of the disorder. If all individuals who have a disease genotype show the disease phenotype, then the disease is said to be "fully penetrant," or to have a penetrance of 100%. Many dominant disorders show age-dependent penetrance. Some conditions show incomplete penetrance (i.e., not all mutation carriers will manifest the disease during a natural lifespan).

Expressivity is the difference in the severity of a disorder in individuals who have inherited the same disease alleles. Many genetic conditions show a striking difference between families (interfamilial variation) and also within families carrying the same mutation (intrafamilial variation). Pleiotropy is when a mutation in a single gene has effects on the body in more than one way (e.g., congenital heart disease and intellectual disability).

The proportion of cases resulting from new (de novo) mutations varies considerably between different AD conditions. In some disorders, the de novo mutation rate is high (nearly 100% of cases), whereas for some other conditions, a new mutation is unusual.

In many AD disorders, reproductive fitness is zero, (i.e., mutation carriers do not reproduce). Such a condition is maintained in the population entirely by new mutations, and the majority of cases are due to de novo mutations (although parental germline mosaicism may sometimes lead to recurrence in a sibling). Many other AD disorders have only modest effects on reproductive fitness.

AUTOSOMAL RECESSIVE DISORDERS

Autosomal recessive (AR) conditions occur when the mutant allele is present in both copies of the gene. Heterozygous individuals are said to be *carriers* for that condition and are asymptomatic (see Fig. 1.5B).

Principles of Autosomal Recessive Inheritance

- Disease is expressed only in homozygotes and compound heterozygotes.
- Parents are obligate carriers.
- Risk to carrier parents for having an affected child is 1 in 4.
- Healthy siblings of affected individuals have a two-thirds risk of being a carrier.
- Males and females are affected equally.

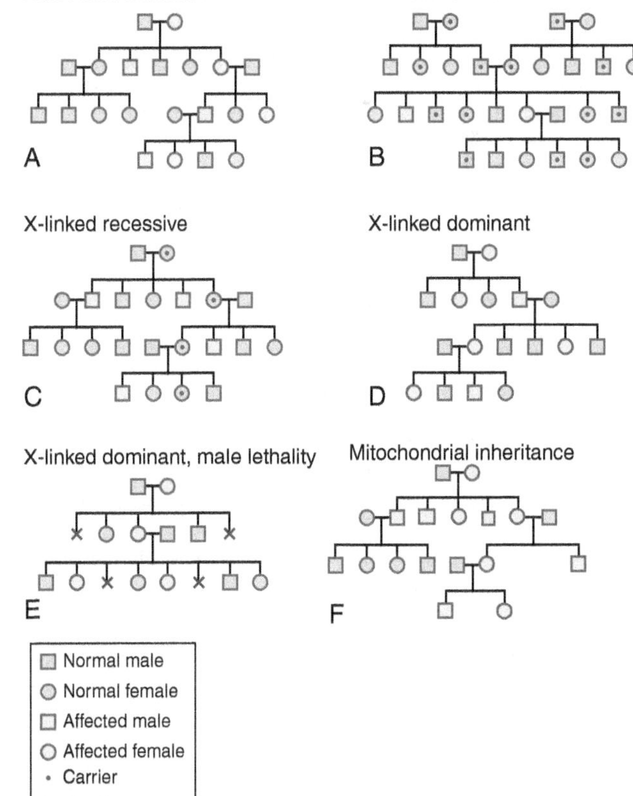

Fig. 1.5 (A–F) Pedigrees for disorders exhibiting the various mendelian and mitochondrial modes of inheritance. These are idealized pedigrees, assuming full penetrance and no new mutations.

Consanguinity is a significant risk factor for AR disorders. The *founder effect* is often responsible for a higher prevalence of a recessive genetic disorder in an isolated population, because multiple individuals of the population are descended from a common ancestor who carried a disease-causing mutation.

X-LINKED RECESSIVE DISORDERS

Principles of X-Linked Recessive Inheritance

See Fig. 1.5C.

- Males carrying the mutation are more severely affected; females carrying the mutation are generally either unaffected or more mildly affected than males, and severity in females depends on the X-inactivation pattern.
- When a carrier female conceives, there are four possible outcomes, each equally likely: a normal daughter, a carrier daughter, a normal son, and an affected son.
- The pedigree shows no male-to-male transmission.
- An affected male transmits the mutation to all his daughters.

X-LINKED DOMINANT DISORDERS

Principles of X-Linked Dominant Inheritance

See Fig. 1.5D.

- Males carrying the mutation are severely affected, often leading to spontaneous pregnancy loss or neonatal death of affected males (see Fig. 1.5E).
- Female heterozygotes are affected but have less severe features than males. X-inactivation patterns determine the degree to which females express the disorder.
- When a heterozygous affected female conceives, there are four genetic possibilities at conception, each equally likely: a normal daughter, an affected daughter, a normal son, and an affected son.
- The pedigree shows no male-to-male transmission.
- When an affected male has a child, all of his daughters will inherit the mutation, and none of his sons will be affected (unless their mother is a carrier).
- Males who are born with features of a severe and usually lethal XLD condition might have Klinefelter syndrome or an additional X chromosome disorder.
- Females with unusually severe features of an XLD disorder may have this as a consequence of:
  - unfavorably X-inactivation,
  - Turner syndrome (45,X), or
  - X-autosome translocation.

MITOCHONDRIAL DISORDERS

PRINCIPLES OF MITOCHONDRIAL INHERITANCE

See Fig. 1.5F

- The condition can only be transmitted by females in the maternal line.
- Males do not transmit mitochondrial inherited disorders, with extremely rare exceptions.
- A mitochondrial inherited condition can affect either sex.
- If the mother is heteroplasmic for a mutation, the proportion of mutant mtDNA in her offspring can vary considerably between offspring and between tissues in the same offspring.

MULTIFACTORIAL DISORDERS

If mutations in two different genes are necessary to cause a phenotype, the inheritance is *digenic*. If a disease is the result of contributions on a few genes, it is *oligogenic*. If a disease is the result of the combination of many genes, it is *polygenic*. If a disease is the result of the combination of many genes and the environment, it is *multifactorial*.

GENETIC DIAGNOSIS

VALUE OF A DIAGNOSIS AND NEED FOR A DIAGNOSIS

Genetic disorders can be classified as Mendelian (monogenic), oligogenic, chromosomal, and multifactorial. In this section, we will limit ourselves to rare diseases. Rare diseases are described as those that affect fewer than 200,000 people in the United States. There are more than 7,000 rare diseases, approximately 80% of which are thought to have a genetic cause.[10] The majority (50% to 75%) of rare diseases affect children.[14] Making an accurate diagnosis is fundamental to good patient care. Molecular diagnoses for patients with rare disorders are important for patients and their families to refine prognosis, management, recurrence risk, and reproductive options; identify other families with the same condition; and participate in research for new sources of support and therapies.[15] It is important to diagnose rare diseases early in the disease course, when the medical and financial burdens to families are fairly minimal, and then proceed with treatment.[16] Increasingly, genomic diagnostic methods are more comprehensive and support more facile diagnoses of genetic conditions.

CLINICAL APPROACH TO CONGENITAL ANOMALIES AND THE DYSMORPHIC CHILD

Dysmorphology is the study of congenital anomalies and developmental disorders. The term is used to describe visible malformations or distinctive structural features of the face or other parts of the body.

A clinical geneticist is often consulted for one or more of the following reasons:

- to examine the patient, gather the clinical and familial information, and plan the genetic tests to order and interpret to make a diagnosis;
- to interpret an existing genetic test result, particularly one that is not definitive;
- to discuss the genetic basis of the condition with the family;
- to recommend studies to evaluate for disease manifestations once a genetic diagnosis is made;
- to consult on the prognosis, management, and therapeutic options;
- to discuss the risk of recurrence and reproductive options;
- to coordinate prenatal/preimplantation genetic testing; and
- to discuss genetic test results with other members of the extended family and arrange for genetic testing for relatives.

PHYSICAL EXAMINATION, FAMILY HISTORY, AND PEDIGREE INFORMATION

A genetic consultation differs in the ability to examine the patient in the prenatal versus neonatal timeframe. In this section, we will focus on how a clinical geneticist evaluates a child. Although the same strategy applies to the prenatal setting, there is less clinical data available in the prenatal setting because the physical examination is limited to ultrasound and magnetic resonance images, and because blood samples cannot be readily obtained.

A genetic consultation includes a review of medical records; interviews with the family to review prenatal exposures; a three-generation family history, including ancestry and any history of consanguinity; and physical examination of the child and, in some cases, the parents. The geneticist will develop a differential diagnosis and order appropriate genetic tests to evaluate the possible conditions. This usually requires a biologic sample from the fetus/neonate and may require samples from the parents for comparison. The genetic testing may yield a definitive diagnosis or, in some cases, will suggest a possible diagnosis for which the geneticist must reassess the patient and determine whether the diagnosis fits the phenotype. If the test does not yield a diagnosis, continued follow-up is important because additional clinical features may become apparent over time and aid in making the diagnosis; in addition, clinical diagnostic lab methods may continue to evolve and improve.

DIAGNOSTIC METHODS IN CLINICAL GENETICS

There are many methods for clinical genetic testing, each of which has been developed for particular clinical scenarios, including carrier screening, non-invasive prenatal testing, newborn screening, and diagnostic testing, with chromosome analyses to detect copy number variants and cytogenetic rearrangement and sequence-based tests.[17]

Many types of chromosomal abnormalities have been clinically and cytogenetically described and are diagnosed using conventional karyotyping, FISH, and chromosomal microarray (CMA). CMA is routinely performed as part of the comprehensive diagnostic testing for patients with unexplained developmental delay/intellectual disability, autism spectrum disorders, or multiple congenital anomalies.[18] CMA is now routinely performed as oligoarrays, with single nucleotide polymorphism (SNP) probes to provide high resolution for copy number variants and identify UPD and long stretches of homozygosity in families with consanguinity.[19]

Sanger sequencing was the primary genetic test for the diagnosis for monogenic disorders due to sequence variants; however, the decreased cost and increased throughput of massive parallel next-generation sequencing has significantly increased the number of conditions that can simultaneously be tested and can now include an entire genome. For conditions that are genetically heterogeneous, rather than selecting a single gene to test, it is now routine to test for a panel of genes causing a particular phenotype/disease. In addition, whole exome sequencing (WES), of all coding segments of almost all genes, and whole genome sequencing (WGS) are feasible and can even be performed within 1 to 2 weeks. As the number of genes assessed increases, the number of genetic variants that could be pathogenic also increases. The laboratory may issue a report with several variants in several genes as possible diagnoses and then rely on the geneticist to further assess the likelihood of the possibilities. Additionally, not all variants are detectable by exome/genome sequencing. Triplet repeats and somatic mutations can be particularly difficult or impossible to detect based upon current sequencing methods and read depth.

As the amount of genetic data generated increases with genetic testing, such as WES and WGS, there is a chance of identifying gene variants of clinical relevance that were not related to the primary indication for testing (incidental findings such as mutations for hereditary cancer or hereditary causes of sudden cardiac death). When the laboratory systematically and intentionally looks for variants in a prespecified set of genes unrelated to the primary indication, these are termed *secondary findings*. The consent process is important to determine which findings the patient would like to receive. Thus the generally accepted approach for incidental findings is to examine the exome/genome data for pathogenic/likely pathogenic variants in 59 genes.[20]

A summary comparing the different clinical genetic testing methods is provided in Table 1.2.

NEED FOR VARIANT REINTERPRETATION OVER TIME

A significant challenge associated with the clinical implementation of next-generation sequencing for large panels and exomes/genomes is the large number of variants identified. Distinguishing which of these variants is pathogenic is difficult since many of the variants identified are rare or novel and little is known about them. In addition, because not all disease genes have yet been identified, a diagnosis may be missed, despite comprehensive exome/genome sequencing, because the condition has not yet been scientifically recognized. Re-evaluation of sequence data over time may clarify the pathogenicity of variants and yield additional diagnoses as scientific understanding of genetic variants and additional genetic conditions advances. Thus reanalyzing and reinterpreting clinical sequence data is inevitable. The ordering healthcare provider, clinical geneticist, clinical laboratory, and patient/family each may have a role regarding reinterpretation of genetic results.[21,22] These expectations should be clearly outlined as part of the informed consent process.

FUTURE DIRECTIONS IN CLINICAL GENETICS

EARLIER DIAGNOSIS, INCREASINGLY PRENATAL

Making a genetic diagnosis earlier in life has a greater impact on medical care and may afford more effective treatment opportunities and minimize harm by decreasing the number of unnecessary diagnostic procedures or ineffective interventions. Rapid diagnosis in the neonatal or even prenatal period allows providers and parents to make more informed decisions about care, obtain more accurate prognostic information, and draw upon experience with the genetic condition. Rapid diagnosis of acutely ill patients in neonatal intensive care unit is increasingly common and decreases costs and length of stay.[23] One of the most common uses of NGS is non-invasive prenatal screening

Table 1.2 Comparison of Clinical Genetic Testing Methods.

	Karyotype	Chromosome SNP Microarray	FISH	Sanger Sequencing	Sequencing Panel	Exome Sequencing	Genome Sequencing
Single nucleotide variations (SNVs)				X	X	X	X
Copy number variations (CNVs)		X	X			+/–	X
Balanced chromosomal rearrangement	X		X				+/–
Identification of new disease genes						X	X
Incidental findings						X	X
Cost	Low	Low	Low	Modest	Modest	High	High

FISH, Fluorescence in situ hybridization; *SNP*, single nucleotide polymorphism.

(NIPS) to noninvasively identify pregnancies with a high likelihood of chromosomal aneuploidies using a maternal blood sample and enriching for and analyzing fragmented fetal DNA within the sample. With an amniocentesis or chorionic villus sample, karyotype, chromosome microarray, single/panel gene tests, WES, and WGS can be used to prenatally diagnose genetic diseases when there is an aberrant ultrasound finding or based upon a family history of a genetic condition, carrier screening, or NIPS result.

FUTURE OF NEWBORN SCREENING

Newborn screening (NBS) is carried out via various large public-health genetic-screening programs. The scope of NBS programs has increased with advances in technology. Current NBS programs in the United States consist of approximately 50 conditions and rely heavily on tandem mass spectrometry to detect inborn errors of metabolism. Molecular methods have been increasingly integrated as second-tier tests for cystic fibrosis or as first-tier tests for immunodeficiencies (TREC assay) and spinal muscular atrophy. In the future, it is possible that NBS will be expanded even further to screen for classes of genetic disorders that can only be diagnosed with sequencing methods such as glucose transport (GLUT1) deficiency syndrome or retinoblastoma. Recent pilot studies of sequencing-based methods are not as sensitive as biochemical screening. Therefore, the utilization of sequence-based methods will first require greater accuracy in variant interpretation in these genes across diverse ethnicities to maximize clinical sensitivity.

THERAPEUTIC APPROACHES FOR MONOGENIC DISEASES

There is an increased demand for therapies of monogenic diseases with the improvement of diagnostic methods described in previous sections. Most of the inborn errors of metabolism rely on dietary changes, enzyme replacement therapies (ERTs), or liver or bone marrow transplant. Transplantation also works for other genetic conditions beyond the inborn error of metabolism (e.g., bone marrow transplant for hematologic conditions and immunodeficiencies). However, therapies are only available for a fraction of genetic diseases.

Therapeutic options for monogenic diseases may significantly expand in the next decade. Gene editing has advanced, specifically with the use of Crispr-Cas9 for gene editing. There is no safe and efficient, approved gene editing for humans yet, but it is an active area of research. Gene therapy trials began in the 1990s but were limited by safety issues, including immunologic responses to viral vectors and genomic integration activating proto-oncogenes, leading to fatal leukemias. With the advent of safer viral vectors without genomic integration and with trophism for a greater range of tissues, there have been significant advances in gene therapy for monogenic diseases (Fig. 1.6). The European Medicines Agency (EMA) and the US Food and Drug Administration (FDA) have approved six gene therapy products since 2016,[24] including gene therapy for spinal muscular atrophy, a common genetic cause of death in infants. In addition to gene replacement or gene addition, there are improving technologies for somatic gene editing. Numerous gene-therapy clinical trials for monogenic diseases, including particularly hematologic, immunologic, and hepatic diseases, are ongoing (Table 1.3). Longer-term outcome studies of safety and durability are still needed, but gene therapy is likely to play a greater role in treatment in the future.

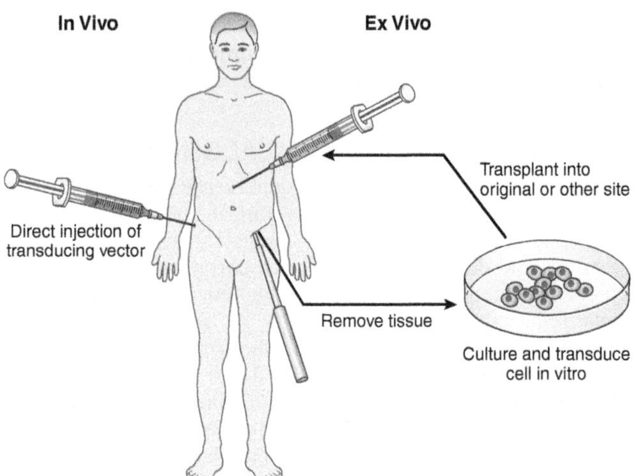

Fig. 1.6 Models for human gene therapy. In vivo gene therapy involves direct introduction of a transducing vector into the patient. Ex vivo gene therapy involves removal of tissue and transduction in vitro.

Table 1.3 Therapeutic Methods for Genetic Diseases.

Method	Example
Dietary for errors of metabolism	PKU and some other inborn errors of metabolism
Enzyme replacement therapy (ERT)	Pompe, CLN2, MPS I, MPS IVA, MPS VIA
Pharmacologic chaperone therapy (PCT)	Pompe, Fabry, Gaucher
Recombinant peptide analog	Achondroplasia (Vosoritide [clinical trial continue] is a C-type natriuretic peptide analog that stimulates enchondral ossification and inhibits the FGFR3-mediated MAPK signaling pathway.)
Gene therapy	Retinal dystrophy (RPE65, AAV vector), SMA (Zolgensma, AAV vector)
Gene editing	Hemoglobinopathies, sickle cell, DMD, immuno-oncology (all in clinical trials)
Antisense and other therapeutic oligonucleotides	SMA (Nusinersen), hATTR amyloidosis (Tegsedi), trinucleotide repeat disorders
Monoclonal antibodies	X-linked hypophosphatemia (XLH) (Burosumab is a fully human monoclonal IgG1 antibody against FGF23 protein.)

CONCLUSION

The Human Genome Project has had a significant impact on medicine and especially neonatology. We routinely use genomic methods and data to diagnose genetic diseases in newborns, especially those associated with congenital anomalies, neurologic conditions, and early organ failure. We are entering the next exciting era, going beyond the diagnosis, toward the treatment of genetic diseases. We need to continue to understand the basic mechanisms of human genes to develop rational treatment strategies. Moreover, transformational platforms to deliver or alter genes may enable the treatment of whole classes of genetic diseases and offer new treatment opportunities to patients.

SUGGESTED READINGS

Nussbaum R, McInnes R, Willard H. *Thompson & Thompson Genetics In Medicine*. 8th ed. Elsevier; 2016.

Turnpenny P, Ellard S. *Emery's Elements of Medical Genetics*. 15th ed. Elsevier; 2017.

Jorde L, Carey J, Bamshad M. *Medical Genetics*. 6th ed. Elsevier; 2019.

Firth H, Hurst J. *Oxford Desk Reference Clinical Genetics and Genomics*. 2nd ed. Oxford University Press; 2017.

REFERENCES

1. Venter JC, Adams MD, Myers EW, et al. The sequence of the human genome. *Science*. 2001;291(5507):1304–1351. https://doi.org/10.1126/science.1058040.
2. Lander ES, Linton LM, Birren B, et al. Initial sequencing and analysis of the human genome. *Nature*. 2001;409(6822):860–921. https://doi.org/10.1038/35057062.
3. Watson JD, Crick FH. Molecular structure of nucleic acids; a structure for deoxyribose nucleic acid. *Nature*. 1953;171(4356):737–738.
4. Tukiainen T, Villani AC, Yen A, et al. Landscape of X chromosome inactivation across human tissues. *Nature*. 2017;550(7675):244–248. https://doi.org/10.1038/nature24265.
5. ENCODE Project Consortium. An integrated encyclopedia of DNA elements in the human genome. *Nature*. 2012;489(7414):57–74. https://doi.org/10.1038/nature11247.
6. Carthew RW, Sontheimer EJ. Origins and mechanisms of miRNAs and siRNAs. *Cell*. 2009;136(4):642–655. https://doi.org/10.1016/j.cell.2009.01.035.
7. Kalousek DK, Vekemans M. Confined placental mosaicism. *J Med Genet*. 1996;33(7):529–533.
8. Soukarieh O, Gaildrat P, Hamieh M, et al. Exonic splicing mutations are more prevalent than currently estimated and can be predicted by using in silico tools. *PLoS Genet*. 2016;12(1):1–26. https://doi.org/10.1371/journal.pgen.1005756.
9. Centers for Mendelian Genomics. Mendelian traits by the numbers. http://mendelian.org/mendelian-traits-numbers. Accessed September 18, 2020.
10. Amberger JS, Bocchini CA, Scott AF, Hamosh A. OMIM.org: leveraging knowledge across phenotype-gene relationships. *Nucleic Acids Res*. 2019;47(D1):D1038–D1043. https://doi.org/10.1093/nar/gky1151.
11. Alkan C, Coe BP, Eichler EE. Genome structural variation discovery and genotyping. *Nat Rev Genet*. 2011;12(5):363–376. https://doi.org/10.1038/nrg2958.
12. Hsu L. *Prenatal Diagnosis of Chromosomal Abnormalities Through Amniocentesis in Genetic Disorders and the Fetus*. 3rd ed. Baltimore: Johns Hopkins University Press; 1992.
13. Lupski JR. 2018 Victor A. McKusick Leadership Award: Molecular Mechanisms for Genomic and Chromosomal Rearrangements. *Am J Hum Genet*. 2019;104(3):391–406. https://doi.org/10.1016/j.ajhg.2018.12.018.
14. European Organisation for Rare Diseases. Rare diseases: understanding this public health priority. *Eurordis*. 2005.
15. Wright CF, FitzPatrick DR, Firth HV. Paediatric genomics: diagnosing rare disease in children. *Nat Rev Genet*. 2018;19(5):253–268. https://doi.org/10.1038/nrg.2017.116.
16. Boycott KM, Rath A, Chong JX, et al. International cooperation to enable the diagnosis of all rare genetic diseases. *Am J Hum Genet*. 2017;100(5):695–705. https://doi.org/10.1016/j.ajhg.2017.04.003.
17. Katsanis SH, Katsanis N. Molecular genetic testing and the future of clinical genomics. *Genomic Precis Med Found Transl Implement Third Ed*. 2016;14(6):263–282. https://doi.org/10.1016/B978-0-12-800681-8.00018-9.
18. Miller DT, Adam MP, Aradhya S, et al. Consensus statement: chromosomal microarray is a first-tier clinical diagnostic test for individuals with developmental disabilities or congenital anomalies. *Am J Hum Genet*. 2010;86(5):749–764. https://doi.org/10.1016/j.ajhg.2010.04.006.
19. Harel T, Lupski JR. Genomic disorders 20 years on-mechanisms for clinical manifestations. *Clin Genet*. 2018;93(3):439–449. https://doi.org/10.1111/cge.13146.
20. Kalia SS, Adelman K, Bale SJ, et al. Recommendations for reporting of secondary findings in clinical exome and genome sequencing, 2016 update (ACMG SF v2.0): a policy statement of the American College of Medical Genetics and Genomics. *Genet Med*. 2017;19(2):249–255. https://doi.org/10.1038/gim.2016.190.
21. David KL, Best RG, Brenman LM, et al. Patient re-contact after revision of genomic test results: points to consider—a statement of the American College of Medical Genetics and Genomics (ACMG). *Genet Med*. 2018;0(0):1–3. https://doi.org/10.1038/s41436-018-0391-z.
22. Bombard Y, Brothers KB, Fitzgerald-Butt S, et al. The responsibility to recontact research participants after reinterpretation of genetic and genomic research results. *Am J Hum Genet*. 2019;104(4):578–595. https://doi.org/10.1016/j.ajhg.2019.02.025.
23. Farnaes L, Hildreth A, Sweeney NM, et al. Rapid whole-genome sequencing decreases infant morbidity and cost of hospitalization. *Npj Genomic Med*. 2018;3(1). https://doi.org/10.1038/s41525-018-0049-4.
24. High KA, Roncarolo MG. Gene therapy. *N Engl J Med*. 2019;381(5):455–464. https://doi.org/10.1056/NEJMra1706910.

Epigenetics 2

William Schierding | Mark H. Vickers | Justin M. O'Sullivan | Wayne S. Cutfield

PRINCIPLES OF EPIGENETICS

INTRODUCTION TO EPIGENETICS

The publication of the majority of the human genome sequence in 2001[1,2] was the precursor to many important discoveries. However, the human genome sequence has not provided researchers with the codex to fully understand the genome's functionality or to predict its response to environmental cues (such as nutritional challenges). One reason why this is the case is that the human genome is more complicated than was originally postulated. Counterintuitively, this complexity partially arises from the finding that the human genome only has approximately one third of the predicted number of genes.[3] Fewer genes means that those genes that are present are more complex, producing multiple different messenger RNAs. As a result, the regulatory processes that control the expression of these genes are complex,[4,5] involving multiple layers of regulation, much of which still remains to be discovered and described.

Traditionally, it had been assumed that inherited genes control gene expression and, ultimately, phenotype. In the early 1940s Waddington introduced the concept of **epigenetics** ("on to top of" or "in addition to" genes) to describe the way in which genes interact with their surroundings to produce a phenotype during the differentiation of cells over the course of development (without a change in gene sequence).[6] Thus, environmental cues can lead to up- or down-regulation of gene activity. This definition leaves out the concept of inheritance, instead emphasizing the effect on the final cell type and how small nongenetic changes in development can lead to measurable differences in adult phenotype. Recently, epigenetics has been redefined, first by Riggs as "the study of mitotically and/or mitotically heritable changes in gene function that cannot be explained by changes in DNA sequence"[7] and more recently by Cavalli and Heard as "the study of molecules and mechanisms that can *perpetuate* alternative gene activity states in the context of the same DNA sequence."[8] Therefore, epigenetics is any element with permanent (or at least semi-permanent) changes in gene expression or cellular phenotype.[9] This encompasses transgenerational inheritance and the persistence of gene activity or chromatin states through extended periods of time. Throughout this chapter we will discuss epigenetics in the context of this more modern definition, but it should be noted that *epigenetics* is a term that has many different definitions, with "mitotically stable" and "epigenetic memory" being points of controversy.

FROM GENETICS TO EPIGENETICS

Double-stranded DNA is an efficient and reliable mechanism to pass information from one generation to another, given that it is stable and there are a number of repair systems that have evolved to maintain it. Thus, genetic changes tend to occur slowly, taking

Box 2.1 Nature Versus Nurture, Genes Versus the Environment

There has been a longstanding debate as to whether health is determined by "nature" or "nurture."[20-22] It is clear that phenotypic traits exist on a continuum, where some are predominantly controlled by genetics (e.g., height) and others by environmental factors (e.g., obesity). However, the influence of genes and environment in the development of phenotypic traits is not mutually exclusive, but rather is a result of their constant interaction. For example, twin studies suggest that genetic factors have a substantial effect on variations in body weight, particularly in children and adolescents. Nonetheless, the fact that obesity is rapidly increasing worldwide shows that environment also plays a significant role in the likelihood of becoming obese. Thus in most cases the resulting manifestation of non-communicable disease is a combination of nature and nurture. Importantly, this interaction between the environment and genetic inheritance is mediated through epigenetics.

many generations for a single mutation to become dominant in a population. By contrast, epigenetic changes can occur in a more rapid timeframe.This means that epigenetics provides a mechanism for rapid responses to environmental changes. Consistent with this, studies have shown that de novo epigenetic "mutation" is one to two orders of magnitude more frequent than de novo somatic DNA mutation.[10] This difference in "mutation rates" is due to a reduction in the fidelity of maintenance of epigenetic features, when compared to genetic features, throughout the cell cycle.[11] For example, the genetic code is copied (replicated) with an error rate of less than 1 base in 10^7 to 10^8 bases copied.[12] By contrast, epigenetic mechanisms, such as methylation, have an error rate that has been estimated to be between 1% and 4%.[4,11,13]

Developmental plasticity is a genotype's or individual's ability to respond to changes in environmental conditions through changes in its phenotypes. All developmental plasticity is, by definition, epigenetic in origin, as the genotype of the responding individual remains unaltered in the process. The plasticity of the epigenome is important for its contribution to the dynamic coordination of the genome's responses to environmental signals. However, changing to suit the present environment can result in a suboptimal phenotype for tomorrow's environment (the mismatch hypothesis).[14] In developmental terms, the epigenome can change to enhance fitness in response to an environmental cue (e.g., reduced placental nutrient supply) during a small window in early development. Subsequent changes to the environmental conditions (e.g., overabundance of high-energy food) mean that the epigenetic changes, which have been stably maintained through the remainder of development, may become detrimental over the course of the individual's lifespan by increasing the risk for metabolic and cardiovascular diseases.[15]

HOW GENES LEARN FROM EXPERIENCE

Twin studies exemplify the epigenetic changes that occur during a lifetime of interactions between the environment and the genome (reviewed in Bell and Spector[16]). In simple terms, genetically identical monozygotic twins are epigenetically indistinguishable when they are born.[17] However, as they age, the twins begin to display differences in the overall phenotype, due to their cumulative individual exposure to environmental signals.[17] As previously mentioned, it is through the epigenetic changes that each individual modifies their phenotype to better suit the environment they have experienced. Collectively, these changes alter the individual twin's risk factors for obesity and a number of non-communicable diseases such as type 2 diabetes mellitus (Box 2.1).[18,19]

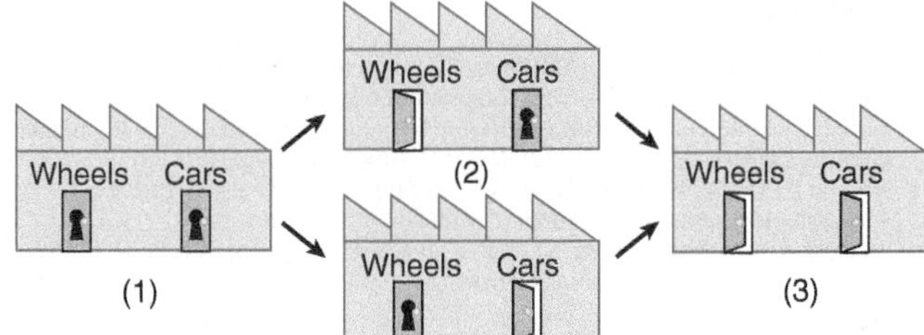

Fig. 2.1 Epigenetic machinery. The following analogy can be used to illustrate this point. Security guards can use keys to lock and unlock doors according to instructions they are receiving from another source. *(1 and 3)* At the beginning and end of each working day, the guards go through their routine of unlocking or locking doors. *(2)* By locking and unlocking doors in a factory, the guards are not changing the structure of the factory, but rather this system is akin to epigenetic modifications that limit the workers' (i.e., the transcription factors, DNA binding proteins, and RNA polymerases) access to the equipment and information within the factory. If there is an error in the unlocking routine for example, part of the factory would remain off-limits to the workers for one cycle of 12 hours. Thus, if the factory is a car assembly line and the section where the wheels are stored (i.e., the gene) remains locked, then no workers are able to access this area and the final product (i.e., the phenotype) is cars without wheels. *(3)* However, when the correct set of keys has opened the correct factory doors, the cars and wheels will both be accessible, and the cars will be made.

THE STRUCTURE OF THE (EPI)GENOME

Eukaryotes use multiple systems to initiate and regulate changes in gene expression. In total, genes are regulated by hundreds of functional DNA elements, controlling when and how much protein is produced. This regulatory control occurs through mechanisms that utilize epigenetic signals to affect nuclear (e.g., transcription and mRNA processing) and cytoplasmic (e.g., translation) processes (Fig. 2.1).These mechanisms include DNA methylation (with or without ubiquitination),[23] histone modifications (i.e., acetylation, phosphorylation, sumoylation, methylation),[24] chromatin folding,[25-30] non-coding RNA (ncRNA and miRNA),[31,32] and prions.[33] Epigenetic effects on transcription are well documented and will therefore form the main focus of the remainder of this chapter.[34-36] A summary of how these various epigenetic processes are analyzed is shown in Table 2.1.

It should be noted that epigenetic effects such as DNA methylation do not turn a gene on or off permanently. Rather, most epigenetic mechanisms lead to semi-permanent changes. As such, epigenetic modifications need to be continually maintained by the recruitment of the required enzymes and proteins to accurately replenish the epigenetic marks, and thus contribute to the maintenance of the appropriate state of transcription.[9] Epigenetic modifications only "contribute to the maintenance of the correct state of transcription"; other factors (e.g., DNA-binding proteins and RNA polymerases) are ultimately responsible for reading and transcribing the gene.

DNA METHYLATION

DNA methylation is a fundamental and evolutionarily conserved epigenetic modification involved in gene regulation and other biologic processes (e.g., see He and colleagues[37]). In mammals, DNA methylation is restricted to sites where a cytosine nucleotide is followed by a guanine nucleotide (CpG, Fig. 2.2). In most mammalian species, 90% to 98% of CpG sites are methylated,[24] and the methylation status and density of CpG sites is associated with gene regulation.[38] Therefore, measuring the methylation status of particular genes within a cell type can provide researchers with information as to which RNA species are likely to be transcribed, albeit there are exceptions to this rule (as will be discussed later.)

Table 2.1 Measuring Epigenetic Profiles.

		Single Locus Analysis			Global (Whole Genome) Analysis		
Epigenetic Process	**Function**	**Platform**	**Cost**	**Time**	**Platform**	**Cost**	**Time**
DNA Methylation	Repress gene activity	Bisulfite conversion followed by various targeted sequencing opt ions	Low	Low	Bisulfite conversion followed by various whole-genome sequencing opt ions	High	High
DNMT1a. DNMTlb	Methylation maintenance (across cell divisions)						
DNMT3a. DNMT3b	De novo DNA methylation						
Historic modifications		Chromatin immunoprecipitation followed by qPCR	Low	Low	Chromatin immunoprecipitation followed by Next Generation Sequencing (ChIP-seq) or hybridization to a microarray (ChIP-chip)	High	High
Post-transcriptional Regulators (miRNA, ncRNA)	Repress gene activity	qRT-PCR, Targeted Sequencing, or Microarray	Low	Low	Microarray or Next Generation Sequencing (RNAseq)	High	High
Chromatin Structure and Function (3D Genome)	10,000× Companion, DNA activity regulation	Chromatin conformation capture (3C, 4C, or GCC) and FISH	Medium	Medium	Global chromatin conformation capture (5C or Hi-C), FISH, and ChIA-PET.	Very high	High

Various techniques are used to characterize epigenetic modifications. The use of antibody precipitation to isolate pieces of DNA that are methylated or unmethylated, or are associated with modified histones is central to many of the techniques that are used to study epigenetic modifications on the local and global scale (e.g., chromatin immunoprecipitation, ChIP-chip ChIP-seq; ChIA-PET; MeDIP).[171] Modifications of methylation of cytosine in CpGs are also studied using bisulfite conversion, which changes the 5me-C residue to a uracil.[172] Finally, chromatin organization (which DNA sequences are nearby or contacting each other within the nucleus) and the effects of epigenetic modifications on this is determined by methods that range from FISH methodologies methodologies,[173,174] differential centrifugation,[175] or chromosome conformation capture based technologies (e.g., 3C 3C,[176] 4C,[177] GCC,[178] or 5C[179]).

Gene activation is typically associated with tracts of largely unmethylated CpG, known as *CpG islands*. The majority (60%) of these CpG islands occur in or near gene promoters.[36,38] Methylation (a mark of down-regulation) inside or within ~2 kb of these CpG islands[39] contributes to the control of gene expression.[24] DNA methylation status is mostly controlled by the family of genes known as *DNA methyltransferases (DNMT)*. Briefly, DNMT1 controls maintenance of methylation (transmission from mother to daughter cells).[40] DNMT 3a and 3b are responsible for de novo methylation (establishment of methylation without a template or changes in methylation state),[41,42] while DNMT3L is largely involved in the methylation of maternally imprinted genes (see later) during oogenesis.[43]

Placental growth and development are regulated in part by epigenetic mechanisms such as DNA methylation. During gestation, embryonic development is associated with the establishment of distinct DNA methylation differences between the trophectoderm and inner cell mass. The trophectoderm (ultimately placenta) becomes significantly less methylated than the inner cell mass (ultimately embryo/somatic tissues). Overall, whole-term placental lysates have 14% to 25% less global DNA methylation when compared to somatic tissues.

For a more exhaustive review on epigenetic marks in development, see the review by Ficz and colleagues.[36]

HISTONE MODIFICATIONS

The most basic unit of chromatin structure is the nucleosome, which consists of approximately 147 base pairs of DNA wrapped 1.67 times around a barrel-shaped histone octamer containing two copies of the core histones H2A, H2B, H3, and H4 (see Fig. 2.2).[44] Nucleosomes are separated by exposed linker DNA that is typically 20 to 50 base pairs in length.[45] Only about 75% to 90% of DNA in eukaryotes is bound within a nucleosome at any time in the cell cycle.[46]

Nucleosomes are the targets of a wide range of post-translational modifications (e.g., acetylation, phosphorylation, sumoylation, and methylation) that combine to form an epigenetic (histone) code.[47] Each of the core histones (H3 and H4) features a long amino acid "tail," where posttranslational modifications may occur to affect gene expression. Enzymes deposit ("write") or remove ("erase") these histone marks of phosphorylation, acetylation, and methylation. Proteins that bind to modified histones ("readers") are part of larger, multisubunit protein complexes that exert downstream functions (note: these complexes often recognize combinations of different histone marks simultaneously).

Post-translational modifications of the histone tails, or to the central histone structure itself,[34] can (1) directly affect the compaction and assembly of the chromatin by regulating the interaction between the DNA and each histone within the nucleosome or the between nucleosomes themselves[46]; or (2) serve as binding sites for recruitment of other proteins that themselves contribute to the regulation of transcription and other nuclear functions.[35] These modifications of the histone residues ("marks") have been correlated with various important genetic elements in the regulation of gene expression. Promoters of transcriptionally active genes are associated with enriched trimethylation on histone H3 lysine 4 (H3K4me3), and lysine

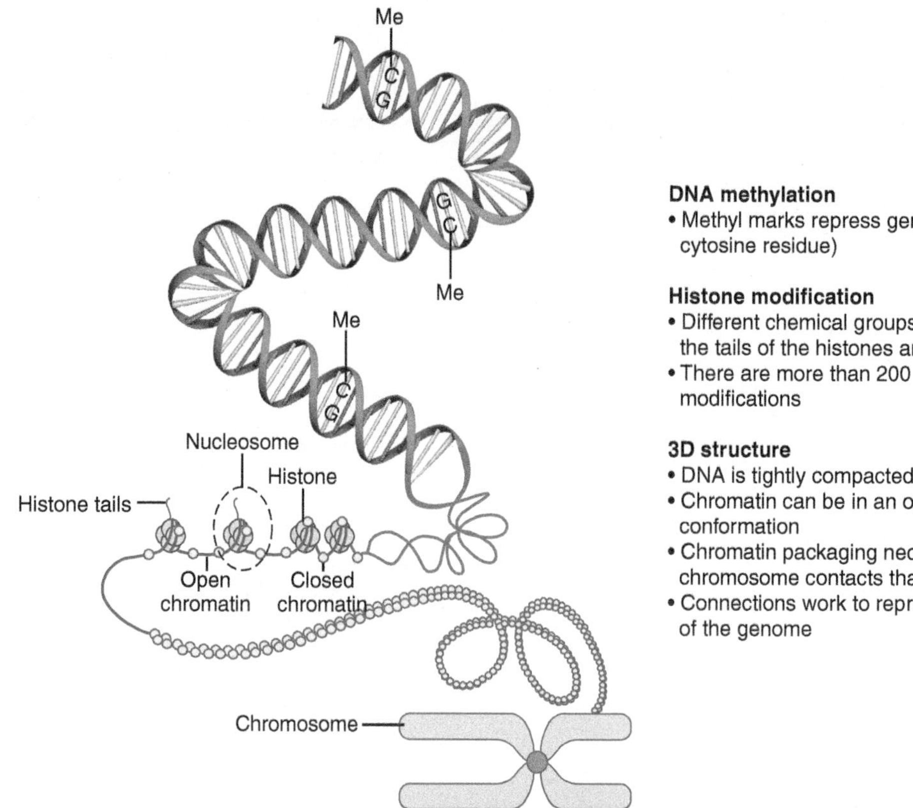

Me
C
G
G
C
Me
Me
C
G
Nucleosome
Histone
Histone tails
Open chromatin
Closed chromatin
Chromosome
DNA methylation
• Methyl marks repress gene activity (usually at a cytosine residue)
Histone modification
• Different chemical groups in combination bind to the tails of the histones and alter DNA activity
• There are more than 200 post-translational modifications
3D structure
• DNA is tightly compacted around histones into chromatin
• Chromatin can be in an open (active) or closed (inactive) conformation
• Chromatin packaging necessitates between- and within-chromosome contacts that are dynamic and non-random
• Connections work to repress or activate certain regions of the genome

Fig. 2.2 Fundamentals of epigenetics.

acetylation (H3K9ac, H3K27ac). For example, an enhancer is a genomic switch that, when activated ("turned on"), increases the likelihood of transcription of a particular gene. These enhancer elements are defined by having both H3K27ac and H3K4me1. Repressed genes have a higher density of nucleosomes (i.e., heterochromatin) and are usually marked by H3K9me, H3K27me3, and H4K20me3.[48]

Polycomb complexes remodel chromatin to maintain developmentally or environmentally programmed expression states. DNA-binding proteins (or noncoding RNAs) recruit polycomb-group proteins to specific regions of the genome for epigenetic silencing of genes. For Polycomb Repressive Complex 2, histone methyltransferase enzyme EZH2 regulates trimethylation of lysine 27 on histone H3 (H3K27me2/3). Processes affected by polycomb complexes include X-chromosome inactivation and Hox gene silencing, through modulation of chromatin structure during embryonic development.[49]

According to the modern definition of epigenetics, epigenetic changes must be mitotically stable. This leads to considerable controversy over the underlying changes that must be present and as to how expression levels of consistently activated genes are maintained when the original activation signal has passed.[46] Some histone modifications (e.g., H3K36 methylation) have not been shown to be "mitotically stable" across several generations, while methylation marks located on H3K4, H3K9, and H3K27 have been shown to be mitotically transmissible.[50] Also, some epigenetic changes are only a transient phenomenon, such as the phosphorylation of a variant of histone H2A (i.e., H2AX) during DNA double-strand breaks.[51] On many levels, this would classify as an epigenetic mark, but it disappears once the break is repaired. Thus, these types of marks will never be classified as stably inherited effects and cannot meet the modern definition of being epigenetic. Therefore, while they are generally called *epigenetic*, not all methylation and histone modifications are epigenetic in the modern definition.[9]

CHROMATIN FOLDING AND 3D STRUCTURE

A non-linear consideration of DNA is important to understand the establishment and maintenance of enhancer-promoter interactions in space and time. Nucleosomes are the lowest form of structural scaffolds for DNA, which, when packaged with other proteins and RNA components, form compacted chromatin structures. The compaction levels for chromatin are not fixed but vary as the cell moves through the cell cycle. This ultimately results in the structures we recognize as chromosomes, in which the DNA has been compacted up to 10,000-fold (see Fig. 2.2).[46]

The dynamic process of changing the compaction level of the DNA within a nucleus is an important component of the regulation of genes.[52,53] At a gross level, chromatin compaction is thought to contribute to the two dominant types of chromatin within eukaryotic cells: (1) heterochromatin, the tightly compacted form of chromatin that is largely transcriptionally silent; and (2) euchromatin, the less condensed, more transcriptionally active form of chromatin.[46] However, closer inspection using new molecular techniques reveals that DNA packaging also creates local chromatin structures that contribute to the establishment of cell-type identity and lineage specificity.[46,54] Briefly, each chromosome folds up into a structure that promotes physical connections between regulatory elements that would be otherwise separated by long distances in the DNA sequence.[55-60]

The organized three-dimensional (3D) chromatin structure within the nucleus (i.e., functional framework between regulatory elements and distant genes) gets substantially reorganized in disease (Fig. 2.3). This restructuring induces an aberrant exposure of gene promoters to inappropriate regulatory elements, resulting in enhanced pro-disease (e.g., oncogenes) or silenced anti-disease genes (e.g., tumor suppressors). In development, Rubinstein syndrome and brachydactyly–mental retardation are both linked to defects in the management of the local chromatin state. In Rubinstein-Taybi syndrome, defects

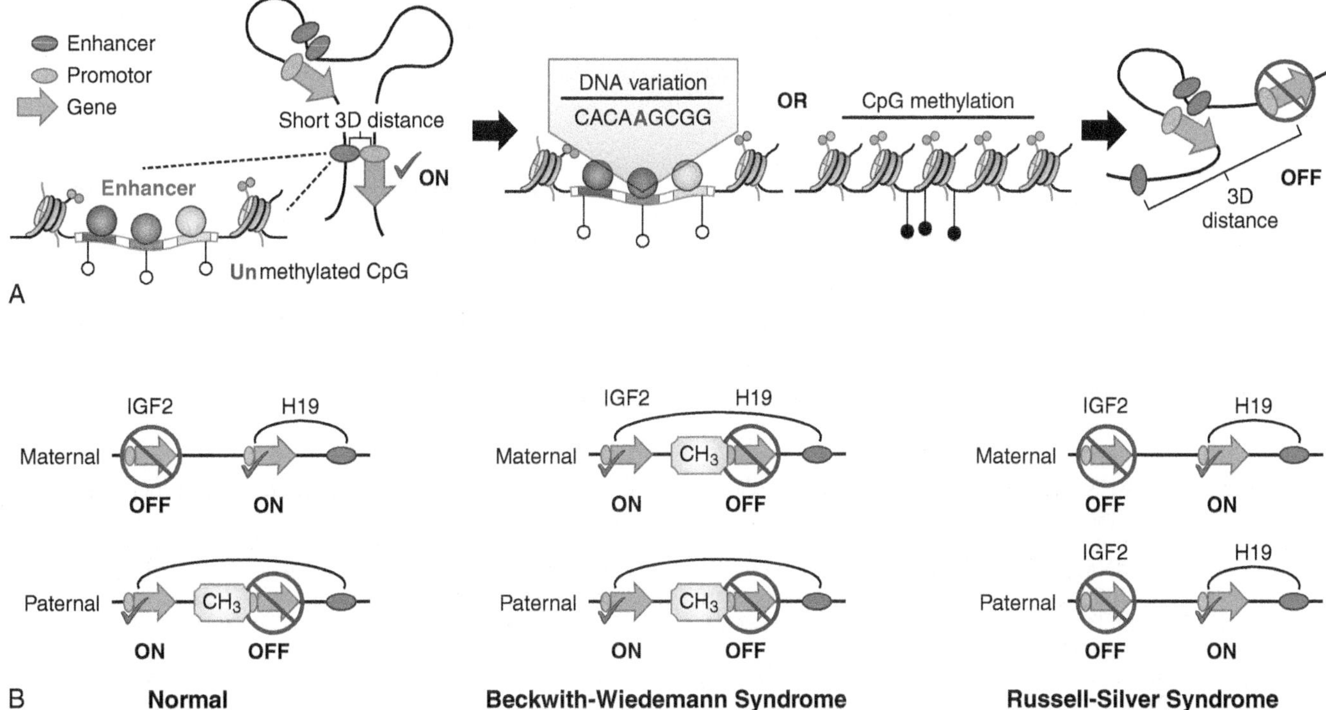

Fig. 2.3 Spatial associations, differential methylation, and imprinting. (A) DNA variation or epigenetic marks can alter the spatial conformation of DNA so that elements normally regulated together are quite far apart. (B) On chromosome 11 (11p15) is a developmentally critical imprinting control region (IGF2 locus). In normal cells, the imprinted IGF2 locus is regulated differently in the maternally and paternally derived chromatin. Hypermethylation of the H19 promotor and loss of imprinting of IGF2 are detectable in 2% to 7% of BWS patients (resulting in over-expression of IGF2). Hypomethylation of the same promoter in RSS patients prevents IGF2 promoter interactions (resulting in under-expression of IGF2).

in genes that encode histone acetyltransferases (i.e., CREBBP and EP300) lead to a deficiency of histone acetylation. This is thought to result in the loss of open chromatin states in critical cell types, ultimately resulting in short stature, broad thumbs, and learning difficulties.[61] In brachydactyly-mental retardation, the opposite problem occurs. Specifically, histone deacetylase 4 (HDAC4) can be mutated. As HDAC4 is an eraser of histone acetylation, mutation of this gene leads to an overabundance of open chromatin states in certain cell types, ultimately leading to skeletal and intellectual abnormalities.[61]

Alterations to long-range chromatin interactions between genes and their regulatory elements also contribute to human disease. For instance, limb formation in mammals is heavily reliant on the spatial co-localization of locus control regions (LCRs) and gene promoters.[62] LCRs are genomic loci located at some distance away on the same chromosome (or even located on another chromosome) that are capable of mediating the activation or repression of one or more promoters (i.e., the LCR contains enhancer or repressor elements; for more on enhancers, see the histone modifications section). LCRs can interact with a specific target gene or with many genes. This allows the coordinated regulation of functionally related genes.[63] Mammalian limb development is controlled by a cluster of genes, termed the *homeobox D genes*, that are partially regulated by an LCR within a 600 kb gene desert (region of the genome devoid of protein-coding genes) on chromosome 2.[62] In cases where the physical interactions between this gene desert and the homeobox D gene are interrupted by translocations, patients develop limb and finger malformations including brachydactyly and syndactyly.[62] Likewise, preaxial polydactyly can develop as a result of an alteration in the long-range interactions between the sonic hedgehog gene (SHH) and an intronic single nucleotide polymorphism (SNP) located 1 Mb away.[64] The mutation in the intron of LMBR1 is incidental to the phenotype, as these elements act as an enhancer for SHH expression, where misexpression of SHH is the cause of the altered limb formation.

NON-CODING RNAS

Non-coding RNA (ncRNA) includes a broad array of RNA species, including microRNA (miRNA), small temporal RNA (stRNA), short interfering RNA (siRNA), short hairpin RNA (shRNA), small nuclear RNAs (snRNA), small nucleolar RNAs (snoRNA), transfer RNAs (tRNA), ribosomal RNAs (rRNA), and long non-coding RNA (lncRNA). All of these ncRNA are important regulators or effectors of RNA expression, and many have been implicated in gene and chromatin structure regulation.[65,66] However, for this review, only ncRNA siRNA, miRNA, and lncRNA will be covered in further detail.

Both siRNA and miRNA are 20 to 25-base-pair-long sequences of RNA that are assembled as single-stranded molecules in the cytoplasm with RNA-induced silencing complexes.[67] These complexes, as their name suggests, result in the inhibition of protein synthesis by silencing the target mRNA(s). The siRNA and miRNA interactions with mRNA are sequence specific, and sometimes hundreds of different mRNA species can be bound by a single type of siRNA or miRNA.[68] While similar in mechanism, siRNA and miRNA differ in how their binding to mRNA causes translational silencing. siRNA primarily acts through mediating the RNA interference pathway, where siRNA has perfect base pair complementarity with the targeted mRNA, resulting in cleaved mRNA.[69] By contrast, miRNA have incomplete base pair complementarity with the target mRNA, leading to translational repression without mRNA degradation.[69] miRNA bind to mRNA molecules and silence their translation into proteins by either: (1) cleaving the mRNA strand into two pieces; (2) destabilizing the mRNA by shortening its poly(A) tail; or (3) altering the mRNA-ribosomal interactions during translation.[31]

miRNA has been identified in different organisms and plays very important roles in the timing of development, particularly in locking down differentiation states.[31] For example, miRNA has important roles in tooth development, controlling size, shape, and the number of teeth.[68] miRNAs have also been linked with

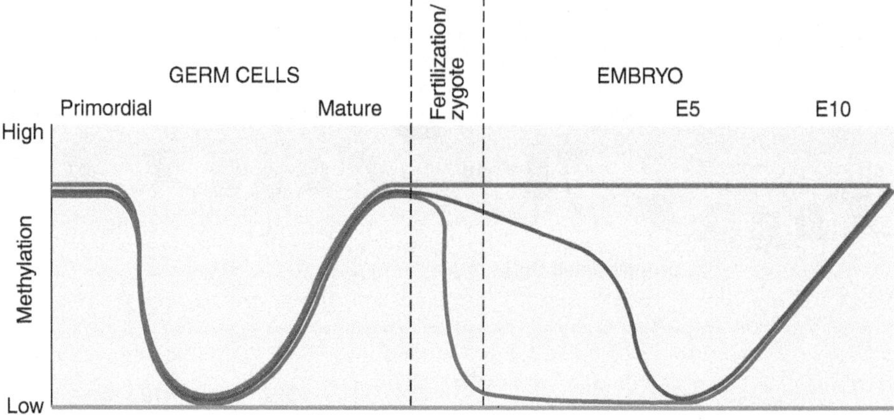

Fig. 2.4 Imprinting methylation levels. The figure shows the level of methylation in methylated *(black)* and non-methylated *(grey)* imprinted genes and non-imprinted sequences (*red*, maternal; *blue*, paternal) during germ-cell and early embryonic development. The horizontal time axis and the vertical axis indicating the relative methylation levels are not to scale. *E*, Embryonic day. (Reprinted with permission from Reik W, Walter J. Genomic imprinting: parental influence on the genome. *Nat Rev Genet*. 2001;2(1):21–32.)

many different disease states, including inflammatory diseases, cancer, Alzheimer disease, cardiovascular disease, type 2 diabetes mellitus, and rheumatoid arthritis.[70]

Long ncRNA (lncRNA) are a "catch-all" for any non-coding RNA species over 200 base pairs in length. The targets of lncRNA are different from those of the short RNA species. These include regulation of chromatin states and folding, epigenetic regulation, X chromosome inactivation, imprinting, establishment of lineage specificity, and formation of anterior-posterior pattern during development. Not surprisingly, because of the range and number of targets, lncRNA have been implicated in a number of developmental processes and diseases, including cancer.[71]

PRIONS

Prions are mis-folded isoform proteins that can serve as transmissible agents of disease.[72] The role of prions in epigenetics is quite different from that of other mechanisms described in this chapter. Prions propagate by transmitting their mis-folded protein state to other proteins.[73] The effect of prions on disease state has been shown to be a robust and transmissible epigenetic phenotype (i.e., that self-propagates and is stably heritable), inducing changes in protein conformations that can profoundly alter its mechanistic properties, resulting in a different cellular phenotype.[46,74] Prions can be inherited, sporadic, or acquired, and may be affected by environmental factors.[72] There is currently debate as to whether more adverse environmental conditions lead to an increase in protein mis-folding and, therefore, more prions, and whether this change could turn out to be beneficial to the fitness of the individual.[74] In humans, exposure to prions by surgery or blood transfusion can transmit diseases such as variant Creutzfeldt-Jakob disease (vCJD).[73] Kuru, the only known epidemic of human prion disease, was transmitted through the ingestion of dead relatives in the Fore tribe of Papua New Guinea.[33] Prions have also been linked to many other human neurodegenerative diseases, including Alzheimer, Parkinson, and Lou Gehrig diseases.[72,73] Finally, there are also inheritable prion diseases in humans, such as familial Creutzfeldt-Jakob disease and Gerstmann-Sträussler-Scheinker disease.[33,74]

SEX-SPECIFIC EPIGENETICS

IMPRINTING

Epigenetic changes can confer either a short-term or a long-term effect on the cell's phenotype, with some modifications needing to be reliably removed or retained across generations. Marks that are used to control the expression of genes in a parent of origin specific manner, across a generation, are imprinted.[11,75]

Within the critical period before birth (gametogenesis through gestation), there are two key points during which the methylation patterns are thought to be set, setting fetal development into vastly different paths (Fig. 2.4).[76] The first is during gametogenesis, when genome-wide demethylation clears most of the parental methylation markings (with a limited amount of methylation occurring just prior to fertilization).[76] The second round of methylation reprogramming occurs in early embryogenesis, when another cycle of genome-wide demethylation occurs.[76] Of note, this second cycle of demethylation is incomplete, leaving room for the early embryo to retain imprinting from the parents.[77] Dysregulation of methylation patterns during these periods is associated with many different diseases, including metabolic syndrome and cancer.[78]

Proper timing of imprinting must happen with each reproductive cycle, as it is crucial for normal growth of the embryo, placental function, and neurobehavioral processes.[75] It is through this incomplete erasure that DNA methylation status (or some key "memory marks" associated with DNA methylation states) of parental origin remains in the offspring.[46] Most of the genes currently known to be under the control of parental imprinting are associated with growth and development, with a number of rare congenital disorders (such as Beckwith-Wiedemann syndrome and Angelman syndrome, discussed later) attributed to faulty imprinting.[79,80] Defects in imprinting during development are also implicated in various forms of later-in-life metabolic and cardiovascular dysfunction, obesity,[78] heavier babies and placentas,[42] premature birth,[42] susceptibility to activation of autoimmune diseases,[81] and neurologic defects.[82,83]

Transmission of epi-alleles to the offspring can be vital, and either the maternal or paternal allele can be imprinted. The *parental conflict hypothesis* was proposed as a way to explain the selection of the imprinted alleles (i.e., maternal or paternal) that are active in the offspring.[84,85] This imprinting "battle" occurs during gametogenesis, while the maternal and paternal genomes are still physically separated. This allows for sex-specific differences between the male and female germlines, through the asynchronous acquisition of methylation marks in genes such as insulin-like growth factor 2 receptor (IGF2R).[86] While maternal epigenetic modifications are more likely to affect future epigenetic patterns in the offspring, paternal epigenetic modifications have also been shown to be imprinted, being passed from the sperm cell during fertilization.[87] The Haig hypothesis argues that the sexual dimorphism in the passage of imprinted genes is the result of different parental interests in the offspring. Specifically, the father's interest is in promoting the success of the offspring (i.e., fetal growth promoting genes, larger offspring) at any cost. By contrast, the maternal interest in reproduction is weighed against that of her own survival (i.e., fetal growth restricting genes, smaller offspring).[84]

Sexual dimorphism in the passage of epigenetic modifications at imprinted genes has important ramifications for the placenta, where imprinted genes are associated with alterations in placental nutrient supply to the developing fetus.[77] Maternally imprinted genes (such as a major fetal growth regulating gene, insulin-like growth factor 2, IGF2) down-regulate placental growth, while paternally imprinted genes (such as Air ncRNA) up-regulate placental growth and affect the efficiency and permeability of placental nutrient supply.[77,88,89] The paternally imprinted Air ncRNA role in placental function is through silencing three genes, including IGF2R, likely through interactions with H3K9 at the genes' promoters.[89] Therefore, in normal births IGF2 and its receptor (IGF2R) are thought to be balanced in this tug-of-war between maternal and paternal imprinting, and imbalanced in disease.[88]

There are many diseases associated with disruptions in normal imprinting. Each of these involves histone modifications (see the section on histone modifications) in and around imprinted genes, resulting in developmental disorders such as Beckwith-Wiedemann, Russell-Silver, Angelman, Prader-Willi, and Rett syndromes.[80,90]

1. Beckwith-Wiedemann syndrome, an overgrowth disorder, is associated with altered methylation imprinting of 11p15, which contains the IGF2 locus and the KCNQ1/LIT1/CDKN1C locus (see Fig. 2.3b).[79]
2. Russell-Silver syndrome, a disorder of severe intrauterine growth restriction (IUGR), is also associated with imprinting defects in 11p15, in particular the paternal hypomethylation at the IGF2 locus.[61] Beckwith-Wiedemann and Russell-Silver syndromes are essentially polar opposites of 11p15 methylation defects.
3. Angelman syndrome is associated with loss of methylation in various imprinted regions on chromosome 15, including the *UBE3A and SNRPN genes (usually disruption of maternal imprinting of these genes).*[80] Prader–Willi syndrome is also associated with imprinting defects in 15q11, but it is the paternal allele that has been faulty in its imprinted state.[61]
4. Rett syndrome is a disorder where development suddenly halts around 6 to 18 months of age, which is associated with loss of function mutations in a methyl CpG binding protein 2 (MeCP2), a protein that is capable of binding to CpG methylated DNA.[61] Both Beckwith-Wiedemann and Angelman syndromes are more likely to occur in individuals born following in vitro fertilization, suggesting a link between an altered early environment and an epigenetic defect, such as loss of methylation of a maternal allele or global hypomethylation.[77,91]

X-CHROMOSOME INACTIVATION

In females, one copy of the X chromosome is inactivated and forms into a Barr body (located at the nuclear envelope or sometimes near the nucleolus).[92] This X chromosome inactivation is understood to occur so that male and female cells have similar expression levels from genes located on the X chromosome, that is as a form of dosage compensation.[93] The process of X chromosome inactivation is regulated primarily by Xist, a 17 kb long lncRNA, which associates with the inactivated X chromosome to control gene silencing.[93] Either the paternally or maternally derived X chromosome can be inactivated early in embryonic development. This inactivation is stable and maintained through the adult somatic and germ cell lines without the further need for Xist.[94]

THE BIOLOGY OF EPIGENETICS

THE BASICS OF THE EPIGENETICS OF DEVELOPMENT

From preconception to birth, development (in particular, human development) is a process carried out largely without changes to the underlying DNA sequence (except for a small somatic mutation rate[4,13]). Instead, development relies on the action of regulatory proteins (e.g., transcription factors) within a genomic environment that is moderated by epigenetics.[11] In this sense, development is a careful orchestration of chemical changes that regulate (activate or deactivate) processes, changing pluripotent cells into the many differentiated cell types present in the human body. These processes are not only time-specific, but also can be quite cell-specific (and sometimes even allele-specific).[4,5,54]

As discussed earlier in this chapter (see imprinting), DNA methylation marks critical changes during embryonic development. The contribution of epigenetics to human development starts at fertilization with the pluripotent cells, where the original transcription factors have predominately originated from the maternal oocyte.[9] Genome-wide DNA methylation marks are early markers of embryonic control during embryogenesis (loss of maternally derived marks). As the pluripotent cells undergo divisions, transcription factors are unevenly distributed between the daughter cells.[4,9] New methylation patterns emerge that ultimately contribute to the eventual suppression and silencing of pluripotent genes, while other processes (e.g., imprinting; see earlier in chapter) confer long-term gene silencing.[11] Through each new round of cell division, these epigenetic modifications combine with external cues from other nearby cells to influence transcription factor profiles, thus promoting the expression of specific gene and starting a feedback cycle.[9]

CRITICAL DEVELOPMENTAL PERIODS

The epigenome is always changing; however it is particularly susceptible to dysregulation at critical periods, particularly during gestation, neonatal development, puberty, and old age.[15,90,95] Each of these periods of development carries a strong association with the future health of the individual. Environmental stressors such as aberrant nutrition during these critical periods may lead to long-term consequences, including the development of metabolic abnormalities and malignancies later in life (Box 2.2).[96]

Box 2.2 Changing the Epigenome

It is important to note that fetal life is not the only period in the lifespan where patterns of epigenetic modifications can be altered, through interactions with environmental cues, with major long-term health consequences. For example, poor dietary choices during adolescence and/or adulthood also play a critical role in the development of metabolic disease. This nutritional effect is often linked to epigenetic modifications[24] and other risk factors (e.g., single nucleotide polymorphisms [SNPs]). For example, SNPs within the methylenetetrahydrofolate dehydrogenase (e.g., rs2236225 in gene *MTHFD1*) or phosphatidyl ethanolamine methyltransferase (e.g., rs12325817 in *PEMT*) or choline dehydrogenase (e.g., rs12676 in *CHDH*) are more sensitive to diets poor in choline, causing greater global hypomethylation in these individuals when choline is not abundant in the diet.[96]

Aging also has an effect on epigenetic regulation beyond the environment. The reliability with which DNA methylation patterns are inherited across cell divisions is ensured by the DNA methyltransferases (DNMTs). Aging is associated with global DNA hypomethylation but with hypermethylation of promoter regions on CpG islands.[97] These epigenetic changes are all typically seen in cancers, suggesting the epigenetic changes attributable to aging might contribute to tumorigenesis.[98] Global DNA hypomethylation with aging is thought to be due to the progressive loss of DNMT1 activity and the subsequent compensatory response of increased DNMT3b activity, leading to promoter region hypermethylation.[99]

Small perturbations in early life have been associated with later-in-life effects for decades. For example, individuals born with either low or high birth weight have an increased risk of metabolic syndrome, specifically obesity, insulin resistance, hyperglycemia, and type 2 diabetes mellitus.[78,96] However, the role of epigenetics in this process is only now becoming clearer. For example, hypermethylation of the RXRα and NOS3 genes in umbilical cord tissue at birth is associated with an increased risk of adiposity at 9 years of age.[100]

Babies born by in vitro fertilization (IVF) are exposed to a manipulated periconceptional environment during a critical developmental phase of early embryo demethylation and remethylation. IVF consists of a variable number of components, any of which could influence epigenetic changes and/or the offspring phenotype. These components include the causes of maternal and/or paternal infertility, maternal treatment with ovulation-inducing drugs, sperm injection into the egg cytoplasm, culture media formulation and incubation duration, bisphenol A exposure to the cultured embryo from plastic culture dishes, use of fresh or frozen embryos, and cultured embryo selection for implantation. IVF is associated with a marked increased likelihood of the following neonatal outcomes: prematurity, low birth weight, and twins.[101] It now appears that there are subtle longer-term changes in IVF offspring. In childhood, IVF is associated with taller stature (notably in girls) with higher serum IGF-I and IGF-II together with a more favorable lipid profile. Interestingly, these changes were more likely to occur in those who were fresh rather than frozen and thawed implanted embryos.[102] Surprisingly there were no changes in imprinted genes from leucocytes found from this cohort.[103] However, the phenotype and epigenotype described of adults born following IVF have been variable and inconsistent.[104]

EPIGENETICS OF FETAL IN UTERO EXPERIENCES AND EXPOSURES

The direct effect of the environment on the development and phenotype of complex diseases might be overstated.[105] Rather, differences within the long-term profiles of epigenetic modifications are often a better explanation for observed differences in phenotype (Fig. 2.5).[105] Hale's original "thrifty phenotype"—and more recently, the predictive adaptive response, PARs—hypotheses postulate that poor fetal and infant nutrition in early life contributes to development of metabolic and cardiovascular disorders in later life.[106,107] Furthermore, the developmental programming hypothesis proposes that the degree of mismatch between the pre- and post-natal environments is a major determinant of subsequent disease risk. Therefore, it is thought that while changes in fetal physiology, in response to environmental cues, may be beneficial for short-term survival in utero and in the immediate postnatal period, they may be maladaptive in later life.[107]

THE EPIGENETICS OF MATERNAL/FETAL DIET

Developmental plasticity involves the adjustment of gene expression to produce a phenotype in utero that will likely be most appropriate for the post-natal environment.[108] However, when there is a mismatch between the expected and actual postnatal environments, the propensity of the individual to develop later disease increases, particularly in the presence of a secondary environmental insult such as a postnatal obesogenic diet.[107] Epigenetic regulation during development undergoes dynamic changes, so that the epigenome is labile, responding and adapting to environmental stressors such as altered nutrition in early life.[109] There is extensive epidemiologic, clinical, and experimental evidence showing a link between altered early-life nutrition and later-life disease risk (preferentially termed as *developmental programming*).[96,110-113] The underpinning epigenetic mechanisms are now being described. For example, maternal carbohydrate intake is associated with epigenetic gene promoter methylation at birth and later adiposity in children, thus suggesting that a component of metabolic disease risk has a prenatal developmental basis.[100] Importantly, this also suggests that analyzing the pattern of epigenetic modifications present during perinatal development may have utility as early biomarkers to identify individual vulnerability to later obesity and metabolic disease.

Maternal Under- or Overnutrition

Maternal malnutrition directly affects fetal growth. When nutrients and/or energy that are vital for growth are lacking, the fetus "switches" into survival mode. This means that sufficient resources are provided to certain organ systems, while other systems that are not essential for short-term survival receive insufficient or no resources.[96] For example, limited maternal protein intake may favor the growth and development of the fetal brain at the expense of growth in skeletal muscle, kidney, or pancreas, leading to alterations in transcription factors that regulate energy homeostasis in skeletal muscle, renal nephrogenesis, or beta-cell development, respectively.[114] Suboptimal nutrition can also affect levels of transcription factors (e.g., hepatocyte nuclear factor 4a [HNF4A]) through alterations to DNA methylation profiles and histone modification.[115]

Early epidemiologic studies demonstrated that fetal growth restriction correlated with adult disease, implying that fetal nutritional deprivation is a strong stimulus for epigenetic

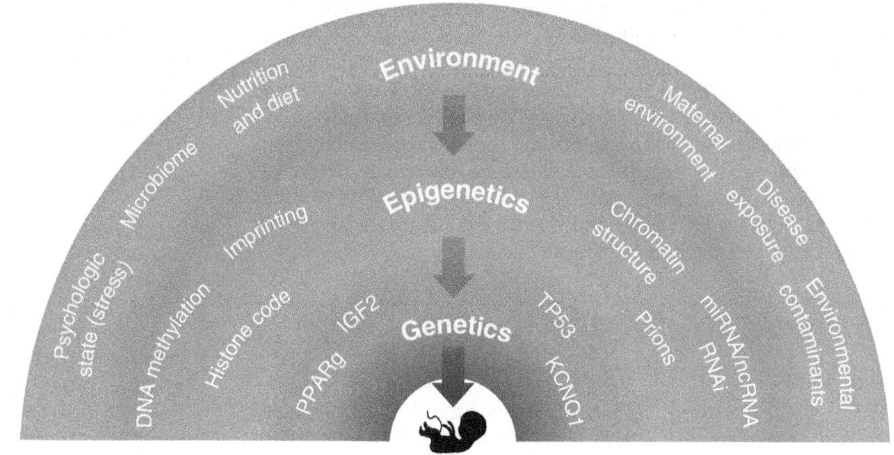

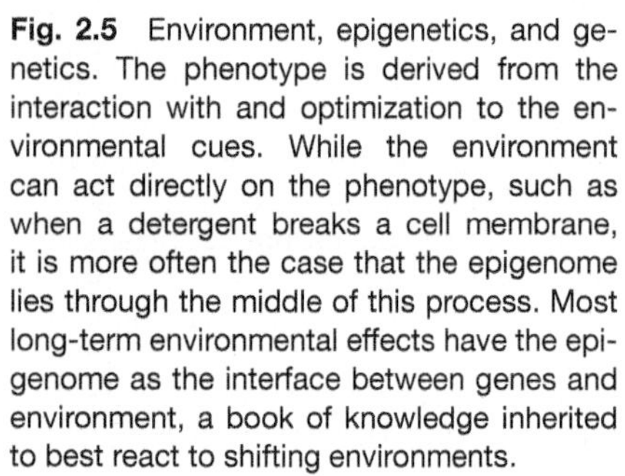

Fig. 2.5 Environment, epigenetics, and genetics. The phenotype is derived from the interaction with and optimization to the environmental cues. While the environment can act directly on the phenotype, such as when a detergent breaks a cell membrane, it is more often the case that the epigenome lies through the middle of this process. Most long-term environmental effects have the epigenome as the interface between genes and environment, a book of knowledge inherited to best react to shifting environments.

programming.[112] In particular, IUGR may arise in late gestation as a consequence of maternal undernutrition, which in rats is associated with a range of metabolic abnormalities in offspring in later life, including insulin resistance and type 2 diabetes mellitus.[96] IUGR has a direct effect on pancreatic epigenetics, being associated with chromatin remodeling and subsequent transcriptional silencing of the pancreatic and duodenal homeobox 1 *(PDX1)* gene in beta cells.[116] Interestingly, neonatal treatment with the glucagon like peptide (GLP)-1 analog Exendin-4 increases histone acetylase activity, reversing epigenetic modifications that silence PDX1 in the growth restricted rat.[117]

In many developed societies, maternal and postnatal caloric intake can be excessive. There is consequently an increasing focus on maternal obesity, given the marked increases in the rates of women entering pregnancy while overweight/obese.[118] Fetuses of obese mothers develop insulin resistance prior to birth.[119] In addition, women who are overweight or obese during pregnancy are more likely to have children born large for gestational age, who are in turn more likely to have higher body mass index later in life.[96] Furthermore, a maternal high-fat diet has been linked to epigenetic changes in the adiponectin promoter region (histone H3K9) and the leptin promoter region (histone H4K20), which cause altered adiponectin and leptin expression in adipose tissue.[120] Moreover, these fetal changes are sex-specific.[121,122]

Notably, both ends of the maternal nutritional spectrum (under- and overnutrition) result in similar long-term phenotypic outcomes in the offspring, thus the relationship is not linear but rather "U" shaped. However, one caveat for models using overnutrition is that, in many cases, human obesity is associated with micronutrient deficiencies. Thus, the phenotypic similarities in the profiles of the epigenetic modifications that are observed in offspring from either undernourished or overnourished mothers may be a consequence of suboptimal nutrient transport. One example of this "obesity malnutrition" has been described in overnourished rat dams that exhibit a reduction in methyl donor availability.[123] Although the mechanisms are yet to be properly defined, it has been hypothesized that prenatal exposures that increase long-term risk for diseases, such as type 2 diabetes, are caused by similar changes to the epigenetic modification profiles.[124]

Beyond DNA methylation and histone modifications, miRNAs are emerging as a focus of research in developmental programming. For example, the miRNA profile of human breast milk has been shown to be altered by a maternal high-fat diet, thus exposing the infant to a different epigenetic load.[125] In male children with low birth weight, suboptimal nutrition in early life increases the expression of miR483-3p in adipose tissue, altering the ability of the adipocytes to store lipids.[126] In experimental models, a maternal high-fat diet has been shown to alter levels of certain hepatic miRNAs concomitant with changes in gene expression, including IGF2, a major fetal growth factor that also plays a key role in islet beta cell survival.[127] Furthermore, a maternal low-protein diet influenced insulin secretion and glucose homeostasis in the offspring through a mechanism that involved a reduction in mTOR expression and increased expression of a subset of miRNAs.[128] Importantly, blockade of these identified microRNAs in these islets restored mTOR and insulin secretion to normal. Therefore, these data suggest that a specific set of miRNAs are important for pancreatic beta-cell differentiation, are essential for the fine-tuning of insulin secretion, and play a crucial role in compensatory beta cell mass expansion in response to insulin resistance.[129,130]

In addition to the role of the maternal diet, it is becoming clearer that the paternal transmission of phenotypic traits is also important.[131] For example, it has been shown in rats that paternal obesity can affect the methylation state of genes and beta-cell dysfunction in the female offspring.[132,133] Clinical data have also now shown that paternal obesity is associated with IGF2 hypomethylation in newborns.[134] Similarly it has been shown that exposure to a low-protein diet in male mice results in sperm that exhibit global hypomethylation concomitant with reduced testicular expression of DNA methylation and folate-cycle regulators as compared to males fed a normal-protein diet.[135]

Macro and Micronutrients in the Maternal and Fetal Diets

Adequate fetal nutrition requires a balanced supply of nutrients in the maternal diet, and altered supplies of various macronutrients have been implicated in developmental problems.[110] Critically, there is evidence of defects in fetal and early-life metabolism when the maternal diet is deficient in methyl donors (i.e., betaine, choline, folic acid, methionine, or vitamin B_{12}), protein, zinc, and/or vitamin D.[136] As an example, increased maternal vitamin B_{12} levels during pregnancy are associated with decreased global DNA methylation in newborns, while increased serum B_{12} levels in newborns are associated with reduced methylation of the insulin-like growth factor-binding protein 3 (IGFBP-3) gene, involved in intrauterine growth.[137]

Existing evidence on the effects of fetal nutrition on developmental programming show that the maternal diet must include foods that contain methyl donors (for a comprehensive review see Dominguez-Salas and colleagues[136] and references therein). Reduced levels of methyl donors within the maternal diet can lead to global genome hypomethylation in the developing fetus, across all cell types. As there are baseline levels of methylation required for normal embryonic development, suboptimal methylation is associated with developmental problems (such as cleft lip and palate or neural tube defects), and very lower levels can be fatal.[40] Without methyl donors, the fetus cannot implement cell-specific methylation patterns.[138] For example, DNA methylation increases with gestational age within at least three differentially methylated regions (DMRs), one near a transcription factor (NFIX), a cyclic AMP binding protein (RAPGEF2), and a methionine sulfoxide reductase B3 (MSRB3) gene.[139] Therefore, preventing the developmental-specific methylation of these loci will impact on a wide range of cellular functions in the fetus.

Diets supplemented with excess methyl donors have also been shown to alter the DNA methylation patterns that are established, causing sex-specific long-term effects such as excessive weight gain, altered immune response, elevated blood pressure, and insulin resistance.[140] This is consistent with epigenetic modifications acting on loci (e.g., IGF2) that are maternally imprinted and have long-term epigenetic differences associated with nutritional or environmental stimuli during fetal growth.[141]

Betaine, folic acid, vitamin B_{12}, and choline are all involved in the synthesis of methionine or in methyl group donation.[24] A deficiency of these nutrients, or SNPs in the enzymes involved in the methyl donor pathway, can lead to clinically relevant phenotypes. Studies have shown that maternal diets poor in vitamins B_{12} or D alter metabolism in the offspring and can lead to low birth weight, higher visceral fat, dyslipidemia, and insulin resistance later in life. The pathways that result in these adverse phenotypic changes are not fully understood. Importantly, in mice, maternal diets with higher folic acid, vitamin B_{12}, choline, or betaine levels have been shown to change the composition of various epigenetic marks in the offspring, including CpG island demethylation in genes responsible for brain development, hippocampal function, and cell cycle.[24,142] Similarly, folic acid supplementation of low-protein diets fed to rat mothers during pregnancy prevented hypomethylation of hepatic peroxisomal proliferator-activated receptor-a (PPARa) and glucocorticoid receptor.[138] Defects in PPARa are associated with dysregulation of fatty acid metabolism (altered lipid levels), resulting in clinical phenotypes such as diabetes and heart disease.[143]

THE EPIGENETICS OF NURTURE

A stressful maternal environment can be associated with major alterations to the epigenetic profile of the fetus.[144] For example, the level of maternal care has been shown experimentally to influence hypothalamic-pituitary-adrenal function through epigenetic modifications of glucocorticoid receptor expression.[145] Moreover, it has been documented that the effects of a stressful environment can be passed on from generation to generation in mice.[144] Higher levels of maternal grooming and care reduce pup anxiety, which was associated with epigenetic modifications at the gene for cortisol receptor (a stress hormone).[146] In addition, these epigenetic modifications at the cortisol receptor were reversible by supplementing the adult diet with methionine or a histone deacetylase inhibitor.[146] On the other hand, a high-stress maternal environment during mouse pregnancy can lead to reduced methylation in the promoters of the offspring genes for central corticotrophin-releasing factor and glucocorticoid receptor.[147]

Similar observations have been made in human studies, where maternal prenatal stress has been linked to methylation in the promoter of the cortisol receptor gene, again reinforcing the concept that early-life events can shape the fetal epigenetic profile, with important consequences across the individual's lifespan.[148] For example, maternal prenatal-stress-related changes at the cortisol receptor were present in the children as late as adolescence.[148] Therefore, the epigenetic programming of prenatal stress can be measured many years later, making it a long-term concern for the individual's health.

THE EPIGENETICS OF EXTERNAL MATERNAL ENVIRONMENT

Environmental agents such as endocrine disruptor chemicals (methoxychlor, polycyclic aromatic hydrocarbons, and bisphenol A [BPA]), diethylstilbestrol, tobacco smoke, and alcohol have all been shown to play a role in shaping the fetal epigenome,[149] with the ultimate result being acute or late-onset diseases in the affected individuals. Methoxychlor has been shown to have transgenerational effects in rats, possibly mediated by increases to DNMT3B activity that leads to hypermethylation in the ovaries.[76] By contrast, prenatal exposure to polycyclic aromatic hydrocarbons is linked to asthma, possibly acting through a mechanism that involves hypomethylation of the genome through early childhood until at least 3 years of age.[76] BPA exposure during development has been associated with a number of diseases, including cancer, abrogation of sexual dimorphism, social behaviors, and memory impairments.[76] For cancer at least, this association has been shown to involve changes to methylation levels in the prostate tissues (reviewed in Perera and Herbstman[76]). Smoking and alcohol intake affect global DNA methylation pathways, leading to increased DNA methylation and reduced DNA acetylation in the brains of subjects exposed in utero.[149,150]

LONG-TERM EFFECTS OF EPIGENETICS

TRANSGENERATIONAL EPIGENETICS

The observation of phenotypic effects across generations is typically assumed to represent a familial aggregation and therefore a genetic cause. However, the transgenerational inheritance of epigenetic modifications has been proposed as means of transmitting phenotypic traits that allow future generations to be maximally competitive in their environment.[151] Under this assumption, adaptive changes to gene expression, or patterns of gene regulation, that are acquired during the parental lifespan may be passed to and persist in the offspring, increasing the fitness of future generations within the same environment. However, if the environment changes, then the evidence suggests that environmental exposures (such as poor early-life nutrition) results in maladaptive parental responses being passed to offspring. Therefore, the transgenerational transmission of epigenetic traits may lead to a population-wide manifestation of a harmful phenotype (i.e., obesity) over several generations.[14,151]

In order for the transmission of epigenetic modifications to be considered truly transgenerational, the effect must be shown to carry across at least four generations, as transmission across three generations can be explained by the environmental exposure acting on the mother (F0), her fetus (F1), and the fetal germ cells (F2), at a single moment in time.[9] In mice, this ability of an environmental exposure to cause an epigenetic change that leads to a persistent phenotypic change through four generations has been proven to exist, in the setting of endocrine disruptors.[152] However, in the context of early-life nutrition, the data from animal models are both limited and varied—in a meta-analysis of nine studies carried through to F3, five failed to show any effect.[153] Therefore, despite transgenerational epigenetic inheritance being established in plants[154] and mice,[155] it remains a controversial area of research in humans and other mammals.[156]

In humans, the best evidence of a transmissible epiallele comes from the comprehensive study of the transgenerational effects of the Dutch Famine cohort. The Dutch famine was caused by food restrictions imposed on the Dutch population by the occupying German forces in 1944–1945. As a result, energy intake by most individuals was far below recommended levels, and ongoing pregnancies during this time were affected by this undernutrition (at the height of the famine intake was between 400 and 800 calories per day).[141] Pregnancies in their first trimester were particularly vulnerable to the effects of maternal undernutrition.[157] Interestingly, the maternal undernutrition not only affected the long-term health of the offspring, but also led to adverse health outcomes that persisted into the next generation (born many years later in a nutritionally replete environment).[158] The long-term effects of the Dutch famine on the subsequent generations have been shown in part to be epigenetic, affecting, among other things, DNA methylation of IGF2.[141] Whether these observed effects are truly transgenerational are not yet known, as the F2 phenotype may simply reflect the impact of the original maternal nutritional insult.

The impact of paternal nutrition in transgenerational epigenetic inheritance has also been reported.[159] Paternal obesity was shown to initiate metabolic disturbances in two generations of mice, albeit with incomplete penetrance to the F2 generation.[159] Diet-induced paternal obesity modulated sperm miRNA content and germ methylation status, which are signals that can program offspring health and initiate the transmission of obesity to future generations. Studies in F1 sperm have suggested a role for altered IGF2 expression in transmission of a phenotype to the F2 offspring.[160] However, not all studies reporting a paternal line transmission have reported epigenetic alterations in the F1 sperm.[161] Recent work in mice has suggested that the paternal diet can program offspring outcomes via both sperm genomic (epigenetic) and seminal plasma (maternal uterine environment) mechanisms.[135] However, despite the "obvious" linkage of these nutritional effects to epigenetic transgenerational inheritance, other studies have shown that the epigenetic reprogramming of imprinting control regions in the germline was not susceptible to nutritional restriction, thus suggesting that mechanisms other than direct germline transmission are responsible.[162]

THERAPEUTIC APPROACHES TO EPIGENETICS

The field of epigenetics represents a relatively new avenue for the discovery of control mechanisms for biologic pathways that are altered in complex disease.[26] Most research to date has been focused on the critical role of epigenetics in mediating the effects of environmental exposure and nutrition. However, one can potentially create a therapy to alter epigenetic markings in a way to silence or activate a gene whose inappropriate expression is linked to the long-term increase in disease risk. Targeting the epigenetic machinery may enable the restoration of balance to a regulatory system that is in disarray.

From a nondevelopmental standpoint, there is a plethora of evidence for epigenetic influences in diseases, including most cancers, asthma, allergy, obesity, type 2 diabetes, coronary heart disease, autism spectrum disorders, bipolar disorder, eating disorders, and schizophrenia (e.g., see Stahl[163]). Within many of these fields of research, there are drugs either on the market or currently in testing that target potential epigenetic modifications.[163] For example, valproic acid (used to treat epilepsy and bipolar mania), carbamazepine (a treatment for epilepsy), and vorinostat (a treatment of cutaneous T cell lymphoma) are known to inhibit histone deacetylases, thus creating open chromatin environments and affecting gene regulation.[164] By contrast, inhibitors of histone acetyltransferases (e.g., curcumin[165] and anacardic acid[166]) could possibly be used to promote the closing of active chromatin states, by reductions in the levels of acetylated histones. Both curcumin and anacardic acid are in clinical trials for human therapy.[61] The antipsychotic drugs clozapine and sulpiride facilitate demethylation of GABAergic promoters[166] and may correct altered gene expression profiles associated with schizophrenia.[167] Likewise, the antidepressant drug amitriptyline acts to induce slight cytosine demethylation without affecting histone acetylation in rat primary astrocytes.[168]

Finally, the manipulation of nutrition itself may be therapeutic for long-term disease outcome in situations where there is a strong epigenetic component. For example, as previously mentioned, experimental models have shown that a range of methyl donor supplements (including glycine, choline, and folic acid) normalize epigenetic profiles and phenotypic outcomes in offspring born to undernourished mothers.[138] Furthermore, neonatal leptin treatment has been shown to be protective against later obesity, via changes in promoter methylation of the hypothalamic pro-opiomelanocortin gene.[169]

CONCLUSION

Early development is characterized by a dynamic process of epigenetic regulation. The sum total of the epigenetic modifications that are present in a cell (i.e., the epigenome) is labile and responds and adapts to environmental stressors that include early-life nutrition.

There are still many questions to be answered about how epigenetic modifications are controlled, established, and remodeled throughout fetal development: (1) How amenable to intervention is the system; (2) which windows of development should be targeted for meaningful therapy; (3) how many generations does it take to reverse epigenetic imprinting; (4) can reliable markers of maladaptive epigenetic profiles be developed for disease prediction? Answering these questions will provide fundamental translatable knowledge for the future development of approaches to take therapeutic advantage of epigenetics.

It should be borne in mind that the link between an altered early-life epigenetic profile and later-life disease risk has been established by epidemiologic, experimental, and clinical studies.[112] However, the contribution and mechanism(s) by which early-life changes to epigenetics make a difference to disease outcomes largely remain to be determined. This is because, in contrast to research on primary DNA sequence, epigenetic modifications are both time- and tissue-specific.[4,5] Moreover, the combinatorial nature of epigenetic modifications means that each grouping can have dramatically different effects on different genes, cells, and ultimately the individual's phenotype. Yet despite being long term, epigenetic processes are potentially reversible and represent a real and viable therapeutic proposition.

GLOSSARY

BIOLOGIC TERMS

Apoptosis: programmed cell death

Cell cycle: the process or series of events that leads to a cell division and duplication, resulting in the production of two daughter cells

Chromatin: the primary basis of DNA packaging, a complex of macromolecules consisting of DNA, RNA, and proteins

Chromosome: consisting of DNA and protein, a chromosome is a packaged and organized form of DNA (chromatin). Healthy humans have 22 pairs of autosomes and 1 pair of sex chromosomes (XX or XY), for a total of 46 chromosomes per cell. Within the mitochondria there also exist hundreds of copies of the mitochondrial genome, sometimes referred to collectively as the mitochondrial chromosome

DNA: deoxyribonucleic acid—the genetic instructions (inherited traits) inside the cell's nucleus that form the basis of the control of cellular replication and function. DNA is composed of four nucleotides, guanine (G), adenine (A), thymine (T), and cytosine (C) in a base-pairing configuration where A pairs with T and C with G through hydrogen bonding

DNA methylation: alkylation with a methyl group, replacing a hydrogen. In humans, this occurs at points in the DNA where a cytosine nucleotide is followed by a guanine nucleotide (CpG)

Epiallele: an allele only different by its epigenetic state. Usually identified as identical genes that differ in the extent of methylation

Epigenetics: the study of heritable traits that are not caused by changes in the DNA sequence

Epigenome: a record or catalog of the epigenetic modifications or states within a cell or individual

Euchromatin: loosely or lightly packaged DNA (chromatin) that is notable for being of high gene concentration and usually high transcription

Gene expression: a process of transcribing DNA gene information into a functional gene product (mRNA or proteins). Most likely to be measured or expressed in terms of levels of mRNA in the cell

Heterochromatin: the opposite of euchromatin. Tightly packaged DNA (chromatin) that is notable for being of low DNA replicative activity

Histone: the main protein component of chromatin and nucleosomes. These proteins package and order the DNA, acting as spools around which DNA winds. Histone modifications play a role in epigenetic gene regulation

Hypomethylation: a decrease or dearth of epigenetic methylation of cytosine residues

Hypermethylation: an overabundance of epigenetic methylation of cytosine residues

Imprinting: an epigenetic (via methylation) phenomenon by which certain genes are expressed in a parent-of-origin-specific manner

Intrauterine growth restriction (IUGR): babies born smaller than expected with a weight below the 10th percentile for their gestational age

Metazoan: any animal that undergoes development from an embryo stage with the ectoderm, mesoderm, and endoderm

Methyl donor: a compound capable of the formation of methionine or of providing a methyl group during a cellular methylation reaction. A good example is dietary folate

Monozygotic and dizygotic twins: twin births can come from a single egg split into two (monozygotic or maternal twins) or from two separate eggs (dizygotic or fraternal twins).

mRNA: messenger RNA—RNA molecules that convey genetic information from DNA to the ribosome, where they specify the amino acid sequence of the protein products of gene expression

Necrosis: traumatic cell death

Nucleosome: approximately 147 base pairs of DNA wrapped 1.67 times around a barrel-shaped histone octamer containing two copies of the core histones H2A, H2B, H3, and H4

Plasticity: the adaptability of an organism to changes in its environment

Pluripotent: a cell that is capable of giving rise to several different cell types. Embryonic stem cells are a good example of pluripotent cells

MEDICAL TERMS

Phenotype: an organism's observable characteristics or traits, such as height or weight

RNA: ribonucleic acid—The major role of RNA is as the molecule of gene expression. DNA is transcribed into mRNA, which is then translated into amino acids, which form proteins. Various regulatory forms of RNA, known broadly as *non-coding RNA*, are epigenetic

Sexual dimorphism: a phenotypic difference between males and females of the same species

SNP: single nucleotide polymorphism—a DNA sequence variation occurring commonly within a population

Transcription: the act of copying DNA into mRNA. The first step of gene expression

A complete reference list is available at www.ExpertConsult.com.

SELECT REFERENCES

1. Lander ES, Linton LM, Birren B, et al. Initial sequencing and analysis of the human genome. *Nature*. 2001;409(6822):860-921. https://doi.org/10.1038/35057062.
2. Venter JC, Adams MD, Myers EW, et al. The sequence of the human genome. *Science*. 2001;291(5507):1304-1351. https://doi.org/10.1126/science.1058040.
3. The human genome. Science genome map. *Science*. 2001;291(5507):1218. https://doi.org/10.1126/science.291.5507.1218.
6. Waddington CH. The epigenotype. 1942. *Int J Epidemiol*. 2012;41(1):10-13. https://doi.org/10.1093/ije/dyr184.
7. Russo VEA, Martienssen RA, Riggs AD, Plainview NY. *Epigenetic Mechanisms of Gene Regulation*. Cold Spring Harbor Laboratory Press; 1996.
8. Cavalli G, Heard E. Advances in epigenetics link genetics to the environment and disease. *Nature*. 2019;571(7766):489-499. https://doi.org/10.1038/s41586-019-1411-0.
12. Kunkel TA, Bebenek K. DNA replication fidelity. *Annu Rev Biochem*. 2000;69:497-529. https://doi.org/10.1146/annurev.biochem.69.1.497.
13. Bird A. Perceptions of epigenetics. *Nature*. 2007;447(7143):396-398. https://doi.org/10.1038/nature05913.
15. Gluckman PD, Hanson MA, Buklijas T, Low FM, Beedle AS. Epigenetic mechanisms that underpin metabolic and cardiovascular diseases. *Nat Rev Endocrinol*. 2009;5(7):401-408. https://doi.org/10.1038/nrendo.2009.102.
17. Fraga MF, Ballestar E, Paz MF, et al. Epigenetic differences arise during the lifetime of monozygotic twins. *Proc Natl Acad Sci U S A*. 2005;102(30):10604-10609. https://doi.org/10.1073/pnas.0500398102.
22. Crews D, Gillette R, Miller-Crews I, Gore AC, Skinner MK. Nature, nurture and epigenetics. *Mol Cell Endocrinol*. 2014;398(1-2):42-52. https://doi.org/10.1016/j.mce.2014.07.013.
23. Gamage TKJB, Schierding W, Hurley D, et al. The role of DNA methylation in human trophoblast differentiation. *Epigenetics*. 2018;13(12):1154-1173. https://doi.org/10.1080/15592294.2018.1549462.
24. Zeisel SH. Epigenetic mechanisms for nutrition determinants of later health outcomes. *Am J Clin Nutr*. 2009;89(5):1488S-1493S. https://doi.org/10.3945/ajcn.2009.27113B.
26. Schierding W, Cutfield WS, O'Sullivan JM. The missing story behind Genome Wide Association Studies: single nucleotide polymorphisms in gene deserts have a story to tell. *Front Genet*. 2014;5:39. https://doi.org/10.3389/fgene.2014.00039.
29. Kempfer R, Pombo A. Methods for mapping 3D chromosome architecture. *Nat Rev Genet*. 2019;21:207-226.https://doi.org/10.1038/s41576-019-0195-2.
30. McCord RP, Kaplan N, Giorgetti L. Chromosome conformation capture and beyond: toward an integrative view of chromosome structure and function. *Mol Cell*. 2020;77(4):688-708. https://doi.org/10.1016/j.molcel.2019.12.021.
31. Chen K, Rajewsky N. The evolution of gene regulation by transcription factors and microRNAs. *Nat Rev Genet*. 2007;8(2):93-103. https://doi.org/10.1038/nrg1990.
35. Chen T, Dent SY. Chromatin modifiers and remodellers: regulators of cellular differentiation. *Nat Rev Genet*. 2014;15(2):93-106. https://doi.org/10.1038/nrg3607.
37. He XJ, Chen T, Zhu JK. Regulation and function of DNA methylation in plants and animals. *Cell Res*. 2011;21(3):442-465. https://doi.org/10.1038/cr.2011.23.
42. Haggarty P, Hoad G, Horgan GW, Campbell DM. DNA methyltransferase candidate polymorphisms, imprinting methylation, and birth outcome. *PloS One*. 2013;8(7):e68896. https://doi.org/10.1371/journal.pone.0068896.
44. Luger K, Mader AW, Richmond RK, Sargent DF, Richmond TJ. Crystal structure of the nucleosome core particle at 2.8 A resolution. *Nature*. 1997;389(6648):251-260. https://doi.org/10.1038/38444.
46. Allis CD, Muir TW. Spreading chromatin into chemical biology. *Chembiochem*. 2011;12(2):264-279. https://doi.org/10.1002/cbic.201000761.
48. Gates LA, Foulds CE, O'Malley BW. Histone marks in the "Driver's Seat": functional roles in steering the transcription cycle. *Trends Biochem Sci*. 2017;42(12):P977-989. https://doi.org/10.1016/j.tibs.2017.10.004.
52. Gibcus JH, Dekker J. The hierarchy of the 3D genome. *Mol Cell*. 2013;49(5):773-782. https://doi.org/10.1016/j.molcel.2013.02.011.
60. French JD, Ghoussaini M, Edwards SL, et al. Functional variants at the 11q13 risk locus for breast cancer regulate cyclin D1 expression through long-range enhancers. *Am J Hum Genet*. 2013;92(4):489-503. https://doi.org/10.1016/j.ajhg.2013.01.002.
61. Fahrner JA, Bjornsson HT. Mendelian disorders of the epigenetic machinery: tipping the balance of chromatin states. *Annu Rev Genomics Hum Genet*. 2014;15:269-293. https://doi.org/10.1146/annurev-genom-090613-094245.
63. Hnisz D, Abraham BJ, Lee TI, et al. Super-enhancers in the control of cell identity and disease. *Cell*. 2013;155(4):934-947. https://doi.org/10.1016/j.cell.2013.09.053.
76. Perera F, Herbstman J. Prenatal environmental exposures, epigenetics, and disease. *Reprod Toxicol*. 2011;31(3):363-373. https://doi.org/10.1016/j.reprotox.2010.12.055.
77. Cutfield WS, Hofman PL, Mitchell M, Morison IM. Could epigenetics play a role in the developmental origins of health and disease? *Pediatr Res*. 2007;61(5 Pt 2):68R-75R. https://doi.org/10.1203/pdr.0b013e318045764c.
80. Butler MG. Genomic imprinting disorders in humans: a mini-review. *J Assist Reprod Genet*. 2009;26(9-10):477-486. https://doi.org/10.1007/s10815-009-9353-3.
88. Haig D, Graham C. Genomic imprinting and the strange case of the insulin-like growth factor II receptor. *Cell*. 1991;64(6):1045-1046. http://www.ncbi.nlm.nih.gov/pubmed/1848481.
90. Jirtle RL, Skinner MK. Environmental epigenomics and disease susceptibility. *Nat Rev Genet*. 2007;8(4):253-262. https://doi.org/10.1038/nrg2045.
92. Riggs AD. X inactivation, differentiation, and DNA methylation. *Cytogenet Cell Genet*. 1975;14(1):9-25. http://www.ncbi.nlm.nih.gov/pubmed/1093816.
96. Duque-Guimaraes DE, Ozanne SE. Nutritional programming of insulin resistance: causes and consequences. *Trends Endocrinol Metab*. 2013;24(10):525-535. https://doi.org/10.1016/j.tem.2013.05.006.
107. Gluckman PD, Hanson MA, Beedle AS, Spencer HG. Predictive adaptive responses in perspective. *Trends Endocrinol Metab*. 2008;19(4):109-110. https://doi.org/10.1016/j.tem.2008.02.002.
109. Jang H, Serra C. Nutrition, epigenetics, and diseases. *Clin Nutr Res*. 2014;3(1):1-8. https://doi.org/10.7762/cnr.2014.3.1.1.
110. McMillen IC, MacLaughlin SM, Muhlhausler BS, Gentili S, Duffield JL, Morrison JL. Developmental origins of adult health and disease: the role of periconceptional and foetal nutrition. *Basic Clin Pharmacol Toxicol*. 2008;102(2):82-89. https://doi.org/10.1111/j.1742-7843.2007.00188.x.
121. Lesseur C, Armstrong DA, Paquette AG, Li Z, Padbury JF, Marsit CJ. Maternal obesity and gestational diabetes are associated with placental leptin DNA methylation. *Am J Obstet Gynecol*. 2014;211(6): 654.e1-9. https://doi.org/10.1016/j.ajog.2014.06.037.
124. Quilter CR, Cooper WN, Cliffe KM, et al. Impact on offspring methylation patterns of maternal gestational diabetes mellitus and intrauterine growth restraint suggest common genes and pathways linked to subsequent type 2 diabetes risk. *FASEB J*. 2014;28(11):4868-4879. https://doi.org/10.1096/fj.14-255240.
131. Hur SSJ, Cropley JE, Suter CM. Paternal epigenetic programming: evolving metabolic disease risk. *J Mol Endocrinol*. 2017;58(3):R159-R168. https://doi.org/10.1530/JME-16-0236.
134. Soubry A, Schildkraut JM, Murtha A, et al. Paternal obesity is associated with IGF2 hypomethylation in newborns: results from a Newborn Epigenetics Study (NEST) cohort. *BMC Med*. 2013;11(1):29. https://doi.org/10.1186/1741-7015-11-29.
136. Dominguez-Salas P, Cox SE, Prentice AM, Hennig BJ, Moore SE. Maternal nutritional status, C(1) metabolism and offspring DNA methylation: a review of current evidence in human subjects. *Proc Nutr Soc*. 2012;71(1):154-165. https://doi.org/10.1017/S0029665111003338.
141. Heijmans BT, Tobi EW, Stein AD, et al. Persistent epigenetic differences associated with prenatal exposure to famine in humans. *Proc Natl Acad Sci U S A*. 2008;105(44):17046-17049. https://doi.org/10.1073/pnas.0806560105.
155. Dolinoy DC. The agouti mouse model: an epigenetic biosensor for nutritional and environmental alterations on the fetal epigenome. *Nutr Rev*. 2008;66(suppl 1):S7-S11. https://doi.org/10.1111/j.1753-4887.2008.00056.x.
162. Radford EJ, Isganaitis E, Jimenez-Chillaron J, et al. An unbiased assessment of the role of imprinted genes in an intergenerational model of developmental programming. *PLoS Genet*. 2012;8(4):e1002605. https://doi.org/10.1371/journal.pgen.1002605.
169. Palou M, Picó C, McKay JA, et al. Protective effects of leptin during the suckling period against later obesity may be associated with changes in promoter methylation of the hypothalamic pro-opiomelanocortin gene. *Br J Nutr*. 2011;106(5):769-778. https://doi.org/10.1017/S0007114511000973.
176. Dekker J, Rippe K, Dekker M, Kleckner N. Capturing chromosome conformation. *Science*. 2002;295(5558):1306-1311. https://doi.org/10.1126/science.1067799.

Basic Embryology

3

David L. Bolender

INTRODUCTION

The human embryo begins as a single large cell, approximately 0.1 mm in diameter, just visible to the unaided eye. During the 266 days of gestation after fertilization, this cell increases in size, weight, and surface area in a rapid and markedly nonlinear fashion. From newly fertilized egg to newborn, length increases by a factor of 5000, surface area by a factor of 61 million, and weight by a factor of nearly 6 billion.[1] During this process the fertilized egg divides and differentiates into more than 200 different morphologically recognizable cell types. Orchestration of the increase in size and specialization in cellular function is a complex process about which much remains unknown. However, it has been argued that the principles of development have been established and that details are missing only at the molecular level.[2] This claim is undoubtedly an overstatement; nevertheless, during the past decade or so, understanding of the molecular control of development has increased substantially. That human embryonic development occurs normally in most pregnancies is a tribute to the design of the control mechanisms that are operating. This chapter presents a brief description of the growth and differentiation of the human embryo, along with a limited discussion of certain factors that play a part in control of these activities.

GAMETES AND THEIR MATURATION

The human egg and sperm are two highly specialized cells that share little in common with the other cells of the adult body. They are different in both form and function. However, like other cells, they must achieve a degree of maturity before they can perform their function (i.e., combining to form the zygote). The steps and the chronology leading to this maturation are quite different in the male and in the female, and such differences reflect the diverse pathways of the two sexes beginning early in human development.[3]

ORIGIN OF THE GAMETES

The human egg and sperm are derived from large, round primordial germ cells that can be identified in the wall of the yolk sac as early as 24 days after fertilization.[4] As the yolk sac begins to be incorporated into the embryo, the germ cells migrate along the dorsal mesentery of the hindgut to the gonadal ridges, which they reach by the end of the fourth or early fifth week (Fig. 3.1). This migration has been observed in vitro in pieces of hindgut, mesentery, and gonadal ridges of mouse embryos.[5] It is facilitated in humans by a striking ameboid shape (which persists even after the cells have reached the gonad[6]) and pseudopodia typical of those found in ameboid cells. The pseudopodia disappear after the migration is complete.[5,7] In humans these cells contain glycogen stores that diminish over time and disappear when the cells have reached their destination in the gonad, suggesting that the glycogen may be the energy source for their journey.[8]

ORGANIZATION OF THE GONAD

The coelomic epithelium covering the medial aspect of the gonadal ridges undergoes proliferation at approximately week 7 of gestation. As the epithelial cells multiply, they grow into the underlying mesenchyme in a series of fingerlike cords of cells called *primitive sex cords*. The primordial germ cells associate with these cords. If the embryo is to become a male, these cords continue to be prominent and eventually develop into the seminiferous tubules and rete testis. The early male gonad can also be recognized by the separation of the cords from their parent epithelial covering by a fibrous connective tissue layer, the tunica albuginea, which forms just under the epithelium. If the gonad is to become an ovary, the primitive sex cords remain rudimentary. The origin of the follicular cells of the ovary remains unclear, but likely candidates are cells from the coelomic epithelium and the mesonephros. The follicular cells associate with the primordial germ cells to form primordial ovarian follicles.[8]

DEVELOPMENT OF THE FEMALE GAMETE (SEE CHAPTER 147)

If the gonad develops into an ovary, the primordial germ cells become oogonia, and mitotic division continues.[9] Mitotic division of these cells has been observed in humans up to the seventh fetal month[10] but ceases sometime shortly before birth. No oogonia form after the birth of the infant after a normal full-term pregnancy.

In both males and females the germ cells form a syncytium while dividing.[11,12] These intercellular connections permit communication and facilitate the high degree of synchrony that has been observed during both mitotic division and meiotic division.[13-15]

By the eighth or ninth week after fertilization, some oogonia enter prophase of meiosis I and become primary oocytes.[9-16] Meiosis begins first deep to the surface of the human ovary and then expands toward the surface. Thus, at an appropriate fetal stage, oogonia are found superficially, oocytes deep to the surface, and small follicles at the inner part of the ovarian cortex.[9] It has been suggested that a diffusible meiosis-activating substance is secreted by rete cells (derived from the mesonephros), which lie in the center of the ovary, and good experimental evidence is available to support this hypothesis.[17-20]

The oocyte goes through the leptotene, zygotene, and pachytene stages of meiosis I, and it then stops at the diplotene stage. At this point the oocyte becomes surrounded by a single, incomplete layer of flat follicular cells[9]; this unit is called a *primordial follicle*. The follicle's large central nucleus is known as the *germinal vesicle*. A crescent-shaped assembly of cellular organelles containing mitochondria, endoplasmic reticulum, the Golgi complex, lysosomes, and annulate lamellae (stacked parallel membrane arrays with pores) remains clustered adjacent to the nucleus.[15,21] Once it has been incorporated into a primordial follicle, the oocyte enters a long period of quiescence, beginning before birth in humans and ending in either atresia or ovulation.

Once sexual maturity is attained, a small number of oocytes begin the process of folliculogenesis, or follicle maturation, during each menstrual cycle.[22] The oocyte grows and eventually becomes one of the largest cells in the human body.[23] The organelles disperse throughout the cytoplasm, and the germinal vesicle (nucleus) enlarges. It increases its complement of nuclear

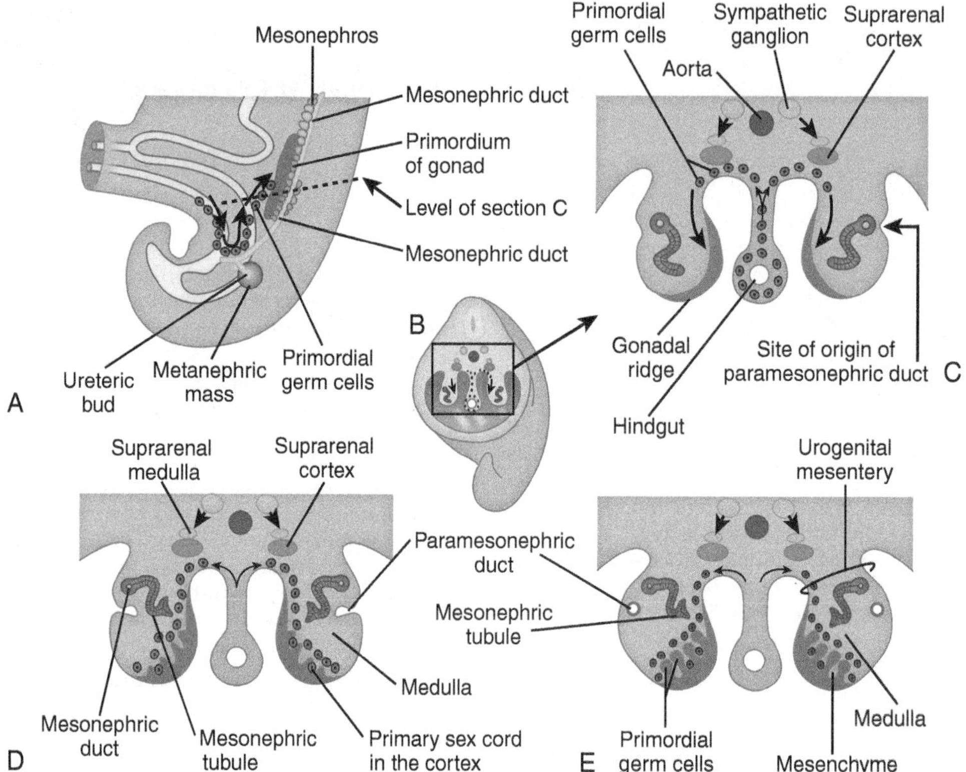

Fig. 3.1 (A) Sketch of a 5-week-old embryo, illustrating the migration of primordial germ cells from the yolk sac. (B) Three-dimensional sketch of the caudal region of a 5-week-old embryo, showing the location and extent of the gonadal ridges on the medial aspect of the urogenital ridges. (C) Transverse section showing the primordium of the suprarenal (adrenal) glands, the gonadal ridges, and the migration of primordial germ cells into the developing gonads. (D) Transverse section through a 6-week-old embryo, showing the primary sex cords and the developing paramesonephric ducts. (E) Similar section at a later stage showing the indifferent gonads and the mesonephric and paramesonephric ducts. (From Moore KL, Persaud TVN. *The Developing Human: Clinically Oriented Embryology.* 5th ed. Philadelphia: WB Saunders; 1993:281.)

pores, facilitating transport of molecules between nucleoplasm and cytoplasm. The follicular cells resume mitosis and increase markedly in size, changing in shape from squamous to cuboidal, and the follicle becomes surrounded by a basement membrane. Those follicles containing an oocyte surrounded by a single layer of cuboidal follicular cells are known as *unilaminar primary follicles,* to distinguish them from cells of earlier or later stages.[3]

During further growth of the primary follicle, a thick, acellular coat, the *zona pellucida,* begins to form between the oocyte and the follicular cells. Mitotic activity increases the number of follicular cell layers, and the follicle is now called a *multilaminar primary follicle.* The expanding follicle compresses the surrounding ovarian stoma, which organizes into a compact layer adjacent to the basement membrane of the follicle. This layer of stromal cells is called the *theca interna,* and its cells have the capacity to produce androgens when stimulated by luteinizing hormone activity (Fig. 3.2). The theca interna is vascularized, but the epithelial layers of follicular cells remain avascular.

The zona pellucida is important in the process of fertilization because it contains sperm receptors, takes part in induction of the acrosome reaction, and becomes a block to polyspermy. It may also act after fertilization as a smooth, slippery envelope to contain the sticky ball of cells of the morula-stage embryo; these cells are free to adhere to the uterine endothelium when the zona breaks down, just before implantation.

The zona pellucida is made up of four separate filamentous glycoproteins, zona pellucida glycoprotein 1 (ZP1) through ZP4, which differ in molecular weight and isoelectric point and account for virtually all protein in the zona pellucida. ZP1 crosslinks these filaments, resulting in a three-dimensional matrix that is permeable to large macromolecules. ZP3 serves as a species-specific sperm receptor and also induces the acrosome reaction in sperm on contact. At or shortly after fertilization, these two characteristics are lost, reducing the likelihood of polyspermy.[24-26] The ZP3 gene has been cloned; it is expressed only in oocytes, and then only during the growth phase of oogenesis.[27] ZP1, ZP2, and ZP3 are located on chromosomes 19, 7, and 5, respectively, while ZP4 is located on chromosomes 11, 16, 7, and 1.[28] The interesting story of these zona pellucida proteins has been the subject of a popularized account[29] and several reviews.[30-32] Radiolabeling studies in mice indicate that all three glycoproteins are synthesized by the oocyte itself, rather than by the follicular cells.[33] Furthermore, immunofluorescence studies show that zona pellucida antigens are present within human oocytes but not in follicular cells.[34] However, studies in species other than the mouse suggest that the granulosa cells that surround the oocyte also may play a role in the synthesis of zona pellucida components.[31]

Numerous cytoplasmic projections of the follicular cells penetrate the zona pellucida to contact the cell membrane of the oocyte. In humans these filopodial extensions of the follicular cell may actually lie deeply buried in the oocyte, in straight invaginations or pits.[35] These pits are lined by the oocyte cell membrane; however, no cytoplasmic continuity exists between the two cell types. Animal studies have demonstrated the presence of gap junctions along the association of these two cell membranes, permitting transfer of small molecules (molecular weight of approximately 1000) between them.[22]

As the primary follicle enlarges, the follicular cells begin to produce follicular fluid, which collects within the intercellular spaces between follicular cells. These spaces coalesce to form a large fluid-filled cavity called the *antrum,* which is characteristic

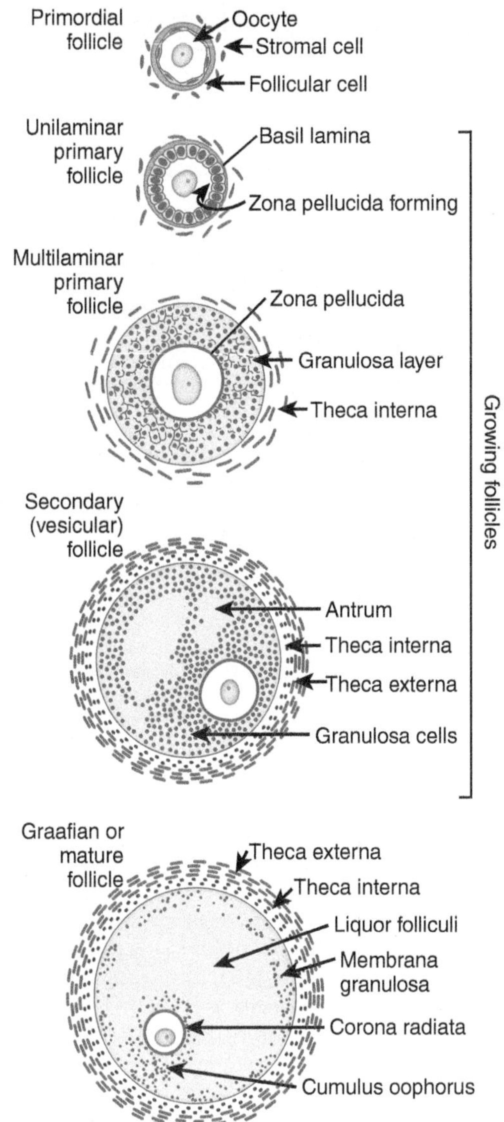

Fig. 3.2 Schematic drawing of development of ovarian follicles, starting with the primordial follicle and ending with mature follicles. (From Junqueira LC, Carneiro J, Kelly RO. *Basic Histology*. 7th ed. Norwalk: Appleton & Lange; 1992.)

of the secondary (vesicular) follicle. The antrum expands, and the oocyte becomes located on one side of the follicle, where it is embedded within a mound of follicular cells known as the *cumulus oophorus.* The layers of follicular cells immediately surrounding the oocyte are termed the *corona radiata.* Because of its increased size, the follicle further compresses the surrounding ovarian stroma. A looser, less organized layer of flattened stromal cells encircles the follicle superficial to the theca interna. This is called the *theca externa,* and its cells have no steroid-secreting activity (see Fig. 3.2). A few days before ovulation, one secondary follicle becomes dominant and inhibits the growth of the remaining secondary follicles. The dominant follicle, now called a *graafian follicle,* can reach several centimeters in diameter. The oocyte is approximately 100 μm in diameter at this stage. Approximately 1 day before ovulation, its nuclear membrane breaks down, the nucleolus disappears, and the first polar body forms, containing one of the two sets of chromosomes. Meiosis I is completed, and the oocyte proceeds to meiosis II, but it again stops on reaching metaphase. In most mammalian species, including humans, meiosis II resumes only after the oocyte has been penetrated by a sperm.[36,37] Completion of meiosis in the fertilized oocyte results in production of the second polar body.

Follicles of any stage can undergo atresia. Atresia begins in the fetus and continues into menopause until all follicles have disappeared. At birth approximately 2 million primordial follicles are present within the two ovaries. It has been estimated that half of the 2 million follicles present at birth are atretic at that time.[10] In humans, follicular growth starts before birth, and the newborn ovary contains multilaminar primary follicles and primordial follicles. Follicular growth and subsequent atresia are continuous during human childhood, and it has been clearly stated that "quiescent ovaries in which follicular growth is absent do not occur in normal children."[38]

Little is known about control of atresia. For example, it is not known whether atresia is initiated by action of the follicular cells, by that of the oocyte, or by both.[22] However, the process of atresia can be manipulated experimentally.[38] Approximately 40,000 follicles are present in the two ovaries of a young adult woman, indicating a reduction to 2% of the pool originally present at birth.[39]

These stages, up to and including the newly fertilized mature ovum, are summarized in Table 3.1. Most or all of the RNA and protein found in a mature oocyte are synthesized during oocyte growth. Those macromolecules present in the oocyte of an atretic follicle are degraded, and the degradation products are subsequently used for new synthesis.[23]

As estimated from an assumed fertility span of 30 years, approximately 400 eggs are shed during a woman's lifetime.[36] Thus approximately 1 in every 100 of the eggs present in a young woman completes maturation and is ovulated; the rest degenerate. A human female has her full complement of eggs, albeit immature, on the day she is born. This is not the case for sperm development in males.

EARLY DEVELOPMENT OF MALE GAMETES (SEE CHAPTER 148)

In male humans the primordial germ cells migrate into the gonadal ridges as outlined earlier (see Fig. 3.1). Once they have reached the gonad, they divide to form a pool of spermatogonia.[40] Both spermatogonia and their supporting cells—the Sertoli cells—can be identified as early as 48 days after fertilization.[41] The germ cells and the supporting cells combine to form seminiferous tubules.

Spermatogonia are located next to the basement membrane of the seminiferous tubule, where they lie quiescent until puberty. Experimental studies with mice have shown that male primordial germ cells are kept in that state by a meiosis-preventing substance, which also can arrest meiosis in female germ cells. Conversely, the female gonad secretes a meiosis-inducing substance, which can induce male germ cells to enter meiosis.[19]

At puberty the spermatogonia begin to differentiate into sperm (spermatogenesis). Spermatogenesis occurs in three phases. In the first phase, the spermatogonia divide mitotically. In the second phase, some spermatogonia differentiate into primary spermatocytes and undergo meiosis. In the third phase, spermatids proceed through spermiogenesis to form spermatozoa. In contrast with women, the cycle of differentiation of gametes in men is essentially continuous throughout life. Studies in which tritiated thymidine was injected into healthy male volunteers indicate that the complete cycle takes approximately 74 days.[42] However, the various stages of spermatogenesis are not synchronized along the length of the coiled seminiferous tubule in humans: different stages are found at different positions.

FERTILIZATION

Development begins with the fusion of the male and female gametes at fertilization, which occurs in the distal third of

Table 3.1 Summary of the Developmental Characteristics of the Human Female Germ Cell.

Name	Approximate First Recognizable Time (After Fertilization)	Location	Approximate Total Number (Both Ovaries)	Size, Shape, Characteristics	Relevant Studies
Primordial germ cell	During wk 4	Caudal yolk sac, among endoderm cells	500	Large, round, 15–20 μm in diameter	Witschi, 1948[4]; Fujimoto et al., 1977[7]
	During wk 5	Dorsal mesentery of hindgut and gonadal ridges	500	Ameboid shape, migrating, with pseudopodia; >20–30 μm in long axis; alkaline phosphatase positive	Witschi, 1948[4]; Fujimoto et al., 1977[7]
Oogonium	During wk 6	Sexually indifferent gonad	100,000	Rapid mitosis increases numbers (mitosis signals name change)	Witschi, 1948[4]; Byskov, 1980[9]
	During wk 7	Gonad recognizable as ovary	100,000	Mitosis continues; almost all primordial germ cells are now in the gonad	Fujimoto et al., 1977[7]; Moore and Persaud, 1998[39]
Oocyte (in primordial follicle)	Wk 8–9	Ovary	?	Meiosis begins; ~19 μm in diameter	Dvorak and Tesarik, 1980[16]
Quiescent oocyte in primordial follicle	Wk 16	Ovary	?	Arrest of meiosis I at diplotene; 50–70 μm; round to ovoid; vitelline body present	Baca and Zamboni, 1967[35]
	2 mo	Ovary	600,000		Baker, 1963[10]
	5 mo	Ovary	6,800,000		Baker, 1963[10]
	7 mo	Ovary		Mitosis of oogonia ceases	Baker, 1963[10]
	Birth	Ovary	2,000,000 (50% atretic)		Baker, 1963[10]; Moore and Persaud, 1998[39]
	7 yr	Ovary	300,000		Baker, 1963[10]
Primary to mature (graafian) follicles	Puberty on	Ovary	40,000 and declining	From oocyte to mature ovum: comes out of meiotic arrest and enters metaphase of meiosis II, then stops again	Moore and Persaud, 1998[39]
Mature ovum	Puberty on	Uterine tube	1 per mo	Meiosis is completed and the second polar body is extruded when penetrated by a sperm	Moore and Persaud, 1998[39]

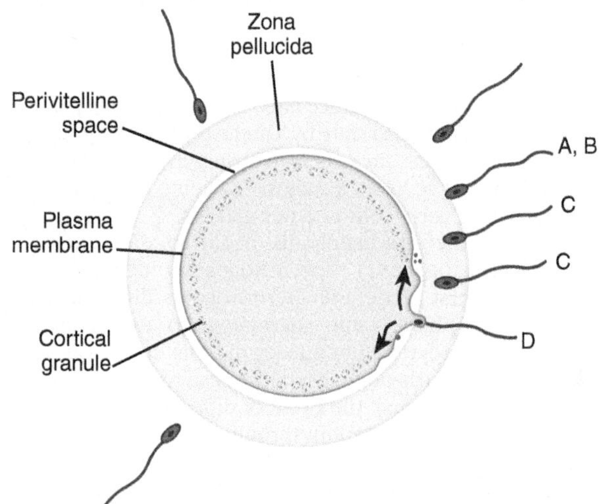

Fig. 3.3 Fertilization pathway. *A* and *B* show sperm binding and the acrosome reaction, exposing the zona pellucida to acrosomal enzymes. *C* depicts penetration of the enzyme-modified zona pellucida by the sperm. *D* shows activation of the egg, including oocyte membrane hyperpolarization and release of enzymes by the cortical granules. (Modified from Wassarman PM. Fertilization in mammals. *Sci Am.* 1988;259:82.)

the oviduct. Although fertilization is an "internal" process in humans and other mammals, the development of culture systems that support fertilization has made detailed study of the sperm-oocyte interaction possible, as well as providing a basis for in vitro fertilization for clinical ends. As a result, the precisely ordered events constituting a "fertilization pathway" have been identified (Fig. 3.3). The mechanisms involved in the fertilization pathway have been the subject of investigation at the molecular level.[29,32,43] Most studies on fertilization have been performed with mice, but comparative data suggest that the pathway is similar in all mammals, including humans.

The fertilization pathway begins with binding of the sperm to the surface of the zona pellucida (see Fig. 3.3). On the surface of every sperm are thousands of copies of an egg-binding protein; these are recognized by thousands of copies of sperm receptors on the zona pellucida.[44] Binding is relatively species-specific and requires a complete plasma membrane (i.e., an acrosome-intact sperm).[45,46] Once bound to the zona pellucida surface, the sperm undergoes a series of dynamic membrane fusions known as the *acrosome reaction* (see Fig. 3.3).[47] During this phase the plasma membrane at the apical end of the sperm fuses with the outer membrane of the acrosome, forming a series of membrane-bound vesicles. These are eventually sloughed, which exposes the inner acrosomal membrane and its complement of enzymes.[32,48]

As a result of enzyme modification of the zona pellucida, the sperm is able to tunnel its way through. The first sperm to penetrate the perivitelline space (between the zona pellucida and the oocyte plasma membrane) and fuse with the plasma membrane triggers activation of the egg (see Fig. 3.3). Oocyte activation is a dynamic, multistep process that includes mechanisms to prevent polyspermy, completion of meiosis by the oocyte, engulfment of the sperm, formation of male and female pronuclei, and initiation of the first mitotic division of the embryo. Prevention of fertilization by more than one sperm (polyspermy—a potentially lethal condition) is thought to be a biphasic reaction, although the first phase is not well documented in humans. The first phase is rapid and consists of hyperpolarization of the oocyte plasma membrane. The second phase may take several minutes and involves the release of enzymes from the cortical granules that alter the structure of the zona pellucida. As a result, the plasma membrane and the zona pellucida become refractory to further penetration by other sperm.

Studies at the molecular level have revealed that a component of the zona pellucida is a key substance in the fertilization pathway. As mentioned earlier, the zona pellucida is an acellular coat that surrounds the oocyte and consists of four glycoproteins—ZP1, ZP2, ZP3, and ZP4—arranged in an interlacing filamentous network.[44,49] ZP3 functions as the sperm receptor, initiates the acrosome reaction, and participates in the zona pellucida reaction.[49] Sperm binding is mediated by a subset of the *O*-linked oligosaccharides associated with ZP3, whereas a segment of the polypeptide backbone is needed to induce the acrosome reaction.[29,50]

Several important events necessary for development of the embryo—initially called a *zygote* after fertilization—are accomplished as a result of fertilization.[39] First, the diploid chromosome number is restored by fusion of the two haploid gametes. Normally, half of the chromosomes come from each parent, and the new complement of chromosomes in the zygote promotes species variation. In addition, the genetic sex of the zygote is determined by the type of sperm that participates in fertilization. Sperm that bear a Y chromosome produce a genetically male zygote (XY), whereas an X-bearing sperm produces a female zygote (XX). Finally, fertilization initiates cleavage, the mitotic division of the zygote. Apposition of the male and female pronuclei results in the formation of a metaphase plate, and the first cleavage soon begins. In contrast with some animal species, the human male and female pronuclei never fuse (i.e., form a complete nucleus). Instead, they immediately enter mitotic metaphase.[51]

Parthenogenesis is activation of the unfertilized oocyte, leading thereafter to various degrees of successful development of the zygote and embryo. In some animal species this process is well known to occur and may even produce viable offspring. However, no verified human cases have been reported in the scientific literature.[39]

MORPHOGENESIS

The mechanisms mediating the transformation of a fertilized oocyte into a three-dimensional embryo are complex and still not completely understood. Studies on human embryos have been, for the most part, limited to observations of static images or serial reconstructions on preserved specimens of different developmental stages. Therefore most knowledge of the mechanisms controlling development has come from animal studies.

During development, cells of different genetic backgrounds are constantly interacting with each other and with a variety of molecules within their extracellular environment. The processes involved in these interactions consist of many well-recognized phenomena of cell biology, including cell division, adhesion, secretion, cytodifferentiation, motility, and cell death. Although the complex interactions that occur during morphogenesis may appear to be unorganized, they are recognized to occur not stochastically but rather in a precisely ordered sequence of events resulting in recognizable patterns of histogenesis and organogenesis. In the past decade an abundance of molecular studies has provided a much clearer picture of the complex signaling activity that controls embryonic development.[8]

As a result of fertilization, the zygote undergoes a series of mitotic divisions termed *cleavage*. The cells derived from these repeated mitotic divisions are called *blastomeres*. The first divisions result in a solid mass of blastomeres that are still surrounded by the zona pellucida. Starting at the 8- to 16-cell stage, intercellular spaces between blastomeres coalesce to form a central cavity. The embryo, now termed a *blastocyst*, consists of a regionalized clump of cells termed the *inner cell mass*, which projects into the blastocyst cavity and is surrounded by an outer layer of trophoblast cells (Fig. 3.4 A and B). Initially the blastocyst floats freely within the uterine cavity. After shedding the zona pellucida, the blastocyst attaches to and implants within the uterine endometrium.[39]

Studies on embryos suggest that the earliest cleavage divisions appear to be driven by maternal messages stored within the oocyte cytoplasm.[52] In mammals (including humans), the embryonic genome is activated by the two- to four-cell stage and begins to synthesize proteins on its own. This functional maturation is reflected in the steady rise in the synthesis of many intracellular proteins, such as actin.[53-55]

During cleavage, several changes fundamental to embryonic development occur at the molecular level. One of the most important processes is the generation of cell diversity. Initially all blastomeres express a specific transcription factor, oct-4, which reflects the undifferentiated state of these cells. If separated from the others at this stage, each of the blastomeres has the capacity to form a complete embryo. By the 8- and 16-cell stage the embryo is a solid mass of cells called a *morula*. At this time the outer cells of the morula are distinguishable from the inner cells because the outer cells no longer express oct-4.[8] The outer cells, now designated the *trophoblast*, also begin to exhibit epithelial polarity.[56] As a result, the first embryonic tissue (trophoblast epithelium) is formed. Subsequent cytodifferentiation of the trophoblast results in a double-layered membrane, which is a progenitor tissue of the chorion, the fetal portion of the placenta (see Fig. 3.4C). The inner cellular layer is called the *cytotrophoblast*, and the outer layer the *syncytiotrophoblast*. The latter structure, which secretes human chorionic gonadotropin and proteolytic enzymes, is critical to implantation.[39]

During the second week of development, the cells of the inner cell mass that face the blastocyst cavity become flattened, forming a second layer of epithelium.[39] The upper layer, located next to the trophoblast, is now designated the *epiblast*, whereas the bottom layer of flattened cells is called the *primary endoderm* or *hypoblast* (see Fig. 3.4C). Cells of the epiblast become organized into an epithelial disk, the progenitor of all embryonic tissues, as well as the extraembryonic mesoderm, amnion, and yolk sac.[54] The cells forming the extraembryonic mesoderm apparently arise from the presumptive caudal end of the epiblast and coat the internal surface of the cytotrophoblast.[57] The extraembryonic mesoderm combined with the trophoblast constitutes the chorion. Even at this early stage of development it is possible to determine that the surface of the epiblast adjacent to the trophoblast represents the dorsal side of the embryo.[58]

Rearrangement of some of the epiblast cells results in the formation of a small amniotic cavity.[59] It is unclear whether the amnion is derived from epiblast cells adjacent to the newly formed cavity[59] or from the cytotrophoblast.[60] Primary endoderm cells of the hypoblast proliferate and migrate onto the inner surface of the cytotrophoblast, forming the yolk sac or umbilical vesicle.[61] Therefore, by the end of the second week of development, the

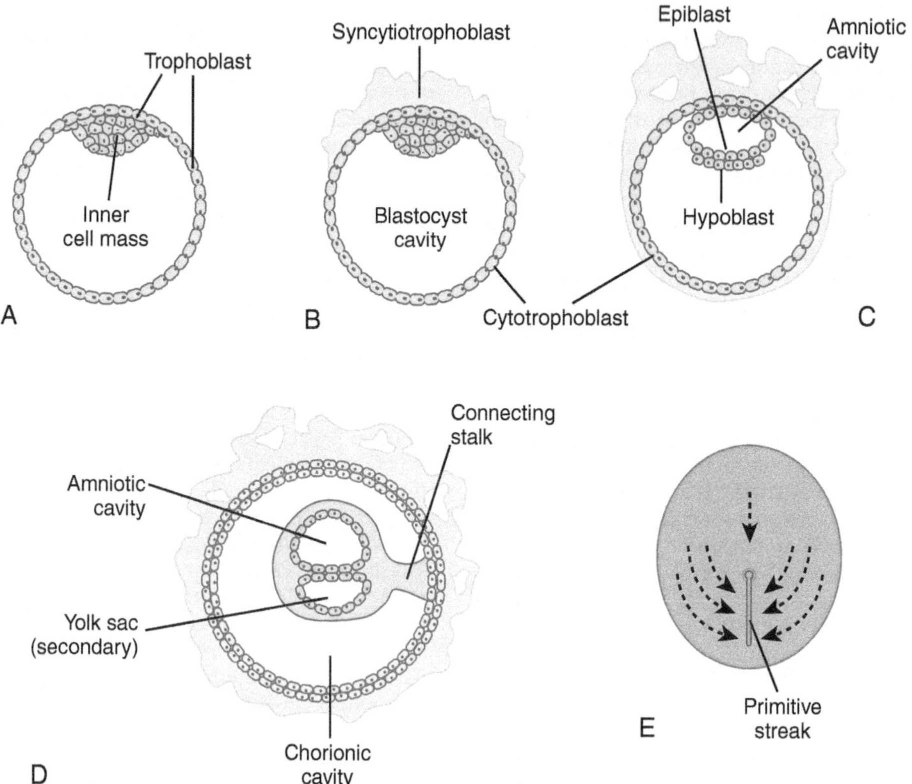

Fig. 3.4 Development of the blastocyst embryonic disk. (A) Blastocyst-stage human embryo, exhibiting the inner cell mass as a regionalized mass of cells projecting into the blastocyst cavity. The cavity is surrounded by trophoblast cells. (B) Blastocyst slightly older than that shown in A. At this time the inner cell mass and trophoblast cells are capped by cells of the syncytiotrophoblast, which are buried in the endometrial stroma (not shown). The cellular layer of trophoblast is now called the *cytotrophoblast*. (C) An older blastocyst-stage human embryo. The cavity is now surrounded by a double-layered membrane, and the inner cell mass has developed into a bilayered embryonic disk capped by a cavity (amniotic cavity). (D) This somewhat older, completely implanted embryo now exhibits cavities both above and below the embryonic disk, the amniotic cavity, and the yolk sac. No axial features are present in the disk at this time; cephalic and caudal regions cannot be discerned. (E) Surface view of the embryonic disk, showing the primitive streak. This midline thickening of epiblast cells occurs during the early part of the third week after fertilization and produces a landmark (the primitive streak) that delineates the midline of the embryo and reveals the future cephalic and caudal ends. The thickening of epiblast cells in the midline (primitive streak) is actually an increased population of cells in this region, resulting from both a high mitotic rate in the midline and migration of a subpopulation of epiblast cells to a midline position. The *arrows* indicate migration of the epiblast cells.

embryo consists of a circular bilaminar disk located between two fluid-filled cavities (see Fig. 3.4C and D). At this time no axial features are visible within the embryonic disk.

At the outset of the third week of development, dynamic cell movements result in extensive rearrangement of the epiblast cells. In most species this period, called *gastrulation,* is characterized by morphogenetic movements and the changes resulting from them. A midline thickening of the now elongated epiblast becomes visible, designating the future posterior end of the embryo.[54] This thickening is the *primitive streak* (see Fig. 3.4E). Cellular activity at the streak results in another fundamental process of morphogenesis, epithelial-mesenchymal transformation. This process begins when some epiblast cells enter the streak while others remain within the epiblast to become the embryonic ectoderm.[62] The transformation from epithelium to mesenchyme consists of a cascade of cellular dynamics, including loss of intercellular connections, cell shape changes, and eventual freedom from the confines of the epiblast. Thus, at the primitive streak, subsets of polarized epithelial cells within the epiblast transform into nonpolarized free cells termed *mesenchyme,* the second embryonic tissue. These events are thought to be mediated by modulation of adhesive molecules located on the cell surface,[63] as well as by cytoskeletal rearrangements. In addition, variable expression of homeobox genes and many other signaling molecules occurs during gastrulation,[8] leading to patterning of axial and nonaxial structures.

The primitive streak provides a means by which subsets of epiblast cells can ingress and be distributed to more ventral regions of the embryo as the endoderm and the mesoderm.[62] The first cells through the streak probably represent the definitive embryonic endoderm. These are followed by a solid cord of cells, the notochordal process, which extends cranially from the streak. These cells form the notochord, which defines the axis of the embryo and plays a significant role in the induction of the nervous system. Studies suggest that the notochord is an important signaling center for organizing the embryo. It secretes several important morphogenetic signaling molecules, such as retinoic acid and Sonic hedgehog.[8,63] Another important signaling center, the prechordal plate, forms just cranial to the notochord. The prechordal plate is an important organizing center for the head of the embryo.[8] Just cranial to the prechordal plate, the endoderm fuses to the overlying ectoderm. This region of fused ectoderm and endoderm is the site of the future mouth.[64] The remainder of the cells that pass through the streak become the intraembryonic mesoderm and come to lie between the endoderm and the ectoderm. Thus the primitive streak provides the embryo with a means to organize epiblast cells, perhaps already partially fate specified, into three primary germ layers—ectoderm, mesoderm, and endoderm.

As a consequence of cleavage and gastrulation, subpopulations of cells in various states of determination are brought together in new spatial relationships, which permits new tissue interactions. Subsequent histogenesis and organogenesis are driven by these tissue interactions, defined as the action of one dissimilar group of cells on another, resulting in the alteration of cell behavior of one of the component groups in a developmentally significant direction.[65] Tissue interactions often result in induction, in which signals from one cell group mediate the change in developmental direction of another group of cells that are competent to respond to the inductive signals. These interactions are mediated by a variety of signaling molecules, such as growth factors, secreted factors, and transcription factors, produced by cells and often concentrated in the extracellular matrix.[8]

EMBRYOLOGY OF THE ORGAN SYSTEMS

The following brief account of the development of some of the major organs provides an overview of some of the complex processes that occur as the embryo is built from raw materials. It is an amazing and precisely timed process. That it happens properly in most conceptions is even more remarkable. For a much more complete account, several other excellent texts are recommended,[8,39,64] as are appropriate chapters elsewhere in this book.

NERVOUS SYSTEM (SEE CHAPTER 124)

The human nervous system begins to form approximately 18 days after fertilization,[65,66] making it the first of the organ systems to initiate development. It begins as a thickening of the ectodermal layer along the craniocaudal axis of the embryo in the area destined to become the cervical region (Fig. 3.5B). This thickening is the result of an increase in the height of the ectodermal cells as they change shape from cuboidal to tall columnar, as well as intercalatory movements within the local population of cells. The result is an oval or keyhole-shaped area of thickened ectoderm known as the *neural plate.* Two ridges of this neural plate on each side of the midline undergo accelerated growth, giving rise to two longitudinal neural folds with a neural groove between. Before this folding, a mesencephalic flexure forms in the cranial portion of the neural plate.[64] This flexure demarcates the future prosencephalon, mesencephalon, and rhombencephalon. These neural folds increase in height, curve toward each other, touch, and fuse to form the rudiment of the neural tube midway along the embryonic axis (see Fig. 3.5B). This fusion then proceeds both cranially and caudally, as if two zipper fasteners were operating simultaneously but in different directions.

The remaining unfused ends of the neural folds at each end of the embryo are called the *cranial* and *caudal neuropores* because the neural tube is open at these sites. The cranial neuropore closes on day 25 and the caudal neuropore on day 27 of development.[65,66] This folding and shaping of the neural tube occur through both intrinsic (cell cycle, cell shape) and extrinsic (proliferation of adjacent tissue) mechanisms.[67,68] Shortly after fusion of the neural folds in a given region of the embryo, the neural tube separates from the ectoderm and becomes buried in the mesenchyme below the surface.

During this process of neural tube formation, an epithelial-mesenchymal transformation occurs, resulting in formation of a group of cells derived from the crests of the neural folds. These neural crest cells come to lie on the superolateral margins of the tube. The neural tube proper goes on to form the central nervous system, which consists of the brain and spinal cord, whereas the neural crest forms much of the peripheral nervous system, consisting of portions of autonomic, cranial, and spinal ganglia and nerves. The lumen of the neural tube becomes the central canal of the spinal cord and the ventricles of the brain.

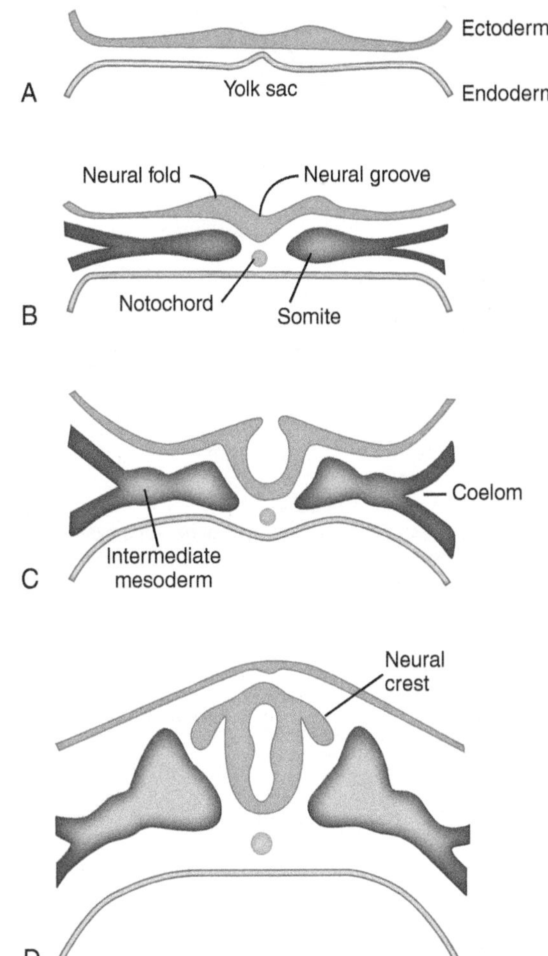

Fig. 3.5 Development of the neural tube. Approximate ages: 15 days (A), 18 days (B), 20 days (C), 23 days (D). All sections are transverse, approximately midway along the embryonic axis. Although the neural tube is completely closed in the section shown in D, the rostral and the caudal neuropores both remain open in an embryo of this age. They do not close until near the end of the fourth week.

FURTHER DEVELOPMENT OF THE CENTRAL NERVOUS SYSTEM

The spinal cord develops from that part of the neural tube caudal to the cervical flexure, one of two unambiguous bends in an embryo approximately 30 days old that give the embryonic axis a C-shaped profile in lateral views (Fig. 3.6). The wall of the tube thickens and soon stratifies into a ventricular zone that borders the central canal, an intermediate zone, and a marginal zone. The intermediate zone is created by migration of neurons from the ventricular zone. These neurons then send out processes that create the marginal zone, later to become the white matter of the spinal cord.

Proliferation of the cells of these zones is greatly influenced by the somites, mesodermal structures that lie lateral to the neural tube along its craniocaudal axis. Later the roof and floor of the neural tube become thin, whereas the lateral walls thicken. Studies in animals show that this particular organization around the circumference of the neural tube is under the influence of an inductive substance from the somites.[69] Experimental manipulation of the number, size, or position of somites influences the cross-sectional profile of the tube, including the keyhole-shaped profile of the neural canal (Fig. 3.7).

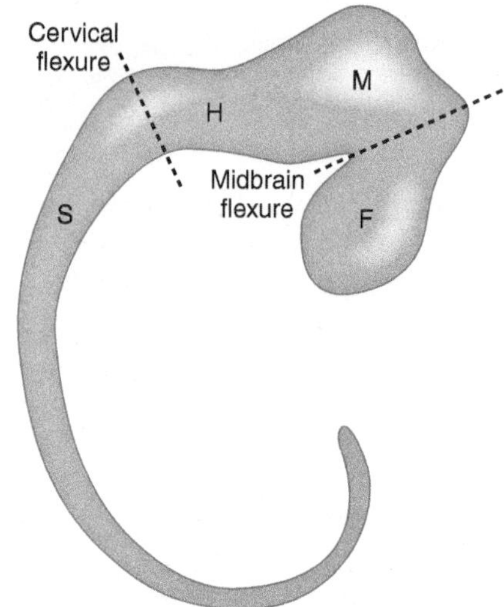

Fig. 3.6 Lateral view of the isolated central nervous system of a 28- to 30-day-old embryo, showing the two flexures *(dotted lines)* and the resulting divisions of the brain and spinal cord at this age. *F,* Forebrain; *H,* hindbrain; *M,* midbrain; *S,* spinal cord.

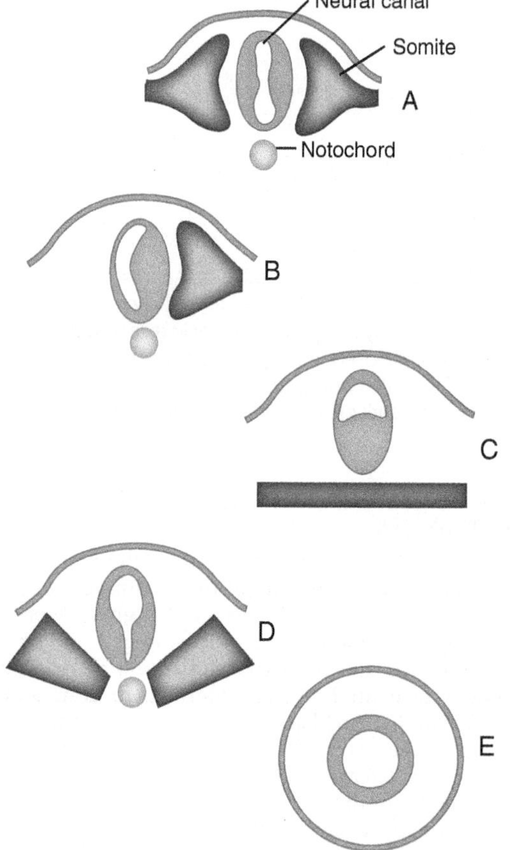

Fig. 3.7 Influence of somite mesoderm *(lightly stippled areas)* on neural tube and neural canal shape. (A) Normal. (B) One somite removed. (C) Somite mesoderm transplanted to the ventral surface of the neural tube. (D) Somite mesoderm transplanted to the ventrolateral surface of the neural tube. (E) Complete absence of somite mesoderm. *Clear areas* between structures contain nonsomite mesoderm. (Modified from Saxen L, Toivonen S. *Primary Embryonic Induction.* London: Logos Press; 1962.)

The sulcus limitans is a groove that divides the more dorsal alar plate from the ventral basal plate. The former develops into the dorsal gray horns associated with sensory (afferent) input. The basal plate gives rise to the ventral and lateral gray horns, which function in motor (efferent) output. The floor plate secretes morphogenetic molecules (e.g., retinoic acid, Sonic hedgehog), which control the patterning of dorsal sensory and ventral motor elements.[8,70]

The spinal cord extends the entire length of the developing vertebral column during the embryonic period. However, the spinal cord grows more slowly than the vertebral column, and so in the fetal period and beyond, these two structures change position with respect to each other. At 24 weeks the spinal cord extends caudally to the level of the first sacral vertebral body. In the newborn it extends to the third lumbar vertebral body, and in the adult it extends to the first lumbar vertebral body. This aspect of spinal development is important clinically with respect to lumbar punctures and other procedures that require knowledge of where the spinal cord ends.

The brain is divided into forebrain (prosencephalon), midbrain (mesencephalon), and hindbrain (rhombencephalon) when the midbrain flexure appears (see Fig. 3.6). These three divisions of the brain quickly become five by the partitioning of the forebrain into telencephalon and diencephalon and the separation of the hindbrain into metencephalon and myelencephalon. The formation of divisions and their adult derivatives are summarized in Table 3.2. Two distinct signaling centers apparently organize the cranial portion of the neural tube. One center organizes the forebrain and the other the hindbrain; each produces its own set of signaling factors. Another important source of signaling molecules for brain regionalization comes from the midbrain-hindbrain signaling center.[8]

THE EYE

At approximately 4 weeks of development two outpouchings of the forebrain (diencephalon) expand laterally to form the optic vesicles (Fig. 3.8A and B), progenitors of the eyes. Inductive interaction occurs between the optic vesicles and the head ectoderm, which lies closest to the vesicles.[71] The first manifestation of this interaction is the formation of a thickened plate in the head ectoderm, the lens placode (see Fig. 3.8B). At approximately the same time the lateral surface of the optic vesicles begins to invaginate to form the double-layered optic cup. The lens placode also invaginates, creating a lens pit (see Fig. 3.8C). The pit continues to deepen as it follows the profile of the increasingly concave optic cup. Finally, the deeply pitted placode pinches off, forming the lens vesicle (see Fig. 3.8D). By this time point (approximately 30 days) the double walls of the optic cup appose each other; fusion of these two layers is completed during the fetal period. The inner layer forms the neural retina, and the outer layer becomes the pigment epithelium of the retina. The peripheral margin of the optic cup forms the iris and ciliary apparatus, whereas the optic nerve is formed from the optic stalk. Mesoderm surrounding the optic cup forms the inner vascular choroid and the fibrous outer sclera.

THE EAR (SEE CHAPTER 135)

The inner ear begins to develop in the fourth week after fertilization as a recognizable thickening of surface ectoderm on either side of the myelencephalon, known as the *otic placode* (Fig. 3.9A). As with the lens vesicle, the otic placode invaginates to form the otic pit (see Fig. 3.9B) and pinches off to form the otic vesicle (see Fig. 3.9C). Small diverticula soon bud from each vesicle to form the endolymphatic sac. As growth of the hollow vesicle proceeds, additional regional morphogenesis yields the

Table 3.2 Brain Vesicles and Their Derivatives.

Early Division	Later Divisions	Wall Derivatives	Lumen Derivatives
Forebrain (prosencephalon)	Telencephalon	Cerebral hemispheres	Lateral ventricles, rostral part of third ventricle
	Diencephalon	Epithalamus, thalamus, hypothalamus, pineal	Most of third ventricle
Midbrain (metencephalon)	Mesencephalon	Midbrain	Cerebral aqueduct
Hindbrain (rhombencephalon)	Metencephalon	Pons, cerebellum	Superior part of fourth ventricle
	Myelencephalon	Medulla	Inferior part of fourth ventricle

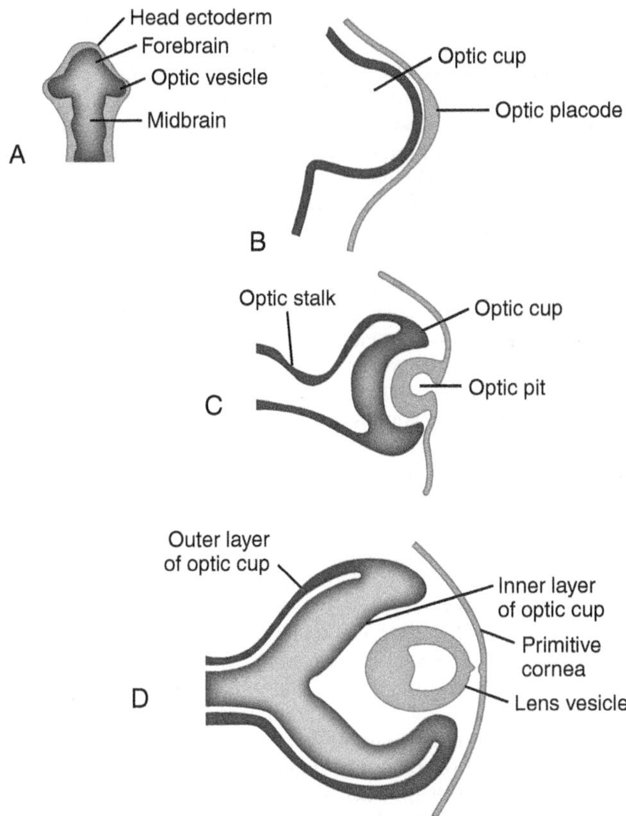

Fig. 3.8 Development of the eye. (A) Dorsal view showing the head, optic vesicles, and overlying head ectoderm. (B–D) Magnified view of the right optic vesicle at successively older stages, illustrating the development of the lens placode, pit, and vesicle, and the optic cup.

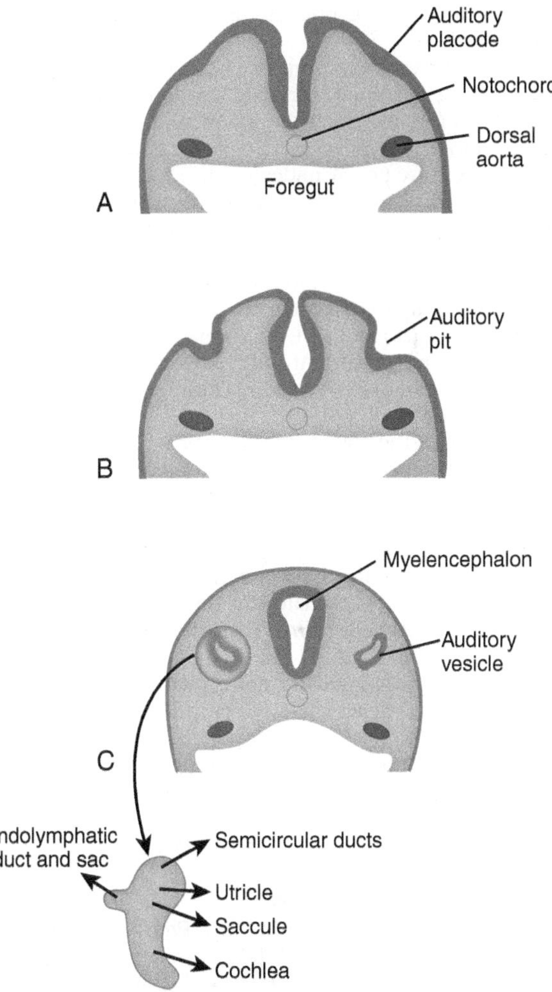

Fig. 3.9 Successively older stages (A–C) showing development of the inner ear from the auditory placode. Derivative adult structures are shown in the *inset* in C.

utricle, semicircular ducts, saccule, and cochlear ducts, as well as other sensory receptors and primary sensory neurons (see Fig. 3.9C).

CARDIOVASCULAR SYSTEM (SEE CHAPTER 45)

HEART

Cells destined to form the primitive heart tube are located within two oval areas of mesoderm (Fig. 3.10) on either side of the midline of the embryo.[72-74] Organized as discrete clusters of cells between the ectodermal and endodermal layers, this precardiac mesoderm migrates cranially and fuses in the midline just cranial to the oral membrane. The cell clusters form two more or less parallel solid cords of cells on reaching the area just forward of the oral plate (see Fig. 3.10). These soon canalize to form endocardial tubes. The tubes swing together because of lateral body folding and fuse to form the primitive heart tube, which then undergoes additional growth, morphogenesis, and changes in position with time. Initially the primitive chambers of the heart tube are arranged in a linear series, with inflow at the caudal end and outflow at the cranial end.

The heart begins beating approximately 22 days after fertilization, and weak circulatory movement of fluid begins in adjacent vessels about 1 day later. At this time the embryo can be compared with an aggregate of cells approximately 1 × 1 × 2 mm. Tissue culture studies indicate that cells in the center of a mass thicker than approximately 0.5 mm die of oxygen deprivation because the simple diffusion of oxygen into the core is not sufficient to support cell metabolism. Thus it appears that the formation of a functional circulatory system is requisite for the continued life of the embryo. Indeed, the circulatory system is the first organ system to become functional in the human embryo.[75,76]

Good evidence from animal experiments indicates that the first contractions of the embryonic heart are initiated by stretching of the heart tube as fluid pressure builds in the developing circulatory system. Isolated hearts do not begin beating on time unless artificially produced fluid pressure is maintained within the lumen of the heart. Moreover, the heart in intact embryos can be induced to begin beating earlier than normal by the introduction of small amounts of fluid into the lumen, thereby increasing intraluminal pressure and causing stretching of the walls of the heart.[77,78]

Almost as soon as the primitive heart tube forms, sulci on its external surface deepen markedly. This begins a process called *cardiac looping,* in which the inflow and outflow regions are brought into approximation. The mechanisms behind the control of looping are poorly understood.

Several concurrent events occur after looping that lead to partitioning of the heart into separate chambers and outflow channels. The sinus venosus, which initially receives all incoming venous blood from the embryo, is remodeled so that all blood enters what will later become the right atrium. Resorption of the sinus venosus results in the formation of the smooth area of the definitive right atrium and contributes to atrial septation. Much of the definitive left atrium is formed by resorption of the pulmonary veins.

Separation of the atria begins during week 5, when a sickle-shaped membrane, the septum primum, grows from the roof of the atrium toward the atrioventricular canal. This canal is simultaneously being divided into right and left channels by the fusion of the enlarging superior and inferior endocardial cushions. The opening between right and left sides of the common atrium, now partially divided by the growing septum primum, is called the *foramen* (or *ostium*) *primum.*

Soon the lower edges of the septum primum fuse with the endocardial cushions, and further growth of both the septum and the cushions closes the foramen primum. However, before it closes completely, several perforations appear in the superior portion of the septum primum. These perforations fuse to form

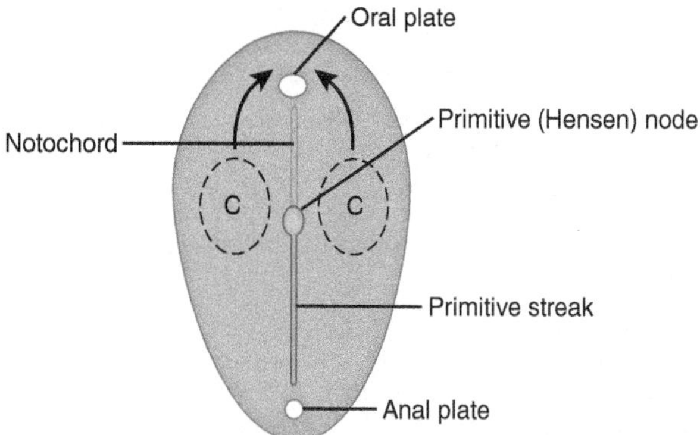

Fig. 3.10 Surface view of an embryo at approximately 16 to 17 days after fertilization. This view is of the ectodermal surface. Structures below the surface are outlined with *dotted lines.* The anal and oral plates are areas in which the ectoderm and endoderm are in tight contact, as in a "spot weld," with no mesoderm between. Mesoderm is present in other areas. At *C* lie the mesodermal cell clusters that migrate *(arrows)* to an area forward of the oral plate, to form the cardiogenic cords. These two *oval areas* contain precardiac mesoderm cells.

the foramen secundum. Thus communication between the right and left atrial cavities is maintained during this complex morphogenetic process.

Another septum (the septum secundum) begins to form at about the time the foramen secundum becomes well defined. This septum forms to the right of the septum primum as a crescentic ridge. Further growth produces a thick membrane, but the oval opening in this membrane persists as the foramen ovale. This arrangement of two parallel septa (septum primum and septum secundum) with offset holes (septum secundum and foramen ovale) produces a flap valve between the two atria, ensuring unidirectional flow of blood from right to left.

Fusion of the endocardial cushions (composed of cardiac mesenchyme) forms the septum intermedium. This structure not only divides the atrioventricular canal into right and left portions but also acts as a central attachment point and reference center for several septation events, as already described. The cushion tissue of the septum intermedium contributes to the formation of the membranous portion of the interventricular septum, as well as to the development of the atrioventricular valves and the fibrous cardiac skeleton. It also serves as a fusion point for the cushion tissue–derived ridges, which divide the proximal outflow region of the heart.

Even though the heart is enlarging while septation proceeds, the dimensions in this central region around the septum intermedium remain constant. A significant enlargement in this region at this time could lead to congenital heart defects.

Partitioning of the ventricle is accomplished primarily by fusion of trabeculae, which form a muscular interventricular septum. Ventricular septation is completed by formation of the membranous portion of the septum from an outgrowth of endocardial cushion tissue. This morphogenetic process occurs simultaneously with division of the proximal outflow area. Initially, no direct communication is present between the right atrium and the right ventricle. Remodeling activities in the inner curvature of the heart create this communication by mechanisms that are still obscure.

Division of the outflow tract is complex and still not completely understood. The proximal portion of the outflow tract is subdivided into the conus and truncus regions, both of which are divided into left and right halves by ridges of endocardial cushion tissue called the *conotruncal* or *bulbar ridges.* Septation of the conus region results in the formation of an outflow segment for each ventricle, whereas in the truncus region distinct aortic and pulmonary valves develop. A portion of the conal septum extends down and attaches to the muscular interventricular septum, partially closing the interventricular foramen. Complete closure of the foramen is accomplished by downgrowth of cushion tissue from the septum intermedium. In the distal outflow tract (the aortic sac), a wedge of mesenchyme (the aorticopulmonary septum) develops between the fourth and sixth aortic arches. This mesenchyme (thought to be of neural crest origin[79]) grows downward and then penetrates and fuses with the conotruncal ridges.

VESSELS

During the third week of development, groups of extraembryonic mesodermal cells in the yolk sac and chorion, known as *angioblasts,* aggregate to form isolated, solid masses called *angioblastic clusters* or *blood islands.* These soon cavitate (Fig. 3.11), and those cells on the periphery of the hollow blood islands differentiate into endothelial cells. Blood cells are formed from those angioblasts remaining in the lumen, as well as by cell division and budding from the primitive endothelial lining. Growth and fusion of the isolated hollow blood islands result in the formation of tubes, and the tubes fuse to form long interconnected channels. Lateral buds from tubes and channels also may extend the developing vasculature into adjacent areas.

This sequence, based on observations of sectioned embryos, constitutes the basic template for how vessels form. It does not explain how the pattern of vessels develops. Little is known concerning how the intricate pattern of anastomosing vessels is established in the early embryo.

THE MUSCULOSKELETAL SYSTEM (SEE CHAPTER 138)

MUSCULAR SYSTEM

The three types of muscle tissue—skeletal, smooth, and cardiac—are largely derived from cells of the mesodermal germ layer. Skeletal muscle forms from paraxial mesoderm, whereas cardiac muscle is a derivative of splanchnic mesoderm. Most smooth muscle is derived from splanchnic mesoderm. However, it seems likely that all mesenchyme, whether derived from mesoderm or from neural crest (as in head mesenchyme), has the potential to form vascular smooth muscle. The dilator and sphincter smooth muscles of the iris and the myoepithelial cells that surround sweat glands and mammary glands are thought to be of neural crest origin.

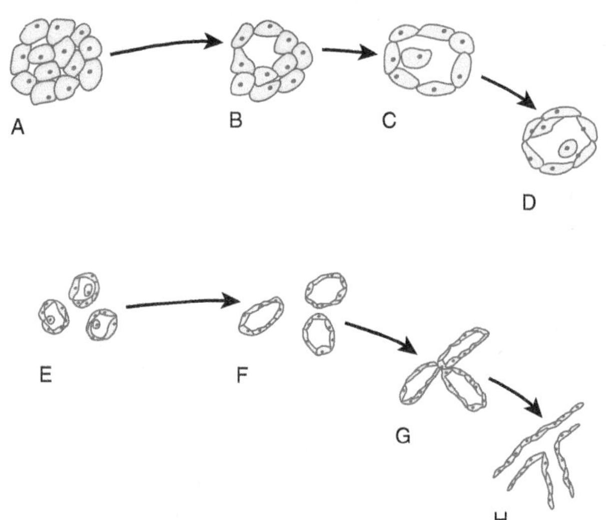

Fig. 3.11 Vasculogenesis. (A–D) Formation of hollow blood islands from solid clusters of angioblasts. (E–H) Formation of a portion of a primitive vascular network by fusion of blood islands. Budding (not shown) also contributes to vascular pattern growth.

Skeletal Muscle

Mesenchyme cells that are to develop into skeletal muscle elongate and lose their multiple processes. The earliest cell that can be identified as a skeletal muscle precursor is a fusiform cell called a *myoblast* (Fig. 3.12). Myoblasts become postmitotic and fuse into cylindric, multinucleated myotubes. These myotubes start producing actin and myosin myofilaments, which increases girth. Growth of myotubes may also occur by fusion of additional myoblasts. The skeletal muscles of the head and neck develop from paraxial mesoderm represented by somitomeres in the early embryo. Trunk musculature is derived from the myotome portion of the somites (Fig. 3.13).

Somites themselves are interesting structures—serially repeated paired blocks of condensed (closely packed) paraxial mesoderm cells. Approximately 44 pairs of somites eventually develop in humans, beginning between day 19 and day 21.[65] These can be seen in a surface view of the embryo because they produce bulges in the overlying sheet of ectoderm. Each member of a pair of somites lies lateral to the neural tube (see Fig. 3.13). Myoblasts of the myotome portion of each somite divide and spread out deep to the embryonic skin, where they form the musculature. Various morphologic processes, including fusion, tangential splitting of layers, reorientation of muscle fibers, and formation of tendon intersections, are responsible for the final morphologic form of the named muscles.

The musculature of the limb is also derived from the myotome portion of the somites. These myoblasts migrate into the elongating limb buds and arrange themselves into dorsal and ventral muscle masses, which later become subdivided into the definitive limb muscles.

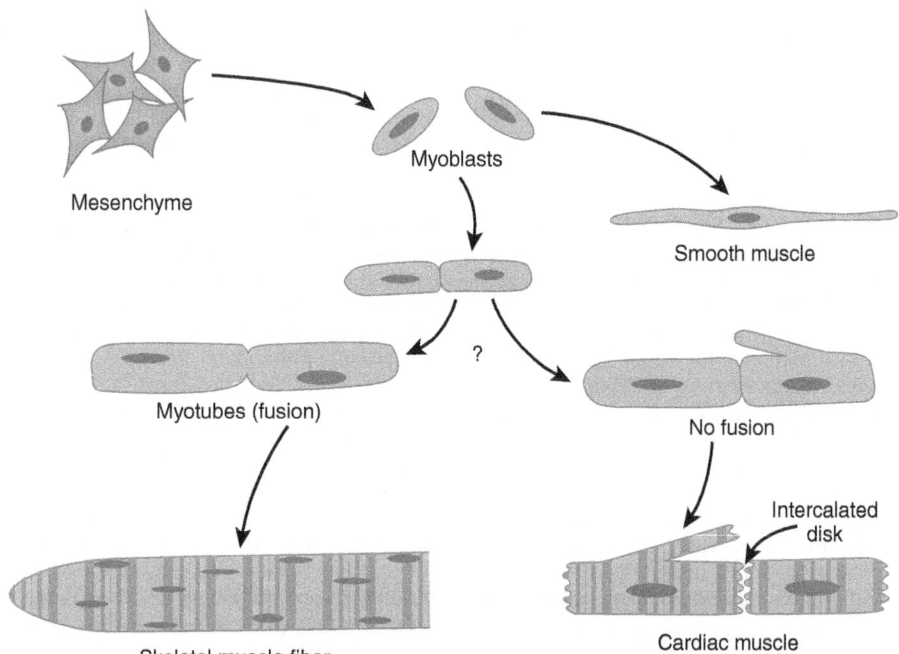

Fig. 3.12 Schematic representation of the development of the three types of muscle cells—skeletal, smooth, and cardiac. A question exists regarding the precursor cells—that is, a current hypothesis is that mesenchyme gives rise to a cell type that develops into cardiac and smooth muscle but that it gives rise to another cell type that develops into skeletal muscle.

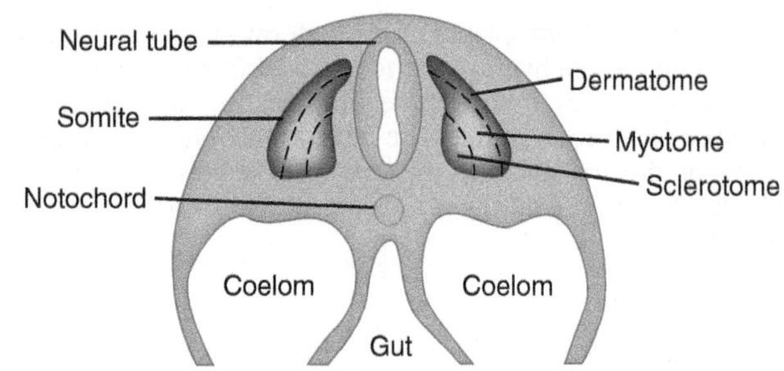

Fig. 3.13 Fate map of the somite, showing regions from which cells developing into dermis, muscle, and cartilage and bone are derived.

Cardiac Muscle

Cardiac muscle develops from splanchnic mesoderm adjacent to the pericardial or transverse portion of the intraembryonic coelom. Myocardial precursor cells undergo mass migration and do not fuse to form myotubes. Rather, the myoblasts differentiate as discrete cells, with closely applied end-to-end junctions, which persist as the adult intercalated disk. They form a layer around the endothelial tube of the heart, which eventually becomes the myocardial or muscular wall of the heart.

Smooth Muscle

Smooth muscle cells form from myoblasts derived primarily from splanchnic mesoderm (see Fig. 3.12).

SKELETAL SYSTEM (SEE CHAPTER 137)

Cartilage develops from mesodermally derived mesenchyme, except in some areas of the head and neck, where it is of neural crest origin. Chondroblasts aggregate, condense, and begin to produce collagen fibers and ground substance. In the embryo, bone tissue is formed in either of two distinct ways, depending on the site and type of bone growth. The first is de novo bone formation, in which mesoderm cells (or, in the case of some skull bones, neural crest cells) first condense (pack) into sheets or membranes. Cells in these sheets then differentiate into osteoblasts, which secrete prebone or osteoid. Osteoid is the extracellular matrix onto which hydroxyapatite crystals (a unique calcium phosphate mineral) form. Once the mineral is present and integrated into the collagen of the matrix, the tissue is considered to be bone. This type of bone formation is called *intramembranous ossification* because the osteogenesis occurs within these sheets or membranes of condensed mesenchyme. Some of the bones of the cranial vault, face, and jaws form in this way.

The second manner in which bone forms in the embryo is called *endochondral ossification*. As implied by the name, bone forms in this case only in sites where preexisting cartilage models are found. The cartilage does not turn into bone. Rather, bone replaces the preexisting cartilage model in a sequence of steps, as follows. Cartilage cells hypertrophy and calcify in an area where bone is to form—that is, they become large and undergo metabolic changes, which lead to infiltration of the surrounding cartilage extracellular matrix with insoluble calcium salts. In this way, the cartilage cells become partitioned from their surroundings by an environment that is presumed to cut off their supply of oxygen and nutrients, and they die. At the same time, local osteoblasts begin to produce osteoid, which then becomes mineralized as described in intramembranous ossification. Once bone has formed in the embryo, it can be remodeled by changes in the balance between addition of more bone by osteoblasts and removal of bone by osteoclasts.

RESPIRATORY SYSTEM (SEE CHAPTER 55)

During the fourth week of development, the embryo forms a C shape, and the primitive gastrointestinal tube is already divided into a foregut, midgut, and hindgut (Fig. 3.14). A groove, the respiratory (laryngotracheal) diverticulum, arises as an evagination of the ventral surface of the foregut, close to the region destined to become the stomach. As the foregut elongates, a wedge of mesoderm, the tracheoesophageal septum, separates the foregut (portion that will become the esophagus) from the future lungs. This early association of developing lung and stomach leads to the occasional finding of ectopic lung and cartilage tissue near the esophagogastric junction.[80]

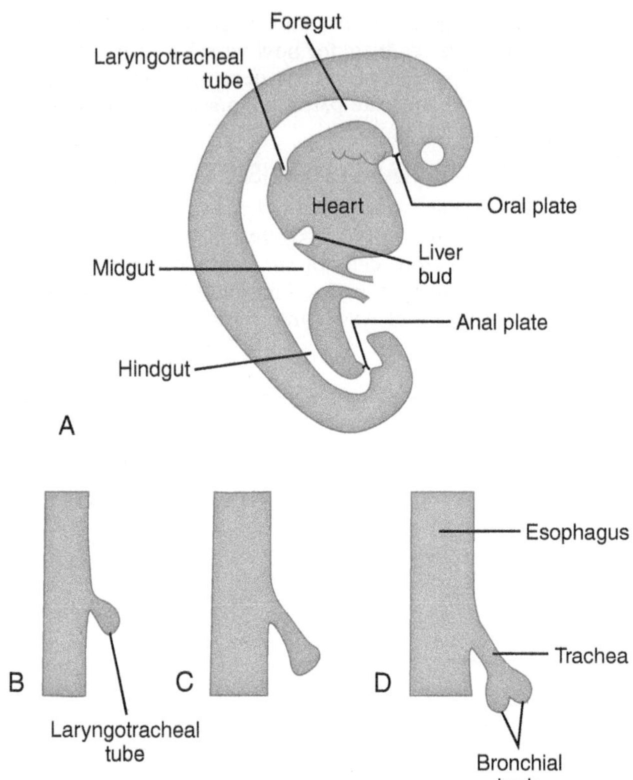

Fig. 3.14 Development of the respiratory system. The laryngotracheal (respiratory) tube buds off from the ventral surface of the foregut, as shown in A. The tube elongates and splits into two bronchial buds (B–D), each of which ultimately gives rise to the epithelial lining of one lung.

The respiratory diverticulum grows caudally and soon splits into two bronchial buds. Each of these buds subdivides to form primitive secondary or lobar bronchi. On the left side, two secondary bronchi supply the developing superior and inferior lobes of the left lung. On the right side, the inferior secondary bronchus divides into two bronchi, providing a total of three secondary bronchi to supply the three lobes on this side. The third-order branches form the bronchopulmonary segments. Altogether, approximately 17 generations of branches form. Differentiation of the respiratory passages begins in the fetal stage and proceeds from distal to proximal along the branches of the respiratory diverticulum. Alveolar formation begins toward the end of the fetal period and continues until the age of 2 to 3 years.[54]

The endoderm of the foregut gives rise to the epithelial lining of the trachea, bronchi, and lungs, including the alveoli. The surrounding splanchnic mesoderm develops into the cartilage and fibrous connective tissue of the larger airways and the blood vessels and supporting tissues of the smaller airways and alveoli.

DIGESTIVE SYSTEM (SEE CHAPTER 82)

The lining of the gastrointestinal tube arises primarily from endoderm, whereas the muscle coats and connective tissue elements are usually derived from splanchnic mesoderm. Toward the end of the third week the embryo folds craniocaudally and laterally, forming an inner gut tube of endoderm that is subdivided into the foregut, midgut (still connected to the degenerating yolk sac), and hindgut.

ORAL CAVITY AND ANAL REGIONS

Throughout most of the developing gastrointestinal tube, the epithelium and derivative glands arise from the endodermal germ layer, which lines the foregut, midgut, and hindgut (see Fig. 3.14). Cranial to the foregut and caudal to the hindgut, the relationship of embryonic structure to adult derivatives is less obvious. For example, the oral membrane, which is a fusion of ectoderm and endoderm, is the cranial boundary of the foregut (in the adult this boundary is at the level of the tonsillar fauces). The oral cavity develops cranial to the oral membrane from an ectodermal depression, the stomodeum, bounded by the first pharyngeal arch and the frontal process. Three groups of salivary glands develop in this region. The sublingual and submaxillary glands develop from endoderm, as might be expected, but the parotid gland is derived from head ectoderm.[39] Similarly, structures below the pectinate line in the adult anal canal are derivatives of the proctodeum, an ectodermal depression in the caudal end of the embryo that is sealed off from the gut tube by the anal plate until the end of the eighth week or beginning of the ninth week. Thus the anal columns (of Morgagni), located above the pectinate line, are of endodermal origin, whereas the anocutaneous (white) line and surrounding epithelial structures are from ectoderm.

LIVER (SEE CHAPTER 88)

The hepatic diverticulum (or liver bud) arises as an outpouching of the lumen of the distal foregut during the fourth week of development (see Fig. 3.14). The liver bud gives rise to the gallbladder and bile ducts, as well as to the parenchyma of the liver. The liver bud grows toward the anterior body wall, at first completely buried in the mesenchyme of the septum transversum. Rapid growth causes the liver bud to bulge into the abdominal cavity, freeing it on all but the cephalic surface. There it remains in contact with the septum transversum as the latter forms part of the diaphragm. After development is complete, this area of contact between the liver and the diaphragm is known as the "bare area of the liver" because it is not covered with capsule or peritoneum.

The liver is connected on its anterior surface to the anterior body wall by the ventral mesentery, which becomes the falciform ligament. The hepatocytes are derived from endoderm, as are the bile canaliculi and the epithelial linings of the intrahepatic biliary ducts. The liver sinusoids, larger blood vessels, and connective tissue stroma of the liver are all derived from the mesenchyme of the septum transversum, which is of mesodermal origin.

PANCREAS (SEE CHAPTER 85)

Most of the pancreas develops from the dorsal pancreatic bud, which arises as an out pouch of the dorsal surface of the future duodenum at the caudal end of the foregut. It grows into the mesenchyme of the dorsal mesentery at this site. The ventral pancreatic bud starts as an outgrowth of the future common bile duct, but it fuses with the dorsal pancreatic bud when rotation of the gut brings these two components of the pancreas into contact. Both exocrine and endocrine (islets of Langerhans) elements of the pancreas are derived from endoderm, whereas the blood vessels and connective tissue components arise from splanchnic mesoderm.

ESOPHAGUS

The esophagus is a short regional specialization of the embryonic foregut tube that elongates with growth of the body. During the middle of the embryonic period, its lumen is obliterated by proliferation of the endoderm-derived lining cells, but cell death (a normal developmental process in many areas of the human embryo) reestablishes the lumen by the 10th to 11th week of development.

STOMACH

The stomach begins as a simple fusiform dilation of the foregut. Growth of the dorsal wall of the stomach surpasses that of the ventral wall, leading to the greater curvature and driving a clockwise rotation of the gut that brings the greater curvature (original dorsal surface) to the left and the lesser curvature (original ventral surface) to the right. As a result of differential growth, the cardiac region (cranial) of the stomach moves inferiorly and to the left, and the pyloric (caudal) end moves superiorly and to the right. Ultimately this rearrangement results in the almost horizontal axis seen in the adult stomach.

DUODENUM

The duodenum develops from both the caudal end of the foregut and the cranial end of the midgut. It rapidly elongates into a loop, the bend of which is toward the ventral body wall. As the stomach rotates to the right, so does the duodenal loop, bringing it to lie against the dorsal wall of the body cavity. There it fuses with the dorsal wall, and most of it comes to lie in a retroperitoneal position. As in the esophagus, the duodenal lumen is transiently obliterated by growth of the endoderm-derived lining cells until about the 9th week of development.

LOWER GASTROINTESTINAL TRACT

Much of the remaining gastrointestinal tube—jejunum, ileum, cecum, ascending colon, and half of the transverse colon—develops from the midgut. The elongating midgut forms a U-shaped loop consisting of a cranial and a caudal limb. The distal end of the loop is closest to the anterior body wall. While herniated, the loop rotates 90 degrees counterclockwise when viewed from the ventral surface of the embryo. Thus the cranial branch of the U-shaped loop moves to the right. At the same time growth and elongation create several additional subloops in the cranial portion of the U-shaped loop; these later give rise to the jejunum and ileum.

The herniated small intestine with its subloops returns to the body cavity first. As the large intestine follows, it rotates an additional 180 degrees, bringing the cecum and appendix to their final position in the lower right quadrant of the abdomen.[81] Little is known about how these complex morphogenetic events are controlled. Nevertheless, thorough knowledge of these events as they occur in a normal embryo can help to explain the numerous anatomic variations and congenital malformations that have been observed. The hindgut contributes to the distal half of the transverse colon, the descending colon, the sigmoid colon, the rectum, and the anal canal down to the white line.

URINARY SYSTEM (SEE CHAPTER 93)

Near the end of the third week after fertilization the intermediate mesoderm appears as a solid cord of condensed mesenchyme just lateral to the paraxial (somite-forming) mesoderm (see Fig. 3.5C). The intermediate mesoderm is bilateral and extends along the length of the body axis as far as the somites do; it gives rise to components of the urinary and genital system.

The intermediate mesoderm is displaced ventrally to a position lateral to the dorsal aorta and notochord when the embryo becomes tubular, owing to growth and formation of the lateral body folds. During this movement the connection between the somites and intermediate mesoderm is broken. Once this connection is lost, the two bars of intermediate mesoderm are called *nephrogenic cords.*

The traditional description of kidney development suggests that three successive sets of kidneys form in the embryo—the pronephros, mesonephros, and metanephros. However, the concept of a pronephros is not relevant in humans.[82] Beginning

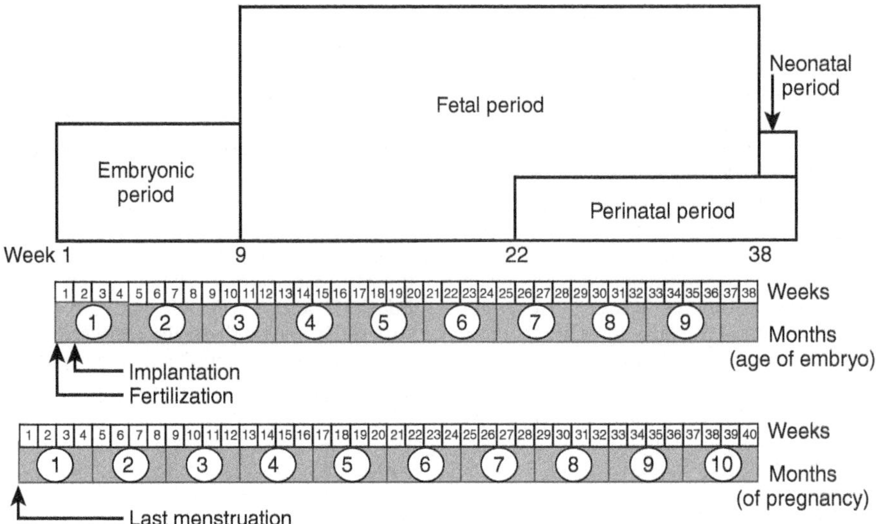

Fig. 3.15 Human development. The *upper portion* of the schematic diagram shows human development divided into periods. The embryonic period extends from fertilization through week 8. The remainder of pregnancy (week 9 through birth) is termed the *fetal period*. The perinatal period extends from prenatal week 22 until 4 weeks after birth. The neonatal period is the first 4 weeks after birth. In the *bottom portion* of the diagram, the ages of the embryo/fetus are shown on two time scales. The lower of the two is a clinical scale, with *pregnancy* counted from the date of the last menstrual period. Above it are weeks and months of *development,* counted from fertilization. Note the 2-week difference, with pregnancy lasting 40 weeks. (Modified from Kaplan S. *Congenital Defects: An Overview: An Introduction to the Principles of Teratology.* Chapel Hill: Health Sciences Consortium; 1981.)

at the level of the eighth or ninth somite,[83] the mesonephric kidney contains primitive tubules associated with glomeruli that empty into a mesonephric (wolffian) duct. The cephalic tubules begin to degenerate even before the more caudal tubules are starting their development. In males the mesonephric duct becomes associated with the primitive gonad and gives rise to the epididymis, ductus deferens, and ejaculatory ducts; some of the mesonephric tubules persist as the efferent ductules. In females the mesonephric duct distal to the ureteric bud degenerates. The mesonephros actively produces urine as early as the sixth week of development, and this continues into the early fetal period.

During the fifth week the metanephros begins as a small diverticulum near the caudal end of the mesonephric duct—the ureteric bud. The mesoderm at the caudal aspect of the nephrogenic cord condenses around the ureteric bud, forming a metanephric blastema. The ureteric bud plus the metanephric blastema form the metanephric or definitive kidney (see Fig. 3.1A). The nephron from the renal corpuscle to the collecting duct is derived from the metanephric blastema, whereas the collecting system and ureter are derived from the ureteric bud. Development of the metanephric kidney depends on mutual inductive signals from the metanephric blastema and the ureteric bud.[69] Signals from the ureteric bud result in mesenchymal-epithelial transformation of the metanephric blastema mesenchyme, leading to formation of an epithelial vesicle. The vesicle remodels itself into a tubule, the proximal end of which attaches to the ureteric bud, whereas the distal end becomes associated with vascular precursors of the glomerulus. Signals from the metanephric mesoderm cause the ureteric bud to branch, forming the collecting system. If for some reason the ureteric bud does not grow to meet the metanephric blastema, the blastema does not develop nephrons, and renal agenesis results. If the blastema is absent, the ureteric bud does not develop into the collecting system of the kidney.[84]

By the end of the first trimester, the fetal kidneys begin to produce urine.[85] At that time they have been displaced from their initial pelvic location to the abdomen, and they lie in a retroperitoneal position close to the adrenal glands. The latter develop from coelomic mesoderm (cortex) and neural crest cells (medulla) that have become associated in the abdominal cavity, cephalic to the final position of the kidneys.

The urogenital sinus is an endoderm-lined cavity from which are derived the epithelium of the urinary bladder, all of the female urethra, and most of the male urethra. The muscular coats and connective tissue elements of all of these structures are of splanchnic mesoderm origin.

GROWTH AND MATURATION OF THE EMBRYO AND FETUS

Human embryonic development is a continuous process that averages 266 days, or 9.5 months, when counted from the day of fertilization. Clinically, one determines the start of gestation by counting from the date of the last menstrual period. Estimated this way, it averages 280 days, or 10 lunar months.[86] Human prenatal development is commonly divided into two periods or phases: the embryonic period and the fetal period (Fig. 3.15). The first 8 weeks after fertilization constitute the *embryonic period.* It has been subdivided into 23 developmental stages (Carnegie stages).[54] During the embryonic period the single-celled zygote is transformed into an embryo. With respect to human embryology, the term *embryo* means "an unborn human in the first 8 weeks" from fertilization.[54] This period is characterized by several developmental milestones, including cell division of the zygote, formation of a blastocyst, implantation, formation of three primary germ layers, segmentation and axis formation, and initial morphogenesis of organ systems.

It is thought that during the first 2 weeks of development the embryo is relatively insensitive to the action of agents that cause congenital malformations (teratogens). Retrospective human studies, as well as studies in animals, suggest that low to medium doses of teratogens will not cause abnormal development during the first 2 weeks but that a large dose will kill the embryo. During this 2-week period, defects may also develop after treatment with the teratogenic agent if for some reason it remains available to the embryo throughout the period—for example, because of slow metabolism or excretion. However, it is during the third to eighth

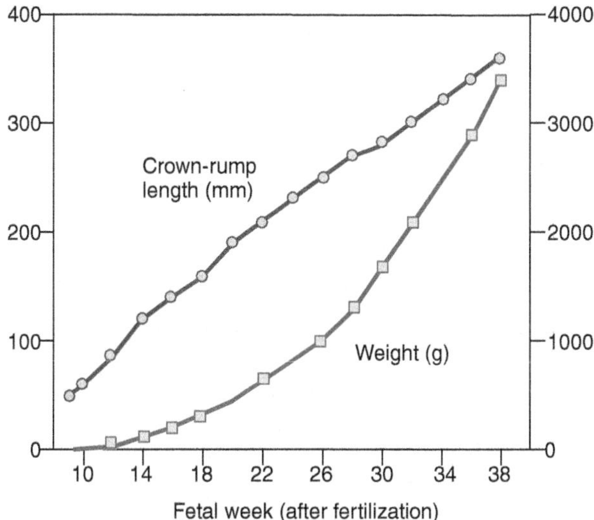

Fig. 3.16 Weight and crown-rump length during human development. (Data from Moore KL, Persaud TVN. *The Developing Human: Clinically Oriented Embryology.* 6th ed. Philadelphia: WB Saunders; 1998.)

week of development that morphogenesis of most organ systems begins and, for many systems, ends. This is the portion of the embryonic period in which the organs, and therefore the embryo as a whole, are most sensitive to the actions of teratogens. For example, a kidney will fail to develop only if, during morphogenesis, the ureteric bud fails to send the proper signals to the metanephric blastema. Moreover, a limb will be abnormally foreshortened only if long bones fail to form during that time when the bony elements are due to undergo their primary morphogenesis. Therefore weeks 3 to 8 of the embryonic period constitute the critical period in human development with regard to the action of teratogenic agents.

During the *fetal period* (beyond the end of the eighth week after fertilization or beyond the 10th week of post-last menstrual period pregnancy; see Fig. 3.15), the fetus becomes increasingly resistant to the action of teratogens. This decreasing susceptibility does not mean that no organ system can become malformed during fetal life. An example of such an organ is the brain, which exhibits the longest developmental period of any organ; it continues both physical and functional development throughout the fetal period and beyond, well after birth.[87] This extended development also prolongs its period of susceptibility; more major congenital defects occur in the brain than in any other organ.[88]

Morphogenesis of organ systems other than the brain continues into the fetal period (e.g., palate, ear, external genitalia, lungs). However, in contrast with the brain, morphogenesis of most other organ systems is essentially complete by the end of the embryonic period.

The fetal period is characterized by rapid increase in the weight and size of the conceptus as a whole (Fig. 3.16), which reflects growth in individual organs. All organs expand and undergo histogenesis, or differentiation of the cell populations of which they are composed, but the particular pattern of the increase in weight may vary from organ to organ. Hematopoiesis begins in the liver during the late embryonic period, making the liver a functional organ relatively early in development.[86] Accordingly, it expands rapidly to make up approximately 10% of total body weight by the beginning of fetal life.[39] Thereafter its growth rate follows that of the whole body, so in proportion to body weight, liver size remains virtually constant.[89]

The same proportional growth pattern is seen in heart and kidney, but growth of the head is quite different. At the beginning of the fetal period the head is approximately half the crown-rump length; at 12 weeks it is approximately one third this value. Thereafter the rate of growth continues to slow in relation to the rest of the body.

An important point is that the establishment of the gross form of an organ does not necessarily correspond to initiation of function. The human fetal gastrointestinal tube closely resembles that of the newborn infant as early as the middle of the sixth month. By contrast, cell differentiation and the development of complex enzyme systems necessary for the digestive process continue through birth and well beyond.[90]

ACKNOWLEDGMENTS

We thank Dr. Stanley Kaplan for his valuable contributions to the previous edition of this chapter.

A complete reference list is available at www.ExpertConsult.com. 

SELECT REFERENCES

1. Corliss CE. *Patten's Human Embryology: Elements of Clinical Development.* New York: McGraw-Hill; 1976.
2. Wolpert L. Do we understand development? *Science.* 1994;266:571.
3. Junqueira LC, Carneiro J, Kelly RO. *Basic Histology.* 7th ed. Norwalk: Appleton & Lange; 1992.
4. Witschi E. Migration of the germ cells of human embryos from the yolk sac to the primitive gonadal folds. *Contrib Embryol Carnegie Inst.* 1948;32:67.
5. Blandau RJ, White BJ, Rumery RE. Observations on the movements of living primordial germ cells in the mouse. *Fertil Steril.* 1963;14:482.
6. Gondos B, Bhiraleus P, Hobel CJ. Ultrastructural observations on germ cells in human fetal ovaries. *Am J Obstet Gynecol.* 1971;110:644.
7. Fujimoto T, Miyayama Y, Fuyuta M. The origin, migration and fine morphology of human primordial germ cells. *Anat Rec.* 1977;188:315.
8. Carlson B. *Human Embryology and Developmental Biology.* 2nd ed. St Louis: Mosby; 1999.
9. Byskov AG. Sexual differentiation of the mammalian ovary. In: Motta PM, Hafez ESE, eds. *Biology of the Ovary.* The Hague: Martinus Nijhoff; 1980:3-15.
10. Baker TG. A quantitative and cytological study of germ cells in human ovaries. *Proc R Soc Lond B.* 1963;158:417.
11. Fawcett DW, Ito S, Slautterback D. The occurrence of intercellular bridges in groups of cells exhibiting synchronous differentiation. *J Biophys Biochem Cytol.* 1959;5:453.
12. Zamboni L, Gondos B. Intercellular bridges and synchronization of germ cell differentiation during oogenesis in the rabbit. *J Cell Biol.* 1968;36:276.
13. Gondos B, Zamboni L. Ovarian development: the functional importance of germ cell interconnections. *Fertil Steril.* 1969;20:176.
14. Peters H. Migration of gonocytes into the mammalian gonad and their differentiation. *Phil Trans R Soc Lond (Biol).* 1970;259:91.
15. Zamboni L. Comparative studies on the ultrastructure of mammalian oocytes. In: Biggers JD, Scheutz AW, eds. *Oogenesis.* Baltimore: University Park Press; 1972:5-45.
16. Dvorak M, Tesarik J. Ultrastructure of human ovarian follicles. In: Motta PM, Hafez ESE, eds. *Biology of the Ovary.* The Hague: Martinus Nijhoff; 1980:121-137.
17. Byskov AG. Does the rete ovarii act as a trigger for the onset of meiosis? *Nature.* 1974;252:396.
18. Byskov AG. The role of the rete ovarii in meiosis and follicle formation in the cat, mink and ferret. *J Reprod Fertil.* 1975;45:201.
19. Byskov AG, Saxen L. Induction of meiosis in fetal mouse testis in vitro. *Dev Biol.* 1976;52:193.
20. Wai-sum O, Baker TG. Initiation and control of meiosis in hamster gonads in vitro. *J Reprod Fertil.* 1976;48:399.
21. Kessel RG. Annulate lamellae (porous cytomembranes): with particular emphasis on their possible role in differentiation of the female gamete. In: Browder LW, ed. *Developmental Biology: A Comprehensive Synthesis.* New York: Plenum Press; 1985:179-233.
22. Schuetz AW. Local control mechanisms during oogenesis and folliculogenesis. In: Browder LW, ed. *Developmental Biology: A Comprehensive Synthesis.* New York: Plenum Press; 1985:3-83.
23. Bachvarova R. Gene expression during oogenesis and oocyte development in mammals. In: Browder LW, ed. *Developmental Biology: A Comprehensive Synthesis.* New York: Plenum Press; 1985:453-524.
24. Van Benedin E. La maturation de l'oeuf, la fecondation et les premieres phases du developpement embryonnaire des mammiferes d'apres des recherches faites le lapin. *Bull Acad Belg Cl Su.* 1875;40:703.
25. Bliel JD, Wassarman PM. Sperm-egg interactions in the mouse: sequence events and induction of the acrosome reaction by a zona pellucida glycoprotein. *Dev Biol.* 1983;95:317.
26. Wassarman PM. Fertilization. In: Yamada KM, ed. *Cell Interactions and Development: Molecular Mechanisms.* New York: John Wiley; 1982:1-27.

27. Dean J, et al. Developmental expression of ZP3, a mouse zona pellucida gene. In: Yoshinga K, Mori T, eds. *Development of Preimplantation Embryos and their Environment*. New York: Alan R Liss; 1989:21-32.
28. Wasserman PM. Zona pellucida glycoproteins. *J Biol Chem*. 2008;283:24285.
29. Wassarman PM. Fertilization in mammals. *Sci Am*. 1988;259:52.
30. Epifano O, Dean J. Biology and structure of the zona pellucida: a target for immunocontraception. *Reprod Fertil Dev*. 1994;6:319.
31. Dunbar BS, et al. The mammalian zona pellucida: its biochemistry, immunochemistry, molecular biology, and developmental expression. *Reprod Fertil Dev*. 1994;6:331.
32. Wassarman PM. The biology and chemistry of fertilization. *Science*. 1987;235:553.
33. Wassarman PM, et al. The mouse egg's extracellular coat: synthesis, structure and function. In: Gall JG, ed. *Gametogenesis and the Early Embryo. 44th Symposium of the Society for Developmental Biology*. New York: Alan R Liss; 1986:371-388.
34. Bousquet D, Léveillé MC, Roberts KD, et al. The cellular origin of the zona pellucida antigen in human and hamster. *J Exp Zool*. 1981;215:215.
35. Baca M, Zamboni L. The fine structure of human follicular oocytes. *J Ultrastruct Res*. 1967;19:354.
36. Shettles LB. Ovulation: normal and abnormal. In: Grady HG, Smith DE, eds. *The Ovary*. Baltimore: Williams & Wilkins; 1963:128-142.
37. Austin CR. *The Mammalian Egg*. Oxford: Blackwell Scientific; 1961.
38. Peters H, McNatty KP. Atresia. In: Peters H, McNatty KP, eds. *The Ovary: A Correlation of Structure and Function in Mammals*. London: Granada; 1980:98-112.
39. Moore KL, Persaud TVN. *The Developing Human: Clinically Oriented Embryology*. 6th ed. Philadelphia: WB Saunders; 1998.
40. Gwatkin RBL. *Fertilization Mechanisms in Man and Mammals*. New York: Plenum Press; 1977.
41. van Wagenen G, Simpson ME. *Embryology of the Ovary and Testis: Homo Sapiens and Macaca Mulatta*. New Haven: Yale University Press; 1965.
42. Heller CG, Clermont Y. Spermatogenesis in man: an estimate of its duration. *Science*. 1963;140:184.
43. Wassarman PM. Early events in mammalian fertilization. *Ann Rev Cell Biol*. 1987;3:109.
44. Wassarman PM, Bleil JD, Florman HM, et al. The mouse egg's receptor for sperm: what is it and how does it work? *Cold Spring Harbor Symp Quant Biol*. 1985;50:11.
45. Anderson E, Hoppe PC, Whitten WK, Lee GS. In vitro fertilization and early embryogenesis: a cytological analysis. *J Ultrastruct Res*. 1975;50:231.
46. Cherr GN, Lambert H, Meizel S, Katz DF. In vitro studies of golden hamster sperm acrosome reaction: completion on the zona pellucida and induction by homologous soluble zonae pellucidae. *Dev Biol*. 1986;114:119.
47. Austin CR, Bishop MWH. Fertilization in mammals. *Biol Rev*. 1957;32:296.
48. Langlais J, Roberts KD. A molecular membrane model of sperm capacitation and the acrosome reaction of mammalian spermatozoa. *Gamete Res*. 1985;12:183.
49. Bliel JD, Wassarman PM. Structure and function of the zona pellucida: identification and characterization of the proteins of the mouse oocyte's zona pellucida. *Dev Biol*. 1980;76:185.
50. Florman HM, Wassarman PM. O-linked oligosaccharides of mouse egg ZP3 account for its sperm receptor activity. *Cell*. 1985;41:313.

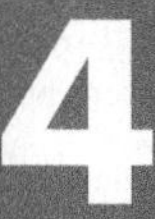

4 Regulation of Embryogenesis

Matt K. Lee | Changgong Li | David Warburton | Parviz Minoo

INTRODUCTION

Embryogenesis results from the divergent proliferation, migration, survival, and differentiation of cells derived from a single cell, the fertilized egg. Regulatory signals, applied to successive generations of cells, establish the architecture of the early embryo. The same processes are recapitulated during the subsequent development of limbs, organs, and craniofacial structures. Consequently, disruption of these reiterative mechanisms distorts seemingly unrelated structures, as observed in human malformation syndromes. Conversely, the same mechanisms guide tissue regeneration following injury. The elucidation of embryonic regulatory mechanisms is therefore of therapeutic importance.

This chapter introduces representative modes of cellular regulation in the context of early embryonic events. The outcome of these mechanisms is modulated expression of proteins that initiate critical developmental events. Protein transcription is controlled by promoters upstream of the coding region and enhancers that lie at a distance from the gene. Promoters and enhancers contain DNA motifs that bind specific transcription factors that then modulate gene transcription. Transcription factors typically bind multiple genes, some of which encode additional transcriptional regulators. Besides its expression, the activity of a transcription factor depends on its posttranslational modifications, its translocation to the nucleus, and the presence or activation of cofactors. The same variables also determine whether that factor increases or decreases the activity of a particular gene. The genes that can be activated at any moment are dependent on whether the chromosomes on which they reside are open and active or whether they are condensed and inaccessible. The state of a cell's chromatin is governed by enhancers and by epigenetic modifications that change during development. Gene expression during embryogenesis is therefore subject to regulation by multiple mechanisms.

EMBRYOGENESIS IS AUTONOMOUSLY REGULATED BY EPIGENETIC IMPRINTING

Regulatory processes may be broadly divided into autonomous and conditional mechanisms. Autonomous mechanisms are internal to the cell, meaning that the regulated behaviors will continue if the cell is moved to a different environment. An example occurs during the implantation of female embryos, when the dividing cells within the morula are segregated into the blastocyst inner cell mass, which becomes the embryo, and the trophoblast, which becomes the placenta (Fig. 4.1). This segregation is determined by the parental origin of the active X chromosome within each cell. Balanced gene expression requires that one of the two X chromosomes within each cell be silenced. This inactivation occurs randomly, and the inactivated X chromosome becomes the Barr body visible in somatic cells. Blastocyst cells containing paternally imprinted active X chromosomes form the trophoblast, while maternally dominated cells become the inner cell mass.[1]

The genes expressed from the active X chromosome differ by parental source. This distinction is conferred by DNA methylation, the covalent addition of methyl groups to cytosine bases within gene promoters. Methylated cytosines are typically located next to guanosines, resulting in the methylation of both DNA strands at diagonally adjacent cytosines. Regulated genes contain clusters of these cytosine/guanosine dinucleotides (so-called *CpG islands*), and their methylation usually reduces gene transcription.[2] The methylation of maternally derived chromosomes differs from those contributed by the sperm, and these patterns can be transferred to daughter cells upon replication. The persistence of paternal methylation also differs from that of the mother; sperm DNA is demethylated within hours of fertilization, whereas the methylation of maternal chromosomes persists into the early morula. The balance between maternally and paternally imprinted chromosomes is critical; a zygote with no maternal DNA (resulting from

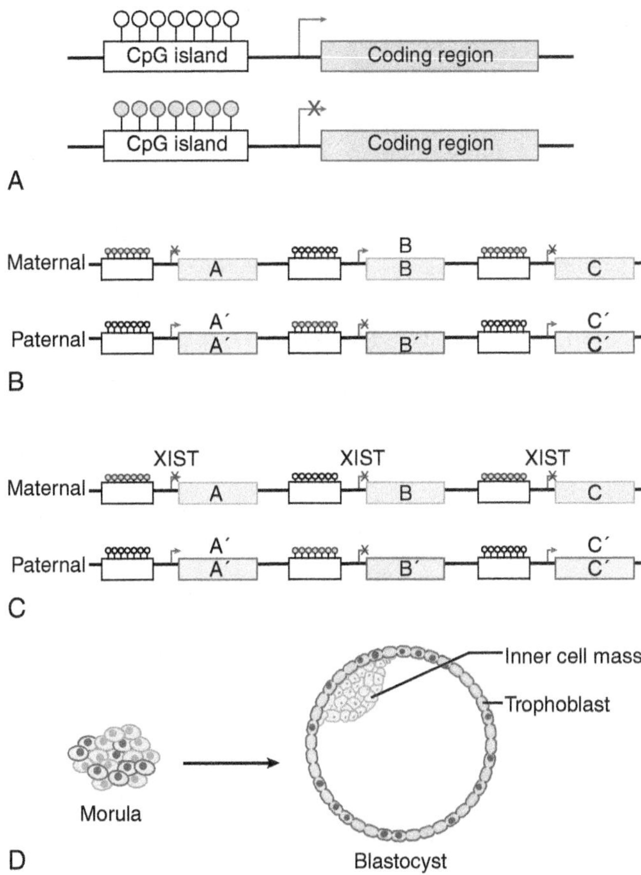

Fig. 4.1 Intrinsic regulation mediates blastocyst differentiation. (A) Regulatory regions are methylated on cytosines, thereby reducing gene transcription. (B) Maternal and paternal genes bear different methylation and hence gene expression patterns. This imprinting is transferred to daughter cells. Here, the maternally derived DNA expresses protein B while its paternal counterpart expresses A′ and C′. (C) Balanced expression requires that in each cell, one X chromosome be randomly inactivated by XIST. Gene expression by that cell is thus dependent on the parental source of the active chromatin. (D) The parental source of the active X chromosome determines whether that cell segregates to the inner cell mass or to the trophoblast.

fertilization of an egg with no nucleus) will form a hydatidiform mole, a dysplastic and occasionally invasive placenta with little or no fetal tissue.[3]

Parental imprinting also contributes to later development, as demonstrated by the expression of UBE3A, a component of the ubiquitin pathway. The maternal allele of UBE3A is almost exclusively expressed in the developing hippocampus and cerebellum, and maternal mutations in UBE3A underlie Angelman syndrome, a disorder characterized by developmental disability, ataxia, and seizures.[4,5] In contrast, paternal mutations in UBE3A result in Prader-Willi syndrome. Although these children also exhibit developmental delay, they are differentiated by hypotonia, obsessive-compulsive behaviors, and insatiable hunger.

EMBRYOGENESIS IS CONDITIONALLY REGULATED BY SECRETED GROWTH FACTORS

In contrast to autonomous regulation, conditional regulation is imposed on cells by environmental factors. The predominance of conditional regulation was demonstrated by Hans Spemann and Hilde Mangold in 1923,[6] who found that implantation of the anterior dorsal lip from one newt embryo into the ventral mesoderm of another induced the formation of a complete second body axis, including a second head. Because most of this material was derived from recipient tissue, it was apparent that the anterior lip, named the *organizer* by Spemann, induced

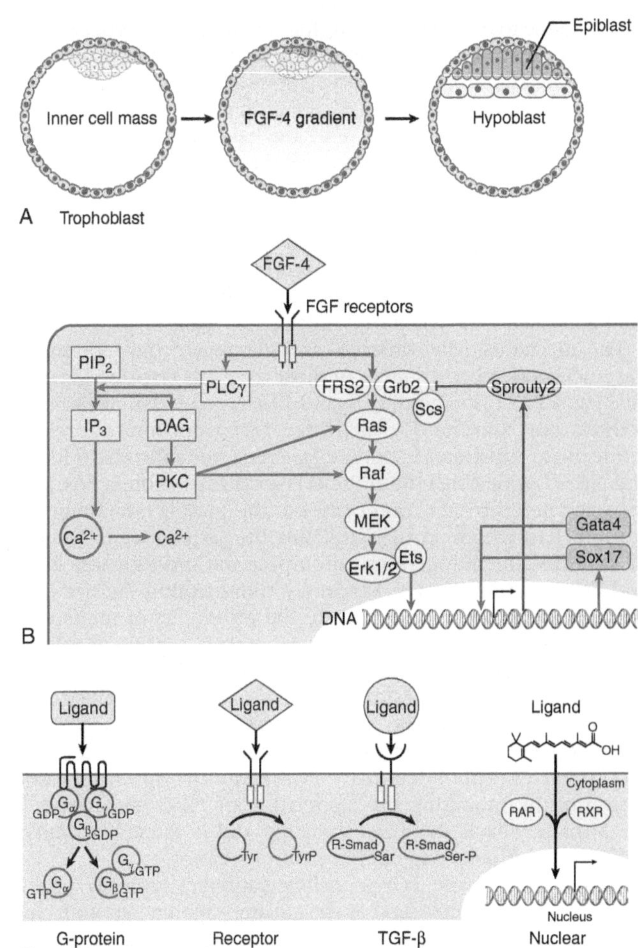

Fig. 4.2 Extrinsic regulation mediates formation of the bilayer germ disk. In the blastocyst (A), production of fibroblast growth factor *(FGF)*-4 by differentiating epiblast cells *(red)* confers extrinsic regulation upon yet undifferentiated cells by inducing them to differentiate into the hypoblast *(blue)*. These receptor families include the seven-transmembrane domain receptors, which activate and release G proteins upon ligand binding; the receptor tyrosine kinases, which phosphorylate intracellular signaling proteins; the transforming growth factor-β (TGF-β) family receptors, whose signals are primarily mediated by serine-threonine phosphorylated Smad proteins; and nuclear receptors that, when complexed with lipid-soluble factors (here, retinoic acid), translocate to nucleus to directly bind DNA promoters. Although receptor families are associated with a dominant pathway, multiple signaling processes are initiated by ligand binding. For example, FGF-4 binds specific receptors to initiate the ERK MAP kinase pathway (B, *green*). This pathway is comprised of the FRS2 and Grb2 adapters, the Sos GTP-exchange protein, and the Ras, Raf, MEK, and ERK1/2 kinases. Ultimately, transcription factors such as Ets are activated to bind regulatory elements that induce the transcription of multiple genes. These genes include Gata4 and Sox17, which induce their own expression (an example of positive feedback) and Sprouty2, an antagonist of FGF signaling (an example of negative feedback). FGF also activates phospholipase C *(PLC)*-γ to initiate protein kinase C *(PKC)* and calcium-mediated signaling processes *(blue)*. Extrinsic regulation is conferred by soluble factors that signal through families of receptors (C).

ventral tissue to undergo dorsal differentiation, which is necessary for neural, heart, kidney, and somite as well as head formation.

In mammals, one of the earliest examples of conditional regulation arises during formation of the bilayer germ disk, during which the inner cell mass differentiates into the epiblast, the pluripotent precursor of the fetal tissues, and the hypoblast, a transient extraembryonic tissue. In some mammals, fibroblast growth factor (FGF)-4 is secreted by primordial epiblast cells to induce the differentiation of as yet uncommitted cells of the inner cell mass into hypoblast (Fig. 4.2A).[7] FGFs comprise a large family of soluble peptides that are secreted into the extracellular environment and bind transmembrane receptors containing tyrosine kinases.

The mechanism by which FGF-4 signals are transmitted to the nucleus is representative of most receptor tyrosine kinases (see Fig. 4.2B). Upon binding ligand, FGF receptors dimerize and activate one another. The activated receptors phosphorylate intracellular substrates including FGF receptor substrate (FRS) 2 and Grb2,[8] which then bind the GTP-exchange protein Sos. The resulting heterotrimer translocates to the plasma membrane to activate Ras, which, in turn, initiates the sequential activation of Raf, MEK, the mitogen-activation protein (MAP) kinases Erk1 and Erk2, and, ultimately, Ets family transcription factors that then enter the nucleus to activate the promoters of numerous genes.[9] Each step in this process represents a node at which the FGF-4 signal may be amplified or attenuated, and the entire process from receptor to transcription factor constitutes a signaling pathway. The FGF pathway also incorporates a negative feedback mechanism; Sprouty2 is a cytosolic protein that, upon phosphorylation by FGF receptors, interrupts Erk activation by inhibiting the association of FRS2 with Grb2.[10] Negative feedback stabilizes signaling and is integral to most biologic and human-engineered control systems.

The activity of the FGF signaling pathways typically peaks within a few minutes and is terminated within an hour by receptor aggregation, internalization, and destruction. However, the resulting transcriptional events may induce sustained changes in the embryo by inducing or interrupting the expression of transcription factors that sustain their own expression. Cells fated to epiblast express the self-sustaining transcription factors Nanog and Oct4, whereas those destined to become hypoblast express Gata4 and Sox17 instead.[11,12]

The many molecules that regulate embryogenesis can be categorized on the basis of their receptors. Besides the fibroblast, epidermal, and insulin-like growth factors that signal through receptor tyrosine kinases, important mediators include members of the transforming growth factor (TGF)-β superfamily that signal through receptor serine/threonine kinases; Wnt and Hedgehog, which signal through G-protein coupled 7-transmembrane domain receptors, and lipid-soluble factors such as retinoic acid and steroids that cross the plasma membrane, complex with nuclear receptors and enter the nucleus to bind DNA directly (see Fig. 4.2C).

Although each receptor type is associated with a canonical pathway, multiple signaling pathways are initiated by each receptor. Besides the ERK pathway, FGF receptors also modulate intracellular calcium by activating phospholipase C gamma (PLCγ), an enzyme that hydrolyzes phosphatidylinositol 4, 5-bisphosphate (PIP_2) into inositol 1,4,5 triphosphate (IP_3).[13] IP_3 receptors embedded in the endoplasmic reticulum release calcium into the cytosol, where it regulates cellular activities as diverse as muscle contraction, nuclear breakdown, and egg fertilization. On the other hand, most intracellular pathways are also activated by multiple receptors; for example, calcium fluxes are also induced by ion channels and G-protein receptors,[14] and Erk signaling is also initiated by receptor serine-threonine kinases.[15] Cell signaling is therefore best described as a network of mutually regulating parallel processes that modulate cell behaviors in a time-dependent and recursive manner.

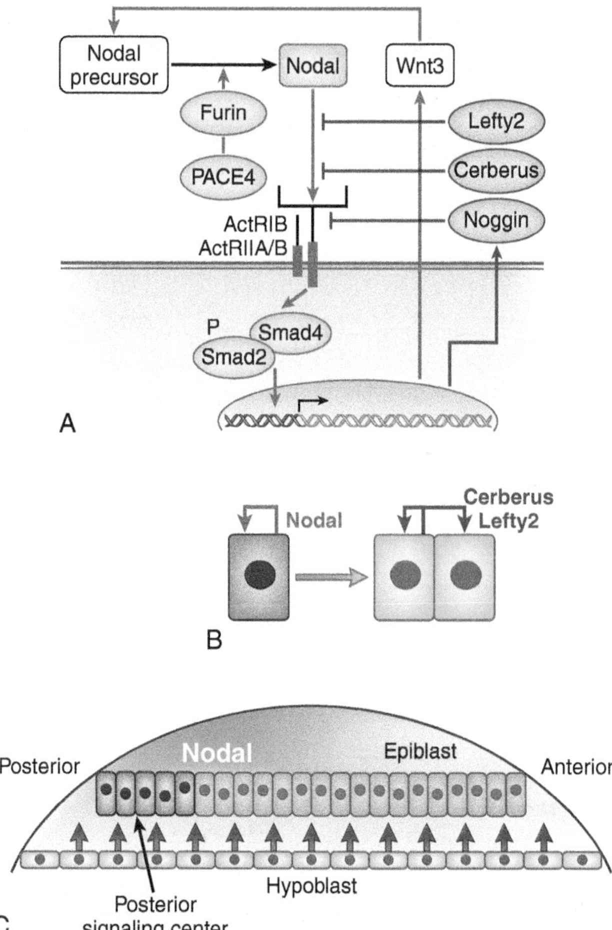

Fig. 4.3 Signaling centers are established by positive and negative feedback. (A) Nodal is a transforming growth factor-β family member that signals through activin type I and II receptors (ActRIB and ActRIIA or ActRIIB). Receptor activation results in the phosphorylation of cytoplasmic Smad3 and Smad4. These then translocate to the nucleus where they bind the promoters of multiple genes. Among the genes induced is Wnt3, which induces Nodal and thereby confers positive feedback on Nodal signaling, and the Nodal inhibitors Lefty2, Cerberus, and Noggin, which represent negative feedback. (B) Nodal effects vary by tissue. Nodal maintains its own expression in the epiblast *(purple)* but induces the expression of Nodal inhibitors in the hypoblast *(light blue)*. (C) The combination of these autoactivation and autoinhibitory effects restricts Nodal expression to a signaling center in the posterior epiblast.

SIGNALING CENTERS ARE ESTABLISHED BY FEEDBACK REGULATION

Signaling proteins can sustain or suppress the activity of their own expression, respectively conferring positive or negative feedback on their own signaling. The autoregulation of TGF-β family signaling peptides contribute prominently to embryonic morphogenesis. Epiblast cells produce Nodal, a member of the TGF-β superfamily that also includes activin and the bone morphogenetic proteins (BMPs). Like other TGF-β family proteins, Nodal is secreted as an inactive precursor into the extracellular space, processed into a mature active dimer by the extracellular enzymes furin and PACE4, and binds complexes of type I and type II cell surface serine-threonine kinase receptors to stimulate targeted cells (Fig. 4.3A).[16]

Upon ligand binding, TGF-β receptor complexes activate cytoplasmic Smad proteins. Of the eight mammalian SMAD proteins, five are receptor activated.[17] One, Smad4, is a cofactor for receptor-activated Smads, and two, Smad6 and Smad7, inhibit Smad signaling. Nodal stimulation causes Smad2 to become phosphorylated and bind Smad4.A cofactor that confers specificity to the complex is also recruited; one such cofactor is the forkhead-family transcription factor FoxH1,[18] which targets the complex to the promoter of *Mix2*, a homeodomain transcription factor (discussed later). Similarly, Smad3 partners with FoxO1, FoxO2, and FoxO3 to up-regulate the cyclin-dependent kinase inhibitor p21Cip1.[19] Nodal thus modulates the transcription of multiple genes that pattern the embryo and slow cell proliferation.

Among the proteins induced by Nodal is *Nodal* itself.[20] Nodal up-regulates Wnt3, which, in turn, maintains Nodal expression in the posterior part of the epiblast (see Fig. 4.3B). Nodal also induces the expression of the Nodal inhibitors Cerberus and Lefty2 in the hypoblast.[21] Together, Nodal autoinduction and autoantagonism restrict its expression to a region termed the posterior signaling center.

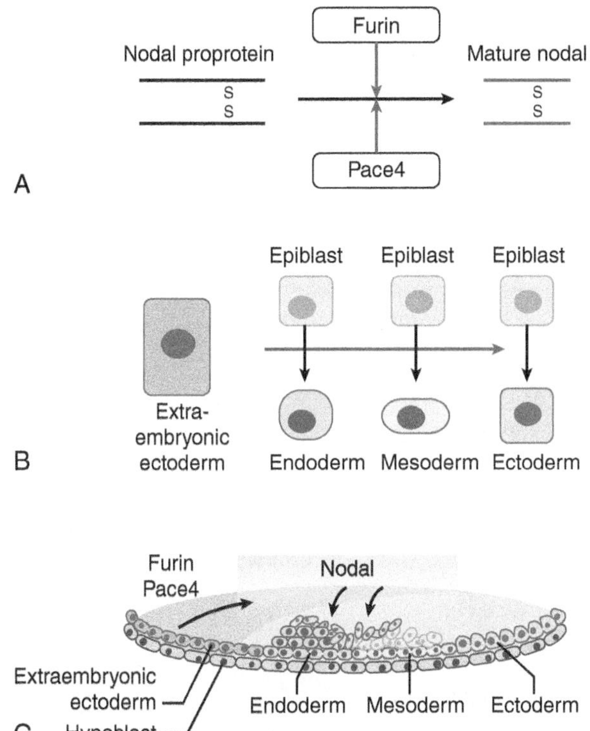

Fig. 4.4 Morphogenic Nodal gradients regulate gastrulation. Morphogens are soluble factors whose actions vary with concentration. Nodal is representative. (A) The inactive Nodal proprotein is processed into its mature active form by the extracellular convertases Furin and Pace4. (B) Nodal proprotein induces the secretion of Furin and Pace4 by the extraembryonic ectoderm. The diffusion and activity of these convertases establish a functional Nodal activity gradient that decreases with distance. Because epiblast transformation into endoderm, mesoderm, and ectoderm are respectively induced by progressively higher Nodal concentrations, the distance from the extraembryonic ectoderm regulates epiblast differentiation. (C) Sagittal section through the mouse gastrula. During gastrulation, epiblast cells undergo epithelial-mesenchymal transformation and migrate towards the midline and the downwards *(black arrows)*, creating the primitive streak. The distance from the extraembryonic ectoderm and determines the whether the transforming epiblast differentiates into endoderm, mesoderm, or ectoderm.

MORPHOGENIC GRADIENTS ARE ESTABLISHED BY SIGNALING CENTERS

As Nodal diffuses away from this source, a concentration gradient is formed. By correlating cell behavior to Nodal activity, induced responses can be restricted to specific locations within the embryo. Such factors are referred to as morphogens, and they represent a powerful mechanism by which complex body plans are specified. An early example occurs during gastrulation, the process by which the bilayered germ disk is transformed into the trilaminar embryo. Gastrulation begins with the formation of the primitive streak. Nodal is required for primitive streak formation; conversely, suppression of Nodal antagonists results in ectopic primitive streaks.[22]

The primitive streak begins as the posterior accumulation of epiblast cells that dissolve their intercellular junctions, acquire pseudopodia, and migrate towards the midline in a process known as epithelial-mesenchymal transition (EMT).[23] EMT is recapitulated during the formation and migration of the neural crest,[24] during wound healing,[25] and pathologically in neoplastic invasion.[26] The passage of epiblast cells through the elongating primitive streak alters their morphology and fate.

In the mouse, the cells that migrate into the streak closest to the extraembryonic ectoderm emerge to become, ultimately, the embryonic endoderm (Fig. 4.4). Cells that accumulate farther away become the mesoderm, and the remaining epiblast cells become the ectoderm. Endodermal and mesodermal differentiation are regulated by a Nodal activity gradient. During gastrulation, Nodal precursor is secreted by the epiblast and processed into its mature form by two extracellular convertases,

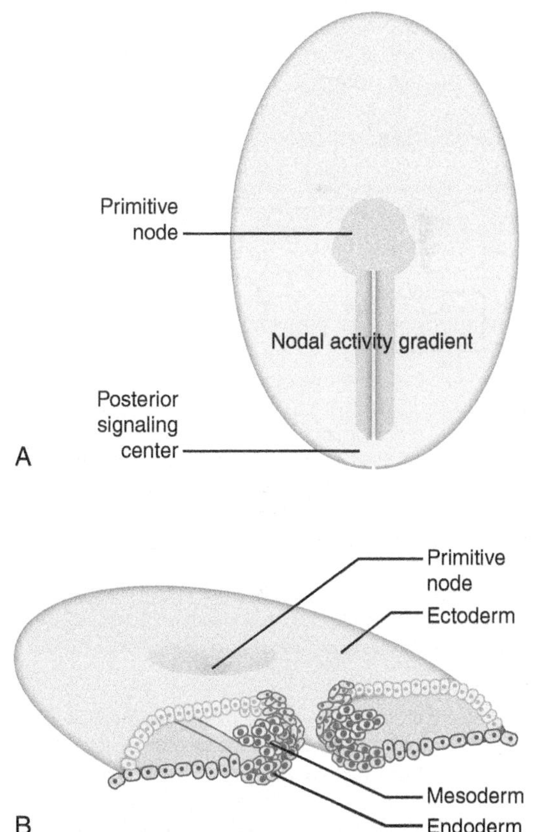

Fig. 4.5 Nodal gradients are established by opposing signaling centers. (A) Nodal produced by the posterior signaling center *(green)* is antagonized by Nodal inhibitors secreted by the primitive node *(red)*. Nodal and its inhibitors combine to establish an anterior-posterior gradient of Nodal activity, depicted in green. (B) Transverse section of gastrulating embryo.

Furin and Pace4, produced by the extraembryonic ectoderm.[27] This establishes a gradient of mature Nodal across the adjacent epiblast.[28] The transforming cells exposed to the highest Nodal concentrations become the endoderm. Cells emerging farther from the extraembryonic ectoderm are subjected to lower Nodal concentrations and become mesoderm.

Nodal also induces the formation and migration of antagonizing signaling centers (Fig. 4.5). Because Nodal induces posterior characteristics, its suppression is necessary for anterior development. Cells at the anterior end of the primitive streak become the primitive node (in birds, Hensen node), which secretes Nodal antagonists such as Lefty and Cerberus. These proteins bind Nodal and/or its cofactors to inhibit its receptor activation.[29,30] The primitive node is necessary for head development and is the mammalian homologue of the Spemann organizer.[31] The primitive node and the posterior signaling center coordinately establish a *Nodal* activity gradient that specifies the anterior-posterior axis of the embryo.[21]

VERTEBRATE LEFT-RIGHT ASYMMETRY IS ESTABLISHED DURING LATE GASTRULATION

Establishment of left-right asymmetry occurs shortly after gastrulation.[32] Left-right asymmetry is initiated by the ventral surface of the primitive node, which forms at the anterior end of the primitive streak and is lined with specialized cilia driven by kinesin motor proteins. The orientation of these cilia and their clockwise rotation establishes a corresponding leftward fluid movement called *nodal flow* (Fig. 4.6).[33] This fluid flow induces asymmetric *Nodal* expression in the left lateral plate mesoderm, and artificial reversal of this flow reverses the orientation of the internal organs.[32,33] Asymmetric Nodal expression is augmented by similarly asymmetric expression of the Nodal inhibitors Lefty1 and Lefty2.[34]

This process also illustrates how defective embryonic regulation can be associated with adult disease. Kartagener syndrome is a congenital condition in which half of the patients have ***situs inversus***, a mirror-image reversal of the internal organs.[35] This phenomenon results from kinesin mutations that impair ciliary motility and nodal flow, with consequent random *Nodal* localization and organ lateralization. Because the same mechanisms are reused throughout life, ciliary akinesis manifests in the adult as immotile sperm and recurrent pneumonias.

DORSAL-VENTRAL AXIS

Nodal also induces another center, the anterior visceral endoderm (AVE), at the rostral end of the hypoblast.[21] This center imparts additional anterior specification by secreting Nodal antagonists.[36] The AVE also specifies the dorsal-ventral axis by secreting Bmp2, another TGF-β family member, which induces the differentiation of the ventral mesoderm[36] and, ultimately, hematopoietic and vascular precursors.[37]

As with anterior-posterior specification, two signaling centers specify dorsal-ventral positioning. In mammals, the second center is the notochord, which condenses in the mesoderm from cells passing anteriorly through the primitive node later during gastrulation (Fig. 4.7).[38] The notochord secretes the BMP inhibitors Flik, Chordin, and Noggin,[39] thereby establishing a dorsal-ventral BMP2 gradient and inducing the differentiation of dorsal mesoderm that will become the somites and, ultimately, the vertebrae, ribs, and axial musculature.

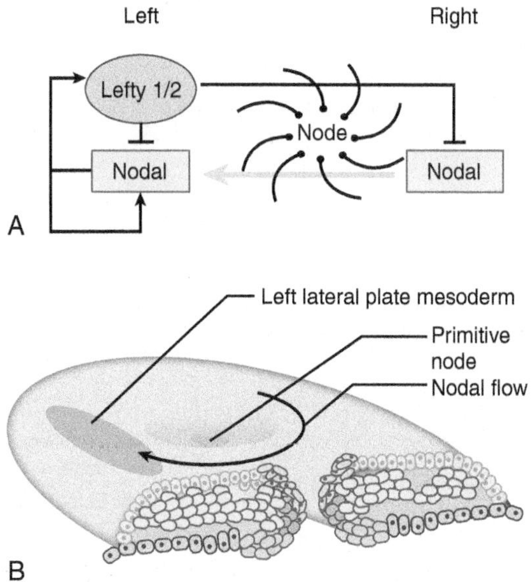

Fig. 4.6 Left-right asymmetry in the mouse is established by ciliary distribution of Nodal. The primitive node becomes visible in late gastrulation at the anterior margin of the primitive streak. (A) The ventral surface of the node is covered with cilia that propel the extraembryonic fluid in a clockwise motion, establishing a higher *Nodal* concentration on the left side of the embryo. Nodal maintains its own expression and also induces the expression of the Nodal inhibitors Lefty 1 and Lefty 2. (B) These positive and negative feedback loops establish and maintain a signaling center in the left lateral plate mesoderm of the late gastrula *(gray)* showing the relationship between the primitive node and the primitive streak.

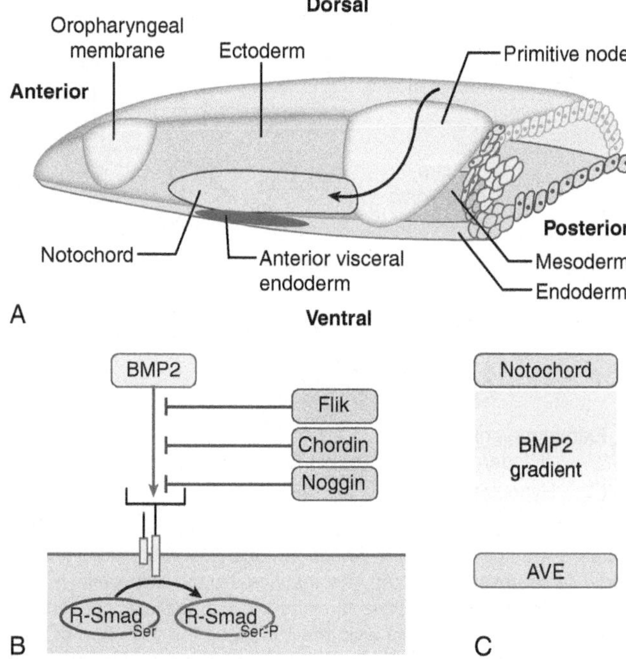

Fig. 4.7 Dorsal-ventral patterning is specified by the notochord and the anterior visceral endoderm *(AVE)*. (A) Sagittal section through a representative gastrulating vertebrate embryo. The notochord forms from epiblast cells that undergo epithelial-mesenchymal transition and pass anteriorly through the primitive node to contact the anterior visceral endoderm. The primitive streak is posterior of the node. (B) The notochord secretes BMP2, a transforming growth factor-β family peptide. In response, the AVE secretes the BMP antagonists Flik, Chordin, and Noggin. (C) Secretion of BMP2 and its antagonists establishes a dorsal-ventral BMP2 activity gradient. *BMP*, Bone morphogenetic protein.

NEURULATION IS INITIATED BY SONIC HEDGEHOG GRADIENTS

Neurulation follows gastrulation and represents the second major embryonic inductive event. The neural plate forms in the ectoderm under the influence of Sonic hedgehog (Shh), a protein expressed by the notochord.[39] Shh signals through a unique mechanism (Fig. 4.8); in its absence, the Patched transmembrane protein prevents activation of Smoothened, a seven-transmembrane domain receptor. In the absence of Smoothened activity, Gli proteins are processed into repressor forms that inhibit gene transcription.[40] Shh binds Patched-1 to allow Smoothened activation, which both activates Gli proteins and attenuates Gli repressor formation.

Dorsal-ventral patterning is imparted to the developing neural tube by Shh secreted from the notochord and BMP4 secreted from the ectoderm.[41] Shh mutations are associated with holoprosencephaly.[42] Cholesterol is added to Shh by posttranslational processing; this modification anchors Shh to cell membranes, slows its diffusion, and possibly enhances its concentration gradient.[43] Shh is used reiteratively to pattern the body, and inborn errors of cholesterol metabolism (as in Smith-Lemli-Opitz syndrome) are associated with limb, heart, brain, and facial dysmorphisms that may be due to disrupted Shh gradients.[44]

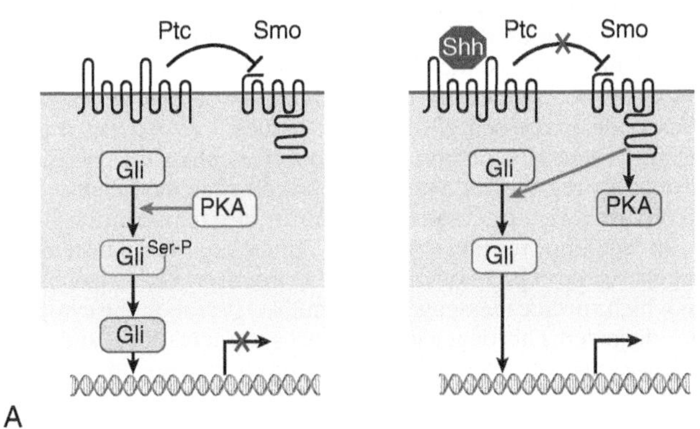

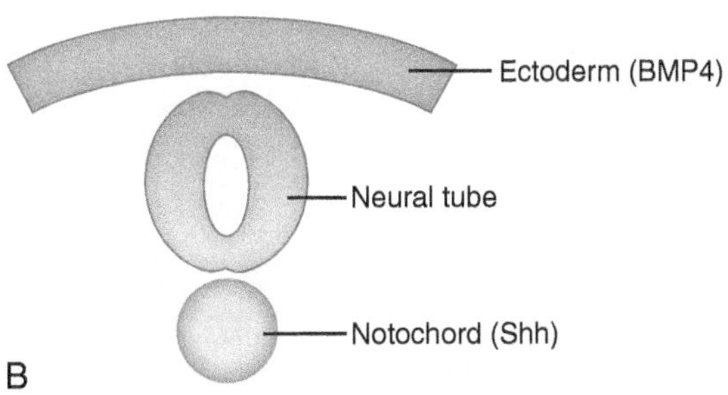

Fig. 4.8 Dorsal-ventral gradients pattern the neural tube. Neurulation is induced by Sonic hedgehog *(Shh)* secreted by the notochord. Shh signals through Patched *(Ptc)*, its cognate receptor, and Smoothened *(Smo)*, a modified G-protein coupled receptor (A). In the absence of Shh, Ptc inhibits Smo, which allows protein kinase A *(PKA)* to phosphorylate Gli transcription factors. This phosphorylation causes Gli to be cleaved into its transcriptional repressor form, thereby attenuating gene transcription. In the presence of Shh, Smo becomes activated. This permits processing of Gli to its activator form and inhibits PKA function. (B) Shh secreted by the notochord *(purple)* imparts ventral specification to the neural tube. An opposing dorsalization gradient is conferred by bone morphogenetic protein *(BMP-4) (gold)*, a TGF-β family peptide secreted from the overlying ectoderm. *TGF*, Transforming growth factor.

SEGMENTATION IS CONTROLLED BY SIGNALING GRADIENTS AND CYCLING GENES

During gastrulation, tissue accumulates anterior to the primitive node to form the prechordal plate, the future location of the mouth. Subsequently, the node and streak regress, or move posteriorly. Somites form in wake of node regression. Signals from the newly differentiated neuroectoderm, the notochord, the surface ectoderm, and the endoderm coordinately induce the condensation of the paired somites from the mesoderm on either side of the midline.[45] Somites will differentiate into the axial musculature, ribs, and vertebrae, and their boundaries regulate the migration of neural crest derivatives including epithelial and neural precursors. Somite size, number, and position are closely regulated, and irregularities in somite formation result in characteristic malformations.[46]

Somitogenesis progresses concomitantly with the regression of the primitive node, beginning at the anterior end and proceeding posteriorly. New somites appear in the presomitic mesoderm at intervals that are characteristic for each species: 30 minutes in zebrafish, 90 for chickens, 120 in mice, and 4 to 5 hours in humans.[47] Somite formation requires two sets of regulatory signals: a maturation wavefront that sweeps through the embryo from anterior to posterior and clock signals that are expressed synchronously throughout the presomitic mesoderm (Fig. 4.9).[48,49] Signaling processes initiated by the advancing maturation wavefront interact with those of the segmentation clock to establish the anterior and posterior margins of each somite.[50]

Segmentation clocks are comprised of signaling pathways that induce oscillating gene expression. Such stable oscillations occur with particular conditions of feedback amplification and latency.[51] The most completely defined pathway centers on Notch, a single-pass transmembrane receptor that mediates signaling between physically adjacent cells; its ligands include Serrate and Jagged, proteins that are expressed on the surface of adjoining cells.[52] Upon binding ligand, Notch is cleaved by proteases embedded in the membrane of the target cell.[52,53] The cleaved cytoplasmic fragment translocates to the nucleus where it associates with the DNA-binding proteins CBF1 and RBPJK, thereby converting them from transcriptional repressors to transcriptional activators. Notch activation is antagonized by the lunatic fringe (Lfng), a short-lived glycosyl transferase whose expression is increased by Notch.[54] Inhibitory feedback conferred by Lfng results in cyclic Notch activation. Notch, in turn, cyclically induces transcription factors, notably members of the Hairy and Enhancer of Split (HES) family of basic helix-loop-helix DNA transcription factors.[55] At least some HES factors are also unstable, and their degradation is necessary for the cyclic expression of Notch.[56]

A second set of molecular oscillators acts through the Wnt pathway. *Wnt* genes encode a large family of secreted lipid-modified proteins with important functions in many developmental contexts.[57,58] Wnt signals are transduced by Frizzled, a receptor with seven transmembrane domains but otherwise has little homology with other G protein–coupled receptors.[59] Frizzled activates the cytoplasmic intermediate, disheveled (Dsh). Dsh antagonizes the ubiquitin-mediated breakdown of β-catenin, which accumulates in the nucleus where it regulates gene transcription. One of the targeted genes encodes axin2, an inhibitor of Wnt signaling whose expression oscillates in parallel with segmentation.[60] Although the two clocks are linked, Wnt cycles out of phase with Notch cycling, and differences in this phase shift regulates the expression of somite boundary markers.[61]

The maturation wavefront appears to be defined by opposing gradients of FGF-8 and retinoic acid. FGF-8 is secreted from the posterior presomitic mesoderm,[62] whereas retinoic acid is produced in the segmented anterior mesoderm and diffuses in a posterior direction to form a gradient that antagonizes FGF signaling.[63] In contrast to Nodal and FGF-8, retinoic acid signaling is not mediated by a membrane-bound receptor. Retinoic acid is a vitamin A derivative, and its receptors belong to the steroid/thyroid hormone nuclear receptor superfamily. Retinoic acid diffuses through the plasma membrane to bind cytoplasmic retinoic acid receptors and retinoid X receptors. Ligand-bound homodimers or heterodimers of these receptors then enter the nucleus to regulate specific promoter response elements.

The antagonism between FGF and retinoic acid signals establishes the maturation wavefront, which moves posteriorly at a constant rate during somitogenesis. The wavefront, in turn, regulates the oscillation of the Wnt clock described earlier.[64] The position of the wavefront at each cycle of the segmentation clock thereby defines the border of each somite. The posterior presomitic mesoderm is comprised of motile mesenchymal cells. The interaction of clock and wavefront signals cause them to assume an epithelial phenotype that solidifies to form the somite's surface.[65]

SEGMENT POSITIONAL IDENTITY IS CONFERRED BY HOMEOBOX GENES

After formation, each segment follows a unique morphogenic pathway that is specified by its position within the embryo. The mechanism by which this identity is conferred was first elucidated in the fruit fly *Drosophila melanogaster*, wherein single mutations resulted in duplication of entire body segments. The genes containing these so-called *homeotic mutations* were recognized as master switches that controlled numerous genes within each segment. Sequencing revealed that these homeotic genes were positioned sequentially on the same chromosome, oriented in the same 5′ to 3′ transcriptional direction, and in the same order as the segments regulated by them.[66] Each gene contained a highly conserved 180-base sequence, termed the homeobox, that encoded a 60-amino acid motif called the *homeodomain*. The homeodomain is a helix-turn-helix DNA-binding motif. The genes themselves were named *homeobox (Hox)* genes.[67]

The mouse and human *Hox* gene complexes are comprised of 38 genes organized in four chromosomal complexes of approximately 120 kb.[68] As in fruit flies, the physical order of the *Hox* genes within these clusters correspond to their expression from anterior to posterior (Fig. 4.10A). However, *Hox* expression boundaries correspond to anatomic regions and not to individual somites[69]; multiple somites may be regulated by a single set of *Hox* genes to assume a similar phenotype. This underlies the similarity, for example, between the seven human cervical vertebrae, relative to the twelve thoracic vertebrae. Moreover, differences in the size and placement of homologous structures (such as the number of cervical vertebrae in mice, humans, and chickens) correspond to differences in the distribution of the analogous *Hox* gene products.

In vertebrates, *Hox* genes are successively activated in the same sequence as their 3′ to 5′ positioning within their respective clusters.[70] *Hox* expression is regulated by several mechanisms. First, early segmentation genes regulate the expression of later ones.[71] This may involve transcription factors encoded by the preceding *Hox* gene[72] (see Fig. 4.10B) or mechanical unpacking of the chromatin that permits transcription factors to associate with the gene.[73] Second, Polycomb and Trithorax proteins antagonistically maintain Hox activation or repression far longer than the initiating signal in an example of epigenetic memory.[74] Third, *Hox* genes regulate one another, with posterior *Hox* genes generally suppressing the activity of anterior ones.[75]

The morphologic development of a somite or anteroposterior region is determined by the combination of *Hox* genes, or the *Hox* code, expressed within those tissues.[76] *Hox* genes regulate arrays of genes by binding Hox-responsive enhancers within DNA regulatory regions. Individual Hox proteins can modulate as many as 68 distinct genes,[77] some of which are also transcription factors.

In addition to transcriptional regulation, *Hox* clusters also regulate gene expression through RNA interference,[78] a mechanism in which specific messenger RNA (mRNA) strands in the cytoplasm are degraded. This degradation reduces the translation and hence expression of the encoded proteins. *Hox* clusters encode precursor microRNA (miRNA) transcripts that contain complementary

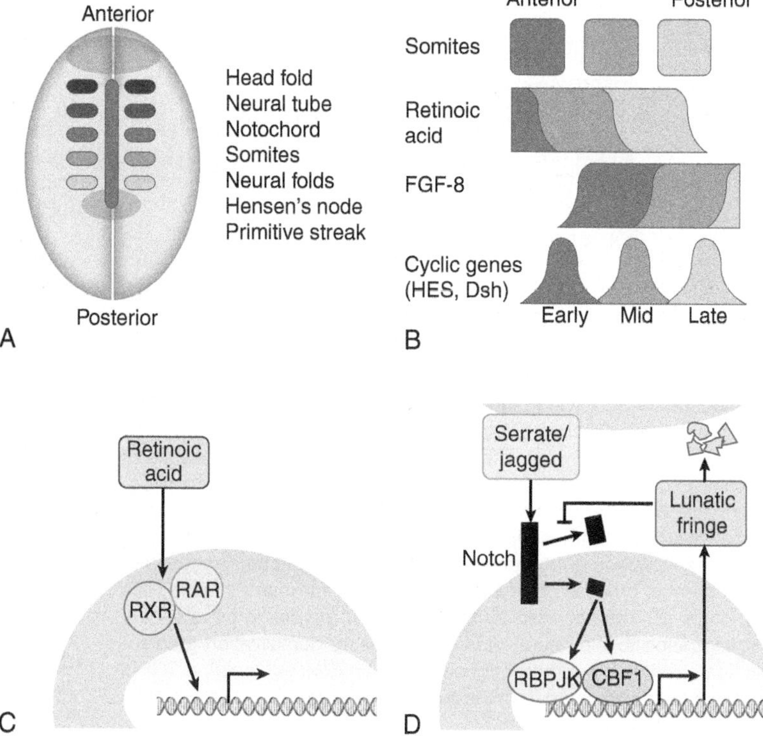

Fig. 4.9 Somitogenesis is regulated by a maturation wavefront and a mesodermal clock signal. Somites arise from paraxial mesoderm at 90-minute intervals in the wake of node regression (A). The boundaries of each somite are established by one or more oscillating genes interacting with a maturational wavefront that is the product of countervailing retinoic acid and fibroblast growth factor *(FGF)*-8 concentration gradients (B). As new somites are formed, the position of this wavefront sweeps posteriorly. Retinoic acid, unlike Nodal or FGF, enters the cytoplasm of targeted cells where it binds homodimers or heterodimers of retinoic acid receptors *(RAR)* or retinoid X receptors *(RXR)* (C). The resulting complex enters the nucleus to bind specific genes. Cyclic genes include components of the Notch pathway (D), which is initiated by Serrate and Jagged expressed on adjoining cells. Upon binding ligand, Notch is cleaved and the cytoplasmic fragment translocates to the nucleus to bind CBF1 and RBPJK and activate gene transcription. One of the induced proteins, the glycosyl transferase lunatic fringe, inhibits Notch cleavage. Lunatic fringe is also short lived, and the resulting oscillating feedback loop results in cyclic Notch activation.

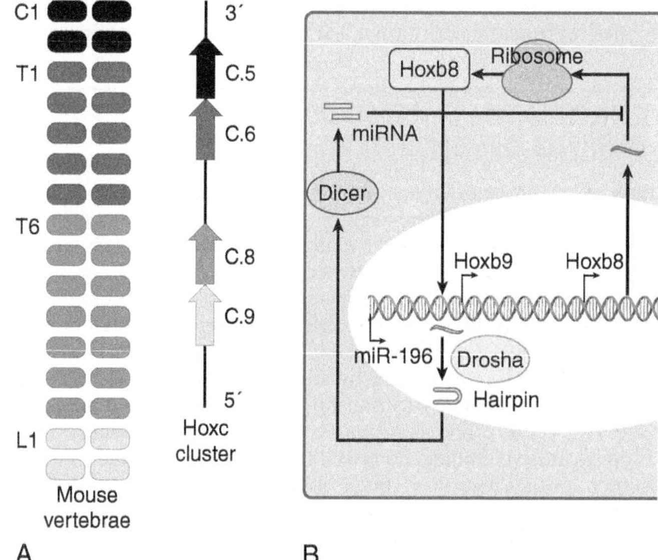

Fig. 4.10 Homeobox *(Hox)* genes confer positional identity to differentiating segments. *Hox* genes are organized in four clusters, and the genes within each cluster are arranged in the same order as they are expressed. (A) The arrangement of genes within the Hoxc cluster is correlated with their expression within a portion of the mouse vertebral column. The *arrows* indicate the direction of transcription. (B) One model of Hox expression is demonstrated wherein one Hox protein, Hoxb8, facilitates the expression of the next, Hoxb9. Also shown is the regulatory function of the miR-196 microRNA sequence embedded within the Hoxb cluster. These sequences are processed by Drosha and Dicer into microRNAs that enable RNA-induced silencing complexes to target and inactivate Hoxb8.

inverted repeat sequences. In addition, it is energetically favorable for such transcripts to fold back on themselves to form hairpin structures that are cleaved within the nucleus by the double-stranded RNA (dsRNA) endonuclease Drosha.[79] The cleavage products are exported to the cytoplasm where they are processed by the dsRNA endonuclease Dicer into approximately 22-base duplexes that are then incorporated into RNA-induced silencing complexes (RISCs) whose specificity is defined by the now single-stranded miRNA. The RISC targets and cleaves mRNA strands that contain sequences complementary to the miRNA, resulting in the posttranscriptional down-regulation of the targeted gene product.

Sequence analyses predict that many *Hox* gene products are targets of the miRNA sequences encoded within *Hox* clusters.[80] Like the *Hox* genes, the miRNAs encoded by the *Hox* cluster have a regional distribution that adds fine resolution control to Hox expression and morphologic development.[81]

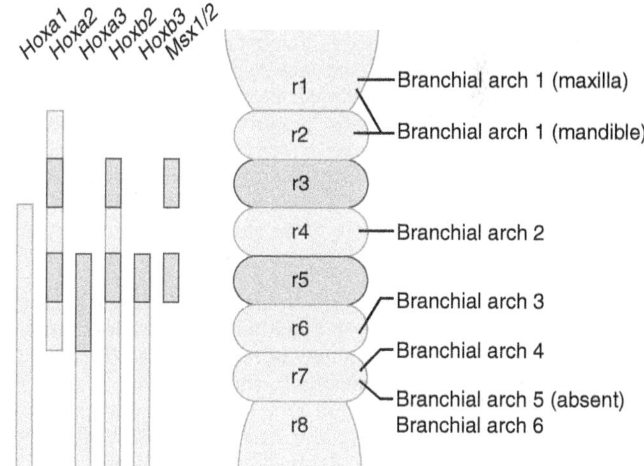

Fig. 4.11 The expression of *Hox* genes within each rhombomere determines the developmental contribution of its derivatives. The distribution of selected Hox genes is shown, together with the branchial arches derived from the migrating neural crest cells of each rhombomere. Many neural crest cells from r3 and r5 *(red)* undergo apoptosis, a process that appears to be initiated by bone morphogenetic protein (BMP)-4 stimulation.

NEUROECTODERMAL REGULATION PATTERNS CRANIOFACIAL STRUCTURES

After neurulation, differentiation of the craniofacial structures begins with invagination of the neural plate to form the neural folds. The subsequent approximation and closure of these folds result in formation of the neural tube.[82] Cells dissociate from the neural folds and undergo epithelial-to-mesenchymal transformation to become the neural crest cells that migrate throughout the embryo along defined routes. The developmental contributions of neural crest cells correlate with their original position, and this identity is conferred by ectodermally secreted Wnt proteins,[83] BMP4, and the BMP antagonists *chordin* and *Noggin* secreted by the anterior mesoderm.[84] BMP4 and its antagonists establish an activity gradient that determines the fate of neuroectodermal derivatives, with the level required for neural crest induction greater than that required for neural plate induction and lower than that required for ectoderm specification.[85] This gradient is associated with regional expression of specific transcriptional regulators[82,86,87]: the zinc-finger transcription factors of the *Zic* family are expressed throughout the neural plate and crest; the homeobox transcriptional repressors Msx1 and Msx2 are expressed in the neural plate border; the paired-box transcriptional activators Pax3 and Pax7 are expressed at the neural plate border; and the transcriptional activators Sox9 and Sox10 localize to premigratory and migratory neural crest, respectively.

After closure, the anterior neural tube differentiates into forebrain, midbrain, and hindbrain components. The hindbrain is of particular clinical interest because hindbrain derivatives are major contributors to facial formation, and craniofacial anomalies comprise one third of all human congenital defects.[88] During early vertebrate hindbrain development, seven transient transverse bulges appear. These divide the hindbrain into eight developmental domains called *rhombomeres*. In contrast to somites, whose numbers vary considerably, the number of rhombomeres is quite stable across vertebrate classes.[89] Like the somites, the divergent differentiation of these rhombomeres is regulated by *Hox* genes whose expression, in turn, is controlled by FGF-8 and retinoic acid.[90,91] Rhombomeres give rise to cranial neural crest cells that migrate out of the neuroectoderm, proliferate, coalesce into the first three branchial arches, and ultimately coalesce into the craniofacial structures (see Fig. 4.8).[92] Subtle differences in rhombomere regulation are reflected in variations in cell migration and proliferation that contribute to each individual's unique facial structure, whereas more

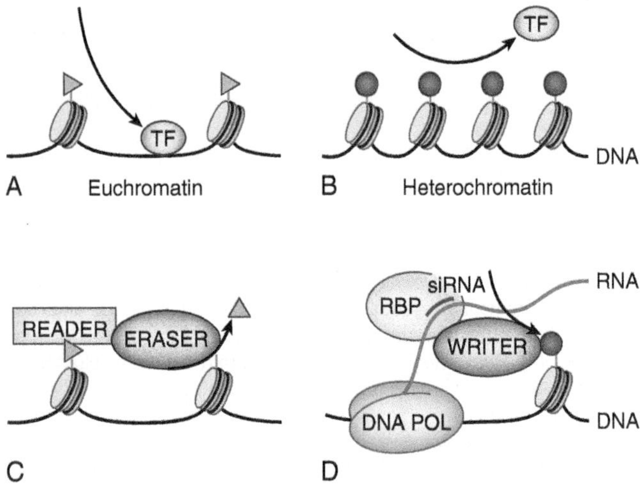

Fig. 4.12 Histone modifications mediate gene expression. Transcription requires that promoters be accessible to transcription factors. When histones bear permissive modifications *(green triangles)*, the associated genomic DNA is loosely packed into euchromatin, which is available to transcription factor *(TF)* (A). Histones bearing restrictive modifications *(red circles)* induce the condensations of DNA into tightly packed heterochromatin that resists transcription factor binding (B). Embryonic chromatin becomes progressively more restrictive with development. To change euchromatin into heterochromatin, permissive markers are first detected by reader proteins and removed by associated eraser enzymes (C). Restrictive modifications are then placed by writer enzymes under the guidance of RNA-binding proteins *(RBPs)* whose specificity is conferred by associated siRNAs. These siRNAs are processed from long noncoding RNAs and are complementary to transcripts emerging from the targeted DNA (D).

disruptive mutations induce overtly dysmorphic features that are often pathognomonic for those mutations. The developmental contribution of each rhombomere is regulated by *Hox* gene expression (Fig. 4.11). For example, rhombomeres 3 and 5 express *Msx2*, and cranial neural crest cells that express this factor undergo apoptosis when stimulated with BMP4.[93] Similarly, Sox9 expression regulates BMP4-mediated chondrogenesis.[94] The profile of *Hox* genes expressed within each rhombomere therefore guides the behavior of its derivatives.

GROWTH FACTOR SIGNALING IS EPIGENETICALLY REGULATED

In these examples, closely related morphogens iteratively pattern the body. Nodal, BMP2, and BMP4 are all TGF-β family members, and all signal through SMAD proteins. New axes of asymmetry can be created without disrupting previously developed axes if different sets of genes respond to these signals. For a gene to be activated, its regulatory elements must be accessible to transcription factors. Genomic DNA is coiled around cores comprised of eight histones to form nucleosomes; the accessibility of the elements therein is determined by where the nucleosomes are placed and how tightly the DNA is wound around them.[95] Packing density is modulated by covalent modification of histone tails protruding from the globular core around which the DNA is spooled; at least nine different modifications (including methylation, acetylation, phosphorylation, and citrullination)[96] have been observed at more than 287 sites.[97] Inactive genes are tightly packed into heterochromatin whose histones bear repressive modifications, whereas genes that are capable of activation are loosely packed into euchromatin whose histones are enriched with permissive modifications (Fig. 4.12A and B).[98] For example, heterochromatin is enriched in histone H3 methylated at Lys 9 (H3K9me). H3K9me is bound by HP1, which in turn recruits transcriptional inactivators to heterochromatin.[99]

CHROMATIN IS REMODELED DURING DEVELOPMENT

How is euchromatin transformed into heterochromatin? Modifications such as H3K9me can be applied ("written") and will persist until actively removed ("erased"). Permissive markers within euchromatin are first identified by sequence-specific reader proteins. These readers are coupled to enzymes that erase permissive marks (see Fig. 4.12C). In a process that is incompletely understood, heterochromatin formation is then induced at specific sites by RNA-binding proteins guided by small interfering RNAs (siRNAs) that are complementary to transcripts from the targeted genome (see Fig. 4.12D). The resulting complex recruits writers that apply repressive modifications to the histones.[100] Heterochromatin is then propagated from these initiation sites by reader-writer complexes largely independently of genomic sequence.

Once established, H3K9 methylation is maintained by noncoding RNAs transcribed from within the heterochromatin. These transcripts are recognized by DNA-binding proteins and siRNA-associated RNA-binding proteins that then recruit histone-lysine-*N*-methyltransferases.[100] Moreover, epigenetic modifications are transmitted to daughter cells, establishing discrete populations with progressively divergent behaviors.

The siRNAs are processed from noncoding RNAs that are often paradoxically expressed from within the heterochromatin. Long noncoding RNAs can induce or maintain the methylation of large groups of genes. In X-inactivation, an entire chromosome is suppressed by the long noncoding RNA Xist.[101,102] Coordinated epigenetic modification establishes chromatin states that are associated with distinct cell behaviors. In general, the open chromatin of pluripotent cells becomes increasingly restrictive with differentiation.[103] Thus the permissive chromatin of the *Xenopus* zygote acquires H3K4me3 as it blastulates, H3K27me3 as it gastrulates, and DNA methylation as it neurulates.[98]

CONCLUSION

Embryonic cells are regulated autonomously by epigenetic imprinting and conditionally by secreted molecules. Morphogens are expressed in signaling centers, from which they diffuse outward to establish concentration gradients that induce tissue differentiation and confer positional identity. Signaling factors may interact cooperatively or antagonistically, and modulate cell behavior by binding receptors with distinct but overlapping functions and specificities. Prominent regulators of embryogenesis include TGF-β receptors (Nodal and BMP), receptor tyrosine kinases (FGF), Notch receptors (Serrate and Jagged), Frizzled receptors (Wnt), and nuclear receptors (retinoic acid). These receptors initiate chains of intracellular kinase reactions that modulate the activity of DNA-binding proteins, thereby activating promoters and enhancers. Certain transcription factors (notably the *Hox* proteins) are master switches that regulate batteries of genes. Regulated genes may themselves encode transcriptional regulators or noncoding RNAs so that dozens of proteins are modulated by a single stimulus, thereby initiating complex cell behaviors. Most signaling pathways incorporate positive feedback loops that maintain and propagate pathway activity and negative feedback loops that stabilize or terminate signaling. Short-lived components within these feedback loops induce oscillations that are exploited to form repeated structures. Conversely, epigenetic regulation persists through generations of replication and permit signaling mechanisms to be reiterated in different contexts to modulate development, homeostasis, and regeneration.

A complete reference list is available at www.ExpertConsult.com.

SELECT REFERENCES

1. Wagschal A, Feil R. Genomic imprinting in the placenta. *Cytogenet Genome Res*. 2006;113:90-98.
2. Suzuki MM, Bird A. DNA methylation landscapes: provocative insights from epigenomics. *Nat Rev Genet*. 2008;9:465-476.
5. Cassidy SB, Dykens E, Williams CA. Prader-Willi and Angelman syndromes: sister imprinted disorders. *Am J Med Genet*. 2000;97:136-146.
6. Spemann H, Mangold H. Induction of embryonic primordia by implantation of organizers from a different species. 1923. *Int J Dev Biol*. 2001;45:13-38.
7. Kuijk EW, van Tol LT, Van de Velde H, et al. The roles of FGF and MAP kinase signaling in the segregation of the epiblast and hypoblast cell lineages in bovine and human embryos. *Development*. 2012;139:871-882.
8. Tsang M, Dawid IB. Promotion and attenuation of FGF signaling through the Ras-MAPK pathway. *Sci STKE*. 2004;2004:e17.
9. Denhardt DT. Signal-transducing protein phosphorylation cascades mediated by Ras/Rho proteins in the mammalian cell: the potential for multiplex signalling. *Biochem J*. 1996;318:729-747.
10. Hanafusa H, Torii S, Yasunaga T, et al. Sprouty1 and Sprouty2 provide a control mechanism for the Ras/MAPK signalling pathway. *Nat Cell Biol*. 2002;4:850-858.
12. Saunders A, Faiola F, Wang J. Concise review: pursuing self-renewal and pluripotency with the stem cell factor Nanog. *Stem Cells*. 2013;31:1227-1236.
14. Berridge MJ, Lipp P, Bootman MD. The versatility and universality of calcium signalling. *Nat Rev Mol Cell Biol*. 2000;1:11-21.
16. Schier AF, Shen MM. Nodal signalling in vertebrate development. *Nature*. 2000;403:385-389.
20. Brennan J, Lu CC, Norris DP, et al. Nodal signalling in the epiblast patterns the early mouse embryo. *Nature*. 2001;411:965-969.
21. Yamamoto M, Saijoh Y, Perea-Gomez A, et al. Nodal antagonists regulate formation of the anteroposterior axis of the mouse embryo. *Nature*. 2004;428:387-392.
23. Lim J, Thiery JP. Epithelial-mesenchymal transitions: insights from development. *Development*. 2012;139:3471-3486.
24. Bronner ME, LeDouarin NM. Development and evolution of the neural crest: an overview. *Dev Biol*. 2012;366:2-9.
26. Nieto MA. Epithelial plasticity: a common theme in embryonic and cancer cells. *Science*. 2013;342:1234850.
30. Piccolo S, Agius E, Leyns L, et al. The head inducer Cerberus is a multifunctional antagonist of Nodal, BMP and Wnt signals. *Nature*. 1999;397:707-710.
33. Zhou X, Sasaki H, Lowe L, et al. Nodal is a novel TGF-beta-like gene expressed in the mouse node during gastrulation. *Nature*. 1993;361:543-547.
34. Hirokawa N, Tanaka Y, Okada Y, et al. Nodal flow and the generation of left-right asymmetry. *Cell*. 2006;125:33-45.
36. Madabhushi M, Lacy E. Anterior visceral endoderm directs ventral morphogenesis and placement of head and heart via BMP2 expression. *Dev Cell*. 2011;21:907-919.
39. Liem Jr KF, Jessell TM, Briscoe J. Regulation of the neural patterning activity of sonic hedgehog by secreted BMP inhibitors expressed by notochord and somites. *Development*. 2000;127:4855-4866.
40. Eaton S. Multiple roles for lipids in the Hedgehog signalling pathway. *Nat Rev Mol Cell Biol*. 2008;9:437-445.
45. Gamse J, Sive H. Vertebrate anteroposterior patterning: the *Xenopus* neurectoderm as a paradigm. *Bioessays*. 2000;22:976-986.
47. Dequeant ML, Pourquie O. Segmental patterning of the vertebrate embryonic axis. *Nat Rev Genet*. 2008;9:370-382.
50. Dubrulle J, Pourquie O. From head to tail: links between the segmentation clock and antero-posterior patterning of the embryo. *Curr Opin Genet Dev*. 2002;12:519-523.
54. Dale JK, Maroto M, Dequeant ML, et al. Periodic notch inhibition by lunatic fringe underlies the chick segmentation clock. *Nature*. 2003;421:275-278.
59. Pierce KL, Premont RT, Lefkowitz RJ. Seven-transmembrane receptors. *Nat Rev Mol Cell Biol*. 2002;3:639-650.
61. Sonnen KF, Lauschke VM, Uraji J, et al. Modulation of phase shift between wnt and notch signaling oscillations controls mesoderm segmentation. *Cell*. 2018;172:1079-1090. e12.
63. Diez dC, Storey KG. Opposing FGF and retinoid pathways: a signalling switch that controls differentiation and patterning onset in the extending vertebrate body axis. *Bioessays*. 2004;26:857-869.
70. Kmita M, Duboule D. Organizing axes in time and space; 25 years of colinear tinkering. *Science*. 2003;301:331-333.
71. Mallo M, Alonso CR. The regulation of Hox gene expression during animal development. *Development*. 2013;140:3951-3963.
74. Steffen PA, Ringrose L. What are memories made of? How Polycomb and Trithorax proteins mediate epigenetic memory. *Nat Rev Mol Cell Biol*. 2014;15:340-356.
78. Pearson JC, Lemons D, McGinnis W. Modulating Hox gene functions during animal body patterning. *Nat Rev Genet*. 2005;6:893-904.
81. Kaschula R, Pinho S, Alonso CR. MicroRNA-dependent regulation of Hox gene expression sculpts fine-grain morphological patterns in a *Drosophila* appendage. *Development*. 2018;145:16.
82. LaBonne C, Bronner-Fraser M. Molecular mechanisms of neural crest formation. *Annu Rev Cell Dev Biol*. 1999;15:81-112.
86. Gammill LS, Bronner-Fraser M. Neural crest specification: migrating into genomics. *Nat Rev Neurosci*. 2003;4:795-805.
88. Trainor PA, Krumlauf R. Patterning the cranial neural crest: hindbrain segmentation and Hox gene plasticity. *Nat Rev Neurosci*. 2000;1:116-124.
95. Klemm SL, Shipony Z, Greenleaf WJ. Chromatin accessibility and the regulatory epigenome. *Nat Rev Genet*. 2019;20:207-220.
96. Tessarz P, Kouzarides T. Histone core modifications regulating nucleosome structure and dynamics. *Nat Rev Mol Cell Biol*. 2014;15:703-708.
98. Bogdanovic O, van Heeringen SJ, Veenstra GJ. The epigenome in early vertebrate development. *Genesis*. 2012;50:192-206.
100. Allshire RC, Madhani HD. Ten principles of heterochromatin formation and function. *Nat Rev Mol Cell Biol*. 2018;19:229-244.
102. Engreitz JM, Pandya-Jones A, McDonel P, et al. The Xist lncRNA exploits three-dimensional genome architecture to spread across the X chromosome. *Science*. 2013;341:1237973.
103. Gokbuget D, Blelloch R. Epigenetic control of transcriptional regulation in pluripotency and early differentiation. *Development*. 2019;146:25.

The Extracellular Matrix in Development

5

Sandra L. Leibel | Martin Post

INTRODUCTION

During embryonic patterning, individual cells divide, migrate, differentiate, and respond to environmental cues. The extracellular matrix (ECM) is effectively involved in all these dynamic processes during development, maintenance, and disease. Cells are continuously connected with the ECM, a latticework of glycoproteins that provides structural support and spatial arrangement and directs tissue morphogenesis. The ECM provides a specialized microenvironment that regulates cell behavior by interacting with cell surface receptors known as integrins. This allows regulation of extracellular and intracellular signaling emanating from extrinsic factors, including growth factors (GFs), hormones, and biomechanical forces. Proteolysis of the ECM also generates neoepitopes that confer functions on cells and tissues distinct from those specified by their nonproteolyzed counterparts. In this chapter, we provide a review of the complex structure of the ECM and its essential role in normal development and pathophysiology, and elaborate on ECM-integrin signaling with tissue-specific examples during embryonic development and adult tissue maintenance.

THE EXTRACELLULAR MATRIX IS STRUCTURALLY DIVERSE

To decipher how the ECM confers numerous different functions, an appreciation of its complex structure is essential. The ECM is an oligomeric, three-dimensional network composed of four major

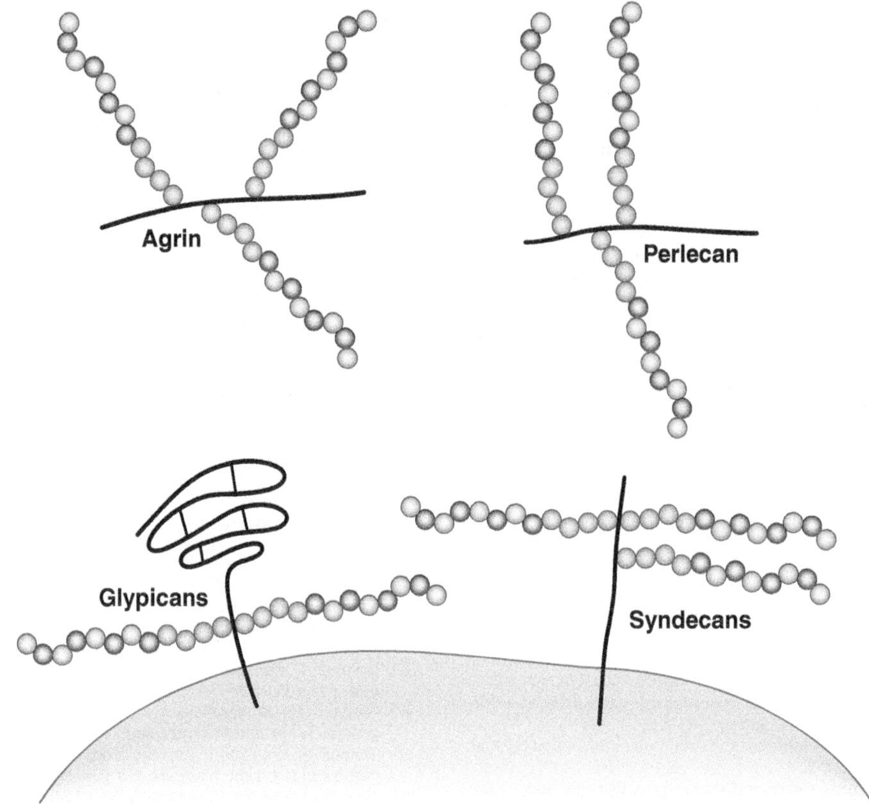

Fig. 5.1 Cell surface and extracellular heparan sulfate (HS) proteoglycans. Glypicans and syndecans are attached to the cell surface via a glycosylphosphatidylinositol anchor. They possess a large globular domain stabilized by conserved di-sulfide (S-S) bonds, and HS chains (represented by chains of *pink*, and *purple circles*). Agrin and perlecan are large multidomain proteoglycans that carry several HS chains and are secreted as different isoforms generated by alternative splicing. (Modified from Poulain FE, Yost HJ. Heparan sulfate proteoglycans: a sugar code for vertebrate development? *Development.* 2015;142:3456–3467.)

protein components: collagens, structural glycoproteins (e.g., fibronectin, laminin, tenascin-C), proteoglycans (e.g., heparan sulfate [HS], chondroitin sulfate, syndecans), and elastic fibers (e.g., elastin, microfibrillar proteins). Matrix proteins are secreted by the epithelial and stromal cells and bind each other as well as cell adhesion molecules.[1] Developmental processes, including the response of unpatterned tissue to morphogen gradients, are regulated by glycosaminoglycans, whereas the surface of most cells and the ECM are decorated by HS proteoglycans (HSPGs).[2] HSPGs are composed of a core protein to which long linear glycosaminoglycan HS chains are covalently linked (Fig. 5.1). They engage in numerous cell-matrix interactions and function by binding and regulating local concentrations of GFs and morphogens, and mediate a wide range of functions in early vertebrate development, for example, left-right patterning and cardiovascular and neural development.[3,4] The distribution and organization of the ECM is both dynamic and tissue-specific. For example, mesenchymal cells are surrounded by an interstitial stromal ECM, which includes type I and type II collagen, fibronectin, and proteoglycans. The basement membrane of endoderm-derived organs such as the lung represents another specialized ECM that is composed predominantly of laminin, type IV collagen, and HSPGs.[5] Alternatively, basement membrane material may separate distinct cell layers, as is the case in the kidney glomerulus, where the basement membrane separating epithelial and endothelial cells also functions as a filter.[6] In the case of elastic tissues such as skin and arteries, the ECM is reinforced with elastin fibers to provide additional structural stability for resilience to mechanical forces. Within these different extracellular matrices, additional structural and functional diversity is generated using alternative gene promoters and RNA splicing, and by posttranslational modifications, including glycosylation and sulfation of newly synthesized matrix proteins. Once secreted into the extracellular space, ECM proteins require integration into a functional network. Identifying binding partners for a specific ECM protein is therefore a prerequisite to ascertaining its biochemical and cell-signaling properties. For example, the ECM glycoprotein tenascin-C (TNC) controls cell adhesion, migration, differentiation, and synthesis of ECM molecules via interacting in a tissue-specific manner with fibronectin, perlecan, neurocan, heparin, phosphacan, syndecan, glypican, and periostin.[7,8] Accordingly, understanding the biology of a single ECM component requires an appreciation of the structure and functions of numerous other affiliated proteins. Because of the number of steps involved in coordinating ECM expression, secretion, and assembly, deciphering how individual ECM proteins contribute to structural morphogenesis during developmental processes has been a challenging task.

THE EXTRACELLULAR MATRIX IS MULTIFUNCTIONAL

Normal development requires precise temporal and spatial coordination of cellular proliferation, migration, differentiation, and apoptosis. Deciding which of these programs a cell will ultimately elect is determined, to a large extent, by the ECM. Promotion or suppression of cellular proliferation by the ECM results in either activation or silencing of genes involved in the regulation of the cell cycle.[9-12] To counteract uncontrolled cellular proliferation and to sculpt or refine developing tissue structures, select cells must be eliminated from developing tissues. To this end, loss of cell contact with the ECM leads to a specialized apoptosis termed *anoikis* during development and cellular differentiation.[13,14] Tissue-specific ECM components also regulate the transcription of genes associated with specialized differentiated functions, including alkaline phosphatase expression in osteoblasts, albumin production in hepatocytes, and intermediate filament protein expression in keratinocytes.[15,16] The critical role of the ECM during heart morphogenesis is apparent by the dependence of precardiac cells' directional movement on a gradient of fibronectin, a matrix protein involved in the active migration of cells across the substratum.[17] Efficient specification to cardiomyocytes is also directly dependent on cell attachment strength and matrix compliance.[18] These observations are supported by the identification of ECM-responsive transcription factors and *cis* elements within gene promoters.[19,20] Moreover, stem cell maintenance, self-renewal, and cell fate determination in adult stem cell populations depend on the ECM.[21-24] For example, matrix-mediated changes in cell adhesion of hematopoietic stem cells in their microenvironment allow for the self-renewal and subsequent differentiation of these multipotent progenitors into blood and other cell types.[25] Therefore, precise cell-matrix interactions act as an important biologic switch that dictates stem cell differentiation or mobilization at specific tissue sites during development and maintenance of adult stem cell populations.

INVESTIGATING EXTRACELLULAR MATRIX FUNCTIONS

Mapping and identifying gene mutations that lead to heritable connective tissue disorders along with generating animal models in which ECM genes have been mutated or ablated have been successfully used to ascertain the functions of individual ECM proteins within specific tissues. Many of the diseases resulting from ECM gene mutations are due to the defective structural integrity of specific tissues. Mutations in collagen type VII, collagen type XVII, and laminin can cause the skin-blistering disease epidermolysis bullosa.[26,27] Mutations in type I collagen genes cause osteogenesis imperfecta,[28] and mutations in both collagen I and tenascin-X genes can cause Ehlers-Danlos syndrome.[29] In addition to gene defects that alter mechanical properties of the ECM, mutations in the fibrillin-1 gene that cause Marfan syndrome appear to increase transforming growth factor (TGF)-β signaling, leading to a cellular disease phenotype.[30]

Although mutations in ECM genes can produce heritable disorders, animal studies suggest that many structural ECM glycoproteins are essential for embryonic or fetal development. As a result, mutations in these genes often cause lethality early in development, complicating the study of gene function in vivo. Inactivation of the fibronectin gene in mice results in embryonic death due to mesodermal, neural tube, and vascular developmental defects[31] and has been shown to be required for normal gastrulation.[32] More targeted studies have provided data on the role of fibronectin in several developmental processes. Injection of inhibitory peptides or antibodies into post-gastrulation embryos prevents fibronectin-cellular interactions and disrupts neural crest migration. In contrast with fibronectin, knockout (KO) of the tenascin-C gene in mice results in viable and fertile adults,[33] suggesting that other ECM proteins may be able to compensate for tenascin-C deficiency. Consistent with this notion, experiments using isolated adult hypertensive pulmonary arteries, in which tenascin-C expression has been suppressed, indicate that osteopontin substitutes for tenascin-C in promoting smooth muscle cell proliferation.[34]

Mutations in ECM component genes may also cause adult-onset phenotypes. Some of these phenotypes may result from abnormalities not visible at birth, and many of these animals have not been analyzed in enough detail to rule out developmental defects. For example, tenascin-C gene-KO mice suffer from several neurologic defects, including hyperactivity, poor sensorimotor coordination, clinging, and freezing behavior, as well as poor performance in passive avoidance tests.[35] Other defects in tenascin-C gene-KO animals have subsequently been detected, including reduced corneal wound healing and hematopoiesis.[36,37] Tenascin-C gene-KO mice also exhibit less severe inflammation in an arthritis model, suggesting that ECM components participate in the inflammatory response.[38]

An alternative approach to genetic manipulation for elucidating the role of matrix proteins during various cellular processes is exposure to agents that perturb protein-cell interactions. Such agents can include small molecules or protein-specific antibodies that will interfere with the matrix protein function. Fibronectin-binding antibody or synthetic peptides have demonstrated the importance of fibronectin-cell interactions during cell migration and normal heart development in the chick.[17] Genetic studies have also been useful in revealing unexpected functions for certain matrix proteins. For example, ablation of the elastin gene was predicted to cause structural defects in the three-dimensional structure of blood vessels. Elastin-null animals, however, die within days of birth as a result of obstructive arterial disease characterized by proliferation of the subendothelial smooth muscle.[39] Thus elastin exerts an unexpected growth-inhibitory role during normal vascular morphogenesis. Elastin haplo-insufficient adult mice are hypertensive, also as a result of abnormal vascular development and remodeling.[40] Results from ECM-mutant animals therefore demonstrate the important roles ECM components play in both normal development and response to injury.

INTEGRINS AS EXTRACELLULAR MATRIX RECEPTORS

Integrins are transmembrane receptors composed of 24 αβ heterodimeric members that link the external ECM environment to the internal cell milieu. Integrin receptors respond to the molecular composition and physical properties of the ECM and integrate both mechanical and chemical signals through direct association with the cytoskeleton. The heterodimers are composed of noncovalently associated 18 α- and 8 β-subunits,[41] with distinct protein functions. The α-subunit determines integrin ligand specificity, and nine of the integrin α chains contain an I domain with a metal ion-dependent adhesive site, which comprises the ligand-binding site. The β-subunit connects to the cytoskeleton and affects multiple signaling pathways. Activation of integrins may stimulate the cell cycle, inhibit apoptosis, and change the shape, polarity, and motility of the cell.[41] The extracellular domain binds to ECM ligands, whereas the cytoplasmic domain binds to adaptor proteins, mediating "outside-in" and "inside-out" signaling (Fig. 5.2).[42] During outside-in signaling, ligand binding leads to separation of the two "legs," allowing the β-subunit cytoplasmic domain to bind intracellular proteins such as talin (Tln) and kindlins. An example of inside-out signaling is the intracellular activation of Tln, leading to its binding the β-subunit and triggering the transition of the integrin heterodimer to a state with high affinity for extracellular ligands.[43] A number of integrins play central roles during fetal and embryonic development, and KO mice have been used extensively to elicit the role of integrins during the development of numerous tissues. During vascular development, α5β1 integrins that recognize the Arg-Gly-Asp (RGD) peptide motifs in fibronectin play a primary role.[44] Mutation of α5 leads to early embryonic lethality due to mesodermal defects and poor vascularization of both the yolk sac and the embryo,[45] whereas a β1 mutation manifests as gastrulation defects and preimplantation mortality.[46] The interaction between integrins and Tlns has also been studied in the KO mouse model of heart disease. Simultaneous loss of both cardiac myocyte Tln1 and Tln2 led to cardiac dysfunction by 4 weeks of life with 100% mortality by 6 months of life. The myocardial abnormalities were secondary to the loss of β1D integrin and other costameric proteins (which connect the sarcomere to the cell membrane) from the cardiac myocytes, compromising membrane integrity leading to myocyte instability.[47]

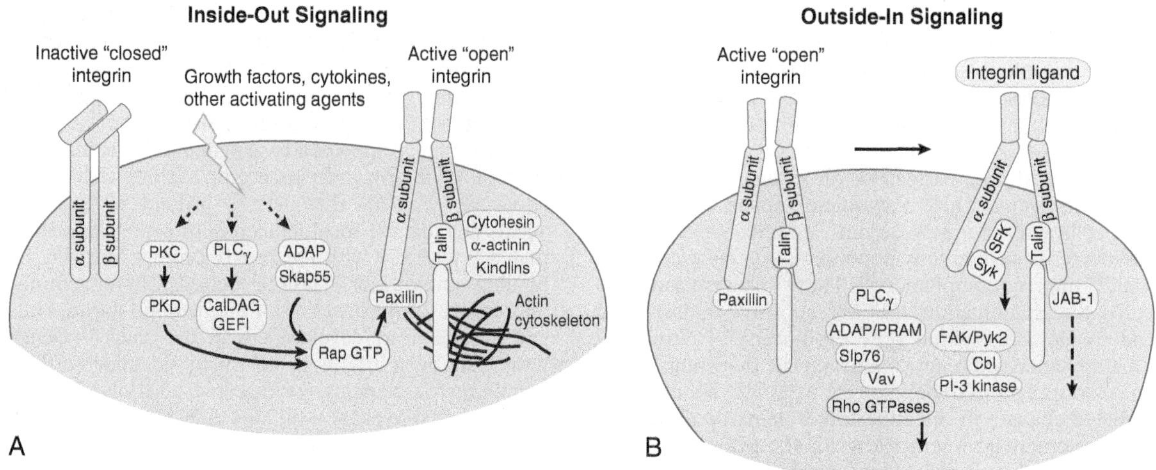

Fig. 5.2 Simplified model of integrin signaling complexes. (A) Ligation of integrins by extracellular matrix proteins leads to linkage to the cytoskeletal network by cytoplasmic proteins (inside-out signaling). (B) Integrins are activated and transmit intracellular signals that affect the polarity, shape, and motility of a cell via members of the Rho family of small GTPases (outside-in signaling). (Modified from Lowell CA, Mayadas TN. *Integrin and Cell Adhesion Molecules: Methods and Protocols 757*. Totowa, NJ: Humana Press; 2011:369–397.)

Integrins play a primary role in linking keratinocytes to the underlying basement membrane during skin development.[48] Conditional deletion of β1 integrins in the epidermis results in severe skin blistering and hair defects, accompanied by massive failure of basement membrane assembly/organization, hemidesmosome instability, and a failure of hair follicle keratinocytes to remodel the basement membrane and invaginate into the dermis.[49] In mice lacking the β1-subunit in neurons, the cortex is completely disorganized, due to a defect between cortical structures and the developing meningeal basement membrane. Conditional deletion of β1 in neural crest cells affects the peripheral nervous system, including failure of normal nerve arborization, delay in Schwann cell migration, and defective neuromuscular junction differentiation. This is thought to be due to defective migration of neural crest cells through the embryonic ECM.[50]

Integrins play an important role during lung development and disease, including branching morphogenesis, epithelial cell polarization, and differentiation. They are found on lung epithelial, endothelial, and fibroblast cells. Early epithelial cells express integrins α3 and α6 pericellularly, but as they mature, they express integrins α3 and α6 basally, suggesting that integrins α3 and α6 might play an important role in lung epithelial maturation, development, and basement membrane organization.[51] Alternately, integrins α5β1, α9β1, and αvβ5 are not expressed in healthy human epithelial cells but are rapidly induced on these cells upon lung inflammation and injury.[52] Integrins have an important role in branching morphogenesis. For example, lack of the α3-subunit in mice manifests in lung and kidney malformations due to aberrant branching morphogenesis.[53]

SIGNALING THROUGH INTEGRINS

There is specificity in the interaction of distinct integrins with regard to their ECM ligands. Certain integrins recognize specific ECM proteins, including fibronectin, vitronectin, and tenascin-C, which contain a small tripeptide sequence designated RGD (Arg-Gly-Asp). By contrast, β4 integrins interacting with α3-, α6-, and α7-subunits recognize laminins, whereas integrins composed of the β1-integrin subunit and the α1-, α2-, α10-, or α11-subunit bind collagen.[42] This apparent redundancy in ligand-binding specificity suggests that integrins might have overlapping functions.

The cytoplasmic domain of the integrins does not possess catalytic activity, and therefore specific adaptors are recruited to the plasma membrane and contribute to signaling events. This is termed the *integrin adhesome* and consists of over 232 components that are divided into intrinsic and transiently associated components. Some of the adhesome molecules are involved in the physical linking of integrins to the actin cytoskeleton, whereas others are involved in adhesion-mediated signaling, which affects multiple cellular downstream targets (Fig. 5.3).[54] This complex promotes the recruitment and activation of several protein kinases such as focal adhesion kinase (FAK) and proto-oncogene tyrosine-protein kinase Src (SRC), leading to the activation pathways involving extracellular signal-regulated kinases (ERK), Jun N-terminal kinase (JNK), or ρ (Rho)-family small guanosine triphosphate (GTP)-ases. These signaling events are crucial for cellular migration, proliferation, survival, and gene expression.[55] Numerous studies suggest that activation of FAK by integrins plays a central role in initiating cell proliferation. For example, mutation of tyrosine residues critical for FAK activation prevents integrin-mediated proliferation. Additionally, oncogenic transformation of cells activates FAK, abolishing the requirement for anchorage-dependent growth. Consistent with this, introduction of a constitutively active FAK mutant leads to cell transformation, anchorage-independent cell division, and suppression of apoptosis.[56] FAK deficiency in mice causes embryonic lethality, with delayed embryonic cell migration, impaired organogenesis, and vascular defects. This phenotype is also reminiscent of fibronectin- and α5-integrin–deficient mice, supporting the notion that ECM, integrins, and FAK are intimately linked. Of interest, a truncated form of FAK is expressed in the brain, a highly differentiated, largely nonproliferative tissue.[56]

Integrin-inactivating proteins have recently been found to be important for the correct balance of integrin activity. Loss of integrin-inactivating proteins manifests in complex phenotypes, demonstrating that integrins do not passively return to their inactive state in the absence of activating proteins. In vitro findings suggest that filamins compete directly with Tln for binding to β-integrins and thereby act as negative functional regulators.[57] This results in the inhibition of cell spreading and cell migration.[58] The inactivation of integrins in Tln-depleted cells is fully restored by the inhibition of filamin expression, suggesting that the switching between Tln and filamin binding to the β-integrin tail is a crucial determinant of integrin activity.[59]

INTEGRINS AND GROWTH FACTORS

The ECM can function as an organizing center for signaling complexes composed of matrix proteins, GFs, and their receptors on the cell surface. Integrins activate several signaling pathways independently but can also act synergistically with GF receptors. They can activate a latent GF by inducing conformational changes

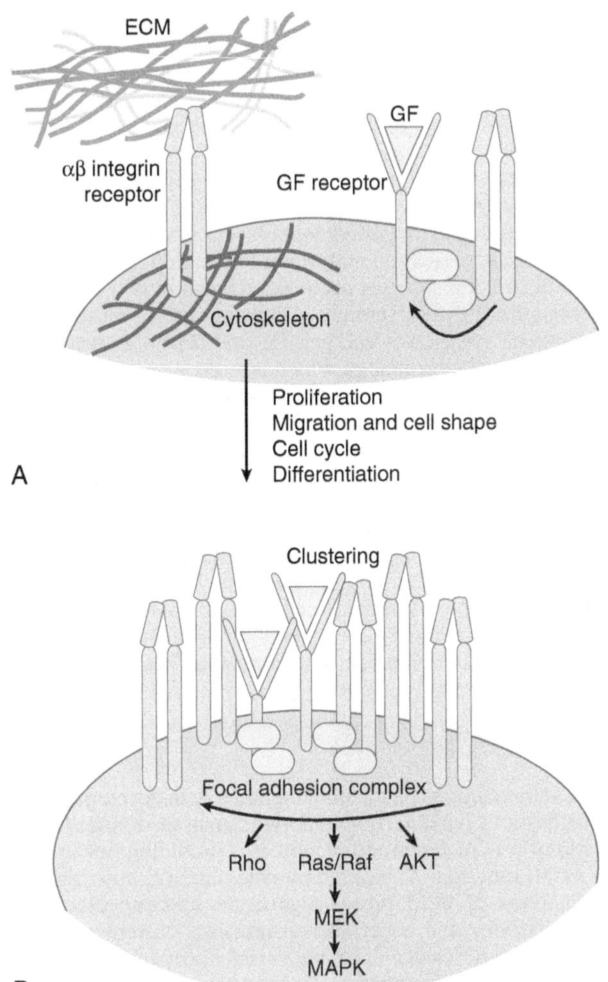

Fig. 5.3 Growth factor signaling regulation by integrins. (A) Tissue stiffness and matrix composition initiate specific signaling pathways that regulate cell behavior. The selection of integrins expressed on the cell surface specifies the signaling pathway due to the differential binding affinity of extracellular matrix *(ECM)* ligands for integrin receptors. Integrins, via their cytoplasmic domain, recruit specific adaptor proteins to the plasma membrane. This in turn can regulate growth factor *(GF)* receptor signaling. (B) Integrins colocalize at focal adhesion sites with growth factor receptors and their associated signaling molecules, in response to GF stimulation. Associated signaling molecules include Src and FAK, as well as cytoskeletal molecules such as paxillin, talin, and vinculin.

or by presenting it to a protease. Integrins assist the binding of a GF to its receptor, whereas GFs have also been shown to activate integrin signaling.[60] GF stimulation can activate FAK, indicating that integrin and GF signaling pathways intersect at focal adhesions (see Fig. 5.3).[59]

Various extracellular GFs regulate cell migration and dynamics by means of integrin-mediated signaling. Consistent with this notion, integrin clustering promotes recruitment and activation of GF receptors within focal adhesion complexes. For example, treatment of endothelial cells with beads coated either with RGD tripeptide or with fibronectin leads to coaggregation of β1 integrins and FAK, as well as with high-affinity fibroblast GF receptors within newly formed focal adhesions.[61] Parallel studies using similar approaches have extended these findings to show that integrin activation can lead to recruitment of a more extensive repertoire of GF receptors, including those for epidermal growth factor (EGF), hepatocyte growth factor (HGF) or Met receptor tyrosine kinase (RTK), vascular endothelial growth factor (VEGF), and platelet-derived growth factor (PDGF).[62]

It is not fully understood how integrin ligation leads to the recruitment of RTKs to the focal adhesion site. However, the fact that high-affinity EGF receptors can directly bind actin, which in turn enhances EGF-dependent autophosphorylation and activation of downstream substrates, indicates a critical role for the F-actin cytoskeleton in coordinating signaling between integrins and GFs.[63,64] Not surprisingly, pharmacologic disruption of the actin cytoskeleton not only prevents focal adhesion formation, but also leads to reduced GF receptor activation.[65] Thus the actin cytoskeleton and associated proteins may act as a solid-state scaffold that spatially and biochemically coordinates crosstalk between integrins and GF RTKs.

In most cases, integrins seem to function as positive regulators of GF receptor signaling. However, α1β1 has a unique negative role in regulating EGFR and VEGFR2 signaling. After binding to collagen, the α1-subunit cytoplasmic tail interacts and activates a nonreceptor protein tyrosine phosphatase, T-cell protein tyrosine phosphatase (TCPTP), resulting in dephosphorylation of EGFR and VEGFR2.[66] The reverse relationship also exists, where some GFs have been found to regulate the endocytosis of integrin ligands. For example, EGFR and EGF have been shown to stimulate β1 internalization. In lymphatic vascular development, α9β1 plays a major role in the assembly of fibronectin bundles in valves of developing lymphatic vessels and is the major binding protein for VEGF-C and VEGF-D.[67] Mutation of α9 leads to a loss of signaling events through these GFs and disordered lymphatic development.

MATRIX METALLOPROTEINASES

Matrix metalloproteinases (MMPs) are a family of 24 proteins. Of these, six are associated with cell membranes or protein transmembrane domains and the remaining are secreted.[68] Cell-associated MMPs are responsible for the majority of ECM degradation activity. They are highly regulated to preserve the integrity of tissues.[69] ECM remodeling is an important mechanism whereby cell differentiation can be regulated; it includes processes such as the establishment and maintenance of stem cell niches, branching morphogenesis, angiogenesis, bone remodeling, and wound repair. For example, in mice, MMP2, MMP14, and an MMP inducer, CD147, are constitutively expressed in all five distinct stages of lung development.[70] In one model of branching morphogenesis, cleft formation is driven by accumulation of TGF-β, which stimulates ECM deposition and directs branching to either side of the accumulated ECM. This process is facilitated by TGF-β-mediated inhibition of MMPs. In support of this hypothesis, TGF-β1 and TGF-β3 inhibit expression of MMP1 and up-regulate expression of TIMP1 in fibroblasts.[71]

Movement of angiogenic endothelial cells through the basement membrane and the perivascular tissue microenvironment also requires catabolism of the ECM. The finding that MMP2-deficient mice show reduced rates of angiogenesis supports this concept.[72] Furthermore, treatment of angiogenic endothelia with a peptide that prevents binding of MMP2 to αvβ3 integrins not only blocks collagenolytic activity, but also inhibits angiogenesis.[73] During angiogenesis, MMP-mediated degradation of ECM reveals neoepitopes that provoke alternative forms of endothelial cell behavior.[74] This mechanism may allow endothelial cells to modify and respond to microenvironmental cues rapidly without de novo gene expression.

MMPs catalytic activity has also been shown to regulate cell mechanics including spreading and motility in invasive cancer cells. Stiffer ECMs allow for enhanced MMP activity, which increases cancer invasiveness. This is attenuated by activating FAK and stabilizing integrins at the cell surface, indicating the importance of interactions between integrins and MMPs.[75]

BIOMECHANICAL FORCES

The developing embryo is exposed to mechanical forces that maintain and modify cell behavior. Integrins can serve as mechanoreceptors that transmit forces between the cytoskeleton and the ECM to maintain structural integrity of tissues.[76] The majority of integrin-mediated attachments between ECM fibers and resting cells are to a bundle of actin filaments in the focal adhesion. Focal adhesions modulate cellular responses to control proliferation, cytoskeletal remodeling, and migration of cells.[77] Cells respond to force on integrin-mediated adhesions by remodeling the ECM. For example, cyclic stretching of fibroblasts and other cell types activates expression of genes for collagens, fibronectin, and metalloproteinases, and stretched cells assemble a dense ECM that is enriched in collagen.[78] Matrix assembly usually occurs in a directional manner according to the applied force.[79] Application of force to integrin α5β1 is required for conversion to a state that can be chemically cross-linked to the fibronectin beneath the cell. Inhibition of cell contractility blocks cross-linking, but can be rescued by application of force from fluid shear stress.[80] In early lymphangiogenesis, interstitial fluid pressure stretches lymphatic endothelial cells, which stimulates integrin-dependent proliferation, and expands the lymphatics.[81]

The idea that integrins detect biomechanical signals is further supported by the finding that FAK is involved in mechanosensing during cell migration.[82] Biomechanical forces also modulate the expression and activities of ECM components and proteases, including tenascin-C and MMP2, positive regulators of angiogenesis.[83] Collectively, these studies indicate not only that biomechanical signals influence the ECM and its receptors but also that downstream signals generated by mechanical force modulate cell adhesion components. Additional studies are clearly needed to determine how local force differentials modulate cell behavior within the developing embryo.

CHANGES IN CELL SHAPE

The ECM has a central role in maintaining and modifying cell morphology within developing, remodeling, and differentiated tissues. It has been shown that the greater the extent of endothelial cell spreading, the greater the extent of proliferation. Subsequently, a role for cell shape affecting integrin-dependent signaling pathways has also been demonstrated in angiogenic endothelia. The proliferation and subsequent survival of endothelial cells require interactions between ECM and αvβ3 integrin. Blocking integrin ECM binding reduces endothelial proliferation and increases apoptosis.[84] If cell spreading is prevented, however, occupation and ligation of αvβ3 integrins using anti-integrin antibodies fail to support endothelial proliferation and survival.[85] Cell rounding may therefore lead to apoptosis because of decreased integrin ligation, with correspondingly less signaling through integrins, FAK, and other downstream components. Integrins also play an important role in leukocyte migration into tissues. When inactive, integrins are unable to bind to ECM or other receptors, an important role for circulating lymphocytes. When activated, they mediate the rolling of cells along the vascular wall and the binding of ligands on the surface of activated endothelial cells, promoting cell arrest.[86] β2-Deficient mice show profound defects in leukocyte migration.[87] To elucidate further how ECM- or integrin-dependent cell shape changes operate, it will be necessary to identify additional proteins that are able to coordinate both intracellular signaling pathways and cell morphology. To this end, the discovery that the Rho family of small GTPases (e.g., RhoA, Rac1, Cdc42) can relay integrin-derived signals and organize the cytoskeleton[88,89] suggests that these proteins are well poised to integrate cell shape and function.

EXTRACELLULAR MATRIX AS A PLATFORM FOR TISSUE ENGINEERING

Stem cell fate is influenced by tightly regulated interactions that include GFs, cell-cell signaling, and cell-matrix interactions. As summarized above, the ECM is a key component in regulating the interactions of secreted factors with cells during the dynamic processes of development. It is not surprising that complex three-dimensional matrices are increasingly used in vitro to replace traditional two-dimensional cultures for recapitulation of tissue-specific microenvironments and to direct differentiation of stem cells. The importance of ECM properties on directing stem cell fate has been demonstrated by the influence of matrix stiffness and elasticity on cell organization and behavior. For example, collagen-coated substrates that are relatively stiff promote maximal cell spreading and drive enrichment of focal adhesions and in turn assembly of a cytoskeleton with stress fiber components, whereas culture of cells on soft gels promotes formation of a diffuse and less organized cytoskeleton.[90] Culturing naïve mesenchymal stem cells on collagen-coated gels for only 24 hours was shown to influence cell morphology, which is suggestive of specific cell lineages.[91] A recent study has demonstrated the capacity of the lung ECM alone for directing the differentiation of stem cell–derived endodermal progenitor cells to functional lung epithelial lineages in vitro.[92] This study and many others using decellularized scaffolds of native organs reveal the feasibility of using the ECM as a natural platform for regenerative medicine purposes.[93] But this use of ECM at the bedside must be done cautiously, as recent studies have shown conflicting reports with regard to rejection of xenogeneic and allogeneic acellular scaffolds, indicating that there may be immunogenic elements on acellular scaffolds that could induce an immune and/or inflammatory response.[94]

CONCLUSION

Cell-ECM interactions play a fundamental role in development, yet many questions remain. The phenotypic analysis of mice bearing mutations in ECM genes and receptors is providing new insights into ECM function. A basic understanding of how different combinations of ECM proteins generate tissue-specific forms of cell behavior will be critical to translate current molecular and cellular knowledge into improved approaches for tissue engineering and regeneration. Regardless of the outcomes of such experiments, the emergence of rapid screening techniques for detection of ECM gene mutations, the development of diagnostic DNA and protein microarrays, and the availability of whole-genome sequencing will aid in determining whether the results gleaned from experimental systems are relevant to defects in human embryogenesis and development.

A complete reference list is available at www.ExpertConsult.com. 

SELECT REFERENCES

1. Kim SH, Turnbull J, Guimond S. Extracellular matrix and cell signalling: the dynamic cooperation of integrin, proteoglycan and growth factor receptor. *J Endocrinol*. 2011;209:139–151.
3. Alberti K, Davey RE, Onishi K, et al. Functional immobilization of signaling proteins enables control of stem cell fate. *Nat Methods*. 2008;5:645–650.
4. Peerani R, Rao BM, Bauwens C, et al. Niche-mediated control of human embryonic stem cell self-renewal and differentiation. *EMBO J*. 2007;26:4744–4755.
5. Thompson SM, Jesudason EC, Turnbull JE, Fernig DG. Heparan sulfate in lung morphogenesis: the elephant in the room. *Birth Defects Res C Embryo Today*. 2010;90:32–44.
6. Lelongt B, Ronco P. Role of extracellular matrix in kidney development and repair. *Pediatr Nephrol*. 2003;18:731–742.
7. Kii I, Nishiyana T, Li M, et al. Incorporation of tenascin-C into the extracellular matrix by periostin underlies an extracellular meshwork architecture. *J Biol Chem*. 2010;285:2028–2039.
9. Streuli CH. Integrins and cell-fate determination. *J Cell Biol*. 2008;122:171–177.
10. Boudreau N, Werb Z, Bissell MJ. Suppression of apoptosis by basement membrane requires three-dimensional tissue organization and withdrawal from the cell cycle. *Proc Natl Acad Sci U S A*. 1996;93:3509–3513.
11. Zhu X, Assoian RK. Integrin-dependent activation of MAP kinase: a link to shape-dependent cell proliferation. *Mol Biol Cell*. 1995;6:273–282.
14. Frisch SM, Screaton RA. Anoikis mechanisms. *Curr Opin Cell Biol*. 2001;13:555–562.
15. Mackie EJ, Ramsey S. Modulation of osteoblast behaviour by tenascin. *J Cell Biol*. 1996;109:1597–1604.
16. Adams JC, Watt FM. Fibronectin inhibits the terminal differentiation of human keratinocytes. *Nature*. 1989;340:307–309.

17. Linask KK, Manisastry S, Han M. Cross talk between cell-cell and cell-matrix adhesion signaling pathways during heart organogenesis: implications for cardiac birth defects. *Microsc Microanal*. 2005;11:200-208.
18. Chen SS, Fitzgerald W, Zimmerberg J, et al. Cell-cell and cell-extracellular matrix interactions regulate embryonic stem cell differentiation. *Stem Cells*. 2007;25:553-561.
20. Jones PL, Jones FS, Zhou B, Rabinovitch M. Induction of vascular smooth muscle cell tenascin-C gene expression by denatured type I collagen is dependent upon a beta-3 integrin-mediated mitogen-activated protein kinase pathway and a 122-base pair promoter element. *J Cell Biol*. 1999;112:435-445.
21. Guilak F, Cohen DM, Estes BT, et al. Control of stem cell fate by physical interactions with the extracellular matrix. *Cell Stem Cell*. 2009;5:17-26.
22. Discher DE, Mooney DJ, Zandstra PW. Growth factors, matrices, and forces combine and control stem cells. *Science*. 2009;324:1673-1677.
23. Chang C, Werb Z. The many faces of metalloproteases: cell growth, invasion, angiogenesis and metastasis. *Trends Cell Biol*. 2001;11:S37-S43.
24. Heissig B, Hattori K, Dias S, et al. Recruitment of stem and progenitor cells from the bone marrow niche requires MMP-9 mediated release of kit-ligand. *Cell*. 2002;109:625-637.
25. Li Z, Li L. Understanding hematopoietic stem-cell microenvironments. *Trends Biochem Sci*. 2006;31:589-595.
26. Bruckner-Tuderman L. Blistering skin diseases: models for studies on epidermal-dermal adhesion. *Biochem Cell Biol*. 1996;74:729-736.
27. Tamai K, Kaneda Y, Uitto J. Molecular therapies for heritable blistering diseases. *Trends Mol Med*. 2009;15:285-292.
28. Basel D, Steiner RD. Osteogenesis imperfecta: recent findings shed new light on this once well-understood condition. *Genet Med*. 2009;11:375-385.
30. Ramirez F, Dietz HC. Extracellular microfibrils in vertebrate development and disease processes. *J Biol Chem*. 2009;284:14677-14681.
31. George EL, Georges-Labouesse EN, Patel-King RS, et al. Defects in mesoderm, neural tube and vascular development in mouse embryos lacking fibronectin. *Development*. 1993;119:1079-1091.
33. Saga Y, Yagi T, Ikawa Y, et al. Mice develop normally without tenascin. *Genes Dev*. 1992;6:1821-1831.
34. Cowan KN, Jones PL, Rabinovitch M. Elastase and matrix metalloproteinase inhibitors induce regression, and tenascin-C antisense prevents progression, of vascular disease. *J Clin Invest*. 2000;105:21-34.
35. Fukamauchi F, Mataga N, Wang YJ, et al. Abnormal behavior and neurotransmissions of tenascin gene knockout mouse. *Biochem Biophys Res Commun*. 1996;221:151-156.
36. Ohta M, Sakai T, Saga Y, et al. Suppression of hematopoietic activity of tenascin-C-deficient mice. *Blood*. 1998;11:4074-4083.
37. Talts JF, Wirl G, Dictor M, et al. Tenascin-C modulates tumor stroma and monocyte/macrophage recruitment but not tumor growth or metastasis in a mouse strain with spontaneous mammary cancer. *J Cell Biol*. 1999;112:1855-1864.
38. Midwood K, Sacre S, Piccinni AM, et al. Tenascin-C is an endogenous activator of toll-like receptor 4 that is essential for maintaining inflammation in arthritic joint disease. *Nat Med*. 2009;15:774-780.
39. Li DY, Brooke B, Davis EC, et al. Elastin is an essential determinant of arterial morphogenesis. *Nature*. 1998;293:276-280.
40. Li DY, Faury G, Taylor DG, et al. Novel arterial pathology in mice and humans hemizygous for elastin. *J Clin Invest*. 1998;102:1783-1787.
41. Hynes RO. Integrins: bidirectional, review allosteric signaling machines. *Cell*. 2002;110:673-687.
42. Lowell CA, Mayadas TN. Overview—studying integrins in vivo. In: Shimaoka M, ed. *Integrin and Cell Adhesion Molecules: Methods and Protocols*. New York: Humana Press; 2011:369-397.
43. Hohenester E. Science direct signalling complexes at the cell-matrix interface. *Curr Opin Struct Biol*. 2014;29:10-16.
44. Astrof S, Hynes RO. Fibronectins in vascular morphogenesis. *Angiogenesis*. 2009;12:165-175.
45. Yang JT, Rayburn H, Hynes RO. Embryonic mesodermal defects in alpha-5 integrin-deficient mice. *Development*. 1993;119:1093-1105.
46. Stephens LE, Sutherland AE, Klimanskaya IV, et al. Deletion of B1 integrins in mice results in inner cell mass failure and peri-implantation lethality. *Genes Dev*. 1995;9:1883-1895.
48. Watt FM. Role of integrins in regulating epidermal adhesion, growth and differentiation. *EMBO J*. 2002;21:3919-3926.
49. Raghavan S, Bauer C, Mundschau G, et al. Conditional ablation of beta1 integrin in skin: severe defects in epidermal proliferation, basement membrane formation, and hair follicle invagination. *J Cell Biol*. 2000;150:1149-1160.
50. Pietri T, Eder O, Breau MA, et al. Conditional beta1-integrin gene deletion in neural crest cells causes severe developmental alterations of the peripheral nervous system. *Development*. 2004;131:3871-3883.
51. Huang XZ, Wu JF, Cass D, et al. Inactivation of the integrin beta-6 subunit gene reveals a role of epithelial integrins in regulating inflammation in the lungs and skin. *J Cell Biol*. 1996;133:921-928.
53. Kreidberg JA, Donovan MJ, Goldstein SL, et al. Alpha 3 beta 1 integrin has a crucial role in kidney and lung organogenesis. *Development*. 1996;122:3537-3547.
54. Winograd-Katz SE, Fassler R, Geiger B, Legate KR. The integrin adhesome: from genes and proteins to human disease. *Nat Rev Mol Cell Biol*. 2014;15:273-288.
55. Zaidel-Bar R, Itzkovitz S, Ma'ayan A, et al. Functional atlas of the integrin adhesome. *Nat Cell Biol*. 2007;9:858-867.
56. Frisch SM, Vuori K, Ruoslahti E, Chan-Hui P. Control of adhesion-dependent cell survival by focal adhesion kinase. *J Cell Biol*. 1996;134:793-799.
57. Calderwood DA, Huttonlocher A, Kiosses WB, et al. Increased filamin binding to beta-integrin cytoplasmic domains inhibits cell migration. *Nat Cell Biol*. 2001;3:1060-1068.
58. Baldassarre M, Razinia Z, Burande CF, et al. Filamins regulate cell spreading and initiation of cell migration. *PLoS ONE*. 2009;4:e7830.
59. Nieves B, Jones CW, Ward R, et al. The NPIY motif in the integrin 1 tail dictates the requirement for talin-1 in outside-in signaling. *J Cell Biol*. 2010;123:1216-1226.
60. Alam N, Goel HL, Zarif MJ, et al. The integrin-growth factor receptor duet. *J Cell Physiol*. 2007;213:649-653.
61. Plopper GE, McNamee HP, Dike LE, et al. Convergence of integrin and growth factor receptor signaling pathways within the focal adhesion complex. *Mol Biol Cell*. 1995;6:1349-1365.
63. den Hartigh JC, en Henegouwen PM, Verkleij AJ, Boonstra J. The EGF receptor is an actin-binding protein. *J Cell Biol*. 1992;119:349-355.
64. Diakonova M, Payrastre B, van Velzen AG, et al. Epidermal growth factor induces rapid and transient association of phospholipase C-gama1 with EGF-receptor and filamentous actin at membrane ruffles of A431 cells. *J Cell Biol*. 1995;108:2499-2509.
65. Abedi H, Zachary I. Vascular endothelial growth factor stimulates tyrosine phosphorylation and recruitment to new focal adhesions of focal adhesion kinase and paxillin in endothelial cells. *J Biol Chem*. 1997;272:15442-15451.
66. Ivaska J, Heino J. Interplay between cell adhesion and growth factor receptors: from the plasma membrane to the endosomes. *Cell Dev Biol*. 2009;339:111-120.
67. Vlahakis NE, Young BA, Atakilit A, Sheppard D. The lymphangiogenic growth factor VEGF-C and D are ligands for the integrin alpha9beta1. *J Biol Chem*. 2005;280:4544-4552.
68. Yong VW. Metalloproteinases: mediators of pathology and regeneration in the CNS. *Nat Rev Neurosci*. 2005;6:931-944.
69. Overall CM, Lopez-Otin C. Strategies for MMP inhibition in cancer: innovations for the post-trial era. *Nat Rev Cancer*. 2002;2:657-672.
70. Fan Q, Kadomatsu K, Uchimura K, Muramatsu T. Embigin/basigin subgroup of the immunoglobulin superfamily: different modes of expression during mouse embryogenesis and correlated expression with carbohydrate antigenic markers. *Dev Growth Differ*. 1998;40:277-286.
71. Eickelberg O, Köhler E, Reichenberger F, et al. Extracellular matrix deposition by primary human lung fibroblasts in response to TGF-beta1 and TGF-beta3. *Am J Physiol*. 1999;276:L814-L824.
72. Itoh T, Tanioka M, Yoshida H, et al. Reduced angiogenesis and tumor progression in gelatinase a-deficient mice. *Cancer Res*. 1998;58:1048-1051.
73. Brooks PC, Silletti S, von Schalscha TL, et al. Disruption of angiogenesis by PEX, a noncatalytic metalloproteinase fragment with integrin binding activity. *Cell*. 1998;92:391-400.
74. Hangai M, Kitaya N, Xu J, et al. Matrix metalloproteinase-9-dependent exposure of a cryptic migratory control site in collagen is required before retinal angiogenesis. *Am J Pathol*. 2002;161:1429-1437.
76. Ingber DE. Cellular mechanotransduction: putting all the pieces together again. *FASEB J*. 2006;20:811-827.
78. Chiquet M, Renedo AS, Huber F, Fluck M. How do fibroblasts translate mechanical signals into changes in extracellular matrix production? *Matrix Biol*. 2003;22:73-80.
79. Nguyen TD, Liang R, Woo SL, et al. Effects of cell seeding and cyclic stretch on the fiber remodeling in an extracellular matrix–derived bioscaffold. *Tissue Eng Part A*. 2009;15:957-963.
80. Friedland JC, Lee MH, Boettiger D. Mechanically activated integrin switch controls alpha5beta1 function. *Science*. 2009;323:642-644.
81. Planas-Paz L, Strilić B, Goedecke A, et al. Mechanoinduction of lymph vessel expansion. *EMBO J*. 2011;31:788-804.
82. Wang HB, Dembo M, Hanks SK, Wang Y. Focal adhesion kinase is involved in mechanosensing during fibroblast migration. *Proc Natl Acad Sci U S A*. 2001;98:11295-11300.
83. Jones PL, Chapados R, Baldwin HS, et al. Altered hemodynamics controls matrix metalloproteinase activity and tenascin-C expression in neonatal pig lung. *Am J Physiol Lung Cell Mol Physiol*. 2002;282:L26-L35.
84. Brooks PC, Clark RAF, Cheresh DA. Requirement of vascular integrin alphaV-beta3 for angiogenesis. *Science*. 1994;264:569-571.
85. Re F, Zanetti A, Sironi M, et al. Inhibition of anchorage-dependent cell spreading triggers apoptosis in cultured human endothelial cells. *J Cell Biol*. 1994;127:537-546.
86. Ley K, Laudanna C, Cybulsky MI, Nourshargh S. Getting to the site of inflammation: the leukocyte adhesion cascade updated. *Nat Rev Immunol*. 2007;7:678-689.
87. Scharffetter-Kochanek K, Lu H, Norman K, et al. Spontaneous skin ulceration and defective T cell function in CD18 null mice. *J Exp Med*. 1998;188:119-131.
88. Nobes C, Hall A. Rho, Rac, and Cdc42 GTPases regulate the assembly of multimolecular focal complexes associated with actin stress fibers, lamellipodia, and filopodia. *Cell*. 1995;81:53-62.
90. Wang MD. Stresses at the cell-to-substrate interface during locomotion of fibroblasts. *Biophys J*. 1999;76:2307-2316.
91. Engler AJ, Sen S, Sweeney HL, Discher DE. Matrix elasticity directs stem cell lineage specification. *Cell*. 2006;126:677-689.
92. Shojaie S, Ermini L, Ackerley C, et al. Acellular lung scaffolds direct differentiation of endoderm to functional airway epithelial cells: requirement of matrix-bound HS proteoglycans. *Stem Cell Reports*. 2015;4:419-430.
93. Song JJ, Ott HC. Organ engineering based on decellularized matrix scaffolds. *Trends Mol Med*. 2011;17:424-432.

6 Angiogenesis

Yalda Afshar | M. Luisa Iruela-Arispe

INTRODUCTION

Embryologically, the cardiovascular system is the first to develop.[1] The vasculature, composed of endothelial cells and their support cells, is critical not only for circulation of blood, but also for the organization, maintenance, and regeneration of multiple organ systems. The embryo forms a primary vascular plexus so that blood vessels first arise through a process called *vasculogenesis*. Further vessels are generated via sprouting and nonsprouting *angiogenesis* and are progressively remodeled into a functional circulatory system.

Vasculogenesis includes the differentiation of angioblastic progenitors from mesenchymal cells and their subsequent organization into primitive channels. This initial process differs from angiogenesis, which refers to the formation of new vessels from existing vessels. The first vascular structures to form emerge in the extraembryonic yolk sac, where mesodermal cells differentiate into angioblast precursors that quickly coalesce into uniform vascular structures.[2] At the same time and place, rounded hematopoietic cells also appear from the yolk sac mesoderm. The coincident emergence of vessels and blood cells in the early embryonic yolk sac gave the impression that a common progenitor, termed the *hemangioblast*, was responsible for both hematopoietic and endothelial lineages.[3] However, the early blood progeny has a limited repertoire and is not capable of long-term adult hematopoiesis. The first hematopoietic stem cells capable of adult engraftment arise later in development from endothelial precursor cells, which are called *hemogenic endothelium*.[4] The angioblasts of the yolk sac coalesce to form a vascular network that is later remodeled. However, the intraembryonic vessels arise from another vasculogenic pool of mesodermal precursors.[5] Within the embryonic mesoderm, angioblast precursors initially form bilateral aortic cords that fuse to form the dorsal aorta, and the rostral bifurcations become the cranial and subclavian vessels, whereas the caudal bifurcation results in the iliac vessels. The terminal expansions of these vascular networks organize an even-sized vascular plexus that later remodels extensively into a hierarchic tree of characteristic arteries, capillaries, and veins.

VASCULOGENESIS AND AORTA FORMATION

Angioblasts from the lateral plate mesoderm in the embryo are arranged in a mirrored fashion, where somite-derived growth factors initiate angioblast specification and formation of paired dorsal aortae. Sonic hedgehog (Shh) signaling is initiated in the midline notochord and endoderm[6] to promote somite induction of vascular endothelial growth factor (VEGF), which is secreted for proper localization of angioblast precursors.[7-9] The aortae remain paired due to antiangiogenic factors secreted by the intervening notochord. These include bone morphogenic protein (BMP) antagonists,[10] as well as negative cues from semaphorins and netrins,[11] imperative to axon guidance.[12] BMP antagonists also play a role in vascular patterning and give the stereotypic structure characteristic of the vascular tree.[13-15] Negative signals from semaphorins also feedback in VEGF signaling, helping to orchestrate vascular patterning.[16] The paired aortae then fuse as midline notochord BMP antagonists are decreased in a rostral to caudal fashion, allowing for the convergence of the paired dorsal aortae into one large aortic vessel (Fig. 6.1).[10]

ENDOTHELIAL SPECIFICATION: ARTERIES, VEINS, AND LYMPHATICS

Before the fusion of the paired dorsal aorta, angioblasts, comprising the two aortic vessels, attain arterial identity through the expression of arterial gene signatures. Somite-derived VEGF signals activate the Notch pathway within the nearby angioblastic chords.[17] The Notch pathway, initially described in *Drosophila* as Notch mutant flies exhibiting "notched" wings,[18,19] is critical for multiple developmental cell fate decisions. In the vasculature, the Notch pathway is responsible for defining arterial and venous identity.[20] The Notch family is composed of Notch receptors (Notch1-4) that bind transmembrane-bound ligands: Delta-like (DLL1, 3, 4) and Jagged (Jag1-2) through either heterotypic or homotypic cell-cell interactions. Upon ligand binding, the Notch receptor undergoes serial proteolytic cleavage steps, resulting in the release of the intracellular domain that in turn binds DNA, regulating downstream gene expression. VEGF signaling in the somites results in Notch1 expression by nearby angiogenic cords, relegating the ensuing vessel as an artery.[17] Accompanying cardinal veins form next to the paired aortae as angioblasts coalesce in a second vessel. Endothelial cells from both the aorta and cardinal vein can remain interchangeable until the establishment of permanent arterial and venous identity.[21-23] As part of the establishment of arterial and venous identity, respective cell forces and polarity cues are established to define arterial and venous system boundaries.

An important repulsive signaling cascade in the vasculature involves the ephrin ligands and Eph receptors.[24] Eph receptors consist of a tyrosine kinase receptor family capable of both forward and reverse signaling in a multitude of cellular contexts.[25] Within the vasculature, EphB4 and ephrinB2 predominate. Designated venous cells express high levels of EphB4 receptor, and alternatively, arterial cells express high levels of ephrinB2.[26,27] Negative regulation between EphB4 and ephrinB2 maintains borders between the arterial and venous circulation to avoid arteriovenous malformations (AVMs).[28] AVMs are a poorly organized mass of arteries and veins that fuse without intervening capillaries to create high-flow arteriovenous shunts. As such, the EphB4 and ephrinB2 signals are essential and also play a role in determining artery and vein size.[29] Abnormal connections between arteries and veins in the form of AVMs are thought to occur when arteries and veins lose their identity markers. Loss of ephrins results in a loss of repulsive cues between the two endothelial cell types and subsequent mixing of circulations. Aberrant Notch signaling can also misidentify arterial and venous endothelial cells, resulting in subsequent AVM formation.[28,30] Arterial mispatterning is seen in diseases such as hereditary hemorrhagic telangiectasia (HHT), when patients have mutations associated with the transforming growth factor (TGF)-β/BMP family of signaling molecules, including its receptors, endoglin (ENG)[31] and Alk1 (ACVRL1),[32] as well as downstream transcriptional mediators of the pathway, including SMAD4.[33] The mechanism leading to aberrant vascular patterning has been

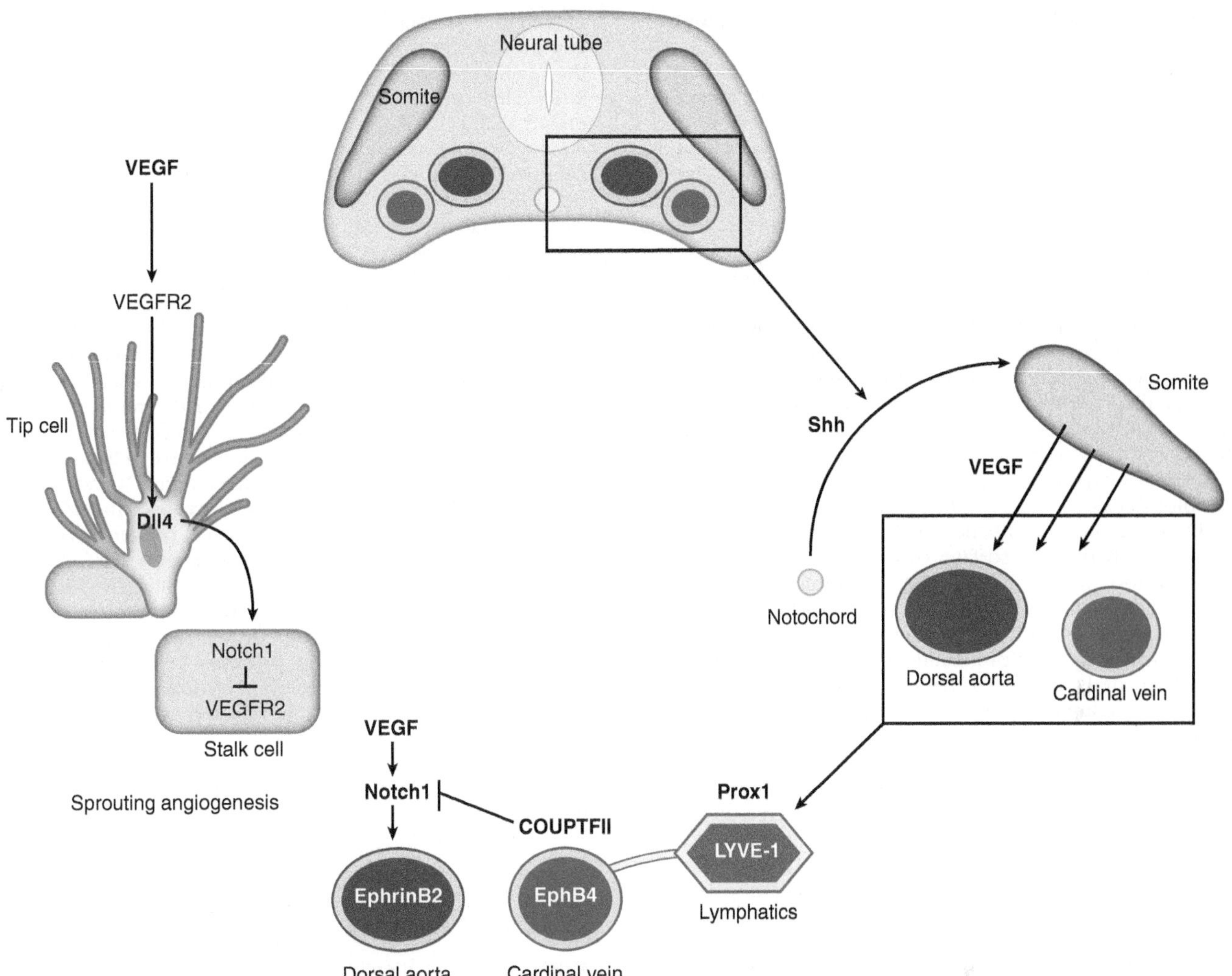

Fig. 6.1 Overview of endothelial development. A transverse section of the developing embryo *(top)* demonstrates local signaling cues that pattern the paired dorsal aorta and cardinal veins *(right)*. Sonic hedgehog *(Shh)* signaling from the notochord activates somite expression of vascular endothelial growth factor *(VEGF)* that signals to developing angioblasts to coalesce and form the respective large vessels of the arterial and venous systems. Increased VEGF signaling *(bottom)* triggers Notch signaling in the aorta, which in turn begins to express the arterial specific marker ephrinB2. The cardinal vein expresses COUPTFII, which represses the VEGF>Notch pathway for venous identity and subsequent expression of ephB4. Similar pathways are activated in tip cell selection *(left),* where high VEGF levels induce high expression of the notch ligand Dll4 in the tip migratory cell via the receptor VEGFR2. Dll4 expression in the migratory tip cell binds to and activates Notch1 receptor signaling in contacting cells. The cells downstream of Dll4 ligand-activated Notch1 repress expression of VEGR2 and become stalk cells.

linked to changes in angiogenic mediators. A connection to the Notch pathway has also been suggested, unifying the similar phenotypes of AVM seen in both Notch pathway mutants and TGF-β pathway mutations.[34] As in all pathology, the contribution of these signals during vascular morphogenesis is necessary to ensure that remodeling of arteries and veins occurs, while separated by interconnecting capillaries.

In addition to arterial and venous circulation, a third circulatory system of lymph vessels develops through the assembly of lymphatic endothelial cells.[35] The first lymphatic endothelial cells originate from the cardinal vein, where a subset of endothelial cells bud off and express Prox1, an early transcriptional regulator of lymphatic fate.[36] These cells then proliferate and migrate to form the lymphatic system, with lymphatic identity defined by Prox1 and LYVE-1 expression.[36,37] Abnormalities in lymphatic identity that are due to Prox1 levels have been associated with chylous-filled lymphatics and adult obesity.[38] Lymphatic dysplasia syndromes in humans have been linked to mutations in *CCBE1*,[39] a gene implicated in lymphatic cell emergence and migration.[40] The connection of the lymphatic system to the circulatory system occurs at the lymphatic duct, the formation of which relies on platelet aggregation and thrombosis to separate the vascular and lymphatic systems.[41] Thus severe thrombocytopenia or platelet disorders during development can lead to blood-filled lymphatics.[41,42]

ANGIOGENESIS

Angiogenesis is the process in which new vessels are made from existing vessels. Angiogenic expansion of a primary capillary plexus, created by vasculogenesis, is essential to the circulatory bed. Specifically, this is the mechanism by which subsequent growth of the vascular tree is achieved in coordination with the physiologic expansion of tissues, in physiology and pathology. The intimate association of growing blood vessels with cellular parenchymal during development also imposes unique heterotypic interactions in distinct organs. These tissue-specific interactions further induce vascular adaptations, resulting in an array of molecular and physiologic variations known as *endothelial heterogeneity*.

In this manner, the liver capillaries are formed by disconnected endothelium and differ significantly from those in the brain, which form highly specialized blood-brain barrier structures to ensure a tight blockade between the blood and the central nervous system (CNS). The underlying cue for endothelial cells to start migrating and form a new vessel begins with the detection of hypoxia and hypoxic cues in adjacent tissue. Hypoxia is sensed by the tissue and triggers cellular production of hypoxia-inducible factor (Hif), a transcription factor that activates many downstream pathways.[43] One of the most important pathways is that of VEGF signaling.[44] As tissue becomes hypoxic, VEGF is secreted and interacts with nearby vessels that express VEGF receptors, particularly VEGFR2. This gradient of VEGF induces the formation of a vascular sprout that migrates toward the region of hypoxia to ensure delivery of oxygen through a newly formed capillary bed.

There is a large repertoire of VEGF receptors that function as receptor tyrosine kinases.[45] VEGFR1 and VEGFR2 are expressed on blood vascular endothelial cells, whereas VEGFR3 is highly expressed on the cell surface of lymphatic endothelial cells. VEGFR3 also plays a role in the formation of blood vessel angiogenic sprouts.[46,47] VEGFR2 is the main receptor on endothelium and coordinates endothelial behavior including migration, survival, and proliferation. VEGFR1 is a receptor that can be secreted or bound to the cell surface; it can bind ligand but is not thought to signal downstream events and hence is thought to be a decoy receptor.[45] To function as a decoy receptor, VEGFR1 binds its ligand (VEGF) and decreases its availability to access the primary functional receptor, VEGFR2. The decoy function is made possible by the increased binding affinity of VEGF to VEGFR1, rather than to the main receptor, VEGFR2. VEGFR1 in secreted form, sVEGFR1, also known as *sFlt1*, is a surrogate biomarker for preterm preeclampsia.[48] Still theoretical, the initiating events of preeclampsia are postulated to include abnormal maternal placental vascular remodeling leading to a compromised hypoxic placenta that sheds sVEGR1 (sFlt1) in high amounts into the maternal systemic circulation. The ensuing hypertension and organ dysfunction (renal, liver, and CNS) are then attributed to a dysregulated hypoxic-angiogenic response.[49]

A variety of VEGF ligands from A to F exists, with VEGFA, B, C, and D having physiologic roles in binding various VEGF receptors. The most prominent VEGF ligand, VEGFA, is the best known and most ubiquitous of the different growth factor subtypes. VEGFA also has multiple splice isoforms of varied size and matrix-binding properties.[50] Once hypoxia sets up a VEGFA source, endothelial cells will migrate toward the gradient of VEGFA that is sensed by the VEGFR2 receptor.

The coordination of angiogenic growth toward a hypoxic source is balanced by vessel stability. Within an endothelial cell monolayer of a vessel, there exists self-selection of which endothelial cell will migrate out of the vessel. The initiating event is a vascular sprout that emerges and is composed of a leading tip cell followed by stalk cells. Tip cell selection occurs by alternate signaling of the Notch pathway in response to VEGF.[51,52] High levels of VEGF signaling activates the expression of Notch ligands in nearby cells, specifically the Notch ligand Dll4.[52] In response to VEGF signaling, the endothelial cell within the existing vessel increases Dll4 expression to a higher extent than its neighbors. It departs from the existing vessel and extends filopodia out toward the VEGF source, becoming a tip cell. An increase in Dll4 correlates with low Notch1 expression in the same tip cell. In turn, Dll4 in tip cells activates Notch in neighboring cells, attenuating the formation of filopodia, becoming stalk cells by default.[53] The ability of the Notch pathway to repress or differentially influence the function of its neighbors is termed *lateral inhibition*.[54] This lateral inhibition is a mechanism by which intersegmental vessel sprouts from the existing vessel.[55] The selection of tip cells is determined by differential expression of Dll4. The process prevents multiple endothelial cells from an established vessel from migrating concurrently toward a hypoxic source and resulting in catastrophic vascular disruption. In this manner, the departing tip cell inhibits its neighbors from migrating, which ensures vascular stability in the preexistent vessel while promoting vascular expansion.

Physiologic retinal angiogenesis occurs postnatally and has a very typified pattern of angiogenic migration via tip and stalk cells, as well as later reorganization and stabilization of the vascular plexus with well-defined arteries and veins. The same programs of artery-vein specification, as well as tip and stalk cell selection, are recapitulated in the retina for proper vascularization. In the neonate, the process of angiogenic sprouting can become deranged or overactive in hypoxic tumor environments or even in the premature retina. It was originally postulated that as premature infants are exposed to higher levels of oxygen, large fluctuations in the retinal oxygen environment trigger a hypoxic cascade, such that overgrowth of the retinal vasculature occurs. This overgrowth can interfere with vision and even result in retinal detachment and blindness, known as *retinopathy of prematurity* (ROP). ROP is now believed to be initiated in a two-step process—a preceding stage of delayed retinal vascular development, followed by a second stage of retinal vasoproliferation triggered by hypoxia and VEGF signaling. Because vasoproliferation is the deleterious factor threatening vision, it is thought to be VEGF driven, and VEGF-blocking antibodies have been introduced in clinical practice, with some success in the treatment of ROP.[56]

THE ROLE OF THE VASCULAR SMOOTH MUSCLE CELLS

Although the formation of the vasculature is driven by the actions of the endothelium, most blood vessels require smooth muscle cells. The association of contractile cells with the primitive vascular tree is critical initially to offer stability to a newly formed vascular bed, but later it is critical to facilitate the propagation of blood flow. The investment of smooth muscle cells around the endothelial tubes provides mechanical resistance against the continuous force imposed by rapid and pulsatile blood flow. The progenitors for these vascular smooth muscle cells are varied, and depending on the location of the blood vessel and the time, they may originate from the neural crest (mostly head vessels) or somatic or lateral mesoderm.[57] During differentiation, smooth muscle cells secrete and organize layers of extracellular matrix (ECM) proteins. The ECM bind with smooth muscle cells to form a highly integrated tissue that is able to respond to and regulate intravascular pressure. The types of ECM proteins (elastic fibers, collagen fibers, and several types of glycoproteins) are distinctly deposited in different vessels.[58,59] For example, the high level of elastin in arteries, in contrast to veins, provides these vessels with the inherent ability to resist pulsatile flow and return to their original size after each intermittent distension.[60]

The molecular regulation that underpins smooth muscle cell investment and differentiation in the vascular tree is less well understood. Part of the difficulty results from the extensive diversity of vascular smooth muscle phenotypes. The vascular smooth muscle cells retain a level of cellular plasticity not observed in other systems.[61] However, it is clear that the Notch signaling pathway also plays a critical role in vascular smooth muscle biology. Notch is required for the development of vascular smooth muscle and the initial association of undifferentiated mesenchymal cells with endothelial tubes.[62,63] In addition,

Notch signaling is necessary to promote differentiation of smooth muscle cells.[62] Continuous Notch signaling, particularly Notch3, is also required for smooth muscle cell viability and survival.[64,65] For example, familiar mutations in NOTCH3 result in cerebral autosomal-dominant arteriopathy with subcortical infarcts and leukoencephalopathy (CADASIL), a syndrome in which progressive degeneration of the vascular smooth muscle results in the clinical phenotype.[66] Thus vascular pathology can result from primary defects in the endothelium, as well as from defective signaling within their support cells, including vascular smooth muscle populations.

ROLE OF THE VASCULATURE IN ORGANOGENESIS

The vascular tree is both critical to the distribution of oxygen and nutrients systemically and as an orchestrator of organ patterning—as a function of heterotypic vascular cell interactions. The developing vasculature provides critical spatial information and differentiation signals to parenchymal cells for proper organ formation. This instructive role of the endothelium has been studied specifically in the pancreas using genetic models that either eliminate or perturb the vascular endothelium.[67] These disturbances result in total or partial impairment of parenchymal development in the pancreas. Liver development is also highly reliant on vascular induction cues. A lack of endothelial cells results in stunted liver bud formation and subsequent liver organogenesis.[68] Later in hepatic development, smooth muscle precursors also play a critical role in organ patterning. In smooth muscle cells, inactivation of Jagged 1, a ligand for Notch receptors, arrests the formation of biliary ducts in the liver and results in liver failure.[69] In this case, the heterotypic interactions are between Notch2 receptors expressed in cholangiocyte progenitors (epithelial cells that form the biliary ducts) and Jagged1 ligands in smooth muscle cells of the portal vein. This molecular crosstalk provides spatial information for the positional location of biliary ducts. In addition, it drives a program of differentiation in cholangiocytes that is critical for their full differentiation into the epithelium of the biliary tree.[69] The resulting phenotype in the mouse resembles the paucity of bile ducts observed in humans with Alagille syndrome, a pediatric disease associated with mutations in JAGGED1[70] and NOTCH2.[71]

CONCLUSIONS

Vascular biology is a fundamental backbone of embryology, developmental biology, and pathology. A well-orchestrated spatiotemporally patterned circulatory system ensures proper nutrient and oxygen delivery for embryonic growth and postnatal development. This coordinated repertoire requires de novo formation of major vessels, vasculogenesis, as well as rapid, organized expansion of vascular beds from preexisting vessels, angiogenesis. Central to a functioning vascular system is the specification of endothelial cells into arterial, vein, and lymphatic endothelial cell lineage and the establishment of their respective circulatory systems. We reviewed the overarching principles governing the formation of the vascular system within the embryo and the signaling mechanisms responsible for its organization. Postnatally, the expansion of the vasculature addresses the needs of growing tissues and promotes repair and regeneration. The Notch pathway, in addition to VEGF and hypoxia, all play integral roles in vascular development and disease. In addition to forming a circulatory system on the organismal level, the regulation and formation of the vasculature are responsible for proper formation and maintenance of specific organs, highlighting the role of the vascular system in organogenesis. The intersection of these pathways, combined with the increased ability to identify environmental cues and human gene and genomic variants, continue to reveal the complex signaling mechanisms in normal vascular formation and function.

A complete reference list is available at www.ExpertConsult.com. 

SELECT REFERENCES

1. Risau W. Mechanism of angiogenesis. *Nature*. 1997;386:671-674.
6. Vokes SA, Yatskievych TA, Heimark RL, et al. Hedgehog signaling is essential for endothelial tube formation during vasculogenesis. *Development*. 2004;131:4371-4380.
7. Leung DW, Cachianes G, Kuang WJ, et al. Vascular endothelial growth factor is a secreted angiogenic mitogen. *Science*. 1989;246:1306-1309.
8. Gerber HP, Hillan KJ, Ryan AM, et al. VEGF is required for growth and survival in neonatal mice. *Development*. 1999;126:1149-1159.
9. Carmeliet P, Ferreira V, Breier G, et al. Abnormal blood vessel development and lethality in embryos lacking a single VEGF allele. *Nature*. 1996;380:435-439.
11. Meadows SM, Fletcher PJ, Moran C, et al. Integration of repulsive guidance cues generates avascular zones that shape mammalian blood vessels. *Circ Res*. 2012;110:34-46.
12. Stein E, Tessier-Lavigne M. Hierarchical organization of guidance receptors: silencing of netrin attraction by slit through a robo/DCC receptor complex. *Science*. 2001;291:1928-1938.
13. Jones CA, London NR, Chen H, et al. Robo4 stabilizes the vascular network by inhibiting pathologic angiogenesis and endothelial hyperpermeability. *Nat Med*. 2008;14:448-453.
14. Fukushima Y, Okada M, Kataoka H, et al. Sema3E-plexinD1 signaling selectively suppresses disoriented angiogenesis in ischemic retinopathy in mice. *J Clin Invest*. 2011;121:1974-1985.
16. Kim J, Oh W-J, Gaiano N, et al. Semaphorin 3E-Plexin-D1 signaling regulates VEGF function in developmental angiogenesis via a feedback mechanism. *Genes Dev*. 2011;25:1399-1411.
20. Lawson ND, Scheer N, Pham VN, et al. Notch signaling is required for arterial-venous differentiation during embryonic vascular development. *Development*. 2001;128:3675-3683.
21. Moyon D, Pardanaud L, Yuan L, et al. Plasticity of endothelial cells during arterial-venous differentiation in the avian embryo. *Development*. 2001;128:3359-3370.
24. Mellitzer G, Xu Q, Wilkinson DG. Eph receptors and ephrins restrict cell intermingling and communication. *Nature*. 1999;400:77-81.
25. Brückner K, Pasquale EB, Klein R. Tyrosine phosphorylation of transmembrane ligands for Eph receptors. *Science*. 1997;275:1640-1643.
26. Adams RH, Wilkinson GA, Weiss C, et al. Roles of ephrinB ligands and EphB receptors in cardiovascular development: demarcation of arterial/venous domains, vascular morphogenesis, and sprouting angiogenesis. *Genes Dev*. 1999;13:295-306.
31. McAllister KA, Grogg KM, Johnson DW, et al. Endoglin, a TGF-beta binding protein of endothelial cells, is the gene for hereditary haemorrhagic telangiectasia type 1. *Nat Genet*. 1994;8:345-351.
32. Johnson DW, Berg JN, Baldwin MA, et al. Mutations in the activin receptor-like kinase 1 gene in hereditary haemorrhagic telangiectasia type 2. *Nat Genet*. 1996;13:189-195.
34. Larrivée B, Prahst C, Gordon E, et al. ALK1 signaling inhibits angiogenesis by cooperating with the Notch pathway. *Dev Cell*. 2012;22:489-500.
45. Ferrara N, Gerber H-P, LeCouter J. The biology of VEGF and its receptors. *Nat Med*. 2003;9:669-676.
47. Tammela T, Zarkada G, Nurmi H, et al. VEGFR-3 controls tip to stalk conversion at vessel fusion sites by reinforcing Notch signalling. *Nat Cell Biol*. 2011;13:1202-1213.
50. Robinson CJ, Stringer SE. The splice variants of vascular endothelial growth factor (VEGF) and their receptors. *J Cell Sci*. 2001;114:853-865.
51. Gerhardt H, Golding M, Fruttiger M, et al. VEGF guides angiogenic sprouting utilizing endothelial tip cell filopodia. *J Cell Biol*. 2003;161:1163-1177.
55. Roca C, Adams RH. Regulation of vascular morphogenesis by Notch signaling. *Genes Dev*. 2007;21:2511-2524.
60. Li DY, Brooke B, Davis EC, et al. Elastin is an essential determinant of arterial morphogenesis. *Nature*. 1998;393:276-280.
61. Yoshida T, Owens GK. Molecular determinants of vascular smooth muscle cell diversity. *Circ Res*. 2005;96:280-291.
62. High FA, Lu M-M, Pear WS, et al. Endothelial expression of the Notch ligand Jagged1 is required for vascular smooth muscle development. *Proc Natl Acad Sci U S A*. 2008;105:1955-1959.
65. Domenga V, Fardoux P, Lacombe P, et al. Notch3 is required for arterial identity and maturation of vascular smooth muscle cells. *Genes Dev*. 2004;18:2730-2735.
66. Joutel A, Corpechot C, Ducros A, et al. Notch3 mutations in CADASIL, a hereditary adult-onset condition causing stroke and dementia. *Nature*. 1996;383:707-710.
69. Hofmann JJ, Zovein AC, Koh H, et al. Jagged1 in the portal vein mesenchyme regulates intrahepatic bile duct development: insights into Alagille syndrome. *Development*. 2010;137:4061-4072.
70. Li L, Krantz ID, Deng Y, et al. Alagille syndrome is caused by mutations in human Jagged1, which encodes a ligand for Notch1. *Nat Genet*. 1997;16:243-251.

7 Prenatal Diagnosis

Laura Smith | Barbara M. O'Brien

INTRODUCTION

The prenatal diagnosis of a fetal genetic disorder or a chromosome abnormality generally requires invasive testing; all of the invasive tests carry small but recognized risks of miscarriage. Accordingly, an important aspect of prenatal care is screening to identify those women who face an increased risk of a pregnancy complicated by aneuploidy, genetic syndrome, or congenital malformation. Screening modalities include review of the clinical history for both the patient and her partner, evaluation of maternal serum markers or noninvasive prenatal screening results, and ultrasound examination in both the first and second trimesters. Ultimately, however, the definitive diagnosis of a genetic condition or chromosome abnormality in the fetus requires fetal nucleic acids obtained by chorionic villus sampling (CVS), amniocentesis, or percutaneous umbilical blood sampling (PUBS). Noninvasive prenatal screening using cell-free DNA (cfDNA) in maternal plasma has been rapidly introduced into prenatal care since it became clinically available in 2011. cfDNA has shown high sensitivity and specificity for common aneuploidies (trisomies 21, 18, 13) and sex chromosome abnormalities.[1,2]

SCREENING

Because women with "positive screens" (risk greater than a predetermined cutoff), which indicates increased risk, often proceed to an invasive prenatal diagnostic test with an inherent risk of miscarriage, screening methods should strive for a high level of detection with the lowest screen-positive rate. Concepts such as *screen-positive rate* (the number of women with an increased risk among those undergoing testing identified on the screening test), *positive predictive value* (the chances of an abnormal result among the screen-positive group), and *detection rate* (number of abnormal fetuses identified from within the screened population) provide useful parameters to compare screening approaches. In addition, knowledge of the gestational age at which screening can be performed is important and may influence pregnancy options.

PARENTAL CLINICAL HISTORY

PARENTAL AGE

A long-recognized increase in aneuploidy as women become older is a cornerstone of prenatal diagnosis. For women who are 35 years of age at delivery, the chance of having a newborn with Down syndrome (trisomy 21) is approximately 1 in 308 pregnancies. Because trisomy 21 is associated with increased risk of miscarriage and stillbirth, for a 35-year-old woman the chance that Down syndrome will be diagnosed is actually higher at amniocentesis (1 in 258) or CVS (1 in 175). Although maternal age was the first screening criterion for Down syndrome, it performs poorly when assessed at a population level. Approximately 15% of women have children at age 35 years or older (screen-positive rate), and the likelihood in this subgroup of women that a pregnancy will be complicated by Down syndrome (positive predictive value) is only 1% to 3%. Furthermore, the detection rate is only approximately 20%; less than one fourth of Down syndrome infants are born to women in this older maternal age subcategory. When evaluated by these screening parameters, the utility of maternal age greater than 35 years alone as an indication for an invasive prenatal diagnostic test has been challenged.[3] Genetic conditions associated with the father's age are more difficult to delineate but include an increased risk of dominant mutations as exemplified by achondroplasia.[4]

REPRODUCTIVE HISTORY

Assessment of the couple's reproductive history may also signal an increased genetic risk for the pregnancy. A history of repeat miscarriages (two or more) is associated with an increased risk of parental balanced translocation (6.8%). Other reproductive outcomes, such as a previous malformed stillbirth along with a single miscarriage, are also associated with an increased risk of a parental balanced translocation (5.4%).[5] A history of three or more consecutive first-trimester abortions carries a 9.6% risk of a parental balanced translocation.[5] Similarly, repeated failure of in vitro fertilization cycles (for more than 10 cycles) attributable to poor implantation is associated with an increased risk of a parental balanced translocation of 2.5%.[6] By comparison, the overall rate of balanced translocations in newborns is 0.2%.[7] A balanced translocation increases the person's risk that offspring may inherit an unbalanced complement of chromosomes, with associated implications for mental and physical delays.

In addition to previous pregnancies, a diagnosis of infertility warrants closer examination of the identified etiologic disorder and the possible recommendation for prenatal diagnostic testing. Balanced translocations and sex chromosome aneuploidy occur in 14.3% and 6.5% of men with absent and low sperm counts, respectively.[8] In addition, with male factor infertility related to obstructive azoospermia, congenital bilateral absence of the vas deferens (CBAVD) is a common diagnosis. Of men with CBAVD, almost two thirds carry at least one mutation in the gene responsible for classic cystic fibrosis (CF) (i.e., the CF transmembrane receptor gene *[CFTR]*). Almost half (54.5%) of the men are double heterozygotes, possessing two mutations for classic CF, although most often the second mutation is a variant specifically associated with infertility and not classic CF.[9] Because men with CBAVD can father children through assisted reproduction using intracytoplasmic sperm injection, carrier screening of the female partner is critical in view of the relatively high carrier frequency—1 in 25 in the white population. Couples in which both members carry a *CFTR* mutation face a 25% risk of having a child with CF; this finding emphasizes the importance of delineating the specifics of male factor infertility.

Female factor infertility also may have an underlying genetic etiology with subsequent risk to the offspring. In particular, poor ovarian reserve and oligomenorrhea or amenorrhea may reflect a premutation of fragile X. Classically, 3% of cases of sporadic premature ovarian failure and 13% of cases of familial premature ovarian failure are associated with a premutation of fragile X.[10] Of significance for female factor infertility, earlier menopause in women with a premutation of fragile X heightens the possibility that these women will seek infertility evaluation and treatment with a diagnosis of poor ovarian reserve.[11] In view of an overall frequency of fragile X premutations in the general population of approximately 1 in 200 women, infertility centers offer screening for fragile X to women. For fragile X premutation carriers, the implications for the offspring reflect the degree of expansion of the fragile X site (as discussed next under family history screening).

FAMILY HISTORY

Finally, review of the clinical history for both parents includes an assessment of family history. Ethnicity and country of origin are now routinely ascertained at preconception and prenatal visits. Various diseases of an autosomal recessive nature occur with increased frequency among specific populations reflecting historical physical or cultural constraints to gene migration. For some disorders, disease distribution is widespread and warrants screening in essentially all individuals. CF is an example of such an autosomal disease. Current recommendations are to offer *CFTR* carrier screening to all women, ideally in the preconception period, with education regarding disease frequency and testing sensitivity within the patient's specific ethnicity (Table 7.1). In persons of Northern European heritage, the carrier frequency is 1 in 25, with screening detecting 88% of carriers. However, in populations in which CF is less common, such as Asians (carrier frequency of 1 in 94), screening detects only 49% of carriers. In any population, screening can reduce but not totally negate the presence of a *CFTR* carrier.

Several autosomal recessive disorders occur more frequently within specific populations, and screening is then specifically directed by the individual patient's race or ethnicity. For example, hemoglobinopathies are more common in people of African, Mediterranean, or Asian origin. The carrier state for sickle cell occurs in approximately 1 in 12 persons of African American ancestry, and hemoglobin electrophoresis is the preferred method of screening. In some populations, further assessment for a hemoglobinopathy is warranted in the presence of a low mean corpuscular volume. β-Thalassemia will be detected by hemoglobin electrophoresis, whereas a low mean corpuscular volume without iron deficiency and with a normal hemoglobin electrophoresis is suggestive of α-thalassemia. Further diagnosis of this carrier state would require molecular diagnostic testing based on the individual patient's country of origin. For persons of Ashkenazi Jewish heritage, the American College of Obstetrics and Gynecology (ACOG) recommends carrier screening for Tay-Sachs disease, CF, Canavan disease, and familial dysautonomia.[12] For each of these disorders, the carrier frequency is sufficiently increased and the molecular diagnostic tests are sufficiently sensitive to meet the criteria for a prenatal screening test. In addition to these four ACOG-recommended screenings, there are expanded carrier screenings that can be considered in patients of Jewish ancestry.[13] As with all autosomal recessive disorders, any offspring would have a 25% chance of inheriting the disease in question if both parents are carriers.

For couples in which only one person is of Eastern European Ashkenazi Jewish heritage, the recommendation remains to offer screening but with the knowledge that in non-Ashkenazi Jewish populations the carrier frequency is lower and is typically not established. Furthermore, among non-Ashkenazi Jewish persons, the sensitivity of the molecular diagnostic tests for specific disease mutations is substantially less. For example, in screening for Tay-Sachs disease carriers in a non-Ashkenazi Jewish population, the recommendation is to use a functional assay with 98% detection, compared with molecular diagnostic tests, which detect only 50% of carriers. Persons of Ashkenazi Jewish heritage also may avail themselves of information regarding additional autosomal recessive diseases (Table 7.2). However, for couples in which only one member is of Ashkenazi Jewish heritage, the constraints of accurate screening in the non-Ashkenazi Jewish person remain; functional assays are available only for Tay-Sachs disease. For couples in which both members are carriers for these autosomal recessive disorders, prenatal diagnosis is possible with use of the same molecular diagnostic tests used for fetal cells obtained by either amniocentesis or CVS.[14]

Of relevance to prenatal diagnosis, a family history of intellectual disability of unknown etiology or significant developmental delay or autism represents a positive screen for fragile X syndrome. Fragile X syndrome is the most common inherited cause of intellectual disability. The specific characteristics result from expansion of the fragile X mental retardation (FMR-1) region on the X chromosome. In most cases, 40 or fewer CGG repeats are present within FMR-1, and the region remains stable when passed from either parent to their offspring. Of note, however, some persons have inherited expansions of this repeat region, either slight (41 to 60—intermediate range) or larger (61 to 200—premutation range).[15] Approximately 1 in 200 women (1 in 113 to 1 in 350) carry a premutation for fragile X syndrome. When this unstable CGG repeat region expands to greater than 200 repeats (full mutation), increased methylation impairs translation, resulting in lack of production of the fragile X mental retardation protein. The size of the maternal premutation allele directly influences whether further expansion occurs during meiosis (Table 7.3).[16] Sons who inherit a full mutation have characteristics of typical fragile X syndrome. In daughters who inherit the full mutation, features of the syndrome are unpredictable because of the normal random silencing of one X chromosome (Lyon hypothesis). As many as two thirds of daughters with a full fragile X mutation may have mild to moderate developmental delay. Although general population screening for the premutation carrier state in women is not currently advocated, given the relatively high frequency of premutation carriers (1 in 200) and implications for disability, judicious review of the family history for characteristics of fragile X syndrome is encouraged.[17]

The family history of both partners also can yield important information regarding adult-onset dominant disorders such as Marfan syndrome, polycystic kidney disease, myotonic dystrophy, and Huntington disease. Such dominant adult-onset disorders may be noted in one or more seemingly remote family members, with no perception of the significance for the current pregnancy. Non-disease-related death of affected persons before disease manifestation and later age at onset of symptoms can cloud the inheritance pattern in a family. In addition, especially in women with myotonic dystrophy, the most common adult-onset muscular dystrophy, the occurrence of congenital myotonic dystrophy with symptoms more severe than those typical of the adult-onset disease should be addressed. Disorders of recessive inheritance

Table 7.1 Cystic Fibrosis Detection and Carrier Rates Before and After Testing.

Racial or Ethnic Group	Detection Rate[a] (%)	Carrier Rate Before Testing	Approximate Carrier Risk After Negative Test Result[b]
Ashkenazi Jewish	94	1/24	1/380
Non-Hispanic white	88	1/25	1/200
Hispanic white	72	1/58	1/200
African American	64	1/61	1/170
Asian American	49	1/94	1/180

[a]Detection rate data based on use of a 23-mutation panel.
[b]Bayesian statistics used to calculate approximate carrier risk after a negative test result.
Modified from ACOG Committee Opinion No. 486: Update on carrier screening for cystic fibrosis. *Obstet Gyncol.* 2011;117(4):1028–1031.

require attention with testing of the individual at risk of the specific DNA mutation known to be segregating within the family. Lack of knowledge of the specific mutation within a family does not prevent testing the person at risk but will limit the assurance of exclusion of the carrier state. For example, in a woman with a brother who has CF arising from the most common mutation, homozygosity for deltaF508, a negative result for the most common CF mutations (including delta508) changes her risk of being a carrier from 2 in 3 (unaffected sibling of a patient with an autosomal recessive disease) to 1 in 208 (background residual risk of any Northern European individual for undetected CF carrier status). By comparison, if her brother had not been tested, perhaps because he died before molecular diagnosis and neither parent was available, then her two-thirds empiric carrier risk could be reduced to only 1 in 15 (as a result of residual undetectable CF mutations in a Northern European person).

CELL-FREE DNA

Cell-free DNA (cfDNA) has become more universally used in prenatal diagnosis of genetic conditions since its introduction in the United States in 2011. Testing has altered genetic counseling and rates of invasive testing among women seeking prenatal counseling. cfDNA screening has a higher sensitivity and lower false-positive rate than conventional screening modalities in detecting fetal aneuploidy (Table 7.4).

cfDNA represents DNA fragments released from the placenta as trophoblasts undergo apoptosis. Maternal blood samples contain maternal and placental cfDNA with the fetal fraction representing the ratio of placental to total cfDNA. The fetal fraction increases throughout pregnancy and typically is

Table 7.3 Maternal Premutation Allele Size and Risk of Expansion to Full Mutation.

	Full Mutation Risk: % (No. of Fetuses Affected)			
Maternal Repeat Size[a]	**Nolin (1996)**	**Pesso (2000)**	**Toledano-Alhadef (2001)**	**Nolin et al. (2003)**
55–59	13 (3/22)	0 (0/11)	0 (0/22)	4 (1/27)
60–69	21 (7/34)	12(1/8)	10 (2/20)	5 (6/113)
70–79	58 (59/102)	50 (1/2)	17 (1/6)	31 (28/90)
80–89	73 (78/107)	50 (1/2)	–	58 (81/140)
90–99	94 (83/88)	100 (1/1)	–	80 (89/111)
100–200	99 (177/179)	75 (3/4)	–	98 (194/197)

[a]With less than 200 repeats.
Data from Nolin SL, Brown WT, Glicksman A, et al. Expansion of the fragile X CGG repeat in females with premutation or intermediate alleles. *Am J Hum Genet*. 2003;72:454–464.

Table 7.2 Autosomal Diseases With Increased Frequency Among Persons of Ashkenazi Jewish Heritage.

		Ashkenazi Jewish		Non-Ashkenazi Jewish	
Disease	**Description**	**Carrier Rate**	**Carrier Detection**	**Carrier Rate**	**Carrier Detection**
Tay-Sachs	Neurologic deterioration, death in early childhood; juvenile- and late-onset forms	1/30	98% by Hex A testing 94% by DNA	1/300	98% by Hex A testing 50% by DNA
Canavan	Neurologic deterioration; death during early childhood, with some survivors into teens	1/40	98% by DNA	Undetermined	60% by DNA
Cystic fibrosis	Chronic pulmonary disease, pancreatic insufficiency, variable survivorship	1/29	97% by DNA	Varies by ethnicity	Varies by ethnicity
Familial dysautonomia	Impairment of sensory and autonomic nervous systems	1/32	99% by DNA	Unknown	Unknown
Fanconi anemia group C	Pancytopenia; developmental delay and failure to thrive	1/89	99% by DNA	Unknown	Unknown
Niemann-Pick type A	Lysosomal storage disease with degenerative course similar to that in Tay-Sachs	1/90	95% by DNA	Unknown	Unique mutations, enzymatic levels poorly discriminate normal and carrier states
Mucolipidosis IV	Neurodegenerative disorder with marked developmental and growth retardation	1/127	95% by DNA	Unknown	Unknown
Bloom	Prenatal and postnatal growth restriction, susceptibility to malignancies	1/100	95% by DNA	Unknown	Unknown
Gaucher	Type 1—variable severity secondary to deposition in spleen, liver, and bones; presentation from chronic illness to asymptomatic	1/15	95% by DNA	Unknown	70% by >30 mutations

Data from ACOG Committee on Genetics: ACOG committee opinion No. 298. Prenatal and preconceptional carrier screening for genetic diseases in individuals of Eastern European Jewish descent. *Obstet Gynecol*. 2004;104:425–428; and Preconception and Prenatal Genetic Screening Pocket Facts. March of Dimes, 20.

detectable at approximately 4%, which corresponds to 10 weeks gestation in the majority of women.[18] Methods for detecting abnormalities use genome sequencing: whole genome, chromosome selective, or single nucleotide polymorphism (SNP). Each method provides similar sensitivities; however, whole genome has been shown to have the lowest failure rate 1.58% in comparison to chromosome selective (3.56%) and SNP (6.39%).[19]

cfDNA screens for trisomies 13, 18, and 21 and sex chromosomal abnormalities. A meta-analysis of detection rates for sex chromosomal abnormalities found that rates were lower than that for trisomies. Table 7.4 provides a summary of the data highlighting monosomy X.[20] The ACOG and Society for Maternal Fetal Medicine (SMFM) have released joint recommendations to offer cfDNA to high risk patients. High-risk pregnancies include those in Table 7.5.[21]

A prospective, blinded study in 2014 demonstrated that the positive predictive value for cfDNA was higher than standard screening for trisomy 21 and 18. Furthermore, cfDNA was shown to be equivalent in low-risk patients as for high-risk patients.[22] Another large study published in 2014 showed similar results.[23]

When reporting results, companies stratify testing as negative or positive. Negative results indicate a decreased risk for the affected conditions; however, this does not completely exclude them. Positive results should prompt referral to a maternal fetal medicine physician or genetic counselor as invasive testing is recommended. Rarely, an alternative result is reported as test failure or "no call," which occurs 0.9% to 8.1% of this time. In this scenario, the fetal fraction may be too low to measure. There are multiple potential causes for "no call" results, including testing methodology, high maternal weight, multigestation, egg donation, and surrogacy. Nonetheless, patients should be counseled that "no call" results have been associated with fetal aneuploidy with some studies demonstrating an odds ratio of 9.2.[24] Current SMFM guidelines recommend genetic counseling and diagnostic testing if cfDNA fails on initial draw.[21]

USE OF CELL-FREE FETAL DNA TO SCREEN FOR RH DISEASE

Use of cfDNA testing for fetal Rh status has become commercially available and has improved care for the isoimmunized patient. Because the mother's genotype is Rh negative, the presence of any Rh-positive DNA in her circulation denotes a fetus with the Rh-positive gene from the father and for whom the risks of isoimmunization exist.[25] The methodology is reproducible and sensitive such that cfDNA is used in the management of Rh disease. When a woman is isoimmunized to Rh antigen and produces antibodies, the Rh status of the fetus becomes an important piece of information in the management of this disease. An Rh-negative fetus would not require the extensive surveillance and testing indicated for the Rh-positive fetus with other risk factors.[26] Before the advent of cfDNA, fetal Rh status could be established only by determining the genotype of the fetal cells, typically obtained by amniocentesis.

PRENATAL ULTRASOUND EXAMINATION

Along with advances in biochemical screening in the 1990s, ultrasound screening for Down syndrome also gained popularity. For the more common aneuploidies, characteristic patterns of ultrasound findings emerged (Table 7.6).[27] Even when isolated malformations exist, the risk of aneuploidy can range from a low percentage to greater than 50% (Table 7.7). Some of the increased risk associated with isolated ultrasonography-detected malformations is attributable to the possibility that further subtle dysmorphia or other minor malformations undetectable even by high-resolution ultrasound will be present in the newborn.

Ultrasound survey in the second trimester has become increasingly used for assessment of structural malformations. Nuchal fold thickness was the first marker introduced and several others followed. "Soft markers" for aneuploidy are increased nuchal fold thickness, echogenic bowel, shortened femur, echogenic cardiac focus, choroid plexus cysts, and renal pelvis dilatation. These findings typically are transient and, if not associated with aneuploidy, have no functional significance in the fetus. The one exception is echogenic bowel, which may be associated with CF or fetal infection (typically cytomegalovirus infection). When ultrasound is used as a screening tool for aneuploidy, the screen-positive rate (based on the presence of any one of these subtle markers as a positive result) is relatively high (13.0%), with a detection rate for Down syndrome of approximately 50%.[28]

Different combinations of markers have been proposed under the term *genetic sonogram*. Genetic sonogram describes any mathematical formula based on second-trimester sonographic markers, which revises an a priori risk of Down syndrome. The goals of the genetic sonogram are to reduce amniocentesis

Table 7.5 Optimal Candidates for Routine Cell-Free DNA Aneuploidy Screening.

- Maternal age 35 years or older at delivery
- Sonographic findings indicating an increased risk of aneuploidy
- History of prior pregnancy with a trisomy detectable by cfDNA screening
- Positive screening results for aneuploidy (first trimester, sequential, integrated, or quadruple screen)
- Parental balanced Robertsonian translocation with increased risk for trisomy 13 or 21

cfDNA, Cell-free DNA.
From Society for Maternal-Fetal Medicine Publications Committee: Society for Maternal-Fetal Medicine Consult Series #36. Prenatal aneuploidy screening using cell-free DNA. *Am J Obstet Gynecol*. 2015;212:711–716.

Table 7.4 Cell-Free DNA Screening Performance Characteristics.

Chromosomal Abnormality	Number of Affected Cases	Detection Rate, % (95% CI)	False Positive Rate, % (95% CI)	Positive Predictive Value[a] 25-Year-Old	Positive Predictive Value[a] 40-Year-Old
Trisomy 21	1963	99.7 (99.1–99.9)	0.04 (0.02–0.07)	51%	93%
Trisomy 18	563	97.9 (94.9–99.1)	0.04 (0.03–0.07)	15%	69%
Trisomy 13	119	99.0 (65.8–100.0)	0.04 (0.02–0.07)	7%	50%
Monosomy X	36	95.8 (70.3–99.5)	0.14 (0.05–0.38)	41%	41%

[a]Positive predictive values obtained using PPV calculator from www.perinatalquality.org/Vendors/NSGC/NIPT/.
CI, Confidence interval.

rates and to increase Down syndrome detection. The presence of a structural malformation or a soft marker increases the probability of Down syndrome.[29] This increase can be expressed as a likelihood ratio, calculated as the ratio of the false-negative rate divided by specificity. Table 7.8 lists the published ratios for trisomy 21 using common second-trimester ultrasound markers.[30]

Studies of the genetic sonogram in the age of cfDNA are lacking. In cases where cfDNA results are positive, the genetic sonogram can be very helpful in determining the true risk. However, although cfDNA has an excellent detection rate, a diagnostic test is still recommended in cases where aneuploidy is suspected and the patient desires a definitive diagnosis.

FIRST-TRIMESTER SCREENING FOR ANEUPLOIDY

With improvements in ultrasound resolution, greater clarity of fetal structures in the first trimester emerged. Between 11 and 14 weeks of gestation, visualization of additional fluid collection at the nape of the fetal neck (nuchal translucency) is a sensitive indicator of aneuploidy in the fetus. In initial studies, 70% detection of Down syndrome was predicted, with only 5% of the population considered screen-positive (increased nuchal lucency >2 standard deviations for gestational age). The addition of maternal serum markers, primarily pregnancy-associated plasma protein-A and human chorionic gonadtropin (hCG), brought the screen-positive rate in line with 5%, with a

Table 7.6 Common Ultrasound Findings in Fetuses With Chromosome Abnormalities.

Abnormality	Ultrasound Findings
Trisomy 21	Ventriculomegaly, brachycephaly
	Nuchal thickening
	Cardiac defect—AV canal
	Duodenal atresia, echogenic bowel
	Renal pyelectasis
	Shortened femur/humerus; clinodactyly involving fifth digit, sandalfoot
Trisomy 18	CNS—agenesis of corpus callosum, meningomyelocele, ventriculomegaly
	Cystic hygroma
	Cardiac anomalies
	Congenital diaphragmatic hernia
	Omphalocele
	Clenched hands with overlapping digits
	IUGR with polyhydramnios
Trisomy 13	CNS—holoprosencephaly, agenesis of corpus callosum, meningomyelocele, microcephaly
	Cleft lip/palate, midface hypoplasia, cyclopia, microophthalmia
	Nuchal thickening
	Cardiac anomalies
	Omphalocele, echogenic bowel
	Echogenic kidneys
	Radial aplasia, polydactyly
Turner	Cystic hygroma
	Cardiac defects (coarctation of the aorta)
	Horseshoe kidneys
	Hydrops
Triploidy	CNS—holoprosencephaly, agenesis of corpus callosum, meningomyelocele, Dandy-Walker malformation
	Hypertelorism, micrognathia
	Syndactyly involving third and fourth fingers
	Cardiac defects
	Omphalocele
	Early-onset IUGR affecting skeleton more than head
	Placental abnormalities—enlarged or small and calcified

AV, Atrioventricular; *CNS*, central nervous system; *IUGR*, intrauterine growth restriction.
Data from Benacerraf B, ed. *Ultrasound of Fetal Syndromes*. New York: Churchill Livingstone, 1998.

Table 7.7 Aneuploidy Risk Among Isolated Major Anomalies.

Anomaly	Risk (%)[a]	Most Common
High-Risk Category		
Cystic hygroma	>50	45,X
Hydrops	>50	13, 21, 18, 45,X
Holoprosencephaly	50	13, 18, 18p–
Complete atrioventricular canal	40	21
Omphalocele	30	13, 18
Duodenal atresia	30	21
Bladder outlet obstruction	20	13, 18
Lower-Risk Category		
Hydrocephaly/ventriculomegaly	10	21, 13, 18, triploidy
Cardiac defects	10	21, 18, 13, 22–, 8, 9
Meningomyeloceles	7	18
Anencephaly	2	
Encephalocele	10	
Limb reduction	8	18
Clubfoot	6	47,XXY, 47,XXX, 18, 21
Facial clefts	1	13, 18, 22q–
Minimal-Risk Category		
Gastroschisis—must be differentiated from ruptured omphalocele		
Hydranencephaly		
Single umbilical artery		

[a]Risk data are estimates, which are influenced by gestational age at detection and the resolution of ultrasound images in reported studies.
Data from Nyberg D, Mahony B, Pretorius D, eds. *Diagnostic Ultrasound of Fetal Anomalies: Text and Atlas*. St Louis: Mosby; 1990; and Sanders R, Hogge W, Spevak P, Wulfsberg E, eds. *Structural Fetal Abnormalities: The Total Picture*. St Louis: Mosby; 2002.

Table 7.8 Published Likelihood Ratios for Trisomy 21 Using Common Second-Trimester Ultrasound Markers.

Marker	Smith-Bindman	Nuberg	Nyberg	Bromley	Agathokleous[a]
None	NA	0.4	0.36	0.22	0.37
Absent or hypoplastic nasal bone	NA	NA	NA	13.94	23.27
Nuchal fold	17	8.6	11	Infinite	23.27
Hyperechoic bowel	6.1	5.5	6.7	NA	11.44
Short humerus	7.5	2.5	5.1	5.8	4.81
Short femur	2.7	2.2	1.5	1.2	3.72
EIF	2.8	2	1.8	1.4	5.83
Pyelectasis	1.9	1.5	1.5	1.5	7.63

[a]Pooled estimate.
EIF, Echogenic intracardiac focus; *NA*, not available.
Data from Odibo AO, Ghidini A. Role of the second-trimester "genetic sonogram" for Down syndrome screen in the era of first-trimester screening and noninvasive prenatal testing. *Prenat Diagn*. 2014;34: 511–517.

detection rate of 80% for trisomy 21 in the fetus.[31] The benefit of screening using ultrasound and noninvasive prenatal testing is that they can be performed in the first trimester, allowing earlier diagnosis. The most recent improvements in the performance of nuchal translucency as a screening tool for trisomies have been based on improved statistical modeling of the data rather than changes in the measurement techniques.[32] Ductus venosus measurements and nasal bone assessments are two additional first-trimester ultrasound parameters that are used to decrease screen-positive rates without loss of detection.[33,34]

Although first-trimester screening with a combination of ultrasound examination and maternal serum screen yields high detection and low screen-positive rates, an alternative approach of so-called *integrated testing* has also been supported. Integrated testing consists of first-trimester ultrasound examination and measurement of serum markers in combination with select second-trimester serum markers. With integrated testing, the screen-positive rate is lower by a few percentage points and the detection rate is greater than 95%.[35] However, this methodology delays screening results until the second trimester. A compromise between first-trimester screening alone and integrated testing is reached with *sequential screening*. Sequential approaches may be stepwise or contingent; both release high-risk screen results in the first trimester. Further screening is done in the second trimester for all (in the stepwise approach) or only a proportion of the women (in the contingent approach).[36,37] Either sequential approach maintains a low screen-positive rate with (<5.0%) with a detection rate for Down syndrome greater than 90%. Currently, ACOG recommends offering women of all ages screening for aneuploidy in pregnancy, with initiation of screening in the first trimester optimal.[3]

The majority of fetuses with increased nuchal translucency but a normal karyotype proceed through gestation without complication. However, as the degree of first-trimester nuchal edema increases, the risk of other structural malformations detected on the second-trimester ultrasound or at birth also increases. Although a relatively low risk of 2.7% is present for fetuses with mild nuchal edema (nuchal translucency 3.0 mm), risk reaches 35.6% for those fetuses with markedly enlarged nuchal translucency (7.0 mm).[38] Although many of the identified abnormalities are cardiac malformations, other disorders such as congenital diaphragmatic hernia, skeletal dysplasias, fetal akinesis, and metabolic storage disease also are reported.[39] Persistence of markedly increased nuchal edema into the second trimester represents the greatest risk, with almost half (40.9%) of fetuses experiencing an adverse outcome such as structural malformation, hydrops, or in utero demise.[40] Conversely, for fetuses with mild increases (2.5 to 3.0 mm) in first-trimester nuchal fold, a majority continue through gestation without adverse outcome, and the risk of structural abnormalities or disability in the newborn period or early childhood is not significantly increased.[41]

A septated cystic hygroma in the first trimester is defined by extensive nuchal thickening extending along the entire length of the fetal back, where septations are clearly visible. This finding is seen in the first trimester and affects 1 in 300 pregnancies. A cystic hygroma is associated with aneuploidy 50% of the time.[42] In the 50% of cases without aneuploidy, there is a 1-in-2 risk of a major structural malformation, typically cardiac or skeletal. If complete prenatal evaluation reveals no evidence of additional abnormalities, the residual risk of an abnormal pediatric outcome ranges from 5% to 25%. Intrauterine demise occurs in 25% of fetuses with a cystic hygroma.[42]

DIAGNOSTIC TESTING

Although use of screening modalities for genetic disease and aneuploidy during pregnancy avoids the risk of miscarriage, none of the available tests provides a definitive answer. For diagnosis, fetal DNA needs to be studied; currently, appropriate samples can be obtained only through invasive testing: the placenta (CVS), amniotic fluid (amniocentesis), or fetal blood (i.e., PUBS) may be used. When patients are counseled regarding each of them, the miscarriage rate is frequently quoted, but other concerns such as procedure-related fetal morbidity and the likelihood of technical complications should also be considered.

CHORIONIC VILLUS SAMPLING

Available from 10 weeks of pregnancy onward, CVS currently affords the earliest diagnostic possibility. Trophoblast cells obtained from the placenta can be studied for specific genetic mutations, as well as chromosome analysis. CVS is performed under ultrasound guidance with the passage of a catheter into the placenta, either transcervically or through the maternal abdomen. Based on large meta-analysis of studies that included a control group, the miscarriage rate is thought to be 0.22% (1 in 455).[43] Concerns related to fetal morbidity include fetal infection (from maternal disease such as human immunodeficiency virus [HIV]), isoimmunization, and fetal damage. With regard to fetal injury, initial reports of higher rates of limb reduction defects among newborns after first-trimester CVS sampling have been extensively investigated. At this time, the risk of such fetal complications is considered rare: 5.2 to 5.7 per 10,000 after CVS compared with 4.8 to 5.97 per 10,000 without CVS.[43] Technical concerns also have surfaced with CVS. Sample procurement is technically different from amniocentesis, and the learning curve is longer. In addition, with multifetal pregnancies, it is possible to ensure sampling of each individual fetus, but this can be more problematic than with amniocentesis. Finally, although both CVS and amniocentesis will provide information concerning the chromosomal makeup of the fetus, CVS may also detect aneuploidy that is confined to the placenta. Occurring in approximately 1% to 2% of CVS samples, confined placental mosaicism reflects a combination of karyotypically normal and abnormal cells. In two thirds of the cases, the abnormal cell line is confined to the placenta; thus further evaluation of the fetus by amniocentesis or PUBS is warranted. An additional outcome associated with confined placental mosaicism is fetal growth restriction, which is likely to be dependent on the specific chromosome abnormality.[44]

STANDARD AMNIOCENTESIS AT 15 WEEKS OR LATER

Amniocentesis for the purpose of genetic diagnosis is typically performed between 15 and 20 weeks gestation. Sterile technique using a 22-gauge spinal needle is used to remove 20 to 30 mL of amniotic fluid under continuous ultrasound guidance. The miscarriage risk of amniocentesis has decreased over time. A recent meta-analysis of miscarriage rate after amniocentesis estimated a loss rate of 0.11% (1 in 900).[43]

Fetal morbidity after amniocentesis also should be considered. In pregnant women who are Rh negative, the combination of an Rh-positive fetus and an invasive diagnostic test carries a small risk of sensitization from fetal-maternal hemorrhage. For this reason, Rho(D) immune globulin is given prophylactically to all Rh-negative women unless the partner is known to be Rh negative or the woman declines it. For women with other red blood cell antigen incompatibilities with their partners, any invasive diagnostic test increases the risk of antibody formation and the effects of isoimmunization in the fetus. These risks also exist for CVS, although they are theoretically lower with amniocentesis, because amniocentesis can avoid the placenta. Similarly, infectious disease in the mother poses a theoretical risk. Transmission of hepatitis B in women who are chronic carriers does not appear to increase the risk of subsequent carriage in their infants. Likewise, although transmission of HIV through amniocentesis remains a theoretical possibility, amniocentesis in women with a low viral load is considered appropriate.

Fetal morbidity is also associated with rupture of membranes occurring after amniocentesis. In approximately 1% of procedures, the amniotic membranes do not promptly reseal, and amniotic fluid leakage occurs. In a majority of such instances (90%), the amniotic fluid will reaccumulate to normal levels, although the mean duration of the recovery period has been reported to be 3 weeks. Amniocentesis-related rupture of membranes with failure to reseal is associated with increased risk of intrauterine growth restriction and prematurity.[45] By contrast, spontaneous rupture of the membranes in the second trimester carries a poor prognosis, with only a limited chance of regaining normal fluid levels.

Technical issues arise with amniocentesis when the genetic diagnosis being pursued relies on molecular genetic studies. All amniotic fluid samples contain a small number of maternal cells, probably obtained as the needle passes through the maternal skin and uterus. When cultured amniotic fluid cells are evaluated, the chance of overgrowth by the maternal cells, with consequent assessment of the karyotype of the mother and not the fetus, is low. Nevertheless, when molecular diagnostic studies are initiated on direct, uncultured amniotic fluid, it is necessary to ensure that the fetal genome is being assessed. This can be accomplished either by (1) clearing the initial 1 or 2 mL from the needle before obtaining the amniotic fluid sample or (2) simultaneously evaluating maternal blood for additional polymorphic markers to ensure that the amniotic fluid sample represents a discretely different genome (maternal cell contamination study).

PERCUTANEOUS UMBILICAL BLOOD SAMPLING

PUBS is performed at 18 weeks or later in gestation by the removal of a blood sample from the umbilical cord under ultrasound guidance. The procedure is accompanied by an approximate 1% to 2% risk of pregnancy loss, which is higher with fetuses with other risk factors such as hydrops. Nevertheless, PUBS can provide rapid and often more extensive information than that obtained by CVS or amniocentesis. Karyotype analysis yields results within 48 hours, because the rapidly dividing peripheral blood cells do not require the extensive (often 2-week) period of culture needed for both CVS and amniocytes. In addition, molecular genetic studies are possible on the extracted DNA, as is functional assessment of the bone marrow, immune system, and hepatic system. Fetal anemia can be diagnosed and treated by umbilical vessel transfusion in situations in which the hematologic suppression is expected to be transitory, such as parvovirus infection. Polymerase chain reaction (PCR) analysis for specific viruses such as parvovirus and cytomegalovirus can also be performed using fetal blood. Altered hepatic or bone marrow function may point to an underlying metabolic disease, guiding more specific molecular testing in the fetus.

PREIMPLANTATION GENETIC DIAGNOSIS

After in vitro fertilization, directed assessment of a single cell from a blastocyst before transfer to the uterus—preimplantation genetic diagnosis (PGD)—can reveal single-gene disorders, as well as chromosome abnormalities. For persons with a balanced chromosome translocation, single blastomeres can be studied with fluorescence in situ hybridization (FISH)—a method to determine copy number for specific, predefined segments of DNA in nondividing cells. With probe combinations designed for the specific translocation carried by the individual, couples proceed through assisted reproduction and in vitro fertilization. On day 3 after fertilization, single cells are removed from each blastocyst and assessed within 12 to 24 hours with the translocation-specific FISH probes. On completion of the FISH analysis, the information obtained is used to guide selection of blastocysts to transfer to the woman. This methodology also allows determination of chromosome copy number and was initially applied as preimplantation genetic screening in women at increased risk related to older maternal age, previous aneuploidy, or repeat miscarriages. Development of the optimal panel of probes remains challenging because increases in the number of chromosomes studied are associated with higher technical error rates and the potential for eliminating from consideration for transfer a blastocyst that may indeed be chromosomally normal.[46] As currently performed, PGD is a screening method to decrease the chance that the pregnancy will be complicated by a chromosome abnormality, but it does not improve outcomes for women of advanced age or habitual miscarriage. Application of comparative genomic hybridization array technology may be helpful in this area.

Various factors can contribute to the approximate 10% error rate, including lack of possibility of retesting owing to use of a single cell, existence of mosaicism in the early blastocyst, and inherent technical difficulties of resolution with FISH probes. Approaches using a molecular approach to chromosome number (such as microarray or PCR methods) are likely to address this concern in the future.

Similarly, individual patients or couples at risk of a single-gene disorder that is inherited in either a recessive or dominant fashion may be candidates for PGD. As the technology continues to progress and the accuracy of PGD improves, current indications range from diagnosis of autosomal recessive disorders associated with childhood lethality to autosomal dominant disorders of adult onset. Areas of ethical controversy in this field are human leukocyte antigen matching for an affected sibling and family balancing.

CHROMOSOMAL MICROARRAY ANALYSIS

In the field of pediatric and adult genetics, chromosomal microarray analysis (CMA) has replaced karyotyping as a first-tier test to detect chromosome abnormalities in the setting of developmental disabilities or congenital anomalies.[47] CMA is able to detect genomic imbalances to within approximately 400 kb. In contrast, routine karyotyping is able to detect genomic imbalances in the 5- to 10-Mb range.[47] In addition, SNP-based microarray testing has the capability to detect regions of homozygosity that may be indicative of uniparental disomy or parental consanguinity. In 2013, ACOG recommended CMA as a first-tier prenatal diagnostic test for fetuses with one or more major structural abnormalities detected by ultrasound, replacing the need for fetal karyotyping. ACOG also stated that either fetal karyotyping or CMA can be performed when invasive testing is done in the setting of a normal ultrasound.[48]

The ACOG guideline was heavily influenced by a 2012 large-scale multicenter National Institute of Child Health and Human Development trial that compared prenatal CMA with traditional standard karyotyping.[49] The results indicated that CMA will detect a finding missed by standard karyotyping in 6% of fetuses with abnormal ultrasound findings and in 1.7% of fetuses with no abnormal ultrasound findings. However, CMA can also lead to counseling challenges because 3.4% of fetuses had a detected copy number variant (CNV) of unknown clinical significance. Just over half of these CNVs (1.8%) were classified as "likely benign" after investigation, with the other half (1.6%) classified as "likely pathogenic."[49] It is important to note that those CNVs that are classified as "likely pathogenic" may be complicated by reduced penetrance, variable expressivity, and delayed onset into adulthood, all of which make phenotyping difficult to predict and complicate counseling.

A recent meta-analysis indicated that when CMA is performed after detection of a structural abnormality by ultrasound, CMA will detect a significant finding missed by routine karyotyping in 10% (95% confidence interval [CI], 8% to 13%) of pregnancies with a variant of unknown significance detected in 2.1% (95% CI,

1.3% to 3.3%) of pregnancies.[50] As CNVs of unknown significance remain one of the greater interpretation challenges of CMA, some authors have advocated not to report them to patients.[51] However, there is no consensus on how to handle the reporting of these CNVs in the clinical setting. Regardless of the reporting strategy in place, pretest counseling and consent are critical components of this process and should include contracting with patients regarding the types of results that can be reported and their potential implications.

CMA can be performed concurrently with standard karyotyping, in place of it, or as a reflex test if standard karyotyping is normal. Cost-benefit analysis favors ordering CMA alone.[52] However, using rapid aneuploidy detection (interphase FISH or qualitative fluorescent PCR) for the most common aneuploidies followed by CMA if this testing is normal and standard karyotyping if this testing is abnormal was not included in this economic analysis and should be evaluated.

FUTURE DIRECTIONS

At this time, noninvasive prenatal screening using cfDNA is limited to the most common aneuploidies. However, there are companies offering cfDNA for single gene disorders. At the writing of this chapter, ACOG does not endorse cfDNA for single gene disorders due to the lack of data. It is not unreasonable to imagine that data will be forthcoming in the near future to detect single gene disorders, such as cystic fibrosis with the use of cell free DNA technology.

Exome sequencing, or sequencing of all the protein coding regions of the genome, is currently standard of care in adult and pediatric practice. This technology is expanding into the prenatal genetic world but with the challenge of how to interpret large datasets and variants of uncertain significance and how to appropriately apply the information in clinical practice.

CONCLUSION

Prenatal genetic diagnosis is currently possible only by means of invasive procedures, with their inherent risk of miscarriage, fetal morbidity, and technical constraints. CVS, amniocentesis, and PUBS can all provide the fetal DNA needed for the assessment of a wide range of genetic and chromosome disorders. A good clinical history, which includes parental ages, reproductive history, and family history, has value in screening for genetic and chromosome risks. During pregnancy, cfDNA, maternal serum markers, and ultrasound examination are productive screening tools used primarily to assess Down syndrome risk. Ideally, such screening should be initiated in the first trimester. Most important, genomics is rapidly changing the field of prenatal screening and diagnosis, and further developments in the use of cfDNA will allow noninvasive prenatal genetic screening for a broad array of conditions from a maternal blood sample and decrease the need for invasive testing.

REFERENCES

1. Palomaki GE, Deciu C, Kloza EM, et al. DNA sequencing of maternal plasma reliably identifies trisomy 18 and trisomy 13 as well as Down syndrome: an international collaborative study. *Genet Med*. 2012;14:296-305.
2. Mackie FL, Hemming K, Allen S, et al. The accuracy of cell-free DNA-based non-invasive prenatal testing in singleton pregnancies: a systematic reviews and bivariate meta-analysis. *BJOG*. 2016;124:32-34.
3. Committee on Practice Bulletins—Obstetrics, Committee on Genetics, and the Society for Maternal-Fetal Medicine. ACOG practice Bulletin No. 163: screening for fetal aneuploidy. *Obstet Gynecol*. 2016;127:e123-e137.
4. Kuhnert B, Nieschlag E. Reproductive functions of the ageing male. *Hum Reprod Update*. 2004;10:327-339.
5. Gadow EC, Lippold S, Otano L, et al. Chromosome rearrangements among couples with pregnancy losses and other adverse reproductive outcomes. *Am J Med Genet*. 1991;41:279-281.
6. Stern C, Pertile M, Norris H, et al. Chromosome translocations in couples with in-vitro fertilization implantation failure. *Hum Reprod*. 1999;14:2097-2101.
7. Hansteen IL, Varslot K, Steen-Johnsen J, Langård S. Cytogenetic screening of a new-born population. *Clin Genet*. 1982;21:309-314.
8. Nagvenkar P, Desai K, Hinduja I, Zaveri K. Chromosomal studies in infertile men with oligozoospermia and non-obstructive azoospermia. *Indian J Med Res*. 2005;122:34-42.
9. De Braekeleer M, Ferec C. Mutations in the cystic fibrosis gene in men with congenital bilateral absence of the vas deferens. *Mol Hum Reprod*. 1996;2:669-677.
10. Conway GS, Payne NN, Webb J, et al. Fragile X premutation screening in women with premature ovarian failure. *Hum Reprod*. 1998;13:1184-1187.
11. Murray A, Ennis S, MacSwiney F, et al. Reproductive and menstrual history of females with fragile X expansions. *Eur J Hum Genet*. 2000;8:247-252.
12. ACOG Committee on Genetics. ACOG Committee Opinion No. 298. Prenatal and preconceptional carrier screening for genetic diseases in individuals of Eastern European Jewish descent. *Obstet Gynecol*. 2004;104:425-428.
13. Carrier screening for genetic conditions. Committee Opinion No. 691129. *Am Col Obstet Gynecol*. 2017:e41-e45.
14. Ferreira JC, Schreiber-Agus N, Carter SM, et al. Carrier testing for Ashkenazi Jewish disorders in the prenatal setting: navigating the genetic maze. *Am J Obstet Gynecol*. 2014;211:197-204.
15. Hagerman PJ, Hagerman RJ. The fragile-X premutation: a maturing perspective. *Am J Hum Genet*. 2004;74:805-816.
16. Nolin SL, Brown WT, Glicksman A, et al. Expansion of the fragile X CGG repeat in females with premutation or intermediate alleles. *Am J Hum Genet*. 2003;72:454-464.
17. Sherman S, Pletcher BA, Driscoll DA. Fragile X syndrome: diagnostic and carrier testing. *Genet Med*. 2005;7:584-587.
18. Bianchi DW, Chiu RWK. 2018. Sequencing of circulating cell-free DNA during pregnancy. *N Engl J Med*. 2018;379:464-473.
19. Yaron Y. The implications of non-invasive prenatal testing failures: a review of an under-discussed phenomenon. *Prenat Diagn*. 2016;36:391-396.
20. Gil MM, Accurti V, Santacruz B, et al. Analysis of cell-free DNA in maternal plasma: recent developments and future prospects. *J Clin Med*. 2014;3:537-565.
21. Society for Maternal-Fetal Medicine Publications Committee. Society for maternal-fetal medicine Consult Series #36. Prenatal aneuploidy screening using cell-free DNA. *Am J Obstet Gynecol*. 2015;212:711-716.
22. Bianchi DW, Parker RL, Wentworth J, et al. DNA sequencing versus standard prenatal aneuploidy screening. *N Engl J Med*. 2014;370:799-808.
23. Pergament E, Cuckle H, Zimmermann B, et al. Single-nucleotide polymorphism-based noninvasive prenatal screening in a high-risk and low-risk cohort. *Obstet Gynecol*. 2014;124:210-218.
24. Yaron Y. The implications of non-invasive prenatal testing failures: a review of an under-discussed phenomenon. *Prenat Diagn*. 2016;36:391-396.
25. Zhong XY, Holzgreve W, Hahn S. Risk free simultaneous prenatal identification of fetal Rhesus D status and sex by multiplex real-time PCR using cell free fetal DNA in maternal plasma. *Swiss Med Wkly*. 2001;131:70-74.
26. Daniels G, Finning K, Martin P, Soothill P. Fetal blood group genotyping from DNA from maternal plasma: an important advance in the management and prevention of haemolytic disease of the fetus and newborn. *Vox Sang*. 2004;87:225-232.
27. Benacerraf B, ed. *Ultrasound of Fetal Syndromes*. New York: Churchill Livingstone; 1998.
28. Weisz B, Pandya PP, David AL, et al. Ultrasound findings after screening for Down syndrome using the integrated test. *Obstet Gynecol*. 2007;109:1046-1052.
29. Benacerraf BR, Figoletto Jr FD, Laboda LA. Sonographic diagnosis of Down syndrome in the second trimester. *Am J Obstet Gynecol*. 1985;153:49-52.
30. Odibo AO, Ghidini A. Role of the second-trimester 'genetic sonogram' for Down syndrome screen in the era of first-trimester screening and noninvasive prenatal testing. *Prenat Diagn*. 2014;34:511-517.
31. Nicolaides KH. Nuchal translucency and other first-trimester sonographic markers of chromosomal abnormalities. *Am J Obstet Gynecol*. 2004;191:45-67.
32. Wright D, Kagan KO, Molina FS, et al. A mixture model of nuchal translucency thickness in screening for chromosomal defects. *Ultrasound Obstet Gynecol*. 2008;31:376-383.
33. Gonce A, Borrell A, Martinez JM, Fortuny A. First-trimester screening for Down syndrome with ductus venosus Doppler studies in addition to nuchal translucency and serum markers. *Prenat Diagn*. 2005;25:901-905.
34. Nicolaides KH. First-trimester screening for chromosomal abnormalities. *Semin Perinatol*. 2005;29:190-194.
35. Wald NJ, Watt HC, Hackshaw AK. Integrated screening for Down's syndrome on the basis of tests performed during the first and second trimesters. *N Engl J Med*. 1999;341:461-467.
36. Wright D, Bradbury I, Benn P, et al. Contingent screening for Down syndrome is an efficient alternative to non-disclosure sequential screening. *Prenat Diagn*. 2004;24:762-766.
37. Wald NJ, Rudnicka AR, Bestwick JP. Sequential and contingent prenatal screening for Down syndrome. *Prenat Diagn*. 2006;26:769-777.
38. Souka AP, Snijders RJ, Novakov A, et al. Defects and syndromes in chromosomally normal fetuses with increased nuchal translucency thickness at 10-14 weeks of gestation. *Ultrasound Obstet Gynecol*. 1998;11:391-400.

39. Bahado-Singh RO, Wapner R, Thom E, et al. Elevated first-trimester nuchal translucency increases the risk of congenital heart defects. *Am J Obstet Gynecol.* 2005;192:1357-1361.
40. Souka AP, Krampl E, Bakalis S, et al. Outcome of pregnancy in chromosomally normal fetuses with increased nuchal translucency in the first trimester. *Ultrasound Obstet Gynecol.* 2001;18:9-17.
41. Senat MV, De Keersmaecker B, Audibert F, et al. Pregnancy outcome in fetuses with increased nuchal translucency and normal karyotype. *Prenat Diagn.* 2002;22:345-349.
42. Malone FD, Ball RH, Nyberg DA, et al. FASTER Trial Research Consortium. First-trimester septated cystic hygroma: prevalence, natural history, and pediatric outcome. *Obstet Gynecol.* 2005;106:288-294.
43. Akolekar R, Beta J, Picciarelli G, Ogilvie C, D'Antonio F. Procedure-related risk of miscarriage following amniocentesis and chorionic villus sampling: a systematic review and meta-analysis. *Ultrasound Obstet Gynecol.* 2015;45:16-26.
44. Wilkins-Haug L, Quade B, Morton CC. Confined placental mosaicism as a risk factor among newborns with fetal growth restriction. *Prenat Diagn.* 2006;26:428-432.
45. Borgida AF, Mills AA, Feldman DM, et al. Outcomes of pregnancies complicated by ruptured membranes after genetic amniocentesis. *Am J Obstet Gynecol.* 2000;183:937-939.
46. Munne S. Preimplantation genetic diagnosis and human implantation—a review. *Placenta.* 2003;24(suppl B):S70-S76.
47. Miller DT, Adam MP, Aradhya S, et al. Consensus statement: chromosomal microarray is a first-tier clinical diagnostic test for individual with developmental disabilities or congenital anomalies. *Am J Hum Genet.* 2010;86:749-764.
48. ACOG Committee on Genetics. ACOG Committee Opinion No. 581. The use of chromosomal microarray in prenatal diagnosis. *Obstet Gynecol.* 2013;1222:1374-1377.
49. Wapner RJ, Martin CL, Levy B, et al. Chromosomal microarray versus karyotyping for prenatal diagnosis. *N Engl J Med.* 2012;367:2175-2184.
50. Hillman SC, McMullan DJ, Hall G, et al. Use of prenatal chromosomal microarray: prospective cohort study and systematic review and meta-analysis. *Ultrasound Obstet Gynecol.* 2013;41:610-620.
51. Brady PD, Delle Chiaie B, Christenhusz G, et al. A prospective study of the clinical utility of prenatal chromosomal microarray analysis in fetuses with ultrasound abnormalities and an exploration of a framework for reporting unclassified variants and risk factors. *Genet Med.* 2014;16:469-476.
52. Harper LM, Sutton AL, Longman RE, Odibo AO. An economic analysis of prenatal cytogenetic technologies for sonographically detected fetal anomalies. *Am J Med Genet.* 2014;164A:1192-1197.

Placental Development

8

Margaret G. Petroff | Helen Jones

INTRODUCTION

For millennia, the remarkable ability of the fetus to derive nourishment and "breath" from within the womb has been a source of wonder for scientists, philosophers, physicians, artists, religious leaders, and lay men and women. That this capability was related to the placenta—an organ of great significance to the fetus, yet no longer used by the neonate—was acknowledged early on, whether it be as the "seat of the external soul," the fetus's "alter ego," or the fetal equivalent of the liver, lung, and kidney, was evident. Indeed, it has long been certain that the fetus is expert at obtaining sustenance from the mother in the form of "uterine milk" and/or maternal blood, and that the placenta must be a key player in this task.

The gradual elucidation of the physiologic role of the human placenta as we understand it today has progressed in stages commensurate with advances in physiology, cell and molecular biology, chemistry, epidemiology, medicine, and importantly, technology. Central to an understanding of exactly how the placenta functions to support fetal life and growth was the anatomic question of how the maternal and the fetal vasculatures are interrelated: does maternal blood flow freely into the fetus, thereby directly sating the young with the "spirits" and nutrients therein, or does the placenta somehow extract nutrients from maternal blood, and if so, by what means? The question is extraordinarily difficult to answer based on gross anatomic features alone: anatomists and physicians disagreed, sometimes vehemently, on this matter. Not helping the situation was the intermittent legality of dissection of human cadavers in medical schools. This central question was, however, finally resolved in the 18th century when the famous experimentalist William Harvey (1578-1657) found that injection of uterine arteries and veins with red and blue wax, respectively, failed to reveal entry of wax into the umbilical vessels or the fetus; likewise, no wax entered the mother upon injection of the umbilical vessels. Further understanding of placental function was enabled with Malphigi's (1628-1694) discovery that capillary beds connect arteries and veins, together with the isolation of elemental oxygen and its exchange with carbon dioxide by Priestly (1733-1804) and Lavoisier (1743-1794), respectively.[1]

Following conception and embryo implantation into the uterus, the placenta is the first organ of the embryo and fetus to become fully functional. Together with the extraplacental membranes and umbilical cord, the placenta is derived entirely extrafetally and is remarkably large. As such, it is essential that placental development occurs early and promptly, so that as the metabolic demands of rapid fetal growth increase, the placenta is ready to deliver. The functions of the placenta are many and include selective delivery of nutrients, immunity, and oxygen to the fetus, return of metabolic waste to the mother for excretion, and serving as a barrier to environmental toxins.

This chapter will begin with a description of the gross appearance of the placenta at term and how it is perfused. We will review in detail how this fully functional structure is the culmination of a developmental plan that starts even prior to conception with hormonal priming of the maternal uterus, allowing implantation and differentiation of extraembryonic structures that make up the placenta.

GROSS ANATOMY AND VASCULAR PERFUSION OF THE MATURE PLACENTA

The term placenta is disc-shaped and large, with a mean diameter of ~220 mm and weight of 470 g in healthy term infants (Table 8.1).[2] It is no wonder that early anatomists faced challenges in elucidating the functional anatomy of the placenta; it can be described on its maternal surface (*basal plate*) as lobular and, inside, spongy, with millions of *chorionic villi*—the functional units of the placenta—stemming from the *chorionic plate* (the fetal-facing surface of the placenta). Obvious vascular connections between the villi, chorionic plate, and umbilical cord are discernable at the gross level only in the latter two, as consecutive branching of vessels within the villi becomes ever smaller. Peripherally attached are the extraplacental membranes that, in utero, reflect away from the maternal surface and around the fetus. The membranes attached to the periphery of the placenta consist of a layer of maternal uterine decidual cells fused with the embryo-derived chorion, connective tissue, and amnion. Owing to the distinct embryologic origins of these layers, the amnion and chorion are easily separable; it can be further appreciated at the gross level that they are avascular.

The basal surface of the term placenta (basal plate) is characterized by 10 to 40 slightly protruding areas called *maternal cotyledons*, *lobes*, or *lobules*.[2] They are minimally separated from each other by the so-called *placental septa* (Fig. 8.1). From the chorionic plate at term, 60 to 70 villous stems (*trunci chorii*) arise. Each of these trunks branches into a villous tree, and at least one tree occupies a maternal cotyledon (see Fig. 8.1). The superficial cotyledonary borderlines are adjacent, to a large extent, to those of a corresponding group of villous trees.

Every maternal cotyledon possesses at least one placentome, that is, the fetomaternal circulatory unit. Each placentome consists of a villous tree and the surrounding intervillous space, which is centrifugally perfused with maternal blood (see Fig. 8.1). The centers of typical placentomes exhibit loosely arranged villi that provide a large intervillous space for maternal arterial inflow. Placentomes are separated by narrow intervillous clefts. Near the chorionic plate and at the border of neighboring placentomes, the villous arrangement provides space for the venous backflow toward the venous openings in the basal plate. Supporting the placentome concept, ultrasonographic technologies have measured flow

Table 8.1 Summary of Mean Data on Placental Development.

Preganancy Week (Postconception)	1–2	3–6	7–10	11–14	15–18	19–22	23–26	27–30	31–34	35–38
Pregnancy month (postmenstruation)	1	2	3	4	5	6	7	8	9	10
Diameter of chorionic sac (mm)	—	5–33	34–65	66–99	—	—	—	—	—	—
Placental diameter (mm)	—	—	—	50–69	75–94	100–119	125–144	150–169	175–194	200–220
Placental weight (g)	—	6	8–26	32–60	70–112	126–180	198–252	270–324	342–396	414–470
Placental thickness (postpartum [mm])	—	—	—	10–12	12–15	15–18	18–20	20–22	22–24	24–25
Placental thickness, including uterine wall, measured by ultrasound in vivo (mm)	—	—	—	—	28	29–34	35–38	39–42	42–44	44–45
Length of the umbilical cord (mm)	2	4–20	33–126	158–240	264–330	350–404	424–464	477–520	530–557	565–585
Fetal weight (g) per g of placental weight	—	0.18	0.25–0.65	0.72–1.00	1.29–2.23	2.54–3.11	3.28–3.97	4.19–4.78	4.97–5.81	6.04–7.23
Villous volume (g) per placenta	—	5	18	28	63	102	135	191	234	273
Villous surface (cm^2) per g of villous tissue	—	166	168	194	235	275	313	377	432	458
Maternofetal diffusion distance (μm)	—	55.9	—	40.2	22.4	21.6	—	20.6	11.7	4.8
Villous trophoblastic thickness (μm)	—	18.9	19.1–21.6	—	11.6	—	9.7	—	5.2	4.1
Fetal vessel lumina per villous volume (%)	—	2.7	3.0–4.0	6.0	6.3–6.6	—	9.1	—	21.3	28.4

From Benirschke K, Burton G, Baergen RN. *Pathology of the Human Placenta*. 6th ed. Berlin: Springer; 2012.

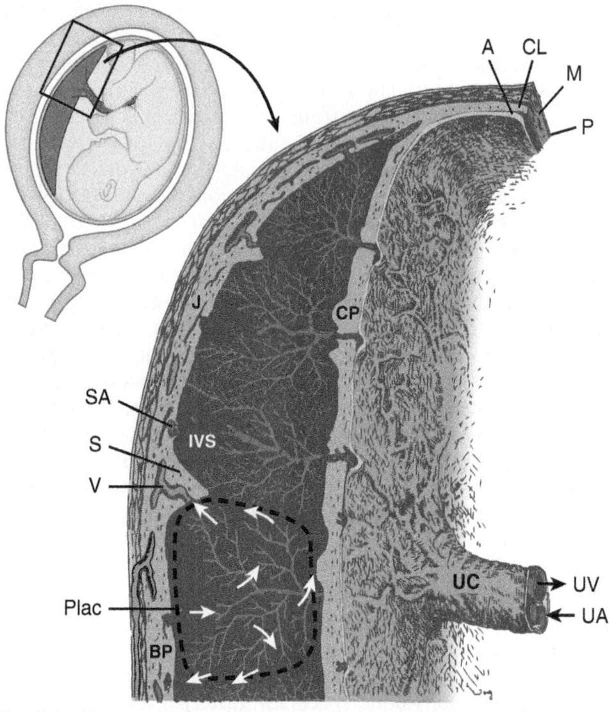

Fig. 8.1 Survey diagram of the mature human placenta in situ. Villous trees arranged around maternal arterial flow from spiral arteries are a central feature of the placenta. Inflowing maternal blood circulates within the intervillous space *(arrows)*, bathing the villous trees, and exits through maternal veins. *A*, Amnion; *BP*, basal plate; *CL*, chorion laeve; *CP*, chorionic plate; *IVS*, intervillous space; *J*, junctional zone; *M*, myometrium; *P*, perimetrium; *Plac*, placentome; *S*, placental septum; *SA*, maternal spiral artery; *UA*, umbilical artery; *UC*, umbilical cord; *UV*, umbilical vein; *V*, maternal vein.

velocities at the spiral artery opening into the intervillous space. Blood flows from typical spiral arteries are described as "jets" that resemble the patterns of flow into the intervillous space that were previously estimated from histologic specimens and simple computational models.[3,4]

Variations within individual villous trees must be kept in mind during histopathologic and functional evaluation of the placenta. The centers of the placentomes act as growth zones of villous trees where new formation and differentiation of villi take place and consist of types of villi called *immature intermediate villi* (see detailed descriptions below). At term, the centers of the placentome are the remainders of immature villous trees from earlier stages of pregnancy and can be observed in at least some placentomes until term. They may disappear completely only in cases of preterm hypermaturity of the placenta.[2] By contrast, the peripheral portions of placentomes represent the metabolically active area in which fetomaternal exchange occurs.

IMPLANTATION AND EARLY PLACENTATION

PREPARATION OF THE UTERUS FOR IMPLANTATION: DECIDUALIZATION

The gross anatomy described above is the culmination of developmental processes that involve a high level of coordination between maternal and fetal elements. Implantation and placental development are critical to pregnancy success; however, so are the series of coordinated events, controlled initially entirely by the mother, called *decidualization*. This prepares the superficial layer of the uterus—that is, the endometrium—into a receptive state that will provide nutrition, trophic support, and immune privilege for the implanting embryo and developing fetus. Early descriptions describe the "union" between the decidua and the chorionic villi of the early placenta, such that these layers function as one.[5]

The endometrium undergoes cyclic decidualization, sloughing, and regeneration under the control of the ovarian hormones estrogen and progesterone. Rising concentrations of estrogen produced by ovarian follicles during the proliferative phase of the menstrual cycle stimulate proliferation of endometrial stromal and epithelial cells, and "prime" the uterus by inducing expression of progesterone receptors in these cells. Following ovulation, progesterone produced by the corpus luteum dominates the endocrine environment, and under its influence the endometrial stromal cells stop proliferating, and instead differentiate. This results in formation of the predecidua late in the menstrual cycle, about 13 days after ovulation. To this end, stromal cells enlarge, accumulating glycogen, glycoproteins, and lipids in their cytoplasm; prolactin and insulin-like growth factor binding protein (IGFBP)-1 also become strongly expressed.[5] These changes are accompanied by increased vascular permeability and leukocyte infiltration; uterine natural killer (uNK) and macrophage cells become particularly abundant, the former eventually comprising about 40% of the total cells of the decidua.

Uterine NK cells will be critical for vascular remodeling at the maternal-fetal interface (discussed in detail below), an event that commences during the first trimester and is complete by the early second trimester of pregnancy. Because these cells recognize human leukocyte antigen (HLA)-C on placental trophoblast cells, they are also believed to play a role in allorecognition of the fetus.[6] Macrophages also accumulate in the decidua and are believed to aid in trophoblast invasion and remodeling of the maternal-fetal interface. Additional changes important to creating an immune-privileged site for the fetus occur: decidual genes for T-cell chemoattractants are epigenetically silenced, and trafficking of dendritic cells between the uterus and draining lymph nodes is blocked.[7]

While decidualization commences with the rise of ovarian progesterone independently of pregnancy, embryo implantation completes the process. This is due to multiple factors produced by the embryo, including interleukin (IL)-1β, cyclooxygenase-2, and matrix metalloproteinases (MMP), all of which promote the functional and morphologic differentiation of endometrial stromal cells. Critically, the decidual endometrial glands begin production of several cytokines, including IL-11 and leukemia inhibiting factor (LIF), which act to bring the uterus into a receptive state, to complete decidualization, and later, to play an indispensable role in allowing embryonic attachment and implantation.[8,9]

As these changes occur, the decidua becomes receptive, but only transiently, to the implanting embryo. During this critical window of implantation, the uterus and embryo are synchronized in maturation and development; lack of synchronicity results in implantation failure. During the implantation window, the embryo becomes apposed to the luminal epithelium, to which a loose, then stronger, adherence is formed; finally, the embryo penetrates the epithelium and invades the stroma. In women, this occurs around days 20 to 24 of the menstrual cycle, or 6 to 10 days after ovulation.

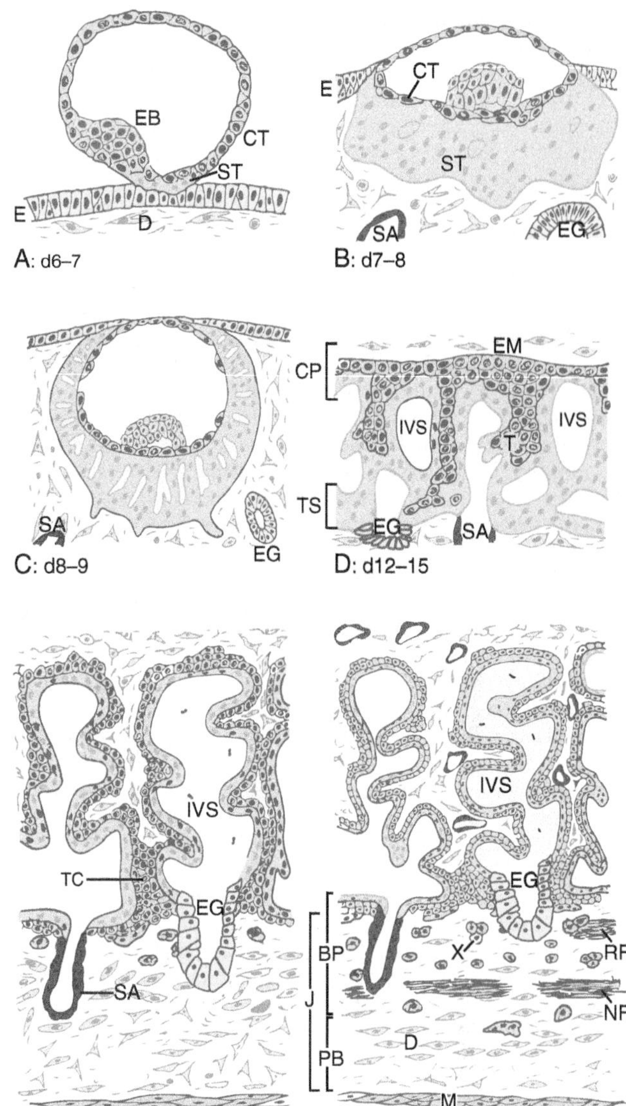

Fig. 8.2 Stages of placental development. (A) Implantation at 6 to 7 days after conception; (B) prelacunar period (7 to 8 days); (C) beginning of lacunar period (8 to 9 days); (D) transition from lacunar period to primary villus stage (12 to 15 days); (E) secondary villus stage (15 to 21 days); and (F) tertiary villus stage (18 days to term). *BP*, Basal plate; *CP*, primary chorionic plate; *CT*, cytotrophoblast; *D*, decidua; *E*, endometrial epithelium; *EB*, embryoblast; *EG*, endometrial gland; *EM*, extraembryonic mesoderm; *EVT*, extravillous trophoblast; *IVS*, intervillous space; *J*, junctional zone; *L*, maternal lacunae; *M*, myometrium; *NF*, Nitabuch fibrinoid; *PB*, placental bed; *RF*, Rohr fibrinoid; *SA*, spiral artery; *ST*, syncytiotrophoblast; *T*, trabeculae; *TC*, trophoblast column; *TS*, trophoblastic shell. (Redrawn and modified from Kaufmann P. Entwicklung der Plazenta. In: Becker V, Schiebler TH, Kubli F, eds. *Die Plazenta des Menschen*. Stuttgart: Thieme Verlag; 1981:13–50.)

IMPLANTATION AND LACUNAR PERIOD

Implantation constitutes the first contact between the developing blastocyst and the uterine mucosa; it begins around 6 to 7 days after conception (Fig. 8.2A). At this contact zone, the placenta develops rapidly and continuously during the course of pregnancy, and from just after implantation the placenta controls fetomaternal exchange of nutrients, gasses, and waste products. While this exchange is common to all placentas, the gross and microanatomic structure, patterns of maternal-fetal interdigitation, and degree of integration of the fetal and maternal layers constituting the placenta vary considerably between mammalian species. The human placenta is of the most invasive type characteristic of those species with interstitial implantation—that is, that in which the blastocyst burrows completely beneath the surface of the uterine epithelium. Placental trophoblast cells invade as far as the myometrium, eroding maternal tissue so extensively that they become completely surrounded by, and in direct contact with, maternal blood. This type of placentation is called *hemochorial*.

Prior to implantation, the blastocyst consists of a single outer layer of epithelium, called the *trophectoderm*, and a cluster of inner cells called the *embryoblast* (see Fig. 8.2A). The trophectoderm is the direct precursor of all the trophoblast cells in the placenta, and ultimately forms the interface between maternal cells, maternal blood, and fetal cells. The embryoblast, on the other hand, contributes placental vasculature and surrounding mesenchyme,[10,11] interior to the trophoblast layers.

The trophectoderm consists of a single layer of trophoblast cells, more specifically called *cytotrophoblast cells*. At implantation, cytotrophoblast cells at the embryonic pole of the blastocyst adhere to the uterine epithelium, proliferate, and the outermost cells begin to fuse with each other (see Fig. 8.2A). This process results in a nascent multinucleated syncytium that, unlike the syncytium of the later chorionic villi, functions as an invasive structure, coordinating the entry of the blastocyst into the decidual stroma. Continued proliferation of the inner trophoblast cells, together with subsequent fusion of daughter cells with the overlying syncytium, is responsible for rapid and enormous increase in volume of the syncytiotrophoblast mass (prelacunar period; see Fig. 8.2B). As the blastocyst becomes more deeply embedded into the decidua, the syncytiotrophoblastic mass rapidly spreads along the outer walls of the blastocyst. Through this action, the blastocyst becomes completely encased within the decidual stroma, below the uterine surface epithelium (see Fig. 8.2C).[12]

The lacunar period of placental development (day 8 to day 13 after conception) begins with the appearance of a system of vacuoles within the syncytiotrophoblastic mass (see Fig. 8.2C). The syncytium erodes maternal capillaries and endometrial glands. As a result, lacunae fill with maternal cell-free blood components and glandular secretions, which together provide histiotrophic nutritional support of the embryo. While it is difficult or impossible to precisely elucidate the precise mechanisms by which the early syncytium coordinates implantation and invasion studies using human embryonic stem cells suggest that these cells do so by production of large quantities of MMPs, tissue inhibitors of matrix metalloproteinases (TIMPs), and through production of its own matrix proteins.[13] Further, these cells likely provide nutritive support to the embryo through transporters that carry ions, water, sugars, amino acids, and lipids across cellular membranes.

The areas of syncytiotrophoblast surrounding the lacunae form trabeculae, and this system of trabeculae and lacunae constitute the antecedents to the primary chorionic villi. Around day 12 after conception, proliferating cytotrophoblast cells start to push into the syncytial trabeculae toward the outermost trophoblast (commonly referred to as the trophoblastic shell) (see Fig. 8.2D). This expansion of cytotrophoblast accounts for longitudinal growth and branching of the trabeculae. Branches that end blindly and protrude into the lacunae are the primary villi (see Fig. 8.2D), while the trabeculae form *anchoring villi*, which connect the villus with the trophoblastic shell and not long afterwards, the decidua. With the appearance of the first primary villi, which remain encased by syncytium, the still-expanding lacunar system is called the *intervillous space*.

TRANSITION FROM THE LACUNAR PERIOD TO THE PRIMITIVE VILLOUS TREE

Around day 14 after conception, extraembryonic mesodermal cells grow out and migrate from the embryoblast and form a loose connective tissue layer above the primary chorionic plate.[11]

These cells begin to spread out from the embryonic disk along the inner trophoblastic surface of the blastocyst cavity, forming a loose network of branching cells, the extraembryonic mesenchyme.[11] This movement of cells thus adds another layer to the primary chorionic plate, which now consists of three layers: (1) the newly added extraembryonic mesoderm, (2) a middle layer of cytotrophoblast, and (3) an outer layer of syncytiotrophoblast facing the intervillous space (see Fig. 8.2D and E).

Between days 15 and 20 after conception, cells of the expanding extraembryonic mesenchyme push into the center of the primary villi, establishing a connective tissue core inside the villi, which were formerly purely trophoblastic. This mesenchymal core establishes them as secondary villi. This mesenchyme never fully reaches the trophoblastic shell: the segments of the anchoring villi that connect them to the trophoblastic shell remain wholly trophoblastic. These trophoblastic segments are called the *trophoblast cell columns* and consist of a voluminous core of proliferating cytotrophoblast cells and an incomplete and interrupted syncytial cover (see Fig. 8.2E). The column cytotrophoblast cells are the main source for longitudinal growth of the anchoring villi. In addition, these cells are the source of invasion: upon contact with the maternal uterine decidua, the trophoblast cells further differentiate and penetrate deeply into the uterus, forming an admixture of maternal and fetal cellular components—the so-called *junctional zone* (see later section, "Extravillous Trophoblast Invasion").

As the placenta continues along its developmental program, the mesenchymal cells constituting the core of the villi give rise to several cell types. In addition to forming fibroblasts, which supply much of the connective tissue of the villous cores, some cells differentiate into macrophages (Hofbauer cells) (see later in this chapter). Others form cords of hemangioblastic cells underlying the trophoblastic epithelium.[14] These endothelial precursors connect via desmosomes or tight junctions and gradually form lumina and vessels. Around day 20 after conception, the first fetal capillaries become apparent, a change that marks the transition from secondary into tertiary villi (see Fig. 8.2F).[15] The villous endothelial cells are of the non-fenestrated type and are linked by junctional complexes including both tight and adherens junctions, suggesting that in early gestation capillaries are highly plastic, permeable, and easily remodeled. Thus, tertiary villi are comprised of the trophoblastic epithelial layers, mesenchyme, and vascular networks: all the basic constituents of the placental barrier.

Concomitantly with the formation of villous capillaries, the vascularized allantois, which arises from embryonic hindgut, comes into contact and fuses with the mesenchyme of the chorionic plate.[2] Allantoic vessels rapidly grow out over the chorionic plate—that is, the fetal side of the placenta. With further branching and growth, these vessels grow into the villi and anastomose with the locally spreading networks of intravillous capillaries. Complete by around the fifth week after conception, these events establish the fetoplacental circulation.[2] In newly formed villous capillaries, continued hematopoiesis can be observed even after this stage.

THE MATERNOFETAL BARRIER

By definition, the maternofetal barrier is that which separates maternal and fetal blood within the intervillous space and placental vasculature, respectively. With the establishment of fetoplacental circulation, the barrier is formed and is composed of the following layers:

1. An outermost, continuous layer of syncytiotrophoblast covering the villi and thus lining the intervillous space.
2. A second layer of cytotrophoblast cells, which is continuous in the first trimester. As growth and branching of villi begin to offset cytotrophoblast proliferation during the second trimester, this layer becomes increasingly discontinuous, such that these cells are comparatively rare by term.
3. A basal lamina upon which the trophoblast layers rest.
4. Connective tissue, fibroblasts, and Hofbauer cells derived from the extraembryonic mesoderm.
5. The innermost fetal endothelium, which by the last trimester is surrounded by an endothelial basal lamina.

Qualitatively, this arrangement of cellular layers remains essentially the same until term. It is important, however, to note that quantitative changes occur over time. The thickness of the two trophoblast layers decreases from more than 15 μm in early pregnancy to a mean of 4.1 μm (see Table 8.1).[2] The cause of this general decrease in thickness is the transition of the trophoblast epithelium from a double- to a single-layered

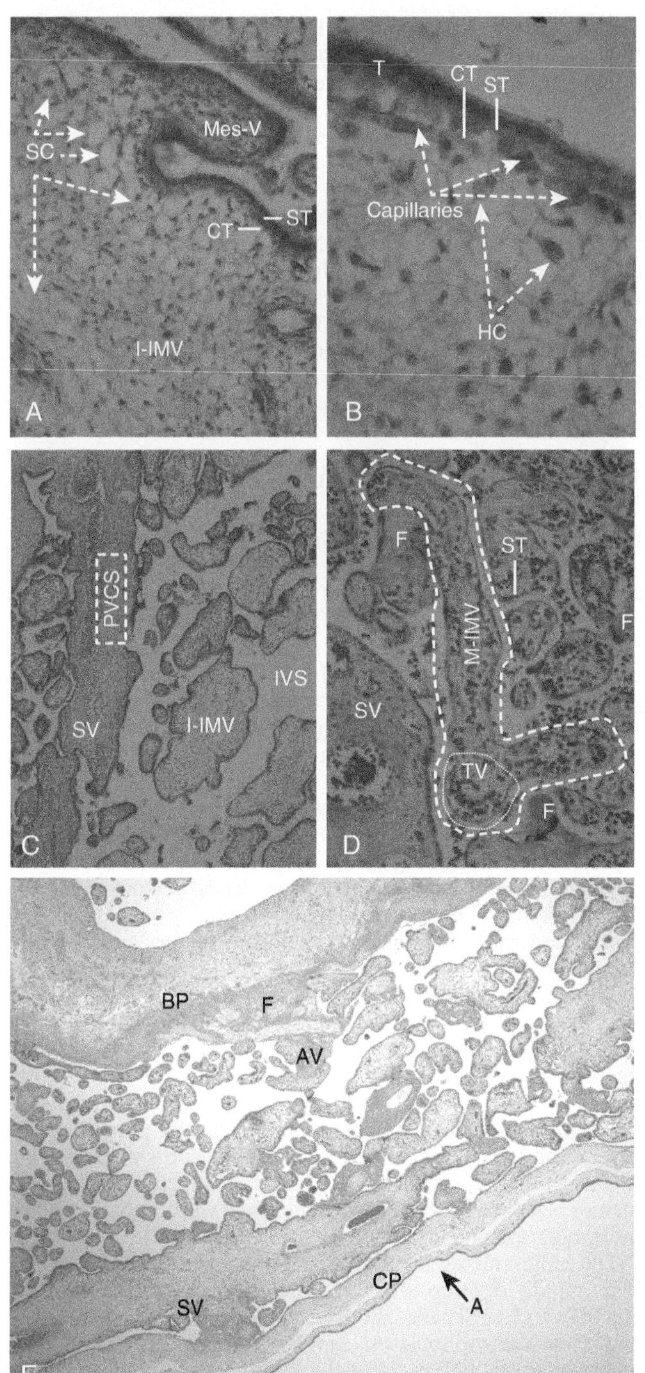

Fig. 8.3 Paraffin sections of placental villi illustrating typical histologic features of villous types. (A) (×200) and (B) (×400) show villi of a placenta of gestational week 10. Immature intermediate villi *(I-IMV)*, a mesenchymal villus *(Mes-V)* branching from an immature intermediate villus, Hofbauer cells *(HC)* inside such stromal channels (SC), the double-layered trophoblast epithelium (*CT*, cytotrophoblast; *ST*, syncytiotrophoblast), and the subtrophoblastic capillary network (capillaries) are labeled. (C) (×70) shows villi in a placenta of gestational week 18. The transition to the mature placental villous tree starts with condensation of the perivascular area of large stem villi *(SV)* originating at the chorionic plate. This new perivascular structure is the perivascular contractile sheath *(PVCS)*. I-IMV with uncondensed perivascular stroma still prevail in the surrounding of the stem villus. *IVS*, Intervillous space. (D) (×250) shows villi of a term placenta. The prevailing villous types are mature intermediate villi *(M-IMV, encircled by black dashed line)* and terminal villi (*TV*, *white dashed line)*, which are loops of sinusoidal capillaries bulging out of the mature intermediate villi thereby kinking these villi. Stem villi of various calibers *(SV)* are also frequent. Patches of fibrinoid *(F)* can occur in various positions. Note the singular layers of ST in the mature placenta. (E) Full-thickness section of a term placenta (×40) showing the basal plate *(BP)*, anchoring villus *(AV)*, SV, and the chorionic plate *(CP)*.

epithelium via increasing singularization of cytotrophoblast in the continually expanding surface of the villous tree (Fig. 8.3A and D). Additionally, regions of vasculosyncytial membranes—thin areas of the placental barrier at terminal villi that are thought to function primarily in gas exchange—appear during the second half of pregnancy (see Fig. 8.3D).

DEVELOPMENT OF THE CHORIONIC VILLOUS TREE

Primary, secondary, and tertiary villi represent the initial stages of growth of villous trees, from the initial appearance of primary villi as sequelae of the lacunar stage, through migration of extraembryonic mesenchyme to form secondary villi, and finally to appearance of vessels resulting in tertiary villi. The mature human placental villus tree (Fig. 8.4) consists of *stem villi*, the largest, central villi that provide mechanical support for the villous tree; *immature intermediate villi*, which give rise to *mesenchymal villi*, which in turn give rise to additional immature intermediate villi as branch points of the tree; *mature intermediate villi*, which branch directly off stem villi; and *terminal villi*, which branch off mature intermediate villi as the final ramifications of the villous tree. Below, we review the features, growth cycles, and functional significance of each type of placental villi, which collectively comprise the villous tree.

PHASE 1: EARLY DEVELOPMENT OF VILLI

Immediately after the appearance of the first tertiary villi (see earlier and Fig. 8.2), the newly formed villi start sprouting.

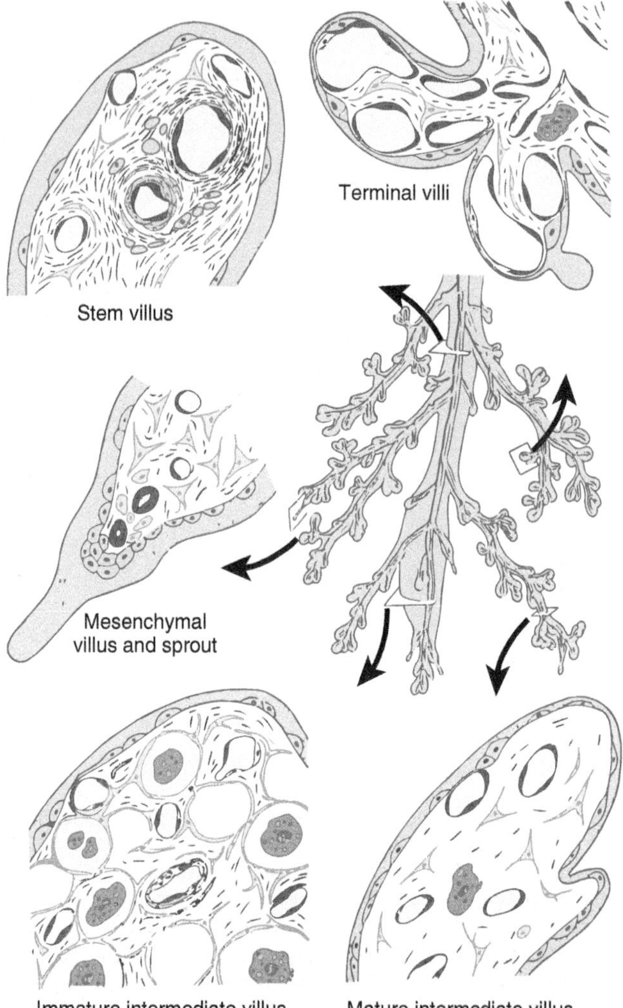

Fig. 8.4 Idealized peripheral part of the placental villous tree and typical cross-sections of the various villous types. Syncytiotrophoblast *(light purple)*, cytotrophoblast *(blue)*, endothelial cells *(red)*, noncontractile stromal cells and mesenchymal cells *(yellow)*, Hofbauer cells in stromal channels *(brown)*, and contractile cells in the arterial media and the contractile perivascular sheath *(orange)* of the stem villus are colored. (Redrawn and modified from Kaufmann P. Influence of ischemia and artificial perfusion on placental ultrastructure and morphometry. *Contrib Gynecol Obstet.* 1985;13:517.)

Trophoblast and underlying mesenchyme form protrusions; these sprouting villi are called *mesenchymal villi* (see Fig. 8.3A) and are the main source of combined trophoblastic-mesenchymal growth of the early villous tree.[16] High-level villi directly originating from the chorionic plate rapidly develop the appearance of *immature intermediate villi*, including numerous stromal channels inside the villi. This establishes the typical composition of the villous tree of the early first trimester: mesenchymal villi originate at various intervals, usually laterally, from immature intermediate villi. The mesenchymal villi themselves regularly develop into immature intermediate villi, which can then either give rise to new mesenchymal villi or mature into stem villi (Fig. 8.5). This cycle of villous growth is established at the transition from the lacunar stage to the villous stage of placental development and drives the first phase of villous maturation, which dominates until around week 20 of gestation.

PHASE 2: VILLOUS MATURATION UNTIL TERM

Starting as early as gestational weeks 15 to 17, the *trunci chorii*—that is, the villi originating directly from the chorionic plate—are the first to see the next wave of maturation, formation of stem villi (see Figs. 8.3C and E, 8.4, and 8.5). The perivascular zone of these large immature intermediate villi progressively loses its stromal channels, and the perivascular fibroblasts differentiate into myofibroblasts to form a contractile sheath, the function of which is not fully understood.[2,17-19] This change progresses in two directions: (1) longitudinally along the axis of the villi from the chorionic plate toward the basal plate, with concomitant loss of stromal channels; and (2) concentrically around their main vessels. In the latter, fibroblasts in the perivascular area differentiate into contractile myofibroblasts.[17-19] This maturation process is most pronounced between gestational weeks 22 and 28, although it can continue until term. At term, immature intermediate villi can persist in the center regions of cotyledons, but generally they are rare.

TYPES OF VILLI AND THEIR FUNCTIONAL SIGNIFICANCE

Human placental villi are classified by the vessels they contain, the thickness of the trophoblast epithelium, and the morphologic features of the villous core—all of which are direct reflections of their developmental stage.[2,20] Fig. 8.4 illustrates an idealized peripheral part of the villous tree containing all villous types mentioned above, and Fig. 8.5 illustrates the processes of villous growth by which they arise. Further, histologic evaluation of villous types in the placenta can be useful clinically to describe possible mismatches between gestational age and villous maturation.[2]

Development of all villi begins with the formation of primitive *mesenchymal villi* (see Figs. 8.3A, 8.4, and 8.5). These villi represent a transient stage of development and can be identified by their slender shape, densely packaged cytotrophoblasts, loosely arranged connective tissue stroma, and poorly developed vasculature that often do not yet show lumina and are thus unperfused.[16]

Mesenchymal villi first form as avascular trophoblastic sprouts via budding of syncytiotrophoblast. This is followed by entry of underlying proliferating cytotrophoblasts, connective tissue, and fetal endothelial cells into the sprouts. During the third to fifth weeks after conception, mesenchymal villi prevail and serve as the main source of trophoblastic-mesenchymal growth of the early villous tree. Very early on, they also perform essential roles in maternal-fetal exchange and endocrine activity.[2,16] In the mature placenta, in contrast, mesenchymal villi are the rarest and most inconspicuous villous type.

The earliest mesenchymal villi that originate from the chorionic plate rapidly develop into the immature intermediate villi (see Fig. 8.3A to C).[16] These villi dominate during the first trimester, and their subtrophoblastic capillary network (see Fig. 8.3B) identifies these villi as the main site of fetomaternal exchange during the first trimester. The typical structural features of immature intermediate villi include central arterioles and venules, accompanied by numerous superficially located capillaries, and a voluminous, reticular connective tissue. In mature placentas, however, immature intermediate villi are generally rare, as most have undergone further differentiation; they can only be found in small, restricted groups located in the centers of the villous trees.

Stromal channels (see Figs. 8.3A and B, and 8.4) are specific features of immature intermediate villi.[21] They are longitudinal spaces filled with extracellular fluid and lined by loosely arranged fibroblasts, which occur in the perivascular region around the central longitudinal axis of the main vessels. Inside, Hofbauer cells frequently occur (see Fig. 8.3B). The dilated characteristic of immature intermediate villi is a consequence of these voluminous perivascular zones with stromal channels. Stromal channels are a normal feature of villous development and should not be interpreted as "villous edema."

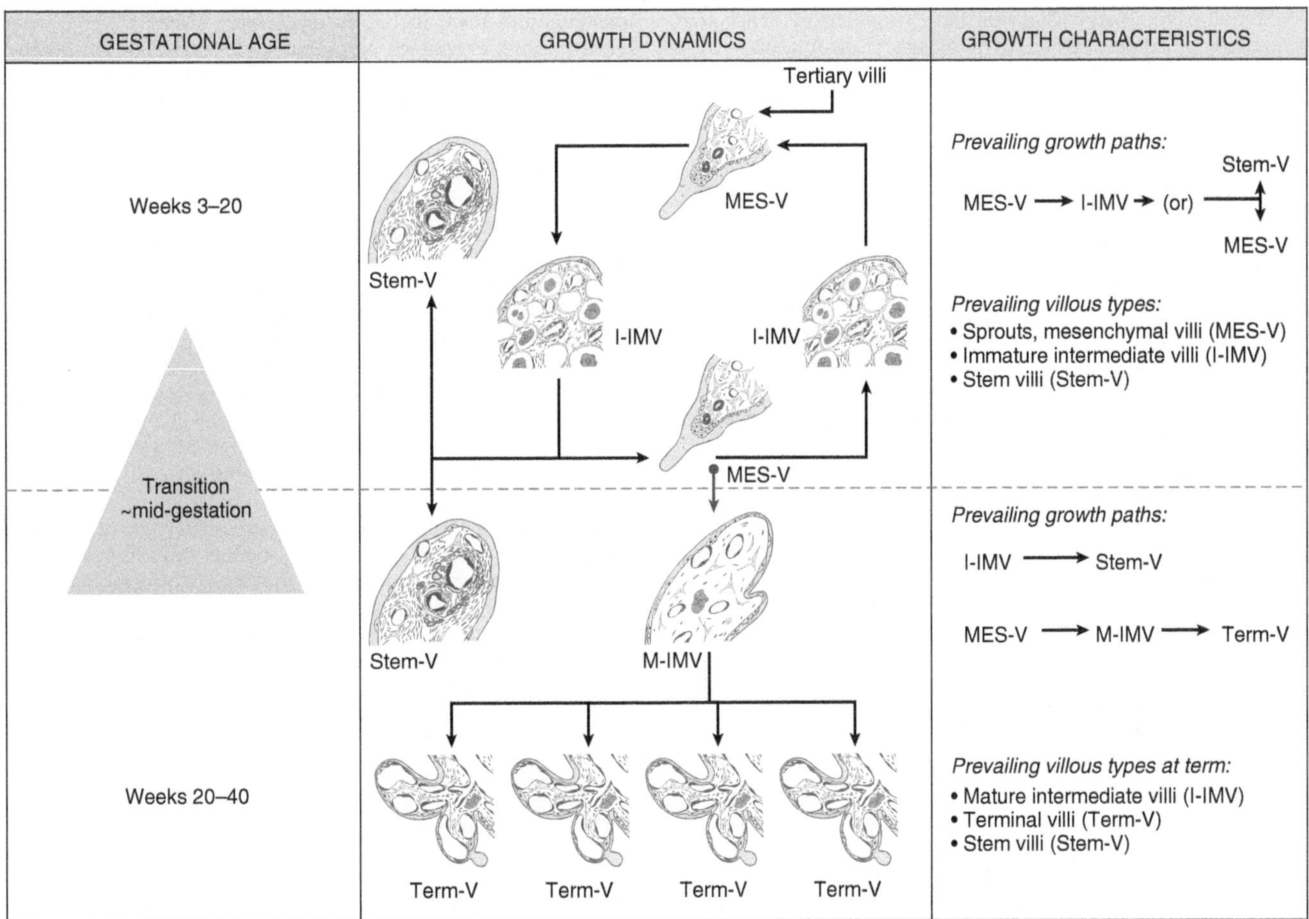

Fig. 8.5 Growth of placental villi throughout pregnancy. The timescale on the *left panel (Gestational Age)* shows the major phases of villous growth from ~3 weeks to term, while the *middle panel (Growth Dynamics)* represents the cyclic growth of villi. After formation of the first tertiary villi around day 18 *(upper panels)*, continuous growth occurs in a cycle based on sprouting of mesenchymal villi *(MES-V)*, differentiation of these villi into immature intermediate villi *[I-IMV]*) intermediate villi, and from these, further sprouting of mesenchymal villi. Some immature intermediate villi differentiate into stem villi *(Stem-V)*. During this early phase, the prevailing villous types *(right panel)* are sprouts and mesenchymal villi, immature intermediate villi, and stem villi. As growth progresses into the second and third trimesters (transition ~ mid-gestation; *lower panels*), increasing numbers of mesenchymal villi differentiate into mature intermediate villi *(M-IMV)* and terminal villi *(Term-V)*, which, along with stem villi, predominate at these stages.

The Hofbauer cells[22] that reside within stromal channels resemble the immunoregulatory phenotype of M2 antiinflammatory macrophages, and studies demonstrate they can be stimulated by multiple cytokines and steroid hormones. These cells play a vital role in placental development including vasculogenesis and angiogenesis. During placental inflammation they may secrete proinflammatory cytokines or mediators leading to villous cellular damage and fibrotic responses.

The immature intermediate villi are the precursors of *stem villi*, into which they are continuously transformed. Once matured, stem villi are characterized by centrally located arteries and veins or larger arterioles and venules surrounded by a stroma rich in connective tissue fibers and highly differentiated myofibroblasts.[18,19,23] Approximately one-third of the total villous volume of the mature placenta consists of stem villi.

Mature intermediate villi are bundles of slender, slightly curved villi that branch directly off stem villi, having also originated as mesenchymal villi (see Figs. 8.3D, 8.4, and 8.5). Most of vessels in these villi are capillaries, some of which are already sinusoidal and between which lie small arterioles and venules. The vessels are embedded in loose connective tissue, with scant fibers and cells. These villi are the main sites of growth and differentiation of terminal villi.[16]

Terminal villi branch off the mature intermediate villi, with a morphologic resemblance to a cluster of grapes. Their bulbous peripheral parts are characterized by numerous dilated capillaries, so-called ***sinusoids***, some of them with diameters up to 40 μm (see Figs. 8.3D, 8.4, and 8.5). The extremely high degree of fetal vascularization and the minimal fetomaternal diffusion distance (<4 μm) point to these villi as key sites of diffusional exchange in the mature placenta.

While the first phase of villous growth is dominated by immature intermediate and mesenchymal villi, the second phase is dominated by stem villi (the direct descendants of immature intermediate villi), mature intermediate villi, and terminal villi (see Fig. 8.5). During the first phase, immature intermediate villi are the hotspots of fetomaternal exchange, while during the second phase, mature intermediate villi and terminal villi take over this function. Regulation of these processes at the transition from gestational week 20 to 28 is considered important and possibly relevant for obstetric complications such as intrauterine growth restriction.

VILLOUS TROPHOBLAST DIFFERENTIATION, MAINTENANCE AND COMMUNICATION

The trophoblastic cover of the villi is the main site for secretory, fetomaternal communication, and maternofetal transfer functions. The villous cytotrophoblast serves as a progenitor cell, proliferating, differentiating, and finally fusing with the syncytiotrophoblast.[2] Quantitative assessments of trophoblast proliferation and syncytial fusion have provided evidence that it exceeds the needs for growth of syncytiotrophoblast by a factor of 5 to 6.[24] The excess production of syncytiotrophoblast is shed into the maternal circulation as extracellular vesicles, including syncytial nuclear aggregates (SNAs), microvesicles, and nanovesicles as mechanisms of disposal and/or communication.[25]

Syncytial fusion is an active process of differentiation, although elements known from the apoptosis cascade and expression of endogenous retroviral proteins make it very unique (Fig. 8.6). Syncytial fusion not only provides proteins and organelles, but likely also pre-transcribed and pre-processed mRNA to the syncytium; this may require high placental concentrations of ribonuclease inhibitor. After fusion, however, and contrary to prior dogma, transcription is maintained in a portion of the nuclei, likely to support the high metabolic and secretory activity this cell type.[26] Once residual transcription ceases, however, the heterochromatin massively aggregates.

The nuclei incorporated by syncytial fusion into the syncytiotrophoblast become aggregated (see Fig. 8.6) into SNAs. Histologically, the definition of these SNAs as knots or sprouts can only be determined by assessing nuclear characteristics, as not all syncytial protrusions containing nuclear aggregates represent SNAs. Rather, many of these structures noted on histologic examination are unavoidable tangential sections of the villous surfaces. Such artificial "trophoblast protrusions" are not only misleading mimics of apoptotic syncytial knots or trophoblastic (proliferative) sprouts in the early placenta. As a rule, true knots or sprouts are rare and section artifacts are frequent.[27]

SNAs are also shed from the placenta and are the largest of the extracellular vesicles released into the maternal circulation from the placenta. SNAs in the blood are likely either unintentional detachment of newly budding mesenchymal villi, or a consequence of the termination of syncytiotrophoblast life. SNAs generated in vitro from both early and term gestation placentas show markers of apoptosis, and it is postulated that this may be important to induce a maternal anti-inflammatory or tolerogenic response to the placenta.[28]

The placenta also releases micro- and nanovesicles into the maternal circulation. Exosomes are ~20 to 100 nm diameter nanovesicles produced by the syncytiotrophoblast and are detectable in the maternal circulation from around 6 weeks of gestation, with an increase in number over the course of pregnancy.[29] Interestingly, the numbers of exosomes in the maternal circulation during pregnancy complications such as preeclampsia or gestational diabetes are elevated compared to uncomplicated pregnancies. Exosome cargoes are comprised of proteins and RNA, including messenger RNA and micro-RNAs. Furthermore, exosomes are capable of regulating the biologic function of the target cell by the transfer of their contents. The potential for placental EVs to be used as a "real time" readout of placental or syncytial health during pregnancy is currently under investigation for many pregnancy complications.

TRANSFER ACROSS THE PLACENTAL BARRIER

The syncytiotrophoblast is a continuous, generally uninterrupted syncytial layer that extends over the surfaces of all villous trees; as such, it completely lines the intervillous space. Physiologic evidence supports the existence of two different routes of transfer across the placental barrier: a transcellular and a paracellular route.[30] The transcellular route involves transfer across the plasma membranes and the cytosol of the syncytiotrophoblast; this subject is reviewed in depth in a later chapter. In addition, there are two paracellular routes for transfer. First, gaps in the syncytiotrophoblast caused by degeneration or by mechanical forces can at least be partially repaired[31] but frequently are bridged by fibrin patches (see Fig. 8.3D). Approximately 7% of the villous surfaces in normal term human placentas show corresponding fibrin spots as replacement of the syncytiotrophoblast. Such areas may serve as paratrophoblastic routes for fetomaternal macromolecule transfer; in vitro, maternally injected horseradish peroxidase (molecular weight, 48,000 Da; molecular radius, 3.0 nm) was shown to pass through the fibrin spots into the fetal villous stroma. Second, transtrophoblastic channels with a diameter of approximately 20 nm provide a paracellular transfer route for smaller molecules.[32] These channels pass through the syncytiotrophoblast as winding and branching membrane-lined tubules from the apical to the basal surface. Morphologic evidence for a basoapical membrane flux along these channels suggests that they are likely to be routes for membrane recycling from the basal to the apical syncytiotrophoblastic plasmalemma.[32]

VILLOUS VASCULATURE DEVELOPMENT

Vasculogenesis begins around day 20 to 21 post-conception by formation of hemangioblastic cords that develop into primitive capillaries containing blood precursor cells. Within immature intermediate villi, the primitive capillaries form a capillary bed that spreads by branching angiogenesis, which dominates during the first trimester. These capillaries, which lie directly below the trophoblast epithelium (see Fig. 8.3B), will eventually connect to the allantoic and umbilical cord vessels around the end of the fifth week. They form a dense meshwork that links the central villous arteries and veins by short anastomosing vessels, and

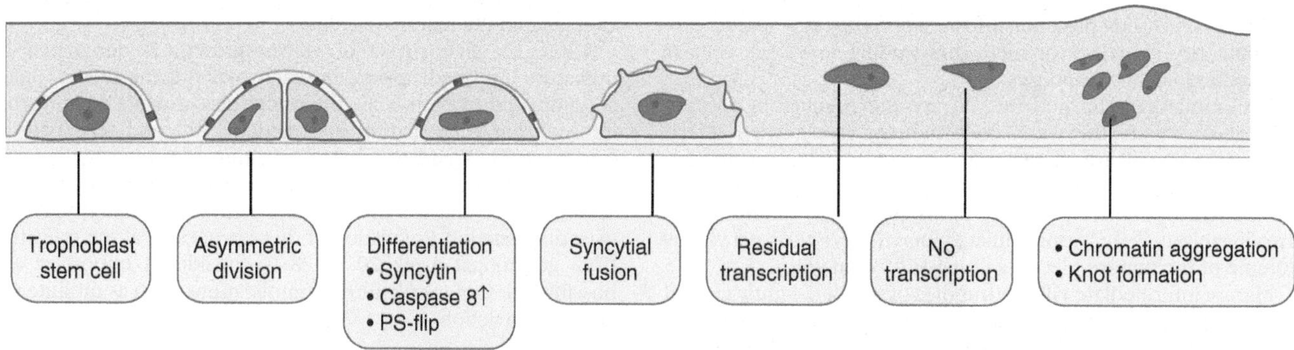

Fig. 8.6 Life cycle of villous trophoblast. From *left to right*: trophoblast stem cells divide, and daughter cells start differentiation along the villous pathway. Preparation for syncytial fusion with syncytiotrophoblast is associated with expression of syncytin, activation of caspase 8, and the flipping of phosphatidylserine to the outer leaflet of the plasma membrane *(PS-flip)*. All materials to be incorporated in the syncytium and required to maintain its full functionality are produced at a high rate prior to fusion. Syncytial fusion imports this cellular package into the syncytium. Transcription persists in the imported nuclei but declines rapidly to low rates. With final aggregation of heterochromatin and ceasing of transcription, the aged nuclear remnants can be aggregated, concentrated in syncytial knots, and extruded in the maternal circulation.

although they are in direct proximity to the subtrophoblastic basal lamina, they usually do not form sinusoidal loops; rather, they occur as small diameter capillaries.

By 4 weeks post conception, the capillaries are connected via the developing umbilical cord to the fetal heart, which has been beating by this time for about 1 week.[14] Despite the presence of an extensive capillary network within the early villi, there is as yet little evidence of an effective chorionic circulation during the first trimester.[33] Instead, the chorionic circulation develops over the second and third month of gestation, coinciding with maternal blood flow into the intervillous spaces. By week 15, large centrally located villi demonstrate regression of peripheral capillaries and remaining central capillaries acquire a tunica media and form arteries and veins.

Previously it was postulated that around week 24 of gestation, there is a definitive switch from branching to non-branching (the formation of capillary loops through elongation) angiogenesis, with non-branching angiogenesis occurring throughout the remainder of gestation.[2] More recently, utilizing novel imaging and reconstruction techniques, the occurrence of blind-ending capillary sprouts in terminal villi has been demonstrated.[34] In addition, the finding of immature endothelial junctional complexes in terminal villi in late pregnancy suggest retention of the capillary plasticity that is seen in the first trimester.[35] Thus, a definitive shift in the type of angiogenesis is questionable; further studies are required to settle this issue.[14]

As mature intermediate villi and terminal villi arise, sinusoidal capillaries and their associated vasculosyncytial membranes appear, becoming typical features of terminal villi (see Fig. 8.3D). Capillary endothelium of these villi is usually continuous, without pores or fenestrations. Macromolecular transfer is restricted to sizes below 20,000 dalton (Da); transfer of macromolecules is also influenced by molecular charge of molecules.[36]

EXTRAVILLOUS TROPHOBLAST INVASION

Characteristic of interstitial implantation is the establishment of placental circulation by means of extensive invasion of trophoblast cells, which occurs concomitantly with formation of villous trees. In the human placenta and in that of other hemochorial species, invasion is both deep and erosive. As soon as the early syncytiotrophoblast of the human blastocyst has invaded through the uterine epithelium, an epitheliochorial placental contact zone, which is typical for many other mammalian species, can no longer be established and is irreversibly lost. This initial invasive process positions the embryo for further penetration of the decidua, uterine glands, and maternal vasculature by trophoblast cells, ultimately functioning to establish uteroplacental circulation.

INTERSTITIAL TROPHOBLAST INVASION

Trophoblast invasion starts from the early trophoblastic shell—the leading edge of the syncytiotrophoblast mass (see Fig. 8.2C and D). From day 12 to 13 after conception onward, cytotrophoblasts enter the trophoblastic trabeculae to form primary villi; many of these cells remain in the villi, where, as described above, they serve as the basis for development and expansion of the villous trees. Other trophoblast cells focally penetrate the syncytiotrophoblast (see Fig. 8.2E), from whence they form columns that connect the villous trees to the basal plate. These villi are now called *anchoring villi*, and the trophoblast cells within their columns produce a matrix-type fibrinoid, which can be observed histologically, which serves to adhere the villi to the basal plate (see Fig. 8.3E).[37,38] Additionally, the trophoblast cells expand laterally to restructure the trophoblast shell to consist of mononuclear extravillous trophoblasts. Some of these cells remain in the shell as nonmigratory, polygonal cells that completely surround the embryo.[2] Other cells at the deepest aspect of the shell break away from each other, acquire an elongated spindle shape, become migratory, and invade the endometrium and myometrium (Fig. 8.7A).

This entry of trophoblast cells into the endometrium results in a mixture of maternal and fetal cells that stretches from the trophoblast shell to the superficial third of the myometrium, where trophoblast cells fuse to form multinucleate giant cells, possibly serving to limit trophoblast invasion. The *junctional zone* is the region of the endometrium where trophoblast cells intermingle with decidual cells and maternal leukocytes—particularly uterine NK cells and macrophages—between endometrial glands (see Fig. 8.7B and C). The superficial part of this zone, called the *basal plate*, consists of 1.0 to 1.5 mm of tissue that adheres to the placenta after placental separation and delivery at term. Those parts that remain in the uterus after delivery are called the *placental bed* and consist mainly of intact and necrotic endometrial tissue.

Trophoblast cells have been compared to cancer cells, as there are clear similarities between trophoblast invasion and tumor metastasis. Both cell types have a high propensity for proliferation and invasion, and they employ closely related mechanisms to accomplish this. Prototypical epithelial-to-mesenchymal transition (EMT) occurs during the shift of trophoblast cells from proliferative to invasive cells, and as tumor cells detach from the primary tumor to invade adjacent tissues. In each case, the cells lose polarity, downregulate E-cadherin, detach from their surroundings, and gain invasive and migratory properties. It has been postulated that to acquire metastatic potential, cancer cells regress to primitive developmental processes that are typical of embryonic cells by commandeering genes used by the embryo.[39] Supporting this postulate, many proteins that are expressed in the fetal-placental unit, including CEACAM1, PLAC1, osteopontin, 5T4, and several cancer-testis antigens, are re-expressed in a variety of cancers. It is important to recognize, however, that both proliferation and invasion in the placental bed halts within a comparatively short distance of the trophoblast shell. Within a few days after delivery of the placenta, extravillous trophoblast cells are eliminated, likely by maternal immune cells. Thus, unlike tumor invasion, trophoblast invasion is a tightly controlled physiologic process.

Fig. 8.8 summarizes important aspects of trophoblast invasion. The integrated network of cell-intrinsic and cell-extrinsic factors that control their migratory activity are complex and incompletely understood, but includes a host of epigenetic alterations, transcription factors, and signaling pathways intrinsic to the cells,[40,41] as well as contact-dependent and -independent mechanisms involving decidual cells and local immune cells.[42-44] Each of these mechanisms involves balances and counterbalances that act to fine-tune trophoblast invasion both regionally and temporally. One mechanism that may limit invasion is syncytial fusion: the limit of the invasive zone near the endometrial-myometrial border is marked by a layer of trophoblastic multinucleate giant cells that are derived from syncytial fusion and show no signs of further invasiveness.[45]

Phenotypically, trophoblast invasion manifests as a truly invasive process during which the trophoblast cells penetrate their host tissue using a combination of migratory and proteolytic activities. Trophoblast cells produce urokinase plasminogen activator, which can activate MMPs. MMPs, along with other matrix-degrading enzymes, are also produced by trophoblast cells, all serving to break down decidual extracellular matrix and make room for migratory trophoblast cells.[43,46] Offsetting this activity, and probably serving to limit trophoblast invasion, are inhibitory enzymes, including plasminogen activator inhibitor (PAI)-1/2 and tissue inhibitors of metalloprotease-1, by both trophoblast and decidual cells.

Alternative expression of cell adhesion molecules appears to be key in regulating the invasive function of trophoblast cells, as

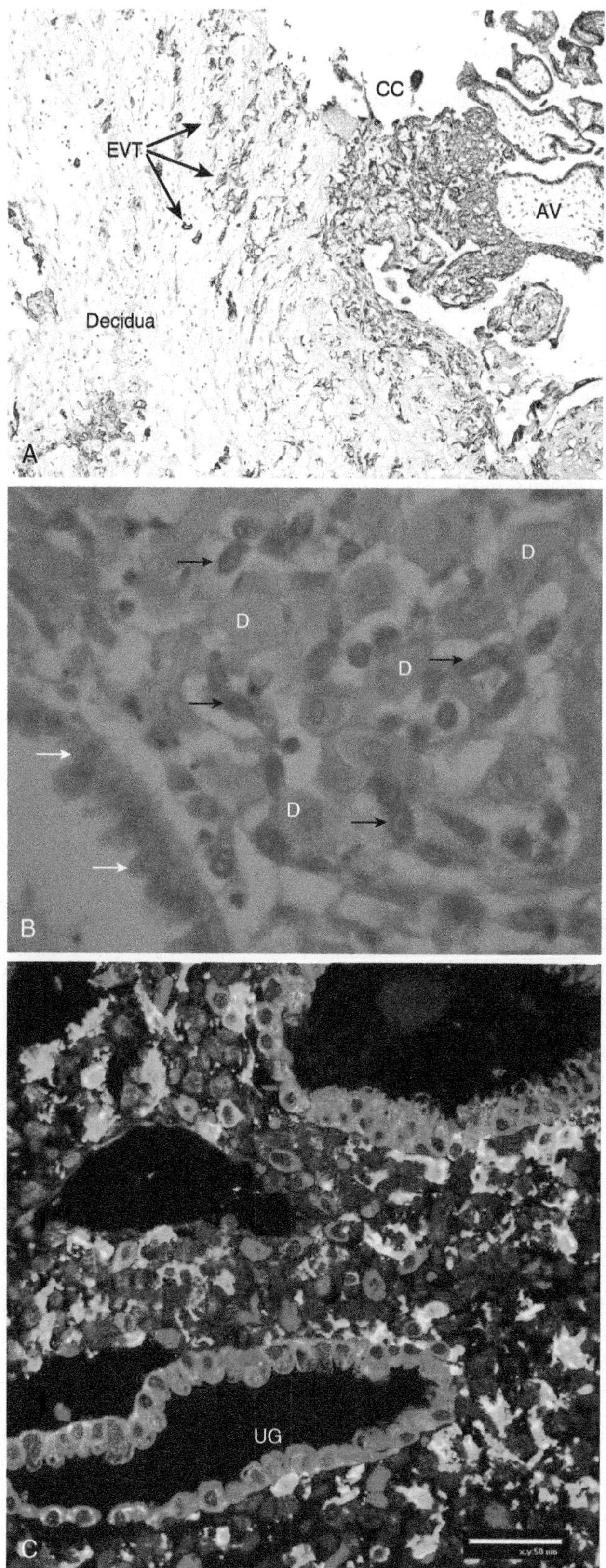

Fig. 8.7 Photomicrographs illustrating apposition between maternal immune and decidual cells and trophoblast cells in the junctional zone. (A) Frozen section of an anchoring villus *(AV)* and trophoblast cell column from a placenta 13 weeks after last menstruation (×100), with trophoblast cells emanating from the cell column *(CC)*. This section was immunostained for cytokeratin7, producing a red-brown stain that marks trophoblast cells as well as uterine gland *(UG)* epithelium. (B) Paraffin section of the junctional zone, week 10 after last menstruation (×400). The prevailing cell types are decidual cells *(D)*, the basophilic, spindle-shaped trophoblast cells *(black arrows)*, and glandular endometrial epithelium *(white arrows)*. (C) Immunofluorescence microscopy showing CD14+ macrophages *(green)* and cytokeratin-7–positive trophoblast and uterine gland epithelial cells *(red)* (enlarged from ×200 image). *EVT*, Extravillous trophoblast. (A, Hunt JS, Petroff MG. Immunologic aspects of pregnancy. In: Kay H, Nelson DM, Wang Y, eds. *The Placenta: From Development to Disease.* Chichester: Wiley-Blackwell; 2010. C, Hunt JS, Petroff MG. IFPA senior award lecture: reproductive immunology in perspective—reprogramming at the maternal-fetal interface. *Placenta*. 2013;34[suppl A]: S52–S55.)

there is a distinctive "switch" in integrin expression by trophoblast cells that likely enables invasive function.[47] Integrin α6β4, which is expressed in villous and proximal column trophoblast cells, is downregulated as the cells approach the decidua, whereas α5β1, absent from villous cytotrophoblast, is up-regulated in distal column cells. Loss of E-cadherin may also contribute to the loss of cell-cell contact and enhanced invasiveness.[48] This pattern of integrin and cell adhesion molecule switching is likely essential for proper invasion of trophoblast cells, as dysregulation of the switch is associated with diseases characterized by placental malinvasion.

Soluble factors produced by decidual cells and uterine NK cells are also key regulators of trophoblast migratory activity. Growth factors and cytokines produced by decidual cells can either promote (for instance, hepatocyte growth factor, epidermal growth factor) or inhibit (interferon-γ, transforming growth factor-β) trophoblast invasion.[43] Uterine NK cells are particularly numerous at the maternal-fetal interface, where they come into close contact with invading trophoblast cells. These cells possess unique properties, including a surface molecular phenotype ($CD56^{hi}CD16^{neg}$) similar to a comparatively rare population of peripheral blood NK cells, reduced killing activity, and a profile of chemokines and growth factors that indicate a trophic rather than a cytotoxic role at the maternal-fetal interface. Uterine NK cell production of CXCL8 and CXCL10 likely promote trophoblast invasion;[49] further, these cells play a critical role in adaptation of uterine spiral arteries for pregnancy (see below). On the other hand, uterine NK cells are suspected to limit trophoblast migration, not by direct killing activity, but rather through their production of soluble factors such as transforming growth factor (TGF)-β, Ang-2, and tumor necrosis factor (TNF).[42] Animal studies in which NK cells are experimentally depleted have also suggested that these cells restrict trophoblast invasion.[50] The unique noncytotoxic properties and growth factor profiles of NK cells can be explained by contact-dependent mechanisms involving expression of HLA-C, -E, and -G by trophoblast cells, and corresponding receptors on uterine NK cells.[51]

Other factors that control trophoblast migration include polarized M2 macrophages; these cells likely play a role in remodeling, control of inflammation, immune privilege, and immune defense at the maternal-fetal interface.[52] Low levels of oxygen that are present in the decidua during early pregnancy are thought to be important for promoting invasion; lack of proper sensing of oxygen levels may predispose the pregnancy to preeclampsia and other pathologies of the placenta.[53] Finally, the intrinsic ability of trophoblast cells to invade changes over the course of gestation is important: those of later gestational ages are much less invasive than those of an earlier gestational time point.[42]

ARTERIAL TROPHOBLAST INVASION

The onset of placental perfusion by maternal blood is one of the most important events of placental growth and occurs between weeks 8 and 12 of pregnancy. Until then, the embryo is nourished primarily via histiotrophic support from glandular secretions. The transition to primarily hemotrophic support is complete when maternal spiral arteries become directly connected with the intervillous space, and this conversion is absolutely critical to provide adequate delivery of nutrients to the rapidly growing fetus. More recently, trophoblast invasion of uterine venules, glands, and lymphatic vessels have been described, although the details of these processes have not been worked out.

To accomplish this, major alterations in maternal arterial vascular structure occur with the assistance of decidual leukocytes and trophoblast cells; this results in the transition of the arteries from narrow, high-resistance, low-flow vasoactive vessels, to low-resistance, high-flow vessels that lack vasoactive control. These alterations include a loss in media smooth muscle cells and elastic elements, and replacement of arterial endothelium by endovascular smooth muscle cells (see Fig. 8.8).[2,44,53-55] Earlier interpretations that these media changes are degenerative in nature are no longer accepted; rather, the dedifferentiated arterial walls redifferentiate into intact media layers within a few days after delivery, with loss of extravillous trophoblast cells.

Spiral artery transformation occurs in several stages, including a trophoblast-independent initial stage that involves swelling of smooth muscle and vacuolation of endothelial cells.[54] This process is thought to involve uterine NK cells and macrophages, which accumulate around the vessels early in pregnancy, possibly using secreted factors to disrupt smooth muscle organization.[42] Studies using mice that lack NK cells have identified a critical role for these cells in smooth muscle breakdown, possibly involving interferon-γ.[56] Although the fate of the smooth muscle cells is not known, a role for apoptosis-inducing factors produced by invading trophoblast cells has been suggested, with macrophages phagocytosing their remains.[42,43]

Inside the spiral artery lumina, extravillous trophoblast cells locally form endovascular plugs, possibly after retrograde migration of these cells into the vessels (see also Fig. 8.8). This process is thought to inhibit uteroplacental blood flow, which serves to maintain low oxygen concentrations in the early placenta, mitigating oxidative stress. By the time these plugs are released (it is not known by what mechanism this occurs), the placenta has increased its capacity to handle reactive oxygen species produced as a result of arterial oxygen brought in by maternal blood, by synthesis of the antioxidant enzymes catalase, glutathione peroxidase, and manganese and copper/zinc superoxide dismutase.[57] Endovascular extravillous trophoblast cells, which replace maternal endothelium, may induce apoptosis of maternal endothelial cells through production of death-inducing TNF family members TRAIL and Fas ligand, with subsequent phagocytosis of the cells by trophoblasts and/or macrophages.[43]

Among others, Moll and colleagues[55] have pointed out that because of the degree of physiologic changes in uteroplacental arteries, these vessels must be released from the vasomotor influences of the mother. This functional separation ensures unrestricted maternal blood supply to the placenta, regardless of maternal attempts to regulate the blood flow distribution within her own body; the mother cannot reduce the nutrient supply to the placenta without decreasing the nutrient supply to her own tissues.

Failure in transformation of spiral arteries results in reduced arterial dilatation and reduced intra-arterial trophoblast invasion, and is regularly observed in pregnancies complicated by preeclampsia, hypertension of pregnancy, and fetal intrauterine growth restriction.[58] By general agreement, failure of adaptation of the uteroplacental arteries to pregnancy, and thus preeclampsia and IUGR, are thought to be closely related to impaired trophoblast invasion. However, several different hypotheses concerning the nature of this impairment have been proposed. The classic view is that the possible mechanism is a general defect of trophoblast invasion,[59] possibly resulting from impaired expression of endothelial adhesion receptors such as vascular endothelial cadherin, platelet endothelial adhesion molecule-1, vascular endothelial adhesion molecule-1, α4 integrins, and αvβ3 integrin.[60] Furthermore, data have shown that interstitial trophoblast invasion may be normal, whereas invasion of vessel walls is inhibited by activated maternal macrophages that secrete TNFα and indoleamine-2,3-dioxygenase, both inducing apoptosis in trophoblast cells approaching the arterial walls.[61] It is especially unclear how the disturbance of invasion—occurring primarily during the first trimester of pregnancy—is connected to the development of the full clinical syndromes (IUGR, preeclampsia, or the combination of both) during the second half of pregnancy: how events occurring in early pregnancy are connected to the

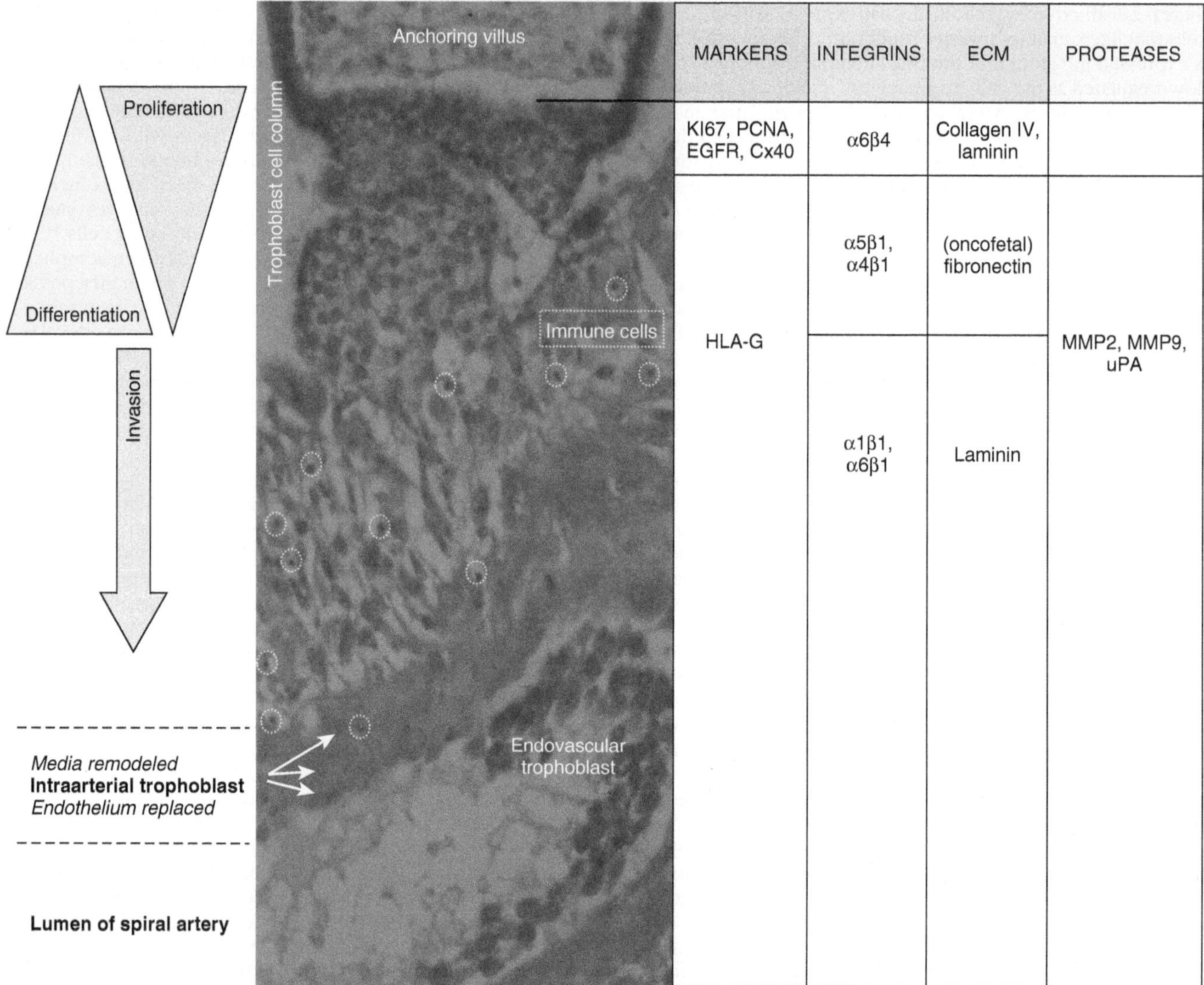

Fig. 8.8 The pathway of extravillous trophoblast differentiation. The middle part shows a microphotograph (×200) of an anchoring villus with attached trophoblast cell column, invasion zone, and a fully remodeled spiral artery. Nuclei of immune cells (lymphocytes, NK-cells) are labeled by *yellow dashed lines* and *circles*. Extravillous trophoblast cells can be found in the former media and lining the lumen of the spiral artery (intraarterial trophoblast). Numerous endovascular trophoblast cells occur in the lumen of the spiral artery. The distribution of proliferation, differentiation, and invasion are marked on the left side of the figure. Corresponding markers are allocated in the table on the right side of the figure. See text for details. *Cx40*, Connexin 40; *ECM*, extracellular matrix; *EGFR*, epidermal growth factor receptor; *HLA-G*, human leukocyte antigen-G; *KI67*, marker of profliferation Ki67; *MMP*, matrix metalloprotease; *PCNA*, proliferating cell nuclear antigen; *uPA*, urokinase plasminogen activator.

manifestation of disease during the second or third trimesters is as yet unknown.

SPECIAL FEATURES OF THE PLACENTA

SEPTA AND CELL ISLANDS

Placental septa and cell islands are oddly shaped conglomerations of fibrinoid, intermingled with groups of trophoblastic and decidual cells. These structures are not vascularized. If they are connected to the basal plate, they are called *septa*. These septa are columnar or sail-like structures rather than real septa. They cannot divide the intervillous space into separate maternally perfused chambers (see Fig. 8.1). They are interpreted as dislocations of basal plate tissue into the intervillous space, caused by lateral movement and folding of the uterine wall and basal plate over each other. Parts of such septa detached from the basal plate and then attached to neighboring villi are called *cell islands*.

Similar islands, without decidual contribution, may be formed from villous tips that have not been opened up by connective tissue and fetal vessels during transition from primary to tertiary villi. In such cases, the cytotrophoblastic core proliferates and subsequently becomes largely transformed into fibrinoid. These cell islands are growth zones for the attached villous stems, comparable to cell columns.[2]

FETAL MEMBRANES

Once the embryo becomes completely encased within the decidua, the processes of formation of the villi and extravillous trophoblast—particularly those comprising the trophoblast shell—occur around the entire chorionic sac. At the pole where umbilical cord is attached to the chorionic plate—that is, the pole deeper within the decidua—villous development occurs more rapidly (see Fig. 8.2C), leaving larger and more developed villi. This side will continue to grow and form the definitive placenta; at the opposite pole, starting around

4 weeks, the newly formed villi will degenerate and the surrounding intervillous space is obliterated. As a consequence, the chorionic plate at this side, including the villous remnants, fuse with the surrounding decidua to form a multilayered compact lamella, the smooth chorion (*chorion laeve*). Formation of the smooth chorion starts opposite to the implantation pole, from where it spreads over approximately 70% of the surface of the chorionic sac until the fourth month of gestation, when the process stops.[2,10] Between weeks 7 and 10 of pregnancy, the expanding amniotic sac comes into contact with the smooth chorion. In most places, the mesenchymal layers of both membranes fuse.

With complete implantation, the decidua recloses over the blastocyst, bulging into the uterine lumen, and is called the *capsular decidua*. With the increasing diameter of the chorionic sac, the capsular decidua locally touches the parietal decidua of the opposing uterine wall. Between weeks 15 and 20 after conception, both decidual layers fuse with each other, thereby obstructing the uterine cavity. From this point onward, the smooth chorion has contact over nearly its entire surface with the decidual surface of the uterine wall and may function as a paraplacental exchange organ. Owing to the absence of fetal vascularization in the smooth chorion and the amnion, all paraplacental material exchanged between fetal membranes and fetus has to pass through the amniotic fluid.

At term, the fetal membranes are structured as follows (see Fig. 8.1).[2] The mean thickness of the membranes, after separation from the uterine wall during labor, is approximately 200 to 300 μm. The innermost layer, the amniotic epithelium, encloses the amniotic fluid. Amniotic epithelium may be involved in the production of the fluid and even partially responsible for its resorption. Moreover, it seems to be involved in pH regulation of the amniotic fluid.[62] Together with the lamina propria, it measures 30 to 60 μm in thickness.

The next layer consists of chorionic connective tissue, which is directly adherent to a cytotrophoblastic layer of variable thickness. Near the placental margin, the thickness increases because persisting ghost villi, embedded in fibrinoid, split the cytotrophoblast into two layers. At the placental margin, these two layers completely disjoin by interposition of the intervillous space, and they become the chorionic and the basal plates (see Fig. 8.1). Attached to the outer surface of the cytotrophoblast is a decidual layer approximately 50 μm thick. The latter finding indicates that the separation of membranes does not take place along the maternofetal interface but instead occurs at a somewhat deeper level.

CHORIONIC PLATE/UMBILICAL CORD

At day 14 after conception, the primary chorionic plate consists of three layers: extraembryonic mesenchyme, cytotrophoblast, and syncytiotrophoblast (see Fig. 8.2D and E). These layers separate the intervillous space from the blastocystic cavity. Between 8 and 10 weeks after conception, the amniotic sac has expanded to such a degree that the amniotic mesenchyme comes into close contact with the mesenchymal surface of the chorionic plate and the smooth chorion. As soon as amniotic and chorionic plate mesenchyme fuse with each other, the definitive chorionic plate is formed (see Figs. 8.1 and 8.3E).

As part of the same process, the expanding amniotic sac surrounds the connective stalk and the allantois and joins them to form the umbilical cord. The allantoic vessels—two arteries and one vein—grow in thickness and length and convert into the umbilical vessels. The allantoic epithelium gradually disappears; small vesicular remnants of the allantois, however, may persist until term. The allantoic mesenchyme differentiates into a complex system of myofibroblasts that probably help in regulating turgor of the cord and avoid bending of the latter, which can have fatal consequences for the fetus.[63] Fusion of the umbilical vessels with the intravillous vessel system establishes a complete fetoplacental circulation at the end of the fifth week after conception. The cord is characterized by a spiral twisting, the number of spiral turns increasing as pregnancy progresses, up to a maximum of 380 turns. In most cases, the twist is leftward, or counterclockwise. The twists have been interpreted to originate with rotary movements of the fetus resulting from asymmetric uterine contractions.[2]

CONCLUSION

The past 40 years have seen a surge of recognition by the scientific community of the placenta and its associated membranes as having great importance to the health of both the mother and the neonate. Maldevelopment of the placenta predisposes the mother to preeclampsia and the fetus to intrauterine growth restriction, life-threatening conditions that occur prior to term pregnancy. Preterm birth is closely tied to health of the placenta and extraplacental membranes, and results from initiation of labor often too early for fetal survival without dramatic intervention. Each of these conditions is associated with long-term sequelae: a relationship between the placenta and developmental origins of health and disease (DOHaD) has become increasingly apparent, the placenta serving as a harbinger for the future health of the child and adult. Finally, the placenta is now recognized as a source of stem cells that offer hope for treatment and cures for immunologic, neurologic, and other diseases. Collectively, these findings have sparked not only a flurry of interest into the basic science of the placenta, but also its recognition as a clinically important organ to heed during pre- and postnatal care.

ACKNOWLEDGMENTS

This chapter is a rewritten and updated form of a chapter appearing in a prior edition of this work, written by Dr. Hans-Georg Frank. Portions of the figures and writing remain Dr. Frank's words. The authors are indebted to Dr. Frank's contribution to the knowledge of placental structure, histopathology, and development as the scientific community understands it today.

A complete reference list is available at www.ExpertConsult.com. 

SELECT REFERENCES

1. Longo LD, Reynolds LP. Some historical aspects of understanding placental development, structure and function. *Int J Dev Biol*. 2010;54:237-255.
2. Benirschke K, Burton GJ, Baergen RN. *Pathology of the Human Placenta*. New York: Springer-Verlag; 2012.
3. Collins SL, Birks JS, Stevenson GN, et al. Measurement of spiral artery jets: general principles and differences observed in small-for-gestational-age pregnancies. *Ultrasound Obstet Gynecol*. 2012;40:171-178.
4. Collins SL, Stevenson GN, Noble JA, Impey L. Developmental changes in spiral artery blood flow in the human placenta observed with colour Doppler ultrasonography. *Placenta*. 2012;33:782-787.
5. Gellersen B, Brosens JJ. Cyclic decidualization of the human endometrium in reproductive health and failure. *Endocrine Rev*. 2014;35:851-905.
6. Colucci F. The role of KIR and HLA interactions in pregnancy complications. *Immunogenetics*. 2017;69:557-565.
7. Erlebacher A. Immunology of the maternal-fetal interface. *Annu Rev Immunol*. 2013;31:387-411.
9. Paiva P, Menkhorst E, Salamonsen L, Dimitriadis E. Leukemia inhibitory factor and interleukin-11: critical regulators in the establishment of pregnancy. *Cytokine Growth Factor Rev*. 2009;20:319-328.
10. Boyd JD, Hamilton WJ. *The Human Placenta*. Cambridge: Heffer; 1970.
11. Enders AC, King BF. Formation and differentiation of extraembryonic mesoderm in the rhesus monkey. *Am J Anat*. 1988;181:327-340.
12. Enders AC. Trophoblast differentiation during the transition from trophoblastic plate to lacunar stage of implantation in the rhesus monkey and human. *Am J Anat*. 1989;186:85-98.
13. Yabe S, Alexenko AP, Amita M, et al. Comparison of syncytiotrophoblast generated from human embryonic stem cells and from term placentas. *Proc Natl Acad Sci U.S.A*. 2016;113:E2598-E2607.
14. Burton GJ, Charnock-Jones DS, Jauniaux E. Regulation of vascular growth and function in the human placenta. *Reproduction*. 2009;138:1470-1626.

15. Demir R, Kaufmann P, Castelluce M, Erbeng T, Kotowsk A. Fetal vasculogenesis and angiogenesis in human placental villi. *Cells Tissues Organs*. 1989;136:190-203.
16. Castellucci M, Kosanke G, Verdenelli F, Huppertz B, Kaufmann P. Villous sprouting: fundamental mechanisms of human placental development. *Hum Reprod Update*. 2000;6:485-494.
18. Graf R, Matejevic D, Schuppan D, et al. Molecular anatomy of the perivascular sheath in human placental stem villi: the contractile apparatus and its association to the extracellular matrix. *Cell Tissue Res*. 1997;290:601-607.
20. Castellucci M, Schepe M, Scheffen I, Celona A, Kaufmann P. The development of the human placental villous tree. *Anat Embryol*. 1990;181:117-128.
21. Castellucci M, Schweikhart G, Kaufmann P, Zaccheo D. The stromal architecture of the immature intermediate villus of the human placenta: functional and clinical implications. *Gynecol Obstet Invest*. 1984;18:95-99.
22. Zulu MZ, Martinez FO, Gordon S, Gray CM. The elusive role of placental macrophages: the hofbauer cell. *J Innate Immun*. 2019;11:447-456.
24. Huppertz B, Frank HG, Kingdom JCP, Reister F, Kaufmann P. Villous cytotrophoblast regulation of the syncytial apoptotic cascade in the human placenta. *Histochem Cell Biol*. 1998;110:495-508.
25. Tong M, Chamley LW. Placental extracellular vesicles and feto-maternal communication. *Cold Spring Harb Perspect Med*. 2015;5(3):a023028.
26. Ellery PM, Cindrova-Davies T, Jauniaux E, Ferguson-Smith AC, Burton GJ. Evidence for transcriptional activity in the syncytiotrophoblast of the human placenta. *Placenta*. 2009;30:329-334.
29. Salomon C, Rice GE. Role of exosomes in placental homeostasis and pregnancy disorders. *Prog Mol Biol Transl Sci*. 2017;145:163-179.
30. Sibley CP, Brownbill P, Glazier JD, Greenwood SL. Knowledge needed about the exchange physiology of the placenta. *Placenta*. 2018;64:S9-S15.
31. Simán CM, Sibley CP, Jones CJP, Turner MA, Greenwood SL. The functional regeneration of syncytiotrophoblast in cultured explants of term placenta. *Am J Physiol Regul Integr Comp Physiol*. 2001;280:R1116-R1122.
32. Kertschanska S, Kosanke G, Kaufmann P. Is there morphological evidence for the existence of transtrophoblastic channels in human placental villi? *Placenta*. 1994;15:581-596.
33. Burton GJ, Jauniaux E. Development of the human placenta and fetal heart: synergic or independent? *Front Physiol*. 2018;9:373.
34. Jirkovská M, Janáček J, Kaláb J, Kubínová L. Three-dimensional arrangement of the capillary bed and its relationship to microrheology in the terminal villi of normal term placenta. *Placenta*. 2008;29:892-897.
35. Leach L, Babawale MO, Anderson M, Lammiman M. Vasculogenesis, angiogenesis and the molecular organisation of endothelial junctions in the early human placenta. *J Vasc Res*. 2002;39:246-259.
36. Firth JA, Bauman KF, Sibley CP. Permeability pathways in fetal placental capillaries. In: *Placental Vascularization and Blood Flow 163-177*. Boston: Springer; 1988.
38. Kaufmann P, Huppertz B, Frank HG. The fibrinoids of the human placenta: origin, composition and functional relevance. *Ann Ana*. 1996;178:485-501.
39. Murray MJ, Lessey BA. Embryo implantation and tumor metastasis: common pathways of invasion and angiogenesis. *Semin Reprod Endocrinol*. 1999;17:275-290.
40. van Dijk M, Oudejans C. Epigenetic control of human trophoblast invasion. *Front Gene*. 2014;5:38.
42. Lash GE. Molecular cross-talk at the feto-maternal interface. *Cold Spring Harb Perspect Med*. 2015;5:a023010.
43. Cartwright JE, Fraser R, Leslie K, Wallace AE, James JL. Remodelling at the maternal-fetal interface: relevance to human pregnancy disorders. *Reproduction*. 2010;140:803-813.
44. Ji L, Brkić J, Liu M, et al. Placental trophoblast cell differentiation: physiological regulation and pathological relevance to preeclampsia. *Mol Aspects Med*. 2013;34:981-1023.
45. Kaufmann P, Castellucci M. Extravillous trophoblast in the human placenta. *Placenta*. 1997;18:21-65.
46. Pollheimer J, Vondra S, Baltayeva J, Beristain AG, Knöfler M. Regulation of placental extravillous trophoblasts by the maternal uterine environment. *Front Immunol*. 2018;9:2597.
47. Damsky CH, Librach C, Lim KH, et al. Integrin switching regulates normal trophoblast invasion. *Development*. 1994;120:3657-3666.
48. Zhou Y, Fisher SJ, Janatpour M, et al. Human cytotrophoblasts adopt a vascular phenotype as they differentiate: a strategy for successful endovascular invasion? *J Clin Invest*. 1997;99:2139-2151.
49. Hanna J, Goldman-Wohl D, Hamani Y, et al. Decidual NK cells regulate key developmental processes at the human fetal-maternal interface. *Nat Med*. 2006;12:1065-1074.
50. Chakraborty D, Karim Rumi MA, Konno T, Soares MJ. Natural killer cells direct hemochorial placentation by regulating hypoxia-inducible factor dependent trophoblast lineage decisions. *Proc Natl Acad Sci U. S. A*. 2011;108:16295-16300.
51. Trowsdale J, Moffett A. NK receptor interactions with MHC class I molecules in pregnancy. *Sem Immunol*. 2008;20:317-320.
52. Yao Y, Xu XH, Jin L. Macrophage polarization in physiological and pathological pregnancy. *Fronti Immunol*. 2019;10:792.
54. Pijnenborg R, Vercruysse L, Hanssens M. The uterine spiral arteries in human pregnancy: facts and controversies. *Placenta*. 2006;9-10:939-958.
55. Moll W, Nienartowicz A, Hees H. Blood flow regulation in the uteroplacental arteries. In: Kaufmann P, Miller R, eds. *Placental Vascularization and Blood Flow*. Boston: Springer; 1988:83-96.
56. Ashkar AA, Di Santo JP, Croy BA. Interferon γ contributes to initiation of uterine vascular modification, decidual integrity, and uterine natural killer cell maturation during normal murine pregnancy. *J Exp Med*. 2000;192:259-270.
57. Hempstock J, Jauniaux E, Greenwold N, Burton GJ. The contribution of placental oxidative stress to early pregnancy failure. *Hum Pathol*. 2003;34:1265-1275.
58. Brosens I. The utero-placental vessels at term—the distribution and extent of physiological changes. In: Kaufmann P, Miller R, eds. *Placental Vascularization and Blood Flow*. Boston: Springer; 1988:61-67.
60. Zhou Y, Damsky CH, Fisher SJ. Preeclampsia is associated with failure of human cytotrophoblasts to mimic a vascular adhesion phenotype: one cause of defective endovascular invasion in this syndrome? *J Clin Invest*. 1997;99:2152-2164.
61. Reister F, Frank H-G, Kingdom JCP, et al. Macrophage-induced apoptosis limits endovascular trophoblast invasion in the uterine wall of preeclamptic women. *Lab Investig*. 2001;81:1143-1152.

9 Regulation of the Placental Circulation

Imran N. Mir | Charles R. Rosenfeld

OVERVIEW

Pregnancy is associated with numerous alterations to the maternal cardiovascular system; however, it is the development of the low-resistance, high-flow placental vascular bed that characterizes this physiologic state. Moreover, this vascular bed is unique in that it is composed of maternal and fetal components separated by several cell layers that differ in structure and function among the mammalian species studied.[1] Although these two vascular beds are intimately associated with each other, they function independently.[2-4] An understanding of the mechanisms that control their vascular tone and the magnitude of blood flow is important in that alterations in either the maternal or the fetal aspect of placental blood flow may modify the delivery of oxygen and/or nutrients to the fetus, as well as affect the removal of carbon dioxide and other fetal metabolic wastes.[5] Thus, the integrity of the maternal uteroplacental and fetal umbilicoplacental vascular beds is essential to fetal growth and development, minute-to-minute fetal well-being, and possibly alterations in fetal programming that contribute to the subsequent occurrence of adult-onset cardiovascular and/or metabolic disease.[6,7]

In view of the importance of the placental vascular beds to fetal well-being and survival of the species, research in this area has been intense since the time of Barcroft's research.[8] Because detailed studies in humans remain problematic and are generally descriptive,[9] current understanding reflects in large part experimental observations in various animal models and, in particular, the pregnant ewe. Thus, conclusions about the relative importance of the mechanisms responsible for the control of blood flow to these vascular beds in the human continue to require careful interpretation.[10] Nonetheless, recent knowledge obtained from animal models—and in particular, sheep—has been replicated in studies of human uterine arteries. Thus, sheep studies provide an excellent basis for characterizing this aspect of pregnancy and improving our understanding of clinical data obtained in Doppler flow velocity studies in women.[11]

DEVELOPMENT OF THE UTEROPLACENTAL AND UMBILICOPLACENTAL VASCULAR BEDS

Although the placenta is of fetal origin and composed solely of fetal cells, its blood supply is derived from the maternal uterine and fetal umbilical arteries, the former serving as the source of placental and fetal oxygen and nutrients. Both vascular beds undergo substantial independent modification throughout pregnancy. For example, the maternal uterine vasculature undergoes remodeling,[12] and the fetal vasculature exhibits ongoing vasculogenesis, angiogenesis, and branching morphogenesis.[13] These changes occur in parallel and are essential in providing the increasing requirements for oxygen and nutrient delivery necessary for the logarithmic fetal growth in the last third of pregnancy, and the increasing endocrine and metabolic functions of the placenta. Understanding these independent, yet parallel, modifications will facilitate our knowledge of fetal growth, maintenance of fetal well-being, and possibly the origins of some pregnancy-related diseases (e.g., preeclampsia).

In women, the uteroplacental vascular bed is composed of cotyledons, lobes, or placentomes similar to those seen in many species.[1] In contrast with their counterparts in the sheep or cow, these structures adhere to each other, rather than existing as separate entities. Nonetheless, they can be identified as individual structures when viewed from the basal or maternal side of the placenta after its delivery. Each placentome receives its maternal arterial blood by way of a ***single*** spiral artery, and alterations in the tone of these and/or more proximal branches of the uterine artery are responsible for modifying the magnitude and distribution of maternal uteroplacental blood flow.[12,14] As in pregnant sheep, a fixed number of placentomes are ultimately available in normal human pregnancy. Therefore, the rise in maternal uterine blood flow during pregnancy is initially due to the development of the placenta (i.e., implantation and growth) and vasodilation of the spiral arteries, allowing for increases in perfusion of the intervillous space.[15]

When maternal uteroplacental blood flow is examined throughout ovine gestation, a complex scenario is observed.[16] Total uterine blood flow (Fig. 9.1B) increases nearly 40-fold during the course of a normal singleton pregnancy, and levels are even higher in multiple gestations. This increase is coincident with a doubling of maternal cardiac output and an increase in the proportion of cardiac output directed to the uterus, increasing from less than 1% of cardiac output in nonpregnant sheep to nearly 25% at term.[17] The pattern of this increase in total ovine uterine blood flow (mL/min) occurs in three phases (see Fig. 9.1B). The first is associated with relatively low absolute

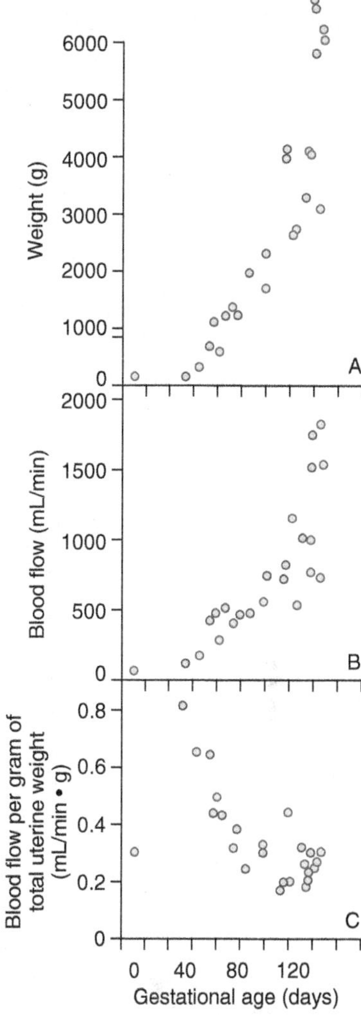

Fig. 9.1 Changes in uterine weight (A), blood flow (B), and blood flow per gram of total uterine weight (C) during ovine pregnancy. Total weight is the sum of all metabolically active tissues. *Blue circle*, twin pregnancy; *red circle*, singleton pregnancy. (From Rosenfeld CR, Morriss FH, Jr, Makowski EL, et al. Circulatory changes in the reproductive tissues of ewes during pregnancy. *Gynecol Invest.* 1974;5:252.)

blood flows, which on the basis of uterine plus conceptus wet weight is actually high, achieving values of 0.8 mL/min•g, compared with 0.3 mL/min•g for the nonpregnant uterus (see Fig. 9.1C). This increase in uterine blood flow is believed to reflect vasodilation secondary to the increased production of maternal ovarian and possibly fetal hormones (e.g., estrogen, progesterone), which may be required for survival of the conceptus before implantation and the initial phase of implantation and placentation.[18,19] In primates and women, this occurs in the first days or weeks of pregnancy. The second phase is associated with the development of the fetal placentomes and in the primate, with the development of the intervillous spaces or the maternal placental vascular bed. At this time, the anatomic maternal placental vascular bed achieves its maximum size. If this does not occur, placentation will be restricted, resulting in a small placenta and a fetus characterized by proportionate growth restriction. In sheep, total uterine blood flow plateaus at this time and averages approximately 500 mL/min; however, blood flow expressed on a weight basis at the same point in gestation (which takes into account metabolically active

Table 9.1 Pathways for Vasoactive Substances That Contribute to the Regulation of the Uteroplacental and Umbilicoplacental Circulations.

	Uteroplacental Circulation	**Umbilicoplacental Circulation**
Angiotensin II (ANG II)	Type 2 ANG II receptor accounts for >80% of binding in UA VSM and decreases ANG II sensitivity, as does reciprocal synthesis of endothelium-derived nitric oxide (NO) and prostacyclin (PGI_2), all contributing to the refractoriness to ANG II in pregnancy.	Type 1 ANG II receptor accounts for >90% of binding, and with advanced functional maturation of umbilical artery, VSM accounts for the increased sensitivity to vasoconstricting effects of ANG II compared to fetal systemic arteries and vascular beds.
Catecholamines	Potent vasoconstrictor effects mediated via VSM α-adrenergic receptors, but in pregnancy is attenuated by substantial increases in endothelium-derived NO.	Refractoriness to the vasoconstrictor effects are poorly studied but may reflect low receptor expression or function and/or high endothelial NO synthesis.
Arginine vasopressin (AVP)	VSM refractoriness to the vasoconstrictor effects, but the mechanisms are unclear. Could reflect alterations in receptor expression and/or function.	VSM is refractory to the vasoconstrictor effects; mechanisms are unclear.
Endothelin-1 (ET-1)	Potent vasoconstrictor mediated via ET-A and ET-B_2 receptors in VSM.	Vasoconstrictor effects mediated via ET-A and ET-B_2 receptors in VSM.
Estrogens	Potent UA vasodilators (E2β>> estrone >> estriol >> E2α) mediated via endothelial estrogen receptor-α (ERα), activation of endothelial and VSM NOS-NO and VSM NO-cGMP-PKG pathway, resulting in increased opening of VSM large conductance calcium-activated potassium channels (BK_{Ca}), which decrease cytosolic Ca^{2+}. Estrogens also increase β1-regulatory subunit expression, which regulates Ca^{2+} entry. Progesterone antagonizes the UA vasodilator effects.	Unclear and poorly studied.
Hydrogen sulfide (H_2S)	Estrogens and pregnancy increase endothelial and VSM cystathionine β-synthase (CBS) expression and activity, thereby increasing H_2S synthesis and UA vasodilation by activating ATP-dependent potassium channels (K_{ATP}) and VSM BK_{Ca} channels.	Unclear and not studied.
Potassium channels	VSM BK_{Ca} channels are activated by NO and estrogens via VSM NO-cGMP-PKG pathway to decrease cytosolic Ca^{2+} (entry and translocation) via effects of β1-regulatory subunits, which increase channel opening and VSM depolarization, resulting in UA vasodilation. In late pregnancy, VSM β1-regulatory subunit expression is increased. K_v channels are more complex and their role in placental circulation is unclear, but their expression may also be estrogen sensitive.	Unclear and not studied.

BK_{Ca}, Large conductance Ca^{2+}-activated K^+ channels; *K_V channels*, voltage-gated K^+ channels; *NO*, nitric oxide; *NOS*, nitric oxide synthase; *PGI_2*, prostacyclin; *UA*, uterine artery; *VSM*, vascular smooth muscle.

tissues) has fallen by 50% to 0.3 to 0.4 mL/min•g, reflecting the ever-increasing weight of the fetus and placenta (see Fig. 9.1C). The final phase in the "growth" of uterine blood flow is exponential and associated with a threefold increase in fetal weight in the last third of pregnancy, or after 110 days in sheep (75% of gestation) and beyond 30 weeks in humans (75%).[16] Because neither the total number of spiral arteries nor that of placentomes changes, this increase in uterine blood flow must be due to vasodilation.

In recent studies, this final stage of vasodilation has been shown to involve activation of large-conductance, calcium-sensitive, potassium channels (BK_{Ca}) in the uterine vascular smooth muscle and membrane hyperpolarization.[20-22] Although the initiating events are unclear, the signaling cascade appears to involve nitric oxide synthase (NOS), nitric oxide (NO), cyclic guanosine monophosphate (cGMP), and cGMP-dependent protein kinase (Table 9.1).[23] Evolving evidence suggests that voltage-regulated K^+ channels (K_V) might also play a role in maintaining basal uterine vascular tone by attenuating the vasoconstrictor effects of angiotensin II (ANG II) and increased sympathetic outflow in response to the fall in maternal systemic vascular resistance. Similar mechanisms appear to exist in women.[24] Of importance, the rise in blood flow in milliliters per minute is proportionate to and parallels the rise in wet weight of the uterus and its metabolically active tissues, which includes the growing fetus, membranes, and placenta. Thus, blood flow per gram of wet weight remains low (0.2 to 0.3 mL/min•g) during the remainder of pregnancy. In the presence of late-onset fetal growth restriction (i.e., after 70% of gestation), blood flow per gram of fetoplacental mass is lower, and nutrient and oxygen delivery is decreased. Fetal growth is attenuated until adaptation has occurred and this ratio is reestablished, at which time a new growth curve is established that lies below the curve for normally growing fetuses.

The dramatic rise in total uterine blood flow during pregnancy actually reflects changes in three separate vascular beds within the gravid uterus: the placentomes, endometrium, and myometrium. The change in distribution of blood flow to these tissues cannot be determined in women but has been

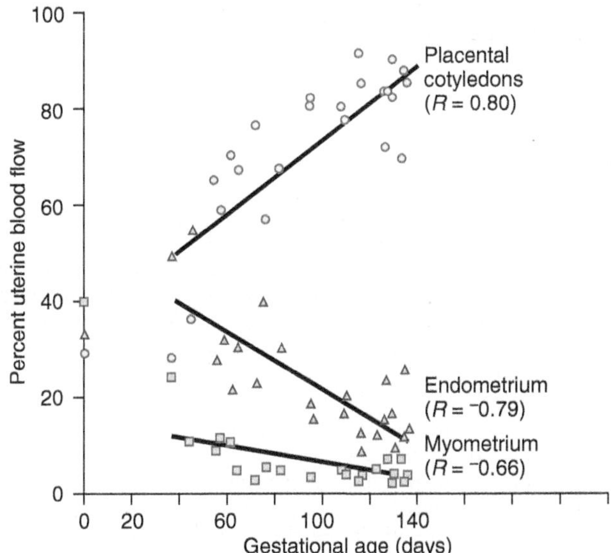

Fig. 9.2 The distribution of uterine blood flow during ovine pregnancy (term is 145 days). Blood flow was determined with the microsphere technique. Correlation coefficients are significant at $P < .01$. *R*, Relative risk. (From Rosenfeld CR. Consideration of the uteroplacental circulation in intrauterine growth. *Semin Perinatol.* 1984;8:42.)

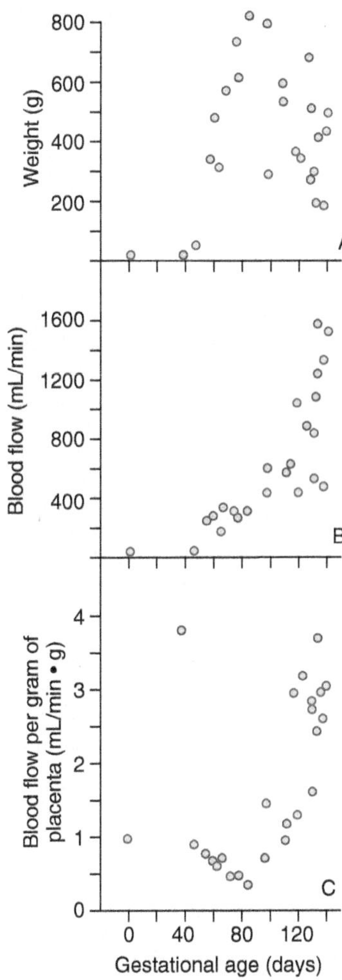

Fig. 9.3 Changes in placental weight (A), blood flow (B), and blood flow per gram of placenta (C). Observations on the nonpregnant animals represent the caruncles or future sites of implantation. Placental weight and blood flow in the twin gestations are the sum for the two placentas. *Blue circle*, twin pregnancy; *red circle*, singleton pregnancy. (From Rosenfeld CR, Morriss FH, Jr, Makowski EL, et al. Circulatory changes in the reproductive tissues of ewes during pregnancy. *Gynecol Invest*. 1974;5:252.)

studied in sheep and other species.[13,25] This limitation is an important consideration because measurement of changes in total uterine blood flow or blood flow in a single, large uterine artery in women by Doppler technology does not necessarily reflect the issue of primary importance—that is, placental perfusion.[9] As illustrated in Fig. 9.2, blood flow to these three tissues is evenly distributed in the nonpregnant uterus, each receiving approximately one third. As pregnancy progresses, a gradual redistribution of uterine blood flow occurs, such that at term the placentomes (cotyledons) receive nearly 90% of total uterine blood flow. Thus in the last third of pregnancy, perfusion of the placentomes accounts for most of the observed increase in uterine blood flow, and it is more likely that measures of Doppler flow in the main uterine artery parallel placental blood flow.

The placentome is the site of nutrient and gas exchange; thus fetal well-being is determined by changes in placental development, growth, and perfusion. Placental weight is relatively unchanged after the middle third of ovine gestation, yet maternal placental blood flow continues to increase exponentially (Fig. 9.3A and B). This discordance in placental growth and blood flow occurs earlier in pregnancy in women and other primates compared with sheep. The pattern of change in absolute blood flow (see Fig. 9.3B) resembles that seen for total uterine blood flow (see Fig. 9.1B). Because placental blood flow accounts for more than 60% of total uterine blood flow in the last two thirds of pregnancy (see Fig. 9.2), it is not surprising that the "patterns" are similar. The principal difference between the two patterns is obvious when blood flow per gram of metabolically active tissue is examined (see Fig. 9.3C). In contrast to the high value for total uterine blood flow early in pregnancy, followed by a fall and leveling off, placental blood flow falls in mid-pregnancy and then progressively increases from about 0.5 mL/min•g to nearly 4 mL/min•g at term—a value 5 times greater than that observed for the total uterus. This increase in placental blood flow is due to progressive vasodilation, because maternal arterial blood pressure (i.e., perfusion pressure) is minimally changed and the number of maternal spiral arteries is *unchanged*.[13,15] The rise in maternal placental blood flow parallels a more general process of functional maturation of the placenta, which involves the simultaneous increase in fetoplacental perfusion[26] and permeability[27]; these physiologic changes are necessary to provide adequate nutrients and oxygen for the rapidly growing fetus. Of note, the volume of placental blood flow greatly exceeds that required for normal fetal growth.[4,5] Thus, there is a substantial "margin" of safety (i.e., an excess of blood flow) that protects the fetus from episodic decreases in uteroplacental blood flow associated with transient increases in maternal plasma levels of vasoconstrictors (e.g., ANG II) or increases in myometrial tone during parturition, which may alter placental perfusion.[15]

Although much has been learned about the functional and anatomic aspects of the maternal uteroplacental circulation, few investigators have tried to describe in detail the pattern of change in umbilicoplacental blood flow over the entire course of pregnancy. This reflects the difficulty in performing such studies, even in an animal model. Nonetheless, many similarities exist between species. For example, a villous stem originating from the fetal side of the placenta contains a distal branch of the umbilical artery and vein. As pregnancy progresses, a villous tree (in the human) or vascular bed originating from this villous stem undergoes angiogenesis and branching morphogenesis throughout pregnancy, providing an ever-enlarging fetal placental vascular bed and surface area for nutrient and gas exchange by term pregnancy. Although the sheep has no villous tree, continued growth of the fetal placental vascular bed occurs as in the human.[1,13] In both species, therefore, the size of the fetal placental vascular bed and the magnitude of umbilicoplacental blood flow increase, the latter increasing exponentially in the last third of normal pregnancy.[26] In contrast with the rise in uteroplacental blood flow, which reflects vasodilation, the rise in umbilicoplacental blood flow is due primarily to vascular growth and, to a lesser extent, vasodilation. Thus, umbilicoplacental blood flow remains approximately 100 to 200 mL/min/kg of fetal weight throughout gestation in most species.[9] Conditions that attenuate the growth of the fetal placental vascular bed in the last third of gestation (e.g., pregnancy-induced hypertension) or increased fetal placental vascular resistance may result in insufficient nutrient delivery and fetal growth restriction. Although this correlation is not well studied, Doppler technology has shown increases in umbilical artery resistance associated with decreased fetal growth.[25]

With the advent of Doppler ultrasound, this has become a routine approach for determining uterine blood flow during pregnancy and has been widely applied to assess blood flow through the maternal uteroplacental circulation noninvasively, at low cost and with high temporal resolution. Doppler ultrasound assesses placental perfusion by measuring impedance to flow in the uterine arteries, which has been reported to increase in pregnancies with preeclampsia and fetal growth restriction.[28] However, Doppler ultrasound measurements of placental perfusion lack sufficient reproducibility and sensitivity, and quantification remains challenging.[29] In contrast, the introduction of magnetic resonance imaging (MRI) produces spatially resolved perfusion images and quantitative assessment. Arterial spin labeling (ASL) is a noninvasive imaging method for measuring tissue perfusion and has extensively been applied in the brain for measurement of cerebral blood flow.[30] While conventional perfusion MRI techniques require infusion of contrast agents, which are contraindicated during pregnancy, ASL utilizes water molecules in arterial blood as an endogenous contrast agent, making it optimal for examining placental perfusion in pregnancy. However, ASL measures the movement of *all* blood within the placenta and thus reflects both maternal and fetal blood flows. As a result, ASL overestimates maternal placental perfusion and complicates the understanding of changes in maternal blood supply and the contributions from the maternal and fetal circulation. Various noninvasive techniques are being examined that might selectively label maternal placental blood flow, including pseudo-continuous ASL[31] and velocity-selective ASL.[32]

VASOCONSTRICTORS

Studies of the factors controlling blood flow through the uteroplacental and umbilicoplacental vascular beds have centered on the effects of endogenous vasoconstrictors, including ANG II, catecholamines, and arginine vasopressin (AVP)—a hypothalamic-pituitary peptide secreted during episodes of fetal stress. This section reviews how these agents may affect placental perfusion and fetal well-being (see Table 9.1).

Normotensive pregnant women are refractory to systemic infusions of ANG II early in the mid-trimester, and this refractoriness is absent in women with hypertension.[33,34] Pregnant sheep and several other species are also refractory to infused ANG II during pregnancy.[35,36] Moreover, the uteroplacental vascular bed in women and sheep is more refractory to ANG II than the systemic vasculature and, as occurs in the peripheral vasculature, this uterine refractoriness is absent in pregnant women with hypertension, possibly increasing the risk for placental hypoperfusion.[37] This difference in sensitivity is seen when the dose-response curves depicting the relative changes in uterine and systemic vascular resistance are compared. As illustrated in Fig. 9.4, at dosages resulting in physiologic blood levels (<1.0 µg/min), infusions of ANG II result in greater relative increases in systemic resistance than in uterine vascular resistance. The rise in perfusion pressure also exceeds that of uterine vascular resistance; thus, uteroplacental blood flow increases throughout this dosage range. These observations suggest that the uteroplacental vascular bed is, in a sense, partially pressure-passive and, importantly, is protected from the vasoconstrictor effects of physiologic levels of ANG II.[36] This protective mechanism is important because plasma ANG II levels rise in normal pregnancy and may intermittently increase further when pregnant women experience episodes of orthostatic hypotension. Importantly, maternal placental blood flow is minimally affected, and the reproductive tissues as a group are more refractory than nonreproductive tissues.[38] The similarity in these responses to ANG II in women and sheep further validates the animal model, as do the studies of BK_{Ca} function cited earlier.[21-24]

This refractoriness of the uteroplacental circulation to ANG II may reflect several mechanisms. Uterine arteries from pregnant ewes demonstrate a threefold rise in the basal synthesis of prostacyclin (i.e., prostaglandin I_2 [PGI_2]), a potent vasodilator and ANG II antagonist, and a further 1.5-fold increase in endothelium-derived PGI_2 synthesis when exposed to ANG II in vivo or in vitro (by activating type 1 ANG II receptors).[36,39-41] This represents a negative-feedback response. Preliminary studies suggest that uterine arteries from normotensive pregnant women respond similarly; however, it is unclear if uterine arteries from hypertensive women are unable to enhance PGI_2 synthesis in

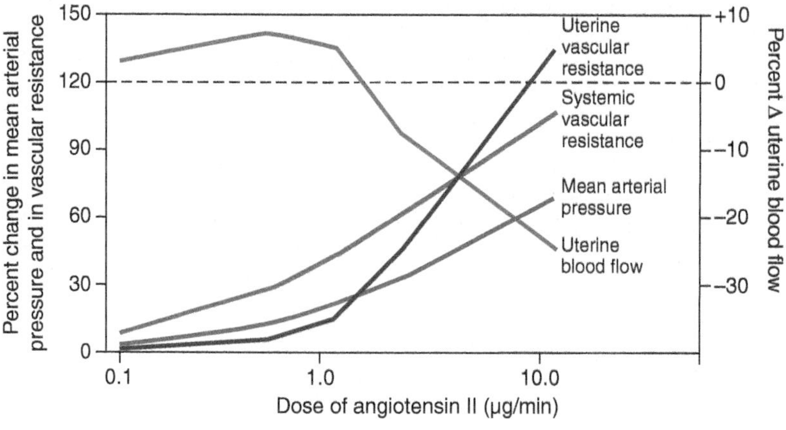

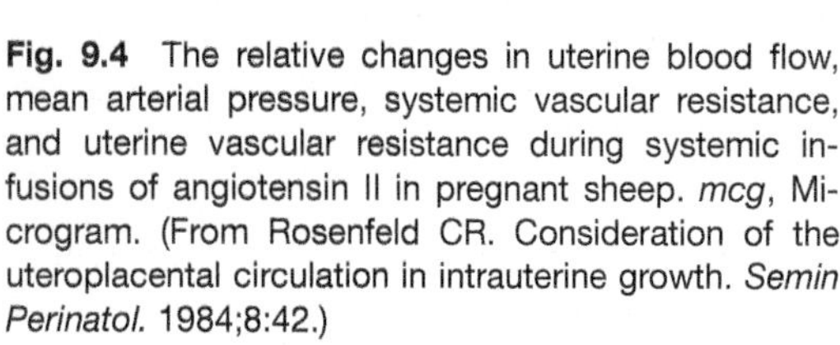
Fig. 9.4 The relative changes in uterine blood flow, mean arterial pressure, systemic vascular resistance, and uterine vascular resistance during systemic infusions of angiotensin II in pregnant sheep. *mcg*, Microgram. (From Rosenfeld CR. Consideration of the uteroplacental circulation in intrauterine growth. *Semin Perinatol.* 1984;8:42.)

the presence of ANG II. Because inhibition of cyclooxygenase activity in the uterine vascular bed of pregnant ewes decreased basal PGI_2 synthesis and enhanced constrictor responses to systemic ANG II infusions, it was believed this mechanism accounted for the attenuated uterine vasoconstrictor responses to ANG II.[36] Although this differential sensitivity to ANG II was not associated with down-regulation of ANG II receptors in uterine vascular smooth muscle, it was subsequently observed that type 2 ANG II receptors, which do not mediate vasoconstriction, account for more than 80% of binding in uterine arteries from nonpregnant and pregnant women and sheep.[36,40,42] Furthermore, uterine intra-arterial infusions of ANG II in pregnant sheep did not increase vascular resistance except at doses that initiated pressor responses before the uterus was affected.[43] It is now clear that the attenuated uteroplacental responses to ANG II are primarily due to the predominance of type 2 receptor expression in uterine vascular smooth muscle. ANG II, however, may exert modest vasoconstrictor effects on the uterine vasculature by activating the few type 1 receptors and/or local, systemic, or central adrenergic mechanisms resulting in the release of an α-agonist, which are antagonized by local PGI_2 and NO synthesis.[36,43-47] In addition, the type 2 receptor may directly attenuate type 1 receptor signaling and activation, but this is not clear.[48] Thus, several local mechanisms contribute to the maintenance of uteroplacental blood flow while permitting adjustments in the peripheral vascular beds during increases in circulating levels of endogenous ANG II in pregnant women. Modifications of these agonist-antagonist interactions likely occur in hypertensive pregnant women, resulting in uteroplacental hypoperfusion and eventually fetal growth restriction.

The pressor responses to infused catecholamines (i.e., epinephrine and norepinephrine) are also attenuated in normal pregnancies[49] and increased in hypertensive pregnant women.[33] The uteroplacental vascular responses to α-agonists, in contrast to ANG II, greatly exceed those seen in the systemic vasculature[49]; that is, increases in uterine vascular resistance exceed simultaneous increases in systemic vascular resistance and perfusion pressure at all doses of infused α-agonists (Fig. 9.5). Moreover, vasoconstrictor effects are several-fold greater than those of ANG II in studies of human and ovine uterine arteries.[45,46] Thus uterine blood flow decreases at doses of α-agonists that minimally alter maternal blood pressure (Fig. 9.6) and are paralleled by decreases in placental blood flow. Thus, the maternal uteroplacental vascular bed is less protected from endogenous α-agonists than from ANG II. These differences are physiologically relevant. It would be senseless to put the fetus at risk for placental hypoperfusion and decreased uterine oxygen delivery each time the pregnant woman rises from the supine position to standing and increases her plasma levels of ANG II. By contrast, in circumstances in which the mother's survival is at risk (e.g., from hemorrhage) and adrenal production and secretion of catecholamines are increased, it is physiologically sound to divert a significant proportion of the excessive volume of uteroplacental blood flow to tissues more relevant to maternal survival. During labor, circulating catecholamine levels are elevated, and this enhanced responsiveness of the placental arteries to catecholamines can potentially endanger the growth-restricted fetus or a normally grown fetus with a small or borderline "margin of safety" by decreasing uterine oxygen delivery to dangerous levels, resulting in fetal heart rate decelerations. This has been noted in Doppler ultrasound studies.[11] Similarly, the use of adrenergic agonists (ephedrine or phenylephrine) in the treatment of hypotensive women after spinal anesthesia may put the fetus at risk. In studies of human uterine arteries[24] and intact pregnant sheep, the BK_{Ca} channel, which modulates basal uterine blood flow, also modifies uterine responses to infused α-agonists.[50] Thus, abnormalities of BK_{Ca} function or expression may contribute to abnormal placental perfusion and increased

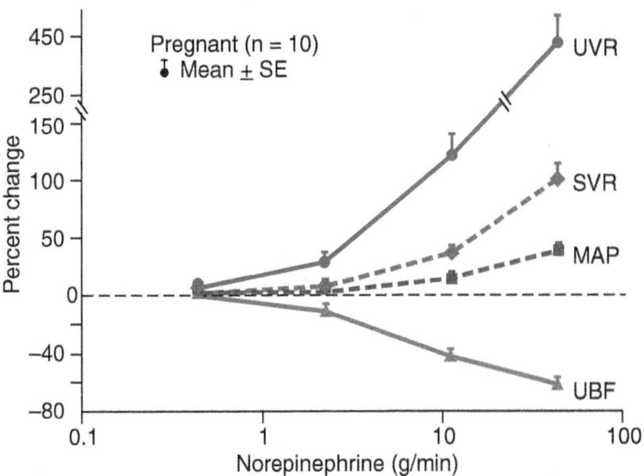

Fig. 9.5 The relative changes in uterine blood flow *(UBF)*, mean arterial pressure *(MAP)*, systemic vascular resistance *(SVR)*, and uterine vascular resistance *(UVR)* during systemic infusions of norepinephrine in pregnant sheep. *SE*, Standard error. (From Magness RR, Rosenfeld CR. Systemic and uterine responses to α-adrenergic stimulation in pregnant and nonpregnant ewes. *Am J Obstet Gynecol*. 1986;155:897.)

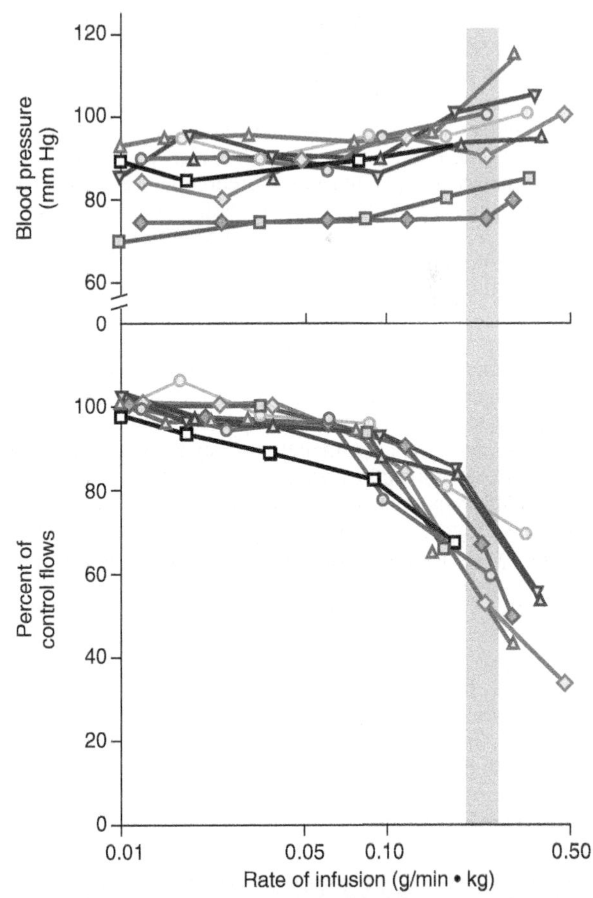

Fig. 9.6 Responses of uterine blood flow and mean arterial pressure to increasing doses of norepinephrine. Uterine blood flow is represented as a percentage of control flows. Different symbols represent responses of separate animals. (From Rosenfeld CR, West J. Circulatory response to systemic infusion of norepinephrine in the pregnant ewe. *Am J Obstet Gynecol*. 1977;127:376.)

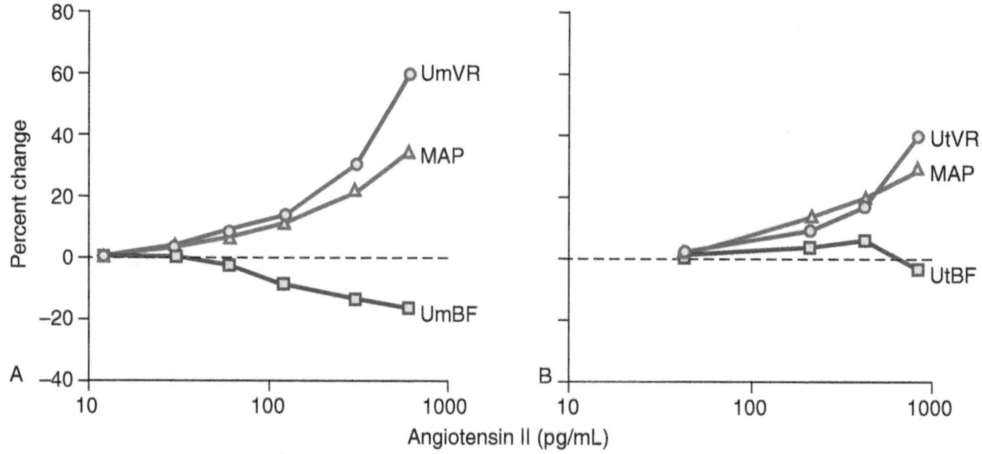

Fig. 9.7 Comparison of the relative changes in blood flow, mean arterial pressure *(MAP)*, and vascular resistance versus plasma levels of angiotensin II in the umbilicoplacental (A) and maternal uteroplacental (B) vascular beds during systemic infusions of angiotensin II. *UmBF*, Umbilical blood flow; *UmVR*, umbilical vascular resistance; *UtBF*, uterine blood flow; *UtVR*, uterine vascular resistance. (From Rosenfeld CR, Gresores A, Roy TA, et al. Comparison of ANG II in fetal and pregnant sheep: metabolic clearance and vascular reactivity. *Am J Physiol.* 1995;268:E237.)

sensitivity to α-agonists seen in hypertensive women.[51,52] This deserves further study.

ANG II is a potent vasoconstrictor in the fetal umbilicoplacental circulation.[53,54] It was previously believed that the fetus was more refractory than the pregnant mother to the effects of ANG II, resulting in the greater circulating levels in the fetus.[55] However, fetal clearance of ANG II is 10-fold greater than that in the mother, and 95% of fetal clearance occurs across the placental vascular bed. Furthermore, the umbilicoplacental vasculature is actually more sensitive to the vasoconstricting effects than the uteroplacental circulation at similar plasma levels of ANG II (Fig. 9.7).[55] This difference between umbilicoplacental and uteroplacental responses is explained by the predominance of type 1 ANG II receptors in the former (>90% of binding), in contrast to type 2 receptors in the latter in both the human and sheep.[40,45,56,57] Moreover, the umbilical artery smooth muscle demonstrates precocious functional maturation compared with fetal systemic arteries,[58] which express primarily the type 2 receptor and exhibit decreased function of contractile proteins.[56] By contrast, catecholamines minimally alter umbilicoplacental blood flow except at super-physiologic doses,[59,60] and these decreases in placental perfusion may actually reflect a fall in fetal cardiac output rather than increases in placental vascular resistance. Thus, fetal responses to catecholamines are associated with the maintenance of umbilicoplacental perfusion, as well as cerebral and myocardial blood flow. In fetal sheep, ANG II-induced modifications in arterial pressure are due primarily to increases in umbilicoplacental resistance mediated by type 1 ANG II receptors.[56,61,62]

AVP is a hypothalamic-pituitary hormone that exhibits increased secretion during episodes of intrauterine hypoxia and asphyxia.[63,64] As with adrenal catecholamines, which mediate the primary fetal responses to intrauterine "stress," umbilicoplacental perfusion is not affected substantially by AVP.[63] Thus, the maternal and the fetal placental vascular beds respond differently to endogenous vasoconstrictors, probably reflecting important mechanisms necessary to ensure adequate fetal oxygen delivery and the survival of the fetus or the mother.

PROSTAGLANDINS

There has been considerable interest in the role of prostanoids in the regulation of uteroplacental and umbilicoplacental blood flows. This interest stems from observations of increased circulating levels of vasodilating prostanoids in normotensive pregnant women and animals.[65,66] In addition, systemic and uterine infusion of cyclooxygenase inhibitors in pregnant sheep increases systemic and uterine responses to infused ANG II.[41] Furthermore, women with pregnancy-induced hypertension exhibit circulating levels of thromboxane (a potent vasoconstrictor) that exceed those of PGI_2, potentially accounting for the increased vascular reactivity seen in these women.[65] Because circulating PGI_2 and thromboxane may be of placental origin, these and other prostanoids could modulate the peripheral and uterine circulations in normotensive and hypertensive pregnant women. This view, however, remains controversial for several reasons. First, prostanoids may not be circulating hormones but rather mediate their effects through paracrine mechanisms. Thus, plasma levels may provide little physiologic information. Second, increases in vessel perfusion or shear stress increase endothelial production of PGI_2.[67] The rise in placental blood flow seen in normal pregnancy, therefore, may be due to another mechanism, and the increase in prostanoid synthesis may be secondary. Third, although cyclooxygenase inhibition enhances systemic and uterine vascular responses to vasoconstrictors in pregnant women and sheep, this effect does not alter basal uteroplacental blood flow commensurate with the fall in plasma prostaglandin levels.[41,68] Finally, pregnancy-induced hypertension is not ameliorated or prevented by low-dose aspirin therapy.[69] This evidence suggests that prostanoids may be a class of stress hormones that antagonize the vascular responses to circulating placental vasoconstrictors, thereby protecting maternal uterine blood flow.

Similar controversy exists regarding the role of prostaglandins in the fetal compartment. PGI_2 is a potent placental vasodilator, while prostaglandin E_2 (PGE_2) is a vasoconstrictor (vs. a vasodilator in the maternal placental circulation). The physiologic role of these two prostanoids, however, remains unclear. It has been suggested that the differential effects of PGE_2 in the two placental vascular beds may act to autoregulate both beds so that when umbilicoplacental blood flow falls, maternal placental perfusion increases to maintain a stable fetal oxygen uptake and delivery. More recently, it has been suggested that PGE_2 may potentiate the vasoconstriction seen with ANG II, whereas PGI_2 antagonizes these effects. These conclusions require further study.

NITRIC OXIDE

NO is the product of at least three isoforms of NOS expressed in endothelium and/or vascular smooth muscle. Total body NO synthesis is increased in normotensive pregnancies and may contribute to normal cardiovascular adaptation and increased cGMP synthesis.[70,71] Furthermore, prolonged administration of an NOS inhibitor to pregnant rats causes hypertension and decreased circulating cGMP levels; however, uteroplacental blood flow is minimally affected. Marked increases in uterine venous cGMP and uterine cGMP synthesis occur in pregnant sheep, suggesting that NO may be essential to the regulation of uteroplacental blood flow.[72] Although uterine artery synthesis of NO increases in pregnancy, it is unclear what proportion of uterine cGMP synthesis is vascular versus placental or nonvascular.[70,73] Furthermore, prolonged uterine NOS inhibition in pregnant sheep decreases uteroplacental perfusion by no more than 30%.[72,74,75] Although studies of NO have focused on the role of endothelium-derived type 3 NOS, type 1 NOS is expressed in uterine artery smooth muscle[76]; however, its role in pregnancy is presently unclear.

Studies of the role of NO in the regulation of umbilicoplacental blood flow are extensive, but it is unclear to what extent NO plays a role.[70] Perfused human umbilical arteries and veins release more NO than PGI_2.[77] Inhibition of NOS increases umbilicoplacental vascular resistance in vitro, and when given to intact fetal sheep, NOS decreases umbilical blood flow by 50%.[78] Increases in NO generation also attenuate constrictor responses to several agonists. Thus, NO may play an important role in both maintaining and modulating umbilicoplacental blood flow. Because inhibition of NOS does not decrease blood flow completely, NO appears to contribute to, but is not totally responsible for, maintaining umbilicoplacental perfusion. Of note, potassium channels are also expressed in umbilical arteries.[79] Their role in regulating umbilicoplacental blood flow is unclear.

STEROID HORMONES

The placenta is a major site of synthesis of maternal and fetal steroid hormones, in particular, estrogens and progesterone. These hormones have profound vascular effects and play important roles in promoting implantation and placentation[19] and modulating placental blood flow and other aspects of maternal cardiovascular adaptation during pregnancy. Unfortunately, few investigators have examined the effects of these hormones on umbilicoplacental blood flow. In sheep, estrogens vasodilate the nonpregnant uterus (increasing blood flow 10-fold to 15-fold) and the pregnant uterus (increasing blood flow by 40% to 50%).[80] Furthermore, maternal and fetal infusions of dehydroepiandrosterone (the fetal adrenal androgen precursor necessary for placental estrogen synthesis) increase production of placental estrogens, which is followed by increases in uteroplacental blood flow.[80] No other naturally occurring substance has an effect of this magnitude on uterine or uteroplacental perfusion. Because the rise in uterine blood flow occurs in the absence of a change in perfusion pressure,[81] this represents true vasodilation. Progesterone can antagonize and modulate these effects of estrogens. Thus, the two steroids appear to coregulate the magnitude of maternal uteroplacental blood flow. The effects of estrogens on uterine blood flow are mediated by estrogen receptors, primarily estrogen receptor α, and involve activation and transcriptional regulation of type 1 and possibly type 3 NOS,[76] resulting in increases in NO synthesis and smooth muscle cGMP levels, activation of protein kinase G (PKG; a cGMP-dependent protein kinase), and phosphorylation and activation of BK_{Ca} in uterine artery smooth muscle in nonpregnant and pregnant sheep.[20,82,83] Importantly, estrogens also up-regulate expression of the BK_{Ca} β_1-regulatory subunit in the uterine artery and can directly activate the channel through the β_1-regulatory subunit, resulting in hyperpolarization.[83,84] BK_{Ca} are expressed in human uterine artery smooth muscle and modulate NO-mediated relaxation and agonist-induced contraction (see Table 9.1).[24]

POTASSIUM CHANNELS

Smooth muscle potassium channels contribute to vascular regulation in all vascular beds examined.[51] They modulate membrane depolarization to regulate vasoconstriction and hyperpolarization so as to regulate relaxation. They also contribute to autoregulation and myogenic responses. As noted earlier, BK_{Ca} are expressed in human and ovine uterine artery smooth muscle. They consist of four pore-forming α-subunits representing a single gene product and upward of four β-regulatory subunits derived from different gene products. In sheep the BK_{Ca} α-subunit is unchanged by estrogens,[83,84] but expression increases during placentation and posttranslational changes have been described.[23] In contrast, the β_1-regulatory subunit is up-regulated several-fold by (1) exogenous estrogens,[83] (2) during the follicular phase of the ovarian cycle in nonpregnant sheep,[84] and (3), in the last third of ovine pregnancy.[22,23] This increases α-β_1 stoichiometry, allowing for changes in channel function (see Table 9.1). Thus, there is a direct relationship between elevated levels of estrogens, expression of the β_1-regulatory subunit, activation of the NO-cGMP-PKG pathway, and enhancement of the direct effects of estrogens on the uterine artery BK_{Ca}. The β_1-subunit also enhances smooth muscle sensitivity to increases in intracellular calcium levels, which in turn inhibits voltage-gated calcium channels. Thus, the β_1-subunit modulates uterine artery vasodilation and sensitivity to vasoconstrictors, supporting a major role in maintaining basal uteroplacental blood flow and attenuating vasoconstrictor responses in women and sheep. The K_V are more complex, as there are at least 70 gene products representing the α-subunit, and they form heterotetradimers with associated β-regulatory subunits. Because of their complexity, the role of K_V in the placental circulation is unclear; however, evolving evidence suggests they may modulate baseline tone, myogenic sensitivity, and vasoconstrictor responses. Thus, K_V may contribute to the uterine refractoriness to vasoconstrictors observed in normotensive pregnant women (see Table 9.1). If this is so, their dysfunction may contribute to the loss of vascular refractoriness to vasoconstrictors seen in hypertensive women. This opens a new area of investigation.

OTHER VASOACTIVE MOLECULES IN THE PLACENTAL CIRCULATION

Hydrogen sulfide (H_2S) is a gaseous signaling molecule that acts as a local fetoplacental vasodilator in humans.[85] Endogenous H_2S production is catalyzed by cystathionine b-synthase (CBS) and cystathionine g-lyase (CSE).[86,87] In intrauterine tissues, there is endogenous H_2S placental production and release, and the presence of placental CSE and CBS in humans.[88] The primary dilator actions of H_2S in the human placenta are mediated via K_{ATP} channels, BK_{Ca} channels, and there is an additional interaction between H_2S and NO that modulates vascular tone (see Table 9.1).[85,89,90] There is decreased placental mRNA expression of CBS in early-onset preeclampsia,[91] and down-regulation of CBS and CSE mRNA and of CBS protein expression in the myometrium during labor.[92] Preeclampsia may also be associated with reduced circulating H_2S, accompanied by downregulation of placental CSE.[85,93] Reduced placental CSE expression at the mRNA and protein levels is associated with abnormal umbilical artery Doppler waveforms in high-risk pregnancies.[85] Thus, decreases in H_2S availability may contribute to the increased umbilical arterial resistance in severe preterm IUGR.[85]

Endothelin (ET) is a 21-amino acid peptide involved in regulating vascular homeostasis. It is present in three isoforms, ET-1, ET-2, and ET-3.[94] ET-1 is the most potent vasoconstrictor known (see Table 9.1)[95-97] and is primarily secreted by vascular endothelial cells.[98] The ET peptides can bind either the ET_A- or ET_B-receptor. In human placentas, ET-1 is involved in constricting fetoplacental blood vessels and is distributed throughout the placental vascular endothelium.[99] The placental expression of ET-1 is increased in preeclamptic women,[100-102] particularly in the placental plate chorion, amnion, and chorion leave.[103] The increase in expression of ET-1 in preeclamptic women could be due to upregulation of endothelin converting enzyme (ECE) activity, an enzyme that cleaves ET into an active form.[104]

CONCLUSION

Fetal growth and well-being depend on the development, growth, and maturation of the placenta, as well as substantial increases in final umbilical and maternal placental blood flows. In the final third of pregnancy, fetal and maternal placental blood flows increase logarithmically, paralleling the increase in fetal weight. In conjunction with increases in placental function and surface area, the rise in blood flows increases the capacity to deliver and transfer oxygen and nutrients to the fetus. Maternal uteroplacental blood flow normally exceeds fetal-placental metabolic needs, providing a large "margin of error"; thus, blood flow may acutely fall by 50% without altering oxygen and nutrient delivery. The maternal placental vasculature is refractory to endogenous and infused vasoconstrictors, including ANG II and catecholamines, protecting it from the increases and variations in circulating levels that occur throughout pregnancy. There also is enhanced local synthesis of vasodilators by the uterine and umbilicoplacental vasculature that not only increase blood flow but may also antagonize vasoconstrictor responses. Thus, several mechanisms, including NO, PGI_2, cGMP, PKG, BK_{Ca}, and maybe K_V, form an interactive complex system that ensures fetal well-being, growth, and propagation of the species. In the presence of maternal hypertension, one or more of these systems may be dysfunctional, placing the fetus at risk for long-term and short-term episodes of hypoxia via increased sensitivity to intracellular calcium and circulating vasoconstrictors. The contribution of each mechanism remains to be determined in order to develop new strategies to maintain placental blood flows and ensure fetal well-being.

ACKNOWLEDGMENTS

Research on which this chapter is based was supported by National Institutes of Health grant HD-008783-39 and the George L. MacGregor Professorship in Pediatrics. I thank the many co-investigators and students who, while in my laboratories, facilitated many of our studies.

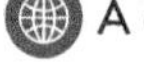 A complete reference list is available at www.ExpertConsult.com.

SELECT REFERENCES

1. King BF. The functional anatomy of the placental vasculature. In: Rosenfeld CR, ed. *The Uterine Circulation*. Ithaca, NY: Perinatology Press; 1989:17-33.
4. Wilkening RB, Anderson S, Martensson L, Meschia G. Placental transfer as a function of uterine blood flow. *Am J Physiol*. 1982;242:H429.
5. Wilkening RB. The role of uterine blood flow in fetal oxygen and nutrient delivery. In: Rosenfeld CR, ed. *The Uterine Circulation*. Ithaca, NY: Perinatology Press; 1989:191-207.
7. Couzin J. Quirks of fetal environment felt decades later. *Science*. 2002;296:2167.
8. Greiss F. Uterine blood flow. An overview since Barcroft. In: Rosenfeld CR, ed. *The Uterine Circulation*. Ithaca, NY: Perinatology Press; 1989:3-16.
9. Battaglia FC, Meschia G. Review of studies in human pregnancy of uterine and umbilical blood flows. *Dev Period Med*. 2013;17:287.
10. Ioannidis JPA. Extrapolating from animals to humans. *Sci Transl Med*. 2012;4:1.
12. Osol G, Mandala M. Maternal uterine vascular remodeling during pregnancy. *Physiology*. 2008;24:58.
13. Teasdale F. Numerical density of nuclei in the sheep placenta. *Anat Rec*. 1976;185:187.
14. Ramsey EM, Corner Jr GW, Donner MW. Serial and cineradioangiographic visualization of maternal circulation in the primate (hemochorial) placenta. *Am J Obstet Gynecol*. 1963;86:213.
16. Rosenfeld CR, Morriss Jr FH, Makowski EL, et al. Circulatory changes in the reproductive tissues of ewes during pregnancy. *Gynecol Invest*. 1974;5:252.
17. Rosenfeld CR. Distribution of cardiac output in ovine pregnancy. *Am J Physiol*. 1977;232:H231-H232.
19. Paria BC, Reese J, Das SK, Dey SK. Deciphering the cross-talk of implantation. advances and challenges. *Science*. 2002;296:2185.
20. Rosenfeld CR, Cornfield DN, Roy T. $Ca2^+$-activated K^+ channels modulate basal and E2β-induced rises in uterine blood flow in ovine pregnancy. *Am J Physiol Heart Circ Physiol*. 2001;281:H22.
21. Rosenfeld CR, Roy T, DeSpain K, Cox BE. Large-conductance $Ca2^+$-dependent K^+ channels regulate basal uteroplacental blood flow in ovine pregnancy. *J Soc Gynecol Invest*. 2005;12:402.
22. Hu X-Q, Xiao D, Zhu R, et al. Pregnancy upregulates large-conductance $Ca2^+$-activated K^+ channel activity and attenuates myogenic tone in uterine arteries. *Hypertension*. 2011;58:1132.
23. Rosenfeld CR, Liu X-T, DeSpain K. Pregnancy modifies the large conductance Ca^{2+}-activated K^+ channel expression and cGMP-dependent signaling pathway in uterine vascular smooth muscle. *Am J Physiol Heart Circ Physiol*. 2009;296:H1878.
24. Rosenfeld CR, Word RA, DeSpain K, Liu X-T. Large conductance Ca2+-activated K+ channels contribute to vascular function in nonpregnant human uterine arteries. *Reprod Sci*. 2008;15:651.
25. Rosenfeld CR. Consideration of the uteroplacental circulation in intrauterine growth. *Semin Perinatol*. 1984;8:42.
26. Meschia G, Cotter JR, Makowski EL, Barron DH. Simultaneous measurements of uterine and umbilical blood flows and oxygen uptakes. *Exp Physiol*. 1967;52:1.
27. Kulhanek JF, Meschia G, Makowski EL, Battaglia FC. Changes in DNA content and urea permeability of sheep placenta. *Am J Physiol*. 1974;226:1257.
33. Chesley LC, Talledo E, Bohler CS, Zuspan FP. Vascular reactivity to angiotensin II and norepinephrine in pregnant and nonpregnant women. *Am J Obstet Gynecol*. 1965;91:837.
36. Rosenfeld CR. Mechanisms regulating angiotensin II responsiveness by the uteroplacental circulation. *Am J Physiol Regul Integr Comp Physiol*. 2001;281:R1025.
37. Erkkola RU, Pirhonen JP. Uterine and umbilical flow velocity waveforms in normotensive and hypertensive subjects during the angiotensin II sensitivity test. *Am J Obstet Gynecol*. 1992;166:910.
39. Magness RR, Rosenfeld CR. Calcium modulation of endothelium-derived prostacyclin production in ovine pregnancy. *Endocrinology*. 1993;132:2445.
40. Cox BE, Rosenfeld CR, Kalinyak JE, et al. Tissue specific expression of vascular smooth muscle angiotensin II receptor subtypes during ovine pregnancy. *Am J Physiol*. 1996;271:H212.
42. Cox BE, Word RA, Rosenfeld CR. Angiotensin II receptor characteristics and subtype expression in uterine arteries and myometrium during pregnancy. *J Clin Endocrinol Metab*. 1996;81:49.
45. Rosenfeld CR, DeSpain K, Word RA, Liu X-t. Differential sensitivity to angiotensin II and norepinephrine in human uterine arteries. *J Clin Endocrinol Metab*. 2012;97:138.
46. Rosenfeld CR, DeSpain K, Xiao-tie L. Defining the differential sensitivity to norepinephrine and angiotensin II in the ovine uterine vasculature. *Am J Physiol Regul Integr Comp Physiol*. 2012;302:R59.
47. Magness RR, Rosenfeld CR, Hassan A, Shaul PW. Endothelial vasodilator production by uterine and systemic arteries. I. Effects of ANG II on PGI2 and NO in pregnancy. *Am J Physiol*. 1996;270:H1914.
48. McMullen JR, Gibson KJ, Lumbers ER, et al. Interactions between AT1 and AT2 receptors in uterine arteries from pregnant ewes. *Eur J Pharmacol*. 1999;378:195.
50. Rosenfeld CR, Hynan LS, Liu X-T, Roy T. Large conductance Ca^{2+}-activated K^+ channels modulate uterine α_1-adrenergic sensitivity in ovine pregnancy. *Reprod Sci*. 2014;21:456-464.
52. Nelson MT, Quayle JM. The β_1 subunit of Ca^{2+}-sensitive K^+ channels protects against hypertension. *J Clin Invest*. 2004;113:955.
54. Yoshimura T, Magness RR, Rosenfeld CR. Angiotensin II and α-agonist. I. Responses of ovine fetoplacental vasculature. *Am J Physiol*. 1990;259:H464.
56. Cox BE, Rosenfeld CR. Ontogeny of vascular angiotensin II receptor subtype expression in ovine development. *Pediatr Res*. 1999;45:414.
57. Knock GA, Sullivan MH, McCarthy A, et al. Angiotensin II (AT1) vascular binding sites in human placentae from normal-term, preeclamptic and growth retarded pregnancies. *J Pharmacol Exp Ther*. 1994;271:1007.
58. Arens Y, Chapados RA, Cox BE, et al. Differential development of umbilical and systemic arteries. II. Contractile proteins. *Am J Physiol*. 1998;274:R1815.
61. Kaiser JR, Cox BE, Roy TA, Rosenfeld CR. Differential development of umbilical and systemic arteries. I. ANG II receptor subtype expression. *Am J Physiol*. 1998;274:R797.
62. Adamson SL, Morrow RJ, Bull SB, Langille BL. Vasomotor responses of the umbilical circulation in fetal sheep. *Am J Physiol*. 1989;256:R1056.

64. Iwamoto HS, Rudolph AM, Keil LC, Heymann MA. Hemodynamic responses of the sheep fetus to vasopressin infusion. *Circ Res*. 1979;44:430.
68. Naden RP, Iliya CA, Arant Jr BS, et al. Hemodynamic effects of indomethacin in chronically instrumented pregnant sheep. *Am J Obstet Gynecol*. 1985;151:484.
69. Italian Study of Aspirin in Pregnancy. Low-dose aspirin in prevention and treatment of intrauterine growth retardation and pregnancy-induced hypertension. *Lancet*. 1993;341:396.
70. Sladek SM, Magness RR, Conrad KP. Nitric oxide and pregnancy. *Am J Physiol*. 1997;272:R441.
71. Weiner CP, Knowles RG, Moncada S. Induction of nitric oxide early in pregnancy. *Am J Obstet Gynecol*. 1994;171:838.
74. Rosenfeld CR, Roy T. Prolonged uterine artery nitric oxide synthase inhibition modestly alters basal uteroplacental vasodilation in the last third of ovine pregnancy. *Am J Physiol Heart Circ Physiol*. 2014;307:H1196.
77. Chaudhuri G, Cuevas J, Buga GM, Ignarro LJ. NO is more important than PGI2 in maintaining low vascular tone in feto-placental vessels. *Am J Physiol*. 1993;265:H2036.
79. Milesi V, Raingo J, Rebolledo A, Grassi de Gende AO. Potassium channels in human umbilical artery cells. *J Soc Gynecol Investig*. 2003;10:339.
82. Rosenfeld CR, White RE, Roy T, Cox BE. Calcium-activated potassium channels and nitric oxide coregulate estrogen-induced vasodilation. *Am J Physiol Heart Circ Physiol*. 2000;279:H319.
83. Nagar D, Liu XT, Rosenfeld CR. Estrogen regulates β_1-subunit expression in Ca^{2+}-activated K^+ channels in arteries from reproductive tissues. *Am J Physiol*. 2005;289:H4147.
84. Khan L, Rosenfeld CR, Liu X, Magness RR. Regulation of the cGMP-cPKG pathway and large-conductance Ca^{2+}-activated K^+ channels uterine arteries during the ovine ovarian cycle. *Am J Physiol Endocrin Metabol*. 2010;298:E222.

Mechanisms of Transfer Across the Human Placenta

10

Rohan M. Lewis | Jane K. Cleal

INTRODUCTION

Transfer of solutes across the placenta is essential for fetal growth and development. Placental transfer occurs in both directions, with maternal nutrients transferred to the fetus and fetal wastes to the mother. A wide range of nutrients and wastes must be transported across the placenta requiring multiple different transport processes. Insufficient placental transfer of nutrients or wastes can impair fetal growth and development. When poor placental function affects fetal development, this can impact health in utero around birth and across the life course.[1]

Placental nutrient uptake from the maternal circulation must be sufficient to meet both placental and fetal metabolic requirements. The fetus needs oxygen, nutrients, and maternal immunoglobulin G (IgG) to sustain its development and prepare for postnatal life. At the same time, the placenta has to clear waste products, such as carbon dioxide, from the fetal circulation. The placenta must also mediate uptake of the metabolites required for its own metabolic demands to support placental functions including nutrient transport and hormone secretion. While there is selective placental transfer of nutrients and wastes, the placenta must also protect the fetus from maternal hormones, metabolites, pharmaceutical drugs, and environmental toxins. The requirements for placental transfer will vary in line with changes in fetal demand across gestation.

Transfer of nutrients and wastes across the placenta can occur by passive diffusion and transporter-mediated processes as well as by endocytosis and transcytosis. Other factors that affect nutrient and waste transfer include placental metabolism, structure, and blood flow. The placenta does not operate in isolation and maternal and fetal physiology and metabolism will affect drivers of placental solute transfer. In particular, maternal and fetal blood flow play a key role in determining the concentrations of substances available for transport and the gradients that may drive their transfer across the placenta. In addition, regulatory signals from the mother or fetus will target the placenta and regulate its function. The way in which these processes interact will also be key in determining what crosses the placenta.[2]

This chapter will address the mechanisms that underpin placental solute transfer and how these mechanisms are regulated. Key determinants of placental transfer include whether an ion or molecule can diffuse across the placenta, whether it can be transported, and whether there are any metabolic processes in the placenta that sequester or degrade it.

PLACENTAL STRUCTURE AND BLOOD FLOW

The structure of the placenta provides the foundations for its function as a barrier and as a mediator of selective transport. It should be noted that placental structure varies across species in terms of both the macro- and micro-architecture.[3]

The term human placenta is typically disc shaped and formed of 15 to 20 functional units called *lobules* or *cotyledons*, each with its own maternal and fetal blood supply. The fetal blood vessels are contained within placental villi, which are tree-like branching structures with an outer surface in direct contact with maternal blood. This hemochorial placentation reduces the diffusion distances and the number of layers that solutes must cross between maternal and fetal circulations.

The villous tree originates from the chorionic plate and is anchored to the basal plate by specialized anchoring villi. Stem villi emerge first and branch into intermediate villi and finally into terminal villi, which mediate the majority of placental solute exchange. Within the villi, arteries and veins are present in stem villi. Venules and arterioles are located in intermediate villi, while capillaries are found in intermediate and terminal villi. The arteries and veins in stem villi contain an outer smooth muscle layer, while arterioles, venules, and capillaries are surrounded by pericytes.

In the first trimester of pregnancy, the embryo implants within the maternal endometrium and villous formation occurs followed by villous vascularization. Maternal blood flow to the placenta does not begin until 10 to 12 weeks of gestation, before which histotrophic nutrition is provided by the uterine glands.[4] In the second trimester, villous branching increases the size and surface area of the placenta, to support increasing fetal demand. In the third trimester, increasing placental efficiency is mediated by dilation of capillaries within the terminal villi. This brings the capillary endothelium into closer contact with the trophoblast and reduces diffusion distances between the maternal and fetal circulations. Placental development across gestation is reviewed in detail elsewhere.[5] Poor placental development in the early stages of gestation, such as villous branching or vascularization, can have a significant impact on later placental structure and function.

BLOOD FLOW IN THE MATERNAL AND FETAL CIRCULATIONS

Maternal blood flow carries nutrients to the placenta and waste products away, whereas the fetal vasculature is important for solute delivery to the fetus and removal of wastes. Blood flow through the maternal and fetal circulations within the placenta maintains the concentration gradients necessary for transfer of many substances.

Maternal blood spills out of maternal spiral arteries into the intervillous space and percolates between the villi until returning to the maternal circulation through venous outflows. The number of spiral arteries per placental lobule and the number and location of decidual veins leaving each lobule have not been clearly established. While the anatomic location of decidual venous outflows is unclear, computer modeling of blood flow suggests that they would be located peripherally for optimal efficiency.[6] Work with Doppler ultrasonography and magnetic resonance imaging (MRI) is leading to a better understanding of maternal blood flow through the intervillous space.[7]

Within the intervillous space there is no fixed direction of maternal blood flow, either between the placental villi or in relation to fetal blood flow within the villous tree. This mixed or multivillous flow pattern differs significantly from the counter current flow system that might exist if the placenta had been designed by an engineer for optimal efficiency.[8] Computer modeling of blood flow in the human placenta based on a multivillous system of flow produces data similar to in vivo experimental data, providing support for this hypothesis.[9]

Maternal blood flow to the placenta may be altered in maternal disease states. In preeclampsia, blood flow to the placenta is believed to be reduced or modified due to impaired spiral artery remodeling. Maternal heart disease is also associated with altered uteroplacental blood flow and a higher incidence of poor fetal outcomes.[10] Impaired maternal flow may reduce the efficiency of nutrient delivery to the fetus, removal of fetal wastes, and the delivery of placental signals (hormones, microparticles, nutrients) back to the mother.

Fetal blood flow is dependent on the capacity of the fetal heart and the resistance of the placental vascular network. Thus the development and maturation of placental villi could affect vascular resistance and therefore blood flow. Impaired placental blood flow will primarily affect the transfer of oxygen and carbon dioxide, whose transport is highly dependent on flow to maintain transplacental partial pressure gradients.

Within the villous tree, fetal arterial blood, which is deoxygenated and depleted in nutrients, will travel up the villi to the capillaries in terminal villi where solute exchange is most efficient. The oxygen- and nutrient-enriched blood will then travel back down the venous system to the fetus. While limited exchange may occur in larger vessels within stem and intermediate villi, the majority is believed to occur in terminal villi. The regulation of feto-placental blood flow and its effects on nutrient transfer is an area that needs further investigation.

The vascular resistance of the feto-placental circulation is determined by the structure of its vascular network and its vascular tone. Placental vascular tone can be regulated by vasoactive drugs and metabolites.[11,12] Interestingly, vascular tone may be regulated in both the arterial and venous vessels, and venous constriction may influence bulk fluid flow between the fetal and maternal circulations.[13] As such, changes in vascular resistance within the fetal circulation may affect both the perfusion of the placenta and bulk flow of fluids between the fetal and maternal circulations.[13] Higher vascular resistance would make it harder for the fetal heart to effectively perfuse the placenta. However, more work is needed to fully understand these dynamics.

THE PLACENTAL BARRIER

In humans, the placental barrier at term consists of three main layers: the trophoblast, connective tissue, and capillary endothelium.

The trophoblast layer consists of a continuous syncytiotrophoblast in contact with maternal blood, overlying a discontinuous layer of cytotrophoblast. The syncytiotrophoblast is a transporting epithelium with a maternal facing microvillous membrane (MVM) and a fetal facing basal membrane (BM). The maternal facing villous surface is covered in microvilli, which are evenly distributed across different regions of villi and increase surface area by fivefold.[14] While the BM is often represented as flat, it does contain highly complex folded regions that indicate that its surface area is larger than generally believed.[15] The syncytiotrophoblast forms the maternal-fetal interface and while it covers the surface of the villi, there are regions of damage where it is replaced by fibrin deposits.[16] At term gestation, the cytotrophoblast lie underneath approximately 30% of the syncytiotrophoblast, as visualized by electron microscopy.[17] The cytotrophoblast are involved in syncytiotrophoblast renewal and continue to fuse with the syncytiotrophoblast until term. Whether the cytotrophoblast play an active role in nutrient transfer is uncertain, although some studies implicate them in lipid transfer.[18]

The trophoblast basal lamina is a layer of dense connective tissue that separates the trophoblast from the villous stroma. The barrier properties of the trophoblast basal lamina are not well characterized, unlike the renal glomerular basement membrane that allows free diffusion of low-molecular-weight molecules and restricts the transfer of larger molecules such as proteins. While the renal glomerular basement membrane effectively stops diffusion of albumin (molecular weight 66.5 kDa), IgG (molecular weight 150 kDa) can cross the trophoblast basal lamina. This suggests that the trophoblast basal lamina may be more permeable than the renal glomerular basement membrane.[19]

The villous stroma consists of a loose connective tissue that is unlikely to provide a significant barrier to the diffusion of hydrophilic molecules. The villous stroma could however provide a more significant barrier to diffusion of hydrophobic molecules (e.g., fatty acids, cortisol), which are normally bound to carrier proteins in plasma. Experimental evidence suggests that placental to fetal transfer of fatty acids and cortisol is much lower than placental to maternal transfer. This is consistent with slower diffusion across the villous stroma; however, further evidence is needed to prove this hypothesis.[20] The fibroblasts and macrophages within the villous stroma may also provide a diffusive barrier and will consume nutrients destined for the fetus. However, the overall effect of stromal cells on solute transfer has not been determined.

The fetal capillary endothelium is the final barrier to nutrient transfer or the initial barrier to waste transfer, depending on the direction of transfer. The fetal capillaries are partially covered by a layer of pericytes in close association with endothelial cells (Fig. 10.1). Transfer across the vascular endothelium can occur by a transcellular route (e.g., oxygen) or by a paracellular route via endothelial cell-cell junctions. The fetal capillary endothelium has a similar diffusive permeability to skeletal muscle.[21] It is assumed that many water-soluble solutes cross the endothelium via the paracellular route; however, there is little direct evidence of this. The endothelial junctions will be less permeable to hydrophobic solutes or larger solutes such as IgG. However, proteins associated with IgG and cholesterol transfer are expressed in the fetal capillary endothelium.[22,23]

Placental metabolism can act as a barrier to placental transfer, for example, the inactivation of maternal cortisol by placental 11β-hydroxysteroid dehydrogenase 2 prevents it from reaching the fetus.[24] Placental metabolism can impact transfer levels across the placenta by consuming nutrients so that they are not

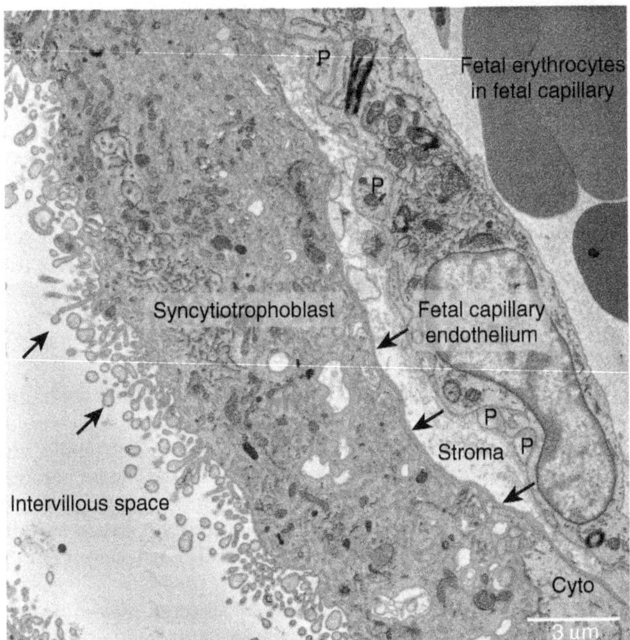

Fig. 10.1 Electron microscopy image showing a cross-section of the human placental barrier at term. The intervillous space is filled with maternal blood, the syncytiotrophoblast forms a continuous barrier across the surface of the villi, the micro villi on the apical plasma membrane are indicated by *white arrows*, and the syncytiotrophoblast basal membrane can be seen abutting the trophoblast basal lamina, which is indicated by *black arrows*. A small region of cytotrophoblast can be seen labeled "cyto" between the syncytiotrophoblast and trophoblast basal lamina. The connective tissue of the villous stroma lies between the trophoblast and the fetal capillaries. The stoma also contains fibroblasts and macrophages, which are not shown here. Pericyte fingers around the fetal capillary are labeled "P." The fetal capillary endothelial cells form the fetal blood vessel.

available to the fetus. Placental metabolism also determines the intracellular concentration of many substrates and therefore their availability to membrane transporters. Nutrients such as amino acids and fatty acids can be sequestered in placental intracellular pools (e.g., protein or phospholipid) with both the uptake and release of these nutrients from the pools affecting their availability for transport out of the placenta.

PASSIVE DIFFUSION

There is diffusion of lipophilic substances across the placenta by a transcellular route and transfer of hydrophilic substances by a poorly defined paracellular route. Oxygen, carbon dioxide, and small lipophilic drugs (such as anesthetics) can readily diffuse across the different layers of the placenta. Because diffusion of these substances across the placenta is rapid, transfer of these substances will be flow limited.

Clear functional evidence for size selective diffusion across the human placenta suggests that there must be a paracellular route; however, the anatomic basis for this remains unclear.[25,26] Transtrophoblastic channels have been proposed to explain the observed diffusion, and while potential channels are seen in human placenta, full width channels have not been directly observed.[27] Alternatively, there is evidence that regions of syncytial damage may provide a route for paracellular diffusion.[16]

MEMBRANE TRANSPORT

Most solutes require transport across the plasma membranes of placental cells including the syncytiotrophoblast and potentially the fetal capillary endothelium. Proteins that facilitate transfer of molecules and ions across plasma membranes include membrane transporters and channels. While the role of these membrane proteins is essential, it is important to recognize that other processes such as metabolism can influence transfer and may also be rate limiting.[28]

MEMBRANE TRANSPORTERS

Membrane transport proteins operate by binding one or more substrates on one side of the membrane, followed by a conformational change that translocates those substrates to the other side of the membrane. Membrane transport proteins can be grouped into transporter families. The P-type ATPase (e.g., sodium potassium ATPase) and ATP-binding cassette protein (ABC, e.g., multi-drug resistance protein) families mediate ATP-dependent active transport, whereas members of the solute carrier family (SLC, e.g., GLUT1/*SLC2A1*) mediate secondary active and facilitate transport.[29,30] The activity of the ATP-dependent transporters, particularly the sodium potassium ATPase, is ultimately responsible for creating the gradients that drive the activity of SLC family members. The ABC transport proteins play a role in transporting solutes such as cholesterol, inorganic ions, as well the efflux of drugs to potentially protect the fetus. The SLC superfamily of transport proteins contain 55 families, although not all are expressed or functional in placenta. The majority of nutrient transporters in the placenta membranes belong to the SLC superfamily.

TRANSPORTER CLASSES

Facilitated transport proteins mediate transport of solutes in both directions across the membrane, with net transport down the concentration gradient. Examples of facilitated transporters in the human placenta include the glucose transporter GLUT1/*SLC2A1*, amino acid transporters (TAT1/*SLC16A10*, LAT3/*SLC43A1*, and LAT4/*SLC43A2*[31]), and monocarboxylate transporters (e.g., MCT1/*SLC16A1* and MCT4/*SLC16A3*[32]).

Exchange transporters, or antiporters, transport one solute into the cell in exchange for another leaving the cell. Examples in the placenta include amino acid transporters (e.g., LAT1/*SLC7A5* and LAT2/*SLC7A8*) and the organic anion transporter (OAT4/*SLC22A11*). Exchange transporter activity will lead to equilibration of the proportions of their different substrates across the membrane with no change to the overall number of molecules. Increasing the number of exchange transporters in the membrane will mean that the equilibrium is reached faster. Therefore increasing exchanger activity will have minimal effect on a system that is already at or near equilibrium.[28]

Active transporters actively pump solutes into or out of cells and can transport against the concentration gradient. These may be primary active transporters that are powered by ATP or secondary active transporters that are driven by previously established membrane gradients. While these transporters can accumulate substrate, biophysical constraints will limit the extent to which they can do this. There is a point at which increasing the number of transporters in the membrane will no longer increase transport across the membrane because the gradient against which they need to pump is too great.

Plasma membrane primary active transporters in the placenta include members of the P-class (sodium potassium ATPase and plasma membrane calcium ATPase [PMCA]) and the ABC transporter superfamily.[30,33] The sodium potassium ATPase is located on both the MVM and BM of the syncytiotrophoblast, with the greatest activity on the MVM.[34] Secondary active transporters in the placenta include co-transporters such as members of the

SLC38 gene family that mediate sodium-dependent amino acid uptake.[35]

ENDOCYTOSIS

Endocytosis is the process whereby solutes or particles are transported into the cell within fluid-filled membrane-bound vesicles that form via invagination of the cell membrane. This is an important active transport mechanism in the placenta that is used to transport essential molecules, such as IgG, to the fetus. Endocytotic processes include phagocytosis, whereby larger particles are engulfed, pinocytosis that transports small solutes and water or receptor-mediated endocytosis. Endocytosis can therefore be nonselective or selective via the receptor-mediated internalization of specific extracellular ligands. Substrates can interact with specific cell surface receptors and form clathrin-coated pits that are released from the membrane into the cytoplasm via dynamin action. IgG, iron, low-density lipoprotein, and vitamin B_{12} are known to be taken up by receptor-mediated endocytosis and other molecules such as vitamin D may also be transported this way.[19,36]

MEMBRANE CHANNELS

Membrane channels provide a selective pore that mediates transfer of substrates, usually ions, across the membrane. Net transport occurs in the direction of the concentration gradient. There are many channels in the placental cell plasma membranes; however, these typically mediate cellular homeostasis rather than transplacental transfer with the exception of aquaporins.

PLASMA DETERMINANTS OF PLACENTAL TRANSFER

The composition of maternal and fetal plasma are important determinants of placental function. Both solute concentration and concentration gradient can be important determinants of placental transport. In addition, the presence of binding proteins may influence availability of solutes for placental uptake.

COMPOSITION OF THE MATERNAL PLASMA

The composition of maternal plasma is determined by maternal dietary intake, nutritional reserves, and metabolic state, as well as maternal lung, liver, and kidney function, for example, maternal plasma oxygen and carbon dioxide levels will be determined by lung function. Maternal metabolism is altered by placental hormones during pregnancy to increase nutrient availability to the fetus. However, maternal metabolic conditions during pregnancy could affect placental transfer, including diabetes mellitus, phenylketonuria, and intrahepatic cholestasis of pregnancy. These conditions may increase the gradient driving placental transfer and may affect the transfer of other substrates by competitive inhibition of their transporters. For instance, high phenylalanine levels with phenylketonuria may impair placental amino acid transport.[28]

Compounds in the maternal blood may also be harmful to the fetus, including pharmaceutical drugs (e.g., metformin, thalidomide), environmental toxins (e.g., phthalates), metabolites or wastes (e.g., bile acids), and maternal hormones. The levels of environmental toxins and pharmaceutical drugs in the maternal blood will be determined by maternal exposure or production versus the clearance of these compounds via the lungs, liver, and kidneys.

COMPOSITION OF THE FETAL PLASMA

The composition of the fetal plasma will be determined by both placental transfer and fetal metabolism. Fetal metabolism will affect placental transfer by controlling the solute gradients driving or opposing transfer. Higher metabolism will increase fetal carbon dioxide levels and reduce fetal glucose levels increasing the gradient driving the transfer of these substances across the placenta. Conversely, reduced fetal metabolism will reduce the gradients driving placental transfer of these solutes. This may provide an autoregulatory mechanism with a decrease in fetal plasma nutrients acting as a "signal" to the placenta to increase transfer to the fetus. Fetal metabolism may also be required to convert wastes into less toxic or more soluble forms to aid their placental transfer away from the fetus. For instance, sulfating many compounds will aid their solubility, and fetal production of urea and glutamate may aid transport of excess nitrogen to the mother.

PLASMA-BINDING PROTEINS

Many substances are transported in the plasma bound to albumin or specific binding proteins such as α-fetoprotein, retinol-binding protein, vitamin D-binding protein, transcobalamin, and corticosteroid-binding globulin. Albumin is the major protein in maternal plasma, and its concentration remains constant around 33 g/L across gestation despite maternal plasma volume expansion.[37] In contrast, vitamin D-binding protein concentrations increase in maternal plasma during pregnancy, suggesting an upregulation to meet fetal demands. Albumin does not cross the placental barrier and receptors such as megalin and cubilin expressed in human placenta may mediate the recycling of albumin back to the maternal circulation.[38]

Maternal plasma-binding proteins play an important role in delivery of their cargos to the placenta and influence the efficiency of placental transfer by acting as donors or acceptors for their substrates. Binding proteins may facilitate receptor-mediated placental uptake of key substrates including free fatty acids, calcium, iron, vitamin A, vitamin D, thyroid hormone, and cortisol. Similarly, many poorly soluble waste products and xenobiotics will need to bind to maternal albumin to be transported away from the placenta.[39]

In fetal plasma, albumin and other binding proteins act as acceptors of substances such as fatty acids and vitamin D and as donors of poorly soluble waste products. Fetal albumin concentrations rise during pregnancy from 16 g/L at 22 weeks to 32 g/L at term, whereas α-fetoprotein concentrations in fetal plasma decline toward term with concentrations of around 0.05 g/L.[40] α-Fetoprotein is a binding protein from the same family as albumin and vitamin D-binding protein. Its exact physiologic role is unclear, but it is known to act as a carrier protein for polyunsaturated fatty acids and bile acids.[41] Although, as in the maternal circulation, it is unclear whether these binding proteins are rate limiting for some or all substances, they need to be considered as part of the transfer system.

PLACENTAL TRANSFER OF SPECIFIC SOLUTES

As outlined earlier, many different factors can affect transfer of nutrients or wastes across the placenta. For some substances, the transplacental gradient will be rate limiting to transfer, while for others transfer may be limited by the actual transport proteins or processes, or by the impact of placental metabolism. Identifying the rate-limiting processes is important because these are most likely to lead to fetal growth restriction. The transfer of specific solutes is summarized in Table 10.1 and different routes of transfer in Fig. 10.2.

Studying placental transfer in humans is complicated by the difficulty of obtaining samples of maternal and fetal blood or placental tissue at different gestational ages. To assess placental transfer directly, four vessel sampling approaches have been used to sample arterial and venous uterine and cord blood alongside Doppler measurements of umbilical and cord blood flow.[42]

Table 10.1 Summary of Placental Solute Transfer Mechanisms.

Solute	Mode of Transfer	Placental Metabolism	Notes	References
Water	Transfer via transcellular and paracellular diffusion		Net diffusion to balance osmotic differences Aquaporins mediate transcellular water transfer	49
Na^+, K^+, Cl^-	Primarily paracellular diffusion		Transfer of Cl^- primarily by diffusion via paracellular route and likely that paracellular transfer exceeds transport for all electrolytes	37, 50
Oxygen	Simple diffusion	Net consumption	Flow limited Lower fetal than maternal partial pressures	45
Carbon dioxide	Simple diffusion	Net production	Flow limited Higher fetal than maternal partial pressures	
Glucose	Facilitated membrane transport	Net consumption of glucose, leading to net production of CO_2, lactate, and pyruvate	Lower fetal than maternal plasma concertation Primarily GLUT1 at term but a range of GLUTs are known to be expressed in placenta	52
Lactate, pyruvate	Facilitated membrane transport by MCT transporters → From placenta to mother and fetus	Net production	In humans transfer is primarily to the mother, but this is different in some other species, e.g., sheep	32
Amino acids	Secondary active membrane transport	Net consumption, interconversion and incorporation and release from placental protein pools	Higher fetal than maternal plasma concentrations Complex interplay of multiple membrane transporters	2
Fatty acids	Facilitated membrane transport and/or passive diffusion	Net consumption, incorporation and release from placental lipid pools	Lower fetal than maternal plasma concertation	80
Vitamin A	Uptake may occur via membrane transport	Placental metabolism	Maternal to fetal transfer	85
Vitamin D	Receptor mediated endocytosis and/or simple diffusion	Synthesis of 1,25 dihydroxyvitamin D and degradation	Low solubility requires plasma-binding protein	97
Folate	Uptake via endocytosis and membrane transport		Higher fetal than maternal plasma concentrations	146
Vitamin B_{12}	Uptake may occur via endocytosis and/or membrane transport		Higher fetal than maternal plasma concentrations Binds transcobalamin in plasma	98
Calcium (Ca^{2+})	Active membrane transport		Higher fetal than maternal plasma concentrations	105
Phosphate	Active membrane transport		Higher fetal than maternal plasma concentrations	147
Iron	Apical endocytosis (Fe^{3+}) and basal transport (Fe^{2+})		Uptake bound to transferrin	148
Sulphate (SO_4^{2-})	Membrane transport		Higher fetal than maternal plasma concentrations	110
Iodine	Membrane transport			112
IgG	Transcytosis		Higher fetal plasma concertation of maternal IgG than in maternal plasma at term	19

Key approaches used to study placental transfer include placental perfusion, villous fragment or explant studies, and trophoblast culture models (Table 10.2).

OXYGEN AND CARBON DIOXIDE TRANSFER

Placental gas transfer is necessary to provide the fetus with oxygen and to remove fetal carbon dioxide. The human placenta is estimated to consume around 40% of the oxygen it takes up,[43] therefore reducing oxygen availability to the fetus and releasing carbon dioxide into both circulations. At altitude, changes in placental glucose metabolism may play a role in prioritizing oxygen for delivery to the fetus.[44] The fetus requires oxygen to sustain metabolism and a mild chronic restriction in oxygen transfer during pregnancy at altitude may constrain fetal growth.[45] An acute decrease in oxygen transfer, for example, with cord occlusion, can cause marked tissue hypoxia. An inability to clear carbon dioxide will result in disturbances in fetal acid base balance and respiratory acidosis.

Oxygen and carbon dioxide are transferred by simple diffusion across the placenta. Transfer will be driven by the size of the transplacental partial pressure gradient for each gas. The partial pressure of oxygen (PO_2) in the maternal blood within intervillous space is only slightly above that in the umbilical vein.[46] The small transplacental PO_2 difference highlights how quickly diffusion leads to near equilibrium conditions and the importance of flow to maintain the necessary pressure gradient.

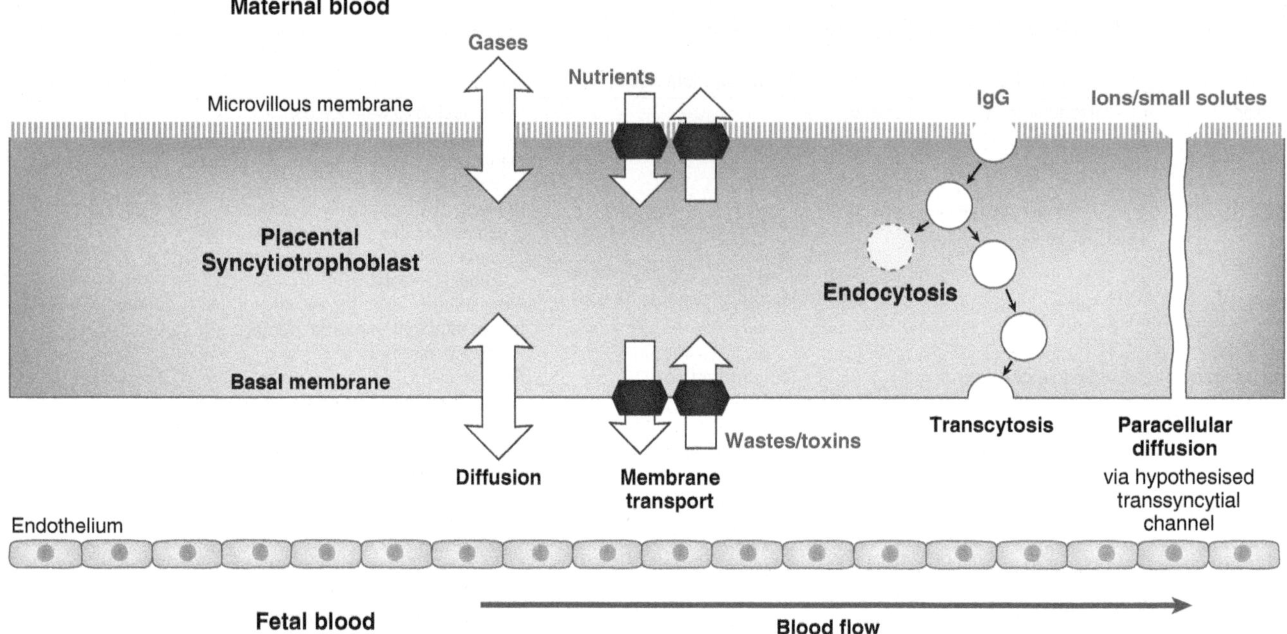

Fig. 10.2 Routes for solute transfer across the placenta. Transfer across the syncytiotrophoblast occurs via diffusion for lipophilic solutes and primarily gasses or by transporter-mediated transport across the microvillous and basal plasma membranes of the syncytiotrophoblast. There is also a paracellular route that allows size-dependent diffusion. Transfer across the villous stroma and endothelium is assumed to be by diffusion, but it is not clear how hydrophobic substances that are usually bound to binding proteins (e.g., cortisol, fatty acids) cross the stroma or how large substances (e.g., IgG) diffuse through capillary endothelial junctions.

Table 10.2 Key Methods Used to Study Placental Transfer.

Method	Description	Limitations	Reference
Placental perfusion	Placental lobule is perfused following delivery	Not blood	149
Villous fragments	Studies carried out on small pieces of fresh villous tissue	No blood flow Limited life in culture	150
Villous explants	Studies carried out on small pieces of fresh villous tissue maintained in culture	No blood flow, integrity of trophoblast needs to be monitored	151
MVM preparations	Purified microvillous membrane	While preparations are enriched for MVM, they may contain contaminants	152
BM preparations	Purified basal membrane	While preparations are enriched for BM, they may contain contaminants	152
Primary trophoblast culture	Cytotrophoblast cells are purified and cultured where they may syncytialize	Limited life in culture, hard to obtain confluent monolayers of syncytialized trophoblast	153
Cell lines (e.g., BeWo, Jeg3)	Easy to maintain	Derived from extra villous trophoblast and may not represent syncytiotrophoblast well	154
Imaging	Real-time uptake of labeled nutrients	Labeled nutrients may behave differently	18
Modeling	Using mathematical modeling to enhance the data generated from the above methods	Availability of good data	80, 155
Knockout mice	Allows knockout of specific genes	Species differences	156

Because diffusion is rapid, the principle rate-limiting factor for transfer will be blood flow; however, mixing of blood within the maternal intervillous space may also be important, especially in localized regions.

Gas transfer will also be influenced by hemoglobin concentrations and the Bohr and Haldane effects. Fetal hemoglobin (two α and two γ chains) has a higher affinity for oxygen than adult hemoglobin (two α and two β chains). The higher oxygen affinity of fetal hemoglobin occurs because it does not interact efficiently with 2,3-bisphosphoglycerate, which binds adult, but not fetal, hemoglobin and decreases its affinity for oxygen.[47]

Fetal blood hematocrit and hemoglobin rise during gestation from a hematocrit of 40% at 22 weeks to over 50% at term.[48] In contrast, maternal hematocrit and hemoglobin concentration fall during pregnancy, in part due to volume dilution, from a hematocrit of around 40% down to 34%.[49] The difference in maternal and fetal blood hemoglobin content means that the oxygen carrying capacity of fetal blood is greater than that of maternal blood.

The properties of circulating hemoglobin are also important for placental oxygen transfer through the Bohr and Haldane effects.

The Bohr effect describes the effect of hydrogen ion concentration on hemoglobin's oxygen affinity. Binding of hydrogen ions to hemoglobin stabilizes deoxyhemoglobin, reducing its affinity for oxygen. As a result, increasing hydrogen ion levels will increase oxygen availability and shift the hemoglobin disassociation curve to the right increasing oxygen availability to tissues. Decreasing hydrogen ion levels will have the reverse effect. The concentration of hydrogen ions is mainly a product of carbon dioxide and water being converted to carbonic acid by carbonic anhydrase and is determined by carbon dioxide concentrations. In the placenta, the effect of the increased carbon dioxide transferred from the fetus makes more maternal oxygen available for transfer to the fetus, while decreasing carbon dioxide concentrations in the feto-placental circulation reduce hydrogen ion binding to hemoglobin and increase its affinity for oxygen.

The Haldane effect describes a property of hemoglobin in which deoxyhemoglobin has a higher affinity for carbon dioxide than for oxyhemoglobin. In the maternal circulation of the intervillous space, loss of oxygen to the fetus will increase the amount of deoxyhemoglobin and increase the carbon dioxide carrying capacity of the blood. In the feto-placental circulation, oxygen arriving from the mother will increase the proportion of oxyhemoglobin and help displace the carbon dioxide, therefore increasing the transplacental carbon dioxide partial pressure gradient.

WATER AND ELECTROLYTE TRANSFER

Keeping the water and electrolyte balance within the fetus is essential to maintain physiologic homeostasis. To remain healthy, cells need to be surrounded by plasma or interstitial fluid of the right osmotic strength. The balance of electrolytes outside and within the cells ensures the electrical gradients necessary to maintain membrane potential and driving secondary active transport. The primary extracellular electrolytes are sodium and chloride ions, while within cells potassium ions predominate.

Water cannot be actively transported across a membrane and its net movement across the placenta will be determined by the net balance of osmotic and hydrostatic forces. It is likely that hydrostatic pressure within the fetal capillary is higher than the surrounding intervillous space, to prevent collapse of these capillaries. However, fetal capillary pressure cannot be too much higher than in the intervillous space because this would drive excessive net movement of fluid out of the fetus. Transfer of water can occur via both para and transcellular routes. Paracellular transfer of water though will be dependent on both osmotic and hydrostatic pressure gradients across the placenta. In contrast, transcellular movement of water mediated by the membrane channels aquaporins will be determined by osmotic rather than hydrostatic gradients. The transcellular transfer of water is mediated by aquaporins 3, 4, 8, and 9 in the trophoblast and aquaporin 1 in the capillaries.[50]

The proportions of placental paracellular versus transcellular water transfer is important because paracellular transfer is likely to be accompanied by small solutes including electrolytes, ions (except those bound to binding proteins), glucose, and amino acids. Electrolytes would be expected to diffuse relatively freely via the paracellular route, as seen for chloride transfer[51] and supported by the fact that sodium and potassium ion concentrations are the same in maternal and fetal plasma.[37] Diffusion of ions across the placenta may also be influenced by the electric potential difference of −2.7 mV across the placental barrier.[52] This may reflect the net transport of ions and charged molecules across the placenta and suggests that diffusion of electrolytes is not so rapid that this cannot be measured. This potential difference may also affect electrolyte diffusion via the transcellular route.

PLACENTAL NUTRIENT TRANSFER

PLACENTAL TRANSFER OF MACRONUTRIENTS

The placenta acts as a selective barrier between the maternal and fetal circulations, mediating transport of macronutrients including glucose, amino acids, and fatty acids to the fetus. Transfer of these substrates is mediated by specific membrane transporter proteins on the MVM and BM of the syncytiotrophoblast and metabolic processes within the placenta may play important roles in regulating transfer.

GLUCOSE TRANSPORT AND METABOLISM

Fetal growth is dependent on the glucose supply from the mother. The maternal to fetal glucose gradient is the major determinant of placental glucose transfer and higher maternal glucose levels drive increased transfer to the fetus.[53,54] Maternal glucose levels are elevated in pregnancy to facilitate placental transfer.[55] However, too much placental glucose transfer can be detrimental to the fetus as observed when maternal diabetes is associated with macrosomic fetuses.

Glucose transfer across plasma membranes is mediated by facilitated glucose transport proteins (GLUTs) on the MVM and BM of the syncytiotrophoblast. The predominant glucose transporter expressed in human placenta is GLUT1,[56] with threefold greater levels on the MVM compared to the BM.[57] While GLUT1 is the primary GLUT isoform in the placental syncytiotrophoblast, expression of GLUT3, GLUT4, GLUT8, GLUT9, GLUT10, and GLUT12 has also been demonstrated.[58] These other GLUT isoforms are likely to be quantitatively less important than GLUT1 in terms of total placental glucose transfer, but may play specific roles in the syncytiotrophoblast or other placental cell types. Insulin is reported to increase GLUT4 levels in the BM of the syncytiotrophoblast, which may increase glucose transfer to the fetus; however, the proportion of glucose flux via this route remains to be determined.[58]

The placenta has a high metabolic demand for glucose, with data from sheep suggesting 55% to 85% of glucose uptake is utilized by the placental tissue.[59] However, in human pregnancies approximately 70% of the maternal uteroplacental glucose uptake was transported to the fetus and approximately 30% was utilized by the placenta.[60] The amount of placental glucose consumption in this in vivo study appears lower than data from human ex vivo perfusion studies and animal studies.[54] Placental glucose consumption is necessary to meet its own metabolic requirements, and any glucose consumed by the placenta will not be available to the fetus. In the ovine placenta, glucose can be oxidized to carbon dioxide (15% to 20%), converted to lactate via glycolysis (30%), and metabolized to fructose via sorbitol (5% to 10%),[61] with lactate and fructose being transported into the maternal and fetal circulations. Under hypoxic conditions at altitude, human placental glucose metabolism is reported to be shifted toward anaerobic metabolism, reducing glucose delivery to the fetus.[44] This may be a mechanism by which fetal growth is reduced at altitude.

Placental release of lactate and pyruvate from glycolysis within the placenta can provide energy substrates to the fetus. It should be noted that there are species differences in placental lactate transport, and in contrast to the human, the sheep primarily transports lactate to the fetus.[62] In humans, placental-derived lactate and pyruvate are preferentially released into the maternal circulation.[53] These are transported by the monocarboxylate transporters MCT1 and MCT4 (*SLC16A1* and *SLC16A4*), which also transport ketone bodies.[32,63] Both transporter proteins are expressed in human placenta in the syncytiotrophoblast MVM and BM: MCT1 expression levels are higher in BM than MVM, and MCT4 levels are higher in MVM than BM. MCT1 on the BM may facilitate removal of excess fetal lactate. MCT1 is usually high in tissues that use lactate as a respiratory fuel and is therefore thought to be important for lactate influx. MCT4 is usually expressed in cells for rapid lactic acid efflux consistent with the observation that placental lactate is primarily released to the maternal circulation.

AMINO ACID TRANSPORT AND METABOLISM

Amino acids must be taken up by the placenta to meet both placental and fetal requirements. Amino acids are required for protein synthesis, as energy metabolites and as biosynthetic precursors in many metabolic pathways. The quantity and composition of amino acids supplied to the fetus are likely to be important determinants of fetal growth. Indeed, reduced placental amino acid transfer to the fetus is associated with poor fetal growth,[64] and studies in animal models suggest that decreased amino acid transport precedes and therefore mediates fetal growth restriction.[65]

There are 20 standard amino acids, and most are transported across the placenta with the notable exception of glutamate for which there is net uptake from the fetal circulation. Transfer of essential amino acids is particularly important as these cannot be made by the fetus. There is evidence for net fetal synthesis of some nonessential amino acids (e.g., glutamate), but any amino acid synthesis requires amino nitrogen, which typically comes from breakdown of other amino acids.

Placental amino acid transport to the fetal circulation is an active process and concentrations of amino acids are higher in fetal than maternal plasma.[2] To reach the fetal circulation amino acids are transported across the MVM and BM of the placental syncytiotrophoblast and are then thought to diffuse through the villous stroma and fetal capillary endothelial junctions into fetal blood.

Placental amino acid transport is mediated by accumulative and exchange transporter proteins working together on the MVM, and facilitated and exchange transporter proteins on the BM.[2] Accumulative transporters on the MVM include members of the SNAT *(SLC38A1-4)*, CAT *(SLC7A1-4),* and EAAT *(SLC1A1-3, 6, 7)* families. These proteins actively transport specific amino acids across the MVM into the syncytiotrophoblast creating transmembrane amino acid gradients to drive uptake of other amino acids via exchangers. The BM-facilitated transporters TAT1 *(SLC16A10)*, LAT3, and LAT4 (*SLC43A1* and *SLC43A2*) provide net amino acid transfer down their concentration gradient into the fetal circulation. These amino acids can then be exchanged for other amino acids via exchangers to ensure all essential amino acids are transferred to the fetus. Amino acid exchangers alter the composition but not the overall quantity of amino acids within the placenta. The exchange transporters on the MVM and BM include the LATs (*SLC7A5* and *SLC7A8*), y^+LATs (*SLC7A6* and *SLC7A7*), and ASCT1 and ASCT2 *(SLC1A4-5)*.[31]

The interdependency of these amino acid transporters can lead to nonintuitive outcomes (e.g., in some cases increased activity of a transporter can decrease overall placental amino acid transfer).[28] Furthermore, the overlap between transporter substrate specificities means that changing transporter activity can affect the transfer of amino acids not transported by that transport protein. For this reason, caution in needed when predicting how changes in individual transporters will affect overall amino acid transport. An important aspect of amino acid transfer is the interplay between different transporter classes and between transporter activity and metabolism. Computer modeling may prove to be an important tool in understanding how these interactions affect amino acid transfer.[28,66]

Within the placenta, amino acids are used for protein synthesis and the interconversion of amino acids,[63] which will change the transmembrane ratios that determine transfer by exchangers.[28] In the human placenta, there is net uptake of fetal glutamate across the BM into the placenta via the highly accumulative EAAT transporters.[67,68] This glutamate uptake leads to high glutamate levels within the placenta, which provide a metabolic substrate for the production of glutamine and provide a gradient to drive uptake of organic anions from the fetus.[67,68] In sheep, the conversion of serine to glycine is also a major pathway, but this is not thought to be the case in humans.[69]

A significant proportion of amino acids taken up by the placenta will be incorporated into placental protein, which needs to be recognized when using tracers to study amino acid transfer.[66] Amino acids incorporated into protein may still be transferred to the fetus when those proteins are broken down, but this will occur over much longer timescales than typical experiments. Therefore, short-term studies may underestimate total placental amino acid transfer.

FATTY ACID TRANSFER

The fetus requires fatty acids for the synthesis of cell membranes, the production of eicosanoid hormones and, in humans but few other species, the deposition of significant adipose deposits before birth.[70] While some fatty acids can be synthesized by the fetus from glucose, others must be transferred across the placenta. In particular, the fetus requires long-chain polyunsaturated fatty acids (LCPUFAs) that it cannot synthesize de novo.[71] These LCPUFAs are important for brain development, membrane fluidity, and eicosanoid synthesis. There is preferential transfer of LCPUFAs across the placenta, reflecting fetal demand for these fatty acids.[72]

Fatty acids are poorly soluble in plasma and are therefore bound to the plasma-binding proteins, albumin in the maternal circulation, and albumin and α-fetoprotein in the fetal circulation. In the ex vivo perfused human placenta the albumin concentration in the perfusion buffer is a major determinant of fatty acid transfer to the fetal circulation.[73] Fetal plasma albumin and total protein levels rise during pregnancy, and this may influence the rates of placental fatty acid transfer.[37]

The placenta can take up non-sterified fatty acids circulating in the maternal blood and fatty acids released from lipoproteins by lipases on the syncytiotrophoblast MVM.[74] Maternal plasma free fatty acids and lipoproteins are elevated during pregnancy, potentially increasing their availability to the fetus.[55] The extent of placental uptake of maternal lipoproteins is unclear, and whether this is a biologically relevant source of fatty acids for the placenta remains to be determined.

The human placenta expresses a number of proteins believed to be involved in fatty acid transport, on both the MVM and BM of the syncytiotrophoblast. These include members of the fatty acid transport protein family (FATP1-6/*SLC27A1-6*), fatty acid translocase (FAT/CD36), and plasma membrane fatty acid-binding protein FABPpm *(GOT2)*.[71] FATP1 *(SLC27A1)* and FAT/CD36 have been localized to both MVM and BM,[75] whereas FATP2 and FATP4 are only expressed on the BM of the syncytiotrophoblast.[76] Cytosolic fatty acid-binding proteins (e.g., FABP3 and FABP1) are also likely to be important and have been shown to play specific roles in LCPUFA transfer in the mouse placenta.[77] Lysophospholipid transporters, such as the major facilitator superfamily member *MFSD2A*, have also been demonstrated in the human placenta.[78] While the functional significance of these transporters is unclear, they may mediate transport of biologically important fatty acids such as docosahexaenoic acid (DHA).[79]

Fatty acids may also be taken up by simple diffusion, although there is no consensus on whether this can occur fast enough to meet biologic demands.[71] As fatty acid concentrations are higher in maternal plasma than in fetal plasma, fatty acid transfer is often portrayed as simple diffusion down a maternal to fetal gradient. However, while some studies suggest greater placental transfer of LCPUFAs with a greater maternal to fetal concentration gradient,[80] other studies of fatty acid transfer do not show this relationship.[81] If fatty acid transfer cannot simply be explained by the concentration gradient, it could be that placental metabolism plays a role. Indeed, fatty acids are rapidly converted to Acyl-CoA, and if this metabolic pathway reduced the placental free intracellular fatty acid concentrations below those in the fetal circulation, then there would not be a continuous transplacental gradient down which diffusion could occur.[71]

Computer modeling of placental fatty acid transfer data suggests that membrane transport is not a rate-limiting factor for placental fatty acid uptake.[81] Although membrane transport may not be rate limiting, FATP transporters have Acyl-CoA synthetase activity, mediating the first step in fatty acid metabolism. Therefore this activity may be more important than the actual transport. Evidence from human placental perfusion experiments suggests that most fatty acids taken up by the placenta are not transported directly to the fetus but are incorporated into lipid pools including phospholipid, triglyceride, and cholesteryl esters.[81] Modeling of these data suggests that metabolism is rate limiting for fatty acid transfer because the placental uptake and release of fatty acids from the placental lipid pools determines both how much nonesterified fatty acid is available and the gradients driving transfer.[81]

CHOLESTEROL TRANSFER

Another lipid that is transported by the placenta is cholesterol, which is important for cell membrane fluidity as well as synthesis of steroid hormones. The placenta requires cholesterol to synthesize progesterone, and fetal dehydroepiandrosterone (DHEA) to synthesize estrogen. The placenta cannot make DHEA as it lacks the correct enzymes, so the fetus makes DHEA from cholesterol, and this is transported to the placenta as DHEA or dehydroepiandrosterone sulphate (DHEAS).[82]

While the fetus is able to make some cholesterol from week 20 of pregnancy, maternal cholesterol is also thought to be transported to the fetus by the placenta.[83,84] There is net placental delivery of cholesterol to the fetus at term, with the level of cholesterol transfer unrelated to maternal serum cholesterol concentrations, suggesting that this is a process regulated by the placenta.[84] The mechanisms of placental cholesterol transfer are not well understood but uptake from the maternal circulation may occur via receptor-mediated endocytosis of lipoproteins. Uptake of lipoproteins has been demonstrated in first trimester and term trophoblast cells via the low-density lipoprotein receptor and scavenger receptor class B type I.[85] Cholesterol efflux transporters are present in villous capillary endothelial cells, which may mediate the final step of cholesterol efflux to the placenta.[22] Because cholesterol and cholesteryl esters are poorly soluble, it is unclear how they are transferred across the villous stroma.

VITAMIN AND MINERAL TRANSFER

Vitamins and minerals are micronutrients that are required in smaller amounts than macronutrients, but any deficiency in the placental transfer of these nutrients will impact fetal growth and development. Key micronutrients include vitamin A, vitamin D, iron, and folate, which are vital during fetal development because they are needed for metabolism, cell proliferation, differentiation, and signaling.

VITAMIN A

Vitamin A is essential for fetal development; however, too much vitamin A is harmful to the fetus.[86,87] Vitamin A is a group of lipid-soluble retinoids including retinol, retinal, and retinoic acid. Vitamin A can be synthesized from carotenoids, principally from β-carotene. In the plasma, vitamin A circulates bound to extracellular retinol-binding protein, and increasing evidence indicates that uptake into cells is mediated by a multi-domain membrane protein that is encoded by the stimulated by retinoic acid 6 *(STRA6)* gene.[88] The STRA6 protein is a transmembrane pore that transports vitamin A between extra- and intracellular retinoid-binding proteins. This is likely to be the case in the placenta that expresses *STRA6*, but other routes cannot be excluded.[86] Vitamin A is stored as inert retinal esters, and the esterification enzymes are expressed in fibroblasts but not trophoblast, suggesting fibroblasts may be a site of vitamin A storage in the placenta.[89]

β-Carotene crosses the human placenta and cord blood levels are correlated with, but lower than, maternal blood levels.[86] While the mechanism is unclear, β-carotene may be taken up when maternal lipoproteins are endocytosed. The extent of β-carotene metabolism to retinoids by the placenta or fetus is not well understood, but the conversion may be upregulated by poor maternal vitamin A status.[90]

VITAMIN D

Maternal vitamin D status during pregnancy is related to adverse pregnancy events such as preterm birth, gestational diabetes, and preeclampsia. Transfer of maternal vitamin D to the fetus is important for both fetal and lifelong health, as positive associations are observed between maternal 25-hydroxyvitamin D levels and fetal bone growth and birth weight[91,92]; these effects persist into postnatal life.[93,94] However, vitamin D transfer across the placenta is relatively poorly understood.

Vitamin D circulates in maternal plasma bound to vitamin D-binding protein or albumin. While vitamin D is seen as a lipid-soluble hormone that can be taken up by simple diffusion, this may not be the case. In the kidney, vitamin D uptake is mediated by receptor-mediated endocytosis via megalin and cubulin.[95] In the placenta, gene expression has been shown to be more closely related to maternal vitamin D-binding protein levels than to vitamin D itself.[96] These findings raise questions about the mechanisms by which vitamin D is transferred across the placenta and suggest that it may be more complicated than simple diffusion.

The placenta expresses many enzymes involved in vitamin D metabolism, and placental metabolism of vitamin D may also determine how much is available for transfer to the fetus. The placenta expresses 1α-hydroxylase *(CYP27B1)* and 24-hydroxylase (*CYP24A1*) indicating that it can mediate conversion of 25-hydroxyvitamin D to the active 1,25-dihydroxyvitamin D as well as break down both these molecules to inactive metabolites.[97] 1,25-dihydroxyvitamin D may modulate placental immunomodulatory function and calcium transport and may play a fundamental role in implantation and placental development.[98]

FOLATE AND VITAMIN B_{12}

Folate and vitamin B_{12} (cobalamin) are water-soluble vitamins that have higher concentrations in fetal blood than in maternal blood.[99] These vitamins facilitate one carbon metabolism, which underpins many biologic processes including DNA synthesis and repair as well as DNA methylation.[100]

During pregnancy, folate requirements are increased to meet the needs of the developing fetus. Risk of folate deficiency is therefore increased during pregnancy, with low maternal folate levels associated with fetal neural tube defects and other congenital abnormalities.[101] Folate uptake on the MVM of the syncytiotrophoblast is thought to be mediated by binding to folate receptor α, followed by endocytosis and uptake into the placenta. It is proposed that the proton-coupled folate transporter (PCFT/*SLC46A1*) mediates the folate efflux from endosomes. Efflux of folate across the BM is then carried out by the reduced folate carrier (RFC/*SLC19A1*).[102]

Maternal vitamin B_{12} deficiency is associated with poor fetal growth and premature birth.[103] Vitamin B_{12} circulates in maternal blood bound to its binding protein, transcobalamin. Uptake of transcobalamin-bound vitamin B_{12} into the placenta is mediated by receptor-mediated endocytosis via the transcobalamin receptor. In mice, there is evidence that vitamin B_{12} transfer can be via both the transcobalamin receptor and the cell surface receptor megalin.[104]

CALCIUM AND PHOSPHORUS

The fetus requires calcium and phosphorus for essential processes including calcium signaling, protein phosphorylation, and third trimester bone mineralization.[105]

Calcium concentrations are higher in the fetal than the maternal circulation, indicating active transport. Uptake of maternal calcium across the MVM of the syncytiotrophoblast is mediated by calcium channels including the transient receptor potential cation channel, subfamily V, and members 5 and 6 (*TRPV5* and *TRPV6*).[106] Transport of calcium from the placenta across the syncytiotrophoblast BM to the fetus is mediated by the ATP-dependent calcium efflux pumps, primarily PMCA1 and PMCA4 (*ATP2B1* and *ATP2B4*) and the sodium/calcium exchanger NCX2 (*SLC8A2*).[106] Once in the fetal circulation, calcium will be present as free ionized calcium and bound to plasma proteins including albumin. The bound calcium fraction will be protected from diffusion via the paracellular route back to the maternal circulation. Placental calcium transport may be regulated by fetal secretion of parathyroid hormone-related protein.[107]

Phosphorus transfer across the placenta is an active process with higher concentrations in the fetal plasma indicating active transport.[105] Phosphorus is transported as phosphate by secondary active transport via sodium-dependent phosphate transporter 1 and 2 (PiT1 and PiT2; *SCL20A1* and *SCL20A2*). The mechanism of phosphorus transport across the syncytiotrophoblast BM remains to be determined.

IRON TRANSFER

The fetus requires iron for the synthesis of heme for hemoglobin and for the function of many enzymes. Iron concentrations are higher in the fetal than the maternal circulation indicating active transport across the placenta. In the maternal circulation, ferric ions (Fe^{3+}) are bound to transferrin, which binds transferrin receptor 1 on the MVM of the placental syncytiotrophoblast initiating endocytosis and uptake into the placenta. Within the placenta, ferric ions are released from transferrin following acidification of the lysosomal vesicle. Ferric ions are reduced to ferrous ions (Fe^{2+}) by a ferroreductase and then transported across the BM by ferroportin (*SLC40A1*).[108] Once transported across the BM, ferrous ions are converted to ferric ions by a ferroxidase. Within the fetal circulation, the majority of ferric ions will be bound by transferrin. Work in mice suggests that placental iron transfer is not mediated by the hormone hepcidin, which regulates iron uptake from the intestinal epithelium.[109]

SULFATE

The fetus requires sulfates for many molecular processes, and sulfation of DHEA to DHEAS allows its transfer to the placenta where it is an essential substrate for estrogen synthesis.[110] Sulfate levels are higher in fetal than maternal plasma suggesting an active transport mechanism.[111] The transporter proteins involved in placental sulfate transport and their localization to the MVM and BM of the syncytiotrophoblast are not well characterized. Directional transfer may be mediated by sodium-dependent sulfate transporters NaS1 and NaS2 (*SLC13A3* and *SLC13A4*), and transfer may be further facilitated by multifunctional anion exchangers (*SLC26A1*, *2*, *6*, *7*, and *11*), which are expressed in placenta. It should be noted that sulfated compounds such as estrone sulfate or DHEAS are transported by different mechanisms, including the organic anion transporters (OATs) and organic anion transporting polypeptides (OATPs).[67,112]

IODINE

Placental iodine transfer is necessary for fetal synthesis of thyroid hormone. While placental iodine transfer is not well understood, several potential iodine transporters are expressed in trophoblast cells. These transporters include the sodium/iodide symporter (*SLC5A5*) and the sodium-dependent multivitamin transporter (*SLC5A6*), which are expressed in placenta and could mediate iodine uptake. The anion exchange protein pendrin (*SLC26A4*) may mediate efflux of iodine to the fetus.[113] Iodine could also be made available within the fetus from deiodination of maternal thyroid hormone.

TRANSFER OF IMMUNOGLOBULIN G, HORMONES, AND WASTES

While the role of the placenta is most often discussed in relation to nutrient transport, placental transfer of other substances including fetal waste products, drugs, selected hormones, and IgG are also essential to support fetal development.

IMMUNOGLOBULIN G TRANSFER

Maternal IgG is the only antibody class that the placenta selectively transfers to the fetus so as to confer passive immunity. There are four IgG subclasses, with IgG1 and IgG4 transported readily across the placenta and IgG2 and IgG3 showing less efficient transplacental transfer.[114] The mechanism of placental IgG transfer is thought to be transcytosis across the syncytiotrophoblast via a specific receptor that binds the fragment crystallizable (Fc) region of IgG: the neonatal Fc receptor (FcRn).[19] As a transcytosis receptor, FcRn is known to bidirectionally transport both IgG and albumin across polarized cellular barriers. The role of FcRn in transplacental transport is supported by ex vivo human placenta transport studies, showing that blocking or increasing the ability of the IgG molecule to bind the FcRn reduces or increases IgG transport, respectively.[114,38]

While the role of FcRn has been most extensively studied, other Fc receptors are expressed in the placenta and may play a role in IgG transfer across the syncytiotrophoblast or subsequently across the endothelium.[115] Indeed, differential transport of IgG subclasses indicate that other factors may be involved in transplacental IgG transport as well as the FcRn. In addition, the transfer of IgG subtypes may be altered in maternal disease states affecting the passive immunity of the fetus.[116]

CORTISOL

Cortisol is a lipid-soluble hormone that can diffuse across the placenta into the fetal circulation. Cortisol circulates in maternal plasma bound to plasma corticosteroid-binding globulin, which may influence its uptake into cells.[117] The placenta protects the fetus from excessive maternal cortisol by enzymatically deactivating cortisol using 11β-hydroxysteroid dehydrogenase 2, which converts cortisol to the inactive metabolite cortisone. In rats, inhibition of 11β-hydroxysteroid dehydrogenase 2 by carbenoxolone, a chemical found in licorice, causes fetal growth restriction and hypertension in the offspring.[118] The placenta itself also forms a barrier to cortisol transfer, with the fact that cortisol cannot freely diffuse across the placenta being as important a barrier as 11β-hydroxysteroid dehydrogenase 2 activity.[24] Cortisol is thought to cross plasma membranes by simple diffusion; however, there is some evidence of transport saturation in the placenta suggesting the possibility of mediated transport.[24]

THYROID HORMONES

Thyroid hormones (thyroxine, T_4, and triiodothyronine, T_3) are important for both the fetus and the placenta. Thyroid hormones can affect placental metabolism, differentiation, and development and can cross the human placenta to regulate fetal development. Evidence for placental transfer comes from the hyperthyroid fetuses where thyroid hormone in fetal blood must have been transferred from the mother.[119] Thyroid hormones in the maternal circulation are bound to the carrier proteins transthyretin, thyroxine-binding globulin, and albumin. Placental transfer of thyroid hormones is not well understood, but both transport processes and metabolism are likely to regulate any placental transfer to the fetus. Specific thyroid hormone transporter proteins have been identified that mediate transfer across the plasma membrane; however, which transporter is functionally important in placenta is not clear.

Studies using the ex vivo perfused placenta indicate transfer of both T_4 and T_3 from the maternal to fetal circulation, with transfer of T_4 limited by its metabolism by the type 3 deiodinase, which converts it to reverse T_3.[120] Thyroid hormones may be taken up by the placenta via the anion exchanger OATP4A1 *(SLCO4A1)* on the syncytiotrophoblast MVM and also by receptor-mediated endocytosis.[111,121] It has been suggested that the placental amino acid transporters LAT1 and LAT2 play a role in placental thyroid transport.[122] The facilitated amino acid transporter TAT1, expressed in human placenta, has also been shown to mediate thyroid hormone transport across the human placenta.[111] TAT1 is a member of the MCT family and is also known as *MCT10*. A further member of this family, MCT8, has also been shown to transport thyroid hormone across the placenta into the fetal circulation.

WASTES AND DRUGS

The placenta must detoxify the fetal blood to remove fetal waste products, drugs, and environmental toxins. This involves many of the transporter proteins that clear wastes into the proximal tubule in the kidney.

Fetal amino acid catabolism leads to synthesis of urea and in the sheep significant quantities of fetal urea are transported across the placenta to the mother. The human placenta expresses a number of facilitated urea transporters. The placenta expresses *SLC14A2*, which codes for several splice variants of urea transporter 2 (UT2).[123] Urea is also transported by aquaporins. Both urea transporters and aquaporins mediate facilitated diffusion of urea down a fetal to maternal gradient.

Wastes and toxins are taken up from the fetal circulation by exchange transporters on the BM, which include members of the OAT, OATP, and organic cation transporter (OCT) families.[124,125] ATP-dependent efflux transporters on the MVM then transport these wastes and toxins to the mother who can clear them through her liver and kidneys.[33] OAT4 *(SLC22A11)* and OATP2A1 *(SLCO2A1)* on the syncytiotrophoblast BM and OATP4A1 *(SLCO4A1)* on the syncytiotrophoblast MVM also play important roles in mediating placental uptake of biosynthetic precursors such as estrone sulfate. Estrone sulfate is an important precursor for the biosynthesis of estrogen by the placenta. High concentrations of the amino acid glutamate within the syncytiotrophoblast will facilitate clearance of wastes and toxins from the fetus as activity of the exchange transporters OAT4 and OATP2B1 is coupled to this gradient.[67]

REGULATION OF PLACENTAL TRANSFER

In order to maintain fetal demand, placental transfer of solutes can be regulated across gestation and in response to changes in the in utero environment. Placental transport is determined by many factors, such as solute concentration gradients, placental blood flow, and metabolism. For nutrients, the expression or activity of the nutrient transporters in the placental syncytiotrophoblast mediates the rate of transfer to the fetus. Changes to the factors regulating placental nutrient transport are seen in pregnancies with abnormal fetal growth. Understanding the regulation of placental nutrient transfer is key to designing effective intervention strategies to modulate fetal growth.

GESTATIONAL CHANGES IN PLACENTAL TRANSFER

Placental transfer capacity must increase across gestation to meet the increasing demands of a growing fetus. This is supported by changes in placental size and structure and may also involve changes in the activity of specific transport mechanisms. Changes in transporter expression, regulation, and activity can be observed across gestation.[126,127] One molecule whose transfer has been measured in vivo across gestation is IgG. At the end of the first trimester, maternal IgG levels in fetal blood are around 10% of the concentration in maternal blood. This rises to 50% of maternal levels by the end of the second trimester, and at term, levels in the fetus often exceed those in the mother.[128]

REGULATORY SIGNALS

The regulation of placental function needs to take into account both fetal demand and maternal capacity to support the pregnancy. In humans, there is evidence for maternal constraint of fetal growth, something that is likely mediated via the placenta. The evidence for maternal constraint in humans includes that twins are typically born smaller than singletons and that birth weight is more strongly related to maternal than paternal weight despite a similar genetic contribution.[129,130]

How the mother signals to the placenta is unclear, but there are correlations between maternal body composition, a factor that mediates the in utero environment, and placental transport function and transporter gene expression.[77,95,131] The exact signaling molecules are unclear but could include nutrients and hormones. Changes in placental structure and transporter gene expression can also be demonstrated in response to maternal disease, diet, and smoking.[95,132,133] Maternal factors have been shown to cause epigenetic changes in the placenta, and these have the potential to change placental function across gestation.[126] Maternal environment and lifestyle factors may therefore modify placental function to match the mother's capacity to support the demands of fetal growth.

How the placenta senses maternal and fetal signals is of great interest. Studies in human primary trophoblast demonstrate how the placenta may respond to stimuli including sensing of nutrient levels and maternal hormones.[134-136] Regulation of fatty acid, amino acid, and glucose transporters in the placenta have all been demonstrated in response to their respective substrates.

Placental sensing of nutrient levels has clearly been demonstrated through the mechanistic target of rapamycin (mTOR) pathway,[134,137,138] which is downregulated in intrauterine growth restriction.[139] This pathway has been shown to regulate the expression of transport proteins and their localization to the syncytiotrophoblast plasma membranes.[140,141] Placental sensing of maternal hormone levels may also be an important regulatory mechanism and transporter protein trafficking to the membrane has been shown to be hormonally regulated.[142] Hormone receptors are present in the maternal facing MVM, and these include receptors for leptin, insulin-like growth factor-1, and insulin, which are factors that stimulate amino acid and glucose transporter activity.[142,143]

Evidence for fetal control of placental function comes from knockout studies in mice where reduced fetal growth is associated with compensatory upregulation of placental transport.[144] Increasing fetal demand may signal indirectly to the placenta by decreasing nutrient levels in fetal blood, which will increase the gradient driving transfer and may also be sensed by placental nutrient sensing mechanisms such as mTOR.

CLINICAL AND HEALTH IMPLICATIONS

The placenta must transport many different nutrients and wastes, and restricted transfer of any one of these could impair fetal development. Altered placental transport may affect overall size of the fetus or specifically alter development of one or more organs. Depending on the extent of placental dysfunction, it may lead to stillbirth, fetal growth restriction, premature birth, or more subtle changes such as a change in nephron number.[118]

In the longer term, the way in which the fetus develops in the womb builds the foundations for lifelong health, and developmental compromises such as the number of nephrons or pancreatic β cells may have implications for health across the life course. From a clinical perspective, placental researchers need to identify the causes of placental dysfunction so as to improve its diagnosis and prevention, as well as to develop effective interventions to optimize placental function when it is already compromised.

An appreciation of how placental transfer operates as an integrated system is important in designing interventions, because a therapy that increases the activity of one transporter may not have the desired effect on placental function if another factor is rate limiting. Identifying the rate-limiting processes within the placenta is not always obvious, and computer modeling may provide key insights here.[2] Given that there may be multiple causes of placental dysfunction, a personalized medicine approach may be necessary with a need to better characterize placental phenotypes and identify accessible biomarkers for this. Just as improving fetal growth may have lifelong benefits, an ill-judged intervention could cause lifelong detriment.[145]

CONCLUSION

By supplying nutrients and clearing wastes from fetal blood, the placenta creates the environment to allow fetal growth and development. The placenta actively mediates transfer processes using specific mechanisms for different classes of nutrients and wastes. Understanding the physiologic basis of placental function and the changes in pathophysiologic states will help develop preventative strategies and new therapeutic interventions.

 A complete reference list is available at www.ExpertConsult.com.

SELECT REFERENCES

1. Burton GJ, Fowden AL, Thornburg KL. Placental origins of chronic disease. *Physiol Rev*. 2016;96(4):1509-1565.
2. Cleal JK, Lofthouse EM, Sengers BG, Lewis RM. A systems perspective on placental amino acid transport. *J Physiol*. 2018;596(23):5511-5522.
4. Burton GJ, Watson AL, Hempstock J, Skepper JN, Jauniaux E. Uterine glands provide histiotrophic nutrition for the human fetus during the first trimester of pregnancy. *J Clin Endocrinol Metabol*. 2002;87(6):2954-2959.
5. Turco MY, Moffett A. Development of the human placenta. *Development*. 2019;146(22).
7. Collins SL, Welsh AW, Impey L, Noble JA, Stevenson GN. 3D fractional moving blood volume (3D-FMBV) demonstrates decreased first trimester placental vascularity in pre-eclampsia but not the term, small for gestation age baby. *PloS One*. 2017;12(6):e0178675.
8. Schroder HJ. Comparative aspects of placental exchange functions. *Eur J Obstet Gynecol Reprod Biol*. 1995;63(1):81-90.
11. Brownbill P, McKeeman GC, Brockelsby JC, Crocker IP, Sibley CP. Vasoactive and permeability effects of vascular endothelial growth factor-165 in the term in vitro dually perfused human placental lobule. *Endocrinology*. 2007;148(10):4734-4744.
13. Brownbill P, Sibley CP. Regulation of transplacental water transfer: the role of fetoplacental venous tone. *Placenta*. 2006;27(6-7):560-567.
15. Jones CJ, Fox H. An ultrastructural and ultrahistochemical study of the placenta of the diabetic woman. *J Pathol*. 1976;119(2):91-99.
16. Brownbill P, Mahendran D, Owen D, et al. Denudations as paracellular routes for alphafetoprotein and creatinine across the human syncytiotrophoblast. *Am J Physiol Regul Integr Comp Physiol*. 2000;278(3):R677-R683.
21. Leach L, Firth JA. Structure and permeability of human placental microvasculature. *Microsc Res Tech*. 1997;38(1-2):137-144.
24. Stirrat LI, Sengers BG, Norman JE, et al. Transfer and metabolism of cortisol by the isolated perfused human placenta. *J Clin Endocrinol Metab*. 2018;103(2):640-648.
29. Hediger MA, Clemencon B, Burrier RE, Bruford EA. The ABCs of membrane transporters in health and disease (SLC series): introduction. *Mol Aspects Med*. 2013;34(2-3):95-107.
31. Cleal JK, Glazier JD, Ntani G, et al. Facilitated transporters mediate net efflux of amino acids to the fetus across the basal membrane of the placental syncytiotrophoblast. *J Physiol*. 2011;589(Pt 4):987-997.
32. Settle P, Mynett K, Speake P, et al. Polarized lactate transporter activity and expression in the syncytiotrophoblast of the term human placenta. *Placenta*. 2004;25(6):496-504.
36. Fisher AL, Nemeth E. Iron homeostasis during pregnancy. *Am J Clin Nutr*. 2017;106(suppl 6):1567S-1574S.
43. Carter AM. Placental oxygen consumption. Part I: in vivo studies–a review. *Placenta*. 2000;21(suppl A):S31-S37.
51. Doughty IM, Glazier JD, Greenwood SL, Boyd RD, Sibley CP. Mechanisms of maternofetal chloride transfer across the human placenta perfused in vitro. *Am J Physiol*. 1996;271(6 Pt 2):R1701-R1706.
53. Day PE, Cleal JK, Lofthouse EM, Hanson MA, Lewis RM. What factors determine placental glucose transfer kinetics? *Placenta*. 2013;34(10):953-958.
59. Vaughan OR, Fowden AL. Placental metabolism: substrate requirements and the response to stress. *Reprod Domest Anim*. 2016;51(suppl 2):25-35.
63. Day PEL, Cleal JK, Lofthouse EM, et al. Partitioning of glutamine synthesised by the isolated perfused human placenta between the maternal and fetal circulations. *Placenta*. 2013;34(12):1223-1231.
65. Jansson N, Pettersson J, Haafiz A, et al. Down-regulation of placental transport of amino acids precedes the development of intrauterine growth restriction in rats fed a low protein diet. *J Physiol*. 2006;576(Pt 3):935-946.
67. Day PE, Cleal JK, Lofthouse EM, et al. Partitioning of glutamine synthesised by the isolated perfused human placenta between the maternal and fetal circulations. *Placenta*. 2013;34(12):1223-1231.
68. Lofthouse EM, Brooks S, Cleal JK, et al. Glutamate cycling may drive organic anion transport on the basal membrane of human placental syncytiotrophoblast. *J Physiol*. 2015;593(20):4549-4559.
71. Lewis RM, Childs CE, Calder PC. New perspectives on placental fatty acid transfer. *Prostaglandins Leukot Essent Fatty Acids*. 2018;138:24-29.
76. Lager S, Ramirez VI, Gaccioli F, Jang B, Jansson T, Powell TL. Protein expression of fatty acid transporter 2 is polarized to the trophoblast basal plasma membrane and increased in placentas from overweight/obese women. *Placenta*. 2016;40:60-66.
81. Perazzolo S, Hirschmugl B, Wadsack C, Desoye G, Lewis RM, Sengers BG. The influence of placental metabolism on fatty acid transfer to the fetus. *J Lipid Res*. 2017;58(2):443-454.
84. Horne H, Holme AM, Roland MCP, et al. Maternal-fetal cholesterol transfer in human term pregnancies. *Placenta*. 2019;87:23-29.
85. Wadsack C, Hammer A, Levak-Frank S, et al. Selective cholesteryl ester uptake from high density lipoprotein by human first trimester and term villous trophoblast cells. *Placenta*. 2003;24(2-3):131-143.
86. Spiegler E, Kim YK, Wassef L, Shete V, Quadro L. Maternal-fetal transfer and metabolism of vitamin A and its precursor beta-carotene in the developing tissues. *Biochim Biophys Acta*. 2012;1821(1):88-98.
88. Kawaguchi R, Yu J, Honda J, Hu J, et al. A membrane receptor for retinol binding protein mediates cellular uptake of vitamin A. *Science*. 2007;315(5813):820-825.
89. Sapin V, Chaib S, Blanchon L, et al. Esterification of vitamin A by the human placenta involves villous mesenchymal fibroblasts. *Pediatr Res*. 2000;48(4):565-572.
91. Harvey NC, Holroyd C, Ntani G, et al. Vitamin D supplementation in pregnancy: a systematic review. *Health Technol Assess*. 2014;18(45):1-190.
96. Cleal JK, Day PE, Simner CL, et al. Placental amino acid transport may be regulated by maternal vitamin D and vitamin D-binding protein: results from the Southampton Women's Survey. *Br J Nutr*. 2015;113(12):1903-1910.
99. Baker BC, Hayes DJ, Jones RL. Effects of micronutrients on placental function: evidence from clinical studies to animal models. *Reproduction*. 2018;156(3):R69-R82.
102. Solanky N, Requena Jimenez A, D'Souza SW, Sibley CP, Glazier JD. Expression of folate transporters in human placenta and implications for homocysteine metabolism. *Placenta*. 2010;31(2):134-143.
104. Arora K, Sequeira JM, Quadros EV. Maternofetal transport of vitamin B12: role of TCblR/CD320 and megalin. *FASEB J*. 2017;31(7):3098-3106.
107. Hayward CE, McIntyre KR, Sibley CP, Greenwood SL, Dilworth MR. Mechanisms underpinning adaptations in placental calcium transport in normal mice and those with fetal growth restriction. *Front Endocrinol (Lausanne)*. 2018;9:671.
115. Martinez DR, Fouda GG, Peng X, Ackerman ME, Permar SR. Noncanonical placental Fc receptors: what is their role in modulating transplacental transfer of maternal IgG? *PLoS Pathog*. 2018;14(8):e1007161.
122. Adu-Gyamfi EA, Wang YX, Ding YB. The interplay between thyroid hormones and the placenta: a comprehensive reviewdagger. *Biol Reprod*. 2020;102(1):8-17.
127. Novakovic B, Gordon L, Robinson WP, Desoye G, Saffery R. Glucose as a fetal nutrient: dynamic regulation of several glucose transporter genes by DNA methylation in the human placenta across gestation. *J Nutr Biochem*. 2012.
134. Rosario FJ, Powell TL, Jansson T. mTOR folate sensing links folate availability to trophoblast cell function. *J Physiol*. 2017;595(13):4189-4206.
135. Aye IL, Jansson T, Powell TL. TNF-alpha stimulates system A amino acid transport in primary human trophoblast cells mediated by p38 MAPK signaling. *Physiol Rep*. 2015;3(10).
137. Rosario FJ, Kanai Y, Powell TL, Jansson T. Mammalian target of rapamycin signalling modulates amino acid uptake by regulating transporter cell surface abundance in primary human trophoblast cells. *J Physiol*. 2013;591(3):609-625.
142. Jones HN, Jansson T, Powell TL. Full-length adiponectin attenuates insulin signaling and inhibits insulin-stimulated amino Acid transport in human primary trophoblast cells. *Diabetes*. 2010;59(5):1161-1170.
144. Dilworth MR, Kusinski LC, Cowley E, et al. Placental-specific Igf2 knockout mice exhibit hypocalcemia and adaptive changes in placental calcium transport. *Proc Natl Acad Sci U S A*. 2010;107(8):3894-3899.
148. McArdle HJ, Andersen HS, Jones H, Gambling L. Copper and iron transport across the placenta: regulation and interactions. *J Neuroendocrinol*. 2008;20(4):427-431.

149. Schneider H. IFPA senior award lecture: energy metabolism of human placental tissue studied by ex vivo perfusion of an isolated cotyledon. *Placenta*. 2015;36(suppl 1):S29-S34.
150. Greenwood SL, Sibley CP. In vitro methods for studying human placental amino acid transport placental villous fragments. *Methods Mol Med*. 2006;122:253-264.
152. Glazier JD, Sibley CP. In vitro methods for studying human placental amino acid transport: placental plasma membrane vesicles. *Methods Mol Med*. 2006;122:241-252.
156. Constancia M, Hemberger M, Hughes J. Placental-specific IGF-II is a major modulator of placental and fetal growth. *Nature*. 2002;417(6892):945-948.

Endocrine and Paracrine Function of the Human Placenta

11

Anna A. Penn

INTRODUCTION

The placenta produces a greater diversity of hormones in greater quantity than any other single endocrine tissue. Near term, steroid hormones (primarily estrogens and progestins) are being made at the rate of 0.5 g/day, and protein hormones (lactogens, growth factors, and other hormones similar to those of the hypothalamic-pituitary-adrenal axis) are being made at more than twice this rate. Although the secretory nature of the placenta was recognized by the early 1900s,[1,2] it was not until the 1950s that the placenta was recognized as part of a highly regulated endocrine system incorporating the fetus and mother. Placental hormones, made either directly by the placenta or dependent on placental synthesis of precursors, are critical for fetal growth and for metabolic adjustments in response to environmental factors of pregnancy in both mother[3] and fetus.[4] These hormones may act as endocrine, paracrine, and autocrine signals that link maternal physiology to fetal development through placental alterations in structure, secretion, or growth.

PLACENTAL STRUCTURE SUPPORTING ENDOCRINE FUNCTIONS

The human hemochorial placenta allows maternal blood to have direct contact with fetal tissue through controlled invasion of the maternal vascular system by fetal trophoblasts. This invasion peaks around 12 weeks gestation[5] although placental maturation continues well into the third trimester. During the initial invasion of the maternal spiral arteries and formation of chorionic villi, trophoblasts differentiate along two major pathways: into invasive extravillous cytotrophoblasts and into a fused layer of syncytiotrophoblasts (Fig. 11.1). Syncytiotrophoblasts are the primary hormone-producing cells in the placenta, making both peptide and steroid hormones, whereas cytotrophoblasts appear to make a limited set of peptide hormones. Additional hormones are made in adjacent fetal and uterine tissues, including amnion, chorion, and decidua. The placenta is not only a producer of hormones but also acts as a barrier to hormone transfer (i.e., thyrotropin-stimulating hormone and insulin) from the mother to the fetus or as a modifier of endocrine signaling through specific metabolism of maternal or fetal hormones.

The human placenta has multiple intrinsic physiologic functions and produces many factors that regulate them. However, the placenta does not act in isolation. Its functions are integrated with those of other intrauterine tissues, such as the maternal uterus, chorion, amnion, decidua, amniotic fluid, and the fetus. These other intrauterine tissues produce or use some of the same hormones and carrier proteins that regulate placental hormone activity. Metabolic signals and precursors, as well as hormones, are carried by maternal and fetal blood or transported from cell to cell from the uterus, decidua, fetal membranes, and amniotic fluid to and from the placenta. Integration of activities across multiple tissues provides the normal physiology of pregnancy, allowing its maintenance and timely parturition.

PLACENTAL HORMONES

This chapter focuses on the major endocrine, paracrine, and autocrine signals made by the placenta; given that the human placenta is capable of synthesizing most of the hormones identified to date, there are many factors that will not be discussed and likely many more will be discovered in the future. Table 11.1 highlights major peptide and steroid factors described in placental endocrine function. Understanding is still limited regarding the roles that many of these hormones play in the local endocrinology of placental development or in the broader regulation of the materno-feto-placental system required for successful pregnancy outcome. This chapter highlights what is currently known about the expression, function, and regulation of the major categories of peptide and steroid placental hormones.

PITUITARY-LIKE HORMONES

HUMAN CHORIONIC GONADOTROPIN

Human chorionic gonadotropin (hCG) is one of the first hormones of pregnancy, produced by trophoblasts even before placenta formation.[6] After placentation, hCG is synthesized primarily by the syncytiotrophoblasts[7] and passes into the maternal circulation via secretion into the intervillous space. hCG can be detected in human serum or urine within a week of conception and is the most frequently used biochemical marker for pregnancy.

The primary biologic role of hCG is to maintain progesterone production by the corpus luteum until this function shifts to the maturing placenta. This transition from ovarian to placental steroid production, required to sustain human pregnancy, is referred to as the *ovarian-placental shift*. This progesterone shift starts at the end of the sixth gestational week and is complete by the ninth week, at least 2 weeks before the level of placental hCG peaks (Fig. 11.2), minimizing the chance of loss of the progestational environment.

hCG is unique to human pregnancy; primate placentas express similar gonadotropins, but the vast majority of placentas from other species do not.[8] hCG is a glycoprotein heterodimer (36 to 40 kDa) composed of an α-subunit and β-subunit encoded by genes on chromosome 6 and chromosome 19, respectively.[9,10] The α-subunit is homologous to pituitary thyroid-stimulating hormone (TSH), luteinizing hormone (LH), and follicle-stimulating hormone (FSH), whereas the β-subunit is homologous to LH. hCG can be immunologically distinguished from LH with use

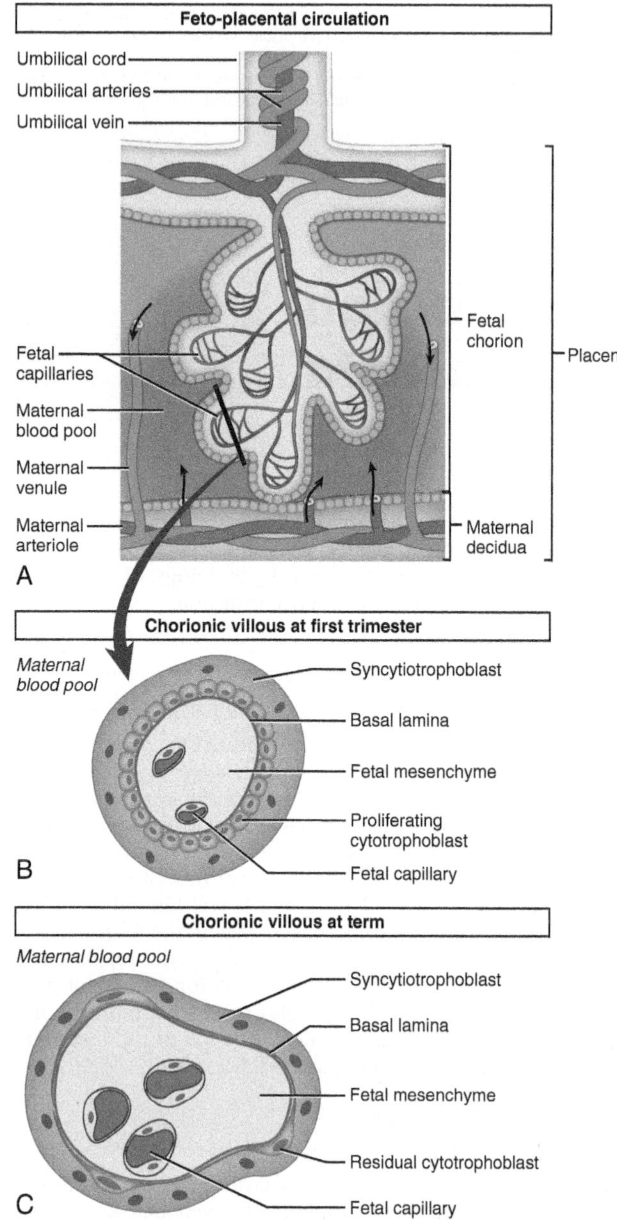

Fig. 11.1 Placental anatomy.

of antisera directed against the C-terminal amino acids of its β-subunit, which are not present in LH. β-subunit hCG–specific antisera is the basis for most current pregnancy tests.

Intact hCG (i.e., having both an α-subunit and a β-subunit) is required for hCG endocrine activities. Because it shares a receptor with LH, the LH chorionic gonadotrophin receptor (LHCGR), hCG mimics the function of LH. Both hormones activate second-messenger pathways, primarily cyclic adenosine monophosphate (cAMP) pathways, via LHCGR. However, the functions of LH and hCG are quantitatively different owing to the longer half-life of hCG and its relatively stable presence in the bloodstream compared with the pulsatile release of pituitary LH.[11]

Variations in both glycosylation and subunit availability appear to regulate hCG activity. A hyperglycosylated form (hCG-H) has been detected in early pregnancy, as well as in choriocarcinoma cells. hCG-H appears to enhance invasive cytotrophoblast activity independently of LHCGR, possibly through a transforming growth factor receptor pathway.[9] hCG-H may be a very early biomarker of placental invasion of the endometrium. A decreased level of hCG glycosylation in very early pregnancy has been correlated with early pregnancy loss, although this measure is not currently used clinically.[9,12,13] Isoform production may also regulate activity. Initially, β-subunit production exceeds α-subunit production, but this ratio rapidly shifts to an excess of the α-subunit, and the ratio increases as gestation progresses. As a result, little free β-hCG is secreted, and circulating hCG is mostly intact hCG or free α-hCG. It has been proposed that the ratios of hCG isoforms (intact hCG, independent subunits, and nicked breakdown products) present in maternal blood and urine might be useful for detection of pregnancy-related disorders because only intact hCG is fully active and abundance of other isoforms may modulate this activity.[14]

Clinically, hCG doubling time may be used in early gestation to predict general pregnancy outcome. After hCG can first be detected, its level increases with a doubling time averaging 2.11 days. It reaches peak levels of approximately 50 international units per milliliter at 9 to 10 weeks from the date of the last menstrual period, declining to 1 IU/mL by mid-gestation (see Fig. 11.2).[15] An abnormally slow doubling time of hCG concentration is considered to be a sign of a poor prognosis for pregnancy outcome, whereas a rising hCG level without detection of an intrauterine embryo suggests an ectopic pregnancy.[16]

Both local and systemic factors can influence hCG production. Locally, hCG expression is regulated by a releasing factor, gonadotropin-releasing hormone (GnRH; isoforms I and II), produced largely in the cytotrophoblasts.[17,18] Additional factors, including neurotransmitters,[19] cAMP,[20] epidermal growth factor (EGF),[21] activin,[22] cytokines,[23] prostaglandins,[23] and hCG itself regulate hCG production. Each of these factors is produced by the placenta, as well as by other trophoblastic tissues. hCG is known to affect placental steroidogenesis by stimulating both progesterone and estrogen formation. Estrogens can inhibit GnRH stimulation of hCG,[24] thereby completing a feedback axis in the paracrine placenta. Other hormones such as inhibin[25] have also been shown to modulate this axis.

Although most of our understanding of hCG expression, function, and regulation comes from studies of its role as an endocrine signal for the maternal corpus luteum, hCG has multiple activities that regulate placental structure and function and modify the intrauterine environment to support implantation and fetal survival. In addition to its well-known endocrine function for the corpus luteum, hCG acts as an autocrine signal in trophoblasts expressing LHCGR. In trophoblasts, hCG regulates the differentiation of cytotrophoblasts into syncytiotrophoblasts, thus amplifying hCG production because it is made primarily by the syncytiotrophoblasts.[19] Phosphorylation of the receptors via this pathway also decreases LHCGR expression in differentiating syncytiotrophoblasts, thus completing a feedback loop.[26]

More recently identified activities of hCG also include roles in endometrial angiogenesis, maintaining uterine quiescence, and enhancing immunotolerance to the fetus.[9,27] In addition, hCG appears to have maternal thyrotropic activity because of its partial homology to TSH. However, recent studies demonstrate that although elevated hCG levels suppress maternal TSH levels, leading to elevation of the levels of free thyroxine, this action is rarely associated with maternal hyperthyroidism.[28] Continued research is required to fully define the wide-ranging effects of this classic human pregnancy hormone given its potential impact on multiple aspects of pregnancy.

PLACENTAL SOMATOTROPINS

A hormone similar to pituitary growth hormone (GH) and prolactin was first extracted from human placenta in the early 1960s.[29,30] This hormone was initially named *human placental lactogen,* but was later renamed *human chorionic somatomammotropin* (hCS), to reflect its GH-like activity and its lactogenic activity; both names remain in use.

Table 11.1 A Subset of Endocrine and Paracrine Hormones and Related Factors Expressed in Human Placenta.[a]

Steroid Hormones	Pituitary-Like Hormones, Including Growth Factors	Hypothalamic-Like Hormones	Neuropeptides	Placental Cytokines	Eicosanoids
Estriol	**hCG**	**CRH**	**Serotonin**	**TNF-α**	**Prostaglandins**
Estradiol	**hCS**	**Urocortins**	**Dynorphin**	**LIF**	**Leukotrienes**
Estrone	**hGH-V**	**GnRH-I, GnRH-II**	**Met-enkephalin**	Interferon-α	**Prostacyclin**
Estetrol	**IGF-I**	**GHRH**	**ANP**	Interferon-β	**Thromboxane**
Progesterone	**IGF-II**	**Somatostatin**	**Leptin**	Interferon-γ	
Allopregnanolone	**Activin**	**TRH**	**Ghrelin**	IL-1	
Pregnenolone5α-DHP	**Inhibin**	**PRH**	**Adiponectin**	IL-2	
Cortisone	**Follistatin**		Neurotensin	**IL-6**	
Testosterone	**β-Endorphin**		Substance P	IL-8	
Androstenedione	**Oxytocin**		Melatonin	IL-10	
DHT	**ACTH**		Cholecystokinin		
DHEA	**MSH**		Galanin		
	Relaxin		Neuropeptide Y		
			Endothelin		
			VIP		

[a]Those mentioned in the text are shown in bold.
5α-DHP, 5α-Dihydroprogesterone; *ACTH,* adrenocorticotropic hormone; *ANP,* atrial natriuretic peptide; *CRH,* corticotropin-releasing hormone; *DHEA,* dehydroepiandrosterone; *DHT,* Dihydrotestosterone; *GHRH,* growth hormone–releasing hormone; *GnRH,* gonadotropin-releasing hormone; *hCG,* human chorionic gonadotropin; *hCS,* human chorionic somatomammotropin; *hGH-V,* human growth hormone variant; *IGF,* insulin-like growth factor; *LIF,* leukemia inhibitory factor; *MSH,* melanocyte-stimulating hormone; *PRH,* prolactin-releasing hormone; *TNF-α,* tumor necrosis factor α; *TRH,* thyrotropin-releasing hormone; *VIP,* vasoactive intestinal peptide.

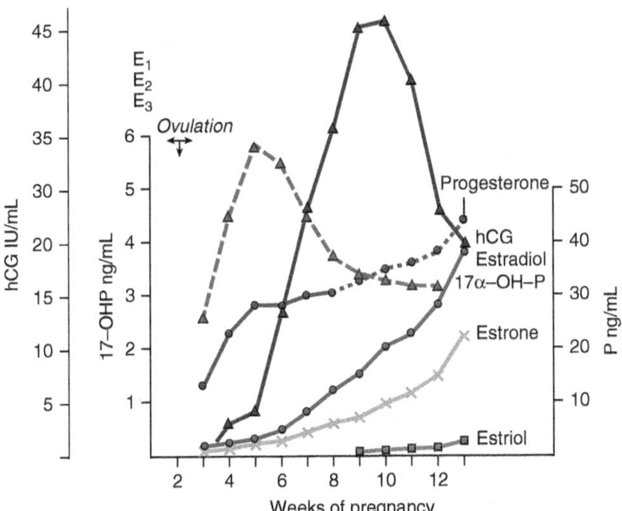

Fig. 11.2 Maternal plasma levels of human chorionic gonadotropin *(hCG)* and steroids during early human pregnancy. *E_1,* Estrone; *E_2,* estradiol; *E_3,* estriol; *17α–OH–P,* 17α-hydroxyprogesterone; *17–OHP,* 17-hydroxyprogesterone; *P,* progesterone. (From Tulchinsky D, Hobel CJ. Plasma human chorionic gonadotropin, estrone, estradiol, estriol, progesterone, and 17 alpha-hydroxyprogesterone in human pregnancy. 3. Early normal pregnancy. *Am J Obstet Gynecol.* 1973;117:884.)

Expression of hCS can first be detected in trophoblast tissue within 10 days of conception and in maternal serum by the third to fourth week of gestation. The hormone is a single 191 amino acid nonglycosylated peptide chain with considerable homology to GH (96%) and prolactin (67%); it is transcribed from a gene cluster on chromosome 17 containing two genes for hCS, one hCS pseudogene, and two GH genes.[31,32] It is synthesized by the syncytiotrophoblasts at a constant rate during gestation, so as placental mass expands, the hCS levels reflect total placental mass and thus gross placental function. By term, hCS is the most abundant placental hormone, produced at more than 1 g/day, representing 10% of total placental protein synthesis.

Despite hCS being so abundant and having been identified more than 50 years ago, understanding of its function in pregnancy remains limited. It is almost exclusively found in maternal rather than fetal circulation. This has led to the hypothesis that the primary role of hCS is to ensure adequate fetal nutrition because, in maternal circulation, it induces metabolic changes such as mobilization of fatty acids, insulin resistance, decreased utilization of glucose, and increased availability of amino acids through decreased maternal use of protein.[33] The levels of circulating maternal glucose and free fatty acids are thus increased. Although glucose readily crosses the placenta, fatty acids cross slowly, thus biasing glucose delivery toward the fetus and use of fatty acids for maternal energy, especially during maternal fasting. hCS is considered one of the major diabetogenic factors of pregnancy, along with placental steroids, placental human GH variant (hGH-V), and maternal cortisol. Within the placenta, hCS may regulate insulin-like growth factor (IGF) I[34] and alter fetal growth through direct action on placental nutrient transport systems. Loss of hCS and hGH-V may result in severe fetal growth restriction,[33] although healthy pregnancies have also been reported in the absence of hCS.[35]

In addition to its metabolic activity, the lactogenic activity of hCS suggests a synergistic role with prolactin and steroids in preparation of the breast for lactation.[36] Most recently, a role for hCS as a placental angiogenic factor has been suggested.[37]

Regulation of hCS release also remains poorly defined. The hypothalamic-like releasing and inhibiting factors found in the placenta do not appear to effect hCS release, in contrast to hypothalamic actions on pituitary GH release. In vitro studies show that hCS can be stimulated by high-density lipoproteins, apolipoproteins,[32-34,36] angiotensin,[38] cAMP,[39] arachidonic acid, insulin, and IGFs,[40] and is inhibited by the prostaglandin E2 (PGE2) and prostaglandin F2α (PGF2α),[41] catecholamines, phorbol esters, and diacylglycerols.[42] Dopaminergic agents may also inhibit hCS release.[43]

PLACENTAL GROWTH HORMONE VARIANT

Placental human GH variant (hGH-V) is encoded by the same gene cluster as hCS and pituitary GH on chromosome 17. In syncytiotrophoblasts, two transcripts are generated from the *hGH-V* gene, one major form and one alternatively spliced version. Secreted hGH-V is translated from the major version and is produced in a highly bioactive 22-kDa non-glycosylated form and to a lesser degree in a 25-kDa glycosylated form.[43] Early in pregnancy, maternal pituitary GH is produced, but from 15 to 20 weeks gestation to term, hGH-V secretion increases, suppressing maternal GH to undetectable serum levels by 24 weeks gestation. The level of hGH-V peaks about 1 month before term delivery and it disappears from the maternal circulation immediately after delivery.[44] hGH-V is not detected in the fetal circulation, but acts as an endocrine factor in the maternal circulation that indirectly affects fetal growth and possibly as a paracrine factor in the placenta.

Much like hCS, hGH-V plays a significant role in modifying maternal metabolism to meet fetal needs. hGH-V primarily appears to control maternal IGF-1 production.[44] In mice overexpressing hGH-V (not normally found in rodents), body weight was increased, IGF-1 levels were elevated, and insulin resistance developed, suggesting that hGH-V strongly contributes to the normal hyperinsulinemia and lack of responsiveness to insulin that characterizes the second half of human gestation.[45] hGH-V expression thus increases the risk for gestational diabetes and other pregnancy-related disorders. This risk is counterbalanced by placental lactogens, hCS, and prolactin, which induce increased insulin secretion by pancreatic β cell expansion. hGH-V itself is not a lactogen. Thus, a combination of pituitary-like GHs is required to support fetal growth while maintaining maternal metabolic homeostasis.

hGH-V secretion is tonic, in contrast to pulsatile pituitary GH secretion, and is not regulated by hypothalamic releasing factors.[44] Secretion is inhibited by elevated glucose levels and mildly increased by hypoglycemia, creating a feedback loop that may ensure constant delivery of nutrients to the developing fetus.

INSULIN-LIKE GROWTH FACTORS

IGF-1 and IGF-2 are highly homologous single-chain polypeptides with similarities to proinsulin. Both are made in human placental tissues.[46] Most of the components of the insulin-IGF system are found in the placenta (IGF-1, IGF-2, and IGF-binding proteins [IGFBPs] 1-6).[47] The exception is insulin, which is not made by the placenta and does not cross the placenta, although insulin has profound indirect effects on fetal growth and well-being. IGFs are the primary somatotrophs in gestation, as GH receptors are expressed at only low levels in fetal tissues. Within the placenta, IGF-1 is expressed predominantly in syncytiotrophoblasts throughout gestation, with some expression in cytotrophoblasts as well. In contrast, IGF-2 is not found in syncytiotrophoblasts but is expressed in cytotrophoblasts with a declining expression level across gestation.[44,46-48] These hormones mediate a variety of metabolic and mitogenic effects by binding to specific receptor tyrosine kinases. At physiologic concentrations, both IGF-1 and IGF-2 bind to IGF-1 receptor (IGF1R). The localization of IGF1R shifts during gestation; initially it is predominantly expressed on the syncytiotrophoblasts (closer to the maternal circulation) and by term it is mainly expressed on the fetal cytotrophoblast side, presumably reflecting the shifting activity from maternal to fetal growth control.[47] The IGF-2 receptor (IGF2R; also known as the *cation-independent mannose 6-phosphate receptor*) controls extracellular IGF-2 concentrations by mediating the endocytosis and degradation of IGF-2 rather than transducing a signal.[49] Mouse experiments suggest that an additional receptor, possibly a variant of the insulin receptor, may mediate some of the fetal growth effects of IGF-2.[49] IGFs are thought to primarily act locally but can circulate, primarily in bound forms. IGF-2 has its highest serum levels in the fetal circulation, although whether the placenta contributes to this circulating IGF-2 is unclear.[47]

Although IGF-2 is often considered the primary fetal GH, IGF-1 plays a significant role in fetal growth as well. Information on the role of IGFs in fetal growth comes from genetic manipulation in mouse models, as well as examination of human tissues, especially in pregnancies having compromised fetal growth.[49] In mice, disruption of the IGF-1, IGF-2, or IGF1R gene retards fetal growth,[50] whereas disruption of the IGF2R gene or overexpression of IGF-2 enhances fetal growth.[51] In humans, IGF-1 or IGF1R mutations are extremely rare, and no IGF-2 deletions have been reported.[49] However, IGF-2 is an imprinted gene normally expressed exclusively from the paternal allele in placenta and fetal tissues. Changes in IGF-2 expression due to abnormal imprinting has been linked to both overgrowth (Beckwith-Wiedemann syndrome) and growth restriction (Russell-Silver syndrome).[49] Whether placentally derived IGFs, as opposed to fetal IGFs, directly contribute to these fetal growth changes is uncertain, as these factors also have paracrine effects in the placenta that determine nutrient transport and placental growth.

Additional roles of IGFs in fetal growth are mediated by their potentiation of EGF activity,[52] stimulation of decidual prolactin production[53] and enhanced progesterone production.[54] In addition, production of placental thromboxane, a potent vasoconstrictor, is specifically inhibited by IGF-1.[55] Thus the production of placental IGFs is thought to be of major importance for normal intrauterine fetal growth.

IGF-1 and IGF-2 play significant, but seemingly distinct, roles in paracrine and/or autocrine signaling in the placenta. The expression of IGF1R in human trophoblasts as noted above also supports paracrine or autocrine effects in the placenta. IGF-1 can regulate the differentiation of cytotrophoblasts into syncytiotrophoblasts, whereas IGF-2 appears not to have this function despite its very early placental expression. Placental mass may also be regulated directly by both placentally produced IGFs. Cytotrophoblast proliferation and survival is mediated by IGFs produced in isolated placental explant cultures.[56] However, in vivo a decreased level of IGF-2 reduces the placental surface area available for gas and nutrient exchange more than loss of IGF-1. Both IGF-1 and IGF-2 alter nutrient transport especially of amino acids.[56,57] The increased amino acid transporter expression caused by increased levels of IGF-1 and IGF-2 in vitro is paralleled by elevated fetal amino acid transport associated with gestational diabetes.[57]

hGH-V concentrations correlate with IGF-1 levels throughout pregnancy, and hGH-V appears to be the critical regulator of placental IGF levels.[34] In addition, IGF-1 and IGF-2 effects are modulated by high-affinity IGFBPs (IGFBP-1 to IGFBP-6) that bind these IGFs with different affinities. IGFBPs are carrier proteins protecting IGF from degradation while blocking its bioactivity. IGFBPs are expressed in human placenta.[46,48,56] In addition to placental IGFBPs, IGFBP-1 is produced by the decidua in large amounts. IGFBPs are themselves regulated by protease activity and posttranslational modifications, adding a further layer of regulatory complexity.

EPIDERMAL GROWTH FACTOR, TRANSFORMING GROWTH FACTOR, AND OTHER GROWTH FACTORS

Additional growth factors have been identified in the placenta and chorionic membranes. The early blastocyst expresses platelet-derived growth factor A, transforming growth factor α, and transforming growth factor β.[58] These factors are thought to be involved in signaling implantation. Other growth factors such as EGF, basic fibroblast growth factor, nerve growth factor β, and granulocyte colony-stimulating factor are not detected in early gestation,[58] but are expressed by the placenta at later gestation stages.[59] Receptors for EGFs, as well as for many other growth factors, have been identified in the placenta and membranes.[60] Most of the EGF receptors in the placenta are localized to the syncytiotrophoblast and correlate with induction of trophoblast differentiation rather than proliferation.[61–63] The finding that EGF stimulates hCG and hCS secretion supports this hypothesis.[61] EGF also stimulates prostaglandin synthesis.[63] Another growth factor, hepatocyte growth factor, also appears to be essential for placental development.[64,65]

INHIBIN, ACTIVIN, AND FOLLISTATIN

Inhibin and activin, so called because they are, respectively, an antagonist and an agonist of pituitary FSH, have also been found in placental cytotrophoblasts, as well as in fetal membranes.[66,67] Activin receptors are expressed in syncytiotrophoblasts but not cytotrophoblasts.[68] Follistatin and follistatin-related gene (activin-binding proteins), which functionally inhibit FSH secretion in the maternal circulation, are also made in the placenta. Inhibin has been shown to inhibit GnRH stimulation of hCG and chorionic GnRH production and reduce progesterone production.[67] Activin potentiates the GnRH-stimulated hCG release and progesterone production.[25] Follistatin can reverse activin potentiation of hCG. Elevated levels of inhibin can be seen in fetal trisomy 21 cases, whereas elevated activin levels have been reported in the setting of preeclampsia and diabetes.[68] During pregnancy these hormones are actively involved in the GnRH-hCG-steroid-prostaglandin axis of the placenta and may serve as potential biomarkers of placental disorders.

PROOPIOMELANOCORTIN HORMONES

Pituitary-like peptides derived from proopiomelanocortin (POMC), including adrenocorticotropic hormone (ACTH), melanocyte-stimulating hormone, β-endorphins, and β-lipoproteins, as well as full-length POMC itself, have been identified in the human placenta.[69,70] POMC is a 31-kDa glycoprotein that is normally cleaved into several peptide hormones that play critical roles in regulation of physiologic stress and behavior. The processing of POMC in the placenta is different from that in the pituitary: POMC is released largely intact from the placenta, whereas it is not detected in the circulation in the nonpregnant state. Placental POMC is not inhibited by glucocorticoids, nor do circulating levels correlate with ACTH or cortisol levels, although they do correlate with corticotropin-releasing hormone (CRH) levels.[70] Chorionic CRH is produced by the placenta and stimulates the release of chorionic ACTH (see later).[71] The physiologic role of chorionic ACTH has not been defined, but it may affect placental cortisol production or maternal resistance of ACTH suppression by glucocorticoids.

HYPOTHALAMIC-LIKE RELEASING AND INHIBITING ACTIVITIES

Every known hypothalamic releasing or inhibiting hormone has a placental analogue,[17,18,72,73] supporting the general hypothesis that the classic hormones of the placenta are produced by means of a controlled paracrine-autocrine system.

GONADOTROPIN-RELEASING HORMONE

Human chorionic GnRH was the first-described placental hormone with hypothalamic-like activity.[17] GnRH is a decapeptide that regulates gonadal steroid production through stimulation of pituitary gonadotropins, LH, and FSH.[73] In the placenta, the GnRH-driven paracrine axis is important for early pregnancy maintenance.

The two isoforms of GnRH (GnRH-I and GnRH-II) are also produced in the human placenta, primarily in cytotrophoblasts.[74,75] GnRH-I is encoded on chromosome 8 as a precursor protein that includes a signal sequence, the GnRH decapeptide, a processing sequence, and a GnRH-associated peptide.[76] GnRH-II is encoded on chromosome 20 and has 70% homology to GnRH-I. Both GnRH-I and GnRH-II signal through the same G protein–coupled receptor, GnRHR-I, which is expressed in the syncytiotrophoblasts.[74] An additional receptor, GnRHR-II, has been found but does not appear to be functional in humans. GnRH-I has a higher affinity for GnRHR-I than does GnHR-II, triggers different conformational changes in GnRHR-I, and may activate different intracellular signaling pathways.[74,77] GnRH-I stimulates cAMP[78] via GnRHR-I, leading to production and secretion of the β-subunit of hCG, with the pattern and degree of hCG response being related to gestational age[79] and steroid levels.[80,81] GnRHR-I levels parallel hCG levels across gestation. Blocking GnRH or GnRHR-I activity can lead to pregnancy failure,[82–85] presumably due to limited hCG production. Early GnRH-I production may also play a role in apoptosis and decidual remodeling during trophoblast invasion.[74,77] GnRH-I and GnRH-II also directly regulate placenta steroid release[81] and regulate prostanoid production from the term placenta.[18,86,87] The release of placental GnRH-I is affected by cAMP, prostaglandins, epinephrine,[88] and inhibin,[29] whereas the expression of GnRHR-I is regulated by GnRH, activin, and inhibin, creating a complex feedback loop.[74] In addition, a placental peptidase that can inactivate GnRH-I and GnRH-II has been isolated and may regulate GnRH levels.[89]

THYROTROPIN-RELEASING HORMONE

Human placenta and membranes also produce a chorionic thyrotropin-releasing hormone (TRH),[90] which has activity similar to that of but is not biochemically identical to its hypothalamic counterpart. Maternal TRH also readily crosses the placenta, but its level is normally low in the maternal circulation. The thyroid-stimulating function of the placenta appears to come from hCG, rather than placental TRH. Pituitary TSH does not cross the placenta nor does the placenta produce it. Similarly, the placenta does not make thyroid hormones itself, but maternal thyroxine and triiodothyronine do cross the placenta. However, placental iodothyronine monodeiodinase enzymes deactivate a significant fraction of triiodothyronine and thyroxine.[91] The placenta produces transthyretin, a carrier protein responsible for passage of thyroxine across the placenta[92]; regulation of transthyretin expression may modulate thyroid hormone transport. Placental iodine transport from the maternal circulation is also critical for adequate thyroid hormone production in the fetus and neonate.[93] In addition, placental estrogen increases the level of thyroid-binding globulin, which lowers the levels of free circulating thyroid hormones.

The role of the placenta in thyroid metabolism has been of considerable recent interest because thyroid disease is common in women of child-bearing age and impacts pregnancy outcomes.[94] Early maternal hypothyroidism appears to be associated with lower IQ in offspring, but there are conflicting reports on the impact of maternal hypothyroidism after the onset of fetal thyroid function in mid-gestation.[94,95] Maternal thyroxine continues to cross from the maternal circulation to the fetal circulation in the second and third trimesters, as demonstrated by 30% to 50% of normal thyroxine levels in umbilical cord blood of neonates who have complete thyroid dysgenesis.[96] Placental endocrine contribution from TRH production, if any, has not been well defined, nor has a specific paracrine mechanism been identified. Placental regulation of thyroid hormone transport and metabolism may play a critical role in fetal well-being.

GROWTH HORMONE–RELEASING HORMONE, SOMATOSTATIN, AND GHRELIN

Regulators of the GH axis, including GH-releasing hormone,[97] somatostatin (also known as *GH-inhibiting hormone*),[98] and ghrelin,[99] the endogenous GH secretagogue, have all been localized to human cytotrophoblasts. They are all potential regulators of hGH-V production or paracrine regulators of

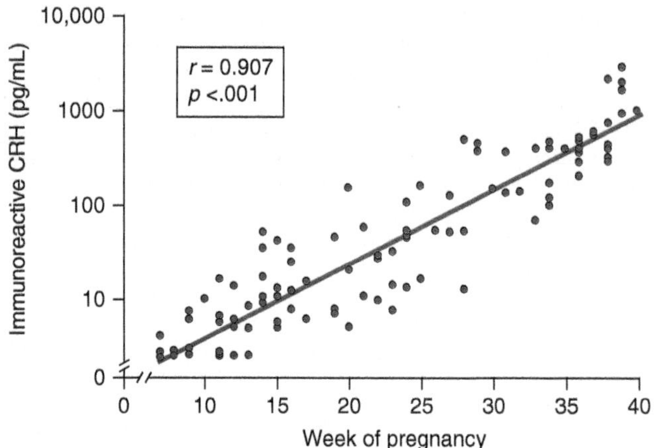

Fig. 11.3 Maternal plasma levels of corticotropin-releasing hormone (*CRH*) during human pregnancy. (From Sasaki A, Shinkawa O, Margioris AN, et al. Immunoreactive corticotropin-releasing hormone in human plasma during pregnancy, labor, and delivery. *J Clin Endocrinol Metab.* 1987;64:224.)

placental differentiation,[100] but their roles in pregnancy have not been defined.

CORTICOTROPHIN-RELEASING HORMONE AND UROCORTINS

Chorionic CRH is another hormone with hypothalamic-like activity identified in the placenta.[101,102] It is a 41 amino acid peptide that has been localized to both the syncytiotrophoblasts and cytotrophoblasts of the placenta and the cytotrophoblasts of the chorion.[103] Multiple CRH receptors types are expressed in the placenta and fetal membranes.[104] Urocortins, members of the CRH family, are also produced in syncytiotrophoblasts and fetal membranes and bind to CRH receptors as well.[105] Early in gestation, CRH family members may promote immune tolerance.[106] As gestation progresses, CRH levels rise (Fig. 11.3), as do the levels of urocortins, but to a lesser degree.[105] Maternal concentrations are greater than fetal levels.[107,108] A rapid increase is seen at term, and levels increase further during labor.

Chorionic CRH and urocortins have been shown to be biologically active in stimulating POMC-derived hormones, including ACTH and β-endorphins, in the placenta.[105,109] CRH-binding protein, which appears to inactivate the biologic activity of circulating CRH, is also produced in the syncytiotrophoblasts and fetal membranes[110] and may regulate these actions in the maternal circulation. Chorionic CRH also stimulates prostaglandin release, potentially activating local myometrial contractions at term.[111] CRH can also stimulate estrogen precursor production by the fetal adrenals,[112] which may contribute to the timing of parturition. Glucocorticoid production can also be stimulated from the fetal adrenals via CRH-stimulated ACTH release. In the placenta, glucocorticoids increase CRH expression,[113] in contrast to glucocorticoid inhibition of CRH in the hypothalamus, thus creating a potential positive feedback loop that amplifies CRH activity.[114]

Because the levels of CRH and related peptides increase across gestation and correlate with the timing of parturition, CRH is often viewed as a *placental clock*.[115] Both CRH and urocortins are under active investigation as potential biomarkers of pregnancy-related disorders. In pregnancies complicated by hypertension, the maternal circulating levels of CRH are already elevated by 28 weeks of pregnancy.[116] Urocortin 1 activity may contribute to local uteroplacental vasculature dilation; it is reduced in preeclampsia, suggesting its importance in blood flow maintenance.[105] Elevated CRH levels are seen in women with preterm labor compared with age-matched controls, suggesting that CRH level might serve as a predictor of preterm delivery,[115,117] but significant clinical utility has not yet been demonstrated.[118,119]

OTHER PEPTIDE HORMONES

OXYTOCIN

Oxytocin is an additional hypothalamic hormone that is also produced in the placenta, as well as in fetal and decidual membranes.[120] Oxytocin is a potent uterotonic hormone, used clinically to induce or speed labor. However, neither the level of circulating maternal oxytocin nor the level of locally produced oxytocin appears to increase markedly before labor; rather uterine response to oxytocin is increased through increases in oxytocin receptor expression and function.[121,122] A local paracrine system within the maternal and fetal intrauterine tissues has been outlined: progesterone suppresses oxytocin receptor signaling[120] and as progesterone activity (although not levels in humans) declines, oxytocin receptor levels rise, making the uterus more responsive to oxytocin. Additionally, placental oxytocinase may play an important role in the regulation of oxytocin levels,[122] although the role in initiation of parturition is unclear. Oxytocin has been shown to increase both prostaglandin[123] and ACTH[109] release from intrauterine tissues as well.

RELAXIN

Relaxin is also synthesized by the membranes, decidua, and placenta.[124] It is a 6-kDa peptide hormone belonging to the insulin family. Receptors for relaxin are present in the syncytiotrophoblast of the placenta.[125] A biologic action for relaxin on the collagenase activity of the chorionic-amnionic membranes has been demonstrated. Relaxin also stimulates prostaglandin release and increases the level of collagenase, the enzyme that degrades collagen.[126] Although these activities suggest a role for relaxin in parturition, most circulating relaxin is made by the corpus luteum and is not detectable in maternal serum in women who become pregnant via egg donation (without a corpus luteum), but these women can experience normal labor.[127] In the placenta, relaxin may be involved in local remodeling via a yet to be defined paracrine mechanism.

ADIPOKINES

Leptin and adiponectin are the major adipokines that are normally secreted by adipocytes to regulate energy balance and insulin actions. Weight gain generally increases serum leptin levels and decreases adiponectin levels. Placental production of leptin is well documented, while placenta production of adiponectin remains controversial.[128-130] In pregnancy the placenta appears to be the primary producer of adipokines synthesized in both cytotrophoblasts and syncytiotrophoblasts.[128] Leptin is proposed to play a role in the cytotrophoblast invasion at the time of implantation and to regulate fetal growth and placental function.[131,132] The precise roles of adipokines in the placenta, mother, or fetus are yet well defined but may differ significantly from the role in the nonpregnant state. For example, leptin levels in pregnancy do not correlate with body mass and elevated levels may not produce satiety because of placental leptin resistance in the second half of pregnancy. Alterations of adipokine production in preeclampsia and gestational diabetes have led to the hypothesis that placental adipokines may play a role in these diseases of pregnancy.[133,134]

ENDOGENOUS OPIOID PEPTIDES

Opioid peptides such as enkephalins[135] and dynorphin[136] have been found in the placenta. Receptors for opiate-like substances are present on the syncytial membrane of the placenta. Dynorphin binds to kappa opiate receptors, the levels of which increase in the placenta at term. The stimulation of these receptors has been shown to modulate acetylcholine[137]

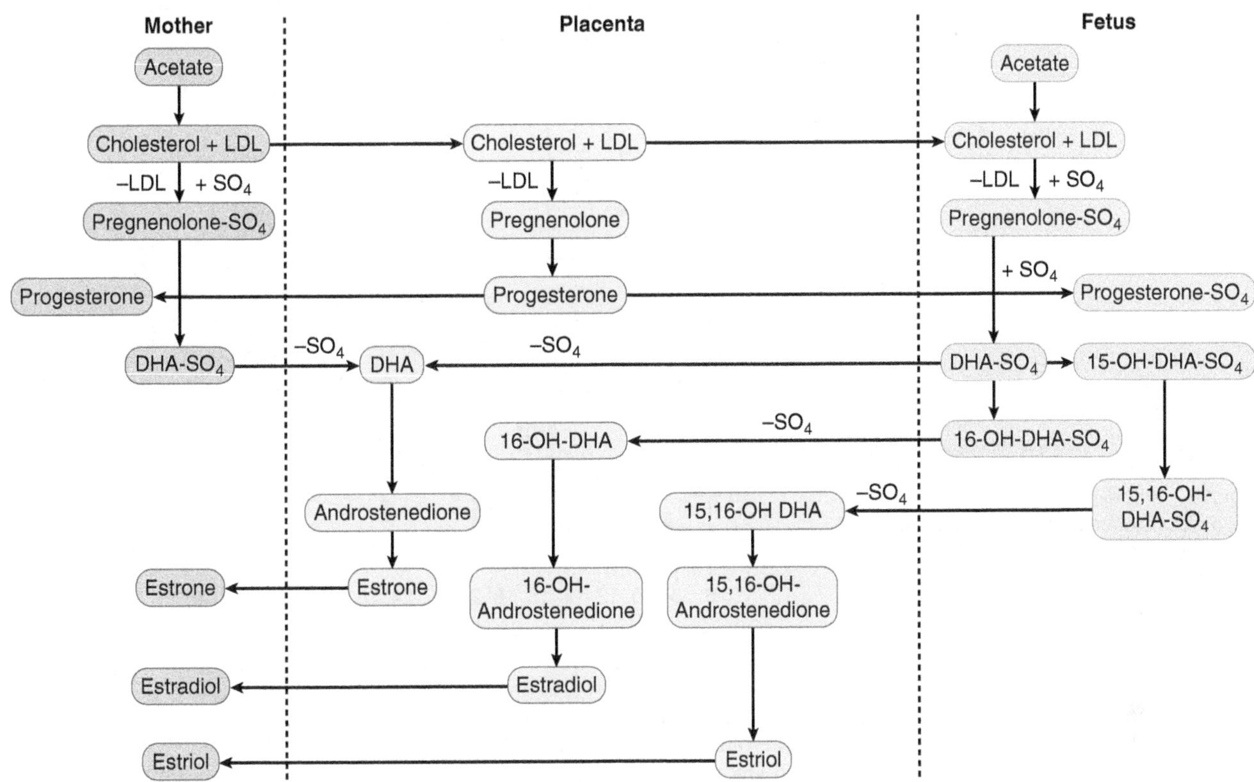

Fig. 11.4 Steroidogenic pathways in the human materno-placentofetal unit. *DHA,* Dehydroepiandrosterone; *DHA-SO₄,* dehydroepiandrosterone sulfate; *LDL,* low-density lipoprotein; *OH,* hydroxy.

and hCG release.[138,139]Adrenergic agonists and antagonists affect placental hCG and prolactin release,[140] whereas dopaminergic receptor stimulation has been shown to lower hCS and increase hCG release.[43]

VASOACTIVE PEPTIDES

The human placenta expresses a number of vasoactive peptides (and their receptors), such as vascular endothelial growth factor, endothelin, angiotensin, and arginine vasopressin. The peptides endothelin-1 and endothelin-3 are produced by the placenta, and both are active and potent vasoconstrictors in the fetal-placental circulation.[141-144] Endothelins also inhibit decidual prolactin release.[141] The angiotensin-renin system has been described in the placenta and is thought to be a factor in the regulation of vascular tone in the placental bed mediated by angiotensin II production and action.[35] Other peptide hormones effecting vascular tone, such as atrial natriuretic peptide and its receptors, have been demonstrated in the placenta.[145] Atrial natriuretic peptide inhibits the vasoconstrictive action of endothelin and angiotensin and induces vasodilatation in the uterus and the placenta. A parathyroid hormone–related protein has been extracted from placental tissues[146] and localized to the cytotrophoblasts.[147] It has been shown to have potent vasodilator activity in the fetal-placental circulation.[148]

PROLACTIN

Although prolactin is primarily made in the maternal pituitary, it is also made in several extrapituitary locations, including the endometrial decidua, although not by the placenta proper.[149]The level of decidual prolactin increases during pregnancy in amniotic fluid.[150] Prolactin may suppress inflammatory cytokines such as IL-6. Recent work suggests that during pregnancy, prolactin supports progesterone activity by repressing 20α-hydroxysteroid dehydrogenase, a hormone that catabolizes progesterone to an inactive form.[149]

STEROID HORMONES

Estrogens, androgens, and progestins are all critical to gestation from implantation to birth; their production and regulation requires integration of the fetoplacental unit with the maternal milieu. Placental synthesis and secretion of steroid hormones increase throughout pregnancy. The placenta was known to be a source of steroid hormones from the early 1900s, but their biosynthetic pathways were not defined until the late 1950s. In 1959, Ryan[151] demonstrated that the placenta could convert dehydroepiandrosterone sulfate (DHEA) to estrogens; 5 years later, Diczfalusy[152] demonstrated the existence of a fetoplacental unit in which fetal and placental enzymes work in concert to produce estrogens. The placenta is an "incomplete" steroidogenic organ and does not express a complete set of enzymes for de novo production of estrogens and progestins. Steroid hormone synthesis in the placenta is dependent on precursors from the mother and the fetus, leading concept of an integrated *materno-feto-placental unit.*[153] Fig. 11.4 shows the tissues and enzymes that participate in the biosynthesis of progestins and estrogens.[154] The concentration of steroid hormones in the maternal circulation increases dramatically throughout gestation (Fig. 11.5).[155]

PROGESTERONE

Maternal cholesterol, derived from low-density lipoprotein, is transported to the placenta and bound to specific low-density lipoprotein receptors on the syncytiotrophoblast, where it is incorporated by endocytosis and hydrolyzed to free cholesterol in the lysosomes. The human placenta lacks any significant 3-hydroxy-3-methylglutaryl-coenzyme A activity and thus cannot produce cholesterol itself. In the syncytiotrophoblasts, maternal cholesterol is converted to pregnenolone and then to progesterone. Cholesterol is converted to pregnenolone in the mitochondria by cytochrome P-450 cholesterol side-chain cleavage enzyme. After transfer to the cytosol, progesterone

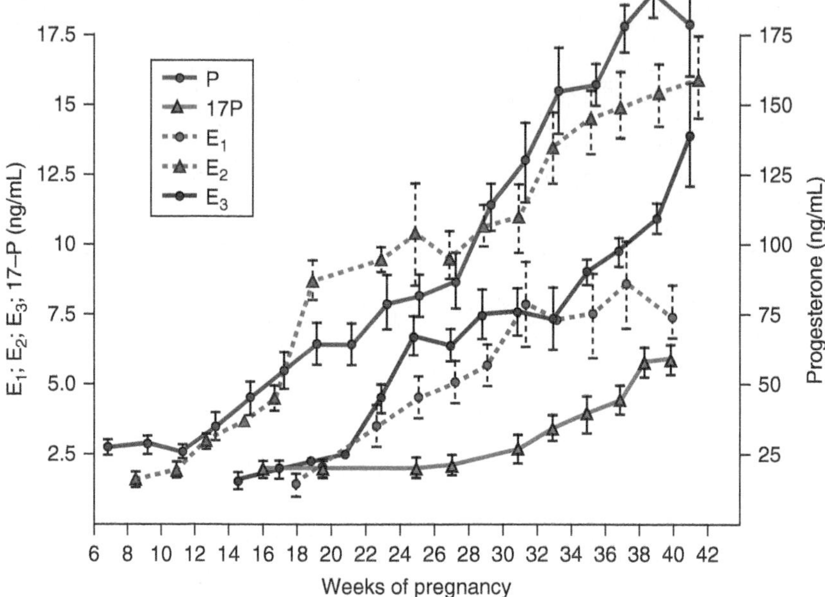

Fig. 11.5 Maternal plasma levels of progesterone *(P)*, 17-hydroxyprogesterone *(17P)*, estrone *(E_1)*, estradiol *(E_2)*, and estriol *(E_3)* across human pregnancy. (From Tulchinsky D, Hobel CJ, Yeager E, et al. Plasma estrone, estradiol, estriol, progesterone and 17-hydroxyprogesterone in human pregnancy: I. Normal pregnancy. *Am J Obstet Gynecol.* 1972;112:1095.)

is produced from pregnenolone by type 1 3β-hydroxysteroid dehydrogenase.[155,156] Approximately 90% of progesterone goes to the mother and 10% goes to the fetus. A limited amount of pregnenolone is also released into the circulation. The fetus has the enzyme activity needed for pregnenolone synthesis but has minimal enzyme to produce progesterone. Thus high levels of circulating fetal progesterone are of placental origin. Circulating progesterone levels thus reflect placental function rather than fetal well-being. The high placental production of progesterone, rather than its metabolism to 17α-hydroxyprogesterone, is not due to lack of further metabolizing enzymes, but is due to the relative efficiency of the enzymes favoring progesterone production. 17α-Hydroxyprogesterone levels rise in the third trimester as progesterone levels peak. Additional progesterone metabolites, particularly 5α-dihydroprogesterone and its metabolite allopregnanolone, are also produced in the syncytiotrophoblasts at increased levels relative to progesterone.[157] These steroids have been hypothesized to play an endocrine role in fetal brain development and provide neuroprotection in the face of hypoxia.[158,159]

Placental steroidogenic capacity is functional early in pregnancy, but not until 35 to 47 days after ovulation can placental progesterone production alone support the maintenance of pregnancy.[160] Before that time, human pregnancy is dependent on the progesterone produced by the corpus luteum of pregnancy or provided by exogenous supplementation. This change in the control locus from the ovary to the placenta is the aforementioned ovarian-placental shift.

Progesterone is required for the maintenance of pregnancy in part by means of its suppressant effect on uterine contractions.[154,160,161] Progesterone inhibits genes that promote contractility[112] and has immunosuppressive activity that may promote uterine quiescence.[161,162] Progesterone counteracts uterine estrogen effects. Unlike the drop in progesterone levels before labor seen in most mammals, there is no progesterone withdrawal per se that occurs before labor in women; however, modulation of progesterone receptor expression in combination with a shift in the progesterone to estrogen balance is presumed to play the same biologic role, but definitive evidence is lacking. Progesterone[163] or a synthetic form of 17α-hydroxyprogesterone[164] is currently offered to women with a history of preterm birth starting in the third trimester and appears to reduce the risk for preterm delivery in this population. The relationship of therapeutic response to normal physiologic mechanisms at work in the materno-feto-placental unit is not yet understood.

ESTROGENS

Unlike progesterone production that relies on maternal precursors, estrogen production relies on fetal precursors. In pregnancy, estrogens are synthesized from C19 steroids,[165] primarily from dehydroepiandrosterone sulfate (DHEA-S) produced in the fetal adrenals. The fetal adrenals rapidly sulfate steroids, resulting in steroid sulfates that are biologically inactive. Pregnenolone is sulfated and then converted to DHEA-S in the fetal adrenal cortex by17α-hydroxylase and 20,21-desmolase.[166] DHEA-S may be hydroxylated in the fetal liver at the 16α or 15α position or at both positions. These biologically inactive androgens are then transferred to the placenta. Placental sulfatases rapidly cleave the sulfate and placental 3β-hydroxysteroid dehydrogenase converts DHEA or hydroxylated DHEA to androstenedione or hydroxylated androstenediones, respectively. These androgens are then primarily aromatized to estrone, 16α-hydroxyestrone, or 15α-hydroxyestrone and then converted to estradiol, estriol, or estetrol, respectively, by the action of the placental 17β-hydroxylation enzyme.[155,156,167] Estriol is the major estrogen of pregnancy, with the majority secreted into the maternal compartment; estrone is the only estrogen preferentially secreted into the fetal compartment. Although maternal DHEA-S serves as 40% of the precursor for estradiol synthesis, estriol and estetrol are formed predominantly from fetal precursors because the maternal liver has limited 5α-hydroxylation or 16α-hydroxylation capabilities.[168] Estriol and estetrol are thus indicators of fetal well-being,[155] although neither is a clinically useful marker because of rapid shifts in circulating levels.

Estrogens influence uterine growth, blood flow, contractility, metabolism, and breast development. However, high estrogen levels are apparently not needed for pregnancy. It has been reported that parturition proceeds normally in the absence of fetal and placental sulfatase[169] or aromatase,[170] although in the latter case both the fetus and the mother are virilized. In either of these deficiencies, there is still circulating estradiol, and there are no reports of pregnancy without detectable estrogen levels, suggesting that a basal level of estrogen is likely required.

The primary function of high estriol levels remains unclear, but they do increase uteroplacental blood flow.[171] Before parturition, an increase in the estrogen-to-progesterone ratio occurs within the intrauterine tissues and may increase prostaglandin and oxytocin activity. As described earlier, steroid hormone production is further influenced by trophic hormones and other factors such as hypothalamic-like releasing or inhibiting hormones. In turn, estrogens affect other endocrine systems (e.g., the renin-angiotensin system)[172] and play a role in organ maturation such as surfactant production in the lung.[173]

ANDROGENS

Maternal serum levels of androgens, including testosterone, dihydrotestosterone (DHT), DHEA, and androstenedione, increase threefold across gestation.[167,174] As noted above, placental androgen synthesis depends the conversion of pregnenolone to progesterone and then to potential androgen precursors. Normally placental androgens are converted to estrogens by placental aromatase (CYP19A1), thus protecting fetuses from excess androgen exposure. However, androgen precursors that are not converted to estrogens can be converted to active testosterone and DHT, as well as less bio-active DHEA and androstenedione, in trophoblasts.[167] While the human placenta does not express important enzymes in standard androgen synthesis (17β-hydroxylase and 17,20-desmolase), it does express 3β-hydroxysteroid dehydrogenase type 1 (HSD3B1), which converts DHEA into androstenedione, and 17β-hydroxysteroid dehydrogenase type 1 (HSD17B1), which can synthesize testosterone from andrestenedione.[167,175]

Studies of maternal serum levels of androgens suggest that levels may be elevated in pregnancy disorders such as preeclampsia and gestational diabetes.[175] Elevated testosterone generated by the placenta has specifically been associated with preeclampsia.[175] Dysregulation of both synthetic enzymes and androgen receptors in the placenta have been implicated in altered androgen levels during pregnancy, as well as the placental response to these levels. For example, placental aromatase expression is decreased in the preeclamptic placenta, diminishing androgen conversion to estrogenic metabolites and increasing androgens in circulation.[175] In addition, since the placenta is a fetal organ, sex may play a role in the production of and response to androgens, and these sex-specific placental responses may in turn have sex-specific impacts on fetal development.[176]

GLUCOCORTICOIDS

In addition to the sex steroids, circulating levels of glucocorticoids and mineralocorticoids are increased in pregnancy.[177] Although the placenta produces ACTH, its action is primarily in the placenta. However, the placenta has the ability to produce cortisol and to convert it to inactive cortisone via 11β-hydroxysteroid dehydrogenase type 2; this enzyme also converts maternal cortisol to cortisone at the placental interface. The activities of these enzymes differ with gestation stage and endocrine milieu.[178] The primary role of this system appears to be to protect the fetus from elevated cortisol exposure, which may play a role in long-term reprogramming of the fetal hypothalamic-pituitary-adrenal axis.[179,180] In addition, the effect of the positive feed-forward axis of cortisol on placental CRH in late gestation described earlier increases fetal adrenal DHEA-S and thus estrogen production, altering the timing of parturition.

CYTOKINES

Cytokines, such as interferons, tumor necrosis factor α, leukemia inhibitory factor, and interleukins,[181-184] are produced by the placenta, and their receptors are expressed in the uteroplacental tissues. Cytokines are expressed in the trophoblasts themselves and are synthesized by endothelial cells and invading macrophages.[185-187] Although successful implantation requires a proinflammatory cytokine environment,[188,189] there is then a shift in the T-cell ratio from T_H1 cells toward T_H2 cells with production of cytokines that suppress the immune response.[190] Before parturition, this balance shifts back toward T_H1 proinflammatory cytokines.[186,187,191] The balance of cytokines and related factors, either proinflammatory or antiinflammatory, may be a key trigger for preterm labor caused by intrauterine infection or other types of inflammation.[28,186] Cytokine expression also regulates trophoblastic and vascular placental function.[190] Cytokines affect these activities by regulation of other cytokines, growth factors, hormones, and prostanoid production.[192-194]

EICOSANOIDS

Eicosanoids, such as thromboxanes, prostaglandins, and leukotrienes, are autocrine or paracrine factors produced in the placenta and fetal membranes.[195] All of these inflammatory mediators are derived from arachidonic acid, which is mobilized (i.e., deesterified from lipoproteins) in cells via two enzymatic pathways: cyclooxygenase and lipoxygenase. Cyclooxygenase metabolism leads to prostaglandins and thromboxanes, whereas lipoxygenase metabolism leads to leukotrienes and other metabolites. Human term placentas convert arachidonic acid primarily to thromboxanes and PGE2, PGF2α, and prostaglandin D2.[195,196] Much like cytokines, they play a role in trophoblast implantation[197] and in parturition.[198,199]

After implantation, these factors, particularly prostacyclin and PGE2, appear to be vasoregulators of the fetoplacental unit.[199-201] PGE2 is a vasodilator of uterine blood flow while constricting the umbilical circulation, whereas PGF2α vasoconstricts both the maternal circulation and the umbilical circulation. Prostacyclin is a potent vasodilator in placental vessels, an inhibitor of platelet aggregation, and a uterine relaxing factor; its loss has been implicated in preeclampsia. Thromboxane A2 opposes prostacyclin and production is increased in preeclampsia; low-dose aspirin preferentially inhibits thromboxanes in the placenta and has had some success in preventing the development of preeclampsia. The role prostanoids and thromboxanes in placental homeostasis and disease has been extensively reviewed.[202]

Factors that are known to stimulate local prostanoid production include CRH, cytokines, and growth factors. Prostanoid production has been proposed as one of the mechanisms through which CRH and cytokines exert their effects in labor. Glucocorticoids, progesterone, and estrogens also effect prostaglandin production,[203] as can GnRH.[78,87]

ENZYMES THAT REGULATE PLACENTAL ENDOCRINE AND PARACRINE ACTIVITIES

Multiple enzymes expressed in the placenta regulate autocrine, paracrine, and endocrine hormones by metabolizing them to other active or inactive products, thus altering their concentrations and activity. Many of these have been mentioned in this chapter, but their role in placental signaling is worth highlighting. The presence of both endocrine factors and modifying enzymatic activity in the placenta provides localized, spatially limited hormone regulation. For example, dual oxidative and reductive enzymatic activity regulates the balance between cortisol and cortisone.[178] In the placenta, oxidation of cortisol to cortisone predominates, whereas in the decidua, the reverse reaction dominates. Differential regulation of these enzymatic systems throughout pregnancy has been demonstrated.[178] When hormones are produced in large quantities but their levels may need to be locally reduced to effect a physiologic transition such as labor initiation, the expression of hormone-degrading enzymes may play a key role. For example, prostaglandin dehydrogenase, oxytocinase, and aminopeptidase have all been implicated in the regulation of parturition.[204-207]

CONCLUSION

The placenta integrates hormonal signals and other indicators of the maternal environment and fetal well-being. In doing so, these signals directly or indirectly shape placental structure and physiology. In turn, the placenta relays current fetal demands to the maternal circulation and signals the fetus regarding resource availability. The placenta is a fetal organ and as such adapts its function to optimize resource allocation to the fetus, but balances maternal homeostatic needs as well, because the fetus is critically dependent on maternal well-being. Placental adaptation can be rapid and brief to adjust to immediate circumstances, such as maternal fasting, or sustained to adjust to ongoing environmental circumstances, such as nutritional shortages or other causes of significant maternal stress.

Newly recognized are some of the ways that the endocrine functions of the placenta can alter development of critical organs, such as the fetal brain. For example, it was recently demonstrated that there are neural pathways that require serotonin produced by the placenta from maternal precursors to form appropriate neural connections early in fetal brain development.[208] Later production of serotonin by the brain itself cannot rescue these lost connections, which may alter long-term behavior in offspring. Besides altering the fetal brain[209] placental hormones can modulate maternal brain circuitry and behavior in preparation for parturition and rearing of offspring (extensively reviewed[210]). In addition, fetal experience in utero that is mediated by the placenta can alter epigenetic information, extending phenotypic alterations in offspring into transmissible genetic traits in future generations.[4,211,212] Dysregulation of placental endocrine, paracrine, and autocrine systems may thus be responsible for disorders of pregnancy as well as long-term programming of human disease. Understanding placental signaling and the complexities of the materno-feto-placental unit promises to lead to an enhanced ability to improve the fetal environment, to develop therapeutics that better maintain pregnancy, and to ensure the well-being of future generations.

 A complete reference list is available at www.ExpertConsult.com.

SELECT REFERENCES

5. Aplin JD. Implantation, trophoblast differentiation and haemochorial placentation: mechanistic evidence in vivo and in vitro. *J Cell Sci*. 1991;99:681-692.
27. Gridelet V, Perrier D'hauterive S, Polese B, et al. Human chorionic gonadotrophin: new pleiotropic functions for an "old" hormone during pregnancy. *Front Immunol*. 2020;11:343.
28. Challis JR, Lockwood CJ, Myatt L, et al. Inflammation and pregnancy. *Reprod Sci*. 2009;16:206-215.
31. Handwerger S, Freemark M. The roles of placental growth hormone and placental lactogen in the regulation of human fetal growth and development. *J Pediatr Endocrinol Metab*. 2000;13:343-356.
44. Newbern D, Freemark M. Placental hormones and the control of maternal metabolism and fetal growth. *Curr Opin Endocrinol Diabet Obes*. 2011;18:409-416.
47. Forbes K, Westwood M. The IGF axis and placental function: a mini review. *Hormone Res*. 2008;69:129-137.
49. Gicquel C, Le Bouc Y. Hormonal regulation of fetal growth. *Hormone Res*. 2006;65(suppl 3):28-33.
59. Morrish DW, Dakour J, Li H. Functional regulation of human trophoblast differentiation. *J Reprod Immunol*. 1998;39:179-195.
62. Marzioni D, Capparuccia L, Todros T, et al. Growth factors and their receptors: fundamental molecules for human placental development. *Ital J Anat Embryol*. 2005;110(2 suppl 1):183-187.
66. Petraglia F. Inhibin, activin and follistatin in the human placenta—a new family of regulatory proteins. *Placenta*. 1997;18:3-8.
68. Florio P, Luisi S, Ciarmela P, et al. Inhibins and activins in pregnancy. *Mol Cell Endocrinol*. 2004;225:93-100.
69. Krieger DT. Placenta as a source of 'brain' and 'pituitary' hormones. *Biol Reprod*. 1982;26:55-71.
71. Reis FM, Fadalti M, Florio P, Petraglia F. Putative role of placental corticotropin-releasing factor in the mechanisms of human parturition. *J Soc Gynecol Investig*. 1999;6:109-119.
73. Pawson AJ, Morgan K, Maudsley SR, Millar RP. Type II gonadotrophin-releasing hormone (GnRH-II) in reproductive biology. *Reproduction*. 2003;126:271-278.
76. Cheng CK, Leung PC. Molecular biology of gonadotropin-releasing hormone (GnRH)-I, GnRH-II, and their receptors in humans. *Endocrine Rev*. 2005;26:283-306.
91. Forhead AJ, Fowden AL. Thyroid hormones in fetal growth and prepartum maturation. *J Endocrinol*. 2014;221:R87-R103.
94. Nathan N, Sullivan SD. Thyroid disorders during pregnancy. *Endocrinol Metab Clin North Am*. 2014;43:573-597.
95. Chan SY, Vasilopoulou E, Kilby MD. The role of the placenta in thyroid hormone delivery to the fetus. *Nat Clin Pract Endocrinol Metab*. 2009;5:45-54.
96. Vulsma T, Gons MH, de Vijlder JJ. Maternal-fetal transfer of thyroxine in congenital hypothyroidism due to a total organification defect or thyroid agenesis. *N Engl J Med*. 1989;321:13-16.
103. Riley SC, Challis JR. Corticotrophin-releasing hormone production by the placenta and fetal membranes. *Placenta*. 1991;12:105-119.
105. Florio P, Vale W, Petraglia F. Urocortins in human reproduction. *Peptides*. 2004;25:1751-1757.
112. Mesiano S, Jaffe RB. Developmental and functional biology of the primate fetal adrenal cortex. *Endocrine Rev*. 1997;18:378-403.
114. Nicholson RC, King BR. Regulation of CRH gene expression in the placenta. *Front Hormone Res*. 2001;27:246-257.
115. McLean M, Smith R. Corticotrophin-releasing hormone and human parturition. *Reproduction*. 2001;121:493-501.
119. Smith R, Nicholson RC. Corticotrophin releasing hormone and the timing of birth. *Front Biosci*. 2007;12:912-918.
120. Gimpl G, Fahrenholz F. The oxytocin receptor system: structure, function, and regulation. *Physiol Rev*. 2001;81:629-683.
131. Hauguel-de Mouzon S, Lepercq J, Catalano P. The known and unknown of leptin in pregnancy. *Am J Obstet Gynecol*. 2006;194:1537-1545.
143. Kingdom J, Huppertz B, Seaward G, Kaufmann P. Development of the placental villous tree and its consequences for fetal growth. *Eur J Obstet Gynecol Reprod Biol*. 2000;92:35-43.
145. VanWijk MJ, Kublickiene K, Boer K, VanBavel E. Vascular function in preeclampsia. *Cardiovasc Res*. 2000;47:38-48.
149. Marano RJ, Ben-Jonathan N. Minireview: extrapituitary prolactin: an update on the distribution, regulation, and functions. *Mol Endocrinol*. 2014;28:622-633.
151. Ryan KJ. Biological aromatization of steroids. *J Biol Chem*. 1959;234:268-272.
152. Diczfalusy E. Endocrine functions of the human fetoplacental unit. *Fed Proc*. 1964;23:791-798.
154. Kallen CB. Steroid hormone synthesis in pregnancy. *Obstet Gynecol Clin North Am*. 2004;31:795-816.
158. Hirst JJ, Kelleher MA, Walker DW, Palliser HK. Neuroactive steroids in pregnancy: key regulatory and protective roles in the foetal brain. *J Steroid Biochem Mol Biol*. 2014;139:144-153.
159. Pasca AM, Penn AA. The placenta: the lost neuroendocrine organ. *NeoReviews*. 2010;11:e64-e77.
165. Siiteri PK, MacDonald PC. Placental estrogen biosynthesis during human pregnancy. *J Clin Endocrinol Metab*. 1966;26:751-761.
166. Benirschke K, Bloch E, Hertig AT. Concerning the function of the fetal zone of the human adrenal gland. *Endocrinology*. 1956;58:598-625.
169. Bradshaw KD, Carr BR. Placental sulfatase deficiency: maternal and fetal expression of steroid sulfatase deficiency and X-linked ichthyosis. *Obstet Gynecol Surv*. 1986;41:401-413.
170. Harada N. Genetic analysis of human placental aromatase deficiency. *J Steroid Biochem Mol Biol*. 1993;44:331-340.
178. Pepe GJ, Albrecht ED. Actions of placental and fetal adrenal steroid hormones in primate pregnancy. *Endocrine Rev*. 1995;16:608-648.
180. Challis JR, Sloboda D, Matthews SG, et al. The fetal placental hypothalamic-pituitary-adrenal (HPA) axis, parturition and postnatal health. *Mol Cell Endocrinol*. 2001;185:135-144.
182. Hauguel-de Mouzon S, Guerre-Millo M. The placenta cytokine network and inflammatory signals. *Placenta*. 2006;27:794-798.
186. Sel'kov SA, Pavlov OV, Selyutin AV. Cytokines and placental macrophages in regulation of birth activity. *Bull Exp Biol Med*. 2000;129:511-515.
189. Loke YW, King A. Immunological aspects of human implantation. *J Reprod Fertil Suppl*. 2000;55:83-90.
190. Keelan JA, Marvin KW, Sato TA, et al. Cytokine abundance in placental tissues: evidence of inflammatory activation in gestational membranes with term and preterm parturition. *Am J Obstet Gynecol*. 1999;181:1530-1536.
208. Bonnin A, Goeden N, Chen K, et al. A transient placental source of serotonin for the fetal forebrain. *Nature*. 2011;472:347-350.
210. Brunton PJ, Russell JA. The expectant brain: adapting for motherhood. *Nat Rev Neurosci*. 2008;9:11-25.
211. Fowden AL, Ward JW, Wooding FP, et al. Programming placental nutrient transport capacity. *J Physiol*. 2006;572(Pt 1):5-15.
212. Murphy VE, Smith R, Giles WB, Clifton VL. Endocrine regulation of human fetal growth: the role of the mother, placenta, and fetus. *Endocr Rev*. 2006;27:141-169.

Intra-Amniotic Infection/ Inflammation and the Fetal Inflammatory Response Syndrome

12

Eunjung Jung | Roberto Romero | Lami Yeo | Piya Chaemsaithong | Nardhy Gomez-Lopez

INTRODUCTION

Infection is the greatest killer in human history. The microbial theory of disease is probably the greatest advance in medicine, for it has made possible the identification of the cause of many diseases, the development of diagnostic modalities (i.e., cultivation of microorganisms), treatment with antimicrobial agents, and the development of vaccines. The achievements of the microbial theory of disease in medicine and public health are unparalleled with regard to any other contribution in medicine. The formulation of the Koch postulates to establish causality between a microbe and a disease provided a major breakthrough that has influenced the philosophy of science. Although during the 20th century some considered that infectious diseases had been conquered, the pandemic of coronavirus disease 2019 (COVID-19), epidemics of acquired immunodeficiency syndrome (AIDS), Ebola virus, swine flu, and the like tell a different story. The recent understanding that infections during pregnancy may predispose to schizophrenia,[1] autism spectrum disorders,[1] and cerebral palsy[2,3] in the offspring suggests that insults occurring during intrauterine life (infection-induced inflammation) can have lasting effects.

Fetal and neonatal physicians and scientists have been interested in intra-amniotic infection as a cause for preterm labor and delivery, neonatal morbidity and mortality, and long-term disorders. This chapter will focus largely on the microbiology, the innate immune response, and the fetal inflammatory response syndrome (FIRS).

BIRTH: TRANSITION FROM A STERILE TO A NONSTERILE ENVIRONMENT

Four major transitions occur at birth: (1) emergence from an aquatic environment where oxygen is acquired through the placenta to a dry environment in which respiratory exchange occurs through the lungs; (2) adaptation from a warm environment in which the fetus has a temperature that is 1°C higher on average than that of the mother to a cooler environment at room temperature; (3) exchange of a continuous supply of nutrients through the placenta for intermittent feedings during the neonatal period; and (4) transition from a sterile bacterial environment to the establishment of the neonatal microbiome (e.g., gut, respiratory tract, skin).[4]

The fetus normally lives in an environment devoid of bacteria, as determined by cultivation and molecular microbiologic techniques of amniotic fluid.[5,6] Therefore, birth represents a critical stage for acquisition of the first microbiota. During labor, the fetus becomes exposed to the vaginal microbiota[7-9] and such bacteria become the pioneer microorganisms that invade the formerly sterile body of the infant[10] to establish the first neonatal microbiota.[11,12] Such microbiota may differ when an infant is born via vaginal or cesarean delivery.[13]

Under pathologic conditions, however, microbial invasion of the amniotic cavity due to bacteria, fungi, and viruses can predispose to fetal infection. Microorganisms can enter the fetus through different sites, including the mucous membranes of the airways, gastrointestinal tract, tympanic membrane, the conjunctiva, or skin. Once bacteria are in contact with the mucous membranes, they can gain access to the fetal circulation and cause bacteremia, which then can lead to sepsis, septic shock, or even death. The fetal immune system, after the second trimester of pregnancy, is capable of mounting both an innate and an adaptive immune response, which play a key role in host defense against infection.[14-18] Indeed, recent studies show that the amniotic fluid harbors innate and adaptive immune cells of fetal origin, which play a central role in host defense against microbes invading the amniotic cavity.[19-27]

Microbial invasion of the amniotic cavity has been causally linked to preterm labor with intact or ruptured membranes.[28-32] One-third of preterm neonates are born to mothers with microbial invasion of the amniotic cavity.[31,33,34] Moreover, the earlier the gestational age at delivery, the greater the frequency of intra-amniotic infection and the greater the burden of disease.[29,35]

NOMENCLATURE: MICROBIAL INVASION OF THE AMNIOTIC CAVITY, INTRA-AMNIOTIC INFLAMMATION, INTRA-AMNIOTIC INFECTION, CLINICAL CHORIOAMNIONITIS, ACUTE HISTOLOGIC CHORIOAMNIONITIS, AND FUNISITIS

Table 12.1 and Fig. 12.1 define terms often used to refer to entities related to intra-amniotic infection. *Microbial invasion of the amniotic cavity* is defined as the presence of organisms in the samples of amniotic fluid retrieved by transabdominal amniocentesis and detected by cultivation methods and/or molecular microbiologic techniques. *Intra-amniotic inflammation* is the presence of an inflammatory response in the amniotic cavity, which can be detected by the presence of inflammatory cells, for instance, white blood cells, in an elevated concentration of an inflammatory mediator, such as interleukin (IL)-6,[36] or in an elevated concentration of matrix metalloproteinase (MMP).[37] Rapid tests that can determine these biomarkers have become available recently as point-of-care tests, and results can be obtained in less than 20 minutes without specialized laboratory equipment.[38-50]

The term *intra-amniotic infection* is used when there is a combination of microbial invasion of the amniotic cavity and intra-amniotic inflammation. Most cases of microbial invasion of the amniotic cavity without evidence of inflammation are due to specimen contamination by skin flora, laboratory bacteria, or reagents. When intra-amniotic inflammation is present in the absence of microorganisms, the condition is referred to as *sterile intra-amniotic inflammation*.[43,51-54] This term should be reserved for samples that are negative for microorganisms detected by both cultivation methods and molecular microbiologic techniques.[43,51-53] Sterile intra-amniotic inflammation has been attributed to "danger signals" (or *alarmins*) that are released during cellular stress or cell necrosis.[55-61]

Clinical chorioamnionitis refers to a syndrome characterized by the presence of a maternal fever (temperature ≥37.8°C or ≥38.0°C) and two or more of the five following clinical signs: (1) maternal tachycardia (heart rate >100 beats/min); (2) fetal tachycardia

Table 12.1 Nomenclature.

Condition	Definition
Microbial invasion of the amniotic cavity	The presence of organisms in the amniotic fluid retrieved by transabdominal amniocentesis and detected by cultivation methods and/or molecular microbiologic techniques
Intra-amniotic inflammation	An increased number of inflammatory cells (white blood cells) or cytokines or matrix metalloproteinase 8 (MMP-8) in amniotic fluid • White blood cell count ≥50 cells/mm³ or amniotic fluid interleukin-6 concentration ≥2.6 ng/mL, or amniotic fluid MMP-8 concentration >23 ng/mL
Intra-amniotic infection	The combination of microbial invasion of the amniotic cavity and intra-amniotic inflammation
Sterile intra-amniotic inflammation	The presence of intra-amniotic inflammation with the absence of microorganisms detected by both cultivation methods and molecular microbiologic techniques
Clinical chorioamnionitis	Maternal fever (temperature ≥37.8°C or ≥38.0°C) and the combination of at least two of the following clinical signs: (1) maternal tachycardia (heart rate >100 beats/min); (2) fetal tachycardia (heart rate >160 beats/min); (3) uterine tenderness; (4) purulent or foul-smelling amniotic fluid or vaginal discharge; and (5) maternal leukocytosis (white blood cells count >15,000/mm³)
Acute histologic chorioamnionitis	The presence of neutrophils in the chorioamniotic membranes or the chorionic plate. This condition represents a maternal inflammatory response
Acute funisitis	Inflammation of the umbilical cord (umbilical vein, umbilical artery, and Wharton's jelly). This condition represents a fetal, not a maternal inflammatory response

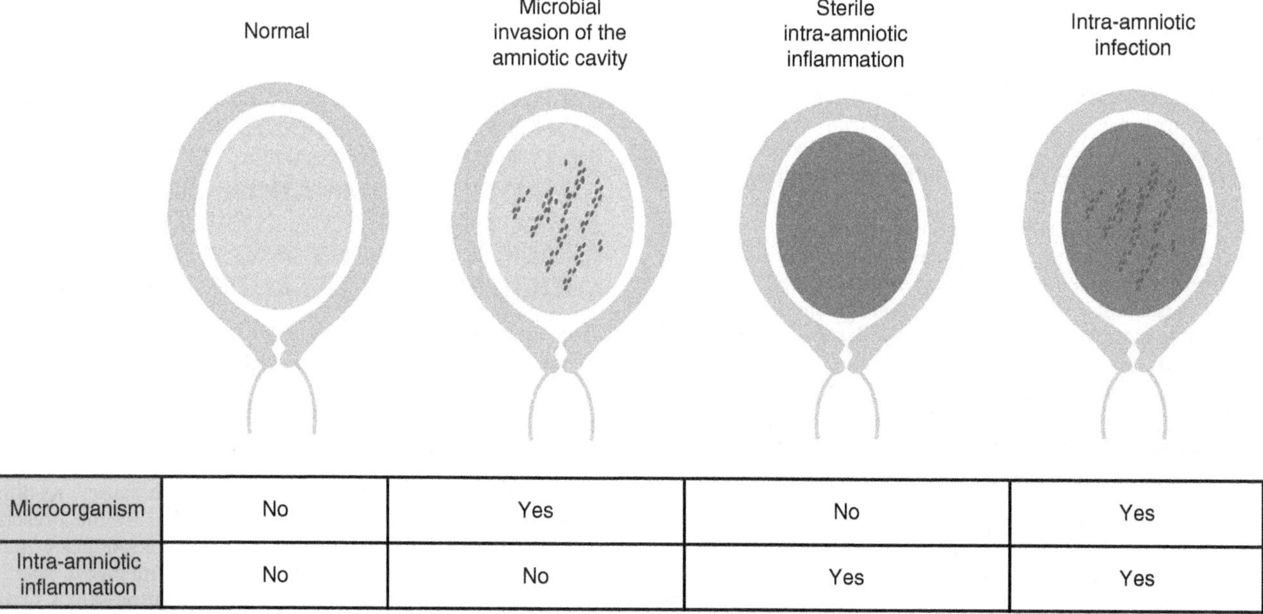

Intra-amniotic inflammation is defined as:

- Amniotic fluid white blood cell count ≥ 50 cells/mm³ or
- An elevated concentration of interleukin-6 (IL-6) ≥ 2.6 ng/mL or
- An elevated concentration of matrix metalloproteinase-8 (MMP-8) > 23 ng/mL

Fig. 12.1 Microbial invasion of the amniotic cavity, intra-amniotic inflammation, sterile intra-amniotic inflammation, and intra-amniotic infection. Microbial invasion of the amniotic cavity is characterized by the presence of microorganisms in the amniotic fluid obtained by transabdominal amniocentesis and detected by cultivation methods and/or molecular microbiologic techniques. Intra-amniotic inflammation is defined by the presence of inflammatory cells (white blood cell count greater than or equal to 50 cells/mm³) or an elevated concentration of a biomarker of inflammation (an interleukin-6 [IL-6] concentration ≥2.6 ng/mL or a matrix metalloproteinase-8 [MMP-8] concentration >23 ng/mL). Sterile intra-amniotic inflammation is defined as the presence of intra-amniotic inflammation in the absence of microorganisms. When intra-amniotic inflammation is accompanied by the presence of microorganisms in the amniotic cavity, this condition is referred to as *intra-amniotic infection.*

(heart rate >160 beats/min); (3) uterine tenderness; (4) purulent or malodorous amniotic fluid or vaginal discharge; and (5) maternal leukocytosis (white blood cell count >15,000/mm³).[62-70]

Clinical chorioamnionitis represents the clinical manifestation of a maternal systemic inflammatory response and is present in only 10% to 20% of all patients with proven intra-amniotic infection. *Acute histologic chorioamnionitis* is the presence of neutrophils in the chorioamniotic membranes or the chorionic plate and represents a maternal host response.[71-82] *Funisitis* is inflammation of the umbilical cord (umbilical vein, artery, and Wharton's jelly) and is a fetal host response.[83,84] *Chorionic vasculitis* consists of inflammation of the fetal vessels on the surface of the chorionic plate and is evidence of fetal inflammation.Acute histologic chorioamnionitis, more common than clinical chorioamnionitis, is the pathologic expression of intra-amniotic inflammation.[72,74,85-92] However, acute histologic chorioamnionitis should not be considered synonymous with intra-amniotic infection, since a fraction of patients with sterile intra-amniotic inflammation have acute histologic chorioamnionitis and, sometimes, funisitis. The term *acute* refers to a specific inflammatory lesion in which the predominant cell is the neutrophil. *Chronic* inflammatory lesions of the placenta are characterized by the infiltration of lymphocytes, plasma cells, and macrophages. Although chronic inflammatory lesions could be due to specific infectious agents (such as viruses), the main cause of chronic inflammatory lesions is *maternal antifetal rejection*,[93-100] and interested readers are referred to a recent review by the authors on this subject.[100]

PATHWAYS FOR INTRA-AMNIOTIC INFECTION

Microorganisms may gain access to the amniotic cavity through three main pathways[101-103]: (1) ascension from the vagina and cervix[85,104-107]; (2) hematogenous dissemination through the placenta (transplacental infection)[86,108-110]; and (3) accidental introduction at the time of invasive procedures, such as amniocentesis, percutaneous fetal blood sampling, chorionic villus sampling, or shunting.[111-118]

The most common pathway of intra-amniotic infection is the ascending route,[101,102,119,120] evidenced as follows:

1. The bacteria isolated in the amniotic fluid of patients with intra-amniotic infection are frequently found in the vagina.[101,107]
2. In twin gestations, acute histologic chorioamnionitis, more common in the first-born twin, is rarely seen in the second twin. Moreover, when intra-amniotic infection is detected, the presenting sac is nearly always involved.[121]
3. In virtually all cases of congenital pneumonia, inflammation of the chorioamniotic membranes is present.[86,119,122]

STAGES OF ASCENDING INFECTION

The stages of ascending infection are listed in Fig. 12.2.[102] *Stage 1* corresponds to a change in the vaginal/cervical microbial flora or to the presence of pathologic organisms (e.g., *Neisseria gonorrhoeae*) in the cervix. Some forms of bacterial vaginosis may be an early manifestation of this initial stage. An abnormal vaginal microbiota (even in the absence of bacterial vaginosis) can correspond to the first stage and predispose to preterm delivery.[123] The specific changes in the vaginal microbiota have been recently described by using sequence-based techniques.[123,124] In *stage 2*, microorganisms gain access to the uterine cavity and reside in the lower pole of the uterus between the membranes and chorion, where they can elicit a localized inflammatory reaction. In *stage 3*, bacteria have penetrated the chorion and the amnion in the lower pole of the uterus into the amniotic cavity, leading to microbial invasion of the amniotic cavity and intra-amniotic infection when an inflammatory response is established in the amniotic fluid. Rupture of the membranes is not a prerequisite for intra-amniotic infection because microorganisms are capable of crossing intact membranes.[125] Finally, in *stage 4*, bacteria may gain access to the fetus through different sites. Aspiration of infected fluid by the fetus may lead to congenital pneumonia. Otitis, conjunctivitis, and omphalitis may occur by the direct spreading of microorganisms from infected amniotic fluid. Seeding from any of these sites to the fetal circulation may result in fetal bacteremia and sepsis.

The traditional concept has been that bacteria invade the decidua from the lower genital tract and, from there, are localized to the space between the chorion and amnion before invading the amniotic cavity.[88,126] However, molecular data bring into question whether most cases of intra-amniotic infection are preceded by a stage in which the infection is in the decidua or in the chorioamniotic space.[127]

MICROBIOLOGY OF INTRA-AMNIOTIC INFECTION

The most common microbial isolates from the amniotic cavity of women with intra-amniotic infection are *Ureaplasma* spp. (*Ureaplasma parvum* and *Ureaplasma urealyticum*), *Fusobacterium* spp., and *Mycoplasma hominis*.[a] These microorganisms are frequently found as members of the vaginal

[a]References 29, 31, 53, 102, 121, 128–136.

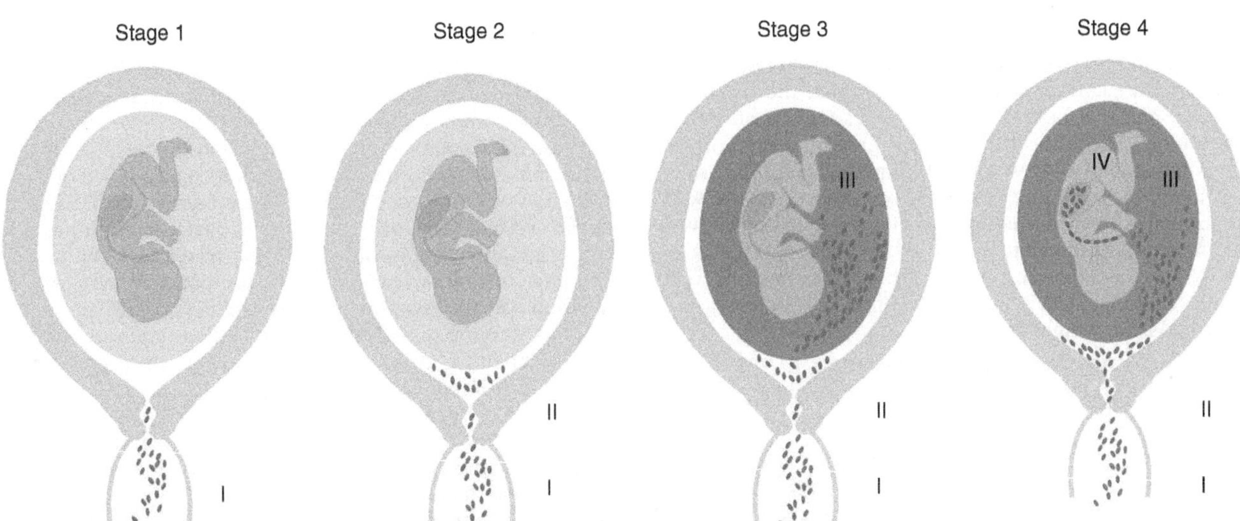

Fig. 12.2 The stages of ascending infection. The first stage corresponds to a change in the vaginal/cervical microbial flora or to the presence of pathologic organisms in the cervix. Once microorganisms gain access to the amniotic cavity, they reside in the lower pole of the uterus between the membranes and the chorion (stage 2). The microorganisms may proceed through the amnion (amnionitis) into the amniotic cavity, leading to an intra-amniotic infection (stage 3). The microorganisms may invade the fetus by different ports of entry (stage 4). (Modified from Fig. 1 in Romero R, Mazor M. Infection and preterm labor. *Clin Obstet Gynecol.* 1988;31:553–584.)

Table 12.2 Microorganisms in the Amniotic Fluid in Patients With Intra-Amniotic Infection.

Ureaplasma urealyticum
Fusobacterium nucleatum
Mycoplasma hominis
Streptococcus agalactiae
Sneathia species
Gardnerella vaginalis
Lactobacillus species
Staphylococcus aureus
Peptostreptococcus species
Streptococcus viridans
Bacteroides species

microbiome in normal pregnant women. Why these specific microorganisms ascend into the amniotic cavity and not others, which are more frequently present, such as *Lactobacilli* spp., is unknown. Table 12.2 displays the most frequent microorganisms found in the amniotic fluid of patients with intra-amniotic infection. Most microorganisms are also found in the lower genital tract of normal pregnant women.

In approximately 50% of patients with intra-amniotic infection, more than one microorganism are isolated from amniotic fluid. The inoculum size differs considerably, and in 71% of cases, more than 10^5 colony-forming units per milliliter are found.[29] *Chlamydia trachomatis* is rarely found in the amniotic fluid.[137]

Viral invasion of the amniotic cavity has been found in 2.2% of women (16 of 729) undergoing second-trimester amniocentesis for genetic indications.[138] Human herpes virus 6 is the most common organism, followed by human cytomegalovirus, parvovirus B19, and Epstein-Barr virus.[138] Studies of the presence of viral genomes in amniotic fluid that used targeted polymerase chain reaction (PCR) approaches showed that viruses are extremely rare in patients with preterm prelabor rupture of the membranes (PROM).[139,140] Characterization of the amniotic fluid virome is a frontier.

FREQUENCY OF MICROBIAL INVASION OF THE AMNIOTIC CAVITY DUE TO BACTERIA

MICROBIAL INVASION OF THE AMNIOTIC CAVITY IN SPONTANEOUS PRETERM LABOR

Preterm labor and preterm PROM account for approximately two-thirds (one-third each) of preterm deliveries, and the remaining third are the result of indicated delivery because of maternal or fetal indications (i.e., preeclampsia, fetal growth restriction).[141] Microbiologic studies suggest that intra-amniotic infection (stage 3 of ascending intra-amniotic infection) occurs in 25% to 40% of preterm births[103]; however, this may be an underestimation because some pathogens are difficult to identify by conventional cultivation methods.[142,143] Indeed, with the use of molecular microbiologic techniques, bacterial DNA has been identified in culture-negative amniotic fluid from women in preterm labor.[133,134,144-146]

MICROBIAL INVASION OF THE AMNIOTIC CAVITY IN PATIENTS WITH PRETERM LABOR AND INTACT MEMBRANES

Approximately 12% of patients presenting with an episode of preterm labor and intact membranes have microorganisms in the amniotic fluid detected by cultivation techniques.[33,36,147,148] Women with amniotic fluid cultures positive for microorganisms generally do not have clinical evidence of infection on presentation (i.e., fever and other signs of clinical chorioamnionitis). However, such patients are more likely to develop clinical chorioamnionitis (37.5% vs. 9%), to be refractory to tocolysis (85.3% vs. 16.3%), and to have spontaneous rupture of the membranes (40% vs. 3.8%) than patients with negative amniotic fluid cultures.[31] Moreover, the earlier the gestational age at preterm birth, the more likely that microbial invasion of the amniotic cavity is present,[35] and at 21 to 24 weeks of gestation, most spontaneous births are associated with acute histologic chorioamnionitis, compared to approximately 10% at 35 to 36 weeks.[35] The rate of neonatal complications is higher in infants born to women with intra-amniotic infection than in those born to women without infection.[35,149,150]

MICROBIAL INVASION OF THE AMNIOTIC CAVITY IN PRETERM PRELABOR RUPTURE OF THE MEMBRANES

The rate of amniotic fluid cultures positive for microorganisms at admission is approximately 32.4% in patients with preterm PROM[33,52]; however, clinical chorioamnionitis is present in only 29.7% of patients with proven microbial invasion.[31,33] The rate of microbial invasion in preterm PROM reported by these studies is probably an underestimation of the true prevalence of intra-amniotic infection. Indeed, available evidence indicates that the frequency of intra-amniotic infection is higher among women with preterm PROM and a severely reduced volume of amniotic fluid than among those without oligohydramnios.[151,152] Because women with oligohydramnios are less likely to undergo an amniocentesis, the bias in these studies is to underestimate the prevalence of infection. In addition, women with preterm PROM admitted in labor generally do not undergo amniocentesis. These patients have a higher rate of microbial invasion of the amniotic cavity than those admitted without labor (39% vs. 25%; $p = .049$).[153] Moreover, of patients who are not in labor at admission, 75% will have an amniotic fluid culture positive for microorganisms when amniocentesis is performed at the onset of preterm labor.[153] This important observation confirms the traditional clinical view that when a patient with preterm PROM goes into labor, this most likely reflects the presence of intra-amniotic infection. Recent studies, utilizing a combination of cultivation methods and molecular microbiologic techniques, indicate that 50% of patients with preterm PROM have microorganisms detected in the amniotic cavity.[134]

MICROBIAL INVASION OF THE AMNIOTIC CAVITY IN ACUTE CERVICAL INSUFFICIENCY AND AN ASYMPTOMATIC SONOGRAPHIC SHORT CERVIX

Women presenting with a dilated cervix, intact membranes, and few, if any, contractions before 24 weeks of gestation are considered to have clinical cervical insufficiency. Of such patients, 51.5% have an amniotic fluid culture positive for microorganisms.[130] The most common microorganism is *U. urealyticum*, which is found in 22.4% of patients with cervical insufficiency.[154] Whether intra-amniotic infection is the cause or a consequence of cervical dilatation or a short cervix has not been determined. Shortening of the cervical canal or silent cervical dilatation with protrusion of the membranes into the vagina may lead to a secondary intra-amniotic infection. The outcomes for patients with microbial invasion of the amniotic cavity are uniformly poor. These patients develop subsequent complications such as rupture of the membranes, clinical chorioamnionitis, or pregnancy loss. The clinical implication of this observation is that it is prudent to assess the microbial state of the amniotic cavity before the placement of a cerclage in patients with cervical insufficiency.

A sonographic short cervix in the second trimester, defined as a cervical length of 25 mm or less, is a powerful predictor of spontaneous preterm delivery.[155,156] Subclinical microbial invasion of the amniotic cavity was detected in 9% of asymptomatic patients with a sonographic cervical length of less than 25 mm.[54,157] Some of these patients have "sludge" in the amniotic cavity, which is often evidence of the presence of a microbial biofilm.[158-163]

MICROBIAL INVASION OF THE AMNIOTIC CAVITY IN TWIN GESTATIONS WITH PRETERM LABOR

Microbial invasion of the amniotic cavity occurs in 11.9% of twin gestations.[121] This finding is in contrast to the 21.6% rate of positive amniotic fluid cultures observed in singleton gestations with preterm labor and delivery.[29] These data suggest that intra-amniotic infection is a possible cause of preterm labor and delivery in twin gestations but they do not support the hypothesis that intra-amniotic infection is responsible for the high rate of preterm delivery observed in twins.[164,165] Moreover, when intra-amniotic infection is detected, the presenting sac is nearly always involved.[121]

MICROBIAL INVASION OF THE AMNIOTIC CAVITY IN CLINICAL CHORIOAMNIONITIS AT TERM

Clinical chorioamnionitis is the most common infection-related pregnancy complication at term[67,69] and is associated with adverse maternal[166,167] and neonatal outcomes.[89,168-181] Neonates born to mothers with clinical chorioamnionitis at term are at an increased risk for cerebral palsy (odds ratio [OR] 9.3, 95% confidence interval [CI] 2.7 to 31.0).[170]

The microbiology of clinical chorioamnionitis was originally described in 1982 by means of cultivation of amniotic fluid obtained with a transcervical catheter. However, such method of amniotic fluid collection is associated with high rates of contamination.[64] Clinical chorioamnionitis is a syndrome in which 60% of patients have proven intra-amniotic infection, 24% have sterile intra-amniotic inflammation, and 15% have no evidence of intra-amniotic infection or inflammation.[53,136,182] The cause of such a systemic inflammatory response in the mother without an intra-amniotic inflammatory response[183] has been attributed to maternal neuroinflammation associated with the administration of epidural anesthesia.[184-198]

Neonates born to mothers with clinical chorioamnionitis at term but without intra-amniotic inflammation often have systemic intravascular inflammation, suggesting that intrapartum fever (maternal systemic inflammation) alters the fetal immune response.[199] Accumulating evidence demonstrates that maternal systemic inflammation can predispose the fetus to neuroinflammation.[200-209]

MICROBIAL INVASION OF THE AMNIOTIC CAVITY AT THE TIME OF GENETIC AMNIOCENTESIS

Compelling evidence from studies of the microbiologic state of the amniotic cavity, using traditional cultivation methods at the time of genetic amniocentesis, suggests that intra-amniotic infection may be chronic in nature. Cassell and colleagues[210] reported the recovery of genital mycoplasmas from 6.6% of amniotic fluid samples (4/61) collected by amniocentesis between 16 and 21 weeks of gestation. Two patients had cultures positive for *M. hominis*, and two had cultures positive for *U. urealyticum.* Subsequently, Gray and colleagues[211] reported a prevalence of cultures positive for *U. urealyticum* of 0.4% (9/2461) in amniotic fluid samples obtained during second-trimester genetic amniocenteses. After exclusion of one patient who had a therapeutic abortion, all patients (8/8) with positive amniotic fluid cultures had either a fetal loss within 4 weeks of amniocentesis (n = 6) or preterm delivery (n = 2). Furthermore, all had histologic evidence of acute histologic chorioamnionitis. A similar finding was reported by Horowitz and colleagues,[212] who detected *U. urealyticum* in 2.8% of amniotic fluid samples (6/214) obtained between 16 and 20 weeks of gestation. The rate of adverse pregnancy outcomes (fetal loss, preterm delivery, and low birth weight) was significantly higher in patients with a positive amniotic fluid culture than in those with a negative one (50% vs. 12%; p = .04). Of interest, patients with a positive amniotic fluid culture were more likely to have an obstetric history that included more than three previous spontaneous abortions than those with a negative culture (33% vs. 4%; p = .03).[212] In a retrospective study of 2718 women undergoing genetic amniocentesis, 1.8% of samples (49/2718) were positive for *Ureaplasma/Mycoplasma;* 34 patients were treated with orally administered erythromycin.[213] Second-trimester pregnancy loss was significantly higher in the untreated group than in the treated group (44.4% vs. 11.4%; p = .04); however, no significant differences were observed between the untreated and treated groups in the rate of preterm delivery (20% vs. 19.4%; p = .7) and adverse pregnancy outcomes (55.6% vs. 28.6%; p = .1).[213] These observations suggest that microbial invasion of the amniotic cavity could be subclinical in the second trimester and that pregnancy loss or preterm delivery may take weeks to occur.

THE RELATIONSHIP BETWEEN CHORIOAMNIOTIC INFECTION AND ACUTE HISTOLOGIC CHORIOAMNIONITIS

Acute inflammation of the chorioamniotic membranes is a non-specific host response to several stimuli, including infection. Fig. 12.3 shows inflammation of the chorioamniotic membranes, and Fig. 12.4 shows the proposed mechanisms implicated in the chemotaxis of neutrophils from the decidua into the chorioamniotic membranes. Traditionally, acute histologic chorioamnionitis has been interpreted to be an indicator of amniotic fluid infection,[72,74,85,88-92,214-216] a view based on indirect evidence. Specifically, there is an association between acute inflammatory lesions of the placenta and the recovery of microorganisms from the subchorionic plate[217,218] and the chorioamniotic space.[219] For example, bacteria have been detected in the subchorionic plate of 72% of placentas with histologic acute chorioamnionitis.[88,218,220] In addition, there is a strong correlation between amniotic fluid cultures positive for microorganisms and acute histologic chorioamnionitis.[74,221] Moreover, Cassell and colleagues[210,222] have reported an association between positive microbial cultures from material obtained from the chorioamniotic space and acute histologic chorioamnionitis. By contrast with acute histologic chorioamnionitis, funisitis is a fetal inflammatory response (Fig. 12.5). However, acute histologic chorioamnionitis and funisitis can be found in cases of sterile intra-amniotic inflammation, suggesting that non-microbial signals can induce inflammation in the chorioamniotic space and even in the fetus.[43,51,52,54]

FETAL INFECTION

The most advanced and serious stage of ascending intra-amniotic infection is fetal infection (stage 4). The mortality rate of preterm neonates with early-onset sepsis is higher than that of nonseptic newborns.[223-227] One study, which focused on infants born before 33 weeks of gestation, found that the mortality rate was 33% for infected fetuses and 17% for uninfected fetuses.[227]

Carroll and colleagues[228] reported that fetal bacteremia (detected by cordocentesis) was found in 33% of fetuses from amniotic fluid cultures positive for microorganisms and in 4% of those with amniotic fluid cultures negative for microorganisms. Furthermore, Goldenberg and colleagues[229] reported in the Alabama Preterm Birth Study that 23% of neonates born between 23 and 32 weeks of gestation have umbilical blood cultures positive for *U. urealyticum* and *M. hominis.* Newborns with a positive blood culture had a higher frequency of the neonatal systemic inflammatory response syndrome, higher umbilical cord serum concentrations of IL-6, and more frequent histologic evidence of acute histologic chorioamnionitis than those with a negative culture.[229] Therefore, subclinical fetal infection (i.e., bacteremia) is far more common than traditionally recognized.

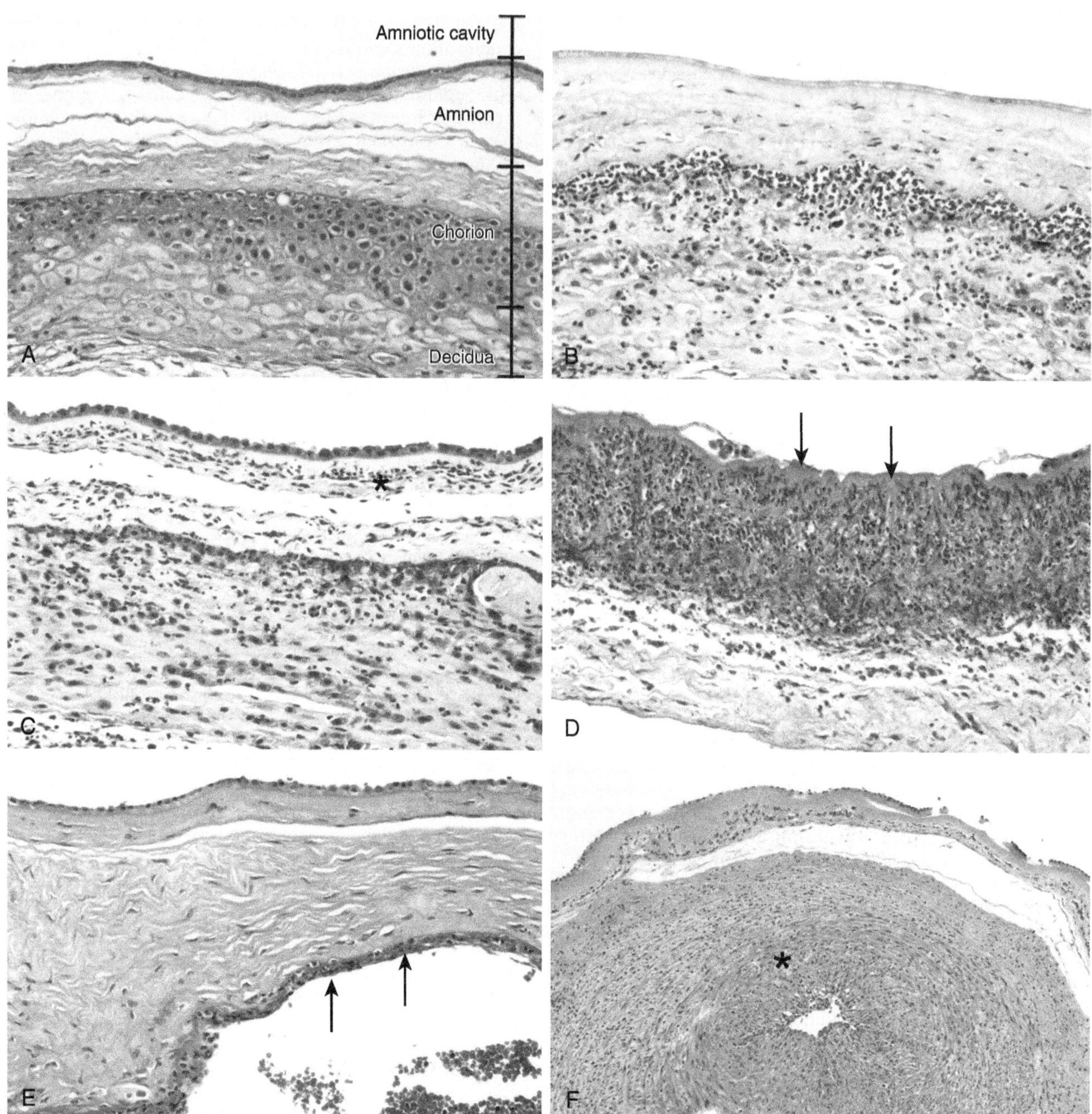

Fig. 12.3 The stages of acute chorioamnionitis. Acute chorioamnionitis of the extraplacental chorioamniotic membranes: (A) Normal chorioamniotic membranes show the absence of neutrophils. (B) Acute chorionitis is defined by stage 1 acute inflammation of the chorioamniotic membranes, in which neutrophilic infiltration is limited to the chorion. (C) Acute chorioamnionitis is defined by stage 2 acute inflammation of the chorioamniotic membranes; neutrophilic migration into the amniotic connective tissue is shown *(asterisk)*. (D) Necrotizing chorioamnionitis is defined by stage 3 acute inflammation of the chorioamniotic membranes, whose characteristic is amnion epithelial necrosis *(arrows)*. Acute inflammation of the chorionic plate: (E) Acute subchorionitis, stage 1 acute inflammation shows neutrophils in the subchorionic fibrin in the chorionic plate *(arrows)*. The area immediately below the arrows represents the intervillous space. (F) Acute chorionic vasculitis *(asterisk)* is a stage 1 fetal inflammatory response. Acute inflammation of the chorioamniotic membranes (A–E) represents a maternal inflammatory response. (Modified from Fig. 5 in Kim CJ, Romero R, Chaemsaithong P, et al. Acute chorioamnionitis and funisitis: definition, pathologic features, and clinical significance. *Am J Obstet Gynecol.* 2015;213(4 suppl):S29–S52.)

INTRA-AMNIOTIC INFECTION AND INFLAMMATION AS A CHRONIC PROCESS

Although intra-amniotic infection has been traditionally considered an acute complication of pregnancy, accumulating evidence suggests that it may be a chronic condition. This finding is derived from studies in which second-trimester genetic amniocenteses were performed, and inflammatory mediators and microbial cultures were obtained. Patients with acute intra-amniotic inflammation (an elevated IL-6 or MMP-8 concentration) are at increased risk for spontaneous preterm delivery.[230–233]

An elevated IL-6 concentration in amniotic fluid is diagnostic of intra-amniotic inflammation and is frequently associated with microbiologic infection in the amniotic fluid or chorioamniotic space.[234–237] Romero and colleagues[238] reported the results of a case-control study in which IL-6 determinations were conducted

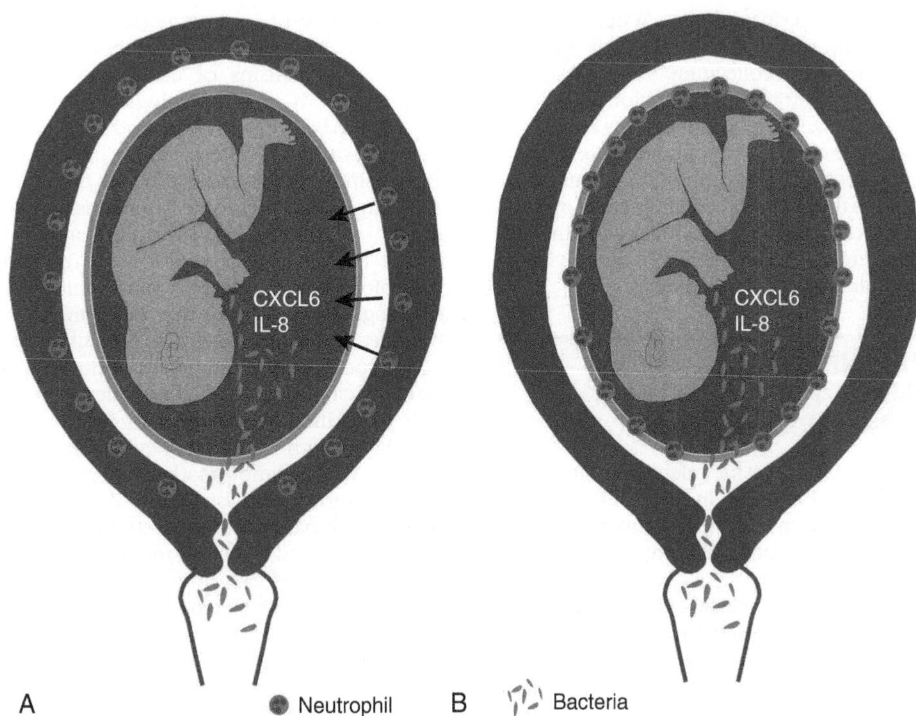

Fig. 12.4 Chemotactic stimuli induce neutrophils to migrate into the fetal membranes. (A) An increase in the amniotic fluid concentrations of chemokines, such as chemokine (C-X-C motif) ligand 6 *(CXCL6)* and interleukin-8 *(IL-8)*, induces neutrophils to migrate toward the amnion *(arrows)*. (B) Consequently, maternal neutrophils infiltrate the chorioamniotic membranes from the decidual vessels. (Modified from Fig. 11 in Kim CJ, Romero R, Chaemsaithong P, et al. Acute chorioamnionitis and funisitis: definition, pathologic features, and clinical significance. *Am J Obstet Gynecol.* 2015;213(4 suppl):S29–S52.)

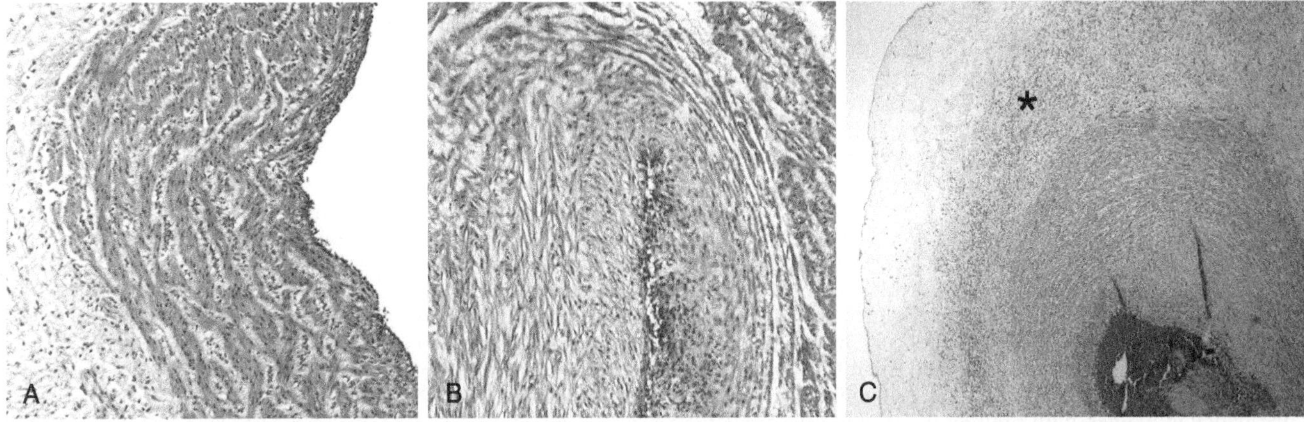

Fig. 12.5 The staging of acute funisitis. (A) Umbilical phlebitis shows an amniotropic migration of fetal neutrophils into the muscle layer of the umbilical vein. Umbilical phlebitis represents stage 1 of fetal inflammation. (B) Umbilical arteritis is a stage 2 fetal inflammatory response. (C) Necrotizing funisitis is considered a stage 3 fetal inflammatory response. Its characteristic feature is a concentric, perivascular distribution of degenerated neutrophils *(asterisk)*. The presence of a thrombus is considered a severe fetal inflammatory response. (Modified from Fig. 6 in Kim CJ, Romero R, Chaemsaithong P, et al. Acute chorioamnionitis and funisitis: definition, pathologic features, and clinical significance. *Am J Obstet Gynecol.* 2015;213(4 suppl):S29–S52.)

in the stored fluid of patients who had a pregnancy loss after a second-trimester amniocentesis and a control group who delivered at term. Patients who had a pregnancy loss had a significantly higher median amniotic fluid IL-6 concentration than those with a normal outcome.[238] Similar findings were reported by Wenstrom and colleagues.[239] Of note, the maternal plasma concentrations of IL-6 were not associated with adverse pregnancy outcomes. Gervasi and colleagues[233] reported similar findings in a cohort study of 796 women who underwent genetic amniocentesis.

The same approach was subsequently used to test the association between markers of inflammation in the second-trimester amniotic fluid samples of asymptomatic women and those with preterm delivery. The concentrations of MMP-8,[230] IL-6,[240–242] and CRP[243] in amniotic fluid obtained during second-trimester amniocenteses were significantly higher in patients who subsequently delivered preterm than in those who delivered at term. Recent observations suggest that intra-amniotic inflammation is heterogeneous and that some patients may have an elevated concentration of the chemokine CXCL-10, rather than IL-6.[244] Such patients are at risk for late spontaneous preterm delivery rather than spontaneous preterm delivery before 32 weeks of gestation.[233]

Collectively, this evidence suggests that a chronic intra-amniotic inflammatory process is associated with both spontaneous abortion and spontaneous preterm delivery. Whether intra-amniotic inflammation can be detected noninvasively remains to be determined. Goldenberg and colleagues[245] demonstrated that the maternal plasma concentration of granulocyte colony-stimulating factor at 24 and 28 weeks of gestation was associated with early preterm birth. To the extent that granulocyte colony-stimulating factor may reflect an intra-amniotic inflammatory process, this finding suggests that a chronic inflammatory process identifiable in the maternal compartment is associated with early preterm birth. However, there are no modalities to identify intra-amniotic inflammation noninvasively at this time.

INTRA-AMNIOTIC INFECTION IS CAUSALLY LINKED TO SPONTANEOUS PRETERM BIRTH

The evidence supporting a causal role for infection follows the criteria outlined by Hill[246] in 1965 and includes: (1) biologic plausibility, (2) temporal relationship, (3) consistency and strength of association, (4) dose-response gradient, (5) specificity, and (6) human experimentation.

Animal experimentation provides clear evidence that the administration of bacterial products (such as endotoxin, a component of the cell wall of gram-negative bacteria) or microorganisms to pregnant animals can lead to preterm labor and delivery.[247-257] Three observations in humans also suggest that infection precedes the spontaneous onset of preterm labor and delivery: (1) subclinical microbial invasion of the amniotic cavity or intra-amniotic inflammation in the midtrimester of pregnancy is frequently associated with spontaneous abortion or preterm delivery; (2) patients with preterm PROM who, on admission, had an amniotic fluid culture positive for mycoplasmas (*U. urealyticum* or *M. hominis*) also underwent a significantly shorter amniocentesis-to-delivery interval than those with sterile amniotic fluid[258] (suggesting that patients with preterm PROM and microbial invasion of the amniotic cavity are more likely to initiate preterm labor than those with a negative amniotic fluid culture); and (3) colonization of the lower genitourinary tract with microorganisms is a risk factor for preterm delivery. These conditions include asymptomatic bacteriuria, bacterial vaginosis, and infection with *N. gonorrhoeae*.[259-268] The consistency and strength of association between infection and preterm delivery have been demonstrated by studies in which amniotic fluid was cultured for microorganisms in patients with preterm PROM[269] and preterm labor with intact membranes.[29] Moreover, the relative risk is high (>2) for preterm delivery in patients with preterm labor and intact membranes and microbial invasion of the amniotic cavity. The hazard ratio is also high for the duration of pregnancy in women with preterm PROM and intra-amniotic infection.

The likelihood of a causal relationship is increased if a dose-response gradient can be demonstrated. Is there a dose-response gradient between the severity of the infection and the likelihood of preterm delivery? Evidence supporting such a relationship includes the following: (1) the median concentration of bacterial endotoxin is higher in patients in preterm labor than in those not in labor[270]; (2) the microbial load is significantly greater in patients with preterm PROM admitted to the hospital with preterm labor than in those admitted to the hospital with preterm PROM but not in labor[153] (this is also the case for patients with preterm labor and intact membranes, in which the number of bacterial genomes relates to the interval-to-delivery in these patients[133,134]); and (3) the rate of abortion or preterm delivery, after the administration of *E. coli* bacterial endotoxin to pregnant mice, exhibits a clear dose-response gradient.[271,272]

One of the criteria for causality that is not met is specificity, meaning that a fraction of patients who deliver preterm do so in the absence of intra-amniotic infection. Today, this is readily recognized because preterm labor is a syndrome caused by multiple mechanisms of disease.[273] However, a high degree of specificity is rare in biologic systems. Although the causal relationship between smoking and lung cancer is widely accepted, it is also nonspecific. Lung cancer occurs in nonsmokers, and of course, smoking can cause diseases other than lung cancer, such as emphysema and chronic bronchitis. Moreover, the formulation of "the necessary and sufficient cause" can inappropriately restrict the analysis of causality. In the case of preterm labor, microbiologic, cytologic, biochemical, immunologic, and pathologic data indicate that preterm labor is a syndrome and that infection is only one of its possible causes.[30,273,274]

An important criterion for causation is whether eradication of the agent can decrease the frequency of outcome or illness. Many trials of antimicrobial treatment for the prevention of preterm birth have been conducted: evidence shows that treatment of patients with asymptomatic bacteriuria will reduce the rates of prematurity and low birth weight,[267] and that antibiotic treatment of patients with preterm PROM prolongs the latency period[275-279] and reduces the rate of maternal and neonatal infection.[276-278,280-282] However, treatment of all patients with preterm labor and intact membranes does not improve pregnancy outcome.[277,283-286] The reason for this outcome is likely related to the syndromic nature of preterm labor with intact membranes. Only a fraction of women with preterm labor present an intra-amniotic infection. Women who do not have an intra-amniotic infection cannot benefit from antimicrobial treatment: this applies to patients presenting with preterm labor and those with bacterial vaginosis.[287,288] In addition, bacterial biofilms make eradication of infection difficult because such bacteria are more resistant to antibiotics.[289-293] The lack of effectiveness of antibiotics in the prevention of preterm delivery, therefore, is related to challenges of treatment and delayed diagnosis.

Patients with intra-amniotic infection and preterm labor have a local "cytokine storm" at the time of presentation, which is instrumental in the mechanisms responsible for preterm labor. In such circumstances, antimicrobial agents are often insufficient to prevent progression of preterm labor to delivery. This phenomenon is akin to what occurs in cases of septic shock, another condition characterized by a local "cytokine storm," in which antibiotics may not prevent death. The lack of effectiveness of antibiotics does not negate the role of infection in the etiology of preterm labor and delivery.

Recent studies suggest that intra-amniotic inflammation or intra-amniotic infection can be eradicated with antimicrobial agents administered to mothers in cases of short cervix,[157] acute cervical insufficiency,[294] preterm labor with intact membranes,[295] and preterm PROM.[279,282,296]

INTRA-AMNIOTIC INFECTION/ INFLAMMATION AND PRETERM LABOR

Normal labor at term, as well as preterm labor, are inflammatory processes.[297-313] Spontaneous labor at term is typically a sterile inflammatory process, except for cases in which there is infection. Evidence supports a role for inflammation in spontaneous labor at term: (1) the concentrations of cytokines[126,314-325] and other inflammatory mediators (such as prostaglandins[326-340] and matrix-degrading enzymes)[341-346] are elevated in the amniotic fluid of women in spontaneous labor at term; (2) unbiased gene expression studies of both the chorioamniotic membranes[304] and myometrium[306,347] have demonstrated an inflammatory signature in patients in spontaneous labor at term without histologic evidence of chorioamnionitis (a signature characterized by an upregulation of cytokines); and (3) the administration of IL-1β, IL-1α, tumor necrosis factor (TNF)-α, and prostaglandins to pregnant animals results in the onset of preterm labor, an effect that can be abrogated by pretreatment with their antagonists.[348]

The mechanisms whereby infection leads to preterm labor require recognition, response, and resolution. *Recognition* refers to pathogens, which, in the case of preterm birth, may involve commensals that have become pathogens, as they are out of place in the amniotic cavity. *Response* refers to the deployment of the cellular and soluble components of the inflammatory response, which culminate in parturition. *Resolution* consists of the expulsion of the infected tissue (delivery of the fetus, placenta, and membranes) and the return of tissue homeostasis.

Microorganisms using an ascending pathway from the lower genital tract can reach the decidua (the lower pole of the uterus), where they can stimulate a local inflammatory reaction and the production of proinflammatory cytokines/chemokines[b] and inflammatory mediators (e.g., platelet-activating factor,[369] prostaglandins,[370-372] leukotrienes,[373] complement,[374,375] reactive oxygen species,[376,377] and nitric oxide[378-380]). If this inflammatory process is not sufficient to signal the onset of labor, microorganisms can pass through intact membranes into the amniotic cavity where they can stimulate the production of inflammatory mediators by host cells. Finally, microorganisms that gain access to the fetus may elicit a systemic inflammatory response syndrome, characterized by increased concentrations of IL-6[381] and other cytokines[382] as well as cellular evidence of neutrophil and monocyte activation.[383]

HOW ARE MICROORGANISMS "RECOGNIZED" BY THE HOST (MOTHER AND/OR FETUS)?

The innate immune system provides the first line of defense against infection. Pattern recognition receptors (PRRs) are mainly expressed by innate immune cells to recognize molecular structures derived from pathogens (i.e., pathogen-associated molecular patterns or PAMPs) or danger signals/alarmins released by cellular stress or necrosis (i.e., damage-associated molecular patterns, DAMPs).[384] PRRs, which are classified according to their function and subcellular localization, include: (1) soluble PRRs, such as the "acute-phase proteins" (i.e., the mannan-binding lectin and CRP), which act as opsonins to neutralize and clear pathogens through the complement and phagocytic systems; (2) transmembrane PRRs, which include scavenger receptors, C-type lectins, and Toll-like receptors (TLR); and (3) intracellular PRRs, including nucleotide-binding oligomerization domain containing protein 1 (NOD1), NOD2, NOD-like receptors (NLRs), retinoic-acid inducible gene 1, and melanoma differentiation–associated protein 5, which mediate recognition of intracellular pathogens (e.g., intracellular bacteria, viruses) as well as danger signals/alarmins.[385-388]

TLRs are a group of transmembrane PRRs,[385,389-391] and 10 different TLRs have been identified in humans.[392] TLR-2 recognizes peptidoglycans, lipoproteins, and zymosan (gram-positive bacteria, mycoplasmas, and fungi)[393]; TLR-4 recognizes lipopolysaccharide (LPS), a major component of the cell wall of gram-negative bacteria; and TLR-3 recognizes double-stranded RNA (viruses).[394-396] TLR engagement results in the activation of nuclear factor (NF)-κB that, in turn, leads to the production of cytokines, chemokines, and antimicrobial peptides.[396] The activation of the TLR pathway also induces surface expression of costimulatory molecules, such as CD80 and CD86, which are required for the full induction of adaptive immune responses mediated by T and B cells. Such T-cell responses are initiated by the recognition of antigenic microbial peptides, which are presented by major histocompatibility complex (MHC) class II proteins expressed by antigen-presenting cells (e.g., dendritic cells and macrophages).[396]

TLRs are crucial for the recognition of microorganisms, and it could be anticipated that defective signaling through these PRRs will impair bacteria-induced preterm labor and birth.[397-402] Indeed, mice with a spontaneous mutation of TLR-4 are less likely than wild-type mice to deliver preterm after intra-amniotic inoculation with heat-killed bacteria or endotoxin administration.[397,403] Moreover, in humans, spontaneous labor at term or preterm with acute histologic chorioamnionitis, regardless of the membrane status (intact or ruptured), is associated with higher mRNA and protein expression of TLR-2 and TLR-4 in the chorioamniotic membranes.[404] These observations support a role for TLRs in sensing bacteria and in the mechanisms leading to preterm labor and birth.

THE INFLAMMATORY RESPONSE TO MICROORGANISMS IS MEDIATED BY CYTOKINES IN PRETERM LABOR

Once microorganisms have been *recognized* by PRRs, the next step is *response*—this is accomplished by the production of chemokines[c] (cytokines that have chemotactic effects, such as IL-8, CXCL6, and CCL20) and proinflammatory cytokines (e.g., IL-1 and TNF- α).[d]

A substantial body of evidence supports participation of the proinflammatory cytokines IL-1 and TNF-α in the mechanisms responsible for preterm labor. Such evidence includes the following: (1) IL-1β and TNF-α stimulate prostaglandin (the mediators of labor) production by the amnion, decidua, and myometrium[405-407]; (2) human decidua can produce IL-1β and TNF-β in response to bacterial products[406,408,409]; (3) the concentrations and bioactivity of IL-1β and TNF-α in the amniotic fluid are elevated in women with preterm labor and intra-amniotic infection[314,349,350]; (4) women with preterm PROM and intra-amniotic infection have higher IL-1β and TNF-α concentrations in the presence of labor[405-407]; (5) IL-1β and TNF-α can induce preterm parturition when administered systemically to pregnant animals[247,410]; (6) pretreatment with the natural IL-1 receptor antagonist before the administration of IL-1 to pregnant animals prevents preterm parturition[348,411,412]; (7) the administration of heat-killed bacteria to pregnant mice lacking the type 1 receptors for IL-1 and TNF is associated with a reduction in the frequency of spontaneous preterm birth[413]; (8) placental tissue obtained from patients in labor, particularly those with chorioamnionitis, produces greater amounts of IL-1β than that obtained from women not in labor[414]; and (9) the concentration of IL-1β and soluble receptors of TNF-α in fetal plasma is elevated in the context of preterm labor with intra-amniotic infection.[415-417]

Considerable redundancy exists, however, in the cytokine network, and blockade of a single factor is insufficient to prevent preterm delivery in the context of infection and inflammation. Indeed, the administration of anti-TNF-α and the natural IL-1 receptor antagonist to pregnant animals with intra-amniotic infection does not prevent preterm delivery.[418] Moreover, results of knockout animal experiments suggest that infection-induced preterm labor and delivery occur in animals that lack a particular cytokine receptor.[419]

IL-1β, as well as TNF-α, can participate in activation of the myometrium, and evidence shows that they involve the participation of cytosolic phospholipase A_2, cyclooxygenase 2,[420,421] mitogen-activated protein kinases,[422] and nuclear factor κβ. The latter transcription factor is responsible for many of the actions of IL-1β and TNF-α in the amnion and may affect uterine

[b] References 44, 221, 234-237, 316, 318, 322, 349-368.

[c] References 316, 321, 351, 352, 355, 357, 359.

[d] References 44, 221, 234-237, 318, 350, 356, 358, 365-367.

function by blocking factors that promote uterine quiescence (e.g., progesterone).[423]

A ROLE FOR THE INFLAMMASOME IN THE MECHANISMS RESPONSIBLE FOR PRETERM LABOR

A central cytokine in the processes of preterm labor is IL-1β; therefore, the molecular mechanisms involved in the processing of this cytokine are worth mentioning. The processing of IL-1β (the transformation of the immature form into the mature/bioactive form) is mediated by the actions of active caspase-1 (CASP-1) that, in turn, is processed by a multi-protein complex termed the *inflammasome*.[424–427] Fig. 12.6 is a schematic representation of the inflammasome complex that contains (1) a pattern recognition receptor or sensor molecule (e.g., NLR Family Pyrin Domain Containing 3 or NLRP3), (2) the adaptor protein ASC (an apoptosis-associated speck-like protein), and (3) pro-caspase-1 (pro-CASP-1). Upon inflammasome activation, active forms of CASP-1 and IL-1β as well as ASC are released into the extracellular space, inducing a pro-inflammatory cell death termed *pyroptosis*, which is largely mediated by the pore-forming protein gasdermin-D (GSDMD).[428–431] The most widely studied of the inflammasomes is NLRP3, since it is activated by multiple PAMPs and DAMPs and, pertinent to this chapter, is involved in the mechanisms responsible for preterm labor and birth.[432]

The following descriptive evidence suggests that the NLRP3 inflammasome is involved in the mechanisms responsible for preterm labor in women with intra-amniotic infection: (1) amniotic fluid concentrations of caspase-1 are higher in women with preterm labor and intra-amniotic infection than in those without this clinical condition[433]; (2) amniotic fluid concentrations of IL-1β[314,318,434–436] and IL-18[437,438] are also elevated in women with preterm labor and intra-amniotic infection; (3) women with preterm labor and acute histologic chorioamnionitis (a histologic sign of intra-amniotic inflammation[74,81]) displayed priming of the inflammasome as evidenced by the upregulation of NLRP3, caspase-1, caspase-4, IL-1β, and IL-18 in the chorioamniotic membranes[439]; (4) women with spontaneous preterm labor and acute histologic chorioamnionitis also show increased concentrations of active caspase-1 and caspase-4 and mature forms of IL-1β and IL-18, as well as enhanced formation of ASC/caspase-1 complexes in the chorioamniotic membranes[439]; (5) amniotic fluid concentrations of the adaptor protein ASC[440] and the effector molecule of pyroptosis GSDMD[441] are increased in women with preterm labor and intra-amniotic infection compared to those without this clinical condition; and (6) both ASC and GSDMD[441] are also overexpressed by the chorioamniotic membranes of women with preterm labor and intra-amniotic infection.

Furthermore, the following mechanistic evidence supports a role for the NLRP3 inflammasome in the pathophysiology of preterm labor: (1) intrauterine administration of peptidoglycan and poly I:C increased the expression of NLRP3 and

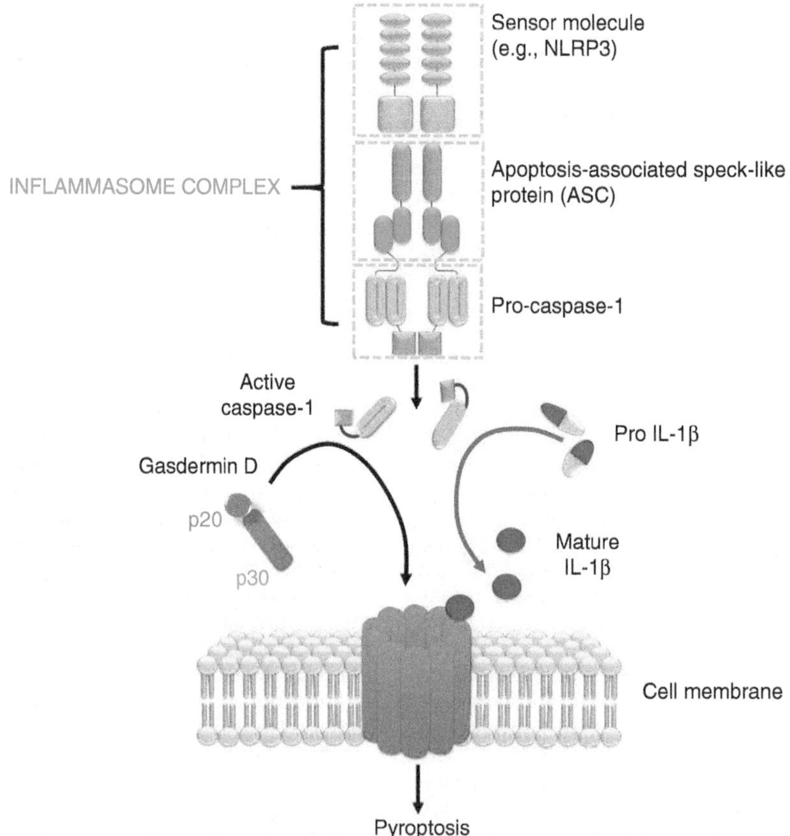

Fig. 12.6 The inflammasome complex. (1) A sensor molecule (NLR Family Pyrin Domain Containing Protein 3 *[NLRP3]*), (2) An apoptosis-associated speck-like protein (the adaptor protein ASC), and (3) Pro-caspase-1. Upon activation, the inflammasome induces the release of active forms of caspase-1 that, in turn, induce the processing of mature interleukin-1β (IL-1β) and interleukin 18 (IL-18) as well as the cleavage of gasdermin D, leading to a pro-inflammatory programmed cell death termed *pyroptosis*. (Originally published in *The Journal of Immunology.* Gomez-Lopez N, Motomura K, Miller D, Garcia-Flores V, Galaz J, Romero R. Inflammasomes: their role in normal and complicated pregnancies. *J. Immunol.* 2019;203:2757–2769. Copyright © 2019 The American Association of Immunologists, Inc.)

caspase-1, as well as increased amounts of active caspase-1, in the uterine tissues[442]; (2) deficiency of *Nlrp3* protects against group B streptococcus-induced preterm birth[443]; (3) the combined injection of MHV-68 and endotoxin induces preterm birth[444,445] by causing exaggerated inflammation in the fetal membranes, which has been suggested to occur, in part, through the activation of the NLRP3 inflammasome[446]; and (4) the ultrasound-guided intra-amniotic administration of endotoxin-induced priming and activation of the NLRP3 inflammasome in the fetal membranes prior to preterm birth, which is ameliorated by blocking the assembly of the NLRP3 inflammasome with a specific inhibitor, MCC950.[447] Collectively, this descriptive and mechanistic evidence supports a role for the NLRP3 inflammasome in the mechanisms responsible for preterm labor in women with intra-amniotic infection.

The NLRP3 inflammasome is also involved in the mechanisms leading to sterile intra-amniotic inflammation-associated preterm labor.[432] The clinical evidence supports this concept in that women with preterm labor and sterile intra-amniotic inflammation have increased concentrations of ASC[440] and GSDMD[441] in the amniotic fluid and the chorioamniotic membranes. These clinical observations led to mechanistic studies in which danger signals or alarmins (molecules that initiate sterile inflammation[448–450]) were used to trigger inflammatory processes in the amniotic cavity and chorioamniotic membranes. For example, the ultrasound-guided intra-amniotic administration of the classical alarmin HMGB1, a molecule present in amniotic fluid of women with preterm labor,[451] induces preterm birth in mice.[452] It was also reported that HMGB1 causes the priming and activation of the NLRP3 inflammasome in the chorioamniotic membranes.[453] Furthermore, the alarmins S100B and IL-1α can induce sterile intra-amniotic inflammation by activating the NLRP3 inflammasome in the fetal membranes prior to inducing preterm birth.[454,455] Importantly, the inhibition of the assembly of this inflammasome, using MCC950, prevented S100B-induced preterm birth.[454] The latter findings have clinical implications given that the use of inhibitors of the NLRP3 inflammasome has been suggested as a therapeutic strategy for the prevention of sterile intra-amniotic inflammation and preterm labor.

ANTIINFLAMMATORY CYTOKINES AND PRETERM LABOR

IL-10, a key cytokine for the maintenance of pregnancy,[456] has been implicated in preterm parturition associated with inflammation.[457] IL-10 expression is reduced in the placental tissues of pregnancies complicated by preterm labor and chorioamnionitis compared to that in the placental tissue from normal controls.[457] IL-10 inhibits cyclooxygenase 2 mRNA expression in cultured placental explants obtained from women who underwent preterm labor/birth, but not in those from women in labor at term, indicating that the mechanisms involved in regulation of the inflammatory response during term and preterm parturition may be different.[457] Further evidence for the role of IL-10 in the down-regulation of the inflammatory response during preterm labor derives from a study in which the administration of dexamethasone or IL-10 to pregnant rhesus monkeys significantly reduced IL-1β-induced uterine contractility. IL-10 treatment also attenuated the concentrations of TNF-α and white blood cells in amniotic fluid.[458] The administration of IL-10 in animal models of infection has been associated with improved pregnancy outcome.[459,460] Moreover, the median amniotic fluid IL-10 concentration was significantly higher in patients with preterm labor who had intra-amniotic infection than in those who did not have intra-amniotic infection.[359]

INFLAMMATORY MEDIATORS IN THE RESPONSE TO MICROORGANISMS: PROSTAGLANDINS AND LIPOXYGENASE PRODUCTS

Prostaglandins are the universal mediators of the onset of labor, and they can induce myometrial contractility[461–464] and changes in the extracellular matrix metabolism associated with cervical ripening,[465–469] as well as decidual and fetal membrane activation.[30]

Evidence supporting the role for prostaglandins in the initiation of human labor includes the following: (1) administration of prostaglandins can induce early or late termination of pregnancy (abortion or labor)[470–477]; (2) treatment with indomethacin or aspirin (prostaglandin inhibitors) can delay the spontaneous onset of parturition in animals[478–480]; (3) prostaglandin concentrations in amniotic fluid abruptly increase before the onset of spontaneous labor at term,[336] and concentrations of prostaglandins in plasma and amniotic fluid increase during labor[326,327,340,370,481–484]; and (4) intra-amniotic injection of arachidonic acid can induce abortion.[485]

Bacteria and their products increase prostaglandin production by the amnion, chorion, or decidua. Amniotic fluid concentrations of prostaglandins (prostaglandin E2 and prostaglandin F2α) and their stable metabolites are significantly higher in women with preterm labor and microbial invasion of the amniotic cavity than in women with preterm labor alone.[326,370,371,483] Similar observations have been reported of patients in labor and with high concentrations of proinflammatory mediators in the amniotic cavity (e.g., IL-1β, TNF-α, IL-6).[314,349,353] Moreover, amnion obtained from patients with histologic chorioamnionitis produces higher amounts of prostaglandins than that obtained from patients without documented chorioamnionitis. In mice, bacteria-induced preterm labor substantially increased the expression of genes involved in prostaglandin synthesis.[486]

Metabolites of arachidonic acid derived through the lipoxygenase pathway, including leukotrienes and hydroxyeicosatetraenoic acids, have also been implicated in the mechanisms for spontaneous preterm and term parturition. The concentrations of 5-hydroxyeicosatetraenoic acid, 15-hydroxyeicosatetraenoic acid, and leukotriene B_4 are higher in the amniotic fluid of women with preterm labor and bacteria in the amniotic fluid cavity than in those without bacteria.[340,487,488] Similarly, the amnion from patients with histologic chorioamnionitis releases more leukotriene B_4 in vitro than the amnion from women who delivered preterm without inflammation.[410,489] Moreover, ovariectomy-induced preterm labor increased the expression of genes involved in lipoxin, leukotriene, and hydroxyeicosatetraenoic acid synthesis.[486] However, the precise role of arachidonate lipoxygenase metabolites in human parturition remains to be determined. 5-hydroxyeicosatetraenoic acid and leukotriene C_4 can stimulate uterine contractility, and leukotriene B_4 is believed to play a role in the recruitment of neutrophils to the site of infection or inflammation and in the regulation of arachidonic acid metabolites of the cyclooxygenase pathway.[490,491] Additionally, leukotriene B_4 has been shown to act as a calcium ionophore (i.e., increases phospholipase activity and enhances the rate of prostaglandin biosynthesis in human intra-amniotic tissues).

MATRIX-DEGRADING ENZYMES: THE EFFECTOR SYSTEM FOR RUPTURED MEMBRANES

The chorioamniotic membranes are fundamentally connective tissue structures, and their tensile strength and elasticity have been attributed to structural extracellular matrix proteins.

Enzymes (matrix metalloproteinases or MMPs, elastase, etc.) that participate in the degradation of extracellular matrix proteins have been implicated in preterm PROM. Compelling evidence shows that preterm PROM is associated with increased availability of MMP-1,[492] MMP-8,[493–495] MMP-9,[341,342,344] and neutrophil elastase,[496] but not MMP-2,[344,345] MMP-3,[346] and MMP-7.[343]

Vaginal bleeding may predispose to membrane rupture by causing a separation between the amniochorion and the decidua, which weakens the fetal membranes.[497] Alternatively, during the formation of a retroplacental clot, thrombin is generated.[498] This enzyme can stimulate the production of MMP-1[499] and MMP-3[498] by the decidual cells and MMP-9 by the chorioamniotic membranes.[500] These MMPs can degrade fibrillar collagen (types I and III) and other components of the extracellular matrix of the chorioamniotic membranes.[501] The mechanisms responsible for defective endometrial hemostasis during pregnancy have not been identified. However, in some cases, the only manifestation of intra-amniotic infection may be vaginal bleeding.[497] This observation links vaginal bleeding in the first and second trimesters of pregnancy, endometrial bleeding/deficient hemostasis, and intra-amniotic infection. This association is important because women with preterm PROM often have clinical or subclinical placental abruption, and histologic examination of the membranes in patients with abruption indicates that acute histologic chorioamnionitis is frequently associated with abruption.[502]

Fig. 12.7 illustrates the cellular and biochemical mechanisms involved in the initiation of preterm labor in cases of intra-amniotic infection.

FETAL INFLAMMATORY RESPONSE SYNDROME

The fetus can deploy an inflammatory response when exposed to bacteria, bacterial products (i.e., endotoxin), viruses, fungi, and protozoa, as well as nonmicrobial stimuli (also known as *danger signals* or *alarmins*). The initial response to microbial invasion or danger signals can be localized to a specific organ, such as the lung; it can then become systemic when the agents inducing inflammation gain access to the fetal circulation.

The term *fetal inflammatory response syndrome* was coined to define a subclinical condition originally describing fetuses of women presenting with preterm labor and intact membranes as well as preterm PROM.[354] The operational definition indicated an elevation of the fetal plasma IL-6 concentration greater than 11 pg/mL.[354] This cytokine was selected as the marker for the definition of FIRS for the following reasons: (1) it is a major mediator of the host response to infection and tissue damage; (2) it is capable of eliciting biochemical, physiologic, and immunologic changes in the host, including stimulation of the production of CRP by liver cells; and (3) many diagnostic criteria proposed for systemic inflammatory response syndrome in adults[503,504] cannot be applied to the human fetus because the vital signs (with the exception of heart rate) cannot be readily determined before birth or in the intrapartum period. By contrast, the proinflammatory cytokine IL-6 is easy to measure and readily detectable in peripheral blood. IL-6 concentration is also elevated in adults with systemic inflammatory response syndrome.[505]

The original work that described FIRS was conducted in samples obtained by cordocentesis (Fig. 12.8).[353,354] In patients with preterm PROM, fetal plasma IL-6 concentrations greater than 11 pg/mL are associated with a shorter cordocentesis-to-delivery interval than that observed with plasma IL-6 concentrations of 11 pg/mL or less (median 0.8 day [range 0.1 to 5 days] vs. 6 days [range 0.2 to 33.6 days], respectively; $p < .05$).[353]

FIRS can also be diagnosed by the demonstration of elevated concentrations of CRP in umbilical cord blood or by histologic examination of the placenta. Funisitis and chorionic vasculitis (inflammation of the umbilical cord or the fetal vessels on the chorionic plate) are the histopathologic landmarks of

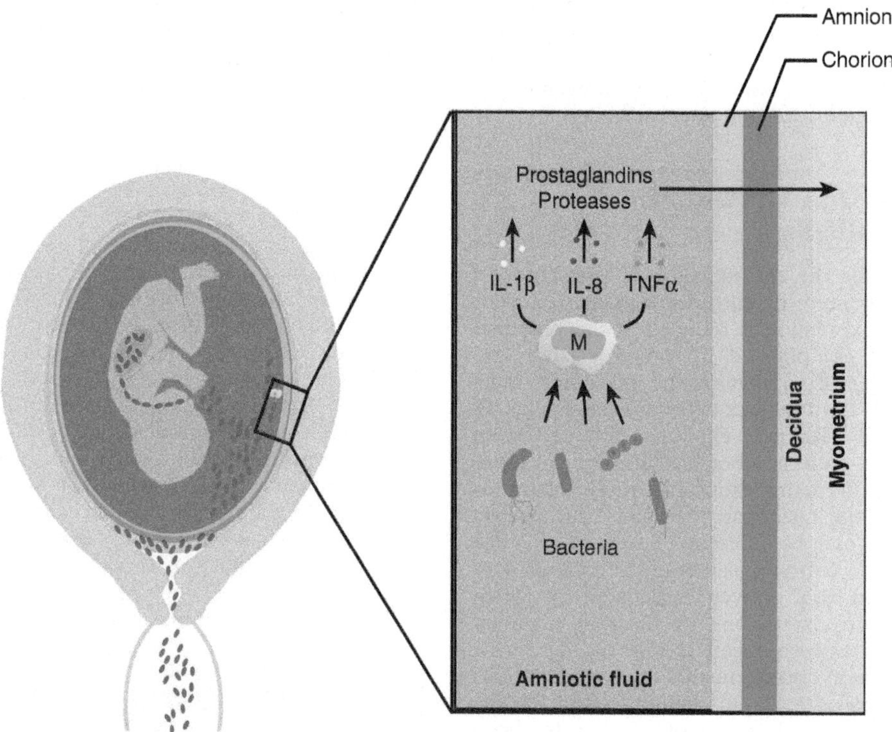

Fig. 12.7 Bacteria from the lower genital tract gain access to the amniotic cavity and stimulate the production of chemokines (interleukin-8 *[IL-8]* and CCL2) and cytokines (interleukin-1β *[IL-1β]* and tumor necrosis factor-α *[TNF-α]*) as well as other inflammatory mediators (prostaglandins and reactive oxygen radicals) and proteases. These products can initiate myometrial contractility and induce membrane rupture. *M,* Macrophage. (Reproduced from fig. 3A in Romero R, Dey SK, Fisher SJ. Preterm labor: one syndrome, many causes. *Science.* 2014;345:760–765.)

		n	Procedure-to-Delivery Interval (Median, Range, Days)
I	AF IL-6 ≤ 7.9 ng/mL FP IL-6 ≤ 11 pg/mL	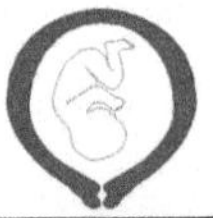 14	5 (0.2–33.6)
II	AF IL-6 > 7.9 ng/mL FP IL-6 ≤ 11 pg/mL	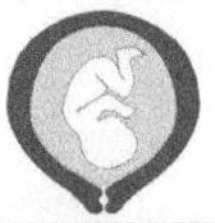 5	7 (1.5–32)
III	AF IL-6 ≤ 7.9 ng/mL FP IL-6 > 11 pg/mL	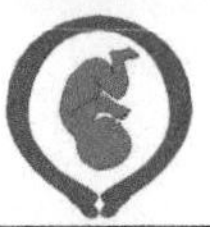 6	1.2 (0.25–2)
IV	AF IL-6 > 7.9 ng/mL FP IL-6 > 11 pg/mL	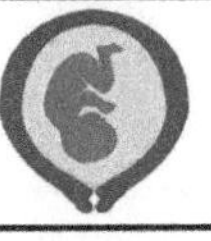 5	0.75 (0.13–10)

Fig. 12.8 Duration of pregnancy according to the presence or absence of intra-amniotic inflammation and fetal systemic inflammation (also known as the *fetal inflammatory response syndrome* [*FIRS*]). The key determinant of pregnancy duration is fetal systemic inflammation regardless of the inflammatory status of the amniotic cavity, as reflected by the procedure-to-delivery interval. The inflammatory status of the amniotic cavity and the fetus was assessed by interleukin-6 (IL-6) concentrations. The fetal image framed by the white background represents no inflammation (defined as fetal plasma *[FP]* IL-6 <11 pg/mL). The fetal image framed by the red background represents fetal systemic inflammation, or FIRS (FP IL-6 >11 pg/mL). The absence of intra-amniotic inflammation from the amniotic fluid compartment is represented in *white*; its presence is represented in *yellow*. The cut-off value for amniotic fluid IL-6 is 7.9 ng/mL. The number of patients in each group is indicated *(n)*. (Modified from Table 2 in Romero R, Gomez R, Ghezzi F, et al. A fetal systemic inflammatory response is followed by the spontaneous onset of preterm parturition. *Am J Obstet Gynecol*. 1998;179:186–193.)

FIRS.[84,506,507] Acute histologic chorioamnionitis, which refers to neutrophil infiltration of the chorioamniotic membranes, is not equivalent to FIRS because inflammation of the membranes is a maternal host response (see Table 12.1 for definitions).

A systematic review and meta-analysis of observational studies has reported that FIRS was a risk factor for adverse neonatal outcomes, including early neonatal sepsis (RR = 3.1), bronchopulmonary dysplasia (RR = 5.9), intraventricular hemorrhage (RR = 4.9), periventricular leukomalacia (RR = 3.3), respiratory distress syndrome (RR = 2.4), and neonatal death (RR = 7.0).[508] In addition, infants born with FIRS are at greater risk for developing retinopathy of prematurity or sensorineural hearing loss.

THE FETAL INFLAMMATORY RESPONSE SYNDROME IS ASSOCIATED WITH MULTI-ORGAN INVOLVEMENT

Fetuses with systemic inflammation (FIRS) have a higher rate of neonatal complications than those without FIRS, after adjustment for gestational age.[508] Multiple organ systems are involved, ranging from the central nervous system to the skin. Fig. 12.9 shows multiple organ involvement in FIRS.

HEMATOPOIETIC SYSTEM

In FIRS, the fetal hematologic profile is characterized by significant changes in granulocyte and red blood cell lineages.[509] Neutrophilia is present in two-thirds of affected fetuses; neutropenia occurs in 5%.[509] The median plasma concentration of granulocyte colony-stimulating factor is significantly higher in FIRS than in the absence of this condition. Granulocyte colony-stimulating factor promotes granulocyte proliferation, maturation, and activation; therefore, it can contribute to the neutrophilia observed in FIRS.[382] FIRS has also been associated with changes in markers of monocyte and neutrophil activation, as shown by flow cytometry.[510] When fetuses of mothers who presented with preterm labor were studied, those delivered within 72 hours of sampling had higher expressions of CD11c, CD13, CD15, and CD67 than those delivered at term, suggesting that activation of the immune system is a feature in preterm parturition.[383] The median nucleated red blood cell count is higher in fetuses with FIRS than in those without FIRS.[509] IL-6 has been implicated in the regulation of the number of fetal nucleated red blood cells.[511]

In experimental models of fetal systemic inflammation, intra-amniotic administration of bacterial endotoxin in sheep increases umbilical cord blood concentrations of IL-6 and IL-8,[512,513] and this indicates that fetal exposure to microbial products recapitulates the key finding used to define FIRS in humans—an elevation of IL-6 concentration in plasma. In addition, intra-amniotic administration of IL-1α or bacterial endotoxin first induces neutropenia, and seven days later, neutrophilia and an increased platelet count can be detected.[512-514] This result suggests that the hematologic response during FIRS changes as a function of time.[383,510]

Exposure of fetal sheep to microbial products or IL-1β increases the size of lymph nodes and the spleen,[513,515,516] and there is an increase in the percentages of CD3, CD4, CD8, and γδ (gamma delta) T cells, demonstrable 48 to 72 hours after exposure.[515,516] Similar observations have been made in fetal rhesus macaques, in which exposure to IL-1β results in a decrease in the percentage of regulatory T cells (CD3+CD4+FOXP3+) in the spleen and lymph nodes (mediastinal and mesenteric).[517] These cells are generally considered to suppress the immune response and are involved in promoting a tolerogenic state. After exposure of fetal rhesus macaques to a single injection of IL-1β, the percentage of regulatory T cells increased after 72 hours. By contrast, the expression of IL-17α, a proinflammatory cytokine, is increased transiently in the same model.[517] Collectively, these data suggest that the immune response of the fetus to microbial products is

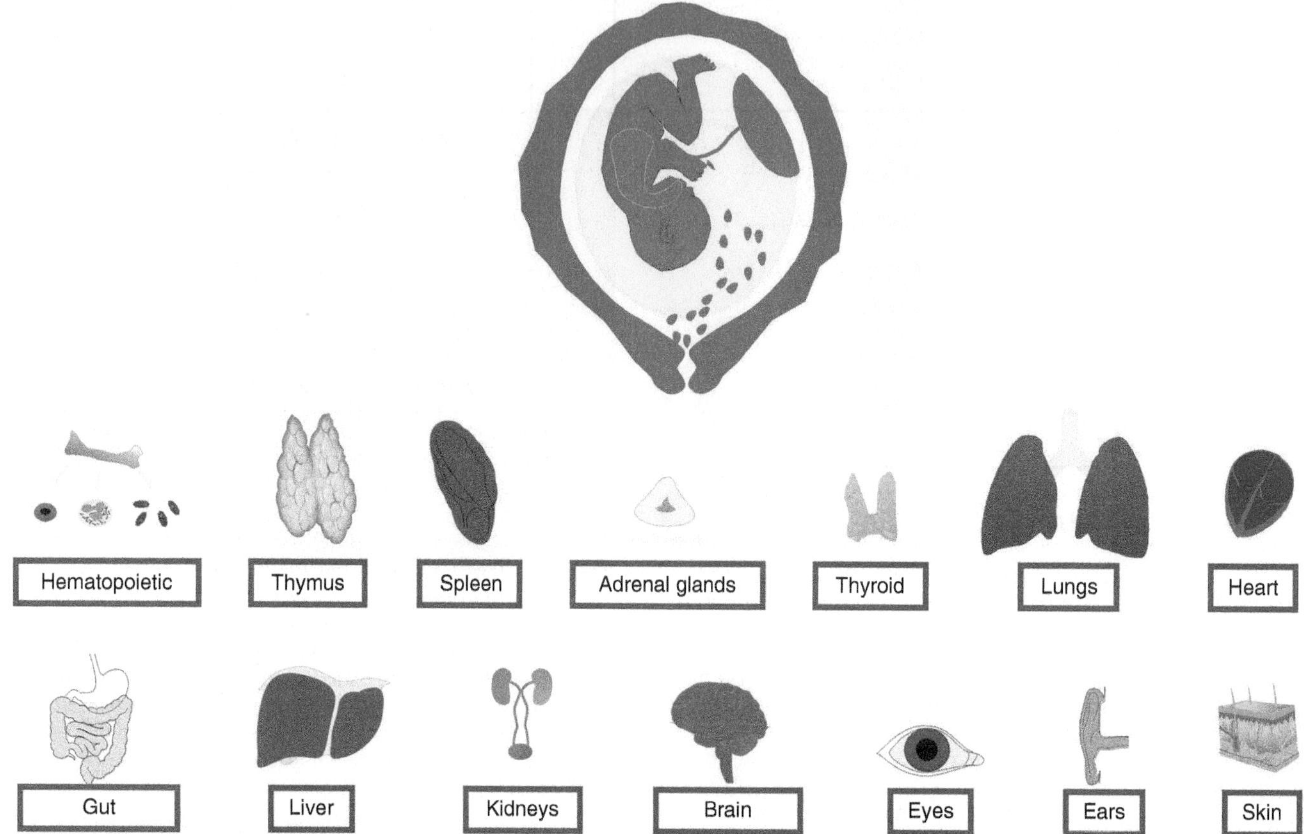

Fig. 12.9 The fetal inflammatory response syndrome (FIRS) is associated with multisystemic involvement. Clinical and/or experimental evidence suggests that there is involvement of the organs displayed in the figure. (Modified from Gotsch F, Romero R, Kusanovic JP et al. The fetal inflammatory response syndrome. *Clin Obstet Gynecol*. 2007;50:652–683.)

complex and is not restricted to the innate limb of the immune response—it also involves the adaptive limb.

Exposure of fetal rhesus macaques to genital mycoplasmas (*U. parvum* or *M. hominis*) (intra-amniotic administration) for 15 days has been associated with diffuse fetal spleen hyperplasia and an increased number of neutrophils, T cells, and plasma cells in the red pulp.[518] However, there was little change in the lymphoid organs 6 days after exposure. Splenic hyperplasia, as reported in these experiments, contrasts with that observed in humans[519]; however, the latter may reflect the end-stage disease associated with perinatal death.

Since intra-amniotic infection may have a chronic course, the laboratories of Jobe and Newnham have explored the potential role of repeated injections of intra-amniotic bacterial endotoxin in fetal sheep.[520] Such repeated exposure was associated with endotoxin tolerance. The weight of the spleen and thymus did not decrease, and there was no change in the proportion of CD8 and γδ T cells.[520]

THYMUS AND IMMUNE SYSTEM

Thymus involution occurs after infection in both the fetus and neonate.[521-526] Subclinical chorioamnionitis has been associated with a small thymus in very low-birth-weight infants,[521] possibly due to an acute fetal[522] and neonatal[522,523] involution. In neonates, thymic involution correlates with the duration of acute illness and with the percentage of lymphocytes in peripheral blood.[523] The mechanism proposed for the development of thymic involution is considered to involve stress (via steroid production) and proinflammatory cytokines.[527-529] Di Naro and colleagues[530] and other investigators[524-526,531] reported that, in the presence of intra-amniotic infection and inflammation, fetuses born to mothers with preterm labor and intact membranes or preterm PROM have a sonographically small thymus. Infants born preterm (before 28 weeks of gestation) with sonographic signs of cerebral white matter damage (white matter echolucencies on postnatal cranial ultrasound scans) have thymic involution more frequently than a control group matched for gestational age.[529]

Intra-amniotic administration of bacterial endotoxin in sheep results in a decrease of thymus weight and the corticomedullary ratio. These effects were observed as early as 5 hours after exposure to endotoxin and documented for five to seven days.[532,533] Increased expression of IL-6 and type I interferons, as well as glucocorticoids, has been implicated in thymus involution.[533-537] In addition, an increase in the percentage of CD3+ cells, but a decrease in the percentages of CD8+ (cytotoxic lymphocytes) and FOXP3+ cells, occurs after exposure to endotoxin.[532,533,538] Such findings suggest that endotoxin exposure has an effect not only in the innate immune response but also in the adaptive immune response. Altogether, FIRS can induce structural, functional, and immunologic changes in the thymus.

Preterm neonates exposed to intra-amniotic infection and/or inflammation have activation of both the innate[383,510,539] and adaptive immune systems.[539-543] The evidence for activation of innate immunity is well established (neutrophil and monocyte activation as determined by flow cytometry, elevated CRP concentration, increased production of reactive oxygen species, etc.). Activation of T cells (members of the adaptive limb of the immune response) has been observed in term and preterm infants born to mothers with clinical chorioamnionitis. These infants have overexpression of CD25, HLA-DR, or CD69 markers in T cells[539] a higher number of memory T cells (CD45RO$^+$), and a decreased number of naïve T cells.[539,540,542,543]

By contrast with the findings in human fetuses/neonates, indicating activation of T cells, studies of fetal rhesus macaques show that such findings are localized to lymphoid tissue. Specifically, the number of regulatory T cells (FOXP3+) is decreased, whereas there is an increase in the number of IL-17-producing (proinflammatory cytokine) cells in lymphoid tissues after intra-amniotic administration of IL-1β.[517] These changes were not observed in fetal blood[517]; however, intra-amniotic exposure to IL-1β is not equivalent to intra-amniotic infection with proliferating bacteria that may invade the human fetus. The differences between results from animal models and humans should be interpreted cautiously, given that in humans the natural infection is observed and that many models in animals have been generated by administration of microbial products.[544] The laboratories of Jobe, Newnham, Gravett, and Novy have reported and are investigating the fetal immune response using such models.[251,518,520,545-549]

ADRENAL GLANDS

Similar to adult patients admitted to intensive care units with burns or pancreatitis, fetuses with FIRS have endocrine evidence of "stress," which is expressed by an elevation of the cortisol and dehydroepiandrosterone sulfate ratio.[550] This endocrine milieu may contribute to the onset of spontaneous preterm labor. Yoon and colleagues[550] reported that in patients with preterm PROM there is a significant association between the fetal plasma cortisol and dehydroepiandrosterone sulfate ratio and a shorter interval from cordocentesis to delivery (hazard ratio 2.9; 95% CI: 1 to 8.4). Patients with preterm PROM who went into spontaneous labor and delivered within 7 days of cordocentesis had a significantly higher median fetal plasma concentration of cortisol than those who delivered after 7 days ($p < .0001$). Fetal plasma cortisol concentration, but not maternal cortisol concentration, was an independent predictor of the duration of pregnancy after adjustment for gestational age and the results of amniotic fluid cultures (hazard ratio 2.9; 95% CI: 1.3 to 6.7). Importantly, a significant correlation was seen between fetal plasma cortisol and fetal plasma IL-6 concentrations ($r = 0.3$; $p < .05$).[550] These endocrine changes may have short-term and long-term implications, given observations about the effect of glucocorticoids in the fetal programming of several metabolic functions.[551-555]

SKIN

Fetal dermatitis can occur during FIRS. Skin samples from fetuses between 21 and 24 weeks of gestation had evidence of epidermal inflammation with overexpression of both TLR-2 and TLR-4.[556] Investigators proposed that microorganisms are recognized by the fetal skin through PRRs; thus, it participates in the fetal inflammatory response to microbial products.[556]

The fetal skin responds robustly to invading microbes by producing antimicrobial peptides, cytokines, and chemokines.[557-559] The administration of intra-amniotic endotoxin and *U. parvum* in sheep can induce production of proinflammatory cytokines (TNF-α, IL-1β, IL-6, and IL-8) and a cellular inflammatory response in the skin.[557] Therefore, both animal and human models demonstrated that skin is an important target of the fetal inflammatory response induced in the context of intra-amniotic inflammation.

KIDNEYS

Human nephrogenesis starts as early as 9 weeks of gestation and continues until the late third trimester (34 to 36 weeks of gestation).[560-562] Fetal urine is the greatest contributor to amniotic fluid volume.[563] Children and adult patients with sepsis typically have oliguria, due to prerenal failure (i.e., hypoperfusion) during the course of a systemic inflammatory response.[564] Similar to the renal response to systemic inflammation in adults, the fetal kidney is one of the target organs involved in FIRS. Yoon and colleagues[152] reported an association between oligohydramnios and a higher rate of fetal infection and inflammation in patients with preterm PROM. Amniotic fluid has natural antimicrobial properties (at least, in part, attributed to defensins).[565,566] Oligohydramnios may reduce this protective effect. It is also possible that oligohydramnios may be the result of a redistribution of blood flow away from the kidneys occurring during the host response to microbial products.[152] After intra-amniotic administration of endotoxin to pregnant sheep, systemic inflammation was associated with a 23% reduction in the nephron number.[567]

HEART

Neonates born to mothers with chorioamnionitis[166,568] are at increased risk for fetal heart rate abnormalities and cardiac dysfunction.[569] Echocardiographic studies have shown that fetuses whose mothers present with preterm PROM and intra-amniotic infection undergo changes in cardiac function that are consistent with a high left ventricular compliance.[570] These changes may reflect a compensatory mechanism similar to that observed in adults with sepsis. In cases of overwhelming fetal sepsis, myocardial depression can lead to fetal death. In the context of FIRS, it is possible that soluble factors, such as bacterial products (e.g., endotoxin) and cytokines, whose concentrations are elevated in the circulation of FIRS, contribute to myocardial depression.[571,572] Fetuses that are unable to modify their cardiac compliance to maintain ventricular stroke volume could exhibit a diminished cardiac output, leading to inadequate brain perfusion, brain ischemia, and brain injury in utero.[573,574] In experimental intra-amniotic inflammation in sheep, fetal exposure to bacterial endotoxin increases cardiac susceptibility to hypoxic injury.[575]

The following evidence shows that microbial products have an effect on the heart: (1) endotoxin impairs myocardial relaxation and contraction, increasing the proportion of isovolumetric relaxation and contraction times[575-577]; (2) mice with a CD14 deletion (CD14 is part of the recognition mechanism for endotoxin) have a protective phenotype against endotoxin-induced left ventricular dysfunction[578]; (3) TLR-4 mRNA and protein are constitutively present in the fetal myocardium[576]; (4) TLR-4-deficient mice do not experience left ventricular diastolic and systolic dysfunction after intraperitoneal injection of endotoxin[579]; (5) endotoxin up-regulates the production of TNF-α and IL-1β mRNA transcripts and protein in the fetal and adult myocardium[576,578]; and (6) intraperitoneal injection of endotoxin in mice induces myocardial mRNA and protein expression of TNF-α, IL-1β, IL-6, and monocyte chemotactic protein 1.[580]

Intra-amniotic inflammation in both the human model and the animal model has deleterious effects on both cardiac function and structure, which may contribute to the increased vulnerability of preterm neonates exposed to intra-amniotic infection/inflammation. However, the long-term consequences remain to be elucidated. Mitchell et al.[581] demonstrated that primates with FIRS had associated changes in the cardiac developmental gene program, involving a disruption in gene networks for morphogenesis and vasculogenesis with consequences later in life.

LUNG

Amniotic fluid and its contents can be inhaled by the fetus and reach the airways. Color Doppler ultrasound imaging demonstrated how the influx and efflux of amniotic fluid can be visualized.[582-585]

The relationship between intra-amniotic inflammation/infection and the development of respiratory complications, such as respiratory distress syndrome and chronic lung disease/bronchopulmonary dysplasia has been the subject of intensive investigation.[586-588] The *Watterberg hypothesis* proposes that intra-amniotic inflammation/infection is associated with a decreased rate of respiratory distress syndrome (RDS) (early protective effect) but an increased rate of bronchopulmonary dysplasia (BPD).[589] A systematic review and meta-analysis reported that there is a significant association between clinical chorioamnionitis and histologic chorioamnionitis and the subsequent development of BPD.[590] However, chorioamnionitis was not a risk factor for the development of RDS.

Watterberg et al.[589] reported that low-birth-weight infants exposed to chorioamnionitis had higher concentrations of IL-1β in tracheal lavage samples and a lower incidence of RDS, but a higher rate of BPD in comparison to the control group. Ghezzi et al.[591] reported that amniotic fluid IL-8 concentrations were higher in women who presented with spontaneous preterm labor (intact or ruptured membranes) and delivered infants at 24 to 28 weeks of gestation who later developed BPD. Indeed, preterm neonates born at 33 weeks of gestation or earlier who developed BPD had median amniotic fluid concentrations of IL-1β and IL-8 that were significantly higher than those in whom BPD did not develop.[592] Collectively, the evidence suggests that exposure to intra-amniotic inflammation is a risk factor for BPD.

Subsequently, Yoon et al.[593] reported that neonates born between 25 and 34 weeks of gestation and in whom BPD developed had a significantly higher median umbilical cord plasma IL-6 concentration in comparison to matched preterm infants without BPD. This finding suggests that the risk for BPD was higher in the offspring of pregnancies in which there was intra-amniotic inflammation as well as fetal systemic inflammation.

Models of intra-amniotic inflammation, such as intra-amniotic administration of endotoxin, the administration of IL-1α, or the inoculation of bacteria in the amniotic cavity, provide solid evidence that inflammation has an effect on surfactant protein production and lung development.[594-597] Bry et al.[594] first reported that intra-amniotic administration of IL-1α to pregnant rabbits increased mRNA and protein expression of surfactant proteins A and B, as well as surfactant lipids, which was accompanied by improved neonatal lung function. Injection of IL-1α also induced preterm labor and delivery; therefore, the effect of inflammation on surfactant production could be interpreted as promoting lung maturation in anticipation of preterm delivery. Subsequently, the laboratories of Jobe and Newnham systematically studied endotoxin-induced fetal lung injury in sheep and rhesus macaques.[514,515,596,598-608] Intra-amniotic administration of endotoxin induced an increase in surfactant production, which was accompanied by structural changes in the developing fetal lungs, such as decreased alveolar numbers, thinning of the alveolar septae, and increased alveolar size.[598] In addition, there was down-regulation of the expression of elastin[607] and several genes involved in vascular development (vascular endothelial growth factor A, vascular endothelial growth factor receptor 2, and endothelial nitric oxide synthase).[602,603] The latter is thought to be implicated in the predisposition to pulmonary hypertension.[609] The structural changes reported after endotoxin administration have also been observed after intra-amniotic inoculation with *U. urealyticum* in sheep and rhesus macques.[516,518,610-612]

Fetal lung inflammation is accompanied by a robust expression of proinflammatory mediators such as IL-1β, IL-8, granulocyte-macrophage colony-stimulating factor, monocyte chemotactic protein 1, and serum amyloid A3 in both sheep and monkeys.[517,596,605,606] It is noteworthy that IL-1β is the major cytokine involved in fetal lung injury as TNF-α and interferon-γ do not elicit the same degree of inflammation.[517,613] Moreover, pretreatment with intra-amniotic injection of an IL-1 antagonist before the administration of bacterial endotoxin prevented lung inflammation and maturation.[604]

In summary, exposure to microbial products and intra-amniotic inflammation induces fetal lung maturity, which favors survival in the context of preterm delivery. However, acceleration of lung maturity is accompanied by dramatic changes in the anatomy of the lung (e.g., reduction in the number of alveoli, impaired microvascular development, and thickening of the arteriolar walls, which collectively resemble changes observed in infants with BPD).[614] Therefore, the short-term gain in lung maturity appears to predispose to the development of chronic lung disease.

BRAIN

A link between exposure to perinatal infection and inflammation and brain injury is well established.[170,615-618] The first observations of this association date back to 1955 when Eastman and DeLeon[619] reported that intrapartum maternal fever conferred a sevenfold increased risk for cerebral palsy. In 1971, Leviton and Gilles[620] reported on the characteristics of perinatal telencephalic leukoencephalopathy (white matter abnormalities in the fetal brain after midgestation) and indicated a potential link to neonatal bacteremia and endotoxin exposure.[621]

Dammann and Leviton[622] proposed that intra-amniotic infection leads to a fetal inflammatory response, which, in turn, contributes to adverse outcomes such as preterm labor and delivery, intraventricular hemorrhage, white matter damage, and neurodevelopment disability (mainly cerebral palsy). Several lines of evidence support this concept: (1) a fetal inflammatory response precedes spontaneous preterm delivery in the context of infection[353,354]; (2) clinical and histologic chorioamnionitis are associated with an increased risk for cerebral palsy[2,170,173,615-617,623-635] (this association has also been reported in near-term infants)[170,636]; (3) a large body of experimental evidence indicates that intra-amniotic infection results in white matter damage and neuronal lesions[637-648]; (4) white matter lesions are associated with intra-amniotic inflammation and infection in women with spontaneous preterm labor[630,649-651]; and (5) elevated concentrations of cytokines in amniotic fluid and fetal plasma[37,617,631,652-656] and fetal vasculitis (chorionic and umbilical cord vessel inflammation)[657-660] are associated with the development of intraventricular hemorrhage, white matter damage, and cerebral palsy.

Leviton[661] proposed that inflammatory cytokines (TNF-α) released during the course of intra-amniotic infection could participate in the pathogenesis of periventricular leukomalacia by four different mechanisms: (1) induction of fetal hypotension and brain ischemia[662]; (2) stimulation of production and release of tissue factor, which, in turn, can activate the hemostatic system and contribute to coagulation necrosis of white matter[663]; (3) induction of the release of platelet-activating factor, which could act as a membrane detergent, resulting in direct brain damage[664]; and (4) a direct cytotoxic effect of TNF-α on oligodendrocytes and myelin.[665,666] Yoon and colleagues[667] proposed that microbial invasion of the amniotic cavity (which occurs in approximately 25% of preterm births) results in congenital fetal infection and inflammation that stimulates fetal mononuclear cells to produce IL-1β and TNF-α. These cytokines promote the passage of microbial products and other cytokines into the brain by increasing the permeability of the blood-brain barrier.[668,669] Interferon-γ and bacterial endotoxin also increase the permeability of the blood-brain barrier. This increase in permeability is, at least in part, dependent on cyclic guanosine monophosphate and nitric oxide.[669] Microbial products activate human fetal microglial cells to produce cytokines such as IL-1 that, in turn, stimulate astrocyte proliferation and TNF-α production. TNF-α damages oligodendrocytes, the cells responsible for the deposition of myelin.

A strong association is recognized between preterm birth and cerebral palsy.[670] Approximately one-third of neonates in whom cerebral palsy develops have a birth weight less than 2500 g.[671] Cerebral palsy is substantially more frequent in newborns with a birth weight less than 1500 g than in neonates of normal birth weight.[671] Extremely preterm neonates, in addition to being exposed to an exaggerated fetal systemic inflammatory response, display a limited ability to buffer the effects of proinflammatory cytokines[618,672-678] generated by intra-amniotic infection and inflammation. It is noteworthy that some studies have not demonstrated an association between histologic chorioamnionitis and cerebral palsy in preterm neonates.[679-683] We have argued that it is necessary to distinguish a maternal inflammatory response from a fetal inflammatory response to gain an understanding of the risk conferred by the latter.

The combination of inflammation and hypoxic-ischemic damage is proposed to have a synergistic role in causing fetal brain injury,[684-686] although some studies suggest that antenatal inflammation may decrease hypoxic-ischemic brain injury.[687,688] Animal models of cerebral palsy have been developed with fetal exposure to endotoxin[689] that has been administered in the uterus in concentrations that are not sufficient to elicit preterm labor. Exposed neonates have evidence of microglial activation, astrogliosis, neuronal damage, and the clinical manifestations of cerebral palsy. A fundamental question with clinical importance is whether it is possible to distinguish the infant exposed to intra-amniotic inflammation/infection who has neuroinflammation from the infant who does not. Studies of positron emission tomography indicate that microglial activation can be detected shortly after birth; therefore, the molecular diagnosis of neuroinflammation is possible.[690-693] This important observation lays the groundwork for the detection of neuroinflammation in humans with the implementation of imaging techniques.

The administration of *N*-acetylcysteine has been demonstrated to restrict brain damage in an animal model that combined inflammation induced by endotoxin and ischemia.[694] This has potential therapeutic effects in humans, given that *N*-acetylcysteine crosses the placenta.[694-697] Evidence suggests that in an animal model of bacterial endotoxin–induced cerebral palsy at term, the administration of *N*-acetylcysteine coupled with nanodevices on the first day of life can reverse the phenotype of cerebral palsy in 5 days. The administration of stem cells can also have powerful effects,[698-703] suggesting that a combination of regenerative medicine and nanotechnology can be used to treat congenital neuroinflammation and prevent long-term disability.[704]

GUT

Neonates born to mothers with intra-amniotic infection are at increased risk for necrotizing enterocolitis (NEC),[705,706] poor nutrient absorption, and late-onset sepsis.[705,707-710] An accumulation of evidence supports that fetuses exposed to intra-amniotic inflammation are at increased risk for developing NEC as newborns. Indeed, a meta-analysis suggests that there is an association between acute chorioamnionitis and funisitis and NEC (OR 3.29; 95% CI: 1.87 to 5.78).[706]

Experimentally, the intra-amniotic administration of IL-1, endotoxin, and *U. parvum* induces fetal gut mucosal inflammation, disruption of the epithelial barrier, enterocyte injury, and subsequent villous atrophy.[711-713] Such inflammatory stimuli can up-regulate mRNA expression of proinflammatory cytokines in the intestinal mucosa (TNF-α, interferon-γ, IL-4, and IL-10) and increase the number of CD3+ and CD4+ T cells. This up-regulation is accompanied by a reduction in the number of antiinflammatory FOXP3+ T cells. This effect on the bowel can be demonstrated for 14 days after exposure to the inflammatory insults after *Ureaplasma parvum* inoculation.[713] The importance of IL-1 in mediating these effects has been demonstrated by the blockade of these biologic effects by the administration of IL-1 receptor antagonists.

EYES

Approximately 2% of preterm birth survivors are diagnosed with blindness,[714-717] and among adolescents born preterm, 50% have vision-related problems that have been attributed to retinopathy of prematurity (ROP).[718] This condition is thought to be a result of an arrest of neural and vascular development, and exposure to inflammation before birth is thought to increase the risk of ROP.

A meta-analysis indicated an association between neonatal sepsis and any stage of ROP (OR 1.57; 95% CI: 1.31 to 1.89) and the severe stage of ROP (OR 2.33; 95% CI 1.21 to 4.51) in infants born preterm.[719] Importantly, infants born to mothers with histologic chorioamnionitis also have an increased risk of any ROP stage (OR 1.39; 95% CI: 1.11 to 1.74), as well as severe ROP (stage 3 or more) (OR 1.63; 95% CI: 1.41 to 1.89).[720] Infants who had a fetal inflammatory response diagnosed by funisitis had a higher risk of ROP than in those with acute histologic chorioamnionitis in the absence of funisitis.[720] The mechanisms whereby intra-amniotic infection/inflammation can lead to ROP are thought to involve either direct effects of cytokines on neovascularization of the retina through vascular endothelial growth factor (VEGF) availability or indirect mechanisms by which decreased systemic blood pressure may decrease retinal perfusion and cause ischemia.[721,722]

EARS

Neonates born preterm are at an increased risk for sensorineuronal hearing loss, and the earlier the gestational age at birth, the greater the risk. Exposure to intra-amniotic inflammation has recently been found to be a risk factor, as elevated concentrations of umbilical cord IL-6 and CRP are significantly associated with neonatal hearing loss.[723] Intra-amniotic infection and inflammation can lead to a congenital otitis media, and this disorder may be inadequately diagnosed and treated in the neonatal period, as otoscopic examination is not part of routine standard care in newborns.

LIVER

Experimental intra-amniotic inflammation induced by bacterial endotoxin administration to pregnant sheep has been reported to lead to intrahepatic inflammation and dysfunction in the neonatal period.[724] The fetal liver inflammatory process is associated with metabolic disturbances that may include increased umbilical cord plasma concentrations of total cholesterol, high-density lipoprotein, low-density lipoprotein, and triglycerides.[724] These effects remain after resolution of the liver inflammatory process, suggesting that there may be long-term consequences in terms of hepatic function and lipid metabolism. Studies in humans are required to determine the frequency and extent of hepatic and metabolic dysfunction in FIRS.

STRATEGIES FOR THE MANAGEMENT OF FIRS

Several approaches can be used to manage the course of FIRS in the context of intra-amniotic inflammation: (1) delivery of the fetus; (2) antibiotic therapy; and (3) immunomodulation of the inflammatory response.[381,725]

Delivery of the fetus provides a rapid exit from a hostile environment. However, preterm delivery places the unborn child at risk for complications of prematurity; therefore, the risks of prematurity and intra-amniotic infection/inflammation must be balanced. Antibiotic treatment can reduce the rate of intra-amniotic infection/inflammation, as well as funisitis in a subset of patients with spontaneous preterm delivery and intact membranes,[295] cervical insufficiency,[294] a sonographic short cervix,[157] and preterm PROM.[279,282,296,381,725]

The use of immunomodulatory approaches in FIRS needs to be considered given recent successful approaches with the treatment of SARS-CoV-2, the virus responsible for COVID-19.[726-732] The success of IL-1 blockage with high-dose anakinra and the blockage of the IL-6 pathway with a recombinant humanized monoclonal antibody suggests that these agents may be useful to manage hyperinflammation in the perinatal period. The subject has been reviewed by Ying Xiong and Pia Wintermark,[733] and recently, by Simone Schüller.[734] Whether these interventions can be extended to the prenatal period is a new frontier. Recent studies suggest that the IL-6 receptor antibody inhibits preterm labor and delivery in a bacterial endotoxin model[735] and that a similar intervention targeting IL-1 may reduce inflammation-induced fetal injury and improve neonatal and developmental outcomes in mice after exposure to bacterial endotoxin during pregnancy.[381,412,725]

A combination of antibiotics and immunomodulatory agents (dexamethasone and indomethacin) has been shown to be effective in nonhuman pregnant primates to eradicate intra-amniotic infection, suppress the local inflammatory response, and prolong gestation in experimental premature labor induced by intra-amniotic inoculation with group B streptococci.[546] In addition, we recently showed that clarithromycin prevents preterm birth and reduces neonatal mortality in mice intra-amniotically injected with *Ureaplasma parvum*.[736] Taken together, this evidence indicates that immunomodulation may be an effective intervention in preventing fetal injury and prolonging gestation among patients with inflammation/infection-induced preterm labor.[381,725]

Given that cells of the immune system are derived from pluripotent hematopoietic stem cells, stem cells have emerged as a promising potential neuroprotective and neuroreparative treatment in the context of the fetal inflammatory response. Many immunomodulatory cells are present in umbilical cord blood, including mesenchymal stem cells and endothelial progenitor cells. In a mouse model of bacterial endotoxin-induced chorioamnionitis, maternal administration of mesenchymal stem cells resulted in a reduced IL-6 concentration in the fetal brain and improved neurobehavioral outcomes.[737] Umbilical cord blood cells have some benefits that support their therapeutic use for infants after birth who are at high risk for brain injury following antenatal or birth complications.[381,725,738-744]

CONCLUSION

Intra-amniotic infection and intra-amniotic inflammation are causally linked to preterm parturition and the development of a fetal systemic inflammatory response syndrome. Systemic inflammation can affect multiple fetal organ systems and predispose to short- and long-term complications, two of the latter being bronchopulmonary dysplasia and cerebral palsy. Modulation of the fetal inflammatory response during pregnancy may have considerable importance for understanding the mechanisms of disease of preterm labor and fetal injury. This approach has substantial potential in the diagnosis, treatment, and prevention of long-term mental and physical disadvantages related to congenital infections.

ACKNOWLEDGMENTS

Research for the preparation of this chapter was supported, in part, by members of the Perinatology Research Branch of the *Eunice Kennedy Shriver* National Institute of Child Health and Human Development, National Institutes of Health, Department of Health and Human Services, and was funded by the Intramural Research Division of the National Institutes of Health.

This chapter has been substantially revised and updated from that published in earlier editions of this book. Nevertheless, we acknowledge the work of the previous authors. In particular, we gratefully acknowledge the intellectual contributions of Maria Teresa Gervasi, Tinnakorn Chaiworapongsa, Nikolina Docheva, and Noppadol Chaiyasit.

A complete reference list is available at www.ExpertConsult.com.

SELECT REFERENCES

29. Romero R, Sirtori M, Oyarzun E, et al. Infection and labor. V. Prevalence, microbiology, and clinical significance of intraamniotic infection in women with preterm labor and intact membranes. *Am J Obstet Gynecol*. 1989;161(3):817-824.
31. Goncalves LF, Chaiworapongsa T, Romero R. Intrauterine infection and prematurity. *J Matern Fetal Neonatal Med*. 2002;8(1):3-13.
35. Watts DH, Krohn MA, Hillier SL, Eschenbach DA. The association of occult amniotic fluid infection with gestational age and neonatal outcome among women in preterm labor. *Obstet Gynecol*. 1992;79(3):351-357.
51. Romero R, Miranda J, Chaiworapongsa T, et al. Prevalence and clinical significance of sterile intra-amniotic inflammation in patients with preterm labor and intact membranes. *Am J Reprod Immunol*. 2014;72(5):458-474.
52. Romero R, Miranda J, Chaemsaithong P, et al. Sterile and microbial-associated intra-amniotic inflammation in preterm prelabor rupture of membranes. *J Matern Fetal Neonatal Med*. 2015;28(12):1394-1409.
53. Romero R, Miranda J, Kusanovic JP, et al. Clinical chorioamnionitis at term I: microbiology of the amniotic cavity using cultivation and molecular techniques. *J Perinat Med*. 2015;43(1):19-36.
81. Kim CJ, Romero R, Chaemsaithong P, Chaiyasit N, Yoon BH, Kim YM. Acute chorioamnionitis and funisitis: definition, pathologic features, and clinical significance. *Am J Obstet Gynecol*. 2015;213(suppl 4). S29-52.
85. Blanc WA. Amniotic infection syndrome; pathogenesis, morphology, and significance in circumnatal mortality. *Clin Obstet Gynecol*. 1959;2:705-734.
88. Hillier SL, Martius J, Krohn M, Kiviat N, Holmes KK, Eschenbach DA. A case-control study of chorioamnionic infection and histologic chorioamnionitis in prematurity. *N Engl J Med*. 1988;319(15):972-978.
89. Hillier SL, Krohn MA, Kiviat NB, Watts DH, Eschenbach DA. Microbiologic causes and neonatal outcomes associated with chorioamnion infection. *Am J Obstet Gynecol*. 1991;165(4 Pt 1):955-961.
100. Kim CJ, Romero R, Chaemsaithong P, Kim JS. Chronic inflammation of the placenta: definition, classification, pathogenesis, and clinical significance. *Am J Obstet Gynecol*. 2015;213(suppl 4). S53-69.
101. Benirschke K. Routes and types of infection in the fetus and the newborn. *AMA J Dis Child*. 1960;99:714-721.
102. Romero R, Mazor M. Infection and preterm labor. *Clin Obstet Gynecol*. 1988;31(3):553-584.
107. Romero R, Gomez-Lopez N, Winters AD, et al. Evidence that intra-amniotic infections are often the result of an ascending invasion - a molecular microbiological study. *J Perinat Med*. 2019;47(9):915-931.
133. DiGiulio DB, Romero R, Amogan HP, et al. Microbial prevalence, diversity and abundance in amniotic fluid during preterm labor: a molecular and culture-based investigation. *PLoS One*. 2008;3(8):e3056.
134. DiGiulio DB, Romero R, Kusanovic JP, et al. Prevalence and diversity of microbes in the amniotic fluid, the fetal inflammatory response, and pregnancy outcome in women with preterm pre-labor rupture of membranes. *Am J Reprod Immunol*. 2010;64(1):38-57.
152. Yoon BH, Kim YA, Romero R, et al. Association of oligohydramnios in women with preterm premature rupture of membranes with an inflammatory response in fetal, amniotic, and maternal compartments. *Am J Obstet Gynecol*. 1999;181(4):784-788.
153. Romero R, Quintero R, Oyarzun E, et al. Intraamniotic infection and the onset of labor in preterm premature rupture of the membranes. *Am J Obstet Gynecol*. 1988;159(3):661-666.
157. Hassan S, Romero R, Hendler I, et al. A sonographic short cervix as the only clinical manifestation of intra-amniotic infection. *J Perinat Med*. 2006;34(1):13-19.
164. Mazor M, Hershkovitz R, Ghezzi F, Maymon E, Horowitz S, Leiberman JR. Intraamniotic infection in patients with preterm labor and twin pregnancies. *Acta Obstet Gynecol Scand*. 1996;75(7):624-627.
170. Grether JK, Nelson KB. Maternal infection and cerebral palsy in infants of normal birth weight. *JAMA*. 1997;278(3):207-211.
221. Hillier SL, Witkin SS, Krohn MA, Watts DH, Kiviat NB, Eschenbach DA. The relationship of amniotic fluid cytokines and preterm delivery, amniotic fluid infection, histologic chorioamnionitis, and chorioamnion infection. *Obstet Gynecol*. 1993;81(6):941-948.
234. Romero R, Avila C, Santhanam U, Sehgal PB. Amniotic fluid interleukin 6 in preterm labor. Association with infection. *J Clin Invest*. 1990;85(5):1392-1400.
237. Yoon BH, Romero R, Kim CJ, et al. Amniotic fluid interleukin-6: a sensitive test for antenatal diagnosis of acute inflammatory lesions of preterm placenta and prediction of perinatal morbidity. *Am J Obstet Gynecol*. 1995;172(3):960-970.
273. Romero R, Dey SK, Fisher SJ. Preterm labor: one syndrome, many causes. *Science*. 2014;345(6198):760-765.
279. Lee J, Romero R, Kim SM, et al. A new anti-microbial combination prolongs the latency period, reduces acute histologic chorioamnionitis as well as funisitis, and improves neonatal outcomes in preterm PROM. *J Matern Fetal Neonatal Med*. 2016;29(5):707-720.
294. Oh KJ, Romero R, Park JY, et al. Evidence that antibiotic administration is effective in the treatment of a subset of patients with intra-amniotic infection/inflammation presenting with cervical insufficiency. *Am J Obstet Gynecol*. 2019;221(2):140.e141-140.e118.
295. Yoon BH, Romero R, Park JY, et al. Antibiotic administration can eradicate intra-amniotic infection or intra-amniotic inflammation in a subset of patients with preterm labor and intact membranes. *Am J Obstet Gynecol*. 2019;221(2):142.e141-142.e122.

296. Kacerovsky M, Romero R, Stepan M, et al. Antibiotic administration reduces the rate of intraamniotic inflammation in preterm prelabor rupture of the membranes. *Am J Obstet Gynecol*. 2020;223(1):114.e111-114.e120.
315. Romero R, Parvizi ST, Oyarzun E, et al. Amniotic fluid interleukin-1 in spontaneous labor at term. *J Reprod Med*. 1990;35(3):235-238.
327. Romero R, Wu YK, Mazor M, Hobbins JC, Mitchell MD. Amniotic fluid concentration of 5-hydroxyeicosatetraenoic acid is increased in human parturition at term. *Prostaglandins Leukot Essent Fatty Acids*. 1989;35(2):81-83.
353. Romero R, Gomez R, Ghezzi F, et al. A fetal systemic inflammatory response is followed by the spontaneous onset of preterm parturition. *Am J Obstet Gynecol*. 1998;179(1):186-193.
354. Gomez R, Romero R, Ghezzi F, Yoon BH, Mazor M, Berry SM. The fetal inflammatory response syndrome. *Am J Obstet Gynecol*. 1998;179(1):194-202.
359. Gotsch F, Romero R, Kusanovic JP, et al. The anti-inflammatory limb of the immune response in preterm labor, intra-amniotic infection/inflammation, and spontaneous parturition at term: a role for interleukin-10. *J Matern Fetal Neonatal Med*. 2008;21(8):529-547.
370. Romero R, Emamian M, Wan M, Quintero R, Hobbins JC, Mitchell MD. Prostaglandin concentrations in amniotic fluid of women with intra-amniotic infection and preterm labor. *Am J Obstet Gynecol*. 1987;157(6):1461-1467.
381. Gotsch F, Romero R, Kusanovic JP, et al. The fetal inflammatory response syndrome. *Clin Obstet Gynecol*. 2007;50(3):652-683.
383. Berry SM, Romero R, Gomez R, et al. Premature parturition is characterized by in utero activation of the fetal immune system. *Am J Obstet Gynecol*. 1995;173(4):1315-1320.
439. Gomez-Lopez N, Romero R, Xu Y, et al. A role for the inflammasome in spontaneous preterm labor with acute histologic chorioamnionitis. *Reprod Sci*. 2017;24(6):934-953.
440. Gomez-Lopez N, Romero R, Panaitescu B, et al. Inflammasome activation during spontaneous preterm labor with intra-amniotic infection or sterile intra-amniotic inflammation. *Am J Reprod Immunol*. 2018;80(5):e13049.
508. Tang Q, Zhang L, Li H, Shao Y. The fetal inflammation response syndrome and adverse neonatal outcomes: a meta-analysis. *J Matern Fetal Neonatal Med*. 2019:1-13.
509. Romero R, Savasan ZA, Chaiworapongsa T, et al. Hematologic profile of the fetus with systemic inflammatory response syndrome. *J Perinat Med*. 2011;40(1):19-32.
512. Kramer BW, Moss TJ, Willet KE, et al. Dose and time response after intraamniotic endotoxin in preterm lambs. *Am J Respir Crit Care Med*. 2001;164(6):982-988.
513. Kallapur SG, Kramer BW, Nitsos I, et al. Pulmonary and systemic inflammatory responses to intra-amniotic IL-1alpha in fetal sheep. *Am J Physiol Lung Cell Mol Physiol*. 2011;301(3):L285-295.
515. Kramer BW, Kallapur SG, Moss TJ, et al. Modulation of fetal inflammatory response on exposure to lipopolysaccharide by chorioamnion, lung, or gut in sheep. *Am J Obstet Gynecol*. 2010;202(1):77.e71-79.
517. Kallapur SG, Presicce P, Senthamaraikannan P, et al. Intra-amniotic IL-1β induces fetal inflammation in rhesus monkeys and alters the regulatory T cell/IL-17 balance. *J Immunol*. 2013;191(3):1102-1109.
520. Lee AJ, Lambermont VA, Pillow JJ, et al. Fetal responses to lipopolysaccharide-induced chorioamnionitis alter immune and airway responses in 7-week-old sheep. *Am J Obstet Gynecol*. 2011;204(4):364.e317-324.
622. Dammann O, Leviton A. Role of the fetus in perinatal infection and neonatal brain damage. *Curr Opin Pediatr*. 2000;12(2):99-104.
630. Leviton A, Paneth N, Reuss ML, et al. Maternal infection, fetal inflammatory response, and brain damage in very low birth weight infants. Developmental Epidemiology Network Investigators. *Pediatr Res*. 1999;46(5):566-575.
651. Dammann O, Kuban KC, Leviton A. Perinatal infection, fetal inflammatory response, white matter damage, and cognitive limitations in children born preterm. *Ment Retard Dev Disabil Res Rev*. 2002;8(1):46-50.
661. Leviton A. Preterm birth and cerebral palsy: is tumor necrosis factor the missing link? *Dev Med Child Neurol*. 1993;35(6):553-558.

Fetal Origins of Adult Disease: A Classic Hypothesis With New Relevance

13

Peter Russell Baker II

INTRODUCTION

In the late 1980s the late Dr. David J. P. Barker used historical birth records to pioneer the concept that the origins of adult disease could be strongly associated with fetal environmental exposures in pregnancy that resulted in low birth weight (BW) and modified both structure and function of tissues regulating human diseases later in life.[1] Over the past several decades the fetal programming or developmental origins of health and disease (DOHaD) hypothesis has been validated epidemiologically and mechanistically using human and animal models. DOHaD has taught us about the role of a mismatch between a constrained prenatal and a plentiful postnatal environment in the pathogenesis of obesity (i.e., the "thrifty" pathway) likely operating in populations undergoing rapid transition. Another developmental pathway to obesity and its comorbidities, more novel evolutionarily and likely more important in Western societies, is developmental overnutrition. This pathway reflects the effects of hypernutrition during fetal and/or early postnatal life and creates the conditions for the later pathophysiologic effects of an obesogenic environment (Fig. 13.1). Both phenomena lead to the same phenotypic ends: adolescent and adult-onset obesity and metabolic syndrome.

Fetal developmental programming can occur fundamentally in two ways: first, via gene-environment interactions that may produce persistent epigenetic events, and secondly, by impacting normal organ development to impart risk for developing chronic disease(s). Data showing that maternal nutritional challenges have epigenetic or molecular effects that underlie chronic metabolic diseases are ongoing. The mechanisms underlying how poor maternal health and diet imparts risk for future metabolic disease beginning in utero remain understudied in humans but are beginning to emerge in nonhuman primate (NHP) models.[1-4] Rodent studies and human clinical data indicate that maternal and early infant nutrition affects multiple organ systems, including the brain, pancreatic islets, liver, adipose, muscle, and the immune system.[5] Human studies suggest that reduced dietary fat intake and improved exercise can slow down the transmission of metabolic risk.[6,7] The effects of modifying adult lifestyle, when formally tested in randomized trials in humans, have been disappointingly small and lack longitudinal results.[8] Importantly, as we move into an era of higher technological capacity, "omics" and "big data" analyses, and larger sample sizes, particularly in longitudinal cohorts, we will be able to discover new pathways and potential nutritional strategies for interventions in high-risk mothers and the next generation of infants.

BIRTH WEIGHT AND CHRONIC DISEASE

Early exploration of the DOHaD hypothesis required systematic studies of BW and adult-onset chronic disease. In Hertfordshire,

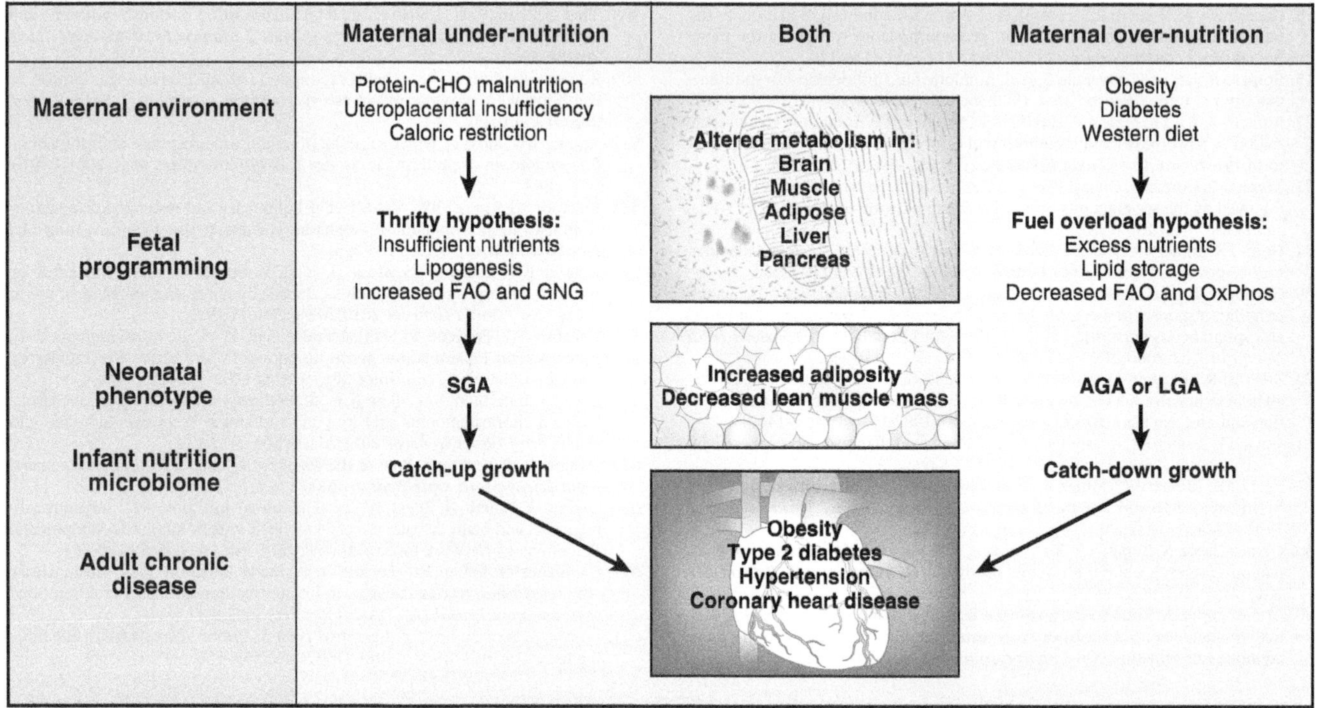

Fig. 13.1 Comparison of maternal undernutrition and overnutrition as causes of chronic adult metabolic disease in offspring. *AGA*, Appropriate for gestational age; *CHO*, carbohydrate; *FAO*, fatty acid oxidation; *GNG*, gluconeogenesis; *LGA*, large for gestational age; *OxPhos*, oxidative phosphorylation; *SGA*, small for gestational age.

United Kingdom, starting in 1911, birthing mothers were attended by midwives, who recorded the BW.[9,10] A health visitor went to the babies' homes at intervals throughout infancy, and weights at 1 year were recorded. Table 13.1 lists the findings for 10,636 men born between 1911 and 1930. Hazard ratios for coronary heart disease increase with decreasing BW. Stronger trends with weight are seen at 1 year. Table 13.2 shows findings for a sample of men following glucose tolerance tests.[11] The percentage with impaired glucose tolerance or type 2 diabetes mellitus increased steeply with decreasing BW. The association between low BW and coronary heart disease has now been replicated among men and women in Europe, North America, and India.[12-15] Low BW has been shown to predict altered glucose tolerance in studies of men and women around the world.[16-18]

The association between coronary heart disease and poor weight gain in infancy, first shown in Hertfordshire, was later confirmed in the Helsinki Birth Cohort.[19] This cohort of 8760 people born in Helsinki during 1934-1944 demonstrated that heart disease developed later in life in boys and girls who were small at birth and remained small in infancy. They experienced accelerated gain in weight and body mass index (BMI) (weight/height^2) after 2 years of age. Heights remained below average, which is consistent with the known association between the disease and short adult stature.[20] Table 13.3 is based on 2997 patients treated for hypertension and 698 patients treated for type 2 diabetes mellitus in the Helsinki Birth Cohort.[21] These two disorders are associated with the same general pattern of growth as for coronary heart disease. Small size at birth is followed by accelerated weight gain in childhood. The highest risk for each disease occurs among men and women who had low BW but were in the highest BMI group at 11 years. As with coronary heart disease, the risk for obesity is determined by body size at birth and BMI in childhood.[16,22] It is the tempo of weight gain in childhood as well as the attained body size that determines risk.

More recent epidemiologic studies have linked *excess* weight gain in utero, as well as exposure to maternal obesity and gestational diabetes, as risk factors for later metabolic dysfunction. Maternal BMI and glucose homeostasis are thought to be the most important determinants of fetal growth,[23,24] and the association between maternal glycaemia and increased BW has been long documented in diabetic pregnancies.[25] However, macrosomia is not uncommon in diabetic pregnancies even with strict glycemic control,[26,27] and among offspring of obese women with normal glucose tolerance.[23,28,29] This suggests that mechanisms other than maternal hyperglycemia contribute to fetal growth. There are clear links between maternal obesity and the risk for early-onset obesity[30,31]; altered immunity,[32]

Table 13.1 Hazard Ratios (95% Confidence Intervals) for Death From Coronary Heart Disease According to Weight at Birth and at Age 1 Year in 10,636 Men in Hertfordshire.

	Death From CHD	
Birth Weight (Pounds)	**Before 65 yr**	**All Ages**
At Birth		
≤5.5	1.50 (0.98–2.31)	1.37 (1.00–1.86)
6.5	1.27 (0.89–1.83)	1.29 (1.01–1.66)
7.5	1.17 (0.84–1.63)	1.14 (0.91–1.44)
8.5	1.07 (0.77–1.49)	1.12 (0.89–1.40)
9.5	0.96 (0.66–1.39)	0.97 (0.75–1.25)
>9.5	1.00	1.00
P-value for trend	.001	.005
Age 1 yr		
≤18	2.22 (1.33–3.73)	1.89 (1.34–2.66)
20	1.80 (1.11–2.93)	1.58 (1.15–2.16)
22	1.96 (1.23–3.12)	1.66 (1.23–2.25)
24	1.52 (0.95–2.45)	1.36 (1.00–1.85)
26	1.36 (0.82–2.26)	1.29 (0.93–1.78)
≥27	1.00	1.00
P-value for trend	<.001	<.001

CHD, Coronary heart disease.

Table 13.2 Percentage of Men Aged 64 Years With Impaired Glucose Tolerance or Type 2 Diabetes According to Birth Weight.

Birth Weight (Pounds)	Men With 2-hr Glucose of ≥7.8 mmol/L (%)	Odds Ratio (95% Confidence Interval)[a]
≤5.5	40	6.6 (1.5–28)
6.5	34	4.8 (1.3–17)
7.5	31	4.6 (1.4–16)
8.5	22	2.6 (0.8–8.9)
9.5	13	1.4 (0.3–5.6)
>9.5	14	1.0
P-value for trend	<.001	

[a]Adjusted for current body mass index.

Table 13.3 Odds Ratios (95% Confidence Intervals) for Hypertension and Type 2 Diabetes According to Birth Weight and Body Mass Index at 11 Years.

Birth Weight (kg)	Body Mass Index (kg/m²) at 11 yr: 15.7	16.6	17.6	>17.6
Hypertension				
≤3.0	2.0 (1.3–3.2)	1.9 (1.2–3.1)	1.9 (1.2–3.0)	2.3 (1.5–3.8)
3.5	1.7 (1.1–2.6)	1.9 (1.2–2.9)	1.9 (1.2–3.0)	2.2 (1.4–3.4)
4.0	1.7 (1.0–2.6)	1.7 (1.1–2.6)	1.5 (1.0–2.4)	1.9 (1.2–2.9)
>4.0	1.0	1.9 (1.1–3.1)	1.0 (0.6–1.7)	1.7 (1.1–2.8)
Type 2 Diabetes				
≤3.0	1.3 (0.6–2.8)	1.3 (0.6–2.8)	1.5 (0.7–3.4)	2.5 (1.2–5.5)
3.5	1.0 (0.5–2.1)	1.0 (0.5–2.1)	1.5 (0.7–3.2)	1.7 (0.8–3.5)
4.0	1.0 (0.5–2.2)	0.9 (0.4–1.9)	0.9 (0.4–2.0)	1.7 (0.8–3.6)
>4.0	1.0	1.1 (0.4–2.7)	0.7 (0.3–1.7)	1.2 (0.5–2.7)

altered stem cell metabolism,[33] increased risk for inflammation and cardiovascular disease,[34,35] and type 2 diabetes mellitus.[36] Strong positive associations between infant BW and later BMI support that larger newborns are more likely to become obese adults,[37] and females born large for gestational age (LGA) (≥90th percentile) have a doubled risk for delivering an LGA infant themselves.[36] Even in normal weight mothers the occurrence of gestational diabetes and potential fetal overnutrition leads to increased risk for both gestational and overt type 2 diabetes mellitus in the offspring as early as the second decade.[38,39]

And so, these two polar opposite maternal conditions lead to similar offspring risk for chronic metabolic disease in adulthood, creating a U-shaped distribution of risk versus infant BW. This potentially indicates two separate mechanisms of fetal programming that lead to metabolic dysfunction. Although the clinical phenotypes seem nearly identical, the biochemistry and effect on cellular functions are likely quite different.

PROGRAMMING AND EPIGENETIC MECHANISMS

Dr. Barker's initial discovery, that people who develop coronary heart disease grew differently than other people during fetal life and childhood, has led to a new "developmental" model for the disease.[40] The interplay between genes and the environment, and an overview of mechanisms involved in fetal programming of adult-onset metabolic disease, can be found in Fig. 13.2. Like other living creatures in early life, human beings are "plastic" and able to adapt to their environment. Phenotypic plasticity is the phenomenon by which one genotype can give rise to a range of different physiologic or morphologic states in response to different environmental conditions during development. Gene-environment interactions are ubiquitous in development. Their evolutionary benefit is that, in a changing environment, they enable the adaptation of phenotypes that are better matched to their in utero environments, which may be much different than encountered in extrauterine environment. To what extent "nutritional mismatch" can account for metabolic disease in adult life is uncertain; however, it is clear that both undergrowth and overgrowth increase the risk for metabolic syndrome.

It may be advantageous, in evolutionary terms, for the body to remain plastic during development. Why this plasticity is ultimately lost in most tissues and systems remains to be fully explained. The fetal/neonatal state may originate in a developmentally regulated epigenetic program, whereas the adult-like epigenetic state may be acquired in some tissues within the first week of life.[41] Other tissues (e.g., the trabeculae of bone) remain epigenetically plastic throughout life.[42] It has been suggested that plasticity during intrauterine life enables animals, and humans, to receive a "weather forecast" from their mothers that prepares them for the type of world in which they will have to live.[43] If the mother is poorly nourished, she signals to her unborn baby that the environment is harsh. The baby responds to these signals by adaptations, such as reduced body size and altered metabolism, which help it to survive a life of food shortage after birth. The transition from the fetal state to adult-like state could be regulated in several possible ways. For example, the fetal tissue precursors may be intrinsically programmed to a defined time in ontogeny. Alternatively, external signals from the maturing environment may promote methylation post birth. In this way some neonatal cells may be poised epigenetically to develop dominant responses based on the stage of ontogeny and the differentiation state of the organism, whereas in some tissues the acquisition of the dynamic phase of DNA methylation is acquired by signals from the maturing environment. What determines "the rules" for programming methylation during neonatal life and the mechanisms underlying these changes have yet to be determined. Whatever the mechanism, this plasticity gives a species the ability to make short-term adaptations, within one generation, in addition to long-term genetic adaptations that may span generations.

Although clinical relationships have been well proven on a population-based scale, the cellular mechanisms by which these plastic changes occur in the fetus, and continue to play out over the life of the organism, has only begun to be investigated.[44] The role of epigenetics in regulating the timing and tissue specific nature of gene expression is paramount. Several well-established mechanisms play a critical role in creating a "cellular memory" of life in utero, which have great bearing on offspring physiology and the development of chronic adult conditions. Histone modification (acetylation, methylation, ubiquitylation, phosphorylation, sumoylation, ribosylation, or citrullination) may inhibit or facilitate transcription by structurally altering chromatin (hypercoiled bundles of DNA that uncoil when transcription of a particular gene is needed).[45] Local DNA modifications like promoter methylation (via enzymes called *demethylases*; e.g., DMNT1) may either silence or activate the expression of a given gene at a given time and place, which extend beyond the traditional regulation of imprinting centers in the human genome.[46–48] Expression of bioactive small RNA molecules also act to regulate and modify gene expression posttranscriptionally.[49] Finally, posttranslational modification of enzymes (e.g., acetylation, sumoylation, and phosphorylation) through enzymes such as sirtuins allows finer regulation of multiple enzymes, including important pathways in mitochondria.[50] We are still trying to understand when these modifications occur in any

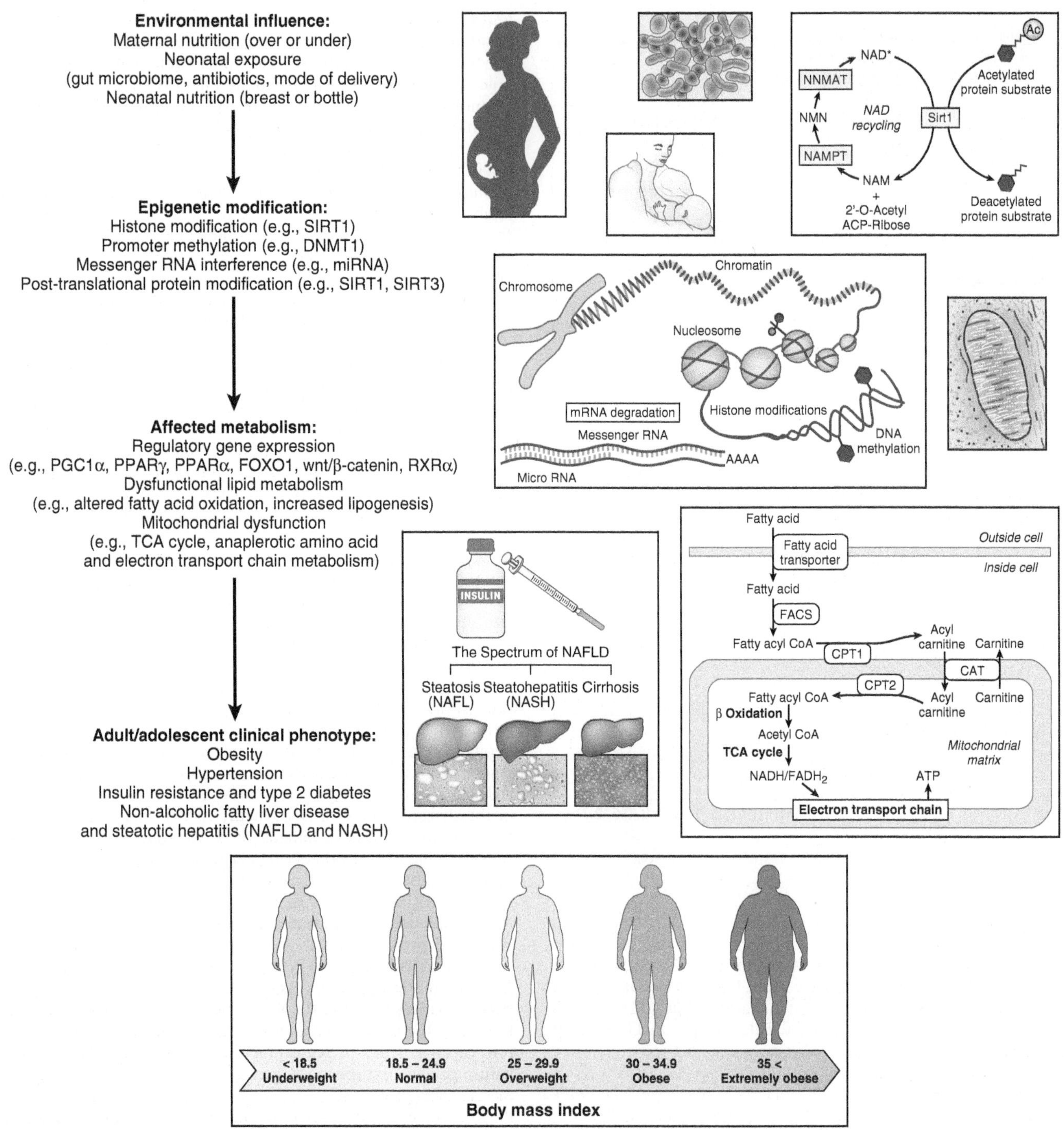

Fig. 13.2 Illustration of the interplay between genes and the environment, and mechanisms of fetal programming of adult onset metabolic disease.

particular tissue, as well as which particular in utero exposures lead to epigenetic changes. As a general rule, unmethylated DNA is largely associated with acetylated histones and active chromatin remodeling.[51] However, the timing and regulation of this plasticity, be they through nearby gene promoters (i.e., CpG shores) or far off (i.e., CpG islands) regions of DNA necessary for regulation of transcription, continue to be discovered.

BIOLOGIC MECHANISMS

FETAL UNDERNUTRITION

When undernutrition during development is followed by improved nutrition, many animals stage accelerated or "catch-up" growth in weight or length. This restores the animal's body size but has long-term costs that include reduced life span.[52] Similarly, when a child who is large for gestational age is maintained on a regular diet for age there is "catch-down" growth. Although anthropometric parameters including body mass and percent body fat appear to normalize by 6 months of age,[53] the lasting effects of early metabolic programming can be observed later in life by earlier-onset and more-severe-onset chronic disease. There are several mechanisms by which reduced fetal and infant growth, followed by accelerated weight gain in early childhood, may lead to later disease. Populations rapidly transitioning from traditional to Westernized lifestyles (e.g., Asia) are particularly vulnerable to the nutritional mismatch paradigm of metabolic disease.[54] Rates of overweight, obesity, and diabetes have risen sharply in populations that move from rural to urban environments.[55-57] Babies who are thin at birth have a lower percentage of lean mass but greater percentage of fat mass—the so-called *thin fat baby*.[58,59] This deficiency arises during the critical period for muscle growth (approximately 30 weeks in utero) and will persist as there is little cell replication after birth.[60] If thin babies develop a high BMI in childhood, fat mass may be disproportionately high. This is associated with the development of insulin resistance.[61]

Muscle and adipose development is intimately involved in metabolic health and is affected in offspring of undernourished mothers. In the fetus with low circulating glucose, skeletal muscle glucose oxidation is decreased in favor of use in neural tissues. Nonglucose substrates need to be used for energy production, including the use of lipids for fatty acid oxidation.[62] This is evidenced by increased fatty acid mobilization in hypoglycemic fetal sheep models.[63] Amino acids including leucine (a key branched chain amino acid), as well as alanine, glutamine, glycine, and lysine are diverted for intermediary metabolism and energy use in hypoglycemic fetal sheep.[64-66] Another important component to skeletal muscle is the number and function of skeletal muscle mitochondria; these are deficient in individuals with type 2 diabetes mellitus and their first-degree relatives.[67] Intrauterine growth restriction is associated with increased reactive oxygen species and mitochondrial dysfunction in skeletal muscle (and pancreatic β cells), which likely plays a key role in the development of metabolic syndrome.[68]

Although lipids are preferentially oxidized in fetal skeletal muscle, they are being programmed for later synthesis and storage in fetal adipocytes. Neonatal rat pups whose mothers were food restricted demonstrated greater circulating lipids and higher capacity for lipid production in primed undernourished adipocytes at birth and at postnatal day 21 despite receiving milk from normally fed mothers.[69] This is regulated by increased levels of PPARγ and SIRT1 and results in adipocyte hyperplasia and hypertrophy,[70] which later predisposes to obesity and metabolic disease.

The liver also plays an integral role in this process. Increases in endogenous glucose production, predominantly of hepatic origin, is a major determinant of fasting glucose levels. The liver remains plastic during its development until the age of approximately 5 years. Its function may be permanently changed by influences that affect its early growth. This includes alterations in lipid metabolism (primarily de novo lipogenic pathways) and glucose homeostasis[71-73] as well as overall alteration of its metabolic capacity and organization.[74] The latter has been explored with cutting-edge "omics" technologies and was found to have profound influence on whole body nutrient homeostasis as well as inflammation and detoxification. Specifically, the physical location of metabolic pathways including the tricaboxylic acid (TCA) cycle, mitochondrial oxidative phosphorylation, lipogenesis, glycogen metabolism, and the urea cycle are all linked to liver zonal organization, which are in turn determined by Wnt/B-catenin pathway signaling early in development.[75]

These data closely align with Dr. Barker's observation that liver development may play an important role in the early pathogenesis of coronary heart disease. Studies of men and women born in Sheffield, England, showed that a smaller abdominal circumference at birth (a measure that reflects reduced liver size and/or abnormal visceral fat distribution) was a stronger predictor of later elevations of serum cholesterol and plasma fibrinogen than any other measure of body size at birth.[76]

FETAL OVERNUTRITION

In animal models it is surprisingly easy to produce lifelong changes in metabolism of a fetus by minor modifications to the diet of the mother before and during pregnancy.[77] For example, maternal Western diet and/or maternal obesity may cause damage to the development of key metabolic systems (liver, muscle and adipose tissue, brain), thereby altering tissue function at the cellular and molecular level in young offspring of obese mothers. Furthermore, the persistence of abnormalities in postnatal animals when switched to a healthy diet suggests that the developmental changes may have permanent epigenetic or molecular effects that alter metabolic outcomes, thereby linking early Western diet exposure to long-term negative effects on other organs.[78]

A westernized lifestyle, which involves a high-energy diet and reduced physical activity, particularly in pregnancy, puts the offspring at particularly high risk of type 2 diabetes mellitus.[13] If the mother is overnourished, as is the case in maternal obesity, the child is at risk for large body size and alterations in visceral fat storage. There are increased circulating nutrients in the mother beginning early in pregnancy[79] that remain high through delivery,[80] which affect the fetal metabolome.[81] This is especially true in the setting of gestational diabetes in which all fuels including carbohydrates, fatty acids, and amino acids may be elevated. In this case, plasticity may act against the best interest of the host. In longitudinal studies of Pima Indians, among whom the prevalence of obesity-associated type 2 diabetes mellitus is very high, offspring of mothers with established disease during pregnancy develop type 2 diabetes mellitus at much younger ages than those born to mothers without diabetes.[82,83] This has now been validated in several other ethnic cohorts and may affect more than just offspring metabolism.[84-86] Metabolic changes in the fetus include but are not limited to increased fuel storage, production of reactive oxygen species, and rapid growth. In the setting of ongoing overnutrition in the mature offspring (via a "Western" high-fat, high-carbohydrate diet) "gasoline is thrown on a smoldering fire." These children are at higher risk for obesity themselves, as well as nonalcoholic fatty liver disease (NAFLD), impaired glucose tolerance, and metabolic syndrome as early as 3 years of age.[87-91] Life-course studies in human infants born to obese mothers, particularly at the molecular and cellular level in tissues relevant to metabolic disease pathways, are currently lacking. Thus the structural and biochemical/molecular changes in tissues that take place just prior to puberty and have direct effects on risk for obesity and type 2 diabetes mellitus later in life are desperately needed. These changes, which have been well studied in animal models, may occur prior to fertilization in the maternal oocyte,[92] during gestation,[93] or after delivery with exposure to maternal lactation.[93]

MOLECULAR MECHANISMS FOR DIFFERENTIATION AND METABOLIC MEMORY

Although molecular mechanisms underlying metabolic risk remains to be elucidated in humans, cells derived from infants and animals at birth have provided some clues. For example, myocytes, as well as adipocytes, osteocytes, and several other cell types, all differentiate from the multipotent fetal mesenchymal stem cell (MSC) population.[94] MSCs, which can be obtained from the umbilical cord at birth, can be differentiated into either adipocytes or myocytes. These processes are governed by threshold levels of adipogenic or myogenic factors[95] that are affected by excess lipid and cellular stressors (e.g., inflammation or oxidative stress). During development, two major regulators of adipogenic and myogenic differentiation are PPARγ and the canonical wnt/β-catenin system.[96] In animal and human models, β-catenin signaling is down-regulated in fetal cells as a result of maternal obesity.[97-99] In humans, another notable example of early epigenetic phenomena involves hypermethylation of the RXRα promoter in umbilical cord DNA of infants born to obese mothers. This change was associated with increased adiposity in the same subjects at 9 years of age.[100] RXRα is one of the endogenous ligands of retinoic acid; RXRα promoter methylation may lead to reduced RXRα content and decreased retinoic acid activity. Consequently, this may favor MSC differentiation shift from myogenesis to adipogenesis and potentiate adipogenic potential throughout the life of the organism, or at least set the stage early in development for postnatal environmental changes to exacerbate a preexisting phenotype.

Once cells have begun differentiating, the "metabolic memory" of tissues appears to be different between offspring of obese and nonobese mothers. Maternal obesity has been shown to affect the capacity for lipid oxidation and allocation of sources for cellular energy metabolism in developing myocytes derived from umbilical cord MSC.[33] Similar metabolic disturbances were found in MSC-derived adipocytes in relation to offspring gain in adiposity in the first months of life.[31] Obese, insulin-resistant humans have been described as "metabolically inflexible."[101-103] This means, in response to influx of nutrients (especially fatty acids), the mitochondrial mechanisms of energy metabolism are overwhelmed, creating a backup of mitochondrial-associated metabolites as well as inflammation, oxidative damage, and a cellular inability to manufacture energy. This metabolic inflexibility is persistent in primary human skeletal muscle derived from obese adults[104,105] and is thought to be regulated at the gene expression level by *PPARα, PGC-1α,* and *FOXO1*, suggesting an epigenetic component to this aspect of skeletal muscle health. Further investigation in rodent models reveals many differences in methylation patterns and expression in skeletal muscle of offspring of obese mothers, including pathways of mitochondrial energy metabolism of fatty acids.[106] Early experiments in NHPs suggest abnormally regulated fatty acid oxidation as well as abnormal mitochondrial function in fetal and juvenile skeletal muscle, influenced not by the current maternal or offspring diet but by maternal obesity and insulin resistant status.[3]

Similarly, fetal and neonatal changes in the liver indicate potentially lasting and detrimental metabolic consequences of maternal obesity and overnutrition despite weaning to a normal diet.[78,90] NAFLD manifests in at least 15% of obese children and predicts chronic, multisystemic, obesity-related disease. In an NHP model, in utero exposure to maternal obesity and insulin resistance alters the normal development of the liver in the third trimester, resulting in increased liver fat and oxidative damage that persists through the first year of life.[78] Using MRI/MRS, human studies have shown that infants born to obese mothers with gestational diabetes have 68% increased liver fat at 2 weeks of age compared with age-matched controls born to normal-weight mothers.[107] Lasting effects into adolescence of infants born to obese mothers have not been investigated in humans, but one recent longitudinal MRI study demonstrated that infants undergo substantial increase (twofold) in liver lipids, along with a doubling of body fat at 2 months of age, regardless of breast- or bottle-feeding.[108] Given that the prevalence of childhood obesity is approximately one in five and NAFLD affects 15% of obese adolescents, gestational exposure to maternal obesity/diabetes might contribute substantially to the overall risk for pediatric NAFLD and progression to the more severe form of nonalcoholic steatohepatitis. The US population prevalence of nonalcoholic steatohepatitis as high as 2% to 3%.[109,110] The propensity of nonalcoholic steatohepatitis to progress to more advanced liver disease is a primary concern. Up to 37% of individuals with nonalcoholic steatohepatitis will progress to fibrosis and cirrhosis with an increased risk of liver cancer.[111] In view of the prevalence of nonalcoholic steatohepatitis, even a low rate of progression to end-stage liver disease has enormous public health implications for both children and adults.

Although the end phenotype of obesity and metabolic disease appear similar, there are mechanistic differences between infants programmed by undernutrition versus overnutrition in utero. Rodent studies show that offspring of undernourished mothers demonstrate decreased acetylation of PGC-1α and increased expression of SIRT1, a major regulator of energy metabolism.[112,113] This is associated with increased lipogenesis, decreased lipolysis, and increased storage of fatty acids in the liver.[114] Hepatic and muscle PPARα is up-regulated specifically with protein restriction,[115,116] as is myocardial carnitine palmitoyl transferase (CPT1), the key transporter of mitochondrial fatty acid to the β-oxidation cycle.[116] β-Oxidation itself is increased as well.[116] The surplus of fatty acids from lipid metabolism deregulation leads to increased oxidative stress and insulin resistance.[117]

In contrast, adult offspring of overfed and obese mothers demonstrated increased PGC-1α acetylation with decreased SIRT1 expression.[112,113] Decreased SIRT1 (an enzyme that deacetylates proteins) is known to increase FOXO transcription factors[118] and acetyl-CoA synthetase[119] expression, and decrease mitochondrial β-oxidation.[120] In the liver, decreased SIRT1 expression is associated with decreased PPARα expression, changes in microRNA expression, and impairment of CPT1, β-oxidation, and mitochondrial complex activity.[121-123] In muscle, there is enhanced fatty acid transporter—CD36 expression increasing intracellular accumulation of fatty acids as well as impaired fatty acid β-oxidation.[124,125] Although mechanistically different from undernourished offspring, this accumulation of fatty acids leads to increased oxidative stress and insulin resistance in adult offspring.[123]

ROLE OF BREAST-FEEDING IN PROGRAMMING

Both small for gestational age (SGA) and LGA infants are at particular risk for later onset metabolic disease. As these babies change rapidly over the first 6 months of life to attain mean weight for age (both catch-up and catch-down growth), care needs to be taken not to introduce interventions at critical stages of development without evidence of short-term and long-term safety and efficacy. In general, breast-feeding is associated with protection against rapid infant weight gain and later obesity.[126-129] However, rapid, excess weight gain during the first 6 months of life has consistently been identified as a predictor of later obesity, even among breast-fed infants.[130-134] The mechanisms responsible likely involve the delivery of bioactive components that regulate infant appetite, metabolism, and weight/adiposity gain.[135]

It is quite likely that bioactive components in human milk including fat composition, adipokine, and cytokine content impact developmental programming paradigm. In one animal study, murine pups born to lean mothers were suckled by an obese mother. Offspring exhibited increased adiposity and reduced insulin sensitivity after weaning.[136] In a separate study pups born to lean mothers were cross-fostered to diet-induced obese mothers. These offspring displayed increased body weight, an NAFLD phenotype, and increased inflammatory cytokines interleukin (IL)-6 and tumor necrosis factor (TNF)-α by 3 months of age.[137] Control murine pups cross-fostered by mothers with gestational diabetes exhibited abnormal hypothalamic programming in the arcuate nucleus post weaning associated with dysregulated appetite, increased food intake, and increased body weight.[138] There are also known associations between maternal high fat diet in rodent models and up-regulation of offspring obesogenic genes (including *PPARα* and *IGF2*)[122]. In human studies, supplementation with n-3 long-chain polyunsaturated fatty acids (LCPUFAs) influenced breast milk fatty acid composition, reducing the n-6 to n-3 LCPUFA ratio, and led to decreased adiposity of offspring in the first year of life.[139]

However, epidemiologic data from humans are not as conclusive. Exclusive breast-feeding at 2 to 4 weeks among gestational diabetic women has been associated with increased infant body weight.[140] However, in 5- and 16-year-old offspring of gestational diabetic mothers, breast-feeding was somewhat protective against obesity in offspring.[141] Maternal BMI factored into that relationship. Obese mothers needed to breast-feed longer to impart protection to offspring.[141] In a separate study, nearly 72,000 children ages 2 to 6 years old were studied over a 4-year period. Maternal BMI and diabetes status were looked at as maternal exposures. The authors found that high offspring BMI was strongly associated with maternal prepregnancy BMI, modestly associated with maternal type 2 diabetes mellitus and gestational diabetes mellitus requiring medication treatment, and only slightly associated with breast-feeding 6 months or less. Gestational diabetes mellitus not requiring medication treatment during pregnancy had little association.[142] There is related support in large populations to suggest that breast-feeding may have little impact on children's BMI.[143]

Finally, the gut flora—the collection of gut microbes (microbiome)—has emerged as a provocative pathway to understanding early changes in both the immune system and energy balance in humans, NHPs, and rodents.[144-146] The postnatal assembly of the human microbiota begins at birth and plays an important role in resistance to pathogen invasion, immune stimulation, and other important developmental cues early in life.[147] Vaginally delivered infants clearly receive a strong input of vaginal and possibly other urogenital microbiota as they pass through and exit the birth canal,[148,149] whereas cesarean-delivered infants display reduced colonization of bacteria early in development.[150,151] The effects of delivery mode may have consequences for infant health; infants delivered by cesarean section delivery tend to be at higher risk for obesity and arguably at greater risk for immune-mediated diseases.[152-155] How these microbial shifts influence the maternal-fetal-infant relationship is not well understood.

The infant gut microbiota, which can be influenced by maternal events in early life such as mode of delivery and feeding and by later life factors such as diet composition and early antibiotic exposure, may also contribute to the risk for obesity and type 2 diabetes mellitus. The gut microbiome is environmentally acquired from birth[156,157]; therefore it may function as an environmental factor that interacts with host genetics (through epigenetic modifications) to shape phenotype.[158-160] Because obesity is associated with altered gut microbial configuration in humans and an obese phenotype can be transmitted via the gut microbiota in animal models of obesity, it is tempting to speculate that the maternal microbiome transmission to the infant may have an important role in energy retention by the infant. Alterations in intestinal microbial composition in the first year of life may last throughout childhood and contribute to the development of obesity.[161,162] Comparisons of the distal gut microbiota of genetically obese mice and lean controls, as well as those of obese and lean humans showed that obesity is associated with changes in the relative abundance of two dominant bacterial divisions—Bacteroidetes and Firmicutes—with obese mice or humans having a higher proportion of Firmicutes to Bacteroidetes. Biochemical analyses show that these proportional changes affect the metabolic potential of the mouse gut microbiota and that the microbiome from obese animals have an increased capacity to harvest energy from the diet. Firmicutes produce more complete metabolism of a given energy source than Bacteroidetes, promoting more efficient absorption of calories and subsequent weight gain. Human studies examining the microbiome of 2-week-old infants have demonstrated lower numbers of important, pioneering Gammaproteobacteria in the offspring of obese versus normal weight mothers.[163] Here, microbiota composition was influenced by breast milk composition, particularly higher concentrations of Gammaproteobacteria and lower concentrations of Firmicutes, correlating with higher levels of insulin in the milk of obese mothers.[163] Interestingly, phenotypic relationships to microbiome composition are transmissible: colonization of germ-free mice with an "obese microbiota" results in significantly greater increase in total body fat[165] and induced liver dysfunction[166] versus colonization with a "lean microbiota." The gut microbiome is environmentally acquired from birth, and along with maternal breast milk composition, antibiotic use, and other early life exposures, it may function as an environmental factor that interacts with the infant and their genome to shape phenotype.

MOTHERS AND BABIES TODAY

In view of the considerable evidence showing that coronary heart disease and related disorders, including stroke, hypertension, and type 2 diabetes mellitus, originate through nutritional influences in utero, protecting the nutrition and health of young women and their babies must be part of any effective strategy for preventing chronic disease. Maintenance of healthy weight during gestation and into early childhood through appropriate diet and exercise, good-quality obstetric, neonatal, and pediatric care, and breast-feeding should be supported, particularly in high-risk (e.g., obese or gestational diabetic) women. Evidence that certain cancers are initiated in fetal life adds to the urgency of this concept.[166-169] The "fetal origins hypothesis" pioneered by Dr. Barker resulted from studies of the geographic association between coronary heart disease and low BW and the recognition that a poor intrauterine environment played a major role in this association.[170] These associations have been extended to high BW and fetal overnutrition based on maternal obesity and insulin resistance. They are currently being defined by biochemical, epigenetic, and regulatory mechanisms to better address the pathophysiology and develop informed strategies of intervention. Dietary modifications for reducing gestational weight gain in gestational diabetes have proven to reduce risk of infant macrosomia and associated morbidity and mortality.[171] Specifically for obese mothers with gestational diabetes, a nonconventional higher-complex carbohydrate, lower-fat diet resulted in improved maternal insulin resistance, reduced maternal inflammation, and most importantly improved infant adiposity.[172,173] Importantly, maternal glucose within the therapeutic targeted range was maintained. Improved maternal weight and diabetes status early in pregnancy and during the postpartum period are effective in improving childhood obesity as well.[174] Some studies have been less definitive about the benefits of acute intervention.[175]

If fetal effects are the result of a lifetime of maternal metabolic dysfunction, then more population-based, childhood interventions should be explored. Direct modification of epigenetic changes may eventually be a potential treatment approach for chronically obese mothers, especially if epigenetic modifications in offspring are present prior to fertilization. Altering methylation by supplementation of folate, vitamin B_{12}, choline, and other nutrients involved in methyl-donor generation have been shown to be effective in mice[59,176,177] and could improve obesity risk in human offspring, although this has not been well studied. Supplements such as Resveratrol, a powerful antioxidant that alters acetylation via modulation of SIRT3, could also help. In an NHP study, Resveratrol was associated with improved placental function and mitochondrial function in offspring of obese mothers.[78] Taurine supplementation has also shown to be beneficial, specifically in altering inflammation, in obese mothers and may also be a viable tool to prevent maternal epigenetic programming effects in offspring.[178] Finally, because the microbiome can be modified for therapeutic applications,[179-182] it constitutes an attractive target for manipulation. Once the interactions between host genetics, diet, and the microbiome are understood, its manipulation could be optimized for a given host to reduce disease risk.

CONCLUSION

Beginning with astute observations based on population data, Dr. David Barker popularized the study of fetal programming in adult chronic disease. Through molecular and biochemical investigation, this has proven to be a complex and intricate process, seemingly dependent on epigenetic mechanisms in utero and influenced by persistent metabolic dysregulation, which may be exacerbated by dietary intake both immediately as well as long after birth.

There are strong rodent and supporting human clinical data to indicate that abnormalities in the development of the brain (appetite control), pancreatic islets (glucose control), liver (gluconeogenesis, lipid metabolism), muscle (main metabolic organ), and/or immune system play critical roles in the development of obesity and are under environmental control. Rodent studies have provided valuable information about specific key systems and factors involved in the complications caused by maternal Western style diet consumption or maternal undernutrition; however, rodents have significantly different developmental ontogeny than humans. Sheep have also provided important insights into the complications of overnutrition or undernutrition during pregnancy on fetal health risks; however, their placental function and ruminant metabolism (particularly fatty acid metabolism) are dramatically different from humans. Although important studies have been conducted in rodent models, the impact of maternal diet on development and function of pancreatic islets, skeletal muscle mitochondria, NAFLD, appetite control, and higher orders of behavior in models that more closely mimic the human condition is critical for developing an understanding of how maternal nutrition affects interorgan metabolism and emergence of disease mechanisms. Thus NHP studies and research using human tissue-like umbilical cord MSCs have been instrumental in uncovering novel mechanistic pathways over the past decade.

Certainly new insights from epigenetic and dietary interventions that examine longitudinal outcomes are needed to address these problems. Dr. Barker's legacy, which has influenced and directed the next century of medicine, will continue to form the framework for investigations in the field of maternal-fetal health and nutrition.

A complete reference list is available at www.ExpertConsult.com.

SELECT REFERENCES

3. McCurdy CE, Schenk S, Hetrick B, et al. Maternal obesity reduces oxidative capacity in fetal skeletal muscle of Japanese macaques. *JCI Insight*. 2016;1:e86612.
4. Wesolowski SR, Mulligan CM, Janssen RC, et al. Switching obese mothers to a healthy diet improves fetal hypoxemia, hepatic metabolites, and lipotoxicity in non-human primates. *Mol Metab*. 2018;18:25-41.
9. Barker DJ, Winter PD, Osmond C, Margetts B, Simmonds SJ. Weight in infancy and death from ischaemic heart disease. *Lancet*. 1989;2:577-580.
10. Osmond C, Barker DJ, Winter PD, Fall CH, Simmonds SJ. Early growth and death from cardiovascular disease in women. *BMJ*. 1993;307:1519-1524.
11. Hales CN, Barker DJ, Clark PM, et al. Fetal and infant growth and impaired glucose tolerance at age 64. *BMJ*. 1991;303:1019-1022.
16. Forsen T, Eriksson J, Tuomilehto J, Reunanen A, Osmond C, Barker D. The fetal and childhood growth of persons who develop type 2 diabetes. *Ann Intern Med*. 2000;133:176-182.
19. Barker DJ, Osmond C, Forsen TJ, Kajantie E, Eriksson JG. Trajectories of growth among children who have coronary events as adults. *N Engl J Med*. 2005;353:1802-1809.
21. Barker DJ, Eriksson JG, Forsen T, Osmond C. Fetal origins of adult disease: strength of effects and biological basis. *Int J Epidemiol*. 2002;31:1235-1239.
22. Eriksson J, Forsen T, Tuomilehto J, Osmond C, Barker D. Fetal and childhood growth and hypertension in adult life. *Hypertension*. 2000;36:790-794.
23. Sewell MF, Huston-Presley L, Super DM, Catalano P. Increased neonatal fat mass, not lean body mass, is associated with maternal obesity. *Am J Obstet Gynecol*. 2006;195:1100-1103.
25. Pedersen J. Weight and length at birth of infants of diabetic mothers. *Acta Endocrinol (Copenh)*. 1954;16:330-342.
31. Baker 2nd PR, Patinkin ZW, Shapiro ALB, et al. Altered gene expression and metabolism in fetal umbilical cord mesenchymal stem cells correspond with differences in 5-month-old infant adiposity gain. *Sci Rep*. 2017;7:18095.
33. Baker 2nd PR, Patinkin Z, Shapiro AL, et al. Maternal obesity and increased neonatal adiposity correspond with altered infant mesenchymal stem cell metabolism. *JCI Insight*. 2017;2:e94200.
35. West NA, Crume TL, Maligie MA, Dabelea D. Cardiovascular risk factors in children exposed to maternal diabetes in utero. *Diabetologia*. 2011;54:504-507.
38. Dabelea D, Snell-Bergeon JK, Hartsfield CL, et al. Increasing prevalence of gestational diabetes mellitus (GDM) over time and by birth cohort: Kaiser Permanente of Colorado GDM Screening Program. *Diabetes Care*. 2005;28:579-584.
39. Dabelea D, Pettitt DJ. Intrauterine diabetic environment confers risks for type 2 diabetes mellitus and obesity in the offspring, in addition to genetic susceptibility. *J Pediatr Endocrinol Metab*. 2001;14:1085-1091.
40. Barker DJ. Fetal origins of coronary heart disease. *BMJ*. 1995;311:171-174.
45. Suter MA, Chen A, Burdine MS, et al. A maternal high-fat diet modulates fetal SIRT1 histone and protein deacetylase activity in nonhuman primates. *FASEB J*. 2012;26:5106-5114.
47. Shock LS, Thakkar PV, Peterson EJ, Moran RG, Taylor SM. DNA methyltransferase 1, cytosine methylation, and cytosine hydroxymethylation in mammalian mitochondria. *ProcNatlAcadSciUSA*. 2011;108:3630-3635.
50. Newsom SA, Boyle KE, Friedman JE. Sirtuin 3: a major control point for obesity-related metabolic diseases? *Drug Discov Today Dis Mech*. 2013;10:e35-e40.
64. Limesand SW, Rozance PJ, Brown LD, Hay Jr WW. Effects of chronic hypoglycemia and euglycemic correction on lysine metabolism in fetal sheep. *Am J Physiol Endocrinol Metab*. 2009;296:E879-E887.
65. van Veen LC, Teng C, Hay Jr WW, Meschia G, Battaglia FC. Leucine disposal and oxidation rates in the fetal lamb. *Metabolism*. 1987;36:48-53.
70. Desai M, Guang H, Ferelli M, Kallichanda N, Lane RH. Programmed upregulation of adipogenic transcription factors in intrauterine growth-restricted offspring. *Reprod Sci*. 2008;15:785-796.
71. Desai M, Crowther NJ, Ozanne SE, Lucas A, Hales CN. Adult glucose and lipid metabolism may be programmed during fetal life. *Biochem Soc Trans*. 1995;23:331-335.
72. Brown LD, Rozance PJ, Bruce JL, Friedman JE, Hay Jr WW, Wesolowski SR. Limited capacity for glucose oxidation in fetal sheep with intrauterine growth restriction. *Am J Physiol Regul Integr Comp Physiol*. 2015;309:R920-R928.
78. Thorn SR, Baquero KC, Newsom SA, et al. Early life exposure to maternal insulin resistance has persistent effects on hepatic NAFLD in juvenile nonhuman primates. *Diabetes*. 2014;63:2702-2713.
79. Borengasser SJ, Baker 2nd PR, Kerns ME, et al. Preconception micronutrient supplementation reduced circulating branched chain amino acids at 12 weeks gestation in an open trial of Guatemalan women who are overweight or obese. *Nutrients*. 2018;10:1282.
80. Sandler V, Reisetter AC, Bain JR, et al. Associations of maternal BMI and insulin resistance with the maternal metabolome and newborn outcomes. *Diabetologia*. 2017;60:518-530.
81. Lowe Jr WL, Bain JR, Nodzenski M, et al. Maternal BMI and glycemia impact the fetal metabolome. *Diabetes Care*. 2017;40:902-910.
89. Lowe Jr WL, Scholtens DM, Kuang A, et al. Hyperglycemia and Adverse Pregnancy Outcome Follow-up Study (HAPO FUS): maternal gestational diabetes mellitus and childhood glucose metabolism. *Diabetes Care*. 2019;42:372-380.
90. Baker 2nd PR, Friedman JE. Mitochondrial role in the neonatal predisposition to developing nonalcoholic fatty liver disease. *J Clin Invest*. 2018;128:3692-3703.
99. Boyle KE, Patinkin ZW, Shapiro AL, Baker 2nd PR, Dabelea D, Friedman JE. Mesenchymal stem cells from infants born to obese mothers exhibit greater potential for adipogenesis: The Healthy Start BabyBUMP Project. *Diabetes*. 2016;65:647-659.
102. Muoio DM, Noland RC, Kovalik JP, et al. Muscle-specific deletion of carnitine acetyltransferase compromises glucose tolerance and metabolic flexibility. *Cell Metab*. 2012;15:764-777.
104. Boyle KE, Zheng D, Anderson EJ, Neufer PD, Houmard JA. Mitochondrial lipid oxidation is impaired in cultured myotubes from obese humans. *IntJObes(Lond)*. 2012;36:1025-1031.

105. Baker 2nd PR, Boyle KE, Koves TR, et al. Metabolomic analysis reveals altered skeletal muscle amino acid and fatty acid handling in obese humans. *Obesity (Silver Spring)*. 2015;23:981-988.
106. Borengasser SJ, Zhong Y, Kang P, et al. Maternal obesity enhances white adipose tissue differentiation and alters genome-scale DNA methylation in male rat offspring. *Endocrinology*. 2013;154:4113-4125.
107. Brumbaugh DE, Tearse P, Cree-Green M, et al. Intrahepatic fat is increased in the neonatal offspring of obese women with gestational diabetes. *J Pediatr*. 2012;162:930-936.e1.
114. Wolfe D, Gong M, Han G, Magee TR, Ross MG, Desai M. Nutrient sensor-mediated programmed nonalcoholic fatty liver disease in low birthweight offspring. *Am J Obstet Gynecol*. 2012;207:308.e1-6.
120. Chen LL, Zhang HH, Zheng J, et al. Resveratrol attenuates high-fat diet-induced insulin resistance by influencing skeletal muscle lipid transport and subsarcolemmal mitochondrial beta-oxidation. *Metabolism*. 2011;60:1598-1609.
122. Zhang J, Zhang F, Didelot X, et al. Maternal high fat diet during pregnancy and lactation alters hepatic expression of insulin like growth factor-2 and key microRNAs in the adult offspring. *BMC Genomics*. 2009;10:478.
134. Young BE, Johnson SL, Krebs NF. Biological determinants linking infant weight gain and child obesity: current knowledge and future directions. *Adv Nutr*. 2012;3:675-686.
146. Ma J, Prince AL, Bader D, et al. High-fat maternal diet during pregnancy persistently alters the offspring microbiome in a primate model. *Nat Commun*. 2014;5:3889.
150. Bennet R, Nord CE. Development of the faecal anaerobic microflora after caesarean section and treatment with antibiotics in newborn infants. *Infection*. 1987;15:332-336.
160. Tims S, Derom C, Jonkers DM, et al. Microbiota conservation and BMI signatures in adult monozygotic twins. *ISME J*. 2013;7:707-717.
163. Lemas DJ, Young BE, Baker 2nd PR, et al. Alterations in human milk leptin and insulin are associated with early changes in the infant intestinal microbiome. *Am J Clin Nutr*. 2016;103:1291-1300.
170. Barker DJ, Osmond C. Infant mortality, childhood nutrition, and ischaemic heart disease in England and Wales. *Lancet*. 1986;1:1077-1081.
172. Hernandez TL, Van Pelt RE, Anderson MA, et al. A higher-complex carbohydrate diet in gestational diabetes mellitus achieves glucose targets and lowers postprandial lipids: a randomized crossover study. *Diabetes Care*. 2014;37:1254-1262.
173. Hernandez TL, Van Pelt RE, Anderson MA, et al. Women with gestational diabetes mellitus randomized to a higher-complex carbohydrate/low-fat diet manifest lower adipose tissue insulin resistance, inflammation, glucose, and free fatty acids: a pilot study. *Diabetes Care*. 2016;39:39-42.

Placental Function in Intrauterine Growth Restriction

14

Jill Chang | Karen Mestan

INTRODUCTION

DEFINITIONS OF INTRAUTERINE GROWTH RESTRICTION

Intrauterine growth restriction (IUGR) remains one of the leading causes of perinatal and neonatal morbidity and mortality worldwide, with significant implications for the short- and long-term health and development of children. IUGR remains an important public health concern in both developing and well-resourced countries. Recent estimates are that IUGR affects 3% to 7% of all newborn infants, with apparently higher incidence during the last decade.[1] IUGR is typically defined as the failure of the fetus to achieve its genetically determined growth potential. Clinically, this individual genetic growth potential is largely unknown and the diagnosis of IUGR relies on proxies, including the estimation of fetal weight in utero and/or measurements of birth weight. The rate and potential for normal growth during pregnancy is also based on the race and gender of the fetus. Small-for-gestational age (SGA) is typically defined as fetal weight or birth weight less than the 10th percentile on standardized weight-for-gestational age growth curves.[2,3] However, only about one-third of infants born at less than 10th percentile have an identified or apparent etiology for pathologic growth restriction,[4] and otherwise healthy, constitutionally small birth weight-for-gestational age infants are usually considered to be at low risk for adverse perinatal or long-term outcomes.

DIAGNOSIS AND TYPES OF INTRAUTERINE GROWTH RESTRICTION

Early, antenatal identification of IUGR is typically achieved with serial assessment of intrauterine growth, using fetal biometric measurements obtained by ultrasound, such as head-to-abdominal ratio and head-to-femur ratio, estimated fetal weight, growth velocity, and abdominal circumference.[5-8] Historically, abdominal circumference less than 10th percentile was considered the most sensitive biometry marker for diagnosis of IUGR[6] with varying thresholds (<3rd or <5th percentiles) to diagnose IUGR and predict fetal compromise in utero.[9] More recently developed growth curves suggest that fetal biometry alone is not sufficient to discriminate constitutionally small fetuses from those at risk for adverse perinatal outcomes.[10] Doppler ultrasound imaging has improved diagnostic accuracy, as pathologic IUGR is often associated with Doppler abnormalities in the uteroplacental and umbilical circulation, whereas constitutionally small fetuses often exhibit normal fetal Doppler measurements.[11-13] Repeated fetal growth estimates from ultrasound imaging showing a deviation from previously established intrauterine growth curves and findings of abnormal blood flow patterns in the fetal circulation, such as increased resistance in the umbilical artery, are indicative of IUGR.[12,13] Amniotic fluid volume, which is believed to reflect placental and fetal renal functions, provides additional information. Low amniotic fluid volume with intact membranes is commonly associated with placental insufficiency.[14]

Two main patterns of IUGR are observed based upon fetal and neonatal assessment. *Symmetric IUGR* is characterized by a proportional lack of growth resulting in small head and abdominal size. The inciting cause is thought to begin early in pregnancy (first or second trimester), with reduced fetal cellular proliferation of all organs. Congenital infections and chromosomal abnormalities are typically associated with symmetric IUGR. In contrast, *asymmetric IUGR* is seen more commonly (70% to 80%) and is characterized by disproportionately larger head size relative to expected abdominal circumference, and is typically associated with failure of nutritional or oxygen supply and/or blood flow in the second half of pregnancy (i.e., placental or maternal vascular factors).[15] In asymmetric IUGR, the growth of the fetal head is relatively spared due to redistribution of cardiac output to preferentially support cerebral blood flow.[16] Changes in placental function have classically been associated with asymmetric IUGR,[2] but with more recent understanding of the role of the placenta in earlier fetal growth and programming, the distinction between symmetric and asymmetric IUGR is not always clear and there is significant overlap between the two groups.

CONSEQUENCES OF INTRAUTERINE GROWTH RESTRICTION

IUGR is associated with increased perinatal morbidity and mortality[17,18] and remains one of the most important risk factors for unexplained intrauterine demise.[19] As the causes of IUGR and stillbirth usually overlap, the risk for stillbirth is directly proportional to the severity of the fetal growth restriction.[20] The risk for stillbirth is 1.5% for fetal weights less than 10th percentile and increases to 2.5% if the fetal weight is below the 5th percentile for gestational age.[21-23] IUGR is also associated with preterm birth, perinatal asphyxia, intraventricular hemorrhage, and infections.[24,25] In the neonatal period, the growth-restricted infant is susceptible to abnormal thermoregulation, hypoglycemia, and other metabolic problems believed to be related to limited glycogen and fat stores.[25]

The adverse consequences of IUGR are not limited to the fetal and neonatal period but can also influence lifelong health by developmental programming.[18] This concept is centered around research of the *fetal origins hypothesis*, which proposes that exposures during gestation have significant impact on the individual's functional capacity, metabolic competence, and responses to the later environment, likely due to epigenetic programming of the fetal phenotype.[26] These concepts have extended to include neurodevelopmental outcomes and cardiopulmonary health. For example, an altered intrauterine environment, accompanied by changes in nutrient availability, is associated with increased risk for chronic diseases, including coronary artery disease, hypertension, and type II diabetes later in life.[27,28] The mechanisms underlying developmental programming remain to be established but may involve epigenetic regulation of key genes or permanent changes in organ structure.[29]

CAUSES OF INTRAUTERINE GROWTH RESTRICTION

Fetal growth and development are the result of complex interactions between the genetic growth potential of the fetus, the maternal environment, and placental function. Primary conditions affecting the mother, fetus, or placenta may interfere with fetal growth and result in IUGR. Common origins of IUGR are therefore typically categorized into three groups: maternal, fetal, and placental causes (Fig. 14.1).

MATERNAL ORIGINS

Certain baseline aspects of prepregnancy maternal health and conditions during pregnancy are known to impact fetal growth. Maternal extremes of age (<16 and >35 years), race/ethnicity, and low socioeconomic status are epidemiologic associations that appear to play a biologic role in IUGR.[15,30] Maternal undernutrition is a major public health concern worldwide and constitutes the most common cause of IUGR in developing countries and remains a significant problem in the United States.[31] Maternal residence at high altitude during pregnancy is associated with IUGR due to exposure to chronic fetal hypoxia.[32] Maternal vascular diseases, such as gestational hypertension, preeclampsia, and chronic hypertension with or without superimposed preeclampsia, are common maternal causes of IUGR.[33,34] Smoking during pregnancy, an example of a modifiable risk factor, increases the risk for growth restriction 3.5-fold.[34] Other maternal conditions include autoimmune disorders, renal disease, exposure to teratogens, and substance abuse.[35-41] Maternal endocrine disorders and internal/extrinsic factors that alter homeostatic mechanisms (e.g., psychosocial stress) have been shown in animal models to impact fetal growth through deviations in maternal cortisol, placental glucocorticoid, and epigenetic processes.[42,43]

FETAL ORIGINS

A wide range of fetal chromosomal and genetic abnormalities are associated with IUGR, with autosomal trisomies 13, 18, and 21 being the most common chromosomal disorders. In addition, fetuses with unbalanced chromosomal translocation or deletion are at increased risk.[16] Even in the absence of a chromosomal or identified genetic disorder, structural congenital abnormalities are associated with IUGR.[44,45] In a population-based study conducted by the Centers for Disease Control and Prevention, more than 20% of infants with structural malformations had IUGR, corresponding to a 2.6-fold higher risk for growth restriction as compared with infants without malformations.[44] Intrauterine infections, in particular rubella, cytomegalovirus, varicella-zoster, toxoplasma, and malaria[46-48] have been estimated to cause 5% to 10% of all cases of IUGR.

PLACENTAL ORIGINS

Changes in placental function, which are often referred to as *placental dysfunction* or *placental insufficiency*, are believed to cause or directly contribute to most cases of asymmetric IUGR;[16] however, percentage estimates are difficult to measure epidemiologically due to complex interaction with maternal and fetal causes (see Fig. 14.1).[49] Defective placentation that results in placental dysfunction is a fundamental pathophysiologic mechanism of IUGR.[50,51] Abnormalities in placental growth and development following early placentation also contribute to IUGR, and these defects may be secondary to maternal and fetal exposures during pregnancy that set the stage for ongoing placental dysfunction. These mechanisms are detailed in this chapter, outlining defects at the various stages and levels of placental development involving structural, cellular, genetic, and epigenetic functions.

STRUCTURAL CHANGES

GROSS PATHOLOGY

Key elements of placental sampling and examination provide valuable information that can help us better understand the mechanisms underlying IUGR. Decreased placental size and weight, usually less than 10th percentile weight-for-gestational age based upon published placental growth curves,[52] is the typical gross placental finding accompanying IUGR. Other macroscopic placental abnormalities include unusual paleness, infarction, and loss of parenchyma. The area of unusual paleness is believed to represent decreased vascularization of chorionic villi, whereas the infarction can be recognized by a pale and indurated region in placental parenchyma.[53]

PLACENTAL HISTOPATHOLOGY

The chorionic villus, the functional unit of the placenta that contains a capillary network derived from fetal circulation, undergoes developmental changes throughout pregnancy. Mediated byprocesses of early spiral artery remodeling and subsequent vascular proliferation and branching, the composition of the placenta shifts from few, large, and poorly vascularized primary villi to numerous, small, and highly vascularized tertiary villi. Histologic lesions accompanying IUGR include those from both vascular and inflammatory domains. The placental domain most commonly associated with IUGR, along with stillbirth and preeclampsia, is *maternal vascular malperfusion of the placental bed*. In 2016,

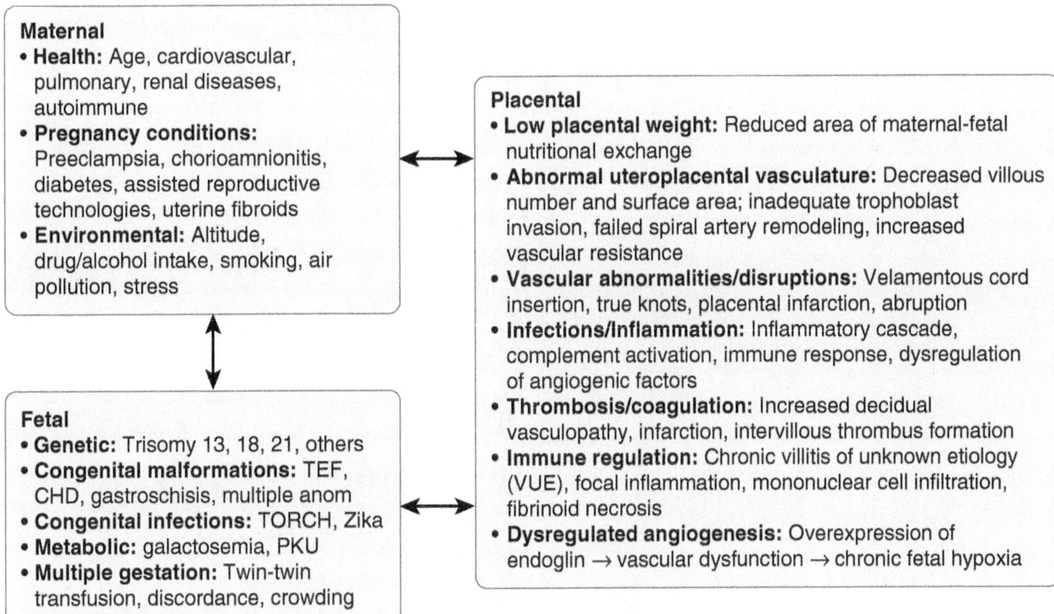

Causes of intrauterine growth restriction
Maternal
• Health: Age, cardiovascular, pulmonary, renal diseases, autoimmune
• Pregnancy conditions: Preeclampsia, chorioamnionitis, diabetes, assisted reproductive technologies, uterine fibroids
• Environmental: Altitude, drug/alcohol intake, smoking, air pollution, stress
Placental
• Low placental weight: Reduced area of maternal-fetal nutritional exchange
• Abnormal uteroplacental vasculature: Decreased villous number and surface area; inadequate trophoblast invasion, failed spiral artery remodeling, increased vascular resistance
• Vascular abnormalities/disruptions: Velamentous cord insertion, true knots, placental infarction, abruption
• Infections/Inflammation: Inflammatory cascade, complement activation, immune response, dysregulation of angiogenic factors
• Thrombosis/coagulation: Increased decidual vasculopathy, infarction, intervillous thrombus formation
• Immune regulation: Chronic villitis of unknown etiology (VUE), focal inflammation, mononuclear cell infiltration, fibrinoid necrosis
• Dysregulated angiogenesis: Overexpression of endoglin → vascular dysfunction → chronic fetal hypoxia
Fetal
• Genetic: Trisomy 13, 18, 21, others
• Congenital malformations: TEF, CHD, gastroschisis, multiple anom
• Congenital infections: TORCH, Zika
• Metabolic: galactosemia, PKU
• Multiple gestation: Twin-twin transfusion, discordance, crowding

Fig. 14.1 Multifactorial causes of intrauterine growth restriction (IUGR). A large majority of IUGR cases are thought to be due to processes of placental insufficiency, but maternal and fetal diseases may also serve as primary or interactive processes contributing to placental dysfunction. *CHD,* Congenital heart disease; *PKU,* phenylketonuria; *TEF,* tracheoesophageal fistula; *TORCH,* toxoplasmosis, other, rubella, cytomegalovirus, and herpes infections.

the Amsterdam workshop recommended renaming this set of criteria from underperfusion to malperfusion; even though many of the effects of inadequate spiral artery remodeling manifest as a spectrum that includes IUGR and preeclampsia,[54] high-velocity malperfusion may be as detrimental as underperfusion to placental function in later pregnancy.[55] While the classic histologic lesions do not reliably distinguish between low- versus high-velocity processes, recent evidence suggests that certain abnormalities in villous architecture may be indicators of dysregulated blood flow more than chronic hypoxia due to persistent underperfusion. For example, three-dimensional reconstruction models of placental intervillous blood flow suggest that increased turbulent jet rates can lead to rupture of anchoring villi, as evidenced by echogenic cystic lesions on ultrasound.[56] Microscopically, high-velocity damage to the villous surface may generate release of syncytial sprouts in early pregnancy and downstream presence of syncytial knots at placental autopsy.[57] Increased shear wall stress at the villous surface has been seen in computer simulation models of turbulent blood flow, combined with elevated blood pressure in the intervillous space.[58] Oxidant stress due to ischemia-reperfusion is another proposed mechanism of villous injury in which retention of smooth muscle predisposes to spontaneous vasoconstriction,[59] leading to high-momentum blood flow entry into the intervillous space and apoptotic changes within the syncytiotrophoblast.

Microscopic findings of maternal vascular malperfusion are indicators of abnormal vascular and villous development involved in the above processes. Decidual arteriopathies, such as mural hypertrophy of membrane arterioles and persistent muscularization of basal plate arteries (Fig. 14.2A), are rare but consistently seen lesions in severe IUGR. Presence of these lesions at placental autopsy represent failed early first trimester spiral artery remodeling with persistence of intramural endovascular trophoblasts in the third trimester. Villous changes include accelerated villous maturation (see Fig. 14.2B) and distal villous hypoplasia (see Fig. 14.2C).[16,55] Placental morphology studies suggest that the presence of more highly branched villi at placental exam of infants with IUGR and ultrasound Doppler evidence of positive end-diastolic flow represent an adaptive response via enhanced branching angiogenesis.[60] In contrast, the pattern of highly branched villi is *not* present in the growth-restricted placenta with absent or reversed end-diastolic flow in the umbilical artery, suggesting failure of the adaptive process.[61,62] Growth-restricted placentas also typically have reduced intervillous space volume, poorly developed peripheral villi, and a thicker trophoblastic epithelium that result in a smaller nutrient exchange area. These changes could also compromise placental oxygen transfer and contribute to fetal hypoxia.[63]

Villitis of unknown etiology (VUE), also known as *nonspecific chronic villitis,* is an inflammatory condition of the placenta characterized by maternal T-cell infiltrates in the villous stroma (see Fig. 14.2D). Despite changes over the years in the classification and nomenclature to define this lesion, VUE continues to be a frequent histologic finding in IUGR and stillbirth[64] and may involve vascular damage when inflammatory cells damage muscular wall vessels.[55] Recent studies of coculture of placental explants with maternal leukocytes resulting in increased leukocytes in villous tissues and elevated cytokine levels support mechanisms by which altered placental inflammation has deleterious effects on placental function.[65] Immunohistochemistry of placentas with chronic villitis has revealed cytokine profiles suggesting a skew toward inappropriate Th1 immune responses.[66]

VASCULAR CHANGES

THROMBOSIS

Normal human pregnancy is characterized by increased thrombin production, resulting in a hypercoagulable state.[67] Coagulation-related lesions such as intraplacental thrombosis are common morphologic findings in growth-restricted placentas; however, whether these changes are causes of or secondary to IUGR remains uncertain.[68,69] The hypercoagulable state and maternal endothelial cell dysfunction can induce platelet activation that leads to vasoconstriction and reduced placental blood flow.[69] The impaired placental circulation, in turn, is believed to enhance coagulation, and this vicious cycle subsequently contributes

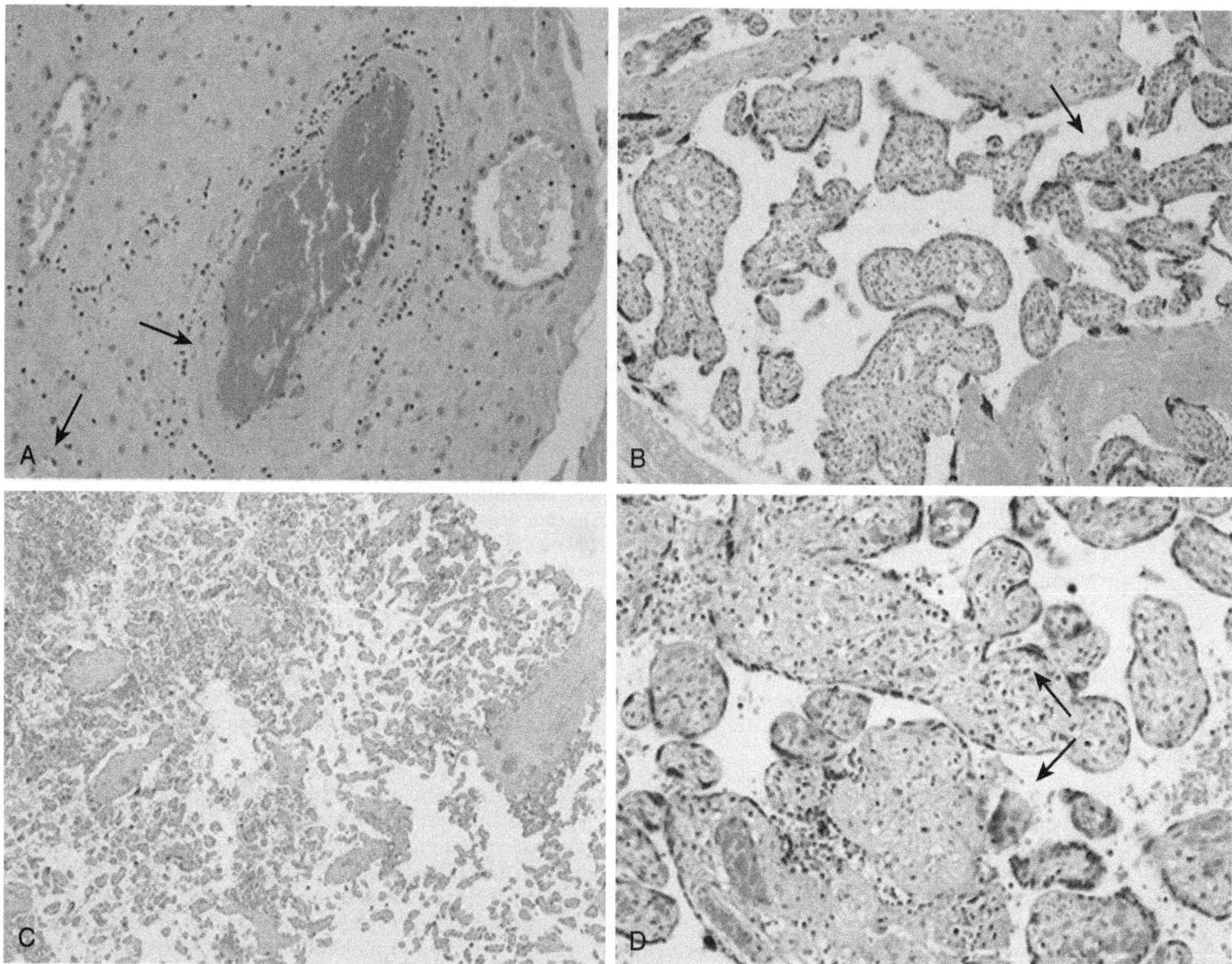

Fig. 14.2 Placental histopathologic lesions accompanying intrauterine growth restriction (IUGR). (A) Decidual arteriopathy of maternal vascular malperfusion: Maternal vessels in the parietal decidua are shown, with persistent muscularization of basal plate arterioles *(arrows)*, which represent failure of the extravillous trophoblast to invade the spiral arteries of the myometrium, with resultant loss of muscular vascular wall. (B) Accelerated villous maturation in a preterm placenta, with areas of increased terminal villi and increased fetal capillaries on the right *(arrow)* as compared with the left. (C) Distal villous hypoplasia: Note the predominance of small, round villi and thin, elongated villi (due to lack of branching), and paucity of villi with wide intervillous spaces. (D) Placenta parenchyma with chronic villitis: Note the reduced vasculature, paucity of villi, and infiltration of lymphocytes and macrophages (Hoffbauer cells). (Images provided courtesy Dr. Jeff Goldstein, Department of Pathology, Northwestern University Feinberg School of Medicine.)

to placental dysfunction and IUGR. Notably, intraplacental thrombosis is uncommon in normal pregnancy, suggesting that factors within the placenta itself may offset normal occurrence of hypercoagulability.[70] Proteoglycans are macromolecules located within vessel walls that contain a core protein with one or more covalently attached glycosaminoglycan chains. The proteoglycans and their glycosaminoglycan side chains play an important role in preventing thrombosis within the placenta.[70,71] Proteoglycan mRNA and protein expression is reduced in IUGR placentas, suggesting that local anticoagulant activity in the intervillous space is reduced.[72,73]

PLACENTAL ANGIOGENESIS

Altered levels of angiogenic factors, resulting in dysregulated placental vascular formation, are believed to play an important role in the development of IUGR. Several growth factors, including vascular endothelial growth factor (VEGF), placental growth factor (PlGF), angiopoietin, and angiostatins are produced within the villi and are involved in placental angiogenesis.[74] VEGF and PlGF act as important paracrine regulators of decidual angiogenesis and autocrine mediators of trophoblast function.[75,76] The expression of VEGF is decreased in the villi of IUGR placentas, whereas PlGF expression has been reported to increase.[77-79] In addition, levels of antiangiogenic growth factors are also altered in pregnancies complicated by IUGR. For example, the protein levels of soluble VEGF receptor 1 (sVEGFR-1), also known as *soluble fms-like tyrosine kinase-1 or sFlt-1*, are increased in IUGR placentas.[80,81] sFlt-1 is a key receptor antagonist for both VEGF and PlGF that inhibits the binding of these growth factors to their receptors, leading to endothelial cell dysfunction through angiogenic imbalance.[80,81]

The expression of VEGF, PlGF, and other angiogenic factors is regulated by oxygen concentrations, largely through HIF-1α and HIF-1β mediated pathways.[82-84] Hypoxia up-regulates VEGF gene expression and inhibits PlGF gene expression.[85] Once the placental vascular network has been established, placental endothelial cells and perivascular cells secrete angiopoietin-2 (Ang-2), the antagonist of Angiopoietin-1 (Ang-1), which promotes the branching of blood vessels by destabilizing newly formed vessel tips. This allows vessels to be responsive to VEGF-induced branching angiogenesis through increased endothelial cell migration.[86] Placental lysates from IUGR pregnancies exhibit decreased Ang-2 protein expression, suggesting premature stabilization of vessels and shift toward non-branching angiogenesis and abnormal development of the villous vasculature.[87] In the absence of VEGF, Ang-2 promotes endothelial cell apoptosis in vitro, and it has been hypothesized that increased Ang-2 may inhibit blood vessel growth and impair exchange.

BLOOD FLOW

In normal pregnancy, villous vascularization shifts from sprouting and branching angiogenesis to nonbranching angiogenesis with advancing gestation, resulting in the formation of a complex vascular network in mature intermediate and terminal villi, which is critical for efficient nutrient and gas exchange across the placental barrier.[88] This gestational change in vascularization is reflected by typical clinical Doppler findings in normal pregnancies characterized by declining resistance, as measured by the pulsatility index and the systolic-to-diastolic ratio, in the umbilical and uterine arcuate arteries (Fig. 14.3A).[89] However, the normal decline of the systolic-to-diastolic ratio may not occur in pregnancies complicated by uteroplacental insufficiency. In IUGR, the placenta is characterized by decreased vascularization, with a reduction in the number of terminal and stem villi capillaries, resulting in an increased resistance and decreased umbilical artery end-diastolic flow velocity.[90-92] With further increase in resistance, end-diastolic flow in the umbilical artery becomes absent (see Fig. 14.3B) and ultimately, reversed (see Fig. 14.3C). These aberrant patterns of umbilical artery Doppler findings are predictive of perinatal and long-term outcomes.[88,93-95]

The degree of villous vascularization as determined morphologically is correlated to umbilical artery Doppler measurements, with a low number of peripheral, highly vascularized villi being linked to absent or reverse end-diastolic flow.[60,88] This altered vascularization is associated with increased placental expression of sVEGFR-1 in IUGR complicated by absent end-diastolic umbilical artery blood flow.[96] Moreover, the underdevelopment of the uteroplacental circulation will increase uterine artery resistance.[97] The uterine artery Doppler waveform in normal pregnancy is characterized by high end-diastolic velocity with continuous forward flow, reflective of a low-impedance circulation. In uteroplacental insufficiency, the changes in uterine artery resistance are reflected by an elevated pulsatility index, an elevated systolic-to-diastolic ratio, and the presence of a diastolic notch in Doppler ultrasonography.[94] These findings can be detected in early gestation but have limited resolution and reliability. Three-dimensional power Doppler ultrasound imaging can detect real-time vascularity and blood flow changes (i.e., vascular density, branching, caliber, and

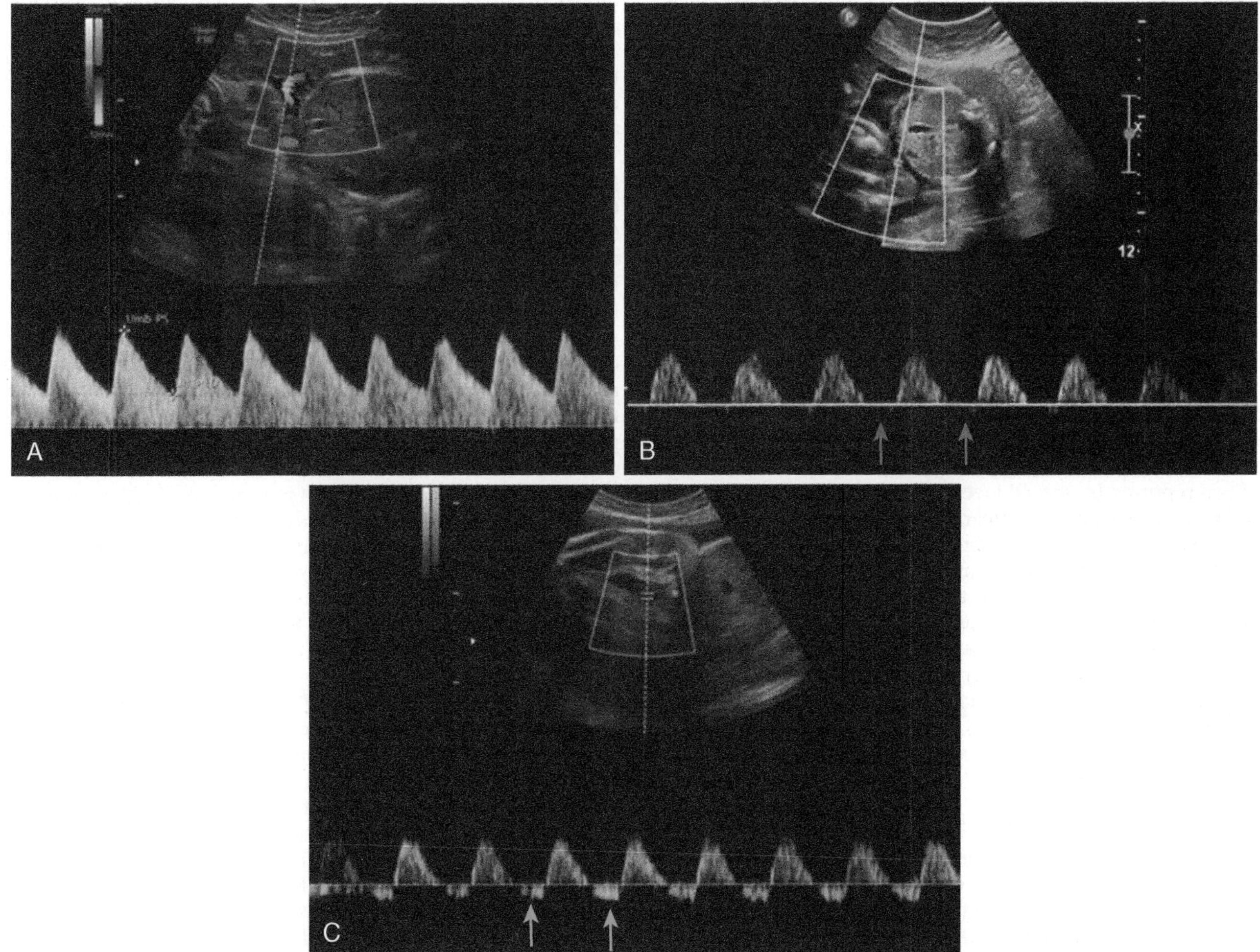

Fig. 14.3 Normal and abnormal Doppler flow velocity patterns in the umbilical artery. (A) Typical ultrasound appearance of normal umbilical artery Doppler flow velocity. (B) Absent end-diastolic flow (AEDF) pattern with no detectable flow in diastole *(red arrows)*. (C) Reversed end-diastolic flow (REDF) velocity as indicated by the *blue arrows*. (Images provided courtesy of Dr. Priya Rajan, Medical Director, Ultrasound. Department of Obstetrics & Gynecology, Division of Maternal-Fetal Medicine, Northwestern University Feinberg School of Medicine.)

tortuosity) beginning in the first trimester with greater detail than conventional ultrasound.[88,98-100] Three-D power Doppler ultrasound features of placentas in cases of severe IUGR include reduced placental vascularity and impaired budding of the villous circulation.[98]

Another re-emerging concept is that the mechanical stimulation of cells by the friction generated from blood flow (shear stress) is a fundamental determinant of vascular homeostasis, regulating vascular remodeling and vasomotor tone. Such mechanisms appear to be key drivers of placental development and function.[101] For example, shear stress generates flow-mediated vasodilation through the release of endothelial nitric oxide, a process vital for adequate placental blood flow.[102] Thus, failed establishment, suboptimal, or disrupted placental blood flow due to a variety of factors may be an early and persistent cause of delayed growth and development of both the placenta and the fetus throughout pregnancy.

ALTERATIONS IN CELL BIOLOGY AND FUNCTION

APOPTOSIS

An increased number of apoptotic nuclei have been observed in IUGR placentas[103-105] and may contribute to placental dysfunction.[106] Apoptosis is characterized by a series of morphologic cell changes including cell shrinkage, membrane blebbing, nuclear fragmentation, chromatic condensation, and chromosomal DNA fragmentation that lead to cell suicide.[107] Increased apoptosis has been observed in IUGR placentas in two distinct gestational periods: Apoptosis in early pregnancy is believed to be associated with impaired vascular remodeling, whereas increased apoptosis in late-gestation IUGR may contribute to impaired villous perfusion and trophoblast function.[105,108] Normal placental development depends on the invasion of maternal decidua by extravillous trophoblasts, followed by remodeling of maternal uterine spiral arteries to ensure anchoring of the placenta and to allow for a rapid increase in maternal-placental blood flow.[109] Decidual leukocytes, particularly uterine natural killer cells and macrophages, participate in the process of vascular smooth muscle cell apoptosis, contributing to vascular remodeling.[110] It has been proposed that exaggerated apoptosis contributes to suboptimal trophoblast invasion within spiral arteries.[108] As a consequence, maternal-placental blood flow fails to increase normally in gestation, contributing to altered placental function.[111,112] Exaggerated villous trophoblast apoptosis in IUGR has been reported by several investigators[105,113,114]; however, the underlying causes remain unclear. It is possible that hypoxia/oxidative stress activates trophoblast apoptotic pathways.[115] Fluctuating oxygen concentrations within the intervillous space caused by intermittent perfusion from the spiral arteries may lead to hypoxia-reoxygenation and villous injury.[116-118] In contrast, some investigators argue that IUGR is associated with placental hyperoxia.[119,120] Nevertheless, both hypoxia and hyperoxia may lead to oxidative stress, which is associated with reduced cytotrophoblast proliferation and increased rate of apoptosis.[59] Increased staining of proapoptotic proteins such as p53 and caspase 3 is observed in IUGR placentas.[114,121]

PLACENTAL CELL SIGNALING: OVERVIEW

The syncytiotrophoblast, the primary endocrine cell of the placenta, integrates a wide array of maternal and fetal signals to balance maternal supply and fetal demand by altering placental growth and function and by secreting signaling molecules, which directly alter maternal and fetal physiology. Although the mechanisms remain to be fully established, emerging evidence suggests that complex trophoblast signaling pathways are involved. In this chapter, we will focus on a few key pathways that have been linked to specific placental functions as illustrated in Fig. 14.4 and detailed below.

INSULIN/INSULIN-LIKE GROWTH FACTOR SIGNALING

Unlike postnatal growth, which is primarily regulated by growth hormone, insulin-like growth factors (IGFs) are the main regulators of fetal growth.[122] The IGF family consists of polypeptide ligands (insulin, IGF-1, and IGF-2), tyrosine kinase receptors (in particular, IGF-1 receptor), and IGF-binding proteins. IGF-1 and IGF-2 not only have mitogenic properties to induce somatic cell growth and proliferation but may also promote glucose and amino acid transport across the placenta.[123] After ligand binding, the IGF-1 receptor activates the mitogen-activated protein kinase/extracellular signal-regulated kinase and protein kinase B pathways, which mediates many of the cellular effects of insulin/IGF-1. Both in vivo and in vitro studies have demonstrated endocrine and autocrine/paracrine functions of IGFs in the regulation of placental function and fetal growth.[124] The IGF-binding proteins modulate IGF function by binding IGFs, thereby limiting the interaction between growth factors and their receptors. Phosphorylation of insulin-like growth factor-binding protein-1 (IGFBP-1) enhances its affinity for IGF-1, decreasing IGF-1 bioavailability and function. Conversely, decreased IGFBP-1 phosphorylation increases IGF-1 bioavailability, resulting in stimulation of amino acid uptake by human trophoblasts in vitro.[125] IUGR has been linked to alterations in the IGF axis both in animal models and in human studies. Placental IGFBP-1 expression[126,127] is increased and circulating levels of fetal[128,129] and maternal total and phosphorylated IGFBP-1[130,131] are increased in IUGR. In addition, it has recently been reported that first trimester maternal plasma IGFBP-1 is hyperphosphorylated in women who later deliver IUGR infants, suggesting its role as an early predictive biomarker.[132] Deletion of IGF-1, IGF-2, or IGF-1 receptor in transgenic mice models is associated with IUGR (Table 14.1).[133-135] In addition, reduced IGF-1 secretion from decidual explants[136] and decreased placental expression of IGF-1 have been reported in human IUGR.[126,137] However, immunohistochemistry and in situ hybridization studies have indicated increased expression of IGF-1 in specific sites of the placenta in IUGR, and this may represent a compensatory mechanism.[138] Overall, the activity of the placental insulin/IGF-1 signaling pathway, as determined by the degree of phosphorylation of key kinases in the signaling pathway, is decreased in human IUGR (see Fig. 14.4).[139,140] Because the insulin/IGF-1 signaling regulates multiple trophoblast functions (including synthesis of hormones such as human placental lactogen, chorionic gonadotrophin, and progesterone)[141] nutrient transport,[142] and protein synthesis (mediated by mTOR signaling, see below), decreased placental insulin/IGF-1 signaling in IUGR is expected to inhibit these functions (see Fig. 14.4).

MECHANISTIC TARGET OF RAPAMYCIN SIGNALING

Mechanistic target of rapamycin (mTOR) is a serine/threonine kinase, which controls cell growth and proliferation through regulation of translation and transcription in response to nutrient availability and growth factor signaling.[116-118] It is highly expressed in the human syncytiotrophoblast[143] and consists of two distinct complexes: mTORC1 contains the accessory protein *raptor*, whereas mTORC2 is associated with *rictor*. Cellular metabolism and growth mediated by regulation of protein synthesis are modulated by mTORC1.[144,145] In addition, mTORC1 is also a positive regulator of amino acid transport systems A and L,[143,146,147] which are critical in mediating transport of nonessential and essential amino acids to the fetus. The downstream effects of mTORC1 are mediated by

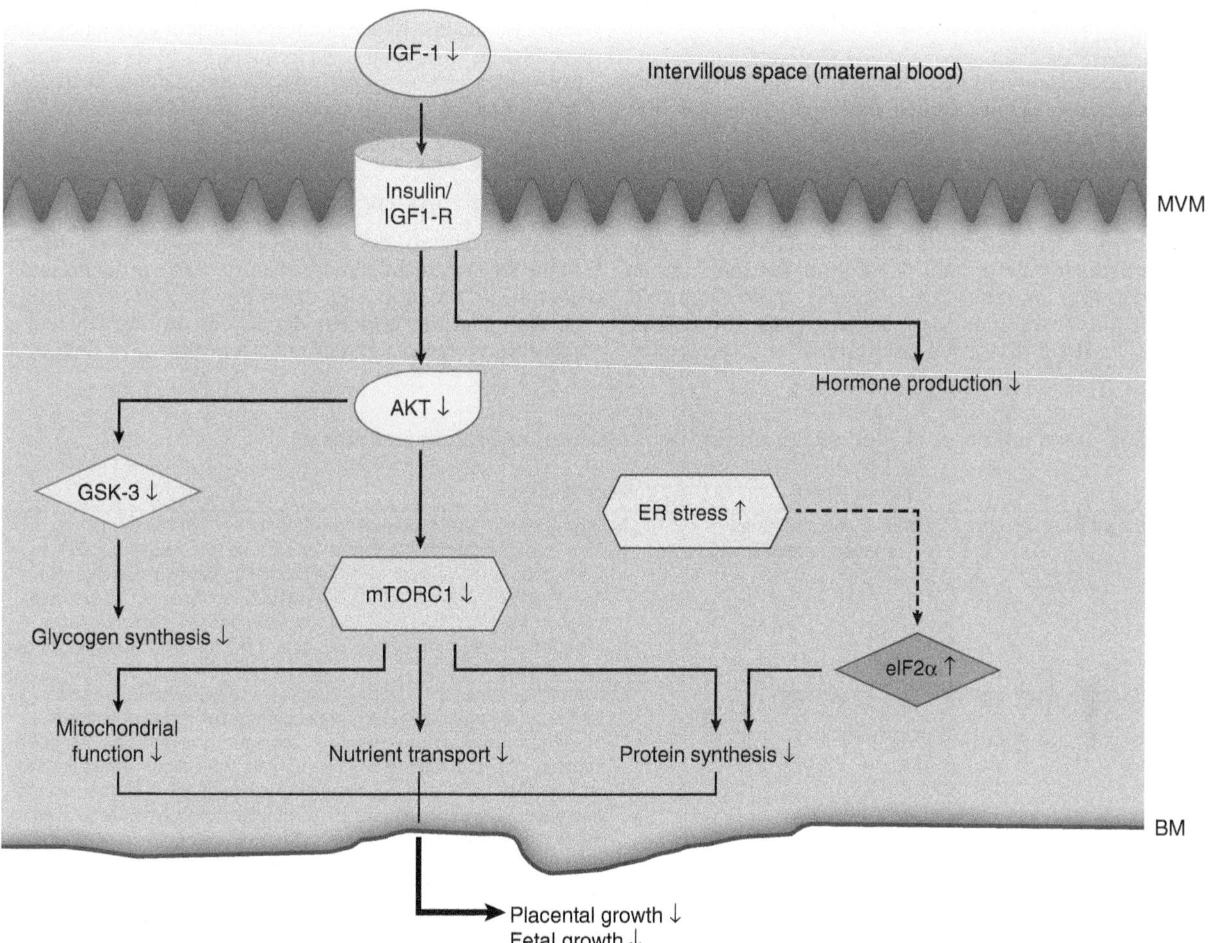

Fig. 14.4 Changes in placental signaling in intrauterine growth restriction (IUGR). Placental insulin/insulin-like growth factor-1 *(IGF-1)* and mechanistic target of rapamycin signaling is inhibited and the endoplasmic reticulum *(ER)* stress pathway is activated in IUGR. For details, see the text. *Solid lines* indicate inhibition in IUGR and *dotted line* indicates activation in IUGR. *AKT,* Protein kinase B; *BM,* basal plasma membrane; *eIF2α,* eukaryotic initiation factor 2α; *GSK-3,* glycogen synthase kinase 3; *IGF1-R,* IGF-1 receptor; *mTORC1,* mechanistic target of rapamycin complex 1; *MVM,* microvillous plasma membrane.

phosphorylation of 4E-binding protein 1 and the ribosomal protein S6 kinase,[148] which promote cap-dependent translation initiation.[149] Further, mTORC1 is stimulated by upstream Ras-related small G-protein Rheb and/or tuberous sclerosis complex 2. The heterodimeric complex of tuberous sclerosis complex 1 and tuberous sclerosis complex 2 stimulates the conversion of Rheb from its GTP-bound active form to a GDP-bound inactive form, thereby inhibiting mTORC1.[150] Growth factors, such as insulin and IGF-1, and cytokines activate mTORC1 by inhibiting tuberous sclerosis complex 2. Thus, mTORC1 activity is controlled directly by cellular nutrient and energy levels and indirectly by systemic nutrient availability and metabolism mediated by hormones and growth factors.[137,151-153] A multitude of signals may impinge on placental mTOR signaling, resulting in inhibition of this signaling pathway in IUGR.[140,143] Recent studies of mTOR signaling have shown that mTORC1 promotes the expression of genes encoding electron transport chain proteins and stimulates oxidative phosphorylation in primary human trophoblast cells by regulating mitochondrial biogenesis.[154] Because mTORC1 is a positive regulator of protein synthesis, nutrient transport, and mitochondrial function, decreased placental mTOR signaling may cause inhibition of these important trophoblast functions in IUGR (see Fig. 14.4). While placental mTORC1 and mTORC2 signaling activities are inhibited in studies of human idiopathic[155-158] as well as malaria-induced IUGR, total protein expression of mTOR varies[140,156,159] and may indicate a regulatory role of these complexes in response to inhibition.

ENDOPLASMIC RETICULUM STRESS SIGNALING

The endoplasmic reticulum (ER) has several specific functions, including synthesis, folding, and transport of membrane and secretory proteins, as well as calcium storage. Disturbances that interfere with ER homeostasis result in ER stress and trigger the unfolded protein response, which initiates homeostatic mechanisms to prevent further damage but can lead to cell death with prolonged unfolded protein response activation.[160] The unfolded protein response comprises three principal signaling pathways with involvement of protein kinase R–like ER kinase, inositol-requiring enzyme 1, and activating transcription factor 6 (ATF6). Recent studies have identified associations between ER stress, autophagy, and protein synthesis inhibition in the placentas of pregnancies complicated by IUGR (see Fig. 14.4).[109,157,158] Specifically, ER stress leads to increased phosphorylation of eukaryotic initiation factor 2α (eIF2α), resulting in inhibition of protein synthesis (see Fig. 14.4).[161] The reduced protein synthesis in the IUGR placenta in response to inhibition of mTOR signaling and activation of ER stress pathways has been proposed to contribute to smaller placental size.

PEROXISOME PROLIFERATOR–ACTIVATED RECEPTOR SIGNALING

Peroxisome proliferator-activated receptors (PPARs), a family of nuclear proteins, are ligand-activated transcription factors that regulate gene expression. Studies in mice and cultured human primary trophoblasts have demonstrated that PPARs are critical for placental development and regulate trophoblast invasion and differentiation.[162,163] Changes in placental PPAR expression have been implicated in the pathophysiology of IUGR.[164,165] PPARγ forms a heterodimer with retinoid X receptor and functions as an insulin sensitizer by regulating fatty acid uptake and lipid storage.[166,167] The observation that placental PPARγ expression is increased in IUGR has been interpreted as a protective response against hypoxia and/or nutrient deficiency caused by insufficient placental development.[164,168,169] Although PPARγ expression appears to vary widely among different studies,[170–172] its compelling role in mediating trophoblast differentiation in hypoxia-induced placental insufficiency makes it a promising therapeutic target for preeclampsia and IUGR.[173,174]

NUTRIENT TRANSPORT: OVERVIEW

The placenta transfers nutrients and oxygen from the maternal to the fetal circulation and transports waste products and carbon dioxide in the opposite direction. Because fetal growth and development are critically dependent on nutrient and oxygen availability, changes in placental transport may directly lead to

Table 14.1 Animal Models of Placental Function and Intrauterine Growth Restriction.

Approach	Animal Models	Main Findings
Maternal nutrient deprivation	Non-human primates (baboon), rats, sheep	Maternal calorie restriction from gestational day 30–165 (term 180–184) inhibits placental insulin/IGF-1, which results in IUGR through down-regulation of mTOR signaling pathways, decreased expression of key placental AA and GLUT isoforms, and lower fetal levels of essential AA.[242] In rats, maternal protein restriction leads to inhibited placental mTOR signaling, and decreased in vitro and in vivo AA transport[181,182,243]
Umbilical or uterine artery ligation	Guinea pig/rats	Unilateral uterine artery ligation (Wigglesworth), allows study of both IUGR and normal-sized pups in the same dam.[244] Uterine artery ligation in mid-pregnancy leads to decreased placental AA transport capacity[245] and in vivo transplacental glucose and AA transport and subsequent IUGR.[246] Fetal circulating levels of IGF-1 and insulin are decreased, IGFBP increased.[247] In rats, ligation is also associated with decreased placental expression of the IGF-1 receptor, reduction in placental lactogen production, and decreased placental glucose and amino acid transport.[248]
Placental embolization	Sheep	Produces placental growth restriction and singleton IUGR. Used to evaluate promising maternal interventions for IUGR: Intra-amniotic IGF-1 treatment,[249] and maternal growth hormone.[250] Most recently used to investigate maternal administration of sildenafil in management of IUGR.[251]
Maternal corticosteroid administration	Mouse	Model of maternal stress: Antenatal administration of synthetic glucocorticoids inhibits placental System A activity leading to reduction in availability of AA to the fetus.[252]
Maternal hyperthermia exposure	Sheep	Elevated maternal body temperature interferes with placental development, causing decreased placental oxygen diffusion and nutrient transport capacity (glucose, leucine, threonine, inhibition of mTOR signaling).[85,253–257] Placental VEGF shows biphasic expression pattern over gestation.[258]
Maternal LPS administration	Sheep, rats	Lipopolysaccharide (LPS) injection from 100 to 112th day of gestation in pregnant ewes induces maternal inflammation and IUGR, via fetal inflammation, reduced B-cell function, and impaired skeletal muscle glucose metabolism.[259] Inflammation-induced IUGR in pregnant rats receiving LPS on days 13.5–16.5 yields altered placental morphometrics.[260] IUGR mediated by TNF-α is associated with deficient trophoblast invasion and spiral artery remodeling, as well as altered uteroplacental hemodynamics.[261]
Maternal hypertension	Mice	Thromboxane A2 (TXA2), a potent vasoconstrictor, induces maternal hypertension and mimics human placental insufficiency-induced IUGR.[262] Growth-restricted pups exhibit white matter injury[263] and intestinal inflammation.[264]
Genetic modification	Mice	The role of the IGF axis has been elucidated by several groups.[135,196,265] Both *igf1*- and *igf2*-mutant mice demonstrate marked IUGR.[134,135] Transgenic mice lacking IGF-1 receptors show altered placental development and IUGR.[133,135] Mice with a placental-specific deletion of *igf2* have placental growth restriction, but placental expression and activity of specific nutrient transporters are up-regulated before IUGR develops[210,211] suggesting that the fetus signals the placenta to upregulate growth and nutrient transport in response to impending IUGR.[211,266]

AA, Amino acids; *GLUT*, glucose transporter; *IGF-1*, insulin-like growth factor-1; *IGFBP*, insulin-like growth factor-binding protein; *IUGR*, Intrauterine growth restriction; *mTOR*, mechanistic target of rapamycin; *TNFα*, tumor necrosis factor-alpha; *VEGF*, vascular endothelial growth factor.

IUGR. The syncytiotrophoblast is the transporting epithelium of the human placenta and constitutes the primary barrier for nutrient and oxygen flux. Because most nutrient transporters must be inserted in the plasma membrane of the cell to mediate transepithelial transport, investigators have compared transporter protein expression and activity in isolated syncytiotrophoblast, specifically the apical or microvillous plasma membrane (MVM), and basal plasma membrane (BM), in IUGR and normal placentas.[175,176] Changes in MVM and BM activity of nutrient transporters with IUGR are summarized in Fig. 14.5 and detailed below.

GLUCOSE

Transplacental glucose transport is mediated by facilitated diffusion through specific GLUTs. A higher density of GLUTs in the MVM, together with the greater surface area, allows rapid glucose uptake into the syncytiotrophoblast and thus provides a maximal gradient for transfer to the fetus across the BM.[177] Several GLUT isoforms are expressed in the human syncytiotrophoblast. GLUT1 is the main isoform mediating glucose transport across the placenta throughout pregnancy.[177] The placental expression of GLUT1 protein and glucose transport activity are unaffected by IUGR, and fetal hypoglycemia in IUGR is unlikely due to changes in placental GLUT expression or activity.[177,178]

AMINO ACIDS

The placental activity of several amino acid transporters is reduced with IUGR. The activity of system A, an Na^+-dependent transporter mediating the uptake of nonessential amino acids, is lower in MVM isolated from IUGR placentas.[179,180] System A activity in MVM is additionally affected by gestational age, as term IUGR fetuses are less affected than preterm IUGR fetuses.[178] Furthermore, the most severe cases of IUGR are associated with the most pronounced decreases in MVM system A activity.[179] It is unclear whether the reduction in placental amino acid transport occurs before fetal growth restriction or as a consequence of reduced fetal needs. In a rodent model of IUGR, a reduction in system A activity has been shown to precede impaired fetal growth,[181,182] suggesting that down-regulation of system. A transporters may be directly contributing to the development of IUGR. The activity of transporters of essential amino acids, including system β (taurine) and system L (lysine and leucine), has also been found to be reduced in the MVM and/or BM of IUGR placentas in vitro.[183,184] This is compatible with findings of reduced placental transfer of the essential amino acids leucine and phenylalanine in IUGR term pregnancies using stable-isotope techniques.[185] Down-regulation of placental amino acid transporters results in the reduction of amino acid transport to the fetus and may account for the low plasma levels of certain amino acids in growth-restricted fetuses.[151,186]

LIPIDS

The activity of lipoprotein lipase, an enzyme responsible for hydrolysis of lipoproteins, is reduced in MVM of IUGR placentas.[187] However, placental lipoprotein lipase mRNA expression is increased in IUGR, possibly representing a

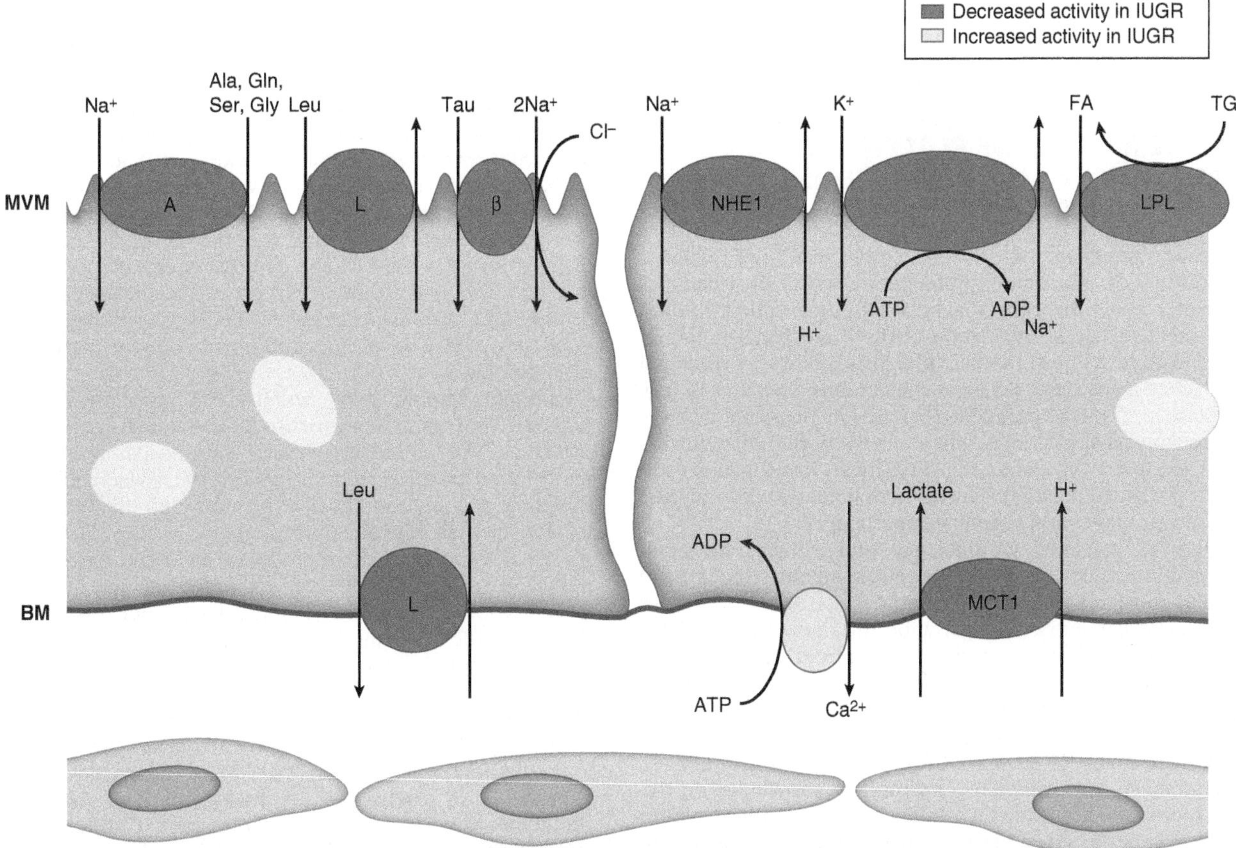

Fig. 14.5 Alterations in placental transport in intrauterine growth restriction (IUGR). Increased *(blue)* and decreased *(red)* transporter activity in syncytiotrophoblast microvillous plasma membrane *(MVM)* and basal plasma membrane *(BM)* isolated from IUGR placentas, as compared with gestational age–matched appropriate-for-gestational-age controls. For details, see the text. *A*, System A; *Ala*, alanine; *β*, system β; *FA*, fatty acid; *Gln*, glutamine; *Gly*, glycine; *L*, system L; *Leu*, leucine; *LPL*, lipoprotein lipase; *MCT1*, monocarboxylate transporter 1; *NHE1*, Na^+-H^+ exchanger 1; *Ser*, serine; *Tau*, taurine; *TG*, triglyceride.

compensatory mechanism or reflecting that MVM lipoprotein lipase activity is not regulated at a transcriptional level.[188] IUGR is associated with reduced placental expression of lipoprotein receptors, low-density lipoprotein, and scavenger receptor class B type-I, the key receptors for cholesterol uptake from maternal low-density lipoprotein and/or high-density lipoprotein.[189] In contrast, MVM fatty acid transport protein-6 expression is increased and long-chain polyunsaturated fatty acids are routed toward cellular storage in triglycerides in the IUGR placenta, possibly representing a protective response to elevated oxidant stress associated with cellular fatty acid accumulation.[190] Collectively, these findings suggest that placental lipid transport may be impaired, which could contribute to the decreased lipid stores in the IUGR fetus.[191]

ION TRANSPORT

Alterations in placental ion transport have been implicated in IUGR. Both the activity and expression of the Na^+-H^+ exchanger, the primary pH-regulating transporter in the syncytiotrophoblast, are reduced, and this could explain the development of acidosis in IUGR neonates resulting from decreased capacity to export metabolically produced protons in the fetus to the maternal circulation.[192] Furthermore, MVM Na^+,K^+-ATPase activity is decreased in IUGR, which may impair the function of all transporters dependent on the Na^+ gradient for energy (see Fig. 14.5).[193] Conversely, BM Ca^{2+}-ATPase is up-regulated in IUGR placentas, possibly because of elevated fetal concentrations of parathyroid hormone–related peptide 38-94, a key regulator of the placental calcium pump.[194] IUGR also affects the placental lactate transporter, which is responsible for clearance of fetal lactate accumulated during hypoxia. Decreased BM lactate transporter activity may contribute to the increased fetal lactate levels associated with IUGR and impair the ability of the IUGR fetus to tolerate stress.[195]

ANIMAL MODELS OF PLACENTAL DYSFUNCTION AND INTRAUTERINE GROWTH RESTRICTION

Enhanced understanding of the molecular and cellular mechanisms of placental dysfunction have provided us with better tools for early diagnosis of, intervention in, and management of IUGR. Elucidation of these mechanisms would not be possible without the use of animal models, as placental studies in humans have significant limitations. Specifically, it is difficult to perform experimental studies in pregnant women, and mechanisms of placental function in liveborn human infants can be explored only after delivery; these investigations are typically restricted to late gestation.These limitations can, at least in part, be circumvented in animal experiments.

Models of placental insufficiency and IUGR have been developed in several animal species and are summarized in Table 14.1. The most commonly used approaches to induce IUGR include maternal nutrient deprivation, uterine artery ligation, placental embolization, maternal corticosteroid administration, and exposure to high ambient temperature.[196,197] Because of extensive similarities in genetics, physiology, and anatomy with humans, non-human primate models, including the baboon, are highly relevant for studies of IUGR.[198] Moreover, studies in pregnant sheep have generated a wealth of knowledge on the fetal responses to placental insufficiency; however, the structure and function of the sheep placenta are distinct from those of the human placenta, somewhat limiting the value of this species in studies of placental physiology. Rodents are also frequently used, a major advantage being their short gestation, allowing affordable studies of placental dysfunction and long-term follow-up of IUGR offspring. In addition, the mouse is the model of choice for mechanistic studies because of well-established techniques for gene targeting in this species. In recent years, the use of CRISPR-Cas9 technology has provided new insights into the contribution of the genome to normal placental development, and demonstrated that far more genes are required for normal placentation than previously appreciated.[199] However, rodents are polytocous, and their metabolism differs significantly from that of the human, which needs to be taken into account when one is extrapolating data obtained in the rodent to pregnant women.

ALTERATIONS IN PLACENTAL GENE EXPRESSION

EPIGENOMICS

Epigenetic regulation, which alters gene expression without changing the underlying DNA sequence and involves processes such as gene methylation and histone modification, has emerged as an important mechanism by which gene expression is modulated by environmental factors such as nutrition and hypoxia.[200-202] Epigenetic regulation has been proposed to constitute a critical link between environmental stimuli and placental development, fetal growth, and later disease.[203,204]

Methylation of genes on cytosine residues by DNA methyltransferases, in particular at CpG islands associated with the promoter region, typically results in decreased transcription. *Genomic imprinting* refers to silencing of one parental allele by methylation, leading to monoallelic expression of the gene.[205] Imprinted genes are critical for placental development and function, thereby influencing fetal growth.[206-208] Two of the most well-studied imprinted genes in the placenta are *IGF2* and *H19*, which are located close to each other at 11p15.5 and have opposite effects on placental growth and function.[209] *IGF2* is an example of a maternally imprinted (paternally expressed) gene, which stimulates placental growth.[210,211] In contrast, *H19* is a paternally imprinted (maternally expressed) gene encoding a regulatory, long noncoding RNA, which has growth-suppressing functions through inhibition of *IGF2* RNA translation.[212] *H19* therefore controls the imprinting of the *IGF2* locus, and deletion of *H19* results in the biallelic expression of *IGF2* and increased fetal and placental growth.[213] In mice, placenta-specific deletion of the *igf2* transcript causes IUGR.[211] In humans, IUGR is associated with loss of imprinting and aberrant methylation of placental *IFG2*.[214]

Although global gene methylation appears not to be different between appropriate-for-gestational-age and IUGR placentas,[215,216] there are several factors that influence DNA methylation patterns in humans (sex, age, tissue and cell types, sampling, and environmental exposures) and that likely account for the lack of reproducibility among studies.[217] Changes in placental expression of microRNAs, including miR-16, miR-21, miR-518b, miR-1323, miR-520h, and miR-519d, may be associated with IUGR.[218,219] There is emerging evidence that these and other microRNA changes may be induced by environmental toxins that compromise placental function.[220,221]

TRANSCRIPTOMICS

Changes in the expression of placental genes may be involved in the pathogenesis of IUGR.With use of microarray technology, expression of thousands of transcripts can be screened simultaneously, facilitating the exploration of differential gene expression in IUGR.A large number of genes have been reported to be up-regulated or down-regulated in the IUGR placenta.[222,223] For example, elevated gene expression of leptin, corticotrophin-releasing hormone, and IGF-binding protein 1 (IGFBP-1) in IUGR placentas supports known mechanisms of IUGR via similarly increased circulating protein levels, and binding of fetal growth factors IGF-1 and IGF-2.[222] Other microarray studies have reported an up-regulation of transcripts for VEGF in IUGR placentas, which is believed to reflect the adaptation of trophoblast cells to hypoxia.[224,225] In contrast, the decrease in mRNA expression of human placental lactogen, predominantly expressed in the syncytiotrophoblast, in IUGR placentas may be due to hypoxia-induced inhibition of trophoblast differentiation.[224]

More recently, RNA-seq approaches have the capacity to detect lower abundance transcripts and a broader dynamic range than microarray, allowing for detection of more differentially expressed genes with higher fold-change. Similar to the limitations in human studies of placental epigenomics, variations and reproducibility of the data rely heavily upon timing and sampling of placental tissues. Emerging single-cell RNA-seq approaches will allow more enhanced resolution. For example, in a recent study of sorted placental cells from first- and second-trimester human placentas, single-cell RNA-seq identified new subtypes of cells of the cytotrophoblast and extravillous trophoblast, and revealed previously unknown functions of the human placenta. Most notable were 102 polypeptide hormone genes found to be expressed by various subtypes of placental cells, suggesting a complex and significant role of these hormones in regulating fetal growth and adaptations of maternal physiology during pregnancy.[226]

METABOLOMICS

Metabolomics, defined as large-scale comprehensive analysis of the downstream metabolites of the transcriptome, is an emerging technology in the era of precision medicine.[227] Its application to the study of the pathophysiology of IUGR is of considerable interest, given the detailed characterization of metabolic derangements that could be linked back to nutritional exchange and metabolic programming mechanisms of the placenta. The placental metabolome appears to vary according to maternal preeclampsia and IUGR status. A recent study using high-resolution magic angle spinning (HR-MAS) nuclear magnetic resonance spectroscopy to phenotype the preeclamptic placenta found several altered metabolic pathways, in particular placental metabolites that correlate with sFlt-1 and triglycerides in maternal serum.[228] These findings have been further validated in recent metabolomics studies of human placentas with none, moderate, and severe dysfunction, in which increased placental sFlt-1 alone could separate pregnancies with and without placental dysfunction.[229] While sFlt-1 is emerging as a precision biomarker for placental dysfunction, levels of maternal and fetal (cord) serum/plasma are highly correlated and may serve as useful clinical markers of IUGR and its sequelae. Similar studies of metabolic profiling and targeted lipidomics in maternal and fetal blood samples are also promising.[230]

INTEGRATED PLACENTAL RESPONSE AND ADAPTATION IN INTRAUTERINE GROWTH RESTRICTION

An incomplete trophoblast invasion resulting in a poor spiral artery remodeling, which restricts the normal increase in uteroplacental blood flow in mid-pregnancy is the most common cause of IUGR in developed countries. Historically, it was often assumed that placental insufficiency (i.e., impaired delivery of nutrients and oxygen to the fetus) was due to a reduced placental blood flow. However, the placental blood flow reduction per se does not adequately explain the impaired placental transfer in IUGR. Oxygen, which is highly lipophilic, diffuses rapidly across the placental barrier, and placental oxygen transfer may therefore be primarily limited by the rate of blood flow, and to some degree by the barrier thickness. In these situations, reduction in uteroplacental and umbilical blood flows is thought to be the primary contributor to fetal hypoxia in IUGR. In contrast, transplacental transport of nutrients is less affected by changes in blood flow because transport across the barrier is the primary limiting factor for effective transfer of these molecules. Thus, placental insufficiency is not just a matter of reduced blood flow or a small placenta. Instead, the complex regulation of multiple placental signaling pathways (see Fig. 14.4) and down-regulation of placental nutrient transporters (see Fig. 14.5) may more directly contribute to the development of IUGR than previously understood.

Widely different causes of IUGR, such as maternal undernutrition, high altitude, and reduced uteroplacental blood flow after suboptimal trophoblast invasion, appear to result in strikingly similar changes in placental histology, signaling, and function.[158,182] This suggests that there are key final common pathways that are regulated in the placenta in response to different perturbations. Jansson and colleagues propose that *placental nutrient sensing* is a function by which the placenta integrates a multitude of maternal and fetal nutritional cues with information from intrinsic nutrient sensing signaling pathways to balance fetal demand with the ability of the mother to support the pregnancy by regulating maternal physiology, placental growth, and nutrient transport.[197,231] Maternal signals conveying nutritional information to the placenta may include metabolic hormones such as cortisol, insulin, leptin, and adiponectin, which are known to reflect maternal nutritional status and regulate placental transport.[181,232] Other maternal signals that may be "sensed" by the placenta are oxygen, nutrient levels, and uteroplacental blood flow. Trophoblast mTOR signaling is one important component of the placental nutrient sensor.[147,233] According to the placental nutrient sensing model, matching fetal growth to maternal resources will produce an offspring that is smaller but that, in most instances, will survive and reproduce. Rather than excess extraction of nutrients from the deprived mother, which would jeopardize the survival of both the mother and her fetus, fetal growth restriction is a necessary evolutionary compromise.[197]

IMPLICATIONS FOR INTERVENTION

Not all placental changes associated with IUGR reflect dysfunction or injury. As described above, they constitute adaptations to fine-tune maternal-fetal resource allocation in response to various maternal and fetal signals. If the initial perturbation is prolonged and severe, placental dysfunction and injury may occur. These may in turn affect various organ systems of the developing fetus, in addition to overall somatic growth. Understanding the mechanisms underlying placental adaptation and dysfunction in IUGR, and their biologic effects on the newborn infant, may help identify new intervention strategies to prevent or alleviate restricted fetal growth and its adverse consequences. For example, maternal IGF-1 administration has been explored in animal models as a strategy to improve placental function and fetal growth in IUGR. IGF-1 has a multitude of effects on placental growth and function, but increased nutrient transfer is believed to be one important mechanism by which IGF-1 treatment may improve outcomes.[234]

Interventions that focus on improving uteroplacental perfusion have also been reported. Aspirin, originally prescribed for its anti-thrombotic properties, was initially reported in the mid-1980s to have efficacy in preventing preeclampsia. During the past several decades, there has been growing evidence that the proangiogenic and anti-inflammatory properties of aspirin may also support placentation.[235] Numerous clinical trials and a recent meta-analysis support its efficacy during early pregnancy.[236] Although the timing and duration of aspirin therapy, as well as its role in preventing IUGR, are still controversial, widespread use in women at risk for preeclampsia is growing.[235] Another established pharmacologic agent is the phosphodiesterase-5 inhibitor, sildenafil citrate, which has been shown to increase fetal abdominal circumference in human IUGR; increased maternal placental blood flow has been proposed as a possible mechanism.[238] Despite promising results in pre-clinical studies, the immediate and long-term side effects of sildenafil administration during pregnancy remain unclear. Relatively newer potential interventions include gene therapies such as adenoviral vectors that mediate overexpression of VEGF in the uterine arteries, which increase uterine artery blood flow in pregnant sheep,[239] but these have yet to be translated into human clinical trials.

In situations of impending fetal demise due to uteroplacental insufficiency, medically indicated delivery remains the mainstay of intervention. Depending upon the severity, timing of onset and diagnosis, IUGR due to placental insufficiency often results in preterm delivery. The risks of complications due to prematurity may increase considerably with lower gestational age and the severity of growth restriction.[240,241] Therefore, interventions tailored to support neonatal growth and development, as well as recovery of organ systems impacted by placental dysfunction, may also improve survival and outcomes of IUGR.

CONCLUSION

The available evidence presented in this chapter illustrate that changes in placental function associated with IUGR represent an adaptive and compensatory response to allocate adequate maternal resources to the developing fetus. Emerging evidence indicates that widely different causes of IUGR appear to result in strikingly similar changes in placental signaling and function.[158,182] These changes are complex and remain poorly understood, highlighting an urgent need for further well-designed and mechanistic research that integrates human studies with animal models. Intervention strategies to alleviate or prevent IUGR must take into account the effects of placental adaptive responses. Interventions targeting maternal health and neonatal management, using the placenta and its correlates as biomarkers to discern individualized pathophysiology, may be promising approaches in future studies to improve the pregnancy outcomes complicated by IUGR.

SUMMARY

IUGR is associated with changes in placental structure and function, as evidenced by alterations in placental development, as well as changes in cell signaling, transport, and epigenetic processes. Structural changes in the IUGR placenta are indicated by gross and microscopic histologic lesions that suggest altered placentation, blood flow, and angiogenesis, as well as inflammatory changes that impact placental regulatory and barrier functions. Functional changes in the IUGR placenta include inhibition of insulin/IGF-I and mTOR signaling; activation of ER stress pathways; decreased activity of transporters for amino acids, protons, and sodium; and increased activity of the calcium pump. These functions may further impact, or be affected by, placental expression of somatic and angiogenic growth factors at the epigenetic or transcriptional level. Widely different causes of IUGR, such as maternal undernutrition, high altitude, and reduced uteroplacental blood flow after suboptimal trophoblast invasion, appear to result in strikingly similar changes in placental signaling and function, suggesting a common placental response to an inability of the maternal supply line to deliver nutrients and oxygen to the fetus. Well-developed animal models indicate that these changes are not a consequence of IUGR but directly contribute to the development of restricted fetal growth. Emerging evidence indicates that the placenta acts as a nutrient sensor to integrate maternal and fetal nutritional cues to match fetal demand with maternal supply by regulating maternal physiology, placental growth, and nutrient transport. Thus, many of the observed placental changes in IUGR may reflect an adaptive response to a compromised maternal supply line rather than primary dysfunction or injury. Intervention strategies to alleviate or prevent IUGR must take into account the effects of the placental adaptive response and its impact on somatic growth and end organ development of the fetus and neonate.

ACKNOWLEDGMENTS

We thank the previous authors, Yi-Yung Chen and Thomas Jansson, for their foundational work and expertise in writing the previous version of this chapter, many of the sections and figures which have been preserved in this revision.

A complete reference list is available at www.ExpertConsult.com. 

REFERENCES

1. Romo A, Carceller R, Tobajas J. Intrauterine growth retardation (IUGR): epidemiology and etiology. *Pediatr Endocrinol Rev*. 2009;6(suppl 3):332–336.
2. Maulik D. Fetal growth compromise: definitions, standards, and classification. *Clin Obstet Gynecol*. 2006;49(2):214–218.
4. Kesavan K, Devaskar SU. Intrauterine growth restriction: postnatal monitoring and outcomes. *Pediatr Clin North Am*. 2019;66(2):403–423.
10. Grantz KL, Hediger ML, Liu D, Buck Louis GM. Fetal growth standards: the NICHD fetal growth study approach in context with INTERGROWTH-21st and the World Health Organization multicentre growth reference study. *Am J Obstet Gynecol*. 2018;218(2S):S641–S655.e628.
13. Detti L, Mari G, Cheng CC, Bahado-Singh RO. Fetal Doppler velocimetry. *Obstet-Gynecol Clin North Am*. 2004;31(1):201–214.
15. Sharma D, Shastri S, Sharma P. Intrauterine growth restriction: antenatal and postnatal aspects. *Clin Med Insights Pediatr*. 2016;10:67–83.
25. Longo S, Bollani L, Decembrino L, Di Comite A, Angelini M, Stronati M. Short-term and long-term sequelae in intrauterine growth retardation (IUGR). *J Matern Fetal Neonatal Med*. 2013;26(3):222–225.
27. Barker DJ, Thornburg KL. Placental programming of chronic diseases, cancer and lifespan: a review. *Placenta*. 2013;34(10):841–845.
46. Maulik D. Fetal growth restriction: the etiology. *Clin Obstet Gynecol*. 2006;49(2):228–235.
49. Burton GJ, Jauniaux E. Pathophysiology of placental-derived fetal growth restriction. *Am J Obstet Gynecol*. 2018;218(2S):S745–S761.
50. Brosens I, Pijnenborg R, Vercruysse L, Romero R. The "Great Obstetrical Syndromes" are associated with disorders of deep placentation. *Am J Obstet Gynecol*. 2011;204(3):193–201.
51. Khong Y, Brosens I. Defective deep placentation. *Best Pract Res Clin Obstet Gynaecol*. 2011;25(3):301–311.
55. Khong TY, Mooney EE, Ariel I, et al. Sampling and definitions of placental lesions: Amsterdam placental workshop group consensus statement. *Arch Pathol Lab Med*. 2016;140(7):698–713.
60. Todros T, Sciarrone A, Piccoli E, Guiot C, Kaufmann P, Kingdom J. Umbilical Doppler waveforms and placental villous angiogenesis in pregnancies complicated by fetal growth restriction. *Obstet Gynecol*. 1999;93(4):499–503.
64. Derricott H, Jones RL, Heazell AE. Investigating the association of villitis of unknown etiology with stillbirth and fetal growth restriction - a systematic review. *Placenta*. 2013;34(10):856–862.
74. Kingdom J, Huppertz B, Seaward G, Kaufmann P. Development of the placental villous tree and its consequences for fetal growth. *Eur J Obstet Gynecol Reprod Biol*. 2000;92(1):35–43.
79. Chen DB, Zheng J. Regulation of placental angiogenesis. *Microcirculation*. 2014;21(1):15–25.
81. Maynard SE, Min JY, Merchan J, et al. Excess placental soluble fms-like tyrosine kinase 1 (sFlt1) may contribute to endothelial dysfunction, hypertension, and proteinuria in preeclampsia. *J Clin Invest*. 2003;111(5):649–658.
85. Regnault TR, de Vrijer B, Galan HL, et al. The relationship between transplacental O2 diffusion and placental expression of PlGF, VEGF and their receptors in a placental insufficiency model of fetal growth restriction. *J Physiol*. 2003;550(Pt 2):641–656.
88. Todros T, Piccoli E, Rolfo A, et al. Review: feto-placental vascularization: a multifaceted approach. *Placenta*. 2011;32(suppl 2):S165–S169.
91. Kuzmina IY, Hubina-Vakulik GI, Burton GJ. Placental morphometry and Doppler flow velocimetry in cases of chronic human fetal hypoxia. *Eur J Obstet Gynecol Reprod Biol*. 2005;120(2):139–145.
94. Cruz-Martinez R, Figueras F. The role of Doppler and placental screening. *Best Pract Res Clin Obstet Gynaecol*. 2009;23(6):845–855.
100. Yamasato K, Zalud I. Three dimensional power Doppler of the placenta and its clinical applications. *J Perinat Med*. 2017;45(6):693–700.
109. Burton GJ, Jauniaux E. The cytotrophoblastic shell and complications of pregnancy. *Placenta*. 2017;60:134–139.

111. Burton GJ, Jauniaux E, Charnock-Jones DS. The influence of the intrauterine environment on human placental development. *Int J Dev Biol*. 2010;54(2-3):303-312.
115. Burton GJ, Jauniaux E. Placental oxidative stress: from miscarriage to preeclampsia. *J Soc GynecolInvestig*. 2004;11(6):342-352.
123. Kniss DA, Shubert PJ, Zimmerman PD, Landon MB, Gabbe SG. Insulinlike growth factors. Their regulation of glucose and amino acid transport in placental trophoblasts isolated from first-trimester chorionic villi. *J Reprod Med*. 1994;39(4):249-256.
132. Gupta MB, Abu Shehab M, Nygard K, et al. IUGR is associated with marked hyperphosphorylation of decidual and maternal plasma IGFBP-1. *J Clin Endocrinol Metab*. 2019;104(2):408-422.
133. Crossey PA, Pillai CC, Miell JP. Altered placental development and intrauterine growth restriction in IGF binding protein-1 transgenic mice. *J Clin Invest*. 2002;110(3):411-418.
137. Calvo MT, Romo A, Gutierrez JJ, Relano E, Barrio E, FerrandezLongas A. Study of genetic expression of intrauterine growth factors IGF-I and EGFR in placental tissue from pregnancies with intrauterine growth retardation. *J Pediatr Endocrinol Metab*. 2004;17(suppl 3):445-450.
140. Yung HW, Calabrese S, Hynx D, et al. Evidence of placental translation inhibition and endoplasmic reticulum stress in the etiology of human intrauterine growth restriction. *Am J Pathol*. 2008;173(2):451-462.
143. Roos S, Jansson N, Palmberg I, Saljo K, Powell TL, Jansson T. Mammalian target of rapamycin in the human placenta regulates leucine transport and is down-regulated in restricted fetal growth. *J Physiol*. 2007;582(Pt 1):449-459.
157. Hung TH, Hsieh TT, Wu CP, Li MJ, Yeh YL, Chen SF. Mammalian target of rapamycin signaling is a mechanistic link between increased endoplasmic reticulum stress and autophagy in the placentas of pregnancies complicated by growth restriction. *Placenta*. 2017;60:9-20.
163. Schaiff WT, Barak Y, Sadovsky Y. The pleiotropic function of PPAR gamma in the placenta. *Mol Cell Endocrinol*. 2006;249(1-2):10-15.
165. Murthi P, Kalionis B, Cocquebert M, et al. Homeobox genes and down-stream transcription factor PPARgamma in normal and pathological human placental development. *Placenta*. 2013;34(4):299-309.
175. Jansson T, Myatt L, Powell TL. The role of trophoblast nutrient and ion transporters in the development of pregnancy complications and adult disease. *Curr Vasc Pharmacol*. 2009;7(4):521-533.
178. Jansson T, Ylven K, Wennergren M, Powell TL. Glucose transport and system A activity in syncytiotrophoblast microvillous and basal plasma membranes in intrauterine growth restriction. *Placenta*. 2002;23(5):392-399.
182. Rosario FJ, Jansson N, Kanai Y, Prasad PD, Powell TL, Jansson T. Maternal protein restriction in the rat inhibits placental insulin, mTOR, and STAT3 signaling and down-regulates placental amino acid transporters. *Endocrinology*. 2011;152(3):1119-1129.
187. Magnusson AL, Waterman IJ, Wennergren M, Jansson T, Powell TL. Triglyceride hydrolase activities and expression of fatty acid binding proteins in the human placenta in pregnancies complicated by intrauterine growth restriction and diabetes. *J Clin Endocrinol Metab*. 2004;89(9):4607-4614.
197. Chassen S, Jansson T. Complex, coordinated and highly regulated changes in placental signaling and nutrient transport capacity in IUGR. *Biochim Biophys Acta (BBA) - Mol Basis Dis*. 2019:165373.
199. Woods L, Perez-Garcia V, Hemberger M. Regulation of placental development and its impact on fetal growth-new insights from mouse models. *Front Endocrinol*. 2018;9:570.
203. Maccani MA, Marsit CJ. Epigenetics in the placenta. *Am J Reprod Immunol*. 2009;62(2):78-89.
224. Roh CR, Budhraja V, Kim HS, Nelson DM, Sadovsky Y. Microarray-based identification of differentially expressed genes in hypoxic term human trophoblasts and in placental villi of pregnancies with growth restricted fetuses. *Placenta*. 2005;26(4):319-328.
228. Austdal M, Thomsen LC, Tangeras LH, et al. Metabolic profiles of placenta in preeclampsia using HR-MAS MRS metabolomics. *Placenta*. 2015;36(12):1455-1462.
231. Gaccioli F, Lager S, Powell TL, Jansson T. Placental transport in response to altered maternal nutrition. *J Dev Orig Health Dis*. 2013;4(2):101-115.
253. Morrison JL. Sheep models of intrauterine growth restriction: fetal adaptations and consequences. *Clin Exp Pharmacol Physiol*. 2008;35(7):730-743.

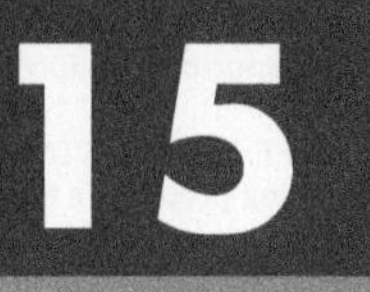

Basic Pharmacologic Principles

Gabriel Altit | Julie Autmizguine | François Duhamel | Sylvain Chemtob

INTRODUCTION

Pharmacology is a science concerned with the interaction of substances (e.g., drugs) with cells, tissues, and organisms. The in vivo efficacy of a drug is guided by two principles of pharmacology, namely pharmacokinetics and pharmacodynamics. Pharmacokinetics deals with the processes of drug concentration in the tissue compartments and therefore involves absorption, distribution, biotransformation, and excretion. Pharmacodynamics applies to the study of mechanisms of action of drugs. Application of these concepts to the newborn requires the practitioner to take into account developmental changes in pharmacokinetics and pharmacodynamics. In this chapter, we present basic pharmacologic principles and introduce how drug disposition and actions can be altered by developmental changes and disorders of the immature subject.

PRINCIPLES OF DRUG ABSORPTION, BIOAVAILABILITY, AND DISTRIBUTION

DRUG ABSORPTION

The majority of drugs administered to the premature newborn are injected intravenously and therefore are not affected by factors that govern systemic absorption. Some agents are administered intramuscularly (e.g., vitamin K, vaccines[1]), given by an enteral route (e.g., thiazides, caffeine, ranitidine,[2] acetaminophen,[3] lansoprazole,[2] sildenafil[4]), or applied topically or by inhalation (e.g., topical antiseptics, anesthetics, nitric oxide, bronchodilators). Regardless of the route of administration, drugs must often cross cell membranes to reach their sites of action. Therefore, the mechanisms that govern the passage of drugs across cell membranes and the physicochemical properties of molecules and membranes are important to consider in drug transfer. Among the most important physicochemical properties of drug molecules are lipid solubility, degree of ionization (pK_a), molecular weight, and protein binding.

Although drugs with molecular weight less than 200 Da cross the cellular lipid membranes by diffusion,[5] many require transporters.[6] The greater the lipid solubility and the lower the degree of ionization, the more easily a drug will transfer across the cell membrane. Furthermore, the binding affinity of drugs to proteins affects their distribution, and therefore their activity. It is the unbound fraction of drugs that exhibits pharmacologic effects, because they have greater access to their site of action.

TRANSPORT MECHANISMS

In addition to physicochemical properties of the drug molecules, there are a number of physiologic transport processes that influence the mechanism by which a drug traverses the cell membrane.[7] Such processes include passive diffusion, active transport, facilitated diffusion, and pinocytosis.

1. *Passive diffusion* is the principal transmembrane process for a number of small drugs. According to Fick's laws of diffusion, drug molecules diffuse from a region of high drug concentration to a region of low drug concentration according to the equation

$$dQ/dt = P\,(C_1 - C_2)$$

where dQ/dt = rate of diffusion, D = diffusion coefficient, K = partition coefficient, A = surface area of membrane, h = membrane thickness, and $C_1 - C_2$ = concentration gradient across the membrane. Because D, A, K, and h are constants under usual conditions, a combined constant P or permeability coefficient may be defined: $P = DAK/h$. Therefore, the previous equation can be simplified to:

$$dQ/dt = P\,(C_1 - C_2)$$

This equation does not take into account the ionization state of the drug molecule, the effect of regional blood flow, or the influence of tissue affinity on drug partitioning. The ionization state is affected by the pH on both sides of the membrane, according to the Henderson-Hasselbalch equation:

$$\mathrm{pH} = \mathrm{p}K_a + \log\,(\text{base/acid})$$

Therefore, acidic compounds, such as salicylic acid and furosemide,[8] diffuse across cell membranes more readily when the environmental pH is low, such as in the stomach, because they are less ionized at low pH. Accordingly, the opposite applies to basic compounds, such as propranolol,[9] that tend to cross membranes more readily in basic environments, such as in the small intestine. Regardless of the acidic or basic nature of drugs, most absorption occurs in the small intestine because of its larger surface area. Regional blood flow also influences the rate of diffusion by altering the delivery and consequently, the local concentration of the drug. Finally, some drugs demonstrate increased affinity for a particular tissue component, which influences the concentration of drug on either side of the membrane. For example, tetracyclines form a complex with calcium in the bones and teeth.

2. *Active transport* is a carrier-mediated transmembrane process that plays an important role in the renal, intestinal, and biliary secretion and absorption of many drugs and metabolites. Active transport is characterized by a transfer of molecules against their concentration gradient. Therefore, energy must be consumed to achieve this process. One example of this transport system is adenosine triphosphate (ATP)-dependent secretion of organic acids in the renal tubule, permitting secretion of indomethacin.[10] Of note, this process, in contrast to diffusion, is saturable and therefore follows Michaelis-Menten kinetics. The Michaelis-Menten equation describes the rates of enzymatic reactions by relating the rate of substrate conversion or uptake by protein (e.g., enzyme, receptor, transporter) to the concentration of the substrate.

3. *Facilitated diffusion* is also a carrier-mediated transport system, in which, in contrast with active transport, molecules move along their concentration gradient. This system does not require energy input but is saturable and selective. Major classes of transporters involved in facilitated diffusion include the solute carrier (SLC) superfamily and the ATP-binding cassette (ABC) superfamily[6,11,12]; examples of drugs transported by these transporters include corticosterone, ethacrynic acid, and captopril.
4. *Pinocytosis* is the process of engulfing large molecules such as immunoglobins.[13]

Membrane Transporters

Transporters are integral membrane proteins that primarily facilitate movement of nutrients and waste products such as amino acids, di- and tripeptides, sugars, nucleosides, vitamins, and bile salts into and out of the cells. Based on their physiologic role, membrane transporters can be classified as uptake transporters (transport solutes into the cell) and efflux transporters (carrying substances out of the cell).[14] In the intestines, it has become increasingly clear that several of these transporters also play a significant role in systemic absorption of xenobiotics, including various pharmacologic agents.

To date, more than 400 genes, encoding membrane transporters, have been identified in human genome[15] and are broadly divided into two superfamilies, SLC and ABC. Members of the SLC superfamily (such as organic anion transporters [OATs] and cation transporters) utilize either facilitated transport (along the electrochemical gradient) or cotransport (against the electrochemical gradient using electrochemical gradient of another solute) mechanisms for import or export of the substance of interest. Sodium and protons are frequently cotransported with the compound of interest in the latter case. Because the activity of such a transporter is a function of the electrochemical gradient driving force, the efficiency of the cotransport is influenced by the activity of the Na^+-H^+ antiporter and that of the Na^+-HCO_3^- symporter. On the other hand, members of the ABC superfamily (such as multidrug resistance-associated protein [MRP] transporters) utilize energy derived from ATP hydrolysis to transport solutes against their electrochemical gradient. The tissue distribution of membrane transporters is diverse and includes liver, kidney, intestine, and blood-tissue barriers (e.g., blood-brain barrier). For description of types and tissue distributions of various membrane transporters, see the review by König et al.[14]

A number of membrane transporters play key roles in drug import, as is the case for SLC members. These include the H^+-dipeptide symporters, facilitative glucose transporter-related proteins, Na^+-glucose cotransporters (SGLTs), Na^+-nucleoside cotransporters (CNTs), amino acid transporters, Na^+-neurotransmitter symporters, organic anion transporting polypeptides (OATPs), and the OATs and organic cation transporters (OCTs).[6,11,12,16] The H^+-dipeptide symporters carry cephalosporins and angiotensin-converting enzyme (ACE) inhibitors (such as captopril and valgancyclovir[17]); OCTs carry antihistamines (such as cimetidine, ranitidine, famotidine, clonidine, dopamine), hormones (such as corticosterone), and β-blockers (such as propranolol)[18-20]; OATPs carry a wide variety of drugs such as antibiotics (ciprofloxacin, penicillin, cephalosporins, rifampicin), β-blockers (sotalol), vasopressin, montelukast, and digoxin.[21,22]

Net absorption is also affected by the activity of exporters (efflux transporters), commonly present on the brush border membrane of luminal epithelial cells (e.g., proximal tubular epithelium of kidney). The MRP and the P-glycoprotein (P-gp) families are prototypes of these transporters. These proteins are ATP-dependent transporters that significantly contribute to the excretion of potentially toxic waste products such as bile salts as well as drugs such as steroids, cyclosporins, and digoxin out of the cells.[23]

These ports of entry across cellular membranes, along with their structural polymorphisms, may pose an additional challenge to pharmacokinetics and drug delivery. For instance, drug-drug interaction affect their activity, such as rifampin induction of P-gp activity, which increase digoxin elimination.[24] Moreover, neonates with an OATP1B1 mutation are at higher risk of developing severe hyperbilirubinemia.[25]Also, efflux pumps may also play an important role in etiopathology of some diseases. For example, mutations of hepatocellular bile salt export pump (BSEP), a type of ABC efflux transporter, have been associated with progressive familial intrahepatic cholestasis (PFIC) type-II.[26]

The distribution of drugs often requires transport across multiple compartments, which affects their concentration at the site of action. Along these lines, P-glycoproteins are major efflux transporters in the blood-brain barrier and, consequently, influence the concentration of various drugs in the central nervous system. Nevertheless, transcellular transport may not be the only function served by P-glycoproteins. Interestingly, they have been localized on intracellular vesicles and more importantly at the inner membrane of the nuclear envelope,[27] suggesting that P-glycoprotein expression at the nuclear envelope may play a role in subcellular distribution of various endogenous substrates and drugs.[28] This intracellular localization is particularly relevant in the context of expression of cognate transmembrane receptors at subcellular organelles, notably on the nuclear envelope.[29-32]

KINETICS OF ABSORPTION

Most pharmacokinetic models assume that drug absorption and elimination follow first-order kinetics (i.e., the rate of change in the concentration of a drug depends on the amount of drug present at that particular time). This process is described in the following equation:

$$dD_B/dt = FK_aD_{si} - K_{el}D_B$$

where dD_B/dt = rate of change of drug in the body (D_B), F = fraction absorbed (bioavailability term), K_a and K_{el} = absorption and elimination constants, and D_{si} = drug concentration at the site of absorption. This equation applies to a single-compartment pharmacokinetic model. In a single-compartment model, the drug rapidly equilibrates with tissues of the body. Therefore, changes in the concentration of the drug in serum or plasma mirror those in the tissues. Although many drugs follow multiple-compartment kinetics, the K_a may still be calculated from a one-compartment model.[33] The importance of the K_a lies in the design of a multiple dosage regimen. Knowledge of the K_a and K_{el} allows for the prediction of the peak and trough steady-state plasma drug concentrations ($C_{ss\ max}$ and $C_{ss\ min}$) following multiple dosing concentrations (see "Clinical Pharmacokinetics" and Fig. 15.1)[34]:

$$Css\ max = (FD_{si} / Vd)\ /\ \left(1 - e^{-Kel\tau}\right)$$

$$Css\ min = Css\ max \bullet e^{-Kel\tau}$$

where τ = dosing interval. From these equations, it is evident that peak and trough concentrations depend on the absorption rate, the volume of distribution, the elimination rate constant, and the dosing interval.

FACTORS THAT AFFECT ABSORPTION OF DRUGS

The systemic absorption of a drug from its site of administration depends on the variables discussed previously, which constitute the physicochemical properties of the drug and those of the membrane. Other factors can also influence the efficiency of drug absorption, including the disintegration, dissolution, and solubility of the compound; the blood flow to the site of absorption; the surface area available for absorption; transit time of the drug through the gastrointestinal tract; export of drugs via P-glycoproteins in

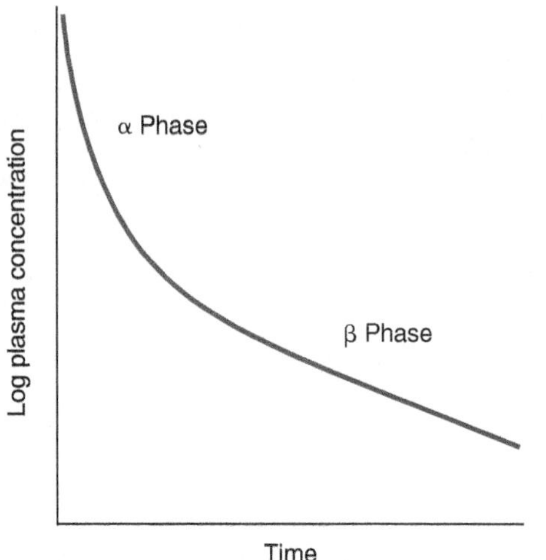

Fig. 15.1 Two-compartment model for serum drug disappearance curve. The α-phase represents the distribution phase, and the β-phase the elimination phase.

enterocytes; and in situ metabolism of the agent, including the first-pass effect. A *first-pass effect* is defined as the rapid uptake and metabolism of an agent into inactive compounds by the liver, immediately after enteric absorption and before it reaches the systemic circulation. Drugs that exhibit a first-pass effect include morphine, isoproterenol, propranolol, and hydralazine. Each of the factors that affect absorption, taken separately or in conjunction, may have profound effects on the efficacy and toxicity of a drug.

Compounds can be administered to newborns via various routes: intravenous, intramuscular, sublingual, oral, enteral, rectal, buccal (submucosal), dermal, inhalational, intravitreal, and conjunctival. Depending on the route, the absorption may be impacted by various factors that are maturational or not. Method of administration can also impact absorption (and bioavailability of the compound of interest), such as the type of intravenous or gavage tubing used, with lipophilic drugs adhering more to the material.[35] While evaluating the absorption of drugs through enteral route in the newborn, the developmental stages of this organ must be taken into account.[36] Gastric acid secretion is lower in premature infants.[37] The increased pH (>4.0) results in a reduced absorption of weak acids (such as phenobarbital) and bases, but may lead to increased absorption of acid-labile drugs (such as penicillin G).[35] By contrast, lipid-soluble drugs (such as methylxanthines) are more easily absorbed in newborns than in older children.[38] Furthermore, the rate of gastric emptying (slower in newborns) and the intestinal motility may be affected by gestational and postnatal age, as well as impacted by the nutritional content (increased with human milk, decreased by rising caloric density and medium-chain triglycerides).[35,39] Bile salt secretion is also diminished in the newborn infant,[40] which can affect micelle formation and enterohepatic recirculation,[35] and secondarily reduce the absorption of fats and lipid-soluble vitamins, such as vitamins D and E[41,42]; on the other hand, vitamin E is adequately absorbed in premature infants,[43] probably due to a lower intake of iron.[44] Gestational and postnatal age, as well as pathologic processes of the newborn, may also affect intestinal surface area and permeability, impacting absorption of enterally administered compounds. In addition, permeability decreases with administration of milk (faster with breast milk compared to formula).[35,45]

Rectal administration, depending upon depth, may result in first-pass enteral metabolism (bypassing metabolism).[39] Specifically, distal rectal exposure leads to absorption via the medium and inferior rectal veins, while deeper rectal absorption proceeds through the superior rectal veins to the liver.[39,46,47] The submucosal buccal route is commonly used with midazolam or fentanyl administration, which may lead to increased and faster absorption compared to the enteral route.[35]

Enzymatic development of the gastrointestinal tract may also alter drug absorption. The elevated activity of β-glucuronidase in the brush border of newborn intestine may cleave drug-glucuronide conjugates,[48] resulting in enhanced reabsorption of free unconjugated drug into the systemic circulation; this may prolong the pharmacologic activity of certain agents, such as indomethacin.[49] In contrast, the presence of P-glycoproteins, highly distributed in the apical brush border of the gastrointestinal tract epithelium as well as in the bile canalicular face of hepatocytes, can reduce drug absorption and bioavailability[50]; lower expression of P-glycoproteins in the immature subject may contribute to variable bioavailability.[51] Although modulators of P-glycoproteins, primarily cyclosporin A and verapamil, have been used with marginal effectiveness to enhance drug action, such as in cancer treatment,[52,53] these drugs exert their own toxicity; selective inhibitors of P-glycoproteins and related MRPs have yet to be developed. Another factor that influences drug absorption and its access to the target organ is the presence of metabolizing enzymes in the intestinal epithelium; this is especially the case for cytochrome P450 enzymes.[54] Depending on their activity, limited or excess bioavailability may be observed.

In comparison with adults, newborn infants also exhibit qualitative and quantitative differences in the bacterial colonization of the gastrointestinal tracts. The development of the intestinal flora has been clearly shown to affect the absorption of vitamin K.[55] The microbiome can also impact the production of bile acids.[56] Therefore, maturation of the gastrointestinal tract may also explain some of the characteristics of intestinal absorption of drugs in the growing child.

Finally, in addition to the physiologic changes in the gastrointestinal tract that occur during development, drug absorption can also be altered by disease processes. Diseases of genetic (e.g., cystic fibrosis), microbial, or circulatory (e.g., necrotizing enterocolitis) origin may alter the intestinal mucosa and result in a reduced absorptive surface. There are a number of developmental differences in the newborn that affect non-enteral absorption. For instance, *topical skin absorption* depends on the dermal thickness, permeability, skin maturation, skin perfusion, and the body surface area to weight ratio (increased in newborns). Stratum corneum maturation accelerates in the immediate weeks of postnatal life, adjusting to extrauterine life and independent of gestational age.[35,57] *Inhalation* is of particular interest in the newborn as numerous drugs are administered via this route as is the case for nitric oxide, inhaled anesthetics, steroids, and endotracheal epinephrine. Neonates have a decreased functional residual capacity but an increased alveolar surface area relative to weight, factors that can affect absorption. Also, they frequently have a bidirectional or right-to-left shunts via an inter-atrial communication or patent-ductus-arteriosus, especially in the first few days of life (or in the context of pulmonary hypertension and/or right ventricular dysfunction). Shunt direction may also impact compound absorption. In the context of pulmonary pathologies, ventilation-perfusion mismatch (such as in meconium aspiration syndrome or bronchopulmonary dysplasia) may also affect impact bioavailability of compounds administered by inhalation. *Conjunctival absorption* may also lead to systemic distribution of drugs; the same applies to intravitreal administration.[35,58] *Intramuscular absorption* is affected by circulation through local capillaries.[35] Following intramuscular administration, there is an early systemic absorption, followed by a delayed release (deep compartment behavior), making it ideal for certain drugs, such as vitamin K for prevention of neonatal bleeding.

BIOAVAILABILITY

Drug *bioavailability* is the fraction of the administered dose that reaches the systemic circulation. For the clinician, the most relevant consideration is the percentage of active drug that reaches the central compartment. Bioavailability does not take into account the rate at which the drug is absorbed but is affected by factors that influence absorption. The absolute availability of a drug may be determined by comparing the respective area under the plasma concentration curves (AUC) after oral and intravenous administration.

$$\text{Absolute availability} = [AUC_{PO} / dose_{PO}] \ / \ [AUC_{IV}/dose_{IV}]$$

This measurement may be performed as long as the volume of distribution (V_d) and the elimination rate constant (K_{el}) are independent of the route of administration.

DISTRIBUTION

The *disposition* of a drug refers to its passage in the body from absorption to excretion. Following absorption, a drug is distributed to various body compartments. This distribution determines its efficacy as well as its toxicity. The *distribution* of drugs is influenced by several factors, including the size of the body-water and lipid compartments, regional hemodynamic features, the degree of binding of drugs to plasma and tissue proteins, and the tissue expression of transporter proteins (importers and exporters). The initial phase of distribution reflects regional blood flow. Organs that are well perfused, such as the brain, the heart, and the kidneys, are first to get exposed to the drug. The second phase of distribution involves a large fraction of the body mass, including muscles and adipose tissue. Therefore, the various distribution compartments form the apparent volume of distribution (V_d), which is expressed by the following equation:

$$V_d = \text{Total drug in the body/Concentration of drug in plasma}$$

Assuming instant equilibration of the drug after administration, V_d can be determined by extrapolating the drug concentration to time zero (C_0) and dividing the dose of drug administered by the concentration of drug at time zero (C_0). This equation, however, can only be applied to a single-compartment model. V_d may also be calculated using the following equation, which is independent of the model used:

$$V_d = \text{Dose} / \text{Kel} \ [AUC]_0^\infty$$

PHYSIOLOGIC AND PATHOLOGIC FACTORS AFFECTING DISTRIBUTION OF DRUGS

The factors that influence the distribution of drugs in the body are subject to developmental changes (weight, body composition, plasma protein concentration, permeability of compartment targeted). The amount and distribution of total body water undergo marked changes in the perinatal period.[59] Total body water and extracellular fluid volume decrease with increasing gestational age. Consequently, the volume of distribution of many drugs has been observed to increase in preterm neonates.[60] This results in increased volume of distribution; accordingly, lipophilic drugs (such as propofol) exhibit decreased volumes of distribution and accumulate with risks of toxicity.[35,39] After birth, free fat mass and total body water decrease and the volume of intracellular fluid increases relative to that of the extracellular fluid. In the term newborn, as well as in the older child,[61] the degree of insensible water loss is linked to the metabolic rate of the infant. In contrast, in the preterm newborn, there is no fixed relationship between metabolic rate and insensible water loss, and in the very low-birth-weight infant, evaporative heat loss is substantially greater than heat produced by the basal metabolic rate.[43,62]

Many disorders of the newborn as well as drugs administered to critically ill newborn infants (such as diuretics[63,64]) can affect total body water and, secondarily, the distribution of drugs. For instance, renal and hepatic dysfunction may have important consequences on both elimination and distribution of xenobiotics. Similarly, diseases that lead to increased total body water (e.g., congestive heart failure, syndrome of inappropriate secretion of antidiuretic hormone) can have profound effects on drug pharmacokinetics and pharmacodynamics. Therefore, any change in either total body water content or the relationship between extracellular and intracellular fluid volume may have significant effects on the distribution of drugs within the body.

The extent and the disposition of the lipid mass in the body also contribute to the distribution of drugs. The adipose tissue mass changes markedly during development. Between 28 and 40 weeks of gestation, the amount of adipose tissue (expressed as a percentage of total body mass) increases from 1% to 15%,[65] and by 1 year of age, it represents approximately 25% of the body mass.

The nervous system contains a high proportion of lipids. Normally, the maximal increment in weight of the human brain occurs in the few weeks preceding term gestation; however, a substantial part of myelination (and lipid deposition) occurs postnatally.[66] The entry of drugs into the central nervous system is generally restricted. In contrast with capillaries elsewhere in the body, endothelial cells of brain capillaries exhibit a predominance of tight junctions, producing nonfenestrated capillaries, which restrict the entry of hydrophilic substances into the brain. Consequently, ionized molecules, such as quaternary amines (e.g., neostigmine), exhibit limited capacity to diffuse into the central nervous system, whereas lipid-soluble compounds, such as cefotaxime and pentobarbital, traverse the blood-brain barrier more readily.

The distribution of drugs into brain and other organs is also dependent on specific transporters of nutrients and endogenous compounds, as described earlier. Furthermore, efflux carriers present in brain endothelium and glia, primarily P-glycoproteins, limit drug concentration in the brain. This is well described for a number of drugs including human immunodeficiency virus (HIV) protease inhibitors, vinca alkaloids, and anthracyclines.[67] Of interest, P-glycoproteins are also present in placenta and function as export transporters to limit fetal exposure to potentially toxic agents. In the newborn, the blood-brain barrier is relatively more permeable than in the older subject.[68] Newborns also display higher cerebral-to-systemic blood flow and greater volume of cerebrospinal fluid, which together increase drug concentrations in the central nervous system.[39,68]

A major determinant of drug distribution is the cardiac output and blood flow to various organs.[69] Marked changes in the neonatal circulation take place during the perinatal period.[70,71] In addition, regional blood flow may also change acutely as a result of congestive heart failure (secondary to patent ductus arteriosus or other congenital heart diseases),[69] as a result of sudden changes in acid-base balance (especially respiratory acidosis), or secondary to the limited ability of the stressed preterm neonate to autoregulate regional blood flow.[72]

Plasma Proteins

The affinity of a drug for plasma proteins is another important variable that affects drug distribution. The degree of binding is inversely related to the volume of distribution, such that increased protein binding tends to maintain the drug within the vascular space. Protein binding affects renal and plasma clearance, the half-life, and the efficacy of the agent at its site of action. Table 15.1 lists the protein binding of some commonly used agents in the neonate.

Several factors modify the binding of drugs to plasma proteins, notably the amount of plasma binding proteins; the number of binding sites; the affinity of the drug for the protein; and pathophysiologic conditions that alter drug-protein binding (such as blood pH, free fatty acids, bilirubin, and disease states, e.g., renal failure, liver failure). Albumin binds principally acidic drugs, whereas basic agents are bound to lipoproteins, β-globulins, and α_1-acid glycoproteins.[73] Albumin contains a few high-affinity and

Table 15.1 Plasma Protein Binding of Commonly Used Drugs in the Newborn.

Drug	Percent Protein-Bound
Ampicillin	~10
Atropine	25
Caffeine	25
Cefotaxime	25–50
Dexamethasone	65
Digoxin	20
Ethacrynic acid	95
Furosemide	95
Gentamicin	45
Hydrochlorothiazide	40
Indomethacin	95
Morphine	30
Phenobarbital	~20
Phenytoin	~80
Theophylline	35

Data from References 73–80.

Box 15.1 Drugs That Cause Significant Displacement of Bilirubin From Albumin In Vitro

Sulfonamides
Ibuprofen
Moxalactam
Fusidic acid
Radiographic contrast media for cholangiography (sodium iodipamide, sodium ipodate, iopanoic acid, meglumine ioglycamate)
Aspirin
Apazone
Tolbutamide
Albumin preservatives (sodium caprylate and *N*-acetyl tryptophan: rapid infusions in vivo)
High concentrations of ampicillin (rapid infusions in vivo)
Long-chain free fatty acids (FFA) at high molar ratios of FFA:albumin

several low-affinity binding sites.[74] In the preterm newborn, both albumin and α_1-acid glycoprotein concentrations and binding affinities are deficient, resulting in an increased fraction of free drug[75] and increased distribution of free drug outside the vascular compartment.[76] Numerous conditions may further reduce the binding of drugs to proteins. For example, a decrease in pH may enhance the dissociation of weak acids from their albumin-binding sites. Therefore, the frequent occurrence of acidosis in premature infants may significantly change the binding of drugs to plasma proteins, especially albumin. The elevated plasma-free fatty acid content of the newborn may also alter drug binding to plasma proteins[77,78]; this effect, however, may be questionable.[79] In a similar fashion, maternal drugs that have crossed placental barrier or other agents (including other drugs) concomitantly administered to the infant may also compete for the same plasma protein-binding sites in the newborn.

The potential interference of endogenous compounds, particularly unconjugated bilirubin, on drug-protein binding has been well addressed.[80] A displacement of bilirubin from its albumin-binding site may result in free circulating unconjugated bilirubin, which can penetrate into the brain and ultimately cause injury. Interestingly, however, bilirubin itself is tightly bound to albumin and may displace drugs from their protein-binding sites.[80] In addition, free bilirubin is only sparingly lipophilic. Thus, the drug-induced displacement of bilirubin from albumin-binding sites possibly plays a minor role in the development of bilirubin-induced encephalopathy. Nonetheless, a few drugs can alter the binding affinity of albumin for bilirubin (Box 15.1).[80]

The volume of distribution of certain compounds is also affected by their binding to proteins outside the vascular space; for example, digoxin exhibits a higher degree of binding to myocardial and skeletal muscle proteins in the newborn than in the adult.[81,82] This results in an increase in the volume of distribution of digoxin. Altogether, in the immature newborn the concentration of albumin is lower and that in the fetus, resulting in decreased binding of weak acids.[39]

In conclusion, numerous factors can influence the distribution of drugs in the body. These factors are themselves affected by development and disease conditions of the newborn infant. Major changes in the distribution of fluids and fat and their proportion relative to body mass occur at the end of gestation and during the neonatal period. Perinatal and neonatal alterations in cardiac output and regional blood flow, secondary to physiologic and disease states, also occur. Furthermore, the degree of drug binding to plasma proteins between the newborn and adult varies for several drugs. These variables should be taken into account when deciding on the appropriate drug dosage for a newborn.

PRINCIPLES OF DRUG ELIMINATION

The relatively high lipophilicity of many drugs does not permit their rapid elimination. After filtration through the glomerulus or passage into the bile, these agents are readily absorbed by the renal tubule or gastrointestinal mucosa. Consequently, the elimination of most drugs from the body requires a step of biotransformation prior to their excretion. This section reviews the different biotransformation processes that take place in the human body, and the mechanisms of renal drug excretion, with particular reference to developmental aspects.

DRUG BIOTRANSFORMATION

Drug *biotransformation* converts drug molecules into more polar derivatives that are less able to diffuse across cell membranes. As a consequence of biotransformation, these converted molecules do not reach their receptors and in addition are not reabsorbed by the renal tubule. Therefore, biotransformation of drugs not only facilitates their excretion from the body but also may diminish their pharmacologic activity.

The metabolism of drugs does not always produce inactive compounds. Initial biotransformation of certain agents results in the formation of active metabolites. For instance, codeine is demethylated to morphine, acetylsalicylic acid is hydrolyzed to salicylic acid, theophylline is methylated to caffeine, propranolol converted to 4-hydroxypropranolol (via hydroxylation), and diazepam is converted to oxazepam.[83,84] Furthermore, oxidation of certain aromatic compounds produces highly reactive (and toxic) electrophiles (compounds that serve as electron acceptors). This latter reaction may be primary (aromatic hydrocarbons) or may be an increasingly active secondary reaction resulting from an inhibited or overwhelmed primary metabolic pathway (as, for example, with an excessive dosage of the agent, such as with acetaminophen overdose). Therefore, biotransformation can produce relatively innocuous metabolites or highly toxic compounds.

The mechanisms that affect the biotransformation of drugs are usually the same as those that metabolize endogenous products (e.g., hormones). Most biotransformation takes place in the liver, but some may occur at other sites, such as the kidneys, intestinal mucosa, and lungs. Biotransformation reactions are classically divided into two phases: phase I, the nonsynthetic reactions, and phase II, the synthetic or conjugation reactions (Table 15.2). Each phase has reactions that can take place in the microsomes or outside of the microsomal system. The great majority of phase I reactions (oxidation, reduction, and hydrolysis) are largely catalyzed by microsomal enzymes, while phase II reactions (other than glucuronidation) are predominantly extramicrosomal.

PHASE I REACTIONS (NONSYNTHETIC REACTIONS)

Microsomal

The microsomal enzymes that metabolize drugs are localized in the smooth endoplasmic reticulum. Oxidative enzymes of this system, called *mixed-function oxidases* or *monooxygenases*, consist of three principal components: an electron transporter, NADPH-cytochrome P450 reductase (a flavoprotein), and multiple cytochrome P450 isoenzymes (oxidase hemoproteins).[85] This system requires both a reducing agent (NADPH) and molecular oxygen (O_2). The end result of cytochrome P450-catalyzed reactions is the incorporation of one oxygen atom into the compound being metabolized (hence the name *monooxygenase*) and formation of water after reduction of the second oxygen atom.

Reactions catalyzed by monooxygenases include aromatic ring and aliphatic side chain hydroxylation, *N*-, *O*-, *S*-dealkylation, deamination, dehalogenation, sulfoxidation, *N*-oxidation, *N*-hydroxylation, nitroreduction, and azoreduction. Epoxides are also formed by monooxygenases, converting aromatic moieties of agents to arene and alkene oxides, which are in turn detoxified by epoxide hydrolases present in endoplasmic reticulum. These electrophilic compounds react avidly with proteins and nucleic acids, exerting potential mutagenic and carcinogenic effects; polychlorinated and polybrominated biphenyls exert their toxicity via their metabolites.[85]

Several drugs, including fluconazole, spironolactone, amiodarone, cimetidine, erythromycin, ciprofloxacin, and metronidazole, can inhibit cytochrome P450 enzyme activity.[86,87] This inhibition reduces the metabolism of potential substrates and secondarily delays their elimination, as seen in fluconazole inhibition of zidovudine elimination.[88] In contrast, other substrates can act as inducers of the cytochrome P450 system. Prototypes of the most extensively studied inducers of cytochrome P450 isozymes are phenobarbital (CYP3A), rifampin (CYP1A, CYP2C), and the polycyclic aromatic hydrocarbon, 3-methylcholanthrene (CYP1A). Other examples of CYP450 inducers are phenytoin and carbamazepine.[86,87]

Approximately 1000 cytochrome P450s are known; only 50 or so are functionally active in humans. Seventeen families and many subfamilies have been sequenced. CYP1, CYP2, and CYP3 families are involved in the majority of drug metabolism reactions; members of the other families are important in the synthesis and degradation of steroids, fatty acids, vitamins, and other endogenous compounds. Individual CYP isoforms tend to have substrate specificities, but overlap is common. CYP3A4 and CYP3A5 are similar isoforms, which together are involved in metabolism of approximately 50% of drugs. CYP2C and CYP2D6 are also involved in the metabolism of many drugs. CYP1A1/2, CYP2A6, CYP2B1, and CYP2E1

Table 15.2 Biotransformation Reactions.

Reaction	Examples of Drug Substrates
Phase I (Nonsynthetic Reactions)	
(a) *Oxidation:*	
Aromatic ring hydroxylation	Phenytoin, Phenobarbital
Aliphatic hydroxylation	Ibuprofen
N-hydroxylation	Acetaminophen
N-, *O*-, *S*-dealkylation	Morphine, codeine
Deamination	Diazepam
Sulfoxidation, *N*-oxidation	Cimetidine
(b) *Reduction:*	
Azoreduction	Prontosil
Nitroreduction	Chloramphenicol
Alcohol dehydrogenase	Ethanol
(c) *Hydrolysis:*	
Ester hydrolysis	Acetylsalicylic acid
Amide hydrolysis	Indomethacin
Phase I (Microsomal Enzymes)	
CYP1A2	Caffeine, theophylline
CYP2A6	Nicotine
CYP2B6	Diazepam
CYP2C9	Warfarin, ibuprofen, indomethacin, phenytoin, sildenafil
CYP2C19	Diazepam, omeprazole, lansoprazole
CYP2D6	Codeine, imipramine, propranolol, timolol, tamoxifen
CYP2E1	Acetaminophen, caffeine, ethanol
CYP3A	Erythromycin, midazolam, 6β-hydroxycortisol, sildenafil
Phase II (Synthetic Reactions: Conjugations)	
(a) Glucuronide conjugation	Morphine, acetaminophen, bilirubin
(b) Glycine conjugation	Salicylic acid
(c) Sulfate conjugation	Acetaminophen, α-methyldopa
(d) Glutathione conjugation	Ethacrynic acid
(e) Methylation	Dopamine, epinephrine
(f) Acetylation	Sulfonamides, clonazepam

Adapted from References 85 and 87.

are not extensively involved in drug metabolism but rather in activation of procarcinogenic agents including aromatic amines and aromatic hydrocarbons.

The cytochrome P450-dependent monooxygenase activity develops in fetal life and significantly increases during the perinatal period, often triggered by parturition.[89] Nonetheless, its activity in the fetal and newborn liver remains considerably lower than in the adult liver.[89,90] The diminished enzyme activity may be clinically important because drugs that are oxygenated slowly by these enzymes (e.g., phenobarbital and phenytoin) can exhibit a prolonged half-life in the young infant[91]; this is especially the case for the CYP1A2, CYP2A6, CYP2B6, CYP2C, CYP2D6, CYP2E1, and CYP3A4 substrates (Table 15.3).[92,93] However, some CYP enzymes, including CYP1A1 and CYP3A7, are expressed in higher levels in the fetal and newborn liver.[89,90,94,95] CYP3A7 expression peaks 1 week after birth and declines thereafter, while CYP3A4, a structurally related isoform, increases concomitantly in the first year of life to become the major isoform in the adult liver.[95] Although substrate specificities overlap between CYP3A4 and CYP3A7, some drugs, such as midazolam, are mainly metabolized by CYP3A4, leading to prolonged half-life in neonates.[96] Of interest, CYP2E1 is induced and metabolized by ethanol in the fetus and has been proposed to be implicated in the development of fetal alcohol syndrome.[97]

Extramicrosomal

A few of the oxidative and reductive reactions are mediated by enzymes in the mitochondria, and cytosol of the liver and other tissues. These enzymes include those involved in oxidation of alcohols and aldehydes; alcohol and aldehyde dehydrogenases; and enzymes that partake in the metabolism of catecholamines, tyrosine hydroxylase, and monoamine oxidase. Although the activity of some of these enzymes can be detected early in gestation, their full activity is reached only in early childhood.[54] However, once again marked ontogenic differences between enzymes are observed. For instance, class I alcohol dehydrogenase, the major ethanol-metabolizing enzyme, tends to be well expressed in fetal liver, whereas class III alcohol dehydrogenase is relatively deficient in the fetus.[98]

PHASE II REACTIONS (SYNTHETIC REACTIONS)

In phase II reactions, molecules that are naturally present in the body are conjugated or combined with the drug or other endogenous compounds. The drug may have first undergone a phase I reaction, or the original drug may be directly conjugated. Conjugation converts drugs into more polar compounds, which are pharmacologically less active and are more readily excreted; an exception applies to acetylation, whereby the metabolite is often less water-soluble. Although it was previously thought that conjugation reactions represented true inactivation and detoxification reactions, it is presently known that certain conjugation reactions (e.g., *N*-acetylation of isoniazid) may lead to the formation of reactive species responsible for hepatotoxicity. Diclofenac biotransformation produces quinoneimine, an over-oxidized metabolite responsible for idiosyncratic hepatotoxicity.[99] The major conjugation reactions are listed in Table 15.2.

Glucuronidation

The formation of glucuronides is the principal conjugation reaction in the body. Natural substrates of this pathway include bilirubin and thyroxine. The same pathway is used by many drugs that contain hydroxyl, amino, carboxyl, thiol, and phenolic groups (e.g., morphine, acetaminophen, phenytoin, sulfonamides, chloramphenicol, salicylic acid, and indomethacin).

The conjugation of a compound with glucuronic acid results in the production of a strongly acidic derivative that is more water-soluble at physiologic pH than the parent compound. This reduces its transfer across membranes, facilitates its dissociation from the receptor, and enhances its elimination in urine or bile. The fate of the glucuronidated drugs in urine or bile depends on their molecular size. Compounds with relatively low molecular weights are almost completely excreted in urine, whereas those with high molecular weights (greater than 500 Da) are eliminated almost entirely in bile.

Glucuronides are eliminated by the kidneys predominantly via glomerular filtration; however, tubular secretion and tubular reabsorption followed by secretion represent alternative pathways. Biliary excretion of drugs conjugated to glucuronic acid occurs by simple diffusion or by active secretion. Once in the intestine, these drugs may be reabsorbed after being deconjugated (hydrolyzed) by glucuronidase, which exhibits an elevated activity in the fetus and newborn.[29]

Drugs or conditions that inhibit formation of glucuronides are likely to prolong the pharmacologic activity of these agents. Inhibition may occur at the level of the synthesis of glucuronic acid (e.g., by certain steroid hormones) or at the level of the UDP-glucuronyl transferase (UGT) activity itself, which consists of 16 different isoforms in humans. In the human fetus and newborn, glucuronide conjugation enzymes often exhibit reduced activity. In this context, fetal underexpression of the 2B isoform is responsible for the gray baby syndrome associated with chloramphenicol intake.[100,101] Postnatal development proceeds relatively rapidly, as occurs with the metabolism of bilirubin.[102,103] In Crigler-Najjar syndrome type 1, a complete hereditary absence of UGT-1 leads to severe neonatal unconjugated hyperbilirubinemia.[104]

Other Synthetic Conjugation Reactions

Other kinds of conjugation reactions that occur in the body are listed in Table 15.2. As with glucuronyl transferase, the activity of the other various transferases is often lower in the fetus and newborn than in the adult (see Table 15.3).[102,103]

Table 15.3 Ontogeny of Human Phase I and II Metabolizing Enzymes.

Enzyme	Fetus	Newborn	Infancy	Adult
Phase I				
CYP1A1	+/–	–	–	–
CYP1A2	–	+/–	+/–	+
CYP2A6	–	NA	NA	+
CYP2B6	–	NA	NA	+
CYP2C9	–	+/–	+	+
CYP2C19	+/–	+/–	+/–	+
CYP2D6	+/–	+/–	+/–	+
CYP2E1	+/–	+/–	+	+
CYP3A4	–	+/–	+/–	+
CYP3A5[a]	+/–	+/–	+/–	+/–
CYP3A7	+	+	–	–
Phase II				
UGT1A1	–	+	+	+
UGT2B7	+/–	+/–	+	+
GST α	+/–	+	+	+
GST μ	+/–	+	+	+
GST π	+	–	–	–
SULT1A1	+/–	+/–	+	+
SULT1A3	+	NA	NA	+/–

UGT, UDP-glucuronosyl transferase; *GST*, glutathione S-transferase; *SULT*, sulfotransferase.
[a]CYP3A5 expression does not vary significantly with age but has a high interindividual variability.
Data from References 89–103.

Available data permit the following generalizations in regard to drug metabolism in the fetus and newborn:

1. The rates of drug biotransformation and overall elimination are slow.
2. The rate of drug elimination from the body exhibits marked interpatient variability.
3. The maturational changes in drug metabolism and disposition as a function of postnatal age are extremely variable and depend on the substrate (or drug) being used.
4. Neonatal drug biotransformation and elimination are vulnerable to pathophysiologic states.
5. Neonates may exhibit activation of alternate biotransformation pathways.

FACTORS AFFECTING BIOTRANSFORMATION IN THE LIVER

Several factors may alter the rate, extent, and type of biotransformation reactions in the liver. The issues of enzyme activity that may be modified by development and by endogenous or exogenous compounds have been addressed. Environmental influences also significantly affect drug metabolism; these include the inducing or inhibitory effects of drugs per se on enzyme activities. For instance, calcium channel blockers, antifungal agents, and macrolide antibiotics are potent inhibitors of CYP3A enzymes, quinidine inhibits CYP2D6, and other compounds such as cimetidine, amiodarone, and fluoxetine reduce activity of many cytochrome P450 enzymes. On the other hand, a number of agents, including anticonvulsants and aromatic hydrocarbons, can induce certain CYP subfamilies and isoforms.

Metabolic enzyme activity is also affected by genetic factors, which is the rule rather than the exception; however, the interplay between ontogeny and genetics remains largely unknown in drug metabolism. There exist approximately 70 single nucleotide polymorphisms (SNPs) and other genetic variants of the CYP2D6 gene, many of which yield diminished enzyme activity; this may impact significantly on drugs metabolized by CYP2D6 such as β-blockers and certain opiates. In the case of CYP3A enzymes, to date, no significant functional polymorphisms have been identified; hence, factors that regulate gene expression are more important to explain the interindividual variability (>10-fold). Because genetic factors and environmental influences exert greater effects on drug metabolism than they do on renal excretion, drugs that are metabolized are considerably more affected by interpersonal differences than those that do not require biotransformation.

Other factors that affect biotransformation include blood flow to the liver, gender, and disease states. For certain drugs (e.g., morphine, meperidine, propranolol, and verapamil), blood flow may be the limiting factor that controls drug elimination. These drugs (often termed *flow-limited* drugs) are so readily metabolized by the liver that hepatic clearance is essentially equal to liver blood flow. By contrast, the biotransformation of *capacity-limited* drugs (e.g., phenytoin, theophylline, diazepam, and chloramphenicol) is determined by the liver's metabolizing capacity rather than by hepatic blood flow.[105] The effect of gender in newborn infants remains unclear but may not be as important as in the adult.

RENAL EXCRETION OF DRUGS

Renal excretion is the most important means for drug elimination in the newborn. The renal processing of drugs and their metabolites occurs via three major processes: glomerular filtration, active tubular secretion, and passive tubular reabsorption. Intracellular enzymatic processing (mainly in proximal tubule) seems to have a minor role in renal drug handling and requires further investigation.[106] Following the entry of a drug into a renal tubule, its elimination is dependent on its lipophilicity and ionization state. Indeed, lipophilic compounds will readily cross membranes and accumulate, thus hampering their elimination by the kidney. Therefore, for their effective renal elimination, lipophilic compounds need to be converted to polar hydrophilic substrates.

The capacity for renal elimination is also influenced by other factors: disease state, gestational and postnatal age (affects renal maturation), hemodynamic transitioning (affects renal perfusion), polypharmaceutical interventions, growth restriction, and genetic polymorphisms.[107] Nephrogenesis is completed at 36 weeks of gestation and can be impacted by the presence of certain maternal medications, maternal disease states that induce growth restriction, fetal obstructive uropathies, as well as intrinsic genetic fetal anomalies.[107] Renal tubular functions are immature in the term newborn due to smaller tubular mass and ongoing maturation of the active transport mechanisms. The different elimination pathways do not mature simultaneously, and one must be vigilant to incorporate ontogenic concepts when addressing renal handling of drugs. Furthermore, differences in elimination of certain drugs by the kidney versus the liver in neonates compared to older subjects needs to be taken into account; for example, this is the case for midazolam, morphine, and tramadol, or drug excipients such as propylene glycol.

GLOMERULAR FILTRATION OF DRUGS

The amount of drug filtered through the glomerulus depends on a molecular size less than that of albumin (molecular weight 69,000 Da), degree of protein binding, and regional perfusion. Hence, nearly all non-protein-bound drugs are filtered. Glomerular filtration rate (GFR) increases during fetal development, but in the newborn it remains far below that observed in the adult.[108-111] Rapid modifications in hemodynamics have an impact on the GFR as a result of the subtle equilibrium maintained between vasodilation at the afferent portion and vasoconstriction at the efferent portion of the glomerulus in the context of relatively low blood pressure in the preterm and term newborn.[107] Therefore, newborns have a very small margin of adaptation in the context of disease states affecting regional perfusion, such as in the case of asphyxia, severe respiratory insufficiency, renal failure, and patent ductus arteriosus. Certain agents (e.g., indomethacin, tolazoline) may hamper their own excretion by reducing GFR.[112-114] In term newborns, GFR is 2 to 4 mL/min or 20 to 45 mL/min/1.73m^2 in the first postnatal month with an increase of 5 to 10 mL/min/1.73m^2/week,[115] and reaches adult values at around 1 year of age.[116] This maturation may also be predicted based on postmenstrual age and weight.[116] Creatinine, often used as a marker of GFR, is largely filtered at the glomerular level and partly secreted at proximal tubular level by the organic cation transporter 2 (OCT2). However, at birth, creatinine values are not a sufficiently precise correlates of GFR and largely reflect maternal creatinemia. Interestingly, certain compounds such as trimethoprim, cimetidine, and ranitidine that are also secreted by OCT2 competitively increase levels of creatinine, without truly decreasing GFR.[106] Some other drugs are largely dependent on GFR for their elimination, such as aminoglycoside and glycopeptide antibiotics, valganciclovir, and sotalol. Hence, renal maturational changes will have great impact on their clearance.[117,118]

ACTIVE TUBULAR TRANSPORT OF DRUGS

In the proximal tubule, active secretion increases the concentration of drug in the renal tubular fluid. A number of transport systems, found in the proximal tubule, are involved in the secretion of organic compounds (endogenous or xenobiotic).[119] Major carriers belonging to the SLC superfamily[21] include the OAT and OCT. OATs act as uptake transporters on drugs conjugated with glucuronic acid, glycine, and sulfates (e.g., penicillins, furosemide, and chlorothiazide). OCTs act on organic cations such as histamine and choline. Some drugs can selectively alter the activity of specific membrane transporters causing drug-drug interactions, consequently, resulting in increased or decreased elimination of compounds using the same transporter for their elimination (e.g., increased vancomycin clearance in the presence of amoxicillin/clavulanic acid,[106] and decreased elimination of digoxin by indomethacin).[106,120] In certain cases, these interactions can be used beneficially, as in the case of inhibited cidofovir renal uptake by co-administration of probenecid, to avoid nephrotoxicity.

The proximal tubule also expresses ABC transporters,[106] which are classified as efflux transporters. Among these ABC efflux transporters are MRPs, of which the 1, 3, 5, and 6 subtypes are localized at the basolateral membrane whereas MRP 2 and 4 are found at the brush-border (apical) membrane of the tubular epithelium.

Secretion of a drug often requires transporters both at the apical and at the basolateral membrane. For example, cationic drugs are transported by OCT2 at the basolateral membrane into the renal tubular cells and are exported out of the cells by the apical multidrug and toxin extrusion proteins MATE1 and MATE2/2K.[121] Similarly, OAT1 and OAT3 will uptake weakly acidic drugs at the basolateral membrane for eventual efflux into the tubular lumen by the apical multidrug resistance-associated proteins, including MRP2.[121]

Members of the proton-coupled oligopeptide transporters (POTs) superfamily, which include PEPT1 (SLC15A1), PEPT2 (SLC15A2), PHT1 (SLC15A4), and PHT2 (SLC15A3), are capable of handling small peptides and peptide-mimetic molecules.[122] PEPT1 and PEPT2 are localized at the apical membrane of renal proximal tubular epithelial cells and operate as influx pumps of peptides. They have the ability for sequence-independent handling of 400 variable dipeptides and 8000 tripeptides.[122]

In the case of organic cation, organic anion, and peptide transporters, cellular import requires an electrochemical gradient especially influenced by Na^+, which is largely maintained by the Na^+/K^+ ATPase pump, whereas MRPs are directly ATP-dependent.[119] Membrane transporters, mainly located in the distal tubule, operate to reabsorb drugs from the tubular lumen back into the systemic circulation. Most such reabsorption occurs by nonionic diffusion. Although polymorphisms of transporters are likely to affect drug disposition, current knowledge about their significance is limited. Ontogeny also affects activity of these transporters; accordingly, tubular secretion of organic anions and cations is lower in newborns than in adults. This developmental characteristic explains the prolonged half-life of certain agents that use this system of elimination, as is the case with furosemide, penicillin, and glucuronidated drugs, in the newborn.

PASSIVE TUBULAR REABSORPTION OF DRUGS

In both proximal and distal tubules, nonionized forms of weak acids and bases undergo net passive reabsorption. Accordingly, this form of renal reabsorption of drugs is regulated by three factors: the concentration gradient across the tubular membrane, the ionization state of the compound in the tubular fluid (which depends on the drug's pK_a and the tubular fluid pH), and the lipid solubility of the drug. Manipulation of these physicochemical properties can be used to enhance or decrease renal excretion. For instance, alkalinization of urine can increase the elimination of salicylic acid by up to sixfold. Weak acids are ionized in the setting of tubular alkalinization, leading to increased excretion. On the other hand, when the tubular content is more acidic, there is a reduction in the ionized form of weak acids and in their excretion. Similarly, one can expect the inverse effects of acidification and alkalinization of urine on excretion of weak bases. Diurnal variations of the urinary pH are not observed in the newborn until the infant reaches age 2 years.[123] As inferred above, the term *passive diffusion* does not exclude specific transporters/exchangers involved in movement across cell membranes and into compartments.

Patterns of renal excretion of drugs can be summarized as follows: (1) renal excretion of lipid-soluble drugs depends largely on urine volume; (2) elimination of polar drugs depends on the GFR; and (3) the renal elimination of drugs that ionize readily is principally dependent on the activity of the tubular secretory systems and the urine pH.

RENAL METABOLISM OF DRUGS

Although the liver is the main organ of drug metabolism, kidneys are also capable of drug biotransformation. For instance, mycophenolic acid, propofol, and 4-methylumbelliferone are metabolized to a greater extent by kidneys than by the liver.[124] The kidneys contain cytochrome P450 isoenzymes in the epithelium (mostly of the proximal tubule); UDP-glucuronosyl-transferases UGT1A5, 1A6, 1A7 and 2B7 have also been found in kidney.[125]

EFFECTS OF DISEASE ON DRUG ELIMINATION

Most pharmacokinetic parameters are determined on healthy or moderately ill individuals. In neonatal intensive care units, drugs are often administered to patients who require very complex care. Life-threatening illnesses produce remarkable variation in pharmacokinetic behavior. Adjustment of drug dosage in the face of a changing disease is critical to avoid toxicity.[36,126] For this reason, an understanding of the pathophysiology of a disease and its pharmacologic consequences becomes of utmost importance for appropriate pharmacologic therapy. This section addresses the issue of diseases as it applies to drug disposition in the newborn.

CARDIOVASCULAR DISEASE

Cardiac output is a major determinant of drug elimination. Heart failure alters the regional distribution of blood flow. Similarly, patients with congenital heart defects and preferential perfusion of the pulmonary or the systemic vasculature will have an impact on pharmaceutical targets. A significant decrease in cardiac output or oxygen delivery can result in adverse effects on liver function and consequently diminish drug metabolism and clearance.[127] Heart failure and conditions with a diastolic steal (such as a hemodynamically significant patent ductus arteriosus) are associated with a reduction in renal blood flow and GFR. This compromise in renal function may contribute to decreased drug elimination. In newborns with congestive heart failure, elevated plasma levels of digoxin have been observed, suggesting a decreased clearance of the drug.

RENAL DISEASE

Alterations in renal function can also significantly influence drug pharmacokinetics.[109] The pharmacologic consequences of renal dysfunction primarily depend on the fraction of drug cleared by the kidneys and on the degree of renal failure. Under these circumstances, drugs, for which the kidneys represent their primary route of elimination (e.g., aminoglycosides, cephalosporins), accumulate in the body; this is especially true when renal drug clearance is greater than 90% of total drug clearance. As GFR falls, there is a decrease in drugs eliminated principally via this route, such as digoxin, aminoglycosides, and cephalosporins. Reduction in tubular function can significantly affect the elimination of compounds, which depend on tubular reabsorption or secretion, such as penicillins and furosemide. In addition, changes in plasma and urine pH can alter the excretion of ionized drugs, especially weak acids and weak bases. The development of uremia may be associated with changes in the cardiac output, liver function, and permeability of blood-brain barrier, all of which can further disturb drug disposition. The clinical significance of drug accumulation depends on whether the unexcreted products are pharmacologically active or toxic. Nomograms have been developed to allow modification of drug dosage in patients with renal failure. However, most nomograms primarily apply to adult and not infant patients and should be used with caution. Notably, the newborn exhibits decreased renal clearance compared to older subjects.[68]

LIVER DISEASE

Because the liver is a major site of drug disposition, hepatic insufficiency is associated with defects in multiple liver functions, many of which have the potential to alter drug excretion. Hepatic insufficiency can affect drug elimination by (1) reducing plasma protein binding, (2) decreasing liver blood flow, and (3) disturbing intrinsic biotransformation reactions. A decrease in plasma protein concentration influences the disposition of drugs extensively bound to proteins. Drugs with liver uptake and metabolism can be categorized into two groups: one dependent on liver blood flow (flow limited) and the other dependent on the liver's metabolic capacity (capacity limited). Drugs that belong to the first group exhibit a more uniform change in drug elimination during hepatic failure. In contrast, drugs dependent on the metabolic activity of the liver exhibit heterogeneic changes in bio-disposition. This results from inconsistent qualitative and quantitative changes in liver enzyme activity in the presence of liver disease of variable severity. Also, there are gestational and postnatal age-dependent changes in the expression of metabolizing enzymes. The expression and activity of CYP450 and conjugation enzymes are different in newborns than in the pediatric and adult population. Expression follows three patterns: high expression during fetal compared to postnatal life, constant levels in the fetal and the postnatal periods, and activation of enzymes in the postnatal life.[128] Therefore, disease state might selectively alter a particular enzyme pathway. As an example, midazolam clearance relies on CYP3A4/5, which is decreased in preterm infants[106] and will increase fivefold in the first postnatal months.

Because of the marked variability in the severity of liver dysfunction, it is difficult to formulate rules for dosage modification. Marked changes in pharmacokinetics (as noted with renal insufficiency) are generally not observed in liver failure.[129] Nonetheless, dosages of drugs eliminated mainly by hepatic biotransformation should be reduced in infants with severe liver disease. The consequences of concurrent disease on the pharmacokinetics and pharmacodynamics of drugs are irrefutably complex. An accurate prediction of drug disposition in the face of interacting, intricate, individual variables is virtually impossible. The relative paucity of information on pharmacokinetics of drugs in infants with cardiac, renal, and hepatic dysfunction and the often changing and transient nature of these disorders render careful clinical observations and appropriate therapeutic monitoring imperative under these circumstances. Of note, the neonate with intrauterine growth restriction expresses less CYP450, thus compromising hepatic drug clearance.[130]

PULMONARY DISEASE

Several cytochrome P450 isoforms, sulfotransferases, UDP glucuronosyl transferases, glutathione S-transferases, esterases, peptidases, and cyclooxygenases are expressed in the lungs. However, their significance in drug handling is yet to be determined.[131] Many conditions of the term and preterm newborn will affect pulmonary functions and/or structure. Pathologies such as pulmonary hypertension, pulmonary hypoplasia, and pulmonary hemorrhage are common in the newborn period. These conditions can impact drug delivery via the inhaled route. In addition, pulmonary hypertension may lead to a concurrent decrease in systemic cardiac output, with all of its consequences on kidney and liver drug handling capacities.

EFFECTS OF SPECIFIC THERAPEUTIC APPLICATIONS ON DRUG DISPOSITION IN THE NEWBORN

Extracorporeal membrane oxygenation (ECMO) is used in newborns with cardiac malformation and failure (veno-arterial approach) or with reversible respiratory insufficiency (usually veno-venous approach). Patients subjected to ECMO therapy are usually very ill and require an abundance of treatments for hemodynamic support, sedation, infection, analgesia, as well as parenteral nutrition. ECMO requires cannulas, polyvinyl chloride tubing, centrifugal pump, and a membrane oxygenator. Properties (size, surface exposed, and material) of the equipment may affect drug sequestration within the circuit, as well as distribution.[132] It should, however, be noted that there is a paucity of data regarding the new biocompatible coatings and polymethylpentene membrane oxygenators.[132] Properties of the priming solution, hemodilution, frequent transfusions or volume repletion, temperature, circuit age, hypoalbuminemia, and clotting may also affect distribution and clearance. ECMO also affects absolute circulatory volume and can also induce an inflammatory cascade leading to capillary extravasation and CYP450 inactivation; in this context, non-pulsatile flow may itself affect renal clearance.[132] In addition, components of ECMO circuits (such as silicone-based or microporous membranes) may impact on drug metabolism and distribution.[128] The distribution of most drugs will increase, and their clearance will decrease.[128] Drugs with a lipophilic profile (midazolam) exhibit a decreased volume of distribution, whereas hydrophilic drugs (gentamicin, cefotaxime, morphine, vancomycin) exhibit a moderate increase.[128] Accordingly, ECMO significantly alters drug distribution and clearance, with the potential to cause either toxicity or subtherapeutic effects.

Therapeutic hypothermia is standard of care treatment for newborns with moderate to severe perinatal asphyxia, as it exerts a neuroprotective effect. Asphyxia, and separately hypothermia, have profound effects on drug metabolism, clearance, and distribution. Newborns with asphyxia often have acute kidney injury with oliguria, liver failure, and cardiac insufficiency. Yet, given the breadth of severity of asphyxia, its effects on renal and hepatic clearance tend to be variable and are rarely predictable.

Hypothermia per se can impact blood composition, circulatory hemodynamics, enzymatic processes, and regional perfusion. Hypothermia, which is associated with decreased cardiac output during attempts to preserve cerebral and cardiac perfusion, will cause decreased volume of distribution of drugs. For instance, distribution of pancuronium, midazolam, gentamicin, and morphine were found to be unchanged or diminished by hypothermia.[128]

CLINICAL PHARMACOKINETICS

Pharmacokinetics is the study of the time course of a drug into the body, which involves the processes of absorption, distribution, metabolism, and excretion. This quantitative science characterizes the relationship between the drug dose and concentration (exposure) over time, mainly in plasma. Safe and effective plasma concentrations or the therapeutic window are determined based on the relationship between plasma concentrations and the concentration at the site of action, as well as the concentration-response relationship (pharmacodynamics). Clinical pharmacokinetics is a key element in determining the right dose to achieve target concentrations and is therefore an important tool in drug development. By guiding dosing regimen, pharmacokinetics also helps with optimizing and individualizing therapy in neonates.

Pharmacokinetics are commonly characterized by representing the body as a system of various compartments into which a drug is distributed and from which it may be eliminated (Fig. 15.2). A compartment is not necessarily a defined physiologic or

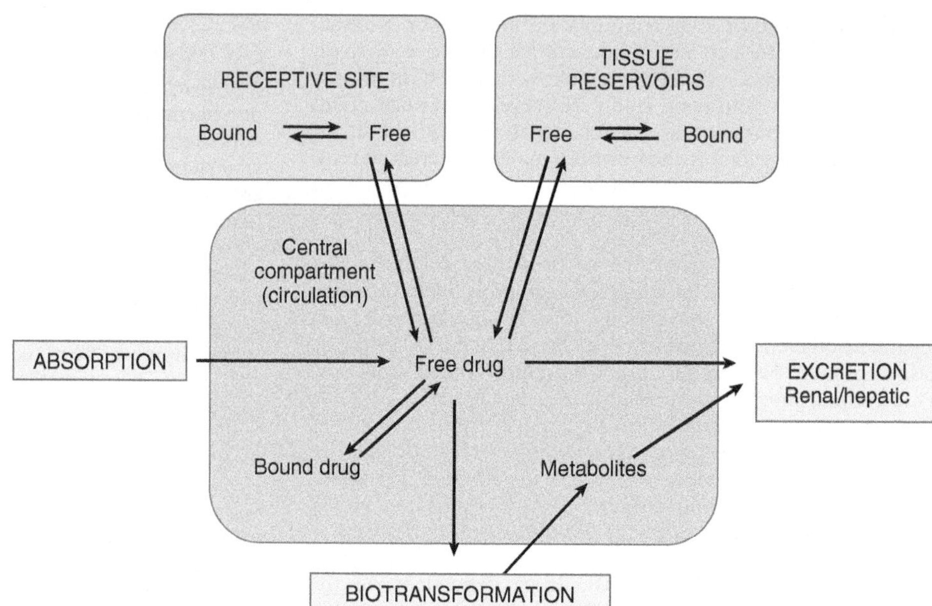

Fig. 15.2 Schematic of possible drug disposition to various compartments in the body.

anatomic site but is considered one or many tissues that exhibit similar affinity for a drug.

The factors that determine the movement of a drug in and out of compartments include absorption, distribution, and elimination. Therefore, the lipophilicity, ionization state, transporters (both influx and efflux carriers), and protein binding of a drug, as well as regional blood flow regulate the extent and rate of passage of an agent into and out of a compartment.

ONE-COMPARTMENT MODEL

The one-compartment model assumes that immediate equilibration of drug concentration is achieved in all major tissues following drug administration. Drugs that are highly hydrophilic, such as aminoglycosides, distribute rapidly in the central compartment. Their pharmacokinetics is therefore well described by a one-compartment model. This simple model allows the clinical application of pharmacokinetics principles for most of the drugs used in clinical practice.

VOLUME OF DISTRIBUTION

The relationship between drug concentration and the amount of drug in the body is defined by the volume of distribution (V_d). When the drug is given intravenously, the amount of drug in the body initially is equal to the dose that was administered (bioavailability of 100%). If the drug is instantaneously distributed throughout the body (one-compartment model assumption), we can express V_d as follows:

$$V_d = C_0 / Dose$$

where C_0 is the plasma concentration at time = 0.

V_d is a proportionality constant and has no defined physiologic meaning. The more a drug is distributed in peripheral tissues, the lower the plasma concentration will be for a given dose, and the higher V_d will be.

For instance, tobramycin is an aminoglycoside commonly used in neonates to treat infections due to aerobic gram-negative bacilli. Its efficacy is concentration-dependent, meaning that antibacterial activity is maximal when the ratio of the peak concentration (C_{max}) to the bacteria minimum inhibitory concentration (MIC) is 10 μg/mL. Tobramycin V_d is higher in more preterm infants (0.70 L/kg vs. 0.54 L/kg in infants <32 weeks of gestational age vs. ≥37 weeks).[133] Preterm infants therefore need a higher dose per kg weight compared with term infants to reach the desired C_{max}. However, due to decreased clearance, this dose is given less frequently (longer dosing interval).

ELIMINATION RATE

In first-order kinetics, the rate of elimination (dX/dt) is the rate at which the drug is cleared and is proportional to the amount of drug present in the body at the time. Thus, the higher the dose, the greater the elimination rate from the compartment. The rate of disappearance of a drug amount can be expressed as:

$$dX/dt = -k * X$$

where X is the amount of drug in the body, and k is the first-order elimination constant, expressed in units of time^{-1} (e.g., h^{-1}).

Based on the relationship between the amount of drug (X) and its concentration (C), we can then express the previous equations as follows:

$$dC/dt = -k * C$$

Integration of this equation yields the concentration at a time, t:

$$\ln C = -kt + \ln C_0 \text{ or } C = C_0 e^{-kt}$$

where C_0 is the drug concentration in the body immediately after an intravenous administration (at $t = 0$), and C is the drug concentration at time t.

Thus, the slope of the natural logarithm of the concentration-time curve is −k and can also be calculated once plasma concentrations at two time points are known:

$$k = [\ln(C_1 / C_2)] / (t_1 - t_2)$$

where C_1 and C_2 are the plasma concentrations at time t_1 and t_2, respectively.

DRUG CLEARANCE

Drug clearance is defined as the volume of blood that is cleared of drug per unit of time (e.g., L/h). Total clearance gives an indication of drug elimination from the central compartment without reference to the mechanism of this process. Clearance by the kidneys is referred to as *renal clearance*, and that by all other organs as *nonrenal clearance*. The latter most often represents clearance by the liver. Total or systemic clearance is the sum of all body clearances.

Table 15.4 Comparative Plasma Half-Lives of Miscellaneous Drugs in Newborns and Adults.

	Plasma Half-Life (Hours)	
	Newborn	**Adult**
Acetaminophen	3.5	2.2
Phenylbutazone	21–34	12–30
Indomethacin	7.5–51.0	6
Meperidine	22	3.5
Phenytoin	21	11–29
Carbamazepine	8–28	21–36
Phenobarbital	82–199	24–140
Caffeine	100	6
Theophylline	30	6
Chloramphenicol	14–24	2.5
Salicylates	4.5–11.5	2.7
Digoxin	52	31–40

Data from References 35, 109, 117, 118, 126, and 133–136.

For drugs that are eliminated by first-order kinetics, clearance is constant. This means that the elimination rate (dX/dt) is proportional to the amount of drug in the body (X). Clearance (Cl) is mathematically defined as the ratio of elimination rate (dX/dt) over plasma concentration (C) and is expressed in volume per unit of time (e.g., L/h).

$$Cl = dX/dt/C$$

Over a given period of time, the previous equation can then be expressed as follow:

$$Cl = \text{Dose}/\text{AUC}$$

where AUC is the area under the concentration-time curve.

After multiple drug dose administrations, and when steady state is achieved, Cl and the dose are the only parameters that determine plasma concentration. The average plasma concentration ($C_{ss\ av}$) at steady state is expressed as:

$$C_{ss\ av} = (\text{Dose}/\tau)/Cl$$

where τ is the dosing interval. This equation illustrates how one can achieve the same $C_{ss\ av}$ with several combinations of doses and dosing intervals for a given drug.

Clearance mechanisms undergo maturation with age, meaning that the drug is eliminated more slowly in younger and more preterm infants. For example, fluconazole clearance doubles between birth and 28 days of age from 0.010 to 0.022 L/kg/h for a 32-week gestation infant.[134] Given that AUC at steady state depends on the dose and the clearance, younger infants need a smaller maintenance dose per kg weight to reach the same target exposure relative to older infants.[134]

DRUG HALF-LIFE

Half-life is another way to characterize drug elimination and is generally more intuitive than Cl and elimination rate to conceptualize in clinical practice. Half-life is not a primary pharmacokinetic parameter, meaning that it can be derived from Cl and V_d estimates. Elimination half-life is the time required for plasma concentration to decrease by one-half when a drug follows first-order elimination kinetics. In first-order kinetics, half-life is constant regardless of the concentrations, meaning that it takes the same time to go from 50 mg/L to 25 mg/L as it takes to go from 5 mg/L to 2.5 mg/L.

From the previous equation, $k = \ln(C_1/C_2)/(t_1 - t_2)$, the first-order half-life can be obtained:

$$t_{1/2} = 0.693/k$$

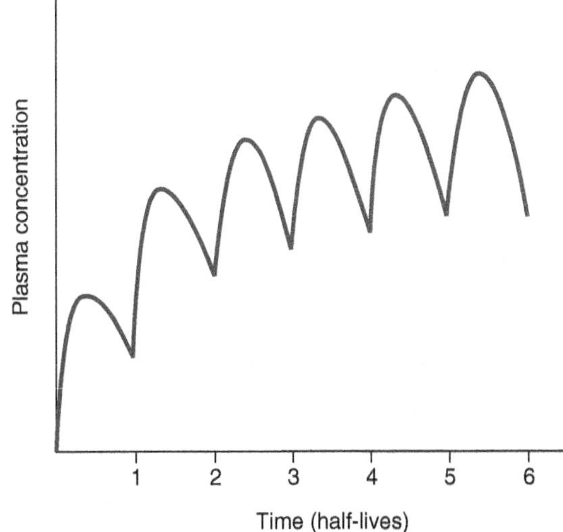

Fig. 15.3 Pharmacokinetic relationships of a multiple dosing regimen. From this graph, it can easily be appreciated that the time required to attain steady-state drug concentrations is equal to approximately five half-lives, when first-order rates of absorption, distribution, and elimination are in process.

where $t_{1/2}$ is the half-life and k is the elimination constant.

Given the exponential decay of concentrations in first-order kinetics, it takes at least 5 half-lives to eliminate the near totality of the drug. In newborns, because the elimination rate is decreased for many drugs, the half-life is often prolonged compared to that of the adult (Table 15.4).

STEADY STATE

After multiple dose administrations, the drug accumulates in the body, because at the time of the next administration, the previous dose is not completely cleared. As drug accumulates, the amount of drug in the body increases, resulting in an increase in the elimination rate in first-order kinetics.

In the context of repeat dose administrations, there are two components to take into account: (1) the input rate: dD/dt (rate of drug administration) and (2) the output rate: dE/dt (rate of drug elimination). Steady state is achieved when the input rate equals the output rate. At this point, the average plasma concentration ($C_{ss\ av}$) is stable.

For any drug following first-order kinetics, it takes 3.3 half-lives to reach 90% of $C_{ss\ av}$, and 5 half-lives to reach 97% of $C_{ss\ av}$ (Fig 15.3). As a result, time to achieve steady state may take several days for drugs with prolonged half-lives. This is especially true in newborn infants who generally clear drugs more slowly, resulting in longer half-lives. Given that target concentrations are generally achieved at steady state, this delay may result in delayed efficacy.

OPTIMAL DOSING

LOADING DOSE

A loading dose (D_L) is considered when time to achieve therapeutic exposure is prolonged. This dose is equal to:

$$D_L = C_{target} * V_d$$

where C_{target} is the desired therapeutic concentration and V_d is the volume of distribution. The need for a loading dose can be illustrated by looking at the fluconazole dosing regimen in infants. A dose of 12 mg/kg/day achieves therapeutic concentrations after 10 days of therapy, which is unacceptable in critically ill infants.[135] This delay may contribute to the high morbidity associated with invasive candidiasis in infants. A loading dose of 25 mg/kg achieves target concentrations within 24 to 48 hours.[135] When V_d increases, as in infants on ECMO (1.3 L/kg vs. 0.93 L/kg), the loading dose needs to be higher (35 mg/kg vs. 25 mg/kg).[135]

MAINTENANCE DOSE

After a loading dose, the dose necessary to maintain this concentration (maintenance dose, D_{ss}) can be calculated from the following equation:

$$D_{ss} = (0.693 \times C_{ss\,av} \times V_d \times \tau)\ / t_{1/2}$$

where τ is the dosing interval and $C_{ss\,av}$ is the average plasma concentration at steady state.

OPTIMAL DOSING SCHEDULE

Knowledge of the elimination constant or the half-life permits the clinician to guide the dosing schedule, having set the maximum and minimum effective steady-state concentrations during a multiple dosing regimen (see Fig. 15.3). Using the same equation to calculate the concentration at a time t ($\ln C = -kt + \ln C_0$), an optimal dosing interval τ can also be determined. By substituting C with $C_{ss\,min}$ and C_0 with $C_{ss\,max}$, the following dosing interval equation is obtained:

$$\ln(C_{ss\,max}/C_{ss\,min})/k \text{ or } \ln(C_{ss\,max}/C_{ss\,min}) * \left(0.693/t_{1/2}\right)$$

where $C_{ss\,max}$ and $C_{ss\,min}$ are the maximum and minimum effective steady-state concentrations, k is the elimination constant, and $t_{1/2}$ is the elimination half-life.

MULTICOMPARTMENT DISTRIBUTION

Many drugs distribute in the body according to the kinetics of a multicompartment model. Consequently, following intravenous administration of the drug, the plasma concentration does not decline linearly on a logarithmic scale (see Fig. 15.1). The first part of the curve with its sharper slope, the α phase, represents the distribution. With time and depending on the affinity of the drug for certain tissues, the agent distributes to the central and peripheral compartments. After equilibration, the tissues are saturated with the drug, and its decline in blood usually occurs via a first-order elimination process, the β phase (see Fig. 15.1). The elimination rate and half-life of drugs that distribute according to a two-compartment model should only be determined during the β phase.

To apply kinetic analysis of a multicompartment model, one assumes that all rate processes for the passage of drug from one compartment to another exhibit first-order kinetics. Therefore, the plasma level-time curve for a drug that follows a multicompartment model is described by the summation of several first-order rate processes. Lipophilic drugs such as benzodiazepines distribute in peripheral compartments and are therefore better described using a multicompartment model.[136]

ZERO-ORDER KINETICS

When elimination processes become saturated, disposition of certain drugs occurs via zero-order kinetics. In contrast to a first-order process, in which the fraction of drug eliminated is constant, in zero-order kinetics the elimination rate itself is constant. Thus the drug is eliminated at a constant rate. Consequently, the clearance decreases as concentration increases. Finally, half-life is not constant but is proportional to the initial amount or concentration of the drug:

$$t_{1/2} = 0.5 * C_0/k_0$$

where k_0 = zero-order rate constant. Many drugs exhibit zero-order kinetics with elevated concentrations, and as these decline, first-order kinetics prevail. Examples of drugs that exhibit saturation kinetics include salicylates, phenylbutazone, phenytoin, diazepam, and chloramphenicol.

The determination of drug pharmacokinetics has not been widely accepted as an essential part of newborn intensive care. The amount of reliable pharmacokinetic data for drugs used in the ill neonate has lagged considerably behind knowledge of pathophysiology. There is little doubt that this information as well as monitoring of plasma levels can optimize drug dosage. When one considers the risks of therapeutic failure and toxicity, the rationale for drug monitoring is obvious. In addition, the many complex development-related and disease-related dynamic processes that take place in the sick newborn provide sufficient justification to measure drug blood levels to obtain an indication of its kinetics.

PRINCIPLES OF PHARMACODYNAMICS: DRUG-RECEPTOR INTERACTION

Pharmacodynamics is defined as the biochemical and physiologic effects of drugs, including mechanisms of their action. This aspect of pharmacology is the *raison d'être* of pharmacotherapeutics. The mechanism of action of drugs at the receptive site has received increased attention over the past three decades. This section reviews some of the basic principles of drug-receptor interaction. The term *receptive site* refers to the molecular entity, with which the drug is presumed to interact.

SITES OF DRUG ACTION

Drugs may act outside the cell, at the cell membrane, or inside the cell. Regardless of cellular localization, the drug action can either be mediated by receptors or independent of receptors. Certain agents do not act on cellular sites but instead on extracellular products of cells. For instance, chelating agents, such as dimercaprol, penicillamine, and desferrioxamine, bind to circulating metals. The action of these agents can be considered truly extracellular. The majority of drugs, however, bind to a specific cellular site. The localization of drug refers both to the drug distribution and to the specificity of drug action. Such specificity implies existence of receptors. Receptors consist of macromolecules that recognize and bind specific ligands and translate this binding into propagation of an intracellular message, either directly (e.g., nicotinic receptor: ion transport) or indirectly via a second messenger (e.g., protein kinase C family of enzymes are activated by a variety of G-protein-coupled receptors on stimulation with respective agonist). These receptor characteristics have led some to suggest the existence of functional domains on the receptor molecule: one or more ligand-binding domains and effector domains. Such conceptualization of the receptor is generally consistent with the mode of action of agonists and antagonists but appears to be a simplified version of complex processes (see below).

Drugs that bind to physiologic receptors and mimic the regulatory effects of the endogenous ligands are termed *agonists*, which may be either non-selective or biased (selective activation of one cellular signaling pathway but not others) in their effects. Partial agonists are drugs that bind to the receptor to produce a submaximal response relative to the full agonist (e.g., endogenous ligand). Compounds that block the effects of endogenous agonists are termed *antagonists*, sometimes referred to as *neutral antagonists* to denote their lack of intrinsic efficacy (i.e., no effect in absence of agonist). Inverse agonists are a class of drugs that stabilize the receptor in its inactive confirmation.[137] By virtue of this property, they neutralize constitutive activity (ability to produce active confirmation in absence of ligand binding) of the receptor. In absence of the constitutive activity, an inverse agonist behaves like a neutral competitive antagonist. In recent years, many drugs that were previously thought to be neutral antagonists have been reclassified as inverse agonists.[138] It is important to note that inverse agonists might be of pharmacologic interest in treatment of diseases that have been shown to be the result of altered constitutive activity of the receptors.[139]

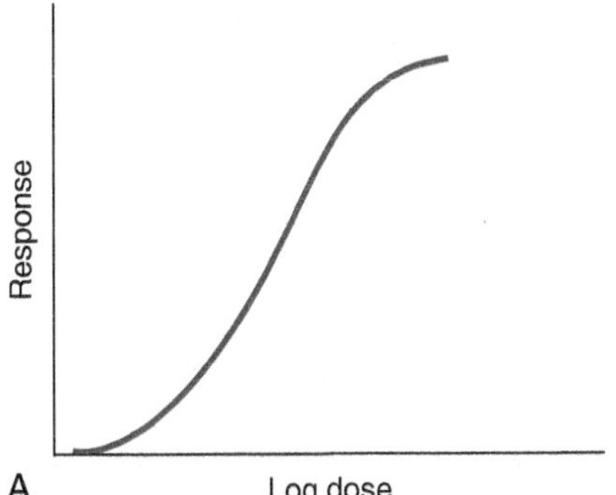

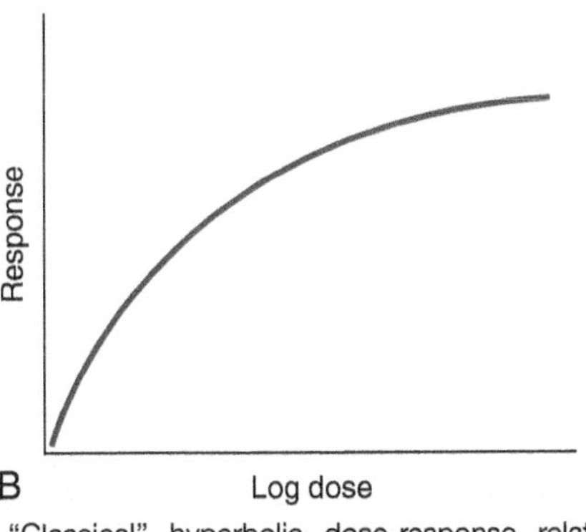

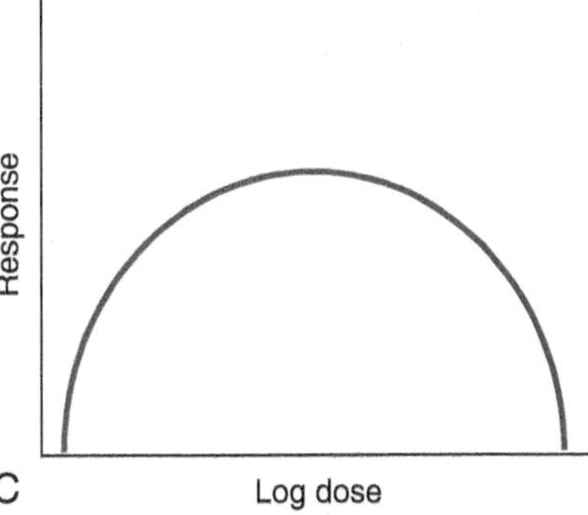

Fig. 15.4 The dose-response relationship. (A) "Classical" hyperbolic dose-response relationship. Examples of complex dose-response relationships: sigmoidal (B) and bell-shaped (C). The slope and shape of the curve reflect the mechanism of action of the drug. The potency is reflected by the position of the curve along the abscissa. The efficacy is reflected by the maximum position of the curve along the ordinate.

RECEPTOR CLASSIFICATION

Receptors have traditionally been classified pharmacologically by their response to specific antagonists. The precise classification of receptors with respect to structure-activity relationship, however, relies on multiple approaches, which include physiologic, biochemical, biophysical, and immunologic techniques. These broadened characteristics delineate more precisely the action of drugs, facilitating the development of therapeutic agents having selectivity for specific receptors. This also provides the clinician with an appropriate basis for therapeutics, by ameliorating efficacy and limiting toxicity.

RECEPTOR REGULATION

The concentration and affinity of receptors are physiologically regulated by ligand-receptor binding and activation. Receptor down-regulation is the process by which the concentration and affinity of receptors are decreased. This regulation of receptor function can be classified on the basis of the time course, short and long term. Short-term regulation occurs in the order of seconds to minutes, and long-term regulation takes place over hours to days. The mechanisms responsible for short-term regulation appear to involve conformational changes, transient intracellular receptor sequestration (e.g., nicotinic and α-adrenergic receptors), and phosphorylation of receptors. Protein phosphorylation is the mechanism by which most receptors are regulated, although myristoylation and palmitoylation are also involved in the regulation of expression of certain receptors. Long-term receptor down-regulation involves initial protein phosphorylation, (myristoylation, palmitoylation, sumoylation, or ubiquitination) followed by internalization and degradation, requiring Rab GTPases.[140]

The term *receptor up-regulation* refers to the process of increasing receptor number. An example of up-regulation is the phenomenon of denervation supersensitivity of nicotinic receptors. The process of up-regulation is less clearly understood. Alterations in transcription of mRNA, translation, or posttranslational modifications seem to contribute to receptor up-regulation. Thus, changes in receptor number and affinity may well explain certain forms of drug tolerance, tachyphylaxis, and desensitization.

Changes in receptor binding, density, and coupling events can also occur with development. For instance, in the brain of the rat and pig, marked ontogenic changes in cholinergic muscarinic, α-adrenergic, and prostaglandin receptor density have been observed.[141-143] In addition, the pathophysiology of diseases such as testicular feminization, pseudohypoparathyroidism, myasthenia gravis, and certain forms of diabetes seems to involve receptor-associated dysfunctions.[144-146] Similarly, mutations of receptors can increase vulnerability to certain conditions and/or accelerate desensitization to receptor agonists as reported for β-adrenoceptor agonists.[147] Thus, developmental and pathologic considerations must be accounted for by the clinician and investigator when evaluating a response.

RELATIONSHIP BETWEEN DRUG DOSE AND RESPONSE

According to the receptor occupancy theory, response is proportional to receptor binding.[148] Thus, maximal response is achieved when all receptors are bound. Although this concept has a degree of practical validity, interpretation of receptor binding is often difficult, particularly when the coupling events encompass a complex sequence of reactions. Such is the case when further receptor occupancy does not produce greater response; this has led to the concept of *spare receptors*, wherein a maximal response is achieved when a relatively small proportion of the receptors is occupied. Other yet more complex receptor-evoked functions involve allosteric modulations and protein interactions.

THE ALLOSTERIC NATURE OF RECEPTOR SIGNALING

The theoretical framework associated with the study of ligand-receptor interactions has adopted the law of mass action—essentially a simple reversible and saturable one-to-one interaction between ligand and receptor (Fig. 15.4A). This classical view has served many pharmacologists in the past. However, insights obtained from research on enzymes, ion channels, and hemoglobin in the last four decades has opened the path to infer more complex interactions between ligands and receptors. Essentially, more than one ligand can interact with a single receptive unit, yielding the concept of "cooperativity." This assumes that conformational changes in the protein of interest (e.g., a receptor) as well as its interaction with adjacent partners results in formation of a dynamic oligomeric complex. Accordingly, one can envisage specific molecules to interact with sites on the receptor, which are distinct and thus remote from the "classical" (or orthosteric) binding site for an endogenous ligand and consequently affect its conformational state; these molecules are termed *allosteric modulators*.[149] This will yield much more complex ligand-receptor interactions than the simple hyperbolic profiles classically observed (see Fig. 15.4A). For example, this may include the ligand-receptor interactions resulting in sigmoidal or bell-shaped dose-response curves (see Fig. 15.4B and C). The slope and shape of the curve reflect the mechanism of action of a drug. The potency describes the location of the curve along the X-axis and is influenced by the inherent affinity of the drug for its receptor and the latter's ability to couple with the post-receptor signaling mechanisms. The efficacy is characterized by the maximum biologic response observed regardless of dose-response profile. In the case of allosteric compounds efficacy and potency often vary depending upon the specific signal and action detected; this variability is further magnified when studying the same signal or action in distinct tissues and organs, resulting from the formation of different oligomeric complexes containing the receptor of interest.[150]

For purposes of illustration, we will briefly elaborate on allosteric behavior using G protein-coupled receptors (GPCRs), which have been the most studied receptors. GPCRs constitute the largest superfamily of cell-surface receptors. In last two decades, a number of GPCRs have been shown to be functional at intracellular locations, including at the nuclear membranes.[29-32] These receptors mediate a plethora of responses. The classical transduction unit of GPCRs is governed by reciprocal allosteric interactions that occur between three elements: (1) a seven transmembrane domain receptor polypeptide that binds the transmitter, (2) a trimeric ($\alpha\beta\gamma$) G protein, and (3) an effector component. Binding of a transmitter to the receptor leads to the exchange of GDP for GTP on the Gα chain. The activated heterotrimeric G protein, either through its α-GTP chain, the $\beta\gamma$ dimer, or both, in turn modulates the effector components, leading to the response. The well-known effectors modulated by GPCRs include enzymes such as adenylyl cyclase and phospholipases C as well as ion channels and antiporters. Moreover, the Erk1/Erk2/p38 MAP/JNK kinase signaling pathways have been shown to be activated by stimulation of G proteins of the Gq, Gi, and Gs family via many distinct signaling pathways.[151-153] In addition to their G protein-mediated effects, GPCRs have also been found to interact directly and modulate the activity of an increasing list of proteins including β-arrestins, NHERF/EBP50, JAK, eNOS, NSF, Rho and Arf, spinophilin, 14-3-3, Nck and Grb2, endophilins, CREB and ATFx, $GABA_A$, and the glutamate NMDA receptors (see Bockaert et al. for a review).[154] The complexity of GPCR signaling is increased further by evidence that suggests same effector molecules can be activated by two or more independent signaling pathways of the receptor. For example, the parathyroid hormone receptor agonist "[Trp^1]PTHrp-(1-36)" results in ERK1/2 activation via G-protein mediated pathway, whereas another agonist "[D-Trp^{12}, Tyr^{34}]PTH-(7-34)" also results in ERK1/2 activation but via β-arrestin mediated signaling.[155] This phenomenon is particularly important in studies that involve "biased" agonists. Moreover, contrary to traditional views, increasing evidence indicates that GPCRs exist as homo- and heterodimers (or even larger oligomeric assemblies) that may have important consequences on their signaling properties.[156,157] It is also worth mentioning that GPCRs can crosstalk with tyrosine kinase receptors, such as epidermal growth factor receptor (EGFR), resulting in transactivation of the latter with the help of transmembrane proteins.[158,159] Although the physiologic importance of many of these interactions needs to be further investigated, the large number of proteins that appear to be involved in GPCR signaling suggest a level of allosteric complexity that was not anticipated just a few years ago.

Classically, orthosteric modulators are thought to bind to the receptor at the same site that is occupied by the endogenous ligand and to promote or to stabilize similar receptor conformations. Allosteric modulators, on the other hand, bind to receptor sites, which are physically remote from that of the orthosteric ligand. By virtue of this binding, specific receptor confirmation (or a small ensemble of confirmations) is stabilized, resulting in the observed effects. These compounds can be classified as positive allosteric modulators (PAMs), which enhance agonist effect and negative allosteric modulators (NAMs), which attenuate agonist response.[160]

One major difference between the orthosteric and allosteric modulators is that the allosteric effect is saturable. This is due to the fact that allosteric modulators also require ligand binding at the orthosteric sites. Once orthosteric sites are occupied by all available ligands, adding more allosteric modulators will not produce more biologic effect.[161,162] It is also important to note that allosteric modulators can produce different effects with respect to different agonists ("probe-dependent" effects).[161]

In the traditional two-state receptor activation model,[163] modulators were believed to control the equilibrium between an active and an inactive GPCR conformer. Increasing evidence indicates that separate ligands can differentially regulate various signaling cascades activated by a given receptor, which suggests that numerous active receptor conformations may exist in dynamic equilibrium and in turn result in different signaling efficacy profiles toward distinct effector systems. One of the most striking illustrations of this phenomenon, known as *agonist trafficking* or *biased agonism*,[164] is the observation that some β-adrenergic ligands, that act as inverse agonists for the adenylyl cyclase pathway, behave as full agonists for the MAPK pathway following binding to the β2-adrenergic receptor.[165] Similar observations have been made for the V2-vasopressin receptor,[165] the histamine receptor,[166] and the angiotensin receptor.[167] This led to the concept that distinct receptor conformations are responsible for the differential allosteric regulation of distinct subsets of signaling partners opening the avenue for the development of compounds that could selectively target only one of the receptor signaling modes. In this context, allosteric regulation of receptor conformations through homo- or heterodimerization or as a result of interactions with various effectors and accessory proteins opens many potential target sites for pharmacologic modulation. Receptors can be seen as allosteric machines of which pharmacologic potential has only been superficially explored; some of the examples of allosteric modulators of receptors include oxytremorine,[168] PDC113.824,[169] SCH-202676,[170] and the anti-interleukin-1 receptor peptide rytvela.[171] Moreover, drugs with allosteric properties have been utilized successfully in the clinical setting, as in anxiety (e.g., benzodiazepines, which act on GABA receptors), arrhythmia (e.g., quinidine, which acts on the Kv1.4 channel), secondary hyperparathyroidism (e.g., cinacalcet, which acts on the calcium-sensing receptor), psychosis (e.g., aripiprazole, which acts on D2 receptor), and HIV infection (e.g., maraviroc, which acts on CCR5 chemokine receptor). The study and exploitation of allosteric phenomena will become progressively of greater importance to drug discovery and development, to enhance pathway selectivity and diminish adverse effects.[172]

RECEPTOR SUBCELLULAR LOCALIZATION AND DRUG ACTION

Another dimension of drug action, which has not been taken into account until recently, refers to the subcellular localization of transmembrane receptors. In this context, a receptor can be functionally localized at the plasma membrane and/or the cell nucleus, where it exerts distinct functions. Interestingly, the signaling machinery necessary for receptor coupling is often already present at the nucleus.[173] This concept was first described for the prostaglandin E_2 receptors[29] and has since been confirmed by others for many different receptors.[174] Moreover, in vivo functionality of a nuclear receptor that complements actions of its congener at the plasma membrane has been reported.[32] Accordingly, targeting a receptor for specific functions based on its cellular localization must be considered in the process of drug discovery, development, and clinical application.

IN VIVO EFFICACY AND POTENCY VERSUS TOXICITY

Regardless of the mode of action of a compound, the main determining factors in the selection of a drug are efficacy and foremost toxicity. In the clinical setting, potency per se should not be a determining factor in the selection of an agent. Under all therapeutic circumstances, the drug chosen should ideally provide the greatest margin of safety. This selectivity has been termed the *therapeutic index*, which is usually defined as the ratio of the median toxic dose to median effective dose (TD_{50}/ED_{50}) and in laboratory studies as the ratio of the median lethal to effective dose (LD_{50}/ED_{50}).

CONCLUSION

Marked differences in drug disposition and action exist between the newborn and adult. Greater differences exist for the ill preterm neonate. These differences must be taken into consideration when applying therapies to newborns. Appropriate application of basic principles in pharmacology as well as adequate drug monitoring allows individualization of drug dosage and ameliorates treatment of neonates by reducing adverse drug effects.[126]

 A complete reference list is available at www.ExpertConsult.com.

SELECT REFERENCES

1. Whittaker E, Goldblatt D, McIntyre P, et al. Neonatal immunization: rationale, current state, and future prospects. *Front Immunol*. 2018;9:532.
2. Malcolm WF, Cotten CM. Metoclopramide, H2 blockers, and proton pump inhibitors: pharmacotherapy for gastroesophageal reflux in neonates. *Clin Perinatol*. 2012;39:99.
3. Cuzzolin L, Antonucci R, Fanos V. Paracetamol (acetaminophen) efficacy and safety in the newborn. *Curr Drug Metab*. 2013;14:178.
4. Abman SH, Hansmann G, Archer SL, et al. Pediatric pulmonary hypertension: guidelines from the American Heart Association and American Thoracic Society. *Circulation*. 2015;132:2037.
5. Schanker LS. Passage of drugs across body membranes. *Pharmacol Rev*. 1962;14:501.
6. Lee VH, Sporty JL, Fandy TE. Pharmacogenomics of drug transporters: the next drug delivery challenge. *Adv Drug Deliv Rev*. 2001;50(suppl 1):S33.
7. Jollow DJ, Brodie BB. Mechanisms of drug absorption and of drug solution. *Pharmacology*. 1972;8:21.
8. Terao T, Matsuda K, Shouji H. Improvement in site-specific intestinal absorption of furosemide by Eudragit L100-55. *J Pharm Pharmacol*. 2001;53:433.
9. Sawada Y, Hanano M, Sugiyama Y, et al. Prediction of the disposition of nine weakly acidic and six weakly basic drugs in humans from pharmacokinetic parameters in rats. *J Pharmacokinet Biopharm*. 1985;13:477.
10. Quamme GA. Loop diuretics. In: Dirks JH, Sutton RAL, eds. *Diuretics: Physiology, Pharmacology and Clinical Use*. Philadelphia: WB Saunders Co; 1986:86-116.
11. Zhang L, Brett CM, Giacomini KM. Role of organic cation transporters in drug absorption and elimination. *Annu Rev Pharmacol Toxicol*. 1998;38:431.
12. Burckhardt G, Wolff NA. Structure of renal organic anion and cation transporters. *Am J Physiol Renal Physiol*. 2000;278:F853.
13. Bode F, Pockrandt-Hemstedt H, Baumann K, et al. Analysis of the pinocytic process in rat kidney. I. Isolation of pinocytic vesicles from rat kidney cortex. *J Cell Biol*. 1974;63:998.
14. König J, Muller F, Fromm MF. Transporters and drug-drug interactions: important determinants of drug disposition and effects. *Pharmacol Rev*. 2013;65:944.
15. Povey S, Lovering R, Bruford E, et al. The HUGO Gene Nomenclature Committee (HGNC). *Hum Genet*. 2001;109:678.
16. Sadee W, Drubbisch V, Amidon GL. Biology of membrane transport proteins. *Pharm Res*. 1995;12:1823.
17. Brandsch M, Knutter I, Bosse-Doenecke E. Pharmaceutical and pharmacological importance of peptide transporters. *J Pharm Pharmacol*. 2008;60:543.
18. Wagner DJ, Hu T, Wang J. Polyspecific organic cation transporters and their impact on drug intracellular levels and pharmacodynamics. *Pharmacol Res*. 2016;111:237.
19. Jonker JW, Schinkel AH. Pharmacological and physiological functions of the polyspecific organic cation transporters: OCT1, 2, and 3 (SLC22A1-3). *J Pharmacol Exp Ther*. 2004;308:2.
20. Koepsell H. Polyspecific organic cation transporters: their functions and interactions with drugs. *Trends Pharmacol Sci*. 2004;25:375.
21. Roth M, Obaidat A, Hagenbuch B. OATPs, OATs and OCTs: the organic anion and cation transporters of the SLCO and SLC22A gene superfamilies. *Br J Pharmacol*. 2012;165:1260.
22. International Transporter C, Giacomini KM, Huang SM, et al. Membrane transporters in drug development. *Nat Rev Drug Discov*. 2010;9:215.
23. Ford JM, Hait WN. Pharmacology of drugs that alter multidrug resistance in cancer. *Pharmacol Rev*. 1990;42:155.
24. Greiner B, Eichelbaum M, Fritz P, et al. The role of intestinal P-glycoprotein in the interaction of digoxin and rifampin. *J Clin Invest*. 1999;104:147-153.
25. Buyukkale G, Turker G, Kasap M, et al. Neonatal hyperbilirubinemia and organic anion transporting polypeptide-2 gene mutations. *Am J Perinatol*. 2011;28:619.
26. Wang L, Soroka CJ, Boyer JL. The role of bile salt export pump mutations in progressive familial intrahepatic cholestasis type II. *J Clin Invest*. 2002;110:965.
27. Maraldi NM, Zini N, Santi S, et al. P-glycoprotein subcellular localization and cell morphotype in MDR1 gene-transfected human osteosarcoma cells. *Biol Cell*. 1999;91:17.
28. Bendayan R, Lee G, Bendayan M. Functional expression and localization of P-glycoprotein at the blood brain barrier. *Microsc Res Tech*. 2002;57:365.
29. Bhattacharya M, Peri KG, Almazan G, et al. Nuclear localization of prostaglandin E2 receptors. *Proc Natl Acad Sci U S A*. 1998;95:15792.
30. Gobeil Jr F, Bernier SG, Vazquez-Tello A, et al. Modulation of pro-inflammatory gene expression by nuclear lysophosphatidic acid receptor type-1. *J Biol Chem*. 2003;278:38875.
31. Gobeil F, Fortier A, Zhu T, et al. G-protein-coupled receptors signalling at the cell nucleus: an emerging paradigm. *Can J Physiol Pharmacol*. 2006;84:287.
32. Joyal JS, Nim S, Zhu T, et al. Subcellular localization of coagulation factor II receptor-like 1 in neurons governs angiogenesis. *Nat Med*. 2014;20:1165.
33. Shargell L, Yu ABC. *Applied Biopharmaceutics and Pharmacokinetics*. New York: Appleton-Century-Crofts; 1980:68-84.
34. Winter ME. *Basic Clinical Pharmacokinetics*. San Francisco: Applied Therapeutics; 1980.
35. Allegaert K, Mian P, van den Anker JN. Developmental pharmacokinetics in neonates: maturational changes and beyond. *Curr Pharm Des*. 2017;23:5769.
36. Bearer CF. The special and unique vulnerability of children to environmental hazards. *Neurotoxicology*. 2000;21:925.
37. Euler AR, Byrne WJ, Meis PJ, et al. Basal and pentagastrin-stimulated acid secretion in newborn human infants. *Pediatr Res*. 1979;13:36.
38. Neese AL, Soyka LF. Development of a radioimmunoassay for theophylline. Application to studies in premature infants. *Clin Pharmacol Ther*. 1977;21:633.
39. Ruggiero A, Ariano A, Triarico S, et al. Neonatal pharmacology and clinical implications. *Drugs Context*. 2019;8:212608.
40. Watkins JB, Szczepanik P, Gould JB, et al. Bile salt metabolism in the human premature infant. Preliminary observations of pool size and synthesis rate following prenatal administration of dexamethasone and phenobarbital. *Gastroenterology*. 1975;69:706.
41. Hillman LS. Absorption and maintenance dosage of 25-hydroxycholecalciferol (25-HCC) in premature infants. *Pediatr Res*. 1979;13:400.
42. Melhorn DK, Gross S. Vitamin E-dependent anemia in the premature infant. II. Relationships between gestational age and absorption of vitamin E. *J Pediatr*. 1971;79:581.
43. Bell EF, Brown EJ, Milner R, et al. Vitamin E absorption in small premature infants. *Pediatrics*. 1979;63:830.
44. Graeber JE, Williams ML, Oski FA. The use of intramuscular vitamin E in the premature infant. Optimum dose and iron interaction. *J Pediatr*. 1977;90:282.
45. Le Huerou-Luron I, Blat S, Boudry G. Breast- v. formula-feeding: impacts on the digestive tract and immediate and long-term health effects. *Nutr Res Rev*. 2010;23:23.
46. Hansen TG, O'Brien K, Morton NS, et al. Plasma paracetamol concentrations and pharmacokinetics following rectal administration in neonates and young infants. *Acta Anaesthesiol Scand*. 1999;43:855.
47. Linakis MW, Roberts JK, Lala AC, et al. Challenges associated with route of administration in neonatal drug delivery. *Clin Pharmacokinet*. 2016;55:185.
48. Yaffe SJ, Stern L. Clinical implications of perinatal pharmacology. In: Mirkin BL, ed. *Perinatal Pharmacology and Therapeutics*. New York: Academic Press; 1976:382-388.
49. Morselli PL, Franco-Morselli R, Bossi L. Clinical pharmacokinetics in newborns and infants. Age-related differences and therapeutic implications. *Clin Pharmacokinet*. 1980;5:485.
50. Matheny CJ, Lamb MW, Brouwer KR, et al. Pharmacokinetic and pharmacodynamic implications of P-glycoprotein modulation. *Pharmacotherapy*. 2001;21:778.

16 Principles of Pharmacokinetics

Robert M. Ward | Kevin M. Watt | Steven E. Kern

INTRODUCTION

Pharmacokinetics describes the absorption, distribution, metabolism, and excretion of drugs. The pharmacokinetic parameters of a drug are used to characterize the drug concentrations reached within the body after a dose and the changes in those concentrations over time.[1] Clinical pharmacokinetics is the discipline that applies pharmacokinetic principles to individualize dosage regimens, optimize the therapeutic effects of a medication, and minimize the chances of an adverse drug reaction. This is accomplished by achieving an effective concentration of unbound drug at the site of action. Clinically important sites of action include receptors, membrane transport systems, intracellular enzymes, interstitial tissues where infections may occur, and many others. Correlations have been made between drug concentrations in the circulation and effective or toxic drug concentrations at various sites of action.[2] Depending upon the strength of those correlations, ranges of effective, toxic, and ineffective circulating drug concentrations have been defined for many drugs. Pharmacokinetics serves as a guide to effective therapy, but achieving specific concentrations is not the goal of therapy. Effective therapy is best judged by improvements in function, not just by reaching the desired peak and trough concentrations in the circulation.

The physiologic processes that transform drugs and remove them from the body were characterized decades ago using simple exponential equations. More modern mathematical approaches provide greater insight into both the rates of these processes and the influence of diverse patient factors upon these rates using nonlinear mixed effects modeling (NONMEM). NONMEM is often combined with the sparse sampling techniques of population-based pharmacokinetics that are critical for measurement of pharmacokinetics in extremely low-birth-weight newborns with limited blood volumes and challenging vascular access. The results of NONMEM analyses can then be used in Monte Carlo simulations to predict the range of concentrations expected from particular dosages in specific patient populations.

PHARMACOKINETIC PROCESSES

The basic physiologic processes involved in pharmacokinetics remain relevant to understanding how to produce optimal concentrations of drugs at the site of action and how to adjust dosages in clinical practice. The change in drug amount within the body can be described by the following general equation in which A is the amount of drug within the body, k is the rate constant of change for A within the body, and n defines the order (e.g., zero, first, second) of the process.[3]

$$\frac{dA}{dt} = -kX^{n} \qquad [16.1]$$

The simplest description begins with the intravenous infusion of a single dose. Infusions are usually carried out with a syringe pump that provides a constant rate of flow (mg/min). Constant rates are described by zero-order exponential equations in which $e^0 = 1$.

$$\text{Dose (mg)} = \text{concentration (mg/mL)} \times \text{infusion rate (mL/min)} \times e^0 \times \text{duration of infusion (minutes)} \qquad [16.2]$$

After a drug enters the circulation composed of red blood cells, proteins, and serum (the water and electrolyte solution), it may remain in that space in the water layer or bind to one of the components of blood, such as albumin, α_1 glycoprotein, or red blood cells, or it may be transported or diffuse across the endothelial membrane out of the circulation. This binding within the circulation is important because only the unbound portion of a drug is free to diffuse across membranes to reach sites of action, sites of metabolism (such as in the hepatocyte), or sites of excretion (such as the renal tubule). Preterm newborns often have reduced total proteins in their circulation, causing a greater percentage of the circulating drug concentration to remain unbound. This can lead to drug toxicity at total circulating concentrations regarded as nontoxic and therapeutic based on studies in adults or older children with higher protein concentrations.

FIRST-ORDER ELIMINATION

Most drugs are eliminated by first-order exponential rates (k) in which a constant fraction of the drug is eliminated per unit of time. If the kinetics are determined by first-order elimination, then the rate of change of drug in the body (dA/dt) is proportional to the amount in the body. Thus at high concentrations a greater amount of drug is eliminated per hour than at low concentrations. For example, if the concentration is 100, it will decrease to 50 in one half-life, a loss of 50, but during the next half-life, only 25 will be removed as the concentration decreases from 50 to 25. This exponential decline in plasma concentration (Fig. 16.1) can be represented by the following equation:

$$C_t = C_0 \times e^{-kt} \qquad [16.3]$$

where C_t is the concentration at some time t, C_0 is the initial concentration at time 0, and e^{-kt} represents the exponential decline in plasma concentration associated with first-order elimination. The exponential decrease in plasma concentration

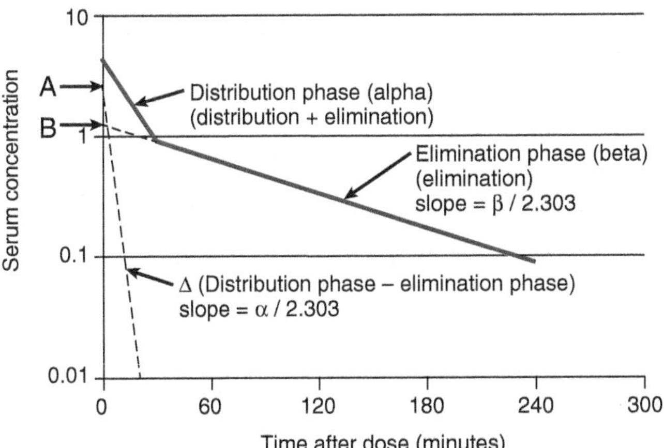

Fig. 16.1 Two-compartment or biexponential kinetics are graphed as a *solid line* on semilogarithmic axes with the initial rapid decrease in concentration resulting from distribution and elimination during the distribution phase (α) followed by the slower decrease in concentration during the elimination phase (β) with a slope of the elimination rate constant of β/2.303. The intercept of the elimination phase, *B*, is extrapolated to time zero with a *dashed line*. The concentration difference between the distribution and elimination phases is graphed with *dashes* in a steeper line with intercept *A* and a slope of the distribution rate constant α/2.303.

with time may be made linear by taking the natural logarithm of each side of Eq. (16.3) to convert this to the equation for a straight line, $y = mx + b$.

$$\text{Ln } C_t = \text{Ln } C_0 - kt \quad [16.4]$$

The slope of this straight line is the elimination rate constant k (time^{-1}), which may be calculated by rearranging Eq. (16.4):

$$k = (\text{Ln } C_1 - \text{Ln } C_2)/\Delta t \quad [16.5]$$

where C_1 is the higher early concentration and C_2 is the lower concentration measured some time later. If the logarithm (base 10) of concentration is graphed versus time, the slope will be k/2.303. The relationship between the elimination rate constant and the half-life for a first-order process may be derived mathematically from Eq. (16.3). For a drug whose initial concentration is 100 mg/L, the concentration at one half-life is 50 mg/L.

$$\text{Ln } 50 = \text{Ln } 100 - kt \quad [16.6]$$

$$kt = \text{Ln } (100/50) \quad [16.7]$$

which can be rearranged to

$$k = \text{Ln } 2/t \quad [16.8]$$

where t represents one half-life; because Ln2 = 0.693, the equation becomes

$$k = 0.693/t_{1/2} \quad [16.9]$$

COMPARTMENTAL ANALYSIS

When circulating concentrations are sampled quickly after intravascular drug infusion, the concentration can be used to estimate the distribution volume within the *central compartment* defined as the volume necessary to describe the change in concentration produced by a specific dose:

$$\text{Concentration (mg/L)} = \text{Dose (mg/kg)}/\text{volume of distribution (L/kg)} \quad [16.10]$$

This volume can be viewed as the volume required to dilute the concentrated dosage formulation to the concentration of drug observed within the body.

For drugs that begin to diffuse out of the circulation soon after administration, the initial drop in concentration due primarily to diffusion is termed the ***distribution phase***. It is generally followed by a phase with a slower decrease in concentration, reflecting elimination by excretion of unchanged drug or by metabolism of the parent molecule that was administered. This produces the familiar biphasic concentration-time graph (see Fig. 16.1) that can usually be fitted to two or occasionally three first-order exponential terms (concentration = $Ae^{-\alpha t} + Be^{-\beta t}$).

The multipliers of time (t), α and β, provide the rate constants for the different rates of drug removal. These rate constants with units of time^{-1} are inversely related to the half-life by the natural logarithm of 2. The rate of distribution is defined by the following equation:

$$t_{1/2}\text{(minutes)} = \text{Ln}2/\alpha\,(\text{minute}^{-1}) = 0.693/\alpha\,(\text{minute}^{-1}) \quad [16.11]$$

Accurate analysis of these rate constants using the older techniques of pharmacokinetics is complicated because both distribution and elimination are occurring simultaneously after the drug enters the circulation. To determine the rate of the distribution phase requires subtracting the change in concentration due to the slower β (elimination) phase (see Fig. 16.1). This procedure is referred to as *curve stripping*.

When there is a third phase after the α and β phases, it is usually attributed to distribution into and out of deep tissue compartments, such as fat or bone, during this third, or γ, phase. In reality these are artificial explanations that may or may not explain the actual movement of the drug within the body, but they do describe the observed changes in concentration. More important, these basic mathematical approaches do not account for factors that may contribute to significant changes in concentration that are especially relevant to neonatal studies. These include factors such as gestational age, urine output, organ dysfunction, and interactions with other drugs. The influence of these factors can be determined using NONMEM, described later in this chapter.

APPARENT VOLUME OF DISTRIBUTION

The *apparent volume of distribution* (V_d) is a mathematical term that relates the total amount of drug in the body to the drug concentration in the circulation. After a rapid intravenous bolus dose, and assuming a one-compartment model, the following equation may be used to relate V_d, dose, and change or increase in circulating concentration:

$$\Delta\ \text{Circulating drug concentration (mg/L)} = \frac{\text{Dose (mg/kg)}}{V_d\ \text{(L/kg)}} \quad [16.12]$$

V_d might be viewed as the volume of dilution into which the dose is added to produce the observed change in concentration. The larger the volume of distribution, the greater the dilution of a dose and the smaller the increase in circulating concentration after administration. V_d does not necessarily correspond to a true physiologic body fluid or tissue volume, hence the designation *apparent* volume of distribution. For drugs that distribute widely into peripheral tissues and leave little drug in the circulation, the V_d derived from changes in concentration within the circulation may be very large. For example, the peripheral V_d of azithromycin in neonates and infants averaged 17.9 L/kg—an anatomic impossibility.[4,5] A large V_d indicates that tissue concentrations of a drug may greatly exceed the concentration in the plasma, often due to protein binding in tissue or fat solubility. Drugs that distribute primarily into extracellular fluid have small V_ds (0.25 to 0.35 L/kg), which can increase significantly in fluid-overload states that lower the circulating drug concentration. In addition, because extracellular water makes up a larger percentage of body weight in the premature and term infant, their V_ds at birth will be proportionally larger for water-soluble drugs. The effect of a decreasing extracellular fluid space on kinetics is illustrated in a study of gentamicin pharmacokinetics by Stolk and colleagues, who found that the V_ds averaged 0.70 L/kg for newborns who were less than 30 weeks' gestation and 0.50 to 0.53 L/kg for those more than 34 weeks' gestation.[6]

To administer a rapid intravenous bolus dose, Eq. 16.12 serves as the basis for other pharmacokinetic calculations because it is easily rearranged to solve for V_d and dose. If a dose is infused over a longer period of time, e.g., 1 to 4 hours, a significant portion of the dose may be cleared from the body during the infusion, especially drugs with short half-lives. Accordingly, a more complex exponential equation that accounts for concurrent drug administration and drug elimination is required to describe the change in concentration. (For a discussion of these calculations, see Lugo et al.[7]) Such equations are needed only when the drug is rapidly eliminated, and the duration of infusion is 40% to 50% of the drug's half-life. In neonates, who often have relatively slow rates of drug elimination, only a small fraction of drug is eliminated during the time of infusion of most drugs, and such adjustments can usually be omitted. Accordingly, a simpler and clinically applicable equation, such as Eq. 16.12, may be used to estimate pharmacokinetic parameters.

CLEARANCE

Clearance represents the capacity for drug removal by various organs and is defined as the volume of blood from which all drug is removed per minute (mL/min). Both clearance and distribution volume are model-independent parameters. Thus plasma drug concentrations are determined by the rate at which drug is administered, its clearance, and V_d. Similarly, the rate of elimination can be determined from clearance (Cl) and V_d.

$$k = \mathrm{Cl}/V_d \qquad [16.13]$$

Drugs can be cleared through numerous pathways. However, most drugs are cleared by some combination of renal clearance ($\mathrm{Cl_R}$), hepatic clearance ($\mathrm{Cl_H}$), and biliary clearance ($\mathrm{Cl_B}$) (Fig. 16.2). The total systemic clearance of a drug ($\mathrm{Cl_S}$) is the sum of all clearances by various mechanisms and can be calculated using the following equation:

$$\mathrm{Cl_s} = \mathrm{Cl_R} + \mathrm{Cl_H} + \mathrm{Cl_B} + \mathrm{Cl_{other}} \qquad [16.14]$$

Because it is seldom possible to calculate each organ's clearance of drug, $\mathrm{Cl_S}$ is often determined by measuring the area under the plasma concentration-time curve (AUC, or area under the curve) after a single dose:

$$\mathrm{Cl_s} = \mathrm{Dose}/\mathrm{AUC} \qquad [16.15]$$

During a continuous infusion, clearance may be easily determined by the relationship between the rate of infusion and the resultant steady-state concentration:

$$\mathrm{Cl} = \text{Rate of drug administration (mg/minute)}/\text{steady-state drug concentration (mg/mL)} \qquad [16.16]$$

FIRST-PASS CLEARANCE

A special situation occurs for some drugs in which dramatic differences in concentrations and effects occur between enteral and parenteral administration due to first-pass effect or presystemic drug clearance. During absorption after enteral dosing, drug passes through the intestinal wall, enters the portal venous circulation, and passes through the liver before reaching the systemic circulation (Fig. 16.2). For some drugs, nearly complete metabolism of a dose may occur in the intestinal wall or the liver (especially for drugs metabolized by cytochrome P450 3A4). When this occurs, the amount of parent drug reaching the systemic circulation is only a small fraction of the dose administered.[8,9] The fraction (F) of the oral dose that reaches the systemic circulation is that which remains after hepatic or intestinal metabolism expressed as the extraction ratio (ER) in the following equation:

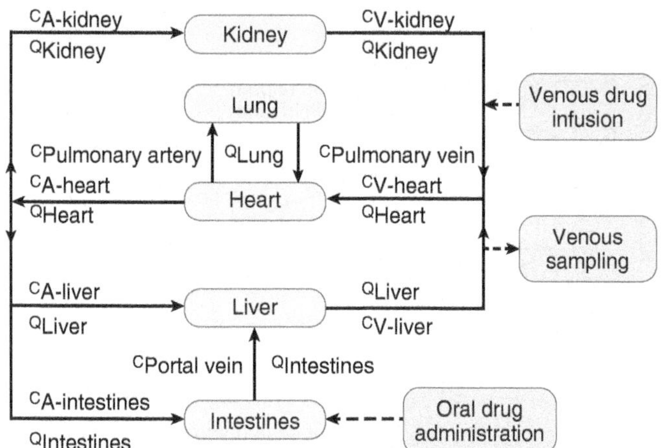

Fig. 16.2 Drug clearance by several organs that combine to produce total body clearance in which C_A is arterial concentration, C_V is venous concentration, and Q is organ blood flow. First-pass clearance may occur during drug absorption from the intestines or during circulation of portal venous blood through the liver before reaching systemic circulation.

$$F = 1 - \mathrm{ER} \qquad [16.17]$$

The ER is determined from the ratio of the AUC after oral administration versus that after intravenous administration. After an intravenous dose of medication infused peripherally, drug enters either the inferior or superior vena caval circulation, returns to the heart, and enters the systemic circulation before perfusing the liver, which receives 25% of the cardiac output. Drugs that undergo almost complete hepatic or intestinal metabolism before reaching the systemic circulation are described as having a high hepatic or intestinal intrinsic clearance. Some drugs used in the care of newborns that exhibit moderate to significant first-pass presystemic clearance are midazolam,[10] morphine,[11] and propranolol.[12]

STEADY STATE

Steady state for a drug exists when the amount of drug removed per unit time is equal to the amount administered per unit time. For drugs administered intermittently, peak and trough concentrations at steady state are the same after each dose. For drugs administered by continuous infusion, serum concentrations will be constant. Constant serum concentrations, however, do not define equilibrium between compartments, because distribution between tissues and circulation may still be occurring.

The time to reach steady state is dependent only on the elimination rate constant and therefore half-life. If a drug is administered repeatedly at a fixed dosing interval, the time to reach greater than 90% of steady state is four or more half-lives, as shown in Table 16.1.

During long-term drug treatment, dose adjustments should be made when concentrations are close to steady state and generally not more often than every three half-lives unless organ dysfunction is altering the half-life or V_d or concentration-related toxicity occurs.

Table 16.1 Percentage of Steady-State Concentration Reached After Drug Administration for 1 to 5 Half-Lives.

Number of Half-Lives Drug Is Administered	Steady-State Concentration (%)
1	50
2	75
3	87.5
4	93.75
5	96.88

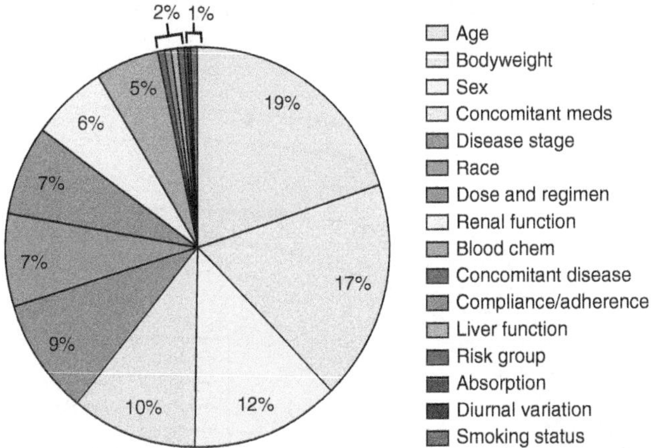

Fig. 16.3 Range of typical covariates that are explored in a population pharmacokinetic analysis for treatment of children with antiretroviral agents. (Redrawn from data in Barrett JS, Labbe L, Pfister M. Application and impact of population pharmacokinetics in the assessment of antiretroviral pharmacotherapy. *Clin Pharmacokinet.* 2005;44:591–625.)

POPULATION PHARMACOKINETICS

The previous sections in this chapter provided guidance on how dosing can be individualized for patients based on pharmacokinetic principles. Measurement of drug concentration values during therapy (at least 2 measurements) can be used to estimate an individual patient's parameter values (e.g., elimination half-life, distribution volume, and clearance). Armed with this insight, the clinician can make adjustments to drug therapy that achieve a desired level of drug exposure and ultimately drug effect for the patient.

For aminoglycoside antibiotics, the ability to measure drug concentration levels is part of standard clinical analytical capability in most institutions so that information can be provided to the clinician to adjust dosage in a timely manner. For most other therapeutics that are used clinically, there is no ability to measure concentrations during the course of clinical care or to adjust an individual patient's therapy. The need for individual adjustment exists because of the variability among individual patients. This variability is due to the range of demographic, anatomic, physiologic, genetic, and biochemical differences among patients that ultimately impacts the pharmacokinetic parameters and influences the concentration profile of a drug at the site of action after a dose is administered.

Population pharmacokinetics estimates the impact of these various differences on pharmacokinetic parameters to provide clinicians with a means to adjust dosage before starting therapy. Based on NONMEM, the population pharmacokinetic approach estimates typical values for pharmacokinetic parameters, such as clearance. By estimating the variability as a separate parameter, factors that contribute to variability can be measured; these factors are referred to as patient covariates.[13] A typical example of a covariate for a drug that is cleared by renal elimination is creatinine clearance as a measure of renal function.

Other typical covariates that can impact pharmacokinetic parameters are factors such as age, body weight or body mass index, genetic variants in drug-metabolizing enzymes, and presence of concomitant disease in a patient. These covariates can be particularly important for adjusting pediatric dosing requirements based on those recommended for adults. An example of the types of variables that are explored as potential covariates to improve the individual estimates of population pharmacokinetic parameters is shown in Fig. 16.3, which shows a range of parameters and their frequency of use for pediatric antiretroviral therapy.[14]

However, caution should be used when extrapolating pediatric parameters from adult parameters when no data exist to confirm that the extrapolation is valid. This occurs most often when dosing is adjusted linearly based on body weight. If a drug has only been studied in a population where the body weight changes are a fraction of the range that occur in the population at large, the impact of the covariate may not be accurately described for populations outside the body weight range that was studied. This occurs often when drugs are studied in relatively healthy adults and dosing is extrapolated to very young or very old patients. If the adjustment is a linear scaling based on weight or age, it can result in underdosing for young patients and overdosing for old patients.[15] It is important that population pharmacokinetic models are determined for the population in which they are intended to inform dosing.

EXAMPLE OF POPULATION PARAMETER ESTIMATION

As defined earlier in this chapter, when a drug is given by infusion, the change in concentration over time is determined by rate of drug infusion, drug clearance, and elimination half-life, if the drug displays one-compartment pharmacokinetics as shown in Eq. (16.16). This equation can be rewritten in terms of volume of distribution and clearance by substituting for the elimination rate constant, $K = Cl/V_d$.

Suppose we conduct a study with six children where drug concentrations are measured in the circulation over a 12-hour period after starting the infusion. The results of this study might look something like Fig. 16.4. The drug concentration rises in each subject to a steady-state concentration level, which differs among the six children. Additionally, the time when steady state occurs varies among them. What is consistent, however, is that each patient's concentration does rise in an exponential manner to a steady-state level. Using population pharmacokinetic modeling, an estimate of the average value for clearance and elimination rate constant can be determined that produces the population-average concentration profile for this group of children.

Individual estimates of the two pharmacokinetic parameters Cl and V_d for each of the six subjects are determined along with the population variability for these parameters. The parameter variability can be explored in many ways. One approach is to plot the residual error between the population estimates of the concentration values against any covariate of interest, such as body weight, sex, creatinine clearance, or other covariates such as those as shown in Fig. 16.3. The residual error is the difference between the measured concentrations and the population-average concentration profile. When the residual error is plotted against a covariate of interest, it should distribute randomly about the line of zero. If this difference plot instead shows a trend in the data that is not equally distributed about the zero line, it suggests that it might

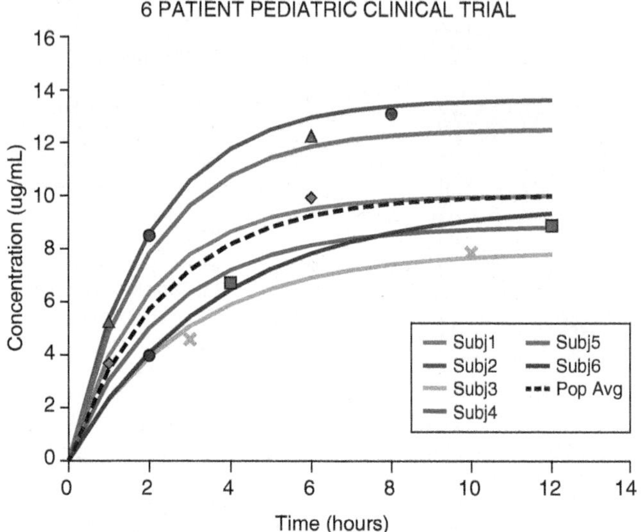

Fig. 16.4 Simulated clinical trial results in six children given a 12-hour infusion of a drug. Each child has a different clearance and volume, which results in different steady-state values and time to reach steady state. The *markers* show the actual measured concentration values. Note that not all children have samples taken at the same times. The population average result for all six children is shown by the *dashed black line*.

be important to incorporate the covariate into the model to reduce the model prediction residual error. A plot of residual error for the six subjects versus their creatinine clearance values and body weight is shown in Fig. 16.5. As can be seen, when the residual error is plotted against body weight, the data are evenly distributed about the line for zero error, but the plot for creatinine clearance shows a decreasing trend with increasing creatinine clearance. Because the residual error plot shows a trend or "structure" versus the creatinine clearance, it indicates that creatinine clearance is likely an important covariate to include in the model.

By plotting the individual subject parameter estimates against a covariate of interest (in this case drug clearance, because creatinine clearance is likely to be directly related to it), an understanding of the relationship between the covariate and model parameter emerges that indicates how it should be included in the model. As Fig. 16.6 shows, the drug clearance increases linearly with creatinine clearance. Therefore the model would be updated to include creatinine clearance as a linear scale factor for drug clearance.

In this example, suppose that a plot of the individual clearance values for the six subjects versus creatinine clearance (CCr) revealed the relationship shown in Fig. 16.6. This clearly shows that drug clearance is linearly related to creatinine clearance with some offset that describes the nonrenal contribution to clearance. Thus we could rewrite the expression for clearance as:

$$Cl = Clnr + Clr \times CCr + \eta \quad [16.18]$$

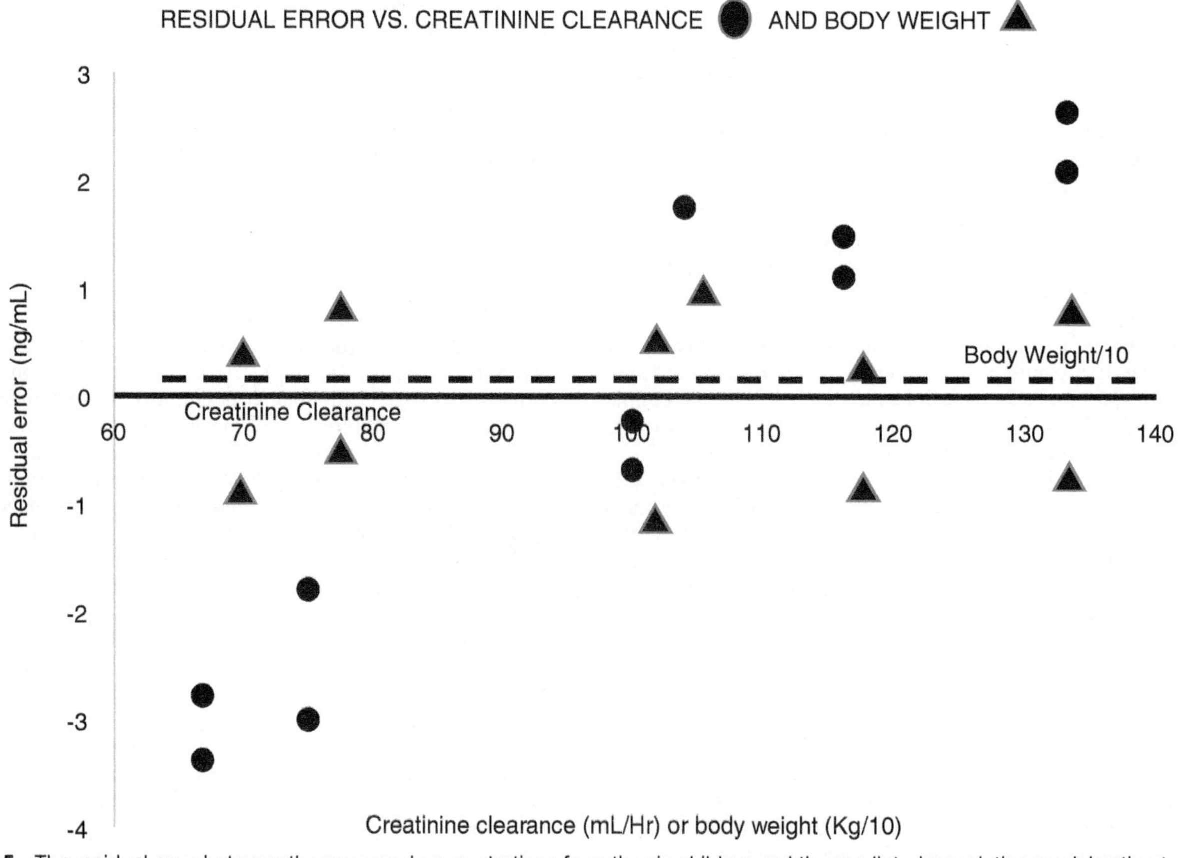

Fig. 16.5 The residual error between the measured concentrations from the six children and the predicted population model estimate plotted against each individual subject's creatinine clearance value and weight. If covariate was not important to consider in the model structure, then the residual error values should sit equally about the line of zero error as shown for weight. Because these residual errors show a strong linear relationship that increases with increasing creatinine clearance, it strongly supports the need to incorporate creatinine clearance into the model equations.

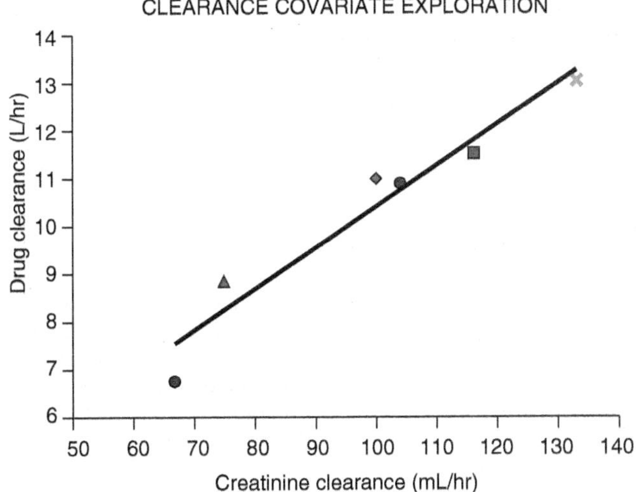

Fig. 16.6 Clearance plotted as a function of creatinine clearance for the six children in the simulated clinical trial. The covariate of creatinine clearance shows a linear relationship against the total clearance value. The model structural parameters for clearance include the intercept, which represents the nonrenal clearance, and the slope, which scales the renal clearance. Deviations from the linear plot indicate residual variability in clearance.

where *Clnr* represents the offset of the linear relationship, the nonrenal clearance; *Clr*, the renal clearance, represents the slope of the curve; and eta (η) represents the variability in the estimates for the individual patient's clearance values. This would represent the range of offset of the actual clearance values from the line.

An advantage to using the population approach is that the sampling times and the number of samples for the different children in the trial does not have to be the same. In essence, because the population approach is fitting the relationship to all the data at the same time, if one subject is missing a sample point, the method uses information from the other samples to infer the likely shape of the curve for the individual. Another advantage is that the population approach identifies important variables that influence pharmacokinetics to guide dosing in a specific population.

UNDERSTANDING POPULATION PARAMETER NOTATION

Population pharmacokinetic modeling uses a unique set of variables to refer to the model parameters. In general, structural parameters (i.e., parameters that describe the main relationship between the concentration profile for the individuals) are designated by the Greek letter theta (θ). The residual variabilities for the parameters are referred to as etas (η). Any remaining residual variability that represents random noise in the concentration versus time relationship is given by epsilon

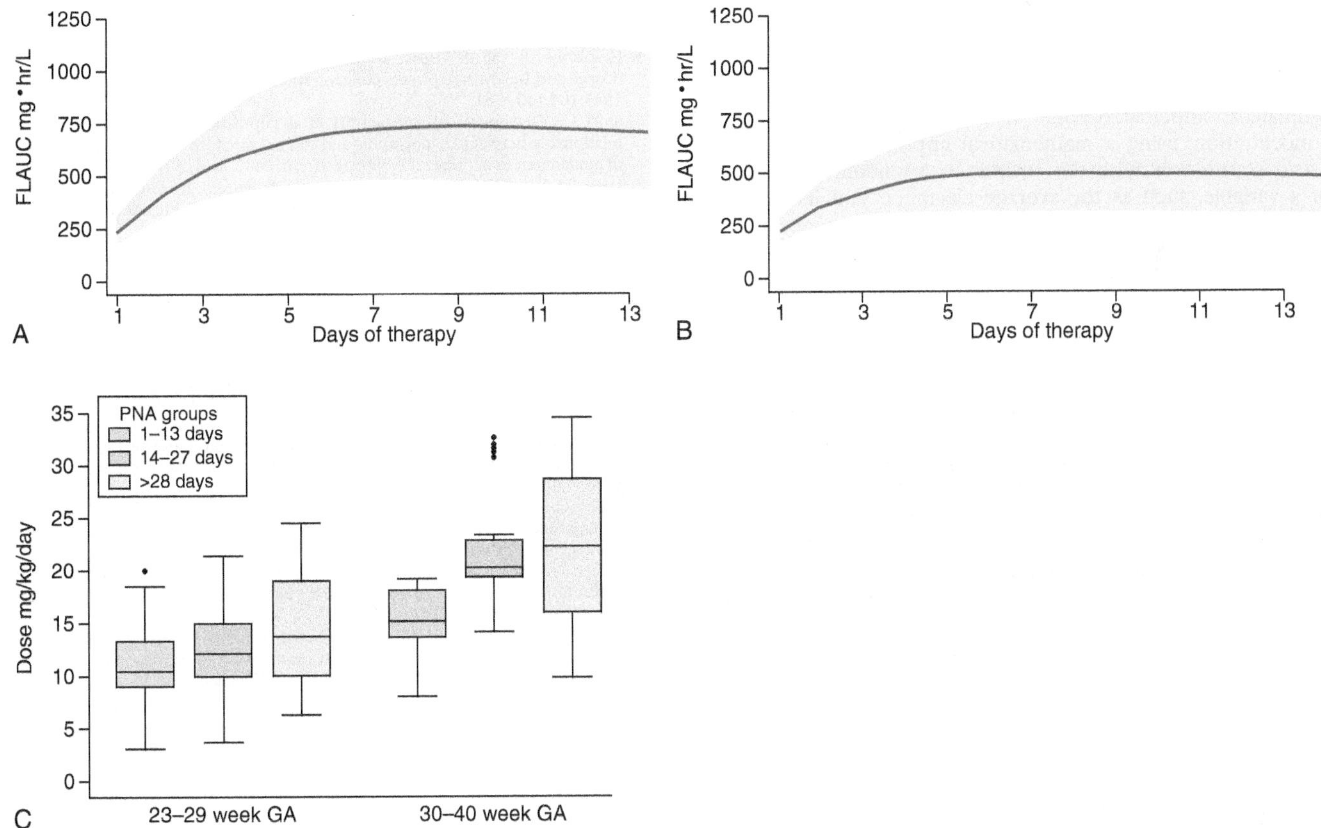

Fig. 16.7 Evaluation of dose exposure relationship. The median *(dark line)* and population predicted interval from the 10th percentile to the 90th percentile *(shaded area)* for fluconazole area under the curve (AUC) from 100 Monte Carlo simulation trials, given the final model and parameters. Simulated 24-hour interval AUC for each day of therapy among A, 23- to 29-weeks' gestation infants or B, 30- to 40-weeks' gestation infants receiving 12 mg/kg/day fluconazole. (C) Median box plot of predicted dose required to achieve steady-state AUC target of 800 mg × hour/L in infants stratified by gestational age *(GA)* and postnatal age *(PNA)*. (From Wade KC, Wu D, Kaufman DA, et al. Population pharmacokinetics of fluconazole in young infants. *Antimicrob Agents Chemother.* 52:4043–4049, 2008. Copyright 2008, American Society for Microbiology. All Rights Reserved.)

(ε). Note that the η and ε define the variation in the parameter values between and within an individual. The actual parameter is assumed to have a mean value of zero for the overall population relationship with nonzero value for the variance. Thus the set of equations that would define our previous clinical trial example would be:

$$C(t) = R/Cli\left(1 - e^{Cli/Vi}\right) + \varepsilon i \quad [16.19]$$

$$Cli = Clnr + Clr \times CCRi + \eta i \quad [16.20]$$

$$Vi = V + \eta j \quad [16.21]$$

And this would be written in population values in terms of θ, η, and ε as:

$$C(t) = R/Cli\left(1 - e^{Cli/Vi}\right) + \varepsilon i \quad [16.22]$$

$$Cli = \theta 1 + \theta 2 + \theta 3 + \eta i \quad [16.23]$$

$$Vi = \theta 4 + \eta j \quad [16.24]$$

This set of relationships can then be used to adjust dosing for a patient based directly on the individual covariates and can improve dosing when it is not feasible to measure concentrations during therapy. It can also provide a means to understand the relationship between adults and children for drugs that have been studied in both groups.

MONTE CARLO SIMULATION

The determination of pharmacokinetic parameters such as clearance and volume of distribution by population pharmacokinetic modeling estimates average values together with the variation for each parameter among a population of patients. These averages and their variation can be used to estimate an anticipated range of outcomes, such as the serum concentration, using a mathematical approach termed *Monte Carlo simulation*. With this technique, a random combination of a variable, such as the average clearance, and its variation among patients are combined to calculate the concentration after a drug dose. This is then repeated hundreds to thousands of times to calculate a range of likely concentrations that will be produced by a particular dosage. An illustrative use of this technique was applied by Wade and colleagues for fluconazole dosed at 12 mg/kg/day for patients 23 to 29 weeks and 30 to 40 weeks of gestational age (Fig. 16.7).[16] It is clear from graphs A and B in Fig. 16.7 that the same dosage will produce lower fluconazole exposures (AUC) as gestational age and clearance increase. The dosages required to meet this developmental increase in clearance with increasing age after birth are shown in Fig. 16.7C. The rapid developmental change in physiology among neonates lends itself to analysis by Monte Carlo simulations to understand the range of possible drug concentrations that are likely to be produced when pharmacokinetic parameters change with maturation or organ dysfunction. This allows prospective selection of optimal dosages based on defined patient covariates.

CONCLUSION

Pharmacokinetics provides tools for optimizing pharmacotherapy in newborns to achieve appropriate drug concentrations at the site of action, to avoid toxicity, and to achieve therapeutic goals. Basic principles of pharmacokinetics are built on the physiologic and pathologic changes encountered in developing and sick newborns. These should become familiar to everyone who provides drug therapy for newborns. The more modern pharmacokinetic approaches to adjusting drug dosages using NONMEN allow prospective design of drug therapy to take into account neonatal physiologic changes related to growth, maturation, and organ dysfunction. When combined with Monte Carlo simulation, these techniques describe ranges of drug concentrations that are likely to be achieved with specific dosages in specific neonatal populations. Using variations among patients that are known and those that are not, these techniques provide useful guidance to dosing and drug concentrations that are likely to be achieved in neonatal pharmacotherapy. When applied to drug concentrations measured during therapeutic drug monitoring, they help guide dosage adjustments to achieve therapeutic goals and avoid toxicity.

REFERENCES

1. Gibaldi M, Perrier D. *Pharmacokinetics*. 2nd ed. New York: Marcel Dekker; 1982.
2. Wilkinson GR. Pharmacokinetics. The dynamics of drug absorption, distribution, and elimination. In: Hardman JG, Limbird LE, Gilman AG, eds. *Goodman & Gilman's the Pharmacological Basis of Therapeutics*. 10th ed. New York: McGraw-Hill; 2001:3–29.
3. Notari RE. In: *Rate Processes in Biological Systems. Biopharmaceutics and Clinical Pharmacokinetics, an Introduction*. 3rd ed. New York: Marcel Dekker; 1980:5–44.
4. Viscardi RM, Othman AA, Hassan HE, et al. Azithromycin to prevent bronchopulmonary dysplasia in ureaplasma-infected preterm infants: pharmacokinetics, safety, microbial response, and clinical outcomes with a 20-milligram-per-kilogram single intravenous dose. *Antimicrob Agents Chemother*. 2013;57(5):2127–2133.
5. Hastreiter AR, van der Horst RL, Voda C, Chow-Tung E. Maintenance digoxin dosage and steady-state plasma concentration in infants and children. *J Pediatr*. 1985;107:140–146.
6. Stolk LM, Degraeuwe PL, Nieman FH, et al. Population pharmacokinetics and relationship between demographic and clinical variables and pharmacokinetics of gentamicin in neonates. *Ther Drug Monit*. 2002;24(4):527–531.
7. Lugo RA, Ward RM. Basic pharmacokinetic principles. In: Polin RA, Fox WW, Abman SH, eds. *Fetal and Neonatal Physiology*. 4th ed. Philadelphia: Elsevier Saunders; 2011:224–230.
8. Paine MF, Shen DD, Kunze KL, et al. First-pass metabolism of midazolam by the human intestine. *Clin Pharmacol Ther*. 1996;60(1):14–24.
9. Heizmann P, Eckert M, Ziegler WH. Pharmacokinetics and bioavailability of midazolam in man. *Br J Clin Pharmacol*. 1983;16(suppl 1):43S–49S.
10. de Wildt SN, Kearns GL, Hop WC, et al. Pharmacokinetics and metabolism of oral midazolam in preterm infants. *Br J Clin Pharmacol*. 2002;53(4):390–392.
11. Penson RT, Joel SP, Roberts M, et al. The bioavailability and pharmacokinetics of subcutaneous, nebulized and oral morphine-6-glucuronide. *Br J Clin Pharmacol*. 2002;53(4):347–354.
12. Borchard U. Pharmacokinetics of beta-adrenoceptor blocking agents: clinical significance of hepatic and/or renal clearance. *Clin Physiol Biochem*. 1990;8(suppl 2):28–34.
13. Pillai GC, Mentre F, Steimer JL. Non-linear mixed effects modeling—from methodology and software development to driving implementation in drug development science. *J Pharmacokinet Pharmacodyn*. 2005;32(2):161–183.
14. Barrett JS, Labbe L, Pfister M. Application and impact of population pharmacokinetics in the assessment of antiretroviral pharmacotherapy. *Clin Pharmacokinet*. 2005;44(6):591–625.
15. Anderson BJ, Holford NH. Mechanism-based concepts of size and maturity in pharmacokinetics. *Annu Rev Pharmacol Toxicol*. 2008;48:303–332.
16. Wade KC, Wu D, Kaufman DA, et al. Population pharmacokinetics of fluconazole in young infants. *Antimicrob Agents Chemother*. 2008;52(11):4043–4049.

The Physiology of Placental Drug Disposition

17

Karel Allegaert | John Nicolaas van den Anker

INTRODUCTION: FROM A PASSIVE FILTER BARRIER CONCEPT TO AN ACTIVE DRUG HANDLING ORGAN

When deconstructed to its basic structure, the placenta is an active ("drug handling") barrier between two separated systems (maternal, fetal) with placental drug disposition driven by differences in concentration-time profiles between both systems, and the maternal and fetal blood flow to and from the filter. This setting is somewhat similar to hemodialysis or extra-corporeal membrane oxygenation, where diffusion will be driven by concentration gradients, characteristics of the membrane, and flows. However, the placenta is an active barrier and transporter. The rate and extent of drug exposure to embryo or fetus are determined by numerous variables, including the drug-related as well as physiology-related characteristics listed in Table 17.1.[1-5]

The placenta is of fetal origin and acts as interface between the maternal and fetal compartments. The major functions of the placenta are to transfer nutrients and oxygen from mother to fetus and to assist in the removal of waste products from fetus to mother. In addition, it plays an important role in the synthesis of hormones (e.g., β-human chorionic gonadotropin, estrogens), peptides, prostaglandins, or steroids that are all vital for a successful pregnancy. The placenta hereby allows tailored transport of nutrients, enables elimination of waste products, and facilitates gas exchange between mother and fetus. Related to these functions, evidence has accumulated that essentially all pharmacologic agents, but also other exogenous substances, are transferred to the embryo and fetus, regardless of whether this transfer is intentional (e.g., medical treatment of the fetus) or unintentional, with possible teratogenic or toxic fetal effects, including aspects such as drug tolerance.[1-5]

It is too simplistic to consider the placenta as an absolute and protective barrier, and the concept of a passive filter function is also not sufficiently sophisticated. This is based on the fact that the placenta is not just an innocent bystander, but an active *regulator* of drug transport (efflux and influx transporters) and metabolism (metabolizing enzymes).[1,2] The "barrier" function of the placenta includes passive diffusion, facilitated diffusion, active transport, and pinocytosis or endocytosis.[3] Besides physicochemical and structural characteristics (such as size) that determine placental permeability, it is important to realize that the placenta is also an active organ (drug accumulation, metabolism, and/or transporters). Placenta drug metabolism can also modify fetal drug exposure.

As concentration gradients also matter, fetal drug exposure may vary according to maternal exposure in addition to placental transfer characteristics. Because of the physiologic modifications occurring during pregnancy, maternal concentration-time profiles commonly differ from nonpregnant women. As a simple illustration, if renal elimination clearance increases significantly during pregnancy, maternal exposure will decrease and so will placental transfer during pregnancy, when the same dose is used for drugs (almost) exclusively cleared by the renal route.[3] Along the same line, fetal drug disposition (metabolism, renal elimination, and/or accumulation) also drives exposure as it may affect the maternal-to-fetal drug gradient.

Finally, exposure will also be determined by maternal arterial uterine blood flow and fetal umbilical blood flow. The rate of blood flow increases 12-fold from 10 weeks' gestation until term (beyond 37 weeks), accounting for about 80% of uterine perfusion at that time.[3] This is still a somewhat underexplored aspect of placental transfer, as maternal (pregnancy-related hypertension; preeclampsia) or fetal (arrhythmia, such as supraventricular tachycardia or heart block; reversed fetal umbilical blood flow) also results in altered maternal or fetal placental blood flow, respectively.

Pregnant women take drugs, and women who take drugs might become pregnant. A relevant number of over-the-counter drugs are taken as self-medication by women who may be unaware of a still-early pregnancy or of possible adverse effects to the fetus. Consequently, requests for public and reliable information are mounting.[6,7] Similarly, young women with medical conditions (e.g., post-transplant, autoimmune disease, hematologic/oncologic diseases, human immunodeficiency virus [HIV], psychiatric diseases, addiction) want to become pregnant. An appreciation of these considerations is important in designing meaningful toxicokinetic and drug disposition studies.[2,3,8] Therefore, a reasonably accurate prediction of placental transfer *before* prescription to pregnant women is needed. To conduct such (in vivo, or computer simulation) studies, the earlier mentioned parameters (see Table 17.1) that drive the extent (total amount) and rate (amount over time) of placental transfer of a specific compound in the human mother-fetus dyad should be considered, to design a study that will generate robust information.

Physiology-based pharmacokinetic (PBPK) models can integrate these different types of information, such as expression data, ontogeny information, and observations obtained from the ex vivo cotyledon perfusion experiments, combined with flow characteristics and the physicochemical characteristics of a given compound. Such a mechanistic modeling framework may leverage the available information and make more reliable predictions on pharmacotherapy during pregnancy (maternal and fetal).[1,2,8] The aim of this chapter is to discuss the physiology of placental drug transfer, but it will commence with a short overview on methods and modeling systems currently applied to investigate placental drug transfer.

Table 17.1 Factors Determining the Rate and Extent of Drug Transfer to and From the Embryo or Fetus.

Transfer Feature	Characteristics: Drug	Characteristics: Maternal-Placental-Fetal Unit
Rate	Lipid solubility	Placental structure, size, and function
	Molecular weight	Maternal, placental, and fetal blood flow
	Structural characteristics	Thickness of placental membranes
	Type of transfer	Passive diffusion, facilitated or active transport, or pinocytosis
	Protein binding	Maternal, placental, or fetal protein binding (albumin, α_1 acid glycoprotein)
Extent	Degree of ionization (pK_a)	Maternal-fetal pH gradient
	Type of transfer	Passive diffusion, facilitated or active transport, or pinocytosis
	Protein binding	Maternal, placental (metabolism, passive diffusion, facilitated or active transport, pinocytosis), and fetal drug handling
Both	Blood flows	Maternal arterial uterine blood flow, cardiac output
		Fetal umbilical blood flow, cardiac output

See References 1–5.

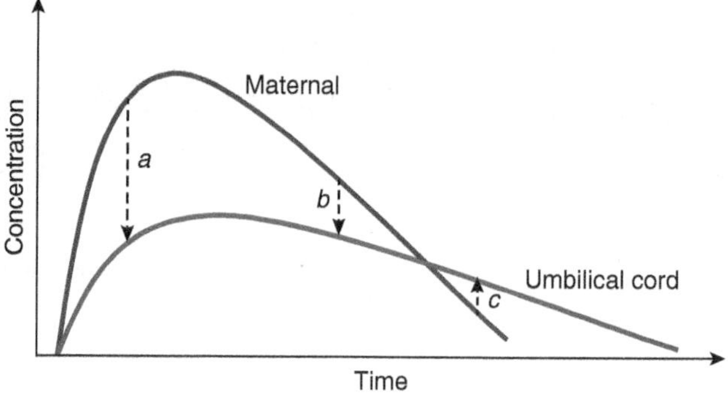

Fig. 17.1 Illustration on the impact of time after maternal administration to assess the maternal/umbilical cord blood ratio of a given compound. Pending on the time of sampling (*a, b,* or *c*) the ratio will be different or even reversed. An area under the curve maternal/umbilical cord blood ratio is more accurate, but necessitates paired observations over time.

METHODS RELATED TO PLACENTAL DRUG RESEARCH

Taking the ethical constraints into account, in vivo quantification of the disposition of clinically indicated drugs in maternal compartments is feasible.[3] In contrast, human fetal sampling is restricted to specific procedures. The most commonly reported approach is paired sampling (umbilical cord and maternal blood) at delivery. There are limitations using this approach, since—depending on the timing of paired sampling—the maternal/fetal ratio will be different, so that a ratio based on the area under the curve (AUC maternal/fetal) is likely more accurate (Fig. 17.1). However, this necessitates pooled data within a broad time interval. Other opportunities to collect samples are ultrasound-guided transfusion, fetal surgery, or termination of pregnancy following timed maternal drug exposure.[2] Serial fetal sampling in the human setting is at present not possible, while in vivo transplacental kinetics are derived from different subjects studied at various times.[2,8] Besides fetal blood, coelocentesis in the first trimester, amniotic fluid (both more commonly used for genetic diagnoses), or quantification of drugs and metabolites in meconium or hair samples (more commonly used for toxicology) after delivery are other matrices to consider.[9-11] However, these methods were initially developed for developmental (environmental, *qualitative* exposure) toxicology, and cannot simply be applied in kinetic models to extrapolate *quantitative* drug transfer to the fetus and estimate subsequent risks. Therefore, we need additional in vivo or in vitro models to estimate an *s* kinetic model (distribution between maternal and fetal circulation).

The use of animal models is helpful, but their relevance may be limited because of difficulties in extrapolating results to humans: *only humans have human placentas*.[2,12,13] Placental structures differ extensively between species. Based on the macroscopic characteristics, a classification of chorioallantoic placentas has been suggested in (1) zonary (carnivore like dogs or cats), (2) diffuse (horses, pigs), (3) cotyledonary (ruminants such as cows, sheep or goats), or (4) discoid (primate and rodents).[2,12,13] Interspecies differences are also defined according to the Grosser classification, which focuses on placental barrier structure and degree of maternal tissue erosion. This classification distinguishes four types in eutherian mammals: syndesmochorial, epitheliochorial, endotheliochorial or hemochorial (human, primates, but also rodents) types. Hemochorial placentation can subsequently be subdivided in three subtypes, based on the number of trophoblastic cells at the villous surface: mono-(human), and di- or trichorial (rodent).[2,12,13]

In vitro models can also contribute to the understanding of placental drug transfer. Such models can mimic the bicompartmental structure by culturing cells—commonly derived from choriocarcinoma cell lines—on a porous filter in a multiwall culture plate. BeWo cell lines hereby result in a cellular monolayer with tight junctions.[14,15] Zhang and colleagues used Caco-2 cell monolayer permeability patterns to predict placental transfer, a model more commonly used to predict intestinal drug permeability.[16,17] A microphysiologic model of the human placental barrier ("placenta on a chip") with co-culture of human trophoblast cells and fetal endothelial cells in a physiologically accurate spatial arrangement has been reported.[18,19]

Human placenta obtained at birth provides an obvious approach to investigate the human placenta using in vitro perfusion studies.[2,20,21] The technique of dual perfusion of the human placental lobule provides potential valuable information on the extent and rate of net transfer of drugs, including placental drug metabolism. Both maternal-to-fetal clearance and fetal-to-maternal clearance can be standardized by comparison with antipyrine clearance, and maternal or fetal flow can be modulated. These tissues can also be used to quantify placental drug metabolism or active transporter processes.[2,20,21] Hutson and colleagues provided a systematic review on performance of the single placental lobule perfusion model to predict placental drug transfer.[22] In their hands, the fetal-to-maternal drug concentration ratios matched well with in vivo samples, commonly taken as single umbilical cord samples at delivery. Once modeling for differences in maternal and fetal/neonatal protein binding and blood pH was established, the perfusion results were able to accurately predict in vivo transfer at steady state ($r = 0.92$). Of the 70 different compounds evaluated, 49 (70%) showed placental transfer (fetal/maternal at least 0.1) in both models, 9 (13%) showed limited transfer (fetal/maternal <0.1), and for 12 (17%) there were discrepancies between in vitro and in vivo observations.[22]

Table 17.2 Compound Specific Observations on Physiology-Based Pharmacokinetic Models to Predict Fetal Exposure Following Maternal Intake.

Reference	Compound	Placental Model	Validation fetal Compartment
Liu et al.[26]	***emtricitabine*** ***acyclovir***, both renal (GFR + tubular)	Ex vivo cotyledon perfusion + apparent Caco-2 cell permeability + OSP estimated permeability (physicochemical characteristics)	Model matched with maternal + umbilical cord blood data
Mian et al.[27]	***acetaminophen*** (UGT1A1 + sulfation + CYP2E1)	Ex vivo cotyledon perfusion + apparent Caco-2 cell permeability + OSP estimated permeability (physicochemical characteristics)	Model matched with maternal + umbilical cord blood data
Freriksen et al.[28]	***dolutegravir*** (UGT1A1 + CYP3A)	Ex vivo cotyledon perfusion.	Model matched with maternal + umbilical cord blood data
Atoyebi et al.[29]	***thalidomide*** (hydrolysis + CYP2C19) ***efavirenz*** (CYP1A2,2A6,2B6,3A)	A priori assumption of bidirectional passive diffusion (Fick's law) for both drugs	Model matched with maternal + umbilical cord blood data for efavirenz
Zhang et al.[17]	***zidovudine*** (UGT2B7) ***theophylline*** (CYP1A1)	Apparent Caco-2 cell line permeability, verification, passive permeability drugs	Model matched with maternal + umbilical cord blood data for both drugs
De Sousa-Mendes et al.[30]	***nevirapine*** (CYP3A4,2D6,2B6)	Ex vivo cotyledon perfusion	Model matched observed umbilical cord blood data
De Sousa-Mendes et al.[31]	***tenofovir*** ***emtricitabine***, both renal (GFR + tubular)	Ex vivo cotyledon perfusion	Model matched with maternal + umbilical cord blood data for both drugs

CYP, Cytochrome P450; *GFR*, glomerular filtration rate; *OSP*, Open Systems Pharmacology software; *UGT*, UDP-glucuronosyl transferase.[17,26-31]

There are also obvious limitations of these models: the experimental period is limited to a few hours; the material is human placenta at delivery (either term or preterm) but not at early gestation, and the model in itself does not fully allow for observation of physiologically relevant parameters, such as blood flow (important for rapidly transferred compounds), plasma protein binding (affects the free concentration), and fluctuations of concentrations in the maternal and fetal compartments.[2,21,22] To further illustrate this, it seems that the equilibrium between the maternal and fetal compartment happens faster in vivo than in the in vitro perfusion model (e.g., morphine 5 minutes versus 120 minutes; bupivacaine 2 to 5 minutes versus 60 minutes).[22] These differences can likely be explained by differences in perfusion rates and differences in the villus surface area, and may reflect some of the limitations of this model.[22]

There are two aspects that need more consideration in future placental studies to better reflect the relevant maternal-fetal setting of women receiving chronic pharmacotherapy. First, placenta tissue accumulation has been described in these in vitro models, for example, tacrolimus or sildenafil in "naïve" unexposed placenta, so that the results may not be simply extrapolated to a chronic setting.[23,24] Second, maternal diseases such as preeclampsia in themselves may affect the permeability characteristics of the placenta (as documented for sildenafil) in addition to maternal blood flow characteristics.[23,25]

Regardless of the model used to estimate placental transfer, integration of the different pieces of information (the *system pharmacology approach, PBPK*) is the way forward to secure further progress. One hereby integrates available in vitro or in vivo observations to guide rational study design or to support dose adjustment for pregnant women.[2,3,8,21] By integrating all physiologic, preclinical, and clinical data, anticipated changes during pregnancy (maternal, fetal, placental) can be quantified using PBPK.[2,8,16] The growing success based on this integrated approach is illustrated in Table 17.2.[17,26-31] The different compounds reflect different clearance pathways (glucuronidation, cytochrome mediated metabolism, renal route), with different approaches to model the placental barrier (ex vivo cotyledon, cell line observations, or estimated permeability based on the physicochemical characteristics), while all were subsequently validated based on umbilical cord blood observations, commonly matched with maternal data. This stresses the relevance of high-quality clinical observational data.

Although such integrated PBPK models are useful tools, we should still be aware that fetal concentration-time profiles are crucial biomarkers of fetal outcome, as clinical pharmacology covers both PK (concentration-time) and pharmacodynamics (concentration-effect).[3] Moreover, (side)-effects do not always necessitate fetal exposure, as (side)-effects can be mediated at the level of the placenta with secondary fetal effects.

PHENOTYPIC PATTERNS OF PLACENTAL MATERNAL-FETAL DRUG EXCHANGE

The rate and extent of drug exchange to embryo or fetus are determined by numerous variables (see Table 17.1), rarely resulting in a "mirror" pattern of concentration-time profiles in both mother and fetus.[17] The combination of these variables results in different archetypical patterns of PK concentration-time profiles in the maternal and fetal compartments (Fig. 17.2).[32-34] Considering these archetypical patterns is a prerequisite for rational interpretation of a dataset. Although "rich" datasets on placental transfer are rare, attempts have been made to assign the kinetics of some drugs, on a tentative basis, to the patterns defined in Fig. 17.2. Examples of drugs with transplacental pharmacokinetics according to the different patterns are listed in Box 17.1.

Pattern A (Fig. 17.2) is applicable for a drug that crosses the placenta rapidly and subsequently distributes rapidly within a single fetal compartment, to quickly attain equilibrium with the maternal compartment. Fetal concentrations rapidly rise to reach maternal plasma concentrations; thereafter, the fetal and maternal curves overlap. This is commonly based on differences in concentration-driven "back leak" from the fetal to maternal circulation. When maternal-fetal exchange is rapid, two additional patterns are possible: as soon as equilibrium between the maternal and fetal compartments has been attained, fetal concentrations may exceed maternal plasma levels (see curve in ***pattern C*** in Fig. 17.2), or they may be less than the corresponding maternal plasma levels (see curve in ***pattern E*** in Fig. 17.2). As discussed later, differential plasma protein binding (total versus free concentration) or a pH gradient in the maternal-to-fetal compartment (pH difference affects ionization) may be responsible for the relatively large (curve in ***pattern C***) or small (curve in ***pattern E***) extent of fetal drug exposure after equilibrium between the maternal and fetal compartment is attained.

When the rate of placental transfer is low, ***pattern D*** (Fig. 17.2) is often applicable for the maternal-fetal unit. The increase in drug concentration in the fetus is slow. However, because the transport of drug from the fetus back to the mother also is slow, fetal concentrations exceed maternal plasma levels after the crossover point of the two curves. Thus, the fetus can be considered as a "deep" compartment. The same is applicable to the amniotic fluid compartment if fetal renal elimination occurs (e.g., cefazolin PK model).[35,36] Protein binding or pH gradient may affect the fetal-maternal concentration gradient once the distribution equilibrium has been reached (***pattern D***). In ***pattern F***, the fetal concentrations never reach the corresponding maternal plasma values because the plasma protein binding or the pH gradient favors higher maternal than fetal concentrations (e.g., differences in protein binding capacity). Alternatively, efficient fetal clearance (e.g., fetal kidney into amniotic fluid) may be responsible for the relatively low fetal drug levels. In ***pattern B***—rarely observed—drug transport is slow from mother to fetus but rapid from fetus to mother. This implies an active or facilitated transport system (efflux transporters).

Considerations in defining patterns may appear of theoretical interest only. However, these patterns reflect the relevance of cautious interpretation of experimental and clinical studies when, for instance, only single-point paired maternal/fetal samples are available. If samples were

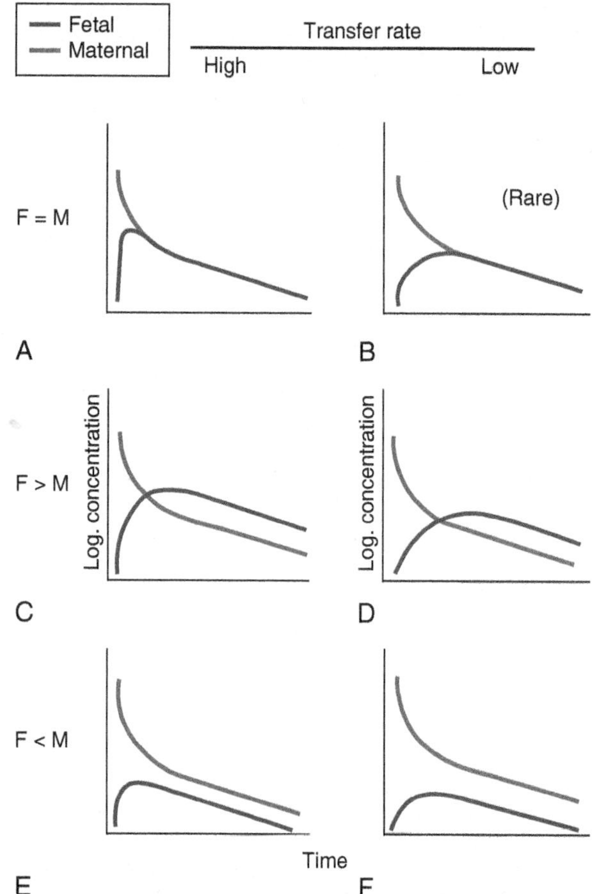

Fig. 17.2 Various patterns of maternal *(M)* and fetal *(F)* plasma concentration-time profiles.[32–34] See text and Box 17.1 for further details.

Box 17.1 Examples of Drugs With Transplacental Pharmacokinetics Reflecting Pattern A to F (see Fig. 17.2)

Pattern A or B	*Pattern C*	*Pattern D*	*Pattern E*	*Pattern F*
Some barbiturates	**Some benzodiazepines**	Ascorbate	**Amide-type local anesthetic agents**	Heparin
Thiopental	Diazepam	Colistimethate[a]	Lidocaine	TCDD
Pentobarbital	Lorazepam	Furosemide	Bupivacaine	**Quaternary ammonium compounds**
Secobarbital	Desmethyldiazepam	Meperidine	**Some β-adrenoreceptor blockers**	Tubocurarine
Antipyrine	Oxazepam	Indomethacin	Propranolol	Succinylcholine
Promethazine	Valproate	**Some cephalosporins**	Sotalol	Vecuronium
Ritodrine	Salicylate	Cephalothin	Labetalol	Pancuronium
Magnesium (sulfate)	Nalidixic acid	Cefazolin	Dexamethasone	Fazadinium
Thiamphenicol	Nicotine	Cephapirin	Betamethasone	Alcuronium
Digoxin	Urea	Cephalexin	Cimetidine	**Elemental ions** (Cd, Hg)
Ketamine	**Some penicillins**	**Some aminoglycosides**	Ranitidine	Fenoterol
Dexmedetomidine	Ampicillin	Gentamicin	Methadone	Chlorthalidone
Acetaminophen	Penicillin G	Kanamycin	Remifentanil	Etozolin (ozolinone)
Nucleoside reverse transcriptase inhibitors	Methicillin	Amikacin	Propofol	Dicloxacillin
(abacavir, lamivudine, stavudine)	Azidocillin		**Some sulfonamides**[b]	Erythromycin
Nevirapine			**Protease inhibitors** (atazanavir, darunavir)	Clarithromycin
				Nitrofurantoin
				Atosiban

[a]Polypeptide antibiotic, molecular weight 1200.
[b]In the first and second trimester.
TCDD, 2,3,7,8-Tetracholorodibenzo-p-dioxin.
Differentiation between models A and B, C and D, or E and F, respectively, is often uncertain because of incomplete data on the initial phase of drug distribution across the placenta, and it is assumed that model B is only rarely applicable.

collected only before crossover (see ***pattern C,*** Fig. 17.2), the wrong conclusion (i.e., relatively low fetal exposure) could be made. It might therefore be prudent to vary sampling times—if feasible—in a naïve pooled dataset ("clever sparse opportunistic sampling") to facilitate concentration-time profiles description.[8,21,35]

For an adequate description of fetal exposure, both maternal and fetal concentration-time curves must be defined, because both the *transfer rate* (high A,C,E, versus low B,D,F) and *the extent* (ratio fetal-to-maternal, A,B to C,D to E,F) matter if the goal is to describe exposure (AUC concept) (see Figs. 17.1 and 17.2).

The placental "barrier" functions include passive diffusion, facilitated diffusion, active transport, and pinocytosis, or endocytosis.[3] Passive diffusion and its mechanisms will be discussed first and will be followed by a section on selective, "non-passive" transporter mechanisms and placental drug metabolism.

MECHANISMS RELATED TO PASSIVE DIFFUSION OF PLACENTAL MATERNAL-FETAL DRUG EXCHANGE

Passive diffusion is primarily driven by the concentration gradient between the maternal and fetal compartments, further modulated by maternal, fetal, and placental blood flow. The rate and extent of drug transfer mainly relates to the physicochemical and structural characteristics of the specific compound, as well as to the physiologic characteristics of the maternal-placental-embryonic-fetal unit.[a] The concept of the placenta as a lipoid membrane is hereby useful to describe and predict the impact of physicochemical characteristics of a specific compound on its placental transfer. For lipophilic drugs, the maternal and fetal blood flow is critical for the rate of placental exchange over the placenta (flow-limited), as opposed to the hydrophilic drugs, which are permeability-limited. In contrast, a drug cannot passively pass the placental barrier in its ionized or charged form.[a]

Most drugs cross the placental membranes by passive diffusion. The rate of diffusion is directly proportional to the surface area of exchange and the maternal-to-fetal concentration gradient across the membrane, and inversely proportional to the membrane thickness. This rate is governed mainly by physicochemical factors according to Fick's law[a]:

$$\text{Rate of diffusion} = D \times \Delta c \times A/d \quad [17.1]$$

where A = area of exchange, d = membrane thickness, Δc = drug concentration gradient across the membrane (e.g., difference between maternal and fetal plasma drug concentrations), and D = diffusion constant for the drug.

This definition reflects the impact of gestational age (area of exchange, membrane thickness), dose, and maternal disease characteristics (area of exchange, membrane thickness) or treatment modalities (e.g., prenatal lung maturation affects placental growth).[b] To further illustrate its application, placental diffusion parameters will be upscaled to the size of the placenta from in vitro cotyledon transfer parameters to placental transfer (see Table 17.2, as reported for emtricitabine, acyclovir, acetaminophen, dolutegravir, nevirapine, tenofovir, emtricitabine).[26-28,30,31] From this equation, it is predicted that a larger area of placental exchange *(A)*, consisting of membranes with limited thickness *(d)*, favors placental bidirectional drug transfer. *A*, *d*, and Δc can be determined in a model; however, *D* is far more difficult to predict because it results from the interactions between membrane and molecule. The resistance within the tissue layers interposed between the maternal and fetal circulations (compartments) limits diffusion, significant for hydrophilic molecules.

In the human placenta, two layers (trophoblast, endothelium) contribute to this diffusional resistance. Hydrophilic molecules either have to cross these layers (i.e., the ***membrane hypothesis***) or find their way through water-filled channels that extend through the trophoblast and communicate with the intracellular channels of the endothelial layer (i.e., the ***aqueous pores hypothesis***). Faster placental transfer relates to better lipid solubility and low ionization and protein binding of drugs with a molecular weight (MW) of less than 500 Da.

The permeability of lipid-soluble substances is much higher. For these substances, the placental transfer rate is limited mainly by availability of drug at the area of exchange, which is ultimately determined by blood flow.[b] Therefore the initial maternal-fetal concentration gradient, Δc, depends on uterine and umbilical blood flow. This mathematical concept has been applied to predict placental barrier permeability using the Quantitative Structure-Activity Relationship (QSAR) method and has been further developed in the meanwhile.[16] Such a QSAR hereby integrates the chemical structures of molecules and the available biologic properties to estimate placental permeability (see Table 17.2, as reported for emtricitabine, acyclovir, and acetaminophen).[17,26-31]

A number of studies have noted that as placental thickness and the number of placental layers decreases and the area of exchange increases during gestation, increased placental transfer occurs.[b] However, in vivo, the placenta barrier cannot fully be described by only anatomic parameters such as area or thickness. Thornburg and Faber[37] found that in rabbit placenta, the fetal endothelium, which is not markedly altered during pregnancy, is the layer defining the transfer rate of many drugs; area of exchange *(A)* and membrane thickness *(d)* apparently are of secondary importance. Maternal-to-fetal transfer occurs across the placental barrier, made up of both the syncytiotrophoblast on the maternal side and the endothelial cell layer on the fetal side.[38] The diffusion of drugs across the hemotrichorial placenta (mouse, rat) often is faster than across the hemomonochorial placenta (monkey, human). The earlier mentioned placenta-on-a-chip approaches will likely generate relevant insights in aspects of interspecies "translation" of such findings.[18,19]

Drugs have the greatest chance of crossing the placenta if they are (1) lipid-soluble, (2) weak acids, and (3) of low MW (<500 Da) (see Box 17.1). Another important covariate is plasma or tissue protein binding.[c] As mentioned earlier, modeling approaches based on—for example, the QSAR method—hereby integrate these different aspects to predict the phenotypic placental barrier permeability pattern and have been integrated in PBPK models (see Table 17.2).[17,26-31]

LIPID SOLUBILITY OF DRUGS

Applying the earlier mentioned basic concepts of passive diffusion (see earlier, Fick's law) through a lipoid barrier, lipophilic drugs (i.e., high lipid-water partition coefficient *K*) will cross the placental barrier fast (panels on the *left* in Fig. 17.2, high transfer rate). The opposite can be anticipated for hydrophilic drugs (i.e., low lipid-water partition coefficient *K* and consequently high water solubility, panels on the ***right*** in Fig. 17.2, low transfer rate).[32-34] Consequently, drugs such as thiopental, methohexital, propofol, or lipophilic opioids (fentanyl, alfentanil, sufentanil) or

[a]References 2, 5, 9, 16, 20, 32-34.
[b]References 2, 5, 9, 16, 20, 32-34.
[c]References 2, 5, 9, 16, 20, 32-34.

other compounds like antipyrine or bisphenol A will cross the placenta extremely rapidly.[17,32,39,40] This pattern has more recently also been confirmed for remifentanil with a fetal/maternal ratio of 0.1 in a sheep model.[41] Along the same concept, cocaine as weak base, further characterized by high lipid solubility, low MW (305 Da), and low plasma protein binding (8% to 10%), quickly equilibrates between the maternal and fetal compartment, as does its metabolite cocaethylene.[42-44] In such setting, it is reasonable to assume that exposure will mainly be driven by maternal arterial uterine blood flow and fetal umbilical blood flow. More polar compounds, such as phenobarbital or the more hydrophilic cocaine metabolite benzoylecgonine, cross the placenta more slowly. The highly lipid-soluble benzodiazepine receptor agonist abecarnil (log $p = 4.6$) reaches higher concentrations in blood of the rabbit fetus than in maternal blood, whereas its more hydrophilic metabolites cannot cross the placental barrier to the same extent.[45]

The relevance of lipophilicity can be illustrated using available data on in vitro maternal-fetal gradients of antibiotics used to treat or prevent perinatal infections (like chorioamnionitis). Despite low plasma protein binding and low MW of clavulanate and ticarcillin (9% and 45%, and 236 and 428 MW, respectively), there is only limited placental transfer to the fetus. In contrast, the equally large but more lipophilic molecule ceftizoxime (30% protein binding, MW 406) reaches higher concentrations in the fetus than in the mother.[46,47] Furthermore, bases such as 2′,3′-dideoxyinosine and 2′,3′-dideoxycytidine and the more lipophilic antiviral drug zidovudine cross the placental barrier rapidly by simple diffusion.[48-50] A zidovudine and PBPK model, including fetal exposure prediction, has recently been described, both using the concept of estimated permeability based on the physicochemical characteristics (bidirectional maternal-placental and fetal-placental unbound transplacental passive diffusion clearance) and the increase in placental villous area over gestational age.[17,18] Therapeutic maternal levels of zidovudine result in fetal levels within the therapeutic range as well. Umbilical cord sample levels ranged as high as 113% to 127% of maternal levels.[17,18] Similar efforts have been reported for different antiviral drugs, with specific focus on drugs used to control HIV infections.[51]

This finding raises the possibility of efficacious preventive treatment for the fetus, but also points to a higher potential for adverse fetal effects. Within the human placenta, zidovudine is metabolized to more polar and still-undefined metabolites, which are not released into the perfusates, probably due to differences in lipid solubility.[18,52] Glucuronidation results in a more polar metabolite that is able to cross the human perfused placenta at approximately half the rate observed for azidothymidine.[52] Tuntland and colleagues[53] proposed models that predict the extent of placental transfer of deoxynucleoside drugs. Predicted fetal-maternal steady-state plasma concentration ratios using their in vitro partition coefficient model deviated from observed values by only 3.9% ± 7.9% (mean ± standard deviation). In vivo and in vitro clearance indices were highly and significantly related to the drug octanol-water partition coefficient.[53]

Another drug in the same group of compounds is acyclovir, which is taken orally by women with recurrent genital herpes simplex infections during late pregnancy to reduce the risk of transmission of herpes simplex to the fetus. As lipophilic compound with low plasma binding (22% to 33%), it also appears to be quickly transferred by simple diffusion.[54] The highest levels of this compound were measured in the amniotic fluid, probably secondary to unchanged renal excretion of the drug by the fetus, providing additional protection against ascending viral infection.[54] We refer to the recently published PBPK on acyclovir that integrated all these findings to quantify maternal and fetal exposure.[26]

Placental transfer of hydrophilic substances is proportional to the coefficient of free diffusion in water, with some evidence of steric restriction of larger molecules.[17,55] The relationship between partition coefficients and placental transfer does not hold true for drugs with rather extreme values (either high or low) for the partition coefficient *K*. If *K* is high, the substance may be so tightly bound to membranes or other cell constituents (proteins, lipids) that it cannot sufficiently cross from the lipid into the aqueous phase. Examples of drugs in this category are cyclosporine and chlorinated aromatics, such as 2,3,7,8,-tetrachlorodibenzo-*p*-dioxin (TCDD), which are extremely lipophilic but are transferred to the embryo and fetus in minute amounts only.[56,57] A similar pattern has recently been reported for tacrolimus with a very high median placental tissue-to-maternal perfusate (113) ratio.[24] These drugs are mainly stored in maternal liver and fat and appear only to a limited extent in the maternal circulation. Placental accumulation of drugs can also be advantageous, such as for spiramycin to treat placental toxoplasmosis infection. This drug will concentrate in the placenta and will reduce maternal-fetal transmission risk of the infection.[58] Furthermore, the low fat content of the fetus is an additional factor limiting the amounts of subsequent fetal accumulation.

Neonatal vitamin K deficiency is another clinically relevant illustration of this aspect of placental transfer. Despite its high lipophilicity, vitamin K_1 is transferred only slowly and in minor quantities through the human placenta.[59] Low-circulating vitamin K_1 levels appear to be common in pregnant women and not limited to women who underwent bariatric surgery or have Crohn's disease or short-bowel syndrome.[60] Vitamin K_1 crosses the placenta slowly and to a limited degree, but data suggest that an adequate lag period (>8 days after intramuscular injection) between maternal supplementation and delivery will enhance maternal-fetal transport of vitamin K_1.[59,60]

Overall, this suggest that lipophilicity is not the only driver of placental transfer; transfer is also in part driven by protein or tissue binding (free fraction concept, cf lower). Another driver that will determine fetal exposure is the maternal and fetal blood flow. Fetal propofol exposure is directly related to the uterine and umbilical blood flows.[61] No particular influence of lipophilicity or other chemostructural properties determines the extent of maternal-fetal transfer of a group of opioids (fentanyl > alfentanil > sufentanil). However, in the event of fluctuation in maternal blood flow, lipophilicity is a covariate of the rate of opioid transfer if compared with that of antipyrine.[62] Related to this, buprenorphine shows marked sequestration to tissues including the placenta, but has only a low rate of transplacental transfer (<10%) in spite of its high lipid solubility, likely due to its high protein binding (to α- and β-globulins, barely to albumin). This may explain why neonates born to mothers treated with buprenorphine during pregnancy less commonly display neonatal abstinence syndrome, compared to methadone.[63]

IONIZATION OF DRUGS

A drug cannot pass the placental barrier in its ionized or charged form. Most drugs are weakly acidic or basic substances and are thus ionized at physiologic pH. The ionized form carries a charge and is polar, so this form cannot simply pass through membranes if based on a passive diffusion. As a clinical illustration, this concept applies for quaternary ammonium compounds, such as neuromuscular-blocking agents, which are fully ionized (e.g., dimethyltubocurarine, pancuronium, succinylcholine).[64-68] Fetal drug levels increase slowly up to levels that are only approximately 10% of corresponding maternal plasma (see ***pattern F*** in Fig. 17.2 and Box 17.1), during both early[64] and late[65] gestation. Transfer of these compounds is confined to water-filled pores within the lipid membranes. Such a mechanism is much less efficient in rate and extent than transfer across lipid membranes.

As a consequence, for fetal surgery, continuous maternal remifentanil can result in fetal narcosis[41] but is combined with fetal intramuscular administration of a neuromuscular blocking agent if fetal immobilization is needed.[69]

Similar to the lipophilicity earlier discussed, this rule does not apply to all highly ionized substances. Weak acids, which constitute an important group of drugs, appear to be rapidly transferred across the placenta. Salicylate[70,71] and valproate (valproic acid VPAk),[72-74] two drugs essentially fully ionized at physiologic pH, are rapidly transported to the fetal compartment (***pattern*** ***C*** in Fig. 17.2 and Box 17.1). Fetal salicylate concentrations reach corresponding maternal levels approximately 1 hour after administration.[71] In mice and rat, transplacental equilibrium of valproic acid between embryonic and maternal compartments was reached in less than 0.5 hour.[75-77] Similar observations have been made for the antibiotics ampicillin and methicillin (***pattern C***).[78] It seems that the small portions of the nonionized fraction are responsible for an efficient transport across the membranes, while the equilibrium between the ionized and nonionized fraction is subsequently rapidly reestablished.

The importance of ionization is supported by in vitro studies using the perfused human placenta model. One of these investigations compared the maternal-fetal clearance ratios of VPA and its glucuronides-β-glucuronidase-susceptible metabolite (VPA-G) and non-β-glucuronidase-susceptible (VPA-GR, in which R denotes *resistant*) metabolite. The glucuronidated acids characterized by partition coefficients of 0.0141 and 0.219 (compared with 1.6 for VPA) were expected to have negative log of dissociation constant (pK_a) values between 3 and 4, resulting in higher degrees of ionization compared with VPA. As expected, the placental transfer was found to be significantly lower for the glucuronides (13% and 17%, compared with 95% for VPA). Furthermore, although transport was positively correlated with the log partition coefficient, no significant dependence on MW was noted.[79] Similar observations were made in vivo, concerning the lower placental transfer of glucuronidated retinoids.[80]

Similar mechanisms may underlie the efficient transfer of some basic substances, such as the tertiary phenothiazines, meperidine, nicotine,[44,81,82] and lysergic acid diethylamide.[83] As noted earlier, the nonionized portion of a drug (in rapid equilibrium with the ionized form) may cross to the fetal compartment. Lead and metallic mercury can be transferred from the blood of occupationally exposed mothers to their fetus.[84,85]

Interestingly, the fetal pH is 0.1 to 0.15 points lower than the maternal pH in late gestation.[2,3,5] This gradient can affect the extent of transfer of acidic and basic drugs. As discussed earlier, only the nonionized form can readily pass the lipoid membranes. Because basic drugs are ionized at the relatively low (acidic) pH of fetal blood to a higher degree than in maternal blood, this class of drugs may accumulate in fetal blood *(ion trapping)* (see ***patterns C and D*** in Fig. 17.2 and Box 17.1). The reverse is true for acidic drugs, which reach lower concentrations in fetal than in maternal blood in late gestation (***patterns E and F*** in Fig. 17.2). The ratio between the fetal and maternal concentrations ($C_{fetal}/C_{maternal}$) for a particular drug can be calculated using the Henderson-Hasselbalch equation from the pK_a of the drug and the fetal and maternal blood pH (Eq. 17.2):

$$\frac{C_{\text{fetal, free}}}{C_{\text{maternal, free}}} = \frac{1 + 10^{(pK_a - \text{pH, fetal})}}{1 + 10^{(pK_a - \text{pH, maternal})}} \quad [17.2]$$

The pH gradient determines the concentration gradient of *free* concentrations, unbound to plasma proteins. The *total* concentrations are determined by the protein-binding gradient across the placenta (see later).

This mechanism has also its clinical relevance. Basic drugs such as amide-type local anesthetic agents are ionized to a greater degree in fetal blood than in maternal blood. Therefore the *free* concentrations of drugs such as lidocaine, bupivacaine, 2-chlorprocaine, ropivacaine, and pethidine accumulate in fetal blood (by a factor of approximately 1.5) even in the normal maternal-fetal pH setting.[86,87] An obvious influence of the fetal pH on maternal-fetal clearance of bupivacaine and ropivacaine has been demonstrated in vitro.[88] Using a human cotyledon perfusion model, Ueki and colleagues documented that placental transfer of amide-type local anesthetics was mainly driven by the basic uncharged free concentration, with the highest fetal/maternal ratios for mepivacaine > lidocaine > bupivacaine = ropivacaine, irrespective of the different pH conditions (fetal/maternal pH conditions 7.4/7.4, 6.9/7.4, and 6.9/6.9, respectively). Based on these observations, the authors suggested that ropivacaine and bupivacaine can be used more safely than mepivacaine if one aims to avoid placental transfer and fetal accumulation.[89] Fetal asphyxia or maternal alkalosis (hyperventilation) may further enlarge the maternal-fetal pH gradient and the subsequent ion trapping. This pattern of pH-driven transfer has been described in a human placental perfusion model for bupivacaine, lidocaine, chloroprocaine, and sufentanil: all were increased when the fetal perfusate pH was lowered to 7.2 (amide anesthetics, ***pattern E*** in Fig. 17.2, Box 17.1, **and** Table 17.3).[90-98] As both pharmacologic effects and side-effects of a drug usually are associated with the free drug concentration, fetal side effects of amide-type local anesthetic agents (cardiac, seizures) are related to the pH gradient across the placenta and not so much the protein-binding gradient.[90]

The reverse would be expected with regard to effects of the fetal-maternal pH gradient on the extent of placental transfer of acidic drugs. In agreement with the pH partition hypothesis, the fetal free concentrations of VPA were lower than the corresponding maternal values (fetal-maternal free concentration gradient was 0.82 ± 0.34 in one study).[99] Again, the concentration gradient of the total levels was quite different. Owing to decreased maternal plasma protein binding (see later), the concentrations in fetal plasma exceeded (factor 1.7) those in maternal plasma.[73,99]

This pattern may also be of relevance for mechanisms related to teratology in early gestation. Little is known on the plasma and embryonic tissue pH during early human gestation. The period between week 3 and weeks 6 to 8 after conception may be particularly important for the formation of major malformations, like those associated with thalidomide or retinoids. The intracellular pH (pH_i), as determined by distribution of the weak acid dimethadione, is surprisingly *high* during early organogenesis.[75,100,101] Embryonic pH_i considerably exceeded corresponding maternal plasma pH at that period and decreased during later developmental periods to approach values similar to those for other tissues. An acidic drug such as VPA would be expected to be ionized to a greater degree in the relatively basic milieu of the early embryo. Based on the pK_a of VPA (4.7), the pH partition hypothesis predicts a concentration of the drug in the embryo twice as high as in maternal plasma, and this has been confirmed experimentally.[74,100] The pH_i of the embryo decreases with advancing gestation; thus, in agreement with the pH partition hypothesis, so does the embryonic-maternal concentration gradient. Salicylate, dimethadione, metabolites of halothane (trichloroacetic acid) and methoxyethanol (methoxyacetic acid), and acidic thalidomide metabolites also accumulate in the early rodent embryo (see Table 17.4).[74,100-102] It has been hypothesized that acidic metabolites formed by hydrolysis of thalidomide within the embryo may become trapped because of their high polarity.[103,104] This pattern suggests that the predominance of acidic drugs in the list of human teratogens may be explained by accumulation and the disproportional high "exposure" *(entrapment phenomenon)* relative to the maternal compartment. The subsequent teratogenic mechanism may involve an alteration of the pH_i of the embryonic cell. This concept is attractive as a mechanism of teratogenesis because pH controls numerous cellular functions, including proliferation and intercellular communication.

PROTEIN BINDING OF DRUGS

Plasma proteins have two functions and exert these functions both in the maternal and fetal circulation: they serve as *vehicles* allowing the drug to be transported, although depending on the affinity of the compound, they may impair subsequent transfer. Conversely, they offer binding sites on the other side of the placental barrier, *acceptors,* potentially facilitating transfer. Only the unbound portion ("free drug") is available for placental transfer, and it therefore may also take additional time to reach distribution equilibrium between the maternal and fetal compartments. As the permeability across the placenta is another rate limiter, the plasma protein-bound fraction can also be considered as a reservoir. Supporting this concept, many lipophilic drugs, commonly highly protein-bound, actually permeate the placenta rapidly. Plasma protein binding is rapidly reversible and may even increase the amount transferred by presenting greater amounts of drug to the placenta. Plasma protein binding may serve as a vehicle especially for drugs with poor water solubility, which otherwise would not reach the maternal side of the placenta in large amounts. An ex vivo cotyledon study documented that increasing fetal circulation of albumin (0.0 to 1 g/dL) enhanced the uptake of steroids to the fetal compartment by freeing them from entrapment to tissue proteins in the placenta.[105] There is still debate to what extent changes in plasma protein binding have clinical relevance.[106]

Albumin and α_1-acid glycoprotein are the most important proteins involved in drug protein binding in plasma. However, protein binding of xenobiotics is not limited to maternal and fetal plasma but also occurs in other tissues. Placental protein binding hereby acts as reservoir to diffuse at a later stage either to the fetus or back to the mother. Maternal and fetal plasma differ and display gestational age-related trends in plasma protein, albumin, and α_1-acid glycoprotein. In Fig. 17.3, we provide trends in total plasma protein and albumin concentration (g/L) in maternal plasma samples as collected in women undergoing fetal surgery at gestational ages between 17 and 34 weeks.[36] At term-equivalent age, the fetal albumin level surpasses the maternal level (fetal/maternal ratio 1.2). In contrast, this is only 0.28 in the first trimester of pregnancy. The α_1-acid glycoprotein concentration remains fairly constant in the maternal circulation throughout pregnancy, with a progressive increase in the fetal circulation, to result in a fetal/maternal ratio of 0.09 in the first trimester and 0.37 at term.[2,3,22,107] Liver disease, preeclampsia, or surgery may further affect maternal plasma composition, while hydrops will affect fetal

Table 17.3 Extent of Transplacental Distribution of Amide-Type Local Anesthetic Agents.

Drug	Measured Fetal (F)-Maternal (M) Total Concentration Ratio (Range)	% Protein Binding		F-M Protein-Binding Ratio	F-M Free Concentration Ratio[a]	F-M Total Concentration Ratio[b]
		M	F			
Lidocaine	0.4–0.7	63	34	0.54	1.4	0.80
		64	24		1.4	0.66
Bupivacaine	0.18–0.56	91	51	0.56	1.5	0.27
		92	72	0.78	1.5	0.42
Etidocaine	0.09–0.37	92	—	—	1.4	—
Mepivacaine	0.5–0.8	5	36	0.65	1.4	0.71
Prilocaine	1.0–1.3	55	—	—	1.4	—
Ropivacaine	0.12 (SD 0.16)	86	—	—	—	—

[a]Predicted according to Equation (17.2).
[b]Predicted according to Equation (17.4).
F, Fetal; *M*, maternal.
Data from References 90–98 and literature citations therein.

Table 17.4 Teratogenicity and Embryo-Maternal (E-M) Concentration Ratios for Acidic and Basic Substances.

Type of Compound	Drug	Species	Placental Transfer		Teratogenic
			Gestation, Duration	E-M Ratio	
Acids	Valproic acid	Mouse	Day 9	1.6–2.3	Yes
	Valproic acid	Rat	Day 11	1.5–1.7	Yes
	Salicylic acid	Rat	Day 10	1.3–1.7	Yes
	Thalidomide (acid metabolite)	Rabbit	Day 8 (blastocyst)	1.2	Yes
	Dimethadione	Mouse	Day 9	1.4–1.7	Yes
		Rat	Day 11		Yes
	Halothane (trichloroacetic acid)	Mouse	Day 11	Accumulation of radioactivity	Yes
	Methoxyethanol (methoxyacetic acid)	Rat	Day 12	2	Yes
		Monkey	Day 28	1	Yes
	Hydrochloric acid (acidified seawater)	Sea urchin embryo, in vitro	5 h (32 cells)	—	Yes
	2-En-valproic acid	Mouse	Day 9	1.2–1.5	No
Basic substances	Nicotine	Mouse	Day 9	3	No
	Doxylamine	Mouse	Day 9	5	No

Data from References 74 and 100–102 and literature citations therein.

plasma composition. Trends in human maternal and fetal albumin and α_1-acid glycoprotein concentrations throughout gestation are summarized in Table 17.5.[36,107,108] After injury or surgery, α_1-acid glycoprotein concentrations may raise as part of an acute phase reaction.[107,109] In contrast, delivery and labor itself does not affect maternal α_1-acid glycoprotein concentrations.[2,3,22,107] Besides the concentration of the protein (like albumin or α_1-acid glycoprotein), protein binding also depends on the binding affinity constant (K_a) and the number of binding sites available *(n)* (Eq. 17.3):

$$B/F = n \times K_a \times P \qquad [17.3]$$

where B/F is the ratio of bound concentration to free concentration of drug.

The importance of protein binding, however, also depends on the degree or extent of binding: a clinically significant effect is expected only when it exceeds approximately 80%.[106] This may account for the failure to detect differences in transplacental transfer between methimazole (no binding to plasma proteins) and propylthiouracil (67% bound to albumin) in vitro.[110] Little information is available on the effects of maternal or fetal hypoproteinemia on placental drug transfer. In a study by Brown and colleagues,[111] fetal (umbilical cord) serum concentrations of the antibiotic cefazolin in human newborns suffering from hydrops fetalis were not different from those obtained from nonhydropic infants. Conversely, no transfer was observed in the presence of low albumin (1 mg/mL) concentrations in the perfused human placental cotyledon.[112] Similarly, low digoxin levels have been observed in hypoproteinemic human fetuses treated transplacentally with digoxin.[113] In vitro, the transplacental transfer of olanzapine (plasma binding in vitro: albumin, 90%; α_1-acid glycoprotein, 77%) was largely dependent on the concentration of acceptor proteins on the opposite side of initial drug placement.[114]

As a consequence, the development of a fetal-maternal plasma protein-binding gradient (and thus the extent of placental transfer) for a particular drug depends greatly on the nature of the binding protein. This is exemplified by a comparison of fetal and maternal protein binding of diazepam,[109] VPA,[115] and propranolol[109] (Table 17.6).[74,109,115] The first two drugs are bound predominantly to albumin. Consequently, protein binding is low in fetal plasma during early to mid-gestation but increases steadily to reach an extent that exceeds maternal binding at term gestation.[116] Propranolol is bound predominantly to α_1-acid glycoprotein. Consequently, protein binding is low in fetal plasma during early and mid-gestation but does not significantly increase during later gestational periods.

Protein binding is defined either as the percentage of drug bound ($C_{bound}/C_{total} \times 100$) or as the unbound (free) fraction ($C_{unbound}/C_{total}$). The fetal-maternal concentration ratio of total drug at post-distributive equilibrium can therefore be predicted as follows (Eq. 17.4):

$$\frac{C_{\text{fetal, total}}}{C_{\text{maternal, total}}} = \frac{\text{Unbound fraction (mother)}}{\text{Unbound fraction (fetus)}} \qquad [17.4]$$

If the drug is an electrolyte, the pH difference between fetal and maternal blood has to be taken into account (Eq. 17.5):

$$\frac{C_{\text{fetal, total}}}{C_{\text{maternal, total}}} = \frac{1 + 10^{(pK_a,\ \text{fetal})}}{1 + 10^{(pK_a - \text{pH, maternal})}} \cdot \frac{\text{Unbound fraction (mother)}}{\text{Unbound fraction (fetus)}} \qquad [17.5]$$

Such predicted fetal-maternal concentration ratios are indeed in strong agreement with those found in clinical studies for numerous drugs (Table 17.7 and Fig. 17.4).[d] Owing to the low fetal albumin concentrations during early pregnancy, fetal *(total)* concentrations of drugs such as VPA are much lower in fetal blood than in maternal plasma (Fig. 17.5).[115]

Competitive binding of other endogenous or exogenous compounds to these proteins may also affect the binding capacity. For example, cefazolin-albumin binding varied between different patient groups (adults, pregnant women, neonates), and these differences could not solely be attributed to alterations in plasma albumin concentrations.[108] This phenomenon is well known for bilirubin in early neonatal life but also applies

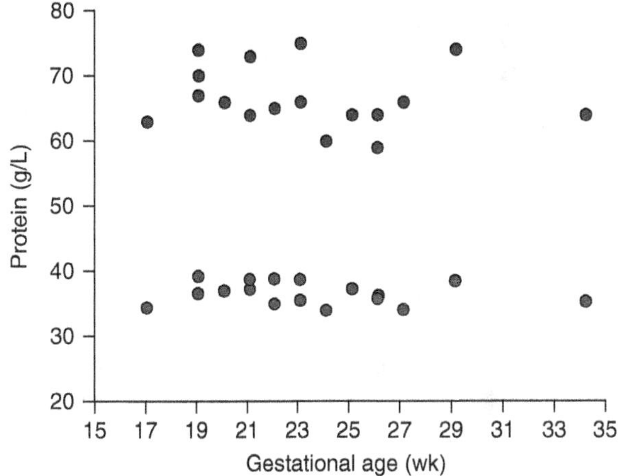

Fig. 17.3 Trends in albumin *(red circles)* and total plasma protein *(blue circles)* concentrations with gestational age as observed in maternal plasma samples. These samples were collected in a study on maternal-fetal amniotic fluid pharmacokinetics of cefazolin. (From Allegaert K, van Mieghem T, Verbesselt R, et al. Cefazolin pharmacokinetics in maternal plasma and amniotic fluid during pregnancy. *Am J Obstet Gynecol.* 2009;200:170.e1–170.e7; and Smits A, Roberts JA, Vella-Brincat JW, et al. Cefazolin plasma protein binding in different human populations: more than cefazolin-albumin interaction. *Int J Antimicrob Agents.* 2014;43:199.)

[d]References 74, 77, 87, 100, 110–115.

Table 17.5 Human Maternal and Fetal Serum Albumin and α_1-Acid Glycoprotein Concentrations During Pregnancy.

	Albumin Concentration (g/L)			α_1-Acid Glycoprotein Concentration (g/L)		
Weeks of Gestation	**Maternal (M)**	**Fetal (F)**	**F-M Ratio**	**M**	**F**	**F-M Ratio**
12–15	28	11	0.28	0.57	0.05	0.09
16–25	34	19	0.66	0.73	0.08	0.11
26–35	28	26	0.97	0.53	0.16	0.24
36–41	29	34	1.20	0.60	0.21	0.37

Data from References 36, 107, and 108 and literature citations therein.

Table 17.6 Dependence of Plasma Protein Binding of Some Drugs on Gestational Age in Humans in Both the Maternal (M) and Fetal (F) Plasma.

		% Bound During Week of Gestation					
		16th Week		23th Week		37th Week	
Drug	Binding Protein	M	F	M	F	M	F
Diazepam	Albumin	90	97	96	97	98.5	97
Valproic acid	Albumin	90	50	85	80	80	90
Propranolol	α_1-acid glycoprotein	63	85	70	85	71	85

Data from References 74, 109, and 115 and literature citations therein.

Table 17.7 Fetal (F)-Maternal (M) Plasma Protein Binding and Total Concentration Ratios of Specific Drugs in Late Human Gestation.

		% Bound		
Drug	Primary Binding Protein	M	F	F-M Primary Ratio Total Plasma Concentration
Betamethasone	AGP	60	41	0.33
Bupivacaine	AGP	91	51	0.27
Lidocaine	AGP	64	24	0.66
Mepivacaine	AGP	55	36	0.71
Phenobarbital	ALB	41	36	1.0
Phenytoin	ALB	87	82	1.0
Salicylate	ALB	43	54	1.2
Diazepam	ALB	97	98.5	1.6
Valproic acid	ALB	73	88	1.7

AGP, Alpha-1 acid glycoprotein; *ALB,* albumin.
Data from references 74, 77, 87, 100, 107, and 110–115 and literature citations therein.

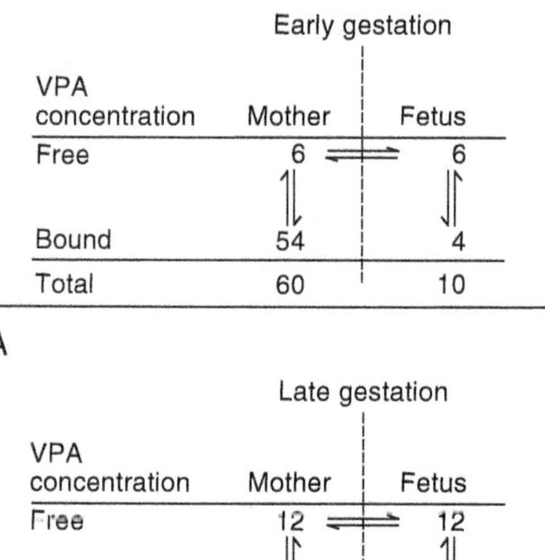

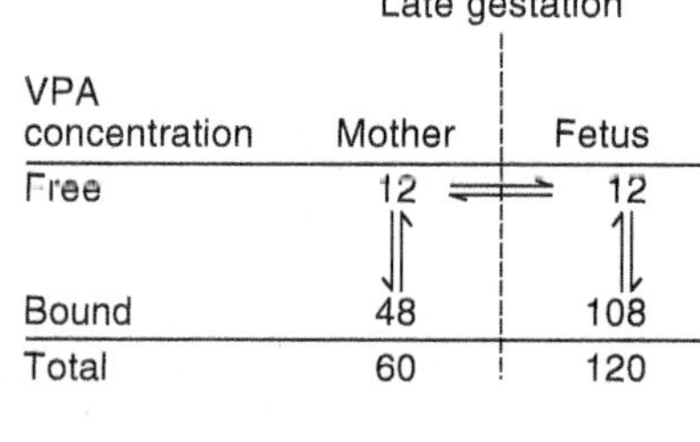

Fig. 17.4 Valproic acid *(VPA)* free and bound concentration gradients in mother and fetus during early (A) and late gestation (B). The *dashed line* represents the placental membranes. Concentrations are measured in mg/L. (From Nau H, Krauer B. Serum protein binding of valproic acid in fetus-mother pairs throughout pregnancy: correlation with oxytocin administration and albumin and free fatty acid concentrations. *J Clin Pharmacol.* 1986;26:215.)

for free fatty acids. This is because free fatty acids also bind to albumin, resulting either in competitive binding or allosteric effects (the regulation of a protein by binding at a site other than the protein's drug-binding site). Free fatty acid concentrations in maternal plasma rise slowly but progressively during pregnancy to end with a three-fold higher concentration at term gestational age.[22] The free fractions of those drugs, which may be displaced from albumin-binding sites, would therefore also be expected to increase during pregnancy. Decreasing maternal albumin concentrations (see Fig. 17.3) further amplify these effects.[108,110] At delivery, maternal plasma free fatty acid concentrations rise sharply to levels two to three times higher than reference concentrations. To illustrate its clinical relevance, free fractions of salicylate,[17,117–119] diazepam,[107,120] or VPA[74] in maternal plasma also increase sharply to values approximately three times those observed for adult control subjects or in cord plasma samples.[109,121–123] Accordingly, the amount of "free" drug available for placental transfer is also increased. In the fetus, the fatty acid concentrations remain at low levels, and binding of these drugs is therefore not compromised by endogenous ligands.[124,125] Consequently, the fetus acts as a reservoir for these drugs, and fetal-maternal plasma concentration gradients for VPA (see Figs. 17.5 and 17.6), diazepam, *N*-desmethyl diazepam, and salicylate[124] are significantly higher than unity. Fetal and neonatal distress may be a result of this unexpectedly high total drug load and its partial displacement after birth. Such adverse effects have been observed in neonates of VPA-treated mothers,[126] as well as in neonates and older infants of mothers who received relatively high doses of diazepam *(floppy infant syndrome).*[127–130] This situation may be especially of relevance for the neonate since increased free drug concentrations may persist longer because of the limited drug clearance capacity in the newborn. This effect may be more pronounced in critically ill and preterm neonates, when free fatty acids can increase, and hyperbilirubinemia may further affect binding capacity.[131]

MOLECULAR WEIGHT OF DRUGS

Placental transfer also relates to the MW. Any molecule with a MW of more than 1000 Da rarely crosses the placenta, those with MW of less than 500 Da readily cross, and the remaining cross at a slower rate (2,4). Accordingly, the high MW of erythropoietin (30 to 34 kDa) is believed to be the reason for its poor placental transfer in the placental perfusion model, and similar conclusions are made for example for insulin, heparin, or low-molecular-weight heparins.[22,132,133] Their absence of placental transfer is commonly used when considering options for maternal pharmacotherapy while avoiding fetal exposure.

The potential clinical relevance can be illustrated by the currently used "low MW" oral hypoglycemic agents, when assessed for their maternal-fetal transport. Using the ex vivo single-cotyledon human placenta model. Glyburide (MW 494 Da) did not cross the human placenta in significant amounts. The glyburide-antipyrine transport ratio was much lower than

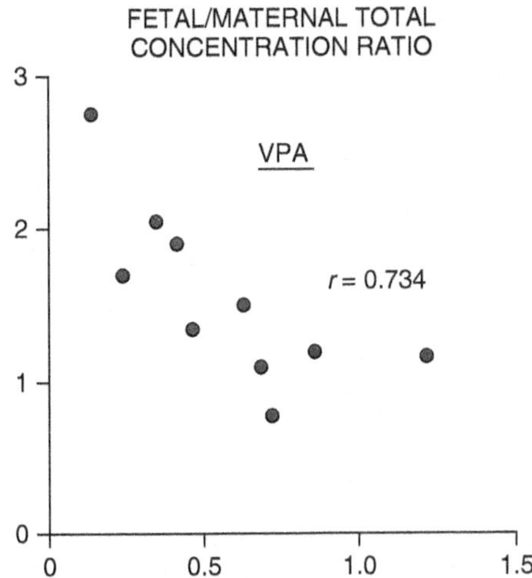

Fig. 17.5 Correlation between valproic acid *(VPA)* total concentration ratio of cord serum to maternal serum at birth and VPA free fraction ratio of cord serum to maternal serum. Accumulation of VPA in the fetus correlates with low free fraction (high protein binding) of this drug in the fetus compared with the mother. (From Nau H, Helge H, Luck W. Valproic acid in the perinatal period: decreased maternal serum protein binding results in fetal accumulation and neonatal displacement of the drug and some metabolites. *J Pediatr.* 1984;104:627.)

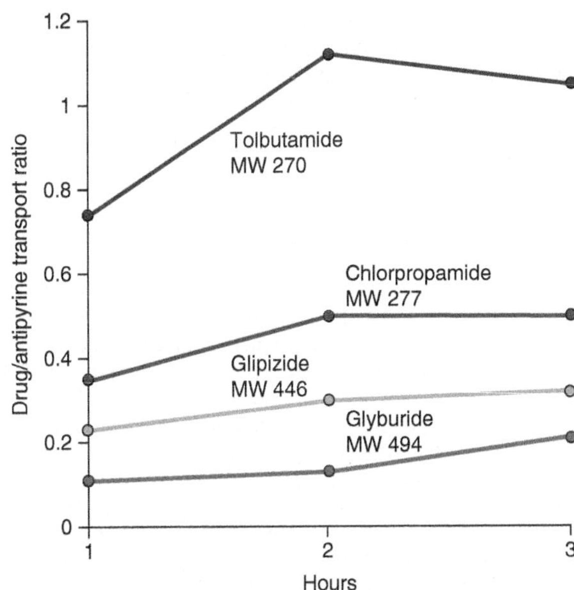

Fig. 17.6 Human placental drug transport for four different oral hypoglycemic agents with different molecular weights *(MWs),* with the drug/antipyrine transport ratio as observed at 1, 2, and 3 hours for 4 different oral hypoglycemic agents compared with the freely diffusible antipyrine (MW= 188, ratio = 1). (Data collected using the single cotyledon human placenta technique as reported by Elliott BD, Schenker S, Langer O, et al. Comparative placental transport of oral hypoglycemic agents in humans: a model of human placental drug transfer. *Am J Obstet Gynecol.* 1994;171:653.)

the tolbutamide-antipyrine transport ratio (see Fig. 17.6).[134] The investigators found a highly significant relationship between the mean drug antipyrine transport ratios obtained in their experiment (tolbutamide MW 270 Da < chlorpropamide MW 277 Da < glipizide MW 446 Da, and < glyburide MW 494 Da) and the independent variables (MW, log partition coefficient, and selected dissociation constants [$R^2 = 0.91$; $P = .0001$]). This relationship was described by the following Equation (17.6):

$$T^d/T^a = -4.90 + 0.5\log\left(P^d\right) + 1.26\,pK_a - 0.0073\,MW^d \qquad [17.6]$$

where T^d = placental transport of the drug, T^a = placental transport of antipyrine, and MW^d = MW of the drug.

The MW is the most important variable in this regression ($F = 61, 75$; $P < .001$) and determined the cumulative percentage of transport of the drugs tested.[134] Neither the log partition coefficient nor the dissociation constant individually provided significant associations by simple regression with either the drug-antipyrine ratio or the cumulative percentage of transport of these drugs. Furthermore, the high plasma protein binding of glyburide (99%) did not account for this finding, as discussed by Koren.[135] However, more recently, the same group reported on in vivo paired maternal/umbilical cord blood samples at delivery in women with gestational diabetes mellitus, treated with glyburide. The mean maternal serum glyburide level at birth was 15.4 ng/mL, and the mean umbilical cord level was 7.5 ng/mL (fetal/maternal ratio = 0.49). However, extensive variability was observed, only partly explained by the maternal glyburide concentration.[136] To further illustrate the clinical relevance of placental transfer, we refer to a case report on fetal macrosomia and neonatal hyperinsulinemic hypoglycemia associated with transplacental transfer of this sulfonylurea (high-dose glyburide, 85 mg/day) in a mother with neonatal diabetes.[137]

In vitro heparin does not cross the human term placenta.[138] No biologic activity and very low fractions of radioactivity used for labeling were found in the fetal circulation in the human perfused placental cotyledon model for unfractionated heparin, low-molecular-weight heparin, and dermatan sulfate.[139] These data are in line with in vivo observations in newborns whose mothers had been treated with unfractionated heparin or low-molecular-weight heparin.[140,141]

STEREOSELECTIVITY

Stereoselectivity refers to enantiomers, meaning that their chemical structure and physical characteristics are identical, but their mirror images are nonsuperimposable. Generally speaking, R- and S-enantiomers are different substances, and in most cases the two enantiomers have different PK. This has also been reported for PK during pregnancy (ketorolac, omeprazole, vigabatrin) with enantiomer specific PK effects of pregnancy.[8] Along this line, it is also to be anticipated that placental transfer also displays stereoselective transport patterns. Stereoselective placental transport has been described for endogenous compounds (e.g., amino acids), drugs (e.g., ketotifen, vigabatrin, fluoxetine), or pollutants. Stereoselectivity is most commonly explained by differences in affinity for protein binding or receptor binding.

Amino acids circulating in the maternal plasma are the primary source for fetal protein synthesis, but also contribute to fetal energy supply. Amino acids are transferred across the placenta against a concentration gradient by active, stereospecific placental transport, which functions unidirectionally from the maternal to fetal side.[142-144]

The chiral nonsteroidal antiinflammatory drug ketotifen is transferred to the fetus with S/R plasma concentrations averaging 2.3 in premature neonates exposed to a racemic formulation of ketoprofen as tocolytic, while maternal S-R plasma concentrations are close to 1. Because the R(−)-enantiomer does not undergo substantial metabolism in humans, another mechanism has to account for this. It appears that stereoselective protein binding results in a higher “free” S(+)-ketotifen concentration with subsequently more effective transfer across the placenta (compared with R(−)-ketotifen).[145] Placental transfer of the water-soluble antiepileptic drug vigabatrin (MW 129) is low and occurs by simple diffusion. In a human case report, however, a slight difference was found between the kinetics of both enantiomers.[146] Significant fluoxetine stereoselectivity with S/R mean AUC ratios averaging 1.65 and 1.73 in ewe and fetus, respectively, after maternal dosing were documented. The authors hereby provided arguments that this is likely due to differential plasma protein binding of the fluoxetine isomers in both the maternal and fetal compartments.[147] Pharmacokinetics and transplacental transfer of fluoxetine enantiomers have more recently been described in the third trimester of pregnancy, and provided evidence on a pregnancy-related effect on its metabolism and placental transfer (predominant transfer of the S-enantiomer).[148]

The placental transport of retinol and related substances (retinoids) is highly structure-specific. Although in the mouse, rat, and rabbit, retinoids with a free carboxyl group in the 13-*cis* configuration are only poorly transferred early in pregnancy,[149-155] a significant increase in transfer has been demonstrated for later gestational periods in the mouse and rat.[101] The β-glucuronide conjugates also show very limited placental transfer (in mouse, rat, rabbit, or monkey).[156] The placental transfer of all-*trans*-retinoic acid (in rat) and all-*trans*-4-oxoretinoic acid (in rabbit) are efficient.[101,156,157] The high affinity of retinoids with the all-*trans* configuration for certain plasma and embryonic cellular binding proteins may be the reason for the efficient transport of these compounds. Binding to plasma albumin cannot explain these differences in transport, because all retinoids with free carboxyl groups bind avidly to albumin and other plasma macromolecules. The increase in glucuronide transfer in later gestational periods may result from the change in the rodent placental structure from a choriovitelline to a chorioallantoic placenta. In the cynomolgus monkey, a relatively efficient transport for 13-*cis*-retinoic acid has been observed once the chorioallantoic placenta has been fully established.[158] This placenta type is functional at earlier developmental stages in the monkey (and presumably in the human) than in the rodent species. This timing may explain the efficient placental transfer and high teratogenicity of 13-*cis*-retinoic acid when it is administered during early primate organogenesis. Enantiomeric ratios were used as indicators of the extent of exposure to dichlorodiphenyltrichloroethane (DDT) and similar pollutants in human placenta, with enantiomer ratios closer to 1 at higher concentrations, reflecting higher exposure.[159]

SELECTIVE TRANSFER MECHANISMS: FACILITATED TRANSFER, ACTIVE TRANSPORT, AND PLACENTAL DRUG METABOLISM

In addition to passive, non-energy taking transport processes, there are a lot of more selective, facilitated placental transfer mechanisms. These include drug transport (facilitated diffusion, active transporters, pinocytosis) mechanisms and drug metabolism[e] These active transport mechanisms can be of relevance for drugs but are obviously also of great importance to transfer endogenous compounds and nutrients, such as amino acids, acetylcholine, vitamin B_{12}, vitamin H (biotin), creatine, and ions such as sodium, potassium, calcium, magnesium, and iron or folate.[160,161]

A folate receptor in the placenta may play a crucial role in the transfer of folate to the fetus.[162] Retinol (vitamin A) is transported to the embryo or fetus at least in part bound to retinol-binding protein.[163-165] This transport mechanism appears to be especially important during early gestation because the early embryo is not able to synthesize its own binding protein.[166] In addition, lipoproteins, as well as retinol-binding protein present in large amounts in the yolk sac, may play a role in placental transport of retinol.[164,165] Water-soluble vitamins are present in higher concentrations in fetal blood than in maternal blood. The most extensive data are available for vitamin B_{12}, a polar molecule of high MW (1355 Da) that is not expected to transfer by simple diffusion. A receptor-mediated endocytosis process has been identified as a carrier mechanism for this compound.[167] In the rabbit placenta, maternal iron is concentrated by a facilitated process as an iron-transferrin complex. This step is followed by a release of iron into the placental cells and return of the apoprotein to the maternal circulation.

The placental transfer of polypeptides is extremely limited, as has been demonstrated for thyroid hormones, growth hormone, corticotropin, chorionic gonadotropin, erythropoietin, oxytocin, interferon, placental lactogen, or protein C.[33,168-172] Maternal hormones therefore cannot simply influence the development of fetal organ systems when the fetus is deficient in synthesis of its own hormones. Although not absolute, this means that the fetal endocrine systems function to a certain extent autonomous and disconnected from the maternal system.[33] Proteins, like insulin complexed to antibodies, however, can be transferred to the fetus.[173] As the transport of insulin-antibody complexes suggests, proteins are transferred from the pregnant woman to her fetus to some extent.[174-176] However, considerable selectivity has been observed in the placental transport of proteins. While polypeptides do not enter the fetal circulation to a significant extent, much larger macromolecules, such as γ-globulins (immunoglobulin G [IgG]), are transported. Relatively small fragments of IgG (with MWs of 20,000 to 50,000) are poorly transported compared with larger fragments (with MWs of 50,000 to 82,000) and intact IgG.[177] Therefore binding of IgG is high, resulting in relatively extensive transport of this protein as compared with other proteins such as albumin, transferrin, IgE, IgM, IgA, insulin, and growth hormone, all of which pass the placental membranes to a much lower extent.[175] The process by which antibodies are transported across the placenta appears to be highly selective, and better understanding becomes more relevant in the era of monoclonal antibodies to treat a variety of diseases.

FACILITATED TRANSPORT

This transport mechanism is rather similar to the earlier discussed passive) diffusion as the transport depends on the existing concentration gradient and does not require energy, but a carrier.[178] In essence, these transporters facilitate transfer of nonlipid-soluble compounds *down* the concentration gradient. Similar to the earlier described relevant factors to passive diffusion, this mechanism is also affected by (non) competitive inhibition, stereoselectivity, or other physiologic aspects like uterine blood flow or placental area. The "solute carrier family" is the most commonly studied family of placental transporters and include organic anion transporters, organic anion transporting polypeptides, organic cation transporters, multidrug and toxin extruding protein 1, and nucleoside transporters.[4,26] Ganciclovir utilizes this mechanism by entering the basolateral side (maternal) into the syncytiotrophoblast to subsequently undergo passive diffusion to reach the fetal circulation.[178] Studies showed the presence of carrier proteins for cephalexin and glucocorticoids. Other compounds that resemble endogenous substances are assumed to be transported by this mechanism as well.[f]

ACTIVE TRANSPORT

Primary active transport is an energy-consuming, ATP-binding cassette (ABC) process potentially against a concentration gradient while a secondary active transport utilizes the energy

[e]References 2, 5, 9, 16, 20, 32-34.

[f]References 2, 5, 9, 16, 20, 32-34.

stored in the electrochemical gradient of a co-transported ion. These transporters have a pivotal role in the exchange of nutrients and waste products from mother to fetus and from fetus to mother respectively.[f] These include P-glycoprotein (P-gp), multidrug resistance proteins (MRPs), and breast cancer resistance protein (BCRP).

The expression and activity of drug transporter proteins in the placenta varies throughout gestation and can be affected by pathophysiologic events, while polymorphisms may also be relevant.[f] However, this variation is not uniform. Based on mRNA expression patterns of 50 ABC proteins in placental samples in the first and third trimester of normal pregnancies, Imperio and colleagues described different trends, either showing increased mRNA expression (ABCA1, ABCA6, ABCA9, ABCC3), or decreased expression (ABCB11, ABCG4) between these trimesters.[179]

P-glycoprotein (P-gp) is mainly retrieved at the apical side facing the maternal circulation, so that its efflux function results in transfer of hydrophobic cations from fetus to mother. P-gp protein expression is twice as high in early pregnancy compared with term pregnancy.[180] In addition to gestational age, other clinical characteristics affecting phenotypic drug transporter activity and subsequent clinical effects include maternal bacterial infection,[181] pharmacogenetics,[166,182] antenatal glucocorticoid therapy,[183] or growth restriction.[183]

To further illustrate its clinical relevance, P-gp-mediated drug interactions were associated with an increased risk of specific anomalies, suggesting that drug-drug interactions at the level of the P-gp transporter (e.g., maternal co-exposure to a P-gp inhibitor) are also of relevance.[184] In the human placenta, the transfer of drugs like vinblastine,[185] vincristine,[185] cyclosporine,[186] and digoxin,[185,187] appears to be regulated by P-gp, presumably protecting the fetus from toxic substances, driven by the efflux transporter mechanisms.[185] Variability in placental opiate transport—including P-gp polymorphisms—is one of the determinants of fetal opiate exposure and subsequent (incidence, severity) neonatal abstinence syndrome.[182] Another study suggests that dexamethasone is actively transported across the placenta. In experimental animals (rat, sheep), fetal levels of dexamethasone are much lower than corresponding maternal values, even after prolonged treatment.[188] This low fetal-maternal concentration ratio also has been observed after fetal administration of dexamethasone, while placental clearance of dexamethasone from fetus to mother is 8.5 times higher than in the reverse direction.[189] The fetal-maternal concentration gradient of betamethasone is also low in humans.[190]

The *multidrug resistance proteins (MRPs)* family plays an essential role in regulating the active transport of substrates in the placenta, with specific emphasis on unconjugated, amphiphilic anions and conjugated lipophilic compounds (glutathione, glucuronate, and sulfate). MRP3 is the most expressed MRP transporter in the placenta and is essential in transport from fetus to mother. Other MRPs are observed on the apical membrane, basolateral membrane, or on fetal endothelial cells.[g] Apical and basolateral localization of MRPs likely reflect a role in transport from fetuses to the mother and from mother to fetus, respectively, like removal of bilirubin from fetus to mother. Several drugs serve as substrates for this transporter family, including anticancer drugs (methotrexate, etoposide, vinca alkaloids, platinum-based compounds), HIV protease inhibitors, acetaminophen, or antibacterial agents, like ampicillin.[1]

Breast cancer resistance proteins display their ATP-dependent transporter activity at the apical side of the syncytiotrophoblast and the fetal endothelial cells, thus have a relevant efflux role.[1,4,5] Among all tissues, BRCP is highest in placental tissue, making it a target for fetal-maternal research. Real time polymerase chain reaction (PCR) analysis

[g]References 2, 5, 9, 16, 20, 32-34.

demonstrated that placental mRNA levels of BCRP remain stable throughout pregnancy, while protein levels increase towards the end of gestation.[191] BCRP is involved in the efflux transport of anticancer drugs (methotrexate, doxorubicin, daunorubicin, mitoxantrone, topotecan, irinotecan), antiretroviral (zidovudine, lamivudine), glyburide, nitrofurantoin, and cimetidine.[1]

Pinocytosis, endocytosis, and exocytosis are receptor-mediated, endocytosis driven processes that facilitate large molecules transfer, like (endogenous) immunoglobulins, or exogenous monoclonal antibodies across the placenta.[5] Particularly, IgG or IgG-based antibodies bind with high affinity to the Fc receptors in the acidic environment (approximately pH 6) of the endosome, with transfer across the trophoblastic layers to be subsequently released into the fetal circulation. These mechanisms of placental transfer are becoming more relevant because of newly emerging treatment approaches, like therapeutic monoclonal antibodies, nano-formulations, or indirect maternal vaccinations to protect against infections in early infancy (RSV, pertussis). However, because of the very effective transport mechanisms, the levels of therapeutic antibodies [infliximab (1.6 factor; adalimumab [1.5 factor)] in umbilical cord blood can even be higher than in the mother at delivery while PEGylation of monoclonal antibodies, like certolizumab, will reduce (0.03 factor) placental transfer (see Fig. 17.2, ***pattern C*** or ***D***).[192] Megalin is another endocytic receptor, well known for reabsorption of aminoglycosides at the level of the renal tubular cell. In a human choriocarcinoma cell line, the expression of megalin was quantified and linked to aminoglycoside uptake.[193]

PLACENTAL DRUG METABOLISM

The placenta can also exert a considerable first-pass metabolism effect. The different enzymatic processes, including phase I (e.g., oxidation, reduction, hydrolysis) and phase II (e.g., glucuronidation, acetylation, sulfation, glutathione-S-transferase), have been documented in the placenta or fetus, indicating that drugs can be metabolized in the fetal-placental compartment. Their expression and activity vary with gestational age. To further illustrate this, mRNA levels were expressed in the placental tissue harvested in the first trimester for CYP1A1, 1A2, 2C, 2D6, 2E1, 2F1, 3A4, 3A5, 3A7, and 4B1, whereas at full term CYP1A1, 2E1, 2F1, 3A3/4, 3A5, and 3A7 mRNA levels were found.[2] Besides gestational age, there are arguments to postulate the impact of other covariates, such as genetic polymorphisms or drug-drug interactions.[h]

OUTLOOK: HOW TO TRANSLATE KNOWLEDGE ON PLACENTAL PHYSIOLOGY TO SUPPORT CLINICAL CARE PRACTICES

Drugs are usually given to pregnant women to treat the mother but may be used to manage pathologic conditions of the fetus (cardiac contractility or rhythm, perinatal infections, lung maturation) or the placenta (sildenafil). Awareness of the principles that govern maternal-fetal pharmacokinetics can hereby tailor our practices to either minimize unnecessary exposure of the fetus to drugs or alternatively, optimize drug delivery to the fetus or placenta.[h]

As discussed in this chapter, placental passage of drugs varies extensively, between compounds as well as throughout the different stages of pregnancy. In a group of drugs with similar pharmacodynamic properties, comparison of lipid solubility, protein binding, ionization, or MW may support clinical decisions on compound selection. This explains why heparin or low-molecular-weight heparins are used instead of warfarin during pregnancy, or why beta- or dexamethasone

[h]References 2, 5, 9, 16, 20, 32-34.

are administered for fetal lung maturation. Oral hypoglycemic agents and biologically active insulin-antibody complexes cross the placental barrier, whereupon they can induce harmful fetal effects such as macrosomia. Newer oral hypoglycemic agents (characterized by a higher MW) only pass the placenta in limited amounts.[134-137] Nanoparticle-mediated targeted drug delivery in pregnancy may be a very novel technique for selective targeting, with minimal risk of off-target effects.[194] A successful reduction in placental transfer of the cytostatic drug cisplatin was achieved by coupling the drug to glycocholic acid.[195] This indicates the possibility of treating certain maternal tumors during pregnancy with a lower risk to the fetus. Liposome encapsulation of VPA reduced placental transfer in the perfused placenta model by 30%, and microencapsulation of chloramphenicol reduced maternal transfer by 85%.[196] To treat intrauterine infection, broad-spectrum antibiotics that cross the placenta and concentrate in the fetus (e.g., the lipophilic ceftizoxime) are desirable.[197,198] In contrast, if only maternal treatment is aimed for, antibiotics with relatively limited placental transfer, such as macrolides, are favored. Another example is treatment for toxoplasmosis. In early pregnancy, spiramycin is preferred because it barely crosses the placenta, where it accumulates.[58] Later, however, when treatment of the fetus is necessary, pyrimethamine is used, because it is efficiently transferred to the fetus. The potential advantage of buprenorphine, because of its placental sequestration on the incidence of neonatal abstinence syndrome, has already been mentioned.[63,182]

Understanding the mechanisms related to placental transport and metabolism is paramount as more pregnant women are receiving medical therapy throughout their pregnancy. Knowledge on these mechanisms should empower clinicians to tailor pharmacotherapy for maternal medical conditions and minimize fetal exposure. In addition, dosing adjustments to some medications can be made to treat fetal conditions and minimize maternal toxicity. Adding to this complexity is the fact that maternal (pregnancy-related) diseases can also contribute to changes in transport expression and may alter physiologic processes.[1]

Data from these experiments can subsequently be leveraged into a mechanistic modeling framework to have impact on our clinical care practices. At best, this understanding should result in predictions, based on the integration of the available pieces (in vivo, in vitro, animal experimental) of information. Integration of the different pieces of information (the *system pharmacology approach, PBPK*) is the way forward to secure further progress. Quantitative pharmacologic tools and PBPK models will provide the framework to facilitate this integration and subsequently test its robustness by comparing predictions to in vivo observations.[i] Table 17.2 hereby serves as an illustration of the progresses made in this field during recent years.

 A complete reference list is available at www.ExpertConsult.com.

SELECT REFERENCES

1. Dallmann A, Liu XI, Burckart GJ, van den Anker J. Drug transporters expressed in the human placenta and models for studying maternal-fetal drug transfer. *J Clin Pharmacol.* 2019;59(suppl 1):S70.
2. Bouazza N, Foissac F, Hirt D, et al. Methodological approaches to evaluate fetal drug exposure. *Curr Pharm Des.* 2019;25:496.
3. Kazma JM, van den Anker J, Allegaert K, et al. Anatomical and physiological alterations of pregnancy. *J Pharmacokinet Pharmacodyn.* 2020;47:271-285.
4. Liu L, Liu X. Contributions of drug transporters to blood-placental barrier. *Adv Exp Med Biol.* 2019;1141:505.
5. Tetro N, Moushaev S, Rubinchik-Stern M, Eyal S. The placental barrier: the gate and the fate in drug distribution. *Pharm Res.* 2018;35:71.
6. Roca C, Sahin L, Yao L. Collaboration in regulatory science to facilitate therapeutic development for pregnant women. *Curr Pharm Des.* 2019;25:609.
7. Van Calsteren K, Gersak K, Sundseth H, et al. Position statement from the European Board and College of Obstetrics & Gynaecology (EBCOG): the use of medicines during pregnancy – call for action. *Eur J Obstet Gynecol Reprod Biol.* 2016;201:89.
8. Dallmann A, Mian P, Van den Anker J, Allegaert K. Clinical pharmacokinetic studies in pregnant women and the relevance of pharmacometric tools. *Curr Pharm Des.* 2019;25:483.
13. Gundling Jr WE, Wildman DE. A review of inter- and intraspecific variation in the eutherian placenta. *Philos Trans R Soc Lond B Biol Sci.* 2015;370(1663):20140072.
16. Zhang Z, Imperial MZ, Patilea-Vrana GI, et al. Development of a novel maternal-fetal physiologically based pharmacokinetic model I: insights into factors that determine fetal drug exposure through simulations and sensitivity analyses. *Drug Metab Dispos.* 2017;45:920.
17. Zhang Z, Unadkat JD. Development of a novel maternal-fetal physiologically based pharmacokinetic model II: verification of the model for passive placental permeability drugs. *Drug Metab Dispos.* 2017;45:939.
19. Pemathilaka RL, Reynolds DE, Hashemi NN. Drug transport across the human placenta: review of placenta-on-a-chip and previous approaches. *Interface Focus.* 2019;9:20190031.
21. Van Hasselt JG, Green B, Morrish GA. Leveraging physiological data from literature into a pharmacokinetic model to support informative clinical study design in pregnant women. *Pharm Res.* 2012;29:1609.
22. Hutson JR, Garcia-Bournissen F, Davis A, et al. The human placental perfusion model: a systematic review and development of a model to predict in vivo transfer of therapeutic drugs. *Clin Pharmacol Ther.* 2011;90:67.
23. Russo FM, Conings S, Allegaert K, et al. Sildenafil crosses the placenta at therapeutic levels in a dually perfused human cotyledon model. *Am J Obstet Gynecol.* 2018;219:e1-619.e10.
24. Freriksen JJM, Feyaerts D, van den Broek PHH, et al. Placental disposition of the immunosuppressive drug tacrolimus in renal transplant recipients and in ex vivo perfused placental tissue. *Eur J Pharm Sci.* 2018;119:244.
25. Hitzerd E, Broekhuizen M, Mirabito Colafella KM, et al. Placental effects and transfer of sildenafil in healthy and preeclamptic conditions. *EBioMedicine.* 2019;45:447.
26. Liu X, Momper JD, Rakhmanina N, et al. Physiologically based pharmacokinetic models to predict maternal pharmacokinetics and fetal exposure to emtricitabine and acyclovir. *J Clin Pharmacol.* 2020;60:240.
27. Mian P, Allegaert K, Conings S, et al. Integration of placental transfer in a fetal-maternal physiologically based pharmacokinetic model to characterize acetaminophen exposure and metabolic clearance in the fetus. *Clin Pharmacokinet.* 2020;59:911-925.
28. Freriksen JJM, Schalkwijk S, Colbers AP, et al. Assessment of maternal and fetal dolutegravir exposure by integrating ex vivo placental perfusion data and physiologically-based pharmacokinetic modeling. *Clin Pharmacol Ther.* 2019;107:1352-1361.
29. Atoyebi SA, Rajoli RKR, Adejuyigbe E, et al. Using mechanistic physiologically-based pharmacokinetic models to assess prenatal drug exposure: thalidomide versus efavirenz as case studies. *Eur J Pharm Sci.* 2019;140:105068.
30. De Sousa Mendes M, Lui G, Zheng Y, et al. A physiologically-based pharmacokinetic model to predict human fetal exposure for a drug metabolized by several CYP450 pathways. *Clin Pharmacokinet.* 2017;56:537.
31. De Sousa Mendes M, Hirt D, Vinot C, et al. Prediction of human fetal pharmacokinetics using ex vivo human placenta perfusion studies and physiologically based models. *Br J Clin Pharmacol.* 2016;81:646.
32. Al-Enazy S, Ali S, Albekairi N, et al. Placental control of drug delivery. *Adv Drug Deliv Rev.* 2017;116:63.
39. Sánchez-Alcaraz A, Quintana MB, Laguarda M. Placental transfer and neonatal effects of propofol in caesarean section. *J Clin Pharm Ther.* 1998;23:19.
40. Sherwin CM, Ngamprasertwong P, Sadhasivam S, et al. Utilization of optimal study design for maternal and fetal sheep propofol pharmacokinetics study: a preliminary study. *Curr Clin Pharmacol.* 2014;9:64.
41. Sato M, Masui K, Sarentonglaga B, et al. Influence of maternal remifentanil concentration on fetal-to-maternal ratio in pregnant ewes. *J Anesth.* 2017;31:517.
42. Schenker S, Yang Y, Johnson RF, et al. The transfer of cocaine and its metabolites across the term human placenta. *Clin Pharmacol Ther.* 1993;53:329.
51. Hodel EM, Marzolini C, Waitt C, Rakhmanina N. Pharmacokinetics, placental and breast milk transfer of antiretroviral drugs in pregnant and lactating women living with HIV. *Curr Pharm Des.* 2019;25:556.
53. Tuntland T, Odinecs A, Pereira CM, et al. In vitro models to predict the in vivo mechanism, rate and extent of placental transfer of dideoxynucleoside drugs against human immunodeficiency virus. *Am J Obstet Gynecol.* 1999;180:198.
57. Bourget P, Fernandez H, Bismuth H, Papiernik E. Transplacental passage of cyclosporine after liver transplantation. *Transplantation.* 1990;49:663.
60. Jans G, Guelinckx I, Voets W, et al. Vitamin K1 monitoring in pregnancies after bariatric surgery: a prospective cohort study. *Surg Obes Relat Dis.* 2014;10:885.
61. Ngamprasertwong P, Dong M, Niu J, et al. Propofol pharmacokinetics and estimation of fetal propofol exposure during mid-gestational fetal surgery: a maternal-fetal sheep model. *PLoS One.* 2016;2016:e0146563.
62. Giroux M, Teixera MG, Dumas JC, et al. Influence of maternal blood flow on the placental transfer of three opioids—fentanyl, alfentanil, sufentanil. *Biol Neonate.* 1997;72:133.
63. Coulson CC, Lorencz E, Rittenhouse K, et al. Association of maternal buprenorphine or methadone with fetal growth indices and neonatal abstinence syndrome. *Am J Perinatol.* 2019;37:28-36.

[i] References 2, 5, 9, 16, 20, 32-34.

79. Fowler DW, Eadie MJ, Dickinson RG. Transplacental transfer and biotransformation studies of valproic acid and its glucuronide(s) in the perfused human placenta. *J Pharmacol Exp Ther*. 1989;24:318.
89. Ueki R, Tatara T, Kariya N, et al. Comparison of placental transfer of local anesthetics in perfusates with different pH values in a human cotyledon model. *J Anesth*. 2009;23:526.
100. Nau H, Scott Jr WJ. Weak acids may act as teratogens by accumulating in the basic milieu of the early mammalian embryo. *Nature*. 1986;323:276.
105. Dancis J, Jansen V, Levitz M. Placental transfer of steroids: effect of binding to serum albumin and to placenta. *Am J Physiol*. 1980;238:E208.
107. Krauer B, Dayer P, Anner R. Changes in serum albumin and α_1-acid glyco-protein concentrations during pregnancy: an analysis of fetal-maternal pairs. *Br J Obstet Gynaecol*. 1984;91:875.
134. Elliott BD, Schenker S, Langer O, et al. Comparative placental transport of oral hypoglycemic agents in humans: a model of human placental drug transfer. *Am J Obstet Gynecol*. 1994;171:653.
138. Simone C, et al. Transfer of heparin across the human term placenta. *Clin Invest Med*. 1995;18:B18.
148. Carvalho DM, Lanchote VL, Filgueira GCO, et al. Pharmacokinetics and transplacental transfer of fluoxetine enantiomers and their metabolites in pregnant women. *Clin Pharmacol Ther*. 2019;105:1003.
158. Hummler H, Hendrickx AG, Nau H. Maternal pharmacokinetics, metabolism, and embryo exposure following a teratogenic dosing regimen with 13- *cis*-retinoic acid (isotretinoin) in the cynomolgus monkey. *Teratology*. 1994;50:184.
166. Daud AN, Bergman JE, Bakker MK, et al. Pharmacogenetics of drug-induced birth defects: the role of polymorphisms of placental transporter proteins. *Pharmacogenomics*. 2014;15:1029.
182. Lewis T, Dinh J, Leeder JS. Genetic determinants of fetal opiate exposure and risk of neonatal abstinence syndrome: knowledge deficits and prospects for future research. *Clin Pharmacol Ther*. 2015;98:309.
183. Hodyl NA, Stark MJ, Butler M, et al. Placental P-glycoprotein is unaffected by timing of antenatal glucocorticoid therapy but reduced in SGA preterm infants. *Placenta*. 2013;34:325.
191. Yeboah D, Sun M, Kingdom J, et al. Expression of breast cancer resistance protein (BCRP/ABCG2) in human placenta throughout gestation and at term before and after labor. *Can J Physiol Pharmacol*. 2006;84:1251.
192. Tun GS, Lobo AJ. Evaluation of pharmacokinetics and pharmacodynamics and clinical efficacy of certolizumab pegol for Crohn's disease. *Expert Opin Drug Metab Toxicol*. 2015;11:317.
194. Keelan JA, Leong JW, Ho D, et al. Therapeutic and safety considerations of nanoparticle-mediated drug delivery in pregnancy. *Nanomedicine*. 2015;10:2229.

Pharmacogenomics

Laura B. Ramsey | Tomoyuki Mizuno | Alexander A. Vinks

INTRODUCTION

Pharmacogenetic variants are DNA variants that influence the metabolism and elimination or the action of medications. Research in pharmacogenetics seeks to understand how these variants influence variability in medication response. For the perinatal pharmacologist, genetic variations that affect drug disposition in the fetus, the mother, and the neonate must be considered as one of many sets of variables, along with developmental changes in fetal and neonatal gene expression,[1] organ maturation, placental transfer and metabolism of drugs, and a host of hormonal and environmental influences, which can combine to produce unique patterns of toxicity in mother and child upon medication exposure. Therefore knowledge of potential genetic contributions to drug-induced toxicity in pregnancy, in utero, and in postnatal life can be important in optimizing dosing of drugs,[2] as well as in understanding adverse drug reactions (ADRs) and preventing their further occurrence in patients.[3]

The field of pharmacogenomics is rapidly expanding, and the number of medications with genetic information in the drug label is increasing. Several actionable gene-drug pairs have been clinically implemented in hospitals across the world. Most pharmacogenetic research has been performed in adults, but many of the associations also could apply to children and neonates that are prescribed the same medications.

There are several resources that provide guidance on pharmacogenetic research and implementation. The first step in pharmacogenetics is defining the variants that influence the medication absorption, distribution, metabolism, elimination, or response. The Pharmacogene Variation Consortium (PharmVar.org) is a repository of pharmacogene variation that focuses on haplotype structure and allelic variation.[4] Pharmacogenetic alleles can contain one or more variants, and sometimes individual variants are included in the definition of more than one allele. Thus, it is very important to have a common terminology for allele nomenclature, which PharmVar provides. The Pharmacogenomics Knowledge Base (PharmGKB.org) is an NIH-funded resource that curates pharmacogenetic literature, including in vitro and in vivo knowledge from medication labels, clinical trials, clinical research, and basic research.[5] Every gene-drug pair in the literature is given a level of evidence based on the association of individual variants with clinical and/or in vitro data.[6] The Clinical Pharmacogenetics Implementation Consortium (CPIC, cpicpgx.org) is a group that publishes evidence-based clinical practice guidelines, facilitating the implementation of pharmacogenetics into clinical care.[7] Currently, there are 23 guidelines that impact 49 medications and involve 18 genes (Table 18.1). CPIC utilizes standard nomenclature for allele functionality and activity[8] and provides guidance on electronic health record integration of pharmacogenetic results.[9]

Most individuals have at least one pharmacogenetic variant but may not receive the medication whose dosing would be informed by that variant.[10,11] This chapter provides an overview and examples of some selected pharmacogenes that influence the pharmacokinetics, pharmacodynamics, and severe adverse reactions to drugs; where possible, these examples were chosen to provide particular relevance to medication use in children.

PHARMACOGENETIC VARIANTS AFFECTING DRUG METABOLISM

The most well-established pharmacogenes are those encoding drug-metabolizing enzymes; variants in these genes affect the exposure by altering the rate of metabolism of the drugs. For example, slow metabolism of a pro-drug would result in decreased exposure to the active metabolite and the potential for inefficacy, but slow metabolism of an active drug into an inactive compound would result in increased exposure to the active drug and the potential for toxicity. The opposite is true for faster metabolism due to genetic variants. For pharmacogenes that influence pharmacokinetics, often the recommendations

Table 18.1 Clinical Pharmacogenetics Implementation Consortium Dosing Guidelines.

Drug	Gene(s)	Guideline	References
Abacavir	*HLA-B*	Do not use in patients with the *HLA-B*57:01* allele	31
Allopurinol	*HLA-B*	Do not use in patients with the *HLA-B*58:01* allele	57, 58
Amitriptyline	*CYP2D6, CYP2C19*	Do not use in CYP2D6 PMs or CYP2D6/CYP2C19 UMs; use 50% lower dose in CYP2C19 PMs	59, 60
Atazanavir	*UGT1A1*	Do not use in PMs	21
Atomoxetine	*CYP2D6*	Use reduced doses in IMs and PMs	61
Azathioprine	*TPMT, NUDT15*	Extreme dose reduction in TPMT or NUDT15 PMs; reduce dose in TPMT or NUDT15 IMs.	18, 62, 63
Capecitabine	*DPYD*	Do not use in homozygous DPYD-deficient patients; use 50% of target dose in heterozygotes	64
Carbamazepine	*HLA-B, HLA-A*	Do not use in carbamazepine-naïve patients with at least one *HLA-B*15:02* or *HLA-A*31:01* allele	65, 66
Citalopram	*CYP2C19*	Do not use in CYP2C19 UMs; reduce starting dose by 50% in PMs	67
Clomipramine	*CYP2D6, CYP2C19*	Do not use in CYP2D6 PMs or CYP2D6/CYP2C19 UMs; use 50% lower dose in CYP2C19 PMs	59, 60
Clopidogrel	*CYP2C19*	Use alternative antiplatelet drugs in CYP2C19 PMs or heterozygotes	68, 69
Codeine	*CYP2D6*	Do not use in CYP2D6 UMs or PMs	13, 70
Desflurane	*RYR1, CACNA1S*	Do not use in patients with risk variants for malignant hyperthermia	71
Desipramine	*CYP2D6*	Do not use in CYP2D6 UMs or PMs; consider a 25% dose reduction in heterozygotes	59, 60
Doxepin	*CYP2D6, CYP2C19*	Do not use in CYP2D6 PMs or CYP2D6/CYP2C19 UMs; use 50% lower dose in CYP2C19 PMs	59, 60
Efavirenz	*CYP2B6*	Decrease dose in CYP2B6 IMs and PMs	72
Enflurane	*RYR1, CACNA1S*	Do not use in patients with risk variants for malignant hyperthermia	71
Escitalopram	*CYP2C19*	Do not use in CYP2C19 UMs; reduce starting dose by 50% in PMs	67
5-Fluorouracil	*DPYD*	Do not use in homozygous DPYD-deficient patients; use 50% of target dose in heterozygotes	64
Fluvoxamine	*CYP2D6*	Reduce starting dose by 25%–50% in CYP2D6 PMs	67
Halothane	*RYR1, CACNA1S*	Do not use in patients with risk variants for malignant hyperthermia	71
Imipramine	*CYP2D6, CYP2C19*	Do not use in CYP2D6 PMs or CYP2D6/CYP2C19 UMs; use 50% lower dose in CYP2C19 PMs	59, 60
Isoflurane	*RYR1, CACNA1S*	Do not use in patients with risk variants for malignant hyperthermia	71
Ivacaftor	*CFTR*	Use only in patients with at least one indicated CFTR variant	73
6-Mercaptopurine	*TPMT, NUDT15*	Extreme dose reduction in TPMT or NUDT15 PMs; reduce dose in TPMT or NUDT15 IMs.	18, 62, 63
Methoxyflurane	*RYR1, CACNA1S*	Do not use in patients with risk variants for malignant hyperthermia	71
Nortriptyline	*CYP2D6*	Do not use in CYP2D6 UMs or PMs; consider a 25% dose reduction in heterozygotes	59, 60
Ondansetron	*CYP2D6*	Do not use in CYP2D6 UMs	74
Oxcarbazepine	*HLA-B, HLA-A*	Do not use in carbamazepine-naïve patients with at least one *HLA-B*15:02* or *HLA-A*31:01* allele	65, 66
Oxycodone	*CYP2D6*	Consider alternative opioids in CYP2C6 UMs and PMs	13, 70
Paroxetine	*CYP2D6*	Consider other drugs for CYP2D6 UMs and PMs; if paroxetine is warranted, reduce starting dose by 50%	67
PEG-interferon α-2a	*IFNL3*	Consider alternate treatments in unfavorable response genotypes rs12979860 T allele carriers	75
PEG-interferon α-2b	*IFNL3*	Consider alternate treatments in unfavorable response genotypes rs12979860 T allele carriers	75
Phenytoin	*CYP2C9, HLA-B*	Reduce dose in CYP2C9 PMs; do not use in patients with the *HLA-B*15:02* allele	76
Rasburicase	*G6PD*	Do not use in G6PD-deficient patients	33
Ribavirin	*IFNL3*	Consider alternate treatments in unfavorable response genotypes rs12979860 T allele carriers	75
Sertraline	*CYP2C19*	Reduce starting dose by 50% in CYP2C19 PMs or consider an alternative drug	67
Sevoflurane	*RYR1, CACNA1S*	Do not use in patients with risk variants for malignant hyperthermia	71
Simvastatin	*SLCO1B1*	Use lower daily doses or consider alternative therapies in patients with 1 or 2 copies of the rs4149056 C allele	25, 77
Succinylcholine	*RYR1, CACNA1S*	Do not use in patients with risk variants for malignant hyperthermia	71
Tacrolimus	*CYP3A5*	Increase starting dose by 50%–100% in patients who are CYP3A5 EMs or heterozygotes	78
Tamoxifen	*CYP2D6*	Consider alternative therapy in CYP2D6 IMs and PMs	79
Tegafur	*DPYD*	Do not use in homozygous DPYD-deficient patients; use 50% of target dose in heterozygotes	64
Thioguanine	*TPMT, NUDT15*	Extreme dose reduction in TPMT or NUDT15 PMs; reduce dose in TPMT or NUDT15 IMs	18, 62, 63
Tramadol	*CYP2D6*	Consider alternative opioids in CYP2C6 UMs and PMs	13, 70
Trimipramine	*CYP2D6, CYP2C19*	Do not use in CYP2D6 PMs or CYP2D6/CYP2C19 UMs; use 50% lower dose in CYP2C19 PMs	59, 60
Tropisetron	*CYP2D6*	Do not use in CYP2D6 UMs	74
Voriconazole	*CYP2C19*	Do not use in CYP2C19 UMs, RMs, and PMs	80
Warfarin	*CYP2C9, VKORC1, CYP4F2*	Calculate dose based on validated pharmacogenetic algorithms for pediatric patients	81, 82

Updated information for each guideline is available at https://cpicpgx.org.
IM, Intermediate metabolizer; *PM,* poor metabolizer; *UM,* ultrarapid metabolizer.

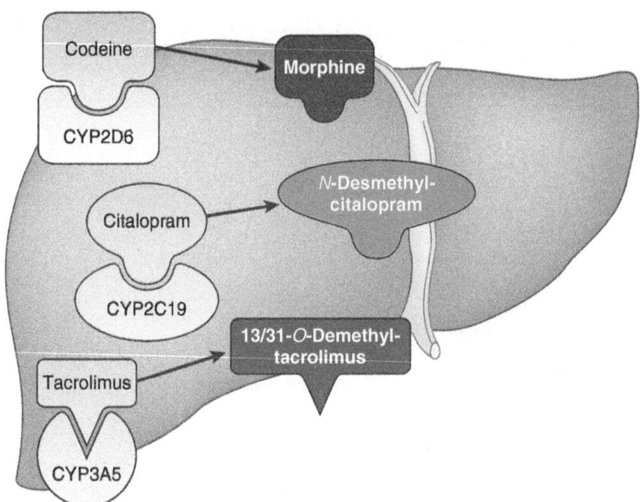

Fig. 18.1 Examples of CYP-mediated oxidation of commonly used medications in the liver.

are to adjust dosage, but for some medications, an alternative medication is recommended. There are two phases of drug metabolism—the first is oxidation or hydrolysis, and the second is conjugation (e.g., glucuronidation). Many drugs are metabolized by oxidation through the cytochrome P450 family of enzymes expressed highly in the liver (Fig. 18.1).

CYP2D6

The first pharmacogene characterized was *CYP2D6*, and to date, more than 130 alleles have been described for this gene (https://www.pharmvar.org/gene/CYP2D6). Approximately 25% of all medications are metabolized by the CYP2D6 enzyme to some degree, and this gene is included on several drug labels and 6 CPIC guidelines, with dosing adjustments or changes in medication recommended. Testing of CYP2D6 is required by the US Food and Drug Administration (FDA) prior to initiation of three medications: eliglustat, pimozide, and tetrabenazine (Table 18.2).

One example of a medication metabolized by this gene with clinical importance to pediatric patients is codeine, which is metabolized to the active drug (morphine) by CYP2D6. Individuals with little or no CYP2D6 activity (poor metabolizers) receive inadequate exposure to morphine with conventional dosing and need alternative analgesic medications to control pain (see Table 18.2).[12,13] Alternatively, those with duplication of the *CYP2D6* gene (ultrarapid metabolizers) are at risk for sedation and respiratory depression from generating high concentrations of morphine. Since the FDA issued a contraindication for codeine use in children younger than 12, many hospitals removed codeine from their formularies or restricted its use. The FDA also issued a warning to mothers that breast-feeding is not recommended when taking codeine due to the risk of serious adverse reactions (excess sleepiness, difficulty breast-feeding, or breathing problems). However, the American College of Obstetricians and Gynecologists does not recommend against using codeine in breast-feeding mothers but recommends counseling mothers on risks and newborn signs of toxicity if codeine-containing medications are selected for postpartum pain control.[14]

CYP2C19

Another pharmacogene that encodes an enzyme that metabolizes many commonly prescribed medications is *CYP2C19*. This gene has alleles with increased function (*17), decreased function, and no function; therefore phenotypes can be ultrarapid, rapid, normal, intermediate, or poor metabolizer.[8] The medications metabolized by CYP2C19 include antidepressants (e.g., escitalopram, sertraline, amitriptyline), clopidogrel, voriconazole, and proton pump inhibitors. Testing of this gene is not required prior to initiating any medications, but it is included in the FDA labels of 22 medications (www.fda.gov/drugs/science-and-research-drugs/table-pharmacogenomic-biomarkers-drug-labeling), usually in the Clinical Pharmacology section, but for citalopram and clobazam, it is included in the dosage and administration section, where dose reductions are recommended in poor metabolizers to avoid adverse reactions (see Table 18.2).

CYP3A5

Tacrolimus is an immunosuppressant that is metabolized by CYP3A5. Variants in *CYP3A5* (e.g., the *3 allele) explain 40% to 50% of the variability in blood concentrations of tacrolimus.[15,16] This is one of the few gene-drug pairs that has been tested in randomized clinical trials to test conventional dosing versus genotype-guided dosing. A trial in pediatric patients receiving a solid organ transplant demonstrated the time to the therapeutic concentration was reached sooner in a genotype-guided group than an unguided group and there were no differences in adverse events.[17] Since CYP3A5 is expressed highly in the liver, in patients receiving a liver transplant, the donor liver must be genotyped in order to provide genotype-guided dosing in these patients.

TPMT AND *NUDT15*

Thiopurines are metabolized by thiopurine methyltransferase (TPMT) into inactive metabolites. Patients receiving normal doses of thiopurines that are TPMT poor metabolizers are at very high risk for acute toxicity and require markedly reduced doses (10-fold lower).[18] *TPMT* variants account for much of the variability in thiopurine intolerance in people of European and African ancestry; however, variants in another gene in the thiopurine metabolism pathway, *NUDT15*, accounts for the majority of the variability in thiopurine intolerance in people of Asian ancestry and have also been found in Hispanic patients.[18] Patients with *NUDT15* no-function alleles also require drastic dose reductions in thiopurines to avoid severe myelosuppression. Adjusting dosages of thiopurines based on *TPMT* genotype has reduced the incidence of adverse effects without compromising efficacy.[19]

UGT1A1

Irinotecan is a chemotherapeutic drug that is metabolized into an active metabolite, SN-38, in the body. This active metabolite then goes through phase 2 metabolism via glucuronidation by UGT1A1. The *UGT1A1**28 allele is an insertion of a TA in the TATA box of the promoter region, which results in decreased transcription initiation of the gene and decreases the function of the enzyme by 70%. The Dutch Pharmacogenetics Working Group recommends reducing the dose of irinotecan by 30% in a patient homozygous for the *28 allele (poor metabolizer).[20] The *UGT1A1* variants also cause Gilbert syndrome, a form of mild unconjugated hyperbilirubinemia. Other medications metabolized by UGT1A1 include atazanavir and nilotinib. If atazanavir is prescribed to a poor metabolizer, there is a high likelihood of developing jaundice that will result in atazanavir discontinuation.[21]

NAT2

This gene was identified as a cause of a bimodal distribution in the plasma concentration of the tuberculostatic drug isoniazid concentrations after a single oral dose in a normal population. Subjects can be classified as "rapid" or "slow" eliminators of the drug based on differences in the rate of isoniazid's N-acetylation taking place through the NAT2 enzyme. Some ADRs are associated with *NAT2* alleles, but the incidence of these adverse reactions are low, and the frequency of the slow acetylation phenotype is

Table 18.2 FDA Labels That Include Pharmacogenomic Biomarkers (Content Current as of 3 Sep 2019).

Drug	Therapeutic Area	Biomarker
Isosorbide Dinitrate	Cardiology	CYB5R
Isosorbide Mononitrate	Cardiology	CYB5R
Nebivolol	Cardiology	CYP2D6
Propafenone	Cardiology	CYP2D6
Metoclopramide (2)	Gastroenterology	G6PD
Metoclopramide (3)	Gastroenterology	CYP2D6
Warfarin (1)	Hematology	CYP2C9
Warfarin (2)	Hematology	VKORC1
Carglumic Acid	Inborn errors of metabolism	NAGS
Eliglustat	Inborn errors of metabolism	CYP2D6
Migalastat	Inborn errors of metabolism	GLA
Sodium Phenylbutyrate	Inborn errors of metabolism	ASS1, CPS1, OTC (urea cycle disorders)
Abacavir	Infectious diseases	HLA-B
Dapsone (3)	Infectious diseases	G6PD
Primaquine (1)	Infectious diseases	G6PD
Tafenoquine	Infectious diseases	G6PD
Amifampridine	Neurology	NAT2
Amifampridine Phosphate	Neurology	NAT2
Clobazam	Neurology	CYP2C19
Deutetrabenazine	Neurology	CYP2D6
Siponimod	Neurology	CYP2C9
Tetrabenazine	Neurology	CYP2D6
Valbenazine	Neurology	CYP2D6
Ado-Trastuzumab Emtansine	Oncology	ERBB2 (HER2)
Afatinib	Oncology	EGFR
Alectinib	Oncology	ALK
Alpelisib (1)	Oncology	ERBB2 (HER2)
Alpelisib (2)	Oncology	ESR (hormone receptor)
Alpelisib (3)	Oncology	PIK3CA
Atezolizumab (1)	Oncology	CD274 (PD-L1)
Belinostat	Oncology	UGT1A1
Binimetinib (1)	Oncology	BRAF
Bosutinib	Oncology	BCR-ABL1 (Philadelphia chromosome)
Brentuximab Vedotin (2)	Oncology	TNFRSF8 (CD30)
Ceritinib	Oncology	ALK
Cetuximab (1)	Oncology	EGFR
Cetuximab (2)	Oncology	RAS
Cobimetinib	Oncology	BRAF
Crizotinib (1)	Oncology	ALK
Crizotinib (2)	Oncology	ROS1
Dabrafenib (1)	Oncology	BRAF
Dabrafenib (3)	Oncology	RAS
Dacomitinib	Oncology	EGFR
Dasatinib	Oncology	BCR-ABL1 (Philadelphia chromosome)
Enasidenib	Oncology	IDH2
Encorafenib	Oncology	BRAF
Erdafitinib (1)	Oncology	FGFR
Erlotinib	Oncology	EGFR
Everolimus (1)	Oncology	ERBB2 (HER2)
Everolimus (2)	Oncology	ESR (hormone receptor)
Exemestane	Oncology	ESR, PGR (hormone receptor)
Gefitinib (1)	Oncology	EGFR
Gilteritinib	Oncology	FLT3
Imatinib (1)	Oncology	KIT
Imatinib (2)	Oncology	BCR-ABL1 (Philadelphia chromosome)
Imatinib (3)	Oncology	PDGFRB
Imatinib (4)	Oncology	FIP1L1-PDGFRA
Irinotecan	Oncology	UGT1A1
Ivosidenib	Oncology	IDH1
Lapatinib (1)	Oncology	ERBB2 (HER2)
Lapatinib (2)	Oncology	ESR, PGR (hormone receptor)
Larotrectinib	Oncology	NTRK
Mercaptopurine (1)	Oncology	TPMT
Mercaptopurine (2)	Oncology	NUDT15
Midostaurin (1)	Oncology	FLT3
Nilotinib (1)	Oncology	BCR-ABL1 (Philadelphia chromosome)
Olaparib (1)	Oncology	BRCA
Olaparib (2)	Oncology	ERBB2 (HER2)
Osimertinib	Oncology	EGFR

Continued

Table 18.2 FDA Labels That Include Pharmacogenomic Biomarkers (Content Current as of 3 Sep 2019).—cont'd

Drug	Therapeutic Area	Biomarker
Panitumumab (2)	Oncology	RAS
Pembrolizumab (2)	Oncology	CD274 (PD-L1)
Pembrolizumab (3)	Oncology	Microsatellite instability, mismatch repair
Pertuzumab (1)	Oncology	ERBB2 (HER2)
Rituximab	Oncology	MS4A1 (CD20 antigen)
Rucaparib (1)	Oncology	BRCA
Talazoparib (1)	Oncology	BRCA
Thioguanine (1)	Oncology	TPMT
Thioguanine (2)	Oncology	NUDT15
Trametinib (1)	Oncology	BRAF
Trastuzumab (1)	Oncology	ERBB2 (HER2)
Vemurafenib (1)	Oncology	BRAF
Aripiprazole	Psychiatry	CYP2D6
Aripiprazole Lauroxil	Psychiatry	CYP2D6
Atomoxetine	Psychiatry	CYP2D6
Brexpiprazole	Psychiatry	CYP2D6
Citalopram (1)	Psychiatry	CYP2C19
Clozapine	Psychiatry	CYP2D6
Iloperidone	Psychiatry	CYP2D6
Pimozide	Psychiatry	CYP2D6
Vortioxetine	Psychiatry	CYP2D6
Azathioprine (1)	Rheumatology	TPMT
Azathioprine (2)	Rheumatology	NUDT15
Celecoxib	Rheumatology	CYP2C9

From US Food and Drug Administration. www.fda.gov/drugs/science-and-research-drugs/table-pharmacogenomic-biomarkers-drug-labeling.

high, indicating that there are additional factors that predispose a patient to these adverse reactions.[22] The slow acetylator phenotype is more common in patients experiencing adverse reactions to sulfonamide antibiotics such as cotrimoxazole (trimethoprim/sulfamethoxazole). This is important from a pediatric perspective, because cotrimoxazole is indicated for the treatment of otitis media in children, and increased adverse effects from the drug have been observed in children who are NAT2 slow acetylators.[23] However, rapid acetylators encounter therapeutic failure more often on treatment with once-weekly isoniazid dosage regimens and require higher doses of hydralazine to control hypertension, or of dapsone for dermatitis herpetiformis.

PHARMACOGENETIC VARIANTS AFFECTING DRUG TRANSPORT

Research has been done to associate variants in transporters with exposure and toxicity of many medications; however, there is only one CPIC guideline for a transporter. One of the best studied transporters for which there are no dosing guidelines is P-gp, encoded by *ABCB1*. P-gp transports many commonly prescribed medications, including simvastatin, ondansetron, opioids, and methotrexate.

SLCO1B1

This gene encodes a transporter expressed in the liver, OATP1B1, which transports many endogenous compounds (e.g., bilirubin) and xenobiotics, including methotrexate and statins. A genome-wide association study identified variants in *SLCO1B1* as associated with simvastatin-induced myopathy,[24] and CPIC recommends a lower dose or alternative statin in patients with the risk allele (see Table 18.1).[25] In children, this variant seems to have a larger effect on simvastatin exposure than it does in adults, potentially due to ontogeny.[26]

PHARMACOGENETIC VARIANTS AFFECTING DRUG RESPONSE (PHARMACODYNAMICS)

There are many pharmacogenes that affect drug response by altering the expression or function of the drug target, especially in oncology.[27] For pharmacogenes influencing expression of the target, dose adjustments are recommended (e.g., warfarin-*VKORC1*) but for the pharmacogenes altering expression or function of the target (e.g., *CFTR*), an alternative medication is recommended.

VKORC1

The target of warfarin is vitamin K epoxide reductase, encoded by the *VKORC1* gene. A variant upstream of the gene influences expression and is associated with warfarin sensitivity. The frequency of the variant varies by race and largely explains the difference in dose requirements among whites, blacks, and Asians. The CPIC warfarin guideline includes ancestry-specific recommendations based on *VKORC1*, *CYP2C9*, *CYP4F2*, and another variant in the *CYP2C* cluster, rs12777823. However, for pediatric patients, CPIC recommends dosing warfarin based on *VKORC1* and *CYP2C9* variants only in those of European ancestry. Our hospital has offered *VKORC1* testing along with *CYP2C9* testing for pediatric patients since 2007.[28]

CFTR

Variants in the *CFTR* gene cause cystic fibrosis, and ivacaftor was developed to treat those with a specific mutation in the gene. Ivacaftor restores function to the CFTR channel, enabling it to transport chloride, but does not work on mutations that keep the CFTR protein from getting to the cell membrane. Thus, testing of *CFTR* is required prior to ivacaftor initiation, and those without the mutations specified in the FDA label should receive alternative medications.

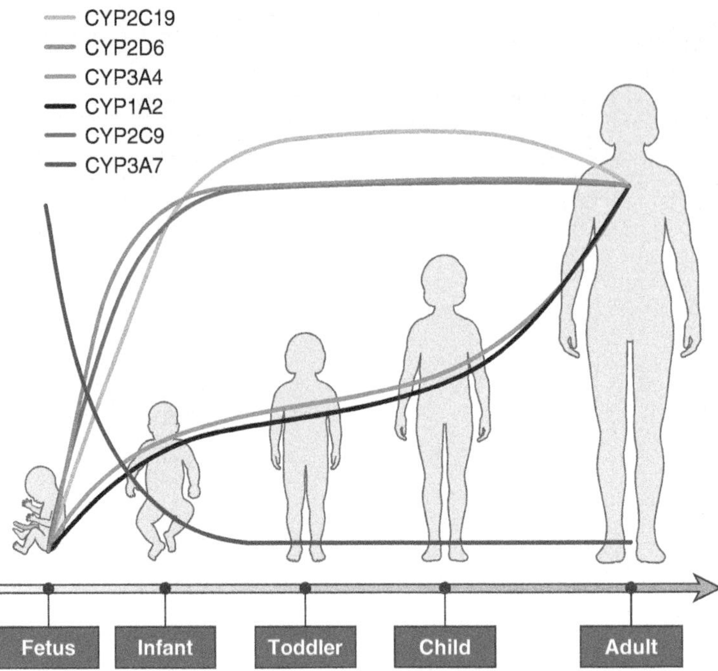

Fig. 18.2 Relative abundance of selected CYP enzymes throughout development. (Adapted from Upreti VV, Wahlstrom JL. Meta-analysis of hepatic cytochrome P450 ontogeny to underwrite the prediction of pediatric pharmacokinetics using physiologically based pharmacokinetic modeling. *J Clin Pharmacol.* 2016;56[3]:266–283.)

PHARMACOGENETIC VARIANTS INCREASING RISK FOR ADVERSE DRUG REACTIONS

A portion of serious ADRs are attributable to immune-mediated responses, including Stevens-Johnson syndrome/toxic epidermal necrosis (SJS/TEN) and hemolytic anemia.

HUMAN LEUKOCYTE ANTIGEN GENES

Carriers of certain human leukocyte antigen (HLA) alleles are at very high risk for SJS/TEN after taking phenytoin, allopurinol, carbamazepine, and oxcarbazepine. The HLA genes encode cell surface proteins that present intracellular antigens to the immune system and are among the most polymorphic genes in the human genome (>4000 HLA-B alleles have been identified).[29] The frequency of the risk alleles for carbamazepine-induced SJS/TEN, *HLA-B*15:02* and *HLA-A*31:01*, are highest in East Asian, Oceanian, and South/Central Asian populations (4.6% to 6.9%). The FDA label for carbamazepine carries a boxed warning about the risk of SJS/TEN in patients positive for the *HLA-B*15:02* allele. The Hong Kong Hospital Authority enacted a policy in 2008 to test patients for *HLA-B*15:02* prior to initiation of carbamazepine, but instead of testing patients, prescribers chose a different antiepileptic medication and the incidence of antiepileptic drug-induced SJS/TEN did not decrease.[30] Additionally, the *HLA-B*57:01* allele is associated with abacavir hypersensitivity reactions. The frequency of this allele also varies by ancestry, with the highest frequency (20%) in Southwest Asian populations, 6% to 7% in European populations, and is lowest in African and Asian populations.[31] The results of a randomized, controlled trial of genetic prescreening for *HLA-B*57:01* prior to abacavir prescriptions prompted the FDA to implement a black box warning in 2008 that recommends screening prior to initiation of the drug.[32] Alternative treatment is recommended in *HLA-B*57:01* carriers.

G6PD

Patients receiving rasburicase for hyperuricemia during chemotherapy that have G6PD deficiency are at high risk for hemolytic anemia. CPIC recommendations are to treat these patients with alternative medications (e.g., allopurinol).[33] There are many variants in *G6PD* that have been described, and since this gene is on the X chromosome, hemizygous males (one variant allele) and homozygous females (two variant alleles) can have G6PD deficiency, depending on the function of the alleles. An enzyme test is often performed to confirm G6PD deficiency.

ONTOGENY OF DRUG-METABOLIZING ENZYMES, TRANSPORTERS, AND TARGETS

The ontogeny of human drug metabolic enzymes has been intensively investigated, especially for the hepatic and intestinal cytochrome P450 (CYP) pathways[34,35] and has been reviewed elsewhere.[36,37] Previous studies suggest that the ontogeny of hepatic metabolizing enzymes appears to follow three typical patterns. The enzymes categorized as the first group (e.g., CYP3A7) are expressed at their highest level during fetal life and are silenced or expressed at low levels within 1 to 2 years after birth.[35] The second group of enzymes (e.g., CYP3A5) are expressed at relatively constant levels throughout gestation with minimal changes after birth. Moderate postnatal increases are observed in CYP2C19 but not in CYP3A5. The third group includes the largest number of enzymes such as CYP1A2, CYP2C9, CYP2D6, and CYP3A4. Those enzymes are not expressed or are expressed at low levels in the fetal liver; however, the expression levels are substantially increased within the first 1 to 2 years after birth, except for some enzymes with delayed ontogeny (e.g., CYP1A2 and CYP3A4, Fig. 18.2).[37-40]

Carboxylesterases (CES) are also important mediators of phase 1 metabolism for various drugs, but ontogeny of these enzymes in humans had been less studied compared to CYPs. Recent studies demonstrated the protein expression patterns for hepatic CES1 and CES2 in infants.[41,42] However, the developmental changes in tissues other than liver remain unclear. Phase 2 metabolism via conjugation (e.g., glucuronidation and sulphate conjugation) are also major metabolic pathways for many drugs. Uridine 5'-diphospho-glucuronosyltransferase (UGT) mediates glucuronidation, which is a major part of phase 2 metabolism. A recent comprehensive proteomic analysis using liquid chromatography-tandem mass spectrometry (LC-MS/MS) has documented the protein abundance of UGT subfamilies in human liver microsomes isolated from children and adults.[43] These proteomics data were integrated into a pediatric physiologically based pharmacokinetic (PBPK) model of zidovudine and improved the prediction of interindividual variability by the PK model.[43]

As the Pediatric Transporter Working Group indicated in their white paper published in 2015,[44] human ontogeny data of transporters are quite sparse, and most available data assess gene expression but not protein abundance, the latter being more relevant to transporter function and effects on drug disposition. In response to the white paper, ontogeny profiles of major transporters have been investigated comprehensively in the intestine,[45] liver,[46-48] and kidney tissues.[49] In several studies, protein abundance has been quantified with a proteomics approach using LC-MS/MS analysis of liver[47,48] and kidney tissues.[49] Protein expression data in the small intestine remain limited.[45] The ontogeny of brain transporters is another important knowledge gap that should be addressed to better predict drug distribution to the brain and its impact on central nervous system-associated efficacy and toxicity, as well as efficacy in children.

In contrast to drug-metabolizing enzymes and transporters, data on human ontogeny of therapeutic target molecules (e.g., receptors) and pathways are very limited. Such data are crucial to characterize the developmental changes in drug effects (pharmacodynamics) that are critical for age-appropriate precision dosing guidelines based on exposure-response data across the age spectrum. For instance, the developmental changes in gene/protein expression of opioid receptors have been investigated in rodents,[50-53] but its translation to humans is lacking. Opioid drugs are increasingly used in critically ill infants—for example, to treat neonatal abstinence syndrome (NAS) or for pain management in the neonatal intensive care unit. Fetal ontogeny of opioid receptors may also be important for a better understanding of development and pathogenesis of NAS as a result of in utero opioid exposure and the severity of NAS symptoms during the first days of life.

A major challenge in the implementation of pharmacogenomics for precision dosing in neonates and infants is to understand relative contributions of ontogeny versus genetic variation. As Leeder et al. described,[54] true genotype-phenotype relationships may not be fully apparent until the gene product is fully expressed. Thus, for enzymes with no or minimal expression during the fetal and early postnatal period, the contributions of genetic variants in infants may be markedly different from those observed in adolescents or adults. For example, different effects of genetic variance in the transporter *OCT1* and morphine pharmacokinetics have been observed between preterm neonates and other pediatric populations.[55,56] In those studies a lower morphine clearance associated with loss of function genetic variants in *OCT1* was observed only in children (term or postterm infants), but not in preterm neonates. These results suggest that the *OCT1* expression level in preterm neonates is insufficient to identify any differences across genotypes.[55] To tease out such complex interactions between pharmacogenetics and ontogeny, integrating high-quality ontogeny data into mechanism-based or physiologically based pharmacokinetic/pharmacodynamic models is critical, and pharmaco-statistical models represent an important in silico platform to bridge ontogeny and pharmacogenetics data to characterize the exposure-response relationship(s).

CONCLUSION

Herein we have provided several examples of pharmacogenes that influence the pharmacokinetics, pharmacodynamics, and severe adverse reactions to drugs. Adjusting medication dose or selection due to genetic variation can help reduce drug-induced toxicity in pregnancy, in utero, and in postnatal life and avoid ADRs. The combination of ontogeny and pharmacogenetics requires further research to understand the contribution of each during childhood and to ultimately develop actionable age-appropriate dosing guidelines.

A complete reference list is available at www.ExpertConsult.com. 

SELECT REFERENCES

3. Rieder MJ, Carleton B. Pharmacogenomics and adverse drug reactions in children. *Front Genet*. 2014;5(APR). https://doi.org/10.3389/fgene.2014.00078.
4. Gaedigk A, Ingelman-Sundberg M, Miller NA, Leeder JS, Whirl-Carrillo M, Klein TE. The Pharmacogene Variation (PharmVar) Consortium: incorporation of the Human Cytochrome P450 (CYP) allele nomenclature database. *Clin Pharmacol Ther*. 2018;103(3):399-401. https://doi.org/10.1002/cpt.910.
5. Caudle KE, Gammal RS, Whirl-Carrillo M, et al. Evidence and resources to implement pharmacogenetic knowledge for precision medicine. *Am J Health Syst Pharm*. 2016;73(23):1977-1985. https://doi.org/10.2146/ajhp150977.
6. McDonagh EM, Whirl-Carrillo M, Garten Y, Altman RB, Klein TE. From pharmacogenomic knowledge acquisition to clinical applications: the PharmGKB as a clinical pharmacogenomic biomarker resource. *Biomark Med*. 2011;5(6):795-806. https://doi.org/10.2217/bmm.11.94.
8. Caudle KE, Dunnenberger HM, Freimuth RR, et al. Standardizing terms for clinical pharmacogenetic test results: Consensus terms from the Clinical Pharmacogenetics Implementation consortium (CPIC). *Genet Med*. 2017;19(2):215-223. https://doi.org/10.1038/gim.2016.87.
13. Crews KR, Gaedigk A, Dunnenberger HM, et al. Clinical pharmacogenetics implementation consortium guidelines for cytochrome P450 2D6 genotype and codeine therapy: 2014 update. *Clin Pharmacol Ther*. 2014. https://doi.org/10.1038/clpt.2013.254.
18. Relling MV, Schwab M, Whirl-Carrillo M, et al. Clinical pharmacogenetics implementation consortium guideline for thiopurine dosing based on TPMT and NUDT15 genotypes: 2018 update. *Clin Pharmacol Ther*. 2019;105(5):1095-1105. https://doi.org/10.1002/cpt.1304.
20. Swen JJ, Nijenhuis M, De Boer A, et al. Pharmacogenetics: from bench to byte an update of guidelines. *Clin Pharmacol Ther*. 2011;89(5):662-673. https://doi.org/10.1038/clpt.2011.34.
21. Gammal RS, Court MH, Haidar CE, et al. Clinical Pharmacogenetics Implementation Consortium (CPIC) guideline for UGT1A1 and atazanavir prescribing. *Clin Pharmacol Ther*. 2016;99(4):363-369. https://doi.org/10.1002/cpt.269.
25. Ramsey LB, Johnson SG, Caudle KE, et al. The clinical pharmacogenetics implementation consortium guideline for SLCO1B1 and simvastatin-induced myopathy: 2014 update. *Clin Pharmacol Ther*. 2014;96(4). https://doi.org/10.1038/clpt.2014.125.
26. Wagner JB, Abdel-Rahman S, Van Haandel L, et al. Impact of *SLCO1B1* genotype on pediatric simvastatin acid pharmacokinetics. *J Clin Pharmacol*. 2018;58(6):823-833. https://doi.org/10.1002/jcph.1080.
28. Ramsey LB, Prows CA, Zhang K, et al. Implementation of pharmacogenetics at Cincinnati Children's Hospital Medical Center: lessons learned over 14 years of personalizing medicine. *Clin Pharmacol Ther*. 2019;105(1):49-52.
31. Martin MA, Klein TE, Dong BJ, Pirmohamed M, Haas DW, Kroetz DL. Clinical Pharmacogenetics Implementation Consortium guidelines for HLA-B genotype and abacavir dosing. *Clin Pharmacol Ther*. 2012;91(4):734-738. https://doi.org/10.1038/clpt.2011.355.
33. Relling MV, Mcdonagh EM, Chang T, et al. Clinical Pharmacogenetics Implementation Consortium (CPIC) guidelines for rasburicase therapy in the context of G6PD deficiency genotype. 2014;96(2):169-174. https://doi.org/10.1038/clpt.2014.97.
35. Hines RN. The ontogeny of drug metabolism enzymes and implications for adverse drug events. *Pharmacol Ther*. 2008;118(2):250-267. https://doi.org/10.1016/j.pharmthera.2008.02.005.
36. Kearns GL, Abdel-Rahman SM, Alander SW, Blowey DL, Leeder JS, Kauffman RE. Developmental Pharmacology — drug disposition, action, and therapy in infants and children. *N Engl J Med*. 2003;349(12):1157-1167. https://doi.org/10.1056/NEJMra035092.
37. Upreti VV, Wahlstrom JL. Meta-analysis of hepatic cytochrome P450 ontogeny to underwrite the prediction of pediatric pharmacokinetics using physiologically based pharmacokinetic modeling. *J Clin Pharmacol*. 2016;56(3):266-283. https://doi.org/10.1002/jcph.585.
43. Bhatt DK, Mehrotra A, Gaedigk A, et al. Age- and genotype-dependent variability in the protein abundance and activity of six major uridine diphosphate-glucuronosyltransferases in human liver. *Clin Pharmacol Ther*. 2019;105(1):131-141. https://doi.org/10.1002/cpt.1109.
44. Brouwer KLR, Aleksunes LM, Brandys B, et al. Human ontogeny of drug transporters: review and recommendations of the pediatric transporter working group. *Clin Pharmacol Ther*. 2015;98(3):266-287. https://doi.org/10.1002/cpt.176.
45. Mooij MG, Schwarz UI, de Koning BAE, et al. Ontogeny of human hepatic and intestinal transporter gene expression during childhood: age matters. *Drug Metab Dispos*. 2014;42(8):1268-1274. https://doi.org/10.1124/dmd.114.056929.
47. Prasad B, Gaedigk A, Vrana M, et al. Ontogeny of hepatic drug transporters as quantified by LC-MS/MS proteomics. *Clin Pharmacol Ther*. October 2016:362-370. https://doi.org/10.1002/cpt.409.
54. Leeder JS, Kearns GL, Spielberg SP, Van Den Anker J. Understanding the relative roles of pharmacogenetics and ontogeny in pediatric drug development and regulatory science. *J Clin Pharmacol*. 2010;50(12):1377-1387. https://doi.org/10.1177/0091270009360533.
55. Hahn D, Emoto C, Euteneuer JC, Mizuno T, Vinks AA, Fukuda T. Influence of OCT1 ontogeny and genetic variation on morphine disposition in critically ill neonates: lessons from PBPK modeling and clinical study. *Clin Pharmacol Ther*. 2019;105(3):761-768. https://doi.org/10.1002/cpt.1249.
58. Hershfield MS, Callaghan JT, Tassaneeyakul W, et al. Clinical pharmacogenetics implementation consortium guidelines for human leukocyte antigen-b genotype and allopurinol dosing. *Clin Pharmacol Ther*. 2013;93(2):153-158. https://doi.org/10.1038/clpt.2012.209.

59. Hicks JK, Swen JJ, Thorn CF, et al. Clinical pharmacogenetics implementation consortium guideline for CYP2D6 and CYP2C19 genotypes and dosing of tricyclic antidepressants. *Clin Pharmacol Ther*. 2013;93(5):402-408. https://doi.org/10.1038/clpt.2013.2.
60. Hicks JK, Sangkuhl K, Swen JJ, et al. Clinical pharmacogenetics implementation consortium guideline (CPIC) for CYP2D6 and CYP2C19 genotypes and dosing of tricyclic antidepressants: 2016 update. *Clin Pharmacol Ther*. 2017;102(1):37-44. https://doi.org/10.1002/cpt.597.
61. Brown JT, Bishop JR, Sangkuhl K, et al. Clinical pharmacogenetics implementation consortium guideline for cytochrome P450 (CYP)2D6 genotype and Atomoxetine therapy. *Clin Pharmacol Ther*. 2019;106(1):94-102. https://doi.org/10.1002/cpt.1409.
64. Caudle KE, Thorn CF, Klein TE, et al. Clinical pharmacogenetics implementation consortium guidelines for dihydropyrimidine dehydrogenase genotype and fluoropyrimidine dosing. *Clin Pharmacol Ther*. 2013;94(6):640-645. https://doi.org/10.1038/clpt.2013.172.
66. Phillips EJ, Sukasem C, Whirl-Carrillo M, et al. Clinical pharmacogenetics implementation consortium guideline for HLA genotype and use of carbamazepine and oxcarbazepine: 2017 update. *Clin Pharmacol Ther*. 2018;103(4):574-581. https://doi.org/10.1002/cpt.1004.
67. Hicks JK, Bishop JR, Sangkuhl K, et al. Clinical Pharmacogenetics Implementation Consortium (CPIC) guideline for CYP2D6 and CYP2C19 genotypes and dosing of selective serotonin reuptake inhibitors. *Clin Pharmacol Ther*. 2015;98(2):127-134. https://doi.org/10.1002/cpt.147.
69. Scott SA, Sangkuhl K, Stein CM, et al. Clinical Pharmacogenetics Implementation Consortium guidelines for CYP2C19 genotype and clopidogrel therapy: 2013 update. *Clin Pharmacol Ther*. 2013;94(3):317-323. https://doi.org/10.1038/clpt.2013.105.
70. Crews KR, Gaedigk A, Dunnenberger HM, et al. Clinical Pharmacogenetics Implementation Consortium (CPIC) guidelines for codeine therapy in the context of cytochrome P450 2D6 (CYP2D6) genotype. *Clin Pharmacol Ther*. 2012;91(2):321-326. https://doi.org/10.1038/clpt.2011.287.
71. Gonsalves SG, Dirksen RT, Sangkuhl K, et al. Clinical Pharmacogenetics Implementation Consortium (CPIC) guideline for the use of potent volatile anesthetic agents and succinylcholine in the context of RYR1 or CACNA1S genotypes. *Clin Pharmacol Ther*. 2019;105(6):1338-1344. https://doi.org/10.1002/cpt.1319.
72. Desta Z, Gammal RS, Gong L, et al. Clinical Pharmacogenetics Implementation Consortium (CPIC) guideline for CYP2B6 and efavirenz-containing antiretroviral therapy. *Clin Pharmacol Ther*. 2019;106(4):726-733. https://doi.org/10.1002/cpt.1477.
73. Clancy JP, Johnson SG, Yee SW, et al. Clinical Pharmacogenetics Implementation Consortium (CPIC) guidelines for ivacaftor therapy in the context of CFTR genotype. *Clin Pharmacol Ther*. 2014;95(6):592-597. https://doi.org/10.1038/clpt.2014.54.
74. Bell GC, Caudle KE, Whirl-Carrillo M, et al. Clinical Pharmacogenetics Implementation Consortium (CPIC) guideline for CYP2D6 genotype and use of ondansetron and tropisetron. *Clin Pharmacol Ther*. 2017;102(2). https://doi.org/10.1002/cpt.598.
75. Muir AJ, Gong L, Johnson SG, et al. Clinical Pharmacogenetics Implementation Consortium (CPIC) guidelines for IFNL3 (IL28B) genotype and PEG Interferon-based regimens. *Clin Pharmacol Ther*. 2014;95(2):141-146. https://doi.org/10.1038/clpt.2013.203.
76. Caudle KE, Rettie AE, Whirl-Carrillo M, et al. Clinical Pharmacogenetics Implementation Consortium guidelines for CYP2C9 and HLA-B genotypes and phenytoin dosing. *Clin Pharmacol Ther*. 2014;96(5):542-548. https://doi.org/10.1038/clpt.2014.159.
78. Birdwell KA, Decker B, Barbarino JM, et al. Clinical Pharmacogenetics Implementation Consortium (CPIC) guidelines for CYP3A5 genotype and tacrolimus dosing. *Clin Pharmacol Ther*. 2015;98(1):19-24. https://doi.org/10.1002/cpt.113.
79. Goetz MP, Sangkuhl K, Guchelaar HJ, et al. Clinical Pharmacogenetics Implementation Consortium (CPIC) guideline for CYP2D6 and Tamoxifen therapy. *Clin Pharmacol Ther*. 2018;103(5):770-777. https://doi.org/10.1002/cpt.1007.
80. Moriyama B, Obeng AO, Barbarino J, et al. Clinical Pharmacogenetics Implementation Consortium (CPIC) guidelines for CYP2C19 and voriconazole therapy. *Clin Pharmacol Ther*. 2017;102(1):45-51. https://doi.org/10.1002/cpt.583.
82. Johnson JA, Caudle KE, Gong L, et al. Clinical Pharmacogenetics Implementation Consortium (CPIC) guideline for pharmacogenetics-guided warfarin dosing: 2017 update. *Clin Pharmacol Ther*. 2017;102(3):397-404. https://doi.org/10.1002/cpt.668.

19 Drug Distribution in Fetal Life

Marianne Garland

INTRODUCTION

Drug distribution and clearance determine the concentration of drug that will be attained at the site of drug action. Drug targets include cell surface receptors, intracellular receptors, enzymes, transcriptional mechanisms, ion channels, and molecular transport systems. These targets may be within the circulatory system, in well-perfused tissues, in less well-perfused tissues, or behind specialized endothelial or epithelial barriers. The fetus lies behind one of these circulatory barriers—the placenta. The placenta is the interface between the maternal and fetal circulations, keeping them separate but bringing them into close apposition for transport of nutritional needs and removal of waste products. In addition, this interface is the major route of drug delivery to and elimination from the fetus. The fetus also has specialized circulatory arrangements designed for intrauterine life that require additional considerations in the understanding of fetal drug distribution. Furthermore, developmental differences in body composition, drug metabolism, renal clearance, and specialized barriers make fetal drug distribution distinct from that in the infant, child, and adult.

Most drug action is predicted on the basis of plasma drug concentrations. It is not easy, even in experimental models, to measure tissue concentrations, particularly when the extracellular versus intracellular concentration warrants consideration. Hence major emphasis is placed on the determinants of fetal plasma concentration. An appreciation of pharmacokinetics requires an understanding of physicochemical properties of drugs, placental transfer of drugs, and fetal clearance of drugs. Many of these concepts also pertain to tissue distribution. Drug delivery to the central nervous system of the fetus is of particular interest and further illustrates concepts relevant to tissue distribution. In considering developmental issues relevant to fetal disposition of drugs, an important point is that drug targets also have complex developmental trajectories. Understanding fetal drug distribution may allow prediction of drug concentration at the site of drug action, but prediction of drug action, which is the true goal, also requires understanding the interaction between the drug and its target.

DETERMINANTS OF FETAL PLASMA CONCENTRATION

The plasma concentration of a drug in the mother is the main factor determining the plasma concentration of drug in the fetus. Fig. 19.1 shows the linear relationship between concentrations of zidovudine measured simultaneously in fetal plasma to those measured in maternal plasma under steady-state conditions in a nonhuman primate.[1] *Steady state* is defined as the condition in which the amount of drug in a compartment does not change with time—that is, the amount of drug being added to the system is the same as that leaving the system.

This linear relationship is the hallmark of first-order kinetics, with the implication that a doubling of the maternal concentration

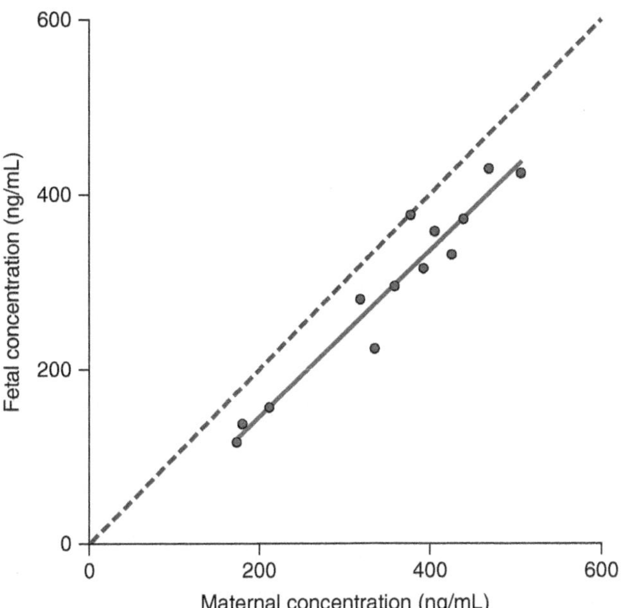

Fig. 19.1 Paired fetal and maternal zidovudine concentrations in plasma samples obtained at steady state in the chronically catheterized baboon infused with 150 to 350 μg/min of zidovudine. *Red dashed line, y = x.*

will double the fetal concentration. In this example of zidovudine infusion to pregnant baboons, the fetal concentration of zidovudine is slightly less than the maternal concentration. This observation is common for many drugs and indicates that other factors also influence the fetal plasma concentration. The focus of this chapter is to review how placental permeability, fetal drug elimination, drug ionization and protein binding, and volumes of distribution affect fetal drug levels.

Once the maternal concentration is known, fetal distribution can be divided into three phases: transfer across the placenta, modification of the fetal plasma concentration, and tissue distribution. An integrated pharmacokinetic approach with graphic representations is used throughout to describe how differences in these various contributors affect fetal drug levels (be it plasma, extracellular, or intracellular).

MATERNAL PLASMA CONCENTRATION

The maternal plasma concentration is the driving force for drug delivery to the fetus. For many drugs, physiologic changes of pregnancy lead to altered drug absorption, distribution, and clearance in the mother, and thus plasma concentrations are different from those seen in the nonpregnant state.[2,3] Generally, plasma drug concentrations tend to be lower in pregnancy. There is an increase in the volume of distribution resulting from an increased plasma volume and increased fat deposition, as well as addition of the fetal compartment. Maternal renal clearance is enhanced owing to increased cardiac output and renal blood flow, or to pregnancy-related changes in renal transporters. Hepatic clearance also may be enhanced as a consequence of increased hepatic blood flow or hormonal stimulation of drug-metabolizing enzymes. In some cases, however, pregnancy hormones may inhibit drug-metabolizing enzymes. Increasingly, comparative data are becoming available for drugs used in pregnancy. For fetal considerations, the physiologic changes of pregnancy that alter maternal drug distribution can be bypassed by measuring the concentration of the drug in maternal plasma.

DRUG TRANSFER ACROSS THE PLACENTA

The placenta is the specialized interface between mother and fetus across which drug distribution occurs. Most drugs are believed to cross the placenta by passive diffusion; accordingly, the surface area provided by the placenta and the nature of the interface, together with drug characteristics, determine placental permeability. Placental transporters are now recognized as an important contributor to fetal drug disposition.

STRUCTURAL DEVELOPMENT OF THE PLACENTA

The following discussion is a synopsis of placental development highlighting the aspects relevant to drug transport, with a focus on the relationship among the maternal and fetal circulations, the surface area of exchange, and the nature of the diffusional barrier.[4]

During implantation, the trophoblastic tissue invades and becomes surrounded by decidua. The placenta develops at the embryonic pole while the trophoblast in contact with the rest of the decidua gradually breaks down. Spaces develop within the expanding trophoblastic tissue to form the lacunae that lie between the villous structures. The uterine spiral arteries supplying the decidua and the veins draining the decidua are invaded by trophoblasts in such a manner that these maternal vessels open directly into the lacunae, and maternal blood bathes the villous structures. Anchoring villi extend the full thickness of the trophoblast layer, whereas other villi project like trees into the villous space (Fig. 19.2A). As pregnancy advances, the placental surface area increases by increasing the number of villi and the number of branches. As with most epithelial transport surfaces, the luminal plasma membrane of the villus trophoblast has microvilli that further increase surface area (see Fig. 19.2C). Later in gestation, the diffusional capacity of the placenta increases mostly by thinning of the trophoblast layer where it overlies fetal vessels within the villi. The villus itself consists of a stromal core to support the fetal blood vessels and is surrounded by a single layer of syncytial trophoblast attached to a basement membrane (see Fig. 19.2B). Cytotrophoblasts and some Hofbauer cells (placental tissue macrophages) lie between the two. The syncytial trophoblast is a multinucleate cellular structure formed by the fusion of trophoblastic cells to form a syncytium. Underlying cytotrophoblastic cells add to the syncytiotrophoblast by fusion, and by term, few cytotrophoblasts are present within the villus. The fetal arterioles branch into a capillary bed, also surrounded by a basement membrane. The capillaries are nonfenestrated and have variably spaced tight junctions between endothelial cells. In the mature placenta, the contact zones between the syncytiotrophoblast and endothelial cells are free of nuclei and are thinner than other regions (see Fig. 19.2B). The layers between maternal and fetal blood over which diffusion occurs are shown in Fig. 19.2C. In addition to the microvillus surface, the luminal membrane of the syncytiotrophoblast (that is in contact with maternal blood) contains clefts. The abluminal membrane also has infoldings. The syncytial nature of the syncytiotrophoblast precludes intercellular spaces through which transport can occur. By contrast, the endothelium does allow some paracellular transport of low-molecular-weight hydrophilic substances. Placental capillaries are less permeable than most other capillaries present in tissues with continuous or nonfenestrated capillaries; however, they are still more permeable, by two orders of magnitude, than those present in the brain.

MODELS OF PLACENTAL TRANSFER OF DRUG

From an anatomic perspective, many placental characteristics are important in the transfer of drug to the fetus. The most striking features are the very large exchange surface and the very thin syncytial-endothelial barrier between the maternal and fetal circulations, supporting passive transfer of substances (see Fig. 19.2). Visualization of the human placental structure suggests a

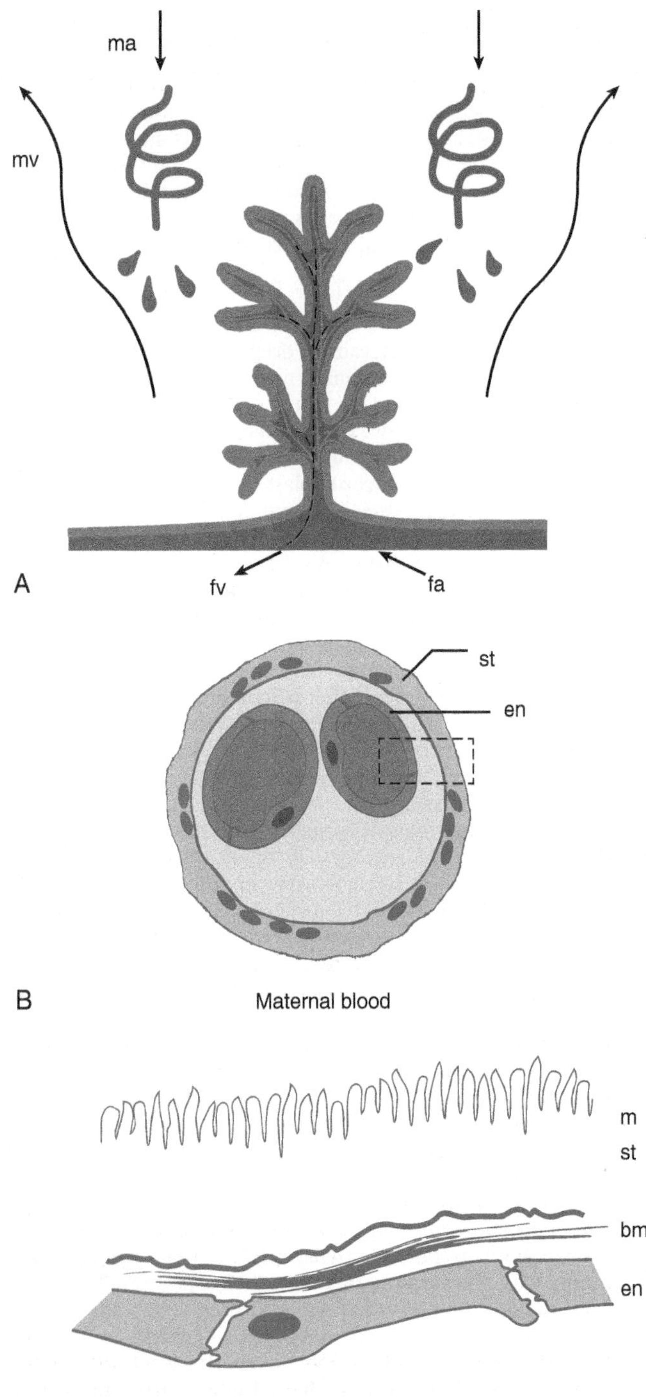

Fig. 19.2 Schematic diagram of mature human placental structure. (A) The placental villus supports vessels from the fetus and is in direct contact with maternal blood. (B) The syncytial trophoblast forms a continuous cellular layer over the fetal villi. Areas in close apposition to fetal capillaries are thinner and lack nuclei. (C) The layers that drugs must cross to transfer from one circulation to the other are depicted. Area surrounded by the *dashed line* is enlarged in the succeeding diagram; *arrows* indicate direction of blood flow. *bm,* Basement membrane; *en,* endothelium; *fa,* fetal artery; *fv,* fetal vein; *m,* microvilli; *ma,* maternal artery; *mv,* maternal vein; *st,* syncytiotrophoblast.

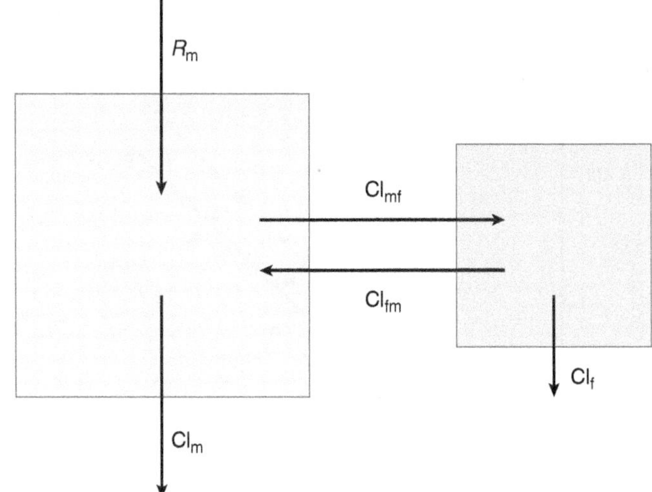

Fig. 19.3 The two-compartment model representation of the maternal-fetal dyad. Drug movement into and out of each compartment is indicated by the *arrows*. Clearance parameters are used to characterize the elimination from or transfer between compartments. *Cl,* Clearance; *f,* fetal; *m,* maternal; *R,* rate of infusion of drug to maternal compartment.

crosscurrent exchange interface; however, experimental data at best support a concurrent model (detailed in Chapter 10).

The simplest and perhaps most illustrative way to view the maternal-fetal dyad with respect to drug distribution is as a two-compartment model (Fig. 19.3).[1,5-7] This model differs from the standard peripheral compartment model in that the fetal compartment includes an elimination route independent of the placenta. In addition, at least in experimental models, this compartment can be sampled. Rate equations for the model describe how the amount of drug in each compartment changes with time and are determined by considering how much drug is entering and leaving each compartment. The amount of drug *(D)* that leaves in a given time period (mass/time) equals the clearance (Cl) (volume/time) multiplied by the mean concentration (*c*, mass/volume) for that time period as follows (see parameter descriptions in Fig. 19.3).

Rate equation for maternal compartment:

$$\frac{dD_m}{dt} = R_m - Cl_m \cdot c_m - Cl_{mf} \cdot c_m + Cl_{fm} \cdot c_f \quad [19.1]$$

Rate equation for fetal compartment:

$$\frac{dD_f}{dt} = Cl_{mf} \cdot c_m - Cl_{fm} \cdot c_f - Cl_f \cdot c_f \quad [19.2]$$

Solutions of these rate equations are used to generate concentration-time plots for each compartment to illustrate the effects of placental permeability and nonplacental fetal elimination on fetal drug distribution, as shown in Figs. 19.4 and 19.5. Fig. 19.4 describes drug administered by an oral bolus, and Fig. 19.5 shows drug administered by continuous infusion to steady state and then stopped. The assumptions for these simplified examples are that drug concentrations are not affected by protein binding or pH effects, and that drug crosses the placenta by passive diffusion such that placental clearance is the same in both directions. In panel *A* of Figs. 19.4 and 19.5, no direct fetal clearance occurs—that is, fetal nonplacental clearance is set at zero. Moving down the panel shows the effect of decreasing placental clearance on the fetal drug concentration-time curve. Placental permeability will affect peak fetal drug concentrations when administered by the bolus (see Fig. 19.4A), but total fetal drug exposure as measured by

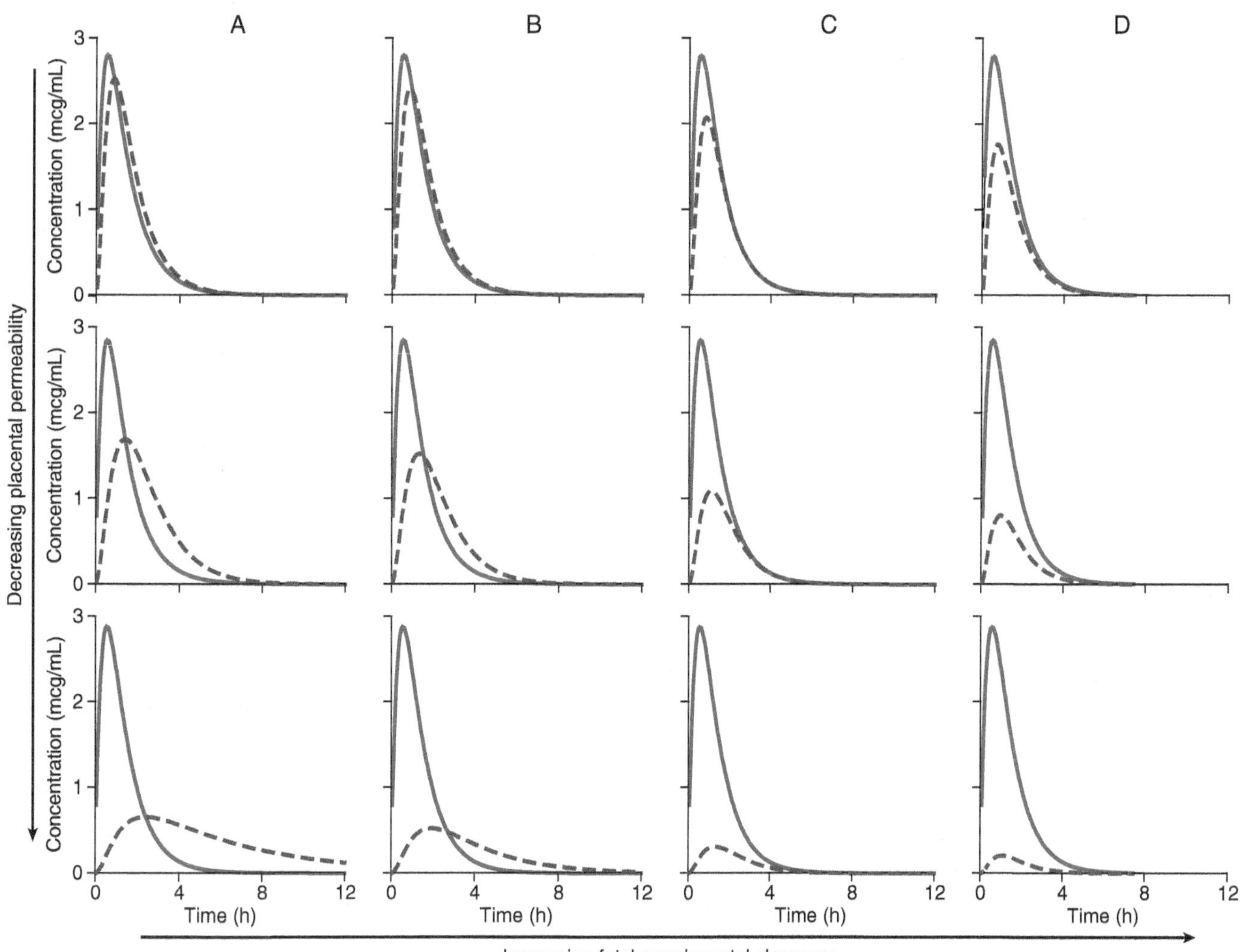

Fig. 19.4 Drug concentration-time curves for mother *(solid blue line)* and fetus *(dashed red line)* after an oral bolus of drug. These plots represent the solutions for the rate equations of a two-compartment model following an oral bolus of drug where placental clearance (a measure of placental permeability) and fetal nonplacental clearance (direct fetal elimination) were varied while all other system parameters remained constant. The general parameters used to make these plots are those obtained experimentally in the pregnant baboon following zidovudine administration.[13] The *top row* represents high placental permeability in that placental clearance is 20% of maternal clearance. In the *middle row,* placental clearance is 5% of maternal clearance (that observed experimentally). The *bottom row* represents limited placental permeability in that only 1% of drug administered to the mother will cross the placenta to the fetus. Levels of direct fetal elimination increase with progression from A to D: (A) no direct fetal clearance; (B) fetal clearance is 1% of maternal clearance (that observed experimentally); (C) fetal clearance is 5% of maternal clearance, as would be the case when fetal metabolic activity expressed per tissue mass is similar to that in the adult; (D) fetal clearance is 10% of maternal clearance, as would occur only when fetal enzyme activity is higher than that in the adult.

the area under the concentration-time curve is the same in each case. With continuous infusion of drug to steady state when there is no direct fetal clearance (see Fig. 19.5A), fetal drug levels will be as high for drugs with low placental permeability as for those that are highly permeable if continued for a sufficient period of time.

A much-debated question was whether fetal drug concentrations could exceed those in the mother with passive placental transfer. During the elimination phase after bolus administration, fetal concentrations are higher than maternal—but the peak fetal concentration will not exceed the peak maternal concentration (see Fig. 19.4A). Even for rapidly transferred substances, the peak concentration will be blunted. During continuous infusion (see Fig. 19.5A), mean steady-state concentrations in the fetus will not exceed maternal concentrations; however, during the elimination phase, fetal concentrations may exceed maternal levels. Moreover, total drug exposure in the fetus will not exceed that in the mother. In Figs. 19.4A and 19.5A, when there is no direct fetal clearance, not only is the area under the curve (measure of total drug exposure) the same in each fetus, but the area under the curve is the same in the mother as in the fetus. In the absence of direct fetal elimination, mean steady-state concentrations (or areas under the concentration time curves) in the fetus are equal to those in the mother. This is an important concept to grasp, because single maternal-fetal drug determinations after bolus drug administration have caused considerable confusion in the understanding of fetal drug exposure. In certain situations, mean active drug concentrations in the fetus can exceed maternal concentrations—for example, in the presence of active transport from the maternal to fetal circulation and after prodrug administration, when active drug metabolite concentrations can be higher in the fetus than in the mother. These circumstances are explored later.

PASSIVE TRANSFER OF DRUG ACROSS THE PLACENTA

It is held that most drugs cross the placenta by passive diffusion. Passive diffusion is the movement of substances in solution

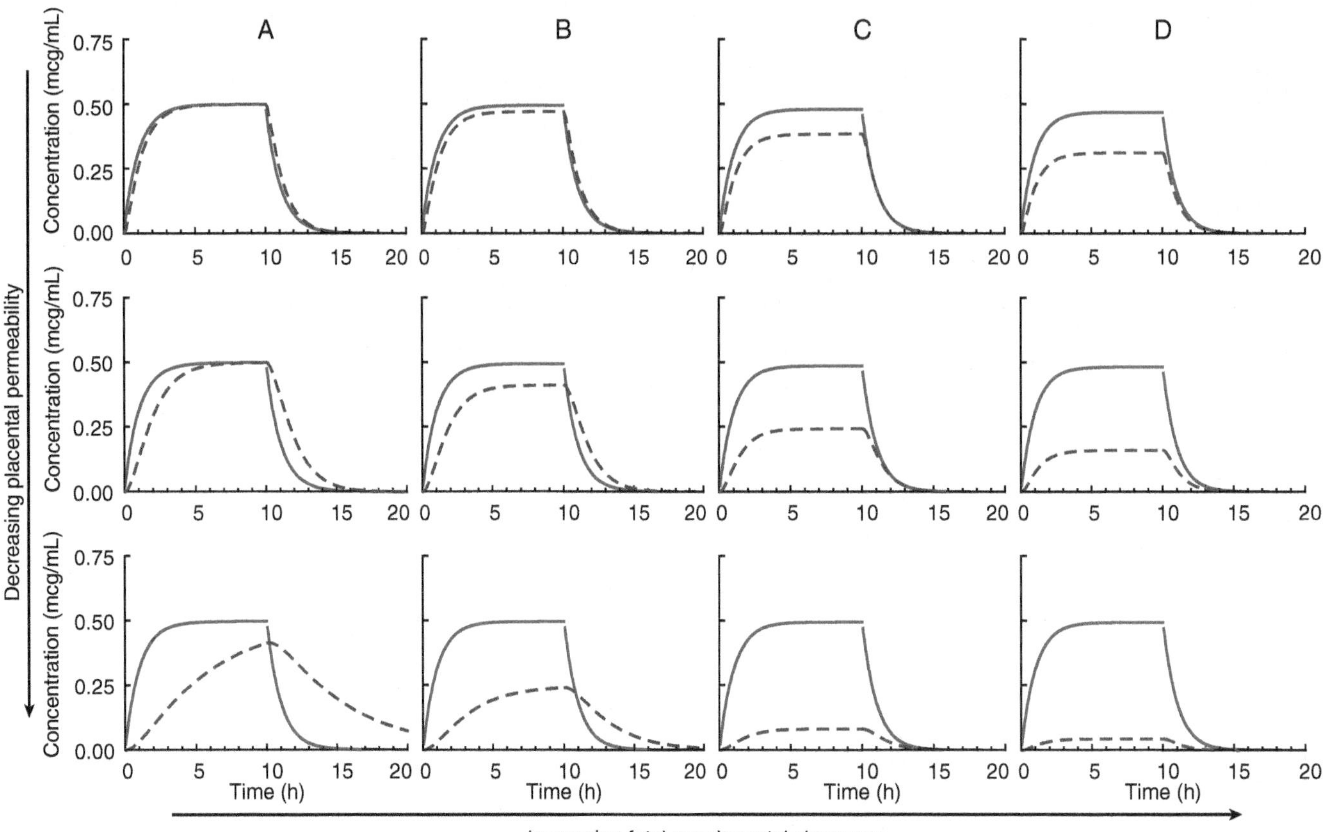

Fig. 19.5 Drug concentration-time curves for the mother *(solid blue line)* and the fetus *(dashed red line)* during and after a constant infusion of drug. These plots represent the solutions for the rate equations of a two-compartment model during and after infusion of drug wherein placental clearance (a measure of placental permeability) and fetal nonplacental clearance (direct fetal elimination) were varied, whereas all other system parameters remained constant. Steady-state concentrations provide a good estimate of fetal exposure in relation to maternal concentrations. See Fig. 19.4 for details on the specific parameter values.

across a semipermeable membrane, in this case, the placenta. This process uses the kinetic energy of the molecules, rather than any energy provided by cellular mechanisms. As molecules bounce around in solution, some will cross to the other side of the membrane. The percentage that crosses is determined by the number of molecules in solution (concentration) and the ease with which molecules cross. Subsequently, as a result of the random movements, a certain percentage of these molecules will in turn cross back to the other side, again dependent on the concentration and ease of transfer. Because the membrane is essentially the same in both directions, more molecules will cross from the side with the higher concentration, and net transfer will be to the side of lower concentration. Once equilibrium is reached, the concentrations on the two sides of the membrane will be the same, with no net transfer. Because net transfer is proportional to the concentration gradient across the membrane, it is not a measure of the permeability of the placenta.

Permeability is the ease with which a molecule (or drug) crosses a membrane and is a function of the membrane itself and properties of the molecules. The placental interface, as described previously, consists of a closely apposed layer of syncytiotrophoblast and fetal endothelial cells. Cell membranes consist of lipid bilayers and allow the passage of small, lipid-soluble molecules relatively easily. Tight junctions between endothelial cells in the placenta minimize paracellular transport. The composition of lipid membranes may alter transport characteristics. Known influences on lipid composition include diet, hormones, and pregnancy.[8]

Permeability can be considered per unit of placental tissue or as the placental unit as a whole. Traditional membrane studies express permeability in terms of surface area and thickness of the membrane. In the placenta, the membrane is very thin, and permeability is much more dependent on surface area. Because it is difficult to estimate placental surface area, permeability usually is expressed per unit of tissue mass or in terms of the whole placenta. For comparisons in different experimental situations, placental perfusion studies often report relative permeability comparing test drugs with known substances, usually antipyrine.[9]

Figs. 19.4 and 19.5 show examples of passive diffusion systems. The concentration of drug in maternal plasma and the initial lack of drug in fetal plasma provide the gradient across the placenta. In the case of bolus administration (see Fig. 19.4), net transfer of drug occurs from mother to fetus, and the fetal concentration increases until the concentration is equal in the maternal and fetal compartments. At this point, net transfer is zero. From this point on, the maternal concentration is less than the fetal concentration, and net transfer is from the fetus to the mother. In the case of a constant infusion (see Fig. 19.5), the fetal concentration increases owing to net transfer from mother to fetus until steady state is achieved Fig. 19.5A. With no elimination from the fetus, an equilibrium is established whereby the fetal and maternal concentrations are equal and no net transfer occurs in either direction. Drug molecules are still randomly crossing back and forth across the placenta as determined by the permeability and drug concentration, but at the same rate in both directions. When the drug infusion is stopped, the maternal concentration will fall, setting up a gradient from fetus to mother. This fundamental process provides the foundation for all distributive properties of drugs.

Rates of transfer from mother to fetus can be determined in experimental models. Using the Fick principle, measuring the change in concentration over either the uterine or umbilical circulations (at specific flow rates) will determine the amount of drug removed from maternal plasma or the amount of drug taken up by fetal plasma. These measurements can be achieved by in situ perfusion of whole placentas of small animals, controlling placental and umbilical blood flows, or in chronically instrumented sheep models using flow probes on uterine and umbilical circulations.[10] In addition, the human placenta can be perfused ex vivo.[9,11,12] When expressed relative to the transplacental gradient, this provides a measure of placental permeability. Of note, this measure has the same units as those for placental clearance (volume/time). This method can also determine the amount of drug eliminated by the placenta.

Another method uses mean steady-state concentrations in the mother and fetus applied to a two-compartment pharmacokinetic model (see Fig. 19.3).[7] This method calculates the placental clearances in both directions across the placenta and is used in sheep and primate models.[13-16] In the absence of active placental transport and placental metabolism, these placental clearances are measures of the permeability of the whole placenta. The advantage of this model is that blood flow measurements are not required. It does require drug administration to steady state (in both compartments) and drug determinations from both circulations. Neither of these methods can be used clinically, so extrapolations from animal and ex vivo placental perfusion studies are required to predict drug concentrations in the human fetus. The two-compartment model under steady-state conditions better reflects long-term drug therapy. In addition, parameters derived under steady-state conditions can be used to model single-dose situations.[6] Most of the equations and graphs in this chapter are generated from this model and provide a framework for understanding the effects that physiologic parameters have on fetal distribution.

Molecular size and solubility are the drug characteristics that determine drug permeability. Lipid-soluble drugs with molecular weights of up to 600 Da are readily transferred across the placenta. Water-soluble drugs up to 100 Da in size also readily cross; larger hydrophilic molecules cross according to their coefficient of diffusion in water.[12] Placental perfusion studies comparing substances of varying sizes and solubilities demonstrate relative permeability rankings that are a combination of the two factors.[9]

ACTIVE DRUG

When drugs are present in plasma, they are often bound to plasma proteins, or, if they are weak acids or bases, they exist in an ionized state. The bulk of the carrier protein or the ionic charge (positive or negative) impedes transfer. Only drug that is unbound and nonionized is available for transfer across the placenta; in this state, it often is referred to as *active* drug. The percentage of drug bound to protein is determined by the number and affinity of binding sites, whereas the percentage of drug ionized is determined by the pK_a (acid dissociation constant) of the drug and the pH of the plasma. In each case, drug will either bind or dissociate from the binding protein or shift between the ionized and nonionized forms of the drug. These chemical shifts occur rapidly. On the maternal side, the active drug concentration decreases as drug is transferred across the placenta to the fetus. Subsequently, drug bound to proteins will dissociate, and ionized drug will shift to a nonionized form; newly formed active drug will then be available for further transfer. On the fetal side, active drug increases in concentration and will bind to proteins and ionize to achieve the appropriate proportions determined by the fetal conditions. If protein-binding attributes and pH were the same in mother and fetus, total drug concentrations in the mother and the fetus would be the same at equilibrium. Because differences exist in protein binding and fetal pH is slightly less than maternal pH, total drug concentrations will be different in the fetal and the maternal compartments, whereas free drug concentrations will be the same.

The two major proteins involved in binding drugs are albumin and α_1-acid glycoprotein, the latter particularly involved in binding basic drugs.[2,3,17,18] During pregnancy, the maternal albumin concentration falls, although total albumin is increased.[17-19] In the fetus, albumin levels increase with gestation and, toward term, exceed those in the mother.[17] α_1-Acid glycoprotein levels tend to be rather variable in both the mother and fetus, but fetal levels are almost always less than maternal levels.[17,20] Protein binding is expressed as percent of drug protein bound. Equation (19.3) and Fig. 19.6 describe the relationship between protein binding in the mother (M) and fetus (F) and the effect on total drug concentration at steady state (C_{ss}).

$$C_{ssF_{total}} = \frac{C_{ssM_{unbound}}/C_{ssM_{total}}}{C_{ssF_{unbound}}/C_{ssF_{total}}} C_{ssM_{total}} \qquad [19.3]$$

Binding differences less than 40% to 60% tend to be insignificant. For drugs with high protein binding, however, a major effect on the fetal-to-maternal difference in total drug may be seen (Fig. 19.6, *right panel*). Although bound drug may seem to be of little relevance because it is not active, it serves as a depot that may prolong fetal or newborn exposure, particularly when affinity is high or when drug clearance in the newborn is poor.

The pK_a of a drug determines the degree of ionization at a specific pH. Usually, only a difference of 0.1 pH units exists between mother and fetus, so the difference in ionization is minimal. The effect of maternal and fetal pH differences on fetal-to-maternal concentration ratios of drugs that are weak acids and bases can be calculated from the Henderson-Hasselbach equation:

The Henderson-Hasselbach equation:

$$pH = pK_a + \log\frac{[base]}{[acid]} \qquad [19.4]$$

For weak acids:

$$C_{ssF_{total}} = \frac{1 + 10^{(pH_F - pK_a)}}{1 + 10^{(pH_M - pK_a)}} C_{ssM_{total}} \qquad [19.5]$$

For weak bases:

$$C_{ssF_{total}} = \frac{1 + 10^{(pK_a - pH_F)}}{1 + 10^{(pK_a - pH_M)}} C_{ssM_{total}} \qquad [19.6]$$

Weak acids are less ionized and weak bases are more ionized at lower pH. As fetal pH decreases below maternal pH, the amount of total drug in the fetus will change (Fig. 19.7); weak acids will decrease in amount, whereas weak bases will increase. As long as the pH differential is maintained, drug effect will not be altered because active drug levels are not affected. In the fetus, transition back to a normal pH is likely to be gradual and placental redistribution will occur without exposure of the fetus to excessive (for basic) or subtherapeutic (for acidic) concentrations of active drug. If at the time of delivery the fetal pH is low, total concentration of basic drugs may be higher than in the mother. Then, as the pH corrects in the newborn, drug quickly returns to an active nonionized state and adverse drug effects may occur. For acidic drugs, drug concentrations in the newborn infant may be less that that required for therapeutic benefit after resolution of fetal acidosis. This effect is well described for lidocaine.[20]

PLACENTAL BLOOD FLOW

The two sides of the placenta are perfused independently. Maternal placental blood flow is about twice that going through the umbilical circulation (see Chapter 10). Experimental

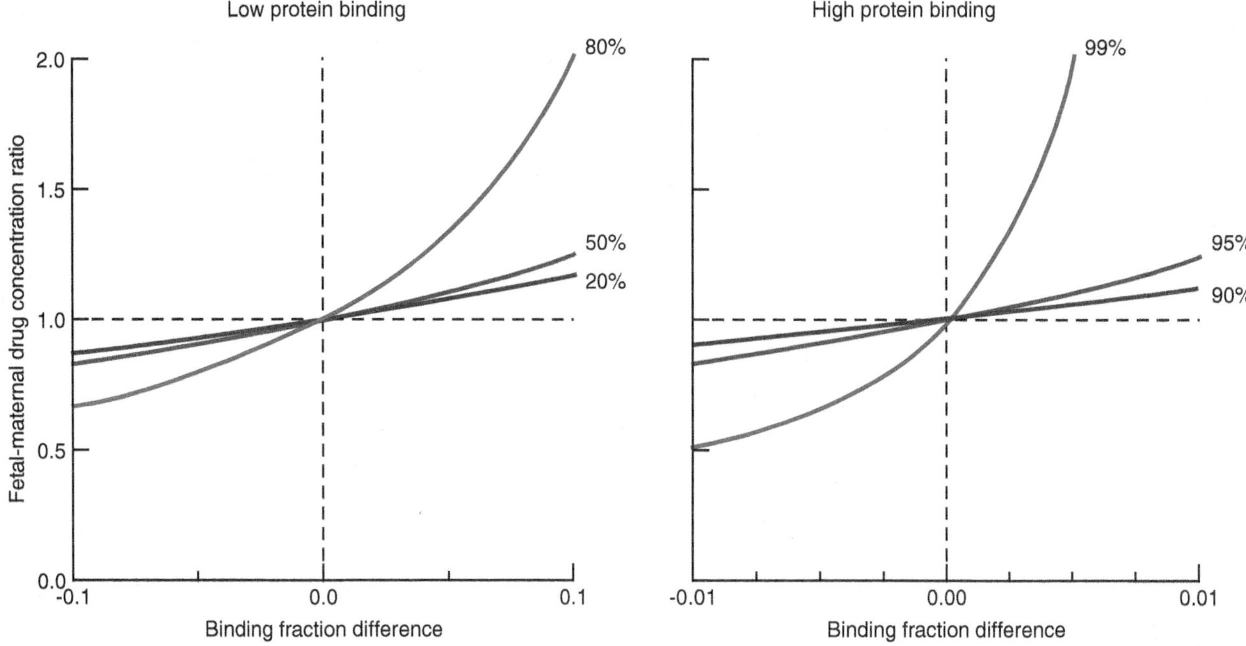

Fig. 19.6 Effect of fetal-maternal differences in protein binding on steady-state fetal-to-maternal total drug concentrations. Recall that unbound drug concentrations will be the same in the fetus as in the mother. Drugs that exhibit low protein binding (up to around 50%) exhibit only small differences in the fetal-to-maternal concentration ratio, even with binding differences up to 10%. As binding increases, more marked effects are seen. For drugs that are highly protein bound, even small differences (<1%) can have marked effects on fetal-to-maternal total drug ratio. Graphs are plotted from Equation (19.3) for various levels of maternal protein binding, with fetal protein binding ±10% of maternal for left-hand graph and ±1% of maternal for right-hand graph.

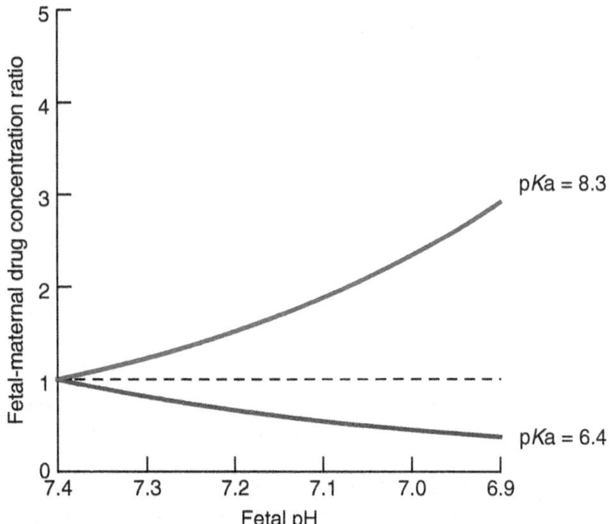

Fig. 19.7 Effect of fetal-maternal pH differences on steady-state fetal-to-maternal total drug concentrations. Recall that non-ionized active drug concentrations will be the same in the fetus as in the mother. Total concentrations of weak acids *(red line)* will be less in the fetus, whereas total concentrations of weak bases *(blue line)* will be higher in the fetus. Graph is plotted from Equations (19.5) and (19.6) with maternal pH set at 7.4.

situations show that decreasing blood flow, particularly in the umbilical circulation, will decrease delivery of freely diffusible drugs across the placenta (flow limited) but will have little effect on drugs that are *permeability limited*. Placental circulations are fairly stable at most times in pregnancy but will show gradual increases over gestation. Fetal compromise and uterine contractions are two clinical entities in which decreased fetal drug transfer has been demonstrated clinically. Changes in blood flow are unlikely to affect steady-state levels achieved, unless the increased blood flow enhances nonplacental clearance mechanisms in the mother or the fetus.

ACTIVE TRANSPORT OF DRUG ACROSS THE PLACENTA

Cell membranes, including those of the syncytiotrophoblast and villous capillary endothelium, contain large numbers of transport proteins that require cellular energy to function.[21,22] The specificity, orientation (into or out of the cell), and position (whether luminal or basal membrane) are important factors in determining the effect placental transporters will have on drug disposition. Few drugs appear to be entirely dependent on active transport for transfer across the placenta to the fetus. Most drugs will cross to the fetus by passive diffusion. However, placental transport proteins may modify the final concentrations achieved.

The transporters involved in drug disposition belong primarily to two classes.[21,22] These are the ATP-dependent binding cassette proteins *(ABC transporters)* and the solute-linked carrier proteins *(SLC transporters)*. In the placenta, ABC transporters cause efflux of drug from the syncytiotrophoblast or fetal endothelium. Energy in the form of ATP is required for activity. ABCB1 (P-glycoprotein) and ABCG2 (breast cancer-related protein [BCRP]) are located in the apical membrane, directing drug toward the maternal circulation. ABCB2 (multidrug-resistant protein 2 [MRP2]) and ABCC1 (multidrug-resistant protein 1 [MRP1]) are on the basolateral membrane and direct drug toward the fetus.[21] Several ABC transporters are present on the fetal endothelium and can direct drug toward the fetus.[21] The SLC transporters are a more diverse group and organic anion transporters (OCT), organic cation transporters (OCT), and novel organic cation transporters (OCTN).[21] They are often found localized to the basolateral membrane. These transporters use the electrochemical gradient of the cell for energy and can transfer substrates in both directions. Although solute exchange is not obligatory, solute exchange can allow transfer against a concentration gradient by using the electrochemical gradient of the co-substrate.

The overall impact of transporters on drug disposition is to protect the fetus from drug exposure.[3,22-24] Studies in placental culture systems, the perfused human placenta, and mouse models wherein P-glycoprotein was inhibited show significant increases in drug levels on the fetal side.[24-27] In mice lacking ABCB1, increases in drug toxicity have been demonstrated in the fetus.[27] Furthermore, placental ABC transporters are differentially regulated by development, hormone concentrations, inflammatory cytokines, and growth factors.[28,29] In the two-compartment model, active transport will be reflected by differences in the maternal-to-fetal and fetal-to-maternal clearances. Active efflux transport from fetus to mother will effectively reduce fetal drug exposure.

OTHER TRANSPORT MECHANISMS

Facilitated diffusion processes are known to occur in the placenta for delivery of nutrients and disposal of waste products, and they also have a role in drug transfer.[21,30] Specific macromolecules are taken up across the placenta by pinocytosis that is often receptor mediated. Immunoglobulin G is transported across the placenta by binding the neonatal Fc receptor present on the syncytiotrophoblast and placental endothelium.[31,32] Recently a monoclonal antibody against this receptor has been shown to reduce placental transfer of IgG and is being investigated as a therapy for immune-mediated diseases of the fetus and neonate.[33] Aquaporins present in the placenta may provide bulk flow channels for small hydrophilic drug molecules.[28]

PLACENTAL METABOLISM

The placenta is a highly metabolic organ, producing and modifying many different hormones. However, the extent to which drugs are metabolized is not well delineated. Several members of the cytochrome P-450 subclasses are present and capable of metabolizing drugs at the maternal-fetal interface, though expression is often less than in other tissues.[34-36] Using sensitive methods, conjugation enzymes have also been detected in the placenta.[37] Again, the extent to which they diminish fetal exposure is unclear. The placenta will act as a first-pass clearance system and decrease drug concentrations reaching the fetus. However, the fetus may well be exposed to metabolites of drugs that are not always harmless.[38] In the two-compartment model with maternal administration, placental metabolism would have the same effect as fetal metabolism.

MODIFIERS OF FETAL PLASMA CONCENTRATION

FETAL CIRCULATION

Streaming of oxygenated blood from the umbilical vein, through the ductus venosus and foramen ovale in the heart, leads to the delivery of better-oxygenated blood to the head and upper extremities. Thus, the concept of having different distribution in separate regions is not new. The high extraction of oxygen from fetal blood maintains this differential across the placenta, and thus the difference in carotid arterial and descending aortic oxygen tensions is able to persist. A similar phenomenon is likely to occur with drugs that cross the placenta, although it has never been clearly documented. This difference will be most pronounced when the umbilical arteriovenous difference is greatest—most likely to occur after bolus administration or for drugs highly metabolized by the fetus.

Another situation in which the fetal circulation affects drug distribution is in the liver.[39-41] The fetal liver is the first organ encountered by fetal blood returning from the placenta. In the healthy fetus at mid-gestation around 27% to 40% of umbilical blood flow is diverted through the ductus venosus, reducing to 15% as term approaches.[39,40] Pathologic conditions can lead to redistribution of umbilical blood flow. In severely growth-restricted fetuses, the ductus venosus shunt in the third trimester is around 90%, with less first-pass fetal drug clearance.[40]

FETAL DRUG CLEARANCE

Thus far the discussion has been limited to systems in which the fetal nonplacental clearance is zero. In the case of zidovudine, fetal steady-state levels were less than those in the mother (see Fig. 19.1). These differences cannot be attributed to differences in protein binding, pH, or active transport.[13] Clear evidence demonstrates that the fetus can metabolize zidovudine to its glucuronide metabolite.[13] Fig. 19.3 and Equation (19.2) include an elimination component by the fetus. The effect of direct fetal clearance on fetal drug concentrations is shown in Fig. 19.4B–D, with oral administration, and in Fig. 19.5B–D, with intravenous administration (see Figs. 19.4 and 19.5). Direct fetal clearance lowers fetal drug concentrations; this decrease is most marked when placental permeability is reduced. Of note, this effect differs from those of protein binding and ionization in that fetal clearance affects active drug concentrations and hence reduces active drug concentrations in the fetus.

THE TWO-COMPARTMENT MODEL AT STEADY STATE

In many of the examples given, the effect of changes in physiologic parameters is best appreciated by comparing steady-state concentrations in the mother and the fetus. A relationship between fetal and maternal plasma concentrations can be deduced from the rate equations for the two-compartment model under steady-state conditions. As noted above, under steady-state conditions the amount of drug in a compartment does not change with time—that is, the amount of drug being added to the system is the same as that leaving the system.

Rate equation for maternal compartment at steady state:

$$\frac{dD_m}{dt} = R_m - Cl_m \cdot c_m - Cl_{mf} \cdot c_m + Cl_{fm} \cdot c_f = 0 \qquad [19.7]$$

Rate equation for fetal compartment at steady state:

$$\frac{dD_f}{dt} = Cl_{mf} \cdot c_m - Cl_{fm} \cdot c_f - Cl_f \cdot c_f = 0 \qquad [19.8]$$

Rearranging the fetal equation gives an expression that relates fetal steady-state plasma concentration to the maternal concentration:

$$\frac{C_{ssF}}{C_{ssM}} = \frac{Cl_{mf}}{Cl_{fm} + Cl_f} \qquad [19.9]$$

This expression shows the interdependence of fetal clearance mechanisms and placental permeability in determining fetal drug exposure. For drugs that cross the placenta by passive diffusion, Cl_{mf} will be equal to Cl_{fm} (clearance being an attribute of the placenta and a measure of placental permeability). When fetal nonplacental clearance and placental clearance are equal, the fetal concentration is half the maternal concentration (see Figs. 19.4 and 19.5C, *middle row*). Furthermore, the same degree of fetal nonplacental clearance will lead to a more marked decrease in fetal plasma concentration when placental clearance (or permeability) is low (see Figs. 19.4 and 19.5C, *bottom row*).

FETAL ELIMINATION MECHANISMS

Drug-metabolizing enzymes are both present and active in the fetal liver, albeit at reduced levels compared with the adult liver for most enzymes.[42-49] As seen in the model in Fig. 19.5, even small amounts of fetal clearance can have marked effects on the fetal-maternal drug ratio, depending on placental permeability. As might be expected, drug-metabolizing capacity will increase as gestation advances; however, placental permeability also increases with advancing gestation. In the sheep, fetal metabolism of acetaminophen increases concordant with growth.[49] In the baboon, fetal morphine metabolism does not appear to change over a similar period of time.[50] Another potential issue is induction of drug-metabolizing enzymes. Maternal smoking is known to induce many placental enzymes, but little is known about corresponding induction of fetal hepatic enzymes prenatally. Phenobarbital has been used successfully near term to reduce hyperbilirubinemia by induction of glucuronosyltransferase UGT1A1.[51]

The products of metabolism also must be considered. These often are inactive; however, some metabolites are known mutagens, some are pharmacologically active, and others are true drugs in that a prodrug was administered.[6,52] Rate equations for metabolite formation can be written for the two-compartment model. The solution for these equations is clearly more complex, even at steady state, but fetal metabolite concentration can be expressed as a function of maternal concentration.[53] In this instance, because the metabolite is being formed in the fetus and because placental clearance for metabolites is often less than for the drug, the tendency is for fetal metabolite concentrations to exceed those in the mother unless other clearance pathways exist.

In adults, the other major route of drug elimination is urinary excretion. The fetal urinary excretion system is unique in that fetal urine, a major component of amniotic fluid, is swallowed by the fetus, thereby providing the potential for any drug excreted in fetal urine to be absorbed back into the fetus through the fetal intestinal tract.[54] The extent to which this occurs is not known. Clearly, not all drugs are reabsorbed in their entirety, because many can be detected in meconium. Under steady-state conditions, drug excreted into urine that is reabsorbed would not contribute to fetal nonplacental clearance; however, drug that becomes sequestered in meconium would contribute to that clearance.

TISSUE DISTRIBUTION

Volume of distribution is a term used to describe the volume a drug appears to occupy based on the plasma concentration; it has little bearing on the physical system. Volumes of distribution vary from drug to drug based on the drug's solubility in different tissues, reflective of the tissues' lipid and water content and binding to tissue proteins. Individual patients also differ in body composition. The fetus has a high water content, so lipid-soluble drugs will not have a large volume of distribution. For water-soluble drugs, the volume of distribution would be expected to be higher (per tissue mass) than in the adult, particularly if the amniotic fluid compartment cannot be separated out. Fat deposition occurs during the last trimester, so during this period the capacity for transfer of lipid-soluble drugs would be greater. Drug would concentrate into fat tissues until steady state is achieved. Because the fetal volume of distribution is small compared with that of the mother, the effect of fetal changes is unlikely to be detectable in maternal plasma concentrations. The total amount of drug delivered to the fetus, however, could be substantially higher.

FETAL BLOOD-BRAIN BARRIERS

The brain has evolved a complex set of protections to shield it from external influences and still provide passage for essential nutrients and communication signals.[55-59] The capillaries that supply the brain are continuous (nonfenestrated), have extremely tight junctions preventing paracellular transport, and are surrounded by astrocytic foot processes.[58] Several transporters are present in the endothelium, transporting drugs among other substances from the endothelium back to the circulation.[58] Pial membranes carry blood vessels across the surface of the brain. Where the pial membrane comes in contact with the ependyma of the ventricular system, choroidal tissue develops.[58] The capillaries within the choroidal tissue are fenestrated; however, the overlying ependyma is highly specialized with very tight junctions; therefore, transfer is essentially all transcellular. Several drug-metabolizing enzymes have been identified in choroidal ependymal tissue and are thought to protect the brain from substrates.[59] In addition, many transporters are present on both luminal and abluminal sides.[55,57] With respect to drugs, P-glycoprotein is on the abluminal side, removing drugs or their metabolites from the ependymal cell back to the capillary. Other transporters are present on the luminal and abluminal membranes, transporting substances into and out of the ependymal cells. The remainder of the ependyma that is in contact with the ventricular system forms a loose network of cells with minimal barrier function. Thus, once in the cerebrospinal fluid, drugs have access to target neurons that lie near brain surfaces. Within the brain itself, certain cells have been identified as containing drug-metabolizing enzymes, although whether their function is protective or activational is not clear.[60,61] Transporters also are present on neuronal cells. Although not all of the details are known at this time, the distribution of drug-metabolizing enzymes and specific transporters at specific sites give some hint of the complexity to unfold.

The fetal blood-brain barrier is more robust than was once thought, although developmental differences are present. Much ongoing research in neonatology is directed toward neuroprotection of the fetal and neonatal brain.[62] Hence understanding brain distribution of potential agents requires prediction of the concentration at the site of action to optimize effectiveness. Again, the plasma concentration is the driving force for drug movement by passive diffusion of drugs down a concentration gradient modulated by metabolism and active transportation.

Box 19.1 Key Points in Fetal Drug Distribution

- The maternal plasma concentration is the driving force for drug delivery to the fetus.
- Drug size and solubility determine a drug's placental (and tissue) permeability.
- Protein binding and ionization of drugs can lead to prolonged exposure for the neonate after birth.
- Fetal elimination mechanisms decrease fetal plasma concentration most markedly for drugs with low permeability.
- Products of fetal metabolism (drug metabolites or active moieties of prodrugs) can reach higher levels in the fetus than in the mother.
- Drug transporters and drug-metabolizing enzymes are important regulators of drug concentrations at the site of action.

CLINICAL APPLICATIONS

Most drugs taken during pregnancy are for the mother's benefit; however, use of drugs for fetal benefit is increasing. Various clinical scenarios can be encountered with ramifications for the patient and the unintentional recipient. Optimally, a drug that achieves therapeutic concentrations in the mother while minimizing fetal concentrations will be selected for maternal treatment, whereas a drug that achieves therapeutic concentrations in the fetus while minimizing maternal adverse effects will be selected for fetal treatment. An appreciation of fetal drug distribution and drug properties (Box 19.1) will allow selection of appropriate drugs to attain these goals. Drugs are developed primarily for use in nonpregnant adults, and desired characteristics include good oral bioavailability, good tissue distribution, and long half-life—properties that generally lend themselves to placental transfer and hence fetal exposure. Furthermore, what may generally be seen as improvements in drug formulation may alter distributive characteristics unfavorably for the fetus.

A complete reference list is available at www.ExpertConsult.com.

SELECT REFERENCES

1. Garland M. Pharmacology of drug transfer across the placenta. *Obstet Gynecol Clin North Am*. 1998;25(1):21-42.
2. TasnifY, Morado J, Hebert MF. Pregnancy-related pharmacokinetic changes. *Clin Pharmacol Ther*. 2016;100(1):53-62.
3. Ward RM, Varner MW. Principles of pharmacokinetics in the pregnant woman and fetus. *Clin Perinatol*. 2019;46(2):383-398.
4. Turco MY, Moffett A. Development of the human placenta. *Development*. 2019;146(22):dev163428.
7. Szeto HH, Umans JG, Rubinow SI. The contribution of transplacental clearances and fetal clearance to drug disposition in the ovine maternal-fetal unit. *Drug Metab Dispos*. 1982;10:382-386.
9. Hutson JR, et al. The human placental perfusion model: a systematic review and development of a model to predict in vivo transfer of therapeutic drugs. *Clin Pharmacol Ther*. 2011;90(1):67-76.
17. Krauer B, Dayer P, Anner R. Changes in serum albumin and alpha 1-acid glycoprotein concentrations during pregnancy: an analysis of fetal-maternal pairs. *Br J Obstet Gynaecol*. 1984;91(9):875-881.
18. Perucca E, Crema A. Plasma protein binding of drugs in pregnancy. *Clin Pharmacokinet*. 1982;7(4):336-352.
19. Whittaker PG, Lind T. The intravascular mass of albumin during human pregnancy: a serial study in normal and diabetic women. *Br J Obstet Gynaecol*. 1993;100(6):587-592.
20. Liu L, Liu X. Contributions of drug transporters to blood-placental barrier. *Adv Exp Med Biol*. 2019;1141:505-548.
23. Dallmann A, et al. Clinical pharmacokinetic studies in pregnant women and the relevance of pharmacometric tools. *Curr Pharm Des*. 2019;25(5):483-495.
32. Leach JL, et al. Isolation from human placenta of the IgG transporter, FcRn, and localization to the syncytiotrophoblast: implications for maternal-fetal antibody transport. *J Immunol*. 1996;157(8):3317-3322.
38. Hakkola J, et al. Xenobiotic-metabolizing cytochrome P450 enzymes in the human feto-placental unit: role in intrauterine toxicity. *Crit Rev Toxicol*. 1998;28(1):35-72.
39. Bellotti M, et al. Role of ductus venosus in distribution of umbilical blood flow in human fetuses during second half of pregnancy. *Am J Physiol Heart Circ Physiol*. 2000;279(3):H1256-H1263.
40. Bellotti M, Pennati G, Ferrazzi E. Re: ductus venosus shunting in growth-restricted fetuses and the effect of umbilical circulatory compromise. *Ultrasound Obstet Gynecol*. 2007;29(1):100-101, author reply 101-2.
41. Rudolph AM. Hepatic and ductus venosus blood flows during fetal life. *Hepatology*. 1983;3:254-258.
44. Matlock MK, et al. A time-embedding network models the ontogeny of 23 hepatic drug metabolizing enzymes. *Chem Res Toxicol*. 2019;32(8):1707-1721.
47. Ring JA, et al. Fetal hepatic drug elimination. *Pharmacol Ther*. 1999;84(3):429-445.
53. Garland M, et al. Maternal-fetal pharmacokinetics: the two-compartment model revisited. *Pediatric Research*. 1996;39(5).
54. Brace RA, Anderson DF, Cheung CY. Regulation of amniotic fluid volume: mathematical model based on intramembranous transport mechanisms. *Am J Physiol Regul Integr Comp Physiol*. 2014;307(10):R1260-R1273.
58. Strazielle N, Ghersi-Egea JF. Physiology of blood-brain interfaces in relation to brain disposition of small compounds and macromolecules. *Mol Pharm*. 2013;10(5):1473-1491.
59. Kratzer I, et al. Developmental changes in the transcriptome of the rat choroid plexus in relation to neuroprotection. *Fluids Barriers CNS*. 2013;10(1):25.
62. Ophelders D, et al. Preterm Brain injury, antenatal triggers, and therapeutics: timing is key. *Cells*. 2020;9(8).

20 Drug Transfer During Breastfeeding

Thomas W. Hale | Kaytlin Krutsch

INTRODUCTION

Since the early 2000s, researchers and clinicians have greatly expanded the knowledge base of drug entry kinetics as they relate to human milk. Most of the physiochemical properties that affect a drug's transfer into milk are well known and understood today.[1,2] For the busy clinician, the National Institutes of Health[3] and others[4] have published reference works that consolidate the evidence supporting the relative safety ratings of common medications. However, many newer drugs have not yet been studied, and usable data related to lactation may be scarce.

Breastfeeding is incredibly important to the health and well-being of infants. Breast-fed infants endure fewer ear infections,[5] have improved cognitive abilities,[6,7] and enjoy a reduced risk of psychiatric disorders as adults.[8-10] The risks of incidental drug exposure in the infant rarely outweigh the benefits of breastfeeding, and a recommendation for complete breastfeeding cessation is almost never required.

PRINCIPLES OF DRUG EXCRETION

THE ALVEOLAR SUBUNIT AND BREAST MILK PRODUCTION

Fig. 20.1 illustrates breast anatomy including the ductal system. Milk ducts extend from the nipple, backward into the breast fat pads, and terminate in extensive, grapelike, lobular-alveolar clusters, as illustrated in Fig. 20.2. Each alveolus is lined with a single layer of polarized, secretory epithelial cells called *lactocytes* that are uniquely capable of synthesizing human milk. A basket-like network of myoepithelium surrounds each alveolus. These specialized smooth muscle cells have receptors for oxytocin and, when stimulated, contract to force milk out of the alveoli and into the terminal ductal system near the nipple.

During pregnancy, circulating maternal hormones (estrogen, progesterone, placental lactogen, prolactin, and oxytocin) induce a substantial increase in the size and number of alveolar complexes. However, plasma progesterone suppresses the lactocytes themselves from making milk, keeping them relatively small in size and poorly functional.[11]

Early in the postpartum period, the initial fluid secreted by the lactocytes is called *colostrum*. Colostrum has limited fat and low volume, averaging less than 60 mL for the first few days. During this early postnatal stage of development, large intercellular gaps exist between the lactocytes, and numerous components from the maternal plasma are able to enter the colostrum. These include immunoglobulins (IgG, IgA, IgM, and IgE), white blood cells, and a variety of other cellular materials from the maternal circulation. Colostrum also provides important gastrointestinal (GI) tract growth factors, such as insulin-like growth factor-1(IGF-1), and maternal antibodies that suppress hazardous bacterial growth. Early breast milk even seeds the infant gut with beneficial microorganisms.[12]

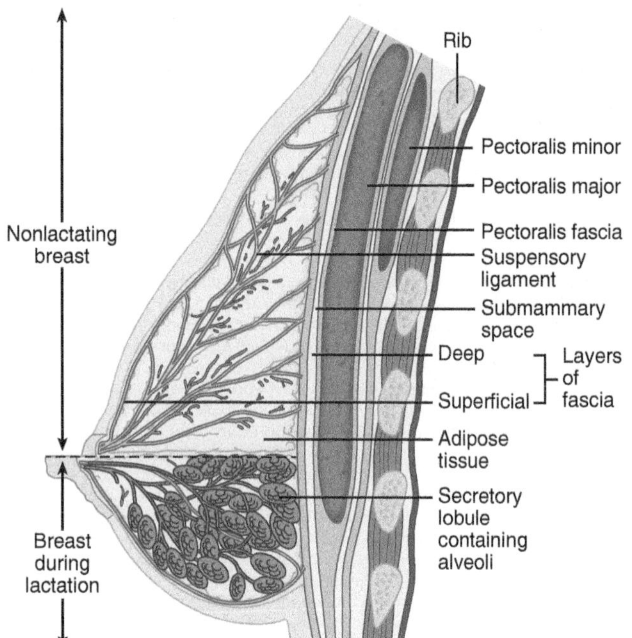

Fig. 20.1 Lactating breast. (Reprinted with permission from Katz VL, Dotters D. Breast diseases: diagnosis and treatment of benign and malignant disease. In: Lentz G, ed. *Comprehensive Gynecology*. Philadelphia; Elsevier: 2013:301–334. © 2013, Figure 15.3.)

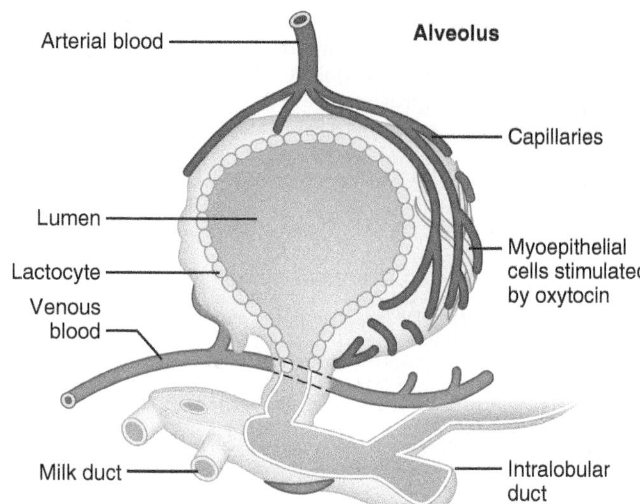

Fig. 20.2 Structure of the alveolar subunit with blood supply and milk-creating lactocytes. (Modified from Vorherr H. *The Breast: Morphology, Physiology and Lactation*. New York: Academic Press; 1974.)

After delivery of the placenta, maternal estrogen and progesterone levels drop to below the pre-pregnancy baseline. Progesterone levels in particular reach a minimum approximately 40 hours postpartum, assuming there are no retained placental fragments. With the inhibitory influence of progesterone removed from the lactocytes, prolactin is free to stimulate copious milk synthesis and release. This is followed by a prolonged maintenance period of galactopoiesis. Thyroid hormones and low levels of estrogen play a role in stimulating milk production, but a consistently high prolactin level is the paramount factor in the maintenance of milk volume. The lactocytes also grow in number and connect to one another via an apical junctional complex that blocks direct paracellular exchange of substances between the maternal plasma and the breast milk. The resulting layer of cells, called the *lactocyte barrier*, has many similarities to the blood-brain barrier in terms of what substances are able to cross. The cell-to-cell junctions persist until lactation ceases, whereupon the lactocytes begin to involute and disappear.

DRUG TRANSFER FROM MATERNAL CIRCULATION INTO BREAST MILK

Once the alveolar lactocytes have established their junctional complexes, the conjoined apical membranes of the individual cells form a cohesive lactocyte barrier able to regulate the transit of substances in and out of the milk compartment. The pathways for drug entry into milk are illustrated in Fig. 20.3. Although there are some notable exceptions, which will be discussed later, drug transfer in and out of human milk is largely a result of a passive diffusion gradient driven by maternal plasma levels.

The concentration of a drug in milk (C_{milk}) determines infant exposure. Clinical trials that assess breastfeeding safety will report the mother's dose and a series of C_{milk} values as samples are collected throughout the trial. This direct measurement of C_{milk} is the most accurate and useful way to estimate the amount of drug that the infant receives. If these studies are not available, as is frequently the case with newer drugs, then a theoretical estimation of C_{milk} is the next best choice. The factors discussed in this section are the tools used to generate that estimate.

MILK/PLASMA RATIO

The ratio of the concentration of a drug in a mother's breast milk to that in her plasma is known as the *milk/plasma* (M/P) *ratio*. M/P is an experimentally determined value for each drug. Because it is the interaction between the lactocyte barrier and the drug's physiochemical properties that determines the M/P ratio, this value for a given drug tends to be fairly consistent in mothers taking the same drug under the same circumstances. Drugs that easily pass through the barrier have high M/P ratios, whereas drugs that cannot pass have low ratios. Note that during periods where the barrier is incomplete, such as the secretory differentiation stage (differentiation of epithelial cells into lactocytes) or late involution stage (death of secretory cells and replacement by adipocytes), drugs cannot be excluded from the milk compartment, and the M/P ratio approaches 1:1. Also, the M/P ratio does not account for active metabolites.

The primary use of the M/P ratio is to give some indication of the underlying mechanisms that affect a drug's transfer into milk. Clinically, it has little to no role in assessing drug safety during breastfeeding unless it is exceedingly low. Many drugs with high M/P ratios still fail to attain clinically relevant doses via breast milk.

ACTIVE TRANSPORT OF MEDICATIONS

There are only a handful of drugs known to enter the milk via an energy-dependent influx transporter. These substances have an M/P ratio significantly higher than what is predicted based on the drug's physiochemical properties alone. The drugs with a hypothesized active transport mechanism are nitrofurantoin (M/P = 6),[13] acyclovir (M/P = 4.1),[14] ranitidine (M/P = 6.7 to 23.77),[15] cimetidine (M/P = 5),[16] and iodine (M/P = 23).[17,18] Although these drugs may be concentrated in milk, they normally do not attain ranges that have a clinical effect and, with the exception of iodine, are quite safe to use in breastfeeding mothers. Iodine is transported so extensively that clinically hazardous ranges have been noted causing hypothyroidism in neonates.[17]

It is also possible that active transport of drugs out of the breast milk compartment exists. For example, the plasma glycoprotein gene is extensively expressed in intestinal

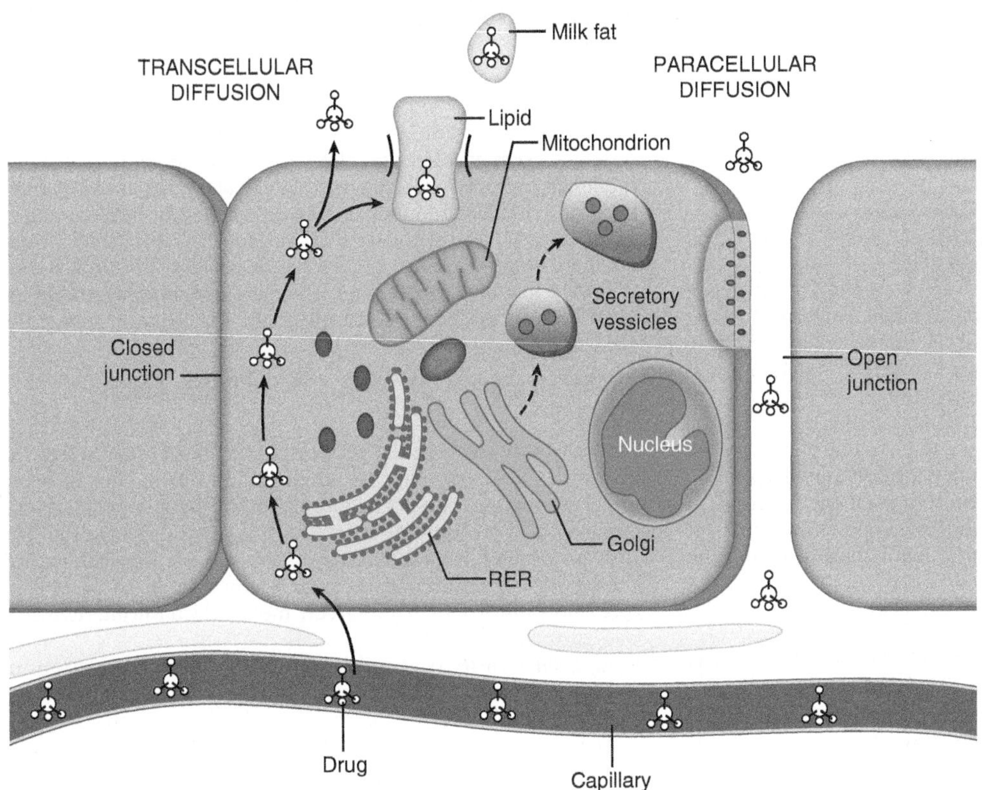

Fig. 20.3 Diagrammatic representation of the various pathways for drug transfer into the human milk compartment. (Reprinted with permission from Hale TW, Kristensen JH, Ilett KF, Hartmann PE. *The Transfer of Medications into Human Milk. Textbook of Human Lactation*. 1st ed. Amarillo: Hale Publishing LP; 2007:465–478.)

epithelium, the blood-brain barrier, hepatocytes, and renal tubules.The plasma membrane protein that this gene encodes is an efflux transporter that actively transports drugs out of cells.[19] Metformin provides an example. Assuming a passive diffusion model, theoretical calculations of the transfer of metformin into human milk would suggest an M/P ratio of 2.9.[20] However, three studies have reported much lower M/P values (0.63, 0.35, and 0.46, respectively) and a flat milk concentration-time profile.[20-22] The lower observed M/P ratios may indicate an active efflux transporter, pumping metformin out of milk and back into the plasma.[23]

MOLECULAR WEIGHT AND PROTEIN BINDING

Molecular weight is the most important determinant of how easily a substance will diffuse across a lipid bilayer, like the lactocyte barrier. Small, nonpolar molecules (<400 Da) are more likely to cross, whereas larger molecules (>800 Da) are unlikely to cross without a dedicated transport mechanism. Many preparations, such as enoxaparin (8000 Da), insulin (6000 Da), and botulism toxin (150,000 Da), are far too large to enter the milk compartment in clinically relevant amounts.Although these drugs have a concerning side-effect profile, due to their near total exclusion from milk, they are considered compatible with breastfeeding.

Most drugs travel in plasma bound to albumin or other plasma-carrier proteins. Those with high binding affinity behave like large-molecular-weight compounds and have difficulty diffusing out of the plasma. Only the free (unbound) drug is available to transfer into milk and other peripheral compartments. For example, small drugs (300 Da), such as warfarin sodium and celecoxib, are found in such low levels in milk as to be clinically irrelevant, mostly because they are 99% protein bound in the plasma.[24] Alternatively, lithium, with no protein binding and a low molecular weight of 6.94 Da, readily enters the milk and can reach high levels.

LIPID SOLUBILITY

The lipid content of milk is high, ranging from 2.3% in foremilk to as high as 8% in hindmilk. In a laboratory setting, the lipophilicity of a drug is measured by its octanol-water partition coefficient ($\log_{10}P$). The more lipid soluble a drug, the better it is able to penetrate through the lactocyte barrier and become concentrated in the milk. Such drugs are often those that penetrate the blood-brain barrier and produce high levels in the central nervous system (CNS).The antidepressant mirtazapine is a classic example.The concentration of mirtazapine in hindmilk (high lipid content) is 2.3 times higher than in foremilk (low lipid content).Thus, if a drug is active in the CNS, it may produce higher levels in breast milk as well.

DRUG DEGREE OF IONIZATION AND MILK TRAPPING

The degree of ionization (pK_a) of a drug is a unique physicochemical property that controls its ionization state when in solution. If the drug's pK_a is the same as the pH of the solution it is dissolved in, then 50% of the drug exists ionized and 50% exists nonionized.As the pH of the solution changes, the state of ionization changes as well. Because the pH of milk (7.2) is lower than that of plasma (7.4), drugs with a pK_a greater than 7.4 will partially ionize in the milk compartment. Ionized compounds are less lipophilic and are less able to pass through a lipid bilayer. The newly ionized form of the drug may have difficulty diffusing back out of the milk. Thus, the ion-trapping phenomenon can significantly elevate C_{milk} above what is expected from passive diffusion alone.[25]

VOLUME OF DISTRIBUTION

A drug's volume of distribution (V_d) is the theoretical amount of water in which a given dose would have to be dissolved to produce an experimentally measured maximum plasma concentration. A dose of a drug that has a high V_d produces a lower plasma concentration than the same dose of a drug with a low V_d. The concentration of a drug in milk is almost exclusively dependent on the concentration of that drug in the mother's plasma; therefore drugs with a high V_d tend to produce lower levels in milk. Drugs with a very high volume of distribution, such as digoxin (V_d = 6 to 7 L/kg) or marijuana, tend to concentrate in the peripheral tissues and do not appear in the milk in clinically relevant amounts after the absorption phase.

TRANSFER OF DRUG FROM BREAST MILK TO THE INFANT

Ultimately, the evaluation of risk to the infant depends on how toxic the drug is and how much of it the infant receives.[26] There are two ways of calculating the infant's dose: the absolute infant dose (AID) and the relative infant dose (RID).[27]

ABSOLUTE INFANT DOSE

The AID is an estimate of the drug concentration in milk (per mL) multiplied by the volume of milk received each day, where C_{max} is equal to the maximum concentration of drug in milk or where C_{ave} is the average concentration of drug in milk throughout the dosing period:

$$\text{AID} = (C_{max} \text{ or } C_{ave}) - (\text{Volume of milk ingested in a day}) \quad (20.1)$$

The use of C_{max} almost always leads to an overestimate of the actual infant dose. When C_{ave} is available, it is more clinically useful. This method assumes that the volume of milk received each day is known. However, many mothers who do not pump do not actually know the volume of milk they feed to the infant each day. Most sources now use a value of 150 mL/kg/day, where kg refers to infant weight, as an estimate of milk delivery to an infant. This estimate only applies to the classic picture of an exclusively breast-fed infant and then only for about the first 4 months postpartum. Toddlers, infants feeding in the colostral period, children supplemented with formula or cereal, and infants of mothers with milk supply problems may receive considerably less than this amount.

RELATIVE INFANT DOSE

The RID (Fig. 20.4) provides an estimate of the weight-normalized dose relative to the mother's dose. If the mother takes 100 mg daily of a drug with an RID of 7%, an exclusively breast-fed infant will receive about 7 mg/day. The RID is the most useful method for assessing drug safety in breastfeeding and is commonly used in many reviews and textbooks.

In 1996, pharmacologist Paul Bennett suggested an RID safety cutoff value of 10%.[28] He considered doses higher than this to be more risky and doses less than 10% to be relatively safer. This level has been widely accepted in the literature as a crude metric for assessing breastfeeding safety. However, each mother's situation is different, and properly evaluating an individual case means looking at several factors in a careful risk-benefit analysis.

RELATIVE INFANT DOSE

$$\text{RID} = \frac{\text{Dose.infant} \left[\dfrac{mg/kg}{day}\right]}{\text{Dose.mother} \left[\dfrac{mg/kg}{day}\right]}$$

Dose.infant = Dose in infant/day

Dose.mother = Dose in mother/day

Fig. 20.4 Relative infant dose *(RID)*.

PREDICTING TOXICITY OF A DRUG TO THE INFANT

LOCAL GASTROINTESTINAL EFFECTS

Some medications do not have to be absorbed systemically in order to exert an effect on the baby. Medications presented to the infant in breast milk can produce local effects in the GI tract, such as irritating the mucosa, disrupting the gut flora, or acting as an osmotic laxative. Diarrhea and constipation are the most common symptoms, but others are possible. If the drug uses a nonoral route of administration, the manufacturer may not report local GI side effects because they did not surface during the clinical trials.

BIOAVAILABILITY OF DRUGS IN MOTHER AND INFANT

Bioavailability refers to the proportion of a dose that reaches the systemic circulation after its administration. Drugs taken orally are absorbed into the portal circulation of the gut, pass through the liver, and are then delivered to the general circulation. The liver sequesters and metabolizes many drugs, often eliminating their systemic effect. This is particularly true of some opiates (e.g., morphine), which are largely metabolized during their first pass through the liver.

Although little is known about the oral absorption or bioavailability of medications in infants, there are apparently many similarities, particularly after the first month of life.[29] Gastric emptying time is delayed in neonates and intestinal absorption is irregular. Slower intestinal absorption tends to be advantageous, because this will keep plasma concentrations of medications lower in the infant.[30] Medications with poor oral bioavailability in adults usually have poor absorption in infants.

Furthermore, drug formulations that are only bioavailable because of special modifications to the tablet or a nonoral route of administration, often produce very low plasma levels after being ingested by a breastfeeding infant.[31] Enoxaparin, for example, is injected into the mother's adipose tissue, passes into her milk, and is then immediately destroyed in the infant's stomach. The proton pump inhibitors (e.g., omeprazole) are similarly vulnerable to stomach acid and have to be taken in an enteric-coated capsule. Because the capsule dissolves in the mother's intestines, the uncoated drug in the breast milk is unlikely to make it past the baby's stomach and into the bloodstream. Recent data suggest that aspirin is not present in human milk, as it is cleared during the first pass by the liver, leaving none in the peripheral circulation to enter breast milk.[32]

Thus, choosing medications with poor oral bioavailability ultimately leads to reduced drug exposure in the infant. Box 20.1 lists some medications that are poorly bioavailable orally.

INFANT RISK FACTORS

An infant's metabolic status determines his or her ability to adjust and maintain homeostasis while exposed to drugs. Infants at low risk of complications are generally older children (6 to 18 months) who can metabolize and handle drugs efficiently. Moderate-risk infants are those younger than 4 months who have additional risk factors, such as complications from the delivery, apnea, GI anomalies, hepatitis, or other metabolic problems. Infants at higher risk are unstable neonates or premature infants or infants with poor renal function.

In summary, the evaluation of the safety of drugs in breast milk depends on four major factors: the amount of medication present in the breast milk, the maternal dose of the medication, the toxicity of the drug, and the ability of the infant to clear the medication if absorbed. Even though there are numerous studies reviewing the levels of drugs in breast milk and their bioavailability, each infant's ability to clear most medications is still highly variable and requires close evaluation by the attending clinician.

CLINICAL IMPLICATIONS OF DRUG EXCRETION DURING LACTATION

The following sections describe the transfer of many drugs and drug classes into human milk. This is not a complete listing of all possible medications, but rather a survey of common and interesting examples. The levels in milk can be approximated using kinetics, but nothing is superior to actual studies in breastfeeding mothers. Many drugs have been studied in the last 30 years, and these data are in part listed below by drug category. In general, drugs with an RID less than 10% are generally considered compatible with breastfeeding.[28] Notable exceptions and illustrative examples are discussed.

A few simple strategies can help to mitigate the risks of drug exposure to the baby:

1. Consider nondrug therapies whenever possible.
2. Substitute formulations with topical or local activity. For example, rectal mesalamine is less systemically absorbed than the oral form and may be equally effective in treating proctitis.
3. Feeding and pumping schedules that avoid the peak plasma concentration can effectively reduce a drug's RID to a more manageable level. This is only useful for drugs that have a short half-life.
4. Diluting the breast milk with donor human milk or hydrolyzed formula can also reduce drug exposure. Donor human milk is preferred because it is closest in composition to the mother's own milk. This works best with short-term, high-dose situations, such as pain control after surgery.
5. Radioisotopes continue to degrade in stored milk samples. In the right circumstances, it may be possible to reduce the risk of toxicity by storing milk for a period of time (technetium-99).

Box 20.1 Examples of Drugs With Poor Oral Bioavailability

Abatacept
Acyclovir
Atorvastatin
Bacitracin
Benzoyl peroxide
Budesonide
Carboplatin
Cefdinir
Ceftriaxone
Chlorothiazide
Chondroitin sulfate
Dalteparin
Sumatriptan
Vancomycin
Daptomycin
Gentamicin
Morphine
Natalizumab

ANALGESICS, OPIATES, AND NONSTEROIDAL ANTIINFLAMMATORY DRUGS

See Table 20.1.

ASPIRIN

Used briefly and in low doses, aspirin (acetylsalicylic acid) probably poses little risk to a breast-fed infant. Reye syndrome, a rare form of hepatic encephalopathy, has been associated with acetylsalicylic acid exposure during a viral illness. Unfortunately, it is not clear how the dosage of aspirin or the age of the infant affects the risk of developing this condition. Most cases of Reye syndrome occur among adolescents using therapeutic doses of aspirin (650 mg or more). Current evidence suggests that low-dose (81 to 325-mg) aspirin is probably compatible with breastfeeding.[32] Aspirin is immediately removed from the plasma during the first pass in the liver, thus no acetylsalicylic acid is found in human milk. As Reye syndrome has been associated with aspirin but not salicylic acid, a brief waiting period of 2 hours to breast-feed following administration of aspirin would likely remove any risk.

ACETAMINOPHEN

Published levels in milk vary enormously but are generally less than 9% of the maternal dose. As acetaminophen is already approved for use in infants, there is little or no concern about the use of this product by breastfeeding mothers.

MORPHINE

The data on morphine levels in breast milk are highly variable. However, the RID matters less than its poor oral bioavailability; less than 25% is orally absorbed due to a high first-pass effect in

Table 20.1 Relative Infant Doses (RIDs) of Selected Analgesic and Antiinflammatory Drugs in Human Milk.

Generic Drug	RID (%)	Lactation Risk	Evidence
Acetaminophen	6–9	Very low	33–38
Acetylsalicylic acid	0	Low Acetylsalicylic acid is undetectable. Only Salicylic acid is found in milk.	32
Celecoxib	<0.7	Low	24, 39, 40
Ibuprofen	<0.7	Very low	41–44
Ketorolac	<0.2	Low	45, 46
Naproxen	3	Low (short term) Moderate (chronic)	47–50
Indomethacin	1	Low	51, 52
Tramadol	3	Low	53
Morphine	9–35	Low	54–56
Hydrocodone	3	Low	57, 58
Oxycodone	1–5	Low	59, 60
Codeine	0.6–8	Moderate	61–63
Fentanyl	3–5	Low	64–67

Table 20.2 Relative Infant Doses (RIDs) of Selected Antibiotics in Human Milk.

Generic Drug	RID (%)	Lactation Risk	Evidence
Amoxicillin	1	Low	69
Cephalexin	0.5–1.5	Low	69–71
Cefotaxime	<0.3	Low	70, 72
Azithromycin	6	Low	73
Ciprofloxacin	0.5–6	Low	74–77
Levofloxacin	11–17	Low	78
Doxycycline	4–13	Low	79–81
Clindamycin	1–2	Low	82–84
Metronidazole	13	Low	85–87
Vancomycin	7	Low	80, 88
Nystatin	Nil	Very low	4, 89
Fluconazole	16–21	Low	90
Sulfamethoxazole	2–3	Low	4, 91
Nitrofurantoin	7	Avoid during hyperbilirubinemia	13, 92
Linezolid	1–16	Low	93, 94

the liver. Morphine is considered compatible with breastfeeding as long as the maternal doses are low to moderate and the infant is stable.

CODEINE AND HYDROCODONE

Both of these analgesics are prodrugs that are metabolized to more pharmacologically active ingredients: codeine to morphine, and hydrocodone to hydromorphone. An individual's expression of the cytochrome P450 enzyme group affects the magnitude of pain relief and side-effect profile of these drugs. At least one infant death has been linked to unusually rapid metabolism of codeine in a breastfeeding mother.[62] In 2017 the US Food and Drug Administration (FDA) issued a warning against the use of codeine in breastfeeding women.[68] Given the rarity of this finding, codeine taken in short courses and at low doses should be safe for the breast-fed infant, but hydrocodone is probably a safer alternative. Only 5% to 6% of hydrocodone is activated to hydromorphone, which has a five- to sixfold higher potency than hydrocodone. Non-metabolizers or poor metabolizers of hydrocodone occur frequently, at a rate of 7%, whereas rapid metabolizers number less than 6 in 1000. With both drugs, the breastfeeding infant should be closely monitored for symptoms of exposure, such as somnolence, apnea, constipation, and poor feeding.

ANTIBIOTICS

See Table 20.2.

TETRACYCLINES

The transfer of tetracycline antibiotics into human milk is very low, but when mixed with the calcium in milk, the bioavailability of these drugs is markedly reduced.[95] However, doxycycline absorption is delayed, but not blocked, and its absorption may be significant over time. Short-term use of these compounds for up to 3 to 6 weeks is permissible and suitable for treatment of many infections. Long-term use, such as for acne, is not recommended for breastfeeding mothers due to the possibility of dental staining in the infant and reduced linear growth rate.

FLUOROQUINOLONES

Use of fluoroquinolones during lactation is somewhat controversial. Pseudomembranous colitis has been reported in one case, although this can occur with any antibiotic.[76] In one group of infants exposed for up to 20 days, a greenish discoloration of the infants' teeth was noted at 12 to 23 months of age.[96] Additionally, fluoroquinolone use in children has been discouraged due to rising resistance and safety concerns of arthralgia and arthropathy.[97] As with the tetracyclines, milk calcium may decrease the bioavailability of ciprofloxacin in the infant. Although the risk of fluoroquinolones may be low to the infant, reasonable alternatives are readily available.

Table 20.3 Relative Infant Doses (RIDs) of Selected Antidepressant Drugs in Human Milk.

Generic Drug	RID (%)	Lactation Risk	Evidence
Duloxetine	0.1–1	Low	23, 101, 102
Paroxetine	1–3	Low	103–109
Fluoxetine	2–15	Low	110–117
Sertraline	0.5–2	Low	118–123
Venlafaxine	7–8	Low	124, 125
Citalopram	3–5	Low	80, 126–131
Escitalopram	5–8	Low	132–134
Bupropion	<0.2–2	Low	135–139
Trazodone	3	Low	140
Amitriptyline	1–3	Low	141–143
Doxepin	0.3–3	High	144–146

METRONIDAZOLE

Although the RID of metronidazole is moderate, the drug is particularly nontoxic and no untoward effects have been reported in infants. It may be responsible for imparting a metallic taste to the milk and making some infants disinclined to feed. Large oral doses, such as the single 2 g dose for treatment of vaginal trichomoniasis, should be followed by a brief interruption of breastfeeding for perhaps 12 hours to avoid the peak plasma concentration.[4]

MACROLIDES

Extensive data now suggest that the use of erythromycin early postnatally increases the risk of hypertrophic pyloric stenosis.[98] Azithromycin or clarithromycin are usually preferred in the early postnatal period for this reason.

FLUCONAZOLE

As much as 21% of the maternal dose of fluconazole transfers into human milk. While the dose in milk exceeds the conventional 10% RID threshold used to determine safety, an infant's dose from milk is still far less than the clinical dose commonly used to treat fungal infections in infants. Fluconazole is commonly used in breastfeeding mothers without detriment to the infant.

ANTIHYPERTENSIVES AND DIURETICS

Of all the antihypertensive agents commonly used postpartum, only a few specific members of the β-blocker family present a significant risk to breast-fed infants. Atenolol and acebutolol have been associated with dangerous cyanosis, bradycardia, and hypotension in breast-fed infants.[99,100] In contrast, other β-blockers, calcium channel blockers, and angiotensin-converting enzyme inhibitors generally produce minimal levels in breast milk, and no untoward effects have been reported in otherwise healthy, breastfeeding infants. Owing to the risk of nephrotoxicity, angiotensin-converting enzyme inhibitors should be used cautiously by mothers with very premature infants, at least until the child is at the gestational age of a full-term infant to allow adequate time for complete nephron development. Angiotensin receptor blockers are less well studied.

Most thiazide diuretics are considered compatible with breastfeeding if doses are kept low. Furosemide is poorly bioavailable, and it is very unlikely that the amount of furosemide transferred into human milk would produce any effects in a nursing infant.

ANTIDEPRESSANTS AND OTHER PSYCHOACTIVE MEDICATIONS

See Tables 20.3 and 20.4.

Table 20.4 Relative Infant Doses (RIDs) of Selected Antimanic and Antipsychotic Drugs in Human Milk.

Generic Drug	RID (%)	Lactation Risk	Evidence
Lithium	0.9–7	High	147–149
Valproate	1–6	High	150–155
Carbamazepine	4–6	Low	155–161
Lamotrigine	9–18	Low	162–165
Haloperidol	0.2–12	Low	166–169
Olanzapine	0.3–2	Low	170–174
Risperidone	3–9	Low	175, 176
Quetiapine	<0.1	Low	177–179
Aripiprazole	1–6	Low	180–182

Using psychoactive medications in the early postpartum period has always been controversial. Concerns about a baby's exposure to drugs that penetrate the CNS during a critical phase of neural development often cast doubt on the decision to use them in the breastfeeding population. These doubts can be difficult to allay given that adverse effects may be subtle or play out over a long period of time. Long-term studies on many of these drugs have failed to show any adverse effects on neurobehavioral development from exposure during lactation.[103,183] Furthermore, information suggests that untreated depression, mania, or psychosis significantly interferes with optimal parenting and results in neurobehavioral delay in infants.[184-186]

SELECTIVE SEROTONIN REUPTAKE INHIBITORS

The selective serotonin reuptake inhibitors (SSRIs) are the drug class most studied in breastfeeding mothers. Neonatal withdrawal symptoms are commonly reported in infants (30%) exposed to SSRIs during pregnancy. Early postnatal symptoms consist of poor adaptation, irritability, jitteriness, and poor gaze control in neonates exposed to paroxetine,[187] sertraline,[188] and less so with fluoxetine.[189,190] In contrast to transfer across the placenta, milk levels of most SSRIs are very low and uptake by the infant is even lower. Many of these drugs are undetectable in the baby's plasma.[103,191]

ANTIPSYCHOTICS

Some typical antipsychotics, such as chlorpromazine, have been associated with neonatal apnea and sudden infant death syndrome (SIDS), and are never preferred in breastfeeding mothers when second generation atypical antipsychotics are available.[192,193] However, the risk of SIDS declines rapidly starting at around 4 months of age. If the mother continues to need additional antipsychotic treatment, the risks should be reevaluated when the infant reaches this age. Even older infants on therapeutic doses of antipsychotics have been affected by apnea, so we cannot discount this risk. If doses exceed two- to three-fold normal studied doses, the added risk to the infant may prohibit safe nursing. Second-generation atypical antipsychotics olanzapine and quetiapine demonstrate low RIDs and are reasonably safe. Symptoms of concern in the infant include sedation, apnea, irritability, and extrapyramidal symptoms. Most second-generation atypical antipsychotics produce hyperprolactinemia in patients, even galactorrhea in males. The one exception to this condition is aripiprazole. This drug is well known to suppress prolactin production in the mother, interfering with the establishment of lactation.[194] Due to a paucity of human lactation data, newer atypical drugs, such as lurasidone and brexpiprazole, are not yet preferred. Although not well documented, antipsychotics may be considered as a cause of withdrawal in infants.

LITHIUM

Relatively high levels in the milk are the result of a small molecular weight and low protein binding. Some toxicity has been reported in infants.[147,148,195] Although plasma levels of lithium in breast-fed infants are moderate, approximately 30% to 40% of the maternal level,[147,196] the situation can change dramatically with the state of hydration. Careful monitoring of plasma lithium levels in both mother and baby is strongly recommended.[149] Routine monitoring of the baby's thyroid function is also appropriate.

VALPROIC ACID

Information suggests that in utero exposure to valproic acid significantly increases the risk of neural tube defects, autism spectrum disorders, and other mental pathologies.[197] Some of these effects could presumably continue during lactation as well.[198] A case of thrombocytopenic purpura has also been associated with valproic acid.[199] This drug should not be the first choice of antimanic or anticonvulsant therapy in a breastfeeding mother.

HORMONAL BIRTH CONTROL

Exogenous estrogen and progesterone may potentially suppress prolactin release and consequently decrease milk supply. Some estrogen is required for milk synthesis, as estrogen-receptor blockers have been found to reduce production.[200] On the other hand, estrogen supplements and birth control pills can also profoundly reduce milk synthesis.[201] Progesterone, the primary inhibitor of lactation during gestation, could theoretically impede the activation of the lactocytes by prolactin if used early in the postnatal period. Women with retained placental fragments often have difficulty in producing breast milk due to the prolonged elevation of progesterone in their blood. Mothers should be advised to avoid progestin-containing products for the first 4 weeks postpartum. The World Health Organization strongly warns against the use of combination oral contraceptives (progesterone + estrogen) by breastfeeding mothers until the baby is 6 months old.[202]

STEROIDS AND OTHER IMMUNOSUPPRESSANTS

CORTICOSTEROIDS

Not only do synthetic steroids transfer poorly into milk, but the amount present is greatly overshadowed by the infant's own endogenous production of corticosteroid.[203-205] Large intravenous doses in adults, such as the 1 to 2 g of prednisone used for severe immune reactions, redistribute into the tissues and plasma levels fall rapidly. A brief breastfeeding interruption of 12 hours should suffice to limit exposure in the milk, even in the most extreme case.[25,206]

Inhaled steroids, such as fluticasone or budesonide, pose no problem for a breastfeeding mother or her infant. These drugs are designed to have potent local effects but minimal to no systemic absorption. Topical steroids are similarly excluded from the plasma. However, significant drug levels are measurable following the use of high-potency topical steroids over a large body surface. A risk-versus-benefit assessment may be required if breastfeeding is to continue under these circumstances.

METHOTREXATE

This drug has an especially low RID (0.1%), and some have suggested that its use should be compatible with breastfeeding.[207] However, animal studies indicate that methotrexate is retained in tissues, particularly in the GI tract of infants, for long periods of time.[208] Epidemiologic studies of pregnant woman have drawn an association between certain fetal malformations and methotrexate use, even if the drug was discontinued 3 months before conception.[209] A more recent study has clearly found that the level of methotrexate in human milk is exceedingly low.[210] Perhaps 24 to 48 hours after use is probably safe to return to breastfeeding. Breastfeeding in women on long-term treatment with this drug should be undertaken only with careful medical oversight, if at all.

T CELL INHIBITORS

Other agents used for immunosuppressive therapy include azathioprine, mycophenolate, cyclosporine, tacrolimus, sirolimus, and everolimus. Both azathioprine and tacrolimus transfer into milk at very low levels, and post-marketing surveillance for these drugs has thus far not identified any serious adverse effects or increase in infection rates among infants exposed through breast milk.[211-222] The data regarding cyclosporine in breast milk are somewhat conflicted. Some studies conclude that the RID is around 1% to 2%, whereas others have identified near-therapeutic plasma levels in infants. Satisfactory studies have not been published for the remainder of the drugs in this class. As always, well-studied drugs with proven safety in breastfeeding should be first line in this population. Careful monitoring of the infant, including laboratory measurement of drug levels, can further reduce the risk of toxicity when mothers receive these medications.

BIOLOGIC THERAPIES

MONOCLONAL ANTIBODIES

Engineered immunoglobulins are commonplace in the treatment of autoimmune and neoplastic diseases. These drugs target specific proteins, such as tumor necrosis factor, while leaving others untouched. The molecules are very large (>100 kDa) and consequently have low RIDs, on the order of 1% to 2%.[223-225] These drugs should also theoretically have poor oral bioavailability due to destruction by proteases. Data suggest that IgG is somewhat resistant to proteolysis. In a study of palivizumab (a recombinant human monoclonal IgG antibody) given orally in infants, survival of the drug was 88% in the stomach, 30% in the small intestine, and 5% in the stool.[226] Thus the overall oral bioavailability of these large proteins as presented in human milk is exceedingly low, even though it is still unknown. Others have postulated that monoclonal antibody drugs might exhibit limited absorption via the immunoglobulin G-transporting neonatal Fc receptor (FcRn) that is expressed in intestinal cells of adults and fetuses.[225] Knowledge in this area continues to evolve, but the current evidence is enough to merit some additional caution when using these products.

Certolizumab is a monoclonal antibody blocking tumor necrosis factor-α receptors cleverly designed without the Fc region of the antibody. It has an exceedingly low RID of 0.04% to 0.30%, and the excision of the Fc region may inhibit infant recycling of any orally bioavailable portion of the antibody from the GI system.[227] These characteristics provide a favorable breastfeeding profile for the infant.

Natalizumab is an unusually long-lasting antibody requiring around 24 weeks to reach a steady-state level in the maternal blood. Over 12 weeks, drug levels in the milk rose to five times the level detected after the first injection.[228] Data on the extended monitoring of this drug after this initial period have not been published, but the implication is that drug levels in the milk may continue to rise, possibly to the point of being hazardous.

A small group of monoclonal medications are designed to antagonize the action of endothelial growth factor. Receptors for this hormone are expressed on the cells of the intestinal lining, leading to the potential for adverse effects without systemic absorption.

ANTINEOPLASTICS

Breastfeeding is contraindicated during treatment with alkylating agents, antimetabolite medications, anthracyclines, topoisomerase inhibitors, and mitotic inhibitors. Although the average dose in milk is generally small, these agents are unusually potent and capable of causing serious, long-term toxicity. As with the tyrosine kinase inhibitors just discussed, breastfeeding cessation for seven half-lives effectively eliminates the risk to the infant. If a combination of chemotherapeutic agents is used, the period of breastfeeding cessation should be based on the agent with the longest half-life.[4]

HERBAL THERAPIES

The FDA does not regulate herbal products, and there can be significant variations in the potency and purity between different products or even between different lots of the same product. Herbs can also interact with each other and with prescription medications. The published literature on the safety of an herb in breastfeeding women is limited and poor, and practically never on combination herbal products. Relevant information about the effectiveness of an herb is more likely to be available. The decision whether or not to take a supplement should include information about both risks and benefits.

VACCINES

As a general rule, vaccines are safe to use while breastfeeding. Dead or inactivated pathogens pose no risk to a breastfeeding infant. Live attenuated viral strains from vaccines have been detected in breast milk, but none has been successfully cultured. The antibodies that the mother produces against these organisms may transfer into the breast milk, but they do not affect the infant's response to the pathogen if he or she is later exposed or vaccinated.[229]

The yellow fever vaccine (live attenuated virus) has been associated with a handful of encephalitis cases in infants younger than 3 weeks of age.[230,231] This vaccine is not recommended for use while breastfeeding. If it is absolutely necessary, then the mother should be advised to avoid breastfeeding for 2 weeks after vaccination. At least 80% of those vaccinated develop neutralizing antibodies by 10 days and 99% develop them by 28 days.[232] The use of some vaccines, such as rotavirus vaccine, in infants born to mothers consuming immunosuppressant monoclonal antibodies before delivery may be risky, as severe diarrhea has been reported in infants receiving the live rotavirus vaccination.

RADIOACTIVE COMPOUNDS

Radiopharmaceuticals are drugs that contain radioactive atoms. They are used as tracers and ablation chemotherapy. Sometimes, the radioisotope is used by itself, but more often it is attached to a "carrier" compound that helps target the organ of interest and speed up elimination of the radioactivity from the body. Each formulation will have two separate half-lives: the biologic half-life that is defined by how quickly the compound is eliminated from the body and the radioactive half-life that measures how quickly the radioactive atom decays into a more stable isotope. These two factors have no influence on each other, but both contribute to the effective reduction of radiation in the patient.

Radiation from the mother reaches the infant in two ways: through ingestion of contaminated breast milk and by direct exposure to radiation emitted from the mother's body. The former is mitigated by breastfeeding cessation, and the latter by restrictions on close contact between mother and child. The amount of radiation that reaches the infant is a function of the half-lives of the compound, the type of radiation emitted, the precautions taken, and the dose administered to the mother (measured in mCi or MBq, 1 mCi = 37 MBq). The Nuclear Regulatory Commission issues guidelines for various radiopharmaceuticals with the intent of delivering an effective dose of less than 1 mSv of radiation (1 mSv = 100 mrem) to the infant for each procedure.[233] Consolidated information based on these guidelines is available from the American Academy of Pediatrics[234] and others.[4]

One product deserves special discussion: radioactive iodine concentrates in the thyroid gland of the adult and infant, and in lactating tissues. Approximately 28% of the total radioactivity is secreted via breast milk.[235] This radioisotope may suppress the infant's thyroid function or increase the risk of future thyroid carcinomas.[4] Even holding the infant close to the breast or thyroid gland for long periods of time can expose the child to harmful gamma rays. Very low doses of radioactive iodine tracers may be compatible with breastfeeding if the affected milk is discarded or stored for an appropriate period of time.[236] Larger doses of I-123 or I-131 or I-125 carry risks that exceed the benefits of breastfeeding.[233] With radioiodine, close contact restrictions are available and should be followed by mothers caring for infants.

RADIOCONTRAST AGENTS

Radiopaque substances are frequently used to enhance imaging techniques, such as magnetic resonance imaging and computed tomography scanning. These substances are not radioactive themselves, but rather they block or absorb radiation to highlight different areas of the body. These products are specifically designed to target certain tissue compartments and do not leak into other areas. Iodinated and gadolinium-based agents in particular exhibit less than 1% excretion via breast milk and less than 1% oral bioavailability in the infant. The American College of Radiologists has issued guidelines stating that these products are compatible with breastfeeding without restriction.[237] That said, data are growing suggesting that gadolinium radiocontrast agents may be sequestered in the brain tissue. While the levels in milk are exceedingly low, the use in newborn infants, or adults, should be minimized.

DRUGS OF ABUSE

Most drugs with the potential for addiction and abuse are psychotropics that readily pass into the CNS. The tendency of a substance to cross the blood-brain barrier is highly correlated with its ability to cross the lactocyte barrier and appear in the milk. No reliable threshold of toxicity in infants has been established for any drug of abuse. Women who wish to breast-feed should not use these drugs. However, the more relevant question of whether a woman who uses these drugs should breast-feed needs to be evaluated on a case-by-case basis. The physiologic and psychologic benefits of breastfeeding may still outweigh the detriments of incidental drug exposure. Issues of drug interactions, contaminants, and addiction all complicate this judgment. Infants may have positive results on drug screens for extended periods of time, even in the absence of observable effects.

ALCOHOL

The M/P ratio is around 1.0, although absolute levels tend to be small. For example, a study of 12 breastfeeding mothers who ingested 0.3 g/kg of ethanol exhibited an average maximum concentration of ethanol in their milk of 320 mg/L.[238] Ethanol has been shown to inhibit oxytocin release and decrease milk delivery to the infant.[239] A woman of average size will reduce her milk alcohol level by 15 to 20 mg/dL/hour, which works out to metabolizing a "standard drink" (14 g of pure ethanol) in about 2 hours.[240]

TOBACCO

The majority of the work done on tobacco exposure in breastfeeding women uses nicotine's main metabolite, cotinine, as a biomarker. Cotinine is pharmacologically active but much less potent than nicotine.[241] Although this is useful for tracking nicotine metabolism, cotinine levels are not necessarily representative of second- and third-hand contact with tobacco residues, the relative safety of using nicotine replacement products, or exposure to the many other dangerous chemicals in tobacco.

Studies have demonstrated a linear relationship between smoking rates in the mother, nicotine levels in the milk, and urine cotinine levels in the breast-fed infant.[242,243] These infants can have urine cotinine levels up to five times greater than infants whose mothers smoke but do not breast-feed.[244] Even second-hand smoke can increase the risk of otitis media, respiratory tract infections, and asthma in the baby.[245] Breastfeeding offsets some of this risk, and the current recommendations are for the mother to continue to breast-feed regardless of her smoking habits but never to smoke in the presence of the infant.[246]

MARIJUANA/CANNABIS

Research is sparse on the effect of marijuana in breast milk. With occasional use, the active ingredient in marijuana (delta-9-tetrahydrocannabinol, or THC) rapidly redistributes from the plasma to the adipose tissue, leaving milk levels low. With chronic or heavy use, THC can accumulate in the breast milk, leading to substantial doses. At least one study has shown significant absorption and metabolism of THC via breast milk.[247] In a more recent study, the transfer of THC into human milk was measured following the smoking of marijuana containing 23.28 mg THC. Milk levels of THC were detected at low concentrations at all the time points beyond time zero.[248] THC was transferred into mother's milk such that exclusively breastfeeding infants ingested an estimated mean of 2.5% of the maternal dose (the calculated RID was 2.5%, with a range of 0.4% to 8.7%). The estimated daily infant dose was 8 micrograms per kilogram per day. Because the oral bioavailability of THC is low (<1% to 6%), the dose absorbed by the infant is likely minimal.

Increasing evidence has begun to emerge suggesting that exposure to THC in pregnancy or chronic use in adolescence and early adulthood may result in changes to the endocannabinoid system in the brain.[249,250] This system is partially responsible for regulating mood, reward, and goal-directed behavior. Adverse neurobehavioral effects have not yet been demonstrated in infants exposed to THC exclusively through breast milk.[247]

HEROIN AND METHADONE

Heroin is diacetyl-morphine, a prodrug that is rapidly converted by plasma cholinesterases to 6-acetylmorphine and more slowly to morphine. Heroin may also transfer directly into breast milk alongside all of its metabolites. As with other opiates, tolerance follows from chronic use, and addicts may end up using extraordinarily large doses. Heavily dependent users should be advised against breastfeeding, and their infants should be transitioned to formula. Methadone is a potent and very long-acting opiate analgesic used primarily to prevent withdrawal in opiate addicts. Unlike heroin, methadone produces only inactive metabolites. A large volume of distribution results in a low RID (2% to 6%), and infant exposure is further reduced by its moderate oral bioavailability.[251-254] Many methadone-maintained women have breast-fed their infants successfully. It is still possible for these infants to have non–life-threatening withdrawal symptoms on discontinuation of breastfeeding.

COCAINE

This potent CNS stimulant exerts its effects only briefly due to rapid metabolism and redistribution out of the brain. Estimates vary significantly regarding the degree of cocaine contamination in the breast milk, ranging from 1% to 10% of the maternal dose.[255,256] Inactive metabolites are excreted in the urine and breast milk for up to 7 days following initial exposure to the drug. Breast milk is likely free of cocaine after 24 hours, but infants can become drug-screen-positive as a result of ingesting these metabolites.

HALLUCINOGENS

There are no high-quality human studies on the transfer of illicit hallucinogens into breast milk. Lysergic acid (LSD) and phencyclidine (PCP) are both detectable in human and animal milk, but definitive levels have not been published.[257-259] Both LSD and PCP are associated with altered levels of consciousness in infants and young children after direct exposure.[260,261] In older patients with larger exposures, more serious effects, including seizures and coma, have been documented. Other hallucinogens, such as dextromethorphan, ketamine, MDMA, gamma hydroxybutyrate, and methamphetamines, produce similar problems with large doses. The signs and symptoms of hallucinogen intoxication have not been described in patients whose sole exposure was through breast milk. Nonetheless, these drugs are all predicted to enter the milk avidly, and mothers abusing these substances should not breast-feed.

DRUGS USED TO ALTER MILK SUPPLY

The most common cause of low milk supply is simply poor lactation management. High-volume milk production depends on frequent and complete emptying of the ducts.[2] Anything that interferes with breast emptying, including blocked ducts or poor infant latching, can lead to a precipitous drop in milk supply. This situation can usually be reversed by nondrug means, but some women will require a galactagogue to maintain adequate milk output.

As discussed previously, milk supply is also dependent on the continual presence of prolactin at levels above the pre-pregnancy baseline (>50 ng/mL).[80] Prolactin is produced and stored in the pituitary gland, but it is blocked from release by the inhibitory effects of dopamine. Dopamine antagonists can function as galactagogues by encouraging the release of prolactin from the pituitary. Dopamine agonists are used to suppress lactation.

METOCLOPRAMIDE

This dopamine antagonist can increase milk production as much as 100% by stimulating the release of prolactin.[262] However, it is difficult to predict which women will respond with elevated milk synthesis. Because the lactocytes' response to prolactin plateaus at a fairly low level, theory would suggest this agent is most useful for mothers whose prolactin levels were originally high but have since dropped.

The prolactin-stimulating effect of metoclopramide appears to be dose-related. The standard oral dose of 10 to 15 mg three times per day can be as much as tripled for maximum effect.[262] Milk production normally responds quickly, with the mother noticing significant increases of milk volume within 24 to 48 hours. The amount of metoclopramide in milk rarely exceeds 160 μg/L, even at the highest maternal doses.[263] In comparison, this drug is regularly prescribed directly to infants at 800 μg/kg/day for other conditions.[264]

Metoclopramide crosses the blood-brain barrier, and a drug-induced depression is a common side effect in mothers who use it. Other problems include extrapyramidal symptoms, gastric cramping, and tardive dyskinesia. Some mothers also experience a rebound drop in milk production if they discontinue the drug without weaning slowly.

DOMPERIDONE

Although not available in the United States, domperidone has been used successfully all over the world to increase milk production.[265-267] This drug is also a dopamine antagonist but, unlike metoclopramide, does not cross the blood-brain barrier. Levels of domperidone in milk are extraordinarily low (around 1.2 ng/mL), and oral bioavailability is less than 20%.[266]

Unfortunately, domperidone is an antagonist to the human *ether-a-go-go-related* gene potassium channel receptor, which is partially responsible for repolarizing cardiac muscle cells. Therefore domperidone may cause arrhythmias. Although this side effect is rare, this drug should not be used in mothers with existing rhythm disorders, especially long QT syndrome.

HERBAL GALACTAGOGUES

A variety of herbal and complementary therapies have historical precedent for their use in increasing milk flow. Examples include fenugreek, goat's rue, asparagus, alfalfa, milk thistle, and fennel. Although many of these plants do contain biologically active compounds, their efficacy in increasing milk production is doubtful. The existing literature in this area is sparse and conflicted.[268]

BROMOCRIPTINE AND CABERGOLINE

These dopamine agonists are effective in inhibiting milk production and reducing the symptoms of engorgement.[269,270] Bromocriptine has been associated with numerous cases of cardiac dysrhythmias, stroke, intracranial bleeding, cerebral edema, convulsions, and myocardial infarction.[271-273] It is no longer approved for use in lactation suppression and has been replaced by cabergoline.[274,275]

CONCLUSION

Most drugs are compatible with breastfeeding, although some will necessitate the use of risk-mitigating strategies. The risk to an infant of using a drug while breastfeeding depends on how toxic the drug is and how much of it the infant receives. Physiochemical properties of a drug that make it more likely to appear in the milk include an active transport mechanism, low molecular weight, low protein binding, high lipid solubility, a tendency to cross the blood-brain barrier, pK_a greater than 7.4, and low volume of distribution. Properties of a drug that make it more likely to be toxic to an infant include high potency, propensity to cause topical effects in the GI tract, high oral bioavailability, long half-life, and a reputation for causing toxic effects in adults. The infant's age, stability, and condition will also impact his or her ability to handle exposure to medications.

Some drug classes are safer than others, and most classes have examples of safe and unsafe drugs within them. In general, drugs with an RID of less than 10% are compatible with breastfeeding, but a risk-versus-benefit assessment is always required before use. In addition to the direct drug-related risks, this assessment should also take into account the efficacy of the drug, the benefits of breastfeeding, and the risks of the untreated disease. Multiple resources[3,4,47] exist to assist with this assessment.

A complete reference list is available at www.ExpertConsult.com. 

SELECT REFERENCES

1. Atkinson HC, Begg EJ. Prediction of drug distribution into human milk from physicochemical characteristics. *Clin Pharmacokinet*. 1990;18(2):151-167.
2. Hale T, Kristensen J, Ilett K. The transfer of medications into human milk. In: Hale TW, Hartmann PE, eds. *Hale & Hartmann's Textbook of Human Lactation*. 1st ed. Amarillo, TX: Hale Pub.; 2007.
3. Tomasulo P. LactMed. *Med Ref Serv Q*. 2007;26(1):51-58.
4. Hale TW. *Hale's Medications & Mothers' Milk™ 2019*. Springer Publishing Company; 2018.
11. Neville MC, McFadden TB, Forsyth I. Hormonal regulation of mammary differentiation and milk secretion. *J Mammary Gland Biol Neoplasia*. 2002;7(1):49-66.
13. Gerk PM, Kuhn RJ, Desai NS, McNamara PJ. Active transport of nitrofurantoin into human milk. *Pharmacotherapy*. 2001;21(6):669-675.
14. Lau RJ, Emery MG, Galinsky RE. Unexpected accumulation of acyclovir in breast milk with estimation of infant exposure. *Obstet Gynecol*. 1987;69(3 pt 2):468-471.
15. Kearns GL, McConnell Jr RF, Trang JM, Kluza RB. Appearance of ranitidine in breast milk following multiple dosing. *Clin Pharm*. 1985;4(3):322-324.
16. Oo CY, Kuhn RJ, Desai N, McNamara PJ. Active transport of cimetidine into human milk*. *Clin. Pharmacol Ther*. 1995;58(5):548-555.
17. Delange F, Chanoine JP, Abrassart C, Bourdoux P. Topical iodine, breastfeeding, and neonatal hypothyroidism. *Arch Dis Child*. 1988;63(1):106-107.
18. Postellon DC, Aronow R. Iodine in mother's milk. *JAMA*. 1982;247(4):463.
19. Raub TJ. P-Glycoprotein recognition of substrates and circumvention through rational drug design. *Mol. Pharm*. 2005;3(1):3-25.
25. Hale T, Ilett K. *Drug Therapy and Breastfeeding. From Theory to Clinical Practice*. London: Parthenon Press; 2002.
26. Ilett KF, Kristensen JH. Drug use and breastfeeding. *Expert Opinion on Drug Safety*. 2005;4(4):745-768.
27. Begg EJ, Duffull SB, Hackett LP, Ilett KF. Studying drugs in human milk: time to unify the approach. *J Hum Lact*. 2002;18(4):323-332.
28. Bennett PN, Jensen AA. *Drugs and Human Lactation: A Comprehensive Guide to the Content and Consequences of Drugs, Micronutrients,*

Radiopharmaceuticals, and Environmental and Occupational Chemicals In Human Milk. 2nd ed. Amsterdam; New York: Elsevier; 1996.

29. Alcorn J, McNamara PJ. Pharmacokinetics in the newborn. *Adv Drug Deliv Rev*. 2003;55(5):667–686.
30. Besunder JB, Reed MD, Blumer JL. Principles of drug biodisposition in the neonate. *Clin Pharmacokinet*. 1988;14(5):261–286.
31. Sandmann BJ, Amiji MM. Solubility, dissolution, and partitioning. In: Amiji MM, Cook TJ, Mobley WC, eds. *Applied Physical Pharmacy, 2e*. New York, NY: McGraw-Hill Education; 2013.
32. Datta P, Rewers-Felkins K, Kallem RR, Baker T, Hale TW. Transfer of low dose aspirin into human milk. *J Hum Lact*. 2017;33(2):296–299.
68. FDA Drug Safety Communication. *FDA restricts use of prescription codeine pain and cough medicines and tramadol pain medicines in children; recommends against use in breastfeeding women [press release]. 4/20/2017*; 2017.
97. Jackson MA, Schutze GE, Committee On Infectious D. The use of systemic and topical fluoroquinolones. *Pediatrics*. 2016;138(5):e20162706.
103. Weissman AM, Levy BT, Hartz AJ, et al. Pooled analysis of antidepressant levels in lactating mothers, breast milk, and nursing infants. *Am J Psychiatry*. 2004;161(6):1066–1078.
105. Hendrick V, Fukuchi A, Altshuler L, Widawski M, Wertheimer A, Brunhuber MV. Use of sertraline, paroxetine and fluvoxamine by nursing women. *Br J Psychiatry*. 2001;179(2):163–166.
149. Moretti ME, Koren G, Verjee Z, Ito S. Monitoring lithium in breast milk: an individualized approach for breast-feeding mothers. *Ther Drug Monit*. 2003;25(3):364–366.
183. Field T. Breastfeeding and antidepressants. *Infant Behav Dev*. 2008;31(3):481–487.
192. Boutroy MJ. Drug-induced apnea. *Biol Neonate*. 1994;65(3-4):252–257.
194. Lozano R, Marin R, Santacruz MJ. Prolactin deficiency by aripiprazole. *J Clin Psychopharmacol*. 2014;34(4):539–540.
198. Meador KJ, Baker GA, Browning N, et al. Breastfeeding in children of women taking antiepileptic drugs: cognitive outcomes at age 6 years. *JAMA Pediatr*. 2014;168(8):729–736.
202. World Health Organization. *Reproductive Health and Research. Medical Eligibility Criteria for Contraceptive Use*. 4th ed. Geneva: Department of Reproductive Health and Research, World Health Organization; 2010.
206. Cooper SD, Felkins K, Baker TE, Hale TW. Transfer of methylprednisolone into breast milk in a mother with multiple sclerosis. *J Hum Lact*. 2015;31(2):237–239.
210. Baker T, Datta P, Rewers-Felkins K, Hale TW. High-Dose methotrexate treatment in a breastfeeding mother with placenta accreta: a case report. *Breastfeed Med*. 2018;13(6):450–452.
225. Fritzsche J, Pilch A, Mury D, Schaefer C, Weber-Schoendorfer C. Infliximab and adalimumab use during breastfeeding. *Journal of Clinical Gastroenterology*. 2012;46(8):718–719.
227. Clowse ME, Forger F, Hwang C, et al. Minimal to no transfer of certolizumab pegol into breast milk: results from CRADLE, a prospective, postmarketing, multicentre, pharmacokinetic study. *Ann Rheum Dis*. 2017;76(11):1890–1896.
228. Baker TE, Cooper SD, Kessler L, Hale TW. Transfer of natalizumab into breast milk in a mother with multiple sclerosis. *J Hum Lact*. 2015;31(2):233–236.
229. National Center for I, Respiratory D. General recommendations on immunization – recommendations of the Advisory Committee on Immunization Practices (ACIP). *MMWR Recomm Rep*. 2011;60(2):1–64.
233. *Regulatory Guide 8.39: Release of patients administered radioactive materials. [press release]*. US Nuclear Regulatory Commission; 1997.
234. Sachs HC, Committee On D. The transfer of drugs and therapeutics into human breast milk: an update on selected topics. *Pediatrics*. 2013;132(3):e796–809.
237. *ACR Manual on Contrast Media*. 10th ed. American College of Radiology; 2020.
238. Mennella JA. Regulation of milk intake after exposure to alcohol in mothers' milk. *Alcohol Clin Exp Res*. 2001;25(4):590–593.
239. Coiro V, Alboni A, Gramellini D, et al. Inhibition by ethanol of the oxytocin response to breast stimulation in normal women and the role of endogenous opioids. *Acta Endocrinologica*. 1992;126(3):213–216.
244. Becker AB, Manfreda J, Ferguson AC, Dimich-Ward H, Watson WTA, Chan-Yeung M. Breast-feeding and environmental tobacco smoke exposure. *Arch Pediatr Adolesc Med*. 1999;153(7):689.
247. Tennes K, Avitable N, Blackard C, et al. Marijuana: prenatal and postnatal exposure in the human. *NIDA Res Monogr*. 1985;59:48–60.
248. Baker T, Datta P, Rewers-Felkins K, Thompson H, Kallem RR, Hale TW. Transfer of inhaled cannabis into human breast milk. *Obstet Gynecol*. 2018;131(5):783–788.
254. Begg EJ, Malpas TJ, Hackett LP, Ilett KF. Distribution of R- and S-methadone into human milk during multiple, medium to high oral dosing. *Br J Clin Pharmacol*. 2002;52(6):681–685.
255. Sarkar M, Djulus J, Koren G. When a cocaine-using mother wishes to breastfeed. *Ther Drug Monit*. 2005;27(1):1–2.
258. Nicholas JM, Lipshitz J, Schreiber EC. Phencyclidine: its transfer across the placenta as well as into breast milk. *Am J Obstet Gynecol*. 1982;143(2):143–146.
261. Schwartz RH, Einhorn A. PCP intoxication in seven young children. *Pediatr Emerg Care*. 1986;2(4):238–241.
266. Brouwers JR, Assies J, Wiersinga WM, Huizing G, Tytgat GN. Plasma prolactin levels after acute and subchronic oral administration of domperidone and of metoclopramide: a cross-over study in healthy volunteers. *Clin Endocrinol (Oxf)*. 1980;12(5):435–440.
268. Therapeutic Research Center. *Natural Medicines Pregnancy & Lactation Comprehensive Database*. Accessed 2020. https://naturalmedicines.therapeuticresearch.com/.

21 Placental and Fetal Circulatory and Metabolic Changes Accompanying Fetal Growth Restriction

Barbra de Vrijer | Giacomo Meschia | Frederick C. Battaglia | Timothy R.H. Regnault | William W. Hay, Jr.

INTRODUCTION

During fetal life, factors associated with maternal, placental, and fetal environments interact to ensure optimal fetal metabolism and growth. However, in 3% to 7% of pregnancies these interactions become suboptimal and growth of the fetus does not align with its in utero genetic growth potential, resulting in a reduced growth trajectory and the outcome at birth often termed *fetal growth restriction (FGR)*. To ensure survival, preservation of fetal development and growth, albeit reduced, lead to significant changes to the fetal circulatory and metabolic systems. The etiology of FGR is multifactorial, and initial insults, responses, and fetal adaptations likely differ across the FGR outcome spectrum, depending on specific causes and adaptations. This chapter summarizes some of the work that has been directed at describing circulatory differences and changes in fetoplacental oxygen and nutrient supply and metabolism in FGR pregnancy, independent of fetal genetic abnormalities or maternal environment (e.g., maternal anemia, respiratory conditions, or altitude), where placental insufficiency arises. This FGR occurs where there is a reduction in the density and size of fetal blood vessels in the placenta, promoting increased vascular resistance in association with reduced oxygen and nutrient exchange. Early foundational work using the sheep model is presented alongside other animal model systems and new and emerging human data. Discussion also focuses on detection of FGR and the clinical implications of abnormal placental development and fetal oxygenation, as well as advances in screening and assessment of abnormal fetoplacental function in FGR.

DEFINING FETAL GROWTH RESTRICTION

FGR is an important clinical problem in obstetrics and has stimulated considerable clinical research that not only has elucidated aspects of the pathophysiology of growth restriction but also has led to a better understanding of normal human biology. A plethora of terms have been used in describing FGR. In part, this potentially confusing terminology has a historical foundation. The first attempts to recognize growth restriction in newborn infants came from studies using gestational age and birth weight information.[1-3] Infants were classified as being small-for-gestational-age (SGA) if their birth weights fell below the 10th percentile. Later reports used terms such as small for dates, basing the definition on standard deviations (SDs) for the birth weight distribution at each gestational age. Many studies identified differences in birth weight-gestational age distribution data among different populations. All of these attempts to define FGR were based on birth weight information that was recorded to establish the norms for populations. However, it was clear from the beginning that preterm birth weights could hardly be considered to represent "normal" in utero growth for a population. It also was clear that growth-restricted infants were not a homogeneous group but instead included some infants who were small but normally grown. The term *intrauterine growth retardation* (IUGR) was used initially to identify SGA infants who had truly grown more slowly in utero because of one or another disease process that usually represented abnormal placental development and function. Later, because of concerns that parents might associate the term *retardation* with mental retardation, this term was modified to *fetal growth restriction*. This latter designation has come to be used more and more widely and interchangeably with IUGR. This chapter will use SGA for fetuses that have growth <10th percentile and FGR to describe the pathologic process of placentally mediated fetal growth restriction whereby genetic growth potential is not obtained.[4] Further to this classification it is important to note that FGR fetuses have often been classified as having an either symmetric or asymmetric body pattern based on the ratio between abdominal circumference (AC) and another reference biometric index (e.g., brain). The rationale underlying this classification is the hypothesis that this pattern may provide information on the etiology of FGR (i.e., constitutional, placental, or intrinsic fetal abnormalities), timing of onset of FGR (early vs. late), duration of FGR, and risk of adverse outcome.[5]

The approach to defining FGR in human pregnancies changed fundamentally once ultrasound techniques permitted in utero determination of fetal body size, a measurement that could be made repeatedly during the pregnancy. This capability removed the necessity to use only birth weight data at the completion of a pregnancy. It also permitted examination of the rate of fetal growth, that is, the change in fetal size with time in normal pregnancy, rather than establishing growth curves based on birth weights of pregnancies that are by definition pathologic because they ended prematurely. This wide application of ultrasound-derived fetal growth curves made possible the early detection of fetuses who were SGA. Currently, the common practice is to use equations derived from population data to calculate an estimated fetal weight, with equations usually relying on ultrasound measurements of head circumference (HC), abdominal circumference (AC), and femur length. Using the 10th percentile as the cutoff to identify SGA, sensitivity has varied among studies between 0% and 10% in low-risk to 72% and 95% in a high-risk populations, while specificity of ultrasound to detect small fetuses ranges from 50% to 95%, with large variability attributed to differences in methodology and the use of either estimated fetal weight (EFW) <10th percentile or only AC <10th percentile as the means to identify SGA.[6,7] High false-positive rates and a measurement inaccuracy of up to 10%[8] have limited the use of ultrasound in normal pregnancy, and there are no guidelines recommending the incorporation of ultrasound for routine screening for FGR in low-risk populations.[9,10]

Distinguishing fetuses who are small but are fulfilling their growth potential (i.e., those who are normally grown) from those with FGR (i.e., those who are growth-restricted as a result of some pathology) is important for a number of reasons: (1) intensive obstetric surveillance can be applied more effectively to the poorly growing fetus, (2) neonatal intensive care can better anticipate problems for affected infants who had FGR, and (3) FGR has important long-term implications for development of the infant, not only through childhood but also into adult life.

However, variability in presentation and difficulties in distinguishing normal fetuses from those with FGR who are at risk for adverse perinatal outcomes has limited the ability of clinicians to prevent all FGR-associated adverse perinatal outcomes. As a result of this inability to detect fetuses most at risk, FGR is still the attributable cause of one-third of stillbirths and perinatal mortality, and is one of the most common causes of spontaneous and iatrogenic preterm births and perinatal morbidity related to birth asphyxia.[11,12]

With only 30% to 50% of SGA fetuses with EFW <10th percentile pathologically growth restricted (FGR) and the remainder of fetuses growing appropriately for maternal ethnicity, parity, and weight,[13] additional measures are needed to distinguish between FGR and the constitutionally SGA fetuses. The addition of measures of asymmetric growth restriction (a small AC to HC ratio) or AC growth velocity may help improve the distinction between FGR and SGA. However, none of these measures has resulted in clinically useful information, and both SGA and FGR remain defined as an EFW and/or AC <10th percentile. Newer modalities such as magnetic resonance imaging (MRI)[14,15], fetal volume, determinations[14,15] and fetal and umbilical blood flow relationships,[16] and the addition of three-dimensional (3D) ultrasound of soft tissue volumes[17] may have the potential to yield better estimates of fetal growth.

Attempts also have been made to sharpen the diagnosis of FGR by the use of standards that incorporate maternal and paternal size. Essentially, this approach seeks to distinguish fetuses that are small because the parents are small from those with growth restriction. Focusing on this approach, Gardosi and colleagues have reviewed this subject extensively,[18] and nomograms for particular countries are available.[19,20] However, there is only limited improvement when maternal factors such as parity, obesity, and ethnic background are accounted for, and all EFW formulas perform less well in fetuses at the extremes of fetal growth and in late gestation.[21,22]

PLACENTAL DEVELOPMENT AND OXYGEN SUPPLY

The human placenta is classified as a discoid haemomonochorial placenta that is dually perfused from the maternal circulation and a separate fetal circulatory system.[23] During pregnancy, the human placenta undergoes two major developmental stages, primarily to expand its surface area and metabolism to support optimal fetal development and growth.[24] The first stage of placental development extends to approximately the 23rd week of gestation. During this stage, maternal blood in the intervillous space (IVS) entering through the uterine arteries and fetal blood are separated by a thick placental endo-epithelial membrane.[25] This layer consists of a monolayer of terminally differentiated trophoblast cells, the syncytialized trophoblast, the underlying layer of progenitor cells, the cytotrophoblast (CTB), and the endothelium of the fetal vasculature.[26] An oxygen gradient exists across this membrane that promotes oxygen diffusion between the uterine and umbilical circulations. This membrane collectively forms what are termed villous trees, and several villous trees might occupy a single placental lobule.[27] The villous trees are extensively branched, commencing with stem villi,[28] and dividing over gestation to form intermediate villi, with the mature type branching off to form the terminal villi in the later part of pregnancy.[29]

Given the placenta's essential roles of hormone production, immunologic protection, waste removal, nutrient production, and nutrient transportation for the developing fetus, there is high oxygen utilization for oxidative metabolism. In fact, the placenta has an extraordinarily high metabolic rate, consuming approximately 40% of the oxygen used by the entire conceptus,[30] and studies in the near-term placenta show that approximately 70% to 75% of the O_2 consumed is used to generate ATP by mitochondrial oxidative phosphorylation to support placental metabolism and subsequent functions. Indeed, it is interesting to note that oxygen consumption rates calculated per kilogram of placenta are of the same order of magnitude in different species with an epitheliochorial placenta and are similar to those of the hemochorial human placenta.[31]

This oxygen consumption by the trophoblast and the stroma of the placental villi is a hindrance to fetal oxygenation, preventing transplacental Po_2 equilibration and enlarging the transplacental Po_2 difference. This hindrance is compensated for by rapid, early growth of uterine blood flow supplying the maternal facing placental membrane. Studies in sheep pregnancies highlight that at mid-gestation, uterine blood flow has already increased to approximately 40% of its near-term value or upwards of 470 mL/min. This high flow is used to oxygenate a fetus whose body weight is only 7% of its near-term value (i.e., 200 vs. 3000 g).[32] The function of a high uterine flow in early pregnancy is to maintain a high Po_2 in the IVS and to counteract the adverse effect of placental structure and oxidative metabolism on the transplacental diffusion of O_2. Attempts to measure IVS Po_2 in early pregnancy indicate a mean value of ~60 mm Hg at 20 weeks gestation.[33] At a Po_2 of 60 mm Hg, human adult blood has an O_2 saturation of approximately 89%. Because maternal arterial O_2 saturation at sea level is ~97%, this observation implies an extremely low (8%) level of uteroplacental O_2 extraction.

The second stage of placental development is from 23 weeks to term, during which there is an exponential growth of fetal O_2 demand that requires the placenta to become more efficient in extracting O_2 from maternal blood. This requirement is met by the exponential growth of the terminal villi and their volume.[29,34,35] These villi grow as short side branches of the villous tree (more exactly, as side branches of the mature intermediate villi) through increased angiogenesis, and each contains a dense capillary network. Some capillaries of this network bulge against a very thin segment of the trophoblastic membrane to form local sites of blood flow limited O_2 transport.[25] These structural adaptations reduce the placental membrane to a diffusion distance of 2 to 3 μm.[27] Accompanying these changes in villous development, there is a synchronous exponential increase of umbilical blood flow, most of which goes to perfuse the expanding capillary bed of the terminal villi.

It is physiologically significant that the intermediate villi continue to be perfused by umbilical blood throughout pregnancy. Even in the term placenta, intermediate villous capillary volume has been estimated to be 18% of the total volume of capillaries in the placental villous tree.[36] This is a manifestation of the fact that respiratory gas exchange is only one of several placental functions, some of which require a substantial fraction of umbilical flow to perfuse the thick, O_2 consuming membrane that maintains a transplacental Po_2 difference. As a consequence, in its last developmental stage, the human placenta fails to attain the maximum level of performance of a venous equilibrator, which would allow umbilical venous Po_2 to become equal to intervillous Po_2. In the last trimester of a normal pregnancy, the Po_2 of maternal blood in the IVS and the uterine veins is approximately 10 mm Hg higher than umbilical venous Po_2 (approximately, 45 vs. 35 mm Hg).[37,38] Additional factors that underscore this imperfect equilibration have come from foundational work using the pregnant sheep. These studies highlight that the umbilical uptake of oxygen is approximately 55% of the total uterine oxygen uptake. The large difference between uterine and umbilical uptakes is due primarily to the large utilization rate of oxygen by the placenta.[39]

The relationships between abnormal placental development and FGR are complex and well-reviewed elsewhere.[24] FGR has many causes, but the majority of cases that are not associated with fetal congenital malformations, fetal genetic anomalies, or infectious etiology are understood to arise from compromise of the uterine circulation to the placenta. The resultant malperfusion induces cell stress within the placental tissues, leading to changes in transcript expression, selective suppression of protein synthesis and reduced cell proliferation and, in more severe cases, infarction, increased fibrin deposition and calcification are observed.[24,40] Correspondingly, within this smaller placenta, there is a reduction in volume, surface area, and vascularization of the intermediate and terminal villi that mediate maternal-fetal exchange,[36,41] and their normal branching to form a dense capillary network is restricted.[25] This maldevelopment of the terminal villi prevents the decrease in resistance to umbilical flow that characterizes normal placental development. Simultaneously, it creates a condition in which the venous return from villous capillaries that carry deoxygenated blood from thick, O_2 consuming portions of the placental membrane becomes an abnormally large fraction of the total umbilical venous effluent. This condition enlarges the Po_2 difference between the uterine and umbilical circulations. It decreases umbilical venous Po_2, as demonstrated in Table 21.1, and increases uterine venous Po_2.[42,43] This increase in the uterine-umbilical oxygen gradient in human FGR pregnancy[44] together with increased placental mitochondrial DNA content and changes in the mitochondrial function of CTB and mesenchymal stromal cells in FGR pregnancy[45-47] confirm that placental oxygen consumption plays a limiting role in the delivery of oxygen to the fetus, and possibly more so in FGR. However, it should be noted that not all FGR and placental mitochondrial reports display an increased mitochondrial DNA content,[48,49] highlighting the need to understand the etiology of the FGR.

In the FGR condition, the increased uterine venous Po_2 represents the failure of the placenta to become more efficient in extracting O_2 from the uterine circulation. Uterine blood flow to the smaller fetoplacental mass is low in absolute terms but is relatively high with respect to O_2 uptake. It has been suggested that a high Po_2 in the IVS of the FGR placenta could inhibit the growth of the terminal villi, that is to say that the initial failure of these villi to grow sets up a self-inhibiting mechanism.[25] Correspondingly, mean umbilical blood flow is significantly lower and increases with FGR severity relative to control pregnancies. However, it is important to note that when umbilical blood flow is normalized to fetal weight, there are no differences between control and FGR umbilical flow rates or relative to the severity of the FGR.[50]

FETAL OXYGENATION

The chronically catheterized pregnant sheep model has permitted the estimation of fetal oxygen consumption by measuring the rate of umbilical blood flow together with the umbilical venous-arterial difference in oxygen content.[51] A unique aspect of prenatal life is that even under normal physiologic conditions, all organs are perfused by blood with a lower level of oxygenation than occurs in the normal neonate after birth. Owing to the structure of the fetal circulation, fetal arterial blood is formed by mixing of oxygenated blood flowing to the fetus via the umbilical vein with deoxygenated blood flowing through the superior and inferior vena cava.[52] In the third trimester, the normal O_2 saturation and Po_2 of the blood perfusing the fetal upper body via the ascending aorta are approximately 65% and 27 mm Hg, respectively. The blood perfusing the lower body via the abdominal aorta is approximately 50% saturated with O_2 and has a Po_2 of 21 mm Hg. The difference between upper and lower body oxygenation is due to preferential streaming of oxygenated blood from the umbilical vein to the left ventricle via the ductus venosus (DV) in the liver and the foramen ovale between the right and left atria of the heart.

In the third trimester, the fetal oxygen consumption rate is approximately 315 μmol/min/kg body weight.[53] This rate is twice that of the maternal body at rest, and virtually equal to that of a newborn infant in a thermo-neutral environment. The main compensatory mechanism that allows the fetus to maintain a high rate of oxidative metabolism in the presence of a low level of oxygenation is a relatively high cardiac output. In the

Table 21.1 Changes in Umbilical Venous Oxygenation With Increasing Severity of Fetal Growth Restriction Grouped According to Pulsatility Index and Heart Rate Abnormalities.

	N	Gestational Age at Study (wk)	Gestational Age at Delivery (wk)	AC Reduction (%)	PI	HR	Birth Weight (g)	Hbg (g/dL)	Umbilical Vein Po_2 (mm Hg)	Umbilical Vein O_2 Saturation (%)	Umbilical Vein pH	Placental Weight (g)
AGA	6	37.4 ± 0.2	39.1 ± 0.6		Normal	Normal	3453 ± 87	13.5 ± 1.0	35.2 ± 1.0	81.4 ± 3.5	7.36 ± 0.01	51.7 ± 16
FGR1	4	34.7 ± 1.0	37.1 ± 0.9	18.2 ± 12.2	Normal	Normal	2285 ± 362	14.6 ± 1.8	32.5 ± 6.0	71.1 ± 10.7	7.33 ± 0.01	332 ± 78
FGR2	5	29.6 ± 1.5	30.3 ± 0.8	14.9 ± 10.2	Abnormal	Normal	982 ± 221	11.9 ± 0.8	24.1 ± 21 (I)	56.5 ± 5.2 (III)	7.34 ± 0.01	169 ± 30
FGR3	5	28.3 ± 0.7	28.6 ± 0.6	18.2 ± 12.2	Abnormal	Abnormal	740 ± 136	11.9 ± 0.8	21.7 ± 1.5 (II)	50.2 ± 4.1 (IV)	7.33 ± 0.01	158 ± 24

FGR vs. AGA: (I) $P = .005$, (II) $P = .001$, (III) $P = .02$, (IV) $P = .007$.

AC, Abdominal circumference; *AGA*, appropriate-for-gestational age; *FGR*, fetal growth restriction; *HR*, heart rate; *PI*, pulsatility index.

Data from Marconi A, Paolini C, Stramare L, et al. Steady state maternal-fetal leucine enrichments in normal and intrauterine growth-restricted pregnancies. *Pediatr Res*. 1999;46:114–119.

third-trimester fetus, the combined output of the two cardiac ventricles is approximately 450 mL/min/kg, giving a biventricular output/O_2 consumption ratio of approximately 1.4 mL/μmol O_2. This ratio is approximately 70% higher than that of an adult mammal of equal body weight at rest.

The most important function of fetal cardiac output is to allow the fetus to maintain a rate of oxidative metabolism that is independent of the O_2 supply rate.[54] The rate at which umbilical venous blood supplies O_2 to the fetus is defined as the product of umbilical blood flow × umbilical venous O_2 content.[55] In the fetal lamb, the normal umbilical venous O_2 supply/O_2 consumption ratio is approximately 3. This ratio is approximately twice the critical value at which O_2 supply begins to limit O_2 consumption. This defines two degrees of fetal hypoxia: mild hypoxia, in which O_2 supply is less than normal but high enough to allow a supply-independent rate of fetal oxidative metabolism, and severe hypoxia in which supply restricts consumption.

Animal and human FGR studies in which the fetus is hypoxic highlight suboptimal placental oxygen diffusion parameters and likely changes in fetal oxygen utilization.[56-60] The adequate transfer of oxygen to the fetus is dependent upon the development of both the uteroplacental and fetoplacental circulations, and as such three categories of fetal hypoxia have been proposed depending on maternal physiologic status and environment and/or adaption to pregnancy.[61] One category is that of *preplacental hypoxia*. This is a situation where both placenta and fetus become hypoxic because of a reduced oxygen content within maternal blood, such as observed with pregnancy at high altitude, maternal anemia, and asthma.[62-64] The second situation, termed *uteroplacental hypoxia,* is where normally oxygenated maternal blood has a restricted entry into the uteroplacental tissues due either to occlusion or failed trophoblast invasion of uteroplacental arterioles, such as in preeclampsia. The third situation termed *post-placental hypoxia* describes the case were normally oxygenated maternal blood enters the IVS, either at a normal or reduced rate, but there is a major defect in fetoplacental perfusion that prevents the fetus from receiving sufficient oxygen, such as in situations of reduced membrane area for exchange and nutrient transporter activity. Being aware of the type of fetal hypoxia is important as differences in fetoplacental adaptative processes likely exist and these may impact differentially upon fetal circulatory and metabolic outcomes, depending on the etiology of the FGR.

Indeed, in an ovine placental insufficiency FGR (PI-FGR) that produces prolonged moderate to severe fetal hypoxia independent of maternal oxygenation, there is a 25% reduction in fetal oxygen uptake, in what is understood to be a post-placental fetal hypoxia situation. Placental oxygen utilization may represent a limiting step in FGR by restricting oxygen delivery to the fetus.[57] In agreement with these animal studies, the human PI-FGR situation displays a similar increase in the uterine-umbilical or transplacental oxygen gradient[42] along with lower rates of umbilical oxygen delivery and uptake, both in absolute values and normalized for fetal body weight.[50]

The development of the placenta as the organ of fetal oxygenation is an autonomous process to which the fetus must adapt. This adaptation is mediated by the fetal adrenal glands. Blood flow to the adrenals[65] and adrenal norepinephrine (NE) output are inversely related to fetal arterial O_2 content.[66,67] The increase in fetal NE blood concentration inhibits pancreatic insulin output and decreases fetal growth rate.[68,69] When sustained over time, the decrease in growth rate generates a "small-for-gestational-age" fetus. In addition, it results in a decrease in the growth of fetal O_2 consumption because in fetal life O_2 consumption is proportional to body weight, and it is clear that this deceleration is the main target of this regulatory mechanism. The low blood O_2 content that stimulates NE output

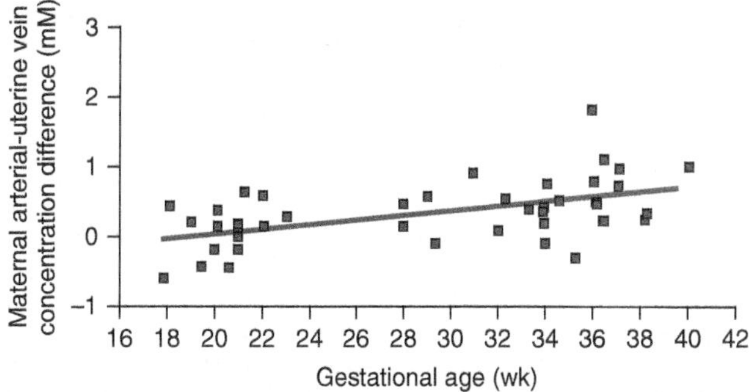

Fig. 21.1 Maternal "arterial"-umbilical venous glucose concentration difference versus gestational age in appropriate for gestational age pregnancies. (From Marconi AM, Paolini C, Buscaglia M, et al. The impact of gestational age and fetal growth on the maternal-fetal glucose concentration difference. *Obstet Gynecol.* 1996;87:937–942.)

is a signal that the placenta is incapable of generating its normal O_2 transport capacity. It is essential for fetal survival to match the growth of fetal O_2 demand to the growth of placental O_2 diffusion. A widening gap between O_2 demand and the ability of the placenta to satisfy that demand leads to a progressive decrease in fetal blood O_2 content.[70] Fetal oxygenation therefore plays an important role in the pathogenesis of all placentally mediated FGR, potentially including those in which there is no evidence of severe hypoxia. The reduced oxygen delivery in FGR fetuses indicates impaired placental oxygen diffusion, whereas reduced oxygen consumption presumably reflects metabolic adaptation to diminished substrate delivery, resulting in slower fetal growth.[57,71]

NUTRIENT TRANSPORT AND METABOLISM

GLUCOSE UPTAKE AND METABOLISM

In animal and human pregnancies, the major carbohydrate the fetus is dependent upon is glucose from the maternal circulation, as there is little fetal gluconeogenesis. Glucose is transported across the placenta by facilitated diffusion, and net transplacental transfer is dependent on the maternal-fetal plasma glucose concentration gradient.[72-77] Placental glucose consumption is high (~30% of uterine glucose uptake) and glucose represents the most important fetal nutrient for energy production. In human pregnancies the glucose/oxygen quotient [(Differnce (uv–ua) glucose concentration (mmol/L)/Difference (uv–ua) O_2 content (mmol/L)] x 6) highlights that if fully oxidized, fetal glucose utilization could account for ≈80% of oxygen uptake.[78] At any one time, however, the percentage of net fetal glucose uptake (utilization) that is oxidized averages approximately 50% to 60%, accounting for only ~30% of the simultaneous net oxygen uptake.[79] The balance of glucose not used immediately for oxidation provides carbon for lactate production, glycogen synthesis and turnover, other metabolic pathways, and in later gestation fat formation.

The glucose gradient across the placenta in normal human pregnancies has been well described by a number of investigators.[72-76] The data described in Fig. 21.1 presents data obtained at the time of cordocentesis for the maternal "arterialized" and fetal umbilical venous glucose concentration differences throughout gestation for normal human pregnancies.[72] It illustrates the fact that the maternal-fetal concentration difference increases with advancing gestation as the fetus develops insulin secretion and insulin sensitive tissue mass (both heart and skeletal muscle), which are also observed in animal model systems.[72,80,81]

In the sheep model of PI-FGR, glucose transport capacity by the placenta is reduced, first because the placenta is smaller, and second because the placenta develops reduced transport capacity, in part due to reduction in selective glucose transporters such as Glut 8.[82,83] In contrast, a study of human placentae with probable FGR showed no reduction in placental Glut 1 transporter expression, which was interpreted as maintenance of glucose transport capacity.[38] However, FGR was defined as infant birth weight <2 SD below the mean for gestational age, indicating that many if not most of the placentae were from normal pregnancies with normal small placentas and fetuses. The proposed FGR group also had only one or two pregnancies complicated by placental disease, such as preeclampsia. Therefore it remains to be determined among human pregnancies with true FGR from true placental insufficiency whether there also might be reductions in glucose transporter expression and related transport capacity.

In FGR pregnancies, glucose uptake into the fetal circulation from the placenta is maintained within the normal range when expressed per kilogram of fetal weight or expressed per gram of placental weight.[84] The maintenance of a normal glucose uptake despite a small placenta is accomplished by an increase in the transplacental glucose gradient, due to the development of lower fetal glucose concentrations. As glucose supply decreases, the fetus increases hepatic glucose production from gluconeogenesis due to specific hepatic insulin resistance,[85] triggered by the low glucose concentrations and potentiation of the gluconeogenic genes by the relative fetal hypoxia.[86-88] Such glucose production protects vital organs such as the brain and heart from potentially damaging or even lethal hypoglycemia. The fetus also maintains weight specific glucose utilization rates from this gluconeogenesis and also the development of increased peripheral glucose and insulin sensitivity.[89-91] Such adaptations have the potential to salvage fetal viability as glucose supply, along with oxygen deficiency, worsens in response to placental insufficiency.

However, in the ovine model of FGR, the maternal-fetal glucose concentration difference is increased significantly in comparison with that in normal pregnancies at the same stage of gestation. Fig. 21.2 illustrates this increase and indicates that the magnitude of the glucose concentration difference correlates with clinical severity of the growth restriction, defined by umbilical artery velocimetry and fetal heart rate (FHR) data.[72] In FGR there are significantly lower umbilical venous and umbilical venoarterial glucose differences, together with a significant reduction (~33%) in umbilical glucose uptake compared with healthy term pregnancy.[50] Umbilical glucose absolute delivery and uptake are significantly reduced, though only glucose uptake is decreased when normalized for fetal body weight.[50] These data support the hypothesis that the human FGR fetus triggers compensatory mechanisms as a survival strategy, principally reducing anabolism, to reduce its metabolic rate, decreasing the proportion of substrate consumption relative to oxygen delivery. The principal compensation is reduced growth rate, since protein synthesis and protein balance are highly energy dependent.[92]

Glucose transport across the placenta is accomplished via insulin independent facilitative glucose transporters grouped collectively as the GLUTs encoded by the *SLC2* genes. GLUT1 *(SLC2A1)*, GLUT3 *(SLC2A3)*, and GLUT8 *(SLC2A8)* have been localized to the placenta. Interestingly, studies of GLUT1 expression in human placentae show no correlation with fetal and placental glucose consumption rates[93] and further, studies in FGR pregnancies have shown that GLUT1 expression is not altered consistent with the foregoing data pointing to the increased transplacental glucose gradient as the primary adaptation to maintain fetal glucose uptake.[94] Reduced glucose transport to the human fetus with FGR therefore is most likely due to the smaller placenta. These findings also are consistent with the hypothesis that GLUT1 expression in the human

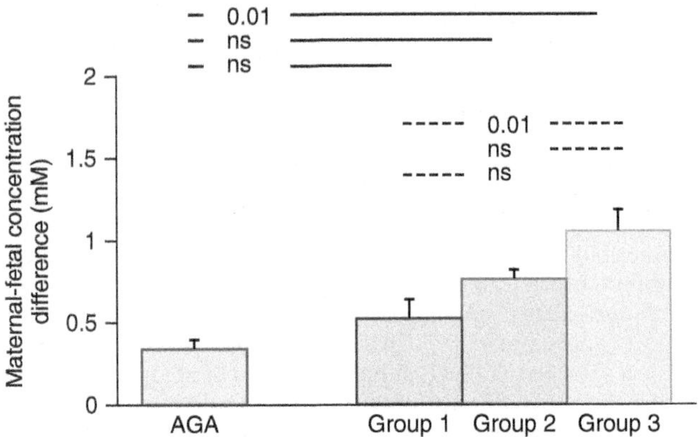

Fig. 21.2 Measured mean ± SD values of maternal "arterial" umbilical venous glucose concentration differences in appropriate-for-gestational age *(AGA)* fetuses and fetal growth restriction *(FGR)* cases with increasing severity (Groups 1, 2, and 3). The *p* values refer to the significance of the differences for the intercepts of AGA versus FGR groups *(solid lines)* and among groups of FGR *(dashed lines)* for the regression analysis of the maternal-fetal difference versus gestational age, because there were no significant differences *(ns)* among the slopes of these regressions. (From Marconi AM, Paolini C, Buscaglia M, et al. The impact of gestational age and fetal growth on the maternal-fetal glucose concentration difference. *Obstet Gynecol.* 1996;87:937–942.)

placenta is altered in type 1 diabetes associated with high maternal glucose concentrations in early pregnancy[95] but not in gestational diabetes, in which maternal glucose concentrations are increased only in late pregnancy.[96]

Another aspect of glucose metabolism in human FGR pregnancies is the question of whether significant gluconeogenesis occurs, as has been documented in FGR sheep. Fig. 21.3 summarizes the normal fluxes into and out of the fetal liver in the ovine fetus in late gestation (control period).[97] Notably in fetal sheep, the fetal liver has a very large uptake of lactate and gluconeogenic amino acids. Despite this large uptake of potential glucose carbon, no significant glucose release from the fetal liver occurs under normal conditions. Instead, carbon leaves the liver primarily as glutamate, and to a lesser extent, as serine, pyruvate, ornithine, and aspartate. It is only when fetal gluconeogenesis is stimulated by a fetal infusion of glucagon that net glucose release from the liver can be found and, in response, glutamate release is virtually shut off. In contrast, long-term fasting producing sustained maternal and fetal hypoglycemia in the pregnant ewe induces fetal glucose production by gluconeogenesis,[98] and this occurs naturally towards the end of gestation in fetal sheep in which FGR was induced by placental insufficiency due to maternal exposure to hyperthermia during mid- and late pregnancy. In this condition, placental glucose transfer capacity was reduced as well as absolute transport based on the smaller size of the placenta. Other models of ovine placental insufficiency do not universally have reduced placental transport capacity.[99] In the sheep maternal hyperthermia model of PI-FGR-induced gluconeogenesis can be enhanced by infusion of amino acids, which might not occur naturally in human FGR, perhaps explaining the lack of gluconeogenesis in human FGR versus ovine PI-FGR.

In human FGR pregnancies, stable isotope-labeled glucose has been infused into the maternal circulation to investigate whether dilution of the fetal plasma glucose enrichment occurs as an indication of fetal glucose production.[100] These measurements were carried out after an overnight fast in a group of pregnant women who had documented small fetuses and other conditions indicating FGR and showed no evidence of dilution of the fetal glucose enrichment, indicating no fetal new glucose production.

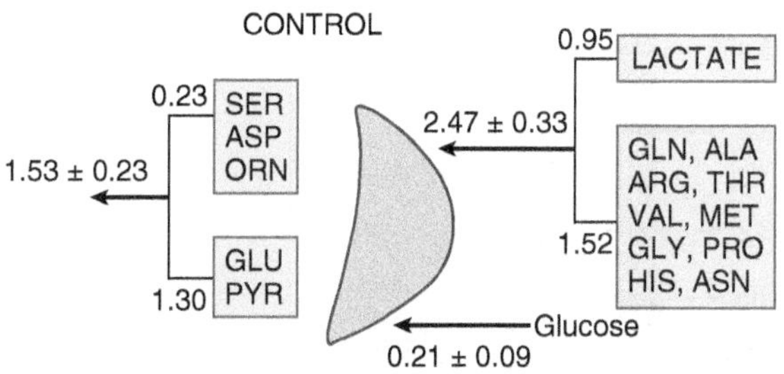

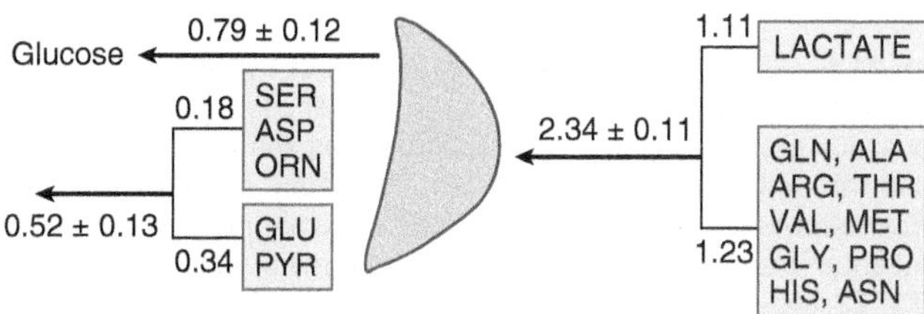

Fig. 21.3 Fetal hepatic uptake and output of glucose carbon and glucogenic substrate carbon under normal conditions (control) and during a glucagon-somatostatin infusion into the fetal circulation. Each number represents a substrate carbon-to-oxygen uptake molar ratio. *ALA,* Alanine; *ARG,* arginine; *ASN,* asparagine; *ASP,* aspartic acid; *GLN,* glutamine; *GLU,* glutamate; *GLY,* glycine; *HIS,* histidine; *MET,* methionine; *ORN,* ornithine; *PRO,* proline; *PYR,* pyruvate; *SER,* serine; *THR,* threonine; *VAL,* valine. (From Teng C, Battaglia F, Meschia G, et al. Fetal hepatic and umbilical uptakes of glucogenic substrates during a glucagonsomatostatin infusion. *Am J Physiol.* 2002;282:542–550.)

Thus, in this study, a human FGR pregnancy did not demonstrate detectable fetal gluconeogenesis, and this highlights the need for further chronic steady state studies. Clearly, fetal glucose production in response to reduced glucose supply is variable among studies and deserves further research into mechanisms that might underlie species differences.

Lactic acidemia, hypoxia, and acidosis are frequent complications of FGR pregnancies, particularly in those with signs of reduced villous vascular development evident through Doppler ultrasound. Considering lactic acidemia and acidosis, it is important to emphasize the unique metabolic characteristics of the fetal liver and placenta with regard to the metabolism and transport of lactate and pyruvate. In animal studies, it has been well established that the fetal liver has a large net output of pyruvate and net uptake of lactate from the fetal circulation. In view of the fact that the fetal liver is perfused with a high percentage of umbilical venous blood, the most-oxygenated blood of the fetus, it is clear that the fetal liver could play an important role in the defense of acid-base balance during fetal hypoxia. Fig. 21.4 presents in graphic form some of the changes in acid-base balance and lactate concentration during severe and persistent fetal hypoxia.[101] The striking finding is that despite persistent, severe fetal hypoxia for 24 hours, the fetal acidosis is largely corrected as reflected in fetal arterial pH, although the lactate concentration is still elevated. This correction of metabolic acidosis occurs because of the continued uptake of lactate and release of pyruvate from the fetal liver. The important finding of continuing uptake of lactate and release of pyruvate by the fetal liver, even during persistent severe fetal hypoxia,[82] was derived from studies carried out on normal pregnancies, which were then made hypoxic. However, in FGR pregnancies in which the DV shunt may be increased, this defense mechanism may be further compromised. It is the reduced hepatic perfusion in some FGR pregnancies that makes the growth-restricted fetus particularly vulnerable to fetal hypoxia.

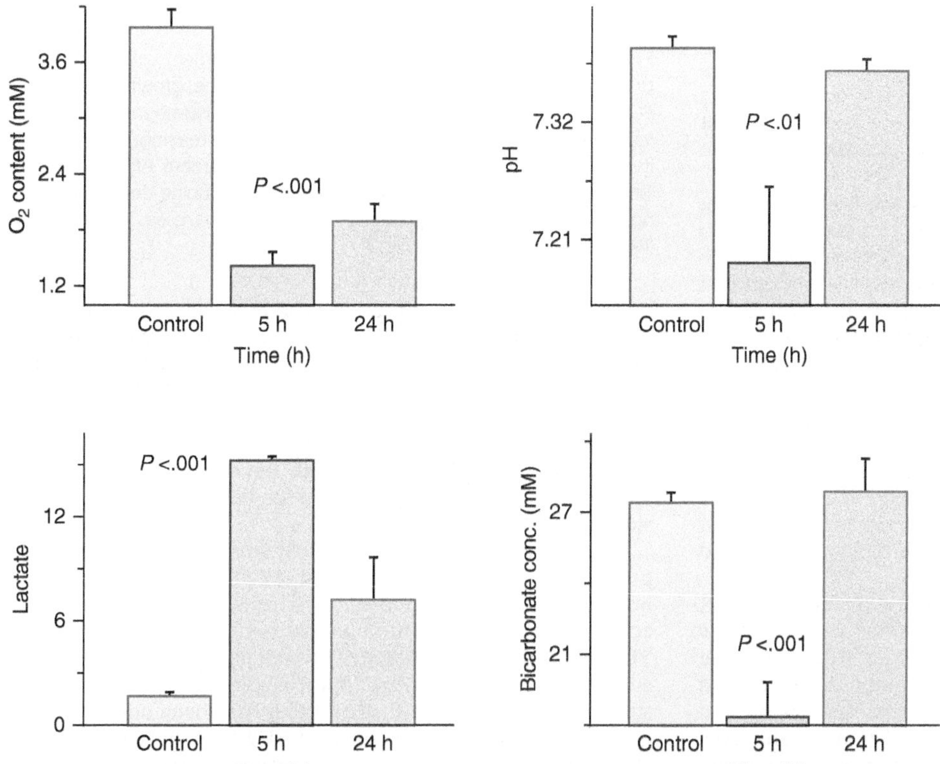

Fig. 21.4 Changes in acid-base balance and lactate concentration during severe and persistent fetal hypoxia. (From Wilkening RB, Boyle D, Meschia G. Fetal pH improvement after 24 h of severe, nonlethal hypoxia. *Biol Neonate.* 1993;63:129–132.)

Scaling of all metabolic data is critically important in studies of FGR pregnancies. Because both the fetus and the placenta are smaller than normal, all of the values for uptake of nutrients and for blood flow will be reduced unless the data are normalized for body size. The smaller conceptus mass significantly reduces the metabolic demand on the mother. In human pregnancies, this issue has been addressed only for glucose.[76] Marconi and co-workers examined the relationship among three variables: (1) maternal plasma glucose disposal rate at steady state, a measure of maternal glucose utilization; (2) conceptus mass (fetal weight plus placental weight); and (3) maternal plasma glucose concentration.[76] These studies highlight the fact that, at comparable maternal glucose concentrations, the smaller the mass of the conceptus, the lower the maternal glucose utilization rate.

AMINO ACID TRANSPORT AND METABOLISM

Placental amino acid transport and metabolism are key determinants of placental and fetal growth, providing essential amino acids for protein synthesis and nonessential amino acids to facilitate the actions of other transporters and metabolic processes.[102-104] Amino acid uptake by all cells, including the trophoblast, is mediated by a large number of transporter proteins, which have been classified into three broad transport systems: accumulative, exchange, and facilitative. These transport systems interact to promote net transfer of amino acids into the placental trophoblast and then, for most of the amino acids, into the fetal plasma against a concentration gradient.[105] The net amino acid flux per unit area of the trophoblast depends on the density of the transporter proteins in the apical (or maternal mircovillous) and basal (fetal-facing) membranes, the metabolic and anabolic demands of the intervening trophoblast cytoplasm, and the rate of blood flow in the uterine and umbilical circulations.[105-107] Studies in animal and human FGR have highlighted multiple differences in placental amino acid transporter expression and activity.[108,109] A key early finding, highlighted in microvesicle preparations from either the apical or basal surface of the trophoblast, is that transport capacity is reduced on both surfaces of the placenta.[100,110,111] This reduction in transport capacity is not present for all of the amino acid transport systems, nor are the reductions the same on each surface of the trophoblast. Furthermore, in vivo changes in amino acid transport in FGR pregnancies can reflect changes not only in membrane transporter activity but also in placental utilization or production of an amino acid and perfusion of the placenta.

The pregnant sheep model has been instrumental is developing a working framework of how these changes in placental amino acid transport occur in human FGR pregnancies. For example, the net uptake of leucine, an essential and nutritionally fundamental amino acid, into the fetal circulation is determined principally by three different fluxes of approximately equal magnitude: (1) the transplacental flux from maternal plasma to fetal plasma, (2) the back flux from the fetal plasma into the placenta, and (3) the leucine flux from placental protein breakdown into the fetal plasma (Fig. 21.5). In a sheep model of FGR, it has been shown for leucine and another essential amino acid, threonine, that the transplacental flux of both are significantly reduced,[112-114] even when the flux is expressed per gram of placenta. In these studies, the fetal adaptation to the reduced transplacental flux is a lower fetal plasma amino acid concentration.

Other sheep FGR studies have shown that the effect of FGR upon fetal amino acid metabolism and plasma concentrations depends on the severity of the FGR. In milder FGR, when fetal growth is still present, amino acid concentrations are reduced due to reduced transport from the placenta and maintained utilization for protein synthesis and oxidation.[115] However, when FGR is severe and fetal growth has stopped, fetal amino acid concentrations appear to be "maintained" because they are

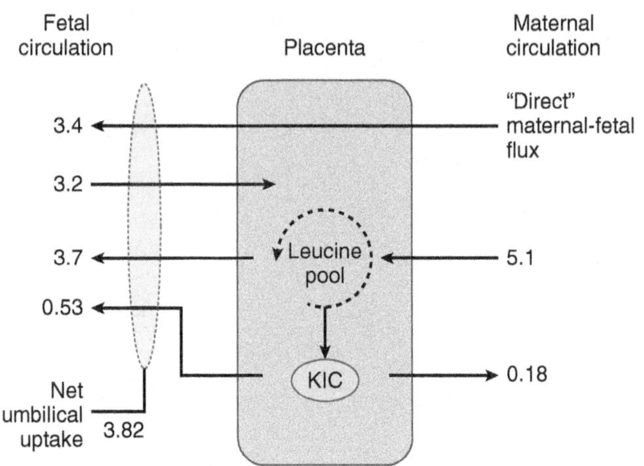

Fig. 21.5 The fluxes of leucine into and out of the placenta (μmol/min/kg fetal weight) measured in vivo under steady-state conditions are presented. The three major fluxes that together determine the umbilical uptake are of approximately equal magnitude. *KIC*, Alpha-ketoisocaproic acid. (From Battaglia FC, Regnault TR. Placental transport and metabolism of amino acids. *Placenta.* 2001;22:145–161.)

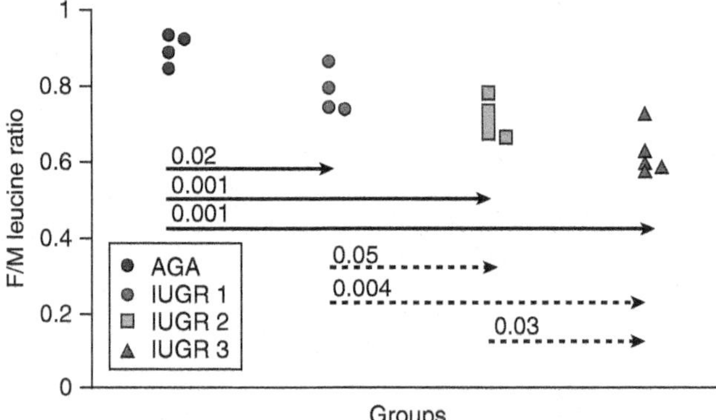

Fig. 21.6 Leucine fetal-maternal *(F/M)* enrichment ratio in appropriate-for-gestational-age *(AGA)* and intrauterine growth restriction *(IUGR)* pregnancies at fetal blood sampling. Numbers indicate *P* values for comparisons between groups for increasing IUGR severity as indicated by adjacent arrows. (From Marconi AM, Paolini C, Stramare L, et al. Steady state maternal-fetal leucine enrichments in normal and intrauterine growth-restricted pregnancies. *Pediatr Res.* 1999;46:114–119.)

no longer used for net protein synthesis and protein balance (growth). This reduced utilization for protein synthesis and balance occurs in conjunction with reduced net oxygen and glucose uptake by the fetus and leads in turn to a lower fetal amino acid oxidation rate and a reduced back-flux into the placenta. These changes tend to divert these amino acids to fetal protein synthesis, even though the overall rate of protein synthesis is reduced (i.e., growth is slowed, but not completely stopped).[57,116,117]

Reduced transplacental amino acid flux in sheep also leads to a significantly lower fetal-maternal (F/M) enrichment ratio for both leucine and threonine when stable isotopes of these amino acids are infused into the maternal circulation in sheep FGR. The fetal enrichment is reduced by endogenous release of amino acids from protein. Similar clinical studies of the F/M ratio of stable isotopes of essential amino acids have been undertaken in normal and FGR human pregnancies (Fig. 21.6).[118] These human studies clearly demonstrate a significant reduction in the F/M enrichment ratio for leucine in FGR pregnancies, presumably

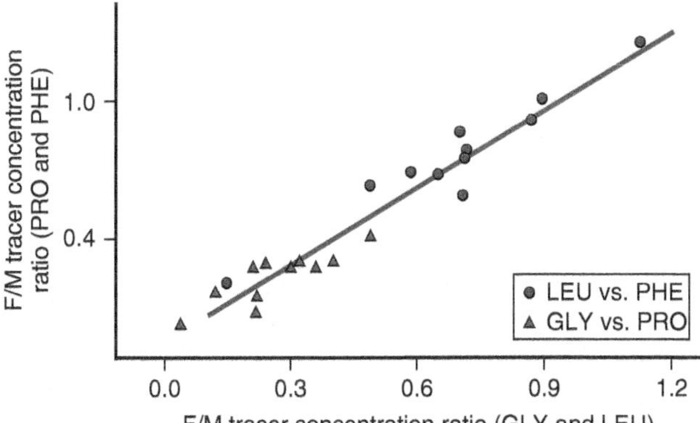

Fig. 21.7 The fetal-maternal *(F/M)* plasma tracer concentration ratios are plotted with the values for glycine *(GLY)* and leucine *(LEU)* along the abscissa and those for proline *(PRO)* and phenylalanine *(PHE)* along the ordinate. The regression is highly significant: (F/M)y = −0.0511 + 1.1274 (F/M)x, $r^2 = 0.94$; $P<.001$. (From Paolini CL, Marconi A, Ronzoni S, et al. Placental transport of leucine, phenylalanine, glycine, and proline in intrauterine growth−restricted pregnancies. *J Clin Endocrinol Metab.* 2001;86:5427–5432.)

reflecting a significant reduction in the maternal-to-fetal transplacental flux. Additionaly, the magnitude of this reduced F/M enrichment correlates with the classification of clinical severity of FGR pregnancies proposed by Pardi and colleagues, which was based on fetal umbilical arterial velocimetry and FHR data.[119]

Using non-steady-state methodologies, the transport rates of the nine essential amino acids have been studied in normal sheep pregnancies.[120] The three branched chain amino acids (leucine, isoleucine, and valine) and phenylalanine and methionine had similar plasma clearances, and their fluxes were directly correlated to their maternal concentrations. Similar methodology has been used in normal and FGR human pregnancies to examine the relative placental transport rates for four amino acids: leucine, phenylalanine, glycine, and proline.[56] Fig. 21.7 compares the F/M plasma enrichment ratio of leucine with phenylalanine and that of glycine with proline. No significant differences in transport rate were found between leucine and phenylalanine, or between glycine and proline. However, leucine and phenylalanine crossed much more quickly than glycine and proline. In human FGR pregnancies, the F/M ratios of leucine and phenylalanine were significantly reduced compared with those in normally grown pregnancies.

Studies in human FGR have shown significant direct relationships between placental weight and fetal oxygenation,[121,122] similar to reports in pregnant sheep.[116] In these human FGR studies, infusion of stable isotopic tracers into the maternal circulation demonstrated that the transplacental fluxes of leucine and phenylalanine were a smaller fraction of the fetal plasma turnover of these amino acids than in normal pregnancy, although the umbilical venous concentrations of these amino acids were not below normal[121,123] values. Sheep studies highlighted that the severe FGR fetuses have a much lower mean umbilical venous O_2 saturation than controls (44.7% vs. 72.5%), in conjunction with an abnormally high impedance to umbilical blood flow, and therefore it is likely that hypoxia decreased the clearance of amino acids from the fetal circulation, resulting in increased F/M ratios with decreased placental weights as observed in the human reports. Together, these data indicate that in the near term FGR fetus, impairment of placental O_2 transport may induce a state of fetal hypoxia that in turn reduces the ability/demand of the fetus to utilize metabolic substrates. Therefore the reduction in amino acid uptake in an FGR pregnancy is not only likely due to reduced placental amino acid transport capacity.[124] but also is the consequence of decreased fetal oxidative metabolism and growth rate, which together reduce fetal amino acid demand.[116,124]

FATTY ACID TRANSPORT AND METABOLISM

Placental transport of fatty acids (FA) is critical for normal fetoplacental function,[125] but their transport across the placenta in FGR pregnancies has not been studied in detail. Studies in food-restricted pregnant baboons as a model of FGR demonstrated increased placental expression of FA binding and transport proteins in late gestation, with fetal plasma FA concentrations that were similar to those of control animals, indicating adaptation of placental transport in this model to maintain delivery of critically needed FAs to the fetus and placenta.[126]

A related study—using human placental tissue from idiopathic FGR and gestational age-matched, appropriately grown fetuses—measured FA binding protein expression of FABP4 and perilipin-2 in placental homogenates and FATPs (2, 4, 6, CD36) in syncytiotrophoblast apical membrane. Apical FATP6 and CD36 expression was significantly increased in FGR. The concentrations of seven *n*-6 and *n*-3 species long-chain polyunsaturated FAs (LCPUFA) were significantly increased in the triglyceride fraction in FGR versus AGA placenta. LCPUFAs were preferentially routed toward cellular storage in triglyceride in the FGR placenta, possibly protecting against oxidative stress associated with cellular FA accumulation. The increased storage of LCPUFAs may have been the result of impaired efflux of FAs across the basal membrane in the FGR placenta.[127]

CLINICAL IMPLICATIONS OF ABNORMAL PLACENTAL DEVELOPMENT AND FETAL OXYGENATION IN FETAL GROWTH RESTRICTION

FETAL UMBILICAL ARTERY BLOOD FLOW VELOCIMETRY

The introduction of Doppler ultrasonography has led to a significant increase in our understanding, diagnosis, and management of placental and fetal changes in FGR. Noninvasive measurements of the pulsatility index (PI), a measure of resistance to flow of fetal blood vessels, have become widely used tools for monitoring the physiologic state of the fetus. In normal pregnancies, umbilical artery (UA) PI starts at high values and then decreases progressively toward term. This indicates that normal placental development entails a progressive decrease in the impedance of the umbilical vascular bed to blood flow. In contrast to the normal pattern of development, in a subset of FGR cases there is a progressive deterioration in the UA velocity wave form, from an abnormally high PI, to absent and subsequently reversed end-diastolic flow.[128] In the human fetus, the two conditions of absent or reversed end-diastolic flow are presumptive evidence of hypoxia, because in association with a decrease in umbilical blood flow, umbilical venous O_2 content is approximately 30% to 40% less than normal[121] (see Table 21.1).

ASSOCIATION OF UMBILICAL ARTERY PULSATILITY INDEX ABNORMALITIES WITH A DECREASE IN UMBILICAL VENOUS OXYGENATION

Sampling of umbilical venous blood via cordocentesis has demonstrated that in FGR, an abnormally high umbilical artery PI is associated with a significant decrease in the Po_2 and O_2 saturation of umbilical venous blood.[37,129] Table 21.1 shows the results of a study that compared 14 FGR cases with six AGA fetuses.[37] The FGR cases were subdivided into three groups according to clinical criteria. The first group (FGR1) consisted of FGR cases having normal UA PI and heart rate variability, the second (FGR2) represented fetuses with abnormally high UA PI and normal heart rate variability, and the third (FGR3) represented cases in which both UA PI and heart rate variability were abnormal. Groups 2 and 3 demonstrated a significant reduction in the oxygenation of umbilical venous blood, while the cord blood pH in FGR remained within normal limits. This is in contrast with the low pH values that are found in acute hypoxia, and in agreement with the observation that fetal lambs re-establish a normal pH within 24 hours from the onset of severe hypoxia.[130]

FETAL RESPONSE TO ABNORMAL OXYGENATION AND UMBILICAL ARTERY DOPPLERS: MIDDLE CEREBRAL ARTERY PULSATILITY INDEX AND BRAIN SPARING

Studies in fetal sheep have demonstrated that cerebral blood flow is inversely related to arterial blood O_2 content.[65] This inverse hyperbolic relationship tends to maintain constant cerebral O_2 delivery (the product of cerebral blood flow × O_2 content). As a result, cerebral vascular resistance to blood flow is decreased in hypoxic conditions, and an abnormally high umbilical PI is often associated with a significantly low middle cerebral artery (MCA) PI. Despite this brain-protective mechanism, fetuses with FGR remain at risk for adverse neurodevelopmental outcomes, regardless of the gestational age at which they are delivered.[131] Human and animal FGR studies have found deficiencies in brain maturation and cortical development, despite the relative increase in cerebral blood flow.[132,133] Associations of abnormal brain development with placental insufficiency and brain sparing have been confirmed using MRI-based technologies.[134] These technologies show promise in assessing the association between placental insufficiency, reduced cerebral oxygenation, and abnormal cerebral growth and maturation noninvasively,[134a] and could be developed into potential tools for antenatal surveillance, clinical management, and improved perinatal outcomes in settings of FGR.

MCA PI increases from mid-gestation to approximately the beginning of the third trimester and then declines. Deterioration of MCA PI or the cerebroplacental ratio (CPR; ratio of MCA PI relative to UA PI) can occur up to 9 weeks before an indication to deliver, sometimes in the absence of other Doppler abnormalities. Alternatively, stillbirth can occur unexpectedly when MCA changes occur closer to the event (median 4 days), and for this reason MCA Dopplers are more useful in guiding the monitoring frequency to screen for more significant signs of fetal deterioration (amniotic fluid volume, abnormal biophysical profile or cardiotocography, DV Dopplers) than in guiding a decision to deliver.[135] A meta-analysis of the value of the assessment of brain sparing concluded that CPR alone or in addition to UA PI adds little to the prediction of adverse perinatal outcomes.[136,137] Despite this, most international guidelines have incorporated MCA Dopplers to guide management of FGR in the third trimester of pregnancy.[138]

Measurement of the MCA PI may be more valuable in the prevention of perinatal morbidity and mortality in situations where risk of fetal compromise is increased despite normal placental development, such as in maternal obesity, pregestational diabetes, and GDM. To meet the requirements of increased fetal growth in GDM,[139] placental blood perfusion and blood volume increase, and vascular resistance decreases.[140] The fetus may experience hypoxia and ischemia, which, it is postulated, occur when fetal oxygen demand exceeds supply. A brain-sparing effect is then triggered, leading to dilation of the MCA.[141] Resistance is reduced and brain development is promoted, reflecting the contribution of the MCA to the head circumference, while the placental circulation is not deficient and changes in UA PI remain absent.[141] These factors may likely contribute to the failure of routine screening for at-risk pregnancies from the measurement of symphysis fundal height or estimated fetal weight, and the failure of UA Dopplers to prevent stillbirth in women with obesity and/or diabetes.[142]

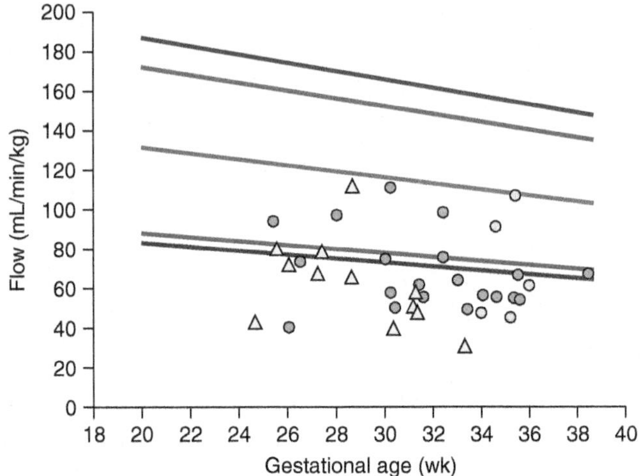

Fig. 21.8 Umbilical vein flow per unit head circumference plotted against gestational age in growth-restricted fetuses. *Purple circle,* Group 1; *gold circle,* group 2; *blue triangle,* group 3. *Continuous lines* represent the 5th, 10th, 50th, 90th, and 95th percentiles from 70 normally grown fetuses. (From Ferrazzi E, Rigano S, Bozzo M, et al. Umbilical vein blood flow in growth-restricted fetuses. *Ultrasound Obstet Gynecol.* 2000;16:432–438.)

FETAL HYPOXIA AND DUCTUS VENOSUS FLOW

In the first DV studies, performed in 137 uncomplicated singleton pregnancies, Bellotti and colleagues[143] reported that the flow through the DV, as a percentage of the umbilical blood flow, decreased from 40% at 20 weeks to approximately 15% at term. Later studies in fetuses with FGR showed that DV flow was significantly increased, with the DV flow exceeding the umbilical flow in 40% of the cases.[144] This increase in DV flow was shown to be due to retrograde flow from the portal vein into the DV. Thus, under conditions of a reduced umbilical flow and an increased DV shunt, the reduction in hepatic flow from the umbilical vein could inhibit normal metabolism of all nutrients, including amino acids, by the fetal liver,[145] thereby adversely impacting fetal liver development and ultimately fetal growth and metabolism.

Ferrazzi and colleagues have shown a significant reduction in umbilical blood flow in FGR pregnancies (Fig. 21.8).[146] This, in itself, would reduce hepatic perfusion, and coupled with an increased ductal shunt hepatic perfusion can be severely effected, resulting in a reduction in hepatic flow from the umbilical vein as large as 80%. When the temporal sequence of changes in eight Doppler indices were studied in FGR fetuses, the changes in the DV were found to occur close to the time fetal heart rate abnormalities were observed,[147] and were considered ominous findings. However, as changes in DV flow are considered a circulatory adaptation to the changes in placental function, these changes in the DV velocity waveforms are only found to occur prior to these abnormal FHR findings in 50% of the cases,[131,148] limiting the clinical utility of DV assessment in the management of FGR pregnancies. It also has been postulated that infants who are delivered for alterations in DV flow velocity rather than changes in FHR are able to maintain brain protection from hypoxia[149] and have better neurodevelopmental outcomes at 2 years of age.[150]

NEW HORIZONS: ASSESSMENT OF ABNORMAL FETOPLACENTAL METABOLISM

Most commonly, FGR screening by ultrasound includes an assessment of estimated fetal weight and adding Dopplers of UA, MCA, and DV if growth is considered abnormal. Whether or not maternal factors and obstetric history, serial measurements, or assessment of body proportions[151] are taken into account, this approach has limitations and antenatal detection of FGR still remains 20% to 50%.[152-154] High false-positive rates are caused by the fact that the majority of thus identified fetuses are healthy and constitutionally small (normal SGA). Limitations in the detection of those fetuses with impaired growth even though EFW is >10th percentile have precluded the use of ultrasound in the screening for FGR in low-risk populations. For this reason, FGR newborns remain at higher risk of stillbirth and neonatal morbidity and mortality. Even in adolescence and adulthood, they often present suboptimal metabolic and cardiovascular outcomes, and there has been a strong push to develop new techniques beyond fetal size and fetoplacental blood flow to assess fetal and placental function and to identify failure to achieve individual growth potential.

New MRI technologies have enabled assessment of tissue concentrations of metabolites (nuclear magnetic resonance), and in vivo blood flow and oxygenation, and have provided promising strategies for further investigations into placental pathology underlying FGR and the fetal response to the placental dysfunction. Blood T2 MRI relaxometry techniques have been used to noninvasively measure fetal oxygenation in near-term sheep and human fetuses, and have shown excellent correlation with invasive O_2 saturation measurements.[155] These techniques, for example, have enabled measurement of the selective streaming of oxygenated umbilical venous blood to the left heart for distribution to brain and coronary arteries, especially when motion-compensating reconstruction algorithms are being used.[155a] Recently, in utero placental shape and textural features computed on 3D MRI have demonstrated high accuracy in healthy and high-risk cohorts.[156] These new imaging technologies are contributing to improved understanding of the processes underlying FGR.

Noninvasive techniques using maternal blood markers provide unique opportunities to address mechanistic aspects of FGR and placental function. In addition to biomarkers, such as placental steroid and peptide hormones, the maternal circulatory system carries bioactive molecules and circulating nucleic acids from the fetoplacental unit, whose concentrations change as gestation progresses. These biomarkers also change in response to stresses and may offer unique signatures in association with suboptimal growth and development patterns in FGR. New and expanding fields in assessing the fetoplacental interactive environment include fetal cell-free RNA/DNA,[157-159] miRNAs,[160,161] proteomic[162] and metabolomic[163,164] profiling, and exosome characterization.[165]

The employment of functional assessments, such as fetal blood vessel oxygenation[154a,167] in conjunction with placental metabolic/function readouts,[164,168] can provide information regarding the association of abnormal fetal growth with pathologic processes in the placenta and fetus. Analysis of metabolic "omic" readouts may provide more detailed information about the pathologic processes in utero and aid in the distinction between constitutional smallness and FGR that could be important for clinical practice. Additional advancements in mathematical and computational models from AI and machine learning will provide new insights into placental physiology.[169-171] Together these new mechanistic approaches are leading to new opportunities to advance clinical management and better outcomes of pregnancies with FGR.

CONCLUSION AND CLINICAL IMPLICATIONS

This chapter has focused on FGR associated with a placental insufficiency that likely is the result of an idiopathic perfusion failure limiting oxygen and nutrient transport to the fetus and the subsequent fetal adaptations to that environment. It is important to remember that understanding the etiology of the FGR is critical to truly assess FGR type specific circulatory and metabolic changes associated with that insult and adaptive processes. In the context of PI-FGR is clear that the fetus experiences deficits in supplies of O_2 and nutrients from a less optimally functioning placenta. Most of these deficits can be attributed initially to maldevelopment of the placenta, which not only is reduced in size but also has structural abnormalities in its vasculature and reductions in diffusion/transport capacity. These changes in the placenta, with the additional factor of chronic fetal hypoxia, can lead to circulatory changes in many fetal vascular beds. Circulatory and metabolic studies have demonstrated a wide range in clinical severity of FGR based on fetal size for gestation. Animal-based studies and human observational studies indicate that the FGR placenta is not always dysfunctional in FGR pregnancies, rather adverse changes in placental diffusion/transport observed in the FGR placenta also represent adaptations to reduced fetal anabolic metabolism and growth in response to an inability of the mother to allocate resources to the fetus. Delineating more homogeneous subsets of FGR pregnancies (e.g., pregnancies from altitude, under or over nutrition, pre-eclampsia) in terms of the type of insult and the severity of the growth restriction, and defining the processes underlying the placental and fetal interactions in FGR add significant potential clinical value; they can (1) help direct optimal timing of delivery in pregnancies that feature severe FGR, (2) form the basis for adjustments in neonatal care of affected infants, and (3) provide the foundation for more focused follow-up studies in both childhood and adulthood.

A complete reference list is available at www.ExpertConsult.com. 

SELECT REFERENCES

1. Battaglia F, Lubchenco L. A practical classification of newborn infants by weight and gestational age. *J Pediatr*. 1967;71:159-163.
2. *Manual of the International Statistical Classification of Diseases. Injuries and Causes of Death. Rev. 6*. Geneva: World Health Organization; 1949.
3. Battaglia F, Frazier T, Ellegers A. Birth weight, gestational age, and pregnancy outcome, with special reference to high birth weight-low gestational age infant. *Pediatrics*. 1966;37:417-422.
18. Gardosi J, Chang A, Kalyan B, et al. Customised antenatal growth charts. *Lancet*. 1992;339:283-287.
19. Altman D, Coles E. Nomograms for precise determination of birth weight for dates. *Br J Obstet Gynaecol*. 1980;87:81-86.
20. Brenner W, Edelman D, Hendricks C. A standard of fetal growth for the United States of America. *Am J Obstet Gynecol*. 1976;126:555-564.
25. Benirschke K, Kaufmann P, Baergen RN. *Pathology of the Human Placenta*. 5th ed. New York: Springer; 2006.
32. Molina RD, Meschia G, Wilkening RB. Uterine blood flow, oxygen and glucose uptakes at mid-gestation in the sheep. *Proc Soc Exp Biol Med*. 1990;195:379-385.
33. Soothill PW, Nicolaides KH, Rodeck CH, et al. Effect of gestational age on fetal intervillous blood gas and acid-base values in human pregnancy. *Fetal Ther*. 1986;1:168.
34. Jackson MR, Mayhem TM, Boyd PA. Quantitative description of the elaboration and maturation of villi from 10 weeks of gestation to term. *Placenta*. 1992;13:357-370.
36. Jackson MR, Walsh AJ, Morrow RJ, et al. Reduced placental villous tree elaboration in small-for-gestational-age pregnancies: relationship with umbilical artery Doppler waveforms. *Am J Obstet Gynecol*. 1995;172:518-524.
37. Marconi AM, Paolini C, Stramare L, et al. Steady state maternal-fetal leucine enrichments in normal and intrauterine growth-restricted pregnancies. *Pediatr Res*. 1999;46:114-119.
38. Fujikura T, Yoshida J. Blood gas analysis of placental and uterine blood during cesarean delivery. *Obstet Gynecol*. 1996;87:133-136.

42. Pardi G, Cetin I, Marconi A, et al. Venous drainage of the human uterus: respiratory gas studies in normal and fetal growth-retarded pregnancies. *Am J Obstet Gynecol*. 1992;166:699-706.
43. Regnault TRH, de Vrijer B, Galan HL, et al. Development of mechanisms of fetal hypoxia in severe fetal growth restriction. *Placenta*. 2007;28:714-723.
52. Dawes GS. *The Foetal Circulation. Foetal and Neonatal Physiology*. Chicago: Year Book Medical Publishers; 1968.
53. Battaglia FC, Meschia G. Review of studies in human pregnancy of uterine and umbilical blood flows. *Dev Period Med*. 2013;12:287-292.
54. Meschia G. Placental respiratory gas exchange and fetal oxygenation. In: Creasy RK, Resnik R, et al., eds. *Creasy & Resnik's Maternal-Fetal Medicine: Principles and Practice*. 7th ed; 2014:163-174.
55. Wilkening RB, Meschia G. Fetal oxygen uptake, oxygenation, and acid-base balance as a function of uterine blood flow. *Am J Physiol*. 1983;244: H749-H755.
65. Peeters LLH, Sheldon RE, Jones Jr M, et al. Blood flow to fetal organs as a function of arterial oxygen content. *Am J Obstet Gynecol*. 1979;135: 637-646.
66. Limesand SW, Rozance PJ, Zerbe GO, et al. Attenuated insulin release and storage in fetal sheep pancreatic islets with intrauterine growth restriction. *Endocrinology*. 2006;147:1488-1497.
67. Rozance PJ, Limesand SW, Barry JS, et al. Glucose replacement to euglycemia causes hypoxia, acidosis, and decreased insulin secretion in fetal sheep with intrauterine growth restriction. *Pediatr Res*. 2009;65:72-78.
68. Bassett JM, Hanson C. Catecholamines inhibit growth in fetal sheep in the absence of hypoxemia. *Am J Physiol*. 1998;274:R1536-R1545.
69. Wilkening R, Boyle D, Meschia G. Fetal pH improvement after 24 h of severe, nonlethal hypoxia. *Biol Neonate*. 1993;63:129-132.
72. Nicolini U, Hubinont C, Santolaya J, et al. Maternal-fetal glucose gradient in normal pregnancies and in pregnancies complicated by alloimmunization and fetal growth retardation. *Am J Obstet Gynecol*. 1989;161:924-927.
73. Bozzetti P, Ferrari M, Marconi A, et al. The relationship of maternal and fetal glucose concentrations in the human from mid-gestation until term. *Metabolism*. 1988;37:358-363.
74. Economides D, Nicolaides KH, Campbell S. Relation between maternal-to-fetal blood glucose gradient and uterine and umbilical Doppler blood flow measurements. *Br J Obstet Gynaecol*. 1990;97:543-544.
75. Marconi A, Davoli E, Cetin I, et al. Impact of conceptus mass on glucose disposal rate in pregnant women. *Am J Physiol*. 1993;264:514-518.
76. Jansson T, Wennergren M, Illsley NP. Glucose transporter protein expression in human placenta throughout gestation and in intrauterine growth retardation. *J Clin Endocrinol Metab*. 1993;77:1554-1562.
82. Thureen P, Trembler KA, Meschia G, et al. Placental glucose transport in heat-induced fetal growth retardation. *Am J Physiol*. 1992;263:578-585.
84. Marconi A, Paolini C, Buscaglia M, et al. The impact of gestational age and fetal growth on the maternal-fetal glucose concentration difference. *Obstet Gynecol*. 1996;87:937-942.
94. Jansson T, Wennergren M, Powell T. Placental glucose transport and GLUT 1 expression in insulin-dependent diabetes. *Am J Obstet Gynecol*. 1999;180: 163-168.
95. Jansson T, Ekstrand Y, Wennergren M, Powell T. Placental glucose transport in gestational diabetes mellitus. *Am J Obstet Gynecol*. 2001;184:111-116.
96. Teng C, Battaglia F, Meschia G, et al. Fetal hepatic and umbilical uptakes of glucogenic substrates during a glucagon-somatostatin infusion. *Am J Physiol Endocrinol Metab*. 2002;282:542-550.
97. Marconi A, Cetin I, Davoli E, et al. An evaluation of fetal glucogenesis in intrauterine growth-retarded pregnancies. *Metabolism*. 1993;42:860-864.
100. Battaglia F, Regnault T. Placental transport and metabolism of amino acids. *Placenta*. 2001;22:145-161.
101. Holcomb RG, Wilkening RB. Hepatic metabolism during acute hypoxia in fetal lambs. *Pediatr Res*. 1998;43:49A.
102. Moe AJ. Placental amino acid transport. *Am J Physiol*. 1995;268:1321-1331.
103. Jansson T. Amino acid transporters in the human placenta. *Pediatr Res*. 2001;49:141-147.
104. Loy G, Quick ANJ, Hay Jr W, et al. Fetoplacental deamination and decarboxylation of leucine. *Am J Physiol*. 1990;259:492-497.
112. Ross JC, Fennessey P, Wilkening R, et al. Placental transport and fetal utilization of leucine in a model of fetal growth retardation. *Am J Physiol*. 1996;270:491-503.
113. Anderson AH, Fennessey PV, Meschia G, et al. Placental transport of threonine and its utilization in the normal and growth-restricted fetus. *Am J Physiol*. 1997;272:892-900.
114. Regnault T, de Vrijer B, Galan H, et al. Umbilical uptakes and transplacental concentration ratios of amino acids in severe fetal growth restriction. *Pediatr Res*. 2013;73:602-611.
115. Marconi A, Paolini C, Stramare L, et al. Steady state maternal-fetal leucine enrichments in normal and intrauterine growth-restricted pregnancies. *Pediatr Res*. 1999;46:114-119.
129. Pardi G, Cetin I, Marconi AM, et al. Diagnostic value of blood sampling in fetuses with growth retardation. *N Engl J Med*. 1993;318:692-696.
130. Wilkening RB, Boyle DW, Teng C, et al. Fetal pH improvement after 24 hrs of severe, nonlethal hypoxia. *Biol Neonate*. 1994;63:129-132.
143. Bellotti M, Pennati G, De Gasperi C, et al. Role of ductus venosus in distribution of umbilical blood flow in human fetuses during second half of pregnancy. *Am J Physiol*. 2000;279:1256-1263.
144. Bellotti M, Pennati G, De Gasperi C, et al. Simultaneous measurements of umbilical venous, fetal hepatic, and ductus venosus blood flow in growth-restricted human fetuses. *Am J Obstet Gynceol*. 2004;190:1347-1358.
146. Ferrazzi E, Bellotti M, Galan H, et al. Investigation in intrauterine growth restriction—from qualitative indices to flow measurements. A review of the experience of a collaborative group. *Ann N Y Acad Sci*. 2001;943:316-325.
147. Ferrazzi E, Bozzo M, Rigano S, et al. Temporal sequence of abnormal Doppler changes in the peripheral and central circulatory systems of the severely growth-restricted fetus. *Ultrasound Obstet Gynecol*. 2002;19:140-146.

22 Endocrine Factors Affecting Neonatal Growth

Kara Kuhn-Riordon | Yvonne K. Lee | Dennis M. Styne

INTRODUCTION

Growth reflects a complex interaction of genetic, epigenetic, endocrine, and nutritional factors that regulate cell division, differentiation, and function (see Meler et al.[1] for a recent compilation of genetic and epigenetic conditions leading to fetal growth restriction). Various phases of growth appear "programmed" to occur within specific time intervals. If missed, growth may not be fully recoverable. Ever-increasing evidence indicates that the pattern and rapidity of fetal and neonatal growth affect the endocrine environment in later life. Thus the role of endocrine factors in modulating growth during this critical epoch of development and the resulting long-term effects are herein reviewed.

PATTERN OF NEONATAL GROWTH

The greatest growth rate occurs during fetal life; in fact, the development of a single fertilized cell into a 3.5-kg neonate entails a 5000-fold increase in length, an increase in surface area of 6×10^6, and an increase in weight of 6×10^{11}. The greatest postnatal growth rate occurs just after birth,[2] followed by slower growth during mid-childhood, only to increase once more in puberty before the final cessation at epiphyseal fusion.

Both longitudinal and cross-sectional studies describe growth rates after birth. The Centers for Disease Control and Prevention (CDC) released the latest version of the commonly used growth charts from birth until the age of 18 years in 2001, using cross-sectional data from the United States. The charts demon-

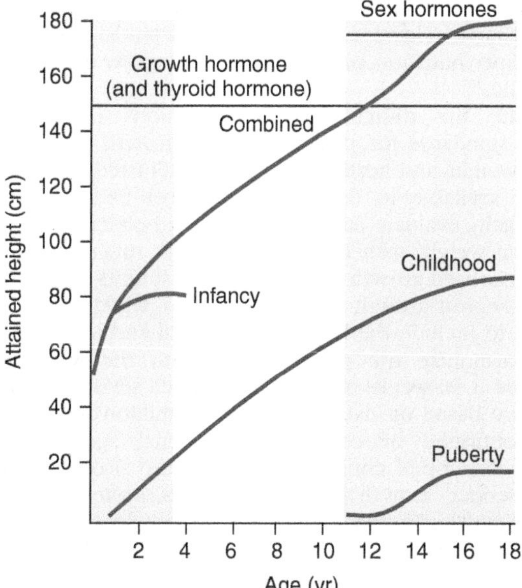

Fig. 22.1 Individual components of the infancy-childhood-puberty growth chart and the combined growth curve that results from the sum of these. (Modified from Karlberg J. On the construction of the infancy-childhood-puberty growth standard. *Acta Paediatr Scand Suppl.* 1989;356:26.)

strate growth between the 3rd to 97th percentiles of length during the first 3 years after birth; the growth charts of the World Health Organization (WHO), which are currently recommended for infants, display the 2nd to the 98th percentiles. Most iterations of the charts show a different color between the 3rd and 97th percentiles. Many versions of the growth charts demonstrate a color change below the lower line of demarcation on the chart. Even though the color change usually found at the 3rd percentile may cause concern in parents of an infant who falls below that line, it is important to recognize that 3% of normal children fall below these lower limits.

Analysis of the factors affecting various phases of growth has led to the development of the infant-childhood-pubertal growth charts,[3] in which the amount of growth for each of three phases of growth (infancy, childhood, puberty) are considered and their sums plotted. Each component of this model can be described by specific mathematical functions (Fig. 22.1).

INFANCY

The slowly decelerating component in infancy occurs as the child has a decrease from the rapid fetal growth phase that starts before birth and falls off by age 3 to 4 years. An infancy-childhood growth spurt starts at 6 to 9 months of age, which originally defined the beginning of the childhood phase, as the infant phase decreases.[4] An update to the original data, based upon a study of 2432 children in a longitudinal study, suggested that the average age of onset of the childhood phase is now 10 months in boys and 9 months in girls.[5] Average total gain in height for Swedish boys (the population from which the plots were originally developed) is 79.0 cm (44.0% of final height) and for girls is 76.8 cm (46.2%) during the infancy period.

Infants undergo a minipuberty, which involves activation of the hypothalamic pituitary gonadotropin axis during the first 3 to 6 months of postnatal life.[6,7] The levels of sex steroids and gonadotropic hormones measured during this period in a longitudinal study of 17 males and 18 females exerted effects on linear growth in boys up to 6 years later.[8] Subsequently, other investigations have been conducted with greater numbers of participants. Another longitudinal study of 45 males and 39 females demonstrated greater height velocity in males than in females up to 6 months of age; the greatest growth velocity difference between the sexes occurred at 1 month of age, which was the time when the highest levels of testosterone, equivalent to those of pubertal boys, were encountered.[9]

MEASUREMENT OF GROWTH

Weight measurements are the standard method of evaluating neonatal growth. Scales used for this purpose may be accurate to within 10 g if calibrated regularly. For a growing 1-kg infant, errors of this magnitude may lead to errors in estimation of growth velocity of up to 2.9 g/kg/day when weights are obtained 1 week apart; with daily weighing, the error may be as much as 20 g/kg/day on any given day.[10] Because the range of variation in measured weights is large relative to the true daily change, weight-gain velocities should be averaged over a period of 5 to 7 days to minimize "noise" in the data.[11] Infants should be weighed naked, ideally disconnected from the ventilator or other respiratory support if feasible and safe, and measurements should be taken at approximately the same time each day.[12] Weight should be plotted on an appropriate growth curve, depending on the infant's age, and the z-score (number of standard deviations from the mean; provided in many growth curves embedded in electronic medical records) should be noted, as it is important to follow the z-score throughout hospitalization and after discharge as a measure of growth trajectory.

The accurate measurement of length at birth is as important as the measurement of weight, because abnormal changes in growth velocity after birth suggest a pathologic condition such as endocrine or genetic disorders.[13] Additionally, length reflects skeletal growth and lean body mass.[12] Unfortunately, accurate and reproducible measurements of neonates and infants are difficult to obtain in clinical practice, and measured lengths of term infants can change over the first 2 days after birth.[14]

A study of the measurement of infants and inanimate dolls showed inaccuracies of up to 25% in length measurements, and weight measurement errors exceeded 10%. Length can be measured accurately if two individuals gently straighten the infant and hold him or her against a calipers-like device such as a Neo-Infantometer (Graham-Field, Inc., Hauppauge, NY) that expands and contracts to measure the linear distance from a perpendicular plate at the top of the head to a perpendicular plate at the bottom of the feet; staff can be trained to perform this with accuracy.[15] Increased flexor tone in term and near-term infants and practitioners reluctant to fully extend the infant's legs can limit accurate measurement. Length should be measured weekly to the nearest millimeter by two people, with one ideally being a parent.[12] As technology becomes more advanced, techniques such as one based on stereoscopic vision may provide a more accurate and precise method for measuring length.[16] Measurement of length is not just a matter of academic interest. Most analyses of infant deaths have been based on birth weight. However, careful analysis of the relationship between birth length and death after premature birth in the Swedish population showed the important effect of length in preterm infants.[17] Careful, accurate measurement of length is critical, as many measures of body composition (such as weight for length ratios, body mass index [BMI], and ponderal index) rely on accurate length measurement, and errors in this measurement are magnified with these indices.[12] Air displacement plethysmography studies are available for neonates and suggest a more direct method of evaluating body composition in neonates and infants.[18-20]

Although low weight or ponderal index at birth have led to a greater risk of early death, those factors at 4 to 5 days of age no longer exerted such a strong effect; however, having a length less than −1 standard deviation (SD) at birth continued to increase the risk of long-term mortality.[17]

Head circumference or occipitofrontal circumference (OFC) reflects brain growth and is an important growth measurement followed in the neonatal intensive care unit (NICU). OFC may decrease by approximately 0.5 cm in the first postnatal week owing to resolving edema and molding. OFCs outside of reference limits may be a variant of normal, and parental OFC should be measured and noted as a percentile or standard deviation from the mean for comparison. OFC should be measured weekly, to the nearest millimeter, using a nonstretchable measuring tape placed at the supraorbital ridges and occipital protuberance. The largest of three measurements should be recorded. Postdischarge head growth measured by OFC seems to better predict cognitive outcomes than does head growth during hospitalization.[12]

Anthropometric measurements are important in the evaluation of neonatal growth and assessment of body composition and nutritional status; thus accurate measurement of weight, length, and head circumference is crucial and can be obtained with extreme care by trained staff.

GROWTH CHARTS

An understanding of normal growth patterns enables the recognition of aberrations in growth that may represent underlying pathology. There are two types of growth charts, and they are to be used and interpreted differently: growth references and growth standards. Growth *references* are typically based on routinely collected data that may have been gathered decades earlier and often have limited quality control/standardization procedures. Growth references describe how subjects have grown at a specific place and time. Growth *standards* use rigorously collected anthropometric measurements that define how a population should grow under optimal conditions. Standards are thought to be universal and independent of time and place.[21]

The CDC's neonatal growth charts for term infants were revised and released in 2001 and are based on cross-sectional data for large numbers of infants; thus they can be assumed to be accurate. However, these are growth *references* that depict how infants grow but do not necessarily describe the ideal growth pattern of healthy infants. In 2006, the World Health Organization (WHO) released new growth *standards* for birth to 5 years derived from an international group of typically developing children raised in optimal environments that maximized growth and nutrition while eliminating confounding variables such as maternal smoking status, poor diet, and infection.[22] The CDC recommends that healthcare providers use the WHO growth charts to monitor growth for infants and children ages 0 to 2 years of age (Fig. 22.2) in the United States and CDC growth charts for children age 2 years and older,[23] as after 2 years of age the charts are quite similar and the latter continue up to 19 years of age. Of note, there are several growth charts that were developed for certain populations; these include growth charts for trisomy 21, achondroplasia, Turner syndrome, Prader-Willi syndrome, and Williams syndrome (among others), which should be used when applicable.

Paralleling advancements in technology, the survival of preterm infants has improved dramatically over the past 2 decades. Unfortunately, the definition of "normal" extrauterine growth is still unknown; thus, growth *standards* for premature infants have been largely unavailable. The American Academy of Pediatrics and the Canadian Pediatric Society recommend that the growth of preterm infants should replicate that of a fetus of the same gestational age. This concept is highly debated among neonatal providers, given that the fetal environment and metabolic responses are very different than those of the preterm infant and many preterm infants experience growth faltering (falling down by one or two marked centile lines between birth and discharge). However, there are recent studies showing that, with proper nutrition, preterm infants may grow near their birth percentile.[20]

Despite the difficulties and limitations in establishing standards for preterm infants, growth references for height, weight, and head circumference adjusted for gestational age are available to determine the most likely appropriate weight gain, evaluate failure to thrive, and observe patterns of excessive weight gain in low-birth-weight infants.[24] The most commonly used growth curves in neonatal units internationally are the Fenton growth curves (Fig. 22.3), which were revised in 2013 to include the best available fetal and infant size data. They harmonize the preterm data with the WHO growth standards at 50 weeks of age.[25] The revised sex-specific growth charts are based on data from nearly 4 million preterm births with confirmed or corrected gestational ages for infants born in developed countries, and they are also based on the recommended growth goal for the fetus, preterm infant, and term infant. The Fenton growth data are not accepted as a good method of assessing size at birth after 36 weeks' gestation owing to concerns regarding discrepancy from intrauterine curves.[26] BMI charts were recently developed for premature babies based on longitudinal data from 68,693 infants.[27]

It has been estimated that up to 50% of preterm labor is associated with intrauterine growth restriction (IUGR);[28] thus using growth data from this population to create a growth reference is problematic. Reference growth charts for preterm infants may underestimate the true prevalence of IUGR.[29] One study examined the prevalence of small for gestational age (SGA) (<10th percentile) utilizing fetal growth standards and found higher rates of 26% to 30% compared with 10% when a neonatal reference chart was used, which is understandable considering that only infants born preterm contribute to the neonatal charts compared with presumably healthy fetuses contributing to the fetal growth charts.[30] Likewise, feeding and postnatal nutritional supplementation practices vary widely between institutions, which further complicates the development of growth references and standards for preterm infants. Many believe that growth standards cannot be produced for preterm infants because babies born prematurely are inherently not normal, given the high proportion of placental insufficiency and other factors that contribute to preterm delivery. The monitoring of postnatal growth had traditionally been based on estimated fetal weight from ultrasounds, size at birth for gestational age, or data from preterm infants taken from longitudinal studies.[31]

Alternate methods to improve the relevance of neonatal growth charts include the use of healthy population standards. A study from Burgundy determined a "healthy-population standard" by using birth weights for preterm infants born to healthy mothers only and compared this with an "entire-population standard" that included all preterm infants.[32] Preterm infants determined to be SGA according to the "healthy-population standard" had a threefold increase in the risk of intraventricular hemorrhage, whereas this association was lost in infants who were deemed to be SGA using the "entire population standard." Therefore growth standards based on healthy maternal populations may better indicate those infants at most risk of complications related to being SGA. Consensus is currently lacking regarding an optimal reference for the growth of premature infants. The INTERGROWTH-21st Project produced prospective, longitudinal, and prescriptive growth standards for fetal and postnatal growth of term and preterm infants up to 2 years of age.[31,33-35] The INTERGROWTH-21st postnatal growth standards serve as a robust tool for monitoring postnatal growth in infants born at 32 or more weeks gestation and can be used up to 6 months postterm.[21] Despite the development of these growth standards, there are concerns that the relatively small sample size of very preterm infants (due in part to the recruitment of low-risk women) makes these growth standards less applicable to the general preterm population.[21] Some argue that it may be useful to consider multiple growth charts and compare the percentiles and SD among the charts.[36]

Longitudinal measurement of length of an infant helps predict childhood growth patterns and other factors in the evaluation of neonates. Although birth length appears to be the most important predictor for adult height, low birth weight is also associated with shorter adult height. The length of a term newborn is closely correlated with the maternal stature, weight,[37] and parity.[38] SGA babies who are born of short or thin mothers have lower risks of perinatal death than those born of primiparous mothers without these characteristics,[39] suggesting that SGA infants born to short or thin mothers may be constitutionally small, whereas SGA infants born to other mothers may be pathologically small. Once free from the constraints of the uterus, the term infant will often adjust growth to reflect the midparental height, and the resulting growth channel should be followed for most of childhood. For children whose birth length percentile is less than their midparental height percentiles, an increase in percentiles occurs sooner after birth and the childhood percentile is reached by 11 to 12 months of age. For children whose birth length percentile is greater than their corrected midparental height percentile, a downward adjustment occurs after the first 3 to 6 months and will allow the child to reach the new lower percentile by a later mean age of 13 months.[40] These changes are gradual, however, and show no abrupt change in growth velocity, which would indicate pathology. Between 3 years of age and the onset of

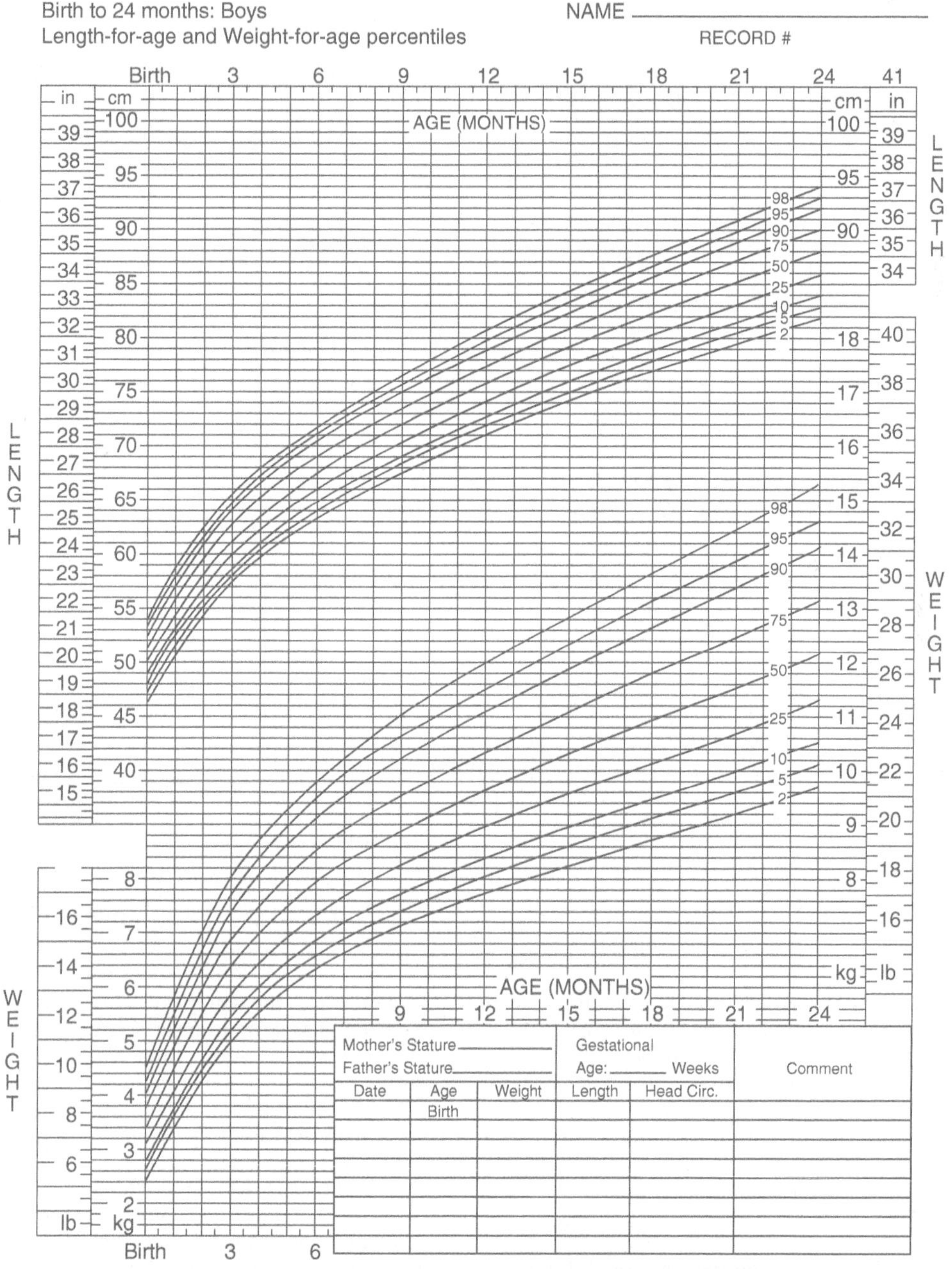

Fig. 22.2 The World Health Organization (WHO) growth standards for boys (A) and girls (B). Released in 2006, these growth standards were derived from an international group of typically developing children raised in optimal environments. The Centers for Disease Control recommends that healthcare providers use these WHO growth standards to monitor growth for children from birth until 2 years of age. (From Centers for Disease Control and Prevention, www.cdc.gov/growthcharts/who_charts.htm.)

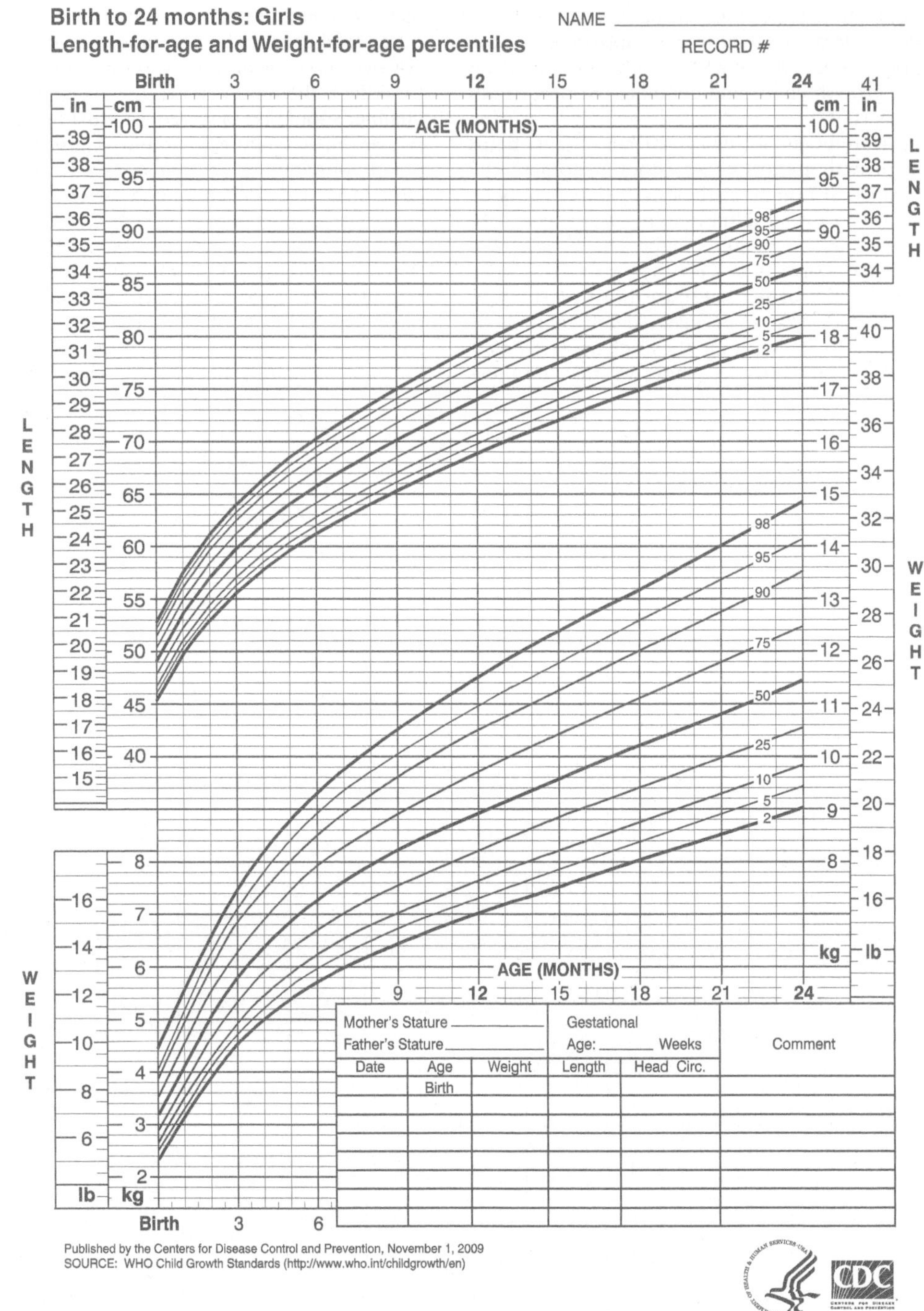

B

Fig. 22.2 cont'd

puberty, normal healthy children will remain close to the same percentile, and a change in standard deviation score (SDS) of more than 0.25/yr is rarely seen. This tendency to maintain a narrow and predictable tract of growth is called "canalization." Accurate data on weight and height velocity, as well as changes in body composition, are available for neonates.[41]

MALNUTRITION

Given the rapidity of growth in the neonatal period, this is a particularly vulnerable time for nutritional deficits, and preterm infants are at the greatest risk. Extrauterine growth restriction (EUGR) is common during the NICU stay, and poor growth postdischarge is also common.[42] The Academy of Nutrition and Dietetics and the American Society for Parenteral and Enteral Nutrition has a consensus statement for the identification of pediatric malnutrition (undernutrition),[43] but these criteria do not apply to preterm neonates or less than 1 month of age. Utilizing the pediatric guidelines, a neonatal practice guideline was created to identify malnutrition in preterm neonates and infants less than 1 month of age.[42] The assessment of change in z-scores for both weight and length is crucial in the assessment of neonatal malnutrition. One study showed that the contraction of extracellular water space that occurs in the first few days after birth causes a permanent change in postnatal growth trajectories, with z-score change of −0.8 from the intrauterine growth percentile.[44] Thus the use of the weight z-scores for the determination of malnutrition takes this into account, in that a decline in weight z-score of 0.8 or more qualifies for malnutrition.[42] Similarly, a decline in length z-score or 0.8 or more, when used in conjunction with another indicator, can signal malnutrition.[42] Growth velocity should be monitored carefully, as this can be another reliable indicator of nutritional adequacy. The generally accepted velocities of 15 g/kg/day or 10 to 30 g/day for weight gain and 1 cm/wk for OFC and length have been shown to fit growth references only for a limited age range and may under- or overestimate appropriate growth outside that range.[45] Rather, utilizing grams per day and centimeters per week to determine growth needed to maintain weight and length z-scores and comparing that to the actual growth velocity has utility in diagnosing malnutrition.[42] Postnatal weight loss and delayed return to birth weight may reflect malnutrition, so the neonatal practice guideline examines days to regain birth weight as an indicator for malnutrition. However, this should be utilized in conjunction with an assessment of nutrient intake.[42] Given that head growth is believed to be spared in periods of undernutrition, faltering head growth (in conjunction with faltering in weight and length growth) may support the diagnosis of moderate to severe malnutrition.[42] Discussing, evaluating, and identifying malnutrition and faltering growth should be a priority during hospitalization, as this period of critical growth can have long-term consequences for an infant's health and neurodevelopment.

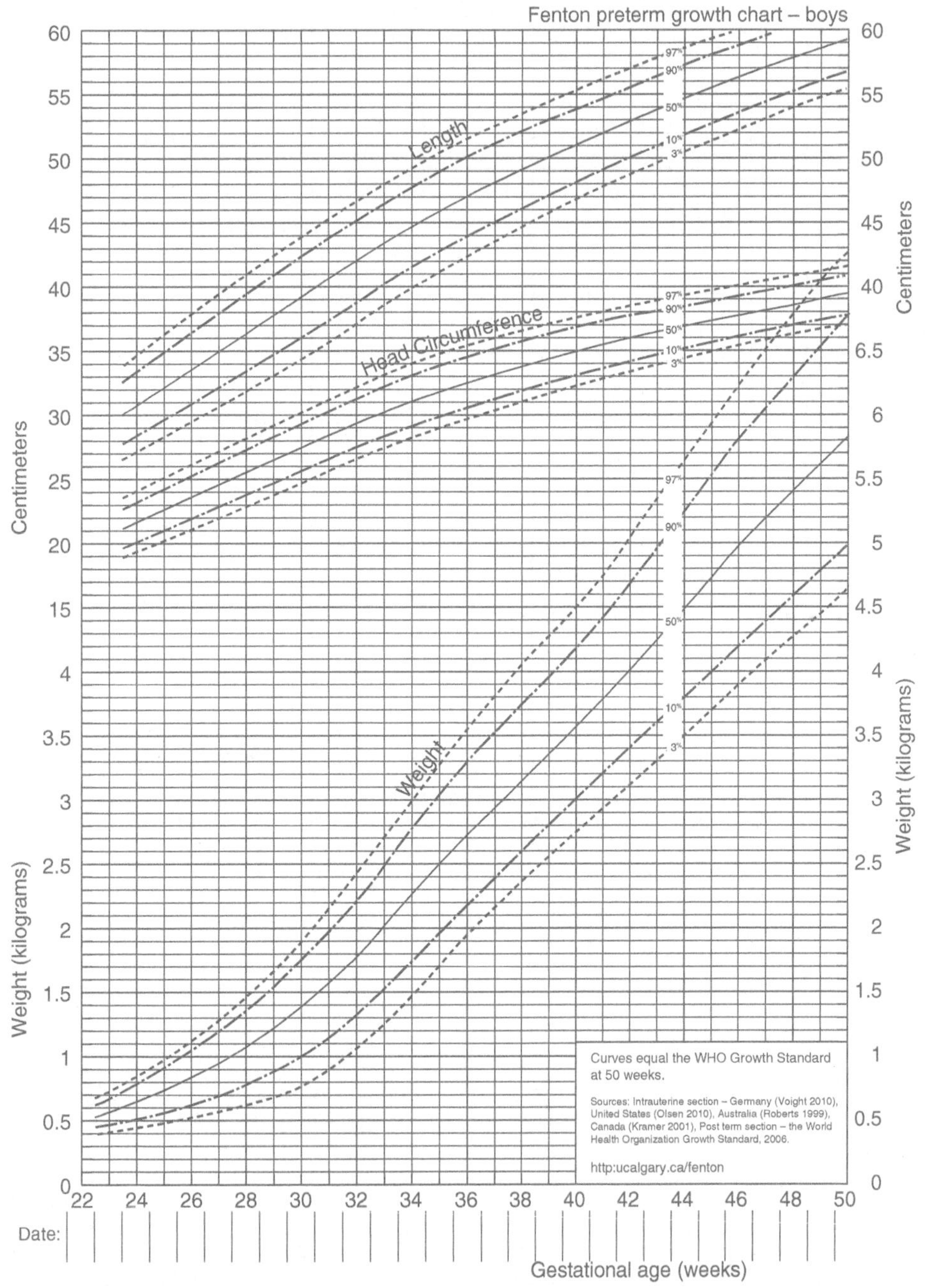

Fig. 22.3 Fenton preterm growth charts for boys (A) and girls (B), updated in 2013. The updated growth curves are gender specific and are based on data from nearly 4 million preterm births, with confirmed or corrected gestational ages in developed countries. They are also based on the currently recommended growth goal for preterm infants, the fetus, and the term infant. They merge smoothly with the World Health Organization's term infant growth standards. (From Fenton TR, Kim JH. A systematic review and meta-analysis to revise the Fenton and growth chart for preterm infants. *BMC Pediatr.* 2013;13:59.)

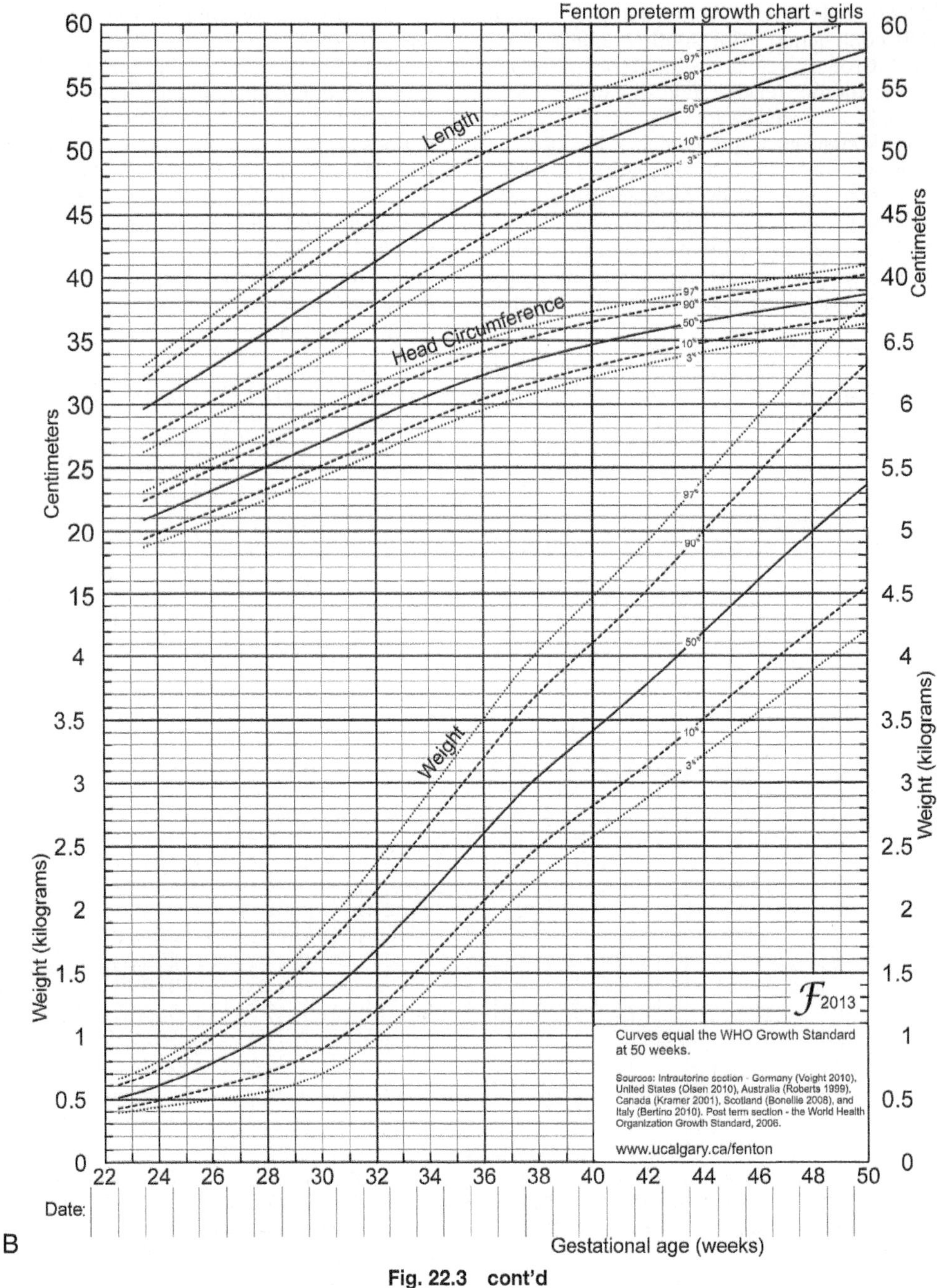

Fig. 22.3 cont'd

PROBIOTICS AND GROWTH

Many studies are beginning to shed light on the role of the intestinal microbiota and their maturation in normal growth and the absence of their maturation in undernutrition.[46] Therapies targeting the microbiota, such as probiotics, are attractive to those attempting to prevent or treat undernutrition. There have been many studies examining how perinatal exposure to probiotics affects fetal and neonatal growth. Probiotics taken during pregnancy and breastfeeding alter the cytokine profile of breast milk and increase secretory immunoglobulin A in infant stool samples. This may help to moderate excessive weight gain in infancy/early childhood.[47] One study examining perinatal probiotic supplementation in addition to dietary counseling examined fetal and infant growth up to 24 months of age. There was no statistically significant difference in weight or length in the groups getting probiotics compared with those receiving placebo plus dietary counseling and the control groups.[48] Studies examining postnatal administration of probiotics have shown mixed results regarding the effects of probiotics on growth. Hartel and colleagues demonstrated that probiotics were associated with improved growth among very low-birth-weight (VLBW) infants who had also received postnatal antibiotics.[49] In another study, extremely low-birth-weight (ELBW) infants given *Lactobacillus reuteri* had improved rate of head growth in the first 28 postnatal days compared with infants who received placebo.[50] Infants given

Bifidobacterium breve and demonstrating colonization with *B. breve* had better growth between 4 and 8 weeks of life.[51] A meta-analysis examining 25 randomized controlled trials demonstrated better weight gain and growth velocity among infants receiving probiotic supplementation.[52] However, there have been several studies showing no clear association between probiotics and growth. The PREMAPRO study, a randomized controlled trial of *Bifidobacterium* probiotics supplements, showed no differences in growth—including measurements of weight, length, and head circumference—compared with infants receiving placebo.[53] A separate randomized controlled trial of *Lactobacillus sporogenes* probiotic in VLBW infants showed no effect on growth.[54] A review of four randomized controlled trials examining the effects of probiotics on growth in formula-fed preterm infants showed no difference in weight gain when compared with controls.[55] Ultimately, the data have been mixed with regard to probiotics and growth and more research is needed; however, probiotics remain a promising target to prevent and treat undernutrition and improve growth among infants.

PREMATURITY, INTRAUTERINE GROWTH RESTRICTION, AND SMALL FOR GESTATIONAL AGE

As reviewed by Saenger and colleagues[56] in 2007, the definitions of IUGR and SGA are often confused; even the medical literature is not always clear. IUGR indicates a documented decrease in intrauterine growth noted by two fetal ultrasound examinations; a baby with IUGR may have a temporary problem that will still allow a normal or near-normal birth weight and length. Thus, the accuracy of fetal ultrasonography becomes an issue in this diagnosis. Because many infants are born with low birth weights, the description of SGA is in fact a proxy for IUGR in many but not all situations.

SGA refers to an infant whose weight and (presumably) length are below some limit. Usually weight or crown-heel length at birth for an SGA infant is at least 2 SD less than the mean for the infant's gestational age, equivalent to the 2.5 percentile, based on data derived from an appropriate reference population. In some of the literature, however, SGA refers to babies with birth weights below the 3rd, 5th, or 10th percentile for gestational age, confusing interpretation of clinical studies during various eras. Furthermore, the difference in percentiles used for diagnosis is of practical importance, because medical insurance companies may adhere to one diagnosis and not cover treatment of children fulfilling other criteria. The WHO defines *low birth weight* as a weight at birth less than 2500 g in an infant of any gestational age; this inclusion of all gestational ages becomes problematic, because long-term outcomes are likely to differ between a baby who was premature but appropriate for gestational age (AGA) and a term infant who is SGA but of the same weight.

A consensus conference on treating SGA babies with growth hormone (GH) suggested a diagnostic criterion of a weight or length more than 2 SD below the mean for gestational age as a definition of SGA[57]; that convention is used in this chapter. SGA may be further classified as SGA with a low birth weight, SGA with a below-normal birth length, or SGA with a low birth weight and below-normal length, and the difference may change the outcomes of therapy. Two other descriptors of IUGR are used: *symmetric IUGR* denotes normal body proportions (a small head and a small body) and may be considered a more severe and long-standing form of IUGR, dating from the second trimester; *asymmetric IUGR* denotes small abdominal circumferences (due mostly to a small liver), decreased subcutaneous and abdominal fat, reduced skeletal muscle mass, and a head circumference in the normal range, probably resulting from stress effects in the third trimester. These definitions do not consider ethnic background, parity, or maternal size, so further classification is possible but not objectively defined, and the clinical utility of such costly and complex growth standards is unknown.[58]

A low ponderal index (birth weight/length^3) is also a marker for asymmetric growth restriction and is associated with an increased risk of cerebral palsy.[59]

Evidence from longitudinal (as well as less powerful cross-sectional) studies shows that up to 90% of term SGA babies catch up in height for age,[60] although often incompletely.[56] In fact, approximately one-fifth of extremely short children have a history of IUGR, which presents at birth as SGA. Although premature infants are expected to have catch-up growth by 2 years, similar to term SGA infants, it is those born after 29 weeks' gestation who exhibit catch-up growth; those born before 29 weeks more likely have a decreased rate of length and weight gain, which may be noted in the first week after birth and lasts up to 2 years.[61] In addition, preterm SGA infants had slower growth velocity for height and weight up to 4 years of age,[62] suggesting that preterm SGA infants did not catch up in growth compared with preterm AGA infants and term SGA infants. One study found that for extremely preterm young adults, height at 2 years of age was a stronger predictor of height at 18 years of age than midparental height,[63] suggesting that medical conditions early on in life influence adult height more than genetic predisposition. A longitudinal study looking at the growth of VLBW infants (birth weight <1500 g) from birth until 20 years of age found that adult males with a history of being VLBW and SGA were significantly more likely to have weights and heights that were more than 2 SD below the mean than those who were VLBW and AGA.[64] This difference was not seen in SGA versus AGA VLBW females. Male and female VLBW infants had similar rates of intrauterine and neonatal growth failure; however, females demonstrated greater catch-up growth than male counterparts, such that females born VLBW did not differ significantly in weight, height, or BMI by 20 years when compared with normal-birth-weight control subjects, suggesting that negative effects of neonatal illness on 20-year height attainment was greater among males. For ELBW infants (birth weight <1000 g), only 60.2% of SGA ELBW infants caught up in height by 2 years corrected age and 72.2% by 5.5 years of age.[65] There were no differences in perinatal characteristics that could explain why some SGA ELBW infants caught up whereas others did not. In summary, it appears that those who are at greatest risk of growth failure are preterm SGA VLBW infant boys and ELBW infants.

It has been demonstrated for decades that catch-up growth can be shown soon after birth for term SGA infants if careful measurements are used.[66] This seems to be a crucial time frame because much of the catch-up growth occurs in this period. Indeed, an acceleration of growth in length is noted in the first 3 months in SGA babies who will catch up.[67] Minimal catch-up growth occurs after 2 years of age; thus those who do not catch up and remain short at 2 years of age have a greater risk for shorter adult stature.[57] In general, children born SGA will achieve an adult height SDS equivalent to their SDS in childhood because skeletal development is normal. Children with a history of SGA at birth without catch-up by 2 years of age may have other conditions that limit growth, such as GH deficiency, thus an endocrine evaluation is warranted.

Longitudinal evaluation of growth in neonates in NICUs demonstrates an almost universal growth impairment.[68] Gestational age is the most important predictor of growth impairment, followed by birth weight and length SDS. The babies born at younger gestational age with higher weights were at greatest risk of both types of growth impairment. However, one recent study reported that optimization of nutritional practices can results in no early postnatal growth failure, demonstrating that such children can grow along their newborn growth percentile without faltering.[20]

A history of very preterm birth and/or VLBW is associated with more neurodevelopmental impairment and lower academic achievement scores.[69,70] Children born preterm with IUGR/SGA appear to have lower cognitive scores than preterm AGA infants, especially preterm IUGR/SGA boys.[71] There is more controversy about long-term effects of SGA on intellectual function in term infants. However, most of the literature has found that even term infants who are SGA have lower neuropsychologic test scores,[72] which appears to be due to IUGR,[73] those who were constitutionally small without a history of IUGR had test scores similar to those of control subjects. These differences in neurocognitive functioning are likely related to the finding of an almost 6% reduction in total brain volume in young adults born term but SGA versus AGA control subjects.[74]

DANGERS OF RAPID OR SLOW NEONATAL GROWTH

Adults born with lower birth weights are at higher risk of impaired glucose tolerance, type 2 diabetes, and cardiovascular death.[75-77] This was initially noted in several studies showing that death rates from cardiovascular disease were inversely related to adult height and paralleled previous geographical history of infant mortality.[75] This original observation grew into the theory of fetal and infant origins of adult disease, also coined the Barker hypothesis. It states that undernutrition in utero and during infancy exerts long-term changes in the cardiovascular, endocrine, and metabolic regulatory systems, leading to poor cardiovascular health in adult life, and that these changes may be transgenerational.[78,79] Thus, the poorly nourished fetus is given a forecast of the nutritional environment following birth, and processes are adapted to survive under conditions of poor nutrition. These adaptations become detrimental when the postnatal environment differs from the forecasted environment and nutrients are normal or excessive, which leads to abnormal growth and obesity, thus increasing the individual's susceptibility to fetal and infant origins of adult disease.[80,81] More recently, this hypothesis evolved into the concept of developmental plasticity—that is, that changes in gene expression during infancy and childhood influenced by environmental forces occur through epigenetic processes such as DNA methylation and histone modification,[82] which can have lifelong consequences.

In addition to SGA status, rapid growth in such children also leads to adult risk of cardiovascular disease and glucose intolerance, as reviewed by Gluckman and colleagues.[76] This tendency is already apparent at 2 to 4 years of age. SGA infants who experience catch-up growth demonstrate a higher degree of insulin resistance than AGA infants.[83] In particular—according to longitudinal studies in Avon, Stockholm, and other sites—weight gain and fat mass accrual[84] during the first months after birth may be more of a risk factor for obesity, insulin resistance, and metabolic syndrome than later weight gain during childhood.[85,86] Infants with the greatest increase in weight and linear growth during the first 2 weeks after birth have endothelial dysfunction up to 16 years later[87] to a degree as significant as that seen with insulin-dependent diabetes mellitus or smoking in adults. Likewise, measures of insulin resistance are higher in those with the greatest weight gain in the postnatal period.[88] Therefore it has been suggested that a degree of slow growth in the postnatal period may not be undesirable.[68] Alternatively, minimizing EUGR of preterm infants, thus removing the need for catch-up growth, may lead to improved neurocognitive outcomes without the potential complications of insulin resistance and metabolic syndrome related to rapid weight gain.[89] It is also postulated that early improvement in postnatal nutrition, especially with protein/amino acids, may have a larger impact on β-cell growth and function leading to less type 2 diabetes mellitus.[90]

Most preterm infants grow poorly during their initial hospital stay,[91] with up to 90% leaving the hospital with weight and length below the 10th percentile for age.[92] This EUGR is associated with poorer neurodevelopment and increased rates of neurologic impairment. Therefore many recommend early aggressive nutrition to minimize caloric and protein deficits and to prevent EUGR and associated negative cognitive and neurodevelopmental outcomes.[92] However, it is difficult to mimic the intrauterine environment for preterm infants, as the extrauterine environment has added stressors that affect growth, including temperature regulation, feeding intolerance, insensible water losses, infectious agents, and medical interventions that increase energy expenditure and nutrient losses.[24]

Preterm birth itself was also found in meta-analyses to be associated with increased risk of decreased insulin sensitivity[93] and type 2 diabetes.[86] Premature babies who are born AGA and demonstrate slow catch-up weight gain nonetheless have postnatal insulin resistance to the same degree as SGA babies. Rapid, excessive weight gain in term neonates also has been correlated with the development of hypertension, obesity, and comorbid illnesses by the age of 30 years.[94,95]

It appears that cardiovascular risk factors are affected differently in preterm girls versus preterm boys.[96] Prematurity is associated with higher blood pressure in adolescent girls and a more atherogenic lipid profile and reduced insulin sensitivity in adolescent boys. The differences in these outcomes strengthened after excluding infants born SGA, suggesting that these differences are not solely due to restricted intrauterine growth. There was also evidence to suggest a dose-response relationship between shorter length of gestation and cardiovascular risk factors.[96]

The effect of prematurity on all features of the metabolic syndrome may not be lifelong. Two meta-analyses found no differences in BMI, waist-to-hip ratio, brachial artery flow-mediated dilation, carotid intimal-medial thickness, high-density lipoprotein levels, and triglycerides in adults born preterm compared with those born at term.[95,97] One meta-analysis demonstrated no difference in percent fat mass in adults born term versus preterm,[95] whereas another found no difference in levels of low-density lipoprotein (LDL).[97] The two meta-analyses did find that blood pressure—including 24-hour ambulatory monitoring—was significantly higher in adults born preterm than in those born at term.[95,97] Parkinson and colleagues found that adults born preterm had significantly higher fasting LDL and total cholesterol.[95] Markopoulou and colleagues found that preterm birth was associated with higher body fat mass, higher fasting glucose and insulin levels, estimated insulin resistance, and higher total cholesterol levels compared with term-born adults.[97] Some have demonstrated that differences in adult blood pressure may be related to gender; 24-hour ambulatory blood pressure measurements were significantly higher in women but not in men born preterm. A separate meta-analysis found that preterm and VLBW status is associated with higher resting systolic blood pressure[98] as well as essential hypertension (blood pressure ≥140/90 mm Hg) later in life versus those born at term.[96]

Low birth weight can affect pubertal development in girls. Girls born with low birth weights extending to the classification of SGA defined previously tend to have early onset of puberty, precocious puberty, or exaggerated precocious adrenarche.[99] In addition, girls with low birth weights have an increased prevalence of insulin resistance by 1 year of age[100] and a tendency toward developing polycystic ovarian syndrome,[101] which is characterized by hyperinsulinemic hyperandrogenism. Girls with average birth weight who display early breast development may have an extended duration of time between breast development and menarche; therefore the age of menarche is relatively stable even if the age of onset of breast development is more variable.[102] However, girls with low birth weight do not demonstrate such an extension of the time between breast development and menarche[103]; treatment with metformin in childhood attenuated this rapid progression. Thus it has been postulated that the hyperinsulinemia characteristic of these girls leads to early menarche. The effect of low birth weight on the reproductive axis in males is not well known, but increased aromatase activity leading to elevated estradiol levels, increased 5-α-reductase activity reflected by elevated dihydrotestosterone, and elevated inhibin B levels reflecting activity of the seminiferous tubules are inversely proportional to birth weight. At present, the effects of these changes are not known.[104]

HORMONAL CONTROL OF NEONATAL GROWTH

The hormones that mediate postnatal growth do not necessarily play the same roles in fetal growth. As noted in Chapter 140, GH is present in very high concentrations in the fetus, in contrast to the limited presence of GH receptors. Although this discrepancy suggests limited activity of GH in the fetus, GH does play a role in fetal growth that is reflected in a mean birth weight 1 SD below the mean in GH-deficient infants. Infants with Laron syndrome (OMIM 262500) (i.e., GH resistance due to reduced or absent GH receptors) have elevated GH and low serum insulin-like growth factor-1 (IGF-1) levels and decreased birth length and weight. However, the small decrease in birth weight does not presage the profound deficit in growth that occurs postnatally with GH or IGF-I deficiency meta-analysis. Thyroid hormone deficiency does not directly affect human birth weight, but prolonged gestation is a feature of congenital hypothyroidism, and this factor will itself increase weight. In contrast, lack of thyroid hormone leads to profound growth failure after birth. Thus, in the postnatal phase, these hormones have important but, in many cases, different roles.

Placental lactogen exerts no apparent effect on birth size in human beings. However, the concentration of placental GH (from the *GHV* gene; see later) is significantly decreased in the serum of a pregnant woman bearing a fetus with IUGR.

GROWTH HORMONE

Human GH is produced as a single-chain 191–amino acid, 22-kDa peptide containing two intramolecular disulfide bonds.[105] A 20-kDa variant of pituitary GH accounts for 5% to 10% of circulating GH.[106] The genes for a family of GH-related proteins share a common structural organization with four introns separating five exons meta-analysis. The gene for GH is located on the long arm of chromosome 17 in a cluster of five genes with evolutionary relationships: *GHN* codes for human GH (a single 191–amino acid polypeptide chain with a molecular mass of 22 kDa), *GHV* codes for a variant GH produced in the placenta, and there are three additional chorionic somatomammotropin genes.[107]

GH is a key mediator of childhood growth and acts primarily through stimulation of hepatic and peripheral IGF-1 production and secretion. GH is released in a pulsatile pattern. These peaks and valleys of GH are under the control of the two hypothalamic regulatory peptides: GH-releasing hormone (GHRH), a meta-analysis stimulatory peptide also released in a pulsatile manner, and somatostatin (or somatotropin release-inhibiting factor), an inhibitory factor.[108] GHRH contains 44 amino acids, but alternative forms have 40 or 37 amino acids; the amino terminus of GHRH must be present for biologic activity. Somatostatin is a 14–amino acid neuropeptide that is secreted by neurons in the periventricular nucleus of the hypothalamus and is delivered to pituitary cells by the portal vascular system. GHRH exerts effects by binding to a G protein–related receptor on the pituitary somatotropes, increasing intracellular cyclic adenosine monophosphate production, leading to calcium influx, and subsequently increasing GH synthesis. Somatostatin, however, regulates the timing and amplitude of the pulses of GH but has no effect on synthesis of GH. In contrast with the action of GHRH on the pituitary, somatostatin inhibits adenylate cyclase activity, which reduces voltage-gated calcium influx and inhibits GH secretion.[109] Pulses of GH secretion occur when a decrease in the release of somatostatin and an increase in the release of GHRH from the hypothalamus occur; however, when somatotropin release-inhibiting factor is released without GHRH, a nadir of the GH pulse occurs.

Release of these hypothalamic factors are regulated by a plethora of neurotransmitters, including serotonin, histamine, norepinephrine, dopamine, acetylcholine, γ-aminobutyric acid, thyroid-releasing hormone, vasoactive intestinal peptide, gastrin, neurotensin, substance P, calcitonin, neuropeptide Y, vasopressin, galanin, and corticotropin-releasing hormone (reviewed by Radovick and colleagues[110]). GH secretion is also affected by physiologic conditions, including stress, sleep stage, hemorrhage, fasting, hypoglycemia, and, at least in older subjects, exercise. GH-stimulatory tests are employed in the evaluation of GH-secretory capacity in neonates if indicated. GH secretion is also influenced by a variety of hormones such as estrogen (which in most cases increases basal and stimulated GH secretion but in excess suppresses GH secretion), androgens (which exert their effect through aromatization to estrogens), thyroid hormone (which is essential in allowing GH secretion), and glucocorticoids (which decrease GH secretion when in excess). Negative feedback from circulating IGF-1 by interaction with pituitary IGF receptors and positive feedback from ghrelin also influence GH release.[111] GH secretagogues are small peptides that regulate GH secretion through pituitary and hypothalamic receptors separate from GHRH and somatotropin release-inhibiting factor.

One such GH secretagogue is ghrelin, a 28-amino-acid peptide mainly secreted from the stomach; it is an orexigenic hormone. Ghrelin receptors are identified in the arcuate and ventromedial nuclei of the hypothalamus.[112] Ghrelin is necessary for triggering the GH response to nutritional deprivation that prevents hypoglycemia and death. Umbilical cord ghrelin concentrations correlate positively with neonatal birth weight and body length and head circumference in infants born of women with normal weight; maternal serum ghrelin levels correlate negatively with neonatal birth weight, body length, and head circumference but positively with chest circumference.[113] In mothers with excessive weight gain during pregnancy, umbilical cord ghrelin concentrations correlate negatively with neonatal birth weight and birth body length. Ghrelin is also decreased in mothers with gestational diabetes and obesity.[114] Ghrelin values at term are negatively correlated to postnatal growth and weight gain.[115] Values increase after birth, peak during the first 2 years after birth, and decrease until the end of puberty.[116] Ghrelin may be particularly important in catch-up growth, with one study finding that ghrelin levels were higher in SGA infants compared with AGA and large-for-gestational-age (LGA) infants and that higher ghrelin levels were associated with more weight gain in SGA infants during the study period (0 to 3 months after birth).[117,118] A longitudinal study found that ghrelin levels rise in neonates with infections and fevers compared to controls, while there is no difference in pancreatic peptide YY (PYY).[119]

GROWTH HORMONE RECEPTOR

The cell membrane GH receptor, a member of the class I cytokine receptor superfamily with 620 amino acids and a molecular mass of 70 kDa, contains an extracellular hormone-binding domain, a single membrane-spanning domain, and a cytoplasmic domain. In human beings, GH receptors exist in two major isoforms, reflecting retention *(GHRfl)* or exclusion *(GHRd3)* of exon 3 of the GH receptor gene. A circulating GH binding protein (GHBP), which has the same amino acid sequence as the extracellular domain of the GH receptor (approximately 55 kDa), is derived from proteolytic cleavage of the extracellular domain of the receptor.[120,121] The major GHBP in human plasma binds GH with high specificity and affinity but with relatively low capacity because only 45% of circulating GH is bound. Levels of GHBP are low in early life, increase through childhood, and plateau during puberty and adulthood. In patients with abnormalities of the GH receptor (e.g., Laron dwarfism), the defect is also reflected in the serum GHBP concentration, such that those with decreased numbers of GH receptors have decreased serum GHBP concentrations.[122] Nutritional state and other factors regulate both GH secretion and GHBP values.

Although serum GH is high in the neonate, GH receptors are decreased, as reflected in the lower serum GHBP. An increase in GHBP occurs at 6 months of age, which just predates the phase of increasing IGF-1 and IGFBP-3 (after approximately 10 months), suggesting a greater GH dependence of GH-responsive factors and GH-dependent growth in the infant of this age and denotes the end of the infancy phase of growth and the beginning of the childhood phase of growth.[123] Nonetheless, even though infants with congenital GH deficiency are of below but close to near-normal length at birth, growth rate decreases soon and even a few months after birth may descend to more than 3 to 7 SD below the mean.[124,125]

Children with Laron syndrome (OMIM 262500) lack GH receptor structure or function; they will not grow when treated with GH and must receive IGF-1 treatment.[126] Serum GHBP is decreased in those with GH receptor deficiency; others have adequate numbers of receptors, which are inactive or have lesser activity, and these children have normal amounts of GHBP. Increased growth was shown in several studies of IGF-1 treatment in such children. IGF-1 is now commercially available for children with primary IGF-1 deficiency, a class of conditions that includes Laron syndrome.[127]

GROWTH HORMONE VALUES AFTER BIRTH

It has long been recognized that a GH surge occurs at birth and decreases during the 2 weeks after birth.[115] Measurements of GH in unstimulated blood samples, if demonstrating a GH value more than 10 μg/L (or 10 ng/mL) in the first few days after birth, eliminate classic GH deficiency; samples taken after the first few days will usually require stimulation by GH secretagogues to test for GH deficiency. Adults exhibit pulsatile GH release, but the sampling blood for analysis of pulsatile GH secretion in neonates has presented technical and ethical difficulties. Safe microsampling techniques, allowing blood withdrawal every 20 to 30 minutes over 12 hours or longer, have been developed.[128] With this technique, all infants demonstrate a pulsatile pattern of GH release, but unlike adults, they have not yet developed entrainment of the GH secretory rhythm with sleep.[129] At 4 days of age, GH secretion and insulin secretion are correlated, which demonstrates a relationship between feeding and GH secretion. On the first day after birth, infants from gestational age 33 to 41 weeks sampled every 20 minutes in 6 hours demonstrated elevated GH released in pulses, with 5 to 6 bursts found in 6 hours leading to a pulse periodicity of 73 minutes and a half-life of 18 minutes.[130] This elevation of GH was due to increased secretion rather than decreased clearance. Prolactin was also high but not released in pulses, and prolactin release was not related to the GH peaks. In another study, sampling term infants every 30 minutes for 12 hours demonstrated higher GH pulse frequency and amplitude soon after birth (8 to 40 hours) compared with later (63 to 85 hours), with no difference between boys and girls.[131] Studies of GH secretion at 1 to 13 days after birth revealed higher values of GH in neonates than in later life, and even higher peaks of GH were found in SGA babies compared with AGA infants.[132-134] Basal mean and peak GH values in AGA and SGA babies were 17 versus 54 and 63 versus 190 μg/L, respectively. The pulse frequency was greater in SGA (5.1 for 12 hours) than in AGA (4.0 for 12 hours) babies, with a pulse periodicity of 180 minutes in AGA and 140 minutes in SGA infants. Premature infants (mean 33 weeks' gestation) sampled every 30 minutes for 12 hours at approximately 40 hours after birth had high basal (24 to 26 μg/L), incremental (20 to 24 μg/L), and peak (45 to 51μg/L) GH values with a frequency of 3 peaks for 12 hours; no difference was seen between male and female infants.[134] Premature infants had higher secretory burst amplitudes, higher production rates, and a higher mass of GH per secretory burst than term infants. The integrated plasma GH concentration exhibited a strong trend toward a higher value in the premature infants.[134] Although serum GH was elevated in SGA infants, values normalized by 1 month of age, and although this elevation was related to the pattern of intrauterine growth, it was not related to postnatal growth.[123] Thus children born SGA have a different profile for GH and IGF-1 from that in infants born at a normal weight; at birth and at 3 days of age, basal GH was high, peak amplitude was low, and frequency of peaks of GH was higher, but serum IGF-1, IGF-binding protein (IGFBP)-3, and leptin were significantly reduced.[135,136] When they were evaluated later in life for GH secretion, however, the children who were SGA at birth showed normal amplitude and normal baseline IGF-1 and IGFBP-3.

Treatment with GH increases growth rate, and catch-up growth proceeds to increase height by 2 years. The *GHRd3* GH receptor isoform is associated with decreased fetal growth but remarkably is associated with increased postnatal growth in height when measured up to adolescence.[137] *GHRd3*, when present in heterozygous or homozygous patterns, is associated with catch-up growth in the SGA neonate as well as increased responsiveness to GH treatment in non–GH-deficient short stature and Turner syndrome.[136] In addition, *GHRd3* appears to modulate hemoglobin A_{1c} levels and thus may play a role in the association between low birth weight and the increased risk of development of insulin resistance later in life.[138] However, in patients with severe isolated GH deficiency treated with GH, adult height is not ultimately increased in those with *GHRd3* compared with those who do not have this isoform, suggesting a temporary effect. The same isoform is associated with decreased third trimester growth in SGA babies[137] and lower placental and birth weights.[139]

CONGENITAL DEFECTS OF THE PITUITARY HYPOTHALAMIC AXIS

Various congenital defects of the pituitary hypothalamic axis lead to deficiency of GH or other pituitary hormones. Defects range from pituitary hypoplasia to other midline defects to holoprosencephaly; any midline defect of the central nervous system area should be suspect as an etiology of hypopituitarism. The pituitary gland resides in the sella turcica near the optic chiasm. A decrease in the size of the sella turcica is an indication of reduced pituitary development. The anterior pituitary and pituitary stalk are often smaller than normal, and a bright spot representing the posterior pituitary is located in the hypothalamus rather than in its normal location. This finding is referred to as an *ectopic posterior pituitary,* but it can be also found as a normal variation in unaffected patients. The appearance of an interrupted pituitary stalk is a finding in congenital hypopituitarism of diagnostic significance. Congenital hypopituitarism is associated with breech birth, forceps delivery, and intrapartum and maternal bleeding. Although nutrition was always of concern in cases of cleft palate or lip, 4% of the cases are associated with GH deficiency; the prevalence rises to 32% if short stature is associated. Rarely, patients have absent anterior pituitary glands and therefore no somatotrophs; loss of ACTH function can be potentially fatal when left untreated.

GENETIC FORMS OF HYPOPITUITARISM

Numerous genes are identified that are involved in pituitary development.[140,141] Depending on the gene involved, mutations can result in different combinations of pituitary hormone deficiencies. For example, a mutation in the pituitary paired like homeodomain transcription factor (PROP1 #262600 pituitary hormone deficiency, combined, 2; CPHD2) causes deficiencies of prolactin, gonadotropins, GH, and thyroid-stimulating hormone (TSH), with evolving ACTH deficiency. However, patients with mutations of the related transcription factor POU1 (#613038 pituitary hormone deficiency, combined, 1; CPHD1) lack GH, prolactin, and TSH but retain ACTH and gonadotropin function (although ACTH deficiency may develop later).

A defect in the function of the pituitary gland is often combined with visual disability in the syndrome of septs-optic dysplasia (OMIM # 182230), in which congenital blindness or nystagmus is an indication of potential pituitary defects. This condition is either sporadic or due to homozygosity of an inactivating mutation of the *Hesx-1* gene.

ISOLATED GROWTH HORMONE DEFICIENCY

Autosomal recessive complete deletions of the *GH1* gene causes isolated GH deficiency (IGHD) type IA (OMIM 262400). This condition leads to the development of antibodies to GH after treatment with GH inhibiting the response to GH treatment. Birth weight is moderately decreased rather than leading to true SGA. Autosomal recessive IGHD type IB results from various sizes and sites of mutations in the GH gene (OMIM 612781), causing low but detectable levels of GH and a less severe form of dwarfism that is usually responsive to GH therapy.

Autosomal dominant IGHD type II (OMIM 173100) is caused by mutations in the *GH1* gene. X-linked IGHD type III (OMIM 307200) is associated with hypogammaglobulinemia and agammaglobulinemia and is thought to be due to mutations in the *BTK* gene, the same gene involved in X-linked agammaglobulinemia. IGHD type IV (IGHD4) (OMIM 618157) is an autosomal recessive disorder caused by mutations in the GHRH-receptor.

INSULIN-LIKE GROWTH FACTORS

The insulin-like growth factors (IGFs) exert important effects on fetal growth.[142] The effects of GH are mediated mainly by the IGFs (reviewed by Cooke and colleagues[110]), originally called the sulfation factor and subsequently nonsuppressible insulin-like activity, somatomedin, and then insulin-like growth factor, or IGF. GH also has direct effects such as lipolysis, increased amino acid transport into tissues, and increased protein synthesis in liver. Two IGFs, IGF-1 and IGF-2, share 45 of a 73-amino-acid sequence and have structures similar to that of the proinsulin molecule (50% homologous with the A and B chains of insulin, with these chains connected by disulfide bonds).[143,144] Both the IGFs and proinsulin have a connecting peptide or a C chain, although the homology is not complete in terms of amino acid structure because the IGF-1 C-peptide region has 12 amino acids and the IGF-2 C-peptide region is 8 amino acids long; neither show homology in amino acid sequence with the C-peptide region of proinsulin. Further, the IGFs have a carboxyl-terminal extension, or D-peptide, unlike proinsulin.

The gene for IGF-1 is located on the long arm of chromosome 12 and contains at least five exons.[145] IGF-1 is produced in most tissues and is exported to neighboring cells to act on them in a paracrine manner or to their cell of origin in an autocrine manner. Thus serum IGF-1 concentrations may not reflect the most significant actions of this growth factor. The liver is a major site of IGF-1 synthesis, and much of the circulating IGF-1 originates in the liver; serum IGF-1 concentrations vary in liver disease with the extent of liver destruction. IGF-1 is a progression factor, so that a cell that has been exposed to a competence factor, such as platelet-derived growth factor, in stage G0 of the cell cycle and has progressed to G1 can, with IGF-1 exposure in G1, undergo division in the S phase of the cell cycle. Aside from the stimulatory effects of IGF-1 on cartilage growth, IGF-1 has stimulatory effects on hematopoiesis, ovarian steroidogenesis, myoblast proliferation and differentiation, and lens differentiation.

The IGF-1 cell membrane receptor (the type I receptor) resembles the insulin receptor in its structure of two alpha and two beta chains.[146] Binding of IGF-1 to type I receptors stimulates tyrosine kinase activity and autophosphorylation of tyrosine residues in the receptor. This leads to cell differentiation or division or both. The type 1 IGF receptor messenger RNA is present in almost all tissues. IGF-1 receptors are downregulated by increased IGF-1 concentrations, whereas decreased IGF-1 concentrations lead to an increase in IGF-1 receptors. The structural similarity of the IGFs and insulin explains why IGFs are able to bind to the insulin receptor and why insulin in excess can bind to the type 1 IGF receptor (in physiologic levels insulin has little binding to the IGF-1 receptor), although the structural differences may explain why insulin cannot bind to the IGFBPs (see later).

One patient with congenital IGF-1 deficiency (OMIM 608747) (not due to GH receptor defects)[147] had a birth length 5.4 SD below the mean and a height 6.9 SD below the mean at age 15 years. Because no IGF-I was found, no feedback to GH secretion occurred and GH values were elevated, similar to those typical for Laron dwarfism. In addition, children with IGF-1 receptor mutations (OMIM 270450) demonstrate intrauterine and postnatal growth retardation, again pointing to the importance of IGF-1 in both periods of growth.[148]

IGF molecules may be bound to one of the IGFBPs, some of which are found in the circulation and others in tissue.[143] IGFBPs may be inhibitory to IGF effects, although some IGFBPs can enhance IGF activity. IGFBP-1 is a 25-kDa protein that inhibits IGF action and is suppressed by insulin but is not affected by GH. IGFBP-1 is present in high concentrations in fetal serum and amniotic fluid. Serum values of IGFBP-1 and IGFBP-2 in blood are inversely proportionate to birth weight, indicating that IGFBP-1 exerts suppressive effect on fetal growth. This suggests that growth is restricted to some degree by elevated IGFBP-1 but that after birth the IGF system becomes more active, increasing the likelihood of catch-up growth.

IGF-1 circulates bound to IGFBP-3 and an acid-labile subunit in a 150-kDa complex, the ternary complex. Serum IGFBP-3 concentrations are directly proportional to GH concentrations, as well as to IGF-1 concentrations and are regulated by nutritional status, as is IGF-1. Thus, in malnutrition, IGFBP-3 and IGF-1 levels fall, whereas GH rises. IGFBP-3 increases with advancing age throughout childhood, with highest values achieved during puberty. In the hippocampus of the mouse, IGF-1–binding protein 2 (IGFBP2) in neurons and astrocytes appears to be important in the development of cognition.[149]

IGFBP proteases (for IGFBP 2 to 5) metabolize the IGFBPs by proteolysis, leading to another level of control of the IGF axis. There is evidence that SGA babies have at least two different proteases, which, by digesting IGFBP-3, increase the effectiveness of IGF-1.[150]

IGF-2 is the primary growth factor involved in embryonic growth, whereas the dominant fetal growth regulator in late gestation is IGF-1.[151] IGF-2 is a 67-amino-acid acidic peptide coded by a gene on the short arm of chromosome 11, close to the gene for preproinsulin.[145] The type 2 IGF receptor preferentially binds IGF-2 and is identical to the mannose 6-phosphate receptor, a single-chain transmembrane protein. The ratio of IGF-2 to IGF2-R (a soluble form of the type 2 IGF receptor that exhibits inhibitory effects on IGF-2 action) is directly related to birth weight and is even more closely related to placental weight.[152,153] Decrease of maternal IGF-2 receptor activity in rodents leads to excessive

IGF-2 availability and placenta and heart overgrowth and increased perinatal lethality; mild maternal expression of IGF-2 receptor exceeds paternal expression with some mutations in the maternal IGF-2 receptor the paternal receptor can rescue the fetus from these changes.[154]

POSTNATAL INSULIN-LIKE GROWTH FACTOR-1 VALUES

Variations in IGF-1 assays lead to difficulty in comparing values between studies; we review the available information to date, although standardized assays improving precision may change the patterns in the future.[155]

IGF-1 in the fetus is regulated by metabolic factors rather than exhibiting significant influence by GH, as is the case in postnatal life (see Chapter 140). One explanation is that there are fewer GH receptors in the fetus than after birth. Thus fetal IGF-1 levels in early gestation are regulated not by GH but by fetal insulin. The GH receptor is first found at about 30 weeks' gestation in human fetuses.[156] GH begins to exert a limited influence after 36 weeks' gestation. In the human fetus, serum GH level decreases during later gestation owing to maturation of central nervous system negative control; serum IGF-1 and IGFBP-3 increase during gestation, demonstrating their differing pattern and independence from GH stimulation. Serum GH level in the last half of gestation decreases, but IGF-1 increases, so do IGF-2 and IGFBP-3 (Fig. 22.4). Premature infants have lower serum IGF-1; these differences were greater with greater gestational age. Decreased IGF-2 is also seen in SGA infants. Preeclampsia decreases DNA methylation at IGF-2 and Gsα-encoding GNAS differentially methylated region (DMR)[157] and lowers cord blood IGF-1 values after correcting for gestational age and for birth weight.[158]

IGF-I levels rise in the second and third trimester at a rate that exceeds the rate of rise after birth.[159,160] The serum values of IGF-1 are 50% or less of adult values; IGF-2 values are approximately 50% of adult values in term neonates. IGF-1 and IGF 2 in cord blood are correlated with weight, length, and OFC.[161,162] IGF-1 concentrations are more highly correlated in monozygotic twins than in same-sex dizygotic twins, indicating a genetic effect on IGF-1 regulation. IGF-1 and IGFBP-3 have a direct relationship to ponderal index; IGF-1, IGFBP-3, and GHBP increased with gestational age, with IGFBP-1 decreased. Inactivating mutations of IGF-I and IGF-I receptors inhibit fetal and postnatal growth. Known mutations in the IGF-I receptor gene are associated also with microcephaly.[163] Likewise paternal inactivation the IGF-2 gene leads to poor fetal and postnatal growth.[164] Alternatively, in LGA infants, products of either diabetic or nondiabetic pregnancies, IGF-1, insulin, and IGFBP-3 were increased but IGFBP-1 was decreased.[165,166] IGFBP-1 is elevated in SGA infants and decreased in LGA infants. There are epigenetic effects on the relationship between IGF-I and fetal growth: methylation at *IGF1* CpG-137 is negatively correlated with birth length.[167]

Growth factor levels are correlated with the development of retinopathy of prematurity (ROP). SGA is a risk factor for any stage of ROP, severe ROP, and treated ROP in preterm infants.[168] While elevated serum GH is not related to growth rate in premature infants, persistent elevation of serum GH has been linked to the development of ROP.[169] However, in a study of 83 infants born before 32 weeks' gestation and at less than 1500 g, greater gains in fat and fat-free mass up to term decreased the risk for stage II retinopathy of prematurity.[170] IGFBP-3 values are associated with retinopathy of prematurity and decreased brain growth; administration of IGF-1 and IGFBP-3 is a potential therapy that was postulated to successfully raise serum values of these moieties.[171] Indeed, there are ongoing studies to determine the effects of continuous infusion of recombinant human IGF-1/recombinant human IGF-binding protein-3 (rhIGF-1/rhIGFBP-3) to determine whether artificially increasing these values will tend to prevent retinopathy of prematurity, developmental

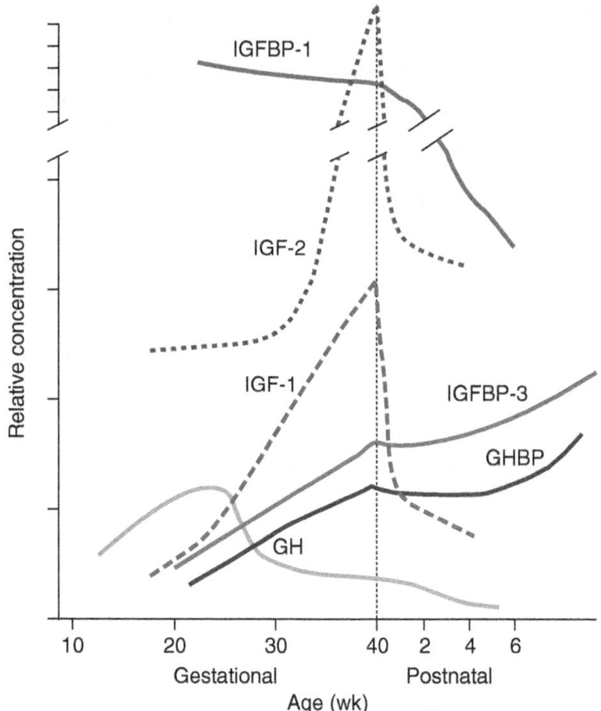

Fig. 22.4 Relative concentrations of growth hormone *(GH)*, GH-binding protein *(GHBP)*, insulin-like growth factor *(IGF)*, and IGF-binding proteins *(IGFBPs)* during gestation and perinatally. (Modified from Wollmann HA. Growth hormone and growth factors during perinatal life. *Horm Res.* 2000;53[suppl 1]:50–54.)

delay, bronchopulmonary dysplasia, and other complications of prematurity.[172] This ongoing study found increased values of interleukin-6 and IGFBP-1 but decreased values of rhIGF-1/rhIGFBP-3, indicating that inflammation or infection can inhibit the effects of this treatment. Another study using such a combination did not find a decrease in ROP but did find a decrease in severe bronchopulmonary dysplasia.[173]

Although GH levels in extremely preterm infants are significantly higher than in term infants, suggesting a degree of GH resistance, serum IGF-1, IGFBP-3, and GHBP are low, but IGFBP-1 and IGFBP-2 levels are higher in extremely preterm infants than in term newborns. IGF-1 levels rise significantly in the third trimester of pregnancy; thus preterm birth in the earlier stages of the third trimester is associated with a loss of maternal sources of IGF-1 and lower levels of serum IGF-1 compared with in utero counterparts as preterm infants grow outside the womb. IGF-1 levels rise slowly after preterm birth compared with the rapid increase that occurs in utero, creating a relative IGF-1 deficiency.[174]

In VLBW infants, IGF-1 and IGFBP-3 concentrations fall in the first week after birth and then begin to rise. In both preterm and term infants, low birth weight is associated with low cord serum IGF-1 and IGFBP-3 and high IGF-1 levels. IGF-1 levels are positively correlated with body weight, body length, and BMI during the first 8 weeks after birth and are not different between AGA and SGA VLBW infants; IGF-1 levels at birth are significantly lower in SGA than in AGA infants,[174] suggesting that intrauterine nutrition may affect IGF-1 levels.

Growth in the first months after birth is mainly regulated by nutrients, insulin, and IGF-1. IGF-1 and insulin are important factors in growth regulation during the first 6 months after birth in both term and preterm infants. IGF-1 and insulin are positively associated with growth until 6 months, but a shift from insulin-dependent toward GH-dependent growth regulation seems to occur at 6 months corrected age.[175] In term infants, growth regulation shifts from the fetal pattern of regulating IGF-1 (insulin/nutrition dependency) at term age toward GH dependency at 6 months postnatal age, when GH receptors increase in number to the extent that GH-dependent growth dominates.[151]

At a mean of 4 days after birth, IGF-1 was higher in AGA than in SGA infants, and peak, mean, and incremental GH and IGFBP-1 were higher in SGA infants. During the first week after birth, IGF-1 decreases in term infants for the first 3 days and then increases at the end of the week, IGF-1 remains stable in preterm infants, and IGFBP-3 and IGF-2 do not change significantly during this first week.[176]

The pattern of change between birth and 1 to 3 months of age in normal-term newborns is one of a decrease in IGFBP-1 and IGFBP-2 and an increase in IGF-2 by 3 months along with a decrease in GH. GHBP values increase at 4 and 6 months of age, but data in the first 3 months are conflicting. Values of IGF-1 and IGFBP-3 remain relatively low in childhood until a peak is reached during puberty, with values higher than at any other time in life. Because the range of IGF-1 is so low in the neonate, it is difficult to determine whether values are below normal. The range of IGFBP-3 values is higher in normal neonates and may be a better indicator of GH deficiency than serum IGF-1. Cord blood IGF-1 correlates with postnatal growth in SGA and AGA infants during the first month.[177] A correlation is found between IGF-1 and IGFBP-3 and catch-up growth for the first year in SGA babies.[176]

Gene manipulation and infusion of growth factors in animals demonstrate the influence that these factors exert on fetal growth. IGF-1 knockout mice (which produce no IGF-1) have reduced late fetal and postnatal growth as well as diaphragmatic muscular hypoplasia (which ultimately causes their death), organ hypoplasia, and delayed ossification of cartilage.[178-180] IGF-2 knockout mice have an earlier fetal growth deficit than IGF-1 knockout mice even though their growth rate is normal later in gestation. This suggests a role for IGF-2 in growth in early gestation and one for IGF-1 in later gestation. Elimination of type 1 receptors (by gene knockout) leads to a more profound growth failure than is found in IGF-1 knockout mice alone, suggesting that factors other than IGF-1 exert effects on fetal growth through the type 1 receptor (IGF-2 is one of these factors).[178]

Artificial elevation of maternal IGF-1 can increase growth in mouse and rat fetuses and overcome the restraint imposed by uterine limitations of litter size.[181] Knockout of the maternal gene for the type 2 receptor leads to high birth weight, generalized organomegaly, and other anomalies, usually leading to rapid postnatal death; the type 2 receptor appears necessary for postnatal life.[182] Transgenic mice overexpressing IGFBP-1 have smaller birth size, lower birth weight, and poorer postnatal weight gain (as well as more frequent postnatal death) with proportional decrease in the size of all organs except the brain, which is much smaller in proportion to other organs; fasting hyperglycemia and impaired glucose tolerance also occur.[182,183] Early postnatal growth restriction occurs in mice experiencing excess IGFBP-1, suggesting an inhibitory role for IGFBP-1 in growth in late gestation and thereafter. Overexpression of IGFBP-3 in mice led to organomegaly of the spleen, liver, and heart, although birth weight was not different from that in wild-type mice. Thus excess IGFBP-1 stunts fetal growth, but excess IGFBP-3 leads to selective organomegaly. IGF-1 exerts prenatal effects in the primate[184]: an increase in spleen, thymus, and kidney weights and an increase in small intestinal length were seen in fetal rhesus monkeys given synthetic IGF-1.

LEPTIN

Leptin is produced in adipose tissue; in older individuals it is correlated with fat mass. Androgens decrease leptin values, so serum levels are higher in females than in males during puberty. Leptin levels in cord blood also correlate with body weight and body fat mass but are best correlated with gestational age, reflecting increasing fat mass with advancing gestation.[185] SGA infants have lower leptin than control subjects because of their lower fat mass.[186] This direct relationship to birth weight is independent of IGF-1 control mechanisms. Leptin levels directly correlate with crown rump length at birth.[187]

Although SGA and control infants follow a similar pattern of BMI change during the first year, BMI is lower in the SGA group. However, in one study during the first 2 years after birth, the customary relationship between leptin and BMI was present in the control infants but not in the SGA infants, and the normal sexual dimorphism was also not found.[188] The higher leptin levels in SGA infants suggests a degree of leptin resistance during this period of catch-up growth or a possible adipocyte defect.

Although lower birth weight is associated with decreased cord blood leptin, weight gain is increased during the first 6 postnatal months and BMI is higher at 3 years of age.[189] However, elevated cord leptin is associated with lower BMI at 3 years. However, higher leptin at 3 months predicts greater BMI at 7 years.[190]

INSULIN

Although insulin is a major regulatory factor for carbohydrate metabolism, many lines of evidence demonstrate its importance in fetal growth as well. Macrosomia is a well-known effect of fetal hyperinsulinism and may be seen in the infant of a mother with diabetes. This appears to be due to the structural similarity of the IGFs and insulin noted earlier, which allows insulin to exert growth effects by binding to the type 1 IGF receptor. These infants have increased body fat at 1 year[191] and by 10 years of age have a higher prevalence of obesity than that seen in nonmacrosomic infants. At the other end of the spectrum is the SGA infant born to a mother with diabetes with vascular disease or who is under extremely tight glucose control or who has eclampsia or preeclampsia; this demonstrates that limited nutrient delivery compromises infant growth. These SGA infants have long-term metabolic defects and severe hypoglycemia (described in Chapter 151).

Infants with Beckwith-Wiedemann syndrome (OMIM #130650) demonstrate increased fetal growth, are macrosomic at birth with congenital malformations, and have elevated insulin concentrations leading to hypoglycemia. This syndrome may result from various mutations of 11p15 containing the genes for IGF-2 and H19, including autosomal dominant inheritance with variable expressivity, contiguous gene duplication at 11p15, and genomic imprinting resulting from a defective or absent copy of the maternally derived chromosome.[192] They have a tendency to develop renal, hepatic, adrenal, and other tumors. Postnatal growth is rapid, but normal rather than tall adult heights are achieved.

Just as increased insulin stimulates fetal growth, syndromes of fetal insulin deficiency—such as congenital diabetes mellitus, pancreatic dysgenesis, or fetal insulin resistance (e.g., Donohue syndrome or leprechaunism, a syndrome of reduced insulin action due to receptor abnormalities [OMIM #246200])—are characterized by IUGR and decreased muscle and fat mass.[193] The ability of insulin to either signal metabolic processes or stimulate growth seems to relate to the ability of insulin to autophosphorylate insulin receptor substrate-1; gene knockout of the insulin receptor substrate-1 leads to a growth-restricted fetal mouse that is born viable but has fetal and postnatal growth deficiency and hyperglycemia (knockout of insulin receptor substrate-2 leads to diabetes).[194] Insulin values are lower in SGA than in normal subjects, but values are elevated in LGA babies.

Two states of decreased insulin effects are known: congenital absence of the insulin receptor as found in Donohue syndrome and congenital absence of insulin in pancreatic aplasia. Infants lacking insulin receptors have severe postprandial hyperglycemia, as expected from the lack of insulin effect. Remarkably, they have preprandial hypoglycemia at first but fasting hyperglycemia months after birth. They are also able to demonstrate some effects of insulin, such as suppression of ketone formation, and the inverse relationship between insulin and IGFBP-1 is maintained, suggesting some insulin effects on the liver.[195] GH is low as well in leprechaunism or the Donohue syndrome (OMIM #246200). It is possible that the insulin effects are caused by the extremely elevated insulin concentration acting through the type 1 IGF receptor. IGF-1 treatment is a successful approach to the hyperglycemia of Donahue syndrome and ameliorates the expected postnatal growth failure.[196] Survival is limited to a matter of months. Other infants with insulin deficiency due to absence of the islets of Langerhans or absence of the pancreas (OMIM #260370) have severe diabetic ketoacidosis in the untreated state and have poor growth, which may be less related to the lack of insulin effects than to the severe illness they experience.

THYROID HORMONE

Thyroid hormone is a major factor in postnatal growth; however, like GH, it has relatively little effect on the fetus's growth in length. The pattern of thyroid function in the fetus is detailed in Chapter 144. After birth, TSH is acutely released in the first 30 minutes postpartum to a peak, followed by a rapid decline during the first 24 hours and a slower decline during the next 5 days. The initial peak of TSH causes an increase in serum T_4 and T_3 (owing to increased conversion from T_4) by a few hours after birth. Thus thyroid hormone values change by the hour and day in the neonatal period. During the next weeks after birth, serum T_4 and T_3 decrease.

CONGENITAL HYPOTHYROIDISM[197,198]

The effects of thyroxine in the neonate and infant are best reflected in the growth of patients with untreated and treated congenial hypothyroidism. Although endemic goiter due to iodine deficiency is the most common cause of hypothyroidism worldwide, in most of the developed world, anatomic or metabolic defects of the thyroid gland, rather than nutritional causes, prevail. Congenital hypothyroidism is found in approximately 1 of 2000 to 4000 infants; defects in the development of the thyroid gland (thyroid dysgenesis) account for 80% of occurrences in infants; approximately one-third of those have complete aplasia,[199] and most of the rest of these neonates have an ectopic location of thyroid tissue.[200] The remaining 20% of infants with congenital hypothyroidism have a normal or enlarged thyroid at birth, caused by a defect of thyroid hormone synthesis,[201] which is usually transmitted in autosomal recessive patterns. The anterior pituitary and hypothalamic deficiency of TSH and thyrotropin-releasing factor (TRF), respectively, were initially thought to be rare—in the range of 1 in 60,000—but studies in the Netherlands suggest that the prevalence may be closer to 1 in 16,000.[202] TSH deficiency may be isolated or may occur in cases of *Pit-1* mutations, leading to combined pituitary hormone deficiency (discussed earlier). Alternatively, blocking antibodies transferred from the mother may suppress the fetal thyroid function. Infants born with resistance to the actions of thyroid hormone may demonstrate elevated T_4 without hyperthyroidism and may have growth failure, as found in hypothyroidism. Screening programs in the United States utilize TSH levels, looking for elevated levels characteristic of primary hypothyroidism. Children who lack TSH or TRF effects will have decreased or normal TSH and therefore will not be identified by the newborn screening programs; TSH or TRF deficiencies are known as *secondary* and *tertiary hypothyroidism*, respectively. The infusion of TRF was recommended as a diagnostic modality to establish the diagnosis of TRF deficiency,[203] because results could provide information regarding any association with multiple pituitary hormone deficiencies. However, TRF has not been available in the United States for several years.

Over the past 20 years, there has been significant progress in understanding the genetic aspects of thyroid dysgenesis and dyshormonogenesis.[204] Five forms of thyroid dysgenesis have been described. Mutations in *PAX8*, *TSHR*, and *NKX2-5* cause nonsyndromic thyroid dysgenesis, and mutations in *FOXE1* (formerly called *TTF2*) and *NKX2-1* (formerly called *TTF1*) lead to Bamforth-Lazarus syndrome (OMIM 241850) and brain-lung-thyroid syndrome (OMIM 610978), respectively. Seven forms of thyroid dyshormonogenesis have been described, including defects in iodide transport (OMIM 274400, thyroid dyshormonogenesis 1) and iodide organification (OMIM 274500, thyroid dyshormonogenesis 2A). However, as stated, mutations in these identified genes account for a small proportion of patients with congenital hypothyroidism.

Infants with congenital hypothyroidism are of normal length or, because gestation is often prolonged, length might even be increased. Careful study of the growth rate demonstrates a decrease in growth in length in the untreated state during the first few weeks after birth, with profound growth failure lasting as long as the infant is not treated. Growth continues to be decreased in congenital hypothyroidism compared with normal controls during the first 2 to 4 weeks of thyroid therapy; this demonstrates that the early dependence of neonatal growth on thyroid hormone lasts for weeks after institution of therapy. A greater decrease in growth rate is seen in those infants most deficient in thyroid hormone in the weeks after onset of therapy.[205] Analysis of infant growth using the infant-childhood-pubertal chart demonstrated a delay in the onset of the childhood component even with early initiation of thyroxine therapy. Thus an effect of thyroxine is exerted on the onset of the childhood component of growth in the last months of the first year after birth.[206] However, diagnosis of congenital hypothyroidism at birth and appropriate treatment soon thereafter will lead to normal height and weight during infancy and is compatible with normal height growth during childhood and normal adult height.[207] If the diagnosis is delayed up to 1 year, the child may still achieve catch-up growth and normal height by 10 months after starting therapy[208-210]; even if thyroxine therapy is started as late as 2 years of age, catch-up growth in length appears to be possible (although IQ will be suboptimal).[211]

There is an inverse relationship between bone age at birth as well as length of time until treatment begins and height at 9 years, demonstrating long-term effects of intrauterine hypothyroidism on long-term postnatal growth.[212] However, adult height is related to genetic potential in early-treated congenital hypothyroidism, because complete catch-up growth occurs in those treated in the first 1 to 2 months after birth.[213]

In addition to a direct effect on epiphyseal cartilage and growth, thyroid hormones have a permissive effect on GH secretion. Individuals with hypothyroidism have decreased spontaneous GH secretion and blunted responses to GH provocative tests. A small study of congenitally hypothyroid infants demonstrated a decrease in GHBP for the first 6 months of therapy with thyroxine, suggesting a degree of GH resistance in congenital hypothyroidism that continues even after replacement therapy.[214] Untreated adult hypothyroid patients have significant reductions in the serum IGF-1 and IGFBP-3.[215] Serum IGF-1 is already so low in normal children that, if the diagnosis is made within the first month after birth, patients with congenital hypothyroidism may appear to have no decrease in IGF-1 and IGFBP-3 at the time of diagnosis.[216,217]

However, if the diagnosis is not made early, the values of IGF-1 and IGFBP-3 decrease below control levels in sensitive assays. With appropriate therapy with thyroxine, the values of IGF-1 and IGFBP-3 increase to age-appropriate levels.[218]

A bone age determination in an infant with congenital hypothyroidism may be performed using radiography of the foot and leg, which normally shows calcification of the distal femoral epiphysis at 40 weeks' gestation, proximal tibial epiphyses at 38 weeks, and cuboid epiphysis at 36 weeks; an infant with severe intrauterine hypothyroidism will have absence of some or all of these. Treatment with thyroid hormone after a long delay results in rapid catch-up growth, which is typically accompanied by rapid skeletal maturation; if doses are excessive, epiphyseal fusion may be overly rapid and adult height may be compromised. Epiphyseal dysgenesis is seen when calcification of the epiphyses progresses with thyroxine treatment after initial delay in development.[219] The normal decrease in the ratio of the upper to lower segment with age is delayed (therefore this ratio elevated) owing to poor limb growth in hypothyroidism in infancy and childhood.

Although some neonatology units have treated extremely premature infants with thyroxine, reasoning that the low levels characteristic of this developmental stage may be detrimental, there is no evidence that this treatment is effective in decreasing complications of prematurity.[220]

Iodine deficiency is a cause of severe hypothyroidism, or cretinism, which leads to profound growth failure. However, chronic iodine excess in breastfed infants was demonstrated to cause poor weight gain and increase in length in children under 4 years of age; therefore the correct balance of iodine intake is essential.[221]

NEONATAL HYPERTHYROIDISM[222]

Neonatal hyperthyroidism is usually temporary and results from the transplacental passage of thyroid-stimulating immunoglobulin from an affected mother to the fetus, causing a transient disorder. The higher the antibodies, the more likely that clinical manifestations will appear.[223] Infants with congenital hyperthyroidism may manifest IUGR. After birth, they have poor weight gain, which will tend to limit growth during the temporary hyperthyroid phase. If nutrition is adequate in older children with hyperthyroidism, increased growth may occur, but this tendency is usually overcome by the hypermetabolic state.

SEX STEROIDS

Gonadal sex steroids exert an important influence on the pubertal growth spurt, but absence of these factors exerts no noticeable effect on prepubertal growth.[224] Even in early life, however, gonadal and adrenal sex steroids in excess can cause a sharp increase in growth rate as well as the premature appearance and progression of secondary sex characteristics. Sex steroids exert a direct effect on the growth of long bones, mainly through conversion to estrogen, and can increase GH secretion once GH receptors are present in adequate supply. Untreated virilizing congenital adrenal hyperplasia is compatible with survival, sometimes for years, if there is no salt losing and as long as severe hypoglycemia or shock does not develop. In those children who have achieved such a state of stability, growth acceleration may occur early in infancy, accompanied by virilization; if the adrenopathy is also of the salt-losing type, the failure to thrive will mask any tendency toward increased growth rate, and the child will grow poorly until treatment is given or the child dies from hyponatremia, hyperkalemia, and hypoglycemic shock. Familial Leydig and germinal cell maturation may also cause increased growth early in the first year. If unabated, increased sex steroids will cause advancement of skeletal age, premature epiphyseal fusion, and short adult stature. Thus, just as growth deceleration requires evaluation, growth acceleration can be abnormal and may be a sign of precocious puberty or virilizing congenital adrenal hyperplasia.

GLUCOCORTICOIDS

Although glucocorticoids are necessary for normal metabolic function, endogenous or exogenous glucocorticoids in excess will quickly decrease or stop growth; this effect occurs more quickly than weight gain. An infant treated with excess glucocorticoids (e.g., incorrect diagnosis) will exhibit a remarkable decrease in growth rate.[225] A multicenter study of 17,621 infants born before 32 weeks of gestation and treated with postnatal glucocorticoids for bronchopulmonary dysplasia demonstrated no ill effects on their weight gain; however, head growth was slower in infants who received glucocorticoids but did not receive mechanical ventilation at 28 days of age.[226] The absence of glucocorticoids has little effect on growth if the individual is clinically well in other respects (i.e., if hypotension and hypoglycemia are absent).

Cord blood cortisol was inversely related to growth achieved in the first 3 months after birth in a preliminary study of normal term infants. When IUGR infants are considered, an inverse relationship between serum cortisol and catch-up growth in the first 6 months of postnatal life is seen.[66]

SOCIOECONOMIC AND NUTRITIONAL FACTORS

Nutrition is a key regulator of prenatal and early postnatal growth.[227] IGF-1 is regulated by nutrition and dietary protein as well as GH; there is a relationship between IGF-1 values and BMI and adiposity. IGF-1 is perhaps the mediator linking weight gain with height gain.[228]

Worldwide, the most common cause of poor growth and short stature is poverty and its effects. Thus, poor nutrition, poor hygiene, and poor health, including infectious disease, influence growth both before and after birth.

VITAMIN D

In the early 1900s, it was noted that improved growth rates in children were associated not only with better nutrition but also with greater exposure to sunlight,[229] which led to the observation that increased growth rates were associated with higher levels of vitamin D. Since then, many have attempted to understand the role that vitamin D plays in growth. However, the association between maternal vitamin D level and birth weight/birth length has been inconsistent, as is the association between antenatal vitamin D supplementation and neonatal growth.

One large-scale multiethnic cohort study found that maternal vitamin D status in the first trimester was inversely related to risk of SGA status at birth.[230] Infants of mothers with first-trimester vitamin D deficiency had accelerated growth in weight and length in the neonatal period, thought to be a rebound effect due to postnatal vitamin D supplementation. Higher risk of SGA birth status was also seen with lower maternal second-trimester vitamin D concentrations.[231] Low maternal vitamin D levels at 28 to 32 weeks' gestation were associated with decreased knee-heel length at birth but not with birth weight or birth length.[232] Other studies found that maternal vitamin D concentration was not correlated with birth indices or infant growth,[233,234] although in one study none of the women had vitamin D deficiency/insufficiency (all 25[OH]D concentrations were >50 nmol/L).[235] Furthermore, others describe a U-shaped rather than a linear association between maternal vitamin D level and SGA birth status in white women but not in black women.[236]

Whereas the association between maternal vitamin D concentration and infant birth parameters or postnatal growth is unclear, it does appear that vitamin D supplementation during pregnancy may improve birth parameters and/or postnatal growth. Vitamin D supplementation during the third trimester resulted in a decrease in risk of SGA birth (incidence of SGA status in the control group was almost twice as high); however, the results were not statistically significant.[237] A randomized placebo-controlled trial conducted in Bangladesh looked at the effect of high-dose vitamin D supplementation during the third trimester of pregnancy on infant growth. Length, weight, head circumference, and femoral length at birth were not significantly different between the two groups; however, length-for-age z-score was significantly higher at 1 year of age for those with maternal vitamin D supplementation.[238] Further breakdown of growth trends identified that the difference in length-for-age z-score resulted from accelerated growth during the first 4 weeks after birth. These findings are similar to a study conducted in London more than 3 decades ago.[239] Another study showed significant increase in birth weight and birth length with antenatal vitamin D supplementation that is sustained in infancy.[240] One randomized control trial of high-dose antenatal vitamin D supplementation in vitamin D–deficient or -insufficient mothers versus standard care found statistically higher neonatal weight, length, and head circumference with supplementation.[241] Another study did not show an association between vitamin D supplementation starting at the beginning of the second trimester until delivery and birth weight, although birth length was not measured.[242]

A Cochrane Review concluded that "the use of vitamin D supplements during pregnancy improves vitamin D concentrations as measured by 25-hydroxyvitamin D at term. However, the clinical significance of this finding is yet to be determined as there is currently insufficient high quality evidence relating to the clinical effects of vitamin D supplementation during pregnancy."[243] Factors that contribute to the variable associations noted between maternal vitamin D status or antenatal vitamin D supplementation include differences in study populations (i.e., ancestry/ethnicity), looking at birth size on a continuum versus size for gestational age, methods (cross-sectional vs. randomized control), measuring vitamin D concentration versus blanket supplementation of an at-risk group, timing of vitamin D assessment, timing of vitamin D supplementation, and dose of vitamin D administered. Furthermore, the maternal/fetal genotype may also play a role, as vitamin D receptor allelic variants may influence intrauterine, early postnatal, and adolescent growth.[236,244,245]

Recently a reappearance of vitamin D–deficient rickets in breastfed infants not supplemented with vitamin D was noted in the United States. This occurs even in sunny areas due to increased (but appropriate) use of sunblock. It can also occur in an infant receiving less than 33.8 oz, or about 1 quart, of vitamin D–supplemented infant formula every day. An infant raised on an inappropriate fad diet deficient in vitamin D or vitamin-deficient formula may develop vitamin D deficiency (this can be considered a form of urban kwashiorkor). Hypocalcemia of vitamin D deficiency can present to such a severe degree that hypocalcemic seizures occur and rickets can appear.

In a study of vitamin D supplementation in VLBW infants in India, treatment with 1000 IU/day rather than 400 IU/day was not only associated with improved biochemical and radiographic indicators of skeletal health but also with increased weight gain and linear growth.[246] Vitamin D deficiency or insufficiency remains a global problem.[247]

EFFECTS OF ENDOCRINE DISRUPTORS ON GROWTH

Endocrine-disrupting chemicals (EDCs) are ubiquitous, natural or human-made chemicals capable of interfering with hormonal action and causing adverse health effects.[209,248] The main offending EDCs that have been investigated regarding growth in infancy are organochlorine (OC) compounds (PCBs, DDT, DDE), poly-and per-fluorinated-alkyl substances—PFAS (PFOA/PFOS), polyhalogenated aromatic hydrocarbons (dioxins, PCDDs, PCDFs), and polycyclic aromatic hydrocarbons (byproducts of smoking and other causes of air pollution). DDEs have antiandrogen affects; dioxins and dioxin-like compounds (DLCs) have antiestrogenic properties. Certain PCBs and dioxin congeners are structurally similar to active thyroid hormones.

Higher prenatal exposure to OC compounds (as measured by cord blood concentrations) is associated with decreased birth weight, length, and head circumference.[249] The effects are seen in particular with DDT and DDEs. Most studies did not find an association between DDT or DDE and postnatal growth.[250] Higher exposure to DLCs in utero was associated with being taller and heavier at 2 years of age and taller at 5 years, but only in females.[251] In addition, females exposed to higher amounts of DLCs in utero had higher IGF-1 levels.[252] Higher in utero exposure of DLCs was also associated with higher IGF-1 levels in males at 5 years of age, but this did not translate to a difference in height. Higher in utero exposure to dioxin and PCB correlated significantly with longer infant length and increased IGF-BP3 levels in females only, but there was no difference in IGF-1 for either males or females.[251] However, a Scandinavian cohort showed that prenatal exposures to PCB, PFOA, and HCB were associated with SGA, although this was noted only in the Swedish cohort; the association was not found to be significant in the Norwegian cohort. Notably, a stronger association was found with male gender; thus certain populations and genders may be more vulnerable to a similar level of exposure.[253] Some studies have shown an association with maternal serum PFOA/PFOS and lower birth weight with inverse association with ponderal index, although not all studies demonstrated this association.[254] A US cohort found that PFOA was negatively associated with birth length.[209] Gestational OC, lead, and PFAS exposures were found to be most strongly associated with lower birth weight.[255] Higher levels of polycyclic aromatic hydrocarbon exposure via air pollution (monitored by personal air monitoring during pregnancy) were associated with increased risk of being born SGA,[256] having reduced birth weight, evidence of delayed fetal growth ratio (correlating well with severity of IUGR),[256] decreased head circumference,[257] and reduced cephalization index (validated marker of severe IUGR) in African American but not Dominican infants. Organophosphate pesticides were also associated with decreased birth weight in African Americans and reduced birth length in Dominicans.[257] To summarize, it appears that EDCs may have an effect on birth parameters and growth, with negative effects seen with most, although positive effects are seen with DLCs. Emerging evidence indicates that DNA methylation, histone modification, and miRNA expression are the mechanisms behind the effects of EDCs.[248,258]

CONCLUSION

Growth reflects a complex interaction of genetic and epigenetic, endocrine, and nutritional factors. Careful measurements are mandatory for accurate monitoring of growth velocity. Deviations of growth velocity from growth standards suggest an underlying disorder and require a comprehensive workup for pathology, including endocrine disorders. Endocrine factors that play a role in neonatal growth include GH, IGFs, insulin, leptin, thyroid hormone, sex steroids, glucocorticoids, and nutritional and socioeconomic factors. The role of vitamin D in neonatal growth is unclear but warrants further investigation. The specific effect and the degree of the effect of EDCs on growth is unclear, although it appears that the possible effects of these compounds are more pronounced in females, perhaps indicating their greater sensitivity to them.

A complete reference list is available at www.ExpertConsult.com. 

SELECT REFERENCES

1. Meler E, Sisterna S, Borrell A. Genetic syndromes associated with isolated fetal growth restriction. *Prenat Diagn*. 2020;40:432–446.
6. Lanciotti L, Cofini M, Leonardi A, et al. Up-to-date review about minipuberty and overview on hypothalamic-pituitary-gonadal axis activation in fetal and neonatal life. *Front Endocrinol (Lausanne)*. 2018;9:410.
7. Johannsen TH, Main KM, Ljubicic ML, et al. Sex differences in reproductive hormones during mini-puberty in infants with normal and disordered sex development. *J Clin Endocrinol Metab*. 2018;103:3028–3037.

9. Kiviranta P, Kuiri-Hanninen T, Saari A, et al. Transient postnatal gonadal activation and growth velocity in infancy. *Pediatrics*. 2016;138:e20153561.
11. Fenton TR, Senterre T, Griffin IJ. Time interval for preterm infant weight gain velocity calculation precision. *Arch Dis Child Fetal Neonatal Ed*. 2019;104:F218-F219.
12. Pereira-da-Silva L, Virella D, Fusch C. Nutritional assessment in preterm infants: a practical approach in the NICU. *Nutrients*. 2019;11:1999.
18. Wiechers C, Kirchhof S, Maas C, et al. Neonatal body composition by air displacement plethysmography in healthy term singletons: a systematic review. *BMC Pediatr*. 2019;19:489.
20. Andrews ET, Ashton JJ, Pearson F, et al. Early postnatal growth failure in preterm infants is not inevitable. *Arch Dis Child Fetal Neonatal Ed*. 2019;104:F235-F241.
21. Villar J, Giuliani F, Barros F, et al. Monitoring the postnatal growth of preterm infants: a paradigm change. *Pediatrics*. 2018;141:e20172467.
27. Williamson AL, Derado J, Barney BJ, et al. Longitudinal BMI growth curves for surviving preterm NICU infants based on a large US sample. *Pediatrics*. 2018;142:e20174169.
30. Boghossian NS, Geraci M, Edwards EM, et al. Neonatal and fetal growth charts to identify preterm infants <30 weeks gestation at risk of adverse outcomes. *Am J Obstet Gynecol*. 2018;219:195 e191-195 e114.
31. Villar J, Giuliani F, Bhutta ZA, et al. Postnatal growth standards for preterm infants: the Preterm Postnatal Follow-up Study of the INTERGROWTH-21(st) Project. *Lancet Glob Health*. 2015;3:e681691.
36. Grantz KL, Hediger ML, Liu D, et al. Fetal growth standards: the NICHD fetal growth study approach in context with INTERGROWTH-21st and the World Health Organization Multicentre Growth Reference Study. *Am J Obstet Gynecol*. 2018;218:S641-S655.e628.
42. Goldberg DL, Becker PJ, Brigham K, et al. Identifying malnutrition in preterm and neonatal populations: recommended indicators. *J Acad Nutr Diet*. 2018;118:1571-1582.
44. Rochow N, Raja P, Liu K, et al. Physiological adjustment to postnatal growth trajectories in healthy preterm infants. *Pediatr Res*. 2016;79:870-879.
45. Fenton TR, Anderson D, Groh-Wargo S, et al. An attempt to standardize the calculation of growth velocity of preterm infants-evaluation of practical bedside methods. *J Pediatr*. 2018;196:77-83.
49. Hartel C, Pagel J, Spiegler J, et al. *Lactobacillus acidophilus/Bifidobacterium infantis* probiotics are associated with increased growth of VLBWI among those exposed to antibiotics. *Sci Rep*. 2017;7:5633.
55. Bertelsen RJ, Jensen ET, Ringel-Kulka T. Use of probiotics and prebiotics in infant feeding. *Best Pract Res Clin Gastroenterol*. 2016;30:39-48.
70. Ostgard HF, Lohaugen GC, Bjuland KJ, et al. Brain morphometry and cognition in young adults born small for gestational age at term. *J Pediatr*. 2014;165:921-927.e921.
79. Carpinello OJ, DeCherney AH, Hill MJ. Developmental origins of health and disease: the history of the barker hypothesis and assisted reproductive technology. *Semin Reprod Med*. 2018;36:177-182.
81. Sharma D, Farahbakhsh N, Shastri S, et al. Intrauterine growth restriction - part 2. *J Matern Fetal Neonatal Med*. 2016;29:4037-4048.
83. Liu C, Wu B, Lin N, et al. Insulin resistance and its association with catch-up growth in Chinese children born small for gestational age. *Obesity (Silver Spring)*. 2017;25:172-177.
88. Li S, Zhang M, Tian H, et al. Preterm birth and risk of type 1 and type 2 diabetes: systematic review and meta-analysis. *Obes Rev*. 2014;15:804-811.
92. Su BH. Optimizing nutrition in preterm infants. *Pediatr Neonatol*. 2014;55:5-13.
97. Markopoulou P, Papanikolaou E, Analytis A, et al. Preterm birth as a risk factor for metabolic syndrome and cardiovascular disease in adult life: a systematic review and meta-analysis. *J Pediatr*. 2019;210:6980 e65.
99. Lee Y, Styne D. Influences on the onset and tempo of puberty in human beings and implications for adolescent psychological development. *Horm Behav*. 2013;64:250-261.
108. Chia DJ. Minireview: mechanisms of growth hormone-mediated gene regulation. *Mol Endocrinol*. 2014;28:1012-1025.
114. Yu X, Rong SS, Sun X, et al. Associations of breast milk adiponectin, leptin, insulin and ghrelin with maternal characteristics and early infant growth: a longitudinal study. *Br J Nutr*. 2018;120:1380-1387.
118. Griffin IJ. Catch-up growth: basic mechanisms. *Nestle Nutr Inst Workshop Ser*. 2015;81:87-97.
126. Laron Z. Epilogue: the future of Laron syndrome - The need for changes. *Growth Horm IGF Res*. 2016;28:79-80.
138. Schreiner F, Gohlke B, Stutte S, et al. Growth hormone receptor d3-variant, insulin-like growth factor binding protein-1 -575G/A polymorphism and postnatal catch-up growth: association with parameters of glucose homeostasis in former extremely low birth weight preterm infants. *Growth Horm IGF Res*. 2010;20:201-204.
142. Hellstrom A, Ley D, Hansen-Pupp I, et al. Insulin-like growth factor 1 has multisystem effects on foetal and preterm infant development. *Acta Paediatr*. 2016;105:576-586.
153. Kadakia R, Josefson J. The relationship of insulin-like growth factor 2 to fetal growth and adiposity. *Horm Res Paediatr*. 2016;85:75-82.
155. Broeren MAC, Krabbe JG, Boesten LS, et al. Impact of the choice of IGF-I assay and normative dataset on the diagnosis and treatment of growth hormone deficiency in children. *Horm Res Paediatr*. 2018;90:181-189.
162. Hawkes CP, Murray DM, Kenny LC, et al. Correlation of insulin-like growth factor-I and -II concentrations at birth measured by mass spectrometry and growth from birth to two months. *Horm Res Paediatr*. 2018;89:122-131.
164. Begemann M, Zirn B, Santen G, et al. Paternally inherited IGF2 mutation and growth restriction. *N Engl J Med*. 2015;373:349-356.
168. Razak A, Faden M. Association of small for gestational age with retinopathy of prematurity: a systematic review and meta-analysis. *Arch Dis Child Fetal Neonatal Ed*. 2020;105:270-278. Epub 2019 Jul 20.
170. Ingolfsland EC, Haapala JL, Buckley LA, et al. Late growth and changes in body composition influence odds of developing retinopathy of prematurity among preterm infants. *Nutrients*. 2019;12:E78.
173. Ley D, Hallberg B, Hansen-Pupp I, et al. rhIGF-1/rhIGFBP-3 in preterm infants: a phase 2 randomized controlled trial. *J Pediatr*. 2019;206:56-65.
175. van de Lagemaat M, Rotteveel J, Heijboer AC, et al. Growth in preterm infants until six months postterm: the role of insulin and IGF-I. *Horm Res Paediatr*. 2013;80:92-99.
189. Mantzoros CS, Rifas-Shiman SL, Williams CJ, et al. Cord blood leptin and adiponectin as predictors of adiposity in children at 3 years of age: a prospective cohort study. *Pediatrics*. 2009;123:682-689.
197. Weiner A, Oberfield S, Vuguin P. The laboratory features of congenital hypothyroidism and approach to therapy. *NeoReviews*. 2020;21:e37-e44.
202. Schoenmakers N, Alatzoglou KS, Chatterjee VK, et al. Recent advances in central congenital hypothyroidism. *J Endocrinol*. 2015;227.R5171.
209. Buck Louis GM, Zhai S, Smarr MM, et al. Endocrine disruptors and neonatal anthropometry, NICHD Fetal Growth Studies - Singletons. *Environ Int*. 2018;119:515-526.
222. Samuels SL, Namoc SM, Bauer AJ. Neonatal thyrotoxicosis. *Clin Perinatol*. 2018;45:31-40.
225. Styne DM. Growth. In: Gardner DG, Shobak D, eds. *Greenspan's Basic and Clinical Endocrinology*. New York: McGraw Hill; 2018:137-170.
226. Zozaya C, Avila-Alvarez A, Garcia-Munoz Rodrigo F, et al. The impact of postnatal systemic steroids on the growth of preterm infants: a multicenter cohort study. *Nutrients*. 2019;11:E2729.
248. Stel J, Legler J. The role of epigenetics in the latent effects of early life exposure to obesogenic endocrine disrupting chemicals. *Endocrinology*. 2015;156:3466-3472.
254. Zheng T, Zhang J, Sommer K, et al. Effects of environmental exposures on fetal and childhood growth trajectories. *Ann Glob Health*. 2016;82:41-99.
258. Bommarito PA, Martin E, Fry RC. Effects of prenatal exposure to endocrine disruptors and toxic metals on the fetal epigenome. *Epigenomics*. 2017;9:333-350.

Human Milk Composition and Function in the Infant

23

Donna Geddes | Zoya Gridneva | Lisa Stinson | Peter Hartmann

INTRODUCTION

Lactation is the defining characteristic of "mammal" and has enabled the wide distribution of more than the 4000 species. The evolution of a large brain that consumes approximately 23% of resting energy has given humankind a significant competitive intellectual advantage over all other mammals. Unlike other mammals, most brain growth in humans occurs after birth and is facilitated by the nutrients present in human milk (HM). The synthesis of HM occurs in the lactating mammary gland, which, similar to the brain, is a very active organ, with the energy in HM representing approximately 30% of resting energy. Its evolution as a secretory organ is closely associated with the innate and acquired immune systems. However, because there is only a small body of basic research on human lactation, evidence-based medical assessment and treatment of lactation difficulties are very limited. Unlike other metabolically equivalent organs in the body, no clinical tests are currently available to assess the normal function of the lactating breast. This is of particular importance when considering the composition of HM and its function in the infant.

After birth, the transfer of nutritional and bioactive components from mother to infant continues through colostrum and milk. The substitution of infant formula for HM deprives the infant not only of nutrients (Table 23.1) that are more accessible from HM than formula (e.g., essential amino acids, casein), but also of many bioactive and immune-protective factors (e.g., oligosaccharides, lactoferrin, lysozyme, leukocytes) directed specifically against pathogens in the infant's environment, thus placing the formula-fed infant at a distinct disadvantage (Table 23.2). HM components also compensate for immature function in the newborn, in whom endogenous production of digestive enzymes, immunoglobulin A (IgA), taurine, choline, nucleotides, and long-chain polyunsaturated fatty acids (LCPUFAs) is insufficient. Furthermore, recent research has revealed the presence of stem cells in HM, some of which are capable of surviving the infant's gastrointestinal tract and integrating into its organs, potentially providing developmental benefits. These nutritional and bioactive components are the reason for the superiority of HM to infant formula.

The composition of HM is indeed spectacular. In addition to viable maternal cells, it contains more than 900 proteins, many bioactive peptides, 200 oligosaccharides, thousands of triacylglycerols (TAGs), approximately 100 known metabolites, hormones, cytokines, and a full complement of minerals and vitamins. Some of these components vary from the beginning to the end of a breast-feed, over the day, with diet, and over the lactation period. Unfortunately, with the notable exception of the growth of breast-fed infants (World Health Organization [WHO] growth charts), there are no reference ranges for normality (predicted values that cover 95% of individuals) for milk production and milk composition. Thus the values given here for the concentration of the components in HM are only a guide to reference ranges for normality.

MILK VOLUME

Daily milk production in women is relatively constant regardless of maternal nutritional status.[1] Exclusively breast-fed healthy infants have a mean daily milk intake of 750 to 800 mL/24 hours from 1 to 6 months of lactation. However, a wide range of intake volumes from 450 to 1200 mL/24 hours has been reported.[2] Despite these differences in milk intake, there is a significant relationship between milk intake and infant growth rate. Milk intake remains consistent from 1 to 6 months. This is not surprising, considering younger infants (1 to 3 months of

Table 23.1 Comparison of Milk Components in Human and Cow Milk.

	Human Colostrum	Human Mature Milk	Cow Mature Milk
Total solids (g/L)	180	124	127
Nonprotein N (g/L)	0.53	0.46	0.29
Protein (g/L)	15.8	9	36
Casein (g/L)	4	3.5	28
α-Lactalbumin (g/L)	3.6	2.7	0.7
sIgA (g/L)	7.8	1	0.03
Lactoferrin (g/L)	5.8	2	Trace
Lysozyme (g/L)	0.36	0.4	0.4 mg/L
IgG (g/L)	0.5	0.05	0.6
Serum albumin (g/L)	2.55	1	0.19
Lactose (mmol/L)	85	185	48
Glucose (mmol/L)	0.2	1.5	0.22
Lipid (g/L)	20	40	43
Zinc (µg/mL)	10	2	4
Citrate	3	2.6	9.2
Copper (µg/mL)	0.6	0.3	0.1
Magnesium (mmol/L)	1.5	1.8	5.1
Calcium (mmol/L)	6.4	7.5	29.4
Phosphorous	1.6	1.8	11.2
Sodium (mmol/L)	18	6.3	25
Chloride (mmol/L)	25	11.6	30.2
Potassium (mmol/L)	18	13.9	34.7
Iron (mmol/L)	0.8	0.3	0.25
Caloric density (kcal/100 g)	68	53	62-72

Table 23.2 Importance of Breastfeeding.

Maternal	Term Infant	Preterm Infant
Rapid uterine involution	Optimal growth and development	Confers passive immunity
More rapid postpartum weight loss	Decreased incidence and severity of infections:	Decreased incidence of late-onset sepsis, NEC
Lactational amenorrhea	• bacterial meningitis	Decreased respiratory infection
Decreased risk of:	• respiratory tract infection	Better cognitive function and academic performance
• breast cancer	• otitis media	Regulation of infant temperature (skin to skin)
• hip fractures and osteoporosis	• urinary tract infection	Psychological benefit for the mother—improved attachment, empowerment, and confidence
• ovarian cancer	Decreased incidence of diabetes (types 1 and 2)	
• rheumatoid arthritis	Decreased incidence of lymphoma	
Significant reduction in:	Better cognitive function and academic performance	
• hypertension	Decreased incidence of leukemia	
• hyperlipidemia	Decreased incidence of obesity	
• cardiovascular disease	Decreased incidence of asthma, atopic dermatitis, and eczema	
• diabetes type 2	Decreased incidence of celiac disease and inflammatory bowel disease	
Increased confidence, attachment to the infant	Reduced risk of sudden infant death syndrome	

NEC, Necrotizing enterocolitis.

age) grow more rapidly than older infants (4 to 6 months of age). Smaller infants also have a larger surface area to volume ratio and therefore have a higher metabolic rate per kilogram of body weight and use more of their nutrient intake for maintenance of body temperature than do older, heavier infants.

Similar levels of milk production have been reported for mothers globally, including in developing countries, although maternal nutritional status may be subject to seasonal variation and may be less than adequate based on industrial country standards. Increasing the intake of fluids does not seem to affect milk production; therefore lactating women should maintain adequate fluid intake, but they should be aware that excess fluids have no impact on milk volume.

The measurement of daily milk production provides an objective measure of mammary gland function and has been shown to be useful to both the clinician and the mother without undermining maternal confidence. In contrast, measurement of milk intake at a single incidence of breast-feeding is of little value because milk intake is controlled by the infant's appetite and can vary greatly from one breast feeding to the next.

MILK COMPOSITION

HM is a unique dynamic fluid that is clearly species specific. It contains nutritional components such as fat, protein, lactose, and micronutrients at levels suitable for optimal growth, as well as bioactive and cellular components that provide protection and promote infant development. These components enter the milk via two different routes; they are either synthesized by the lactocytes that line the mammary alveoli, or they are transferred directly from the maternal circulation and/or modified within the lactocyte after uptake from the blood.[3]

FAT

The fat content of milk accounts for approximately 50% to 60% of the caloric intake of the term infant. The average fat content is 41 g/L, with a threefold variation within and between women (from 22 to 62 g/L).[2] Fat content increases from the beginning to the end of a feed and is associated with the volume of milk in the breast. Factors influencing milk fat content include gestation, stage of lactation, parity, maternal age, diet, and nutritional status. Specifically, low caloric intake and high margarine intake are associated with increased palmitic acid (C16) and trans-fatty acids, respectively.

The emulsified fat globule is secreted by the lactocyte and consists of a core composed almost entirely of TAGs (98% to 99%) and of an outer membrane of phospholipids, cholesterol, glycolipids, proteins, and glycoproteins. The TAGs are either saturated or unsaturated fatty acids esterified to a glycerol backbone.[4] The fatty acids are short-, medium-, or long-chain fatty acids (LCFAs). Short-chain fatty acids (SCFAs) (<10-carbon chain) and medium-chain fatty acids (MCFAs) (10- to 14-carbon chain) are synthesized by the lactocyte. LCFAs (16- to 24-carbon chain) and LCPUFAs, including the omega-3 fatty acid docosahexaenoic acid (DHA) and the omega-6 fatty acid arachidonic acid (AA), are derived from the maternal circulation. LCFAs dominate (85%) by weight, followed by MCFAs (13%) and the remainder LCPUFAs and SCFAs. The mean concentrations of DHA and AA are 0.32% (by weight; range: 0.06% to 1.4%) and 0.47% (range: 0.24% to 1.0%), respectively.

Maternal diet has a minimal effect on the total fat content. However, fatty acid composition responds to maternal diet in that women who consume a diet high in fish have milk with a high concentration of DHA compared with those with low fish intake.[5] In addition, women who consume a low-fat, high-carbohydrate diet have higher concentrations of MCFAs in their milk. Absorption of fat from HM is greater than that from milk of other species, likely because of innate differences such as the structure of the TAGs and action of bile salt-stimulated lipase (BSSL).

NUTRITIONAL FUNCTIONS

Interestingly, evidence suggests that fat intake in the first 2 years of life appears to have little to no effect on later overweight and obesity. This is in contrast to studies of protein, where increased protein intake is associated with detrimental effects on growth. Furthermore, no relationship has been found between fat intake in the first 2 years of life and later development of noncommunicable diseases.[6] A small recent study has even suggested that higher fat intake may be protective against adult overweight. Fat also provides a vehicle for transfer of fat-soluble vitamins to the infant.

DEVELOPMENTAL FUNCTIONS

DHA and AA preferentially accumulate in the lipid membranes of the infant retina and brain and are important for neural function.[5] Indeed, breast-fed infants exhibit higher plasma levels of DHA and AA; at autopsy, higher levels of DHA have been detected in their gray and white matter, as well as the brain cortex compared with formula-fed infants. Improved visual function[7] and higher IQ out to 15 years of age have also been reported in those who were breast-fed as infants compared with their formula-fed counterparts. These advantages have been postulated to be due to the unique fatty acid composition of HM.

IMMUNE FUNCTIONS

Selected fatty acids have also been shown to protect against lipid-coated microorganisms in vitro. For example, myristic acid (14:0) has antimicrobial actions. The concentration of *n*-6 polyunsaturated fatty acids (*n*-6 PUFAs) in HM has an inverse relationship with the risk of mother-to-child transmission of human immunodeficiency virus (HIV), suggesting a protective role of *n*-6 PUFA.[8] Evidence from rodent studies suggests that maternally derived SCFAs may protect the infant from developing asthma/atopy via their effects on regulatory T cell biology.[9]

PROTEIN

The nitrogen content of HM (1.71 ± 0.31 g/L) consists of protein and nonprotein (approximately 25%; 0.42 ± 0.10 g/L) components.

Nonprotein nitrogen is derived from a number of components such as free amino acids, peptides, creatine and creatinine, nucleic acids and nucleotides, urea, uric acid, ammonia, amino sugars, polyamines, carnitine, and other compounds. A number of these components have functions for the infant; for example, nucleotides and nucleosides become semiessential during periods of high physiologic growth such as in the preterm infant, with evidence suggesting their involvement in lymphocyte production and regulation of gut development. Carnitine is also essential for fatty acid metabolism and is involved in lipolysis, ketogenesis, and thermogenesis. Similarly, taurine is involved in fat absorption, bile acid secretion, hepatic function, and retinal function.

Protein levels in HM are relatively low, constituting 0.8% to 0.9% by weight; nevertheless, they are highly bioavailable to the infant. Protein content fluctuates during lactation with high levels during early lactation (15.8 ± 4.2 g/L) that gradually decline to a relatively stable level in mature milk (6.9 ± 1.2 g/L).

Three distinct groups of protein exist in HM: caseins as micellar structures, whey water-soluble proteins, and mucins, which are associated with the milk fat globule membrane.

Caseins are a major protein in mammalian milk. Casein micelles consist of several casein subunits, calcium phosphate, and other ionic constituents and give bovine milk its characteristic white appearance. Caseins are less abundant in HM, which accounts for its distinctive pale blue appearance. The functions of caseins are largely nutritive, providing essential amino acids and minerals to the infant. For example, the casein micelle is the main source of calcium and phosphorous for the infant and is essential for bone mineralization. Intrinsic protease activity in the breast and in the infant's stomach creates casein-derived peptides that have a myriad of effects, including antimicrobial (e.g., casecidin), immunomodulatory, antithrombic (e.g., casopiastrin), antihypertensive, opioid (β-casomorphins), and gastrointestinal functions. HM has low casein content: less than 10% total protein content of colostrum, 40% in transitional milk, and 50% in mature milk. Low levels of casein result in soft curds formed in the infant's stomach, which are easily digested, facilitating gastric emptying, and are therefore more compatible with frequent feeding. In comparison, the concentration of casein in bovine milk is more than 10 times that of HM, resulting in the formation of harder curds in the infant's stomach, the effects of which may be offset to some degree by addition of whey protein to bovine-based formula. Lower casein content is also commensurate with the slow growth rate of human infants compared with the offspring of other mammals.

Whey proteins account for the major proportion of protein content in HM (90% of the total protein content in colostrum, 60% in mature milk, and 50% in late lactation). Whey is a complex protein fraction comprising a large number of proteins. Several proteins are abundant in the whey portion; however, there are many lower abundant proteins that have yet to be well characterized. The major immunologic proteins present in the whey fraction are lactoferrin, lysozyme, and secretory IgA (sIgA), α-lactalbumin and BSSL.

sIgA is the most abundant immunoglobulin in HM, accounting for more than 90% of immunoglobulins and up to 25% of total protein content. The sIgA concentration is higher in early lactation (1 to 2 g/L) and lower in later lactation (0.5 to 10 g/L).[10] Adaptive immunity is achieved by IgA via the enteromammary pathway, in which IgA-producing lymphocytes in the maternal intestine are transferred to the mammary gland during lactation. sIgA is resistant to digestion, thereby boosting the infant's immature immune system. Protection is afforded mainly against pathogens from the intestine.

Lactoferrin, another major protein in HM, is present at 305 g/L in colostrum, falling to 1.9 g/L as milk production is established. Each molecule of lactoferrin has the capability to bind two ferric ions, and binds most of the iron in HM is bound by lactoferrin. Sequestering of iron contributes to lactoferrin's bacteriostatic properties. Proteolysis of lactoferrin in the infant stomach produces lactoferricins that possess diverse functions. In vitro studies in cultured human intestinal cells also show that lactoferrin facilitates the uptake of iron due to a lactoferrin receptor specific to enterocytes.[11]

α-Lactalbumin comprises 10% to 20% of the total protein in HM and has 40% gene similarity to lysozyme, implying that it was intimately entwined in the evolution of the mammary gland from the innate immune system.[12] α-Lactalbumin binds Ca^{2+} and Zn^{2+} and is involved in lactose synthesis. Furthermore, the amino acid composition of HM α-lactalbumin is similar to the infant's requirements for amino acids. Although supplementation of infant formula with bovine α-lactalbumin increases absorption of zinc and iron in infant rhesus monkeys,[13] the effect on mineral absorption in breast-fed infants has not been investigated.

Lysozyme, one of the major three proteins in HM, is found in particularly high concentrations in HM compared with the milk of other species. It is thought to be synthesized by the mammary epithelial cells. The HM form of lysozyme is considered identical in structure to lysozyme in other bodily fluids such as pancreatic juice and saliva. It possesses bacteriostatic properties by lysis of gram-positive and some gram-negative bacteria.

BSSL levels are relatively low in HM (1% to 2% of total milk proteins), but BSSL has an important role in efficient digestion of dietary fats. It is present in bovine milk but is lost from infant formula during the manufacturing process. In the intestinal lumen, activation by bile salts enables BSSL to hydrolyze lipid substrates, such as short- and long-chain triacylglycerides, diacylglycerides, monoacylglycerides, cholesteryl esters, retinol esters, and *p*-nitrophenyl esters. BSSL is unfortunately inactivated by heat pasteurization, resulting in reduced fat absorption in preterm infants. A novel method of pasteurization with ultraviolet (UV)-C radiation has been shown to retain almost all of the BSSL activity when compared with raw milk,[14] but this has yet to be tested clinically to determine whether fat absorption is improved in infants fed with UV-C–pasteurized milk.

NUTRITIONAL FUNCTIONS

The quality and quantity of protein intake during the first 2 years of life influence infant growth, neurodevelopment, and long-term health. Evidence suggests that a high-protein intake during the first 2 years of life may have a negative impact on long-term health.[15] Not only is the protein intake of formula-fed infants greater than that of breast-fed infants, but the composition of protein is also markedly different, particularly in terms of its amino acid content. This has compelled formula companies to produce lower-protein formulas to mimic the growth rates of breast-fed infants, because high-protein formulas result in higher infant weight gains and body mass index (BMI). HM contains approximately 5% of energy as protein (PE%), which meets the 5.6 PE% mean protein requirement for 6-month-old infants. During the next few years of life, the PE% needed to meet physiologic needs decreases to a mean PE% of 3.8 with a safe upper level of 5.2 PE%. The acceptable range for 1- to 3-year-old children is 5% to 20% PE%. Average protein intake is typically 3 to 4 times higher than the requirements with large variation. One of the major sources of protein during this period is whole bovine milk, which has a PE% of 20%.[16]

IMMUNE FUNCTIONS

A number of proteins and products of their digestion play important roles in the protection of the infant via both defense against pathogenic viruses and bacteria and support of the immune system.[10] Typically, many of these components either have multiple functions or work synergistically with other proteins in HM.

Lactoferrin possesses antimicrobial properties due in part to sequestering of iron and thus depriving iron-dependent pathogens. However, it has also been shown to have potent effects on pathogens not dependent on saturation of lactoferrin. This activity has been largely attributed to lactoferricin, which is released during the digestion of lactoferrin. Lactoferricin has powerful antimicrobial and weak antiviral activity, as well as antitumor activity.

α-Lactalbumin has not been extensively studied in relation to antimicrobial activity. However, three polypeptide fragments generated after exposure of α-lactalbumin to proteases from the gastrointestinal tract do have antimicrobial activity against *Escherichia coli*, *Klebsiella pneumoniae*, *Staphylococcus aureus*, *Staphylococcus epidermis*, streptococci, and *Candida albicans*.

Lysozyme is one of three major proteins that dominate the whey fraction of milk. Its functions are largely immunologic and include degradation of the outer cell wall of gram-positive bacteria, inactivation of gram-negative bacteria in the presence of lactoferrin, inhibition of amoeba, and anti-HIV activity.

DEVELOPMENTAL FUNCTIONS

Human lactoferrin stimulates intestinal cell differentiation and proliferation in vitro. Furthermore the ability to eliminate bacteria with no inflammation suggests that it is plays a role in the development of the gut microbiome. Similarly animal models show sIgA prevents translocation of aerobic bacteria from the neonatal gut to the lymphatic system and that no exposure to maternal sIgA resulted in a vastly different gut microbiome.[17] Lactoferrin has also been implicated in neurologic and cognitive development in animal models.[18]

GROWTH FACTORS

HM growth factors have multiple roles that include the growth and maturation of multiple organs including the neonatal gastrointestinal tract via gut immunity and proliferation and differentiation of intestinal cells. The main growth factors include neuronal, vascular endothelial (VEGF), hepatic (HGF), epidermal (EGF), and insulin-like growth (IGF) factors. Neuronal growth factors such as brain-derived neurotrophic factor, S-100B protein, and glial cell line–derived neurotrophic factor work together in the development and maintenance of the nervous system. HGF is not only involved in liver development but also the kidney, lung, mammary gland, teeth, muscle, and neuronal tissues. EGF is integral to normal intestinal cell development and is implicated in reduction of necrotizing enterocolitis. IGF include IGF-1 and IGF-2, which are controlled amino acid and overall energy intake. IGF-1 has a role in protecting enterocytes and enhancing erythropoiesis and also synergizes with VEGF in angiogenesis.[19]

CARBOHYDRATES

Lactose is the main carbohydrate in HM, accounting for 30% to 40% of its energy content. Lactose concentration is lower in colostrum (19 g/L), rising to 54 g/L at secretory activation (onset of copious milk production), and is related to milk volume produced.[20] Lactose is digested by lactase into the monosaccharides glucose and galactose. Galactose is converted to glucose in the liver. Glucose is the primary fuel for living cells.

HM oligosaccharides (HMOs) are the third most abundant component in milk. In contrast to lactose, their concentration is highest in colostrum (20 to 25 g/L) and decreases in term milk (5 to 20 g/L). More than 200 HMOs have been identified in HM, with women having a range of 23 to 130 different HMOs.[21] The HMO composition is classified into four major groups: secretors and nonsecretors, and Lewis positive or Lewis negative. HMOs are largely indigestible by the infant's gut, with only a small proportion absorbed into the circulation and excreted in the urine. Not surprisingly, HMOs possess many nonnutritive functions such as protection from disease and promotion of growth of intestinal *Bifidobacteria*.[20]

NUTRITIONAL FUNCTIONS

Both galactose and glucose are used by the brain. In particular, galactose is involved in formation of galactolipids essential for rapid brain development. Lactose also improves infant absorption of calcium and aids bacterial colonization of the infant intestine. HMOs have also been linked to infant cognitive and body composition development.

IMMUNE FUNCTIONS

HMOs provide protection from infection via an antiadhesive antimicrobial action. HMOs provide protection from pathogenic diarrhea-causing organisms such as *E. coli*, *Campylobacter pylori*, *Campylobacter jejuni*, norovirus, and rotavirus. In general, the higher the consumption of HMOs, the lower the risk of any diarrheal disease in infants. HMOs have also been implicated in reduced transmission of HIV, protection from specific protozoa such as *Entamoeba histolytica*, and lower risk of necrotizing enterocolitis and respiratory or urinary tract infections. This is likely due to their prebiotic and bifidogenic function, providing a competitive advantage to commensal bacteria in preference to potential pathogens.

DEVELOPMENTAL FUNCTIONS

Because sialic acid is prominent in gangliosides and glycoproteins involved in infant brain development and cognition, it has been postulated that sialylated HMOs, which are sialic acid carriers, may be required for optimal infant brain development. Sialic acid concentrations are significantly higher in the brains of breast-fed infants compared to formula-fed infants. HMOs also have prebiotic effects and thereby influence bacterial colonization of the infant gut. Indeed, they have been shown to enhance growth of bifidobacteria and lactobacilli.

VITAMINS AND MINERALS

HM provides both vitamins (water and fat soluble) and minerals, including trace minerals for the infant.[1] The vitamin content of HM is dependent on the maternal vitamin status, with water-soluble vitamins being more responsive than fat-soluble vitamins to maternal intake. In particular, there should be sufficient amounts of thiamin, riboflavin, vitamins B6 and B12, vitamin A, iron, and iodine in the diets of lactating women. The concentrations of some minerals and vitamins in milk are independent of maternal diet (e.g., calcium [250 mg/L] and phosphorus [150 mg/L]).

Vitamin D is a steroid hormone produced by skin exposure to ultraviolet light. Vitamin D is important in the regulation of calcium and phosphorus absorption and therefore bone health. It also plays a role in the innate and adaptive immune system. HM concentrations of vitamin D (25-hydroxyvitamin D) are positively related to maternal intake and serum concentrations but are not consistent.[20] Recent recognition of high rates of maternal vitamin D deficiency combined with a resurgence in the reported cases of rickets has raised concern about the adequacy of vitamin D in HM. Although there is evidence that maternal vitamin D supplementation has a direct effect on HM concentration and infant 25-hydroxyvitamin D status, the American Academy of Pediatrics currently recommends that all breast-fed infants should be supplemented with 400 IU/day of oral vitamin D from birth.

Iron in milk is highly bioavailable to the infant, so it is widely considered that infant supplementation is generally not required in the first 6 months. However, special consideration must be given to certain infants, such as low-birth-weight infants and those born to diabetic mothers, whose low iron stores at birth are often not accounted for. In line with this, a study has surprisingly found that 36% of healthy fully breast-fed infants have iron deficiency or iron deficiency anemia at 5 months of age. Friel and colleagues[21a] showed that breast-fed infants (1 to 6 months) supplemented with 7.5 mg/day of elemental iron as ferrous sulfate had higher hemoglobin concentrations and higher mean corpuscular volumes at 6 months of age than those who were not supplemented. Supplemented infants also exhibit better visual acuity and higher Bayley Mental and Psychomotor Developmental Indices at 13 months. On this basis, the American Academy of Pediatrics recommends that exclusively breast-fed term infants and those receiving more than half of their daily feeds as HM be given oral iron supplementation of 1 mg/kg/day from 4 months of age.[21b]

Zinc deficiency is common (>20%), and 50% of those deficient are infants and children younger than 5 years of age. Symptoms include growth retardation, altered immune function, and gastrointestinal effects such as diarrhea. Those with high requirements for zinc due to rapid growth and tissue synthesis are at highest risk and are therefore typically infants and children, particularly those consuming a combination of HM and predominantly plant-based diet of low zinc content (i.e., premature and low-birth-weight infants). Because the zinc content of HM is independent of maternal zinc status and has high bioavailability to the infant, zinc intake from HM should also

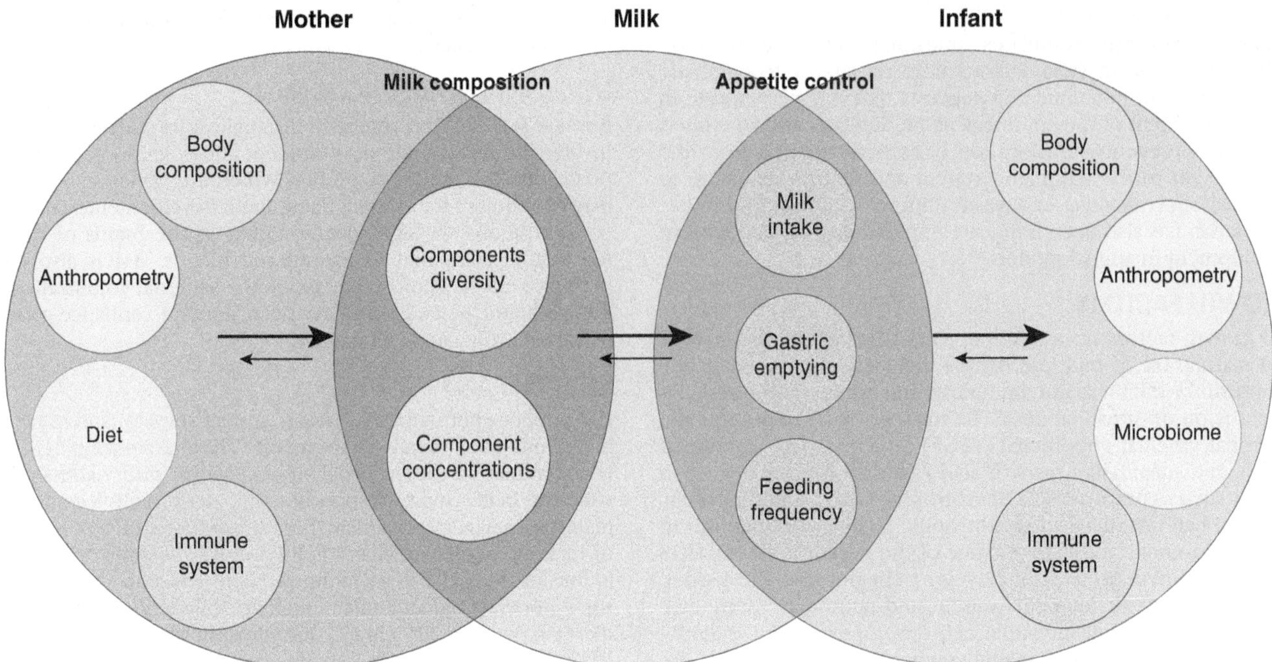

Fig. 23.1 Framework for possible interconnecting pathways of lactocrine programing of the infant body composition. (Reproduced by permission and modified from Gridneva Z, Kugananthan S, Hepworth AR, et al. Effect of human milk appetite hormones, macronutrients, and infant characteristics on gastric emptying and breastfeeding patterns of term fully breastfed infants. *Nutrients.* 2017;9:15.)

be sufficient, provided that HM volume is adequate.[20] However, zinc supplements are indicated if complementary foods are low in zinc or in poor resource settings.

A multitude of trace elements are present in HM (copper, zinc, barium, cadmium, cesium, cobalt, cerium, lanthanum, manganese, molybdenum, nickel, lead, rubidium, tin, strontium), and these are also highly bioavailable. Unfortunately, no reference values exist, and many of these trace elements are affected by maternal diet.

IMPACT OF MATERNAL BODY COMPOSITION ON HUMAN MILK COMPOSITION

Maternal body composition has been linked to concentrations of HM components, indicating the potential to influence development of infant body composition (Fig. 23.1). Increased maternal adiposity is related higher total protein and whey protein[22] HM concentrations. Furthermore, milk leptin concentration is also modified by maternal adiposity, with higher concentrations reported in mothers with increased fat mass.[23] Thus maintenance of healthy maternal adiposity preconception and during pregnancy and lactation may ensure appropriate levels of total protein and leptin supply to the infant, supporting the optimal programing of appetite control and body composition in infancy.

INFANT BODY COMPOSITION

Breast-fed infants are at 15% to 20% reduced risk of obesity and obesity-related disease later in life, although the protective mechanisms of HM and breast-feeding are not fully elucidated. The plasticity of HM composition in part explains programing of infant growth and development. Bioactive agents in HM (including hormones, growth factors, neuropeptides, and antiinflammatory and immune-modulating agents) influence the growth, development, and function of organs and tissues during early infancy.[24] HM likely enhances infant programing, reduces obesity, and results in lower incidence of late metabolic diseases, such as type 2 diabetes.Although milk volume is associated with infant growth rate,[25] information on the effect of specific HM components on infant body composition or, specifically, fat-free and fat mass is limited.

MILK COMPOSITION AND INFANT BODY COMPOSITION

Studies that measure intakes of HM components with respect to infant body composition are rare, with majority analyzing the relationships with concentrations, which should be taken with caution, given the variations in milk intake volumes that infants receive.[2]

FAT

Fat intake is positively associated with weight gain and fat-free mass gain, in term breast-fed infants at 3 and 6 months.[26] Interestingly, there is an inverse association between fat intake at 2 years of age and body fat and serum leptin concentration at 20 years of age,[27] suggesting that an early diet with higher fat intake may benefit the development of infant body composition. Because fat concentration in HM is inversely related to milk intake,[28] it is plausible that infants ingesting milk with lower fat concentrations consume larger volumes of HM, and hence higher amounts of protein and carbohydrate, to reach satiation and thus increase their body weight. Indeed, milk fat concentrations at 4 to 8 weeks postpartum are negatively associated with infant delta weight (3 to 12 months), delta skinfolds (3 to 12 months), and delta BMI (3 to 12 months), as well as BMI and skinfolds at 12 months.[29]

PROTEIN

Total protein intake is positively associated with infant weight gain[26] and fat-free mass gain[26] in breast-fed infants. Furthermore,

HM total protein concentration at 4 to 8 weeks postpartum is positively associated with infant BMI at 12 months.[30] Specific proteins may also play a critical role in shaping infant body composition, with intake of casein being the most significant contributor.[22] Daily intakes of casein relate differentially to infant body composition: positively to fat mass and negatively to fat-free mass. Higher breast-feeding frequency is also related to higher casein intakes, leading to higher infant milk intake and adiposity but lower fat-free mass.[31] Casein also influences infant gastric emptying; higher casein-to-whey ratios in lower HM volumes are associated with faster gastric emptying in exclusively breast-fed infants.[32] Thus casein may influence infant body composition via breast-feeding frequency, gastric emptying, and modulation of milk intake.

Immunologic proteins such as both administered and HM lysozyme have been shown to improve weight gain in preterm infants, and daily intakes of lysozyme are positively associated with term breast-fed infant adiposity during the first year of lactation. Because lysozyme is involved in the protection of gastrointestinal tract against chronic inflammation and in the homeostasis of cartilage and bone growth, the effect on HM lysozyme on infant body composition is logical. Lysozyme may contribute to the optimal fat mass development during infancy, resulting in a beneficial adipose phenotype of breast-fed infants that is associated with a reduced risk of obesity.

CARBOHYDRATES

Carbohydrate/lactose intakes are also lower in breast-fed infants compared with formula-fed infants. Higher estimated carbohydrate daily intake is positively related to weight gain and fat-free mass gain.[26] Studies of the effect of carbohydrate concentrations show conflicting relationships with infant body composition. However, concentrations of individual HMOs show differing associations with infant body composition.[33] HMOs are speculated to exert effects on body composition by enhancing the growth of beneficial gut bacteria, as the gut microbiome has been implicated in the development of obesity. Indeed one study reported multiple associations between various carbohydrates (total carbohydrates, lactose, and HMOs) and infant body composition, showing complicated differential relationships for concentrations and intakes of these components with infant fat and fat-free mass, as well as anthropometry over the first 12 months of lactation.[34] Daily intakes of HM total carbohydrates and lactose were positively associated with infant adiposity and negatively with fat-free mass. Furthermore, higher total carbohydrates and lactose intakes were reported for infants that fed more frequently. Lactose likely influences infant body composition via gastric emptying and breast-feeding frequency, in turn modulating the milk intake.

GROWTH FACTORS

Several growth factors have been studied in regard to infant body composition. For example, lower EGF concentrations have been reported in milk of mothers with obese infants.[35] In addition, IGF-1 has been associated with higher infant weight gain,[36] interleukin-6 (IL-6) with reduced growth and adiposity in infants, and tumor necrosis factor (TNF)-α with lower infant fat-free mass.[37] TNF-α is implicated in bone mineral content, with results differing depending on either infant sex or the time post partum[38]; it may play a role in bone health and modeling process, thus affecting infant body composition through bone accretion rate and/or through immune system pathways.

APPETITE HORMONES

HM contains multiple growth-, appetite- and metabolism-regulating hormones, which are also implicated in development of infant body composition. Hormones such as leptin and adiponectin, resistin, ghrelin, obestatin, motilin, and insulin appear to play important roles in regulation of energy conversion, appetite control, and development of infant body composition. The two most studied adipokines, leptin and adiponectin, may contribute to the regulation of infant food intake, weight, and adiposity, decreasing risk of obesity.

In breast-fed infants, associations between HM concentrations of leptin and infant weight gain,[39] BMI,[39] and weight and/or adiposity are predominantly negative.[39] The only study that measured daily intakes of HM leptin and infant body composition over several time points during first 12 months of lactation showed no associations with leptin concentrations but reported positive associations between daily intakes of leptin and infant adiposity.[40]

Adiponectin, an appetite-stimulating hormone, is present in HM at considerably higher concentrations than leptin. In term exclusively breast-fed infants, consumption of higher doses and concentrations of HM adiponectin resulted in longer gastric emptying times,[32] which may in part explain the growth-regulating effect of adiponectin in early months of life. Adiponectin has also been reported to have differential age-related effects on infant body composition, downregulating growth in early development and upregulating growth later in infancy, promoting a growth pattern thought to be responsible for the modification of the risk of adult obesity. Indeed, adiponectin intakes in breast-fed infants during the first 12 months of lactation are associated negatively with lean body mass and positively with adiposity.[40] There is a potential to improve infant outcomes through interventions such as the continuation of breast-feeding during the first year of life and beyond, which may facilitate optimal developmental programing and reduced risk of obesity later in life.

HUMAN MILK MICROBIOME

HM contains an array of live microorganisms that play important roles in both maternal and infant health and disease. The origins of the HM microbiota have not been experimentally demonstrated; however, influx from the maternal gut, breast/nipple skin, and infant oral cavity are likely.

Bacteria are the most heavily studied component of the HM microbiome. This community can be highly diverse between individuals and within an individual at different stages of lactation.[41] Nonetheless, a "core microbiome" of *Staphylococcus* species and *Streptococcus* species has been identified across a range of populations by numerous investigators. These two genera are broadly present in HM samples and make up 29% to 79% of the HM bacterial community.[42] HM bacteria contribute to the seeding the infant gut microbiome. In fact, breast-feeding is the primary factor that shapes the composition and function of the infant gut microbiome,[43] likely due to transfer of live microorganisms as well as microbiome-shaping factors such as HMOs. The early-life establishment of the gut microbiome is important for life-long health, and aberrations to this process have been associated with the development of a wide range of noncommunicable diseases.[44] Transfer of commensal bacteria to the infant gut also contributes to immune tolerance and maturation, as well as intestinal epithelial barrier function.[45,46] *Bifidobacteria* are a notable member of the HM bacterial community. Although this genus makes up a small fraction of the HM microbiome, it is a major feature of the gut microbiome of breast-fed infants, where it plays important roles in shaping the infant gut bacterial community via glycan cross-feeding and in programing health via its probiotic effects.[47]

Viruses are also present in HM and are vertically transferred to the infant via breast-feeding. Bacteriophages (viruses that infect bacteria) are the most abundant form of viruses in both HM and the infant gut. Bacteriophages are likely to play important roles in protecting the infant from pathogenic bacterial infections and

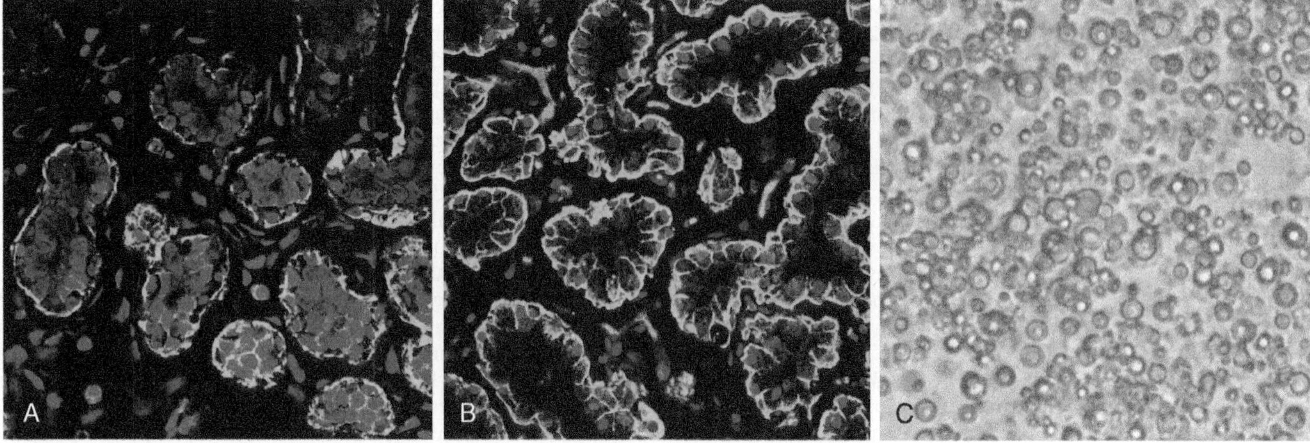

Fig. 23.2 Cells in the mammary gland and in breast milk. (A) Resting human breast. (B) Lactating human breast. (C) Cells isolated from fresh breast milk. Blue (DAPI [4′,6-diamidino-2-phenylindole]) stains nuclei. Green stains EPCAM (epithelial cell adhesion molecule). Scale bars: 20 μm.

in controlling the bacterial portion of the infant gut microbiome. Fungi have also been identified in HM samples; however, they do not appear to be universally present, nor have they been shown to be vertically transmitted to the infant gut. There is also some evidence that archaea may be present at low abundances in HM, but evidence on this point is conflicting.

CELLS IN HUMAN MILK

HM contains a variety of cells, including white blood cells, leukocytes (T cells, macrophages, lymphocytes), mammary epithelial cells (lactocytes and myoepithelial cells), and progenitor and stem cells. Although the majority (13% to 70%) of colostrum cells are leukocytes, the number of them in mature milk drops dramatically (0% to 2%) but increases if either mother or infant have an infection.[48] HM leukocytes provide active immunity and promote development of immunocompetence in the breast-fed infant via phagocytosis and secretion of antimicrobial factors. They also may play a role in protecting the mammary gland from infection. Stem cells found in HM appear to be nontumorigenic and therefore have potential uses in regenerative medicine.[49] A small proportion of HM stem cells enter the offspring's bloodstream[50] and migrate to different organs and tissues (microchimerism), where they may potentially provide immunity or boost infant development early in life.[51]

HM is a dynamic fluid, changing in response to the needs of the infant and the status of the mammary gland. A number of factors are known to influence the cellular content of HM, including the health status of both mother and infant, breast fullness, lactation stage, and development of the mammary epithelium.[48,52] New knowledge has come to light on the cells in milk, their properties, and their potential significance for the mother and infant (Fig. 23.2). They represent a wide spectrum of functions and stages of development and the health status of the lactating mammary gland and also of the infant. Their noninvasive availability warrants further investigations of the potential of these cells to be used in medicine, as well as to improve our understanding of the normal biology of the mammary gland and its pathologies.

CONCLUSION

The species-specific advantages offered by HM for human infants are unquestionable. It is a living dynamic fluid that provides the necessary nutritional components and protective factors for optimal infant development and protection. The myriad of HM components include appetite regulating hormones, microbes that inoculate the infant's gastrointestinal tract with beneficial bacteria, and live cells of different types (including leukocytes responding to both maternal and infant infection). It is likely that synergies between components contribute to the importance of HM with respect to both short- and long-term health outcomes.

REFERENCES

1. Prentice AM, Roberts SB, Prentice A, et al. Dietary supplementation of lactating Gambian women. I. Effect on breast-milk volume and quality. *Hum Nutr Clin Nutr*. 1983;37:53–64.
2. Kent JC, Mitoulas LR, Cregan MD, et al. Volume and frequency of breastfeedings and fat content of breast milk throughout the day. *Pediatrics*. 2006;117:e387–e395.
3. McManaman JL, Neville MC. Mammary physiology and milk secretion. *Adv Drug Deliv Rev*. 2003;55:629–641.
4. Innis SM. Dietary triacylglycerol structure and its role in infant nutrition. *Adv Nutr*. 2011;2:275–283.
5. Innis SM. Human milk: maternal dietary lipids and infant development. *Proc Nutr Soc*. 2007;66:397–404.
6. Agostoni C, Caroli M. Role of fats in the first two years of life as related to later development of NCDs. *NutrMetab Cardiovasc Dis*. 2012;22:775–780.
7. Makrides M, Neumann MA, Byard RW, et al. Fatty acid composition of brain, retina, and erythrocytes in breast- and formula-fed infants. *Am J Clin Nutr*. 1994;60:189–194.
8. Villamor E, Koulinska IN, Furtado J, et al. Long-chain n-6 polyunsaturated fatty acids in breast milk decrease the risk of HIV transmission through breastfeeding. *Am J Clin Nutr*. 2007;86:682–689.
9. Thorburn AN, McKenzie CI, Shen S, et al. Evidence that asthma is a developmental origin disease influenced by maternal diet and bacterial metabolites. *Nat Commun*. 2015;6:7320.
10. Goldman AS. The immune system of human milk: antimicrobial, antiinflammatory and immunomodulating properties. *Pediatr Infect Dis J*. 1993;12:664–671.
11. Suzuki YA, Lonnerdal B. Characterization of mammalian receptors for lactoferrin. *Biochem Cell Biol*. 2002;80:75–80.
12. Vorbach C, Capecchi MR, Penninger JM. Evolution of the mammary gland from the innate immune system? *Bioessays*. 2006;28:606–616.
13. Kelleher SL, Chatterton D, Nielsen K, et al. Glycomacropeptide and alpha-lactalbumin supplementation of infant formula affects growth and nutritional status in infant rhesus monkeys. *Am J Clin Nutr*. 2003;77:1261–1268.
14. Christen L, Lai CT, Hartmann B, et al. Ultraviolet-C irradiation: a novel pasteurization method for donor human milk. *PloS One*. 2013;8:e68120.
15. Michaelsen KF, Larnkjaer A, Molgaard C. Amount and quality of dietary proteins during the first two years of life in relation to NCD risk in adulthood. *NutrMetab Cardiovasc Dis*. 2012;22:781–786.
16. Michaelsen KF, Greer FR. Protein needs early in life and long-term health. *Am J Clin Nutr*. 2014;99:718S–722S.
17. Rogier EW, Frantz AL, Bruno ME, et al. Secretory antibodies in breast milk promote long-term intestinal homeostasis by regulating the gut microbiota and host gene expression. *Proc Natl Acad Sci U S A*. 2014;111:3074–3079.
18. Wang B. Molecular determinants of milk lactoferrin as a bioactive compound in early neurodevelopment and cognition. *J Pediatr*. 2016;173(suppl):S29–S36.

19. Gila-Diaz A, Arribas SM, Algara A, et al. A review of bioactive factors in human breastmilk: a focus on prematurity. *Nutrients*. 2019;11:1307.
20. Dror DK, Allen LH. Overview of nutrients in human milk. *Adv Nutr*. 2018;9:278S-294S.
21. German JB, Freeman SL, Lebrilla CB, et al. Human milk oligosaccharides: evolution, structures and bioselectivity as substrates for intestinal bacteria. *Nestle Nutr Workshop Ser Pediatr Program*. 2008;62:205-218; discussion 218-222.
21a. Friel JK, Aziz K, Andrews WL, et al. A double-masked, randomized control trial of iron supplementation in early infancy in healthy term breast-fed infants. *J Pediatr*. 2003;143(5):582-586.
21b. Baker RD, Greer FR. Diagnosis and prevention of iron deficiency and iron deficiency anemia in infants and young children (0-3 years of age). *Pediatrics*. 2010;126(5):1040-1050.
22. Gridneva Z, Tie WJ, Rea A, et al. Human milk casein and whey protein and infant body composition over the first 12 months of lactation. *Nutrients*. 2018;10:1332.
23. Khodabakhshi A, Ghayour-Mobarhan M, Rooki H, et al. Comparative measurement of ghrelin, leptin, adiponectin, EGF and IGF-1 in breast milk of mothers with overweight/obese and normal-weight infants. *Eur J Clin Nutr*. 2015;69:614-618.
24. Goldman AS. Modulation of the gastrointestinal tract of infants by human milk. Interfaces and interactions. An evolutionary perspective. *J Nutr*. 2000;130:426S-431S.
25. Mitoulas LR, Kent JC, Cox DB, et al. Variation in fat, lactose and protein in human milk over 24 h and throughout the first year of lactation. *Br J Nutr*. 2002;88:29-37.
26. Butte N, Wong W, Hopkinson J, et al. Infant feeding mode affects early growth and body composition. *Pediatrics*. 2002;16:1355-1366.
27. Rolland-Cachera MF, Maillot M, Deheeger M, et al. Association of nutrition in early life with body fat and serum leptin at adult age. *Int J Obesity*. 2013;37:1116-1122.
28. Nommsen LA, Lovelady CA, Heinig M, et al. Determinants of energy, protein, lipid, and lactose concentrations in human milk during the first 12 mo of lactation: the DARLING Study. *Am J Clin Nutr*. 1991;53:457-465.
29. Prentice P, Ong KK, Schoemaker MH, et al. Breast milk nutrient content and infancy growth. *Acta Paediatr*. 2016;105:641-647.
30. Prentice P, Ong KK, Schoemaker MH, et al. Breast milk nutrient content and infancy growth. *Acta Paediatr*. 2016;105:641-647.
31. Gridneva Z, Rea A, Hepworth AR, et al. Relationships between breastfeeding patterns and maternal and infant body composition over the first 12 months of lactation. *Nutrients*. 2018;10:45.
32. Gridneva Z, Kuganathan S, Hepworth AR, et al. Effect of human milk appetite hormones, macronutrients, and infant characteristics on gastric emptying and breastfeeding patterns of term fully breastfed infants. *Nutrients*. 2017;9:15.
33. Alderete TA, Autran C, Brekke BE, et al. Associations between human milk oligosaccharides and infant body composition in the first 6 mo of life. *Am J Clin Nutr*. 2015;102:1381-1388.
34. Gridneva Z, Rea A, Tie WJ, et al. Carbohydrates in human milk and body composition of term infants during the first 12 months of lactation. *Nutrients*. 2019;11:1472.
35. Khodabakhshi A, Ghayour-Mobarhan M, Rooki H, et al. Comparative measurement of ghrelin, leptin, adiponectin, EGF and IGF-1 in breast milk of mothers with overweight/obese and normal-weight infants. *Eur J Clin Nutr*. 2015;69:614-618.
36. Kon IY, Shilina NM, Gmoshinskaya MV, et al. The study of breast milk IGF-1, leptin, ghrelin and adiponectin levels as possible reasons of high weight gain in breast-fed infants. *Ann Nutr Metab*. 2014;65:317-323.
37. Fields D, Demerath E. Relationship of insulin, glucose, leptin, IL-6 and TNF-a in human breast milk with infant growth and body composition. *Pediatric Obesity*. 2012;7:304-312.
38. Casazza K, Hanks LJ, Fields DA. The relationship between bioactive components in breast milk and bone mass in infants. *BoneKEy Rep*. 2014;3:577.
39. Miralles O, Sanchez J, Palou A, et al. A physiological role of breast milk leptin in body weight control in developing infants. *Obesity*. 2006;14:1371-1377.
40. Gridneva Z, Kuganathan S, Rea A, et al. Human milk adiponectin and leptin and infant body composition over the first 12 months of lactation. *Nutrients*. 2018;10:1125.
41. Cabrera-Rubio R, Collado MC, Laitinen K, et al. The human milk microbiome changes over lactation and is shaped by maternal weight and mode of delivery. *Am J Clin Nutr*. 2012;96:544-551.
42. Lackey KA, Williams JE, Meehan CL, et al. What's normal? Microbiomes in human milk and infant feces are related to each other but vary geographically: the INSPIRE Study. *Front Nutr*. 2019;6:45.
43. Stewart CJ, Ajami NJ, O'Brien JL, et al. Temporal development of the gut microbiome in early childhood from the TEDDY study. *Nature*. 2018;562:583-588.
44. Stinson LF. Establishment of the early-life microbiome: a DOHaD perspective. *J Dev Orig Health Dis*. 2019;11:1-10.
45. Toscano M, De Grandi R, Grossi E, et al. Role of the human breast milk-associated microbiota on the newborns' immune system: a mini review. *Front Microbiol*. 2017;8:2100.
46. Latuga MS, Stuebe A, Seed PC. A review of the source and function of microbiota in breast milk. *Semin Reprod Med*. 2014;32:68-73.
47. Milani C, Duranti S, Bottacini F, et al. The first microbial colonizers of the human gut: composition, activities, and health implications of the infant gut microbiota. *Microbiol Mol Biol Rev*. 2017;81:e00036-17.
48. Hassiotou F, Hepworth AR, Metzger P, et al. Maternal and infant infections stimulate a rapid leukocyte response in breastmilk. *Clin Transl Immunology*. 2013;2:e3.
49. Hassiotou F, Hepworth AR, Beltran AS, et al. Expression of the pluripotency transcription factor OCT4 in the normal and aberrant mammary gland. *Front Oncol*. 2013;3:79.
50. Ghosh A. Breast milk stem cells survive in the neonate's gut, enter into the neonate circulation and are adapted into the body. *Curr Stem Cell Res Ther*. 2019;14.
51. Aydin MS, Yigit EN, Vatandaslar E, et al. Transfer and integration of breast milk stem cells to the brain of suckling pups. *Sci Rep*. 2018;8:14289.
52. Twigger AJ, Hepworth AR, Lai CT, et al. Gene expression in breastmilk cells is associated with maternal and infant characteristics. *Sci Rep*. 2015;5:12933.

Physiology of Lactation 24

Jayne F. Martin Carli | Jenifer Monks | James L. McManaman

FUNCTIONAL ANATOMY OF THE BREAST

The human female breast is composed of a tubuloalveolar parenchyma embedded in a connective and adipose tissue stroma. The glandular component of the mature breast is composed of radially organized lobes, each connected to the nipple by a single milk duct. Each lobe is composed of multiple lobules containing the alveolar structures responsible for milk production and an associated network of small ducts that join to form larger ducts that drain into the milk duct. Most textbooks describe the mature breast as containing 15 to 20 lobes on the basis of cadaver dissections; however, more recent ultrasound measurements put this number at approximately 9, with some individuals having as few as 4 and others as many as 14.[1] Development of the lobuloalveolar units (referred to as terminal duct lobular units, or TDLUs, by pathologists), starting with organogenesis, begins in the 18- to 19-week fetus, at which time a bulb-shaped mammary bud can be discerned extending from the epidermis into the dense sub-epidermal mesenchyme (Fig. 24.1A).[2] A nipple forms in the epidermal portion of the structure, and ducts invade the fat-pad precursor, branching and canalizing to form the rudimentary system that is present at birth.[2,3] The formation of the nipple and rudimentary glandular structures is regulated by paracrine interactions between mesenchymal and epithelial cells that are guided in part by the actions of parathyroid hormone–related protein (PTHrP) and members of the Wnt and bone morphogenic protein signaling pathways.[4,5] It is possible for limited milk secretion to occur in the infant after birth because of changes in maternal hormones. The immature gland remains a nipple with a set of small branching ducts that grow in parallel with the child until puberty.

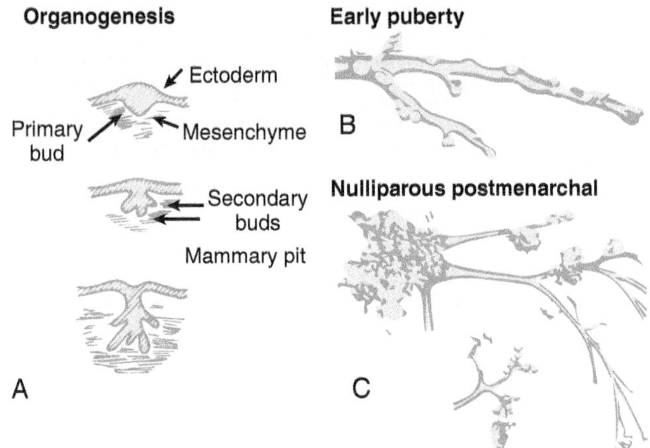

Fig. 24.1 Human mammary development. (A) (Embryogenesis) A thickening of the ectoderm called the *placode* pushes branches into the underlying stroma to produce the rudimentary mammary gland with the nipple present at birth in both sexes. (B) (Virgin) At the onset of puberty, ductal structures branch and elongate into the fat pad. (C) (Virgin) With the onset of the menstrual cycles, progesterone secretion during the luteal phase brings about budding of alveolar complexes called *terminal duct lobular units (TDLU)* from the sides and ends of the ducts.

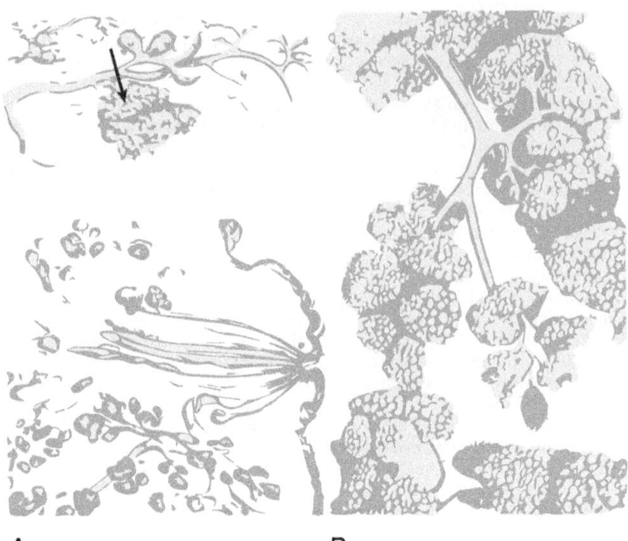

Fig. 24.2 (A) Pregnancy. (B) Lactating. The TDLU undergo extensive development during pregnancy. (The camera lucida drawings of sections of the human breast are from Dabelow A. Die postnatale Entwicklung der menschlichen Milchdruse und ihre Korrelationen. *Morphol J.* 1941;85:361–416; used with permission for publication from Springer-Verlag.)

At puberty, estrogen secreted by the ovary, growth hormone secreted by the pituitary, and insulin-like growth factor-1 (IGF-1) secreted by the liver and adipose tissue, combine to stimulate the further elongation and branching of the mammary ductal system by regulating proliferation of cells located within specialized structures termed *terminal end buds*.[5] In early puberty, bare ducts course through the fat pad (see Fig. 24.1B). With the onset of menses and ovulatory cycles, the progesterone secreted by the ovary during the luteal phase brings about some lobular development (see Fig. 24.1C). The lobular clusters are dynamic structures that increase in size and complexity during each luteal phase but tend to regress with the onset of the menses and the loss of hormonal support.[6] The hormones of pregnancy, particularly the ovarian hormone progesterone and the pituitary hormone prolactin, bring about expansion and functional differentiation of alveoli (termed *lactogenesis*) through paracrine actions mediated by members of the rank (RANKL) ligand and the JAK/STAT signaling pathways.[5,7] By mid-pregnancy, the gland has developed extensive lobular clusters (Fig. 24.2A), and, indeed, small amounts of secretion product are formed. However, maturation of the cells producing milk continues until parturition, with full secretion being inhibited by the high circulating concentrations of progesterone. The onset of copious milk secretion occurs by a process termed *secretory activation* that takes place during the first 4 days postpartum in humans (see Fig. 24.2B). A major volume increase that occurs around 40 hours postpartum is often referred as the "coming in" of the milk. Both the fall in progesterone, resulting from loss of the placenta, and maintenance of prolactin secretion from the pituitary gland are necessary for milk secretion.

The later parts of this developmental program are repeated during each pregnancy because the glandular epithelium responsible for the secretion of milk regresses after weaning to a state resembling that found in mammary glands in the pre-pregnant state. Involution of the mammary gland takes place when regular extraction of milk from the gland ceases or (in many but not all species) when prolactin is withdrawn. Like lactogenesis, this stage involves an orderly sequence of events that include cessation of milk secretion, apoptosis of alveolar epithelial cells,[8,9] and remodeling of the gland[10] to a morphologic and functional state closely resembling, but not identical to, that of prepregnancy.[11]

LACTATION

Lactation is the physiologic process of milk secretion; it will continue as long as milk is removed from the gland on a regular basis. The pituitary hormones prolactin and oxytocin are required to maintain milk secretion, with prolactin maintaining synthesis of milk products and oxytocin stimulating the letdown response that allows the infant to extract milk from the gland. An example of the swollen ducts and alveoli that occur when milk is not removed from the gland is shown in Fig. 24.2B. The actual volume of milk secreted is adjusted to the requirements of the infant and is regulated, in part, by a neuronal reflex loop linking suckling stimuli to hypothalamic regulation of prolactin and oxytocin production.

SECRETORY ACTIVATION

The most critical time in the establishment of lactation is its onset during the transition from pregnancy to lactation, a period now referred to as *secretory activation* (previously termed *lactogenesis stage II*). Secretory activation takes place after birth in women, in contrast to many animal species where it occurs concomitantly with parturition.[12] Most lactation problems arise during this period as the result of stress of childbirth, obesity and/or diabetes, or problems with the mechanics of suckling. If unresolved, these problems can lead to lactation failure.

MILK VOLUME AND COMPOSITION DURING THE FIRST WEEK POSTPARTUM

Fig. 24.3A shows milk volumes in 11 American women who weighed their infants before and after every feeding for the first week postpartum. Although there is wide variation among individuals, the trend is revealed by the averaged data in Fig. 24.3B: volumes of breast secretion of less than 100 mL per day

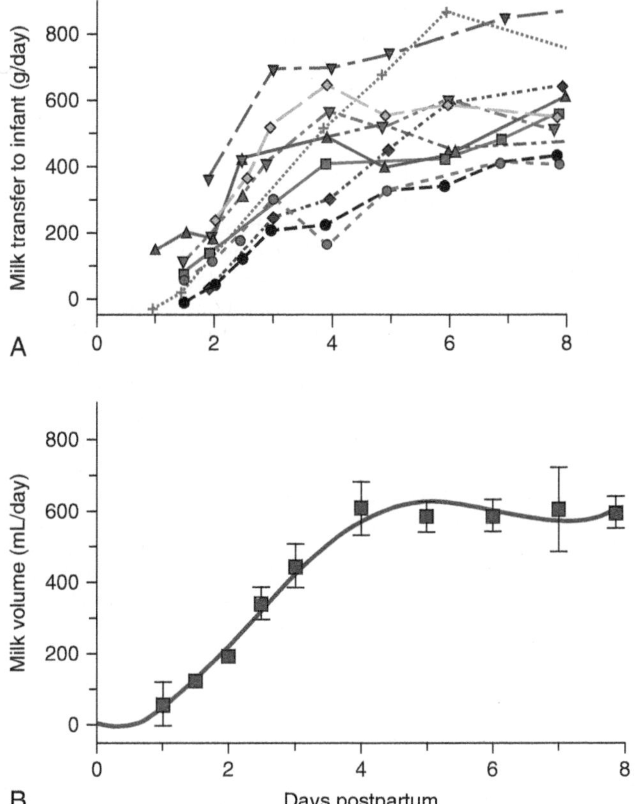

Fig. 24.3 Milk volumes during the onset of lactation in American women. (A) Eleven multiparous women weighed their infants before and after every feed for 7 to 8 days postpartum. Milk output was averaged by 0.5-day intervals for the first 3 days and then daily for the remainder of the experiment. All women had successfully breast-fed at least one previous infant. Note the extensive variation in the volumes of milk produced. All these women breast-fed successfully for at least 6 months. (B) Mean output in the women shown in (A). (Plotted from Neville MC, Keller RP, Seacat J, et al. Studies in human lactation: milk volumes in lactating women during the onset of lactation and full lactation. *Am J Clin Nutr*. 1988;48:1375–1386; Graphs from Neville MC. Lactogenesis in women: a cascade of events revealed by milk composition. In: Jensen RD, ed. *The Composition of Milks*. San Diego: Academic Press; 1995:87–98. Used with permission.)

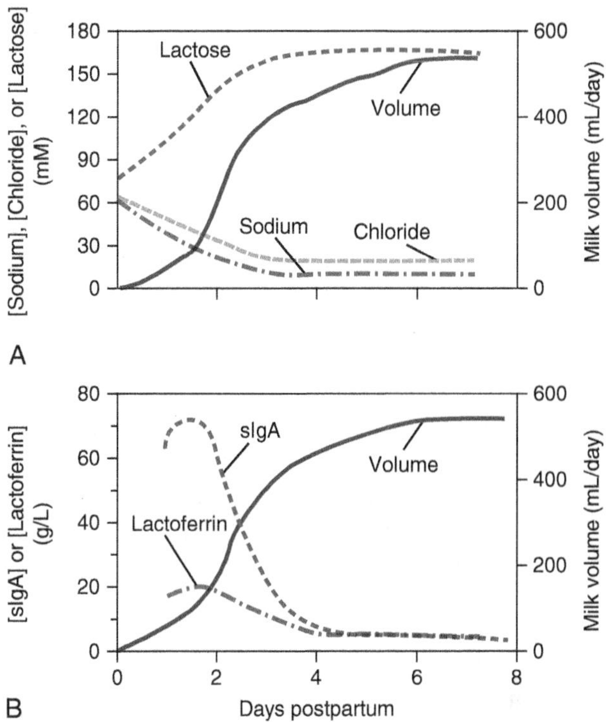

Fig. 24.4 Changes in the concentration of certain milk components during the first week postpartum. (A) Time course of changes in the lactose, chloride, and sodium concentrations contrasted with the mean milk volume transfer to the infant. Changes in these milk components begin immediately postpartum and are complete at least 24 hours before achievement of a steady state in milk volume. As described in the text, the decrease in sodium and chloride and increase in lactose concentration reflect closure of the tight junctions between the mammary epithelial cells. (B) Changes in the concentration of secretory immunoglobulin A *(sIgA)* and lactoferrin during the onset of lactation in women. (A, Data from Neville MC, Allen JC, Archer PC, et al. Studies in human lactation: milk volume and nutrient composition during weaning and lactogenesis. *Am J Clin Nutr*. 1991;54:81–92. B, Data replotted from Dils R, Clark S, Knudsen J. Comparative aspects of milk fat synthesis. In: Peaker M, editor. *Comparative Aspects of Lactation*. London: Academic Press; 1977:43–55; Figure modified from Neville MC, et al. *Pediatr Clin North Am*. 2001;48:35. Used with permission.)

characterize the first 2 days postpartum, after which a rapid increase in milk volume leads to production of an average of 600 mL/day by the fourth day postpartum. A detailed study of milk composition over this period reveals a carefully programmed cascade of events that leads to a mammary secretion product with a composition close to that of mature milk. Although the secretion product in the first few days is usually called *colostrum*, we avoid that term here because it implies a secretion product with a fixed composition. In fact, as we shall see, milk composition changes dramatically during the first 3 to 4 days postpartum. The first compositional change to occur after delivery is a fall in the sodium and chloride concentrations in the milk and an increase in lactose levels (Fig. 24.4A). These modifications commence immediately after delivery and are largely complete by 72 hours postpartum.[12] They precede the rapid increase in milk volume by at least 24 hours and can be explained by closure of the tight junctions that block the paracellular pathway during lactation. With the paracellular pathway closed, lactose, produced by the epithelial cells, can no longer pass into the plasma, and sodium and chloride can no longer pass directly from the interstitial space into the milk space and must be secreted by the cellular route.

The next changes to occur are increases in the concentrations of serum immunoglobulin (Ig) A and lactoferrin (see Fig. 24.4B). The concentrations of these two important protective proteins remain high for the first 48 hours postpartum, the two together comprising as much as 10% by weight of the milk before they decrease rapidly after day 2 postpartum, as a consequence of both dilution as milk volume increases and an actual decrease in the rate of secretion, particularly in the case of immunoglobulins. By day 8 postpartum, these protective proteins together comprise less than 1% of the total weight of the milk; however, their secretion rate is still substantial, amounting to 2 to 3 g/day for each protein. Concentrations of oligosaccharides in milk are also high in the early secretion product of the mammary gland, amounting to as much as 2% of milk weight on day 4 postpartum. These complex sugars are also considered to have substantial protective effect against a variety of infections, including human immunodeficiency virus.[13-15] Finally, 36 to 48 hours postpartum, milk secretion begins in earnest (Fig. 24.4). This volume increase is perceived by the parturient woman as the coming in of the milk, and reflects a massive increase in the rates of synthesis and secretion of almost all the components of mature milk, including but not limited to lactose, protein, lipid, calcium, sodium,

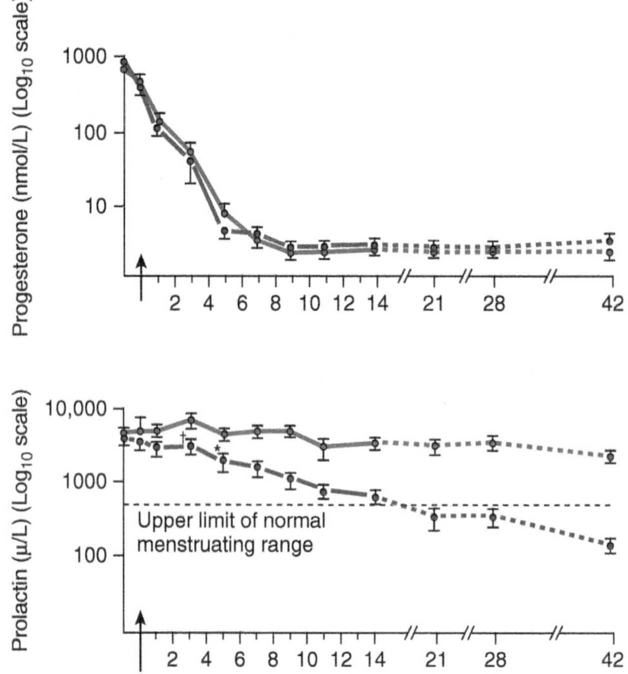

Fig. 24.5 Maternal hormone levels after parturition in breastfeeding and non-breastfeeding women. Breastfeeding subjects (n = 10; *blue*); non–breastfeeding subjects (n = 9; *red*). P <0.02. (From Martin RH, Glass MR, Chapman C, et al. Human alpha-lactalbumin and hormonal factors in pregnancy and lactation. *Clin Endocrinol (Oxf)*. 1980;13:223–230, Reprinted with permission.)

magnesium, and potassium. Reference ranges of some of the mentioned milk components have recently been described for normal human lactation to allow for objective efforts to identify potential abnormalities.[16]

HORMONAL REQUIREMENTS FOR SECRETORY ACTIVATION

It has been clear for nearly three decades that the major inhibitor of milk production during pregnancy is progesterone.[12] Once birth occurs, a developed mammary epithelium, the continuing presence of high levels of prolactin, and a fall in progesterone are necessary for the onset of copious milk secretion. The levels of these hormones are shown in Fig. 24.5. Evidence is clear for the inhibitory effect of progesterone during pregnancy in women. Thus removal of the placenta, the source of progesterone during pregnancy in humans, has long been known to be necessary for the initiation of milk secretion.[17] Conversely, retained placental fragments with the potential to secrete progesterone have been reported to delay secretory activation.[18] The conundrum that progesterone does not inhibit established lactation was solved when Haslam and Shyamala[19] showed that progesterone receptors are lost in lactating mammary tissues. In most species, high levels of plasma prolactin also appear to be essential for secretory activation; although the level declines with continued lactation, some prolactin is thought to be necessary for active milk secretion. In women, bromocriptine and other analogues of dopamine, drugs that effectively prevent prolactin secretion, inhibit the onset of lactation when given in appropriate doses.[20] Conversely, an older hypothesis that a prolactin surge is the trigger for secretory activation is probably incorrect. Although a biphasic rise in prolactin is associated with the stress of parturition in women,[21] it precedes the onset of copious milk secretion by 2 days.

DELAYS IN SECRETORY ACTIVATION

A delay in the onset of milk secretion is a significant problem for the initiation of breastfeeding in a large number of women. The timing of secretory activation for normal women has been determined carefully from milk volume or composition in a few studies of middle-class white women.[22] Most of these data are in reasonable accord, but some do suggest that either parity or previous lactation experience may influence the timing of secretory activation. Various practices and conditions have been reported to be associated with delayed secretory activation in women, including maternal educational attainment, breastfeeding education, smoking, cesarean section, diabetes, obesity, and stress during parturition.[23,24] Much progress has been made to improve maternal access to lactation support, but many questions remain regarding physiologic barriers to lactation. The role of cesarean section has been controversial, historically, but an international meta-analysis has shown an association between cesarean section—in particular, elective cesarean section—with a lower rate of early breastfeeding.[25] Women with obesity and/or diabetes are known to have poor lactation outcomes, including delayed secretory activation and early termination of exclusive and any lactation, compared to normal weight women and/or those with normal glucose tolerance.[26-28] Insulin resistance is a likely driver of this impairment for women with both conditions, although the precise nature of this relationship is not yet clear. Insulin signaling may affect mammary development during puberty and pregnancy and/or function during lactation. Additionally, obesity impairs lactation independently of insulin sensitivity status,[29,30] for reasons that are still unknown. Challenges in study design have yet to lead to meaningful interventions to improve lactation outcomes for women who have obesity and/or diabetes.[31,32] These factors require serious investigation in the future.

CELLULAR MECHANISMS FOR MILK SYNTHESIS AND SECRETION

Milk components are secreted into the alveolar lumina by five distinct pathways, as illustrated diagrammatically in Fig. 24.6.[33] Four secretory processes are synchronized in the alveolar cell: (1) exocytosis, (2) fat synthesis and secretion, (3) secretion of ions and water, and (4) transcytosis of immunoglobulins and other substances from the interstitial space. These processes are summarized briefly here, followed by an introduction to the role of a fifth pathway, the paracellular pathway, in determining the composition of the mammary secretion.

EXOCYTOSIS

Most components of the aqueous phase of milk are secreted by the exocytotic pathway (see pathway I, see Fig. 24.6). The basic mechanisms of exocrine secretion, worked out for the pancreas more than 40 years ago by Palade,[34] are thought to apply essentially to all exocrine cells, including milk-secreting cells. Like the exocytotic pathway in all cells, exocytosis in the mammary gland ultimately begins in the nucleus with the synthesis of messenger RNA molecules specific for milk proteins. The mature messenger RNA serves as a template for protein synthesis. The protein molecules are transported into the endoplasmic reticulum where they are folded and transported through the Golgi system to take part in secretory vesicle formation. In the Golgi, molecules destined for release are packaged in vesicles as a highly condensed granule matrix visible in the electron microscope as electron-dense structures. Distinct mechanisms appear to exist for concentrating proteins in secretory granules.[35] Pancreatic exocrine granules, for example, exhibit pH-dependent aggregation of granular proteins and require Ca^{2+} for stability, whereas caseins, the major type of protein found in milk, are packaged into electron-dense granules as micellar aggregates that are cross-linked by colloidal calcium phosphate.[36] Once formed, secretory vesicles move to the apical

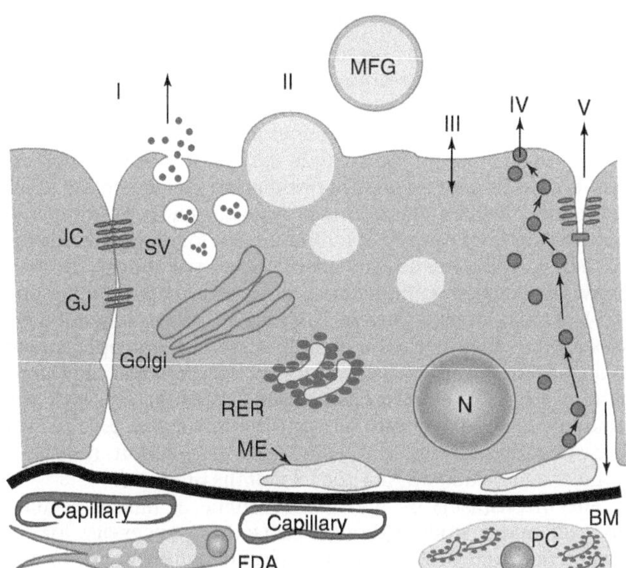

Fig. 24.6 Cartoon of a mammary epithelial cell showing pathways for milk secretion. *Pathway I,* Exocytotic pathway for secretion of milk proteins, lactose, calcium, and other components of the aqueous phase of milk. *Pathway II,* Milk fat secretion with formation of cytoplasmic lipid droplets that move to the apical membrane to be secreted as a membrane-bound milk fat globule *(MFG)*. *Pathway III,* Transporters for the direct movement of monovalent ions, water, and glucose across the apical membrane of the cell. *Pathway IV,* Vesicular transcytosis of proteins such as immunoglobulins from the interstitial space. *Pathway V,* The paracellular pathway for plasma components and leukocytes. Pathway V is open only during pregnancy, involution, and in inflammatory states such as mastitis. *BM*, Basement membrane; *FDA*, fat-depleted adipocyte; *GJ*, gap junction; *JC*, junctional complex containing the tight and adherens junctions; *ME*, myoepithelial cell; *RER*, rough endoplasmic reticulum; *N*, nucleus; *PC*, plasma cell; *SV*, secretory vesicle. (Redrawn from Neville MC, Allen JC, Watters C. The mechanisms of milk secretion. In: Neville MC, Neifert MR, editors. *Lactation: Physiology, Nutrition and Breast-Feeding*. New York: Plenum Press; 1983:50. Used with permission.)

membrane, where they discharge their contents into the alveolar lumen by exocytosis. Several specialized reactions within this pathway give the composition of milk its final form. For example, in addition to this pathway's secretion of milk proteins such as casein, lactose and the oligosaccharides, comprising together almost 8% of the weight of human milk, are synthesized and secreted by this pathway as well. In mammary glands of most species, lactose is an important regulator of the osmotic movement of water into milk and maintenance of iso-osmolarity. Lactose is synthesized in the Golgi from uridine diphosphate-galactose and glucose, which enter from the cytoplasm, by the enzyme β-1,4-galactosyltransferase 1, with α-lactalbumin acting as a cofactor. The high concentration of lactose present in the Golgi during lactation osmotically stimulates the influx of water that contributes to the fluidity of milk.[35] The importance of this mechanism in the maintenance of milk fluidity was established by the observation that α-lactalbumin-deficient mice produce highly viscous milk.[37]

LIPID SYNTHESIS AND SECRETION

The majority of lipid in milk exists as triacylglycerols (98%).[38] Milk triacylglycerols are synthesized from precursor fatty acids and glycerol by enzymes of the smooth endoplasmic reticulum membrane of the mammary alveolar cell. Fatty acids used for synthesis of milk lipids are derived from the diet, by mobilization from lipids stored in adipose tissue, and by de novo synthesis in alveolar epithelial cells. Fatty acid synthesis in mammary alveolar cells differs from that found in other cell types in that in mammary alveolar cells the fatty acid synthase complex contains a distinct medium-chain acyl-thioesterase (thioesterase II) that cleaves nascent fatty acyl chains to produce mainly medium-chain products (C8, C10, and C12) rather than long-chain fatty acids (C14, C16, and C18) produced by thioesterase I found in the fatty acid synthase complex of other mammalian cell types.[39] Overall, however, milk lipid composition is largely driven by genetics and diet.[40] In particular, enrichment of medium-chain fatty acids occurs during consumption of diets high in carbohydrate, when de novo lipogenesis is upregulated in the mammary gland.[41] Medium-chain fatty acids are more readily absorbed in the infant intestine, and their enrichment may benefit neonatal energy metabolism in infants with fat malabsorption disorders.[42]

Triacylglycerols undergo assembly into protein and phospholipid-coated structures referred to as *cytoplasmic lipid droplets* by mechanisms that are still poorly understood.[43] After transport to the apex of the cell (see pathway II, see Fig. 24.6), these droplets become enveloped by the apical plasma membrane and are released into milk as plasma membrane bilayer-coated structures (milk fat globules) by a process that is distinct from the classical secretory pathway used for lipid secretion by hepatocytes and enterocytes.[44] The occasional inclusion of a crescent of cytoplasm within the membrane-bound globule[45] enables any substance contained in the cytoplasm to enter milk. The membrane surrounding the milk fat globule is the primary dietary source of phospholipids for the breast-fed infant and serves to prevent the triglyceride globules from coalescing into large fat droplets that might interfere with milk removal. In addition, this membrane may enhance the uptake of lipid and lipid-soluble vitamins by the neonatal intestine.[46] Investigations into the effects of milk lipids on infant growth, development, and health are ongoing and have revealed roles for the milk fat globule in immune modulation and cognitive development.[42]

TRANSPORT OF SMALL MOLECULES ACROSS THE APICAL MEMBRANE

Unlike other pathways for milk secretion, the pathways for the direct transport of substances across the apical membrane of the mammary alveolar cell are poorly understood (see pathway III, see Fig. 24.6). Linzell and Peaker[47] devised a clever technique to determine which molecules could use this pathway, infusing isotopes of small molecules up the teat of a goat and calculating how much of the substance left the milk and entered the blood. They found that sodium, potassium, chloride, and certain monosaccharides, as well as water, directly permeated this membrane, but calcium, phosphate, and citrate did not. Although the mechanisms are not understood, it is clear that apical membrane transport pathways are limited to a modest number of small molecules that also include glucose and possibly amino acids. It has now become clear that calcium is also transported across the apical membrane to the lumen by a well-studied transporter called plasma membrane $Ca2^{+}$ ATPase 2 (PMCA2), a plasma membrane calcium adenosine triphosphatase.[48,49]

TRANSCYTOSIS OF INTERSTITIAL MOLECULES

Intact proteins in the interstitial space surrounding the basal and lateral surface of the mammary alveolar cell can cross the mammary epithelium in two possible ways: by transcytosis and through the paracellular pathway. Because the paracellular pathway is closed during lactation, plasma proteins must enter milk through transcytosis (pathway IV, see Fig. 24.6). The best-studied molecule in this regard is IgA.[50] IgA is synthesized by plasma cells that reside in the interstitial spaces of the mammary gland or elsewhere in the body. Dimeric IgA binds to receptors on the basal surface of the mammary alveolar cell, after which the entire IgA-receptor complex is endocytosed and transferred to the apical membrane, where the extracellular portion of the receptor is cleaved and secreted together with the IgA. Other plasma proteins, including serum albumin, insulin, prolactin, IGF1, and possibly other growth factors, also undergo transcytotic transport into milk by similar but much less well-studied pathways. In addition, specific transcytosis pathways exist for the transfer of trace elements, including iron, copper, and zinc, from the serum into milk.[51]

THE ROLE OF THE PARACELLULAR PATHWAY IN MILK SECRETION

Pathway V (see Fig. 24.6) involves passage of substances between epithelial cells, rather than through them, and for this reason is designated the paracellular pathway. During lactation the passage of even low-molecular-weight substances between alveolar cells is impeded by a gasket-like structure called the *tight junction* that joins the epithelial cells tightly, one to another.[52] Although immune cells apparently can exhibit diapedesis between epithelial cells to reach the milk,[53] the junctions seal tightly behind them and leave no permanent gap. During pregnancy, and probably mastitis, these tight junctions are leaky and allow components of the interstitial space to pass unimpeded into the milk. At the same time, milk components can enter the plasma. This leakiness is useful during these periods, inasmuch as secretion products are allowed to leave the gland and inflammatory cells can enter. It is not clear when junctions open during involution, but when milk volume drops below approximately 400 mL/day, the concentration of sodium and chloride in the mammary secretion increases, suggesting a change in the permeability barrier.[54] When the junctions are open, mammary secretions have a high concentration of sodium and chloride, a fact that is sometimes useful in diagnosing breastfeeding problems.[55]

REGULATION OF MILK SYNTHESIS, SECRETION, AND EJECTION

Milk is synthesized continuously and secreted into the alveolar lumen where it is stored until it is ejected from the breast by a letdown reflex. This means that two levels of regulation must exist: regulation of the rate of synthesis and secretion and regulation of milk ejection. Although both processes ultimately depend on sucking by the infant or other stimulation of the nipple, the mechanisms involved, both central and local, are very different. Prolactin mediates anterior pituitary regulation of milk secretion, but its influence is greatly modified by local factors that depend on milk removal from the breast. Oxytocin, on the other hand, participates in a neuroendocrine reflex that results in stimulation of the myoepithelial cells that surround the alveoli and ducts. When these cells contract, milk is forced out of the alveoli to the nipple. Only then does it become available to the suckling infant. If the letdown reflex is inhibited, milk cannot be removed from the breast and local mechanisms bring about an inhibition of milk secretion. With consistent partial removal of milk, these local factors adjust milk secretion to a new steady-state level.[56] If milk removal ceases altogether, involution sets in and the gland loses its competency to secrete milk within days to weeks, depending on the species.

MILK VOLUME PRODUCTION IN LACTATING WOMEN

A meta-analysis of the volume of milk secreted by exclusively breastfeeding women showed that milk volume at 6 months postpartum is remarkably constant at about 800 mL/day in populations throughout the world.[56] Milk volume is approximately 5% to 15% higher in women with very low body fat because of secretion of milk with reduced lipid content, which has a caloric density of up to 15% lower than milk with normal fat content. This observation illustrates the important principle that milk volume secretion in lactating women is regulated by infant demand. Thus, when the milk has a lower caloric density, increased sucking by the infant is thought to result in increased emptying of the breast, in turn bringing about an increase in milk secretion. Mothers of twins, and occasionally even triplets, are able to produce volumes of milk sufficient for complete nutrition of their multiple infants. Studies of wet nurses done in the 1930s show that at least some women are capable of producing up to 3.5 L of milk per day. Conversely, if infants are supplemented with foods other than breast milk, milk secretion is proportionately reduced. For example, in countries such as Peru and the Gambia, where infants' diets are customarily supplemented with small amounts of food at mealtimes, but the infants are given several breastfeedings a day, the daily milk production remains at approximately 600 mL/day for 12 months or longer.

The mechanisms by which the volume of milk is regulated are still under study. Although prolactin is necessary for milk production, and prolactin levels are consistently above baseline for the duration of lactation,[57] they are not proportional to milk volume secretion. Local mechanisms, including autocrine and stretch, have been implicated in the regulation of milk volume production.[58-60] Definitive evidence in support of either mechanism remains elusive. However, cellular transduction of stretch responses remains an attractive mechanism for regulating milk production, because stretch is a known regulator of signal transduction and gene expression in physiologic systems affected by mechanical tension,[61,62] and stretch-dependent effects on gene expression have been reported for mammary epithelial cells.[63,64]

OXYTOCIN, MILK EJECTION, AND SUCKLING

Milk removal from the breast is accomplished by the contraction of myoepithelial cells, the processes of which form a basketlike network around the alveoli where milk is stored. When the infant suckles, afferent impulses from sensory stimulation of nerve terminals in the areolae travel to the central nervous system where they promote release of oxytocin from the posterior pituitary. In the woman, oxytocin release is often associated with such stimuli as the sight or sound, or even the thought, of the infant, indicating a significant psychological component in this so-called neuroendocrine reflex. The oxytocin is carried through the bloodstream to the mammary gland, where it interacts with specific receptors on myoepithelial cells, initiating their contraction and expelling milk from the alveoli into the ducts and subareolar sinuses. The process by which milk is forcibly moved out of the alveoli is called *milk ejection* or *letdown* and is essential to milk removal from the lactating breast. During correct suckling, the nipple and much of the areola are drawn well into the mouth so that a long teat reaching nearly to the infant's soft palate is formed.[65] The mammary sinuses extend into this teat. Milk is removed not so much by suction as by the stripping motion of the tongue against the hard palate. This motion carries milk through the teat into the baby's mouth. The sinuses refill as the continued action of oxytocin forces milk from the alveoli into the ducts. It has been known for some time that psychological stress or pain decreases milk output. The basis for this finding was shown by Ueda and colleagues[66] to be inhibition of oxytocin release. In relaxed, undisturbed women suckling their infants, oxytocin release begins with the onset of suckling, or even before suckling when the infant cries or becomes restless. When the suckling women were asked to carry out difficult mental calculations or were fed traffic noise through earphones while nursing the infant, the number of oxytocin pulses was significantly reduced. Interestingly, the prolactin response to suckling was not impaired by psychological stress, implicating different neural pathways in the release of the two hormones.

Alcohol and drugs of abuse may have effects on milk letdown. Building on earlier studies showing that ethanol inhibits milk ejection in a dose-dependent manner, Coiro and colleagues[67] measured plasma oxytocin concentrations in response to breast stimulation in nonlactating women and found that 50 mL of ethyl alcohol completely abolished the rise in oxytocin levels. Minor effects of long-term maternal ethanol consumption on motor development of breast-fed infants in a well-controlled study in humans[68] were attributed to alcohol transfer to the infant rather than suppression of milk secretion. A potent effect of morphine on oxytocin release has been described in rats,[69] but while research has illuminated the effects of opioids and other drugs of abuse on infant outcomes,[70-73] their effects on milk production have not been studied in women.

EFFECTS OF LACTATION ON THE MOTHER

NUTRITIONAL EFFECTS

In many species such as dairy cattle and laboratory mice, a large portion of the metabolic output is directed to milk synthesis, so careful management of nutrient intake is critical for lactation success. In humans the energetic costs of milk production are estimated to be about 700 kcal/day,[74,75] which can represent as much as a third of a woman's metabolic output. Typically the increased energy requirements of lactation are met by relatively small increases in food intake or decreased metabolic rate in healthy individuals.[76] Nonetheless, it is important to remember that, as already stated, the amount of milk produced is almost entirely regulated by infant demand. If a woman breast-feeds twins, she will produce double the usual volume of about 800 mL/day.[56] Under these circumstances nutritional demands may be substantial and attention should be paid to nutritional intake, particularly in malnourished women, so that maternal nutrient depletion does not result. One maternal effect that seems clear is that lactating women whose menses have not yet returned have a significant loss of calcium from their bones.[77] Both secretion of parathyroid hormone (PTH)-related peptide from the mammary epithelium and the lack of estrogen caused by postpartum amenorrhea may be involved. That PTH-related peptide plays an active role in mobilizing bone calcium during human lactation is suggested by findings that plasma calcium and alkaline phosphatase are elevated in lactating women and that the calcium regulatory hormone PTH is decreased.[77] After weaning, bone calcium levels return to normal.

EFFECTS OF LACTATION ON REPRODUCTION

The most marked maternal effect of lactation is on fertility. In the early postpartum period, secretions of the ovarian follicle remain suppressed for a period of time, the duration of which depends to a substantial extent on the pattern of suckling.[78] In non-breastfeeding women, fertility returns about 6 weeks postpartum as pulsatile secretion of gonadotropin-releasing hormone returns to normal.[79] In breastfeeding women who suckle their infants at regular intervals, follicle-stimulating hormone secretion returns to normal follicular phase levels during the course of lactation, but pulsatile secretion of luteinizing hormone tends to remain in a suppressed state, so that the preovulatory surge of luteinizing hormone does not occur. The contraceptive effects of lactation may also reflect effects of breastfeeding intensity on maternal metabolism and associated reproductive hormone suppression.[80] Postpartum suppression of fertility is thought to play a significant role in birth spacing on a population basis in developing countries where prolonged breastfeeding may be the rule and the use of supplementary feedings delayed. In developed countries, women who wish to ensure against pregnancy during lactation are usually advised to use other contraceptive means, often progesterone-containing compounds that do not interfere with milk secretion.[20]

CONCLUSION

Milk secretion is a robust process that is assumed to go according to plan in most women. However, true rates and reasons for lack of success in breastfeeding are not well understood because it is easy to substitute formula when infants fail to thrive on the breast, at least in Western societies. It has been estimated that as many as 10% to 15% of women fail to produce milk and 40% to 90% of women are concerned with poor milk supply.[81] Although this is not the place to discuss possible pathologic mechanisms, it should be noted that breastfeeding failure usually takes place in the first week or so postpartum, and a much better understanding of the mechanisms by which milk secretion is initiated during this period may help us to understand why some women have serious problems with lactation. Other areas that require attention are the behavioral correlates of breastfeeding and the transfer of drug and toxins into milk. The latter may have a long-term impact on infant health and should receive additional attention.

A complete reference list is available at www.ExpertConsult.com. 

SELECT REFERENCES

1. Ramsay DT, Kent JC, Hartmann RA, et al. Anatomy of the lactating human breast redefined with ultrasound imaging. *J Anat*. 2005;206:525-534.
2. Pechoux C, Clezardin P, Dante R, et al. Localization of thrombospondin, CD36 and CD51 during prenatal development of the human mammary gland. *Differentiation*. 1994;57:133-141.
3. Russo J, Russo IH. Development of the human mammary gland. In: Neville MC, Daniel CW, eds. *The Mammary Gland*. New York: Plenum; 1987:67-96.
4. Cowin P, Wysolmerski J. Molecular mechanisms guiding embryonic mammary gland development. *Cold Spring Harb Perspect Biol*. 2010;2:a003251.
5. Macias H, Hinck L. Mammary gland development. *Wiley Interdiscip. Rev Dev Biol*. 2012;1:533-557.
6. Anderson E, Clarke RB, Howell A. Estrogen responsiveness and control of normal human breast proliferation. *J Mammary Gland Biol Neoplasia*. 1998;3:23-35.
7. Shin HY, Hennighausen L, Yoo KH. STAT5-driven enhancers tightly control temporal expression of mammary-specific genes. *J Mammary Gland Biol Neoplasia*. 2019;24:61-71.
8. Watson CJ. Key stages in mammary gland development - involution: apoptosis and tissue remodelling that convert the mammary gland from milk factory to a quiescent organ. *Breast Cancer Res*. 2006;8:203.
11. Dos Santos CO, Dolzhenko E, Hodges E, et al. An epigenetic memory of pregnancy in the mouse mammary gland. *Cell Rep*. 2015;11:1102-1109.
12. Neville MC, McFadden TB, Forsyth I. Hormonal regulation of mammary differentiation and milk secretion. *J Mammary Gland Biol Neoplasia*. 2002;7:49-66.
13. Newburg DS. Oligosaccharides and glycoconjugates of human milk: their role in host defense. *J Mammary Gland Biol Neoplasia*. 1996;1:271-283.
15. German JB, Freeman SL, Lebrilla CB, et al. Human milk oligosaccharides: evolution, structures and bioselectivity as substrates for intestinal bacteria. *Nestle Nutr Workshop Ser Pediatr Program*. 2008;62:205-218;discussion 218-222.
18. Neifert MR, McDonough SL, Neville MC. Failure of lactogenesis associated with placental retention. *Am J Obstet Gynecol*. 1981;140:477-478.
19. Haslam SZ, Shyamala G. Effect of oestradiol on progesterone receptors in normal mammary glands and its relationship with lactation. *Biochem J*. 1979;182:127-131.
21. Rigg LA, Yen SS. Multiphasic prolactin secretion during parturition in human subjects. *Am J Obstet Gynecol*. 1977;128:215.
22. Neville MC, Keller RP, Seacat J, et al. Studies in human lactation: milk volumes in lactating women during the onset of lactation and full lactation. *Am J Clin Nutr*. 1988;48:1375-1386.
23. Rasmussen KM, Hilson JA, Kjolhede CL. Obesity may impair lactogenesis II. *J Nutr*. 2001;131:3009-3011.

24. Cohen SS, Alexander DD, Krebs NF, et al. Factors associated with breastfeeding initiation and continuation: a meta-analysis. *J Pediatr*. 2018;203:190-196.
26. Nommsen-Rivers LA. Does insulin explain the relation between maternal obesity and poor lactation outcomes? An overview of the literature. *Adv Nutr*. 2016;7:407-414.
28. Turcksin R, Bel S, Galjaard S, et al. Maternal obesity and breastfeeding intention, initiation, intensity and duration: a systematic review. *Matern Child Nutr*. 2014;10:166-183.
29. Matias SL, Dewey KG, Quesenberry Jr CP, et al. Maternal prepregnancy obesity and insulin treatment during pregnancy are independently associated with delayed lactogenesis in women with recent gestational diabetes mellitus. *Am J Clin Nutr*. 2014;99:115-121.
31. Fair FJ, Ford GL, Soltani H. Interventions for supporting the initiation and continuation of breastfeeding among women who are overweight or obese. *Cochrane Database Syst Rev*. 2019;9:CD012099.
33. Neville MC. Anatomy and physiology of lactation. *Ped Clin N Amer*. 2001;48: 1-34.
35. McManaman JL, Reyland ME, Thrower EC. Secretion and fluid transport mechanisms in the mammary gland: comparisons with the exocrine pancreas and the salivary gland. *J Mammary Gland Biol Neoplasia*. 2006;11:249-268.
37. Stinnakre MG, Vilotte JL, Soulier S, et al. Creation and phenotypic analysis of alpha-lactalbumin-deficient mice. *Proc Natl Acad Sci U S A*. 1994;91:6544-6548.
38. Dils R, Clark S, Knudsen J. Comparative aspects of milk fat synthesis. In: Peaker M, ed. *Comparative Aspects of Lactation*. London: Academic Press; 1977:43-55.
39. Libertini LJ, Smith S. Purification and properties of a thioesterase from lactating rat mammary gland which modifies the product specificity of fatty acid synthetase. *J Biol Chem*. 1978;253:1393-1401.
40. Miliku K, Duan QL, Moraes TJ, et al. Human milk fatty acid composition is associated with dietary, genetic, sociodemographic, and environmental factors in the CHILD Cohort Study. *Am J Clin Nutr*. 2019;110:1370-1383.
42. Lee H, Padhi E, Hasegawa Y, et al. Compositional dynamics of the milk fat globule and its role in infant development. *Front Pediatr*. 2018;6:313.
43. Mather IH, Masedunskas A, Chen Y, et al. Symposium review: intravital imaging of the lactating mammary gland in live mice reveals novel aspects of milk-lipid secretion. *J Dairy Sci*. 2019;102:2760-2782.
44. McManaman JL. Milk lipid secretion: recent biomolecular aspects. *Biomol Concepts*. 2012;3:581-591.
45. Huston GE, Patton S. Factors related to the formation of cytoplasmic crescents on milk fat globules. *J Dairy Sci*. 1990;73:2061-2066.
46. Bezelgues JB, Morgan F, Palomo G, et al. Short communication: milk fat globule membrane as a potential delivery system for liposoluble nutrients. *J Dairy Sci*. 2009;92:2524-2528.
47. Linzell JL, Peaker M. Mechanism of milk secretion. *Physiol Rev*. 1971;51:564-597.
48. VanHouten JN, Wysolmerski JJ. Transcellular calcium transport in mammary epithelial cells. *J Mammary Gland Biol Neoplasia*. 2007;12:223-235.
50. Hunziker W, Kraehenbuhl JP. Epithelial transcytosis of immunoglobulins. *J Mammary Gland Biol Neoplasia*. 1998;3:287-302.
52. Nguyen D-AD, Neville MC. Tight junction regulation in the mammary gland. *J Mammary Gland Biol Neoplasia*. 1998;3:233-246.
53. Seelig Jr LL, Beer AE. Transepithelial migration of leukocytes in the mammary gland of lactating rats. *Biol Reprod*. 1981;22:1157-1163.
54. Neville MC, Allen JC, Archer PC, et al. Studies in human lactation: milk volume and nutrient composition during weaning and lactogenesis. *Am J Clin Nutr*. 1991;54:81-92.
55. Morton JA. The clinical usefulness of breast milk sodium in the assessment of lactogenesis. *Pediatrics*. 1994;93:802-806.
56. Neville MC. Volume and caloric density of human milk. In: Jensen RG, ed. *Handbook of Milk Composition*. San Diego: Academic Press, Inc.; 1995:101-113.
57. McNeilly AS, Robinson IC, Houston MJ, et al. Release of oxytocin and prolactin in response to suckling. *Br Med J Clin Res*. 1983;286:257-259.
63. Schischmanoff PO, Yaswen P, Parra MK, et al. Cell shape-dependent regulation of protein 4.1 alternative pre-mRNA splicing in mammary epithelial cells. *J Biol Chem*. 1997;272:10254-10259.
64. Stewart TA, Davis FM. Formation and function of mammalian epithelia: roles for mechanosensitive PIEZO1 ion channels. *Front Cell Dev Biol*. 2019;7:260.
65. Ardran GM, Kemp FH, Lind J. A cineradiographic study of breast feeding. *Br J Radiol*. 1958;31:156-162.
66. Ueda T, Yokoyama Y, Irahara M, et al. Influence of psychological stress on suckling-induced pulsatile oxytocin release. *Obstet Gynecol*. 1994;84:259-262.
75. Dewey KG. Energy and protein requirements during lactation. *Annu Rev Nutr*. 1997;17:19-36.
77. Kalkwarf HJ. Hormonal and dietary regulation of changes in bone density during lactation and after weaning in women. *J Mammary Gland Biol Neoplasia*. 1999;4:319-329.
78. McNeilly AS. Lactational control of reproduction. *Reprod Fertil Dev*. 2001;13:583-590.
81. Lee S, Kelleher SL. Biological underpinnings of breastfeeding challenges: the role of genetics, diet, and environment on lactation physiology. *Am J Physiol Endocrinol Metab*. 2016;311:E405-E422.

Fetal and Neonatal Iron Metabolism

25

Harry J. McArdle | Michael K. Georgieff

INTRODUCTION

Iron is the fourth most abundant element and constitutes approximately 0.0075% of human body composition. It is a cofactor in some of the most basic biologic reactions, yet its beneficial effects are tempered by the fact that iron can be highly toxic, particularly in its unbound state since it participates in the generation of reactive oxygen species (ROS). An average normal newborn has a total body iron content of 75 mg/kg body weight, 55 mg/kg of which is complexed in hemoglobin.[1] In addition to its predominant role in erythropoiesis, iron is important for normal growth and function of all rapidly developing organ systems. An important principle of iron biology is that rapidly dividing cells require more iron to support their metabolism. Thus the rapidly growing fetus and neonate has higher iron requirements on a body weight basis than do older children and adults.

The clinical signs of iron deficiency are highly variable because iron-containing proteins are important in many facets of human biology. These processes include cellular energetics, DNA replication, tissue oxygenation, neurotransmitter synthesis, maintenance of thyroid status, white cell function, and fatty acid synthesis. The signs and symptoms of iron deficiency result not only from the hypoxia of anemia but the effect of tissue-level iron deficiency in the heart, skeletal muscle, gastrointestinal tract, and brain.

Negative iron balance occurs most commonly during three time periods in child development: the late fetal–early neonatal period (up to 6 months postnatal age), 6 to 24 months of age, and the teenage years. The acute clinical effects and long-term hematologic and nonhematologic sequelae of iron deficiency in the fetal and neonatal period have received intense study in the past 15 years. The previous lack of investigation in this field was a consequence of the misperception that neonatal iron deficiency occurs only secondary to severe maternal iron deficiency. The incidence of fetal iron deficiency anemia as a consequence of maternal iron deficiency anemia is relatively low in high-income countries because most mothers are supplemented with iron during pregnancy and because of prioritization of iron to the fetus by active placental iron transport (see further on). Nevertheless, the rate of maternal iron deficiency with or without anemia in high-income countries is 40% to 50%.[2] The rate approaches 80% among mothers in low- and middle-income countries.[3] Maternal iron deficiency during pregnancy is associated with an increased risk of adverse pregnancy outcome as defined by increased rates of prematurity and intrauterine growth failure.[4] Moreover, a relatively high incidence of reduced iron stores and frank iron deficiency has been found in specific groups of infants born to otherwise iron-sufficient mothers.[5] Iron deficiency in these groups is due to reduced placental iron transport (e.g., maternal hypertension or cigarette smoking) or to increased fetal iron demand that exceeds the capacity of placental iron transport (e.g., maternal glucose intolerance).[5]

Iron overload is also a potential in the fetus and neonate. This condition is rarely due to nutritional iron overload but can result from excessive red cell transfusions, congenital hemochromatosis, or reperfusion injuries. Iron overload of any cause is dangerous because free iron reacts with oxygen to create ROS. Iron overload has been proposed to play a role in neonatal diseases characterized by oxidative injury such as bronchopulmonary dysplasia, necrotizing enterocolitis, and retinopathy of prematurity.[6,7]

This chapter begins with a review of the biochemistry of iron-containing proteins, their biologic functions, and the regulation of cellular iron accretion. The subsequent discussion of fetal iron balance emphasizes the mechanisms of maternal-fetal iron transport with particular attention to the relative contributions of maternal and fetal iron status to regulating placental iron transport proteins. The section on postnatal iron balance addresses the various sources of iron and the overall iron requirements of term and preterm infants. Finally, the potential physiologic consequences of fetal and neonatal iron deficiency and iron excess are discussed.

GENERAL PRINCIPLES OF IRON METABOLISM

THE BIOLOGY OF IRON

Iron is a ubiquitous mineral that exists in trace conditions in humans. It is vital for the proper function of multiple proteins and is incorporated into their structures, typically as heme moieties or iron-sulfur clusters. The greatest amount of iron in the human neonate is found within red cells in the hemoglobin molecule.[1] Hemoglobin is prototypical of hemoproteins whose function is to carry oxygen or transfer electrons. Closely related compounds (because of their iron-containing porphyrin ring) include the cytochromes that are necessary for electron transport during oxidative phosphorylation and the generation of adenosine triphosphate (ATP). Iron therefore participates in the most basic aspects of cellular respiration during aerobic metabolism. In addition, iron-containing proteins reside in crucial pathways for detoxification (cytochrome P-450), neurotransmitter and hormone synthesis (tyrosine hydroxylase), and fatty acid production. Consequently, iron deficiency manifests as dysfunction of multiple organ systems including red blood cells, white blood cells, brain, heart, and skeletal muscle. Although iron deficiency anemia can produce classic signs and symptoms of fatigue, lethargy, and growth failure, most clinical manifestations are due to primary failure of nonhematologic organ systems dependent on iron-containing proteins and enzymes.

Iron is not only a necessary element whose deficiency produces symptomatology but also a highly toxic metal whose excess can cause severe organ damage through its interaction with oxygen (in the Fenton reaction) to generate ROS, which cause lipid membrane peroxidation. The Fenton reaction to generate ROS is as follows:

$$Fe^{2+} + H_2O_2 \rightarrow Fe^{3+} + OH^- + OH^\bullet$$

Iron is generally found in the ferric (Fe^{3+}) or ferrous (Fe^{2+}) state, but in either case it is always meant to be protein bound, whereby the structure of the protein physically shields the iron, effectively keeping it from reacting with oxygen. Multiple degenerative disorders and reperfusion injuries are postulated to be caused in part by free iron-mediated ROS, including Alzheimer disease, Parkinson disease, brain injury after stroke, and myocardial injury after infarction. Investigators of neonatal states have explored potential deleterious roles for free iron in the pathogenesis of birth asphyxia, necrotizing enterocolitis, bronchopulmonary dysplasia, and retinopathy of prematurity.[6,7]

REGULATION OF CELLULAR IRON HOMEOSTASIS AND IRON TRANSPORT

Iron is a highly necessary but potentially toxic mineral that requires tight regulation to maintain its concentration in a therapeutic range. An elegant posttranscriptional system regulates the expression of proteins involved in cellular iron uptake, storage, and export. All cells need iron to survive. Most take up iron specifically for utilization within themselves. These cells require a mechanism for iron uptake but typically do not express proteins that excrete iron. Others—such as duodenal epithelial cells, mammary epithelial cells, endothelial cells in the blood-brain barrier, and syncytiotrophoblasts—also take up iron in order to transport it from one compartment to another (Table 25.1). These cells require proteins not only for iron uptake but also for its excretion. Details on the mechanism of transfer of maternal-fetal iron across the placenta are given below.

Within the cell, cytoplasmic iron that is not immediately used for cellular functions—which can be referred to as the labile iron pool—is stored in the form of cytoplasmic ferritin. Ferritin is a nonheme iron protein complex consisting of a protein shell (apoferritin) made up of 24 protein subunits. In human tissue, two important subunits have been identified, designated as H (heavy) and L (light). These subunit chains form a shell into which iron can bind reversibly and be stored. Under various conditions, apoferritin can store up to 270 atoms of elemental ferric iron to form ferritin.[8] The greatest concentrations of fetal ferritin are located in the cells of the reticuloendothelial system in the liver, placenta, and spleen. Iron in these cells serves as a reservoir for iron used for other fetal organ systems. Late in fetal life, a major shift of iron (and erythropoiesis) from the liver to the bone marrow occurs. Ferritin is also present in all other cells, which serve as a short-term storage depot for unused cytoplasmic iron. However, cellular concentrations in most tissues outside the reticuloendothelial system are small.[8]

The regulation of cellular iron accretion and storage has been elucidated in erythrocyte, hepatocyte, placental trophoblast, and mammary epithelial cell lines.[9] A tightly controlled regulatory mechanism is necessary to ensure adequate availability of cytoplasmic iron while also guaranteeing efficient removal of potentially toxic excess cellular iron. This dual process is accomplished by coordinated regulation of the synthesis of the transferrin receptor-1 (TfR-1) and divalent metal transporter-1 (DMT-1), responsible for the uptake of iron by cells, and of ferritin, responsible for the conversion of excess cytoplasmic iron into its storage form. The simultaneous regulation of the iron uptake proteins and the iron storage protein occurs through posttranscriptional modification of TfR-1 and ferritin messenger RNAs (mRNAs). TfR-1, DMT-1, and ferritin mRNAs have specific binding sites known as *iron-responsive elements (IREs)*. These represent conserved palindromic mRNA stem loops with a specific six-base sequence 5′-CAGUGN-3′. One IRE is found on the 5′ untranslated sequence of ferritin mRNA, whereas five are found in the 3′ region of TfR-1 and DMT-1 mRNA.[10] These structurally and functionally identical sets of IREs are able to competitively bind iron-sensitive-specific cytoplasmic mRNA binding proteins known as *iron regulatory proteins (IRPs)*. Two IRPs are recognized. IRP-1 is constitutively expressed but changes its conformation and binding affinity for the IREs based on whether its iron-sulfur cluster is in its iron-deficient Fe_3S_4 or its iron-sufficient Fe_4S_4 form. The Fe_3S_4 form has higher affinity for the IRE.[10] IRP-2 is more classically regulated, with increased mRNA expression in response to iron deficiency. When cellular iron concentrations are low, the IRPs bind the IREs found in the 3′ untranslated region of TfR-1 and DMT-1 mRNA, stabilizing it and producing more copies. At the same time, IRP binding of the IRE in the 5′ untranslated region of ferritin mRNA prevents ribosomal binding. The combination results in increased synthesis of the iron importers and decreased synthesis of ferritin. High cytoplasmic iron concentrations lead to reduced IRP binding to the IREs on both mRNAs. This decreased binding leads to destabilization of the mRNAs of the importers while improving the binding of ferritin mRNA to ribosomes, increasing apoferritin synthesis, and promoting of storage of cytoplasmic iron.[10] Once iron has been internalized by the cell, chaperone proteins such as poly rC-binding proteins 1 and 2 deliver iron to the ferritin molecule and nuclear receptor coactivator 4 (NCOA4) to regulate ferritin release of iron back to the cytoplasmic pool for utilization in iron-containing proteins.[11]

REGULATION OF MATERNAL IRON UPTAKE AND PLACENTAL IRON TRANSPORT

The onset of pregnancy heralds an impending iron deficient state. The rapid expansion of the maternal blood volume coupled with the increasing iron needs of the fetus throughout pregnancy creates a large iron requirement for the mother.[12] The documented high incidence of iron deficiency during pregnancy supports this notion. An additional 1 g of iron, roughly equally distributed between mother's blood volume and the growing fetus, will be required during the pregnancy. Transferrin saturation decreases

Table 25.1 Vectoral Iron Transport Across Single-Cell Membrane Barriers.

Tissue	Source	Single Cell Barrier	Destination
Intestine	Lumen	Intestinal epithelium	Blood
Placenta	Maternal blood	Syncytiotrophoblast	Fetal blood
Mammary gland	Maternal blood	Mammary epithelium	Milk
Brain			
Vascular	Blood	Vascular epithelium	Parenchyma/astrocyte
Choroid plexus	Blood	Choroid epithelium	CSF
Ventricular ependyma	CSF	Ependymal cell layer	Parenchyma

CSF, Cerebrospinal fluid.

as these demands increase during pregnancy, blocking synthesis of hepcidin. Hepcidin levels are very low, providing a mechanism for increased iron absorption from the diet and release of iron from the reticuloendothelial system by the mother.[12,13]

Iron is carried bound to transferrin in the maternal plasma. The Fe-Tf complex binds to the TfR1 on the syncytiotrophoblast membrane (see Fig. 25.1).[14] The dimeric TfR-1 has a molecular weight of approximately 180 kDa and contains *O*-linked and three *N*-linked carbohydrate chains with a disulfide bridge in its extracellular domain. The extracellular, carboxy terminal component is large, approximately 140 kDa in size. For optimal binding to occur, the receptor must be fully glycosylated, with an intact disulfide bridge that binds the two monomers close to the cell membrane surface. TfR-1 isolated from cytosolic membranes demonstrates a lower binding affinity for transferrin[15] because of a presumably immature or incomplete glycosylation pattern. Similarly, truncation of the oligosaccharide side chains, particularly at Asn137, reduces the binding affinity for diferric transferrin.[15] The complex is internalized in clathrin coated pits and acidified by a H-ATPase. The Fe^{3+} is reduced by STEAP4 and is released from the transferrin. The reduced iron effluxes from the vesicle, presumably through DMT-1, although there is some doubt about this being the only pathway. From the cytoplasm, it is transferred to the basolateral side of the syncytium. How this is accomplished is not known. In the case of copper, which also has the potential to generate electrons, the metal is bound to carrier proteins termed chaperones. Over the last few years, iron chaperones have also been identified.[11] Termed Pcbp1 and Pcbp2, these proteins are members of the hnRNP K family and bind iron in a 1:3 ratio. Expression of these genes has been identified in placenta,[16] although how, when, and where they are expressed has not yet been determined.

Iron effluxes from cells through an iron channel termed ferroportin. Ferroportin-1 has been localized to the duodenal epithelium, the basal (fetal facing) surface of the syncytiotrophoblast, and the blood-brain barrier.[17,18] Mutations of ferroportin-1 resulting in iron overload of these transporting cells have been identified.[19] The mechanism by which ferroportin transports ferrous iron across the basal or basolateral membrane remains unclear. The iron is still as Fe^{2+} when it is released and is oxidized to Fe^{3+} by a ferroxidase called *zyklopen*.[20] This is a copper protein, similar to ceruloplasmin and hephaestin, which fulfil the same function at the liver and basolateral side of the gut, respectively (see Fig. 25.1). Ferroportin expression, and thus iron transport activity, are negatively regulated by the liver protein hepcidin.[21] When cells are iron sufficient or iron overloaded, hepcidin concentrations increase, repressing ferroportin-mediated iron transport. Of interest, inflammation induces a similar increase in hepcidin activity, which may explain the observation that during inflammatory states, iron is sequestered in the reticuloendothelial system (as ferritin) and therefore is not available in the circulation for cellular accretion and erythropoiesis, leading to the anemia of inflammation.[9,22] Thus it may be worth considering that the chronic anemia seen

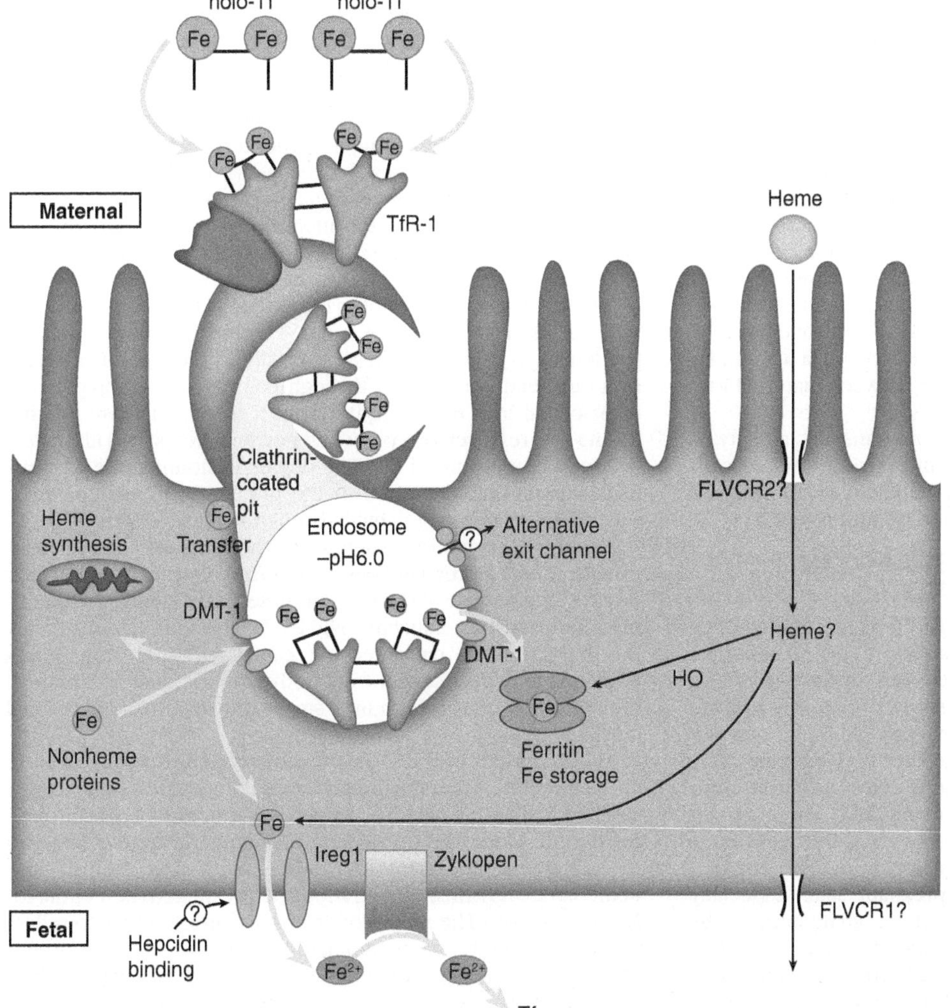

Fig. 25.1 Iron transport across the syncytiotrophoblast. Diferric transferrin is bound to transferrin receptor-1 (TfR-1) at the apical (maternal facing) membrane. Ferrous iron is transported out of the endosome into the cytoplasm by the divalent metal transporter-1 (DMT-1). Iron export at the basal (fetal facing) membrane is mediated through ferrous iron transport by ferroportin-1. See text for details. *FLVCR,* Feline leukemia virus receptor; *HO,* heme oxygenase. (Adapted from McArdle HJ, Lang C, Hayes H, Gambling L. The role of the placenta in regulation of iron status. *Nutr Rev.* 2011;69:S17–S22.)

in premature infants despite normal or elevated iron stores may be due in part to chronic inflammatory states common in this group of infants.

In the placenta, DMT-1 may not be the only exit mechanism from the vesicles. Andrews and colleagues generated mice with the *DMT-1* gene silenced. The mice with this mutation were anemic when born but were born alive and did have significant iron levels, showing that there was an alternative efflux mechanism or that another iron delivery mechanism is operating in tandem with the transferrin-mediated pathway.[23]

Such a pathway has been suggested by O'Brien and coworkers,[24] who proposed that heme iron can be transferred across the placenta. Heme in plasma is largely derived from senescent red blood cells and is carried on a protein called *hemopexin*. It has been suggested that the protein encoded by the feline leukemia virus receptor 1 *(FLVCR1)* and *FLVCR2* can bind hemopexin and take heme into the cell or efflux heme from the cell. Both these genes are expressed at high level in placenta, and it is hypothesized that this forms an alternative delivery system for iron to the fetus (see Fig. 25.1).[24,25] Recently, further indirect support has been provided for this hypothesis. LRP1 is also thought to be a hemopexin receptor. Heme in maternal plasma is carried on hemopexin, and levels of LRP1 increase in placentas of adolescent girls who have low iron status.[24]

When the maternal iron status and fetal iron demand are normal, TfR-1 expression is inversely related to placental nonheme iron content.[26] Placental nonheme iron is found largely in the form of ferritin in fetal cells, including Hofbauer cells. These macrophage-derived cells may constitute a form of placental iron storage, much as the Kupffer cells are major iron storage cells in the liver. Placental nonheme iron concentrations are closely correlated with cord blood serum ferritin concentrations and calculated total body storage iron at birth.[12] In clinical studies, the placental nonheme iron status (as well as the fetal storage iron content) correlates inversely with syncytiotrophoblastic TfR-1 expression in both iron-sufficient and iron-deficient fetuses.[27] This finding suggests that increased fetal iron demand can also positively influence TfR-1 expression.

In the gut, iron uptake is regulated by a small protein called hepcidin.[9] This peptide, produced by the liver, is regulated by many factors other than iron, which indicates the central role the nutrient plays in so many biologic processes. In pregnancy, iron absorption and metabolism seem largely to be controlled by fetal hepcidin, at least in rodents.[25,26] In humans, the data are similar, but it is difficult to study the relationship between maternal iron status and fetal hepcidin.

Ferroportin expression, and thus iron transport activity, is negatively regulated by the liver protein hepcidin.[9] When cells are iron-sufficient or iron-overloaded, hepcidin concentrations increase, repressing ferroportin-mediated iron transport.

FETAL IRON ACCRETION AND THE RELATIONSHIP OF MATERNAL AND FETAL IRON STATUS

The normal human fetus contains 70 to 75 mg/kg of elemental iron during the third trimester of gestation.[1] This represents a fetal accretion rate of 1.9 mg/day between 24 and 40 weeks of gestation. The iron is distributed between erythrocyte hemoglobin (50 to 55 mg/kg), liver, spleen, bone marrow, and kidney storage ferritin and hemosiderin (10 mg/kg), and nonstorage tissue iron such as hemoproteins and iron-sulfur proteins, found in virtually all tissues (7 mg/kg).[1] The pregnant woman is the source of iron for the fetus, and the placenta is the delivery system. Pregnant women will require increased iron over amounts adequate for the nonpregnant state, especially during the second and third trimesters, characterized by significant fetal growth and maternal blood volume expansion.[12]

Conditions that reduce maternal-fetal iron transport (e.g., maternal iron deficiency anemia or placental vascular disease) and those characterized by increased fetal iron demand (e.g., chronic fetal hypoxemia) threaten the normal accretion and distribution of fetal iron (Box 25.1).[5] Neonatal iron status is a function of the duration of gestation, fetal sex, maternal iron status, efficiency of placental iron transport, fetal iron demand, fetal growth rate, and duration of umbilical cord clamping.[28] Fetal iron stores as indexed by cord serum ferritin concentrations increase with advancing gestational age.[5] A meta-analysis has determined that the mean ferritin concentration for term infants is 134 μg/L, with 5th and 95th percentiles of 40 and 309 μg/L, respectively.[5] Preterm infants have lower values, with a mean of 115 μg/L and 5th and 95th percentiles of 35 and 267 μg/L, respectively.[5]

Fetal iron status correlates poorly with maternal iron status when the mother is iron-sufficient. The fetus accretes iron against a concentration gradient through active transport by the syncytiotrophoblast, resulting in higher ferritin concentrations in the fetus than in the mother. With progressive degrees of maternal deficiency, fetal iron stores are initially spared,[29] with compromise of those stores occurring later. Infants born to mothers with frank iron deficiency anemia have low cord blood ferritin and serum iron concentrations.[30] Typically, the risk to the fetus increases when the maternal hemoglobin is less than 100 g/L[31] or a maternal serum ferritin is less than 13.4 μg/L.[30] These findings suggest that the fetus can accumulate iron normally in the face of maternal iron deficiency, most likely through compensatory upregulation of placental iron transport, but with a threshold effect, so that during severe maternal iron deficiency, fetal iron status ultimately becomes compromised.[29,30] The degree of nonheme (e.g., brain, heart) tissue iron depletion in the human fetus resulting from severe maternal iron deficiency is unknown.

Despite maternal iron sufficiency, the fetus also can become iron-deficient in pregnancies characterized by placental vascular disease or in those in which increased iron demand exceeds placental transport capacity (Fig. 25.2).[5] In both circumstances, the reduction in measured or calculated fetal iron stores reflects a true decrease in total body iron, not just an intrafetal redistribution of iron from liver stores into an expanded red cell mass.[5,32]

An increased prevalence of reduced cord serum ferritin concentrations occurs in pregnancies complicated by placental vascular disease,[5] most often associated with intrauterine growth restriction. Moreover, up to 50% of infants of appropriate size for gestational age born to mothers with preeclampsia also demonstrate ferritin concentrations below the fifth percentile for gestational age.[5] The reduction in hepatic iron is likely to reflect the lack of iron transport adequate to fill the iron storage pool.

Increased fetal iron demand also can lead to abnormal iron distribution and iron deficiency at the tissue level. Fetal iron demand increases most markedly when erythropoiesis is

Box 25.1 Risk Factors to Fetal/Neonatal Iron Status

Risks for Iron Deficiency
Moderate to severe maternal iron deficiency anemia
Intrauterine growth restriction due to placental insufficiency
Poorly controlled maternal diabetes during pregnancy
Maternal obesity during pregnancy
Maternal smoking
Premature delivery
Twin-twin transfusion (donor)
Premature cord clamping

Risks for Iron Overload
Congenital hemochromatosis
Fetal viral infection
Twin-twin transfusion (recipient)

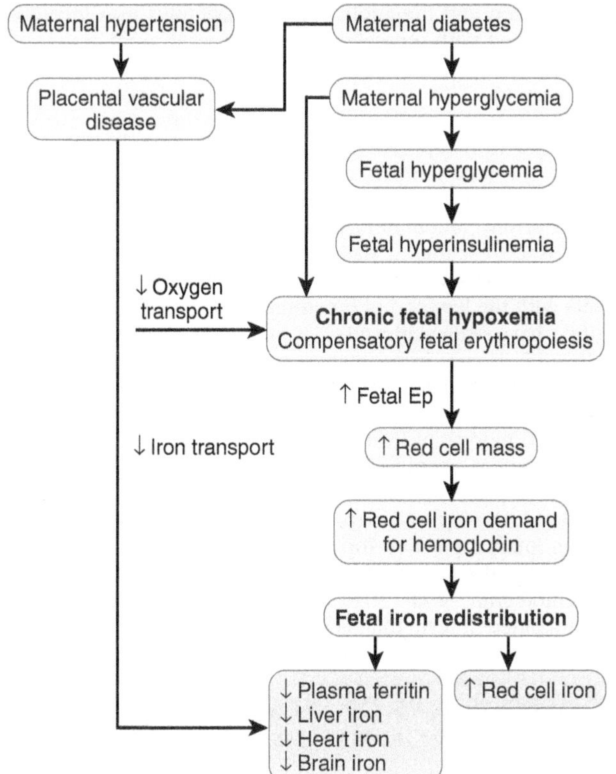

Fig. 25.2 Pathophysiology of fetal iron deficiency in pregnancies complicated by maternal hypertension and diabetes mellitus. (Modified from Krebs NF, Domellof M, Ziegler E. Balancing benefits and risks of iron supplementation in resource-rich countries. *J Pediatr.* 2015;167[Suppl]:S20–S25.)

augmented by chronic fetal hypoxemia, especially when it is accompanied by rapid fetal growth. Clinically, this sequence commonly is seen during pregnancies complicated by diabetes mellitus.[5,32] An autopsy study of large-for-gestational-age infants born to diabetic mothers demonstrated that hepatic iron concentrations were 7% of those in control (normal) infants, implying complete depletion of the iron storage pool.[32] Brain and heart iron concentrations were reduced to 61% and 46% of control levels, respectively. The reduction in nonstorage tissue iron is consistent with conventional iron deficiency theory in that storage iron must be reduced to less than 25% of normal before nonstorage tissue iron concentrations are compromised.

The causes of tissue iron deficiency in pregnancies complicated by diabetes mellitus and chronic fetal hypoxia have been studied in preclinical models (see Fig. 25.2). Chronic fetal hyperinsulinemia and hyperglycemia, which are characteristic of poorly controlled diabetic pregnancies, increased fetal cellular oxygen consumption in a relatively oxygen-limited environment.[32] The resultant chronic fetal hypoxemia stimulates erythropoietin release, with consequent expansion of the red cell mass by up to 40%.[32] The red cell mass may be further expanded by the rapid growth of the fetus with the attendant increase in the vascular volume.

The hypoxic fetus has two potential sources for iron to supply this rapidly expanded red cell mass: increased maternofetal iron transport and mobilization of endogenous fetal hepatic iron stores. When hepatic iron is depleted to less than 10% of control levels, fetal heart and brain iron concentrations fall (see Fig. 25.2).[32] The status of TfR-1 during diabetic pregnancies characterized by fetal iron deficiency has also been studied.[27] TfR-1 mRNA and IRP-1 activity are both increased by 40% in iron-deficient diabetic placentas, supporting the hypothesis that upregulation is possible and is probably controlled by fetal iron demand.[27] However, the lack of complete compensation due to abnormal binding of maternal transferrin to TfR-1 forces a redistribution of fetal iron toward the red cell mass and away from vital organs such as the heart and brain (see Fig. 25.2). These findings illustrate the fundamental principle that iron is prioritized to red blood cells at the expense of the brain and other tissues when iron supply does not meet iron demand in the fetus and neonate. Thus, brain iron deficiency with its risk for acute and long-term neurobehavioral sequelae occurs before anemia is present. Protection of the fetal and neonatal brain from iron deficiency requires screening tools that assess change in iron status before the onset of anemia.[33]

POSTNATAL IRON BALANCE

Iron deficiency in full-term infants born with normal iron stores (i.e., ferritin concentration) during the first 6 postnatal months has been of minimal concern as long as postnatal growth is not excessive.[34] An abundance of hemoglobin and accretion of storage iron during fetal life generally ensures an adequate source of iron for the first 6 months as the red cell mass breaks down in postnatal life. This supply is likely to be particularly abundant if the infant has received a transfusion of red cells from the placenta through delaying cord clamping for up to 2 minutes. The higher partial pressure of oxygen in arterial blood (Pa_{O_2}) of postnatal life reduces the need for the hemoglobin-mediated oxygen-carrying capacity; thus, the first 6 to 8 postnatal weeks are characterized by declining hemoglobin concentrations with subsequent liberation of heme iron. Because this iron is not lost from the body, the healthy term newborn infant is well supplied with iron for the first 4 to 6 postnatal months. After 6 months, as the infant grows and the blood volume expands, the iron necessary for hemoglobin synthesis continues to be derived from the reticuloendothelial stores and from the absorption of dietary iron. The estimated daily dietary iron requirement for the term infant is 1 mg/kg per day, but the percent absorption from the intestine varies inversely with the iron status of the individual infant.

The serum ferritin concentration is a reasonable reflection of iron stores, with each 1 μg/L of serum ferritin thought to represent 8 to 10 mg of stored iron.[5] Serum ferritin concentrations (and iron stores) are higher in newborn infants than in older infants, children, and adults. Ferritin concentrations decrease precipitously by the age of 6 months,[35] as storage iron is used for the rapidly expanding blood volume of the growing infant in lieu of the low amount of dietary iron found in human milk. Although studies assessing iron status of breast-fed infants are difficult to perform because of multiple confounding variables, the bulk of the data support the concept that infants fed human milk exclusively for 6 months have a normal iron status at 6 months.[34] Recently, concerns have been raised that unabsorbed iron following enteral iron supplementation may negatively impact the intestinal microbiome, a condition termed intestinal dysbiosis.[34] The relationship of the intestinal microbiome to acute and long-term disease risk is a subject of intensive investigation.

Dietary iron is absorbed by the duodenum and proximal jejunum through a process mediated by hepcidin-ferroportin. The postnatal and postconceptional ages at which intestinal iron absorption becomes as well regulated as it is in older children and adults is not known, although the proteins involved in regulation are present in preterm infants. Absorption is modulated not only by iron demand but also by the dietary source of the iron. Heme iron, in the form of hemoglobin and myoglobin, is enhanced by the ingestion of meat and inhibited by calcium. Nonheme iron, which represents the major portion of dietary iron, is absorbed more avidly in the presence of ascorbic acid. Its absorption is inhibited by calcium, phytates (found in soy protein–based formulas), manganese, and polyphenols.

Infant formulas fortified with at least 4 mg/L of iron are most likely to prevent depletion of iron stores and iron deficiency, although infants fed formulas with this amount of iron demonstrate lower ferritin and higher TfR-1 concentrations than those measured in infants fed formulas with higher iron contents.[36] This observation suggests that 4 mg/L may be close to the minimum concentration of iron content that can support iron sufficiency. Most iron-fortified formulas in the United States contain 10 to 12 mg/L. Low-iron formulas are defined by the US Food and Drug Administration (FDA) as containing less than 6.7 mg/L of elemental iron. Current low-iron formulas contain 4 mg/L of iron or more and appear to present sufficient dietary iron to the young infant who does not have additional risk factors for early iron deficiency.

The iron status of the preterm infant is at higher risk of perturbation than that of the term infant (Box 25.2). Preterm infants with intrauterine growth restriction are at risk for further reductions in iron stores owing to placental insufficiency and poor placental iron transfer.[5]

Based on estimates of third-trimester fetal iron accretion, iron stores at birth are lower for all preterm infants[5] and postnatal estimated daily iron needs per kilogram of weight are greater than those of full-term infants.[1,37] The iron balance of preterm infants can be markedly affected by the management of their hematologic status (i.e., how often they are phlebotomized, whether they receive red cell transfusions or recombinant human erythropoietin). Iron intake can be compromised because of delayed onset of enteral feedings and a reluctance to give intramuscular or intravenous iron.

Preterm infants become anemic partly because of the amount of iron they lose through phlebotomy.[38] Evaluation of iron deficiency in preterm infants is difficult, but iron deficiency may contribute to the magnitude and duration of anemia of prematurity. In previous eras, supplemental iron was administered to preterm infants indirectly through repeated blood transfusions. Many neonatologists now use restricted red blood cell transfusion protocols, and the number of transfusions per infant has declined in recent years.[38] The unintentional effect of this change in management has been to decrease the total body iron content of preterm infants, stimulating a fresh look at red cell transfusion thresholds and the dietary iron requirements of preterm infants.

The use of erythropoietin in preterm infants also results in increased iron requirements because each gram of newly synthesized hemoglobin requires an additional 3.46 mg of elemental iron. Trials of recombinant human erythropoietin to prevent or modify the anemia of prematurity have shown that the young preterm infant is capable of mounting an erythropoietic response.[38] The stress of augmented erythropoiesis on the iron axis of the preterm infant is considerable[39] and may be rate-limiting in the erythropoietic response.[39] Because these infants receive fewer red cell transfusions, their total body iron is likely to be reduced and their reliance on exogenous iron increased. Infants treated with recombinant human erythropoietin require at least 6 mg/kg/day to maintain adequate serum ferritin concentrations.[39] The percent of absorbed iron incorporated into hemoglobin varies with the degree of erythropoietic pressure. To this end, iron supplementation enhances the erythropoietic response to recombinant erythropoietin therapy in preterm infants.[39]

The current recommendation for iron intake for preterm infants is 2 to 4 mg/kg daily.[37] Use of either fortified human milk or preterm formula at 150 mL/kg/day will provide preterm infants with the low end of recommended iron intake when goal feedings have been achieved.

After discharge, iron intakes of 2 to 3 mg/kg daily are recommended.[40] Breast-fed infants may meet this requirement through the use of multivitamin supplements with iron, which provide 10 mg/mL of iron. However, most infants will outgrow this dose before supplemental foods (such as cereal) are added. Formula-fed preterm infants meet this requirement when taking in 120 calories/kg of body weight. Gestationally less mature preterm infants may develop iron deficiency anemia before the age of 6 months, and evaluation of iron status by measurement of hemoglobin and ferritin concentrations sooner than recommended in term infants is prudent.

Box 25.2 Risks to Postnatal Iron Status in Preterm Infants

Risks for Negative Iron Balance

Low endowment (intrauterine growth restriction)
Rapid postnatal growth rate
Delayed onset of iron therapy (>2 months)
Low iron dose (<2 mg/kg body weight daily)
Recombinant human erythropoietin therapy
Phlebotomy

Risks for Iron Overload

Red blood cell transfusion
Parenteral iron therapy
Reperfusion Injuries (nonnutritional)

CONSEQUENCES OF FETAL AND NEONATAL IRON DEFICIENCY

The nonhematologic consequences of fetal and neonatal iron deficiency are significant. When fetal iron is in short supply (as with maternal iron deficiency anemia or uteroplacental insufficiency) or when fetal iron demand is increased (as with chronic fetal hypoxemia), prioritization of available fetal iron will occur.[33] This prioritization takes place among organs and among iron-containing compounds within organs. The process preserves tissue oxygen delivery. For example, iron is prioritized to red blood cells over all nonheme tissues including the brain and heart.[33]

The potential short-term and long-term physiologic consequences of fetal and neonatal iron deficiency must be considered for each of the organ systems. No direct physiologic effects of reduced hepatic storage iron are known. Nevertheless, infants born with low iron stores (infants of diabetic mothers, infants with intrauterine growth restriction) are likely to be at higher risk for postnatal iron deficiency, particularly if the low stores are not due to sequestration of iron in an expanded red cell mass. Thus infants with low serum ferritin concentrations and normal or low hemoglobin concentrations at birth may be at highest risk for an earlier onset of postnatal iron deficiency.[41]

The physiologic consequences of a postnatal deficiency in cardiac and skeletal muscle iron are well described.[42] Myopathies of both organ systems are characterized by decreased contractile force and easy fatigability, contributing to the clinical picture of weakness and lethargy. The biochemical basis for these findings is unknown, although it has been speculated that reduced cytochrome *c* concentrations result in decreased ATP generation and that reduced myoglobin levels result in reduced oxygen delivery and greater dependence on anaerobic glycolysis. These findings are clearly independent of the presence and degree of anemia. Furthermore, although newborn infants of diabetic mothers are frequently lethargic and cardiomyopathic, the role of iron deficiency in these conditions has not been defined. The possibility exists that the inability of iron-deficient tissue to withstand hypoxic and hypoglycemic stress contributes to the higher rates of fetal distress and intrauterine death seen in diabetic pregnancies.

The biochemical, anatomic, and neurochemical effects of perinatal brain iron deficiency have been extensively characterized in mice, rats, pigs, sheep, and nonhuman primate preclinical models.[33]

Perinatal iron deficiency in rodents causes reduced oxidative metabolism in the hippocampus and frontal cortex, elevated intracellular glutamate concentrations, reduced dopamine concentrations in the striatum, altered fatty acid profiles, and central nervous system hypomyelination.[43] Development of the brain is impaired, with truncation of dendritic arbors, particularly in the hippocampus.[44] Specific hippocampal synaptic plasticity genes—such as brain-derived neurotrophic factor (BDNF) as well as gene networks that underlie diseases such as autism, schizophrenia, and mood disorders—are altered acutely by fetal/neonatal iron deficiency and remain altered in adulthood.[45,46] Nonanemic, neuronal-specific iron deficiency in genetic mouse models confirm that the short- and long-term molecular, cellular, structural, metabolic, electrophysiologic, and behavioral effects of neonatal iron deficiency are due to the lack of brain iron and not to anemia.[45] The behavioral deficits these rodents display are consistent with targeted areas of the brain including trace recognition memory, procedural memory, and spatial navigation.[45,46] The effects last well beyond the period of iron deficiency, suggesting the possibility of long-term iron deficiency–induced alterations in brain structure, gene regulation, and function.[46] The effects on energy metabolism, dendritic structure, monamine metabolism, and myelination all appear to work together to alter brain processing, particularly in memory domains.[43,46]

Growth-restricted infants, infants of poorly controlled diabetic mothers, and preterm infants are at increased risk for poorer long-term developmental outcomes. Although the etiology of cognitive impairments in these groups of children is likely to be multifactorial, the relationship of developmental outcomes to perinatal iron status may be of importance because an iron-deficient brain may be less likely to tolerate hypoxic or hypoglycemic events.

Developmental outcomes as a function of iron status have been assessed after fetal and neonatal iron deficiency.[47-51] Low maternal intake at the time of conception is associated with an increased risk of autism,[47] and low intake in midgestation increases the risk of schizophrenia[48] in the offspring. These epidemiologic findings map remarkably onto gene networks that are perturbed by gestational/neonatal iron deficiency in rodents.[46] Preterm infants with cord blood serum ferritin concentrations less than 76 μg/L have slower conduction velocities on auditory brain-stem evoked responses, indicating delayed neurotransmission or hypomyelination.[49] Term infants of diabetic mothers with serum ferritin concentrations less than 40 μg/L have poorer auditory recognition memory at birth, implicating abnormal fetal hippocampal development.[50] Tamura and colleagues reported findings from a large study of infants born at term, correlating umbilical cord serum ferritin concentrations and results of cognitive testing at 5 years of age. Infants in the lowest quartile of umbilical cord ferritin concentration (<76 ng/dL) had poorer scores on language comprehension, fine motor skills, attention, and tractability than children with umbilical cord ferritin concentrations in the two median quartiles.[51] These short- and long-term neuropathologies are consistent with animal models of fetal/neonatal iron deficiency that demonstrate acute (i.e., while iron deficient) and long-term abnormalities of neurotransmission, myelination, learning, and memory.[43-46] These interdisciplinary research findings may explain at least in part the poorer neurodevelopmental outcomes of populations at risk for fetal/neonatal iron deficiency, including infants born to anemic mothers, intrauterine growth-restricted infants, infants of diabetic mothers, and premature infants.[5]

POTENTIAL IRON TOXICITY IN THE FETUS AND NEONATE

Iron deficiency is not the only iron-related problem that may affect the developing human. The newborn infant also is theoretically at greater risk for iron toxicity. Newborn infants in general are at higher risk for oxidant injury as a consequence of immature antioxidant systems (e.g., vitamin E, selenium, superoxide dismutase) and the increased sensitivity of rapidly growing tissues to free radicals.[7] The vitamin C system matures after the age of 2 weeks, so antioxidant abilities improve thereafter.[7] Free radical formation is less likely to occur when iron is tightly bound and hidden by the three-dimensional protein structure of hemoglobin, myoglobin, transferrin, or ferritin. Non–protein bound or loosely bound iron, however, can generate free radicals through the Fenton reaction, potentially resulting in serious tissue damage from the effects of oxidant stress on cell membranes.[7] Because newborn infants have low levels of iron-binding proteins, rapid infusions of iron may result in oversaturation of the iron-binding capacity, potentially resulting in liberation of free serum iron. Rapid influx of free iron is more likely to occur following intravenous iron administration or lysis of transfused red blood cells than following enteral iron therapy. Newborn term and preterm infants are prone to hypoxic-ischemic events, which may result in tissue reperfusion injury and iron deposition. Birth asphyxia resulting in hypoxic-ischemic encephalopathy increases non–protein bound iron (NPBI) and thio-barbituric-acid-reactive species in cord blood. Increased NPBI in cerebral spinal fluid correlates with Sarnat stage (reviewed in Perrone et al.[7]). Tissue reperfusion after hypoxia-ischemia in the neonatal rodent model potentiates the likelihood of the Fenton reaction and, consequently, the possibility of iron-related oxidant activity.[52] Indeed, iron deposition has been noted in perivascular areas of the brain associated with neuronal loss in animal models of hypoxia-ischemia.[50] These roles of iron in reperfusion injuries, however, could be considered a nonnutritional effect of the metal.

Although these considerations have raised considerable concern about the oxidant properties of iron, only indirect evidence is suggestive of clinical effects of possible iron toxicity in newborn infants. In theory, the highest-risk situation would arise with rapid intravenous boluses of iron, either via parenteral iron infusions or by transfusions of senescent blood cells that hemolyze and release iron. Blood transfusions have been associated with increased free iron levels and an increased risk of chronic lung disease in preterm infants.[6,7] These findings were not associated with lipid peroxidation; accordingly, the study investigators were not able to provide evidence that blood transfusions or iron toxicity results in oxidative injury to the lung.

Regarding the use of oral iron supplements, it is theoretically possible that high doses of enteral iron may be sufficient to result in non–protein bound serum iron, oxidative stress, and increased risk of diseases such as bronchopulmonary dysplasia.[6,7] These are difficult subjects to investigate in preterm babies because of the many potential confounding variables involved and the lack of biomarkers of tissue oxidative damage. Available research suggests that doses of iron up to 18 mg/kg daily given to preterm infants do not result in an increase in oxidant stress markers in the serum.[53] Overall, the relationship among iron toxicity from enteral iron intake, serum or urine markers of oxidant stress, and oxidant organ damage in preterm infants has been inadequately studied.

A related consideration is iron overload in the newborn term infant. Primary iron overload in adults occurs in the hereditary hemochromatosis syndromes, which are not seen in the newborn infant and are rare even during childhood. Neonatal hemochromatosis previously was thought to be a syndrome of primary iron overload. However, the biochemical abnormalities found in neonatal hemochromatosis also have been shown to occur nonspecifically in severe liver disease, and the patterns of organ injury in neonatal hemochromatosis are not consistent with juvenile or adult forms of hemochromatosis.[54] Although the full-blown disease is generally fatal, a few survivors have been described who have resolution of their liver disease and who do not have ongoing manifestations of hemochromatosis. It is now postulated that iron deposition is a consequence rather than a cause of the liver disease. According to some evidence, the primary inciting factor in many patients may be an alloimmune process targeting an antigen present on fetal hepatocytes.[54] Intravenous immune globulin has been given to fetal siblings conceived after the birth of an affected infant. Nearly all treated infants have shown biochemical evidence of neonatal hemochromatosis but with reduction in clinical symptoms and no deaths.[54]

Secondary iron overload syndromes have been described in which infants with Rh disease had undergone multiple fetal transfusions. Affected infants show severe liver disease, marked elevation of serum ferritin concentrations, and iron overload on liver biopsy. Resolution of symptoms occurs after treatment with the iron chelator deferoxamine.

ANEMIA OF CHRONIC DISEASE

The interrelated roles of iron and inflammation have been well studied in adults and children[9] but not extensively in neonates. Nevertheless, hepcidin appears to be actively regulated in maternal-fetal iron transport, and it is likely that the neonate also has a responsive system. It is not unusual to encounter neonates in the neonatal intensive care unit that are anemic and have low reticulocyte counts and high serum ferritins, particularly in the setting of infection and inflammation. Hepcidin's role in iron regulation is to reduce enteral iron absorption and sequester iron in the reticuloendothelial system,[9] which effectively reduces iron availability to siderophilic bacteria. However, long-term iron sequestration associated with chronic infectious or inflammatory diseases could result in long-term anemia and reduced availability of iron for organ development. Although it is clear that the proteins involved in this iron regulatory system are present in the fetus, placenta, and neonate, further research is necessary to understand how well regulated this system is in this developmental time period. Understanding this regulation will be particularly useful in driving decision making with respect to iron therapy in preterm and term neonates.

CONCLUSION

Iron sufficiency is important for the normal growth, development, and function of fetal and neonatal organ systems. The regulation of maternal-fetal iron transport and intracellular iron accretion, trafficking, and storage continues to be investigated with the recent discovery of additional IRPs. Certain pregnancy subgroups are associated with an increased risk for fetal and neonatal iron deficiency, either because of inadequate maternal-fetal iron transport, in the case of maternal anemia or intrauterine growth retardation, or because of excessive iron demand, as seen in diabetic pregnancies. In the neonatal period, preterm infants treated with recombinant human erythropoietin and receiving fewer red cell transfusions appear to be at greatest risk for early depletion of iron stores. Iron excess may also play a role in certain neonatal disease processes through the peroxidation of lipid membranes. It is important to document the short- and long-term physiologic consequences of iron imbalances in all of these settings.

ACKNOWLEDGMENTS

Preparation of this chapter was supported by grants from the National Institutes of Health (NICHD) and the Scottish Government (Rural and Environmental Scientific and Analytical services, RESAS).

A complete reference list is available at www.ExpertConsult.com.

SELECT REFERENCES

1. Oski FA. The hematologic aspects of the maternal-fetal relationship. In: Oski FA, Naiman JL, eds. *Hematologic Problems in the Newborn*. 3rd ed. Philadelphia: WB Saunders; 1982:32-33.
2. Auerbach M, Abernathy J, Juul S, Short V, Derman R. Prevalence of iron deficiency in first trimester, nonanemic pregnant women. *J Matern Fetal Neonatal Med*. 2019;3:1-4.
3. WHO. *Iron Deficiency Anaemia. Assessment, Prevention, and Control. A Guide for Programme Managers*. Geneva, Switzerland: World Health Organization; 2001.
4. Dewey KG, Oaks BM. U-shaped curve for risk associated with maternal hemoglobin, iron status, or iron supplementation. *Am J Clin Nutr*. 2017;106(suppl): 1694S-702S.
5. Siddappa AM, Rao R, Long JD, et al. The assessment of newborn iron stores at birth: a review of the literature and standards for ferritin concentrations. *Neonatology*. 2007;92:73-82.
6. Patel RM, Knezevic A, Yang J, et al. Enteral iron supplementation, red blood cell transfusion, and risk of bronchopulmonary dysplasia in very-low-birth-weight infants. *Transf usion*. 2019;59:1675-1682.
7. Perrone S, Tataranno ML, Negro S, et al. Early identification of the risk for free radical-related diseases in preterm newborns. *Early Hum Dev*. 2010;86: 241-244.
8. Harrison PM, et al. In: Ponka P, Schulman HM, Woodworth RC, eds. *Iron Transport and Storage*. Boca Raton, FL: CRC Press, Ferritin; 1990:81-101.
9. Coffey R, Ganz T. Iron homeostasis: an anthropocentric perspective. *J Biol Chem*. 2017;292:12727-12734.
10. Anderson CP, Shen M, Eisenstein RS, Leibold EA. Mammalian iron metabolism and its control by iron regulatory proteins. *Biochim Biophys Acta*. 2012;1823:1468-1483.
11. Philpott CC, Jadhav S. The ins and outs of iron. Escorting iron through the mammalian cytosol. *Free Rad Biol Med*. 2019;133:112-117.
12. Fisher A, Nemeth E. Iron homeostasis during pregnancy. *Am J Clin Nutr*. 2017;106(suppl):1567S-74S.
13. Sangkhae V, Fisher AL, Wong S, et al. Effects of maternal iron status on placental and fetal iron homeostasis. *J Clin Invest*. 2020;130(2):625-640.
14. McArdle HJ, Lang C, Hayes H, Gambling L. The role of the placenta in regulation of iron status. *Nutr Rev*. 2011;69:S17-S22.
15. Williams AM, Enns CA. A region of the C-terminal portion of the human transferrin receptor contains an asparagine-linked glycosylation site critical for receptor structure and function. *J Biol Chem*. 1993;268:12780.
16. Van Dijk M, Visser A, Buabeng KM, et al. Mutations within the LINC-HELLP non-coding RNA differentially bind ribosomal and RNA splicing complexes and negatively affect trophoblast differentiation. *Human Mol Genet*. 2015;24:5475-5485.
17. Donovan A, Brownlie A, Zhou Y, et al. Positional cloning of zebrafish ferroportin 1 identifies a conserved vertebrate iron exporter. *Nature*. 2000;403:776-781.
18. Bradley J, Leibold EA, Harris ZL, et al. The influence of gestational age and fetal iron status on IRP activity and iron transporter protein expression in third trimester human placenta. *Am J Physiol*. 2004;287:R894-R901.
19. Donovan A, Lima CA, Pinkus JL, et al. The iron exporter ferroportin/Slc40a1 is essential for iron homeostasis. *Cell Metabol*. 2005;1:191-200.
20. Chen H, Attieh ZK, Syed BA, et al. Identification of zyklopen, a new member of the vertebrate multicopper ferroxidase family, and characterization in rodents and human cells. *J Nutr*. 2010;140:1728-1735.
21. Nemeth E, Tuttle MS, Powelson J, et al. Hepcidin regulates cellular iron efflux by binding to ferroportin and inducing its internalization. *Science*. 2004;306:2090-2093.
22. Roy CN, Andrews NC. Anemia of inflammation: the hepcidin link. *Curr Opin Hematol*. 2005;12:107-111.
23. Gunshin H, Fujiwara Y, Custodio AO, DIrenzo C, Robine S, Andrews NC. Slc11a2 is required for intestinal iron absorption and erythropoiesis but dispensable in placenta and liver. *J Clin Invest*. 2005;115:1258-1266.
24. Cao C, Pressman EK, Cooper EM, Guillet R, Westerman M, O'Brien KO. Placental heme receptor LRP1 correlates with the heme exporter FLVCR1 and neonatal iron status. *Reproduction*. 2014;148:295-302.
25. McArdle HJ, Gambling L, Kennedy C. Iron deficiency during pregnancy: the consequences for placental function and fetal outcome. *Proc Nutr Soc*. 2014;73:9-15.
26. Gambling L, Lang C, McArdle HJ. Fetal regulation of iron transport during pregnancy. *Am J Clin Nutr*. 2011;94:1903S-1907S.
27. Petry CD, Wobken JD, McKay H, et al. Placental transferrin receptor in diabetic pregnancies with increased fetal iron demand. *Am J Physiol*. 1994;267:E507-E514.
28. Georgieff MK, Krebs NF, Cusick SE. The benefits and risks of iron supplementation in pregnancy and childhood. *Annu Rev Nutr*. 2019;39:121-146.
29. Chang SC, O'Brien KO, Nathanson MS, Mancini J, Witter FR. Hemoglobin concentrations influence birth outcomes in pregnant African-American adolescents. *J Nutr*. 2003;133:2348-2355.
30. Shao J, Lou J, Rao R, et al. Maternal serum ferritin concentration is positively associated with newborn iron stores in women with low ferritin status in late pregnancy. *J Nutr*. 2012;142:2004-2009.
31. Erdem A, Erdem M, Arslan M, et al. The effect of maternal anemia and iron deficiency on fetal erythropoiesis: comparison between serum erythropoietin, hemoglobin and ferritin levels in mothers and newborns. *J Matern Fetal Neonatal Med*. 2002;11:329-332.

32. Petry CD, Eaton MA, Wobken JD, et al. Iron deficiency of liver, heart and brain in newborn infants of diabetic mothers. *J Pediatr*. 1992;121:109-114.
33. Georgieff MK. Iron assessment to protect the developing brain. *Am J Clin Nutr*. 2017;106(S):1588S-1593S.
34. Krebs NF, Domellof M, Ziegler E. Balancing benefits and risks of iron supplementation in resource-rich countries. *J Pediatr*. 2015;167(suppl):S20-S25.
35. Ziegler EE, Nelson SE, Jeter JM. Iron supplementation of breastfed infants from an early age. *Am J Clin Nutr*. 2009;89:525-532.
36. Lonnerdal B, Hernell O. Iron, zinc, copper and selenium status of breast-fed infants and infants fed trace element fortified milk-based infant formula. *Acta Pediatr*. 1994;83:367-373.
37. Domellof M. Meeting the iron needs of low and very low birth weight infants. *Ann Nutr Metab*. 2017;71(suppl 3):16-23.
38. Widness JA. Pathophysiology of anemia during the neonatal period, including anemia of prematurity. *NeoReviews*. 2008;1:e520.
39. Carnielli VP, Da Riol R, Montini G. Iron supplementation enhances response to high doses of recombinant human erythropoietin in preterm infants. *Arch Dis Child Fetal Neonatal Ed*. 1998;79:F44-F484.
40. Domellof M, Georgieff MK. Postdischarge iron requirements of the preterm infant. *J Pediatr*. 2015;167:S31-S35.
41. Zhao G, Guobin X, Zhou M, et al. Prenatal iron supplementation reduces maternal anemia, iron deficiency, iron deficiency anemia in a randomized clinical trial in rural China, but iron deficiency remains widespread in mothers and neonates. *J Nutr*. 2015;145:1916-1923.
42. Blayney L, Bailey-Wood R, Jacobs A, et al. The effects of iron deficiency on the respiratory function and cytochrome content of rat heart mitochondria. *Circ Res*. 1976;39:744-758.
43. Lozoff B, Georgieff MK. Iron deficiency and brain development. *Semin Pediatr Neurol*. 2006;13:158-165.
44. Bastian TW, von Hohenberg WC, Mickelson DJ, Lanier LM, Georgieff MK. Iron deficiency impairs developing hippocampal neuron gene expression, energy metabolism and dendrite complexity. *Dev Neurosci*. 2016;38:264-276.
45. Fretham SJB, Carlson ES, Wobken J, Tran PV, Petryk A, Georgieff MK. Temporal manipulation of transferrin receptor-1 dependent iron uptake identifies a sensitive period in mouse hippocampal neurodevelopment. *Hippocampus*. 2012;22:1691-1702.
46. Tran PV, Kennedy BC, Pisansky MT, et al. Prenatal choline supplementation diminishes early-life iron deficiency induced preprogramming of networks associated with behavioral abnormalities in the adult rat hippocampus. *J Nutrition*. 2016;146:484-493.
47. Schmidt RJ, Tancredi DJ, Krakowiak P, et al. Maternal intake of supplemental iron and risk of autism spectrum disorder. *Am J Epidemiol*. 2014;180:890-900.
48. Insel BJ, Schaefer CA, McKeague IW, et al. Maternal iron deficiency and the risk of schizophrenia in offspring. *Arch Gen Psychiatry*. 2008;65:1136-1144.
49. Amin SB, Orlando M, Eddins A, MacDonald M, Monczynski C, Wang H. In utero iron status and auditory neural maturation in premature infants as evaluated by auditory brainstem response. *J Pediatr*. 2010;156:377-381.
50. Siddappa A, Georgieff MK, Wewerka S, et al. Iron deficiency alters auditory recognition memory in newborn infants of diabetic mothers. *Pediatr Res*. 2004;55:1034-1041.

Fetal and Neonatal Calcium, Phosphorus, and Magnesium Homeostasis

26

Karen M. O'Callaghan | Daniel E. Roth

INTRODUCTION

Calcium, phosphorus, and magnesium are essential minerals that function in their physiologically active ionic forms in a wide range of cellular processes, and as key components of the bone mineral matrix. In utero, calcium, phosphorus, and magnesium are readily transferred from maternal to fetal circulations, and fetal mineral stores are predominantly accrued in the third trimester. In the postnatal period, the newborn must rapidly adapt to the cessation of the continuous transplacental supply of these nutrients by enabling homeostatic mechanisms that regulate intestinal absorption, bone deposition/resorption, and renal reabsorption of calcium, phosphate, and magnesium. Transcellular and paracellular transport pathways are regulated by a shared set of hormones including vitamin D, parathyroid hormone (PTH), fibroblast growth factor 23 (FGF23), and calcitonin. However, as detailed later, distinct mechanisms govern the homeostatic control of each of these three minerals in the fetus and newborn.

CALCIUM

BODY DISTRIBUTION AND MEASUREMENT OF CALCIUM

Calcium is a highly abundant and essential mineral in the human body. Although calcium is most widely recognized for its role as the major inorganic constituent of bone, it exerts countless other physiologic effects by serving as a cellular signal involved in gene expression, synaptic transmission, muscle contraction, and embryogenesis.[1] Every cell in the human body relies on the specific decoding of calcium signals for its normal function and survival, and therefore is sensitive to minute variations in the calcium concentration within the cell and in its microenvironment. Because the intracellular calcium concentration is about 10,000-fold lower than the surrounding extracellular fluid (ECF), individual cells rely on active transport mechanisms to maintain a concentration gradient.[2]

All tissues depend on the systemic regulation of calcium availability by a complex, interconnected series of feedback loops involving the bones, intestinal tract, and kidneys; in utero, the role of the intestines is essentially substituted by the placenta (Fig. 26.1). Over 99% of total body calcium is in the skeleton. Bone contains a variety of calcium salts, of which hydroxyapatite is the least soluble and, thus, the most important structural component that integrates with collagen fibrils to form the bone matrix.[2] However, other salts such as amorphous calcium phosphate are relatively abundant on the crystal surfaces of the bone matrix, where the calcium is in equilibrium with the ECF, constituting an *exchangeable pool* of calcium (about 1% of the calcium in bone)[3]—a critical resource for maintenance of a physiologic serum calcium concentration.[2,4]

The remaining 1% of total body calcium is contained in all of the nonskeletal tissues, including soft tissues, blood (including serum/plasma), and other ECFs. Serum (or plasma) calcium is solubilized in three forms: 50% as the free ion, termed *ionized calcium* (iCa^{2+}); 40% bound to plasma protein (of which, 80% is bound to albumin and the remainder to globulins); and approximately 10% as diffusible complexes of calcium bound to anions such as bicarbonate, phosphate, or citrate.[3] Ionized calcium is the only physiologically active fraction in blood; therefore tight regulation of the iCa^{2+} concentration is a major focus of calcium homeostasis. Because of the substantial fraction of total plasma calcium that is bound to albumin, alterations in

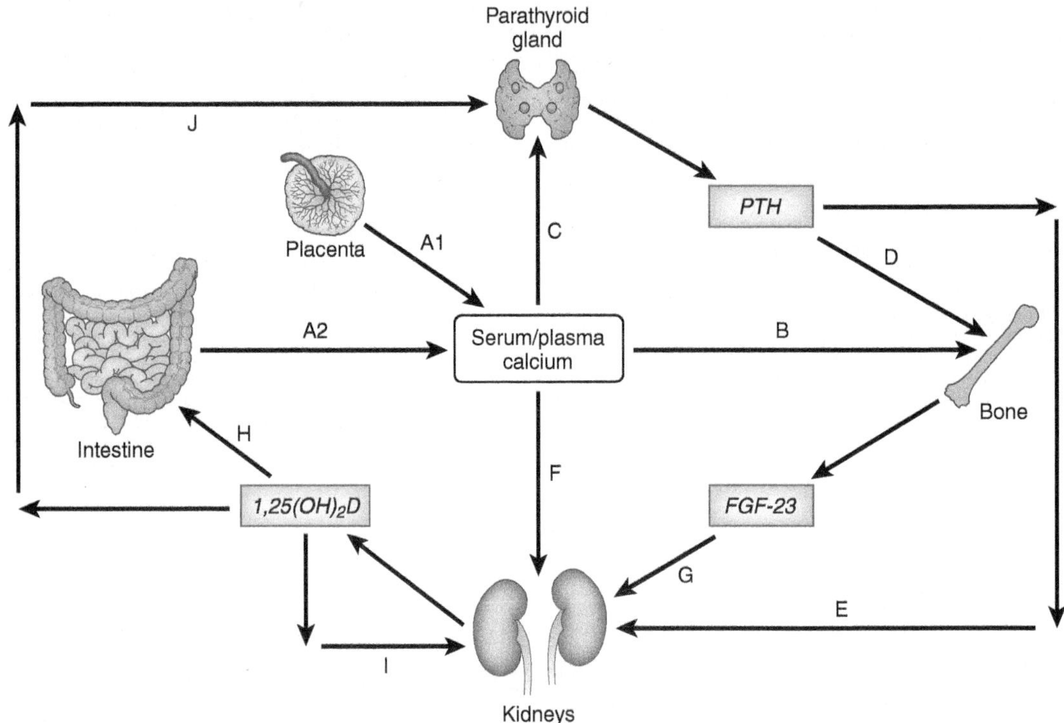

Fig. 26.1 Schematic representation of the sources and actions of major regulatory hormones that influence fetal-neonatal calcium accrual and maintenance of the serum/plasma calcium concentration. Calcium is transferred transplacentally against a concentration gradient into the fetal circulation *(A1)* or absorbed from the intestinal lumen in the neonate *(A2)*; net calcium retention enables bone mineralization and skeletal growth *(B)*; increases in serum calcium are detected by calcium-sensing receptors in the parathyroid gland, leading to inhibition of parathyroid hormone *(PTH)* release *(C)*; PTH acts on bone to stimulate calcium release *(D)*, and acts on the kidney to stimulate renal calcium reabsorption and renal 1,25-dihydroxyvitamin D synthesis *(E)*; an increase in the serum calcium concentration promotes urinary excretion *(F)*; fibroblast growth factor 23 *(FGF23)*, produced in bone, acts on kidneys to promote phosphate excretion and inhibit $1,25(OH)_2D$ synthesis *(G)*; $1,25(OH)_2D$, which is produced from 25-hydroxyvitamin D by renal *CYP27B1*, acts on the intestinal epithelial cells to promote calcium absorption *(H)*, feedback inhibits its own synthesis in the kidneys *(I)*, and suppresses PTH release by the parathyroid gland *(J)*. (Adapted from Goltzman D, Mannstadt M, Marcocci C. Physiology of the calcium-parathyroid hormone-vitamin D axis. *Front Horm Res*. 2018;50:1–13; and Pike JW, Christakos S. Biology and mechanisms of action of the vitamin D hormone. *Endocrinol Metab Clin North Am*. 2017;46:815–843.)

the plasma concentration of albumin can affect the measured total serum or plasma calcium concentration. Sudden changes in the concentration of albumin can change the iCa^{2+} concentration (as observed upon rapid addition of albumin to neonatal serum in vitro[5]), but in vivo, this effect is transient[6] and modest.[7] Over the long term, iCa^{2+} is relatively less affected by albumin concentrations compared to total calcium.[3] Therefore the total calcium concentration (which includes all fractions) is often a poor predictor of the iCa^{2+} concentration. The propensity for calcium to bind to proteins is reduced at acidic pH, such that iCa^{2+} varies inversely with blood pH.[3] Laboratory methods to quantify calcium concentrations in body fluids vary widely, and some studies have shown poor correlation of values generated by different automated chemistry platforms.[8] Furthermore, published pediatric reference intervals may not reflect the expected pattern of decline and then recovery of serum/plasma calcium concentrations in the first week of life (Fig. 26.2A).

In the clinical context, measurement of an individual's serum/plasma total calcium or iCa^{2+} provides insights into the extent to which homeostasis is intact and operational. Since these values are expected to be maintained in narrow physiologic ranges, high or low values (hypercalcemia or hypocalcemia, respectively) indicate a perturbation or failure of homeostatic mechanisms. Therefore, it is essential to recognize that serum/plasma calcium measurements do not provide a reliable measure of calcium intake or calcium status (i.e., the extent to which an individual is in an appropriate calcium balance).

HOMEOSTATIC REGULATION OF CIRCULATING AND TISSUE DISTRIBUTIONS OF CALCIUM

Calcium homeostasis is primarily controlled by two interacting hormones—vitamin D and PTH. The integrated effects of PTH on distal renal tubular calcium reabsorption (within minutes) and bone resorption (over hours), and the effects of the active metabolite of vitamin D on intestinal calcium absorption (over days), serve two primary goals in the fetus and newborn—to ensure appropriate accrual of calcium to enable skeletal growth and development, and to maintain the serum calcium concentration within a narrow physiologic range (see Fig. 26.1).

PARATHYROID HORMONE

PTH is a peptide hormone released by the parathyroid glands in response to decreases in the serum ionized calcium concentration detected by calcium-sensing receptors (CaSR) on parathyroid cells.[9] PTH mobilizes calcium by binding the type 1 PTH receptor (PTH1R) in its two primary target tissues—bone and kidney. PTH directly stimulates bone resorption through a variety of putative mechanisms, including the upregulation of the receptor activator of nuclear factor κB (NF-κB) ligand (RANKL), which leads to the differentiation of osteoclasts, and downregulation of osteoprotegerin, a RANKL inhibitor.[10] In the kidney, PTH reduces urinary excretion of calcium by its actions in the distal nephron, and promotes the synthesis of 1,25-dihydroxyvitamin D [1,25(OH)$_2$D] from 25-hydroxyvitamin D [25(OH)D] by upregulating the expression of the *CYP27B1* 1-alpha-hydroxylase in proximal renal tubular epithelial cells (see Fig. 26.1).[4]

VITAMIN D

Vitamin D is a steroid hormone precursor that has an essential role in calcium and bone mineral metabolism at all life stages. Vitamin D is obtained from two sources—endogenous production from cutaneous 7-dehydrocholesterol in response to ultraviolet B (UVB) radiation exposure of the skin, or absorption from the intestinal tract following ingestion of foods (including breast milk) or dietary supplements that contain vitamin D.[11] To attain its final biologically active state as 1,25(OH)$_2$D, the parent vitamin

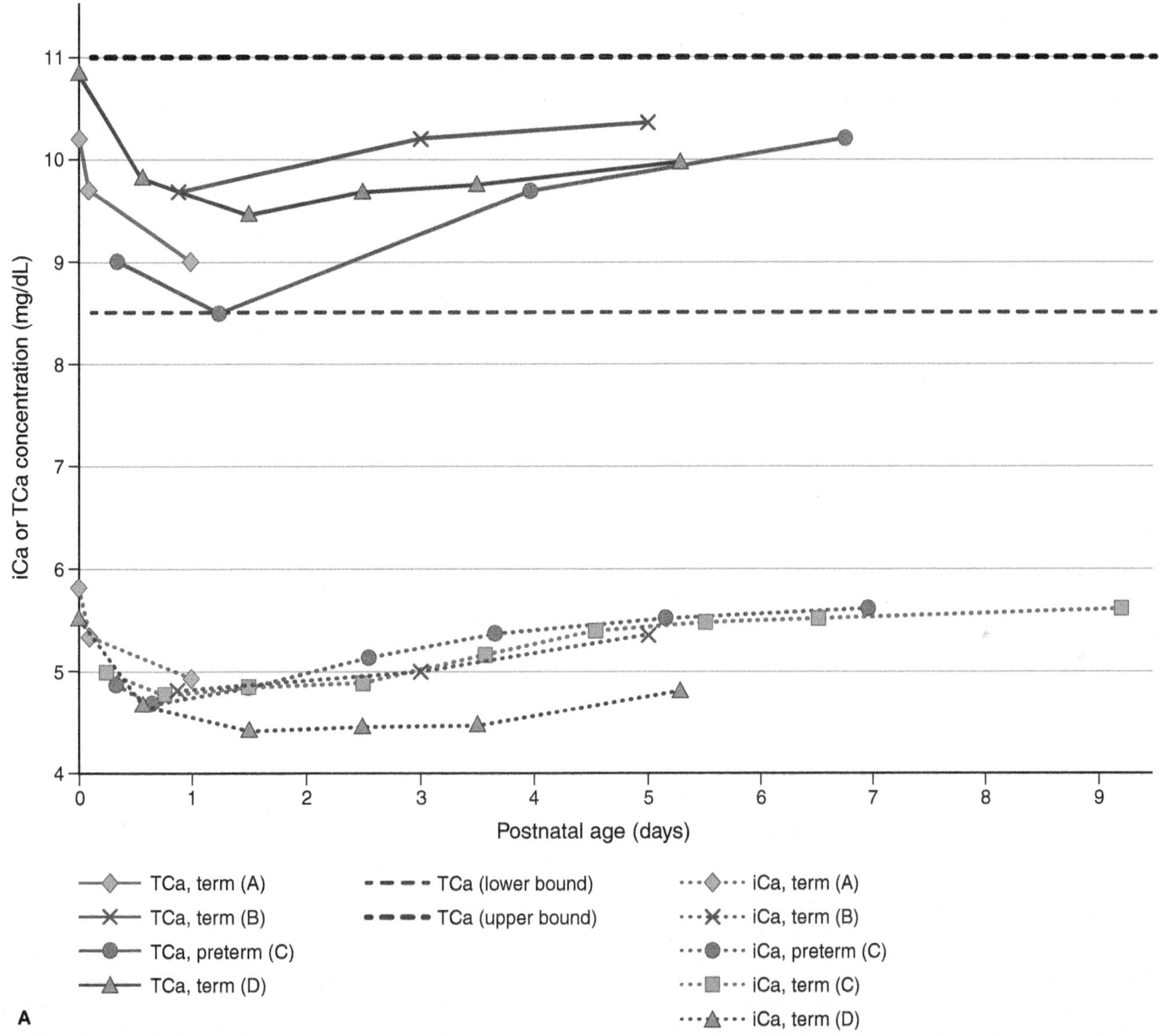

Fig. 26.2 (A) Neonatal whole blood ionized calcium (iCa; *dotted lines*) and serum/plasma total calcium (TCa; *solid lines*) concentrations or (B) serum/plasma magnesium (Mg; *dotted lines*) and phosphate (PO$_4$; *solid lines*) concentrations in the first week of life. Each line connects mean values for a group of term or preterm infants from one of three studies: Loughead and colleagues 1988 (study A; ◆ term), Nelson and colleagues 1987 (study B; × term), Wandrup and colleagues 1988 (study C; ● preterm, ■ term), David and Anast 1974 (study D; ▲ term). Means at 0 days represent cord blood concentrations (studies A and D). Otherwise, means are plotted at the midpoints of reported age ranges. Horizontal dashed lines indicate the lower and upper limits of the pediatric laboratory reference intervals for TCa, PO$_4$, and Mg from the CALIPER study (Colantonio and colleagues 2012). (Data from Loughead JL, Mimouni F, Tsang RC. Serum ionized calcium concentrations in normal neonates. *Am J Dis Child*. 1988;142[5]:516–518; Nelson N, Finnstrom O, Larsson L. Neonatal reference values for ionized calcium, phosphate and magnesium. Selection of reference population by optimality criteria. *Scand J Clin Lab Invest*. 1987;47[2]:111–117; Wandrup J, Kroner J, Pryds O, et al. Age-related reference values for ionized calcium in the first week of life in premature and full-term neonates. *Scand J Clin Lab Invest*. 1988;48[3]:255–260; David L, Anast CS. Calcium metabolism in newborn infants. The interrelationship of parathyroid function and calcium, magnesium, and phosphorus metabolism in normal, "sick," and hypocalcemic newborns. *J Clin Invest*. 1974;54[2]:287–296; and Colantonio DA, Kyriakopoulou L, Chan MK, et al. Closing the gaps in pediatric laboratory reference intervals: a CALIPER database of 40 biochemical markers in a healthy and multiethnic population of children. *Clin Chem*. 2012;58:854–868.)

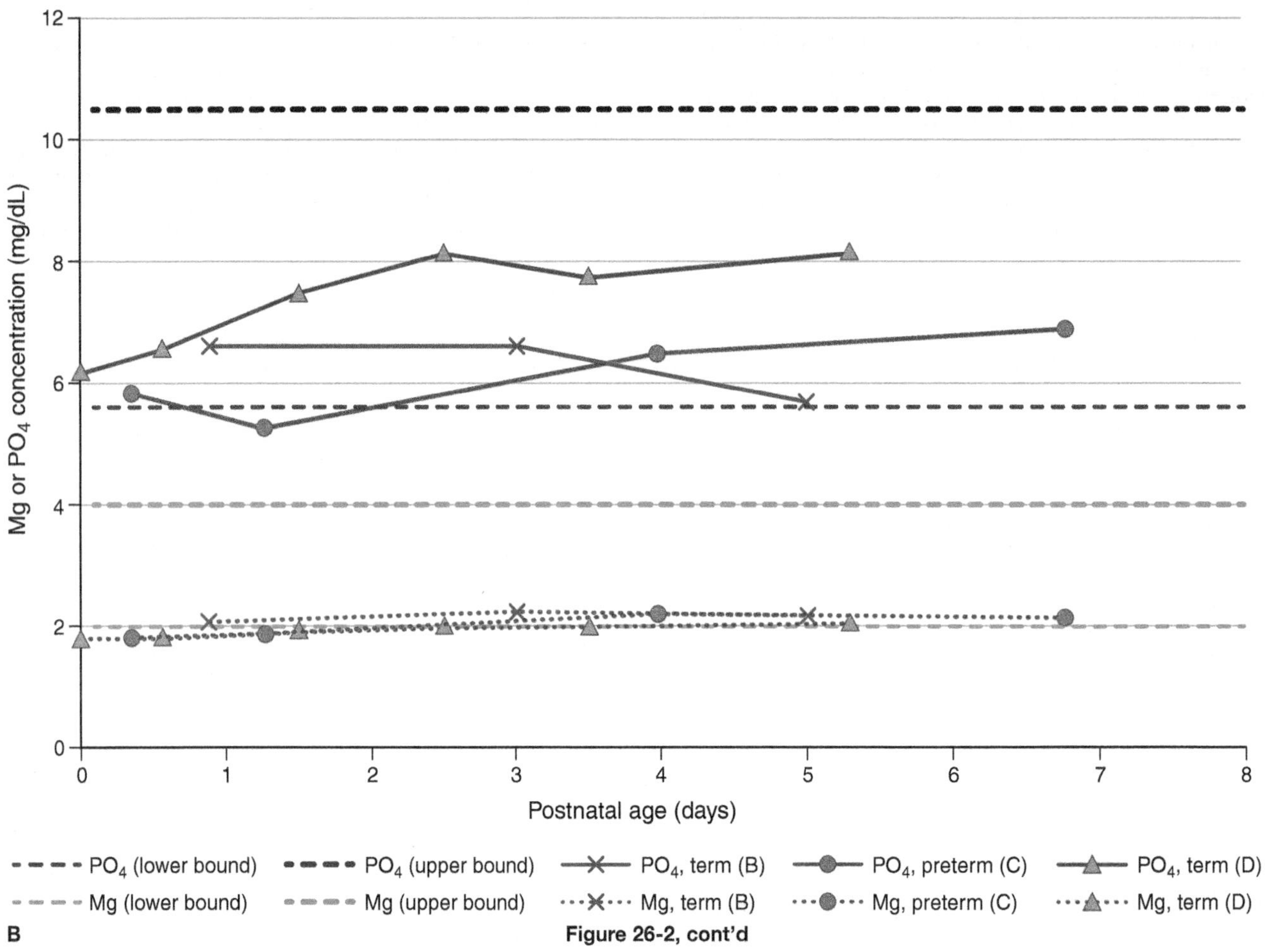

Figure 26-2, cont'd

D molecule (cholecalciferol or ergocalciferol) undergoes a series of two hydroxylation reactions: first, 25-hydroxylation is catalyzed primarily (though not exclusively) by the cytochrome P450 enzyme *CYP2R1* in a relatively unconstrained reaction in the liver, yielding 25(OH)D; then, 25(OH)D circulates to the kidney where the mitochondrial enzyme *CYP27B1* catalyzes the 1-alpha-hydroxylation reaction that generates $1,25(OH)_2D$. In contrast to 25-hydroxylation, the synthesis and activity of renal *CYP27B1* are tightly controlled by the enhancing effect of PTH (as mentioned earlier) and the downregulatory effects of FGF23, a phosphaturic hormone described in more detail below, and by $1,25(OH)_2D$ itself in a classical feedback loop (see Fig. 26.1).[11,12]

Vitamin D activity in target tissues is primarily mediated by the high-affinity binding of $1,25(OH)_2D$ to the vitamin D receptor (VDR), which is widely distributed. Numerous genes include VDR-binding sites and are responsive to $1,25(OH)_2D$-regulated gene transcription.[11] Vitamin D metabolites are primarily catabolized and rendered relatively inactive by 24-hydroxylation catalyzed by *CYP24A1*, which is downregulated by PTH and upregulated by FGF23.[11,13] The major circulating vitamin D metabolite is 25(OH) D, a well-established primary biomarker of vitamin D status at all life stages due to its relatively long serum half-life and its empirical responsiveness to recent vitamin D inputs, regardless of route.[14] Although the bulk of the clinical and epidemiologic evidence supporting the use of serum/plasma 25(OH)D as a biomarker is based on studies of adults, there is nonetheless abundant evidence from prenatal and infant vitamin D trials to support its utility in the perinatal period,[15] and in preterm[16-18] and term infants.[19] Although serum 25(OH)D reflects vitamin D status insofar as it is a measure of recent endogenous and exogenous vitamin D inputs, it is otherwise of limited value in providing information about the downstream effects of vitamin D, such as calcium absorption or bone mineral metabolism. There is insufficient evidence to establish serum 25(OH)D reference ranges specific for cord blood or early infancy; however, the lower limits of adequacy that are widely used in adults (25 or 30 nmol/L) are generally applied at all life stages, including the perinatal period.[20,21] Severe vitamin D deficiency, typically manifesting as serum 25(OH)D well below 25 nmol/L, causes vitamin D-deficient rickets (often referred to as *nutritional rickets*), for which the primary clinical manifestations are due to defects in growth plate function and bone mineralization.[22] To prevent infantile rickets, many organizations and national health agencies recommend routine oral vitamin D supplementation of breastfed term and preterm infants.[16,20]

The primary biologically active vitamin D metabolite, $1,25(OH)_2D$, may also be readily measured in serum or plasma, but due to its short half-life and tightly regulated production, $1,25(OH)_2D$ is not an appropriate clinical indicator of systemic vitamin D status or intake.[23] In infancy, measurement of serum/plasma $1,25(OH)_2D$ may be useful in the diagnosis of inborn errors of vitamin D metabolism, such as vitamin D 1-alpha-hydroxylase deficiency caused by mutations in *CYP27B1*,[24] or other rare disorders of calcium handling.[23]

Vitamin D, 25(OH)D, and $1,25(OH)_2D$ in circulation are bound by the vitamin D binding protein (DBP), or to albumin, or exist at very low concentrations as free steroids. DBP, which has much higher affinity for 25(OH)D than albumin, binds about 85% of 25(OH)D compared to 15% bound to albumin and less than 0.1% as the free form. DBP-bound 25(OH)D may be preferentially endocytosed by renal tubular epithelial cells, rendering it available as a substrate for 1-alpha-hydroxylation.[13] Moreover, variability in DBP concentrations and genetic polymorphisms in the gene encoding DBP may contribute to population variability in 25(OH)D concentrations. However, the essential role of DBP in vitamin D metabolism has been questioned, and there is emerging interest in the functional significance of "free" (unbound) 25(OH)D.[13]

Numerous tissues, including the placenta,[25] express both the VDR and the *CYP27B1* 1-alpha-hydroxylase, suggesting local autocrine/paracrine vitamin D functions.[12,26] Placental expression of *CYP2R1, CYP27B1, VDR,* and other genes related to vitamin D metabolism are believed to contribute to the regulation of placental immunomodulation and may influence systemic maternal prenatal vitamin D status[27,28]; however, there is little evidence to suggest an important effect of vitamin D metabolites of *placental* origin on fetal-neonatal calcium homeostasis. Vitamin D (parent compound) itself does not readily cross the placenta, and $1,25(OH)_2D$ in fetal circulation is assumed to be mainly of fetal origin.[29,30] Conversely, maternal 25(OH)D is readily transferred across the placenta, and maternal and cord blood concentrations are highly correlated,[29,31] although possibly to a lesser extent in preterm deliveries.[32] Therefore 25(OH)D of maternal origin is considered to be the major contributor to fetal and early neonatal vitamin D status, outweighing genetic factors.[33] Accordingly, cord blood 25(OH)D concentrations are affected by the same factors that determine maternal vitamin D status, including characteristics that influence the mother's endogenous production of vitamin D (e.g., season, sunlight exposure, latitude, skin pigmentation) and maternal prenatal vitamin D intake from diet and supplement use.[34-36]

Numerous prenatal vitamin D supplementation trials have proven that improvements in maternal vitamin D status are associated with concordant increases in neonatal vitamin D stores, as reflected by cord blood or early neonatal 25(OH)D concentrations.[15,21,37] However, the effect of maternal-fetal 25(OH)D transfer is transient, as infant vitamin D status is largely dependent on postnatal inputs by about 2 months of age.[38] In the postnatal period, cutaneous production and oral intake contribute to vitamin D status, similar to older children and adults. Breast milk was traditionally assumed to be a poor source of vitamin D, but it is now accepted that the breast milk vitamin D metabolite content (primarily the concentration of vitamin D itself) is a function of maternal vitamin D intake, such that relatively high maternal intakes of vitamin D can maintain physiologic 25(OH)D concentrations in breastfeeding infants.[39] Newborns, including those born preterm, have full capacity to absorb vitamin D and carry out the serial hydroxylation reactions that convert vitamin D to 25(OH)D and $1,25(OH)_2D$, even in the first few days of postnatal life.[18] Thus physiologic immaturity of the vitamin D metabolic pathway is not usually considered to be a factor that impairs early neonatal calcium handling.

There has been considerable interest in C3-epimers of 25(OH)D and $1,25(OH)_2D$ (C3-epi-25(OH)D and C3-epi-$1,25(OH)_2D$, respectively) based on the observation of relatively high concentrations of C3-epi-25(OH)D in infants compared to other life stages.[40] Maternal prenatal C3-epi-25(OH)D increases through pregnancy,[41] but does not appear to efficiently cross the placenta, such that fetal C3-epi-25(OH)D is generated primarily within the fetal-placental unit from maternally derived 25(OH)D; however, neither maternal nor fetal C3-epi-25(OH)D accounts for the relatively high concentrations of infant C3-epi-25(OH)D, suggesting neonatal generation of the epimer from infant 25(OH)D or epimerized vitamin D.[42] C3-epimers of vitamin D can be metabolized analogously to their corresponding non-epimeric forms, but bind the VDR relatively weakly; therefore C3-epi-$1,25(OH)_2D$ may lack some of the conventional functional attributes of $1,25(OH)_2D$.[40]

OTHER HORMONE REGULATORS OF CALCIUM HOMEOSTASIS

Calcitonin was historically portrayed as a major factor in bone mineral homeostasis, but this has not been supported by accumulated evidence in humans. In the early newborn period, calcitonin was found to be unresponsive to changes in serum calcium.[43] Conversely, there has been substantial interest in the calcium-regulating role of FGF23, a phosphaturic factor produced by bone (described in detail later in relation to phosphate homeostasis). The secretion of FGF23 is upregulated by $1,25(OH)_2D$, and its primary target organ is the kidney, where FGF23 acts to increase urinary phosphate excretion and inhibit renal $1,25(OH)_2D$ synthesis. Data suggest that FGF23 may also interfere with $1,25(OH)_2D$-mediated intestinal calcium absorption[44]; however, the physiologic relevance of this effect in humans is unknown.

FETAL CALCIUM ACCRETION AND HOMEOSTASIS

Fetal calcium accrual occurs throughout gestation but is particularly important in the third trimester, not only because accrual is a direct function of total body weight, but also because total body calcium becomes a progressively greater fraction of fetal body weight at later gestational ages.[45,46] The rate of skeletal calcium deposition peaks at about 35 weeks of gestation, reaching approximately 130 mg/kg/day.[47] About 26 to 30 g of calcium are accrued by the time of term delivery.[45,48]

The increase in the rate of fetal calcium accrual during gestation is paralleled by a gradual increase in the calcium concentration in fetal circulation (as indicated by cord blood serum concentrations) (Fig. 26.3).[49] Fetal (umbilical cord blood) serum calcium concentrations are correlated with—but consistently higher than—their corresponding maternal concentrations in both preterm and term infants (Fig. 26.4). The existence of a steep concentration gradient underscores the necessary presence of active transport mechanisms responsible for efficient maternal-fetal calcium transfer. The regulation of active transplacental calcium transport has been the subject of long-standing inquiry, particularly with respect to its responsiveness to maternal and fetal vitamin D status. Evidence from animal models suggests

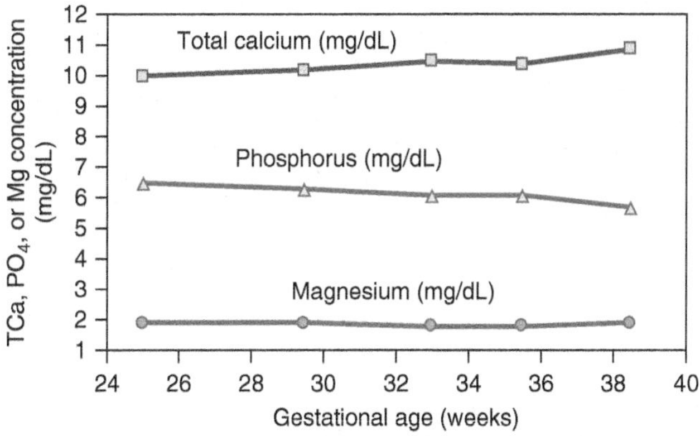

Fig. 26.3 Mean cord blood serum concentrations of total calcium, phosphate, and magnesium by gestational age. Values are plotted at the midpoints of the reported gestational age range across which data were aggregated. (Data from Fenton TR, Lyon AW, Rose MS. Cord blood calcium, phosphate, magnesium, and alkaline phosphatase gestational age-specific reference intervals for preterm infants. *BMC Pediatr.* 2011;11:76.)

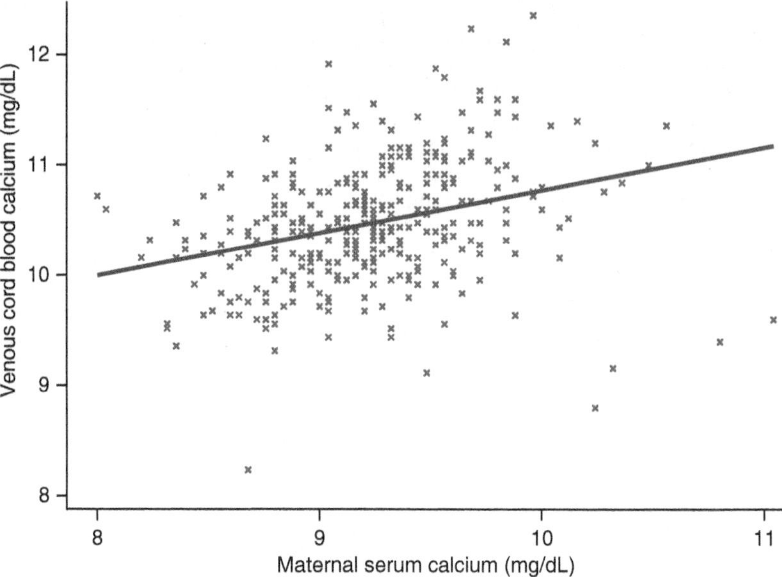

Fig. 26.4 Venous umbilical cord blood and maternal prenatal serum calcium concentrations in mother-infant pairs for whom maternal blood samples were collected within 6 hours preceding delivery (n = 335), from a vitamin D trial cohort in Dhaka, Bangladesh. Mean (standard deviation) calcium concentration was 10.4 (0.56) mg/dL in cord blood and 9.2 (0.44) mg/dL in maternal samples. The solid line represents the linear fit; maternal-cord correlation coefficient, r = 0.31. Among term and preterm infants (n = 315 and 20, respectively), 98% and 95%, respectively, had higher cord serum calcium concentrations than the corresponding maternal sample. Findings were similar when analyses were limited to participants in the placebo group (not shown). (Data from Roth DE, Morris SK, Zlotkin S, et al. Vitamin D supplementation in pregnancy and lactation and infant growth. *N Engl J Med.* 2018;379:535–546.)

that both parathyroid-hormone related protein (PTHrP) and PTH regulate transplacental calcium flux via their binding to the PTH/PTHrP receptor.[50-52] Accordingly, animals and human neonates with inactivating PTH/PTHrP receptor mutations develop severe chondrodysplasias in utero.[53] Endogenous fetal PTH is capable of regulating fetal calcium concentrations, but its expression is normally suppressed by the relatively high fetal calcium concentration, mediated by the CaSR.[54] However, the regulation of placental mineral transport by PTH or PTHrP has not been well characterized in humans, and newer evidence suggests that fetal serum calcium concentrations may be further directly influenced by other PTH-independent mechanisms of calcium influx into fetal bone.[55]

The presumed mechanism of active transplacental calcium transport is remarkably similar to that involved in intestinal calcium absorption (described below), in that it is a three-step process involving uptake of calcium by the trophoblasts via the transient receptor potential vanilloid type 6 (TRPV6) cation channel,[56] intracellular shuttling of calcium through the trophoblast by calbindin-D9k, and extrusion at the basolateral aspect into the ECF by a Ca^{2+}-ATPase (Fig. 26.5; Table 26.1). Skeletal abnormalities in fetuses with *TRPV6* mutations suggest a dominant role for this calcium-selective channel in third trimester transplacental calcium transport in humans.[57] The similarities between intestinal and transplacental calcium transport mechanisms raise the possibility that active transplacental transfer would be responsive to maternal-fetal vitamin D status, as in the intestine. However, rodent studies generally do not support the direct dependency of transplacental calcium transport, fetal calcium homeostasis, or fetal skeletal development on fetal VDR or 1,25(OH)$_2$D expression.[30,58] Moreover, findings from animal models are consistent with observations of relatively normal skeletons and serum calcium concentrations in newborns with mutations in *VDR* or *CYP27B1*.[24]

Maternal vitamin D metabolites may affect fetal calcium balance by mechanisms that are independent of fetal VDR expression.[30] VDR-independent effects of 1,25(OH)$_2$D on fetal trophoblast expression of TRPV6 or Calbindin-D9k[30,58,59] remain to be fully characterized, but may occur via 1,25(OH)$_2$D binding of protein disulfide isomerase family A member 3 (PDIA3), also known as the *1,25D3-membrane associated, rapid response steroid binding protein (1,25D3-MARRS)*.[30] In addition, vitamin D in the maternal circulation appears to influence the extent to which circulating maternal calcium is rendered available for transfer to the fetus. In humans, some randomized controlled trials of high-dose maternal vitamin D supplementation in pregnant women have demonstrated that vitamin D slightly increases cord blood calcium concentrations.[60,61] Consistent with animal models, this effect seems to be attributable to increases in maternal serum calcium availability, rather than a direct effect of vitamin D on the rate of transplacental calcium flux.[61] Notably, even if vitamin D can directly or indirectly increase transplacental calcium flux, human fetuses appear to be protected against hypercalcemia, even in the context of maternal hyperparathyroidism and elevated fetal 25(OH)D.[60]

CALCIUM HOMEOSTASIS IN THE IMMEDIATE POSTNATAL PERIOD

At birth, the abrupt termination of the maternal-to-fetal calcium supply chain via the placental and umbilical cord necessitates an urgent transition to postnatal mechanisms that serve to maintain serum calcium in a physiologic range as well as promote bone growth and mineralization. Numerous longitudinal studies have described the typical pattern of changes in serum ionized and total calcium that occur in most preterm and term infants during the first several days of lifean initial decline in the first 48 hours, followed by a rebound and then stabilization over the rest of the first week of life (see Fig. 26.2A).[18,61-65] Some otherwise healthy infants do not experience the classic postnatal nadir and therefore may appear to have unusually high serum calcium values by the end of the first week of life, but this usually normalizes by the second or third week.[61] Most infants mount an effective PTH response to the natural first-week nadir in serum calcium, as demonstrated by a spiking increase in the PTH concentration in the immediate postnatal period, which attenuates as the calcium concentration stabilizes.[66] Even in very low-birth-weight (VLBW) infants (<32 weeks; <1500 g), PTH increased as calcium declined in the first few days of life, and the pattern was reversed following a bolus infusion of calcium.[43] Impaired parathyroid gland responsiveness may therefore account for the exaggerated postnatal hypocalcemia (which may be symptomatic) that occurs in some newborns.[65,67,68] The reason for blunted PTH responses in these infants is unknown but has been related to severe maternal vitamin D deficiency.[67,69] In contrast to the uncertain

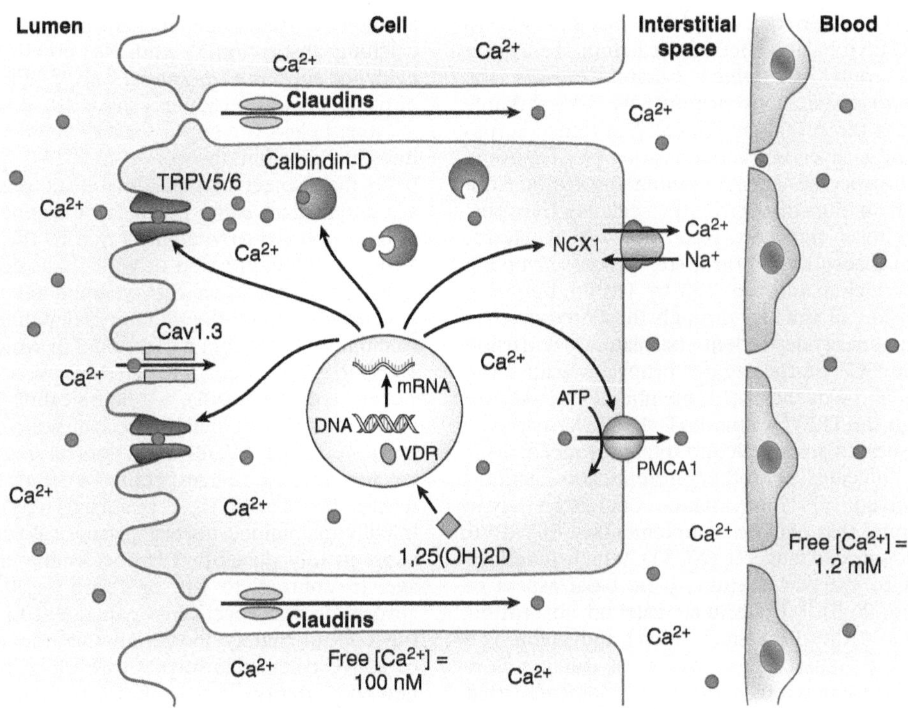

Fig. 26.5 Schematic representation of active transcellular calcium transport mechanisms in the placenta, intestine, and kidney. In all three organs, active transcellular transport is a three-step process involving apical surface uptake of calcium into the cell (trophoblast, enterocyte, or renal tubular epithelial cell), shuttling through the cell by a carrier protein, and extrusion at the basolateral surface into the interstitial space. Paracellular pathways described in the intestine and nephron are also shown. *1,25(OH)₂D*, 1,25-dihydroxyvitamin D; *ATP*, adenosine triphosphate; *Cav1.3*, L-type apical calcium channel; *NCX1*, sodium-calcium exchanger 1; *PMCA1*, plasma membrane Ca2+-ATPase 1; *TRPV5/6*, transient receptor potential vanilloid 5 and 6; *VDR*, vitamin D receptor. (Adapted from Nijenhuis T, Hoenderop JGJ, Bindels RJM. TRPV5 and TRPV6 in Ca2+ (re)absorption: regulating Ca2+ entry at the gate. *Pflugers Arch—Eur J Physiol.* 2005;451:181–192; and Diaz de Barboza G, Guizzardi S, Tolosa de Talamoni N. Molecular aspects of intestinal calcium absorption. *World J Gastroenterol.* 2015;21[23]:7142–7154.)

Table 26.1 Overview of Calcium, Phosphorus, and Magnesium in Serum/Plasma and Their Principal Ion Transport Mechanisms.

	Serum/Plasma Fractions (%)			Circulating Free Ions in Serum/ Plasma	Active Transport			
Mineral	**Protein-Bound**	**Salt Complexes**	**Free Ions**		**Cellular Uptake**	**Intracellular Transit**	**Basolateral Extrusion**	**Passive Transport**
Calcium	40	10	50	Ca^{2+}	TRPV5 TRPV6 Cav1.3	Calbindin-D9k	PMCA1 NCX1	Claudin-2 Claudin-5 Claudin-15
Phosphorus	15–17	33–35	50	HPO_4^{2-} $H_2PO_4^-$	NaPi-IIa NaPi-IIb NaPi-IIc PiT2	Undefined	Undefined	Unspecified tight junction proteins
Magnesium	20–30	5–15	55–70	Mg^{2+}	TRPM6 TRPM7	Undefined	Undefined	Claudin-16 Claudin-19

NaPi-II, Sodium-phosphate transporter type II; *NCX1*, sodium-calcium exchanger 1; *PiT2*, sodium-phosphate transporter type III; *PMCA1*, plasma membrane Ca^{2+}-ATPase 1; *TRPM*, transient receptor potential melastatin; *TRPV*, transient receptor potential vanilloid.

role of vitamin D in calcium homeostasis in utero, there is strong evidence that vitamin D plays a critical role in regulating serum calcium homeostasis in the immediate postnatal period.[18] In fact, randomized controlled trials of maternal prenatal vitamin D supplementation have consistently demonstrated that higher newborn vitamin D status attenuates the physiologic postnatal infant nadir in serum calcium in the first week of life, without an apparent increase in the risk of infantile hypercalcemia.[60,61,70] It remains unclear whether this early postnatal effect of vitamin D is primarily a result of the rapid mobilization of calcium from bone or direct effects of vitamin D on intestinal calcium absorption.

INTESTINAL CALCIUM ABSORPTION

CELLULAR MECHANISMS OF CALCIUM ABSORPTION

Beginning in the postnatal period, the gastrointestinal tract assumes its major importance in calcium homeostasis by providing the only physiologic route of calcium intake, as well as by regulating the relative balance between calcium absorption and excretion. The routes by which calcium crosses the intestinal mucosa into systemic circulation have a remarkably similar architecture as those that govern calcium transit across the placental trophoblast layer, as described earlier (see Fig. 26.5). Two major transport processes enable calcium absorption from the intestinal lumen in humans: active transcellular transport and passive paracellular transport (see Table 26.1). Active transcellular calcium absorption is a three-step process involving the apical entry of calcium into the cell by TRPV6, buffering and facilitated diffusion of calcium through the enterocyte by calbindin-D9k, and energy-dependent basolateral extrusion of calcium into the ECF of the lamina propria—against the electrochemical gradient—by the plasma membrane Ca^{2+}-ATPase 1 (PMCA1). Although the TRPV6-calbindin-D9k-PMCA1 pathway is the most well-described active calcium transport mechanism, emerging evidence indicates that other proteins and channels are also likely involved.[71,72] These include Cav1.3, an L-type apical calcium channel that may be complementary to TRPV6, and the sodium-calcium exchanger 1 (NCX1), which functions similarly to PMCA1 to extrude calcium at the basal aspect of enterocytes (see Fig. 26.5).[73] Paracellular calcium absorption, which predominates in the distal small bowel and colon, is a passive diffusional and nonsaturable process of calcium flow via tight junctions.[71,74] Numerous studies have indicated that paracellular calcium absorption may be regulated; for example, claudins are intercellular components of tight junctions that modulate paracellular permeability and calcium transport, and their expression may be modulated by vitamin D.[71,73]

In older children and adults, the duodenum displays the highest rate of intestinal calcium absorption as it primarily expresses the cellular machinery for active transport of calcium from the lumen to the extracellular space; yet, due to its longer length, the distal small bowel (primarily the ileum) is likely where the majority of ingested calcium is absorbed. Nonetheless, there remains considerable uncertainty about the relative contributions of transcellular (active) versus paracellular (passive) routes, or proximal versus distal sites of calcium uptake, particularly in early infancy. Early evidence suggested that calcium absorption in preterm infants is primarily a nonsaturable function of calcium intake, and thus primarily dependent on paracellular mechanisms,[75] whereas active transport mechanisms are underdeveloped at birth and mature in the early postnatal period.[76,77] However, studies of a piglet model suggested that active transport mechanisms are indeed present in the immediate postnatal period, but are vitamin D-independent.[78,79] More recent insights into the age-related dynamics of calcium absorption were revealed by a mouse study showing that transcellular transport mediated by TRPV6 and Cav1.3 was present in the distal small bowel rather than the duodenum prior to weaning; notably, the pattern was reversed after weaning age, when the duodenum acquired—and the distal small bowel lost—the capacity for active TRPV6-mediated transcellular transport.[72] However, the extent to which these findings are applicable to humans remains unknown.

REGULATORS OF CALCIUM ABSORPTION IN THE NEWBORN

Vitamin D in its activated form—$1,25(OH)_2D$—upregulates all three steps of the TRPV6-calbindin-D9k-PMCA1 active transport mechanism, therefore serving as a primary pathway by which vitamin D exerts direct effects on calcium homeostasis in humans (see Fig. 26.5). The VDR is expressed throughout the small and large intestine, suggesting the plausibility of $1,25(OH)_2D$-regulated calcium absorption in distal as well as proximal bowel segments.[71,74] Moreover, local conversion of 25(OH)D to $1,25(OH)_2D$ in the intestinal mucosa may represent an autocrine/paracrine mechanism by which vitamin D regulates calcium absorption.[80] And, as noted previously, additional evidence supports a potential role of vitamin D in the regulation of paracellular diffusion of calcium.

Nonetheless, the importance of vitamin D in the regulation of intestinal calcium absorption in the early newborn period has been the subject of considerable debate. Animal studies have suggested that early postnatal intestinal calcium absorption is unresponsive to vitamin D due to the initial absence of the VDR, the full expression of which was not found to occur until 4 weeks postnatal in the weaning rat pup.[81] Schroeder and colleagues studied the vitamin D-dependency of early neonatal calcium absorption in a pig model in which renal production of $1,25(OH)_2D$ is absent, referred to as pseudo-vitamin D-deficiency rickets, type I (PVDRI).[78,79] Significantly increased net calcium fluxes across duodenal mucosal samples were observed in both newborn PVDRI and control piglets, indicating active calcium absorption irrespective of the availability of $1,25(OH)_2D$ during the first 3 to 4 postnatal weeks. The PVDRI piglets initially maintained normal plasma calcium concentrations, but subsequently developed hypocalcemia and rickets at weaning age. In contrast to the newborn period, active net calcium absorption was absent in weaned PVDRI piglets but present in the control piglets, indicating that the vitamin D-dependency of active calcium absorption develops beyond the immediate newborn period.[78,79] In both rodents and humans with a congenital absence or defect of the VDR,[82,83] signs of rickets appear in the post-weaning period (mice) or at variable ages after the newborn period (humans), indicating that either vitamin D-mediated calcium absorption is non-essential in the immediate postnatal period or that vitamin D acts by VDR-independent mechanisms during this early period. Humans may have the capacity for vitamin D-dependent active calcium absorption at an earlier age than suggested by rodent studies. Yet, few human studies have directly examined calcium absorption in response to varying intakes of vitamin D in the preterm or newborn periods. In a study of preterm infants (mean gestational age at birth of 32 weeks), Senterre and Salle found that both human milk- and formula-fed infants who received supplementary vitamin D had greater fractional calcium absorption at 2 to 4 weeks of age compared to infants without vitamin D supplements, supporting the presence of vitamin D-dependent transport mechanisms even before term age[84]; however, a later study did not corroborate this effect of vitamin D.[75] Therefore, although the early postnatal responsiveness of calcium absorption to vitamin D—and its essentiality—in human newborns remains unclear, it is nonetheless evident that vitamin D has an important overall role in the newborn's ability to regulate serum calcium concentration during the period of rapid transition from placental to intestinal sourcing of calcium.

Calcium absorption may be influenced by a wide range of other hormones, drugs, and intraluminal components (Table 26.2).[85-87] Variation in such factors likely contributes to the substantial age-related changes and between-infant variability in intestinal calcium absorption, but few in vivo studies have clarified the physiologic relevance of these factors in newborns. Early studies suggested that fractional calcium absorption was higher in breast milk- versus formula-fed preterm infants[77,84]; however, this has not been a consistent finding.[88,89] Understanding these potential differences is challenged by the multitude of dissimilarities between human milk and formula, including the current standard of incorporating relatively high concentrations of calcium in commercial formulas.

There has been substantial interest in the potential modifying effects of dietary carbohydrates and lipids on calcium bioavailability in infancy. In one trial, the presence of lactose in infant formula was shown to significantly increase fractional and total calcium absorption in healthy, full-term infants 8 to 12 weeks

Table 26.2 Promoters and Inhibitors of Intestinal Calcium Absorption.

	Promoters	Inhibitors
Hormones and drugs	• Vitamin D • Growth hormone • Estrogen • Prolactin	• Glucocorticoids • FGF23 • Theophylline • Neurotoxins (e.g., tetrodotoxin)

Dietary and intraluminal factors	• Amino acids
	• Carbohydrates
	  ◦ Monosaccharides (glucose, galactose)
	  ◦ Disaccharides (lactose)
	  ◦ Oligosaccharides
	• Bile salts
	  ◦ Ursodiol (ursodeoxycholic acid)
	  ◦ Lithocholic acid (indirect effect by preventing the inhibitory effect of sodium deoxycholic acid)
		• Iron
		• Tannin
		• Phytate
		• Oxalate
		• Fructose
		• Bile salt: sodium deoxycholic acid
		• Palm olein (compared to other long-chain triglycerides)

FGF23, Fibroblast growth factor 23.
Data from Fleet JC, Schoch RD. Molecular mechanisms for regulation of intestinal calcium absorption by vitamin D and other factors. *Crit Rev Clin Lab Sci.* 2010;47:181–195; and Christakos S, Dhawan P, Porta A, et al. Vitamin D and intestinal calcium absorption. *Mol Cell Endocrinol.* 2011;347:25–29.

of age.[90] The putative mechanism by which lactose influences calcium absorption is unclear but may involve the stimulation of active transcellular transport mechanisms[91] or a phenomenon known as *solvent drag*, whereby intraluminal molecules that increase osmolality, such as carbohydrates, drive paracellular fluid shifts in which calcium is an incidental passenger.[85] Partial substitution of long-chain triglycerides with medium-chain triglycerides in infant formula was not found to affect calcium absorption.[92] However, some evidence indicates that the long-chain fatty acid composition of infant formula affects calcium absorption or retention; in particular, palm olein (a form of palmitic acid added to many infant formulas) has been shown to decrease calcium retention, possibly due to the formation of insoluble and indigestible palmitic acid-calcium complexes.[93] Bile salts appear to affect calcium absorption, but the direction of effect depends on the specific salt (see Table 26.2).[94]

Apart from the type or composition of the milk, feeding strategies may also influence calcium absorption and/or retention in the early postnatal period. For example, in a randomized controlled trial of different methods of introducing early feeds in preterm VLBW infants, Schanler and colleagues found that early gastrointestinal priming (i.e., introducing human milk or formula at 20 mL/kg/day from days 4 to 14) was associated with higher calcium retention (104 mg/kg/day) compared to the group that had received only parenteral nutrition until day 14 (78 mg/kg/day); these differences were evident at 6 weeks of age but attenuated by 9 weeks of age.[95] The mechanism for this transient effect is unknown, but the authors proposed that it may reflect a form of "early programming" of mineral absorption.[95]

CALCIUM BALANCE IN NEWBORNS

Calcium balance refers to the aggregated effects of calcium intake, absorption, and excretion.[48] During fetal and infant growth, the balance should always be positive, reflecting the net calcium retention that enables bone accretion. Abrams and others have applied a straightforward, yet empirically useful, model to understand calcium balance in infants that takes into account the amount of oral calcium ingested, the fractional absorption (i.e., proportion of ingested calcium that is absorbed by the intestine), endogenous fecal excretion (i.e., calcium that is secreted into the intestinal lumen, apart from the ingested calcium that remains unabsorbed), and urinary calcium excretion (Fig. 26.6). The net amount of calcium retained is assumed to be deposited in the skeleton, and bone resorption at this age is considered to be negligible.[88,96]

To accommodate rapid skeletal growth rates during early infancy, newborn calcium requirements are relatively high compared to older age groups, with an adequate intake (AI) of 200 mg/day recommended for the term infant, based on estimated average intake from breast milk.[48] For the preterm VLBW infant, 150 to 220 mg/kg/day is recommended by the American Academy of Pediatrics (AAP) (see Fig. 26.6),[47] although the requirement is lower (120 to 140 mg/kg/day) according to the European Society for Paediatric Gastroenterology, Hepatology, and Nutrition (ESPGHAN).[97]

Several studies have yielded estimates of average fractional calcium absorption rates of 50% to 60% in healthy preterm and term infants.[88,89,96] Accounting for losses due to endogenous secretion into the intestine and urinary excretion (both of which are greater in early infancy compared to adults), average overall retention is slightly less than 50% of the ingested amount.[47] Therefore, in preterm infants, intakes of more than 200 mg/kg/day may be required to achieve the in utero calcium accretion requirements of over 100 mg/kg/day.[47] However, there is considerable unexplained between-infant variation in the efficiency of calcium absorption, intestinal secretion, and net retention.[77,88] In theory, the physiologic need for calcium drives the homeostatic regulation of fractional calcium absorption, intestinal secretion, and urinary excretion in response to variations in calcium intake. Yet, studies of preterm infants have not concluded that fractional calcium absorption or intestinal secretion respond in a predictable manner to changes in oral calcium intake. Using dual tracer stable isotope methods, Abrams and colleagues[88] and Hillman and colleagues[77] demonstrated that net calcium retention in preterm infants is primarily a function of the total amount of calcium absorbed, and that increases in intake did not lead to substantial decreases in fractional absorption.

A study of children aged 3 to 14 years found that endogenous fecal calcium excretion averaged 1.4 ± 0.4 mg/kg/day and was lower than urinary calcium excretion.[98] In contrast, in LBW infants fed a high-calcium formula, Abrams and colleagues found that endogenous fecal calcium excretion averaged 15 ± 9 mg/kg/day (7.2% ± 4.1% of intake) and was greater than concurrent urinary calcium excretion.[88] Similarly, Hillman and colleagues found that endogenous fecal calcium excretion in LBW infants

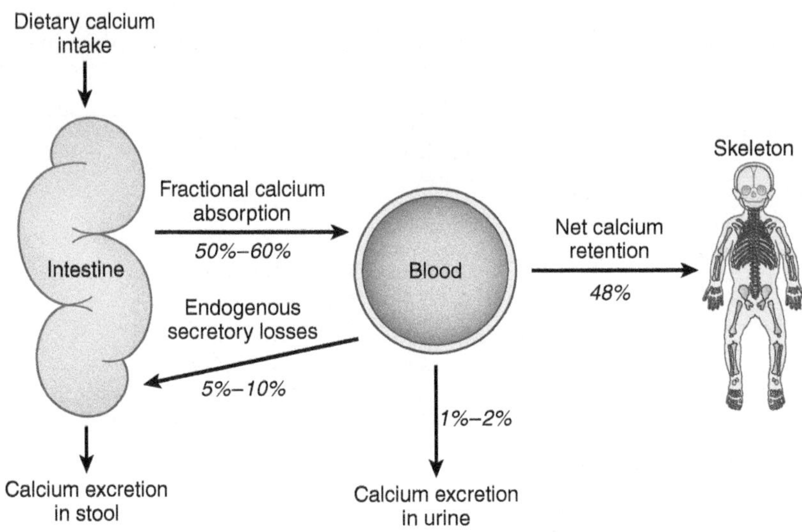

Fig. 26.6 Conceptual model of calcium balance in the newborn. To maintain the equivalent of the estimated rate of third-trimester in utero calcium accretion (approximately 100 to 130 mg/kg/day), a preterm infant would require an estimated dietary intake of up to approximately 220 mg/kg/day elemental calcium.[47] (Figure and estimates based on data from Abrams SA, Esteban NV, Vieira NE, et al. Dual tracer stable isotopic assessment of calcium absorption and endogenous fecal excretion in low birth weight infants. *Pediatr Res.* 1991;29:615–618; Abrams SA. Calcium absorption in infants and small children: methods of determination and recent findings. *Nutrients.* 2010;2:474–480; and Hicks PD, Rogers SP, Hawthorne KM, et al. Calcium absorption in very low birth weight infants with and without bronchopulmonary dysplasia. *J Pediatr.* 2011;158:885–890.)

fed preterm formula with differing calcium contents ranged from 6.9 to 19.0 mg/kg/day, compared to an average excretion rate of 5.1 mg/kg/day in infants fed human milk.[77] Both studies found that endogenous fecal calcium excretion was not related to the amount of calcium ingested or absorbed, suggesting that intestinal secretion may not function as a homeostatic mechanism of adapting to an unnecessarily high calcium intake in preterm infants; and, in both studies, intestinal secretion was a minor contributor to variations in net retention, although the individual factors that govern intestinal secretion remain unclear.[77,88]

In both preterm and term newborns, urinary calcium excretion is initially very low but increases rapidly in the second week of life and remains stable thereafter for several months, at higher levels than is observed in older children after adjusting for glomerular filtration rate (GFR).[99,100] Compared to older children and adults, renal calcium reabsorption is relatively undeveloped in newborns, particularly in preterm and VLBW infants.[76] Consequent hypercalciuria is therefore an important contributor to the elevated incidence of nephrocalcinosis in preterm infants.[101]

Urinary calcium excretion is tightly regulated but may not greatly contribute to overall calcium balance in infancy. Most of the calcium that enters the nephron is reabsorbed through paracellular routes in the proximal tubule (70%) and thick ascending limb (20%), and the remainder in the distal nephron.[76] Mechanisms of transcellular and paracellular calcium reabsorption in the distal nephron are remarkably similar to those involved in transplacental transport and intestinal absorption; and, similar to the intestine, active transport in the distal convoluted tubule is upregulated by vitamin D and PTH (see Fig. 26.5). However, in the distal renal tubule, the transient receptor potential vanilloid 5 (TRPV5) is probably the dominant apical calcium channel,[102] whereas TRPV6 appears dominant in the intestine.

PHOSPHORUS

BODY DISTRIBUTION AND MEASUREMENT OF PHOSPHORUS

Phosphorus is a widely distributed element in intra- and extracellular compartments of the human body and, among minerals, is second only to calcium in terms of its overall abundance.[103] In newborns, phosphorus constitutes approximately 0.5% of total body weight, which increases to 1% in adults.[104,105] Phosphorus is an essential structural component of the nucleotides that comprise DNA and RNA, phospholipids that form the lipid bilayer of cell membranes (e.g., phosphatidylcholine), and the mineral matrix that, with calcium, provides stability and strength to bones and teeth.[104] Phosphorus is involved in numerous important biochemical processes, including energy storage and transfer (primarily as adenosine triphosphate [ATP]), cell signaling and regulation (i.e., protein phosphorylation), and intracellular buffering that is essential for the maintenance of physiologic acid-base balance in blood.[104] Whereas phosphorus is the name of the element itself, the term phosphate (PO_4^{3-}) refers to a free inorganic phosphorus-containing anion that exists in an approximate 4:1 ratio of HPO_4^{2-} to $H_2PO_4^-$ in blood at a normal pH of 7.4.[106]

Similar to calcium, the majority (approximately 85%) of total body phosphorus is found in the bone matrix as hydroxyapatite and, to a lesser extent, as amorphous bone crystals formed by more loosely complexed calcium-phosphate salts.[105] Skeletal integrity is therefore dependent upon the simultaneous homeostatic regulation of calcium and phosphorus. The remaining 14% of total body phosphorus is widely distributed throughout the soft tissues, and approximately 1% is present in blood and ECF. Serum (or plasma) phosphate concentrations therefore reflect only a limited portion of total body phosphorus and may not be a reliable indicator of total body phosphorus stores.[106,107] Intracellular phosphate is present in organic compounds such as ATP, or as free monovalent and divalent inorganic phosphate anions ($H_2PO_4^-$ and HPO_4^{2-}), whereas cell membrane phosphorus exists predominately as organic phosphate esters (e.g., membrane phospholipids).[107] About half of all phosphorus in serum/plasma is in the form of free inorganic phosphate ions, about one-third is a component of sodium, calcium, and magnesium salts, and the remaining 15% to 17% is bound to plasma proteins.[108,109]

As phosphorus is present in many forms, and the ratio of HPO_4^{2-} to $H_2PO_4^-$ in serum/plasma is dependent on blood pH, measured phosphate is typically expressed as the mass of elemental phosphorus (i.e., millimoles per liter or milligrams per deciliter), rather than milliequivalents per liter (mEq/L).[106] Serum inorganic phosphate, the most widely measured indicator of phosphate status, is found in relatively high concentrations of 5.6 to 10.5 mg/dL (1.8 to 3.4 mmol/L) in the first 2 weeks after birth compared to the rest of infancy (≥15 days to end of first year), when the reference range is 4.8 to 8.4 mg/dL (1.6 to 2.7 mmol/L).[110] Though typically not reflective of dietary phosphate intake, fasting measurements are recommended where possible to limit the within-individual fluctuations caused by diurnal variations.[107] In the preterm infant, lower phosphorus stores are associated with higher risks of metabolic bone disease of prematurity[111] and hyperglycemia in neonates of extremely LBW.[112] Umbilical cord concentrations do not differ by sex,[113] but phosphate concentrations in both term and preterm infants often fluctuate in the initial days after birth (see Fig. 26.2B).[18,65,114] In contrast to the rapid postnatal response of serum calcium to PTH, the relationship between serum phosphate and PTH is inconsistent.[65,67,68] Rather, intra- and interindividual variations in serum phosphate may reflect an adaptation to feeding practices and/or the mineral composition of parenteral feeds[115-117]; as for calcium, these short-term dynamics are not reflected in published pediatric reference values.[110]

HOMEOSTATIC REGULATION OF PHOSPHORUS

Homeostatic regulation of phosphorus is primarily achieved by three mechanisms: intestinal uptake, bone recycling, and renal reabsorption—collectively forming a gastrointestinal-bone-renal network that operates via negative feedback loops involving PTH, FGF23, Klotho (co-receptor of FGF23), and vitamin D.[118,119] As such, the endocrine regulation of phosphorus is closely integrated with that of calcium, functioning to maintain an optimal calcium-phosphate balance.

PARATHYROID HORMONE

PTH is the most well-characterized of the known hormonal regulators of phosphate homeostasis. PTH adjusts renal phosphate clearance by regulating the abundance of sodium-dependent transport proteins that control phosphate transit and proximal tubular reabsorption. Elevations in PTH induce the internalization of NaPi-IIa at the brush border to sub-apical compartments by means of a clathrin-mediated endocytotic pathway that ultimately leads to transporter degradation by lysosomes.[120] As such, reabsorption of phosphate is inhibited at high levels of circulating PTH, resulting in increased urinary phosphate excretion. The tubular maximum for phosphate reabsorption (TmP) is inversely related to PTH; increased phosphate excretion due to elevated PTH is, therefore, a function of a reduction in the TmP.[104]

Earlier evidence for the direct regulation of PTH by serum phosphate was shown in a study of weanling rats, in which hypophosphatemia induced by a low dietary phosphorus intake led to a reduction in PTH mRNA levels in parathyroid cells, and a lower concentration of circulating PTH, even under conditions of normal serum calcium and $1,25(OH)_2D$ concentrations.[121] Further studies demonstrated that the effect of phosphate on PTH mRNA is a post-transcriptional effect; phosphate stabilizes PTH mRNA by promoting the binding of cytosolic proteins to its 3′-untranslated terminus; in contrast, calcium inhibits binding of PTH mRNA to parathyroid proteins, accelerating its degradation and, therefore, reducing the synthesis of PTH.[122]

FIBROBLAST GROWTH FACTOR 23

Belonging to the peptide-hormone family known as *phosphatonins*, FGF23 is a 251-amino acid glycoprotein[123] that is biologically active in its intact form and plays a key role in bone mineral metabolism.[124] Now considered a major contributor to the postnatal bone-renal regulation of phosphate homeostasis,[124,125] FGF23 was first identified as the underlying cause of autosomal dominant hypophosphatemic rickets (ADHR), a rare disorder caused by an inheritable *gain-of-function* mutation of the gene encoding FGF23, which inhibits its inactivation.[123] FGF receptors (FGFRs) are present in numerous tissues, primarily in bone (osteoclasts and osteoblasts),[126] but downstream intracellular signaling is governed by a co-receptor, the transmembrane protein Klotho.[127] Functioning in a negative feedback loop, release of FGF23 from bone is triggered by high levels of $1,25(OH)_2D$; FGF23 acts on *CYP27B1* and *CYP24A1* to downregulate renal $1,25(OH)_2D$ activation and upregulate $1,25(OH)_2D$ catabolism, respectively (see Fig. 26.1).[11,13] The interplay of PTH and FGF23 controls the renal handling of phosphate by inhibiting sodium-dependent transport in the proximal tubule.[128] However, in chronic phosphorus deficiency, the prolonged calcium-phosphate imbalance is insufficient to yield adequate mineralization of the osteoid. The disruption of the calcium-phosphate balance is a shared characteristic of heritable FGF23-mediated phosphate wasting disorders, of which X-linked hypophosphatemia is the most common heritable form of rickets and osteomalacia.[129] Previously referred to as *vitamin D resistant rickets*, X-linked hypophosphatemia results from mutations in the *PHEX* (phosphate-regulating endopeptidase homolog, X-linked) gene. Expressed primarily in bone, loss of *PHEX* induces an increased expression of FGF23.[130] X-linked hypophosphatemia is characterized by elevations in circulating FGF23, hyperphosphaturia, and low or normal $1,25(OH)_2D$ concentrations; its clinical manifestations present in early life and include skeletal deformities and linear growth faltering. Novel human monoclonal antibodies that directly inhibit FGF23 show promising results in the treatment of X-linked hypophosphatemia, as evidenced by improvements in growth velocity and biochemical markers of bone turnover (including increased serum phosphorus, renal phosphate reabsorption, and serum $1,25(OH)_2D$), relative to conventional therapy.[131]

Beyond its interactions within the vitamin D-calcium endocrine system, FGF23 also has an important direct down-regulatory effect on phosphate reabsorption that is independent of PTH and $1,25(OH)_2D$.[125,132] In 2012 Andrukhova and colleagues[133] showed that binding of intact FGF23 to FGFR-Klotho complexes in the renal proximal tubule results in the phosphorylation of extracellular signal-regulated kinase (ERK1/2), which activates the downstream signaling of serum/glucocorticoid-regulated kinase (SGK)-1; phosphorylation of the Na^+/H^+ exchange regulatory cofactor (NHERF-1) by SGK-1 reduces the apical membrane abundance of NaPi-IIa/ NHERF-1 complex. Degradation of NaPi-IIa by lysozymes causes a subsequent rise in urinary phosphate excretion (Fig. 26.7).[133] The characteristics of Klotho deficiency mirror that of FGF23-null young mice (6 weeks), presenting as hyperphosphatemia and a corresponding elevation in serum calcium and $1,25(OH)_2D$.[127]

As with calcium, the skeleton acts as a phosphate reservoir that can be mobilized in response to low phosphate in ECF. Following prolonged phosphate deprivation, NaPi-IIb knockout mice show greater osteoclast activity and a reduction in bone mineral density,[134] such that bone resorption appears to partially compensate for inadequate dietary phosphate. During skeletal formation, alkaline phosphatase (ALP)—an ectoenzyme of osteoblasts—cleaves phosphate from phosphate esters in the plasma membrane to provide free inorganic phosphate to the osteoblast for mineralization of the bone matrix.[119,135] The activity of *bone-specific* ALP is determined by the intracellular need for phosphate in bone cells and is inhibited by calcium and skeletal growth factors, including insulin-like growth factors I and II.[135] Bone-specific ALP (rather than total ALP) is therefore reflective of the rate of bone turnover when monitored over a given time period. In hypophosphatasia, rare *loss-of-function* mutations of the gene encoding the tissue-nonspecific isoenzyme of ALP (TNSALP)[136] lead to an accumulation of inorganic pyrophosphate (an inhibitor of bone matrix mineralization), thereby preventing the formation of hydroxyapatite crystals.[137] The blocked entry of minerals into bone results in irregular calcification, which can manifest in utero in extreme cases.[138] Infantile hypophosphatasia typically presents early in life (<6 months of age) as classical rachitic signs of demineralized bone but, in contrast to nutritional rickets, is accompanied by an elevation in both serum phosphate and calcium.[136,139]

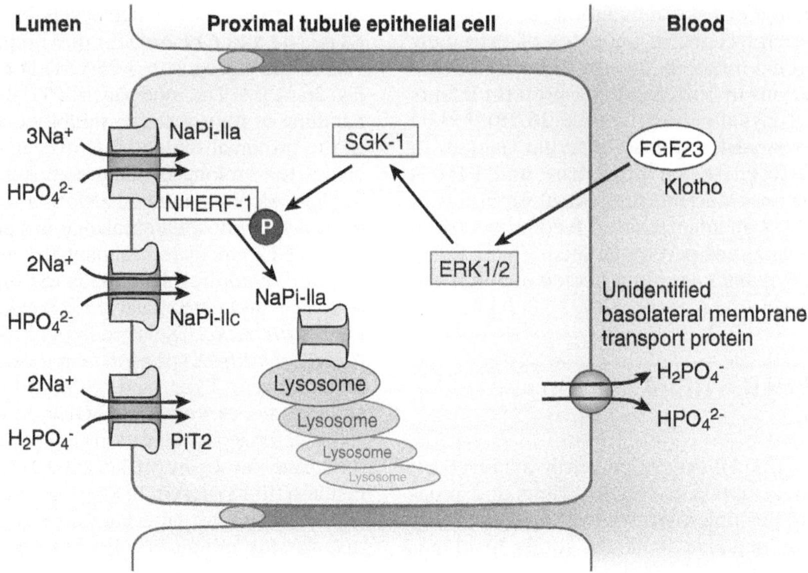

Fig. 26.7 Sodium-dependent transport of phosphate in renal proximal tubule. Active transcellular transport of inorganic phosphate from the luminal filtrate into epithelial cells is mediated by the sodium-phosphate co-transporters NaPi-IIa, NaPi-IIc, and PiT2, and extrusion into the peritubular capillaries by an unidentified basolateral membrane transport protein. Binding of FGF23 to its co-receptor Klotho results in the phosphorylation of ERK1/2 and subsequent activation of SGK-1. Internalization and degradation of NaPi-II- NHERF-1 complexes inhibits phosphate reabsorption. *ERK1/2*, Extracellular signal-regulated kinase; *FGF23*, fibroblast growth factor 23; *NHERF-1*, Na^+/H^+ exchange regulatory cofactor 1; *SGK-1*, serum/glucocorticoid-regulated kinase 1. (Adapted from Wagner CA, Rubio-Aliaga I, Hernando N. Renal phosphate handling and inherited disorders of phosphate reabsorption: an update. *Pediatr Nephrol*. 2019;34[4]:549–559; Blaine J, Chonchol M, Levi M. Renal control of calcium, phosphate, and magnesium homeostasis. *Clin J Am Soc Nephrol*. 2015;10[7]:1257–1272; and Andrukhova O, Zeitz U, Goetz R, et al. FGF23 acts directly on renal proximal tubules to induce phosphaturia through activation of the ERK1/2-SGK1 signaling pathway. *Bone*. 2012;51[3]:621–628).

The complex interplay of PTH, $1,25(OH)_2D$, and FGF23 regulates renal phosphate reabsorption, and these hormones are therefore the central drivers of phosphorus homeostasis. The extent to which other hormones such as glucocorticoids,[134] growth hormone, and insulin (and/or insulin-like growth factors) contribute to renal phosphate handling is unclear[140–142]; glucocorticoids are considered to influence serum concentrations by facilitating mobilization of phosphorus from bone,[134] whereas growth hormone and insulin promote renal phosphate retention and transcellular redistribution, respectively.[106]

FETAL PHOSPHORUS ACCRETION AND HOMEOSTASIS

As with calcium, approximately 80% of the total body phosphorus in term infants is accumulated during the last trimester of pregnancy, at a rate of approximately 75 mg/kg fetal weight/day.[46] Phosphorus accretion is approximately half that of calcium,[46] with the whole body molar ratio of calcium to phosphorus estimated to range between 1.4:1 and 1.9:1. At term, total body phosphorus content is estimated at 16 g.[143] Fetal phosphorus accretion increases with gestational age and is proportional to birth weight, such that total body phosphorus content of a full term neonate weighing 3.2 kg is approximately fivefold higher than an early preterm, extremely LBW (500 g) infant.[46]

Fetal phosphorus accretion is mediated by the transplacental transport of inorganic phosphate against a concentration gradient.[144] Expression of sodium-phosphate transporters in the placental tissue of mice support their involvement in the maternal-fetal phosphorus exchange,[145] but the factors controlling their regulation are unknown. In the placenta, syncytiotrophoblasts are considered to be the main site of soluble α-Klotho expression, which accounts for the finding of higher umbilical cord blood concentrations of α-Klotho in comparison to maternal and neonatal (first week of life) serum.[146] The lower circulating intact FGF23 in cord blood, compared to the maternal circulation,[146,147] is suggested to contribute to the higher serum phosphate concentrations in newborns relative to maternal values.[146] However, despite the expression of FGF23 in the placenta and fetal kidneys, murine models suggest FGF23 may not be essential during fetal development, since both FGF23 and Klotho knockout mice show normal serum phosphate concentrations and similar placental phosphate transport to wild-type mice.[145] Serum α-Klotho concentrations are higher in term-born than premature infants and increase with advancing postnatal age,[148] which may be related to the decline in serum phosphate concentrations that occurs during the newborn period.

RENAL PHOSPHORUS REABSORPTION

In the kidney, phosphate is freely filtered at the glomerulus and then reabsorbed in a tightly regulated, energy-dependent transcellular process that occurs predominantly in the proximal tubule of the nephron (80% to 85%).[149] There is some evidence to support a minor amount of phosphate reabsorption at more distal sites in the nephron (approximately 5%).[150] Overall, renal phosphate reabsorption is highly efficient, such that retention of dietary phosphate intake during hypophosphatemia results in minimal urinary phosphate excretion.[106] During infancy, phosphate excretion, as reflected by the urinary phosphate/creatinine ratio, shows wide intra- and interindividual variation, and is estimated to reach an upper limit (95th percentile) of 5.2 mg/mg in the first 1 to 6 months of life, before declining towards adult values throughout infancy and early childhood.[151] Evidence to define specific reference values for preterm infants is limited, but available data suggest a relatively higher 95th percentile (7.3 mg/mg) than term infants.[152] Phosphate excretion in the initial days after birth varies with feeding practices (i.e., lower in infants receiving parenteral nutrition) and increases due to the age-related decrease in fractional renal tubular reabsorption in the preterm infant in the second week after birth.[116,152]

Renal phosphate transport into tubular cells occurs via a family of sodium-dependent phosphate co-transporter channels that govern the balance between phosphate reabsorption and excretion. Conversely, paracellular flux of phosphate is believed to be of negligible importance.[153] Transport of inorganic phosphate from the luminal filtrate into epithelial cells is therefore dependent on the energy generated by movement of sodium down its concentration gradient (see Fig. 26.7).[149] At least two types of sodium-phosphate co-transporters are expressed in the kidney and facilitate phosphate reabsorption in the proximal tubule: NaPi-IIa and NaPi-IIc (Na-Pi type II transporters encoded by the *SLC34A1* and *SLC34A3* genes, respectively), and PiT2 (NaPi type III transporters encoded by the *SLC20A2* gene). Phosphate uptake in the proximal tubule represents the rate-limiting step in the reabsorption process,[119] and is determined by the relative expression of these transporters at the apical brush border.[154-156] Murine models have shown that increases in phosphate reabsorption parallel the upregulation of renal sodium-phosphate co-transporters and correspond to a decrease in urinary phosphate excretion.[156] Conversely, high dietary phosphate downregulates co-transporter expression[156,157] to conserve the serum calcium-phosphate balance. *Loss-of-function* mutations in renal phosphate transporters result in excess urinary phosphate excretion, secondary $1,25(OH)_2D$-induced hypercalciuria and impaired bone mineralization that often presents in infancy.[158,159]

Both NaPi-IIa- and NaPi-IIc-mediated transport are important in humans, despite animal studies showing only a modest role for NaPi-IIc in renal phosphate handling.[160] While there are no reported disorders of phosphate handling related to mutations in PiT2,[161] mutations in type II co-transporters have been documented as causes of renal phosphate wasting in patients with hereditary hypophosphatemic rickets, Fanconi syndrome, or idiopathic infantile hypercalcemia.[158,159,162,163] Whereas NaPi-IIc facilitates the transport of divalent phosphate anions (HPO_4^{2-}) via an electroneutral transport cycle (i.e., two sodium cations are transported with one divalent phosphate anion resulting in a 2:1 Na^+:P_i stoichiometry),[164,165] NaPi-IIa co-transporters function by an electrogenic transport cycle that involves the net translocation of one positive charge per cycle (3:1 Na^+:P_i stoichiometry).[165] The different sensitivities of the transporters to protons directly affect transport kinetics; as PiT2 shows higher substrate affinity for $H_2PO_4^-$ anions, efficiency of PiT2-mediated transport is considered greater at lower pH, whereas type II transporters operate at neutral body pH of ~7.0 to 7.4.[166] In juvenile rats (6 to 8 weeks), upregulation of PiT2-mediated transport observed during metabolic acidosis indicates a pH-induced adaptation to renal phosphate regulation, while the increased expression of PiT2 in response to low dietary phosphate suggests a compensatory mechanism for maintaining phosphate homeostasis during phosphate deprivation.[160] However, the overall extent to which PiT2 can offset a dysfunction of type II transporters in humans is so far incompletely understood.

The mechanism by which phosphate is extruded from the proximal tubular cells into the peritubular capillaries has not yet been identified (see Fig. 26.7).[149] The Retrovirus Receptor XPR1 has been suggested as a candidate basolateral membrane protein responsible for transport of phosphate into the blood,[167] but its function and regulation in humans remain to be fully characterized.

Dietary phosphate intake regulates renal tubular reabsorption by promoting the expression of type II co-transporters during phosphate restriction and downregulating their expression in response to a high phosphate load.[161] In vivo studies of weanling rodents (mice[154] and rats[168]) fed low-phosphorus diets demonstrated that upregulation of NaPi-II expression was attributable to an increased transcriptional rate[154] or mRNA stability,[168] thereby enabling a compensatory increase in renal phosphate reabsorption. However, in a study of juvenile rats (6 to 8 weeks old) who switched from a high- to low-phosphate diet, there was a rapid increase in NaPi-II abundance in the proximal tubular brush border membrane prior to an increase in mRNA levels, suggesting a posttranslational mechanism of rapid adaption to low-phosphate intake.[157] The 2020 study by Motta and colleagues showed that NaPi-IIb mRNA expression in adult mice is unaffected by acute or chronic changes in phosphate intake, corroborating the earlier finding that renal adaption to dietary phosphate occurs at a post-transcriptional level.[169]

Tubular reabsorption is a saturable process, such that phosphorus homeostasis is maintained by excretion of phosphate into the urine when serum phosphate concentrations surpass the renal threshold. The renal reabsorptive capacity of phosphate (often expressed as a ratio of the tubular maximum reabsorption rate of phosphate to GFR, or TmP/GFR) is dependent on the systemic phosphorus need; for example, the relatively high TmP/GFR in newborns (1.43 to 3.43 mmol/L) reflects increased mineral requirements for growth, which gradually decrease throughout childhood and adolescence.[170] Abnormalities in renal phosphate handling (i.e., hypo- or hyperphosphaturia) are important causes of inadequate or excess total body phosphorus, for which monitoring of the TmP/GFR may be a useful indicator of phosphate reabsorption.[170]

INTESTINAL PHOSPHORUS ABSORPTION

In contrast to its predominant role in the regulation of calcium, the intestine has a relatively minor role in phosphate homeostasis. Intestinal phosphate absorption is highly efficient, such that absorption in neonates typically exceeds 80% of total phosphate intake.[171-174] Absorption occurs primarily in the proximal small intestine by paracellular (passive) and transcellular (active) pathways (see Table 26.1). Passive diffusion of phosphate in the small intestine occurs through tight junctions, dependent upon electrochemical gradients; however, the underlying mechanisms that govern paracellular phosphate absorption remain unclear.[175] Transcellular phosphate absorption relies on sodium-dependent active transport mechanisms at the enterocyte brush border membrane and is considered an adaptive mechanism that responds to changes in dietary phosphate intake.[175] In contrast to the dominant role of NaPi-IIa and NaPi-IIc co-transporters in the renal tubule, murine models have demonstrated that expression of NaPi-IIb in the small intestine is primarily responsible for active intestinal phosphate transport and is regulated independently by both dietary phosphate intake and $1,25(OH)_2D$.[176-178] Transcellular absorption of phosphate via sodium-dependent channels in humans occurs predominantly in the duodenum and ileum, whereas expression of NaPi-IIb in the jejunum is minimal.[179] In mice, low dietary phosphate induces a reciprocal upregulation of NaPi-IIb in the jejunum and ileum, alongside increased transcriptional activity of NaPi-IIb mRNA across the entire small intestine, suggesting that NaPi-IIb-mediated absorption of phosphorus is particularly relevant at low dietary phosphate intakes.[176] However, corresponding to the proposed translocation mechanisms in renal tubular cells, more recent observations in weanling pigs suggests the response of intestinal sodium-dependent transport to dietary phosphate restriction involves a posttranslational mechanism, whereby an elevation in the abundance of the NaPi-IIb at the enterocyte brush border facilitates increased phosphate absorption.[180] Despite the relative importance of NaPi-IIb-dependent transport in animals, mutations of *SLC34A2* (gene encoding NaPi-IIb) in humans tend to present in childhood or later, with characteristic pulmonary pathology rather than features of hypophosphatemia,[181] indicating that NaPi-IIb is not essential for phosphate homeostasis, possibly due to compensation by another transporter such as NaPi-IIa.[182]

Since hypophosphatemia induces renal 1,25(OH)$_2$D production, regulation of intestinal phosphate absorption via NaPi-IIb was originally considered a function of crosstalk between renal and intestinal homeostatic pathways. Earlier studies described an increase in phosphate uptake following stimulation with 1,25(OH)$_2$D in the presence of a sodium concentration gradient. The saturable, sodium-dependent influx of phosphate into epithelial cells was therefore considered to be dependent upon the renal *CYP27B1*-induced upregulation of 1,25(OH)$_2$D.[183] In later studies, however, the upregulation of both renal NaPi-IIa and intestinal NaPi-IIb in VDR and 1-alpha-hydroxylase knockout mice in response to low dietary phosphate suggested the mechanism for active phosphate absorption is independent of 1,25(OH)$_2$D.[178]

Although the type III NaPi transporters, PiT1 and PiT2, are expressed in the small intestine, their relative contribution to phosphate absorption in humans is unknown. Similar to the compensatory upregulation of PiT2 co-transporters in the renal proximal tubule, rodent studies suggest both PiT1 and PiT2 proteins are present in the intestinal brush border membrane, but there is conflicting evidence for an increase in their expression during phosphate deprivation.[184,185] The site-specific action of these proteins (i.e., ileum, duodenum, or jejunum) and time-course of response (i.e., acute vs. chronic dietary phosphate deficiency) in humans have not been clearly established.[175]

Other physiologic regulators of intestinal phosphorus absorption have been suggested, including epidermal growth factor,[186] estrogen,[187] and others.[119] However, their relative importance under normal conditions of phosphate intake and handling (i.e., in the absence of related disease states) is not well characterized. Despite the high efficiency of intestinal phosphate absorption, nutrient-nutrient interactions (e.g., reduced intestinal phosphate absorption at high calcium intakes[188]) and elemental phosphate complexes (i.e., the phosphate matrix) are important determinants of phosphate bioavailability in infants at risk of phosphate depletion, specifically those who require specialized nutritional support.

PHOSPHORUS BALANCE IN THE NEWBORN AND EARLY INFANT PERIOD

Unlike the phosphorus equilibrium maintained in later life (i.e., when urinary phosphorus excretion equals that of intestinal phosphorus absorption),[170] growth periods require a positive phosphate balance to support bone mineral accretion and soft tissue formation.[104] Dietary recommendations for phosphate are therefore age-dependent and closely related to calcium, considering a molar calcium-to-phosphorus intake ratio of 1.4:1 to 1.9:1; the highest net requirements (mg/kg/day) correspond to peak growth phases during infancy.[104,107] Although the phosphate concentration of human milk is relatively low, breast milk phosphate is highly bioavailable, and therefore phosphorus deficiency is not generally a concern in otherwise healthy, exclusively breastfed, vitamin D-replete infants.[104] Dietary recommendations for phosphate in early infancy (0 to 6 months) were established according to a mean phosphate content of breast milk of 124 mg/L and an assumed breast milk intake of 780 mL/day, corresponding to an AI of 100 mg/day.[104] To reduce the risk of metabolic bone disease, ESPGHAN recommendations for the premature VLBW infant are 60 to 90 mg/kg/day, to achieve a calcium-to-phosphorus ratio of 1.5:1 to 2.0:1.[97] Although a slightly higher intake range of 75 to 140 mg/kg/day is recommended by the AAP,[47] both European and North American guidelines for enteral nutrition in the preterm infant advise that the calcium-to-phosphorus intake ratio be maintained below 2.1:1 to optimize mineral retention. For parenteral nutrition, 2018 guidelines by ESPGHAN advise a lower molar calcium-to-phosphorus ratio for preterm infants in the first few days of life to reduce risk of early postnatal hypophosphatemia and hypercalcemia.[189]

There are minimal differences in phosphate concentration of breast milk between mothers of pre- and term-born infants[190]; however, dietary requirements in preterm infants are dependent on the need to compensate for the under-mineralization of bone in utero, and hence phosphate fortification of breast milk or specialized infant formulas is required to reduce the risk of metabolic bone disease of prematurity.[111] Early studies showed a high efficiency of intestinal phosphate absorption in both pre- and full-term neonates (approximately 80% to 95%),[171-174] but uptake is dependent on the phosphate matrix. Dietary organic phosphorus requires enzymatic hydrolysis to release phosphate ions and is less readily absorbed than inorganic phosphorus salts.[107,191] Phosphorus in early soy-based formulas had low bioavailability as it was primarily bound within phytate/phytic acid complexes and, therefore, unavailable for absorption. Concerns raised in the 1980s about poor bone mineralization in infants receiving soy-based formulas[192,193] have been allayed by subsequent changes in commercial soy formula compositions.[194,195]

MAGNESIUM

BODY DISTRIBUTION AND MEASUREMENT OF MAGNESIUM

Magnesium is the 11th most abundant element in the human body and second most abundant intracellular cation (after potassium). Acting as a cofactor for more than 300 enzymatic reactions, magnesium is required in numerous processes related to cell growth and proliferation.[196] For example, through its involvement in ATP synthesis, magnesium contributes to the regulation of energy storage and transfer.[197] In addition, magnesium facilitates the active transport of calcium and potassium across cell membranes, thereby serving a key role in muscle and nerve function.[198]

Total body magnesium is widely distributed in bone (approximately 50%) and as an intracellular constituent of muscle (approximately 30%) and soft tissues (approximately 20%), with less than 1% in the ECF, mostly in serum and red blood cells.[199] In bone, magnesium is present within the mineral matrix and on the crystal surface of hydroxyapatite. Compared to calcium, a substantial fraction (about one-third in adults) of the magnesium in bone is in the surface pool and therefore freely exchangeable with extracellular magnesium.[200] The decrease in the size of this exchangeable pool from early infancy likely reflects changes in the rate of bone turnover and skeletal formation.[201] Endogenous losses in urine and feces govern whole body magnesium balance; in the absence of mineral wasting disorders, a positive magnesium balance in infants supports normal growth and development. Irrespective of mode of feeding, fecal excretion is higher than urinary magnesium output in both healthy preterm and term infants and is therefore a major determinant of overall magnesium retention.[202]

Serum magnesium exists in three forms: as the free ionized Mg^{2+} cation (55% to 70%), which is the physiologically active form; bound to protein (20% to 30%); or as magnesium-anion complexes, including magnesium-phosphate salts (5% to 15%).[196] The majority (~60% to 70%) of protein-bound magnesium is coupled to albumin, and the remaining fraction is bound to serum globulins.[203] In adults, albumin and magnesium are directly related to one another at low- and high-albumin concentrations, but uncorrelated when albumin is in the physiologic range of 39 to 45 g/L.[203]

Despite being widely measured in clinical practice, the serum magnesium concentration does not predictably respond to changes in magnesium intake (thereby putting in question its use for deriving dietary reference values[204]), shows variable agreement between commercially available laboratory assays,[8] and is generally considered an unreliable biomarker of overall magnesium status.[205] As magnesium concentrations are higher in red blood cells than serum, hemolysis may artifactually increase serum magnesium concentrations.[196] Serum concentrations in newborns are highly variable, but generally fall within the adult reference interval (1.82 to 2.33 mg/dL[206]). The Canadian Laboratory Initiative on Paediatric Reference Intervals (CALIPER) study found that the upper limit of the pediatric reference interval was elevated in the first 2 weeks of life (1.99 to 3.94 mg/dL), and overall the range in children was slightly higher than for adults[110]; however, reference intervals remain undefined for extremely- and very-preterm infants.[207] Serum magnesium concentrations in umbilical cord blood are similar to (and correlated with) their corresponding maternal values[207] but are not consistently associated with gestational age (see Fig. 26.3).[207,208] Magnesium concentrations of neonates whose mothers received prenatal magnesium supplementation are higher than those without supplementation, consistent with the higher maternal concentrations in supplemented women.[207] In both preterm and term infants, serum magnesium has been observed to increase slightly in the first 3 days after birth and stabilize thereafter (see Fig. 26.2B).[63-65,208-210] Urinary excretion of magnesium follows a circadian rhythm[211]; therefore, urinary magnesium excretion over 24 hours may be a useful indicator of magnesium wasting.[196,199]

HORMONAL REGULATION OF MAGNESIUM HOMEOSTASIS

Similar to calcium and phosphorus, homeostatic control of magnesium is based on the relative influx and efflux of magnesium in the intestinal tract, kidneys, and skeleton by both passive and active transport (see Table 26.1).[212] However, the hormonal mechanisms involved in the systemic regulation of serum magnesium are less clearly understood than for calcium and phosphorus.

PARATHYROID HORMONE

Regulation of PTH by magnesium mirrors the calcium-induced inhibition of PTH by activating the CaSR, a G-protein-coupled receptor that is sensitive to both calcium and magnesium ions.[213] Magnesium therefore directly influences PTH secretion, albeit at a lower potency than extracellular calcium. Urinary magnesium excretion is increased at low PTH and is induced by hypermagnesemia.[214] As serum magnesium concentrations tend to remain normal in primary hyper- or hypoparathyroidism, additional physiologic factors must compensate for disturbances in PTH-meditated regulation of renal magnesium handling.[214] In cases of severe hypomagnesemia, a "paradoxical block" in PTH secretion has been observed,[215] resulting in a rare disorder of secondary hypocalcemia that may present in early infancy and which is reversible upon administration of magnesium.[216,217]

VITAMIN D

In contrast to its central role in calcium and phosphorus homeostasis, vitamin D appears to have a minor role in the regulation of serum magnesium concentrations. Based on site-specific perfusion studies, administration of $1,25(OH)_2D$ to healthy adults increased jejunal but not ileal magnesium absorption.[218] Kladnitsky and colleagues in 2015 showed that claudin-mediated renal tubular transport of magnesium, both in vivo and in vitro, was inhibited by $1,25(OH)_2D$.[219] The authors suggest the renal response to $1,25(OH)_2D$ is a compensatory mechanism by which the kidney adapts to increased intestinal magnesium absorption,[219] such that the net effect of $1,25(OH)_2D$ on magnesium balance is likely minimal. In extremely preterm infants (≤32 weeks' gestation) with refractory hypocalcemia, serum magnesium and calcium were unrelated, and unaffected by intramuscular treatment with $1,25(OH)_2D$. Conversely, there is some evidence that magnesium affects vitamin D metabolism. In vitro analyses have shown activation of the major hydroxylase enzymes involved in vitamin D metabolism (1-alpha-hydroxylase, and 24-hydroxylase) are influenced by magnesium, such that serum $1,25(OH)_2D$ is reduced in the context of magnesium deficiency.[220-222] Albeit limited, some clinical trial data also support a direct influence of magnesium supplementation on circulating 25(OH)D.[223]

CALCITONIN

Although its role in calcium homeostasis is minor, calcitonin is suggested as a major regulator of fetal magnesium homeostasis. In a murine knockout model for genes encoding both calcitonin and calcitonin gene-related peptide-alpha, McDonald and colleagues in 2004 demonstrated that an absence of maternal calcitonin leads to fetal hypomagnesemia and a reduction in skeletal magnesium accretion,[224] but this did not appear to be a result of increased fetal urinary mineral excretion in utero.[224]

FETAL MAGNESIUM ACCRETION AND HOMEOSTASIS

The rate of fetal magnesium accretion gradually increases over the latter half of gestation (weeks 24 to 40 of gestation).[225] Reported fetal accrual rates for magnesium are approximately 5 to 7.5 mg/day[204] (or 3 to 5 mg/kg/day[225]) in the third trimester, resulting in a neonatal total body magnesium content of approximately 0.76 g at term.[143] Circulating magnesium is maintained at similar (or higher) concentrations in umbilical cord (fetal) compared to maternal blood[207] consistent with the existence of an active transport mechanism, as suggested by in vitro perfusion studies of human placentae.[226] To date, the dynamics of the maternal-fetal magnesium exchange remain poorly understood.[227] As noted earlier, transplacental magnesium flux may be regulated by calcitonin,[224] which is expressed in the placenta along with its receptor,[228] but the hormonal regulation of magnesium transfer to the fetus has not been well characterized. The transcellular pathway is dependent upon transient receptor potential melastatin (TRPM) channels, a family of kinase-coupled nonspecific cation channels; in particular, TRPM6 and TRPM7 have been shown to be involved in magnesium transport. In mouse models, active transcellular transport of magnesium is supported by the expression of *TRPM6* mRNA in placental syncytiotrophoblasts and the endoderm cells of the yolk sac.[229] Placental histology of these mice show TRPM6 activity is restricted to syncytiotrophoblasts I (SynT I) cells and is not expressed in SynT II cells, indicating direct active transport from the maternal blood to the fetus. Magnesium depletion in *TRPM6*-null mouse embryos supports a central role for TRPM6-mediated transport of magnesium in utero.[229] However, hypomagnesemia due to human genetic mutations in *TRPM6* is not present at birth but develops in the newborn period or later in infancy,[230,231] suggesting that transplacental magnesium exchange in humans may be maintained adequately by paracellular pathways.[232] TRPM6 activity in trophoblasts is reliant on the formation of a heteromeric complex with TRPM7; whereas TRPM6 is readily inhibited by physiologic intracellular concentrations of magnesium and magnesium bound to ATP (and TRPM7 is inhibited by elevated magnesium-ATP), the TRPM6/TRPM7 complex appears to operate constitutively irrespective of intracellular magnesium or magnesium-ATP concentrations.[233] TRPM6 and

TRPM7 therefore operate collectively to facilitate fetal magnesium uptake by creating a more robust, heteromeric ion channel.[229,233] Some evidence from mouse models suggests deleterious mutations in *TRPM7* disrupt embryonic development in a manner unrelated to magnesium uptake.[234]

INTESTINAL MAGNESIUM ABSORPTION

Similar to calcium and phosphorus, intestinal magnesium absorption involves both passive and active transport mechanisms. Passive (paracellular) absorption in the distal small intestine is determined by the luminal magnesium concentration and is the primary means of intestinal magnesium uptake, whereas the active transport of magnesium is a tightly regulated, saturable process induced at low magnesium intakes and usually reflects only a modest component of overall dietary absorption.[149] Paracellular uptake is mediated by the transepithelial electrical voltage and is dependent upon the permeability of tight junctions.[149,235] As with calcium, the claudin family of tight junctional proteins are believed to play an integral role in magnesium absorption; however, the detailed mechanisms of paracellular magnesium transport in the intestine have not been well characterized.[235] Unlike in the nephron, claudin-16 and claudin-19 are not expressed in the intestine and therefore do not control intestinal magnesium flux.[236]

In contrast to the small intestine, comparatively little magnesium absorption occurs in the colon, where it is mainly an active rather than passive process.[149] Active transcellular transport of magnesium follows a similar three-step pattern to calcium, involving receptor-mediated apical entry, intracellular transit, and basolateral extrusion. The precise mechanism of basolateral extrusion of magnesium in the intestine is unknown but is believed to rely on a magnesium-sodium exchange system. Uptake at the apical brush border of enterocytes is mediated by the TRPM6 and TRPM7 divalent cation transport channels,[235] which form complementary heteromeric complexes to facilitate magnesium influx.[237] *TRPM6*-knockout mice show higher fecal magnesium excretion compared to wild-type mice, which is not accompanied by a compensatory increase in magnesium reabsorption. The lower skeletal magnesium content in *TRPM6*-knockout mice is therefore considered a function of reduced magnesium uptake from the colon, rather than excess renal loss.[229] However, in both humans and mice, magnesium supplementation can overcome effects of loss of TRPM6 function,[229] likely by relying on passive mechanisms of absorption.

Hereditary mutations in the *TRPM6* gene result in impaired intestinal magnesium absorption as well as renal reabsorption, causing severe hypomagnesemia that manifests in early infancy.[230,231,238] Prolonged magnesium depletion is accompanied by a decline in serum calcium that may be a result of hypomagnesemia-inhibited release of PTH.[239] Though rare, more than 30 *loss-of-function* mutations in the *TRPM6* gene have been identified, including stop, frame-shift, and splice-site mutations, as well as deletions of exons, which collectively underlie the autosomal recessive disorder termed *familial (primary) hypomagnesemia with secondary hypocalcemia (HSH)*.[231,232,240]

Mouse models have shown TRPM7 to be essential for normal early postnatal intestinal absorption of magnesium and other divalent cations, including both calcium and zinc.[241,242] Given the lack of known mutations in humans, the distinct relevance of TRPM7 in humans has not been confirmed. However, targeted blocking of the TRPM6/TRPM7 complex in human colonic epithelial cell lines leads to inhibition of magnesium uptake, highlighting the interdependence of TRPM6 and TRPM7 in intestinal magnesium absorption.[243] Hormonal (e.g., insulin, estrogen, and epidermal growth factor) and nonhormonal (e.g., ATP) influences on TRPM expression and channel activity have been proposed, but the precise mechanisms of TRPM6/TRPM7 regulation remain to be determined.[244,245]

RENAL REABSORPTION OF MAGNESIUM

Both pre- and full-term infants show high efficiency of renal magnesium reabsorption, with no evidence to suggest immaturity of tubular reabsorption even in the VLBW infant.[246] In contrast to calcium and phosphorus, the majority (approximately 70%) of renal magnesium reabsorption occurs in the thick ascending limb of the loop of Henle where it is a passive rather than active pathway. Relatively little magnesium is reabsorbed in the proximal tubule (approximately 15%).[212] Despite only modest total magnesium reabsorption occurring in the distal tubule (approximately 10%), renal regulation via TRPM divalent cation channels at this site is considered a principal regulator of magnesium homeostasis.

Proximal tubular reabsorption occurs via the paracellular pathway, mediated by a sodium-dependent concentration gradient that promotes an increased luminal magnesium concentration and luminal-positive electrochemical charge to facilitate transport across epithelial cells.[149] In the loop of Henle, paracellular magnesium reabsorption is driven by the lumen-positive voltage and is regulated by the tight junction membrane proteins, claudin-16 and claudin-19.[149] In patients with familial hypomagnesemia with hypercalciuria and nephrocalcinosis (FHHNC), a rare autosomal recessive disorder, *loss-of-function* mutations in the genes encoding claudins-16 and -19 (*CLDN16* and *CLDN19*, respectively) result in renal wasting of both calcium and magnesium, and subsequent hypomagnesemia and nephrocalcinosis.[247,248] Both in vitro (human embryonic kidney cells) and in vivo (juvenile/young adult mice) models have shown the claudin-16-mediated paracellular transport of magnesium is dependent on magnesium load; reabsorption is upregulated in response to low dietary magnesium.[219,249] Juvenile (8-week-old) mice exposed to parenteral treatment with $1,25(OH)_2D$ showed an increase in urinary magnesium excretion attributed to inhibition of *Cldn16* transcription in the renal tubule that persists even at low magnesium intakes.[219]

Following the passive reabsorption in the proximal tubule and loop of Henle, the remainder of magnesium reabsorption in the distal convoluted tubule occurs predominantly by active transcellular transport. Although mouse models suggest that TRPM6 function is essential in the intestine but may be relatively unimportant in the kidney,[229,250] human *TRPM6* mutations are associated with inappropriately elevated urinary magnesium losses, indicating an essential role of TRPM6 in renal regulation of magnesium balance in humans.[230,238,244] In contrast to TRPM6, luminal uptake of magnesium ions via TRPM7 channels in the distal tubule have been narrowly studied to date and remain incompletely understood.[245] TRPM7 is expressed in the mouse kidney but is not considered essential for renal magnesium reabsorption.[242] In contrast to CLDN16, *TRPM6* transcriptional activity is not influenced by $1,25(OH)_2D$, suggesting the effect of vitamin D on renal magnesium absorption is specific to the paracellular, rather than transcellular, pathway.[219]

While there is currently no known intracellular shuttling mechanism, mitochondria may play a role in buffering intracellular magnesium in the distal convoluted tubule, for which the uptake and extrusion of magnesium in mitochondria is considered to be facilitated by the mitochondrial RNA splicing 2 (MRS2) and solute carrier family 41 A3 (SLC41A3) transport proteins, respectively.[245] Basolateral extrusion of magnesium from the distal tubule may be mediated by a member of the solute carrier family 41 channel, SLC41A1. Though previously considered to operate as a sodium-magnesium cation (Na^+-Mg^{2+}) exchanger,[251] more recent evidence from studies of zebrafish suggested SLC41A1-mediated magnesium transport functions independently of extracellular sodium concentrations.[252]

MAGNESIUM BALANCE IN THE NEWBORN AND EARLY INFANT PERIOD

Efficiency of intestinal magnesium absorption is greater in the newborn period than later life, but is highly variable, ranging from 60% to 85% in studies of term and preterm infants.[253,254] In adults, fractional absorption is inversely related to magnesium intake, displaying a curvilinear absorption-intake relationship that has greatest efficiency at very low intakes.[255] Although a similar relationship has been suggested in infancy (4 to 11 months),[201] labeled isotope studies have not reported the fractional absorption across a range of magnesium doses in the neonatal period.

Intestinal absorption is also dependent upon the solubility of magnesium in the intestine; animal studies show high calcium and phosphate diets result in the formation of insoluble mineral complexes that reduce magnesium bioavailability and absorption,[256] but this is thought to be of minor concern for infants.[253,257,258] Although earlier evidence suggests greater magnesium retention in formula-fed infants,[254] more recent data have shown net magnesium retention (3 to 4 mg/kg/day) in breastfed term-born infants to be almost as high as infants receiving commercial formula,[202] which may reflect changes in formula composition over time. Despite the considerably lower magnesium content in breast milk, lower relative fecal and urinary losses contributed to an overall similar rate of net magnesium retention, irrespective of mode of feeding.[202] Retention as a percentage of intake was therefore shown to be higher in breastfed term infants (approximately 67%) relative to those receiving formula (approximately 41%). Similarly, reduced urinary and fecal output accounted for greater magnesium retention rates in formula-fed preterm (approximately 49%) compared to term infants, with elemental formula composition resulting in the highest overall retention.[202] Like calcium, the type and composition of milk may therefore contribute to the wide variability in magnesium absorption and retention during infancy. However, the limited evidence for interactions between magnesium and other dietary components stems primarily from studies in older children and adults, and the physiologic relevance of these interactions to overall magnesium balance is poorly understood.[259]

As for calcium and phosphorus, dietary magnesium requirements for the healthy term infant are estimated based on mean intakes from breast milk, corresponding to an AI of 30 mg/day.[104] For the preterm VLBW infant receiving enteral nutrition support, a daily intake of 8 to 15 mg/kg was recommended by ESPGHAN.[97]

CONCLUSION

A network of interconnected mechanisms facilitates bone mineral accrual and maintains circulating concentrations of calcium, phosphate, and magnesium in the fetus and newborn. Calcium is primarily controlled by the interactions of vitamin D and PTH, whereas phosphate is also potently regulated by FGF23/Klotho. Although considered to be a minor player in bone mineral metabolism, calcitonin may regulate the transplacental transfer of magnesium. Healthy preterm and term newborns are able to rapidly engage the necessary physiologic mechanisms to safely transition to the postnatal environment, exemplified by functional vitamin D metabolic pathways, the surge in PTH in response to the early postnatal decline in serum calcium, and relatively efficient rates of intestinal absorption and renal reabsorption. Failure of essential feedback mechanisms leads to inappropriately elevated or reduced circulating mineral concentrations that may precede radiologic or morphologic signs of skeletal abnormalities, as bones are progressively resorbed to compensate for insufficient circulating and intracellular mineral stores. Characterizations of numerous inborn errors of metabolism have greatly improved our understanding of the underlying molecular mechanisms of bone mineral homeostasis in humans, thereby complementing insights from animal models. Yet, there remain critical knowledge gaps related to the endocrine regulation of transcellular and paracellular transport of calcium, phosphorus, and magnesium in the placenta, kidneys, and intestines. And, although bone is well recognized as the principal mineral reserve at all life stages, much remains to be learned about the mechanisms by which the skeleton can dynamically respond to mineral requirements and fluctuations in circulating ion concentrations in the growing infant.

A complete reference list is available at www.ExpertConsult.com. 

SELECT REFERENCES

4. Goltzman D, Mannstadt M, Marcocci C. Physiology of the calcium-parathyroid hormone-vitamin D axis. *Front Horm Res.* 2018;50:1-13.
9. Brown EM, Pollak M, Seidman CE, et al. Calcium-ion-sensing cell-surface receptors. *N Engl J Med.* 1995;333(4):234-240.
10. Huang JC, Sakata T, Pfleger LL, et al. PTH differentially regulates expression of RANKL and OPG. *J Bone Miner Res.* 2004;19(2):235-244.
11. Pike JW, Christakos S. Biology and mechanisms of action of the vitamin D hormone. *Endocrinol Metab Clin North Am.* 2017;46(4):815-843.
15. Roth DE, Leung M, Mesfin E, et al. Vitamin D supplementation during pregnancy: state of the evidence from a systematic review of randomised trials. *BMJ.* 2017;359:j5237.
19. Gallo S, Comeau K, Vanstone C, et al. Effect of different dosages of oral vitamin D supplementation on vitamin D status in healthy, breastfed infants: a randomized trial. *JAMA.* 2013;309(17):1785-1792.
27. O'Brien KO, Li S, Cao C, et al. Placental CYP27B1 and CYP24A1 expression in human placental tissue and their association with maternal and neonatal calcitropic hormones. *J Clin Endocrinol Metab.* 2014;99(4):1348-1356.
39. O'Callaghan KM, Taghivand M, Zuchniak A, et al. Vitamin D in breastfed infants: systematic review of alternatives to daily supplementation. *Adv Nutr.* 2020;11(1):144-159.
43. Venkataraman PS, Blick KE, Fry HD, et al. Postnatal changes in calcium-regulating hormones in very-low-birth-weight infants. Effect of early neonatal hypocalcemia and intravenous calcium infusion on serum parathyroid hormone and calcitonin homeostasis. *Am J Dis Child.* 1985;139(9):913-916.
47. Abrams SA. Calcium and vitamin D requirements of enterally fed preterm infants. *Pediatrics.* 2013;131(5):e1676-e1683.
49. Fenton TR, Lyon AW, Rose MS. Cord blood calcium, phosphate, magnesium, and alkaline phosphatase gestational age-specific reference intervals for preterm infants. *BMC Pediatr.* 2011;11:76.
52. Kovacs CS, Lanske B, Hunzelman JL, Guo J, Karaplis AC, Kronenberg HM. Parathyroid hormone-related peptide (PTHrP) regulates fetal-placental calcium transport through a receptor distinct from the PTH/PTHrP receptor. *Proc Natl Acad Sci U S A.* 1996;93(26):15233-15238.
57. Suzuki Y, Chitayat D, Sawada H, et al. TRPV6 variants interfere with maternal-fetal calcium transport through the placenta and cause transient neonatal hyperparathyroidism. *Am J Hum Genet.* 2018;102(6):1104-1114.
58. Kovacs CS, Woodland ML, Fudge NJ, Friel JK. The vitamin D receptor is not required for fetal mineral homeostasis or for the regulation of placental calcium transfer in mice. *Am J Physiol Endocrinol Metab.* 2005;289(1):E133-E144.
62. Loughead JL, Mimouni F, Tsang RC. Serum ionized calcium concentrations in normal neonates. *Am J Dis Child.* 1988;142(5):516-518.
63. Nelson N, Finnstrom O, Larsson L. Neonatal reference values for ionized calcium, phosphate and magnesium. Selection of reference population by optimality criteria. *Scand J Clin Lab Invest.* 1987;47(2):111-117.
64. Wandrup J, Kroner J, Pryds O, Kastrup KW. Age-related reference values for ionized calcium in the first week of life in premature and full-term neonates. *Scand J Clin Lab Invest.* 1988;48(3):255-260.
65. David L, Anast CS. Calcium metabolism in newborn infants. The interrelationship of parathyroid function and calcium, magnesium, and phosphorus metabolism in normal, "sick," and hypocalcemic newborns. *J Clin Invest.* 1974;54(2):287-296.
66. Salle BL, Delvin EE, Lapillonne A, Bishop NJ, Glorieux FH. Perinatal metabolism of vitamin D. *Am J Clin Nutr.* 2000;71(suppl 5): 1317S-24S.
67. Ashraf A, Mick G, Atchison J, Petrey B, Abdullatif H, McCormick K. Prevalence of hypovitaminosis D in early infantile hypocalcemia. *J Pediatr Endocrinol Metab.* 2006;19(8):1025-1031.
72. Beggs MR, Lee JJ, Busch K, et al. TRPV6 and Cav1.3 mediate distal small intestine calcium absorption before weaning. *Cell Mol Gastroenterol Hepatol.* 2019;8(4):625-642.

75. Bronner F, Salle BL, Putet G, Rigo J, Senterre J. Net calcium absorption in premature infants: results of 103 metabolic balance studies. *Am J Clin Nutr*. 1992;56(6):1037–1044.
80. Balesaria S, Sangha S, Walters JR. Human duodenum responses to vitamin D metabolites of TRPV6 and other genes involved in calcium absorption. *Am J Physiol Gastrointest Liver Physiol*. 2009;297(6):G1193–G1197.
88. Abrams SA, Esteban NV, Vieira NE, et al. Dual tracer stable isotopic assessment of calcium absorption and endogenous fecal excretion in low birth weight infants. *Pediatr Res*. 1991;29(6):615–618.
89. Hicks PD, Rogers SP, Hawthorne KM, Chen Z, Abrams SA. Calcium absorption in very low birth weight infants with and without bronchopulmonary dysplasia. *J Pediatr*. 2011;158(6). 885–90.e1.
96. Abrams SA. Calcium absorption in infants and small children: methods of determination and recent findings. *Nutr*. 2010;2(4):474–480.
97. Agostoni C, Buonocore G, Carnielli VP, et al. Enteral nutrient supply for preterm infants: commentary from the European Society of Paediatric Gastroenterology, Hepatology and Nutrition Committee on Nutrition. *J Pediatr Gastroenterol Nutr*. 2010;50(1):85–91.
107. EFSA Panel on Dietetic Products, Nutrition and Allergies. Scientific opinion on dietary reference values for phosphorus. *EFSA Journal*. 2015;13(7):4185.
110. Colantonio DA, Kyriakopoulou L, Chan MK, et al. Closing the gaps in pediatric laboratory reference intervals: a CALIPER database of 40 biochemical markers in a healthy and multiethnic population of children. *Clin Chem*. 2012;58(5):854–868.
111. Chinoy A, Mughal MZ, Padidela R. Metabolic bone disease of prematurity: causes, recognition, prevention, treatment and long-term consequences. *Arch Dis Child Fetal Neonatal Ed*. 2019;104(5): F560–f6.
120. Bacic D, Lehir M, Biber J, Kaissling B, Murer H, Wagner CA. The renal Na^+/phosphate cotransporter NaPi-IIa is internalized via the receptor-mediated endocytic route in response to parathyroid hormone. *Kidney Int*. 2006;69(3):495–503.
125. Shimada T, Hasegawa H, Yamazaki Y, . FGF-23 is a potent regulator of vitamin D metabolism and phosphate homeostasis. *J Bone Miner Res*. 2004;19(3):429–435.
128. Weinman EJ, Steplock D, Shenolikar S, Biswas R, et al. Fibroblast growth factor-23-mediated inhibition of renal phosphate transport in mice requires sodium-hydrogen exchanger regulatory factor-1 (NHERF-1) and synergizes with parathyroid hormone. *J Biol Chem*. 2011286:37216–37221;.
129. Carpenter TO, Imel EA, Holm IA, Jan de Beur SM, Insogna KL. A clinician's guide to X-linked hypophosphatemia. *J Bone Miner Res*. 2011;26(7):1381–1388.
130. Liu S, Guo R, Simpson LG, Xiao ZS, Burnham CE, Quarles LD. Regulation of fibroblastic growth factor 23 expression but not degradation by PHEX. *J Biol Chem*. 2003;278(39):37419–37426.
133. Andrukhova O, Zeitz U, Goetz R, Mohammadi M, Lanske B, Erben RG. FGF23 acts directly on renal proximal tubules to induce phosphaturia through activation of the ERK1/2-SGK1 signaling pathway. *Bone*. 2012;51(3):621–628.
149. Blaine J, Chonchol M, Levi M. Renal control of calcium, phosphate, and magnesium homeostasis. *Clin J Am Soc Nephrol*. 2015;10(7):1257–1272.
166. Wagner CA, Rubio-Aliaga I, Hernando N. Renal phosphate handling and inherited disorders of phosphate reabsorption: an update. *Pediatr Nephrol*. 2019;34(4):549–559.
170. Payne RB. Renal tubular reabsorption of phosphate (TmP/GFR): indications and interpretation. *Ann Clin Biochem*. 1998;35(Pt 2):201–206.
175. Marks J. The role of SLC34A2 in intestinal phosphate absorption and phosphate homeostasis. *Pflugers Arch*. 2019;471(1):165–173.
190. Gidrewicz DA, Fenton TR. A systematic review and meta-analysis of the nutrient content of preterm and term breast milk. *BMC Pediatr*. 2014;14:216.
202. Sievers E, Schleyerbach U, Schaub J. Magnesium balance studies in premature and term infants. *Eur J Nutr*. 2000;39(1):1–6.
207. Rigo J, Pieltain C, Christmann V, et al. Serum magnesium levels in preterm infants are higher than adult levels: a systematic literature review and meta-analysis. *Nutr*. 2017;9(10):1125.
219. Kladnitsky O, Rozenfeld J, Azulay-Debby H, Efrati E, Zelikovic I. The claudin-16 channel gene is transcriptionally inhibited by 1,25-dihydroxyvitamin D. *Exp Physiol*. 2015;100(1):79–94.
224. McDonald KR, Fudge NJ, Woodrow JP, et al. Ablation of calcitonin/calcitonin gene-related peptide-alpha impairs fetal magnesium but not calcium homeostasis. *Am J Physiol Endocrinol Metab*. 2004;287(2):E218–E226.
229. Chubanov V, Ferioli S, Wisnowsky A, et al. Epithelial magnesium transport by TRPM6 is essential for prenatal development and adult survival. *Elife*. 2016;5:e20914.
242. Mittermeier L, Demirkhanyan L, Stadlbauer B, et al. TRPM7 is the central gatekeeper of intestinal mineral absorption essential for postnatal survival. *Proc Natl Acad Sci U S A*. 2019;116(10):4706–4715.
245. Schaffers OJM, Hoenderop JGJ, Bindels RJM, de Baaij JHF. The rise and fall of novel renal magnesium transporters. *Am J Physiol Renal Physiol*. 2018;314(6):F1027–f1033.
248. Perdomo-Ramirez A, Aguirre M, Davitaia T, Ariceta G, Ramos-Trujillo E, Claverie-Martin F. Characterization of two novel mutations in the claudin-16 and claudin-19 genes that cause familial hypomagnesemia with hypercalciuria and nephrocalcinosis. *Gene*. 2019;689:227–234.

27 Zinc in the Fetus and Neonate

Nancy F. Krebs | K. Michael Hambidge

INTRODUCTION

In a remarkably short time, the general perception of zinc has progressed from that of a rather obscure essential trace mineral of doubtful significance for human health to that of a micronutrient of exceptional biologic and public health importance. This is most evident in relation to early development, both prenatal and postnatal. Space allotted to an overview of trace minerals other than iron and zinc in previous editions of this book is therefore devoted entirely to zinc in this edition, and the reader is referred to other texts for information on other trace minerals.[1] The principal focus of this chapter is on the complex biology of zinc, which underlies its clinical importance.

BIOCHEMISTRY AND BIOLOGY OF ZINC

The abundance of zinc in the human body (approximately 2 g in the adult female and 2.5 g in the adult male) is second only to that of iron among those trace elements for which a nutritional requirement has been established in humans. In contrast to iron and iodine, however, zinc is distributed relatively evenly throughout the body, being found as a component of thousands of zinc metalloproteins or zinc-binding proteins and also of nucleic acids. This wide distribution of the element, along with the tight homeostatic control within tissues over a wide range of dietary intakes, makes assessment of zinc status particularly challenging.[2] With an atomic weight of 65.39, zinc is near several first-row transition elements of biologic importance, yet its biochemical properties are very different from those of other elements of similar atomic weight. One of the properties of the zinc atom that has proved to be of outstanding value in biology is its ability to participate in strong but readily exchangeable ligand binding.[3] Coupled with this feature is the notable flexibility of the coordination geometry of this metal. These two properties are responsible for its unique ability to interact with a wide range of organic ligands and thus to be incorporated into myriad biologic systems. The principal amino acids supplying ligands that bind with zinc are histidine, glutamic acid, aspartic acid, and cysteine. Structural zinc sites have four protein ligands, with cysteine being preferred. Zinc affects tertiary and quaternary protein structure, and the resulting scaffolding of these zinc coordination spheres is important for the function and reactivity of the metal atom.

Zinc can participate in oxidation-reduction (redox) reactions,[4] specifically through the combined biochemistry of zinc, metallothionein, and glutathione. In contrast to iron and copper, however, the zinc atom has no oxidant properties; it exists virtually entirely in the divalent state, an attribute that simplifies the safe transport of Zn^{2+}, both extracellularly and intracellularly, and its incorporation into biologic systems.

The biologic roles of zinc are now recognized in protein structure and function, including those for enzymes, transcription factors, hormonal receptor sites, and biologic membranes. Zinc has numerous central roles in DNA and RNA metabolism, and it is involved in signal transduction, gene expression, and apoptosis.

First to be appreciated were the catalytic properties of zinc, a function of its biochemistry outlined earlier. The number of zinc metalloenzymes with known three-dimensional structures exceeds 200. Although zinc also has a structural role in numerous enzymes, its primary importance is as an active component of the catalytic site. Zinc metalloenzymes have been identified in each of the six major enzyme classifications. Several of the key enzymes involved in nucleic acid metabolism, cellular proliferation, differentiation, and growth are either zinc metalloenzymes or zinc-dependent enzymes. A major advance in the understanding of the biology of zinc was the identification of proteins that contain a *zinc finger motif*.[5] Structurally, the zinc finger motif is a recurring pattern of amino acids with conserved cysteine and histidine residues at the base to which zinc binds in a tetrahedral arrangement. Subsequently, hundreds of zinc finger motifs were identified. More than 1000 genes in the human genome encode members of three protein families with zinc finger domains alone: C2H2 zinc fingers, RING fingers, and LIM domains. The number of genes containing zinc finger domains exceeds 3% of all identified human genes. Although all zinc fingers are quite similar, they differ in their precise conformation. Steroid hormone receptors, for example, have several such domains that are involved in the structure itself, and one each for binding to DNA and RNA polymerases. Among the identified zinc transcription factors are several involved in early intrauterine development.

The numerous transcription factor proteins with the zinc finger motif gives this metal a broad role in gene expression. This role has perhaps been best characterized by the self-regulation of this metal of its own metabolism[6] and that of metallothionein, with which zinc is so closely associated. Gene expression in this context is considered later, in the discussion of zinc metabolism.

Zinc is an important regulator of apoptosis. This micronutrient has cytoprotective functions that suppress major pathways leading to apoptosis and also directly influences apoptotic regulators, especially the caspase family of enzymes.[7] In airway epithelial cells, zinc is colocalized with the precursor forms of caspase 3, mitochondria, and microtubules. A decline in intracellular zinc concentration may trigger pathways leading to caspase activation. An early and direct effect of zinc deficiency, not only on proliferation and differentiation but also in inducing apoptosis, has been demonstrated in growth plate chondrocytes of the chick.

There is evidence of a direct signaling function of zinc at all levels of signal transduction.[7] Zinc can modulate cellular signal recognition, second-messenger metabolism, and protein kinase and protein phosphatase activities. In the brain, zinc is sequestered in the presynaptic vesicles of zinc-containing neurons, from which zinc is released into the cleft and is then recycled into the presynaptic terminal. Synaptically released zinc functions as a conventional synaptic neurotransmitter or neuromodulator but, analogous to calcium, also functions as a transmembrane neural signal. The best-established physiologic role of this vesicular zinc is the tonic modulation of brain excitability. Vesicular-rich regions such as the hippocampus are responsive to dietary zinc deprivation, which causes brain dysfunction, including learning impairment and susceptibility to epileptic seizures. Normal neuronal function is dependent on normal zinc homeostasis in the brain.

The biology of zinc is closely linked with that of metallothionein, a unique small intracellular protein of less than 7 kDa that is strongly conserved across species. Of the 61 to 68 amino acids in the protein, more than one-third are cysteine. Metallothionein occurs in all tissues, including those of the conceptus, and is especially abundant in liver and also in pancreas, intestine, and kidney. The metallothioneins have a high affinity for zinc and are critical for maintaining cytoplasmic zinc pools to protect against cytotoxicity.[8] Zinc is the major physiologic inducer of metallothionein. Its synthesis is also stimulated by cytokines, especially the interleukins (IL)-1 and IL-6, tumor necrosis factor-α, and stress hormones (glucocorticoids and catecholamines), supporting a key role for zinc in the inflammatory response as well as in zinc metabolism.[9] Zinc binds directly and reversibly to the zinc finger domains of metal response element–binding transcription factor 1 (MTF-1), which functions as a cellular zinc sensor. As a result of this binding, MTF-1 assumes a DNA-binding conformation and translocates to the nucleus, where it binds to metal-response elements of the metallothionein gene, thereby initiating transcription. MTF-1 provides zinc responsiveness to many genes and acts as a master regulatory transcription factor for microRNA genes. involved in gene expression, including of zinc transporters.[10] Null mutation of the *MTF-1* gene is lethal in embryonic mice.

Factors that increase the induction of maternal hepatic metallothionein during early pregnancy may divert zinc from the conceptus to the maternal liver, potentially resulting in a conceptus that is deficient in zinc. Curtailment of fetal zinc uptake can occur with maternal ingestion of alcohol, a mechanism that may be important in the origin of fetal alcohol syndrome.[11] Close similarities have been recognized between the teratogenicity of maternal zinc deficiency and alcohol administration to mice in early gestation, and this effect can be diminished by parenteral administration of zinc. Cytokines cause a similar disturbance of maternal zinc metabolism and also are teratogenic in rodents.

PHYSIOLOGY OF ZINC

INTRACELLULAR ZINC METABOLISM

Zinc metabolism is tissue and organ specific. Although this specificity is important for an understanding of zinc metabolism, the following discussion is limited to selected aspects of more universal intracellular zinc metabolism. The intracellular concentration of unbound "free" Zn^{2+} is extremely low. In conjunction with metallothioneins, the distribution, storage, and intra- and extracellular concentrations of Zn are tightly controlled. An elaborate homeostatic system of protein transporters regulates cellular Zn^{2+} distribution by the control of influx and efflux and also perhaps by control of a hierarchy of zinc-dependent functions. To date, over 20 mammalian transporters have been identified, with two major families of genes, the Zn transporter (ZnT)/SLC30A family, which export zinc across cellular membranes, and the Zrt/Irt-like protein/solute carrier family 39 (ZIP/SLC39A), which import zinc.[10] The expression of the transporters' genes is regulated by both transcriptional and posttranscriptional mechanisms to orchestrate zinc homeostasis in response to numerous stimuli, such as hormonal changes, cytokine release, oxidative stress, and hypoxia. Tremendous expansion has emerged in the understanding of the specific roles of each of the zinc transporters and of the pathophysiologic effects on numerous systems with disruption of their expression and/or function. Much remains to be learned, however, regarding how the molecular regulation of zinc metabolism and homeostasis responds to variations in dietary zinc intake and observations at the whole-body level.

GENETICALLY BASED ZINC DEFICIENCY

Mutations of two specific zinc transporter genes are linked to distinct conditions of severe zinc deficiency. Acrodermatitis enteropathica (AE)—classically associated with characteristic dermatitis, alopecia, and diarrhea—is an autosomal recessive disorder linked to mutations of the *ZIP4 (SLC39A4)* gene, which results in a partial block in intestinal zinc absorption. Untreated, this is a lethal condition; lifelong treatment with high doses of zinc results in an excellent prognosis.[12] The availability of genetic testing has now revealed numerous distinct alterations of the gene, and as many as 50% of phenotypic AE cases do not present with the classic signs or with detectable mutation in the *ZIP4* gene.[13,14] Global incidence rate of AE has been estimated to be 1 per 500,000 newborns.[15]

The other recognized genetic condition associated with severe zinc deficiency is due to abnormally low zinc concentrations in breast milk secondary to mutations in the *ZnT-2 (SLC30A2)* gene.[16,17] Multiple missense mutations and single nucleotide polymorphisms (SNPs) have now been identified, resulting in 10% to 75% reductions milk zinc concentrations at all stages of lactation. Infants who are breast-fed by mothers with this transporter defect typically display the classic phenotype of AE by approximately 2 months postnatal age. Infants with the clinical syndrome respond rapidly and completely to an initial oral zinc supplement of 2 mg/kg body weight per day, progressing to a smaller maintenance dosage while breast-feeding continues. The defect lies solely in the mammary gland's ability to transfer zinc. The recipient infant's presentation with classic signs of severe zinc deficiency, including dermatitis, is secondary to low intake but with no absorptive defect. This condition has been termed *acquired zinc deficiency of lactogenic origin* or *transient neonatal zinc deficiency (TNZD)*. The exact prevalence is unknown, but emerging evidence suggests that it is not rare, with recent estimates of at least 1 in 2334 newborns being susceptible.[18] Early observations[19] suggested that the primary vulnerability was in premature infants, which has been confirmed,[20] but it is now clear that term infants are also susceptible.[21-23]

MATERNAL, PLACENTAL, FETAL, AND MAMMARY GLAND ZINC METABOLISM

MATERNAL METABOLISM

A plethora of studies in animal models have documented abnormal embryogenesis, including lethal defects, due to mutations or knockouts of several zinc transporters.[24] Severe to moderate zinc deficiency has been associated with abnormal placental morphogenesis, impaired maternal cardiovascular responsiveness,[25] multiple fetal malformations and growth restriction, as well as maternal complications during pregnancy and labor.[26] However, comparable physiologic data from zinc-deficient pregnant women are essentially unavailable, although global estimates suggest that a majority of pregnant women consume inadequate amounts of zinc. Systematic reviews have identified only a reduction in preterm birth as a benefit of maternal zinc supplementation during pregnancy.[27] This may in part be due to homeostatic adjustments to enhance absorption in late pregnancy, thus averting deprivation to the fetus despite marginal maternal intake.[26,28] A physiologic increase in maternal hepatic metallothionein concentration in pregnancy has been documented; this increase may provide a maternal store of zinc that is readily available to the conceptus. It is only when zinc is abnormally diverted to the maternal liver, as with alcohol ingestion, that the inappropriately large shift of zinc from the plasma compartment is potentially deleterious to the embryo or fetus. A progressive physiologic decline in maternal plasma zinc also occurs as pregnancy advances,[29] but it is only when this decline is excessive because of maternal zinc deprivation or disturbed metabolism that the embryo or fetus is at risk.

PLACENTAL AND FETAL METABOLISM

Uptake of Zn^{2+} into the placental villous syncytiotrophoblast is the first step in the transfer of this metal from the mother to the fetus, and it is the rate-limiting process.[30] This zinc is thought to be derived from the low-molecular-weight maternal plasma zinc pool, probably by a carrier-mediated process, and also from zinc bound to serum protein, possibly by an endocytic mechanism.[31] Zinc uptake capacity in human placenta is influenced both by gestational age and by low levels of maternal serum zinc, findings consistent with ensuring an adequate maternal-fetal zinc transfer. Fetal plasma zinc concentrations are higher than maternal concentrations. Short-term changes in fetal zinc status do not influence placental zinc transfer, suggesting that no ready mechanism is available for adjustment to fetal zinc deprivation when (or if) it occurs.[32] As gestation progresses, there are marked increases in fetal hepatic zinc concentration, which then declines during the third trimester. The increase in hepatic zinc concentration early in the third trimester appears to be secondary to hepatic metallothionein induction rather than its cause.[33]

Metallothionein has been found in fetal amniotic cells, syncytial trophoblasts, and villous interstitial cells.[34] The mammalian embryo is surrounded by cells that actively express metallothionein 1 and metallothionein 2 genes, suggesting that metallothionein has a functional role in the establishment as well as the maintenance of normal pregnancy.[35] Metallothionein 3 and 4 messenger RNAs are abundant in the maternal decidua, in contrast with fetal tissues, and these genes are refractory to induction by either zinc or inflammation in the decidua.[36] Additional research is needed to determine how the roles of these and other factors, such as zinc transporters, are integrated to achieve regulation of placental Zn^{2+} transport. Only then will it be possible to understand how regulation, and hence the zinc status of the embryo or fetus, may be compromised, especially early in gestation.

MAMMARY GLAND METABOLISM

ZnT-1 (present in serosal membrane), ZnT-2, and ZnT-4 (present intracellularly) have been identified in the mammary gland.[17] Milk zinc concentrations decline sharply from parturition through approximately the first 6 months postpartum and gradually thereafter; this pattern is physiologic and independent of maternal zinc status or intake.[37,38] Although this pattern is undoubtedly regulated through coordination among the mammary gland zinc transporters, exact regulatory mechanisms have not been elucidated. In addition to zinc secretion into milk, recent work has established that zinc also has critical functional roles for mammary gland proliferation, differentiation, and secretion, all of which are critical to the success of lactation.[39]

WHOLE-BODY ZINC HOMEOSTASIS

Postnatally, the gastrointestinal tract, specifically the small intestine and pancreas, has the major role in maintaining whole-body zinc homeostasis. Zinc transporter expression is a major component of homeostatic regulation, including regulation of zinc absorption by the small intestine and excretion of zinc through both the pancreas and the small intestine. Multiple zinc transporters have been identified in these organs. When dietary zinc intake is reduced, ZIP4 is upregulated at the apical surface of the small intestine. As described earlier, this transporter is defective in classic AE. The quantity of zinc ingested rather than zinc status is the principal factor triggering regulation of expression of the transporters involved with zinc absorption into and through the enterocyte.[2]

Zinc absorption is a saturable transport process. Therefore fractional absorption declines with increasing zinc intake and vice versa. Passive paracellular diffusion also occurs in animal models but has not been detectable in models of human zinc absorption. When data are adjusted for differences in the length of the small intestine, the term infant can absorb ingested zinc as efficiently and with the same capacity as the adult.[40] This also appears to be true for the preterm infant at 33 weeks after conception,[41] suggesting that the synthesis of zinc transporters and other zinc-containing molecules in the enterocyte is mature by this stage of development, although no absorption studies are available for more prematurely born infants. However, the small intestine is shorter; consequently, absorption of adequate zinc to meet the high requirements is a challenge in the premature infant.[42]

Regulation of the quantity of intestinal endogenous zinc excreted has a major role in maintaining whole-body zinc homeostasis in most circumstances. The zinc exporters ZnT-1 and ZnT-2 exhibit progressive downregulation, most notably in the pancreas, when the level of dietary zinc is chronically reduced. The ability to regulate endogenous zinc losses through the intestine appears to be well developed in early postnatal life in the term infant.[43,44] In the premature infant, the rate of endogenous zinc excretion is also positively correlated with the quantity of zinc absorbed, as in term infants, but the premature infant may be unable to regulate intestinal excretion of endogenous zinc as efficiently as the term infant. Endogenous zinc losses through the kidneys, although small in comparison with intestinal losses, are also relatively high in the very low-birth-weight infant on a body weight basis.

In addition to high demands for zinc to support growth, the premature infant is also born with relatively low tissue zinc levels. Model-based compartmental analysis of zinc metabolism in the adult has identified several pools of zinc that intermix with zinc in plasma within 3 days. The combined size of these pools (exchangeable zinc pool [EZP]) can be estimated from what appears as a single exponential between 3 and 9 days after administration of a stable-isotope zinc tracer and from urine enrichment with this tracer.[45] On a body weight basis, the size of the EZP is approximately sevenfold higher in premature infants at 33 weeks after conception than in adults. This finding may be attributable in part to the higher concentrations of metallothionein in the fetal liver earlier in the third trimester.[46] This is also consistent with EZP sizes, measured within 24 hours of birth, being elevated relative to body weight. Small-for-gestational-age infants were reported to have a lower EZP for comparable degrees of prematurity, suggesting particular vulnerability to zinc deficiency.[47] These and other available data confirm a strong susceptibility of premature infants to zinc deficiency.[42]

ACQUIRED ZINC DEFICIENCY FROM CONCEPTION TO PREMATURE DELIVERY

EMBRYOGENESIS

An adequate supply of maternal zinc is critically important for the oocyte and embryo.[48,49] The teratology in rodents resulting from maternal zinc deficiency is quite exceptional.[50] Consequences include a high mortality rate and congenital malformations affecting nearly all organ systems. Relevant data in the human are very limited; prospective trials of zinc supplementation in carefully selected population groups encompassing the perinatal period will be required to clarify this issue. Suggestive evidence points to a causal association between severe maternal zinc deficiency resulting from suboptimally treated AE and congenital malformations, including neural tube defects.

FETAL DEVELOPMENT

Maternal zinc restriction during fetal development is associated with intrauterine growth retardation in rodent models. However, results are conflicting regarding the effects of maternal zinc supplementation on fetal loss, fetal growth, and birth weight; as noted earlier, reduction of preterm delivery was the only significant benefit of supplementation.[27] Multicenter, carefully designed, prospective intervention studies will be required to resolve questions of optimal timing and dose of supplementation and whether maternal zinc deficiency contributes to low birth weight by reducing the duration of gestation or the rate of growth in utero. Perhaps unexpectedly, more consistent evidence suggests that maternal zinc supplementation starting in the second trimester and discontinued at delivery is associated with decreased infectious disease morbidity during the first 6 months of the infant's life.[51] This effect, which presumably is mediated through an effect of fetal zinc status on the developing immune system, is itself an important reason for ensuring optimal maternal zinc intake.

NEONATAL ZINC DEFICIENCY IN VERY LOW-BIRTH-WEIGHT PREMATURE INFANTS

Recognition of and concern regarding the occurrence of zinc deficiency in low-birth-weight and especially very low-birth-weight infants has grown with the increasing recognition of the health benefits of zinc supplementation of the very low-birth-weight infant. As early as 1993, Friel and colleagues[52] observed greater growth with zinc supplementation in the first 6 months and evidence of favorable neurodevelopment even in formula-fed very low-birth-weight infants. Yet reports of severe zinc deficiency in premature infants continue to appear regularly in the literature, especially (but not exclusively) in cases of very premature/very low birth weight and in infants receiving primarily human milk.[53-56] Since the classic dermatitis of severe zinc deficiency is a late finding, it is quite plausible that mild to moderate zinc deficiency may be relatively common in this population, manifesting with such nonspecific signs as growth impairment and impaired immune function, which could increase the risk for common morbidities. Furthermore, as the use of donor human milk for the prevention of necrotizing enterocolitis has become more routine in neonatal intensive care units (NICUs), the risk of zinc deficiency may further increase because donor human milk tends to come from mothers who are several months postpartum, when zinc concentrations are much lower than age-matched mother's own milk.[57] In many of the aforementioned reports of zinc deficiency, zinc supplementation or fortification regimens had been followed, suggesting that current recommendations may be insufficient.

The challenges of assessing zinc status[2] are evident in the NICU population, and the prevalence of zinc deficiency in this high-risk population is simply unknown. To address this and to potentially improve outcomes, a number of trials of zinc supplementation have been undertaken. In one trial, a generous zinc supplement (>2 mg elemental Zn/kg/day) was associated with a significantly lower mix of neonatal morbidities involving the pulmonary, gastrointestinal, immune, and central nervous systems.[58] A systematic review to examine the effect of zinc as an adjunct to antibiotic therapy for treatment of neonatal sepsis included four randomized controlled trials (RCTs), three of which focused on preterm infants and used doses of 3 mg/kg/day. The results indicated a significant reduction in mortality without an impact on duration of hospital stay.[59] Another supplementation trial in preterm neonates reported improved postnatal neurologic development.[60] A prospective observational study in a US NICU found that zinc intake at ~14 days postnatal age ranged widely—from 0.4 to 1.8 mg/kg/day; intake was positively associated with weight gain and growth in head circumference.[61] Although all of these trials have limitations, they add to the plausibility that current recommendations for zinc intake may be insufficient and that zinc deficiency is not rare in the modern NICU. Clearly, adequately powered RCTs are needed to rigorously assess the potential role of zinc deficiency in commonly observed suboptimal outcomes in preterm infants.

CONCLUSION

The emergence of the impressive biology of zinc and recognition of the public health implications of zinc deficiency in infants and young children are now alerting the scientific and medical communities to the need for special attention to this trace element. This need is more apparent in the very low-birth-weight infant than in any other population group. From a practical standpoint, the most pressing issue is to delineate the zinc requirements of infants born very or extremely prematurely, including, as a special subgroup, those with intrauterine growth retardation.

A complete reference list is available at www.ExpertConsult.com.

SELECT REFERENCES

1. Krebs NF, Hambidge KM. Trace Elements. In: Duggan C, Watkins JB, Koletzko B, Walker WA, eds. *Nutrition in Pediatrics*. 5th ed. Vol 1. Connecticut: People's Medical Publishing House-USA; 2016:95-116.
2. King JC, Brown KH, Gibson RS, et al. Biomarkers of Nutrition for Development (BOND)-Zinc review. *J Nutr*. 2016;14(suppl 6):858S-885S.
3. Williams RJP. An introduction to the biochemistry of zinc. In: Mills CF, ed. *Zinc in Human Biology*. London: Springer-Verlag; 1989:15-31.
4. Maret W. The function of zinc metallothionein: a link between cellular zinc and redox state. *J Nutr*. 2000;130(suppl 5s):1455S-1458S.
5. Miller J, Mclachian AD, Klug A. Repetitive Zn-binding domains in the protein transcription factor IIIA from *Xenopus* oocytes. *EMBO J*. 1985;4:1609-1614.
6. Andrews GK. Cellular zinc sensors: MTF-1 regulation of gene expression. *Biometals*. 2001;14(3-4):223-237.
7. Wessels I, Maywald M, Rink L. Zinc as a gatekeeper of immune function. *Nutr*. 2017;9(12):1-44.
8. Colvin RA, Holmes WR, Fontaine CP, Maret W. Cytosolic zinc buffering and muffling: their role in intracellular zinc homeostasis. *Metallomics*. 2010;2(5):306-317.
9. Coyle P, Philcox JC, Carey LC, Rofe AM. Metallothionein: a multi-purpose protein. *Cell Mol Life Sci*. 2001;59:1-21.
10. Hara T, Takeda TA, Takagishi T, Fukue K, Kambe T, Fukada T. Physiological roles of zinc transporters: molecular and genetic importance in zinc homeostasis. *J Physiol Sci*. 2017;67(2):283-301.
11. Gaither LA, Eide DJ. Eukaryotic zinc transporters and their regulation. *Biometals*. 2001;14(3-4):251-270.
12. Kharfi M, El Fekih N, Aounallah-Skhiri H, et al. Acrodermatitis enteropathica: a review of 29 Tunisian cases. *International Journal of Dermatology*. 2010;49(9):1038-1044.
13. Ricci G, Ferrari S, Calamelli E, Ricci L, Neri I, Patrizi A. Heterogeneity in the genetic alterations and in the clinical presentation of acrodermatitis enteropathic: case report and review of the literature. *Int J Immunopathol Pharmacol*. 2016;29(2):274-279.
14. Kury S, Kharfi M, Schmitt S, Bezieau S. Clinical utility gene card for: acrodermatitis enteropathica. *European Journal of Human Genetics*. 2012;20(3).
15. Jagadeesan S, Kaliyadan F. Acrodermatitis enteropathica. In: *StatPearls*. Treasure Island: FL; 2019.
16. Chowanadisai W, Lonnerdal B, Kelleher SL. Identification of a mutation in SLC30A2 (ZnT-2) in women with low milk zinc concentration that results in transient neonatal zinc deficiency. *Journal of Biological Chemistry*. 2006;281(51):39699-39707.
17. McCormick NH, Hennigar SR, Kiselyov K, Kelleher SL. The biology of zinc transport in mammary epithelial cells: implications for mammary gland development, lactation, and involution. *J Mammary Gland Biol Neoplasia*. 2014;19(1):59-71.
18. Golan Y, Lehvy A, Horev G, Assaraf YG. High proportion of transient neonatal zinc deficiency causing alleles in the general population. *J Cell Mol Med*. 2019;23(2):828-840.
19. Zimmerman AW, Hambidge KM, Lepow ML, Greenberg RD, Stover ML, Casey CE. Acrodermatitis in breast-fed premature infants: evidence for a defect of mammary zinc secretion. *Pediatrics*. 1982;69(2):176-183.
20. Watson L, Cartwright D, Jardine LA, et al. Transient neonatal zinc deficiency in exclusively breastfed preterm infants. *J Paediatr Child Health*. 2018;54(3):319-322.
21. Murthy SC, Udagani MM, Badakali AV, Yelameli BC. Symptomatic zinc deficiency in a full-term breast-fed infant. *Dermatol Online J*. 2010;16(6):3.
22. Tang T, Lam JM. Unique presentation of transient zinc deficiency from low maternal breast milk zinc levels. *Pediatr Dermatol*. 2018;35(2):255-256.
23. Mohammed J, Mehrotra S, Schulz H, Lim R. Severe infant rash resistant to therapy due to zinc deficiency. *Pediatr Emerg Care*. 2017;33(8):582-584.
24. Hojyo S, Fukada T. Zinc transporters and signaling in physiology and pathogenesis. *Arch Biochem Biophys*. 2016;611:43-50.
25. Wilson RL, Leemaqz SY, Goh Z, et al. Zinc is a critical regulator of placental morphogenesis and maternal hemodynamics during pregnancy in mice. *Sci Rep*. 2017;7(1):15137.
26. Donangelo CM, King JC. Maternal zinc intakes and homeostatic adjustments during pregnancy and lactation. *Nutr*. 2012;4(7):782-798.
27. Chaffee BW, King JC. Effect of zinc supplementation on pregnancy and infant outcomes: a systematic review. *Paediatr Perinat Epidemiol*. 2012;26(suppl 1):118-137.
28. Hambidge KM, Miller LV, Mazariegos M, et al. Upregulation of zinc absorption matches increases in physiologic requirements for zinc in women consuming high- or moderate-phytate diets during late pregnancy and early lactation. *J Nutr*. 2017;147(6):1079-1085.
29. Mas A, Sarkar B. Binding, uptake and efflux of 65Zn by isolated human trophoblast cells. *Biochim Biophys Acta*. 1991;1092(1):35-38.
30. Bax CM, Bloxam DL. Two major pathways of zinc(II) acquisition by human placental syncytiotrophoblast. *J Cell Physiol*. 1995;164(3):546-554.
31. Aslam N, McArdle HJ. Mechanism of zinc uptake by microvilli isolated from human term placenta. *J Cell Physiol*. 1992;151(3):533-538.
32. Lindsay Y, Duthie LM, McArdle HJ. Zinc levels in the rat fetal liver are not determined by transport across the placental microvillar membrane or the fetal liver plasma membrane. *Biol Reprod*. 1994;51(3):358-365.
33. Goyer RA, Huast MD, Cherian MG. Cellular localization of metallothionein in human term placenta. *Placenta*. 1992;13(4):349-355.
34. De SK, McMaster MT, Dey SK, Andrews GK. Cell-specific metallothionein gene expression in mouse decidua and placentae. *Development*. 1989;107(3):611-621.
35. Liang L, Fu K, Lee DK, Sobieski RJ, Dalton T, Andrews GK. Activation of the complete mouse metallothionein gene locus in the maternal deciduum. *Mol Reprod Dev*. 1996;43(1):25-37.
36. Huber KL, Cousins RJ. Maternal zinc deprivation and interleukin-1 influence metallothionein gene expression and zinc metabolism of rats. *J Nutr*. 1988;118(12):1570-1576.
37. Krebs NF, Reidinger CJ, Hartley S, Robertson AD, Hambidge KM. Zinc supplementation during lactation: effects on maternal status and milk zinc concentrations. *Am J Clin Nutr*. 1995;61(5):1030-1036.
38. Brown KH, Engle-Stone R, Krebs NF, Peerson JM. Dietary intervention strategies to enhance zinc nutrition: promotion and support of breastfeeding for infants and young children. *Food Nutr Bull*. 2009;30(1 Suppl):S144-171.
39. Lee S, Kelleher SL. Molecular regulation of lactation: the complex and requisite roles for zinc. *Arch Biochem Biophys*. 2016;611:86-92.
40. Davidson AJ, Melinkovich P, Beaty BL, et al. Immunization registry accuracy: improvement with progressive clinical application. *Am J Prev Med*. 2003;24(3):276-280.
41. Jalla S, Krebs NF, Rodden D, Hambidge KM. Zinc homeostasis in premature infants does not differ between those fed preterm formula or fortified human milk. *Pediatr Res*. 2004;56(4):615-620.
42. Krebs NF. Update on zinc deficiency and excess in clinical pediatric practice. *Annals of Nutrition and Metabolism*. 2013;62(suppl 1):19-29.
43. Ziegler EE, Serfass RE, Nelson SE, et al. Effect of low zinc intake on absorption and excretion of zinc by infants studied with 70Zn as extrinsic tag. *J Nutr*. 1989;119(11):1647-1653.
44. Krebs NF, Reidinger CJ, Miller LV, Hambidge KM. Zinc homeostasis in breast-fed infants. *Pediatr Res*. 1996;39(4 Pt 1):661-665.
45. Miller LV, Hambidge KM, Naake VL, Hong Z, Westcott JL, Fennessey PV. Size of the zinc pools that exchange rapidly with plasma zinc in humans: alternative techniques for measuring and relation to dietary zinc intake. *J Nutr*. 1994;124(2):268-276.
46. Zlotkin SH, Cherian MG. Hepatic metallothionein as a source of zinc and cysteine during the first year of life. *Pediatr Res*. 1988;24(3):326-329.
47. Krebs NF, Westcott JL, Rodden DJ, Ferguson KW, Miller LV, Hambidge KM. Exchangeable zinc pool size at birth is smaller in small-for-gestational-age than in appropriate-for-gestational-age preterm infants. *Am J Clin Nutr*. 2006;84(6):1340-1343.
48. Hurley LS. Teratogenic aspects of manganese, zinc, and copper nutrition. *Physiol Rev*. 1981;61(2):249-295.
49. Keen CL, Hurley LS. Effects of zinc deficiency on prenatal and postnatal development. *Neurotoxicology*. 1987;8(3):379-387.
50. Record IR, Dreosti IE, Tulsi RS, Manuel SJ. Maternal metabolism and teratogenesis in zinc-deficient rats. *Teratology*. 1986;33(3):311-317.

Vitamin A Metabolism in the Fetus and Neonate

28

Libo Tan | A. Catharine Ross

INTRODUCTION

Vitamin A *(retinol)* is an essential nutrient for all vertebrates. It was discovered in 1913 as an ether-soluble fraction present in certain fats and tissues, such as butter and egg yolk, that young rats required for growth and survival.[1] Early in the history of vitamin A research, investigators demonstrated some of the fundamental properties of vitamin A, namely its indispensability for proper vision, immunity, reproduction, and epithelial cell differentiation. The chemical nature of vitamin A was elucidated in the 1930s as all-*trans*-retinol, which is mainly in the form of retinyl esters (RE) in tissues. β-Carotene was shown to have the same qualitative activity as retinol, and metabolic studies demonstrated that β-carotene can be converted to retinol in the intestine and thus have same biologic activity as dietary retinol or RE. In the 1940s, the acid form of vitamin A, *retinoic acid,* was synthesized[2] and shown to have essentially all of the properties of retinol, except in vision.[3] By the 1950s, the essential role of 11-*cis*-retinaldehyde, also known as 11-*cis-retinal*, in vision was demonstrated, leading to a Nobel Prize for this research.[4]

FORMS PRESENT IN THE DIET AND IN TISSUES

DIET

There are two major forms of vitamin A in the human diet. The first is preformed vitamin A, comprised of retinol (Fig. 28.1A) and RE, which are present in foods of animal origin such as whole milk, eggs, meat, and liver. The second is provitamin A, mostly as β-carotene (see Fig. 28.1B) but also including α-carotene and β-cryptoxanthin; these forms are present in yellow, orange, and leafy green vegetables and orange-fleshed fruits. The provitamin A carotenoids are partially converted to retinol during intestinal absorption.

TISSUES

Vitamin A and its metabolites are referred to collectively as retinoids. Within plasma and tissues, there are 4 predominant forms of retinoids: (1) all-*trans*-retinol, which circulates in plasma bound to retinol-binding protein (gene name *RBP4*), by which it is delivered to most tissues for further metabolism to other forms; (2) RE, the major storage form, which is derived from the intracellular esterification of retinol with long-chain fatty acids; (3) retinal, which exists in small amounts as the metabolic intermediate all-*trans*-retinal, and at much higher concentrations as 11-*cis*-retinal (see Fig. 28.1C) in the rod and cone cells of the retina; and (4) all-*trans*-retinoic acid (see Fig. 28.1D), a quantitatively minor but physiologically important metabolite of retinol that is formed intracellularly through oxidative metabolism.

In addition to these principal forms of vitamin A, there are numerous other related molecules. However, their function is either unclear or they may be side and/or end-products of metabolic processes. 9-*cis*-RA (see Fig. 28.1E) is believed to function as a ligand for the nuclear receptors of the RXR family, but its in vivo relevance is still being debated.[5,6] 13-*cis*-RA (see Fig. 28.1F) does not function as a receptor ligand but is found in plasma as a retinoid metabolite,[7] and it is used as a drug (see "The Retinoid Analogue, Isotretinoin" section). Glucuronides of retinol or retinoic acid, exemplified in Fig. 28.1G, are water-soluble compounds due to the glucuronide moiety; they are present in blood[8,9] and bile and readily excreted.[10]

The metabolism of vitamin A is carried out by numerous proteins that function as chaperones, transport proteins, enzymes, and receptors, and together they can be considered the "machinery" for vitamin A metabolism. They also serve to assure that vitamin A is stored in the relatively inert form of RE, and to eliminate excess retinol and retinoic acid when the levels of these forms become elevated. An overview of the vitamin A biochemical pathways discussed below is shown in Fig. 28.2. Not all reactions occur in all cells and the transport of metabolites through plasma provides a means of intertissue communication. An overview of the metabolic interrelationships among vitamin A during its metabolism in the intestine, liver, and other organs is illustrated in Fig. 28.3.

DIGESTION, ABSORPTION, AND CHYLOMICRON METABOLISM

In the digestive process, RE, the primary form of vitamin A in foods, must first be solubilized and hydrolyzed to liberate unesterified retinol. Micelle formation is required to solubilize the RE, and therefore the diet must contain adequate dietary fat. Hydrolysis is catalyzed by pancreatic lipases present in the intestinal lumen and by RE hydrolases associated with the brush border of enterocytes.[11-14] Once the micelle containing the released retinol traverses the unstirred water layer[15] and reaches the apical surface of the enterocyte, retinol is transported across the apical brush border membrane. Most retinol is absorbed in the upper small intestine. Overall, the absorption efficiency of retinol is high, as approximately 70% to 90% of a dose of vitamin A was absorbed in adult rats[12] and nearly 100% in neonatal rats.[16] However, the absorption efficiency can be compromised in diseases such as cystic fibrosis and other lipid malabsorption syndromes.[17] In the enterocyte, most of the retinol becomes bound to a relatively abundant cytosolic protein, cellular retinol-binding protein (CRBP) type 2.[18-20] The concentration of CRBP2 is lower in the small intestine of immature fetuses relative to that in the mature newborn and adult rat.[21] Retinol is then transferred to the enzyme lecithin:retinol acyltransferase (LRAT), which esterifies the retinol. LRAT is present in the membranes of intestinal enterocytes as well as in other vitamin A-storing tissues. The esters formed are mostly retinyl palmitate, stearate, oleate, and linoleate,[22,23] which are very hydrophobic. The newly formed RE are packaged into the lipid core of nascent chylomicrons as they are assembled in the enterocytes. Chylomicron vitamin A content directly reflects the vitamin A content of the recent meal, or dose of supplemental vitamin A, that is being absorbed, and therefore it can be highly variable, from a trace to larger amounts, although still low in comparison to dietary fat.

Carotenoids are generally far less bioavailable than preformed vitamin A. Their bioavailability depends significantly on the type of food in which they are present. β-Carotene in milk, butter,

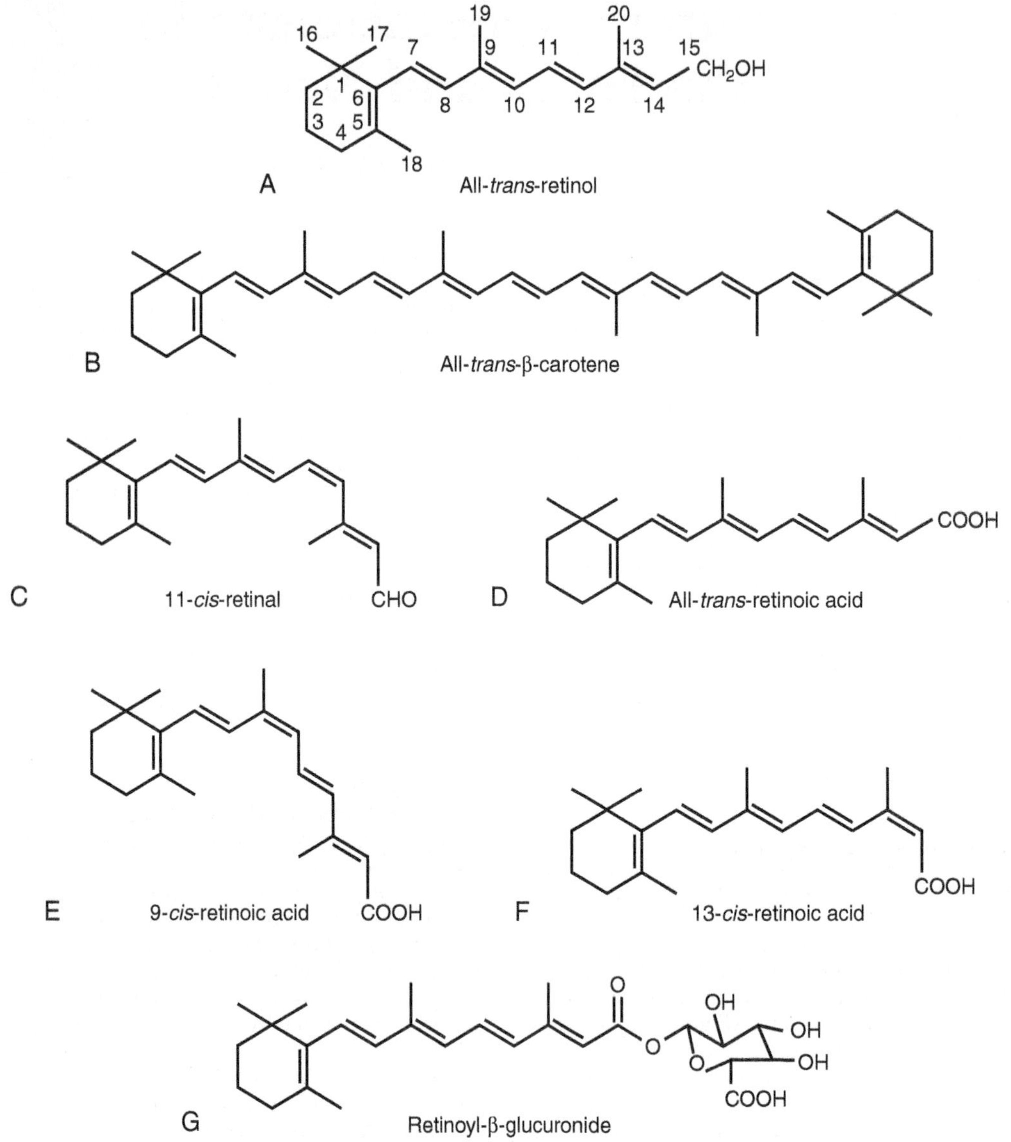

A All-*trans*-retinol

B All-*trans*-β-carotene

C 11-*cis*-retinal CHO

D All-*trans*-retinoic acid COOH

E 9-*cis*-retinoic acid COOH

F 13-*cis*-retinoic acid COOH

G Retinoyl-β-glucuronide

Fig. 28.1 Retinol and metabolites produced during its metabolism.

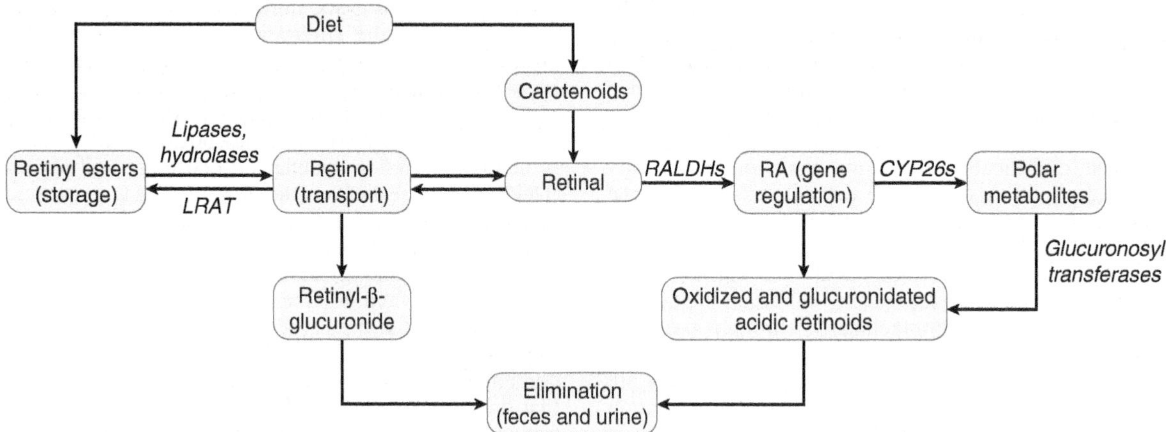

Fig. 28.2 Biochemical pathways of vitamin A utilization and oxidation. *LRAT,* Lecithin:retinol acyltransferase.

Absorptive phase

RE synthesis and CM assembly in enterocytes

Release of CM to lymphatics

Transport of CM to systemic circulation

LPL-mediated delipidation cascade

CM remnant uptake (hepatic and EH) and cellular retinol metabolism

Distributive phase

Retinol-binding protein production in liver and EH tissues

Secretion of holo-RBP

Uptake of retinol from RBP into most tissues

Intracellular metabolism, or recycling of retinol back to plasma

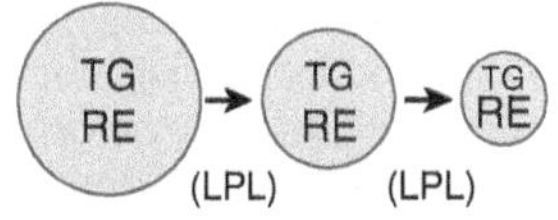

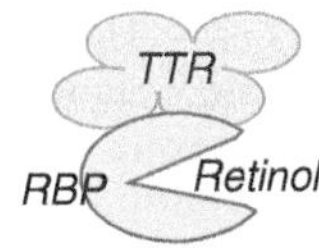

Fig. 28.3 Main characteristics of the absorptive, postprandial phase of chylomicron vitamin A incorporation and metabolism and the distributive phase of vitamin A transport to target tissues by retinol-binding protein. Target tissues include eyes, immune system, reproductive organs, and other epithelial tissues including the intestine and liver. *CM,* Chylomicron; *EH,* extrahepatic; *LPL,* lipoprotein lipase; *RBP,* retinol-binding protein; *RE,* retinyl ester (the main form of VA in CM); *TTR,* transthyretin; *VA,* vitamin A. (Figure reproduced from Tan L, Green MH, Ross AC. Vitamin A kinetics in neonatal rats vs. adult rats: comparisons from model-based compartmental analysis. *J Nutr.* 2014;145:403–410, 27, by permission of Oxford University Press.)

and dietary supplements is relatively soluble and absorbed with higher efficiency than β-carotene, or other provitamin A carotenoids, that are present within fibrous foods, such as green leafy vegetables. In these foods, they are bound within membranes and must first be liberated from the food matrix through the intestinal digestive process before the carotenoids can be solubilized into micelles and absorbed. The absorption process utilizes a scavenger receptor class B type I transporter in the brush border membrane.[24] Once within the enterocytes, β-carotene may undergo cleavage by the enzyme known as β-carotene oxygenase-1 (BCO-1), which cleaves β-carotene into retinal. The retinal is then enzymatically reduced to retinol and esterified by LRAT to RE. Although this is the major route for the intestinal metabolism of β-carotene in humans, some lesser portion of the newly absorbed β-carotene becomes incorporated directly into the chylomicron core and is absorbed intact. Chylomicrons containing RE and/or β-carotene are secreted into the lymphatic vessels. Additionally, small amounts of retinol or β-carotene may also be oxidized within the intestine, presumably in enterocytes, to form retinoic acid. Retinoic acid is secreted into the portal circulation, bound to albumin.[25]

POSTINTESTINAL METABOLISM

In tissues that express lipoprotein lipase (LPL), most of the chylomicron triglyceride is digested, leaving the majority of RE in the chylomicron remnant. However, in some extrahepatic tissues, such as adipose tissue, skeletal muscle, heart, lungs, and kidneys, LPL may also be able to hydrolyze RE.[26] Additionally, during lactation the mammary gland takes up significant amounts of chylomicron RE, in proportion to the RE content of the chylomicron.[26] The ability of these tissues to take up chylomicron RE postprandially may account for their accumulation of vitamin A in a dietary dose-dependent manner. Nevertheless, in adults, the majority of chylomicron RE, as well as the β-carotene in chylomicrons, remain within the chylomicron remnant and are cleared into the liver. Because the processing of chylomicron triglycerides takes place very rapidly, the half-life of chylomicron remnant RE in plasma is very short, on the order of minutes, and thus dietary RE circulate in postprandial plasma very transiently. As compared to adult animals, extrahepatic tissues in neonatal rats[16,27] and piglets[28] play a significantly greater role in the clearance of chylomicron RE from plasma, especially after supplementation with vitamin A.

Studies in adult humans have shown that a fraction of the absorbed β-carotene may undergo a slow conversion to retinol over many days after the main peak of β-carotene absorption.[29] This suggests that tissues besides the intestine (most likely the liver) can generate vitamin A. Although the *BCO-1* gene is expressed mainly in the intestine, its mRNA is also present in other tissues although at lower levels,[30] consistent with a possible capacity for extrahepatic metabolism of β-carotene to retinol after intestinal absorption. Various single nucleotide polymorphisms (SNPs) in the human *BCO-1* gene have been implicated in alterations in the efficiency of carotene cleavage. Interestingly, the distribution of BCO1 SNPs differs among ethnic groups,[31] and, although still unproven, this may correlate with the variability in β-carotene conversion to vitamin A that has been observed among human subjects.[32]

HEPATIC PROCESSING

RE contained within chylomicron remnants is cleared into the liver, specifically hepatocytes, which it enters via receptor-mediated endocytosis,[33] where it is rapidly hydrolyzed.[34] In both the adult and neonate, the liver accumulates vitamin A as RE when vitamin A intake exceeds the body's requirements. Under conditions of vitamin A sufficiency, most of the released retinol is transferred from hepatocytes to hepatic stellate cells, where retinol is bound to CRBP type I and reesterified by LRAT and then stored as RE within cytoplasmic lipid droplets.[35] Storage also serves as a detoxification mechanism, removing excess "free" retinol. When peripheral tissues require retinol, these stored esters are hydrolyzed, and retinol is mobilized back to hepatocytes. Hepatocytes are also the major site of synthesis of RBP. The newly released retinol combines with apo-RBP to form the holo-RBP complex that is released from the liver into the circulation. In the condition of vitamin A deficiency, apo-RBP is still synthesized, but it accumulates in the liver without retinol bound to it.[36] If vitamin A is ingested or injected, the holo-RBP complex is then rapidly released from liver to plasma.[36]

TRANSPORT OF VITAMIN A IN PLASMA

Due to the short half-life of chylomicrons in plasma, RE is present in plasma transiently after meals. In contrast, retinol bound to RBP as holo-RBP is present continuously. In the fasted state, holo-RBP constitutes nearly all (>95%) of total plasma retinol. RBP is a 21-kDa protein with a single binding site for all-*trans*-retinol, and the concentrations of both in plasma are highly correlated. Although RBP is synthesized mostly in hepatocytes, *RBP4* mRNA is present in measurable amounts in several extrahepatic tissues, including the kidney. Therefore these tissues might also contribute RBP, or holo-RBP, to plasma.[37] Within plasma, holo-RBP circulates in association with another plasma protein, transthyretin (TTR, previously known as *prealbumin*). The complex of holo-RBP and a tetrameric TTR protein has a molecular mass of approximately 55 kDa. The increased size of holo-RBP-TTR, as compared to holo-RBP alone, is believed to limit the filtration rate of the complex in the kidney and thereby to reduce the loss of holo-RBP in urine. In contrast, apo-RBP has a reduced affinity for TTR, and consequently, it is rapidly filtered and excreted in the urine.

Retinoic acid, the acidic form of vitamin A, circulates in plasma at generally low concentrations (5 to 20 nM).[38,39] The concentration of retinoic acid does not correlate well with plasma retinol,[38] but it is increased in plasma after a high-vitamin A meal such as animal liver.[40] In addition, minor quantities of other retinoid compounds are present in plasma, including *cis*-isomers of retinoic acid and small amounts of water-soluble metabolites such as the glucuronide adducts of retinol, retinoic acid, and their oxidation products.

PLASMA RETINOL CONCENTRATION

The concentration of retinol in plasma is quite stable and regulated within a relatively narrow range, so long as there is adequate vitamin A for its secretion as holo-RBP from liver. Conversely, plasma retinol, and RBP with which it is closely correlated, decreases when hepatic stores of RE are too low. The figure of 20 µg total retinol/g liver (equal to 70 nmol/g) is generally considered a value below which hepatic secretion of holo-RBP is impaired.[41] In adult animals and humans, plasma retinol concentrations above 1.05 µM are generally accepted as indicating vitamin A adequacy; levels between 0.7 and 1.05 µmol/L as indicating vitamin A-marginal status; and levels less than 0.7 µmol/L as indicating vitamin A deficiency.[42] Whether these same numerical criteria are also appropriate in newborn and infants, however, is unknown. In general, serum retinol levels are lower in infants than in children, even when vitamin A intakes are adequate, suggesting that this is a physiologically determined level that may be appropriate for age. Serum retinol concentrations tend to increase with age, reaching a plateau after puberty that is slightly higher in boys than girls.[43] Plasma retinol is usually lower in preterm infants than in full-term infants.[44,45] Retinol concentrations in plasma and serum are nearly identical, and either can be used for analysis.

RBP is a negative acute phase protein whose rate of synthesis in the liver decreases in states of infection or inflammation.[46–48] Thus, a reduction in RBP concentration, and therefore also of retinol secretion as holo-RBP, may reflect inflammation rather than a deficiency of vitamin A, although the retinol concentrations cannot be distinguished.[49] For example, plasma retinol may be low, and urinary retinol loss increased, in children with diarrheal disease.[50] After inflammation is resolved, and if vitamin A storage is adequate, plasma retinol can return to previous normal values as RBP synthesis increases again. Other rare causes of low serum retinol are transport defects due to mutations in the genes for *RBP4* or *TTR*.[51] Average plasma retinol concentrations tend to be lower in low-income countries than in developed countries, but whether this is due to differences in nutrition, higher rates of inflammation, or other causes is not certain. The use and interpretation of serum retinol distributions to evaluate the impact of vitamin A supplementation in public health programs is discussed in Palmer et al.[52]

CAROTENOIDS

In the fasting state, β-carotene is transported in low- and high-density lipoproteins.[53] Its concentration varies with carotenoid intake and may also co-vary with plasma lipid and lipoprotein concentrations.

UPTAKE OF RETINOL FROM PLASMA AND RETINOL RECYCLING

A plasma membrane-spanning receptor protein, Stimulated by Retinoic Acid 6 (STRA6), has been shown to bind the holo-RBP-TTR complex.[54] STRA6 is expressed in several types of cells; it appears to be necessary for the normal uptake of retinol by retinal pigment epithelium cells.[55] It may also play a role in other tissues, such as lung[56] and spleen,[57] in which its expression is up-regulated by retinoic acid. When STRA6 protein as expressed in cultured cells, it catalyzes retinol release from holo-RBP, retinol loading into apo-RBP, and retinol exchange between retinol- binding proteins, and therefore it transports retinol both into and out of the cell.[54,58,59] In transfected cells, the coexpression of STRA6, CRBP, and LRAT facilitated the uptake and retention of retinol by the cell, likely by binding the internalized retinol and trapping it intracellularly as RE.[60]

Recycling of retinol between plasma, liver, and peripheral tissues has been demonstrated in studies of retinol kinetics analyzed by mathematical modeling. In adult humans, the average retinol molecule recirculated between plasma and tissues greater than 3 times before undergoing irreversible degradation.[61] The recycling number was even higher in rats, with 12 to 13 passages before irreversible retinol disposal,[62] and it was higher still in neonatal rats.[63] These data suggest that retinol circulates in a highly dynamic state, with rapid bidirectional transfer between plasma and tissue compartments. Although the liver expresses very little STRA6, another structurally similar transmembrane protein, referred to as RBPR2, has been described in liver,[64] where it may be suited to taking up plasma retinol as it recycles from peripheral tissues. The kidney also plays a role in retinol recycling and conservation through the reuptake of holo-RBP from the renal filtrate.

VITAMIN A METABOLISM IN LIVER AND PERIPHERAL TISSUES

RETINOL STORAGE IN LIVER

The distribution of vitamin A in various tissues of the body depends on vitamin A status. In the vitamin A–adequate state, as much as 90% of the total body reserves are stored in the adult liver in most animal species, mainly in lipid droplets in hepatic stellate cells.[35,65] The liver vitamin A concentration ranges from 100 to 300 µg total retinol/g in healthy human adults[41] and varies with age in children, being low during infancy compared to later childhood.[66,67]

RETINOID HOMEOSTASIS AND OXIDATIVE METABOLISM

Retinoids are metabolized in most tissues, many of which express one or more retinoid-binding proteins. A generally accepted view is that cellular retinoid metabolism is coordinated by these proteins, which serve to chaperone the bound retinoid to specific enzymes that, in turn, maintain cellular retinoid homeostasis through the processes of retinol esterification, oxidation, and recycling. The specific types of cellular retinoid-binding proteins and retinoid-metabolizing enzymes differ by cell type. LRAT and CYP26 each play important roles in vitamin A homeostasis.[68] Their levels of expression are tightly regulated by vitamin A status and in many cases specifically by retinoic acid, especially in the liver and lungs.[68] The levels of LRAT and CYP26 mRNA are down-regulated in vitamin A–deficient tissues;[69,70] this reduced level of expression may serve to maintain the availability of unesterified retinol, for secretion or metabolism, as long as possible. Conversely, the expression of these genes is rapidly up-regulated when vitamin A or retinoic acid is administered. The difference is especially strong for CYP26A1,[71,72] which catabolizes excess retinol and retinoic acid and thereby limits retinoid accumulation. The response of LRAT and CYP26, especially in the liver, to changes in dietary vitamin A intake, and hence vitamin A status, is an autoregulatory mechanism that helps to control whole-body retinol homeostasis and to avoid, to the extent that is possible, either vitamin A deficiency or retinoid toxicity.[73]

Many types of cells are capable of producing retinoic acid through oxidative metabolism. The oxidation of retinol to retinal is a reversible process in which the forward and reverse reactions are catalyzed by members of the alcohol dehydrogenase family (ADH)[74,75] and other enzymes.[76] The second step, the oxidation of retinal to retinoic acid, is irreversible. This process is catalyzed by enzymes of the aldehyde dehydrogenase (ALDH1A) family.[76] The isoform known as *ALDH1A2 (RALDH2)* is critical for normal embryonic development, as shown in studies in mice.[77] ALDH1A1 and ALDH1A3 were shown to regulate cellular function in tumor-initiating stem-like cells, promoting tumor growth and resistance to drugs and radiation.[78] Many cells contain cellular retinoic acid-binding proteins (CRABP1 or -2). These proteins have been implicated in controlling the flow of retinoic acid to the nucleus, where it may bind to nuclear receptors of the retinoic acid receptor (RAR) family.

Furthermore, retinoic acid bound to a CRABP molecule can be directed to enzymes that metabolize the retinoic acid into polar and less active metabolites, such as 4-oxo-retinoic acid, 4-hydroxy-retinoic acid, 18-hydroxy-retinoic acid, and 5,18-epoxy-retinoic acid,[75,79] produced by members of the CYP26 family as well as other oxidative enzymes. CYP26A1, B1, and C1[80-82] are expressed in specific patterns with respect to timing and location during embryonic development, when they are significant for establishing the body pattern of the embryo.[83,84] In adults, CYP26 genes are expressed in several tissues where they appear to prevent, to the extent possible, the accumulation of retinol and other retinoids. All-*trans*-retinoic acid acts as both inducer of CYP26A1[85,86] and CYP26B1 expression,[71] and as the principal substrate of the enzymes produced by these genes.

NUCLEAR ACTIVITY OF RETINOIC ACID

Three isoforms of the nuclear RAR, termed *RARα, -β, -γ*, are expressed in temporal- and tissue-specific patterns beginning early in development and continuing throughout life. RARs form heterodimers with member of the RXR gene family for which, as with RARs, there are also three different isomers—RXR-*α*, -*β*, -*γ*—that are expressed in distinct patterns. The binding of all-*trans*-retinoic acid to RAR in a RAR-RXR heterodimer serves to activate the transcription factor complex that, when bound to specific retinoic acid response elements (RARE) in target genes, serves to recruit additional protein factors that activate or repress gene expression. The activity of the RARs is further modulated by posttranslational modifications, for example by phosphorylation and sumoylation.[87,88] Physiologically, several hundred genes respond as targets of retinoic acid, but precise mechanisms for their induction are known for only a few of them.[89] Some of these genes are crucial for normal embryonic development, cell differentiation, and immune function, and others control aspects of vitamin A's own metabolism.

EXCRETION

The excretory end products of vitamin A metabolism are derived from the metabolism of both retinol and retinoic acid.[90] Retinoic acid is excreted in bile partly in the ester form as retinoyl-*β*-glucuronide, and is subject to reabsorption.[91] Enterohepatic circulation of retinoic acid serves as a means to conserve this biologically active form of vitamin A. The remainder of the retinoic acid is excreted largely in the urine as inactive metabolites. The oxidized end products of retinol and retinoic acid are excreted similarly.

Holo-RBP in the circulation is filtered into the renal glomerulus. However, most of the retinol is recovered from the tubules and recycled. Megalin, the major endocytic receptor of proximal tubules, plays a crucial role in the reuptake of retinol, and in its absence a significant amount of retinol is lost in the urine.[92] Under these conditions, retinol must be mobilized from liver at a faster rate in order to maintain a normal plasma retinol concentration.[93]

VITAMIN A IN THE FETAL AND NEONATAL PERIODS

Vitamin A plays critical roles in prenatal and perinatal development. In the form of retinoic acid, vitamin A is required for normal embryonic development, for example, for specification of the body plan and organogenesis of the nervous system, heart, kidney, lung, and axial skeleton; and for hematopoiesis, immune response, metabolism, and growth and differentiation of many types of cells.[94,95] Vitamin A plays an important role in both innate and adaptive immunity, and therefore it is essential to infants and neonates, who are at high risk of infectious diseases. Vitamin A-deficient children are at increased risk of mortality and morbidity from infectious diseases; for example, measles and diarrheal diseases have been reported to be more severe in areas of the world in which children are most likely to be vitamin A deficient.[96] As noted below in the "Vitamin A and the Lung" section, vitamin A is also critical for normal postnatal alveolarization.[97-100]

FETAL ACQUISITION OF VITAMIN A

Vitamin A is transferred from the mother to the fetus during pregnancy, particularly in late gestation in most animal species, although the quantity is limited.[101,102] Transplacental transport of maternal retinol-RBP complex appears to be the predominant route for providing vitamin A to the fetus in early gestation.[101-103] *β*-carotene is also transported across the placenta.[104] Transplacental transfer of vitamin A in humans has been studied by analyzing paired samples of maternal and fetal or cord blood at various gestational ages.[105-108] The ratio of maternal to fetal concentrations of plasma vitamin A in healthy human pregnancies is approximately 2:1. In conditions in which the mother's vitamin A status is marginal or deficient, the fetal plasma vitamin A concentration often is maintained within normal limits and may exceed the maternal concentration.[109-111] Conversely, in studies involving maternal vitamin A supplementation, the cord blood vitamin A concentration in the supplemented cohort remained similar to that in unsupplemented control infants.[110,112,113] Thus the plasma vitamin A concentration in the fetus appears to be maintained within a normal range despite variations in maternal vitamin A status and intake. The regulatory mechanism(s) by which this homeostasis is achieved remains unclear. Nor is it known whether such mechanisms can compensate successfully for extremes of maternal vitamin A deprivation or excess.

In late gestation, RBP is synthesized by the fetal liver, beginning around gestational day 16, and may be involved in extracting vitamin A from the placental circulation.[103] Swallowing of amniotic fluid containing vitamin A and transfer of maternal lipoproteins containing REs are other possible means for the fetus to acquire vitamin A.[102,114]

VITAMIN A METABOLISM IN FETUS/NEONATES

A number of factors required for vitamin A metabolism are expressed early in life. The mRNAs for all the retinoid nuclear receptors (RARα, *β* and *γ*, and RXR*α*, *β* and *γ*), CRBP1 and CRBP2, and two of the enzymes able to convert retinol to retinal [retinol dehydrogenase 5 (RDH5) and ADH4] were detected in mouse embryos dissected as early as 7.5 days post-coitum.[115] RALDH-2, an enzyme capable of oxidizing the final step in all-*trans*-retinoic acid synthesis, was also detected.[115] These genes are expressed during embryonic development in temporally and spatially regulated patterns.[116,117] Genes required for *β*-carotene metabolism are also expressed during gestation.[104] In addition, as studied in a rat model, levels of important proteins involved in intestinal RE formation, including CRBP2 and LRAT, were detectable by gestational days 18 to 19, increasing at birth, reaching high levels in the middle of the suckling period, and then declining after weaning to adult levels. CRBP1 was present on day 16 of gestation, declined by 70% at birth, and then was maintained to adulthood.[118] RBP is detectable in liver of the fetal rat around gestational day 16.[103] LRAT, CYP26, and STRA6 are expressed in lung and liver of the neonatal rat,[56] while LRAT and megalin are expressed in neonatal kidneys.[119] The activity of LPL, the enzyme required for chylomicron RE clearance, in rat lung, skeletal muscle, heart, and brown adipose tissue emerges substantially during the first 24 h after birth, and LPL activity in brown adipose tissue and skeletal muscle is highest during the period of suckling.[120] As a result, despite the immaturity of the neonate, the stage is well set before birth for important processes in retinol trafficking and metabolism.

VITAMIN A STATUS AT BIRTH

Comparisons of vitamin A levels in plasma, liver, and extrahepatic tissues in newborns with those in adults have consistently shown lower levels in neonates. In healthy newborns, plasma retinol concentration, the most commonly used biochemical marker of vitamin A status, is approximately 50% of that in the corresponding maternal plasma.[121,122] Plasma RBP concentration, another biochemical marker of vitamin A status, also equals approximately 60% of adult values.[107] A liver retinol level of less than 10 μg/g tissue was reported[123] in an autopsy study of otherwise healthy infants who died at 0 to 1 month of age from sudden infant death syndrome as well as other causes. Such a low level would be considered an indicator of vitamin A deficiency in older children and adults, but whether this low value has the same meaning in neonates needs further validation.

Most preterm infants are born with low liver vitamin A stores,[124-127] probably because of a shortened period of transplacental vitamin A supply.[44,128] Higher cord blood vitamin A levels were observed with increasing birth weight of the newborn as well as with gestational age and maturity.[129] Vitamin A levels of term infants (median 0.71 μM) were higher than those of infants born preterm (median 0.35 μM).[130] Concentrations of RBP in cord blood were also found to be lower before 37 weeks gestation than at term,[128] which might impair the mobilization of vitamin A stores. Studies in a neonatal rodent model demonstrated that a high dose of vitamin A given to neonates raised under vitamin A–marginal conditions increased vitamin A concentrations in plasma and various tissues, but the effect is transient.[131] Indirect vitamin A supplementation through enriching the maternal diet, however, provided a sustained effect on neonatal VA status.[132]

VITAMIN A KINETICS IN NEONATES VERSUS ADULTS

Retinol kinetics studied in neonatal and adult rodent models and analyzed by mathematical modeling revealed both similarities and differences.[133] Similarities include the capacity for an efficient absorption of vitamin A; a high-response system, in which the retinol turnover rate is much higher than the disposal rate; extensive retinol recycling between plasma and tissues; and comparable vitamin A disposal rates. Differences between neonatal and adult models include that, in neonates, retinol turnover is faster and retinol recycling is more extensive, especially in neonatal rats treated with supplements containing vitamin A;[134] extrahepatic tissues, including the lungs, the intestine, and the brain, play a greater role in the uptake of chylomicron vitamin A.[16,135] These differences may reflect an adaption to the lower vitamin A status found in neonates as compared with adults.

VITAMIN A AND THE LUNG

Although the liver is the principal storage site for vitamin A, other organs, including the developing lung, are capable of storing vitamin A.[34,98,136] Vitamin A stores are high in fetal lung and decrease toward term, and are almost depleted in newborns.[136,137] Depletion of these stores continues into early postnatal period, suggesting that the developing lung may depend on these local stores of vitamin A during the period of active growth and differentiation that is associated with rapid alveolarization. Evidence from animal models of postnatal vitamin A supplementation suggests the rapid uptake of chylomicron REs into the lung,[138] as well as uptake of retinol from holo-RBP.[133] STRA6 is expressed in lung tissue and modestly upregulated after treatment with retinoic acid.[56] CRBP1 is also expressed,[139] as is LRAT, which likely accounts for the significant capacity of the lung to store RE.[56] Following cellular uptake, retinol is bound to CRBP1 and deposited for storage in a cell type similar to the stellate cells in the liver, known as lipid interstitial cells or lipofibroblasts,[140] or it may be further oxidized to form retinal and retinoic acid through the actions of retinol and retinaldehyde dehydrogenases, respectively. Excess or unutilized retinoic acid can be further oxidized to polar metabolites for excretion by CYP26 enzymes, particularly CYP26B1 in lung tissue.[56,141]

Prematurely born animals, deprived of adequate stores of vitamin A in the lungs, may be susceptible to the adverse pulmonary effects of vitamin A deficiency. The fetal lung stores of vitamin A can be augmented by prenatal maternal vitamin A supplementation.[142] Conversely, prenatal interventions, such as maternal glucocorticosteroid treatment, can deplete the lung's vitamin A.[143] In rodent models, retinoid deficiency caused by dietary restriction of the mother or offspring results in impaired alveolar septation, as well as altered pulmonary tissue composition and elasticity.[144,145]

Retinoic acid is needed for proper lung development, maintenance, and repair.[146] Lung-specific genes regulated at least in part by retinoids include growth factors, homeobox genes, and extracellular matrix genes that activate cellular differentiation, regulate axial patterning, and promote secondary septation of alveoli, respectively. This ultimately leads to alveolarization and vascularization necessary for increasing lung surface area for optimal gas exchange.[147,148] Retinoic acid treatment of neonatal rats exposed to hypoxia or treated with dexamethasone, both of which cause alveolar simplification, resulted in improved septation, suggesting an important role for retinoic acid in postnatal lung maturation.[148-150]

In preterm and low-birth-weight (LBW) infants, poor vitamin A status may contribute to the development of chronic lung disease, such as bronchopulmonary dysplasia (BPD), which is a major cause of morbidity in preterm infants, associated with exposure to high oxygen concentrations, mechanical ventilation, and inflammation, and predisposing to chronic lung disease.[147,151] Poor vitamin A status (plasma retinol concentrations <0.35 μmol/L) during the first month of life in LBW infants was reported to be related to increased risk of developing BPD and long-term respiratory disability.[152] Retinol therapy slightly but significantly improved outcomes in extremely LBW infants.[153,154]

VITAMIN A DEFICIENCY AND TOXICITY

DEFICIENCY

Depending on its severity, vitamin A deficiency during gestation can result in fetal malformations, often of the neural cord, limbs, and craniofacial structures, or in death and fetal resorption. Interestingly, these outcomes are similar to those produced by excess vitamin A, suggesting that either a deficiency or excess of retinol or its products at critical periods of develop are teratogenic.[155-158] Vitamin A deficiency also affects growth and survival in neonates and young children. An important role for vitamin A apart from its well-known requirement for vision has been demonstrated by randomized clinical trials in which vitamin A supplementation to children (6 months to 5 years of age) has been shown to reduce child mortality by 23%, with reductions in all-cause as well as measles- and diarrhea-associated mortality.

Despite public health programs aimed at eradicating nutritional blindness, vitamin A deficiency is still a leading cause of nutrition-related blindness.[159,160] Administration of vitamin A can be sight- and life-saving in situations of impending vitamin A deficiency. A high dose of vitamin A is typically given orally in the form of concentrated retinyl palmitate, at a dose of 50,000 to 200,000 IU (equal to 15 to 60 mg RAE, depending on age, given once or more).[159] The use of vitamin A in measles is discussed in the section "Vitamin A as Enteral and Parenteral Therapy."

In the United States, few healthy children are severely vitamin A deficient, but the 5th percentile of children 4 to 8 years and 9 to 13 years of age, respectively, in National Health and Nutrition Examination Survey (NHANES) fell below less than 1.05 μmol/L,[43] while a serum retinol concentration from 0.7 to 1.05 μmol/L is generally interpreted as an indicator of mild vitamin A deficiency.[161] Thus, it is recommended to question all pediatric patients about their intake of vitamin A-containing foods (e.g., whole milk or fortified low-fat milk, eggs, orange or yellow cheeses, fortified cereals, and dark-green leafy or yellow and orange vegetables), and nutritional supplements, to ensure that intakes are adequate.

TOXICITY

Vitamin A toxicity, also called *hypervitaminosis A*, is a serious and even life-threatening condition. Toxicity is dose-dependent; it may be acute and even fatal with very high doses of vitamin A, while with lower but still excessive intakes over a longer time, onset is likely to be slower but symptoms may still be severe. Signs of acute vitamin A toxicity include hydrocephalus, anorexia, anemia, rough and dry skin, and bone pain. A prolonged elevation of vitamin A may lead to irreversible organ damage. Manifestations of vitamin A toxicity in the reproductive period include teratogenic birth defects, including malformations of the face, nervous system, heart, and thymus.[162] Hypervitaminosis A occurs when plasma retinol exceeds the availability of RBP to bind it, leading to unbound and elevated levels of free retinol in plasma, and formation of excess retinoid metabolites. Although there is no antidote, hypervitaminosis A may be slowly reversible by restriction of VA consumption, with remediation of symptoms within a few hours to a few months. However, a patient with chronic hypervitaminosis A was reported to still experience hydrocephalus and elevated serum retinol and RBP levels almost 2 months after cessation of vitamin A supplementation.[163] Dietary vitamin E has displayed some therapeutic benefit in treating vitamin A toxicity,[164] and 2-hydroxypropyl-β-cyclodextrin has shown to be safe and has been used to solubilize vitamin A, which allows for urinary excretion.[165] However, more research is needed to provide therapeutic interventions for chronic hypervitaminosis A.

DIETARY RECOMMENDATIONS FOR VITAMIN A

RECOMMENDED DIETARY ALLOWANCE AND TOLERABLE UPPER INTAKE LEVEL

Dietary advice is provided by the Institute of Medicine in terms of the estimated average requirement (EAR), the recommended dietary allowance (RDA), which defines a level of intake sufficient to cover the requirements for greater than 97% of the healthy population, and the tolerable upper intake level (UL), which describes the highest intake that does not pose a risk, whereas for intakes of retinol above the UL there is uncertainty, or risk is known to increase. Values for age and sex groups are shown in Table 28.1. The RDA for vitamin A is based on a factorial model that allows for adequate storage, determined in adults and then scaled for body weight in children and adolescents.[166] For the UL, criteria are also based on adult data, scaled by extrapolation for children and adolescents. These criteria include irreversible teratogenic effects in females of reproductive age and liver damage.[166] It is important to note that the RDA can be met by consuming either preformed retinol or provitamin A carotenoids, or a combination of both, whereas the UL refers only to preformed vitamin A.

Table 28.1 Recommended Dietary Allowances and Tolerable Upper Intake Levels for Vitamin A by Life Stage.

	RDA (μg RAE/day)		UL (μg retinol/day)	
0–6 mo	400		600	
7–12 mo	500		600	
Children	**Boys**	**Girls**	**Boys**	**Girls**
1–3 yr	300	300	600	600
4–8 yr	400	400	900	900
9–13 yr	600	600	1700	1700
14–18 yr	900	700	2800	2800
Adults	**Men**	**Women**	**Men**	**Women**
19 yr and older	900	700	3000	3000
Pregnancy				
14–18 yr	750		2800	
19–50 yr	770		3000	
Lactation				
14–18 yr	1200		2800	
19–50 yr	1300		3000	

The observed average or experimentally determined intake by a defined population or subgroup. The AI is used if sufficient scientific evidence is not available to derive an estimated average requirement.

AI, Adequate intake; *RAE*, retinol activity equivalents; *RDA*, recommended daily allowance; *UL*, upper intake level.

CAROTENOIDS

There is no specific nutritional requirement for carotenoids, although dietary guidelines to consume more fruits and vegetables would naturally result in increased intakes of carotenoids. There is no evidence that a high intake of β-carotene causes toxicity (thus its omission from the UL). Persons who consume a persistently high dietary intake of carotenoids in foods or supplements may experience yellowing of the skin, especially the palms of the hands, but this condition is considered benign. A case report of a 1-½ year old Indian boy fed carrot juice equivalent to 2 carrots/day illustrates the yellowing of the palms; by 3 months after feeding was stopped the discoloration disappeared. The safe use of carotene as a source of vitamin A is also discussed in Grune et al.[167]

VITAMIN A AS ENTERAL AND PARENTERAL THERAPY

ENTERAL NUTRITION

The vitamin A value of a diet is expressed in μg equivalents of retinol, termed *retinol activity equivalents (RAE)*.[166] An older unit, the international unit (IU), is still sometimes used; 1 IU is equal to 0.3 μg of retinol. The vitamin A content of human milk is variable and influenced by several factors including mother's age, parity, and socioeconomic status, which may affect diet, and the volume and fat content of the milk. The vitamin A concentration is higher in human colostrum (above 333 IU/dL) than in mature milk, which ranges from 110 to 257 IU/dL.[168–172] The vitamin A concentration of preterm milk is lower than that of term milk during the first week of lactation, but is higher thereafter.[172–174] More than 90% of the vitamin A in milk of human, cow, and other species is in the form of RE contained in the core of the milk fat globules.[171,175–177] Various infant formulas have been designed to meet the nutritional needs of a preterm infant. The vitamin A content of these formulas varies, ranging from approximately 296 to 1000 IU/dL.[178]

Preterm infants receiving full enteral feedings often are given multivitamin supplements. The vitamin A content of a typical multivitamin supplement is 1500 IU/dL, also generally in the form of RE, which confers greater stability but must be hydrolyzed before absorption.[178] The efficiency of use of vitamin A in a neonate fed human milk or an infant formula with or without a multivitamin supplement depends largely on the ability of the infant's gastrointestinal tract to process RE.

Vitamin A is also used therapeutically in the prevention of nutritional blindness and treatment of measles, as has been discussed above. A typical dose for a child greater than 6 months of age is 200,000 IU, equal to 60 mg RAE. Current practice is based on findings that this large amount, given once or twice, will support vitamin A-dependent functions and reduce risk of disease-related mortality.[179-182] The Committee on Infectious Diseases of the American Academy of Pediatrics also recommends vitamin A supplementation for children who are hospitalized with measles or who have additional risk factors.[183] However, studies investigating vitamin A supplementation in 1- to 5-month-old infants did not show any survival benefits. Also, vitamin A supplementation to newborns has produced mixed results, with reduced mortality in some trials but not in others, but most failed to provide a clear indication of benefit.[184,185] As a result, at present, neonatal vitamin A supplementation (within 0 to 28th day of life) is not recommended as an intervention to reduce infant morbidity and mortality. Studies in rodent models have also indicated potential roles of vitamin A in treating necrotizing enterocolitis (NEC), the most devastating gastrointestinal disease in preterm newborns.[186-188] Vitamin A was shown to improve the condition via regulating intestinal flora, attenuating inflammation, and enhancing the intestinal epithelial barrier,[186] while all-*trans*-retinoic acid modulated lymphocyte balance[187] and alleviated inflammation as well as oxidative stress.[188]

PARENTERAL NUTRITION

Preterm infants requiring intravenous nutrition are often fed a protein-dextrose solution and a lipid emulsion prepared for intravenous nutrition. The vitamin A concentration of the protein-dextrose solution is estimated at approximately 930 IU/dL.[189] A newborn infant fed by total parenteral nutrition and receiving the protein-dextrose solution at a conventional rate of 120 to 135 mL/kg/day is, therefore, expected to receive vitamin A intakes from 1116 to 1256 IU/kg/day. Several reports have been published regarding loss of vitamin A due to photodegradation, and/or binding to the plastic of the bag or intravenous tubing,[190-194] which render the intravenous administration of vitamin A inefficient. Alternative methods of vitamin A administration, such as by intramuscular route,[195,196] may be necessary to optimize the vitamin A status of neonates on long-term parenteral nutrition.

THE RETINOID ANALOGUE, ISOTRETINOIN

The acidic form of vitamin A, typically in the form of 13-*cis*-retinoic acid, commonly known as *isotretinoin* and first marketed as Accutane, is an approved drug for the treatment of severe intractable nodular acne and other serious skin conditions, some of them relatively common in the adolescent years. Due to the known teratogenicity of retinoids, the FDA has issued a Risk Evaluation and Mitigation Strategy, known as *iPLEDGE*, to monitor the prescription by physicians and the use by patients of isotretinoin (https://www.fda.gov/drugs/postmarket-drug-safety-information-patients-and-providers/isotretinoin-marketed-accutane-capsule-information). One clinical study reported that memory and executive function were unchanged or even improved,[197] and another that isotretinoin did not reduce learning and memory and may improve specific aspects of hippocampal learning and memory.[198] One study conducted in adolescent acne vulgaris patients demonstrated an improvement for neurocognitive functions in patients receiving isotretinoin.[199] Retinoic acid is known to affect the expression of the dopamine receptor D2R in the brain and pituitary gland.[200] Further research under appropriate clinical conditions and dose ranges may be revealing regarding the relationship of isotretinoin treatment in relation to cognitive and behavioral outcomes. Retinoids may also have a role in treatment of pediatric neuroblastoma.[201]

ACKNOWLEDGMENTS

We wish to acknowledge NIH grant HD066982 for support for our research mentioned in this chapter and Dr. Sarah A. Owusu for contributions to an earlier version of this chapter.

A complete reference list is available at www.ExpertConsult.com. 

SELECT REFERENCES

5. Blomhoff R, Blomhoff HK. Overview of retinoid metabolism and function. *J Neur*. 2006;66:606-630.
6. Gutierrez-Mazariegos J, Schubert M, Laudet V. Evolution of retinoic acid receptors and retinoic acid signaling. *Subcell Biochem*. 2014;70:55-73.
16. Tan L, Wray AE, Green MH, et al. Compartmental modeling of whole-body vitamin A kinetics in unsupplemented and vitamin A-retinoic acid-supplemented neonatal rats. *J Lipid Res*. 2014;55:1738-1749.
24. Harrison EH. Mechanisms involved in the intestinal absorption of dietary vitamin A and provitamin A carotenoids. *BiochemBiophys Acta*. 2012;1821: 70-77.
27. Tan L, Green MH, Ross AC. Vitamin A kinetics in neonatal rats vs. adult rats: comparisons from model-based compartmental analysis. *J Nutr*. 2014;145:403-410.
45. Woodruff CW, Latham CB, Mactier H, et al. Vitamin A status of preterm infants; correlation between plasma retinol concentration and retinol dose response. *Am J Clin Nutr*. 1987;46:985-988.
50. International Life Science Institute Research Foundation. *Reduction In Serum Retinol And Urinary Loss Of Vitamin A In Children With Acute Diarrhea. Virtual Elimination Of Vitamin A Deficiency: Obstacles And Solutions For The Year 2000*. Washington, DC: ILSI Human Nutrition Institute; 1996:83.
56. Wu L, Ross AC. Acidic retinoids synergize with vitamin A to enhance retinol uptake and STRA6, LRAT, and CYP26B1 expression in neonatal lung. *J Lipid Res*. 2010;51:378-387.
68. Ross AC. Retinoid production and catabolism: role of diet in regulating retinol esterification and retinoic acid oxidation. *J Nutr*. 2003;133:291S-296S.
88. Wei LN. Retinoid receptors and their coregulators. *Ann Rev Pharmacol Toxicol*. 2003;43:47-72.
89. Balmer JE, Blomhoff R. Gene expression regulation by retinoic acid. *J Lipid Res*. 2002;43:1773-1808.
94. Clagett-Dame M, DeLuca HF. The role of vitamin A in mammalian reproduction and embryonic development. *Ann Rev Nutr*. 2002;22:347-381.
97. Geevarghese SK, Chytil F. Depletion of retinyl esters in the lungs coincides with lung prenatal morphological maturation. *BiochemBiophysi Res Commun*. 1994;200:529-535.
98. Shenai JP, Chytil F. Vitamin A storage in lungs during perinatal development in the rat. *Biol Neonate*. 1990;57:26-32.
99. McGowan SE, Harvey CS, Jackson SK. Retinoids, retinoic acid receptors, and cytoplasmic retinoid binding proteins in perinatal rat lung fibroblasts. *Am J Physiol Lung Cell Mol Physiol*. 1995;269:L463-L472.
100. Maden M, Hind M. Retinoic acid in alveolar development, maintenance and regeneration. *Philos Trans R Soc Lond B Biol Sci*. 2004;359:799-808.
101. Moore T. Vitamin A transfer from mother to offspring in mice and rats. *Int J VitamNutr Res*. 1970;41:301-306.
102. Ismadi S, Olson JA. Dynamics of the fetal distribution and transfer of Vitamin A between rat fetuses and their mother. *Int J VitamNutr Res*. 1981;52: 112-119.
103. Takahashi YI, Smith JE, Goodman DS. Vitamin A and retinol-binding protein metabolism during fetal development in the rat. *Am J Physiol*. 1977;233:E263-E272.
104. Spiegler E, Kim Y-K, Wassef L, et al. Maternal-fetal transfer and metabolism of vitamin A and its precursor β-carotene in the developing tissues. *BBA-Mol Cell Biol L*. 2012;1821:88-98.
110. Berggren Söderlund M, Fex GA, Nilsson-Ehle P. Concentrations of retinoids in early pregnancy and in newborns and their mothers. *Am J Clin Nutr*. 2005;81:633-636.
112. Lewis J, Bodansky O, Lillienfeld M, et al. Supplements of vitamin A and of carotene during pregnancy: their effect on the levels of vitamin A and carotene in the blood of mother and of newborn infant. *Am J Dis Child*. 1947;73:143-150.
113. Barnes A. The placental metabolism of vitamin A. *Am J Obstet Gynecol*. 1951;61:368-372.
114. Wallingford J, Milunsky A, Underwood B. Vitamin A and retinol-binding protein in amniotic fluid. *Am J Clin Nutr*. 1983;38:377-381.
117. Mark M, Ghyselinck NB, Chambon P. Function of retinoid nuclear receptors: lessons from genetic and pharmacological dissections of the retinoic acid

signaling pathway during mouse embryogenesis. *Ann Rev Pharmacol Toxicol.* 2006;46:451–480.

119. Owusu SA, Ross AC. Retinoid homeostatic gene expression in liver, lung and kidney: ontogeny and response to vitamin A-retinoic acid (VARA) supplementation from birth to adult age. *PLoS One.* 2016;11:e0145924.
121. Yeum K-J, Ferland G, Patry J, et al. Relationship of plasma carotenoids, retinol and tocopherols in mothers and newborn infants. *J Am Coll Nutr.* 1998;17:442–447.
124. Olson JA, Gunning DB, Tilton RA. Liver concentrations of vitamin A and carotenoids, as a function of age and other parameters, of American children who died of various causes. *Am J Clin Nutr.* 1984;39:903–910.
127. Shenai JP, Chytil F, Stahlman MT. Liver vitamin A reserves of very low birth weight neonates. *Pediatr Res.* 1985;19:892–893.
129. Agarwal K, Dabke A, Phuljhele N, et al. Factors affecting serum vitamin A levels in matched maternal-cord pairs. *Indian J Pediatr.* 2008;75:443–446.
131. Hodges JK, Tan L, Green MH, et al. Vitamin A supplementation transiently increases retinol concentrations in extrahepatic organs of neonatal rats raised under vitamin A-marginal conditions. *J Nutr.* 2016;146:1953–1960.
132. Tan L, Babbs AE, Green MH, et al. Direct and indirect vitamin A supplementation strategies result in different plasma and tissue retinol kinetics in neonatal rats. *J Lipid Res.* 2016;57:1423–1434.
135. Hodges JK, Tan L, Green MH, et al. Vitamin A supplementation redirects the flow of retinyl esters from peripheral to central organs of neonatal rats raised under vitamin A-marginal conditions. *Am J Clin Nutr.* 2017;105:1110–1121.
138. Ross AC, Ambalavanan N, Zolfaghari R, et al. Vitamin A combined with retinoic acid increases retinol uptake and lung retinyl ester formation in a synergistic manner in neonatal rats. *J Lipid Res.* 2006;47:1844–1851.
148. Massaro D, Massaro GD. Lung development, lung function, and retinoids. *N Engl J Med.* 2010;362:1829–1831.
152. Spears K, Cheney C, Zerzan J. Low plasma retinol concentrations increase the risk of developing bronchopulmonary dysplasia and long-term respiratory disability in very-low-birth-weight infants. *Am J Clin Nutr.* 2004;80:1589–1594.
153. Tyson JE, Wright LL, Oh W, et al. Vitamin A supplementation for extremely-low-birth-weight infants. National Institute of Child Health and Human Development Neonatal Research Network. *N Engl J Med.* 1999;340:1962–1968.
154. Guimarães H, Guedes MB, Rocha G, et al. Vitamin A in prevention of bronchopulmonary dysplasia. *Curr Pharm Des.* 2012;18:3101–3113.
172. Thomas MR, Pearsons MH, Demkowicz IM, et al. Vitamin A and vitamin E concentrations of the milk from mothers of preterm infants and milk of mothers of full term infants. *Acta Vitaminol Enzymol.* 1981;3:135–144.
173. Chappell JE, Francis T, Clandinin MT. Vitamin A and E content of human milk at early stages of lactation. *Early Hum Dev.* 1985;11:157.
176. Vahlquist A, Nilsson S. Mechanisms for vitamin A transfer from blood to milk in rhesus monkeys. *J Nutr.* 1979;109:1456–1463.
177. Ross AC, Davila ME, Cleary MP. Fatty acids and retinyl esters of rat milk: effects of diet and duration of lactation. *J Nutr.* 1985;115:1488–1497.
179. Shenai JP. Vitamin A supplementation in very low birth weight neonates: rationale and evidence. *Pediatrics.* 1999;104:1369–1374.
183. Committee on Infectious Diseases. Vitamin A and measles. *Pediatrics.* 1993;91:1014–1015.
184. Gogia S, Sachdev HS. Vitamin A supplementation for the prevention of morbidity and mortality in infants six months of age or less. *Cochrane Database Syst Rev.* 2011: CD007480.
185. Haider BA, Sharma R, Bhutta ZA. Neonatal vitamin A supplementation for the prevention of mortality and morbidity in term neonates in low and middle income countries. *Cochrane Database Syst Rev.* 2017; 2: CD006980.
186. Xiao S, Li Q, Hu K, et al. Vitamin A and retinoic acid exhibit protective effects on necrotizing enterocolitis by regulating intestinal flora and enhancing the intestinal epithelial barrier. *Arch Med Res.* 2018;49:1–9.
188. Ozdemir R, Yurttutan S, Sari FN, et al. All-trans-retinoic acid attenuates intestinal injury in a neonatal rat model of necrotizing enterocolitis. *Neonatology.* 2013;104:22–27.
190. Hartline JV, Zachman RD. Vitamin A delivery in total parenteral nutrition solution. *Pediatrics.* 1976;58:448.
196. Ambalavanan N, Tyson JE, Kennedy KA, et al. Vitamin A supplementation for extremely low birth weight infants: outcome at 18 to 22 months. *Pediatrics.* 2005;115:E249–E254.

29 Vitamin E Nutrition in Pregnancy and the Newborn Infant

Karla Danielly da S. Ribeiro | Débora Gabriela Fernandes Assunção | Natália Carlos Maia Amorim | Priscila Gomes de Oliveira

INTRODUCTION

Vitamin E, a micronutrient with antioxidant functions, has important actions in both intrauterine and postnatal life. Even in pregnant women with adequate vitamin stores, it seems that there is a transplacental barrier that limits its transfer to the fetus. Thus, physiologic concentrations of vitamin E are lower at birth, which makes newborns (especially premature infants) more susceptible to development of vitamin E deficiency (VED). This nutritional deficiency can have repercussions in the neonatal period (retinopathy, intraventricular hemorrhage, and others), or later, as evidenced by its adverse impact on cognitive performance in childhood. Thus, in this chapter we will discuss vitamin E and its role in pregnancy and lactation, to understand the repercussions of vitamin E for the health of the newborn.

VITAMIN E: STRUCTURE AND FUNCTION

Vitamin E is an antioxidant that reacts with free radicals, preventing lipid peroxidation of cell membranes. This nomenclature represents eight forms synthesized by plants (four tocopherols and four tocotrienols) that vary according to the number of methyl groups in the chromanol ring, being trimethyl (α-), dimethyl (β- or γ-), or monomethyl (δ-).[1] Tocopherols are characterized by a saturated side chain attached to the chromanol ring, while tocotrienols have three unsaturated bonds in the side chain at carbons C (3′), C (7′), and C (11′) (Fig. 29.1). Of the eight naturally occurring forms, α-tocopherol is the most abundant isomer of vitamin E found in human plasma and tissues and is therefore the most studied.

All tocopherols that occur naturally in food have RRR- conformation on the side chain, while the synthesized α-tocopherol (racemic) contains eight stereoisomers [RRR, RSR-, RSS-, and RRS- (form 2R-) and SRR-, SRS-, SSR-, SSS-]. The various forms of vitamin E are not interconvertible in humans and therefore do not have the same metabolism.[2]

The main function of vitamin E is to be a potent antioxidant, capable of neutralizing free radicals by donating electrons from its chromanol ring, regardless of the presence of cofactors.[1] It protects polyunsaturated fatty acids (PUFAs, mainly arachidonic acid [ARA; 20:4 ω-6] and docosahexaenoic acid [DHA; 22:6 ω-3])

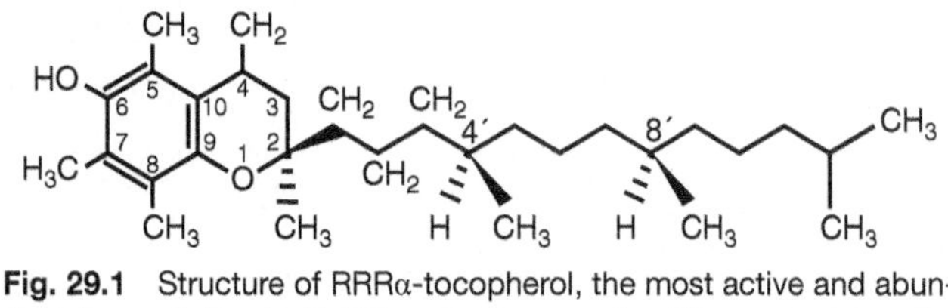

Fig. 29.1 Structure of RRRα-tocopherol, the most active and abundant form of vitamin E. This schema uses the RS nomenclature for specifying configuration at the three chiral centers at carbon 2′, 4′, and 8′. *R*, Clockwise (right-handed) orientation; *S*, counterclockwise *(left-handed)* orientation; *solid triangles,* in front of the plane of the paper; *lined triangles,* behind the plane of the paper.

from the lipid peroxidation chain reaction by reducing peroxyl radicals as they are formed,[3] so it is essential in any life cycle. In the presence of vitamin E, peroxyl radicals (ROO•) react more quickly with the vitamin (hydroxyl tocopherol, or vit E-OH) than with PUFAs, to form the corresponding hydroxide and the tocopheroxyl radical (vit EO•),[4] as shown below:

$$\text{ROO} \bullet + \text{vit E-OH} \rightarrow \text{ROOH} + \text{vit E-O} \bullet$$

The resulting tocopheroxyl radical reacts with vitamin C or other electron donors to return to its reduced state (recycling of vitamin E).[5]

Vitamin E is known for its important role in reproduction, making a major contribution to fetal antioxidant capacity, since other antioxidant enzyme systems are still developing in the embryonic phase.[6] In addition to prevention of oxidative damage to DNA, proteins, and lipids, other research suggests that adequate levels of vitamin E may be required for optimal intrauterine growth.[7,8]

Thus, for both fetus and newborn, adequate body reserves of α-tocopherol are important, particularly at the critical moment of birth, which abruptly increases oxidative stress. The transition from the relatively hypoxic intrauterine environment to the relative hyperoxia of postnatal life favors imbalance between production of free radicals and antioxidant, especially in situations of prematurity.[9-14]

Other functions attributed to vitamin E are believed to be—at least in part—consequences of its antioxidant role in maintaining the integrity of cell membranes.[4] Vitamin E is essential in brain functioning, protecting neuronal membranes against lipid peroxidation, which could result in neuronal loss, DNA damage, and decline in memory and learning.[15-18] This function has been supported by clinical or observational studies documenting benefits of vitamin E on cognitive development and neurodegenerative diseases.[19-22] Vitamin E also has antiinflammatory activities,[23-25] and α-tocopherol appears to suppress expression of adiponectin in neonates.[26]

Specific cellular functions have been attributed to α-tocopherol that are independent of its antioxidant capacity. These actions complement the vitamin's role in several processes, such as protein C kinase inhibition and transcriptional gene modulation through direct effects on gene transcription.[27,28]

RECOMMENDATIONS FOR VITAMIN E INTAKE

Although gamma-tocopherol (γ-tocopherol) is the predominant form of the vitamin in the diet,[1,29,30] the Institute of Medicine of the USA in 2000 advised that nutritional requirements for vitamin E in humans should be met only by the RRR-α-tocopherol form in foods or by 2R-α-tocopherol isomers present in fortified foods or supplements.[2] This decision was based on the specific affinity of the liver protein α-tocopherol transfer protein (α-TTP) for α-tocopherol, which primarily secretes this form into the circulation with consequent uptake by tissues, while the other vitamin counterparts are preferentially metabolized and excreted. In addition, at that time, scarcity of scientific knowledge about the other elements of vitamin E and their health benefits also contributed to this determination.

Table 29.1 Recommendations for Vitamin E Intake by Age or Population Group From the Institute of Medicine.

Life-Stage Group	AI	EAR	RDA	UL
Infants				
Preterm (<37 wk gestation)				21[a]
0–6 mo	4			
7–12 mo	5			
Children				
1–3 yr		5	6	200
4–8 yr		6	7	300
9–13 yr		9	11	600
14–18 yr		12	15	800
Adults ≥ 19 yr		12	15	1000
Pregnancy 14–50 yr		12	15	1000
Lactation		16	19	1000

[a]From Brion LP, Bell EF, Raghuveer TS. Vitamin E supplementation for prevention of morbidity and mortality in preterm infants. *Cochrane Database Syst Rev*. 2003;(4):CD003665.
Institute of Medicine (U.S.). *Panel on dietary antioxidants and related compounds: Dietary reference intakes for vitamin c, vitamin e, selenium, and carotenoids: A report of the panel on dietary antioxidants and related compounds, subcommittees on upper reference levels of nutrients and of interpretation and use of dietary reference intakes, and the standing committee on the scientific evaluation of dietary reference intakes, food and nutrition board, institute of medicine.* Washington, DC: National Academy Press; 2000.
mg/day of 2R-α-tocopherol. *AI*, Adequate intake; *EAR*, estimated average requirement; *UL*, tolerable upper intake level.

The reference values for nutrient intake are established according to characteristics of sex and stage of life of healthy individuals. Currently, the Dietary Reference Intakes (DRIs) provide four categories of suggested nutrient intake recommendations to assess the food consumption of individuals or population groups, among other applications.[2] The recommendations for nutrient intake for vitamin E are shown in Table 29.1. These vitamin E intake recommendation categories were established based on observations of reversal of deficiency symptoms in humans using supplements containing 2R-α-tocopherol, the amounts of α-tocopherol needed to correct erythrocyte hemolysis in vitro, or serum concentrations of α-tocopherol needed to prevent peroxide-induced erythrocyte hemolysis. The estimated average requirement (EAR) was based on experiments with individuals with VED resulting from prolonged insufficient vitamin E consumption. The recommended dietary allowance (RDA) was estimated to meet the needs of a nutrient for 97% to 98% of healthy individuals. For lactating women, it was defined based on the average amount of vitamin E secreted in human milk each day (4 mg/780 mL) plus the EAR for nonlactating women (12 mg), which totals 16 mg/day of α-tocopherol.

As it derives from EAR, this recommendation does not apply to neonates and children under 1 year of age. Because of the lack of functional criteria to establish reversal of VED symptoms in infants, intake recommendations are based on the adult EAR only for infants and children over 1 year of age. For neonates and children under 1 year of age, recommendations are formulated in terms of adequate intake (AI), based on estimates of vitamin E intake of breastfeeding children (0 to 6 months of age).

The vitamin E AI for children from 0 to 6 months of exclusive breastfeeding was defined based on the average volume of breast milk consumed by children of this age (780 mL/day), regardless of the gestational age of delivery, with an estimated content of 4 mg of α-tocopherol.[2] Finally, the tolerable upper intake level (UL) defines the highest value of prolonged daily intake of a nutrient that poses no apparent risk of adverse health effects in almost all individuals of any stage of life or sex. For premature and very low-birth-weight children (<37 gestational weeks and <1500 g), the intake limit of 21 mg/day has been adopted, due to evidence demonstrating that excess vitamin E supplementation at this stage of life may increase the risk of sepsis.[31]

Insufficient consumption of vitamin E can result in a nutritional status of inadequacy or deficiency, especially during stages of life characterized by increasing requirements. It is therefore essential to identify risk situations to support future intervention strategies to combat nutritional deficiencies.

FOOD SOURCES AND BIOAVAILABILITY OF VITAMIN E

Although the various forms of vitamin E are found in foods, α-tocopherol is the main form to be evaluated in the chemical composition tables of foods, being found in foods that are sources of fats, including vegetable oils (such as olive oil, sunflower, and canola), wheat germ, sunflower seeds, nuts (such as hazelnut, peanut, Brazil nut, almond, pistachio), dark green leaves (such as spinach and kale), and some fruits (Table 29.2).[32]

The absorption of vitamin E is strongly influenced by the amount of fat available in the meal. Because of its fat-soluble nature, intestinal absorption occurs through solubilization in micelles, which reach the liver through the remaining chylomicrons.[4,33] Vitamin E's bioavailability appears to be greater when it is found in long-chain triglyceride emulsions than when it is in medium-chain triglyceride emulsions.[34] The addition of milk and iron does not seem to alter the bioavailability of α-tocopherol.[35]

A high intake of vitamin A can reduce bioavailability of vitamin E, reflecting the antioxidant role of vitamin E in protecting vitamin A during absorption.[36-38] Other nutrients may also interfere with bioavailability of vitamin E. Intestinal α-tocopherol transporters—such as scavenger proteins class B type I (SR-BI), CD36 molecule (CD36), NPC1-like transporter 1 (NPC1L1), and ATP-binding cassettes A1 and G1 (ABCA1 and ABCG1)—are also carriers of cholesterol, γ-tocopherol, vitamin D, vitamin K, and carotenoids, among other nutrients and phytochemicals, which could lead to competition and reduced transport. However, more research is needed to answer questions that permeate bioavailability and recommendations for vitamin E intake.[39]

Table 29.2 Vitamin E Food Composition.

Food	Vitamin E (α-Tocopherol) mg/100 g[a]
Sunflower oil	41.08
Nuts, almonds	25.63
Olive oil	14.35
Canola oil	17.46
Soy oil	8.18
Brazil nuts	7.14
Peanut	6.91
Canned tuna	2.50
Mango	1.11

[a]USDA.[32] Nutrient Database for Standard Reference.

VITAMIN E METABOLISM

As previously anticipated, digestion and absorption of vitamin E is closely associated with the same steps as fats. Dietary vitamin E (mainly α- and γ-tocopherol) requires bile salts and pancreatic secretions to form micelles, with consequent uptake by intestinal epithelial cells (distal part) and release into the circulation in chylomicrons.[36,40] Chylomicrons are rapidly hydrolyzed by lipoprotein lipase (LPL), producing chylomicron remnants. Although this stage is not limited by the absence of fat or by fasting, it is enhanced by fat ingestion, suggesting that the absorption of α-tocopherol is highly dependent on the chylomicron assembly processes.[41]

The vitamin E molecules released during chylomicron hydrolysis are transferred directly to peripheral tissues, while those remaining in the chylomicron remnants are endocytosed by liver cells through a receptor-mediated mechanism.[40] Other forms of the vitamin are efficiently absorbed and supplied to the liver in chylomicrons, but little of that material is captured into newly secreted lipoproteins for the supply to peripheral tissues.[2] Intestinal fat can also modulate the physiology of α-tocopherol, sequestering it from circulation and decreasing the bioavailability of the vitamin to the liver.[42]

In the liver, these lipoproteins are hydrolyzed and vitamin E released. The α-tocopherol is captured and transported by α-TTP (α-tocopherol transport protein) to the cell membrane, where it is secreted into the circulation by the ABCA1 receptor and incorporated by very low-density lipoproteins (VLDLs). α-TTP is a small hepatic cytoplasmic protein with differential affinity for α-tocopherol, also expressed in other tissues such as the brain and placenta. It is largely responsible for the intracellular transport of α-tocopherol and mediates its secretion into plasma, which explains why α-tocopherol is the most abundant form of the vitamin in the circulation.[43,44] Haga and colleagues[45] demonstrated that the liver plays a central role in the regulation of α-tocopherol, with high expression of at least six genes related to blood concentration, distribution, transport, and metabolism of α-tocopherol, including afamin (AFM); class B receiver scavenger, type I (SCARB1); tocopherol-associated protein (SEC14L2)[46]; *α-TTP* gene; ABCA1; and cytochrome P450 family 4, subfamily F, polypeptide 2 (CYP4F2).[47]

Similarly to chylomicron particles, VLDL triacylglycerols are catabolized by LPL on the surface of peripheral tissues, which results in the transfer of α-tocopherol to adjacent tissues and to high-density lipoprotein (HDL) particles. VLDL particles (or intermediate density lipoproteins, IDL) with remaining α-tocopherol are removed by the liver. Some vitamin is transferred to other peripheral tissues during catabolism of LDL.[4]

Depending on the metabolism of lipoproteins, exchanges between LDL and HDL favor the transport of α-tocopherol in the circulation and its transfer to reproductive and other tissues, especially the liver, lung, brain, placenta, and mammary gland. The acquisition of α-tocopherol by these tissues appears to be mediated by an SR-BI receptor, located on the surface of cells and capable of binding HDL and LDL to capture lipids.[48]

The largest body store of α-tocopherol is in adipose tissue (about 90%), but it seems that its mobilization is weak in response to dietary VED in adults,[49,50] probably due to the redistribution of α-tocopherol from other tissues to fat cells.[51] It is not known how this reserve behaves during lactation.

The body's ability to sustain high plasma concentrations of α-tocopherol is limited, apparently not because of reduced absorption but due to increased excretion.[52] Fairus and colleagues[53] demonstrated that plasma levels of α-tocopherol peak at 6 to 8 hours after oral supplementation, with return toward baseline after that period. Levels of circulating α-tocopherol are maintained through mechanisms associated with those that control the circulation of lipids, with a positive correlation being found between plasma levels and half-life of α-tocopherol and serum total lipid levels in individuals without dyslipidemia.[54] These findings raise the question of whether this relationship is due to greater vitamin E consumption for antioxidant protection against lipid peroxidation or if it is due to a lower catabolism of circulating lipoproteins that also carry vitamin E.

The main route of elimination is through the feces, resulting from incomplete absorption, secretion by mucus cells, and excretion along with bile salts. In the liver, the other forms of vitamin E (δ-, β- and γ-) and the excess of α-tocopherol are excreted in the bile or metabolized by side-chain degradation via initial enzymatic degradation of cytochrome P450 (ω-oxidation) and subsequent β-oxidation to form carboxyethyl hydroxychromanol (CEHC).[55,56] Finally, this main metabolite of tocopherols is largely excreted in the urine, especially in situations of increased dietary intake of vitamin E (>12.8 mg/day) and high circulating α-tocopherol levels.[57,58]

TRANSFER OF TOCOPHEROL TO TISSUES

INTRAUTERINE PHASE

The mechanism of vitamin E delivery across the placenta is still unknown. Several studies have been carried out analyzing the concentration of α-tocopherol in maternal serum, umbilical cord, placental tissue, and expression of α-TTP in the placenta.[6,14,59-63] There is relationship between maternal and newborn vitamin E, but the cord values are less than one-third of the maternal levels, suggesting that adequacy of maternal vitamin E nutritional status in pregnancy is protective against low fetal concentrations at birth and that placental transfer to the fetus during pregnancy may be limited.[7,64,65] It was believed that there was a placental "barrier" associated with this difference in the maternal-fetal vitamin, but evidence has shown that levels of vitamin E in the placenta and in the maternal serum were similar and strongly associated,[62] and that lower fetal levels were proportionate to lower total serum lipid levels, indicating that the lower levels in the neonate are attributable to less efficient distribution of vitamin E from the placenta to fetal blood.

Studies with other animal models (mice, pigs) reveal that this placental-fetal uptake is closely related to lipid metabolism and can be mediated by lipoprotein receptors on the placental membranes (VLDL, LDL, SRB1-HDL receptor), lipase activity lipoprotein, and presence of α-TTP in the placenta. In humans, LDL and VLDL fractions are the main sources of vitamin E for the fetus, but in umbilical cord blood, HDL is the predominant carrier of vitamin E. Placental expression of α-TTP increases toward the end of pregnancy, a period in which fetal accumulation of vitamin E is also greater.[7,14,43,66-69] Thus, lower α-tocopherol concentrations in the neonate may be caused by the reduced fetal expression of α-TTP and/or the scarcity of circulating lipids in the fetus and neonate (triglycerides, phospholipids, total cholesterol), since lipid metabolism is also immature and the concentration of vitamin E has been associated with an increase in the fetus's lipid body mass.[7,62]

This maternal-fetal transfer is believed to be more effective with γ-tocopherol and δ-tocopherol than with α-tocopherol.[70] It is proposed that vitamin E is delivered to the placenta mainly by LDL and VLDL and transported to the fetal side by a tocopherol-binding protein, which selectively transfers the 2R form to umbilical venous blood. As in the postnatal situation, vitamin E and its congeners are taken up by the fetal liver, and isomers other than α-tocopherol are ultimately returned to the maternal circulation.[66] This is corroborated by the studies demonstrating expression of enzymes capable of metabolizing α-tocopherol in the fetal liver and sheep placenta.[71] In a novel study, Didenco and colleagues found a higher ratio of the vitamin E metabolite α-carboxyethyl hydroxychromanol (α-CEHC) to α-tocopherol metabolite in cord blood compared to that in the maternal blood, and hypothesized that lower cord blood α-tocopherol levels may be attributable to higher fetal hepatic metabolism of the vitamin.[57] This hypothesis needs to be further explored since it was not possible to determine whether the metabolite was produced by the fetus or originated from maternal metabolism and was preferentially captured by the placenta.

LACTATION PHASE

As with placental transfer, the mechanism for transferring α-tocopherol to milk through the mammary glands is not fully understood. There are reports of transport of α-tocopherol from plasma to tissues through lipid transport proteins such as phospholipid transfer protein (PLTP), LDL receptors, or even selective transport through the scavenger receptor class B, type I (SRBI) lipoprotein receptor, which is responsible for cellular uptake of HDL and is present in membranes of mammary cells.[72,73] It is also suggested that during lactation there is a greater participation of LPL, an enzyme that hydrolyzes chylomicrons allowing the cellular transfer of α-tocopherol. LPL activity and concentrations of α-tocopherol were higher in the mammary glands of pregnant rats when compared to nonpregnant rats, with no differences observed in adipose tissue,[63] suggesting specific adaptations to prioritize transfer of the vitamin into breast milk at the expense of storage in adipose tissue. Another form of transfer may be through the α-TTP receptors present on the membrane of the mammary glands.[74]

Some researchers found changes in expression of genes related to transfer and metabolism of α-tocopherol in the pre- and postpartum period in the liver and mammary glands of cows around calving, suggesting genetic regulation of transfer of α-tocopherol from maternal blood to colostrum and milk. After calving, expression of *α-ttp* gene tocopherol-associated protein *(SEC14L2)*, afamin, and albumin in the liver decreased, while expression of *α-ttp* mRNA peaked and *SEC14L2* mRNA reached a nadir in mammary tissue.[75] High expression of the *α-ttp* gene may explain the high concentration of α-tocopherol in colostrum in the first postpartum week.

In humans so far, such analyses are not available, but some studies already reflect some transport mechanisms. Rebouças and colleagues[76] reported that maternal supplementation with 800 IU vitamin E increased the concentration of α-tocopherol in breast milk, regardless of baseline vitamin values, which suggests that membrane receptors present in breast tissue are not modulated by prior concentration of α-tocopherol in milk. Consequently, supplemental vitamin E intake is able to increase its concentration in breast milk.

Therefore, evidence indicates that in the pre- and postpartum period, the body undergoes adaptations that may include expression of genes for proteins involved in vitamin E metabolism. The consequent alterations of transport protein concentrations and uptake of α-tocopherol by the mammary glands favor secretion of vitamin E into breast milk and mobilization of body reserves of α-tocopherol.

CURRENTLY AVAILABLE VITAMIN E BIOMARKERS

Measurements of the α-tocopherol content of serum, plasma, or red blood cells are the indicators most used to assess vitamin E nutritional status in neonates, both in the umbilical cord blood and in postnatal samples.[77,78] Its concentration naturally increases from birth to 1 year of age.[79] Levels are strongly controlled by mechanisms that are still not very clear, remaining stable even during periods of low dietary intake.[80]

The classification of vitamin E inadequacy or deficiency was based on in vitro experiments showing erythrocyte hemolysis induced by peroxides. For premature and low-birth-weight neonates, serum α-tocopherol concentrations below 500 μg/dL (<11.6 μmol/L) in umbilical cord blood were associated with increased lipid oxidation.[81,82] However, use of this classical cut-off can overestimate rates of vitamin E inadequacy at birth, as it is similar to the threshold for adults (<517 μg/dL or <12 μmol/L) and physiologic serum vitamin E levels are one-third to one-quarter of those in adults.[64] In 2014, Traber[80] gathered information on α-tocopherol from children with low vitamin E intake and associated diseases, and suggested reference values for assessing vitamin E nutritional status in childhood, with deficiency considered when serum levels are below 388 μg/dL (<9 μmol/L) (Table 29.3).

Breast milk vitamin E concentration is not considered a biomarker for vitamin E sufficiency. However, milk concentrations may more reliably estimate the vitamin supply to the infant, as breast milk vitamin concentrations may decline throughout lactation, without corresponding reduction in maternal serum concentrations.[83,84] The probable supply of the vitamin is estimated by analyzing α-tocopherol composition in breast milk, multiplying by the volume of milk ingested per day, and compared with AI for infants, equivalent to 4 mg/day.[2,84–89] It is important to consider the differences in volume of milk ingested per day between full-term (≥37 weeks) and preterm (<37 weeks) newborns. Thus, for colostrum, daily intake can be estimated to be 254 mL and 396 mL preterm and term, respectively; for transition milk (7 to 15 days postpartum), 500 mL for preterm and 780 mL for term neonates; and for mature milk (>15 days postpartum), 780 mL can be estimated for both groups.[2,90]

Other markers have been suggested to assess vitamin E nutritional status, since there is no consensus on the relationship between dietary vitamin intake and serum levels of α-tocophe rol.[30,80,91] Measurement of the vitamin E metabolite α-CEHC in urine or serum has been proposed as a biomarker of the adequacy of micronutrient intake, since its excretion is increased after the dietary adequacy of the vitamin requirement.[57,58,92] However, further investigations are still needed, because formation of α-CEHC differs according to the origins of the vitamin (food or supplements).[93]

Analysis of vitamin E in stool samples from preterm neonates has also been suggested as an indicator of vitamin bioavailability.[94] Those authors themselves express some reservations about this method, mainly due to the quantity and quality of the samples, including variation in composition of the feces caused by interactions between food components and gastrointestinal secretions.

Table 29.3 Summary of Biomarkers and Classification for Vitamin E Status.

Classification	α-Tocopherol (μg/dL)
Infants[a]	
Low level (α-tocopherol serum)	<500
Probable inadequate intake (α-tocopherol in breast milk)	<4 mg/day[b]
Children and Adolescents[c]	
Vitamin E deficiency (α-tocopherol serum)	<388
Marginal level (α-tocopherol serum)	388–517
Adequate level (α-tocopherol serum)	>517
Adults[d]	
Vitamin E deficiency (α-tocopherol serum)	<517

[a]Gutcher et al.[82]
[b]Rodrigues.[85]
[c]Traber.[80]
[d]Institute of Medicine.[2]

VITAMIN E AND PREGNANCY

ROLE OF VITAMIN E IN REPRODUCTION

Maintenance of reproductive health is strongly associated with the balance between reactive oxygen species and antioxidants,[95] highlighting the essential role of vitamin E in this period. Oxidative stress, resulting from the imbalance in the production of free radicals and their removal by antioxidants, causes the peroxidation of cell membranes that can occur with smoking, alcohol use, extremes of body weight, exposure to environmental toxins, and advanced maternal age. This can impair physiologic processes such as oocyte maturation, ovulation, luteolysis, and follicular atresia. This can lead to infertility or conditions that reduce fertility, such as polycystic ovary syndrome (PCOS) and endometriosis.[96]

Vitamin E can antagonize oxidative stress caused by oxygen free radicals and antioxidant imbalance, inhibiting the activity of phospholipase A and lipoxygenase to stabilize cell membranes and regulate the normal physiologic function of the reproductive system. Studies during the periconceptional period showed that the placenta may be the main source of free radicals due to the high metabolic rate and increased mitochondrial activities.[97,98]

In addition to the impact on women's reproductive health, lipid peroxidation in men can alter the fluidity and integrity of cell membranes, causing increased permeability and decreased motility of sperm and inhibiting membrane fusion events (acrosome reaction and sperm-oocyte interaction) and viability, also affecting reproduction.[99]

Thus, vitamin E in women and men can impact the results of in vitro fertilization, not only reducing the time to achieve pregnancy in women, possibly via improving the endometrial environment due to its antioxidant effects, but also by improving sperm motility and reduction of associated oxidative damage,[100] demonstrating the necessity for adequate vitamin E status during pregnancy.

VITAMIN E SUPPLEMENTATION DURING PREGNANCY: EVIDENCE AND RECOMMENDATIONS

Vitamin E acts on embryo development, implantation, placental maturation, and protection of the fetus against oxidative stress.[7] As oxidative stress is associated with adverse pregnancy outcomes, and vitamin E has powerful antioxidant properties, vitamin E status in pregnancy has a potential effect on pregnancy outcomes.

During pregnancy, maternal vitamin E supplementation caused an improvement in the vasoreactivity of the middle cerebral artery (MCA) in premature fetuses.[101] Léger and colleagues[102] supplemented pregnant women with a daily dose of 1 g DL-α-tocopherol acetate for 3 days before delivery, demonstrating an increase in α-tocopherol in the circulation of women associated with postpartum lipidemia, but found no effect in the neonates, suggesting that the peculiarities in lipid transport in the neonate were the possible cause for the restriction of the circulating vitamin. Surprisingly, vitamin E supplementation has also been associated with an increased risk of low birth weight, probably due to insufficiency of insulin-like growth factor 1 (IGF-1).[103,104]

There is also evidence that vitamin A supplementation may cause disorders in the uteroplacental circulation, manifested by development of small-for-gestational-age fetuses and erythrocytosis, by inhibition of free-radical processes due to the excess of the vitamin E.[105] Supplementation with 400 IU RRR-α-tocopherol in pregnant women with pre-eclampsia also did not reduce respiratory complications in children in the long term.[106]

This evidence suggests that supplementation should be carefully evaluated during pregnancy, as the safe dose is not known. It is important to encourage adequate vitamin E consumption via diet, as it is recognized as a crucial factor that influences maternal, fetal, and child health. In practice, the possibility of nutritional deficiencies may be reduced by strengthened monitoring of vitamin status, developing early prevention and intervention strategies, emphasizing nutritional education in the perinatal period, and guiding pregnant women on food and on the safe use of nutritional supplements.[107]

VITAMIN E AND NEONATE

NEONATAL VITAMIN E STATUS AND PREMATURITY

Physiologically, newborns have lower α-tocopherol serum concentrations compared with their mothers, probably due to low placental transfer or high production of free radicals resulting from the relative hyperoxia of the extrauterine environment.[7,68] There is also evidence of excessive fetal vitamin E metabolism due to the high quantities of vitamin E metabolite present in the circulation of the fetuses of women given high vitamin E supplementation during pregnancy. It is suggested that absorption of this vitamin by the preterm fetus is limited due to immaturity, with lower expression of α-TTP protein contributing to lower vitamin E levels at birth.[57]

Another hypothesis to explain lower vitamin E concentrations in the neonate, especially preterm neonates, is its association with low levels of circulating lipids and the concordance between accumulation of fetal α-tocopherol and the period of greatest fetal growth and accumulation of adipose tissue reserve in the third trimester. Since about 90% of vitamin E in the body is located in adipose tissue, premature delivery also impairs the total body reserves.[108]

These inadequate α-tocopherol reserves make preterm neonates more susceptible to problems resulting from VED, such as mortality, hemolytic anemia, retinopathy of prematurity, intracranial hemorrhage, and bronchopulmonary dysplasia.[109] VED has been defined by low plasma α-tocopherol concentrations (below 500 μg/dL or 11.6 μmol/L) accompanied by a low tocopherol-lipid ratio or increased erythrocyte hemolysis.[110]

In 15 preterm neonates, weight of 1190 g and gestational age of 30 weeks, Schwalbe and colleagues[111] found mean serum α-tocopherol levels of 8 μmol/L. In 35 preterm infants with gestational age ranging from 28 to 34 weeks and weight of 940 to 1980 g, Wu and Chou[112] found mean umbilical cord blood concentrations of 4 μmol/L, well below the recommended (>11.6 μmol/L). A study carried out in Tunisia found VED in 71% of preterm newborns with low birth weight. In Thailand, this proportion reached 77% of those evaluated, in Brazil it reached more than 90% of premature and term neonates.[64,81,113-115] Because lower levels of vitamin E are physiologic in newborns, however, caution should be exercised when evaluating VED using these classical cutoff points in neonates, since these approximate the values used for adults (see Table 29.3). Therefore, it is important to correlate low serum levels with other biomarkers of vitamin E insufficiency, such as clinical signs of VED, the vitamin E content in breast milk, or the infant's dietary intake.

After birth, α-tocopherol levels increase regardless of the type of dietary intake, with a parallel reduction in cases of deficiency.[81,113,116-118] However, preterm infants may still have lower concentrations of α-tocopherol at 90 days.[85]

INTERVENTION STRATEGIES FOR VITAMIN E STATUS IN NEONATES

Intravenous vitamin E supplementation in preterm neonates is contraindicated, even in those with intrauterine growth restriction and clinical signs and symptoms of deficiency. The basis for this decision lies in a meta-analysis carried out by Brion and collaborators,[31] which demonstrated unacceptable side effects including increased risks of necrotizing enterocolitis, neonatal sepsis, and mortality; it was hypothesized that these effects may be due to pro-oxidant effects of excessive quantities of the vitamin. Another study did not find inadequacy of circulating α-tocopherol in breastfed newborns after 6 weeks of age, suggesting that routine vitamin E supplementation is not indicated.[110]

Daily supplementation with 5 IU (5 mg) of d-(L)-tocopherol acetate in term or preterm newborns, breastfed with formula or milk, produced an increase in circulating levels of α-tocopherol at 3 months of age.[116,119] In a randomized clinical trial using a single enteral dose of 50 IU/kg (50 mg/kg) of d-(L)-α-tocopherol acetate in preterm neonates, serum α-tocopherol levels were increased at 7 days post-supplementation, but a substantial proportion (30%) of treated infants still met criteria for VED (α-tocopherol level <500 μg/L) at 24 hours and all infants were vitamin E sufficient (α-tocopherol level >500 μg/L) by 7 days.[81]

Breastfeeding is a strategy to increase vitamin E reserves in neonates. Kositamongkol and colleagues[113] observed that low consumption of human milk was one of the factors associated with prolonging post-birth VED. In addition, it appears that the maternal vitamin E status is also an explanatory and protective factor for the child's vitamin status during lactation.[85] Maternal supplementation with vitamin E in its natural form (RRR-d-(L)-α-tocopherol)[120] produced a greater increase in α-tocopherol in colostrum than the racemic form. Supplementation with 400 IU (400 mg) of RRR-d-(L)-α-tocopherol, in a single dose, in premature or term postpartum women, increased the vitamin E concentration in breast milk up to 15 days postpartum, but this increase was not sustained after this period.[121,122] Increasing the dose to 800 IU (800 mg) resulted in a more effective transfer of the vitamin to breast milk, representing a 124% increase after supplementation.[76]

Lira[123] applied two protocols for maternal vitamin E supplementation and demonstrated that supplementation with 400 UI of α-tocopherol in the immediate postpartum period and repeated on the 20th postpartum day was able to guarantee higher concentrations of α- tocopherol in milk until the 60th day of lactation. This milk had a better vitamin supply profile for the infant, when compared to the milk of women who did not receive the supplement and those who received a single dose in the postpartum period, demonstrating that supplementation with higher doses of vitamin may be necessary to obtain a more effective intervention.

Despite the well-established impact on quantities in milk, the tendency for vitamin concentration in milk to decrease during lactation, and naturally low vitamin E reserves in the premature newborn,[124] there is still no evidence of a favorable impact of maternal supplementation in their infants. Therefore, it is important to assess how (and if) maternal vitamin E supplementation impacts the prevention and/or treatment of VED in breastfed preterm neonates.

VITAMIN E AND LACTATION

VITAMIN E COMPOSITION OF BREAST MILK AND ASSOCIATED FACTORS

The concentration of vitamin E (α-tocopherol) in breast milk decreases during lactation, accompanied by an increase in fatty acids, with colostrum (milk produced from the beginning of lactation until the 4th or 6th postpartum day) having the highest concentration, declining in transitional milk (produced from the 7th to the 21st postpartum days), until reaching lower concentrations in mature milk (produced after the 21st postpartum day

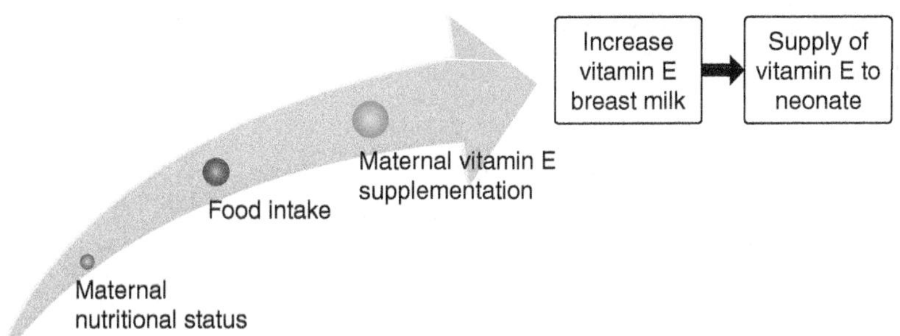

Fig. 29.2 Summary of recommendations to improve α-tocopherol concentration in breast milk and the supply to infants.

until the end of lactation).[124-127] Colostrum has α-tocopherol concentrations between 56 and 86 μmol/L, in transition milk between 33 and 38 μmol/L of α-tocopherol,[128,129] while vitamin concentrations in mature milk were between 7 and 9 μmol/L.[83,88,130,131] Even with this reduction in vitamin E content of milk, breastfeeding is considered an effective form of prevention of and intervention for VED. Breast milk, especially colostrum, represents concentrated source of this nutrient, with a high capacity for absorption. Vitamin E is an important contributor to the oxidative stability of human milk.[7,110,132] Higher values were observed in studies in lactating women who used supplements, with an average α-tocopherol concentration of 18 μmol/L,[128,129] which shows that high intake of vitamin E can influence its concentration in breast milk.

Studies that estimated the vitamin E supply through analyzed milk found adequate values only in colostrum and transitional milk (>4 mg/780 mL),[a] even without changes in maternal vitamin E intake between these stages of lactation. Without supplementation, dietary intakes of vitamin E by breastfeeding women are typically less than recommended (16 mg/day).[2] Similar low intakes have been observed across populations of different countries,[76,83,84,88,128] with average intakes ranging from 4 to 8 mg of vitamin E per day and inadequate intakes in up to 100% of breastfeeding women.

Despite the dietary inadequacy of vitamin E in lactating women and the low vitamin values in mature milk, studies have found no direct effect between vitamin consumption and its composition in milk, except in situations of α-tocopherol supplementation.[61,76,84,83] The vitamin E content of milk can be affected by other dietary factors, however, such as a positive association with dietary fat intake[88,131] and inverse relationship with high vitamin A intake.[37] A very recent study[134] of the impact of consumption of ultra-processed foods—those industrially manufactured products that are produced through several processing steps and techniques and are labeled as ready to eat, drink, or heat—on composition of breast milk demonstrated that a greater proportions of such foods in the maternal diet were associated with an inadequate vitamin E profile in milk; this is likely due to the type of vitamin E (racemic form) added to these foods by the food industry, which is less bioavailable.

Other factors associated with the concentration of α-tocopherol in breast milk include gestational age at delivery, with higher values being observed in the breast milk of lactating women after preterm delivery (<37 gestational weeks) compared to those who deliver at term (≥ 37 weeks),[85] as well as with prepregnancy excess weight and cesarean delivery.[124,135] Lower vitamin E contents were found in the milk of women who smoke and in those from low-income populations.[133,136]

[a]References 64, 83, 84, 128, 129, 133.

CONCLUSION

The essential role of vitamin E is evident both in intrauterine and postnatal life, mainly due to its antioxidant action in combating lipid peroxidation. Placental transfer of the vitamin appears to be limited, resulting in serum or plasma levels in newborns one-fourth to one-third of those in their mothers. This gradient may be associated with the similarly lower concentrations of lipids in the fetal circulation. Because of this difference, caution should be exercised in the use of serum levels as a biomarker for the status of the vitamin, since the cutoff point adopted is very similar to that of adults. As there is no evidence concerning the dose and safe frequency of supplementation during pregnancy and in the newborn, maternal supplementation may be an alternative to contribute to the newborn's vitamin E reserves (Fig. 29.2). This strategy produces an increase in the concentration of vitamin E in milk, but clinical research is still needed to assess the effect of this strategy on the vitamin E status of neonates.

A complete reference list is available at www.ExpertConsult.com. 

SELECT REFERENCES

1. Traber MG. Vitamin E. In: Ross CA, Caballero B, Cousins R, Tucker K, Ziegler T, eds. *Org: Modern Nutrition in Health and Disease*. 11th ed. Philadelphia: Wolters Kluwer/Lippincott Williams; 2014:293–304.
2. Institute of Medicine (U.S.). *Panel on Dietary Antioxidants and Related Compounds: Dietary Reference Intakes for Vitamin C, Vitamin E, Selenium, and Carotenoids: A Report of the Panel on Dietary Antioxidants and Related Compounds, Subcommittees on Upper Reference Levels of Nutrients and of Interpretation and Use of Dietary Reference Intakes, and the Standing Committee on the Scientific Evaluation of Dietary Reference Intakes, Food and Nutrition Board, Institute of Medicine*. Washington, DC: National Academy Press; 2000.
6. Jauniaux E, Cindrova-Davies T, Johns J, et al. Distribution and transfer pathways of antioxidant molecules inside the first trimester human gestational sac. *J Clin Endocrinol Metab*. 2004;89(3):1452–1458. https://doi.org/10.1210/jc.2003-031332.
7. Debier C. Vitamin E during pre- and postnatal periods. *Vitam Horm*. 2007;76:357–373. https://doi.org/10.1016/S0083-6729(07)76013-2.
9. Lee YS, Chou YH. Antioxidant profiles in full term and preterm neonates. *Chang Gung Med J*. 2005;28(12):846–851.
11. Negi R, Pande D, Kumar A, Khanna RS, Khanna HD. In vivo oxidative DNA damage and lipid peroxidation as a biomarker of oxidative stress in preterm low-birthweight infants. *J Trop Pediatr*. 2012;58(4):326–328. https://doi.org/10.1093/tropej/fmr078.
13. Robles R, Palomino N, Robles A. Oxidative stress in the neonate. *Early Hum Dev*. 2001;65(suppl):S75–S81. https://doi.org/10.1016/s0378-3782(01)00209-2.
19. Kitajima H, Kanazawa T, Mori R, Hirano S, Ogihara T, Fujimura M. Long-term alpha-tocopherol supplements may improve mental development in extremely low birthweight infants. *Acta Paediatr*. 2015;104(2):e82–e89. https://doi.org/10.1111/apa.12854.
31. Brion LP, Bell EF, Raghuveer TS. Vitamin E supplementation for prevention of morbidity and mortality in preterm infants. *Cochrane Database Syst Rev*. 2003;4:CD003665. https://doi.org/10.1002/14651858.CD003665.
33. Reboul E. Vitamin E bioavailability: mechanisms of intestinal absorption in the spotlight. *Antioxidants*. 2017;6(4):95. https://doi.org/10.3390/antiox6040095.
37. Grilo EC, Medeiros WF, Silva AG, Gurgel CS, Ramalho HM, Dimenstein R. Maternal supplementation with a megadose of vitamin A reduces colostrum level of

α-tocopherol: a randomised controlled trial. *J Hum Nutr Diet*. 2016;29(5):652–661. https://doi.org/10.1111/jhn.12381.

39. Reboul E. Vitamin E intestinal absorption: regulation of membrane transport across the enterocyte. *IUBMB Life*. 2019;71(4):416–423. https://doi.org/10.1002/iub.1955.
40. Gagné A, Wei SQ, Fraser WD, Julien P. Absorption, transport, and bioavailability of vitamin E and its role in pregnant women. *J Obstet Gynaecol Can*. 2009;31(3):210–217. https://doi.org/10.1016/s1701-2163(16)34118-4.
41. Traber MG, Leonard SW, Ebenuwa I, et al. Vitamin E absorption and kinetics in healthy women, as modulated by food and by fat, studied using 2 deuterium-labeled alpha-tocopherols in a 3-phase crossover design. *Am J Clin Nutr*. 2019;110:1148–1167.
44. Kono N, Arai H. Intracellular transport of fat-soluble vitamins A and E. *Traffic*. 2015;16(1):19–34. https://doi.org/10.1111/tra.12231.
49. El-Sohemy A, Baylin A, Ascherio A, Kabagambe E, Spiegelman D, Campos H. Population-based study of alpha- and gamma-tocopherol in plasma and adipose tissue as biomarkers of intake in Costa Rican adults. *Am J Clin Nutr*. 2001;74(3):356–363. https://doi.org/10.1093/ajcn/74.3.356.
54. Traber MG, Leonard SW, Bobe G, et al. α-Tocopherol disappearance rates from plasma depend on lipid concentrations: studies using deuterium-labeled collard greens in younger and older adults. *Am J Clin Nutr*. 2015;101(4):752–759. https://doi.org/10.3945/ajcn.114.100966.
57. Didenco S, Gillingham MB, Go MD, Leonard SW, Traber MG, McEvoy CT. Increased vitamin E intake is associated with higher alpha-tocopherol concentration in the maternal circulation but higher alpha-carboxyethyl hydroxychroman concentration in the fetal circulation. *Am J Clin Nutr*. 2011;93(2):368–373. https://doi.org/10.3945/ajcn.110.008367.
59. Gordon MJ, Campbell FM, Dutta-Roy AK. alpha-Tocopherol-binding protein in the cytosol of the human placenta. *Biochem Soc Trans*. 1996;24(2):202S. https://doi.org/10.1042/bst024202s.
60. Johnston PC, McCance DR, Holmes VA, Young IS, McGinty A. Placental antioxidant enzyme status and lipid peroxidation in pregnant women with type 1 diabetes: the effect of vitamin C and E supplementation. *J Diabetes Complications*. 2016;30(1):109–114. https://doi.org/10.1016/j.jdiacomp.2015.10.001.
61. de Lira LQ, Lima MS, de Medeiros JM, da Silva IF, Dimenstein R. Correlation of vitamin A nutritional status on alpha-tocopherol in the colostrum of lactating women. *Matern Child Nutr*. 2013;9(1):31–40. https://doi.org/10.1111/j.1740-8709.2011.00376.x.
62. Martinez FE, Goncalves AL, Jorge SM, Desai ID. Vitamin E in placental blood and its interrelationship to maternal and newborn levels of vitamin E. *J Pediatr*. 1981;99(2):298–300. https://doi.org/10.1016/s0022-3476(81)80482-9.
64. Ribeiro KDS, Lima MS, Medeiros JF, et al. Association between maternal vitamin E status and alpha-tocopherol levels in the newborn and colostrum. *Matern Child Nutr*. 2016;12(4):801–807. https://doi.org/10.1111/mcn.12232.
65. Weber D, Stuetz W, Bernhard W, et al. Oxidative stress markers and micronutrients in maternal and cord blood in relation to neonatal outcome. *Eur J Clin Nutr*. 2014;68(2):215–222. https://doi.org/10.1038/ejcn.2013.263.
68. Debier C, Larondelle Y. Vitamins A and E: metabolism, roles and transfer to offspring. *Br J Nutr*. 2005;93(2):153–174. https://doi.org/10.1079/bjn20041308.
69. Schenker S, Yang Y, Perez A, et al. Antioxidant transport by the human placenta. *Clin Nutr*. 1998;17:159–167. https://doi.org/10.1016/S0261-5614(98)80052-6.
70. Hanson C, Lyden E, Furtado J, et al. Vitamin E status and associations in maternal-infant Dyads in the Midwestern United States. *Clin Nutr*. 2019;38(2):934–939. https://doi.org/10.1016/j.clnu.2018.02.003.
75. Haga S, Miyaji M, Nakano M, et al. Changes in the expression of α-tocopherol-related genes in liver and mammary gland biopsy specimens of periparturn dairy cows. *J Dairy Sci [Internet]*. 2018;101(6):5277–5293. https://doi.org/10.3168/jds.2017-13630.
76. de Sousa Rebouças A, Costa Lemos da Silva AG, Freitas de Oliveira A, et al. Factors associated with increased alpha-tocopherol content in milk in response to maternal supplementation with 800 IU of vitamin. *E. Nutrients*. 2019;11(4):900. https://doi.org/10.3390/nu11040900.
80. Traber MG. Vitamin E inadequacy in humans: causes and consequences. *Adv Nutr*. 2014;5(5):503–514. https://doi.org/10.3945/an.114.006254.
81. Bell EF, Hansen NI, Brion LP, et al. Serum tocopherol levels in very preterm infants after a single dose of vitamin E at birth. *Pediatrics*. 2013;132(6):e1626–e1633. https://doi.org/10.1542/peds.2013-1684.
83. da Silva AGCL, de Sousa Rebouças A, Mendonça BMA, Silva DCNE, Dimenstein R, Ribeiro KDDS. Relationship between the dietary intake, serum, and breast milk concentrations of vitamin A and vitamin E in a cohort of women over the course of lactation. *Matern Child Nutr*. 2019;15(3):e12772. https://doi.org/10.1111/mcn.12772.
84. Machado MR, Kamp F, Nunes JC, El-Bacha T, Torres AG. Breast milk content of vitamin A and E from early- to mid-lactation is affected by inadequate dietary intake in Brazilian adult women. *Nutrients*. 2019;11(9):2025. https://doi.org/10.3390/nu11092025.
85. Rodrigues KDSR. *Estado nutricional em vitamina e de mães e crianças pré-termo e termo do nascimento aos 3 meses pós-parto. [Tese doutorado]*. Natal: Centro De Biociências, Universidade Federal do Rio Grande do Norte; 2016.
88. Antonakou A, Chiou A, Andrikopoulos NK, Bakoula C, Matalas AL. Breast milk tocopherol content during the first six months in exclusively breastfeeding Greek women. *Eur J Nutr*. 2011;50(3):195–202. https://doi.org/10.1007/s00394-010-0129-4.
89. Garcia L, Ribeiro K, Araújo K, Pires J, Azevedo G, Dimenstein R. Alpha-tocopherol concentration in the colostrum of nursing women supplemented with retinyl palmitate and alpha-tocopherol. *J Hum Nutr Diet*. 2010;23(5):529–534. https://doi.org/10.1111/j.1365-277X.2010.01063.x.
92. Stone Jr C, Qiu Y, Kurland IJ, et al. Effect of maternal smoking on plasma and urinary measures of vitamin E isoforms in the first month after extreme preterm birth. *J Pediatr*. 2018;197:280–285.e3. Epub 2018 Feb 2. https://doi.org/10.1016/j.jpeds.2017.12.062.
105. Ivanova AS, Peretyatko LP, Sitnikova OG, Nazarov SB. Changes in the mother-placenta-fetus system under the effect of α-tocopherol in albino rats with normal pregnancy. *Bull Exp Biol Med*. 2015;159(4):517–519. https://doi.org/10.1007/s10517-015-3006-6.
106. Greenough A, Shaheen SO, Shennan A, Seed PT, Poston L. Respiratory outcomes in early childhood following antenatal vitamin C and E supplementation. *Thorax*. 2010;65(11):998–1003. https://doi.org/10.1136/thx.2010.139915.
107. Sámano R, Martínez-Rojano H, Hernández RM, et al. Retinol and α-tocopherol in the breast milk of women after a high-risk pregnancy. *Nutrients*. 2017;9(1):14. https://doi.org/10.3390/nu9010014.
108. Woods Jr JR, Cavanaugh JL, Norkus EP, Plessinger MA, Miller RK. The effect of labor on maternal and fetal vitamins C and E. *Am J Obstet Gynecol*. 2002;187(5):1179–1183. https://doi.org/10.1067/mob.2002.127131.
113. Kositamongkol S, Suthutvoravut U, Chongviriyaphan N, Feungpean B, Nuntnarumit P. Vitamin A and E status in very low birth weight infants. *J Perinatol*. 2011;31(7):471–476. https://doi.org/10.1038/jp.2010.155.
114. Silva ABD, Medeiros JFP, Lima MSR, et al. Intrauterine growth and the vitamin E status of full-term and preterm newborns. *Rev Paul Pediatr*. 2019;37(3):291–296. https://doi.org/10.1590/1984-0462/;2019;37;3;00003.
116. Delvin EE, Salle BL, Claris O, et al. Oral vitamin A, E and D supplementation of pre-term newborns either breast-fed or formula-fed: a 3-month longitudinal study. *J Pediatr Gastroenterol Nutr*. 2005;40(1):43–47. https://doi.org/10.1097/00005176-200501000-00008.
121. Pires Medeiros JF, Ribeiro KD, Lima MS, et al. α-Tocopherol in breast milk of women with preterm delivery after a single postpartum oral dose of vitamin E. *Br J Nutr*. 2016;115(8):1424–1430. https://doi.org/10.1017/S0007114516000477.
124. Lima MS, Dimenstein R, Ribeiro KD. Vitamin E concentration in human milk and associated factors: a literature review. *J Pediatr*. 2014;90(5):440–448. https://doi.org/10.1016/j.jped.2014.04.006.
125. Wu K, Zhu J, Zhou L, et al. Lactational changes of fatty acids and fat-soluble antioxidants in human milk from healthy Chinese mothers. *Br J Nutr*. 2020;123(8):841–848. https://doi.org/10.1017/S0007114520000239.
131. da Mata AMB, da Silva AGCL, Medeiros JFP, et al. Dietary lipid intake influences the alpha-tocopherol levels in human milk. *J Pediatr Gastroenterol Nutr*. 2020;70(6):858–863. https://doi.org/10.1097/MPG.0000000000002668.
133. Whitfield KC, Shahab-Ferdows S, Kroeun H, et al. Macro- and micronutrients in milk from healthy Cambodian mothers: status and interrelations. *J Nutr*. 2020;150(6):1461–1469. https://doi.org/10.1093/jn/nxaa070.
134. Amorim NCM. *Influência do consumo de alimentos ultraprocessados em indicadores nutricionais de vitamina E de mulheres lactantes. [Dissertação defendida, em fase de publicação]*. Natal: Universidade Federal do Rio Grande do Norte; 2020.

Vitamin K Metabolism in the Fetus and Neonate

30

Martin J. Shearer | Paul Clarke

INTRODUCTION

In his classic studies in the 1930s, Henrik Dam identified vitamin K as an essential fat-soluble antihemorrhagic factor.[1] Later studies pinpointed the bleeding disorder caused by a dietary deficiency of vitamin K to a lack of four coagulation proteins, namely *prothrombin (factor II)* and *factors VII, IX,* and *X,* all of which are synthesized in the liver.[1] Descriptions of a bleeding syndrome in newborns that had the hallmarks of vitamin K deficiency first appeared in 1894.[2] This syndrome was originally called *hemorrhagic disease of the newborn* but was renamed in the 1990s as *vitamin K deficiency bleeding (VKDB) of early infancy* to clarify both its etiology and that it often occurs beyond the immediate newborn period.[3] In 1974 it was established that vitamin K serves as a cofactor for a microsomal enzyme, γ-glutamyl carboxylase (GGCX), which catalyzes the conversion of specific peptide-bound glutamate (Glu) residues to γ-carboxyglutamate (Gla) residues.[1] This posttranslational modification of Glu to Gla is essential for the biologic activity of vitamin K–dependent proteins (VKDP); hence they are often known as *Gla proteins.* Other significant discoveries in the 1970s were that γ-glutamyl carboxylation was intimately linked to the enzyme vitamin K epoxide reductase (VKOR) and that this enzyme was inhibited by vitamin K antagonists (VKA) such as warfarin.[1] The discovery of γ-glutamyl carboxylation led to the identification of a plethora of Gla proteins. Among them are proteins C and S, which together play an anticoagulant role in the negative feedback control of coagulation. Other Gla proteins are known or suspected to play roles in processes as diverse as bone and cardiovascular mineralization, energy metabolism, immune response, brain metabolism, and the growth, survival, and signaling of cells.[1,4] In the context of the fetus and neonate, the only clinical syndrome firmly connected to a noncoagulation function of vitamin K is an embryopathy belonging to the chondrodysplasia punctata spectrum of disorders that are characterized by abnormal calcium deposition during endochondral bone formation.[5] Vitamin K–related factors identified in the etiology of chondrodysplasia punctata include maternal dietary deficiency, or exposure to VKA, fetal mutations of key enzymes involved in vitamin K metabolism (GGCX or VKOR), and mutations of matrix Gla protein (MGP), which is a known inhibitor of calcification.[5] Bleeding due to dietary vitamin K deficiency is extremely rare in adults. In contrast, a window exists from birth to approximately 6 months of age when the human infant is exposed to a small but potentially life-threatening risk for VKDB.[3] Three subtypes of VKDB are recognized according to the age of presentation, namely *early* (first 24 hours), *classic* (between days 2 and 7), and *late* (between day 8 and 6 months). Late VKDB, with a peak incidence between 3 and 8 weeks, is generally regarded as the most insidious type because it typically presents as intracranial bleeding.[3] Classic and late VKDB are primarily syndromes of breast-fed infants but are preventable by ensuring that newborns receive vitamin K prophylaxis.

SOURCES OF VITAMIN K

CHEMISTRY AND OCCURRENCE IN NATURE

Vitamin K is the family name for a series of lipophilic isoprenoid quinones that possess a common 2-methyl-1,4-naphthoquinone ring structure (menadione) and a variable alkyl side chain at the 3-position (Fig. 30.1). The major dietary form phylloquinone (vitamin K_1) has a phytyl side chain and is synthesized by photosynthetic tissues of plants. Another subfamily of menaquinones (vitamin K_2) are predominately synthesized by bacteria and have multiprenyl side chains, the number of prenyl units being indicated by a suffix (i.e., menaquinone-n, abbreviated MK-n). Menadione has no cofactor activity per se but can be prenylated in vivo to the biologically active menaquinone-4 (MK-4).[1] An important discovery is that the menadione precursor required for MK-4 biosynthesis can be derived from phylloquinone catabolism in the intestine.[6–8]

NUTRITIONALLY IMPORTANT FORMS OF VITAMIN K TO NEONATES

Vitamin K occurs in breast milk mainly as phylloquinone and MK-4 (at approximately half the concentrations of phylloquinone) with trace concentrations of the longer side forms, MK-6 to MK-8.[9,10] Using standardized sampling techniques, mean concentrations of phylloquinone in colostrum and mature human milk were 2 μg/L and 1 μg/L, respectively.[11] MK-4 in breast milk is derived from maternal dietary phylloquinone, either selectively taken up or synthesized by the mammary gland.[10] An important determinant of neonatal vitamin K status lies in the large disparity in the daily intakes of phylloquinone in breast-fed and formula-fed infants that typically average 1 μg/day and 50 μg/day, respectively.[12] The relevance of MK synthesized by gut microflora to vitamin K nutrition is controversial, but the weight of evidence suggests that they do make a significant contribution to hepatic requirements.[1,13]

INTESTINAL ABSORPTION AND TRANSPORT TO TISSUES

A schematic illustration of the metabolic processes and pathways that lead from the intestinal absorption of dietary vitamin K to its plasma transport and entry into cells is shown in Fig. 30.2. Most of the available data pertain to phylloquinone and have been reviewed in detail.[13–15] The physicochemical principles governing the intraluminal phase of intestinal absorption of dietary vitamin K were established in the 1970s and share several common features with other fat-soluble vitamins.[16] Thus, in the upper intestine, dietary vitamin K is emulsified by bile salts and incorporated into mixed micelles containing the products of pancreatic hydrolysis (2-monoglycerides and fatty acids).[16] These mixed micelles are taken up by enterocytes and packaged into chylomicrons (CM) before being secreted into the lymph and entering the blood via the thoracic duct.[13–16] Once within the blood, CM follow the well-delineated pathway of metabolism, of which a major feature is the gradual loss of their triglyceride content to generate chylomicron remnants (CR). The stripping of triglyceride from CM is catalyzed by lipoprotein lipase on the surface of endothelial cells lining the capillary beds within muscles and adipose tissue. This conversion of CM to CR is accompanied by the acquisition of apolipoprotein E (apo E) and the loss of apo A and apo C. The importance of CR to all fat-soluble vitamins is that they provide a vehicle for their delivery to the liver and to

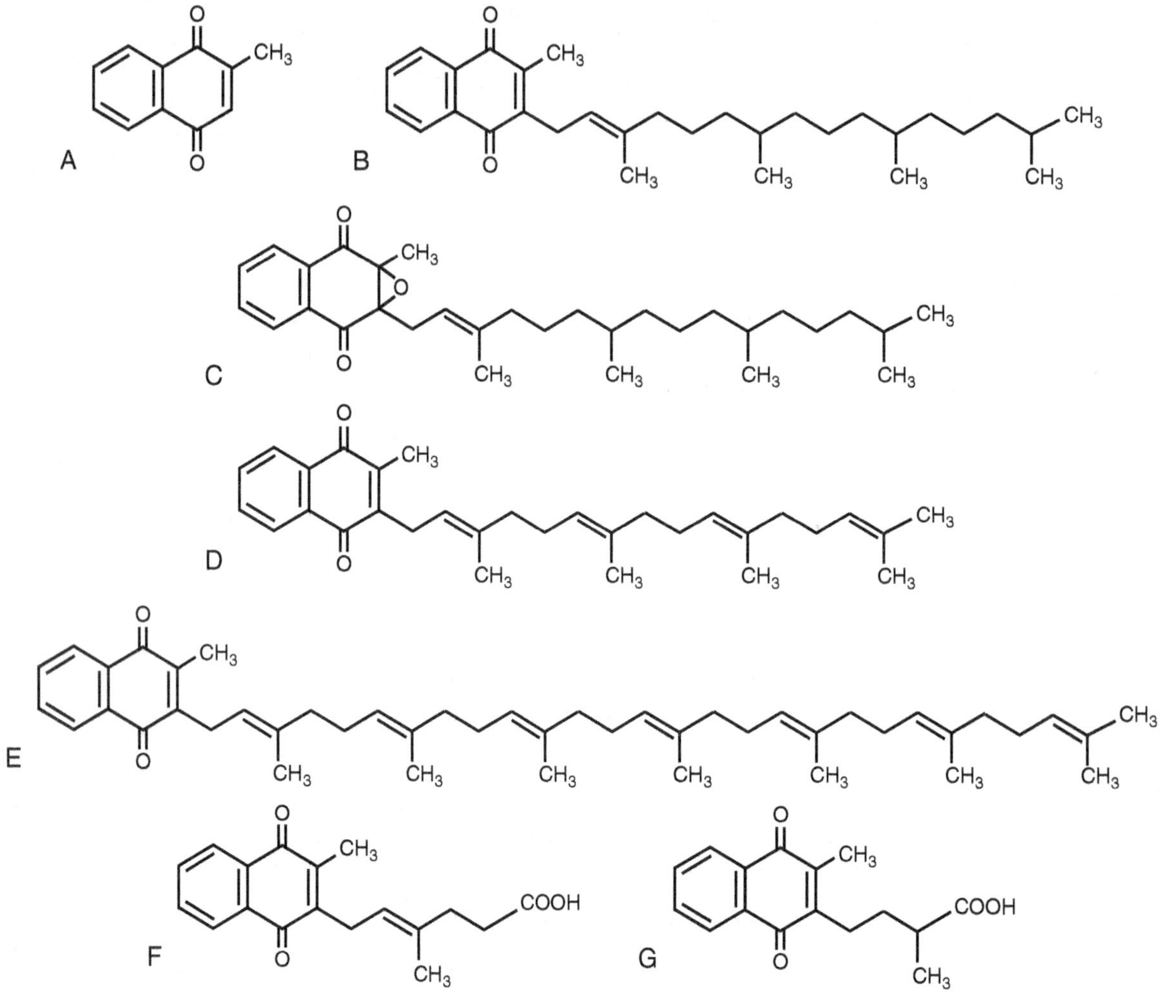

A = 2-methyl-1,4-naphthoquinone (menadione; K_3)
B = 2-methyl-3-phytyl-1,4-naphthoquinone (phylloquinone; K_1)
C = 2-methyl-3-phytyl-1,4-naphthoquinone-2,3-epoxide (phylloquinone epoxide; K_1>O)
D = 2-methyl-3-geranyl-geranyl-1,4-naphthoquinone (menaquinone-4; MK-4)
E = 2-methyl-3-farnesylgeranyl-geranyl-1,4-naphthoquinone (menaquinone-7; MK-7)
F = 2-methyl-3-(5′-carboxy-3′-methyl-2′-pentenyl)-1,4-naphthoquinone
G = 2-methyl-3-(3′-carboxy-3′-methyl propyl)-1,4-naphthoquinone

Fig. 30.1 Chemical structures of some K vitamins and metabolites.

extrahepatic tissues. For vitamin K, there is still a lack of knowledge of the molecular sequences and mechanisms whereby the various lipoprotein fractions acquire and lose their cargo of different molecular forms of vitamin K, so our current knowledge is limited to extrapolations from studies of plasma kinetics and analysis of the vitamin K content of different lipoprotein fractions. The molecular form of vitamin K with the highest concentrations in blood is phylloquinone. In both postprandial and fasting states, the bulk of phylloquinone in plasma is carried by triglyceride-rich lipoproteins (TRL) comprising CR and very low-density lipoproteins (VLDL).[17,18] The remainder is approximately equally distributed between low-density lipoproteins (LDL) and high-density lipoproteins (HDL). Different molecular forms of vitamin K exhibit marked differences in their plasma kinetics.[17] In general, phylloquinone and MK-4 are cleared rapidly from the circulation, whereas long-chain MK are cleared much more slowly.[13,17] A comparison of the lipoprotein distribution of phylloquinone, MK-4, and MK-9 showed that during the first 4 hours after a meal, all molecular forms were predominately associated with TRL.[17] Thereafter, there was divergence in lipoprotein distribution. MK-4 appeared very early in LDL and HDL, and by 8 hours 80% of MK-4 was carried by LDL. In contrast, MK-9 was not found in HDL at any time point and did not appear in LDL until after 8 hours; thereafter the proportion of MK-9 in LDL increased as its proportion in TRL declined. By 24 hours, approximately 50% of MK-9 was present in the LDL fraction, and this increased to greater than 90% at 48 hours.[17] Other studies suggest that the slow plasma clearance of MK-7 also results from its transfer to LDL.[13]

CELLULAR UPTAKE OF VITAMIN K

Although early studies had showed that uptake of phylloquinone from the proximal intestine was saturable and required energy, the identification and roles of specific transport pathways is only

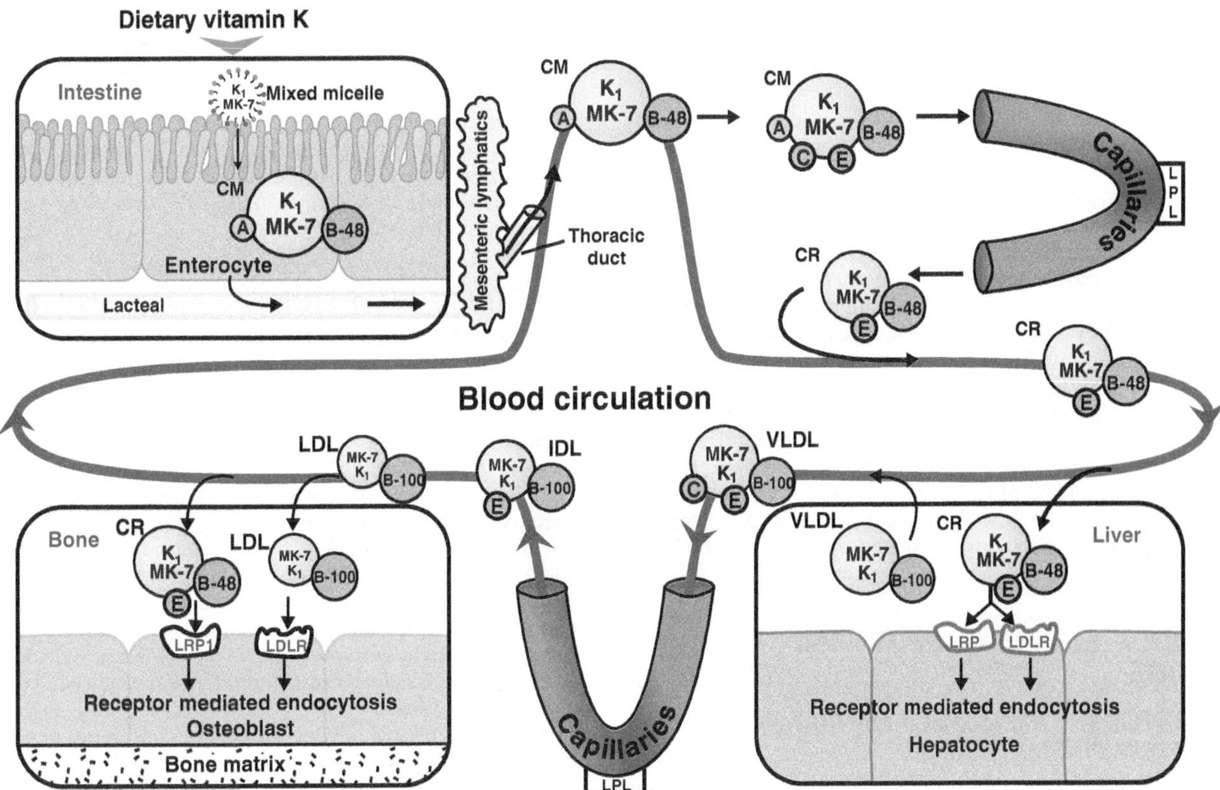

Fig. 30.2 Schematic representation of the absorption, transport, and cellular uptake of dietary phylloquinone *(K_1)* and menaquinone-7 *(MK-7)*. Key processes shown are: *Intestinal absorption and entry into circulation:* After digestion, dietary vitamin K and the products of pancreatic hydrolysis of triglycerides (TG) are emulsified by bile salts to form mixed micelles that are taken up by the enterocytes of the intestinal epithelium and processed into nascent chylomicrons *(CM)* that contain apolipoprotein A (apo A) and apo B-48. CM are then secreted into the lacteals within the intestinal villi. The lacteals drain into larger lymphatic vessels eventually emptying into the blood circulation via the thoracic duct. Once in the blood, CM acquire apo C and apo E from high-density lipoproteins *(HDL)*. In the capillaries of muscle, adipose tissues, etc., CM are stripped of their TG by the action of lipoprotein lipase *(LPL)* that lines the capillaries. The resultant smaller chylomicron remnants *(CR)* reenter the circulation having lost much apo A and apo C but retaining vitamin K in the lipophilic core. *Uptake by liver:* In the liver, CR enter hepatocytes by binding to low-density lipoprotein receptor *(LDLR)* and low density lipoprotein receptor-related protein 1 *(LRP1)* followed by receptor-mediated endocytosis. Their lipids are repackaged into very low-density lipoproteins *(VLDL)* that contain apo B-100 and then return to the circulation where they acquire apo C and apo E. Further TG is removed by LPL in the capillaries resulting in VLDL remnants called *intermediate-density lipoproteins (IDL)*. Subsequent metabolism and loss of apo C and apo E from IDL gives rise to smaller LDL particles containing almost exclusively apo B-100. Vitamin K is presumed to be still located in the lipophilic core. *Uptake by bone:* Circulating lipoproteins such as CR and LDL can deliver lipids to osteoblasts that are attached to the surfaces of bone matrix. Osteoblasts express lipoprotein receptors such as LDLR and LRP1 that can interact with CR and LDL, allowing receptor-mediated endocytosis of the particles and their cargoes of vitamin K. Evidence suggests that osteoblasts obtain most of their K_1 via the CR pathway and most of their MK-7 via the LDL pathway. (Republished with permission from Shearer MJ, Newman P. Metabolism and cell biology of vitamin K. *Thromb Haemost*. 2008;100:530–547.)

just emerging. To date, three candidate transporter proteins for the uptake of phylloquinone by the gut have been identified. They include two members of the class B scavenger receptor family (SR-B1 and CD36) and Niemann-Pick C1-like 1 protein (NPC1L1) that were already known to play key roles in cholesterol transport. Evidence for their role in the cellular uptake of phylloquinone by intestinal enterocytes has been reviewed.[15] Of the three transporter proteins, NPC1L1 is associated with the strongest evidence for a physiologic role in human vitamin K absorption.[15] This evidence is based on cell culture models, in vivo studies in normal and transgenic animals, and studies of the interaction between specific inhibitors of both NPC1L1 (ezetimibe) and vitamin K recycling (warfarin).[15] The inhibitor evidence includes a clinical study in patients taking warfarin.[15] The relevance of this finding to the human neonate is that certain mutations and polymorphisms in the human *NPC1L1* gene are known to influence cholesterol absorption and LDL concentrations. Therefore genetic variants that reduce cholesterol absorption are also likely to reduce vitamin K absorption. Although reduced cholesterol absorption may be beneficial in adults, the reduction of vitamin K absorption in infants is likely to adversely affect their already fragile vitamin K status in the first 6 months of life.

Kinetic studies demonstrate that the liver is the primary target organ for the uptake of newly absorbed vitamin K, which forms a small fraction of the lipid cargo carried by TRL in the immediate postabsorptive state.[13,16] In the absence of direct evidence, the initial stage of the hepatic uptake of vitamin K is thought to follow the well-established pathway for TRL uptake. Essentially this involves a series of interactions of TRL with apo E and hepatic lipase (both anchored by proteoglycan ligands to the hepatocyte microvillar membrane) with high-affinity cell surface lipoprotein receptors. Apo E serves as the predominant ligand for the high-affinity binding of TRL.

Interest in the role of vitamin K in bone health has stimulated research into the cellular uptake of vitamin K by osteoblasts that are responsible for the synthesis of Gla proteins such as osteocalcin. In this respect, unlike the indirect evidence for the mechanism of vitamin K uptake by hepatocytes, there is direct experimental evidence that the uptake of phylloquinone by human osteoblasts is facilitated by heparan sulfate proteoglycans on the cell surface and by apo E in lipoprotein particles.[19] It was also established that the LDL receptor–related protein 1 plays a predominant role in the uptake of phylloquinone from CR that represent the major lipoprotein delivery vehicle to bone.[20] Experiments using an in vivo murine model revealed that fluorescently labeled CR localized with the sinusoidal endothelial cells in bone and that these cells served as a docking site to concentrate CR in the bone marrow.[21] In summary, the available evidence suggests that CR travel through the endothelial fenestrae to the subendothelial space where, after enrichment with osteoblast-derived apo E, they interact with osteoblast receptors and are internalized.[21] Support for a physiologic functional role of CR in delivering phylloquinone to bone was obtained by showing that the γ-carboxylated fraction of osteocalcin in the circulation increased significantly within 4 hours of injecting mice with phylloquinone-loaded CR.[21] Although there are no comparable studies for the uptake of phylloquinone by the liver, the general mechanism of uptake of CR by hepatocytes is well described and is analogous to the receptor-mediated process described for bone.[13,14]

VITAMIN K STATUS OF FETUS AND NEONATE

METHODS FOR THE ASSESSMENT OF VITAMIN K STATUS FROM PLASMA SAMPLES

Traditional coagulation screening tests for vitamin K deficiency such as the prothrombin time are nonspecific and insensitive. More selective and sensitive tests of vitamin K status are based on the immunologic detection of abnormal, functionally defective molecules of VKDP that are released into the bloodstream at an early stage of vitamin K insufficiency. These abnormal molecules comprise a heterogeneous spectrum of undercarboxylated molecules of different VKDP collectively known as *proteins induced by vitamin K absence or antagonism (PIVKA)*. A raised PIVKA for a given VKDP is indicative of a functional vitamin K deficiency in the tissue in which it is synthesized. Thus measurements of undercarboxylated factor II (PIVKA-II), osteocalcin, and MGP reflect the vitamin K status of liver, bone, and vessel wall, respectively. There are problems associated with interpretation of osteocalcin and MGP assays, so only PIVKA-II measurements are in widespread use for the assessment of the vitamin K status of neonates. The major circulating form of vitamin K is phylloquinone, which is the only isoprenologue that is routinely measured. Plasma concentrations of phylloquinone are responsive to dietary restriction and supplementation and represent a useful indicator of tissue stores, although interpretation is hampered by an association with plasma lipids.[22]

PLASMA CONCENTRATIONS OF PIVKA-II: A MARKER OF VITAMIN K COAGULATION FUNCTION

Newborn infants represent the only healthy population in which a raised PIVKA-II concentration is a relatively common finding. Although this indicates that the liver stores of vitamin K are insufficient to fully γ-carboxylate factor II, for the great majority of infants the extent of γ-undercarboxylation is minor and has no impact on hemostasis. PIVKA-II is often raised in cord blood. Using assays with a comparable high sensitivity, the prevalence of detectable PIVKA-II was approximately 20% in surveys from Japan[23] and Thailand.[24] A similar prevalence (23%) was reported in preterm infants in England.[25] In the Thai study of 693 cord/maternal pairs, approximately 1.5% of cord plasma samples had a PIVKA-II concentration that would have been expected to be associated with a clinically significant lengthening of the prothrombin time.[24] Without adequate vitamin K prophylaxis, PIVKA-II prevalence increases during the first week after birth,[23,26] confirming the temporary dip in vitamin K status reported in early coagulation studies.[27] In breast-fed infants, this early decline of vitamin K status is associated with ingestion of low volumes of milk.[26] The concentrations and prevalence of PIVKA-II are significantly reduced in infants who receive vitamin K prophylaxis[23,28,29] or are fed with supplemented milk formulas.[26,28]

PLASMA CONCENTRATIONS OF VITAMIN K: A MARKER OF TISSUE STORES

In adult populations, mean fasting concentrations of phylloquinone are approximately 0.5 μg/L (1.0 nmol/L).[18,22] Concentrations of phylloquinone in cord plasma of healthy newborns are difficult to measure and below the level of detection of all but the most sensitive assay methodologies.[22] In reviewing the literature, Shearer concluded that cord plasma concentrations of phylloquinone were less than 0.05 μg/L (<0.10 nmol/L).[22] There is a paucity of data regarding the plasma concentration gradient for circulating phylloquinone between mothers and newborns at the time of delivery, but concentration gradients of between 20:1 and 40:1 have been reported and may be higher.[22] Despite lack of exactitude, this barrier to placental transport of phylloquinone (and as far as is known to MK of bacterial origin) is clearly much greater than that seen for other fat-soluble vitamins.[22]

Endogenous plasma phylloquinone concentrations begin to be measurable in breast-fed infants at approximately 12 to 24 hours after delivery and by 3 to 4 days of age are within the same range as adults.[22] Phylloquinone intakes in infants fed with a typical phylloquinone-supplemented formula milk are approximately 50-fold higher than those in breast-fed infants.[22] This results in plasma concentrations that are approximately 25- to 50-fold higher than those in breast-fed infants and explains why formula-feeding protects against VKDB.[3,22] Thus, in a comparative longitudinal study in neonates between 6 and 20 weeks of life, Greer and colleagues reported that plasma phylloquinone concentrations averaged 5 μg/L (10 nmol/L) in infants fed with a phylloquinone-supplemented cows' milk formula compared with 0.1 to 0.2 μg/L (0.2 to 0.4 nmol/L) in exclusively breast-fed infants.[12]

LIVER RESERVES OF VITAMIN K

The liver is the only known site of synthesis of the Gla-containing procoagulant proteins, so maintaining adequate vitamin K stores in this organ is essential for the maintenance of normal hemostasis. In adults, the hepatic profile of vitamin K differs from that of other tissues in that phylloquinone is a minor constituent (typically representing 10% of the total content) with the majority comprising MK, typically with long side chains ranging from MK-7 to MK-13.[30,31] A substantial proportion of this MK fraction comprises MK-10, 11, and 12, which are low constituents of most human diets[32] but are synthesized by anaerobic bacteria in the large intestine including *Escherichia coli* and *Bacteroides* species.[33] The average total liver pool of vitamin K in adults is of the order of 200 to 300 nmol but with wide interindividual variation.[30,31] In contrast to adults, MK are undetectable in fetal livers and build up slowly over several weeks.[30] Phylloquinone is detectable in fetal liver throughout gestation; at birth, the median hepatic concentration in preterm and term infants was 1.4 ng/g (3.1 pmol/g) and 1.0 ng/g (2.2 pmol/g), respectively.[30] Hepatic concentrations of phylloquinone in infants at birth are approximately one-fifth of those found in adults,[30] but in the absence of MK, total reserves of vitamin K represent only 2% of those found in adults. The implication of these findings is that the needs of the human fetus and neonate are met largely by phylloquinone.

VITAMIN K-EPOXIDE CYCLE

The *vitamin K-epoxide cycle* refers to a metabolic cycle that seems to have evolved to conserve the available tissue stores of vitamin K, not only in the liver but also in extrahepatic tissues. In essence, the cycle serves to regenerate vitamin K that is converted to vitamin K 2,3 epoxide (K>O) during the γ-carboxylation of VKDP in the endoplasmic reticulum (Fig. 30.3).[1,13-15] The key enzyme in the cycle is VKOR, which converts K>O to the native quinone form while a reductase activity converts the quinone to its active cofactor form, vitamin K hydroquinone (KH_2). Vitamin K is present in foods in its stable oxidized quinone form, so that before dietary vitamin K can function it must undergo reduction to KH_2, either before or after entry into the vitamin K cycle.

It is well documented that the VKOR is the target of VKA that are used in clinical practice for the prevention and treatment of thromboembolic disorders.[1] When VKA inhibit the VKOR, the ability to reuse K>O is diminished, thus reducing the efficiency of γ-carboxylation of VKDP and their biologic activities. In their pioneering work, Reidar Wallin and colleagues also identified an alternative warfarin-insensitive pathway that enables reduction of vitamin K to KH_2 given a sufficient supply of exogenous vitamin K.[34] The identity of the microsomal enzyme(s) responsible for this antidotal activity is still unknown.

Studies in VKOR-knockout mice have provided significant insights into the biologic role of the vitamin K-epoxide cycle. A major finding is that animals without VKOR cannot maintain normal hemostasis without being fed supraphysiologic doses of vitamin K.[35] Thus, although homozygous *VKOR*$^{-/-}$ mice appeared to be normal at birth, all died within 2 to 20 days from extensive bleeding (mainly in the brain) due to severe depletion of factors II, VII, IX, and X. Importantly, newborn *VKOR*$^{-/-}$ mice could be rescued by then giving supraphysiologic oral doses of phylloquinone directly, but not indirectly via the breast milk from their supplemented mothers. In addition, the length of the calcified regions of the long bones of VKOR-deficient mice was shorter than in wild-type control mice.[35] This skeletal phenotype resonates with cases of chondrodysplasia punctata observed in human newborns with homozygous mutations of VKOR or after in utero exposure to VKA.[5]

IN VIVO CONVERSION OF PHYLLOQUINONE TO MENAQUINONE-4

One area of vitamin K metabolism that has seen rapid and significant advances in the past 10 years is an endogenous biosynthetic pathway that is able to convert dietary phylloquinone to MK-4.[13-15] This pathway, first described in the 1950s, is present in both invertebrates and vertebrates; because menadione is also a substrate, the prevailing concept was that this was a two-step reaction in which the side chain of phylloquinone was first cleaved and the geranylgeranyl side chain of MK-4 was then added in a separate prenylation step.[13] Comparative studies of the tissue concentrations of phylloquinone and MK-4 in mammals, including humans, reveal a tissue selective pattern, some tissues being phylloquinone rich (e.g., liver, heart) and others MK-4 rich (e.g., brain, kidney, pancreas).[36]

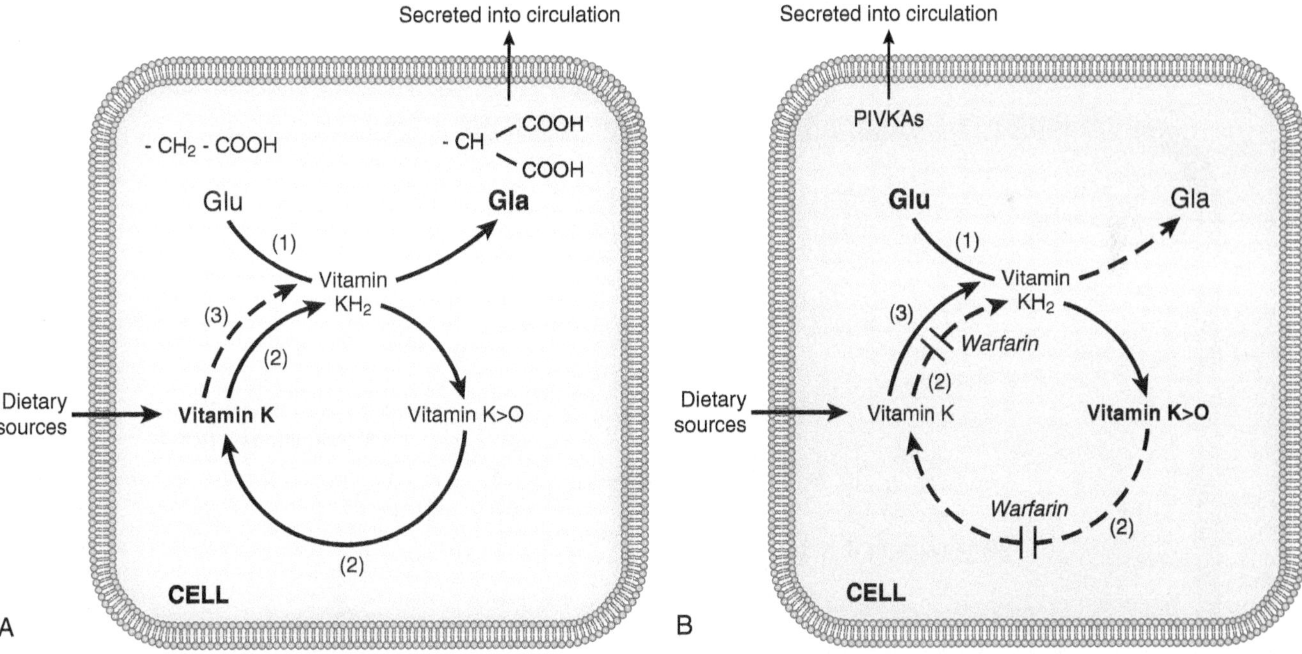

Fig. 30.3 Scheme showing the vitamin K-epoxide cycle in the absence (A) and presence (B) of warfarin. (A). Posttranslational conversion of peptide-bound glutamic acid *(Glu)* to γ-carboxyglutamic acid *(Gla)* residues and its linkage to the recycling of vitamin K by a pathway known as the *vitamin K-epoxide cycle.* Enzyme activities shown are *(1)* γ-glutamyl carboxylase *(GGCX)*, *(2)* vitamin K epoxide reductase *(VKOR)* and *(3)* NAD(P)H-dependent quinone reductase(s). The active cofactor form of vitamin K required by GGCX is the reduced form vitamin K quinol *(KH_2)*. During γ-glutamyl carboxylation, KH_2 becomes oxidized to vitamin K epoxide *(K>O)*, which in turn undergoes reductive recycling, first to the vitamin K quinone (K) and then to KH_2. Only VKOR can carry out the reduction of K>O to K, but there are several candidate quinone dehydrogenases for activity *(3)*. Under conditions of optimal vitamin K status, only the carboxylated substrates (Gla proteins) are secreted into the circulation. (B) Metabolic inhibition and consequences of a vitamin K antagonist such as warfarin. These drugs block the activity of the VKOR *(2)*, leading to an accumulation of K>O in the cell. Given a sufficient supply of vitamin K (e.g., from the diet) an alternative hepatic quinone reductase activity *(3)* can bypass the warfarin inhibition of the VKOR to provide the KH_2 substrate for the carboxylase enzyme and overcome the inhibitory action of warfarin, even under extreme blockade. In the presence of warfarin, or in states of nutritional vitamin K deficiency, species of undercarboxylated forms called *PIVKAs* are secreted into the circulation. (Republished with permission from Shearer MJ, Gorska R, Harrington DJ, et al. Vitamin K. In: Herrmann W, Obeid R, eds. *Vitamins in the Prevention of Human Diseases*. Berlin: De Gruyter; 2011:515–560 [chapter 12].)

Evidence suggests that tissue distribution of MK-4 is determined by local synthesis of MK-4 rather than by its uptake from blood.[6–8] In 2010, Okano and coworkers made a major breakthrough when a search for candidate prenyltransferase enzymes in the human genome database led to the discovery of the gene that encodes for a novel human MK-4 biosynthetic enzyme known as *UbiA prenyltransferase-containing domain 1 (UBIAD1)*.[7] Although this enzyme was clearly identified as the prenyltransferase that catalyzed the conversion of menadione to MK-4, its role in the side-chain cleavage of phylloquinone is unclear. Several lines of evidence suggest that side-chain cleavage of phylloquinone only occurs during intestinal absorption and that the menadione product is transported into the blood via the lymphatic absorption pathway.[6–8,15] After delivery to target tissues, the precursor menadione is then converted to MK-4 by the enzyme UBIAD1.[7,8,15] Historically, the connection between UBIAD1 (also known as *TERE1*) and human health emerged from independent observations of either gene mutations linked to the eye disease Schnyder corneal dystrophy or to a reduced gene expression in bladder and prostate cancer. These diseases are linked by a deregulation of cholesterol synthesis or metabolism and characterized by elevated extracellular or intracellular cholesterol. However, there is no evidence to date of a causal link between the diseases associated with UBIAD1 and the biosynthesis of MK-4 even though this is the only clearly identified function of the enzyme.[15]

The strategic importance of the UBIAD1 pathway for the synthesis of MK-4 to the functions of vitamin K is presently unclear, but one hypothesis is that the UBIAD1-driven pathway delivers a cellular pool of MK-4 that is locally available as a cofactor for γ-carboxylation or other putative biologic effects specific to MK-4. With respect to the latter, MK-4 has been shown to be capable of regulating gene expression either through binding and activation of the steroid and xenobiotic receptor (SXR) or through a protein kinase A-dependent mechanism (Fig. 30.4).[15]

CATABOLISM AND EXCRETION OF VITAMIN K

Phylloquinone, the major dietary form of vitamin K, has a much faster turnover than vitamins A, D, and E. In early radioisotopic studies, healthy adults excreted approximately 60% to 70% of a single oral dose of vitamin K within 3 days.[16] The production of catabolites occurs exclusively in the liver and the amount excreted by the biliary route is approximately double that excreted in the urine.[16] Importantly, the same 60% to 70% losses to the body were observed regardless of whether the administered dose was within the dietary range (45 μg) or in the low pharmacologic range (1 mg). This extensive excretion of phylloquinone explains the rapid turnover and depletion of hepatic phylloquinone observed in patients placed on a low vitamin K diet.[31] The unchanged hepatic reserves of long-chain MK observed in the same study[31] is consistent with their slower turnover as was also observed from plasma kinetics.[17]

The degradative pathway of phylloquinone and MK results in the shortening of the polyisoprenoid side chains to the same two major carboxylic acids with side-chain lengths of 7- and 5-carbon atoms, respectively (see Figure 30.1 for chemical structures).[16,37] Most of the enzymologic steps have not been studied in detail but, by analogy to similar isoprenoids including vitamin E, would proceed by an initial ω-hydroxylation followed by a progressive side-chain shortening via the β-oxidation pathway.[38] In fact, a member of the cytochrome P-450 family

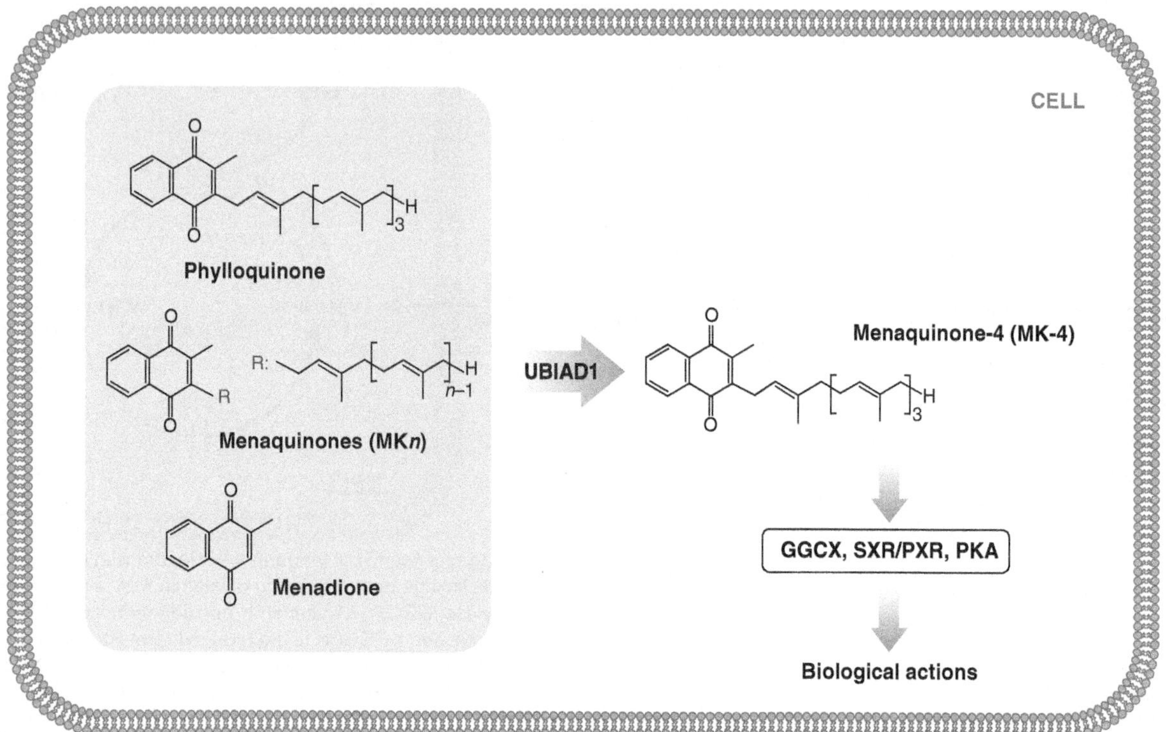

Fig. 30.4 Overview of synthesis and cellular functions of menaquinone-4 *(MK-4)*. The enzyme UbiA prenyltransferase domain–containing protein 1 *(UBIAD1)* mediates the in vivo tissue conversion of vitamin K forms to MK-4 in extrahepatic tissues. Besides its canonical role as a cofactor for *GGCX*-mediated synthesis of VKD-proteins, MK-4 has been shown to modulate gene expression and signal transduction. Examples shown are those initiated by binding to nuclear receptors such as the steroid and xenobiotic receptor *(SXR)*, also known as the pregnane X receptor *(PXR)*, or through activation of protein kinase A *(PKA)*. (Modified with permission from *The Annual Review of Nutrition*, Volume 38 © 2018 by Annual Reviews, http://www.annualreviews.org.)

(CYP4F2) known to catalyze the ω-oxidation of tocopherols has been shown to catalyze conversion of phylloquinone to ω-hydroxy-phylloquinone.[39] Excretion of the terminal 5C- and 7C-side-chain metabolites occurs mainly as glucuronides with the 5C-side-chain metabolite normally predominating.[16,38,40] Supraphysiologic doses of phylloquinone may overload the pathway leading to a greater excretion of less extensively metabolized aglycones.[38]

In adults, excretion of 5C- and 7C-metabolites responds relatively slowly to dietary depletion but rapidly to dietary repletion.[40] Both term and preterm infants have the same capacity as adults to produce the same 5C- and 7C-urinary catabolites and to excrete them in urine[41] and feces.[42] As in adults, the 5C-metabolite predominates in term infants and in the majority of preterm infants both before and after vitamin K prophylaxis.[41] The finding that the rate of total metabolite excretion in infants was some 25-fold lower in neonates than adults probably reflects the low vitamin K stores at birth but does not discount an immaturity of the enzymic pathway for vitamin K catabolism.[41]

VITAMIN K PROPHYLAXIS FOR NEONATES

Prevention of VKDB has had a long and checkered history, but there is currently a consensus throughout the world that vitamin K prophylaxis is both necessary and effective. Phylloquinone is the form of vitamin K used in nearly all countries. Recommendations are guided by the fact that, unlike other vitamin deficiencies, the onset is sudden and potentially catastrophic.

Regimens of vitamin K prophylaxis vary widely with respect to the dose, route of administration, and formulation.[3,43] Although there was a trend in some countries towards oral prophylaxis in the 1990s, the failures of some oral regimens, or in some cases their relative expense and lack of convenient formulations, has led the trend back to giving a single intramuscular injection at birth.[3,43]

Although there are no known clinical manifestations of toxicity from phylloquinone prophylaxis in neonates, it is theoretically possible that the high doses needed to prevent VKDB might adversely affect some metabolic processes. Studies in term and particularly in preterm infants show that post prophylaxis, the majority of infants have prolonged, supraphysiologic plasma phylloquinone concentrations irrespective of dose, route, or formulation.[43,44] In one study, a subgroup of preterms was identified who, after receiving phylloquinone prophylaxis, mainly excreted the less extensively processed 7C-metabolite instead of the usual 5C-metabolite.[41] This subgroup also had the highest serum phylloquinone concentrations and raised concentrations of K_1>O, which is normally undetectable. This combination of increased excretion of the 7C-metabolite, high serum phylloquinone, and detectable K_1>O is indicative of a metabolic overload of both vitamin K recycling and catabolic pathways. The intramuscular doses of 0.2 or 0.5 mg phylloquinone (0.1–0.4 mg/kg) that the preterms received in metabolite study[41] were below or at the lower end of the dose range of 0.5 to 1.0 mg recommended by the American Academy of Pediatrics for preterms.[45] In conclusion, preterm infants may not be able to efficiently metabolize current prophylactic doses of phylloquinone.[43,44]

CONCLUSION

Compared with adults, the vitamin K sufficiency status of the fetus and breast-fed neonates is poor.[3] The causes lie partly with a marginal nutritional supply of vitamin K and partly with metabolic factors. The main metabolic factor influencing the low vitamin K liver stores found in the fetus seems to be a placental barrier that limits the passage of phylloquinone and blocks the passage of long-chain MK. Despite this, the risk to the fetus of maternal vitamin K deficiency is very low, but when it does occur, it can result in fetal bone defects at early stages of pregnancy[46] or fetal bleeding at later stages.[47] It is often said that the reason why exclusive breast-feeding is a known risk factor for VKDB is because breast milk contains low concentrations of vitamin K. However, phylloquinone contents of breast milk from mothers who had been exclusively breast-feeding infants who had suffered VKDB were found to be in the normal range.[48] Rather, the cause of VKDB often lies with an undiagnosed metabolic disorder in the infant, most commonly of the hepatobiliary system resulting in cholestasis and malabsorption of vitamin K.[3] Knowledge of metabolism can inform and promote best practice for vitamin K prophylaxis. For example, a major reason for the failure of some oral regimens is that vitamin K is poorly absorbed in infants with cholestasis, a group at major risk for VKDB.[3,49] Also because phylloquinone has a rapid turnover, multiple oral doses are required for full protection. The reason for the greater effectiveness of the intramuscular route over intravenous or oral routes is probably because the muscle forms a slow-release depot.[50] This is supported by findings that showed that the rate of urinary excretion of vitamin K catabolites in preterms over 24 hours is much lower after intramuscular injection than after intravenous injection.[41]

REFERENCES

1. Suttie JW. *Vitamin K in Health and Disease*. 1st ed. Boca Raton, FL: CRC Press (Taylor & Francis Group); 2009.
2. Townsend CW. The haemorrhagic disease of the newborn. *Arch Pediatr.* 1894;11:559–565.
3. Shearer MJ. Vitamin K deficiency bleeding (VKDB) in early infancy. *Blood Rev.* 2009;23:49–59.
4. Booth SL. Roles for vitamin K beyond coagulation. *Annu Rev Nutr.* 2009;29:89–110.
5. Irving MD, Chitty LS, Mansour S, Hall CM. Chondrodysplasia punctata. A clinical diagnostic and radiological review. *Clin Dysmorphol.* 2008;17:229–241.
6. Thijssen HHW, Vervoort LMT, Schurgers LJ, Shearer MJ. Menadione is a metabolite of oral vitamin K. *Br J Nutr.* 2006;95:260–266.
7. Nakagawa K, Hirota Y, Sawada N, et al. Identification of UBIAD1 as a novel human menaquinone-4 biosynthetic enzyme. *Nature.* 2010;468:117–121.
8. Hirota Y, Tsugawa N, Nakagawa K, et al. Menadione (vitamin K_3) is a catabolic product of oral phylloquinone (vitamin K_1) in the intestine and a circulating precursor of tissue menaquinone-4 (vitamin K_2) in rats. *J Biol Chem.* 2013;288:33071–33080.
9. Indyk HE, Woollard DC. Vitamin K in milk and infant formulas: determination and distribution of phylloquinone and menaquinone-4. *Analyst.* 1997;122:465–469.
10. Thijssen HHW, Drittij M-J, Vermeer C, Schoffelen E. Menaquinone-4 in breast milk is derived from dietary phylloquinone. *Br J Nutr.* 2002;87:219–226.
11. von Kries R, Shearer M, McCarthy PT, et al. Vitamin K_1 content of maternal milk: influence of the stage of lactation, lipid composition, and vitamin K_1 supplements given to the mother. *Pediatr Res.* 1987;22:513–517.
12. Greer FR, Marshall S, Cherry J, Suttie JW. Vitamin K status of lactating mothers, human milk, and breast-feeding infants. *Pediatrics.* 1991;88:751–756.
13. Shearer MJ, Newman P. Metabolism and cell biology of vitamin K. *Thromb Haemost.* 2008;100:530–547.
14. Shearer MJ, Newman P. Recent trends in the metabolism and cell biology of vitamin K with special reference to vitamin K cycling and MK-4 biosynthesis. *J Lipid Res.* 2014;55:345–362.
15. Shearer MJ, Okano T. Key pathways and regulators of vitamin K function and intermediary metabolism. *Annu Rev Nutr.* 2018;38:127–151.
16. Shearer MJ, McBurney A, Barkhan P. Studies on the absorption and metabolism of phylloquinone (vitamin K_1) in man. *Vitam Horm.* 1974;32:513–542.
17. Schurgers LJ, Vermeer C. Differential lipoprotein transport pathways of K-vitamins in healthy subjects. *Biochim Biophys Acta.* 2002;1570:27–32.
18. Lamon-Fava S, Sadowski JA, Davidson KW, et al. Plasma lipoproteins as carriers of phylloquinone (vitamin K_1) in humans. *Am J Clin Nutr.* 1998;67:1226–1231.
19. Newman P, Bonello F, Wierzbicki AS, et al. The uptake of lipoprotein-borne phylloquinone (vitamin K_1) by osteoblasts and osteoblast-like cells: role of heparan sulfate proteoglycans and apolipoprotein E. *J Bone Miner Res.* 2002;17:426–433.
20. Niemeier A, Kassem M, Toedter K, et al. Expression of LRP1 by human osteoblasts. A mechanism for the delivery of lipoproteins and vitamin K_1 to bone. *J Bone Miner Res.* 2005;20:283–293.
21. Niemeier A, Niedzielska D, Secer R, et al. Uptake of postprandial lipoproteins into bone *in vivo*: impact on osteoblast function. *Bone.* 2008;43:230–237.
22. Shearer MJ. Vitamin K metabolism and nutriture. *Blood Rev.* 1992;6:92–104.

23. Motohara K, Endo F, Matsuda I. Effect of vitamin K administration on acarboxy prothrombin (PIVKA-II) levels in newborns. *Lancet*. 1985;2:242-244.
24. Chuansumrit A, Plueksacheeva T, Hanpinitsak S, et al. Prevalence of subclinical vitamin K deficiency in Thai newborns: relationship to maternal phylloquinone intakes and delivery risk. *Arch Dis Child Fetal Neonatal*. 2010; 95:104-108.
25. Clarke P, Mitchell SJ, Wynn R, et al. Vitamin K prophylaxis for preterm infants. A randomized, controlled trial of 3 regimens. *Pediatrics*. 2006;118:1657-1666.
26. von Kries R, Becker A, Göbel U. Vitamin K in the newborn: influence of nutritional factors on acarboxy-prothrombin detectability and factor II and VII clotting activity. *Eur J Pediatr*. 1987;146:123-127.
27. Aballi AJ, de Lamerens S. Coagulation changes in the neonatal period and in early infancy. *Pediatr Clin North Am*. 1962;9:785-817.
28. Widdershoven J, Lambert W, Motohara K, et al. Plasma concentrations of vitamin K_1 and PIVKA-II in bottle-fed and breast-fed infants with and without vitamin K prophylaxis at birth. *Eur J Pediatr*. 1988;148:139-142.
29. Motohara K, Endo F, Matsuda I. Vitamin K deficiency in breast-fed infants at one month of age. *J Pediatr Gastroenterol Nutr*. 1986;5:931-933.
30. Shearer MJ, McCarthy PT, Crampton OE, Mattock MB. The assessment of human vitamin K status from tissue measurements. In: Suttie JW, ed. *Current Advances in Vitamin K Research*. New York: Elsevier; 1988:437-452.
31. Usui Y, Tanimura H, Nishimura N, et al. Vitamin K concentrations in the plasma and liver of surgical patients. *Am J Clin Nutr*. 1990;51:846-852.
32. Schurgers LJ, Vermeer V. Determination of phylloquinone and menaquinones in food. Effect of food matrix on circulating vitamin K concentrations. *Haemostasis*. 2000;30:298-307.
33. Ramotar K, Conly JM, Chubb H, Louie TJ. Production of menaquinones by intestinal anaerobes. *J Infect Dis*. 1984;150:213-218.
34. Wallin R, Patrick SD, Martin LF. Vitamin K_1 reduction in human liver. Location of the coumarin-drug-insensitive enzyme. *Biochem J*. 1989;260:879-884.
35. Spohn G, Kleinridders A, Wunderlich FT, et al. VKORC1 deficiency in mice causes early postnatal lethality due to severe bleeding. *Thromb Haemost*. 2009;101:1044-1050.
36. Thijssen HHW, Drittij-Reijnders MJ. Vitamin K status in human tissues. Tissue specific accumulation of phylloquinone and menaquinone-4. *Br J Nutr*. 1996;75:121-127.
37. Harrington DJ, Soper R, Edwards C, et al. Determination of the urinary aglycone metabolites of vitamin K by HPLC with redox-mode electrochemical detection. *J Lipid Res*. 2005;46:1053-1060.
38. McBurney A, Shearer MJ, Barkhan P. Preparative isolation and characterization of the urinary aglycones of vitamin K_1 (phylloquinone) in man. *Biochem Med*. 1980;24:250-267.
39. McDonald MG, Rieder MJ, Nakano M, et al. CYP4F2 is a vitamin K_1 oxidase. An explanation for altered warfarin dose in carriers of the V433M variant. *Mol Pharmacol*. 2009;75:1337-1346.
40. Harrington DJ, Booth SL, Card DJ, Shearer MJ. Excretion of the urinary 5C- and 7C-aglycone metabolites of vitamin K by young adults responds to changes in dietary phylloquinone and dihydrophylloquinone intakes. *J Nutr*. 2007;137:1763-1768.
41. Harrington DJ, Clarke P, Card DJ, et al. Urinary excretion of vitamin K metabolites in term and preterm infants: relationship to vitamin K status and prophylaxis. *Pediatr Res*. 2010;68:508-512.
42. Card DJ, Gorska R, Cutler J, Harrington DJ. Vitamin K metabolism. Current knowledge and future research. *Mol Nutr Food Res*. 2014;58:1590-1600.
43. Clarke P. Vitamin K prophylaxis for preterm infants. *Early Hum Dev*. 2010;86:17-20.
44. Costakos DT, Greer FR, Love LA, et al. Vitamin K prophylaxis for premature infants: 1 mg versus 0.5 mg. *Am J Perinatol*. 2003;20:485-490.
45. American Academy of Pediatrics Committee on Fetus and Newborn. Controversies concerning vitamin K and the newborn. *Pediatrics*. 2003;112: 191-192.
46. Menger H, Lin AE, Toriello HV, et al. Vitamin K deficiency embryopathy: a phenocopy of the warfarin embryopathy due to a disorder of embryonic vitamin K metabolism. *Am J Med Genet*. 1997;72:129-134.
47. Minami H, Furuhashi M, Minami K, et al. Fetal intraventricular bleeding possibly due to maternal vitamin K deficiency. *Fetal Diagn Ther*. 2008;24:357-360.
48. von Kries R, Shearer MJ, Göbel U. Vitamin K in infancy. *Eur J Pediatr*. 1988;147:106-112.
49. van Hasselt PM, de Koning TJ, Kvist N, et al. Prevention of vitamin K deficiency bleeding in breast-fed infants: lessons from the Dutch and Danish biliary atresia registries. *Pediatrics*. 2008;121:857-863.
50. Loughnan PM, McDougall PN. Does intramuscular vitamin K_1 act as an unintended depot preparation? *J Paediatr Child Health*. 1996;32:251-254.

Maternal-Fetal Transfer of Lipid Metabolites

31

Emilio Herrera | Miguel Angel Lasunción

INTRODUCTION

Changes in maternal lipid metabolism during gestation control the availability of lipid metabolites to the fetus, even though some components do not directly cross the placental barrier. This is the case with maternal plasma lipoproteins, the profile of which differs markedly during pregnancy from that seen in nonpregnant subjects. Although no evidence exists for the transfer of maternal lipoproteins to the fetus, placental cells have lipoprotein receptors that allow their uptake and the subsequent release of their lipid components to the fetus. However, other products of maternal lipid metabolism, such as nonesterified fatty acids (NEFAs), glycerol, ketone bodies, and cholesterol, are able to cross the placenta and become available to the fetus without prior modification. Although the efficiency of transfer across the placenta differs for each of these metabolites, the major force controlling their actual transfer is the maternal-fetal concentration gradient.

HYPERLIPOPROTEINEMIA IN PREGNANCY AND ITS ROLE AS A SOURCE OF FATTY ACIDS FOR THE FETUS

Maternal hypertriglyceridemia is one of the most striking changes that takes place in lipid metabolism during gestation. The increase in plasma triglycerides during pregnancy is greater than the increases in phospholipids and cholesterol,[1,2] and more triglycerides are found in all of the lipoprotein fractions.[3,4] As shown in Fig. 31.1, although both triglycerides and cholesterol in very low-density lipoproteins (VLDLs), low-density lipoproteins (LDLs), and high-density lipoproteins (HDLs) are higher in pregnant women in the third trimester of gestation than in the same women during the postlactation period, the triglyceride-cholesterol ratio remains stable in VLDLs despite significant increases in both LDLs and HDLs. An examination of different HDL subclasses indicates that the rise in triglyceride-enriched HDL_{2b} is mainly responsible for the changes in HDL levels, whereas the small HDL_3 fractions become less abundant.[5] The increase in triglycerides per LDL particle is accompanied by a decrease in cholesterol and phospholipid content,[6] which causes reductions in LDL particle size,[7] although increases in the most buoyant of the LDL subfractions, LDL_1, have been reported with advancing gestation.[6]

The mechanisms responsible for these changes in the maternal lipoprotein profile during pregnancy are summarized in Fig. 31.2. The increased adipose tissue lipolytic activity during late gestation[8,9] (which is mediated by an insulin-resistant condition[10]) enhances the availability of substrates for triglyceride synthesis in the liver. The triglycerides thus produced become pooled with the lipid components derived from the uptake of chylomicron remnants. These actions, together with the stimulating effect of estrogen on VLDL production[11] and the decreased extrahepatic lipoprotein lipase (LPL) activity,[5,12] are responsible in part for the augmented levels of circulating maternal VLDL in late pregnancy. The change in LPL activity corresponds to its decrease in adipose tissue, which is the body tissue that normally has the highest LPL activity and is the only tissue that shows a marked decrease during late gestation.[13,14] The decreased adipose tissue LPL activity is also a consequence of the insulin-resistant state characteristic of late pregnancy.[10,15]

The specific enrichment in triglycerides seen in LDL and HDL seems to be the result of two mechanisms (see Fig. 31.2): (1) augmented activity of the cholesteryl ester transfer protein (CETP),[5,16] which mediates the transfer of esterified cholesterol from LDL and HDL_{2b} to VLDL in exchange for triglycerides, therefore contributing to the enrichment of triglycerides in the higher-density lipoproteins, LDL and HDL_{2b}; and (2) decreased activity of hepatic lipase (HL),[5,12] therefore reducing the conversion of triglyceride-rich HDL_{2b} into the lipid-poor HDL_3. The decreased HL activity during late gestation may be a response to the increase in estrogens, because these hormones are known to inhibit both HL activity and messenger RNA (mRNA) expression.[12,17,18]

The events just summarized together with the changes in other hormones and cytokines that take place during late pregnancy are responsible for the maternal insulin-resistant condition[19-21] and for the sustained maternal hyperlipoproteinemia. Despite the impermeability of the placenta to lipoproteins, their lipid components do become available to the fetus; therefore the changes actively contribute to fetal development. In fact, reducing maternal hyperlipoproteinemia in rats by treatment with hypolipidemic drugs has detrimental effects on fetal development.[22,23]

Essential fatty acids (EFAs) and long-chain polyunsaturated fatty acids (LCPUFAs) derived from the maternal diet are transported mainly in their esterified form in maternal plasma lipoproteins, rather than in their NEFA form,[24,25] and must become available to the fetus despite the lack of a direct placental transfer of maternal lipoproteins. The transfer occurs thanks to the presence of lipoprotein receptors in the placental trophoblast cells that lie at the interface with maternal blood. These cells are therefore positioned to bind maternal lipoproteins and mediate their metabolism and the subsequent transfer of the fatty acids they carry to the fetal circulation. VLDL/apolipoprotein E (apo E) receptor (VLDLR) and LDL, HDL, and scavenger receptors are expressed in human placental tissue.[26-34] Furthermore, placental tissue has different lipolytic activities, including endothelial lipase (EL)[35], LPL,[36-38] and phospholipase A_2,[39-41] and intracellular lipase activities.[42,43] Consequently, esterified fatty acids of maternal plasma lipoproteins are hydrolyzed either extracellularly before uptake or intracellularly after receptor mediated endocytosis. After uptake they are reesterified before eventual release (see later). Using cultured placental trophoblast cells, it has been shown that esterified lipids provide a reservoir of fatty acids that can be released into the experimental medium.[44] The placenta also has different fatty acid transport and binding proteins that actively contribute to the transfer of those fatty acids to the fetal circulation.[45,46]

The mechanism by which placental fatty acids are released into the fetal circulation is not completely understood. One

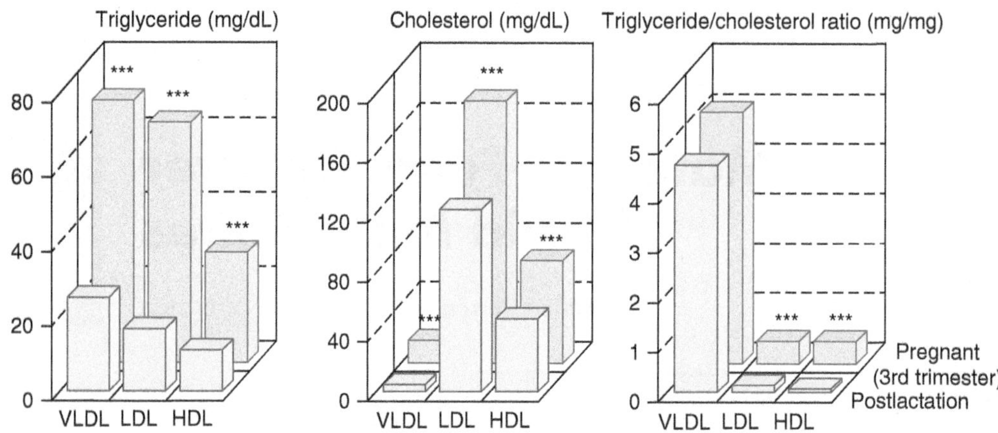

Fig. 31.1 Plasma lipoprotein lipids in women in the third trimester of pregnancy and after lactation. *Asterisks* indicate significant differences between the two groups. *HDL,* High-density lipoprotein; *LDL,* low-density lipoprotein; *VLDL,* very low-density lipoprotein. (From Montelongo A, Lasunción MA, Pallardo LF, et al. Longitudinal study of plasma lipoproteins and hormones during pregnancy in normal and diabetic women. *Diabetes.* 1992;41:1651.)

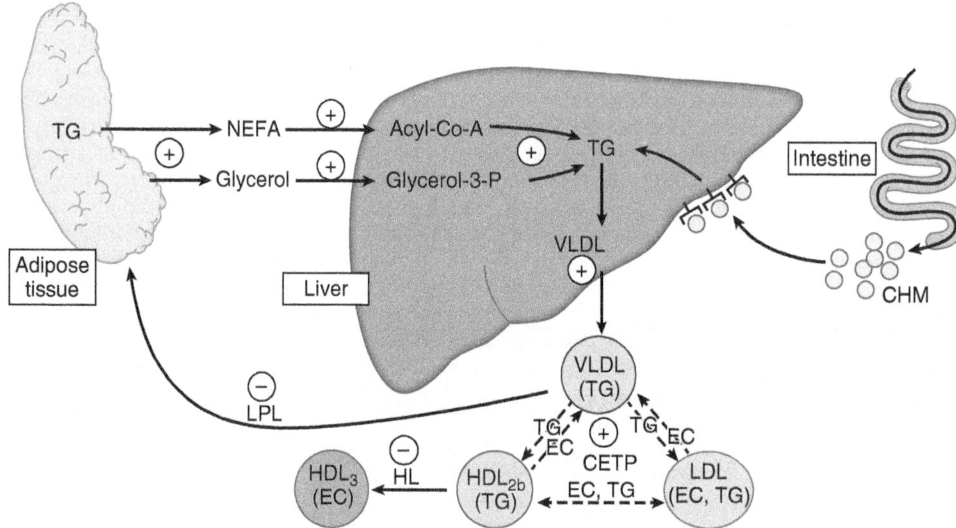

Fig. 31.2 Proposed control of major lipoprotein metabolic pathways during late pregnancy. *CETP,* Cholesteryl ester transfer protein; *CHM,* chylomicrons; *EC,* esterified cholesterol; *HDL,* high-density lipoproteins; *HL,* hepatic lipase; *LDL,* low-density lipoproteins; *LPL,* lipoprotein lipase; *NEFA,* nonesterified fatty acids; *TG,* triglycerides; *VLDL,* very low-density lipoproteins.

possibility is in the form of NEFA after the intracellular hydrolysis of esterified fatty acids in the placenta. In the fetal circulation these NEFAs would bind to a specific oncofetal protein, α fetoprotein,[47-49] and be rapidly transported to fetal liver. Fatty acids taken up by fetal liver are esterified and released back into circulation in the form of VLDL-triglycerides. Another possibility is release to the fetal circulation in their esterified form associated with specific lipoproteins. This mechanism is consistent with the report that rat yolk sac can synthesize apo B-containing lipoproteins[50] and that the placenta can express apo B[51]; similar findings have also been reported in mouse yolk sak[52,53] and in the human placenta.[54] Both of these possibilities are consistent with the findings that the concentrations of certain polyunsaturated fatty acids (PUFAs) in maternal plasma triglycerides during late gestation in humans are significantly and positively correlated with their concentrations in cord plasma triglycerides[55] and that the concentration of all individual fatty acids in serum during late pregnancy were lower in cord serum than in maternal serum.[56] It also agrees with the finding that concentrations of esterified fatty acids were higher than those of NEFAs in venous cord plasma after the oral administration of different fatty acids to pregnant women at term before elective caesarean section.[57] A linear correlation has also been found between maternal and fetal plasma triglycerides and PUFAs in the rat.[58,59] This relationship may have important implications for newborn weight because a direct relationship between maternal triglycerides and newborn weight has been found in humans.[60-62]

MATERNAL LIPID METABOLISM AND PLACENTAL TRANSFER OF FREE FATTY ACIDS, GLYCEROL, AND KETONE BODIES TO THE FETUS

During the first part of gestation, the maternal body accumulates fat[63,64] as the result of combined effects of hyperphagia,[65] enhanced lipogenesis,[66] and unmodified or even increased extrahepatic LPL activity.[5,14,67] The tendency to accumulate fat ceases during late gestation[64,68] because maternal lipid metabolism changes to a catabolic condition. This is evidenced by increased adipose tissue lipolysis[9,14] and reduced uptake of circulating triglycerides,[69] secondary to the reduction in adipose tissue LPL activity.[5,12,14] These changes, together with very active hepatic production of triglycerides[70,71] and the increased absorption of dietary lipids[72] are responsible for the marked progressive increase in maternal circulating triglycerides occurring during late gestation.[3,5] The major changes in the maternal lipid metabolism are summarized in Fig. 31.3, which depicts the changes in adipose tissue, liver, and intestinal activity that are responsible for the physiologic increase in circulating

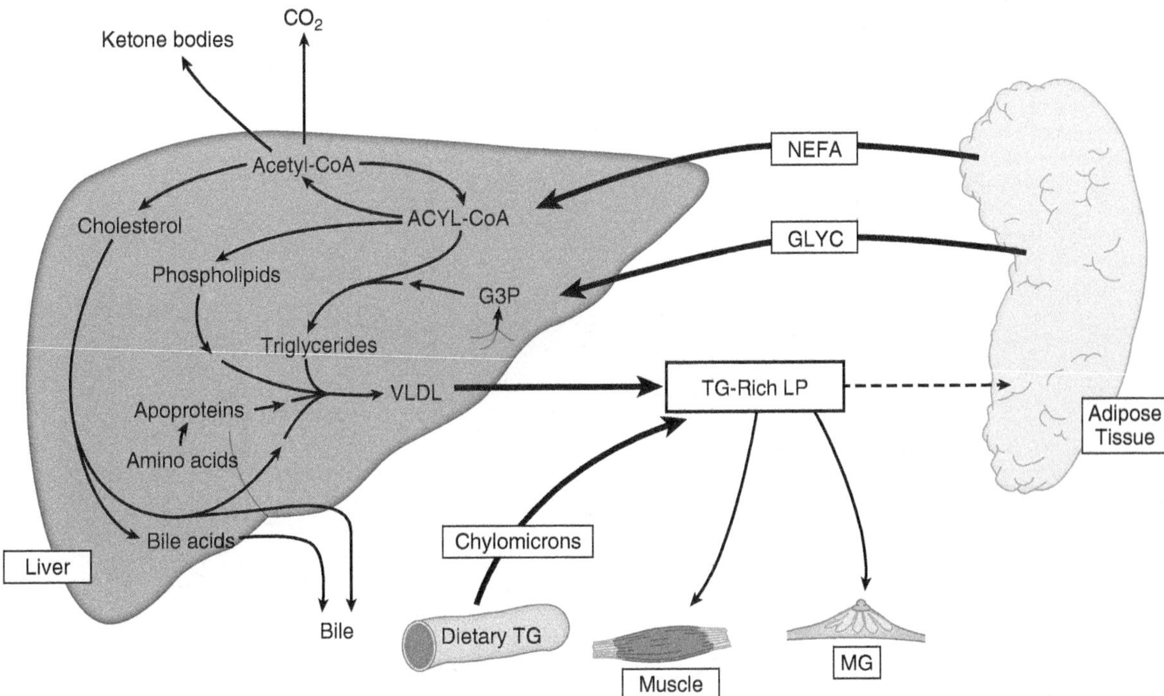

Fig. 31.3 Summary of major changes in maternal lipid metabolism at late gestation. *CoA,* Coenzyme A; *G3P, sn*-glycerol 3-phosphate; *Glyc,* glycerol; *MG,* mammary gland; *NEFA,* nonesterified fatty acids; *TG,* triglycerides; *TG-RICH LP,* triglyceride-rich lipoproteins; *VLDL,* very low-density lipoprotein. (From Herrera E, Gómez-Coronado D, Lasunción MA. Lipid metabolism in pregnancy. *Biol Neonate.* 1987;51:70.)

NEFA, glycerol, and triglyceride-rich lipoproteins (VLDLs and chylomicrons). Under fed conditions, the frequency of maternal ketosis is not different from that in nonpregnant subjects, but it increases markedly under fasting conditions.[73,74]

With the exception of glycerol used in gluconeogenesis[75,76] and the LPL-mediated uptake of circulating triglycerides by the mammary gland before labor,[72,77,78] no part of the increase in circulating lipid components in the fed mother during late gestation seems to benefit her own metabolic needs directly. However, the increase may benefit the fetus because this gestational period coincides with the state of maximal fetal accretion, a time when the substrate, metabolic fuel and essential component requirements of the fetus are particularly prominent. The lipid component also may constitute a "floating" fuel store for both mother and fetus, easily accessible under conditions of food deprivation; this may explain the increased ketogenesis in the mother seen under fasting conditions.[73,79]

The enhanced availability of ketone bodies to maternal tissues under fasting conditions allows them to be used as metabolic fuels, sparing other, more limited and essential substrates, such as amino acids and glucose, for transport to the fetus. Augmented lipolytic activity also increases maternal circulating glycerol levels.[13,75] Glycerol can be used by the mother as an efficient gluconeogenic substrate,[75,76,80] contributing to the maintenance of glucose production for fetal and maternal tissues. Metabolic adaptations found in the mother during starvation are summarized in Fig. 31.4. The transfer of glucose, ketone bodies, and amino acids is emphasized in this figure because quantitatively, they are the major substrates crossing the placenta in periods of starvation.

An understanding of fatty acid, glycerol, and ketone body placental transfer and their subsequent metabolic fates in the fetus provides an insight into the effect on the fetus of the persistently elevated maternal circulating lipid levels. Fig. 31.5 compares plasma levels of these metabolites in virgin and in 24-hour-fasted late-pregnancy rats and their fetuses. It can be seen that although fetal NEFA and glycerol levels are much lower in the fetuses than in their mothers, the concentrations of ketone bodies are similar. These maternal-fetal concentration differences probably reflect the efficiency or magnitude of the placental transfer process.

Maternal-fetal nutrient transfer through the placenta may be accomplished by different mechanisms, including facilitated diffusion, active transport, and simple diffusion.[81,82] The rate of transfer by simple diffusion is a direct function of the concentration gradient and decreases with the molecular size and hydrosolubility.[83] However, in the case of placental transfer, other factors also play a role[84,85]: uterine and umbilical blood flows, intrinsic placental metabolism, and structural characteristics. As might be expected, some of these factors, such as blood flow, contribute analogously to the transfer of any nutrient, but other factors differ with each nutrient and require specific consideration.

FATTY ACIDS

The fetus requires not only EFAs from the mother, to support growth and brain development,[86] but also nonessential fatty acids, which—stored in fetal body fat—constitute an important substrate during early postnatal life.[87] This storage pool is especially important in species such as the guinea pig and human, in which body fat at term represents a substantial percentage of body weight (10% in guinea pigs and 16% in humans),[88] and where fatty acid synthesis by fetal tissues de novo cannot fulfill fetal requirements.

NEFAs bound to albumin and esterified fatty acids transported in lipoproteins are both potential sources of the maternal fatty acids that will cross the placenta. Early studies in sheep[89] measured venous-arterial differences across the umbilical circulation of the fetus in utero and across the maternal uterine circulation and showed that no significant passage of NEFA to the fetus had occurred and led to the conclusion that NEFAs did not appear to constitute a significant part of the metabolic fuel

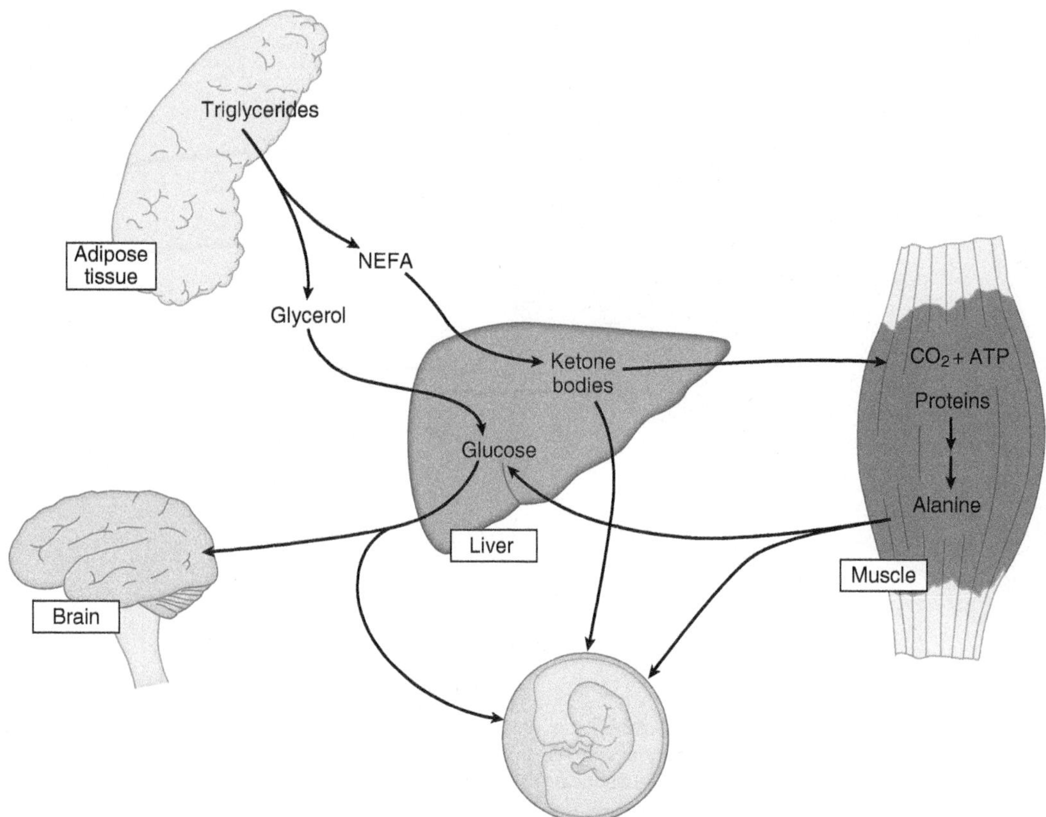

Fig. 31.4 Maternal response to starvation. More active adipose tissue lipolysis increases the availability in the liver of glycerol to be used as a preferential substrate for gluconeogenesis and of nonesterified fatty acids *(NEFAs)* for ketone body synthesis. By this mechanism, the mother conserves other gluconeogenic substrates, such as alanine, and ensures the adequate availability of fuels and metabolites to the fetus. *ATP*, Adenosine triphosphate. (From Herrera E, Gómez-Coronado D, Lasunción MA. Lipid metabolism in pregnancy. *Biol Neonate.* 1987;51:70.)

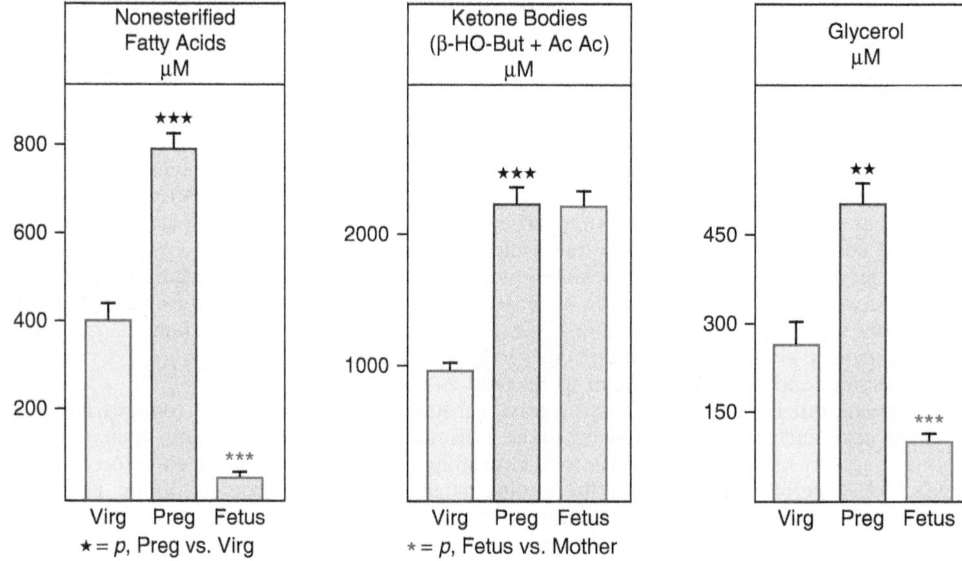

Fig. 31.5 Concentrations of nonesterified fatty acids, ketone bodies, and glycerol in plasma of 48-hour starved virgin (Virg) and 19-day pregnant (Preg) rats and their fetuses. *AcAc,* Acetoacetate; *β-HO-But,* β-hydroxybutyrate. (From Herrera E, Gómez-Coronado D, Lasunción MA. Lipid metabolism in pregnancy. *Biol Neonate.* 1987;51:70.)

supplied by the mother.[89] However, later studies demonstrated that the net flux of fatty acids from mother to fetus across the placenta varies greatly among species. For example, in species with both maternal and fetal layers in the placenta, such as the sheep, pig, and cat, the net transfer of fatty acid to the fetus generally is small.[90-92]

In humans, as mentioned earlier, LCPUFAs in maternal circulation are mainly carried as their esterified form in plasma lipoproteins rather than as NEFAs,[24,25] although there are also proposals that NEFAs could be also an important source of PUFAs to the fetus.[93,94] Current evidence suggests that cellular uptake of NEFA occurs through a process of facilitated membrane translocation involving a plasma membrane fatty acid–binding protein ($FABP_{pm}$).[95,96] It has been shown that $FABP_{pm}$ and the fatty acid transfer proteins (FAT/CD36 and FATP) are present in human placental membranes,[97,98]

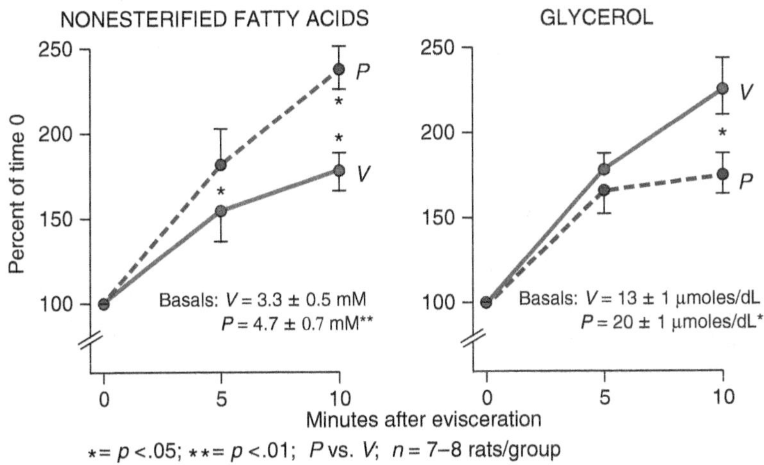

Fig. 31.6 Effect of hepatectomy-nephrectomy on plasma nonesterified fatty acids and glycerol in virgin *(V)* and 20-day pregnant *(P)* rats. (From Mampel T, Villarroya F, Herrera E. Hepatectomy-nephrectomy effects in the pregnant rat and fetus. *Biochem Biophys Res Commun.* 1985;131:1219))

but the precise way in which membrane-associated FABPs facilitate transmembrane passage of fatty acids is still a matter of speculation.[99] The preference for human placental fatty acid transfer from the maternal to the fetal circulation has been reported as docosahexaenoic > α-linolenic > linoleic > oleic > arachidonic acid.[100] However, arachidonic acid was the fatty acid that accumulated most in the placenta,[100] and it has been shown that the process of arachidonic uptake by placental syncytiotrophoblast membranes is highly dependent on adenosine triphosphate (ATP) and sodium,[101] implying an active transport mechanism for this fatty acid. A selectivity in the LCPUFA placental transfer also may be exerted at the level of cellular metabolism: a certain proportion of arachidonic acid is converted to prostaglandins and other eicosanoids,[94] a selective incorporation of certain fatty acids into phospholipids has been found in the ovine placenta,[102] and even selective placental fatty acid oxidation[103,104] and lipid synthesis[105,106] may occur.

The combination of all of these processes determines the actual rate of placental fatty acid transfer and its selectivity. The placenta selectively transports arachidonic acid and docosahexaenoic acid from the maternal to the fetal compartment, resulting in a proportional enrichment of these LCPUFAs in the circulating lipids of the fetus,[107,108] although their actual concentrations are lower in fetal than in maternal circulation.[56] This transport occurs during the third trimester, when the fetal demands for neural and vascular growth are greater.[109,110]

Although, as just described, current evidence indicates that fatty acids are selectively transferred across the placenta, EFAs and nonessential fatty acids also may use a common transfer mechanism. Using guinea pig or rabbit placentas perfused in situ, several investigations have demonstrated that, within the physiologic range, the net NEFA transfer to the fetus correlates with maternal plasma levels of NEFA and that this transfer is regulated by the transplacental concentration gradient.[111,112] Furthermore, during maternal fasting, increased amounts of maternal NEFA cross the placenta into fetal circulation and are incorporated into fetal stores.[113] These observations suggest that the transfer of several NEFAs across the placenta is mainly by diffusion. Other factors affecting this transfer process are the uterine and umbilical blood flow rates[111,112] and the concentration of fetal serum albumin.[111,114,115] In this respect, the increase in albumin levels throughout the third trimester in the human fetus[116] may increase its NEFA supply.

GLYCEROL

As a result of the lipolytic activity of maternal adipose tissue, glycerol levels in plasma are consistently elevated during late gestation.[14,75,76] Values for plasma glycerol therefore generally are higher in the mother than in the fetus as seeing in humans[117] and in rats (see Fig. 31.5).

Although the molecular characteristics of glycerol (a low-molecular-weight uncharged molecule) should facilitate easy placental transfer, its transfer is notably lower than for other metabolites with similar molecular characteristics, such as glucose or L-alanine.[118-120] Placental glycerol transfer is accomplished by simple diffusion.[121] In humans, it has not been possible to detect a transfer of glycerol from mother to fetus despite its favorable gradient.[122] In rats, the fetal-placental unit has been demonstrated to convert glycerol into lactate and lipids[123]; this rapid use may contribute to maintaining the high glycerol gradient found between maternal and fetal blood.[119,120,122]

Accelerated turnover of maternal glycerol seems to be influenced by the high liver glycerol kinase activity, which facilitates its rapid phosphorylation and subsequent conversion into glucose.[75,76,80] Although this mechanism indirectly benefits the fetus by providing glucose (see Fig. 31.4), it may limit the availability of enough glycerol molecules for transfer to the fetus. Fig. 31.6 summarizes studies that support this hypothesis. In rats, hepatectomy results in increased plasma glycerol levels because of a reduction in glycerol use secondary to the absence of the liver, which is the major site for uptake and further metabolism of glycerol.[124] In pregnant rats, hepatectomy and nephrectomy produce significant increases in plasma glycerol levels but smaller than those seen in nonpregnant animals. This difference cannot be interpreted as reduced lipolytic activity in the pregnant rat because plasma NEFA, the other lipolytic product, increases more than in nonpregnant animals (see Fig. 31.6). However, the smaller increase of glycerol may reflect an augmented transfer of glycerol to the fetus, because glycerol levels in fetal plasma increase significantly after maternal hepatectomy and nephrectomy.[125]

Therefore placental glycerol transfer seems to be limited by its rapid use for gluconeogenesis by the liver and renal cortex of the mother. Although the fetal-placental unit actively uses glycerol, its quantitative and physiologic roles in the fetus, except as the preferred substrate for fetal liver glyceride-glycerol synthesis,[123] seems to be relatively minor under normal conditions.

IMPLICATIONS OF PLACENTAL LIPID TRANSFER ON NEONATAL BODY WEIGHT AND FAT MASS

In normal pregnancies, although glucose is the compound crossing the placenta in greatest quantities, during late pregnancy there is a positive correlation between maternal serum glucose, NEFA and glycerol, but not triglycerides, with those in cord blood.[117] Nevertheless, of those compounds, only maternal glucose levels correlated with neonatal fat mass and body weight, but linear correlations were found between cord serum glucose, NEFA, and triglycerides with either neonatal fat mass or birth weight.[117] As summarized in Fig. 31.7, it is proposed that under conditions of increased fetal glucose levels as result of maternal hyperglycemia there is a consequent increased fetal insulin levels, as it is the case in gestational diabetic pregnancies,[117] and liver lipogenesis and triglyceride synthesis must be stimulated. Moreover, maternal hyperlipidemia and subsequent increased transfer of maternal fatty acids to the fetal circulation would facilitate the uptake of NEFA by fetal liver and their use for triglyceride synthesis. It is hypothesized that those liver triglycerides are released into fetal circulation as components of VLDL. From previous studies,[126,127] it can be concluded that LPL is present in fetal adipose tissue from early intrauterine life. Because insulin appears to increase in human adipose tissue both the LPL activity[128] and lipogenesis,[129,130] it can be also hypothesized that under conditions of fetal hyperinsulinemia both LPL activity and lipogenesis in adipose tissue are actively enhanced contributing to the fetal fat mass accumulation that take place during the last weeks of intrauterine life.[131,131a]

KETONE BODIES

Although plasma levels of ketone bodies in the fed pregnant mother late in gestation are unchanged under physiologic, fasting,[73,79,132,133] or diabetic[3,134] conditions, they are greatly elevated as a result of increases in both adipose tissue lipolytic activity and delivery of NEFA to the liver. Maternal ketone bodies can cross the placental barrier and be used as fuels and lipogenic substrates by the fetus.[135-137]

Maternal ketonemia in the pregnant patient with poorly controlled diabetes, with or without acidosis, has been associated with an increased stillbirth rate, an increased incidence of congenital malformations, and impaired neurophysiologic development in the infant.[136,138,139] These effects are thought to be secondary to placental transfer of maternal ketone bodies to the fetus.[140]

In all species studied (human,[132,133,141] rat,[79,142] and sheep[140]), increments in maternal ketone bodies are accompanied by increments in fetal plasma levels, indicating efficient placental transfer; fetal liver ketogenesis is negligible.[143]

Placental transfer of ketone bodies occurs either by simple diffusion or by a low-specificity carrier-mediated process,[121,144] the efficiency of which varies among species. Although the maternofetal ratio for ketone bodies is higher than 10 in sheep,[140] in humans it is approximately 2[122] and in rats it is close to 1[79,142] (see Fig. 31.5), indicating that the amount of ketone bodies crossing the placenta is much smaller in ruminants than in nonruminant species. It has even been proposed that in the fasting condition, the contribution of ketone bodies to the fetal oxidative metabolism accounts for only 2% to 3% of total oxygen consumption in the case of sheep.[145] In the rat, 3-hydroxybutyrate adequately replaces the glucose deficit in the placenta, fetal brain, and liver during fasting hypoglycemia.[137] This finding suggests a much greater contribution of ketone bodies to the fetal oxidative metabolism in the fasted nonruminant.

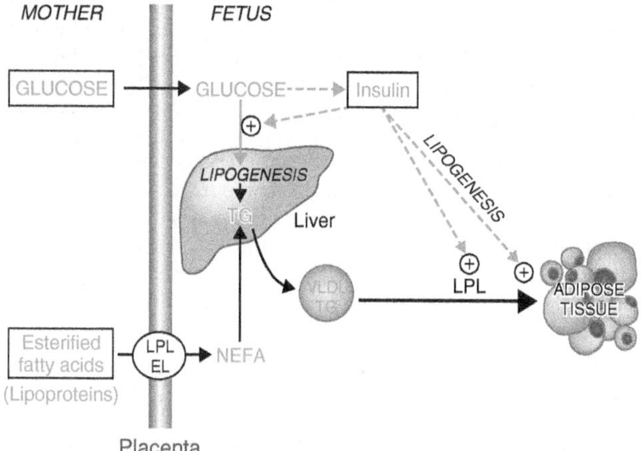

Fig. 31.7 Proposed mechanism for the development of fetal fat mass during late gestation. Details are described in the text. *EL*, Endothelial lipase; *LPL*, lipoprotein lipase; *NEFA*, nonesterified fatty acids; *TG*, triglycerides; *VLDL TG*, very low-density lipoprotein triglycerides.

Key enzymes for ketone body use—3-hydroxybutyrate dehydrogenase (EC 1.1.1.30), 3-oxoacid-coenzyme A (CoA) transferase (EC 2.8.3.5), and acetyl-CoA acetyltransferase (EC 2.3.1.9)—have been found in the brain and other tissues in both the human and the rat fetus.[135,146] Both the rat and human brain[136,137] oxidize 3-hydroxybutyrate in vitro in a form that is dependent on substrate concentration and not on the maternal nutritional state. Other fetal tissue types known to oxidize ketone bodies are kidney, heart, liver, and placenta.[147,148] Some tissues are even known to use ketone bodies as substrates for fatty acid and cholesterol synthesis, as has been shown in the rat brain, liver, placenta, and lung after administration of 3-hydroxybutyrate to pregnant animals in vivo.[149] The activity of ketone body-metabolizing enzymes in fetal tissues (brain, liver, and kidney) can be increased by conditions that result in maternal hyperketonemia, such as starvation during the last days of gestation[150] or high-fat feeding.[151] Such a change is especially evident in the fetal brains from starved late-pregnant rats[150] and may represent an important fetal adaptation to guarantee brain development under these conditions because fetal brain weight is better preserved than other fetal organ weights.

In conclusion, evidence obtained in nonruminant species is suggestive of efficient placental ketone body transfer and of fetal use of these materials as substrates for both oxidation and lipogenesis. Because both the placental transfer and the use of ketone bodies are concentration dependent, their quantitative contribution to fetal metabolism is important only under conditions of maternal hyperketonemia (e.g., starvation, high-fat diet, diabetes).

CHOLESTEROL IN THE FETUS

ROLE OF CHOLESTEROL AND RELATED COMPOUNDS IN DEVELOPMENT

Cholesterol plays an important role in fetal development and in the general physiology of the organism. First, it is an essential component of cell membranes. By interacting with phospholipids and sphingolipids, cholesterol contributes to the characteristic physicochemical properties of membranes, mainly fluidity and passive permeability.[152] Cholesterol is not homogeneously distributed in the membrane; rather, it is concentrated in structures such as rafts and caveolae, where it modulates the function of different integral proteins and receptors. Cholesterol is the precursor of both bile acids and steroid hormones; in the fetus, glucocorticoids are intensely synthesized by the adrenal gland in the last part of development. Cholesterol and its oxidized derivatives—oxysterols—are also key regulators of different metabolic processes, both by modulating the proteolytic activation of sterol response element-binding protein (SREBP) and by acting as ligands of nuclear receptors, such as liver X receptor (LXR).[153,154] Active SREBP and LXR are transcription factors that regulate the expression of multiple genes implicated in intracellular lipid homeostasis and lipoprotein metabolism.[153,155]

Other important actions of cholesterol, which have special relevance for the fetus because they are related to development, embryogenesis, and differentiation, have also become apparent.[156]

Cholesterol is essential for cell proliferation, not only for membrane formation but also for the activation of regulatory proteins involved in cell cycle progression.[157-159] Cholesterol plays important roles in differentiation and cell-to-cell communication; in fact, it has been demonstrated to be a key factor in synaptogenesis.[160] Finally, cholesterol is essential in embryonic patterning in both vertebrates and invertebrates.[161] This patterning is attained mainly by activation of hedgehog proteins (i.e., sonic hedgehog [Shh] in humans), which are involved in cell differentiation.[161]

It is therefore conceivable that defects affecting cholesterol availability will have deleterious consequences in fetal development. In fact, congenital defects in cholesterol biosynthesis or the reduction of cholesterol synthesis with xenobiotics result in severe malformations and dysfunctions, mainly affecting the craniofacial organs and the central nervous system, respectively, alterations that are similar to those caused by Shh deficiency.[161-163]

In pigs, fetal weight is directly correlated with plasma cholesterol concentration in the fetus at late gestation.[164] Similarly, neonatal pigs from lines with genetically low cholesterol levels are smaller at birth and grow more slowly, but the growth rate improved when they were fed with cholesterol.[165,166] An increase in neonatal survival is noted with supplementary dietary fat for the peripartal sow.[167] Thus cholesterol is essential to body growth and the development of the central nervous system, and fetal requirements must be met either by efficient endogenous cholesterol biosynthesis or transfer from the mother.

CHOLESTEROL BIOSYNTHESIS AND CONGENITAL DEFECTS

Cholesterol biosynthesis is a multienzymatic pathway that uses acetyl-CoA as precursor, ATP, O_2, and NADPH. In the first part, three molecules of acetyl-CoA are successively condensed by the action of acetyl-CoA acetyltransferase and cytosolic 3-hydroxy-3-methylglutaryl (HMG)-CoA synthase to form HMG-CoA, which is then reduced with the loss of CoA, generating mevalonate, a six-carbon compound (Fig. 31.8).[168] This complex reaction is catalyzed by HMG-CoA reductase, which is present in the endoplasmic reticulum and is the rate-limiting enzyme in cholesterol biosynthesis. In the next series of reactions, mevalonate is converted into isopentenyl diphosphate and then squalene (see Fig. 31.8), which is the immediate precursor of sterols. The first sterol formed is lanosterol, which contains 30 carbons. The transformation of lanosterol into cholesterol occurs in the endoplasmic reticulum and involves at least seven different enzymes (Fig. 31.9).

In humans, several genetic defects in the cholesterol biosynthesis pathway have been identified. Excellent reviews on this subject are available.[163,169-173] Mevalonic aciduria is caused by missense mutations in mevalonate kinase, which impair the formation of both isoprenoids and sterols (see Fig. 31.8). The patients show dysmorphias and failure to thrive. Milder mutations of the enzyme also underlie hyperimmunoglobulinemia D and periodic fever syndrome. The rest of the disorders are due to defects in the postsqualene segment of the pathway (see Fig. 31.9). Deficiency of lanosterol 14α-demethylase causes synostosis in multiple bones leading to malformations and deformities of the skeleton. Greenberg skeletal dysplasia, which is associated with short-limb dwarfism, is probably caused by mutations in Δ^{14}-reductase. Mutations in *NSDHL* or *SC4MOL* genes, which affect the C4-demethylation of sterols, cause CHILD (congenital hemidysplasia with ichthyosiform erythroderma and limb defects) syndrome and SC4MOL deficiency, respectively. Conradi-Hünermann-Happle syndrome (or human X-linked dominant chondrodysplasia punctate, CDPX2) is caused by deficiency of $\Delta^{8,7}$-isomerase (also named emopamil-binding protein, EBP). Desmosterolosis is an extremely rare disorder due to the deficiency of Δ^{24}-reductase; the infants affected died shortly after birth and suffered from multiple malformations and dysmorphias. Among these disorders, the best known and most widely studied is the Smith-Lemli-Opitz syndrome (SLOS), caused by mutations in Δ^7-reductase, which most prominent anomalies are microcephalia and facial dysmorphias. All affected patients accumulate 7-dehydrocholesterol in plasma and tissues, but the clinical severity is best correlated to the 7-dehydrocholesterol/cholesterol ratio. In general, these congenital alterations show the important role of cholesterol and its immediate precursors in morphogenesis and fetal development.

SOURCES OF FETAL CHOLESTEROL

The demands for cholesterol in the fetus are relatively high, especially during the last third of gestation, when fetal growth is extremely rapid. The fetus may obtain cholesterol from both endogenous biosynthesis and the mother blood through the yolk sac and placenta. In humans, the yolk sac is responsible for maternal-fetal nutrient exchange during the first 8 weeks approximately, by transporting molecules from the exocoelomic cavity to the fetal circulation through a thin line of cells.[174,175] Thereafter, once the placenta has been fully developed, nutrients circulating in the maternal blood must cross two layers: the placental syncytiotrophoblasts and then the fetal capillary epithelium. The first one, which is made up of polarized cells with two clearly distinguished membranes: apical microvillous and basal plasma, respectively, appears to function as the rate-limiting step of this transport.[174,175]

Several lines of evidence demonstrate the transfer of maternal sterols to the fetus (see reviews[175-180]): (1) radioactivity-labeled sterols injected into the maternal blood readily appear in the fetus; (2) cholesterol concentration in the umbilical vein blood is higher than that in the umbilical artery[175,181]; (3) cholesterol is detected in fetuses unable to synthesize cholesterol due to genetic mutations[182,183]; and (4) phytosterols, which must necessarily come from the maternal blood, are detected in the fetus.[184] Nevertheless, differences in the relative importance of these two sources of cholesterol among different mammals and changes throughout pregnancy have been recognized.

By tracking the appearance of radioactivity in the fetus, early experiments demonstrated the placental transfer of maternal cholesterol to the fetus in several species.[185-187] In those studies, the estimated contribution of maternal cholesterol to the fetus varied widely. Measurements of [^{3}H]-water incorporation into cholesterol revealed that the rate of cholesterol synthesis in fetal tissues is several times higher than in maternal tissues in different species when calculated per unit of mass.[188-194] This is especially high in the fetal brain, which appears almost completely autonomous in cholesterol accretion, and the liver, which secretes the excess of cholesterol into the plasma for uptake by other developing fetal organs.[191,192] These findings are consistent with the near-maximal expression at the level of mRNA of different enzymes involved in cholesterol biosynthesis[193] and the high activity of HMG-CoA reductase—the rate-limiting enzyme of cholesterol biosynthesis—in fetal tissues.[194,195]

In the rat, endogenously synthesized cholesterol appears to account for practically all fetal cholesterol,[191,192] meaning that a maternal source is less significant, at least during the later stages of gestation. Belknap and Dietschy[189] found that although the rat placenta did take up [^{125}I]-cellobiose-labeled lipoprotein from maternal circulation, neither the apo nor cholesterol was transferred in any appreciable amount to the fetus. Maneuvers directed to modify cholesterol homeostasis in the mother had no significant effects on cholesterol levels or cholesterol synthesis rates in the fetus. Thus feeding rats with cholesterol, which resulted in an increase in plasma cholesterol concentration and reduced cholesterol synthesis in the maternal compartment, did not affect any of these parameters in the fetus.[188,189,196] Conversely, treatment with cholestyramine—a bile acid sequestrant that

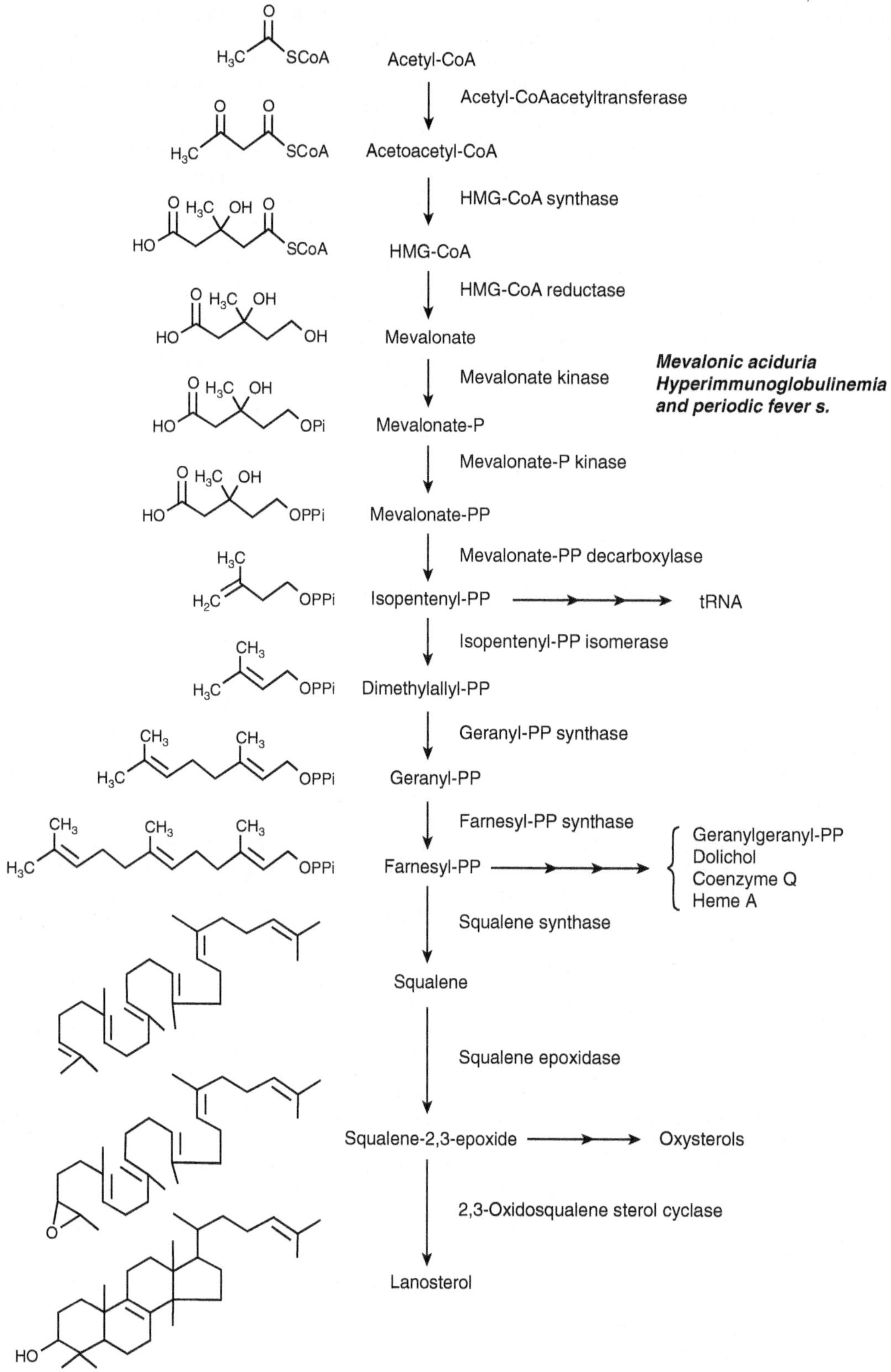

Fig. 31.8 Biosynthesis of lanosterol from acetyl-CoA. Aside from the route leading to the formation of lanosterol, the first sterol in the cholesterol biosynthesis pathway, the alternative use of isopentenyl-PP for the derivation of certain transfer RNA *(tRNA)* and farnesyl-PP for several isoprenoids is shown. *Multiple-headed arrows* indicate several reactions. The name of a human inherited disorder is shown *(bold, italics)* beside the affected enzyme. *CoA,* Coenzyme A; *HMG,* 3-hydroxy-3-methylglutaryl; *PP,* pyrophosphate.

interferes with intestinal cholesterol absorption and consequently stimulates cholesterol biosynthesis in maternal tissues—did not alter cholesterol accretion in the fetus.[197] All of these findings led to the notion that in the rat, fetal cholesterol originates mainly from endogenous de novo synthesis.

In the early stages of gestation, however, maternal cholesterol may make a significant contribution to the fetal cholesterol pool. Thus treatment of rats with AY 9944—an inhibitor of Δ^7-reductase—resulted in fetal teratogenesis, and the simultaneous oral administration of cholesterol early in gestation completely prevented the characteristic holoprosencephalic brain malformations.[160,198,199] By contrast, the anomalies of fetal masculinization caused by AY 9944 administered late in gestation are not prevented by compensatory administration of cholesterol to the mother.[160] These results firmly suggest that maternal cholesterol reaches the fetal compartment early in gestation and is of significant physiologic relevance in the rat.

In mice, by injecting [^{13}C]-cholesterol into the maternal circulation at different stages of pregnancy, it was demonstrated that maternal cholesterol is transferred through the yolk sac and the placenta to the embryo and fetus, respectively.[200] By measuring the different sterols by GC-MS in *Dhcr7* knockout mice, which are unable to synthesize cholesterol, Tint and colleagues confirmed that early in gestation, most fetal sterols are of maternal origin, but as the fetus develops, the endogenous synthesis becomes increasingly important, and by birth, approximately half of newborn sterols have been synthesized by the fetus.[201]

In other species too, maternal cholesterol appears to be an important, quantitative source for the fetus. In the golden Syrian hamster, Woollett found that endogenous biosynthesis accounted for only 40% of the fetal cholesterol, suggesting that the placenta or the yolk sac, or both, contributed the remainder.[190] Actually, in hamsters fed increasing amounts of cholesterol, the cholesterol concentration in the fetal tissues was found to be linearly correlated with the maternal plasma cholesterol concentration, whereas cholesterol synthesis decreased in the reverse way.[202] In line with this, the uptake of maternal LDL and quantitatively more important HDL by both the placenta and the yolk sac were increased in diet-induced hypercholesterolemic dams compared with controls, as determined by using [^{3}H]-cholesteryl oleate-labeled lipoproteins.[203] In the guinea pig, fetal cholesterol homeostasis was found to be relatively insensitive to maternal, diet-induced hypercholesterolemia, yet maternal hypocholesterolemia induced by cholestyramine resulted in a slight increase in cholesterol synthesis in the fetus, demonstrating that fetal cholesterol homeostasis may respond to changes in maternal plasma lipoprotein concentrations during late gestation.[188] In the rhesus monkey, Pitkin and colleagues calculated that an average of 43% of the serum cholesterol in the fetus at term originated from the maternal blood.[187]

Data in humans are more limited, and cholesterol biosynthesis in fetal tissues has not been directly determined for obvious reasons. However, by using different approaches several studies have demonstrated the transport of maternal sterols to the fetus in humans. In a woman who was 3 months' pregnant and administered a tracer dose of [^{14}C]-cholesterol before undergoing a therapeutic abortion 13 days later, Lin and colleagues[204] estimated that 21% of the fetal cholesterol was derived from the maternal circulation. Parker and associates measured cholesterol levels in the umbilical venous and the umbilical arterial plasma in deliveries at term and found a highly significant difference between paired HDL, LDL, and total cholesterol concentrations, venous levels being 8% to 13% higher than those in arterial plasma.[205] More recently, by sampling both the maternal and the fetal vessels, a significant uteroplacental uptake of total and HDL cholesterol and a fetal uptake of HDL, LDL, and total cholesterol was demonstrated.[181] Moreover, phytosterols, which must necessarily come from the maternal blood, were detected in the fetus at the time of delivery,[84] and although the phytosterols concentration in the umbilical cord is 20% lower than in maternal blood, a positive and significant correlation between these pairs was observed.[206] Finally, in fetuses with SLOS, significant amounts of cholesterol were detected in fetal tissues.[182,183] Of note, cholesterol was as abundant as 7-dehydrocholesterol in the fetal liver but practically unappreciable in the brain, an organ that relies on endogenous biosynthesis. This further indicates the maternal origin of cholesterol in this condition.[182]

These data were indicative of the delivery of cholesterol from the placenta to the fetus, which could either be synthesized in the placenta or derived from the maternal plasma, but its relative contribution to the fetal demands in the normal physiologic condition is unclear. Studies comparing maternal lipoprotein-cholesterol levels with those in mixed umbilical cord blood, reported either a positive correlation[207,208] or no correlation between these values[181,205,209,210] Again, the gestational stage could influence these results.[211,212] In fact, fetal cholesterol levels show a strong inverse correlation with fetal age, being two-fold higher in 5-month than in 7-month fetuses, suggesting that the requirements of cholesterol are relatively greater in the younger, more immature fetuses.[213] Of interest, in fetuses younger than 6 months but not in older fetuses, plasma cholesterol levels are significantly, directly correlated with maternal levels.[213] Therefore available results in humans strongly suggest that maternal cholesterol substantially contributes to fetal cholesterol accretion early in gestation, whereas it seems to be of minimal quantitative importance at term.[205]

PROTEINS AND MECHANISMS INVOLVED IN THE TRANSFER OF CHOLESTEROL TO THE FETUS BY THE YOLK SAC AND THE PLACENTA

The yolk sac and the placenta, in addition to synthesizing cholesterol, are able to remove cholesterol from the maternal circulation and to export it into the fetal circulation. In humans, the yolk sac is vestigial while it appears to play an important role in fetal nutrition in rodents.[180] This is sustained by the expression of a number of lipoprotein receptors and cholesterol transporters and by the ability to secrete newly formed lipoproteins to the fetal circulation.[180,214] Later in gestation, the placenta becomes functional and takes the control of human nutrition. To reach the fetal circulation, maternal cholesterol has to cross several placental barriers, depending on the species. In the human, the syncytiotrophoblast must first take lipoprotein cholesterol from the lacunae; then cholesterol must be transferred to the endothelial cells and secreted to the fetal vessels, either forming part of newly synthesized lipoproteins or effluxed to acceptors present in the fetal blood.[176,177] The ability of trophoblast from different species to take up LDL and HDL cholesterol is well demonstrated.[34,177,201,215-217]

The expression of LDL receptor (LDLR) at both mRNA and protein levels in the placenta and the yolk sack are well known.[26-30,32,215] Several other proteins or receptors that mediate the uptake of lipoprotein cholesterol were also detected in placental preparations. These include the following: CLA-1/SR-BI (CD36 and LIMPII analogous-1/scavenger receptor type B class I),[215,218-220] which mediate the selective uptake of cholesteryl esters from HDL and LDL; megalin/glycoprotein 330,[215,221,222] a protein related to the LDLR; cubilin,[223] a protein that binds HDL and acts in conjunction with megalin to mediate HDL endocytosis; LDLR-related protein (LRP)[221] and apo ER2,[224,225] which bind to and mediate the uptake of VLDL. Epithelial cells of the visceral yolk sac also express several receptors able to mediate lipoprotein-cholesterol uptake, such as LDLR,[215] CLA-1/SR-BI,[215,226] megalin,[221] and cubilin.[227,228] The uptake of free cholesterol by the placenta through receptor-independent mechanisms could not be ruled out,[217,229] but

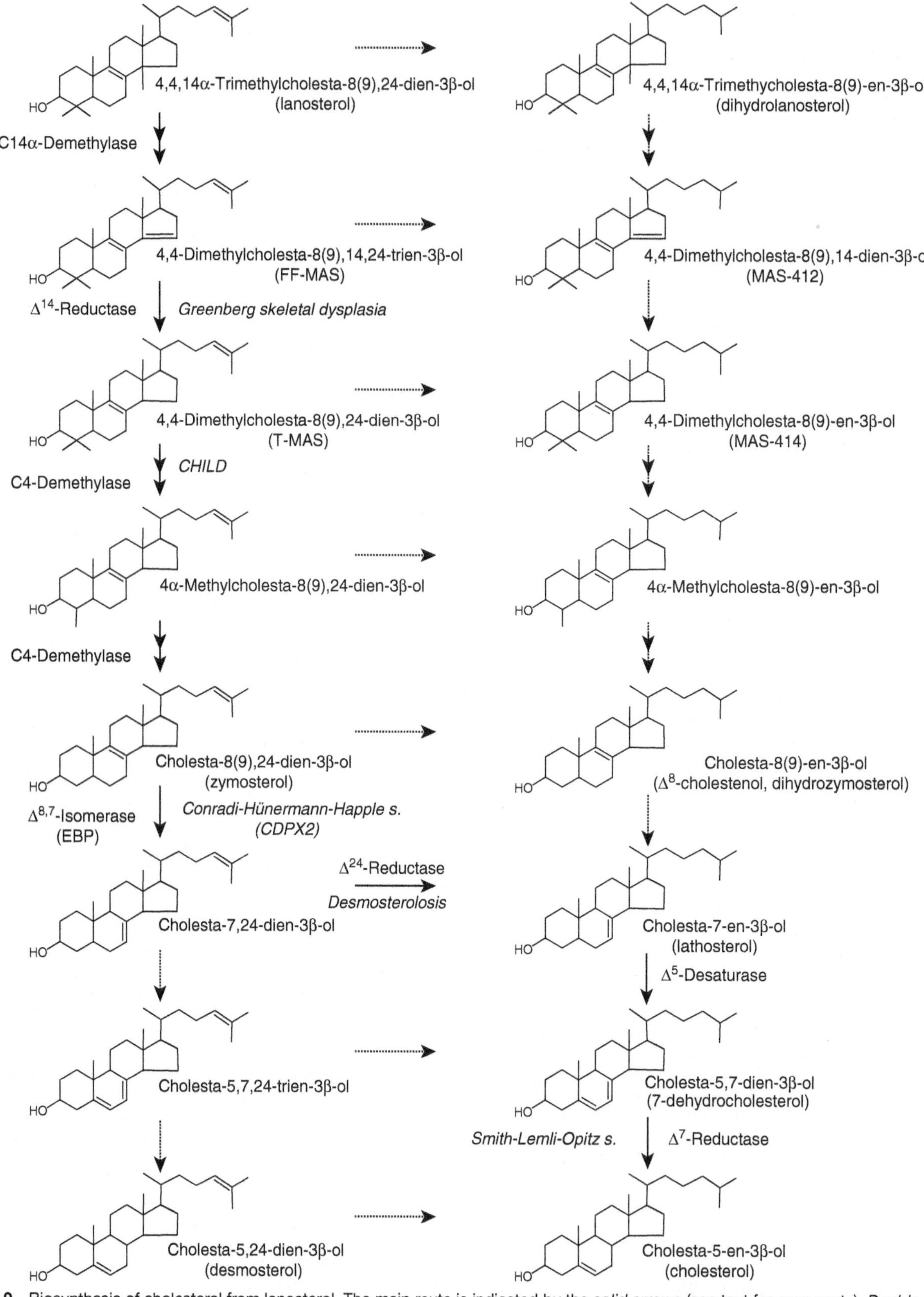

Fig. 31.9 Biosynthesis of cholesterol from lanosterol. The main route is indicated by the *solid arrows* (see text for comments). *Double-headed arrows* indicate several reactions. The names of the human inherited disorders are shown *(bold, italics)* beside the affected enzymes. *CHILD*, Congenital *h*emidysplasia with *i*chthyosiform erythroderma and *l*imb *d*efects; *CDPX2*, human X-linked dominant chondrodysplasia punctate; *EBP*, emopamil- binding protein; *FF-MAS*, follicular fluid-MAS; *MAS*, meiosis-activating sterol; *s.*, syndrome; *T-MAS*, testis-MAS.

the relative contribution of the different mechanisms in the maternofetal cholesterol transport is unclear.

The involvement of SR-BI in the transfer of maternal cholesterol to the fetus was demonstrated by the findings showing that mouse embryos lacking SR-BI contain less cholesterol[230] and take up less cholesterol from their mothers.[231] The use of maternal LDL as a source of cholesterol for progesterone synthesis by the placenta is also well known.[216,217] However, the finding that women with homozygous familial hypercholesterolemia, bearing inactivating LDLR mutations, become pregnant and reached delivery uneventfully,[232] firmly suggests that mechanisms other than the LDLR are operative in the uptake of cholesterol from maternal lipoproteins by the placenta. At this regard, in placental explants from healthy pregnant women at delivery, it was found that HDL_2 cholesterol stimulated placental progesterone secretion to a greater extent than LDL did, by a mechanism that did not involve the LDLR.[217] Further evidence on the role of maternal HDL as an exogenous source of fetal cholesterol comes from studies in apo A-I–deficient mice. These animals have markedly reduced HDL cholesterol levels in plasma, and cholesterol accretion in the fetus was diminished, although fetal cholesterol synthesis was not affected.[233] These results were in line with previous observations by Knopp and associates,[234] describing apo A-I concentration in maternal plasma as a significant positive predictor of birth size, and also with studies in mice with varying levels of apo A-I gene dose.[235] Taken together, the results suggest that cholesterol or some other HDL component may facilitate fetal growth.

How trophoblast or yolk sac cholesterol reaches fetal circulation is another issue to be considered. In biopsy specimens from human term placentas, both apo B and microsomal triglyceride transfer protein (MTTP) mRNAs were detected, and on incubation in vitro, secretion of newly formed apo B–containing lipoproteins was demonstrated.[54] Similar findings were reported for human choriocarcinoma BeWo cells[236] and the yolk sac in rodents.[50,237] Whether these newly formed lipoproteins efficiently reach the fetal circulation is still under investigation. It is intriguing that no abnormalities of conception and embryonic lethality have been reported in humans who inherit genetic deficiencies of either of these proteins, whereas in mice bearing knockouts of either apo B[238,239] or MTTP,[240] early embryonic lethality is characteristic. This difference may reflect a greater dependence of the mouse embryo on lipoproteins from placental or yolk sac origin for development.

Another mechanism that allows the delivery of placental cholesterol to the fetus is the specific efflux to lipoproteins and acceptors already present in the fetal circulation.[176,177] Placental tissue is able to synthesize apo A1[241] and apo E,[242] but both are preferentially secreted to the maternal side, as determined in human perfused placenta.[243] Moreover, the ATP-binding cassette transporters, ABCA1 and ABCG1, known to mediate the efflux of cholesterol to apo A-I and HDL, respectively, are present in the placenta, in both the trophoblast and the endothelial cells of the fetal vessels.[244-247] Interestingly, ABCA1 is localized to the apical membrane (maternal) of the syncytiotrophoblast, while ABCG1 is predominantly expressed in the basolateral membrane.[244,248] The observation that genetic ablation of *Abca1* in mice decreased fetal weight and increased fetal death suggested a prominent role for this protein in fetal development.[244] By determining the maternal-fetal transfer of [^{14}C]-cholesterol in mice, Lindegaard and collaborators found that disruption of *Abca1* decreased cholesterol transfer by approximately 30%, whereas *Abcg1* ablation had no apparent effect.[231] In human primary trophoblast, silencing *ABCA1* decreased, while activation with LXR increased cholesterol efflux to apo A-I.[249] When the directionality of the cholesterol efflux was determined in syncytiotrophoblast monolayers from human term placentas, it was found that it occurs predominantly at the apical side and is stimulated by LXR, concluding that the apo A-I/ABCA1 pathway acts in transporting cholesterol back to the mother.[248]

A role, although smaller, of the ABCG1-mediated pathway in the cholesterol transfer to fetus cannot be ruled out. In BeWo cells grown on transwells, radiolabeled free cholesterol and LDL cholesteryl esters given to the apical side were transported to the basolateral surface of the cells and then effluxed to lipid acceptors present in the fetal side, including HDL and phospholipid vesicles but not apolipoprotein A-I.[250] Moreover, endothelial cells from human term placenta (HPEC) released cholesterol to both lipid-free apo A-I and HDL, and specific inhibition of ABCA1 or ABCG1 markedly decreased cholesterol efflux to apo A-I and HDL_3, respectively.[245] Conversely, up-regulation of ABCA1 and ABCG1 with LXR increased cholesterol efflux from HPEC to those acceptors.[247] In this final step, secretion of phospholipid transfer protein (PLTP) by the placental endothelium may cooperate in the formation of fetal HDL particles.[251]

Based on these findings, a model for maternal-fetal cholesterol transport in the placenta has been proposed.[176,177,180,252] In this model, LDLR, LRP, and SR-B1 present in the apical cell membrane of the syncytiotrophoblast are involved in the uptake of LDL and HDL cholesterol from maternal blood. Once cholesterol is internalized by endocytosis or selective or passive transfer, it incorporates to the placental cholesterol pool and is mainly used for steroid synthesis. Some cholesterol is secreted back to the mother either as nascent lipoproteins or directly to plasma apo A-I by means of ABCA1. A smaller proportion but physiologically important for the fetus, especially in early gestation, moves to the basal membrane via vesicular trafficking and sterol carriers and is delivered to the placental endothelial cells. Then, this cholesterol is effluxed to HDL, apoA-I, and/or phospholipids present in the fetal blood by the action of ABC transporters present in the luminal membrane of fetal endothelial cells.

Taken together, the available data demonstrate the ability of both the yolk sac and the placenta to synthesize and take up cholesterol from maternal lipoproteins and deliver it to the fetus. The extent to which it is exported in the different stages of pregnancy and the factors that regulate this process are not completely clarified.

SUMMARY

During gestation, both triglyceride and cholesterol increase in all lipoprotein fractions and are associated with an increase in the triglyceride-cholesterol ratio in LDL and HDL. The increase in HDL corresponds mainly to triglyceride-enriched HDL_2. The presence of lipoprotein receptors in the placenta ensures the availability of essential lipoprotein components to the fetus and provides a teleologic reason for maternal hyperlipoproteinemia.

Sustained maternal hyperlipidemia during late pregnancy is of pivotal importance in fetal development, especially during the stage of maximal fetal accretion. Besides using transferred fatty acids, the fetus also benefits from two other products of maternal lipid metabolism: glycerol and ketone bodies. Although only a small proportion of maternally derived glycerol crosses the placenta, it is quantitatively important as a substrate for maternal gluconeogenesis. Because fetal oxidative metabolism is preferentially sustained by maternal glucose crossing the placenta, the use of glycerol for glucose synthesis actively contributes to the fetal glucose supply.

In nonruminant species, maternal ketone bodies are readily transferred to the fetus, where they can be efficiently used as carbon fuels for oxidative metabolism or as lipogenic substrates. Because all of these processes are concentration dependent, they become relevant only under conditions of maternal hyperketonemia. Under healthy physiologic conditions, they constitute an important support for fetal metabolism when the availability of other substrates is more limited (e.g., during periods of maternal starvation). Under conditions of sustained maternal hyperketonemia, such as high-fat feeding, fetal metabolism also adapts to an increased consumption of ketone bodies.

Experimental studies have demonstrated the transport of maternal cholesterol to the fetus, which is especially important but not restricted to the first third of gestation. In addition, several of the potential mechanisms have been elucidated. Defects in the involved proteins may affect the cholesterol supply to the fetus in critical stages, with dramatic consequences. On the other side, stimulation of proteins involved in the placental transfer of cholesterol has been shown to increase the affluence of maternal cholesterol to the fetus in some instances, which has opened the possibility to treat fetal cholesterol biosynthesis deficiency syndromes in utero.

ACKNOWLEDGMENTS

The authors thank pp-science-editing.com for editing and linguistic revision of the manuscript. Preparation of this chapter was carried out in part with grants from the Universidad CEU—San Pablo, and the Ministerio de Economía y Competitividad (SAF2015-70747-R) of Spain. CIBEROBN is an initiative of the Instituto de Salud Carlos III (ISCIII), Spain.

 A complete reference list is available at www.expertconsult.com.

SELECT REFERENCES

3. Montelongo A, Lasuncion MA, Pallardo LF, Herrera E. Longitudinal study of plasma lipoproteins and hormones during pregnancy in normal and diabetic women. *Diabetes*. 1992;41(12):1651-1659.
5. Alvarez JJ, Montelongo A, Iglesias A, Lasuncion MA, Herrera E. Longitudinal study on lipoprotein profile, high density lipoprotein subclass, and postheparin lipases during gestation in women. *J Lipid Res*. 1996;37(2):299-308.
6. Winkler K, Wetzka B, Hoffmann MM, et al. Low density lipoprotein (LDL) subfractions during pregnancy: accumulation of buoyant LDL with advancing gestation. *J Clin Endocrinol Metab*. 2000;85(12):4543-4550.
10. Ramos P, Herrera E. Reversion of insulin resistance in the rat during late pregnancy by 72-h glucose infusion. *Am J Physiol*. 1995;269(5 Pt 1):E858-863.
13. Herrera E, Lasuncion MA, Gomez-Coronado D, Aranda P, Lopez-Luna P, Maier I. Role of lipoprotein lipase activity on lipoprotein metabolism and the fate of circulating triglycerides in pregnancy. *Am J Obstet Gynecol*. 1988;158(6 Pt 2): 1575-1583.
16. Iglesias A, Montelongo A, Herrera E, Lasuncion MA. Changes in cholesteryl ester transfer protein activity during normal gestation and postpartum. *Clinical Biochem*. 1994;27(1):63-68.
24. Herrera E. Lipid metabolism in pregnancy and its consequences in the fetus and newborn. *Endocrine*. 2002;19(1):43-55.
34. Wadsack C, Hammer A, Levak-Frank S, et al. Selective cholesteryl ester uptake from high density lipoprotein by human first trimester and term villous trophoblast cells. *Placenta*. 2003;24(2-3):131-143.
41. Varastehpour A, Radaelli T, Minium J, et al. Activation of phospholipase A2 is associated with generation of placental lipid signals and fetal obesity. *J Clin Endocrinol Metab*. 2006;91(1):248-255.
52. Terasawa Y, Cases SJ, Wong JS, et al. Apolipoprotein B-related gene expression and ultrastructural characteristics of lipoprotein secretion in mouse yolk sac during embryonic development. *J Lipid Res*. 1999;40(11):1967-1977.
54. Madsen EM, Lindegaard ML, Andersen CB, Damm P, Nielsen LB. Human placenta secretes apolipoprotein B-100-containing lipoproteins. *J Biol Chem*. 2004;279(53):55271-55276.
56. Ortega-Senovilla MH, Schaefer-Graf, U., Herrera, E. Pregnant women with gestational diabetes and with well controlled glucose levels have decreased concentrations of individual fatty acids in maternal and cord serm. *Diabetologia*. 2020;63(4):864-874.
57. Pagan A, Prieto-Sanchez MT, Blanco-Carnero JE, et al. Materno-fetal transfer of docosahexaenoic acid is impaired by gestational diabetes mellitus. *Am J Physiol Endocrinol Metab*. 2013;305(7):E826-833.
58. Herrera E. Implications of dietary fatty acids during pregnancy on placental, fetal and postnatal development-a review. *Placenta*. 2002;23(suppl A). S9-19.
66. Palacin M, Lasuncion MA, Asuncion M, Herrera E. Circulating metabolite utilization by periuterine adipose tissue in situ in the pregnant rat. *Metabolism*. 1991;40(5):534-539.
72. Argiles J, Herrera E. Appearance of circulating and tissue 14C-lipids after oral 14C-tripalmitate administration in the late pregnant rat. *Metabolism*. 1989;38(2):104-108.
77. Ramirez I, Llobera M, Herrera E. Circulating triacylglycerols, lipoproteins, and tissue lipoprotein lipase activities in rat mothers and offspring during the perinatal period: effect of postmaturity. *Metabolism*. 1983;32(4):333-341.
78. Carrascosa JM, Ramos P, Molero JC, Herrera E. Changes in the kinase activity of the insulin receptor account for an increased insulin sensitivity of mammary gland in late pregnancy. *Endocrinology*. 1998;139(2):520-526.
98. Campbell FM, Dutta-Roy AK. Plasma membrane fatty acid-binding protein (FABPpm) is exclusively located in the maternal facing membranes of the human placenta. *FEBS letters*. 1995;375(3):227-230.
99. Haggarty P. Fatty acid supply to the human fetus. *Annu Rev Nutr*. 2010;30:237-255.
110. Uauy R, Mena P, Wegher B, Nieto S, Salem Jr N. Long chain polyunsaturated fatty acid formation in neonates: effect of gestational age and intrauterine growth. *Pediat Res*. 2000;47(1):127-135.
118. Lasuncion MA, Lorenzo J, Palacin M, Herrera E. Maternal factors modulating nutrient transfer to fetus. *Biol Neonate*. 1987;51(2):86-93.
125. Mampel T, Villarroya F, Herrera E. Hepatectomy-nephrectomy effects in the pregnant rat and fetus. *Biochem Biophys Res Commun*. 1985;131(3):1219-1225.
131. Herrera E, Ortega-Senovilla H. Implications of lipids in neonatal body weight and fat mass in gestational diabetic mothers and non-diabetic controls. *Curr Diab Rep*. 2018;18(2):7.
137. Shambaugh GEI, Metzger BE, Radosevich JA. Nutrient metabolism and fetal brain development. In: Herrera E, Knopp RH, eds. *Perinatal Biochemistry*. Boca Raton: CRC Press; 1992:213-231.
153. Brown MS, Goldstein JL. The SREBP pathway: regulation of cholesterol metabolism by proteolysis of a membrane-bound transcription factor. *Cell*. 1997;89(3):331-340.
156. Lasuncion MA, Martin-Sanchez C, Canfran-Duque A, Busto R. Post-lanosterol biosynthesis of cholesterol and cancer. *Curr Opin Pharmacol*. 2012;12(6):717-723.
157. Martinez-Botas J, Suarez Y, Ferruelo AJ, Gomez-Coronado D, Lasuncion MA. Cholesterol starvation decreases p34(cdc2) kinase activity and arrests the cell cycle at G2. *FASEB J*. 1999;13(11):1359-1370.
160. Roux C, Wolf C, Mulliez N, et al. Role of cholesterol in embryonic development. *Am J Clin Nutr*. 2000;71(suppl 5):1270S-1279S.
161. Mann RK, Beachy PA. Cholesterol modification of proteins. *Biochim Biophys Acta*. 2000;1529(1-3):188-202.
163. Moebius FF, Fitzky BU, Glossmann H. Genetic defects in postsqualene cholesterol biosynthesis. *Trends Endocrinol Metab*. 2000;11(3):106-114.
171. Porter FD, Herman GE. Malformation syndromes caused by disorders of cholesterol synthesis. *J Lipid Res*. 2011;52(1):6-34.
173. Kanungo S, Soares N, He M, Steiner RD. Sterol metabolism disorders and neurodevelopment-an update. *Dev Disabil Res Rev*. 2013;17(3):197-210.
176. Palinski W. Maternal-fetal cholesterol transport in the placenta: good, bad, and target for modulation. *Circ Res*. 2009;104(5):569-571.
177. Woollett LA. Review: transport of maternal cholesterol to the fetal circulation. *Placenta*. 2011;32(suppl 2):S218-221.
190. Woollett LA. Origin of cholesterol in the fetal golden Syrian hamster: contribution of de novo sterol synthesis and maternal-derived lipoprotein cholesterol. *J Lipid Res*. 1996;37(6):1246-1257.
191. Jurevics HA, Kidwai FZ, Morell P. Sources of cholesterol during development of the rat fetus and fetal organs. *J Lipid Res*. 1997;38(4):723-733.
196. Munilla MA, Herrera E. A cholesterol-rich diet causes a greater hypercholesterolemic response in pregnant than in nonpregnant rats and does not modify fetal lipoprotein profile. *J Nutr*. 1997;127(11):2239-2245.
200. Yoshida S, Wada Y. Transfer of maternal cholesterol to embryo and fetus in pregnant mice. *J Lipid Res*. 2005;46(10):2168-2174.
201. Tint GS, Yu H, Shang Q, Xu G, Patel SB. The use of the Dhcr7 knockout mouse to accurately determine the origin of fetal sterols. *J Lipid Res*. 2006;47(7):1535-1541.
216. Winkel CA, MacDonald PC, Simpson ER. The role of receptor-mediated low-density lipoprotein uptake and degradation in the regulation of progesterone biosynthesis and cholesterol metabolism by human trophoblasts. *Placenta Suppl*. 1981;3:133-143.
217. Lasuncion MA, Bonet B, Knopp RH. Mechanism of the HDL2 stimulation of progesterone secretion in cultured placental trophoblast. *J Lipid Res*. 1991;32(7):1073-1087.
231. Lindegaard ML, Wassif CA, Vaisman B, et al. Characterization of placental cholesterol transport: ABCA1 is a potential target for in utero therapy of Smith-Lemli-Opitz syndrome. *Hum Mol Genet*. 2008;17(23):3806-3813.
248. Kallol S, Huang X, Muller S, Ontsouka CE, Albrecht C. Novel insights into concepts and directionality of maternal(-)fetal cholesterol transfer across the human placenta. *Int J Mol Sci*. 2018;19(8):2334.
250. Schmid KE, Davidson WS, Myatt L, Woollett LA. Transport of cholesterol across a BeWo cell monolayer: implications for net transport of sterol from maternal to fetal circulation. *J Lipid Res*. 2003;44(10):1909-1918.

Brown Adipose Tissue: Development and Function

32

Jan Nedergaard | Barbara Cannon

INTRODUCTION

Mammals such as humans are exposed to their greatest temperature-related shock at birth. Coming from a protected and thermoneutral environment, the newborn infant is suddenly exposed to "cool" surroundings, where survival depends on self-generation of sufficient heat to keep warm. The development of the ability to regulate body temperature regardless of the temperature of the surroundings (and through this to ensure that activity of the organism is constant and high) apparently was a necessary step in the evolution of so-called *higher animals*. A requirement for this development was that newborns be endowed with a physiologic ability to produce the heat essential for survival. To accomplish this, an organ was developed without parallel in ectothermic animals, an organ endowed with the function of producing heat exactly when required, not least around the time of birth. This organ is brown adipose tissue.

Thus, in evolutionary terms, brown adipose tissue is a rather new organ. Even in the scientific community, brown adipose tissue is rather new. Its function as a heat producer in the cold[1] and in newborns[2,3] was first described only 60 years ago. However, during subsequent years, understanding has grown about the events responsible for the heat production in that tissue,[4-10] and at present, researchers are actively elucidating mechanisms underlying the recruitment processes in brown adipose tissue (i.e., those processes that, during perinatal development, are responsible for the growth and differentiation of the tissue).

One of the most important accomplishments in research on brown adipose tissue thermogenesis has been the recognition that the ability to produce heat resides in the fact that brown adipose tissue mitochondria are endowed with a unique protein—the original uncoupling protein-1 (UCP1), also known as *thermogenin*. This protein functions as a regulated protonophore through the mitochondrial membrane. The identification of this protein consolidated, in many ways, research on brown adipose tissue. Thus, a description of the function and fate of this protein must be a central issue in a review on the perinatal recruitment of brown adipose tissue.

DEVELOPMENT OF BROWN ADIPOSE TISSUE IN HUMAN INFANTS AND OTHER NEWBORNS

BROWN ADIPOSE TISSUE IN ADULT HUMANS

Although it was earlier accepted that brown adipose tissue was found only in young mammals, it has been convincingly demonstrated (reviewed by Nedergaard and colleagues[11]) that brown adipose tissue is indeed present in most adults, where it has a thermogenic function and is regulated just as in experimental animals. These realizations came from investigations using positron emission tomography (PET) with ^{18}F-fluorodeoxyglucose (FDG) as the radioactive tracer. Extensive uptake of FDG occurred occasionally in some fatty depots. It became apparent that if patients were feeling cold at the time of the examination, then areas in the neck and supraclavicular area took up significant amounts of tracer. Retrospective studies from hospital archives showed random occurrence of uptake in these depots as the environmental conditions were not controlled. More recent studies have used healthy subjects under controlled conditions and show correlations between FDG uptake in brown adipose tissue and nonshivering thermogenic capacity,[12] with chronic environmental temperature,[13,14] with degree of obesity,[15] and inversely with aging.[16] While this method provides significant information, it is inappropriate to use frequently in healthy subjects. The only other available methods to determine the presence of brown adipose tissue (but not its acute activity) are invasive and therefore also inappropriate for extensive studies. Magnetic resonance imaging and infrared thermography techniques are now being evaluated and will hopefully provide more suitable means of study in the near future.

BROWN ADIPOSE TISSUE IN NEONATAL AND YOUNG HUMANS

Retrospective analyses of PET scans of young children have also been performed from hospital archive material. However, although such investigations can provide some information on tissue abundance,[17,18] they have obviously not been performed under optimal conditions for brown adipose tissue detection, so there is a large information deficit here. There are reports suggesting certain levels of abundance in children, but these are unable to give reliable information, since the environmental temperature has not been suitable for optimizing the visibility of brown adipose tissue. Thus, these give only minimal levels and should not be viewed otherwise. The ethical aspects of using PET to study children preclude attaining further information until a reliable alternative method becomes available.

PERINATAL BROWN ADIPOSE TISSUE FUNCTION

Experiments describing the function of brown adipose tissue in the perinatal animal have generally been performed in rat fetuses and rat pups, and if not specifically stated, the animal referred to here is the rat.

Significant differences in perinatal development of brown fat (and many other characteristics) have been documented among newborns of different species.[19-23] Broadly speaking, three different groups of newborns can be distinguished: altricial newborns, so-called true immature newborns, and precocial newborns.[19]

The *altricial* (literally, nest-dependent) newborns are often born as members of litters of more than five pups. They are poorly developed at birth, have no fur, are blind, and move poorly, if at all. To keep warm, they huddle together. As discussed later on, development of brown adipose tissue in these newborns is a slow process that starts just before birth and reaches its maximum some days after birth. The main driving force for this recruitment is probably the (comparatively) low environmental temperature coupled with the attempt by these newborns to activate processes to oppose hypothermia. Rat and mouse pups belong to this group. The morphologic and ultrastructural development of the tissue in these animals has been described.[24-29]

The *immature* (not to be confused with premature) *neonate* is not able to respond to the environmental temperature at birth and is truly poikilothermic. In species with immature newborns, the recruitment process in brown adipose tissue starts only when the central control system has developed, after which processes occur that seem similar to those elicited immediately after birth in the altricial newborns. Hamster pups[30] and possibly the newborns of marsupials[31,32] belong to this group. (However, it is unlikely that marsupials at any stage of development have thermogenically active brown adipose tissue, despite the presence of a UCP1 ortholog.)[33]

The *precocial* newborns are normally born singly or in small litters. They are very well developed, their eyes are open, they are furred, and they can walk around shortly after birth. These newborns are born with well-developed brown adipose tissue, which tends to atrophy postnatally. It is unknown how this intrauterine recruitment of brown adipose tissue is accomplished. Certain small newborns, such as the guinea pig,[34] belong to this group, but more obvious members are the newborns of many larger species, such as lambs,[35-37] goats,[38] calves,[39,40] and musk oxen.[41]

Classification of the human infant (or other primate infants[42]) into one or the other of these groups is not self-evident. Although born in a somewhat developed state, the human infant has several traits of immaturity and probably is most akin to the altricial newborns—specifically, human perinatal brown adipose tissue development has similarities to that found in the newborn rat pup.

HOW MANY ADIPOSE TISSUES EXIST?

Experiments concerning the function of most body organs are helped from a practical standpoint by the fact that most organs are anatomically well-defined entities with a single localization in the body and with structurally homogeneous and stable cells. Unfortunately, such characteristics do not pertain to brown adipose tissue.

Brown adipose tissue is found in many depots within the body; six major depots have been identified in the human infant and constitute 90% of the total brown fat. These include the perirenal depots, interscapular and cervical depots, and periaortic depots. The remaining 10% is found in seven other sites.[43,44]

Distinguishing between white and brown fat is not straightforward. When activated, brown adipose tissue can be distinguished from white by its ability to express UCP1. However, because the potential ability to express UCP1 in a given cell (in a given physiologic situation) may not have been invoked at the moment of study, it is likely that each anatomically defined depot contains cells that are genuinely "white," as well as cells that are only visually disguised as white but that still carry the potential to be brown-like. Leptin is well expressed in white adipose tissue, but it is not expressed in recruited (i.e., activated) brown adipose tissue.[45] However, it is expressed in nonactive brown adipose tissue, and its expression in both adipose tissues is inhibited by sympathetic stimulation.[46]

Morphologically, even epididymal white adipose tissue can be altered by an intense cold stress to visually resemble brown adipose tissue and to have brown fat-like mitochondria.[47,48] However, not even under these extreme circumstances was it originally possible to detect UCP1 as a protein immunologically.[48] More recently, the use of quantitative polymerase chain reaction has allowed the detection of UCP1 messenger RNA (mRNA) in epididymal fat depots,[49] although its functional significance is unclear and thermogenically limited. Thus, within this depot, apparently mainly "true" white fat cells are present, with few potentially brown-like precursors. By contrast, in the parallel female tissue, the parametrial fat pad, good evidence has emerged for the presence of genuine brown-like fat cells (i.e., those containing UCP1).[50]

In certain species, the subcutaneous adipose tissue (which is generally believed to have storage and insulatory properties) can be or become brown-like. As indicated by a functional analysis of the mitochondria in the subcutaneous adipose tissue of newborn seals[51] and in dog pups treated with sympathomimetics,[52] the presence of UCP1 in subcutaneous tissue can be readily discerned.[53] In these species, the subcutaneous adipose tissue could even work as an "electric blanket." Even in mouse strains where UCP1 is fairly well expressed in inguinal adipose depots, the total thermogenic capacity is nonetheless only a fraction of that in the total brown depots.[54] Thus, although certain fat depots apparently lack a significant capacity for conversion to brown-like fat, most depots have this potential to some degree, and UCP1 may be expressed under certain physiologic or pharmacologic circumstances.

As a general rule, more visible brown adipose tissue depots are present in the newborn than in the adult, even the cold-acclimated adult. It has been stated that in some newborn species, all adipose tissue is brown, and these depots are converted to white adipose tissue in the adult. However, in cell biologic terms, the meaning of this statement is vague.[55] It is now clear that the adipocytes in certain classic brown depots have a close lineage relation with a skeletal muscle lineage.[56-59] However, the brown-like depots, also termed beige or brite (brown-like in white), may or may not be muscle-related depending on localization.[60] Some brown-like depots are related to smooth muscle.[61] Certainly, the behavior of certain depots that look white in the adult is functionally close to that of brown adipose tissue in the newborn, and the fat in these depots retains some potential to again become brown-like.[62]

UCP1 AND THERMOGENESIS

Heat production may result from shivering or nonshivering thermogenesis. In the newborn infant and in the adult animal, the first resource used for extra heat production is nonshivering thermogenesis. Only after this capacity is used does shivering begin. In an adult living in a warm environment, with little active brown adipose tissue, shivering is initially the dominant source of extra heat production. However, in the infant, the ability to shiver sufficiently to produce substantial amounts of heat does not seem to be fully developed, so brown adipose tissue is the sole source of heat production.

Most heat produced during nonshivering thermogenesis results directly from the activity in brown adipose tissue of the unique mitochondrial UCP1 (i.e., thermogenin); in the absence of this protein, no heat is produced in brown fat cells.[63,64] Heat production is governed by signals from the hypothalamus. These signals are relayed through the sympathetic nervous system and transmitted to the cell as a norepinephrine stimulus leading to a series of events within the cell (for an overview, Fig. 32.1). Sympathetic innervation to the tissue is dense. One system of fibers, which contains co-stored neuropeptide Y, innervates the numerous blood vessels entering the tissue, and another system innervates the adipocytes.[65] The neuropeptides calcitonin gene-related peptide (CGRP) and substance P also are found in the tissue, the latter in afferent nerves; however, the localization of CGRP is currently not completely understood, and the functions of these neuropeptides are unknown.[66]

UCP1, THERMOGENIN

Considerable research by several groups of investigators led to the identification of UCP1 as the key enzyme in nonshivering heat production. UCP1, discussed earlier as thermogenin or as the nucleotide-binding protein, the 32-kDa protein of brown fat, or the guanosine diphosphate (GDP)-binding protein, has also been referred to as the proton conductance pathway of brown adipose tissue mitochondria. Much is known today about this protein (Fig. 32.2A). It has been sequenced both as a protein and from complementary DNA (cDNA) clones corresponding to

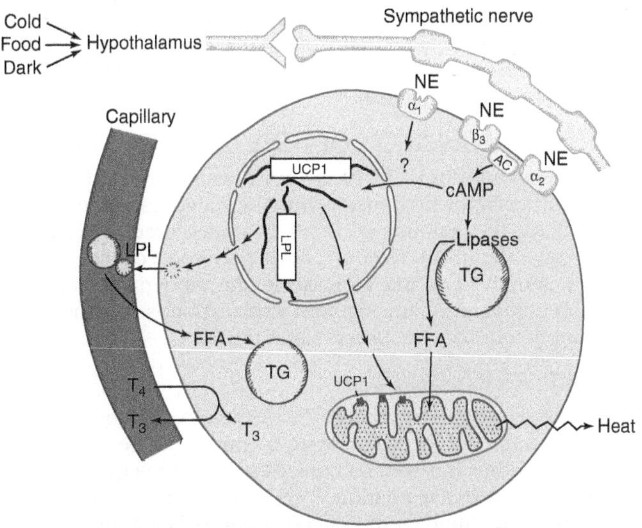

Fig. 32.1 Function of the brown fat cell: an overview. When postnatal cold is perceived, the sympathetic nervous system is activated. Norepinephrine *(NE)* released interacts with adrenergic receptors, leading to release of fatty acids, which undergo combustion in the mitochondria. This combustion is possible as a result of the presence of uncoupling protein-1 *(UCP1)*. Further substrate is provided by the action of lipoprotein lipase *(LPL)*. Brown adipose tissue also may produce triiodothyronine *(T_3)* from thyroxine *(T_4)*, leading to local and systemic effects. Dietary factors and darkness also activate centers in the hypothalamus in a manner analogous to that of norepinephrine. *AC,* Adenylyl cyclase; *cAMP,* cyclic adenosine monophosphate; *FFAs,* free fatty acids; *HSL,* hormone-sensitive lipase; *TG,* triglycerides.

the UCP1 mRNA. The amino acid sequence is known for many species of mammals.[67-70] The amino acid sequence of the human protein is 79% homologous to that of the rat protein, allowing considerable immunologic cross-reactivity between human UCP1 and rodent UCP1.[71] The human *UCP1* gene has also been isolated[72,73] and its organization analyzed.

UCP1 is a member of the superfamily of mitochondrial carrier proteins (see Fig. 32.2B).[74-76] Most closely related to UCP1 are two more recently identified but evolutionarily more ancient proteins known as UCP2 and UCP3 because of their extensive homology with UCP1.[77] The functions of these proteins remain unclear. However, they are not responsible for any thermoregulatory thermogenesis.[64] Other proteins (e.g., UCP4, UCP5) are not closely related to UCP1; therefore functional relationships cannot be expected.

From analysis of the amino acid sequence, it has been proposed that UCP1 may constitute three membrane-spanning Us (see Fig. 32.2A). When functionally inserted into the brown fat mitochondrial inner membrane, UCP1 endows these mitochondria with a series of unique properties, including a high rate of respiration in the absence of adenosine diphosphate or uncoupler addition, a high proton conductivity, and a high Cl^- conductivity.

THE *UCP1* GENE

The *UCP1* gene is found on chromosome 8 in mice[78] and on chromosome 4 in humans.[79] Only one copy of the gene is present.[72]

An interesting functional and evolutionary connection between the exon-intron pattern of the *UCP1* gene and the suggested transmembrane structure of the protein has been described. Each of the six proposed membrane-spanning segments is represented by one exon.[70,79,80] This pattern is also found in the other *UCP* genes.

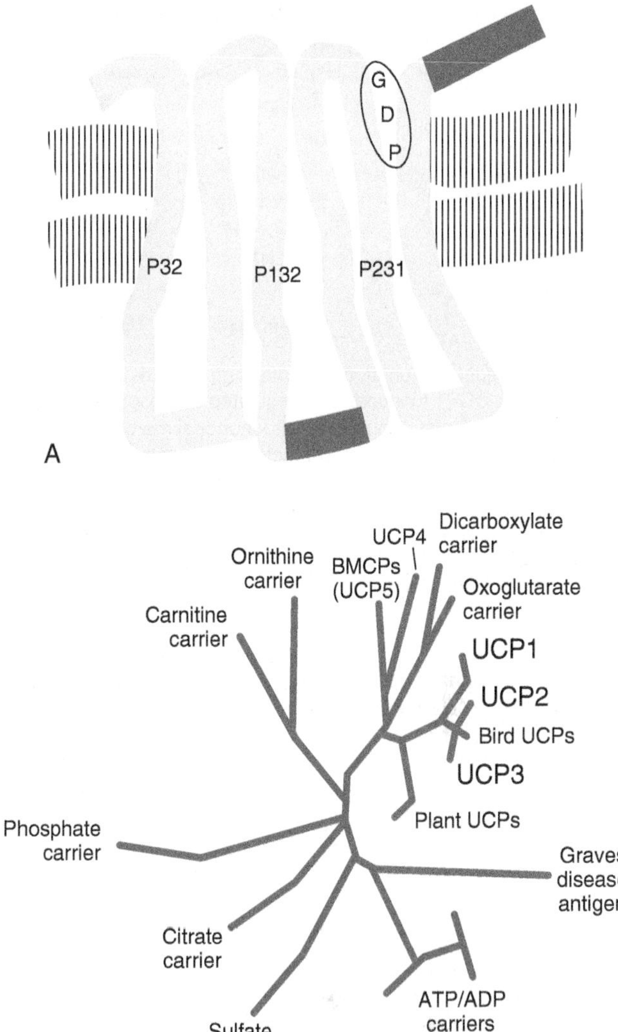

Fig. 32.2 (A) Suggested structure of uncoupling protein-1 *(UCP1)*. The tripartite transmembrane structure is common to members of the mitochondrial carrier protein superfamily. P32, P132, and P231 indicate proline residues conserved among all family members, and GDP denotes the general area in which nucleotide binding occurs. (B) Rootless dendrogram showing similarity between members of the mitochondrial carrier protein superfamily. *ADP,* Adenosine diphosphate; *ATP,* adenosine triphosphate; *BMCPs,* brain mitochondrial carrier proteins; *GDP,* guanosine diphosphate. (A, Modified from Nedergaard J, Golozoubova V, Matthias A, et al. UCP1: the only protein able to mediate adaptive non-shivering thermogenesis and metabolic inefficiency. *Biochim Biophys Acta.* 2001;1504:82. B, From Borecký J, Maia IG, Arruda P. Mitochondrial uncoupling proteins in mammals and plants. *Biosci Rep.* 2001;21:201.)

ACUTE REGULATION OF UCP1 ACTIVITY

The function of UCP1 in the mitochondrial membrane is depicted in simplified form in Fig. 32.3. UCP1 acts as the equivalent of a proton translocator, allowing dissipation of the proton gradient that has arisen from the functioning of the respiratory chain.

UCP1 cannot be constantly active, because such activity would lead to constant high heat production in the tissue, irrespective of the environmental (or ambient) temperature. In experiments with isolated mitochondria, it has been observed that the activity of UCP1 can be inhibited by the addition of purine nucleotides.[81,82] Traditionally, GDP has been the nucleotide of choice for such experiments, and thus UCP1 has been known

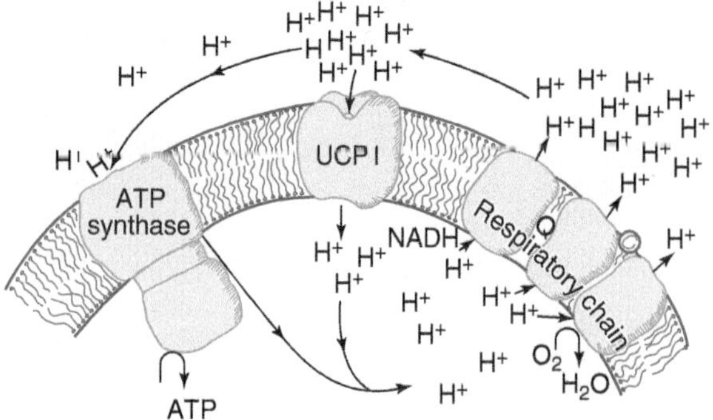

Fig. 32.3 Suggested function of uncoupling protein-1 *(UCP1)* in the brown fat cell. UCP1 functions as a regulated translocator of protons (or proton equivalents) through the mitochondrial membrane, thereby allowing dissipation of the proton gradient built up by the respiratory chain, as a consequence of the oxidation of substrate, such as nicotinamide adenine dinucleotide. Thus respiration can proceed unlimited by the turnover of adenosine triphosphate *(ATP)*. (Based on descriptions in Nicholls DG. The bioenergetics of brown adipose tissue mitochondria. *FEBS Lett.* 1976;61:103.)

as the *GDP-binding protein*. This protein is not related to the G-proteins in signal transduction or to the ribosomal guanosine triphosphate (GTP)-binding proteins. The term may be considered to be physiologically misleading, because adenosine triphosphate (ATP) is as good as or better than GDP for both binding and inhibiting respiration.[83,84] Because ATP is present in much higher concentrations in the cytosol of brown fat cells than is GDP,[85] ATP is the physiologically relevant nucleotide that binds to UCP1 and inhibits thermogenesis when thermogenesis is not physiologically required.

The affinity of UCP1 for ATP is so high that the binding site would probably always be saturated with ATP and thermogenesis inhibited if this were the only agent that interacted with UCP1. Thus, it is necessary to postulate the existence of a physiologic activator of UCP1.[82] The nature of this "positive" modulator continues to be investigated. A detailed analysis of the problem is outside the scope of this chapter, but a few main points can be summarized here.

Among the many suggestions, the simplest hypothesis for the nature of this modulator is that it is produced during the release of fatty acids, occurring as an effect of stimulation of the cell. Within this framework, several alternatives have been proposed. The positive modulator could be the free fatty acids themselves.[82,86,87] The most telling experiments that indicate a direct effect of free fatty acids are those of Rial and colleagues.[88] More recent experiments support this theory.[89,90] Alternatively, fatty acids have been suggested to have a catalytic function, although in this case a positive modulator may be involved.[91,92] Another hypothesis along the same line has suggested that palmitoyl-coenzyme A (CoA) may interact directly with UCP1.[93,94] Each postulate has advantages and problems. Although conclusive experiments have been published that the modulator is downstream of lipolysis, general agreement on the mechanism has not yet been reached.

POSSIBLE SEMI-ACUTE REGULATION OF UCP1 ACTIVITY

Under certain conditions, apparently no direct correlation has been established between the amount of UCP1 (e.g., as measured immunologically) and the activity of UCP1 (as estimated by GDP binding or proton or Cl^- translocation). When the level of activity is found to be lower than expected, the phenomenon has been termed *masking* of UCP1.[95] UCP1 is thus typically masked when it is inactive (as is probably the case in utero) but becomes *unmasked* when called into function. Accordingly, it is reasonable to speculate that the rapid increase in GDP-binding capacity seen shortly after birth in guinea pigs[34] may be due to this unmasking mechanism.[96]

ADAPTIVE REGULATION OF UCP1 AMOUNT

The total amount of UCP1 in the newborn is expected to be the rate-limiting factor for nonshivering thermogenesis. In newborns and adults, the amount of UCP1 is under precise regulation. Although a significant temporal delay between a change in UCP1 mRNA and the ensuing increase in the amount of UCP1 has been documented,[97] the simplest explanation is that the mRNA amount determines the protein amount.

RECEPTORS INVOLVED

The major stimulus for *UCP1* gene expression is from the sympathetic nervous system through the release of norepinephrine. It is well recognized that β-adrenergic receptors are involved in this regulation.[98-100] Furthermore, some evidence indicates that simultaneous α-stimulation is necessary in vivo.[99] Perhaps this α-stimulation is of a permissive nature.

PERINATAL UCP1 EXPRESSION

ALTRICIAL SPECIES

The amount of UCP1 increases around the time of birth (in mice and rats).[11,28] This increase is caused by a concomitant increase in the amount of UCP1 mRNA (Fig. 32.4A and B).[100-103] The cause of the postnatal recruitment in brown adipose tissue (and increase in UCP1 mRNA) could be either ontogenic or an effect of the cold stress experienced by the pups at birth.[19] No postnatal increase in UCP1 mRNA occurs in the absence of a postnatal cold stress (see Fig. 32.4C); therefore, in these species, the postnatal brown adipose tissue recruitment is presumably a response to the cold stress experienced by the newborn.[102] This correlation indicates that the increase is mediated by sympathetic activation, as in adults.

IMMATURE NEWBORN SPECIES

In immature-type newborns, the increase in UCP1 occurs rather late.[30,31] It is conjectured that when the ability to react to environmental cues has developed in these animals, the recruitment of brown adipose tissue takes place in the same way as described previously for altricial species.

PRECOCIAL NEWBORN SPECIES

In species with precocial newborns, UCP1 is expressed in the fetal state.[34,39,104] Because fetal production of excessive heat would be potentially lethal, it follows that a uterine inhibitor of thermogenesis must exist, which still allows transmission of the signal for gene expression to occur but inhibits a thermogenic response. Without such an inhibitor, the activation signal would presumably trigger fetal heat production in utero. In experiments in which the umbilical cord has been sectioned, some indications for the existence of such an inhibitor have been observed.[105-108]

The central signal that leads to sympathetic stimulation of the tissue in utero is unknown. It cannot be a cold stimulus and could hardly be a food stimulus. The only other documented pathway for sympathetic stimulation of brown fat recruitment is through short day length,[109] probably mediated by the pineal gland and melatonin. It could be argued that the fetus lives its life in darkness, and that newborns are more sensitive to the day's elapsed length.[110] Whether such a mechanism could function in precocial species is doubtful, and most available data indicate that it is merely the dam's level of melatonin that is reflected in the fetal blood level.

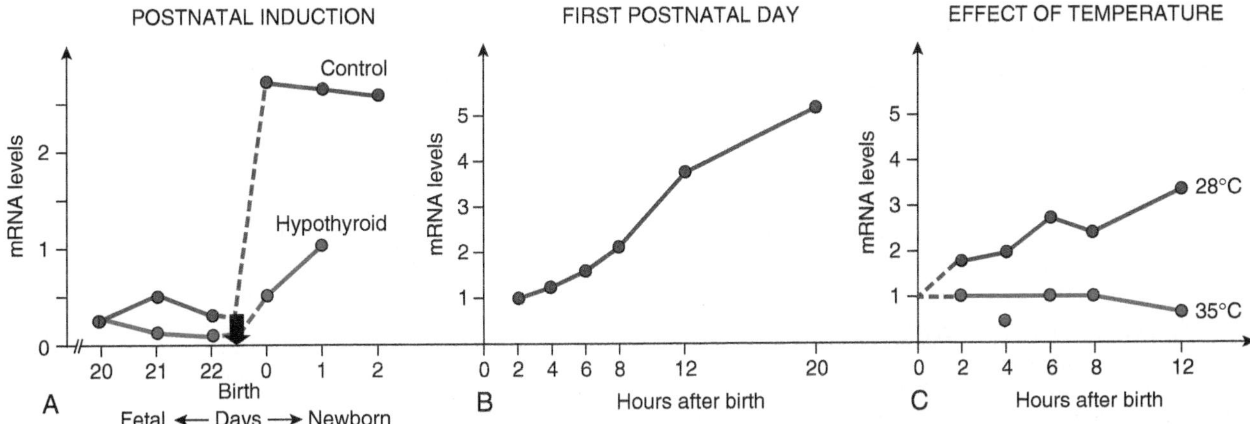

Fig. 32.4 Postnatal increase in uncoupling protein-1 (UCP1) messenger RNA *(mRNA)*. (A) Prenatal to postnatal transition; note the effect of hypothyroidism. (B) Time resolution of the first postnatal day. Pups remained with their dams. (C) Effect of temperature on the postnatal increase in UCP1 mRNA. Pups were exposed individually to the indicated environmental temperatures. (Modified from Obregón MJ, Jacobsson A, Kirchgessner T, et al. Postnatal recruitment of brown adipose tissue is induced by the cold stress experienced by the pups: an analysis of mRNA levels for thermogenin and lipoprotein lipase. *Biochem J.* 1989;259:341.)

Alternatively, another mechanism of recruitment, independent of sympathetic stimulation, may be postulated: specifically, it is possible that activators of peroxisome proliferator-activated receptor (PPAR)-γ are formed and stimulate UCP1 expression without concomitant thermogenesis.[111]

THE HUMAN NEWBORN

Because the classification of the human newborn as precocial or altricial is not fully clear, it is not evident which animal neonate is the best experimental model applicable to the human infant. Human brown adipose tissue is not only present in considerable quantities at term gestation but also demonstrates a postnatal increase.[112] The amount of UCP1 is high in children, and it can be found in adults.[11,113-116]

SUBSTRATES FOR THERMOGENESIS

INTRACELLULARLY DERIVED FATTY ACIDS

During the initial acute phase of thermogenesis, the supply of fatty acids for combustion comes from triglyceride droplets found within the tissue. The release of fatty acids for combustion is caused by a series of events similar to those known to occur in white fat cells, leading to a release of fatty acids in the circulation. Thus, stimulation of β-receptors leads to an increase in intracellular levels of cyclic adenosine monophosphate (cAMP),[117] which results in activation of the cAMP-dependent protein kinase (see Fig. 32.1). Both of these events can be observed during postnatal development: cAMP is elevated in brown adipose tissue,[118,119] and the activity ratio of cAMP-dependent protein kinase increases from 0.3 in fetal tissue to 0.7 after birth.[120]

DIFFERENT ADRENERGIC RECEPTORS

A β-adrenergic receptor is the adrenergic receptor type involved in the increase in cAMP in fully differentiated brown adipocytes. In rodents, it is the β_3-receptor that is predominantly involved, but the situation in human brown fat is less clearly understood.[121-126] The effects of β-receptor activation on cAMP levels may be counteracted by α_2-adrenergic receptors, which are also found in brown adipose tissue of fetuses and newborns.[127-129] Adenosine, acting through A1 receptors, may also counteract β-stimulation.[130] However, it has been proposed that it could activate brown adipose tissue through A2A receptors.[131]

Brown fat cells also are endowed with α_1-adrenergic receptors.[132] Although some of their intracellular actions are known,[133-135] their significance for thermogenesis is not fully understood. During in vitro experiments, only a small fraction of thermogenesis resulting from adrenergic stimulation can be demonstrated to result from stimulation of α_1-adrenergic processes. Nonetheless, a large fraction of nonshivering thermogenesis can be inhibited in vivo by α_1-blockade[136] in the newborn rabbit. This effect may be secondary to cardiovascular phenomena. In isolated cells, α_1-adrenergic stimulation may enhance the effectiveness of cAMP.[137]

PROTEIN KINASE A AND ACTIVATION OF TRIGLYCERIDE LIPOLYSIS

One substrate for the activated cAMP-dependent protein kinase is perilipin, found around lipid droplets in the tissue. It is heavily phosphorylated by protein kinase A, which presumably allows the cofactor CGI-58 to gain access to and activate the main adipose triglyceride lipase (ATGL).[138] Subsequently, the diglycerides formed are degraded by hormone-sensitive lipase, which is also phosphorylated by protein kinase A.[139] The fatty acids released probably undergo immediate combustion in the mitochondria, whereas glycerol probably is released to the circulation. The decrease in triglyceride droplet size after birth can be seen on electron micrographs.[26]

Whether a physiologically significant release of fatty acids from brown adipose tissue into the circulation occurs is still unconfirmed. It was originally suggested that brown fat (unlike white fat) did not release any fatty acids to the circulation,[140] but isolated brown fat cells break down more triglycerides to fatty acids than can be subject to combustion within the cells and release fatty acids in vitro.[141] Investigations of the effluent blood from brown adipose tissue have yielded somewhat variable results,[142,143] but a capacity for export is likely.

Also unknown is whether increases in plasma levels of fatty acids found in cold-stressed animals may be due to an increased release from brown fat and thus reflect the activity of this tissue. Tissue ablation experiments have indicated that this may be the case,[144] especially in newborns in whom a large fraction of the adipose tissue found is in the form of brown adipose tissue.

FATTY ACIDS FROM THE CIRCULATION

The brown fat cell is endowed with a store of triglycerides that can be used in any situation in which thermogenesis is required. However, this store is limited; in newborn rabbits, the amount of stored triglycerides is sufficient for only 3 days of heat production. After this time, unfed rabbits die as a result of hypothermia.[145] Similar observations can be made in premature human infants.[146] To ensure a constant supply of substrate for combustion, additional substrate must be supplied by the circulation. Only under conditions of starvation before cold stress has it been reported that the uptake of circulating free fatty acids is significant.[147] The quantitatively most important source of lipid substrate is that found in chylomicrons, which are formed from ingested food. Fatty acids in chylomicron triglycerides are released to the brown fat cells by the enzyme lipoprotein lipase. Circulating very low-density lipoproteins are also a substrate for lipoprotein lipase.

REGULATION OF LIPOPROTEIN LIPASE

In contrast to the situation in white adipose tissue, brown adipose tissue lipoprotein lipase activity is increased by adrenergic stimulation.[148,149] (In this respect, the tissue is similar to that of the heart.) This stimulation is mediated by β-adrenergic receptors, resulting in an increase in cAMP and an ensuing increase in the expression of the gene for lipoprotein lipase.[149-152] This is a comparatively slow process, requiring several hours to reach full effect, because the lipase must be synthesized and transported to the capillaries. Thus, the tissue cannot rely on this process to generate an acute thermogenic response.

Insulin can also stimulate lipoprotein lipase activity.[153-155] This insulin stimulation does not seem to be mediated through central effects and the sympathetic nervous system; instead, it seems to be a direct effect of insulin on tissue in states of proper nutrition. Insulin stimulation is also mediated through an increased expression of the lipoprotein lipase gene.[151,152]

PERINATAL RECRUITMENT OF LIPOPROTEIN LIPASE

Lipoprotein lipase activity is low in the fetus but increases postnatally (Fig. 32.5A).[156] This postnatal increase also can be seen in premature pups. It is not known whether the increased activity is an effect of suckling, temperature change, or release of an inhibitor transferred through the umbilical cord.

When this "birth-induced" increase in activity is evaluated in the context of measurements of lipoprotein lipase mRNA, an enigma arises (see Fig. 32.5B). Lipoprotein lipase mRNA is not increased (possibly owing to an inhibitory factor in the colostrum).[157] To explain the discrepancy between lipoprotein lipase mRNA level and lipoprotein lipase activity, a transfer of lipoprotein lipase across gut membranes has been suggested.[102] This hypothesis requires further investigation. However, under conditions of mild cold stress in the absence of the dam, lipoprotein lipase mRNA levels within brown adipose tissue increase, apparently through processes similar to those described in the adult (see Fig. 32.5C).

One effect of this postnatal activation of lipoprotein lipase on the fatty acid composition of tissue triglycerides is that fatty acids become more unsaturated and, in this respect, reflect the composition of the diet (i.e., the mother's milk).[158-160]

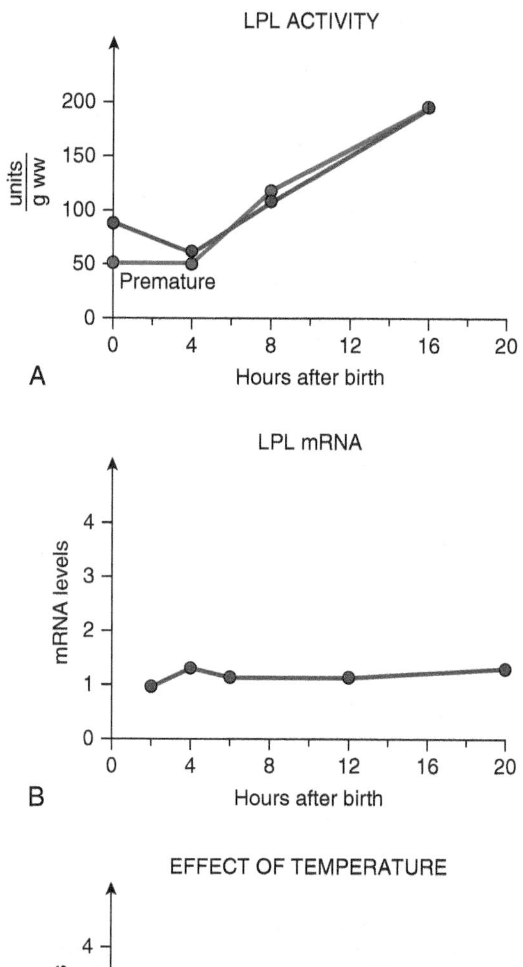

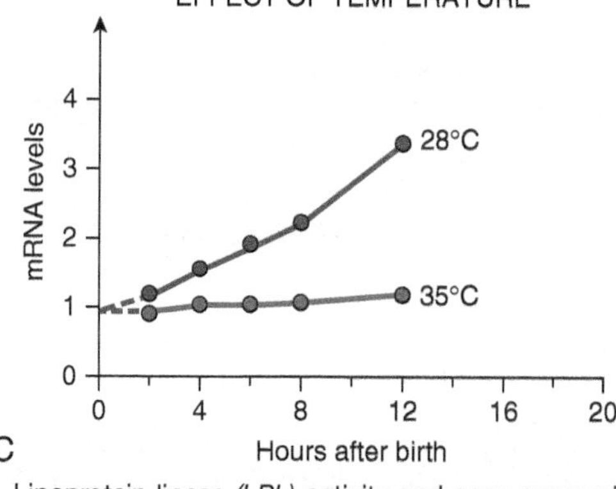

Fig. 32.5 Lipoprotein lipase *(LPL)* activity and gene expression. (A) LPL activity in newborns staying with their dams. (B) LPL messenger RNA *(mRNA)* levels in newborns staying with their dams. (C) LPL mRNA levels in individual pups exposed to the indicated environmental temperatures. (A, Modified from Cryer A, Jones HM. Developmental changes in the activity of lipoprotein lipase (clearing factor lipase) in rat lung, cardiac muscle, skeletal muscle and brown adipose tissue. *Biochem J.* 1978;174:447. B and C, Modified from Obregón MJ, Jacobsson A, Kirchgessner T, et al. Postnatal recruitment of brown adipose tissue is induced by the cold stress experienced by the pups: an analysis of mRNA levels for thermogenin and lipoprotein lipase. *Biochem J.* 1989;259:341.)

PATHOLOGY

No pathologic state that involves activity of lipoprotein lipase in human brown adipose tissue is known, but a genetic disease in mice, combined lipase deficiency (the mutation is therefore designated *cld/cld*), leads to the synthesis of an inefficient lipoprotein lipase.[161] The absence of lipoprotein lipase activity has the expected effect of reducing the amount of fat droplets in brown adipose tissue.[162]

GLUCOSE

Uptake of glucose was originally documented in brown adipose tissue in the newborn rabbit.[147] On the basis of in vitro experiments, it may be envisaged that glucose uptake may increase the catabolic capacity of the citric acid cycle through the action of pyruvate carboxylase.[163] The marked ability of brown adipose tissue to take up glucose under cold conditions forms the basis for the detection of brown adipose tissue with PET scanning. This stimulation is sympathetically mediated through norepinephrine, rather than insulin. Norepinephrine increases glucose uptake by increasing the synthesis and translocation of GLUT1 and, correspondingly, glucose uptake rates.[164-167] Brown adipose tissue shows insulin-sensitive glucose transport through redistribution of the GLUT4 glucose transporter from intracellular vesicles to the plasma membrane.[168]

Glucose can be combusted in active brown adipose tissue, converted to and stored as glycogen, participate in glyceroneogenesis, or take part in lipogenesis (which is discussed in the following sections).

FATTY ACID SYNTHESIS

The significance of lipogenesis in brown adipose tissue has been discussed. The capacity for lipogenesis in brown adipose tissue is high.[169,170] Lipogenesis has also been observed in human infants.[171] However, strong evidence suggests that this lipogenesis is not of quantitative or qualitative significance for thermogenesis. Rather, it could be considered to represent a "refilling" reaction that occurs in the tissue after cessation of the thermogenic stimulus. Thus, during the perinatal period, the activity of lipogenesis is low when thermogenesis is high. This reverse correlation is probably due to the effect of suckling (i.e., a change from a carbohydrate "diet" in the fetal state to a high-lipid diet). A direct inhibitory effect of increased sympathetic stimulation on lipogenesis also has been postulated.[19] Weaning, which not only reintroduces a high-carbohydrate diet but also coincides with a reduced demand for thermogenesis, is associated with an increase in lipogenesis.

The so-called *lipogenic enzymes* (in addition to the fatty acid synthase complex) include pyruvate dehydrogenase, the citrate cleavage enzyme (ATPcitrate lyase), acetyl-CoA carboxylase, glucose-6-phosphate dehydrogenase, 6-phosphogluconate dehydrogenase, and malic enzymes. All of these enzymes generally follow the same perinatal pattern: levels are high in the fetal state and much reduced during suckling, returning toward high fetal values as suckling ends.[19] For malic enzyme, it has been demonstrated that this phasic pattern is due to a change in the amount of enzyme (not a change in activity of existing enzyme).[172]

The activities of the glycolytic enzymes increase after weaning,[173] indicating that during the time when the diet consists of milk alone, it is those fatty acids that supply brown adipose tissue and are spent in combustion. Only after weaning to a diet rich in carbohydrates does glycolysis contribute to fatty acid synthesis.

AMINO ACID UPTAKE

The possibility that amino acid uptake occurs has been investigated. It is generally believed that this pathway is of minor importance for the functioning of brown adipose tissue.[174] Several amino acids have propionyl-CoA as the end product of oxidation. This three-carbon fatty acid cannot be degraded through the normal β-oxidation pathway for fatty acid derivatives, so its accumulation could result in sequestration of all mitochondrial CoA, with consequent inhibition of thermogenesis. This effect may explain why the mitochondria have a high activity level of a propionyl-CoA hydrolase with unusual regulatory properties.[175-177] This hydrolase could function to recover the CoA otherwise bound up in propionyl-CoA.

5′-DEIODINASE AND THYROID HORMONE

In brown adipose tissue, high activity of thyroxine 5′-deiodinase, which produces the active thyroid hormone triiodothyronine (T_3), has been described (Fig. 32.6).[147] The 5′-deiodinase found in brown adipose tissue has been classified as a type II deiodinase (distinguished from type I by its insensitivity to propylthiouracil in vitro[178] and by its being induced by hypothyroidism in vivo[179]). The gene has been cloned.[180] It is probably localized to the endoplasmic reticulum. The presence of 5′-deiodinase has been demonstrated in human, lamb, and rodent brown fat.[178,181,182]

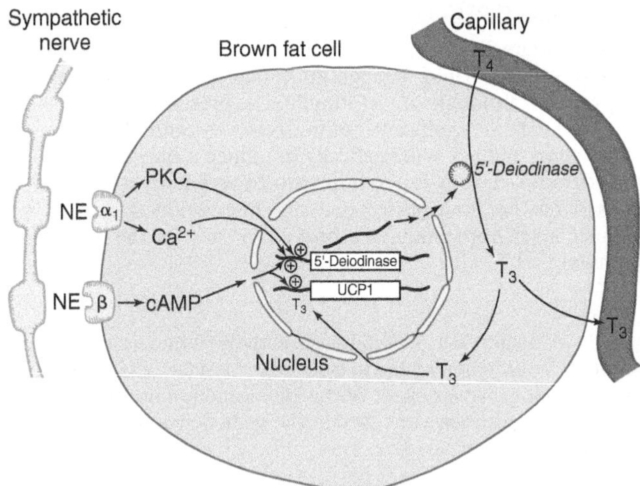

Fig. 32.6 The regulation and action of 5′-deiodinase in brown adipose tissue. *cAMP,* Cyclic adenosine monophosphate; *NE,* norepinephrine; *PKC,* protein kinase C; *T_3,* triiodothyronine; *T_4,* thyroxine; *UCP1,* uncoupling protein-1.

INTERNAL ACTION

It is believed that the activity of the 5′-deiodinase to generate T_3 is important for both the normal development of brown adipose tissue and the rapid increase in brown fat during the perinatal period. The T_3 produced probably binds to T_3 receptors found within the tissue[183,184] (see Fig. 32.6) and in this way influences expression of the *UCP1* gene through binding to sequences in the promoter region.[185] Indeed, hypothyroidism leads to a decreased expression of UCP1 in both rats and lambs (see Fig. 32.4A).[101,181] However, in mice in which the nuclear thyroid hormone-binding receptors are ablated, UCP1 expression is high, confirming that the hormone is required primarily to relieve a repression of gene expression, rather than to cause activation.[186,187] Studies indicate that T_3 causes at least some of its actions on brown adipose tissue activity through a central action in the hypothalamus.[188]

SYSTEMIC ACTION

The possibility has also been considered that brown adipose tissue 5′-deiodinase is of systemic physiologic significance in that it could release T_3 from brown fat into the circulation.[189] Indeed, such release has been substantiated in the newborn rat.[190]

T_3 could be responsible for the small increase in basal metabolism sometimes found in conditions in which brown fat is stimulated, but experiments in which brown fat is removed to investigate this possibility are not technically possible currently.

In addition to the metabolic effects of T_3, thyroid hormone also may have an important role in promoting differentiation. Some interesting, but unconfirmed, observations suggest that removal of brown adipose tissue at a young age affects development of other bodily functions in later life. Thus, in several studies, Jankovic and colleagues implied the presence of such a brown adipose tissue effect on the development of the immune response,[191-193] but so far these observations have not been independently verified.

REGULATION OF BROWN ADIPOSE TISSUE DEIODINASE ACTIVITY

The activity of 5′-deiodinase is rapidly induced under conditions in which brown adipose tissue is recruited. This increase in activity is due to an increased synthesis of the enzyme.[194,195]

ADRENERGIC REGULATION

It was originally suggested that the increase in deiodinase activity was mediated through an α_1-adrenergic mechanism.[196] Apparently, although an α_1-stimulus is presumably necessary to produce a significant stimulation, α- and β-adrenergic stimulation interact synergistically to induce a maximal increase in 5′-deiodinase activity. From in vitro experiments with isolated cells, it has been suggested that this interaction occurs at the cellular level, apparently at a post-cAMP step in the activation pathway.[197,198]

INSULIN

Insulin can increase 5′-deiodinase activity when injected into animals[195] and when added to isolated brown fat cells.[199] Neither the physiologic significance of this phenomenon nor the specific intracellular pathways involved in the gene activation events has been characterized.

PERINATAL RECRUITMENT OF 5′-DEIODINASE

The perinatal pattern of development of 5′-deiodinase is unusual: the deiodinase activity rises markedly before birth, after which it spontaneously declines (Fig. 32.7).[200-202] The regulation of this activity and its significance for brown fat recruitment are of interest, but no experimental evidence concerning these questions is available at present.

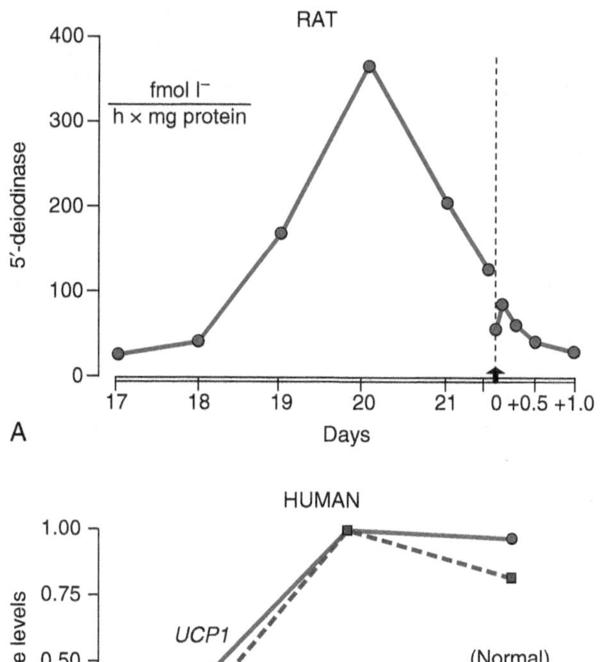

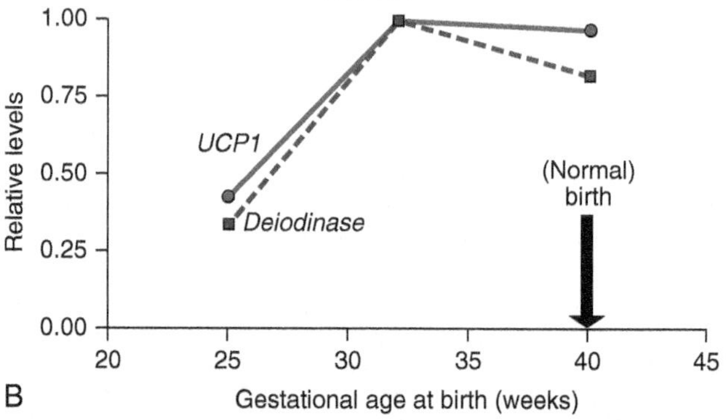

Fig. 32.7 5′-Deiodinase activity in the perinatal period. *UCP1,* Uncoupling protein-1. (Data in A based on rat studies from Giralt M, Martin I, Mampel T, et al. Evidence for a differential physiological modulation of brown fat iodothyronine 5′-deiodinase activity in the perinatal period. *Biochem Biophys Res Commun.* 1988;156:493. Supported by similar data from Obregón MJ, Ruiz de Oña C, Hernandez A, et al. Thyroid hormones and 5′-deiodinase in rat brown adipose tissue during fetal life. *Am J Physiol.* 1989;257:E625. Human data in B from Houstěk J, Vízek K, Pavelka S, et al. Type II iodothyronine 5′-deiodinase and uncoupling protein in brown adipose tissue of human newborns. *J Clin Endocrinol Metab.* 1993;77:383.)

REGULATION OF RECRUITMENT OF THE TISSUE

The capacity of brown adipose tissue thermogenesis is limited by the amount of UCP1 in the tissue, and this level is governed by the activity of the sympathetic nervous system and norepinephrine. To increase the amount of UCP1 in the tissue, two principal strategies may be used. In the first, the amount of UCP1 per brown adipocyte is increased. In the second, an increase in cell proliferation (i.e., in the number of adipocytes) occurs, but each individual adipocyte maintains an unchanged capacity. Although different species appear to use more or less of either the first or the second modality, both seem to be operative in all species studied. The situation has not been studied for the human neonate.

The tissue retains a potential proliferative capacity, even in adulthood. Preadipocytes in culture can be stimulated to increase their proliferation by the addition of norepinephrine, and the stimulation is through β_1-receptors and cAMP-coupled mechanisms.[203] This mechanism is in contrast with the norepinephrine stimulation of *UCP1* gene expression in mature brown adipocytes, which, while also using cAMP as the intracellular messenger, couples to the adenylyl cyclase through β_3-receptors.[204]

Various transcription factors might be expected to be involved in control of cell proliferation, and many are currently being studied. Of note, an important adipose-related factor, CCAAT/enhancer binding protein α (C/EBPα), is transiently decreased as proliferation begins.[205] Other fat-related transcription factors such as members of the PPAR family and the coactivator PGC1α (PPAR-γ coactivator 1) also appear to be of importance.[206] A more comprehensive study of the roles of these transcription factors is required to elucidate the complex control of cell proliferation, both in utero and postnatally. It is evident that in the fetal state, growth factors, such as insulin-like growth factor-1,[207,208] are important for cell growth.

CLINICAL IMPLICATIONS

Considerable evidence suggests that one of the major problems with temperature regulation in small premature infants is that the lipid supply to brown adipose tissue and its mechanism of recruitment are not sufficiently developed. This deficiency, combined with the larger surface-to-volume ratio characteristic of small premature infants that promotes rapid heat loss, places them at increased risk for hypothermia. Therefore, the main problem resulting from the incomplete development of brown adipose tissue in premature newborns was solved through the introduction of the incubator.[209]

EFFECTS OF ENVIRONMENTAL TEMPERATURE

Convincing evidence from animal experiments indicates that the postnatal environmental temperature has a substantial effect on brown adipose tissue development (see Figs. 32.4 and 32.5).[19] Indeed, some anecdotal evidence suggests that children who live in relatively cold environments will acquire or maintain an improved cold tolerance, probably through persistent brown adipose tissue function.

ANESTHESIA IN INFANTS

During general anesthesia, body temperature regulation is disturbed, an effect more marked in young infants. Although effects on central mechanisms controlling body temperature may also be observed, it is now apparent that the commonly used inhalation anesthetics halothane and its derivatives are potent inhibitors of brown adipose tissue thermogenesis.[210-213] This effect is of particular significance in young infants, in whom the activity of brown adipose tissue is crucial for body temperature regulation.

EFFECTS OF MALNUTRITION

The effects of pre- or postnatal malnutrition have been investigated in experimental animals. In general, food restriction reduces the function of brown adipose tissue,[214,215] although paradoxical observations have been reported.[216] Adverse effects of more specific dietary restrictions (e.g., riboflavin, protein) have also been reported.[217,218] In scattered reports in the literature, malnutrition has been implicated as a cause of hypothermia in human newborn infants, presumably owing to a lack of substrate available for thermogenesis.[219]

OVERFEEDING

The presentation of a palatable, so-called *cafeteria diet* to adult rats results in overfeeding. However, these animals do not gain weight to the extent anticipated by the degree of overfeeding. The brown adipose tissue of such animals is markedly recruited, and it has been suggested that the decrease in the animals' whole-body efficiency (as indicated by lower weight gain than anticipated) could result from increased thermogenesis in brown adipose tissue.[220,221] Postnatal overfeeding in rats (induced by a reduction in the number of pups per litter) also leads to the activation of brown adipose tissue.[222] However, postnatal overfeeding may lead to decreased brown fat thermogenesis in the adult.[223]

It can be posited that also in the human infant, overfeeding may cause an activation of brown adipose tissue, leading to increased thermogenesis.

GENETICALLY OBESE ANIMALS

In genetically obese animals (the fa/fa rat and the ob/ob and db/db mice, all of which have problems in the leptin system), the postnatal recruitment process in brown adipose tissue is blunted, before any signs of obesity become evident.[224-226] This inactivity of brown adipose tissue has been discussed to constitute at least one cause of developing obesity. This correlation was apparently confirmed by studies in which brown adipocytes were molecularly ablated from mice.[73] For these experiments, transgenic animals were produced in which the UCP1 promoter region was coupled to the gene for the diphtheria toxin A chain. This A chain inhibits protein synthesis, thereby killing the cells in which it is expressed (e.g., primarily brown adipocytes). The transgenic animals developed obesity and other manifestations of pathophysiology associated with obesity, such as insulin resistance. However, mice with an ablation in the *UCP1* gene and thus possessing thermogenically incompetent brown fat did not become manifestly obese.[227] These mice therefore seemed competent to regulate food intake to compensate for a decreased ability to combust food substrates. However, of note, if animals are kept at thermoneutral temperatures, at which thermogenesis is not needed to defend body temperature, the absence of UCP1 can lead to increased adiposity.[228,229]

It is unclear whether some humans may be subject to the same forces as in these genetically obese animals. Although the potential to develop obesity is known to have a strong genetic component, to what extent brown adipose tissue inactivity contributes to development of obesity in children remains undetermined.

DISEASES AFFECTING BROWN ADIPOSE TISSUE

In fever, some of the heat necessary for the increase in body temperature comes from brown adipose tissue, at least in young experimental animals.[230,231] It also is clear that brown adipocytes are not only responsive to cytokines released during infections that cause fever but also can synthesize such cytokines.[232,233] A relatively rare benign tumor, the hibernoma, can occur even in neonates.[234] Also of note is that treatment with prostaglandin E_1 for palliation of neonatal congenital heart disease results in calcific brown fat necrosis, which can resolve over time.[235,236] In a number of diseases—such as Duchenne progressive muscular dystrophy,[237] subcutaneous fat necrosis of the newborn,[238] and sudden infant death syndrome[239-241]—a role for brown adipose tissue has been suggested. In sudden infant death syndrome, a link with gestational magnesium deficiency has been proposed.[242] However, at present, no direct evidence has emerged to show causative involvement of brown adipose tissue in any of these syndromes.[243]

CONCLUSION

Brown adipose tissue is a uniquely mammalian tissue that protects neonatal body temperature around the time of birth by combusting triglycerides in the numerous mitochondria to emit heat. The process can occur because of the presence in the mitochondrial inner membrane of the UCP1, which transports proton (equivalents) across the membrane to dissipate the proton gradient formed during substrate oxidation. Well-developed neonates already possess active brown adipose tissue at birth, while less mature species develop brown adipose tissue upon the cold exposure that follows birth. During this period, the body temperature of the offspring is primarily defended by the mother. UCP1 is found primarily in classic depots of brown adipose tissue, notably periaortic, cervical, interscapular, and perirenal, in the human infant. Smaller amounts can be found in other adipose depots normally considered white, although their contribution to total heat production is rather minor. The heat production is regulated by release of norepinephrine from the sympathetic nerves innervating the tissue, when skin receptors and central thermal receptors experience cold exposure. This results initially in the breakdown and combustion of intracellular triglycerides and thereafter uptake and combustion of circulating substrates—primarily lipids and glucose. It is now accepted that brown adipose tissue is found to some extent in the majority of adult humans throughout the greater part of life and influences not only cold sensitivity, but also body weight regulation.

A complete reference list is available at www.ExpertConsult.com. 

SELECT REFERENCES

1. Smith RE. Thermogenic activity of the hibernating gland in the cold-acclimated rat. *Physiologist*. 1961;4:113.
3. Dawkins MJ, Hull D. Brown adipose tissue and the response of new-born rabbits to cold. *J Physiol*. 1964;172:216.
9. Cannon B, Nedergaard J. Brown adipose tissue: function and physiological significance. *Physiol Rev*. 2004;84:277.
11. Nedergaard J, Bengtsson T, Cannon B. Unexpected evidence for active brown adipose tissue in adult humans. *Am J Physiol*. 2007;293:E444.
12. van der Lans AA, Hoeks J, Brans B, et al. Cold acclimation recruits human brown fat and increases non-shivering thermogenesis. *J Clin Invest*. 2013;123:3395.
13. Saito M, Okamatsu-Ogura Y, Matsushita M, et al. High incidence of metabolically active brown adipose tissue in healthy adult humans: effects of cold exposure and adiposity. *Diabetes*. 2009;58:1526.
14. Vosselman MJ, Vijgen GH, Kingma BR, et al. Frequent extreme cold exposure and brown fat and cold-induced thermogenesis: a study in a monozygotic twin. *PloS One*. 2014;9:e101653.
15. Saito M. Brown adipose tissue as a regulator of energy expenditure and body fat in humans. *Diabetes Metab J*. 2013;37:22.
16. Yoneshiro T, Aita S, Matsushita M, et al. Age-related decrease in cold-activated brown adipose tissue and accumulation of body fat in healthy humans. *Obesity*. 2011;19:1755.
17. Zukotynski KA, Fahey FH, Laffin S, et al. Constant ambient temperature of 24 degrees C significantly reduces FDG uptake by brown adipose tissue in children scanned during the winter. *Eur J Nucl Med Mol Imaging*. 2009;36:602.
18. Hong TS, Shammas A, Charron M, et al. Brown adipose tissue 18F-FDG uptake in pediatric PET/CT imaging. *Pediatr Radiol*. 2011;41:759.

19. Nedergaard J, Connolly E, Cannon B. Brown adipose tissue in the mammalian neonate. In: Trayhurn P, Nicholls DG, eds. *Brown Adipose Tissue*. London: Edward Arnold; 1986:152-213.
24. Barnard T. The ultrastructural differentiation of brown adipose tissue in the rat. *J Ultrastruct Res*. 1969;29:311.
25. Suter ER. The fine structure of brown adipose tissue. II. Perinatal development in the rat. *Lab Invest*. 1969;21:246.
30. Sundin U, Herron D, Cannon B. Brown fat thermoregulation in developing hamsters (*Mesocricetus auratus*): a GDP-binding study. *Biol Neonat*. 1981;39:141.
33. Jastroch M, Withers KW, Taudien S, et al. Marsupial uncoupling protein 1 sheds light on the evolution of mammalian non-shivering thermogenesis. *Physiol Genomics*. 2008;32:161.
37. Lomax MA, Sadiq F, Karamanlidis G, et al. Ontogenic loss of brown adipose tissue sensitivity to beta-adrenergic stimulation in the ovine. *Endocrinology*. 2007;148:461.
40. Smith SB, Carstens GE, Randel RD, et al. Brown adipose tissue development and metabolism in ruminants. *J Anim Sci*. 2004;82:942.
43. Merklin RJ. Growth and distribution of human fetal brown fat. *Anat Rec*. 1974;178:637.
49. Suarez J, Rivera P, Arrabal S, et al. Oleoylethanolamide enhances beta-adrenergic-mediated thermogenesis and white-to-brown adipocyte phenotype in epididymal white adipose tissue in rat. *Dis Model Mech*. 2014;7:129.
54. Shabalina IG, Petrovic N, de Jong JM, et al. UCP1 in brite/beige adipose tissue mitochondria is functionally thermogenic. *Cell Rep*. 2013;5:1196.
57. Timmons JA, Wennmalm K, Larsson O, et al. Myogenic gene expression signature establishes that brown and white adipocytes originate from different lineages. *Proc Natl Acad Sci U S A*. 2007;104:4401.
58. Seale P, Bjork B, Yang W, et al. PRDM16 controls a brown fat/skeletal muscle switch. *Nature*. 2008;454:961.
59. Sanchez-Gurmaches J, Guertin DA. Adipocyte lineages: tracing back the origins of fat. *Biochim Biophys Acta*. 2014;340:1842.
60. Sanchez-Gurmaches J, Guertin DA. Adipocytes arise from multiple lineages that are heterogeneously and dynamically distributed. *Nat Commun*. 2014;5:5099.
61. Long JZ, Svensson KJ, Tsai L, et al. A smooth muscle-like origin for beige adipocytes. *Cell Metab*. 2014;19:810.
63. Matthias A, Ohlson KB, Fredriksson JM, et al. Thermogenic responses in brown fat cells are fully UCP1-dependent: UCP2 or UCP3 do not substitute for UCP1 in adrenergically or fatty-acid induced thermogenesis. *J Biol Chem*. 2000;275:25073.
64. Golozoubova V, Hohtola E, Matthias A, et al. Only UCP1 can mediate adaptive non-shivering thermogenesis in the cold. *FASEB J*. 2001;15:2048.
89. Shabalina IG, Jacobsson A, Cannon B, Nedergaard J. Native UCP1 displays simple competitive kinetics between the regulators purine nucleotides and fatty acids. *J Biol Chem*. 2004;279:38236.
90. Fedorenko A, Lishko PV, Kirichok Y. Mechanism of fatty-acid-dependent UCP1 uncoupling in brown fat mitochondria. *Cell*. 2012;151:400.
111. Petrovic N, Walden TB, Shabalina IG, et al. Chronic peroxisome proliferator-activated receptor gamma (PPARgamma) activation of epididymally derived white adipocyte cultures reveals a population of thermogenically competent, UCP1-containing adipocytes molecularly distinct from classic brown adipocytes. *J Biol Chem*. 2010;285:7153.
112. Karlberg P, Moore RE, Oliver Jr TK. The thermogenic response of the newborn infant to noradrenaline. *Acta Paediatr*. 1962;51:284.
124. Arch JRS, Kaumann AJ. β_3 and atypical α-adrenoceptors. *Med Res Rev*. 1993;13:663.
131. Gnad T, Scheibler S, von Kugelgen I, et al. Adenosine activates brown adipose tissue and recruits beige adipocytes via A2A receptors. *Nature*. 2014;516:395.
138. Young SG, Zechner R. Biochemistry and pathophysiology of intravascular and intracellular lipolysis. *Genes Dev*. 2013;27:459.
147. Hardman MJ, Hull D. Fat metabolism in brown adipose tissue *in vivo*. *J Physiol*. 1970;206:263.
166. Dallner O, Chernogubova E, Brolinson KA, Bengtsson T. Beta$_3$-adrenergic receptors stimulate glucose uptake in brown adipocytes by two mechanisms independently of glucose transporter 4 translocation. *Endocrinology*. 2006;147:5730.
167. Olsen JM, Sato M, Dallner OS, et al. Glucose uptake in brown fat cells is dependent on mTOR complex 2-promoted GLUT1 translocation. *J Cell Biol*. 2014;207:365.
187. Golozoubova V, Gullberg H, Matthias A, et al. Depressed thermogenesis but competent brown adipose tissue recruitment in mice devoid of all hormone-binding thyroid hormone receptors. *Mol Endocrinol*. 2004;18:384.
188. Lopez M, Varela L, Vazquez MJ, et al. Hypothalamic AMPK and fatty acid metabolism mediate thyroid regulation of energy balance. *Nat Med*. 2010;16:1001.
203. Bronnikov G, Houstěk J, Nedergaard J. β-Adrenergic, cAMP-mediated stimulation of proliferation of brown fat cells in primary culture: mediation via β_1 but not via β_3 receptors. *J Biol Chem*. 2006;267:1992.
204. Rehnmark S, Néchad M, Herron D, et al. α- and β-adrenergic induction of the expression of the uncoupling protein thermogenin in brown adipocytes differentiated in culture. *J Biol Chem*. 1990;265:16464.
211. Dicker A, Ohlson KB, Johnson L, et al. Halothane selectively inhibits non-shivering thermogenesis: possible implications for thermoregulation during anesthesia of infants. *Anesthesiology*. 1995;82:491.
215. Luz J, Griggio MA, Vieira LV. Impact of maternal food restriction on cold-induced thermogenesis in the offspring. *Biol Neonate*. 2003;84:252.
220. Rothwell NJ, Stock MJ. A role for brown adipose tissue in diet-induced thermogenesis. *Nature*. 1979;281:31.
223. Xiao XQ, Williams SM, Grayson BE, et al. Excess weight gain during the early postnatal period is associated with permanent reprogramming of brown adipose tissue adaptive thermogenesis. *Endocrinology*. 2007;148:4150.
227. Enerbäck S, Jacobsson A, Simpson EM, et al. Mice lacking mitochondrial uncoupling protein are cold-sensitive but not obese. *Nature*. 1997;387:90.
229. Feldmann HM, Golozoubova V, Cannon B, Nedergaard J. UCP1 ablation induces obesity and abolishes diet-induced thermogenesis in mice exempt from thermal stress by living at thermoneutrality. *Cell Metab*. 2009;9:203.
233. Burysek L, Houstek J. β-Adrenergic stimulation of interleukin-1α and interleukin-6 expression in mouse brown adipocytes. *FEBS Lett*. 1997;411:83.
234. Baskurt E, Padgett DM, Matsumoto JA. Multiple hibernomas in a 1-month-old female infant. *AJNR Am J Neuroradiol*. 2004;25:1443.

33 Lipids as an Energy Source for the Premature and Term Neonate

Emilio Herrera | Henar Ortega-Senovilla

INTRODUCTION

In utero, the fetus receives a continuous supply of substrates for growth and oxidative metabolism, and produces large quantities of heat and carbon dioxide.[1,2] Based on experiments with rats and various other animal species, it is thought that the continuous placental transport of glucose and amino acids represents over 80% of the energy supply during late intrauterine life. At birth there is an abrupt termination of these major fetal fuels and a switch to intermittent feedings with breast milk, which contains a high proportion of lipids, meaning that about 50% of neonatal energy supply comes from the oxidation of fatty acids.[1,3,4]

However, several laboratories have reevaluated the role of mitochondrial fatty acid oxidation (FAO) in human placental and fetal metabolism.[5-8] Using a variety of approaches it has been shown that mRNA expression and activity of FAO enzymes are both present in substantial proportions in several human fetal tissues and in placenta[7,9] leading to the conclusion that FAO is an important component of fetal and placental energy production.

Before breast-feeding is established, the newborn infant must produce glucose to meet the needs of the central nervous system.[10] The human neonate is capable of producing sufficient glucose to meet cerebral energy needs,[11] initially by glycogenolysis. However, glycogen stores last for only about 10 to 12 hours in a term infant,[12] and gluconeogenesis becomes the principal source of hepatic glucose production soon after birth,[13] but daily glucose production alone can barely satisfy the whole-body metabolic requirements in the first day of life.[14] Therefore during early postnatal life, there is an absolute need for other oxidizable endogenous substrates to meet the infant's energy demands. Near term, the human fetus has an increased accumulation of adipose tissue,[15,16] attaining fat stores of around 15% of body weight at birth.[17,18] Immediately after birth, there is an increase in adipose tissue lipolysis with an intense increase in plasma nonesterified fatty acids (NEFA).[19-22] A fall in the respiratory quotient (RQ) takes place,[23] indicating that mobilized fatty acids become the primary source of energy. Thus, FAO becomes an important supply of energy for the newborn infant. Ketone bodies are formed in liver from the end product of β-oxidation[24] and become an alternative energy substrate for the neonatal brain.[12] Lipolysis of adipose tissue triglycerides (TG, more formally known as *triacylglycerols*) also releases glycerol into the circulation, which can be converted into glucose in the gluconeogenic pathway.[25,26] These metabolic interactions explain the decrease in plasma glucose concentration of the newborn infant immediately after birth, which lasts approximately two hours, followed by a rise to reach its steady state a few hours after birth.[4,27]

In this chapter the importance of lipids as a fuel for oxidative metabolism in premature and full-term neonates is discussed.

FATTY ACID UTILIZATION AS ENERGY SOURCE DURING INTRAUTERINE LIFE

During pregnancy, the fetus is continuously supplied through the placenta with a diet rich in carbohydrates and amino acids and poor in fat.[2] In fact, from animal studies, the fetus is considered to be primarily dependent on glucose oxidation for energy production[28] because (1) glucose is quantitatively the main substrate supplied by the mother to the fetus, (2) mRNA expression and activity of FAO enzymes in fetal heart and liver are low with a rapid rise after birth,[29-31] and (3) the high utilization of glucose by the fetus results in the conversion of acetyl-CoA to malonyl-CoA by acetyl-CoA carboxylase, and the resultant inhibition of the carnitine palmitoyl-CoA transferase 1 (CPT1), the key enzyme controlling the entry of long-chain fatty acids into the mitochondria and consequently their oxidation.[32]

Based on the evidence above, one of the dogmas in fetal and perinatal medicine has been that the fetus depends upon the constant supply of glucose transported to and across the placenta from the maternal circulation to generate all placental and fetal energy needs, using glycolysis and the tricarboxylic acid (TCA) cycle, for essential functions.[28] However, immediately after birth the newborn infant has to withstand a brief period of starvation before being fed at intervals with milk. In human mature milk, the lactose content is higher (7 g/100 g) than that of fat (4 g/100 g),[33] although it depends on the stage after delivery, colostrum having a lower lactose and a higher fat content.[34-36] Around 95% of that fat is in the form of TG[33] and represents more than 60% of the energy intake in the neonate. Thus, the fetal-to-neonatal transition implies a very rapid switch from glucose to fat as the major source of energy.

Several reports have characterized recessively inherited disorders in the more than 20 genes of the mitochondrial FAO pathway that cause early morbidity and mortality.[37,38] The majority of the affected infants are premature and show phenotypes of growth restriction, fasting-induced hypoketotic hypoglycemia, and hepatic encephalopathy, and may progress to coma and death.[6,39,40] Two pathogenic mechanisms for FAO disorders have been proposed: first, a lack of sufficient energy production, and second, the accumulation of fatty acid intermediates that enter the maternal circulation in toxic concentrations. Data to support both hypotheses exist, and it has been shown that FAO enzyme disorders in the affected fetus may cause significant maternal morbidity and mortality, including acute fatty liver of pregnancy (AFLP), the HELLP (hemolysis, elevated liver enzymes, and low platelets) syndrome, placental floor infarction, and pre-eclampsia.[39-44] Furthermore, a higher frequency of prematurity, intrauterine growth retardation (IUGR), and intrauterine death have been described, in association with deficiencies in enzymes involved in the FAO pathway like long-chain 3-hydroxyacyl-CoA dehydrogenase (LCHAD) or the mitochondrial trifunctional protein (MTP) (see below),[40,45,46] which is a protein with fatty acyl-CoA dehydrogenase activity. All these findings suggest that FAO plays an important role in the human fetal-placental unit, in contrast to the results obtained in animal studies and to the widely accepted view that embryologic development depends on glucose as the major source of metabolic energy.

Fig. 33.1 shows the mitochondrial long-chain FAO pathway. The process starts with the uptake of fatty acids and carnitine (3-hydroxyl-4-trimethylamino-butanoic acid) into the cell. Long-chain fatty acid transport is facilitated by membrane associated transporters such as specific fatty acid transport proteins (FATPs), fatty acid-binding protein ($FABP_{pm}$), and fatty acid translocase CD36/FAT,[47-49] whereas carnitine uptake is mediated by its transporter OCTN2.[50] Intracellular long-chain fatty acid is activated to fatty acyl-CoA by the action of fatty acyl-CoA synthase (FACS) in a reaction that consumes the equivalent of two adenosine triphosphates (ATPs). Activated fatty acyl-CoA are converted to carnitine esters by the action of CPT1, and then transferred by carnitine-acylcarnitine translocase (CACT) across the mitochondrial membranes, where fatty acyl-CoA is reconstituted by carnitine palmitoyl-CoA transferase 2 (CPT2). Once inside the mitochondria, the FAO process (usually called *β-oxidation*) brings about the breakdown of a long-chain acyl-CoA molecule to a number of acetyl-CoA molecules, the number of which depends on the length of the fatty acid's carbon chain. The process involves a variety of enzymes, the four main ones of which are acyl-CoA dehydrogenase, enoyl-CoA hydratase, hydroxyacyl-CoA dehydrogenase, and ketoacyl-CoA thiolase.[51] In each β-oxidation cycle, an acetyl-CoA, an acyl-CoA two carbons shorter, one NADH, and one $FADH_2$ are formed. Acetyl-CoA may be used for steroidogenesis, enter the TCA cycle for oxidation and energy production, or become transformed into ketone bodies in the liver; the electrons derived from NADH and $FADH_2$ are used by the respiratory chain eventually leading to the production of energy as ATP. The β-oxidation enzymes have different isoforms with affinities for different fatty acid chain lengths (e.g., there is a very-long-chain acyl-CoA dehydrogenase [VLCAD], a medium-chain acyl-CoA dehydrogenase [MCAD], and a short-chain acyl dehydrogenase [SCAD]). The enoyl-CoA hydratase, hydroxyacyl-CoA dehydrogenase, and ketoacyl-CoA thiolase isoforms specific for long-chain fatty acids form an enzyme complex in the inner mitochondrial membrane that is named the MTP. The activity of several FAO enzymes and different acylcarnitines have been found in human embryo, fetus, and placenta, showing that the mitochondrial FAO enzymes are metabolically active.[6,52]

The activities of the enzymes of FAO are subject to feedback inhibition by the products of their own reaction,[53] so that any buildup of acyl-CoA product will inhibit the specific β-oxidation enzyme that produced it.[54] Moreover, the proteins involved in fatty acid β-oxidation are regulated by both transcriptional and post-transcriptional mechanisms. There are a number of transcriptional factors that regulate the expression of these proteins, the best known being the peroxisome proliferator-activated receptors (PPARs) and a transcription factor coactivator PGC-1α.[55]

In animal studies, the ablation of genes encoding enzymes of the FAO pathway is associated with reduced fertility, fetal demise, and fetal growth restriction,[39,56,57] and the ablation or inactivation of genes encoding for the transcription factors involved in the regulation of FAO like PPARs cause embryonic lethality as well as the failure of the syncytiotrophoblast to develop and sustain pregnancy.[58-60]

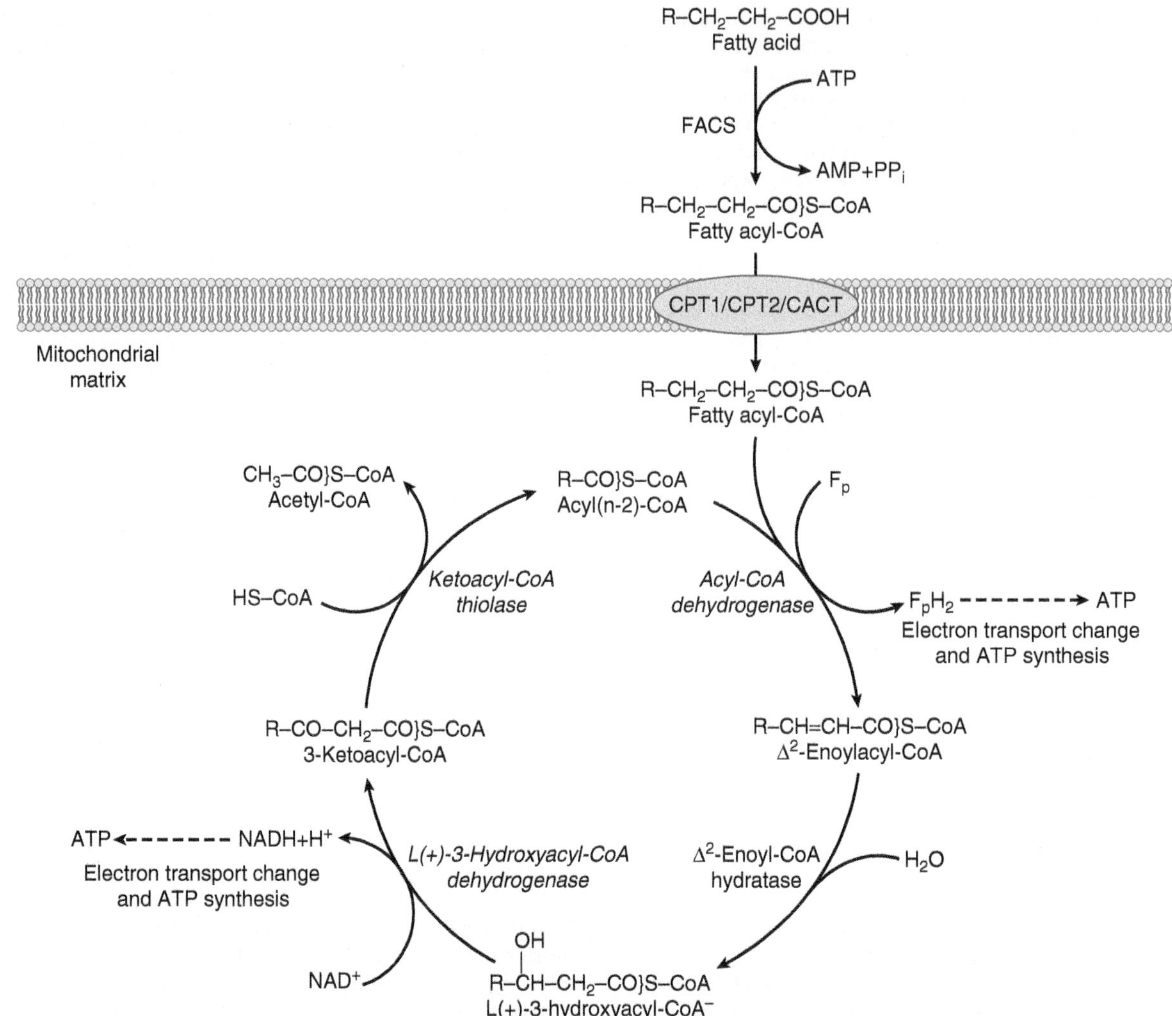

Fig. 33.1 Pathway of fatty acid β-oxidation in the mitochondria. Once inside the cell, the fatty acyl-CoA synthase *(FACS)* adds a coenzyme-A to the fatty acid forming fatty acyl-CoA. Carnitine palmitoyltransferase 1 *(CPT1)* converts fatty acyl-CoA to fatty acylcarnitine, which is transported across the inner mitochondrial membrane by the carnitine translocase *(CAT)*. An inner mitochondrial membrane carnitine palmitoyltransferase 2 *(CPT2)* then converts the fatty acylcarnitine back to fatty acyl-CoA, which enters the β-oxidation pathway that results in the production of one acetyl-CoA from each cycle. The acetyl-CoA formed enters the TCA cycle, and the NADH and reduced flavoprotein (FpH_2, $FADH_2$) produced by both fatty acid β-oxidation and the TCA cycle are used by the electron transport chain for ATP synthesis.

It may be therefore concluded that FAO plays an essential role in the fetoplacental unit, where it is critical for placental function and fetal development.

CARNITINE IN PERINATAL FAT METABOLISM

Carnitine is used to facilitate the transport of fatty acids across the inner mitochondrial membrane, which is impermeable to coenzyme A derivatives. Consequently, the liver needs to maintain sufficient carnitine concentrations to enable mitochondrial FAO and ketogenesis. During human pregnancy there is a decrease in maternal plasma carnitine concentrations, values being lowest at term,[61-64] and maternal-fetal placenta carnitine transfer has been shown to be in excess of the estimated fetal carnitine requirements.[65] More recently it has been shown that the human placenta and fetal kidney, liver, and spinal cord have the capacity to synthesize carnitine,[66] suggesting that in circumstances of limited maternal carnitine supply carnitine biosynthesis by the fetal-placental unit may supply sufficient carnitine for placental and fetal metabolism.

Cord blood carnitine concentrations are higher in premature than in full-term infants,[67] and a positive correlation has been found between calculated carnitine intake and total carnitine concentrations in premature infants.[68] For example, premature infants receiving total parenteral nutrition that contains no carnitine have decreased plasma carnitine concentrations in spite of an adequate supply of the amino acid precursors of carnitine biosynthesis.[69-71] However, preterm infants receiving total parenteral nutrition supplemented with L-carnitine have normal or elevated plasma carnitine concentrations and an increased ability to utilize fatty acids.[72,73] This indicates that premature infants have a reduced capacity for carnitine biosynthesis, explaining their impaired FAO, but that carnitine supplementation successfully ameliorates the disturbances in fat metabolism.

ENERGY ADAPTATIONS AT BIRTH

At birth, the assured continuous transplacental supply of energy substrates is abruptly disrupted and the neonate has to make severe adjustments to adapt to extrauterine life. The transplacental nutrient flow, rich in carbohydrates, is terminated and replaced by a high fat, lower carbohydrate milk diet that is cyclically interrupted by periods of nutrient deprivation.[74]

Successful adaptation and survival in the extrauterine environment depends on a complex metabolic regulation that ensures a continuous supply of energy fuels, coordinating the endogenous production of substrates with the enteral feeding and assimilation of nutrients. Hormonal changes in this transition mainly consist of an endocrine stress response that control these challenges, but the pattern of the metabolic and hormonal changes differs according to the gestational maturity, intrauterine growth characteristics, and postnatal feeding.

LIPIDS AS A SOURCE OF ENERGY AT BIRTH

Following cessation of placental transfer of nutrients from the mother to the newborn infant, the requirement for energy by the neonate remains. Before the start of enteral feeding, which represents an intermittent high-fat energy supply, newborn infants have to produce their own glucose, particularly to meet the needs of the central nervous system. Thus, neonatal metabolism shifts from predominant anabolism to catabolism, releasing the energy stored in late gestation, including glucose from fetal hepatic glycogen and fatty acids from fetal fat stores,[2] which become the main sources of energy during the first postnatal hours and days. Hepatic glucose output through glycogenolysis and gluconeogenesis provides the only source of glucose until feeding is established. During the first hours after birth, blood glucose concentrations fall due to the high glucose utilization rates and the limited glycogen stores, which become depleted within hours of birth.[12] In turn, this results in a fall in the plasma insulin/glucagon ratio that increases the expression and activity of rate-limiting enzymes of gluconeogenesis like phosphoenolpyruvate carboxykinase (PEPCK), glucose-6 phosphatase, and fructose-1,6-bisphosphatase,[75,76] which together with an increased availability of gluconeogenic precursors (lactate, alanine, and glycerol) ensure the production of glucose after birth.

In spite of the above, there is still insufficient glucose to supply the newborn infant with energy; in fact, glucose utilization is thought to support only 70% of the neonatal brain's energetic needs, and additional substrates are required to supply the balance.[74] Within hours of birth, the RQ falls and there is evidence of competition between fatty acids and glucose for oxidation and carbon dioxide production.[77] Immediately after birth, before breastfeeding has started, there is an acute elevation of epinephrine, glucagon, cortisol, and thyroid hormone (with a peak in thyroid stimulating hormone [TSH]) and a decrease in the secretion of insulin. Besides triggering neonatal glucose production,[78] the hormonal status just described stimulates the mobilization of fat depots that were accumulated during the last weeks of intrauterine life.[16] This results in an increase in circulating fatty acids and glycerol concentrations, leading to an increased hepatic β-oxidation of fatty acids[39] and to the preferential use of glycerol for gluconeogenesis.[79]

In the preterm infants, abnormalities in the metabolic adaptations at birth are customary. These neonates have very limited glycogen stores and delayed maturation of the gluconeogenic pathways,[80] so they are particularly dependent on external glucose for energy supply to their brains. In addition, prematurity precludes the appropriate acquisition of adipose tissue by the fetus, which has lower values of total body fat than a term infant and considerably more visceral than subcutaneous adipose tissue.[81,82] However, in spite of limited fat depots, preterm neonates are capable of lipolysis, generating glycerol within the range of mature newborn infants, and have the ability to convert part of it to glucose.[83]

Although immaturity of the enzymatic pathways in preterm infants could explain most of the metabolic differences between preterm and term neonates, there are also other factors that can contribute to the differences between them. The mode of delivery is one of these factors. Stress hormones such as epinephrine and cortisol, as well as TSH, are major inducers of lipolysis in the neonatal period.[84,85] The concentration of these hormones, mainly cortisol, increases in the fetal circulation several days prior to the onset of delivery, and there is a further marked rise during labor[86,87] in response to hypoxia and hypoglycemia.[88] As well as increasing neonatal lipolysis, the augmented concentration of cortisol is important in the expression of genes associated with gluconeogenesis.[89-91] Newborn infants delivered by cesarean section normally show lower levels of cortisol than those that are delivered spontaneously[92]; therefore the reduced concentration of circulating cortisol in preterm infants (more often born by cesarean section), as well as immaturity of their adrenal glands, contribute to lower lipolysis and gluconeogenesis, making them more vulnerable to developing hypoglycemia. However, although cortisol production normally increases from 32 weeks of gestation,[93] some preterm infants of 33 to 36 weeks gestational age have high cord blood cortisol concentrations,[94] reducing severity and duration of their hypoglycemia.

REGULATION OF ENERGY HOMEOSTASIS IN THE PERINATAL PERIOD BY ADIPOKINES

In addition to the already-mentioned hormonal signals that regulate the metabolic adaptations in the newborn infant, there are several peptides in the umbilical and neonatal circulations that are produced mainly in adipose tissue and known as *adipokines*, which play critical roles in energy substrate production. Most of them target liver, brain, pancreas, and the immune system and directly or indirectly affect glucose and lipid metabolism, as well as insulin sensitivity.[95] This explains the interest in carrying out longitudinal studies to evaluate the effects of these adipokines on the regulation of energy homeostasis in the perinatal period and more especially in preterm infants.

Leptin is produced by both adipose tissue and placenta, and its concentration in neonatal blood increases at delivery,[96] probably induced by the higher concentration of cortisol.[97,98] Circulating leptin concentrations directly reflect the amount of energy stored in adipose tissue and are proportional to the body adipose tissue mass as shown in Fig. 33.2. Leptin also acts as a negative feedback adipostatic signal by promoting fat oxidation and inhibiting lipogenesis.[99] Interaction of leptin with its receptor increases the phosphorylation and activity of a critical energy sensor, AMP-activated protein kinase (AMPK),[100] resulting in inhibition of lipogenesis and activation of lipolysis.[101,102] Accordingly, as shown in Fig. 33.3, in newborn infants there is a linear correlation between the concentrations of plasma leptin and glycerol. Moreover, as a result of such increased lipolysis, there is also an increase in liver CPT1 and FAO,[103] which reinforces the role that leptin plays in the regulation of energy homeostasis[104] by increasing energy provision at delivery.[105] In fact, the observation of a surge in leptin soon after birth suggests that there is a critical neonatal moment, in which leptin could stimulate the development of hypothalamic pathways involved in the regulation of energy balance and appetite.[106-108] However, neonatal leptin concentrations usually decline in the first week after birth[96,109,110]; this postnatal decrease in leptin may be of physiologic advantage to both term and preterm infants by limiting their body energy expenditure and conserving nutritional reserves for subsequent growth and development.[111,112] In postnatal life, it seems that leptin does not affect food consumption,[113] in contrast to its anorexigenic effect in adults,[114] therefore contributing to the rapid growth and weight gain of the newborn infant.

Adiponectin is also expressed and secreted by adipose tissue, although during pregnancy it is also produced by the placenta.[115] During its secretion, adiponectin self-associates to form multimeric structures, with a molecular weight above 360 kDa, which cannot be transported through the placenta.[116] Thus, maternal and fetal adiponectin are not interchangeable. In contrast to leptin, adiponectin reduces energy expenditure

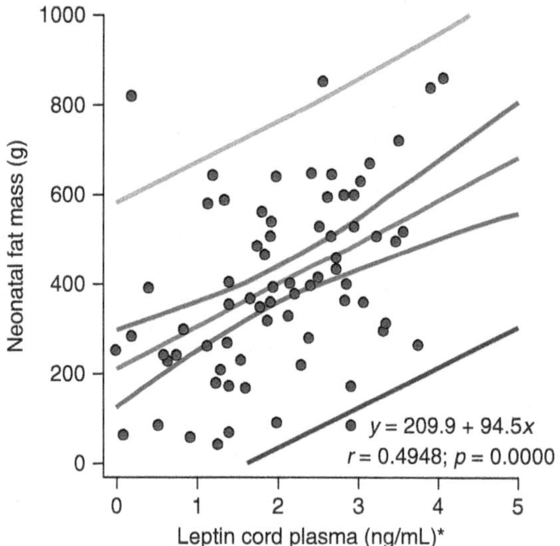

Fig. 33.2 Correlation between leptin levels in cord blood plasma and fat mass in control neonates derived from Battaglia and Meschia[1] and Ortega-Senovilla et al.[87] *Log-transformed for statistical comparisons.

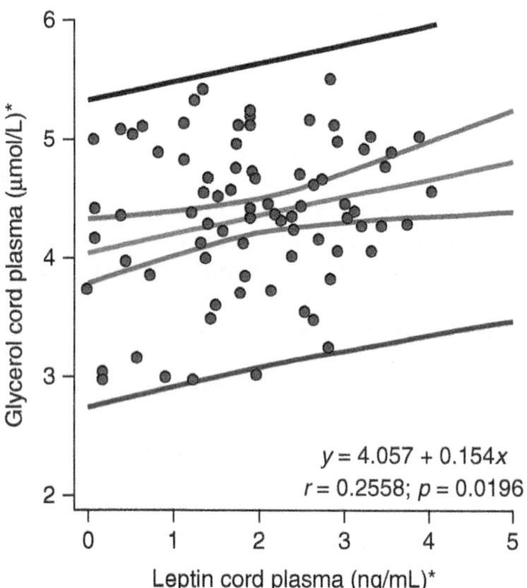

Fig. 33.3 Correlation between leptin and glycerol levels in cord blood plasma in control neonates derived from Battaglia and Meschia[1] and Ortega-Senovilla et al.[87] *Log-transformed for statistical comparisons.

and enhances energy conservation.[117] Therefore, adiponectin induces lipid accumulation in adipose tissue by increasing adipocyte differentiation and suppressing lipolysis.[116,118,119] Moreover, this adipokine plays an important role in carbohydrate metabolism, favoring insulin sensitivity and reducing hepatic glucose production.[120,121] Recently, it has been shown that in preterm infants adiponectin may affect short-term growth,[122] mainly due to intrauterine maldevelopment of adipose tissue.[123] Furthermore, in full-term neonates during the first days of life, circulating adiponectin is higher than in adolescents or adults[124] and is positively correlated with neonatal adiposity,[125] presumably due to its insulin sensitizing action.

Resistin is another adipokine expressed in adipose tissue, but also in non-fat cells such as endothelial or vascular smooth cells, mononuclear cells, and placental cells.[126,127] In humans, serum resistin concentrations are positively correlated with the amount of body fat, but there is controversy regarding the association between resistin, insulin resistance, and obesity, observed in animal models.[128] High concentrations of resistin in umbilical cord plasma samples have been reported,[129,130] with a significant relationship between resistin and anthropometric indices, suggesting a role for this adipokine in the regulation of fetal energy homeostasis. However, to date there is not sufficient evidence of a role for resistin in the increased fuel availability during the perinatal period.[129,131] Moreover, resistin has a proinflammatory effect and has been proposed as a sepsis biomarker, because higher concentrations of resistin have been found in preterm infants with severe sepsis and among those who needed mechanical ventilation.[132]

In preterm infants, serum concentrations of leptin, adiponectin, and resistin are lower than in full-term infants,[130,133-135] which could contribute to their delayed metabolic adaptation to the extrauterine life.

LIPID METABOLIC ADAPTATIONS IN THE POSTNATAL PERIOD

Enteral feeding at birth marks a shift from a low-fat to a high-fat diet. Human breast milk is the best source of nutrients for the newborn infant, and it is sufficient as the sole source of energy for the infant until around 6 months of age. Although the fat and fatty acid content of human milk is highly variable and dependent on maternal nutrition, there are no major differences between full-term and preterm human milk in terms of total fat or type of fatty acids. The proportion of palmitic acid (PA) is high,[136] but human milk also supplies the two essential fatty acids, linoleic acid (LA) and alpha-linolenic acid (LNA), as well as their long-chain derivatives arachidonic acid (ARA) and docosahexaenoic acid (DHA), respectively. The content of ARA and DHA is similar in preterm and in full-term infants indicating that they depend more on maternal diet than on gestational age.[137] One difference is that compared to term milk, preterm milk may contain a slightly higher proportion of medium- and intermediate-chain fatty acids, which may be advantageous for fat and calcium absorption in preterm infants.[138] Saturated fatty acids are found in high proportions at the *sn*-2 position of milk TG, while *sn*-1 and *sn*-3 positions are mainly occupied by unsaturated fatty acids such as oleic[139] and omega-6 fatty acids.[140]

Subsequent to their digestion and uptake in the intestine by the neonate, TG and phospholipids are synthesized by the enterocyte and assembled with other lipids and $apoB_{48}$ in chylomicrons,[141] a TG-rich lipoprotein that transports these diet-derived lipids from the intestine to the liver, where TG are hydrolyzed and their fatty acids are used to provide energy via mitochondrial oxidation.[142]

As schematically summarized in Fig. 33.4, the onset of enteral nutrition together with the initial mobilization of lipid from adipose tissue after birth result in increased concentrations of circulating NEFA and enhanced neonatal hepatic β-oxidation and ketogenesis. Early studies showed that the activity and expression of hepatic mitochondrial and peroxisomal enzymes of FAO are low in the fetus and increase rapidly after birth,[143,144] consistent with the onset of feeding the high-fat milk. During the first hours after birth, newborn infants have low plasma ketone bodies concentrations despite adequate concentrations of NEFA, but once suckling begins, circulating concentrations of ketones quickly increase.[145,146] Ketone bodies are water-soluble fatty acid derivatives that have the unique capacity to replace glucose for the energy needs during physiologic states characterized by limited carbohydrate supply.[147] For neonatal bioenergetic homeostasis, ketone body oxidation spares glucose utilization in peripheral tissues, which reduces the requirement for hepatic gluconeogenesis.[148] Thus, neonatal brain (which cannot use fatty acids for energy) metabolizes ketone bodies much more effectively than the adult brain, and their oxidation can support an important proportion of total basal energy requirements.[149] Furthermore, since the neonatal diet has high

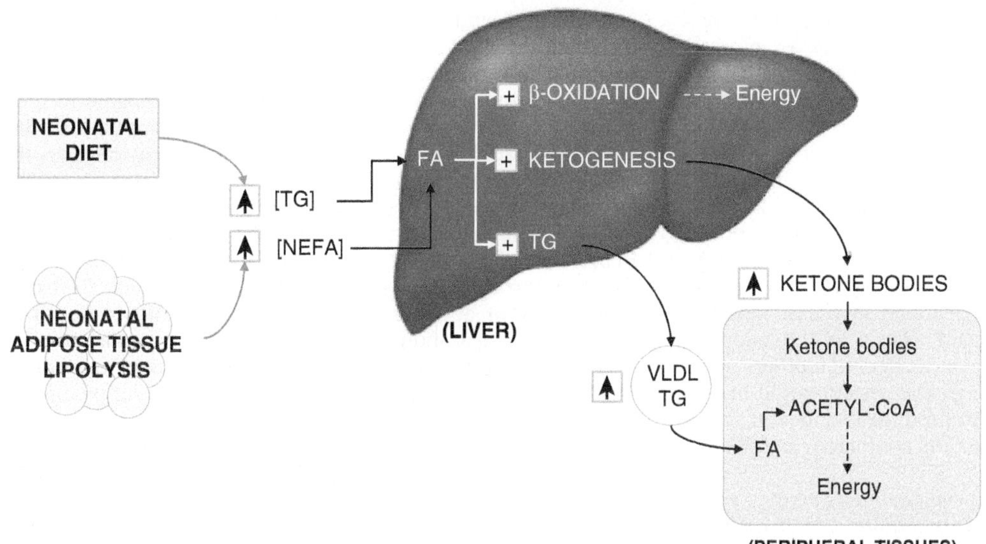

Fig. 33.4 Schematic representation of neonatal metabolic adaptations at birth. Neonatal diet and enhanced adipose tissue lipolysis increases the availability of fatty acids *(FA)* in the liver, where it is used as a source of energy through β-oxidation, and to the synthesis of hepatic ketone bodies and triglycerides *(TG)*, that could be used as a source of energy by peripheral tissues. *VLDL,* Very low-density lipoproteins.

lipid content, ketogenesis provides a discharge pathway for excess FAO and prevents buildup of acetyl-CoA.[150,151] Therefore, preservation of bioenergetic homeostasis during the transition from the carbohydrate-rich fetal diet to the high-fat, low-carbohydrate neonatal diet requires the induction of hepatic FAO, gluconeogenesis, and ketogenesis.[151]

The fatty acids that are not metabolized in the manner above are re-esterified in the liver and assembled to form very low-density lipoproteins (VLDL), which are released into the circulation to transport TG and other hepatic lipids to peripheral tissues. Lipoprotein lipase (LPL) is an enzyme present in the tissue vascular bed and catalyzes the hydrolysis of plasma TG carried in the TG-rich lipoproteins, chylomicron and VLDL; it is the key enzyme for their metabolic clearance.[152] In adults, LPL activity is only present in extrahepatic tissues, being especially high in adipose tissue.[153] However, in newborn rats, which are born with a proportionally much lower adipose tissue mass than humans, LPL expression and activity has been found in liver,[154,155] contributing to their liver hydrolysis and uptake of circulating TG and controlling the use of their fatty acids for FAO and ketogenesis.[156,157]

In human fetuses it is not known whether LPL is expressed in liver. However in newborn infants, post-heparin lipolytic activity (PHLA) has been used as a measure of LPL,[158-160] although the measure represents its presence in all of the different tissues. It has been found that PHLA activities were similar in newborn infants and adults,[160] suggesting that clearance of fat from circulation is as effective in newborn infants as in adults. PHLA activity in newborn infants has been found to correlate positively with birth weight.[161] Based on the fact that LPL activity in adipocytes correlates with fat tissue weight,[162] these interactions point to the association between the PHLA activity and fat depots that occurs during the last weeks of intrauterine life.[16] However, in both infants who are small for gestational age and in those of very low birth weight, PHLA activity was lower than in the infants of appropriate weight.[158,159,161] These findings agree with those showing that the clearance of fat in infants less mature than 32 weeks of gestation or those small for gestational age is slower than in infants of appropriate weight.[163] In fact, poor clearance of fat infused to preterm infants results in triglyceridemia, the extent of which is in inverse proportion to gestational age.[163,164]

The activity of LPL is regulated by several factors, among others by members of the angiopoietin-like (ANGPTL) protein family[165-167] such as ANGPTL4, which irreversibly inhibits LPL activity, impairing clearance of TG-rich lipoproteins from blood. There is no relationship between the concentration of ANGPTL4 and TG in cord plasma at birth. Nevertheless, an increased concentration of TG and a decreased concentration of ANGPTL4 in maternal plasma at term in pregnant women whose newborn infants had high fat mass has been reported, suggesting the existence of a maternal-fetal TG gradient and a lower concentration of the LPL inhibitor that could facilitate a greater fatty acid placental transfer that would contribute to the higher fat accumulation in the fetus.[87]

Palmitic and oleic acid contained in maternal human milk are important energy substrates,[168] but omega-3 and omega-6 fatty acids present can also be used for energy production in the perinatal period. In rats, it has been shown that giving diets rich in omega-3 fatty acids during the first days of lactation led to a higher concentration of eicosapentaenoic acid (EPA) and DHA in the offspring's liver, increased FAO, and a reciprocal decrease in glucose oxidation.[169] In human neonates, administration of omega-3 PUFAs is associated with an increased liver FAO and hypotriglyceridemia, which may ameliorate tissue lipid accumulation and increase insulin action.[170]

From studies in rats, it has been proposed that large doses of omega-3 fatty acids in the neonatal period may provide long-term health benefits[171] beyond energetic use, but in humans there are also meta-analyses that do not show clear benefits of higher administration of omega-3 fatty acids on neurodevelopment in preterm infants.[172,173] Consequently, most professional organizations and expert panels recommend not exceeding the maximum concentrations of DHA and ARA found in breast milk, equivalent to 84 and 45 mg/kg/day, respectively, which should be sufficient to compensate for intestinal malabsorption, DHA and ARA oxidation, and early deficiencies in preterm infants.[138]

LONG-TERM EFFECTS OF BREAST-FEEDING

It has been reported that breast-feeding could confer not only short-term health benefits but also be beneficial over the long-term in adult life.[174,175] One of the most characterized is the association between breast-feeding and a lower risk of childhood obesity compared with formula feeding.[176] Although breast-feeding infants can self-control the amount of milk they consume, and so may self-regulate their energy intake better than formula-fed infants,[177] there are several components in breast milk that could be responsible for its beneficial effect of avoiding later obesity. The question of whether the effects result from the nutritional composition of breast milk or from the amount consumed remains open. Several studies support the finding that formula-fed infants consume a higher volume and more energy-dense milk than breast-fed babies leading to faster growth, especially in the first weeks of life.[178-180] Thus, it appears that the first weeks of newborn life are particularly critical for long-term outcomes, and faster postnatal weight gain during this early life stage may be especially critical for the risk of later obesity.[181]

It has also been proposed that the differences in growth pattern and body composition between breast-fed and formula-fed infants might be because of a different endocrine response to feeding or to the presence of beneficial bioactive substances in breast milk.[182] Leptin, adiponectin, visfatin, ghrelin, resistin, and other adipokines have been identified in breast milk,[183-188] which appears to be their main source in the neonatal circulation, contributing to the beneficial effect of mothers' milk. Not surprisingly, immaturity of the gastric system could impair the function of these adipokines in preterm infants and could explain the differences in their action compared to full-term infants.[189]

In conclusion, the metabolic adaptations taking place after birth in human newborn infants require a high body fat content, adipokines, and hormonal settings that can facilitate appropriate fat mobilization, allowing maintenance of normal blood glucose concentrations even after prolonged starvation.[190] However, during the first hours after birth premature infants and other small for gestational age infants that have limited fat stores at birth have low plasma NEFA, glycerol, and ketone bodies concentrations,[191,192] have low lipolytic activity, develop severe hypoglycemia after a short fast,[192-194] and show delayed maturation of the gluconeogenic pathway.[193] Thus, lipids play a key role as energy source for both intrauterine and postnatal life, and alterations in the FAO pathway or in the capacity for adipose tissue development by the fetus are associated with major disorders during the perinatal stage of life.

CONCLUSION

Current wisdom holds that during pregnancy the fetus is continuously supplied through the placenta with a diet rich in glucose and amino acids and poor in fat, and is primarily dependent on glucose oxidation for energy production. However, several recessively inherited disorders in genes of the mitochondrial FAO, that cause higher frequency of prematurity, IUGR, and intrauterine death, have been characterized. The pathogenic mechanism is a lack of sufficient energy production, indicating that development of the embryo depends also on fatty acids as a major source of metabolic energy. Carnitine is needed to facilitate the transport of fatty acids across the inner mitochondrial membrane for FAO and ketogenesis. The placental transfer of carnitine has been shown to exceed the fetal carnitine requirements, and the placenta and several fetal tissues have the capacity to synthesize carnitine. Premature infants receiving parental nutrition have decreased plasma carnitine levels but increased carnitine levels and ability to utilize fatty acids when supplemented with L-carnitine. The LPL catalyzes the hydrolysis of plasma TG controlling their clearance. In contrast to adults, LPL expression and activity has been found in the liver of newborn rats, where it controls the use of fatty acids from circulating TG for FAO and ketogenesis. In humans, PHLA is used as a measure of LPL, it is associated to fat depot accumulation during the last weeks of intrauterine life, and it correlates positively with birth weight. Neonatal metabolism shifts to a catabolic condition to release energy stores like glucose from hepatic glycogen and NEFA from fetal fat stores, which become the main source of energy during the first postnatal hours and days. Preterm infants have low fat stores, in spite of which they increase lipolysis at birth generating glycerol, which is mainly converted into glucose. Decreased concentrations of stress hormones, mainly cortisol, are found in preterm babies, caused by several factors including the mode of delivery, which normally is by cesarean section. These hormonal changes contribute to the lower rate of lipolysis and gluconeogenesis in preterm compared to term newborn infants. In the newborn circulation there are several adipokines from adipose tissue that play critical roles in the energy substrate production. In newborn infants the high-fat milk diet and increased adipose tissue lipolysis results in increased circulating concentrations of NEFA and in ketogenesis. In preterm infants, dietary lipids also provide most of the energy they need to achieve a postnatal growth rate similar to that of a normal fetus at the same gestational age. The composition of infant formula should be similar to human milk although preterm infant formula should have high concentrations of medium-chain TG. These formulas are currently supplemented with LCPUFA, which in the case of omega-3 acids are associated with increases in liver FAO and hypotriacylglycerolemia, which may ameliorate tissue lipid accumulation and enhance insulin action. However, infant formulas do not contain any of the adipokines and hormones present in maternal milk, and this difference could account for the differences in growth pattern between breast-feeding and formula-feeding infants. In any case, the immature gastric system in preterm infants could impair the function of those adipokines and hormones present in breast milk explaining the differences in their action when compared to full-term infants.

ACKNOWLEDGMENTS

The authors thank Dr. Peter Dodds for editing and linguistic revision of the manuscript. Preparation of this chapter was carried out in part with grants from the Universidad San Pablo—CEU, the Fundación Ramón Areces (CIVP16A1835) of Spain, and the Spanish Ministry of Science and Innovation (SAF2012-39273).

A complete reference list is available at www.ExpertConsult.com. 

SELECT REFERENCES

2. Girard J, Ferre P, Pegorier JP, et al. Adaptations of glucose and fatty acid metabolism during perinatal period and suckling-weaning transition. *Physiol Rev.* 1992;72:507-562.
7. Oey NA, den Boer ME, Ruiter JP, et al. High activity of fatty acid oxidation enzymes in human placenta: implications for fetal-maternal disease. *J Inherit Metab Dis.* 2003;26:385-392.
8. Strauss AW. Surprising? Perhaps not. Long-chain fatty acid oxidation during human fetal development. *Pediatr Res.* 2005;57:753-754.
12. Bougneres PF. Stable isotope tracers and the determination of fuel fluxes in newborn infants. *Biol Neonate.* 1987;52(Suppl 1):87-96.
18. Widdowson EM. Chemical composition of newly born mammals. *Nature.* 1950;166:626-628.
20. Novak M, Melichar V, Hahn P. Postnatal changes in the blood serum content of glycerol and fatty acids in human infants. *Biol Neonat.* 1964;7:179-184.
23. Senterre J, Karlberg P. Respiratory quotient and metabolic rate in normal full-term and small-for-date newborn infants. *Acta Paediatr Scand.* 1970;59:653-658.
26. Sunehag A, Gustafsson J, Ewald U. Glycerol carbon contributes to hepatic glucose production during the first eight hours in healthy term infants. *Acta Paediatr.* 1996;85:1339-1343.
36. Saint L, Smith M, Hartmann PE. The yield and nutrient content of colostrum and milk of women from giving birth to 1 month post-partum. *Br J Nutr.* 1984;52:87-95.
38. Bennett MJ, Rinaldo P, Strauss AW. Inborn errors of mitochondrial fatty acid oxidation. *Crit Rev Clin Lab Sci.* 2000;37:1-44.
47. Dutta-Roy AK. Cellular uptake of long-chain fatty acids: role of membrane-associated fatty-acid-binding/transport proteins. *Cell Mol Life Sci.* 2000;57:1360-1372.
54. Eaton S. Control of mitochondrial beta-oxidation flux. *Prog Lipid Res.* 2002;41:197-239.
65. Schmidt-Sommerfeld E, Penn D, Sodha RJ, et al. Transfer and metabolism of carnitine and carnitine esters in the in vitro perfused human placenta. *Pediatr Res.* 1985;19:700-706.
66. Oey NA, van Vlies N, Wijburg FA, et al. L-carnitine is synthesized in the human fetal-placental unit: potential roles in placental and fetal metabolism. *Placenta.* 2006;27:841-846.
74. Ward Platt M, Deshpande S. Metabolic adaptation at birth. *Semin Fetal Neonatal Med.* 2005;10:341-350.
79. Gustafsson J. Neonatal energy substrate production. *Indian J Med Res.* 2009;130:618-623.

83. Sunehag A, Ewald U, Gustafsson J. Extremely preterm infants (< 28 weeks) are capable of gluconeogenesis from glycerol on their first day of life. *Pediatr Res.* 1996;40:553–557.
86. Vogl SE, Worda C, Egarter C, et al. Mode of delivery is associated with maternal and fetal endocrine stress response. *BJOG.* 2006;113:441–445.
87. Ortega-Senovilla H, Schaefer-Graf U, Meitzner K, et al. Decreased concentrations of the lipoprotein lipase inhibitor angiopoietin-like protein 4 and increased serum triacylglycerol are associated with increased neonatal fat mass in pregnant women with gestational diabetes mellitus. *J Clin Endocrinol Metab.* 2013;98:3430–3437.
92. Ortega-Senovilla H, Schaefer-Graf U, Meitzner K, et al. Lack of relationship between cord serum angiopoietin-like protein 4 (ANGPTL4) and lipolytic activity in human neonates born by spontaneous delivery. *PLoS One.* 2013;8:e81201.
96. Kyriakakou M, Malamitsi-Puchner A, Militsi H, et al. Leptin and adiponectin concentrations in intrauterine growth restricted and appropriate for gestational age fetuses, neonates, and their mothers. *Eur J Endocrinol.* 2008;158:343–348.
100. Minokoshi Y, Kim YB, Peroni OD, et al. Leptin stimulates fatty-acid oxidation by activating AMP-activated protein kinase. *Nature.* 2002;415:339–343.
101. Harris RB. Direct and indirect effects of leptin on adipocyte metabolism. *Biochim Biophys Acta.* 2014;1842:414–423.
103. Shirwany NA, Zou MH. AMPK: a cellular metabolic and redox sensor. A minireview. *Front Biosci.* 2014;19:447–474.
105. Gautron L, Elmquist JK. Sixteen years and counting: an update on leptin in energy balance. *J Clin Invest.* 2011;121:2087–2093.
109. Wang LJ, Mu SC, Cheng I, et al. Decreased leptin concentration in neonates is associated with enhanced postnatal growth during the first year. *Kaohsiung J Med Sci.* 2012;28:521–525.
110. Bozzola E, Meazza C, Arvigo M, et al. Role of adiponectin and leptin on body development in infants during the first year of life. *Ital J Pediatr.* 2010;36:26–33.
111. Ng PC, Lam CW, Lee CH, et al. Leptin and metabolic hormones in preterm newborns. *Arch Dis Child Fetal Neonatal Ed.* 2000;83:F198–F202.
115. Chen J, Tan B, Karteris E, et al. Secretion of adiponectin by human placenta: differential modulation of adiponectin and its receptors by cytokines. *Diabetologia.* 2006;49:1292–12302.
119. Qiao L, Kinney B, Schaack J, et al. Adiponectin inhibits lipolysis in mouse adipocytes. *Diabetes.* 2011;60:1519–1527.
130. Ng PC, Lee CH, Lam CW, et al. Resistin in preterm and term newborns: relation to anthropometry, leptin, and insulin. *Pediatr Res.* 2005;58:725–730.
133. Nakano Y, Itabashi K, Sakurai M, et al. Preterm infants have altered adiponectin levels at term-equivalent age even if they do not present with extrauterine growth restriction. *Horm Res Paediatr.* 2013;80:147–153.
136. Lapillonne A. Enteral and parenteral lipid requirements of preterm infants. *World Rev Nutr Diet.* 2014;110:82–98.
141. Demignot S. Beilstein F, Morel E. Triglyceride-rich lipoproteins and cytosolic lipid droplets in enterocytes: key players in intestinal physiology and metabolic disorders. *Biochimie.* 2014;96:48–55.
142. Dallinga-Thie GM, Franssen R, Mooij HL, et al. The metabolism of triglyceride-rich lipoproteins revisited: new players, new insight. *Atherosclerosis.* 2010;211:1–8.
147. McGarry JD, Foster DW. Regulation of hepatic fatty acid oxidation and ketone body production. *Annu Rev Biochem.* 1980;49:395–420.
148. Williamson DH. Ketone body metabolism during development. *Fed Proc.* 1985;44:2342–2346.
151. Cotter DG, Ercal B, d'Avignon DA, et al. Impact of peripheral ketolytic deficiency on hepatic ketogenesis and gluconeogenesis during the transition to birth. *J Biol Chem.* 2013;288:19739–19749.
156. Ramirez I, Llobera M, Herrera E. Circulating triacylglycerols, lipoproteins, and tissue lipoprotein lipase activities in rat mothers and offspring during the perinatal period: effect of postmaturity. *Metabolism.* 1983;32:333–341.
157. Grinberg DR, Ramirez I, Vilaro S, et al. Starvation enhances lipoprotein lipase activity in the liver of the newborn rat. *Biochim Biophys Acta.* 1985;833:217–222.
165. Kersten S. Regulation of lipid metabolism via angiopoietin-like proteins. *Biochem Soc Trans.* 2005;33:1059–1062.
170. Drevon CA. Fatty acids and expression of adipokines. *Biochim Biophys Acta.* 2005;1740:287–292.
171. Ryan AS, Astwood JD, Gautier S, et al. Effects of long-chain polyunsaturated fatty acid supplementation on neurodevelopment in childhood: a review of human studies. *Prostaglandins Leukot Essent Fatty Acids.* 2010;82:305–314.
174. Lucas A. Scientific evidence for breastfeeding. *Nestle Nutr Inst Workshop Ser.* 2019;90:1–12.
176. Arenz S, Ruckerl R, Koletzko B, et al. Breast-feeding and childhood obesity–a systematic review. *Int J Obes Relat Metab Disord.* 2004;28:1247–1256.
177. Brown A, Lee M. Breastfeeding during the first year promotes satiety responsiveness in children aged 18-24 months. *Pediatr Obes.* 2012;7:382–390.
182. Savino F, Fissore MF, Liguori SA, et al. Can hormones contained in mothers' milk account for the beneficial effect of breast-feeding on obesity in children? *Clin Endocrinol (Oxf).* 2009;71:757–765.
186. Weyermann M, Beermann C, Brenner H, et al. Adiponectin and leptin in maternal serum, cord blood, and breast milk. *Clin Chem.* 2006;52:2095–2102.
187. Savino F, Nanni GE, Maccario S, et al. Breast-fed infants have higher leptin values than formula-fed infants in the first four months of life. *J Pediatr Endocrinol Metab.* 2004;17:1527–1532.

Ketone Body Metabolism in the Neonate

34

Baris Ercal | Peter A. Crawford

INTRODUCTION

The metabolism of ketone bodies is evolutionarily conserved among all the domains of life on Earth.[1-3] In mammals, ketone bodies are predominantly synthesized in the liver from acetyl coenzyme A (CoA) derived from fatty acid oxidation and are then transported to peripheral tissues for oxidation during physiologic states consisting of limited carbohydrate and surplus fatty acid availability (reviewed by Robinson and Williamson,[4] McGarry and Foster,[5] and Cotter and colleagues[6]; Fig. 34.1A and B). During the neonatal period, starvation, and adherence to low-carbohydrate diets, ketone body oxidation contributes significantly to energy metabolism within numerous extrahepatic tissues (Fig. 34.2). In these carbohydrate-limiting states, circulating ketone body concentrations can increase from approximately 50 μmol/L in a normal fed mature human to up to 7 mmol/L. In neonatal humans, or after a prolonged fast in healthy adults, circulating ketone body concentrations can rise to approximately 1 mmol/L. In certain pathologic states such as diabetic ketoacidosis, ketone body concentrations can reach as high as 20 mmol/L if the state is left untreated.[2,4,7] Although ketone bodies often serve energetic roles, ketone body metabolism also provides substrates for de novo lipogenesis and sterol biosynthesis in many tissues, including the developing brain, lactating mammary gland, and liver (see Fig. 34.1C).[8-11] Within the mitochondria, hepatic ketogenesis converges with the fundamental metabolic pathways of fatty acid β-oxidation, the tricarboxylic acid (TCA) cycle, and gluconeogenesis (Fig. 34.3). In various disease states, including infantile ketoacidosis and type 1 diabetes, dysfunctional ketone body metabolism is observed and may even play a role in pathogenesis. Ketone body metabolism also shifts over the course of normal development and aging.[12-20] The dynamic role of ketone body metabolism in the neonatal period will be the primary focus of this chapter.

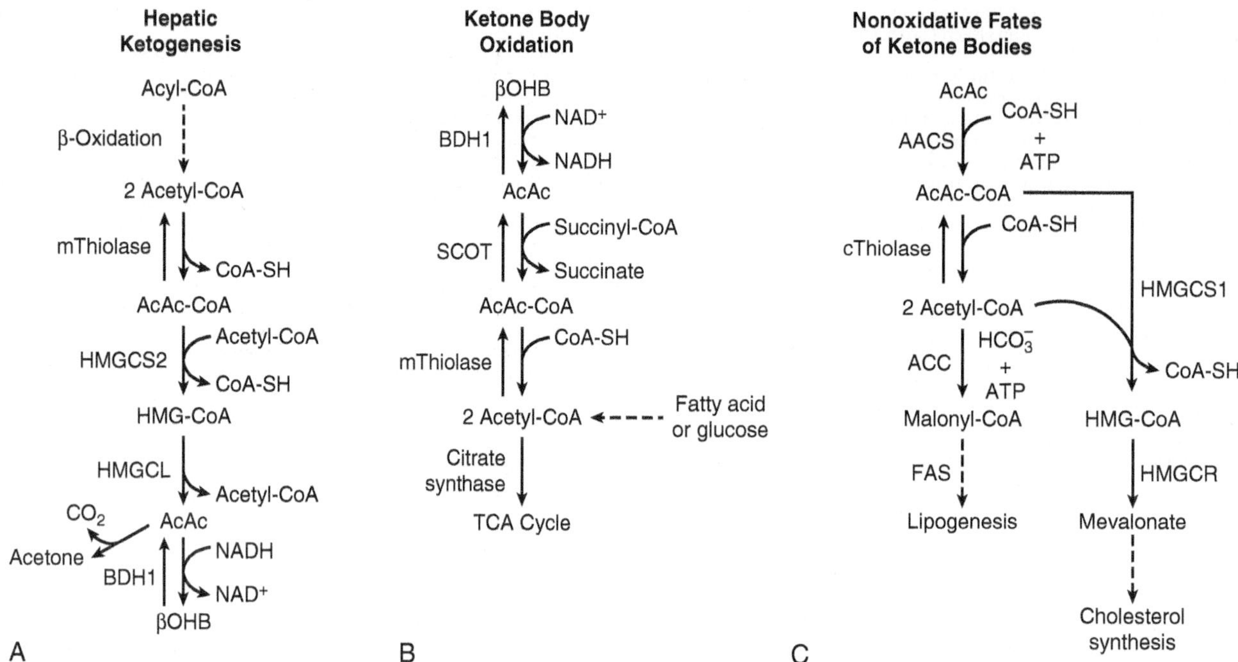

Fig. 34.1 Pathways of ketone body metabolism. (A) Hepatic pathway of mitochondrial ketogenesis via 3-hydroxy-3-methylglutaryl coenzyme A *(HMG-CoA)* synthase 2 *(HMGCS2)*. (B) Oxidation of ketone bodies within mitochondria of peripheral tissues via succinyl coenzyme A:3-oxoacid coenzyme A transferase *(SCOT)*. Substrate competition with acetyl coenzyme A (acetyl-CoA) derived from glycolysis or fatty acid oxidation is also shown. (C) Nonoxidative metabolic fates of ketone bodies including cytoplasmic lipogenesis and cholesterol synthesis. *AACS,* Acetoacetyl coenzyme A synthetase; *AcAc-CoA,* acetoacetyl coenzyme A; *ACC,* acetyl coenzyme A carboxylase; *ATP,* adenosine triphosphate; *BDH1,* β-hydroxybutyrate dehydrogenase 1; *βOHB,* β-hydroxybutyrate; *CoA,* coenzyme A; *CoA-SH,* free coenzyme A; *FAS,* fatty acid synthase; *HMGCL,* HMG-CoA lyase; *HMGCS1,* HMG-CoA synthase 1; *HMGCR,* HMG-CoA reductase; *NAD+,* oxidized nicotinamide adenine dinucleotide; *NADH,* reduced nicotinamide adenine dinucleotide; *PDH,* pyruvate dehydrogenase; *TCA,* tricarboxylic acid; *cThiolase,* cytoplasmic thiolase; *mThiolase,* mitochondrial thiolase.

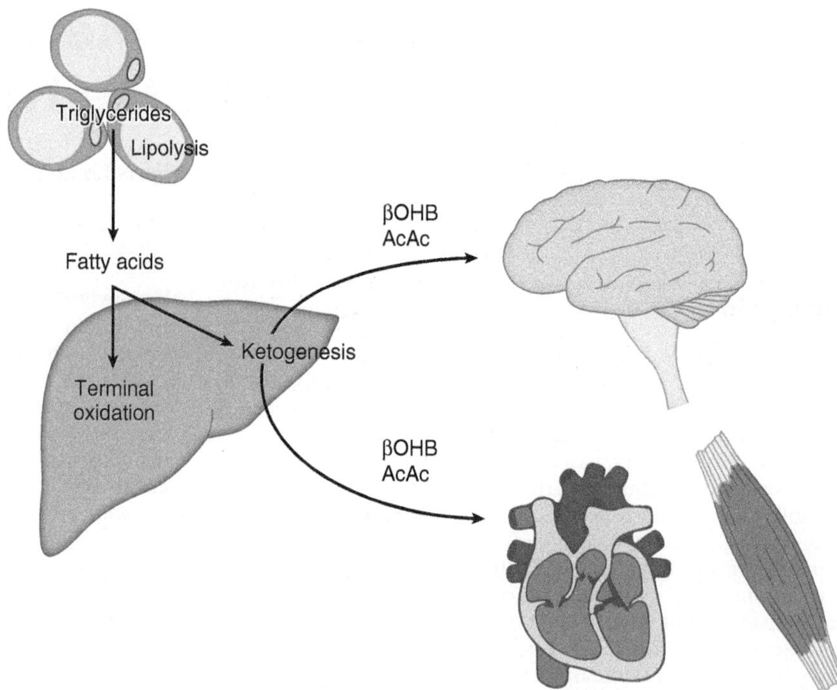

Fig. 34.2 Integrative physiology of ketone body metabolism. Intertissue coordination of hepatic ketogenesis and peripheral disposal of ketone bodies. *AcAc,* Acetoacetate; *βOHB,* β-hydroxybutyrate.

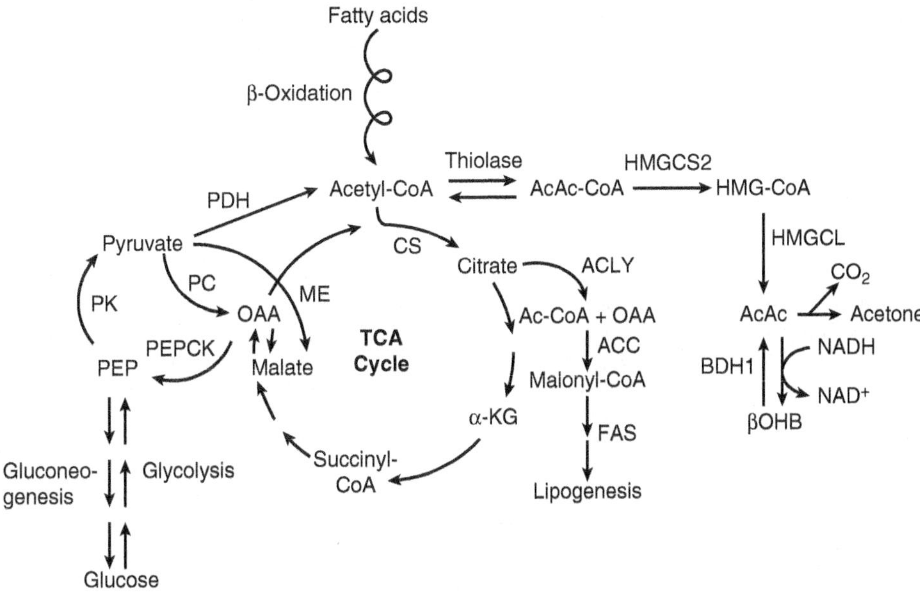

Fig. 34.3 Integration of ketogenesis with hepatic mitochondrial metabolism. Ketogenesis is shown here interfacing with the hepatic mitochondrial metabolic pathways, including the tricarboxylic acid *(TCA)* cycle, lipogenesis, anaplerosis, cataplerosis, and glucose metabolism. *AcAc,* Acetoacetate; *ACC,* acetyl coenzyme A carboxylase; *ACLY,* adenosine triphosphate citrate lyase; *BDH1,* β-hydroxybutyrate dehydrogenase 1; *βOHB,* β-hydroxybutyrate; *CoA,* coenzyme A; *CS,* citrate synthase; *FAS,* fatty acid synthase; *HMG,* 3-hydroxy-3-methylglutaryl; *HMGCL,* 3-hydroxy-3-methylglutaryl coenzyme A lyase; *HMGCS2,* 3-hydroxy-3-methylglutaryl coenzyme A synthase 2; *α-KG,* α-ketoglutarate; *ME,* malic enzyme; *NAD+,* oxidized nicotinamide adenine dinucleotide; *NADH,* reduced nicotinamide adenine dinucleotide; *OAA,* oxaloacetate; *PC,* pyruvate carboxylase; *PDH,* pyruvate dehydrogenase; *PEP,* phosphoenolpyruvate; *PEPCK,* phosphoenolpyruvate carboxykinase; *PK,* pyruvate kinase.

AVAILABILITY OF KETONE BODIES

Under physiologic conditions, the rate of utilization of ketone bodies is directly proportional to their concentration in the circulation, which in turn represents a balance between production (ketogenesis) by the liver and disposal by peripheral tissues (ketolysis). Ketone bodies are excreted in the urine (ketonuria) when the renal reabsorption threshold is exceeded. The relationship between production and disposal can be disturbed if the utilization of ketone bodies is inhibited by drugs,[21,22] with congenital absence of key enzymes required for ketone body utilization,[23] or in insulin-deficient states secondary to a metabolic defect in utilization.[24]

The concentration of ketone bodies in the blood is extremely sensitive to alterations in the physiologic state. The balance of ketone body production and disposal determines the steady-state circulating concentration of ketone bodies, and although it is inappropriate to apply the definitions universally among all individuals, in general terms, in humans *normoketonemia* is characterized by a serum total ketone body concentration of less than 0.2 mmol/L, ***ketonemia*** is characterized by a serum total ketone body concentration of greater than 0.2 mmol/L, and ***ketoacidosis*** is characterized by a serum total ketone body concentration of greater than 7 mmol/L.[25] In adult humans, small but characteristic diurnal changes in blood ketone body concentrations have been observed.[26] Larger increases in concentration occur with fasting (in both humans and rats), with consumption of a high-fat diet, after exercise, in late pregnancy, and during suckling (Table 34.1). In pregnancy, blood ketone bodies are available to the fetus in prevailing concentrations because the placenta appears to be freely permeable to the ketone bodies acetoacetate (AcAc) and β-hydroxybutyrate (βOHB).[27,28]

Table 34.1 Range of Blood Ketone Body Concentrations in Humans and Rats.

Clinical/Experimental Condition	Ketone Body Concentration (mmol/L)[a]	
	Human	**Rat**
Fed normal diet	~0.1	≤0.3
Fed high-fat diet	≤3	4–5
Fasted: 12–24 h	≤0.3	1–2
Fasted: 48–72 h	2–3	2–3
After exercise	≤2	≤2
Late pregnancy	≤1	≤0.3
Late pregnancy after 48-h fast	4–6	6–15
Neonate: 0–1 day	0.2–0.5	0.2
Neonate: 5–10 days	0.7–1.0	0.5–1.1
Hypoglycemia	1.5–5	–
Untreated diabetes mellitus	≤25	≤10

[a]Concentrations of total ketone bodies (acetoacetate plus 3-hydroxybutyrate measured by enzyme assay) in whole blood.

KETONEMIA IN PREGNANCY

The major substrate of the mammalian fetus is glucose supplied by the mother.[28] However, the concentration of ketone bodies in maternal blood is increased in the last trimester of pregnancy,[25,27] and high concentrations are attained during delivery, particularly if it is prolonged (ketosis of labor).[27,28] This increase in the concentration of blood ketone bodies may be related in part to the decrease in food intake around parturition because hyperketonemia develops more rapidly with fasting in women in the second trimester of pregnancy than in nonpregnant control subjects.[29,30] Poorly controlled diabetes during pregnancy (including gestational diabetes) leads to wide fluctuations in the concentrations of blood ketone bodies.[31]

KETONEMIA IN THE NEONATAL PERIOD

During the suckling period the neonate is presented with a relatively high-fat and low-carbohydrate diet. Both humans and rats have marked hyperketonemia in the early suckling period, compared with the respective adult fed values (see Table 34.1). By contrast, the concentrations of ketone bodies are not increased to the same extent in the blood of puppies,[32] piglets,[33] and lambs.[34] Fatty acids (both long-chain fatty acids [LCFAs] and medium-chain fatty acids [MCFAs]) are the major precursors of ketone bodies, and one contributing reason for the species differences in neonatal ketonemia may be the fat content of the maternal milk (rat milk contains 14.8 g fat/100 g; sheep milk contains 5.3 g fat/100 g). Some mammalian species, including pigs, do not leverage ketogenesis as a high-capacity conduit for disposal of excess acetyl-CoA, instead using acetate to export acetyl-CoA carbons.[35,36]

Neonatal hyperketonemia in humans is a physiologic event; thus any marked deviation in blood ketone body concentration likely indicates underlying disease.[37] Increased concentrations of ketone bodies may accompany the hypoglycemia associated with inborn errors of metabolism, and a decrease may occur in hyperinsulinism. It is therefore advisable to measure blood ketone body concentrations by a specific enzymatic method[38] in neonates presenting with hypoglycemia or any other abnormality in the concentration of circulating substrates. For example, infants born small for their gestational age have increased blood concentrations of gluconeogenic substrates, in association with decreased blood ketone body concentrations.[37,39] The latter is due to defective development of the ketogenic capacity of the liver and decreased availability of peripheral adipose tissue to supply the key ketogenic substrate nonesterified fatty acids (see later).

REGULATION OF KETOGENESIS

Insight into the regulation of ketogenesis has increased dramatically with the use of novel genomic, proteomic, and metabolomic analyses. Earlier investigations were based mainly on studies in rats—in particular, during the fed-to-starved transition, as well as from work on perfused livers or isolated hepatocytes from adult rats. Consequently, in the review of regulation of ketogenesis in the adult presented in this section, comparison is made with the neonate or fetus whenever information is available. Further details are available in more detailed reviews.[5,6,40-43]

EXTRAHEPATIC REGULATION

Regulation of ketogenesis is both extrahepatic and intrahepatic (see Fig. 34.2). The major precursors of ketone bodies in the postabsorptive state are LCFAs, and in all physiologic situations associated with hyperketonemia, including those of the neonatal period, the plasma concentrations of LCFAs are increased (see Table 34.1).[44-47] Extraction of LCFAs by the liver is concentration dependent, and a direct relationship between their concentration and the rate of ketogenesis exists in both rats and humans.[48]

ADIPOSE TISSUE LIPOLYSIS

In the adult, a key factor in determining the supply of LCFAs to the liver is their rate of release (lipolysis) from adipose tissue triacylglycerol stores. Lipolysis is initiated by activation of adipose tissue lipases, adipose triglyceride lipase, and hormone-sensitive lipase.[49] Glucagon, epinephrine, norepinephrine, and thyroxine increase enzyme activity, whereas insulin (as well as some prostaglandins) has the opposite effect.[50] Isolated human adipocytes from neonates are very sensitive to the lipolytic effects of thyrotropin,[51] which increases in concentration immediately after birth and may therefore be involved in the regulation of lipolysis in the perinatal period. A decrease in blood glucose concentration (e.g., in starvation, fat feeding) along with a concomitant decrease in plasma insulin concentration leads to an increase in lipolysis and efflux of nonesterified fatty acids from adipose tissue. Carbohydrate provision increases insulin concentrations and thereby inhibits lipolysis. The rate of ketogenesis can therefore respond in a reciprocal way to the availability of glucose in the circulation, so an alternative fuel for the brain is provided when needed (see Fig. 34.2). During suckling in the rat, the plasma insulin-to-glucagon ratio is decreased, favoring lipolysis.[52,53]

Ketone bodies regulate their own formation by feedback mechanisms on adipose tissue to decrease lipolysis. Current evidence suggests there are two mechanisms: (1) direct inhibition of lipolysis by ketone bodies via binding to the G protein–coupled niacin receptor GPR109A and (2) an indirect effect mediated by stimulation of insulin secretion.[4,54,55] Work with the perfused rat pancreas suggests that ketone bodies increase insulin secretion only at concentrations greater than 1 mmol/L.[56] These feedback mechanisms have not been investigated in neonates.

In the suckling neonate, the MCFAs (i.e., 12 or fewer carbons) of maternal milk are an important source of precursors for ketogenesis.[57] These are in the form of triacylglycerols (one MCFA and two LCFAs per triacylglycerol) and are hydrolyzed by the action of lingual lipase. They are rapidly absorbed from the stomach into the portal venous system[58] and are therefore directly available to the liver, unlike LCFAs derived from milk lipids, which are transported as triacylglycerols (within chylomicrons) by way of the lymphatic system and initially enter the peripheral circulation. In the neonatal period, chylomicrons may provide a direct source of LCFAs for the liver, as suggested by the presence of lipoprotein lipase (responsible for the hydrolysis of triacylglycerols contained in chylomicrons to LCFAs) in neonatal rat liver.[59] However, the total lipoprotein lipase activity in liver constitutes only a small percentage (3%) of that in the whole body,[57] the rest being contributed by muscle and adipose tissue.

INTRAHEPATIC REGULATION

The liver is the primary tissue capable of synthesis and release of ketone bodies into the circulation, primarily due to the relatively hepatocyte-specific expression of the fate-committing ketogenic enzyme mitochondrial 3-hydroxy-3-methylglutaryl (HMG)-CoA synthase 2 (HMGCS2). Ketone bodies can also be formed by the intestinal mucosa of neonatal rats via enterocyte-derived HMGCS2.[60,61] Expression of HMGCS2 in intestinal mucosa is suppressed in weaned suckling rats but is regulated by the gut microbiome.[62-64] The rate of intestinal ketogenesis is less than 10% of that in liver of suckling animals, but this mechanism does provide an additional strategy for supplying ketone bodies to developing tissues.[57]

HEPATIC FATTY ACID CATABOLISM

LCFAs hydrolyzed from triacylglycerols in adipose tissue are transported in the plasma bound to albumin, cross the cell membrane as free fatty acids, and then bind again to cytosolic binding proteins.[4] Within the liver, the LCFAs either can be reesterified to form triacylglycerols (for subsequent secretion as very-low-density lipoprotein) and phospholipids or can enter the mitochondria by way of the carnitine palmitoyltransferase (CPT) system to undergo β-oxidation. The resulting yield of acetyl-CoA can (1) be converted to the ketone bodies AcAc and βOHB via a series of four mitochondrial enzymatic reactions referred to as the HMG-CoA pathway (see Fig. 34.1A),[65-68] (2) enter the TCA cycle, where it can undergo terminal oxidation, or (3) pass out of mitochondria as citrate to be used as a cytosolic substrate for fatty acid or sterol biosynthesis (see Figs. 34.2 and 34.3).[69] By contrast, MCFAs are not converted to triacylglycerols in mammalian liver and directly traverse the inner mitochondrial membrane, bypassing the CPT system. Within the mitochondrial matrix, the MCFAs are converted to the corresponding acyl-CoA derivatives by acyl-CoA synthetases and undergo β-oxidation. Ketone bodies efflux from hepatocytes via SLC16 members of the monocarboxylate transporter (MCT) family, enter the circulation, are transported into cells of extrahepatic tissues through MCT-dependent mechanisms, and are ultimately oxidized.[70] Mechanisms of ketone body transport into and out of mitochondria have not been definitively established.

MITOCHONDRIAL 3-HYDROXY-3-METHYLGLUTARYL COENZYME A SYNTHASE REGULATION

The mitochondrial matrix enzyme HMGCS2 catalyzes the formation of HMG-CoA from acetoacetyl-CoA and acetyl-CoA. A cytosolic HMG-CoA synthase, HMG-CoA synthase 1 (HMGCS1), catalyzes the same reaction in the sterol biosynthetic pathway (see Fig. 34.1C). *HMGCS2* diverged from *HMGCS1* between 400 million and 900 million years ago, and this occurred, in part, to support the emergence of early vertebrates and the development of larger brains.[71] In the 1960s, HMGCS2 was proposed by Williamson and colleagues[72] to be the fate-committing enzyme of hepatic ketogenesis, and subsequent experiments by separate groups confirmed this.[73]

Expression of the *Hmgcs2* gene and the encoded protein is dynamically regulated throughout various physiologic contexts, including the transition to extrauterine life, starvation, diabetes, aging, and during adherence to ketogenic diets.[2,12,74-77] Transcriptional regulation of *Hmgcs2* includes methylation of its 5′ regulatory sequences, which silences *Hmgcs2* transcription in fetal liver as well as in nonketogenic adult tissues.[78] At birth these regulatory regions of hepatic *Hmgcs2* become hypomethylated, allowing it to respond to circulating hormones.[78-80] Insulin and glucagon regulate *Hmgcs2* transcription via sequestration of forkhead box A2 (FOXA2) from the nucleus or activation of cyclic adenosine monophosphate (cAMP) regulatory element binding protein, respectively.[64,67,76,79,81] Free fatty acids induce *Hmgcs2* expression in a peroxisome proliferator–activated receptor α (PPARα)-dependent manner.[82,83] Inhibition of mammalian target of rapamycin complex 1 signaling has been identified as a primary mechanism responsible for relieving repression of PPARα transcriptional activity and thus inducing ketogenesis during the fasting period.[12,84] HMGCS2 may translocate to the nucleus and play a role as a transcriptional cofactor for PPARα and induce its own gene transcription.[85,86]

Using an established PPARα-knockout mouse model, a study assessed the impact of the loss of this transcription factor specifically in the livers of neonatal mice. Livers of neonatal PPAR-knockout mice exhibited surprisingly normal terminal fatty acid oxidation, despite decreased expression of acyl-CoA dehydrogenases. However, PPARα-deficient neonates exhibited impaired ketogenesis, with associated decreases in messenger RNA (mRNA) and protein abundances of both HMGCS2 and βOHB dehydrogenase 1 (BDH1). These knockout mice accumulated a substantial amount of triacylglyerols in their livers, thus implicating ketogenic deficiency in defective hepatic lipid metabolism.[87] PPARα-dependent regulation of ketogenesis during the neonatal period and starvation is mediated via hepatic fibroblast growth factor 21, an important circulating biomarker and signaling molecule involved in glucose and lipid metabolism in a variety of tissues.[82,88-90] HMGCS2 also appears to regulate fibroblast growth factor 21 in a positive feedback loop, although this observation requires further experimental evaluation.[91]

Since the resolution of the crystal structure of human HMGCS2,[92] ongoing investigations have addressed the role of posttranslational modifications in regulating enzyme catalytic activity and the subsequent impact on ketogenesis among other cellular metabolic pathways. Studies have demonstrated that HMGCS2 is regulated by lysine acetylation and succinylation, as well as via serine phosphorylation. Two members of the sirtuin family of oxidized nicotinamide adenine dinucleotide dependent deacylases, sirtuin 3 and sirtuin 5, were further shown to deacetylate and desuccinylate HMGCS2, respectively. Lysine deacetylation and desuccinylation, and serine phosphorylation all increase HMGCS2 catalytic activity.[93-96] Although these posttranslational modifications alter HMGCS2 activity in vitro, their roles and effects in vivo have yet to be determined.

A transgenic mouse model of hepatic HMGCS2 overexpression revealed augmented ketogenesis, normoglycemia, normal plasma triglyceride concentrations, diminished concentrations of circulating fatty acids, and hyperketonemia.[97] Unfortunately, this model was not explored in neonatal, dietary, or metabolic contexts other than the adult fed state. A more recent study revealed the roles of HMGCS2 in carbohydrate-laden, non-classically ketogenic states using an antisense oligonucleotide-based approach to knockdown *Hmgcs2* to generate ketogenesis-insufficient mice. This model revealed alterations in TCA cycle activity and increased glucose and fatty acid synthesis in ketogenesis-insufficient animals, indicating redirection of acetyl-CoA handling. When given a high-fat diet, adult ketogenesis-insufficient mice exhibited features of nonalcoholic steatohepatitis, including liver damage, inflammation, and severely dysfunctional mitochondrial metabolism. These findings reveal unexpected roles for ketogenesis as a regulator of substrate flux through mitochondrial and cytosolic metabolic pathways even during physiologic states that are not classically ketogenic.[98] Partial ketogenic insufficiency was also induced in neonatal mice. Even with modest reductions in HMGCS2 levels and the circulating levels of ketone bodies, a sixfold increase in hepatic triglyceride content was observed in mildly ketogenic-insufficient animals. This striking discrepancy reinforces ketogenesis as a potential target in dysfunctional fat metabolism during the neonatal period.

KETOGENIC ADAPTATIONS OF NEONATAL LIVER

Livers of fetal rats have a low capacity for fatty acid catabolism and ketogenesis, but these functions rapidly increase after birth. Available evidence indicates that the capacity of the liver for LCFA catabolism increases in the suckling period. A number of the key enzymes show higher activities,[99-101] particularly CPT I, the concentration of which increases at birth and attains values 3 to 6 times higher than those of the adult within a few days of parturition; it then declines rapidly on weaning.[101] Increases in enzyme activity[99-103] are paralleled by higher rates of ketogenesis from LCFAs in isolated hepatocytes from suckling rats than in cells from adult rats.[102,104] These enzymatic changes also correlate with nutrient supply. During the prenatal period there is a steady supply of carbohydrates and protein via the placenta, whereas free fatty acids are either unable to cross this barrier or are unable to be metabolized by fetal tissues. After birth a short-term starvation (which in human neonates stimulates lipolysis of peripheral adipose stores) precedes the suckling period, which is marked by ingestion of the high-fat, low-carbohydrate diet of maternal milk. These dietary changes correspond to hormonal levels, gene expression patterns, and ultimately substrate utilization during the fetal and neonatal periods (as reviewed by Girard and colleagues[77]). The rate of ketogenesis from MCFAs is not increased in hepatocytes from suckling rats compared with that in cells from adult animals.[102] Increased ketogenesis from LCFAs during the neonatal period is connected with either their esterification or their entry into the mitochondria via CPT.

MALONYL COENZYME A

In adult liver, CPT I is regulated by short-term changes in the concentration of carnitine (a cosubstrate) and malonyl-CoA, which is a potent inhibitor of CPT I.[5] Malonyl-CoA is a key intermediate in the conversion of carbohydrate to fat, and the hepatic concentration is directly correlated with the rate of lipogenesis (de novo fatty acid synthesis).[105] In liver, a major lipogenic precursor is pyruvate, formed from lactate returning to the liver as a product of glycolysis in peripheral tissues or from hepatic glucose through glucose uptake or glycogenolysis and then glycolysis. Therefore the rate of lipogenesis and the concentration of malonyl-CoA generally indicate the carbohydrate status of the liver: a high rate of lipogenesis is associated with an elevated malonyl-CoA concentration, inhibition of CPT I, and a decreased rate of ketogenesis. Conversely, a decrease in lipogenesis secondary to lack of substrate or hormonal inactivation of the malonyl-CoA–synthesizing enzyme acetyl-CoA carboxylase (ACC)[106] results in a decrease in malonyl-CoA concentration and stimulation of ketogenesis due to increased entry of long-chain acyl-CoA into the mitochondria. In addition, the sensitivity of CPT I to inhibition by malonyl-CoA is affected by a change in the physiologic state.[107-111]

The rate of lipogenesis in isolated hepatocytes from suckling animals[102] or livers of suckling animals in vivo[112] is low, partially due to dietary alterations but mainly due to the decrease in the activities of key lipogenic enzymes (e.g., ACC,[113] fatty acid synthase[114]), a pattern that is rapidly reversed on weaning. Hepatic malonyl-CoA concentration is very low during suckling. This fact, together with the decreased sensitivity of CPT I to inhibition by malonyl-CoA,[110,111] suggests that in the suckling neonate, regulation of ketogenesis depends on substrate supply, increased capacity of the mitochondria for fatty acid catabolism, particularly the entry of LCFA, and an increased expression of the key catalytic enzymes of ketone body production. Still to be determined is the nature of the signal or signals that bring about the stimulation of ketogenesis immediately after birth.[77,80,115] One contributor is the sharp and rapid decrease in the insulin-to-glucagon ratio,[53,77] but observations also suggest that fatty-acid-ligand-activated PPARα-dependent DNA demethylation regulates the fatty acid β-oxidation genes in the postnatal liver.[116]

INSULIN AND GLUCAGON

Hormones regulate the supply of LCFAs to the liver, and insulin and glucagon can also act directly on the liver. Glucagon or dibutyryl cAMP—its second messenger—stimulates ketogenesis from LCFAs in perfused livers[117,118] and isolated hepatocytes[102] from adult rats. Dibutyryl cAMP or glucagon does not increase ketogenesis from MCFAs,[119,120] suggesting that the site of action of glucagon is at the disposition of long-chain acyl-CoA between the pathways of esterification and β-oxidation. A possible mechanism for the effects of glucagon on ketogenesis is suggested by the finding that the hormone (or cAMP) inhibits hepatic lipogenesis in vivo[121] and in vitro[121,122] and consequently decreases the concentration of malonyl-CoA.[105] The site of inhibition is ACC, which is inactivated by glucagon through increased phosphorylation of the protein.[106] A separate mechanism by which glucagon regulates ketogenesis is via direct activation of HMGCS2 by it desuccinylating the enzyme and thus relieving it of this inhibitory modification.[66,67] Glucagon was also found to induce the acetylation and activation of the transcription factor FOXA2, inducing a gene expression profile of increased fatty acid oxidation and ketogenesis.[123]

Decreased esterification of LCFAs by microsomal fractions isolated from livers of fed rats perfused with dibutyryl cAMP has been reported.[124] Activation of CPT I by glucagon (or cAMP) has been described.[125] In hepatocytes from suckling rats, dibutyryl cAMP has no effect on ketogenesis.[102] This lack of effect may be due to the elevation of cAMP concentration in neonatal hepatocytes[28] and the consequent maximal stimulation of ketogenesis. Additional evidence that hepatocytes from neonatal rats are maximally stimulated is the finding that starvation of neonatal rats, in contrast with adult rats, does not further increase the rate of ketogenesis from LCFA in vitro.[104]

By analogy to its potent antilipolytic effect on adipocytes, insulin likely exerts a direct antiketogenic effect on the liver. Unlike glucagon, the mechanism of insulin-mediated suppression of ketogenesis remains incompletely delineated. Insulin stimulates the de novo synthesis of fatty acids, in part by activation of acetyl-CoA mediated by a change in LCFA supply to the liver.[126] In addition, insulin-mediated sequestration of the transcription factor FOXA2 from the nucleus, resulting in decreased expression of fatty acid oxidation and ketogenic genes, including *Hmgcs2*.[81] Livers of suckling rats[55] and human neonates[127] are resistant to the suppressive effects of insulin on glucose production, and this resistance may also extend to its effects on lipid metabolism. None of the putative direct hepatic actions of glucagon or insulin discussed earlier are likely to affect MCFA metabolism, which appears to be favored over LCFA metabolism in livers of suckling rats.[128] This predilection may be important in the formulation of infant feedings.[129] Thus a number of changes favor a high rate of ketogenesis in the suckling neonate (Table 34.2), which are reversed on weaning the neonate to a high-carbohydrate diet.

Table 34.2 Changes That Favor Ketogenesis in Suckling Rats.

Factor	Change[a]
Plasma insulin concentration[52,53,77]	Decreased
Plasma glucagon concentration[52,53,77]	Increased
Insulin-to-glucagon ratio[52,53,77]	Decreased
Plasma concentration of LCFAs[46]	Increased
Hepatic carnitine palmitoyltransferase I activity[101]	Increased
Sensitivity of carnitine palmitoyltransferase I to malonyl-CoA inhibition[110,111]	Decreased
Hepatic carnitine concentration[207]	Increased
Hepatic lipogenesis[102,112]	Decreased
Hepatic malonyl-CoA concentration	Decreased[b]

[a]Reported changes are relative to determinations in the adult fed rat, which has a low rate of ketogenesis.
[b]Malonyl-CoA has not been measured in neonatal rat liver, but a reasonable assumption is that its level is low.
Data from cited references.
CoA, Coenzyme A; *LCFA,* long-chain fatty acid.

KETONE BODY UTILIZATION

With availability of sufficient ketone bodies in the circulation, their rate of utilization is to a large extent regulated by the circulating concentration.[130] Transport of ketone bodies through the plasma membrane or mitochondrial inner membranes is not considered to limit their utilization in muscle because the tissue concentration is linearly related to the plasma concentration.[131] However, this may not be true for brain, because the ketone body concentrations in rat brain[132] and human cerebrospinal fluid[133] are considerably less than those in blood in hyperketonemic states. Within the cell, the metabolism of ketone bodies depends on the activities of the "initiating" enzymes, which allow their entry into the metabolic pathways of the cell. The acetyl-CoA formed from ketone bodies either is completely oxidized in the TCA cycle to provide energy (adenosine triphosphate) or can be used along with ketone bodies themselves as precursors of fatty acid or sterol (cholesterol) synthesis (see Fig. 34.1). More detailed reviews of ketone body metabolism in peripheral tissues are available.[4,6]

MITOCHONDRIAL PATHWAY

The major sites of ketone body utilization are the mitochondria. Before transport to mitochondria, ketone bodies must transverse the plasma membrane. MCT1 and MCT2 facilitate the uptake of ketone bodies from the circulation into cells, including across the blood-brain barrier.[134,135] Once in the mitochondria, the primary circulating ketone body, D-(−)-βOHB, is oxidized to AcAc by BDH1, along with conversion of oxidized nicotinamide adenine dinucleotide to its reduced form. The reaction is reversible, but the equilibrium is in favor of AcAc reduction to D-(−)-βOHB, and thus mass action favors BOHB oxidation. BDH1 is tightly bound to the inner mitochondrial membrane. The initiating enzyme for AcAc metabolism is the mitochondrial matrix enzyme succinyl-CoA:3-oxoacid-CoA transferase (SCOT; encoded by nuclear *Oxct1*), succinyl-CoA is derived from the TCA cycle, and because succinate is returned to the cycle, no loss of cycle intermediates occurs. The equilibrium of the reaction is in favor of AcAc formation, but mass action drives AcAc conversion to acetoacetyl-CoA, particularly in the setting of high citrate synthase activity (see Fig. 34.1B). K_m (approximately 0.2 mmol/L) of SCOT for AcAc and its kinetic properties are similar in different rat tissues.[136] SCOT of rat tissues is inhibited by AcAc at concentrations in excess of 5 mmol/L, which may suppress ketone body utilization in severely hyperketonemic, highly ketogenic states.[137] To limit futile cycling, expression of SCOT is selectively excluded in hepatocytes, possibly due to specific silencing of *Oxct1* mRNA via hepatic expression of the microRNA miR-122.[138]

Acetoacetyl-CoA formed by the SCOT reaction is cleaved by acetoacetyl-CoA thiolase to yield two molecules of acetyl-CoA (see Fig. 34.1B). The equilibrium of this reaction is strongly in favor of acetyl-CoA formation, and when this reaction is coupled with that of SCOT, utilization of AcAc is favored. Acetoacetyl-CoA thiolase, unlike SCOT, is present in both the mitochondrial matrix and the cytosol (see Fig. 34.1B and C).[139]

Unlike the hepatic HMG-CoA pathway for synthesis of ketone bodies, the mitochondrial utilization pathway is reversible, and thus utilization of ketone bodies depends on the prevailing concentrations of βOHB and AcAc and the rate of removal of acetyl-CoA. The latter depends on the activity of the TCA cycle and on the rate of acetyl-CoA formation from other substrates, mainly oxidation of fatty acids. This alternative acetyl-CoA source explains why it is possible to demonstrate net formation of ketone bodies in vitro when kidney slices are incubated with fatty acids.[140] Thus in certain tissues, the free reversibility of the pathway can be viewed as a means of "buffering" the mitochondrial acetyl-CoA pool. Of course, the concentrations of cosubstrates (succinyl-CoA, succinate) and cofactors (CoA, oxidized nicotinamide adenine dinucleotide, reduced nicotinamide adenine dinucleotide) also influence the utilization of ketone bodies.

To explore the role of this pathway in the neonate, *Oxct1*$^{-/-}$ mice, which exhibit a congenital and global loss of SCOT, were generated. After use of stable isotopic tracers and nuclear magnetic resonance (NMR) spectroscopy had confirmed that SCOT deficiency abrogated ketone body oxidation, it was revealed that these mice are born normal but develop severe hyperketonemic hypoglycemia after the onset of suckling and invariably die within 48 hours of birth. Unlike most states of hyperketonemia, these knockout mice displayed very high AcAc-to-βOHB ratios. Brains of neonatal SCOT-deficient mice exhibited increased concentrations of markers of cellular autophagy and oxidation of glucose, whereas skeletal muscle in these animals had increased lactate oxidation as a compensatory means of attempting to maintain metabolic homeostasis.[141] Loss of extrahepatic SCOT was found to ultimately impact intermediary metabolism in the livers of neonatal mice that have fed after birth. On postnatal day 1, the livers of germline SCOT-deficient mice engage a gluconeogenic transcriptional program, but exhibit dysfunctional fatty acid oxidation, and demonstrate impaired de novo βOHB production, resulting in an oxidized hepatic redox potential (due to a high circulating AcAc-to-βOHB ratio), all of which occur in response to the ingestion of high-fat milk from the mother.[142] These mice could not be completely rescued long term with carbohydrate feeding, although some benefit was achieved.[141]

CYTOSOLIC PATHWAY

After efflux from mitochondria, ketone bodies contribute to key anabolic pathways in the cytosol as well. Ketone bodies serve as substrates for lipogenesis and sterol biosynthesis in developing brain, lactating mammary gland, and in the liver after the enzymatic activation of AcAc to AcAc-CoA by acetoacetyl-CoA synthetase (AACS) (see Fig. 34.1C).[8–11] Although AACS enzyme activity is at most 10% that of SCOT, it has a high affinity (K_m = 50 μmol/L) for AcAc and can be readily saturated even in the fed state. AcAc-CoA acts as a direct substrate for HMGCS1, the cytoplasmic HMG-CoA synthase, which catalyzes the fate-committing step of sterol biosynthesis. However, entry of AcAc-CoA into lipogenesis requires a thiolytic cleavage reaction to yield acetyl-CoA, which can then be carboxylated via ACC to form the lipogenic substrate malonyl-CoA.[9,69,143–145] Studies support the physiologic importance of ketone bodies as anabolic substrates. By use of in vivo and in vitro AACS-knockout models, lack of cytosolic ketone body metabolism was found to lower total blood cholesterol concentration in mice, impair differentiation of primary mouse embryonic neuronal cells in culture, and inhibit adipocyte differentiation in immortalized cells.[146–148] Although the anabolic fates of ketone bodies have been shown to serve important metabolic roles, these pathways are not essential for the disposal of ketone bodies because SCOT deficiency alone causes severe hyperketonemia.[141,149–152] Further studies using genetic and functional disruption of AACS are warranted to thoroughly assess the physiologic roles for nonoxidative fates of ketone bodies in various cell and organ systems.

L-(+)-β-HYDROXYBUTYRATE

Although hepatic ketogenesis produces only D-(−)-βOHB, the physiologic substrate used for oxidation, L-(+)-βOHB is measurable in ketolytic tissues but not in the circulation. L-(+)-βOHB is generated from the hydrolysis of the β-oxidation intermediate L-(+)-βOHB-CoA but is not a BDH1 substrate.[153–156] SLC16A transporters in rat myocytes do not demonstrate stereoselectivity for βOHB.[157] In brains of suckling rats, L-(+)-βOHB can be used for synthesis of fatty acids and sterols.[91,92] These observations may be important when racemic DL-βOHB is administered to humans or used for experiments.

SIGNALING ROLES OF KETONE BODIES

Evidence has solidified the notion that metabolic status plays a crucial role in regulating cellular functions via signaling, transcriptional, and epigenetic pathways. As mentioned earlier, βOHB has been identified as an endogenous ligand for the niacin receptor GPR109A, which is not stereoselective for βOHB.[54,158] Through an unknown mechanism, βOHB also modulates autonomic nervous system activity through GPR41, expressed primarily in sympathetic ganglia.[159]

βOHB inhibits class I histone deacetylases. Providing exogenous βOHB to mouse tissues led to increased histone acetylation, which was correlated with the induction of antioxidant gene expression, ultimately leading to improved handling of oxidative stress.[160] βOHB supplementation has also been implicated in extending life span in *Caenorhabditis elegans*,[161] as well as promoting neuroprotection, potentially via activation of a specific macrophage population.[162,163]

Finally, βOHB modulates macrophage signaling by inhibiting the NLRP3-dependent inflammasome, through incompletely defined mechanisms.[164] The various mechanisms through which βOHB may act as a signaling metabolite via extracellular receptors or by ultimately altering epigenetic regulation of gene expression are explored in a review by Newman and Verdin.[165] Although it remains possible that redox alterations or oxidative metabolism of βOHB may account for part of these signaling effects, the results are promising and pave the way for further understanding of the signaling roles ketone bodies may serve.

EFFECTS OF KETONE BODIES ON GLUCOSE METABOLISM

GLUCOSE UTILIZATION

Physiologic concentrations of AcAc and βOHB decrease glucose utilization in a number of adult rat tissues, including heart, soleus muscle, kidney, brain, and lactating mammary gland.[4] These tissues all exhibit high rates of glycolysis and utilization of the pyruvate formed from glucose 6-phosphate. Consequently, if glucose metabolism were not inhibited in conditions associated with relative carbohydrate deficit, the animal would rapidly become hypoglycemic. The mechanism for the inhibition of glucose metabolism by ketone bodies was established in studies by Randle and colleagues[166] and involves inhibition of the enzymes phosphofructokinase and hexokinase and inactivation of pyruvate dehydrogenase. The overall effect is decreased glucose utilization. In addition, a higher proportion of any glucose that still undergoes glycolysis leaves the tissue as lactate and pyruvate and returns to the liver for gluconeogenesis. Neonatal SCOT-deficient mice exhibit increased glycolysis and glucose oxidation in the brain despite high circulating levels of ketone bodies, suggesting other regulatory mechanisms at the substrate flux level that may be independent of glycolytic enzyme inhibition.[141,167] However, in normal children, an inverse correlation has been noted between glucose flux and the degree of ketonemia.[168] This observation supports the view that glucose and ketone body interactions operate at the whole-body level.

GLUCOSE PRODUCTION

Ketone bodies can alter hepatic glucose production by their effects on the supply of two important precursors, glycerol and alanine. Ketone bodies decrease the flux of glycerol to the liver by their antilipolytic action on adipose tissue and apparently also on muscle triacylglycerol stores.[169] Hypoalaninemia is present in a number of conditions associated with hyperketonemia, including starvation, diabetes, and ketotic hypoglycemia of childhood, and can be induced by infusion of βOHB.[170] The mechanism by which ketone bodies decrease muscle release of alanine has not yet been established. Two possibilities are recognized: (1) inhibition of muscle glycolysis decreases pyruvate availability to form alanine by transamination or (2) a direct inhibition of muscle proteolysis.

ROLES OF KETONE BODIES IN NEONATAL BRAIN

Ketone bodies are the primary alternative fuel source for cerebral metabolism when glucose is unavailable. This is due primarily to the brain's poor ability to oxidize fatty acids, attributable in part to the low activity of 3-ketoacyl-CoA-thiolase in the brain.[171] Permeability of the blood-brain barrier to ketone bodies depends on MCT1. In rats, permeability of the blood-brain barrier to βOHB increases by a factor of 7 during suckling before falling again after they have been weaned. This rise in permeability has been shown to be associated with a 25-fold increase in MCT1 expression while they are suckling compared with adult levels. In addition, there is regional variation in uptake and use of ketone bodies in the brain,[10,172] and it appears that the telencephalon uses the most ketone bodies and the hind brain uses the least.[172,173]

Arteriovenous difference measurements across the brain of adult and suckling rats have shown that for a given arterial concentration of ketone bodies, the extraction by suckling rat brain is 3 to 4 times higher than that by adult brain.[132,174] This finding is in agreement with the higher activities of the enzymes of ketone body utilization in suckling rat brain. A similar increase in ketone body extraction by brain has been demonstrated when human neonates and adults have been compared.[175,176] However, no appreciable increase in the activities of the enzymes of ketone body utilization has been demonstrated in human neonatal brain.[176,177] Therefore the increased utilization in the human neonatal brain is likely to be due to increased cerebral permeability to ketone bodies, as demonstrated in neonatal rat brain.[178]

The major route of ketone body utilization by brains of suckling rats is terminal oxidation via TCA cycle and electron transport chain activity for high-energy phosphate generation,[179] which spares glucose. However, a portion of the carbon (5% to 10%) is converted to fatty acids and cholesterol.[179-183] The newborn brain, which consumes up to 70% of the total energy expenditure at birth, is capable of oxidizing ketone bodies at a rate at least fourfold greater than that of adult brain, with ketone bodies accounting for as much as 12% of the cerebral oxygen consumption in neonates.[2,184] Therefore studies of animal models congenitally deficient for ketone body oxidation in brain were expected to reveal metabolic abnormalities. Although germline SCOT-knockout mice exhibit hyperketonemic hypoglycemia and die in the first 2 days of life, tissue-specific SCOT-knockout models resulted in relatively normal development to adulthood and metabolic homeostasis. SCOT was selectively knocked out in neurons, cardiomyocytes, or skeletal myocytes, three tissues that most avidly oxidize ketone bodies for energetic needs. Mice from each of these tissue-specific knockout strains grew to adulthood, tolerated starvation with moderate hyperketonemia but not hypoglycemia, and were overtly normal. Neonatal neuron-specific SCOT-deficient mice exhibited altered glucose handling, exhibiting increased glycolysis and glucose oxidation in the brain.[6] Together with the analysis of mice with congenital but global SCOT deficiency, these studies reveal an essential role for whole-body utilization of ketone bodies during neonatal development that cannot be attributed to any one particular ketolytic tissue, but that selective loss of ketone body oxidation forces metabolic adaptations that could lead to deficiencies in select environmental conditions.

HUMAN KETONE BODY ENZYME DEFICIENCIES

The increasing availability and decreasing cost of genomic sequencing opens the possibility of personalized medicine. Inborn errors of metabolism can have devastating consequences if left untreated, and potential mutations in the enzymes of ketogenesis and ketone body oxidation should be included in this category.

SCOT DEFICIENCY

SCOT deficiency was first reported in 1972, with the postmortem tissue analysis of a 6-month-old child who had died after periods of persistent ketonemia and recurring bouts of severe ketoacidosis.[23] In the following decades, numerous clinical cases of SCOT deficiency have been reported. These patients exhibit recurring attacks of ketoacidosis secondary to dysfunctional peripheral utilization of circulating ketone bodies. Most patients were neonates or young children who presented with hyperketonemia and metabolic acidosis of unknown cause, occasionally with concomitant hypoglycemia and cardiomyopathy. Enzyme activity assays and sequencing analysis ultimately revealed various mutations in the *OXCT1* gene that rendered the encoded SCOT dysfunctional.[150-152,185-190]

MITOCHONDRIAL 3-HYDROXY-3-METHYLGLUTARYL COENZYME A SYNTHASE 2 DEFICIENCY

Mutations in the fate-committing ketogenic enzyme HMGCS2 have been characterized in more than a dozen clinical cases in young patients. In each of these cases, the patient typically presents within the first few years of life with hypoketotic hypoglycemia, commonly after a prolonged fast secondary to a gastrointestinal tract infection. Urinary organic acid and plasma acylcarnitine profiles are frequently nonspecific or normal.[191-197] A description of human HMGCS2 deficiency identified a number of novel and known circulating biomarkers to assist in confirming the diagnosis. By retrospectively examining urine organic acid profiles, Pitt and colleagues[198] concluded that a cutoff of adipic acid of more than 200 μmol/mmol creatinine and 4-hydroxy-6-methyl-2-pyrone of more than 20 μmol/mmol creatinine generated a positive predictive value of 80% for HMGCS2 deficiency.

3-HYDROXY-3-METHYLGLUTARYL COENZYME A LYASE DEFICIENCY

HMG-CoA lyase is a ketogenic enzyme in the liver that catalyzes the formation of AcAc from HMG-CoA within the mitochondria. However, it also plays a prominent role in the catabolism of the amino acid leucine. Because of this, HMG-CoA lyase deficiency not only causes hypoketotic hypoglycemia similar to that caused by HMGCS2 mutations but also leads to organic acid accumulation and metabolic acidosis due to altered leucine metabolism. This disorder also occurs in childhood and can be mistaken for Reye syndrome because of the overlapping symptoms, including vomiting, lethargy, and convulsions.[199-202]

MITOCHONDRIAL β-KETOTHIOLASE DEFICIENCY

Similarly to HMG-CoA lyase, mitochondrial β-ketothiolase functions as both an enzyme of ketone body metabolism and in the processing of the amino acid isoleucine. Mitochondrial β-ketothiolase is involved in the conversion of acetoacetyl-CoA to acetyl-CoA in the ketolytic pathway. Mitochondrial β-ketothiolase deficiency is an autosomal recessive disorder that occurs in young childhood with vomiting, hyperketonemic hypoglycemia, and accumulation of isoleucine breakdown products in the blood and urine, including 2-methylacetoacetate, 2-methyl-3-hydroxybutyrate, and tiglylglycine.[203-207]

KETONE BODY TRANSPORTER DEFICIENCY

A study analyzed the genome of a patient with severe ketoacidosis, suspecting a defect in the extrahepatic ketolytic machinery, and discovered a homozygous mutation in the gene encoding MCT1 *(SLC16A1)*. Numerous patients were subsequently found to have inactivating mutations in *SLC16A1*, all of whom presented with ketoacidosis after a period of fasting or infection in early childhood. Intravenous administration of glucose or dextrose with bicarbonate quickly reversed the ketoacidosis, while avoidance of fasting prevented future ketoacidotic episodes.[70]

SUMMARY

Ketone body metabolism serves an essential metabolic role in the development of the neonate. Although ketone bodies are important energetic substrates, particularly in highly oxidative tissues such as the brain, the pathways of hepatic ketogenesis and peripheral ketolysis are dynamically regulated mitochondrial processes that impact cellular signaling and metabolic functioning in myriad ways. Disruption of ketone body metabolism in model organisms and in humans has severe clinical consequences, including steatohepatitis, ketoacidosis, and death in the neonatal period. Clinical assessment of metabolic abnormalities in the neonatal period should usually interrogate this pathway, and ongoing investigation will elucidate the mechanisms involved in how ketone body metabolism may ameliorate or exacerbate pathologic conditions.

ACKNOWLEDGMENTS

The authors are most grateful to previous edition contributors to this chapter, including Paul S.Thornton, whose leadership and input on the chapter's themes and data (particularly within the tables) were invaluable.

A complete reference list is available at www.ExpertConsult.com. 

SELECT REFERENCES

1. Aneja P, Dziak R, Cai GQ, et al. Identification of an acetoacetyl coenzyme A synthetase-dependent pathway for utilization of L-(+)-3-hydroxybutyrate in *Sinorhizobiummeliloti*. *J Bacteriol*. 2002;184:1571-1577.
2. Cahill Jr GF. Fuel metabolism in starvation. *Annu Rev Nutr*. 2006;26:1-22.
3. Krishnakumar AM, Sliwa D, Endrizzi JA, et al. Getting a handle on the role of coenzyme M in alkene metabolism. *Microbiol Mol Biol Rev*. 2008;72:445-456.
4. Robinson AM, Williamson DH. Physiological roles of ketone bodies as substrates and signals in mammalian tissues. *Physiol Rev*. 1980;60:143-187.
5. McGarry JD, Foster DW. Regulation of hepatic fatty acid oxidation and ketone body production. *Annu Rev Biochem*. 1980;49:395-420.
6. Cotter DG, Schugar RC, Crawford PA. Ketone body metabolism and cardiovascular disease. *Am J Physiol Heart Circ Physiol*. 2013;304:H1060-H1076.
7. Johnson RH, Walton JL, Krebs HA, et al. Post-exercise ketosis. *Lancet*. 1969;2:1383-1385.
8. Freed LE, Endemann G, Tomera JF, et al. Lipogenesis from ketone bodies in perfused livers from streptozocin-induced diabetic rats. *Diabetes*. 1988;37:50-55.
9. Endemann G, Goetz PG, Edmond J, et al. Lipogenesis from ketone bodies in the isolated perfused rat liver. Evidence for the cytosolic activation of acetoacetate. *J Biol Chem*. 1982;257:3434-3440.
10. Morris AA. Cerebral ketone body metabolism. *J Inherit Metab Dis*. 2005;28:109-121.
11. Robinson AM, Williamson DH. Utilization of D-3-hydroxy[3-14C]butyrate for lipogenesis *in vivo* in lactating rat mammary gland. *Biochem J*. 1978;176:635-638.
12. Sengupta S, Peterson TR, Laplante M, et al. mTORC1 controls fasting-induced ketogenesis and its modulation by ageing. *Nature*. 2010;468:1100-1104.
13. Soeters MR, Sauerwein HP, Faas L, et al. Effects of insulin on ketogenesis following fasting in lean and obese men. *Obesity (Silver Spring)*. 2009;17:1326-1331.
14. Neely JR, Rovetto MJ, Oram JF. Myocardial utilization of carbohydrate and lipids. *Prog Cardiovasc Dis*. 1972;15:289-329.
15. Lommi J, Kupari M, Koskinen P, et al. Blood ketone bodies in congestive heart failure. *J Am Coll Cardiol*. 1996;28:665-672.
16. Kupari M, Lommi J, Ventila M, et al. Breath acetone in congestive heart failure. *Am J Cardiol*. 1995;76:1076-1078.
17. Lommi J, Koskinen P, Naveri H, et al. Heart failure ketosis. *J Intern Med*. 1997;242:231-238.
18. Pittman JG, Cohen P. The pathogenesis of cardiac cachexia. *N Engl J Med*. 1964;271:403-409. CONTD.
19. Fery F, Balasse EO. Ketone body production and disposal in diabetic ketosis. A comparison with fasting ketosis. *Diabetes*. 1985;34:326-332.
20. Hall SE, Wastney ME, Bolton TM, et al. Ketone body kinetics in humans: the effects of insulin-dependent diabetes, obesity, and starvation. *J Lipid Res*. 1984;25:1184-1194.
21. Stacpoole PW, Moore GW, Kornhauser DM. Metabolic effects of dichloroacetate in patients with diabetes mellitus and hyperlipoproteinemia. *N Engl J Med*. 1978;298:526-530.
22. Williamson DH, Wilson MB. The effects of cyclopropane derivatives on ketone-body metabolism *in vivo*. *Biochem J*. 1965;94:19C-20C.
23. Tildon JT, Cornblath M. Succinyl-CoA. 3-ketoacid CoA-transferase deficiency. A cause for ketoacidosis in infancy. *J Clin Invest*. 1972;51:493-498.
24. Sherwin RS, Hendler RG, Felig P. Effect of diabetes mellitus and insulin on the turnover and metabolic response to ketones in man. *Diabetes*. 1976;25:776-784.
25. Williamson D. The production and utilization of ketone bodies in the neonate. In: Jones CT, ed. *Biochemical Development of the Fetus and Neonate*. Amsterdam: Elsevier Biomedical Press; 1982:621-650.
26. Wildenhoff KE, Johansen JP, Karstoft H, et al. Diurnal variations in the concentrations of blood acetoacetate and 3-hydroxybutyrate. The ketone body peak around midnight and its relationship to free fatty acids, glycerol, insulin, growth hormone and glucose in serum and plasma. *Acta Med Scand*. 1974;195:25-28.
27. Paterson P, Sheath J, Taft P, et al. Maternal and foetal ketone concentrations in plasma and urine. *Lancet*. 1967;1:862-865.

28. Sabata V, Wolf H, Lausmann S. The role of free fatty acids, glycerol, ketone bodies and glucose in the energy metabolism of the mother and fetus during delivery. *Biol Neonat*. 1968;13:7-17.
29. Felig P, Lynch V. Starvation in human pregnancy: hypoglycemia, hypoinsulinemia, and hyperketonemia. *Science*. 1970;170:990-992.
30. Kim YJ, Felig P. Maternal and amniotic fluid substrate levels during caloric deprivation in human pregnancy. *Metabolism*. 1972;21:507-512.
31. Persson B, Lunell NO. Metabolic control in diabetic pregnancy. Variations in plasma concentrations of glucose, free fatty acids, glycerol, ketone bodies, insulin, and human chorionic somatomammotropin during the last trimester. *Am J Obstet Gynecol*. 1975;122:737-745.
32. Spitzer JJ, Weng JT. Removal and utilization of ketone bodies by the brain of newborn puppies. *J Neurochem*. 1972;19:2169-2173.
33. Gentz J, Bengtsson G, Hakkarainen J, et al. Metabolic effects of starvation during neonatal period in the piglet. *Am J Physiol*. 1970;218:662-668.
34. Varnam GC, Jeacock MK, Shepherd DA. Hepatic ketone-body metabolism in developing sheep and pregnant ewes. *Br J Nutr*. 1978;40:359-367.
35. Lin X, Adams SH, Odle J. Acetate represents a major product of heptanoate and octanoate beta-oxidation in hepatocytes isolated from neonatal piglets. *Biochem J*. 1996;318(Pt 1):235-240.
36. Duee PH, Pegorier JP, Quant PA, et al. Hepatic ketogenesis in newborn pigs is limited by low mitochondrial 3-hydroxy-3-methylglutaryl-CoA synthase activity. *Biochem J*. 1994;298(Pt 1):207-212.
37. Hawdon JM, Ward Platt MP, Aynsley-Green A. Patterns of metabolic adaptation for preterm and term infants in the first neonatal week. *Arch Dis Child*. 1992;67:357-365.
38. Williamson DH, Mellanby J, Krebs HA. Enzymic determination of D(-)-beta-hydroxybutyric acid and acetoacetic acid in blood. *Biochem J*. 1962;82:90-96.
39. Haymond MW, Karl IE, Pagliara AS. Increased gluconeogenic substrates in the small-for-gestational-age infant. *N Engl J Med*. 1974;291:322-328.
40. Fukao T, Lopaschuk GD, Mitchell GA. Pathways and control of ketone body metabolism: on the fringe of lipid biochemistry. *Prostaglandins Leukot Essent Fatty Acids*. 2004;70:243-251.
41. Sugden M, Williamson D. Short-term hormonal control of ketogenesis. In: Hue L, Van de Werve G, eds. *Short-term Regulation of Liver Metabolism*. Amsterdam: Elsevier/North Holland Biomedical Press; 1981:291-309.
42. Zammit VA. Regulation of hepatic fatty acid oxidation and ketogenesis. *Proc Nutr Soc*. 1983;42:289-302.
43. Zammit VA. Mechanisms of regulation of the partition of fatty acids between oxidation and esterification in the liver. *Prog Lipid Res*. 1984;23:39-67.
44. Dahlquist G, Persson U, Persson B. The activity of D-β-hydroxybutyrate dehydrogenase in fetal, infant and adult rat brain and the influence of starvation. *Biol Neonate*. 1972;20:40-50.
45. Novak M, Melichar V, Hahn P, et al. Release of free fatty acids from adipose tissue obtained from newborn infants. *J Lipid Res*. 1965;6:91-95.
46. Page MA, Krebs HA, Williamson DH. Activities of enzymes of ketone-body utilization in brain and other tissues of suckling rats. *Biochem J*. 1971;121:49-53.
47. Persson B, Gentz J. The pattern of blood lipids, glycerol and ketone bodies during the neonatal period, infancy and childhood. *Acta Paediatr Scand*. 1966;55:353-362.
48. Garber AJ, Menzel PH, Boden G, et al. Hepatic ketogenesis and gluconeogenesis in humans. *J Clin Invest*. 1974;54:981-989.
49. Nielsen TS, Jessen N, Jorgensen JO, et al. Dissecting adipose tissue lipolysis: molecular regulation and implications for metabolic disease. *J Mol Endocrinol*. 2014;52:R199-R222.
50. Belfrage P. Hormonal control of lipid degradation. In: Cryer A, Van R, eds. *New Perspectives in Adipose Tissue: Structure, Function and Development*. London: Butterworths; 1985:121-144.

35 Long-Chain Polyunsaturated Fatty Acids in Neurodevelopment

Kathleen M. Gustafson | John Colombo | Susan E. Carlson

INTRODUCTION

The brain and retina contain large quantities of long-chain (20 and 22 carbon) *n*-3 and *n*-6 polyunsaturated fatty acids (LCPUFAs), particularly docosahexaenoic acid (DHA; 22:6*n*-3) and arachidonic acid (AA; 20:4*n*-6).[1,2] During the last intrauterine trimester[3,4] and the first 18 months of postnatal life, DHA and AA accumulate in neural tissue at a high rate, supported by selective placental transfer of DHA and AA from mother to fetus,[5,6] transfer of preformed DHA and AA from human milk consumption,[7,8] and synthesis of DHA and AA from the dietary essential fatty acids, α-linolenic acid (18:3*n*-3) and linoleic acid (18:2*n*-6), respectively.[9-12] The first studies of infants fed formulas, which, at that time, did not contain DHA or AA, found lower levels of DHA and AA in red blood cell (RBC) and plasma lipids[7,8] and lower levels of DHA in brain,[13,14] compared with infants fed human milk. This finding suggested that synthesis of these fatty acids might not meet the needs for DHA and AA in the developing retina and brain and that a dietary source was important. Furthermore, infants born preterm had lower brain DHA than infants born at term,[15] reinforcing the importance of the last intrauterine trimester for postnatal DHA status.

DOCOSAHEXAENOIC ACID ACCUMULATION AND SYNTHESIS

These studies are evidence that formulas containing α-linolenic acid, the 18-carbon precursor of DHA, did not compensate for the DHA accumulation that occurs in RBCs, plasma, and brains of infants fed even small amounts of DHA[13-17] with functional consequences.[17,18] In the months after birth, infants fed formulas that contain α-linolenic acid but no DHA have progressively lower RBC DHA,[16] whereas infants fed formulas with DHA have higher RBC DHA.[16,19] Preterm-born infants are especially vulnerable to receiving a diet without DHA. The third-trimester fetus is estimated to accumulate approximately 40 to 60 mg of DHA per kg each day,[20] whereas Carnielli and colleagues[21] quantified DHA synthesis in 1-month-old infants born preterm and showed that they could synthesize only approximately 13 mg/kg/day. Their synthesis fell dramatically to approximately 3 mg/kg/day by 3 months of age. The rate of endogenous synthesis of LCPUFA from their precursors is further dependent on genetics,[22] balance of fatty acids,[23] and amount of DHA consumed.[24]

EARLY CLINICAL TRIALS IN INFANTS

Randomized studies of DHA and AA supplementation in preterm infants were conducted early in the history of the field to test the hypotheses that (1) erythrocyte DHA and AA were biomarkers for DHA and AA status, (2) lower status could have functional consequences, and (3) neurodevelopmental function could be improved or optimized by DHA and AA supplementation. The functional outcomes chosen for early study were those linked to lower brain DHA in animals: retinal electrophysiology,[25-27] visual acuity,[28] and various measures of cognition.[29-37] We now have evidence that the effects of DHA on development include positive effects on blood pressure,[38] response to stress,[39] and autonomic nervous system (ANS) development.[40] The latter is discussed in this chapter. The beneficial effects observed in these realms are most certainly related to increased DHA accumulation in the central nervous system and ANS.

A critical difference between preclinical animal models and human studies was that animals were fed diets lacking α-linolenic acid, the essential fatty acid precursor for DHA, whereas infant formula contained α-linolenic acid. In most animal models, brain DHA was extremely depleted over several generations and replaced by *n*-6 docosapentaenoic acid (22:5*n*-6).[36,41] In contrast, brain DHA in studies of human term and preterm infants fed formulas without LCPUFA were respectively reduced to only 20% and 50% compared with human milk–fed infants.[13,15]

In the first studies of preterm infants, researchers found that DHA-supplemented formula (there were no sources of AA available at the time) produced higher visual acuity and more mature retinal physiology.[18,42] These results led to larger randomized trials in which the growth and neurodevelopment of term and preterm infants fed formulas supplemented with DHA and AA were compared with those fed formulas without DHA and AA. These studies have been reviewed previously elsewhere.[43-51]

Single-cell oil sources of DHA and AA were added to commercially available term formula in the United States beginning in 2002, after the Food and Drug Administration gave single-cell oils generally recognized as safe (GRAS) status.[52] DHA and AA were added to preterm formulas somewhat later. Before DHA and AA were added to formulas, infants had to rely on synthesis for any additional postnatal DHA accumulation; as noted previously, synthesis is likely inadequate as a source for optimal levels of DHA.

The Docosahexaenoic Acid Intake and Measurement of Neural Development (DIAMOND) trial, the only randomized, controlled dose-response study of infant formula LCPUFA, was initiated in 2002 soon after the addition of DHA to infant formula in the United States became routine. All three DHA-containing formulas included the same amount of AA. The primary outcome of this study was to determine the effects of LCPUFA on visual acuity of term infants at 12 months of age. The study included additional aims to study child development at the individual study sites in Dallas and Kansas City. Results from the trial out to age 9 years are discussed in the section on LCPUFA and the developing human infant.

MATERNAL INFLUENCE ON OFFSPRING DOCOSAHEXAENOIC ACID STATUS

INTRAUTERINE DOCOSAHEXAENOIC ACID TRANSFER

Intrauterine DHA accumulation is variable, as evidenced by (1) a large range of normative values for DHA in cord RBC phospholipids of infants born preterm,[53] (2) a progressive increase in maternal phospholipid DHA throughout the last intrauterine trimester,[54] (3) variable brain DHA content among infants born at the same gestational age,[3] and (4) variable fetal concentration of DHA in adipose tissue.[55]

Variable maternal DHA intake is one well-known reason for this variability, which in turn influences the amount of DHA transferred to the fetus.[6] A review by Haggarty[56] illustrates the influence of maternal DHA intake and gestation duration on fetal DHA accumulation, with most accumulation in fetal adipose tissue at term. However, Kuipers and colleagues question the basis for some of Haggarty's estimates of adipose tissue DHA concentrations.[55] Although these authors confirm an overall trend to adipose DHA accumulation in the last trimester of gestation, they found extreme variability in individual DHA accumulation at all gestational ages from 25 and 42 weeks. The size of the adipose tissue pool of DHA at birth could be a variable influencing postnatal DHA status.[56]

A large multicountry comparative study included pregnant women from the Netherlands, Hungary, Finland, England, and Ecuador. In the results of this study, researchers reported significant differences among countries in the concentrations of DHA in maternal plasma, most likely due to differences in DHA intake across these locations.[57] As mentioned previously,[5,6] there is selective transfer of DHA and AA across the placenta and much is known about the specifics of fatty acid transport. Despite the relationship between maternal DHA status and newborn DHA status[6,57,58]; however, only 25% of the variance in DHA status of newborns is predicted by maternal DHA status.[59] Gestational age is also a predictor of cord blood DHA, but no predictor has been found for the majority of variance in cord blood DHA.[60]

Pregnancy itself has been shown to influence the amount of DHA in circulating blood lipids and RBC phospholipids. Al and colleagues[61] observed that phospholipid DHA in maternal plasma and RBCs increases in early pregnancy, regardless of the initial levels of RBC DHA. These data suggest that DHA is mobilized during pregnancy for transfer to the fetus. However, the same group of investigators reported increased maternal 22:5*n*-6 relative to DHA, from which they concluded that pregnant women's systems lag behind with respect to DHA production and transfer to the fetus.[62] Van Houwelingen and colleagues[63] observed similar relative increases in the ratio of 22:5*n*-6 to DHA in infants born preterm, further suggesting that an increase in the ratio of 22:5*n*-6 to DHA indicates inadequate DHA synthesis or accumulation. Thus, even though it appears that DHA is mobilized during pregnancy, the amount transferred may not provide for optimal fetal development when maternal DHA status is low. The number of prior pregnancies is inversely related to maternal DHA status, suggesting that maternal DHA stores are depleted by repeated pregnancy and/or lactation.[64]

The *FADS* complex contains the genes that govern the rate-limiting enzymes of the fatty acid metabolic pathways. Studies show the relation between single nucleotide polymorphisms (SNPs) in the *FADS* gene complex and AA and/or DHA status.[22,65-67] Maternal DHA supplementation improves DHA status in all women; however, minor allele carriers of *FADS*1rs174553 and *FADS*2rs174575 experienced a significant drop in AA status with DHA supplementation.[67]

HUMAN MILK PROVIDES DOCOSAHEXAENOIC ACID POSTNATALLY

Just as women's DHA status during pregnancy affects transfer of DHA to the fetus, it influences DHA transfer in human milk. Connor and colleagues[68] and Harris and colleagues[69] first showed that higher maternal DHA intake increases the amount of DHA in breast milk and, in turn, increases the DHA status of their infants. The DHA content of human milk as a percentage of total fatty acids varies within and among populations. The extremes of milk DHA that have been reported are 0.02% in vegans[70] and 2.4% in women from China who consume a diet high in ocean fish.[71] Human milk DHA in most groups tends to fall on the lower side of this range.[72,73]

Like DHA, the reported average amount of AA in human milk varies across cultural groups, from 0.2% to 1.2%.[74] However, the average AA in the milk of most populations falls within the range of 0.4% to 0.6%, and the average linoleic acid content between 10% to 17% of total fatty acids.[64,73-75] Women homozygous for minor alleles of some *FADS* SNPs appear to have limited transfer of DHA to human milk. Molto-Puigmarti and colleagues[76] linked lower milk DHA content to genetic polymorphisms of two *FADS* SNPs, *FADS*1 rs174561 and *FADS*2 rs174575. In a randomized controlled study of DHA supplementation, women assigned to DHA and homozygous for the minor allele *FADS*2 rs174575 had lower DHA in milk compared with other genotypes, although their circulating DHA was increased by supplementation.[67,77]

We have reported that DHA supplementation reduces RBC phospholipid AA in women with minor alleles of *FADS1/FADS2*,[67] suggesting that alterations in the balance of *n*-3 and *n*-6 LCPUFA with DHA intake are greater in minor allele carriers. The implications of this are not known and deserve further study.

CLINICAL TRIALS OF DOCOSAHEXAENOIC ACID SUPPLEMENTATION IN PREGNANCY

Because maternal DHA status during pregnancy and lactation can influence fetal and infant DHA accumulation, studies of the effects of DHA supplementation during pregnancy and lactation on cognitive and other brain-related functions in childhood have been needed. Several trials of supplementation during pregnancy completed since the last edition have measured offspring neurodevelopment. The results are included in the next section.

LCPUFA AND THE DEVELOPING HUMAN INFANT

EFFECT OF DIETARY LCPUFA ON INFANT LCPUFA STATUS

The addition of DHA from fish oil,[16,42,78,79] egg phospholipids,[80] and single-cell oils[51] increases DHA in circulating phospholipids of infants, evidence that these sources increase DHA availability for accumulation in brain and other tissues. As noted previously, infant formulas with α-linolenic acid (but no DHA) do not prevent a gradual postnatal decline in RBC DHA; infants consuming such formulas show low DHA in circulating phospholipids for at least a year.[16,81]

After birth, there is an apparent physiologic decline in AA in plasma and RBC phospholipids. AA is higher in preterm than in term cord blood, and even after 4 to 6 months of breast-feeding, infants born at term had much lower RBC AA than seen at preterm delivery (8.8% vs. 15.7%).[8] AA in the brain and liver also declines during the last intrauterine trimester.[82] However, breast-fed infants have more AA in RBC and plasma phospholipids than do infants fed formulas without LCPUFAs, and infants fed formulas with *n*-3 LCPUFAs have even lower phospholipid AA levels than those fed formulas without *n*-3 LCPUFAs.[83]

CONTROVERSY: DO INFANTS REQUIRE ARACHIDONIC ACID DURING INFANCY?

A European Food Safety Authority (EFSA) opinion stated that there is no need to require AA in formula for infants older than 6 months of age.[84] Regulatory standards adopted for the European Union stipulate that, from February 2020, infant and follow-on formulas marketed in the European Union must contain the equivalent of 0.5% to 1% of fatty acids as DHA but do not require the addition of AA.[85] The opinion has been contested[86,87]; although it is true that many studies emphasize questions about DHA, most interventions combine DHA with AA, and so any benefits shown must be attributed logically to both LCPUFA. There are other reasons to provide a balance of these fatty acids in infant formula, including the fact that AA concentration exceeds that of DHA in most human milk and in brain phospholipids.[4,13,14]

AA is the source of metabolically important prostaglandins and leukotrienes. Researchers report significant correlations between AA levels with both intrauterine growth[54] and growth in the first year of life.[19,88] In formula-fed infants, dietary DHA or total *n*-3 LCPUFAs are related to lower AA and subsequently an altered balance of *n*-3 and *n*-6 LCPUFAs in RBC phospholipids.[83] Three randomized trials found some reduction in growth of infants born preterm who consumed infant formula that contained fish oil DHA and no AA.[19,88,89] In one study, the effect was limited to a lower weight for length at several ages in the first year.[89] Researchers have not found slower growth in either term infants fed formula containing DHA or in preterm infants fed formula with both AA and DHA.[90]

Long-term feeding of *n*-3 LCPUFAs without AA could decrease the accumulation of *n*-6 LCPUFA in brain and thus affect the developing central nervous system. The consumption of high concentrations of α-linolenate[91] decreased brain AA accumulation in rats. Wainwright and colleagues[92] reported lower brain and body weights in mice beginning approximately 2 weeks after birth when they were suckled by dams fed a very low *n*-6/*n*-3 ratio (0.32) created by feeding DHA but no AA. Arbuckle and associates[93] reported that piglets fed a diet with 4% of fatty acids as α-linolenic acid (compared with 1% α-linolenic acid) had lower brain weights and lower levels of AA in membranes of synaptosomes.

Studies in human and nonhuman primates also suggest that AA intake is needed to balance DHA intake early in development: AA concentration exceeds that of DHA in the cortex as a whole in infants who died from crib death[4,13,14] and in young children in which fractions of phospholipids have been analyzed.[94,95] AA and its 22-carbon product, 22:4*n*-6 (adrenic acid), exceeded DHA in the hippocampus and occipital cortex of infant baboons, except when DHA was fed in excess of AA (e.g., formula containing 0.96% DHA and 0.64% AA).[96] Infants in the DIAMOND trial fed the same formula had a reduction in blood AA and showed consistently reduced cognitive benefit in early childhood relative to those who received the two lower DHA intakes.[97]

Therefore, despite the lack of direct experimental evidence for adding AA to the diet of formula-fed infants, several lines of evidence suggest it is prudent to balance the addition of DHA to infant formulas with AA as has happened with LCPUFA-supplemented formulas in the United States and most of the world.

NEURODEVELOPMENTAL OUTCOMES AFTER DOCOSAHEXAENOIC ACID SUPPLEMENTATION

RETINAL FUNCTION AND VISUAL ACUITY

DHA is the predominant fatty acid in the retina, and the essentiality of DHA for retinal function is well established from studies in nonhuman primates fed diets deficient in *n*-3 fatty acids.[98] Lower retinal and visual development were noted first in primates fed low α-linolenic acid-containing diets,[28] which led to low retinal DHA accumulation in monkeys[98] and piglets.[93] Retinal function was evaluated in an early preterm trial comparing formulas with low or higher α-linolenic acid or with DHA. Retinal electrophysiology was abnormal but became normal within weeks after birth even in infants fed an α-linolenic acid (and DHA)-deficient formula.[99] In infants fed formulas with α-linolenic acid, retinal DHA is similar to retinal DHA in human milk-fed infants.[14] However, developing infants appear to acquire adequate retinal DHA even when fed diets that contain little omega-3 fatty acids. This does not appear to be the case for the brain.

Visual acuity has been assessed by both behavioral (Teller Acuity Card) and electrophysiologic (visual evoked potential [VEP]) procedures. Visual acuity was the most common neurodevelopmental measure in most early infant studies.[17,18,80,100,101] Although studies have found higher visual acuity with DHA supplementation with these procedures, a study in term infants that measured visual acuity with both procedures found significantly higher visual acuity following DHA supplementation only with VEP.[14,80]

In addition to the methodologic differences between the acuity tests, the cortical regions responsible for processing the visual stimuli are different and mature at different rates; the primary visual cortex begins myelination at 3 to 4 months, and higher-order visual processing regions mature later.[102] Electrophysiologic methods rely on time-locked activity in the primary visual cortex, in response to black-white gratings alternating at a specific temporal frequency. Teller acuity cards require a behavioral response, requiring input from higher-order visual association cortex and other brain regions that influence visual behavior. Functional studies of DHA supplementation during pregnancy suggest that in utero brain DHA accumulation is important for optimal performance on visual tasks in infancy[103-105] and out to at least 5.5 years.[106]

The first interventions in which DHA was added to infant formula were designed for infants born preterm since these infants were the most likely to benefit from supplementation in the absence of in utero maternal transfer. Early randomized trials of DHA supplementation in preterm infants involved relatively small samples (*n*/group = 20 to 30), and all were conducted in the United States. All found higher visual acuity with DHA at some age in the first year of life when comparing formula without DHA to a formula with DHA.[17,18,89,107] The DHA for Neurodevelopment of Preterm Infants (DINO) trial was conducted in Australia and includes the largest group of infants born preterm studied in a single randomized controlled trial. In this study, the control group received approximately 0.3% of total fatty acids as DHA (like the amount currently in most US formulas) and the experimental group received 1% DHA. At 4 months corrected age, the group fed the higher amount of DHA had significantly higher visual acuity, suggesting that preterm infants may benefit from more DHA than is provided in current preterm formulas.[101]

Two additional studies in term infants found persistent effects of supplementation after postnatal DHA supplementation is discontinued.[108,109] The DIAMOND trial found higher visual acuity at 12 months of age in infants supplemented from birth to 12 months of age with DHA (0.32%, 0.64%, and 0.96%) and AA (0.64%) compared with those fed a control formula without DHA and AA.[51] Two large multicenter trials of LCPUFA-supplemented formulas found no effect of DHA and AA supplementation on visual acuity,[110,111] but the formulas used in these studies contained much less DHA than the formulas used by Birch and colleagues.[51,108,109] Although only approximately half of the studies find higher visual acuity in term infants with addition of DHA to infant formula, it should be noted that there is wide variation among studies in the environments of the populations assessed, the duration of supplementation, and the sources of LCPUFA. In addition, many of these studies lack appropriate statistical power.[112]

In contrast to postnatal DHA and AA supplementation, large randomized trials of prenatal DHA supplementation conducted in several countries have not found a benefit of maternal DHA supplementation in the range of 400 to 800 mg/day for visual acuity in infancy.[113,114]

AUTONOMIC DEVELOPMENT

The developing ANS is sensitive to the uterine environment and is thus a target for fetal programing effects. The transition from fetal to newborn life requires an integrated, flexible, and adaptive ANS to regulate and coordinate basic physiologic functions such as heart rate variability, blood pressure, and respiration. Furthermore, the ANS also supports basic cognitive domains of arousal, orienting, attention, and more advanced regulative functions such as impulse control and adaptation to stress.

HEART RATE VARIABILITY

Fetal autonomic development has been shown to be sensitive to maternal DHA intake. Researchers found more mature fetal heart rate variability at 36 weeks gestation in a small study of prenatal DHA supplementation (600 mg/day beginning before 20 weeks and ending at birth).[115] A secondary analysis, featuring a more comprehensive systems-biology approach, revealed that DHA supplementation led to more rapid ANS maturation, indexed by increased periods of vagal function and greater sympathovagal integration.[116] Similarly, higher maternal *n*-3 status during pregnancy was associated with lower infant heart rate and higher heart rate variability at 2 weeks and 4 and 6 months of age, whereas the inverse was found for maternal *n*-6 status.[117]

INFANT SLEEP

The ANS plays an important role in sleep, regulating both heart rate variability and respiration during sleep onset and transition through different sleep states. With infant maturation, there is an increase in quiet sleep, a decrease in active sleep, increased wakefulness, and a more marked transition from sleep to wake. Lammi-Keefe and colleagues[118] reported an association between maternal plasma phospholipid DHA and brain maturation in newborn infants based on differences in sleep patterns at birth. These researchers noted inverse relationships between maternal DHA status and maturity of sleep patterns (i.e., less active sleep, and a lower active sleep-to-quiet sleep ratio, more time awake, and less transition time between sleep and wake). In a subsequent randomized study, the same group provided pregnant women with a DHA-containing functional food (300 mg/day beginning at 24 weeks of gestation) and found evidence of a benefit of maternal DHA supplementation for more mature infant sleep/wake states in the first 48 hours of life.[119]

These effects on infant sleep/wake states suggest that higher DHA is associated with a more mature ANS. The underlying effect of DHA on the ANS could be due to effects of DHA supplementation on the endocannabinoid system as shown in a mouse model.[120] However, other potential mechanisms of action for DHA in the brain exist.[121-123] For example, the effects of DHA exposure on neurotransmitters[124-126] may have long-term programing effects on brain function. More work in this area is needed to determine if the beneficial effects of pregnancy supplementation are prolonged into infancy (i.e., if increased intrauterine DHA exposure has long-term effects on autonomic and central nervous system function).

COGNITIVE DEVELOPMENT

BRAIN PROCESSES UNDERLYING COGNITIVE DEVELOPMENT

The acquisition of information (including the speed and efficiency of information processing) and the retention of (i.e., memory for) that information are major indicators of cognitive development.[127] As DHA is concentrated at the synapses,[128] it may improve synaptic efficiency and neuronal transmission speed. DHA has also been implicated in processes that are integral to the laying down of a memory trace, such as long-term potentiation in the hippocampus.[129] Thus measurement of specific cognitive processes such as attention, processing speed, and memory is warranted in studies of the effects of DHA supplementation on the development of the child. We have elsewhere argued that the integration of memory and attention underlie and drive the development of the higher-order cognitions known as *executive functions*.[127] Executive functions include cognitive processes such as inhibitory control, problem solving, behavioral regulation, and planning/strategic behavior. These functions are widely accepted to be attributed to development of the frontal lobes, which mature at a more protracted rate relative to the rest of the brain. Although such integrated cognition is initiated at the end of the first year, these abilities are not reliably evident until the early preschool period (e.g., 3 to 4 years of age).

The frontal lobes accumulate significant amounts of DHA during development,[130] and the neurotransmitter dopamine appears to modulate working memory and attentional control.[131] Frontal dopamine is decreased in DHA-depleted rats,[125,126] and these DHA-depleted rats do not do as well on executive function types of tasks as DHA-adequate rats.[35,132] Moreover, the adverse effects of reduced brain DHA during development are not reversible if brain DHA is not remediated by DHA supplementation at weaning[124]; thus poor perinatal DHA status may program long-term brain structure and function. It seems reasonable to posit that the effects of DHA supplementation in infancy may also be manifest in the development of executive function.

White matter (i.e., myelin) quantity or quality may be another mechanism by which LCPUFA influences cognitive outcomes. White matter quality, as measured by diffusion tensor imaging (DTI), is related to cognition,[133,134] executive function and processing speed,[135] verbal fluency,[136] inhibitory control,[137] and improvement of hyperactive/impulsive symptoms.[138] Martinez and colleagues were the first to identify the link between brain myelination and DHA when they supplemented children with generalized peroxisomal disorders (DHA synthesis requires normal peroxisome function) with DHA and found improved brain myelination and function.[139,140] A report from Peters and colleagues[141] associated brain white matter development from childhood to adulthood with a *FADS* haplotype that predicts higher *n*-3 and *n*-6 LCPUFA in blood.

LANGUAGE DEVELOPMENT

Many studies have sought to establish whether various indices of language development vary as a function of DHA supplementation. Innis and colleagues[142] found that several indicators of DHA status (plasma phospholipid DHA, RBC phosphatidylcholine DHA, and phosphatidylethanolamine DHA) in breast-fed infants were significantly correlated with the preservation of plasticity in speech perception (i.e., the ability to discriminate nonnative language at 9 months) and with a parent-report measure of vocabulary comprehension and production at 14 months of age.[143] O'Connor and colleagues[80] found higher 14-month vocabulary comprehension in preterm infants from English-speaking families who were fed formulas with DHA and AA, compared with a placebo. Australian infants born at term and provided a fish oil supplement with 250 mg DHA/day from birth to 6 months showed higher performance on communicative gestures at 12 and 18 months on the Macarthur Bates Communicative Development Inventory (MBCDI), but they did not find differences between the groups in total words understood or spoken.[144]

There are three reports of apparent negative effects of DHA on early vocabulary: Lower scores on the MBCDI were observed at 14 months of age in a DHA-supplemented group relative to a control group in the United States,[145] although this difference in vocabulary did not persist at 3 years of age when the same children were administered a standardized expressive language assessment.[146] Similarly, Lauritzen and colleagues[147] found a lower language ability at 12 months of age in Danish breast-fed infants whose mothers had received DHA supplements compared with those who had not, but again these differences did not persist when children were reassessed at 2 years of age. Finally, in an extension of the DIAMOND study with the Dallas sample, Drover and colleagues[148] found that infants supplemented with LCPUFA at 0.32% and 0.96% levels performed worse than controls on the Peabody Picture Vocabulary Test (PPVT) at 2 years of age, but it should be noted that administration of the PPVT at this age is questionable; indeed, the scores obtained for children at age 2 in both supplemented and control groups fell at least one standard deviation below normal. These differences were no longer present when the test was repeated at 3.5 years of age.

Mulder and colleagues[149] reported on language assessments administered between 14 and 18 months of age in children whose mothers were randomly assigned to a placebo or 400 mg DHA/day beginning at approximately 16 weeks of gestation until birth. Results were analyzed in terms of risk for language delay, and DHA supplementation was observed to reduce this on measures of words understood, words produced, and sentences produced on the MBCDI. Differences were also observed on expressive language items measured on the Bayley Scales of Infant Development (BSID)-III at 18 months.

Two reports show positive effects of higher perinatal DHA exposure on language functions in 5-year-old children. In one of these, data from an observational study in the Seychelles (where fish consumption is very high) had led researchers to conclude that language in 5.5-year-old children was associated with maternal methylmercury exposure from seafood.[150] Reanalysis of data controlling for maternal serum DHA and AA obtained early in the third trimester and at delivery led to the conclusion that maternal DHA was actually responsible for significantly higher total language score and verbal ability on the Preschool Language Scale-Revised Edition and significantly higher verbal knowledge on the Kaufman Brief Intelligence Test.[151]

In a randomized controlled trial, all groups (control and LCPUFA groups) performed similarly on the MBCDI at 18 months of age in the Kansas City DIAMOND trial cohort, but at 5 years of age the groups of children randomly assigned to LCPUFA supplemented formulas in infancy (DHA 0.32%, 0.64%, or 0.96%; AA 0.64%) scored significantly higher on the PPVT-III. At 6 years of age, the supplemented groups scored higher than the control group on the verbal IQ subscale of the Weschler Preschool Primary Intelligence Scale (WPPSI)-III.[152]

Children from this trial were invited to return for fMRI studies at approximately 9 years of age. Children who were supplemented with LCPUFA (0.32% and 0.64% DHA with 0.64% AA) in infancy had in an increased percentage of white matter relative to controls, and the percentage of white matter was correlated with verbal IQ.[153] Taken together, the results of all published trials indicate that higher LCPUFA exposure in the perinatal period is a positive predictor of language function at school age.

VISUAL ATTENTION: RECOGNITION MEMORY AND ATTENTION

Attention is a fundamental component of information processing that is commonly measured in infancy. Attention reflects brain processes that are involved in learning, and infants' attention to a novel stimulus after repeated exposure to a familiarized one is a longstanding index of recognition memory. Research suggests that early attention is modestly correlated with more sophisticated measures of cognitive function at school age.[127,154,155] Several studies in infants born preterm compared visual recognition memory and/or the duration of attention in infants fed formulas with or without DHA or DHA and AA.[80,107,156] As noted previously, both novelty preference and shorter look duration in infancy are modestly correlated with higher cognitive function later in childhood.[157] In two randomized trials involving very small preterm infants (~28 weeks gestation and ~1000 g birth weight), infants fed control and DHA-supplemented formulas had similar recognition memory performance but supplemented infants had a shorter look duration at 6, 9, and 12 or at 12 months corrected age,[107,156] indicative of more rapid stimulus processing. These results are analogous with those reported in *n*-3-sufficient compared with *n*-3-deficient monkeys, in that higher DHA status was associated with shorter look duration.[37] Both the nonhuman primate and human studies are consistent with the idea that higher brain DHA accumulation enhances the speed or efficiency of visual processing.

O'Connor and colleagues[80] conducted a much larger multicenter trial and took the same measures on two groups of preterm infants whose diets were supplemented with DHA and AA (fish/fungal and fish/egg triglyceride), compared with a control group of infants whose diets were not supplemented. Neither recognition memory nor attention varied among groups at 6 and 9 months of age. Compared with the two earlier reports, these infants had longer gestations, less chronic lung disease, and higher birth weight, which might explain the lack of different outcomes for look duration.

Look duration declines sharply across the first year of life, as infants' ability to process information improves. This decline was accelerated in infants born at term whose mothers had higher RBC phospholipid DHA.[158] The difference in look duration dissipated by 8 months of age but reemerged as longer sustained attention at 12 and 18 months of age with the administration of more sophisticated tasks.[155,159] Given that infants were not provided DHA supplementation after birth and toddler DHA intake in the United States is very low,[160] the data are consistent with the possibility that higher DHA accumulation during intrauterine life was responsible for more mature infant and toddler attention.

Experimental studies that manipulate maternal DHA status during pregnancy have tested this hypothesis. Gould and colleagues[161] reported no overall benefit of DHA supplementation during pregnancy (DOMInO trial) on childhood attention in Australian children at 2.3 years of age using single-object and distractibility tasks; however, on multiple-object attention tasks supplemented toddlers showed slightly fewer episodes of inattention.

In the Kansas City DIAMOND cohort, infants who were supplemented with DHA (either 0.32%, 0.64%, or 0.96%) and AA (0.64%) had higher proportions of sustained attention (a measure derived from a combination of looking and heart rate deceleration) during looking compared to infants who were consuming the control formula.[104] This cohort of children was tested every 6 months on further specific measures of cognitive function out to age 6 (see "Targeted Measures of Cognitive Development in Infants and Young Children" later). Finally, in the Kansas University DHA Outcomes Study (KUDOS), a large randomized trial involving prenatal DHA supplementation with 600 mg/day or a placebo, infants from mothers who were supplemented during pregnancy showed a maintenance of sustained attention across the first year; sustained attention in infants from mothers assigned a placebo declined over the same period.[105]

GLOBAL MEASURES OF DEVELOPMENT IN INFANTS AND YOUNG CHILDREN

The BSID,[162] currently in its 4th edition, is a standardized assessment that provides indices of developmental status relative to group norms. Because standardized tests like this one are more familiar to pediatricians, they are frequently used as outcome measures in DHA supplementation trials. The BSID was initially developed to identify infants at risk for later delayed development, but over the years, scores from the scale have been increasingly interpreted as a continuous measure of developmental status. It measures broad categories of function in different behavioral domains, and while the test is certainly useful, its limitations are widely acknowledged.[163] The results from global assessments such as the BSID in LCPUFA supplementation studies are decidedly mixed. Some have found that supplementation with DHA resulted in higher standardized scores,[164-167] whereas others, including several larger and appropriately powered trials, have found no effect. There could be several reasons for these mixed results; for example, differences in samples, supplementation, and administration could confound the results. We have argued[168] that the effects of LCPUFA supplementation may be specific to certain cognitive components; if that is the case, global tests such as the BSID may not possess the level of granularity that would make it sensitive to LCPUFA status. Because most studies of infants and toddlers rely such global measures, meta-analyses and systematic reviews rely heavily on outcomes like the BSID. We strongly suggest that these meta-analyses be interpreted with caution.[168]

The BSID Mental Developmental Index was higher in the combined groups supplemented with DHA and AA compared with the control group in the Dallas DIAMOND cohort[169] but not in the Kansas City DIAMOND cohort.[152] Morales and colleagues[170] found that LCPUFA supply during pregnancy and lactation linked to the maternal *FADS* and *ELOVL* genes were related to performance on the BSID II at 14 months of age. The effects of breast-feeding were modified by the child's *FADS* and *ELOVL* genotype. In infants born preterm, Sabel and colleagues[171] observed a positive relationship between performance on the BSID II in relation to infant plasma DHA and AA at 1-month corrected age. Infants had been fed their mother's milk, with variable DHA and AA. They were evaluated at several ages in infancy and again at 18 months. Thus the global assessments may have utility in studies of at-risk children such as those with preterm histories or studies in the hypothesis-building stages such as the current state of the genetic work.

TARGETED MEASURES OF COGNITIVE DEVELOPMENT IN INFANTS AND YOUNG CHILDREN

Researchers who have used targeted measures of cognitive development in infants and very young children more consistently find benefits, compared with researchers who have used global measures. As noted previously, infants fed formula supplemented with DHA or DHA and AA are better able to detect novelty,[80] show faster visual processing,[89,107,172] and have better problem solving[173,174] compared with infants fed control formula without LCPUFA. As previously mentioned, infants whose mothers had DHA levels greater than the sample median at the time of their births had enhanced information processing performance, as well as more mature orienting and attentional abilities.[158]

PRENATAL LCPUFA AND COGNITIVE OUTCOMES IN CHILDHOOD

At the time of the previous edition, there were a few observational reports of cognitive function in children in relation to maternal DHA status and a couple of reports from randomized clinical trials that provided DHA or AA during the perinatal period. Since publication of the previous edition, Gustafsson and colleagues[175] reported that DHA levels in colostrum were significantly related to IQ at 6.5 years of age. As noted in the section on language development, higher maternal DHA during pregnancy in the Seychelles was linked to higher language scores at 5 years of age on a test of preschool language development.[151] Another study from the Seychelles found beneficial effects of maternal *n*-3 LCPUFA but not *n*-6 LCPUFA on the BSID-II Psychomotor Developmental Index (PDI) at 9 months of age.[176] Both maternal DHA and AA during pregnancy had a significant positive effect on IQ at 8 years of age in another large cohort ($n = 2839$).[177]

Analogous to work done in the Seychelles, Jacobson and colleagues sought to untangle the adverse effects of environmental pollutants from the possible beneficial effects of *n*-3 LCPUFA on cognitive function in a high-fish consuming population in Arctic Quebec. In children at a mean age of 11.3 years, they found shorter brain F400 latency and enhanced amplitude (both suggesting greater brain maturation) as well as higher performance on a task assessing memory in relation to the DHA level measured at birth in cord blood.[178] In another study, higher DHA intake during pregnancy was linked to performance on a task measuring search for a novel object at 22 months of age.[179] In yet another study, researchers assessed neurologic development at 4 and 5.5 years of age in children of pregnant women enrolled in Spain, Germany, and Hungary. Similar to the findings reported by Mulder and colleagues,[149] the odds of optimal neurologic development increased with each unit increase in cord blood, maternal plasma, and maternal erythrocyte phospholipid DHA at birth.[180]

Several randomized clinical trials that provided DHA or a placebo during pregnancy have reported on cognitive function of the offspring. In an Australian trial by Dunstan and colleagues,[181] there was no effect on hand-eye coordination in the supplemented group at 2.5 years of age, but hand-eye coordination scores were significantly related to n-3 PUFA levels in cord blood erythrocytes. Helland and colleagues[182] found higher IQ on a standardized test at 4 years of age in Norwegian children whose mothers received a very large fish oil supplement during pregnancy and the first several months of lactation. At 7 years of age, children of women assigned to placebo did not differ from those assigned to fish oil during pregnancy, but maternal DHA during pregnancy was associated with higher scores on the Kaufman Assessment Battery for Children (K-ABC) sequential processing index.[183] No effect of LCPUFA supplementation was found on the outcomes measured during infancy.

Maternal DHA and EPA supplementation during pregnancy did not affect working memory at 2.3 years in the Australian DOMInO trial.[161] At 4 and 7 years of age, the DHA-supplemented group in that trial still showed no cognitive benefit, while parents reported more behavior problems in the supplemented group on subscales of the Behavior Rating Inventory of Executive Function-Preschool.[184,185] Campoy and colleagues[186] reported that fish oil supplementation during pregnancy did not affect K-ABC scores, although higher maternal erythrocyte DHA at birth was associated with scores greater than the 50th percentile on the Mental Processing Composite Score. In the KUDOS, supplementation with 600 mg/day of DHA compared with placebo resulted in improved early visual attention during infancy[104]; however, there were only a few positive effects of supplementation noted through age 6, and they occurred in the first 3 years of life.[187] Infants of mothers whose DHA status improved did have higher IQ scores at 5 and 6 years, but the effect was confounded by socioeconomic status. No significant effects of DHA supplementation on parent reported behavior (Behavioral Assessment Scale for Children [BASC-2]) were found.[187]

POSTNATAL LCPUFA AND COGNITIVE OUTCOMES IN CHILDHOOD

The Southampton Women's Survey Study Group compared full scale and verbal IQ of 4-year-old children fed formulas with or without LCPUFA during infancy. Although both full scale and verbal IQ were higher in the LCPUFA-formula fed group, investigators found no effect of LCPUFA supplemented formula when they controlled for maternal IQ and education in this nonrandomized study.[188] Jensen and colleagues[189] randomly assigned US women to consume 200 mg/day of DHA from a single-cell oil during lactation. The toddlers of the women who received supplements had higher scores on a standardized test of motor function at 30 months of age[189] and longer sustained attention at 5 years of age.[190] The average milk DHA content was 0.35% of total fatty acids (equivalent to most US formulas).[189]

Three reports provide results for older children randomly exposed to LCPUFA-supplemented formula for a short period of time (2 to 4 months) after birth. Willatts and colleagues[191] reported that 6-year-old children supplemented with formula containing DHA and AA for the first 4 months of life showed faster information processing but no overall effect on IQ or attention control. The Groningen LCPUFA study provided a supplemented formula for only 2 months after term birth and found an interaction between LCPUFA supplementation and maternal smoking with regard to child IQ at 9 years of age; specifically, children of women who smoked during pregnancy had significantly higher verbal IQ and learning memory scores on the Weschler Abbreviated Scale of Intelligence and the Children's Memory Scale, respectively, if they received LCPUFA.[192] On the other hand, the control group performed better than the LCPUFA group on verbal IQ and verbal memory in children of women who did not smoke during pregnancy.[192] No effect of early LCPUFA supplementation was found on the Neurological Optimality Score at 9 years of age.[193]

Cognitive performance of 7-year-old Danish children was not influenced by maternal fish oil consumption during the first 4 months of lactation; however, the mean maternal n-3 LCPUFA intake in the control group was 260 mg/day,[194] approximately five times that of most US adult women. The fish oil-supplemented group had a mean intake of 1.59 grams/d of n-3 LCPUFA. There was a trend for lower prosocial score in the supplemented group (a potential adverse effect of maternal fish oil consumption), which post hoc analysis demonstrated to be related to a higher prosocial score in males whose mothers were in the control formula compared with the scores of children whose mothers were in the LPCUFA group. The authors suggest the post hoc result should be regarded with caution because the study was not designed to look at sex effects.

Cognitive function has been evaluated in both Dallas and Kansas City cohorts of the DIAMOND trial. As mentioned earlier, the DIAMOND study was a randomized, controlled DHA dose-response study of DHA and AA supplemented infant formula with infants provided the study formulas from birth to 12 months of age. The DIAMOND cohort studied in Kansas City was evaluated on attention and memory in infancy and on age-appropriate tests of cognitive function every 6 months beginning at 18 months and ending at 6 years of age. At preschool age, the children who were supplemented with LCPUFA during infancy scored significantly higher on tests of inhibitory control (Stroop, Dimensional Change Card Sort) and on tests of verbal IQ.[152] Unlike the Dallas cohort, no benefit of LCPUFA was observed at 18 months of age on the MBCDI or BSID-II[152] when analyzed by intervention group. However, Drover and colleagues[169] evaluated performance on the BSID-II in toddlers and reported significantly higher performance in the combined LCPUFA-supplemented groups with DHA intake ranging from 0.32% to 0.96% of total fatty acids (see "Global Measures of Development in Infants and Young Children").

BRAIN ELECTROPHYSIOLOGY AND IMAGING

Studies of brain structure and function have helped to elucidate the role of DHA in the developing brain. Healthy boys aged 8 to 10 years were randomized to placebo oil, low-dose (400 mg/day) or high-dose (1200 mg/day) DHA for 8 weeks,[117] then underwent functional magnetic resonance imaging (fMRI) during the performance of a visual sustained attention task. Supplementation resulted in a dose-dependent increase in RBC DHA that, in turn, was positively associated with functional cortical activity and negatively related to reaction time during performance of the task. This was the first study to provide brain-imaging evidence suggesting a role for DHA in the neural networks underlying attention. The same research group performed a cross-sectional study of 8- to 10-year-old boys, using a median split to divide groups into "low DHA" and "high DHA" based on RBC DHA as an indicator of DHA status.[195] Boys performed the same visual attention task, and like the results in the previously described controlled dose-response trial, the low-DHA group had reduced functional connectivity and slower reaction times. Investigators also measured brain metabolites in this cohort using proton magnetic resonance spectroscopy and found significantly lower myo-inositol, N-acetyl aspartate, choline, and creatine concentrations in the anterior cingulate cortex in the low-DHA group.

Multi-modal brain imaging was used in the long-term follow-up of 9-year-old children who participated in the DIAMOND trial.[153] The study was designed to determine whether there were long-term effects of DHA-arachidonic acid (ARA) exposure during infancy and included fMRI to a Flanker task, resting state MRI, anatomic structural MRI, and proton magnetic resonance spectroscopy. There were significant group differences, confirming that early life DHA-ARA has long-term effects on brain structure, function, and neurochemical concentrations in brain regions associated with attention and inhibition. Further, like previously reported studies of DHA status in boys, brain metabolites associated with neuronal integrity (N-acetyl aspartate) and brain cell signaling (myo-inositol) were higher in children who received supplemented formula in the first year of life.

Another study reported greater dorsal anterior cingulate cortex activation during successful inhibition of a No-Go response in 11- to 13-year-old children with lower self-reported dietary omega-3 index (a summation of reported EPA and DHA intakes).[196] This finding differs from Lepping and colleagues,[153] who found greater activation in the anterior cingulate cortex during inhibition to the Flanker in 9-year-old children who received DHA-ARA supplemented formulas throughout the first year of life but a freely chosen diet that was likely similar to the low US intake of EPA and DHA in childhood.[197]

Studies of brain function using electrophysiology (e.g., event-related potentials [ERPs]) have also increased understanding of long-term effects of early life LCPUFA supplementation. ERPs are recorded during the performance of a specific task, often requiring recognition memory, rule following, and conflict resolution. For example, the Flanker task requires a different response to congruent versus incongruent conditions, whereas the Go/No-Go task requires subjects to press a button to one stimulus (Go) but inhibit the response to another (No-Go). For the Go/No-Go task, the test is designed to favor the Go condition to induce a prepotent response weighted towards pressing the button. Behavioral responses such as reaction time, correct and incorrect responses, and brain electrophysiology are simultaneously recorded. Components of the averaged waveform are stimulus specific. Relevant to this discussion are the P2 and N2 components. P2 is thought to represent endogenous attention orienting, an action that facilitates the visual process of identification, comparing and analyzing the target stimuli. As such, P2 amplitude indicates improved performance on visual tasks. N2 is a marker of inhibitory control and amplitude is typically greater to the No-Go than the Go condition; the "condition difference" is greater in subjects with greater inhibitory control.

A large study of Inuit children found evidence of long-term beneficial effects of prenatal and childhood LCPUFA on visual recognition memory and ERP components related to recognition memory when the children were tested at age 11 years. The larger amplitude ERP components were specifically related to higher umbilical cord plasma concentrations of DHA.[198]

Children in the DIAMOND study underwent ERP testing when they were 5.5 years of age, performing an age-appropriate Go/No-Go task.[199] There was no effect of supplementation on behavior other than a trend for faster reaction time. Compared with children in the control group who were randomized to formula with no added LCPUFA, those children who received supplemented formulas the first year of life had greater P2 amplitude. This finding is especially important because children receiving the supplemented formula also had improved visual attention over the first year of life. These children also had the typical N2 amplitude condition difference associated with greater inhibition, whereas children randomized to control formula failed to show this difference. Secondary analysis of the ERP microstates (i.e., transient, semistable patterns of the electroencephalogram (EEG) lasting a few milliseconds) revealed a novel microstate in supplemented children, linked to the time range of active visual processing and decision making prior to pressing the button. Importantly, the microstate to the No-Go condition had a longer duration and, like the N2 condition difference, was missing in the children who did not receive DHA-ARA in infancy.

The same Go/No-Go ERP was used to test the long-term effects of prenatal supplementation. Women were randomized to either placebo or 600 mg DHA during the second and third trimesters of pregnancy. When children were 5.5 years of age, they performed the ERP task.[106] Prenatal DHA resulted in a sex difference for response accuracy (correct Go trials) in that males in the supplemented group were most accurate. Response inhibition (correct No-Go trials) was improved by prenatal DHA supplementation, although for DHA females, this inhibitory effect carried over to the Go trials. Like the postnatal study, P2 amplitude was greater in the DHA group and N2 amplitude was greater in DHA males.

MOTOR DEVELOPMENT

Agostoni and colleagues reported earlier achievement of sitting without support in infants who received a daily DHA supplement of 20 mg in infancy[164]; however, they did not find a benefit of later motor milestones in infancy (crawling, standing, walking). Ninety-eight percent received some human milk in infancy, which would have provided DHA. Hadders-Algra and her collaborators in The Netherlands[180,200-203] published several reports of LCPUFA during pregnancy on motor milestones and quality of movement in infants and toddlers. A 2011 report linked better motoric outcomes at 5.5 years to higher cord RBC and plasma phospholipid DHA.[180] Another research group from The Netherlands associated movement quality at 7 years of age with higher umbilical plasma DHA (signifying higher intrauterine DHA exposure).[204]

SOCIOEMOTIONAL DEVELOPMENT

The LISAplus Study conducted in Germany linked higher cord blood serum DHA, AA, and total LCPUFA to parental assessment of less difficult behavior on the Strengths and Difficulties Questionnaire. In particular, they found fewer total difficulties, less hyperactivity/inattention, and fewer emotional symptoms at 10 years of age.[205] In another study of problems from Germany, DHA in midpregnancy was associated with higher (favorable) scores on combined parent and teacher assessment of emotional and behavioral problems at 6 years of age while AA was associated with lower (less favorable) scores.[206] In contrast to these reports, a randomized trial conducted in Australia with 800 mg DHA/day (and 100 mg EPA/day) during pregnancy found more total difficulties and more hyperactivity in the DHA-supplemented group compared with the placebo group.[184] As noted previously, parents of children in DOMInO reported more behavioral problems[184,185]; however, prenatal DHA supplementation was unrelated to child behavior in KUDOS.[187]

A COMMENTARY ON INFANT SUPPLEMENTATION TRIALS

Although there have been several meta-analyses and systematic reviews of LCPUFA supplementation of infants, this type of analysis is not well suited to studies of nutrients where there are large differences in intake among populations. DHA and AA are nutrients, and the goal of good nutrition is for diet (or dietary supplements) to provide a safe and adequate amount of nutrients for optimal health. A fundamental flaw of meta-analyses and systematic reviews for studies of nutrients is that they pool results from studies conducted in different cultures with very different LCPUFA intakes. With respect to DHA, this leads to a bias toward a conclusion of no effect for supplementation, because most trials have been conducted in fish-eating populations, rather than in world populations with low DHA intakes. However, a number of trials have been conducted in the United States, where dietary DHA intake of adults is very low (~48 mg of DHA per day).[207]

If the results of meta-analyses were solely used to define public policy, the result might well be harm to individuals and populations who have inadequate intake of that nutrient. We have also expressed our concern about the primary outcomes on which meta-analyses/systematic reviews on this topic have been based.[168] The need to study groups that are deficient in a nutrient is beginning to be accepted[208]; indeed, one study in particular illustrates the presence of differences in DHA status within a cohort of pregnant women and relates status to functional outcomes in the perinatal period.[149] To truly understand the effects of fatty acids, future research should focus on controlling variables not previously considered, such as genetics, nutrient balance, and synergistic effects of nutrients, when considering whether supplementation of the infant diet with fatty acids has a positive effect on development. For example, Cheatham and coworkers found synergistic effects of DHA and choline in human milk on infant recognition memory.[209] Most importantly, samples chosen for study should have an initial, fundamental need for supplementation. Quite simply put, if remediation is not needed, supplementation should not be expected to have an effect.

CONCLUSION

In 2002, DHA and AA began to be added to formulas in the United States. The last published randomized trial of LCPUFA supplemented formula began in 2003 and was the only dose-response study of LCPUFA conducted.[51] The Kansas City cohort from that trial was studied out to 10 years of age, and the results demonstrate clear benefits of LCPUFA supplementation, ranging from longer sustained attention and better memory in infancy to higher verbal IQ and ability to inhibit behavior at school age. These findings are supported by brain electrophysiology at 5.5 years (evoked response potentials) and multimodal brain imaging at 9 to 10 years (higher density white matter; and a higher percentage of white compared with gray matter that correlates with verbal IQ).

Although this is one of the more intensely and comprehensively evaluated cohorts of children randomized to variable LCPUFA in the perinatal period, there are several reports of cognitive outcomes at school age and beyond from cohorts exposed to perinatal (prenatal or postnatal) DHA or DHA and AA. At the time of the last edition, results in children exposed to higher DHA during the perinatal periods were very limited; available reports showed higher IQ at 4 years of age[182] and longer sustained attention at 5 years of age.[190] These two early studies encouraged other investigators to follow cohorts of children into childhood, because they provided the first evidence that perinatal exposure to LCPUFA could program the developing brain with long-term benefit to cognition.

It is now clear that (1) LCPUFA are needed for optimal fetal and neonatal development; (2) some samples received inadequate supplementation in the perinatal period; and (3) the presence of LCPUFA in the perinatal period appears to confer a long-term benefit (i.e., programs) later brain function. Evidence suggests that changes in the ratio of white to gray matter and white matter quality long after LCPUFA exposure are linked to this programing. Animal studies have already shown that DHA is a factor in neuronal development. In addition, there are other possible mechanisms through which LCPUFA program the developing brain and influence later brain outcomes. For example, animal studies have shown programing of neurotransmitter systems occur very early in development in relation to DHA supply.

Although the importance of DHA in infant development is becoming increasingly obvious from human and animal work, the optimal and maximum levels of DHA intake for pregnant women and infants have not yet been determined. Likewise, the optimal balance of DHA and AA is unknown, and optimal balance may be different during pregnancy compared with postnatally. Progress in these areas is to be expected in the future because several large trials are currently ongoing around the world. However, these studies are taking place at the same time as DHA intake from supplements, foods with added DHA, and formula with LCPUFA may be changing the background DHA exposure of women, infants, and children. Variable DHA exposure in control groups will be a potential confounder of new studies of DHA supplementation. Studies of infant behavior will need to control for maternal prenatal and background diet postnatal LCPUFA intake and/or use some biochemical measure of LCPUFA status such as RBC or plasma phospholipid concentrations. In addition, the evidence of a confounding effect of maternal and offspring genetics is amassing. The presence of minor alleles in the *FADS* gene complex may predispose an individual to a higher need for exogenous DHA because the enzymes for the metabolism of the precursors may be less functional. Researchers must consider the genetic make-up of the mothers and babies, as well as background diet to fully elucidate the effects of LCPUFA on human development.

A complete reference list is available at www.ExpertConsult.com. 

SELECT REFERENCES

14. Makrides M, Neumann MA, Byard RW, et al. Fatty acid composition of brain, retina, and erythrocytes in breast- and formula-fed infants. *Am J Clin Nutr.* 1994;60:189–194.
18. Carlson SE, Werkman SH, Rhodes PG, et al. Visual-acuity development in healthy preterm infants: effect of marine-oil supplementation. *Am J Clin Nutr.* 1993;58:35–42.
42. Birch DG, Birch EE, Hoffman DR, et al. Retinal development in very-low-birth-weight infants fed diets differing in omega-3 fatty acids. *Invest Ophthalmol Vis Sci.* 1992;33:2365–2376.
51. Birch EE, Carlson SE, Hoffman DR, et al. The DIAMOND (DHA Intake and Measurement of Neural Development) Study: a double-masked, randomized controlled clinical trial of the maturation of infant visual acuity as a function of the dietary level of docosahexaenoic acid. *Am J Clin Nutr.* 2010;91:848–859.
54. Leaf AA, Leighfield MJ, Costeloe KL, et al. Long chain polyunsaturated fatty acids and fetal growth. *Early Hum Dev.* 1992;30:183–191.
55. Kuipers RS, Luxwolda MF, Offringa PJ, et al. Gestational age dependent changes of the fetal brain, liver and adipose tissue fatty acid compositions in a population with high fish intakes. *Prostaglandins Leukot Essent Fatty Acids.* 2012;86:189–199.
66. Koletzko B, Lattka E, Zeilinger S, et al. Genetic variants of the fatty acid desaturase gene cluster predict amounts of red blood cell docosahexaenoic and other polyunsaturated fatty acids in pregnant women: findings from the Avon Longitudinal Study of Parents and Children. *Am J Clin Nutr.* 2011;93:211–219.
67. Scholtz SA, Kerling EH, Shaddy DJ, et al. Docosahexaenoic acid (DHA) supplementation in pregnancy differentially modulates arachidonic acid and DHA status across FADS genotypes in pregnancy. *Prostaglandins Leukot Essent Fatty Acids.* 2015;94:29–33.
72. Henderson RA, Jensen RG, Lammi-Keefe CJ, et al. Effect of fish oil on the fatty acid composition of human milk and maternal and infant erythrocytes. *Lipids.* 1992;27:863–869.
79. Carlson SE, Rhodes PG, Rao VS, et al. Effect of fish oil supplementation on the n-3 fatty acid content of red blood cell membranes in preterm infants. *Pediatr Res.* 1987;21:507–510.
84. EFSA NDA Panel (EFSA Panel on Dietetic Products). Scientific opinion on the essential composition of infant and follow-on formulae. *EFSA J.* 2014;12:3760.
86. Koletzko B, Carlson SE, van Goudoever JB. Should infant formula provide both omega-3 DHA and omega-6 arachidonic acid? *Ann Nutr Metab.* 2015;66:137–138.
87. Koletzko B, Bergmann K, Brenna JT, et al. Should formula for infants provide arachidonic acid along with DHA? A position paper of the European Academy of Paediatrics and the Child Health Foundation. *Am J Clin Nutr.* 2020;111:10–16.
95. Svennerholm L. Distribution and fatty acid composition of phosphoglycerides in normal human brain. *J Lipid Res.* 1968;9:570–579.
96. Hsieh AT, Anthony JC, Diersen-Schade DA, et al. The influence of moderate and high dietary long chain polyunsaturated fatty acids (LCPUFA) on baboon neonate tissue fatty acids. *Pediatr Res.* 2007;61:537–545.
102. Sampaio RC, Truwit CL. Myelination in the developing human brain. In: *Handbook of Developmental Cognitive Neuroscience.* Cambridge, MA: MIT Press; 2001:35–44.
103. Ramakrishnan U, Stinger A, DiGirolamo AM, et al. Prenatal docosahexaenoic acid supplementation and offspring development at 18 months: randomized controlled trial. *PloS One.* 2015;10:e0120065.
104. Colombo J, Carlson SE, Cheatham CL, et al. Long-chain polyunsaturated fatty acid supplementation in infancy reduces heart rate and positively affects distribution of attention. *Pediatr Res.* 2011;70:406–410.
105. Colombo J, Gustafson KM, Gajewski BJ, et al. Prenatal DHA supplementation and infant attention. *Pediatr Res.* 2016;80:656–662.
106. Gustafson KM, Liao K, Mathis NB, et al. Prenatal docosahexaenoic acid supplementation has long-term effects on childhood behavioral and brain responses during performance on an inhibitory task: prenatal DHA and childhood inhibitory performance. *Nutr Neurosci.* 2020;1–11.

113. Smithers LG, Gibson RA, Makrides M. Maternal supplementation with docosahexaenoic acid during pregnancy does not affect early visual development in the infant: a randomized controlled trial. *Am J Clin Nutr*. 2011;93:1293–1299.
114. Stein AD, Wang M, Rivera JA, et al. Auditory- and visual-evoked potentials in Mexican infants are not affected by maternal supplementation with 400 mg/d docosahexaenoic acid in the second half of pregnancy. *J Nutr*. 2012;142: 1577–1581.
116. Hoyer D, Schmidt A, Schneider U, et al. Fetal developmental deviations reflected in a functional autonomic brain age score. In: *Computing in Cardiology Conference (CinC)*. Maastricht, The Netherlands: IEEE; 2018:23–26.
129. Itokazu N, Ikegaya Y, Nishikawa M, et al. Bidirectional actions of docosahexaenoic acid on hippocampal neurotransmissions in vivo. *Brain Res*. 2000;862:211–216.
131. Nieoullon A. Dopamine and the regulation of cognition and attention. *Prog Neurobiol*. 2002;67:53–83.
140. Martinez M, Vazquez E. MRI evidence that docosahexaenoic acid ethyl ester improves myelination in generalized peroxisomal disorders. *Neurology*. 1998;51:26–32.
141. Peters BD, Voineskos AN, Szeszko PR, et al. Brain white matter development is associated with a human-specific haplotype increasing the synthesis of long chain fatty acids. *J Neurosci*. 2014;34:6367–6376.
142. Innis SM, Gilley J, Werker J. Are human milk long-chain polyunsaturated fatty acids related to visual and neural development in breast-fed term infants? *J Pediatr*. 2001;139:532–538.
150. Davidson PW, Myers GJ, Cox C, et al. Effects of prenatal and postnatal methylmercury exposure from fish consumption on neurodevelopment: outcomes at 66 months of age in the Seychelles Child Development Study. *J Am Med Assoc*. 1998;280:701–707.
151. Strain JJ, Davidson PW, Thurston SW, et al. Maternal PUFA status but not prenatal methylmercury exposure is associated with children's language functions at age five years in the Seychelles. *J Nutr*. 2012;142:1943–1949.
152. Colombo J, Carlson SE, Cheatham CL, et al. Long-term effects of LCPUFA supplementation on childhood cognitive outcomes. *Am J Clin Nutr*. 2013;98: 403–412.
158. Colombo J, Kannass KN, Shaddy DJ, et al. Maternal DHA and the development of attention in infancy and toddlerhood. *Child Dev*. 2004;75:1254–1267.
161. Gould JF, Makrides M, Colombo J, et al. Randomized controlled trial of maternal omega-3 long-chain PUFA supplementation during pregnancy and early childhood development of attention, working memory, and inhibitory control. *Am J Clin Nutr*. 2014;99:851–859.
173. Willatts P, Forsyth JS, DiModugno MK, et al. Effect of long-chain polyunsaturated fatty acids in infant formula on problem solving at 10 months of age. *Lancet*. 1998;352:688–691.
175. Gustafsson PA, Duchen K, Birberg U, et al. Breastfeeding, very long polyunsaturated fatty acids (PUFA) and IQ at 6 1/2 years of age. *Acta Paediatr*. 2004;93:1280–1287.
177. Steer CD, Lattka E, Koletzko B, et al. Maternal fatty acids in pregnancy, FADS polymorphisms, and child intelligence quotient at 8 y of age. *Am J Clin Nutr*. 2013;98:1575–1582.
180. Escolano-Margarit MV, Ramos R, Beyer J, et al. Prenatal DHA status and neurological outcome in children at age 5.5 years are positively associated. *J Nutr*. 2011;141:1216–1223.
182. Helland IB, Smith L, Saarem K, et al. Maternal supplementation with very-long-chain n-3 fatty acids during pregnancy and lactation augments children's IQ at 4 years of age. *Pediatrics*. 2003;111:e39–e44.
184. Makrides M, Gould JF, Gawlik NR, et al. Four-year follow-up of children born to women in a randomized trial of prenatal DHA supplementation. *J Am Med Assoc*. 2014;311:1802–1804.
187. Colombo J, Shaddy DJ, Gustafson K, et al. The Kansas University DHA Outcomes Study (KUDOS) clinical trial: long-term behavioral follow-up of the effects of prenatal DHA supplementation. *Am J Clin Nutr*. 2019;109:1380–1392.
188. Gale CR, Marriott LD, Martyn CN, et al. Breastfeeding, the use of docosahexaenoic acid-fortified formulas in infancy and neuropsychological function in childhood. *Arch Dis Child*. 2010;95:174–179.
190. Jensen CL, Voigt RG, Llorente AM, et al. Effects of early maternal docosahexaenoic acid intake on neuropsychological status and visual acuity at five years of age of breast-fed term infants. *J Pediatr*. 2010;157:900–905.
191. Willatts P, Forsyth S, Agostoni C, et al. Effects of long-chain PUFA supplementation in infant formula on cognitive function in later childhood. *Am J Clin Nutr*. 2013;98:536s–542s.
192. de Jong C, Kikkert HK, Fidler V, et al. Effects of long-chain polyunsaturated fatty acid supplementation of infant formula on cognition and behaviour at 9 years of age. *Dev Med Child Neurol*. 2012;54:1102–1108.
195. Almeida DM, Jandacek RJ, Weber WA, et al. Docosahexaenoic acid biostatus is associated with event-related functional connectivity in cortical attention networks of typically developing children. *Nutr Neurosci*. 2017;20:246–254.
178. Boucher O, Burden MJ, Muckle G, et al. Neurophysiologic and neurobehavioral evidence of beneficial effects of prenatal omega-3 fatty acid intake on memory function at school age. *Am J Clin Nutr*. 2011;93:1025–1037.
199. Liao K, McCandliss BD, Carlson SE, et al. Event-related potential differences in children supplemented with long-chain polyunsaturated fatty acids during infancy. *Dev Sci*. 2017;20:10.
204. Bakker EC, Hornstra G, Blanco CE, et al. Relationship between long-chain polyunsaturated fatty acids at birth and motor function at 7 years of age. *Eur J Clin Nutr*. 2009;63:499–504.
205. Kohlboeck G, Glaser C, Tiesler C, et al. Effect of fatty acid status in cord blood serum on children's behavioral difficulties at 10 y of age: results from the LISAplus Study. *Am J Clin Nutr*. 2011;94:1592–1599.
209. Sheppard KW, Cheatham CL. The balance between n-6 and n-3 and its relation to executive function. In: Watson R, Preedy V, eds. *Omega Fatty Acids in Brain and Neurological Health*. New York: Academic Press; 2019:43–62.

SECTION VII Carbohydrate Metabolism

Glucose Metabolism in the Fetus and Newborn, and Methods for Its Investigation

Sarah A. Wernimont | Andrew W. Norris

INTRODUCTION

Glucose metabolism has been studied extensively in the fetus and newborn, in both animal and human models. The study of glucose metabolism is enabled by the availability of (1) the chronic fetal preparation in large animals, in which fetal blood sampling and physiologic monitoring can be done without causing major changes in the state of the fetus; (2) isotopic tracers, especially stable, nonradioactive ones; (3) molecular biology techniques and transgenic animals; and (4) human molecular genetics. In this chapter, glucose metabolism in the fetus and newborn is discussed. The classic physiology experiments—especially glucose tracer work, which provide core understandings—are reviewed along with recent developments. Throughout the chapter, emphasis is placed on the available data in humans, supplemented when necessary with animal data.

METHODS FOR STUDYING GLUCOSE METABOLISM IN THE FETUS AND NEWBORN

ISOTOPIC TRACERS

Beginning in the 1980s, improvements in the synthesis of metabolites labeled with stable isotopes and sensitive mass-spectrometric methods have allowed investigators to examine glucose metabolism in the human fetus and newborn. In addition, improved synthetic techniques have increased the number of isotopic tracers that can be used simultaneously, allowing investigators to answer more complex questions. By combining novel tracer methods with measurements of energy consumption, the metabolic fate of fuel substrates (e.g., glucose, amino acids, fatty acids) can be quantified along with their contribution to overall fuel economy. To help localize these processes, imaging techniques have been developed to interrogate fetal usage of fuel substrates in a visuospatial and quantitative manner.

Isotopic tracers have proved invaluable in understanding the details of fuel metabolism. They can be used in vivo to quantify rates of metabolic turnover including the appearance and disappearance of a substrate, to quantify the utilization and metabolic fate of a substrate, to determine the contribution of a substrate to another compound, and/or to determine tissue-specific aspects of metabolism. The isotopic labels employed in tracers can be either stable or radioactive, with each having differing merits. The obvious advantage of stable isotopic tracers is that they are nonradioactive. However, another major advantage is that they often can be designed to carry positional information that delineates how specific portions of a molecule are metabolically transformed. Mass spectrometry is used to detect stable isotopic tracers. One disadvantage of stable isotopes is that they are typically less sensitive than radioactive tracers, owing in part to a higher natural abundance, and thus greater amounts of tracer are often required than for radioactive tracers. This point highlights a major advantage of radioactive tracers, in that even very small amounts can be detected. Another advantage of certain radioactive tracers, especially those that emit positrons, is that they can be imaged to determine their location in the body in real time.[1-4] An example of imaging a glucose uptake tracer during pregnancy in rats is shown in Fig. 36.1 (experimental details are described by Sawatzke and colleagues[5]). However, a disadvantage of radioactive tracers is that they do not provide molecular positional information as readily compared to stable isotope tracers. Additionally, their radioactivity limits their use in human studies. Isotopic tracer experimentation is not only a complex subject with various pitfalls but also an opportunity for savvy and informative designs as highlighted in recent reviews.[5-7]

MEASUREMENTS OF ENERGY EXPENDITURE

Measurements of energy expenditure have become integral components of metabolic studies. There are several experimental approaches to measure energy expenditure, and the two most commonly employed techniques are indirect calorimetry and doubly labeled water. Additionally, studies using carbon-labeled tracers can be used to estimate the isotopic enrichment of CO_2 either in the blood or in the expired CO_2 to quantify the oxidation rate of that particular labeled substrate.[8,9]

INDIRECT CALORIMETRY

Energy expenditure can be estimated from the rate of oxygen consumption and carbon dioxide production by an infant. In this system, a hood or canopy is placed over the subject's head, and a pump is used to draw air through the hood. The air exiting from the hood is thoroughly mixed. The concentration of O_2 and CO_2 is measured in the mixed air as is the total flow of air through the system. From this information, energy expenditure can be estimated.[10-14] This general approach has been used over many years in a large number of studies in adults, children, and newborn infants,[10,15-17] and its limitations have been examined.[10,18]

DOUBLY LABELED ($^2H_2{}^{18}O$) WATER

Doubly labeled water contains the stable isotopes deuterium and ^{18}O, and can be used to measure energy expenditure by

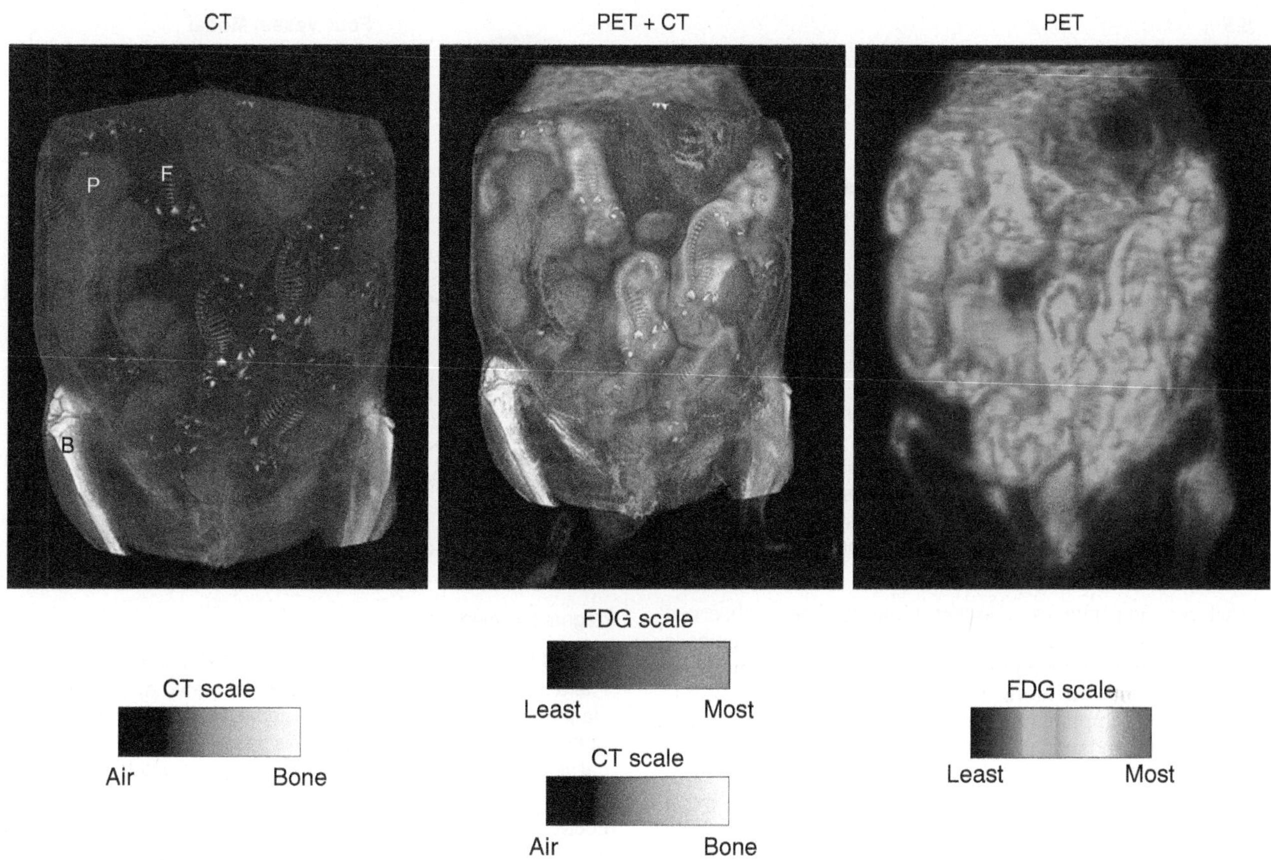

Fig. 36.1 Visuospatial localization of glucose uptake in the pregnant rat using positron emission tomography/computed tomography *(PET/CT)*. Images show the abdomen of a pregnant rat near term gestation. CT with intravenous contrast was used to help identify abdominal structures. "*P*" identifies one of the several placentae, which contain contrast and have an appearance similar to jellyfish. "*F*" identifies one of the several fetuses, with ribs easily seen. The contrast material does not cross the placenta, so fetal structures are darker (other than fetal bones). "*B*" shows one of the maternal bones. The PET imaging used ^{18}F-fluorodeoxyglucose *(FDG)* tracer. FDG is a non-metabolizable glucose analog that cannot be exported from most cells, except those that express glucose-6-phosphatase (mainly the postnatal liver). Hence FDG is considered a glucose uptake tracer and accumulates in glucose-avid tissues. The glucose-avid nature of placenta and fetus is apparent. FDG also accumulates in urine, so the maternal bladder and kidney have been subtracted from the image. The middle panel shows co-registration of the CT and PET images, using a different PET color scale.

enabling estimation of the rate of CO_2 elimination from the body. Its advantages include that it can be applied to free-living individuals, that CO_2 elimination is measured over hours to days providing an integrated measure of energy consumption, and that the method is relatively simple and noninvasive. It requires administration of a single dose of doubly labeled H_2O and a few subsequent samples of urine, saliva, or blood to be obtained to measure the changes in isotopic enrichment over several days. The underlying general principle is that the deuterium in doubly labeled water is eliminated as water (^2H_2O), whereas the oxygen (^{18}O) is eliminated with water ($H_2{}^{18}O$) and with carbon dioxide ($CO^{18}O$), owing to the rapid equilibrium between H_2O and CO_2 in the body. Thus the difference in turnover rates between the ^{18}O and ^2H of water represents the CO_2 elimination rate.[19] Use of doubly labeled water to study energy metabolism has been extensively evaluated in humans, both adults and newborns.[20-29]

GLUCOSE METABOLISM IN THE FETUS

MATERNAL-FETAL GLUCOSE RELATIONSHIP

In most mammalian species, including humans, the fetal blood glucose concentration is significantly lower than that measured in a blood sample obtained simultaneously from the mother.[30,31] A significant linear relationship has been observed between glucose levels in the mother and the fetus.[32,33] In humans, fetal blood samples had originally been obtained mostly at term gestation from fetal scalp blood or from a segment of doubly clamped umbilical cord at the time of cesarean delivery.[32-34] However, because of the effects of labor and delivery on maternal and fetal circulation, these data were questioned in regard to their representation of fetal metabolism. The technique of percutaneous umbilical blood sampling permits access to fetal circulation, though there are risks of pregnancy loss associated with this procedure and its use in clinical and human subjects research practice has decreased. Historically, fetal blood samples have been obtained in midgestation (18 to 21 weeks) by fetoscopy or late in gestation by ultrasound visualization of the umbilical vessels to interrogate fetal metabolic status.[30,31]

A significant correlation between maternal arterialized venous blood glucose and fetal umbilical venous glucose concentrations has been observed in fetuses examined across gestation.[31,35] In these studies, the fetal glucose concentration was generally lower than that in the mother, more so as gestation progressed. By later in gestation, as shown in Fig. 36.2, most investigators observe a close linear relationship between maternal and fetal glucose concentrations whether the samples were obtained by percutaneous umbilical blood sampling, by scalp sampling during labor, or from umbilical vessels at the time of elective cesarean delivery.[32-34,36,37] This linear relationship between

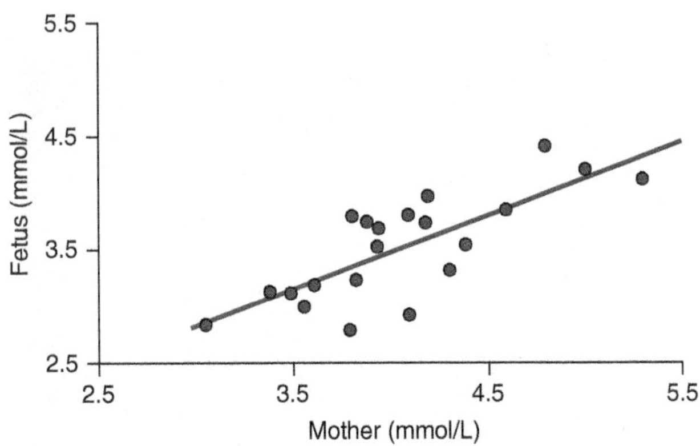

Fig. 36.2 Relationship between maternal and fetal glucose concentrations. Maternal venous and umbilical venous blood samples (via percutaneous umbilical blood sample) were obtained simultaneously in the third trimester of pregnancy. (Data from Ashmead GG, Kalhan SC, Lazebnik N, et al. Maternal-fetal substrate relationships in the third trimester in human pregnancy. *Gynecol Obstet Invest*. 1993;35:18.)

maternal and fetal glucose concentrations has been observed during euglycemia, during hyperglycemia induced by glucose infusion into the mother, and during hypoglycemia induced by insulin infusion into the mother.

The 4-vessel sampling approach was developed to study human placental and fetal glucose uptake in vivo (Fig. 36.3).[38,39] In this approach, women undergoing cesarean delivery have simultaneous blood samples taken from the maternal radial artery and uterine vein, umbilical vein, and umbilical artery. By incorporating data on uterine and umbilical blood flow, rates of uptake are determined.[40] With this information, the maternal-fetal gradient, uteroplacental uptake, and placental consumption may be calculated as follows:

- Maternal-fetal gradient = $[\text{Glucose}]_{\text{maternal radial artery}} - [\text{Glucose}]_{\text{fetal umbilical artery}}$
- Uteroplacental uptake = $([\text{Glucose}]_{\text{radial artery}} - [\text{Glucose}]_{\text{uterine vein}}) \times$ Uterine blood flow
- Fetal consumption = $([\text{Glucose}]_{\text{fetal umbilical vein}} - [\text{Glucose}]_{\text{fetal umbilical artery}}) \times$ Umbilical vein blood flow
- Placental consumption = Uteroplacental uptake − Fetal consumption

Using this technique, the relationships between maternal glucose delivery, uteroplacental uptake, fetal glucose consumption and outcomes such as birth weight are interrogated. Overall, the studies find that fetal glucose consumption, not simply the concentration of maternal arterial or fetal umbilical vein glucose, is the primary contributor to birth weight. Further, they demonstrate that fetal glucose consumption may be modulated by placental glucose consumption.[40] For example, the placenta extracted approximately 6% of the available glucose in perfusing maternal blood while the fetus extracted approximately 10% of available glucose from blood flowing in the fetal-placental circulation.[39] While these studies demonstrate a correlation between maternal arterial glucose concentration and umbilical vein concentration, as seen in prior studies, there is no correlation between maternal arterial glucose and fetal uptake (defined by difference in umbilical vein and umbilical artery glucose concentrations). This suggests that the fetal glucose uptake is not regulated solely by maternal glucose delivery. Additionally, the four-vessel studies find that fetal birth weight is correlated with fetal uptake of glucose driven by fetal insulin concentration, not simply the concentration of glucose in the umbilical vein. In more recent work that incorporates both uterine and umbilical artery flow into models, placental glucose consumption is identified as a key modulator of fetal glucose consumption.[40] Specifically, these

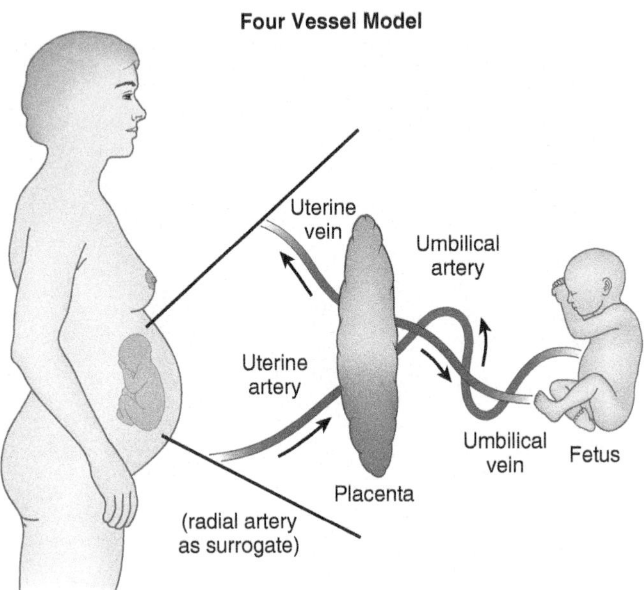

Fig. 36.3 Four vessel model for assessing maternal-fetal metabolic interactions at the placenta. Sampling of maternal arterial circulation via the radial artery and maternal uterine vein allows determination of utero-placental nutrient uptake. This can be compared to fetal umbilical vein and artery sampling to determine fetal uptake.

recent studies find a significant negative correlation between placental glucose consumption and fetal glucose consumption, suggesting that high placental glucose requirements would limit the glucose available for fetal delivery and consumption. The regulation and mechanisms by which glucose is partitioned within the placenta to manage its own versus fetal needs remains unclear.

There are ongoing efforts to better understand the impact of the placenta on regulating maternal nutrient supply to match fetal needs. Investigations into placental nutrient sensing[41] have identified several key regulators of placental development that impact fetal growth, including the mechanistic target of rapamycin (mTOR) and insulin-like growth factor (IGF). mTOR is expressed in the human placenta and responds to changes in maternal oxygen levels and nutrient status by altering placental nutrient transport (reviewed in Dimasuay and colleagues[42]). mTOR activity is decreased during hypoxia or decreased nutrient availability,[43] and its expression is increased by maternal overnutrition.[44] IGF-2 is also increasingly recognized to regulate placental growth, development, and nutrient transport and is thought to be dysregulated in cases of fetal growth restriction (reviewed in Sferruzzi-Perri and colleagues[45]). Ongoing work seeks to better define the role of the placenta in responding to fetal nutrient needs and how these processes may be dysregulated in the context of fetal growth restriction and fetal overgrowth.

GLUCOSE TRANSPORT ACROSS THE PLACENTA

From in vivo studies in animals and isolated perfused placenta, it can be concluded that glucose is transported across the placenta along a concentration gradient by a facilitated, carrier-mediated diffusion.[46,47] This process is facilitated by the presence of glucose transporter (GLUT) transporters on the syncytiotrophoblast, a multinucleated cell that separates maternal from fetal circulation,[48,49] as schematized in Fig. 36.4. GLUT1 is thought to be the predominant transporter involved in placental glucose transport, with three-fold higher expression on the maternal-facing microvillous membrane compared to the basal membrane.[50,51] Although glucose transport between the fetal and maternal

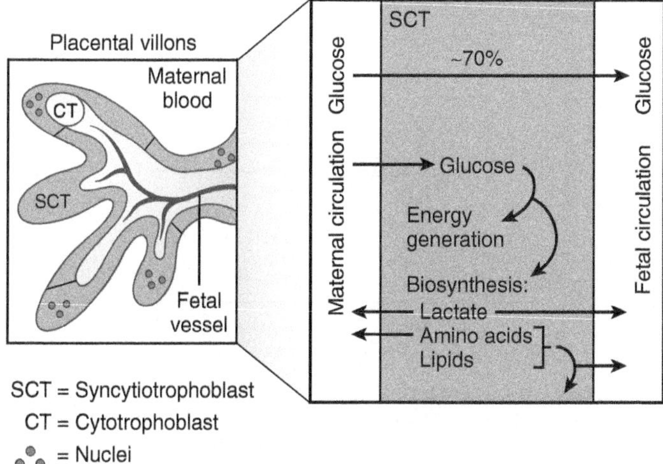

Fig. 36.4 Placental transport and metabolism of glucose. The smallest functional unit of the human placenta is the villus, which is bathed in maternal blood and facilitates the transfer of nutrients to fetal circulation. The syncytiotrophoblast is a giant multinucleated cell that directs nutrient transfer between the two circulations. Approximately 70% of glucose that makes it to the placenta is transferred to the fetus whereas 30% remains in the placenta. Glucose remaining in the placenta is thought to contribute not only to adenosine triphosphate synthesis, but also to biosynthesis of other molecules such as lactate, amino acids, and lipids for placental utilization and possibly export for fetal use.

blood is bidirectional, it is asymmetric such that transfer from maternal fetal circulation is greater than in the other direction, as demonstrated in placental explants.[52,53] This is consistent with greater GLUT1 expression on the maternal facing surface of the syncytiotrophoblast.[54] In addition, the explant studies suggest that at least a fraction of glucose may be transported via a paracellular route, though this has not been demonstrated in vivo.

Studies of human placenta perfused in vitro have shown that placental glucose uptake from the maternal perfusate and glucose transfer to the fetal perfusate is linearly correlated with maternal glucose concentration up to 20 mmol/L. Beyond this level, glucose is transferred to the fetal perfusate by simple diffusion.[55] Metabolically, the placenta is a very active organ, using approximately 50% to 60% of delivered glucose in early ex vivo studies.[56] More recent, in vivo data suggests that 30% of delivered glucose is taken up by the utero-placental unit.[40] How glucose is partitioned to placental or fetal use remains uncertain, as does the ultimate fate of this placentally directed glucose. Glucose within the placenta is thought to contribute to adenosine triphosphate generation through oxidative phosphorylation, with consequent lactate production.[56-59]

As gestation advances, an increase in uterine blood flow results in an increased delivery of glucose to the fetus.[60] In the presence of a constant blood glucose concentration in pregnant sheep, a reduction of uterine blood flow (from 600 to 300 mL/min/kg of fetus) did not have any effect on fetal glucose uptake or fetal arterial glucose concentration.[61] However, any further decrease in uterine blood flow decreased fetal glucose uptake and caused variable fetal arterial glucose concentrations. Conversely, a reduction in umbilical blood flow by ligation of one of the umbilical arteries decreased fetal glucose uptake and caused fetal growth restriction.[62]

SOURCES OF GLUCOSE FOR THE FETUS IN UTERO

Maternally supplied glucose is considered the primary source of glucose for the developing fetus in utero. This is partially inferred by simultaneous changes in fetal glucose concentration corresponding to changes in maternal glucose concentration. To determine whether the fetus can regulate glucose metabolism, ^{13}C-labeled glucose has been infused into women prior to cesarean delivery and isotopic enrichment in maternal and fetal compartments examined.[36] As shown in Fig. 36.5, the [^{13}C] glucose enrichment in the maternal vein, umbilical cord vein, and umbilical cord artery was similar in healthy women and women with gestational diabetes. These data indicate that the fetal glucose pool was in equilibrium with the maternal glucose pool and that maternal glucose was the only source of glucose

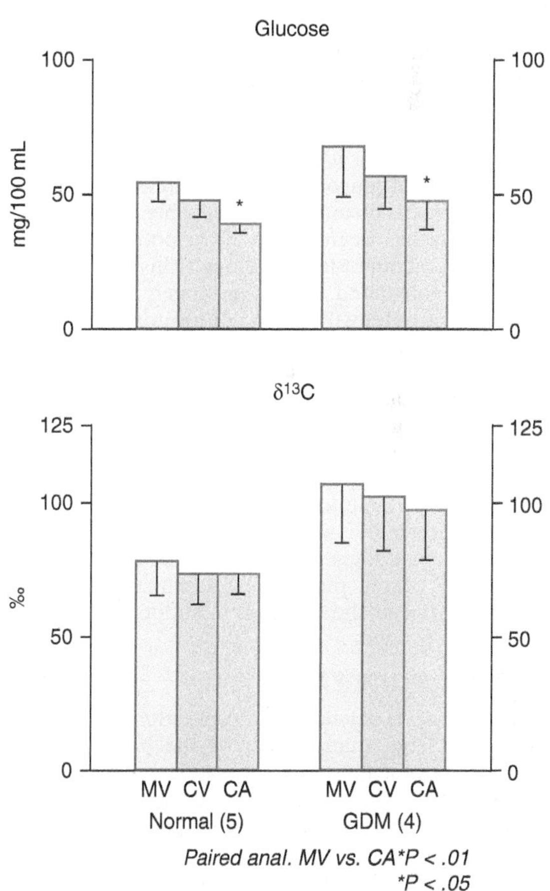

Fig. 36.5 Glucose tracing at term. Plasma glucose and glucose-^{13}C enrichment during [1-^{13}C] glucose infusion in maternal venous *(MV)*, umbilical cord arterial *(CA)*, and umbilical cord venous *(CV)* blood. [1-^{13}C] Glucose tracer was infused into five healthy mothers and four mothers with gestational diabetes *(GDM)* for at least 2 hours before elective cesarean delivery. Simultaneous maternal venous and umbilical blood samples were obtained at delivery. (Reproduced with permission from Kalhan SC, D'Angelo L, Savin SM, et al. Glucose production in pregnant women at term gestation: sources of glucose for the human fetus. *J Clin Invest.* 1979;63:388. Copyright American Society for Clinical Investigation.)

for the human fetus at term gestation after a brief overnight fast. If the fetus had been producing glucose, a lower [^{13}C]glucose enrichment would have been seen in the fetal blood.

Marconi and colleagues[63] examined whether the fetus could produce glucose in nine subjects with pregnancy complicated by intrauterine growth restriction between 29 and 35 weeks gestation. They administered [^{13}C]glucose tracer to the mother and measured the isotopic enrichment in the maternal blood and in the fetal blood obtained by cordocentesis. No difference in tracer enrichment in the maternal and fetal compartments was found, confirming that even in pregnancies with fetal growth restriction, maternal glucose is the only source of glucose for the fetus.

However, these results do not unequivocally indicate that the fetus cannot mobilize hepatic glycogen or complete gluconeogenesis. While some animal studies[64-67] have suggested a potential role of fetal gluconeogenesis in maintaining fetal glucose homeostasis, methodologic concerns related to fasting duration and ruminant feeding behaviors have made this challenging to confirm. The key gluconeogenesis enzymes, pyruvate carboxylase, phosphoenolpyruvate carboxykinase (PEPCK), and fructose diphosphatase, have been demonstrated to some degree from early fetal life onward in humans.[68,69] However, the presence of these enzymes does not necessarily correlate with gluconeogenic activity. Recent work in the ovine model demonstrates that hypoxic conditions may prime fetal expression of gluconeogenic regulators but does not result in increased endogenous glucose production.[70] Thus in the mammalian species studied, even though the potential for hepatic gluconeogenesis exists, the gluconeogenic capacity is not expressed in utero under unperturbed circumstances, and the contribution of gluconeogenesis from lactate, pyruvate, or alanine to glucose is quantitatively negligible.[71]

The placenta has been proposed to potentially contribute to fetal glucose homeostasis,[72] though this has not yet been definitely demonstrated. While glycogen is noted within placental villi, a potential role in contributing to fetal glucose homeostasis has not been clearly identified.[73] Gluconeogenic enzymes including PEPCK[74] are expressed in term human placentae; however, due to the lack of expression of glucose-6-phosphatase,[75] gluconeogenesis is not thought to occur. However, more recent work suggests that gluconeogenesis may occur in the placenta, potentially facilitated by other potential isoforms of glucose-6-phosphatase, though this has not been definitively shown,[76,77] and glucose analog tracing imaging experiments in rats suggest that there is no functional glucose-6-phosphatase in rat placenta.[5] Additional work clarifying the potential role of the placenta in supporting fetal glucose homeostasis is needed.

FETAL GLUCOSE UTILIZATION

Quantitative aspects of fetal glucose utilization have been studied extensively in large animals, such as sheep.[67,71,78-81] In ovine models, fetal glucose utilization rates are estimated at ~30 μmol/min/kg (5.4 mg/kg/min),[82] and limited human data suggest a similar rate of fetal glucose utilization in human pregnancies.[40] Whether such a magnitude of glucose uptake can account for the oxidative metabolism of the fetus has been examined by calculation of the glucose and O_2 quotient.[83,84] The glucose and O_2 quotient represents the fraction of the total fetal O_2 consumption required to metabolize aerobically and completely the glucose acquired by the fetus across the placental circulation and is calculated as follows: glucose and O_2 quotient = 6 × [umbilical vein − umbilical artery difference of glucose (millimoles)]/[umbilical vein − umbilical artery difference of O_2 (millimoles)]. The fetal glucose and O_2 quotient has been estimated to be approximately 0.5 in fed sheep[85] and approximately 0.8 in humans.[83] These data suggest that the maternally acquired glucose is not sufficient for the entire oxidative metabolism of the fetus, and that other substrates, such as lactate and amino acids, also may be used by the fetus in utero for its energy needs.

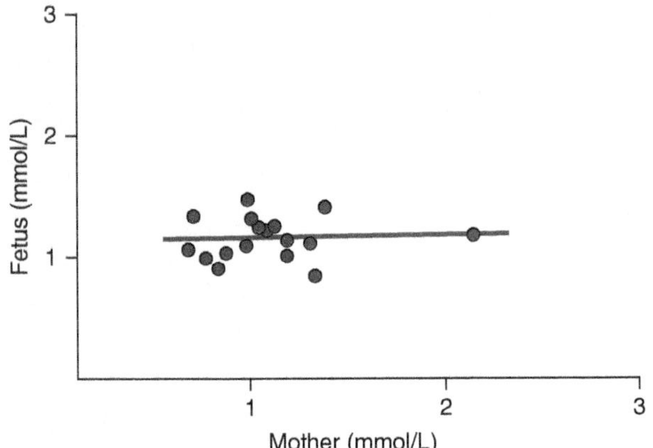

Fig. 36.6 Lack of relationship between maternal and fetal blood lactate concentrations. The fetal samples were obtained by percutaneous umbilical blood sampling late in gestation. (Data from Ashmead GG, Kalhan SC, Lazebnik N, et al. Maternal-fetal substrate relationships in the third trimester in human pregnancy. *Gynecol Obstet Invest.* 1993;35:18.)

UTILIZATION OF OTHER SUBSTRATES BY THE FETUS

Because glucose does not appear to account for the total O_2 uptake by the fetus, attention has been focused on the utilization of other substrates, especially lactate and amino acids, by the fetus. Studies of quantitative aspects of lactic acid metabolism by the fetus are confounded by the rapid changes in the concentration of lactic acid in response to small perturbations in the fetus. Therefore, particularly in humans in whom previous blood samples had been obtained only at the time of vaginal or elective cesarean delivery, the umbilical arterial concentration of lactate has been observed to be higher than the simultaneously obtained umbilical venous and maternal venous blood concentrations.[86] These data suggest fetal production and placental clearance of lactate but are subject to criticism because of a lack of a steady state and the effect of labor on fetal metabolism. Even in a relatively unperturbed state in which percutaneous umbilical blood samples have been obtained from the fetus in utero, the fetal blood lactate concentrations were found to be similar to the simultaneously obtained maternal venous blood concentrations.[30] However, in a subsequent study in which fetal blood samples were obtained by cordocentesis late in gestation, no correlation between maternal and fetal blood lactate concentrations was observed (Fig. 36.6).[37]

In contrast to the data in humans, stable chronic preparations in the sheep fetus provide near-optimal conditions to study the maternal-fetal lactate relationship. As shown in Fig. 36.7, the umbilical venous and uterine venous concentrations of lactate have been shown to be higher than the simultaneously measured umbilical arterial and uterine arterial lactate concentrations.[58] These data, which have been confirmed by Char and Creasy,[59] indicate uteroplacental production and maternal and fetal utilization of lactate. The metabolic fate of the lactate produced by the uteroplacental unit and used by the fetus was not examined in these studies. However, estimation of the lactate and O_2 quotient suggested that complete oxidation of lactate could account for 25% of fetal O_2 consumption.[58] These studies are of interest in that the lactate derived from the placenta could potentially be used by the fetus for both oxidative purposes and nonoxidative purposes, such as glycogen synthesis.

Amino acids are actively transported across the human placenta from the mother to the fetus, and, in addition to glucose and lactate, they are an important source of energy, as well as substrates for glycogen synthesis.[87-89] It is suggested

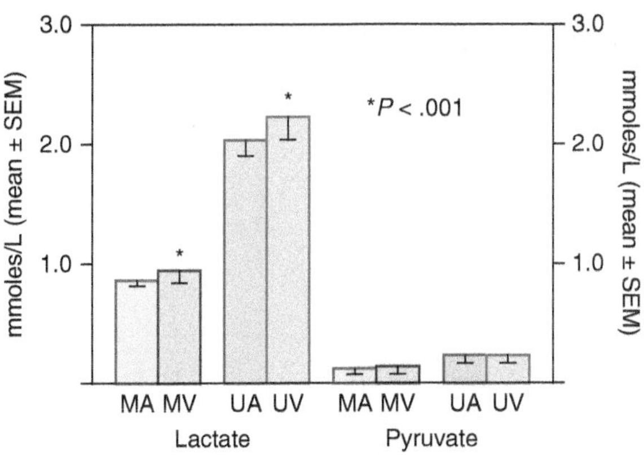

Fig. 36.7 Maternal-fetal lactate and pyruvate gradients in the sheep, late in gestation. *MA,* Maternal artery; *MV,* maternal vein; *SEM,* standard error of the mean; *UA,* umbilical artery; *UV,* umbilical vein. (Reprinted by permission from Burd LI, Jones MD Jr, Simmons MA, et al. Placental production and foetal utilisation of lactate and pyruvate. *Nature.* 1975;254:710. Copyright Macmillan Magazines Ltd.)

that a significant amount of amino acids taken up by the fetus is oxidized. Gresham and colleagues[90] estimated that up to 25% of the total fetal O_2 consumption in the sheep fetus could be accounted for by the oxidation of amino acids. In the human, on the basis of urea concentration gradients across the umbilical circulation, it can be assumed that the human fetus in utero catabolizes amino acids to some degree and synthesizes urea.[91]

Holm and colleagues evaluated differences in amino acid concentrations using the 4-vessel sampling approach at the time of elective cesarean delivery.[92] Comparing 19 amino acid concentrations determined by liquid chromatography and tandem mass spectrometry, they calculated the uteroplacental arteriovenous difference as the difference between the concentration in the maternal radial artery and uterine vein and the umbilical venoarterial-difference as the difference in concentration between the umbilical vein and umbilical artery. Uniquely, this study corrected for net passage of water to the placenta or fetus and incorporated samples from both maternal arterial and venous compartments. Using this method, they calculated both uteroplacental and fetal uptake and release of amino acids. While the maternal artery and umbilical vein amino acid concentrations are correlated, they did not find a correlation between amino acid uptake by the uteroplacental unit and the concentration in the fetal vein. This suggests that more than simply transporting amino acids to fetal circulation, the placenta itself may synthesize amino acids to supply fetal circulation. Similar to prior work,[93] they found that the concentration of alanine is greater in the umbilical vein compared to the maternal artery, similar to many other amino acids. They further identified alanine as the amino acid with the greatest uptake from the fetal circulation, suggesting its importance in fetal metabolism. While alanine enrichment in the umbilical vein is conventionally attributed to increased placental transport of amino acids, it is notable that alanine can be produced following transamination of pyruvate, the end product of glycolysis. It is possible that alanine is synthesized within the placenta, which expresses aminotransferases,[94,95] thus providing a potential link between glucose and protein metabolism within the placenta. Notably, pregnancies complicated by gestational diabetes have approximately 30% higher concentrations of alanine in the umbilical vein despite similar concentrations in maternal circulation. To potentially explain this, we speculate that placental alanine synthesis may be increased in response to the presumed increase in placental pyruvate derived from excess maternal glucose.[96]

Overall, while maternally derived glucose is thought to be the primary fetal fuel, further work is needed to determine how the presence of lactate and amino acids contribute to fetal metabolism. These investigations may provide insights into how fetal growth may be normalized in pregnancies complicated by maternal diabetes in the presence of well-controlled maternal blood glucose levels.

REGULATION OF UMBILICAL GLUCOSE UPTAKE AND FETAL GLUCOSE UTILIZATION

Fetal uptake of glucose is closely regulated by the maternal plasma glucose concentration because the fetal glucose concentration closely follows the maternal glucose concentration in humans. Likewise, in studies of fetal sheep, when the maternal glucose concentrations are decreased by fasting[97] or acute insulin infusion,[78] there is diminished maternal-to-fetal glucose transfer and decreased fetal glucose concentration. Insulin is a potent regulator of glucose homeostasis, and insulin levels are similar in the maternal and fetal circulations.[39] While insulin regulates maternal glucose levels, maternal insulin levels are not associated with fetal glucose consumption, placental glucose consumption, or birth weight in human studies.[40] However, fetal insulin levels are positively correlated with fetal glucose consumption and birth weight, suggesting that fetal insulin is a critical regulator of fetal glucose utilization.[40] In ovine models, injection of streptozotocin, a pancreatic β-cell toxin, into fetal circulation[98] results in a 66% decrease in fetal glucose consumption. However, no change in uteroplacental uptake was noted, suggesting that fetal insulin regulates fetal, not placental, glucose consumption.

Investigations suggest that stressors, such as maternal hypoxia and corticosteroids, impact uteroplacental glucose consumption but not necessarily fetal glucose consumption. For instance, uterine artery constriction to decrease oxygen delivery and glucose delivery to the placenta does not decrease fetal glucose consumption[99] but does decrease uteroplacental glucose consumption. By altering placental glucose metabolism, it is hypothesized that oxygen delivery to the fetus is preserved during periods of relative hypoxia.

Maternal glucocorticoid infusions also impact placental glucose metabolism and alter fetal glucose consumption in the ovine mode. Following infusion of physiologic dosages of cortisol in sheep, increased maternal insulin, glucose, and lactate levels are noted, although there is no change in fetal cortisol levels.[100] Maternal cortisol infusions increase uteroplacental glucose uptake and placental lactate synthesis and decrease fetal glucose consumption. This suggests that maternal corticosteroids can regulate placental glucose metabolism, thereby altering the amount and potentially type of carbohydrates available for fetal consumption.

GLYCOGEN METABOLISM AND SOURCES OF GLYCOGEN IN THE FETUS

The hepatic glycogen content in the human fetus is low early in gestation. As measured by Čapková and Jirásek,[101] the glycogen content of the fetal liver between 51 and 60 days (average, 8 weeks) of gestation was 3.4 mg/g. A slow continuous increase in hepatic glycogen content occurred, such that between 121 and 130 days of gestation it had reached 24.6 mg/g. In preparation for birth, a rapid steep increase appears to occur at around 36 weeks of gestation. As shown by Shelley and Neligan,[102] in the human fetus at 40 weeks of gestation, the hepatic glycogen content approaches 50 mg/g net weight (Fig. 36.8). Fetal glycogen levels can be regulated by hypoxia and also altered by fetal hormones.[103] In ovine models, restricting uterine blood flow results in reduced fetal liver glycogen and decreased glycogen phosphorylase and glucose-6-phosphatase activity. Additionally, fetal thyroidectomy decreases fetal glycogen levels, whereas prepartum T3 or cortisol administration increases fetal liver glycogen content prior to

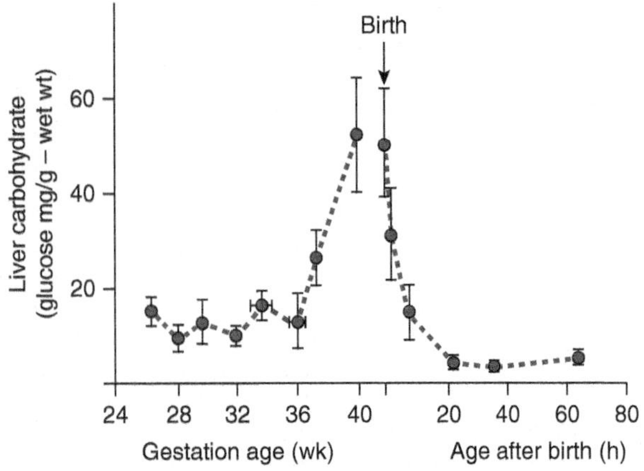

Fig. 36.8 Changes in liver glycogen concentration in the human during fetal life and after birth. (Modified from Shelley HJ, Nelligan GA. Neonatal hypoglycaemia. *Br Med Bull.* 1966;22:34.)

delivery.[104] Overall, this suggests that changes in the uterine environment and fetal hormonal milieu impact the availability of glycogen after delivery.

SUMMARY OF FETAL GLUCOSE CONSUMPTION

In utero, the fetus relies upon maternally supplied glucose. By virtue of high expression of glucose transporters, the placenta enables facile diffusion of glucose from mother to fetus. This transport relies on the maternal-fetal glucose concentration gradient. As a result, fetal glucose levels are modulated by maternal glycemia, placental glucose consumption, and fetal metabolic needs. In addition to transporting maternal glucose to the fetus, the placenta metabolizes glucose for its own energetic and biosynthetic needs, and may play an important role in exporting glucose-derived fuels, especially lactate, to the fetus. In late gestation, the fetus accumulates hepatic glycogen in preparation to maintain glucose homeostasis following delivery. In the next section, the singular glucose source for the fetus will be contrasted with the pleiotropic sources of glucose in the newborn (Box 36.1).

Box 36.1 Major Sources of Glucose for Fetus and Neonate

- Fetus
  - Maternal glucose
- Neonate
  - Oral intake
  - Glycogenolysis
  - Gluconeogenesis

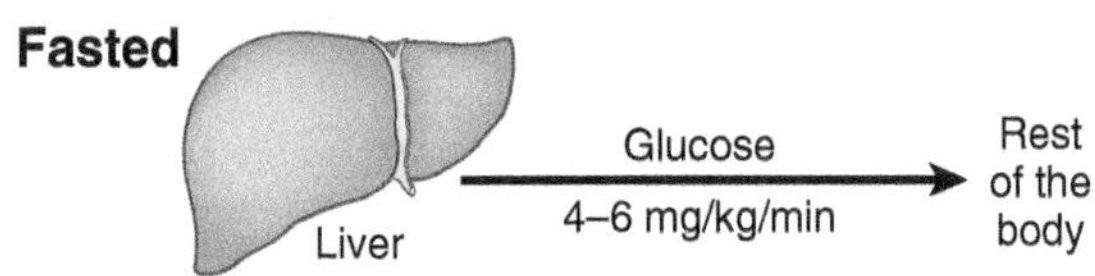

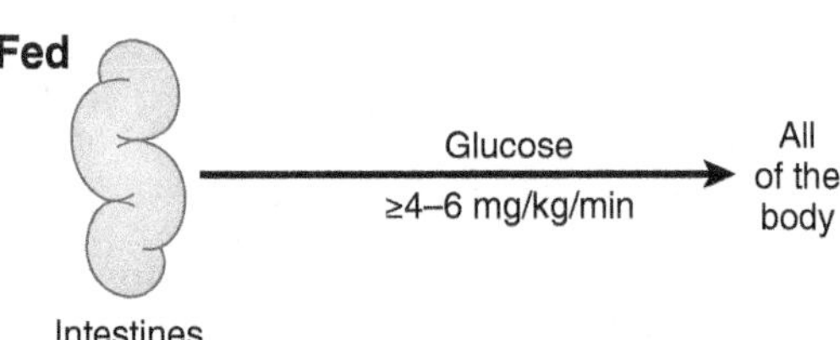

Fig. 36.9 Simple overview of glucose metabolism in newborns. In the fasted state, hepatic glucose production supplies appoximately 4 to 6 mg/kg/min of glucose to the rest of the body. In the fed state, lactose is converted to glucose to supply the glycemic needs of the body. Hepatic glucose production is suppressed during the fed state.

GLUCOSE METABOLISM IN THE NEWBORN

A TIME OF MARKED TRANSITION

At birth the newborn must adapt to a markedly different metabolic environment, including abrupt cessation of umbilical nutrient supply, unfamiliar cold stress, increased systemic oxygen tension, and the initiation of nutritional boluses via the gastrointestinal tract. Umbilical glucose delivery from the maternal circulation ceases, but yet energetic needs increase. Widespread but well-orchestrated endocrine and metabolic changes occur to successfully meet these postnatal glycemic challenges. When these responses are impaired, there is significant risk of neonatal hyperglycemia and/or hypoglycemia. The immediate postnatal period is marked by increases in the plasma concentrations of counterregulatory hormones epinephrine, norepinephrine, growth hormone, and glucagon, whereas the concentration of insulin decreases.[105-111] Thyroxine concentrations also surge after birth.[112] The net effect of these changes is mobilization of glycogen,[113] stimulation of gluconeogenesis,[114] and increases in lipolysis and fatty acid oxidation.[107,108] After birth in healthy human newborns, glucose concentrations become more variable and can decline for several hours, but typically stabilize by 48 to 72 hours at normal childhood levels.[114-118] Newborn blood glucose levels do vary with clinical practice regarding nutritional management of the newborn; for example, breastfed newborns tend to have lower blood glucose levels than formula fed newborns.[114] The neonatal period is a time of increased risk for hypoglycemia and hyperglycemia, which can constitute a significant problem in the clinical management of the infant. The risks of abnormal glucose levels are greater in the premature newborn and in the presence of fetal growth restriction.

GLUCOSE KINETICS DURING FASTING

The rates of glucose production and utilization in the human newborn during fasting—that is, 3 to 4 hours after birth, before feeding, or 8 to 9 hours after the last feeding—have been estimated to be between 4 and 6 mg/kg/min (Fig. 36.9).[119-121] The rates of glucose production per body weight measured in the newborn are significantly higher than those observed in adults and reflect the higher metabolic rate and the higher brain-body weight ratio of the newborn—the brain being the major glucose-using organ. As the newborn grows, the rate of glucose production per unit body weight decreases; therefore, by adolescence, the rates of glucose production approximate the rates in adults, which are half to one-third those seen in the newborn.[120]

To better understand glucose metabolism in newborns, tracer studies have combined infusion of ^{13}C-uniformly labeled glucose with indirect respiratory calorimetry.[121,122] In the fasted newborn state, only 53% (range, 40.9% to 68.1%) of glucose produced was oxidized to CO_2, and oxidation of plasma glucose contributed up to 38% of the total calorie expenditure.[121] Administration of glucose to newborns increases metabolic rate, glucose utilization, and glucose oxidation.[122]

In adult humans, the brain derives almost all its energy from glucose.[123,124] The O_2 consumption rate of the brain in the newborn human has been determined to be 104 μmol/100 g brain tissue per minute.[125] If the average weight of the brain in newborn infants is 360 g,[126] glucose at a rate of approximately

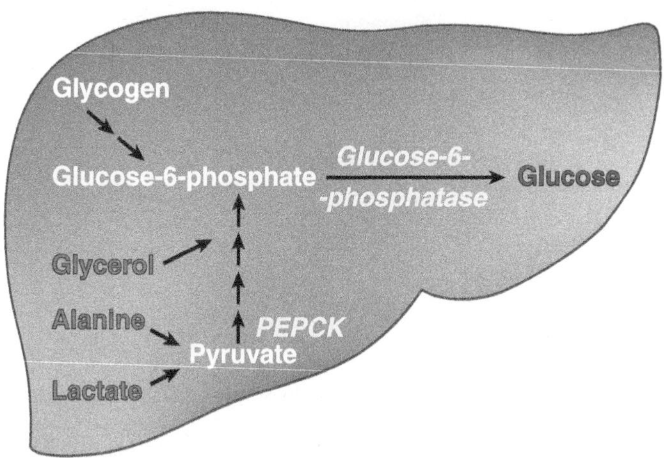

Fig. 36.10 The two components of hepatic glucose production. Glycogenolysis is the process by which glycogen is converted to glucose *(top section)*. Gluconeogenesis is the process by which lactate, select amino acids such as alanine, or glycerol are converted to glucose *(lower section)*. Circulating fuels are shown in blue, whereas fuels that remain primarily in the liver are shown in white. Key enzymes are shown in yellow, namely phosphoenolpyruvate carboxykinase *(PEPCK)* and glucose-6-phosphatase. Note that the final step to produce glucose from glucose-6-phosphate is common to both processes.

3.7 mg/kg/min would be required to meet the metabolic needs of the brain. Thus, the measured rates of glucose oxidation in the human newborn will supply only approximately 70% of the energy needs of the brain.[121] These data, at the time, were taken to suggest that in the human newborn, especially during fasting, the energy requirements of the brain were supported in part by fuels other than glucose. Indeed, there is now strong evidence that the brain of newborns is more facile than the adult brain in using fuels other than glucose, including ketone bodies, lactate, select amino acids, and select fatty acids.[127] Circulating ketone body levels climb for the first 48 hours after birth,[128] providing one possible alternative fuel. The stress of delivery induces a degree of catabolism, the mobilization of amino acids with flux of gluconeogenic amino acids to lactate, which can also be used as an alternative fuel.[129] In many infants at risk for hypoglycemia, ketone levels are often also low, whereas lactate levels are not diminished, suggesting that in some newborns lactate is an important alternative fuel for the brain.[130] However, the degree to which these alternative fuels can compensate for hypoglycemia and the long-term consequences to the brain of prolonged compensation are largely unknown.

GLUCOSE PRODUCTION IN THE NEWBORN

During fasting, blood glucose levels are determined by the balance between total body glucose utilization and endogenous glucose production. The latter occurs mainly in the liver and is often termed hepatic glucose production. Hepatic glucose production occurs via two distinct processes: glycogenolysis and gluconeogenesis (Fig. 36.10). Hepatic glucose production is governed by a myriad of hormonal, metabolic, and neuronal inputs, both direct and indirect, that have been extensively studied in adults and animal models.[131] In brief, insulin action diminishes hepatic glucose production, whereas glucagon, cortisol, and/or epinephrine stimulate hepatic glucose production.[131,132] Furthermore, hyperglycemia suppresses glycogenolysis by directly facilitating the inhibition of glycogen phosphorylase.[131] The final steps of each process employ the same mechanisms, namely dephosphorylation of glucose-phosphate by glucose-6-phosphatase and then export of glucose from the hepatocyte.

REGULATION OF HEPATIC GLUCOSE PRODUCTION IN NEWBORNS

There are several hormonal regulators of hepatic glucose production, especially insulin, glucagon, epinephrine, and cortisol (Fig. 36.11). Neonatal pancreatic islets are capable of secreting the major glucoregulatory hormones, insulin, and glucagon, in response to glycemic levels. Newborns and modestly premature infants exhibit insulin secretion in response to intravenous and oral glucose,[133] although the degree of insulin secretion is less well-regulated in newborns than in children.[134] Glucagon levels in newborns are higher when glucose levels are low,[135] and glucose infusion suppresses glucagon levels in newborns.[136] Cortisol levels surge in the initial hours after birth,[137] with higher levels observed after vaginal compared to cesarean delivery.[138] Likewise, catecholamines surge with parturition and likely contribute to acute stimulation of glycogenolysis, and longer-term increases in circulating substrates for gluconeogenesis, such as lactate.[139] As noted earlier, functional PEPCK levels are relatively low before birth, but climb rapidly after birth, reaching mature levels within 1 to 2 days postpartum[71,140] to help enable robust gluconeogenesis. Hepatic levels of another enzyme important to hepatic glucose production, glucose-6-phosphatase, are also low before birth, but climb rapidly after birth reaching mature levels by approximately 3 days postpartum.[139] All of these changes with birth are supportive of increased hepatic glucose production, especially when blood glucose levels are low, insulin levels suppressed, and glucagon levels elevated. Of the two components of hepatic glucose production, it appears that glycogenolysis is primed to be available immediately upon birth. Glycogen levels in the liver climb as gestation progresses, to the point that by term levels exceed that of adults. Glycogen levels then drop dramatically in the hours after birth,[141,142] and eventually climb several days thereafter. Gluconeogenesis capability ramps up after birth and eventually becomes a sizable contributor to glucose production in newborn infants.[71,143]

The above hormonal and regulatory changes at birth enable robust hepatic glucose production via glycogenolysis and gluconeogenesis. Because glycogenolysis is limited to available glycogen stores, which run low within a few hours of birth, gluconeogenesis can become a critical source of hepatic glucose production in fasted newborns. However, for gluconeogenesis to proceed, it must have a carbon source from which to build glucose (see Fig. 36.11). Several compounds commonly can serve as such, especially glycerol, lactate, and select glucogenic amino acids. Glycerol levels rise within minutes after birth,[144] making glycerol a newborn gluconeogenic carbon source. To assess this, gluconeogenesis from glycerol has been quantified in healthy term infants by simultaneous infusion of carbon-labeled glycerol along with labeled glucose. The appearance of tracer carbon in glucose is used to quantify the contribution of glycerol to glucose.[145-147] These data show that gluconeogenesis from glycerol is active in the healthy term infant immediately after birth, accounting for approximately 5% to 20% of glucose production. Because the primary source of glycerol is from adipose tissue lipolysis, these data also show that this process (lipolysis) is also active in the newborn.

All gluconeogenic carbon sources other than glycerol traverse through pyruvate. To ascertain this component, gluconeogenic

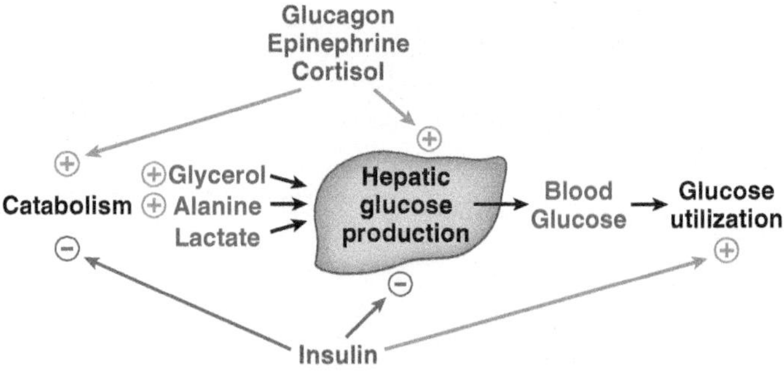

Fig. 36.11 Hormonal control of blood glucose. Hormones in brown, circulating fuels in blue. While fasting, blood glucose is controlled by the balance between hepatic glucose production and glucose utilization by the rest of the body. Glucagon, epinephrine, and cortisol stimulate hepatic glucose production and promote catabolism to supply glycerol and amino acid that can provide the carbon substrates that are used by gluconeogenesis to form glucose. These actions raise blood glucose levels. In contrast, insulin suppresses catabolism, inhibits hepatic glucose production, and stimulates the utilization of glucose. These insulin actions serve to lower blood glucose.

flux through pyruvate has been estimated using deuterium labeling of body water and mass isotopomer distribution analysis examining the appearance of glucose deuterium labeled on carbon-6. This approach has found that 31% of glucose appearance in healthy term fasted newborns proceeds via pyruvate.[143] The major carbon sources that can traverse through pyruvate to supply gluconeogenesis are lactate and amino acids. As noted earlier, lactate levels climb soon after birth, allowing this fuel to also potentially serve as a carbon source to support newborn gluconeogenesis. To measure this contribution, the rates of appearance of glucose and lactate have been quantified by the use of [6,6-$^2H_2$]glucose and [$^{13}C_3$]lactate, respectively, showing that lactate accounts for approximately 27% of hepatic glucose production in fasted (3 to 4 hours) newborns.[143] The contribution of alanine, a major gluconeogenic amino acid, to total newborn glucose production has been measured at roughly 9% by using infusion of [2,3-$^{13}C_2$]alanine into fasted term infants on the first day of life.[148] In summary, the newborn is capable of substantive gluconeogenesis shortly after birth from a variety of circulating carbon sources.

INSULIN ACTION IN THE NEWBORN

The actions of insulin to impact glucose metabolism have been less well studied in newborns than has hepatic glucose production. Direct study of insulin's glycemic actions has been accomplished in preterm human infants.[149] The infants were 32 to 33 weeks of gestational age, of appropriate size for gestation, not critically ill, and studied at age 12 to 72 hours while fasted for 3 hours. The responses to continuous insulin infusion were examined using glucose tracer. Interestingly, on one hand the infants exhibited a more robust response than adults in terms of insulin stimulating clearance of glucose from the bloodstream into tissues.[149] On the other hand, insulin failed to fully suppress hepatic glucose production, unlike in adults.[149] Similar conclusions were derived from a different study design examining the responses to glucose infusion in fasting preterm and term infants while tracing glucose.[150] In term infants, glucose infusion increased insulin levels and led to robust suppression of hepatic glucose production. By contrast, in preterm infants, although glucose infusion stimulated an increase in insulin levels, it failed to suppress hepatic glucose production in one study[150] but not in a separate study.[151] Similar to the former result, a study in premature infants receiving parenteral nutrition found that insulin and glucose failed to suppress hepatic glucose production.[152] Taken together, these three studies indicate that in newborns, insulin acts robustly to stimulate tissue utilization of blood glucose, but that in preterm infants the ability of insulin and glucose to suppress hepatic glucose production is often partially impaired.

PREMATURITY AND GLUCOSE METABOLISM

Infants born prematurely are at increased risk of glycemic instability, including both hypoglycemia and hyperglycemia. Although feeding intolerance contributes to this risk, there are a myriad of other contributing factors. While premature infants secrete insulin in response to hyperglycemia, the response curve is shifted and broadened such that a greater degree of hyperglycemia is required to provoke higher levels of insulin secretion.[134] With regard to gluconeogenesis, although on average premature infants exhibit normal levels of gluconeogenesis, this is highly variable from infant-to-infant.[143] In other words, some premature infants have excess gluconeogenesis while others have insufficient gluconeogenesis, thus presumably putting those premature infants with extremes of gluconeogenesis at risk of dysglycemia. Furthermore, premature infants have additional risk factors for dysglycemia. In premature infants, lower liver glycogen content, lower glucose-6-phosphatase content, reduced catecholamine responses, and sometimes impaired cortisol responses are factors that can contribute to hypoglycemia risk,[139] whereas high glucagon levels and lack of insulin suppression of hepatic glucose production contribute to hyperglycemia risk.[153]

NEONATAL HYPOGLYCEMIA

Transient, nonsevere hypoglycemia is common for the first 48 to 72 hours after birth among otherwise healthy term infants, affecting up to 10% to 30% depending on definition, conditions, and population.[114-118] The ideal glycemic threshold to distinguish normal versus pathologic hypoglycemia in healthy newborns this age remains controversial despite ongoing intensive study.[118,154,155] Nonetheless, most healthy newborns with mild hypoglycemia respond simply to feeding and/or brief administration of glucose. By contrast, some newborns develop more serious hypoglycemia that is prolonged, refractory, recurrent, occurs beyond 48 to 72 hours, extremely low, and/or symptomatic. There are numerous risk factors for neonatal hypoglycemia (Box 36.2).[156,157] The box is organized by presumed pathophysiology, although there are few detailed studies, except as noted for prematurity and small for gestation infants. Polycythemia is often listed as a risk factor for neonatal hypoglycemia, but recent data suggest that it is not an independent risk factor.[158]

ABERRANT INSULIN SECRETION IN NEWBORNS

Several genetic diseases lead to under- or over-secretion of insulin in newborns, leading to dramatic hyperglycemia or hypoglycemia, respectively. The severe nature of these conditions highlights the dominant importance of insulin in regulating neonatal glucose levels. The hypoglycemia induced by neonatal hyperinsulinism can be striking, incurring substantial requirements for continuous glucose infusion that exceeds 10 mg/kg/min to achieve euglycemia. Even then, in severe hyperinsulinism, blood glucose levels tend to be unstable and can become intermittently low despite ongoing glucose infusion. There are multiple causes of neonatal hyperinsulinemic hypoglycemia, but these can be divided into genetic versus environmental causes (Box 36.3). In most centers, the environmental forms are more common than genetic forms and include fetal growth restriction, birth asphyxia, and intrauterine exposure to maternal diabetes.[159] These environmental forms are usually transient, with a variable resolution speed ranging from hours to months. The genetic forms of neonatal hyperinsulinemic

Box 36.2 Risk Factors for Serious Neonatal Hypoglycemia, Categorized by Presumed Etiology

- Decreased fuel supply
  - Prematurity
  - Small for gestational age
  - Perinatal stress (sepsis, asphyxia)
  - Inadequate feeding
  - Hypopituitarism
  - Cortisol deficiency
  - Inborn errors of metabolism
  - Liver failure
- Increased glucose utilization
  - Infant of diabetic mother
  - Large for gestational age
  - Hyperinsulinemia
  - Polycythemia

This list is not exhaustive and merely presents major categories. It includes risk factors associated with either transient or long-lasting hypoglycemia risk.

Box 36.3 Causes of Neonatal Hyperinsulinemic Hypoglycemia

- Genetic (by gene symbol)
  - *ABCC8*
  - *KCNJ11*
  - *GCK*
  - *GLUD1*
  - *HADH*
- Environmental
  - Prematurity
  - Intrauterine growth restriction
  - Birth asphyxia
  - Infant of diabetic mother

Genetic forms that generally do not present until after the first week of life are excluded, although later presentation is possible for these forms. This list is not exhaustive.

hypoglycemia are often permanent and often cause fetal overgrowth. The causative genetic loci are generally involved in β-cell function, and some cases are in imprinted regions yielding complex but powerful molecular diagnostics. Readers interested in more depth are referred to an excellent recent review.[159] The converse of genetic neonatal hyperinsulinemic hypoglycemia is neonatal diabetes. In fact, there are several genes causative for both conditions but involving opposing mutational types (e.g., activating versus inactivating). Neonatal diabetes is almost always due to genetic lesions (Box 36.4). The genetic defects causing neonatal diabetes lead to impaired insulin secretion. Because transient neonatal hyperglycemia is relatively common, especially among ill and/or preterm infants, it can be difficult to initially distinguish from neonatal diabetes. Neonatal diabetes manifestations can include small for gestational age, failure to thrive, and/or diabetic ketoacidosis. Interestingly, a portion of cases will remit over the span of weeks, and a portion of these will recur years later. Some genetic forms of neonatal diabetes are associated with nonglycemic manifestations, including neurologic issues, polycystic kidney disease, and exocrine pancreatic insufficiency, among others. Interested readers are referred to recent reviews.[160,161]

Box 36.4 Selected Genes for Which Specific Mutations Cause Neonatal Diabetes Mellitus

- Impaired β-cell function
  - *KCNJ11*
  - *ABCC8*
  - *GCK*
- Pancreatic hypoplasia or aplasia
  - *PDX1*
  - *PTF1A*

Genetic forms that generally do not present until after the first week of life are excluded, although later presentation is possible for the above forms. This list is not exhaustive.

CONCLUSION

Several decades of investigation have led to a better understanding of fetal and newborn glucose metabolism. Metabolic tracer experiments employing both stable and radioactive isotopes have been crucial to gaining this deeper insight. In general, the fetus is dependent upon glucose supplied by the maternal circulation via the placenta. As term approaches, hepatic glycogen accumulation and incipient enzymatic expression prepare for the abrupt cessation of the glucose supply from the maternal circulation. Feeding, glycogenolysis, and gluconeogenesis then maintain newborn blood glucose levels. The newborn period carries risk for both hypoglycemia and hyperglycemia.

ACKNOWLEDGMENTS

The authors thank Satish C. Kalhan, MD, as we adapted portions of the text and several figures from his version of this chapter in the prior edition. Dr. Sarah Wernimont was supported by grant T32 DK112751. Dr. Andrew Norris and the previously unpublished data shown in this chapter were supported by grants R01 DK115791, R24 DK96518, and R01 DK097820.

A complete reference list is available at www.ExpertConsult.com. 

SELECT REFERENCES

5. Sawatzke AB, Norris AW, Spyropoulos F, et al. PET/CT imaging reveals unrivaled placental avidity for glucose compared to other tissues. *Placenta*. 2015;36(2):115-120.
10. Bell EF, Johnson KJ, Dove EL. Effect of body position on energy expenditure of preterm infants as determined by simultaneous direct and indirect calorimetry. *Am J Perinatol*. 2017;34(5):493-498.
16. Marks KH, Coen P, Kerrigan JR, Francalancia NA, Nardis EE, Snider MT. The accuracy and precision of an open-circuit system to measure oxygen consumption and carbon dioxide production in neonates. *Pediatr Res*. 1987;21(1):58-65.
18. Kalhan SC, Denne SC. Energy consumption in infants with bronchopulmonary dysplasia. *J Pediatr*. 1990;116(4):662-664.
22. Guilfoy VM, Wright-Coltart S, Leitch CA, Denne SC. Energy expenditure in extremely low birth weight infants near time of hospital discharge. *J Pediatr*. 2008;153(5):612-615.
25. Roberts SB, Coward WA, Ewing G, Savage J, Cole TJ, Lucas A. Effect of weaning on accuracy of doubly labeled water method in infants. *Am J Physiol*. 1988;254(4 Pt 2):R622-R627.
31. Bozzetti P, Ferrari MM, Marconi AM, et al. The relationship of maternal and fetal glucose concentrations in the human from midgestation until term. *Metabolism*. 1988;37(4):358-363.
33. Tobin JD, Roux JF, Soeldner JS. Human fetal insulin response after acute maternal glucose administration during labor. *Pediatrics*. 1969;44(5):668-671.
34. Coltart TM, Beard RW, Turner RC, Oakley NW. Blood glucose and insulin relationships in the human mother and fetus before onset of labour. *BMJ*. 1969;4(5674):17-19. https://doi.org/10.1136/bmj.4.5674.17.
35. Marconi AM, Paolini C, Buscaglia M, Zerbe G, Battaglia FC, Pardi G. The impact of gestational age and fetal growth on the maternal-fetal glucose concentration difference. *Obstet Gynecol*. 1996;87(6):937-942.

36. Kalhan SC, D'Angelo LJ, Savin SM, Adam PA. Glucose production in pregnant women at term gestation. Sources of glucose for human fetus. *J Clin Invest*. 1979;63(3):388-394.
37. Ashmead GG, Kalhan SC, Lazebnik N, Nuamah IF. Maternal-fetal substrate relationships in the third trimester in human pregnancy. *Gynecol Obstet Invest*. 1993;35(1):18-22.
38. Holme AM, Holm MB, Roland MCP, et al. The 4-vessel sampling approach to integrative studies of human placental physiology in vivo. *J Vis Exp*. 2017;(126):e55847. https://doi.org/10.3791/55847.
39. Holme AM, Roland MCP, Lorentzen B, Michelsen TM, Henriksen T. Placental glucose transfer: a human in vivo study. *PLoS One*. 2015;10(2):e0117084.
40. Michelsen TM, Holme AM, Holm MB, et al. Uteroplacental glucose uptake and fetal glucose consumption: a quantitative study in human pregnancies. *J Clin Endocrinol Metab*. 2019;104(3):873-882.
42. Dimasuay KG, Boeuf P, Powell TL, Jansson T. Placental responses to changes in the maternal environment determine fetal growth. *Front Physiol*. 2016;7:12.
43. Kavitha JV, Rosario FJ, Nijland MJ, et al. Down-regulation of placental mTOR, insulin/IGF-I signaling, and nutrient transporters in response to maternal nutrient restriction in the baboon. *FASEB J*. 2014;28(3):1294-1305.
44. Jansson N, Rosario FJ, Gaccioli F, et al. Activation of placental mTOR signaling and amino acid transporters in obese women giving birth to large babies. *J Clin Endocrinol Metab*. 2013;98(1):105-113.
48. Illsley NP, Baumann MU. Human placental glucose transport in fetoplacental growth and metabolism. *Biochim Biophys Acta Mol Basis Dis*. 2020;1866(2):165359.
50. Barros LF, Yudilevich DL, Jarvis SM, Beaumont N, Baldwin SA. Quantitation and immunolocalization of glucose transporters in the human placenta. *Placenta*. 1995;16(7):623-633.
51. Jansson T, Wennergren M, Illsley NP. Glucose transporter protein expression in human placenta throughout gestation and in intrauterine growth retardation. *J Clin Endocrinol Metab*. 1993;77(6):1554-1562.
52. Day PE, Cleal JK, Lofthouse EM, Hanson MA, Lewis RM. What factors determine placental glucose transfer kinetics? *Placenta*. 2013;34(10):953-958.
55. Hauguel S, Desmaizieres V, Challier JC. Glucose uptake, utilization, and transfer by the human placenta as functions of maternal glucose concentration. *Pediatr Res*. 1986;20(3):269-273. https://doi.org/10.1203/00006450-198603000-00015.
58. Burd LI, Douglas Jones M, Simmons MA, Makowski EL, Meschia G, Battaglia FC. Placental production and foetal utilisation of lactate and pyruvate. *Nature*. 1975;254(5502):710-711. https://doi.org/10.1038/254710a0.
59. Char VC, Creasy RK. Lactate and pyruvate as fetal metabolic substrates. *Pediatr Res*. 1976;10(4):231-234.
63. Marconi AM, Cetin I, Davoli E, et al. An evaluation of fetal glucogenesis in intrauterine growth-retarded pregnancies. *Metabolism*. 1993;42(7):860-864. https://doi.org/10.1016/0026-0495(93)90060-2.
64. Goodner CJ, Conway MJ, Werrbach JH. Relation between plasma glucose levels of mother and fetus during maternal hyperglycemia, hypoglycemia, and fasting in the rat. *Pediatr Res*. 1969;3(2):121-127. https://doi.org/10.1203/00006450-196903000-00003.
68. Marsac C, Saudubray JM, Moncion A, Leroux JP. Development of gluconeogenic enzymes in the liver of human newborns. *Neonatology*. 1976;28(5-6):317-325. https://doi.org/10.1159/000240833.
73. Akison LK, Nitert MD, Clifton VL, Moritz KM, Simmons DG. Review: alterations in placental glycogen deposition in complicated pregnancies: current preclinical and clinical evidence. *Placenta*. 2017;54:52-58.
75. Barash V, Riskin A, Shafrir E, Waddell ID, Burchell A. Kinetic and immunologic evidence for the absence of glucose-6-phosphatase in early human chorionic villi and term placenta. *Biochim Biophys Acta*. 1991;1073(1):161-167.
83. Morriss jr FH, Makowski EL, Meschia G, Battaglia FC. The glucose/oxygen quotient of the term human fetus. *Neonatology*. 1974;25(1-2):44-52.
99. Hooper SB, Walker DW, Harding R. Oxygen, glucose, and lactate uptake by fetus and placenta during prolonged hypoxemia. *Am J Physiol*. 1995;268(2 Pt 2):R303-R309.
114. Güemes M, Rahman SA, Hussain K. What is a normal blood glucose? *Arch Dis Child*. 2016;101(6):569-574.
118. Dani C, Corsini I. Guidelines for management of neonatal hypoglycemia: are they actually applicable? *JAMA Pediatr*. 2020. https://doi.org/10.1001/jamapediatrics.2020.0632.
119. Kalhan SC, Savin SM, Adam PAJ. Measurement of glucose turnover in the human newborn with glucose-1-13C. *J Clin Endocrinol Metab*. 1976;43(3):704-707. https://doi.org/10.1210/jcem-43-3-704.
120. Bier DM, Leake RD, Haymond MW, et al. Measurement of "true" glucose production rates in infancy and childhood with 6,6-dideuteroglucose. *Diabetes*. 1977;26(11):1016-1023. https://doi.org/10.2337/diabetes.26.11.1016.
121. Denne SC, Kalhan SC. Glucose carbon recycling and oxidation in human newborns. *Am J Physiol Endocrinol Metab*. 1986;251(1):E71-E77. https://doi.org/10.1152/ajpendo.1986.251.1.e71.
122. Sauer PJJ, Van Aerde JEE, Pencharz PB, Smith JM, Swyer PR. Glucose oxidation rates in newborn infants measured with indirect calorimetry and [U-13C]glucose. *Clin Sci*. 1986;70(6):587-593. https://doi.org/10.1042/cs0700587.
128. Hawdon JM, Ward Platt MP, Aynsley-Green A. Patterns of metabolic adaptation for preterm and term infants in the first neonatal week. *Arch Dis Child*. 1992;67(4 Spec):357-365.
129. Platt MW. Lactate, glucose and the neonatal brain: it's time to challenge the paradigm. *Arch Dis Child Fetal Neonatal Ed*. 2015;100(2):F96-F97.
139. Hume R, Burchell A, Williams FLR, Koh DKM. Glucose homeostasis in the newborn. *Early Hum Dev*. 2005;81(1):95-101.
143. Kalhan SC, Parimi P, Van Beek R, et al. Estimation of gluconeogenesis in newborn infants. *Am J Physiol Endocrinol Metab*. 2001;281(5):E991-E997.
147. Sunehag A, Gustafsson J, Ewald U. Glycerol carbon contributes to hepatic glucose production during the first eight hours in healthy term infants. *Acta Paediatr*. 1996;85(11):1339-1343. https://doi.org/10.1111/j.1651-2227.1996.tb13921.x.
148. Frazer TE, Karl IE, Hillman LS, Bier DM. Direct measurement of gluconeogenesis from [2,3]13C2]alanine in the human neonate. *Am J Physiol Endocrinol Metab*. 1981;240(6):E615-E621. https://doi.org/10.1152/ajpendo.1981.240.6.e615.
150. Cowett RM, Oh W, Schwartz R. Persistent glucose production during glucose infusion in the neonate. *J Clin Invest*. 1983;71(3):467-475.
152. Chacko SK, Ordonez J, Sauer PJJ, Sunehag AL. Gluconeogenesis is not regulated by either glucose or insulin in extremely low birth weight infants receiving total parenteral nutrition. *J Pediatr*. 2011;158(6):891-896.
153. Mitanchez D. Glucose regulation in preterm newborn infants. *Horm Res*. 2007;68(6):265-271.
154. Thornton PS, De Leon DD, Sperling MA. Treatment threshold for neonatal hypoglycemia. *N Engl J Med*. 2020;382(23):2272.
155. van Kempen AAMW, Eskes PF, Nuytemans DHGM, et al. Lower versus traditional treatment threshold for neonatal hypoglycemia. *N Engl J Med*. 2020;382(6):534-544.
156. Thompson-Branch A, Havranek T. Neonatal hypoglycemia. *Pediatr Rev*. 2017;38(4):147-157.
157. Alsaleem M, Saadeh L, Kamat D. Neonatal hypoglycemia: a review. *Clin Pediatr*. 2019;58(13):1381-1386.
159. Lord K, De León DD. Hyperinsulinism in the Neonate. *Clin Perinatol*. 2018;45(1):61-74.
160. Dahl A, Kumar S. Recent advances in neonatal diabetes. *Diabetes Metab Syndr Obes*. 2020;13:355-364.

37 Oxygen Consumption and General Carbohydrate Metabolism of the Fetus

Anthony F. Philipps

INTRODUCTION

This chapter reviews a number of factors that are involved in control of fetal metabolism, with reference to relationships between fetal energy balance and substrate uptake during the last trimester. This information relies heavily upon research data obtained from a variety of experiments in animals as well as some theoretical considerations. Data from human studies are now also becoming more available than in previous years and are incorporated here when applicable. Because hospitalization of neonates younger than 30 weeks gestation who were very recently in utero is common in newborn intensive care units, understanding of those factors involved in determining fetal metabolic needs may be of use in these settings. The term *metabolism* (derived from the Greek *metabole*, a change) is used in this context to describe a number of biochemical reactions that illustrate chemical processes in the fetus that alter carbon-containing substrates to synthesize tissue (accretion/growth) or provide energy needed for basic homeostasis (fuel/energy).

HISTORY AND FETAL ENERGY REQUIREMENTS

The consumption of oxygen is closely tied to the resting metabolic rate, which, as we will see later, varies with mass in nongrowing adult mammals but not in the fetus or newborn. The first individual who gained insight into the process of metabolism was John Mayow (1640–1679), who noted that the consumption of an undefined substance in air was similar when measured in breathing mammals in a sealed container or during combustion of inert materials.[1] It was not until almost 100 years later that the substance consumed was discovered and named. The discovery of oxygen is attributed to Carl Wilhelm Scheele in 1771 ("fire air"), although both Joseph Priestly (1774, "extra pure air") and Antoine Lavosier (1775) are also credited.[1-3] However, it was Lavoisier who named the gas oxygen (from the Greek *oxys* [sharp acid] and *gène* [produces]) and demonstrated that in human respiration, oxygen was taken up and converted into another substance he called "fixed air" as part of the metabolism of nutrients. Joseph Black (1775) is credited with the discovery of carbon dioxide shortly thereafter. The fetus was not thought to have any independent metabolism of its own, but in 1786 the surgeon and scientist John Hunter showed that fetal and maternal circulations within the placenta were distinct from each other. Shortly thereafter, Erasmus Darwin, Charles Darwin's grandfather, surmised correctly in his text *Zoonomia* (1794) that at least one of the functions of the placenta was to supply the fetus with this newly discovered gas, oxygen, for its own separate metabolic demands.[4]

However, it was not until the late 1800s that fetal blood was demonstrated to contain oxygen derived from mother's blood,[5,6] and only in the 1930s did it become possible for the fetal blood oxygen content and hemoglobin saturation to be accurately measured.[6] Fetal oxygen consumption was found to be similar to that of the newborn animal and a maternofetal gradient for oxygen was demonstrated. Even so, mammalian fetuses were thought to live in hypoxic environments[6,7] because human and animal umbilical venous blood had significantly lower partial pressures than adult arterial blood. This finding led to the "Mount Everest in utero" concept attributed to Sir Joseph Barcroft,[8] and attempts were then made to understand how the fetus adapted to such conditions. Because of the leftward shift in the oxyhemoglobin dissociation curve,[9,10] elevated levels of fetal (vs. adult) hemoglobin, and increased circulating red cell mass, relatively normal umbilical venous oxygen content (measured by the standard of milliliter or millimole of oxygen per milliliter of blood) was found to be the case.

Parenthetically, it has been demonstrated that acquiring hemoglobin concentrations of 16 to 18 g/dL, similar to those found in the fetus, also appears to confer significant survival advantage for some adults living at high altitude (i.e., 3800 m),[11] another condition placing constraints on arterial blood oxygen tension, although no shifts in the hemoglobin-oxygen dissociation curve have been found in these populations.[12] This predominantly genetic adaptation is also likely to spare cardiac work (i.e., obviating the need to increase cardiac output, which is somewhat limited in the fetus). In addition, it has recently been shown that in these high-altitude populations, presumably due to genetic adaptation, pregnancy induces increases in uterine artery diameter and uteroplacental blood flow and thus oxygen delivery to the fetoplacental unit.[13]

The other major factor not often considered in discussions of maternofetal oxygen transport is the effect of the Bohr effect on both oxygen loading (fetal umbilical venous blood) and unloading (maternal uterine arterial to venous blood). Zhang and colleagues studied the theoretical shifts in hemoglobin affinity for oxygen in five mammalian species.[10] Their study concluded that oxygen delivery to fetal tissues by fetal hemoglobin was found to be more efficient than that of adult hemoglobin, as was the theoretical ability of hemoglobin to load oxygen at the placental level, due to the Bohr effect on pH (Fig. 37.1). The

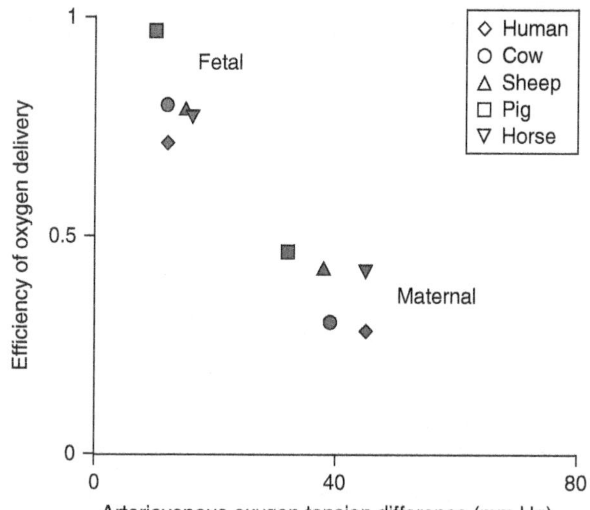

Fig. 37.1 Enhanced efficiency of oxygen delivery of fetal versus maternal blood in five mammalian species. Efficiency is calculated as the ratio of the arteriovenous saturation difference (ΔS) associated with the observed arteriovenous partial pressure difference (ΔP) for an oxyhemoglobin dissociation curve at physiologic P_{50} to the maximum saturation change achievable for the same ΔP for dissociation curves for which P_{50} is allowed to vary arbitrarily. Efficiency–that is, $(\Delta S_{P_{(a-v)}O_2}(\text{Phys}P_{50}) / \max\Delta S_{P_{(a-v)}O_2})$–is then plotted as a function of the arteriovenous partial pressure difference for oxygen ($\Delta P_{(a-v)}O_2$). Values much closer to 1 for fetal blood indicate that the physiologic P_{50} for fetal blood is more nearly optimal for oxygen delivery at physiologic arterial and venous oxygen tensions. *Brown symbols:* fetal, *blue symbols:* maternal. (Data from Zhang Y, Kobayashi K, Kitazawa K, et al. Contribution of cooperativity and the Bohr effect to efficient oxygen transport by hemoglobins from five mammalian species. *Zoolog Sci.* 2006;23:49.)

developmental and species-specific differences in hemoglobin gene regulation have been reviewed elsewhere.[10,11] Thus, overall, in both human cord blood and umbilical venous samples from fetuses of a number of species, fetal oxygen delivery as measured by blood oxygen content (not Po_2 [i.e., the partial pressure of oxygen in blood]) is adequate for aerobic metabolic needs.[14]

It follows that fetal mammals, under steady-state, or unstressed, conditions, ought to achieve adequate oxygen delivery (the product of umbilical venous blood oxygen content and umbilical venous blood flow) and should not exhibit evidence of hypoxia (low tissue oxygen availability), unless specific organ or total blood flow falls dramatically or fetal blood oxygen content declines below a critical level. Studies of fetal acid-base or lactate balance indirectly test this hypothesis. The consensus is that no evidence exists to support a hypoxic fetal milieu because (1) umbilical cord blood pH values of unstressed fetal humans, pigs, monkeys, and sheep are all similar to one another and to the normal adult range of 7.35 to 7.45; (2) venoarterial H^+ concentration differences in cord blood of these species are only modest, suggesting relatively small fetomaternal H^+ transfer, inconsistent with hypoxia-induced lactic acid production; (3) both in vitro and in vivo, the placenta has been shown to deliver lactate into the fetal circulation, where it is taken up, particularly by the fetal liver, for purposes of accretion and oxidation[15-17]; and (4) experimental production of maternal and relative fetal hyperoxia in the sheep is not associated with an increase in fetal oxygen consumption.

Thus, in the unstressed fetus, energy processes use oxidative pathways, and estimation of fetal oxygen consumption may be used as a direct indicator of the fetal metabolic rate.[14,18,19] Although rates of substrate uptake and carbon dioxide production provide alternate measurements of fetal metabolic activity, the calculation

Table 37.1 Fetal Oxygen Consumption in Various Species.

Species	Measurement	$\dot{V}O_2$ (mL/kg/min)
Human at term[25-28]	B	6.8
Rhesus monkey[159]	F	7.0
Sheep[24]	F	7.9
Cow[160]	F	6.7
Horse[161]	F	7.0
Guinea pig[162]	B	8.8

B, Bohr principle measurement; *F*, Fick principle measurement.

of each requires a significant number of assumptions. In the case of substrate utilization, the relative partitioning of carbon uptake by the fetus for use as fuel (oxidative needs) or growth (accretion needs) must be considered. Measurement of CO_2 production must also take into account the relative contributions of carbon from the oxidative metabolism of carbohydrates, amino acids, and fats toward carbon dioxide generation, which may be less than equimolar depending upon the fetal diet.[14,20]

FETAL OXYGEN CONSUMPTION

MEASUREMENT

Fetal oxygen consumption ($\dot{V}O_2$) has been estimated using a variety of techniques. Two methods have been used to gauge fetal oxygen consumption in vivo. Because the fetus has little stored oxygen, the vast majority of fetal requirement for oxidative metabolism of substrate is met by transfer of oxygen to the fetus via the placenta and umbilical venous circulation. Negligible transfer is thought to occur across the fetal membranes. The earliest known method for measuring fetal $\dot{V}O_2$ accurately in the intact animal was that derived by Christian Bohr (circa 1900). By measuring $\dot{V}O_2$ before and after intermittent umbilical occlusion in pregnant guinea pigs (or in subsequent studies by others before and after delivery of other fetal mammals), fetal $\dot{V}O_2$ could be calculated as follows:

$$\text{Fetal } \dot{V}O_2 = \text{Predelivery maternal } \dot{V}O_2 - \text{Predelivery maternal } \dot{V}O_2 \quad [37.1]$$

Fetal $\dot{V}O_2$ is usually expressed as either mL or mmol O_2/kg/min. As shown in Table 37.1, estimates for fetuses of several species, including humans, are available.

The major assumption in these studies is that the act of delivery (or cord occlusion) does not measurably alter maternal, uterine, or placental $\dot{V}O_2$. Such assumptions are likely not entirely accurate due to parturition-induced changes in fetal, placental, and maternal rates of metabolism and/or blood flow, but the results of these studies provide a framework for estimates obtained using other methods.

The second technique for measuring fetal $\dot{V}O_2$ relies on the principle originally derived by Adolf Fick (circa 1870), whereby uptake of substrates or oxygen for the whole organism can be calculated as the product of cardiac output and the arteriovenous difference in substrate or oxygen content. In the case of specific fetal organ uptake (or in this case, the whole fetus), the product may be transposed as organ or whole fetal blood flow multiplied by the arteriovenous or venoarterial concentration difference of the substance in question across the organ or umbilical circulation, respectively. (See review by Carter.[11])

Thus, for oxygen consumption of the mammalian fetus, the principle may be restated according to Eq. 37.2:

$$\text{Fetal } \dot{V}O_2 = F_{umb} \times C_{(v-a)O_2} \quad [37.2]$$

where F_{umb} = umbilical blood flow (mL/min or mL/kg/min) and $C_{(v-a)O_2}$ = the venoarterial difference in O_2 content (mL or mmol of O_2/100 mL blood) across the umbilical circulation. The advantages of the Fick method over the original Bohr technique include (1) the ability to perform serial studies in the same animal during late gestation, (2) the ability to measure uptake and excretion of potential fetal metabolites simultaneously with the uptake of oxygen, and (3) the ability to observe changes in metabolic rate before and after experimental manipulation.

Noninvasive methods for determination of animal and human fetal $\dot{V}O_2$ are being developed, such as blood oxygenation level-dependent (BOLD) magnetic resonance imaging (MRI),[21,22] near-infrared spectroscopy (NIRS), and intensity-modulated optical spectroscopy (IMOS; a modification of NIRS).[23] Fig. 37.2 demonstrates the use of BOLD to assess oxygenation in placenta, brain, and liver of two groups of fetuses (normal [AGA] and growth restricted [SGA]) during maternal normoxia and hyperoxia. Changes in signal intensity (R2*, a measure of hemoglobin saturation in tissues) did not differ between groups in the study, but responses to hyperoxia varied among those organs. These techniques make use of the differences observed in either image density or spectroscopic patterns between saturated and desaturated hemoglobin and may be particularly useful for assessing specific organ (i.e., liver, brain, placenta) oxygen requirements or abnormalities of metabolic function due to maternal or fetal disease states.[22]

EXPERIMENTAL DATA

The difficulties involved in obtaining Fick principle estimates of fetal $\dot{V}O_2$ include the necessity of obtaining samples of umbilical venous and umbilical or distal aortic blood for oxygen content analysis, which requires use of a relatively large fetus (i.e., sheep, cow, pig) for catheter placement, or in humans, sampling from the umbilical cord at the time of delivery (usually cesarean section) and the requirement of a reliable estimate of umbilical blood flow. The former problem in animal experiments has been overcome by the implantation of fetal catheters[14] for serial measurements under nonstressed conditions. The latter problem in animals has been overcome by the development of several methods for the accurate measurement of umbilical blood flow, which include the use of laser-Doppler, ultrasonic, or electromagnetic flow transducers; radiolabeled microspheres; or steady-state diffusion of substances such as antipyrine, ethanol, or tritiated water across the placenta. For human studies, F_{umb} has been estimated using ultrasound and Doppler as the product of the umbilical vein cross-sectional diameter and umbilical vein blood flow velocity. However, technical difficulties in obtaining consistent measurement of both of these parameters have produced published estimates of F_{umb} varying by more than 20%.[11,24]

As can be seen in Table 37.1, when corrected for fetal weight, fetal $\dot{V}O_2$ as measured in a variety of animal species is remarkably consistent, with a range of 6.7 to 8.8 mL O_2/kg/min. Despite the aforementioned caveats regarding F_{umb}, in recent studies of fetal $\dot{V}O_2$ obtained in term human fetuses,[25-28] values of 5.4 to 6.9 mL/kg/min fit well within the range observed for other species. As an example, a noninvasive study of human fetuses near term using MRI/Doppler flow determined $\dot{V}O_2$ to be 6.9 ± 1.7 mL/kg/min with O_2 extraction of 34 ± 8%.[29]

DETERMINING FACTORS

Factors that control fetal energy expenditure are not fully understood, but one main tenet is that there is a relatively consistent relationship between mass and metabolic rate across species in the adult. Although it had been known for many years that body weight correlates with metabolic rate, Kleiber[30] formulated the seminal allometric scaling relationship in comparative physiology:

$$\text{Metabolic rate} \propto \text{Mass}^{3/4} \quad [37.3]$$

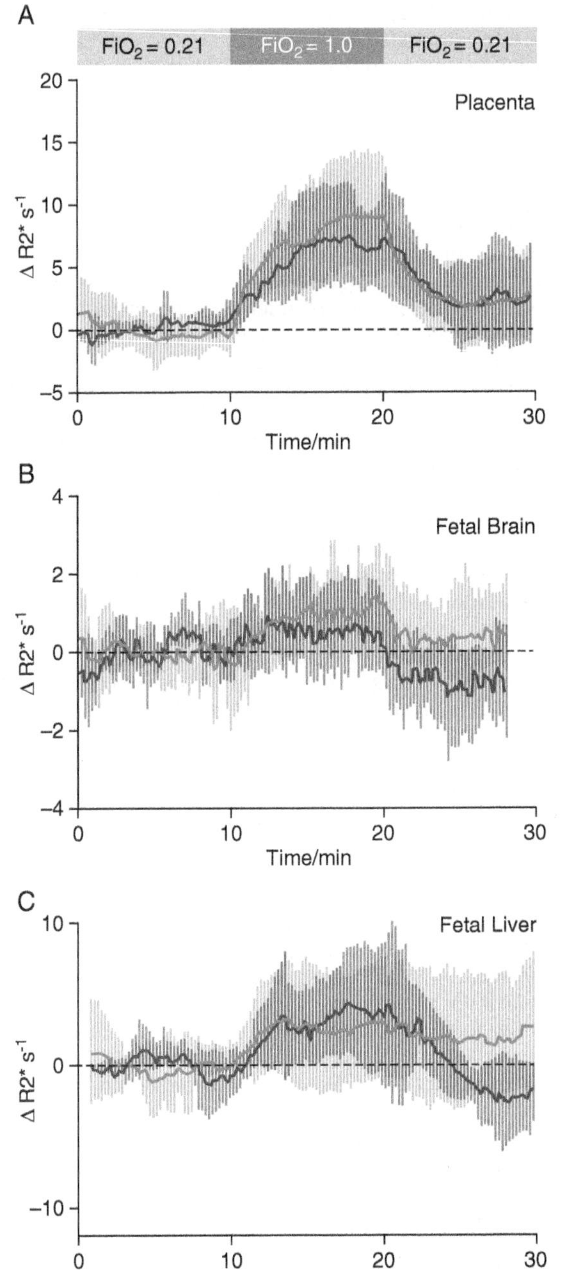

Fig. 37.2 Changes in R2* (an indicator of regional hemoglobin saturation) relative to baseline in placentas and organs of AGA *(green)* and SGA *(red)* twin pairs (mean and standard deviation), before, during, and after maternal hyperoxia. (A) placentas, (B) fetal livers, (C) fetal brain. (Data from Luo J, Turk EA, Bibbo C, et al. *In vivo* quantification of placental insufficiency by BOLD MRI: a human study. *Sci Rep.* 2017;7:3713, 1–10, Fig. 5.)

In this relationship, it is important to point out that metabolic rate is expressed in kcal/day (not kcal/kg/day, which would be nonallometric), so daily energy expenditure is proportional to $(mass)^{3/4}$. Since Eq. 37.3 was first formulated, this basic principle has been extended and is reasonably predictive of the aerobic metabolic rates not only for a variety of mammals and other vertebrates, but also for the metabolic rates of single cells, mitochondria, and even for the turnover rate for substrates in the respiratory enzyme chain within mitochondria.[31] However, newer work suggests that the actual scaling ratio between mass (M) and metabolic rate (Rm) may be somewhat greater or less, depending on the species (Fig. 37.3). Factors that might alter this relationship have been explored by several recent research groups, and the reader is directed there for further review.[32,33]

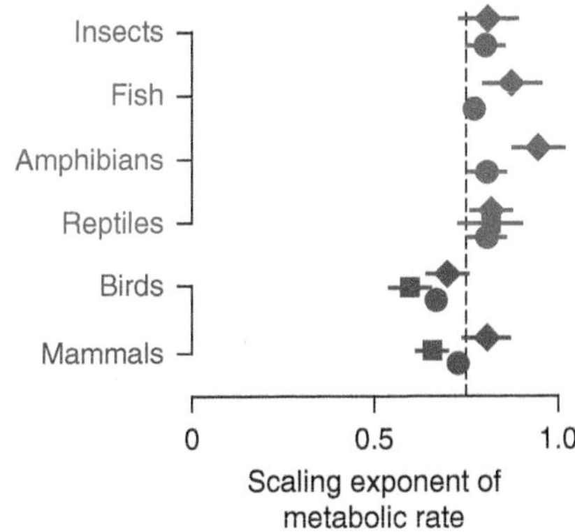

Fig. 37.3 Estimates of empirical scaling exponents of R_m for a range of species measured at rest *(circles),* while free living *(squares)* or during intense activity *(diamonds),* shown ± 95% confidence intervals. Groups that are predominantly endothermic are colored *red,* while groups that are predominantly ectothermic are colored *blue.* The vertical dashed line represents the scaling exponent of ¾ predicted by several metabolic theories. (Data from White CR, Marshall DJ, Alton LA, et al. The origin and maintenance of metabolic allometry in animals. *Nat Ecol Evol.* 2019;3:598–603.)

The aforementioned general relationship may be predicted theoretically due to the basic limitations of nutrient and oxygen transport placed on respiring cells that relates to the geometry of branching networks, such as blood vessels or mitochondrial cristae. The caveats in such a relationship are that the metabolic rate is measured (classically as $\dot{V}O_2$) (1) in the resting state and (2) in nongrowing adults (i.e., not in subjects that are actively growing, such as the fetus or newborn).[31]

To reiterate, as suggested by Kleiber,[30] if nonallometric basal metabolic rate (kcal/kg/time unit) is used, the relationship between mass and metabolic rate becomes an inverse one, with smaller adult nongrowing animals having relatively larger mass-specific metabolic rates. However, there exists a relative constancy of fetal $\dot{V}O_2$ across species lines when corrected for fetal weight under standard conditions. Among species whose fetal weights differ by as much as a factor of 300, weight-specific fetal $\dot{V}O_2$ estimates (mL/kg/min) differ by only 15% with a mean value of 7.4 mL/kg/min (see Table 37.1).[14] The most frequently studied steady-state data remain available from the fetal lamb, which, in one review of data from 162 near-term sheep,[24] the mean fetal $\dot{V}O_2$ was 354 ± 45 μmol/kg/min (7.93 ± 1.01 mL/kg/min).

The observation that the inverse scaling principle does not apply to fetal mammals has led to the speculation that confounding factors such as the rapid rate of growth in late perinatal life and changes in membrane lipid composition[34] may be important. In addition, it has been hypothesized that another reason for the apparent inconsistency is that the fetus is relatively free from the "adult" oxidative demands of temperature homeostasis and, to a lesser extent, gravity and muscular activity, all of which are dependent on body mass and surface area.

During and after the transition from fetus to newborn, there is a gradual increasing ratio between weight and mass-specific metabolic rate. Predominantly due to diminished needs for such metabolic functions as heat control, $\dot{V}O_2$ in late fetal life is somewhat closer to the weight-specific metabolic rate for the adult (Fig. 37.4).[35,36] Postnatally, metabolic rate rises significantly

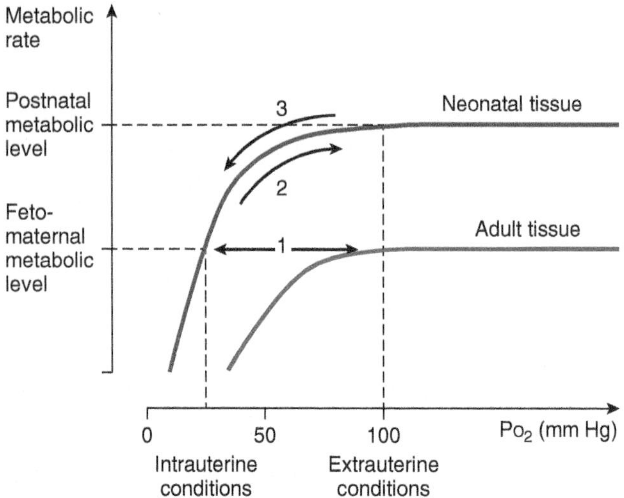

Fig. 37.4 Left-shift of Po_2/metabolic rate relationship in neonatal mice as compared with adult tissue. Microcalorimetric data were recorded on mouse heart tissue slices under various oxygenation conditions. The same metabolic adaptation that enables the fetus at low Po_2 to maintain a metabolic rate similar to the adult at high Po_2 *(arrow 1)* may lead to the metabolic increase with increasing Po_2 at birth *(arrow 2)* and to "hypometabolism" being observed under hypoxic conditions *(arrow 3)*. (Data from Schneider H. Oxygenation of the placental-fetal unit in humans. *Respir Physiol Neurobiol.* 2011;178:51–58. Reprinted from Singer [2004].)

greater than that of the adult, with a slow decline thereafter.[34-36] Studies in human infants have concluded that the relationship between body mass and $\dot{V}O_2$ declines back to "adult" levels by approximately 18 months of age, or at a body weight of approximately 12 kg.[37]

At the cellular level, the control of metabolic rate has not been clearly elucidated but involves complex interactions between a number of factors, including (1) the concentration of adenosine triphosphate (ATP; the product of mitochondrial oxidative phosphorylation); (2) the ratio of intracellular adenosine diphosphate (ADP) to ATP, (3) rates of intracellular protein synthesis, and (4) the generation of proton (H^+) gradients by respiratory enzymes across the mitochondrial and cell membranes.[18,38] It has been estimated that approximately 15% of $\dot{V}O_2$ of the term fetus might be spent on total active transport processes.

One general assumption has been that metabolic rate is not influenced by oxygen availability unless the diffusion of oxygen is severely limited. Justification for this view stems from the observation that several mammalian tissues (i.e., heart, liver, and kidney) have similar in vivo and in vitro rates of oxygen consumption, suggesting an intrinsic regulatory mechanism. For example, in exteriorized artificially ventilated premature lambs, mitochondrial respiratory activity in heart, kidney, and muscle was no different from control animals.[39] However, some contradictory in vivo studies in mammals genetically adapted to living at high altitude (the South American Andean llama)[40-42] and in sheep recently acclimatized to high altitude[43] have shown that prolonged exposure to relative fetal hypoxemia can induce long-standing protective changes. These changes include, in addition to the well-known compensatory increase in hemoglobin concentration, changes in glucocorticoid signaling, depression of cerebral Na^+, K^+-ATPase pump activity, reduced expression of at least two Na channel proteins, decreased cerebral heat production, altered cerebral vasculature anatomy, and decreased cerebral $\dot{V}O_2$ without apparent biochemical or histologic evidence of brain damage.[40,44,45] At least some of these changes appear to be mediated by endothelin-1 and intrinsic nitric oxide (NO), both potent mediators of vascular tone, as well as by vascular endothelial growth factor (VEGF) and endogenously produced carbon monoxide (CO).[42,46] Studies of two distinct human populations living at high altitude for many centuries (Andeans and Tibetans) suggest that a broad range of genetic adaptations, including divergent hypoxia-inducible factor (HIF)-1 responses (see later), have evolved to deal with the challenge of oxygen delivery under these conditions.[47,48] Furthermore, the use of microarray genomic techniques are beginning to elucidate even more information about cellular responses to chronic hypoxic stimuli. Such studies have important implications for understanding the manner in which the fetus might be protected against sudden changes in oxygen delivery.

However, at sea level, classic studies have shown the characteristic fetal blood flow (and consequent oxygen) redistribution during graded maternal hypoxia, in which blood flow and oxygen delivery are preferentially shunted to brain and away from carcass.[49] Interestingly, in vitro studies have shown that tissues such as fetal muscle[50] do decrease $\dot{V}O_2$ in response to change in media Po_2. Similar findings have been observed in other fetal organs such as liver and kidney.[51]

A series of studies have also shown that brief fetal hypoxia induces a number of changes in regulatory genes, particularly in the fetal hypothalamus and pituitary.[52] More prolonged hypoxia causes stimulation of HIF-1, 2, and 3,[53,54] potent gene transcriptional factors.[55] Hypoxic response elements (HREs), which bind HIFs, are intrinsic to a number of genes that are developmentally regulated[54,56,57] and control synthesis of several protective proteins such as VEGF, erythropoietin (Epo), platelet-derived growth factor and metabolic enzymes that induce increases in anaerobic ATP production via increased mitochondrial glycolysis.[58]

Furthermore, activation of carotid body chemoreceptors, specifically the adenosine A_{2A} receptor, plays a significant role in defending against fetal hypoxia by helping to maintain brain blood flow.[59,60] Activation of specific calcium channel receptors[61] such as RyR1 may act to stimulate local organ intravascular synthesis of the intrinsic vasodilator NO, thereby increasing local blood flow and therefore oxygen delivery during times of relative hypoxemia. Fetal hemoglobin appears to facilitate this change in delivery by at least twice that of adult hemoglobin.[46]

INTEGRATION OF FETAL METABOLIC RATE

Under a wide variety of conditions, changes in O_2 delivery to the fetus are met by changes in O_2 extraction to meet metabolic demands.[11] In the fetal sheep, O_2 extraction may be calculated as the ratio between O_2 consumption (see Eq. 37.2) and O_2 delivery (the product of umbilical blood flow and umbilical venous O_2 content). In the steady state, this ratio is usually approximately 0.4 in the fetal sheep, meaning that only 40% of the oxygen delivered to the fetus via the placental circulation is extracted. The ratio during experimental hypoxemia in animals may rise to some extent (to 0.5 to 0.6) without serious adverse effects.[11] Measurements in healthy human fetuses[29] were in this range, but during delivery, extraction ratios of 0.57 to 0.7 have been observed.[16,27] At high altitude, ratios even higher than these were observed. Confirming earlier work in animals, extraction was inversely related to oxygen delivery.[62]

However, in human fetuses with intrauterine growth restriction who were excreting significant amounts of lactate (and presumably had relative fetal hypoxia), no increase in extraction was observed, suggesting a relative maximum in extraction efficiency had been reached in that population.[16,29]

Of those factors influencing fetal $\dot{V}O_2$, several are particularly prominent (Box 37.1). "Specific organ metabolism" refers to those various cellular processes common to most tissues. It is, of course, well known that it is chemical energy provided by oxygen and a variety of carbon-containing substrates including glucose that is the actual fuel underpinning all forms of homeostasis.[1] In adults only approximately 20% of this energy is converted to support basal cellular metabolism, with the remainder used to produce heat.[30,63] Regarding cellular homeostasis, virtually all mitochondrial and plasma membrane ion pumps require energy in the form of ATP and are thus heavily dependent on cellular respiratory activity. Such pumps consist of F-type H^+ pumps (mitochondria), V-type H^+ pumps (lysosomes, storage granules), or P-type Na^+, K^+, or H^+ pumps (plasma membranes).[63,64] Although it has thus far been difficult to estimate the contribution of such processes to the fetal metabolic rate, it is probable that in many tissues, pump activity is vital in determining intraorgan $\dot{V}O_2$. For example, in one estimate,[65] ouabain (via inhibition of Na^+, K^+-ATPase pump activity) caused a decline in fetal sheep liver and placental $\dot{V}O_2$, which accounted for 20% and 34% of whole organ $\dot{V}O_2$ in those organs, respectively. Similarly, in the newborn rat, approximately 50% of liver metabolism was due to activity of the sodium pump, followed by a significant decline in infancy.[66]

Other metabolic processes, such as protein synthesis and attendant energy-dependent chemical reactions such as transamination and decarboxylation, have metabolic costs, but the contributions of these to fetal $\dot{V}O_2$ have not been determined. Fetal work (i.e., muscle oxidative requirements to perform such activities as fetal breathing and limb movements) also accounts for a significant fraction of the total fetal $\dot{V}O_2$. For example, striated muscle activity (excluding cardiac work), as assessed in the fetal sheep, has been estimated to account for as much as 15% of the total fetal $\dot{V}O_2$, which agrees with an in vitro measurement of approximately 20 μmol/100 g/min, assuming muscle mass in the term fetal lamb of 25% fetal wet weight. If specific cardiac $\dot{V}O_2$, as also measured in the lamb, is added, slightly greater than 20% of the fetal requirement for oxygen is necessary for normal striated muscle activity.

Unfortunately, further information of tissue-specific oxygen needs in the fetus is limited to several accessible organs in animals, predominantly sheep, although some in vitro tissue data from prematurely delivered humans are available for comparison.[67] Lastly, the energy cost of growth (i.e., the energy necessary to synthesize new tissue) has been estimated to be approximately 10% of the caloric value of new tissue, which is equivalent to approximately 6% of the fetal $\dot{V}O_2$.

In summary, it can be seen that approximately 50% of the measured fetal $\dot{V}O_2$ is attributable to metabolism in fetal brain, liver, kidney, and intestine (Table 37.2). In the sheep fetus, approximately 83% of the fetal $\dot{V}O_2$ can be accounted for in the resting state. It is assumed that measurement of $\dot{V}O_2$ in other tissues (e.g., bone marrow, lung, adrenal gland, cartilage, skin) and underestimation of fetal tissue pump activity and limited thermogenesis would provide for the remaining 17% of whole fetus oxygen needs.

Several factors may further influence the fetal metabolic rate (see Box 37.1). Interestingly, other than active fetal cooling, such potential adverse stimuli such as mild hypoxemia or other experimental manipulations such as maternal exercise[68] or severe maternal starvation[69] do not appear to depress overall fetal metabolic activity. Although not well studied, maternally administered drugs that cross the placenta and have a depressive effect on fetal activity are likely to decrease fetal $\dot{V}O_2$. For example, experimental skeletal muscle paralysis in the fetal lamb causes a 10% to 15% decrease in fetal $\dot{V}O_2$.[70] Significant depression of fetal respiratory or body movement have been noted after maternal exposure to ethanol, antidepressants, cigarette smoking, hypoxemia, or steroids.[71,72] The fetal metabolic rate can be stimulated by such factors as change in fetal sleep state,[71] excessive fetal muscular activity, maternal fever, and possibly external stimuli such as sound.[73]

Studies regarding changes in human fetal behavior are now possible using fetal ultrasound to gauge fetal movement and breathing. Using these techniques, it has also been shown that fetal breathing is more prominent after maternal food intake[71] or glucose infusion[74] and by maternal drug abuse (cocaine,

Box 37.1 Factors Influencing Fetal Oxygen Consumption

Specific organ metabolism[a]
Activity
Fetal breathing
Fetal limb movement
Fetal cardiac activity
Fetal sleep state
Fetal growth
Substrate uptake
Maternal exercise
Fetomaternal temperature gradient
Fetal hormonal status
Thyroid hormones
Catecholamines
Insulin

[a]Including ion pump activity and other processes necessary for cellular homeostasis.

Table 37.2 Tissue-Specific Oxygen Needs in the Fetus.

	$\dot{V}O_2$/100 g Tissue	$\dot{V}O_2$/kg Body Weight	
	μmol/100 g Tissue/min	μmol/kg Body Weight/min	% Total $\dot{V}O_2$
Whole fetus	—	360 (8.0)	100.0
Brain[134,135,148]	190	30 (0.7)	8.8
Heart[15,41,163]	400	25 (0.6)	7.5
Liver[164]	174	67 (1.5)	18.0
Intestine[49,67]	100	40 (0.9)	11.3
Kidneys[14]	100	8 (0.2)	2.5
Adrenal	68	2	0.05
Muscle[a,14,50,165]	20	50 (1.1)	14.0
Other Growth[14]	—	20 (0.45)	5.6
Activity[a,70]	—	54 (1.2)[a]	15.0
Total	—	296 (6.6)	83.0

[a]Data for muscle (in vitro) and activity (in vivo) must reflect both sedentary and active states of striated muscle respiration.

methadone).[72] In addition, one recent study using a fetal accelerometer sensor to monitor human fetal movement over longer epochs during maternal sleep showed that gross human fetal movement declines normally during the last trimester of pregnancy from 17% of time studied at 28 weeks to 6% near term.[75]

The hormonal milieu also plays a significant role in setting the background for the fetal metabolic rate at rest and during changes in the fetal environment. The interplay between the hypothalamic-pituitary-adrenal axis, catecholamines, and other fetal hormones also influences cellular respiration and metabolic rate. Fetal concentrations of thyroxine (T_4) and triiodothyronine (T_3) are crucial to accretion of fetal mass and regulation of fetal $\dot{V}O_2$.[76] The control of circulating levels of these hormones is a complicated balance between activation of synthesis and endogenous secretion, peripheral conversion of T_4 to T_3, uptake into peripheral tissues, and, in some species including humans, transplacental transfer from mother to fetus. Fetal thyroid ablation has been shown to cause a 20% to 30% reduction in fetal metabolic rate, mostly related to effects on skeletal muscle and fat.[76] These observations may have important implications for such disease states as fetal thyrotoxicosis or maternal diabetes. Other hormones such as insulin and catecholamines also play roles in control of fetal $\dot{V}O_2$. For example, although fetal insulin deficiency does not alter resting umbilical $\dot{V}O_2$,[77,78] maternal and subsequent fetal hypoglycemia have been shown to lower $\dot{V}O_2$ by as much as 30%.[79] As noted in the following sections, both fetal hyperinsulinemia and hyperglycemia appear to have independent effects upon accelerating fetal $\dot{V}O_2$.

FETAL ENERGY SUBSTRATES

As noted in the previous sections, fetal $\dot{V}O_2$ in most mammals, including humans, is approximately 7 to 8 mL/kg/min or approximately 11.5 L of oxygen per kg body weight per day. Assuming a "fetal diet" (see further on) relatively low in fat oxidation for most species and a conversion factor of approximately 4.8 to 4.9 kcal energy generated per liter of oxygen consumed, the energy requirement (caloric value of substrate used for oxidation) by the fetus would be equivalent to approximately 55 kcal/kg/day. Because fetal energy requirements dictate a significant source of carbon uptake, it has been useful to determine the relative uptakes of potential substrates across the fetal circulation. This has been accomplished both by classic Fick principle physiologic methods and by radioisotope infusion studies (e.g., ^{14}C-labeled glucose, lactate). Although the latter method has been more completely defined in fetal sheep, transfer studies are also available in small mammals such as the guinea pig, rabbit, and rat.[80,81] Recently, investigators using doubly clamped umbilical vessels in human fetuses delivered by cesarean section in term pregnancies[82] have shown umbilical glucose uptake to be approximately 5.4 mg/kg/min, but with a relatively wide range from 3 to 7.5 mg/kg/min. Differences in blood flow were determined by Doppler ultrasound and an estimate of vessel cross-sectional area, which may add some complexity and uncertainty to these estimates.

METHODS AND TERMINOLOGY

UPTAKE

Uptake of a substrate such as glucose may be calculated using the equation derived for fetal $\dot{V}O_2$:

$$U_{substrate} = F_{umb} \times [substrate]_{(v-a)} \qquad [37.4]$$

where $U_{substrate}$ = the umbilical uptake of a particular substrate in mmol or mg/kg/min and $[substrate]_{(v-a)}$ = the umbilical vein-distal aortic concentration difference of substrate in mmol or mg/mL. Note that U does not necessarily measure fetal uptake because, theoretically, endogenous production of a particular substrate (such as glucose or lactate) from other substrates must be taken into account. Therefore U measures net umbilical uptake and provides only a minimum estimate of fetal uptake. Another limitation of this method for estimating fetal substrate utilization is the sensitivity of the method used to assay substrate concentration (usually colorimetric or spectrophotometric methods) relative to the percentage extracted from the circulation. For example, in the fetal sheep, the umbilical venous concentration of glucose is approximately 30 mg/dL (1.7 mmol/L), and the extraction coefficient ([uptake/delivery] × 100) ranges from 10% to 15%. The coefficient of variation of the glucose assay is approximately 3%, and thus it is possible to measure umbilical glucose uptake with accuracy. By contrast, the umbilical venous concentration for the amino acid serine is 700 μmol/L with a coefficient of variation of the assay of 1%.[83] However, in this case the extraction coefficient of serine is only 0.6% of the delivery rate. It is therefore obvious that for substances with small extraction coefficients, accuracy in measuring umbilical uptake using the Fick principle is problematic.

OXYGEN QUOTIENT

Previously it was difficult to determine directly whether specific fetal substrates were taken up by the umbilical circulation and oxidized completely. The concept of substrate-oxygen quotient was adapted for the fetus,[14] predominantly using sheep to address this question. To estimate the maximum fraction of fetal oxygen consumption accounted for by the oxidation of any given substrate, the following equation is applied:

$$\text{Substrate: } O_2 \text{ quotient} = F_{umb} \times [substrate]_{(v-a)} \times n / \left(F_{umb} \times [O_2]_{(v-a)}\right) \qquad [37.5]$$

where F_{umb} = umbilical blood flow, $[substrate]_{(v-a)}$ and $[O_2]_{(v-a)}$ = venoarterial differences in substrate and oxygen concentrations (mol/L), respectively, and n = the number of moles of oxygen required for the complete oxidation of substrate:

Substrate	n
Glucose	6.0
Lactate	3.0
Glycerol	3.5
Palmitic acid	23.0
β-Hydroxybutyrate	4.5
Acetoacetate	4.0

Using Eq. 37.5 and assuming steady-state conditions, the blood flow terms in the numerator and denominator (F_{umb}) cancel out, leaving the ratio of the venoarterial concentration differences of substrate versus oxygen. Thus, as adapted for fetal metabolic studies under steady-state conditions, this method of estimating substrate requirements for energy has the advantage of not requiring measurement of umbilical blood flow or fetal mass. The demonstration of a substrate-oxygen quotient near or equal to 1.0 suggests that if the particular substrate measured was completely oxidized, it could provide 100% of the carbon necessary for the measured fetal $\dot{V}O_2$. A substrate-oxygen quotient significantly less than 1.0 would indicate the requirement for other carbon sources to be used to sustain metabolic rate even if the measured substrate were completely oxidized. It then follows that substrate-oxygen quotients greater than 1.0 indicate use of a significant portion of measured substrate for purposes other than energy production

Table 37.3 Umbilical Glucose Uptake and Glucose-Oxygen Quotient.

Species	Umbilical Glucose Uptake (mg/kg/min)	Umbilical Glucose-O_2
Sheep[88,140]	6.4	0.45
Cow[160]	5.2	0.57
Horse[161]	6.8	0.69
Human[88,93,138]	5.0	0.80

(i.e., for synthesis or transformation into other substrates). In fetal sheep, substrate-oxygen quotients measured under steady-state conditions include glucose, 0.5; total amino acids, 0.25; and lactate, 0.25, with negligible fatty acid uptake.[14] In other species, including humans, estimates vary from 0.5 to 0.8 (Table 37.3) for glucose-oxygen quotients.

Although useful conceptually and in situations in which steady-state umbilical blood flow is difficult or impossible to determine, substrate-oxygen quotients that have been measured have had limited usefulness. Major limitations to their interpretation include (1) the inability to trace metabolic pathways of degradation or transformation and (2) the necessity for conditions of steady state (i.e., no change in metabolic rate or blood flow) to be fulfilled to determine venoarterial differences accurately. The latter has been particularly problematic in estimating quotients for human fetuses when mothers were in labor or at time of caesarian section, particularly if mothers were receiving intravenous dextrose, the usual circumstances under which such measurements have been reported.[28]

RESPIRATORY QUOTIENT

In the adult mammal, the ratio between generated carbon dioxide and consumed oxygen, the RQ, may provide some indirect information regarding the relative oxidation rates of carbohydrates, fats, and proteins. For example, the RQs of adult subjects oxidizing either carbohydrates or fat are 1.0 or 0.7, respectively, with those who are on a mixed diet having an RQ of 0.85. In the resting state, the RQ of the fetal lamb is approximately 0.94, suggesting little fetal oxidation of fat. The inequality between carbon uptake and excretion across the umbilical circulation invalidates this method as providing a sensitive measure of differential substrate utilization by the rapidly growing fetus.

SUBSTRATE UTILIZATION

Use of radioactive and nonradioactive isotope methodology[84] has provided useful insights into fetal metabolic processes and added substantially to the body of knowledge obtained from interpreting substrate-oxygen quotients and substrate umbilical uptakes via the Fick method. Fetal infusion of ^{13}C- or ^{14}C-labeled substrates such as glucose or lactate[85] have been performed and the fluxes of both radioactive and nonradioactive substrates then measured across the umbilical circulation. In addition, the transformation into other metabolites or carbon dioxide can be quantified, and fetal glucose utilization (i.e., glucose used for oxidation and storage from exogenous and endogenous sources) can also be measured in the steady state. As discussed later, under nonstressed conditions in ruminants, uptake studies are either in agreement with (glucose) or underestimate (lactate, amino acids) actual fetal utilization. Limited data have also become available[86,87] in humans using stable isotopes, particularly related to fetal gluconeogenesis (see later).

GLUCOSE UPTAKE AND UTILIZATION

In most species studied, there is a significant relationship between maternal and fetal levels of glucose, the most abundant carbohydrate in fetal blood.[88] Other carbohydrates, such as fructose (ruminants) or galactose, are present in fetal blood but appear to play relatively minor roles in oxidative metabolism during fetal life. Because of estimates of fetal RQ approaching 1.0 as well as the relatively high concentrations of glucose in fetal blood, it was previously thought that a significant net fetal uptake of glucose occurred across the umbilical circulation. To test this hypothesis, a number of investigators measured glucose uptake in the fetus using classic Fick principle techniques (net umbilical uptake, Eq. 37.2) as well as radiolabeled glucose transfer (fetal uptake and utilization). In one comparison of the two methods, Hay and colleagues[88] reported essentially identical results—measured net umbilical uptake of glucose was similar to the rate of fetal glucose utilization in the sheep, and both were related to the maternal glucose concentration. These results in the sheep fetus imply negligible endogenous fetal glucose production in the resting nonstressed state (see later discussion).

As noted earlier, maternal to fetal transfer of glucose has been best studied (although not exclusively so) in ruminant species, in which determinants of transfer include (1) the maternal glucose concentration, (2) the maternal to fetal glucose gradient, (3) the fetal endocrine milieu (specifically fetal insulin, glucagon, cortisol and thyroxin secretion), and (4) the degree of placental metabolism of glucose. In several other species, including humans, these general determinants of glucose transfer also appear to be applicable. In humans, since the advent of percutaneous blood sampling (PUBS), fetomaternal substrate relationships have been examined more closely,[28,82] and such studies have documented that in both mid-gestation and late-gestation human pregnancies there is a high degree of correlation between maternal and fetal blood glucose concentrations under steady-state conditions. Assuming that in the steady state, fetal "consumption" is close to, or at least mirrors umbilical "uptake," it has been shown in humans, just as in the fatal sheep, that glucose uptake was also highly correlated with birth weight and placental weight, as well as with the maternofetal glucose gradient.[28,82] Marconi and associates[89] have also demonstrated in humans that the maternal to fetal glucose gradient increases with advancing gestational age in normal pregnancies (Fig. 37.5) and that this difference is more pronounced in growth-restricted fetuses. Using ^{13}C-labeled glucose injected before cesarean section or PUBS, or by other means, fetal glucose utilization has been estimated in humans.[90-92] Although the measured glucose disposal rate (i.e., the amount of glucose taken up by tissues for oxidation, storage, and other metabolic transformations) of the human conceptus necessarily included both the placenta and fetus, glucose disposal rate was related to the maternal plasma glucose concentration and increased with increasing conceptus mass. Studies in a variety of species, including humans, show that net umbilical glucose uptake near term is between 4 and 7 mg/kg/min (22 to 39 μmol/kg/min). This equates to approximately 6 to 10 g glucose/kg/day or approximately 32 kcal/kg/day in potential energy production. However, it is significantly less than the energy estimated to be required by the measured fetal $\dot{V}O_2$, which is approximately 55 kcal × kg/day. In fact, in estimates of umbilical glucose-oxygen quotients obtained in several ruminant species, the complete oxidation of glucose accounted for at best 50% of the fetal $\dot{V}O_2$ (i.e., umbilical glucose-oxygen ratio = 0.5; see Eq. 37.5). These estimates, as noted previously, represent only the maximum percentage of the fetal $\dot{V}O_2$ accounted for by complete oxidation of glucose, which therefore is an overestimate of the actual fraction if any significant glucose conversion or storage (such as transformation to glycogen, fatty acids, or triglycerides) occurs. Some studies in humans are available for comparison (see Table 37.3)[89,93] and are remarkably similar to data obtained in animals. Thus, although glucose represents a quantitatively significant source of fetal energy (fuel), it probably does not supply enough carbon to support the total oxidative demands

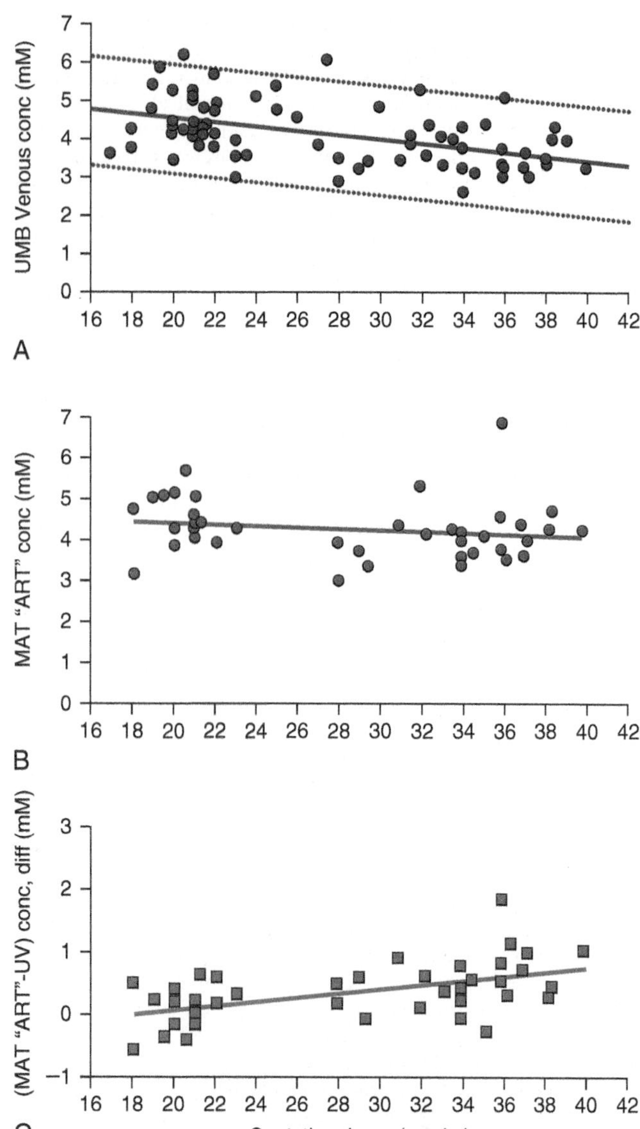

Fig. 37.5 Human maternal versus fetal blood glucose concentration changes during gestation. (A) Umbilical venous glucose versus gestational age in normal fetuses, (UV = 5.66 − 0.56 × GA). (B) Maternal arterial glucose versus gestational age. (C) Maternal-fetal glucose difference versus gestational age. (Data from Marconi AM, Paolini C, Buscaglia M, et al. The impact of gestational age and fetal growth on the maternal-fetal glucose concentration difference. *Obstet Gynecol.* 1996;87:937.)

of late fetal life, the remainder being met by lactate and amino acids.

Studies suggest that at least 80% of measured fetal glucose uptake can be accounted for by oxidation by brain and striated skeletal and, to a lesser extent, cardiac muscle. Parenthetically, the late gestation fetal heart appears to reduce glucose uptake considerably in favor of other substrates such as lactate. Increasing mitochondria number in humans also appears to set the stage for postnatal oxidation of fatty acids.[94] Although the fetal liver consumes and oxidizes glucose, net consumption as measured in the sheep is small,[95,96] with significant concomitant hepatic outputs of pyruvate, lactate, and glutamate.[97] For example, Thorngren-Jerneck and associates,[98] using PET scans, have determined that the global cerebral glucose metabolic rate (rate of intracellular cellular glucose phosphorylation) in near-term fetal lambs was 37.8 μmol/min/100 g. Calculation of the cerebral glucose/O_2 quotient from Table 37.3 and Eq. 37.5 yields a value of 1.1, similar to previous estimates measured more directly. Unfortunately, similar measurements of glucose uptake and oxidation are not available in other species. However, less-direct data in other animals[81,99] are in agreement with these estimates. In the human, demonstration of glucose uptake and utilization by fetal brain, liver, and placenta have also been documented. Direct measurements of overall glucose uptake and oxidation are necessarily limited in the human conceptus (fetus and placenta). However, in one study measuring maternal glucose disposal and extrapolating fetal and placental glucose utilization, the authors estimated similar values (5 mg/kg/min or 28 μmol/kg/min) to those in the term sheep.[92]

MATERNOFETAL GLUCOSE TRANSPORT

The molecular basis for understanding placental glucose transport has been expanded with the discovery of two families of specific membrane associated carrier proteins: the glucose transporter proteins (GLUTs), also known as *SCL2A proteins*, now labeled GLUT1 to 14, and sodium-dependent glucose transporter (SGLT) 1 and 2.[100,101] Specifically, the GLUT1 isoform, known also as the *brain erythrocyte glucose transporter*, is expressed on both the maternal and the fetal-facing sides[102] of human placentas. Although the density of transporters on the maternal side (microvillus membranes) remains constant after the first trimester, the concentration of transporters on the fetal-facing (basal) side increases at least two-fold after the first trimester. Furthermore, measured rates of placental glucose uptake in vitro match the density of placental GLUT1 transcripts. In addition, GLUT1 expression is inhibited by glucose but is not regulated by insulin.[79] Structural characteristics and specific molecular folding of GLUT1 and other GLUTs have been demonstrated that specifically allow for one-way transport.[101]

In both humans and sheep, it has been estimated that glucose transport capacity is considerably higher than necessary, given the normal range for maternal serum glucose concentrations. For example, in human fetuses at term, glucose uptake was 22% of umbilical delivery.[28] This suggests that changes in fetal and maternal glucose concentration or metabolism are the key factors in determining fetal glucose transport. Within certain tissues, GLUT expression is important for determining the overall contribution of glucose as a major substrate for the fetus. In addition, various factors including insulin and glucose concentrations may modify synthesis of these transport proteins. As an example, acute hyperinsulinemia or hyperglycemia in the sheep fetus leads to an increase in muscle GLUT-4 expression, with a commensurate increase in hindlimb glucose uptake.[103] However, chronic hyperglycemia in the sheep fetus promotes a state of relative insulin resistance, presumably due to a depression of muscle GLUT4.[79] The complex roles and interactions of other tissue-specific GLUTs in regulation of fetal glucose utilization and metabolic rate are not yet fully understood.

The placenta metabolizes glucose derived from both mother and fetus.[102] The rate of placental glucose consumption is not static and appears to be related to the fetal glucose concentration as studied in the fetal sheep and in human fetuses at term.[82] The placental contribution to total uterine glucose uptake is significant and approximates 50% of uterine glucose uptake when measured in the sheep.

In addition to concentration gradient, a number of studies have documented that the fetus is capable of exerting some hormonal control over glucose uptake, at least in the last trimester. Studies in sheep and humans[82,104] have shown that fine control of glucose uptake under steady-state conditions is also mediated by changes in the endogenous fetal insulin concentration. In addition, surgical or chemical ablation of fetal insulin release induces relative hyperglycemia and a decline in umbilical glucose uptake and fetal glucose utilization.[78,79] As noted earlier, Hay and colleagues[79] have shown conclusively that changes in circulating insulin concentration act as the principal regulator of glucose oxidation (vs. other potential substrates in the fetus) but that regulatory control is more related to the combined factors of glucose and insulin concentrations than either taken separately. Other potential glucose regulatory hormones, such as glucagon, cortisol, and thyroid hormones, also have been studied in the fetus. In the absence of maternal or fetal disease, such as starvation, hypoxia, or diabetes, changes in physiologic concentrations of these hormones in fetal blood do not seem to be major factors in regulating steady state fetal glucose uptake until late gestation. It is highly likely that they are important coregulators of glucose metabolism during parturition, particularly fetal cortisol,[17] and may also be very important in providing glucose homeostasis during times of stress.

GLUCOSE STORAGE

GLYCOGEN

In the fetus, as in the adult, the major storage form of glucose is glycogen, a glucose polymer stored intracellularly as a precipitate, with an average molecular weight of 500,000 daltons or greater. In fetal life, glycogen is stored in significant concentration in liver, skeletal and cardiac muscle, kidney, intestine, brain, and placenta. From the work of Shelley,[105] it is apparent that fetal glycogen storage in most species reaches a maximum concentration at term gestation in organs such as liver and skeletal muscle. In the sheep, fetal glycogen content near term is approximately 30 mg glucose/g liver or almost 3 g of glucose per whole liver.[106] The factors responsible for glycogen synthesis and induction of enzymes necessary for glycogen production are complex (Fig. 37.6) and are reviewed elsewhere.[107,108] However, delineation of the synthetic process is becoming better understood with the identification of several structural proteins needed for actual building of the molecule, including the primer protein, glycogenin, and other associated glycogen-related proteins, laforin and malin.[108] Developmental changes in the genes controlling these key proteins in the developing fetus have not yet been studied. The following generalizations may be made regarding fetal glycogen:

1. Activity of the major enzyme necessary for glycogen synthesis (glycogen synthase) correlates well with the relative presence or absence of glycogen in fetal tissues.
2. Fetal liver glycogen synthesis appears to be regulated predominantly by endogenous fetal insulin production, thyroid function, and intactness of the fetal pituitary-hypothalamic-adrenal axis.[17,78,109] Regarding proof for the latter assumption, an absence of hepatic glycogen accumulation has been observed in decapitated fetal rats or rabbits, with little effect on glycogen synthesis in other organs.[110]
3. Significant fetal glycogen turnover with active degradation probably occurs to a limited extent in the last trimester but with relative net accumulation in tissues such as liver.
4. Certain organs, such as the placenta, accumulate glycogen in response to maternal stimuli such as human placental lactogen or insulin with little response to changes in fetal hormonal levels.[111]

Maternal nutritional sufficiency and normoglycemia play major roles in late fetal glycogen deposition. For example, when studied in the goat or sheep, significant maternal malnutrition or stress caused a decrease in fetal hepatic glycogen.[112–115] Interestingly, leptin infusion in late gestation fetal sheep was shown to inhibit glycogen storage and enzymes of gluconeogenesis, suggesting an important role for leptin in control of fetal glucose homeostasis.[116] Maternal circadian rhythms may also play a role as changes in "clock gene" regulation have been shown to disturb hepatic glucoregulatory enzymes during pregnancy.[117]

Regarding other potential substrates for glycogen synthesis, in the sheep fetus[109] a significant portion of glycogen is synthesized not from glucose, but from precursors of gluconeogenesis, such as lactate and pyruvate, similar to what has been observed in adult humans. Another potential pathway for glycogen production via transformation of glycolytic intermediates through serine has been documented in fetal hepatocytes.[118] This pathway allows for bypass of the gluconeogenic step oxaloacetate to phosphoenolpyruvate (which is rate-limiting because of the developmental lag in fetal gluconeogenic enzyme synthesis). It has been estimated that this alternative serine pathway may account for up to 25% of synthesized glycogen. In addition, serine and glycine are known to cycle between fetal liver and placenta,[83] providing yet another convenient source of precursor for fetal glycogen deposition.

Glycogenolysis with resultant availability of glucose for use as a fuel substrate is an obvious important factor contributing to glucose homeostasis during the perinatal period. Regulation of activity of the enzyme involved (glycogen phosphorylase) is reciprocal to that of synthase. Thus, when one is stimulated (as when phosphorylase expression is stimulated by catecholamines or glucagon), the other (synthase) is inhibited. In fetal tissues such as liver and kidney, glycogen breakdown may be induced by such hormones as catecholamines or glucagon or by stimuli such as cold stress or hypoxia. In these tissues the presence of glucose-6-phosphatase allows for glucose dephosphorylation, net glucose exit from intracellular stores, and thus free glucose release into peripheral circulation for use at sites (e.g., brain) distant from the original storage tissue. Glucose-6-phosphatase has recently been found to be present in placental tissue, but its functional significance is not known.[83,119] In other organs such as fetal lung and myocardium, phosphorylase, but not glucose-6-phosphatase, is present, and stored glycogen is available only for intracellular consumption within the storage site. However, central nervous system glycogen storage in fetal life is minimal.

In the late-gestation fetus it is possible to demonstrate glycogenolysis in response to pharmacologic doses of such secretagogues as glucagon.[120] However, in malnourished or hypoglycemic sheep, as in humans with intrauterine growth restriction, inconsistent evidence exists as to whether significant glucose production may occur from stored glycogen.[89,109,113] However, growth-restricted rat fetuses[121] have been shown to have markedly diminished glycogen synthesis because of deficiencies in pyruvate oxidation and mitochondrial ATP generation.

MATERNAL DISORDERS: FETAL EFFECTS

In common clinical situations that affect the maternal milieu, fetal metabolic changes often occur as well. Effects of three of the most common are included in the following discussion: (1) fetal hypoxemia induced by maternal hemorrhage and/or by maternal hypoxemia, (2) fetal hyperglycemia as a consequence of maternal diabetes, and (3) fetal hypoglycemia due to maternal malnutrition or insulin therapy. The majority of information available was derived from studies performed in animals under steady-state conditions, although some human data are also available. Such studies, in addition to clinical observations, have allowed for some insight into adaptive mechanisms by which the fetus may protect against potential injury by altering metabolic rate.

FETAL HYPOXEMIA

A variety of adverse events may lead to a fall in umbilical venous oxygen content. The predominant factors responsible

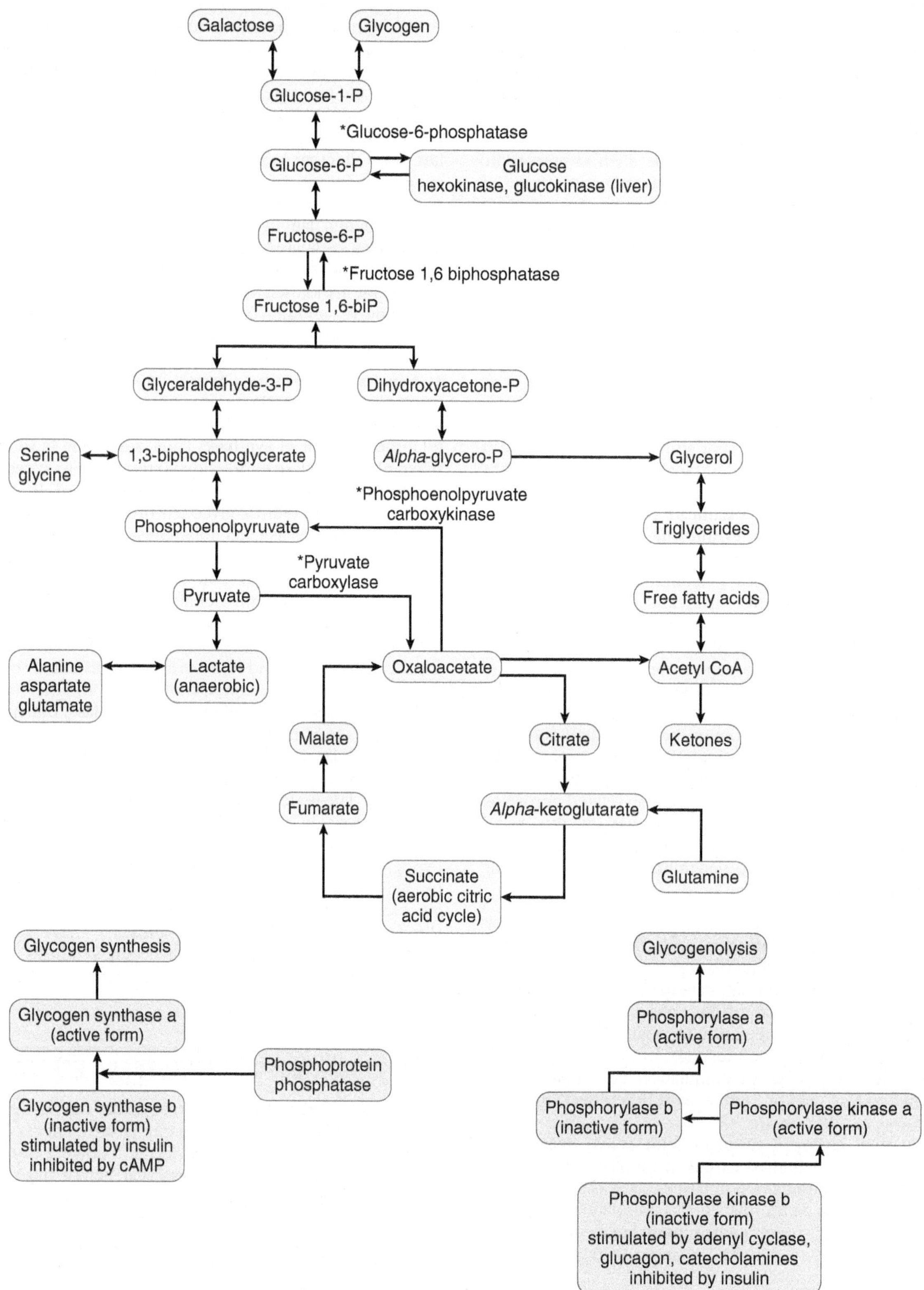

Fig. 37.6 Metabolic pathways involving fetal metabolic substrates. Key gluconeogenic enzymes *(*)* include (1) glucose-6-phosphatase, (2) fructose-1,6-biphosphatase, (3) phosphoenolpyruvate carboxykinase, and (4) pyruvate carboxylase*(top)* and the metabolic pathways involved in glycogen synthesis and degradation *(bottom)*. (Redrawn after Pagliara AS, Karl IE, Haymond M, et al. Hypoglycemia in infancy and childhood. I. *J Pediatr.* 1973;82:365; Milner RDG. In: Beard RW, Nathanielsz PW, eds. *Fetal Physiology and Medicine.* New York: Marcel Dekker; 1984. Reprinted courtesy Marcel Dekker, Inc. and Harris RA. Carbohydrate metabolism I: major metabolic pathways and their control. In: Devlin TM, ed. *Textbook of Biochemistry*. 6th ed. Hoboken, NJ: Wiley-Liss; 2006.)

Box 37.2 Fetal Response to Hypoxemia or Ischemia

Redistribution of blood flow
To: Brain
Myocardium
Adrenal
From: Gastrointestinal tract
Skin
Muscle
Increased umbilical O_2 extraction
Decreased fetal movement
Selective decrease in $\dot{V}O_2$ (muscle)
Bradycardia
Selective shift toward increased anaerobic glycolysis

for oxygen transport across the placenta include uterine and umbilical blood flow, the maternal-fetal oxygen tension difference, and differences in hemoglobin affinities for oxygen between the circulations and their hemoglobin concentrations.[12] Thus clinically relevant abnormalities that could affect fetal oxygenation include (1) abnormal uterine or placental blood flow, as may occur in hypertensive diseases of pregnancy, abruptio placentae, cord occlusion, or after nicotine or cocaine use; (2) maternal hypoxemia as a result of maternal pulmonary or cardiac disease, seizures secondary to eclampsia, anemia, or living at high altitude; and (3) fetal disorders such as sepsis, hemorrhage, anemia, or heart block and certain other tachyarrhythmias or bradyarrhythmias.

Acute fetal hypoxemia is known to produce a variety of circulatory adaptations that may improve the chances for fetal survival (Box 37.2).[11,29,49,122] These fetal responses include the development of reflex bradycardia, hypertension, redistribution of blood flow (toward central nervous system, myocardium, and adrenals and away from intestine and muscle), depression of fetal breathing and skeletal muscle activity, and increase in fetal oxygen extraction from umbilical blood. Some of these processes are mediated by endothelial NO[46,123] and may be even noted in relatively immature fetuses.[124] In addition, researchers[125] have demonstrated that in fetal sheep, hemoglobin concentration rises rapidly by as much as 10% to 15% during controlled cord occlusion. This increase could not be explained on the basis of newly generated red cells or splenic sequestration. Such an increase could work to ameliorate the concomitant reduction in transplacental oxygen transport. Fetal hypoxemia also induces changes in fetal metabolic processes, particularly if it is acute. Theoretically, depression of oxygen delivery to respiring tissues increases the ADP-ATP ratio, stimulating glycolysis (the Pasteur effect), with subsequent increase in anaerobic ATP production. Thus acute hypoxia would be expected to produce relatively high rates of glucose uptake and lactic acid production in most fetal tissues. If hypoxia is severe, both hypoglycemia and metabolic acidosis with ultimate tissue necrosis result. However, several factors appear to lessen the effect of hypoxemia on fetal metabolic processes. When oxygen transport is limited experimentally in the sheep fetus, by partial occlusion of uterine blood flow[126] or by mild maternal hypoxemia,[127] redistribution of blood flow occurs, but little change in fetal $\dot{V}O_2$ is noted. However, in sheep fetuses exposed to more severe hypoxemia, fetal oxygen consumption declined by 25% to 40%.[49,125,126] Because, as mentioned earlier, the metabolic rate of fetal muscle is related to the ambient oxygen tension, it is not surprising that carcass $\dot{V}O_2$ declines more than that of the whole fetus and that fetal growth restriction is a frequent result.[128] It is likely that the decline in overall fetal oxygen consumption is due to depressed metabolism in other nonessential organs as well, such as fetal intestine, liver, and kidney, and that decreased metabolic work of skeletal muscle (decreased activity) and myocardium (bradycardia)[49,125] also plays a role. Interestingly, in one recent study, depressed nutrient transport to the fetus due to maternal hypoxia was gender specific.[129]

Chronic fetal hypoxemia, as demonstrated in both simulated and true high-altitude animal experiments, induces an acclimatization, with increases in fetal erythropoiesis, cerebral blood flow, and oxygen extraction, at the expense of a significant decrease in blood flow to carcass and other organs, a decrease in fetal growth rate,[36] and a modest fall in cerebral metabolic rate at very low oxygen tensions.[41,43,126] The acclimatization of fetal cerebral arteriolar structure and changes in sensitivity[130] to adrenergic agents both allow for stable cerebral oxygen delivery. The aforementioned responses of the fetus to a superimposed potentially hypoxic environment are in contrast to those of animals apparently genetically adapted to living at high altitude,[40] where hypoxic stimuli superimposed on high altitude do produce more significant changes in fetal cerebral $\dot{V}O_2$. In both human and animal studies at high altitiude,[44,131] significant metabolic changes in both fetus and placenta appear to occur. Best studied in a species adapted to high altitude for centuries (llama), these differences include decreases in placental and fetal glucose uptake, relative down-regulation of oxidative metabolism with a greater emphasis on anaerobic glycolysis and inhibition of mitochondrial $\dot{V}O_2$. All of these are suggested to be part of long-term metabolic reprograming of the fetoplacental unit. Lastly, such studies have also shown that newborn llamas from these high-altitude pregnancies have an inherent protection against pulmonary hypertension that is modulated by NO-induced vasodilatation[132] as well as an increase in pulmonary-generated carbon monoxide. It has also been hypothesized that the elevation of circulating Epo levels due to relative hypoxemia may not only stimulate erythropoiesis, but also have tissue protective effects.[133]

Unlike the studies performed at high altitude, at sea level, fetal cerebrum and myocardium appear relatively protected from generalized acute fetal hypoxemia because of the increase in blood flow to these organs, probably induced by catecholamine secretion as outlined earlier. In studies of hypoxemia in fetal guinea pigs[134] and sheep,[135] relatively small changes in cerebral $\dot{V}O_2$ occur (at the expense of other organs). An increased rate of anaerobic glycolysis can also be demonstrated, allowing for the ongoing production of high-energy phosphates such as ATP. It has also been suggested that elevated levels of adenosine 5-monophosphate (AMP) (the precursor for adenosine) constitute an important regulator of blood flow in brain and heart (i.e., that increased levels of AMP and ADP result in increased local concentrations of adenosine, a potent vasodilator). Several investigators have documented a greater dependence of fetal compared with adult myocardium on energy supplied via glycolysis.[20] Another factor that provides protection against the effects of hypoxia is an increased fetal availability of glucose, particularly during late gestation. Hypoxia and concomitant secretion of catecholamines and cortisol are major stimuli for glycogenolysis. In fetal lambs and monkeys at term, hypoxia causes a fall in hepatic glycogen content and concomitant rise in blood glucose concentration.[105] In fetal lambs exposed to severe hypoxemia, the net fetal glucose uptake doubles within 30 minutes, as hepatic glucose output rises to equal umbilical glucose uptake, and suggests active fetal glycogenolysis. However, in more chronic states of hypoxemia, replenishment of glycogen stores appears unlikely. For example, in the rat fetus exposed to maternal hypoxia, fetal hepatic glycogen synthase mRNA levels fall to approximately 60% of control with a concomitant 50% fall in hepatic glycogen content.[136] Using adult rat hepatocytes raised in tissue culture, studies have demonstrated a link between gene expression of key glucogenic enzymes, such as phosphoenolpyruvate carboxykinase (PEPCK), and specific nuclear-modifying transcription factors, such as HREs and normoxia regulatory elements (NREs).[53,56,137] For example, the gene regulating PEPCK has been shown to contain an oxygen-sensing element that modulates action of glucagon in stimulation of gluconeogenesis.Although not yet proven, it is likely that HREs and other transcription factors play significant roles in modulating fetal responses to stress, possibly also affecting those responses noted earlier due to high altitude fetal hypoxemia.[47,50,138]

Lastly, in states of chronic maternal hypoxemia, such as may occur in a variety of clinical situations such as at high altitude, fetal growth restriction is not uncommon.[138] Depression of potent fetal growth factors such as insulin-like growth factor-1 during hypoxic states may have an important protective effect by conserving fetal substrate for energy as opposed to accretion needs.

MATERNAL HYPERGLYCEMIA

Diabetes in pregnancy is associated with a number of placental, fetal, and neonatal abnormalities, some structural and some metabolic. The development of fetal hyperglycemia as a result of excessive maternal-fetal glucose transfer has been well documented in a number of species, including the human, and appears to be the major but not sole factor in the development of such neonatal complications as macrosomia, hyperinsulinemia, and postnatal hypoglycemia.[139] Evidence in sheep[79,140] and monkeys[141] suggests that fetal hyperglycemia or hyperinsulinemia may accelerate fetal metabolism. Resultant fetal hyperinsulinemia has also been hypothesized to accelerate maternal-fetal glucose transfer by widening the glucose gradient between these compartments.[142] As noted earlier in the fetal sheep, changes in the circulating concentrations of glucose and insulin appear to have independent stimulatory effects on fetal $\dot{V}O_2$ and glucose oxidation.[79] In relatively short-term studies, direct fetal glucose infusion over 3 to 4 days caused increases in fetal insulin concentrations, fetal glucose and lactate uptake, placental lactate production and a 20% to 30% increase in fetal $\dot{V}O_2$, all suggestive of a significant increase in fetal metabolic rate.[140,143] These findings are all consistent with possible glucose-induced hypoxia. However, in other work by Hay and coworkers,[79,143] prolonged maternal glucose infusions (2 to 5 weeks) that were performed in sheep induced similar levels of fetal glycemia to those of the more acute studies. These investigators observed lower fetal plasma insulin concentrations during the study but no significant changes in fetal $\dot{V}O_2$, despite large increases in glucose uptake and uteroplacental lactate production. In another study, also in fetal sheep, pulsatile maternal glucose infusions produced significant fetal glucose-stimulated hyperinsulinemia, as well as elevated lactate levels, but no consistent changes in fetal oxygenation.[144]

The differences in fetal metabolic responses between the acute and more chronic studies are not clearly understood. Blunting of fetal insulin response to more prolonged glycemia may be due to an increase in fetal adrenergic activity[145] or to the difference between glucose infusions given directly to the mother or fetus. One other conclusion would be that intermittent, repetitive glycemic (or pulsatile) insults to the late gestation fetus, such as may occur during human diabetic pregnancy, might be more injurious than chronic sustained hyperglycemia.

In humans, fetuses and infants of diabetic mothers have been thought to exhibit signs of in utero oxygen deprivation, such as late fetal demise, increased hematopoiesis occasionally leading to polycythemia, and neonatal hyperbilirubinemia. In addition, cord blood from infants of diabetic mothers[146] exhibit changes highly suggestive of in utero hypoxemia that mirror those seen in experimental models of fetal hyperglycemia. Lastly, newborns of diabetic women have been shown to have increased evidence of oxidative stress in cord blood.[147] However, conclusive proof of a link between maternal and fetal hyperglycemia and in utero oxygen deficiency remains speculative. It is presumed that the increase in fetal fuel needs for sustaining the increased $\dot{V}O_2$ are met by increased uptake of glucose, placentally derived lactate, and perhaps amino acids and ketones.

Factors responsible for the increase in fetal metabolic rate noted in some studies are unclear, although as mentioned, both glucose and insulin appear to be codependent factors.[79] Fetal hyperglycemia is known to increase the rate of fetal breathing movements in sheep and humans,[74] which might serve to increase muscular work and thus increase the $\dot{V}O_2$. In addition, specific organ responses to accelerated substrate influx or hyperinsulinemia, particularly in liver and brain, may play important roles. For example, fetal glucose infusion in the sheep may accelerate cerebral $\dot{V}O_2$ by as much as 70%; with a concomitant increase in cerebral blood flow and glucose entry and changes in fetal electrocortical activity.[148] Fetal catecholamine secretion[145] is likely to be responsible for at least some of these changes.

MATERNAL HYPOGLYCEMIA

Because the major factor responsible for placental glucose transport to the fetus is the maternal-fetal glucose concentration gradient,[102] it follows that falling maternal blood glucose levels should ultimately depress fetal glucose uptake. Clinical maternal hypoglycemia, of course, may occur as a result of a number of clinically relevant problems, including acute or chronic malnutrition, poor placental transfer, or due to certain drugs, such as after insulin or insulin mimetic therapies for maternal diabetes. Fetal defenses against such changes in circulating glucose concentrations have been best studied in animal models, although limited information is also available in humans.

In the sheep, maternal hypoglycemia induced by fasting is associated with a fall in fetal plasma glucose concentration and in depression of both umbilical glucose uptake and fetal glucose utilization.[84] Similar findings have also been shown in other animals such as the rat.[149] Chronic fetal hypoglycemia induced by infusing pregnant sheep with insulin or by making the fetus anemic[106] is associated with fetal endogenous glucose production, fetal stunting, marked increases in fetal expression of key hepatic enzymes of gluconeogenesis, depression of fetal insulin secretion, and elevation of key counter-regulatory hormones (cortisol, glucagon).[84,106,113] In addition, fetal hypoglycemia induced by experimental maternal hypoglycemia also induces chronic changes in fetal pancreatic and β cell mass not improved by fetal insulin infusion.[150] In human fetal growth restriction presumably due to maternal hypertension and/or placental dysfunction,[16,28] depressed glucose uptake, and delivery were also observed.

Because fetal $\dot{V}O_2$ does not change during experimental hypoglycemia induced by maternal fasting or maternal insulin infusion,[97] it is likely that other fuel sources, particularly amino acids and endogenously produced glucose and lactate, are used instead. For example, myocardial lactate uptake alone in the fetus may account for the majority of oxygen consumption in this organ,[151] even in steady state. Fetal muscle and brain also have the capacity to use ketones.[152] In addition, endogenous glucose production has been demonstrated in hypoglycemic fetal sheep, probably secondary to hepatic glycogenolysis and gluconeogenesis[113] under such circumstances. During hypoglycemia of short duration, intracellular stores of glycogen, particularly in myocardium, liver, and kidney, clearly offer an available source of glucose for cellular metabolic processes. However, more prolonged chronic hypoglycemia caused by malnutrition may deplete cellular stores of glycogen in a variety of organs, particularly the brain, liver, and heart.[112] Although not completely analogous, in studies of human fetal growth restriction, depression in both fetal O_2 uptake and consumption have been shown.[28]

Lastly, expression of GLUTs[132] (see Maternofetal Glucose Transport) such as GLUT1 in placenta and GLUT4 in muscle may also up-regulate in response to changes in circulating glucose (and insulin) concentration and act to increase the cellular uptake of glucose during relative glucose deprivation.

During induction of maternal hypoglycemia, evidence also suggests that other fetal counter-regulatory mechanisms may blunt the fall in fetal blood glucose. For example, as noted previously, in sheep fetuses whose mothers were made hypoglycemic either by fasting[104] or by insulin infusion,[153] endogenous fetal insulin levels fell significantly. In the latter case, chronic fetal hypoglycemia appears also to render the fetus less sensitive to later challenges of glucose or arginine, suggesting a state of insulin resistance. In the fetal rat exposed to insulin-induced maternal hypoglycemia, catecholamine levels rise rapidly[154] and may be elevated in some newborn humans with hypoglycemia. These effects act to stimulate both fetal glycogenolysis and gluconeogenesis. The role that other potential glucose regulatory hormones, such as glucagon, growth hormone, or cortisol, play in defense against fetal hypoglycemia is not known but seems more limited in scope. The use of some corticosteroids during pregnancy has been associated with significant neonatal (and possibly fetal) hypoglycemia as a result of fetal adrenal suppression.[155,156]

The effect of fetal hypoglycemia on fetal organ metabolism, particularly fetal cerebral metabolism, has not been studied in great depth. As the principal cerebral substrate, glucose is of major importance in maintaining neuronal and white matter integrity. Postnatal hypoglycemic brain damage and resultant neuronal and white matter necrosis have been well documented. Theoretically, similar damage should result from sustained fetal hypoglycemia as well. However, in sheep, modest hypoglycemia of 2 to 4 hours duration produces no changes in fetal cerebral metabolic rate or in cerebral glucose uptake.[157] Lactate, fatty acids, and ketone bodies are probably used as alternate substrates for fetal cerebral oxidative needs during such times.[158]

CONCLUSION

Regulation of fetal metabolic rate and the factors that influence it in times of stress are the topics of this chapter. Included are basic concepts of how metabolic studies are performed (and interpreted) in the fetus, with examples and a summary of information derived from data of both individual organs and the whole fetus. Relevant information from studies in a variety of mammals, including humans, has been presented, although both species differences and different experimental designs provide only generalizations of cause and effect in some cases. The chapter also includes a brief review of general carbohydrate metabolism with reference to the fetus and also several clinically relevant disorders that may affect maternal and fetal metabolism. The basic theme of this chapter is that the fetus in late gestation is able to partition and control energy needs under most circumstances through a variety of interconnected means to maintain homeostasis when the maternal milieu is altered.

A complete reference list is available at www.ExpertConsult.com.

SELECT REFERENCES

1. Taylor NAS, et al. Foundational insights into the estimation of whole-body metabolic rate. *Eur J Appl Physiol*. 2018;118:867-874.
2. Bell MS. *Lavoisier in the Year One*. New York: WW Norton; 2005.
3. Hulbert AJ, Else PL. Mechanisms underlying the cost of living in animals. *Ann Rev Physiol*. 2000;62:207-235.
7. Meschia G. Evolution of thinking in fetal respiratory physiology. *Am J Obstet Gynecol*. 1978;132:806.
9. Malte H, Lykkeboe G. The Bohr-Haldane effect: a model-based uncovering of the full extent of its impact on O_2 delivery to and CO_2 removal from tissues. *J Appl Physiol*. 2018;125:916-922.
10. Zhang Y, et al. Contribution of cooperativity and the Bohr effect to efficient oxygen transport by hemoglobin from five mammalian species. *Zoolog Sci*. 2006;23:49-55.
11. Carter AM. Placental gas exchange and the oxygen supply to the fetus. *Compr Physiol*. 2015;5:1381-1403.
14. Battaglia FC, Meschia G. *An Introduction to Fetal Physiology*. New York: Academic Press; 1986.
22. Luo, et al. *In vivo* quantification of placental insufficiency by BOLD MRI: a human study. *Sci Rep*. 2017;7:3713.
24. Battaglia FC, Meschia G. Review of studies in human pregnancy of uterine and umbilical blood flows. *Dev Period Med*. 2013;17:287-292.
26. Raedelli T, et al. Estimation of fetal oxygen uptake in human term pregnancies. *J Matern Fetal Neonatal Med*. 2012;25:174-179.
28. Cetin I, Taricco E, Mando C, et al. Fetal oxygen and glucose consumption in human pregnancy complicated by fetal growth restriction. *Hypertension*. 2020;75:748-754.
29. Zhu MY, et al. The hemodynamics of late-onset intrauterine growth restriction by MRI. *Am J Obstet Gynecol*. 2016;214:367.e1-17.
30. Kleiber G. *The Fire of Life: An Introduction to Animal Energetics*. Huntington, NY: RE Krieger; 1975.
31. West GB, Brown JH. The origin of allometric scaling laws in biology from genomes to ecosystems: towards a quantitative unifying theory of biological structure and organization. *J Exp Biol*. 2005;208:1575-1592.
32. White CR, et al. The origin and maintenance of metabolic allometry in animals. *Nat EcolEvol*. 2019;3:598-603.
35. Singer D, Mühlfeld C. Perinatal adaptation in mammals: the impact of metabolic rate. *Comp Biochem Physiol*. 2007;148:780-784.
36. Schneider H. Oxygenation of the placental-fetal unit in humans. *Respir Physiol Neurobiol*. 2011;178:51-58.
46. Liu T, et al. The role of gasotransmitters in neonatal physiology. *Nitric Oxide*. 2020;95:29-44.
47. Storz JF. Genes for high altitudes. *Science*. 2010;329:40-41.
48. Moore LG. Measuring high-altitude adaptation. *J Appl Physiol*. 2017;123:1371-1385.
52. Wood CE, et al. Transcriptomics modeling of the late-gestation fetal pituitary response to transient hypoxia. *PloS One*. 2016;11(2):1-16.
53. Semenza GL. Pharmacological targeting of hypoxia-inducible factors. *Annu Rev Pharmacol Toxicol*. 2019;59:379-403.
60. Koos BJ. Adenosine A_{2a} receptors and O_2 sensing in development. *Am J Physiol Regul Integr Comp Physiol*. 2011;301:R601-R622.
64. Pederson SF, Counillon L. The SLC9A-C mammalian Na^+/H^+ exchanger family: molecules, mechanisms and physiology. *Physiol Rev*. 2019;99:2015-2113.
66. Else PL. Oxygen consumption and sodium pump thermogenesis in a developing mammal. *Am J Physiol Regul Integr Comp Physiol*. 1991;261:1575-1578.
70. Rurak DW, Gruber NC. The effect of neuromuscular blockade on oxygen consumption and blood gases in the fetal lamb. *Am J Obstet Gynecol*. 1983;145:258-262.
76. Forhead AJ, Fowden AL. Thyroid hormones in fetal growth and prepartum maturation. *J Endocrinol*. 2014;221:87-103.
78. Fowden AL, Forhead AJ. Insulin deficiency alters the metabolic and endocrine responses to undernutrition in fetal sheep near term. *Endocrinology*. 2012;153:4008-4018.
79. Hay WW. Recent observations on the regulation of fetal metabolism by glucose. *J Physiol*. 2006;572:17-24.
82. Michelson TM, et al. Uteroplacental glucose uptake and fetal glucose consumption: a quantitative study in human pregnancies. *J Clin Endocrinol Metab*. 2019;104:873-882.
85. DiGiacomo JE, Hay WW. Fetal glucose and oxygen consumption during sustained hypoglycemia. *Metabolism*. 1990;39:193-202.
88. Hay Jr WW, et al. Fetal glucose uptake and utilization as functions of maternal glucose concentration. *Am J Physiol*. 1984;246:237-242.
89. Marconi AM, et al. The impact of gestational age and fetal growth on the maternal-fetal glucose concentration difference. *Obstet Gynecol*. 1996;87:937-942.
90. Tchirikov M, et al. Glucose uptake in the placenta, fetal brain, heart and liver related to blood flow redistribution during acute hypoxia. *J Obstet Gynaecol Res*. 2011;37:979-985.
97. Houin SS, et al. Coordinated changes in hepatic amino acid metabolism and endocrine signals support hepatic glucose production during fetal hypoglycemia. *Am J Physiol Endocrinol Metab*. 2015;308:E306-E314.
98. Thorngren-Jerneck K, et al. Reduced postnatal cerebral glucose metabolism measured by PET after asphyxia in near term fetal lambs. *J Neurosci Res*. 2001;66:844-850.
101. Yan N. A glimpse of membrane transport through structures-advances in the structural biology of the GLUT glucose transporters. *J Mol Biol*. 2017;429:2710-2725.
104. Philipps AF, et al. Insulin secretion in fetal and newborn sheep. *Am J Physiol*. 1978;235:467-474.
106. Culpepper C, et al. Chronic anemic hypoxemia increases plasma glucagon and hepatic PCK1 mRNA in late-gestation fetal sheep. *Am J Physiol Regul Integr Comp Physiol*. 2016;311:R200-R208.

109. Forhead AJ, et al. Developmental regulation of hepatic and renal gluconeogenic enzymes by thyroid hormones in fetal sheep during late gestation. *J Physiol*. 2006;548:941-947.
115. Zhou X, et al. Evidence for liver energy metabolism programming in offspring subjected to intrauterine undernutrition during midgestation. *Nutr Metab*. 2019;16:20.
128. Rozance PJ, et al. Skeletal muscle protein accretion rates and hindlimb growth are reduced in late gestation intrauterine growth-restricted fetal sheep. *J Physiol*. 2018;596:67-82.
129. Cuffe JSM, et al. Mid-to late term hypoxia in the mouse alters placental morphology, glucocorticoid regulatory pathways and nutrient transporters in a sex-specific manner. *J Physiol*. 2014;592:3127-3141.
132. Reyes RV, et al. The role of nitric oxide in the cardiopulmonary response to hypoxia in highland and lowland newborn llamas. *J Physiol*. 2018;596:5907-5923.
138. Illsley NP, et al. Placental metabolic reprogramming: do changes in the mix of energy-generating substrates modulate fetal growth? *Int J Dev Biol*. 2010;54:409-419.
140. Philipps AF, et al. Effects of chronic fetal hyperglycemia upon oxygen consumption in the ovine uterus and conceptus. *J Clin Invest*. 1984;74:279.
143. Hay Jr WW, et al. Effects of glucose and insulin on fetal glucose oxidation and oxygen consumption. *Am J Physiol*. 1989;256:704-713.
144. Carver TD, Anderson SM, Aldoretta PW, et al. Effect of low-level basal plus marked "pulsatile" hyperglycemia on insulin secretion in fetal sheep. *Am J Physiol*. 1996;271:E865-E871.
158. Lust WD, et al. Changing metabolic and energy profiles in fetal, neonatal, and adult rat brain. *Metab Brain Dis*. 2003;18:195-206.

38 Role of Glucoregulatory Hormones in Hepatic Glucose Metabolism During the Perinatal Period

Kathryn Beardsall | Amanda Ogilvy-Stuart | Myat Su Win

INTRODUCTION

After birth, the newborn must rapidly become capable of balancing glucose deficiency with glucose excess to maintain euglycemia.[1-3] Development of carbohydrate homeostasis is essential to avoid both hypoglycemia and hyperglycemia, to which neonates (especially the sick, preterm, and growth restricted) are vulnerable. Both hypoglycemia and hyperglycemia contribute to adverse outcomes in compromised neonates, infants, and older children.[4-10] Hypoglycemia or hyperglycemia may result from alterations in glucose production and utilization, disturbances in insulin secretion, or disruption of peripheral homeostatic mechanisms in tissues that are responsive to the effects of insulin, such as muscle and fat. This chapter describes the metabolic pathways in the perinatal period that maintain glucose homeostasis and the role of regulatory hormones, such as insulin, the insulin-like growth factor (IGF) axis, and the counter-regulatory hormones including catecholamines, corticosteroids, and glucagon.

PRENATAL GLUCOSE REGULATION

The growing and developing fetus has a high energy requirement, which is predominantly met by glucose oxidation. Glucose is also a precursor for other carbon-containing compounds, including protein and glycogen, and for fat synthesis.[11] Fetal glucose utilization rates average 5 mg/kg/min, nearly double the adult requirement of 2 to 3 mg/kg/min. The placenta and fetal liver are the principal organs that maintain supply and production to meet these high fetal requirements.[11,12] In healthy pregnancies, transplacental glucose transport from mother to fetus is well regulated, with a direct relationship between maternal and fetal glucose levels.[13] The fetus is not generally exposed to rapid fluctuations in glucose levels, with the placenta playing a key role in glucose delivery and buffering acute fluctuations in maternal glucose levels.

FETAL METABOLISM IN HEALTHY PREGNANCIES

During the first trimester, maternal insulin sensitivity is increased, which results in maternal fat deposition. This is reversed in later pregnancy, when increasing insulin resistance allows mobilization of these stores.[14,15] The gravid mother increases glucose production by 15% to 30% in late gestation to provide for the increasing needs of the growing fetus. Fetal glucose uptake from the placenta is equivalent to fetal glucose utilization, and fetal glucose levels are maintained at about 70% of maternal levels.[16] The fetal liver and kidneys do not normally produce glucose, but in adverse conditions such as placental insufficiency or maternal starvation the fetal liver and kidney adapt from their normal focus on the anabolic processes of glycogen and lipid storage with upregulation of enzymes for gluconeogenesis (GNG) (Fig. 38.1).[17] The fetus maintains oxidative phosphorylation in the face of a relatively low oxygen tension. Although energy is produced predominantly by aerobic metabolism, the fetus has the potential for a significant level of anaerobic metabolism and can use lactate efficiently.[18] Ketone bodies can be used as an alternative source of fuel by the fetus as well as providing precursors for glucose production (see Fig. 38.1).[14,17,19]

FETAL HORMONAL SECRETION

Glucocorticoids and insulin mediate the rate of glycogen accumulation in fetal life, with 40% of glucose taken up by the fetus being converted to glycogen or lipid. Insulin and glucagon are detected in most species early in gestation, with a high insulin to glucagon molar ratio in the fetus, promoting growth.[20] The pancreatic islet cells contain three cell types that support glucose regulation. β Cells, which make up 60% to 80% of the islets, can be detected from 14 weeks of gestation and secrete insulin from 18 weeks. Fetal insulin secretion increases during the last trimester of pregnancy in humans and is critical for normal fetal growth, with increased insulin concentrations leading to increased rates of protein synthesis and increased glucose uptake. Insulin has a positive correlation with plasma glucose and amino acid levels after 20 weeks of gestation. The high insulin to glucagon ratio appears to be important in maintaining glycogen synthesis while suppressing GNG during fetal life. The secretion of insulin and glucagon is regulated by ATP-sensitive potassium channels and voltage-gated calcium channels in the islet cells and is dependent on the blood glucose level. Glycogen is synthesized from the ninth week of gestation and stored in the liver, lung, heart, skeletal muscle, kidney, intestine, and brain. Glycogen synthesis increases with gestation and is activated by insulin and induced by glucocorticosteroid. The healthy term baby has two to three times the adult level of glycogen stores. α Cells make up 15% to 20% of the islet cells and secrete glucagon, which increases GNG.

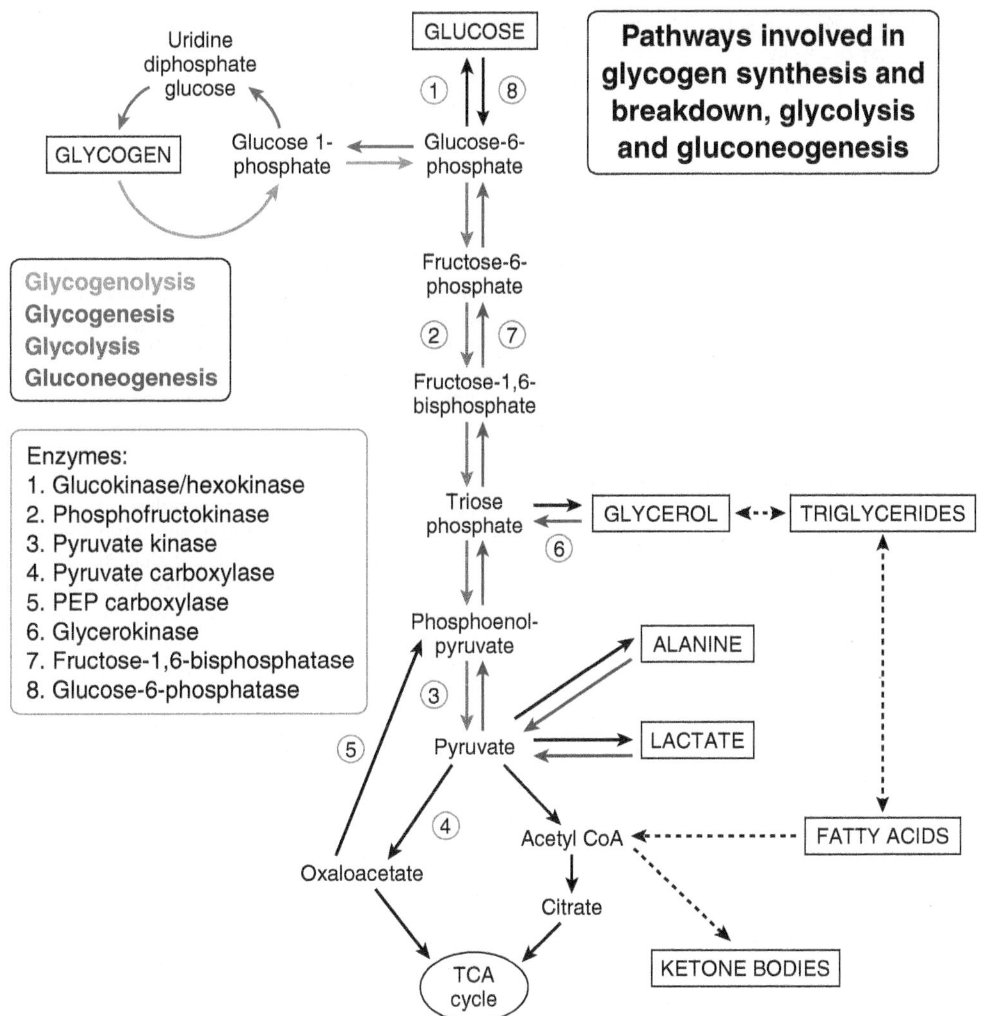

Fig. 38.1 Pathways in glucose metabolism. *PEP*, phosphoenolpyruvate; *TCA*, tricarboxylic acid cycle. (With permission from Ogilvy-Stuart A, Midgley P. Hypoglycemia. In: *Practical Neonatal Endocrinology*. Cambridge, UK: Cambridge University Press; 2006:15, Fig. 2.2.)

Glucagon can be detected in fetal plasma by 15 weeks' gestation and peaks at 24 to 26 weeks' gestation. The remaining delta cells (5% to 10%) release somatostatin and a small number of cells release incretins.

DISRUPTIONS TO FETAL PHYSIOLOGY

Acute changes in glucose levels that would lead to significant changes in either insulin or glucagon secretion in adults do not produce this effect in the fetus. However, chronic hyperglycemic exposure in pregnancies complicated by maternal diabetes increases fetal insulin secretion and β-cell hyperplasia. Chronic hyperglycemia then leads to increased fetal glycogen and fat deposition and fetal macrosomia. Furthermore, this chronic exposure to hyperglycemia throughout early pregnancy with β-cell hyperplasia has more impact on newborn glucose control than the acute effects of maternal glucose levels immediately before delivery.[21,22]

Insulin has indirect actions on growth through its regulation of IGF-1 and by increasing the cellular availability of glucose. Both IGF-1 and IGF-2 are the primary endocrine regulators of fetal growth as levels of both isoforms increase gradually until about 33 weeks of gestation and then increase two- to threefold until term.[23] IGFs have roles in cell proliferation, differentiation, and metabolism and are found in the circulation by 15 weeks' gestation, but activity is regulated by a family of binding proteins, which are developmentally and nutritionally regulated.[24,25]

In contrast, with reduced glucose delivery to the fetus, such as in pregnancies complicated by placental insufficiency, insulin levels are low and growth and fat deposition are reduced. Reduced plasma IGF-1 and IGF-2, a consequence of low insulin levels, play key roles in the regulation of fetoplacental growth, with cord blood insulin and C-peptide as well as IGF-1 levels correlating with size at birth. The fetal insulin to glucose ratio is lower in small for gestational age fetuses compared with those where growth is appropriate for gestational age.[26] Cord blood levels correlate with birth weight, and low levels of IGF-1 are found following fetal growth restriction.[24,25]

Polymorphic variation in the fetal genome, in particular in fetal growth and imprinted genes, can lead to maternal metabolic alterations.[27] Alterations in the imprinted H19 gene and IGF-2 control element leads to pups that are heavier than their unaffected litter mates,[28] with increased circulating glucose concentrations in late pregnancy in comparison with those of genetically matched controls.[29] Similarly, associations have been shown in humans between SNP alleles from 15 fetal imprinted genes and maternal glucose concentrations in late pregnancy.

NEONATAL TRANSITION

Increasing gestational age and the birth process itself have maturational effects on enzyme systems, glucose transporter levels, and hormone and hormone receptor levels. These effects, combined with substrate availability, clinical morbidities, and clinical interventions all impact on glucose levels during the transition to independent life. In the first 4 to 6 hours after birth glucose values fall and then stabilize at about 50 to 60 mg/dL (2.8 to 3.3 mmol/L) in healthy newborn babies. The fall in glucose

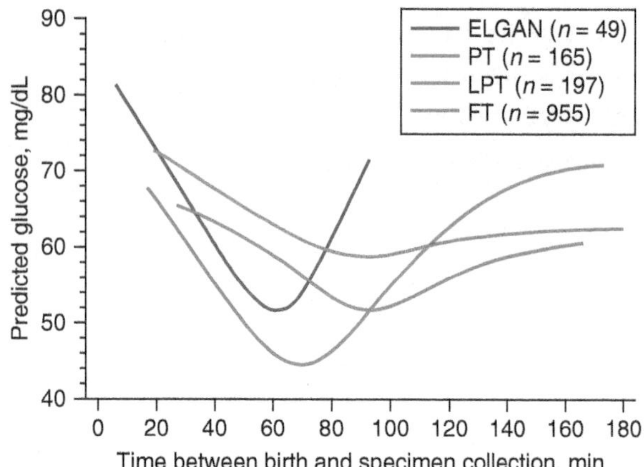

Fig. 38.2 Predicted pattern of glucose concentrations during the first 3 hours after birth by gestational age groups. *ELGAN*, Extremely low gestational age; *FT*, full term; *LPT*, late preterm; *PT*, preterm. (With permission from Kaiser JR, Bai S, Rozance PJ. Newborn plasma glucose concentration nadirs by gestational-age group. *Neonatology.* 2018;113:353–359.)

levels can be influenced by maternal glucose infusions during labor and is earlier and more pronounced in preterm and small for gestational age infants (Fig. 38.2).[30] By 2 to 3 days of age, plasma glucose levels average 70 to 80 mg/dL (3.9 to 4.4 mmol/L) in healthy term neonates.[31]

ENDOCRINE RESPONSE AT BIRTH

Gradually rising cortisol levels in the fetus in the last trimester lead to maturation of enzymes for GNG and increased pancreatic sensitivity to glucose. These changes are thought to prepare the fetus to be able to regulate glucose control after delivery. Clamping the umbilical cord interrupts the maternal glucose supply, and this, along with transient hypoxia and cold exposure, generates a stress response. This leads to increased plasma levels of catecholamines, glucagon, and cortisol and to suppression of plasma insulin levels resulting in a reduced insulin to glucagon ratio.

These changes led to an increase in phosphoenolpyruvate carboxykinase (PEPCK) and pyruvate carboxylase expression. The activity of the hepatic enzyme glucose 6-phosphatase (G6P), which catalyzes the last step of both GNG and glycogenolysis, rises rapidly to adult levels in the first week after birth. This is thought to be dependent on the postnatal drop in plasma glucose levels and the high glucagon to insulin ratio.[32] This promotes glycogenolysis, lipolysis, and GNG, which supply lactate moieties and ketones that are oxidized as alternative fuels in the early neonatal period. The elevated glucagon and noradrenaline levels activate adenylate cyclase, which causes an increase in intracellular cyclic adenosine monophosphate (cAMP) and promotes glycogenolysis, lipolysis, and GNG to maintain euglycemia postnatally. There is a decrease in glycogen synthetase activity and an increase in glycogen phosphorylase activity, which is mediated by enzyme phosphorylation and activated by cAMP. Glycogenolysis is critical in maintaining glucose levels; however, liver glycogen stores are rapidly diminished within 2 to 3 hours of birth, almost completely depleted by 12 hours and remain low for several days. Glucocorticoids also promote lipolysis and protein breakdown increasing the availability of gluconeogenic substrates for healthy term infants who mobilize free fatty acids and oxidize ketones to maintain their blood glucose levels.

GNG maintains glucose levels during this period and is dependent on the availability of gluconeogenic precursors, as well as activation of the enzymes for GNG. Hepatic glucagon receptors are upregulated and linked to cyclic 3,5 adenosine monophosphate protein kinase, and there is induction of the key enzymes for GNG, PEPCK, and G6P. The low blood glucose levels and increased cortisol levels at birth stimulate hepatic G6P activity. Hepatic G6P activity is low before birth but rises rapidly after birth in term infants, reaching adult levels by 3 days of age. In addition, the reduced insulin levels result in the reversal of the insulin to glucagon ratio, which induces PEPCK (the rate-limiting enzyme in GNG). The concentration of PEPCK continues to increase during the first week after delivery irrespective of gestational age. Together these adaptations lead to increased hepatic glucose release from GNG, maintaining glucose supplies to vital organs. Mobilization of muscle stores of glycogen is a much longer process, and those stores can only be used by the muscles themselves. Lactate formed by glycolysis can leave the muscle and be converted into glucose in the liver or oxidized by other tissues. Animal studies have demonstrated that stimulation of the vagus nerve increases activation of hepatic glycogen synthetase, whereas stimulation of the splanchnic nerve induces glycogen phosphorylase and increases glycogenolysis.

Kinetic studies of glucose production and the plasma concentrations of insulin and glucagon suggest that the insulin to glucagon ratio may be more important than the absolute concentration of insulin in controlling glucose metabolism in the newborn.[33] In a small study of 4 neonates with severe hypoglycemia, hepatic glucose production rates were low (less than 20% of normal), and plasma insulin concentration was greater than 12 µU/mL, with half of the neonates having a low plasma glucagon concentration. However, glucagon infusion restored the glucose production rate toward normal, and in one neonate diazoxide further depressed plasma insulin concentration from 4.2 to 1.6 µU/mL.

Studies comparing the impact of vaginal delivery with elective cesarean section on immediate postnatal adaptation have demonstrated that neonates delivered vaginally exhibit higher catecholamine and glucose concentrations at birth than those delivered by Cesarean section.[34] Despite the marked differences in catecholamine concentrations, there were relatively small differences in glucose levels, leading to the speculation that the metabolic response to sympathoadrenal stimulation is attenuated at birth. The relationship between thyroid status at birth and the endocrine response to insulin-induced hypoglycemia has been studied in a neonatal rat model.[35] This demonstrated that in the euthyroid rat, insulin-induced epinephrine secretion increased during the first 10 days of postnatal life. In contrast, hypothyroidism slowed the development of this response and hyperthyroidism accelerated the response. After insulin-induced hypoglycemia, recovery was slower for the hyperthyroid animal than for the hypothyroid or euthyroid animal.

POSTNATAL METABOLISM

Postnatally, the newborn has to adapt to be able to maintain independent glucose homeostasis after feeding and when fasting. Because of the relatively large brain to body weight ratio (13% in the newborn compared with 2% in the adult), newborn glucose requirements are high, as the brain is primarily dependent on glucose as its energy source. Steady-state glucose utilization in the term newborn is two- to threefold higher than in the adult (relative to body weight) at 4 to 6 mg/kg/min. Preterm and growth-restricted babies have even higher glucose requirements (6 to 8 mg/kg/min). Hypoxia, hyperinsulinism, respiratory distress, and cold stress all increase glucose utilization.[36,37]

In the healthy term newborn, blood glucose levels vary greatly compared with the tight glycemic control in healthy adults. There remains significant controversy as to the definitions and clinical significance of glucose levels that may be referred to as hypoglycemia. This is in part because in newborns the clinical signs of hypoglycemia are nonspecific and difficult to identify. The use of continuous glucose monitoring has helped to better characterize the pattern of glucose control in this period.[38,39] Furthermore, low glucose levels may play a role in the induction of enzymes involved in GNG. On the basis of historical neurophysiologic and neurodevelopmental outcome studies, hypoglycemia in the newborn is usually defined as less than 46 mg/dL (<2.6 mmol/L), although this threshold remains controversial and some have suggested a lower "operational" threshold.[40-42] The neonatal brain is able to use alternative fuels, such as ketones and lactate, and is therefore thought to be resistant to relatively low glucose levels that could be harmful. Ketone levels are high in the perinatal period related to increased hepatic ketogenesis and rate of turnover (12 to 22 μmol/min).[43,44] However, in many babies such as the preterm and growth restricted, there is limited availability of substrates or altered metabolism and inability to produce these alternative fuels. This has the potential to put these babies at risk of long-term neurodevelopmental impairment.[45]

The definition of hyperglycemia in the newborn is also controversial. In utero and in healthy term infants, blood glucose levels are rarely greater than 126 mg/dL (>7 mmol/L). In contrast, preterm infants commonly have high blood glucose levels that are a result of both prematurity and the response to critical illness.[46] Persistent glucose dysregulation has also been reported in preterm babies once they have established full feeds and may be a precursor of longer-term glucose dysregulation.[47] While most neonatologists would not intervene to treat blood glucose levels until they rose to greater than 180 to 216 mg/dL (>10 to 12 mmol/L), early hyperglycemia is linked with both mortality and morbidity. It is yet to be established whether this relationship is simply an association or is causal,[48] but the use of insulin to treat hyperglycemia has been associated with reduced mortality and morbidity.[49]

GLUCOSE PRODUCTION

Substrate availability plays a key role in glucose regulation with the availability of gluconeogenic precursors including lactate being important in adults and childhood.[46,50,51] It is estimated that 20% to 50% of glucose requirements of the newborn baby, providing approximately 6.1 g/k/day of glucose, comes from the hydrolysis of lactose from milk. Of the remaining gluconeogenic substrates, galactose provides the largest amount with smaller amounts available from lactate, amino acids, and glycerol. Galactose from milk is mainly converted to glucose by glucose-6-phosphate dehydrogenase (G6PD). Uptake is independent of insulin concentrations, and clearance is very rapid compared with that of glucose (6.9% per minute disappearance compared with 1.4% per minute). Glycerol accounts for approximately 10% to 20% of glucose production. The first step of GNG from glycerol is not influenced by glucagon, insulin, or glucocorticoids (which regulate the rate of GNG from nonglycerol precursors) but is related to changes in blood glycerol concentration. In healthy full-term newborns, GNG via pyruvate contributes significantly to glucose appearance rates (31%), with rates similar to those seen in fasted healthy adults. GNG from lactate contributes approximately 30% of the total glucose production in the healthy term newborn, with the rate of lactate turnover almost two-fold higher than the rate of glucose turnover. This contrasts with the finding in adult studies where lactate turnover is much lower than the rate of glucose turnover. Alanine also contributes to glucose production in the human newborn, providing approximately 9% of blood glucose at 8 hours of age.[52] Breastfed babies have lower blood glucose levels but higher ketones compared with formula-fed babies, and this is thought to be neuroprotective.[53]

GLUCOSE UPTAKE

Glucose uptake is dependent on a family of developmentally regulated facilitated glucose transporters, each having a specific tissue distribution. GLUT1 is the predominant isoform during fetal and early neonatal life with levels decreasing after birth. GLUT1 has a high affinity for glucose, is insulin-independent, and is responsible for basal glucose uptake.[54-56] It is found in most tissues but particularly abundant in the brain and maintains glucose transport across the blood-brain barrier. GLUT1 appears to be downregulated by high glucose concentrations and upregulated by low glucose concentrations.[57] The other isoforms—GLUT2 in the liver, GLUT3 in the brain and GLUT4 in the muscle—increase after birth.[55,57] GLUT2 is the major glucose transporter isoform expressed in hepatocytes, pancreatic β cells, and the kidney. This isoform is a low-affinity, high-turnover transporter and forms part of a glucose-sensing apparatus that responds to subtle changes in blood glucose levels with alterations in the rate of glucose uptake into the cell. GLUT4 is expressed in adipocytes and muscle cells. These are the ***insulin-sensitive*** cell types, as they respond to insulin with a rapid increase in glucose transport and are important for the maintenance of whole-body glucose homeostasis.[58] GLUT4 is usually found in intracellular vesicles, but in adults, insulin stimulates the migration of GLUT4 to the plasma membrane.[59] In the newborn, however, upregulation of GLUT4 in muscle is only modestly responsive to insulin.[60]

GLUCOSE UTILIZATION

Rates of glucose utilization in the newborn can far exceed that of adults, as has been demonstrated by the effect of increasing dextrose or insulin infusions.[61] The mean glucose oxidation rate in the term newborn has been estimated to be 6 mg/kg/min (3.8 to 9.7 mg/kg/min) compared with an adult rate of 3 mg/kg/min.[62,63] Glucose oxidation rates have also been reported to be high in preterm infants ranging from 2.9 to 7.9 mg/kg/min.[2,64] There is a change during the first week of life in the percentage of total energy expenditure utilized for oxidative compared with non-oxidative glucose metabolism, with an increase in nonoxidative disposal. This marks the change from a catabolic to an anabolic state.[56] Nonoxidative glucose disposal through lipogenesis, glycogenesis, and protein synthesis is stimulated by increasing insulin levels, which impacts growth both directly and indirectly through the regulation of IGF-1 and IGF binding protein one (IGFBP-1).[65-67]

INSULIN SECRETION

Insulin is the primary hormonal regulator of glucose uptake and utilization in the newborn, and its secretion is under the influence of neural and enteroendocrine mechanisms. Glucoreceptor neurons are present in the ventromedial hypothalamic nucleus and the portal vein causing an increase in insulin secretion in response to hyperglycemia.[68] Insulin secretion is linked to the enteric supply of milk and release of incretins.[69-71] However, in the newborn, this insulin response to glucose is initially blunted but matures in the weeks after birth.[72,73]

Studies of insulin secretion and sensitivity in the newborn are limited, but impaired glucose homeostasis in the neonate has been postulated as secondary to either a decreased insulin secretion or to increased insulin resistance compared with that in the adult.[74,75] To determine developmental changes in insulin secretion and clearance, studies have been undertaken using [^{131}I]insulin as a tracer in preterm compared with term lambs and in 4- to 5-month-old sheep.[76] After a 7-hour fast, animals received 0.45% saline or glucose (5.7 mg/kg/min) for 6 hours, followed by the tracer insulin infusion for 11 minutes. Posthepatic insulin secretion rates and metabolic clearance rates did not differ between the groups either after infusion of 0.45% saline or after dextrose infusion. This suggested that, at these relatively low rates of glucose infusion, the inability to regulate glucose control may be explained by hepatic unresponsiveness to insulin rather than secretory capacity of the pancreatic β cell.[76] In contrast, King and colleagues studied postnatal development of insulin secretion in term and preterm neonates (born at 26 to 30 weeks of gestation) after birth. Insulin levels were measured before and 30 minutes after administration of glucose parenterally or enterally.[73] The term neonates secreted more insulin than preterm infants. The increase in insulin secretion in response to glucose administration in preterm infants gradually increased postnatally, taking up to 18 weeks to develop a fully mature response. Studies have also shown that in preterm infants there is immature processing of insulin from proinsulin resulting in high proinsulin to insulin ratios. As proinsulin is 10 times less active than mature insulin, this can add to the picture of insulin deficiency.[77]

There is evidence from animal studies of pancreatic remodeling after birth that is associated with weaning and increased apoptosis and β-cell neogenesis, which can be influenced by nutritional intake.[78-80] There is similar postmortem evidence of β-cell apoptosis in humans with a new population of β cells compensating for the perinatal loss.[80] It is thought that this may be important in perinatal adaptation to the change from continuous placental glucose delivery to the intermittent enteral supply of nutrients. The secretion of incretins may be necessary for the remodeling of a new population of β cells that are better suited to metabolic control in postnatal life. In rats this period of apoptosis occurs at the same time as a significant fall in levels in IGF-2 expression, and overexpression of IGF-2 leads to a reduction in apoptosis, suggesting a protective role for IGF-2.[81] This may be a critical window for pancreatic development, with any interference with remodeling impacting on the ability of the pancreas to meet requirements for insulin secretion later in life.[82]

INSULIN SENSITIVITY AND PERIPHERAL GLUCOSE UTILIZATION

In both neonate and adult there is a strong positive linear correlation between plasma insulin concentration and glucose utilization rates, although basal glucose production rates, glucose utilization rates, and plasma insulin concentrations are quite different. In human neonatal studies, increases in insulin infusion from basal rates of 2 and 4 mU/kg/min led to significant increases in peripheral glucose utilization,[61] but because a plateau was not reached, the maximal effect on glucose utilization was not defined. In these studies, the neonatal glucose utilization rate, even at a lower plasma insulin concentration, far exceeded that reported as the maximal response in the adult.[83] This increase in glucose utilization occurred at a higher insulin concentration than was required to reduce the rate of glucose production (Fig. 38.3). These data support a strong positive correlation between plasma insulin concentration and glucose utilization.[32,61,83-86]

Animal studies using the euglycemic hyperinsulinemic clamp in 3- to 6-day-old lambs and 31- to 35-day-old sheep demonstrated that the younger animals needed a higher rate of glucose infusion to maintain euglycemia compared with the older animal group receiving the same amount of insulin.[87] Although endogenous glucose production persisted in both groups, the percent decrease within insulin infusion was greater in the younger (neonatal) lambs compared with the adult sheep. The younger animals exhibited greater glucose utilization than that seen in the older animals (Fig. 38.4). As in the human neonate, endogenous glucose production was not completely suppressed in the lamb, despite very high plasma insulin concentrations.

These data are consistent with findings in human preterm neonates, who exhibited persistent glucose production and greater peripheral sensitivity to insulin. If insulin sensitivity is calculated at euglycemia (i.e., not confounded by non-insulin-mediated glucose utilization),[88] it is apparent that the neonate has a greater peripheral sensitivity to insulin than the adult. This increased sensitivity may result from a higher receptor concentration and affinity, provided that the postreceptor cascade is intact peripherally.

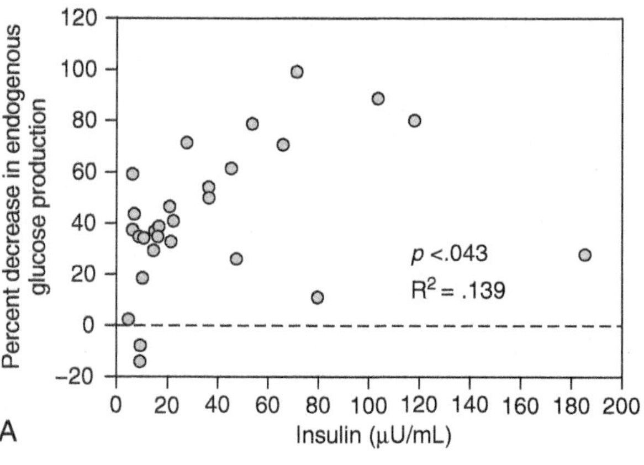

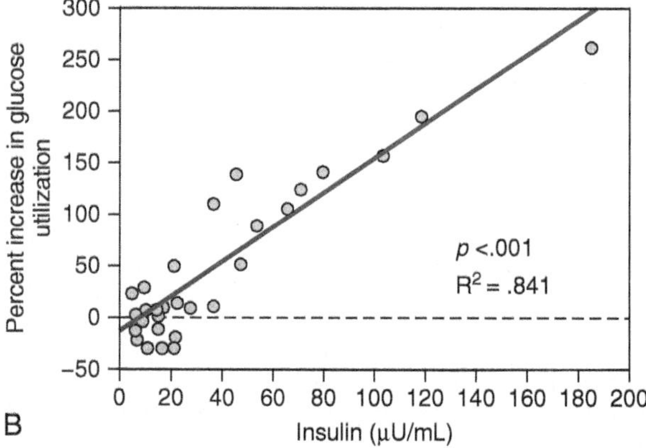

Fig. 38.3 (A) Regression correlating the percent decrease in endogenous glucose production relative to plasma insulin concentration in the neonate. (B) Regression correlating the percent increase in glucose utilization relative to plasma insulin concentration in the neonate. (From Farrag HM, Nawrath LM, Healey JE, et al. Persistent glucose production and greater peripheral sensitivity to insulin in the neonate vs. the adult. *Am J Physiol.* 1997;272:86.)

INSULIN RESISTANCE AND PERSISTENT GLUCOSE PRODUCTION

In term neonates, infants of diabetic mothers, and preterm neonates, persistent endogenous glucose production greater than 1.0 mg/kg/min has been reported despite administration of exogenous glucose infusions. Unlike the adult, complete suppression of glucose production is not achieved in the human neonate.[61] Early animal studies using the euglycemic hyperinsulinemic clamp model to generate a dose-response curve to a graded increase in insulin infusion rates demonstrated an 80% suppression of glucose production in the newborn puppy compared with adults.[89,90] This lack of complete suppression of glucose production in the neonate demonstrated hepatic resistance to insulin and persistent GNG.

Insulin resistance is a combination of insulin insensitivity and/or insulin unresponsiveness. With *insulin insensitivity* there is a shift to the right of the insulin dose-response curve such that a higher concentration of insulin is necessary to produce a lower effect but with a maximal effect achieved eventually. This shift in the dose-response curve is usually the result of decreased affinity or a decreased concentration of insulin receptors. In contrast, with *insulin unresponsiveness,* all responses to insulin are reduced (including the maximal response), but the dose-response relationship remains normal (i.e., the insulin concentration required to produce a half-maximal response is normal) and is the result of a postreceptor defect.[91] In the newborn, a

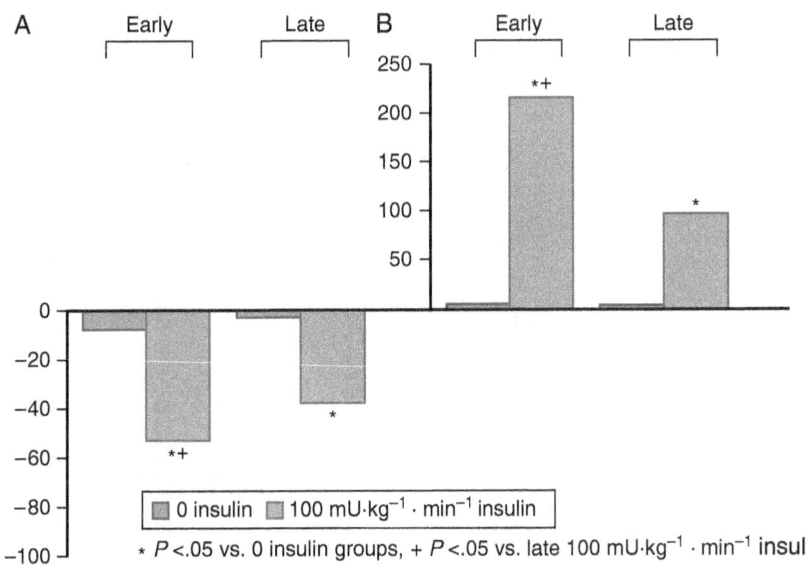

Fig. 38.4 The percent decrease in endogenous glucose production (A) and the percent increase in glucose utilization (B) during the clamp period in the early and late groups. (From Gelardi NL, Rapoza RE, Renzulli JF, et al. Insulin resistance and glucose transporter expression during the euglycemic hyperinsulinemic clamp in the lamb. *Am J Physiol.* 1999;277:1142.)

combination of both may exist simultaneously so that a higher insulin concentration is required to produce an effect and the maximal effect is reduced compared with a normal response.[92,93]

Basal glucose production rates in the newborn are two to three times higher than in the adult.[94,95] In animal models to investigate insulin sensitivity, persistent glucose production is seen when using the euglycemic hyperinsulinemic clamp technique,[96] the glucose clamp,[56] or glucose and amino acid infusion.[56] The lack of control of endogenous glucose production in response to glucose infusions have shown this response to be poorly developed in the newborn.[94,97] Hepatic insulin sensitivity studies of rates of endogenous glucose production in response to glucose infusions of 0, 5, 6, 11.7, or 21.7 mg/kg/min in newborn lambs demonstrated that both newborn and adult animals maintained a constant plasma glucose concentration.[50] However, glucose production rates persisted in term newborn lambs until an infusion rate of 21.7 mg/kg/min was reached. In contrast, the glucose production rate was reduced with a glucose infusion rate of only 5.7 mg/kg/min in adult sheep. At the point when the glucose production rate was significantly reduced, the plasma insulin concentration in the newborn lamb was five times greater than in the adult. The blunted hepatic responsiveness to insulin appeared to be a major factor explaining the inefficiency in glucose homeostasis.

Cowett and colleagues studied neonatal lambs using radiolabeled glucose for isotope-based measurement of glucose production.[98] To isolate the contribution of glucose, a baseline glucose infusion rate of 8.5 mg/kg/min was combined with somatostatin to block insulin, glucagon, and growth hormone release; metyrapone to block cortisol release; phentolamine to block α-adrenergic release; and propranolol to block β-adrenergic release. With an increase in glucose infusion at a rate 49% greater than the basal rate, the endogenous glucose production persisted, showing that glucose alone did not control neonatal glucose homeostasis.

The independent roles of hyperglycemia and hyperinsulinemia were explored by studies varying the concentrations of glucose and insulin in newborn lambs to produce steady-state euglycemia and hyperinsulinemia.[99] Glucose production rates and GNG from lactate were measured. Increasing the rate of glucose infusion without administering insulin (groups II and III in Fig. 38.5) produced a stepwise increase in plasma glucose and insulin concentrations when compared with controls (group I). Elevation of the plasma insulin concentration induced by hyperglycemia was associated with a significant reduction in the glucose production rate but was seen only when marked hyperglycemia and hyperinsulinemia were achieved (group III). With insulin administration, a significant and stepwise increase in plasma insulin concentration was observed, depending on the dose of insulin administered. By simultaneous glucose infusion, a state of euglycemia or hyperglycemia was produced with concomitant hyperinsulinemia. With a slight increase in plasma insulin (group IV), a significant reduction in GNG was noted together with a slight but insignificant reduction in the rate of glucose production. When hyperinsulinemia was moderate to marked (groups V and VI, respectively), there was a significant reduction of GNG and the rate of glucose production. Insulin is known to inhibit glycogenolysis and GNG, and it suppresses glucose production in the adult.[100,101] These data suggest that a moderate elevation of plasma insulin concentration effectively reduces GNG (groups II and IV) but does not influence the endogenous glucose production. The latter was reduced only when a much higher insulin concentration was achieved (groups II, V, VI). These data suggest that insulin, rather than glucose, controlled the rate of glucose production in newborn lambs but that there is relative central insulin resistance.

IMPACT OF COUNTER-REGULATORY HORMONES

In sheep, increases in glucose production rate and plasma glucose concentration in response to epinephrine has been reported to be smaller in newborn lambs than in mature animals.[102,103] However, catecholamine infusions tend to lead to hyperglycemia, and stopping adrenaline increases the risk of hypoglycemia. This imprecise effect of counter-regulatory hormones on neonatal glucose control mirrors the imprecise control by insulin and appears to be developmentally regulated.[104] Glucocorticoids play an important role in preparing the fetus for extrauterine life, as they effect glucose transport mechanisms. Glucocorticoids upregulate GLUT1 and 3 expression in human endothelial cells and in extrauterine life glucocorticoid treatment causes a rise in blood glucose concentration and insulin resistance.

INCRETINS

The gut hormones, or incretins, which include glucagon-like peptide (GLP)-1, gastric-inhibitory polypeptide (GIP), amylin, and peptide YY (and pancreatic polypeptide), play a major role in adult glucose homeostasis, but their roles in term and preterm neonates are not clear. GIP and GLP-1 are produced from duodenal K-cells and intestinal L-cells, respectively, as a response to food intake, bind to specific receptors and increase

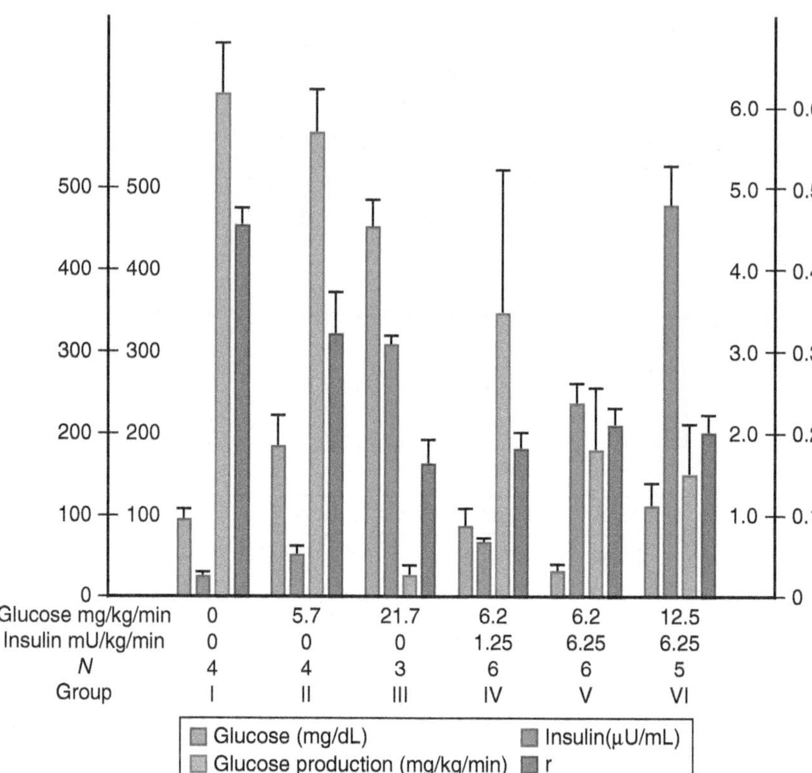

Fig. 38.5 Plasma glucose and plasma insulin concentrations, glucose production rates, and ratio of U-[^{14}C]lactate to D-[6-^{3}H]glucose for all groups. (From Susa JB, Cowett RM, Oh W, et al. Suppression of gluconeogenesis and endogenous glucose production by exogenous insulin administration in the newborn lamb. *Pediatr Res.* 1979;13:594.)

the level of intracellular cyclic adenosine. Both GIP and GLP-1 have insulinotrophic effects on β cells by promoting their proliferation and inhibiting apoptosis, but GIP also enhances glucagon secretion while GLP suppresses it. These incretins not only have actions on the pancreas but also on bone, the brain, and regulate lipid metabolism and decrease intestinal motility. GLP-1 and GIP levels are highest between 3 and 4 weeks of age; premature infants <30 weeks gestational age have particularly high GLP-1 levels. The fasting GLP-1 level of premature infants (>34 weeks) at 4 to 10 days is four times higher than that in adults. GLP-1 leads to an increase in the conversion of glucose to lipids and promotes energy storage in lipids with enteral feeding eliciting an increase in GLP-1 secretion.

The roles of leptin and ghrelin in neonatal glucose regulation are not clear. In adults, leptin has been shown to have a number of effects including suppressing production of glucagon and corticosterone and inhibiting hepatic glucose output. Serum leptin levels are positively related to gestational age and birth weight, and vary according to the amount of adipose tissue, but decline from the first week until 6 weeks of age. Ghrelin is a peptide hormone produced mainly in the stomach that increases glucose levels via a variety of mechanisms in adults. The role of ghrelin in the newborn is not well defined, but higher ghrelin levels are associated with greater catch-up growth in SGA infants.

PRETERM INFANT STUDIES

It is clear that the preterm infant has reduced homeostatic mechanisms to moderate glucose control both in the first days of life and toward term.[10,105] Better understanding of the underlying mechanisms would allow us to improve the management of these babies in whom supporting nutritional intake to optimize growth is challenging.

Stable isotope methodology has enabled kinetic studies in human neonates.[106] Fig. 38.6 depicts the glucose production rate for preterm and term neonates compared with adults, with 5 of 13 preterm and 2 of 7 term neonates showing persistent glucose

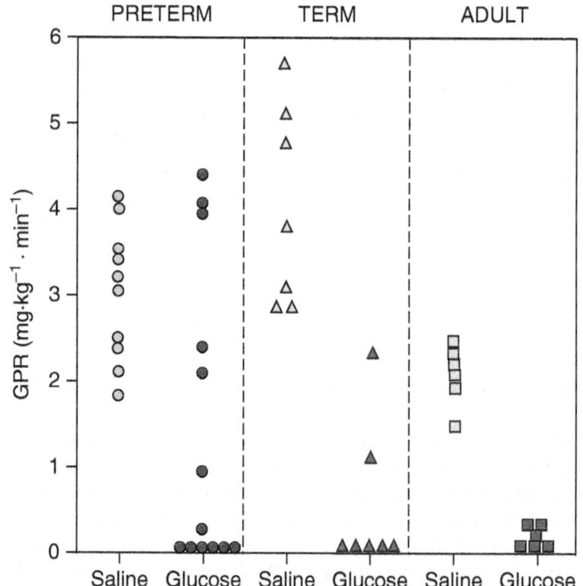

Fig. 38.6 Glucose production rate *(GPR)* during saline or glucose infusion in preterm and term infants and adults. Plotted values are for individual patients. (From Cowett RM, Oh W, Schwartz R. Persistent glucose production during glucose infusion in the human neonate. *J Clin Invest.* 1983;71:467.)

production rates (>1 mg/kg/min) during glucose infusion, in contrast to complete suppression of glucose production in adults. No correlation was found between plasma glucose concentration and the glucose production rate (Fig. 38.7). However, there was a correlation between the plasma insulin concentration and the glucose production rate but with considerable variability in the neonate (Fig. 38.8). These data point to significant developmental differences in neonatal glucose homeostasis and reaffirmed that

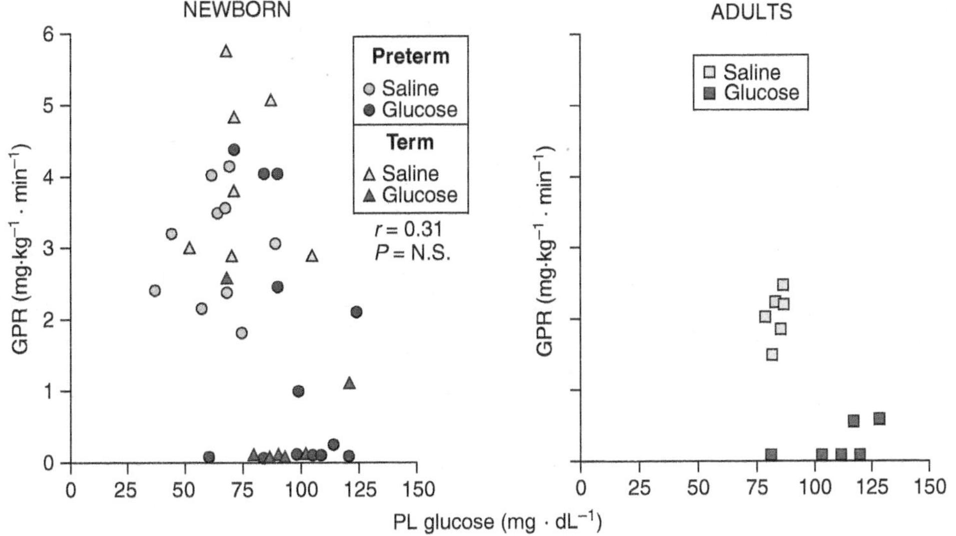

Fig. 38.7 Correlation between plasma *(PL)* glucose concentration during the turnover period and glucose production rate *(GPR)* in neonates and adults. *N.S.*, Not significant. (From Cowett RM, Oh W, Schwartz R. Persistent glucose production during glucose infusion in the human neonate. *J Clin Invest*. 1983;71:467.)

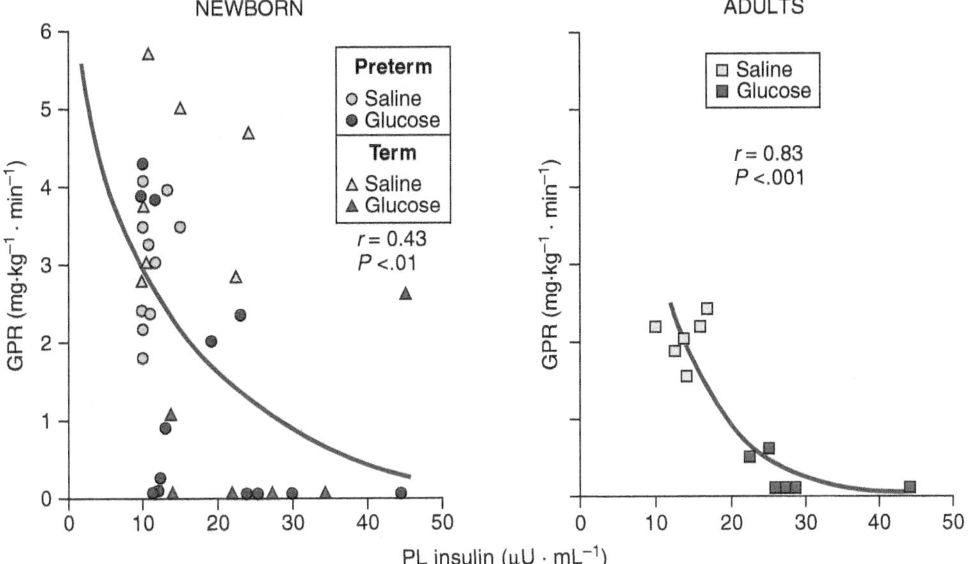

Fig. 38.8 Correlation between peripheral plasma *(PL)* insulin concentration during the turnover period and glucose production rate *(GPR)* in neonates and adults. (From Cowett RM, Oh W, Schwartz R. Persistent glucose production during glucose infusion in the human neonate. *J Clin Invest*. 1983;71:467.)

insulin is important in neonatal hormonal control of glucose production.

The contribution of GNG to glucose production was evaluated in eight preterm neonates (26.5 ± 0.5 weeks gestational age) who were receiving parenteral nutrition that administered glucose at a rate exceeding the usual neonatal glucose production rate. Stable isotope kinetics were used to measure glucose production and GNG rates. GNG and glycogenolysis were not affected by the total glucose infusion rate, the glucose concentration, the gestational age, or birth weight.[107] Potential factors regulating GNG were also studied by decreasing the rate of glucose infusion over a period of 11 hours while measuring glucose production rate and GNG. GNG and glucose production rates remained unchanged while the rate of glucose infusion was decreased in the face of decreased glucose and insulin concentrations.[108]

In studies of preterm babies, moderate rates of dextrose infusion (8 mg/kg/min) were insufficient suppress glucose production.[109] This finding is further supported by data showing that no endogenous glucose production was noted with combined infusions of glucose at 6.8 mg/kg/min with intravenous amino acids and fat emulsion.[110] In addition, the relative role of each of these substrates as a secretagogue for insulin is unknown. These physiologic findings are supported by larger clinical studies where the prevalence of hyperglycemia is not clearly associated with the rates of glucose or insulin infused, adding to many challenges in maintaining glucose control in the preterm infant.[46,48,111]

Persistent endogenous glucose production (i.e., ≥1 mg/kg/min or <80% decrease in the rate of glucose appearance [Ra]) in response to glucose infusion is evidence of a transitional homeostatic state in the neonate during the first days after birth. To determine when an adult-like response developed, Ra was measured in 11 preterm babies (33 ± 0.3 weeks) at 2 to 5 weeks after birth. In these paired studies, a 4 μg/kg/min D-[U-^{13}C] glucose tracer was infused by prime constant infusion to determine Ra during saline or glucose infusion (5.3 ± 0.2 mg/kg/min). In comparison with the saline infusion turnover period, the plasma glucose concentration increased significantly during the glucose infusion turnover period. Plasma insulin concentration remained unchanged (12 ± 5 μU/mL vs. 8 ± 3 μU/mL). Ra was heterogeneous during glucose infusion, and persistent Ra was present in 6 of 11 neonates (Fig. 38.9). Of the five infants with decreased Ra during glucose infusion, three received glucose at a rate exceeding basal Ra. Of the remaining six infants who exhibited persistent Ra during the glucose infusion, three received glucose at a rate equal to or in excess of basal Ra.

Others have reported an approximate 50% reduction in glucose production in response to an exogenous glucose infusion rate of 4 to 6 mg/kg/min, which is similar to the basal glucose production rate in the neonate and resulted in a plasma insulin concentration of approximately 19 mU/mL.[112,113] Whether this reduction in glucose production is primarily a response to a higher plasma insulin concentration or plasma glucose concentration remains controversial. A high glucose infusion rate (i.e., 9.5 mg/kg/min) was shown to completely suppress glucose production in stable, extremely premature infants, while significantly increasing both plasma glucose and insulin concentrations.[32] At a similar plasma insulin concentration, a 41% reduction in glucose production was noted, suggesting that the combined effect of glucose and insulin is necessary for complete suppression of glucose production. By contrast, an infusion of glucose at a rate of 5.5 mg/kg/min resulted in a 90% suppression of glucose production when administered with or without lipid.[114] Suppression was achieved at a glucose concentration of approximately 90 mg/dL and an extremely low insulin concentration of approximately 6 μU/mL.

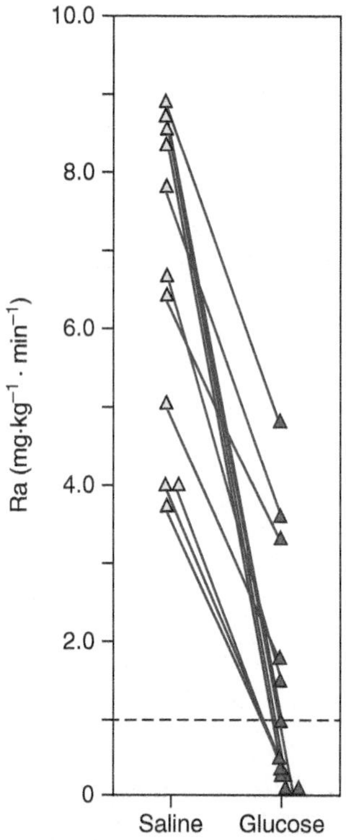

Fig. 38.9 Endogenous glucose production rate *(Ra)* during saline and glucose infusion. (From Cowett RM, Andersen GE, Maguire CA, et al. Ontogeny of glucose homeostasis in low birth weight infants. *J Pediatr.* 1988;112:462.)

Most studies have evaluated the insulin effect on plasma glucose concentration in the hyperglycemic, stressed neonate.[115-121] Fewer studies have evaluated the effects of insulin (or glucose) on glucose production in the healthy term or preterm neonate.[106,113,122] When the euglycemic hyperinsulinemic clamp was used in human preterm neonates to evaluate insulin sensitivity, hepatic glucose production was reduced at relatively low insulin concentrations (Fig. 38.10).[61] Hepatic glucose production did not change with increases in insulin infusion rates to achieve up to 10-fold higher plasma insulin concentrations. Endogenous glucose production was reduced from between 41% and 58% of basal rates, but persistent glucose production was noted throughout the study. This lack of complete suppression of glucose production demonstrates a central insulin resistance in the preterm infant.[84]

This mechanism may include factors at the membrane level (aside from receptor concentration and affinity) such as the state of the receptor, its ability to interact with other membrane proteins required for signal generation, or a variety of intracellular factors, including effects of insulin on glucose transporters or key enzymes in the glycolytic, glycogenolytic, or gluconeogenic pathways. Decreased receptor concentration or affinity has been suggested to be an unlikely explanation, but these findings were based on a higher insulin receptor concentration and affinity in cultured cord lymphocytes in comparison with adult lymphocytes.[85]

The indirect effect of insulin on endogenous glucose production has been evaluated, including the effect of inhibition of lipolysis and reduction of free fatty acid concentrations.[86] These indirect effects of insulin were shown to suppress hepatic glucose production; however, the limited amount of adipose

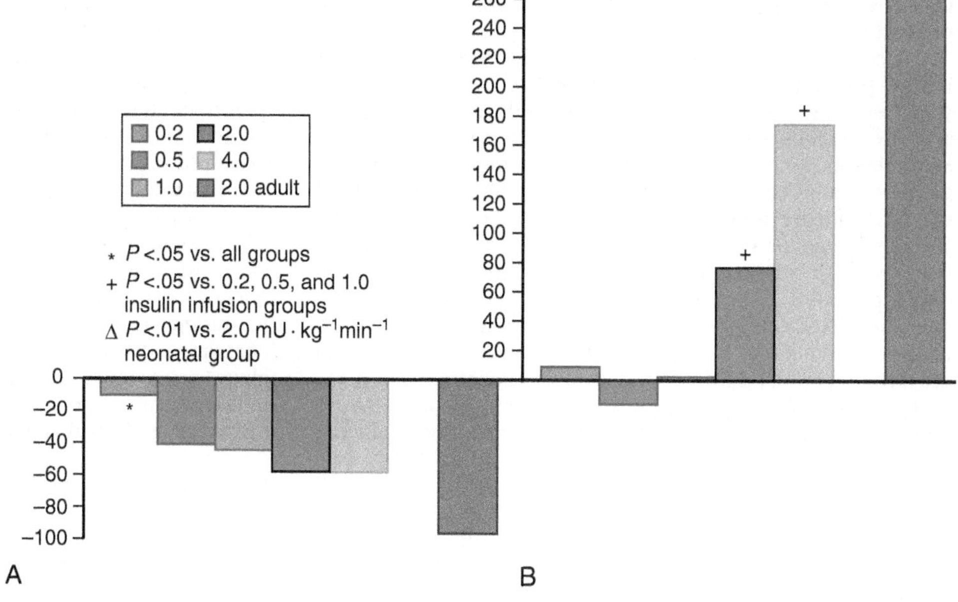

Fig. 38.10 The percent decrease in endogenous glucose production and the percent increase in glucose utilization for the various insulin infusion rates of administration in the neonate as well as the insulin rate of administration in the adult (2 mU/kg/min). (From Farrag HM, Nawrath LM, Healey JE, et al. Persistent glucose production and greater peripheral sensitivity to insulin in the neonate vs. the adult. *Am J Physiol.* 1997;272:86.)

tissue in the preterm neonate may alter this indirect effect of insulin on endogenous glucose production. An attenuated response to insulin in the very low-birth-weight neonate has been suggested as the reason for the occurrence of hyperglycemia and attributed to insulin resistance, rather than lack of the β-cell response.[117] However, high insulin infusion rates and plasma insulin concentrations appear to provide sustained improvement in glucose tolerance.[115-121,123]

Preterm infants are heterogeneous in their metabolic status and the mechanisms explaining differences between infants may relate to a combination of relative energy requirements and coexisting pathologies, including both chronic factors, such as growth restriction, or acute effects, as with infection. Furthermore, it is clear that the development of glucose homeostasis is in transition throughout the neonatal period and that differences in preterm babies from 22 weeks to term evolves over time.[112] These differences are increasingly being demonstrated by the use of continuous glucose monitoring, which allows detailed data on glucose control to be collected for prolonged periods without the need for multiple blood tests, and a more proactive approach to management as fluctuations in glucose levels can be detected earlier.[124]

The multiplicity of factors that influence development and maintenance of glucose control and homeostasis in the neonatal period has also led to attempts to model neonatal glucose metabolism.[125,126] Le Compte and associates reported on their use of a metabolic system computer model to determine insulin infusion rates in the very low-birth-weight neonate. In a pilot study, the combination of such a computer model with continuous glucose monitoring has been shown to better target glucose control in these babies.[123] Although these models have been shown to clinically support glucose control, further studies will be important to determine the optimal targets for glucose control in these babies and the best strategies to achieve them.

LONG-TERM CONSEQUENCES

Epidemiologic data in humans and studies in animals indicate that during critical periods of prenatal and postnatal development, nutrition and other environmental stimuli influence developmental pathways inducing permanent changes in metabolism and chronic disease susceptibility via epigenetic programming. Adverse consequences of altered intrauterine environments can be passed from first generation to second generation offspring. Transient environmental influences can have permanent effects on the developmental establishment of epigenetic gene regulation. Physiologic adaptation to the in utero and postnatal environment related to reduced or excess nutrient delivery can alter organ development and endocrine function. While this adaptation may be advantageous for the physiologic environment at the time of the insult, it may not be beneficial for a different environment in later life and can lead to altered glucose, insulin, and lipid metabolism. Hence, a baby subjected to an adverse in utero environment but an increased postnatal nutrient supply as reflected by excessive postnatal weight gain is at future risk of developing the metabolic syndrome with increased adiposity and insulin resistance, hypertension, and type-2 diabetes.

Animal models have shown pancreatic remodeling of the pancreas after birth, as reflected by increased apoptosis and β-cell neogenesis in association with hypoinsulinemia. IGF-1 is associated with increased proliferation of precursor β cells, and the period of apoptosis occurs at the same time as a significant fall in the levels of IGF-2 expression. Overexpression of IGF-1 and IGF-2 can reduce apoptosis, suggesting a protective role. Postmortem studies in humans have shown similar increases in apoptosis in the early postnatal period. In addition, the secretion of incretins in response to enteral feeds may influence β-cell neogenesis with the establishment of a nonproliferative population of cells that are better suited to metabolic control in postnatal life. There are adaptive changes in insulin secretion with alteration in the neonatal diet. The perinatal period may therefore be a critical time for programming of the endocrine pancreas. Interference with this process of remodeling may have a significant impact on the ability of the pancreas to meet the requirements for insulin secretion both in the perinatal period and in later life.

CONCLUSION

The transition from fetal to independent life requires rapid metabolic adaptation to ensure glucose homeostasis, and consequently the perinatal period is one when glucose levels are more variable than in later life. The healthy baby is prepared for these challenges with sufficient glycogen stores and fat to tolerate fasting and a healthy stress response with the suppression of insulin secretion and promotion glycogenolysis, lipolysis, and GNG ensuring glucose and alternative fuels are available to the newborn while feeding is established. In contrast, many babies born following pregnancies complicated by maternal diabetes or placental insufficiency or who are born preterm are not well prepared to respond to these metabolic challenges. Determining optimal management for each of these babies requires better measurement of glucose itself, as well as alternative fuels and the metabolic environment. Furthermore, longer-term follow-up of these babies is also imperative if we are to truly understand the long-term consequences, both neurologic and metabolic.

ACKNOWLEDGMENTS

The authors wish to thank Richard M. Cowett, MD, for his valuable contributions to this chapter in the fifth edition.

A complete reference list is available at www.ExpertConsult.com. 

SELECT REFERENCES

1. Cowett R. *Principles of Perinatal-Neonatal Metabolism*. 2nd ed. New York: Springer-Verlag; 1998.
2. Farrag HM, Cowett RM. Glucose homeostasis in the micropremie. *Clin Perinatol*. 2000;27:1-22.
10. Pertierra-Cortada A, Ramon-Krauel M, Iriondo-Sanz M, et al. Instability of glucose values in very preterm babies at term postmenstrual age. *J Pediatr*. 2014;165:1146-1153.
11. Hay Jr WW, Sparks JW. Placental, fetal, and neonatal carbohydrate metabolism. *Clin Obstet Gynecol*. 1985;28:473-485.
19. Bougneres PF, Lemmel C, Ferre P, et al. Ketone body transport in the human neonate and infant. *J Clin Invest*. 1986;77:42-48.
22. Yamamoto JM, Corcoy R, Donovan LE, et al. Maternal glycaemic control and risk of neonatal hypoglycaemia in type 1 diabetes pregnancy: a secondary analysis of the CONCEPTT trial. *Diabet Med*. 2019;36:1046-1053.
26. Bazaes RA, Salazar TE, Pittaluga E, et al. Glucose and lipid metabolism in small for gestational age infants at 48 hours of age. *Pediatrics*. 2003;111:804-809.
27. Petry CJ, Mooslehner K, Prentice P, et al. Associations between a fetal imprinted gene allele score and late pregnancy maternal glucose concentrations. *Diabetes Metab*. 2017;43:323-331.
30. Kaiser JR, Bai S, Rozance PJ. Newborn plasma glucose concentration nadirs by gestational-age group. *Neonatology*. 2018;113:353-359.
34. Hagnevik K, Faxelius G, Irestedt L, et al. Catecholamine surge and metabolic adaptation in the newborn after vaginal delivery and caesarean section. *Acta Paediatr Scand*. 1984;73:602-609.
36. Boardman JP, Hawdon JM. Hypoglycaemia and hypoxic-ischaemic encephalopathy. *Dev Med Child Neurol*. 2015;57(suppl 3):29-33.
38. Beardsall K. Real time continuous glucose monitoring in neonatal intensive care. *Early Hum Dev*. 2019:104844.
41. Ogilvy-Stuart AL, Harding JE, Beardsall K. Thresholds for hypoglycaemic screening-a cause for concern? *Arch Dis Child Educ Pract Ed*. 2019;104:33-34.
42. Levene I, Wilkinson D. Identification and management of neonatal hypoglycaemia in the full-term infant (British Association of Perinatal Medicine-Framework for Practice). *Arch Dis Child Educ Pract Ed*. 2019;104:29-32.
45. McKinlay CJD, Alsweiler JM, Anstice NS, et al. Association of neonatal glycemia with neurodevelopmental outcomes at 4.5 years. *JAMA Pediatr*. 2017;171:972-983.

46. Beardsall K, Vanhaesebrouck S, Ogilvy-Stuart AL, et al. Prevalence and determinants of hyperglycemia in very low birth weight infants: cohort analyses of the NIRTURE study. *J Pediatr*. 2010;157:715-719.
49. Zamir I, Tornevi A, Abrahamsson T, et al. Hyperglycemia in extremely preterm infants-insulin treatment, mortality and nutrient intakes. *J Pediatr*. 2018;200:104-110.
51. Antonowicz I, Lebenthal E. Developmental pattern of small intestinal enterokinase and disaccharidase activities in the human fetus. *Gastroenterology*. 1977;72:1299-1303.
52. Frazer TE, Karl IE, Hillman LS, et al. Direct measurement of gluconeogenesis from [2,3]13C2]alanine in the human neonate. *Am J Physiol*. 1981;240:E615-621.
56. Cowett RM, Farrag HM. Selected principles of perinatal-neonatal glucose metabolism. *SeminNeonatol*. 2004;9:37-47.
57. Sadiq HF, Das UG, Tracy TF, et al. Intra-uterine growth restriction differentially regulates perinatal brain and skeletal muscle glucose transporters. *Brain Res*. 1999;823:96-103.
59. Slot JW, Geuze HJ, Gigengack S, et al. Translocation of the glucose transporter GLUT4 in cardiac myocytes of the rat. *Proc NatlAcad Sci USA*. 1991;88:7815-7819.
61. Farrag HM, Nawrath LM, Healey JE, et al. Persistent glucose production and greater peripheral sensitivity to insulin in the neonate vs. the adult. *Am J Physiol*. 1997;272. E86-93.
65. Iniguez G, Ong K, Bazaes R, et al. Longitudinal changes in insulin-like growth factor-I, insulin sensitivity, and secretion from birth to age three years in small-for-gestational-age children. *J Clin Endocrinol Metab*. 2006;91:4645-4649.
66. Fant ME, Weisoly D. Insulin and insulin-like growth factors in human development: implications for the perinatal period. *SeminPerinatol*. 2001;25:426-435.
67. Woods KA, Camacho-Hubner C, Savage MO, et al. Intrauterine growth retardation and postnatal growth failure associated with deletion of the insulin-like growth factor I gene. *N Engl J Med*. 1996;335:1363-1367.
68. Heijboer AC, Pijl H, Van den Hoek AM, et al. Gut-brain axis: regulation of glucose metabolism. *J Neuroendocrinol*. 2006;18:883-894.
69. Amin H, Holst JJ, Hartmann B, et al. Functional ontogeny of the proglucagon-derived peptide axis in the premature human neonate. *Pediatrics*. 2008;121: e180-186.
71. Aynsley-Green A. The endocrinology of feeding in the newborn. *Baillieres Clin Endocrinol Metab*. 1989;3:837-868.
73. King RA, Smith RM, Dahlenburg GW. Long term postnatal development of insulin secretion in early premature infants. *Early Hum Dev*. 1986;13:285-294.
75. Teng C, Battaglia FC, Meschia G, et al. Fetal hepatic and umbilical uptakes of glucogenic substrates during a glucagon-somatostatin infusion. *Am J Physiol Endocrinol Metab*. 2002;282:E542-550.
81. Agudo J, Ayuso E, Jimenez V, et al. IGF-I mediates regeneration of endocrine pancreas by increasing beta cell replication through cell cycle protein modulation in mice. *Diabetologia*. 2008;51:1862-1872.
83. Rizza RA, Mandarino LJ, Gerich JE. Dose-response characteristics for effects of insulin on production and utilization of glucose in man. *Am J Physiol*. 1981;240:E630-639.
86. Rebrin K, Steil GM, Getty L, et al. Free fatty acid as a link in the regulation of hepatic glucose output by peripheral insulin. *Diabetes*. 1995;44:1038-1045.
91. Kahn CR. Insulin resistance, insulin insensitivity, and insulin unresponsiveness: a necessary distinction. *Metabolism*. 1978;27:1893-1902.
93. Arslanian SA, Bacha F, Saad R, et al. Family history of type 2 diabetes is associated with decreased insulin sensitivity and an impaired balance between insulin sensitivity and insulin secretion in white youth. *Diabetes Care*. 2005;28:115-119.
96. Fowden AL, Gardner DS, Ousey JC, et al. Maturation of pancreatic beta-cell function in the fetal horse during late gestation. *J Endocrinol*. 2005;186:467-473.
99. Susa JB, Cowett RM, Oh W, et al. Suppression of gluconeogenesis and endogenous glucose production by exogenous insulin administration in the newborn lamb. *Pediatr Res*. 1979;13:594-598.
100. Clark MG, Filsell OH, Jarrett IG. Gluconeogenesis in isolated intact lamb liver cells. Effects of glucagon and butyrate. *Biochem J*. 1976;156:671-680.
101. Curnow RT, Rayfield EJ, George DT, et al. Control of hepatic glycogen metabolism in the rhesus monkey: effect of glucose, insulin, and glucagon administration. *Am J Physiol*. 1975;228:80-87.
102. Cowett RM. Decreased response to catecholamines in the newborn: effect on glucose kinetics in the lamb. *Metabolism*. 1988;37:736-740.
103. Cowett RM. Alpha-adrenergic agonists stimulate neonatal glucose production less than beta-adrenergic agonists in the lamb. *Metabolism*. 1988;37:831-836.
104. Cowett RM, Rapoza RE, Gelardi NL. Insulin counterregulatory hormones are ineffective in neonatal hyperinsulinemichypoglycemia. *Metabolism*. 1999;48:568-574.
109. Lafeber HN, Sulkers EJ, Chapman TE, et al. Glucose production and oxidation in preterm infants during total parenteral nutrition. *Pediatr Res*. 1990;28:153-157.
110. Yunis KA, Oh W, Kalhan S, et al. Glucose kinetics following administration of an intravenous fat emulsion to low-birth-weight neonates. *Am J Physiol*. 1992;263:E844-849.
111. Morgan C. The potential risks and benefits of insulin treatment in hyperglycaemic preterm neonates. *Early Hum Dev*. 2015;91:655-659.
112. Cowett RM, Andersen GE, Maguire CA, et al. Ontogeny of glucose homeostasis in low birth weight infants. *J Pediatr*. 1988;112:462-465.
113. Kalhan SC, Oliven A, King KC, et al. Role of glucose in the regulation of endogenous glucose production in the human newborn. *Pediatr Res*. 1986;20:49-52.
114. Denne SC, Karn CA, Wang J, et al. Effect of intravenous glucose and lipid on proteolysis and glucose production in normal newborns. *Am J Physiol*. 1995;269:E361-367.
115. Ostertag SG, Jovanovic L, Lewis B, et al. Insulin pump therapy in the very low birth weight infant. *Pediatrics*. 1986;78:625-630.

39 Cell Glucose Transport and Glucose Handling During Fetal and Neonatal Development

Rebecca A. Simmons

INTRODUCTION

Glucose is the primary substrate for the growing and developing fetus, and in normal human pregnancies there is little fetal gluconeogenesis. Glucose is required by most cells for oxidative and nonoxidative adenosine triphosphate (ATP) production and serves as a precursor for other carbon-containing compounds. It is the primary fuel used for several specialized cells and is the major fuel used by the brain. Its storage in the liver as glycogen provides a means by which glucose homeostasis can be maintained, particularly during the neonatal period. Glycogen stores also represent the primary source of energy for muscle tissue during exercise in postnatal life. Because of the diverse metabolic roles played by glucose, defects in its uptake or metabolism can alter cellular functions and can lead to significant morbidity and mortality. This chapter focuses on the molecular biology and regulation of glucose transporters (GLUTs) in the fetus and newborn.

The plasma membranes of most mammalian cells, except those of the proximal kidney and small intestine, have a passively mediated transport system for glucose. Facilitative entry of glucose into the cell is controlled by GLUTs, structurally related proteins that are encoded by a gene family[1-7] and are expressed in a tissue-specific manner. A different family of proteins, sodium (Na^+)-coupled transporters (SLGTs), actively transport glucose across the apical membranes of polarized intestinal and renal epithelial cells.[8-13] The driving force for active glucose absorption is the electrochemical Na^+ gradient across the membrane.

Most cells contain at least one GLUT isoform, and many contain more than one (Table 39.1). Furthermore, there are changes in distribution during development (Table 39.2). In most cell types, GLUTs mediate a net uptake of glucose. Under some circumstances, glucose is transported out of the cell. For example, the Na^+-coupled transporter actively transports glucose into epithelial cells of the small intestine, and a facilitative transporter mediates the efflux of glucose from the cell into the interstitium.

Table 39.1 Tissue Distribution of Known Glucose Transporters.

GLUT (Gene Name)	Chromosomal Localization	Tissue Localization	Substrate Specificity
GLUT1 *(SLC2A1)*	1p35-31.3	Ubiquitous distribution in tissues and culture cells	Glucose/galactose
GLUT4 *(SLC2A4)*	17p13	Muscle, fat, heart	Glucose, not galactose
GLUT3 *(SLC2A3)*	12p13.3	Brain and nerve cells	Glucose/galactose
GLUT14 *(SLC2A14)*		Testis	Glucose/galactose
GLUT2 *(SLC2A2)*	3q26-1-q26.2	Liver, islets, kidney, small intestine	Glucose/galactose/fructose
GLUT5 *(SLC2A5)*	1p36.2	Intestine, kidney, testis	Fructose/glucose
GLUT7 *(SLC2A7)*	1p36.22	Small intestine, colon, testis	Glucose/fructose, not galactose
GLUT9 *(SLC2A9)*	4p16-p15.3	Liver, kidney	Glucose/fructose, not galactose
GLUT11 *(SLC2A11)*	22q11.2	Heart, muscle	Glucose/fructose, not galactose
GLUT6 *(SLC2A6)*	9q34	Spleen, leucocytes, brain	Glucose
GLUT8 *(SLC2A8)*	9q33.3	Testis, blastocyst, brain, muscle, adipocytes	Glucose/fructose
GLUT10 *(SLC2A10)*	20q13.1	Liver, pancreas	Glucose/galactose, not fructose
GLUT12 *(SLC2A12)*	6q23.2	Heart, prostrate, mammary gland	Glucose/galactose/fructose
HMIT *(SLC2A13)*	12q12	Brain	Myoinositol

GLUT, Glucose transporter; *HMIT*, H+/myoinositol cotransporter.

Table 39.2 Ontogeny of Glucose Transporters.

Embryo	Placenta	Postnatal Brain	Postnatal Lung	Postnatal Liver	Postnatal Muscle
GLUT1[a] Trophectoderm, inner cell mass	GLUT1 syncytiotrophoblast, fetal endothelial cell	GLUT1[a] Vasculature, meninges, ependyma, choroid plexus, glial cells	GLUT1	GLUT1	GLUT1
GLUT2 Trophectoderm, 8-cell embryo	GLUT3 vascular endothelium	GLUT2 cerebellum		GLUT2[a]	GLUT4[a]
GLUT3[a] trophectoderm		GLUT3 cerebellum			
GLUT8 Blastocele					

[a]Major glucose transporters.
GLUT, Glucose transporter.

In hepatocytes, facilitative GLUTs are responsible for the uptake of glucose from the portal circulation and for the release of glucose generated by glycogenolysis or gluconeogenesis. Thus GLUTs ensure efficient tissue uptake and distribution of glucose.

SODIUM-DEPENDENT GLUCOSE TRANSPORTERS

It has long been known that dietary sugars are actively absorbed from the small intestine; however, only recently has the molecular mechanism been elucidated. Active absorption of glucose across epithelial cells of the small intestine and the kidney proximal tubule is accomplished by Na^+-glucose cotransporters located in the brush border membranes. Transport of each glucose molecule is coupled to the cotransport of two Na^+ ions (SGLT1) or of one Na^+ ion (SGLT2). This transport system uses the energy from an extracellular to intracellular Na^+ ion electrochemical gradient, generated by Na^+,K^+-ATPases, to drive the accumulation of glucose into the cell. These transporters belong to a major class of membrane proteins called *cotransporters* (or *symporters*) and exist in bacteria, plants, and animal membranes, and they actively transport sugars, amino acids, carboxylic acids, and some ions (chloride, phosphate, sulfate, iodide) into cells.

SGLT1 is a hydrophobic integral membrane protein with approximately 12 membrane-spanning domains. The gene encoding the human intestinal SGLT has been localized to the q11.2-qter region of chromosome 22.[14] SGLT1 is a high-affinity, low-capacity transporter protein and is abundantly expressed in the brush border of the small intestine and at lower levels in kidney, lung, heart, pancreas, eyes, tongue, prostate, uterus, salivary glands, and liver.[15-19]

Clinical interest in the intestinal brush border Na^+-glucose cotransporter has focused on diarrhea and malabsorption. Glucose-galactose malabsorption is a rare autosomal recessive disorder characterized by onset of severe, watery diarrhea in the newborn period. Unless glucose and galactose are eliminated from the diet, death rapidly ensues. Wright and colleagues demonstrated that a single missense mutation in the gene encoding the intestinal Na^+-glucose cotransporter is sufficient to cause life-threatening diarrhea.[20]

SGLT2 complementary DNA (cDNA) was originally isolated by Hediger and colleagues from a human cDNA library.[8] The SGLT amino acid sequences are approximately 60% identical to those of SGLT1, and the proteins have the same predicted secondary structure. The expression of this cotransporter is restricted to the renal cortex and is located in epithelial cells of proximal tubule S1 segments. It is generally thought that the bulk of the filtered glucose is reabsorbed in the proximal convoluted tubule by a low-affinity, high-capacity SGLT2 and that the remainder is reabsorbed by the high-affinity cotransporter SGLT1.

Familial renal glycosuria is an autosomal dominant disorder (an autosomal recessive mode of inheritance has not been excluded in all cases) affecting 0.2% to 0.6% of the general population and is characterized by the excretion of large amounts of glucose into the urine in the presence of normal blood glucose concentrations. The molecular basis of benign renal glycosuria has not been determined. It is possible that mutations in the low-affinity Na^+-glucose cotransporter SGLT2 may be responsible for the defect in renal absorption of filtered glucose.

Na^+-glucose cotransporters appear to be active prenatally, and, as a consequence, the intestine is ready to absorb the first ingested glucose.[21] The cloned cDNAs and specific antibodies for the different Na^+-glucose cotransporters will be valuable tools for identifying the specific cells in the intestine and kidney that express these proteins and for studying the regulation of their expression during development and in altered metabolic states such as diabetes mellitus or pregnancy.

There has been a great deal of interest in the development of novel agents to inhibit SGLT2 as a means to control glucose levels and augment calorie-wasting leading to weight loss in adults with type 2 diabetes.[22] However, to date, there are no studies on the safety and efficacy of this class of drugs in pregnancy.

FACILITATED GLUCOSE TRANSPORTERS

The energy-independent process of transporting glucose across the cell membrane occurs by facilitative diffusion. Transport of glucose is saturable, stereoselective, and bidirectional. The kinetics of glucose transport inward and outward are not necessarily identical,[23] and, in fact, in the erythrocyte, the rate of exchange flux for glucose is faster than net flux. The primary function of the facilitative GLUTs is to mediate the exchange of glucose between blood and the cytoplasm of the cell. This may involve a net uptake or output of glucose from the cell, depending on the type of cell in question, its metabolic state, and the metabolic state of the organisms. In most cells, cytoplasmic glucose is rapidly phosphorylated by hexokinase or glucokinase, levels of glucose-6-phosphatase are low, and therefore there is little intracellular free glucose. These cells are involved only in net uptake and metabolism of blood glucose. The hepatocyte is also a net producer of glucose in the postabsorptive state. Glycogenolysis and gluconeogenesis increase intracellular free glucose to levels greater than its concentration in the blood and result in net efflux of glucose from the cell. In the postprandial state, glucose is transported into the hepatocyte to replenish glycogen stores.

The facilitative GLUTs comprise a family of structurally related proteins. Six facilitated GLUT isoforms have been identified and are designated GLUT, and the gene name is *SLC2A*.[2,3,24-28] Several additional GLUTs (see Table 39.1) have been identified.[29-33] Isoforms are expressed in a tissue-specific manner, reflecting the unique glucose requirements of various tissues.

These proteins vary in size from 492 to 524 amino acids. They exhibit 39% to 68% sequence identity and 50% to 76% sequence similarity in pairwise comparisons.[1,3,25,26,34-39] A topology map of the GLUTs has been proposed based on analysis of the primary amino acid sequence of GLUT1.[26] Each isoform consists of 12 membrane-spanning domains, an intracytoplasmic hydrophilic loop, and an exofacial loop bearing a single *N*-glycosylation site. Both the amino and carboxy terminals are exposed intracellularly (Fig. 39.1). Comparisons among the different isoforms have revealed that the sequences of the transmembrane segments and the short cytoplasmic loops connecting these transmembrane regions are highly conserved. Most likely, these regions are responsible for the transport of glucose. The NH_2 and COOH-terminals are unique for each of the different isoforms and may contribute to isoform-specific properties, such as kinetics, hormone sensitivity, and subcellular localization.[1,3,24-26,28,35-39]

STRUCTURE AND PROPERTIES OF FACILITATIVE GLUCOSE TRANSPORTERS

GLUCOSE TRANSPORTER 1 (SLC2A1)

GLUT1 was the first GLUT to be cloned. Antibodies were raised against the purified erythrocyte GLUT to screen antigen-expression cDNA libraries from RNA from a human hepatoblastoma cell line (HepG2). The amino acid sequence of GLUT1 is highly conserved. There is 98% identity between the sequences of human and rat GLUT1 and 97% identity between the sequences of human and mouse, rabbit, or pig. This high degree of sequence conservation implies that all domains of this 492-residue protein are functionally important.

GLUT1 is the most ubiquitously distributed of the transporter isoforms. It is found in virtually all tissues of the fetus and in many tissues and cell types of the adult.[40-47] GLUT1 has a very high affinity for glucose. These properties make it likely that GLUT1 is responsible for constitutive glucose uptake. In many organs, GLUT1 is concentrated in endothelial cells of blood-tissue barriers. Thus one of the specialized roles of GLUT1 is to shuttle glucose between blood and organs that have limited access to small solutes via passive diffusion.

GLUT1 is the predominant isoform of the fetus. This transporter is also expressed in fetal tissues that fail to express it significantly in the adult. Most fetal cells exhibit rapid growth and differentiation necessitating an increased supply of energy-producing substrates. This may be the reason for the prevalence of GLUT1 in fetal tissues. After birth, GLUT1 decreases, and other isoforms such as GLUT2 in the liver and GLUT4 in the muscle increase.[40,41,46,49] The signals responsible for the decline in GLUT1 expression during the neonatal period are not known. It is hypothesized that the switch from a carbohydrate to a fat source of fuel may induce this change in some organs.[46]

Most of the studies concerning the regulation of GLUT1 have been carried out in cultured cells and cell lines from humans and rodents. GLUT1 expression is induced by growth factors. Growth factors and hormones such as insulin, insulin-like growth factor-1 (IGF-1), growth hormone, glucose, estrogen, transforming growth factor-β, thyroid hormone, cyclic adenosine monophosphate, fibroblast growth factor, and oncogenes increase GLUT1 expression in many different cell types.[47-57] Few studies have examined the regulation of GLUT1 in vivo, and data regarding GLUT1 regulation in the human fetus are scarce. These reports are discussed later.

GLUCOSE TRANSPORTER 2

GLUT2 is the major transporter isoform expressed in adult liver, pancreatic β cells, and epithelial cells of the intestinal mucosa and kidney.[35-37] Levels of this isoform are quite low in the fetus. GLUT2 has 55% amino acid identity with sequences of GLUT1, and it has a similar structure and orientation in the plasma membrane. In contrast to GLUT1, whose sequence is highly conserved, there is only 81% identity between the sequences of human and rat GLUT2. The most characteristic feature of this isoform is its low affinity for glucose. GLUT2 and glucokinase form a glucose-sensing apparatus in hepatocytes and β cells that responds to subtle changes in blood glucose concentrations by altering the rate of glucose transport into the cell. The transport capacity of GLUT2 is in excess of the glucokinase trapping reaction, thus making phosphorylation of glucose the rate-limiting step for glucose uptake in hepatocytes and β cells. In the intestine and kidney, the high-capacity, low-affinity system is necessary to transport glucose under conditions of large transepithelial substrate fluxes that occur after meals.

Expression of GLUT2 appears to be developmentally regulated. β Cell content of GLUT2 protein in the fetus is approximately

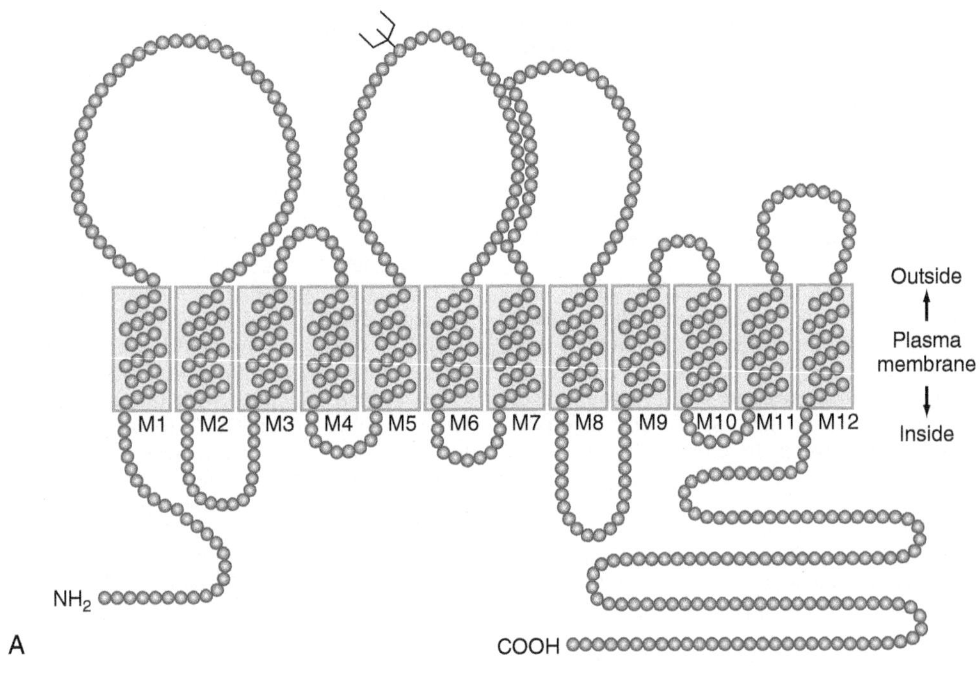

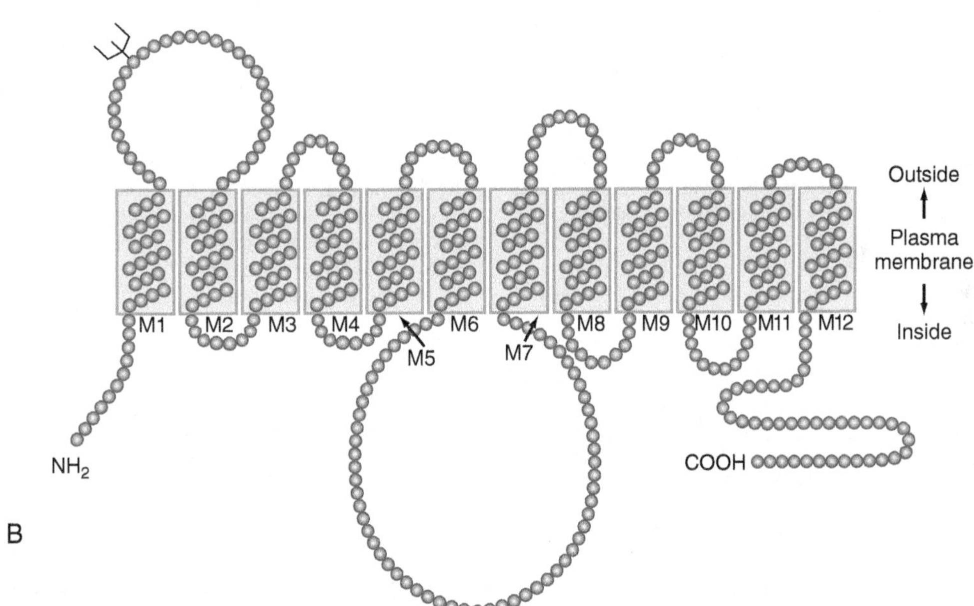

Fig. 39.1 Models for the orientation of the human sodium/glucose cotransporter SGLT1 (A) and members of the facilitative glucose-transporter family (GLUT1 to GLUT5) in the plasma membrane (B). The 12 potential membrane-spanning α-helices are shown as *boxes* and are numbered M1 to M12.

half that of the adult rat.[58] Despite the reduction in GLUT2 content, the blunted insulin secretory response seen in fetal islet cells is not the result of a limitation of glucose transport. At least a 10-fold decrease in transport activity would be required to reduce metabolism of glucose sufficient to perturb glucose-induced insulin secretion.[59,60] Other factors appear to be responsible for the blunted insulin secretory response observed in the fetus.

Studies done in fetal rats have demonstrated that GLUT2 levels are markedly diminished in fetal hepatocytes compared with the adult.[61-64] Shortly after birth, GLUT2 protein content dramatically rises and increases again, coinciding with the newborn pup's weaning from high-fat maternal milk.[57,58] Although an altered hormonal or substrate milieu is often implicated etiologically in the metabolic maturation associated with birth, the mechanism of this change is still unknown.

GLUCOSE TRANSPORTER 3

GLUT3 was first isolated from human fetal skeletal muscle.[65] Human GLUT3 has 64% and 52% identity with human GLUT1 and GLUT2, respectively, with an 83% amino acid sequence identity between the sequences of human and mouse GLUT3. Thus, as with GLUT2, the sequence of GLUT3 is not as highly conserved among species as that of GLUT1. GLUT3 messenger RNA (mRNA) is present at variable levels in all human tissues and is most abundant in brain, kidney, and placenta. The ubiquitous distribution of GLUT3 in human tissues suggests that it, together with GLUT1, may be responsible for basal glucose transport. In other animals such as rats, monkeys, and mice, the pattern of expression of GLUT3 is much different from that observed in humans.[3] In these animals, GLUT3 is abundant only in brain. The expression of GLUT3 in brain indicates that two facilitative GLUTs are involved in the uptake of glucose. GLUT1 is primarily responsible for transport of glucose across the blood-brain barrier, and GLUT3 controls the uptake of glucose into the neuron.

There is relatively little information available about the regulation of GLUT3. Studies done in fetal rat brain suggest that glucose concentrations do not regulate expression of this transporter isoform.[66] This finding is in contrast to GLUT1, in which high levels of glucose down-regulate GLUT1 protein and mRNA abundance.[50] In contrast to glucose, chronic hypoxia increases GLUT3 mRNA expression in embryonic (day 14) rodent brain.[67]

GLUCOSE TRANSPORTER 4

GLUT4 is primarily expressed in adult tissues that exhibit insulin-stimulated glucose transport, such as adipose tissue and skeletal and cardiac muscle.[50] Low levels are also expressed in fetal rat brain.[67] Compared with the adult, little GLUT4 is expressed in fetal muscle[50] and brown fat,[68] and levels do not increase until well after birth.[44,46,68] The sequence of human GLUT4 is highly conserved, and there is 95% and 96% identity between the sequences of human and rat or mouse GLUT4.[69]

Insulin causes a rapid and reversible increase in glucose uptake in adipocytes and skeletal muscle. This increase results primarily from translocation of a latent pool of GLUTs from intracellular vesicles[70] to the plasma membrane. Glucose transport in the insulin-sensitive tissues has received considerable attention because of the importance of this process in the maintenance of whole-body glucose disposal. The transport step is rate limiting for glucose uptake into fat and muscle under most conditions.[71,72]

GLUCOSE TRANSPORTER 5

GLUT5 is the most divergent member of the GLUT family.[28] Human GLUT5 shares 42%, 40%, 39%, and 42% identity with human GLUT1, GLUT2, GLUT3, and GLUT4, respectively.[73] GLUT5 is expressed at high levels in the apical membrane of intestinal enterocytes and mature spermatocytes in adults. Fructose is transported across intestinal epithelial cells by passive transport. There is also a high rate of fructose utilization by testes. In view of these findings, it seems likely that GLUT5 is the major mammalian fructose transporter.

GLUT5 is also found in smaller quantities in adult human kidney, brain, muscle, and adipose tissue.[74,75] The physiologic significance of GLUT5 in these tissues is unknown.

NOVEL GLUCOSE TRANSPORTERS

The facilitative GLUTs GLUT1 to GLUT4 have considerable sequence similarity and different tissue distributions. Other similar sequences have also been cloned. GLUT6, a pseudogene, is not thought to encode a functional glucose transport protein.[34] GLUT7, originally cloned from a rat liver library, had been proposed to encode an endoplasmic reticulum protein that would facilitate the glucose produced by glucose-6-phosphatase produced in the endoplasmic reticulum lumen to reach the cytosol.[76] However, more recent studies from the same laboratory were unable to demonstrate that neither rat nor human liver RNA normally contains mRNA equivalent to the clone termed *GLUT7*.[77]

Although the diverse tissue distribution and the specific functions of GLUT1 to GLUT5 appear to indicate that these genes are sufficient to control glucose uptake in all mammalian tissues, it is likely that additional sugar transport facilitators exist. By searching the expressed sequence tag (EST) databases and taking advantage of the conserved sugar transporter signatures, several novel GLUT-like genes have been identified.

GLUT8 exhibits significant sequence similarity with the GLUT1 (29.4%).[29,30] In human tissues, it is predominantly found in testis, and lower amounts are detected in most other tissues, including skeletal muscle, heart, small intestine, and brain.[29,30] GLUT8 is expressed in testis only from adult, not from prepubertal, rats, and expression is markedly inhibited by estrogen treatment.[29] Thus GLUT8 may be involved in the provision of glucose required for DNA synthesis in male germ cells. GLUT8 has also been found to be the GLUT responsible for insulin-stimulated glucose uptake in the blastocyst.[30]

GLUT9 (44.8% amino acid identity with GLUT8) is detected in human spleen, peripheral leukocytes, and brain.[31,32] GLUT10 (35% sequence identity with human GLUT1 to GLUT8) is the latest member of the GLUT to be cloned and is expressed in human heart, lung, brain, liver, skeletal muscle, kidney, and placenta.[33] It is also detected in fetal brain and liver.[33] Table 39.1 shows the distribution of identified glucose tranporters to date.

LOCALIZATION AND REGULATION OF FACILITATIVE GLUCOSE TRANSPORTERS

EMBRYO

Reverse transcriptase polymerase chain reaction, immunofluorescence, and immunoelectron microscopy techniques have confirmed that GLUT1 is expressed in all stages of embryonic development of the mouse, rat, rabbit, cow, and human, including the oocyte and the blastocyst. It is readily detectable in trophectoderm and inner cell mass cells of the mouse blastocyst, and it is associated with intracellular membranes and plasma membranes of all cell types.[78-81] It helps in the implantation of the embryo by its increased expression in the endometrium and the basolateral surface of the polarized trophectodermal cells and the inner cell mass under the influence of the hormones estrogen and progesterone.[82] During organogenesis in the rat embryo, GLUT1 is localized to the neural tube, as well as the heart tube, gut, and optic vesicle.[83]

GLUT2 also appears to be an important mediator of glucose uptake in the early embryo and is essential for embryonic survival.[84] GLUT2 can transport the amino sugar glucosamine, and maternally derived glucosamine is needed for biomass accumulation by the embryo.[84] GLUT2 is expressed as early as the eight-cell blastocyst stage. It is located on trophoectoderm membranes facing the blastocyst cavity.[78,80]

Expression of GLUT3 appears by day 4 of gestation (in rat), and it is found on the apical membranes of trophoectoderm cells and seems to be responsible for the uptake of maternal glucose.[83,85] GLUT8 is primarily expressed within vesicles in the cells lining the blastocoele.[30] Insulin and IGF-1 stimulate translocation of GLUT8 to the plasma membrane of these cells via binding to the IGF-1 receptor.[30] Studies suggest that GLUT8 expression and translocation in response to insulin are critical for blastocyst survival.[86] However, the physiologic role that insulin-regulated GLUTs play in vivo in the human blastocyst remains to be determined.

One of the characteristics displayed by preimplantation embryos is the metabolic shift from a dependence on the tricarboxylic acid cycle during the precompactation stages to a metabolism based on glycolysis after compactation.[87] This change in substrate utilization is coincident with the rapid proliferation that occurs during this developmental stage. Similar changes in substrate preference occur in numerous other cells as the undergo proliferation. Therefore high-affinity GLUTs such as GLUT1 and GLUT3 are required for glucose uptake.

Pregnant women with diabetes are at increased risk for both first trimester spontaneous abortions and major fetal malformations. Data suggest that hyperglycemia-induced apoptosis in the embryo may contribute to early pregnancy loss.[88,89] Preimplantation studies have shown that maternal hyperglycemia down-regulates GLUT1, GLUT2, and GLUT3 at the blastocyst stage of development,[90] which is associated with increased apoptosis.[88] Only 40% of the cells showed evidence of apoptosis, which has been shown to result in neural tube defects, limb abnormalities, and abdominal wall malformations, similar to malformations seen among infants of diabetic women.[91]

PLACENTA

In the human placenta, placental villi are in direct contact with maternal blood. The surface of the placental villi is covered with a single syncytiotrophoblast layer, formed by the fusion of the underlying cytotrophoblast elements. Fetal capillaries lie directly beneath the syncytiotrophoblast. Transfer of glucose from maternal to fetal blood occurs via the placental villi and is most likely mediated by GLUT1. It has been recently reported that approximately 70% of the glucose taken up from maternal blood is allocated to the fetus and approximately 30% is consumed by the placenta suggesting that fetal glucose consumption is balanced against the placental needs for glucose and that placental glucose consumption is a key modulator of maternal-fetal glucose transfer in women.[92] Interestingly, in this in vivo study GLUT1 expression was not positively correlated with birth weight, fetal glucose consumption, and glucose in the umbilical vein suggesting that fetal glucose consumption is not affected by basal membrane GLUT1 expression in normal pregnancies. However, they did observe a positive correlation between basal membrane and microvillous membrane GLUT 1 expression and umbilical artery glucose concentrations, providing some support for the concept that the abundance of GLUTs in the placental barrier contributes to transplacental glucose transport.[92]

GLUT1 is abundantly expressed in the plasma membranes of both the basal and apical sides of the syncytiotrophoblast. GLUT1 may facilitate the entry of glucose into the cytoplasm of the syncytiotrophoblast from maternal blood, whereas GLUT1 at the basal plasma membrane may aid in the exit of glucose from the cytoplasm of the syncytiotrophoblast to the pericapillary space of the fetus. GLUT1 on the endothelial cell of the capillary then transfers glucose into the fetal circulation.[93-96] Protein and mRNA levels of GLUT1 increase in the placenta as the fetus matures, thus underscoring the importance of this transporter in fetal development.[85]

GLUT3 is distributed throughout placental villous tissue and decreases during gestation.[94,96-98] Although GLUT3 mRNA is abundantly expressed in villous tissue, GLUT3 protein is primarily localized to the vascular endothelium. GLUT3 may play a role in transporting glucose from mother to fetus after transsyncytial transport.

There are limited data regarding the regulation of GLUT expression in human placenta. A study in the JEG-3 human choriocarcinoma cell line, which resembles a first-trimester placental model, showed that GLUT3 expression is regulated by mTORC1, but because these studies were performed in a transformed cell line, it remains to be determined how GLUT3 expression is regulated in vivo in the human.[99]

A few studies have been carried out in placentas from pregnancies complicated by intrauterine growth retardation and diabetes. Growth-retarded fetuses are often hypoglycemic, and impaired placental glucose transport has been implicated as a pathophysiologic mechanism. Growth-retarded fetuses have a reduced umbilical venoarterial concentration difference in glucose and lower fetal weight-specific umbilical volume flow.[100,101] A decrease in placental GLUT1 expression has been shown in intrauterine growth restriction (IUGR) concomitant with reduced fetal growth.[102]

The levels of placental GLUT3 expression appear to be altered by maternal diabetes and IUGR in humans. GLUT3 is increased in human IUGR placenta.[103] In rodents, there is a reduction of placental GLUT3 levels in IUGR in mice.[104] Furthermore, birth weight corresponded to placental weight, indicating that the total amount of GLUT3 is increased in macrosomia and reduced in IUGR.[105]

Gestational diabetes is associated with placenta overgrowth and an increase in transplacental glucose transfer to the fetus. Levels of GLUT1 protein are increased in the basal membranes and lead to an increase in glucose transport activity of syncytial basal membranes.[106,107] Microvillous expression and activity are unaffected by hyperglycemia.[95,96] Likewise, levels of GLUT4 are not altered in placentas of women with diabetes during pregnancy.[105,108] Thus it appears from these studies that increased glucose transport to the fetus of the diabetic mother is facilitated by increased levels of GLUT1. Illsley proposed that this process leads to fetal hyperglycemia, which, in turn, stimulates the production of IGF-1 leading to excess fetoplacental growth.[109]

BRAIN

Brain glucose utilization accounts for approximately 80% of whole-body glucose disposal in humans.[110] Furthermore, there is heterogeneity in glucose utilization among different regions of the brain. Circulating glucose crosses the blood-brain barrier and enters brain parenchyma cells via facilitative GLUTs. Most studies of GLUT expression in the nervous system of the developing animal have been performed in the rat. Before the formation of the blood-brain barrier, GLUT1 is abundant in the germinal neuroepithelium, which gives rise to both neurons and neuroglia.[111] Just before birth, GLUT1 is abundant in the brain vasculature, meninges, ependyma, and choroid plexus. After birth, GLUT1 is also found in glial cells.[111,112] GLUT1 is developmentally regulated in rat and rabbit brain.[41-43] Its expression is highest in adult brain, followed by fetal and neonatal brain, respectively.

Few localization studies have been done in the human fetus. One report has demonstrated that the localization of GLUT1 in the mid-gestation to late-gestation human fetus is similar to the rat; that is, it is primarily located in the microvascular endothelial cells that constitute the blood-brain barrier.[113] However, a more recent study suggested a much wider distribution of GLUT1 in the developing brain.[112] From 10 to 21 weeks of gestation, GLUT1 is expressed in all regions of the fetal brain and is primarily present in the endothelial cells of the brain capillaries, in the epithelial cells of the choroid plexus, and in neurons.[112] GLUT2 is not expressed until mid-gestation (21 weeks), and at that time it is highly expressed in the granular layer of the cerebellum.[112] No study to date has been able to detect GLUT3 or GLUT4 in human fetal brain.

After birth, GLUT3 is found in the cerebellum in neurofilament-positive cellular transverse fibers, cell bodies of Purkinje cells, and other neuronal elements in close proximity to the Purkinje layer.[113] This region-specific pattern of GLUT3 expression may reflect the differing glucose needs of anatomically distinct regions of the brain. Localization of GLUT3 is similar to the distribution of glucose utilization, which during early infancy is mainly infratentorial and later in development occurs in supratentorial structures as well.[114,115]

Regulation of glucose transport in the fetal brain is uniquely different from that in the adult. Before birth, low levels of glucose (in vivo or in vitro) fail to up-regulate glucose transport in whole fetal rat brain[66] or isolated glial cells. However, after birth, hypoglycemia induces a marked increase in GLUT1 expression[116] in whole rat brain isolated glial cells. Furthermore, glucose transport in the fetal brain does not respond to insulin or IGF-1,[48] two hormones that increase GLUT1 expression in glial cells of older animals.[117-118] The mechanisms underlying these differences in regulation of glucose transport that occur with maturation are unknown. In contrast to glucose, hypoxia during gestation does induce a marked increase in GLUT3 levels in fetal rat brain.[67] In contrast, experimentally induced growth restriction in the ovine fetus is associated with a reduction of GLUT1 immunoreactivity in vascular endothelium in fetal brain.[119]

LUNG

Glucose is an important metabolic substrate for the lung and provides carbon moieties for energy production and synthesis of surfactant. In adult lung, transport of glucose across the apical membrane of the type II pneumocyte occurs by Na^+-coupled transport,[120-122] and it occurs across the basolateral membrane by facilitative glucose transport. To date, GLUT1 is the only isoform found to be expressed in type II pneumocytes of fetal rats and humans.[123] It is hypothesized that SGLT1 is also expressed in type II pneumocytes; however, no study has thus far been able to localize this transporter in fetal lung.

GLUT1 is abundantly expressed in the fetal lung when compared with that of the juvenile and adult rat.[41] Glucose utilization and levels of GLUT1 mRNA and protein dramatically decline as the animal matures.[47,124] By day 14 of life, GLUT1 is undetectable in rat pups. The factors responsible for this significant decrease in the synthesis of GLUT1 are unknown.

Insulin and IGF-1 are important modulators of glucose transport in type II pneumocytes of fetal rats. Physiologic levels of insulin and IGF-1 stimulate glucose transport,[47] whereas higher levels of insulin inhibit glucose uptake.[125] Several animal studies suggest that hyperinsulinemia, through its inhibitory effects on glucose transport, contributes to the decrease in surfactant synthesis observed in infants of diabetic mothers. In a model that somewhat mimics human gestational diabetes, diabetes is induced in pregnant rats by streptozotocin. Fetal rats are hyperglycemic, hyperinsulinemic, and large for gestational age. Type II pneumocytes from these animals exhibit markedly diminished glucose uptake and GLUT1 expression.[126] It is possible that the decrease in glucose uptake diminishes the supply of glucose available for surfactant synthesis. This could be one factor that increases the risk of respiratory distress syndrome in infants of diabetic mothers. Similarly, in a sheep model of maternal late gestation overnutrition, there was a decrease in the numerical density of surfactant protein positive cells, as well as a reduction in mRNA expression of surfactant proteins (SFTP-A, -B, and -C) and GLUT1 in the fetal lung.[127]

Male fetuses exhibit delayed lung maturation and surfactant production in comparison with female fetuses. This delay may be related to sex hormone effects: estrogen enhances and androgens delay lung development. The uptake of glucose, an important precursor for surfactant synthesis, appears to be differently affected by estrogen and androgens. In vitro studies performed in fetal rat have shown that estradiol and dehydrotestosterone differentially regulate glucose uptake in fetal rat lung tissue. This regulation of substrate supply (glucose) by estradiol and dehydrotestosterone may be another mechanism for the sexual dimorphism observed in lung development and surfactant synthesis.[128]

LIVER

Transport of glucose across the hepatocyte does not appear to be rate limiting for glucose metabolism. However, glucose transport is developmentally regulated in the human and rat, and glucose transport contributes to the changes in glucose metabolic capacity from fetal to extrauterine life. The major GLUT in the adult hepatocyte is GLUT2. GLUT1 is expressed only in perivenous hepatocytes.

In contrast, in the fetus, GLUT1 and GLUT2 are abundantly expressed in hepatocytes.[61,62,64] During the fetal to neonatal transition, there is a shift from abundant GLUT1 in the hepatocyte to an adult pattern of little GLUT1 expression.[40,63] Many metabolic and hormonal factors dramatically change during the perinatal period. The factors responsible for the switch in GLUT1 expression remain to be delineated.

Similar to other tissues, substrate availability and hormones such as cortisol have been shown to regulate hepatic glucose metabolism. For example, hepatic chronic fetal hypoglycemia (produced by maternal insulin infusion) results in a reduction in liver GLUT1 protein levels.[129]

MUSCLE

Most of the studies regarding glucose transport in muscle have been carried out in adults. As described earlier, GLUT4 is the predominant isoform expressed in adult muscle. In response to insulin, this transporter isoform significantly increases the transport of glucose into the myocyte. In contrast to the marked insulin responsiveness observed in the adult, fetal muscle only modestly responds to insulin. Insulin and IGF-1 increase GLUT1 expression 1.5-fold in normal fetal rat muscle explants,[48] compared with the 20-fold increase observed in adult muscle.[130,131] Insulin does not stimulate GLUT1 expression in isolated myoblasts from fetal rats,[46] a finding suggesting that stimulation of glucose transport by insulin requires tissue-specific additional factors.

GLUT1 is localized to the myoblast, and levels are quite high in the fetal and newborn rat pup. GLUT1 in fetal muscle is regulated by glucocorticoids, hypoxemia, decreased substrate, and increased substrate availability.[132-134]

GLUT1 decreases significantly during weaning.[46,135] It appears that the switch from GLUT1 to GLUT4 expression during this period is secondary to dietary factors. If rats are weaned to a diet rich in fat, the normal increase in GLUT4 is prevented.[46,135,136] The molecular mechanisms responsible for this observation are unknown.

KIDNEY

The kidney, small intestine, and liver can all release glucose during periods of decreased glucose availability. Although the liver is the principal supplier of glucose during short fasts, the kidney also produces glucose during prolonged starvation. The Na^+-glucose cotransporter SGLT1 transports glucose into the brush border cell of the proximal tubule of the kidney. GLUT2, localized on the basolateral membrane of epithelial cells lining renal tubules, is involved in the net release of glucose into the blood during absorption of renal glucose.

No data are available concerning the regulation of glucose transport in the fetal kidney, and only a few reports have described the ontogeny of renal glucose transport. SGLT1 is expressed in lower quantities in fetal compared with adult kidney. GLUT2 is also present in the fetal kidney, and its expression increases with maturation.

CONCLUSION

GLUTs have acquired distinct physiologic and biochemical properties that allow them to serve specific functions in the tissues in which they are expressed. An understanding of the mechanisms underlying tissue-specific expression of these transporters will facilitate an understanding of in vivo glucose utilization and clearance processes that occur normally and in disease states. Although studies in adults provide insight into the regulation of glucose transport, similar studies are required in the fetus and newborn to understand fully the role of the GLUT in fetal and neonatal development.

A complete reference list is available at www.ExpertConsult.com. 

SELECT REFERENCES

1. James DE, et al. Molecular cloning and characterization of an insulin-regulatable glucose transporter. *Nature*. 1989;333:83-87.
2. Fukumoto H, et al. Sequence, tissue distribution, and chromosomal localization of mRNA encoding a human glucose transporter-like protein. *Proc Natl Acad Sci USA*. 1988;85:5434-5438.
3. Kayano T, et al. Evidence for a family of human glucose transporter-like proteins: sequence and gene localization of a protein expressed in fetal skeletal muscle and other tissues. *J Biol Chem*. 1988;263:15245-15248.
5. Lodish HF. Anion-exchange and glucose transport proteins: structure, function, and distribution. *Harvey Lect*. 1988;82:19-46.
6. Gould GW, Bell GI. Facilitative glucose transporters: an expanding family. *Trends Biochem Sci*. 1990;15:18-22.
8. Hediger MA, et al. Expression, cloning and cDNA sequencing of the Na^+/glucose cotransporter. *Nature*. 1987;330:379-381.
14. Hediger MA, et al. Assignment of the human intestinal Na^+/glucose gene (SGLT 1) to the q 11.2-q ter region of chromosome 22. *Genomics*. 1989;4:297-300.
20. Wright EM, et al. Molecular genetics of intestinal glucose transport. *J Clin Invest*. 1991;88:1435-1440.
23. Carruthers A. Facilitative diffusion of glucose. *Physiol Rev*. 1990;70:1135-1176.
24. Birnbaum MJ. Identification of a novel gene encoding an insulin-responsive glucose transporter protein. *Cell*. 1989;57:305-315.
25. Birnbaum MJ, et al. Cloning and characterization of cDNA encoding the rat brain glucose-transporter protein. *Proc Natl Acad Sci USA*. 1986;83:5784-5788.
26. Mueckler M, et al. Sequence and structure of a human glucose transporter. *Science*. 1985;229:941-945.
27. Bell GI, et al. Structure and function of mammalian facilitative sugar transporters. *J Biol Chem*. 1993;268:19161-19164.
28. Kayano T, et al. Human facilitative glucose transporters: isolation, functional characterization, and gene localization of cDNAs encoding an isoform (Glut 5) expressed in small intestine, kidney, muscle, and adipose tissue and an unusual glucose transporter pseudo-gene-like sequence (Glut 6). *J Biol Chem*. 1990;265:13276-13282.
30. Carayannopoulos MO, et al. GLUT 8 is a glucose transporter responsible for insulin-stimulated glucose uptake in the blastocyst. *Proc Natl Acad Sci USA*. 2000;97:7313-7318.
31. Phay JE, et al. Cloning and expression analysis of a novel member of the facilitative glucose transporter family, SLC2A9 (GLUT 9). *Genomics*. 2000;6:217-220.
33. Dawson PA, et al. Sequence and functional analysis of GLUT10: a glucose transporter in the type 2 diabetes-linked region of chromosome 20q12-13.1. *Mol Genet Metab*. 2001;74:186-199.
38. Fukumoto H, et al. Cloning and characterization of the major insulin-responsive glucose transporter expressed in human skeletal muscle and other insulin-responsive tissues. *J Biol Chem*. 1989;264:7776-7779.
40. Werner H, et al. Developmental regulation of rat brain/Hep G2 glucose transporter gene expression. *Mol Endocrinol*. 1989;3:273-279.
41. Sadiq F, et al. The ontogeny of the rabbit brain glucose transporter. *Endocrinology*. 1990;126:2417-2424.
42. Sivitz W, et al. Regulation of the glucose transporter in developing rat brain. *Endocrinology*. 1989;124:1875-1880.
43. Devaskar S, et al. Developmental regulation of the distribution of rat brain insulin-insensitive (Glut 1) glucose transporter. *Endocrinology*. 1991;129:1530-1540.
44. Santalucia T, et al. Developmental regulation of Glut 1 (erythroid/Hep2) and Glut 4 glucose transporter expression in rat heart, skeletal muscle, and brown adipose tissue. *Endocrinology*. 1992;130:837-846.
46. Leturque A, et al. Nutritional regulation of glucose transporter and adipose tissue of weaned rats. *Am J Physiol*. 1991;260:E588-E593.
47. Simmons RA, et al. Glut 1 gene expression in growth-retarded juvenile rats. *Pediatr Res*. 1994;35:382A.
48. Simmons RA, et al. The effect of insulin and IGF-I upon glucose transport in normal and small for gestational age fetal rats. *Endocrinology*. 1993;133:1361-1368.
50. Simmons RA, et al. Glucose regulated Glut 1 function and expression in fetal rat lung and muscle in vitro. *Endocrinology*. 1993;132:2312-2318.
51. Hart CD, et al. Modulation of glucose transport in fetal rat lung by estrogen and dihydrotestosterone. *Pediatr Res*. 1995;37:335A.
55. Leuthner SR, et al. Regulation of Glut 1 gene expression by cAMP in fetal rat brain. *Pediatr Res*. 1994;35:382A.
59. Meglasson MD, Matschinsky FM. Pancreatic islet glucose metabolism and regulation of insulin secretion. *Diabetes Metab Rev*. 1986;2:163-214.
61. Lane RH, et al. Localization and quantification of glucose transporters in liver of growth retarded fetal and neonatal rats. *Am J Physiol*. 1998;276:E135-E142.
62. Lane RH, et al. Measurement of GLUT mRNA in liver of fetal and neonatal rats using a novel method of quantitative polymerase chain reaction. *Biochem Mol Med*. 1996;59:192-199.
63. Postic C, et al. Development and regulation of glucose transporter and hexokinase expression in rat. *Am J Physiol*. 1994;266:E548-E559.
64. Levitsky LL, et al. Glut 1 and Glut 2 mRNA, protein, and glucose transporter activity in cultured fetal and adult hepatocytes. *Am J Physiol*. 1994;267:E88-E94.
65. Yano H, et al. Tissue distribution and species difference of the brain type glucose transporter (Glut 3). *Biochem Biophys Res Commun*. 1991;174:470-477.
66. Simmons RA, et al. Glucose regulates Glut 1 function and gene expression in fetal rat brain. *Pediatr Res*. 1993;35:71A.
67. Royer C, et al. Effects of gestational hypoxia on mRNA levels of GLUT3 and GLUT4 transporters, hypoxia inducible factor-1 and thyroid hormone receptors in developing rat brain. *Brain Res*. 2000;856:119-128.
69. James DE, et al. Insulin-regulatable tissue express a unique insulin sensitive glucose transport protein. *Nature*. 1988;333:183-185.
73. Bell GI, et al. Molecular biology of mammalian glucose transporters. *Diabetes Care*. 1990;13:198-208.
74. Bell GI, et al. Structure and function of mammalian facilitative sugar transporters. *J Biol Chem*. 1993;268:19161-19164.
77. Burchell A. A re-evaluation of GLUT7. *Biochem J*. 1998;331:973.
83. Matsumoto K, et al. Abundant expression of Glut 1 and Glut 3 in rat embryo during the early organogenesis period. *Biochem Biophys Res Commun*. 1995;209:95-102.
84. Jung JH, et al. Embryonic stem cell proliferation stimulated by altered anabolic metabolism from glucose transporter 2-transported glucosamine. *Sci Rep*. 2016;6:28452.
90. Moley KH, et al. Maternal hyperglycemia alters glucose transport and utilization in mouse preimplantation embryos. *Am J Physiol*. 1998;275:E38-E47.
118. Werner H, et al. Regulation of rat brain/HepG2 glucose transporter gene expression by insulin and insulin-like growth factor-I in primary cultures of neuronal and glial cells. *Endocrinology*. 1989;125:314-326.
123. Simmons RA, et al. Intrauterine growth retardation: fetal glucose transport is diminished in lung but spared in brain. *Pediatr Res*. 1992;31:59-63.
124. Simmons RA, Charlton VE. Substrate utilization by the fetal sheep lung during the last trimester. *Pediatr Res*. 1988;23:606-611.
126. Simmons RA, et al. The effect of maternal diabetes on glut 1 function and expression in fetal lung. *Pediatr Res*. 1992;31:182A.
128. Hart CD, et al. Modulation of glucose transport in fetal rat lung: a sexual dimorphism. *Am J Respir Cell Mol Biol*. 1998;19:63-70.
129. Hay WW. Recent observations on the regulation of fetal metabolism by glucose. *J Physiol*. 2006;572:17-24.

General Concepts of Protein Metabolism

Chris H.P. van den Akker | Johannes (Hans) B. van Goudoever | Dwight E. Matthews

INTRODUCTION

This chapter describes the methods used to evaluate dynamic changes in protein metabolism in the newborn infant. Throughout life, proteins not only form the key structural components of cells but also have key physiologic roles as, for example, transporters, immune mediators, receptor proteins, enzymes, and hormones. In a consideration of the relevant kinetics, the fundamental point of interest is that amino acids—the building blocks of protein—differ from carbohydrates and fats *only* by the inclusion of a nitrogen (N) atom in its molecule. Alanine without its single N atom is pyruvate, which is half a glucose molecule. Similar to carbohydrates, amino acids yield 4 kcal/g if not used for protein synthesis but are oxidized to ammonia and CO_2 instead.

Proteins consist of polymers of 20 different available amino acids that vary in length from two (dipeptide) to thousands of amino acids. Proteins are synthesized after transcription and translation from DNA and RNA, respectively. Amino acids, in turn, are classified as nonessential (dispensable), essential (indispensable), or conditionally essential (Table 40.1). This distinction depends on whether they can be synthesized de novo (nonessential amino acids) or whether they can only be derived from dietary sources (essential amino acids), or whether their enzymatic synthesis capacity is suboptimal to meet total requirements during stress, disease, or otherwise increased demands (conditionally or semi-essential amino acids). If the dietary intake of any essential amino acid is too low, protein synthesis is limited by the availability of that amino acid, giving an excess of all other amino acids that would normally be integrated into protein. Those excess amino acids that are not incorporated into new protein synthesis are then oxidized.

Besides considering total protein intake, it is therefore important to acknowledge dietary protein quality as well. This relates to the amount of each essential amino acid from dietary intake (parenteral or enteral). Parenteral amino acid solutions for infants have for example higher relative amounts of (conditionally) essential amino acids as compared with solutions for adults, because of their higher growth rate and immature enzymatic systems.[1] Regarding enteral nutrition, the highest-quality source of proteins for term infants is from breast milk.

All proteins undergo a continuous process of synthesis and subsequent degradation into separate amino acids. This process can serve to replace damaged or defective proteins or to regulate the amount of a specific protein (e.g., an active enzyme). Proteins have a range of life spans from only minutes (enzymes), to slow turnover rates of up to weeks or months (e.g., muscle structural proteins and collagen), or to practically never (protein in neurons and the lens of the eye). The total amount of protein that is broken down and reconstituted every day is several times higher than the amount of protein that is derived from the diet. The net difference between protein degradation and synthesis determines whether an individual is catabolic or anabolic, leading to cachexia or growth, respectively.

Box 40.1 lists the methods used to measure protein and N metabolism in humans. Most of them will be elaborated upon later.

STUDYING GROWTH: ANTHROPOMETRY AND N BALANCE TECHNIQUES

Early nutritional studies investigated anthropometric changes (growth) to determine efficacy of the level and quality of protein in the diet of infants. However, these methods require prolonged periods of study diet and may be unethical and inaccurate.

The most widely used method to follow changes in body protein is the N balance method. This method defines the difference of N between that is going in and that coming out of the body and for long has been the standard modality for defining minimum levels of dietary protein and essential amino acid intake in humans of all ages.[2-4] This determination is done by carefully recording all food consumed and collecting all material excreted: urine, feces, sputum, and so on during at least 12 to 24 hours in neonates but preferably longer. The N from aliquots of each food, urine, and fecal collection is tediously converted to ammonia by boiling the specimens in concentrated acid. The ammonia content is determined, and N intake and excretion are calculated. In practice, N losses are routinely *underestimated* because of incomplete collections of urine and feces and insensible losses through skin, sweat, and so on, and N intake is routinely *overestimated* because of variable content or availability of protein in foods consumed, inaccurate recording of ingested amounts, and so forth.[2]

Although measures of anthropometry or N balance often have been used to study infant nutrition,[3,5] both methods require weeks or days, respectively, to measure effects. Neither method provides any information concerning the turnover of N *within* the body. For example, an infant may be receiving adequate protein but insufficient energy intake for growth. Owing to this restricted intake, the child will not grow and has a N balance of zero. When more calories are provided, the infant starts growing and shows a positive N balance. How does the child's body respond to produce this effect? N balance and growth measurements do not provide this information.

Fig. 40.1 shows four possible responses to the original clinical situation. Case 0 is the starting zero N balance. Positive N balance could be obtained by increasing protein synthesis (*case A* in the figure), decreasing protein breakdown *(case C),* increasing both protein synthesis and breakdown but with a

Table 40.1 Amino Acids Classified as Essential, Semi-essential, or Nonessential in Infants.

Essential	Semi-essential	Nonessential
Histidine	Arginine	Alanine
Isoleucine	Cysteine	Asparagine
Leucine	Glutamine	Aspartic acid (aspartate)
Lysine	Glycine	Glutamic acid (glutamate)
Methionine	Proline	Ornithine
Phenylalanine	Taurine[a]	Serine
Threonine	Tyrosine	
Tryptophan		
Valine		

[a]Not an α-amino acid (not incorporated in proteins).

Box 40.1 Methods for Measuring Protein and Nitrogen Metabolism in Humans

- Growth assessment
- Nitrogen balance method
- End-product method
- Turnover of individual components
- Essential amino acids (index of protein breakdown)
- Nonessential amino acids (de novo synthesis and gluconeogenesis)
- Urea (protein oxidation)
- Arteriovenous measurement of amino acid concentrations across a tissue bed
- Protein synthesis of a specific protein by following tracer incorporation
- Protein degradation of a specific protein by following disappearance of tracer from the protein

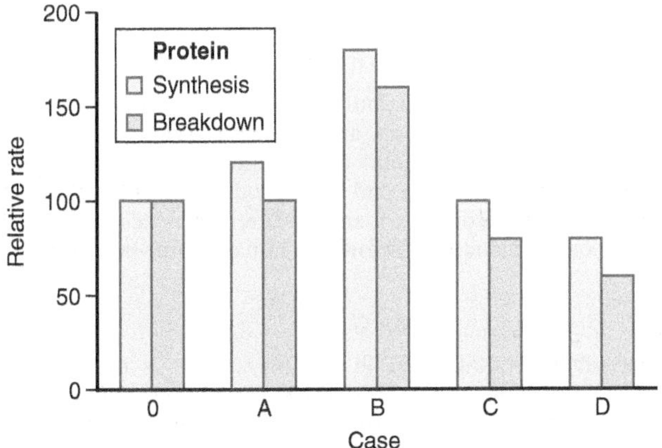

Fig. 40.1 Four different hypothetical responses to a change from a zero balance (case 0) to a positive nitrogen balance (cases A to D). A positive nitrogen balance can be obtained by increasing protein synthesis, as in case A; by increasing synthesis more than breakdown, as in case B; by decreasing breakdown, as in case C; or by decreasing breakdown more than synthesis, as in case D. The nitrogen balance method does not distinguish among any of the four possibilities.

greater increase in protein synthesis *(case B)*, or decreasing both but with a greater decrement in protein breakdown *(case D)*. The effect is a positive N balance for all four scenarios, but the energy implications are considerably different. Because protein synthesis costs energy, cases A and B are more "expensive," whereas cases C and D require less energy than in the starting scenario *(case 0)*. Investigation of these possible mechanisms requires direct assessment of rates of protein breakdown, protein synthesis, and amino acid turnover within the body. Such assessment can be accomplished with the use of stable isotope or radiolabeled tracers, although the latter technique is not used for studying the pediatric population. Underneath we will explain several of the stable isotope techniques that can be used to study neonatal nutrition and metabolism. These methods have also been elaborated on more in detail elsewhere.[6-8]

STABLE ISOTOPE MODELS FOR MEASURING PROTEIN METABOLISM IN HUMANS

The simplest approach to the study of amino acid and protein kinetics is to hypothesize a single, free pool of amino acid N, with *two inflows*—amino acid from dietary protein and amino acid released from protein breakdown—and *two outflows*—amino acid oxidation to end products (CO_2 and ammonia, which is subsequently metabolized into urea) and amino acid uptake for protein synthesis (Fig. 40.2). This model can be considered either for whole-body protein turnover, in which the pool is the total free amino acid pool (see Fig. 40.2), or for the kinetics of a single amino acid, in which the pools are for a particular amino acid (illustrated for a ^{13}C essential amino acid stable isotope tracer in Fig. 40.3). The difference between the two approaches is related to how the system is viewed: on the one hand, looking at protein turnover versus, on the other hand, looking at the kinetics of a specific amino acid from which inferences to whole-body protein turnover are drawn.

However, lumping all body protein into a single entity is of course a gross oversimplification. Each of the many different tissues of the body is made up of a wide range of proteins with different turnover rates. Obviously, following the individual rates of hundreds of proteins would be impracticable. However, because most of the important stores of N in the body turnover at similarly slow rates, it is possible to simplify the system into a conceptual model of clinical and experimental utility.

Changes in amino acid metabolism for a specific tissue can be inferred by measuring the difference between the amino acids delivered to the tissue (arterial blood levels) and the amino acids released from the tissue (venous blood levels). In animals and adults, this technique has been applied to studies of forearm, leg, liver, kidney, and brain metabolism.[9-11] In pregnant animals and women, this model has been important in dissecting fetal and placental metabolism.[12-14] However, measuring an arteriovenous substrate concentration difference across a tissue bed is similar to the N balance technique—it provides information about the balance but tells nothing about the mechanism within the tissue affecting the balance. Most exciting is the combination of tracer infusion with the measurement of amino acid balance across the tissue bed. This technique allows for a complete solution of the various pathways operating in the tissue for each amino acid tracer used and can measure tissue-specific rates of protein synthesis and balance.[15-17] However, the use of arterial and venous catheters restricts the applicability of this method primarily to animal models.[12,18-24] Yet, a limited number of investigations have addressed human fetal amino acid metabolism by infusing amino acid tracers into the mother before delivery and obtaining cord blood at delivery to determine fetal metabolism.[25-28] Alternatively, specific tissue amino acid metabolism in human neonates across the splanchnic tissues may be assessed with the simultaneous use of different enteral and intravenous tracers. First-pass amino acid metabolism of the small intestine and liver is measured by comparison of the tracer enrichments of both tracers in plasma.

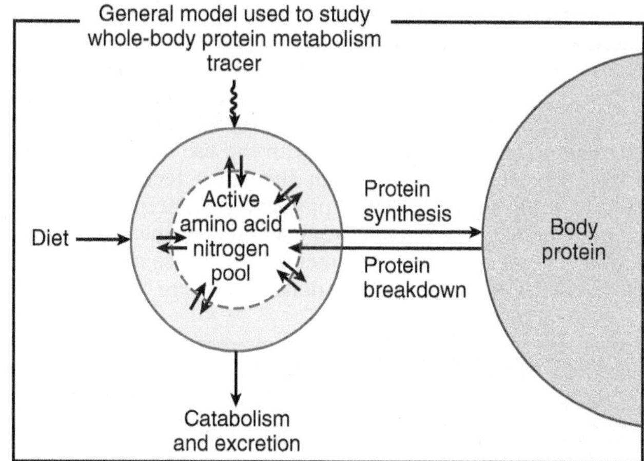

Fig. 40.2 Single-pool amino acid model for whole-body protein metabolism. The model is applied without requiring definition of individual pools. All free amino acid nitrogen is lumped together. The *shaded outer circle* indicates interchange of free amino acids with various intracellular free amino acid pools and with incorporation into and release from faster-turnover proteins. Slower-turnover protein, such as muscle protein, appears as an exit from the system for free amino acid by way of protein synthesis and as a source of free amino acid entry by way of protein breakdown. Amino acids also leave the system by oxidation to the end products (carbon dioxide, urea, and ammonia) and can enter through absorption of dietary protein or amino acids. (From Matthews DE. In: Duncan WP, Susan AB, eds. *Synthesis and Applications of Isotopically Labeled Compounds.* Amsterdam: Elsevier; 1983:279–284.)

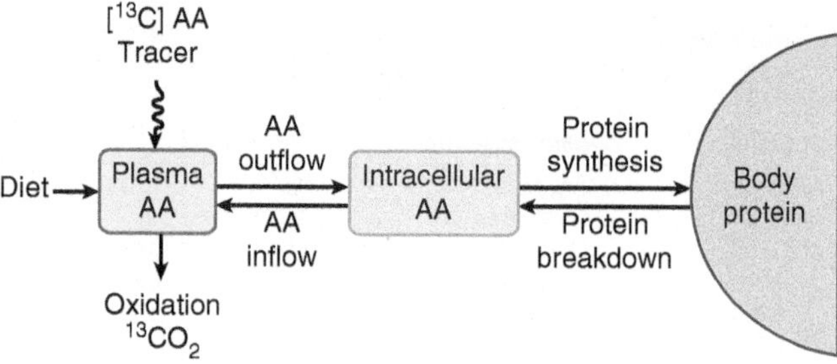

Fig. 40.3 Simplified model for following the kinetics of an individual essential amino acid (AA) using a ^{13}C label. The ^{13}C-labeled amino acid is infused intravenously. The tracer equilibrates with the free amino acid in plasma and in intracellular compartments. Amino acid is taken up from and released into the intracellular compartment through protein synthesis and breakdown. Amino acid oxidized intracellularly to form CO_2 is released into plasma as bicarbonate, and then into exhaled breath as CO_2. (From Bier DM, Matthews DE, Young VR. Interpretation of amino acid kinetic studies in the context of whole-body protein metabolism. In: Garrow JS, Halliday D, eds. *Substrate and Energy Metabolism in Man*. London: John Libbey; 1985:27–36.)

The plasma enrichment of the enteral administered tracer will be lower than that of the intravenously infused tracer by the amount of tracer sequestered by the gut and liver on the first pass during enteral absorption of the tracer. The ratio between the enrichment of the intravenously administered tracer and that of the enterally administered tracer is used to calculate the first-pass uptake.[29]

END-PRODUCT APPROACH TO MEASUREMENT OF PROTEIN METABOLISM

Because glycine is the only amino acid without an optically active α-carbon center, [^{15}N]glycine is the easiest labeled amino acid to synthesize and was the earliest tracer used for measuring protein turnover in the body dating back more than 70 years ago.[30] However, this single-pool compartmental analysis was overly simplistic and limiting. In 1969 Picou and Taylor-Roberts[31] proposed a significant improvement, removing the need for kinetic equations by viewing the system in a stochastic fashion.[32] When [^{15}N]glycine tracer is given, the label mixes (scatters) in the free amino acid pool and it is diluted with unlabeled amino acids entering from protein breakdown and from dietary intake. Using the rate of ^{15}N infusion and after measuring the dilution of ^{15}N in the free amino acid pool, the rate of unlabeled N appearance is readily calculated:

$$Q = 100 \cdot i/E \qquad [44.1]$$

where Q is the free amino acid N pool turnover rate (typically expressed as mg N/kg/day), i is the rate of [^{15}N]glycine infusion (mg ^{15}N/kg/day), and E is the ^{15}N enrichment in urine (dilution of ^{15}N by unlabeled N, expressed as *atom* or *mole% excess*). The 100 factor converts mole% to mole fraction. The dilution of the ^{15}N-glycine tracer (i.e., enrichment in the free amino acid N pool) is measured indirectly via its enrichment in urinary urea and/or ammonia end products. According to the standard precursor-product relationship,[32] a product (i.e., urinary urea or ammonia) formed from a single precursor will have an enrichment equal to the precursor (i.e., the free amino acid N pool).

The rate of whole-body protein breakdown *(B)* is determined from the turnover *(Q)* by subtracting the rate of dietary N intake *(I)*:

$$B = Q - I \qquad [44.2]$$

In these calculations, the standard value of 6.25 g protein = 1 g N is used to interconvert protein and N. Attention to the units (g of *protein* versus g of *N*) is important, because both units often are used concurrently in the literature.

Like most of the kinetic methods, the end-product method assumes steady-state conditions with respect to the free pool (i.e., the free N pool is neither expanding nor contracting). Obviously, the free pool does both, but over the period of most measurements, increases cancel decreases so that the steady-state assumption is reasonable. When *inflows* equal *outflows*,

$$Q = I + B = C + S \qquad [44.3]$$

where the outflows are amino acid N oxidation *(C)* to end products urea and ammonia, and *(S) is the* amino acid N uptake for protein synthesis. Amino acid N oxidation is simplified by the sum of the ammonia and urea production rates, which are estimated by measuring urinary N excretion as described in the section on N balance. Therefore the rate of whole-body synthesis is:

$$S = Q - C \qquad [44.4]$$

Occasionally encountered in the literature[33] is the term *net protein balance* or *net protein gain,* which refers to the difference between the measured synthesis and breakdown rates (*S–B*). Rearranging the balance equation for *Q* shows that:

$$S - B = I - C \qquad [44.5]$$

and $I - C$ is simply the difference between intake and excretion (i.e., *N balance*). Therefore the $S - B$ term is a misnomer in that it is based solely on the N balance measurement and not on the administration of the ^{15}N tracer.

The overwhelming advantage of the end-product method of Picou and Taylor-Roberts[31] is that it is noninvasive. Accordingly, it became the cornerstone method for protein metabolic research in pediatrics. However, this method is not without its problems. When the [^{15}N]glycine tracer is given orally at short intervals (e.g., every 3 hours), it takes approximately 60 hours to reach a

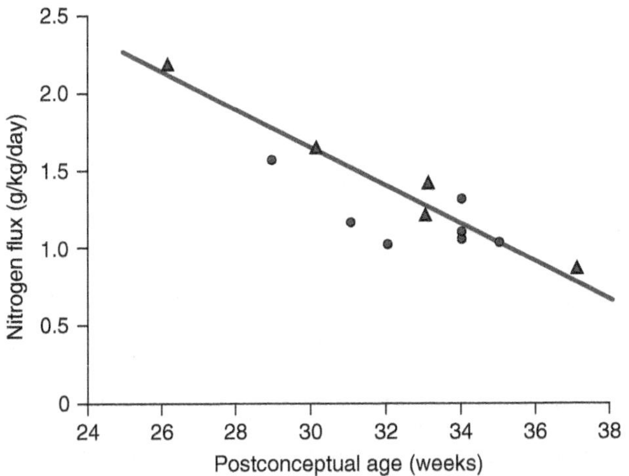

Fig. 40.4 Whole-body nitrogen flux versus conceptual age measured using a single dose of [^{15}N]glycine given intravenously to eight infants. (From Nissim I, Yudkoff M, Pereira G, Segal S. Effects of conceptual age and dietary intake on protein metabolism in premature infants. *J Pediatr Gastroenterol Nutr.* 1983;2:507–516.)

plateau for urinary [^{15}N]urea or ammonia, regardless of whether adults,[34] children, or infants[35-37] are studied. Alternatively, a single [^{15}N]glycine bolus technique has been described, followed by very precise urine collections during a shorter duration of for example 24 hours. By using the single bolus end-product method, protein turnover was nicely shown to be negatively correlated to conceptual age (Fig. 40.4).[38] However, whether the single bolus or the steady-state method gives more precise results is not known.[7,39,40]

Another clue to difficulties with the end-product method is that the urinary [^{15}N]ammonia enrichment usually is different from the urinary [^{15}N]urea enrichment,[37,41,42] because the amino acid ^{15}N precursor for ammonia synthesis is of renal or muscle origin, whereas the amino acid ^{15}N precursor for urea synthesis is of hepatic origin. It has therefore been suggested to take the arithmetic or harmonic average as this could reflect whole-body metabolism most accurately.[39]

In three studies,[37,43,44] an interesting observation was reported after receiving [^{15}N]glycine. Although [^{15}N]ammonia could be measured in urine, urinary [^{15}N]urea enrichment was too low to detect in some preterm infants, especially those with intrauterine growth restriction. This suggests that either these patients are better able to spare N from oxidation and subsequent urea synthesis[44] or that glycine may be inadequate in the diet of the preterm infant to meet growth requirements.[43] This event could happen only if glycine synthesis was limiting (i.e., if glycine was conditionally essential).[2,45] Alternatively, the amount of [^{15}N] glycine given could have been too low to produce detectable levels of ^{15}N greater than the natural abundance in urea. However, other groups of investigators[46,47] have had no difficulty measuring ^{15}N enrichment in urinary urea when [^{15}N]glycine was administered to infants with glycine intake in excess of their requirements,[48] suggesting that glycine can be considered an essential amino acid for preterm and possibly small for gestational age infants.

TURNOVER OF INDIVIDUAL COMPONENTS OF N METABOLISM

An alternative to studying the turnover of whole-body protein metabolism by the end-product method is to measure the kinetics of individual amino acids (see Fig. 40.3). Essential amino acid kinetics can then be extrapolated to rates of protein metabolism. An essential amino acid enters the free pool only from dietary intake (I_{aa}) and protein breakdown (B_{aa}); it disappears from the free pool by oxidation (C_{aa}) and uptake for protein synthesis (S_{aa}). These are the same components (I, B, C, and S) discussed previously but cast in terms of the turnover, or *flux*, of a specific individual amino acid:

$$Q_{aa} = I_{aa} + B_{aa} = C_{aa} + S_{aa} \quad [44.6]$$

The turnover rate (or flux, Q_{aa}) of a metabolite is measured by the tracer dilution measured directly in the free pool. Typically, a tracer of an essential amino acid is infused until isotopic steady state (constant dilution) is reached in the blood free amino acid pool. Knowing the tracer enrichment and infusion rate and measuring the tracer dilution in blood from samples taken at plateau allow determination of the rate of unlabeled metabolite appearance (Q_{aa}):

$$Q_{aa} = i_{aa} \cdot (E_i / E_p - 1) \quad [44.7]$$

where i_{aa} is the infusion rate of tracer with enrichment E_i (mole% excess), and E_p is the plasma amino acid enrichment.[49-51]

For a ^{13}C-labeled tracer, the amino acid oxidation rate can be measured from the rate of $^{13}CO_2$ excretion.[49,50] This approach assumes that the label is *quantitatively* released with the oxidation of the amino acid. For example, the ^{13}C of a L-[1-^{13}C] leucine tracer is removed at the first irreversible step of leucine catabolism (Fig. 40.5),[51] and leucine oxidation is determined directly from $^{13}CO_2$ excretion. Even phenylalanine, for which the pathway to oxidation is not direct, has been used to define phenylalanine-tyrosine oxidation.[52-54]

To measure amino acid kinetics, the amino acid tracer is infused into the blood and sampled from the blood, but the metabolic action takes place within cells. Amino acids do not freely pass through cells as does urea; amino acids are transported.[55,56] For the neutral amino acids, which are leucine, isoleucine, valine, phenylalanine, and tyrosine, transport into and out of cells is rapid, with only a small concentration gradient between plasma and intracellular milieus.[50] Still, the intracellular enrichment of leucine, as measured by plasma α-ketoisocaproate (KIC), which is formed from intracellular leucine after transamination and then released into plasma (Fig. 40.6), is approximately 20% lower than plasma leucine enrichment.[57] Using the plasma leucine enrichment to calculate leucine turnover thus underestimates whole-body flux by approximately 20%. The plasma KIC enrichment can be used during the leucine tracer infusion to resolve the question of intracellular leucine enrichment for calculating leucine kinetics. For amino acids such as glutamate and glutamine, which have extremely large intracellular to extracellular gradients, very little intracellular glutamate or glutamine exchanges with plasma, and the sampled plasma amino acid enrichment reflects primarily interorgan transport of amino acid, rather than whole-body flux.[58,59] The partitioning of amino acid between intracellular and extracellular milieus must therefore be considered carefully for every individual amino acid studied.

Determining an amino acid flux does not require a ^{13}C label per se. Any label (e.g., ^{15}N, ^{2}H, ^{18}O) can be used, but the caveat is that the label must follow the metabolic pathway expected. For example, a deuterium label in the tail of leucine or any ^{13}C label will trace leucine metabolism through the critical, irreversible second step of catabolism (see Fig. 40.5), but a [^{15}N]leucine tracer is removed with transamination.[60] Because more than 70% of the leucine transaminated to KIC is immediately reaminated to leucine,[60] the ^{15}N label measures a leucine N turnover rate that is considerably faster than the leucine carbon flux. Therefore the [^{15}N]leucine tracer cannot be used to follow leucine carbon metabolism. For all metabolites to be studied, the biochemistry of the tracer must be carefully considered when choosing an isotopic label.

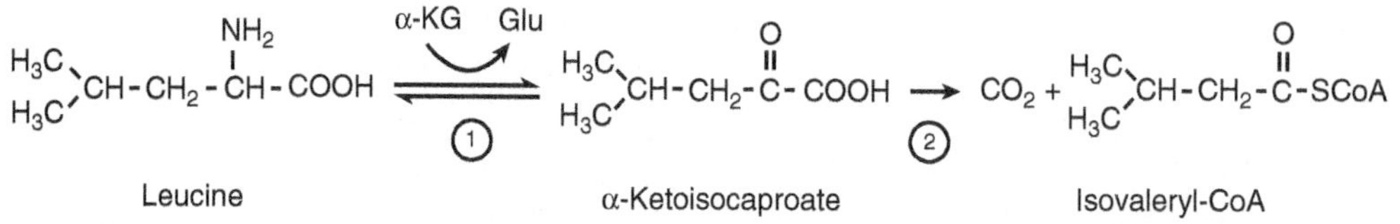

$$\underset{\text{Leucine}}{(H_3C)_2CH\text{-}CH_2\text{-}CH(NH_2)\text{-}COOH} \underset{①}{\overset{\alpha\text{-KG} \quad Glu}{\rightleftharpoons}} \underset{\alpha\text{-Ketoisocaproate}}{(H_3C)_2CH\text{-}CH_2\text{-}C(=O)\text{-}COOH} \underset{②}{\longrightarrow} CO_2 + \underset{\text{Isovaleryl-CoA}}{(H_3C)_2CH\text{-}CH_2\text{-}C(=O)\text{-}SCoA}$$

Fig. 40.5 Leucine metabolism. *1,* Leucine is first transaminated to α-ketoisocaproate. This reaction is rapid and reversible. *2,* The ketoacid is then decarboxylated, releasing a CO_2 and an organic acid, which is further oxidized. The other two branched-chain amino acids, valine and isoleucine, also are metabolized by the same enzymes in these first two metabolic steps. *CoA,* Coenzyme A; *Glu,* glutamate; *KG,* ketoglutarate.

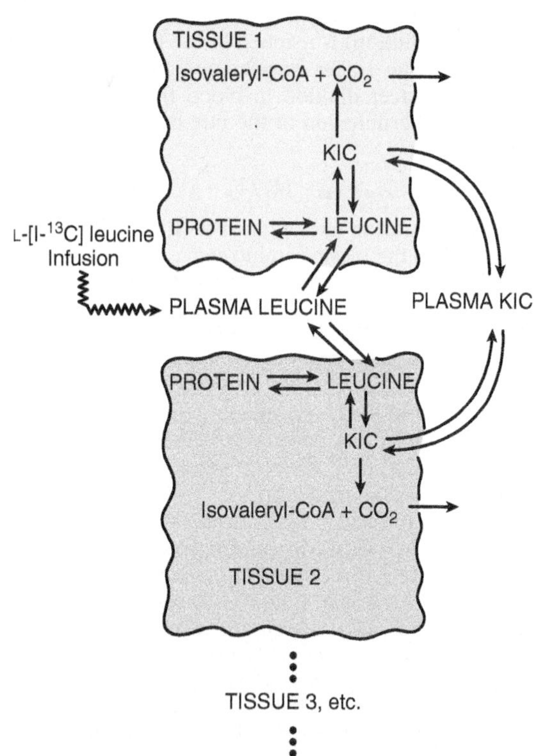

Fig. 40.6 Multitissue model of whole-body leucine metabolism. Leucine is transported into and out of cells of various tissues in the body (e.g., muscle, kidney, liver, adipose tissue). α-Ketoisocaproate *(KIC)*, formed within cells from leucine by transamination, is released into plasma. During an infusion of [1-^{13}C]leucine, the plasma KIC ^{13}C enrichment is the weighted average of the intracellular leucine ^{13}C enrichment of those tissues releasing KIC. *CO_2,* Carbon dioxide; *CoA,* coenzyme A. (From Matthews DE, Schwarz HP, Yang RD, et al. Relationship of plasma leucine and alpha-ketoisocaproate during a l-[1-13C]leucine infusion in man: a method for measuring human intracellular leucine tracer enrichment. *Metabolism.* 1982;31:1105–1112.)

The rates of amino acid release from protein breakdown (B_{aa}) and uptake for protein synthesis (S_{aa}) are calculated by subtracting dietary intake and oxidation from the flux, respectively, just as is done with the end-product method. The primary distinction is that the measurements are for a specific amino acid, not protein. Flux components typically are determined in units of μmol/kg/h and then extrapolated to whole-body protein kinetics by dividing the amino acid rates by the assumed concentration of the amino acid in body protein (μmol of amino acid/g of protein).

The principal *advantages* of following individual metabolite kinetics are that (1) the results are specific, improving confidence in the measurement, and (2) the turnover time of the free pool usually is fast. With use of a priming dose to reduce the time required to come to isotopic steady state, the tracer infusion study can be completed in less than 4 hours.

The principal *disadvantages* are that (1) the method is invasive (in terms of infusing tracer and sampling blood at least twice during steady state, total sampled volume usually <1 mL), (2) the true intracellular precursor pool usually is not sampled but plasma instead, and (3) dietary intake often is through a route different from that of the tracer. Catheters may already be in place in the seriously ill infant, but invasive procedures are not warranted for studying healthy infants. Yet it is in the healthy infant that the tracer techniques offer the greatest tool for defining normal metabolism and nutritional requirements.

An alternative to invasive blood sampling is sampling amino acids from urine.[61] Small amounts of amino acids are continually filtered through kidney and normally appear in the urine. Because urinary amino acids are derived from blood, they should be a reasonable substitute for blood amino acids measured by means of tracer enrichment under isotopic steady-state conditions. De Benoist and colleagues[61] demonstrated in 1984 that urinary leucine enrichments in infants were nearly identical to plasma leucine enrichments during infusion of [1-^{13}C]leucine, indicating that the urinary leucine came directly from plasma and was not contaminated significantly with unlabeled renal-derived leucine. Since then, several applications using this technique have been described in the literature.[46,62,63] However, in some commercial preparations of stable isotopically labeled L-amino acid tracers, D-amino acid tracer also will be present in variable amounts. Because D-amino acids are not metabolized by the same pathways as for L-amino acids, and usually are removed by kidney and excreted in the urine, D-amino acid tracer may accumulate in urine, resulting in distortion of L-amino acid tracer measurements in urine. This problem can be avoided by using a chiral column to separate the D and L forms before measurement of amino acid tracer enrichment using a mass spectrometer.[64]

Other and new model stable isotope models are constantly being developed and improved. The tracer pulse approach is one such model.[65] Although it may have several experimental benefits, its practicability in small infants is limited because of the requirement of at least five plasma samples to measure decay of the enrichment curve.

STUDYING SPLANCHNIC UPTAKE AND METABOLISM

Because a significant portion of human milk N is urea N, urea represents a potentially important N source. The bioavailability of dietary urea N has been determined in infants noninvasively by adding [^{15}N]urea tracer to the feeding solution and collecting and measuring the tracer in the urine.[66-68] The purpose of the studies using this technique was to determine what fraction of the urea N was retained in the body, rather than passing into the urine. Retention of urea N would reflect gut microorganism hydrolysis of the urea and incorporation of the resulting ammonia (presumably by the liver) into other N-containing compounds, including essential amino acids. This result has been demonstrated in both adults[69] and infants.[70] Because the major portion of the [^{15}N]urea consumed by infants is recovered in the urine, not much of the urea N will be bioavailable.

In terms of nutrition, many of the questions to be addressed in infants are related not only to parenteral nutrition, but also to or enteral feeding. However, the fed state complicates calculating kinetics more than by just adding a dietary intake term to the flux equation. Any dietary amino acid oxidized or taken up for protein synthesis by either gut or liver during absorption of food will not have mixed with the systemic circulation in which the tracer is administered. The flux of amino acid released from protein breakdown will therefore be underestimated by an amount equal to that amino acid sequestered on the first pass through the splanchnic bed. It is possible under some circumstances to have a *negative* protein breakdown after dietary amino acid inflow has been subtracted from the flux. This problem is negated if the tracer is administered with the food, given orally or by intragastric tube feeding.[61] However, oral feeding will not provide a constant flow of tracer into the system unless tube feeding is used.[61]

Addition of the tracer to the enteral feeding solution solves the problem of following the metabolism of the constituent amino acids. However, an enteral tracer does not necessarily help when the goal is to compare the effects of parenteral and enteral feeding regimens. For those kinds of studies, the tracer may be administered intravenously with the parenteral nutrition solution or enterally with the enteral formula. The use of two different administration routes for delivery of the amino acid tracer yields data that do not allow direct comparison—the proverbial apples and oranges.[46] A more elaborate design is required for comparing enteral and parenteral feeding regimens. For example, if two tracers of the same amino acid are available that give identical measures of metabolism (e.g., [1-^{13}C]leucine and [5,5,5-$^{2}H_3$] leucine), they can be administered simultaneously by both enteral and intravenous routes.[29,50] This approach gives direct measurement of tracers by both routes simultaneously during both parenteral and enteral feeding regimens.[18,71,72] More recent studies have shown that turnover rates may vary up to 80%, depending on the route of tracer.[73-76] Enterally administered tracer will yield a much higher turnover rate, reflecting first-pass removal by gastrointestinal tract and liver.

FREE, EXTRINSICALLY LABELED, OR INTRINSICALLY LABELED AMINO ACIDS

Almost all tracer studies have been performed using labeled amino acids as *free* amino acids, rather than amino acid tracers incorporated into proteins. When amino acids and proteins are given enterally, differences in the time course of hydrolysis and absorption of the amino acids and small peptides have been documented.[77] Although it takes time to hydrolyze enterally delivered proteins to peptides, peptides are absorbed more rapidly than free amino acids.[78] Thus an enterally delivered labeled free amino acid will have different absorption kinetics from those for the corresponding protein-bound amino acids it is meant to trace.

Metges and coworkers[79] measured the prandial metabolic fate of ^{13}C-labeled dietary leucine when it was ingested either as an intrinsically labeled component (incorporated into casein protein) or as a free amino acid (extrinsically labeled) in a mixture of crystalline free amino acids which simulated the casein amino acid pattern. To serve as control data, leucine kinetics also were measured when free labeled leucine was given together with the intact casein. Leucine oxidation was higher for the free [^{13}C]leucine tracer combined with a free amino acid mixture than for an intrinsically [^{13}C]leucine-labeled casein. This result, together with the finding of a higher uptake of leucine for protein synthesis with the intrinsically labeled casein, suggests that protein-bound leucine was better used for whole-body protein synthesis than as a free amino acid. Such studies have not yet been performed in neonates but may prove to be important in defining infant formulas in terms of amino acid and protein composition.

REQUIREMENTS FOR SPECIFIC AMINO ACIDS

Dietary recommendations for essential amino acids have historically been based on N balance studies and short-term growth studies. In the past few decades, the indicator amino acid oxidation (IAAO) method has been developed to establish specific amino acid requirements throughout life including pregnancy[80] and validated extensively in animal models of infancy.[81,82] The results of the IAAO method have been incorporated into recommendations of amino acid requirements not only for adults, but also for children and infants.[2,83] This technique is based on the partitioning essential amino acid outflow under steady-state conditions between oxidation and protein synthesis ($Q_{aa} = C_{aa} + S_{aa}$, as defined earlier). When a single essential amino acid is present in limited quantity in the diet, the amount of protein that can be synthesized likewise is curtailed. With an essential amino acid in limited supply, the use of all other dietary amino acids for protein synthesis also will be limited, and the body will have no choice but to oxidize the excess amounts of these amino acids. If the dietary amount of the limiting amino acid is increased, protein synthesis will increase and so will the utilization of the other dietary amino acids—which in turn reduces their oxidation. Once the requirement for the limiting amino acid is reached, further increases in its dietary intake will cause no further increase in protein synthesis, nor decrease in the oxidation of the other essential amino acids.

The IAAO method works on this principle.[84-86] Subjects are given a series of diets containing various amounts of the amino acid for which the requirement is to be determined. The amounts vary below and above requirement. All other amino acids are furnished at constant amounts ***above*** requirement. At the end of each diet period, a dose of another essential amino acid with a ^{13}C label (the indicator amino acid) is given, and its oxidation is measured. The oxidation of the labeled indicator amino acid will decrease as the amount of test amino acid increases, until requirement is reached, and then the oxidation will plateau. As shown in Fig. 40.7, plotting the oxidation of the labeled indicator amino acid against test amino acid intake should show a breakpoint at the requirement level for the test amino acid. More recent studies have used the IAAO technique to determine sulfur (methionine and cysteine) amino acid requirements for neonates both in a piglet model[87,88] and in human infants.[89] Providing preterm infants with different intakes of cysteine while methionine (the sulfur donor of cysteine) and serine (the carbon donor of cysteine) were supplied in adequate amounts did not influence the oxidation rate of the indicator amino acid, suggesting that cysteine can be adequately synthesized from serine and methionine and is not conditionally essential.[89] A different indirect technique yielded similar results, demonstrating that glucose carbon (labeled with ^{13}C) is incorporated into cysteine. This finding indicates that cysteine synthesis is not limited by serine availibility.[90]

This method has been used extensively in the past few years, yielding the exact amino acid requirements for term (and preterm) neonates.[91-97] This enables the development of a new concept of infant formula, reducing the protein intake and thereby possibly reducing the risk for development of obesity later on in life.[98,99]

SYNTHESIS OF SPECIFIC PROTEINS

Most of the preceding stable isotope models describe protein metabolism at a whole-body level. However, one may also be able to study the synthesis rates of specific proteins or peptides provided the compound of interest can be sampled and isolated.

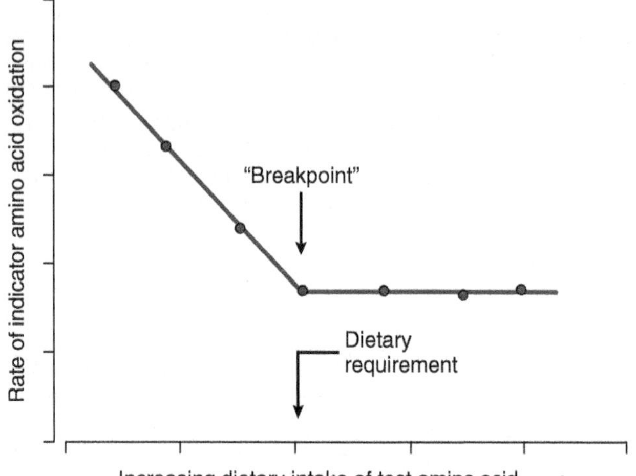

Fig. 40.7 The rate of oxidation of an indicator amino acid in response to various dietary intakes of a test amino acid. The inflection or breakpoint in the rate of indicator oxidation represents the physiologic requirement of the test amino acid for the individual patient. (From Brunton JA, Ball RO, Pencharz PB. Determination of amino acid requirements by indicator amino acid oxidation: applications in health and disease. *Curr Opin Clin Nutr Metab Care.* 1998;1:449–453.)

Lipoproteins, albumin,[100,101] and glutathione[102-104] are examples that are obtained from blood; muscle or liver protein can be obtained by biopsy although this is practically impossible in pediatric studies. A protein synthesis rate can be determined directly from the rate of tracer incorporation into the protein of interest if multiple samples are taken.[6-8] For proteins with slow turnover (e.g., muscle protein or albumin), incorporation of tracer is linear with time during the first several hours of tracer infusion.[4,105-107] If the tracer infusion was continued for several half-lives of turnover, the tracer concentration in the protein would rise exponentially to match that of its precursor, the intracellular amino acid enrichment.[108,109] For proteins with slower turnover, then, it is more convenient to measure the synthesis rate from the initial rate of tracer incorporation into the protein.

The disadvantage of this method can be that multiple samples must be taken. To circumvent this, a staggered infusion protocol can be applied, so that multiple tracers are infused starting at different times after which a single sample can be taken.[110] This principle has been adapted so that for example albumin synthesis rates could be determined in the human fetus after infusing multiple tracers in a staggered fashion to pregnant women prior to delivery.[26]

To convert the initial rate of tracer incorporation in protein into a protein synthesis rate requires knowledge of the intracellular amino acid precursor enrichment for synthesis. For muscle protein synthesis, L-[1-^{13}C]leucine often is used as the tracer[111] because plasma [^{13}C]KIC enrichment approximates the intracellular muscle leucine enrichment. Various other schemes have been used to estimate intracellular liver amino acid tracer enrichment.[112-114]

For proteins such as very low-density lipoprotein apolipoprotein B for which turnover occurs within the period of tracer infusion (typically 4 to 8 hours), tracer incorporation into the protein rises exponentially to a plateau. If the tracer enrichment in the protein does not reach plateau during the time course of the tracer infusion, curve fitting usually can predict the plateau. If the enrichment plateau can be defined, then the precursor enrichment (the enrichment of the intracellular free amino acid from which the protein was made) will now have been measured directly.[112] Several groups of investigators have used plateau enrichment of tracers in apolipoprotein B as a surrogate measure of intracellular hepatic tracer enrichment in both a piglet model[20,115,116] and human infants.[90]

Garlick and colleagues have proposed an alternative method to measure protein synthesis of slow turnover proteins.[117] Their method is to administer a "flooding dose" of tracer amino acid, producing a large momentary concentration gradient between the extracellular and intracellular spaces. The gradient pushes the amino acid rapidly into cells, "flooding" them with the tracer. This scheme is meant to force the intracellular tracer enrichment (which cannot be readily measured) to equalize with the extracellular enrichment (which can be measured), thereby removing the uncertainty of what is the precursor enrichment for protein synthesis.[117-121] An obvious drawback is that the administered dose is a *pharmacologic* dose of material that may alter metabolism and induce secretion of various hormones (e.g., insulin) and factors that are known to regulate protein metabolism. Nevertheless, the flooding dose approach is a convenient method for determining protein synthesis of slow-turnover proteins, which can be sampled readily in a short period of time.

DEGRADATION OF SPECIFIC PROTEINS

Measurement of protein degradation is much more difficult. It usually requires prelabeling a protein and following its disappearance over time. The first problem arises with prelabeling the protein. This can be done for plasma proteins by using radioactive iodine and following its disappearance from the system, but this technique is not suitable for infants. Alternatively, if a protein is prelabeled by first incorporating one or more stably labeled amino acids into it, a problem emerges due to recycling of amino acid tracer. As the protein degrades, the newly released amino acids can again be taken up for new protein synthesis. That is, some of the labeled amino acids are *reused* or recycled back into protein. This recycling greatly complicates interpretation of the labeled protein data.

A few amino acids cannot be reused for protein synthesis. For example, proline is hydroxylated and both histidine and lysine are methylated after protein synthesis by a posttranslational process that occurs in very specific proteins (i.e., hydroxyproline in collagen and 3-methylhistidine in actin and myosin). When these proteins degrade, these modified amino acids are not reused. Hydroxyproline has been used to follow collagen kinetics,[122] and 3-methylhistidine has been used extensively to follow myofibrillar protein breakdown.[123,124] Although most of the myofibrillar protein is in muscle, 3-methylhistidine also is present in gut actin. Although the gut actin pool is very small relative to muscle protein, protein turnover within the gut is rapid and therefore can be a significant contributor to urinary 3-methylhistidine output, warranting cautious interpretation.[125]

A method was developed to measure the fractional breakdown rates of slow turnover proteins by the use of deuterated water as a label donor.[126] Deuterium oxide was built into alanine that was subsequently incorporated into body proteins. The rate of disappearance of deuterated alanine from the proteins allowed for the quantification of fractional breakdown rate.

CONCLUSION

Amino acids are the building blocks of protein and differ from carbohydrates and fats by the inclusion of an amino N group. Anabolism is defined by a positive N balance, as catabolism is characterized by a negative N balance. Interventions aimed at improving anabolic state are hampered by the methodology to quantify N metabolism as N intake is usually overestimated, whereas N excretion is underestimated. However, the N balance method does not offer insights into the actual processes of protein synthesis and breakdown that produces the N balance change. Stable isotope labeled amino acids do provide these insights, and by using those, we are able to determine specific protein synthesis rates, intermediary metabolism, and uptakes and metabolism of splanchnic tissues. Furthermore, these techniques allow us to determine amino acid and protein requirements under different circumstances. Those measurements provide the basis for determining optimal nutrition of the neonate, and subsequently determine later health.[127]

A complete reference list is available at www.ExpertConsult.com.

SELECT REFERENCES

1. Embleton ND, van den Akker CHP. Protein intakes to optimize outcomes for preterm infants. *Semin Perinatol*. 2019;43(7):151154.
2. FAO/WHO/UNU. *Protein and Amino Acid Requirements in Human Nutrition, Vol Technical Report Series #935*. Geneva: World Health Organization; 2007:1-265.
6. Schierbeek H, Van den Akker CH, Fay LB, et al. High-precision mass spectrometric analysis using stable isotopes in studies of children. *Mass Spectrom Rev*. 2012;31(2):312-330.
7. Liu G, Li ZG, Wu HW. Pediatric protein metabolism techniques - a review. *Eur Rev Med Pharmacol Sci*. 2017;21(suppl 4):9-12.
8. Schierbeek H. *Mass Spectrometry and Stable Isotopes in Nutritional and Pediatric Research*. Hoboken, New Jersey: Wiley; 2017.
14. Holm MB, Bastani NE, Holme AM, et al. Uptake and release of amino acids in the fetal-placental unit in human pregnancies. *PloS One*. 2017;12(10):e0185760.
20. Stoll B, Burrin DG, Henry JF, et al. Dietary and systemic phenylalanine utilization for mucosal and hepatic constitutive protein synthesis in pigs. *Am J Physiol Gastrointest Liver Physiol*. 1999;276:49-57.
25. Chien PF, Smith K, Watt PW, et al. Protein turnover in the human fetus studied at term using stable isotope tracer amino acids. *Am J Physiol Endocrinol Metab*. 1993;265:31-35.
26. van den Akker CH, Schierbeek H, Rietveld T, et al. Human fetal albumin synthesis rates during different periods of gestation. *Am J Clin Nutr*. 2008;88:997-1003.
27. van den Akker CH, Schierbeek H, Dorst KY, et al. Human fetal amino acid metabolism at term gestation. *Am J Clin Nutr*. 2009;89:153-160.
28. Van den Akker CH, Schierbeek H, Minderman G, et al. Amino acid metabolism in the human fetus at term: leucine, valine, and methionine kinetics. *Pediatr Res*. 2011;70:566-571.
29. Matthews DE, Marano MA, Campbell RG. Splanchnic bed utilization of leucine and phenylalanine in humans. *Am J Physiol Endocrinol Metab*. 1993;264:109-118.
32. Bier DM. Intrinsically difficult problems: the kinetics of body proteins and amino acids in man. *Diabetes Metab*. 1989;5:111-132.
39. Duggleby SL, Waterlow JC. The end-product method of measuring whole-body protein turnover: a review of published results and a comparison with those obtained by leucine infusion. *Br J Nutr*. 2005;94(2):141-153.
49. Wolfe RR, Chinkes DL. *Isotope Tracers in Metabolic Research: Principles and Practice of Kinetic Analysis*. 2nd ed. Hoboken: Wiley-Liss; 2004:1-488.
51. Matthews DE, Motil KJ, Rohrbaugh DK, et al. Measurement of leucine metabolism in man from a primed, continuous infusion of l-[1-13C]leucine. *Am J Physiol Endocrinol Metab*. 1980;238:473-479.
59. Brosnan JT. Interorgan amino acid transport and its regulation. *J Nutr*. 2003;133(6 suppl 1):2068S-72S.
60. Matthews DE, Bier DM, Rennie MJ, et al. Regulation of leucine metabolism in man: a stable isotope study. *Science*. 1981;214:1129-1131.
65. Engelen M, Ten Have GAM, Thaden JJ, et al. New advances in stable tracer methods to assess whole-body protein and amino acid metabolism. *Curr Opin Clin Nutr Metab Care*. 2019;22(5):337-346.
66. Fomon SJ, Matthews DE, Bier DM, et al. Bioavailability of dietary urea nitrogen in the infant. *J Pediatr*. 1987;111:221-224. 1987.
70. Millward DJ, Forrester T, Ah-Sing E, et al. The transfer of 15N from urea to lysine in the human infant. *Br J Nutr*. 2000;83:505-512.
71. Beaufrère B, Fournier V, Salle B, Putet G. Leucine kinetics in fed low-birth-weight infants: importance of splanchnic tissues. *Am J Physiol Endocrinol Metab*. 1992;263:214-220.
73. Corpeleijn WE, Riedijk MA, Zhou Y, et al. Almost all enteral aspartate is taken up in first-pass metabolism in enterally fed preterm infants. *Clin Nutr*. 2010;29:341-346.
74. van der Schoor SR, Schierbeek H, Bet PM, et al. Majority of dietary glutamine is utilized in first pass in preterm infants. *Pediatr Res*. 2010;67:194-199.
76. van der Schoor SR, Wattimena DL, Huijmans J, et al. The gut takes nearly all: threonine kinetics in infants. *Am J Clin Nutr*. 2007;86:1132-1138.
77. Boirie Y, Dangin M, Gachon P, et al. Slow and fast dietary proteins differently modulate postprandial protein accretion. *Proc Natl Acad Sci U S A*. 1997;94:14930-14935.
79. Metges CC, El-Khoury AE, Selvaraj AB, et al. Kinetics of L-[1-13C]leucine when ingested with free amino acids, unlabeled or intrinsically labeled casein. *Am J Physiol Endocrinol Metab*. 2000;278:1000-1009.
80. Elango R, Ball RO. Protein and amino acid requirements during pregnancy. *Adv Nutr*. 2016;7(4):839s-844s.
84. Brunton JA, Ball RO, Pencharz PB. Determination of amino acid requirements by indicator amino acid oxidation: applications in health and disease. *Curr Opin Clin Nutr Metab Care*. 1998;1:449-453.
85. Elango R, Ball RO, Pencharz PB. Indicator amino acid oxidation: concept and application. *J Nutr*. 2008;138:243-246.
86. Elango R, Levesque C, Ball RO, et al. Available versus digestible amino acids - new stable isotope methods. *Br J Nutr*. 2012;108(suppl 2):S306-S314.
87. Shoveller AK, Brunton JA, House JD, et al. Dietary cysteine reduces the methionine requirement by an equal proportion in both parenterally and enterally fed piglets. *J Nutr*. 2003;133:4215-4224.
89. Riedijk MA, van Beek RH, Voortman G, et al. Cysteine: a conditionally essential amino acid in low-birth-weight preterm infants? *Am J Clin Nutr*. 2007;86:1120-1125.
91. Hogewind-Schoonenboom JE, Zhu L, Zhu L, et al. Phenylalanine requirements of enterally fed term and preterm neonates. *Am J Clin Nutr*. 2015;101:1155-1162.
92. de Groof F, Huang L, van Vliet I, et al. Branched-chain amino acid requirements for enterally fed term neonates in the first month of life. *Am J Clin Nutr*. 2014;99:62-70.
93. Huang L, Hogewind-Schoonenboom JE, van Dongen MJ, et al. Methionine requirement of the enterally fed term infant in the first month of life in the presence of cysteine. *Am J Clin Nutr*. 2012;95:1048-1054.
98. Weber M, Grote V, Closa-Monasterolo R, et al. Lower protein content in infant formula reduces BMI and obesity risk at school age: follow-up of a randomized trial. *Am J Clin Nutr*. 2014;99:1041-1045.
99. Kouwenhoven SMP, Antl N, Finken MJJ, et al. A modified low-protein infant formula supports adequate growth in healthy, term infants: a randomized, double-blind, equivalence trial. *Am J Clin Nutr*. 2019.
101. Vlaardingerbroek H, Schierbeek H, Rook D, et al. Albumin synthesis in very low birth weight infants is enhanced by early parenteral lipid and high-dose amino acid administration. *Clin Nutr*. 2016;35(2):344-350.
103. Rook D, TeBraake FW, Schierbeek H, et al. Glutathione synthesis rates in early postnatal life. *Pediatr Res*. 2010;67:407-411.
106. Wagenmakers AJ. Tracers to investigate protein and amino acid metabolism in human subjects. *Proc Nutr Soc*. 1999;58:987-1000.
110. Dudley MA, Burrin DG, Wykes LJ, et al. Protein kinetics determined in vivo with a multiple-tracer, single-sample protocol: application to lactase synthesis. *Am J Physiol*. 1998;274(3):G591-G598.
112. Cayol M, Boirie Y, Prugnaud J, et al. Precursor pool for hepatic protein synthesis in humans: effects of tracer route infusion and dietary proteins. *Am J Physiol Endocrinol Metab*. 1996;270:980-987.
118. Davis TA, Fiorotto ML, Nguyen HV, Burrin DG. Aminoacyl-tRNA and tissue free amino acid pools are equilibrated after a flooding dose of phenylalanine. *Am J Physiol Endocrinol Metab*. 1999;277:103-109.
119. Garlick PJ, McNurlan MA, Essén P, Wernerman J. Measurement of tissue protein synthesis rates in vivo: a critical analysis of contrasting methods. *Am J Physiol Endocrinol Metab*. 1994;266:287-297.
120. Garlick PJ, McNurlan MA. Measurement of protein synthesis in human tissues by the flooding method. *Curr Opin Clin Nutr Metab Care*. 1998;1:455-460.
121. Reeds PJ, Davis TA. Of flux and flooding: the advantages and problems of different isotopic methods for quantifying protein turnover in vivo: I. Methods based on the dilution of a tracer. *Curr Opin Clin Nutr Metab Care*. 1999;2:23-28.
126. Holm L, O'Rourke B, Ebenstein D, et al. Determination of steady-state protein breakdown rate in vivo by the disappearance of protein-bound tracer-labeled amino acids: a method applicable in humans. *Am J Physiol Endocrinol Metab*. 2013;15:895-907.
127. Hoffer LJ. Human protein and amino acid requirements. *JPEN J Parenter Enteral Nutr*. 2016;40(4):460-474.

41 Placental Transfer and Fetal Requirements of Amino Acids

Laura D. Brown | Rohan M. Lewis | William W. Hay, Jr. | Timothy R.H. Regnault

INTRODUCTION

Placental uptake, metabolism, and transfer of amino acids to the fetus are critical for both placental and fetal development and growth to produce a successful pregnancy. Placental amino acid transfer is mediated by active transport and is performed by over 20 distinct amino acid transport systems that are present on the maternal facing apical, microvillous, and fetal facing, basal plasma membranes of the placental syncytiotrophoblast. The transport systems are made up of proteins that are members of the solute carrier (SLC) superfamily. These SLCs exhibit a degree of specificity for certain classes of amino acids, but there also is overlap among the systems. Expression of the amino acid transporters is time dependent across gestation and is regulated by a host of factors including hormones, adipokines, and cytokines and is influenced by adverse in utero conditions. These systems can operate as accumulative transporters, exchangers, or facilitative transporters. Placental amino acid transfer requires the interplay of all three types of transporters. The interplay of these systems in conjunction with an increase in their number and activity rates over the course of placental development during gestation promote an adequate amino acid supply for placental and fetal metabolism and growth. This chapter focuses on describing the protein systems associated with placental amino acid transport as well as examining aspects of placental and fetal amino acid metabolism in animals and humans.

PLACENTAL AMINO ACID SUPPLY

Amino acid supply to the placenta and the fetus involves active, energy-dependent transport of amino acids across the placental membranes that is mediated by transport proteins (Fig. 41.1). The transport of amino acids is altered qualitatively and quantitatively by membrane transporter location and activity, competition among circulating amino acids for transporters, placental metabolism of amino acids, and relative concentrations of the amino acids in maternal and fetal plasma. Furthermore, changes in the overall placental surface area and architecture of the placental tissues also impact placental amino acid supply.

The placental membranes through which amino acids are transported into the placenta and into the fetus are the maternal and fetal surfaces of the syncytial epithelium of the human placenta, or the *syncytiotrophoblast,* a polarized multinucleate epithelium (see Fig. 41.1). The maternal-facing, apical surface of this epithelium has a microvillus membrane (MVM); the basal surface facing the fetus is termed the basal membrane (BM). The transport of amino acids across the syncytiotrophoblast involves three steps: (1) uptake from the maternal circulation across the MVM, (2) movement through the trophoblast cytoplasm, and (3) transport out of the trophoblast across the BM into the placental villous stroma (see Fig. 41.1).

Amino acids must diffuse across the villous stroma before crossing the fetal capillary endothelium into the umbilical circulation. It is not clear whether amino acid transfer across the capillary endothelium is primarily mediated through the paracellular routes (via cell-cell junctions) or a transcellular transporter mediated route. For most of the amino acids and in all mammalian species that have been studied, transport across the trophoblast membranes from maternal to fetal plasma occurs against a concentration gradient and involves energy-dependent transport proteins.[1-6] The major membrane transport proteins and their location for amino acid supply to the placenta are discussed below and are reported in Table 41.1.[4,6-9]

PLACENTAL AMINO ACID SOLUTE CARRIER PROTEINS

Amino acid transporters are found to operate as accumulative transporters, exchangers, or facilitated transporters and placental amino acid transfer requires the interplay of all three types of transporters. Accumulative transporters mediate uptake of amino acids into the cell and can operate against the concentration gradient by coupling transport to electrochemical gradients, primarily the Na^+ gradient. Exchanger systems take up one amino acid while mediating the efflux of a second, while facilitated transporters mediate both uptake and efflux. Historically, these amino acid transporters were described in terms of systems that were based on common substrates (e.g., system L that transported leucine).[9a,9b] More recently, the ability to clone, sequence, and study the expression of individual transporter proteins has led to an explosion of data defining the molecular basis of amino acid transporter systems that are all members of the SLC superfamily.[9]

SLC1

The SLC1 family contains the accumulative anionic amino acid transporters that form System X_{AG} and the neutral amino acid exchangers comprising the System ASC (alanine, serine, and cysteine). Through System X_{AG} proteins, the amino acids glutamate and aspartate are taken up into the placenta by the highly accumulative excitatory amino acid transporters (EAATs; SLC1A1-3, 6, and 7). The EAATs mediate sodium-coupled uptake of anionic amino acids and are found on both the MVM and BM of the placenta.[10,11] The rat BM preparation is reported to have a higher maximal velocity,[11] an observation that is consistent with the predominant flux of glutamate from the fetus to the placenta, as has been demonstrated in the sheep and human.[12,13] EAAT-1, EAAT-2, and EAAT-3 have been detected in human placental tissue.[14] The regulation of these proteins appears to be under the control of growth hormone (GH) and insulin-like growth factor (IGF) family members,[15] both of which are regulated by nutrient supply, as shown in rodent cell line culture nutrient deprivation studies.[11,16]

ASCT1 (SLC1A4) and ASCT2 (SLC1A5) mediate sodium-dependent exchange of small neutral amino acids—alanine, serine, and cysteine—originally termed the ASC transport proteins. These transporters have been found in the MVM and in the BM.[17-18a] Hypoxia is reported to inhibit or limit their expression,[19] and levels are reduced in placentae with growth-restricted fetuses.[20] Both ASCT1 and ASCT2 are expressed in placental tissue[21,22] and play additional critical roles in cytotrophoblast fusion[23] into the syncytiotrophoblast.

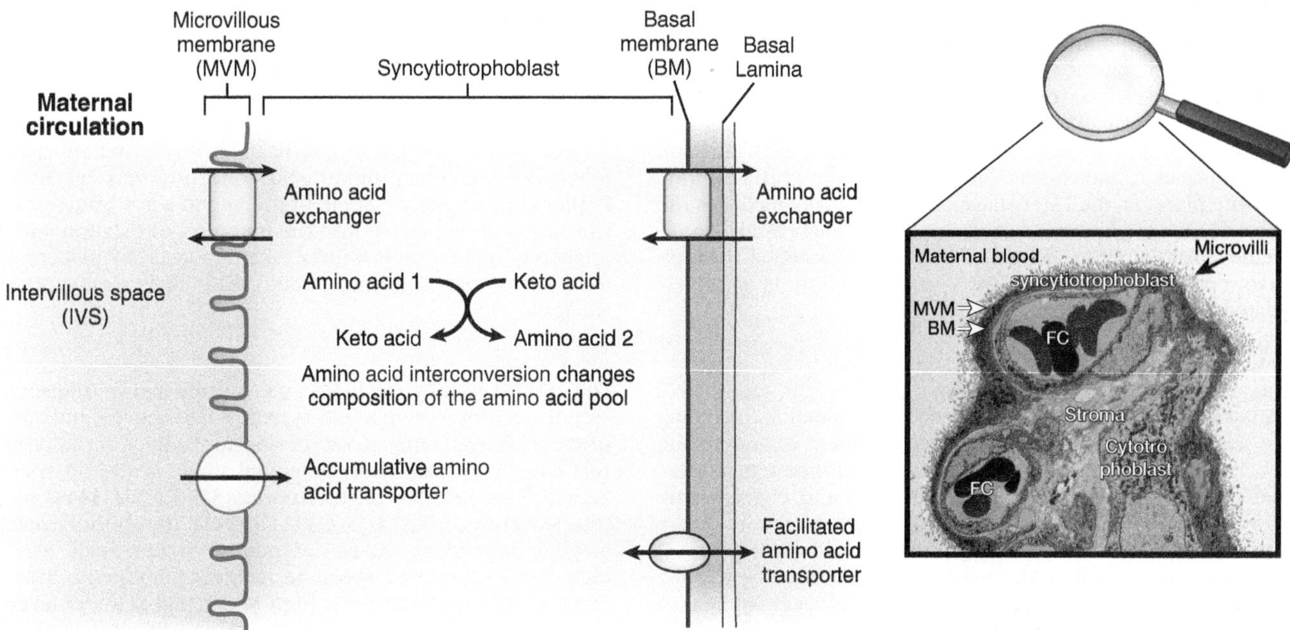

Fig. 41.1 The location of transporter systems upon the microvillous membrane *(MVM)* and basal membrane *(BM)* of the placental syncytiotrophoblast, amino acid conversions occurring within the placenta and amino acid transfer within the uteroplacental unit. The transmission election micrograph shows a cross section of a placental villus. The villus is surrounded by the syncytiotrophoblast, which is covered in microvilli, increasing the surface area for exchange, and is in direct contact with the maternal blood surrounding the villi. Fetal erythrocytes can be seen within the fetal capillaries within the villi. *FC*, Fetal capillary.

Table 41.1 Characteristics of the Primary Amino Acid Transporters Expressed in Placenta.

Gene/Protein (Traditional System)	Mechanism	Predominant Substrates	Reported Localization in the Syncytiotrophoblast
SLC1A1/EAAT3 (System X^{AG})	$3Na^+/1H^+$/AA co-transport/$1K^+$-antiport	E, D	MVM, BM
SLC1A2/EAAT2 (System X^{AG})			
SLC1A3/EAAT1 (System X^{AG})			
SLC1A4/ASCT1 (System ASC)	Na^+ dependent amino acid exchange	A, S, C, T	ASC activity on the BM
SLC1A5/ASCT2 (System ASC)	Na^+ dependent amino acid exchange	A, S, C, T, Q, N	
SLC7A1/CAT1 (System y^+)	Facilitated but highly trans-stimulated	R, K, H	CAT activity on MVM, BM
SLC7A2/CAT2B System y^+	Facilitated	R, K, H	
SLC7A3P/CAT3 (System y^+)	Facilitated	R, K, H	
SLC7A5/LAT1 (System L)	Exchanger	Large neutral L-amino acids	MVM, BM
SLC7A8/LAT2 (System L)	Heterodimerize with 4F2hc *(SLC3A2)*	Neutral L-amino acids	MVM, BM
SLC7A7/y^+LAT1 (System y^+L)	exchanger, Heterodimerize with 4F2hc *(SLC3A2)*	Cationic amino acids and Na^+-dependent transfer of neutral AA	MVM
SLC7A6/y^+LAT2 (System y^+L)	Exchanger, Heterodimerize with 4F2hc *(SLC3A2)*	Favor efflux of cationic amino acids	MVM, BM
SLC7A10/Asc1 (System asc)	Exchanger Heterodimerize with 4F2hc *(SLC3A2)*	Small neutral amino acids	MVM
SLC16A10/TAT1	Facilitated diffusion	F, Y, W	BM
SLC38A1/SNAT1 (System A)	Na^+/AA co-transport	Q, A, N, C, H, S	MVM/BM
SLC38A2 /SNAT2 (System A)	Na^+/AA co-transport	A, N, C, Q, G, H, M, P, S	MVM/BM
SLC38A4/SNAT4 (System A)	Na^+/AA co-transport	A, N, C, G, S, T	MVM BM
SLC38A3 /SNAT3 (System N)	Na^+/AA co-transport - H antiport	Q, H, A, N	Localization unclear
SLC38A5/SNAT5 (System N)	Na^+/AA co-transport - H antiport	Q, N, H, S	MVM
SLC43A1/LAT3	Facilitated diffusion	L, I, V	BM
SLC43A2/LAT4	Facilitated diffusion	L, I, V	BM

BM, Basal membrane; *EAAT,* excitatory amino acid transporter; *MVM,* microvillus membrane; *SLC,* solute carrier.

Based on Cleal JK, Lofthouse EM, Sengers BG, Lewis RM. A systems perspective on placental amino acid transport. *J Physiol.* 2018;596(23):5511–5522 and the series introduced by Hediger, MA, Clémençon B, Burrier RE, Bruford EA. The ABCs of membrane transporters in health and disease (SLC series): introduction. *Mol Aspects Med.* 2013;34(2–3):95–107.

SLC6

The taurine transporter (TAUT) (SLC6A6) has been found in MVM placental tissue and is thought to be important in maintaining the high intracellular concentrations of taurine observed in the human placenta.[24] Taurine is essential for fetal growth and is thought to be important in maintaining osmotic balance and functioning as an antioxidant.[25] In addition to transporting taurine into the placenta, the TAUT transporter potentially mediates the bilateral release of taurine into maternal and fetal circulations.[26] Studies examining the impact of obesity on placental function have reported that placental TAUT activity at term is negatively related to maternal body mass index (BMI).[27]

SLC7

The SLC7 family contains a large number of amino acid transporters that are relevant to placental function, including the transporters that constitute System L, System y^+, and System y^+L. LAT1 (SLC7A5) and 2 (SLC7A8) are exchange transporters that mediate transfer of neutral amino acids and, characteristic of System L, mediate transfer of the L-system-specific substrate 2-aminobicyclo-(2,2,1)-heptane-2-carboxylic acid (BCH). These[28] transporters, especially LAT2, have a broad substrate specificity for the neutral amino acids. Functional System L activity occurs through specific light chain proteins associated with 4F2hc.[29-30a] System L activity is reported on both the MVM and BM.[31-33] Immunologic and functional studies suggest that at term gestation, the light chain LAT1 is located predominantly in the MVM.[34,35] Furthermore, the L transport system phenotype associated with the MVM occurs when the LAT1 catalytic subunit is coexpressed with the 4F2hc, not LAT2.[36,37] Human LAT2 mRNA also has been reported in human choriocarcinoma BeWo cells and placental villous tissues.[38-41] Placental BM studies concerning the inhibition of specific amino acid and/or synthetic amino acid uptake have determined that the BM L transport system phenotype is associated with the coexpression of LAT2 and 4F2hc, and not LAT2, as observed to occur in the MVM.[30,40,42] Furthermore, regulation of placental System L activity does not seem to be under the control of hypoxia,[43] although evidence exists that it may not be the case in other cell preparations.[44,45] Although evidence is lacking in placental preparations, IGF-1 appears to regulate System L activity where chronic infusions of IGF-1 have corrected impaired transport of leucine in the brush border of the rat intestine.[46] Additionally, in a mouse model of intrauterine growth restriction (IUGR), System L remained at control levels after Ad-hIGF-1 administration.[47]

The transport of cationic amino acids occurs through the CAT and the y^+LAT transporters. The cationic amino acid transporter (CAT) activity is associated with System y^+ activity and in placental cell culture and human placental studies, CAT 1 (SLC7A1), 2B (SLC7A2), and 3 (SLC7A3) are expressed.[2,48] In contrast to the other SCL7 family transporters the CATs do not require a heavy chain for their activity.[37,49] CAT activity has been extensively studied in the rodent and human placenta.[50-52] In human preparations, CAT activity has been localized to the MVM and BM, although conflicting data exist as to y^+ activity in the BM.[48,53]

System y^+L activity is mediated by the transporters y^+LAT1 (SLC7A7) and y^+LAT2 (SLC7A6).[30a,53a,53b] y^+LATs are exchangers for cationic amino acids and sodium dependent exchangers for neutral amino acids. The effect of this selective Na-dependence is that they preferentially mediate efflux of cationic amino acids (as intracellular sodium concentrations are low, precluding efflux of neutral amino acids). y^+LAT activity is localized to both the MVM and BM.[2,48,37] This system may play an essential role in supplying cationic amino acids to the fetus by exchanging cationic amino acids within the trophoblast for neutral amino acids from the fetal circulation.[49,54,55]

SLC16

TAT1 (SLC16A10) is a facilitative transporter on the BM of the syncytiotrophoblast that mediates efflux of aromatic amino acids to the fetus. Placental expression of this transporter is positively associated with measures of fetal growth.[56] Unlike exchangers that take up one amino acid in exchange for each amino acid they release, facilitative transporters mediate transport in both directions. While this transporter can mediate transfer in both directions, it typically mediates net efflux to the fetus, as intracellular amino acid concentrations are typically higher than in plasma. Some of the amino acids transported in this way will be carried into the umbilical circulation and into fetal cells, while others will be taken up again by placental BM exchangers allowing other amino acids to be transported to the fetus.

SLC38

The SLC38 family includes the accumulative transporters responsible for system A and system N-like activity and are one of the more well understood transporter families of the placenta that take up a broad range of neutral amino acids.[57,58] System A activity is mediated by the transporters SNAT1 (SLC38A1), SNAT2 (SLC38A2), and SNAT4 (SLC38A4). These transporters mediate sodium dependent uptake of neutral amino acids and the characteristic System A substrate, methyl-aminobutyric. System A activity has been demonstrated in MVMs and at lower levels on the BMs. It is important to note that BM SNATs take fetal amino acids up into the placenta and do not typically transport amino acids into the fetus.[17,31,59] The SNAT1 isoform is expressed in the placenta, and is responsible for the transport of small, short-chain neutral amino acids, such as alanine, serine, methionine, asparagine, and glutamine.[60] The functional characteristics of SNAT2 are similar to those of SNAT1, although it is found in a wider range of tissues, including the placenta.[60,61] SNAT4 is reported to be present in both microvillus and BMs, and similarly to SNAT1 and SNAT2, it is expressed in the human placenta from early pregnancy onwards.[62]

SNAT transporters have been shown to be regulated by a number of factors, including angiotensin II,[63] phosphatidylinositol 3-kinase (PI3K), mechanistic target of rapamycin (mTOR), p70S6 kinase-dependent pathways, hypoxia, cortisol,[43,64-66] and IGF[47] through the mitogen-activated protein (MAP) kinase-dependent and independent pathways.[67] In mice, the *Slc38a4* gene is imprinted and potentially regulated by fetal nutrient demands. In studies using the placental-specific *Igf2* transcript (P0) knockout, placental growth is compromised, although fetal growth is not immediately affected, which is the result of an up-regulation of transporter genes *Slc2a3* (glucose transporter) and the imprinted gene, *Slc38a4*.[68,69] When fetal demands for nutrients are reduced through removal of the fetal *Igf2*, the up-regulation does not occur, providing evidence for regulation of placental transport activity via fetal growth demand genes. Both the *Igf2* and *Slc38a4* are paternally expressed, and this interaction is seen as a display of paternally inherited genes maximizing placental and fetal extraction of maternal nutrients.[68]

SNAT3 and SNAT5 mediate the activity attributed to System N. These transporters mediate uptake of sodium dependent amino acids in exchange for a proton.[70] Major SNAT3 and 5 substrates include histidine, glutamine, and asparagine. System N activity has been localized in the MVM in human placenta,[13,71] and SNAT3 (SLC38A3) is associated with this activity.[72]

In terms of amino acid movement into and out of trophoblast cells, it is interesting to note that the System A transport proteins, SNAT1 and SNAT2, are sodium coupled and function under physiologic conditions as influx transporters. In contrast, SNAT3 and its other System N isoform, SNAT5 (SLC38A5), are coupled to a sodium gradient and a proton gradient. They mediate a transport process in which sodium and glutamine move in one direction and H^+ moves in the opposite direction; this system has been highlighted as being responsible for cellular glutamine release in certain cell types.[73,74]

SLC43

LAT3 (SLC43A1) and LAT4 (SLC43A2) mediate facilitated transport of a restricted group of substrates including the branched chain amino acids (BCAA; leucine, isoleucine, and valine). While these transporters can mediate transfer in both directions, they typically mediate net efflux to the fetus, as intracellular amino acid concentrations are typically higher than in plasma. In the placenta these transporters are found on the BM of the syncytiotrophoblast and mediate net efflux of amino acids from the placenta to the fetus.[56] Placental LAT3 mRNA is positively associated with measures of fetal growth and has an important role in the net efflux of amino acids across the BM into the fetus and also in fetal development.[75,76]

As pregnancy advances, the increasing nutrient demands of the developing conceptus must be met through an appropriate increase in placental nutrient transport capacity. This enhanced performance, as it relates to amino acid transport, is facilitated through increased placental perfusion, including increased uteroplacental blood flow and membrane exchange area, together with changes in amino acid transporter concentrations and activity within the plasma membrane (see Box 41.1).

In conjunction with the dramatic increases in uteroplacental blood flow over gestation (human[77] and sheep[78]), the developing surface area of the trophoblast is an important factor regulating total placental nutrient transport. Between week 16 and term gestation, human fetal weight increases approximately 20-fold, whereas the peripheral placental villous surface area increases only 9-fold.[79–81] The demonstrated increases in total surface area of the placenta[82,83] alone cannot account for the rapid fetal growth occurring over this period. Fetal growth also is supported by changes in concentrations and activities of specific amino acid transporter proteins on the trophoblast cell membrane surface.

As amino acids require active transport, they fit into the category of substances transported by the placenta according to diffusion-limited clearance. Placental transport rates of amino acids are thus not affected by moderate fluctuations in uterine or placental blood flow. More severe reductions in uterine or placental blood flow could potentially affect amino acid transport, but this has not been observed. If reduced flow contributes to this process, the mechanisms may be mediated through altered placental energetics and ion gradients rather than by a direct reduction of flow-mediated delivery. Furthermore, changes in uterine or placental blood flow may alter transport of certain amino acids more than others, potentially leading to changes in the relative proportions of amino acids delivered to the fetus.[84] Such highlighted energetics and ion gradient deficiencies may be more important than amino acid delivery as the means by which amino acid uptake and transport are reduced by relatively decreased placental blood flow.

In addition to flow-mediated and placental exchange surface area changes, the capacity for placental amino acid transport also is affected by the differing expression and transport parameters of transport systems over gestation.[48,59,85–87] For example, in first-trimester and term human MVM preparations, L-arginine transport occurs through both y^+ and y^+L systems, whereas in the BM, transport may be restricted at term to only the y^+LAT system.[48] In addition, the kinetic properties of transport systems also may change as gestation advances. First-trimester MVMs have increased y^+LAT transport activity compared with term placenta vesicles,[85] and CAT activity appears to increase with gestational age.[50] Additionally, 4F2hc protein levels differ between early gestation and term placentae.[48] Such studies highlight the complex interactions that occur between developing MVM and BMs, within the trophoblast, and between the two circulations, to facilitate an increase in nutrient delivery to the growing fetus as gestation advances.

Box 41.1 Factors Affecting Placental Amino Acid Transfer

1. Transporter proteins in the trophoblast membranes: ontogeny, location (maternal-facing microvillus, fetal-facing basal, or both), regulation by local or circulating factors
2. Ion channel activity, ion gradients: Na^+, K^+-ATPase; Na^+, H^+, Cl^- gradients (e.g., inward Na^+ gradient with System A co-transport)
3. Transport capacity, measured by V_{max} (maximum transport rate, affected by number of active transporters, the number of transporters per unit membrane area, and total membrane surface area)
4. Transporter-substrate binding affinity, measured by K_m (plasma amino acid concentration at half V_{max})
5. Placental disease (e.g., fetal growth restriction and preeclampsia)
6. Intracellular concentrations of amino acid, maternal amino acid concentrations, fetal amino acid concentrations, maternal-fetal amino acid concentration gradients leading to competition for transporters among amino acids
7. Turnover of transporters (rates of synthesis, degradation, or both)
8. Metabolism of amino acids by the trophoblast (e.g., oxidation of glutamate, conversion to other amino acids or substrates such as serine to glycine and leucine to ketoisocaproic acid, protein synthesis, deamination-producing NH_3)
9. Uterine/umbilical blood flows: absolute rates (substrate delivery), the ratio of their flows (substrate delivery versus uptake and transport capacity), and the role of vasoactive substances (local or circulating) that alter uterine and/or umbilical blood flow (e.g., reduction in flow with epinephrine, enhancement of flow with nitric oxide)
10. Circulating hormone concentrations, placental receptors, and second messengers (e.g., hormone stimulation of cyclic adenosine monophosphate (AMP)-responsive increase in calcium channel and intracellular calcium release, activating amino acid metabolism and transporter activity)
11. Diffusional leaks into or out of cells or via paracellular pathways
12. Inhibitory effects of drugs (e.g., alcohol, nicotine, cocaine)

CHANGES IN AMINO ACID SUPPLY IN ADVERSE CONDITIONS IN UTERO

Data collected from IUGR pregnancies show reduced total amino acid placental concentrations,[88,89] reduced amino acid transporter activities,[90,91] and reduced amino acid transport.[92] Additionally, plasma amino acid concentrations are reported to be lower in growth-restricted fetuses, whether the measurements were made at the time of term delivery or many weeks before term.[88] Furthermore, fetal amino acid concentrations are lower in pregnancies with IUGR, even if the fetuses have normal fetal heart rate and velocimetry monitoring, indicating that the decreases in amino acid concentrations likely preceded other clinically significant pathologic changes in these pregnancies.[93,94]

Although reduced, circulating amino acid concentrations in the fetus have been used to interpret reduced placental supply; these values actually represent a balance among the rates of amino acid supply, synthesis into protein, release by protein catabolism, and oxidation. As such, reliance on concentration data alone in assessing the transport capacity of a placenta may not be entirely accurate. For example, more recent studies of fetal plasma amino acid concentrations in well-defined groups of human fetuses with IUGR, where samples were derived from fetal blood sampling, have not repeated earlier observations of reduced values for fetal amino acid concentrations.[95] Similarly, studies in models of sheep with IUGR have not shown reductions in all of the fetal plasma amino acid concentrations, especially the branch chain amino acids (BCAA) noted by the earlier studies.[96,97] Placental amino acid transport studies in human and sheep IUGR, using radioactive and stable tracer techniques, do support the earlier conclusions of reduced placental transport, but together they highlight that tissue uptake and fetal metabolism of amino acids might also be impaired in IUGR, as there appear to be conditions in which fetal concentrations are maintained despite decreased placental transport.[98] Mechanisms might include reduced fetal cellular amino acid uptake, reduced protein synthesis rates, and increased protein breakdown rates. Indeed, work in IUGR fetal sheep has shown evidence for reduced fetal utilization of amino acids as a result of decreased skeletal muscle protein synthesis rates and reduced demand for growth.[94,99]

In vitro observations, in which MVM vesicles from neonates who were appropriate-for-gestational-age (AGA) and small-for-gestational-age (SGA) were prepared, have demonstrated markedly lower activity (by 63%) of the System A transporters in the SGA neonates.[100] Several investigations have reported that System A membrane activity per milligram of MVM is reduced in IUGR placentae, indicating a positive association between fetal growth and System A activity.[86,101,102] In addition, the sodium-dependent and sodium-independent transport of taurine from maternal to fetal circulation also is reduced in IUGR pregnancies, thereby reducing fetal taurine concentration.[103]

Regarding the essential amino acids, the uptake of leucine in both MVM and BMs of the human IUGR placenta is reduced, indicating decreased concentration or activity of the placental L-transport system.[104] In these studies, BM uptake was also reduced, indicating that the changes in the BM could be an important adaptive response by the trophoblast to limit back flux of leucine from the fetal circulation to the placenta, which would otherwise further reduce fetal anabolic capacity. In vivo studies of sheep IUGR placental transport have indeed shown a reduced back flux of leucine (and threonine) from the fetal circulation to the placenta.[96,97] In addition, under steady-state conditions, the fetal-maternal enrichment ratio of leucine in normal human pregnancies is approximately 0.8, a much higher ratio than that of 0.4 in sheep.[97,105] However, in both species, this ratio is significantly lower in pregnancies with fetal growth restriction, indicating similarly reduced placental transport and metabolism characteristics. Clinical studies have shown that the fetal-maternal leucine enrichment ratio is significantly lower in human pregnancies with growth-restricted fetuses compared with normal pregnancies.[105] Furthermore, the magnitude of its reduction correlates with a clinical classification of IUGR severity based on a completely different set of clinical data, namely, fetal arterial velocimetry and fetal heart rate data.[93] Interestingly, the uptake of another essential amino acid, lysine, is not altered in placental preparations with growth-restricted fetuses.[104] This amino acid uses the CAT amino acid transporters and further studies confirm that the CAT and y^+LAT transporter activities are not altered in IUGR placental vesicles.[50] By way of additional species comparison, studies in rats in which IUGR was induced through maternal protein deprivation also have demonstrated a down-regulation of placental amino acid transport systems, including the CAT, SNAT, and EAAT systems.[106,107]

Another component of change in IUGR that relates to placental amino acid transport is that of surface area,[82,83,100] indicating that morphometric changes also are likely to contribute to the overall reduction in placental amino acid transport capacity. Thus, it currently appears that both reductions in surface area for exchange and reductions in specific transporter activity and/or number contribute to the reduction in amino acid transport in pregnancies with IUGR.

Despite considerable knowledge about amino acid transport differences in pregnancies with fetal growth restriction, understanding of how these systems are modulated in relation to maternal body composition is now rapidly advancing. In humans, placental System A transporter activity has been positively correlated with maternal muscle mass and negatively correlated with obesity.[108,109] At the mRNA level the placental expression of ASCT1 and 2 have been related to increased maternal adiposity.[110,111] Studies indicate that a maternal high-fat (HF) diet in pregnant rats causes up-regulation of placental nutrient transporters (GLUT1 and SNAT2), which is associated with fetal overgrowth.[112] Much of the work concerned with placental function and obesity is currently focused around System A. Activation of System A activity in placentae from obese mothers is associated with increased cytokine levels and reduced maternal adiponectin levels. Physiologic concentrations of the proinflammatory cytokines interleukin (IL)-6 and tumor necrosis factor (TNF)α are found to stimulate the activity of amino acid transporter System A but not System L in cultured human primary trophoblast cells,[113] whereas adiponectin appears to negatively impact insulin-stimulated System A amino acid transport.[114] Elevated circulating fatty acids are also associated with maternal obesity and have been postulated to play a regulatory role. Oleic acid in trophoblast culture is found to significantly up-regulate trophoblast System A activity.[115] Other observations indicate that maternal obesity-associated activation of insulin/IGF-1 and mTOR signaling pathway also may activate System A,[116] highlighting the possibility that fetal overgrowth that is associated with maternal obesity is the result of a complex interaction of factors culminating in the increased activity of System A in the placenta. In contrast, other studies have reported that System L is not increased with maternal obesity, opening the question of how other placental amino acid transport systems are affected by maternal obesity and what maternal factors in obese pregnant mothers account for such regulation.[117]

UTERINE AND PLACENTAL UPTAKE AND METABOLISM OF AMINO ACIDS

Uterine and placental amino acid uptake and metabolism have been studied extensively in the sheep model and also in human preparations using the placental perfusion model.[13,118,119] In sheep studies, net uptake rates of amino acids by the uterus have been difficult to measure because of small uterine arteriovenous concentration differences and relative inaccuracies in the determination of the high rate of uterine blood flow (from as low as 600 to as high as 1600 mL/min in late gestation pregnant sheep). Despite these measurement limitations, uterine arteriovenous concentration differences in pregnant sheep are positive, indicating net uptake by the uterus for all amino acids tested except glutamate.[119a] Furthermore, the ratio of umbilical-uterine arteriovenous differences (1.9:1) in late gestation when placental growth has slowed but fetal growth is maximal is approximately equal to the uterine-umbilical blood flow ratio.[120] This evidence indicates that in late gestation most uterine amino acid uptake is transported to the fetus and that uterine requirements for amino acids are small relative to those of the fetus.

In contrast, the placenta of the sheep in early gestation is highly active in amino acid utilization and metabolism, particularly for leucine, threonine, glycine, alanine, and glutamate.[12,97,121-123] Early in gestation, the placental-fetal weight ratio is several-fold higher than at term, and placental growth (by increase in surface area relative to weight or by absolute increase in mass, depending on species and gestational age) is greatest at this period, indicating that placental amino acid metabolism might be quantitatively significant relative to that of the fetus. Lemons and associates[124] estimated that placental growth over gestation would require 10.6 g of nitrogen (or 66 g of protein).[124] Additionally, infusions of certain radioactively labeled amino acids (lysine, leucine, glycine, and aspartate) into the in situ perfused guinea pig placenta showed that 12% to 16% of the label was incorporated into placental proteins. This process was inhibited (by 81% to 96%) by cycloheximide, demonstrating that an active process of placental synthesis of proteins was, in fact, occurring.[125] In human placentae, a study of phenylalanine uptake indicated that an even higher proportion of phenylalanine was incorporated into protein, and this had a major effect on amino acid transfer.[126]

The near-term placenta contains a large variety of enzymes that are capable of metabolizing amino acids through pathways such as gluconeogenesis, glycogen synthesis, protein synthesis, amino acid oxidation, and the production of ammonia.[124] Amino acid oxidation by human placental mitochondria has been demonstrated for alanine, aspartate, glutamate, and glycine, and ammonia is produced in vivo in the placentae of sheep, rabbits, and guinea pigs.[127-130] Other amino acid requirements include synthesis of secreted protein products (e.g., hormones, such as human chorionic gonadotropin, luteinizing hormone, and placental lactogen).

Studies in the human placenta suggest that a large proportion of amino acids taken up by the placenta are rapidly incorporated into placental protein.[126] This prevents them from reaching the fetus immediately, but as these proteins are recycled the amino acids will again become available for transfer to the fetus. The amino acids transferred to the fetus will be a mixture of those recently taken up from the maternal circulation and those released from placental protein breakdown.

The placenta and fetus interact in a variety of ways to ensure amino acid supply to vital developmental, metabolic, and signaling processes that are unique to fetal growth and development (see Fig. 41.1).[131] For example, alanine is consumed by the sheep placenta.[123] Placental metabolism of alanine may contribute to placental lactate production[132] and to placental carbon oxidation. Furthermore, in the sheep model, maternal plasma alanine entering the placenta is metabolized and exchanged for placentally derived alanine. In fact, most of the alanine delivered to the fetus is of placental origin.[123]

Given that the placenta actively metabolizes amino acids, it produces ammonia, which is delivered into both the uterine and umbilical circulations.[129,133] This process appears to be normal and occurs over a large part of gestation. For example, in sheep, the absolute rate of uteroplacental ammonia production (approximately 25 μmol/min) at mid-gestation is similar to rates measured near term,[134] as negligible urea cycle activity occurs in sheep placental tissue.[133,135] This relatively high placental ammonia production rate in mid-gestation probably accounts for the higher concentration of ammonia (approximately two-fold) in fetal blood. At that stage of development, fetal weight and the capacity of the fetus to clear ammonia are markedly reduced relative to term.[136] As the fetus matures, fetal hepatic urea cycle enzyme activity and production rates increase, approaching 0.4 g of nitrogen excretion/kg/day.[129] The higher ratio of ammonia production to urea excretion rate that occurs earlier in gestation may be an advantage to the smaller fetus, providing nitrogen for reincorporation into amino acids and amines essential for rapid fetal growth.[137,138] A fraction of the net umbilical ammonia uptake is extracted by fetal tissues in sheep, perhaps contributing to hepatic urea formation and to other specific metabolic pathways. However, the ammonia taken up by the fetal sheep liver near term (approximately 6.5 μmol/min) is 1.5 to 1.8 times that taken up by the umbilical circulation, demonstrating considerable fetal endogenous ammonia production,[139] which contributes to positive nitrogen balance across the fetal hindlimb.[140]

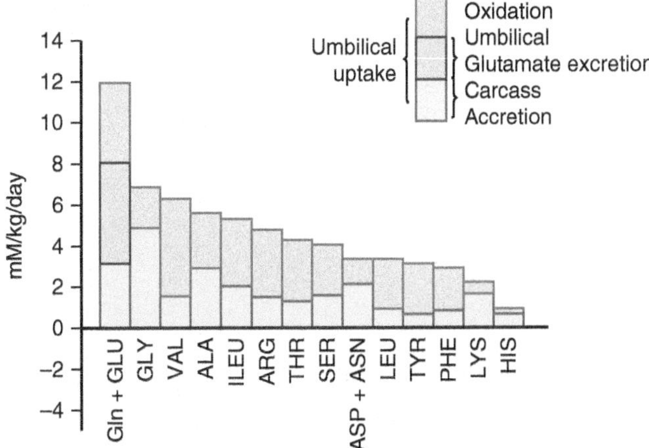

Fig. 41.2 Umbilical uptake of individual amino acids by the late gestation fetal sheep, partitioned into amino acid utilization for carcass accretion *(lower, green portion of bar)* and that presumably used for oxidation *(upper, orange portion of bar)*. There was a net excretion to the placenta from the fetus for glutamate in this study. *ALA*, Alanine; *ARG*, arginine; *ASN*, asparagines; *ASP*, aspartate; *Gln*, glutamine; *GLU*, glutamate; *GLY*, glycine; *HIS*, histidine; *ILEU*, isoleucine; *LEU*, leucine; *LYS*, lysine; *PHE*, phenylalanine; *SER*, serine; *THR*, threonine; *TYR*, tyrosine; *VAL*, valine. (From Lemons JA, Adcock EW 3rd, Jones MD Jr. Umbilical uptake of amino acids in the unstressed fetal lamb. *J Clin Invest.* 1976;58:1428.)

UMBILICAL (FETAL) AMINO ACID UPTAKE

The net uptake of amino acids by the umbilical circulation represents the dietary or nutritional supply of amino acids for fetal growth and protein metabolism. Although net protein uptake by the fetus has been observed, this additional amount of protein supply to the fetus probably provides little nutritional value over free amino acid uptake. However, protein molecules across a range of molecular weights can either diffuse across the placenta or cross by receptor mediated transcytosis.[141,142]

The uptake of amino acids by the fetus via the umbilical circulation has been studied most extensively in fetal sheep because this well-characterized large animal model has allowed for accurate quantification of plasma amino acid concentrations in both the umbilical artery and vein. Umbilical uptake rates of amino acids can be calculated by application of the Fick principle, whereby the product of umbilical blood flow times the umbilical venous-arterial blood concentration difference for each amino acid yields the *net* uptake of each amino acid by the fetus.[5] Fig. 41.2 illustrates the net uptake for each amino acid in fetal sheep studied during the last 20% of gestation (net uptake equals the total height of each bar). Several studies in late gestation fetal sheep have found total fetal umbilical nitrogen uptake rates that range from 0.91 to 1.2 g nitrogen/kg/day.[139,143,144] This range of values does not differ from the calculated total fetal nitrogen requirement of approximately 1 g nitrogen/kg/day based on nitrogen accretion data and estimated fetal urea production rates in near-term fetal sheep.[5] Fig. 41.2 also shows, in the solid portion of the bars, the net accretion of each amino acid in the fetal carcass. The net fetal uptake of most of the basic amino acids exceeds their net accretion by considerable amounts. In contrast, the net uptakes of the two basic amino acids, lysine and histidine, and the uptake of the neutral amino acid glycine barely exceed net accretion. Similarly, the combined accretion of asparagine and its product aspartate and the combined accretion of glutamine

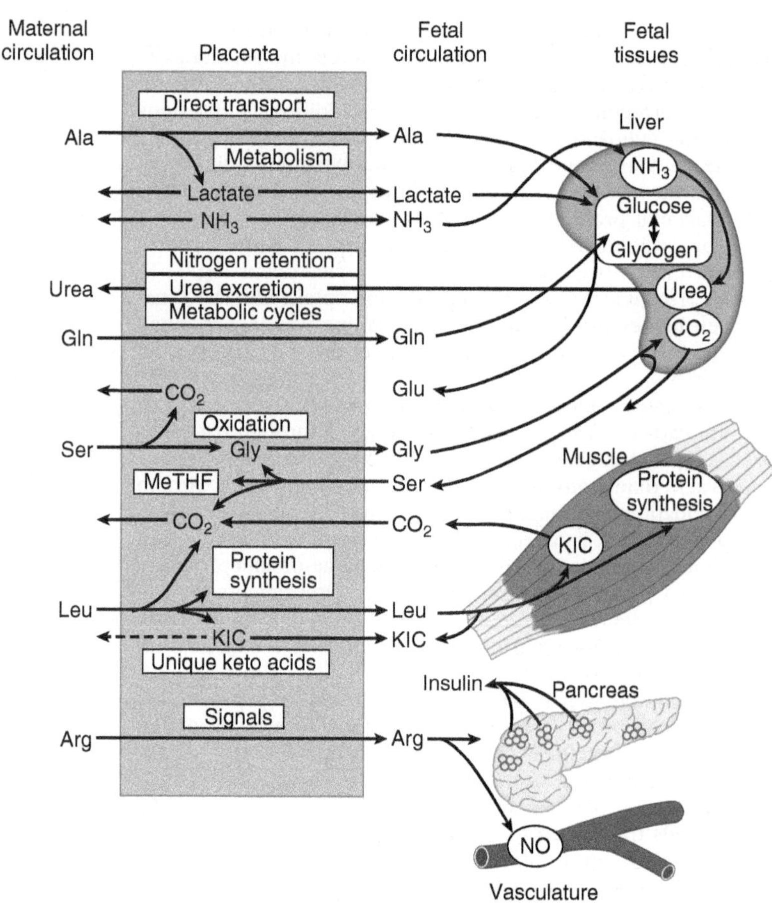

Fig. 41.3 Schematic representation of a variety of placental-fetal metabolic interactions with respect to amino acid uptake by the placenta, metabolism in the trophoblast cells, direct transfer to the fetus, signaling of fetal vascular and metabolic processes, and utilization in fetal tissues. *Ala,* Alanine; *Arg,* arginine; *Gln,* glutamine; *Glu,* glutamate; *Gly,* glycine; *KIC,* α-ketoisocaproic acid; *Leu,* leucine; *MeTHF,* methyltetrahydrofolate; *NH_3,* ammonia; *NO,* nitric oxide; *Ser,* serine. (From Hay WW Jr. Metabolic interrelationships of placenta and fetus. *Placenta.* 1995;16:19.)

and its product glutamate are very close to the net uptakes of asparagine and glutamine, respectively. For these amino acid pairs, no net uptake of the acidic forms, glutamate and aspartate, occurs. This is true not only in sheep[139] but also in primates[145] and in humans.[146] Glutamate and aspartate are derived in the fetus from deamination. It is very likely that limitation of supply of these five amino acids (lysine, histidine, glycine, glutamine, and asparagine) would lead to reduced protein accretion and growth.

PLACENTAL-FETAL AMINO ACID CYCLING

The placenta also contributes to fetal amino acid and nitrogen balance in sheep through selective interorgan cycling, although it is not clear that this occurs in humans (Fig. 41.3).[147,148] Measurements of umbilical and hepatic concentrations of amino acids in fetal sheep have demonstrated reciprocal relationships among three pairs of amino acids: glutamine and glutamate, serine and glycine, and asparagine and aspartate.[147,149,150] Based on studies that show net release of serine, glutamate, and aspartate from the fetus to the placenta, it is clear that fetal requirements for some amino acids are met by net production within fetal tissues, mainly the fetal liver.[139]

Sheep studies have shown interorgan cycling of serine and glycine. Glycine is released by the placenta into the fetal circulation, taken up by the fetal liver, converted to serine, and serine, in turn, is taken up by the placenta.[151,152] Tracer studies in near-term fetal sheep show no direct transplacental transport of maternal plasma serine to the fetal circulation. Rather, maternal plasma serine is used within the uteroplacental tissues to produce glycine, which is then taken up by the fetus.[122,153] Further studies have shown that the fetal liver is the major site of serine synthesis from plasma glycine.[151,152] Fetal hepatic glycine oxidation and serine production from glycine are linked by the enzymes, glycine oxidase and serine hydroxymethyl transferase.[154] However, glycine entry into the fetal pool is principally derived from umbilical uptake (30%) and from protein breakdown (56%). Glycine production in the placenta utilizes serine derived from both maternal and fetal circulations.[153] A byproduct of placental glycine production is methylene tetrahydrofolate (MeTHF), which is involved in a variety of methylation reactions within the placenta.[153,155]

In contrast, in humans the activity of the serine hydroxyethyl transferase enzyme, that mediates conversion of serine to glycine, was 24-fold lower than in the sheep.[148] The human umbilical venous-arterial difference for glycine also is small, evidence that this pathway, that is prominent in sheep is not a primary feature of human placental metabolism. The alternative pathway for glycine synthesis is the amino transferase reaction, but this is not observed in human placenta either.[156]

Another example of placental-fetal amino acid cycling involves glutamine and glutamate.[149] In sheep and primates, very little transport of glutamate directly from the maternal to the fetal circulation occurs.[139,145] Consistent with these findings, glutamate concentrations are lower in the umbilical vein than in the umbilical artery in humans at delivery.[146,157] However, glutamine is delivered directly from the placenta into the fetal circulation. Net fetal glutamine uptake and fetal glutamate transfer back to the placenta are directly correlated, certainly in the sheep pregnancy.[158] In the human placenta, glutamate is taken up from the maternal and fetal circulations, and more than 90% of this fetal derived glutamate is transported to the maternal circulation.[13,157] In the sheep placenta, almost 100% of fetal glutamate production is accounted for by fetal hepatic production from glutamine, as 45% of the glutamine taken up by the liver is released as glutamate.[159] Tracer studies in late gestation fetal sheep show that the placenta extracts almost 90% of the tracer glutamate carried by the umbilical circulation, representing a remarkably high placental clearance of fetal glutamate.[12] Of the glutamate taken up from the umbilical circulation, 70% to 80% is oxidized, which is the major pathway for disposal.[12] The sheep placenta also contains glutamine synthetase, which allows a small fraction of glutamate taken up by the placenta from the fetal circulation to be synthetized into glutamine and returned to the fetus.

Uterine uptake rates of BCAA are higher than their umbilical uptake rates.[160] This finding, in conjunction with relatively high concentrations and activities of BCAA aminotransferases in the placenta (sheep, human),[161,13] supports significant BCAA deamination within the placenta to their respective ketoacids. Studies in sheep show that 10% to 15% of leucine carbon transferred to the fetus is in the form of ketoisocaproic acid (KIC).[162,163] The deamination of BCAA provides the placenta with ammonia (as a nitrogen source) that, in addition to other placental metabolic functions, is used to sustain a high rate of glutamate production.[134] Thus the sheep placenta receives two major influxes of glutamate: the placental uptake of fetal plasma glutamate at approximately 4.8 µmol/kg/min and the placental production of glutamate from deamination of BCAA at 3.2 µmol/kg/min.[160,163] Placental oxidation of glutamate serves as its principal pathway of disposal. In addition to maintaining nitrogen production and excretion within the placenta, placental glutamate oxidation also provides nicotinamide adenine dinucleotide phosphate (NADPH), which is required for placental lipid metabolism and steroidogenesis, particularly that of progesterone.[159]

The release of glutamate and serine from the fetal liver could be a direct reflection of the uncoupling of gluconeogenesis from amino acid oxidation. No significant liver gluconeogenesis has been demonstrated in the normally growing fetus, as the fetus relies on facilitated transport of glucose down a concentration gradient from mother to fetus.[164,165] Thus the shuttling of glutamate from fetus to placenta provides an energy-efficient pathway for the fetal liver to divert the products of amino acid metabolism (carbon, nitrogen) to the placenta instead of producing glucose. This hypothesis is supported by a study in late gestation fetal sheep, which showed that fetal hepatic glucose production induced by a glucagon infusion was mirrored by an equivalent reduction in hepatic output of pyruvate and glutamate.[166] At birth this pattern shifts, so that with the loss of the placenta and the development of net hepatic production of glucose, glutamine carbon can be shunted directly to gluconeogenesis.

HUMAN INTRAUTERINE GROWTH AND PROTEIN ACCRETION

As it is not possible to obtain direct measurements of human fetal growth and fetal body composition, fetal growth rates have been estimated by inference from cross-sectional data of anthropometric measurements of infants born at different gestational ages. Data on chemical composition are based on studies of infants who died close to birth but appeared normally grown at autopsy. The better of these studies have excluded obviously abnormal infants and have involved defined, relatively homogeneous populations. Even with such precautions, there has been no assurance that infants born preterm had grown normally in utero; therefore, it is not known for certain whether their weights represent those of normally growing fetuses. Furthermore, anthropometric measurements have their own inherent range of accuracy, and cross-sectional, static size-for-gestational-age groupings of neonates may not accurately reflect the dynamics of fetal growth.[167] In addition, population means of fetal growth rate do not necessarily reflect growth of a given fetus or the changes in body composition with growth that occur with

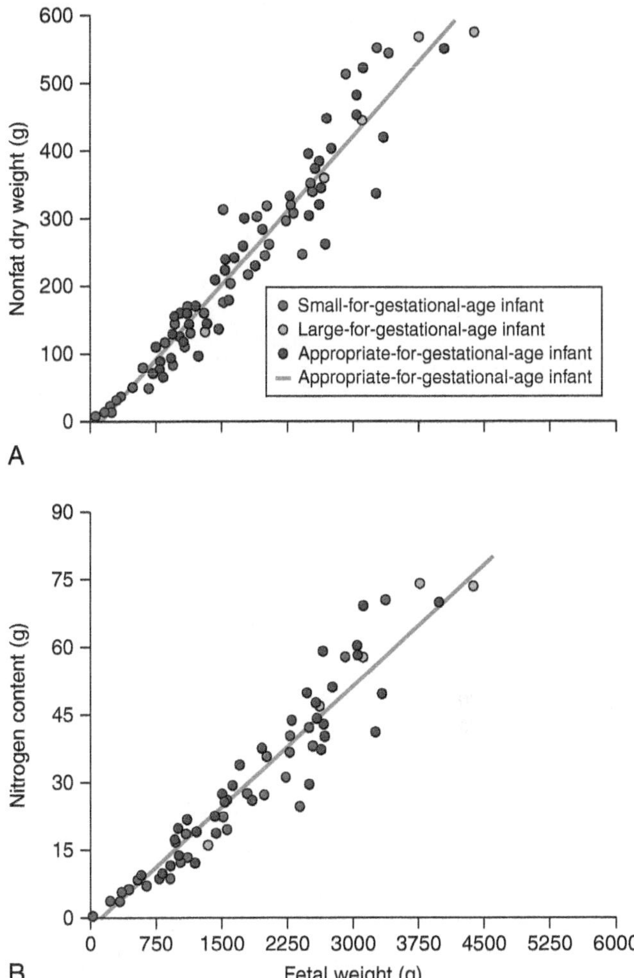

Fig. 41.4 (A) Relationship of nonfat dry weight (NFDW) to fetal weight in 169 human fetuses. NFDW = 0.0589 g. (B) Relationship of nitrogen (N) content to fetal weight in the same infants. *N* = 0.00665 g. (From Sparks JW. Human intrauterine growth and nutrient accretion. *Semin Perinatol.* 1984;8:74.)

advancing gestational age.[168] Because of these potential concerns with using cross-sectional newborn data to approximate fetal growth, fetal growth references also have been published based on prospective serial ultrasound measurements of fetuses who were born to healthy women with low-risk pregnancies from across the world[169,170] and for different racial and ethnic groups in the United States.[171]

Despite such concerns about the reliability of data, most composite evaluations of human fetal growth based on neonatal anthropometric measurements at birth are relatively similar.[172] Most mean percentiles among the many different growth curves differ by ±5% or less and can be accounted for primarily by factors such as suboptimal pregnancy dating, adverse maternal and/or fetal medical and obstetric complications of pregnancy, and variations in male-female proportions, maternal race, ethnicity, socioeconomic status, altitude, and diet. In the more recent studies that have accounted for many of the factors that can affect fetal growth and fetal size, fetal weight gain appears to be a linear function of gestational age from approximately 26 weeks gestation through to about 36 weeks gestation (15 to 18 g/day), with only slight increases for male versus female sex and for maternal obesity.[173-176] In contrast, estimated weight gain per kg body weight per day is highest (20 to 23 g/kg/day) in extremely low-birth-weight infants (500 to 1000 g) and slowly

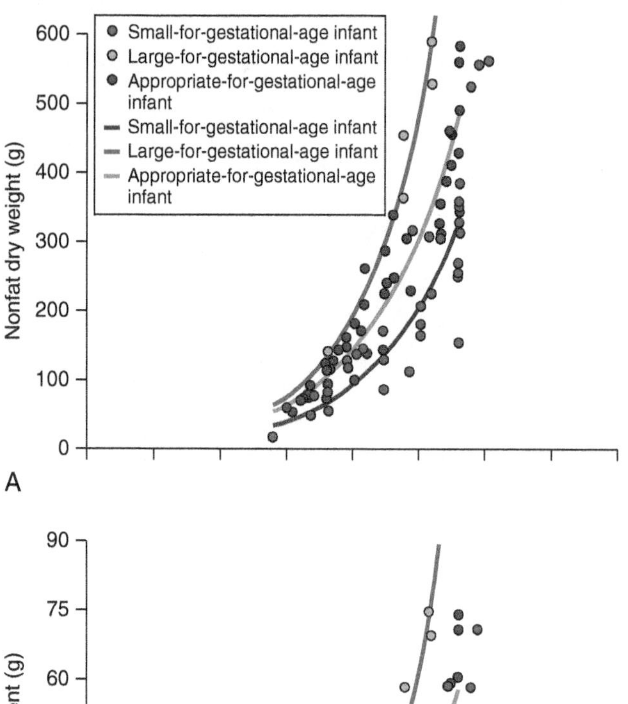

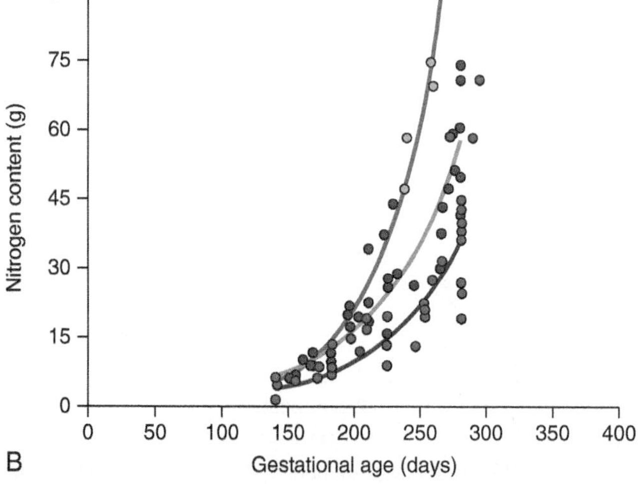

Fig. 41.5 (A) Relationship of nonfat dry weight (NFDW) to gestational age in 97 human fetuses. Increase in NFDW:LGA-NFDW (g) = 4.78, $e^{(0.0184.GA)}$, $r = 0.9869$; AGA-NFDW (g) = 6.38, $e^{(0.01548.GA)}$, $r = 0.9511$; SGA-NFDW (g) = 3.60, $e^{(0.0161.GA)}$, $r = 0.9380$. (B) Relationship of nitrogen content to gestational age in the same infants. Increase in total body nitrogen (N); LGA-N (g) = 0.227, $e^{(0.0225.GA)}$, $r = 0.9870$; AGA-N (g) = 0.703, $e^{(0.0157.GA)}$, $r = 0.9385$; SGA-N (g) = 0.377, $e^{(0.0163.GA)}$, $r = 0.9351$. *AGA,* Appropriate-for-gestational-age; *LGA,* large-for-gestational-age; *SGA,* small-for-gestational-age. (From Sparks JW. Human intrauterine growth and nutrient accretion. *Semin Perinatol.* 1984;8:74.)

declines as birth weight increases towards 2000 to 2500 g (12 to 14 g/kg/day).

Information regarding chemical composition is based on several older studies that included relatively few cases. Sparks reviewed data from 15 studies with a combined 207 infants.[168] Based on these data, nonfat dry weight and nitrogen content (both reasonably good predictors of protein content) show a linear relationship with fetal weight (Fig. 41.4) and an exponential relationship with gestational age (Fig. 41.5).[168] However, at each gestational age, a variety of fetal weights are observed. Thus, nonfat dry weight and nitrogen content for a given fetus can also be compared with the "average" fetus. When these comparisons are made, larger fetuses grow faster than smaller fetuses at the same gestational age; protein accretion and therefore protein nutritional requirements follow accordingly.

Tables 41.2 and 41.3 present nitrogen, protein, and selected amino acid composition and accretion rates, respectively, in reportedly normal human fetuses.[177] However, according to data from sheep and guinea pigs, 80% of the nitrogen content of the fetus in these species is found in protein; the remainder largely occurs in urea, ammonia, and free amino acids. The data for human fetal protein content and accretion in these tables may be high because they are based solely on nitrogen content. Additional nitrogen requirements for urea excretion (and for other possible nitrogen excretion products) are not known for human fetuses. Several items of comparative chemical and physical growth in six species are summarized in Table 41.4.[178] Variation among certain parameters is considerable; for example, growth rate variation is 20-fold and weight-specific content of fat at term varies 16-fold among different species. In contrast, nonfat dry weight and protein weight specific contents (as a percentage of total weight) at term are constant. Limited chemical analyses at different gestational ages indicate that fetal protein content and requirements are linearly related to fetal weight.

DIRECT MEASURES OF FETAL AMINO ACID METABOLISM AND ACCRETION

Table 41.5 summarizes the contributions of amino acids to fetal carbon, calories, and nitrogen balance compared with other known substrates in late-gestation fetal sheep.[179-181] Studies in the fetal sheep have demonstrated that the net uptake of amino acids by the fetus exceeds the requirements for growth. This observation implies that the excess portion of amino acid uptake is used for oxidation. More direct evidence for the fetal oxidation of amino acids comes from two observations: the high fetal urea production rate[182,183] and the direct measurement of labeled carbon dioxide production and excretion during fetal infusions of carbon-labeled amino acids.[184] Estimates of fetal urea production rate range from 0.4 mg/min/kg in humans,[185] horses,[186] and rhesus monkeys[127] to 0.7 mg/min/kg in sheep.[182] The urea production rate in sheep could account for approximately 0.36 g/kg/day of nitrogen excretion (or 25% of fetal nitrogen uptake in amino acids) and 0.2 g/kg/day of carbon (or 2% of total fetal carbon uptake and 6% of fetal carbon uptake in amino acids). Such fetal urea production rates are large, exceeding neonatal and adult body weight–specific rates, indicating relatively rapid protein turnover and oxidation in the fetus.

Direct measurement of fetal amino acid oxidation with carbon-labeled isotopic tracers of selected amino acids quantifies oxidation as the net excretion of labeled carbon dioxide from the fetus via the umbilical circulation relative to the plasma labeled amino acid specific activity (SA).[187] Central to this methodology has been the documentation that, at least in the fetal lamb, almost 100% of fetal carbon dioxide production (as measured by fetal infusion of $NaH^{14}CO_3$) is excreted via the umbilical circulation.[187] Further measurements of organ-specific carbon dioxide production can be obtained in fetal sheep from measurements of labeled blood carbon dioxide content from catheterized hepatic (liver) and femoral (hind limb) veins after amino acid tracer infusion.[99,152] Several ^{13}C or ^{14}C-labeled amino acids have been infused into the fetus in vivo, documenting $^{13}CO_2$ or $^{14}CO_2$ production (leucine, lysine, alanine, glycine, serine, threonine, glutamate).[a]

At mid-gestation, leucine oxidation is at least as great as it is at term, indicating that amino acids provide carbon for fetal oxidative metabolism over a large part of gestation.[190] Fetal sheep demonstrate the ability to increase leucine oxidation rates by nearly 50% when amino acid supply is increased by direct intravenous infusion of mixed amino acids.[191] In addition, net fetal glucose uptake rates and glucose-oxygen quotients decrease

[a]References 12, 97, 121, 151, 188, 189.

Table 41.2 Increments per Day of Nutrients in the Fetal Body at Selected Intervals During Gestation.

Fetal age range (wk) Weight range (kg)	12–16 0.02–0.1	16–20 0.1–0.3	20–24 0.3–0.75	24–28 0.75–1.35	28–32 1.35–2.0	32–36 2.0–2.7	36–40 2.7–3.4
Increments of Nitrogen (N) and Protein in Fetal Body/24 h							
Total N	29	93	243	326	386	504	714
Protein (g) (N × 6.25)	0.18	0.58	1.52	2.04	2.41	3.15	4.46
Increments of Individual Acids in Fetal Body (mg/day)							
ILE	6	26	53	71	82	109	148
LEU	13	43	111	151	174	231	330
LYS	13	41	107	145	167	222	313
MET	4	11	28	39	44	59	92
PHE	7	23	61	83	95	127	184
TYR	5	17	44	59	68	91	127
THR	7	23	61	83	95	127	184
ARG	14	43	114	154	177	236	340
HIS	5	15	39	53	61	81	112
ALA	13	41	107	145	167	222	319
ASP	17	52	136	183	211	281	392
GLU	23	74	195	263	303	403	568
GLY	21	68	177	240	276	367	513
PRO	15	48	125	168	194	258	300
SER	5	25	66	89	102	136	191

ALA, Alanine; *ARG*, arginine; *ASP*, aspartate; *GLU*, glutamate; *GLY*, glycine; *HIS*, histidine; *ILE*, isoleucine; *LEU*, leucine; *LYS*, lysine; *MET*, methionine; *PHE*, phenylalanine; *PRO*, proline; *SER*, serine; *THR*, threonine; *TYR*, tyrosine.
From Widdowson EM. Chemical composition and nutritional needs of the fetus at different stages of gestation. In: Aebi H, Whitehead R, eds. *Maternal Nutrition During Pregnancy and Lactation*. Beme: Hans Huber; 1980:39–48.

Table 41.3 Body Composition of the Human Fetus.

Fetal age (wk) Weight (kg)	12 0.02	16 0.1	20 0.3	24 0.75	28 1.35	32 2.0	36 2.7	40 3.4
Total Nitrogen (N) and Protein in Fetal Body								
Total N (g)	0.18	1.0	3.6	10.4	19.6	30.2	44.3	64.3
Protein (g) (N × 6.25)	1.1	6.3	22.5	65	123	189	227	402
Content of Individual Amino Acids in Fetal Body (g)								
ILE	0.04	0.22	0.77	2.3	4.2	6.5	9.6	13.7
LEU	0.08	0.46	1.7	4.8	9.0	13.9	20.3	29.6
LYS	0.08	0.44	1.6	4.6	8.6	13.3	19.5	28.3
MET	0.02	0.12	0.42	1.2	2.3	3.5	5.2	7.8
PHE	0.05	0.25	0.91	2.6	4.9	7.6	11.1	16.3
TYR	0.04	0.18	0.65	1.9	3.5	5.4	8.0	11.5
THR	0.05	0.25	0.91	2.6	4.9	7.6	11.1	16.3
VAL	0.05	0.28	1.0	3.0	5.6	8.7	12.8	18.6
ARG	0.08	0.47	1.7	4.9	9.2	14.1	20.7	30.3
HIS	0.03	0.16	0.59	1.7	3.2	4.9	7.2	10.4
ALA	0.08	0.44	1.6	4.6	8.6	13.3	19.5	28.5
ASP	0.10	0.56	2.0	5.8	10.9	16.8	24.7	35.7
GLU	0.14	0.80	2.9	8.3	15.7	24.2	35.5	51.4
GLY	0.14	0.73	2.6	7.6	14.3	22.0	32.3	46.6
PRO	0.09	0.51	1.8	5.3	10.1	15.5	22.7	33.2
SER	0.05	0.27	0.97	2.8	5.3	8.2	12.0	17.3

ALA, Alanine; *ARG*, arginine; *ASP*, aspartate; *GLU*, glutamate; *GLY*, glycine; *HIS*, histidine; *ILE*, isoleucine; *LEU*, leucine; *LYS*, lysine; *MET*, methionine; *PHE*, phenylalanine; *PRO*, proline; *SER*, serine; *THR*, threonine; *TYR*, tyrosine; *VAL*, valine.
From Widdowson EM. Chemical composition and nutritional needs of the fetus at different stages of gestation. In: Aebi H, Whitehead R, eds. *Maternal Nutrition During Pregnancy and Lactation*. Beme: Hans Huber; 1980:39–48.

as a result of the amino acid infusion, suggesting a shift in substrate oxidation patterns to favor amino acids over glucose when the amino acids are in excess supply in normally growing fetal sheep. When amino acid supply was similarly increased in IUGR fetal sheep, leucine oxidation rates also increased by about 30%, although there was no simultaneous decline in net fetal glucose utilization rates or glucose-oxygen quotients.[192] One possible explanation for this observation is that excess amino acid supply was used to support gluconeogenesis, a process that is prematurely activated in the IUGR fetus.[193] Direct measurement of amino acid metabolism in the fetus using chronic catheterization of the fetal lamb will become even more important as efforts persist to increase nitrogen intake as a therapy for fetal growth disturbances.

Table 41.4 Growth Characteristics and Chemical Composition at Term of Selected Mammals and a Representative Human Fetus.

	Human	Monkey	Sheep	Guinea Pig	Rabbit	Rat
Gestation (days)	280	163	147	67	30	21.5
Number of fetuses	1	1	1	3–5	4–6	10–12
Growth rate (g/kg/day)	15	44	60	70	300	350
Fetal weight (g)	3500	500	4000	100	60	5
Dry weight (g/%)	1050/30	125/25	760/19	25/25	9/15	0.2/4
Nonfat dry weight (g/%)	490/14	–	640/16	14/14	–	–
Protein (g/%)	490/12	–	480/12	12/12	7.2/12	0.6/12

From McCance RA, Widdowson EM. Glimpses of comparative growth and development. In: Falkner F, Tanner JM eds. *Human Growth*. 2nd ed. New York: Plenum Press; 1985:139.

Table 41.5 Metabolic Balance for the Late Gestation Fetal Sheep.

Carbon-Caloric Balance	(g/kg/day)	(kcal/kg/day)
Requirement		
Accumulation in carcass	3.2	32
Excretion as CO_2	4.4	0
Excretion as urea	0.2	2
Excretion as glutamate	0.3	2
Heat (O_2 consumption)	0.0	50
Total	8.1	86
Uptake		
Amino acids	3.9	45
Glucose	2.4	17
Lactate	1.4	14
Fructose	1.0	7
Acetate	0.2	3
Total	8.9	86
Nitrogen Balance Requirement		
Urea nitrogen excretion	0.4	
Nitrogen accretion	0.6	
Total	1.0	
Uptake (in amino acids)	1.0	
Total	1.0	

From Battaglia FC, Meschia G. Fetal nutrition. *Annu Rev Nutr*. 1988;8:43; Meier P, Teng C, Battaglia FC, et al. The rate of amino acid nitrogen and total nitrogen accumulation in the fetal lamb. *Proc Soc Exp Biol Med*. 1981;167:463; and Battaglia FC, Meschia G. *Fetal and Placental Metabolism: Part I. Oxygen and Carbohydrates. An Introduction to Fetal Physiology*. Orlando, FL: Academic Press; 1986:49–99.

In the growing fetus, net protein synthesis exceeds net protein degradation, although both processes continue simultaneously. Protein synthetic rate equals the sum of the rates of protein accretion and protein degradation, where protein accretion has been measured in fetuses by whole carcass protein analysis at different gestational ages. The protein synthetic rate has been determined using isotopic tracers of various amino acids. The rate of incorporation of tracer amino acid into proteins is the difference between infusion rate and the combined loss of tracer to catabolic pathways (oxidation) and diffusional loss to the placenta.[194] Such tracer methodology is limited by the fact that it calculates a whole-body protein synthetic rate, which does not address the markedly different rates of growth and protein synthesis that occur among individual organs. Newer methodology using staggered start time of isotopomers of phenylalanine and a single muscle biopsy have enabled the measurement of fractional protein synthetic rates in fetal skeletal muscle.[99] Several studies performed in preterm infants receiving intravenous amino acids in addition to intravenous glucose using a [1-^{14}C]leucine tracer have found that amino acid administration primarily increases leucine oxidation and increases protein synthesis, with less of an effect on proteolysis.[195-197] However, in term human infants, administration of amino acids suppresses proteolysis in addition to increasing amino acid oxidation, indicating differences in the regulation of protein turnover by amino acids at different stages in early development.[198]

The fractional protein synthetic rate (K_S, or the fraction of body proteins that are synthesized/unit time) can be calculated and compared with fractional growth rate (K_G). K_S is calculated by infusing an amino acid tracer until a plateau SA in proteins and in the plasma is reached[180]; thus $K_S = SA_{proteins}/(SA_{plasma} \times$ time of infusion). The accuracy of this calculation can be improved by calculating the rate at which steady-state SA is obtained and by accounting for the recycling of tracer from degradation of newly synthesized (tracer-containing) proteins. In the fetal lamb, K_S and K_G have been compared using two tracers, [1-^{14}C]leucine and [1-^{14}C]lysine, at different gestational ages.[190,199] Fig. 41.6 is a composite of data from these studies, demonstrating that both K_S and K_G decrease with gestational age, but the decline in K_S is greater. The higher protein synthetic rate in the mid-gestation fetus compared to near term is proportional to higher amino acid nitrogen uptake rate, the higher metabolic rate, and the greater glucose uptake and utilization rates at that stage of gestation. Estimates of amino acid requirements at mid-gestation in fetal sheep range from 3.5 to 4.5 g/kg/day, rates, which, when scaled to human fetal growth rates, compare favorably with that of 4 g/kg/day determined by the factorial method.[200] Thus protein synthesis per millimole of oxygen consumed is essentially constant from mid-gestation until term.[190]

The decline in K_S and K_G with gestational age indicate that the reduced rate of fetal growth toward term is an intrinsic quality of fetal development and not the result of placental limitation of nutrient supply. However, even the term fetus demonstrates fetal protein synthesis rates higher than protein breakdown rates, reflecting an anabolic state with considerable net amino acid uptake and accretion.[201] At least a partial explanation can be derived from the changing proportion of body mass contributed by the major organs (Table 41.6). Based on the relatively increased mass of skeletal muscle (which has a relatively lower fractional synthetic rate in late gestation), it is logical that the whole body fractional synthetic rate should decrease. However, it is clear that a direct, causal relationship with anabolic endocrine-paracrine factors, (e.g., insulin, pituitary and placental GH, placental lactogen, IGFs, epidermal growth factors) cannot be proposed because most studies suggest an increasing concentration or secretion of these substances with advancing gestation.[168]

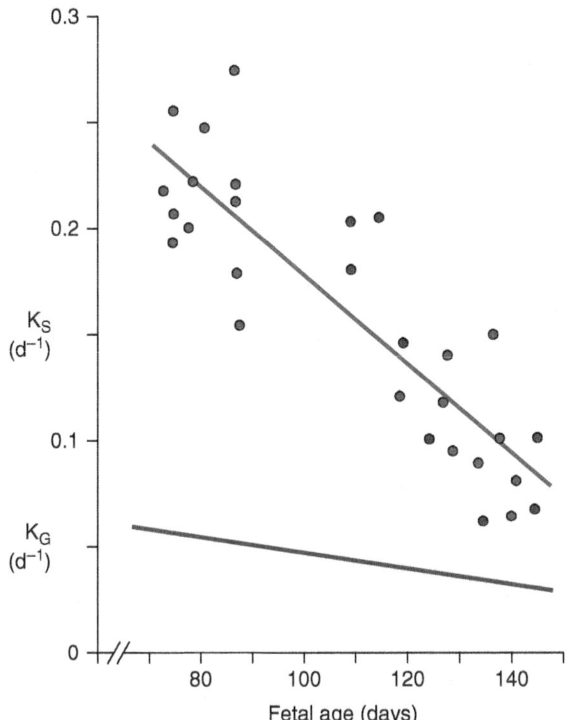

Fig. 41.6 Fractional rate of protein synthesis (K_S; *blue line*) over gestation in fetal sheep studied with leucine *(blue circles)* and lysine *(red circles)* radioactive tracers compared with fractional rate of growth (K_G; *red line*) in the lower portion of the figure. (From Battaglia FC, Meschia G. Fetal and placental metabolism: part II. Amino acids and lipids. In: Battaglia FC, Meschia G, eds. *An Introduction to Fetal Physiology.* Orlando: Academic Press; 1986:120; Kennaugh JM, Bell AW, Teng C, et al. Ontogenetic changes in the rates of protein synthesis and leucine oxidation during fetal life. *Pediatr Res.* 1987;22:688; and Meier PR, Peterson RG, Bonds DR, et al. Rates of protein synthesis and turnover in fetal life. *Am J Physiol.* 1981;240:320.)

Table 41.6 Fractional Synthetic Rates Among Organs in Early Postnatal Life.

Organ	Percent Synthesis/Day (K_s)	
Liver	57.0	±12.0
Kidney	50.0	±10.0
Brain	17.0	±3.0
Heart	18.5	±4.0
Skeletal muscle	15.2	±2.8

From Waterlow JL. *Protein Turnover in Mammalian Tissues and in the Whole Body.* Amsterdam: Elsevier/North-Holland Biomedical Press; 1978.

ROLE OF FETAL GROWTH HORMONES IN FETAL AMINO ACID METABOLISM

Insulin and IGFs are important anabolic hormones for the fetus. All studies have shown that a reduction in fetal insulin concentration, from genetic defects in human infants that produce pancreatic agenesis[202] to experimental surgical removal of the pancreas,[203] decreases the rate of fetal growth. Growth still occurs in all of these conditions, just at a slower rate. Conversely, experimental manipulation of maternal or fetal concentrations of insulin and IGF-1 by direct infusion or transgenic overexpression increases fetal weight.[204] One of the primary actions of insulin in the fetus is to increase amino acid uptake by the cells, promoting direct amino acid synthesis into protein and, when energy is deficient, into oxidative metabolism and energy production. In adults, insulin consistently increases protein accretion by decreasing protein breakdown.[205,206] However, in the fetus and the preterm newborn, the anabolic effects of insulin on protein kinetics have not been as consistent and depend on many variables, including adequacy of circulating amino acid supply and glucose availability. When amino acid concentrations fall during an exogenous insulin infusion in late gestation fetal lambs and preterm newborns, insulin has been shown to suppress protein breakdown, but protein synthesis rates were also lower, resulting in no net protein gain.[207,208] In contrast, insulin may be anabolic and induce a net gain in protein balance in the fetus and preterm infant of the same gestational age when euglycemia and euaminoacidemia are maintained.[144,209-210] Effects of insulin are organ specific as well, as insulin has been shown to increase the fractional protein synthetic rate in fetal skeletal muscle, but not fetal albumin synthesis.[210]

IGF-1 also has been shown to have anabolic effects on protein metabolism in the fetus. Mutations in the IGF-1 and IGF-1 receptor in humans result in IUGR,[211,212] as do heterozygous and homozygous *igf1* knockouts in mice.[213,214] A series of studies in late gestation fetal sheep have shown that fetal IGF-1 infusion suppresses whole fetal protein breakdown and amino acid oxidation, resulting in net fetal protein accretion.[215] The effect of IGF-1 on the suppression of proteolysis was dose-dependent.[216] When combined with an insulin infusion, both hormones resulted in increased fetal protein synthesis.[210]

Both insulin and IGF-1 regulate protein synthesis through well-recognized intermediates in their signal transduction pathways, including mTOR and the eukaryotic initiation factors (Fig. 41.7),[217] which are active in all cells throughout their life span, even in the fetal period. mTOR is an evolutionary-conserved protein that consists of two multiunit complexes: mTORC1 and mTORC2. mTORC1 functions as a sensor for growth factors, nutrients, energy, and stress, and coordinates these signals to regulate cell growth and proliferation and mTORC2 highlighted as a major regulator of Akt activity.

Insulin, via a well-described cascade of serine/threonine phosphorylation events, activates mTORC1 and its downstream targets.[218] Activated mTORC1 phosphorylates eukaryotic translation initiation factor 4-binding protein (4E-BP1), releasing it from one of the eukaryotic initiation factors, eukaryotic translation initiation factor 4E (elF4E). This enables elF4E to form the elF4E translation initiation complex, which binds mRNA and the ribosome to initiate protein synthesis. mTORC1 also phosphorylates ribosomal protein p70S6 kinase, which in its phosphorylated (activated) form will increase the translation of 5′-TOP mRNAs that encode for ribosomal proteins and other translation factors. Insulin also activates the Ras/extracellular signal-regulated kinases (ERK) pathway, leading to both inhibition of tuberous sclerosis protein 1/2 (TSC1/2) and activation of p70S6 kinase.[219] Acute fetal infusions of insulin and IGF-1 have been shown to phosphorylate 4E-BP1, p70S6 kinase[143,217] and ERK[220] in fetal skeletal muscle, promoting protein synthesis.

Amino acids, and particularly leucine, also function as direct-acting nutrient signals that activate mTORC1.[221] Leucine can stimulate mTORC1 independently of insulin or IGF-1 by binding to leucyl-tRNA synthetase and activating RAG GTPase proteins, thus bringing RHEB (Ras homolog enriched in brain) to the surface of the lysosome.[222] When both insulin and amino acids were infused to the late gestation sheep fetus, phosphorylation states of ERK and p70S6 kinase were increased three-fold and four-fold, respectively. However, amino acids alone did not activate the phosphorylation of any of these proteins. Thus, insulin appears to be a more effective regulator of the mTORC1 signaling pathway in the fetus, at least when administered acutely.[209]

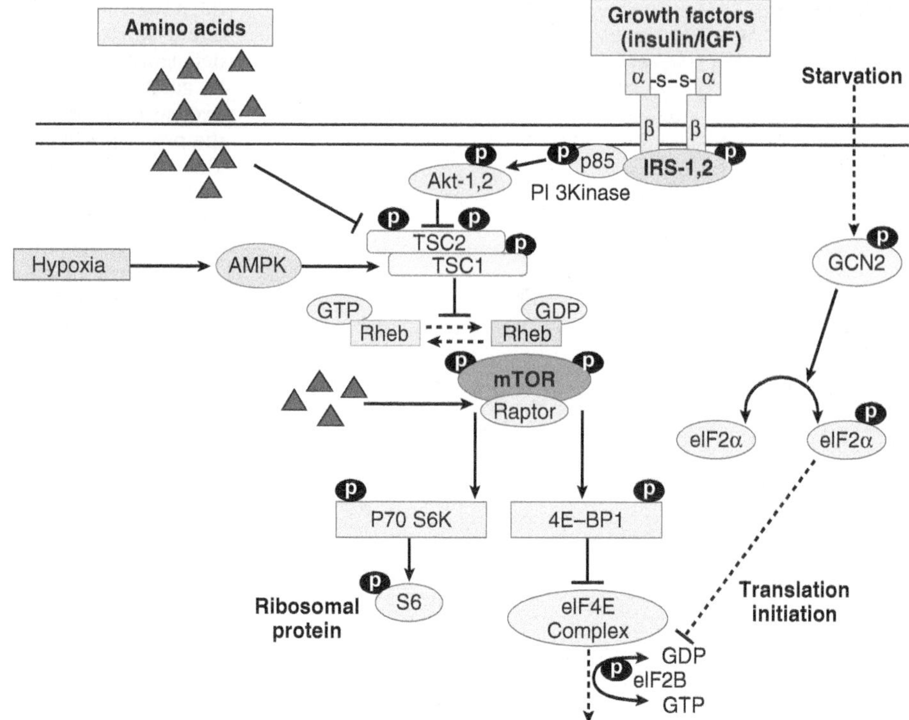

Fig. 41.7 Schematic representation of the cellular signal transduction pathways of regulatory proteins leading from stimulation by amino acids, growth factors such as insulin and IGF, or energy substrate supply to protein synthesis. *4E-BP1*, Factor 4-binding protein; *AMPK*, adenosine monophosphate-activated protein kinase; *eIF4E*, eukaryotic translation initiation factor 4E; *GCN*, guanosine cyclic nucleotide; *GDP*, guanosine diphosphate; *GTP*, guanosine triphosphate; *IGF*, insulin-like growth factor; *IRS*, insulin receptor substrate; *mTOR*, mechanistic target of rapamycin; *TSC*, tuberous sclerosis protein.

FETAL PROTEIN METABOLISM IN RESPONSE TO ADVERSE INTRAUTERINE ENVIRONMENTS

As protein synthetic and growth rates are high in fetal life, it is appropriate that a number of investigators have studied changes in fetal protein and amino acid metabolism in response to maternal conditions that either restrict or increase amino acid supply, energy supply, or both to the fetus, resulting in fetal undergrowth (e.g., in placental insufficiency-induced IUGR) or overgrowth (e.g., in maternal obesity).

One of the most common causes of reduced nutrient supply to the human fetus is placental insufficiency.[223] Placental insufficiency is a condition in pregnancy whereby a poorly functioning and/or smaller than normal placenta restricts nutrient and oxygen supply to the fetus, leading to IUGR.[97] In a sheep model of placental insufficiency, both glucose and leucine flux from mother to fetus are reduced compared to normal term gestation placentae.[97,98,143,224] Similarly, amino acid transport across the placenta is impaired in the third trimester of a human pregnancy with IUGR, and this is associated with reduced amino acid transporter activity.[89,95,225] Protein and energy deficits in the growth-restricted fetus adversely affect the growth and development of individual organs. Chronic and progressive nutrient restriction to the fetus results in less skeletal muscle mass,[226] fewer nephrons,[227,228] evidence for prematurely activated gluconeogenesis, decreased pancreatic beta cell function,[229,230] and a propensity to develop later life metabolic syndrome (obesity, insulin resistance, glucose intolerance, diabetes mellitus, and cardiac disease) in infants with IUGR.[231]

Long-standing conditions of chronic and progressive placental insufficiency compared to shorter-term maternal fasting and/or maternal hypoglycemia show both similarities and differences in the fetal protein metabolic response. In a sheep model of chronic and progressive placental insufficiency induced by exposure of the pregnant ewe to elevated ambient temperatures during gestation, fetal skeletal muscle mass is reduced as a result of lower muscle protein synthesis rates, as opposed to increased protein breakdown rates.[99] However, in acutely glucose-deprived and hypoglycemic fetal sheep and rats, fetal protein breakdown rates increase.[189,232,233] When maternal malnutrition with both energy and protein restriction was more prolonged in rats, decreased protein synthesis and proteolysis was observed, but protein synthesis rates were reduced to a greater extent.[234] Thus it appears that in more acute fasting conditions and conditions of selective energy restriction (e.g., glucose), the fetal response is to increase proteolysis; with more chronic and prolonged nutrient restriction, the adaptation is to reduce protein synthesis rates, at least in skeletal muscle. In cases of both maternal fasting and prolonged placental insufficiency, the fetal hindlimb releases both alanine and glutamine,[140,235] major potential sources of gluconeogenesis, and amino acid oxidation rates are either maintained or increased, reflecting energy-sparing adaptations.[184,189]

Attempts to restore protein accretion in the IUGR fetus by increasing protein intake in the maternal diet have not been successful and, in fact, have adversely affected the fetal condition (worsening growth failure and even increased mortality) when protein delivery was not balanced by a concurrent increase in carbohydrate (energy) supplementation.[236-238] The mechanisms to explain these findings are beginning to be elucidated and are likely to involve the potential inability to increase amino acid transfer from mother to fetus by increased maternal amino acid concentrations, reduced essential amino acid active transport with insufficient energy supply, and/or competitive inhibition of amino acids across the placenta—all of which could lead to insufficient and/or imbalanced delivery of amino acids, especially the essential amino acids, to the fetus.[239,240,241] In the IUGR fetal sheep, a prolonged amino acid infusion directly to the fetus similarly did not increase protein accretion rates but did potentiate glucose-stimulated insulin secretion and β-cell mass in the pancreas.[192,242] In terms of a supplementation strategy, the most promising results have come from chronic, low-dose IGF-1 infusions into growth-restricted fetal sheep, either by direct fetal intravenous infusion or by intraamniotic supplements, both of which improved fetal organ growth.[243,244]

As noted, it is difficult to produce increased net fetal amino acid uptake from higher protein in the maternal diet or amino acid infusions into the maternal circulation. Augmented maternal diets have largely involved excess energy, both carbohydrates and lipids, and such diets have produced fatter, more macrosomic fetuses and newborn infants.[245-248] Maternal medical conditions, such as obesity and/or diabetes, also increase fetal energy delivery, and their fetuses also suffer from fat overgrowth leading to a greater frequency of macrosomic infants.[249] Interestingly, children born to obese mothers and those women with gestational diabetes are also more likely to develop obesity and metabolic disease in adulthood,[250,251] similar to the IUGR infant, further supporting the link between the intrauterine environment and long-term health risk. As discussed previously, placental amino acid transport capacity is increased in maternal obesity[252] and diabetic pregnancies,[253] and this has included positive correlations between placental amino acid transporter expression, notably for System A, and birth weight in both human pregnancies and in murine models of maternal obesity in pregnancy.[254] The fetal amino acid uptake and metabolism in response to increased amino acid delivery from the placenta has been less well studied compared to the IUGR condition, in part due to the difficulty in experimentally achieving obesity in sheep where the fetus can be catheterized for direct measurement of amino acid kinetics. Those studies that have assessed body composition in offspring of obese mothers and mothers with diabetes reproducibly show increased adiposity, which may be one of the reasons why the fetus who has experienced overgrowth in utero is at risk for later life obesity.[255] The response in lean mass growth to both maternal obesity and maternal diabetes is not as clear. LGA infants born to nondiabetic mothers have accelerated growth of lean mass during the early postnatal period.[256] Increased lean mass has been reported in the hyperinsulinemic infant of a diabetic mother,[257] but lean mass also has been reported to be reduced after in utero exposure to gestational diabetes.[258] Body composition that reflects reduced lean mass and increased fat mass as a result of the intrauterine environment may significantly contribute to developmental programming of obesity and diabetes risk.

CONCLUSION

Amino acid supply to the fetus by the placenta is quantitatively large and qualitatively unique. Individual amino acids are actively transported into the fetal circulation at relatively high rates to meet the rapid growth and energy needs of the fetus through an array of active transport protein systems. The active transport also produces amino acid concentrations in the fetal circulation that are higher than those in the maternal circulation. The relative concentrations of amino acids achieved in the fetal circulation are also unique. This occurs as a combined result of unique transport characteristics for each amino acid and for groups of amino acids in the placenta, unique rates of placental metabolism of amino acids, and unique placental-fetal amino acid metabolic cycles. The majority of amino acid transporters at the fetal-placental interface have now been characterized at the molecular level. Animal and human placental preparation studies are building on these data to determine how these transporters work together in vivo in an integrated way to mediate transepithelial transfer across the placenta,[126,259] and how these amino acid transfers promote fetal protein accretion and growth in the normal and the adverse in utero environment.[99,235]

A complete reference list is available at www.ExpertConsult.com.

SELECT REFERENCES

1. Eaton BM, Yudilevich DL. Uptake and asymmetric efflux of amino acids at maternal and fetal sides of placenta. *Am J Physiol*. 1981;241:106-112.
2. Eleno N, Deves R, Boyd CA. Membrane potential dependence of the kinetics of cationic amino acid transport systems in human placenta. *J Physiol*. 1994;479:291-300.
3. Hill PM, Young M. Net placental transfer of free amino acids against varying concentrations. *J Physiol*. 1973;235:409-422.
4. Jansson T. Amino acid transporters in the human placenta. *Pediatr Res*. 2001;49:141-147.
5. Lemons JA, Adcock 3rd EW, Jones Jr MD, et al. Umbilical uptake of amino acids in the unstressed fetal lamb. *J Clin Invest*. 1976;58:1428-1434.
6. Moe AJ. Placental amino acid transport. *Am J Physiol*. 1995;268:1321-1331.
7. Battaglia FC, Regnault TR. Placental transport and metabolism of amino acids. *Placenta*. 2001;22:145-161.
17. Hoeltzli SD, Smith CH. Alanine transport systems in isolated basal plasma membrane of human placenta. *Am J Physiol*. 1989;256:630-637.
21. Fukasawa Y, Segawa H, Kim JY, et al. Identification and characterization of a Na(+)-independent neutral amino acid transporter that associates with the 4F2 heavy chain and exhibits substrate selectivity for small neutral D- and L-amino acids. *J Biol Chem*. 2000;275:9690-9698.
31. Johnson LW, Smith CH. Neutral amino acid transport systems of microvillous membrane of human placenta. *Am J Physiol*. 1988;254:773-780.
38. Pineda M, Fernandez E, Torrents D, et al. Identification of a membrane protein, LAT-2, that co-expresses with 4F2 heavy chain, an L-type amino acid transport activity with broad specificity for small and large zwitterionic amino acids. *J Biol Chem*. 1999;274:19738-19744.
39. Segawa H, Miyamoto K, Ogura Y, et al. Cloning, functional expression and dietary regulation of the mouse neutral and basic amino acid transporter (NBAT). *Biochem J*. 1997;328:657-664.
43. Nelson DM, Smith SD, Furesz TC, et al. Hypoxia reduces expression and function of system A amino acid transporters in cultured term human trophoblasts. *Am J Physiol Cell Physiol*. 2003;284:310-315.
48. Ayuk PT, Sibley CP, Donnai P, et al. Development and polarization of cationic amino acid transporters and regulators in the human placenta. *Am J Physiol Cell Physiol*. 2000;278:1162-1171.
54. Mastroberardino L, Spindler B, Pfeiffer R, et al. Amino-acid transport by heterodimers of 4F2hc/CD98 and members of a permease family. *Nature*. 1998;395:288-291.
55. Pfeiffer R, Rossier G, Spindler B, et al. Amino acid transport of y+L-type by heterodimers of 4F2hc/CD98 and members of the glycoprotein-associated amino acid transporter family. *EMBO J*. 1999;18:49-57.
59. Novak DA, Beveridge MJ, Malandro M, et al. Ontogeny of amino acid transport system A in rat placenta. *Placenta*. 1996;17:643-651.
60. Wang H, Huang W, Sugawara M, et al. Cloning and functional expression of ATA1, a subtype of amino acid transporter A, from human placenta. *Biochem Biophys Res Commun*. 2000;273:1175-1179.
61. Hatanaka T, Huang W, Wang H, et al. Primary structure, functional characteristics and tissue expression pattern of human ATA2, a subtype of amino acid transport system A. *Biochim Biophys Acta*. 2000;1467:1-6.
62. Desforges M, Lacey HA, Glazier JD, et al. SNAT4 isoform of system A amino acid transporter is expressed in human placenta. *Am J Physiol Cell Physiol*. 2006;290:305-312.
64. Christie GR, Hyde R, Hundal HS. Regulation of amino acid transporters by amino acid availability. *Curr Opin Clin Nutr Metab Care*. 2001;4:425-431.
65. Jones HN, Ashworth CJ, Page KR, et al. Expression and adaptive regulation of amino acid transport system A in a placental cell line under amino acid restriction. *Reproduction*. 2006;131:951-960.
66. Jones HN, Ashworth CJ, Page KR, et al. Cortisol stimulates system A amino acid transport and SNAT2 expression in a human placental cell line (BeWo). *Am J Physiol Endocrinol Metab*. 2006;291:596-603.
68. Constancia M, Angiolini E, Sandovici I, et al. Adaptation of nutrient supply to fetal demand in the mouse involves interaction between the Igf2 gene and placental transporter systems. *Proc Natl Acad Sci U S A*. 2005;102: 19219-19224.
69. Constancia M, Hemberger M, Hughes J, et al. Placental-specific IGF-II is a major modulator of placental and fetal growth. *Nature*. 2002;417:945-948.
139. Marconi AM, Battaglia FC, Meschia G, et al. A comparison of amino acid arteriovenous differences across the liver and placenta of the fetal lamb. *Am J Physiol*. 1989;257:909-915.
167. Demerath EW, Fields DA. Body composition assessment in the infant. *Am J Hum Biol*. 2014;26:291-304.
168. Sparks JW. Human intrauterine growth and nutrient accretion. *Semin Perinatol*. 1984;8:74-93.
172. Fenton TR, Kim JH. A systematic review and meta-analysis to revise the Fenton growth chart for preterm infants. *BMC Pediatr*. 2013;13:59.
173. Clark RH, Olsen IE, Spitzer AR. Assessment of neonatal growth in prematurely born infants. *Clin Perinatol*. 2014;41:295-307.
174. Fenton TR, Nasser R, Eliasziw M, et al. Validating the weight gain of preterm infants between the reference growth curve of the fetus and the term infant. *BMC Pediatr*. 2013;13:92.
175. Nahum GG, Stanislaw H, Huffaker BJ. Fetal weight gain at term: linear with minimal dependence on maternal obesity. *Am J Obstet Gynecol*. 1995;172: 1387-1394.

176. Olsen IE, Groveman SA, Lawson ML, et al. New intrauterine growth curves based on United States data. *Pediatrics*. 2010;125:214-224.
177. Widdowson EM. Chemical composition and nutritional needs of the fetus at different stages of gestation. In: Aebi H, Whitehead R, eds. *Maternal Nutrition during Pregnancy and Lactation*. Bern, Switzerland: Hans Huber; 1980:39-48.
178. McCance RA, Widdowson EM. Glimpses of comparative growth and development. In: Falkner F, Tanner JM, eds. *Human Growth*. New York: Plenum Press; 1985:131-151.
239. Bertran J, Magagnin S, Werner A, et al. Stimulation of system y(+)-like amino acid transport by the heavy chain of human 4F2 surface antigen in Xenopus laevis oocytes. *Proc Natl Acad Sci U S A*. 1992;89:5606-5610.

Temperature Control in Newborn Infants

42

Rakesh Sahni

INTRODUCTION

This chapter is an updated revision of Dr. Kurt Brück's comprehensive treatise on neonatal thermal regulation presented in earlier editions; it is not an original synthesis by the current author. Dr. Brück remains the senior contributor despite his death in 1995 in recognition of and with immense admiration for his many contributions to our understanding of the physiology of human neonates. His classic study of temperature regulation[1] provided fundamental knowledge that was validated and refined in subsequent years. Using continuous measurements of heat production and cutaneous blood flow, before, during, and after discrete and timed environmental cold stress, Brück defined the fundamental features of the neonatal response to chilling and its dependence on gestational and postnatal ages. These important observations concerning the basic responses of infants to cold—increased heat production and decreased heat loss, as well as the timing of these events and their development pattern—remain central to our understanding of how best to care for human neonates.

CURRENT MODELS AND TERMINOLOGY

It is useful to model the temperature control system of newborn infants using the basic biocybernetic concept of a passive (i.e., controlled) system, the temperature of which depends on metabolic heat production and heat transfer to the environment. The controller consists of sensor, integrator, and effector components (Fig. 42.1). Current understanding is that various central and peripheral thermal sensors monitor information about heat storage and heat gradients within the body continuously. These multiple inputs are transmitted to an integrating neural control network, located in the hypothalamus and limbic systems, which, in turn, is linked by means of efferent neuronal pathways to effector mechanisms that are capable of controlling heat storage. The earlier concept that the controlled variable is a single temperature at a single site within the body has been refined to take into account evidence that temperatures at multiple sites provide important input to the controller.[2-5]

For clarity, the following discussion is structured according to this controller model, reviewing information about the sensors, integrator, and effectors as separate components followed by a consideration of how the integrated control system functions in response to environmental thermal transients, how the system changes during development, and how it operates under special circumstances, such as fever, heart failure, and hypoxia.

PRINCIPLES OF PHYSIOLOGIC TEMPERATURE REGULATION

The maintenance of a stable body temperature that is much warmer than the environmental temperature is a property of the two higher classes of the animal kingdom: birds and mammals. These classes form the group of *homeothermic* beings; all others are designated as *poikilothermic*. A prerequisite of homeothermy is a basal rate of metabolism several times higher than that in poikilothermic animals. The former are thus referred to as *tachymetabolic* and the latter as *bradymetabolic* organisms. Furthermore, homeothermy requires a balance among heat production, skin blood flow, sweating, and respiration in such a way that changes in heat loss or gain from the environment are precisely compensated.

METABOLISM AND HEAT PRODUCTION

Metabolic processes that provide energy for maintenance of homeostasis and physical exercise are closely linked with heat production. The overall efficiency of energy transformation in homeotherms is only on the order of 10% to 25%, meaning that most of the energy transformed during metabolic activities is liberated as heat and must either be eliminated or stored depending on the needs of the organism. For organisms that are tachymetabolic (including human neonates), the metabolic rate at rest is sufficient to increase body temperature by several degrees Celsius greater than the ambient temperature. The metabolic rate at rest is of great importance for the state of the controlled system.

STANDARD METABOLIC RATE

The at-rest metabolic rate depends on several factors, including physical activity, environmental temperature, feeding, thermic effect of food, diet-induced thermogenesis (formerly called *specific dynamic action*), time of day (diurnal rhythmicity), age, and growth rate. By convention, the conditions used for the measurement of at-rest metabolic rate have been standardized: (1) subjects must be awake and have fasted at least 12 hours; (2) they must be fully relaxed; and (3) thermoneutral conditions should be maintained.

Metabolic rate measured under these standard conditions is termed the *basal metabolic rate* (BMR). Neonates are unlikely to fulfill the first and second standard conditions at the same time; thus, special conditions for measurement must be defined. The following conditions have been suggested[6]:

1. The infant should remain on a normal feeding schedule (this suggestion is not unreasonable because the maximum increase in energy metabolism in infants is only 4% to 10% after an ordinary feeding).
2. The measurements must be made in a period of 5 to 10 minutes, during which the infant is fully relaxed (in contrast with the BMR standard conditions, the infant does not have to be awake). The metabolic rate determination may even be made during postprandial sleep.[7]
3. The measurements must be made under thermoneutral conditions.

The minimum metabolic rate measured in this way is called the *standard metabolic rate (SMR)* or *minimum observed metabolic rate*.[8] The designation BMR should be used only

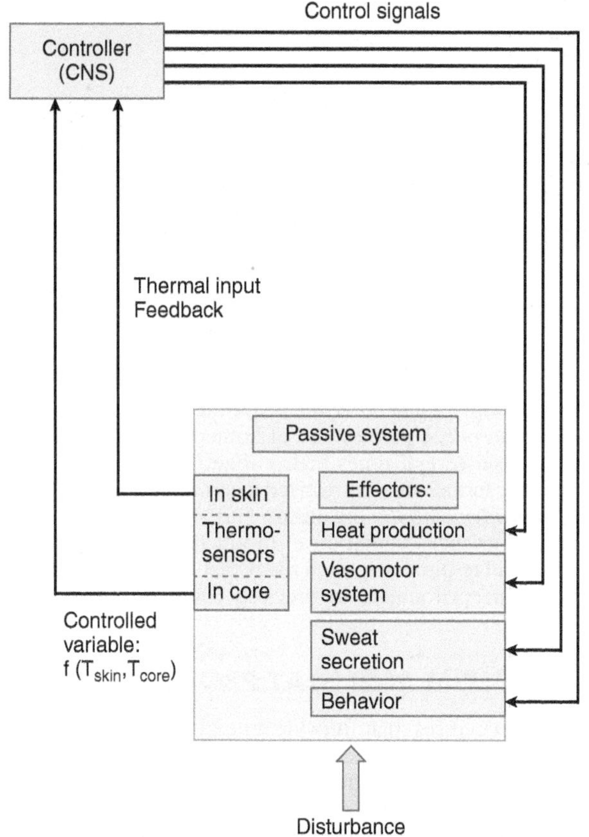

Fig. 42.1 Diagram representing the biocybernetic concept of temperature regulation in humans. Temperature is sensed at various sites of the body, and the temperature signals are fed into the central controller (multiple-input system). *CNS*, Central nervous system.

for determinations performed under standard conditions as employed in adults. Depending on why the metabolic rate is being measured, longer periods of observation (i.e., 3 to 6 hours) are required.[9,10]

STANDARD METABOLIC RATE IN RELATION TO BODY MASS AND AGE

Total heat production is related to body size; for example, the overall metabolic rate of sheep is greater than that of rabbits. Because body temperatures of homeothermic species are close to one another at similar preferred environmental temperatures, it can also be anticipated[11] that the metabolic rate per kilogram of body mass will be larger in a rabbit than in a sheep. In fact, there is a close correlation between the logarithm of body weight and the logarithm of at-rest metabolic rate (oxygen consumption) with a slope of 0.75 for adult animals of various sizes. This means that the metabolic rate per (kilogram body weight)$^{3/4}$ of at-rest animals of different sizes, including adult humans, is independent of body size. This relationship has been termed the *law of metabolic reduction* by Kleiber[11] and has been found useful by some observers for cross-species comparisons of the physiology of metabolism.

Although the Kleiber equation can be useful for predicting metabolic rates when comparing different species, attempts to predict metabolic rates within a group of individual organisms of the same species but of different body sizes reveals its limited applicability. Several deviations from the law of metabolic reduction must be introduced. Age, sex, body shape, and body composition affect metabolic rate. The age dependency of metabolic rate makes it impossible to predict the metabolic rates of neonates and adults from an individual species with a single exponential function of weight, even if a higher exponent than Kleiber's is used.[1]

As illustrated in Fig. 42.2, newborn infants to 1 week of age have an SMR that is lower than that predicted by Kleiber's equation—that is, the SMR is lower in a 3-kg human newborn than in a 3-kg rabbit. Conversely, in the weight range of 5 to 20 kg, the SMR is higher in human infants than in adult animals of the same weight. During this period of growth, the SMR demonstrates a nearly linear relationship to body weight. Mathematically, this relationship can be expressed by an exponent of $b = 1$ in the equation SMR = $a \times m^b$ where a is age and m is mass. During the period that corresponds to the weight range of 20 to 70 kg, the SMR approaches data in Kleiber's curve.

An exponent close to 1, or somewhat larger than 1, should also be used to calculate the SMR for infants weighing between 1 and 4 kg. This means that during the neonatal period, the SMR/body mass unit is almost independent of weight, whereas a decrease would be expected with increasing weight according to Kleiber's equation (see Fig. 42.2). These SMR values demonstrate a relatively large amount of scatter during the first day of life. A survey of these data and a discussion of the possible reasons for the scattering may be found elsewhere.[7,12] Given these limitations, attempts to refer observations of the metabolism of human neonates to standards derived for other mammals should be avoided.

Certain quantitative changes in the SMR during early postnatal development are worth keeping in mind:

1. Immediately after birth, the SMR/kg body mass is lower in human infants than in adult animals of the same weight (see Fig. 42.2).
2. After birth, the SMR/kg body weight increases and eventually attains a value that is up to 50% higher in infants than in adult animals of the same body mass. The time course of this process appears to be variable. It may take 2 days to a few weeks (particularly in premature infants) to attain values that are characteristic of the post-neonatal period.[7,12]

The seeming violation of the law of metabolic reduction (see Fig. 42.2) during the early neonatal period may be only a fictitious problem if one takes into account the considerable change in extracellular water content (extracellular fluid [ECF]) that occurs from the early fetal to the adult stage. Sinclair and colleagues[13] have suggested using body weight minus ECF as the reference value in metabolic reference standards. According to their calculations, ECF composes as much as 44% of body weight in a 4000-g newborn infant and 58% in a 1000-g premature neonate. The corresponding average value for ECF in the adult is only 20%. Because the ECF does not participate in oxidative metabolism, the expression "body weight—ECF" may be considered representative of the active tissue mass. Thus, it seems theoretically justified to relate metabolic rate to this active tissue mass rather than to total body weight. In contrast, the lean body mass (i.e., total body mass—fat mass) has not been found to be a suitable reference value.

One can also relate metabolic rate in a neonate to the expression "active tissue mass + adult ECF"—that is, to a body mass that corresponds in composition to that of the adult organism. Metabolic rates related to this calculated value closely approximate Kleiber's curve, whereas the metabolic rate related to the actual body weight remains less than the predicted values.[7]

METABOLIC RATE IN RELATIONSHIP TO BODY TEMPERATURE

All chemical reactions in an organism are temperature dependent and obey the van't Hoff law. According to this law, oxygen uptake and body temperature of a poikilothermic animal are expected to decrease with decreasing environmental temperature. This decrease has, in fact, been demonstrated in frogs, reptiles, and other poikilothermic animals without exception. The ratio of the reaction rates at temperatures differing by 10°C is called the Q_{10}. In general, the Q_{10} for the metabolic rate in poikilothermics is approximately 2 to 3. van't Hoff's law applies to homeotherms in the same way but is masked by regulatory processes.

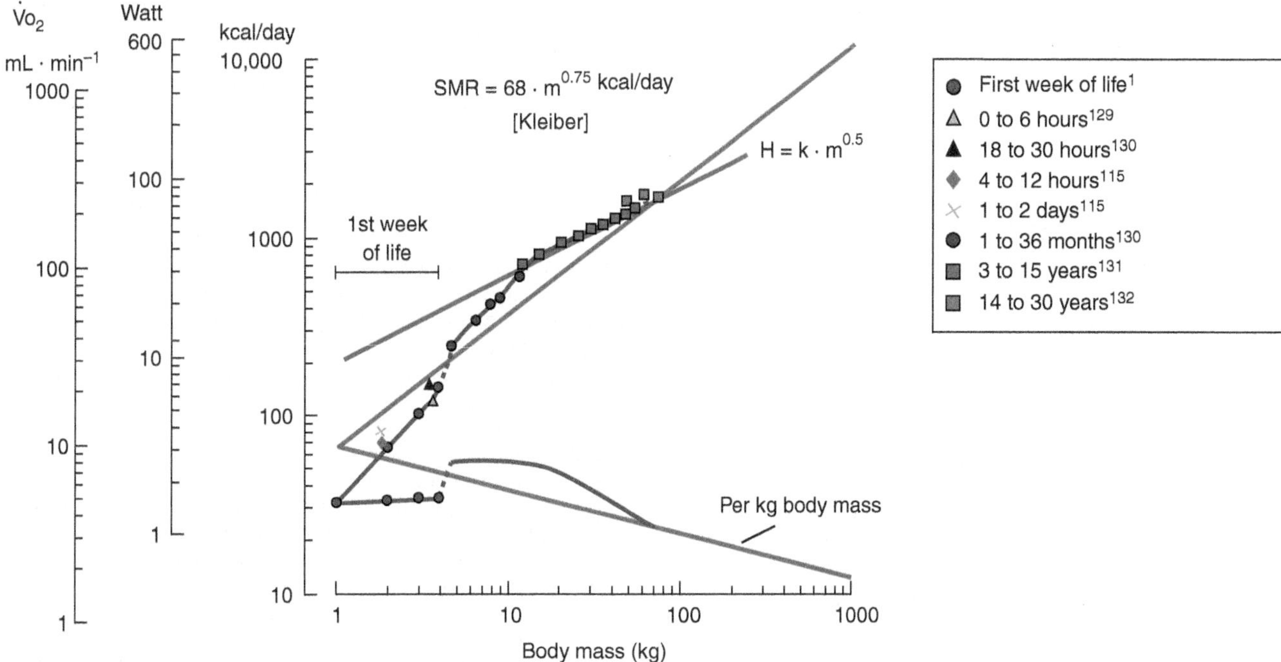

Fig. 42.2 Relationship of standard metabolic rate *(SMR)* to body mass and age. Top curve, SMR and the corresponding $\dot{V}O_2$ in relationship to body mass. Bottom curve, the same data but expressed in relation to unit of body mass = SMR according to Kleiber's equation; heat production that would yield equal temperature differences between body core and environment. (See text for further discussion.) (Modified from Brück K. Heat production and temperature regulation. In: Stave U, ed. *Perinatal Physiology*. New York: Plenum Publishing; 1978:455–498.)

Thus, in the intact homeothermic organism, the metabolic rate increases initially with decreasing body temperature (Fig. 42.3, *top curve*). This *regulatory metabolic rise* can be blunted or prevented by pharmacologic intervention, in particular by moderate or deep anesthesia (see Fig. 42.3, *middle* and *bottom curves*). In fully anesthetized dogs, metabolic rate decreases with decreasing body temperature *(bottom curve)*, obeying van't Hoff's law. The slope of the curve corresponds to a Q_{10} of 2 to 3. At body temperatures below 30°C, the metabolic rate drops steeply to the basal curve (*solid lines* in Fig. 42.3) because the thermoregulatory drive generated in the thermointegrative areas of the central nervous system vanishes with increasing hypothermia. The body temperature at which this reduction occurs may be species dependent.

Before describing the response of the integrated system to changes in environmental temperature, we review what is known about the individual components of the biocybernetic model.

THERMAL SENSORS: THERMORECEPTIVE STRUCTURES AND THE THERMOAFFERENT SYSTEM

LOCATION AND PROPERTIES OF CUTANEOUS THERMAL RECEPTORS

The cutaneous thermal receptors are a group of structures that function as temperature sensors in the temperature control system (the term *sensor* is gaining preference to *receptor* to avoid confusion with chemical structures reacting with specific substances; both terms are used interchangeably within this section). It is generally agreed that the cutaneous thermosensors in the thermoregulatory system are identical with those mediating thermal sensation. The distribution of the cutaneous thermoreceptors can thus be studied in adult humans by stimulation of so-called *warm* and *cold spots* using fine temperature probes. There is scarcely any area of the skin that does not respond to cold stimulation, although the number of cold spots/cm^2 may vary between 1 and 5 on the palm of the hand and more than 15 on the face. The number of warm spots/cm^2 is much less in all skin areas (0.3 to 1.7). This agrees with the better spatial resolution of cold stimuli, but it does not mean that cutaneous warm sensitivity is any less developed than is cold sensitivity. In fact, with larger stimulus areas (using thermodes of 10- to 100-cm^2 contact areas), warm sensitivity can be demonstrated on all skin areas with few exceptions (cornea, glans penis).[14] Employing electrophysiologic methods (recording single-receptor activity from nerves), warm and cold receptors have been demonstrated on the faces of cats and other species and on the lower arms and legs of monkeys.[14] By inserting fine metal electrodes through the intact skin into a branch of the radial nerve, it has even been possible to record the activity of single warm and cold receptors in humans in response to thermal stimulation on the skin of the back of the hand.[15]

The morphologic correlate of cold sensors is the fine unmyelinated nerve endings penetrating into the basal layer of the epidermis.[16] These endings contain numerous mitochondria, providing energy for a temperature-sensitive Na^+, K^+ pump, which seems to be part of the transduction of the cold stimulus into an electrical signal.[17]

Fig. 42.4 illustrates the average response characteristics of cold and warm receptors from different species (including humans) under static conditions (i.e., after the temperature of the skin had been constant for several minutes). Minimum activity occurs at a skin temperature of 35°C. The maximum discharge frequency of cold receptors is found between 35°C and 20°C, and that of warm receptors takes place between 40°C and 45°C. At temperatures above 45°C, warm-receptor activity decreases. At temperatures lower than approximately 25°C, the activity of cold receptors may also be reduced.

Sensor activity during temperature changes is noteworthy in that receptor discharges may reach frequencies that are two- to three-fold greater than under static conditions. Irrespective of the initial temperature, a warm receptor will always show an overshoot of its discharge on sudden warming and a transient inhibition on cooling, whereas a cold receptor will respond in the

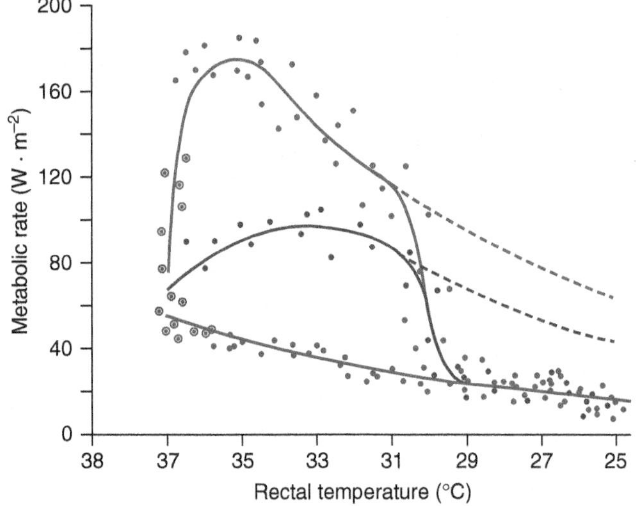

Fig. 42.3 Relationship between metabolic rate and rectal temperature in anesthetized dogs, the body temperatures of which were manipulated by intravascular heat exchangers. *Top curve, blue circles*: Light anesthesia; thus a marked cold-induced increase in heat production with decreasing body temperature was observed. *Middle curve, red circles*: Moderate anesthesia; the response of heat production to cooling is reduced. *Lower curve, green circles*: Deep anesthesia; there is no cold defense reaction. *Black circles*: Baseline values before initiation of cooling. After having reached a maximum, thermoregulatory heat production follows van't Hoff's law. Note that the upper and middle curves tend to approach the lower curve as soon as the rectal temperature drops below a critical temperature (about 30°C). (From Behmann FW, Bontke E. Regulation of heat formation in artificial hypothermia. I. Experimental studies on the effects of depth of anesthesia. *Pflügers Arch.* 1958;266:408.)

opposite way (with an inhibition on warming and an overshoot on cooling). Correspondingly, sensitivity to temperature changes is amplified and increases with the size of the exposed area. With exposure of larger areas (e.g., the whole hand), a temperature change of less than 0.01°C/s may evoke a thermal sensation[18] and probably a regulatory reaction.

In summary, thermoregulatory responses elicited through cutaneous thermoreceptors are determined by the average skin temperature (T_{skin}), the rate and direction of temperature change ($\Delta Tskin/\Delta t$), and the size of the stimulated area.[14,18] Because of the temperature discharge characteristics (see Fig. 42.4), warm receptors may contribute to the stimulation of heat dissipation actions only when mean skin temperature is considerably higher than normal levels.

LOCATION AND PROPERTIES OF INTERNAL THERMOSENSITIVE STRUCTURES

Evidence for the existence of deep body thermosensors has been obtained in three ways: (1) by demonstrating that there is poor correlation between body temperature and the action of the final control elements if only skin temperature is taken into consideration,[19] (2) by observing thermoregulatory actions after heating and cooling of circumscribed areas within the body using implanted thermodes and vascular heat exchangers,[20] and (3) by recording the activity of single units of the central nervous system and relating these responses to their own local temperatures.[21]

HYPOTHALAMUS

According to thermal stimulation studies (using thermodes implanted on a long-term basis), deep body thermosensors are located in the preoptic area and the anterior hypothalamus. Local warming of this region stimulates heat-dissipating mechanisms (i.e., vasodilation, panting, sweating), whereas it inhibits heat production (i.e., metabolic reactions [Fig. 42.5] and vasoconstriction). Inversely, cooling evokes heat production and vasoconstriction, whereas heat dissipation mechanisms are inhibited.

Thermal stimulation does not permit discrimination between internal cold and warm receptors (e.g., the effects of local cooling might be ascribed to actuation of central cold receptors and to the

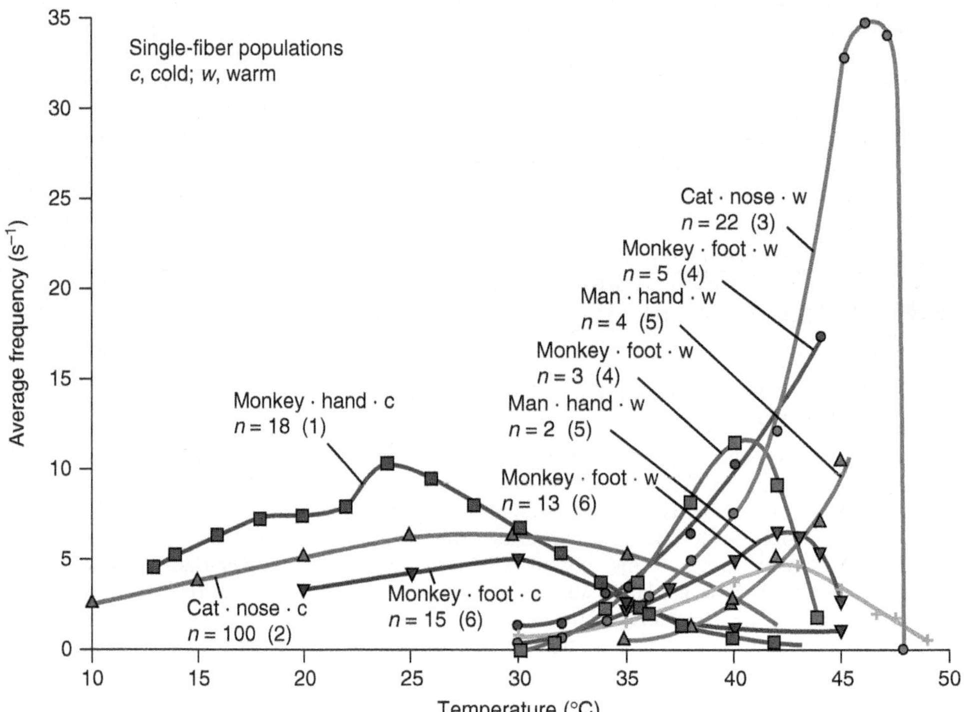

Fig. 42.4 Average static discharge frequency of populations of cutaneous cold and warm receptors as a function of skin temperature obtained from various species and body sites by several authors. (From Hensel H. *Thermoreception and Temperature Regulation.* New York: Academic Press; 1981.)

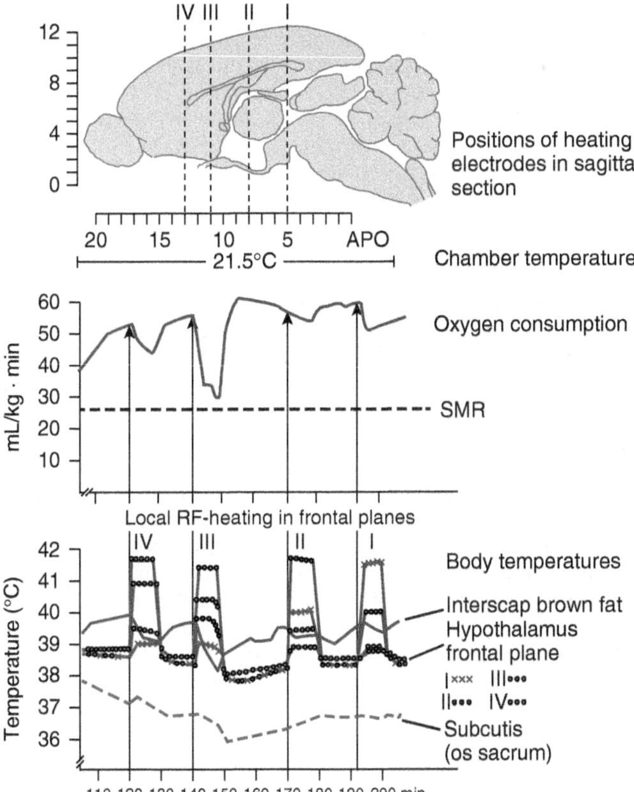

Fig. 42.5 Effect of local radio frequency *(RF)* heating in different frontal planes of the hypothalamus on nonshivering thermogenesis (NST) induced by external cooling in a newborn guinea pig (for these small animals, an ambient temperature of 21.5°C is below neutral temperature). The upper part of the figure shows the projection of the four implanted electrodes on the sagittal section of the brain. The different frontal planes were locally heated in succession. Only heating of plane III, corresponding to the preoptic area and anterior hypothalamus, resulted in an almost complete suppression of the cold-induced NST (note reduction of the temperature within the interscapular brown fat). *APO,* Apomorphine; *SMR,* oxygen uptake corresponding to standard metabolic rate. (From Zeisberger E, et al: In: Jansky L, ed. *Depressed Metabolism and Cold Thermogenesis.* Prague: Charles University; 1981:182–187.)

inhibition of central warm receptors). Here further clarification is obtained from single-unit studies.[21] As shown in Fig. 42.6, warming of the preoptic area results in markedly increased activity of one single unit and leads to an increase in respiratory frequency (panting). Units like this are considered to be warm sensors.

In vitro studies of hypothalamic slices[22] and of cell cultures[23] have addressed the question of whether hypothalamic thermosensitivity is tied to individual thermosensitive ganglion cells or is based on the temperature dependence of synaptic transmission between afferent and efferent neurons (Fig. 42.7). After synaptic transmission is blocked by electrolyte solutions with a low Ca^{2+} content and a high Mg^{2+} content, the structures in question remain sensitive to thermal stimuli. This implies the existence of thermosensitive cells within the preoptic region and anterior hypothalamus. Both areas contain not only warm-sensitive cells but also thermosensitive and cold-sensitive cells, the latter two being less numerous than the warm-sensitive cells.

LOWER BRAIN STEM AND SPINAL CORD

Thermosensitive structures have also been demonstrated in the lower brain stem (midbrain and medulla oblongata), and thermoregulatory reactions can be initiated by local warming of these areas.[24] However, the thermosensitivity of this region is distinctly less than in the preoptic region and anterior hypothalamus.[20] In contrast, the spinal cord is extremely thermosensitive. When the temperature of the spinal cord is raised only a few tenths of a degree along its entire length in dogs and other animals, the results include panting, vasodilation, and inhibition of thermogenesis.[20,25] Cooling of the spinal cord elicits shivering, but in this case a greater temperature change is required. In newborn and young guinea pigs, a local temperature change in the region of the cervical cord suffices to trigger thermoregulatory reactions.[3]

OTHER THERMOSENSORS

Quantitative considerations suggest that thermoreceptive structures exist outside the central nervous system and the skin.[20] Experimental evidence for the presence of thermosensors in the region of the dorsal wall of the abdominal cavity and in the musculature exists. Evidence for the existence of subcutaneous thermosensors has also been confirmed.[26]

AFFERENT THERMOSENSITIVE PATHWAYS

The cutaneous thermoreceptors are served by thin myelinated and unmyelinated axons belonging to the slowly conducting group III and group IV nerves. Warm fibers are mostly unmyelinated (group IV). The axons run within the afferent cutaneous nerve bundles,

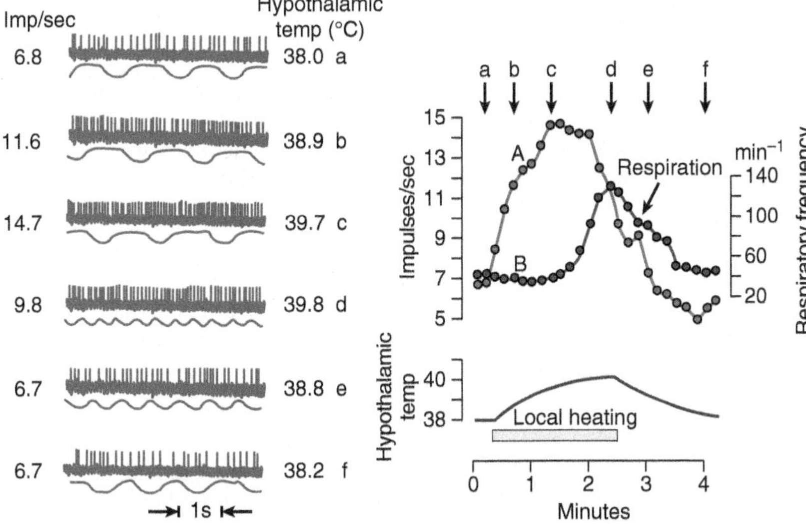

Fig. 42.6 Left, Sections of original records of impulse frequency of a hypothalamic neuron and respiratory rate in relation to hypothalamic temperature. *Right,* Discharge of a warm-sensitive neuron in the preoptic region *(curve A)* and simultaneous record of respiratory rate during local heating of the hypothalamus. *Arrows* marked with lowercase letters designate time at which the original record *(left)* was taken. (From Nakayama T, Hammel HT, Hardy JD, et al. Thermal stimulation of electrical activity of single units of the preoptic region. *Am J Physiol.* 1963;204:1122.)

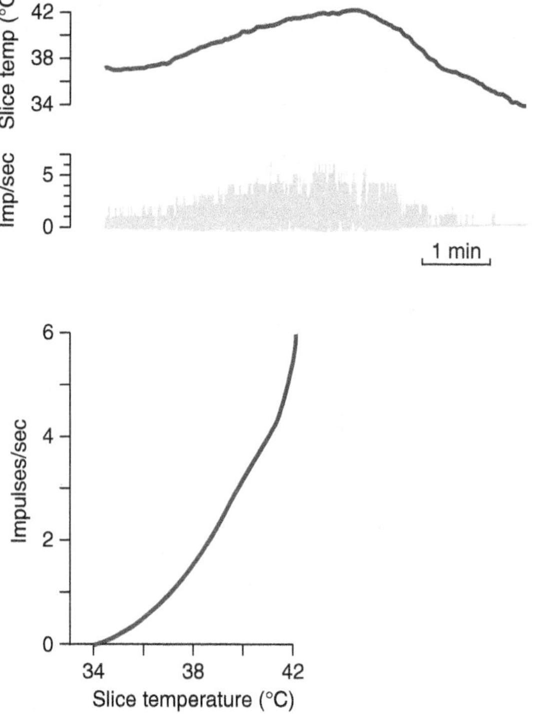

Fig. 42.7 *Top,* Original record of a single warm-sensitive unit. *Bottom,* Thermal response curve of the same warm-sensitive unit located in the preoptic area of a slice preparation of the rat hypothalamus. (From Hori T, Nakashima T, Hori N, et al. Thermo-sensitive neurons in hypothalamic tissue slices *in vitro*. *Brain Res.* 1980;186:203.)

and they enter the spinal cord through the segmental dorsal root ganglia. Those axons cross over to the contralateral side and ascend within the spinothalamic tract in the anterolateral section of the spinal cord. On their way to the thalamus, the ascending thermal fibers join the medial lemniscus and are accompanied by the afferents coming from the trigeminal region. From the medial lemniscus, collaterals diverge and project to the hypothalamus through a pathway not definitively described. Evidence has been obtained that part of the cutaneous thermal input is conveyed through the spinoreticular pathway to the reticular formation; from there, it is projected to the hypothalamus through the raphe nuclei and the ventral noradrenergic system, which passes the subcerulean area.[24,27-29]

The spinal cord thermal sensors are connected to the posterior hypothalamus through axons running in an anterolateral pathway of the spinal cord, as has been shown in young guinea pigs[30] and cats.[31,32] The thermosensors of the preoptic area also end in the posterior hypothalamus; however, these short pathways have not yet been identified.

INTEGRATION OF THERMAL INPUTS

INTEGRATION OF MULTIPLE THERMAL INPUTS

The theoretic concepts of thermoregulation require the demonstration of some elements that "process" the thermal information originating at the receptors in various sites of the body (multiple-input system) and that transform these inputs from the sensors into effector outputs.

There are many experimental studies implicating the hypothalamus (especially the posterior hypothalamic area, which has no appreciable thermosensitivity) as an integration center for thermoregulation. This premise is further supported by electrophysiologic findings. For example, neurons exist in the posterior hypothalamic area, the activity of which (discharge rate) is influenced by local thermal stimulation in either the preoptic region or the cervicothoracic part of the spinal cord.[33] At the boundary between the anterior and posterior hypothalamus, neurons have been found that respond to changes in the skin temperature on the limbs and trunk.[24] The posterior hypothalamus, therefore, is characterized by the presence of thermoresponsive cells (i.e., cells that respond to changes in the temperature of distant structures but are not sensitive to changes in their own temperature). However, there is no absolute spatial separation of receptive and integrative functions. In the preoptic region and anterior hypothalamus, cells shown to be thermosensitive have also been found to be affected by skin temperature changes and thus are simultaneously thermoresponsive.[4,34]

A special feature of biologic thermoregulation (compared with the familiar simple technical system) is that two kinds of sensors in different locations (the cold and warm receptors) interact antagonistically. The cutaneous cold receptors are activated when the temperature decreases to less than the lower limit of the thermoneutral zone. This reaction is counteracted by heat-activated internal thermosensors when the body temperature increases as a result of overshooting cold-protective mechanisms or after bodily activity. This circuitry enables the protective mechanisms to be set in motion rapidly in case of external cooling, long before the core temperature has begun to decrease and internal thermoreceptors can be influenced.

Conversely, heat dissipation processes (vasodilation, sweating) may be activated by internal warm receptors, which are primarily stimulated when body core temperature increases. This effect is counteracted by cold activation of the cutaneous cold receptors. When the body is heated externally, sweat secretion is stimulated by the combined action of cutaneous and internal warm receptors.

Fig. 42.8 shows a simplified model of the neuronal circuitry underlying the central nervous system integrative processes. Three kinds of neuronal elements are distinguished: (1) efferent neurons located in the hypothalamus, the axons of which activate the peripheral controlling elements (Fig. 42.9) either directly or, more probably, by way of a chain of interneurons; (2) facilitative and inhibitory interneurons within the hypothalamus; and (3) thermal afferents, arising in part from the cutaneous thermoreceptors and in part from internal receptors (e.g., those of the preoptic region).

Cold receptors directly activate the effectors for thermogenesis. The inhibitory action on the efferents to heat loss effectors is exerted through interneurons. Activation of warm receptors excites the efferents to the heat loss effectors, simultaneously inhibiting (through interneurons) the efferents to the effectors for heat production. The various effector neurons may receive different combinations of thermal afferents. Thus, as shown in studies of newborn guinea pigs, nonshivering thermogenesis is driven by cutaneous cold receptors and is inhibited by hypothalamic warm receptors, whereas the inhibitory influence of shivering is exerted mainly by spinal cord warm-receptive structures (Fig. 42.10). The cervical spinal cord is the region that preferentially receives (through vascular connections) the heat that is generated in the interscapular brown adipose tissue (BAT).[3,7,35] As a result of this "meshed control" of the two heat-generating mechanisms, shivering remains suppressed in neonates so long as sufficient heat is supplied from the interscapular BAT to the spinal cord warm-sensitive structures and intrathoracic organs.

PRINCIPLES GUIDING THE ACTIONS OF THE INTEGRATOR

Given that the thermosensitive structures are distributed over the entire body, the thermoregulatory effector actions (see Fig. 42.9) cannot be described as a function of a single local temperature

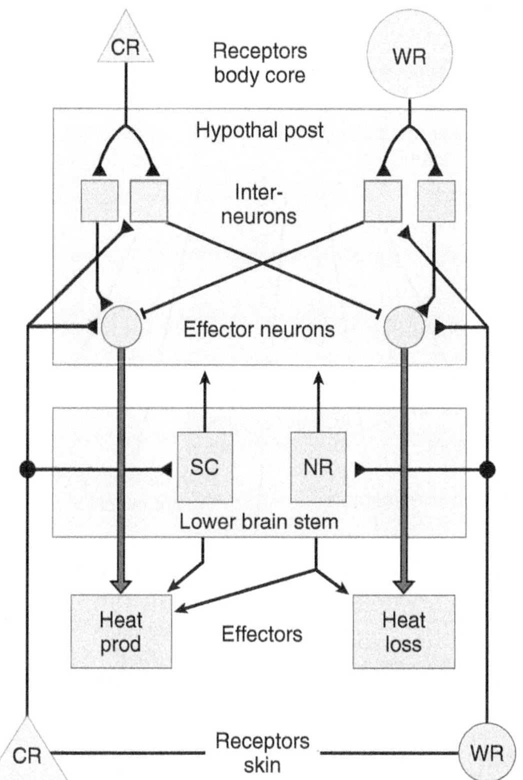

Fig. 42.8 Highly simplified model of the connections between thermal afferents and the efferent neuronal networks that control the thermoregulatory effector elements. Shaded areas represent the thermointegrative regions of the hypothalamus (mainly the posterior hypothalamus) and the lower brain stem, which contain crucial structures for the processing of thermal information from the skin (*NR*, raphe nuclei; *SC*, subceruleus region). The inhibitory neurons shown *(blue squares)* mediate the reciprocal inhibition of the heat-losing and heat-generating processes. The symbols for neurons represent not single neurons but neuron pools. Some details of the connections in the SC, NR, and hypothalamus are known but are not within the scope of this diagram. The arrows pointing down from the lower brain stem represent pathways to mononeurons and dorsal horn neurons in the spinal cord; the latter can suppress input from the warm afferents. *CR*, Cold receptors; *WR*, warm receptors (size of the symbols indicates roughly the difference in numbers); activating; inhibitory synaptic connections. (Data from Brück K, Hinckel P. Thermoafferent systems and their adaptive modifications. *Pharmacol Ther.* 1982;17:357.)

(e.g., the rectal temperature). Thus, the goal of thermophysiology is to describe thermoregulatory actions as a function of as many as possible of the temperatures associated with various thermosensitive parts of the body. Systems of equations with several variables are required for such a description. The data must be collected by experiments on animals in which spatially circumscribed temperature changes are produced by means of thermodes and heat exchangers[20]; in humans, limited opportunity exists for experimental manipulation of local temperature while the temperature of the rest of the body is kept constant. Only an approximate description is possible; the thermoregulatory parameters are presented as a function of two temperatures, the temperature of the interior of the body (measured at a representative site) and the mean skin temperature.[2,28,36] Shivering and sweating threshold temperatures, as well as the temperature pairs yielding equal magnitudes of shivering and sweating, are represented by contour lines in a coordinate system with mean skin temperature and core temperature as the coordinates (Fig. 42.11). Blood flow through the skin follows similar contour lines located between shivering and sweating threshold lines.[37] The contour plots portrayed in Figs. 42.11 and 42.12, although involving only two temperatures, are good semiquantitative illustrations of the performance of the multiple-input control system. Note that the relative impact of the sensors increases as temperatures become increasingly "out of range," and that the whole contour plot depends on other attributes such as the warm/cold adapted state of the animal. Within a certain range of temperatures (i.e., near the set point), at which the contour lines can be approximated by straight lines, it is possible to express the effector responses and the threshold temperature conditions for the elicitation of effector responses in terms of a weighted mean body temperature, T_b, calculated with the following linear equation:

$$T_b = a \times T_{\text{core}} + b \times T_{\text{skin}} \qquad [42.1]$$

Data from human adults can be best fitted if values of 0.9 and 0.1 are chosen for the coefficients a and b, respectively.[28] Fig. 42.12 shows the shivering threshold contour lines of adult humans, rabbits, goats, and young (4-week-old) guinea pigs. In addition, the threshold contour line for nonshivering thermogenesis in newborn guinea pigs is given. The curvilinear contour lines in small animals do not allow the use of arithmetic mean body temperature except for small sections of the temperature ranges that may be approximated by straight lines.

SET POINT AND NORMAL BODY TEMPERATURE

In a multiple-input system, the control actions of the thermoregulatory system can be ineffective at various combinations of temperatures. For instance, shivering remains suppressed so long as the combination of body surface and body core temperatures stays at or greater than the threshold contour line (see Figs. 42.11 and 42.12). Conversely, heat dissipation actions will be ineffective so long as the combination of surface and internal temperature values remains less than the heat dissipation threshold hyperbola (see Fig. 42.11).

Under environmental conditions that allow the control actions to reach ineffective levels, the deep body temperature will stabilize at a value typical for the species (if enough time is allowed to attain steady-state heat flow). This temperature, whether measured within the tympanic canal, the rectum, the esophagus, or elsewhere, may then be called the *normal body temperature*. Deviations of such a representative temperature from an empirically attained normal value may be described as a set-point displacement or, more specifically, as a deviation of the threshold temperatures for the respective control actions.

EFFECTOR RESPONSES OF THE THERMOREGULATORY SYSTEM

The effector outputs of the thermoregulatory controller restore the system to the desired set point by regulating both heat production and heat loss. After a brief review of the relationship between metabolic rate and environmental temperature, control of heat production and heat loss are discussed separately.

METABOLIC RATE AND ENVIRONMENTAL TEMPERATURE

The cold-induced increase in metabolic rate (see Fig. 42.3) is the most characteristic feature of homeothermic organisms. In the neonates of all homeothermic species studied thus far (except for the ground squirrel and golden hamster, which are hibernators), a cold-induced increase in metabolic rate has been demonstrated immediately after birth. Although this response may be small

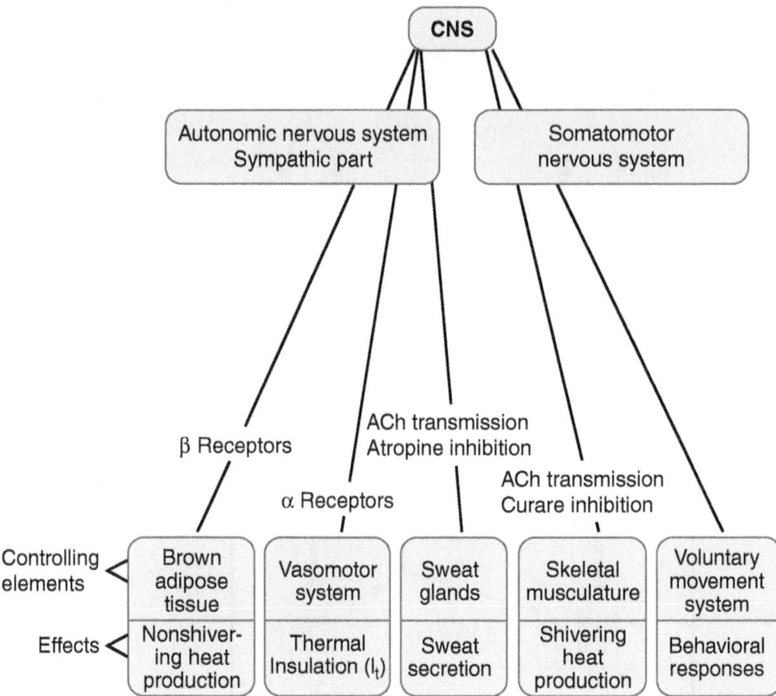

Fig. 42.9 Schematic representation of the neural control of the thermoregulatory effector systems. *CNS*, Central nervous system. (From Brück K. In: Schmidt RF, Thews G, eds. *Human Physiology.* Berlin: Springer; 1983:531–547.)

during the first hours of life, neonates should not be considered poikilothermic.

The influence of postnatal age on cold-induced thermogenesis is shown in Fig. 42.13. As demonstrated by several investigators, oxygen uptake (directly proportional to thermogenesis) is distinctly greater at 28°C ambient temperature than at 32°C to 35°C, even during the first few hours of life. At an ambient temperature of 23°C, oxygen consumption is even greater. Depending on the species, this cold-induced metabolic response increases to a greater or lesser extent during the first week of life. Preterm and small-for-date infants also increase their metabolic rate with cooling, and on average their response is not much less than that in term infants (see Fig. 42.13). Oxygen uptake values of 15 mL/kg/min measured at an ambient temperature of 23°C[1] and of 16.8 mL/kg/min measured at 26°C[38] appear to represent the maximum (summit) metabolic response to cold in 1-week-old term infants. For comparison, in well-trained young adults, summit oxygen consumption may increase to five times the level at rest—that is, to 17 to 20 mL/kg/min, when the environmental temperature is maintained at 0°C to 5°C.

The maintenance of constant body temperature requires that heat loss and heat production be equal in the steady state. Fig. 42.14 illustrates the possible ways in which body temperature can be kept constant when the environmental temperature changes. According to Newton's law, dry (nonevaporative) heat loss is proportional to the temperature difference between the body core and the surroundings. Therefore, in humans, heat loss should be nonexistent at an ambient temperature of 37°C, and it should increase linearly with decreasing ambient temperature. Because heat loss also depends on heat conduction and convection within the body, and thus on peripheral blood flow, two heat loss curves may be generated (see Fig. 42.14), one for peripheral vasodilation and another for vasoconstriction. Within the thermoneutral zone, heat production (corresponding to the at-rest [basal] metabolic rate) is in equilibrium with heat loss only if skin blood flow is progressively reduced as the temperature decreases from the upper end of the thermoneutral zone (T_3) to its lower end (T_2). At temperatures less than T_2, body temperature can be kept constant only if heat loss is exactly compensated for by

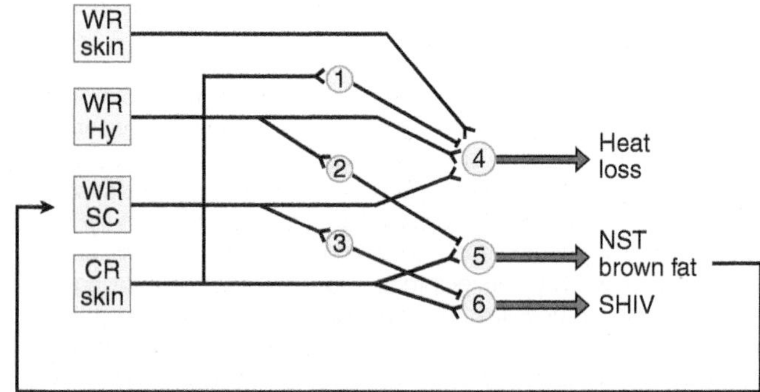

Fig. 42.10 Schematic representation of the presumed neuronal circuitry underlying the control of heat loss and thermogenesis. Note that nonshivering thermogenesis *(NST)* and shivering *(SHIV)* are differentially controlled. It must be inferred from experimental evidence that with increasing age, connections are being formed between WR_{Hy} and the number 6 effector neurons. *ACh,* Acetylcholine; *CR,* cold receptors; *Hy,* hypothalamus; *SC,* spinal cord; *WR,* warm receptors; *1, 2, 3,* inhibitory interneurons; *4, 5, 6,* effector neurons.

increasing thermoregulatory heat production (cold-induced thermogenesis). The maximum thermogenesis (which amounts to three to five times the BMR in adults but only two to three times the SMR in neonates) determines the lower limit of the thermoregulatory range (T_1 in Fig. 42.14). The value for T_1 is approximately 5°C in adults and 23°C in term neonates.[1] When this limit is exceeded, hypothermia ensues.

At temperatures greater than T_3, thermal equilibrium can be achieved only by an additional heat loss mechanism—the secretion and evaporation of sweat. It is not possible for the organism to down-regulate the BMR. In Fig. 42.14, point T_4 indicates the upper limit of the range of regulation, which is determined by the sweat rate capacity. Between points T_3 and T_4, body temperature inevitably increases because of a load error typical for a proportional control system, resulting in an increasing metabolic rate according to van't Hoff's rule.

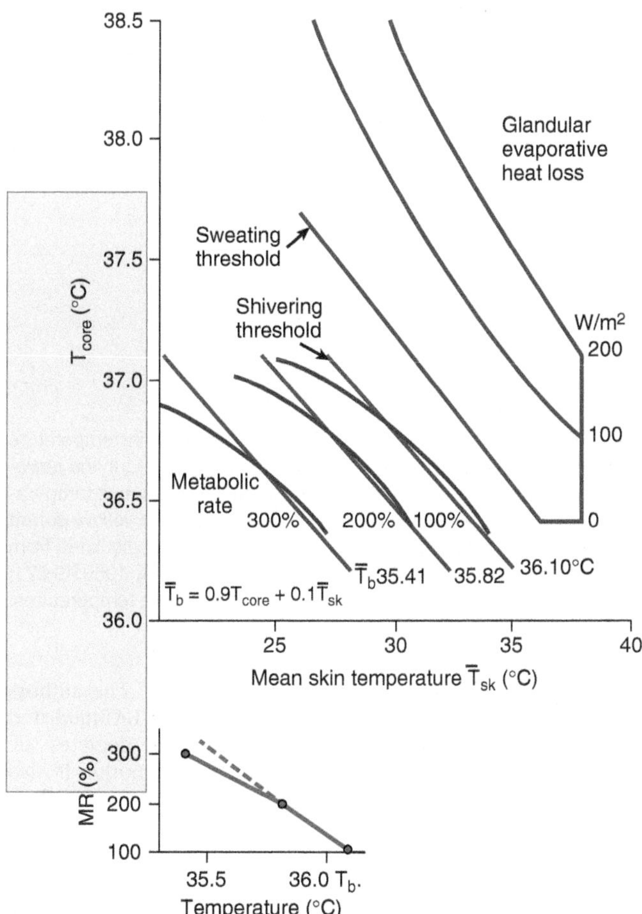

Fig. 42.11 Contour plot of metabolic rate and sweat rate (glandular evaporative heat loss) as a function of core temperature and mean skin temperature. The *curved lines* for metabolic rate were approximated by *straight lines* (and so might be the 100 and 200 W curves for evaporative heat loss). Each *straight line* represents all pairs of core and skin temperature with equal T_b calculated from the inset equation. *Green area* indicates range of mean skin temperatures relevant for the comparison of shivering threshold values. Percentage metabolic rate *(MR)* in relation to T_b is shown at the bottom of the figure. (Data from human adults in Benzinger TH. Heat regulation: homeostasis of central temperature in man. *Physiol Rev.* 1969;49:671; and Nadel ER, Bullard RW, Stolwijk JA. Importance of skin temperature in the regulation of sweating. *J Appl Physiol.* 1971;31:80.)

The term *thermoneutral zone* was originally defined solely with respect to metabolic rate, and some problems arose concerning its use in perinatal physiology.[39] The thermoneutral zone is now defined as "the range of ambient temperature at which metabolic rate is at a minimum, and within which the temperature regulation is achieved only by control of sensible ("dry" or "nonevaporative") heat loss—that is, without regulatory changes in metabolic heat production or evaporative heat loss."[8] This range is delineated by the symbols T_2 and T_3 in Fig. 42.14. In unclothed adults at rest, the lower range limit of the thermoneutral zone (T_2) is 26°C to 28°C (50% relative humidity, still air); however, it is 32°C to 35°C (operative temperature, 50% relative humidity, still air) in naked term newborn infants.[1,39] This difference is of importance because it shows that environmental temperature conditions that do not require any thermoregulatory effort in adults may seriously overtax the metabolic thermoregulatory system of neonates.

In small premature infants (1 kg), the lower limit of the thermoneutral zone may be as high as 35°C.[39] The lower end of the thermoneutral zone may change with postnatal development as body size increases[39] and as small changes in the sensitivity of the thermoregulatory system occur. It is thus extremely difficult to provide exact standard values for the thermoneutral zone in neonates.

CONTROL OF HEAT PRODUCTION

MODES OF EXTRA HEAT PRODUCTION

The ability to produce extra heat in a cool environment is one of the characteristic features of homeothermy. Three principal modes of heat production are responsible for the increase of heat production with decreasing environmental temperature: (1) voluntary muscle activity, (2) involuntary tonic or rhythmic muscle activity (the latter may be manifest as shivering or may be invisible and detectable only by electromyography), and (3) nonshivering thermogenesis. The existence of nonshivering thermogenesis was originally evidenced by the demonstration of a cold-induced increase in oxygen uptake that persisted after neuromuscular blockade with curare.

SHIVERING AND NONSHIVERING THERMOGENESIS

In adult humans and in larger adult mammals, shivering is quantitatively the most important involuntary mechanism of thermoregulatory heat production. In contrast, nonshivering thermogenesis is an important and effective mechanism of heat production in the neonates of many mammalian species, including human infants. In comparison with nonshivering thermogenesis, shivering is a less economical form of heat production in that it inevitably increases convective heat loss because of the body oscillations. Moreover, shivering interferes with body movement. This economical aspect becomes more important in smaller organisms (high surface-to-mass ratio) with poorer thermal insulation. Thus, it is satisfying from a teleologic point of view to find that the maximum extent of nonshivering thermogenesis available in one species is inversely related to its order of body size (Fig. 42.15). Extrapolating the regression line in Fig. 42.15, one can conclude that subjects with body weights heavier than 10 kg lack the capacity for nonshivering thermogenesis.

LOSS OF NONSHIVERING THERMOGENESIS

In relatively mature newborns, such as guinea pigs, the extent of nonshivering thermogenesis is greatest at the time of birth and vanishes within a few weeks (Fig. 42.16). This involution of nonshivering thermogenesis can be retarded and partly inhibited by rearing the animals in a cold environment. After nonshivering thermogenesis has been extinguished through exposure to a warm environment, it can again be evoked by exposing older guinea pigs to a cool environment. In human neonates, no experimental data are available to document the process of the disappearance of nonshivering thermogenesis. It may be assumed that nonshivering thermogenesis is the prevailing mechanism of thermoregulatory heat production during the first 3 to 6 months of life.[12] By contrast, in rats, the extent of nonshivering thermogenesis increases during the postnatal period.[40,41] Such behavior may be expected to occur in other altricious neonates that, like rats, are born in a relatively immature stage. This would explain the gradual increase in the maximum cold-induced heat production that can be observed during the first few weeks of life in premature infants.[1]

LACK OF NONSHIVERING THERMOGENESIS

At least one example exists of a species in which the neonates, although small, do not possess nonshivering thermogenesis—pigs. Piglets shiver vigorously when exposed to cold, even on the first day of life.[42] Miniature piglets have no demonstrable nonshivering thermogenesis even when they are reared for a

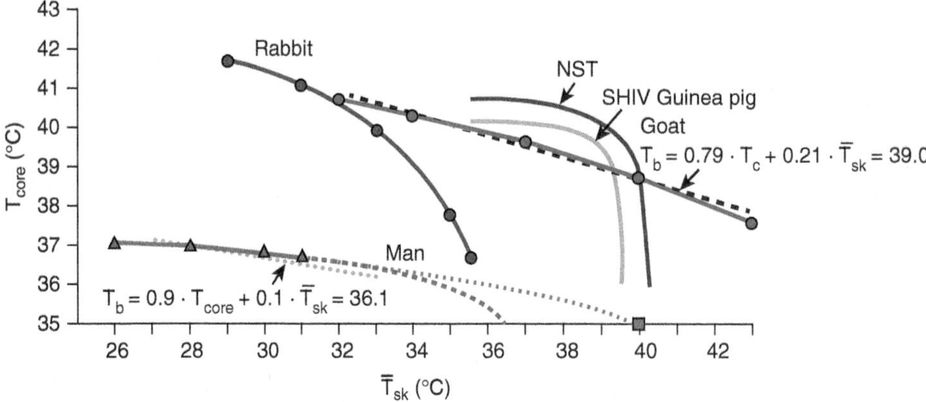

Fig. 42.12 Thresholds for shivering *(SHIV)* and nonshivering thermogenesis *(NST)* as a function of core *(T_{core})* and mean skin temperature *($\bar{T}_{sk}$)*. Shivering threshold contour lines from adult humans, rabbits,[133] goats,[20] and 4-week-old guinea pigs,[3] as well as the contour line representing threshold conditions for NST in newborn guinea pigs, are compared.[134] Note that core temperature is the local hypothalamus temperature in the case of rabbits and newborn guinea pigs and the spinal cord temperature in the case of 4-week-old guinea pigs. The *yellow-dotted* and *black-dashed straight lines* represent pairs of T_{core} and T_{sk} with equal weighted mean body temperature T_b, 36.1 and 39, as calculated from the respective inset equations. (Data from Benzinger TH. Heat regulation: homeostasis of central temperature in man. *Physiol Rev.* 1969;49:671; and Hayward JS, Eckerson JD, Collis ML. Thermoregulatory heat production in man: prediction equation based on skin and core temperatures. *J Appl Physiol.* 1977;42:377.)

few weeks in a cold environment.[43] In agreement with the data depicted in Fig. 42.15, similarly calves (a larger neonate) have no metabolic response to norepinephrine, indicating lack of nonshivering thermogenesis.[44]

SITES OF NONSHIVERING THERMOGENESIS

For many decades, the liver, other intestinal organs, white subcutaneous adipose tissue, and the skeletal musculature were suggested as sites of nonshivering thermogenesis. During the early 1960s it was suggested that BAT was the primary site of nonshivering thermogenesis.[40,45-47]

PHYSIOLOGY OF INFANT BROWN ADIPOSE TISSUE

In modern eutherian (placental) mammals, BAT evolved as a specialized thermogenic organ that is responsible for adaptive nonshivering thermogenesis through conversion of chemically stored energy, in the form of fatty acids and glucose, into heat. For nonshivering thermogenesis, energy metabolism of BAT mitochondria is increased by activation of uncoupling protein 1 (UCP1), which dissipates the proton motive force as heat. The collective data from studies of BAT in human fetuses and infants indicate that the tissue is widely distributed during these developmental stages, and that the tissue is particularly developed in the axillae, neck, and upper back regions as well as deep internally, around important structures such as the kidneys.[48-50] The thermogenic capacity of the tissue, as measured by its UCP1 content, develops with gestational age and reaches its maximum in infancy and early childhood when the demands for thermogenesis can be expected to be especially high. When subjected to cold, human infants lack a sufficiently developed skeletal muscle mass for maintaining body temperature through shivering thermogenesis. Instead, they respond to cold exposure by inducing nonshivering thermogenesis. As the response is associated with increased lipolysis in BAT, and induction of heat production in regions harboring the tissue, it is reasonable to assume that the cold-induced thermogenesis occurs in BAT. Recently, Hu and colleagues used magnetic resonance imaging (MRI) to study a group of newborns who had been subjected to hypothermia therapy as a treatment for hypoxic-ischemic encephalopathy and found that the fat-signal fraction was significantly lower in the supraclavicular BAT depots of the hypothermia-treated infants as compared to those in the untreated control group, suggesting a lower triglyceride content in the BAT of the cold-exposed group.[49] The authors concluded that the hypothermia therapy triggers BAT-mediated nonshivering thermogenesis, which subsequently depletes the tissue of its intracellular triglyceride stores. This notion is also supported by numerous animal studies that additionally have shown that thermogenesis in BAT is essential for maintaining a stable core body temperature in a cold environment.

Over the last years, our knowledge of rodent BAT[51-53] and factors that affect its recruitment and activation have increased substantially. However, despite these advances, little is still known about the human tissue on a molecular level. Importantly, the infant data that are available imply that humans, like rodents, harbor two types of thermogenic adipocytes, the classical brown and the beige adipocytes. Further evaluations of the molecular features of the human cells would benefit from establishing clonal cell lines from the different fetal and infant BAT depots. Such clonal cell lines would also be useful tools in studies aiming to identify factors with the capacity of activating and/or expanding the thermogenic potential of human BAT; that is, factors that would pose potential targets for therapy against obesity and obesity-related diseases such as type 2 diabetes.

SHIVERING

Newborn animals and newborn infants rarely shiver in response to cooling, though the metabolic rate is considerably increased. As shown in Fig. 42.17, no muscle activity is demonstrable by electromyography on day 2 of life in the cold-stressed guinea pig. In contrast, on day 12 of life, exposure to the same ambient temperatures (16°C and 8°C) evokes bursts of electrical muscle activity that are accompanied by visible muscle oscillations. This does not mean, however, that the shivering mechanism is not developed in the immediate postnatal period. To the contrary, shivering can be elicited in the guinea pig on the first day of life when nonshivering thermogenesis is blocked by a β-receptor blocker (Fig. 42.18) and body temperature is thereby allowed to fall. One may conclude, therefore, that the shivering mechanism is well developed at the time of birth but is normally suppressed by nonshivering thermogenesis. Shivering has also been observed in human neonates with severe hypothermia after birth. It has thus been concluded that the shivering threshold is displaced in neonates to a lower body temperature in comparison with the adult.

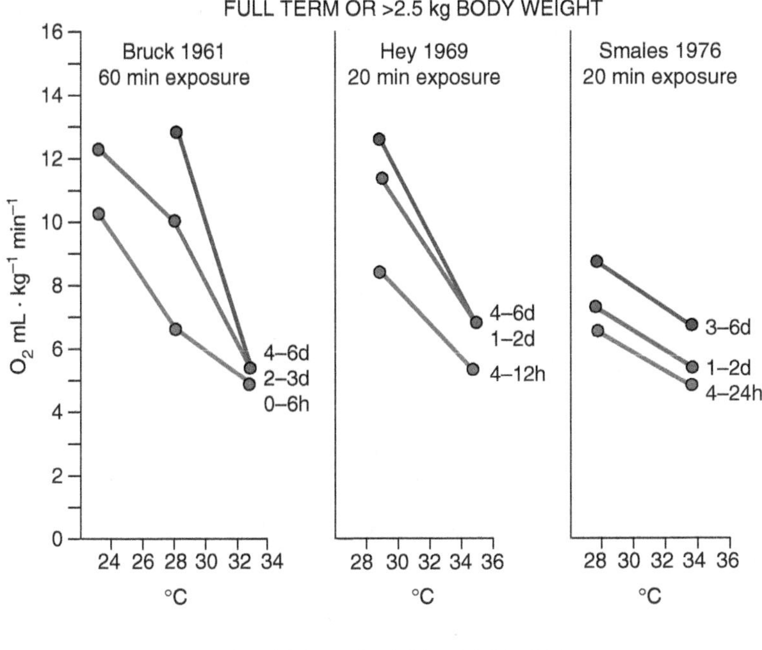

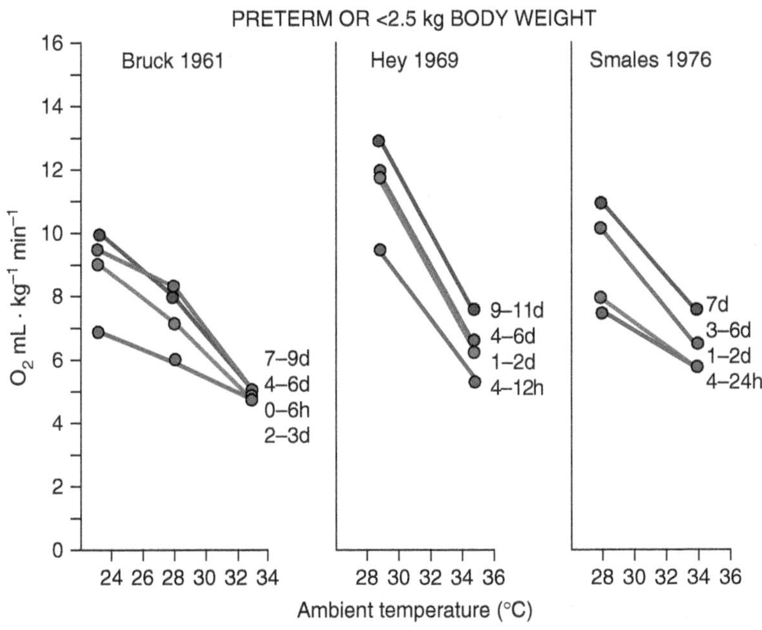

Fig. 42.13 Average rates of oxygen consumption of mature *(top panels)* and premature infants *(bottom panels)* at different ages and different ambient temperatures as measured by Brück,[1] Hey,[38] and Smales.[135] (From Hull D, Smales ORC. Heat production in the newborn. In: Sinclair JC, ed. *Temperature Regulation and Energy Metabolism in the Newborn*. New York: Grune & Stratton; 1978:129–156.)

The control of the thermoregulatory effector responses (thermogenesis, skin blood flow changes, sweat secretion, and behavioral responses) is predominantly exerted by the nervous system (see Fig. 42.9); hormonal transmission has a role only in long-term modifications of the thermoregulatory system. Two neuronal systems participate in thermoregulation: (1) the somatomotor system and (2) the sympathetic system.

METABOLIC RESPONSES: NEURAL CONTROL OF SHIVERING AND NONSHIVERING THERMOGENESIS

Shivering is controlled by means of the somatomotor system. The descending axons of the central shivering pathway project from the posterior hypothalamus to the reticular formation of the midbrain and pons. There they contact the supraspinal pathways and descend to the motor neurons in the anterior horns of the spinal cord. From there the musculature is rhythmically actuated through the motor nerves that leave through the anterior roots.

Nonshivering thermogenesis is controlled from the hypothalamic ventromedial nucleus[54] through the sympathetic nervous system. The transmitter in the target system (in particular, BAT) is norepinephrine, which acts on adrenergic β-receptors located in the cell membranes. Nonshivering thermogenesis can thus be blocked by β-receptor-blocking agents (see Fig. 42.18). The norepinephrine released at the nerve endings liberates free fatty acids from the lipid droplets and stimulates their subsequent oxidation.

CONTROL OF HEAT LOSS

VASOMOTOR RESPONSES

Thermoregulatory control of blood flow varies regionally.[55] At least three functionally different regions can be distinguished: (1) acral areas (e.g., fingers, hands, ears, lips, and nose), (2) trunk and proximal limbs, and (3) head and brow. Blood flow through the acral areas is controlled exclusively through noradrenergic sympathetic nerves. An increase in sympathetic tone causes vasoconstriction, and a decrease in tone results in vasodilation. In

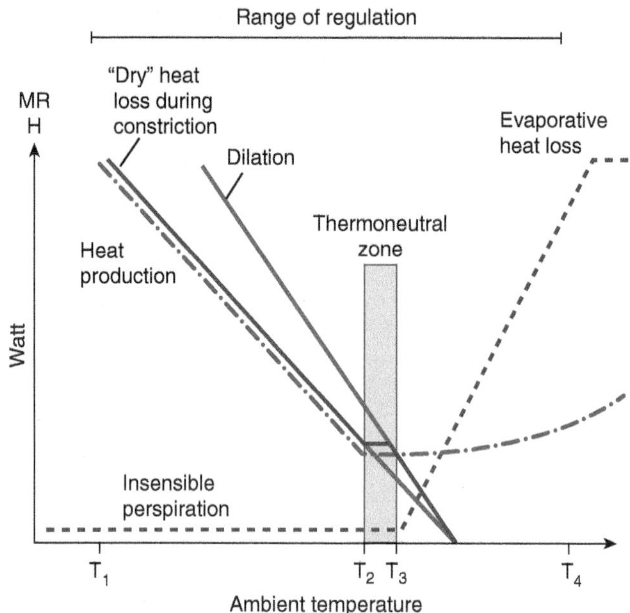

Fig. 42.14 Schematic representation of thermal balance in a homeothermic organism. In the range between T_1 and T_3, heat loss is matched by heat production; between T_3 and T_4, evaporative heat loss matches heat production plus heat gain from the environment. In the range T_2 to T_3 (thermoneutral zone), heat loss can be matched to at rest heat production by vasomotor adjustments. Less than T_1, heat loss exceeds the thermogenetic capacity. Greater than T_4, the production and influx of heat exceed the capacity for evaporative heat loss. *H,* Heat loss; *MR,* metabolic rate. (For further discussion, see text.)

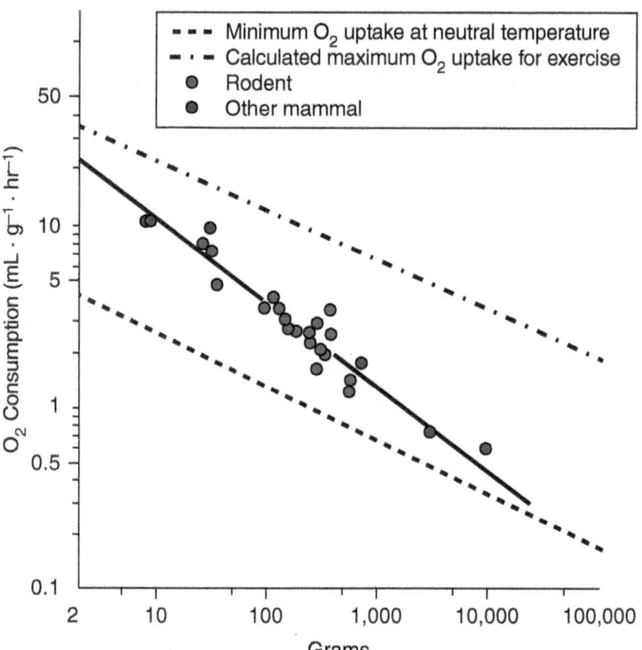

Fig. 42.15 Maximum amount of nonshivering thermogenesis, measured as increase in O_2 uptake after norepinephrine injection, in relation to body mass (various species in the adult age). (From Heldmaier G. Zitterfreie wärmbildung und Körper-größe bei Säugetieren. *Z Vergl Physiol.* 1971;73:222.)

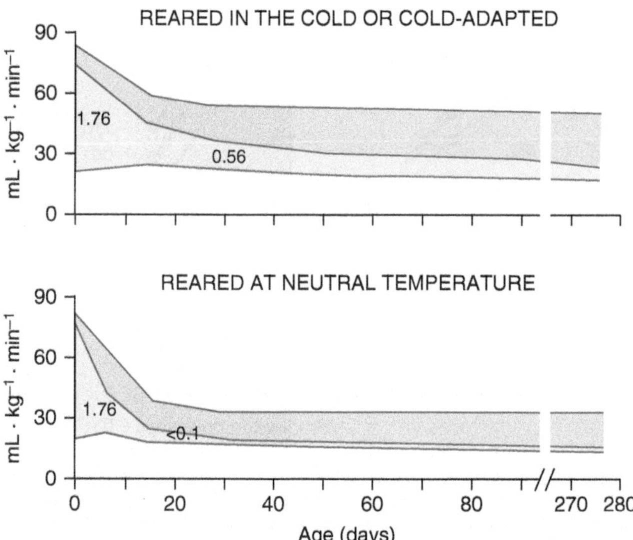

Fig. 42.16 Reduction of the maximum extent of nonshivering thermogenesis (NST) with increasing age and the dependence of this process on the environmental temperature at which the guinea pigs were reared. *White area,* Minimal oxygen consumption; *green area,* NST; *blue area,* shivering. The inset figures indicate the percentage mass of interscapular brown adipose tissue, which is closely related to the maximum extent of NST. Based on data from Zeisberger et al.[136] (From Brück K: Heat production and temperature regulation. In: Stave U, ed. *Perinatal Physiology*. New York: Plenum Publishing; 1978:455–498.)

contrast to the distal extremities, heat-induced reflex vasodilation in the trunk and proximal limbs results in a much larger blood flow than that observed after sympathectomy.[56] It has been suggested that in these areas there are specific vasodilator nerves that inhibit the vascular smooth muscles (active vasodilation).[56] Conversely, additional vasodilation has been ascribed to an enzyme secreted in sweat that catalyzes the formation of a vasoactive mediator, possibly bradykinin. The latter concept is supported by the frequent occurrence of a second phase of vasodilation coinciding with the onset of sweat secretion in the forearm (Fig. 42.19) and by the observed lack of substantial vasodilation in people congenitally lacking sweat glands.[45] Vasomotor nerves exert only a slight effect on the forehead, and practically no vasoconstriction occurs in response to cold stress; however, vasodilation does occur in these regions along with sweat secretion in response to heat stress. Well-developed vasomotor responses to environmental temperature changes have been demonstrated in term and premature newborn infants.[7]

SWEAT SECRETION

Apocrine sweat glands, as found in various mammals such as the *Bovidae* and *Equidae*, are controlled by an adrenergic sympathetic mechanism. However, in humans, apocrine sweat glands are controlled by cholinergic sympathetic fibers.[57,58] Consequently, sweat secretion can be inhibited by atropine. Acetylcholine, pilocarpine, and other parasympathetic drugs evoke sweat secretion.

BEHAVIORAL REGULATION

Behavioral measures must not be neglected in considering the constancy of body temperature. In adults of various species, particularly humans, behavioral measures may have a more important part in temperature constancy than do the autonomic reactions, and under some circumstances they may be the only way to maintain thermal comfort. A civilized human is rarely seen to shiver; he or she would rather increase the set temperature of the air conditioning system, or decrease it before perspiration begins.

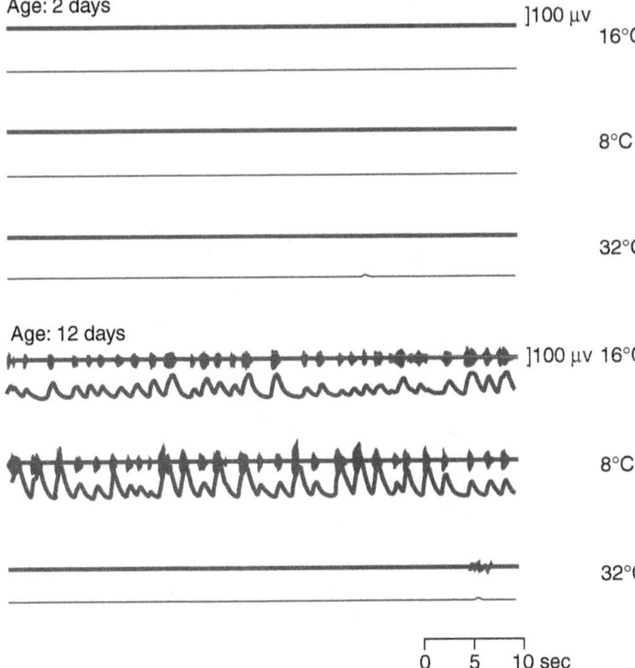

Fig. 42.17 Electromyograms from a guinea pig examined on days 2 and 12 postnatally at three different environmental temperatures (indicated on the *right side*). The lower traces on each record represent the integrated electrical muscle activity. Note that no shivering occurred on day 2 (although oxygen uptake was increased to three times standard metabolic rate). (From Brück K. In: Linneweh F, ed. *Fortschritte der pädologie*. Berlin: Springer; 1965:96–108.)

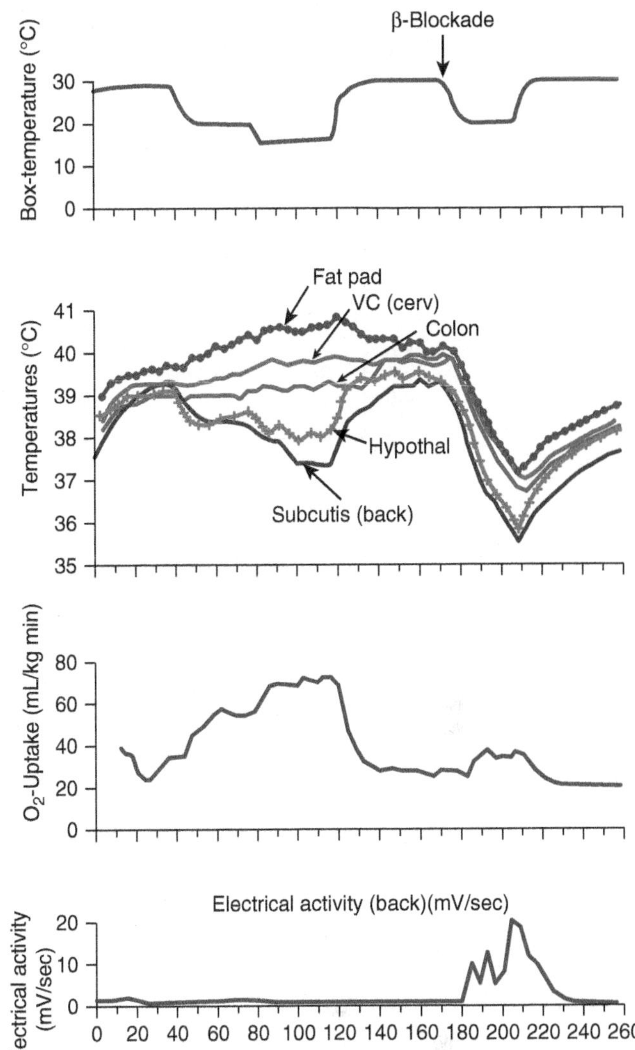

Fig. 42.18 Demonstration of shivering and nonshivering thermogenesis (NST) in a newborn guinea pig, age 0 days, body mass 101 g. In the first part of the experiment, only NST occurs during cold exposure. After administration of a β-receptor blocker and blockade of NST, shivering takes place and can be recognized by the increased electrical activity of the back muscles. Note: Increasing temperature in the area of the interscapular adipose tissue (Fat pad) and in the cervical part of the vertebral canal (*VC* [cerv]) occurs before, but parallel decrease of all temperatures occurs after blockade of NST. (For further explanation, see text.) (Adapted from Brück K, Wünnenberg W. Beziehung zwischen Thermogenese im "brounen" Fettgewebe, Temperatur im cervicalen Anteil des VertebralKanals und Kgiltezittem. *Pflügers Arch.* 1966;290:167.)

Behavioral regulation has been generally looked on as a highly developed type of thermoregulation in comparison with the autonomic regulatory measures described previously. More recent studies, however, have shown that behavioral regulation is, from a phylogenetic point of view, the more primitive state of thermoregulation. Behavioral thermoregulatory actions may even be manifested in a species that is not at all able to respond by autonomic effector actions. Thus, numerous fish species have been shown to seek out a preferred water temperature when they are given a choice, thereby stabilizing body temperature at a certain level. The "sunbathing" of reptiles is another well-known behavioral thermoregulatory response by which the body temperature is increased to, and precisely maintained at, a level comparable with that of homeothermic animals.[59]

Neonates also make considerable use of behavioral measures. Both piglets and newborn rabbits[60] reduce heat loss by huddling together. Moreover, when newborn rabbits are put into a temperature-gradient environment (a tube with steadily increasing temperature from one end to the other), they will move to a section of the tube warm enough to cause their body temperatures to stabilize near the adult level.[61-63]

In human neonates, postural reactions against overheating have been described.[64] Moreover, babies may cry to signal "thermal discomfort." This would represent another type of behavioral thermoregulation, namely, one mediated by the parents.

ADAPTIVE AND DEVELOPMENTAL CHANGES IN THERMOREGULATION

Unlike engineered physical regulatory systems, thermoregulation by living organisms is not invariant; its properties are influenced by thermal loading itself—its duration, frequency, and intensity. Some of the so-called *long-term thermoadaptive phenomena* may be traced to changes in the thermoregulatory system. As for the "passive system" (see Fig. 42.1), heat insulation may change with development because of an increase in the size of the subcutaneous fat layer or growth of a fur coat. The capacity of the effector systems (nonshivering and shivering thermogenesis) and some regulatory characteristics (namely, alterations in the threshold and gain of the relationship between effector response and body temperature)[28,65] can also undergo changes with development. As a consequence of these thermoadaptive modifications, the range of regulation (see Fig. 42.14) may increase, and the thermal discomfort evoked by thermal stress may be relieved.

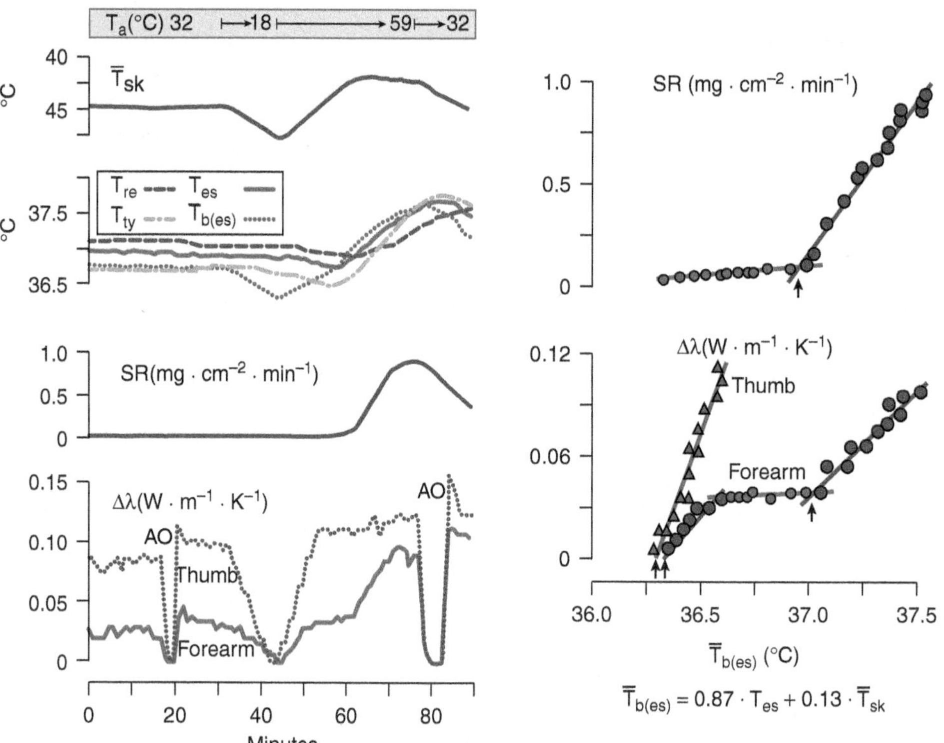

Fig. 42.19 Temperature-induced changes in skin blood flow and local sweat secretion (chest) in an adult. Left, Before body heating, ambient temperature *(T_a)* was decreased from 32°C to 18°C for establishing initial skin vasoconstriction (skin blood flow estimated from heat conductivity increment [Δλ]); thereafter T_a was raised to 59°C. Right, Skin blood flow and sweat secretion in relation to mean body temperature, $T_{b(es)}$ (calculated from esophageal temperature *[T_{es}]* and mean skin temperature *[T_{sk}]* as shown previously). Note second vasodilation on forearm *(arrow)* coinciding with onset of sweat secretion. *AO*, Arterial occlusion at upper arm; *SR*, local sweat rate (chest); T_{re}, rectal temperature; T_{ty}, tympanic temperature. (Adapted from Hessemer V, Brück K. Influence of menstrual cycle on shivering, skin blood flow, and sweating responses measured at night. *J Appl Physiol.* 1985;59:1902.)

ACCLIMATION VERSUS MATURATION

So long as the neonatal temperature control system was considered merely as deficient, it was thought that thermal acclimation, in addition to maturational processes, improved this system postnatally. With regard to nonshivering thermogenesis, however, the capacity of this cold defense mechanism is already maximized at birth in some species (see Fig. 42.16). Only a narrow margin exists for improving cold resistance by adaptive modifications in the metabolic system during the neonatal period.

In neonates born in a less mature state, development of nonshivering thermogenesis and BAT may proceed postnatally (even at thermoneutral conditions) and contribute to an improvement in temperature regulation. Thus the increasing summit metabolic rate in response to cold during the first few days of life in term and premature infants (see Fig. 42.13) may be due to postnatal development of nonshivering thermogenesis and an increase in BAT. In hamsters and rats (altricious animals), which are born in a rather immature state, guanosine diphosphate binding (as a measure of the thermogenic concentration) has also been shown to increase postnatally.[41,66]

LONG-TERM THRESHOLD TEMPERATURE DISPLACEMENT

Modifications in the threshold temperature for the elicitation of thermoregulatory effector actions have been demonstrated in animals other than humans. In guinea pigs reared in the cold, the shivering threshold is shifted to a temperature level about 1°C lower than in controls reared at neutral temperature (Fig. 42.20).[28,65] This shift enables these animals to make full use of nonshivering thermogenesis before the less economical shivering mechanism is evoked. A similar shift in the shivering threshold can be produced in adult humans by repeated short-term cold exposure (Fig. 42.21). Linked with the change in shivering threshold in humans is a shift in the threshold temperature for the experience of thermal discomfort, estimated by the subjects being studied on the basis of a subjective rating scale.[67] This type of adaptation has been called *tolerance adaptation*—that is, larger deviations in body temperature are tolerated before actuation of the appropriate thermoregulatory effectors occurs. In other words, the precision in temperature regulation is reduced, but at the same time cold discomfort is diminished.

Repeated heat exposure has been known to decrease the sweating threshold, that is, a sensitization occurs in the course of repeated heat exposure rather than development of tolerance. The load error of the thermoregulatory system is thereby diminished, that is, a tendency occurs to keep body temperature at less than a critical level. As the sweating threshold shift occurs during heat adaptation, it is accompanied by similar changes in the threshold temperatures for shivering and vasodilation (Fig. 42.22). Such concurrent shifts of the thresholds for all autonomic effector systems correspond to a resetting of the set point of the thermoregulatory control system.[28,68] In some instances, the threshold deviation may be accompanied by alterations in the gain of the temperature-response relationship.

SHORT-TERM THRESHOLD TEMPERATURE DISPLACEMENT

In addition to the described threshold changes that occur during repeated or continuous cold-heat exposures for several days or weeks, threshold deviations developing on the order of minutes have been demonstrated in humans, as well as in animals. Short-term shivering threshold displacement in men exposed twice to a low climatic chamber temperature with an interposed 20-minute

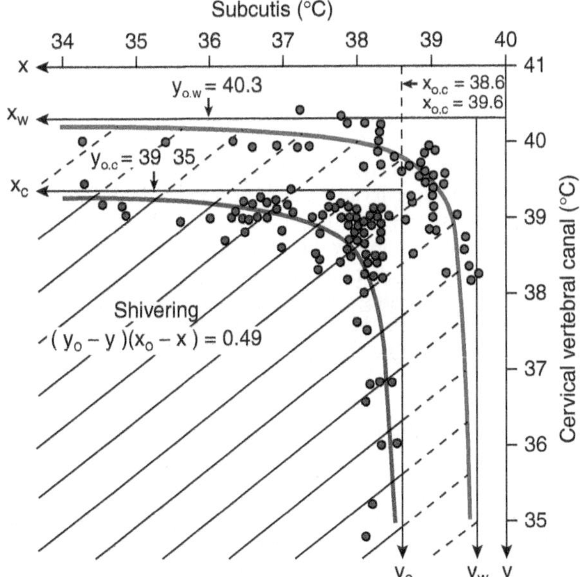

Fig. 42.20 Shivering threshold curves for two groups of guinea pigs (aged 4 to 8 weeks) reared in different environmental temperatures. The values were obtained by independent changes of the body surface temperature and the temperature in the cervical vertebral canal. The diagram shows, for instance, that at a certain body surface temperature, which corresponds to a subcutaneous temperature of 37°C, shivering begins in warm-adapted animals *(blue circle)* when the hypothalamic temperature drops below 40°C. In the cold-adapted animals *(red circle),* however, shivering does not occur until the hypothalamic temperature has reached a value slightly below 39°C. (From Brück K, Wünnenberg W. Meshed control of two effector systems: nonshivering and shivering thermogenesis. In: Hardy JD, Gagge AP, Stolwijk JAJ, et al., eds. *Physiological and Behavioral Temperature Regulation.* Springfield, IL: Charles C. Thomas; 1970:562–580.)

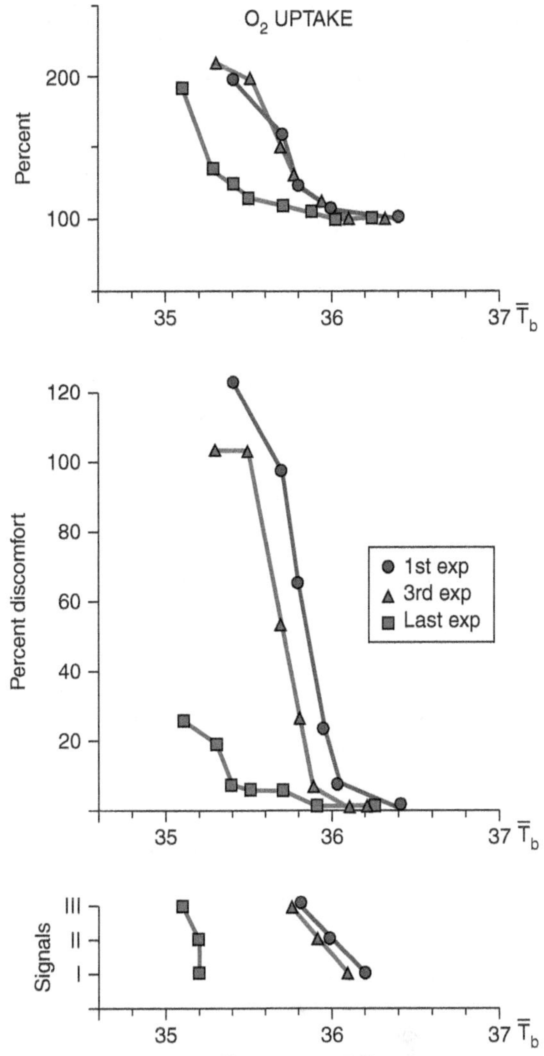

Fig. 42.21 Responses of a young man wearing only shorts on exposure to cold (ambient temperature decreasing from 28°C to 5°C in 45 minutes) in the course of an acclimatization series. Note that shivering threshold (onset of increase in VO_2) and discomfort threshold were shifted to lower mean body temperatures at the last (sixth day of the acclimatization period) exposure. *Signals* indicate subjective rating of cold sensation: *I,* Cool; *II,* cold; *III,* very cold. (From Brück K, Baum E, Schwennicke HP. Cold-adaptive modifications in man induced by repeated short-term cold-exposures and during a 10-day and 10-night cold-exposure. *Pflügers Arch.* 1976;363:125.)

rewarming period has been observed. During the second cooling phase, shivering occurred at a 0.4°C lower mean body temperature; in contrast, the slope of the temperature-response relationship was unchanged. In addition, the thresholds for skin blood flow and for sweating were shifted to lower values when the subjects were exposed to cold before they started an exercise test; this shift led to vasodilation and sweating. Thus a short cooling period causes a concurrent displacement of the threshold temperatures for all autonomic thermoregulatory responses in adult humans. In animals that are adapted to normal room temperature (21°C), this phenomenon of short-term acclimation is even more pronounced.

Previous observations in premature infants who were maintained at ambient temperatures so low as to yield steady-state body core temperatures near 35°C without arousing any cold defense have been ascribed to such short-term acclimation. In a subsequent study of a group of premature infants (weighing <1500 g), minimal oxygen uptake was compatible with rectal temperatures in the range of 35°C to 36°C. As judged from the time spent in quiet sleep, these babies did not show any signs of thermal discomfort.[69] Thus, the discomfort threshold can also shift to a lower level of body temperature. Moreover, the infants in this study exhibited a slight tendency toward vasodilation, indicating a decreased threshold for vasomotor responses. However, these effects may be related to postnatal maturation.

MATURATION

Although the control system (passive system; see Fig. 42.1) undergoes considerable alteration during ontogenesis, the thermoregulatory system tends to maintain deep body temperature from birth onward at a value typical for the species. This maintenance requires a number of adjustments by the thermoregulatory system to the smaller body size of neonates. These adjustments may be mediated by an increased thermogenic capacity, an additional heat production mechanism (nonshivering thermogenesis), and special changes in threshold conditions for eliciting effector responses. Conversely, modifications developing during thermal adaptation may consist of intrinsic mechanisms functioning in a neonatal organism that has not been stimulated by any environmental factor. These same mechanisms may serve to adjust the regulatory system either to body size or to special environmental conditions.

STABILITY OF DEEP BODY (CORE) TEMPERATURE DURING ONTOGENESIS

As shown in Fig. 42.23, colon temperature in newborn guinea pigs or rabbits is maintained close to the adult level, even during severe cold exposure. Remarkably, thermostability seems to be even greater during the first few days of life than it is later on. In guinea pigs, this enhanced stability can be accounted for by a greater metabolic response in the younger and smaller animal (Fig. 42.24). As shown in Fig. 42.16, newborn guinea pigs maintain body temperature mainly by nonshivering thermogenesis. In other species (e.g., pigs or miniature pigs), nonshivering thermogenesis does not occur. In these species, shivering supplies the extra heat for stabilizing body temperature at ambient temperatures as low as 20°C in neonates.[43] In human neonates exposed to ambient temperatures of 33°C to 23°C, the thermoregulatory effort is much larger than in adults for a given ambient temperature (Fig. 42.25). The metabolic increase is mainly due to nonshivering thermogenesis.

CHANGES IN THE PASSIVE SYSTEM

The neonatal passive system is characterized by a large body surface area-to-volume ratio and by decreased heat insulation

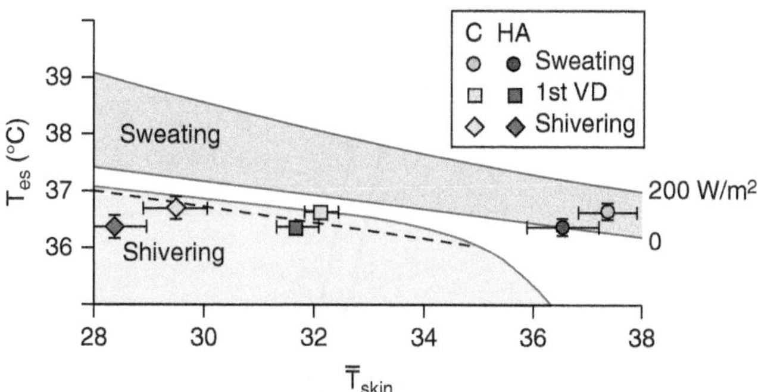

Fig. 42.22 Concurrent shift of the threshold temperatures of all autonomic thermoregulatory effectors to lower body temperatures in the course of a 5-day heat adaptation series. Means of seven subjects. Each subject was exposed to heat for approximately 90 minutes daily. Shivering threshold was determined 1 day before and 1 day after the 5 heat-exposure days. (For explanation of lines, see Fig. 42.12.) *C,* Control studies before acclimation; *HA,* after heat acclimation; *1st VD,* first vasodilation (see text). (Data from Hessemer V, Zeh A, Brück K. Effects of passive heat adaptation and moderate sweatless conditioning on responses to cold and heat. *Eur J Appl Physiol Occup Physiol.* 1986;55:281.)

resulting from the smaller absolute thickness of the body shell. With growth, the surface area-to-volume ratio decreases by a factor of 2.7. Comparison of data from neonates[70] and adults[71] indicates that overall insulation (I_{a+t}) (Fig. 42.26) increases by a factor of 1.8 as body mass increases from 3.5 to 70 kg. In a cool environment, maximum tissue insulation (I_t) changes by a factor of 3, and air insulation (I_a) increases by a factor of 1.2 because of the change in the curvature radii of the trunk and extremities.

The heat production (H) required for equilibrium heat flow at any given overall temperature difference would therefore have to be nearly five times as large in neonates as in adults (per unit of body mass). From the preceding data, an equation is derived that predicts heat loss in relation to body mass (m) at a given temperature difference between body core and environment (see Fig. 42.2):

$$H = k \times m^{0.5} \quad [42.2]$$

The SMR is actually lower in the neonates of various species than heat loss predicted from the preceding equation. It even falls short of Kleiber's equation, in which metabolic rate is related to body mass to the 0.75th power (see Fig. 42.2). In humans, beginning with the second year of life (corresponding to a body mass of more than 10 kg), the SMR is a function of body mass to the 0.5th power. In the first year of life (and especially during the first week of life), the SMR in relation to body mass is only 1.5 to 2 times larger than in adults. This means that the overall temperature difference (ΔT) that can be maintained in term neonates under the condition of SMR is less than half that of adults (and even less in premature infants) (Fig. 42.27). At an ambient temperature below 33°C, deep body temperature will drop unless heat production is increased. In fact, metabolic rate is increased at such high ambient temperature that the lower limit of the neutral temperature range is shifted to a higher level of ambient temperature.

ADJUSTMENT OF EFFECTOR THRESHOLD TEMPERATURES

Because of the small amount of tissue insulation, the difference between core and mean skin temperature is considerably smaller in neonates than in adults. Thus, cold defense reactions should be elicited at higher mean skin temperatures than in the adult to maintain core temperature at the adult level (Fig. 42.28). In other

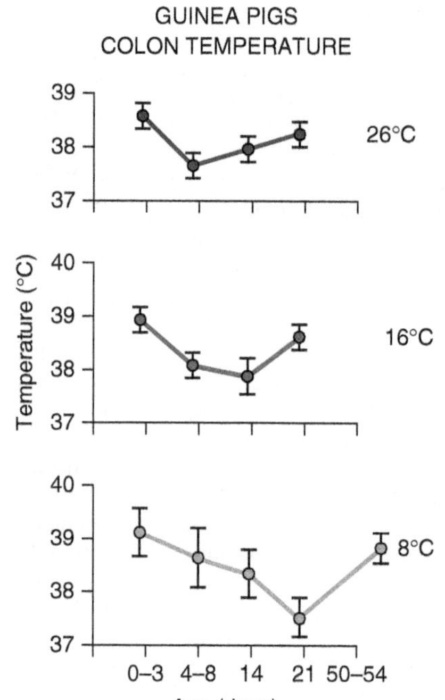

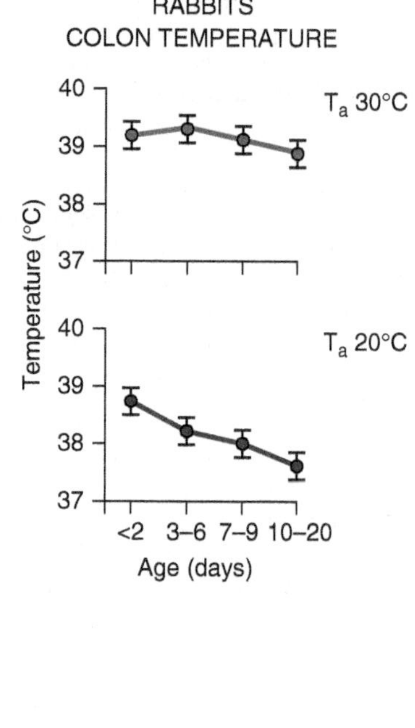

Fig. 42.23 Colon temperatures In guinea pigs and rabbits in relationship to age and ambient temperature (T_a). (Data from Brück K, Wünnenberg B. Über die Modi der Thermogenese beim neugeborenen Warmblüter. Untersuchungen am Meerschweinchen. *Pflügers Arch.* 1965;282:362; and Várnai I, Farkas M, Donhoffer S, et al. Thermoregulatory heat production and the regulation of body temperature in the new-born rabbit. *Acta Physiol Acad Sci Hung.* 1970;38:299.)

words, the threshold for increasing vasoconstrictor tone and for the metabolic reactions is shifted to a higher level in neonates, thereby adjusting the thermoregulatory system to the smaller body size.

The displacement of the neonatal threshold temperature can be explained in two ways. First, because of the increased body surface area to body mass quotient, the number of cutaneous cold receptors/unit body mass is increased (assuming that the density of the distribution of cold receptors is the same in adults and neonates). Second, the central processing of thermal input signals (see Figs. 42.1 and 42.8) in neonates is different from that in adults. The increased cutaneous sensitivity is a prerequisite for enabling newborn infants to maintain core temperature (within a limited range of environmental temperature) at the same level and with the same accuracy as occurs in the adult.

STAGE OF MATURITY OF THE THERMOREGULATORY SYSTEM AT BIRTH

Temperature regulation is frequently referred to as immature at the time of birth. However, one should be cautious in asserting immaturity of the thermoregulatory mechanisms even though neonates show greater fluctuations in body temperature than adults. Greater fluctuations of body temperature are to be expected in smaller organisms because of their large surface area-to-volume ratio, the relatively small insulating body shell, and the smaller body mass that acts as a heat buffer in large organisms. Because of these peculiarities in body size and shape, a reduced range of regulation (see Fig. 42.14) should be expected in neonates.

The degree of maturity of the thermoregulatory system should be evaluated according to the following three criteria:

1. What is the capacity of the effector system (a) in comparison with adults and (b) in relation to body size?
2. What is the qualitative and quantitative (threshold, gain) responsiveness of the effector systems to thermal stimuli?
3. Are there qualitative or quantitative differences in the central thermointegrating system between adults and neonates?

Regarding the first criterion, the capacity of the metabolic system in full-sized human neonates is comparable with that of an adult system when the metabolic rate is related to body mass, but it is too small to compensate for heat loss in as wide a range of ambient temperatures as in adults. Therefore, the tolerated ambient temperature range (range of regulation) (see Fig. 42.14) is

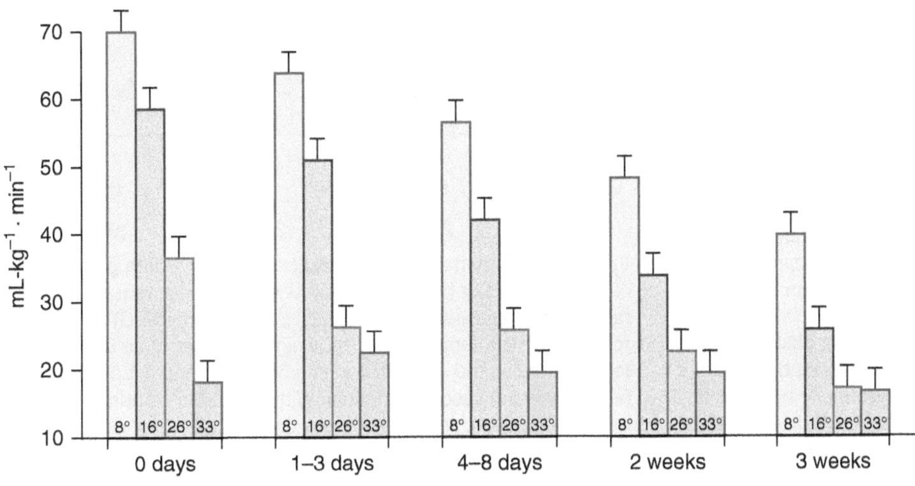

Fig. 42.24 Heat production (expressed as oxygen uptake) in relationship to ambient temperature (°C) and age in guinea pigs. (From Brück K, Wünnenberg B. Über die Modi der Thermogenese beim neugeborenen Warmblüter. Untersuchungen am Meerschweinchen. *Pflügers Arch.* 1965;282:362.)

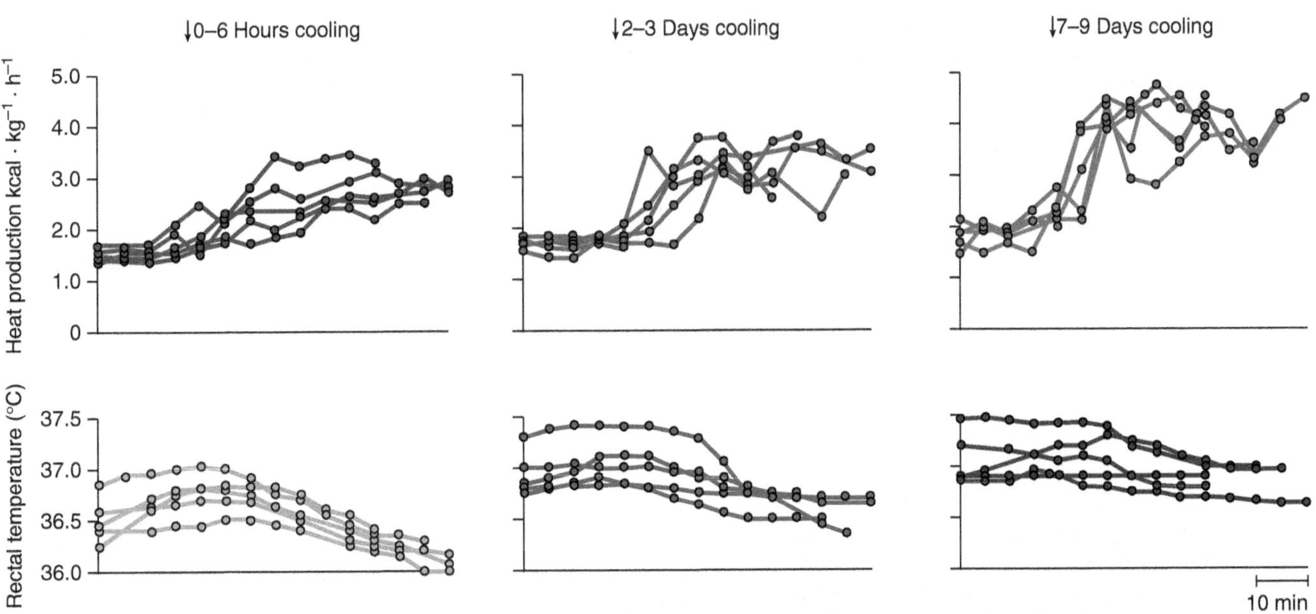

Fig. 42.25 Course of rectal temperatures and heat production in term newborn infants. Ambient temperature to the left of downward-pointing arrow 33°C, then a quick drop to 23°C. (From Brück K. Temperature regulation of the newborn infant. *Biol Neonate.* 1961;3:65.)

reduced. Term neonates are, at best, able to maintain a stable body temperature at an ambient temperature as low as 23°C (Fig. 42.29), at which point maximum thermogenesis is required for thermal balance. In adults, by contrast, maximum thermogenesis (although smaller/unit body weight) is sufficient to balance heat loss at an ambient temperature as low as 0°C to 5°C. It is notable that adults and neonates can maintain thermal balance under these extreme conditions only for restricted periods (30 to 60 minutes). More extended exposure results in exhaustion of the metabolic system and hypothermia. In neonates born at term gestation, the lower limit of the range of regulation (see Fig. 42.14; T_l) comes closer to that of adults than it does in preterm neonates.

Regarding the second criterion, the threshold and gain for the metabolic reactions are adjusted to the smaller body size of neonates (see Fig. 42.28). The sweating threshold is comparable with that in adults, except in premature and small-for-gestational-age neonates[72] in whom the threshold is shifted upward. Even in the very small premature infant, metabolic and vasomotor control responses are developed at birth,[1,73] although the threshold for elicitation of these responses may not be appropriately adjusted to body size. In addition, the capacities of the effector systems may be smaller than in adults. In neonates, maximum evaporative heat loss is in the range of the SMR.[72,74] In contrast, it is five times the SMR in adults.

As for the third criterion, no substantial neuronal or hormonal differences have yet been described between the neonatal and adult thermoregulatory systems.

According to these criteria, one may distinguish three groups of mammals according to their functional stage of temperature regulation immediately after birth. The first group exhibits a thermoregulatory system more or less completely adjusted to a smaller body size. The body temperature is stable within a certain control range. This range is narrower, however, than in adults. Members of this group include term human neonates, guinea pigs,[75] pigs,[42] miniature pigs,[43] lambs,[76] and larger mammals such as calves.[77]

The second group of mammals has the following characteristics: thermoregulatory responses can be evoked at birth, but the capacity of the effector systems, the threshold temperatures, or both are not sufficiently adjusted to the smaller body size. Body temperatures drop on exposure to environmental temperatures slightly less than thermal neutrality. Mammals in this group include low-birth-weight human newborns,[1] kittens, rabbits,[78] puppies,[79] and rats.[80]

In the third group, thermoregulatory responses are not evocable, and oxygen uptake does not increase with decreasing environmental temperatures. Instead, it follows van't Hoff's law (see Fig. 42.3). These animals (e.g., ground squirrels[79] and golden hamsters[66,81]) behave as poikilothermic animals do. This group is presumably restricted to the neonates of hibernators.

PATHOPHYSIOLOGY

SUDDEN INFANT DEATH SYNDROME

A possible role for hyperthermia in sudden infant death syndrome (SIDS) has been hypothesized because some victims

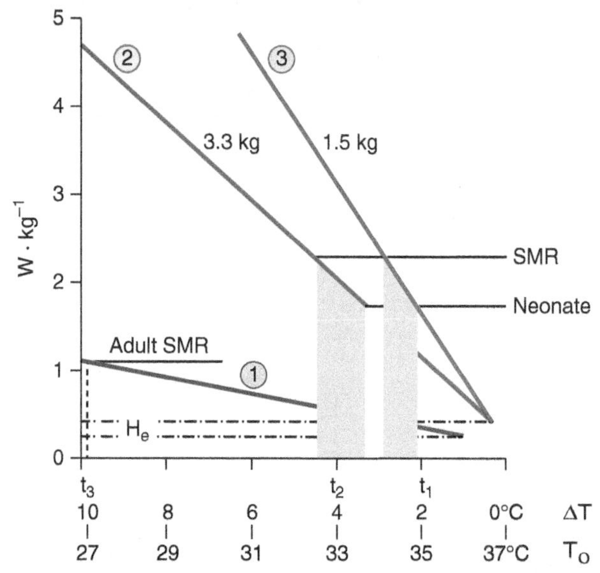

Fig. 42.27 Schematic representation (based on data given in Figs. 42.2 and 42.26) of heat production/unit body mass required to maintain the temperature differences (ΔT) in body core (37°C) and environment (operative temperature, T_O, weighted mean of air and radiation temperature) in the adult *(1)* and in a 3.3-kg *(2)* and a 1.5-kg *(3)* infant (with maximum vasoconstriction). With the actual standard metabolic rate *(SMR)* given, the temperature differences t_1, t_2, and t_3 can be maintained under conditions of thermal neutrality; conversely, the neonates require an environmental temperature of about 33°C *(2)* or even 34°C to 35°C *(3)* to maintain a deep body temperature of 37°C. In contrast, this level is much lower in the adult, 27°C *(1)*. H_e, minimum evaporative heat loss. (From Brück K. Heat production and temperature regulation. In: Stave U, ed. *Perinatal Physiology.* New York: Plenum Publishing; 1978:455–498.)

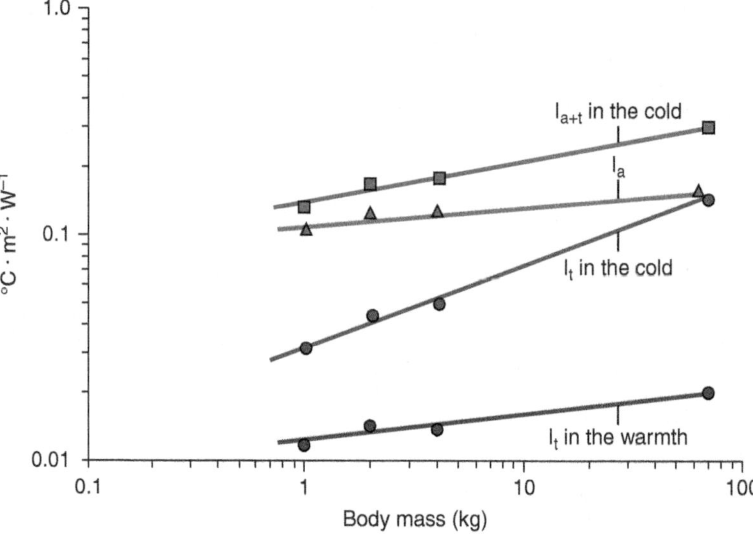

Fig. 42.26 Tissue insulation *(I_t)* under cold and warm environmental conditions, ambient insulation *(I_a)*, and total insulation *(I_{a+t})* in relation to body mass in humans. (From Brück K. Heat production and temperature regulation. In: Stave U, ed. *Perinatal Physiology*. New York: Plenum Publishing; 1978:455–498.)

are found in unusually warm environments, are warm and sweating when found dead, are wrapped tightly in clothing or bedding, have a history of febrile illness before death, or have high rectal temperatures at examination or autopsy.[82,83] Given the association between SIDS and another important risk factor, prone body positioning,[84] investigators have recently begun to examine the relationships in body position, body temperature, state of sleep, and cardiorespiratory activity. Infants sleeping prone have a higher peripheral skin temperature.[85,86] Heat loss is lower in infants sleeping prone than in those sleeping supine, perhaps because of less heat loss from the head. Thus prone infants take longer than supine infants to reach the lower rectal temperature that occurs after the onset of sleep and rectal temperature remains higher during sleep.[87,88] The weight of evidence obtained from term and low-birth-weight infants and infants a few months old also suggests that prone positioning is associated with reduced heat production. Even so, heart rate,[89,90] blood pressure,[91] and absolute skin temperatures[85,86] are higher and temperature gradients from central to peripheral skin are narrower.[92] Taken together, these data suggest that, despite attempts to eliminate heat through adjustments in the peripheral circulation (narrowing central-peripheral gradients), infants are unable to maintain set-point temperature(s). Alternatively, the prone position may be linked to an elevation in the set point. Either way, the evidence points toward probable differences in autonomic control of metabolism and cardiorespiratory function in the prone versus the supine position.

FEVER

It is well known that newborn infants may suffer severe infection without increased body temperature. In contrast, clinical reports show body temperature elevations higher than 38°C to 39°C in newborn infants with septicemia, purulent meningitis, and pneumonia.[93] Experimental studies suggest that some peculiarities of fever mechanisms exist during the neonatal period. Newborn lambs fail to respond with fever after the administration of bacterial pyrogen or leukocyte pyrogen during the first few days of life.[94] Newborn guinea pigs have been shown to react to adult doses of pyrogen no sooner than a few days after birth, but they do respond with fever immediately after birth when this pyrogen is administered at much higher doses than in the adults.[93] If one takes certain precautions (e.g., providing an ambient temperature that does not overwhelm thermogenesis, sufficient nutrition, and so on), a pyrogen fever comparable with that of adults may be evoked in neonates of many species. However, many species-related differences in the pattern of the febrile response exist. For example, newborn guinea pigs demonstrate a biphasic response when endotoxin is administered intraperitoneally (Fig. 42.30). In contrast, 0- to 3-day-old rabbits exhibit a short-lasting monophasic fever, and 3- to 6-day-old kittens show a more sustained monophasic fever. A hypothermic response is commonly observed in 8- to 10-day-old rats.[93] In most cases, pyrogen administration causes heat production to increase; as in thermoregulation, nonshivering thermogenesis is a prevailing mechanism of extra heat production during febrile response.

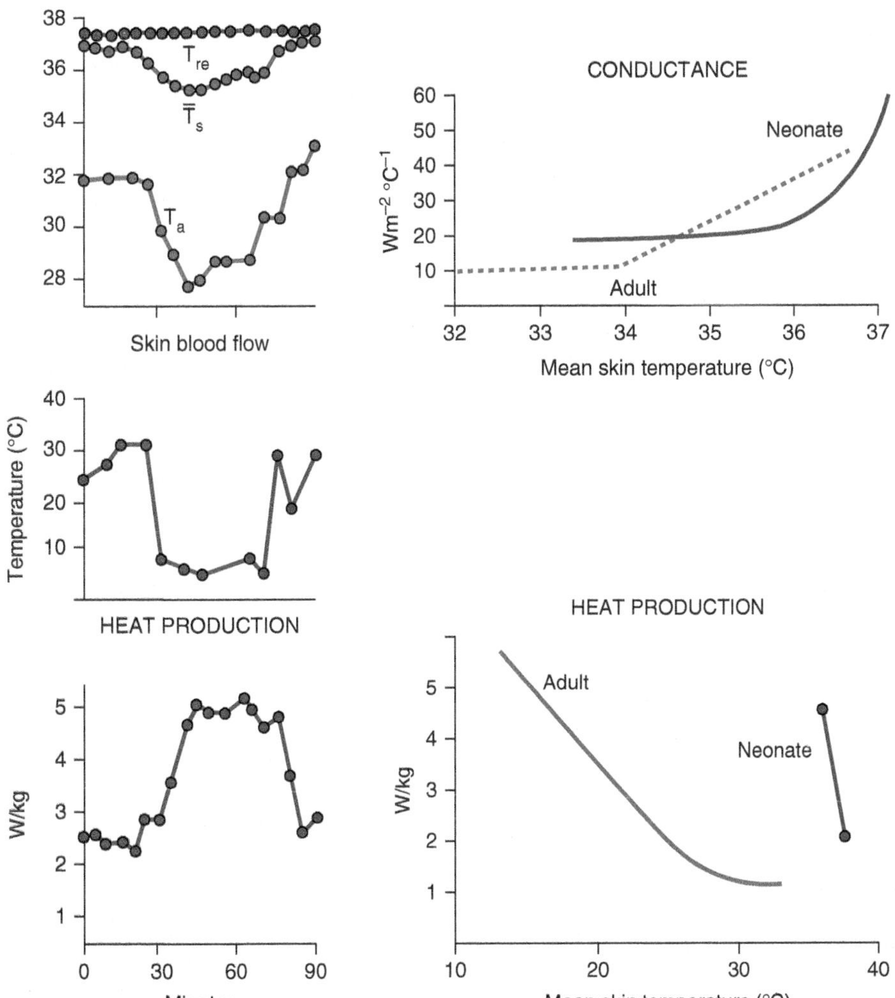

Fig. 42.28 Left, Simultaneous response of skin blood flow (heel) and heat production to a slight drop in mean skin temperature (T_s) evoked by a decrease in ambient temperature (T_a) from 32°C to 28°C. Study in a 7-day-old infant, 3290 g. Right, Relationship of and heat production in adults[137] and newborn infants[1] and thermal conductance (peripheral blood flow) in relationship to mean skin temperature in neonates[138] and adults.[139] Note onset of responses at higher body temperatures in the neonate. T_e, Rectal temperature. (From Brück K. Heat production and temperature regulation. In: Stave U, ed. *Perinatal Physiology*. New York: Plenum Publishing; 1978:455–498.)

MECHANISM OF FEVER

Set-Point Displacement

Fever develops as a result of an activation of cold defense reactions as they normally occur when an organism is exposed to cold. Generally, the process begins with peripheral vasoconstriction and is followed by enhanced thermogenesis. In adults, the latter response is accompanied by shivering, whereas in neonates, nonshivering thermogenesis prevails. With increasing body temperature, these thermoregulatory effector actions, thermogenesis and vasoconstriction, are diminished just as if the organism aimed to reach a new target temperature. Recovery from the fever is induced by the activation of heat dissipation mechanisms—vasodilation and sweating. During the constant fever phase, thermal disturbances (see Fig. 42.1) are compensated for by the appropriate control processes. It appears from this description that the thermoregulatory effector system remains completely functional but that the organism aims to assume and sustain a higher body temperature during fever. This phenomenon has been termed *set-point displacement,* thereby excluding other conceivable interpretations—for example, a toxic effect on one or more effector systems (see Fig. 42.9). Current fever research is focusing on the question of how bacterial and viral toxins (exogenous pyrogens) act to finally affect the thermointegrative system (see Fig. 42.8) in such a way that body temperature is shifted to a higher level.

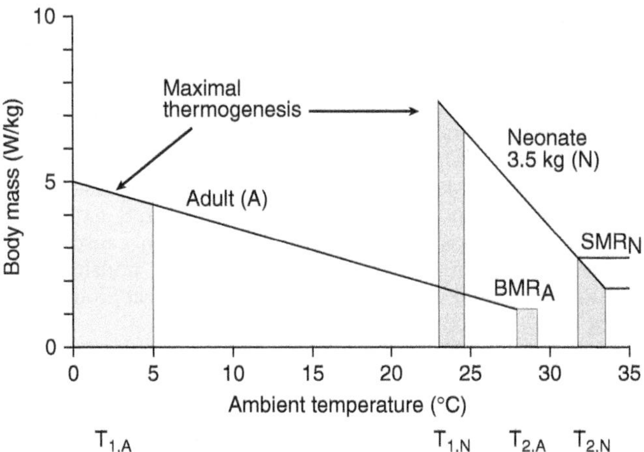

Fig. 42.29 Minimal (basal or standard) and maximum metabolic rate in relation to ambient temperature in neonates *(N)* and adults *(A)*. The inflection point of each curve marks the lower limit of the thermoneutral zone *(T_2)*, which is shifted to a higher temperature in neonates because of relatively low standard metabolic rate *(SMR)*. As the SMR increases during the first few days of life, $T_{2,N}$ shifts to lower ambient temperature. The lower limit of the range of regulation, T_1 (see Fig. 42.14), is determined by the maximal rate of heat production and is about 23°C in newborns and 0°C to 5°C in adults. *BMR*, Basal metabolic rate. (Data from Brück K. Heat production and temperature regulation. In: Stave U, ed. *Perinatal Physiology*. New York: Plenum Publishing; 1978:455–498.)

PATHOGENESIS OF FEVER

Fever is considered an immunoreactive process.[95,96] Certain fever-producing substances of external origin (e.g., exogenous pyrogens), such as the heat-stable lipopolysaccharides of bacterial membranes (endotoxins), stimulate granulocytes and macrophages of the reticuloendothelial system to produce a heat-labile peptide called *endogenous pyrogen*. Endogenous pyrogen is identical to the cytokine interleukin-1. Microinjection of endogenous pyrogen into small regions of the hypothalamus triggers typical fever reactions that are not observed when it is injected into other parts of the brain. Endogenous pyrogen initiates a cascade of processes by activating phospholipase A_2, which then converts phospholipids in cell membranes to arachidonic acid. This compound may then be converted to prostaglandins.

One of the prostaglandins, prostaglandin E_2 (PGE_2), has a pyrogenic action when injected into the hypothalamus in minute amounts.[97] PGE_2 produces the set-point shift already described by interacting with thermosensitive, integrative structures (see interneurons; Fig. 42.8), or both in the hypothalamus. Antipyretics (e.g., acetylsalicylic acid) inhibit cyclooxygenase activity and thus prostaglandin formation. However, PGE_2 is not the only fever mediator because specific PGE_2 antagonists do not prevent pyrogen-initiated fever.[98] Evidence suggests that endogenous pyrogen may penetrate, in minute amounts, into the hypothalamus through a special transport system located in the organon vasculosum of the upper brain stem,[97] which belongs to the so-called *circumventricular system*. Based on evidence that PGE_2 appears before the increase in plasma cytokine concentration and the increases in related enzymatic activity, it has been suggested that rapid neural pathways may be involved in the pyrogenic sensing and signaling.[99] A more complex model

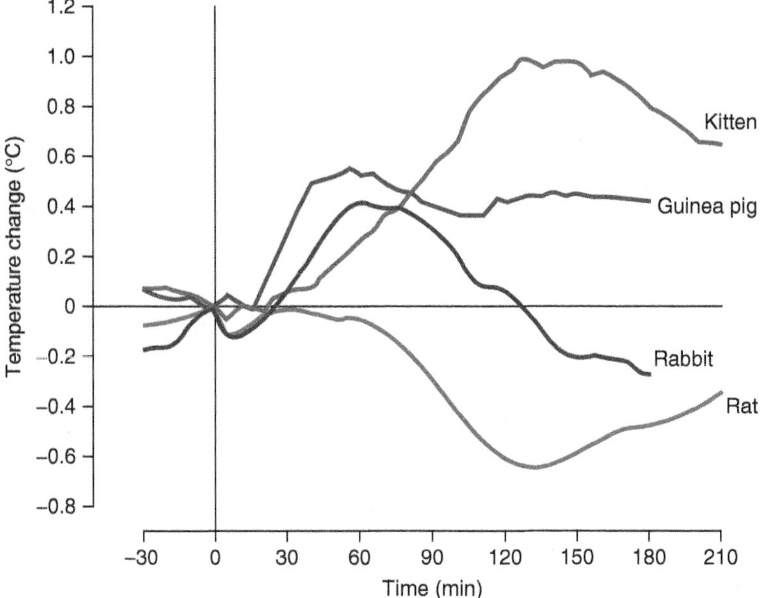

Fig. 42.30 Average body temperature changes in the newborn of four species after two intraperitoneal injections of 20 μg/kg *Escherichia coli* endotoxin at the individual thermoneutral ambient temperature. (From Szeákely M, Szeleányi Z. The pathophysiology of fever in the neonate. In: Milton AS, ed. *Pyretics and Antipyretics*. Berlin: Springer; 1982:479–528.)

for the genesis of fever is warranted, and a search is under way for other fever mediators, particularly circulating products of oxidative stress and their interactions with nitric oxide (NO) and the thermointegrative networks.[100] Interest in the role of NO in body temperature control is expanding. This ubiquitous molecule appears to mediate both peripheral (vasomotor tone and brown fat metabolism) and central (set-point) responses of the thermal control system to a variety of stimuli, including exogenous pyrogens, psychologic stress, and exercise.[101] Studies based on intradermal administration of nitric oxide synthase (NOS) inhibitors via microdialysis probes during hyperthermia have found that active vasodilation during heat stress was significantly attenuated by NOS inhibition.[102,103] These studies suggest that an active vasodilator requires functional NOS to achieve full expression. Alternatively, Farrell and Bishop[104] noted that nitroprusside could restore the vasodilation inhibited by previous NOS blockade during hyperthermia in rabbit ears, but the same dose of nitroprusside infused into the ear circulation in normothermia did not raise ear blood flow. This implies that active vasodilation in rabbit ears requires both NO production and activation of the vasodilator nerves and suggests a "permissive" role of NO in active vasodilation. Human studies based on NO breakdown products during hyperthermia have shown that both skin blood flow and bioavailable NO concentrations begin to increase at the same core temperature. This indicates that NO could well be an active effector of cutaneous vasodilation during heat stress.[105,106] In addition, Shibasaki and colleagues[107] have shown that acetylcholine-mediated NO production via muscarinic receptor activation was only possible early in heat stress, and then only before occurrence of substantial cutaneous vasodilation. Although both neuronal NOS and endothelial NOS have been detected in human skin,[108,109] it is unclear which isoform produces the increased NO required for active vasodilation. Wong and colleagues[110] reported that H_1 histamine receptors may play a role in the generation of NO during cutaneous active vasodilation in hyperthermia. The source of histamine remains to be identified; however, work by Wilkins and coworkers[111] suggests that (1) vasoactive intestinal peptide-induced release of histamine from mast cells could be involved and (2) vasoactive intestinal peptide and histamine have NO-dependent components to their vasodilatory effects. Thus, several pathways may be involved in the generation of NO in the skin during hyperthermia.[107,110,111]

BEHAVIORAL FEVER

In newborn rabbits, which are born in a very immature state, the thermogenic response to a standard pyrogen dose may be weak or even lacking. Nevertheless, these animals have been shown to experience fever when they are put into a temperature-gradient tube in which they are able to move to an area so hot as to cause their body temperatures to increase.[62] This response has been termed *behavioral fever* in contrast to the fever produced by the activity of the autonomous thermoregulatory effectors (see Fig. 42.9).

TEMPERATURE REGULATION IN HEART FAILURE

Thermal instability is a common accompaniment of cardiac disease in newborns, often leading to unnecessary treatment for infection. It should be remembered that circulatory changes are central to control of body temperature and thus dependent on cardiac function. Cardiac-dependent changes are noted within and outside the thermoneutral zone, and these alterations are likely to differ with the severity and etiology of heart failure. Unfortunately, there are limited studies addressing this issue, particularly during the neonatal period. The upper boundary of the zone of hypothermia is elevated to include environments that, at worst, are only mildly chilling for normal patients but induce shivering in patients with heart failure. The cardiac stress associated with the onset of shivering is likely to be compounded by increased thermal stress through enhanced rate of decline of core temperature and a further stimulus to shivering.[112] In the neutral zone, where core temperature is maintained by control of skin blood flow, pharmacologic interventions have the potential to deprive the individual of the ability to vasodilate appropriately and could lead to a 2°C decline in core temperature.[113] In the zone of hyperthermia, both skin and core temperatures are likely to increase. Thermal steady states are possible when reflex sweating and cutaneous vasodilation are adequate to achieve thermal balance. The vasodilator component of this response is undoubtedly influenced by the physiologic changes and pharmacologic interventions associated with heart failure and its treatment. Interestingly, a vasodilator response has been shown experimentally to result in improvement of cardiac function because of afterload reduction,[114] similar to that observed with pharmacologic vasodilator treatment. In this situation, the increase in cardiac output is entirely diverted to the cutaneous vasculature. Although it has not been well studied, monitoring central and peripheral temperatures would likely provide useful information about the adequacy of cardiac reserve of children with congenital heart disease.

HYPOXIA

ACUTE AND CHRONIC HYPOXIA

Considerable impairment of temperature regulation should be anticipated if the oxygen supply is critically reduced to the tissues subserving thermoregulatory heat production (skeletal tissues, musculature, and BAT). Anaerobic metabolic processes are quantitatively insufficient to provide enough heat for thermoregulation. In fact, a reduction of oxygen content in the inspired gas to 10% has been shown to completely block thermogenesis in newborn kittens exposed to an ambient temperature that is lower than neutral.[115,116] As a result, body core temperature drops. Remarkably, the at-rest metabolic rate as measured at neutral temperature remains unaffected by this degree of hypoxia. Similar results have been obtained in newborn lambs,[117] rhesus monkeys,[118] guinea pigs,[115] and rabbits.[119] By contrast, in larger adult organisms that do not possess nonshivering thermogenesis (e.g., adult humans[120] and dogs[121]), cold-induced thermogenesis (shivering) is only transiently reduced by hypoxia. With sustained hypoxia, shivering thermogenesis appears to be almost unimpaired. Thus, nonshivering thermogenesis appears to be more vulnerable to the effect of hypoxia.

This view is supported by a study in newborn rabbits.[119] As shown in Fig. 42.31, oxygen uptake increases on cold exposure without shivering. Offering a 10% oxygen gas mixture immediately abolishes the cold-induced nonshivering thermogenic response. In the subsequent hours, however, oxygen uptake steadily increases and is accompanied by shivering. Because the interscapular BAT is a major site of thermogenesis and the heat produced in this organ inhibits shivering through cervicospinal warm-sensitive structures, the appearance of shivering during hypoxic blockade of nonshivering thermogenesis is understandable. With prolonged hypoxia, the capacity for nonshivering thermogenesis may more or less recover. Normal thermogenic responses without obvious shivering have been observed in some neonates and infants with cyanotic congenital heart disease in whom arterial oxygen contents range from 10 to 20 mL/dL (Fig. 42.32). Even with arterial oxygen content as low as 5 mL/dL, thermogenic responses can be evoked, although they are reduced in magnitude. These results suggest that in chronic hypoxia, adjustments take place that restore the capacity for nonshivering thermogenesis.

As for the mechanism of the hypoxic reduction of cold-inducible thermogenesis, two possibilities have been suggested: (1) reduced oxidative capacity from the lowered oxygen tension at the level

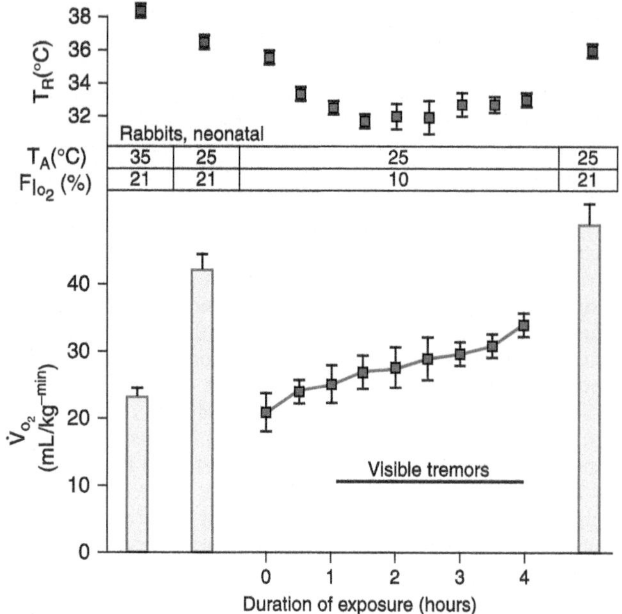

Fig. 42.31 Effect of cold and hypoxia on the oxygen consumption and colonic temperature of unanesthetized newborn rabbits. Exposure to 25°C in air caused an increase in oxygen consumption, which was produced without shivering. This increase was abruptly abolished when the inspired oxygen content was decreased to 10%. During the next 4 hours, oxygen consumption gradually increased. Visible shivering developed after 1 hour and persisted into the posthypoxic period. (From Blatteis CM. Shivering and nonshivering thermogenesis during hypoxia. In: Smith RE, ed. *Bioenergetics. Proceedings of the International Symposium on Environmental Physiology.* Bethesda, MD; 1988: 151–160.)

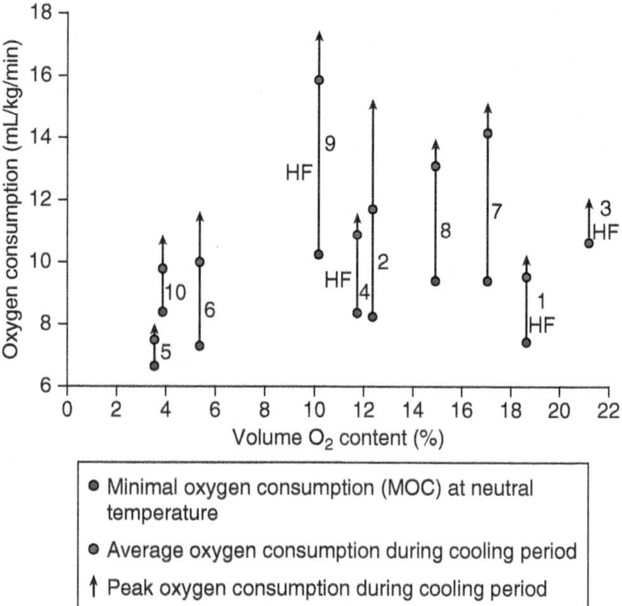

Fig. 42.32 Responses of oxygen consumption on cold exposure (ambient temperature drop from 32°C to 28°C) in relation to arterial oxygen content. Three infants with heart failure *(HF)* had severe heart failure. Note that oxygen consumption increased on cooling even in infants with arterial oxygen content as low as 5% vol. (From Brück K, Adams M. Temperature regulation in infants with chronic hypoxemia. *Pediatrics.* 1962;30:350.)

of mitochondria in the organs involved in thermogenesis (BAT, skeletal musculature) and (2) central inhibition of the effector systems. As shown by Blatteis,[119] the effect of norepinephrine infusion on nonshivering thermogenesis is abolished or grossly reduced during hypoxia. This would support the first hypothesis.

In hibernators, hypoxia and hypercapnia have been shown to displace the threshold for the elicitation of cold defense reactions to a lower body temperature level through a central action.[122,123] In a study in conscious adult cats,[124] hypoxia caused by inspiration of 11% oxygen reduced shivering. This suppression of shivering was partially reversed, however, when the end-tidal carbon dioxide concentration was returned to normal by addition of carbon dioxide to the inspired gas. These data would argue against the first possibility, at least with regard to moderate grades of hypoxia. Thus Gautier and colleagues concluded that "brain hypoxia lowers the regulated body temperature during cold stress."[124] More recent observations suggest that, as in the case of fever, molecular mediators of the central effector response are likely to be important. Murine hypoxic hypometabolism and associated hypoventilation have been ameliorated by inhibitors of NOS.[125] Depending on the experimental design and species under study, various, often contradictory effects of NO have been reported. Overall, the evidence points toward a fundamental, but complex, role for NO in the control of metabolism, cardiorespiratory function, and temperature during hypoxia.

EFFECTS OF FETAL HYPOXIA ON NEONATES

Fetal hypoxia has been shown to increase the plasma norepinephrine concentration. This, in turn, results in peripheral vasoconstriction and circulatory centralization of cardiac output.[126] Moreover, increased norepinephrine levels have been shown in guinea pigs to cause a downward displacement of the shivering threshold temperature.[127,128] Neonates who had fetal asphyxia may thus display a delayed metabolic response to cold exposure, as well as a delayed cutaneous vasodilation on heat exposure. This has been demonstrated in neonates who have undergone severe asphyxiation during delivery.[1]

CONCLUSIONS

Adaptive changes of the thermoregulatory system include morphologic and functional modifications. The morphologic modifications such as changes in body shape and insulation need months to years to develop, unless they are genetically fixed and appear seasonally. In general, they are preceded by functional modifications, including changes in capacity of the effector systems and changes in regulatory characteristics, which need much less time to develop. These early changes in regulatory characteristics, which can be defined as deviations in threshold and gain of the thermoregulatory responses, have been described. On the basis of insights into the organization of the thermoregulatory system and on evaluation of experimental evidence from electrophysiologic, neuropharmacologic, and neuroanatomic studies, it can be concluded that the monoaminergic brain systems are involved in adaptive modifications. Receiving information from several sensory systems, they seem to deliver additional modulatory signals, which may interfere with the processing of specific thermal information at several sites. Theoretically, the central monoamines may participate in the control of thermal input, in the central integration of thermal signals, and in the modification of output signals to thermoregulatory effectors. Best documented is their modulatory action on thermosensitive and thermointegrative hypothalamic neurons. There, the monoamines 5-hydroxytryptamine and noradrenaline act as antagonists, which enhance or diminish the effects of thermal afferents mediated by other transmitters. Moreover, the antagonistic monoaminergic systems are interconnected and can influence each other at the level of the lower brain stem. The activity in central monoaminergic systems can also be modified by neurohumoral feedback mechanisms from the periphery. By means of these interrelations the vegetative responses of the organism can be corrected and optimized. These interrelations can also explain some cross-adaptive changes in the thermoregulatory threshold for shivering evoked by nonthermal factors such as food intake.

ACKNOWLEDGMENT

Based on a previous chapter by Karl Schulze, MD.

 A complete reference list is available at www.ExpertConsult.com.

SELECT REFERENCES

1. Brück K. Temperature regulation in the newborn infant. *Biol Neonate*. 1961;3:65.
2. Brown AC, Brengelmann GL, et al. The temperature regulation control system. In: Hardy JD, ed. *Physiological and Behavioral Temperature Regulation*. Springfield, IL: Charles C.Thomas; 1970:684–702.
3. Brück K, Wünnenberg W, et al. Meshed control of two effector systems: non-shivering and shivering thermogenesis. In: Hardy JD, ed. *Physiological and Behavioral Temperature Regulation*. Springfield, IL: Charles C. Thomas; 1970:562–580.
4. Hensel H, Brtick K, Raths P. Homeothermic organisms. In: Precht H, Christophersen J, Hensel H, Larcher W, eds. *Temperature and Life*. Berlin: Springer-Verlag; 1973:503–761.
5. Stolwijk JAJ, Hardy JD. Temperature regulation in man—a theoretical study. *Pflügers Arch*. 1966;291:129.
6. McCance RA, Strangeways WMB. Protein catabolism and oxygen consumption during starvation in infants, young adults and old men. *Br J Nutr*. 1954;8:21.
7. Brück K. Heat production and temperature regulation. In: Stave U, ed. *Perinatal Physiology*. New York: Plenum Publishing; 1978:455–498.
8. Glossary of Terms for Thermal Physiology. Ed 2. Revised by the Commission for Thermal Physiology of the International Union of Physiological Sciences (IUPS Thermal Commission). *Pflügers Arch*. 1987;410:567.
9. Schulze K, Stefanski M, Masterson J, et al. An analysis of the variability in estimates of bioenergetic variables in preterm infants. *Pediatr Res*. 1986;20:422.
10. Bell EF, Rios GR, Wilmoth PK. Estimation of 24-hour energy expenditure from shorter measurement periods in premature infants. *Pediatr Res*. 1986;20:646.
11. Kleiber M. *The Fire of Life: An Introduction to Animal Energetics*. New York: John Wiley & Sons; 1961.
12. Hull D, Smales ORC. Heat production in the newborn. In: Sinclair JC, ed. *Temperature Regulation and Energy Metabolism in the Newborn*. New York: Grune & Stratton; 1978:129–156.
13. Sinclair JC, Scopes JW, Silverman WA. Metabolic reference standards for the neonate. *Pediatrics*. 1967;39:724.
14. Hensel H. *Thermal Sensations and Thermoreceptors in Man*. Springfield, IL: Charles C.Thomas; 1982.
15. Konietzny F, Hensel H. The neural basis of the sensory quality of warmth. In: Kenshalo DR, ed. *Sensory Functions of the Skin of Humans*. New York: Plenum Press; 1979:241–259.
16. Hensel H, Andres KH, von Düring M. Structure and function of cold receptors. *Pflügers Arch*. 1974;352:1.
17. Schäfer K, Braun HA, Hensel H. Temperature transduction in the skin. In: Hales JRS, ed. *Thermal Physiology*. New York: Raven Press; 1984:1–11.
18. Hensel H. Die Intracutane Temperaturbewegung bei Einwirkung äußere Temperaturreize. *Pflügers Arch*. 1950;252:146.
19. Benzinger TH. Heat regulation: homeostasis of central temperature in man. *Physiol Rev*. 1969;49:671.
20. Jessen C. Thermal afferents in the control of body temperature. *Pharmacol Ther*. 1985;28:107.
21. Nakayama T, Hammel HT, Hardy JD, et al. Thermal stimulation of electrical activity of single units of the preoptic region. *Am J Physiol*. 1963;204:1122.
22. Kelso SR, Boulant JA. Effect of synaptic blockade on thermosensitive neurons in hypothalamic tissue slices. *Am J Physiol*. 1982;243:R480.
23. Baldino F, Geller HM. Electrophysiological analysis of neuronal thermosensitivity in rat preoptic and hypothalamic tissue cultures. *J Physiol*. 1982;327:173.
24. Brück K, Hinckel P. Thermoafferent systems and their adaptive modifications. *Pharmacol Ther*. 1982;17:357.
25. Simon E, Pierau FK, Taylor DC. Central and peripheral thermal control of effectors in homeothermic temperature regulation. *Physiol Rev*. 1986;66:235.
26. Ivanov K, Konstantinov V, Danilova N, et al. Thermoreceptor localization in the deep and surface skin layers. *J Therm Biol*. 1982;7:75.
27. Brück K, Hinckel P. Thermal afferents to the hypothalamus and thermal adaptation. *J Therm Biol*. 1984;9:7.
28. Brück K, Zeisberger E. Adaptive changes in thermoregulation and their neurophysiological basis. *Pharmacol Ther*. 1987;35:163.
29. Hinckel P, Schröder-Rosenstock K. Central thermal adaptation of lower brain stem units in the guinea-pig. *Pflügers Arch*. 1982;395:344.
30. Wünnenberg W, Brück K. Studies on the ascending pathways from the thermosensitive region of the spinal cord. *Pflügers Arch*. 1970;321:233.
31. Simon E. Temperature regulation: the spinal cord as a site of extrahypothalamic thermoregulatory functions. *Rev Physiol Biochem Pharmacol*. 1974;71:1.
32. Simon E, Iriki M. Sensory transmission of spinal heat and cold sensitivity in ascending spinal neurons. *Pflügers Arch*. 1971;328:103.
33. Wünnenberg W, Hardy JD. Response of single units of the posterior hypothalamus to thermal stimulation. *J Appl Physiol*. 1972;33:547.
34. Hensel H. *Thermoreception and Temperature Regulation*. New York: Academic Press; 1981.
35. Brück K. Non-shivering thermogenesis and brown adipose tissue in relation to age, and their integration in the thermoregulatory system. In: Lindberg O, ed. *Brown Adipose Tissue*. New York: American Elsevier Publishing; 1970:117–154.
36. Nadel ER, Bullard RW, Stolwijk JA. Importance of skin temperature in the regulation of sweating. *J Appl Physiol*. 1971;31:80.
37. Wenger CB, Roberts MF, Nadel ER, et al. Thermoregulatory control of finger blood flow. *J Appl Physiol*. 1975;38:1078.
38. Hey EN. The relation between environmental temperature and oxygen consumption in the new-born baby. *J Physiol*. 1969;200:589.
39. Hey EN. Thermal neutrality. *Br Med Bull*. 1975;31:69.
40. Jansky L. Non-shivering thermogenesis and its thermoregulatory significance. *Biol Rev Camb Philos Soc*. 1973;48:85.
41. Sundin U, Cannon B. GDP-binding to the brown fat mitochondria of developing and cold-adapted rats. *Comp Biochem Physiol*. 1980;65B:463.
42. Mount LE. *The Climatic Physiology of the Pig*. London: Edward Arnold; 1968.
43. Brück K, Wünnenberg W, Zeisberger E. Comparison of cold-adaptive metabolic modifications in different species with special reference to the miniature pig. *Fed Proc*. 1968;28:1035.
44. Jenkinson DM, Noble RC, Thompson GE. Adipose tissue and heat production in the newborn ox (*Bos taurus*). *J Physiol*. 1968;195:639.
45. Brück K. Non-shivering thermogenesis and brown adipose tissue in relation to age, and their integration in the thermoregulatory system. In: Lindberg O, ed. *Brown Adipose Tissue*. New York: American Elsevier Publishing; 1970:117–154.
46. Dawkins MJR, Hull D. Brown adipose tissue and the response of newborn rabbit to cold. *J Physiol*. 1964;172:216.
47. Smith RE, Horwitz BA. Brown fat and thermogenesis. *Physiol Rev*. 1969;49:330.
48. Hu HH, Yin L, Aggabao PC, et al. Comparison of brown and white adipose tissues in infants and children with chemical-shift-encoded water-fat MRI. *J Magn Reson Imaging*. 2013;38:885–896.
49. Hu HH, Wu TW, Yin L, et al. MRI detection of brown adipose tissue with low fat content in newborns with hypothermia. *Magn Reson Imaging*. 2014;32:107–117.
50. Lidell ME, Betz MJ, Dahlqvist Leinhard O, et al. Evidence for two types of brown adipose tissue in humans. *Nat Med*. 2013;19:631–634.

43 Structure and Development of the Skin and Cutaneous Appendages

David H. Chu | Cynthia A. Loomis

INTRODUCTION

Skin is a complex organ that comprises many different cells and cell types; it forms a critical physical barrier that protects the body and maintains fluid homeostasis, temperature regulation, and sensation. Skin cells derive from both embryonic mesoderm and ectoderm, and development from these precursors is tightly regulated. Perturbations in the developmental process, either from genetic anomalies or as a result of exogenous (e.g., teratogenic) agents, can result in severe abnormalities that have important consequences in the care of infants. Understanding the normal progression of molecular and cellular events that underlie the development and differentiation of skin allows for a more rational approach to infants who have defects in these processes. For clinicians, this knowledge will direct the diagnosis, therapy, and parental counseling necessary for care of the patients.

As with all organs, organogenesis of the skin proceeds through three distinct but overlapping stages, from early embryonic through fetal and neonatal development.[1,2] These stages are (1) *specification,* in which portions of superficial ectoderm and lateral plate mesoderm become distinct from other portions of the body wall; (2) *morphogenesis,* in which the specific structural and biochemical characteristics of skin begin to appear; and (3) *differentiation,* in which the skin tissue further develops to its mature form and postnatal stem cell niches are established.[3-5]

For the sake of clarity, we have organized the discussion of the developmental progression of the skin to follow each component sequentially, first with a discussion of the epidermis, followed by the dermis and subcutaneous tissue, the dermal-epidermal junction (DEJ), and finally, epidermal appendages. Each of these sections discusses the structural and biochemical changes that occur during the particular stage of development, followed by a discussion of related clinical syndromes and genetic disorders that are related to defects in this developmental progression.[6] However, all these tissues of the skin are, in fact, developing in parallel, and in some cases they require interaction with adjacent tissues for development. A timeline is included to illustrate the sequence of events that are occurring simultaneously (Fig. 43.1).

EPIDERMIS

OVERVIEW

The mature adult *epidermis* is a stratified squamous epithelium that develops from the ectoderm. Keratinocytes form 80% of the cellular composition. The germinative keratinocytes reside in the deepest portion of the epidermis, known as the *basal layer,* and these cells are known as *basal cells.* As differentiation of the basal cells proceeds, these cells migrate to more superficial cell layers and become progressively flattened; they also begin to express large insoluble proteins that ultimately become crosslinked along the exterior of the cell to form an insoluble shell or brick, known as the *cornified cell envelope.* The human epidermis self-renews every 40 to 56 days, and the constant turnover is credited to the interfollicular epidermal stem cells that reside in the basal layer.[3] These cells are also critical for generating sufficient progeny to re-epithelialize the surface of a wound. It remains controversial as to whether most basal cells or only a select subpopulation of basal cells have stem cell self-renewal capabilities.

Above the basal cell layer rests the spinous layer, or stratum spinosum. The "spines" seen in this layer result from the abundance of desmosomes, specialized regions of the keratinocyte cell surface that promote adhesion between these cells in a calcium-dependent manner. Desmosomal proteins include plakoglobin, desmoplakins I and II, keratocalmin, desmoyokin, band 6 protein, and the cadherins—desmogleins 1 and 3 and desmocollins 1 and 2.[7,8]

The cell layer superficial to the stratum spinosum is the stratum granulosum.[9,10] Granular cells begin to express some of the components that will contribute to the cornified cell envelope, a protein-lipid polymer that is found on the outer boundary of terminally differentiated keratinocytes. The cornified cell envelope serves a critical role in the barrier function of the epidermis. Keratohyalin granules, found within the granular cells, are principally composed of two proteins, loricrin and profilaggrin. Profilaggrin undergoes sequential proteolytic cleavage into filaggrin oligomers and finally monomers, as well as dephosphorylation, during its processing. This process is initiated at the time of formation of the granular layer and continues even after its eventual extrusion from the cornified cell. Loricrin, another major component of the cornified envelope, is also initially localized to the keratohyalin granules. Lamellar granules, which are also abundant in the granular cell layer, contain the lipid components that will be extruded from the cells and crosslinked to the cornified cell envelope. Other proteins that contribute to the cornified envelope include involucrin, small proline-rich proteins, annexin, elafin, desmoplakin, envoplakin, periplakin, repetin, and trichohyalin. Modifying enzymes such as transglutaminases are important in the final crosslinking of the cornified envelope components. Mutations in either the structural proteins or the enzymes involved in protein crosslinking and lipid and steroid metabolism can have clinically significant outcomes in genetic skin disease.[11]

The stratum corneum contains the terminally differentiated keratinocytes, flattened dead "squames" that lack nuclei and other organelles.[10] These cells are composed primarily of keratin filaments, tightly packed within the crosslinked cornified envelopes. Some specialized components within the epidermis maintain its architecture. Keratins are some of the

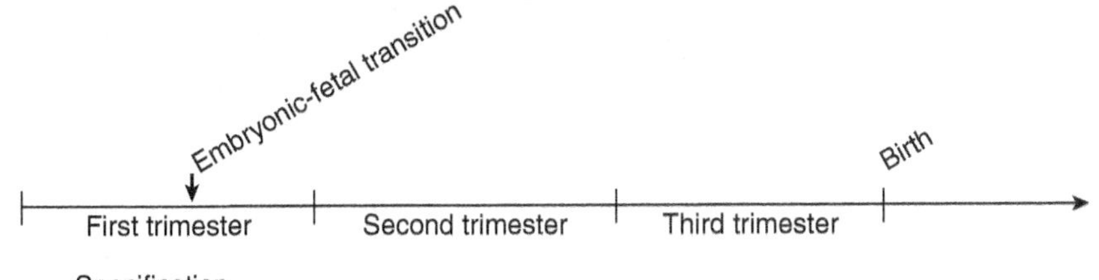

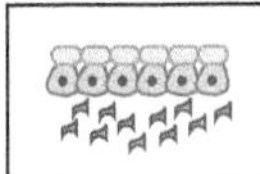

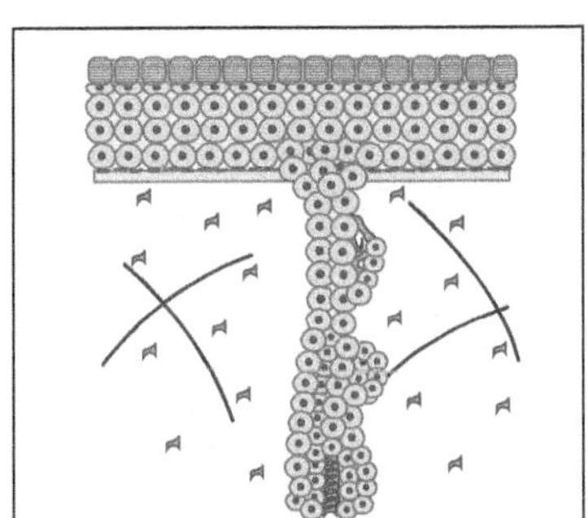

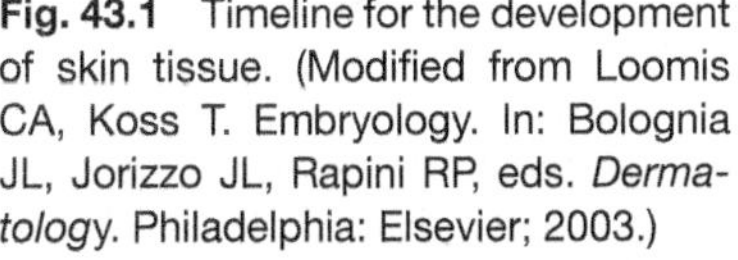

Fig. 43.1 Timeline for the development of skin tissue. (Modified from Loomis CA, Koss T. Embryology. In: Bolognia JL, Jorizzo JL, Rapini RP, eds. *Dermatology*. Philadelphia: Elsevier; 2003.)

most important structural proteins within the epidermal cells. They assemble as filaments composed of "basic" and "acidic" keratin peptides, which form *obligate heterodimers*—that is, different keratins are found to associate with a limited number of partners.[12,13] Their expression is regulated in a tissue-specific and developmentally selective manner. Mutations in these genes often exhibit clinical phenotypes that reflect the tissue expression of the specific keratin gene. For example, whereas basal cells express K5 and K14, suprabasilar keratinocytes express K1 and K10 (K1 and K9 in palmoplantar epidermis).

Other critical structural elements of the epidermis are the cell-cell and cell-matrix adhesion systems.[7,8] The major cell-cell adhesion junctions of the epidermis are desmosomes. The proteins in these complexes include specialized adhesion proteins (cadherins, calcium-dependent adhesion molecules), as well as intracellular plaque and adaptor proteins. An analogous adhesion structure, the hemidesmosome, attaches basal cells to the basement membrane at the DEJ. Although the proteins in the hemidesmosome are distinct from those of the desmosome, the plaque proteins have similar amino acid sequences, and both are tightly associated with the keratin filament network. Gap junctions form important intercellular bridges that allow small molecules to pass from one keratinocyte to another. These specialized junctions are formed by proteins known as *connexins*. Mutations in any of these molecules have effects on the normal formation of the epidermis that can result in certain genodermatoses, many of which have manifestations from birth.

SPECIFICATION

Gastrulation of the embryo occurs during the third week after fertilization. This is a critical process that results in the generation of the three primary embryonic germ layers: endoderm, mesoderm, and ectoderm. The ectoderm then is further divided into the neuroectoderm and the presumptive epidermis. The epidermis is then subsequently specified into distinct regional domains, such as palmoplantar skin, scalp skin, and mammary skin.

The earliest presumptive epidermis consists of a basal cell layer, which covers the embryo.[14,15] By 6 weeks estimated gestational age (EGA), the surface ectoderm consists of two layers: basal cells and more superficial periderm cells. The periderm layer does not give rise to any portion of the definitive epidermis, and as such it serves as a transient embryonic covering that protects the underlying basal cells and prevents interepidermal adhesions.[16,17] This layer is ultimately sloughed during late gestation and contributes to the vernix caseosa, which covers the newborn.

MORPHOGENESIS

The process of *morphogenesis* begins at approximately 8 weeks EGA, the classic transition between embryonic and fetal development, when hemopoietic production shifts to the bone marrow. At this point, the epidermis begins its process of stratification, by forming an intermediate layer between the basal cell and the periderm layers. This intermediate layer remains highly proliferative, and more layers are added as development proceeds over the next several weeks. In mice, it has been shown that this process of epidermal stratification requires the *TP63* genes.[18] In humans, partial loss of function mutations in *TP63* have been seen in various ectodermal dysplasias.

DIFFERENTIATION

Maturation of the epidermal layers includes keratinization, which results in the *differentiation* of granular and stratum corneal layers and the formation of a water-impermeable barrier. Accompanying this stage of development is the sloughing of the periderm. Keratinization occurs first in the skin appendages between 11 and 15 weeks EGA, followed by the interfollicular epidermis between 22 and 24 weeks EGA.[13,14,19]

The process of keratinization involves the production of certain proteins, including filaggrin and loricrin.[10,20] Posttranslational modification of the crosslinked proteins and production of specialized lipid and steroid components contribute to the water-impermeable matrix formed in the mature cornified layer. Structurally, the third-trimester stratum corneum is similar to that of an adult, but functional studies have shown that it is much less effective at preventing water loss and is more permeable than the mature epidermis. It is actually not until the third week of life that the barrier function of a newborn's stratum corneum is comparable to that of an adult.

CLINICAL RELEVANCE

Human mutations that inhibit the process of specification in the epidermis have not been reported, most likely because such mutations would be incompatible with further development of the embryo. However, experiments in animals have suggested that a group of proteins—the bone morphogenetic proteins (BMPs), as well as the Engrailed-1 *(En1)*, Lmx1b, and Wn7a—may play an important early role in specifying distinct skin domains on the distal limb.[21] Similarly, only a few mutations in humans have been found that affect epidermal morphogenesis. RIPK4 and IRF6, the genes defective in Bartsocas-Papas syndrome and popliteal pterygium syndrome, have been shown to be critical for early periderm formation and function, preventing inappropriate interepithelial fusions.[17] Subsequent stratification of the definitive epidermis depends on a functional *TP63* gene.[18,22]

In contrast to the relative lack of mutations that affect epidermal specification and morphogenesis, mutations that have an important impact on epidermal differentiation are quite numerous.[23] In general, these genes are not required for development in utero, but they become critical for effective barrier function of the epidermis after birth. Thus defects in these genes can often cause significant postnatal morbidity.

Two groups of such diseases include the palmoplantar keratodermas and ichthyoses. The *palmoplantar keratodermas* are a diverse group of disorders that share a common presentation of hyperkeratosis of the palms and soles. These disorders are also commonly associated with other cutaneous, as well as noncutaneous, findings. The genetic bases of many of these disorders have been discovered, and they include defects in connexins, differentiation keratins, and desmosomal components.

Table 43.1 Summary of Ichthyoses.

Disease	Inheritance	Defective Protein(s)
Ichthyosis vulgaris	AD	Filaggrin
X-linked ichthyosis	XLR	Steroid sulfatase
Lamellar ichthyosis	AR	Transglutaminase 1
NBCIE	AR	Transglutaminase 1; ALOX12B; ALOXE3; CGI58
Bullous congenital ichthyosiform erythroderma	AD	Keratin 1; keratin 10
Harlequin fetus	AR	ABCA12
Sjögren-Larsson syndrome	AR	Fatty aldehyde dehydrogenase
Refsum syndrome	AR	Phytanoyl-CoA hydroxylase
Conradi-Hünermann syndrome	XLD	Emopamil binding protein
CHILD syndrome	XLD	NSDHL (NAD(P) H steroid dehydrogenase-like protein)
Netherton syndrome	AR	LEKTI (lymphoepithelial Kazal-type–related inhibitor)
Erythrokeratodermia variabilis	AD	Connexin 31, connexin 30.3
KID syndrome	AD	Connexin 26

AD, Autosomal dominant; *AR*, autosomal recessive; *CHILD*, congenital hemidysplasia with ichthyosiform erythroderma and limb defects; *KID*, keratitis-ichthyosis-deafness; *NBCIE*, nonbullous congenital ichthyosiform erythroderma; *XLD*, X-linked dominant; *XLR*, X-linked recessive.

The *ichthyoses* are another diverse group of diseases that often present around the time of birth with diffuse scaly skin and defective epidermal barrier function.[24] These conditions differ in both pattern and morphology of scaling, as well as extracutaneous features. Ichthyosis vulgaris, lamellar ichthyosis, and X-linked ichthyosis have phenotypes predominantly restricted to the skin (Table 43.1). Ichthyoses can also be a cause of erythroderma (e.g., in bullous and nonbullous congenital ichthyosiform erythroderma). Neurologic abnormalities can be associated with the skin condition, as in Sjögren-Larsson syndrome, Refsum syndrome, or Tay syndrome (IBIDS: ichthyosis, brittle hair, intellectual deficit, decreased fertility, and short stature). In X-linked dominant ichthyoses, female children inheriting the relevant mutation can develop asymmetry of limbs, as in congenital hemidysplasia with ichthyosiform erythroderma and limb defects (CHILD) syndrome or chondrodysplasia punctata (Conradi-Hünermann disease). Interestingly, mutations in several genes required for barrier formation and normal epidermal desquamation also confer susceptibility to development of atopic dermatitis-like inflammatory skin diseases, including the genes encoding the cornified envelope protein filaggrin, the serine protease inhibitor SPNK1 (LEKT1), and the adhesion molecule desmoglein 1 (DSG1).[20,25]

One of the earliest phenotypic presentations of a group of these disorders is known as *collodion baby*, in which an infant is born encased in a parchment-like membrane. Over the next few days to weeks, the membrane is shed, eventuating in lamellar ichthyosis, nonbullous congenital ichthyosiform erythroderma, Netherton syndrome, Tay syndrome (IBIDS), Conradi-Hünermann disease, and occasionally, a normal baby.

In contrast to the relatively benign outcome for collodion babies, the so-called *harlequin fetus* usually dies soon after birth. These babies are born encased in restrictive plates of thick, armor-like scale that have extremely poor barrier function, often resulting in fluid derangements, infections, sepsis, and death. Mutations in the gene *ABCA12*, which encodes an adenosine-5′-triphosphate (ATP) binding cassette transporter, have recently been discovered to be responsible for this condition.[24] Milder mutations with protein function cause a less severe congenital ichthyosis (lamellar ichthyosis or congenital ichthyosiform erythroderma).

NONKERATINOCYTES IN THE EPIDERMIS

MELANOCYTES

Although keratinocytes are the most abundant cell type that makes up the epidermis, other cell types migrate there early in development. Among these are the neural crest-derived melanocytes, which synthesize and distribute pigment to the epidermis.[26,27] Melanocyte precursors exit the dorsal region of the neural tube, migrate through the superficial mesenchyme, and ultimately come to reside in the epidermis by 7 weeks EGA. Melanocyte stem cells reside in the lower bulge and subbulge region of the hair follicle; they are positive for the markers Pax3 and TYRP2 but are negative for KIT, tyrosine, and TYRP1.[28]

LANGERHANS CELLS

Langerhans cells are another migratory cell population that enters the epidermis before the embryonic-fetal transition and in the adult facilitate the adaptive immune response to pathogens invading the skin. Lineage labeling studies in mice indicate Langerhans cells are derived from two embryonic sources: yolk sac precursors and early fetal hematopoietic stem cells.[29,30] Langerhans cells remain relatively undifferentiated until the embryonic–fetal transition, at which time they begin to express CD1 on their cell surface and begin to produce their characteristic Birbeck granules, tennis racket–shaped intracellular vesicles that form during the processing of membrane-bound antigens. The density of Langerhans cells remains low until the third trimester, when they undergo robust proliferation. Postnatally, Langerhans cells self-renew and differentiate within their resident epidermal niche, with contribution from bone marrow–derived cells only in response to intense inflammatory events.[29]

MERKEL CELLS

The third type of specialized cell within the epidermis is the Merkel cell, a highly innervated neuroendocrine cell type involved in mechanoreception. These cells are first detectable around 8 to 12 weeks in volar skin and slightly later in interfollicular skin. They are often associated with skin appendages. Merkel cells express both neural-specific markers and epithelial-specific proteins, such as keratins. Recent lineage tracing experiments in mice have demonstrated that Merkel cells are derived from a pluripotent epidermal cell progenitor and not neural crest cells.[31]

CLINICAL RELEVANCE

Many mutations have been identified that are critical for melanoblast migration and survival and for melanocyte differentiation and function (summarized in Table 43.2).[26,27,32-34] Defects in these genes result in disorders of pigmentation, which can be detected at an early age.

One of the most common abnormalities is that of albinism. There are variations in severity of depigmentation and associated abnormalities. These differences depend on the particular gene affected and its global function.

Defects in melanin synthesis result in oculocutaneous albinism (OCA), a set of disorders characterized by absent pigment in the skin, hair, and eyes at birth. Often associated with the skin findings are neurologic and ophthalmologic findings of nystagmus, photophobia, and visual disturbances, reflecting the neuroectodermal derivation of melanocytes. In OCA type 1, mutations in the enzyme tyrosinase, critical for the conversion of tyrosine to melanin (either null or partial loss of function alleles), are responsible. In OCA type 2, tyrosinase functions normally (tyrosinase-positive albinism), but the *P* gene, a putative tyrosine transporter, is defective. This subtype can be distinguished from OCA type 1 because a child's skin and eyes begin to darken with age. The children usually have white, yellow, or red hair. OCA type 3 results from defects in tyrosinase-related protein-1. This condition is also known as *brown OCA,* featuring minimal to light brown skin pigmentation in some persons of African descent.

Other genes result in a patchier distribution of pigmentation defects, as in the white forelock (poliosis) seen in both piebaldism and Waardenburg syndrome. These diseases occur as a result of defective melanocyte specification, migration, or survival. The gene responsible for piebaldism is *c-KIT*, a growth factor receptor and protooncogene. Waardenburg syndrome subtypes can be caused by defects in transcription factors Pax3, Sox10, MITF and in endothelin receptor B and endothelin 3 ligand. In Waardenburg syndrome, depending on the subtype, neural tube defects, heterochromia iridis, deafness, and Hirschsprung disease may be associated with depigmentation.

Finally, defects in melanosome production result in the entities Hermansky-Pudlak, Chédiak-Higashi, and Griscelli syndromes.

Table 43.2 Disorders of Pigmentation.

Disorder	Mutant Gene	Defective Protein/Function
Melanocyte Specification, Migration, or Survival		
Piebaldism	*c-KIT*	Growth factor receptor, protooncogene
Waardenburg Syndrome		
Types 1 and 3	*HuP2*	Pax3 transcription factor
Type 2	*MITF*	Transcription factor
Type 4	*EDNRB*	Endothelin receptor B
	EDN3	Endothelin 3
	Sox 10	Sox-10 transcription factor
Melanin Biosynthesis		
Oculocutaneous Albinism		
Type 1	Tyrosinase, null alleles	Rate-limiting enzyme of pigment production
Type 1b	Tyrosinase, partially functional alleles	Rate-limiting enzyme of pigment production
Type 2	P gene	Putative tyrosine transporter
Type 3	*TRP-1*	Tyrosinase-related protein-1
Melanosome Production		
Hermansky-Pudlak syndrome	*HPS1*	Putative membrane component of various organelles
	AP3	Putative component of endocytic protein trafficking pathway
Chédiak-Higashi syndrome	*LYST*	Putative involvement in protein trafficking
Griscelli syndrome	*RAB27A*	Guanosine triphosphate-binding protein involved in membrane fusion and protein trafficking

Patients with Hermansky-Pudlak syndrome have mutations in the *HPS1* gene, which is a putative transmembrane component of a number of cytoplasmic organelles, or the *AP3* gene, which is a protein subunit involved in the sorting of proteins in the exocytic-endocytic pathway. Patients present with creamy, light skin tones, dysfunctional platelets (prolonged bleeding time), pulmonary fibrosis, granulomatous colitis, and ceroid lipofuscinosis in phagocytic cells. Chédiak-Higashi syndrome is characterized by nystagmus, decreased visual acuity, skin and respiratory infections, light skin tones, and silvery yellow to brown hair. Giant melanosomes are found in white blood cell smears and hair, and giant lysosomal inclusion granules are found in all leukocytes. The defect is in LYST, a protein proposed to be important in intercellular protein trafficking. Griscelli syndrome also features hair shafts with large pigment granules and hypopigmentation with silver-gray hair. Patients have hemophagocytic syndrome and experience episodes of massive lymphocyte and leukocyte activation and organ infiltration. Polymorphonuclear leukocytes are morphologically normal, unlike in Chédiak-Higashi syndrome. The defect is in a guanosine triphosphate-binding protein involved in vesicular fusion and trafficking, *RAB27A*.

Langerhans cell function is critical for skin pathogen surveillance and subsequent antigen presentation to T cells in the draining lymph nodes. Langerhans cell dysfunction is implicated in the development of atopic dermatitis and other skin inflammatory disorders, such as psoriasis.[35] Recently, BRAF mutations in Langerhans cells has been identified in congenital, benign Langerhans cell histiocytosis.[36]

DERMIS AND SUBCUTIS

OVERVIEW

Unlike the epidermis, which is derived exclusively from ectoderm, the *dermis* originates from different tissues depending on the specific body site.[5] Dermal mesenchyme of the face and anterior scalp comes from neural crest ectoderm, whereas that of the back is derived from the dermomyotome of the embryonic somite. Dermal mesenchyme of the limbs and ventral trunk, conversely, is likely derived from the lateral plate mesoderm.

Early fetal mesenchyme is highly cellular, containing few fibrillar elements. These fetal mesenchymal cells are thought to be pluripotent, able to give rise to adipose tissue, cartilage, and dermal fibroblasts. The superficial mesenchyme becomes visibly distinct from underlying skeletal elements by 60 days EGA. By 12 to 15 weeks, the different characteristics of the dermis can first be observed—the papillary dermis has a finer weave than the thicker reticular dermis. Collagen and elastic fibers begin to be assembled in the latter half of pregnancy, and a more rigid, fibrillar meshwork gradually forms.

Dermal repair shifts from nonscarring to scarring by the end of the second trimester. At birth, the dermis is thick and well organized but is still more cellular than in adults.

A distinct region identifiable as the subcutis can be seen by 50 to 60 days EGA. It is separated from the dermis by a plane of thin-walled vessels. By the end of the first trimester, the distinction between the fibrous dermis and the sparse matrix of the subcutis can be seen. Preadipocytes arising from a variety of undifferentiated mesenchymal lineages at different anatomic sites[37] begin to mature and accumulate lipids by the second trimester. By the third trimester, the more differentiated adipocytes begin to aggregate into lobules separated by fibrous septa. Although the initial events leading to the commitment of mesenchymal cells to become white or brown adipocytes are not well understood, numerous regulators of later preadipocyte-adipocyte differentiation have been identified, including the hormone leptin.[38]

BLOOD VESSELS, LYMPHATICS, AND NERVES

Blood vessels and lymphatics begin to develop early in gestation but do not evolve into those of adults until a few months after birth.[39] Initially, these vessels form horizontal plexuses within the subpapillary and deep reticular dermis, which are interconnected by groups of vertical vessels. This vascular framework has been shown to be in place by 45 to 50 days EGA. By the fifth month of EGA, arterioles and venules are able to be distinguished. Capillary loops, which supply the developing epidermal appendages and maintain thermoregulation, are established at the time of rete ridge formation at the DEJ. During the period of embryonic and fetal development, this framework changes constantly, depending on many factors, including site of the body and presence of associated adnexal structures.

Accumulating evidence suggests that lymphatics originate from endothelial cells that bud from veins, and the pattern of embryonic lymphatic vessel development parallels that of blood vessels.[40] Studies using newly discovered molecular markers specific for lymphatics have allowed a more detailed understanding of lymphangiogenesis. Defects in some of the genes encoding some of these proteins have been found to result in congenital disorders of the lymphatic system.[41]

Nerves, like blood vessels and lymphatics, are also present in early embryonic skin and continue to develop after birth. Nerves begin as large trunks at the dermal-subcutaneous boundary that branch into fibers and extend into the dermis. They form networks distinct from the cutaneous vasculature, although they become more closely juxtaposed in the fetal dermis. At 70 days EGA, an arrangement of nerves that is similar to the adult configuration can be detected, although the density and final distribution of fibers continue to be modified until after birth. Sensory receptors such as the pacinian and meissnerian corpuscles begin to develop in the fourth month of EGA. Although meissnerian corpuscles are fully developed only after birth, pacinian corpuscles are completed and are found in plantar and palmar skin in neonates.

CLINICAL RELEVANCE

Few human mutations have been identified that result in generalized defective dermal specification, most likely because such mutations would be incompatible with life. However, experiments in animal model systems have suggested that the genes *Lmx1b*, *Wnt7a*, and *En1* are important in specifying dorsal and ventral (palmoplantar) mesenchyme as distinct tissues.

Restrictive dermopathy is a clinical entity in which the dermis is universally abnormal, now found to be caused by mutations in *LMNA* and *ZMPSTE24*.[33] Several mosaic conditions also show localized defects in dermal development, most notably focal dermal hypoplasia (Goltz syndrome), as well as Proteus syndrome.[42–44] Goltz syndrome is X linked, and dermal hypoplasia occurs in Blaschkoid patterns in affected females. It is caused by mutations in PORCN, an effector of the Wnt signaling pathway that is critical for normal dermal development. Proteus syndrome results from somatic activating mutations in AKT1, which promotes local tissue overgrowth. The disorder is characterized by subcutaneous masses, lipomas, capillary malformations, plantar and palmar hyperplasia, varicose veins, and asymmetric soft tissue and bony hypertrophy of the hands, feet, and limbs.

Connective tissue disorders are caused by mutations in genes encoding differentiation products of mature dermal fibroblasts and other mesenchymal cells.[45] Ehlers-Danlos syndrome has many clinical subtypes, caused by a variety of mutations in genes affecting collagen types I, III, and V, collagen-modifying enzymes, and other important structural proteins (Table 43.3).[36,37] Mutations in the genes encoding elastin and the latent transforming growth factor-β (TGF-β) binding protein-4 gene (*LTBP4*), which is an extracellular matrix protein that controls the bioavailability of TGF-β, leads to defective elastic fiber assembly in cutis laxa. Cutis laxa is characterized by loose,

Table 43.3 Ehlers-Danlos Syndrome Classification.

Type	Clinical Findings	Inheritance	Gene Defect(s)
Classic (I/II)	Skin and joint hypermobility, atrophic scars, easy bruising	AD	*COL5A1, COL5A2*
Hypermobility (III)	Joint hypermobility, pain, dislocations	AD	*COL3A1*
Vascular (IV)	Thin skin, arterial or uterine rupture, easy bruising, small joint hyperextensibility	AD	*COL3A1*
Kyphoscoliosis (VI)	Scoliosis, joint laxity, ocular fragility and retinal detachment, skin laxity, muscle hypotonia	AR	Lysyl hydroxylase
Arthrochalasia (VIIA, VIIB)	Joint hypermobility, mild skin laxity, bruising, scoliosis	AD	*COL1A1, COL1A2*
Dermatosparaxis (VIIC)	Severe skin fragility, cutis laxa, bruising	AR	*ADAMTS2* (procollagen N-peptidase)
Other			
X-linked EDS (V)	Skin laxity, bruising	XL	Lysyl oxidase
Periodontitis (VIII)	Periodontitis, blue sclerae, atrophic scarring, bruisability	AD	?
Fibronectin-deficient (X)	Striae distensae, joint laxity, skin laxity, scarring, bruisability, bleeding (platelet) disorder (petechiae)	?	?
Familial hypermobility (XI)	Recurrent joint dislocation, joint laxity	AD	?
Progeroid	Progeroid facies, short stature, osteopenia, skin laxity, atrophic scarring, hypermobile joints	?	*XGPT-1*

AD, Autosomal dominant; *AR*, autosomal recessive; *EDS*, Ehlers-Danlos syndrome; *XL*, X linked.

redundant skin, a syndrome that can be complicated by lung hypoplasia, diaphragmatic hernias, gastrointestinal diverticula, bladder diverticula, and emphysema.[38] Osteogenesis imperfecta is characterized by multiple fractures in utero, beaded ribs, crumpled humeri and femora, limb avulsion during delivery, kyphoscoliosis, blue sclerae, and easily bruisable skin. Although frequently caused by defects in collagen type I components, osteogenesis imperfecta is genetically heterogeneous and can result from alterations in a variety of proteins that impact on collagen structure and physiology. Marfan syndrome results from mutations in fibrillin, which codes for a vital component of the microfibrillar elastic tissue network, resulting in defects in ocular, cardiovascular, and musculoskeletal systems.[40]

Defects in angiogenesis lead to a diverse and complex set of vascular malformations, and many of the underlying genetic causes have been identified.[46] Hereditary hemorrhagic telangiectasia (Osler-Weber-Rendu syndrome) is a vascular dysplasia that leads to telangiectasis and arteriovenous malformations of skin, mucosa, and viscera. Mucosal involvement often results in epistaxis and gastrointestinal bleeding. Visceral involvement includes that of the lung, liver, and brain. Mutations in endoglin, as well as activin receptor-like kinase 1, have been shown to cause this disease. TIE2 is a tyrosine kinase, mutations in which have been shown to result in a dominantly inherited syndrome of venous malformations.

Work on lymphangiogenesis has uncovered genetic mutations in some forms of hereditary lymphatic anomalies and lymphedema.[41] The most common form of primary hereditary lymphedema, Milroy disease, is caused by mutations in vascular endothelial growth factor receptor 3. This disease is characterized by severe edema, especially below the waist.[45] Mutations in MFH1 (FOXC2), a transcription factor, have been implicated in lymphedema-distichiasis syndrome, featuring late-onset lymphedema and a double row of eyelashes (distichiasis).

DERMAL-EPIDERMAL JUNCTION

The DEJ is a key interface for inductive interactions during early skin organogenesis. Defects in this region are also responsible for many well-studied congenital blistering diseases, the group of diseases known as *epidermolysis bullosa (EB)*.[47,48] This zone includes the adhesive structural elements along the basal surface of the basal keratinocyte plasma membrane, as well as the extracellular matrix proteins of the basal lamina and the most superficial fibrillar structures of the papillary dermis.

The most primitive form of the DEJ can be seen between the epidermis and the dermis by 8 weeks EGA. Laminin, collagen type IV, heparan sulfate, and proteoglycans, components common to all basal lamina, can be found at this stage. The more specific molecules that make up the basal lamina of stratified epithelia, such as hemidesmosomal components, begin to be detected at the time when the presumptive epidermis begins to stratify. It is at this time that such proteins as integrins ($\alpha6$ and $\beta4$) become properly localized to the DEJ, even though the expression of some can be detected at earlier times.

CLINICAL RELEVANCE

As alluded to earlier, several congenital disorders characterized by severe blistering occur as a result of mutations in the genes encoding the components of this region (Table 43.4).[47,48] The severity of the disorder, the plane of tissue separation, and the involvement of noncutaneous tissues depend on the specific proteins affected by the mutations. These diseases carry with them a high degree of morbidity and mortality, and as such they are frequent candidates for prenatal testing.

The most superficial of these phenotypes is EB simplex.[49] Keratins 5 and 14, the proteins defective in this disease subtype, are expressed by basal keratinocytes. Because of loss of adhesion at the level of the basal keratinocyte, the epidermis is fragile, and bullae develop. Depending on the particular mutation, the blistering phenotype can be more or less severe. These blisters can involve the mucous membranes and can result in a hoarse voice. One specific subtype of EB simplex is associated with muscular dystrophy. The mutation for this disease is within a protein called *plectin*, involved in adhesion within the hemidesmosome.

Junctional EB variants form bullae within the lamina lucida, the superficial portion of the DEJ. Affected patients have been found to have defects in laminin 5. One form of junctional EB, the Herlitz variant, is more severe: in addition to blistering, laryngeal and respiratory edema can be associated with the disorder, as well as anemia and hypoproteinemia. The non-Herlitz variant is less life-threatening, although, in this case, bullae heal with atrophic scarring. Nails and hair can also be affected. Another subtype is associated with pyloric atresia, which is caused by mutations in the $\alpha6$ and $\beta4$ integrins.

Table 43.4 Disorders of the Dermal-Epidermal Junction.

Location	Disorder	Defective Protein(s)
Basal cell adhesion complex	Epidermolysis bullosa (EB) simplex	K5, K14
	EB with muscular dystrophy	Plectin
Basal lamina	Generalized atrophic benign EB	BPAG2 (collagen type XVII)
	EB with pyloric atresia	β4 subunit of α6 and β4 integrins
	Junctional EB, lethal and less severe forms	Laminin 5 subunits
Superficial dermis	Dystrophic EB (dominant and recessive)	Collagen type VII

The most disfiguring form of EB is termed *dystrophic EB*. Because the blisters in this variant affect the superficial dermis, with defects in collagen type VII, they heal with scarring. In the more severe forms, extensive scarring can lead to digital fusions and so-called mitten deformities of the hands and feet, flexion contractures, mucous membrane scarring, dental abnormalities, and hematologic disorders.

SKIN APPENDAGES

Skin appendages include hair, nails, and sweat and mammary glands. These structures are derived from both an epidermal component and a dermal component. The epidermis contributes the physical structure of the unit, whereas the dermis provides signals for the unit's differentiation. During embryogenesis, interactions between the dermis and the epidermis are critical for normal development of these structures, disruption of which often results in defects in the formation of skin appendages.

HAIR

Between 75 and 80 days EGA, dermal signals instruct the basal cells of the scalp epidermis to cluster together at regularly spaced intervals.[2] This initial group is known as the *follicular placode* or *anlage*.[50-52] Although the specific mediators of this first "dermal signal" are not definitively identified, β-catenin has been implicated as a candidate gene based on its molecular localization.

From the scalp, the follicular placodes develop ventrally and caudally and eventually cover the skin. The epidermal placodes then signal back to the underlying dermis to form a dermal condensate, which occurs at 12 to 14 weeks EGA. The communication between the epidermis and dermis at this stage and the morphogenetic development are considered to be a balance between placode promoters and placode inhibitors.[48] Wnt family signaling molecules are proposed to mediate placode promoting effects via the molecules LEF and β-catenin, as well as fibroblast growth factor, TGF-β2, Msx1 and 2, and ectodysplasin A (EDA) and EDA receptor (EDAR). BMP family molecules, conversely, act as inhibitors of follicle formation. In model systems, ectopic expression of this family of molecules tends to suppress the formation of follicles. In mice, EDAR and β-catenin expression are required for expression of BMP4 and sonic hedgehog (Shh), a finding implicating these molecules in early follicular morphogenesis. Furthermore, EDAR may be important for lateral inhibition of cells surrounding the follicles.

The dermal papilla forms as a result of epithelial cell instructions transmitted to the underlying mesenchyme. Molecular candidates for this signal include platelet-derived growth factor and Shh. The dermal cells, in turn, instruct the epidermal cells to proliferate and invade the dermis. The dermal cells differentiate into the dermal papilla; the involved epithelial cells become the inner root sheath and hair shaft of the mature follicle.

In addition to the widened bulge at the base of the mature hair follicle, two other bulges form along the length of the developing follicle. The uppermost bulge is the presumptive sebaceous gland, whereas the middle bulge serves as the site for insertion of the arrector pili muscle. Accumulating evidence also suggests that there are multiple sets of stem cells within the middle part of the hair follicle in the bulge, and the known markers are α 6 and β 1 integrins, keratin 15, CD200, PHLDA1, follistatin, frizzled homolog1, and LRG5, among others.[53,54] These important multipotent cells are able to differentiate into any of the cells of the hair follicle and to help reconstitute the entire epidermis after wound healing, which has been reported in cases of extensive surface wounds or burns.[50-53]

Although bulge cells from the hair follicle are capable of adopting all these different cell fates, recent work suggests that under normal homeostatic conditions, these cells restrict their contributions to the hair follicle.[51,54]

By 19 to 21 weeks EGA, the hair canal has completely formed, and fetal scalp hair becomes visible. These hairs continue to lengthen until 24 to 28 weeks, at which time they shift from the active growth (anagen) phase to the degenerative phase (catagen), then to the resting phase (telogen), thus completing the first hair cycle. With subsequent hair cycles, hairs increase in diameter and coarseness. During adolescence, vellus hairs of androgen-sensitive areas mature to terminal-type hair follicles. As in development, many of the postnatal changes are directed by signaling from the specialized mesenchymal cells in the hair dermal papilla.[55,56]

SEBACEOUS GLANDS

Sebaceous glands, as mentioned earlier, mature during the course of follicular differentiation, beginning at 13 to 16 weeks EGA.[57] At this time, the presumptive sebaceous gland is the most superficial bulge in the developing hair follicle. As the sebaceous gland develops further, the outer cells differentiate and proliferate, giving rise to cells that accumulate lipids and sebum. These differentiated cells ultimately disintegrate to release their contents into the upper portion of the hair canal, contributing to the vernix caseosa. The production of sebum is responsive to hormonal influences, including maternal steroids during the second and third trimesters and at adolescence, a finding suggesting a factor contributing to the increased incidence of acne at this age. Although stem cells residing within the glands are known to replenish the terminal differentiating sebocytes, their precise location and unique molecular marker status have not been defined.[4]

NAIL DEVELOPMENT

The earliest nail structures begin to appear on the dorsal digit tip at 8 to 10 weeks EGA, slightly earlier than the initiation of hair follicle development.[58,59] The first sign is the delineation of the flat surface of the future nail bed. The proximal nail fold is formed from a portion of ectoderm that buds inward at the proximal boundary of the early nail field. The presumptive nail matrix cells ultimately differentiate to become the nail plate; these cells are present on the ventral side of the proximal invagination. At 11 weeks EGA, the dorsal nail bed surface begins to keratinize. By the fourth month of gestation, the nail plate grows out from the proximal nail fold and completely covers the nail bed by the fifth month.

ECCRINE AND APOCRINE SWEAT GLAND DEVELOPMENT

Eccrine glands begin to develop on the volar surfaces of the hands and feet, beginning as mesenchymal pads at 55 to 65 days EGA.[2,60] By 12 to 14 weeks EGA, parallel ectodermal ridges overlay these mesenchymal pads. The eccrine glands arise from the ectodermal ridge. By 16 weeks EGA, the secretory portion of the gland becomes detectable. The dermal duct is complete by this time, but the epidermal portion of the duct is not canalized until 22 weeks EGA. Dermatoglyphics are formed by the curvilinear patterns of the epidermal ridges, and these become visible on the volar surfaces of the digits by 5 months EGA.

Interfollicular eccrine and apocrine glands, in contrast to volar glands, do not begin to bud until the fifth month of gestation. Apocrine sweat glands usually bud from the upper portion of the hair follicle. By 7 months EGA, the cells of the apocrine glands become distinguishable, composed of both clear cells and mucin-secreting dark cells. Apocrine glands become transiently functional during the third trimester, but eccrine glands are not functional until the postnatal period. Both glands continue to mature postnatally, with the apocrine glands increasing secretory activity in puberty in response to androgens. Overall, cellular turnover in the mature glands is low, but upon wounding, eccrine glands and likely apocrine glands contribute progeny to facilitate re-epithelialization.[60] Recent lineage tracing experiments in mouse-paw skin (the only sweat gland–containing skin in mice) have demonstrated two distinct unipotent stem cell populations in the mature gland: one that gives rise only to luminal cells and one that gives rise to basal myoepithelial cells.

CLINICAL RELEVANCE

As has been described in some of the genetic diseases affecting development of the skin, genes that affect cutaneous appendage formation can also have effects on noncutaneous tissues; findings suggest an early role for these factors or a more global role in development and differentiation.[52,61,62]

Certain genetic syndromes with prominent hair defects, often associated with other ectodermal appendageal abnormalities, have been identified. Menkes kinky hair syndrome is an X-linked recessive syndrome featuring pili torti (twisted hair) that is sparse and brittle with a "steel wool" quality. The skin is doughy, and patients have skeletal abnormalities and general failure to thrive. The defect for this disease is an ATP-dependent copper transporter, ATP7A. Argininosuccinic aciduria is an autosomal recessive disorder, resulting from defective argininosuccinate lyase; it may present neonatally with trichorrhexis nodosa and short, broken scalp hairs, neurologic deficits including lethargy and mental retardation, hepatomegaly, and failure to thrive. The mechanism responsible for the hair defects is not known.

Other defects occur in the structural proteins of hair, such as hair keratins.[63] Monilethrix is caused by defects in hair cortex keratins 1, 3, and 6 (HB1, HB3, and HB6), which result in beaded hair and brittle nails. Diseases such as pachyonychia congenita present primarily with cutaneous and ectodermal appendageal defects, including hyperkeratotic nails, palmoplantar keratoderma, follicular hyperkeratosis, and steatocystoma multiplex. These defects have been found to be mutations in typical "soft" keratin genes: *K6a*, *K6b*, *K16*, and *K17*. Trichothiodystrophy, or Tay syndrome, presents as short, brittle hair with alternating dark and light "tiger-tail" bands, as well as trichoschisis. Nails are dystrophic, skin is ichthyotic, and patients exhibit photosensitivity, short stature, intellectual impairment, and decreased fertility. Two genes have been identified that are involved in DNA repair and are identical to the genes mutated in the xeroderma pigmentosum complementation groups B and D. The reasons for the cutaneous manifestations of this disease are not clear, but the hair and nail phenotypes have been proposed to be a result of low cysteine content.

Mutations in critical developmental regulatory genes, such as those encoding DNA binding proteins and growth factors, have also been found in congenital syndromes affecting skin appendage formation.[60] Hypohidrotic ectodermal dysplasia—a defect in either EDA or EDAR—features sparse hair, nail dystrophy, as well as hypohidrosis or anhidrosis, which can lead to poor thermoregulation. In contrast, hidrotic ectodermal dysplasia, which presents with sparse hair, dystrophic nails, palmoplantar keratoderma, and tufting of terminal phalanges, is associated with defects in connexin 30. Mutations in p63 affect nail development in syndromes such as ankyloblepharon, ectodermal defects, and cleft lip and ectrodactyly-ectodermal dysplasia clefting.[18] Functional p63 is required for the formation and maintenance of the apical ectodermal ridge, an embryonic signaling center essential for limb outgrowth and hand plate formation. The secreted factor Wnt7a and the transcription factor Lmx1b are important for dorsal limb patterning, including nail formation. Nail-patella syndrome results from mutations in *LMX1B*. In contrast, the transcription factor En1 is required for ventral limb patterning and eccrine gland formation. Other regulatory molecules important in appendage development include the secreted factor Shh, which is required for hair follicle formation but not nail plate formation, and the transcription factor MSX1, which is required for tooth and nail formation. *Hoxc13* is an important homeodomain-containing gene for later stages of follicular and nail differentiation, at least in murine models.[62]

PRENATAL DIAGNOSIS

Identification of the genes involved in early cutaneous development and determination of associated mutations responsible for disease have allowed prenatal diagnosis of life-threatening or debilitating cutaneous disease.[62,64] Some techniques have been devised for such testing, such as chorionic villous sampling, which can be performed at 8 to 10 weeks EGA, or amniocentesis, which can be done at 16 to 18 weeks EGA. These diagnostic procedures can be performed earlier and are associated with less fetal morbidity and mortality than the only previously available technique—fetal skin biopsy—performed 19 to 22 weeks EGA. Candidates for prenatal testing include fetuses with an affected sibling or family member.

ACKNOWLEDGMENT

The editors wish to thank authors David H. Chu and Cynthia A. Loomis for their excellent contribution to this text in the fifth edition. This chapter has been reproduced here in the sixth edition essentially unchanged.

A complete reference list is available at www.ExpertConsult.com. 

SELECT REFERENCES

2. Holbrook KA. Structure and function of the developing human skin. In: Goldsmith L, ed. *Physiology, Biochemistry, and Molecular Biology of the Skin*. Oxford, UK: Oxford University Press; 1991:63-110.
3. Hsu YC, Li L, Fuchs E. Emerging interactions between skin stem cells and their niches. *Nat Med*. 2014;20:847-856.
4. Kretzschmar K, Watt FM. Markers of epidermal stem cell subpopulations in adult mammalian skin. *Cold Spring Harb Perspect Med*. 2014;4:a013631.
5. Driskell RR, Watt FM. Understanding fibroblast heterogeneity in the skin. *Trends Cell Biol*. 2015;25:92-99.
6. Online Mendelian Inheritance in Man (OMIM). *McKusick-Nathans Institute of Genetic Medicine*. Baltimore, MD: Johns Hopkins University School of Medicine; 2016. Available at: http://www.ncbi.nlm.nih.gov/omim.
7. Peltonen S, Raiko L, Peltonen J. Desmosomes in developing human epidermis. *Dermatol Res Pract*. 2010;2010:698761.
8. Sumigray KD, Lechler T. Cell adhesion in epidermal development and barrier formation. *Curr Top Dev Biol*. 2015;112:383-414.
9. Eckhart L, Lippens S, Tschachler E, et al. Cell death by cornification. *Biochim Biophys Acta*. 1833:3471-3480. 2013.
10. Matsui T, Amagai M. Dissecting the formation, structure and barrier function of the stratum corneum. *Int Immunol*. 2015;27:269-280.

11. Natsuga K. Epidermal barriers. *Cold Spring Harb Perspect Med*. 2014;4:a018218.
12. Homberg M, Magin TM. Beyond expectations: novel insights into epidermal keratin function and regulation. *Int Rev Cell Mol Biol*. 2014;311:265-306.
13. Pan X, Hobbs RP, Coulombe PA. The expanding significance of keratin intermediate filaments in normal and diseased epithelia. *Curr Opin Cell Biol*. 2013;25:47-56.
16. Richardson RJ, Hammond NL, Coulombe PA, et al. Periderm prevents pathological epithelial adhesions during embryogenesis. *J Clin Invest*. 2014;124:3891-3900.
18. Koster MI. p63 in skin development and ectodermal dysplasias. *J Invest Dermatol*. 2010;130:2352-2358.
20. Thyssen JP, Kezic S. Causes of epidermal filaggrin reduction and their role in the pathogenesis of atopic dermatitis. *J Allergy Clin Immunol*. 2014;134:792-799.
22. Botchkarev VA, Flores ER. p53/p63/p73 in the epidermis in health and disease. *Cold Spring Harb Perspect Med*. 2014;4:a015248.
23. Lopez-Pajares V, Yan K, Zarnegar BJ, et al. Genetic pathways in disorders of epidermal differentiation. *Trends Genet*. 2013;29:31-40.
24. Richard G, Choate K, Milstone L, et al. Management of ichthyosis and related conditions gene-based diagnosis and emerging gene-based therapy. *Dermatol Ther*. 2013;26:55-68.
25. Samuelov L, Sprecher E. Peeling off the genetics of atopic dermatitis-like congenital disorders. *J Allergy Clin Immunol*. 2014;134:808-815.
26. Mort RL, Jackson IJ, Patton EE. The melanocyte lineage in development and disease. *Development*. 2015;142:620-632.
27. Yamaguchi Y, Hearing VJ. Melanocytes and their diseases. *Cold Spring Harb Perspect Med*. 2014;4:a017046.
29. Collin M, Milne P. Langerhans cell origin and regulation. *Curr Opin Hematol*. 2016;23:28-35.
31. Woo SH, Stumpfova M, Jensen UB, et al. Identification of epidermal progenitors for the Merkel cell lineage. *Development*. 2010;137:3965-3971.
32. Kamaraj B, Purohit R. Mutational analysis of oculocutaneous albinism: a compact review. *BioMed Res Int*. 2014;2014:905472.
33. Bonaventure J, Domingues MJ, Larue L. Cellular and molecular mechanisms controlling the migration of melanocytes and melanoma cells. *Pigment Cell Melanoma Res*. 2013;26:316-325.
34. Baxter LL, Pavan WJ. The etiology and molecular genetics of human pigmentation disorders. *Wiley Interdiscip Rev Dev Biol*. 2013;2:379-392.
35. Haniffa M, Gunawan M, Jardine L. Human skin dendritic cells in health and disease. *J Dermatol Sci*. 2015;77:85-92.
37. Sanchez-Gurmaches J, Guertin DA. Adipocytes arise from multiple lineages that are heterogeneously and dynamically distributed. *Nat Commun*. 2014;5:4099.
38. Ma X, Lee P, Chisholm DJ, et al. Control of adipocyte differentiation in different fat depots; implications for pathophysiology or therapy. *Front Endocrinol*. 2015;6:1.
39. Kume T. Specification of arterial, venous, and lymphatic endothelial cells during embryonic development. *Histol Histopathol*. 2010;25:637-646.
40. Chen H, Griffin C, Xia L, et al. Molecular and cellular mechanisms of lymphatic vascular maturation. *Microvasc Res*. 2014;96:16-22.
41. Brouillard P, Boon L, Vikkula M. Genetics of lymphatic anomalies. *J Clin Invest*. 2014;124:898-904.
45. Vanakker O, Callewaert B, Malfait F, et al. The genetics of soft connective tissue disorders. *Annu Rev Genomics Hum Genet*. 2015;16:229-255.
46. Blatt J, Powell CM, Burkhart CN, et al. Genetics of hemangiomas, vascular malformations, and primary lymphedema. *J Pediatr Hematol Oncol*. 2014;36:587-593.
47. Bruckner-Tuderman L, Has C. Disorders of the cutaneous basement membrane zone—the paradigm of epidermolysis bullosa. *Matrix Biol*. 2014;33:29-34.
48. Has C, Nystrom A. Epidermal basement membrane in health and disease. *Curr Top Membr*. 2015;76:117-170.
49. Toivola DM, Boor P, Alam C, et al. Keratins in health and disease. *Curr Opin Cell Biol*. 2015;32:73-81.
50. Biggs LC, Mikkola ML. Early inductive events in ectodermal appendage morphogenesis. *Semin Cell Dev Biol*. 2014;25-26:11-21.
51. Ahn Y. Signaling in tooth, hair, and mammary placodes. *Curr Top Dev Biol*. 2015;111:421-459.
52. Duverger O, Morasso MI. To grow or not to grow: hair morphogenesis and human genetic hair disorders. *Semin Cell Dev Biol*. 2014;25-26:22-33.
53. Purba TS, Haslam IS, Poblet E, et al. Human epithelial hair follicle stem cells and their progeny: current state of knowledge, the widening gap in translational research and future challenges. *Bioessays*. 2014;36:513-525.
54. Markeson D, Pleat JM, Sharpe JR, et al. Scarring, stem cells, scaffolds and skin repair. *J Tissue Eng Regen Med*. 2015;9:649-668.
55. Morgan BA. The dermal papilla: an instructive niche for epithelial stem and progenitor cells in development and regeneration of the hair follicle. *Cold Spring Harb Perspect Med*. 2014;4:a015180.
56. Driskell RR, Clavel C, Rendl M, et al. Hair follicle dermal papilla cells at a glance. *J Cell Sci*. 2011;124:1179-1182.
57. Niemann C, Horsley V. Development and homeostasis of the sebaceous gland. *Semin Cell Dev Biol*. 2012;23:928-936.
60. Lu C, Fuchs E. Sweat gland progenitors in development, homeostasis, and wound repair. *Cold Spring Harb Perspect Med*. 2014;4(2):a015222.
61. Harel S, Christiano AM. Genetics of structural hair disorders. *J Invest Dermatol*. 2012;132:E22-E26.
62. Lemke JR, Kernland-Lang K, Hortnagel K, et al. Monogenic human skin disorders. *Dermatology*. 2014;229:55-64.
63. Schweizer J, Langbein L, Rogers MA, et al. Hair follicle-specific keratins and their diseases. *Exp Cell Res*. 2007;313:2010-2020.
64. DeStefano GM, Christiano AM. The genetics of human skin disease. *Cold Spring Harb Perspect Med*. 2014;4:a015172.

44 Physiologic Development of the Skin

Marty O. Visscher | Vivek Narendran

INTRODUCTION

Human skin is a complex structure with unusual functional diversity.[1,2] Topologically, the skin is continuous with the lung and intestinal epithelia. The lung and gut are generally viewed as exchange surfaces for gases and nutrients; the skin is more commonly considered a barrier.[1,3,4] The concept of an integumental barrier emphasizes the role of the skin as a protective boundary between an organism and a potentially hostile environment. This protective role is evident at birth as the fetus abruptly transitions from a warm, wet, sterile, protected sphere to a cold, dry, microbe-laden world filled with physical, chemical, and mechanical dangers. Focusing only on the barrier properties of the skin, however, minimizes the critical role of the skin in social communication, perception, and behavioral interactions. The skin, as the surface of an organism, is both a cellular and a molecular structure, as well as a perceptual and psychological interface.[5] This dual functionality befits a true boundary and must be kept in mind to fully appreciate the dynamic organization of the skin and its close kinship with the nervous system.[6]

The skin also provides the physical scaffold that defines the form of an animal.[7] A wide variety of strategies have been devised by animals to cope with different habitats (Table 44.1).[8] Arthropods have a largely inflexible body surface, covered with an exoskeleton. Many vertebrates, such as amphibians, live on land but are confined to humid or wet microhabitats. Reptiles and fish have a skin surface covered predominantly with scales; birds have evolved feathers; and most mammals are covered with a protective mantle of fur. Among primates, humans are unique in possessing a non-furred skin with a thick stratified interfollicular epidermis and a well-developed stratum corneum.

The question of the presumptive advantage of losing a protective and insulating coat of fur has long intrigued evolutionary biologists and physical anthropologists.[9] Three of the most distinctive physical features distinguishing humans are (1) a non-furred skin surface, (2) a large, versatile, highly complex brain, and (3) opposable thumbs. The close embryologic connection between the epidermis and the brain (both are ectodermal derivatives) supports the contention that these peculiar structural aspects of human development have coevolved.[6] We often overlook the direct participation of the

Table 44.1 Animal Body Covering.

Type	Biologic Example
Simple membrane	Earthworm
Simple stratified epidermis, often mucus secreting[258,259]	Frog, toad
Exoskeleton	Insects, crustaceans
Scales	Reptiles, fish
Feathers	Birds
Fur	Most mammals (including all primates except humans)
Nonfurred Complex Stratified Epidermis	
Thick interfollicular epidermis with separate functional strata and well-developed stratum corneum	Humans
Lipid droplets in stratum corneum	Dolphins

skin in higher-level functions, such as perception and behavioral interactions. Cutaneous attributes form the basis for many readily observed biologic distinctions (age, race, sex), as well as multiple, overlapping sociocultural characteristics (tattooing, cosmetics, tanning). During recovery from illness, the skin forms a critical interface linking a patient with caregivers and a nurturing environment.

In this chapter, specific aspects of the physiologic development of fetal and neonatal skin are highlighted, focusing particularly on the development of the epidermal barrier and the functions subserved by the outermost layer of the skin, the stratum corneum. Where relevant, new areas of skin biology pertinent to a fetus and a newborn are emphasized. Areas of active research and unanswered questions will be identified in the hope of spurring new investigation of this highly accessible but extraordinarily complex interface.

DEVELOPMENT OF THE EPIDERMAL BARRIER

Human epidermis consists of several renewing structures, including the interfollicular epidermis, the hair follicle, the sweat gland, and the sebaceous gland.[1,10] The major component is the dermis, composed of collagen and elastin fibers embedded in a hydrated glycosaminoglycan matrix and containing blood vessels and most of the cutaneous nerve endings. Dermal and subcutaneous fat cells (e.g., fibroblasts and adipocytes) derive from embryonic mesoderm. Epidermal appendages (i.e., hair follicles, sweat glands, sebaceous glands, and the interfollicular epidermis) derive from embryonic ectoderm.[6]

The epidermis consists of multiple cell types, including keratinocytes, melanocytes, Merkel cells, and antigen-presenting Langerhans cells derived from mesoderm.[11,12] The epidermis is traditionally segmented into four separate structural and functional compartments (Fig. 44.1): (1) *stratum basale*, responsible for keratinocyte proliferation and epidermal renewal; (2) *stratum spinosum*, with tightly packed keratinocytes linked via desmosomal connections; (3) *stratum granulosum*, responsible for barrier lipid synthesis and corneocyte production via programmed cell death; and (4) *stratum corneum* (SC), the anucleated outermost layer, forming the physical environmental interface.[13,14] As discussed later, the SC is markedly deficient in preterm infants.[15-18] Protective functions of the SC are listed in Table 44.2.

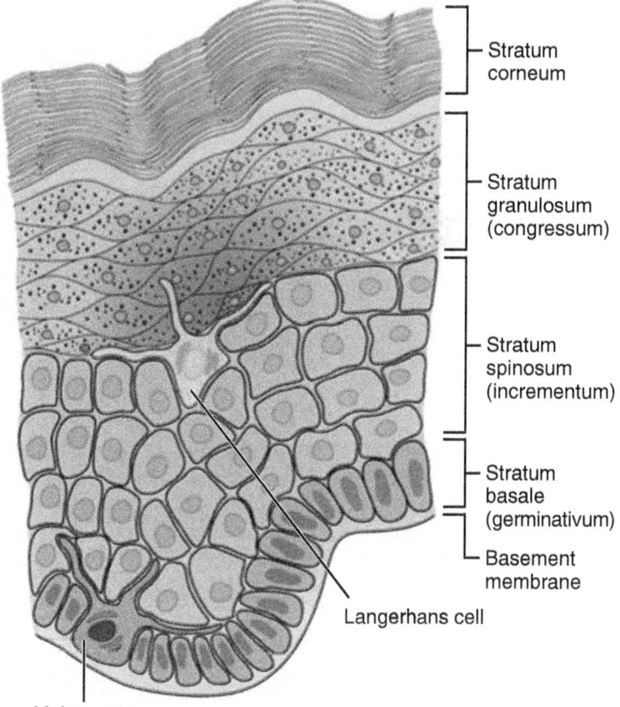

Fig. 44.1 Organization of human epidermis. The interfollicular epidermis is traditionally considered to be a tetratomic identity incorporating four separate structural and functional epidermal strata. In humans the epidermis between the hair follicles is much thicker than in furred animals. The epidermis is composed primarily of keratinocytes but includes other epidermal cells such as melanocytes, Langerhans cells, and Merkel cells (latter not shown). The outermost stratum, the stratum corneum, incorporates the transition from living, nucleated keratinocytes to terminally differentiated corneocytes. This diagram is schematic only and does not illustrate the important intercellular connections (desmosomes) converting single cells into integrated membrane structures. (Modified from Hoath SB, Leahy DG. The human stratum corneum as extended, covalently cross-linked biopolymer: mathematics, molecules, and medicine. *Med Hypotheses.* 2006; 66(6):1191–1198.)

CORNIFIED ENVELOPE AND EPIDERMAL LAMELLAR BODIES

During later gestation, epithelial surfaces at environmental interfaces undergo structural and functional changes, including complex proteolipid synthesis. These highly coordinated events can be influenced by gender and prenatal hormone exposure (rat model), for example, maternal glucocorticoids.[19-24] The three stages of fetal skin development are stratification, follicular keratinization, and interfollicular epidermal keratinization.[6] Interfollicular keratinization occurs in a rostrocaudal and dorsoventral fashion, beginning at 23 to 24 weeks of GA,

Table 44.2 Protective Functions of the Stratum Corneum.

Functions	Structural Basis	Biochemical Mechanisms
Mechanical integrity/resilience	Cornified envelope, cytosolic filaments	Crosslinked peptides (e.g., loricrin, keratin filaments)
Xenobiote defense	Lamellar bilayers, extracellular matrix	Acidic pH; free fatty acids; antimicrobial peptides
Antioxidant defense	Corneocytes and extracellular matrix	Keratins; sebaceous gland–derived vitamin E and other antioxidants
Cytokine signaling	Corneocyte cytosol	Storage and release of interleukins; serine proteases
Permeability barrier	Lamellar bilayers	Hydrophobic lipids
Hydration	Lamellar bilayers, corneocyte cytosolic matrix	Sebaceous gland–derived glycerol; filaggrin breakdown products (natural moisturizing factors)
Waterproofing/repellency	Lamellar bilayers	Keratinocyte and sebum-derived lipids
Cohesion/desquamation	Corneodesmosomes	Acidic pH serine proteases
UV protection	Corneocyte cytosol	Structural proteins; urocanic acid; light scattering/absorption

Modified from Chuong CM, Nickoloff BJ, Elias PM, et al. What is the "true" function of skin? *Exp Dermatol.* 2002;11:159.[7]

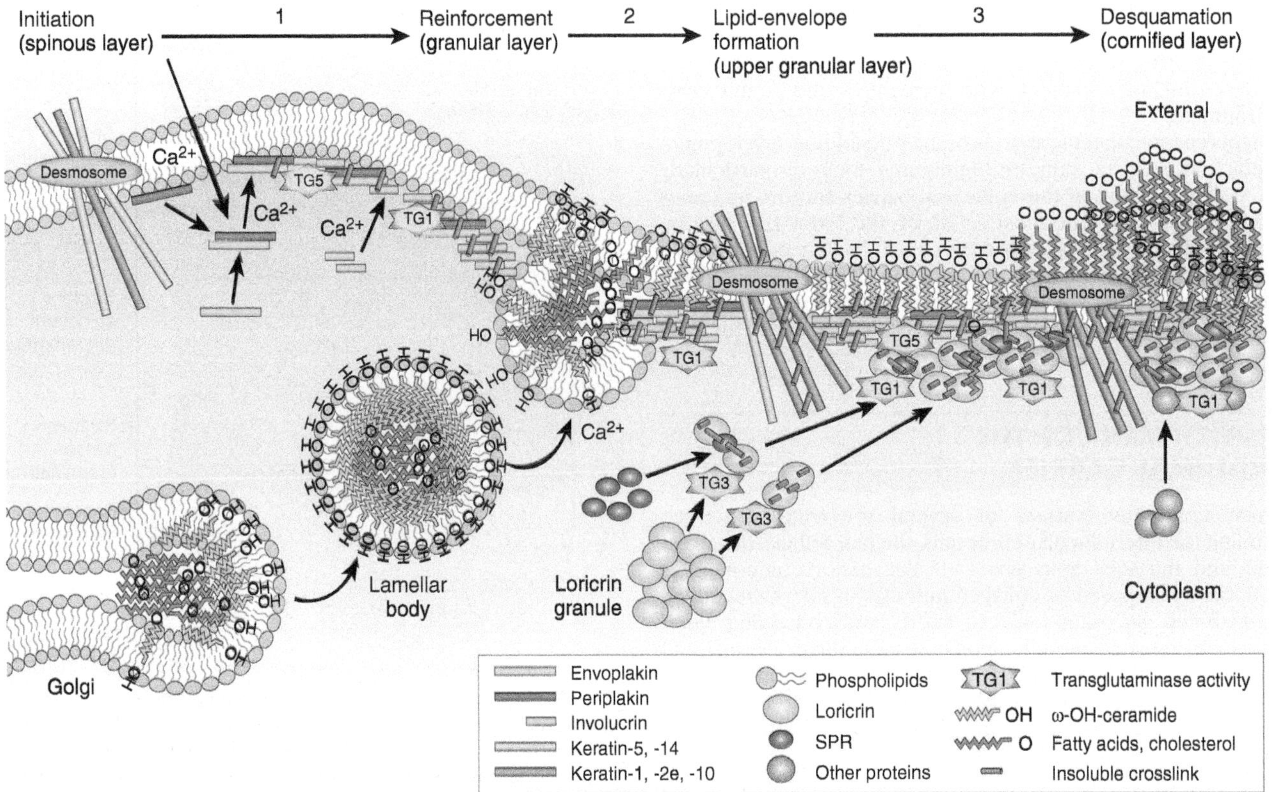

Fig. 44.2 Stages in the assembly of the cornified envelope in human stratum corneum. *1,* In the upper layers of the epidermis, rising levels of intracellular Ca^{2+} lead to expression of envoplakin, periplakin, and involucrin, as well as transglutaminase 1 with subsequent covalent cross-linking of the structural proteins along the inner surface of the plasma membrane. *2,* Synthesis, packaging, and extrusion of barrier lipids (free fatty acids, cholesterol, ceramides) in the form of lamellar bodies are accompanied by replacement of the plasma membrane with covalently bound ceramides that serve to interdigitate with and organize the extracellular lipids into the characteristic lamellar pattern. *3,* Covalent cross-linking of intracorneocyte proteins, including keratins, loricrin, and small proline-rich *(SPR)* peptides, occurs via mediation of transglutaminase 1 and transglutaminase 3. The end product is the transformation of nucleated keratinocytes in the uppermost granular layer of the epidermis into a network of interlinked, terminally differentiated corneocytes embedded in a matrix of structured lipid lamellae, collectively called the *stratum corneum.* The stratum corneum provides the vital barrier to water loss and infection necessary for life after birth. *TG,* Transglutaminase. (Modified from Candi E, Schmidt R, Melino G. The cornified envelope: a model of cell death in the skin. *Nat Rev Mol Cell Biol.* 2005;6:328.[26])

coinciding roughly with the time of postnatal viability.[25] The formation of a barrier to water loss and infection is essential for extrauterine survival. Fig. 44.2 illustrates the SC cornified envelope assembly.[26-28] Synthesis and secretion of epidermal barrier lipids occurs as lamellar bodies, similar to a parallel process in the developing lung (Table 44.3). The intracellular lamellar body fuses with the plasma membrane and extrudes barrier lipids, consisting of free fatty acids, cholesterol, and ceramides, to form the primary barrier to transepidermal water loss (TEWL); the barrier lipids form a regular, bilayer structure that further ensures impermeability to outside agents (see Table 44.3).[3] Covalent cross-linking of structural proteins (e.g., keratins) by intracellular transglutaminases and ceramides forms the insoluble, cornified SC envelope,[26,27] essentially a huge macromolecule.[14,28-31]

Table 44.3 Comparison of Lamellar Bodies of Epidermal and Pulmonary Origins.

	Epidermis	Lung
Cell type	Spinous and granular keratinocytes	Type II alveolar cell
Size/structure	Ovoid (0.25–0.5 μm) Disklike lamellations	Spheroid (1.2–1.6 μm) Lamellated sacs with amorphous core
Lipid content	40% phospholipids 20% glycosphingolipids 20% free sterols 20% other neutral lipids	85% phospholipids 10% free sterols 5% other neutral lipids
Protein content	Acid phosphatase Glycosidases Proteases Lipases	Acid phosphatase Proteases Glycosidases Surfactant apoproteins
Function	Delivery of lipids to form extracellular matrix of stratum corneum Skin permeability barrier	Delivery of surfactant lipid to alveolar spaces Lower alveolar surface tension

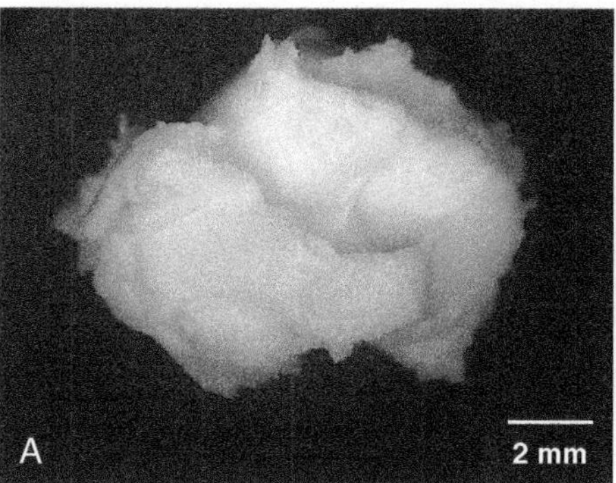

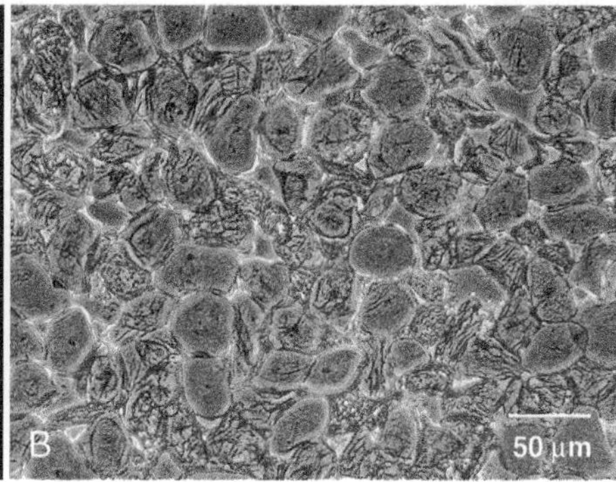

Fig. 44.3 Vernix caseosa. Macroscopically, vernix is a thick, viscous, white paste (A). The phase contrast image of native vernix (B) reveals a dense packing of fetal corneocytes. Vernix consists primarily of thin, hydrated, polygonal, terminally differentiated, fetal corneocytes embedded in a nonlamellar lipid matrix. The cells are heterogeneous in size and structure. Many nuclear ghosts are evident.

This cross-linked assembly forms the scaffolding for the highly ordered lamellar lipid matrix (see Chapter 43). The cells within the stratum spinosum and stratum granulosum are attached to each other in all directions by desmosomes, protein-based materials that provide mechanical integrity (see Fig. 44.2).[31]

THE BIOLOGY OF VERNIX

Scientifically, the development of epidermal barrier function has many similarities to surfactant production and lung development (see Table 44.3). Both epidermal keratinocyte and type II alveolar cells are lipid-synthesizing cells that secrete barrier lipids as lamellar bodies. Both ultimately interface with a gaseous environment and are under similar hormonal control at similar periods of development. The mechanisms by which the lung develops a functionally mature epithelial surface ready for air adaptation and skin surface matures under total aqueous conditions for terrestrial adaptation to a dry environment are analogous. An unanswered question, however, is by which mechanism the epidermal barrier forms under total aqueous immersion. Prolonged exposure of the skin to water in adults is harmful.[32] Vernix caseosa, a complex proteolipid cellular cream, forms during the last trimester, interacts with the epidermis, and facilitates the SC formation (Fig. 44.3).[33-35]

The barrier forms initially in the region of the pilosebaceous apparatus.[25,36] This finding strongly supports the hypothesis that vernix caseosa (partly from sebaceous secretions) participates in "waterproofing" the skin surface, allowing cornification initially in the hair follicles and then over the interfollicular skin,[37] perhaps analogous to skin culture systems raised to an air-liquid interface for cornification.[38] Sebaceous glands excrete sebum, a complex nonpolar lipid mixture synthesized de novo by the glands.[39] Sebaceous glands are multiacinar, holocrine-secreting structures that occur over the skin.[39] Their development is closely related to hair follicle differentiation. In neonates, sebaceous glands are hyperplastic and visible in areas such as the nose. The timing of vernix production and the developing pilosebaceous apparatus supports a mechanism by which the surge in sebaceous gland activity leads to production of vernix overlying the developing SC.[39] Sebaceous gland hyperplasia in term infants is putatively secondary to androgenic stimulation from hyperplastic fetal adrenal glands,[15] providing a testable model integrating hyperplasia of sebaceous and adrenal glands during later gestation (Fig. 44.4). This hypothesis explains other clinical observations, such as turbidity of amniotic fluid during the last trimester of pregnancy.[40] In vitro, the addition of physiologically relevant amounts of pulmonary surfactant leads to emulsification and release of immobilized vernix (i.e., a test tube coated with native vernix). This finding is consistent with a mechanism by which the outermost portion of the vernix coating is "removed" from the fetal skin surface by lung-derived surfactant contained in the amniotic fluid (see Fig. 44.4).[41] The fetus subsequently swallows the detached vernix (see Fig. 44.4). Vernix contains branched chain fatty acids (BCFA), which are trophic and protective factors for the developing gut.[42,43] A diet enriched with vernix-like BCFA significantly reduced necrotizing enterocolitis in the neonatal rat model[43] and BCFA-enriched vernix-monoacylglycerol decreased inflammatory markers in human enterocytes.[44] Vernix contains antimicrobial agents, including lactoferrin and lysozyme, and antioxidants, providing additional protection at birth.[45] When vernix is retained on the skin surface at birth, the skin is more hydrated and has a lower surface acidity than when it is removed.[46]

SKIN TRANSITIONS AT BIRTH

Few events are as physiologically abrupt as birth. The skin must immediately perform multiple functions vital to the survival

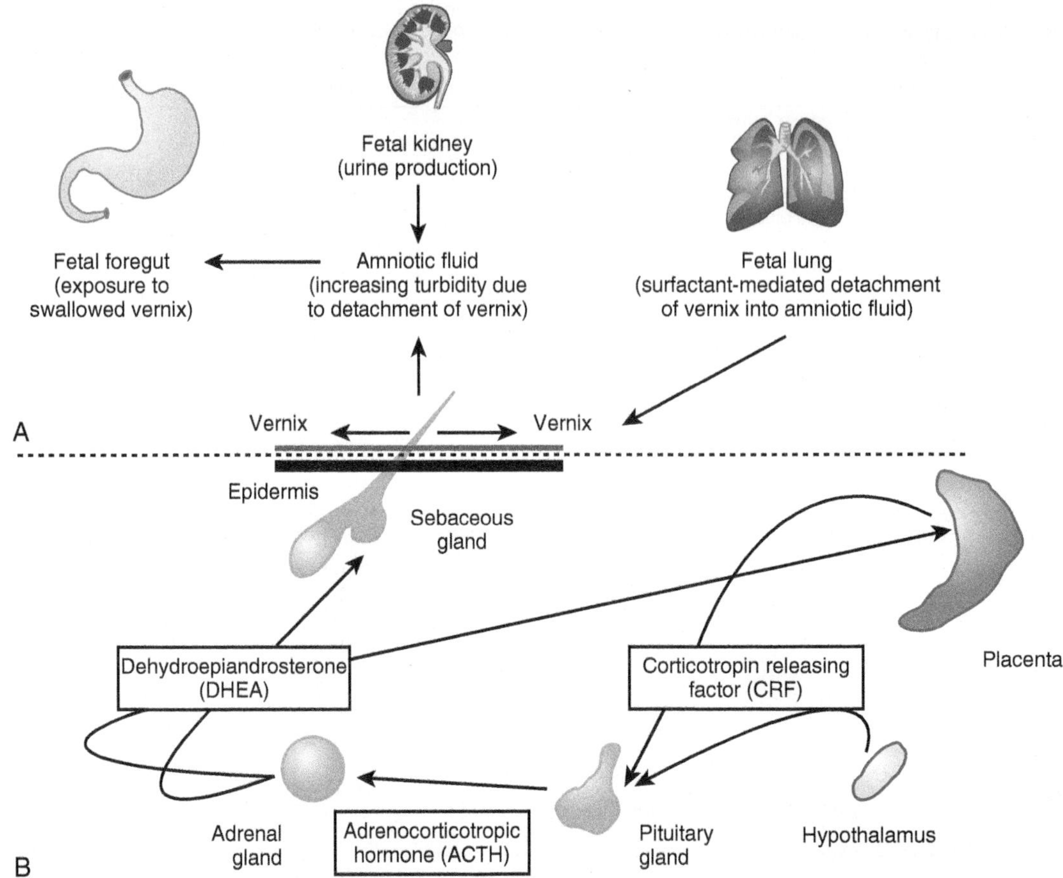

Fig. 44.4 (A) Proposed mechanism for pulmonary surfactant–mediated vernix detachment. The fetal kidney contributes significantly to amniotic fluid production. During the third trimester, vernix covers the developing epidermis, and the fetal lung produces and secretes increasing amounts of pulmonary surfactant into the amniotic fluid. Vernix on the skin surface builds up and detaches into the surrounding milieu, leading to amniotic fluid turbidity.[43] Vernix within the amniotic fluid is subsequently swallowed by the fetus, with potential effects on the fetal foregut and/or systemic absorption of vernix components. (B) Endocrine-based model for vernix production and epidermal barrier maturation. In this working model, corticotropin-releasing factors from either the placenta or the hypothalamus act to initiate adrenocorticotropic hormone release from the pituitary gland. Adrenocorticotropic hormone stimulation of the adrenal cortex promotes synthesis and release of androgenic steroids such as dehydroepiandrosterone *(DHEA)*, which are subsequently converted enzymatically within the sebaceous gland to active androgens. Production of superficial lipid film (sebum) in the immediate vicinity of the hair follicle modulates the transepidermal water gradient with putative effects to facilitate cornification of the underlying epidermis.[36] Desquamation of corneocytes into the overlying lipid matrix results in formation of vernix. The findings of Ito and colleagues[253] that human hair follicles synthesize cortisol and exhibit a functional equivalent of the hypothalamic-pituitary-adrenal axis raise interesting questions regarding local versus systemic control mechanisms in the schema. (Modified and expanded from Zouboulis C, Fimmel S, Ortmann J, Turnbull J, Boschankow A. Sebaceous glands. In: Hoath SB, Maibach H, eds. *Neonatal Skin: Structure and Function.* 2nd ed. New York: Marcel Dekker; 2003:59–88.[39])

(Box 44.1). Epidermal physiologic mechanisms in the epidermis activate eccrine sweating,[47] important for thermoregulation and bacterial homeostasis and sebum production.[15] The neutral pH rapidly develops an acid mantle.[48,49] The epidermis and the SC remain in balance via cornification and desquamation.[3,50-52] Transepidermal water flux regulates DNA and lipid synthesis.[53-55] SC hydration is necessary for normal desquamation.[56,57]

Postnatally, lipid synthesis and metabolism subserve multiple functions, including SC structure formation, sebum, and adipose tissue for biomechanical support (Table 44.4).The epidermis and the brain contain unusually high concentrations of ceramides,[58-60] supporting the embryologic and functional connection between two ectodermal derivatives.[6]

Box 44.1 Multiple Physiologic Roles of the Skin at Birth

- Barrier to water loss
- Thermoregulation
- Infection control
- Immunosurveillance
- Acid mantle formation
- Antioxidant function
- Ultraviolet light photoprotection
- Barrier to chemicals
- Tactile discrimination
- Attraction to caregiver

WATER LOSS, TEMPERATURE CONTROL, AND BLOOD FLOW

A dry environment necessitates protection against dehydration. Barrier formation against TEWL is a function of gestational age (Fig. 44.5),[61,62] decreasing dramatically and approximating adult values near term.[63] This critical function resides almost entirely in the outermost 20 μm of the skin surface—in the SC.[3] Heat exchange occurs between infant skin and the environment via evaporation, radiation, conduction, and convection.[65] Evaporative heat loss is the primary mode of temperature instability in not only in very low-birth-weight preterm but in all infants and is the primary mode of heat loss at birth. It is important to distinguish between evaporative heat loss from standing water or amniotic fluid on the skin surface and evaporative heat loss secondary to a poorly developed epidermal barrier, which occurs after delivery in very low-birth-weight preterm infants. Evaporative heat and fluid loss are ongoing and are exacerbated in non-humidified, radiant-heated environments.

The periphery is important in temperature control in newborn infants (Fig. 44.6).[66] Given the critical importance of limiting evaporative water and heat loss in temperature control, it is surprising how little attention is given to the role of the SC in thermoregulation. The strategic position of the SC is taken for granted, and focus is placed on more central mechanisms for maintaining body temperature, yet it is essential in organizing, maintaining, and guiding central nervous system development. At 4 hours of age, oxygen consumption is not simply a function of central body temperature, as might be expected with warm-blooded endothermic organisms, but is largely a function of heat exchange at the skin-environment interface, as central homeothermic mechanisms are not well developed at birth. Preterm infants are more vulnerable to environmental heat loss due to a higher surface area to mass ratio, lower endogenous heat generation (e.g., brown adipose tissue), an incompetent epidermal barrier, and inability to self-regulate with flexural positioning.[15] Central control of body temperature requires autonomic mechanisms such as eccrine sweating and vasodilatation/vasoconstriction, which are not well-established at birth.[47] Newborn infants may exhibit vasoconstriction of the extremities (acrocyanosis) and have widely variable hematocrits and blood volumes. Peripheral cooling results in increased blood viscosity and decreased blood flow. In the first 3 months, the cutaneous vascular bed undergoes reorganization, with development of a subpapillary plexus (Fig. 44.7). The formation of a superficial vascular plexus is associated with increased convolution in the epidermis (rete peg formation) a hallmark of the mature epidermis. Abnormal cutaneous vascular development and the role of associated growth factors have been reviewed elsewhere.[67,68]

FULL-TERM NEONATAL SKIN ADAPTATION

At birth, full-term skin is well-developed and protective, despite having been in a wet environment during gestation. An appropriate level of moisture (hydration) is necessary for flexibility with movement, desquamation of the outer layers during SC self-renewal, and other functions. The level of skin hydration depends upon presence or vernix, environmental temperature, and body site.[46,69] Hydration decreases rapidly during postnatal day one then increases significantly over the next 2 weeks (Fig. 44.8),[70] but the skin remains drier than older infants and their mothers.[71-73] Low hydration is likely caused by a delay in the production of water-binding materials, including

Table 44.4 Sources, Composition, and Presumed Functions of Skin Lipids in Neonates.

Source	Composition	Functions
Stratum corneum	Ceramides, cholesterol sulfate, neutral lipids (free and esterified sterols, free fatty acids, triglycerides)	Permeability barrier, cohesion/desquamation, antibacterial
Sebaceous glands	Triglyceride, wax/sterol esters/squalene	Antibacterial, moisturizing
Adipose tissue	Triglyceride	Systemic energy reservoir

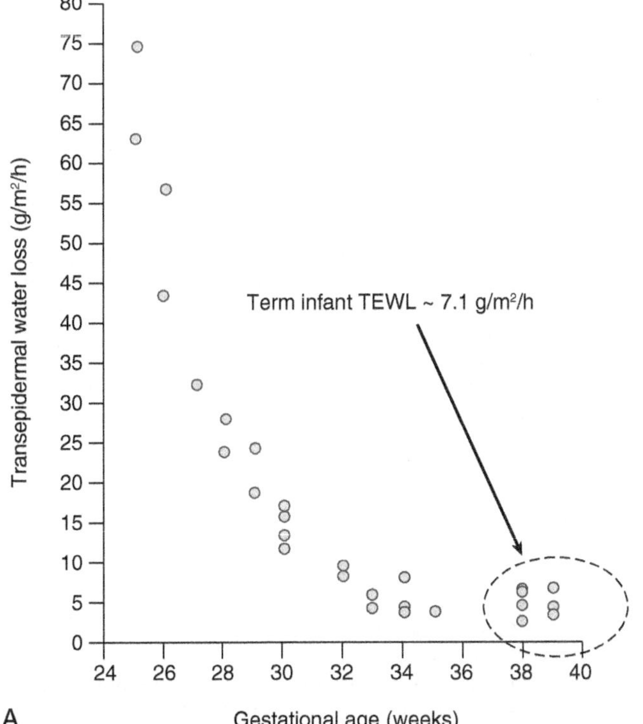

Fig. 44.5 (A) Transepidermal water loss *(TEWL)* as a function of gestational age.[61] Very low-birth-weight preterm infants have extraordinarily high TEWL in the range of 50 to 70 g/m²/h. A large study by Kelleher and colleagues[64] of more than 1000 term infants showed a low TEWL, approximately 7 g/m²/h, which is comparable with adult values. Such normative values may prove important in future studies of conditions other than prematurity, which are also characterized by a defective epidermal barrier (e.g., atopic dermatitis).

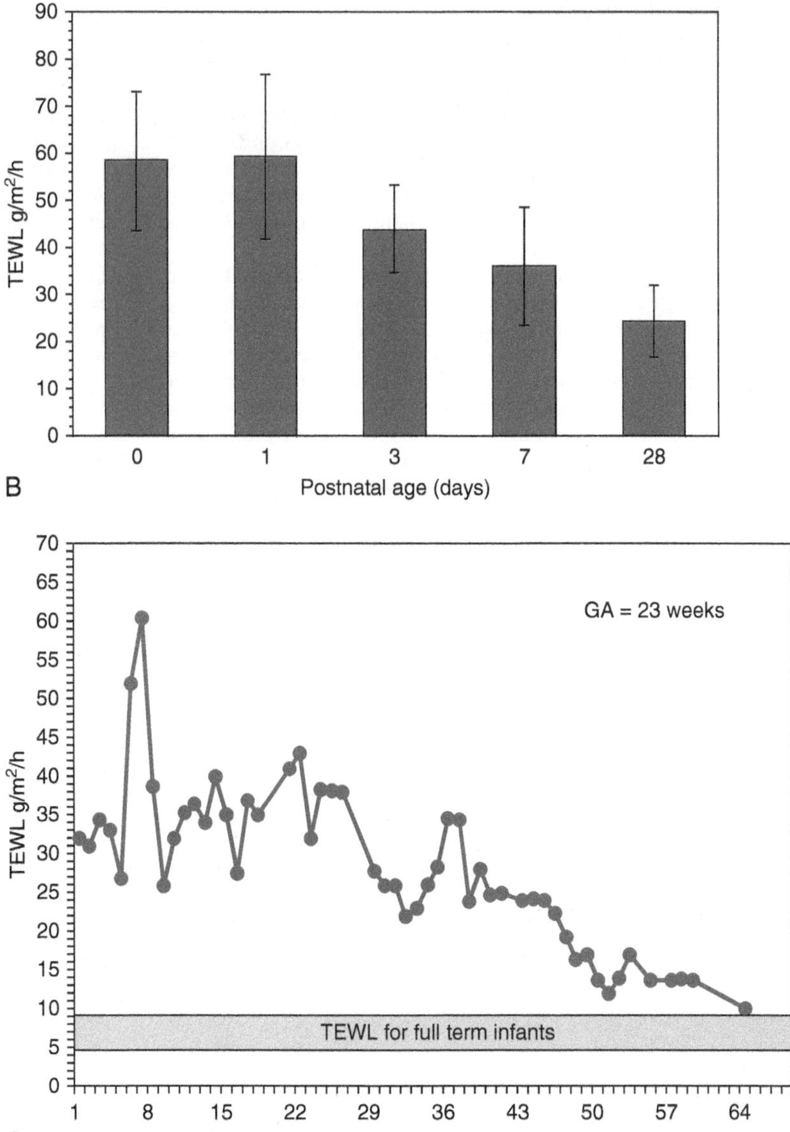

Fig. 44.5, cont'd (B) TEWL over 1 month for infants of 24 to 25 weeks gestational age *(GA)*. TEWL was measured and corrected to 50% relative humidity in 13 premature infants of 24 to 25 weeks GA. Values decreased but at one month of life they remained considerably higher than readings for full-term neonates.[62] (C) Transepidermal water loss profile for a 23-week gestational age infant over time from birth. The epidermal barrier of premature infants is functionally compromised for several weeks after birth with estimates of full maturation time varying from 2 to 9 weeks postnatal age.[81] The factors that influence the rate/pattern of SC maturation are currently unknown.

amino acids, from enzymatic proteolysis of filaggrin in the outer SC layers. These processes are delayed under high humidity in utero[74] and are activated in the drier extrauterine environment.[57]

IMPACT OF PREMATURE BIRTH: AN INEFFECTIVE EPIDERMAL BARRIER

Without the prevention of water and heat loss provided by the SC, life in a terrestrial environment is impossible. Very premature neonates have an underdeveloped epidermal barrier with few SC layers,[75,76] increasing their risk for water loss, electrolyte imbalance, thermal instability, exposure to toxins, increased permeability, delayed skin maturation, and infection.[75-77] The dermis is also deficient and susceptible to skin stripping and tears/splits.[78] The SC is nearly absent at 23 weeks GA with TEWL of 75 g/m²/h (see Fig. 44.5A).[61] Even at one month of age, TEWL is higher in preterms than full-terms (see Fig. 44.5B).[62] By week 26, a few cornified layers have formed (TEWL of ~ 45 g/m²/h), corresponding essentially to wounded skin.[75,76] At 29 weeks, TEWL is 17 g/m²/h, still markedly higher than full-term values. The time of completion of SC maturation is largely unknown, but may be as late as 9 weeks postnatal age (see Fig. 44.5C).[62,79-81] Exposure to the dry environment promotes rapid SC maturation (Fig. 44.9).[82,83] The sticky, wet, translucent skin of a very low birth-weight infant rapidly transitions to the dry, opaque stratum of corneum, and excessive scaling/desquamation often occurs.

New SC sampling methods and analytical techniques facilitate investigations of neonatal skin development. Selected biomarkers of innate immunity differed for premature versus full-terms and adults.[84] Infants 32 weeks GA or younger had higher levels of involucrin, albumin, and proinflammatory cytokines (interleukin [IL]1β, IL6, MCP1, and IL8) than full-terms and adults. All infants had higher IL1α concentrations and lower keratin 1,10,11 and tumor necrosis factor-α than adults. Involucrin was higher in full-terms than adults and inversely related to GA.

Immature preterm skin is permeable, and care is required to avoid toxic transdermal exposures.[85,86] The permeable barrier allows the efflux of carbon dioxide[87] and the influx of oxygen[88] in a manner similar to that of water vapor. Gaseous movement across the skin surface, facilitated by local skin heating, is the

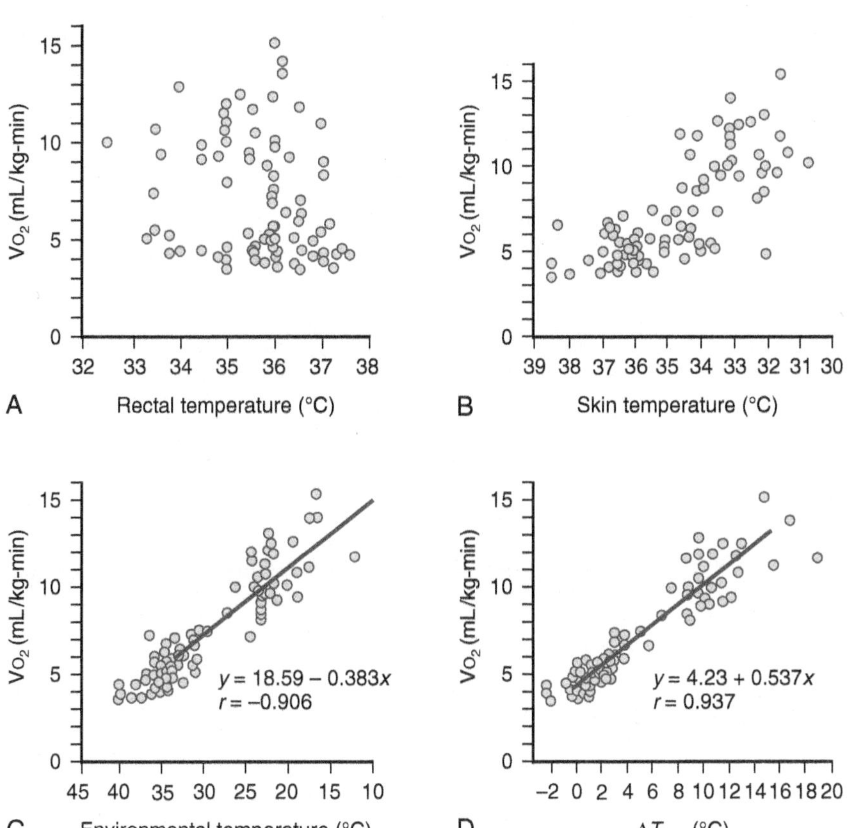

Fig. 44.6 Oxygen consumption of term newborn human infants approximately 4 hours after birth. Systemic oxygen consumption correlates best with the skin-environment gradient (D), indicating the importance of peripheral heat flux in regulating body temperature in neonates rather than core temperature (A). (From Adamsons K, Gandy G, James L. The influence of thermal factors upon oxygen consumption of the newborn human infant. *J Pediatr.* 1965;66:495.[66])

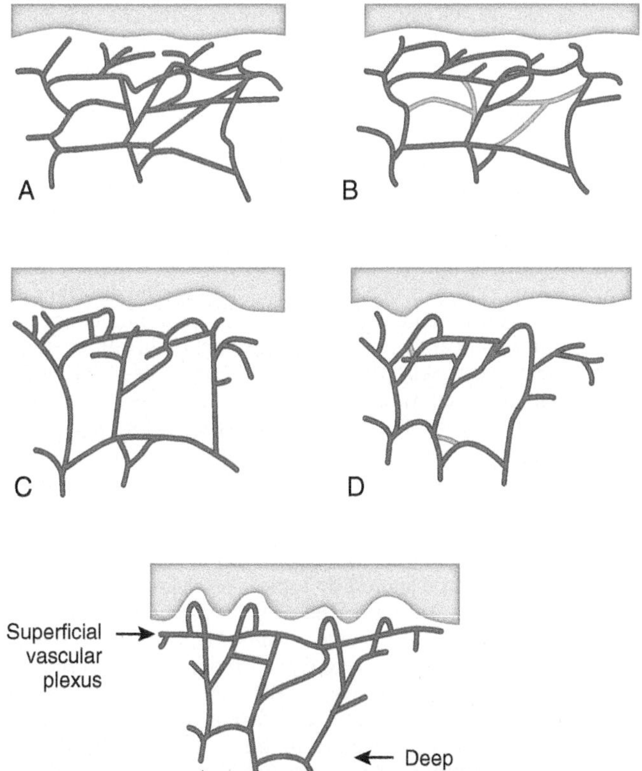

Fig. 44.7 The blood supply at birth. The gradual development of papillary buds and organization of the subpapillary plexus from birth (A) to 3 months of age (B–D) and the vascular pattern at 3 months of age (E). The arrows (E) show the direction of blood flow for arteriolar and venous systems. (Modified from Perera P, Kurban A, Ryan T. The development of the cutaneous microvascular system in the newborn. *Br J Dermatol.* 1970;82[suppl 5]:86.[254])

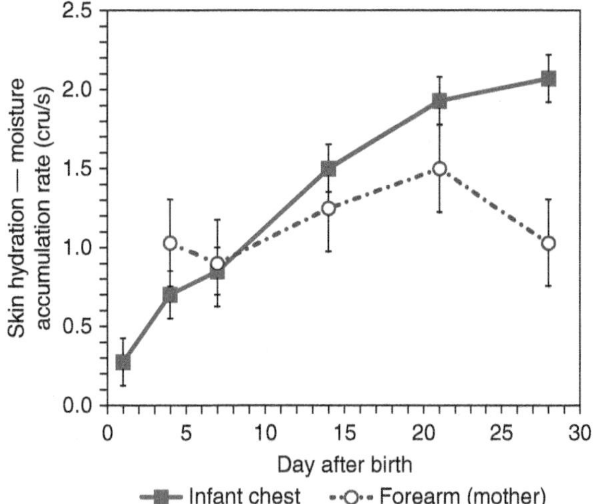

Fig. 44.8 Skin barrier water handling properties during postnatal month one. Skin hydration in full-term infants is very low shortly after birth, lower than adult (mother) forearm skin. Hydration increases rapidly during the first two weeks of life as it adapts to the dry environment.[70] The initial low hydration is likely due to reduced proteolysis of filaggrin to form water binding natural moisturizing factor that occurs at high humidity[89] and/or until the surface is sufficiently dry to activate filaggrin.[57] (Modified from Visscher MO, Chatterjee R, Munson KA, et al. Changes in diapered and nondiapered infant skin over the first month of life. *Pediatr Dermatol.* 2000;17:45–51.[70])

basis for the use of transcutaneous gas electrodes in clinical practice.

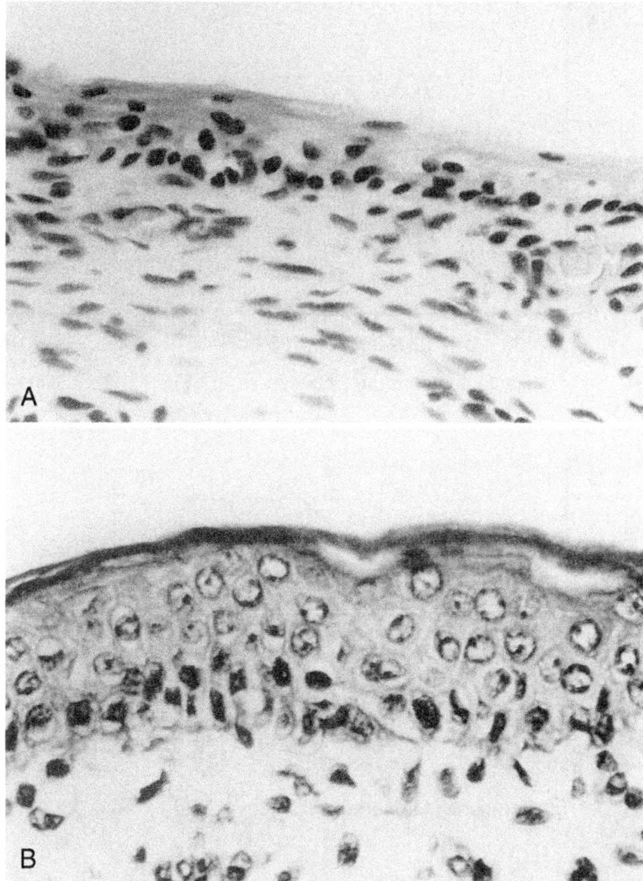

Fig. 44.9 Rapid development of the epidermal barrier after exposure to the ambient environment (xeric stress) in very low birth-weight preterm infants. (A) The epidermis of a 26-week gestational age infant on day 1 of life. No stratum corneum is present and the nucleated epidermis is thin. (B) The epidermis of a 26-week gestational age infant on postnatal day 10. (Reproduced from Rutter N. Percutaneous drug absorption in the newborn: hazards and uses. *Clin Perinatol.* 14:911, 1987.[255])

DEVELOPMENT OF THE ACID MANTLE

A number of physiologic protective, skin-based mechanisms are triggered at birth, as they were unnecessary during gestation. The skin surface of full-term infants has a neutral pH at birth. However, an acid skin surface, known as the acid mantle, is necessary for effective barrier function. Multiple mechanisms are responsible for acid mantle development. The lamellar bodies in the stratum granulosum (see Fig. 44.1) contain phospholipids that are hydrolyzed to free fatty acids that lower skin pH.[90] Activity of the sodium-hydrogen antiporter NHE-1, located at the stratum granulosum/SC interface, is responsible for pH reduction.[91] The protein filaggrin aggregates keratin proteins in the stratum granulosum and SC and plays a key role in skin barrier function. Filaggrin is hydrolyzed by skin enzymes to form lower molecular weight compounds, collectively known as natural moisturizing factor (NMF). The components of NMF (1) bind water in the upper SC to hydrate and plasticize the tissue and (2) lower the skin surface pH.[90] An acidic surface pH enhances SC formation, for example, lipid metabolism and structure, and SC integrity, cohesion, desquamation, and homeostasis.[92–96] An acidic pH facilitates skin colonization with appropriate bacteria, that is, *S. epidermidis* attachment to the skin,[95] antimicrobial peptide activity, microbiome diversity,[96] and inhibition of pathogenic bacterial such as *S. aureus*.[97–99] In contrast, increased skin pH activates enzymes that damage SC integrity, enhances susceptibility to mechanical trauma, and increases the amount of pathologic flora.[99–101]

FACTORS INFLUENCING NEONATAL SKIN PH

Full-term skin pH is neutral at birth, decreases markedly over days 1 to 4 and continues to decline for as long as 3 months after birth.[70,102,103] For example, NMF levels were very low at birth in full-term infants but increased over the first postnatal month,[104,105] contributing to the acid mantle. Vernix plays a role in this process. Full-term skin pH was lower when vernix was retained at delivery than when vernix was removed at 4 or 24 hours after birth.[46]

In low-birth-weight infants, skin pH decreased rapidly over days 1 to 3, more slowly over days 4 to 7, and declined further up to day 28.[106] Individually, GA and day of life did not influence the skin pH but significantly impacted the reduction in combination. A rapid decrease in skin pH occurred in infants 24 to 34 weeks GA during postnatal week 1 then was more gradual. Infants weighing less than 1000 g had a higher skin pH for longer than infants weighing more than 1000 g.[107] Unlike full-term neonates, premature infants less than ~29 weeks GA have little vernix on the skin surface at birth. Consequently, the premature skin barrier may not experience the benefits of reduced pH and increased hydration observed in full-term infants.[46]

The skin pH can be altered by topical products and items. For example, the pH of skin under the diaper was higher than a nondiapered site in neonates and older infants (Fig. 44.10).[70,102] Higher diaper skin pH was related to greater irritant contact dermatitis and hydration (wetness).[108] Higher pH may increase the risk of mechanical damage in vulnerable infants (e.g., friction, cleaning)[101] and increase skin permeability to toxins.[109] Higher skin pH may predispose development of inflammatory skin diseases of infancy, including atopic dermatitis and seborrheic dermatitis.[92]

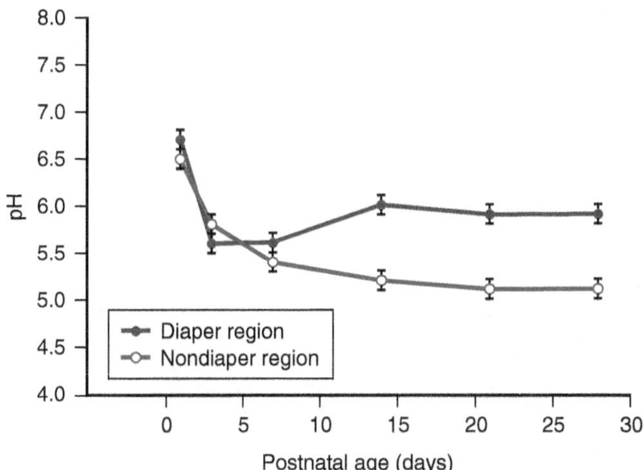

Fig. 44.10 Postnatal development of the acid mantle in term newborn infants—effect on body site. Skin pH was measured with a flat-surface electrode (model 900, pH meter, Courage and Khazaka, Cologne, Germany) in male and female infants born at 37 to 42 weeks of gestation. Values are means ± the standard error. (Data from Visscher M, Munson K, Pickens W, et al. Changes in diapered and nondiapered infant skin over the first month of life. *Pediatr Dermatol.* 2000;17:45.[70])

Box 44.2 Common Skin Microorganisms Colonizing Newborn Skin

Micrococcaceae

- Coagulase-negative staphylococci
- Staphylococcus epidermidis
- Staphylococcus hominis
- *Staphylococcus saprophyticus* (perineum)
- *Staphylococcus capitis* (sebum-rich areas)
- *Staphylococcus auricularis* (ear canal)
- *Peptococcus* species
- *Micrococcus* species

Diphtheroids

- Corynebacterium (moist intertriginous areas)
- *Brevibacterium* (toe webs)
- *Propionibacterium* (hair follicles, sebaceous glands)

Gram-Negative Bacilli

- *Acinetobacter* (moist, intertriginous areas, perineum)
- Rarely *Klebsiella*, *Enterobacter*, *Proteus*

Yeast

- *Malassezia* species

BACTERIAL COLONIZATION AND CUTANEOUS MICROBIOME DEVELOPMENT

The paramount skin function is prevention of infection. Before birth, a fetus resides in a relatively sterile environment. Colonization of newborn skin begins on first exposure to the external world.[110,111] Human skin is the largest interface for microbiome interaction given the extensive surface area of hair follicles and eccrine ducts.[112] In adults, one cm^2 of skin (total 1.8 m^2) has one million bacteria.[113] *Actinobacteria* are the majority, with significant Gram-negative bacteria, for example, *Propionibacteria*, *Staphylococcus*, and *Corynebacteria*.[114] Box 44.2 lists the commonly cultured, clinically relevant, skin-colonizing bacteria. Epidermal barrier properties, specifically lipid composition and molecular components, impact the adult skin microbiome.[115] The skin microbiome of neonates delivered vaginally was similar to the maternal vaginal microflora while the microbiome of infants delivered by C-section was similar to maternal skin microflora.[116] Full-term skin was populated by *Lactobacillus*, *Propionibacterium*, *Streptococcus*, and *Staphylococcus* regardless of body site but differed by site 6 weeks later.[117] *Corynebacterium* and *Staphylococcus* populated the skin, similar to maternal skin and independent of delivery mode.

Skin microbiotas contribute to innate immunity in response to inflammation via the cytokine IL1α.[118] They regulate levels of antimicrobial peptides (AMPs), including β-defensins and cathelicidins, made by sebocytes and keratinocytes (Fig. 44.11). Microbes including *S. epidermidis* and *Cutibacterium* may stimulate production of other AMPs.[113] The skin barrier contains a network of 50 plasma and membrane proteins that collectively moderate inflammation and immunity upon exposure to microbes. When this network is blocked, gene expression for AMPs, proinflammatory mediators, and pattern recognition receptors decrease.[119] *S. epidermidis* and *hominis* together generate AMPs that are toxic to *S. aureus*.[120,121] IL-17$^+$CD8$^+$T cells are stimulated by *S. epidermidis* and cause keratinocytes to generate AMPs to help prevent skin infection.[122] Lipoteichoic acid from *S. epidermidis* mitigated inflammation from skin injury by preventing keratinocytes from releasing cytokines via a toll-like receptor 2 process.[123] *S. epidermidis* interfered with the formation of a biofilm by *S. aureus*.[124] Triglycerides from the sebaceous glands (sebum) are hydrolyzed to glycerin and free fatty acids by skin bacteria and yeasts.[101] Free fatty acids contribute to the SC surface pH and have antimicrobial properties.[114]

Since the skin barrier adapts after birth in full-term infants and further matures in premature infants, dynamic alterations in the skin microbiome are expected.[125] Infant skin bacterial composition and diversity are influenced by barrier properties including pH, hydration, dryness, and sebum content. The microbiome is unstable in infancy, increasing the potential for inflammation such as diaper dermatitis and vulnerability to pathogens and allergens.[126] The dry areas of buttock skin are typically colonized by Actinobacteria (*Propionibacterium* and *Corynebacterium*), Proteobacteria, Firmicutes (*Staphylococcus* spp.), and Bacteroidetes.[126] The diaper skin microbiota is impacted by intestinal tract bacteria including *Clostridium* spp. and increased *Bacteroides*.

Pammi et al. examined premature infants of 24 to 32 weeks GA over 2 weeks after birth and full-term (mean 39 weeks) infants over 4 weeks post birth.[125] Microbial richness decreased then increased in preterms but changes over time were not significant for either group. Hierarchical cluster analysis of all infants indicated Firmicutes (40%), Bacteroidetes (30%), Proteobacteria (11%), and Actinobacteria (7%) with Firmicutes being higher than Bacteroidetes in preterms and *Staphylococcus* dominating the Firmicutes. Both GA and corrected age were significantly related to operational taxonomy units (OTUs) and Shannon diversity index.

Despite the beneficial effects of *S. epidermis* on skin function, it can be pathogenic, especially in premature infants.[127,128] *Staphylococcus epidermidis* is the most common cause of nosocomial sepsis and bacterial colonization within indwelling devices such as intravenous catheters.[129-131] Virulence has been attributed to *S. epidermis* extracellular polymers (e.g., polysaccharide intercellular adhesion), enzymes (e.g., protease SepA, endopeptidase ESP, lipases GehD and GehC), toxins (e.g., phenol-soluble modulins, enterotoxins), antigens (e.g., teichoic acid), and AMP sensors.[132] Soeorg et al. compared the skin and intestinal microbiome in preterms 30 weeks GA or younger and full-terms and found different forms of *S. epidermidis* versus those in maternal breast milk.[133] Full-term subtypes became similar to

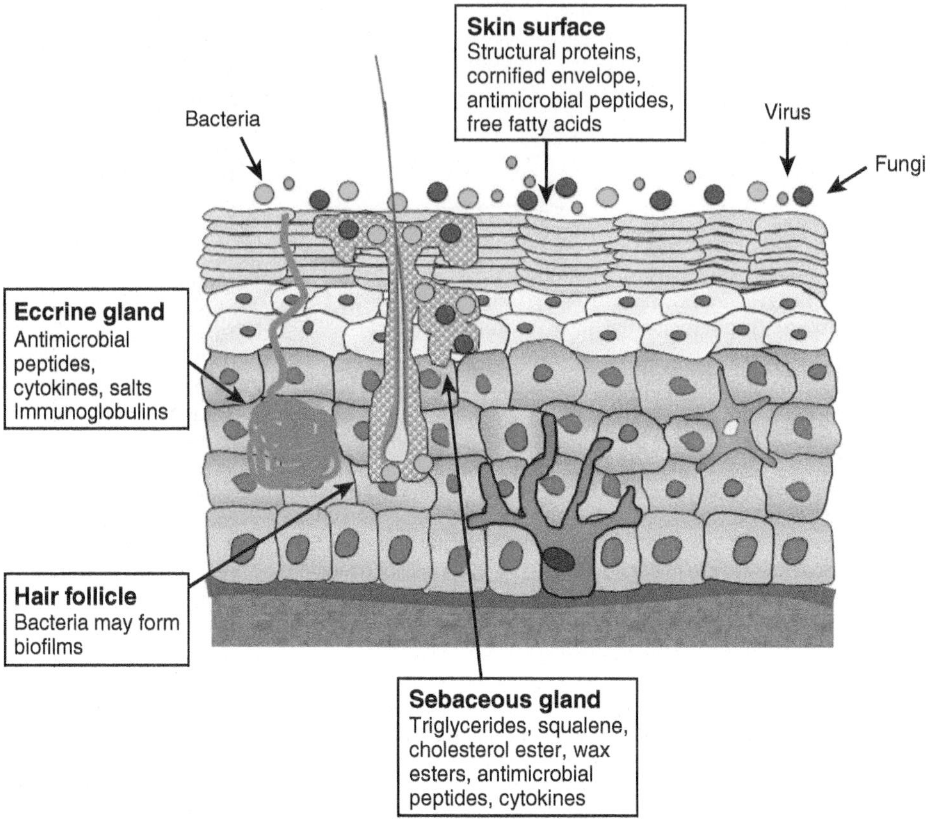

Fig. 44.11 Interactions among skin microbiota and the epidermal barrier. Various microbes, that is, bacteria, virus, fungi, colonize the skin surface, hair follicles, and eccrine glands. Certain lipids have antimicrobial properties. Microbes cause the skin to make beneficial agents including fatty acids from metabolism of triglycerides, and antimicrobial peptides. The components within the epidermis cause keratinocytes to make immune mediators and interact with other microbes to inhibit pathogenic bacteria and cause keratinocytes to make immune mediators.[113,121] (Adapted from Chen YE, Fischbach MA, Belkaid Y. Skin microbiota-host interactions. *Nature.* 2018;553:427–436.[121])

those in breast milk with time. *S. epidermidis* in preterm infants were more virulent and resistant at 1 month of life. Exploration of potential causes for the pathogenic behavior of *S. epidermidis* in premature infants suggested that exposure to chorioamnionitis resulted in monocytes that could not appropriately respond.[134]

CUTANEOUS IMMUNITY

The skin has a well-developed immune system.[111,135-137] The skin colonization mechanisms involve rapid growth of commensal organisms, acid mantle development, and local microenvironmental factors.[138] Innate immune function in term infants appears to be well developed, whereas it is poor in preterm infants.[111,139] Cutaneous immunity develops through a balance of pro- and anti-inflammatory cytokines, immune proteins, surface lipids, antigen presenting cells, and an impermeable physical barrier, the SC, which is in contact with the external environment (Fig. 44.12). The sebaceous glands secrete a mixture of squalene, triglycerides, and wax monoesters, that is, the sebum, onto the skin surface. Sapienic and lauric fatty acids are generated from triglyceride hydrolysis and both have antibacterial properties.[140] Dermcidin, an antimicrobial peptide, is produced in the eccrine sweat glands during sweating.[141] Dermcidin causes keratinocytes to secrete cytokines and chemokines, presumably to activate an immune response.[142] Differentiating keratinocytes produce human β-defensins (HBD) and cathelicidins, two classes of AMPs.[141] Their levels increase markedly with epidermal damage, for example, wounding or infection. LL37, a degradation product of cathelicidin (hCAP18), and HBD2 are associated with the lamellar body lipids in the granular layer.[143] The AMPs RNase 7, human β-defensin 3, and psoriasin are expressed in the epidermis as early as the second trimester of gestation.[144] A partial list of AMPs in human skin is given in Fig. 44.12. Cationic peptides may be elaborated in the skin with direct antimicrobial effects on the bacterial side of the cytoplasmic membrane.[145] Lysozyme and lactoferrin are two antimicrobial proteins present in newborn SC at levels 5 times higher than adults.[146] Vernix contains multiple AMPs, including lactoferrin and lysozyme.[45,147-149] Synthesis and release of skin-derived antimicrobials may be an important defense measure against fetal infections such as maternal chorioamnionitis.[150] The SC acid mantle is part of the innate immune system via regulation of enzymes required for proper desquamation.[92] The SC barrier lipids include fatty acids that provide multiple functions in the innate immune system.These components of sebum contribute to acid mantle formation and promotion of epidermal keratinocyte differentiation and hair follicle development.[151]

Keratinocytes have been reported to internalize bacteria, leading to bacterial death and containment of infection.[152,153] The epidermis also contains Langerhans cells, migratory dendritic cells associated with antigen presentation.[11,154] Their density and function within preterm epidermis have not been extensively explored.

STRATEGIES FOR EPIDERMAL BARRIER MATURATION AND REPAIR

The immature, ineffective epidermal barrier of prematurely born infants necessitates the implementation of strategies to facilitate maturation and repair of compromised skin. This section discusses several approaches.

HUMIDITY

Prematurity and infection are leading worldwide causes of neonatal morbidity and death, particularly in developing countries during the first postnatal week, when 50% to 70% of life-threatening illnesses occur.[131,155] Therapies for preventing bacterial and fungal infections assume high priority for improving neonatal outcomes.[155,156]

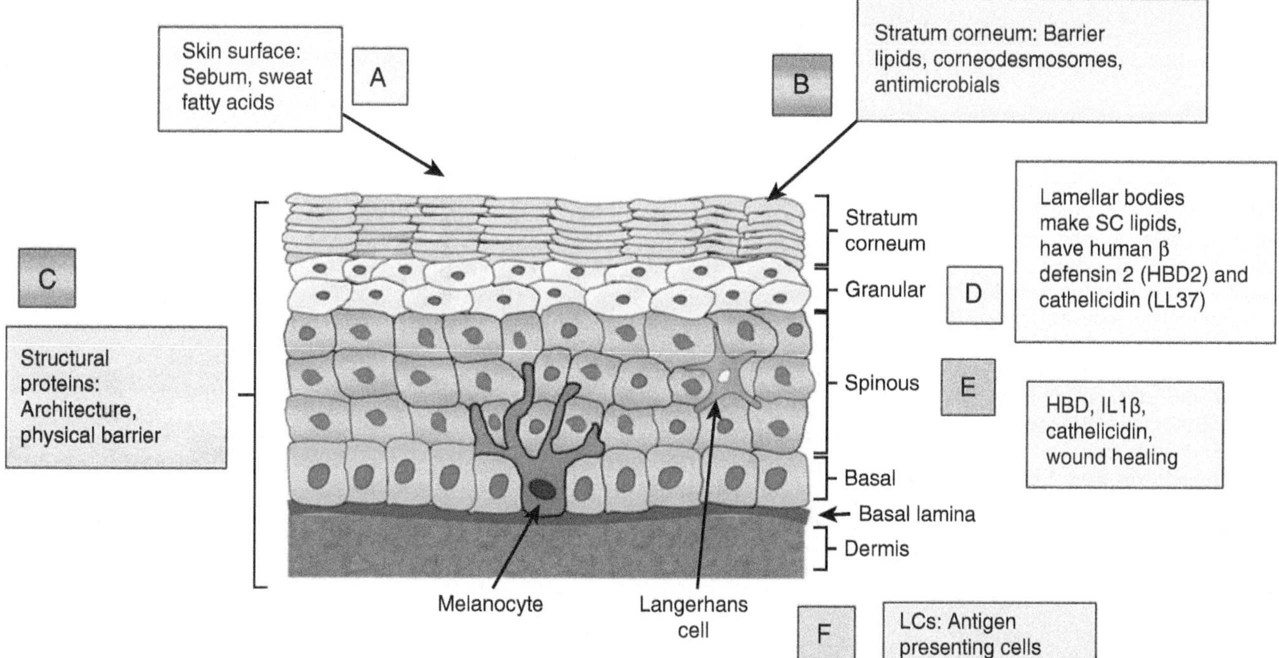

Fig. 44.12 The epidermal innate immune system. The epidermis provides innate immunity by several strategies. (A) Surface sweat, sebum, and fatty acids function as antimicrobials. (B) The stratum corneum itself provides structural integrity in the form of epidermal barrier lipids, corneodesmosomes (hold adjacent cells together), and antimicrobials lysozyme and lactoferrin. (C) Structural proteins throughout the skin form the highly structured physical barrier and include integrin (2), transglutaminases (3), desmoplakin (4), keratin 1,10 (5), involucrin (6), filaggrin (7), loricrin (8), as well as collagen in the dermis (1). (D) The lamellar bodies contain lipids that compose the *stratum corneum (SC)* lipids. (E) Differentiating keratinocytes produce cytokines and proteins that provide antimicrobial and wound repair properties. (F) The Langerhans cells *(LC)* defend the organism if the SC barrier is breached. *HBD*, Human β-defensins.

One of the earliest methods of improving outcomes was the provision of a thermal neutral environment with increased ambient humidity.[157-159] Ambient humidity is inversely related to TEWL as a function of gestational age. Increasing the convective incubator humidity lessens TEWL. However, incubators with high humidity (e.g., >80%) may experience "rain-out" with obscuration of the infant. Warm, wet environments carry increased infection risk. Radiant warming devices increase TEWL secondary to the low humidity of the overlying air and direct drying due to the effects of infrared radiation and require increased fluid replacement.[160]

The use of polyethylene films on premature infants at delivery reduced the evaporative water loss leading to better temperature stability and decreased mortality in extremely low-birth-weight infants.[161] Incubator humidity reduction is a potential strategy for facilitating skin barrier maturation. After 7 days at 85% relative humidity (RH), infants of 23 to 27 weeks GA were housed at either 75% or 50% for 3 weeks. TEWL was significantly lower for infants nursed at lower RH (day 28), that is, TEWL of 22 g/m²/h at 75% versus 13 g/m²/h at 50%.[83] Reduction from high to low humidity upregulates DNA synthesis and epidermal barrier repair,[54] a mechanism that may explain the more effective barrier at 50% RH.

TOPICAL EMOLLIENTS

Application of topical lipid-rich skin emollients has emerged as a potential strategy to enhance barrier function and thereby reduce newborn mortality.[162-164] The emollient may provide a physical barrier, provide material for active epidermal lipid metabolism, and/or reduce inflammation.[165,166] Reduction in premature infant nosocomial infections and mortality by sunflower seed oil (SSO) application in hospital settings was attributed to improved barrier function, that is, reduced SC dryness.[162-164] Infections were reduced only in the absence of skin compromise, for example, dryness.[167] However, in another trial,[168] premature infants who received SSO massage every 3 to 4 hours for 10 days had increasing TEWL from day 1 to day 11, but TEWL remained steady for the untreated infants. These results suggest that application of SSO may have delayed postnatal skin barrier maturation.

The reduction in infection with topical application of sunflower oil in the hospital setting prompted a large-scale trial of two oils, that is, either sunflower or mustard oil, for repeated routine massage among premature and full-term infants in the community setting of rural Nepal.[169] Skin pH decreased more quickly for SSO than MO in the first week, but erythema and rash worsened by day 14 then improved, with no differences between the topical treatments (Fig. 44.13).[169] Miliaria was observed with the highest frequency on day 14,[170] perhaps due to sweat duct occlusion from the oils[171] or sweating from the high temperature and humidity (mean 75% RH, similar to incubator levels used for premature infants in other settings).[172] The parent trial for the Nepal study included over 29,000 premature and full-term infants and found no effects of oil on mortality or morbidity. Taken together, the study results varied making it difficult to recommend the use of sunflower oil for enhancing skin barrier function in neonates.

Coconut oil versus no treatment in preterms resulted in lower sepsis rates, higher occurrence of intact skin, and greater time to infection.[173] Twice daily coconut oil among very premature infants produced lower skin scores versus no treatment[174] and reduced sepsis.[175] In moderately preterm infants, petrolatum application improved barrier function and reduced the rate of nosocomial infections.[176] However, a multicenter trial of twice daily petrolatum treatment (Aquaphor) versus conventional skin care in premature infants found that nosocomial blood stream infections were significantly higher in infants 501 to 750 g receiving daily emollient.[177] There was no difference in mortality. A meta-analysis of seven studies in moderately preterm infants in low-resource

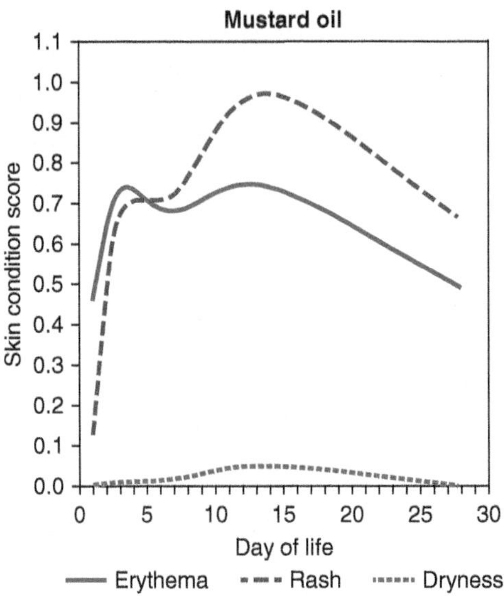

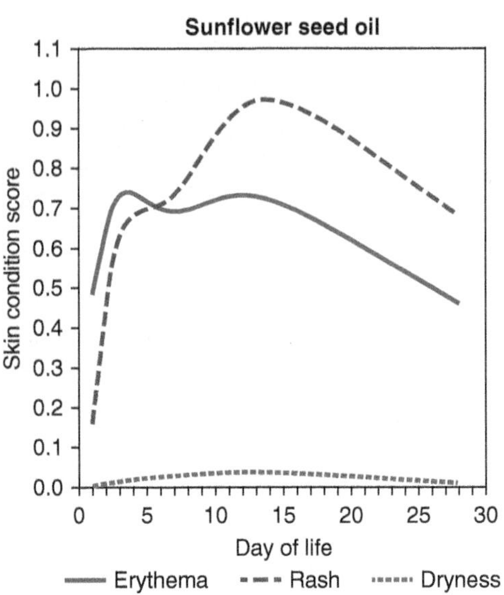

Fig. 44.13 Effect of multiple daily routine massage with topical oils on neonatal skin. A randomized controlled trial of sunflower (n = 495, *SSO*) and mustard (n = 500, *MO*) oils for routine, repeated massage in rural Nepal among premature and full-term infants showed that skin pH decreased more quickly for SSO than MO in the first week.[169] Erythema, rash, and dryness worsened over days 1 to 14 then decreased by day 28, with no oil differences.

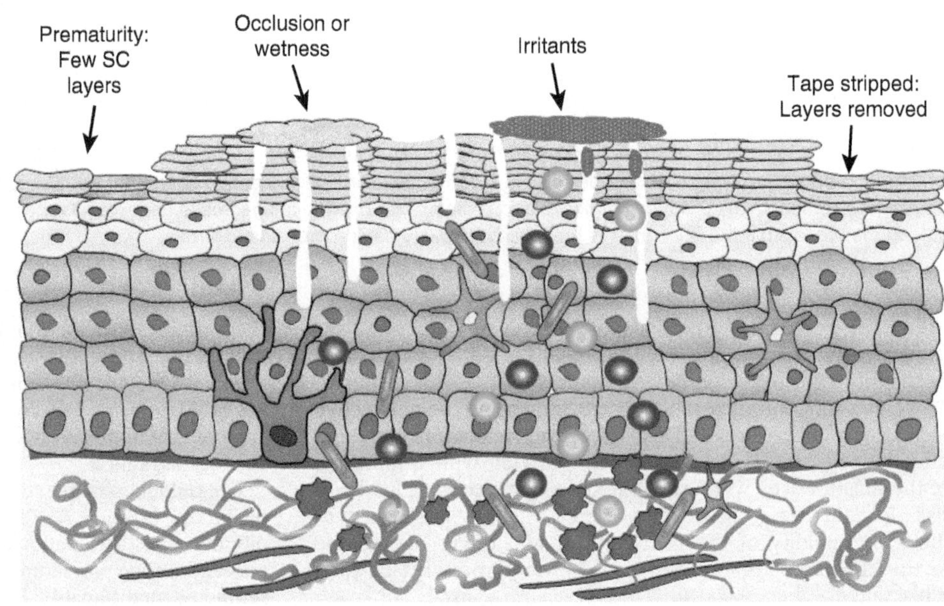

Fig. 44.14 Occlusion of the skin barrier with water-impermeable dressings, tapes, and devices allows transepidermal water to accumulate in the *stratum corneum (SC)*. This can cause disruption of the lipid bilayer structure thereby allowing topical agents, including irritants and microbes, to penetrate into the viable epidermis. Irritants cause inflammation, for example, via cytokines, and upregulation of barrier repair processes and Langerhans cell activation. Combinations of effects, such as increased hydration and exposure to fecal enzymes, can create more severe compromise and allow microbes to access the lower epidermis and dermis. Premature birth allows access to the viable epidermis because the SC is not fully formed, that is, fewer layers. Skin stripping from adhesives (dressings, tapes, electrodes) can remove all or part of the SC creating access to the tissues below.

countries concluded that topical emollients significantly reduce infection and mortality and improve weight gain.[178]

Therapeutic strategies may result from a combination of individual methods optimized for a specific infant.[15] Prenatal steroid administration coupled with optimal delivery room management and a seamless transition to a controlled neonatal intensive care unit environment using physiologic emollients and minimal adhesive injury may provide the optimal therapeutic interface between the preterm infant and the care environment. Many questions remain unanswered. Nonetheless, an attractive concept to investigate is that clothing or bedding material, in addition to wound dressings, may contain physiologic emollients and growth factors for facilitation of epidermal barrier development.

PREMATURE INFANT SKIN CARE CHALLENGES AND PRACTICES

OCCLUSION

Skin damage can occur when "topical products," including tapes, electrodes, dressings, and devices, are fully occlusive, that is, no or low water vapor permeability to normal transepidermal SC water movement (Fig. 44.14). Consequently, water that would normally bind to the upper layers and/or evaporate from the skin surface becomes trapped in the SC. Even occlusion for short periods (4 hours), as within a diaper or underneath a tape, results in water damage to the SC lipid layers and integrity to cause maceration.[32,179,180] If the damage is sufficient, materials contacting the skin surface may penetrate and cause further epidermal damage, for example, inflammation.[181] At a cellular level, hydration (water) causes corneocytes to swell, increases lipid membrane fluidity, enhances molecular transport, increases permeability to exogenous materials, and increases friction that may exacerbate mechanical damage.[182-184]

DIAPER DERMATITIS

Irritant diaper dermatitis results from multiple factors including overhydration, irritants (urine, feces, enzymes, bile salts), friction (skin-to-diaper, skin-to-skin), skin pH, diet (fecal composition), urinary frequency, gestational age (barrier maturation), antibiotic therapy, diarrhea, and medical conditions.[108,185-190] Damaged skin allows penetration of localized microflora, including *Candida albicans* and *Staphylococcus aureus*, into the epidermis.[126,191,192] β-Hemolytic *Streptococcus* species, *E. coli*, and *Bacteroides* species, *Candida tropicalis*, *C. parapsilosis*, and *C. glabrata* have also been associated with diaper dermatitis.[193] Diapered skin pH was higher than non-diapered skin.[70] Fecal enzyme (proteases, lipases) activity increased at higher pH values.[194] Higher skin pH altered the normal skin flora and increased the risk of infection by common skin species including *Staphylococcus*, *Streptococcus*, and *Candida*.[195]

The incidence of perianal dermatitis in a Level IV neonatal intensive care unit (NICU) was 28.5% among patients without neonatal abstinence syndrome (NAS) and substantially higher (86%) for NAS infants.[196] The onset, time course, and severity of diaper skin compromise, starting at birth, have not yet been described for premature infants (23 – <37 weeks GA).The effects of stool composition (e.g., pH, enzyme activity),[108,186-188,193] stool consistency, medication (e.g., antibiotics), and feeding/nutrition variables are unknown, particularly among infants younger than 29 weeks GA.

DRESSINGS AND TAPES

A protective layer of dressing, or underlying dressing with low adhesive, may be used to shield the skin from stripping when tapes are used to secure other devices, for example, endotracheal tube or central lines. Dressings should be permeable to water vapor, that is, not fully occlusive, if they are to remain in place for long periods (days). In contrast, the dressing adhesive and moisture accumulation under fully occlusive tapes can cause skin damage known as maceration. Signs of maceration are erythema and rash, indicative of inflammation. Once dressings are removed, the skin may lighten or darken, indicating post-inflammatory changes in pigmentation.

Removal of tapes and dressings can strip the skin, creating superficial wounds. A single tape strip can remove 70% to 90% of the epidermis, especially in the most premature infants, and increase skin permeabilty.[197] The extent of skin stripping varies with adhesive type. Pectin and plastic adhesive tapes created significantly higher damage than hydrogel tapes in NICU patients.[198] Silicone adhesives can be considered as they may remove significantly less skin than either hydrocolloid or acrylic adhesives.[199,200]The management of life-saving tapes and adhesives is a significant challenge in neonatology since adhesives designed to secure devices are likely to create more damage upon removal. This remains an area where innovation is essential.

ANTISEPSIS AND CHLORHEXIDINE GLUCONATE

The use of chlorhexidine gluconate (CHG) is continuously debated. Safe levels have not been established in any premature infant population. Skin compromise, including contact dermatitis and significant chemical burns have been reported, particularly in premature infants.[201] Use of CHG for umbilical cord care found higher CHG levels in preterms that increased from day 5 to 9. Among 29 premature infants, 10 (all ≤34 weeks GA) had CHG in the blood at days 5 and/or 9.[202] Infants ≥27 and <32 weeks GA had CHG blood levels of 0 to 214 ng/mL on postnatal days 0 to 28.[202-204]There were no infants of 23 to 26 weeks GA in this study. Seventy percent of infants (36 to 48 weeks) receiving biweekly CHG baths had CHG absorption of 100 ng/mL (blood) resulting in study termination by the FDA after 10 patients were treated.[205] Povidone iodine is an alternative, but thyroid dysfunction and skin compromise need to be monitored.[206] Systemic toxicity of CHG in premature infants is currently unknown and, consequently, remains a safety concern in this population.

PRESSURE INJURY, DEVICES

Pressure injuries can develop from the surface or below, particularly with repeated ischemia/reperfusion. In neonates, 80% were from devices versus 20% from conventional pressure, and device injuries occurred at younger ages.[207] Forty-two percent on neonatal CPAP developed nasal erosions.[208]

THE SKIN AS A NEURODEVELOPMENTAL INTERFACE

In all vertebrates, touch is the first sense to develop, followed closely by vestibular or position sensing.[209] Human neonates, compared with neonates of other species, are relatively helpless in motor capabilities and relatively precocious in sensory capabilities.[210] Sensory and affective information is necessary for body orientation and the spatial organization required for proper motor output. Evaluation of sensory competency is difficult; however, studies in newborn infants typically use developmental scoring systems, which rely heavily on tests of motor skills or behavior. The idea that the sensory system is precocious in early human development places the skin in a strategic location to affect subsequent development.[5,211] As an interface between the body and the environment, the skin provides a link to the developing brain, on the one hand, and to external environment (light, heat, fabrics, and the interactions of caregivers and parents), on the other hand. Neonatal animals, such as kittens and rodents, have proved to be useful models to study the effect of sensory inputs on central nervous system development.[212-216] These models clearly suggest that sensory signals are required during critical developmental windows for proper central nervous system maturation. In humans, clinical studies have demonstrated various effects of tactile stimulation during infancy. Field and colleagues showed that massage of hospitalized preterm infants results in greater weight gain, shorter length of hospital stay, and improved behavioral scores.[217]

CUTANEOUS RECEPTORS AND ELECTRICAL MATURATION

A useful concept for interpreting the functional role of the skin surface is the idea from engineering sciences of a "smart material" interface.[218]The SC has many attributes of a smart material.[5,14] It is strategically positioned as part of a larger functional system and adapts readily to changes in the environment. This material is self-cleaning, self-assembling, and possesses sensing and actuating properties putatively secondary to the piezoelectric and piezomechanical properties of the contained keratin filaments.[219] In its role as the limiting surface of the body, the SC simultaneously forms the perceived surface of the organism and the biologic boundary with the environment.

Most textbooks on neurophysiology consider sensory signal processing to be mediated initially by specialized nerve endings (Fig. 44.15). Nerve endings, however, never directly touch the environment. Interfacing with the environment is a function of the material in which the nerve endings are embedded. This perspective applies an engineering view to the material properties of the skin surface and is important for understanding innovative approaches to interactions between the skin and the central nervous system as suggested by Ansel and colleagues.[220] Thus the SC and the epidermal/dermal matrix are potential mediators of sensory signal processing.[221] After birth the physical properties of the epidermis change rapidly during adaptation to a gaseous environment. Biophysical properties of the skin can be easily measured with noninvasive instrumentation.[166,222] These properties include skin viscoelasticity, hydrophobicity, thermal conductivity, color, TEWL, and pH. In particular, study of the electrical properties of the skin may be relevant for very low-birth-weight preterm infants.[82] Table 44.5 shows the measured electrical resistance to direct current in human skin (adult) and various commonly used animal models.[223] Only newborn rats have an electrical resistance comparable with that seen in adult

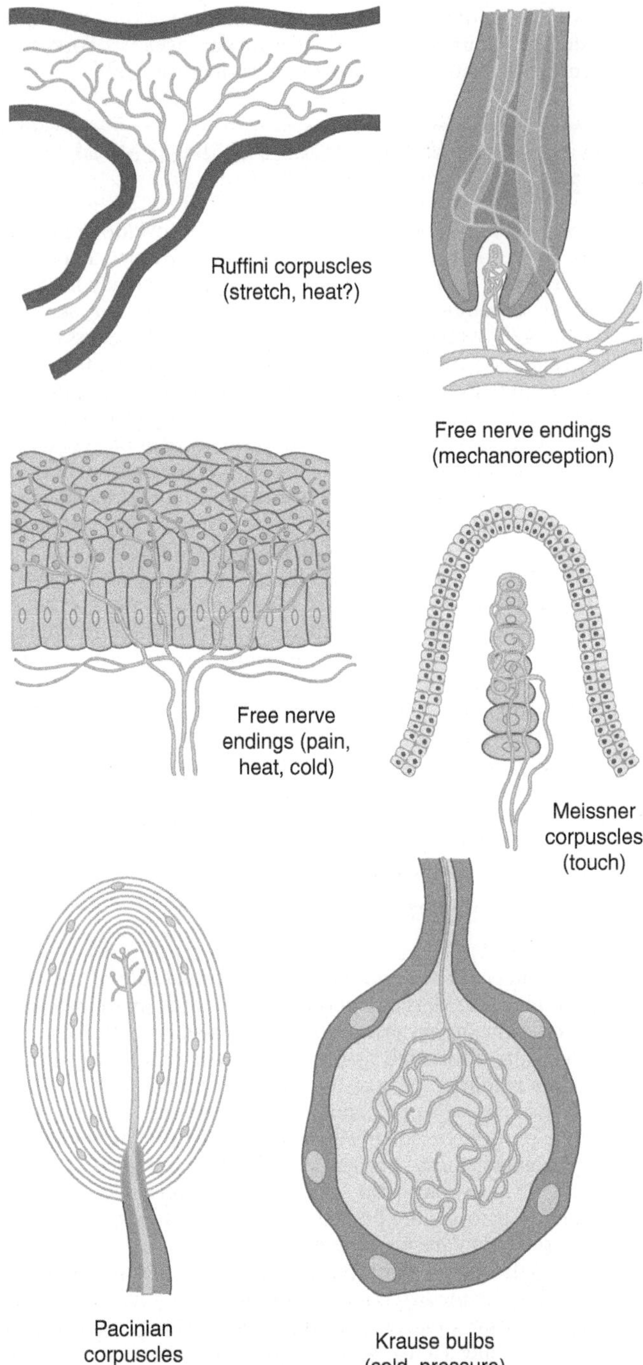

Fig. 44.15 Types of cutaneous nerve endings. Ruffini organs are deep, slowly adapting structures for stretch and/or warmth sensing. Free nerve endings are associated with crude touch, itch, pain, and temperature sensations. Krause end bulbs are particularly associated with the perception of cold. Pacinian corpuscles are deep cutaneous receptors for crude touch, pressure, and vibration on both hairy and glabrous skin. Meissner corpuscles are superficially located, rapidly adapting organs modulating light touch and vibration on primarily glabrous skin. Free sensory nerve endings are also tightly associated with hair follicles and mediate movement and mechanoreception. Of note, all nerve endings are embedded in a material biomatrix and never touch the environment. The biomatrix surrounding the nerve endings directly contacts the environment and modulates the signal received.

Table 44.5 Electrical Resistance to Direct Current in Skin.

Skin Specimens	Effective Resistance (kΩ/cm²)
Excised human skin	135 ± 54.0 (*n* = 40)
Newborn rat (day 0)	124 ± 24.2 (*n* = 18)
Infant rat (day 6)	27.7 ± 8.9 (*n* = 9)
Adult rat	28.3 ± 6.8 (*n* = 4)
Hairless mouse	9.3 ± 5.3 (*n* = 10)

Data from Shivanand P. Electrical and transport properties of neonatal rat skin. PhD thesis. Division of Research and Advanced Studies, College of Pharmacy, Cincinnati, OH: University of Cincinnati; 1995:173.[223]

humans. By contrast, the electrical resistance of the epidermal barrier in very low-birth-weight preterm infants is likely to be low owing to relative deficiency of vernix and SC.

Wakai and colleagues[224] demonstrated the development of a high electrical impedance barrier in utero during the last trimester of pregnancy. During the first half of gestation, the amplitude of the fetal electrocardiogram can be measured directly from the surface of the maternal abdomen. After 26 to 27 weeks of gestation, the amplitude gradually disappears, concomitant with the intrauterine development of an epidermal barrier consisting of vernix caseosa and the SC. Thus the gradual disappearance of the fetal electrocardiogram from the maternal skin surface is secondary to a film of high electrical impedance developing between the fetus and amniotic fluid. This process presumably reflects growing fetal autonomy with electrical isolation of the fetus from the mother.

After birth, the electrical resistance of the skin of the term newborn is relatively high.[225] Surface electrical measurements are a common form of noninvasive monitoring in NICUs. New advances, such as evoked potential testing of the brain, hold great promise for the assessment of multiple clinical conditions such as birth asphyxia.[226-229] In contrast to commonly performed electrocardiographic measurements, however, evoked potential testing of the electrical activity of the brain requires measurement of low-amplitude voltages (microvolts versus millivolts), which are greatly affected by the skin-electrode contact surface.[223] It is common practice for electrical signals to be obtained after abrasion of the skin surface with a gritty contact paste. From a practical standpoint, the field of evoked potential testing in newborns could be improved by focus on the electrode-skin interface and the development of a seamless electrical contact, which avoids wounding the skin.

SKIN AS AN INFORMATION-RICH SURFACE

Development of the immature central nervous system depends on sensory input during the immediate postnatal period. Experimental interference with several sensory modalities, such as vision, touch, and hearing, results in profound anatomic, functional, and biochemical impairment of the central nervous system structures that regulate such modalities. In newborn rats, tactile stimulation is an important regulator of somatic growth. Schanberg and colleagues[214-216,230] have studied the link between tactile stimulation and the molecular regulation of internal cellular growth-promoting enzymes, such as ornithine decarboxylase, which is a sensitive index of the maturation and growth of internal organs such as the heart, liver, and brain. Brain, liver, and heart ornithine decarboxylase levels are decreased by 35%, 81%, and 53%, respectively, when rat pups are removed from their mothers for periods as short as 1 hour. Restoration of the pups to the litters rapidly normalizes enzyme activity. This normalization is specific for touch. Other potential mediators, such as nutrition, have no effect.

Tactile stimulation of neonates influences circulating levels of lactate, an important energy substrate for brain metabolism.[212] In both newborn rats and human infants, lactate levels are high immediately after birth and decrease rapidly after the first few hours after birth.[212,231] When newborn rat pups are removed from maternal contact and receive light tactile stimulation by rostral-caudal stroking with a camel hair brush, lactate levels increase significantly and the elevations persist for up to 30 minutes after cessation of the tactile stimulus. These same stimuli fail to elicit an increase in serum lactate levels at 1 week of age. These results are noteworthy because the brain of the early suckling rat uses lactate in preference to other metabolic fuels such as glucose and 3-hydroxybutyrate.[232] Moreover, lactate levels increase without development of metabolic acidosis. This experiment demonstrates, in an animal model, that sensory interaction between the organism and the environment is a potential regulator of the availability of cerebral energy substrates. Such studies have yet to be performed in humans.

The concept that the human newborn infant is precocious in terms of sensory capabilities and relatively helpless in terms of motor capabilities[210] provides a conceptual framework to investigate the complex maturation of sensorimotor feedback loops. Preterm infants exhibit an age-dependent neurophysiologic response pattern similar to that of newborn rats insofar as the threshold for eliciting a motor response (flexor withdrawal) progressively increases with advancing gestational age.[233] This finding is usually attributed to increased inhibition of the reflex arc by central nervous system structures. The cutaneous flexor response is elicited by stimulation of the foot with nylon filaments (von Frey hairs) of graded thickness. In addition to maturation of central nervous system structures, the material properties of the interface (dermis, epidermis/SC) are changing concomitantly and may contribute to the increasing threshold for the motor response with advancing gestational age. The accessibility of the skin surface and the availability of multiple biomedical instruments for noninvasive measurement provide an open area for skin-based research in neonatology, with potential relevance for central nervous system organization and control. The concept of a smart material interface presumes that changes in the biophysical properties of the skin surface will have a direct influence on adaptive environmental interfacing and sensorimotor response loops.[217,218]

An area in which noninvasive monitoring of the skin surface may reveal important information on central nervous system response and behavioral state involves skin conductance measurements in newborn infants associated with eccrine (emotional/nonthermal) sweating.[47] Sweating is commonly viewed as secondary to the need for thermoregulation and evaporative cooling. It also occurs in response to arousal and pain, in addition to temperature. This "emotional" sweating is easily measured from the palm or sole with a skin evaporimeter[234] but is usually estimated indirectly by measurement of skin electrical conductance or resistance.[235] The presence of sweat within the eccrine ducts of the epidermis, and to a lesser extent, the circumferential hydration of the SC surrounding the sweat glands, lowers the electrical resistance of the skin and raises its electrical conductance. Instruments are available for directly, simply, and noninvasively measuring skin surface conductance at the bedside.[222,236] This technique has been widely used in psychological research but has yet to be systematically applied in neonatology.

Skin conductance increases after a painful stimulus.[235] A heel prick was administered to the foot, followed by skin conductance measurement over the sole of the other foot. Peak values are reached approximately 1 minute after the heel prick. This response is characteristic of the change in skin conductance caused by arousal in a neonate. Confirmatory measurements can also be made using different techniques, such as TEWL. Palmar water loss in crying infants varies from 25 to 41 weeks of gestational age.[47,237] Of note, the profile for palmar water loss is *inversely* related to TEWL over the same age range (see Fig. 44.5A). This inverse relationship deserves further investigation. Storm and Fremming[236,238,239] used conductance measurements of the skin surface to study behavioral state changes and developmental effects. This skin-based method, combined with sensory evoked potential testing, offers a new technique for assessment of central nervous system functioning in developing preterm infants.

Studies of epidermal barrier function may exhibit not only short-term responses secondary to autonomic nervous system activation of eccrine sweating, but also long-term consequences related to stress and glucocorticoid secretion. Denda and colleagues[240,241] showed that stressful events such as immobilization, overcrowding, and abrupt change in physical environment can result in impaired epidermal barrier function in murine skin. Similarly, Garg and colleagues[242] demonstrated a delay in recovery of epidermal barrier function after induced trauma in psychologically stressed graduate students. These studies indicate a link between physiologic stress and epidermal barrier function. A very low-birth-weight preterm infant exhibits compromised barrier function up to 28 days after delivery.[62] Whether this increased TEWL is secondary to stress-related events is unclear.

The idea of the skin as an information-rich surface can be extended to the intensive care setting.[243,244] Cardiorespiratory and thermal monitoring, as well as transcutaneous blood gas measurements, are skin-based systems of clinical data retrieval. Given the ready accessibility of the skin surface and the plethora of noninvasive measurement techniques that have yet to be applied to the study of newborn physiology,[166] it seems reasonable to assume that a number of innovative and useful skin-based sensing systems will be designed for clinical decision making in the future. This concept extends Kligman's idea of "invisible dermatology"[245] to the neonatal intensive care unit; early, objectively measured changes in the physical properties of the skin may herald illness in the term or preterm infant before such illness is apparent to the caregiver. De Felice and colleagues,[246] for example, used skin colorimetry to provide a significant quantitative predictor of illness severity in hospitalized newborns. This work supports the hypothesis that noninvasive measurements of skin physical properties directly reflect the pathophysiologic state of infants. Such measurements can be used as objective adjuncts to clinical decision making and bedside assessment.

Given the close embryologic connection of the skin and the brain, it is not surprising that there is a strong functional overlap between perception of the body surface and correlative neurobehavior. This overlap is particularly evident in the determination of gestational age. The most commonly used clinical assessment tool for determining gestational age (i.e., the Ballard score) relies on a graded, quantitative battery of physical findings and neurologic signs which en toto provide a score indicative of gestational age between 20 and 44 weeks.[247] The physical scores shown in Table 44.6 are primarily markers of cutaneous development. Best estimates of gestational age are important for prediction of clinical outcomes and as a guide for physiologic development and expectant management by the newborn caregiver.

Finally, recent advances in three-dimensional/four-dimensional fetal ultrasound imaging have resulted in an unprecedented ability to image the body surface in utero. Enhanced software capabilities add color and shadowing to reconstructed serial three-dimensional images. Four-dimensional reconstruction allows temporal visualization of fetal behavior such as yawning and response to external stimuli such as touch. This technology

Table 44.6 Determination of Gestational Age by Physical Signs.

	Maturity Score						
	−1	0	1	2	3	4	5
Skin (general)	Sticky friable transparent	Gelatinous red translucent	Smooth pink visible veins	Superficial peeling and/ or rash, few veins	Cracking pale areas, rare veins	Parchment, deep cracking, no vessels	Leathery, cracked, wrinkled
Lanugo	None	Sparse	Abundant	Thinning	Bald areas	Mostly bald	
Plantar surface	Heel-toe 40–50 mm −1, <40 mm −2	>50 mm no crease	Faint red marks	Anterior transverse crease only	Creases anterior 2/3	Creases over entire sole	
Breast	Imperceptible	Barely perceptible	Flat areola, no bud	Stippled areola, 1–2 mm bud	Raised areola, 3–4 mm bud	Full areola, 5–10 mm bud	
Eye/ear	Lids fused loosely −1, tightly −2	Lids open, pinna flat, stays folded	Slightly curved pinna; soft; slow recoil	Well-curved pinna; soft but ready recoil	Formed and firm instant recoil	Thick cartilage, ear stiff	
Genitals (male)	Scrotum flat, smooth	Scrotum empty, faint rugae	Testes in upper canal, rare rugae	Testes descending, few rugae	Testes down, good rugae	Testes pendulous, deep rugae	
Genitals (female)	Clitoris prominent and labia flat	Prominent clitoris and small labia minora	Prominent clitoris and enlarging labia minora	Labia majora and labia minora equally prominent	Labia majora large, labia minora small	Labia majora cover clitoris and labia minora	

Skin-based scores used in the Ballard examination for the determination of gestational age in premature and term infants. The physical criteria reflect developmental maturation of the skin and cutaneous appendages. When combined with neurologic signs (not shown) based primarily on regional muscle tone, the result provides a useful estimate of gestational age between 20 and 44 weeks.

Adapted from the scoring system from Ballard JL, Khoury JC, Wedig K, et al. New Ballard score, expanded to include extremely premature infants. *J Pediatr.* 1991;119(3):417–423.[247]

forms the basis for a new prenatal correlate of the postnatal Ballard score (i.e., Kurjak's antenatal neurodevelopmental test, the "KANET") for assessing normal fetal neurobehavior.[248] The physical signs of the KANET are primarily based on observation of selected neurobehavior exhibited using whole-body surface imaging with four-dimensional fetal ultrasonography (Box 44.3). These technologic advances point to a possible new frontier in fetal skin research and correlative neurobehavior.

NEWEST DEVELOPMENTS

While rapid changes occur after birth, the kinetics of neonatal epidermal maturation to a fully functional, protective barrier are largely unknown. We recently investigated skin barrier maturation and integrity as a function of GA for 61 neonates (NICU setting) and compared it to 34 adults.[249] Outcomes were measured within 5 days from birth (designated T1) and about 10 weeks later (designated T2) when the infants were of similar post-gestational ages. Total protein, protein biomarkers, and filaggrin proteolysis products were quantified from skin surface samples and TEWL, hydration, pH, and were measured.

Skin barrier integrity was greater (TEWL lower) in full-term infants versus preterms soon after birth. Visual skin scaling was greater for preterm and full-term infants versus adults at T1 and higher for full-term infants vs. adults 10 weeks later. Skin pH was lower for full-term infants versus adults at T2. Protein amounts were higher in full-term infants than preterms and adults at T1, indicating lower skin cohesion. Protein amounts were higher for all infants than adults at T2.

In full-term infants, 40 and 46 protein biomarkers were differentially expressed (upregulated) versus adults soon after birth and 10 weeks later, respectively. For preterm infants, 12 and 54 proteins were differentially expressed versus parents soon after birth and 10 weeks later. The upregulated proteins were involved in (1) processing filaggrin to form NMF, (2) protease inhibition/enzyme regulation, (3) antimicrobials, (4) keratins, (5) lipids, and (6) cathepsins. Eight proteins were downregulated in preterm infants versus full-terms soon after birth with no differences at T2, 10 weeks later.

Importantly, the neonatal epidermal barrier exhibited a markedly different array of protein biomarkers shortly after birth and 2 to 3 months later compared versus adult skin. Not surprisingly, the stratum corneum of preterm infants younger than 34 weeks GA is deficient in expression of certain biomarkers, that is, downregulated, versus full-term infants. The stratum

Box 44.3 Physical Signs of the Kurjak Antenatal Neurodevelopmental Test[248]

- Isolated head anteflexion
- Cranial sutures and head circumference
- Isolated eye blinking
- Facial alteration (grimace or tongue expulsion)
- Mouth opening (yawning or mouthing)
- Isolated hand movement
- Isolated leg movement
- Hand to face movements
- Finger movements
- Gestalt perception of general movements

These in utero assessments are scored individually and the compiled score yields a determination of neurobehavioral well-being.[248] All assessments are based on observation of the fetal body surface (i.e., skin) as determined by four-dimensional ultrasonography.[248,256–258]

Box 44.4 Aspects of the Skin as a Primary Care Interface

- Surface of interaction with soaps, surfactants, disinfectants, and bacteria
- Support for tapes and other adhesives
- Interface for bedding, clothing, and the environment
- Site of action of topical anesthetics and analgesics
- Surface for wound and ostomy care
- Barrier for transdermal drug delivery
- Site of most laboratory blood drawing
- Platform for percutaneous catheters
- Boundary for noninvasive monitoring and skin-based sensing techniques
- Medium of interaction in kangaroo care and massage therapy
- Basis for initial clinical evaluation of patient well-being (appearance)

corneum changes over time with varying patterns depending upon GA. The biomarker differences for filaggrin processing were manifested functionally, namely as increases in NMF over time regardless of GA. Many of the differentially expressed proteins are involved in late differentiation and cornification. PI3 (elafin) and other proteins upregulated inhibit various proteases, regulate enzymes, have antimicrobial properties, and process filaggrin to generate NMF and decrease skin pH. The presence of multiple antimicrobial proteins suggests redundancy in an adaptive and/or maturational defense against pathogenic bacteria. The production of higher NMF levels (than adult amounts) suggests that mechanisms for acid mantle formation, capability to respond to microbial threats, and protection against early desquamation are critical for premature and full-term infant development. This understanding of the early life epidermal barrier changes by proteomic and instrumental endpoints is key to improving neonatal skin care practices.

FUTURE DIRECTIONS AND SUMMARY

A better understanding of fetal and neonatal skin physiology and use of quantitative measures of skin structure and function is an essential goal for perinatal medicine.[52] Every patient care encounter involves the skin in some practical way (Box 44.4). Importantly, the skin as a primary patient care interface creates an opportunity for parental satisfaction and collaborative practice between nursing and medicine.[250] The dual nature of the skin as a boundary interfacing cellular and molecular domains with psychological and perceptual domains is a fundamental assumption of neurodevelopment consistent with this approach. A better understanding of skin barrier development, especially the role of the epidermal barrier and infection control, has global implications for improving infant care.[164,169,170,251]

Finally, the life-saving critical role of the epidermal barrier, the plethora of AMPs in innate immune function, and early events in neonatal sensory transduction place the epidermis, an ectodermal derivative like the brain, front and center in the translation of molecular biology to clinical bedside care.

 A complete reference list is available at www.ExpertConsult.com.

SELECT REFERENCES

6. Hoath SB, Mauro TM. Fetal Skin Development. In: Eichenfield LF, Frieden IJ, Zaenglein A, Mathes E, eds. *Neonatal and Infant Dermatology*. 3 ed. London: Sanders; 2015.
10. Holbrook KA. Structure and function of the developing human skin. In: Goldsmith L, ed. *Physiology, Biochemistry, and Molecular Biology of the Skin*. Oxford: Oxfore University Press; 1991:63-110.
13. Hoath S, Leahy D. Formation and function of the stratum corneum. In: Marks E, Leveque JL, Voegeli R, eds. *The Essential Stratum Corneum*. London: Martin Dunitz; 2002:31-40.
15. Hoath SB, Maibach H, eds. *Neonatal Skin: Structure and Function*. 2 ed. New York: Marcel Dekker; 2003:153-178.
22. Okah FA, Pickens WL, Hoath SB. Effect of prenatal steroids on skin surface hydrophobicity in the premature rat. *Pediatr Res*. 1995;37(4 Pt 1):402-408.
25. Hardman MJ, Moore L, Ferguson MW, Byrne C. Barrier formation in the human fetus is patterned. *J Invest Dermatol*. 1999;113(6):1106-1113.
26. Candi E, Schmidt R, Melino G. The cornified envelope: a model of cell death in the skin. *Nat Rev Mol Cell Biol*. 2005;6(4):328-340.
36. Hardman MJ, Sisi P, Banbury DN, Byrne C. Patterned acquisition of skin barrier function during development. *Development*. 1998;125(8):1541-1552.
38. Supp AP, Wickett RR, Swope VB, Harriger MD, Hoath SB, Boyce ST. Incubation of cultured skin substitutes in reduced humidity promotes cornification in vitro and stable engraftment in athymic mice. *Wound Repair Regen*. 1999;7(4):226-237.
43. Ran-Ressler RR, Khailova L, Arganbright KM, et al. Branched chain fatty acids reduce the incidence of necrotizing enterocolitis and alter gastrointestinal microbial ecology in a neonatal rat model. *PloS one*. 2011;6(12):e29032.
44. Akinbi HT, Narendran V, Pass AK, Markart P, Hoath SB. Host defense proteins in vernix caseosa and amniotic fluid. *Am J Obstet Gynecol*. 2004;191(6):2090-2096.
45. Visscher MO, Narendran V, Pickens WL, et al. Vernix caseosa in neonatal adaptation. *J Perinatol*. 2005;25(7):440-446.
53. Denda M, Sato J, Tsuchiya T, Elias PM, Feingold KR. Low humidity stimulates epidermal DNA synthesis and amplifies the hyperproliferative response to barrier disruption: implication for seasonal exacerbations of inflammatory dermatoses. *J Invest Dermatol*. 1998;111(5):873-878.
59. Hoeger PH, Schreiner V, Klaassen IA, Enzmann CC, Friedrichs K, Bleck O. Epidermal barrier lipids in human vernix caseosa: corresponding ceramide pattern in vernix and fetal skin. *Br J Dermatol*. 2002;146(2):194-201.
62. Agren J, Sjors G, Sedin G. Transepidermal water loss in infants born at 24 and 25 weeks of gestation. *Acta Paediatr*. 1998;87(11):1185-1190.
70. Visscher MO, Chatterjee R, Munson KA, Pickens WL, Hoath SB. Changes in diapered and nondiapered infant skin over the first month of life. *Pediatr Dermatol*. 2000;17(1):45-51.
71. Minami-Hori M, Honma M, Fujii M, et al. Developmental alterations of physical properties and components of neonatal-infantile stratum corneum of upper thighs and diaper-covered buttocks during the 1st year of life. *J Dermatol Sci*. 2014;73(1):67-73.
72. Nikolovski J, Stamatas GN, Kollias N, Wiegand BC. Barrier function and water-holding and transport properties of infant stratum corneum are different from adult and continue to develop through the first year of life. *J Invest Dermatol*. 2008;128(7):1728-1736.
77. Rutter N. Clinical consequences of an immature barrier. *Semin Neonatol*. 2000;5(4):281-287.
81. Kalia YN, Nonato LB, Lund CH, Guy RH. Development of skin barrier function in premature infants. *J Invest Dermatol*. 1998;111(2):320-326.
82. Okah FA, Wickett RR, Pickens WL, Hoath SB. Surface electrical capacitance as a noninvasive bedside measure of epidermal barrier maturation in the newborn infant. *Pediatrics*. 1995;96(4 Pt 1):688-692.
83. Agren J, Sjors G, Sedin G. Ambient humidity influences the rate of skin barrier maturation in extremely preterm infants. *J Pediatr*. 2006;148(5):613-617.
84. Narendran V, Visscher MO, Abril I, Hendrix SW, Hoath SB. Biomarkers of epidermal innate immunity in premature and full-term infants. *Pediatr Res*. 2010;67(4):382-386.
89. Scott IR, Harding CR. Filaggrin breakdown to water binding compounds during development of the rat stratum corneum is controlled by the water activity of the environment. *Dev Biol*. 1986;115(1):84-92.
90. Elias PM. The how, why and clinical importance of stratum corneum acidification. *Exp Dermatol*. 2017;26(11):999-1003.
98. Elias PM. The skin barrier as an innate immune element. *Semin Immunopathol*. 2007;29(1):3-14.
102. Hoeger PH, Enzmann CC. Skin physiology of the neonate and young infant: a prospective study of functional skin parameters during early infancy. *Pediatr Dermatol*. 2002;19(3):256-262.
104. McAleer MA, Jakasa I, Raj N, et al. Early-life regional and temporal variation in filaggrin-derived natural moisturizing factor, filaggrin-processing enzyme activity, corneocyte phenotypes and plasmin activity: implications for atopic dermatitis. *Br J Dermatol*. 2018;179(2):431-441.
105. Visscher MO, Barai N, LaRuffa AA, Pickens WL, Narendran V, Hoath SB. Epidermal barrier treatments based on vernix caseosa. *Skin Pharmacol Physiol*. 2011;24(6):322-329.
106. Green M, Carol B, Behrendt H. Physiologic skin pH patterns in infants of low birth weight. The onset of surface acidification. *Am J Dis Child*. 1968;115(1):9-16.
107. Fox C, Nelson D, Wareham J. The timing of skin acidification in very low birth weight infants. *J Perinatol*. 1998;18(4):272-275.
113. Belkaid Y, Segre JA. Dialogue between skin microbiota and immunity. *Science*. 2014;346(6212):954-959.

115. Baurecht H, Ruhlemann MC, Rodriguez E, et al. Epidermal lipid composition, barrier integrity, and eczematous inflammation are associated with skin microbiome configuration. *J Allergy Clin Immunol.* 2018;141(5):1668-1676. e1616.
121. Chen YE, Fischbach MA, Belkaid Y. Skin microbiota-host interactions. *Nature.* 2018;553(7689):427-436.
122. Naik S, Bouladoux N, Linehan JL, et al. Commensal-dendritic-cell interaction specifies a unique protective skin immune signature. *Nature.* 2015;520(7545):104-108.
125. Pammi M, O'Brien JL, Ajami NJ, Wong MC, Versalovic J, Petrosino JF. Development of the cutaneous microbiome in the preterm infant: A prospective longitudinal study. *PloS one.* 2017;12(4):e0176669.
140. Drake DR, Brogden KA, Dawson DV, Wertz PW. Thematic review series: skin lipids. Antimicrobial lipids at the skin surface. *J Lipid Res.* 2008;49(1):4-11.
146. Walker VP, Akinbi HT, Meinzen-Derr J, Narendran V, Visscher M, Hoath SB. Host defense proteins on the surface of neonatal skin: implications for innate immunity. *J Pediatr.* 2008;152(6):777-781.
164. Darmstadt GL, Saha SK, Ahmed AS, et al. Effect of topical treatment with skin barrier-enhancing emollients on nosocomial infections in preterm infants in Bangladesh: a randomised controlled trial. *Lancet.* 2005;365(9464):1039-1045.
169. Summers A, Visscher MO, Khatry SK, et al. Impact of sunflower seed oil versus mustard seed oil on skin barrier function in newborns: a community-based, cluster-randomized trial. *BMC Pediatr.* 2019;19(1):512.
176. Nopper AJ, Horii KA, Sookdeo-Drost S, et al. Topical ointment therapy benefits premature infants. *J Pediatr.* 1996;128(5 Pt 1):660-669.
188. Berg RW, Buckingham KW, Stewart RL. Etiologic factors in diaper dermatitis: the role of urine. *Pediatr Dermatol.* 1986;3(2):102-106.
197. Hoath S, Narendran V. Adhesives and emollients in newborn care. *Seminars in Neonatology.* 2000;5:289-296.
210. Brazelton T. Behavioral competence. In: Avery G, Fletcher M, MacDonald M, eds. *Neonatology: pathophysiology and management of the newborn.* Philadelphia: JB Lippincott; 1994:289-300.
211. Hoath S. The skin as a neurodevelopmental interface. *NeoReviews.* 2001;2(12):e292-e301.
249. Visscher MO, Carr AN, Winget J, et al. Biomarkers of neonatal skin barrier adaptation reveal substantial differences compared to adult skin. *Ped Res.* 2020;89(5):1208-1215.

Cardiovascular Development 45

Maurice J.B. van den Hoff | Andy Wessels

INTRODUCTION

The formation and subsequent development of the heart is a complex process that involves multiple cell populations, a plethora of molecular regulatory mechanisms, and intrinsic, complicated spatiotemporal remodeling events. When all the developmental steps have been properly concluded, the fully septated four-chambered heart will beat a few billion times during the individual's life span, thereby sustaining three interdependent blood circulations (systemic, pulmonary, and coronary). Although this chapter can only scratch the surface of all the aspects associated with the formation of the cardiovascular system, we believe that it provides relevant insights into the most important events in that system's development.

DEVELOPMENT OF THE HEART-FORMING REGION

Cardiovascular development about 3 weeks after ovulation (or at 3 weeks of development)[a] when, during the process of gastrulation, the three germ layers (ectoderm, mesoderm, and endoderm) become established. During this process, cells from the embryonic epiblast undergo epithelial-to-mesenchymal transformation (EMT) and migrate to the primitive streak, a visible groove that begins at the caudal end of the embryo and extends cranially. The mesenchymal cells enter the streak uncommitted as to their developmental potential but become committed to their mesodermal phenotype and migratory pathways after leaving the primitive streak. Once this process has been completed, the mesoderm occupies the space between the ectoderm and the endoderm. A part of the mesoderm is induced by the hypoblast and endoderm to enter the precardiac lineage. This involves molecular signaling by, for instance, the Wnt/β-catenin, fibroblast growth factor (FGF), bone morphogenetic protein (BMP), and activin/nodal signaling pathways.[1] The mesoderm differentiates into the chorda and the paraxial, intermediate, and lateral plate mesoderm. Two precardial mesodermal cell population contributing to the formation of the primitive heart tube are located laterally in the embryo and are referred to as the heart-forming regions.[2] As a result of the formation of the intraembryonic coelomic cavity, the lateral plate mesoderm splits into two layers: a splanchnic layer, located directly above the endoderm, and a somatic layer, found directly below the ectoderm. The region of splanchnic mesoderm expressing precardiac markers is now known as the *first heart field (FHF)*.[3] Molecular markers used to identify the precardiac mesoderm include the transcription factors ISL1, NKX2.5, MEF2C, HAND1, HAND2, GATA4, and TBX5.[4–8]

With folding of the embryo, the two heart-forming regions meet anterior to the developing head region, thereby forming a horseshoe-shaped structure. Continuation of the fusion process in an anteroposterior direction brings the left and right legs of the horseshoe together along the embryonic midline (Fig. 45.1A–C).

FORMATION OF THE TUBULAR HEART

As the heart fields are fusing, a subset of the precardiac mesodermal cells undergo EMT. The mesenchymal cells differentiate into endocardial cells, which then form a network of tiny channels that remodel into a single endocardial channel with ongoing folding. Concomitantly, this endocardial tube becomes surrounded by a mantle of cardiomyocytes, which express characteristic sarcomeric proteins such as atrial and ventricular myosin heavy chain and cardiac troponin. Between the endocardial and myocardial layers an acellular, extracellular matrix (ECM)–rich substance known as *the cardiac jelly* is accumulating. Together, these three components form the linear primary heart tube.

The cardiomyocytes of the tubular heart do not proliferate. The heart tube grows and increases in length primarily by the addition of newly differentiated cardiomyocytes to both the anterior and posterior pole of the heart tube. The mesodermal cells that are added to the lengthening tube are referred to as the anterior or second heart field (AHF/SHF).[9–11] Molecular markers for the SHF include the transcription factors TBX1, ISL1, FGF8, and FGF10. It is beyond the scope of this chapter to discuss in detail the importance of the FHF and SHF in the development of each single structure of the heart. Suffice it to note that numerous cell fate studies have established that, as far as the myocardial components are concerned, the FHF contributes mainly to the left ventricle and most of the myocardial tissues of the left and right atria. The SHF contributes mainly to the outflow tract (OFT), the right ventricle, the ventricular septum, and the dorsal mesenchymal protrusion (DMP) at the venous pole of the heart (Fig. 45.2).[12–14]

FORMATION AND GROWTH OF THE TUBULAR HEART

After its initial formation, the tubular heart is initially tethered over its entire length to the rest of the embryo by the dorsal mesocardium. As the heart tube starts to lengthen and loop, the dorsal mesocardium disintegrates in its center portion, leaving the heart attached to the rest of the embryo by its

[a]For consistency with the embryology literature, weeks of development (postovulatory age) is used throughout this chapter, rather than postmenstrual or gestational age.

arterial and venous poles. This partial disintegration of the dorsal mesocardium is crucial, as it enables the process of cardiac looping during lengthening of the tube (Fig. 45.3).

Cardiac looping is a somewhat ill-defined term that refers in the most general sense to the bending of the heart tube before septation.[15,16] The initial bend results in a C-shaped structure, with the outer loop of the C positioned to the right side of the embryo (see Fig. 45.1D and E). Within the C-shaped heart, inner and outer curvatures can be distinguished. As the heart continues to remodel, the myocardium of the outer curvature differentiates and starts to proliferate. From this myocardium, the primitive left and right ventricles emerge—a process that has been described as *ballooning*.[17] It is noteworthy that each ventricle has its own molecular identity. Much of the patterning of the primitive and ventricular myocardial molecular identities is linked to the expression of T-box gene family members such as *TBX1, TBX2, TBX3, TBX5,* and *TBX20*.[18-23] At the junction between the developing ventricles and atria, the atrioventricular (AV) myocardium maintains its "primitive" molecular characteristics. In addition, the right AV junctional myocardium has additional molecular features that are associated with the development of the AV conduction system. As the heart continues to grow, its shape changes significantly and becomes more complex. Once it has assumed an S shape (see Fig. 45.1E), the respective compartments of the heart more or less assume their final position in relation to each other, even though all compartments are essentially still connected in series as one long tube. It is at this stage that the atria start to appear at the venous pole.

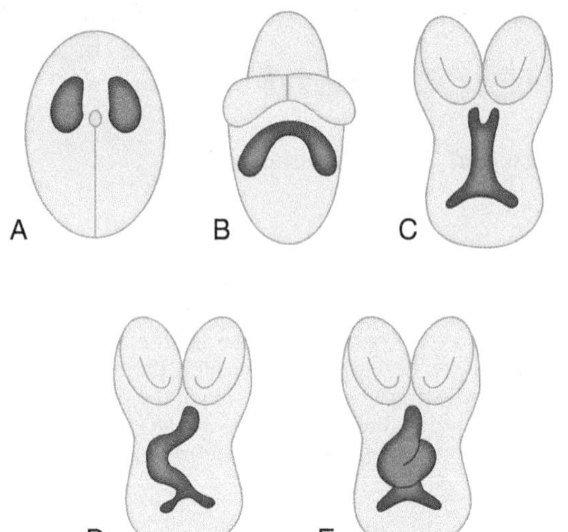

Fig. 45.1 The early stages of heart development. This figure shows in simplified cartoons five crucial stages in early heart development. (A) Bilateral heart fields form from precardiac mesoderm after migration from the primitive streak. (B) The cardiac crescent is formed after fusion of the heart fields at the cranial end of the embryo. (C) The linear heart tube is formed from fusion of the cardiac crescent in a cranial-to-caudal direction. (D) Elongation of the heart tube and regression of the dorsal mesocardium results in the formation of a C-shaped structure and permits further looping. (E) The S-shaped primitive heart formed on the completion of looping. (Modified from Snarr BS, Kern CB, Wessels A. Origin and fate of cardiac mesenchyme. *Dev Dyn*. 2008;237:2804–2819.)

LEFT-RIGHT DETERMINATION

Left-right (L/R) axis determination is a critical element in vertebrate body design.[24] As is the case with most internal organs (e.g., liver, lungs, stomach), the cardiovascular system shows distinct L/R asymmetry. For instance, the pulmonary veins (PuVs) enter the left atrium, whereas the systemic veins enter the right atrium. The absence of correct establishment of the L/R axis typically results in complex abnormalities, as seen in patients with heterotaxy syndromes.[25-27] The hearts of patients in which L/R laterality has been developmentally perturbed typically show severe abnormalities in atrial, AV, and OFT morphology. The ventricular chambers are typically less severely affected.[28,29]

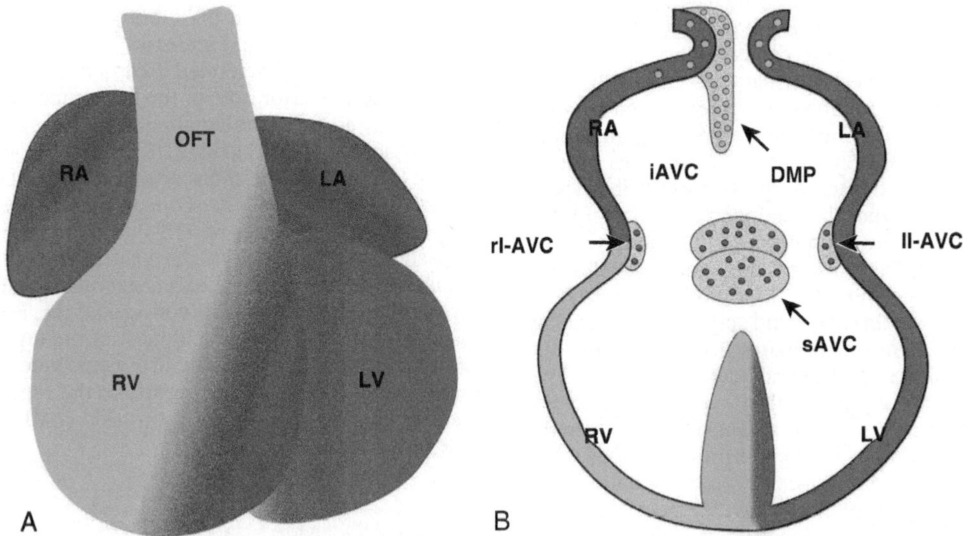

Fig. 45.2 Contribution of the first and second heart fields to the developing heart. This figure shows schematically the contribution of the first heart field (FHF, *red*) and second heart field (SHF, *green*) to the respective components of the developing heart. (A) After looping has completed, the FHF contributes primarily to both atria and the left ventricle. (B) In a four-chamber cross-sectional view of the heart, the contribution of the SHF to the right ventricle, the ventricular septum, and the dorsal mesocardium is highlighted. Note that the mesenchyme of the respective atrioventricular cushions is derived from the FHF. *DMP*, Dorsal mesenchymal protrusion; *iAVC*, inferior atrioventricular cushion; *LA*, left atrium; *ll-AVC*, left lateral atrioventricular cushion; *LV*, left ventricle; *OFT*, outflow tract; *RA*, right atrium; *rl-AVC*, right lateral atrioventricular cushion; *RV*, right ventricle; *sAVC*, superior atrioventricular cushion.

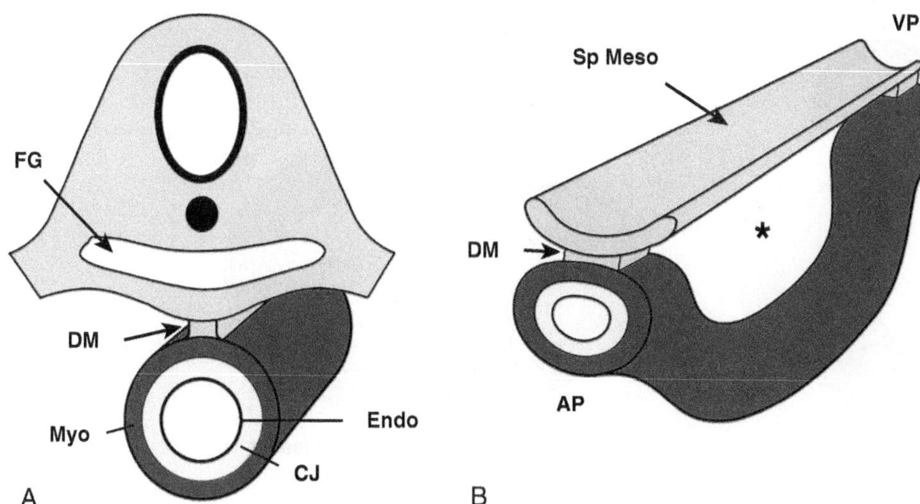

Fig. 45.3 Involvement of the dorsal mesocardium in heart development. (A) The heart tube is suspended along its length from the embryo by the dorsal mesocardium *(DM)*. (B) After regression of the DM along the midsection *(asterisk)*, the heart tube remains connected to the embryo by the arterial pole *(AP)* and venous pole *(VP)* attachments of the DM. The DM is continuous with the splanchnic mesoderm *(Sp Meso)*, which lies ventral to the foregut *(FG)*. *CJ*, Cardiac jelly; *Endo*, endocardium; *Myo*, myocardium. (Modified from Snarr BS, Kern CB, Wessels A. Origin and fate of cardiac mesenchyme. *Dev Dyn*. 2008;237:2804–2819.)

Laterality becomes established very early in embryonic development. Studies to determine the underlying mechanisms have historically been conducted on animal models. Experiments in mouse embryos have shown that the oriented motion of cilia on cells in the Hensen node,[30] located at the cranial tip of the primitive streak, is critical in determining the L/R axis.[31] FGF is an important factor in this process, as it plays a role in ciliary growth.[32] The ciliary activity leads to asymmetric calcium transients[33] and asymmetric expression of laterality genes, including nodal, sonic hedgehog, lefty,[34-36] and the homeodomain transcription factor PITX2C.[37,38] As is true in general for developmental processes, most of the molecules involved in determining L/R signaling play a role across different species. Interestingly, in an intriguing twist on that theme, some of the molecules required for left sidedness in mice are determinants of right sidedness in birds.[39] Many of the genes that have been found to control L/R determination in animal models are candidate genes involved in the pathogenesis of heterotaxy syndromes.[36]

The anteroposterior (craniocaudal) body axis is also established during gastrulation. Retinoid signaling pathways are critical to normal anteroposterior axial patterning in general and for cardiac development in particular.[39,40] Furthermore, retinoids are also implicated in the regulation of SHF differentiation.[41] Failure of formation of atrial chambers and the systemic venous connections with the heart is observed in conditions of retinoid deficiency. Excess retinoids create cardiac malformations, often involving the OFT, and result in the ventricular expression of several genes that are normally largely restricted to the atria at the equivalent stages of normal development.[42,43]

DEVELOPMENT OF THE ATRIOVENTRICULAR VALVES

The formation of the AV valves is critically dependent on the proper development of their precursors, the AV cushions. During cardiac looping, the accumulation of cardiac jelly in the subendocardial space between the endocardium and myocardium at the AV junction leads to the formation of the two initially acellular ECM-rich major AV cushions. The inferior AV cushion (iAVC) is attached to the dorsal wall of the AV canal, whereas the superior AV cushion (sAVC) is attached to the ventral wall. After their initial development, the cushions become populated by cells derived from an endocardial-to-mesenchymal transformation (endMT) of the endocardial lining, a process in which cells delaminate from the endocardium and migrate as mesenchymal cells into the cardiac jelly.[40] The process of EMT in the major AV cushions has been thoroughly studied, and much is known about the molecular mechanisms regulating this process. Key molecular players include TGFβ2, BMP2, and Notch.[41-43] Later in development, two smaller cushions emerge on the wall of the AV canal between the major cushions. These are known as the right and left lateral AV cushions (Fig. 45.4A). Like the major AV cushions, they also initially become populated by endocardially derived cells (ENDCs), but studies have shown that after this initial migration of ENDCs into the cushions, significant numbers of epicardially derived cells (EPDCs) start to populate the lateral AV cushions (Fig. 45.5).[44] As the major cushions fuse, they separate the common AV canal into left and right AV canals. The mitral and tricuspid valves will develop in these orifices. Each AV cushion plays a specific role in valve formation (see Fig. 45.4B). The fused major cushions contribute to the valve leaflets that are attached to the ventricular septum, whereas the lateral AV cushions give rise to the leaflets that are attached to the left and right ventricular free wall.[45-47] In the human, the tricuspid valve begins to form around the fifth week of development. The AV cushions are actively reconfiguring at this time. Despite the overall advanced stage of cardiac morphogenesis at this point, the leaflets are still very primitive in appearance and not freely mobile. The inferior leaflet is fully delaminated by the end of the 8th week of development, the anterior leaflet by the 11th week, and the septal leaflet in the 12th week. The commissure separating the anterior and septal leaflets is not complete until the septal leaflet is fully delaminated.[48] Proper development of the mitral valve is dependent on the fusion of the inferior and sAVC and the formation of the left lateral cushion, which is the precursor to the posterior or mural leaflet; it is visible by the 7th week of development. At about this time, initial delamination of the mitral valve structures becomes detectable and continues until the 10th week. Between the 10th and 14th weeks of development, myocardial elements of the leaflets are eliminated by apoptosis. Furthermore, to support the function of the mitral valve leaflets, two mitral papillary muscles evolve at approximately 5 weeks of development from an enlarged trabecular complex. With the formation of a free motile valve leaflet, the papillary muscles also achieve their adult appearance, with chordae tendineae connecting the valve leaflets with the tip of the papillary muscle.[46] Molecularly, a pathway linking FGF4 signaling to the expression of scleraxis and transcriptional activation of tenascin has been described in chick limb tendon[49] and is proposed to be active in the normal formation of chordae tendineae.[50-52] With subsequent development, the valve leaflets further mature and become organized in three layers: atrialis, spongiosa, and fibrosa. Each layer comprises specific ECM compositions and valve interstitial cells that are essential for proper function of the leaflets.

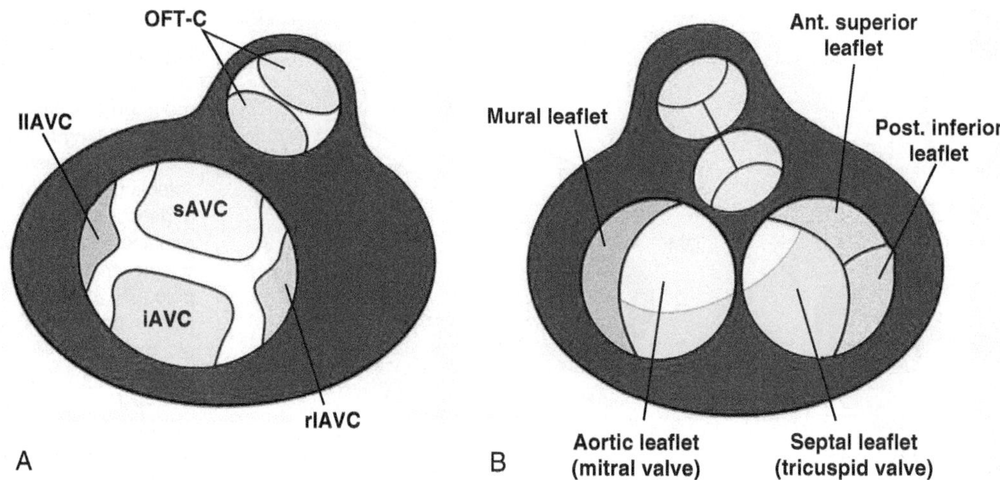

Fig. 45.4 Fate map of the atrioventricular (AV) and outflow endocardial cushions. (A) The major AV cushions consist of the superior AV cushion *(sAVC)* and the inferior AV cushion *(iAVC)*. (B) The sAVC predominantly gives rise to the aortic leaflet of the mitral valve, whereas the iAVC gives rise to the septal leaflet of the tricuspid valve. The right lateral AV cushion *(rlAVC)* contributes to the anterosuperior and posteroinferior leaflets of the tricuspid valve. The left lateral AV cushion *(llAVC)* contributes to the mural leaflet of the mitral valve. The outflow tract cushions *(OFT-Cs)* give rise to the semilunar valves. *Ant.*, Anterior; *Post.*, posterior. (Modified from Snarr BS, Kern CB, Wessels A. Origin and fate of cardiac mesenchyme. *Dev Dyn.* 2008;237:2804–2819.)

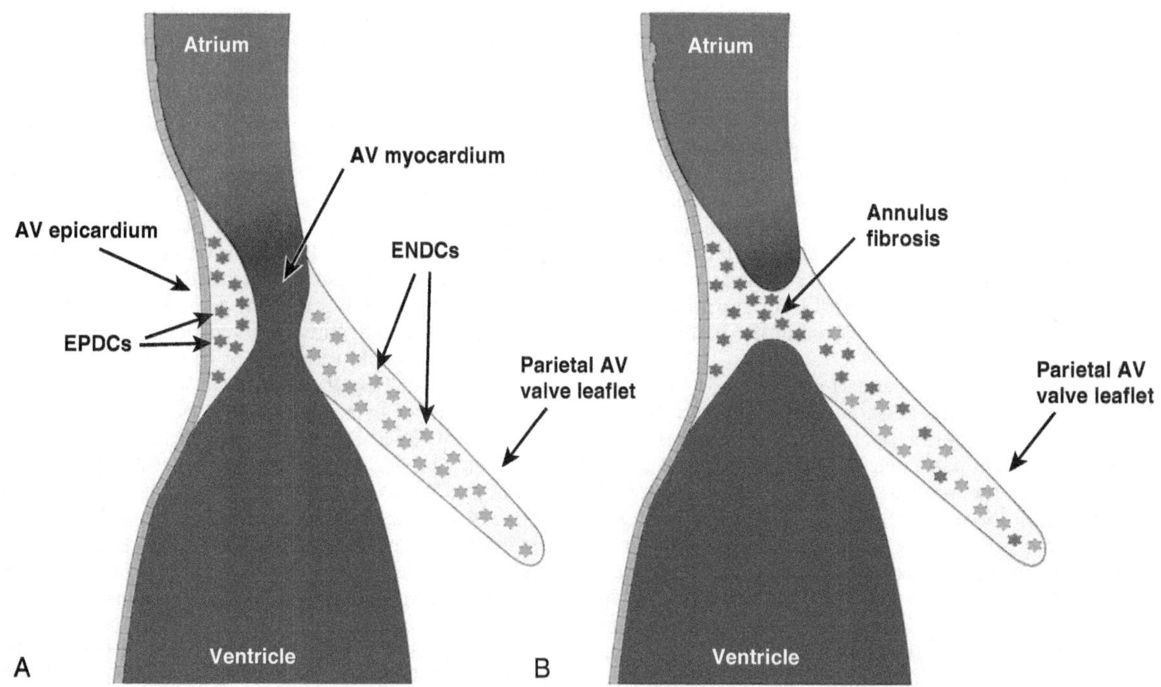

Fig. 45.5 Role of the epicardium in the development of the atrioventricular junction. (A) In early stages of development, atrial and ventricular myocardia are in continuity through the atrioventricular *(AV)* myocardium. In the AV groove, epicardially derived cells *(EPDCs)* are accumulating, whereas the developing AV valve leaflets are being populated by endocardially derived cells *(ENDCs)*. (B) At later stages of development, the EPDCs penetrate the AV junctional myocardium, establish the annulus fibrosus, and populate the parietal AV valve leaflets. (From Lockhart MM, Phelps AL, van den Hoff MJB, et al. The epicardium and the development of the atrioventricular junction in the murine heart. *J Dev Biol.* 2014;2:1–17)

SEPTATION OF THE CARDIAC CHAMBERS

Proper septation of the left and right chambers of the postnatal heart is essential for keeping separate the deoxygenated blood in the right part of the heart (RA and RV) from the oxygenated blood in the left part (LA and LV). In this process, the AV mesenchymal complex (AVMC) plays a crucial role (Fig. 45.6). The AVMC is composed of the mesenchymal tissues of the AV cushions, the mesenchymal cap on the leading edge of the primary atrial septum (pAS), and the DMP. Earlier, the development of the AV cushions was described. The mesenchyme of the atrial septal cap (ASC) is just like that of the AV cushions derived from an endMT. Compared with the development of the cushions, very little work has been done on the development of this structure; hence little is known about the mechanisms that regulate this process. The third critical component of the AVMC is the DMP. The DMP is a mesenchymal structure that derives from the SHF[14] and gains access to the atrial cavity using the dorsal mesocardium at the venous pole as its portal of entry (at about the level of the lung buds).

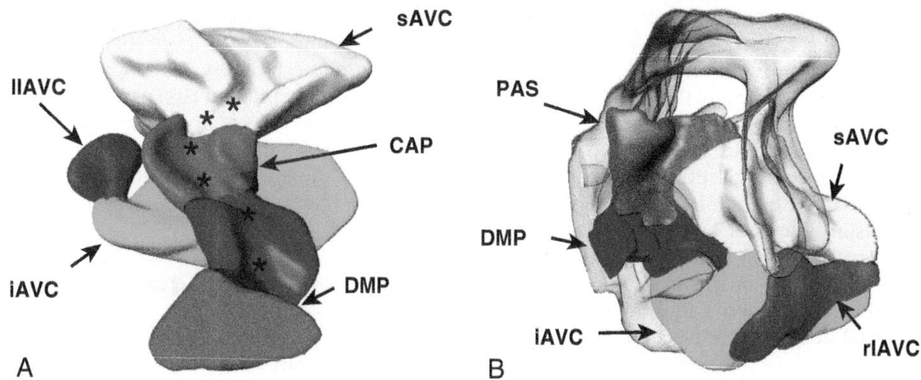

Fig. 45.6 The atrioventricular mesenchymal complex. The contribution of the respective components of the atrioventricular mesenchymal complex is best demonstrated by three-dimensional reconstruction of these tissues at different stages of development. (A) A three-dimensional rendering showing a dorsal view of the dorsal mesenchymal protrusion (DMP, *blue*) and the other components of the AVMC at embryonic day 11.5 in the mouse. The *asterisks* in A indicate where the myocardial part of the primary atrial septum (which was not included in this reconstruction) is located. (B) The atrioventricular mesenchymal tissues at embryonic day 13. At this stage, the mesenchymal tissues have fused and the mesenchymal cap on the primary atrial septum cannot any longer be recognized at a separate entity. *CAP*, Mesenchymal cap on the primary atrial septum; *DMP*, dorsal mesenchymal protrusion; *iAVC*, inferior atrioventricular cushion; *ll-AVC*, left lateral atrioventricular cushion; *PAS*, primary atrial septum; *rl-AVC*, right lateral atrioventricular cushion; *sAVC*, superior atrioventricular cushion

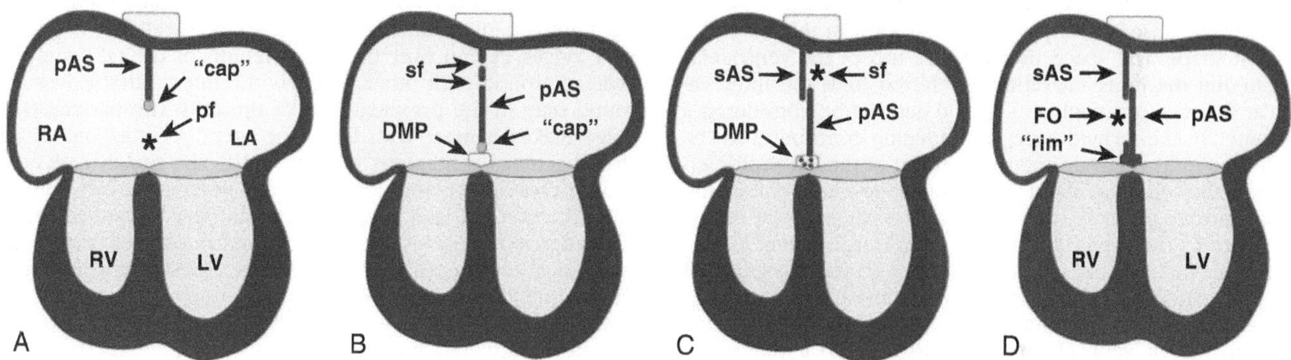

Fig. 45.7 Atrial septation. This figure illustrates the different phases in the development of the atrial septal complex. (A) The first step in this process is the formation of the primary atrial septum *(pAS)* with a mesenchymal cap *(green)* on its leading edge. (B) Fusion of the pAS and associated dorsal mesenchymal protrusion (*DMP*, *yellow*) with the atrioventricular cushions closing the primary foramen *(pf)* between the left and right atria (*LA* and *RA*). At this stage, the secondary foramen *(sf)* appears in the upper part of the pAS. (C) The secondary atrial septum *(sAS)* is forming in the roof of the RA and is closing off the secondary foramen. The DMP derived from the second heart field is undergoing myocardial differentiation. (D) The muscularized DMP has developed into the base of the atrial septum and formed the muscular rim. *FO*, Foramen ovale; *LV*, left ventricle; *RV*, right ventricle. (From Burns T, Yang Y, Hiriart E, et al. The dorsal mesenchymal protrusion and the pathogenesis of atrioventricular septal defects. *J Cardiovasc Dev Dis*. 2016;3:29)

ATRIAL SEPTATION

In the initial phase of atrial development, there is no separation between the future left and right atria. Atrial septation is the process that leads to the physical and functional separation of both chambers. Atrial separation is characterized by a series of complicated interrelated spatiotemporal events (Fig. 45.7).[53] The first step in this process is the formation of the pAS (or septum primum), which emerges from the atrial roof as a myocardial sheath resulting from directed myocardial proliferation (see Fig. 45.7A). Based on cell-fate tracing, at least part of the myocardial septum appears to be derived from the SHF. On the leading edge of the pAS is located the mesenchymal ASC. The development of the pAS is intrinsically related to the development of the DMP. As the DMP develops, it is contiguous with the ASC and the iAVC.[54] Proper fusion of the major AV cushions, the ASC, and the DMP leads to the formation of the AVMC and results in closure of the primary interatrial foramen (or foramen primum).[54,55] In contrast to its endocardially derived counterparts, the DMP eventually undergoes a mesenchymal-to-myocardial differentiation, thereby forming the myocardial base of the septum primum.[1] The importance of the DMP in cardiac septation is demonstrated by studies showing that abnormal DMP development is associated with the pathogenesis of atrioventricular septal defects (AVSDs).[13,14,55-60]

As the primary interatrial foramen is closing, a second communication between the left and right atria is created when the secondary interatrial foramen (or foramen secundum) forms in the body of the pAS close to the atrial roof (see Fig. 45.7B). In humans, this process is initiated by the appearance of small fenestrations that increase in number and size until they coalesce into a definitive secondary foramen (the foramen secundum, also known as the *fossa ovalis* or *foramen ovale*).[53] During the fetal stages, before a pulmonary circulation is established, this secondary foramen allows the oxygenated blood from the placenta arriving in the right atrium to flow into the left atrium.

In the final phase of atrial septation in the human, the secondary atrial septum (sAS, or septum secundum) forms as an infolding of the right atrial myocardium between the left venous valve and the pAS, this marking the site of the left atrial–right atrial myocardial boundary.[61,62] The sAS folds into the atrial lumen and, by doing so, covers the secondary interatrial foramen (see Fig. 45.7C and D). After birth, when the lungs become functional and oxygenated blood arrives via the PuVs in the left atrium, the pressure in the left atrium forces the pAS against the sAS, thereby functionally closing the interatrial communication. In roughly two-third of the human population, the two septa will eventually physically fuse, thereby creating a permanent barrier. However, in one out of three individuals, this fusion does not take place, leading to a condition known as *patent foramen ovale (PFO)*, which is sometimes linked to stroke.[63] Failure of the sAS to completely cover the secondary interatrial foramen can lead to a more serious secondary atrial septal defect (septum secundum defect).

VENTRICULAR SEPTATION

Early formation of the ventricular septum and enlargement of the ventricular chambers are closely linked processes.[64] The development of the septum is intrinsically related to the overall process of ventricular growth. The primitive ventricular septum appears to be the product of apposition of compact myocardium produced during the growth of the ventricles. Lineage studies show that, just like that of the OFT and RV, the myocardium of the muscular septum is largely derived from the SHF.[59-61]

The distal rim of primitive ventricular septum initially has a crescent shape. The space between the top of the ventricular septum and the inner curvature is referred to as the interventricular foramen, although this should actually be considered a misnomer. In the formed heart, this opening contributes to the inlet of the right ventricle and to the outlet of the left ventricle.

When they fuse at about 6 weeks of development in the human, the two major AV cushions as well as the septal OFT ridge contribute to the septation of the ventricular foramen. Except for the part that becomes the membranous septum, a significant part of the fused mesenchymal tissues subsequently becomes myocardialized. This septum has an AV component, located between the left ventricle and right atrium, and a ventricular component, situated between the left and right ventricles.[65]

DEVELOPMENT OF THE ATRIOVENTRICULAR JUNCTION

During the early stages of development, the developing atria and ventricles are in myocardial continuity at the AV junction by means of the junctional AV myocardium.[66] This AV myocardium has a number of unique molecular and functional characteristics that are essential for the sequential contraction of atria and ventricles. As the heart continues to grow and is in the process of developing a pattern of coordinated contraction to allow sequential filling and emptying of the atrial and ventricular chambers, it is essential that the myocardial continuity between atrium and ventricle is interrupted to ensure electrical insulation between the working myocardium of atria and ventricles. This separation is accomplished by the formation of a layer of fibrous tissue (annulus fibrosus) between the AV and the ventricular myocardium (see Fig. 45.5). The formation of the annulus fibrosus results from the ingrowth of epicardially derived cells (AV-EPDCs).[44,67] The AV EPDCs that establish the electrical separation of atrial and ventricular myocardium come from the AV epicardial sulcus, which has formed in the AV groove on the external surface of the AV junction as a result of an epicardial EMT (or epiMT), a process likely regulated by BMP signaling.[44,68] The role of the epicardium in heart development is discussed later in this chapter. Interruption of the myocardial continuity begins in the eighth week of human development and is normally "completed" around the fourth month.[45] As a result, the AV myocardium eventually becomes incorporated into the atrial walls.[45] It is important to note that there is one area where the AV myocardial continuity does not become interrupted, where the penetrating bundle of His (or AV bundle), which forms part of the AV conduction system, connects the AV node, located in the right atrium, with the ventricular components of the conduction system (i.e., the left and right bundle branches and the network of Purkinje fibers).

DEVELOPMENT OF THE OUTFLOW TRACT

The fact that the myocardial OFT is a relatively late addition to the primary heart tube was initially indicated by experiments in which cell-fate mapping was conducted by placing carbon particles on specific spots in developing chicken embryos. Subsequently, with the emergence of transgenic mouse models that allow cell-fate tracing using molecular tools, it was confirmed that the OFT is a derivative of the SHF. As the OFT develops, two elongated cushions develop in a process reminiscent to the formation of the AV cushions. These are known as the *parietal and septal ridges* and are the two major cushions in the OFT. As is the case with the AV cushions, these OFT ridges also become colonized by ENDCs as the result of endMT. Similarly, in between the parietal and septal ridges of the OFT, two smaller ridges—the right and left intercalated ridges—develop as well. The two large OFT ridges extend over the entire length of the OFT and are twisted around each other, whereas the intercalated ridges are found only in the proximal part of the OFT. The parietal OFT ridge makes contact with the right lateral AV cushion, which itself becomes continuous with the sAVC. The septal ridge ends on the crest of the ventricular septum, where it makes contact with the iAVC. At later stages, a large number of cardiac neural crest-derived cells (CNDCs) originating from the cardiac neural crest migrate into the OFT from its distalmost end. The origins of the endocardial cushion of the outlet septum and much of the ventricular septum are not apparent on inspection of the mature heart owing to the replacement of cushion mesenchyme by myocardium in a process known as *myocardialization*.[69,70]

DEVELOPMENT OF THE SEMILUNAR VALVES

Semilunar valve development begins shortly after septation. As studied in mice, the initial process is outgrowth of unexcavated cusps of tissue corresponding to the future leaflets from the arterial surface of the distal OFT ridges and intercalated cushions.[71] Valve sinuses are formed by active endothelial excavation of the outlet surface of the leaflets.[72] The initial valve leaflets are thickened structures filled with abundant ECM and densely populated with endocardial- and neural crest-derived mesenchymal cells,[47] bordered by a cuboidal endothelium on the arterial surface and a flattened, streamlined endothelium on the ventricular surface. After the sinuses have been fully excavated, the leaflets remodel into the delicate fibrous tissue characterizing mature semilunar valves.[73] Valve remodeling is a slow process that may be histologically incomplete at the time of birth.[74] The molecular biology of semilunar valve development shares many features with AV valve development.[75,76]

DEVELOPMENT OF THE PHARYNGEAL ARCH ARTERIES

The embryonic arterial circulation is initially bilaterally symmetric and consists of six pairs of pharyngeal arch arteries (PAAs) connecting the aortic sac to the paired dorsal aortas.

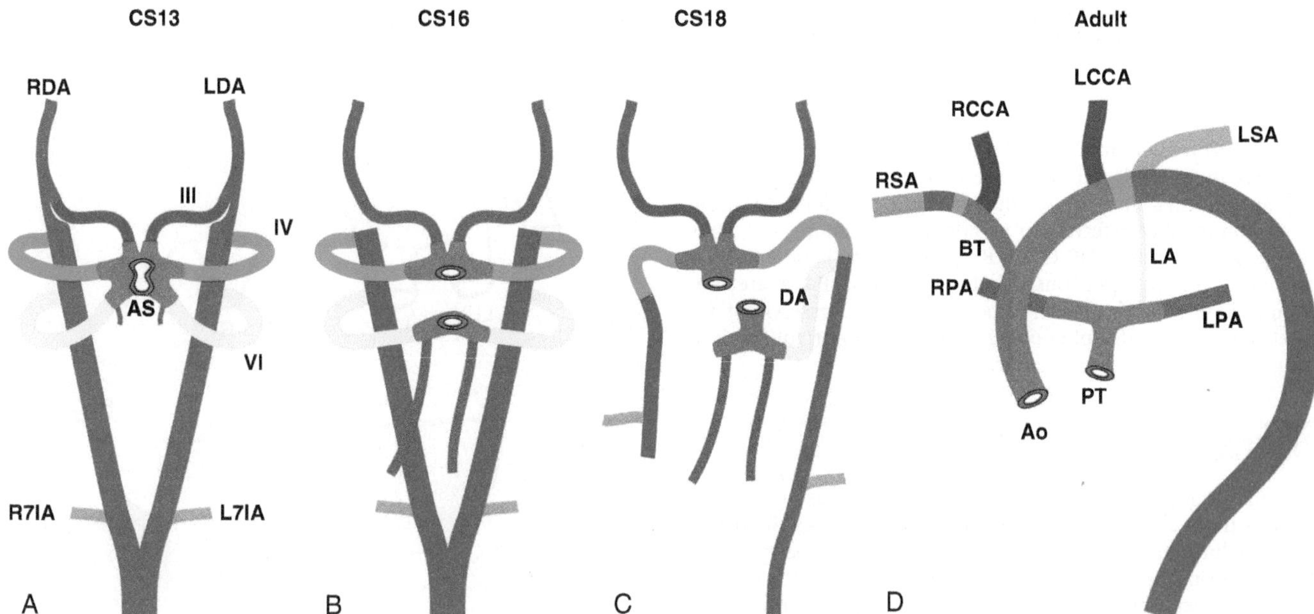

Fig. 45.8 Development of the pharyngeal arch arteries. Schematic representation of the remodeling of the pharyngeal arch arteries at 4.5 (A), 5.5 (B), 6 (C), and 8 (D) weeks of development (CS13, CS16, CS18, and CS23, respectively). The different colors depict the different vessels and their contribution in subsequent stages of development. *Ao*, Aorta; *AS*, aortic Sac; *BT*, brachiocephalic trunk; *CS*, Carnegie stage; *DA*, ductus arteriosus; *III*, third pharyngeal arch artery; *IV*, fourth pharyngeal arch artery; *LA*, ligamentum arteriosum; *PT*, pulmonary trunk; *R/L7IA*, right/left seventh intersegmental artery; *R/LCCA*, right/left common carotid artery; *R/LDA*, right/left dorsal aorta; *R/LPA*, right/left pulmonary artery; *R/LSA*, right/left subclavian artery; *VI*, sixth pharyngeal arch artery. (Modified from Sylva M, van den Hoff MJB, Moorman AFM. Development of the human heart. *Am J Med Genet A*. 2014;164A[6]:1347–1371.)

The right and left dorsal aortas fuse into a single vessel distally and progress retrograde to the seventh somite. As development proceeds, the paired first, second, third, fourth, and sixth PAAs and their connections to the dorsal aortas undergo an intricate series of transformations (Fig.45.8). The paired fifth PAAs immediately regress at their formation in the human but persist in lower vertebrates. The first and second aortic arch vessels largely regress, remaining patent only as capillary structures in the upper and lower jaw regions. Both the left and right portion of the dorsal aortas between the third and fourth PAAs (the carotid duct) regresses completely, leaving no remnant; as a result, the paired third PAAs become the only conduit of blood flow from the aortic sac to the embryo's head. This third PAA pair is the precursor of the definitive right and left common carotid arteries. The right dorsal aorta completely regresses between the right seventh intersegmental artery and at the confluence of left and right dorsal aortas; as a consequence, the right fourth PAA and remaining part of the right dorsal aorta become part of the right subclavian artery in the adult. Both the right and left sixth partially PAAs regress; the proximal parts become part of the pulmonary arteries, the right distal part regresses, and the left distal part becomes the ductus arteriosus, allowing most blood to bypass the nonfunctional lungs during intrauterine development. The left dorsal aorta distal to the fourth left PAA remains widely patent throughout its length but remodels, so that the definitive left fourth aortic arch vessel, the ductus arteriosus, and the left seventh intersegmental artery (future left subclavian artery) all connect to the left dorsal aorta within a very short span.

The vertebral arteries are derived from anastomoses that form between the seven cervical intersegmental arteries. After continuity has been established between the intersegmental arteries, their connections to the dorsal aorta regress with the exception of the connection of the seventh intersegmental vessel (as noted previously, the seventh intersegmental artery becomes the subclavian artery), creating the subclavian origin of the definitive vertebral arteries.

NEURAL CREST AND MOLECULAR REGULATION OF AORTIC ARCHES

During the formation of the neural tube, a set of mesenchymal cells is set apart lateral of the neural tube. These mesenchymal cells are referred to as neural crest cells. The neural crest cells migrate through specific pathways to specific structures.[77] The cells that reach the OFT of the early heart migrate through the third, fourth, and sixth pharyngeal arches and are referred to as cardiac neural crest cells. A role for the neural crest in cardiac development was recognized in 1983 through the work of Kirby.[78,79] The patterning of the PAA is greatly influenced by the migration of neural crest cells into the pharyngeal arches. Studies in animal models have shown that expression of the receptor for endothelin 1 in neural crest cells is necessary for interaction with endothelial cells of the arch arteries.[80] Definitive pharyngeal arch formation is the product of complex signaling interactions among neural crest cells, SHF cells, and pharyngeal mesoderm.[22,80,81]

DEVELOPMENT OF THE PULMONARY VEINS

At the start of the fifth week of development, an endocardial indentation in the dorsal roof marks the spot where the primitive PuV is connected to the common atrium. The PuV is initially a midline structure located in the dorsal mesocardium and will eventually connect to the vascular plexus forming in the developing lung. The incorporation of the pulmonary orifice into the left atrium is the result of a series of events. It starts with the development of the DMP and the associated pAS on the right margin of the PuV and is followed by the myocardial differentiation of the accumulated SHF-derived mesenchyme bordering the PuV.[62,82] In this process, Semaphorin 3d (SEMA3D) appears to play an important role. SEMA3D is expressed in the mesothelial cells covering the dorsal mesocardium and as such flanking the tissue through which the pulmonary vessel is formed. SEMA3D is thought to act as a repulsive guidance molecule to constrain and direct the endothelial cells from the developing pulmonary plexus toward the atrium, an event in which neuropilin 1 (NRP1), expressed on the endothelial cells, is thought to be involved. In SEMA3D-null mice, the pulmonary endothelial cells display abnormal invasion of the dorsal mesocardium, resulting in an abnormality referred to as abnormal pulmonary venous connection or return (APVC/APVR).[83] Interestingly, the muscular walls of proximal portions of the individual PuVs are not composed of smooth muscle (as are most other vessels) but are instead of a myocardial phenotype, a clinically important factor in the cause and management of atrial fibrillation.[84,85]

DEVELOPMENT OF SYSTEMIC VEINS

The embryonic systemic veins are also formed by vasculogenesis. Initially, there are three bilaterally symmetric venous drainages: the vitelline, umbilical, and cardinal venous systems. The vitelline veins drain the embryonic gastrointestinal tract and gut derivatives. The umbilical veins bring oxygenated blood to the heart from the placenta. The cardinal venous system returns blood from the embryonic head, neck, and body wall. All three of these drainages enter via the left and right sinus horns into the sinus venosus of the primitive heart tube. The adult venous return is established through a complex process of regression, remodeling, and replacement of the embryonic venous systems and their connections to the sinus venosus (Fig. 45.9).

In the human, the connections of the left-sided cardinal, vitelline, and umbilical veins with the left horn regress. This results in the coronary sinus remaining as the primary structural derivative of the left sinus horn in the formed heart and draining in the right atrium. The left superior cardinal vein, contributing in the adult to the left internal jugular vein, drains via the brachiocephalic vein into the superior caval vein, which originates from the right superior cardinal vein. The regressed confluence of the left superior and inferior cardinal veins remains as the ligament of Marshall. A small remnant of the inferior cardinal veins on the surface of the heart persists as a passage of coronary venous blood to the coronary sinus and is known as the *oblique vein of the left atrium*. When the left cardinal system persists, it is recognized as persistence of the left superior vena cava.

The right horn of the sinus venosus normally accommodates the entirety of the systemic venous drainage. After the left vitelline vein loses connection with the left horn of the sinus venosus, it regresses. However, because the right and left vitelline veins are distally connected to each other through a plexus of veins that becomes the liver sinusoids, the entire venous system of the embryonic gut drains to the heart through the right vitelline vein. The connection of the right vitelline vein to the adult heart persists as the terminal portion of the inferior vena cava (IVC). The left umbilical vein also loses its connection with the left sinus horn. Distally, the left umbilical vein forms anastomoses with the ductus venosus (derived from the liver plexus of the vitelline veins), allowing the oxygen and nutrient-rich placental venous blood to bypass the liver and drain into the heart through the IVC. In the adult, there are no derivatives of the embryonic umbilical venous drainage that connect to the heart or persist after closure of the ductus venosus. The right cardinal system persists and is postnatally represented by the superior and inferior venae cavae as well as the smooth-walled part of the right atrium in between their entrance into the right atrium, the sinus venarum. The posterior cardinal veins are the only portion of the embryonic venous drainage that is destined to have a symmetric fate. Both posterior cardinal veins will regress throughout most of their length and lose their direct connections with the sinus venosus. The posterior cardinal veins originally drain the body wall, gonadal, and renal structures. Their function in venous drainage of the body wall is supplanted by the supracardinal venous plexus, whereas the gonadal and renal venous drainage is captured by the subcardinal venous plexus.

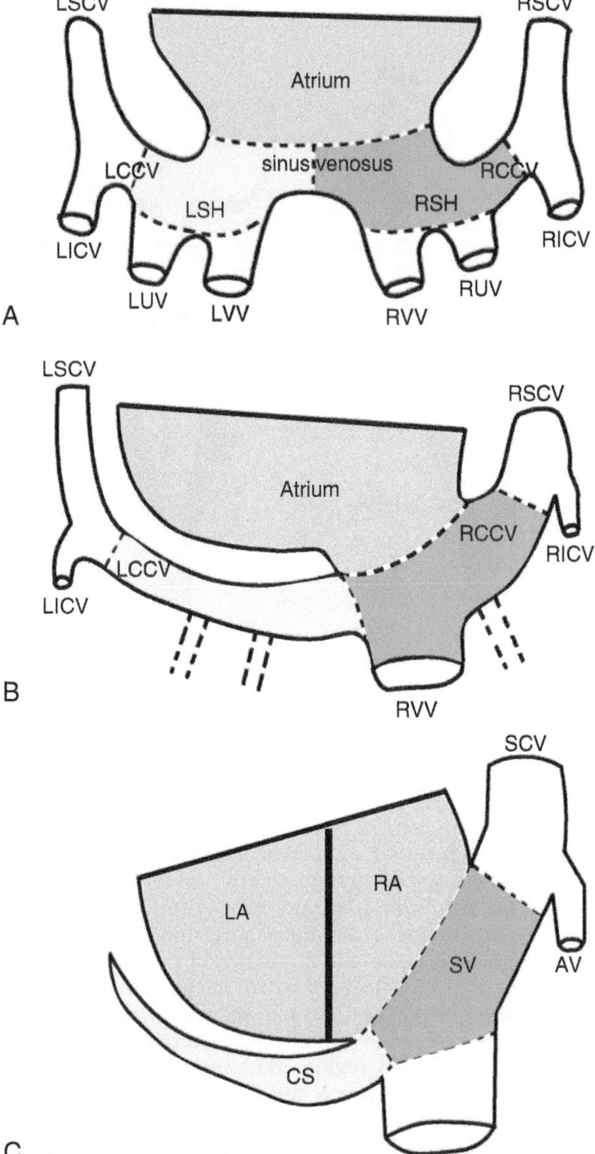

Fig. 45.9 Development of the cardiac venous pole. Schematic representation of the developing inflow tract of the human heart. (A) The inflow tract at 4 weeks of development. The sinus venosus and common atrium basically form one common chamber. (B) At 7 weeks of development, the sinoatrial communication shifts to the right atrium. (C) At 8 weeks of development, the left common cardinal veins and associated vessels largely regress, leading to the formation of the coronary sinus. *AV*, Azygos vein; *CS*, coronary sinus; *ICV*, inferior caval vein; *L/RA*, left/right atrium; *L/RCCV*, left/right common cardinal vein; *L/RICV*, left/right inferior cardinal vein; *L/RSCV*, left/right superior cardinal vein; *L/RSH*, left/right sinus horn; *L/RUV*, left/right umbilical vein; *L/RVV*, vitelline vein; *SCV*, superior caval vein; *SV*, sinus venarum. (Modified from van den Hoff MJB, Kruithof BP, Moorman AFM. Making more heart muscle. *BioEssays.* 2004;26:248–261.)

The posterior cardinal, supracardinal, and subcardinal venous beds contribute the segments that form the definitive IVC to the level of the vitelline vein-derived segment connecting to the right atrium. Remnants of the posterior cardinal veins in the fetal and adult circulation are limited to the most distal portion of the IVC (formed by anastomosis of the right and left posterior cardinal veins) and the common iliac veins. The IVC derived from the posterior cardinal vein connects with the supracardinal segment of the IVC. The supracardinal venous system is the site of origin of the azygos and hemiazygos veins, which ordinarily connect to the IVC between the renal veins and the common iliac veins. The supracardinal segment of the IVC connects to the subcardinal segment of the IVC, which receives the drainage of the gonadal veins and renal veins before connecting with the vitelline venous channel to the heart.

THE EPICARDIUM

Epicardial development starts with the formation of the proepicardium, a cluster of mesothelially derived cells in the region of the septum transversum.[86-89] Cells from the proepicardium then travel through from the proepicardium to the myocardial surface of the heart by a mechanism that appears to be slightly different between avian and mammalian species.[90,91] After attaching to the myocardium of the looping heart, the attached cells flatten out, spread out as an epithelium, and migrate over the myocardial surface.[90,92] The normal development of the epicardium and subepicardial mesenchyme is dependent on cell-cell interactions with the underlying myocardium. Gene knockout studies in mice show that the absence of expression of genes such as vascular cell adhesion molecule 1 *(VCAM1)*, the transcription factor "friend of GATA2" *(FOG2)* in the myocardium, Wilms tumor suppressor 1 *(WT1)*, and α_4 integrin in the epicardium will produce a similar phenotype of abnormal coronary development and in some models ventricular myocardial hypoplasia.[90]

After the epicardium has formed, ECM accumulates between the epicardium and myocardium in a process similar to the formation of the cardiac jelly at the AV junction and in the OFT. Through a process of epithelial-to-mesenchymal transformation of the epicardium (epiMT), EPDCs are generated that subsequently populate the subepicardial space. This epiMT process is regulated by transcription factors such as Slug and Snail as well as members of the transforming growth factor-β superfamily.[68,93] A subset of EPDCs migrate into the myocardial wall, where they differentiate into cardiac fibroblasts and coronary vascular smooth muscle cells.[94-97] EPDCs have also been reported to play a role in the formation of coronary endothelium and to contribute to subpopulations of myocardium, but these are still contentious topics.[98-102]

During valvuloseptal development, relatively large numbers of EPDCs accumulate in the AV groove. In addition to contributing to the formation of the coronaries in the AV sulcus, these AV-EPDCs will also form the annulus fibrosus, the fibrous insulating ring between the atria and the ventricles,[44,67,94,103] and will substantially contribute to the cell population of the AV valve leaflets that derive from the lateral AV cushions (see Fig. 45.5).[44,104] Mice in which AV-EPDCs are prevented from migrating into the lateral AV cushions develop, later in life, myxomatous AV valves that look similar to those observed in patients with myxomatous valve disease (MVD), a condition that often leads to mitral valve prolapse (MVP).[68]

CONCLUSION

This chapter has reviewed the major developmental events associated with the formation of the heart, a number of which were initially reported many years ago. Insight into some other aspects of cardiovascular development has resulted from advancements in transgenic mouse technology, molecular biology, and imaging techniques. Therefore our knowledge of the mechanisms leading to the formation of a healthy human heart and our insights into the pathogenesis of congenital and acquired heart diseases is constantly evolving. For instance, it was only about 30 years ago that the importance of the cardiac neural crest in OFT development became clear, 20 years ago that the SHF was discovered, and less than 10 years ago that the role of the epicardium in AV valve development was discovered. New techniques, such as single cell RNA sequencing, will continue to generate new information on the molecular mechanisms that drive heart development. This new information, in combination with good "old-fashioned" descriptive approaches to put the molecular finding in proper context, will undoubtedly lead to future chapters, like this one, in which the content will look just a bit different.

A complete reference list is available at www.ExpertConsult.com. 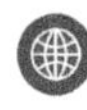

SELECT REFERENCES

3. Dyer LA, Kirby ML. The role of secondary heart field in cardiac development. *Dev Biol*. 2009;336:137-144.
5. Bodmer R, Venkatesh TV. Heart development in drosophila and vertebrates: conservation of molecular mechanisms. *Dev Genet*. 1998;22:181-186.
6. Srivastava D. Hand proteins: molecular mediators of cardiac development and congenital heart disease. *Trends Cardiovasc Med*. 1999;9:11-18.
8. Stennard FA, Harvey RP. T-box transcription factors and their roles in regulatory hierarchies in the developing heart. *Development*. 2005;132:4897-4910.
9. Mjaatvedt CH, Nakaoka T, Moreno-Rodriguez R, et al. The outflow tract of the heart is recruited from a novel heart-forming field. *Dev Biol*. 2001;238:97-109.
10. Kelly RG, Buckingham ME. The anterior heart-forming field: voyage to the arterial pole of the heart. *Trends Genet*. 2002;18:210-216.
11. Waldo KL, Hutson MR, Ward CC, et al. Secondary heart field contributes myocardium and smooth muscle to the arterial pole of the developing heart. *Dev Biol*. 2005;281:78-90.
12. Verzi MP, McCulley DJ, De Val S, et al. The right ventricle, outflow tract, and ventricular septum comprise a restricted expression domain within the secondary/anterior heart field. *Dev Biol*. 2005;287:134-145.
13. Briggs LE, Phelps AL, Brown E, et al. Expression of the bmp receptor alk3 in the second heart field is essential for development of the dorsal mesenchymal protrusion and atrioventricular septation. *Circ Res*. 2013;112:1420-1432.
14. Snarr BS, O'Neal JL, Chintalapudi MR, et al. Isl1 expression at the venous pole identifies a novel role for the second heart field in cardiac development. *Circ Res*. 2007;101:971-974.
15. Manner J. Cardiac looping in the chick embryo: a morphological review with special reference to terminological and biomechanical aspects of the looping process. *Anat Rec*. 2000;259:248-262.
17. Moorman AF, Christoffels VM. Cardiac chamber formation: development, genes, and evolution. *Physiol Rev*. 2003;83:1223-1267.
18. Hoogaars WM, Barnett P, Moorman AF, Christoffels VM. T-box factors determine cardiac design. *Cell Mol Life Sci*. 2007;64:646-660.
19. Boukens BJ, Christoffels VM, Coronel R, Moorman AF. Developmental basis for electrophysiological heterogeneity in the ventricular and outflow tract myocardium as a substrate for life-threatening ventricular arrhythmias. *Circ Res*. 2009;104:19-31.
21. Moskowitz IP, Pizard A, Patel VV, et al. The t-box transcription factor tbx5 is required for the patterning and maturation of the murine cardiac conduction system. *Development*. 2004;131:4107-4116.
23. Takeuchi JK, Bruneau BG. Directed transdifferentiation of mouse mesoderm to heart tissue by defined factors. *Nature*. 2009;459:708-711.
25. McQuinn TC, Miga DE, Mjaatvedt CH, et al. Cardiopulmonary malformations in the inv/inv mouse. *Anat Rec*. 2001;263:62-71.
26. Seo JW, Brown NA, Ho SY, Anderson RH. Abnormal laterality and congenital cardiac anomalies. Relations of visceral and cardiac morphologies in the iv/iv mouse. *Circulation*. 1992;86:642-650.
27. Franco D, Campione M. The role of pitx2 during cardiac development. Linking left-right signaling and congenital heart diseases. *Trends Cardiovasc Med*. 2003;13:157-163.
30. Hamada H, Meno C, Watanabe D, Saijoh Y. Establishment of vertebrate left-right asymmetry. *Nat Rev Genet*. 2002;3:103-113.
31. Gros J, Feistel K, Viebahn C, et al. Cell movements at Hensen's node establish left/right asymmetric gene expression in the chick. *Science*. 2009;324:941-944.
37. Ai D, Liu W, Ma L, et al. Pitx2 regulates cardiac left-right asymmetry by patterning second cardiac lineage-derived myocardium. *Dev Biol*. 2006;296:437-449.
39. Schlueter J, Brand T. Left-right axis development: examples of similar and divergent strategies to generate asymmetric morphogenesis in chick and mouse embryos. *Cytogenet Genome Res*. 2007;117:256-267.

40. Bolender DL, Markwald RR. Epithelial-mesenchymal transformation in chick atrioventricular cushion morphogenesis. *Scan Electron Microsc*. 1979:313-321.
44. Wessels A, van den Hoff MJ, Adamo RF, et al. Epicardially derived fibroblasts preferentially contribute to the parietal leaflets of the atrioventricular valves in the murine heart. *Dev Biol*. 2012;366:111-124.
45. Wessels A, Markman MW, Vermeulen JL, et al. The development of the atrioventricular junction in the human heart. *Circ Res*. 1996;78:110-117.
47. de Lange FJ, Moorman AF, Anderson RH, et al. Lineage and morphogenetic analysis of the cardiac valves. *Circ Res*. 2004;95:645-654.
51. Lincoln J, Alfieri CM, Yutzey KE. BMP and FGF regulatory pathways control cell lineage diversification of heart valve precursor cells. *Dev Biol*. 2006;292:292-302.
54. Snarr BS, Wirrig EE, Phelps AL, et al. A spatiotemporal evaluation of the contribution of the dorsal mesenchymal protrusion to cardiac development. *Dev Dyn*. 2007;236:1287-1294.
55. Briggs LE, Kakarla J, Wessels A. The pathogenesis of atrial and atrioventricular septal defects with special emphasis on the role of the dorsal mesenchymal protrusion. *Differentiation*. 2012;84:117-130.
56. Briggs LE, Burns TA, Lockhart MM, et al. Wnt/beta-catenin and sonic hedgehog pathways interact in the regulation of the development of the dorsal mesenchymal protrusion. *Dev Dyn*. 2016;245:103-113.
57. Goddeeris MM, Rho S, Petiet A, et al. Intracardiac septation requires hedgehog-dependent cellular contributions from outside the heart. *Development*. 2008;135:1887-1895.
58. Hoffmann AD, Peterson MA, Friedland-Little JM, et al. Sonic hedgehog is required in pulmonary endoderm for atrial septation. *Development*. 2009;136:1761-1770.
62. Wessels A, Anderson RH, Markwald RR, et al. Atrial development in the human heart: an immunohistochemical study with emphasis on the role of mesenchymal tissues. *Anat Rec*. 2000;259:288-300.
65. de la Cruz MV, Markwald RR, Krug EL, et al. Living morphogenesis of the ventricles and congenital pathology of their component parts. *Cardiol Young*. 2001;11:588-600.
67. Zhou B, von Gise A, Ma Q, et al. Genetic fate mapping demonstrates contribution of epicardium-derived cells to the annulus fibrosis of the mammalian heart. *Dev Biol*. 2010;338:251-261.
68. Lockhart MM, Boukens BJ, Phelps A, et al. Alk3 mediated bmp signaling controls the contribution of epicardially derived cells to the tissues of the atrioventricular junction. *Dev Biol*. 2014;396:8-18.
69. Kruithof BP, van den Hoff MJ, Wessels A, Moorman AF. Cardiac muscle cell formation after development of the linear heart tube. *Dev Dyn*. 2003;227:1-13.
70. van den Hoff MJ, Kruithof BP, Moorman AF, et al. Formation of myocardium after the initial development of the linear heart tube. *Dev Biol*. 2001;240:61-76.
76. Combs MD, Yutzey KE. Heart valve development: regulatory networks in development and disease. *Circ Res*. 2009;105:408-421.
82. Mommersteeg MT, Brown NA, Prall OW, et al. Pitx2c and nkx2-5 are required for the formation and identity of the pulmonary myocardium. *Circ Res*. 2007;101:902-909.
83. Degenhardt K, Singh MK, Aghajanian H, et al. Semaphorin 3d signaling defects are associated with anomalous pulmonary venous connections. *Nat Med*. 2013;19:760-765.
85. Haissaguerre M, Jais P, Shah DC, et al. Spontaneous initiation of atrial fibrillation by ectopic beats originating in the pulmonary veins. *N Engl J Med*. 1998;339:659-666.
92. Vrancken Peeters MP, Mentink MM, Poelmann RE, Gittenberger-de Groot AC. Cytokeratins as a marker for epicardial formation in the quail embryo. *Anat Embryol (Berl)*. 1995;191:503-508.
94. Dettman RW, Denetclaw Jr W, Ordahl CP, Bristow J. Common epicardial origin of coronary vascular smooth muscle, perivascular fibroblasts, and intermyocardial fibroblasts in the avian heart. *Dev Biol*. 1998;193:169-181.
97. Gittenberger-de Groot AC, Vrancken Peeters MP, Mentink MM, et al. Epicardium-derived cells contribute a novel population to the myocardial wall and the atrioventricular cushions. *Circ Res*. 1998;82:1043-1052.
98. Red-Horse K, Ueno H, Weissman IL, Krasnow MA. Coronary arteries form by developmental reprogramming of venous cells. *Nature*. 2010;464:549-553.
100. Zhou B, Ma Q, Rajagopal S, et al. Epicardial progenitors contribute to the cardiomyocyte lineage in the developing heart. *Nature*. 2008;454:109-113.
103. Pérez-Pomares J, Phelps A, Sedmerova M, et al. Experimental studies on the spatiotemporal expression of wt1 and raldh2 in the embryonic avian heart: a model for the regulation of myocardial and valvuloseptal development by epicardially derived cells (epdcs). *Dev Biol*. 2002;247:307-326.

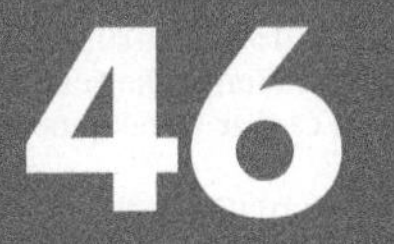

46 Developmental Electrophysiology in the Fetus and Neonate

Janette F. Strasburger | Annette Wacker-Gussmann | Michael A. Schellpfeffer

INTRODUCTION

In this chapter, the physiology of both impulse formation and conduction in the developing heart is discussed. Significant developmental or age-related changes in the ionic currents are responsible for the generation of cardiac action potential, as well as changes in the microscopic and macroscopic anatomic and neural substrates that govern the physiology of cardiac depolarization and repolarization during health and disease. Recently, important breakthroughs in clinical fetal electrophysiology have emerged, thanks to new imaging techniques and new genetic studies of arrhythmias. These have furthered our understanding of fetal anatomic substrates, fetal demise, and the response of the fetal conduction system to disease, medication, and other stressors. These new insights emphasize the need for research into diagnostic and management strategies that promote fetal survival. Rhythm and conduction will be integrated into the overall assessment of the high-risk pregnancy in the future, using tools such as fetal magnetocardiography, fetal and neonatal electrocardiography, and fetal magnetic resonance imaging, alongside existing echocardiographic assessment of anatomy and function.

NORMAL CONDUCTION

CARDIAC ACTION POTENTIAL

The cardiac action potential is a transient reversible electromagnetochemical wavefront responsible for the generation of the cardiac impulse. It is based on a complex series of transmembrane ion fluxes that result in a net flow of electric current across the cell membrane.[1,2] First, there is an unequal distribution of electrically charged sodium, potassium, and calcium ions across the lipid bilayer cell membrane (Table 46.1). These ion gradients are established and maintained largely as a result of energy-expending membrane ion pumps (sodium-potassium adenosine triphosphatase [ATPase]) and ion exchange complexes (the sodium-calcium exchanger). Second, under appropriate biophysical conditions, complex polypeptide pores known as *ion channels,* embedded within the cell membrane, are opened, thereby allowing the passage of charged ions through the cell membrane. The detailed molecular structure of many of these ion channels is understood, and defects in ion channel transcription lead to significant levels of fetal and neonatal demise (Fig. 46.1).[3-5]

Table 46.1 Intracellular and Extracellular Ion Distributions in the Cardiac Cell.

	Na^+	K^+	Cl^-	Ca^{2+}
Extracellular fluid	145 mM	4 mM	120 mM	2 mM
	Cell membrane			
Intracellular fluid	15 mM	145 mM	5 mM	10^{-4} mM

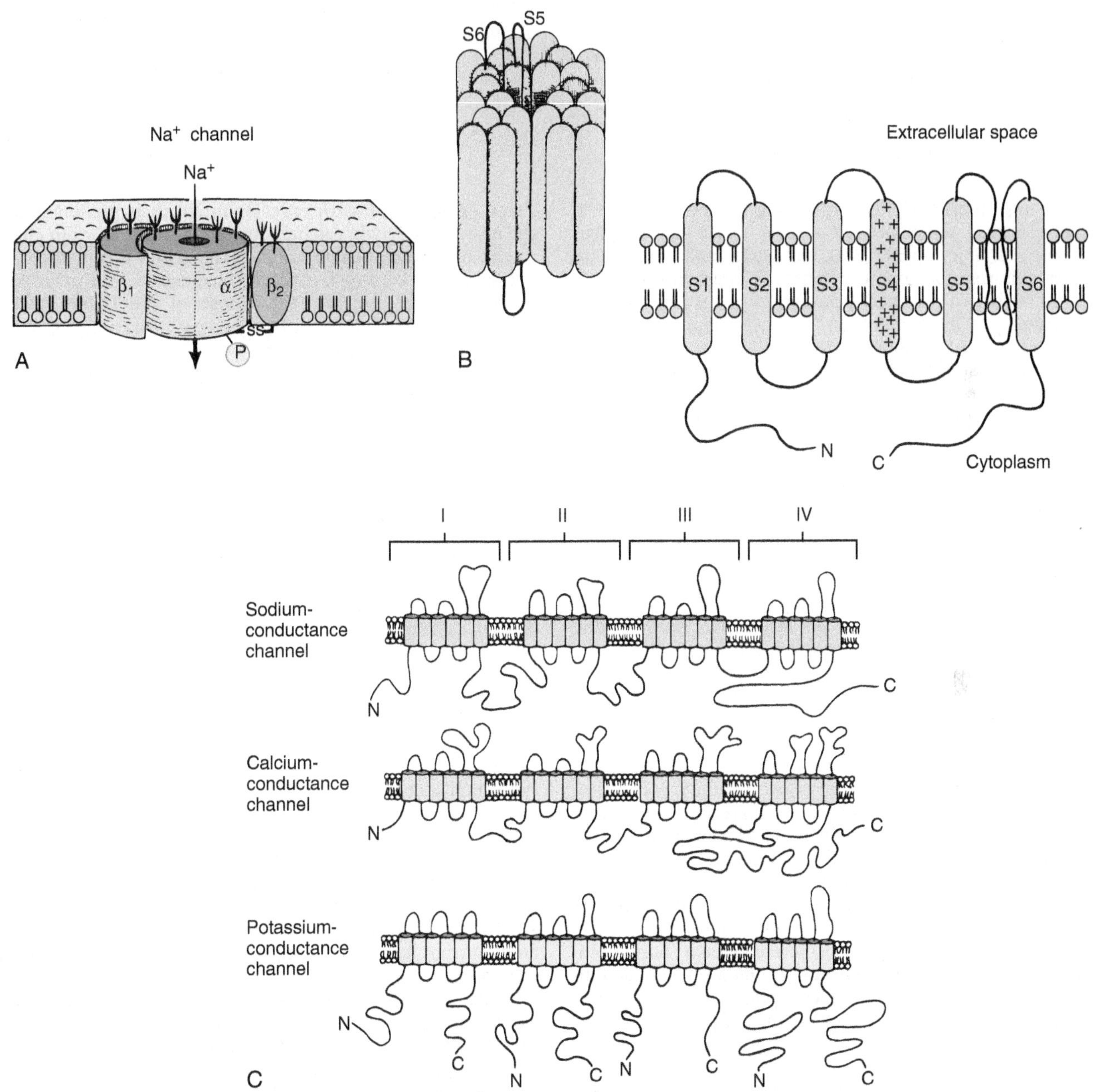

Fig. 46.1 (A) Three-dimensional representation of a sodium channel from mammalian brain. The ion channel consists of the α-subunit, with two smaller protein subunits (β_1 and β_2) associated with the main channel. The β_1-subunit is found only in cardiac sodium channels and is thought to stabilize the channel. The treelike (cactuslike) structures are glycosylation sites. (B) The ion channel is composed of four domains of a protein complex that consists of six separate transmembrane segments (S1–S6). The topographic arrangement of one such domain is shown on the *left.* The peptide loops between S5 and S6 are thought to be the central pore of the channel. Subunit S4 is a highly charged protein segment that is thought to serve as the voltage sensor of the ion channel. (C) The sodium channel, calcium channel, and potassium channel. In sodium and calcium channels, there is covalent linkage of the four domains (I–IV). (Each domain consists of the six transmembrane segments S1–S6 already described.) Potassium channels consist of single domains. There is no covalent linkage between domains. *P,* Phosphorylation sites; *SS,* disulfide bond. (A, Modified from Shih H-T. Anatomy of the action potential in the heart. *Tex Heart Inst J.* 1994;21:30. B, From Brown AM. Ion channels in action potential generation. *Hosp Pract (Off Ed).* 1992;27:129. Illustration by Alan D. Iselin. C, Modified from Catterall WA. Structure and function of voltage-sensitive ion channels. *Science.* 1988;242:50. Copyright 1988 American Association for the Advancement of Science.)

Table 46.2 Action Potential Characteristics in Cardiac Cells.

	SA Node	Atrium	AV Node	His-Purkinje	Ventricle
Resting Potential (mV)					
Action potential	250–260	280–290	260–270	290–295	280–290
Amplitude (mV)	60–70	110–120	70–80	120	110–120
Overshoot (mV)	0–10	30	5–15	30	30
Duration (ms)	100–300	100–300	100–300	300–500	100–200
$\dot{V}_{max}$ (V/s)	1–10	100–200	5–15	500–700	100–200
Conduction velocity (m/s)	<0.05	0.3–0.4	0.1	2–3	0.3–0.4

AV, Atrioventricular; *SA,* sinoatrial.
Modified from Sperelakis N. Origin of the cardiac resting potential. In: Berne RM, Sperelakis N, eds. *Handbook of Physiology, Vol 1. The Cardiovascular System.* Bethesda, MD: American Physiological Society; 1979:187–267.

At rest, the interior of the typical cardiac cell exhibits a negative electrical potential with respect to the extracellular space. For Purkinje fibers (PFs) and atrial and ventricular myocytes, this transmembrane potential is approximately −90 mV. In the sinoatrial (SA) and atrioventricular (AV) nodes, it is approximately −60 mV (Table 46.2). The energy-requiring ATPase pump maintains a high intracellular concentration of potassium ions and a low intracellular sodium ion concentration relative to the extracellular space. The unequal exchange rate of positive ions (2 K^+ ions incorporated, 3 Na^+ ions extruded) results in a net negative charge of the intracellular space due to high potassium ion permeability (relative to that for sodium ions and anions).

When the resting potential of the cardiac cell is made less negative, either as a result of the cell exhibiting spontaneous depolarization (SA or AV node automaticity) or as a result of an advancing wave of electric current (Purkinje cells or cardiac myocytes), the cell reaches a level of depolarization called the *activation threshold.* The ensuing rapid influx of positively charged sodium ions *(phase 0 of the action potential)* rapidly depolarizes the cell to potentials close to +20 to 30 mV (Fig. 46.2). The maximal rate of rise of the action potential phase 0, $\dot{V}_{max}$, in ventricular and atrial muscle approaches 200 V/s; in Purkinje fibers, even higher rates of change in membrane potential can be observed ($\dot{V}_{max}$ of approximately 500 V/s) (see Table 46.2). The amplitude and rate of rise of phase 0 of the action potential are key determinants of conduction velocity in the myocardium and specialized conduction system, with greater conduction velocities resulting from action potentials of greater amplitude and greater $\dot{V}_{max}$. Phase 0 is triggered by the change in membrane potential that results from the sodium channel changing from a conformationally specific "rest" state to an active or "open" channel configuration (Fig. 46.3).[3]

After the completion of phase 0, there is often a short, rapid repolarization phase, which creates a notch in the action potential. This notch, which represents *phase 1 of the action potential*, and the resulting spike-and-dome appearance of the initial portion of the action potential plateau, are most notable in epicardial ventricular muscle cells and Purkinje fibers (Fig. 46.4A). There are two principal charge carriers responsible for this phase 1 notch. One is a transiently activated outward potassium current, referred to as I_{to}, and the second is an inward chloride current (I_{to2}).[6]

The cardiac action potential is unique in its long duration when compared with ion channels in skeletal muscle and neurons. The plateau of the action potential, *phase 2,* which accounts for this length (see Fig. 46.2), can persist for hundreds of milliseconds and reflects the delicate balance of both inward and outward currents on a high-resistance membrane. The most important of the inward currents during the action potential plateau is the inward calcium current. L-type (*L* for *long-lasting*, *large*) and T-type (*T* for *tiny, transient*) calcium channels predominate in the heart.[7] The L-type calcium current ($I_{Ca\text{-}L}$) is the main charge carrier responsible for maintaining the action potential plateau during phase 2.[8] T-type calcium channels, which activate at potentials more negative than those of the L-type calcium channels, may primarily contribute to pacemaker activity in the heart.[7] The slow inward current, $I_{Ca\text{-}L}$, is also the major current responsible for phase 0 of the action potential in the sinoatrial and AV nodes, which lack a rapid inward sodium current (see Fig. 46.2, *right side*), and is characterized by a very slow $\dot{V}_{max}$ of approximately 10 V/s. The action potentials recorded from these regions are therefore referred to as *slow response action potentials.*

Balancing the inward depolarizing plateau currents is a family of repolarization currents, largely outward potassium currents that drive the membrane potential back towards the resting potential (see Fig. 46.2).[9] I_K begins to activate relatively late during the action potential plateau, as the time-dependent slow calcium current $I_{Ca\text{-}L}$ begins to inactivate. In humans, there are two principal components of the delayed rectifier potassium current, a fast (I_{Kr}) and a slow (I_{Ks}) component.[10]

Phase 3 of the action potential represents the phase of rapid repolarization of the cell towards the resting membrane potential. Phase 3 occurs as the result of decay in the inward calcium current and the activation of (several) outward potassium currents. The ion current responsible for the terminal portion of this phase of the action potential, as well as the current responsible for maintaining the resting potential, is an outward potassium current activated at negative membrane potentials, referred to as the *inward rectifier,* or I_{K1}.[11] An additional outward potassium repolarization current called I_{Kur} (*ur* for *ultrarapid*) is identified in the human atrium. This atrial current is a rapidly activating, noninactivating potassium current.[12]

Other outward potassium currents have been described that can become important under specific conditions. For example, the ATP-dependent potassium current, $I_{K(ATP)}$, activates strongly under conditions of depleted intracellular stores of ATP.[13] This outward current may become important under hypoxic conditions.

Under normal conditions, spontaneous automaticity is generally confined to the pacemaker cells of the sinoatrial node, which entrain all subsidiary pacemakers with each systole. In these cells, microelectrode recordings of atrial tissue have revealed a slow spontaneous depolarization of the membrane potential during *phase 4 of the action potential,* from the maximal diastolic potential towards the activation, or threshold, potential (Fig. 46.5). Atrial myocytes, AV junctional cells, and His-Purkinje cells can all exhibit spontaneous diastolic depolarization, at slower rates than the sinoatrial node. These subsidiary natural pacemaker

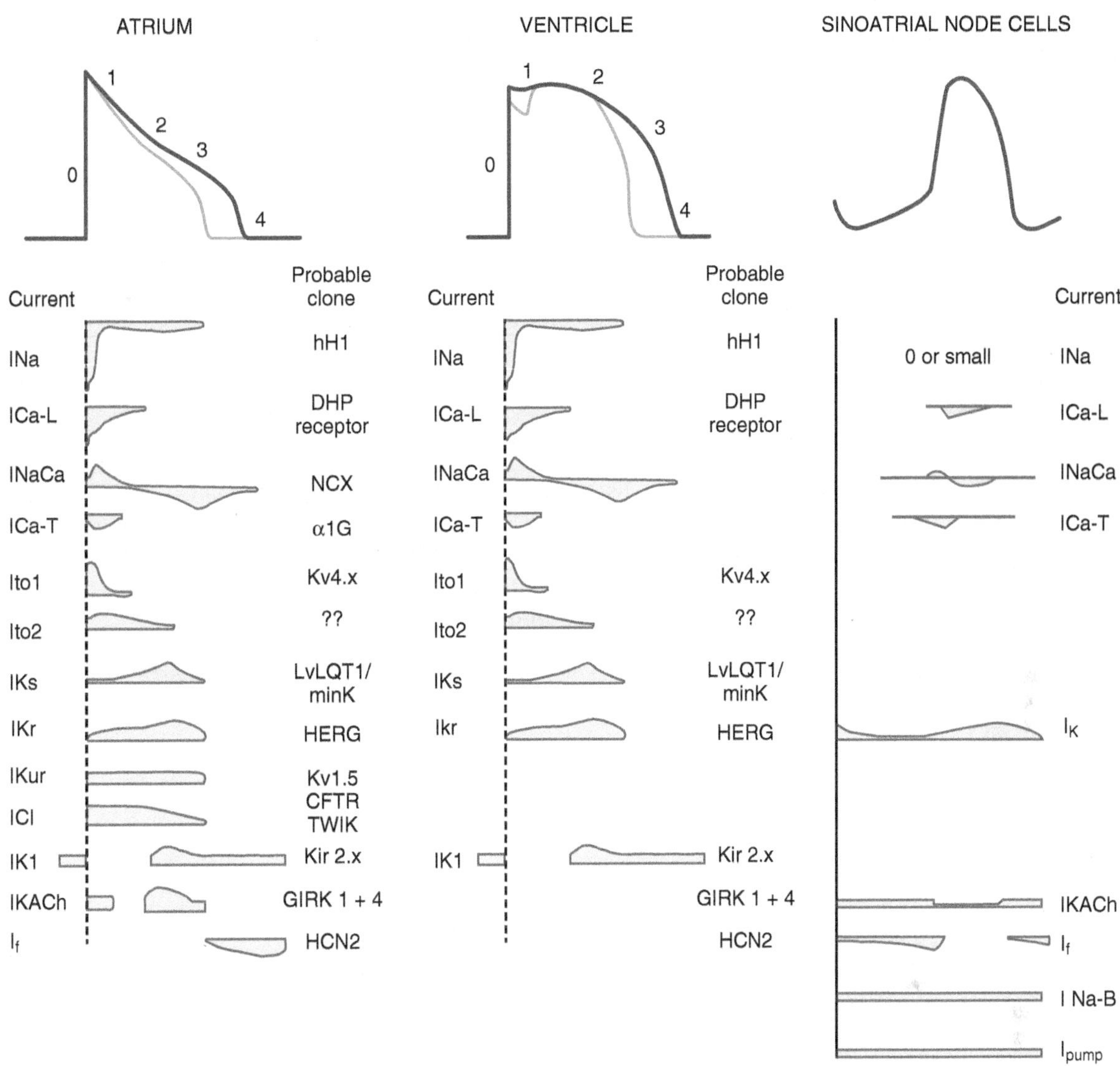

Fig. 46.2 The atrial, ventricular, and sinoatrial node action potential. (For atrial and ventricular action potentials, the action potentials depict changes in action potential morphology that have been associated with the failing heart.) The major ion currents and ion pumps involved in the generation of the action potentials are depicted. For each of the currents, the direction of current flow is indicated (downward indicating an inward current, upward indicating an outward current), as is the approximate time course of activation and inactivation. Gene products *(probable clone)* that are associated with each current are shown. Relative current amplitudes are not depicted. *INa* represents the inward sodium current, *ICa-L* represents the large, long-lasting slow inward calcium current, *ICa-T* represents the tiny, transient calcium current, and *INaCa* represents the current generated by the action of the sodium-calcium exchanger. Outward potassium currents depicted include I_{K1} (IK1), the inward rectifier current; I_K, the delayed rectifier current; I_{to}, the transient outward current (of which there are two components, represented by *Ito1* and *Ito2*); and, limited to the atrium, I_{Kur} (IKur). *IKACh* represents the receptor-activated potassium channel (activated by acetylcholine and adenosine). I_f represents the "funny" pacemaker current, a current carried by both sodium and potassium. All these currents are discussed further in the text. Not discussed but presented here for completeness are I_{Cl} *(ICl)*, a chloride current; I_{pump}, an ion pump current; and $I_{Na\text{-}B}$ *(I Na-B)*, an inward background current thought to be present in sinoatrial node cells. (Modified from The Sicilian gambit: a new approach to the classification of antiarrhythmic drugs based on their actions on arrhythmogenic mechanisms. Task Force of the Working Group on Arrhythmias of the European Society of Cardiology. *Circulation.* 1991;84:1831, by permission of the American Heart Association; and modified from Fuster V, Alexander RW, O'Rourke RA. *Hurst's the Heart*. 11th ed. New York: McGraw-Hill; 2004.)

cells have an important function in maintaining viability in the fetus that develops complete heart block due to AV nodal damage from certain maternal antibodies associated with systemic lupus erythematosus (SSA and SSB), or in complex congenital heart disease. The rates of these "escape" pacemakers are determined by their location, with atrium greater than ventricle. It is now believed that spontaneous automaticity may result from a combination of factors, including a decline in an outward potassium current (possibly a decline in I_K or in AV node cells, I_{K1}), increases in both L-type and T-type calcium currents, and a transient background Na^+ current.[14,15] Spontaneous automaticity contributes to "parasystolic foci," which are premature ventricular contractions (PVCs) that can maintain a regular rhythmic pattern despite the SA node influence, and may also explain many ectopic beats. When rhythmic, abnormal spontaneous automaticity can result in tachyarrhythmia, such as sinus tachycardia and atrial ectopic tachycardia. Another inward current, carried partly by potassium and partly by sodium and termed I_f (*f* for *funny*), has been described and is believed to be an important pacemaker current in relatively hyperpolarized cells.[16]

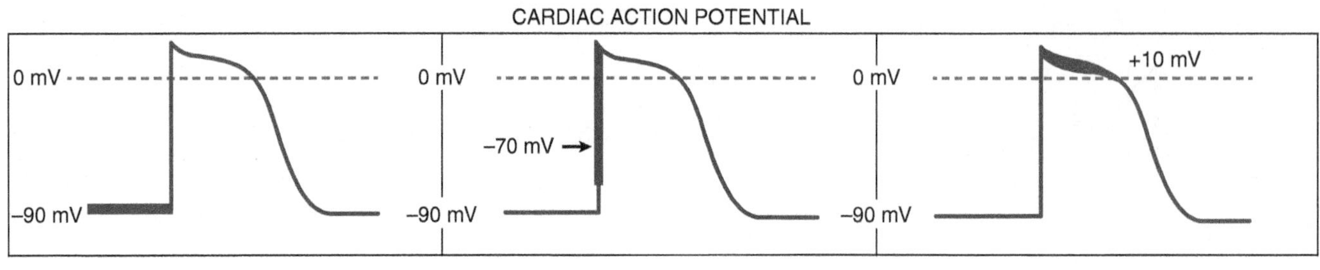

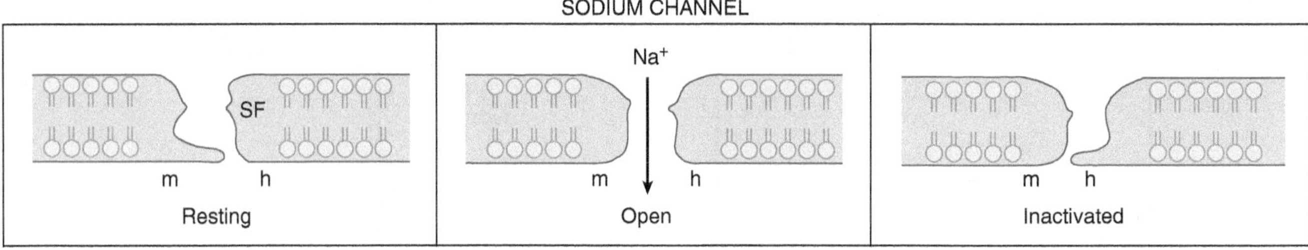

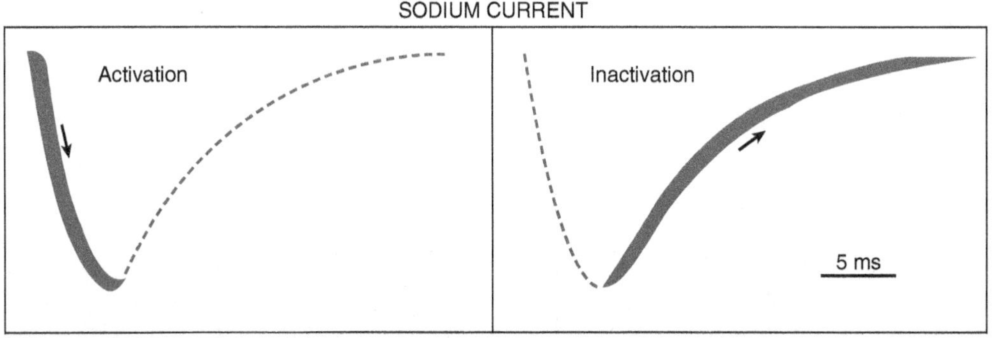

Fig. 46.3 Three conformational states of the sodium channel. Illustration of the changes in transmembrane action potential *(top row)*, changes in the conformational state of the sodium channel *(middle row)*, and corresponding activation and inactivation of the sodium current *(bottom row)*. At rest, the membrane potential is approximately −90 mV *(left)*. At this membrane potential, the sodium channel exists primarily in the rested state. The *m* gate of the sodium channel is closed. (*SF* denotes the selectivity filter of the ion channel.) As the cell membrane depolarizes (phase 0 of the action potential), the sodium channel changes to the open conformation, associated with opening of the *m* gate *(middle)*. The sodium current rapidly activates because sodium ions can now pass through the ion channel. As the membrane potential becomes more positive, the sodium channel enters into its third conformational state, the inactivated state. This occurs as a result of closure of the inactivation gate *h (right)*. The sodium current rapidly inactivates, or decays, back towards zero current.

DEVELOPMENTAL CHANGES IN ACTION POTENTIAL MORPHOLOGY AND TRANSMEMBRANE ION CURRENTS

Changes in action potential morphology and corresponding changes in ion current physiology occur throughout the course of development.

RESTING MEMBRANE POTENTIAL

Increase in sodium-potassium ATPase activity noted during development may in part result from expression of different isoforms of the sodium-potassium ATPase pump,[17] resulting in a more negative resting membrane potential.

An increase in membrane permeability to potassium with development also contributes to the more negative resting potential observed with maturation. Specific increases in the current density of the inward rectifier current, I_{K1}, the main outward potassium current responsible for maintenance of the resting membrane potential, have been reported in animal studies.[18–23]

In the human fetus at mid-gestation (about 20 weeks), and in young infants undergoing heart surgery, resting membrane potentials are similar to values reported in adults.[24,25]

ACTION POTENTIAL UPSTROKE, PHASE 0

Increases in action potential phase 0 amplitude and $\dot{V}_{max}$ with maturation have been documented and are only partly the result of the increases in the resting membrane potential already described. Developmental changes in the structure or function of the ion channel or channels responsible for the upstroke of the action potential appear to contribute.[26,27]

PHASE 1 OF THE ACTION POTENTIAL

Maturation of the spike-and-dome appearance in Phase 1 correlates with the messenger RNA expression of genes associated with the transient outward current I_{to}, specifically, *KCNIP2* and *KCND3* (which encodes Kv4.3).[28] The maturation of the transient outward current is also associated with the development of the phenomenon of "cardiac memory," which refers to changes in repolarization that occur with, and that persist after, a period of chronic pacing. In human atrial cells, an absence of the typical spike-and-dome shape of the action potential has been reported in infant tissue, and is believed to reflect a paucity of the transient outward current. However, I_{to} current was subsequently identified in some cells isolated from young infants undergoing heart surgery,[29,30] significant changes in current density and in recovery

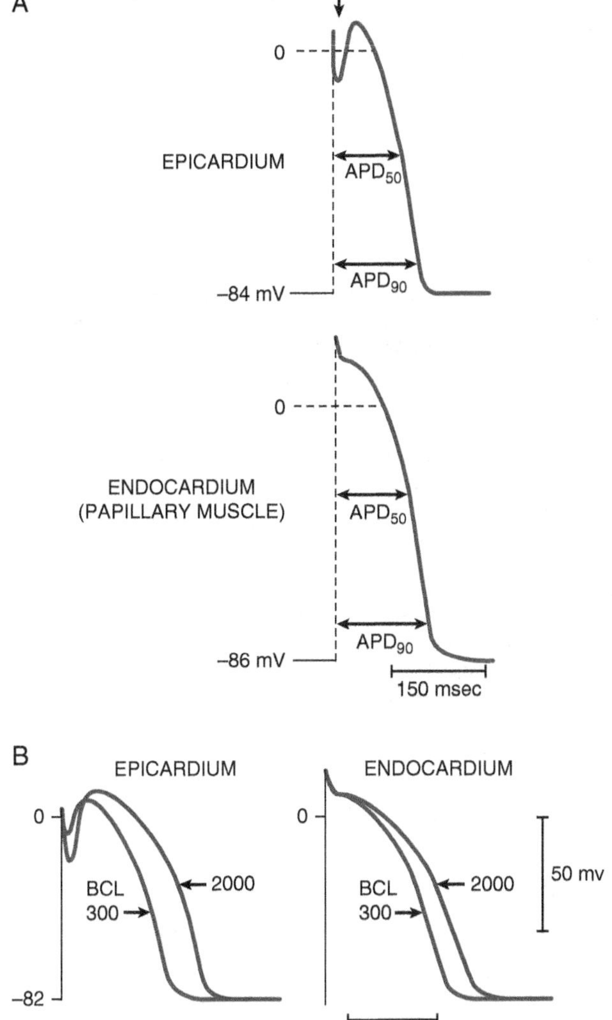

Fig. 46.4 (A) Representative action potentials from ventricular endocardium and epicardium. In the epicardium, there is a prominent spike-and-dome appearance of the action potential plateau *(arrow)*. This spike-and-dome appearance is the result of a prominent transient outward current, carried by potassium, which is present in the epicardium and separates phases 1 and 2 of the action potential. This is much less pronounced in action potentials recorded from the endocardium. (B) Demonstration of the rate-dependent behavior of the transient outward current in canine ventricular myocardium. In epicardium, decreasing basic cycle length *(BCL)* (i.e., increasing heart rate) from 2000 to 300 msec markedly diminishes the spike-and-dome appearance of the action potential plateau and causes marked shortening of action potential duration. This is due to rate-dependent reduction of the transient outward current at faster heart rates (due to incomplete recovery from inactivation). This is not seen in endocardium, where the transiently activated outward potassium current (I_{to}) is negligible, resulting in little or no change in action potential duration in response to increases in heart rate. (Note the effects of the rate-dependent decreases in I_{to} on action potential duration are variable. In some species and preparations, action potential duration increases; in others, it decreases.) *APD_{50}*, Action potential duration to 50% repolarization; *APD_{90}*, action potential duration to 90% repolarization. (A, Modified from Litovsky SH, Antzelevitch C. Transient outward current prominent in canine ventricular epicardium but not endocardium. *Circ Res*. 1988;62:116, by permission of the American Heart Association. B, From Litovsky SH, Antzelevitch C. Rate dependence of action potential duration and refractoriness in canine ventricular endocardium differs from that of epicardium: role of the transient outward current. *J Am Coll Cardiol*. 1989;14:1053. Reprinted with permission from the American College of Cardiology.)

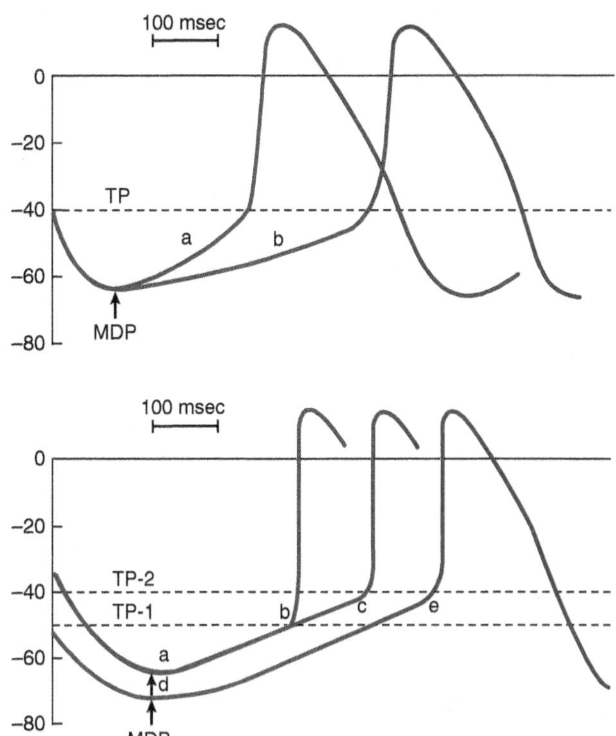

Fig. 46.5 Mechanisms of modulation of cardiac pacemaker rate. *Top panel*, Two sinoatrial node action potentials are illustrated. The threshold potential *(TP)* for both action potentials is −40 mV. The maximal diastolic potential *(MDP)* is approximately −60 mV. If the slope of spontaneous depolarization decreases *(b)*, the pacemaker firing rate is delayed. *Bottom panel*, Three sinoatrial node action potentials are shown. A decrease in the TP (i.e., less negative, TP-1 to TP-2) results in a delay in firing rate (*c* vs. *b*). Pacemaker firing rate can also be delayed (*e* vs. *c*) by an increase in the MDP (i.e., a more negative diastolic potential) (*a* vs. *d*), with the slope of spontaneous depolarization and the TP remaining constant. (From Hoffman BF, Cranefield PF. *Electrophysiology of the Heart*. New York: McGraw-Hill; 1960:109.)

kinetics have been reported with maturation to adulthood. A larger current density, faster inactivation, and slower recovery from inactivation of I_{to} in the neonate has been described and are believed to be a function of the differences in the relative expression of *KCNIP2* and *KCND3*.[31] Thus there appear to be consistent age-related increases in I_{to}, the transient outward current (Fig. 46.6). The functional significance of the increase in the transient outward current is not fully understood, nor are the mechanisms that lead to the increased expression of the transient outward current in postnatal life, although augmentation of I_{to} may be linked to postnatal increases in oxygen tension.[32]

ACTION POTENTIAL PLATEAU AND REPOLARIZATION, PHASES 2 AND 3

The slow inward calcium current ($I_{Ca\text{-}L}$) contributes importantly to the sustained depolarization that constitutes the action potential plateau. Shifts occur in the relative contributions of L-type and T-type calcium channels, which accounts for the calcium transient in early embryonic development.

In the rabbit, progressive increases in myocardial calcium current density and kinetics have been described from fetal to adult life.[19,33] Inactivation of the calcium current occurs at less-negative membrane potentials in fetal myocytes compared with adult myocytes. In addition, recovery from inactivation occurs over a longer time in immature cells. Because of the more prolonged time course of recovery from inactivation

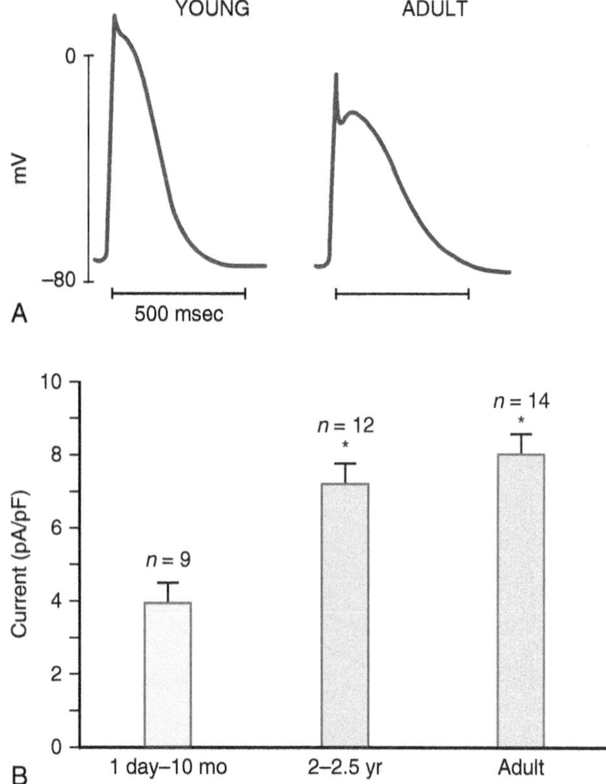

Fig. 46.6 (A) Comparison of human atrial action potentials. Note that in the adult atrial action potential, there is a prominent spike-and-dome appearance to the plateau phase of the action potential. This is presumed to reflect a prominent transient outward current (I_{to}) in the adult. This spike-and-dome shape of the atrial action potential is absent in the recording from a young infant. (B) Relationship between age and I_{to} amplitude in human atrial myocytes. Note that the I_{to} amplitude *(pA/pF)* is significantly less *(asterisk,* $P < .05$) in atrial cells isolated from infants younger than 2 years. (A, From Escande D, Loisance D, Planche C, et al. Age-related changes of action potential plateau shape in isolated human atrial fibers. *Am J Physiol.* 1985;249:H843. B, From Crumb WJ Jr, Pigott JD, Clarkson CW. Comparison of I_{to} in young and adult human atrial myocytes: evidence for developmental changes. *Am J Physiol.* 1995;268:H1335.)

in immature cells, the calcium current becomes inhibited to a greater extent at faster stimulation frequencies in the fetus and newborn. This inhibition of the calcium current at faster heart rates may place the immature heart at a potential disadvantage for excitation-contraction coupling (a process that is dependent on transsarcolemmal calcium transport, predominantly through the Na^+-Ca^{2+} exchanger but also to some extent through the L-type calcium channel).[34,35] On a clinical basis, this explains the hypotension and bradycardia seen (prior to the use of adenosine) when neonates were administered verapamil, a calcium channel blocker, to terminate supraventricular tachycardia (SVT). Finally, it has been reported that calcium current density is equivalent in atrial myocytes of newborn and adult humans.[36]

IMPULSE FORMATION (PHASE 4) AND INTRA-ATRIAL AND ATRIOVENTRICULAR CONDUCTION IN THE EMBRYO, FETUS, AND NEONATE: MORPHOLOGIC AND PHYSIOLOGIC CONSIDERATIONS

In the chick embryo, spontaneous cardiac electrical depolarizations can be detected by voltage-sensitive dyes at about the seventh somite stage, well before contractions become evident.[37] These studies, as well as direct microelectrode recordings,[38] have demonstrated that, although contraction is first noted in the primitive ventricle of the chick embryo (somite stage 10), pacemaker activity evolves simultaneously in both atrial and ventricular sites, and later becomes confined to atrial sites. There is little information concerning the specific ion currents responsible for cardiac automaticity during development. Very early in embryonic life, before the development of true pacemaker ionic currents, "shuttling" of calcium in and out of the sarcoplasmic reticulum, through an inositol triphosphate-dependent mechanism, may be responsible for pacemaker activity at the earliest stages of development.[39] Embryonic stem cell–derived cardiomyocytes depend on a functional ryanodine receptor to differentiate into contracting myocytes with a progressively increasing beating rate.[40] Murine embryonic stem cells, or *pacemaker nodes,* are characterized by the expression of the genetic molecular marker *GATA6*.[41] It has been suggested that the so-called funny inward pacemaker current, I_f, which normally activates at hyperpolarized membrane potentials, may also contribute importantly to cardiac automaticity in very early embryonic life.[42,43]

The genetic and environmental factors that contribute to pacemaker formation are largely unknown. It is known that cardiac mesenchymal tissues that are destined to form specific regions of the embryonic heart beat at predetermined, characteristic rates.[44] Genetically determined differences in ion channel populations and kinetics of ion channel function are believed to be important in determining these programmed beating rates. Defects in *NKX2-5*, *SCN5A*, and *HCN4* lead to sinoatrial node dysfunction, which can manifest itself in the human before birth or later. That environmental cues can also modulate pacemaker development and function is demonstrable, in that transplantation of mesenchymal tissue from "fast" sinoatrial regions into "slow" regions results in a gradual decrease in the rate of spontaneous firing of the transplanted tissue.[45] With exposure to cold, automaticity also diminishes.[46] Physical contact between myocardial cells and nonmyocardial elements may also contribute to the induction of pacemaker cell aggregates.[47] In vivo, looping of the heart may bring the sinoatrial region of the heart into close contact with nonmyocardial mesenchyme and thereby induce formation of the sinoatrial pacemaker. In the human embryo, a sinoatrial node is first identified shortly after the looping process is completed. The sinoatrial node, an epicardial structure, is positioned at the junction of the superior vena cava and the right atrium. It is relatively larger in the fetus than in the adult and is horseshoe-shaped rather than having the spindle shape observed in the adult.[48]

CONDUCTION OF THE IMPULSE FROM THE SINOATRIAL NODE TO THE ATRIOVENTRICULAR NODE

The existence of specialized "internodal" conduction pathways within the right atrium, linking the sinoatrial and AV nodes, has been proposed.[49] These putative specialized conduction pathways are located laterally, along the terminal crest of the right atrium, and medially, along the posterior and anterior rims of the fossa ovalis. Although such internodal pathways have been demonstrated histologically and by immunochemistry (including in the developing heart[50,51]), a lack of true specialized cell types and lack of insulation from surrounding myocardium have been cited by some researchers as evidence against true specialized internodal conduction pathways.[52,53]

Whether or not true specialized internodal pathways exist, intra-atrial conduction tends to propagate as waves of excitation within the atrium along directions that roughly follow the anatomic courses of the putative internodal pathways. This preferential conduction, along the terminal crest and the anterior and posterior interatrial septum, may be the result of a more uniform, longitudinal alignment of atrial myocytes in these anatomic locations, rather than being the result of specialized conduction pathways.[54]

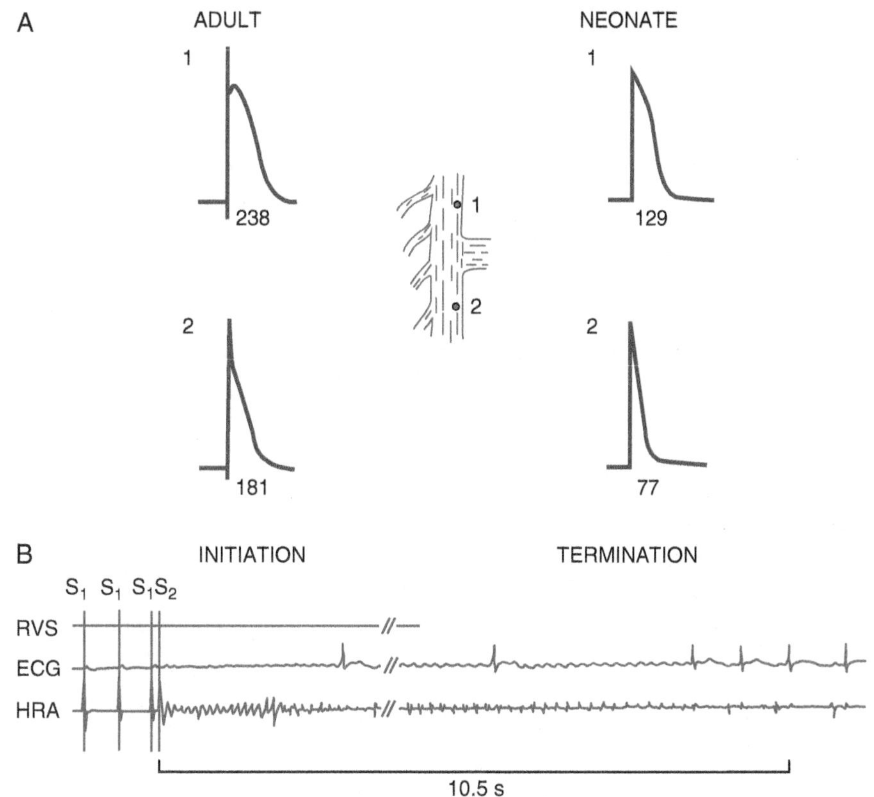

Fig. 46.7 (A) Atrial action potentials recorded from roughly similar locations along the terminal crest in adult and newborn dogs. Note that neonatal action potentials are characterized by little or no action potential plateau and shorter action potential durations (indicated beneath each action potential, in milliseconds) compared with adult action potentials. (B) The effect of premature atrial simulation during vagal stimulation in the newborn dog. Right vagal stimulation *(RVS)* indicates the period of stimulation of the right vagus nerve, S_1 refers to a basic paced drive train, and S_2 refers to a single premature atrial paced beat. Surface electrocardiogram lead II and intracardiac recordings of atrial activity from the right atrium *(HRA)* are shown. Note that with the introduction of the premature beat *(S_2)*, a long train of atrial fibrillation-flutter is induced. (Similar but shorter runs of atrial fibrillation-flutter are induced in the atrium of the newborn in the absence of vagal stimulation.) *ECG*, Electrocardiogram. (A, Modified from Spach MS, Dolber PC, Anderson PA. Multiple regional differences in cellular properties that regulate repolarization and contraction in the right atrium of adult and newborn dogs. *Circ Res.* 1989;65:1594, by permission of the American Heart Association. B, Modified from Pickoff AS, Stolfi A. Modulation of electrophysiological properties of neonatal canine heart by tonic parasympathetic stimulation. *Am J Physiol.* 1990;258:H38.)

Electrophysiologic differences in atrial action potential morphology and intra-atrial conduction have been described during the course of development.[55] Atrial action potential durations (APDs) tend to be significantly more uniform in the human fetus, and shorter in the human newborn compared with the adult (Fig. 46.7A).[25,55–57] Shorter APDs result in shorter refractory periods in the neonatal atrium compared with the adult atrium, which may facilitate the development of intra-atrial reentry (see Fig. 46.7B).[58,59] It is possible that the occurrence of atrial flutter in the fetus and newborn with an otherwise structurally normal heart results in part from these shorter atrial refractory periods.[58,60] Atrial flutter may also be triggered because of reentry over an accessory AV pathway, with a very short coupling interval. Finally, in addition to developmental changes in the electrophysiology of the developing atrial myocyte, growth of nonmyocardial elements within the atrium is believed to contribute to developmental differences noted in propagation patterns within the atrium. For example, in the neonatal heart, impulses are conducted directly from the superior rim of the terminal crest to the adjacent atrial myocardium, whereas in the adult, atrial conduction proceeds inferiorly first, before activation of the myocardium adjacent to the superior terminal crest.[55]

ATRIOVENTRICULAR CONDUCTION BEFORE THE FORMATION OF THE SPECIALIZED ATRIOVENTRICULAR CONDUCTION SYSTEM

In the prelooped, preinnervated rat heart, as well as in the chick embryo, AV delay appears to originate in cell populations corresponding to the endocardial cushions or AV canal.[61] Shortly after looping (Fig. 46.8), a synchronization of ventricular wall motion is observed, coupled with a 10-fold increase in conduction velocity.[61] These changes are highly correlated with expression of the major gap junction protein, connexin 43.[62] Gap junctions are the specialized protein channels that connect adjacent myocytes (Fig. 46.9A–C).[63] These channels allow not only the passage of electric current through a low-resistance pathway from cell to cell but also the exchange of larger molecules between cells.[64] In the human heart, connexin 40 is initially diffusely up-regulated with its expression largely confined to the atrium, whereas connexin 43 becomes the dominant isoform expressed in the ventricular myocardium.[62,65] The differential regulation of expression of connexins within the developing heart may be altered by factors such as exposure to hypoxia and tumor necrosis factor (TNF)-α.[66,67] A study[68] demonstrated the importance of chronic electrical stimulation in the expression of connexin 43, expression of certain β-subunits such as Kv11.1 and Kv4.2, cell

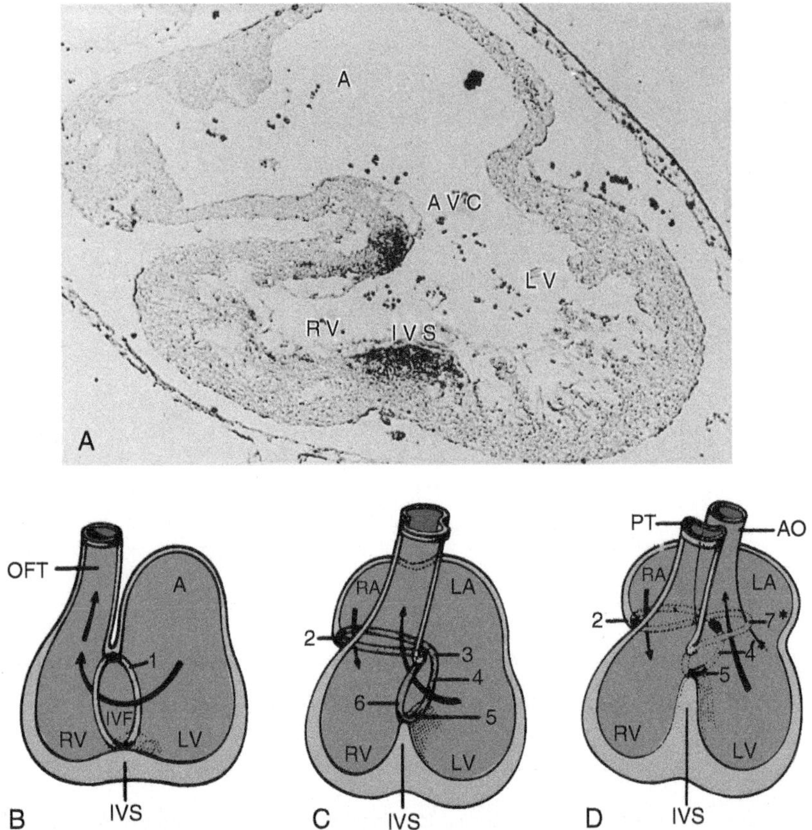

Fig. 46.8 (A) Immunohistochemical staining of the embryonic precursor of the atrioventricular (AV) conduction system in the human heart (Carnegie stage 14). A single ring of tissue, stained for the ganglion nodosum (GLN) antigen, is seen surrounding the interventricular foramen. It is from this single ring of tissue that the entire AV conduction system forms. This includes the AV node, the bundle of His, and the right and left bundle branches. (B–D), Formation of the AV conduction system. (B) The single GLN ring surrounds the interventricular foramen (IVF) in the looped heart (Carnegie stage 14). At this stage of development, the primitive atrium connects solely with the left ventricle *(LV)*. (C) At Carnegie stages 15 to 17, there is rightward expansion of the GLN ring, as the right atrium *(RA)* and tricuspid orifice form over the right ventricle *(RV)*. Note the interventricular septum *(IVS)* rising from the floor of the ventricles. The AV node forms at position *3,* the bundle of His at position *4,* and the bundle branches at position *5.* (D) At Carnegie stages 18 to 23, there is further development of the IVS. Involution of much of the original GLN ring now occurs, leaving the newly formed AV conduction system. *A,* Atria; *AO,* aorta; *AVC,* atrioventricular canal; *LA,* left atrium; *OFT,* outflow tract; *PT,* pulmonary tract. (From Wessels A, Vermeulen JLM, Verbeek FJ, et al. Spatial distribution of "tissue-specific" antigens in the developing human heart and skeletal muscle. III. An immunohistochemical analysis of the distribution of the neural tissue antigen G1N2 in the embryonic heart; implications for the development of the atrioventricular conduction system. *Anat Rec.* 1992;232:97, by permission of Wiley-Liss, Inc., a subsidiary of John Wiley & Sons.)

length, and cell alignment, leading to shortening of the APD to 50% repolarization (APD50) and cell maturation. The critical role of connexins for normal cardiac conduction, as well as normal cardiac development, is demonstrated by reports of abnormal, sometimes lethal, intracardiac conduction abnormalities, and of abnormal anatomic development, in hearts of mice with absent or diminished expression of specific connexins.[69,70]

In the developing embryo, the newer regions of fast conduction remain flanked by persisting zones of slow conduction, including the AV canal region and the outflow tract. These regions are characterized by continued expression of both atrial and ventricular myosin heavy chain isoforms and very scarce gap junction protein.[71] Two-dimensional optical mapping in the chick embryo has shown a switch from an "immature" base-to-apex activation pattern to the "mature" apex-to-base activation pattern.[72-75]

FORMATION OF THE SPECIALIZED ATRIOVENTRICULAR CONDUCTION SYSTEM

The specialized AV conduction system (AV node, bundle of His, right and left bundle branches) forms after the looping process of the heart is completed. This process normally occurs at 25 days of gestation in the human, at which point a typical adult-like electrocardiographic pattern of conduction is seen.[76]

Multiple immunohistochemical markers have been used to delineate and track the development of the specialized conduction system in the human heart. These molecular markers are mainly of neural tissue (e.g., ganglion nodosum, human natural killer-1 [HNK-1]). However, the conduction system is derived from multipotential mesenchymal precursors and not from neural precursors. The sinoatrial node, AV node, and bundle of His are derived from the embryonic primary myocardium of the heart tube. The more distal ramifications of the conduction system or bundle branches are formed from embryonic secondary myocardium, specifically prechamber trabecular myocardium. The latter is genetically distinct from the adjacent embryonic compact myocardium.[77] Derivatives of the secondary myocardium are characterized by the expression of atrial natriuretic factor (ANF), connexin 40, and connexin 43.

Cardiomyogenic precursor cells may be induced by regional cues to express genetic programs. One crucial signaling molecule is endothelin 1.[78,79] The genetic programs promote differentiation to the specialized cells of the cardiac conduction system (CCS). The inducers may also include neural crest cells, which migrate

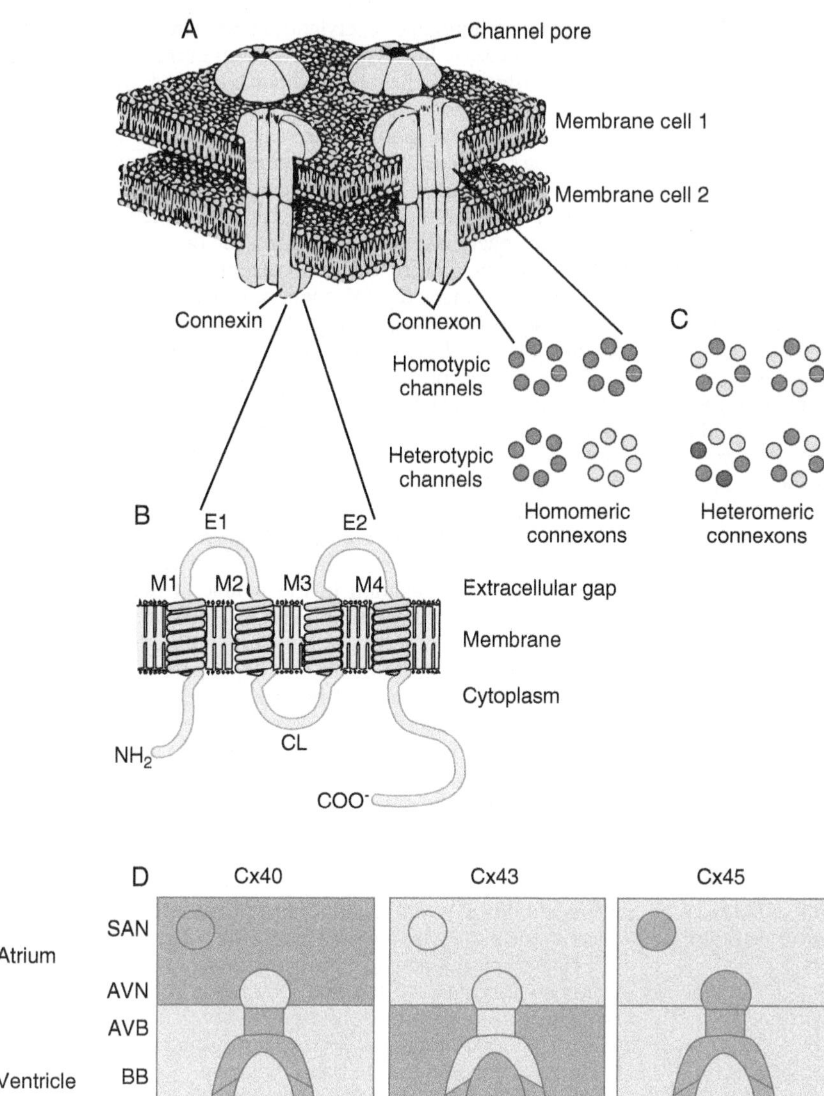

Fig. 46.9 Ultrastructure of cardiac gap junctions. Gap junctions occur as "plaques" of multiple intercellular channels. (A) Portion of a gap junction plaque demonstrating the structure of the intercellular channels, which join cell membranes from two adjacent cardiac myocytes (membrane cell 1, membrane cell 2). Each cell membrane contributes half of the channel structure, called a *connexon.* Each connexon consists of six connexin proteins. (B) Secondary structure of a single connexin protein. (C) Connexons formed from identical sets of connexins are termed *homomeric connexons.* Those formed from dissimilar connexin isoforms are termed *heteromeric connexons.* These then combine to form either homotypic or heterotypic intercellular channels. (D) Expression of the major connexin isoforms, connexin 40 (Cx40), connexin 43 (Cx43), and connexin 45 (Cx45), in the mammalian myocardium and specialized conduction system. *AVB,* Bundle of His; *AVN,* atrioventricular node; *BB,* bundle branches; *PF,* Purkinje fibers; *SAN,* sinoatrial node. (From van Veen TA, van Rijen HVM, Opthof T. Cardiac gap junction channels: modulation of expression and channel properties. *Cardiovasc Res.* 2001;51:217.)

into the central CCS, as well as into the epicardium-derived cells. This process might influence the differentiation of the more distal ramification of the Purkinje network.[78,80,81] Neural crest cells entering the heart may add to the differentiation of the conduction system: entering by the arterial pole may contribute to the differentiation of the bundle branches, whereas entering through the venous pole may influence the induction of sinoatrial node and AV node cell development.[82]

The transcriptional regulation of the differentiation of cardiomyogenic precursor cells into cells of the specialized CCS has been investigated intensively. GATA6, Nkx2-5, members of the T-box family (Tbx2, Tbx3, Tbx5), and homeodomain-only protein seem to be the most important factors in the differentiation, formation, and function of the CCS.[83-88] Mutations of transcription factors can result in congenital heart defects, conduction disturbances, and arrhythmias.[89,90] Cardiomyopathy has also been described.[91]

ANF is an amino acid polypeptide hormone secreted mainly by the atria of the heart in response to atrial stretch. The promoter region of ANF contains multiple binding sites for several cardiac transcription factors that are important in the development or function of the CCS, including Nkx2-5, GATA4, and Tbx5.[92-94] It is speculated that chamber-specific working myocardium gene expression is repressed in the nodal myocardium (sinoatrial node, AV node, and bundle of His), secondary to an inhibition of ANF expression, as a result of the binding of Tbx2 and Nkx2-5 to the ANF promoter region.[95] Elements of the bundle branches do express ANF and connexin 40. Therefore with differentiation the specialized CCS expresses a molecular pattern that is distinct from the surrounding atrial and ventricular myocardium.[82]

In humans, immunohistochemical studies have demonstrated that the entire AV conduction system develops from a single ring of specialized tissue. This ring, stained for ganglion nodosum antigen, surrounds the interventricular foramen, which connects the primitive left and right ventricles. After the looping of the heart has occurred, the atrium is connected only with the left ventricle. With further development the rightward expansion of the ring is observed, because the atrium expands rightward to form the tricuspid orifice. As the interventricular septum (IVS) extends, the lower part of the ring raises superiorly. After the contact between the rising IVS and the lesser curve of the looped heart, the AV node and bundle of His have formed.

In the normal heart, the AV node is located in the triangle of Koch. This triangular area is located on the septal wall of the right atrium, between the tricuspid valve, coronary sinus orifice, and tendon of Todaro, and marks the site of the AV node. Histologically, the AV node consists of a loose and transitional zone and a compact region. Extension of this compact zone is believed to be a normal variant.

The AV bundle arises from the compact node and penetrates the central fibrous body of the heart, branching into the right and left bundle branches. The left bundle branch has a subendocardial location over the left ventricular septal surface, and it further subdivides into anterior and posterior fascicles. The right bundle branch is intramyocardial, within the right septal surface. It is more cordlike and emerges onto the endocardial surface of the right ventricle beneath the medial papillary muscle, descending to the apex of the right ventricle along the moderator band and across to the free border of the right ventricle.

PHYSIOLOGY OF ATRIOVENTRICULAR CONDUCTION

The characteristics of the AV node in the neonatal heart are poorly understood. Reasons include a lack of information on the structure and physiology of the AV node in the immature myocardium.[96] However, it is known that the AV node can be subdivided functionally and histologically into the inferior nodal extension, compact node, and lower nodal bundle.[96] The refractory period of the AV conduction system in the neonate is significantly longer than the ventricular refractory period. The AV node serves as the primary site of conduction slowing in both neonatal and adult animals.[97]

In clinical settings, normal fetal AV conduction intervals have been demonstrated by fetal echocardiography from about 11 weeks of gestation, and by fetal magnetocardiography from about 15 weeks of gestation onwards.[98-100]

AUTONOMIC INNERVATION-MODULATION OF CARDIAC AUTOMATICITY AND CONDUCTION

In considering developmental cardiac electrophysiology, maturation of the autonomic nervous system and its effect on the electrophysiologic properties of the heart must also be considered. Changes in autonomic tone profoundly affect pacemaker impulse generation, as well as AV conduction and myocardial refractoriness.

PARASYMPATHETIC NERVOUS SYSTEM

Progressive increases are seen in choline acetyltransferase concentration, and in the uptake of the parasympathetic neurotransmitter precursor cholinewithdevelopment.[101] In the mammalian heart, muscarinic receptors are present before actual innervation of the heart. Acetylcholinesterase is also demonstrable before innervation.[102] Progressive cholinergic innervation of the heart becomes denser in the regions of the sinoatrial and AV nodes and throughout the atria. In the human newborn, moderate cholinesterase activity is found in association with the sinoatrial and AV nodes.[103] Little or no cholinesterase staining of the bundle branches is observed in the newborn infant. Postnatal maturation of innervation to include the remainder of the conduction system occurs, reaching a maximal density in childhood.[104,105] Developmental changes in the expression and function of ion channels of intracardiac neurons have been described.[106]

Muscarinic receptor density and production of phosphoinositol (a secondary muscarinic messenger) is greater in the immature heart.[107] Muscarinic receptor subtypes may differ in the immature heart and may have different physiologic responses to acetylcholine stimulation.[108]

The primary actions of acetylcholine on cardiac ion channels include an increase in outward potassium currents, resulting in hyperpolarization of the cell, and with marked shortening of the atrial action potential.[109] Hyperpolarization, coupled with muscarinic inhibition of the inward calcium current, accounts for the slowing of the cardiac pacemaker rate that is characteristic of muscarinic stimulation. It has also been shown that acetylcholine inhibits I_f, the funny pacemaker current, which contributes to cardiac pacemaker slowing caused by acetylcholine.[110] Inhibition of the inward calcium current, primarily within the nodal or N region of the AV node, reduces the amplitude and rate of rise of the slow-response AV nodal action potential. This accounts for the slowing of conduction through the AV node. The refractoriness of the AV node is also markedly increased by muscarinic stimulation. In ventricular myocardium, a slight but significant increase in ventricular refractory periods occurs with vagal stimulation. Evidence is increasing that this is a direct effect of acetylcholine.[111]

Maturation of parasympathetic control of cardiac electrophysiology is evident from studies of heart rate variability, as well as the effects of muscarinic blockade, vagus nerve transection, and vagus nerve stimulation in the course of development. In the human fetus, the increase in heart rate observed in response to a maternal dose of atropine increases with advancing gestation.[112] In the premature infant (32.3 ± 1.3 weeks), analyses of the respiratory component of heart rate variability, a surrogate of vagal activity, suggest that respiratory vagal activity increases during the first postnatal month.[113] In the fetal lamb, vagal stimulation causes a greater slowing of the heart rate as gestation progresses.[114,115] The response to brief trains of vagal stimuli, which experimentally mimics how the vagus nerve actually fires in vivo, also changes with development. In the adult the degree of prolongation of sinus cycle length (as well as the degree of prolongation of AV nodal conduction) progressively *increases* as a brief vagal train is delivered progressively later in the cardiac cycle. This typical phase-response relationship is not observed in the newborn (Fig. 46.10). Full maturation of the response to brief vagal stimuli is not observed until about 1 to 2 months of age.[116,117] Thus although parasympathetic responses and reflexes are clearly present in utero and in the preterm infant, it is incorrect to consider the parasympathetic nervous system as being fully mature at birth. Significant maturation occurs in both the magnitude and the type of responses elicited by parasympathetic stimulation in postnatal life.[115]

SYMPATHETIC NERVOUS SYSTEM

Evidence of functional β-adrenergic receptor modulation of calcium channel currents is observed in the early mammalian heart, before the time of sympathetic innervation.[118] However, in many mammalian species, including the human, rat, and dog, it is believed that the sympathetic nervous system is not as well developed as the parasympathetic nervous system at the time of birth. Rapid maturation occurs within the first postnatal months. Evidence of sympathetic innervation of the atrium, sinoatrial and AV nodes, and the ventricular epicardium is first observed at mid-gestation and progressively increases, reaching full maturity only after 2 months of age.[119-122]

Maturation of sympathetic innervation is associated with profound changes in the electrophysiologic responses of the developing heart to catecholamine stimulation.[123] It has been shown that the conversion of the chronotropic response to α-adrenergic stimulation from the neonatal response (increase in automaticity in Purkinje fibers) to the adult response (decrease in automaticity) is contingent on the process of sympathetic innervation. Two separate subtypes of α_1-adrenergic receptors appear to mediate the positive and negative chronotropic responses. One subtype is antagonized by an analogue of clonidine and is linked to the neonatal positive chronotropic response.

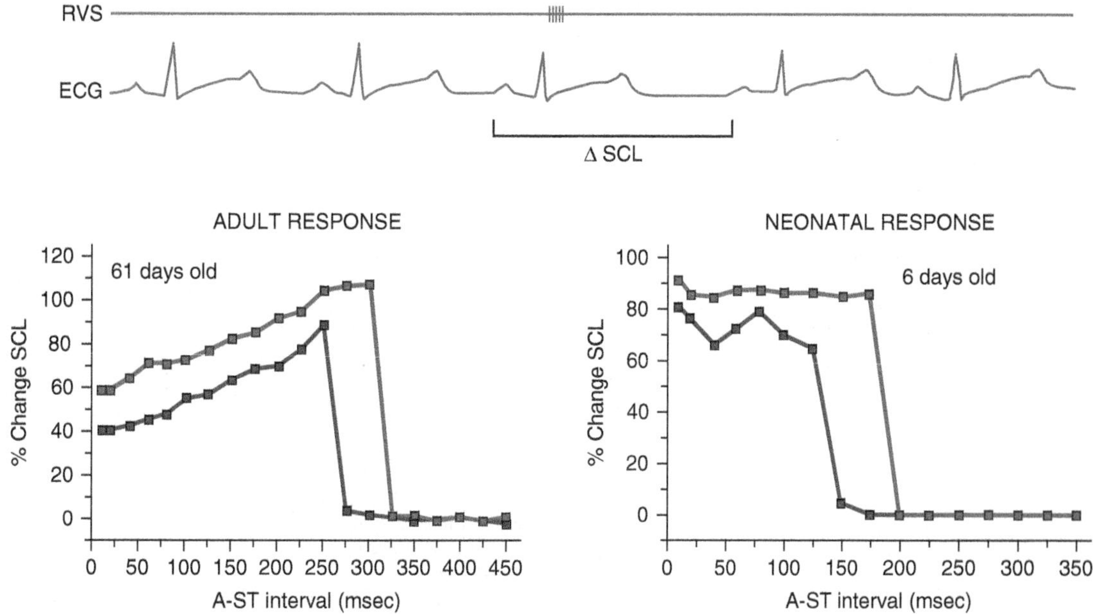

Fig. 46.10 The response of heart rate to brief vagal stimulation. A short train of vagal stimulation is delivered once, at different times, within the cardiac cycle. The effect of each brief, critically timed vagal train on sinus cycle length *(SCL)* is determined, and a phase-response curve is generated. *Left,* A typical adult-type vagal phase-response curve, obtained in experiments performed on a 2-month-old puppy. As the vagal train is delivered at progressively later times after the last atrial depolarization *(A-ST interval)*, the change in SCL (percentage change of SCL) evoked by that vagal stimulation train progressively increases. Eventually the vagal train is delivered too late in the cardiac cycle to affect SCL. *Right,* A typical phase-response curve in a newborn. In contrast to in the older puppy, in the neonate, the vagal response remains flat as the vagal train is advanced through the cardiac cycle. *Closed squares* indicate right vagal stimulation *(RVS)*; *open squares* indicate left vagal stimulation. (Phase-response curves are from Pickoff AS, Rios R, Stolfi A, et al. Postnatal maturation of the response of the canine sinus node to critically timed, brief vagal stimulation. *Pediatr Res.* 1994;35:55.)

The other subtype is linked to the adult negative chronotropic response.[124] In the neonatal rat, α_1-adrenergic activation increases the L-type calcium current, $I_{Ca\text{-}L}$, one of the currents responsible for automaticity. This α_1-adrenergic-mediated increase in calcium current is not observed in the adult heart. This suggests that there is also a developmentally determined switching of the coupling of α_1-adrenergic receptors with respect to calcium channels during development.[125]

In contrast to the cardiac electrophysiologic effects of parasympathetic stimulation, which exhibit rapid kinetics, the kinetics of sympathetic stimulation are more prolonged. The maximal effects of adrenergic stimulation on heart rate, myocardial refractoriness, and conduction tend to develop over several seconds, in contrast to the nearly instantaneous effects of vagal stimulation. The dominant electrophysiologic actions of sympathetic stimulation in the heart are mediated by the β_1 receptor, although β_2 receptors do coexist on the cardiac myocyte. The main electrophysiologic effects of β-adrenergic stimulation include an increase in sinoatrial node automaticity, which is in part mediated by an increase in the rate of diastolic depolarization (phase 4 of the action potential). There is also an increase in the maximal diastolic potential of the sinoatrial node, which serves to increase the activity of the I_f pacemaker current. In the AV node, conduction velocities are increased and refractory periods are shortened; the increases in AV nodal action potential amplitude and $\dot{V}_{max}$ account for the increase in conduction velocity. In the myocardium, β-adrenergic stimulation increases the height of the action potential plateau by increasing the inward calcium current; it also increases the speed of repolarization by increasing outward potassium currents. Overall, these effects tend to shorten myocardial refractoriness. The increase in the maximal diastolic potential, observed in the sinoatrial node and in the working myocardium, is likely caused by an adrenergic-mediated increase in the activity of the sodium-potassium pump. These primary effects of β-adrenergic stimulation are mediated through a membrane-bound stimulatory guanine nucleotide binding protein, G_s (Fig. 46.11B). The effects of sympathetic stimulation on the heart of the newborn and young infant are qualitatively similar to those in the adult, but quantitatively may be less.[115] The increase in response to sympathetic stimulation with maturation is probably multifactorial. As mentioned previously, the density of sympathetic innervation continues to increase postnatally. Furthermore, the stimulatory effect of β-agonists on adenylate cyclase increases postnatally.[126–129]

SYMPATHETIC-PARASYMPATHETIC INTERACTIONS

Several complex interactions between the two branches of the autonomic nervous system have been described.[130,131] At the postsynaptic level, the precise basis for interaction between the sympathetic and parasympathetic nervous systems is still somewhat speculative but may involve a muscarinic-mediated stimulation of phosphatases (enzymes), which results in a reversal of the adrenergic-stimulated phosphorylation of key intracellular proteins, such as the calcium channel.[132] Nitric oxide, a derivative of L-arginine, has also been implicated as a mediator of the cholinergic inhibition of β-adrenergic responses.[133,134]

There have been few studies of interactions between the two branches of the autonomic nervous system during development. Although not present in the neonate, prominent sympathetic-vagal interactions in the control of heart rate can be demonstrated, with sympathetic effects becoming more attenuated with higher levels of background vagal stimulation.[135] Studies of beat-to-beat variability in AV nodal conduction in the premature infant during the first postnatal month (measured as variability in the PR interval of the surface electrocardiogram [ECG]) provide evidence for accentuated sympathetic modulation of AV nodal conduction.[113]

It is known that in addition to the classic autonomic neurotransmitters, acetylcholine and norepinephrine, a family of "neuropeptides" also appears to innervate the human heart.

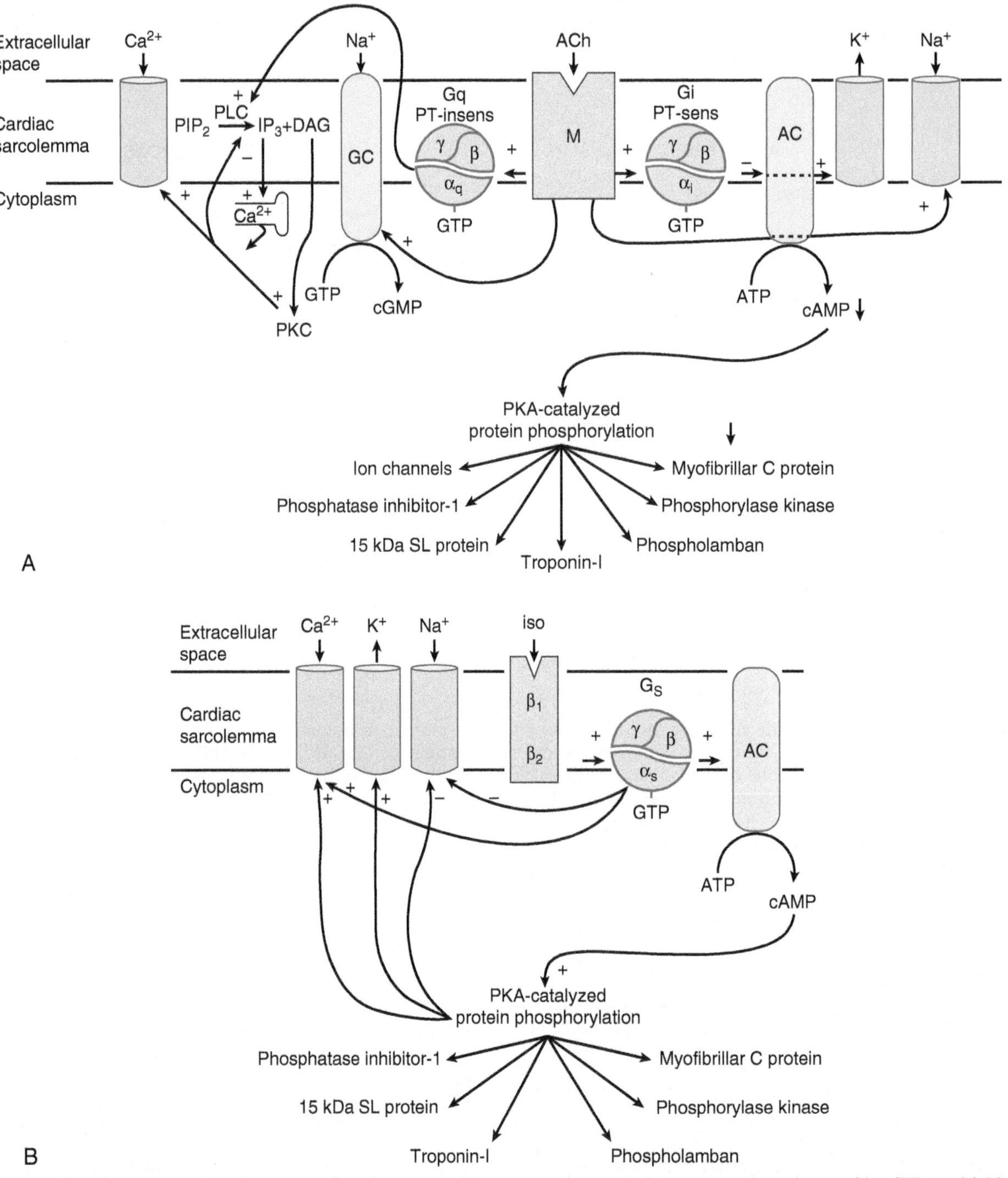

Fig. 46.11 (A) Cholinergic receptor-effector coupling. The muscarinic receptor is coupled to a pertussis toxin–sensitive (PT-sens) inhibitory G protein (Gi). When activated, the α_i-subunit of the G protein dissociates and causes an inhibition of adenylate cyclase *(AC)* and a fall in intracellular cyclic adenosine monophosphate *(cAMP)* levels, with a resultant decrease in protein kinase A *(PKA)* phosphorylation of cellular proteins, including cardiac ion channels. It is by this mechanism that muscarinic stimulation decreases the inward calcium current. Direct activation of potassium channels by the G protein is also known to occur. There is also a pertussis toxin-insensitive *(PT-insens)* G protein *(Gq)* that is linked to the muscarinic receptor. This G protein stimulates phospholipase C *(PLC)* production, which stimulates the production of diacylglycerol *(DAG)* and inositol 1,4,5-trisphosphate *(IP$_3$)*. DAG stimulates protein kinase C *(PKC)*, which phosphorylates and stimulates sarcoplasmic reticulum receptors, causing intracellular release of calcium. IP$_3$ directly stimulates release of calcium from the sarcoplasmic reticulum. (B) β-Adrenergic receptor-effector coupling. The β-adrenergic receptor is coupled to the stimulatory trimeric G protein *(G$_S$)*. In the presence of guanosine triphosphate *(GTP)*, this G protein dissociates, and the α_s-subunit results in direct activation of AC. This increases intracellular cAMP concentration and stimulates PKA. This enhances phosphorylation of cellular proteins, including cardiac ion channels. *ACh,* Acetylcholine; *ATP,* adenosine triphosphate; *cGMP,* cyclic guanosine monophosphate; *PIP2,* phosphatidylinositol 4,5-bisphosphate. (From Fleming JW, Wisler PL, Wantanabe AM. Signal transduction by G proteins in cardiac tissues. *Circulation.* 1992;85:420, by permission of the American Heart Association.)

These peptides include neuropeptide Y, vasoactive intestinal peptide, calcitonin gene-related peptide, somatostatin, and substance P.[136] These neuropeptides exist, either co-localized with the classic neurotransmitters within neurons of the sympathetic or parasympathetic nervous system, or confined to neurons that appear to be separate from the two major branches of the autonomic nervous system. In the human fetal heart, peptide (primarily neuropeptide Y) -immunoreactive nerves first appear at about 10 weeks of gestation, or 3 weeks after the appearance of cardiac ganglia and nerves, first in atrial cells and then in ventricular cells.[137,138] Vasoactive intestinal peptide and somatostatin appear localized primarily within the atrium and are first observed at 10 to 12 weeks of gestation. Substance P and calcitonin gene-related peptide do not appear in the fetal heart until somewhat later, at 18 to 24 weeks of gestation.[139]

Although the precise function and mechanisms of action of this peptidergic neurotransmission system remain to be fully elucidated, it is clear that at least two of these peptides, vasoactive intestinal peptide and neuropeptide Y, may exert significant direct or indirect (or combined) effects on cardiac automaticity and conduction. Vasoactive intestinal peptide can be shown to increase sinoatrial node automaticity directly and to enhance AV nodal conduction in both the adult dog[140,141] and the newborn canine.[142] In the adult dog, vasoactive intestinal peptide shortens atrial refractoriness,[140] an effect not observed in the neonatal atrium.[142] Vasoactive intestinal peptide may be responsible for the acceleration in heart rate observed with vagal stimulation in the presence of autonomic blockade.[143] Neuropeptide Y appears to function as a sympathetic co-transmitter, being localized with norepinephrine within adrenergic neurons.[144-146] Stellate stimulation, however, causes only a small inhibition of cardiac vagal response in the neonate, suggesting that the neuropeptide Y-sympathetic-parasympathetic autonomic interaction is immature at birth. The magnitude of the neuropeptide Y-autonomic interaction increases dramatically within the first postnatal month, probably as a result of the general postnatal maturation of adrenergic innervation (Fig. 46.12C).[147]

ANATOMY AND EMBRYOLOGY OF THE FETAL/ NEONATAL CONDUCTION SYSTEM

Embryologically, certain congenital heart defects, especially those related to the development of the AV canals and the IVS, are particularly prone to be associated with congenital cardiac arrhythmias. There are also embryologic variations of the CCS that create accessory pathways of conduction. The most common of these conditions is Wolff-Parkinson-White syndrome, where an accessory bundle of the CCS develops called the *bundle of Kent*. Clinically, this disorder demonstrates a specific electrocardiographic change called a *delta wave*. The disorder predisposes affected individuals to certain significant cardiac arrhythmias during their lifetime. Also, many regions of the heart muscle are anatomically distinct from, but embryologically connected to the definitively developed embryonic CSS. It is thought that remodeling of these tissues with age and certain cardiac diseases also predisposes individuals to significant cardiac arrhythmias (Table 46.3).[148,149]

As previously described, the SA node and the intra- and inter-atrial conduction fibers, which extend from the SA node throughout both atria over three distinct main bands of intra-atrial conduction tissue as well as an interatrial band of conduction tissue (Bachman's bundle), act to synchronize right and left atrial contractions, but under pathologic conditions or following injury or scarring from surgery, can result in routes for stable intra-atrial reentry known as *atrial flutter*.

The AV node is another collection of specialized cardiomyocytes that act to delay conduction to the ventricles enabling sequential synchronized atrial and ventricular contractions to optimize cardiac output. The AV node is located in posterior-inferior aspect of the intra-atrial septum near the opening of the coronary sinus. The AV bundle (bundle of His) is a collection of conduction fibers insulated by a portion of the fibrous skeleton of the heart as it passes through the membranous and then the muscular portions of the IVS. The fibrous skeleton isolates the AV bundle fibers from the contractile cardiomyocytes to prevent premature activation of the ventricular portion of the CCS.

Finally, the ventricular portion of the CCS is divided into a left and right ventricular fascicule or bundle (Purkinje fibers) that extends from the AV bundle along the endocardium of the ventricles to activate coordinated contraction of both ventricles. These CCS fibers also allow for coordinated contraction of the right ventricle (Fig. 46.13)[150] Anderson and colleagues[151,152] has a much more detailed discussion the anatomy of the CCS.

CLINICAL EVALUATION OF FETAL AND NEONATAL CARDIAC CONDUCTION

Fetal cardiac rhythm assessment has been done for several centuries as a part of normal prenatal care with the aid of a special stethoscope (fetoscope) auscultating through the mother's abdomen the fetal heart rate and its regularity after 20 weeks of gestation. With the advent of portable hand-held Doppler devices this same assessment can be undertaken as early as 10 weeks gestation. Today, this is the primary clinical modality with which the majority of fetal arrhythmias are initially identified.

With the evolution of abdominal and then transvaginal ultrasound imaging technology fetal arrhythmias and other abnormal patterns of conduction can be identified and classified in all three trimesters of pregnancy. Visualization of the fetal heart is accomplished with real-time or B-mode ultrasound, often combined with Doppler (Fig. 46.14A). Arrhythmias are then further classified with the use of M-mode ultrasound imaging (one dimensional imaging with respect to time), which can simultaneously view the atrial and ventricular chambers (Fig. 46.14B). With the aid of pulse wave spectral Doppler ultrasound (an image of the waveform of blood velocity and direction with respect to time) even more information can be obtained by observing the velocity waveforms in systole and diastole (Fig. 46.14C). Finally, a detailed evaluation of cardiac anatomy and function, fetal echocardiography, is used to identify congenital cardiac structural defects which accompany fetal arrhythmias.[153]

The human fetal ECG has not, historically, been easily obtained due to the weak fetal electrical signal transmitted through the maternal abdomen and the insulating effect of the vernix caseosa. In 1974, Kariniemi[154] first obtained a fetal magnetocardiogram (fMCG) using the magnetic field signals emanating from the fetal heart. The magnetic analog of the ECG signal is not as attenuated and after mid-gestation can be consistently recorded. By the early 1990s this technology improved to the point where all components of the ECG were consistently obtainable.[155-158] These technologic improvements allowed for more specific diagnoses and classification of fetal arrhythmias. The normal values for the components of a fMCG are listed below Table 46.4.[156] Note that there are distinct differences in the fMCG that are gestation dependent. Until recently, superconducting quantum interference device (SQUID) magnetometry, which required expensive cryogenics, had made little inroads into common usage; however, newer optically pumped magnetometers (OPM) will soon be available at lower cost.

During the labor and delivery, and with more advanced prenatal testing (the nonstress test and the contraction stress test), the fetal heart rate is continuously monitored using external continuous wave Doppler technology similar to the devices used in obtaining fetal heart rates in the prenatal setting.[159] An ECG tracing measuring the R-R intervals can also be obtained using a transvaginal fetal scalp electrode placed on the fetal scalp after rupture of the amniotic membrane in the labor process. Both

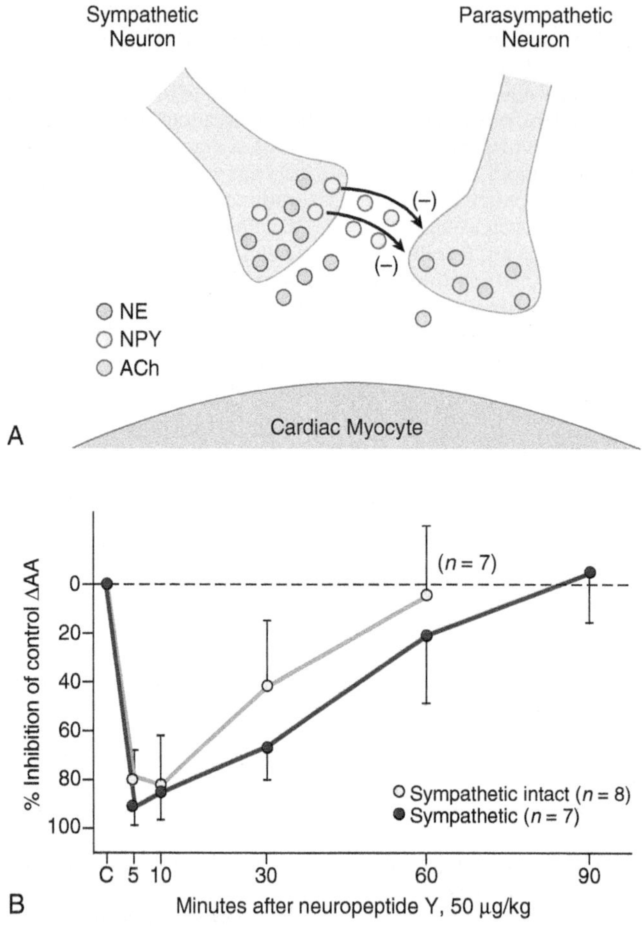

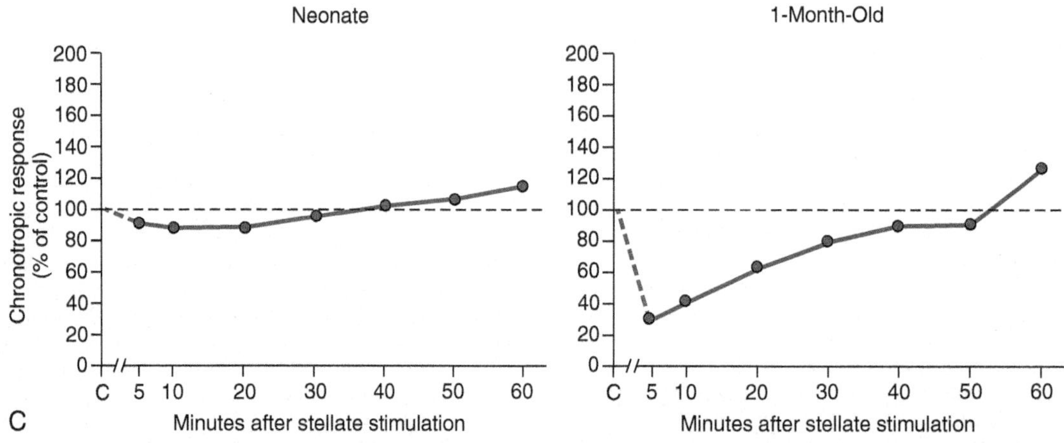

Fig. 46.12 (A) The neuropeptide Y *(NPY)*-mediated sympathetic-parasympathetic interaction. NPY is stored within neuronal vesicles, along with norepinephrine *(NE)*, in sympathetic nerve endings. When released, NPY can bind to receptors on the parasympathetic nerve terminals and inhibit the release of acetylcholine *(ACh)*. (B) The effects of an intravenous injection of NPY (50 μg/kg) on the vagal response of heart rate to vagal stimulation in sympathetically intact and sympathectomized newborn dogs. In both groups, NPY causes a profound (nearly 100%) and long-lasting (nearly 60 minute) inhibition of the change in sinus cycle length caused by vagal stimulation (percentage inhibition of control ΔAA). *C,* Control (before NPY administration). (C), The effects of right stellate ganglion stimulation (10 Hz, 5 minutes) on cardiac vagal chronotropic responses in young puppies. In these graphs, 100% represents the control (*C*; i.e., prestellate stimulation) vagal response. In the neonate *(left)*, stellate stimulation causes little change in the magnitude of elicited vagal responses. In contrast, in the 1-month-old puppy *(right)*, 5 minutes of stellate stimulation causes a profound, long-lasting inhibition of the cardiac vagal response. This occurs, presumably, as a result of the release of NPY during stellate stimulation. *ACh*, Acetylcholine. (A and C, From Rios R, Stolfi A, Campbell PH, et al. Postnatal development of the putative neuropeptide-Y-mediated sympathetic-parasympathetic autonomic interaction. *Cardiovasc Res.* 1996;31:E96, with permission of Elsevier Science. B, From Yamasaki S, Stolfi A, Mas MS, et al. Rapid attenuation ("fade") of the chronotropic response during vagal stimulation in the canine newborn. Evidence for a prominent neuropeptide Y effect. *Circ Res.* 1991;69:406, by permission of the American Heart Association.)

Table 46.3 Anatomic Locations of Common Focal Arrhythmias and Their Relationship With the Embryologic Development of the Cardiac Conduction System.

Arrhythmia	Location	Embryologic Origin	Embryologic Markers of CCS	Nodal Similarities
Focal atrial tachycardia	Crista terminalis	Right horn of sinus venosus	HNK1 Tbx3 CCS-lacZ Cx43-negative	• Small cell diameter • Exhibit independent pacemaker activity • Similar ion channel and gap junction protein expression
	Interatrial groove (septum)	Left horn of sinus venosus	HNK1 Tbx3 CCS-lacZ Cx43-negative	• HCN4 • Cx45 • Small nodal-like cells
	Coronary sinus ostium	Left horn of sinus venosus	HNK1 Tbx3 CCS-lacZ Cx43-negative	Not previously studied
	Tricuspid annulus	Atrioventricular canal	HNK1 Tbx3 CCS-lacZ Cx43-negative	• Small cell diameter • Nodal-type action potentials • Reduction of action potential amplitude with adenosine
	Superior mitral annulus	Atrioventricular canal	Tbx3 CCS-lacZ Cx43-negative	• Small cell diameter • Nodal-type action potentials • Reduction of action potential amplitude with adenosine
	Retroaortic node	Atrioventricular canal	HNK1 Tbx3	• HCN4 • Cx45
Atrial fibrillation	Pulmonary veins	Unknown	Transient HNK1 CCS-lacZ	• Clear cytoplasm, round mitochondria/few myofibrils • P cells/transitional cells/Purkinje cells
Normal heart tachycardia	Right ventricular outflow tract	Primitive outflow tract	minK-lacZ Cx45	• Cells embedded in connective tissue • Lack expression of Nav1.5, Cx43, and Kir2.1

CCS, Cardiac conduction system; *HNK*, Human natural killer.
The anatomic location of common focal arrhythmias and evidence for their association with the developing CCS and their nodal-like properties.

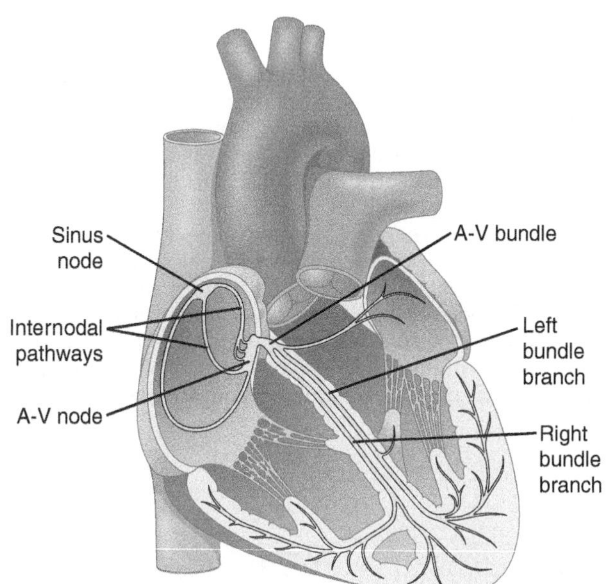

Fig. 46.13 Sinus node and the Purkinje system of the heart, showing also the atrioventricular *(A-V)* node, atrial internodal pathways, and ventricular bundle branches. (From Hall JE, Hall ME. Rhythmical excitation of the heart. In: Hall JE, eds. *Guyton and Hall Textbook of Medical Physiology*. 14th ed. Philadelphia: Elsevier; 2016:124, fig. 10.1.)

of these devices only record the fetal heart rate with respect to time, but they can identify fetal arrhythmias during labor. More recently, a more sophisticated fetal scalp electrode has been developed to obtain a more detailed and precise fetal ECG. This technology is called *STAN (ST segment analysis)* and is used to identify fetuses at risk for fetal acidosis and hypoxic ischemic encephalopathy.[159] The ultimate utility of the STAN technology, however, still remains unclear.[160]

The neonatal ECG is quite similar to the adult ECG with several important exceptions. Normative values of the neonatal ECG are listed in Table 46.5.[161-163] In transition from fetal to neonatal life many significant changes occur within the heart, lungs, and the associated vasculature. These events are discussed in detail in Chapter 50 of this book. In concert with these cardiovascular changes there are changes that occur, as well, with the CCS. The principal factors are changes in pulmonary vascular resistance and intracardiac pressures within the right and left sides of the heart at birth. Subsequently in the neonatal period more vascular and cardiac changes occur with closure of the two right-to-left cardiovascular shunts, the foramen ovale and the ductus arteriosus.

Certain fetal diseases can create changes in the CCS in fetuses and neonates. Premature infants are noted to have delay in maturation of the autonomic nervous system in postnatal life,[164] as well as cardiac repolarization abnormalities.[164-168] These issues may also be present in the late-term premature infants[169] and may persist into the neonatal period. In fetuses with intrauterine growth restriction, changes in cardiac time intervals and fetal heart rate variability, as well as in the maturation of sinus rhythm dynamics, have been reported.[170-173] Lastly, infants exposed to certain medications in utero, including illicit drugs,[174,175,] appear to have cardiac repolarization abnormalities and other cardiac arrhythmias in fetal and postnatal life. It is speculated that cardiac arrhythmias may be a possible cause of the increased risk of intrauterine fetal demise and postnatal sudden infant death syndrome (SIDS) in 10% to 15% of this population of fetuses and infants.[176-182]

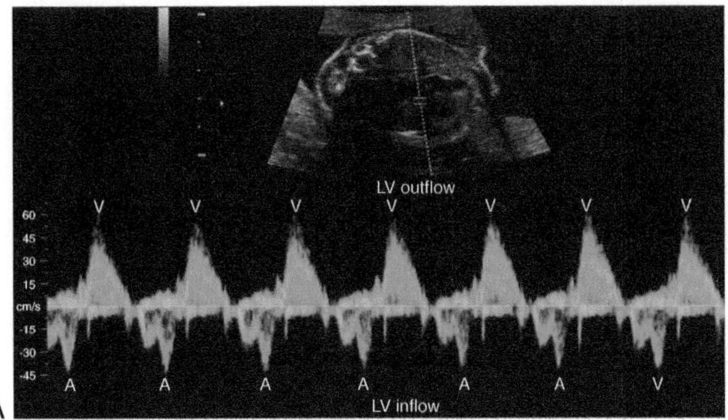

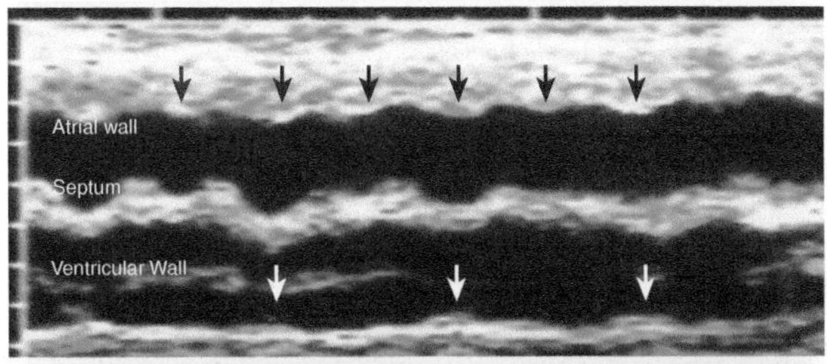

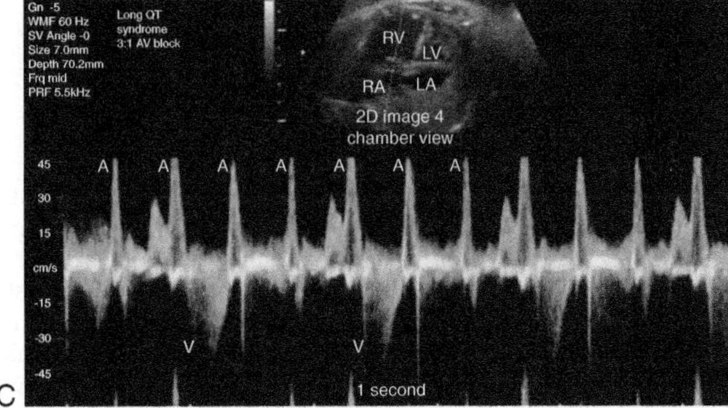

Fig. 46.14 (A) Two-dimensional and Doppler tracing of left ventricle *(LV)* inflow and outflow. This is the most utilized view for assessing fetal arrhythmias. (B) M-mode tracing of the 3:1 AV block with atrial *(black arrows)* and ventricular *(white arrows)* wall contractions are. (C) Doppler tracing of LV inflow and outflow showing three atrial systolic velocities *(A)* for every 1 ventricular systolic velocity *(V)*. This severe presentation of long QT syndrome is often associated with ventricular arrhythmias as shown in Fig. 46.15.

Neonatal ECGs are routinely performed for a variety of indications after the birth of a child. Most commonly ECGs are done for abnormalities of the neonatal heart rate or rhythm, or as a part of a medical evaluation for a suspected congenital heart defect. Detailed electrophysiologic and ablation studies can be performed in more complicated cardiac conditions that specifically diagnose and also treat drug-refractory neonatal cardiac tachyarrhythmias. These procedures are generally of last resort, since the AV groove contains the coronary arteries, which can be injured due to close proximity to the ablation sites in the coronary sinus in infants. Recently, electrophysiologic studies and pacemaker placements in animals have been performed in utero as a possible way to better diagnose and potentially treat complete heart block with hydrops.[183] To date, successful long-term treatment has not, however, been possible in any fetus. For life-threatening ventricular tachyarrhythmias due to long QT syndrome, defibrillators have been placed in the very young; however, medical treatment with standard pacing is preferred.[184,185]

ABNORMAL CARDIAC CONDUCTION IN THE HUMAN FETUS AND NEONATE

Fetal and neonatal arrhythmias are quite common in the human during development and are seen commonly in neonatal ICUs. The frequency has been reported to be about 1% to 3% for atrial or ventricular ectopy, with atrial ectopy about 10 times more common than ventricular ectopy. Transient sinus bradycardia that resolves in the first week of life is likely due to hypervagotonia, perhaps due to neck stretch during birth, head compression, or other cause. These have been reported to be benign as long as associations, such as long QT syndrome, have been ruled out. About 1:2500 fetuses have SVT, and approximately 1:10,000 have AV block. AV block can be associated with either congenital heart defects that displace the AV node or isoimmune damage to the AV node by SSA auto-antibodies. Rare arrhythmias such as atrial ectopic or junctional ectopic tachycardia, ventricular tachycardia, and accelerated ventricular rhythm occur. PVCs may be a marker for more malignant disease such as ventricular aneurysms, tumors, or myocarditis. In a recent study, we found that in addition to these associations, 10% had maternal ectopy as well. premature ventricular contractions (PACs) are often related to the patulous nature of the septum primum flap in the atrium, which can abut the atrial septum or even become aneurismal and approach the mitral valve. In the neonate, the more common cause for arrhythmias is iatrogenic due to intravascular catheter migration. In both the fetus and neonate atrial ectopy can trigger atrial flutter or SVT due to shortening of the cardiac cycle refractory period. Therefore, the fetus should have fetal heart rate monitoring no less than once weekly during periods of PACs, to detect development of SVT-related hydrops fetalis.

It has long been recognized that acquired electrophysiologic abnormalities mediated through ischemia or inflammation can result in profound physiologic changes in conduction leading to fetal demise. The contribution to fetal demise from

Table 46.4 Fetal Waveform Intervals Versus Gestational Age.

Gestational Age (wk)		RR (ms)	P (ms)	PR (ms)	QRS (ms)	QT (ms)	QTc (ms)
	N	Mean	Mean ± SD	Mean ± SD	Mean ± SD	Mean ± SD	Mean ± SD
15–24	53	408	39.5 ± 7.7	93.3 ± 10.1	44.4 ± 6.0	254.0 ± 30.5	398.4 ± 50.1
24–29	71	409	41.3 ± 7.1	95.3 ± 11.7	46.5 ± 6.7	250.5 ± 35.3	392.1 ± 55.1
29–35	63	432	45.7 ± 8.0	99.3 ± 12.1	49.2 ± 6.0	263.5 ± 31.5	401.5 ± 47.1
35–40	48	434	49.6 ± 9.3	101.5 ± 12.3	51.0 ± 7.5	249.8 ± 34.2	377.7 ± 46.9
15–40	235	420	43.8 ± 8.7	97.2 ± 11.9	47.6 ± 6.9	254.5 ± 33.5	393.0 ± 51.0

Table 46.5 Normal Neonatal ECG Standards.

Age group	Heart rate (beats × min^{-1})	Frontal plane QRS axis[a] (degrees)	P wave amplitude (mm)	P-R interval[a] (s)	QRS duration[a] V_5	Q III[c] (mm)	QV_6[c] (mm)	RV_1[b] (mm)	SV_1[b] (mm)	R/S V_1[c]	RV_6[b] (mm)	SV_6[b] (mm)	R/S V_6[c]	SV_1 + RV_6[c] (mm)	R + SV_4[c] (mm)
0–1 days	93–154 (123)	+59 to +192 (135)	2·8	0·08–0·16 (0·11)	0·02–0·08 (0·05)	5·2	1·7	5–26	0–22·5	9·8	0–11	0–9·8	10	28	52
1–3 days	91–159 (123)	+64 to +197 (134)	2·8	0·08–0·14 (0·11)	0·02–0·07 (0·05)	5·2	2·1	5–27	0–21	6	0–12	0–9·5	11	29	52
3–7 days	90–166 (129)	+77 to +187 (132)	2·9	0·08–0·14 (0·10)	0·02–0·07 (0·05)	4·8	2·8	3–24	0–17	9·7	0·5–12	0–9·8	10	25	48
7–30 days	107–182 (149)	+65 to +160 (110)	3·0	0·07–0·14 (0·10)	0·02–0·08 (0·05)	5·6	2·8	3–21·5	0–11	7	2·5–16	0–9·8	12	22	47
1–3 mo	121–179 (150)	+31 to +114 (75)	2·6	0·07–0·13 (0·10)	0·02–0·08 (0·05)	5·4	2·7	3–18·5	0–12·5	7·4	5–21	0–7·2	12	29	53

[a]2nd–98th percentile (mean).
[b]2nd–98th percentile (1 mm = 100 μV).
[c]98th percentile (1 mm = 100 μV).
From Schwartz PJ, Garson A Jr, Paul T, et al. Guidelines for the interpretation of the neonatal electrocardiogram. *Eur Heart J.* 2002;23:1329–1344, table 1. doi:10.1053/euhj.2002.3274.

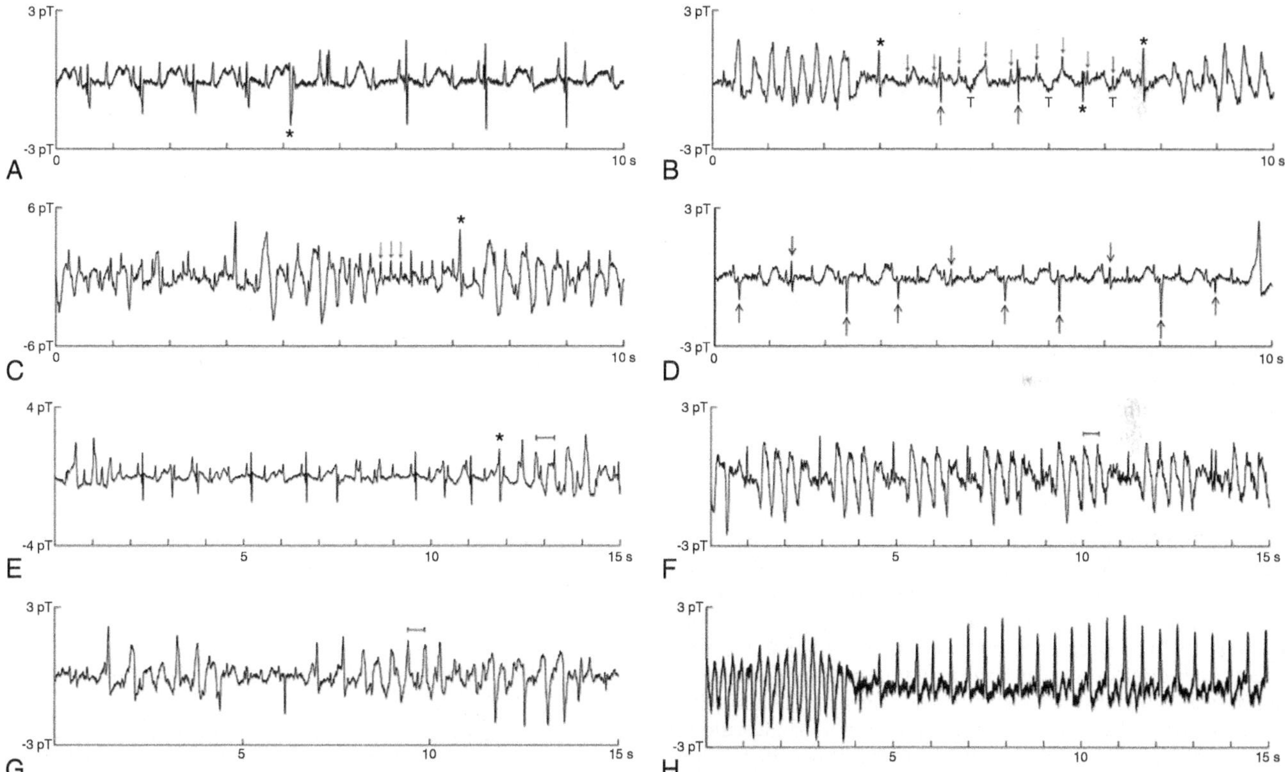

Fig. 46.15 Novel long QT syndrome (LQTS) rhythm patterns. (A) Transition from 2:1 to 3:1 atrioventricular (AV) block in a 33 4/7–weeks gestation fetus. A premature ventricular contraction (PVC; *) occurs at the transition, followed by an aberrantly conducted beat and a relatively short QT interval that progressively lengthens. In 2:1 AV block, the T waves are notched, which is commonly seen in LQT2. In 3:1 AV block, the QRS complexes change morphology and become narrower. (B and C) Complex rhythm with torsade de pointes (TdP) and PVCs: (B) periods of AV block in a 3:1 or 2:1 conduction ratio (C) atrial flutter (26-week fetus). Sinus beats *(upward arrows)* were relatively rare due to AV block, PVCs *(*)*, and the prevalence of TdP. P waves are indicated by *downward arrows*. The T waves (T) show a negative-positive biphasic morphology. TdP was usually initiated by a PVC. Atrial flutter (330 bpm) was seen approximately 25% of the time and occurred with and without the presence of TdP. (D) QRS alternans in 2:1 atrioventricular block in a 26 0/7–week fetus. The QRS complexes *(arrows)* are narrow and on time but show marked beat-to-beat variation in amplitude and polarity. Normally, QRS alternans occurs during 1:1 atrioventricular conduction in an every-other-beat (AB-AB) pattern and is characterized by modest variation in QRS amplitude and prominent variation in QRS morphology. (E–G) TdP with a cycle length similar to that of sinus rhythm in three separate fetuses of 33 4/7, 21, and 26 weeks gestation. *Horizontal bars* indicate the duration of the PP intervals. (H) Transition from typical TdP to a slow ventricular tachycardia with a rate of 127 bpm in a 31-week fetus. (Modified from Strand S, Strasburger JF, Cuneo BF, Wakai RT. Complex and novel arrhythmias precede stillbirth in fetuses with de novo long QT syndrome. *Circ Arrhythm Electrophysiol.* 2020;13(5):e008082. https://doi.org/10.1161/CIRCEP.119.008082. Epub 2020 May 18.)

genetic causes of electrophysiologic disorders, called *inherited arrhythmia syndromes*, was recognized only relatively recently.[186-189] Increasing evidence suggests that fetal demise in some cases can be the culmination of changes in fetal physiology and electrophysiology that lead to sudden cardiac arrest. Crotti and colleagues[187] have shown that in molecular autopsies of unexplained fetal demise cases, 3% harbor a known ion channelopathy gene defect, and 8.8% have polymorphisms that altered channel function under stress. Plant and colleagues[190] showed that in African American infants with a common S1105Y polymorphism of *SCN5A*, the sodium channels behave differently when exposed to acidosis. They speculated that the disproportionate incidence of SIDS among African American infants may relate to this alteration in repolarization, when combined with fetal acidosis.

A number of investigators, using new and advanced recording techniques, such as fetal magnetocardiography, have documented life-threatening fetal arrhythmic events not unlike those seen postnatally (Fig. 46.15) and have challenged the concept that the final common pathway to death in the fetus is bradycardia or asystole.[184,191,192] Better means of evaluating conduction in the fetus, such as with fetal magnetocardiography, may allow recognition and analysis of repolarization abnormalities in the human fetus during the second and third trimesters. Because many fetuses with inherited arrhythmia syndromes will present with heart rates below the third percentile, recognizing this marker may identify the fetus at risk. Gestation-specific fetal heart rate algorithms are available to clinicians.[156,184] Parents with familial long QT syndrome have an eightfold higher risk of stillbirth and a twofold higher risk of miscarriage than the general population.[184,191]

Congenital long QT syndrome is an important contributor to fetal demise and SIDS. There are multiple types of long QT syndrome. Some of the long QT syndrome types are more likely than others to manifest themselves as life-threatening arrhythmias in the human fetus; these include LQT2 (defects in *KCNH2*, also known as *HERG*), LQT3 *(SCN5A)*, double mutations or dominant negative single mutations in LQT1 *(KCNQ1)*, or other rare mutations (LQT4-LQT8, RYR2, etc.).[193]

Torsades de pointes (see Fig. 46.15) has been diagnosed between 19 to 34 weeks of gestation and has been effectively treated in utero. Life-threatening manifestations are much more common in *de novo* gene defects; 82% of de novo defects manifest at least one LQTS rhythm (Torsades, second degree AV block, or QRS or T wave alternans) compared to only 22% of those with familial long QT syndrome. PVCs in this setting are a particularly ominous sign and are only seen in those fetuses with symptoms and QTcs greater than 600 ms. In these cases, 5 of 11 were stillborn. For *SCN5A* gene defects presenting in utero or in the first month of life, the long-term mortality is so high that neonatal cardiac transplantation may be a consideration.[184] Sinus bradycardia, a more minor manifestation of LQT, occurs in LQT1. Persistent fetal bradycardia may be a helpful marker in determining in whom neonatal electrocardiographic screening may be most useful and cost-effective. At present, in the United States, neonatal screening is not routine; however, it is used in Japan, Italy, and other countries.

CONCLUSION

Our understanding of human fetal electrophysiology is evolving. Increasing access to advanced recording technologies such as fetal magnetocardiography promises to allow a hands-on assessment of human fetal electrophysiology and disease response, which until recently was not possible. Further research into the basic mechanisms of cellular automaticity, genetics, physiology, and autonomic control, using research techniques such as cardiac organoids, animal models, and use of new fetal imaging techniques, is needed to understand complex interactions during pre- and postnatal development. Optimal management of arrhythmias clinically relies on a solid understanding of the fundamental changes and their timing in the development of the human fetus and infant. Many of these processes are still being elucidated through vital developmental research.

A complete reference list is available at www.ExpertConsult.com. 

SELECT REFERENCES

4. Roden DM, Balser JR, George Jr AL, et al. Cardiac ion channels. *Annu Rev Physiol.* 2002;64:431-475.
5. Crotti L, Tester DJ, White WM, et al. Long QT syndrome-associated mutations in intrauterine fetal death. *J Am Med Assoc.* 2013;309(14):1473-1482.
8. Anderson ME. Ca^{2+}-dependent regulation of cardiac L-type Ca^{2+} channels: is a unifying mechanism at hand? *J Mol Cell Cardiol.* 2001;33:639-650.
9. Nerbonne JM. Regulation of voltage-gated K^+ channel expression in the developing mammalian myocardium. *J Neurobiol.* 1998;37:37-59.
10. Wang Z, Fermini B, Nattel S. Rapid and slow components of delayed rectifier current in human atrial myocytes. *Cardiovasc Res.* 1994;28:1540-1546.
14. Kodama I, Nikmaram MR, Boyett MR, et al. Regional differences in the role of the Ca^{2+} and Na^+ currents in pacemaker activity in the sinoatrial node. *Am J Physiol.* 1997;272:H2793-H2806.
16. DiFrancesco D. Current i_f and the neuronal modulation of heart rate. In: Zipes DP, Jalife J, eds. *Cardiac Electrophysiology. From Cell to Bedside.* Philadelphia: WB Saunders; 1990:28-35.
24. Gennser G, Nilsson E. Excitation and impulse conduction in the human fetal heart. *Acta Physiol Scand.* 1970;79:305-320.
31. Wang Y, Xu H, Kumar R, et al. Differences in transient outward current properties between neonatal and adult human atrial myocytes. *J Mol Cell Cardiol.* 2003;35:1083-1092.
34. Chin TK, Friedman WF, Klitzner TS. Developmental changes in cardiac myocyte calcium regulation. *Circ Res.* 1990;67:574-579.
36. Roca TP, Pigott JD, Clarkson CW, et al. L-type calcium current in pediatric and adult human atrial myocytes: evidence for developmental changes in channel inactivation. *Pediatr Res.* 1996;40:462-468.
40. Yang HT, Tweedie D, Wang S, et al. The ryanodine receptor modulates the spontaneous beating rate of cardiomyocytes during development. *Proc Natl Acad Sci U S A.* 2002;99:9225-9230.
46. Sarre A, Maury P, Kucera P, et al. Arrhythmogenesis in the developing heart during anoxia-reoxygenation and hypothermia-rewarming: an *in vitro* model. *J Cardiovasc Electrophysiol.* 2006;17:1350-1359.
50. Gittenberger-de Groot AC, Wenink AC, et al. The specialized myocardium in the foetal heart. In: Van Mierop LH, ed. *Embryology and Teratology of the Heart and the Great Arteries.* The Hague: Leiden University Press; 1978:15-24.
63. van Veen AA, van Rijen HV, Opthof T. Cardiac gap junction channels: modulation of expression and channel properties. *Cardiovasc Res.* 2001;51:217-229.
67. Zeevi-Levin N, Barac YD, Reisner Y, et al. Gap junctional remodeling by hypoxia in cultured neonatal rat ventricular myocytes. *Cardiovasc Res.* 2005;66:64-73.
70. Kirchhoff S, Kim JS, Hagendorff A, et al. Abnormal cardiac conduction and morphogenesis in connexin40 and connexin43 double-deficient mice. *Circ Res.* 2000;87:399-405.
77. Moorman AF, Christoffels VM, Anderson RH. Anatomic substrates for cardiac conduction. *Heart Rhythm.* 2005;2:875-886.
78. Gittenberger-de Groot AC, Blom NM, Aoyama N, et al. The role of neural crest and epicardium-derived cells in conduction system formation. *Novartis Found Symp.* 2003;250:125-134, discussion 134-141, 276-129.
84. Ismat FA, Zhang M, Kook H, et al. Homeobox protein Hop functions in the adult cardiac conduction system. *Circ Res.* 2005;96:898-903.
86. van Weerd JH, Badi I, van den Boogaard M, et al. A large permissive regulatory domain exclusively controls *Tbx3* expression in the cardiac conduction system. *Circ Res.* 2014;115:432-441.
88. Arnolds DE, Liu F, Fahrenbach JP, et al. TBX5 drives Scn5a expression to regulate cardiac conduction system function. *J Clin Invest.* 2012;122:2509-2518.
91. Pashmforoush M, Lu JT, Chen H, et al. Nkx2-5 pathways and congenital heart disease; loss of ventricular myocyte lineage specification leads to progressive cardiomyopathy and complete heart block. *Cell.* 2004;117:373-386.
98. Kato Y, Takahashi-Igari M, Inaba T, et al. Comparison of PR intervals determined by fetal magnetocardiography and pulsed Doppler echocardiography. *Fetal Diagn Ther.* 2012;32:109-115.
100. Zhao H, Chen M, Van Veen BD, et al. Simultaneous fetal magnetocardiography and ultrasound/Doppler imaging. *IEEE Trans Biomed Eng.* 2007;54:1167-1171.
104. Chow LT, Chow SS, Anderson RH, et al. Autonomic innervation of the human cardiac conduction system: changes from infancy to senility—an immunohistochemical and histochemical analysis. *Anat Rec.* 2001;264:169-182.
106. Adams DJ, Harper AA, Hogg RC. Neural control of the heart: developmental changes in ionic conductances in mammalian intrinsic cardiac neurons. *Auton Neurosci.* 2002;98:75-78.

107. Birk E, Riemer RK. Myocardial cholinergic signaling changes with age. *Pediatr Res*. 1992;31:601-605.
115. Mace SE, Levy MN. Neural control of heart rate: a comparison between puppies and adult animals. *Pediatr Res*. 1983;17:491-495.
150. Hall J. *Rhythmical Excitation of the Heart*. 13th ed. Philadelphia: Guyton and Hall Textbook of Medical Physiology; 2016:124. Figure 10.1.
152. Anderson RH, Yanni J, Boyett MR, Chandler NJ, Dobrzynski H. The anatomy of the cardiac conduction system. *Clin Anat*. 2009;22(1):99-113.
153. Donofrio MT, Moon-Grady AJ, Hornberger LK, et al. Diagnosis and treatment of fetal cardiac disease: a scientific statement from the American Heart Association. *Circulation*. 2014;129(21):2183-2242.
156. Strand SA, Strasburger JF, Wakai RT. Fetal magnetocardiogram waveform characteristics. *Physiol Meas*. 2019;40(3):035002.
158. Wacker-Gussmann A, Plankl C, Sewald M, Schneider KM, Oberhoffer R, Lobmaier SM. Fetal cardiac time intervals in healthy pregnancies - an observational study by fetal ECG (Monica Healthcare System). *J Perinat Med*. 2018;46(6):587-592.
159. Intrapartum fetal heart rate monitoring: nomenclature, interpretation, and general management principles. *ACOG Prac Bull Clin Prac Guide Obstet Gynecol*. 2009;106:192-202.
162. Brockmeier K, Nazal R, Sreeram N. The electrocardiogram of the neonate and infant. *J Electrocardiol*. 2016;49(6):814-816.
163. Davignon A. ECG standards for children. *Pediatr Cardiol*. 1980;1(2):133-152.
173. Schneider U, Fiedler A, Liehr M, Kahler C, Schleussner E. Fetal heart rate variability in growth restricted fetuses. *Biomed Tech*. 2006;51(4):248-250.

Developmental Biology of the Pulmonary Vasculature

47

Cristina M. Alvira | Shazia Bhombal | Marlene Rabinovitch

INTRODUCTION

This chapter discusses the changing morphology of the developing fetal, neonatal, and postnatal pulmonary vascular bed. Studies have focused on structural and functional alterations in endothelial cells during postnatal development and have addressed the phenotypic heterogeneity of the vascular smooth muscle cells (SMCs) in the perinatal period. There are new insights into mechanisms regulating endothelial migration and angiogenesis, SMC proliferation, hypertrophy, and migration. These studies have also provided novel therapeutic targets whereby progression of pulmonary vascular disease may be slowed or prevented and regression induced.

MORPHOLOGY OF THE DEVELOPING PULMONARY CIRCULATION IN THE FETUS

Primitive pulmonary vessels arise from the sixth aortic arch in the 5-week human embryo to supply the upper poles of the right and left lung, and a pair of intersegmental arteries arising from the dorsal aorta penetrate upward through the diaphragm to supply the lower poles. At this stage, the parenchymal blood vessels of the developing lung are largely localized to the interlobular septa. Between 5 and 8 weeks of gestation it is likely that numerous paired dorsal intersegmental arteries supply the emerging blood vessels developing alongside the branching bronchi in the lung parenchyma. Once the true central pulmonary arteries form from the aortopulmonary trunk and anastomose with the intrapulmonary arteries, the primitive pulmonary arteries arising from the aorta and the primitive intersegmental arteries involute. By 9 weeks of gestation, the developing bronchial system is observed as one or two small vessels extending from the dorsal aorta, subsequently extending to the lung periphery as the airways increase in size.[1] At each airway generation, the airway acquires an accompanying artery, in addition to numerous supernumerary arteries, branching at frequent but irregular intervals to enter the lung parenchyma from the pulmonary arterial branches running alongside the bronchi.[2] By 16 weeks of gestation, development of the preacinar airways and accompanying arteries is complete. Thereafter, as the acini (terminal and respiratory bronchioles, alveolar ducts, and alveoli) develop, so do the accompanying and supernumerary arteries.[3,4] Experimental evidence shows that branching morphogenesis of the large preacinar airways provides cues to regulate branching morphogenesis of the preacinar arterial tree, whereas the intraacinar vessels regulate the development of the alveoli (this is discussed later).

Antenatal disruption of pulmonary vascular development occurring as a result of congenital heart disease and other intrauterine factors may present with respiratory difficulties soon after birth. For example, persistent pulmonary hypertension of the neonate has been reported in association with pulmonary arterial maturational arrest at the fifth week of gestation (Fig. 47.1).[5] Infants with pulmonary atresia and ventricular septal defect frequently have persistence of the intersegmental arteries (aortopulmonary collaterals) that can serve as a source of blood supply to a lobe or lobar segment (Fig. 47.2).[6] Alternatively, a dual circulation with intersegmental arteries anastomosing to arteries can be traced back to a central pulmonary artery origin. In these infants there can also be multiple indirect aortopulmonary collaterals arising from branches of aortic branches (e.g., from subclavian, intercostal, and coronary arteries). Because these indirect collaterals can be observed in the absence of direct collaterals, they probably represent the sequelae of pulmonary atresia when it occurs later in development. Finally, in some cases of pulmonary atresia, there is supply by anastomotic vessels that arise from true bronchial arteries. Pulmonary vascular abnormalities are also observed with absence of the pulmonary valve.[7] In those patients who present with severe respiratory problems from birth, abnormal branching of the vessels has been observed with tufts of intersegmental pulmonary arteries arising in a weeping willow or squidlike fashion, encircling and compressing the intrapulmonary airways (Fig. 47.3).

MICROSCOPIC FEATURES

The normal morphologic development of the pulmonary circulation has also been studied at the microscopic level. In the fetus, the preacinar arteries and those at the level of the terminal bronchioles are muscular, whereas the intraacinar arteries (i.e., those accompanying respiratory bronchioles) are either partially muscular (surrounded by a spiral of muscle) or nonmuscular. Arteries at alveolar duct and alveolar wall levels are also nonmuscular. The preacinar arteries are thick walled and change

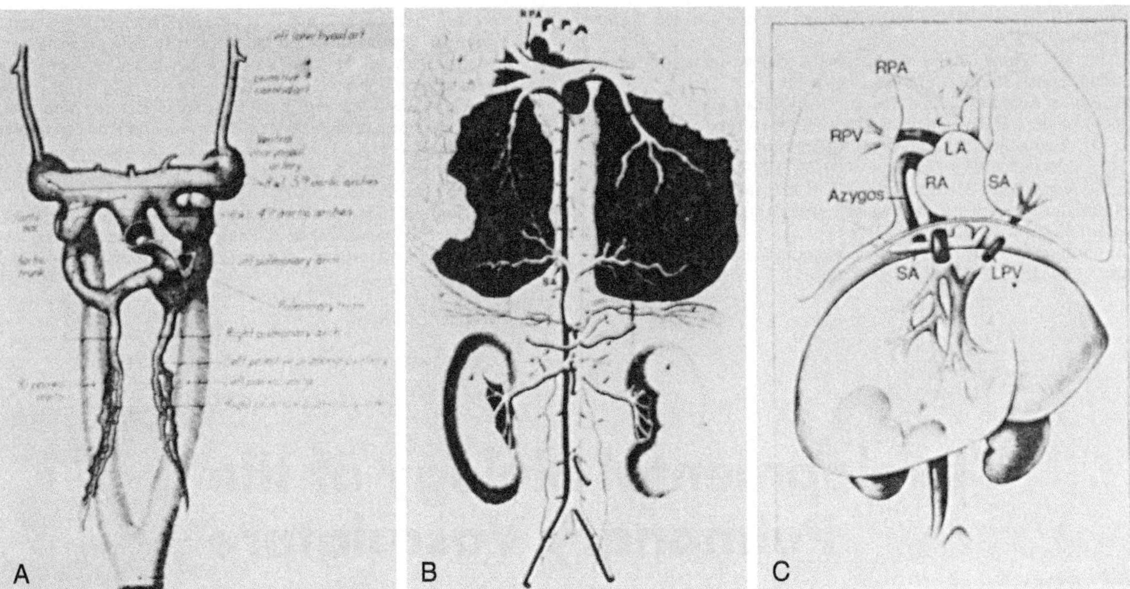

Fig. 47.1 (A) Early embryologic development shows normal disparity between the large main pulmonary artery and narrow right and left branch pulmonary arteries at 5 weeks. (B) Only the arterial system is shown. The bilateral systemic arteries arising from a single trunk supply the lower lobes. (C) An infant with persistent pulmonary hypertension and developmental arrest at 5 weeks gestation. *LA,* Left atrium; *LPV,* left pulmonary vein; *RA,* right atrium; *RPA,* right pulmonary artery; *RPV,* right pulmonary vein; *SA,* systemic arteries. (A, From Congdon ED. Transformation of the aortic-arch system during the development of the human embryo. *Contrib Embryol.* 1922;14:47. B, From Maugars A. *J Med Chir Pharm Paris* 1802;3:453. C, Reprinted by permission of the publisher from Goldstein JD, Rabinovitch M, Van Praagh R, et al. Unusual vascular anomalies causing persistent pulmonary hypertension in a newborn. *Am J Cardiol.* 1979;43:962. Copyright 1979 by Excerpta Medica.)

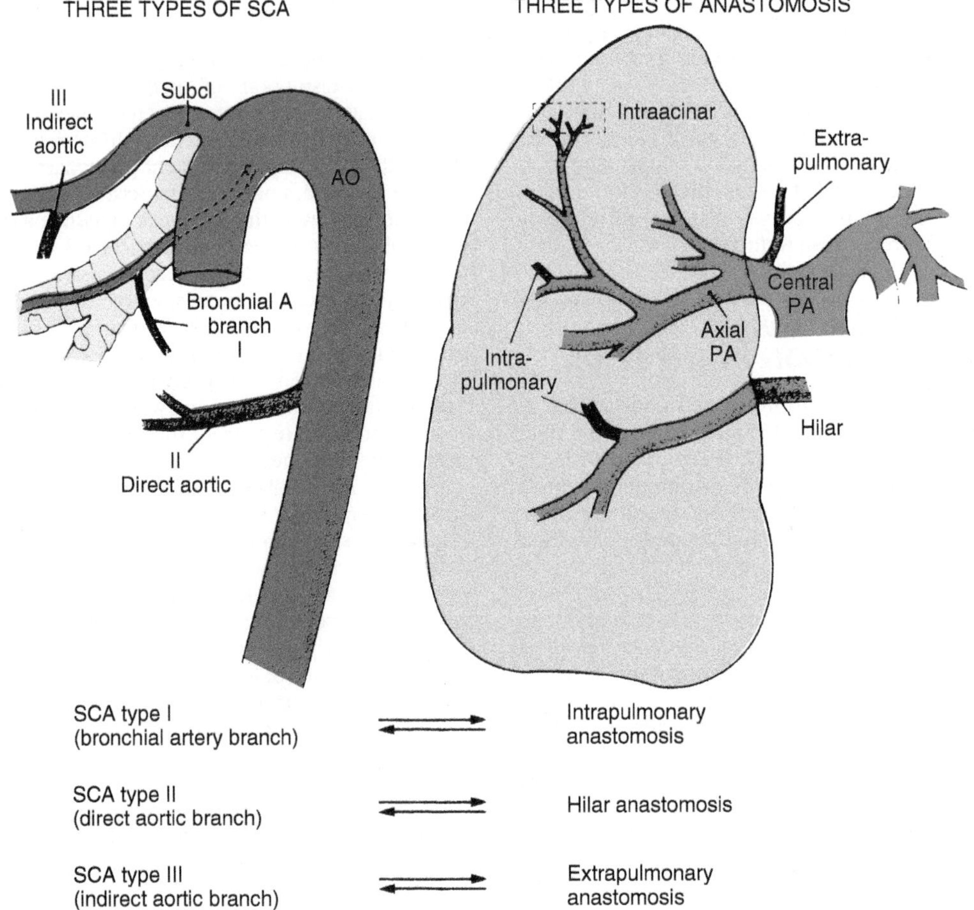

Fig. 47.2 The three types of systemic collateral artery *(SCA)* and the three types of anastomosis with the pulmonary artery *(PA)*. The characteristic pattern of anastomosis for each type of SCA is given. *AO,* Aorta; *Subcl,* subclavian. (From Rabinovitch M, Herrera-deLeon V, Castaneda AR, et al. Growth and development of the pulmonary vascular bed in patients with tetralogy of Fallot with or without pulmonary atresia. *Circulation.* 1981;64:1234.)

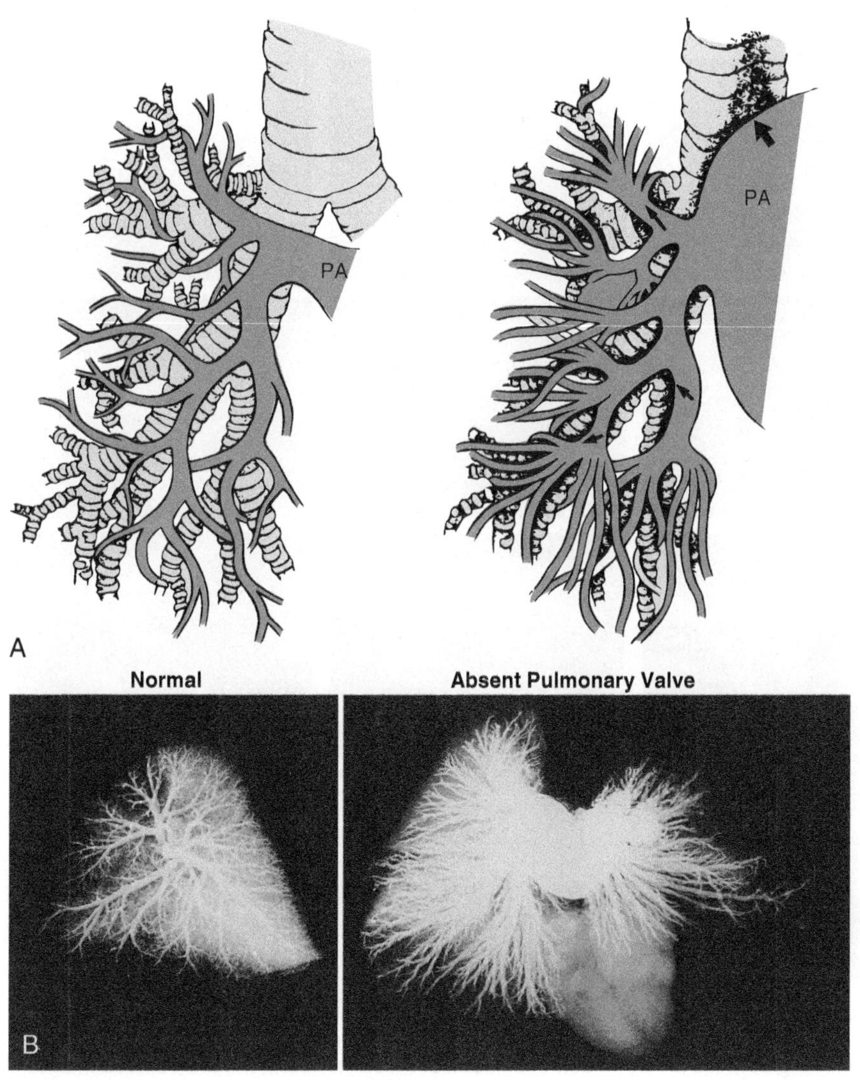

Fig. 47.3 (A) Diagrammatic representation of normal pulmonary artery *(PA)* branching and the abnormal pattern seen in cases of absent pulmonary valve syndrome—tufts of vessels emerging at the segmental artery level that entwine the bronchi. *Arrows* denote large right pulmonary artery compressing right mainstem bronchus. (B) Postmortem arteriograms from a 4-day-old normal infant *(left)* following severe cardiorespiratory failure and from a 4-day-old patient with absent pulmonary valve syndrome associated with a ventricular septal defect and D-transposition of the great arteries *(right)*, showing tufts of vessels in both lungs. (Reprinted by permission of the publisher from Rabinovitch M, Grady S, David I, et al. Compression of intrapulmonary bronchi by abnormally branching pulmonary arteries associated with absent pulmonary valves. *Am J Cardiol.* 1982;50:804. Copyright 1982 by Excerpta Medica, Inc.)

little in wall thickness relative to external diameter throughout the fetal period. Experimental studies[8] suggest that the immediate postnatal period is characterized by rapid recruitment of small alveolar duct and wall vessels that appear to be functionally and structurally closed in the prenatal period. There is also progressive dilation of muscular arteries. Within a few days the smallest muscular arteries (<250 μm) dilate, and their walls thin to adult levels; by 4 months of age this process has included the largest pulmonary arteries at the hilum. As intraacinar arteries increase in external diameter during maturation, muscularization extends peripherally. Nonmuscular arteries first become partially muscular and become fully muscularized with postnatal age. For example, alveolar duct arteries are still largely nonmuscular in infancy, but become partially muscularized in childhood, and can be fully muscularized in adulthood.[9] In contrast, alveolar wall arteries remain largely nonmuscular, even in the adult.

Clinical and experimental studies have suggested that the muscularization of peripheral pulmonary arteries involves the differentiation of pericytes and recruitment of fibroblasts.[10,11] However, more recent studies using fate mapping indicate that strategically located resident SMCs dedifferentiate and migrate to muscularize peripheral arteries (Fig. 47.4).[12] Arteries proliferate through early infancy, accompanying the proliferation of alveoli. Therefore, vessel density or the alveoli-to-artery ratio can be used as a measure of arterial growth, with the ratio decreasing from 20:1 in the newborn to 8:1 by early childhood (Fig. 47.5). The growth and development of the pulmonary circulation may also be influenced by the trophic effects of neuropeptides with growth-factor-like properties released from neuroendocrine cells and neuroendocrine bodies[13] associated with accompanying airways (Fig. 47.6).

Experimental studies have indicated how changes in connective tissue, especially elastin and collagen,[14,15] and cellular arrangement[16] modulate the normal adaptation to postnatal life. The endothelial cells in peripheral arteries increase elastin deposition to form an intact elastic lamina. Similar changes occur in the central pulmonary arteries, and elastin remodeling in the subendothelium is prominent in the early neonatal period.[15] In contrast, elastin synthesis, as judged by messenger RNA (mRNA) levels, appears to be less prominent in the outer media and adventitia (Fig. 47.7). Subpopulations of vascular SMCs with differing proliferative potentials and specialized functions, characterized by expression of specific cytoskeletal proteins, become more distinct during late fetal and early neonatal development.[17] For example, metavinculin-positive SMCs are relatively resistant to proliferation, yet the high proliferative potential demonstrated in neonatal bovine pulmonary artery SMCs is reflective of a difference in activation of protein kinase C.[18]

CELLULAR MECHANISMS

The cellular and molecular mechanisms that regulate growth and development of the fetal vasculature have been extensively

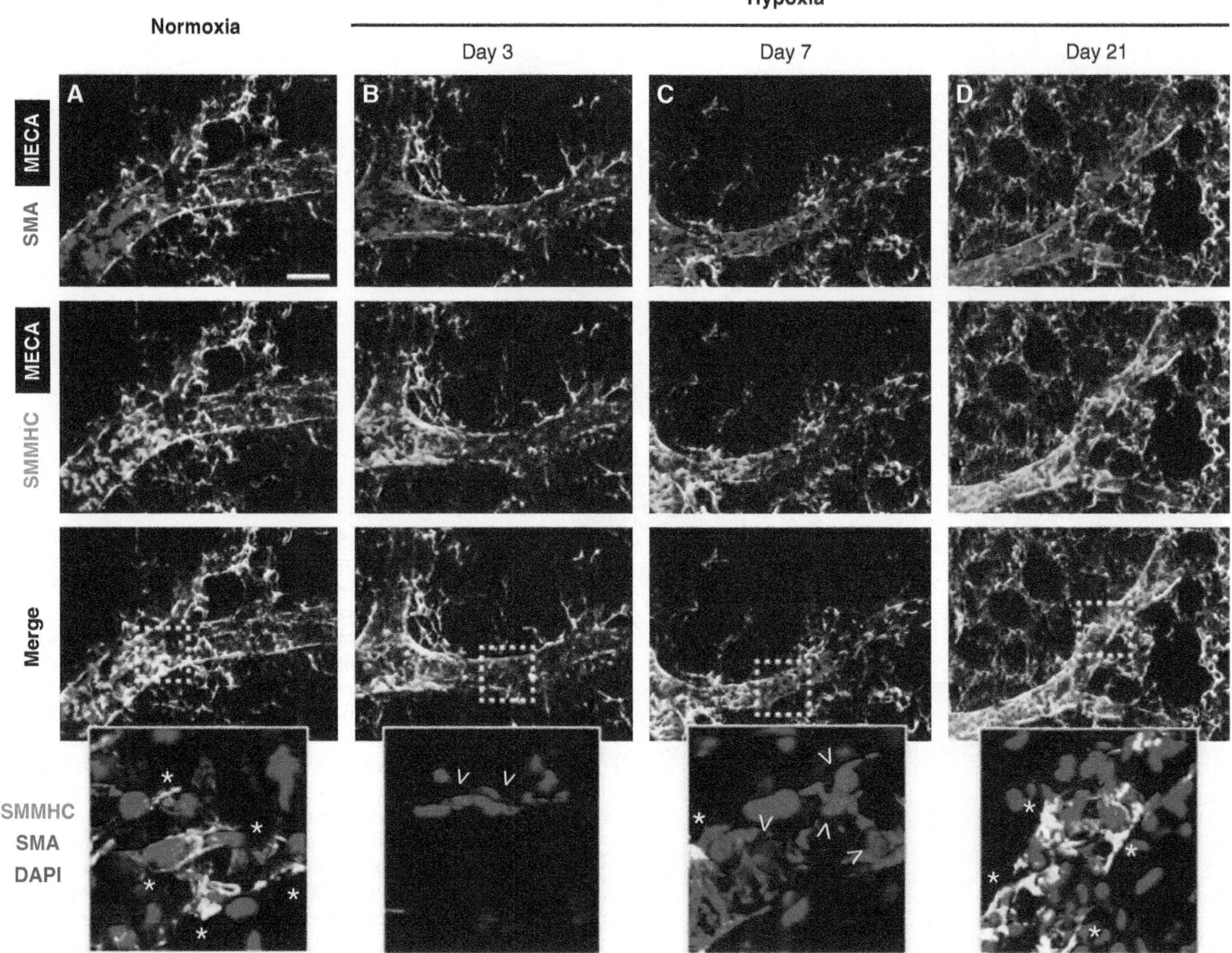

Fig. 47.4 Dynamic and distinct expression of smooth muscle actin (SMA) and smooth muscle myosin heavy chain (SMMHC) during hypoxia-induced distal pulmonary arteriole muscularization. (A–D) Adult mice were exposed to normoxia or to hypoxia for 3, 7, and 21 days as indicated, and then left lungs were stained for SMA *(red)*, SMMHC *(green)*, MECA-32 *(white)*, and nuclei (DAPI, *blue*). Representative confocal images of arteriole beds located in proximity to L.L1.A1 airway branches. The boxed regions in the merged images are shown as close-ups below with *asterisks* and *open arrowheads* representing SMA$^+$SMMHC$^+$ and SMA$^+$ cells, respectively. Note the transitory down-regulation of SMMHC in SMA$^+$ cells in the distal arteriole at 3 and 7 days of hypoxia. Scale bar, 25 μm. (From Sheikh AQ, Lighthouse JK, Greif DM. Recapitulation of developing artery muscularization in pulmonary hypertension. *Cell Rep*. 2014;6:809–817.)

studied.[19] A summary of key molecules that influence pulmonary vascular growth and remodeling is presented in Table 47.1. Cell adhesion molecules, such as vascular cell adhesion molecule 1 (VCAM-1)[20] and platelet cell adhesion molecule (PECAM)[21] (Fig. 47.8), and the β_1[22] and β_3 families of integrin receptors, particularly $\alpha_v\beta_3$[23] direct interactions between endothelial and SMCs and the extracellular matrix. Perturbations of those interactions may lead to malformation of the pulmonary and systemic arteries. The β_1 integrins bind fibronectin; the β_3 family binds fibronectin, as well as a host of matrix molecules, but especially tenascin, osteopontin, and vitronectin, many of which govern vascular cell migration (e.g., fibronectin)[24-27] and proliferation (e.g., tenascin).[28]

In addition, a variety of growth factors also appear to be responsible for the orderly growth and branching morphogenesis of the lung and blood vessels. These include vascular endothelial growth factor (VEGF),[29] particularly VEGF-A, and angiopoietin-1,[30] as well as acidic and basic fibroblast growth factor (FGF-1 and FGF-2).[31] Epithelial production of VEGF is essential for angiogenesis, and blockade of VEGF-A mediated angiogenesis represses epithelial proliferation, suggesting that blood vessel formation promotes alveolar formation.[32-34] The endothelium also appears to influence alveolar development via the production of angiocrine signals such as hepatocyte growth factor (Fig. 47.9).[35] In an experimental model of neoalveolarization induced by unilateral pneumonectomy, endothelial derived matrix metalloproteinase-14 drives expansion of epithelial progenitors by increasing the availability of ligands for the epidermal growth factor (EGF) receptor.[36] In addition, endothelial nitric oxide synthase (eNOS) regulates distal vascular and alveolar growth, based on studies in transgenic mice with eNOS deleted. Growth factors also promote vascularization by inducing the chemokine stromal-derived factor-1,[37] and also its receptor CXCR4 on endothelial cells. Interactions between members of the Wingless (Wnts) and bone morphogenetic protein families (BMPs) regulate lung branching morphogenesis,[38-41] as well as endothelial and SMC survival, proliferation, and migration. Wnt7b[42] has specifically been implicated in vascular development, particularly in regulating the investment of SMCs around the endothelial framework (Fig. 47.10).

Downstream effects of growth factors are mediated through specific tyrosine kinase receptors, such as FLT1, FLK1, TEK, and TIE,[43-45] as well as the activin receptor-like kinase (ALK1)[46] and numerous BMP receptors. ALK-1 has been implicated in the late vasculogenesis, and mutations in *ALK1* are associated with hereditary hemorrhagic telangiectasia,[47] whereas BMP receptor (*BMPR*) 2 mutations are associated with primary pulmonary

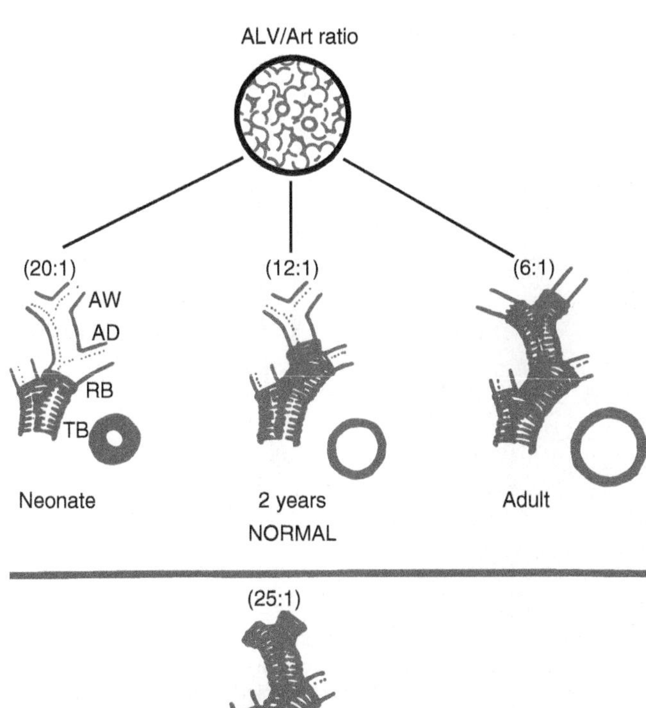

Fig. 47.5 Schema showing peripheral pulmonary arterial development through morphometric changes: extension of muscle into peripheral arteries, percent wall thickness, and artery number (alveolar-arterial ratio), as they relate to age. *Top panel*, Normal development. *Bottom panel*, Abnormalities in all three features in a 2-year-old child with a hypertensive ventricular septal defect *(VSD)*. *AD,* Artery accompanying an alveolar duct; *ALV/Art,* alveolar-arterial; *AW,* artery accompanying an alveolar wall; *RB,* artery accompanying a respiratory bronchiole; *TB,* artery accompanying a terminal bronchiole. (From Rabinovitch M, Haworth SG, Castaneda AR, et al. Lung biopsy in congenital heart disease: a morphometric approach to pulmonary vascular disease. *Circulation.* 1978;58:1107.)

hypertension.[48] Using a murine *Flk1* reporter construct, Schachtner and colleagues[49] found lung vascular development occurred at all stages of development and corresponded with overall lung growth. Notch and Jagged1 interaction are associated with early stages of lung vascular development.[50]The transcription factor TAL1[51] is implicated in vasculogenesis from precursor cells of the hematopoietic lineage. Sox17 was identified as a major requirement for normal pulmonary vascular morphogenesis[52] (Figs. 47.10 and 47.11); NFκB is critical in neonatal angiogenesis and control of alveolar growth[53]; and Prx1 is critical to extracellular matrix production and vascular smooth muscle investment of endothelial cells during embryonic lung growth.[54]

Matrix components (especially elastin and collagen) are regulated by insulin-like growth factor-I[55,56] and transforming growth factor-β (TGF-β).[57] Insulin-like growth factor-1 and its receptor act in concert with VEGF to stimulate fetal vascular growth through the same intracellular signaling pathways.[56] Lack of elastin leads to extensive proliferation of SMCs in pulmonary arteries. The balance between proteases and anti-proteinases also regulates growth factor interactions with cell surface molecules. Plasmin, thrombin,[58,59] and elastases, including leukocyte and endogenous vascular elastase (EVE),[60] release active growth factors from storage sites in the extracellular matrix. Also, numerous endogenously expressed inhibitors of proteinases and elastases, such as plasminogen activator inhibitor[61] and elafin,[62] control growth and development, and other classes of molecules are known to control angiogenesis, such as angiostatin, a molecule derived from plasminogen.[63]

The expression of vasoactive peptides in the lung during development also may play a role in the development of the pulmonary vasculature. Endothelin has been associated with cell proliferation and nitric oxide (NO) with the suppression of SMC growth.[64] Early expression of NOS[65] likely regulates vasculogenesis in addition to vascular tone.

ABNORMAL LUNG GROWTH

Underdevelopment of the lung parenchyma and the associated pulmonary vasculature[3] are frequent correlates of congenital diaphragmatic hernia (CDH),[66] genetic diseases such as Trisomy 21, scimitar syndrome, and oligohydramnios secondary to renal agenesis and dysplasia. Pulmonary hypoplasia is also a feature of prematurity, absence of the phrenic nerve, asphyxiating thoracic dystrophy, Rh isoimmunization, and, experimentally, amniocentesis[67] and smoking.[68]

Pulmonary artery hypertension and right-to-left shunting at birth can occur as a result of pathologic pulmonary vascular remodeling, heightened pulmonary vascular tone, or hypoplasia of the pulmonary vascular bed. In addition to the structural changes in the vessels, impaired gas exchange (hypoxia, hypercapnia) may cause pulmonary vasoconstriction, heightening pulmonary vascular resistance. In infants with CDH, reversal of pulmonary hypertension has been achieved with the use of vasodilators,[69] extracorporeal membrane oxygenation (ECMO),[70] high-frequency ventilation, prostacyclin and prostacyclin analogs,[71] and inhaled NO (iNO) alone or in combination with phosphodiesterase inhibitors.[72] Infants with CDH and hypoplastic lungs who were refractory to iNO prior to initiation of ECMO receive a beneficial effect from iNO after ECMO initiation.[69] Optimal lung recruitment may also improve the response to iNO in patients who initially appear non-responsive.[73,74] Strong experimental data suggest that pharmacologic reduction in pulmonary artery resistance will stimulate growth of the pulmonary arteries and regression of vascular remodeling, but this has not yet been substantiated in controlled trials.

The major determinant of mortality in infants who underwent attempted repair of CDH was a striking decrease in the number of alveoli and associated arteries (Fig. 47.12). This, combined with the pulmonary venous hypertension from left ventricular hypoplasia or dysfunction that occurs in some patients with CDH, may limit success in reversing severe pulmonary hypertension with NO in this group.[75-77] Inflation of the lungs in utero via occlusion of the trachea has been proposed to help mature the lung.[78,79] Further, in a nitrofen-induced model of CDH, vitamin A stimulated lung maturation. In an experimental lamb model of CDH, soluble guanylate cyclase activity is decreased and pulmonary hypertension was reduced by endothelin A receptor blockade but not by endothelin B receptor stimulation.[80,81] In fact, guanylate cyclase activation has been successful in reversing experimental neonatal pulmonary hypertension.[82]

Future strategies to improve lung vascular growth may come from understanding underlying transcription factor pathways that are repressed, such as the Sonic hedgehog pathway.[83] Studies have also focused on the possible contribution of resident, bone marrow-derived, or engineered stem cells.[84,85] Hyperoxia represses the expansion of these cells and of endothelial progenitor cells.[86,87] It is interesting that conditioned media from endothelial colony-forming cells[88] or from mesenchymal stem cells[89] can promote angiogenesis in experimental bronchopulmonary dysplasia via microRNAs in exosomes.[90] In lungs studied postmortem from infants with pulmonary hypoplasia or dysplasia, the number of arteries is reduced, but in proportion to the reduced number of

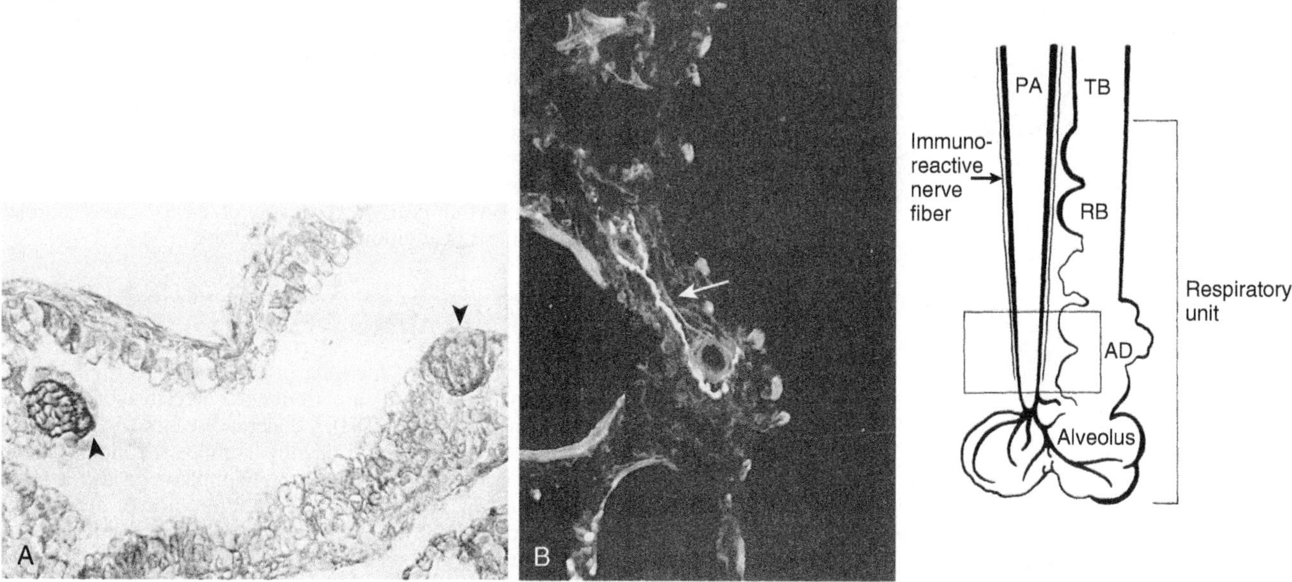

Fig. 47.6 (A) Neuroepithelial bodies *(arrowheads)* are seen as dark-staining regions (immunoreactive for serotonin) in the airway of a newborn infant. (B) Tyrosine hydroxylase immunoreactive perivascular nerve fibers *(arrow)* at the adventitial-medial border of an alveolar duct artery in a child age 2.5 years. Diagram on the *right* shows terminal bronchiole *(TB)* and airways of respiratory unit accompanied by an innervated pulmonary artery *(PA)*. *AD,* Alveolar duct; *RB,* respiratory bronchiole; square indicates area shown in (B). (A, From Rabinovitch M. Pathophysiology of pulmonary hypertension. In: Emmanouilides GC, et al. eds. *Moss and Adams' Heart Disease in Infants, Children, and Adolescents Including the Fetus and Young Adult*. Baltimore: Williams & Wilkins; 1995:1659–1695. Original supplied by E. Cutz, Hospital for Sick Children. B, From Allen KM, Wharton J, Polak JM, et al. A study of nerves containing peptides in the pulmonary vasculature of healthy infants and children and of those with pulmonary hypertension. *Br Heart J.* 1989;62:353.)

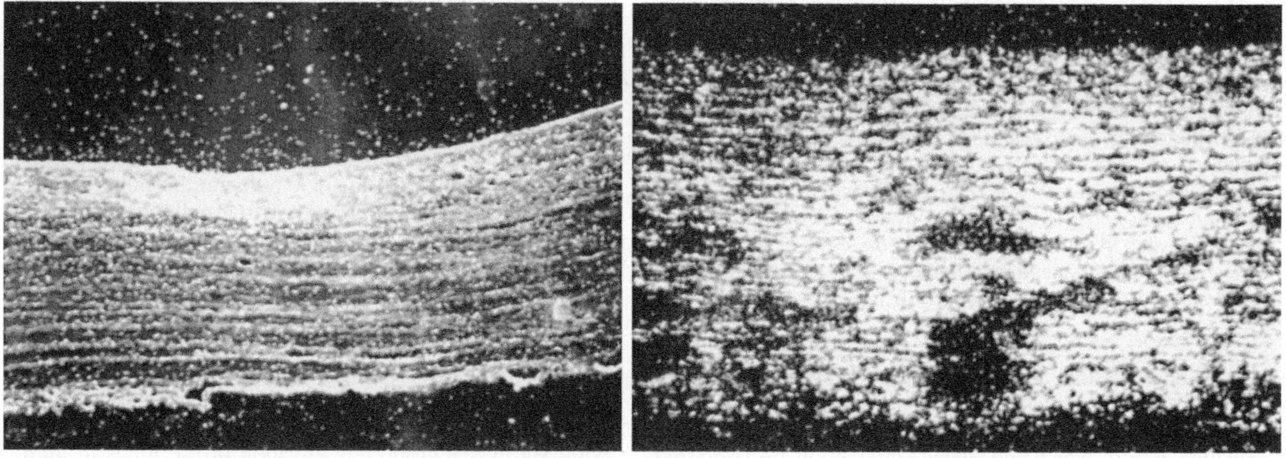

Fig. 47.7 In situ hybridization localization of tropoelastin messenger RNA (mRNA) in control and hypertensive vessels from neonatal calves. White staining over areas indicates tropoelastin mRNA labeling. In normotensive vessels *(left)*, labeled cells (^{35}S-labeled T66-T7) were confined to the inner media. Minimal signal is noted in the outer vessel wall. In vessels from hypertensive animals (14 days of hypoxia) *(right)*, intense autoradiographic signal was observed throughout the media, albeit in a patchy distribution. (From Prosser IW, Stenmark KR, Suthar M, et al. Regional heterogeneity of elastin and collagen gene expression in intralobar arteries in response to hypoxic pulmonary hypertension as demonstrated by *in situ* hybridization. *Am J Pathol.* 1989;135:1073.)

alveoli (see Fig. 47.12). The arteries are also generally small but not inconsistent with the size of the lung. The arteries, both centrally and peripherally, may be more muscular than normal, as in CDH, or have hypoplasia of the pulmonary musculature, as in renal agenesis. Dysplasia of the lung associated with persistent pulmonary hypertension of the newborn (e.g., alveolar capillary dysplasia) (Fig. 47.13)[91] is so refractory to treatment that a diagnostic biopsy should be done to guide clinical management. In newborn lambs and rabbits, heparin stimulates remodeling and accelerates maturation of the pulmonary circulation, as evidenced by an increase in the number of peripheral pulmonary arteries relative to alveoli.[92] This therapeutic strategy might prove clinically useful in inducing the growth of peripheral arteries and thereby reducing pulmonary vascular resistance.

Mechanical ventilation, another factor that contributes to arrested arterial and alveolar development, has been studied in the fetal lamb[93] and the neonatal mouse.[94] The latter study showed that genes that regulate arterial and alveolar growth are suppressed by mechanical ventilation. Dysregulation of elastin with mechanical ventilation appears to play a critical role in impairing the formation of the distal lung vasculature and alveoli, and the elastase inhibitor elafin protects against ventilator-induced lung injury.[95,96]

FAILURE TO REVERSE ELEVATED PULMONARY VASCULAR RESISTANCE

Perinatal stress (e.g., hemorrhage, hypoglycemia, aspiration, or hypoxia) may result in failure of dilation of normally muscular

Table 47.1 Cellular Mechanisms Regulating Pulmonary Vascular and Parenchymal Growth.

Molecule	Function
Cell Adhesion Molecules	
VCAM-1	Binds $\alpha_4\beta_1$ integrins. Deletion results in embryonic lethality with defective placental vascularization and cardiac development.
PECAM	Promotes EC-EC and EC-matrix adhesion.
β_1 and β_3 integrins	Allows binding to fibronectin and other matrix components (e.g., tenascin, osteopontin, and vitronectin). Regulates vascular cell migration and proliferation.
Growth Factors, Chemokines, and Vasoactive Peptides	
VEGF-A	Signals through receptor FLT-1 and FLK-1 to promote EC survival and proliferation. Deletion in mice results in embryonic lethality in association with complete absence of blood vessel formation.
Angiopoetin-1	Ligand for TIE2. Promotes blood vessel maturity and stability. Deletion in mice results in embryonic lethality in association with impaired vascular remodeling and complexity.
FGF-2	Promotes autocrine expression of VEGF by EC and increases expression of alpha and beta-integrins.
HGF	Angiocrine factor produced by EC that promotes development of primary septae.
MMP-14	Endothelial derived factor that drives expansion of epithelial progenitors by liberating ligands for the EGF receptor.
SDF-1α	Induced by VEGF and FGF. Chemoattractant for EC expressing CXCR4. Pro-angiogenic.
WNT7b	Activates canonical Wnt signaling to promote lung branching and vascular smooth muscle cell differentiation and survival.
BMP4	Regulates proximal-distal patterning of the lung. Promotes EC and VSMC migration and proliferation.
IGF-1	Promotes elastin expression and EC survival. Stabilizes nascent blood vessels.
NO	Promotes pulmonary vasodilation during the fetal-neonatal transition. Promotes angiogenesis downstream from VEGF.
Endothelin-1	Induces vasoconstriction. Promotes VSMC proliferation and may lead to pulmonary vascular remodeling.
Transcription Factors	
TAL1	Expressed by endothelial progenitor cells during vasculogenesis.
Sox17	Required for normal pulmonary vascular morphogenesis. Deletion is mesenchymal cells results in dilation of macrovasculature but diminished complexity of microvasculature.
NFκB	Promotes pulmonary EC survival, proliferation, and migration during alveolarization.
Prdx1	Promotes VSMC differentiation by regulating ECM stiffness and TGFβ signaling.
Matrix Components, Proteinases, Elastases	
Elastin	Prevents excessive VSMC proliferation.
Endogenous vascular elastase	Release FGF-2 from the ECM to promote VSMC proliferation.
Plasmin	Serine proteinase that cleaves ECM proteins. Generates the antiangiogenic protein angiostatin.

BMP4, Bone morphogenetic protein 4; *CXCR4,* C-X-C chemokine receptor type 4; *EC,* endothelial cell; *ECM,* extracellular matrix *FGF,* fibroblast growth factor; *HGF,* hepatocyte growth factor; *IGF-1,* insulin-like growth factor-1; *MMP-14,* matrix metalloproteinase-14; *NFkB,* nuclear factor kappa-B; *NO,* nitric oxide; *PECAM,* platelet cell adhesion molecule; *Prdx1,* peroxiredoxin; *SDF*-1a, stromal cell derived factor-1 alpha; *Sox17,* transcription factor SOX-17; *TAL1,* T-cell acute lymphocytic leukemia protein 1; *TGF-β,* transforming growth factor-β; *TIE2,* tyrosine-protein kinase receptor TEK; *VCAM-1,* vascular cell adhesion molecule 1; *VEGF-A,* vascular endothelial growth factor-A; *VSMC,* vascular smooth muscle cells.

vessels and left ventricular dysfunction, both contributing to persistent pulmonary hypertension. The use of inhaled NO in clinical studies,[97] L-arginine in experimental studies,[98] gene transfer of endothelial NOS,[99] and inhibition of phosphodiesterases[100] have proved effective in lowering pulmonary artery pressure. Because increased production of endothelin may underlie the pathophysiology of persistent pulmonary hypertension of the newborn,[101] the use of endothelin receptor blockade or endothelin-converting enzyme inhibition[102] was predicted to be beneficial.[103] Although early retrospective studies indicated a potential benefit of bosentan, an oral endothelin-1 receptor antagonist,[104] for infants with PPHN, a more recent multicenter, randomized controlled trial found that bosentan did not improve oxygenation or other outcomes.[105]

INDUCTION OF VASCULAR ABNORMALITIES

IN UTERO

Postmortem studies of the lung in fatal cases of meconium aspiration suggest that antecedent pulmonary vascular abnormalities exacerbate postnatal pulmonary hypertension.[106] The most striking feature is the muscularization of small, peripheral arteries that are normally nonmuscular. The muscle cells are surrounded by darkly stained elastic laminae, suggesting that they formed several weeks before death and therefore in utero. Early clinical studies suggested a relationship between maternal ingestion of prostaglandin synthetase inhibitors and subsequent persistent pulmonary hypertension.[107] However, a large number of women take aspirin or indomethacin during pregnancy, and the incidence of persistent pulmonary hypertension in their newborn infants is low. Further, in the majority of infants with persistent pulmonary hypertension, there is no history of maternal ingestion of these compounds. Yet, experimental studies in lambs have shown that prostaglandin synthetase inhibitors constrict the ductus arteriosus in utero. Chronic indomethacin treatment in pregnant rats produces structural changes in the pulmonary vascular bed of the newborn.[108] Thus it seems likely that, in an occasional susceptible human fetus, there may be a relationship between prostaglandin synthetase inhibitors and persistent pulmonary hypertension.

Disturbances in oxygen tension, alterations in placental blood flow, and inflammation may also perturb development of the pulmonary vasculature and induce pathologic remodeling. Although chronic maternal hypoxemia in guinea pigs does not reproduce the structural and physiologic changes of pulmonary hypertension,[109] relatively short periods of hypoxia in the fetal lamb result in sustained elevation of pulmonary artery pressure

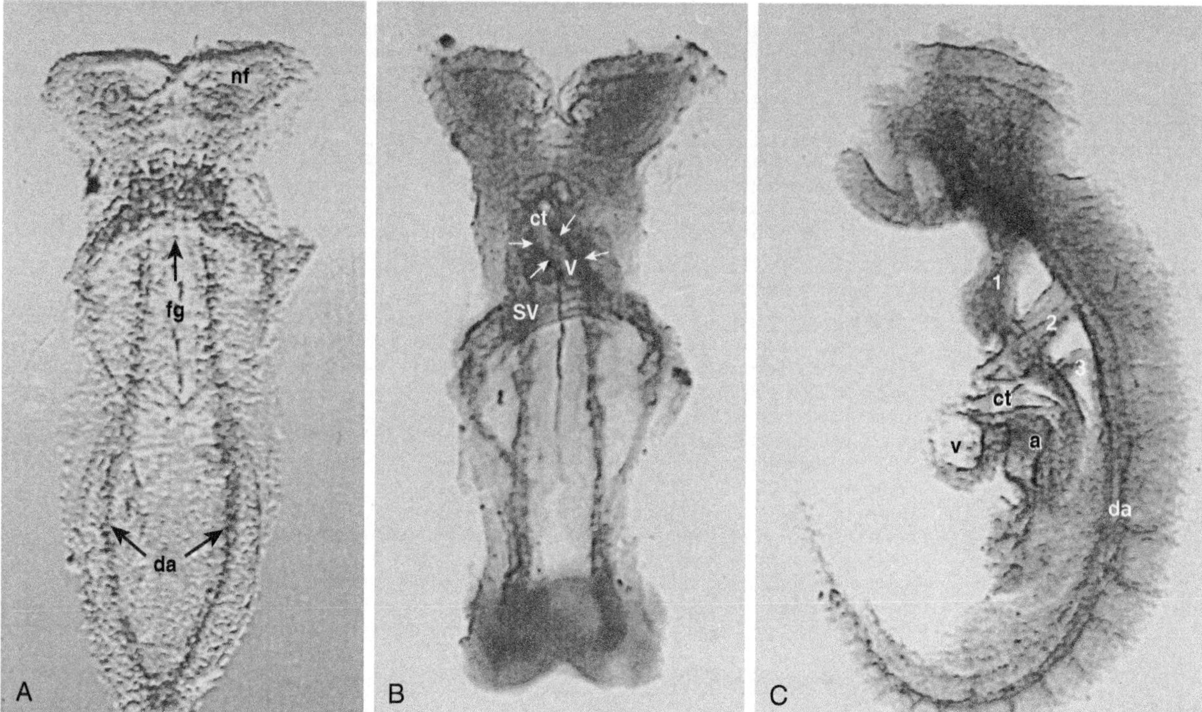

Fig. 47.8 Early vascular development in the mouse embryo as defined by whole-mount in situ hybridization with platelet cell adhesion molecule (PECAM)-1 (CD31) riboprobes. (A) Day-7.5 mouse embryo (4 somites) showing a neural fold *(nf)* and an organized bilateral dorsal aorta *(da)* with initial formation of a vascular plexus in the cardiogenic crescent just cranial to the developing foregut *(fg)*. (B) Sequential organization of the endocardial cell of the vascular plexus *(arrows)* in the 8.5-day embryo (6 to 8 somites) into a lumen forming the sinus *(sv)*, ventricle *(v)*, and conotruncus *(ct)*. (C) Definitive organization of endothelial cells into the vascular template for the embryo, including clearly defined endocardium of the atrium *(a)*, ventricle *(v)*, and conotruncus *(ct)*, as well as the pharyngeal arches 1 to 3 and dorsal aorta *(da)*. (From Baldwin HS. Early embryonic vascular development. *Cardiovasc Res.* 1996;31:E34, with permission of Elsevier Science-NL.)

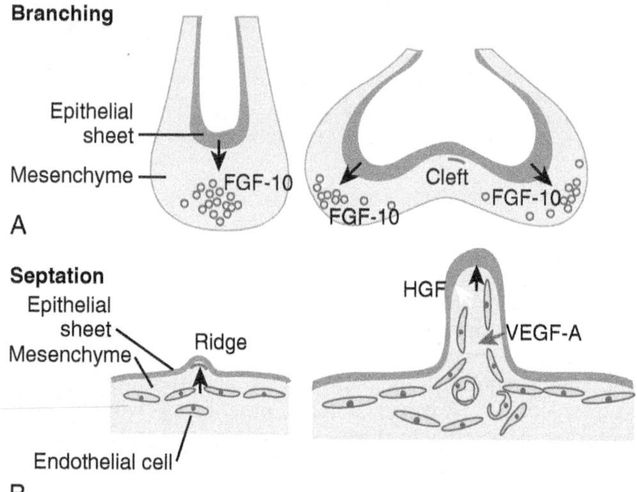

Fig. 47.9 Model for septation in comparison to branching morphogenesis. (A) During branching morphogenesis, epithelial tubes grow toward a chemoattractive source such as fibroblast growth factor *(FGF)*-10 in the mesenchyme. On redistribution of the chemoattractive source, the epithelial tube bifurcates to grow toward the new sources and a cleft is formed at the previous tip, causing branching. (B) During septation, the epithelial sheet is pushed up to form a ridge or crest by underlying endothelial cells. Capillary angiogenesis stimulated by epithelium-derived vascular endothelial growth factor-A *(VEGF-A)*, coupled with growth of epithelial cells induced by endothelium-derived paracrine factors such as hematocyte growth factor *(HGF)*, causes formation and growth of the septae. (From Yamamoto H, Jun Yun E, Gerber HP, et al. Epithelial-vascular cross talk mediated by VEGF-A and HGF signaling directs primary septae formation during distal lung morphogenesis. *Dev Biol.* 2007;308:44–53.)

and structural changes in the pulmonary arteries. In lambs, pulmonary hypertension can also be induced by administration of a cytokine associated with inflammation (i.e., tumor necrosis factor-α).[110] Chronic placental insufficiency in a lamb model of IUGR decreases both alveolar and vascular growth.[111] The role of chronic fetal hypoxia-ischemia and the risk for bronchopulmonary dysplasia or pulmonary hypertension is also being elucidated in clinical studies of pregnancies exhibiting maternal vascular underperfusion (MVU) of the placental bed.[112,113] Cord blood angiogenic factors such as VEGFA, granulocyte-colony stimulating factor (GCSF), and placental growth factor (PIGF) are decreased in premature infants exposed to placental MVU, and decreased cord blood GCSF and PIGF are also associated with a higher risk of developing bronchopulmonary dysplasia and pulmonary hypertension.[114]

In utero closure or constriction of the ductus arteriosus also induces the structural changes and the initial hemodynamic profile of persistent pulmonary hypertension.[115,116] An intriguing association between increased superoxide generation and pulmonary hypertension has been established in this model,[117] suggesting a potential for treatment with superoxide dismutase.[118] This also helps explain the refractoriness of this particular group of patients to NO[119] and is in keeping with the elevated levels of soluble guanylate cyclase and phosphodiesterase.[120] The association between increased soluble VEGFR1 (sFLT1) in amniotic fluid and impaired lung growth may link preeclampsia to bronchopulmonary dysplasia and pulmonary hypertension.[121,122]

Although the mechanism is not established, changes in the balance of vasodilators and vasoconstrictors may also play a role in disease pathogenesis. Given that NO induces angiogenesis and endothelin is a mitogen for SMCs,[123] one might speculate that increased production of endothelin or reduced production of nitric oxide in utero might lead to an increase in muscularity

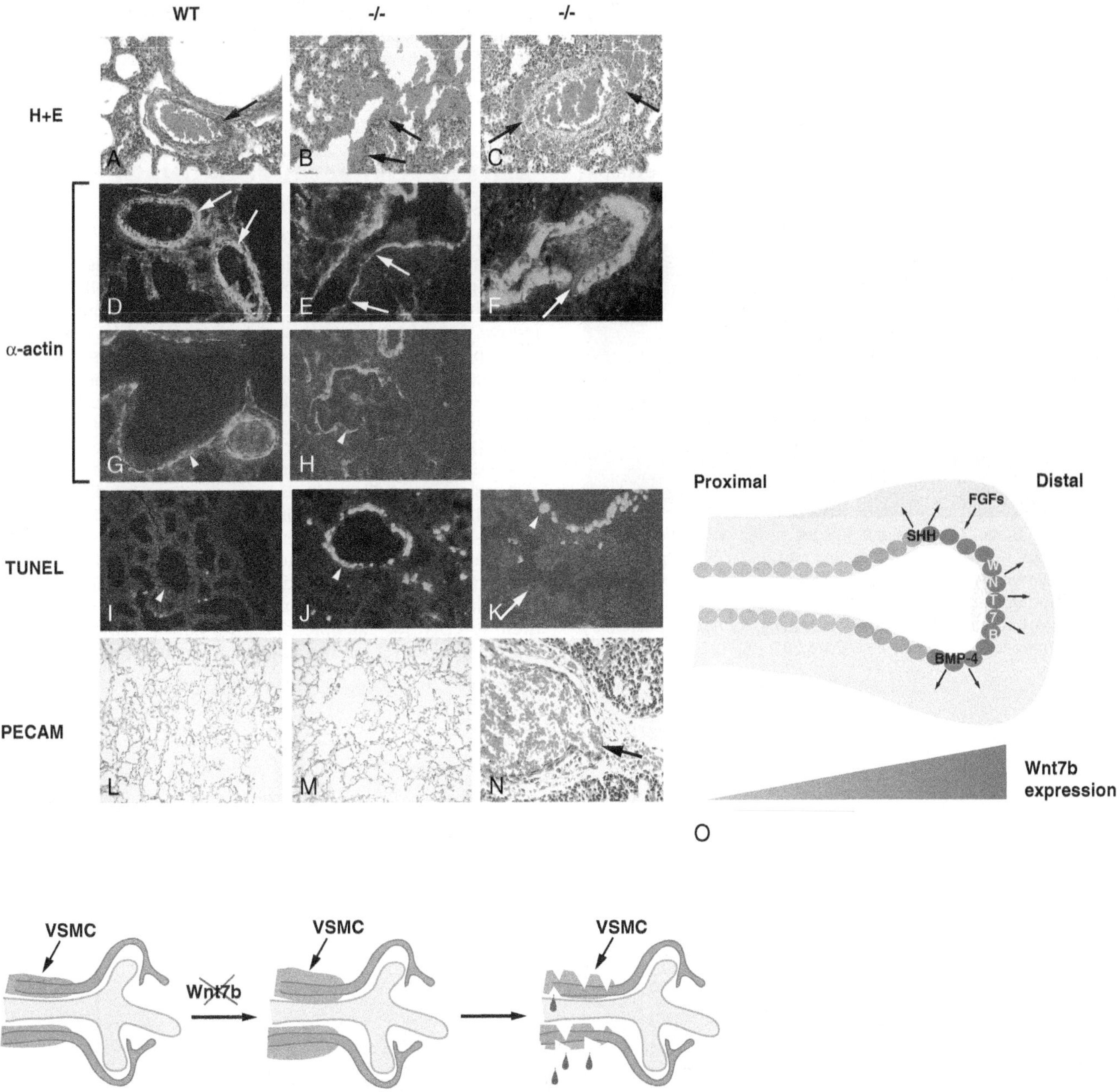

Fig. 47.10 Defective smooth muscle integrity in Wnt7b$^{lacZ-/-}$ embryos and mice. Close examination of blood vessels in wild-type (A, *arrow*) and Wnt7b$^{lacZ-/-}$ P0 neonates (B and C) reveals several breaches in the vessel wall in Wnt7b$^{lacZ-/-}$ mice. In some instances, very little of the structure of the wall is left (B, *arrows*), whereas in others a thicker vessel wall with several ruptures is observed (C, *arrows*). Staining of sections with an antibody against smooth muscle α-actin shows robust staining surrounding blood vessels in wild-type *(WT)* neonates (D, *arrows*). Smooth muscle α-actin staining shows reduced staining, suggesting degradation of smooth muscle surrounding some vessels in Wnt7b$^{lacZ-/-}$ neonates (E, *arrows*), whereas other vessels show frank breaches in the hypertrophic vessel wall (F). Bronchial smooth muscle appears normal in both wild-type (G, *arrowhead*) and Wnt7b$^{lacZ-/-}$ neonates (H, *arrowhead*). TUNEL staining shows an increase in TUNEL-positive cells in the smooth muscle of the blood vessel wall in Wnt7b$^{lacZ-/-}$ neonates (J, *arrowhead*) but not in bronchial smooth muscle (K, *arrow*). This is not observed in wild-type littermates (I, *arrow*) PECAM staining reveals a normal endothelial network in wild-type (L) and Wnt7b$^{lacZ-/-}$ neonates (M). Many large blood vessels showed rupture of the smooth muscle layer, with herniation of the intact endothelial cell layer (N, *arrow*). (O) A model for the role of Wnt7b in lung development. Wnt7b is expressed at the distal tips of the airway epithelium in a pattern similar to that observed with BMP4 and overlapping that of sonic hedgehog (SHH). In addition, Wnt7b is expressed in an increasing gradient from the proximal-to-distal airway epithelium. FGFs are expressed in the mesenchyme and are known to regulate epithelial branching and proliferation. However, because BMP-4 and SHH expression are unchanged in Wnt7b$^{lacZ-/-}$ embryos and Wnt7b expression is unchanged in *Shh*-null mice, Wnt7b regulates mesenchymal proliferation and differentiation through a unique pathway. (P) Lung vasculature is composed of both endothelium *(red)* and vascular smooth muscle *(VSMC, blue)*, and develops in parallel with the airways *(green)*. Loss of Wnt7b function results in defects in vascular smooth muscle differentiation and/or survival, leading to a hypertrophic response (change from *dark blue* to *light blue*), degradation of the vessel wall, and eventual rupture of the weakened vessels. *BMP*, Bone morphogenetic protein; *FGF*, fibroblast growth factor; *H+E*, hematoxylin and eosin (stain); *PECAM*, platelet cell adhesion molecule; *TUNEL*, terminal deoxynucleotidyl transferase dUTP nick-end labeling. (From Shu W, Jiang YQ, Lu MM, et al. Wnt7b regulates mesenchymal proliferation and vascular development in the lung. *Development*. 2002;129:4831.)

of peripheral pulmonary arteries and a reduction in their number.

As previously discussed, SMCs with differences in potential for proliferation and for production and accumulation of extracellular matrix components may also be differentially responsive to stimuli that perturb the pulmonary vasculature. Conversely, structural remodeling of the pulmonary circulation affects the responsivity to vasodilator stimuli. For example, increased adventitial thickening, as observed in hypoxia-induced neonatal pulmonary hypertension, may prevent the access of NO to the vascular SMCs.[124] The heme oxygenase pathway is an alternative pathway that might be equally important in reducing vascular tone and in suppressing the propensity to vascular inflammation.[125]

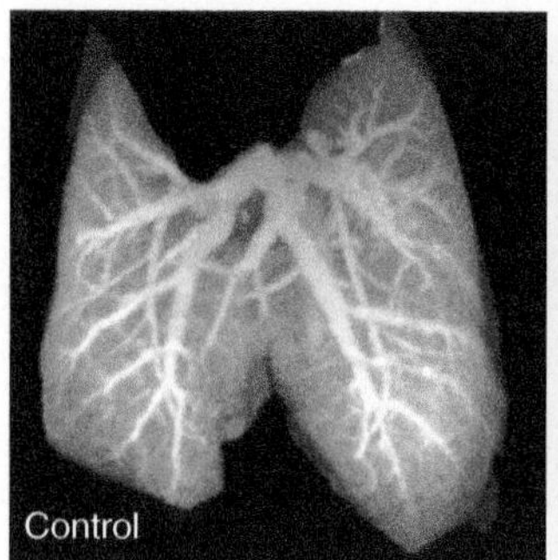

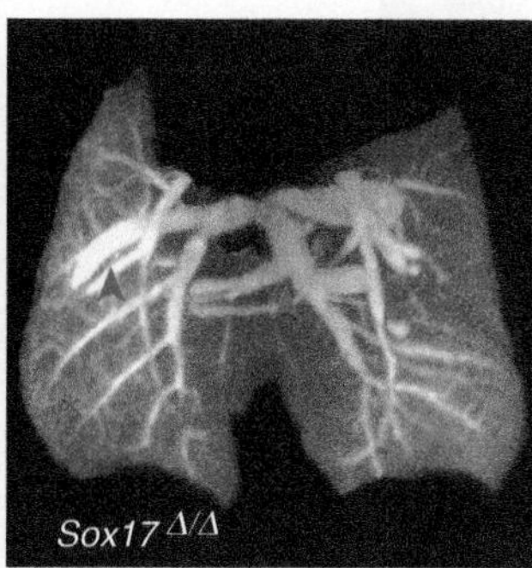

Fig. 47.11 Static 3-dimensional images of the developing pulmonary vascular network in E18.5 control and *Sox17*$^{\Delta/\Delta}$ lungs showing dilated pulmonary blood vessels *(arrowheads)* and reduced staining of the peripheral microvasculature *(asterisks)*. (From Lange AW, Haitchi HM, LeCras TD, et al. Sox17 is required for normal pulmonary vascular morphogenesis. *Dev Biol.* 2014;387:109–120.)

ALTERED POSTNATAL PULMONARY VASCULAR DEVELOPMENT

Hypoxia, hyperoxia, toxins, or alterations in pulmonary blood flow also affect the postnatal structural development of the pulmonary vascular bed in infancy and childhood. We have shown in clinical studies that high flow and pressure induce increasing pulmonary hypertension in association with progressive vascular abnormalities.[126] First, there is extension of muscle into peripheral, normally nonmuscular arteries (morphometric grade A). This is followed by medial hypertrophy of muscular arteries (grade B = Heath-Edwards grade I)[127] and reduced arterial concentration (morphometric grade C), associated with increased pulmonary artery pressure and resistance.[126] There is also the concomitant development of neointimal formation. This is initiated by cellular changes (Heath-Edwards grade II), which further progress to occlusive fibroproliferative lesions (grade III) and culminate in plexiform networks of obstructed and dilated vessels (grade IV). The potential for reversibility of these changes is dictated by their severity; for example, grade I-B almost always regresses following removal of the abnormal hemodynamic stimulus,

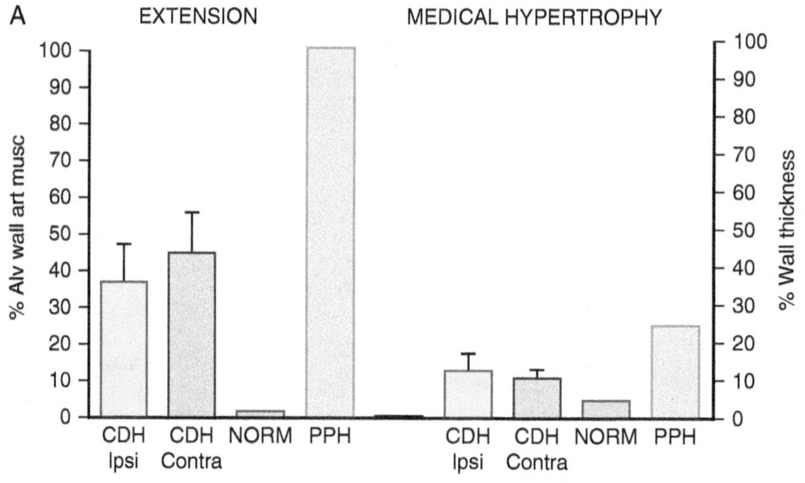

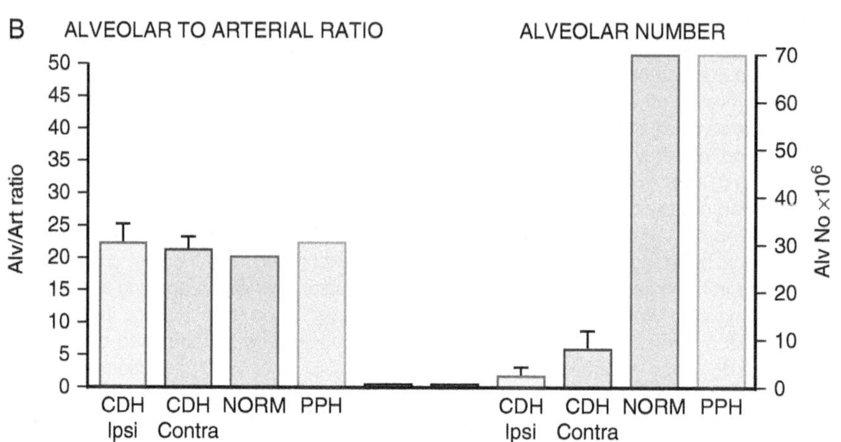

Fig. 47.12 (A) Morphometric data from nine patients with congenital diaphragmatic hernia *(CDH)*, compared with published values in normal neonates and in infants with idiopathic persistent pulmonary hypertension of the newborn *(PPH)*. Infants with CDH had greater smooth muscle extension into peripheral arteries and increased medial hypertrophy than normal *(NORM)* infants but less than infants with PPH. (B) Morphometric data from six infants with CDH compared with normal neonates and infants with PPH. Alveolar-arterial *(Alv/Art)* ratio was similar to that in normal infants, but total alveolar number was severely reduced in both ipsilateral and contralateral lungs. (From Bohn D, Tamura M, Perrin D, et al. Ventilatory predictors of pulmonary hypoplasia in congenital diaphragmatic hernia, confirmed by morphologic assessment. *J Pediatr.* 1987;111:423.)

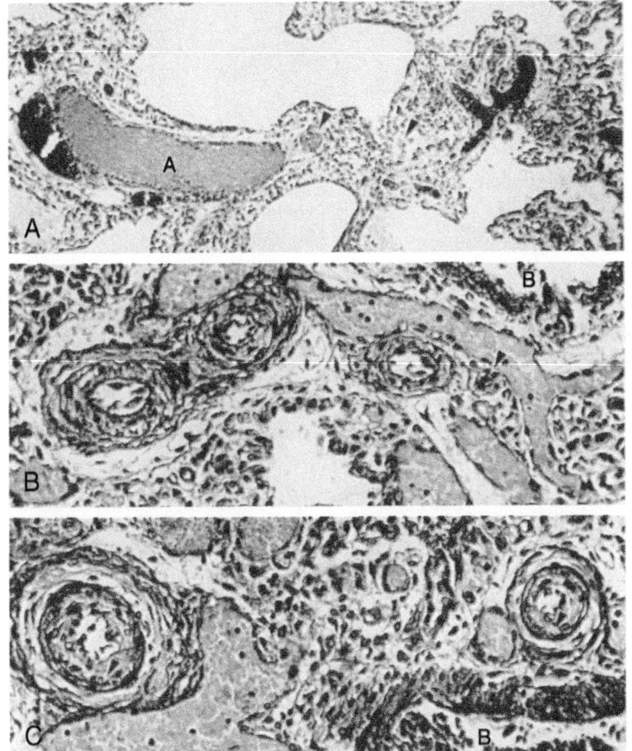

Fig. 47.13 Lung micrographs from the left (A) and right (B and C) lungs of a patient with alveolar capillary dysplasia. (A) Barium distends the lumen of a preacinar artery *(A)* but does not enter the anomalous vein to the left of the artery. Intraacinar arterial branches that contain barium are identified *(arrowheads),* but intraacinar veins and venules are distended with red blood cells, presumably forced ahead of the barium by the postmortem angiogram. Air spaces are lined by cuboidal epithelium, and no luminal capillaries are seen, all vessels lying centrally in the air space walls. (Hematoxylin-eosin, ×90.) (B) Intraacinar pulmonary arteries showing medial muscular thickening that forms a continuous layer even in the smallest branch *(arrowhead),* which is 20 μm in external diameter. Media is demarcated by external and internal elastic laminae, stained black in this elastic stain. A bronchiole *(B)* is identified (Elastic-van Gieson, ×220). (C) Intraacinar arteries, the smaller measuring 60 μm in external diameter, with concentric intimal fibrosis; the latter is overlaid by *arrowheads* that mark the internal elastic laminae. The media is narrow in these branches but note that the lumen (containing festooned endothelial cells) is the same size as in the similar-sized arteries seen in (B) (Elastic-van Gieson, ×220). (From Cullinane C, Cox PN, Silver MM, et al. Persistent pulmonary hypertension of the newborn due to alveolar capillary dysplasia. *Pediatr Pathol.* 1992;12:499. Reproduced with permission. All rights reserved.)

whereas the loss of arteries (grade C) and the higher Heath-Edwards grades generally regress or remain functionally insignificant only if the hemodynamic insult is relieved in early infancy (first 8 months after birth).[128]

To investigate the cellular mechanisms that control the pulmonary vascular abnormalities in congenital heart defects, we applied electron microscopy to the study of lung biopsy tissue. Endothelial changes were observed on scanning and transmission electron microscopy, suggesting a potential for altered interaction with circulating blood elements, such as platelets and leukocytes.[129] Functional abnormalities also were reflected in increased production of von Willebrand factor.[130,131] In addition, alterations in the subendothelium, reflected in fragmentation of elastin, suggested that an elastolytic enzyme might be stimulating the remodeling process.[129]

EXPERIMENTAL PATHOPHYSIOLOGY OF PULMONARY HYPERTENSION

Significant insight into the molecular mechanisms underlying neonatal pulmonary hypertension has been gained from high-flow models of neonatal pulmonary hypertension produced by constricting or closing the ductus arteriosus prenatally. Chronic intrauterine hypertension decreases expression of Ca^{2+} sensitive potassium channels that mediate vasodilation of the pulmonary vascular bed during the perinatal transition[132] and disrupts the ability of the pulmonary circulation to appropriately sense changes in oxygen tension.[133] Additional studies using this model indicate that postnatal inhibition of PPAR-γ[134] and increased Nox4-derived hydrogen peroxide and reactive oxygen species may play critical roles in adverse vascular remodeling.[135,136]

In experimental rodent models, exposure to low oxygen (equivalent to 10% FiO_2), hyperoxia (80% to 100% FiO_2), or the toxin monocrotaline also induce abnormal muscularization of peripheral arteries, medial hypertrophy of muscular arteries, and reduced arterial relative to alveolar density.[3] Although the pulmonary vascular abnormalities induced by changes in ambient oxygen appear largely reversible, monocrotaline-induced changes progress in the adult animal but not in the infant, suggesting developmental differences in the remodeling response. Hyperoxia is especially associated with a failure of normal lung compliance and growth, whereas monocrotaline induces only alveolar abnormalities when given to neonatal rats.

Experimentally, the induction of structural changes in pulmonary arteries is related to increased activity of the EVE.[137,138] Levels of EVE are increased in rat pulmonary arteries several days after exposure to hypoxia or injection of monocrotaline, and serine elastase inhibitors effectively prevent the development or progression of pulmonary vascular changes and pulmonary hypertension.[137,139] The induction of elastase activity appears to be related to a loss of endothelial barrier function, potentially allowing serum or endothelial factors to access the subendothelium and induce the release of a serine elastase from pulmonary vascular SMCs.[140] This elastase can subsequently liberate biologically active SMC mitogens, such as basic fibroblast growth factor 2 (FGF), from extracellular matrix stores.[60]

The resulting SMC hyperplasia contributes to the hypertrophy of the arterial wall. Release of other growth factors, such as TGF-β, induce increased synthesis of elastin and collagen, likely contributing to the thickening. There is also induction of the matrix glycoprotein tenascin, which cooperates with growth factors such as EGF and basic FGF to induce a proliferative response in the vessel wall (Fig. 47.14).[141] Experimental data demonstrating the prevention of hyperoxia-induced pulmonary hypertension and altered lung compliance in newborn rats with elastase inhibitors[142] prompted a clinical trial with promising results in preventing and reducing the severity of bronchopulmonary dysplasia in premature infants.[143] Experimental studies have also shown that elastase inhibitors can reverse established pulmonary vascular disease produced by the toxin monocrotaline, including muscularization of distal arteries, medial hypertrophy of muscular arteries, and loss of small vessels (Fig. 47.15).

The knowledge that elastase was critical in maintaining survival signals through EGF receptors (EGFRs) motivated studies to block EGFR, resulting in the reversal of progressive pulmonary arterial hypertension (PAH) that was sustained even 1 month after cessation of treatment.[144] Similarly, the use of a PDGF receptor blocker to reverse PAH in this experimental model[145] prompted a case report showing the successful use of the tyrosine kinase inhibitor imatinib in a patient with advanced pulmonary vascular disease[146] and motivated several clinical trials. However, although a randomized controlled trial

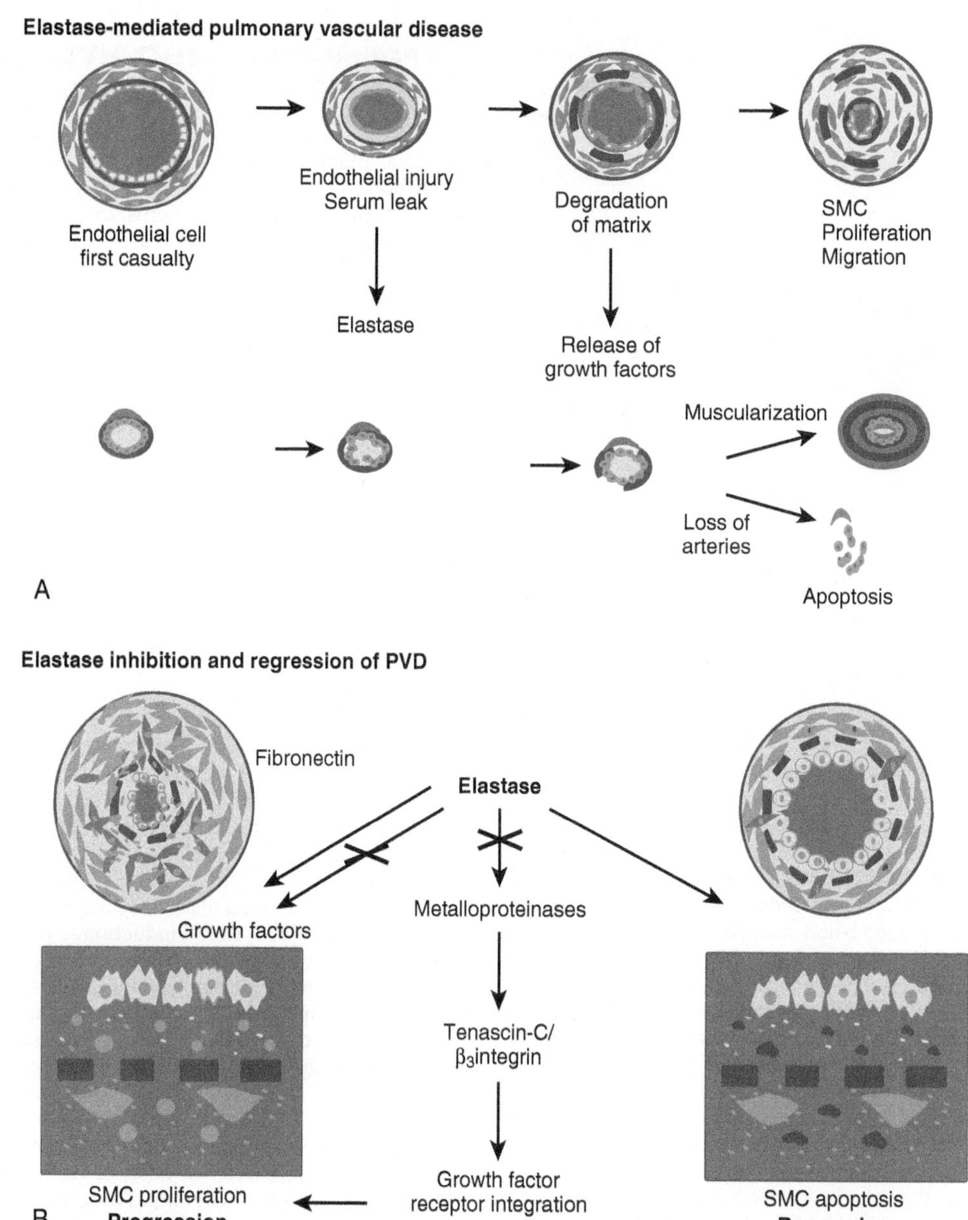

Fig. 47.14 Schema describing relationship of elastase to pulmonary vascular disease *(PVD)*. We speculated, based on our studies in cultured cells and in experimental animals, as to how a stimulus could induce activity of an elastolytic enzyme and how this might stimulate the remodeling process. (A) In response to an injurious stimulus, the first "casualty" is the endothelial cell. As a result of structural and functional alterations in endothelial cells, some of the barrier function would be lost, allowing a leak into the subendothelium of a serum factor normally excluded from this region. The serum factor could induce activity of an endogenous vascular elastase. This enzyme released from precursor or mature smooth muscle cells *(SMCs)* would activate growth factors normally stored in the extracellular matrix in an inactive form, which are known to induce smooth muscle hypertrophy and proliferation and increases in connective tissue protein (e.g., collagen and elastin) synthesis. The growth factors could also result in the differentiation of precursor cells to mature smooth muscle related to the muscularization of normally nonmuscular small peripheral arteries. Elastase activity could also contribute to the loss of small arteries. (B) As a result of elastase activity, a proteolytic cascade could be amplified through the activation of matrix metalloproteinases. We have shown that proteolysis of the matrix leads to the induction of tenascin-C, which in clustering to β_3 integrins results in the clustering and activation of growth factor receptors that send important survival and growth signals to the cells. Continued elastase activity causes migration of SMCs in several ways. The elastin peptides or degradation products of elastin can stimulate fibronectin, a glycoprotein that is pivotal in altering SMC shape and in switching them to the motile phenotype. Inhibition of elastase activity could lead to SMC apoptosis and regression of vascular disease. (From Rabinovitch M. Pathobiology of pulmonary hypertension. *Annu Rev Pathol Mech Dis.* 2007;2:369–399.)

demonstrated improved exercise tolerance and hemodynamics with imatinib,[147] serious adverse events and side effects were common, resulting in the majority of the patients withdrawing from the study and limiting its widespread use for PAH.[147,148] Others have used simvastatin[149] or endothelial eNOS gene therapy in association with endothelial progenitor cell administration (Fig. 47.16)[33,150] to reverse PAH in a monocrotaline-pneumonectomy model. The study by Drake and colleagues[165] is important in showing recovery of the distal vasculature using this strategy. It is interesting that loss of

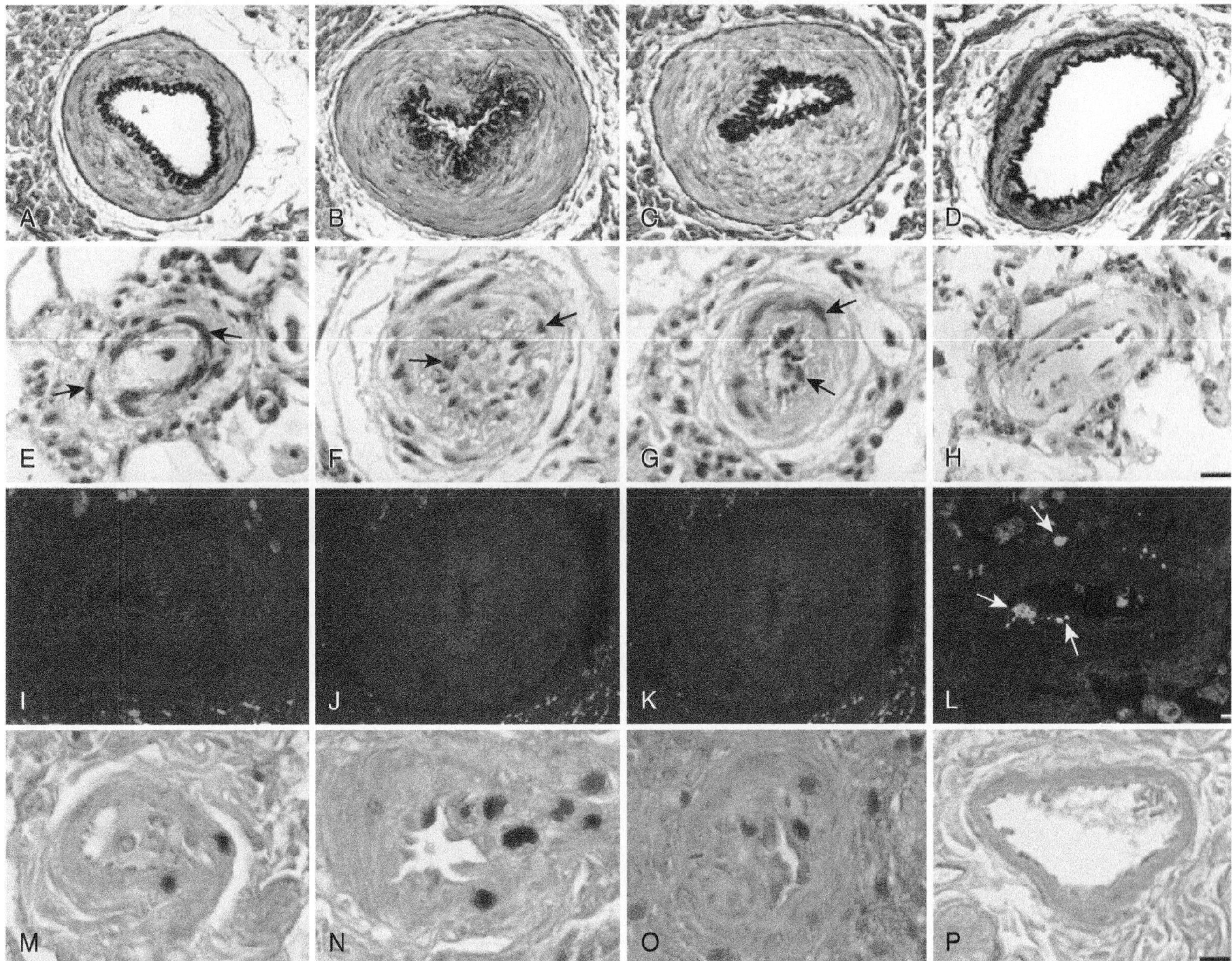

Fig. 47.15 Cellular mechanism responsible for reversal of pulmonary artery muscularity. Elastase inhibition arrests tenascin-C accumulation and proliferation and induces apoptosis and loss of extracellular matrix (such as elastin). (A–P) Days refer to time after injection of monocrotaline: (A, E, I, M) day 21; (B, F, J, N) day 28; (C, G, K, O) day 28; (D, H, L, P) day 28. (A–D) Saline-perfused pulmonary arteries stained with Movat pentachrome stain. (E–H) Pulmonary arteries after tenascin-C immunohistochemistry. *Arrows* indicate positive brown peroxidase staining. (I–L) In situ TUNEL assays identifying apoptosis. *Arrows* indicate TUNEL-positive vascular cells. (M–P) Proliferating vascular cells, shown by immunohistochemistry for proliferating cell nuclear antigen (PCNA); dark nuclei are PCNA-positive cells. *TUNEL,* Terminal deoxynucleotidyl transferase dUTP nick-end labeling. (From Cowan KN, Heilbut A, Humpl T, et al. Complete reversal of fatal pulmonary hypertension in rats by a serine elastase inhibitor. *Nat Med.* 2000;6:698–702.)

endothelial cells plays a key initiating role in the pathogenesis of PAH and severe remodeling.[151]

Gene therapy with survivin[152] or angiopoietin-1,[153] inhibition of the serotonin transporter (SERT),[154] adrenomedullin,[155] and the rho kinase inhibitor fasudil[156] have all been used to reverse experimental pulmonary vascular disease. Potassium channel dysfunction is implicated in the pathogenesis of pulmonary vascular disease,[157] and gene therapy restoring K channel function has been used effectively to suppress[158] and reverse experimentally induced pulmonary vascular abnormalities. Our ability to prevent progression or reverse advanced pulmonary vascular disease in patients and restore the normal growth of blood vessels may require further identification of the cause of the SMC and fibroblast proliferative response and the initial endothelial cell susceptibility to apoptosis.[159-162] Recent attention has focused on reversing pulmonary hypertension by activating BMPR2 receptor signaling, because there is evidence that even in the absence of a mutation in BMPR2, there is reduced expression of this receptor in all forms of pulmonary hypertension. Strategies to activate BMPR2 receptor signaling and to reverse pulmonary hypertension include treatment with FK-506,[163] the elastase inhibitor elafin (Fig. 47.17),[164] ataluren and chorloquine,[165] and BMP9.[166] More recent studies suggest that rare variants in the T-box transcription factor 4 *(Tbx4)* gene appears to be an emerging cause of pulmonary hypertension specific to the neonatal and pediatrics population.[168,169] Therefore, *Tbx4* may represent an additional promising therapeutic target.

DECREASED GROWTH OF THE PULMONARY VASCULAR BED

Reduced pulmonary blood flow and pressure may also result in reduced growth of the pulmonary vascular bed with relative hypomuscularity of vessels that are decreased in size and number. This can be further aggravated by suppressed growth of the lung parenchyma, which can also be a feature of low pulmonary blood supply.[6]

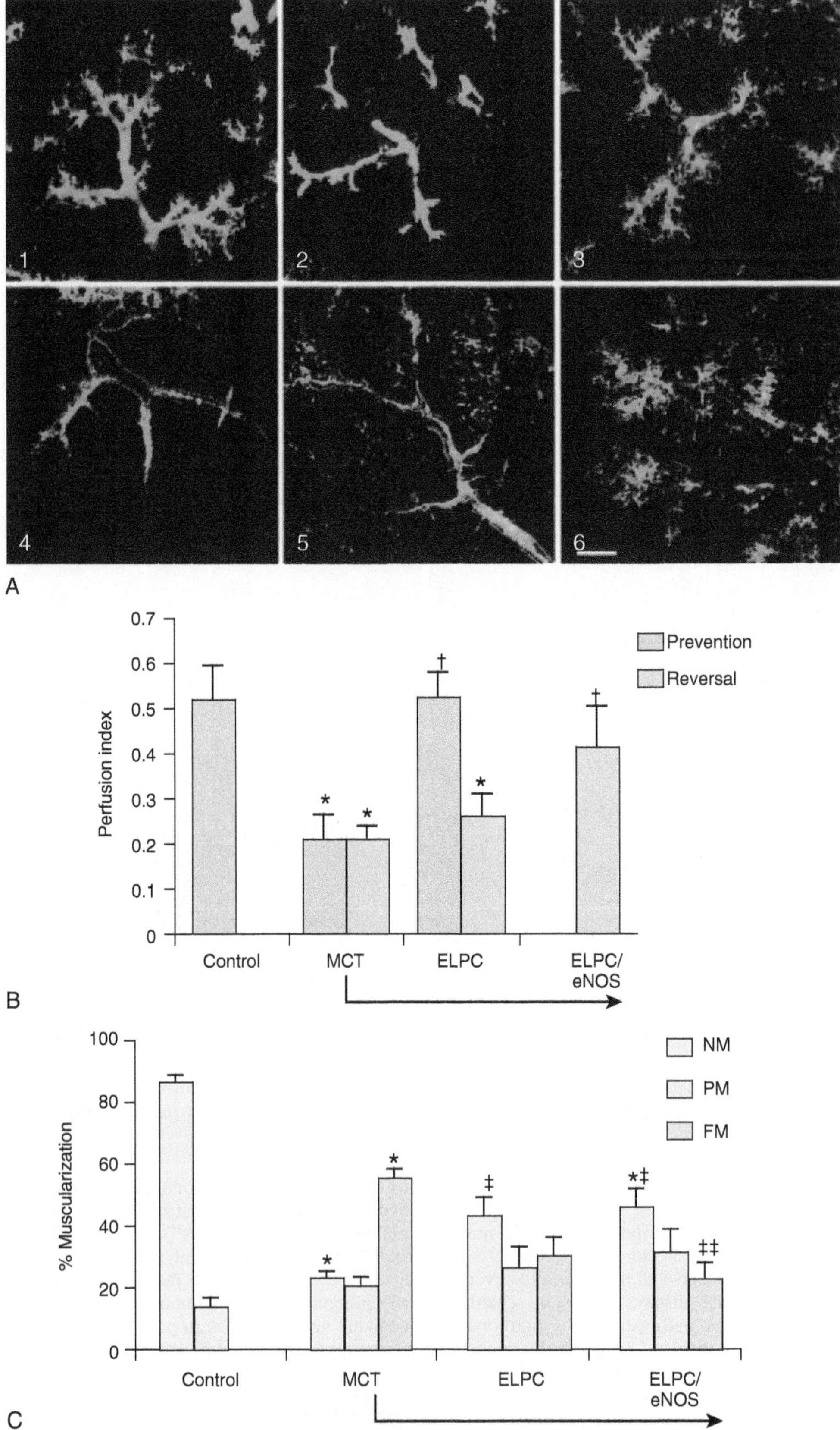

Fig. 47.16 (A) Representative confocal projection images of lung sections perfused with fluorescent microspheres *(green)* suspended in agarose (i.e., fluorescent microangiography) and immunostained for α-smooth muscle actin *(red)*. Normal filling of the microvasculature was observed in control rats *(1)*, whereas rats treated with toxin monocrotaline *(MCT)* showed a marked loss of microvascular perfusion and widespread precapillary occlusion 21 days *(2)* and 35 *(4)* days after MCT injection. In the prevention model, animals receiving endothelial progenitor cells *(ELPCs)* displayed improved microvascular perfusion and preserved continuity of the distal vasculature *(3)*. In the reversal model, endothelial nitric oxide synthase *(eNOS)*-transduced ELPCs dramatically improved the appearance of the pulmonary microvasculature *(6)*, whereas progenitor cells alone resulted in more modest increases in perfusion and little noticeable reduction in arteriolar muscularization *(5)*. (B) Summary data for pulmonary microvasculature perfusion for animals treated in the prevention *(red bars)* and reversal *(blue bars)* protocol. (C) Proportion of small pulmonary arterioles that are nonmuscularized *(NM)*, partially muscularized *(PM)*, or fully muscularized *(FM)* in the various treatment groups of the reversal protocol. (From Zhao YD, Courtman DW, Deng Y, et al. Rescue of monocrotaline-induced pulmonary arterial hypertension using bone marrow-derived endothelial-like progenitor cells: efficacy of combined cell and eNOS gene therapy in established disease. *Circ Res.* 2005;96:442–450.)

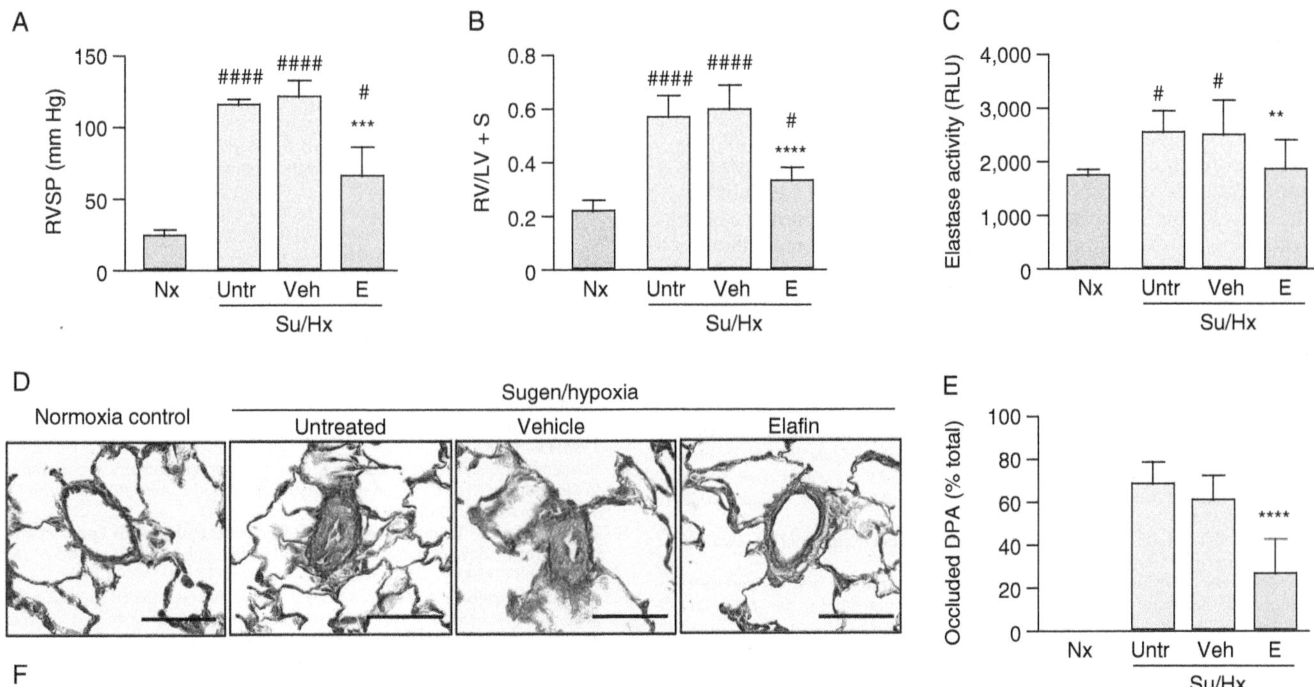

Fig. 47.17 Elafin reversed pulmonary hypertension, heightened elastase activity, obstructed distal pulmonary arteries, and increased vessel number and lung expression of endothelial nitric oxide synthase and apelin in Su/Hx rats. Rats were exposed to room air only (normoxia, *Nx*, *n* = 6) or to the Sugen hypoxia (Su/Hx) protocol. The Su/Hx rats were then divided into three groups: no intervention (*Untr, n* = 6), 0.9% saline vehicle (*Veh, n* = 6), or elafin treatment (*E, n* = 9). (A) Right ventricular systolic pressure *(RVSP)*. (B) Right ventricular *(RV)* hypertrophy, defined by the Fulton index, weight of RV/left ventricle + septum *(LV+S)*. (C) Elastase activity was measured in whole lung lysate by the DQ elastin assay. *RLU,* Relative luminescent units. (D) Representative histology of distal pulmonary arteries *(DPA)* from Nx, Su/Hx (Untr, Veh and E) rats; scale bar 50 μm. (E) Number of occluded alveolar duct and wall DPA. Bars represent mean ± standard error of the mean, $^{**}p < .01$, $^{***}p < .001$, and $^{****}p < .0001$ versus Veh, $^{\#}p < .05$ and $^{\#\#\#\#}p < .0001$ versus Nx, by one-way ANOVA and Bonferroni's post test. (From Nickel NP, Spiekerkoetter E, Gu M, et al. Elafin reverses pulmonary hypertension via caveolin-1 dependent bone morphogenetic protein signaling. *Am J Respir Crit Care Med.* 2015;191:1273–1286. Reprinted with permission of the American Thoracic Society. Copyright © 2015 American Thoracic Society.)

PULMONARY VENOUS ABNORMALITIES

Pulmonary vascular abnormalities associated with pulmonary venous hypertension have been noted in patients with and without structural heart disease. Interruption of normal lung vascular and parenchymal growth as a result of premature birth and development of bronchopulmonary dysplasia is increasingly recognized as a risk factor for pulmonary vein stenosis and pulmonary hypertension.[169-171] The etiology of pulmonary venous stenosis in this population is likely multifactorial; patients with a history of intrauterine growth restriction, exposure to prolonged mechanical ventilation, or factors associated with impaired pulmonary vascular development appear particularly at risk.[93,94,111,171]

Structural diseases including mitral valve or left ventricular dysfunction and anomalous pulmonary venous return can also lead to vascular abnormalities due to pulmonary venous hypertension. Pulmonary vein abnormalities resulting from congenital heart disease largely regress following correction of the anatomic or physiologic abnormality, although in the initial postoperative period the abnormally muscularized vasculature[172,173] may be reactive. Focal stenoses of pulmonary veins (particularly if intraparenchymal) are difficult to correct with current surgical or interventional cardiologic approaches. In a neonatal piglet model of progressive pulmonary venous obstruction, altered compliance of the veins is reflected in increased pulmonary arterial pressure.[174] Elevation in pulmonary venous pressure occurred later when the vessel lumen was compromised by the intimal lesion. At this stage, there was a disproportionate increase in collagen in the vessel wall, which likely further contributes to the hemodynamic abnormality and the resistance to successful intervention. Pathologic specimens of pediatric pulmonary vein stenosis have identified neointimal proliferation of myofibroblast-like cells with increased tyrosine kinase receptor activity.[175,176] Clinical trials using agents to target these receptors including imatinib and the VEGF receptor inhibitor, bevacizumab, combined with standard intervention, were well-tolerated and increased survival to 18 months in a small, heterogeneous population.[177] Further trials are needed to establish approach to therapy.

CLINICAL IMPLICATIONS

Reduced growth of the pulmonary circulation may pose a contraindication for surgery using the Fontan principle.[172] Also, consideration of patients for cavopulmonary anastomoses in preparation for a final-stage Norwood operation must take into account evidence of regression of the left-sided obstructive lesion-induced vascular changes—that is, the increased muscularity of pulmonary arteries and veins that are associated with heightened pulmonary vascular reactivity. Future studies aimed at accelerating the structural maturation of the lung to induce both dilation and recruitment of small vessels may prove of benefit in allowing surgical correction of even complex congenital heart disease in the newborn infant. Increasing knowledge of the genes that control vascular cell phenotype and differentiation and their regulation in development will lead to new and fruitful directions in preventing or reversing abnormal structural development of the lung.

SUMMARY

We are learning more about lung vascular development by using novel techniques such as cell fate mapping and transcriptomics applied to single cells and by relating abnormalities in fetal and neonatal pulmonary vascular pathology such as PAH to genetic and epigenetic changes. This new knowledge will help inform the development of new targeted therapies aimed at both regression of vascular pathology and also at lung regeneration that is closely coupled with lung vascular growth.

 A complete reference list is available at www.ExpertConsult.com.

SELECT REFERENCES

1. Rabinovitch M. Pathophysiology of pulmonary hypertension. In: Allen HD, Driscoll DJ, Shaddy RE, et al., eds. *Moss and Adams' Heart Disease in Infants, Children, and Adolescents, Including the Fetus and Young Adult.* 7th ed. Vol. 2. Philadelphia: Lippincott Williams & Wilkins; 2008: 1322-1354.
2. Hislop A, Reid L. Intra-pulmonary arterial development during fetal life—branching pattern and structure. *J Anat.* 1972;113:35-48.
3. Goldstein JD, Rabinovitch M, Van Praagh R, et al. Unusual vascular anomalies causing persistent pulmonary hypertension in a newborn. *Am J Cardiol.* 1979;43:962-968.
4. Rabinovitch M, Herrera-deLeon V, Castaneda AR, et al. Growth and development of the pulmonary vascular bed in patients with tetralogy of Fallot with or without pulmonary atresia. *Circulation.* 1981;64:1234-1249.
5. Rabinovitch M, Grady S, David I, et al. Compression of intrapulmonary bronchi by abnormally branching pulmonary arteries associated with absent pulmonary valves. *Am J Cardiol.* 1982;50:804-813.
6. Hall SM, Haworth SG. Normal adaptation of pulmonary arterial intima to extrauterine life in the pig: ultrastructural study. *J Pathol.* 1986;149:55-66.
7. Hislop M, Reid L. Pulmonary arterial development during childhood: branching pattern and structure. *Thorax.* 1973;28:129-135.
8. Meyrick B, Reid L. Ultrastructural findings in lung biopsy material from children with congenital heart defects. *Am J Pathol.* 1980;101:527-537.
9. Jones R. Ultrastructural analysis of contractile cell development in lung microvessels in hyperoxic pulmonary hypertension: fibroblasts and intermediate cells selectively reorganize nonmuscular segments. *Am J Pathol.* 1993;141:1491-1505.
10. Sheikh AQ, Lighthouse JK, Greif DM. Recapitulation of developing artery muscularization in pulmonary hypertension. *Cell Rep.* 2014;6:809-817.
11. Prosser IW, Stenmark KR, Suthar M, et al. Regional heterogeneity of elastin and collagen gene expression in intralobar arteries in response to hypoxic pulmonary hypertension as demonstrated by *in situ* hybridization. *Am J Pathol.* 1989;135:1073-1088.
12. Durmowicz AG, Parks WC, Hyde DM, et al. Persistence, re-expression, and induction of pulmonary arterial fibronectin, tropoelastin, and type I procollagen mRNA expression in neonatal hypoxic pulmonary hypertension. *Am J Pathol.* 1994;145:1411-1420.
13. Allen K, Haworth SG. Human postnatal pulmonary arterial remodeling. Ultrastructural studies of smooth muscle cell and connective tissue maturation. *Lab Invest.* 1988;59:702-709.
14. Frid MG, Moiseeva EP, Stenmark KR. Multiple phenotypically distinct smooth muscle cell populations exist in the adult and developing bovine pulmonary arterial media *in vivo*. *Circ Res.* 1994;75:669-681.
15. Das M, Stenmark KR, Dempsey EC. Enhanced growth of fetal and neonatal pulmonary artery adventitial fibroblasts is dependent on protein kinase C. *Am J Physiol.* 1995;269:L660-L667.
16. Baldwin HS. Early embryonic vascular development. *Cardiovasc Res.* 1996;31:E34-E45.
17. Kwee L, Baldwin HS, Shen HM, et al. Defective development of the embryonic and extraembryonic circulatory systems in vascular cell adhesion molecule (VCAM-1) deficient mice. *Development.* 1995;121:489-503.
18. Baldwin HS, Shen HM, Yan HC, et al. Platelet endothelial cell adhesion molecule-1 (PECAM-1/CD31): alternatively spliced, functionally distinct isoforms expressed during mammalian cardiovascular development. *Development.* 1994;120:2539-2553.
19. Drake CJ, Davis LA, Little CD. Antibodies to beta 1-integrins cause alterations of aortic vasculogenesis, *in vivo*. *Dev Dyn.* 1992;193:83-91.
20. Drake CJ, Cheresh DA, Little CD. An antagonist of integrin alpha v beta 3 prevents maturation of blood vessels during embryonic neovascularization. *J Cell Sci.* 1995;108:2655-2661.
21. Ffrench-Constant C, Hynes RO. Patterns of fibronectin gene expression and splicing during cell migration in chicken embryos. *Development.* 1988;104: 369-382.
22. Drake CJ, Davis LA, Walters L, et al. Avian vasculogenesis and the distribution of collagens, I, IV, laminin, and fibronectin in the heart primordia. *J Exp Zool.* 1990;155:309-322.
23. Boudreau N, Turley E, Rabinovitch M. Fibronectin, hyaluronan, and a hyaluronan binding protein contribute to increased ductus arteriosus smooth muscle cell migration. *Dev Biol.* 1991;143(2):235-247.
24. Roman J, McDonald J. Expression of fibronectin, the integrin VLA-5 and a smooth muscle actin in lung and heart development. *Am J Respir Cell Mol Biol.* 1992;6:472-480.
25. Jones P, Rabinovitch M. Tenascin-C is induced with progressive pulmonary vascular disease in rats is functionally related to increased smooth muscle cell proliferation. *Circ Res.* 1996;79:1131-1142.
26. Drake CJ, Little CD. Exogenous vascular endothelial growth factor induces malformed and hyperfused vessels during embryonic neovascularization. *Proc Natl Acad Sci U S A.* 1995;92:7657-7661.
27. Chinoy MR, Graybill MM, Miller SA, et al. Angiopoietin-1 and VEGF in vascular development and angiogenesis in hypoplastic lungs. *Am J Physiol Lung Cell Mol Physiol.* 2002;283(1):L60-L66.
28. Klein S, Giancotti FG, Presta M, et al. Basic fibroblast growth factor modulates integrin expression in microvascular endothelial cells. *Mol Biol Cell.* 1993;4:973-982.
29. Balasubramaniam V, Tang JR, Maxey A, et al. Mild hypoxia impairs alveolarization in the endothelial nitric oxide synthase-deficient mouse. *Am J Physiol Lung Cell Mol Physiol.* 2003;284:L964-L971.
30. Zhao L, Wang K, Ferrara N, et al. Vascular endothelial growth factor co-ordinates proper development of lung epithelium and vasculature. *Mech Dev.* 2005;122:877-886.
31. Thebaud B, Ladha F, Michelakis ED, et al. Vascular endothelial growth factor gene therapy increases survival, promotes lung angiogenesis, and prevents alveolar damage in hyperoxia-induced lung injury: evidence that angiogenesis participates in alveolarization. *Circulation.* 2005;112:2477-2486.
32. Yamamoto H, Jun Yun E, Gerber HP, et al. Epithelial-vascular cross talk mediated by VEGF-A and HGF signaling directs primary septae formation during distal lung morphogenesis. *Dev Biol.* 2007;308:44-53.
33. Han RN, Stewart DJ. Defective lung vascular development in endothelial nitric oxide synthase-deficient mice. *Trends Cardiovasc Med.* 2006;16:29-34.
34. Salcedo R, Wasserman K, Young HA, et al. Vascular endothelial growth factor and basic fibroblast growth factor induce expression of CXCR4 on human endothelial cells: *in vivo* neovascularization induced by stromal-derived factor-1alpha. *Am J Pathol.* 1999;154:1125-1135.
35. Wang Z, Shu W, Lu MM, et al. Wnt7b activates canonical signaling in epithelial and vascular smooth muscle cells through interactions with Fzd1, Fzd10, and LRP5. *Mol Cell Biol.* 2005;25:5022-5030.
36. De Langhe SP, Sala FG, Del Moral PM, et al. Dickkopf-1 (DKK1) reveals that fibronectin is a major target of Wnt signaling in branching morphogenesis of the mouse embryonic lung. *Dev Biol.* 2005;277:316-331.
37. Cardoso WV, Lu J. Regulation of early lung morphogenesis: questions, facts and controversies. *Development.* 2006;133:1611-1624.
38. Shu W, Guttentag S, Wang Z, et al. Wnt/beta-catenin signaling acts upstream of N-myc, BMP4, and FGF signaling to regulate proximal-distal patterning in the lung. *Dev Biol.* 2005;283:226-239.
39. Shu W, Jiang YQ, Lu MM, et al. Wnt7b regulates mesenchymal proliferation and vascular development in the lung. *Development.* 2002;129:4831-4842.
40. Dumont DJ, Fong GH, Puri MC, et al. Vascularization of the mouse embryo: a study of flk-1, tek, tie, and vascular endothelial growth factor expression during development. *Dev Dyn.* 1995;203:80-91.
41. Shalaby F, Rossant J, Yamaguchi TP, et al. Failure of blood-island formation and vasculogenesis in FLK-1 deficient mice. *Nature.* 1995;376:62-66.
42. Fong GH, Rossant J, Gertsenstein M, et al. Role of the Flt-1 receptor tyrosine kinase in regulating the assembly of vascular endothelium. *Nature.* 1995;376:66-70.
43. Lamouille S, Mallet C, Feige JJ, et al. Activin receptor-like kinase 1 is implicated in the maturation phase of angiogenesis. *Blood.* 2002;100:4495-4501.
44. Trembath RC, Harrison R. Insights into the genetic and molecular basis of primary pulmonary hypertension. *Pediatr Res.* 2003;53:883-888.
45. Thomson JR, Machado RD, Pauciulo MW, et al. Sporadic primary pulmonary hypertension is associated with germline mutations of the gene encoding BMPR-II, a receptor member of the TGF-beta family. *J Med Genet.* 2000;37:741-774.
46. Schachtner SK, Wang Y, Scott BH. Qualitative and quantitative analysis of embryonic pulmonary vessel formation. *Am J Respir Cell Mol Biol.* 2000;22:157-165.
47. Taichman DB, Loomes KM, Schachtner SK, et al. Notch1 and Jagged1 expression by the developing pulmonary vasculature. *Dev Dyn.* 2002;225:166-175.
48. Thomson JR, Machado RD, Pauciulo MW, et al. Sporadic primary pulmonary hypertension is associated with germline mutations of the gene encoding BMPR-II, a receptor member of the TGF-beta family. *J Med Genet.* 2000;37:741-774.
49. Schachtner SK, Wang Y, Scott BH. Qualitative and quantitative analysis of embryonic pulmonary vessel formation. *Am J Respir Cell Mol Biol.* 2000;22:157-165.
50. Taichman DB, Loomes KM, Schachtner SK, et al. Notch1 and Jagged1 expression by the developing pulmonary vasculature. *Dev Dyn.* 2002;225:166-175.

Development of the Gastrointestinal Circulation in the Fetus and Newborn

48

Upender K. Munshi | David A. Clark

INTRODUCTION

The intestine is a complex series of tissues, each with a specific role in digestion and excretion. For a mature intestine to function properly, it must protect its component cells from other organisms, including bacteria, viruses, and parasites, as well as from toxic substances. In addition, the intestine, in partnership with the liver and pancreas, disassembles potential nutrients and presents them (sugars, fats, proteins, vitamins, and minerals) to the liver for organization and distribution. Rapid cellular growth of the fetal intestine requires sufficient energy and a means for clearance of metabolic waste products. This is accomplished by a rapid and proportional growth of the intestinal circulation. As the solid intestine hollows and motility develops, amniotic fluid components—primarily the whey-like proteins—may be an additional source of substrate for growth of the proximal intestine.

Although anatomic and histologic studies have been performed on salvaged human fetal intestines, lack of availability of samples and autolysis has precluded detailed and systematic studies of the physiology of the developing gastrointestinal circulation. Therefore much of the information presented in this chapter is derived from controlled studies in animals. In addition, the most reliable data involve only that portion of the alimentary tract below the diaphragm, namely, the gastrointestinal and colonic circulation.

Several principles of gut development have an impact on intestinal blood flow. The cephalic portion of the embryonic intestinal tract develops and matures more rapidly than the caudal region.[1] As the intestinal lining rapidly grows, the embryonic ileum is obliterated and eventually recanalizes. Although the intestine begins as a straight tube, differential growth rates result in the contrasting calibers of various gut segments and in the rotation and final positioning of various components.[2]

The arterial supply to the intestine matures in response to its rapid growth. The majority of the intestinal tract mucosa, along with the liver parenchyma and pancreas, is derived from endoderm. In contrast, the connective tissue and muscular components are derived from splanchnopleuric mesoderm. Oral and anal epithelium is derived from the ectoderm of the stomatodeum and proctodeum, respectively. Progressing from the germ cell stage, the intestine is divided into three primary portions: the foregut, midgut, and hindgut.[2-4] The foregut includes all structures distal to the tracheal diverticulum from the esophagus through the first half of the duodenum. The midgut is composed of structures distal to the second portion of the duodenum, including the jejunum, ileum, and proximal two thirds of the transverse colon. The hindgut consists of the distal transverse colon and the proximal two thirds of the anal canal.

DEVELOPMENT OF INTESTINAL CIRCULATION

Early somite embryos have an extensive vascular network on the yolk sac. In the process of vasculogenesis, vascular endothelial precursor cells (angioblasts) migrate to the location of future vessels, coalesce into cords, differentiate into endothelial cells, and ultimately form patent vessels. When the primary vascular bed is formed, additional capillaries and vessels are added by angiogenesis, which is controlled by vascular endothelial growth factor (VEGF) and other stimulants such as transforming growth factor-β (TGF-β) and platelet-derived growth factor (PDGF).[5] Erythropoietin stimulates vasculogenesis in neonatal rat mesenteric microvascular endothelial cells.[6] Unpaired ventral branches of the dorsal aorta (vitelline arteries) pass to the yolk sac, allantois, and chorion. The network drains by way of the vitelline veins to the heart. During the fourth week, the primitive gut is formed as the dorsal portion of the yolk sac is incorporated into the embryo. Three vitelline arteries persist to supply the foregut (celiac artery), midgut (superior mesenteric artery), and hindgut (inferior mesenteric artery).[2]

The vessels distributed to the foregut fuse and form a single vessel, the celiac artery. With a downward migration of the viscera, the aortic attachment of the celiac artery moves caudally. It divides into the hepatic artery, splenic artery, and left gastric branches to supply the stomach and duodenum. The liver, pancreas, and related mesodermal spleen receive their blood supply from these branches. At the vascular division between the foregut and midgut is the anastomosis between the superior pancreaticoduodenal and the inferior pancreaticoduodenal arteries.[4]

The embryonic vitelline arteries fuse and form a superior mesenteric trunk, which reaches the midgut by passing through the mesentery. Terminal branches of this trunk supply the yolk sac. The various branches distal to the intestine are obliterated when the ileum separates from the yolk sac and vitelline stalk. However, the superior mesenteric artery remains and supplies the intestinal circulation from the second part of the duodenum through the proximal two thirds of the transverse colon.[3,4]

The ventral branches of the aorta supplying the hindgut fuse to form a single inferior mesenteric trunk. Its final distribution includes the distal one third of the transverse colon and the entire descending colon and sigmoid. The inferior mesenteric trunk anastomoses with the middle colic artery, which is a branch of the superior mesenteric artery. Distal to this is an anastomosis to branches of the inferior and middle rectal arteries from the internal iliac trunk.[2,3]

VENOUS DRAINAGE OF THE GASTROINTESTINAL TRACT

The venous drainage of the intestine is much more variable than is the arterial blood supply. The low-pressure venous drainage in the embryo is plexiform, and therefore patency is based somewhat on blood flow. In addition, blood has a tendency to seek the most direct route of flow due to hydrodynamic factors.

The vitelline veins initially pass along each side of the anterior intestinal portal vein. They form an anastomotic plexus around the developing duodenal loop in the tissue of the septum transversum. Cords of liver cells extend into the septum transversum and divide the vitelline plexus into the primitive hepatic sinusoids. Anterior stems of the vitelline veins enter the

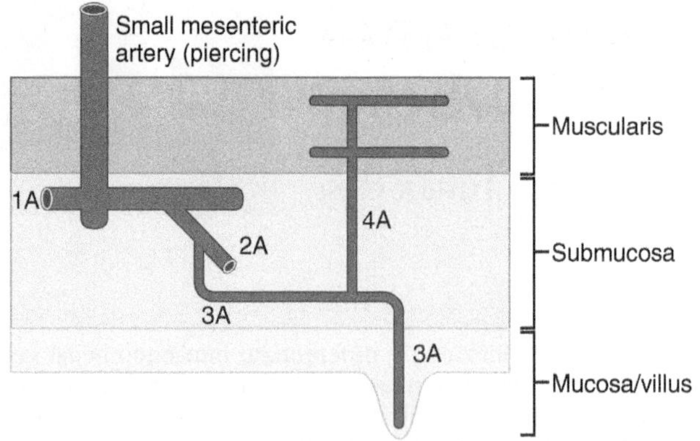

Fig. 48.1 Schematic representation of the intestinal microcirculation: Small mesenteric arteries from the mesenteric arcade pierce the muscularis layers and terminate in the submucosa, where they give rise to first order arterioles *(1A)*, which further give rise to second order *(2A)* arterioles in submucosa. Third order arterioles *(3A)* arise from 2A and enter each villus before giving off fourth order *(4A)* arterioles that enter the muscularis layer.

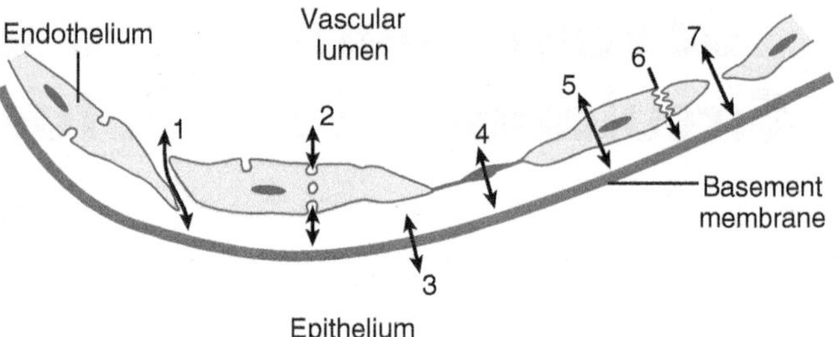

Fig. 48.2 Transport pathways in intestinal capillaries. *Arrow* represents potential direction of movement of fluid and solids. Intercellular junction *(1)*, pinocytosis *(2)*, basement membrane *(3)*, fenestrae with diaphragms *(4)*, cell membrane *(5)*, transendothelial channel *(6)*, and open fenestrae *(7)*.

primitive sinus venosus. As the stomach, duodenum, and small intestine elongate and rotate from their original midsagittal position to the adult position, blood flow develops along the most direct route to the liver, cutting from one vitelline vein to another through the connecting plexus. Consequently, the portal venous system does not develop in a spiral fashion around the developing intestine but instead evolves short and straight with the duodenum and intestine around it.[2,3]

In embryos of less than 5-mm crown-rump length (<5 weeks), blood from the paired umbilical veins passes into the liver, at which point it communicates with the vitelline sinusoids. At a 7-mm crown-rump length (33 to 34 days), the right umbilical vein atrophies and disappears.[2] As a result, all the placental blood entering the embryo enters through the left umbilical vein and empties into the hepatic sinusoids. As the right side of the sinus venosus elaborates, an enlargement of the hepatic sinusoidal communication occurs between the right hepatocardiac channel and the left umbilical vein forming the ductus venosus.[4] Thus blood entering from either the umbilical or vitelline systems can pass by way of the ductus venosus to the right atrium or into the liver sinusoids. The venae advehentes, connecting the umbilical and vitelline systems to the hepatic sinusoids, become the branches of the portal vein in the liver. In addition, the venae revehentes connecting the sinusoids to the right hepatocardiac channel become the tributaries to the hepatic veins. After birth the left umbilical vein and the ductus venosus are obliterated and become the ligamentum teres and the ligamentum venosum, respectively.[3]

THE INTESTINAL MICROCIRCULATION

The microscopic anatomy of the intestinal circulation varies from species to species. In rabbits and humans, villus arterioles ascend from the submucosal arterioles into the villus. Distribution of blood flow within the intestinal wall is not uniform but appears to follow a pattern of functional importance of the tissue layer (Fig. 48.1). At a resting stage without feeding, the mucosal layer (the primary site of absorption) receives approximately 70% of the intestinal blood flow, while the muscular and serosal layer receives approximately 25% and the submucosa receives 5%.[7] As the arteriole reaches the villus tip, it divides into a diffuse capillary network, which then drains into a centrally located villus venule originating in the distal one third of the villus.[5] In most mammals, the capillaries of the intestinal villus are fenestrated. Just as the villus and the microvillus are exposed to a large solute and water load, so the villus capillaries must be capable of handling the absorbed nutrients. The endothelium of the capillary facing the epithelium is very thin and usually contains fenestrae, with the greatest number at the villus tips and in the crypts.

Water and solutes are transported into the capillary by a number of different pathways (Fig. 48.2). Low-molecular-weight nonpolar substances and lipid-soluble substances such as oxygen and carbon dioxide may cross directly through the cell membrane. The bulk of absorbed materials passes through fenestrae, which are numerous circular openings of up to 30 nm in the capillary endothelium and may be either opened or diaphragmed.[7] At least 60% of the fenestrae have a diaphragm. Although the porosity is not known, these diaphragms limit the movement of molecules. Much less commonly, water and solutes move slowly by pinocytosis. In this process, vesicles are formed that move through the cell to the opposing side before releasing their contents. On rare occasions, transendothelial channels may be formed when several vesicles simultaneously open and bridge the cell. These occurrences are relatively infrequent and do not have a major impact on total absorptive capacity. Intercellular junctions are impermeable to solutes of 2-nm diameter in the arteriole and capillary but may play a limited role in venule absorption.

CONTROL OF BLOOD FLOW

Intestinal blood flow varies by gestational age and species. For example, in fetal sheep, mesenteric vasoconstriction predominates in late-preterm gestation.[8] Numerous factors impinge on the maintenance of intestinal blood flow. They can be grouped into at least four major categories: cardiovascular status, neural control, humoral substances, and local control.[9-11] Although specific data regarding the fetal intestine in these areas are sparse, certain principles can be inferred to be operative in the fetus.

CARDIOVASCULAR FUNCTION

Adequate perfusion of any tissue in the body is dependent on the maintenance of sufficient cardiac output and mean arterial blood pressure. Reduction in cardiac output or systemic arterial pressure within a physiologic range leads to compensatory vasodilation of the regional circulation to maintain relatively constant tissue blood flow, a process termed as pressure-flow autoregulation. Autoregulation of intestinal blood flow guarantees the preservation of continuous blood flow to the intestine while large fluctuations are occurring in the arterial perfusion pressure.[9,11] Although superior mesenteric circulation autoregulation has been well established in canine, porcine, and feline circulations, the mechanism for this regulation is controversial.[12] The capacity to autoregulate the intestinal blood flow is a function of gestational maturation. However, in the presence of profound hypotension, net vasoconstriction occurs and intestinal blood flow decreases. In newborn swine, moderate systemic arterial hypoxemia causes vasodilation and increase in gut perfusion, whereas severe hypoxemia (PO_2 <40 mm Hg) causes vasoconstriction and gut ischemia. Intestinal perfusion and oxygenation are profoundly reduced in puppies made polycythemic by exchange transfusion. Fortunately, few neonates have polycythemia and most escape intestinal damage. Both of these factors are influenced by blood volume.The proportion of cardiac output destined for the intestine is altered in newborns with cyanotic congenital heart disease and vascular malformations, such as coarctation of the aorta, which limits blood flow to the intestinal tract. In the fetus, systemic circulatory needs are maintained even with severe left ventricular obstruction. However, fetal asphyxia and acidosis can be associated with reduced myocardial contractility and tricuspid regurgitation, limiting cardiac output and consequently reducing intestinal flow.

Intestinal oxygen uptake and blood flow increase dramatically after birth to sustain rapid growth of the mucosa and oxidative demands of enteral nutrition (secretion, absorption, motility).[12] Postnatally, the splanchnic circulation accounts for 20% of cardiac output; however, splanchnic blood flow increases by 30% to 130% after a meal, known as *postprandial hyperemia*.[11] Glucose and solubilized long-chain fatty acids increase jejunal blood flow. In preterm infants, dietary nucleotides increased the superior mesenteric artery blood flow velocity, peaking at 30 minutes postprandial and having a sustained effect for 90 minutes.[13] Bile and bile salts may double ileal blood flow. Volatile fatty acids (acetic, butyric, propionic) derived from fermentation of undigested carbohydrates by microflora increase colonic blood flow and serve as a metabolic substrate for colonic enterocytes.[9]

NEURAL CONTROLS

The gastrointestinal tract is extensively innervated by the autonomic and enteric nervous system.[8,12] Enhanced sympathetic tone elicits arterial smooth muscle contraction, which raises intestinal vascular resistance and decreases blood flow. This effect is mediated through the α-adrenergic receptors in the vascular smooth muscle. However, this vasoconstrictor response is short lived, and decreased vascular resistance and improved blood flow rapidly return by stimulation of α-adrenergic receptors.[10,14,15] Thus sympathetic stimulation may produce a variable response (Box 48.1). Although acetylcholine causes vasodilation through an endothelium-dependent mechanism,[15-17] the effects of acetylcholine on intestinal blood flow are also variable. Acetylcholine has the ability to initiate intestinal smooth muscle contraction, which can impede blood flow by increasing transmural pressure.

Marginal tissue oxygenation antagonizes the sympathetic response by inducing vasodilation. Furthermore, intestinal wall relaxation resulting from sympathetic stimulation decreases the resistance of the vessels and allows increased blood flow to the stomach and intestines. The adrenal medullary catecholamines and angiotensin II, formed locally in response to renal renin, constrict vascular smooth muscle in the gastrointestinal circulation and therefore decrease local blood flow.[18-20] However, this effect may be temporary and can be readily overridden by local metabolic control.

The majority of extrinsic nerves innervating the intestine are afferents. They contain two important polypeptides, substance P and calcitonin gene-related peptide (CGRP), which are released by noxious chemical and mechanical stimulation. These agents induce local vasodilation and contribute to neurogenic inflammation by mast cell degranulation and altering vascular permeability.[20]

HUMORAL CONTROLS

Numerous humoral substances have been demonstrated to alter gastrointestinal blood flow in experimental animals. Some are circulating substances, whereas others are released locally. Boxes 48.1 and 48.2 summarize the agents that have been well demonstrated to increase or decrease intestinal blood flow. Gastrointestinal hormones released during various phases of digestion may dilate the gastrointestinal circulation. Glucagon and cholecystokinin increase both intestinal blood flow and pancreatic flow.[20-22] Gastrin specifically increases blood flow to the gastric mucosa.[20,22]

Box 48.1 Agents That Increase Intestinal Blood Flow

Acetylcholine[15,18,20,40]; motlin[9,11,21]
Adenosine[9]; neurotensin[11]
Adrenergics[17] nitric oxide[25,27,41,42]
Isoproterenol
Salbutamol peptide hormones
Cholecystokinin[20–22]
Aminophylline[1]; gastrin[20–22]
Glucagon[43,44]
Bradykinin[22,45]; vasoactive intestinal polypeptide[46]
Calcium antagonists[47]; platelet-activating factor (directly)[16,48]
Carbon dioxide[15]; potassium low dose[17,21,24]
Dietary nucleotides[14]; prostaglandins[9,45,49]
PGD_2, PGE_1, PGE_2
Histamine[18,43]
Serotonin[9]
Magnesium[17,23]
Methionine-enkephalin[46]; substance P[19]

Box 48.2 Agents That Decrease Intestinal Blood Flow

Adrenergic[9,17]; peptide hormones
Dopamine angiotensin II[9]
Epinephrine vasopressin[22,50]
Methoxamine
Norepinephrine physostigmine[9]
Phenylephrine
Potassium high dose[17,22]
Calcium[17,24,47]
Endothelin[35,36]; prostaglandin F_2a[40]
5-Hydroxytryptamine[1]; somatostatin[50]
Leukotrienes D4[38,39]; thromboxane A2[49]
Methacholine[44]; tyramine[1]

LOCAL CONTROLS

The local extracellular environment is altered by the increased metabolic activity of the gastrointestinal parenchymal cells, for example, during digestion.[11] An increased metabolic demand may lead to relative tissue hypoxia and consequently the release of many vasodilators (e.g., K^+, Mg^{2+}, histamine [mast cells], polypeptides [bradykinin, vasoactive intestinal polypeptide], prostaglandins, carbon dioxide, and adenosine).[9,15-17,23,24] Cells with an increased metabolic rate are likely to produce greater quantities of dilator metabolites, which ensure the provision of more substrate by increasing blood flow.

Role of Nitric Oxide

Basal vascular resistance, which determines the regional gastrointestinal blood flow, depends upon the delicate balance between the constrictor and dilator forces that are acting upon the vascular smooth muscle. Nitric oxide is the major dilator that counterbalances the constrictive effect of the endothelin 1 and the intrinsic contractile response of smooth vascular muscle. Under basal conditions, nitric oxide is continuously produced from L-arginine by endothelial cell nitric oxide synthase (constitutive isoform). It relaxes vascular smooth muscle by decreasing cytosolic free calcium via increased cyclic guanosine monophosphate (cGMP).[25] In rats, acute administration of a nitric oxide synthase inhibitor (L-NNA) reduces basal intestinal blood flow.[26] Nitric oxide production can increase markedly following chemical or mechanical stimulation of nitric oxide synthase (induced or stimulated isoform). Methylene blue, a guanylate cyclase inhibitor, abolishes intestinal vasodilation resulting from administration of sodium nitroprusside, a nitric oxide donor.[27] After ischemia with reperfusion, exogenous nitric oxide sources (SIN-1, CAS-754, and nitroprusside) and L-arginine reduce mucosal barrier dysfunction without improving intestinal blood flow, suggesting that nitric oxide may have modulating effect on microvascular permeability.[28]

The fetal circulation has an increased basal production of nitric oxide compared with the adult.[29] In late gestation sheep fetus, nitric oxide was shown to play important role in contributing to low vascular resistance and increased blood flow throughout the gastrointestinal tract, as well as in redistribution of intestinal blood flow between intestinal segments.[30] Inhibition of endogenous nitric oxide in mid-gestation fetal sheep results in substantial blood flow reduction across all segments of gastrointestinal tract, implying that nitric oxide plays a major vasodilator role at such an early stage of development of gastrointestinal circulation.[31] Sustained inhibition of nitric oxide synthase in utero results in vasoconstriction of fetal blood vessels, but no evidence of injury to the gastrointestinal tract exists.[32] A lack of nitric oxide synthesis appears to be causative in neonatal hypertrophic pyloric stenosis,[33] but this effect is mediated by the neuronal not the endothelial isoform of nitric oxide synthase based on gene knockout studies.[34]

Endothelin 1

Endothelin 1 is a vasoactive and mitogenic polypeptide synthesized and secreted by endothelial cells.[16] It acts on specific receptor ET_A on vascular smooth muscle, causing sustained powerful vasoconstriction, whereas binding to ET_B receptors on endothelial cells causes release of nitric oxide with resultant vascular relaxation. Although cord blood levels are higher than any other values reported in humans, little information is available about its role in the splanchnic circulation of the fetus and newborn.[35] Hypoxia and shear stress stimulate endothelin 1 secretion.[36] Preterm neonates born to mothers with preeclampsia have increased circulating levels of endothelin 1 and reduced superior mesenteric artery blood flow velocity, possibly due to fetal hypoxia.[37]

Local Inflammatory Mediators. Systemic or local activation of polymorphonuclear cells has been demonstrated to be a component of the pathophysiology of a variety of altered blood flow states. Activated neutrophils and other granulocytes adhere to vascular endothelium and may damage or occlude the vessel. Secondary release of vasoconstrictors (leukotrienes) and substances that increase permeability (platelet-activating factor [PAF], leukotrienes) may further compromise tissue perfusion.[38,39]

PAF is a phospholipid synthesized by many types of cells including endothelium, macrophages, and granulocytes.[27] Although PAF is a vasodilator, it may cause paradoxical vasoconstriction and ischemic injury to the intestine as a consequence of its ability to activate leukocytes. PAF-activated leukocytes may plug postcapillary venules and release vasoconstrictors (e.g., leukotriene C_4).[39]

CONCLUSION

Virtually no study has examined the human fetal and neonatal intestinal blood flow in vivo. It may be inferred from various animal models that some of the clinical conditions encountered in critically ill neonates may result from compromise of the gastrointestinal circulation. Limitation of blood flow as local tissue metabolism increases may result in malabsorption. The early-onset form of necrotizing enterocolitis (in the first week of life) is often associated with perinatal asphyxia, arterial catheterization, or the polycythemia-hyperviscosity syndrome. In each of these conditions, poor tissue perfusion may result in ischemic necrosis of the intestine.

With gene expression techniques it may be possible to trace the ontogeny of systems regulating the gastrointestinal circulation (neural and humoral) in the developing human and experimental animals. These approaches may circumvent the technical problems of directly assessing the splanchnic circulation in the perinatal period. Insights drawn from these molecular approaches may guide improvements in the therapeutic management of the fetus and newborn.

REFERENCES

1. Edelstone DI, Holzman IR. Fetal and neonatal circulations. In: Shepard AP, Granger DN, eds. *Physiology of the Intestinal Circulation*. New York: Raven Press; 1984:179-190.
2. Moore KL, Persaud TVN. *The Developing Human*. Philadelphia: WB Saunders Co; 1993.
3. Langman J. *Medical Embryology*. Vol. 4. Baltimore: Williams & Wilkins; 1981.
4. Nankervis CA, Giannone PJ, Reber KM. The neonatal intestinal vasculature: contributing factors to necrotizing enterocolitis. *Semin Perinatol*. 2008;32:83-91.
5. Ashley RA, Dubuque SH, Dvorak B, et al. Erythropoietin stimulates vasculogenesis in neonatal rat mesenteric microvascular endothelial cells. *Pediatr Res*. 2002;51:472.
6. Matheson PJ, Wilson MA, Garrison RN. Regulation of intestinal blood flow. *J Surg Res*. 2000;93:182-196.
7. Watkins DJ, Besner GE. Role of the intestinal microcirculation in necrotizing enterocolitis. *Semin Pediatr Surg*. 2013;22:83-87.
8. Nair J, Gugino SF, Nielsen LC, Caty MG, Lakshminrusimha S. Fetal and postnatal ovine mesenteric vascular reactivity. *Pediatr Res*. 2015;79:575-582.
9. Crissinger KD, Granger DN. Characterization of intestinal collateral blood flow in the developing piglet. *Pediatr Res*. 1988;24:473.
10. Jacobson ED. The splanchnic circulation. In: Johnson LR, ed. *Gastrointestinal Physiology*. Vol. 4. St. Louis: Mosby-Year Book; 1991.
11. Parks DA, Jacobson ED. Mesenteric circulation. In: Johnson LR, ed. *Physiology of the Gastrointestinal Tract*. New York: Raven Press; 1987:1649-1670.
12. Perry MA, Jacobson ED. Physiology of the splanchnic circulation. In: Kvietys PR, Barrowman JA, Granger DN, eds. *Pathophysiology of the Splanchnic Circulation*. Vol. 1. Boca Raton, FL: CRC Press; 1987:1-56.
13. Svanik J, Laudgren O. Gastrointestinal circulation. In: Crane R, ed. *Gastrointestinal Physiology II. Baltimore, International Review of Physiology*. Vol. 12. University Park Press; 1972:1-34.
14. Reber KM, Nankervis CA, Nowicki PT. Newborn intestinal circulation, physiology and pathology. *Clin Perinatol*. 2002;29:23.
15. Carver JD, Sosa A, Saste M, et al. The effects of dietary nucleotides on intestinal blood flow in preterm infants. *Pediatr Res*. 2002;52:425.
16. Caplan MS, Mackendrick W. Inflammatory mediators and intestinal injury. *Clin Perinatol*. 1994;21:235.
17. Chou CC, Gallavan RH. Blood flow and intestinal motility. *Fed Proc*. 1982;41:2090.
18. Jacobson ED, Brobmann GF, Brecher GA. Intestinal motor activity and blood flow. *Gastroenterology*. 1970;58:575.
19. Chaaban H, Stonestreet B. Intestinal hemodynamics and oxygenation in perinatal period. *Semin Perinatol*. 2012;36:260-268.
20. Sharkey KA, Parr EJ. The enteric nervous system in intestinal inflammation. In: Sutherland LR, ed. *Inflammatory Bowel Disease: Basic Research Clinical Implications and Trends in Therapy*. Boston: Kluwer Academic Publishers; 1994:40-60.
21. Bowen JC, Pawlik W, Fang WF, Jacobson ED. Pharmacologic effects of gastrointestinal hormones on intestinal oxygen consumption and blood flow. *Surgery*. 1975;78:515.
22. Fasth S, Filipsson S, Hultén L, Martinson J. The effect of the gastrointestinal hormones on small intestinal motility and blood flow. *Experientia*. 1973;29:982.
23. Schuurkes JAJ, Charbon GA. Motility and hemodynamics of the canine gastrointestinal tract: stimulation by pentagastrin, cholecystokinin and vasopressin. *Arch Int Pharmacodyn Ther*. 1978;236:214.

24. Chou CC, Grasmick B. Motility and blood flow distribution within the wall of the gastrointestinal tract. *Am J Physiol*. 1978;235:H34.
25. Dabney JM, Scott JB, Chou CC. Effects of cations on ileal compliance and blood flow. *Am J Physiol*. 1967;212:835.
26. Alemayehu A, Lock KR, Coatney RW, Chou CC. NAME L, Nitric oxide and jejunal motility, blood flow and oxygen uptake in dogs. *Br J Pharmacol*. 1994;111:205.
27. Ignarro LJ. Biological actions and properties of endothelium-derived nitric oxide formed and released from artery and vein. *Circ Res*. 1989;65:1.
28. Pawlik WW, Gustaw P, Thor P, et al. Microcirculatory and motor effects of endogenous nitric oxide in the rat gut. *J Physiol Pharmacol*. 1993;44:139.
29. Andriantsitohaina R, Suprenant A. Acetylcholine released from Guinea-pig submucosal neurons dilates arterioles by releasing nitric oxide from endothelium. *J Physiol*. 1992;453:493.
30. Kubes P, Granger DN. Nitric oxide modulates microvascular permeability. *Am J Physiol*. 1992;262:H611.
31. Pierce RL, Pierce MR, Liu H, Kadowitz PJ, Miller MJ. Limb reduction defects after prenatal inhibition of nitric oxide synthase in rats. *Pediatr Res*. 1995;38(6):905.
32. Fan WQ, Smolich JJ, Wild J, et al. Nitric oxide modulates the regional blood flow differences in the fetal gastrointestinal tract. *Am J Physiol*. 1996;271:G598.
33. Fan WQ, Smolich JJ, Wild J. Major vasodilator role for nitric oxide in the gastrointestinal circulation of the mid-gestation fetal lambs. *Pediatr Res*. 1998;44:344.
34. Bustamante SA, Pang Y, Romero S, et al. Inducible nitric oxide synthase and the regulation of central vessel caliber in fetal rat. *Circulation*. 1996;94:1948.
35. Voelker CA, Miller MJ, Zhang XJ, et al. Perinatal nitric oxide synthase inhibition retards neonatal growth by inducing hypertrophic pyloric stenosis in rats. *Pediatr Res*. 1995;38(5):768.
36. Huang PL, Dawson TM, Bredt DS, et al. Targeted disruption of the neuronal nitric oxide synthase gene. *Cell*. 1993;75:1273.
37. Ekblad H, Arjamaa O, Vuolteenaho O, et al. Plasma endothelin-1 concentrations at different ages during infancy and childhood. *Acta Paediatr*. 1993;82:302.
38. Masaki T. Possible role of endothelin-1 in endothelin regulation of vascular tone. *Annu Rev Pharmacol Toxicol*. 1995;35:235.
39. Weir JF, Ohlsson A, Fong K, et al. Does endothelin-1 reduce superior mesenteric artery blood flow velocity in preterm neonates? *Arch Dis Child Fetal Neonatal Ed*. 1999;80:F123.
40. Pawlik WW, Gustaw P, Sendur R, et al. Vasoactive and metabolic effects of leukotriene C4 and D4 in the intestine. *Hepato-Gastroenterology*. 1998;35:87.
41. Wallace JL, MacNaughton WK. Gastrointestinal damage induced by platelet-activating factor: role of leukotrienes. *Eur J Pharmacol*. 1988;151:43.
42. Oh W. Neonatal polycythemia and hyperviscosity. *Pediatr Clin North Am*. 1986;33:523.
43. Walus KM, Fondacaro JD, Jacobson ED. Hemodynamic and metabolic changes during stimulation of ileal motility. *Dig Dis Sci*. 1981;26:1069.
44. Stark ME, Szurszewski JH. Role of nitric oxide in gastrointestinal and hepatic function and disease. *Gastroenterology*. 1992;103:1928.
45. Schwaiger M, Fondacaro JD, Jacobson ED. Effects of glucagon, histamine and perhexiline on the ischemic canine mesenteric circulation. *Gastroenterology*. 1979;77:730.
46. Walus KM, Jacobson ED. Relation between intestinal motility and circulation. *Am J Physiol*. 1981;241:G1.
47. Fasth S, Hultén L. The effect of bradykinin on intestinal motility and blood flow. *Acta Chir Scand*. 1973;139:699.
48. Eklund S, Jodal M, Lundgren O, Sjöqvist A. Effects of vasoactive intestinal polypeptide on blood flow, motility and fluid transport in the gastrointestinal tract of the cat. *Acta Physiol Scand*. 1979;105:461.
49. Walus KM, Fondacaro JD, Jacobson ED. Effects of calcium and its antagonists on the canine mesenteric circulation. *Circ Res*. 1981;48:692.
50. Zipser RD, Patterson JB, Kao HW, et al. Hypersensitive prostaglandin and thromboxane response to hormones in rabbit colitis. *Am J Physiol*. 1985;249:G457.

49 Physiology of Congenital Heart Disease in the Neonate

†Thomas J. Kulik | Philip T. Levy

INTRODUCTION

Understanding the cardiovascular physiology of a neonate with a cardiac malformation requires consideration of many factors, including myocardial systolic and diastolic function; intravascular volume; cardiac and vascular transmural pressures; the pattern of intracardiac blood flow with shunting lesions; and arterial and pulmonary venous oxygen (O_2) content.[1] Any description taking into account only these variables would be incomplete, however, because cardiac lesions affect somatic physiology in various indirect ways (e.g., sympathetic nervous system activation). Indeed, such alterations account for many of the clinical manifestations of cardiac lesions.[2,3] The net physiologic effects result from complex interactions of (1) cardiac and vascular anatomy and function; (2) lung function; (3) O_2 carrying capacity, O_2 release, and delivery; and (4) other factors, such as cellular metabolism, O_2 consumption ($\dot{V}O_2$), neurohormonal mechanisms, lymphatic structure and function, and yet others, too many to mention.

Anatomic cardiac lesions are physiologically complex for other reasons as well. With cardiac structural anomalies, more than one type of physiologic derangement may be operative. For example, with a large patent ductus arteriosus (PDA), the left ventricle (LV) may have both an increased volume load and reduced myocardial perfusion, the latter due to decreased aortic diastolic pressure. The consequences of multiple anatomic abnormalities may be additive, or conversely, may offset each other. Additionally, subtle differences in physiology may result in variable clinical phenotypes in anatomically identical patients. For example, the arterial O_2 saturation (Sao_2) in neonates with d-transposition of the great arteries after balloon atrial septostomy is variable and unpredictable, apparently related to subtle differences in physiology.[4]

Second, physiologic variables change over time. Some factors affecting cardiovascular physiology have effects over months, especially those causing anatomic changes (as in pressure-related remodeling of myocardium or pulmonary blood vessels), whereas others are relevant over seconds or minutes (e.g., those related to changes in vascular tone). The physiology of a given cardiac defect thus reflects multiple contributing factors. Assessment of cardiovascular physiology has improved with noninvasive imaging, such as echocardiography, magnetic resonance imaging, and other strategies; however, precise determination of relevant pressures, blood flows, and ventricular function can be challenging when using noninvasive approaches and may occasionally require the selective use of invasive approaches, especially cardiac catheterization.

This chapter focuses on congenital *anatomic* cardiovascular lesions; nonanatomic abnormalities (e.g., arrhythmia, intrinsic myocardial muscle dysfunction) are not discussed. The biology of specific elements related to cardiovascular function (e.g., cardiac mechanics) and structural alterations caused by cardiac lesions (e.g., ventricular hypertrophy with pressure overload) or anatomic details of the malformations are also beyond the scope of this chapter.

Understanding congenital cardiac malformations requires an appreciation of normal fetal and neonatal physiology,[5,6] the physiology and pharmacology of the pulmonary circulation,[7-9] and general principles of cardiac hemodynamics.[10] The following are discussed in this chapter: (1) how congenital cardiac lesions

†Deceased.

affect the phenotype of the neonate; (2) select basic hemodynamic concepts necessary for understanding these malformations; (3) the effect of intracardiac shunting on the clinical phenotype; and (4) nonshunting anatomic abnormalities (e.g., abnormal valves) commonly seen in neonates.

HOW CONGENITAL HEART LESIONS ALTER THE CLINICAL PHENOTYPE OF THE NEONATE

A congenital anatomic lesion may affect a neonate's phenotype in one of three ways.

NO APPRECIABLE EFFECT

Some anatomic lesions, such as a small ventricular septal defect (VSD) may *never* have any appreciable physiologic consequences. In other cases, a lesion destined to later have a significant impact may have few manifestations in the immediate postnatal period but become relevant later. The classic example is a large VSD, which has little impact at birth yet causes congestive heart failure (CHF) a few weeks later. The clinical phenotype changes partly because the relatively high neonatal pulmonary vascular resistance (PVR) falls over time, increasing left-to-right shunting and hence the LV volume pumped,[11] and partly because of other changes, such as the normal postnatal decline in hematocrit.[12] Lesions that cause higher than normal right ventricular (RV) pressure (especially if the pressure is no higher than roughly systemic[13]; e.g., pulmonary stenosis) usually have little impact on ventricular function in the newborn because the neonatal RV is generally well-adapted to pumping at systemic pressure.[6] Ductal-dependent left-sided obstructive lesions (e.g., severe coarctation of the aorta) may also have only subtle clinical manifestations in the first few days of life if the ductus remains widely patent.

REDUCTION OF SYSTEMIC OXYGEN TRANSPORT

Cardiac lesions may reduce systemic arterial blood O_2 tension *(hypoxemia)* or *systemic blood flow* ($\dot{Q}s$) and thus decrease systemic O_2 transport (systemic O_2 transport [SOT] = arterial O_2 content × $\dot{Q}s$).[14] Resting SOT may be adequate in some patients, but the ability to increase SOT with agitation, fever, or even spontaneous ventilation may be limited, resulting in clinical signs of disease (e.g., poor peripheral perfusion, dyspnea).

REDUCTION OF SYSTEMIC O_2 TRANSPORT DUE TO HYPOXEMIA

Hypoxemia may be the only manifestation of some lesions (e.g., tetralogy of Fallot), or it may occur with defects that also cause reduced $\dot{Q}s$ (e.g., severe Ebstein anomaly). The neonate may tolerate a lower Po_2 better than older infants or children,[15] and moderate hypoxemia, as an isolated abnormality, generally has little short-term physiologic effect. Increased O_2 extraction, redistribution of blood flow to organs of high O_2 need, and perhaps increased $\dot{Q}s$ help to maintain systemic $\dot{V}O_2$ with hypoxemia.[16,17] For example, when conscious lambs younger than 1 week old were subjected to acute alveolar hypoxia (fraction of inspired O_2 [Fio_2] = 0.12; arterial Po_2 = 35 mm Hg), $\dot{V}O_2$ did not change and acidosis did not occur.[17] More severe hypoxia (Fio_2 <0.10; arterial Po_2 approximately 25 mm Hg) reduced $\dot{V}O_2$ but may not be enough to cause significant acidosis in conscious newborn lambs.[16,17] Multiple variables (e.g., hematocrit, half-saturation O_2 pressure [P_{50}] of hemoglobin, environmental temperature, $\dot{Q}s$, $\dot{V}O_2$, and whether the organism is spontaneously ventilating) determine the physiologic impact of hypoxemia.[14–17]

The quantitative relationship between hypoxemia and organ dysfunction or damage in the *human* neonate is unknown. One study found an Fio_2 of 0.15 caused $\dot{V}O_2$ to fall significantly in human infants, albeit without obvious detrimental effect.[18] Perhaps the clearest evidence that neonates can tolerate substantial hypoxemia with modest or no long-term consequences comes from experience treating infants with d-transposition of the great arteries, a lesion that usually causes considerable hypoxemia, especially before balloon septostomy is performed. A total of 129 such neonates were operated on in the first week of life at the Boston Children's Hospital; the mean lowest preoperative arterial Po_2 was approximately 24 mm Hg. Even though these infants had undergone a period of substantial hypoxemia (before operation), the hospital survival rate for these patients was more than 98%.[19] Neuropsychologic evaluation and psychiatric assessment at 16 years of age revealed that these patients are at increased neurodevelopmental and psychiatric risk,[20] but it is likely that at least some of the observed decrement in neurologic function was related to aspects of the patient's treatment and clinical course distinct from the hypoxemia.

REDUCTION OF SYSTEMIC O_2 TRANSPORT DUE TO REDUCTION OF SYSTEMIC BLOOD FLOW

Congenital heart lesions may also decrease SOT by decreasing $\dot{Q}s$. As is the case for hypoxemia, modest reductions of $\dot{Q}s$ may not affect tissue oxygenation. For example, Fahey and Lister[21] found that $\dot{Q}s$ could be reduced to approximately 42% of the resting value before $\dot{V}O_2$ fell in conscious 2-week-old lambs; increased fractional extraction of O_2 from the blood maintained O_2 delivery. Most congenital cardiac lesions that reduce $\dot{Q}s$ do so by one or more of three mechanisms: (1) abnormally low systemic ventricular output, (2) abnormal arterial connection between the heart and peripheral tissues (e.g., interruption of the aortic arch), and (3) recirculation of previously oxygenated blood to the lungs (see later). Only limited quantitative data regarding $\dot{Q}s$ in the human neonate with heart disease are available.

NEUROHUMORAL AND OTHER EFFECTS OF ABNORMAL HEMODYNAMICS

Symptoms occur in infants with a heart lesion not attended by a reduction in SOT. For example, infants with CHF resulting from a large VSD generally have $\dot{Q}s$ within or near the normal range[11,22,23] (but see references[12,24]). The symptoms of "CHF" are a consequence of *neurohumoral alterations* related to the physiologic abnormality, not reduced resting SOT[2,3,25] (although limitation in increasing $\dot{Q}s$ with stress is likely also important). These alterations help to maintain adequate blood pressure and tissue perfusion in part by augmenting myocardial contractility (sympathetic nervous system activation),[26,27] increasing systemic vascular resistance (SVR), and activating the sympathetic nervous system, the renin-angiotensin-aldosterone system,[25,28,29] and release of vasopressin. Ventricular output is also increased (via the Frank-Starling principle) through fluid retention (and therefore increased ventricular filling) caused by activation of the renin-angiotensin-aldosterone system and other mechanisms.[2,3,25]

These factors help to maintain adequate SOT, but they also have *unfavorable consequences*. For example, vasoconstrictors increase SVR and ventricular afterload; the clinical result is decreased peripheral perfusion. Increased catecholamines increase $\dot{V}O_2$.[30] Fluid retention causes edema[31] and increases lung water and the work of breathing. Failure to thrive is the culmination of these and perhaps other physiologic derangements caused by structural defects. It is these secondary manifestations of abnormal cardiovascular function, rather than critically reduced resting SOT per se, that affect most symptomatic infants with cardiac lesions.

HEMODYNAMICS: VASCULAR RESISTANCE, FLOWS, AND SHUNTS

PULMONARY VASCULAR RESISTANCE

The *resistance to blood flow through the lungs* is an important determinant of the physiologic effects (ventricular work and Sao_2) of many cardiac lesions with shunting. A useful, albeit simplified,[10,32] way to conceive of PVR is PVR = (PAP − LAP) / $\dot{Q}p$, where PAP is mean pulmonary arterial pressure (mm Hg), LAP is mean left atrial pressure (mm Hg), and $\dot{Q}p$ is pulmonary blood flow (which, for pediatric patients, is usually indexed—L/m²/minute). SVR is calculated in an analogous way. Because PVR is primarily a reflection of resistance to flow through the pulmonary microcirculation, it is sometimes referred to as pulmonary *arteriolar* resistance. The calculated PVR can be low, but total resistance to flow through the lungs and into the heart can be high, with obstruction to systemic ventricular inflow (e.g., mitral stenosis) or poor systemic ventricular compliance. The concept of *total pulmonary resistance* (total pulmonary resistance = mean PAP/ $\dot{Q}p$) takes into account all resistance to flow from the central pulmonary arteries to the ventricle, although the term is misleading because some of the resistance to flow resides outside the lungs.

PVR is much higher than SVR in the fetus,[8,33] but PAP normally decreases to approximately one-half systemic arterial pressure in the first 24 hours of life (presuming the ductus is not widely patent) and reaches essentially mature levels by 1 to 2 weeks after birth.[34] The postnatal decline in PVR is slower with cardiac lesions that maintain elevated PAP (e.g., a large VSD or PDA).

RATIO OF PULMONARY TO SYSTEMIC BLOOD FLOW

The *$\dot{Q}p/\dot{Q}s$ ratio* provides an estimate of the volume pumped by the ventricles and an estimate of the $\dot{Q}p$ (and hence of PVR if the PAP is known). It can be calculated by using blood oximetry values: $\dot{Q}p/\dot{Q}s = (SaO_2 - S\bar{v}O_2)/(SpvO_2 - SpaO_2)$, where Sao_2 is the systemic arterial O_2 saturation, $S\bar{v}O_2$ is the mixed venous O_2 saturation, $Spvo_2$ is the pulmonary venous O_2 saturation, and $Spao_2$ is the pulmonary arterial O_2 saturation. The superior vena caval O_2 saturation is generally taken as representative of the $S\bar{v}O_2$ when there is left-to-right intracardiac shunting. This formula can be used to calculate $\dot{Q}p/\dot{Q}s$ with any sort of lesion, if the relevant O_2 saturations can be measured. If there is no right-to-left shunt, $Spvo_2 = Sao_2$. This formula cannot be used when multiple sources of pulmonary or systemic flow are present, with each source having a different O_2 saturation. For example, with right-to-left ductal shunting, Sao_2 levels in the ascending aorta and transverse arch differ from those in the descending aorta, making calculating $\dot{Q}p/\dot{Q}s$ impossible.

EFFECTIVE VERSUS INEFFECTIVE BLOOD FLOW

Left-to-right shunting occurs when blood that has traversed the lungs is recirculated to them without having first crossed the systemic capillary bed. Such pulmonary flow is termed *ineffective,* because little additional O_2 is picked up with more than one pulmonary passage. ($\dot{Q}p$ composed of systemic venous blood is *effective* pulmonary flow.) Ineffective $\dot{Q}p$ represents volume pumped by the heart to no useful end. Similarly, blood that has traversed the lungs before it is pumped to the systemic circulation is *effective* $\dot{Q}s$, whereas systemic venous blood that enters the systemic arterial circulation without passage through the lungs (right-to-left shunting) is *ineffective* $\dot{Q}s$. The concepts of effective and ineffective blood flow can help in thinking about complex cardiac physiology, such as that in d-transposition of the great arteries (see later).

LEFT-TO-RIGHT SHUNTING AT THE VENTRICULAR OR GREAT ARTERY LEVEL

Since the ventricle only pumps blood that enters during diastole, left-to-right shunting at the ventricular or great artery level imposes a volume load on the *systemic* ventricle (LV in an otherwise normal heart). (Actually, with a large VSD, because some pulmonary venous blood enters the RV during diastole, the RV volume pumped is also somewhat increased.[35,36])

If the connection between the systemic and pulmonary circulations (e.g., VSD or PDA) is large enough so that the systolic pressure in the two circuits is equal, the communication is said to be *unrestrictive*. With an unrestrictive defect, the *$\dot{Q}p/\dot{Q}s$ is primarily determined by the ratio of total PVR to SVR*. (With a small defect, the pressure difference between the ventricles and the size of the communication are usually the primary determinants of the shunt magnitude.) Factors that affect $\dot{Q}p/\dot{Q}s$ include the cross-sectional area of the pulmonary microcirculation, *all* resistances to flow the size of the central pulmonary arteries and large pulmonary veins, any atrioventricular valve dysfunction, and the systemic ventricular compliance. The $\dot{Q}p/\dot{Q}s$ can vary because systemic and PVR can change with physiologic, pharmacologic, and other perturbations.[8,37]

In an anatomically normal heart, PAP is a function of $\dot{Q}p$ and total pulmonary resistance. However, the *systolic PAP will always essentially be the same as the ventricle or artery to which it is connected* regardless of the $\dot{Q}p$ or the resistance to flow. Therefore, with an unrestrictive VSD or PDA, systolic PAP is essentially the same as aortic pressure, regardless of the magnitude of flow or PVR. In neonates with unrestrictive ventricular or great vessel communications, PVR falls after birth (and a large shunt develops), but the systolic PAP remains elevated. High PVR with unrestrictive communications is reflected by a low $\dot{Q}p/\dot{Q}s$, not the pulmonary arterial *systolic* pressure. (But pulmonary arterial *diastolic* pressure *is* a reflection of PVR with a large VSD; i.e., relatively low diastolic PAP generally implies low PVR.) Thus pulmonary arterial systolic hypertension and increased PVR are related but distinct concepts.

Other factors besides PVR and SVR also influence cardiovascular physiology with shunting lesions. For example, Jarmakani and colleagues[38] demonstrated that infants younger than 2 years old with a PDA had greater LV end-diastolic pressure and end-diastolic wall stress than patients with a VSD and comparable magnitude of shunt. The reason for this is unclear, but it may be related to differences in LV stroke work with the two lesions.[38] *Diastolic runoff* into the pulmonary arteries with connections between the aorta and pulmonary artery may decrease aortic diastolic pressure and hence reduce coronary perfusion.[39] *Streaming* of blood can affect whether pulmonary venous blood ends up in the aorta or in the pulmonary artery. For example, with double-outlet RV, the location of the VSD (subpulmonary vs. subaortic) will influence the *effective* $\dot{Q}p$ (with a subpulmonary VSD, pulmonary venous blood tends to be recirculated to the lungs rather than into the aorta).[40] Left-to-right shunting from the *LV to the right atrium* can occur, usually through a defect in the tricuspid valve. The magnitude of an LV-to-RA shunt is primarily determined by the effective size of the LV–right atrial communication; PVR and right atrial pressure are largely irrelevant.

LEFT-TO-RIGHT ATRIAL SHUNTING

Left-to-right shunts across an atrial septal opening increase the volume of blood pumped by the pulmonary ventricle. With a small defect, left atrial pressure is usually substantially different from the right atrium, and shunting is primarily the result of this pressure difference. With a large defect (where the mean atrial pressures are essentially equal), the shunt magnitude is generally ascribed to the relative compliances of the left atrium–pulmonary veins–LV and the RA–vena cava–RV: blood tends to flow into the

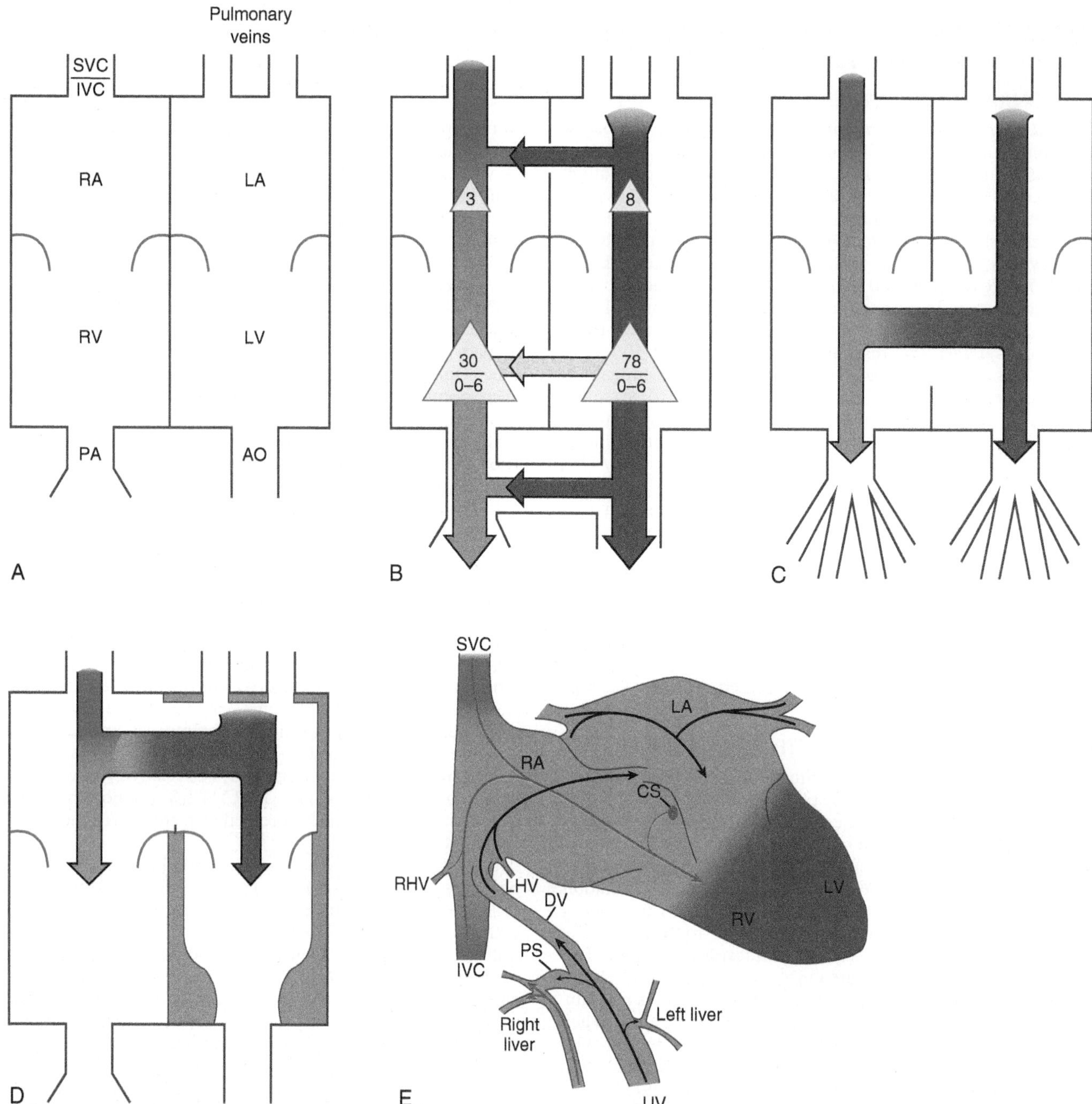

Fig. 49.1 Factors that influence where blood goes with structural heart lesions. (A) General scheme of box diagrams. (B) Blood moves from high pressure to low. Shunting at the atrial, ventricular, and great vessel levels can result from a pressure gradient between communicating structures if the communication is small enough to be pressure restrictive. (C) When two vascular beds differing in resistance to flow are connected to a source of flow, more blood finds its way into the lower-resistance circuit than into the higher-resistance circuit. With an unrestrictive ventricular septal defect and low pulmonary vascular resistance, systolic pressures are essentially the same in both the aorta and the pulmonary artery, yet there is more flow to the pulmonary artery. (D) When two chambers differing in resistance to filling (compliance) are connected by a large defect, more blood finds its way into the chamber with the greater compliance. (E) Streaming can influence the chamber or vessel to which the blood flows. As depicted here, in the fetus umbilical venous blood preferentially crosses the foramen ovale, and therefore the most highly oxygenated blood tends to go to the organs of greatest need. Streaming can also take place at the ventricular and great vessel levels. *AO,* Aorta; *CS,* coronary sinus; *DV,* ductus venosus; *IVC,* inferior vena cava; *LA,* left atrium; *LHV,* left hepatic vein; *LV,* left ventricle; *PA,* pulmonary artery; *PS,* portal sinus; *RA,* right atrium; *RHV,* right hepatic vein; *RV,* right ventricle; *SVC,* superior vena cava; *UV,* umbilical vein. Numbers in *triangles* indicate pressure. (E, From Teitel DF, et al. *Moss and Adams' Heart Disease in Infants, Children, and Adolescents*. Vol 1. 5th ed. Baltimore: Williams & Wilkins; 1995:49.)

venous chamber or ventricle that most readily accepts it (Fig. 49.1).[41] Hence, left-to-right shunting occurs in older patients, because the RV is thinner than the LV and more compliant. Because substantial atrial shunting can occur in the neonate,[42,43] whose RV and LV have similar compliances, Rudolph[44] proposed that such shunting may be a function of *differential ejection* of blood from the two ventricles, given that RV afterload is less than that of the LV. Left-to-right atrial shunting also occurs with *partial anomalous pulmonary venous connection* to the right side of the circulation. Assuming no defect in the atrial septum, the shunt is determined by the fraction of $\dot{Q}p$ going to the lobes of the lungs anomalously connected, which is a function of the total resistance to blood flow through those lobes relative to the normally connected lobes. Atrial level shunts in *children*—even if the $\dot{Q}p$ is very large—are seldom associated with significant pulmonary hypertension.[45] However, in the *neonate*, the capacity for flow-related dilation or recruitment in the pulmonary vascular bed is limited, and large *atrial* level shunts (e.g., unobstructed total anomalous pulmonary venous connection, and intracranial arteriovenous malformations) are often accompanied by considerably increased PAP.[46–49]

RIGHT-TO-LEFT SHUNTING

Right-to-left shunting occurs when systemic venous blood enters the systemic arterial circulation without having passed through the pulmonary capillaries. Although isolated right-to-left shunting can occur (e.g., tetralogy of Fallot), both right-to-left and left-to-right shunting are present in many congenital heart defects.

DETERMINANTS OF SYSTEMIC ARTERIAL OXYGEN SATURATION WITH RIGHT-TO-LEFT SHUNTING

With right-to-left shunting, Sao_2 is primarily a function of four variables:

1. The *fraction of systemic arterial blood composed of systemic venous blood.* No matter how complex the pattern of intracardiac shunting is, with right-to-left shunting a certain portion of the aortic blood will not have crossed the lungs, which reduces Sao_2. The greater the fraction of systemic arterial blood bypassing the lungs, the lower the Sao_2.
2. $S\bar{v}O_2$. The O_2 saturation of venous blood that reaches the aorta affects the Sao_2. Because the $S\bar{v}O_2$ reflects what O_2 remains in the blood after crossing the systemic capillary bed, this value is influenced by the following:
   a. Hematocrit. The greater the O_2 carrying capacity of the blood, the greater the SOT, and given a fixed quantity of O_2 unloaded to the tissue, the greater the $S\bar{v}O_2$.
   b. $\dot{Q}s$. Given a fixed amount of O_2 unloaded into the tissues, the greater the quantity of O_2 transported, the greater the $S\bar{v}O_2$.
   c. $\dot{V}O_2$. The greater the quantity of O_2 consumed, given a fixed amount transported, the lower the $S\bar{v}O_2$.
   d. *The O_2 dissociation characteristics of hemoglobin.* With a leftward shift of the O_2 dissociation curve, *less* O_2 is unloaded from hemoglobin at any given Po_2. Therefore, for any given end-capillary Po_2, the $S\bar{v}O_2$ will be a function of the P_{50} of the hemoglobin. With a right-to-left shunt, a leftward shift of the curve will increase the $Spvo_2$ and therefore *increases* the $S\bar{v}O_2$, all other things being equal.
3. *Pulmonary venous O_2 saturation.* For obvious reasons, the lower the $SpvO_2$, the lower the SaO_2.

SYSTEMIC O_2 TRANSPORT WITH RIGHT-TO-LEFT SHUNTING

With *right-to-left* shunting lesions, SOT and O_2 delivery to the tissues are not strictly proportional to SaO_2. For example, a leftward shift in the hemoglobin-O_2 dissociation curve is associated with a higher SaO_2 at any PaO_2 (which will be low with right-to-left shunting); however, this higher saturation does not imply an increase in O_2 delivery to the tissue, because less O_2 is released at any given tissue Po_2. In addition, with admixture lesions, SOT actually *declines* as SaO_2 increases beyond a certain point (see later). *Maximum* $\dot{V}O_2$ = maximum O_2 uptake in the lungs, which is a function of $\dot{Q}p$, PaO_2, SpaO2, and the O_2 capacity of the blood. Hence, if effective $\dot{Q}p$ is severely reduced, SOT will be compromised, regardless of $\dot{Q}s$ or any other factors.

ISOLATED RIGHT-TO-LEFT SHUNTING

Isolated right-to-left shunting occurs at the *ventricular level* with a VSD when resistance to $\dot{Q}p$ (from obstruction in the RV outflow tract or points beyond) exceeds resistance to flow into the systemic vascular bed, thus shunting desaturated (RV) blood into the aorta. Right-to-left *ductal* shunting occurs when total pulmonary resistance is greater than SVR, most often due to increased PVR, but this can also be caused by pulmonary venous hypertension. Right-to-left ductal shunting also occurs when the descending aorta is mostly or entirely supplied by the RV, such as severe coarctation of the aorta. (In such cases there is usually a component of left-to-right shunting—at the atrial or ventricular level—as well.) The magnitude of right-to-left shunting with ventricular or arterial communications is determined by the ratio of resistance to flow into and through the pulmonary circuit relative to the systemic circuit. Because SVR and PVR (and sometimes even the degree of RV outflow tract obstruction, as in tetralogy of Fallot) may fluctuate, the magnitude of right-to-left shunting is variable. Right-to-left shunting across an atrial defect most commonly results from reduced RV compliance, relative to that of the LV, usually because of RV hypertrophy or hypertension (see Figs. 49.1 and 49.2).

BIDIRECTIONAL SHUNTING

Bidirectional shunting is present in various cardiac lesions. For example, a patient with severe aortic stenosis (and severely reduced LV ejection) with an open ductus arteriosus (DA) will often have a left-to-right atrial shunt, and a right-to-left shunt across the ductus into the aorta. Right-to-left atrial shunting can also occur simultaneously with a left-to- RV shunt (e.g., with an atrioventricular septal defect).

With *total anomalous connection of the pulmonary veins*, all pulmonary veins connect to the systemic veins or right atrium; thus a fraction of both the pulmonary and systemic venous return must cross the atrial septum to supply the LV. The variables that influence $\dot{Q}p$ (the systemic and pulmonary venous blood that finds its way into the RV) and $\dot{Q}s$ (the systemic and pulmonary venous blood entering the LV) include the size of the atrial opening,[49] the relative ventricular compliances, and possibly any preferential streaming of venous blood. Whether streaming of venous blood actually affects $\dot{Q}p$ per se is unclear, but it can affect the Sao_2[46,49] because pulmonary venous return from the inferior vena cava (with infradiaphragmatic connections) can preferentially stream across the foramen ovale into the left atrium. With total anomalous pulmonary venous connection (assuming no other communication between the pulmonary and systemic arterial circuits), PVR affects only the pattern of intracardiac shunting insofar as it influences RV pressure and therefore RV compliance and systolic function. (Another physiologic consequence of obstructed pulmonary venous connection is pulmonary edema, which interferes with gas exchange and reduces lung compliance.) The shunting physiology with cerebral arteriovenous malformations is similar in many ways (see Fig. 49.2).[48]

CARDIAC ADMIXTURE LESIONS

Lesions that cause complete mixing of systemic and pulmonary venous blood are sometimes termed *admixture lesions.* All malformations with a single functional ventricle (e.g., hypoplastic left heart syndrome, tricuspid atresia) have this physiology, as well as some two-ventricle defects (e.g., tetralogy of Fallot with pulmonary atresia). Actually, preferential streaming of pulmonary or systemic venous blood into one or the other great artery can occur in some lesions with mixing of pulmonary and systemic venous blood (e.g., truncus arteriosus), but unless the quantity of "streamed" blood is significant, the physiology is best understood as admixture.

DETERMINANTS OF SYSTEMIC ARTERIAL OXYGEN SATURATION WITH ADMIXTURE LESIONS

With admixture lesions, Sao_2 is a function of all the variables outlined earlier. The fraction of aortic blood composed of

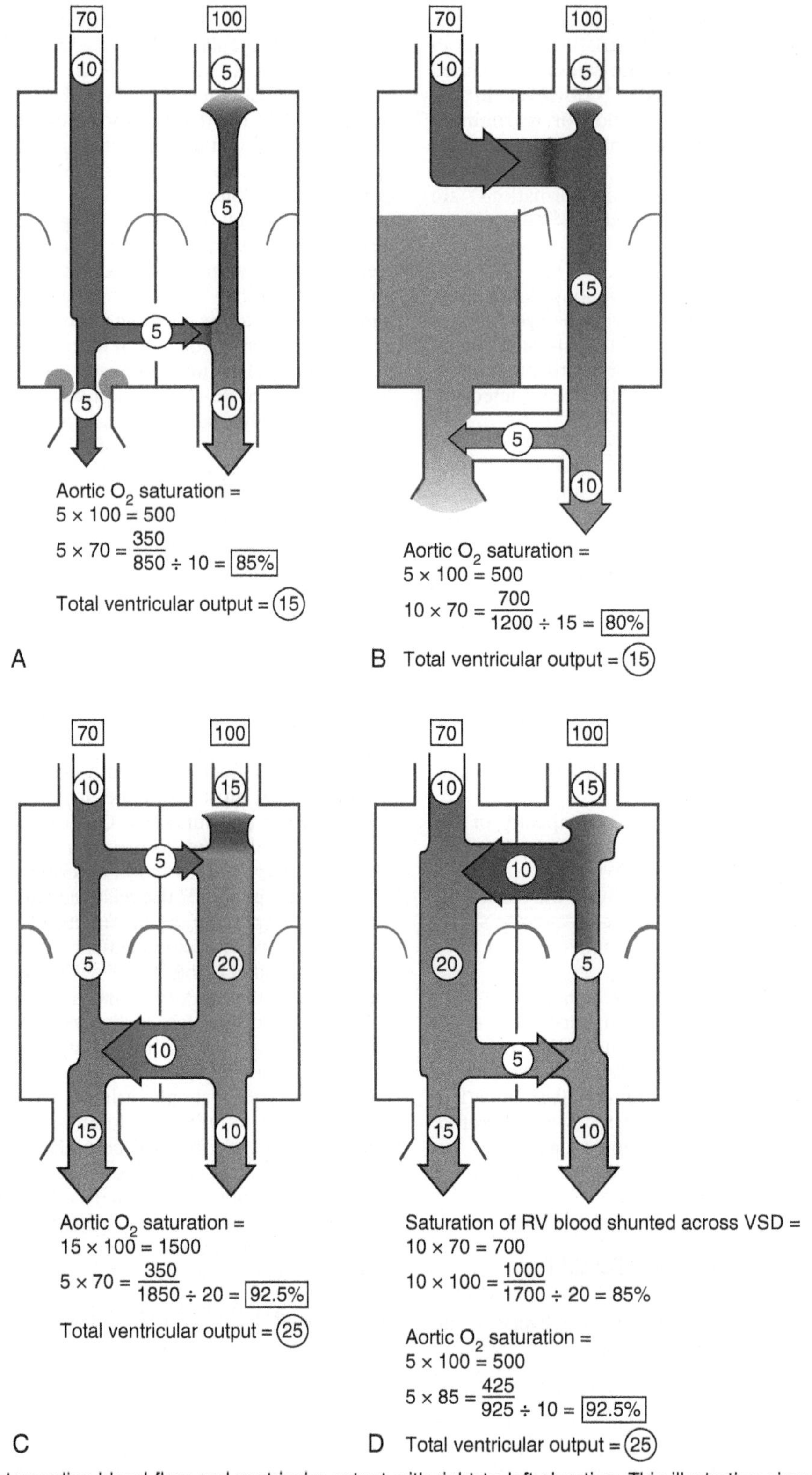

Fig. 49.2 Patterns of intracardiac blood flow and ventricular output with right-to-left shunting. This illustration aims to provide a conceptual understanding of the relationship among intracardiac shunting, ventricular output, and oxygen (O_2) saturation, but it is a simplified view relative to cardiac physiology; for example, given a fixed O_2 consumption, it would be unrealistic to expect systemic venous saturation to remain constant, because systemic O_2 transport varies. Numbers in *boxes* indicate blood O_2 saturation; numbers in *circles* indicate the relative amount of blood flow. (A) With an isolated right-to-left shunt (e.g., tetralogy of Fallot), all pulmonary blood flow is effective, and combined ventricular output is normal. (B) With admixture physiology, there is ineffective pulmonary blood flow, and therefore systemic arterial saturation is less, for a given amount of ventricular output, than for a lesion with isolated right-to-left shunting. (C and D) With bidirectional shunting, equal volumes of right-to-left shunting at either the atrial or ventricular level will result in equal systemic arterial O_2 saturation and equal ventricular output. The relationship between systemic arterial O_2 saturation and ventricular output depends on the volume of ineffective pulmonary blood flow (left-to-right shunt). *RV,* Right ventricular; *VSD,* ventricular septal defect.

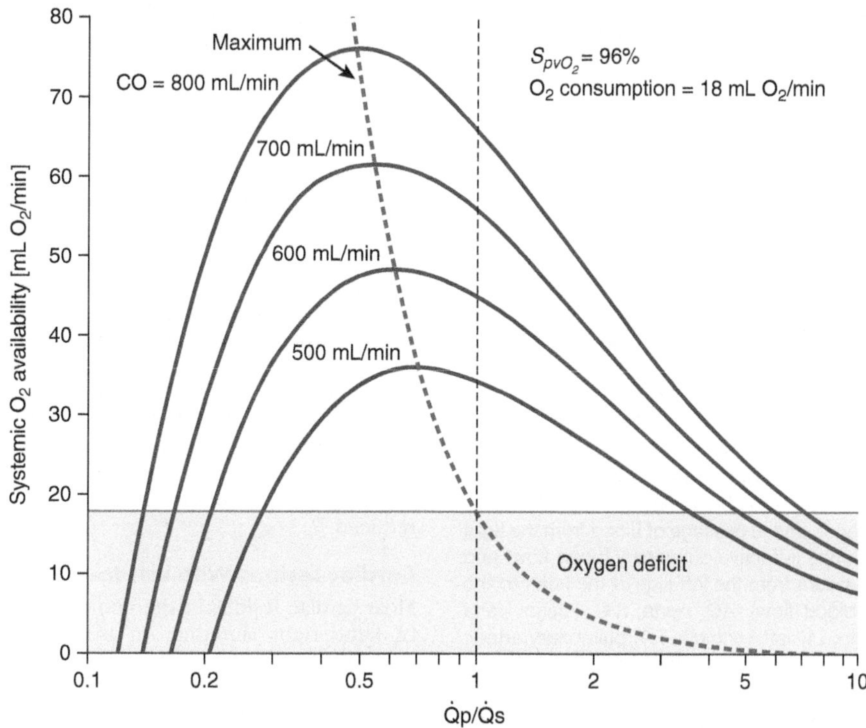

Fig. 49.3 The relationship between systemic oxygen availability (transport) and the ratio of pulmonary to systemic blood flow *(Q̇p/Q̇s)* with cardiac admixture lesions. Barnea and colleagues[50] used a mathematical model to determine systemic oxygen (O_2) transport (SOT) for a patient with a single ventricle, with the aorta and pulmonary artery in communication, assuming the O_2 capacity of the blood to be 22 mL O_2 per deciliter, pulmonary venous O_2 saturation *($Spvo_2$)* to be 96%, and O_2 consumption ($\dot{V}O_2$) to be 18 mL O_2 per minute (the normal mean value for a 3-kg neonate). SOT is a function of both cardiac output and Q̇p/Q̇s. Maximum SOT occurs with a Q̇p/Q̇s of less than 1, a value lower than that typical of most patients with hypoplastic left heart syndrome and probably most patients with a "single-ventricle" lesion. (From Barnea O, Austin EH, Richman B, Santamore WP. Balancing the circulation: theoretic optimization of pulmonary/systemic flow ratio in hypoplastic left heart syndrome. *J Am Coll Cardiol.* 1994;24:1376.)

pulmonary venous blood is determined by the *Q̇p/Q̇s:* because all the pulmonary venous blood mixes with all the systemic venous blood, the ratio of "blue" and "pink" blood greatly influences Sao_2. When the systemic and pulmonary arterial circuits are in unrestricted communication, the Q̇p/Q̇s is primarily determined by the ratio of total PVR to SVR. With *atrial* mixing of venous blood and separate systemic and pulmonary arterial circulations (e.g., total anomalous pulmonary venous connection), Q̇p/Q̇s may be largely determined by other factors (see earlier) (see Fig. 49.2).

SYSTEMIC ARTERIAL OXYGEN SATURATION VERSUS SYSTEMIC OXYGEN TRANSPORT IN ADMIXTURE LESIONS

The variables that determine systemic arterial O_2 *transport* in admixture lesions (usually more relevant to tissue oxygenation than Sao_2 per se) are more complex. At any given ventricular output, every milliliter of blood pumped to the lungs is one less milliliter going to the systemic circulation. Therefore, assuming that the total ventricular output is fixed, as the Q̇p/Q̇s (and Sao_2) *increases*, Q̇s *falls*. SOT is therefore a function of total ventricular output, hematocrit, $Spvo_2$, $\dot{V}O_2$, and Q̇p/Q̇s; the relationship between Q̇p/Q̇s and SOT is complex (Fig. 49.3).[50-52]

TRANSPOSITION PHYSIOLOGY

With d-transposition of the great arteries, the aorta arises from the RV and the pulmonary artery from the LV. Because systemic and pulmonary venous blood enters the right and left atria, respectively, the systemic and pulmonary circulations function in parallel rather than in series. Systemic venous blood, largely depleted of O_2, entering the RV is pumped out again to the body, whereas oxygenated pulmonary venous blood is ejected into the lungs.[53] Without any communication between the two circuits, all blood flow would be ineffective, and life would cease shortly after birth. As it happens, communications between the systemic and pulmonary circuits usually exist at one or more levels (atrial septum, ventricular septum, DA) and, if of sufficient size, usually allow for enough *mixing* of systemic and pulmonary venous blood for adequate Sao_2 (Fig. 49.4). (Note, however, that communication at the ductal or ventricular level alone is typically not sufficient—atrial level mixing is usually required for adequate Sao_2.)

The essence of mixing is (in a steady-state system) that for every milliliter of systemic venous blood that crosses from the right side of the heart, or the aorta, into the left side of the heart or pulmonary artery (and then into the lungs, constituting effective Q̇p), 1 mL of pulmonary venous blood must cross from the left side of the heart into the right side of the heart and into the aorta (becoming effective Q̇s). Were more blood to flow in one direction than the other, one of the two circulations would become depleted of blood. That is not to say that the volumes of blood pumped by the LV and RV need to be equal, but rather the average amount of blood crossing from left to right must equal the amount moving from right to left.[53] In the neonate the LV volume pumped is similar to normal, but it is considerably greater than normal by about 6 months of age.[54,55]

Echocardiography demonstrates that infants with d-transposition and an atrial septal opening shunt from the left to the right atrium during systole and right-to-left during diastole.[56] The factors determining mixing are unclear, although it is known that Q̇p is strongly positively related to the Sao_2.[57] Thus a PDA increases

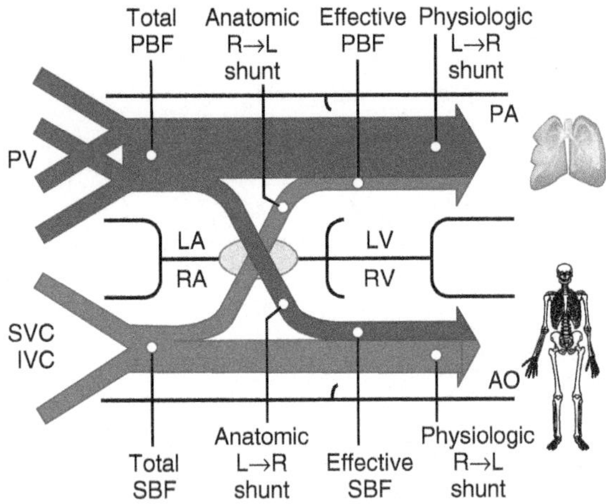

Fig. 49.4 Intracardiac blood flow with d-transposition of the great arteries. Most pulmonary and systemic blood flow is ineffective. Systemic oxygen delivery depends on the passage of blood from the right side of the heart into the lungs (effective pulmonary blood flow) and the passage of an equal amount from the left side of the heart to the aorta (effective systemic blood flow). *AO*, Aorta; *IVC*, inferior vena cava; *L*, left; *LA*, left atrium; *LV*, left ventricle; *PA*, pulmonary artery; *PBF*, pulmonary blood flow; *PV*, pulmonary vein; *R*, right; *RA*, right atrium; *RV*, right ventricle; *SBF*, systemic blood flow; *SVC*, superior vena cava. (From Paul MH, Wernovsky G. Transposition of the great arteries. *Moss and Adams' Heart Disease in Infants, Children, and Adolescents*. Vol 2. 5th ed. Baltimore: Williams & Wilkins; 1995:1166–1170.)

mixing by increasing $\dot{Q}p$.[58] Conversely, increased PVR in neonates with d-transposition can markedly reduce the Sa_{O_2}.[59] The number of mixing sites also plays a role, with Sa_{O_2} increasing with the number of sites.[57]

Whereas cyanosis is usually the key physiologic feature of this lesion (although some neonates with d-transposition and a large VSD are not cyanotic), CHF can develop with d-transposition and a large PDA or VSD.[58,60] With a large VSD, the pattern of blood flow has not been fully elucidated, but there appears to be increased volume pumped by both ventricles,[61] and the $\dot{Q}p/\dot{Q}s$ can be very large. The latter may be associated with *reduced* $\dot{Q}s$, so increasing SaO_2 may be a warning sign rather than an indication of physiologic improvement.

SHUNTING AND THE CLINICAL PHENOTYPE

LEFT-TO-RIGHT SHUNTING

How Much Volume Reserve Does the Neonatal Heart Have?

The neonatal ventricle is capable of pumping considerably more blood than normal under certain circumstances. Tabbutt and colleagues[62] measured the $\dot{Q}p/\dot{Q}s$ in 10 anesthetized and hemodynamically stable neonates with hypoplastic left heart syndrome and found that the mean $\dot{Q}p/\dot{Q}s$ was approximately 3.4:1. Because neither actual $\dot{Q}p$ nor $\dot{Q}s$ was measured, the output from the (single) RV could not be determined. However, if one assumes that $\dot{Q}s$ was only 50% of usual (likely an underestimate), the single ventricle (RV) in these patients pumped 2.2 times as much blood as normal.

Animal data are conflicting regarding how much extra volume can be pumped without compromising $\dot{Q}s$. In one study of mechanically ventilated preterm newborn lambs, relevant blood flows were measured with the DA open and closed; an approximately 60% increase in LV output resulting from opening the ductus was associated with a significant fall in $\dot{Q}s$.[63] A similar study, however, showed no fall in $\dot{Q}s$ even with a 100% increase in LV output with ductal opening.[64] Both studies were conducted over an hour or two and may not be reflective of long-term physiology. The newborn *human* with a PDA can have an LV output greater than 150% of normal,[65-68] but information regarding $\dot{Q}s$ in these neonates is limited. Data from a few neonates with a PDA suggest that LV output of more than three times normal may be generated with $\dot{Q}s$ greater than 3 L/m^2/minute,[65,67] although accurate measurement of $\dot{Q}p$ in this setting is difficult. Infants (generally >1 month old) with a VSD may have an LV output of three to four times normal, assuming that normal cardiac output = 4.2 ± 1.2 L/m^2/minute,[68,69] while still maintaining $\dot{Q}s$ greater than 3 L/m^2/minute.[11,22,23]

Notwithstanding the capacity of the neonatal LV to pump considerably more blood than normal, left-to-right shunts of sufficient size cause CHF. In addition to those previously mentioned, other physiologic perturbations may attend lesions that cause left-to-right shunting: (1) with a large communication between the aorta and pulmonary artery, diastolic pressure and hence myocardial perfusion may be reduced[39]; and (2) with shunting lesions attended by increased PAP lung compliance is reduced.[70]

Cardiac Lesions With Left-to-Right Shunting

Most cardiac lesions in the neonate have at least a component of left-to-right shunting. An isolated *VSD* causes left-to-right shunting, although as noted earlier, symptoms of CHF usually do not develop for a few weeks. However, *premature babies* with a large VSD can have symptoms within 1 to 2 weeks of age, in part because PVR declines more rapidly than in the term infant,[33] and possibly preterm ventricles have less capacity to accommodate volume loading. A large PDA is usually associated with a large left-to-right shunt, especially in premature infants (Fig. 49.5).

It is also very unusual, but well described,[43] for left-to-right atrial level shunting through an isolated *atrial septal defect* to cause symptoms in the first few months of life. Left-to-right atrial shunting across the foramen ovale may be substantial in neonates with left-sided obstructive lesions (e.g., aortic stenosis, coarctation).[71] (This shunting is actually helpful, because the LV may have a limited capacity to accept pulmonary venous return—especially with critical aortic stenosis and hypoplastic left heart syndrome—and without an atrial opening, pulmonary venous pressures are high and pulmonary blood flow limited.)

RIGHT-TO-LEFT SHUNTING

In the neonate, mildly to moderately reduced Sa_{O_2} may have little detectable impact on physiology. However, it is unclear where to draw the line between moderate hypoxemia (with little or no short-term physiologic impact) and severe hypoxemia (which impairs organ function) in the neonate. As previously noted, other determinants of SOT (especially $\dot{Q}s$ and hematocrit) and $\dot{V}O_2$ undoubtedly influence what level of hypoxemia is compatible with aerobic metabolism, and there must be intraindividual variation as well. It seems that an arterial P_{O_2} in the mid-20 mm Hg range (and possibly even somewhat lower) can be tolerated for at least hours or days in most patients, *presuming that other factors influencing SOT are acceptable*, although the long-term CNS and other effects of such hypoxia are unknown. A lack of metabolic acidosis is often taken as an indication that SOT (and hence P_{O_2}) is acceptable, but whether a lack of acidosis with hypoxemia correlates with a lack of long-term sequelae (especially central nervous system dysfunction) is unknown.

Cardiac Lesions With Right-to-Left Shunting

Hypoxemia is usually the primary or sole physiologic manifestation of most lesions with *reduced* $\dot{Q}p$ (e.g., tetralogy of Fallot or severe valvar pulmonary stenosis) (Fig. 49.6). When some or all $\dot{Q}p$ is provided by a ductus with a right-sided

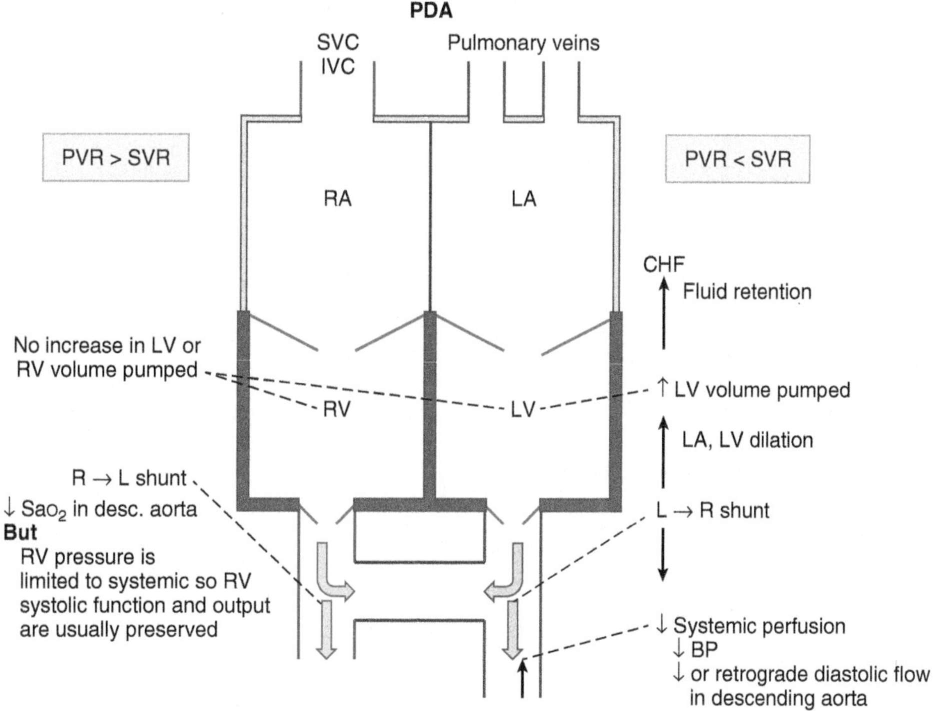

Fig. 49.5 Patent ductus arteriosus *(PDA)*. *BP*, Blood pressure; *CHF*, congestive heart failure; *IVC*, inferior vena cava; *L*, left; *LA*, left atrium; *LV*, left ventricle; *PVR*, pulmonary vascular resistance; *R*, right; *RA*, right atrium; *RV*, right ventricle; *Sao_2*, systemic arterial O_2 saturation; *SVC*, superior vena cava; *SVR*, systemic vascular resistance.

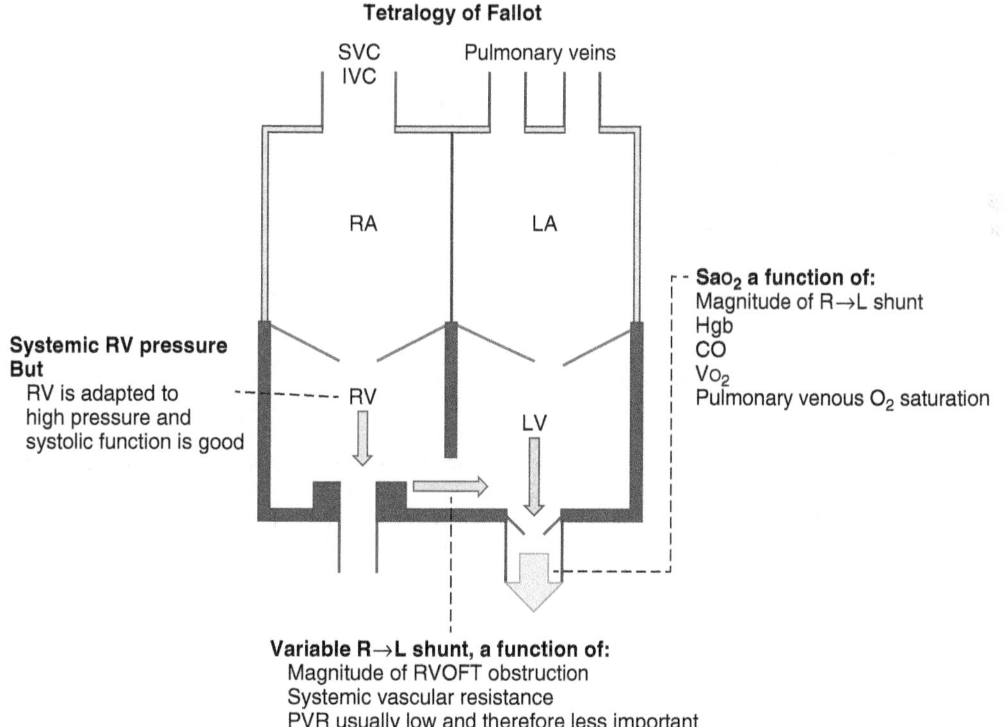

Fig. 49.6 Tetralogy of Fallot. *CO*, Cardiac output; *Hgb*, hemoglobin; *IVC*, inferior vena cava; *L*, left; *LA*, left atrium; *LV*, left ventricle; *PVR*, pulmonary vascular resistance; *R*, right; *RA*, right atrium; *RV*, right ventricle; *RVOFT*, right ventricular outflow track; *Sao_2*, systemic arterial O_2 saturation; *SVC*, superior vena cava; *$\dot{V}O_2$*, O_2 consumption.

obstructive lesion, there is ineffective $\dot{Q}p$ and therefore increased volume pumped by the ventricle, but this volume load is usually modest, presumably because the ductus is usually restrictive with those lesions. Patients with lesions with *admixture physiology* and an unrestrictive communication between the systemic and pulmonary circulations (e.g., single-ventricle lesions without significant pulmonary stenosis) usually have only mild hypoxemia (presuming that PVR falls normally postnatally), but commonly manifest CHF due to increased volume load. Single-ventricle lesions with limitation of $\dot{Q}p$ resulting from increased PVR or

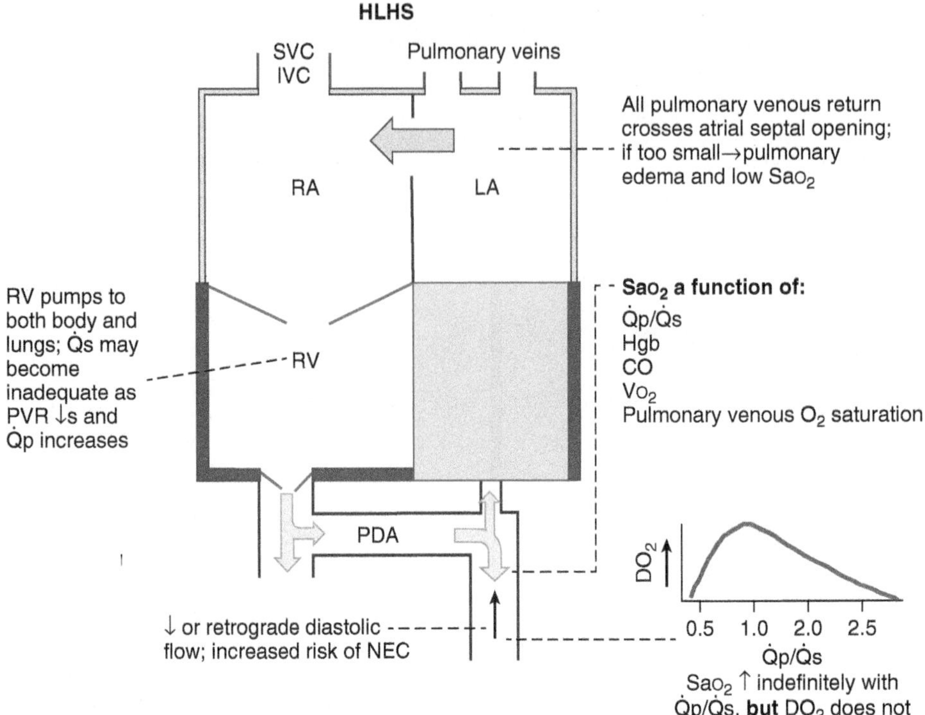

Fig. 49.7 Hypoplastic left heart syndrome *(HLHS)* as an example of a single-ventricle cardiac malformation. *CO,* Cardiac output; *Do_2,* O_2 delivery; *Hgb,* hemoglobin; *IVC,* inferior vena cava; *LA,* left atrium; *NEC,* necrotizing enterocolitis; *PDA,* patent ductus arteriosus; *PVR,* pulmonary vascular resistance; *$\dot{Q}p$,* pulmonary blood flow; *$\dot{Q}p/\dot{Q}s$,* pulmonary to systemic flow ratio; *$\dot{Q}s$,* systemic blood flow; *RA,* right atrium; *RV,* right ventricle; *Sao_2,* systemic arterial O_2 saturation; *SVC,* superior vena cava; *$\dot{V}O_2$,* O_2 consumption.

anatomic restriction (e.g., tricuspid atresia with a restrictive VSD) can be well- balanced and have adequate Sao_2 without CHF.

SINGLE-VENTRICLE PHYSIOLOGY

Multiple factors affect the physiology of neonates with complete mixing of systemic and pulmonary venous blood due to communication at the level of the ventricle or great arteries (Fig. 49.7). See "Cardiac Admixture Lesions" for determinants of SaO_2 and SOT. Note especially the following:

1. With single-ventricle physiology, *volume work is increased for the ventricle,* which can be considerable (see later and Fig. 49.2).
2. With left-sided obstructive lesions and an unrestrictive PDA (e.g., hypoplastic left heart syndrome), the $\dot{Q}p$ tends to be large, especially as PVR falls perinatally, and hence *$\dot{Q}s$ tends to be reduced,* as discussed earlier. This is less the case for right-sided obstructive ductal-dependent lesions (e.g., pulmonary atresia with intact ventricular septum) because the ductus is usually restrictive.
3. Lesions with aortic diastolic runoff into the pulmonary circuit can have *decreased diastolic pressure* and therefore decreased coronary perfusion,[39] although quantitative information regarding the impact of this on myocardial performance or reserve is lacking. In term infants with congenital cardiac malformations, *diastolic retrograde flow away from the mesenteric arteries,* perhaps in combination with reduced SOT, appears to increase the risk of *necrotizing enterocolitis.*[72,73]

The concurrence of these factors, especially in infants with high $\dot{Q}p$, often leads to CHF and sometimes even substantially reduced SOT. For example, some babies with truncus arteriosus have severe CHF and even die in the neonatal period,[74] because of the combination of large ventricular volume load, cyanosis, and reduced myocardial perfusion.

NONSHUNT ANATOMIC AND PHYSIOLOGIC ABNORMALITIES

AFTERLOAD

The term *afterload* is used here to denote the resistance against which the heart pumps. This is an incomplete way to think of afterload (e.g., resistance to ventricular ejection imposed by small blood vessels is different than that caused by semilunar valve stenosis, and arterial capacitance is not accounted for), but a useful simplification for the purposes of the following discussion.

INCREASED AFTERLOAD

The amount of blood ejected by the ventricle is inversely related to the afterload against which it ejects.[75,76] Although the normal heart can to some extent maintain its output in the presence of *acutely* increased afterload,[76,77] this reserve is limited, especially for a dysfunctional ventricle. Because the neonatal heart has less contractile reserve than the more mature one,[78] this is especially pertinent. Furthermore, because the major determinant of myocardial $\dot{V}O_2$ is pressure work,[79,80] the ventricle's ability to respond to an increase in afterload is dependent on coronary perfusion pressure[81]; when increased afterload occurs with normal or decreased aortic pressure (e.g., severe valvar aortic stenosis) or reduced Sao_2, myocardial O_2 supply may be inadequate.

Chronically increased afterload causes myocardial hypertrophy, which is usually adequate to maintain ventricular systolic function. Whereas hypertrophy is adaptive insofar as it normalizes wall stress,[82] *ventricular compliance* is reduced, as manifested in *increased atrial pressure* (absent an interatrial communication). Left atrial hypertension can cause pulmonary edema, left-to-right shunting, and "reflex" pulmonary vasoconstriction,[83-85] thereby increasing PAP beyond that accounted for by the elevation in LAP alone. Pressure overload of the RV can also cause increased *right atrial pressure* and systemic venous congestion. However, because the foramen ovale is usually nonrestrictive to right-to-left flow in neonates, a reduction in RV filling is usually reflected by a right-to-left atrial shunt, rather than by systemic venous hypertension. Finally, *subendocardial ischemia* from severe chronic pressure overload can lead to endocardial fibrosis and papillary muscle dysfunction, or infarction and hence mitral regurgitation, especially in the fetus.[86]

CARDIAC LESIONS CAUSING INCREASED AFTERLOAD

The effects of increased afterload are clearly manifest in neonates with severe valvar *aortic stenosis*.[86] LV output is reduced,[87] sometimes so much so that adequate systemic perfusion requires a PDA to allow the RV to contribute to $\dot{Q}s$. Left atrial hypertension causes a left-to-right atrial shunting, pulmonary edema, and pulmonary arterial hypertension. Relief of the increased afterload by aortic balloon dilation immediately decreases (but does not normalize) LAP,[88,89] but LV systolic function remains abnormal for some time—at least days and probably weeks.[90] *Severe coarctation of the aorta* also causes LV systolic and diastolic dysfunction and output, and left-to-right atrial shunting. PAP is increased, partly because of left atrial hypertension.[91]

Because the fetal RV operated at (and is therefore well adapted to) systemic pressure,[6] *increased RV pressure* usually has little measurable impact on RV systolic performance in a neonate, as long as it is approximately at or lower than systemic blood pressure.[13] However, neonates with *severe valvar pulmonary stenosis* with suprasystemic RV pressure have reduced RV output and an atrial right-to-left shunt.[92] Right-to-left atrial shunting, often enough to cause substantial arterial desaturation, may persist for weeks after reduction of RV afterload by balloon dilation, reflecting the relatively slow pace of normalization of RV compliance.[93]

DECREASED AFTERLOAD

Because pressure is a function of vascular resistance and flow, inappropriately *low* SVR causes hypotension unless $\dot{Q}s$ is increased. Lower-than-normal SVR (resulting from dilation of systemic arterioles) occurs in some settings (e.g., with sepsis), but it does not seem to be an inherent feature of congenital cardiac malformations. It is important to recognize when hypotension is due to low SVR rather than low systemic flow because the therapy is different: in the case of the former, agents that increase SVR (e.g., arginine vasopressin or alpha adrenergic agonists) may be more useful than other forms of therapy.

In lesions in which the systemic arterial circulation is in unrestricted communication with the venous circulation (e.g., arteriovenous malformation)[48] or pulmonary circulation (e.g., large VSD or PDA), outflow resistance to systemic ventricular ejection is reduced (at least if PVR is lower than SVR, in the case of the latter). This does not generally have a clinically significant impact on blood pressure because total blood flow into the systemic and pulmonary circuits is usually sufficient to maintain normal blood pressure. However, relatively low blood pressure with a large PDA in the premature infant[94,95] suggests that total (systemic plus pulmonary) flow is insufficient to compensate for the low total vascular resistance resulting from inclusion of the pulmonary circuit.

VALVAR INSUFFICIENCY

Semilunar and atrioventricular valve regurgitation perturb cardiac mechanics and biology somewhat differently. For example, acute mitral regurgitation increases LV systolic and diastolic wall tension much less than aortic regurgitation does.[96] The magnitude of regurgitation is primarily influenced by the degree of valve deformity, the heart rate, resistance to ventricular ejection (for atrioventricular valves), and PVR or SVR (for pulmonary and aortic valves, respectively). Mild regurgitation minimally affects the physiology, but more severe degrees may be attended by CHF, atrial hypertension, and even reduced $\dot{Q}s$. *Aortic valve regurgitation,* by reducing coronary perfusion pressure, may also compromise myocardial perfusion.[39] *Pulmonary valve regurgitation* may be more pernicious in neonates than older patients because PVR is likely to be higher in the newborn.

CARDIAC LESIONS WITH VALVE REGURGITATION

Atrioventricular valve regurgitation is uncommon in the neonate, although it can occur in isolation, with cardiac malformations,[86,97,98] or with papillary muscle dysfunction caused by neonatal asphyxia.[99] Aortic valve regurgitation is exceedingly unusual (absent intervention on the aortic valve) but occurs with (the rare) aorto-left ventricular tunnel. With absent pulmonary valve syndrome (tetralogy of Fallot with absent pulmonary valve), there is pulmonary regurgitation, but its effect on the neonate is unclear because these patients also have a large VSD and RV outflow tract obstruction. With this condition, the clinical phenotype is substantially determined by large airway abnormalities.[100]

RESTRICTION OF VENTRICULAR FILLING

The heart can eject only what it receives, and ventricular filling is largely a function of transmural filling pressure. Impaired flow into the heart can reduce ventricular output, but more commonly adequate output is maintained at the expense of venous hypertension, which causes third spacing (pulmonary edema, systemic edema, effusion, body wall edema). This can be a serious liability, especially in neonates, and tends to beget more of the same: chest wall edema and effusions increase mean airway pressure (in the mechanically ventilated patient), compress abdominal venous return, or directly compress the heart, leading to yet more fluid accumulation.

CARDIAC LESIONS WITH RESTRICTION OF FILLING

Isolated obstruction to ventricular inflow is very unusual in the neonate; when the tricuspid or mitral valve is small, the corresponding ventricle is usually reduced in volume. When filling of the RV is impeded (e.g., pulmonary atresia with intact ventricular septum), right-to-left flow across the foramen ovale is rarely obstructed; hence right atrial pressure is usually normal. With mitral stenosis or atresia and hypoplasia of the LV (hypoplastic left heart syndrome), the atrial septal opening is usually large enough so that pulmonary venous return is only modestly obstructed (although the opening usually becomes smaller over the first few weeks of life). Occasionally, the atrial septal opening is very small, with resulting severe left atrial hypertension and increased total pulmonary resistance, reducing $\dot{Q}p$. Pulmonary edema further reduces $Sa{O_2}$ by interfering with gas exchange and by reducing lung compliance. $\dot{Q}s$, however, may actually be increased, because systemic venous return to the RV is not obstructed, and the increased total PVR reduces the fraction of RV output that goes to the lungs.

Isolated mitral stenosis with adequate LV size is rare in the neonate.[101] Obstruction to pulmonary venous return can occur with *total anomalous pulmonary venous connection, cor triatriatum, and stenosis of the individual pulmonary veins,* the latter two being very rare (Fig. 49.8). Pulmonary artery hypertension, reduced RV compliance and output, and pulmonary edema are the primary physiologic manifestations of pulmonary venous hypertension.

Rarely, one *massively enlarged chamber encroaches* on the other and inhibits ventricular filling, such as LV encroachment by the right atrium or RV with a severe Ebstein anomaly[98] (Fig. 49.9). There are other impediments to ventricular filling, such as pericardial effusion, that are not congenital malformations per se.

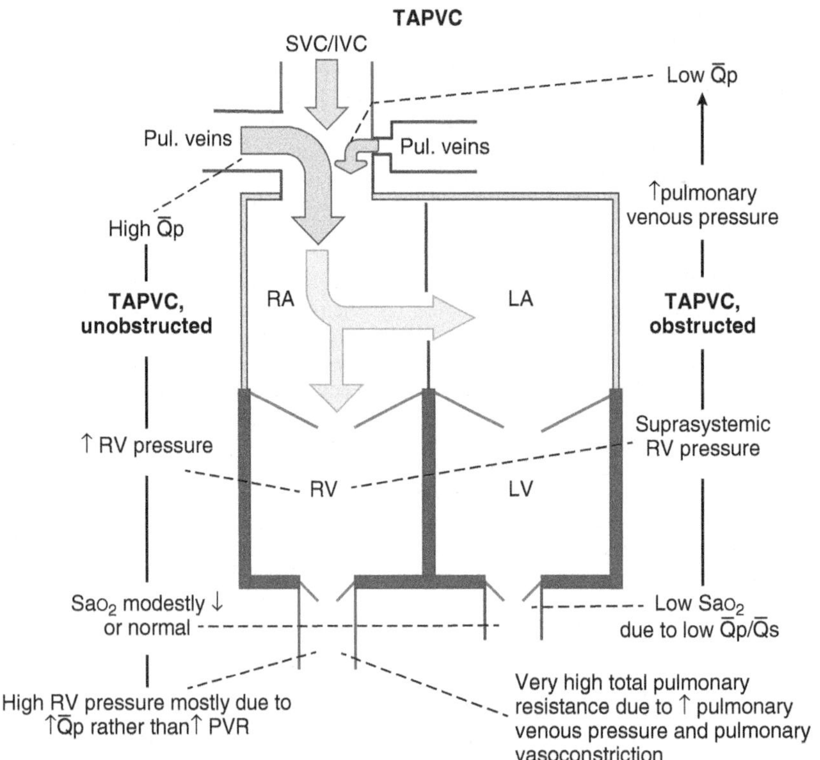

Fig. 49.8 Total anomalous pulmonary venous connection *(TAPVC)*, with and without obstruction. In addition to reduced pulmonary blood flow *($\dot{Q}p$)* and intracardiac shunting, with obstructed TAPVC pulmonary edema impairs lung function, further compromising oxygenation and ventilation. *IVC,* Inferior vena cava; *LA,* left atrium; *LV,* left ventricle; *PVR,* pulmonary vascular resistance; *$\dot{Q}p/\dot{Q}s$*, pulmonary to systemic flow ratio; *RA,* right atrium; *RV,* right ventricle; *Sao_2*, systemic arterial O_2 saturation; *SVC,* superior vena cava.

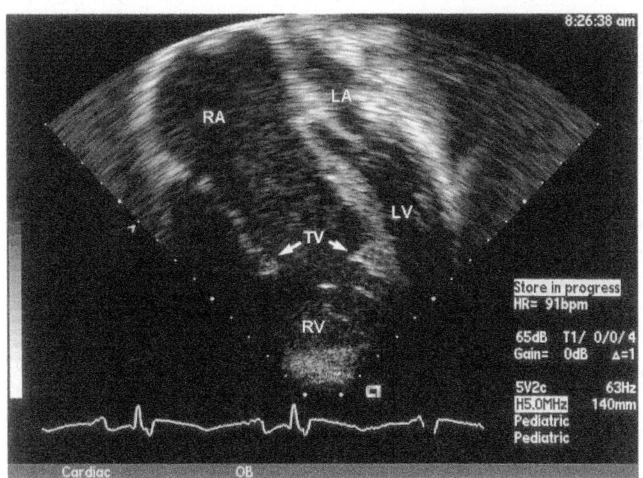

Fig. 49.9 A cardiac ultrasound scan of a patient with Ebstein anomaly. The dilated right-sided structures impinge on the much smaller left ventricle *(LV)*. *LA,* Left atrium; *RA,* right atrium; *RV,* right ventricle; *TV,* tricuspid valve.

THE DUCTUS ARTERIOSUS IN NEONATES WITH CRITICAL CONGENITAL CARDIAC DEFECTS

The DA has a biologic role in neonates with heart defects that ranges from physiologic and supportive to pathologic.[102] Found in nearly every neonate at birth, the DA plays a role in sustaining the fetal circulation and typically undergoes spontaneous closure after assisting a normal circulatory transition in term and preterm infants.[103] A small subset of patients is born without a DA because it closed prematurely in utero or never developed (e.g., truncus arteriosus).A patent DA (PDA) is a DA that remains open past the natural history, which varies based on gestational age at birth. With a hemodynamically significant DA it not only remains patent (occurring more often in low-birth-weight infants), but the volume of the shunt is sufficiently large that cardiovascular compromise may ensue. But in neonates with CHD, ductal patency may be critical to supporting the circulation. An understanding of the role of the DA in neonates with CHD is therefore mandatory for the neonatologist.

Neonates with CHD and ductal dependency can be categorized into three broad groups: (1) right-sided obstructive lesions with ductal-dependent pulmonary circulation, (2) left-sided obstructive lesions with ductal-dependent systemic circulation, and (3) d-transposition of the great arteries (and similar malformations) where ductal patency is often required for adequate mixing of the pulmonary and systemic venous blood, mostly in the atria (Table 49.1).[104]

With anatomic obstruction to $\dot{Q}p$, infants present as cyanotic and possibly hypoxic, with oxygen saturations generally between 75% and 85% but sometimes lower or higher. In the absence of a PDA, hypoxia develops due to inadequate $\dot{Q}p$. The hypoxemia may compromise organ function and, if severe enough, lead to death; a PDA is required until surgical intervention or catheter palliation provides an alternate source of $\dot{Q}p$.

With anatomic obstruction to $\dot{Q}s$, the DA maintains adequate systemic perfusion. These ductal-dependent lesions present with signs of poor perfusion in the presence of a constricting or closed DA. Other signs and symptoms include hypotension, weak or absent pulses, acidosis, and shock. With critical coarctation of the aorta, a patent ductus widens the pathway from the aortic isthmus to the descending aorta and allows the RV to provide descending aortic blood flow. With interruption of the aortic arch, the ductus allows the RV to supply all (excepting that provided by any collaterals) descending aortic flow. With critical aortic stenosis, the RV provides much or nearly all $\dot{Q}s$; with

Table 49.1 The Ductus Arteriosus in Congenital Cardiac Defects.

Role of DA	Examples of CHD	Physiologic Affect	Clinical Presentation
DA required for adequate pulmonary blood flow	• Two ventricle malformations with severe obstruction to $\dot{Q}p$ (e.g., tetralogy of Fallot, critical pulmonary stenosis) • Single ventricle malformations with significant obstruction to $\dot{Q}p$ (e.g., tricuspid atresia with obstruction from LV to the pulmonary artery) • Severe Ebstein malformation with pulmonary atresia, or inadequate RV pressure generation to propel blood into the lungs	$\dot{Q}p$ is inadequate without a patent DA	Postnatal constriction of the DA causes cyanosis, hypoxemia, and related symptoms
DA required for adequate systemic blood flow	• Any malformation with critical narrowing between systemic ventricle and the aorta (e.g., hypoplastic left heart syndrome, interrupted arch, coarctation of the aorta, critical aortic stenosis)	$\dot{Q}s$ is inadequate without a patent DA	Postnatal constriction of the DA causes tachycardia, poor perfusion, hypotension, weak or absent pulses, shock
DA required for aorta-to-pulmonary shunt for adequate atrial level mixing	• D-Transposition of the great arteries • Double-outlet right ventricle with subpulmonary VSD	Inadequate mixing of pulmonary venous and systemic venous blood with resulting hypoxemia without a patent duct	Infant may present with early profound hypoxia, especially in presence of restrictive PFO

CHD, Congenital heart defects; *DA*, ductus arteriosus; *PFO*, patent foramen ovale; *RV*, right ventricle; *VSD*, ventricular septal defect.

hypoplastic left heart syndrome the RV supplies the entire $\dot{Q}s$ (and $\dot{Q}p$). With most left-sided ductal-dependent lesions the RV is either the systemic pump or augments flow from the LV, but not always. For example, in tricuspid atresia and transposition of the great arteries, with obstruction to systemic flow, the LV is the systemic pump.

The DA may also be beneficial in lesions with parallel circulations and poor mixing, the vast majority of which are d-transposition of the great arteries (d-TGA). In these malformations a PDA (assuming PVR is less than SVR) increases $\dot{Q}p$ and increases atrial mixing. Not all babies with d-TGA require an open duct for mixing, but many do. (But note that in a minority of babies with d-TGA and PDA, the ductal shunt is large enough to cause hemodynamic instability.)

Finally, there are a few other ductus-related considerations. Patients with total anomalous pulmonary venous connection with obstruction may have supra-systemic resistance to flow through the lungs; a PDA will allow shunting from the PA into the aorta, hence *reducing* $\dot{Q}p$ and systemic arterial O_2 saturation. Also, as physiology changes, so too may the role of a PDA. For example, a neonate with critical aortic stenosis may have so little LV output that a PDA is beneficial in allowing the RV to supplement $\dot{Q}s$. But after balloon dilation of the valve, LV output increases and a PDA now serves only to allow left-to-right shunting through the lungs. Finally—although this is not related to cardiac malformations—a PDA may be helpful when PVR exceeds SVR by limiting RV pressure to systemic levels and thereby helping to preserve RV function; babies with congenital diaphragmatic hernia are one such example.

CONCLUSIONS

Structural cardiac malformations have a variety of effects that, depending upon the defect(s), include (1) increased ventricular volume load (left-to-right intracardiac shunting, valve regurgitation); (2) right-to-left intracardiac shunting (due to obstruction of pulmonary arterial flow or mixing of systemic and pulmonary venous blood); (3) increased ventricular afterload (semilunar valve stenosis, coarctation, pulmonary arterial hypertension); and (4) impeded ventricular filling (atrioventricular valve stenosis, hypoplasia of the ventricle). Other variables influence the defect-driven physiology in important ways (e.g., systemic and PVR, ventricular systolic and diastolic function, hematocrit, $\dot{V}O_2$, lung function, pulmonary and body wall edema). SOT is sometimes significantly or even critically impaired as a result of reduced $\dot{Q}s$, hypoxemia, or both. In others, resting SOT is preserved, but reduced cardiovascular reserve, and CHF (including failure to thrive) are the major phenotypic manifestations. Determining the impact of a cardiac defect on the clinical phenotype can usually be accomplished by estimating or measuring intracardiac pressures and blood flows using echocardiography, although occasionally cardiac catheterization is required.

A complete reference list is available at www.ExpertConsult.com. 

SELECT REFERENCES

1. Sylvester JT, Goldberg HS, Permutt S. The role of the vasculature in the regulation of cardiac output. *Clin Chest Med*. 1983;4:111.
2. Chatterjee K. Neurohormonal activation in congestive heart failure and the role of vasopressin. *Am J Cardiol*. 2005;95(suppl):8B.
3. Schrier RW, Abraham WT. Hormones and hemodynamics in heart failure. *N Engl J Med*. 1999;341:577.
4. Turley K, Ebert PA. Transposition of the great arteries in the neonate: failed balloon septostomy. *J Cardiovasc Surg*. 1985;26:564.
5. Rudolph AM. Congenital cardiovascular malformations and the fetal circulation. *Arch Dis Child Neonatal Ed*. 2010;95:F132.
6. Rudolph AM. Fetal circulation and postnatal adaptation. In: Rudolph AM, ed. *Congenital Diseases of the Heart: Clinical-Physiological Considerations*. 2nd ed. Armonk, NY: Futura Publishing; 2001:3–44.
7. Fineman JR, Soifer SJ, Heymann MA. Regulation of pulmonary vascular tone in the perinatal period. *Annu Rev Physiol*. 1995;57:115.
8. Abman SH, Stevens T. Perinatal pulmonary vasoregulation: implications for the pathophysiology and treatment of neonatal pulmonary hypertension. In: Haddad GG, Lister G, eds. *Tissue Oxygen Deprivation: From Molecular to Integrated Function*. New York: Marcel Dekker; 1996:367–432.
9. Rabinovitch M. Developmental biology of the pulmonary vasculature. In: Polin RA, Fox WW, Abman SH, eds. *Fetal and Neonatal Physiology*. 4th ed. Philadelphia: Saunders; 2011:757–772.
10. Vargo TA. Cardiac catheterization: hemodynamic measurements. In: Garson Jr A, Bricker JT, Fisher DJ, Neish SR, eds. *The Science and Practice of Pediatric Cardiology*. 2nd ed. Baltimore: Williams & Wilkins; 1998:961–993.
11. Hoffman JIE, Rudolph AM. The natural history of ventricular septal defects in infancy. *Am J Cardiol*. 1965;16:634.
12. Lister G, Hellenbrand WE, Kleinman CS, Talner NS. Physiologic effects of increasing hemoglobin concentration in left-to-right shunting in infants with ventricular septal defects. *N Engl J Med*. 1982;306:502.

13. Kulik TJ, Rhein LM, Mullen MP. Pulmonary hypertension in infants with chronic lung disease: will we ever understand it? *J Pediatr*. 2010;157:186.
14. Lister G, Moreau G, Moss M, Talner NS. Effects of alterations of oxygen transport on the neonate. *Semin Perinatol*. 1984;8:192.
15. Rudolph AM. Hypoxia: historical and unresolved issues. In: Haddad GG, Lister G, eds. *Tissue Oxygen Deprivation: From Molecular to Integrated Function*. New York: Marcel Dekker; 1996:5-11.
16. Sidi D, Kuipers JR, Teitel D, et al. Developmental changes in oxygenation and circulatory responses to hypoxia in lambs. *Am J Physiol*. 1983;245:H674.
17. Moss M, Moreau G, Lister G. Oxygen transport and metabolism in the conscious lamb: the effects of hypoxia. *Pediatr Res*. 1987;22:177.
18. Cross KW, Tizard JP, Trythall DA. The gaseous metabolism of the new-born infant breathing 15% oxygen. *Acta Paediatr*. 1958;47:217.
19. Newburger JW, Jonas RA, Wernovsky G, et al. A comparison of the perioperative neurologic effects of hypothermic circulatory arrest versus low-flow cardiopulmonary bypass in infant heart surgery. *N Engl J Med*. 1993;329:1057.
20. Bellinger DC, Wypij D, Rivkin MJ, et al. Adolescents with d-transposition of the great arteries corrected with the arterial switch procedure: neurological assessment and structure brain imaging. *Circulation*. 2011;124:1361.
21. Fahey JT, Lister G. Postnatal changes in critical cardiac output and oxygen transport in conscious lambs. *Am J Physiol*. 1987;253:H100.
22. Beekman RH, Rocchini AP, Rosenthal A. Hemodynamic effects of nitroprusside in infants with a large ventricular septal defect. *Circulation*. 1981;64:553.
23. Beekman RH, Rocchini AP, Rosenthal A. Hemodynamic effects of hydralazine in infants with a large ventricular defect. *Circulation*. 1982;65:523.
24. Berman Jr W, Yabek SM, Dillon T. Effects of digoxin in infants with a congested circulatory state due to a ventricular septal defect. *N Engl J Med*. 1983; 308:363.
25. Weber KT. Aldosterone in congestive heart failure. *N Engl J Med*. 2001; 345:1689.
26. Lees MH. Catecholamine metabolite excretion of infants with heart failure. *J Pediatr*. 1966;69:259.
27. Ross RD, Daniels SR, Schwartz DC, et al. Plasma norepinephrine levels in infants and children with congestive heart failure. *Am J Cardiol*. 1987;59:911.
28. Baylen BG, Johnson G, Tsang R, et al. The occurrence of hyperaldosteronism in infants with congestive heart failure. *Am J Cardiol*. 1980;45:305.
29. Scammell AM, Diver MJ. Plasma renin activity in infants with congenital heart disease. *Arch Dis Child*. 1987;62:1136.
30. Barrington K, Chan W. The circulatory effects of epinephrine infusion in the anesthetized piglet. *Pediatr Res*. 1993;33:190.
31. Brace RA. Fluid distribution in the fetus and neonate. In: Polin RA, Fox WW, eds. *Fetal and Neonatal Physiology*. 2nd ed. Philadelphia: Saunders; 1998:1711.
32. Mitzner W. Resistance of the pulmonary circulation. *Clin Chest Med*. 1983;4:127.
33. Rudolph AM. Prenatal and postnatal pulmonary circulation. In: Rudolph AM, ed. *Congenital Diseases of the Heart: Clinical-Physiological Considerations*. 2nd ed. Armonk, NY: Futura Publishing; 2001:121-152.
34. Dawes GS. Sudden death in babies: physiology of the fetus and newborn. *Am J Cardiol*. 1968;22:469.
35. Levin AR, Spach MS, Canent Jr RV, et al. Intracardiac pressure-flow dynamics in isolated ventricular septal defects. *Circulation*. 1967;35:430.
36. Graham Jr TP, Atwood GF, Boucek Jr RJ, et al. Right ventricular volume characteristics in ventricular septal defect. *Circulation*. 1976;54:800.
37. Reddy VM, Liddicoat JR, Fineman JR, et al. Fetal model of single ventricle physiology: hemodynamic effects of oxygen, nitric oxide, carbon dioxide, and hypoxia in the early postnatal period. *J Thorac Cardiovasc Surg*. 1996;112:437.
38. Jarmakani MM, Graham Jr TP, Canent Jr RV, et al. Effect of site of shunt on left heart-volume characteristics in children with ventricular septal defect and patent ductus arteriosus. *Circulation*. 1969;40:411.
39. Hoffman JIE. Transmural myocardial perfusion. *Prog Cardiovasc Dis*. 1987; 29:429.
40. Bernhard WF, Dick 2nd M, Sloss LJ, et al. The palliative mustard operation for double outlet right ventricle or transposition of the great arteries associated with ventricular septal defect, pulmonary arterial hypertension, and pulmonary vascular obstructive disease. *Circulation*. 1976;54:810.
41. Levin AR, Spach MS, Boineau JP, et al. Atrial pressure-flow dynamics in atrial septal defects (secundum type). *Circulation*. 1968;37:476.
42. Hoffman JI, Rudolph AM, Danilowicz D. Left to right atrial shunts in infants. *Am J Cardiol*. 1972;30:868.
43. Hunt CE, Lucas RV. Symptomatic atrial septal defect in infancy. *Circulation*. 1973;67:1042.
44. Rudolph AM. Atrial septal defect: partial anomalous drainage of pulmonary veins. In: Rudolph AM, ed. *Congenital Diseases of the Heart: Clinical-Physiological Considerations*. 2nd ed. Armonk, NY: Futura Publishing; 2001:253-254.
45. Kulik TJ. Pulmonary blood flow and pulmonary hypertension: is the pulmonary circulation flowophobic or flowophilic? *Pulm Circ*. 2012;2:327.
46. Gathman GE, Nadas AS. Total anomalous pulmonary venous connection: clinical and physiologic observations of 75 pediatric patients. *Circulation*. 1970;62:143.
47. Delisle G, Ando M, Calder AL, et al. Total anomalous pulmonary venous connection: report of 93 autopsied cases with emphasis on diagnostic and surgical considerations. *Am Heart J*. 1976;91:99-122.
48. Cumming GR. Circulation in neonates with intracranial arteriovenous fistula and cardiac failure. *Am J Cardiol*. 1980;45:1019.
49. Ward KE, Mullins CE, Huhta JC, et al. Restrictive interatrial communication in total anomalous pulmonary venous connection. *Am J Cardiol*. 1986;57:1131.
50. Barnea O, Austin EH, Richman B, Santamore WP. Balancing the circulation: theoretic optimization of pulmonary/systemic flow ratio in hypoplastic left heart syndrome. *J Am Coll Cardiol*. 1994;24:1376.

50 Regulation of Cardiovascular Function During Fetal and Newborn Life

Dino A. Giussani | Jeffrey L. Segar

INTRODUCTION

The regulation of cardiovascular function in the fetal and newborn periods is mediated through interacting neural, endocrine, and metabolic mechanisms acting at central, systemic, and local levels. The role of the central nervous system, in particular, is critical for cardiovascular homeostasis, including maintenance of blood pressure within normal limits.[1,2] Sympathetic outflow to the heart and blood vessels is continuously modulated by an array of peripheral sensors, including arterial baroreceptors and chemoreceptors located in the aortic arch and carotid bifurcation, as well as mechanoreceptors located in the heart and lungs.[3] Cardiovascular responses triggered through neural reflexes can then be maintained or modified by endocrine and local redox responses. Although these basic mechanisms likely exist in the fetus and newborn, differential rates of maturation of these systems influence the ability of the developing individual to maintain adequate perfusion pressure and organ blood flow.

NEURAL MODULATION OF BASAL CARDIOVASCULAR FUNCTION

Tonic discharge of spinal vasoconstrictor neurons is an important regulator of vasomotor tone and, ultimately, maintenance of arterial pressure within its physiologic range.[4] Studies in sheep, which to date have served as the most common model for studying integrative developmental cardiovascular physiology, show that the contribution of the autonomic nervous system on cardiovascular homeostasis clearly changes during development. Both α-adrenergic and ganglionic blockade produce greater decreases in blood pressure in term, than preterm, fetal sheep.[5,6] The hypotensive effect following α-adrenergic and ganglionic blockade is less in newborn lambs than term fetuses and continues to decline with postnatal development.[7] Sympathetic nerve efferents co-release norepinephrine and neuropeptide Y (NPY) from sympathetic varicosities, both of which exert potent pressor and peripheral vasopressor effects in fetal sheep.[8,9] The peripheral vasoconstrictor effect resulting from sympathetic outflow is likely fine-tuned in the late gestation fetus by an opposing vasodilator influence, such as nitric oxide (NO). For instance, treatment of fetal sheep in late gestation with NO synthase inhibitors during basal conditions leads to generalized peripheral vasoconstriction and a pronounced increase in fetal arterial blood pressure.[10,11] Combined, these findings suggest that sympathetic noradrenergic and peptidergic tone is pronounced in fetal life late in gestation, and that this is balanced by a NO dilator tone to provide the appropriate maintenance of fetal arterial pressure.

Maturational changes in parasympathetic function, particularly related to governance of heart rate, also exist.[12] Cholinergic blockade produces no consistent effect in heart rate in premature fetal sheep, a slight increase in heart rate in term fetuses, and the greatest effect in lambs beyond the first week of life.[6,7] Longitudinal studies in preterm and term infants of spectral indices of heart rate variability reveal parasympathetic modulation of heart rate increases over the first 6 months of life, though preterm infants exhibit less parasympathetic modulation at similar postnatal ages.[13,14]

Within a physiologic range, arterial pressure displays a naturally occurring variability, the degree of which is similar in fetal and postnatal life.[15-18] In the adult rat, ganglionic blockade increases arterial pressure variability,[15,19] suggesting that a component of arterial pressure lability is peripheral or humoral in origin and is buffered by autonomic functions. In contrast, ganglionic blockade in term fetal sheep significantly attenuates heart rate and arterial pressure variability.[17] Oscillations in basal sympathetic tone, as recorded from the renal sympathetic nerve, have been shown to be positively correlated with normal fluctuations in heart rate and arterial pressure, and appear to be related to changes in the behavioral state of the fetus.[17,20-22] Although fetal electrocortical and sympathetic activity were not recorded simultaneously in early studies, electrocortical activity appeared to mediate changes in both sympathetic and parasympathetic tone.[22,23] More recently, it has been confirmed that the near-term sheep fetus shows marked sleep-state-dependent changes in hemodynamics and resting renal sympathetic nerve activity (RSNA).[24] Moreover, there appears with advancing age an emergence of sleep-state-dependency on RSNA, as well as an increase in the basal level of RSNA.[25] Consistent with these findings, basal heart rate, arterial pressure, and catecholamine levels are highest during periods of high-voltage low-frequency electrocortical activity.[21,26,27] Other physiologic variables, including organ blood flows, regional vascular resistances, and cerebral oxygen consumption, are also dependent on electrocortical state and likely reflect changes in autonomic activity.[26,28,29]

THE ARTERIAL BAROREFLEX DURING DEVELOPMENT

ONTOGENY OF BAROREFLEX FUNCTION

Short-term changes in vascular stretch related to arterial pressure modify the discharge of afferent baroreceptors fibers located in the carotid sinus and aortic arch.[2] This, in turn, results in alterations in parasympathetic and sympathetic nerve activities that influence heart rate and peripheral vascular resistance and serve to buffer changes in arterial pressure.[30,31] Studies in sheep demonstrate the arterial baroreflex is functional during fetal and early postnatal life.[12,18,32,33] Investigators disagree, however, about the magnitude of the baroreflex early in development and the influence of these reflexes on controlling heart rate and arterial pressure. Early studies indicated that the threshold for baroreceptor activity is above the normal range of arterial pressure during fetal and neonatal life, and that baroreceptors may not be loaded during fetal life.[34,35] Other studies in fetal sheep demonstrate that sino-aortic denervation (SAD) produces marked fluctuations in fetal arterial pressure and heart rate,[18,33] suggesting that the arterial baroreflex plays an important role in maintaining cardiovascular homeostasis. Evidence for the presence of functional baroreceptors in the immature animal is provided by single fiber recordings of baroreceptor afferents in the carotid sinus and aortic depressor nerves.[36-39] In fetal and newborn animals carotid sinus nerve activity is phasic and pulse synchronous while activity increases with a rise in arterial or carotid sinus pressure.[37,38,40] Basal discharge of baroreceptor afferents does not change during fetal and postnatal maturation, despite a considerable increase in mean arterial pressure during this time.[37] These findings are consistent with those demonstrated in developing rabbits[39] and indicate that baroreceptors reset during development, such that they continue to function within the physiologic range for arterial pressure. Furthermore, the response of carotid baroreceptor activity to increases in carotid sinus pressure is greater in fetal than in newborn and 1-month-old lambs.[37] The threshold for carotid baroreceptor discharge is lower and the sensitivity of the baroreceptor is also greater in newborn, compared to adult, rabbits.[39] Although parasympathetic influence on heart rate early during development is limited,[32,41-44] results obtained from direct recording of baroreceptor afferents[37,39] demonstrate that the sensitivity of the baroreceptors is greater during early development and resets at a lower level as arterial pressure increases during fetal and postnatal life. These findings suggest that reduced heart rate responses to changes in arterial pressure during fetal life are not due to underdeveloped afferent activity of baroreceptors but to differences in central integration and efferent parasympathetic nerve activity.

The mechanisms regulating the changes in sensitivity of the baroreceptors early in development have not been investigated, but may be similar to those proposed in the adult.[45-47] In younger animals, the carotid sinus is more distensible, resulting in an increase in the degree of mechanical deformation of nerve endings and, ultimately, in a greater strain sensitivity.[45] Alternatively, ionic mechanisms,[46,48] such as activation of the sodium pump that may operate at the receptor membrane to cause hyperpolarization of the endings, and substances released from the endothelium, including prostacyclin[49] and NO,[50-52] may modulate baroreceptor activity during development. Blockade of cyclooxygenase with indomethacin reduces carotid baroreceptor sensitivity in newborn, but not adult, sheep.[53] Along these lines, prostaglandin E_2 and I_2 levels within carotid sinus tissues are sixfold higher in newborn than adult sheep.[53] Whether such influences on baroreceptor activity are present during fetal development has not been investigated.

Arterial baroreflex function and sensitivity are equally dependent on the efferent limb of the reflex, including sympathetic and parasympathetic nerve activity and end organ neuroeffector responsiveness. The arterial baroreflex during fetal and postnatal maturation has primarily been investigated by examining the relationship between the increase in arterial pressure and the fall in heart rate.[33,35,42,54,55] Baroreflex control of fetal heart rate is dominated by changes in cardiac vagal tone, although integrity of the reflex is dependent upon both sympathetic and parasympathetic pathways.[56] A number of studies describe a relatively reduced heart rate response to alterations in arterial pressure in fetal and newborn animals, and in human infants.[35,43,44,57] Recording reflex bradycardia in response to increased blood pressure induced by balloon inflation, Shinebourne and colleagues[43] found that baroreflex activity is present as early as 0.6 gestation in fetal lambs, and that the sensitivity of the reflex increased up to term. Studies in sheep[44] and other species[58,59] have similarly found increasing baroreflex sensitivity with postnatal age. In addition to changes in the sensitivity, or slope of the relationship between change in blood pressure and change in heart rate that occur with maturation, the

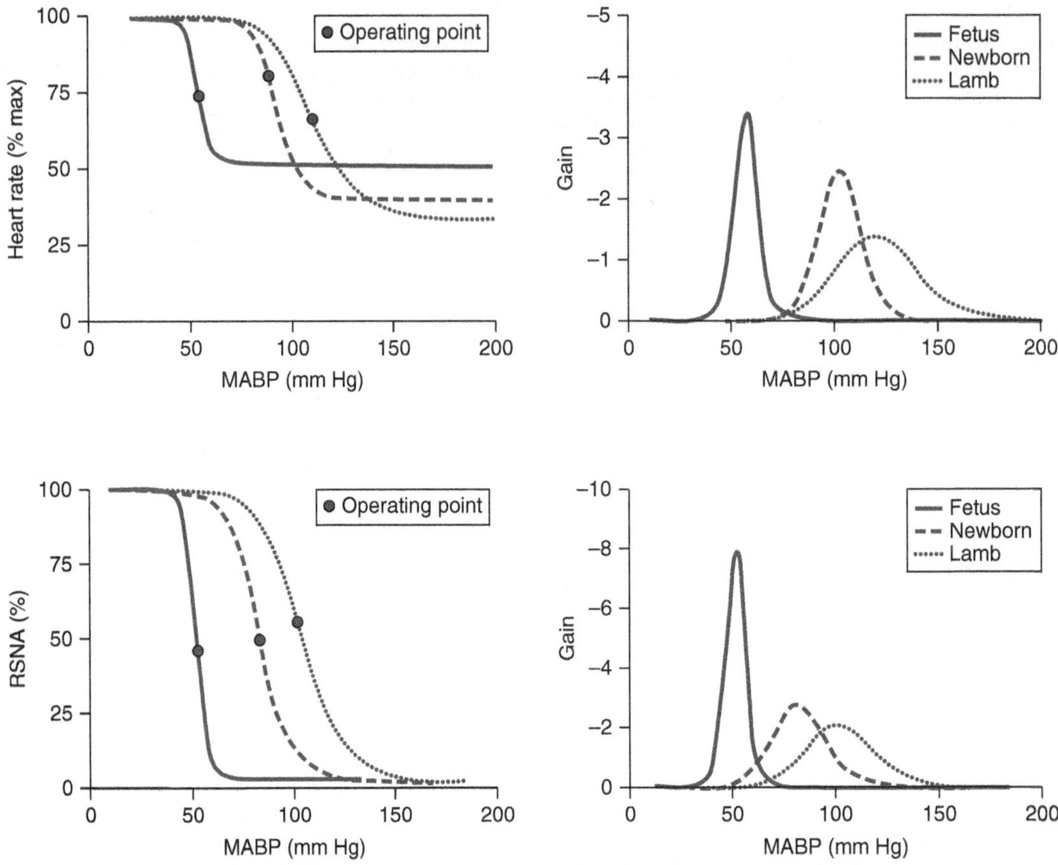

Fig. 50.1 Ontogeny of baroreflex responses during early development. Baroreflex function curves relating heart rate *(top)* and renal sympathetic nerve activity (RSNA, *bottom*) to mean arterial blood pressure *(MABP)* in near-term fetal, newborn (7 days old), and 4- to 6-week old lambs. Heart rate and RSNA are expressed as % of maximum response elicited during hypotension induced by nitroprusside infusion. Gain of curve reflects the sensitivity, as measured by slope, over the range of MABP, and is derived by taking the first derivative of the baroreflex curve. •, Operating point, representing basal values relative to curves. (From Segar JL, Hajduczok G, Smith BA, et al. Ontogeny of baroreflex control of renal sympathetic nerve activity and heart rate. *Am J Physiol.* 1992;263:H1819–H1826, with permission.)

response time of heart rate changes to hypotension are markedly slower in preterm compared to term fetus.[60] Maturational changes continue to occur during postnatal life. For example, reflex bradycardia in response to carotid sinus stimulation is absent during the first week of life in the piglet, although vagal efferents exert a tonic action on the heart at this stage of development.[58] Age-related changes in heart rate in response to phenylephrine are also greater in 2-month old piglets than in 1-day old animals.[59] On the other hand, several studies suggest that the sensitivity of the cardiac baroreflex is, in fact, greater in the fetus than in the newborn and decreases with maturation.[55,61] For example, studies in the fetal horse have reported that fetal cardiac baroreflex sensitivity decreased with advancing gestational age.[62]

Developmental changes in control of efferent RSNA in response to increases and decreases in blood pressure over the last third of gestation and after birth have been examined.[60,63,64] These studies demonstrate that baroreceptor activity regulates sympathetic outflow as well as heart rate during fetal life, that functional baroreflex control of RSNA shifts toward higher pressures during development, and that the sensitivity of the RSNA baroreflex function curve is greatest in the late term fetus and decreases following the transition from fetal to newborn life (Fig. 50.1). Although cardiac baroreflex function is present in the preterm sheep fetus (0.7 of gestation), there is no significant baroreflex control of RSNA at this stage of development.[60] It is likely that attenuated cardiac and RSNA responses to hypotension described in these animal studies may contribute to blood pressure instability in the preterm infant.

Several reasons for reported differences in the sensitivity of baroreflex function early in development are apparent. First, there is interspecies variability in the maturation of sympathetic and parasympathetic activity and function, including maturity of the central and efferent components of the reflex.[59] For example, a functional baroreflex is not present in rats until three weeks of age,[65] while baroreceptor sensitivity in newborn pigs and dogs is low, increasing with postnatal age.[44,59] Second, there have been differences in experimental design and analysis of baroreflex responses. Investigators have studied baroreflex responses to alterations in blood pressure using either pharmacologic agents[33,55] or intravascular balloon inflation,[43,55] and analyzed responses using derived sigmoidal baroreflex curves or linear slopes.[63] These considerations are important, particularly as it has now become clear that—in addition to interspecies differences—there may be differential maturation of the vagal and sympathetic components mediating cardiac baroreflex responses that would not be appreciated from complete sigmoidal autonomic baroreflex curve analysis.

Resetting of the arterial baroreflex is defined as a change in the relation between arterial pressure and heart rate; or between pressure and sympathetic and parasympathetic nerve activities.[46,47] As noted earlier, a number of studies demonstrate that the sensitivity of the baroreflex changes with maturation and shifts or resets toward higher pressures.[63,66,67] This shift occurs during fetal life, is present immediately after birth, and continues with postnatal maturation, paralleling the naturally occurring increase in blood pressure.[68] The mechanisms regulating developmental changes in baroreflex sensitivity and controlling the resetting of the baroreflex are poorly understood. Changes in the relationship between arterial pressure and sympathetic activity or heart rate can occur at the level of the baroreceptor itself (peripheral resetting) or from altered coupling within the central nervous system of afferent impulses from baroreceptors to efferent sympathetic or parasympathetic activities (central resetting).[46] Locally produced factors, such as NO; circulating hormones and neuropeptides such as angiotensin II (ANG II), vasopressin (AVP), and serotonin; and activation of additional neural reflex pathways likely modulate the changes in arterial baroreflex set-point and sensitivity during development.[46,69,70]

HORMONAL INTERACTIONS ON BAROREFLEX FUNCTION

The arterial baroreflex not only modulates heart rate and the peripheral vascular tone by altering autonomic activity, the baroreflex also regulates the release of vasoactive hormones, such as ANG II and AVP.[69,71] Changes in the levels of these circulating hormones, in turn, may influence neural regulation of cardiovascular function by acting at several sites along the baroreflex arc.[69] In the adult, ANG II facilitates activation of sympathetic ganglia and enhances the release and response of norepinephrine at the neuroeffector junction.[72] Within the central nervous system, ANG II stimulates sympathetic outflow and alters baroreceptor reflexes by acting on ANG II type 1 (AT_1) receptors located within the hypothalamus, medulla, and circumventricular organs.[73-75]

Endogenous ANG II participates in regulating arterial baroreflex responses during early development. The absence of rebound tachycardia after reduction in blood pressure by angiotensin converting enzyme (ACE) inhibitors is well described in fetal and postnatal animals,[76] as well in human adults and infants.[77] In the newborn lamb, ACE inhibition or angiotensin II type 1 (AT_1) receptor blockade decreases RSNA and heart rate and resets the baroreflex toward lower pressure.[70,78] Resetting of the reflex is independent of changes in prevailing blood pressure. Lateral ventricle administration of an AT_1 but not AT_2 receptor antagonist also lowers blood pressure and resets the baroreflex toward lower pressure in newborn and 8-week-old sheep at doses that have no effect when given systemically.[78] Converting enzyme inhibition has no effect on baroreflex control of RSNA in fetal sheep.[70] However, when enalapril is administered to the fetus immediately prior to delivery, baroreflex control of RSNA and heart rate in the newly born lamb is shifted toward lower pressures.[70] Two- to fourfold higher levels of ANG II in the newborn than in fetal or adult sheep may help explain these observations.[79]

The effects of exogenous ANG II on reflex control of fetal heart rate have been studied. In the sheep fetus, a rise in arterial blood pressure produced by ANG II administration produces little or no cardiac slowing,[79,80] though dose-dependent decreases in heart rate have been reported.[42,61] The bradycardic and sympathoinhibitory responses to given increase in blood pressure is less for ANG II than that produced by other vasoconstrictor agents.[70] As in adults, ANG II is likely to act centrally (primarily within the area postrema) to interfere with the cardiac baroreflex through suppression of vagal efferents.[42,81,82]

In adults of several species, vasopressin has also been reported to modulate parasympathetic and sympathetic tone, ultimately regulating cardiovascular and baroreflex function.[69,83,84] Administration of AVP evokes greater sympathoinhibition and bradycardia than other vasoconstrictors for a comparable increase in blood pressure.[69,84] This modulation of the baroreflex has been attributed to AVP enhancing the gain of the reflex as well as resetting the reflex to a lower pressure.[69,84] There is disagreement, however, regarding the type of vasopressin receptor that mediates the action of the peptide on the baroreflex. Several studies suggest that activation of AVP type 1 (V_1) receptor enhances the inhibitory effect of the arterial baroreflex on heart rate and sympathetic outflow, whereas others conclude that V_2 receptors are involved.[84,85]

Studies during fetal and newborn life demonstrate that AVP secretory mechanisms are well developed early in life, and that AVP increases fetal arterial pressure and decreases heart rate in a dose-dependent manner.[86,87] However, endogenous AVP appears to have little effect on baroreflex function during early development. Administration of a V_1-receptor antagonist has no measurable effects on resting hemodynamics in fetal sheep or on basal arterial blood pressure,[88] heart rate, RSNA, or baroreflex response in newborn lambs.[89] This lack of baroreflex modulation by AVP may facilitate the pressor response to AVP in fetuses and newborns during stressful situations such as during hypoxia and hemorrhage. In this way, AVP could play a particularly important role in maintaining arterial pressures during these conditions early in development. For example, vasopressin V_1 receptor antagonism impaired the maintenance of arterial blood pressure in the fetus during an acute hypoxic challenge.[89-91]

Though not regarded as a classic neurotransmitter or neurohumoral factor, NO plays an important role in autonomic control of systemic hemodynamics early in development. In vivo studies demonstrate that NO attenuates the sensitivity of the cardiac baroreflex during fetal life, while pharmacologic blockade of NO synthase abolishes age-related differences in baroreflex control of heart rate in 1- and 6-week-old lambs.[52,91] The site of action for NO has not been identified, although NO synthase immunoreactivity has been shown in multiple locations along the central baroreflex pathway and in preganglionic sympathetic neurons, and appears to be developmentally regulated in sheep brain stem.[92-94]

Accumulating evidence shows that both endogenous and exogenous glucocorticoids during early development can have significant effects on the set-point and gain of the arterial baroreflex, similar to that shown in adult animals.[95,96] In adrenalectomized fetal sheep, restoring circulating cortisol levels to the prepartum physiologic range shifts the fetal and neonatal heart rate and RSNA baroreflex function curves toward higher pressure without altering the slope of the curves.[97] Treatment of preterm fetal sheep with low doses of dexamethasone induced a parallel rightward shift in the pulse interval—arterial blood pressure relationship, indicating an increase in set-point but not in the sensitivity of the cardiac baroreflex.[98] Other studies found antenatal administration of betamethasone decreases the sensitivity of baroreflex-mediated changes in heart rate in preterm fetuses and premature lambs.[99] Of interest, adult sheep exposed to antenatal betamethasone display increased blood pressure and decreased baroreflex sensitivity compared to age-matched controls. The impairment of baroreflex sensitivity precedes the elevation in blood pressure and appears to involve an imbalance in renin-angiotensin–dependent cardiovascular regulation.[100]

In sheep, treatment of ewes with dexamethasone for 48 hours at the end of the first month of pregnancy, induces an increase in basal arterial blood pressure in lambs at 3 months of age.[101] Interestingly, newborn lambs exposed in utero to this early course of dexamethasone display a shift in the cardiac baroreflex towards higher pressures without a concomitant increase in resting blood pressure.[102] Taken together, these findings suggest that inappropriate exposure to glucocorticoids in early life may contribute to the programming of an increased risk of hypertension in later life as a result of induced changes in baroreflex setting and sensitivity. Of interest, 2-week-old human newborns born from mothers treated with dexamethasone had higher mean blood pressure than newborns from mothers who received a placebo.[103] However, 30-year follow-up of over 500 adults whose mothers participated in a randomized trial to receive antenatal betamethasone for prevention of respiratory distress syndrome failed to identify differences in blood pressure or history of cardiovascular disease.[104]

THE ARTERIAL CHEMOREFLEX DURING DEVELOPMENT

ONTOGENY OF CHEMOREFLEX FUNCTION

Acute hypoxia evokes integrated cardiovascular, metabolic, and endocrine responses that likely facilitate fetal survival. The fetal cardiovascular responses include transient bradycardia, an increase in arterial blood pressure, and an increase in peripheral vascular resistance.[105,106] The bradycardia reduces oxygen consumption by the fetal heart.[107,108] The increase in peripheral vascular resistance contributes to the maintenance of arterial blood pressure and the redistribution of the fetal cardiac output away from peripheral circulations and towards essential vascular beds, such as those perfusing the brain.[106] The bradycardia is mediated by parasympathetic efferents, as it can be blocked by atropine,[108] while the peripheral vasoconstriction triggered by the chemoreceptor stimulation results from increased sympathetic tone and can be prevented with α-adrenergic antagonists.[109,110]

In the adult and fetus, discrete chemoreceptor sites are located in the carotid and the aortic bodies. Recordings from carotid chemoreceptors in fetal sheep demonstrated responses to natural stimuli from ca. 90 days of gestation.[37,111] For example, chemoreceptor units increased discharge when exposed to CO_2– saturated saline. Blanco and colleagues[111] concluded that in the fetus the carotid chemoreceptors were active and responsive to hypoxia, but only to changes in PaO_2 within the fetal range. Furthermore, the position of the response curve of the chemoreceptors to hypoxia was shifted to the left and the sensitivity to an absolute change of arterial PO_2 was less compared to that of the adult.

The rise in arterial pressure and the fall in fetal heart rate seen in intact fetuses during hypoxemia are absent in fetuses following SAD (achieved by stripping of carotid sinus and cutting aortic and superior laryngeal nerves), suggesting that arterial chemoreceptor afferents in these structures mediate the responses.[112] Denervation of the aortic and carotid bodies not only abolished the fetal bradycardia and the increase in arterial pressure seen in intact fetuses but also attenuated peripheral vasoconstriction.[113] Compared to that in intact fetuses, redistribution of blood flow during hypoxia was attenuated after vagotomy (to disrupt aortic chemoreceptors) or vagotomy with carotid sinus-denervation, although the effects of combined vagotomy and carotid sinus denervation were greater than those of vagotomy alone, suggesting a greater role for the carotid chemoreceptors during acute fetal hypoxia.[114] More recently, it has been demonstrated that carotid sinus nerve denervation alone prevented fetal bradycardia and the initial increase in femoral vascular resistance during acute hypoxia, whereas selective aortic denervation did not (Fig. 50.2).[109,115] Thus, it appears that the carotid, and not the aortic, chemoreceptors principally trigger the fetal cardiovascular defense to an episode of oxygen deprivation.

Although chemoreceptors are active and responsive in the fetus and newborn, studies in sheep and human infants suggest that chemoreceptor sensitivity and activity is reduced immediately after birth.[111,116] This decreased sensitivity persists for several days until the chemoreceptors adapt and reset their sensitivity from the low oxygen tension of the fetus to that seen postnatally.[116,117] The mechanisms involved with this resetting are not known, although the postnatal rise in PaO_2 appears crucial as raising fetal PaO_2 produces a rightward shift in the response curve of carotid chemoreceptors to differing oxygen tension.[118] Holgert and colleagues[119] hypothesized that developmental changes in dopamine turnover within the carotid body contribute to the postnatal resetting of the arterial chemoreceptors. Studies of carotid chemoreceptor cells isolated from neonatal and adult rabbits suggest differences in intracellular calcium mobilization during hypoxia may also be an important component of chemoreceptor maturation.[120]

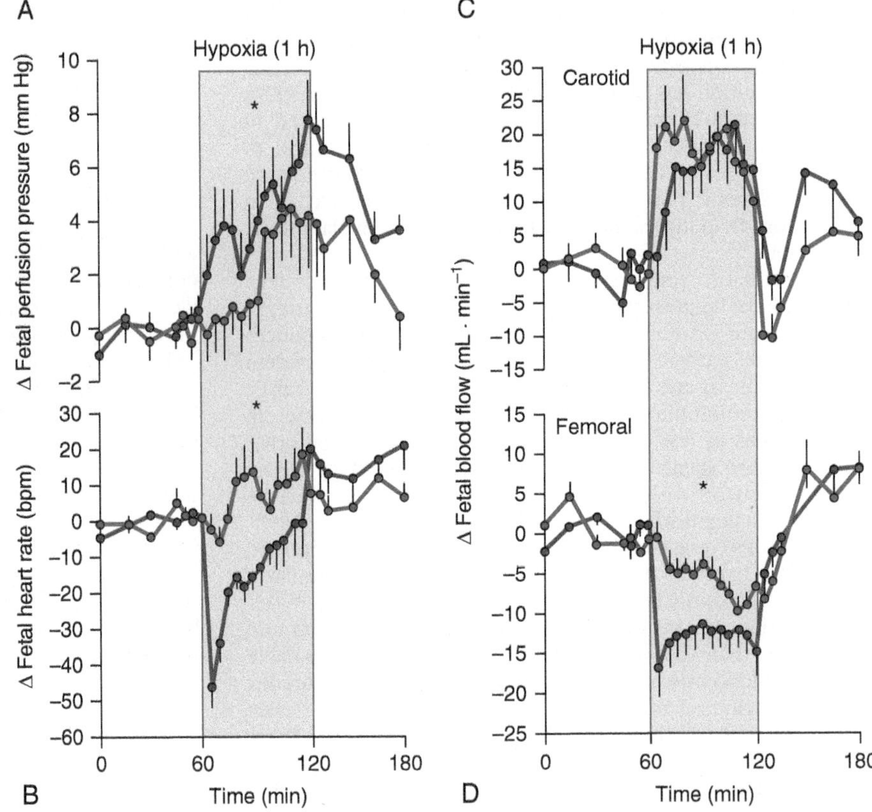

Fig. 50.2 Fetal cardiovascular responses to acute hypoxia. The data show mean ± SE for the change in fetal perfusion (arterial-venous) pressure (A), fetal heart rate (B), carotid blood flow (C), and femoral blood flow (D) in intact (*red*, *n* = 14) and carotid body denervated (*blue*, *n* = 12) chronically instrumented sheep fetuses at 0.8 of gestation during a 1 hour episode of acute hypoxia (PaO_2 reduced from *ca.* 23 to 13 mm Hg, *shaded box*). Carotid body denervation delays the increase in fetal perfusion pressure, prevents the bradycardia, and impairs the fall in femoral blood flow without affecting the increase in carotid blood flow in response to acute hypoxia. **P* <.05, intact vs. denervated. (Redrawn from Giussani DA, Spencer JA, Moore PJ, et al. Afferent and efferent components of the cardiovascular reflex responses to acute hypoxia in term fetal sheep. *J Physiol*. 1993;461:431–449, with permission.)

The purine nucleoside adenosine appears to play an important role in chemoreceptor-mediated responses as adenosine receptor blockade abolishes hypoxia-induced bradycardia and hypertension in fetal sheep.[121-123] Treatment with an adenosine receptor antagonist or carotid sinus denervation prior to acute fetal hypoxia also prevents an increase in plasma epinephrine and markedly reduces the increase in plasma norepinephrine.[124,125] Thus, adenosine receptor blockade may act via chemoreceptor-dependent mechanisms to abolish circulatory and adrenergic responses to acute hypoxia in fetal sheep, although chemoreflex-independent mechanisms also likely exist. In postnatal animals, adenosine increases carotid body afferent discharge, whereas hypoxia-induced increases in afferent activity are attenuated by adenosine receptor antagonists.[126] The adenosine A_{2A} receptor gene is expressed in the carotid body, suggesting adenosine may act in this location to regulate chemoreceptor responses to hypoxia.[127]

Once the efferent limb of the chemoreflex is initiated, the peripheral vasoconstriction is maintained by the release of constrictor agents into the fetal circulation, such as catecholamines, vasopressin, and NPY.[106,128] The influence on the peripheral vasoconstrictor response of local agents, in particular NO, independent of neuroendocrine control has gathered increasing attention.[10,129] Studies have shown that fetal chemoreflex and endocrine constrictor mechanisms mediating peripheral vasoconstriction can be opposed by increased NO bioavailability during acute hypoxemia, since fetal treatment with a NO synthase inhibitor enhanced the magnitude of the fetal peripheral constrictor response.[10] Furthermore, increased generation of reactive oxygen species during acute hypoxia can interact with NO, providing an oxidant tone to the fetal vasculature.[129-131] Therefore, the fetal peripheral vasoconstrictor response to acute hypoxia designed to redistribute the fetal cardiac output towards essential vascular beds while maintaining fetal arterial blood pressure is an aggregate of carotid chemoreflex activation, humoral constrictor influences, and local redox modulation of vascular tone, itself determined by the ratio of NO:O^- in the fetal circulation.[106]

HORMONAL INTERACTIONS ON CHEMOREFLEX FUNCTION

As with fetal baroreflex function, there is evidence that fetal chemoreceptors are involved in modifying the release of hormones into the fetal circulation. In turn, there is evidence that the endocrine milieu, in particular fetal exposure to glucocorticoids, can influence the pattern and magnitude of fetal chemoreflex responses. In the fetus, sympathetically mediated release of catecholamines during acute hypoxia may be triggered by a carotid chemoreflex, in addition to the direct effect of hypoxia on the adrenal gland. Transection of the carotid sinus nerves in the sheep fetus delays the increase in plasma catecholamine concentrations during acute asphyxia.[125] Similarly, neural control of adrenocortical function is also evident in the late gestation fetus as section of either the carotid sinus nerves or the splanchnic nerves affects the steroidogenic response without affecting the increase in adrenocorticotropic hormone (ACTH) during acute hypoxic or acute hypotensive stress.[132-134] These studies suggest the presence of a carotid chemoreflex mediated by splanchnic nerve efferents that act to trigger the release of cortisol, as well as sensitize the fetal adrenal cortex to ACTH delivery. Conversely, carotid sinus nerve section does not affect the release of vasopressin[135] or of angiotensin[136] into the fetal circulation, suggesting these effects are not mediated by carotid chemoreceptors.

The pattern and the magnitude of the fetal cardiovascular defense response to acute hypoxia change as the fetus approaches term, in close association with the prepartum increase in fetal plasma cortisol. With advancing gestation, the magnitude and persistence of bradycardia and vasoconstriction in response to hypoxemia become more pronounced (Fig. 50.3).[128] The more sustained bradycardia in the term relative to preterm fetus results from maturation of carotid body chemoreflex responses and the reciprocal maturational changes in the fetal cardiac responsiveness to autonomic agonists. Similarly, the greater

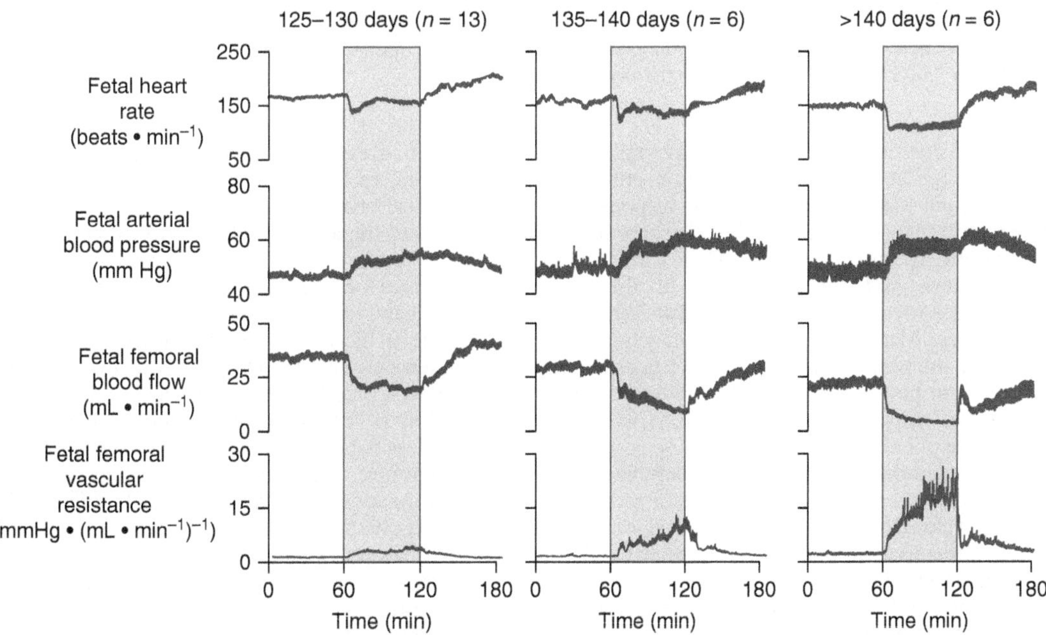

Fig. 50.3 Ontogeny of the fetal cardiovascular responses to acute hypoxia. The data show mean ± SE calculated every minute for the fetal heart rate, fetal arterial blood pressure, fetal femoral blood flow, and fetal femoral vascular resistance during a 1 hour episode of acute hypoxia *(shaded box)* in 13 fetuses between 125 and 130 days of gestation, 6 fetuses between 135 and 140 days of gestation, and 6 fetuses more than 140 days (term is ca. 145 days). Note that basal fetal heart rate and basal fetal femoral blood flow decreases with advancing gestation. In addition, the bradycardia becomes persistent and the femoral vasoconstriction is more intense as the fetus approaches term. (Redrawn from Fletcher AJW, Gardner DS, Edwards CM, et al. Development of the ovine fetal cardiovascular defense to hypoxemia towards full term. *Am J Physiol Heart Circ Physiol.* 2006;291:H3023–3034, with permission.)

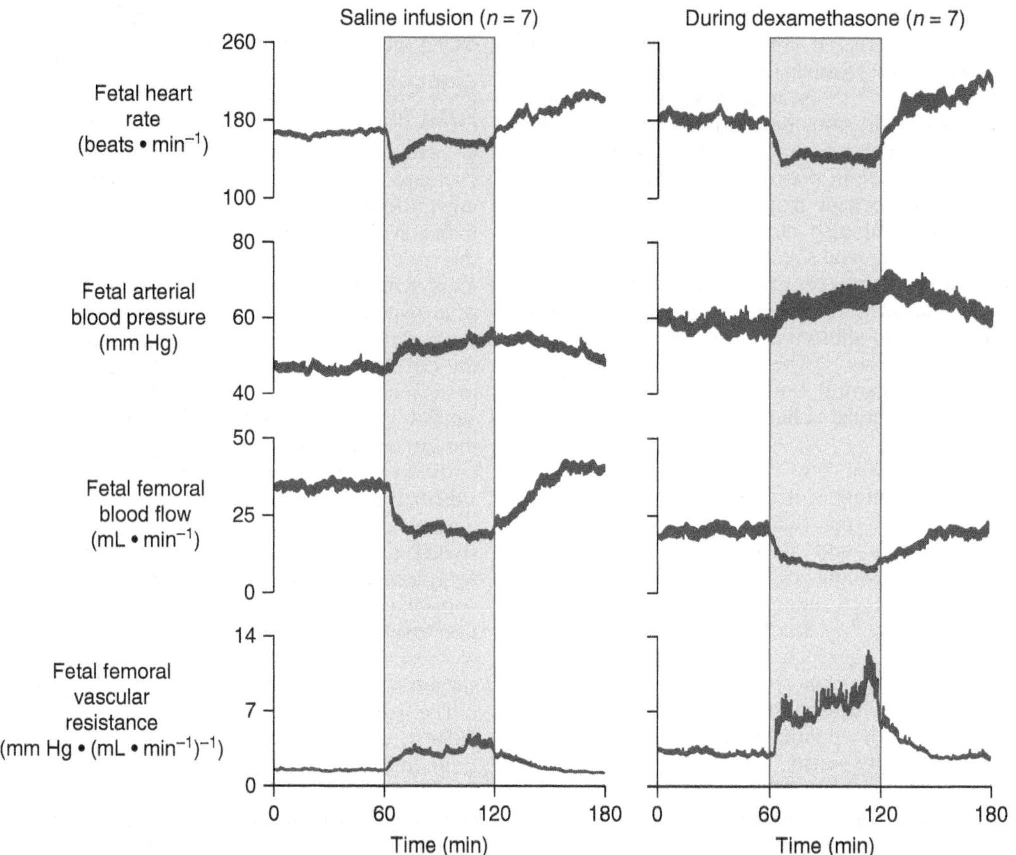

Fig. 50.4 Antenatal dexamethasone and maturation of the fetal cardiovascular responses to acute hypoxia. The data show mean ± SE calculated every minute for the fetal heart rate, arterial blood pressure, femoral blood flow, and femoral vascular resistance during a 1-hour episode of acute hypoxia (box) in 14 fetuses at 127 ± 1 day of gestation (term ca. 145 days) following 2 days of continuous fetal intravenous infusion with saline or with dexamethasone treatment. Note that fetal treatment with dexamethasone switches that pattern and the magnitude of the fetal heart rate and femoral vascular resistance responses to acute hypoxia towards those seen in fetuses close to term (see Fig. 50.3). This indicates accelerated maturation of the fetal cardiovascular defense to acute hypoxia by antenatal glucocorticoid treatment. (Redrawn from Fletcher AJW, Gardner DS, Edwards CM, et al. Cardiovascular and endocrine responses to acute hypoxaemia during and following dexamethasone infusion in the ovine fetus. *J Physiol.* 2003;549[Pt 1]:271–287 with permission.)

peripheral vasoconstrictor response to acute hypoxia with advancing gestational age in the fetus results from enhanced chemoreflex and plasma vasopressin and NPY responses.[128] Exposure of the preterm sheep fetus to synthetic glucocorticoids, such as dexamethasone, in doses of human clinical relevance, can modify the pattern and the magnitude of the fetal cardiovascular responses to acute hypoxia in similar fashion to advancing gestational age. Maternal intramuscular injection with dexamethasone or fetal intravenous infusion with dexamethasone at 0.7 to 0.8 of gestation both switch the fetal bradycardic and femoral vasoconstrictor responses to acute hypoxia from the immature to the mature phenotype (Fig. 50.4).[137]

Little is known regarding central chemoreceptors, their associated neuronal networks, and the influence of circulator function early in development. While there is evidence for central medullary chemoreceptor function in utero, which appear to govern breathing movement to a greater extent than systemic hemodynamics,[138-141] the precise location and the role of these sensors in fetal life remain largely unknown.

MODULATION OF BAROREFLEX AND CHEMOREFLEX FUNCTION BY ADVERSE INTRAUTERINE CONDITIONS

Despite growing recognition and acceptance of the science of developmental programming of disease, investigations of the effects of adverse intrauterine conditions on fetal reflex function and during early development remain limited. Several different techniques have been used, primarily during ovine pregnancy, to simulate impaired nutrient and oxygen delivery to the fetus that may occur during high-risk pregnancies.[142] The majority of studies have focused on effects of adverse intrauterine conditions on fetal basal cardiovascular function, reporting changes in fetal basal arterial blood pressure, fetal heart rate, and in the distribution of the fetal cardiac output.[143-145] Few investigations have studied the effects of adverse intrauterine conditions on the neural regulation of cardiovascular function during a superimposed acute stress. Nonetheless, a consensus is beginning to emerge that fetal exposure to prolonged or repeated periods of hypoxia of varying duration can have dramatically different, and sometimes opposing, effects on fetal chemoreflexes[138] and differential effects on fetal baroreflex and chemoreflex function. For instance, fetal exposure to sustained hypoxia (SH), defined as lasting from a few hours to days, usually enhances the magnitude of fetal chemoreflex but desensitizes the baroreflex. Conversely, fetal exposure to chronic hypoxia (CH), defined as that occurring for weeks or months, imposes a depressive effect on fetal chemoreflex responses.[146,147] Studies of chronically instrumented fetal sheep, grouped according to postsurgical PaO_2, found fetuses that had been hypoxic for a few days (SH) with a baseline PaO_2 of 17.3 ± 0.5 mm Hg displayed greater increases in arterial blood pressure and femoral vascular resistance than control fetuses (baseline PaO_2 22.9 ± 1.0 mm Hg), in response to a superimposed 1 hour episode of acute hypoxia.[105] Functional chemoreflex analysis performed by plotting the change in PaO_2 against the change in heart rate and femoral vascular resistance[109,115] revealed that the slopes of the cardiac and vasoconstrictor chemoreflex curves were enhanced in hypoxic fetuses relative to controls.[105] Similarly, greater cardiovascular chemoreflex responses to a 1 hour episode of acute hypoxia are seen in fetal sheep exposed to 1 to 2 days of reduced uterine blood flow (SH) compared to controls.[148] Conversely, studies with novel isobaric hypoxic chambers able to maintain ovine pregnancies under significant hypoxic conditions for most of gestation (CH) are beginning to show that the fetal bradycardia and the increase in femoral vascular resistance in response to a 30-minute period of acute hypoxia are almost absent in late gestation pregnancies exposed to hypoxic conditions for longer than 10 days (CH) (personal communication). This switch in fetal cardiovascular chemoreflex strategy is remarkably similar to the change from sensitization to desensitization of chemoreflex responses to acute episodes of hypoxia in postnatal animals and humans exposed to either sustained or CH. For example, exposure of cats and goats to 48 hours of hypoxia (SH) enhances carotid body discharge and their ventilatory response to an acute episode of isobaric hypoxia.[149] In contrast, it is established that the chemoreflex ventilator response to acute hypoxia is markedly blunted in residents at high altitude (CH).[150] While the physiologic mechanisms responsible for this switch from sensitization to desensitization in either the fetal cardiovascular chemoreflex responses or the postnatal ventilatory chemoreflex responses are unknown, the change in the phenotype of the responses likely represents a switch in homeostatic strategy to either enhance defenses during shorter periods of hypoxic stress or to minimize energy requirements during longer periods of hypoxic stress.

CARDIOPULMONARY REFLEXES DURING DEVELOPMENT

In the adult, extracellular fluid (ECF) volume remains remarkably constant despite day-to-day variations in dietary intake of salt and water.[151] The integrity of this system is essential to preserve circulatory performance and to insure appropriate fluid and electrolyte homeostasis. Contrary to the steady-state condition of ECF volume in the adult, significant changes in total body water and in the partition of body water between intracellular and extracellular compartments occur during fetal and postnatal development.[152,153] It is likely that the changes in body water during development are, in part, linked to ontogenic changes in the sensing and effector mechanisms regulating ECF volume, including cardiopulmonary receptors. These receptors are sensory endings located in the four cardiac chambers, in the great veins, and in the lungs.[154] In the adult, the volume sensors mediating reflex changes in cardiovascular and renal function are believed to be primarily those residing in the atria[155,156] and the ventricles,[154] with the ventricular receptors being of utmost importance during decreases in cardiopulmonary pressures.[154,157] The majority of ventricular receptor vagal afferents are unmyelinated C-fibers that can be activated by exposure to chemical irritants (chemosensitive) and changes in pressure or strength (mechanosensitive receptors).[158,159] These receptors have a low basal discharge rate that exerts a tonic inhibitory influence on sympathetic outflow and vascular resistance,[154] and regulates plasma AVP concentration.[160] Interruption of this basal activity results in increases in heart rate, blood pressure, and sympathetic nerve activity, whereas activation of cardiopulmonary receptors results in reflex bradycardia, vasodilation, and sympathoinhibition.[154]

Characterization of the cardiopulmonary reflex during the perinatal and neonatal period was initially performed by stimulation of chemosensitive cardiopulmonary receptors.[59,161,162] These studies[161,162] demonstrate that the heart rate, blood pressure, and regional blood flow responses to stimulation of chemosensitive cardiac receptors are smaller early during development than later in life, and are in fact absent in premature fetal lambs[161] and in piglets under 1 week old.[162]

Indirect evidence suggests that cardiopulmonary mechanoreceptors are functional early during development and respond to changes in blood volume by eliciting reflexes that influence both renal and cardiac function. Inhibition of vagal afferents during slow and non-hypotensive hemorrhage blocks the normal rise in plasma vasopressin but does not alter the rise in plasma renin activity in near-term fetal sheep.[163] Fetal heart rate also increases in response to non-hypotensive hemorrhage[164] or to a decline in central venous pressure following furosemide administration.[165] With direct recording of renal sympathetic activity in fetal and newborn sheep, the role of cardiac mechanoreceptors in modulating sympathetic outflow and circulatory function during development has been more clearly defined. Stimulation of cardiopulmonary receptors with volume expansion has no effect on basal renal nerve activity in the fetus, but significantly reduces RSNA in newborn and 8-week-old sheep.[166,167] However, in these studies, stimulation of carotid sinus and aortic arterial baroreceptors may have contributed to the sympathoinhibitory and natriuretic responses observed during volume expansion. To clarify this issue, studies were repeated in newborn and 6- to 8-week-old sheep following SAD.[168] The decrease in RSNA in response to volume expansion was totally abolished in SAD newborn lambs but was not affected by SAD in 6- to 8-week-old sheep. These results indicate that cardiopulmonary reflexes are not fully mature early in life, and that stimulation of sino-aortic baroreceptors plays a greater role than cardiopulmonary mechanoreceptors in regulating changes in RSNA in response to changes in vascular volume early during development.

Developmental changes in cardiovascular and autonomic responses to blood volume reduction also exist. Gomez and colleagues[164] found that the systemic hemodynamic responses to fetal hemorrhage were dependent upon the maturational state of the animal. Hemorrhage produced a significant decrease in arterial blood pressure without accompanying changes in heart rate in fetuses less than 120 days gestation, whereas blood pressure remained stable and heart rate increased in near-term fetuses. However, other investigators[163,169] found the hemodynamic response to hemorrhage to be similar in immature and near-term fetuses, this being reductions in both heart rate and blood pressure. In newborn lambs, cardiovascular responses to hemorrhage are dependent upon intact renal nerves, which in turn modulate release of AVP.[170]

When input from cardiopulmonary receptors is removed by section of the cervical vagosympathetic trunks, the decrease in fetal blood pressure in response to hemorrhage is similar to that in intact fetuses,[171] whereas vagotomy with SAD enhances the decrease in blood pressure.[163] Therefore, it is likely that activation of fibers from the carotid sinus (arterial baroreceptors and chemoreceptors), but not vagal afferents (cardiopulmonary baroreceptors and chemoreceptors), is involved in the maintenance of blood pressure homeostasis during fetal hemorrhage. Cardiopulmonary receptors also appear to have a diminished role in early postnatal life as reflex changes in newborn lamb RSNA during nonhypotensive and hypotensive hemorrhage are dependent upon the integrity of arterial baroreceptors but not cardiopulmonary receptors.[172] Factors responsible for the decreased sensitivity of the cardiopulmonary reflex early in development may involve maturational changes in the mechanoreceptor organ itself, the mechanical properties of the tissue in which the baroreceptor is located, the vagal afferent fibers, the central neural processing of afferent input, and/or efferent sympathetic fibers. In addition, alterations in neuroendocrine control of cardiopulmonary reflex activity may contribute to the attenuated sympathetic and cardiovascular responses to volume expansion in SAD newborn lambs. Indirect evidence suggests that atrial natriuretic peptide (ANP) plays an important role in the regulation of the autonomic nervous system during fetal life and that its role changes with maturation.[173] The sympathoinhibition seen in older lambs but not newborn SAD lambs may therefore be due to either a greater sensitivity to the central actions of ANP or a consequence of the larger increase in circulating ANP concentration in older lambs,[168] or both.

The RSNA responses to vagal afferent nerve stimulation are similar in sino-aortic denervated fetal and postnatal lambs,[174] suggesting that delayed maturation of the cardiopulmonary reflex is not secondary to incomplete central integration of vagal afferent input. On the other hand, the decreased sensitivity of the cardiopulmonary reflex early in development in the face of a hypersensitive arterial baroreflex response (as outlined above) is intriguing. One may suggest that there is an occlusive interaction between these two reflexes during development. In support of this hypothesis, studies in adults[175,176] have shown that activation of arterial baroreceptors may impair the reflex responses to activation of cardiopulmonary receptors.

BAROREFLEX AND CHEMOREFLEX FUNCTION IN THE HUMAN NEONATE

In the human neonate, neural control of the circulation has been assessed most often by recording alterations in the heart rate in response to postural changes, though recent use of noninvasive continuous blood pressure systems have extended our understanding of cardiovascular regulation. Several studies demonstrated in healthy term and preterm infants that head-up tilting (to unload arterial baroreceptors) produces a significant heart rate response,[177,178] and that the magnitude of the response is proportional to the degree of tilting.[178] In contrast, others have been unable to demonstrate a consistent response of heart rate to tilting and concluded that the heart rate component of the baroreflex is poorly developed during the neonatal period.[179] Using venous occlusion plethysmography, Waldman and colleagues[179] found in otherwise healthy preterm and term infants that 45 degrees head-up tilting produced, on average, a 25% decrease in limb blood flow, suggestive of an increase in peripheral vascular resistance, although no significant tachycardia was observed.

Spectral analysis of heart period or systolic blood pressure in the time or frequency domain has been used in human adults,[180] infants,[181-184] and fetuses[185] to evaluate the contribution of the autonomic nervous system in maintaining cardiovascular homeostasis and determine sympathovagal interactions, as well as regulation of baroreflex sensitivity during sleep conditions and following postural changes. Studies of fetal electrocardiogram tracings have shown that younger fetuses have a greater total energy of the power spectrum compared with more mature fetuses, consistent with the evolution of a stable and mature autonomic nervous system.[185] Maturational changes in the power spectra of HR variability have also been shown by comparing preterm to term infants.[181,182] There is a progressive decline in the low-frequency/high-frequency (LF/HF) power ratio associated with both increasing postnatal and gestational age, indicating an increase in parasympathetic contribution to control resting HR with maturation. Clairambault and colleagues[182] found that changes in the HF component of the spectrum were greater at 37 to 38 weeks, suggesting a steep increase in vagal tone at this age.

Power spectral analysis has also been used to characterize developmental changes in sympathovagal balance in response to arterial baroreceptor unloading in preterm infants beginning at 28 to 30 weeks post-conceptional age.[186] By longitudinally examining changes in heart rate power spectrum on a weekly basis, Mazursky and coworkers[186] found that in infants at 28 to 30 weeks the LF/HF ratio did not change with head-up postural change, whereas with increasing postnatal age the LF component of the spectrum increased with head-up tilt. Longitudinal study of healthy term infants over the first 6 months of life found baroreflex sensitivity, in response to head-up tilt, was decreased in the prone compared to supine position during quiet but not active sleep.[184] Sensitivity was also positively correlated with postnatal age. Similar studies in preterm infants found postnatal age had no significant effect on baroreflex sensitivity regardless of sleep state, though preterm birth was associated with impaired maturation of the response, resulting in a reduction in baroreflex sensitivity at 5 to 6 months chronologic age.[183]

Comparatively few studies have investigated chemoreflex function in the human neonate and the investigations available have focused on ventilatory rather than on cardiovascular chemoreflexes. In fact, interactions of multiple reflexes make such study difficult. While the primary cardiac effect of chemoreceptor stimulation is bradycardia, concomitant increases in ventilatory drive, lung stretch, and resultant hypocapnic effects on central neurons result in tachycardia.[187] In otherwise healthy term infants, ages 2 to 82 days, heart rate declined during hyperoxia (Fio_2 1.0), and rose during hypoxia (Fio_2 0.15) and hypercapnia (3% CO_2).[187] The percent change in heart rate was positively correlated with the percent change in ventilation. Examination of induced reflex respiratory responses to breath-by-breath alternations of fractional inspired oxygen in full-term human infants, delivered either vaginally or by cesarean section, found that the magnitude of the respiratory response increased with postnatal age, likely reflecting postnatal increases in the hypoxic sensitivity of the peripheral arterial chemoreceptors.[188] In infants with bronchopulmonary dysplasia, the chemoreflex respiratory response is blunted, likely as a result to pre-exposure to CH.[189]

Combined, therefore, the available studies in human infants suggest that baroreflex and chemoreflex regulation undergoes changes with maturation, becoming more functional with postnatal development and that the set-point and gain of these reflexes are also subject to modulation by adverse intrauterine conditions.

SYMPATHETIC ACTIVITY AT BIRTH

The transition from fetal to newborn life is associated with numerous hemodynamic adjustments, including changes in heart rate and peripheral vascular resistance and a redistribution of blood flow.[190,191] Although the mechanisms regulating these changes are not fully understood, the striking increases in circulating catecholamine levels at birth[192,193] have led investigators to suggest that activation of the sympathetic nervous system is vital for cardiovascular adaptation at birth.[191] In sheep, arterial pressure and cardiac function, including heart rate and cardiac output, are depressed by ganglionic blockade in newborn (1 to 3 days) but not older lambs,[194] suggesting that sympathetic tone is high during the immediate postnatal period. In support of this hypothesis, RSNA increases nearly 250% following delivery of term fetal sheep by cesarean section and parallels the rise in arterial pressure and heart rate.[68] This increase in sympathetic outflow is sustained for at least 6 hours after birth, significantly longer than are catecholamine levels.[68] Delivery appears to produce near maximal stimulation of renal sympathetic outflow since further increases cannot be elicited by small decreases in blood pressure.[68] This finding may help explain the inability of the newborn to further increase cardiac output in response to normal physiologic challenges.[195,196] Furthermore, reflex inhibition of this increase in RSNA could not be achieved by arterial baroreceptor stimulation, as seen in fetal and 3- to 7-day-old lambs,[63] suggesting that central influences exist which override the arterial baroreflex and that the maintenance of a high sympathetic tone is vital during this transition period. A similar pattern of baroreceptor reflex gating has been well described in adult animals as part of the defense reaction.[197] The cardiovascular component of this group of behavioral responses, characterized by sympathetic nerve-mediated tachycardia, increased cardiac contractile force, vasoconstriction, and hypertension, mimics the physiologic changes that occur at birth.[198]

The factors mediating the large increase in sympathetic outflow at birth are unclear. Removal of the placental circulation, the onset of spontaneous respiration, and exposure to a cold environment are factors occurring at birth that may stimulate changes in sympathetic activity.[199,200] In utero ventilation studies of fetal sheep have shown that rhythmic lung inflation increases plasma catecholamine concentrations,[199,201] although there are no consistent effects on blood pressure and heart rate. Fetal RSNA increases only 50% during in utero ventilation, while oxygenation and removal of the placental circulation by umbilical cord occlusion produces no additional effect.[202] Such studies demonstrate that lung inflation and an increase in arterial oxygen tension contribute little to the sympathoexcitation process at birth. The increases in heart rate, mean arterial blood pressure, and RSNA following delivery are similar in intact and sino-aortic denervated plus vagotomized fetal lambs,[203] suggesting that afferent input from peripheral chemoreceptors and mechanoreceptors also contribute little to the hemodynamic and sympathetic responses at delivery.

The change in environmental temperature at birth may play an important role in the sympathoexcitatory response at birth. Cooling of the near-term fetus, both in utero and in exteriorized preparations, results in an increase in heart rate, blood pressure, and plasma norepinephrine concentration, consistent with sympathoexcitation.[200,204] Conversely, exteriorization of the near-term lamb fetus into a warm water bath does not produce the alterations in systemic hemodynamics or catecholamine values typically seen at birth.[200] Fetal cooling, but not ventilation or umbilical cord occlusion, also initiates nonshivering thermogenesis via neutrally mediated sympathetic stimulation of brown adipose tissue.[205] In utero cooling of fetal lambs also produces an increase in RSNA of similar magnitude to that at delivery by cesarean section,[179] suggesting that cold-stress plays a role in the activation of the sympathetic nervous system at birth. These changes occur before a decrease in core temperature and are reversible with rewarming. Taken together, these results suggest that the increase in sympathetic nerve activity seen with cooling is neurally mediated by sensory input from cutaneous cold-sensitive thermoreceptors, rather than in response to a change in core temperature. The increases in heart rate, mean arterial blood pressure, and RSNA that normally occur at birth are absent in animals subjected to transection of the brain stem at the level of the rostral pons prior to delivery. These data suggest that supramedullary structures are involved in mediating the sympathoexcitation seen at birth. Additional studies, also in fetal sheep, demonstrate the paraventricular nucleus of the hypothalamus plays a vital role in regulating postnatal increases in sympathetic outflow and baroreflex function.[206] Given the known role of the hypothalamus in temperature and cardiovascular regulation,[198] one may suggest that this structure is intimately involved in the regulation of circulatory and autonomic functions during the transition from fetal to newborn life.

The hemodynamic and sympathetic responses at birth are markedly different in prematurely delivered lambs (0.85 of gestation) compared to those delivered at term.[207] Postnatal increases in heart rate and blood pressure are attenuated, and the sympathoexcitatory response, as measured by RSNA, is absent.[207] This impaired response occurs despite the fact the descending pathways of the sympathetic nervous system are intact and functional at this stage of development, as demonstrated by a large pressor and sympathoexcitatory response to in utero cooling.[207] Antenatal administration of glucocorticoids, which has been shown to improve postnatal cardiovascular as well as pulmonary function, augments hemodynamic and sympathetic responses at birth in premature lambs and decreases the sensitivity of the cardiac baroreflex (Fig. 50.5).[207] Taken together, these data

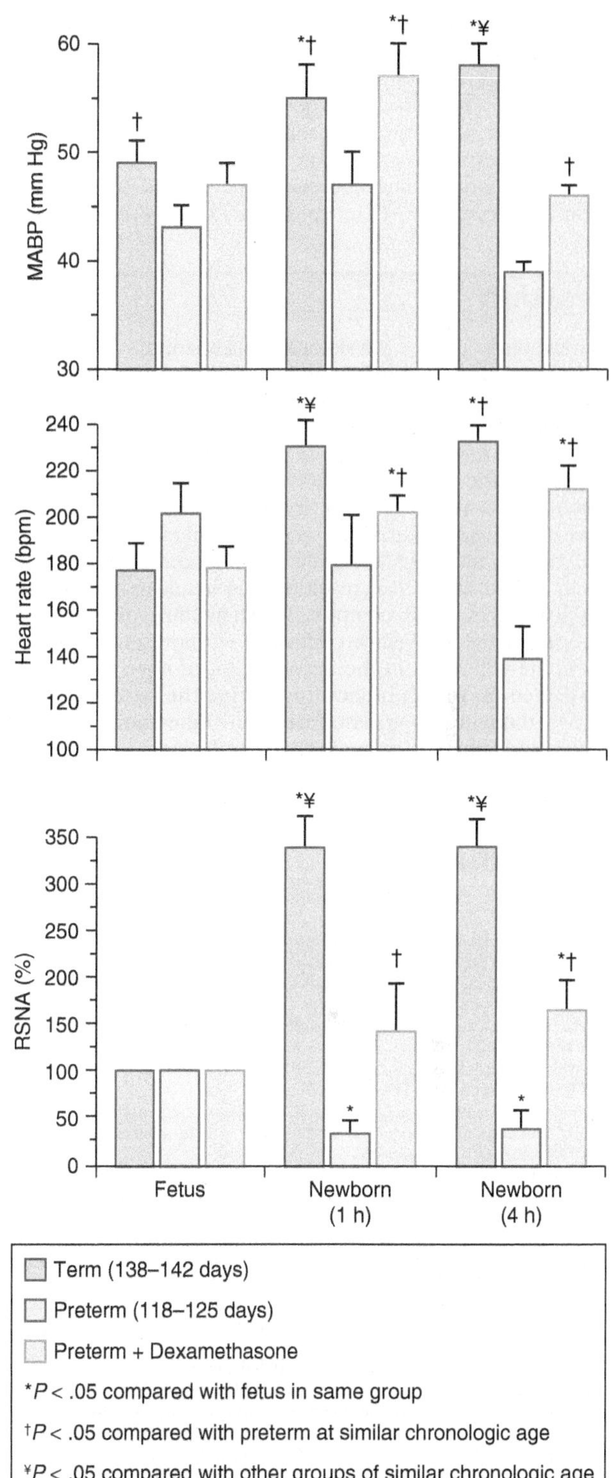

Fig. 50.5 Changes in renal sympathetic nerve activity *(RSNA)* and systemic hemodynamics at birth in term, preterm, and dexamethasone (Dex)-treated preterm lambs delivered by cesarean section. All animals were mechanically ventilated following birth. Exposure to dexamethasone prior to birth resulted in a maturational effect of the sympathetic and hemodynamic responses after birth. Term ca. 145 days gestation. *bpm*, Beats/min; *MABP*, mean arterial blood pressure. (From Segar JL, Lumbers ER, Nuyt AM, et al. Effect of antenatal glucocorticoids on sympathetic nerve activity at birth in preterm sheep. *Am J Physiol.* 1998;274:R160–R167, with permission.)

suggest exogenous corticosteroids have a maturational effect on the sympathetic response at birth, which may be one mechanism by which maternal steroid administration improves postnatal cardiovascular homeostasis. The mechanisms for antenatal glucocorticoid administration augmenting cardiovascular and sympathetic responses at birth are unclear, although stimulation of the peripheral renin-angiotensin system and activation of systemically accessible AT_1 receptors are not involved.[208]

SUMMARY

Understanding the physiologic mechanisms regulating sympathetic tone, baroreflex and chemoreflex function is of particular significance to the appropriate maintenance of arterial blood pressure during basal and stressful conditions in the fetus and the newborn. Evidence also suggests that autonomic reflexes and the sympathetic activity are important regulators of blood pressure and circulatory changes occurring at birth. Failure to regulate arterial pressure, peripheral resistance, and blood volume may lead to significant variations in organ blood flow and substrate delivery, resulting in ischemic or hemorrhagic complications. A more complete understanding of the neural, endocrine, and local redox control of cardiovascular function early in life will result in the development of novel therapeutic strategies to prevent complications during the perinatal period that are thought to be associated with alterations in blood pressure and failure to maintain tissue perfusion.

A complete reference list is available at www.ExpertConsult.com.

SELECT REFERENCES

1. Kirchheim HR. Systemic arterial baroreceptor reflexes. *Physiol Rev*. 1976; 56:100-177.
2. Persson P. Cardiopulmonary receptors and "neurogenic hypertension." *Acta Physiol Scand Suppl*. 1988;570:1-53.
3. Spyer KM. Annual review prize lecture. Central nervous mechanisms contributing to cardiovascular control. *J Physiol*. 1994;474:1-19.
4. Calaresu FR, Yardley CP. Medullary basal sympathetic tone. *Annu Rev Physiol*. 1988;50:511-524.
5. Nuwayhid B, Brinkman 3rd CR, Su C, et al. Development of autonomic control of fetal circulation. *Am J Physiol*. 1975;228:337-344.
6. Woods Jr JR, Dandavino A, Murayama K, et al. Autonomic control of cardiovascular functions during neonatal development and in adult sheep. *Circ Res*. 1977;40:401-407.
7. Vapaavouri EK, Shinebourne EA, Williams RL, et al. Development of cardiovascular responses to autonomic blockade in intact fetal and neonatal lambs. *Biol Neonate*. 1973;22:177-188.
8. Fletcher AJ, Edwards CM, Gardner DS, et al. Neuropeptide Y in the sheep fetus. effects of acute hypoxemia and dexamethasone during late gestation. *Endocrinology*. 2000;141:3976-3982.
9. Sanhueza EM, Johansen-Bibby AA, Fletcher AJ, et al. The role of neuropeptide Y in the ovine fetal cardiovascular response to reduced oxygenation. *J Physiol*. 2003;546:891-901.
10. Morrison S, Gardner DS, Fletcher AJ, et al. Enhanced nitric oxide activity offsets peripheral vasoconstriction during acute hypoxaemia via chemoreflex and adrenomedullary actions in the sheep fetus. *J Physiol*. 2003;547:283-291.
11. van Bel F, Sola A, Roman C, et al. Role of nitric oxide in the regulation of the cerebral circulation in the lamb fetus during normoxemia and hypoxemia. *Biol Neonate*. 1995;68:200-210.
12. Walker AM, Cannata J, Dowling MH, et al. Sympathetic and parasympathetic control of heart rate in unanaesthetized fetal and newborn lambs. *Biol Neonate*. 1978;33:135-143.
13. Patural H, Barthelemy JC, Pichot V, et al. Birth prematurity determines prolonged autonomic nervous system immaturity. *Clin Auton Res*. 2004;14:391-395.
14. Yiallourou SR, Witcombe NB, Sands SA, et al. The development of autonomic cardiovascular control is altered by preterm birth. *Early Hum Dev*. 2013;89:145-152.
15. Alper RH, Jacob HJ, Brody MJ. Regulation of arterial pressure lability in rats with chronic sinoaortic deafferentation. *Am J Physiol*. 1987;253:H466-H474.
16. Barres C, Lewis SJ, Jacob HJ, et al. Arterial pressure lability and renal sympathetic nerve activity are dissociated in SAD rats. *Am J Physiol*. 1992;263:R639-R646.
17. Segar JL, Merrill DC, Smith BA, et al. Role of sympathetic activity in the generation of heart rate and arterial pressure variability in fetal sheep. *Pediatr Res*. 1994;35:250-254.
18. Yardley RW, Bowes G, Wilkinson M, et al. Increased arterial pressure variability after arterial baroreceptor denervation in fetal lambs. *Circ Res*. 1983;52:580-588.
19. Robillard JE, Nakamura KT, DiBona GF. Effects of renal denervation on renal responses to hypoxemia in fetal lambs. *Am J Physiol*. 1986;250:F294-F301.
20. Davidson SR, Rankin JH, Martin Jr CB, et al. Fetal heart rate variability and behavioral state: analysis by power spectrum. *Am J Obstet Gynecol*. 1992;167:717-722.
21. Mann LI, Duchin S, Weiss RR. Fetal EEG sleep stages and physiologic variability. *Am J Obstet Gynecol*. 1974;119:533-538.
22. Zhu YS, Szeto HH. Cyclic variation in fetal heart rate and sympathetic activity. *Am J Obstet Gynecol*. 1987;156:1001-1005.
23. Walker AM. Development of reflex control of the fetal circulation. In: Kunzel W, Jensen A, eds. *The Endocrine Control of the Fetus . Physiologic and Pathophysiologic Aspects*. Berlin, New York: Springer-Verlag; 1988:108-120.
24. Lumbers ER, Yu ZY, Crawford EN. Effects of fetal behavioral states on renal sympathetic nerve activity and arterial pressure of unanesthetized fetal sheep. *Am J Physiol Regul Integr Comp Physiol*. 2003;285:R908-R916.
25. Booth LC, Bennet L, Guild SJ, et al. Maturation-related changes in the pattern of renal sympathetic nerve activity from fetal life to adulthood. *Exp Physiol*. 2011;96:85-93.
26. Clapp 3rd JF, Szeto HH, Abrams R, et al. Physiologic variability and fetal electrocortical activity. *Am J Obstet Gynecol*. 1980;136:1045-1050.
27. Reid DL, Jensen A, Phernetton TM, et al. Relationship between plasma catecholamine levels and electrocortical state in the mature fetal lamb. *J Dev Physiol*. 1990;13:75-79.
28. Jensen A, Bamford OS, Dawes GS, et al. Changes in organ blood flow between high and low voltage electrocortical activity in fetal sheep. *J Dev Physiol*. 1986;8:187-194.
29. Richardson BS, Patrick JE, Abduljabbar H. Cerebral oxidative metabolism in the fetal lamb: relationship to electrocortical state. *Am J Obstet Gynecol*. 1985;153:426-431.
30. Abboud F, Thames MD. Interaction of cardiovascular reflexes in circulatory control. In: Shepherd JT, Abboud FM, eds. *Handbook of Physiology. Section 2*. Vol III. Bethesda, MD: American Physiological Society; 1983:675-753. Part 2.
31. Persson PB, Ehmke H, Kirchheim HR. Cardiopulmonary-arterial baroreceptor interaction in control of blood pressure. *News in Physiological Sciences*. 1989;4:56-59.
32. Brinkman 3rd CR, Ladner C, Weston P, et al. Baroreceptor functions in the fetal lamb. *Am J Physiol*. 1969;217:1346-1351.
33. Itskovitz J, LaGamma EF, Rudolph AM. Baroreflex control of the circulation in chronically instrumented fetal lambs. *Circ Res*. 1983;52:589-596.
34. Bauer DJ. Vagal reflexes appearing in asphyxia in rabbits at different ages. *J Physiol*. 1939;95:187-202.
35. Dawes GS, Johnston BM, Walker DW. Relationship of arterial pressure and heart rate in fetal, new-born and adult sheep. *J Physiol*. 1980;309:405-417.
36. Biscoe TJ, Purves MJ, Sampson SR. Types of nervous activity which may be recorded from the carotid sinus nerve in the sheep foetus. *J Physiol*. 1969;202:1-23.
37. Blanco CE, Dawes GS, Hanson MA, et al. Carotid baroreceptors in fetal and newborn sheep. *Pediatr Res*. 1988;24:342-346.
38. Downing SE. Baroreceptor reflexes in new-born rabbits. *J Physiol*. 1960;150: 201-213.
39. Tomomatsu E, Nishi K. Comparison of carotid sinus baroreceptor sensitivity in newborn and adult rabbits. *Am J Physiol*. 1982;243:H546-H550.
40. Ponte J, Purves MJ. Types of afferent nervous activity which may be measured in the vagus nerve of the sheep foetus. *J Physiol*. 1973;229:51-76.
41. Gootman PM, Buckley NM, Gootman N. Postnatal maturation of neural control of the circulation. In: Scarpelli EM, Cosmi EV, eds. *Reviews in Perinatal Medicine*. New York, NY: Raven Press; 1979:1.
42. Ismay MJ, Lumbers ER, Stevens AD. The action of angiotensin II on the baroreflex response of the conscious ewe and the conscious fetus. *J Physiol*. 1979;288:467-479.
43. Shinebourne EA, Vapaavuori EK, Williams RL, et al. Development of baroreflex activity in unanesthetized fetal and neonatal lambs. *Circ Res*. 1972;31:710-718.
44. Vatner SF, Manders WT. Depressed responsiveness of the carotid sinus reflex in conscious newborn animals. *Am J Physiol*. 1979;237:H40-H43.
45. Andresen MC. Short- and long-term determinants of baroreceptor function in aged normotensive and spontaneously hypertensive rats. *Circ Res*. 1984;54: 750-759.
46. Chapleau MW, Hajduczok G, Abboud FM. Mechanisms of resetting of arterial baroreceptors: an overview. *Am J Med Sci*. 1988;295:327-334.
47. Chapleau MW, Hajduczok G, Abboud FM. Resetting of the arterial baroreflex. Peripheral and central mechanisms. In: Zucker IH, Gilmore JP, eds. *Reflex Control of the Circulation*. Boca Raton, FL: CRC Press; 1991:165-194.
48. Heesch CM, Abboud FM, Thames MD. Acute resetting of carotid sinus baroreceptors. II. Possible involvement of electrogenic Na+ pump. *Am J Physiol*. 1984;247:H833-H839.
49. McDowell TS, Axtelle TS, Chapleau MW, et al. Prostaglandins in carotid sinus enhance baroreflex in rabbits. *Am J Physiol*. 1989;257:R445-R450.
50. Jimbo M, Suzuki H, Ichikawa M, et al. Role of nitric oxide in regulation of baroreceptor reflex. *J Auton Nerv Syst*. 1994;50:209-219.

Nutritional and Environmental Effects on the Fetal Circulation

51

Lucy R. Green | Mark A. Hanson

INTRODUCTION

The fetus depends on its cardiovascular system for growth and development. Vascular growth is closely linked to tissue growth, and the fetal heart must develop in relation to the venous return (preload), primarily from the umbilical vein, and the similar arterial pressures in the pulmonary trunk and the aortic arch (afterload). This matching of cardiovascular function to growth is important in late gestation when the fetus may need to cope with placental insufficiency.[1,2] But the matching is also important for the way in which the fetus responds and adapts to many aspects of the environment, like changes in fetal nutrition (e.g., glucose, amino acid, or micronutrient provision).

The unborn baby is adaptable to many aspects of maternal modifiable environment, and this provides plausible new explanations, aside from adult lifestyle or inherited genes, for risk of noncommunicable diseases (NCDs), such as the cardiovascular diseases (CVDs) that caused death for an estimated 17.9 million people worldwide in 2016.[3] It is now widely acknowledged by scientists and nongovernment agencies that the first 1000 days of development (conception to 2 years old) is a period of high susceptibility to the environment, and this period will influence an individual's response to their adult environment and lifestyle, hence influencing in part their risk of disease.[4] It might explain why not all individuals have the same risk of NCDs, even if they are in the same environment. Poverty, insecurity, and environmental toxins are some of the threats to the nutritional status of women before and during pregnancy,[5] whether that makes the mother underweight, overweight, or obese. These pose potential health challenges for mothers and their children over their life course.

This chapter explores what is known about the effect of prenatal nutrition on cardiovascular developmental mechanisms in relation to growth and puts this into a life course perspective that could impact how pregnancies are managed clinically.

EPIDEMIOLOGIC OBSERVATIONS

Considerable evidence has now accumulated that small or disproportionate size at birth is associated with increased risk of coronary heart disease, hypertension, and stroke in later life. The studies of Barker and colleagues[6] in adult men and women showed that the standardized mortality ratio for coronary artery disease increased in a graded manner across the normal birth weight range. Numerous studies have linked low birth weight to metabolic syndrome[7] or to its components (defined as fasting plasma glucose concentration more than 6 mmol/L [108 mg/dL], blood pressure more than 130/85 mmHg, fasting plasma triglyceride concentration greater than 1.7 mmol/L [150 mg/dL], plasma high-density lipoprotein cholesterol concentration less than 1.1 mmol/L [40 mg/dL], and, in men, waist measurement greater than 102 cm). A meta-analysis of the blood pressure effect suggests that a 1-kg increase in birth weight is associated with a decrease of 2 mm Hg in systolic blood pressure in later life.[8] Inevitably, the size and nature of these studies differ enormously, and the effect of study size has been questioned[9] because larger studies (where birth weight is more likely to have been self-reported than actually measured) show weaker associations between birth weight and blood pressure than do smaller studies. Nonetheless, the direction of the effect (small size at birth predicting higher blood pressure in later life) is not under question, even if the magnitude of the effect is debated. Thus a major part of an individual's predisposition to CVD appears to be established during early development in response to the environment, the so-called Developmental Origins of Health and Disease (DOHaD) concept.[10]

Birth size is a measure of the fetal environment but does not give a full picture of fetal growth. Importantly, some effects of maternal diet on the offspring's cardiovascular system (e.g., carotid intima-media thickness[11]) are not necessarily associated with low birth weight, suggesting that the processes operate across the normal birth weight range. For these reasons, it is vital that physiologic studies are conducted to understand the mechanisms underlying the priming of cardiovascular function by life events in utero. Moreover, it is highly unlikely that appropriate intervention measures to prevent the progression to disease (i.e., metabolic syndrome) in susceptible individuals can be developed without an understanding of the mechanisms underlying the development of the disease. Interventions may have enormous implications for public health; calculations based on epidemiologic studies conducted in Finland[12] suggest that if all male offspring could be prevented from being thin at birth and thin and short at 1 year of age, the incidence of coronary arterial disease would be halved. The implications are not confined to high-income societies because the phenomenon exists in low-to-middle-income societies across the normal birth weight range, which averages 1 kg less than in developed societies.[13] The problem is also more acute in low socioeconomic position groups in high-income countries.

In many populations worldwide, a substantial proportion of women of reproductive age are obese or overweight (>50% in the United Kingdom). Gestational diabetes mellitus and maternal obesity/weight gain are associated with long-term adverse consequences in the offspring and subsequent generations. These implications include increased offspring obesity, which tracks from intrauterine into adult life, and poor health in later life, including CVD risk.[13-19] Human data suggest that although gestational weight gain is associated with adverse cardiovascular risk factors at 9 years, pre-pregnancy weight has a greater overall impact.[15] Guidelines on pregnancy weight management issued in 2010 aim to break the cycle of obesity and reduce the incidence of CVD.[20] Probably those at greatest risk throughout the world belong to transitional societies, in which, for example, children from agrarian societies in the developing world move to cities as adolescents. These considerations may explain the epidemic in coronary arterial disease and in type 2 diabetes that is developing in the Indian subcontinent, for example.[13]

Developmental responses by the fetus to overabundant or lean maternal environments, such as the cardiovascular responses explored in this chapter, might be immediate coordinated responses that are good for survival. However, later in this chapter we will also describe the idea that under some circumstances fetal adaptive responses could give offspring a survival advantage in the postnatal environment in which they predict that they will live.

GENES VERSUS ENVIRONMENT

Many reasons exist for believing that the high prevalence of NCDs is not purely genetic in origin. The most obvious is that changes in the incidence of metabolic syndrome within a generation cannot be due purely to genetic (heritable) traits. Moreover, the maternal and paternal genetic contributions to fetal growth and to outcome measures such as systolic blood pressure in adulthood are highly dissimilar; in a study of adults in Preston, United Kingdom, systolic pressure was inversely related to maternal but not to paternal birth weight.[21]

The processes most likely involved in mediating the maternal versus paternal genomic effects on development involve imprinting. Of the range of genes that are imprinted, the *H19/IGF2* cluster has received particular attention.[22] The insulin-like growth factor (IGF)-2 peptide, which is paternally expressed, is a potent stimulator of fetal cell division and differentiation—showing how the paternal genome drives growth in various key tissues, such as the fetal liver and growth and nutrient transport in the placenta.[23] The type 2 IGF receptor, which is maternally expressed, serves as a clearance receptor that modulates IGF-2 peptide action in the tissues—showing how the maternal genome can down-regulate growth in accordance with the maternal body habitus. This observation is consistent with the concept of maternal constraint of fetal growth, which was highlighted by the pioneering studies of Hammond and Walton,[24] in which Shire horses were crossed with Shetland ponies, and confirmed by more recent studies in horses and humans.[25,26] It is therefore clear that the trajectory of growth in early life is determined by maternal and environmental factors acting to regulate the gene expression of the early embryo. First-trimester growth in the human sets the trajectory for later fetal growth and predicts the risk of low birth weight.[27]

Imprinting processes are a subset of the broader epigenetic processes that are now believed to provide a mechanism whereby undernutrition during development can influence gene expression and the cardiovascular or metabolic phenotype into mature adulthood (see "Mechanisms of Fetal Cardiovascular Response to the Environment"),[28,29] ideas consistent with those of the Encyclopedia of DNA Elements (ENCODE) Consortium, which is looking beyond the exome to the function of all other parts of the human genome.[30] Of importance, these processes involve not simply imprinted genes but a much wider range of the genome, which appears to be under graded epigenetic control throughout development.[31] Numerous processes have been discovered that modify gene expression, and the production of the proteins that confer the phenotype on the organism. These go beyond genetic processes (e.g., single-nucleotide polymorphisms, deletions, or multiple repeats) to epigenetic modifications such as DNA methylation, changes in histone structure, posttranscriptional regulation by small noncoding RNAs, and also the many transcription factors that act to modify gene transcription and the processes that control the half-life of messenger RNA. So this is a way for aspects of the early developmental environment, such as nutrition, to have a persistent lifelong effect without changing the inherited DNA sequence. The effect might not be immediate; instead, it could set up later life responses by genes to transcription factors. This idea is explored further later in this chapter.

ENVIRONMENTAL STIMULI

In investigating the interaction between gene and environment, one should take a life course perspective in considering the influence of maternal diet, body composition, social status, smoking, exposure to environmental toxicants,[32] the effect of the tubal and uterine fluid environment on the early embryo, the development of the placenta, fetal adaptations, and postnatal effects that may exacerbate the problem. A growing area of research also highlights that environmental toxicant or nutritional effects on the father, via seminal plasma or the sperm, can effect male reproductive function and cardiovascular function across successive generations of offspring.[33,34]

TIMING

The first 1000 days of life, from conception to the age of two, is a period of life when the child is most susceptible to the environment around it, as acknowledged in a United Nations political declaration[4] and the World Health Organization's Global Strategy for Women's, Children's and Adolescents' Health (2016–2030).[5] Each organ has a timetable for development, so it is not surprising that the timing of environmental stimuli will influence the effects on the offspring phenotype. In adults who were in utero at the time of the Dutch Winter Famine (an abrupt-onset 5-month period of malnutrition in 1944–1945), exposure during early gestation was associated with increased incidence of coronary arterial disease[35,36] and increased blood pressure response to stress;[37] exposure to famine in mid-gestation was associated with microalbinuria in adults, possibly indicative of hyperfiltration injury as a result of fewer nephrons.[38] Mid-gestation to late-gestation undernutrition was associated with reduced glucose tolerance in adulthood.[39] Sheep are widely used as an animal model for studying the DOHaD phenomenon, not least because, as in humans, the full complement of cardiomyocytes and renal glomeruli are formed prenatally. Studies support the concept that the early-gestation nutrient environment is important in determining later cardiovascular control,[40-43] whereas nutrition in the late-gestation period may be important in determining later metabolic function and endocrine control.[44-46] However, evidence suggests that despite no overt effect of maternal undernutrition in mid-gestation to late gestation on endothelium-dependent relaxation of fetal sheep coronary arteries, the mechanisms that mediate the vessel's responses may be different.[47] The rat model has been widely used for studying programming phenomena (reviewed by Brawley and colleagues[48] and Armitage and colleagues[49]). Most previous studies with this model involved administration of the diet for the whole of pregnancy (approximately 21 days), and now a range of studies show that offspring of rats fed a low-protein diet during pregnancy have altered endothelial function (e.g., the degree of relaxation to the endothelium-dependent vasodilator acetylcholine). However, Kwong and colleagues[50] have also shown that administration of a low-protein diet to rat dams in the first 4 days of gestation (i.e., preimplantation) produces blastocysts that have altered allocation of cells to the trophectoderm and inner-cell mass and offspring, with permanently increased blood pressure in adult life. Similarly in mice, a maternal low-protein diet in the preimplantation period led to elevated blood pressure and impaired in vitro arterial vasodilation in 5-month-old offspring,[51] and elevated blood pressure was still present at approximately 1 year of age.[52] One study suggests that feeding mouse dams this low-protein diet exclusively during oocyte maturation leads to altered behavior and cardiovascular control in postnatal life.[53] Further observations in the mouse have shown that embryos transferred to recipient females developed elevated blood pressure in adult life.[54] Apart from demonstrating the importance of the early-preimplantation embryonic environment in the programming of the subsequent phenotype, these studies raise important questions about the long-term effects of reproductive technologies increasingly used in humans.[55] Additional evidence from animal studies suggests that even the pre-pregnancy maternal nutrient environment can influence cardiovascular function,[56,57] and better preconceptional care is widely considered to be a core part of the solution to getting pregnancies off to the best possible start to ensure health across the life course for the next generation.[58]

NUTRIENTS

The relative contribution of specific macronutrients or micronutrients in determining the balance between supply and demand during fetal growth has not yet been resolved. The fetal requirements in late gestation for the amino acid glycine are greater than those for any other amino acid, even though glycine is not normally considered to be essential. Glycine provision, with the availability of the micronutrient cofactor folate, is important in a range of biologic processes that may alter cardiovascular function (Fig. 51.1). It is involved in the synthesis of DNA and RNA, which is important for cell growth and differentiation. It provides a source of methyl groups for the methylation of CpG dinucleotides, which silences gene transcription and thus the transition from the genotype to the phenotype.[28] An example of such methylated genes with an important role in the pathogenesis of CVD is estrogen receptor α, which is linked to the risk of atherosclerosis. Finally, glycine is important in the interconversion of homocysteine to methionine, such that its deficiency (or of the balance of folate to vitamin B_{12}) leads to accumulation of homocysteine in the plasma and associated vascular damage. The offspring of low protein-fed rat dams have elevated plasma homocysteine levels. In rats, the addition of glycine, or indeed folic acid, to the low-protein diet prevents the elevation of blood pressure in the offspring and the development of vascular dysfunction in these offspring.[59,60] In the liver, hypomethylation of glucocorticoid receptor (GR) and peroxisome proliferator-activated receptor α (PPAR-α) promoters was also prevented by addition of folic acid to the diet.[28]

The major provision of fetal glycine is not by direct transport from the mother. Placental glycine production from the conversion of serine by serine hydroxymethyltransferase is now thought to be important in sheep, but not in humans, in whom serine hydroxymethyltransferase activity is low.[61] The serine itself enters the placenta from the maternal and fetal circulation via system A and alanine/cysteine/serine transporter systems.[62,63] Placental size relates not only to fetal growth but also to blood pressure in later life.[64] However, relatively few studies have been performed on placental transport function (see Chapter 10) in relation to fetal growth and outcome.[23] Placental gene expression of facilitated amino acid transporters TAT-1 and LAT-3 increased with increased fetal growth.[65] It is of interest that placental system A activity increases with reductions in birth weight in the normal range,[65] although an association exists between reduced system A activity and intrauterine growth retardation.[66] Current work deepening our understanding of the complex mechanisms by which amino acids are transferred is important.[65] This includes the regulation of amino acid transport by other aspects of the modifiable maternal environmental like vitamin D status and relates to the expanding knowledge on how vitamin D transported by the placenta can itself play a role in fetal cardiovascular development and growth.[67,68] Recent identification of air pollutant carbon particles on the fetal side of the placenta in humans is notable[69] and part of important areas of newer work concerning how environmental toxicants c(airborne or other) are affecting the developing baby.[70]

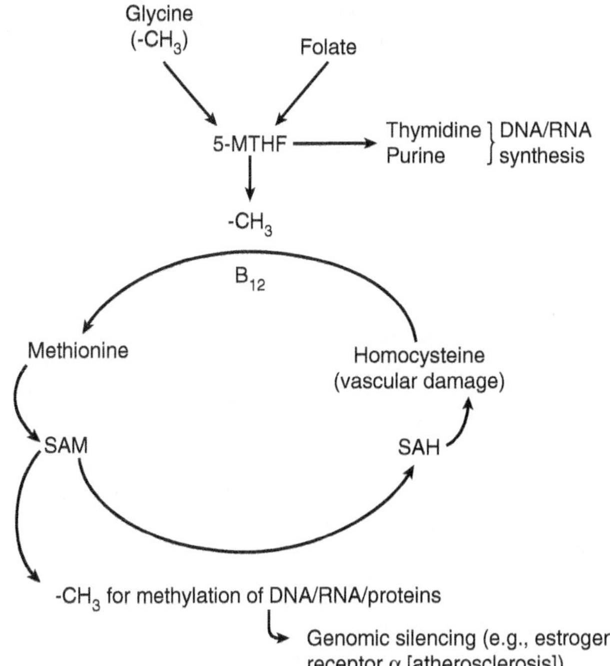

Fig. 51.1 The importance of glycine and folate in the processes that may underlie atherosclerosis. *B_{12}*, vitamin B_{12}; *5-MTHF*, 5-methyltetrahydrofolate; *SAH*, *S*-adenosyl-L-homocysteine; *SAM*, *S*-adenosyl-L-methionine.

FETAL ADAPTIVE RESPONSES

Evidence of fetal adaptive responses to perturbed nutrition comes from a relatively small number of human and sheep studies. The incidence of singleton pregnancies in sheep allows the comparison of fetal growth patterns with human pregnancies, and their size and tolerance of surgery permit cardiovascular and growth measurements to be made over several weeks of gestation. Current knowledge of late gestation fetal cardiovascular control is based on the concept that the mechanisms of such control will be best revealed when the system is challenged with a stimulus and the resulting response is measured. The stimulus most widely used is hypoxia, which has permitted the development of a fairly complete picture of a temporal and functional hierarchy of reflex, endocrine, and local mechanisms operating during acute hypoxia (see Chapter 50).[71] Such mechanisms change in the course of gestation,[72,73] in the face of repeated acute or sustained hypoxia,[74-76] and in species adapted to life in the hypoxia of altitude.[77-80]

Most evidence of fundamental fetal adaptive responses comes from hypoxic fetuses in which the "brain-sparing" cardiovascular phenomenon has been demonstrated, whereby a higher percentage of the combined ventricular output is directed to the brain at the expense of the developing fetal body. Such brain-sparing is associated in the human fetus with late-gestation asymmetric growth retardation, and the supposition has been that if any of these fetuses are not hypoxic, the response must be due to reduced nutrition. The rapid phase of the vasoconstrictor component of the response to hypoxia is mediated by the carotid bodies; therefore it is of great interest that these chemoreceptors are also responsive to a reduction in plasma glucose concentration in adults,[81] and data suggest that the differential fetal organ growth effects of maternal undernutrition are dependent on carotid sinus innervation.[82] Of course, it is more than likely that not all features and mechanisms induced by oxygen will be the same for other nutrients. Indeed, in fetuses of hypoxic pregnant rats there was fetal aortic thickening without changes in cardiac volumes, but in fetuses of undernourished pregnant rats fetal cardiac morphology was affected without changes in aortic structure, and fetal aortic vascular reactivity was differentially affected by hypoxia or undernutrition.[83]

Understanding of the fetal redistribution in response to changes in nutrition requires consideration of effects on individual organs, and one of particular interest is the developing fetal liver. Blood supply to the liver comes from a range of sources, primarily the oxygenated and highly nutritious blood from the umbilical vein. However, this blood entirely supplies the left lobe of the liver and to a lesser extent supplies the right lobe, which also receives blood from the hepatic portal veins and the hepatic arteries (which is less well oxygenated and nutritious). A proportion of oxygenated umbilical blood is shunted through the ductus venosus toward the foramen ovale and through into the left atrium. The degree of shunting of this blood changes during gestation and is altered by challenges such as acute hypoxemia.[84] It is now known that the degree of shunting is also increased in late-gestation fetuses of mothers with a high pre-pregnancy body mass index or skinfold thickness[85] (Fig. 51.2) and that low maternal weight gain is associated with preferential blood supply to the fetal left liver lobe and with higher birth weight and neonatal ponderal index.[86] This therefore fits with the notion that women with greater fat stores, or with altered endocrine status leading to increased body fat mass, produce fetuses with a more rapid trajectory of growth, at least in early gestation. If this growth imposes demands on the developing placenta that cannot be met, fetal cardiovascular redistributions must occur. Whether such processes operate in early gestation is not known.

Preliminary data in these fetuses indicate a redistribution of combined ventricular output in late gestation because baseline femoral blood flow tends to be lower and baseline carotid blood flow tends to be elevated (Green and Hanson, unpublished observations). The fetus can make immediate cardiovascular adaptations to hypoglycemia with a redistribution of blood flow away from organs such as the liver and skeletal muscle and toward the adrenal gland, as in hypoxia. Specific early-gestation moderate (30%) reduction of maternal protein intake markedly exacerbated the vascular dysfunction of isolated mid-gestation fetal resistance vessels[87] (Fig. 51.3), indicating the importance of nutrient balance (see above).

In spite of the association between early-life nutrition and later risk of coronary artery disease,[35,36] there is limited information from animals on the impact of early-gestation undernutrition on the fetal heart. Maternal undernutrition around the time of conception alters the abundance of genes that regulate cardiac growth in late-gestation fetal sheep,[88] and early-gestation to mid-gestation undernutrition caused ventricular hypertrophy in the late-gestation sheep fetus.[89] In contrast, moderate (30%) maternal total or specific-protein restriction in the first half of gestation did not affect mid-gestation fetal heart size or heart rate as assessed by Doppler echocardiography.[87] Moreover, in guinea pigs the impact of early-gestation maternal undernutrition on offspring left ventricular wall thickening persists into the next generation.[46] Obesity in pregnancy is a particular issue in higher income populations (>50% women in UK) and numerous rodent studies have linked pregnancy consumption of a high fat or high sucrose diet to offspring later-life cardiovascular dysfunction.[90-93] It is less well characterized, but these effects appear to start during fetal life since in sheep greater maternal weight gain is linked to altered fetal organ growth consistent with a redistribution of nutrient provision in favor of the liver.[82] Also, maternal obesity in humans, sheep, and guinea-pigs was associated with altered cardiac contractility and structure, and vascular dysfunction.[94-96]

The extent to which concomitant changes in cardiovascular control and growth result from perturbations in the fetal nutrient supply line is unclear. Reduced maternal body condition at mating results in an elevated fetal blood pressure trajectory in late-gestation fetuses,[97] and the normal developmental increase in arterial pressure during late gestation in sheep is perturbed in small fetuses.[98] Restricted fetal nutrient supply by removal of placental caruncles before conception perturbs cardiovascular development and function in late-gestation fetuses—with or without growth restriction.[99] Moreover, mild-to-moderate (15% to 30%) reduction in maternal nutrient intake for the first half of gestation lowered blood pressure in late-gestation fetuses,[100] impaired vascular function in vitro,[101] and enhanced the increase in peripheral vascular resistance in the hindlimb in response to acute hypoxia,[40] with no change in fetal organ or body weight. However, these sorts of associations are likely not to reflect changes at the tissue level, for example studies in sheep show that either peri-implantation or late-gestation maternal undernutrition decreases late-gestation fetal myofiber density and that this is associated with decreased capillary density (Fig. 51.4), and in the late-gestation nutrient-restricted group with altered molecular markers of glucose uptake,[102] and these changes are specific to the muscle bed.

The prevailing glycemic environment of the fetus can influence its cardiovascular response to acute hypoxia,[74] and lower circulating blood glucose concentration in late gestation is associated with greater vasoconstrictor activity in isolated vessels.[103] Moreover, the decrease in blood flow to the femoral bed during this maternal hypoglycemia is heightened by previous exposure to a restricted maternal diet around the time of implantation.[104] Undernutrition of a greater intensity leads to decreased fetal size, but the response depends on the rate at which growth is occurring: the growth of a rapidly growing fetus is slowed, whereas slow-growing fetuses fail to respond.[105] Such fetuses may have adapted to an earlier-gestation insult, such as periconceptional undernutrition,[106] thereby protecting them from a subsequent late-gestation challenge. These observations suggest that cardiovascular adaptations may be able to buffer changes in growth when there is an altered nutrient supply. But

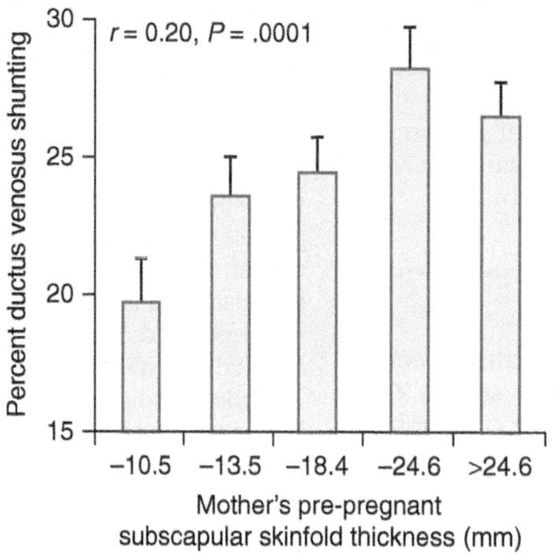

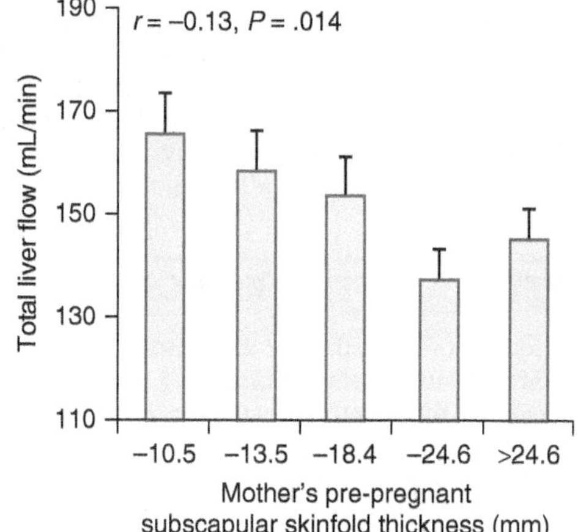

Fig. 51.2 Data from 381 fetuses at 26 weeks of gestation showing lower ductus venosus shunting and greater total liver blood flow in those mothers who had lower skinfold thicknesses before pregnancy. Maternal subscapular skinfold thickness is grouped into strict fifths of the distribution for presentation purposes; correlation analyses are based on continuously distributed variables. (From Haugen G, Hanson M, Kiserud T, et al. Fetal liver-sparing cardiovascular adaptations linked to mother's slimness and diet. *Circ Res.* 2005;96:12.)

it may be that when the upper limit in this buffering capacity has been reached, a change in growth will result.

In sheep, moderate total calorific restriction in early gestation did not alter the size at birth, but it did cause a faster growth rate in the first 12 weeks after birth.[107] This is consistent with the epidemiologic observations that adult blood pressure is inversely related in a graded manner across the normal birth weight range[8] (see earlier) while also highlighting that postnatal growth needs to be considered. This concept is explored further in the next section of this chapter.

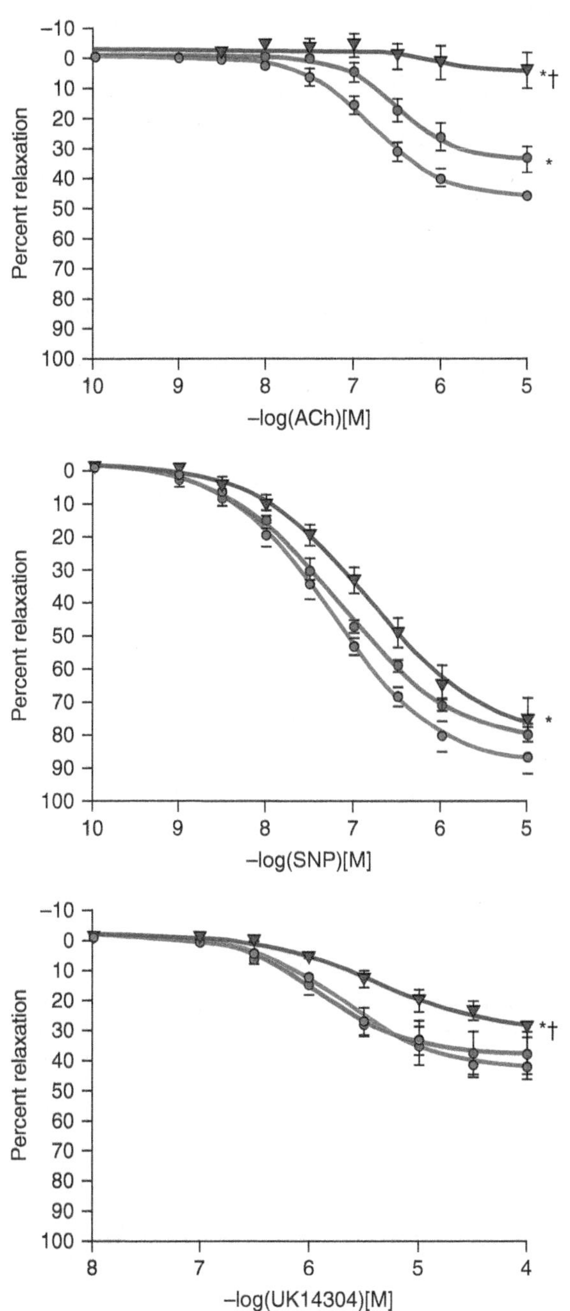

Fig. 51.3 Vasorelaxation in response to acetylcholine *(ACh)*, sodium nitroprusside *(SNP)*, and UK14303 (an α2-adrenoceptor agonist) in femoral arteries of fetuses from control and nutrient-restricted ewes. Data are expressed as a percentage of the initial preconstriction values. Values are the mean ± standard error of the mean in control *(orange circles)*, 70% global *(green circles)*, and 70% protein *(red triangles)* fetuses. *Asterisk*, $P < .05$ (ANOVA), significantly different from the control group. *Dagger*, $P < .05$ (ANOVA), significantly different from the global group. (From Nishina H, Green LR, McGarrigle HH, et al. Effect of nutritional restriction in early pregnancy on isolated femoral artery function in mid-gestation fetal sheep. *J Physiol.* 2003;553:637.)

PRENATAL AND POSTNATAL ENVIRONMENTAL MISMATCH

From the previous section it is apparent that a coordinated fetal cardiovascular adaptive response, designed to get nutrients where they are really needed, can be made to cues (e.g. nutrient supply, maternal stress) from the environment. The redistribution of the cardiovascular resources could preserve the growth of some organs at the expense of others. There are also likely to be limits to the extent that the fetus can cope through cardiovascular or growth adaptations (stretched to the limit by duration or severity of challenge), at which point the cue from the maternal environment becomes "disruptive."[108] Certainly, several serious clinical conditions originate during fetal life, including neurologic impairment, premature birth, fetal growth restriction (FGR), and pulmonary hypoplasia.

Another way in which fetal cardiovascular and growth adaptations might be viewed as disruptive is if the adaptation or "channeling of development" does do not suit the postnatal environment and results in poor responses of the cardiovascular system (or other body systems) after birth, with longer-term health problems. The cardiovascular responses made by the fetus to maternal obesity are less well investigated but are likely to be "nonadaptive" or disruptive. After all, the modern Western diet is a relatively recent problem for which humans are unlikely to have evolved such protective adaptive mechanisms.[108]

Importantly, the window of opportunity for priming of cardiovascular function in early life does not stop at birth. A study from Helsinki[12] showed that the effect of low ponderal index at birth on the risk of coronary arterial disease in adulthood in men was amplified by an increase in body mass index during the first 12 years of life. Considerable interest exists concerning the effects of obesity in childhood (which in Western societies may affect 20% of children younger than 12 years of age and in the United Kingdom may affect one in four children younger than 16 years by 2050[109]) on the risk of later disease. Indeed, in female sheep, early postnatal nutrient restriction (12 weeks of moderate intensity) improved later glucose handling through increased insulin sensitivity.[45] In rodents, severe undernutrition during fetal life leads to offspring that are hyperphagic, obese, insulin resistant, and demonstrate reduced physical activity.[110,111] This suggests a compounding of fetal effects by postnatal adaptations to an unhealthy lifestyle (unbalanced diet, reduced physical activity, smoking, and excessive alcohol consumption), including during childhood.

Relatively few studies have tested directly the concept that such a mismatch between the in utero and childhood nutritional environments increases risk of CVD. In male sheep, this postnatal undernutrition altered cardiovascular function, but not if they were also exposed to a poor nutritional environment in early gestation.[43,112] In rats, dietary manipulation to minimize the mismatch between pre-weaning and post-weaning nutrition minimizes endothelial dysfunction, low heart rate, and the disruption of mechanisms regulating appetite and energy expenditure in offspring.[113,114] In sheep and rats, a greater prenatal and postnatal dietary mismatch worsened the liver function and metabolic profile in offspring,[115] and in rats decreased life span.[116] In pigs, the coronary atherosclerotic effects of a high-fat diet were prevented by previous feeding of a similar diet to the pregnant mother.[117] Together, these studies support the concept that a greater mismatch between

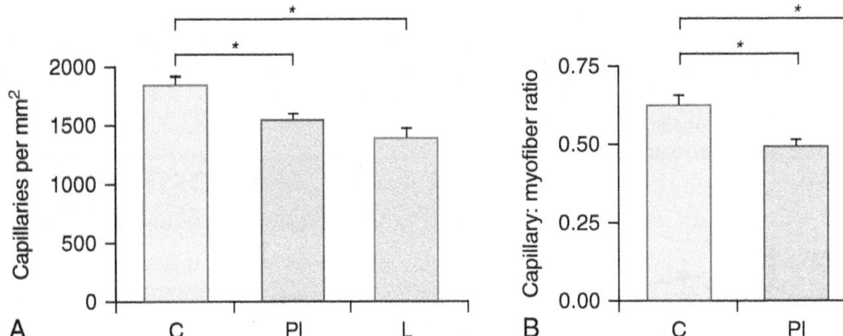

Fig. 51.4 Capillary density and capillary-to-myofiber ratio in the triceps brachii muscle of late-gestation fetuses. Capillary density (A) and capillary-to-myofiber ratio (B) in control (*C*; $n = 6$), peri-implantation nutrient-restricted (*PI*; $n = 9$), and late-gestation nutrient-restricted (*L*; $n = 6$) groups. *Asterisk*, $P < .05$. (From Costello PM, Rowlerson A, Astaman NA, et al. Peri-implantation and late gestation maternal undernutrition differentially affect fetal sheep skeletal muscle development. *J Physiol.* 2008;586:2371.)

the prenatal and the postnatal nutrient environment increases the risk of later disease, including disease of the cardiovascular system, in an individual.

TRANSMITTING ENVIRONMENTAL CUES TO THE FETUS

MATERNAL ADAPTATIONS

Cardiovascular adaptations of the mother to pregnancy provide another potential route whereby dietary or endocrine stressors may be transmitted to her fetus. The increase in blood volume and cardiac output during pregnancy[118] involves a redistribution of cardiac output in favor of the reproductive tract. In humans this is mediated primarily by a dramatic decrease in resistance in the spiral arteries supplying the endometrium, but there is an additional component of vasodilation in the uterine bed provided by vascular endothelial growth factor/nitric oxide (NO) mechanisms.[119] Ahokas and colleagues[120] observed that with dietary restriction in the rat dam (50%), maternal liver blood flow was maintained at the expense of the pregnant uterus. In sheep, 40% restriction of maternal nutrition decreased uterine artery blood flow.[121] In the low protein-diet rat model, Itoh and colleagues[122] found an impaired vasodilator response to vascular endothelial growth factor in late-pregnancy uterine arteries in vitro. Similarly, in hypertensive rat offspring of protein-restricted dams, Brawley and colleagues[123] found a blunting of mesenteric vasodilator responses to acetylcholine. This effect clearly persists in the female offspring when they become pregnant, despite their adaptations to pregnancy, and even though they had not been exposed to any dietary challenge during postnatal life or pregnancy itself (unlike their mothers).[124] But dietary supplementation with folic acid (a key player in gene methylation) or the conditionally essential amino acid glycine during pregnancy was subsequently found to ameliorate the offspring hypertension and maternal and offspring vascular dysfunction by a caused by a low protein diet.[60]

THE PLACENTA

Placental development and transport functions are contained in Section II. But it is important to mention here that the maternal environment affects the number of cells that are allocated to the trophectoderm (which forms the placenta) relative to the inner cell mass (which forms the fetus).[125] Then when the placenta is formed, its size and function are affected by numerous hormones and nutrients from the mother and fetus. Interestingly, in humans maternal upper-arm muscle mass before pregnancy (an index of lean mass) is positively associated with activity of the amino acid transporter system A in the term placenta; this provides a mechanism by which maternal environmental signals might be transmitted to the fetus.[126] Human and animal studies suggest that the placenta can adapt its vascular structure and transport function in response to changes in nutrients or even a specific deficiency in vitamin D,[68,127] and that it does this in accordance with both the fetal drive for growth and the maternal ability to supply the required nutrients.[128]

STRESS

Glucocorticoids are administered routinely during pregnancy to treat complications and medical disorders. Their less desirable effects on the fetus have been studied extensively, including reduced growth and altered hypothalamo-pituitary-adrenal (HPA) axis function. Their administration in specific early-gestation periods leads to postnatal hypertension, which persists into mature adulthood.[129-131]

Glucocorticoids may also mediate effects of altered maternal nutrition, including via interaction with the expression of other genes, NO signaling pathways, and effects on DNA methylation.[132-135] Indeed, there is some evidence that nutrient restriction in guinea pigs elevates maternal plasma cortisol concentration[136] and a high-fat diet in rats is associated with stimulation of the HPA axis.[137] Findings suggest that maternal cortisol concentration is lower during undernutrition in early gestation;[138,139] however, and it has not been shown unequivocally in animals that altered maternal nutritional balance alters the level of plasma glucocorticoid in fetal life.[140,141] Even in the absence of an elevation in maternal glucocorticoid concentration, the nutrient-challenged fetus may be exposed to greater levels of steroid as a result of a reduction in the level of placental 11β-hydroxysteroid dehydrogenase type 2,[142] which inactivates cortisol. That being said, in sheep late-gestation fetal plasma cortisol levels were not altered after early-gestation maternal nutrient restriction and fetal HPA axis responsiveness was reduced, rather than being enhanced as predicted.[40] However, these observations are coupled to a reduction in glucocorticoid receptor messenger RNA levels in the pituitary in "programmed" late-gestation sheep fetuses,[143] and the implied reduction in feedback inhibition of the HPA axis is consistent with the hyperresponsiveness of the HPA axis seen in offspring from this sheep cohort at 3 months of age[40] and in adult men who were of low birth weight.[144]

Similarly in rodents, altered components of the HPA axis consistent with exposure to greater levels of active steroid in certain tissues and altered expression of glucocorticoid-responsive genes (e.g., Na^+,K^+-ATPase) have been observed in offspring of mothers fed a low-protein diet.[145]

MECHANISMS OF FETAL CARDIOVASCULAR RESPONSE TO THE ENVIRONMENT

NEURONAL, HORMONAL, AND LOCAL VASCULAR FACTORS

Unraveling the relative contribution of the key mechanisms by which the fetal cardiovascular system responds to dietary imbalance in pregnancy is likely to be complicated, but is informed by several decades of work on mechanisms of the fetal cardiovascular control under baseline conditions and during hypoxemia (see Chapter 50); such mechanisms include carotid chemoreflexes, hormonal factors (e.g., catecholamines, arginine vasopressin, adrenocorticotropic hormone, cortisol, angiotensin, the IGF system), and local mechanisms such as NO and endothelin 1.[71] There is now evidence that the fetal cardiovascular system can respond to changes in nutrients other than oxygen, although the mechanisms mediating these responses are still being worked out.

The carotid chemoreceptors, which mediate the rapid fetal cardiovascular adaptations to hypoxia, are also responsive to reductions in circulating plasma glucose concentration.[81,82] Common mechanisms of detection of changes in substrate (e.g., glucose) and oxygen levels may exist. Evidence from cultured rat hepatocytes indicates that regulation of glucagon receptor, insulin receptor, and L-type pyruvate kinase gene expression by glucose and oxygen may be due to crosstalk between hypoxia-inducible factor-1 and glucose-responsive transcription factors at the glucose response element and hypoxia response element.[147] An additional consideration is that multiple genes and proteins may respond simultaneously to altered nutrition—analogous to the 14-protein "stimulon" induced by glucose depletion in *Escherichia coli*.[148] As the available evidence indicates, the expression of a variety of genes implicated in cardiovascular control and growth during fetal life can be modulated by the direct action of nutrients; for example, IGF-2 gene expression in cultured β cells is regulated by glucose.[149] During fetal life, glucose appears to regulate IGF-2 directly, but its effect on IGF-1 is likely to be mediated by insulin.[150] Glucose activation of plasminogen activator inhibitor 1 gene expression in cultured rat vascular smooth muscle cells,[151] and of the osteopontin gene,[152] may be of relevance to vascular complications in patients with diabetes. High glucose concentration stimulates angiotensinogen gene expression in rat kidney proximal tubular cells, mediated in part by the generation of reactive oxygen species.[153]

Likely candidates mediating the fetal cardiovascular response include components of the HPA axis, the renin-angiotensin system, and the IGF axis. Similarly to the HPA axis (see "Stress" earlier), evidence exists that the fetal and postnatal renin-angiotensin system and IGF axis are primed by altered substrate supply during pregnancy.[154-159] It is possible that there are common control mechanisms, such as angiotensin II, IGF-1, and cortisol, that integrate cardiovascular control and growth in a graded manner in the face of altered nutrient supply.[71] (See "Fetal Adaptive Responses".) The role of the kidney is uncertain because its structure or function in late-gestation sheep is unaltered by early or late gestation undernutrition,[157,161] but fetal kidney development in later life function is altered by gestation-long protein restriction in rats,[162] early-gestation protein restriction in sheep,[163,164] or pharmacologic doses of dexamethasone in early-gestation sheep.[165]

In animal studies, the mechanisms by which altered maternal nutrient environment after birth changes peripheral vascular function are becoming clearer. The observation that small-resistance vessel responses to endothelium-dependent vasodilators, such as acetylcholine and bradykinin, are impaired in offspring of rat dams fed a low-protein diet during gestation is supported by our finding that both basal and acetylcholine-stimulated NO release are reduced in the mesenteric arteries of such offspring.[123,166] In a rat model using global undernutrition during pregnancy, Franco and colleagues[167] have shown that the adult offspring have reduced endothelial NO synthase activity and messenger RNA expression in the aorta. Feeding rat dams a diet high in soy isoflavones improves endothelial function and increases endothelial NO synthase and antioxidant gene expression in offspring.[168] Estrogen, through its estrogen receptor α, has a well-established vascular protective role mediated in part by its effects on NO production.[169] Endothelial responsiveness mediates flow-mediated vasodilation in many vascular beds, and this can be studied in humans by techniques such as forearm plethysmography.[170] Such methods have demonstrated reduced flow-mediated vasodilatation with lower birth weight in adults[171] and an effect that is comparable to that of smoking. Similarly, endothelium-dependent vasodilator responses in the leg are reduced in obese persons with type 2 diabetes compared with control subjects.[172] Disorders of endothelial function predispose affected persons to atherosclerosis and hypertension. In sheep, enhanced vasoconstrictor tone after peri-implantation undernutrition was mediated in part by increased expression of myosin light-chain kinase, and the effect was minimized when the mismatch between the prenatal and postnatal nutrient environments was minimized.[43]

THE NEXT GENERATION AND EPIGENETIC MODIFICATIONS

In this chapter we have already raised the idea that changes in the mother's nutrient environment can still have an impact on the cardiovascular system of her grandchildren. For example, the grandchildren of women exposed to a dietary impairment during pregnancy also show impaired vasodilator function through defects in endothelium-derived hyperpolarizing factor or NO-mediated mechanisms.[124,173] In fact, the legacy of the mother's environment may be even longer, affecting multiple generations even in the absence of additional dietary or other stressors. Similar transgenerational programming of risk of diabetes has been demonstrated for the male lineage.[174]

Mounting evidence suggests that epigenetic alterations may underlie many of the persistent effects of changes in the early nutrient environment on the later cardiovascular phenotype. The idea is that altering gene expression by stable methylation marks on the genome, without changing DNA sequence, could set up responses to transcription factors. The impact of this may not become apparent until later life, perhaps when an additional challenge is received. In sheep, depletion of B vitamins (B_{12} and folate) and methionine within normal ranges from the periconceptional diet of ewes led to widespread altered DNA methylation in the liver of adult offspring, with associated elevation of blood pressure.[175] In sheep fetuses periconceptional undernutrition altered epigenetic regulatory mechanisms (i.e., histone acetylation and methylation) in hypothalamic proopiomelanocortin and *GR* genes, which influence food intake, energy expenditure, and glucose homeostasis in later life.[176] In the baboon, moderate maternal undernutrition in mid-gestation was associated with less methylation of the PCK1 gene promotor in the fetal liver.[177] In sheep, prenatal and postnatal undernutrition altered methylation of imprint control regions of imprinted gene clusters *DLK1/MEG3* and *IGF-2* in adult offspring liver in a sex-specific manner[178] and is linked to an altered metabolic and growth offspring phenotype. In rats, maternal protein restriction in pregnancy caused increased methylation and decreased expression of genes (e.g., *PPARγ* and *GR*) that regulate cardiovascular and metabolic function. These effects can be prevented by maternal dietary folate supplementation and can be transmitted to the F2 generation.[28] Also, evidence is emerging that gestational dietary effects on angiotensin receptor expression in rats may be mediated via altered methylation in the promoter region.[179]

The evidence is clear that epigenetic modifications provide a plausible mechanism by which environmental influences on cardiovascular control, metabolism, and growth might be integrated into a life course response, starting from very early in development. Important emerging work from international human cohorts and trials shows links between maternal diet and body composition and epigenetic changes; for example, low maternal carbohydrate diet in early pregnancy was associated with methylation of one CpG in the *RXRA* gene at birth and child's adiposity in 6- and 9-year-old children,[180] and obesity is an established risk factor for CVD. Other work shows that altered CpG methylation on the ANRIL promoter from umbilical cords may predict childhood CVD risk.[181] So the goal of using these markers to predict early individuals who are at risk of later disease, and even reverse the process, is in sight.

CONCLUSION

The fetus can adapt to its environment, whether that is to cues of oxygen, other nutrients, or toxin levels. This is not just at extremes, where a severe deficiency might be disruptive to normal development (i.e., "pathophysiologic") and result in potentially serious clinical conditions like neurologic handicap, premature birth, FGR, or pulmonary hypoplasia. The work in this field and DOHaD concepts suggest that the broad spectrum of cues from the environment may "channel" rather than "disrupt" development of the fetus in a way that optimizes the individual for the environment that it is born into. The responses that the fetus can make in cardiovascular control or modification of growth may have their limits, or perhaps the environment after birth may not be as predicted—either or both of these scenarios could result in an individual being more susceptible to adult NCDs.[108]

Knowledge has advanced on the mechanisms of detection and response used by the fetus to respond to its environment, from neuronal and hormonal pathways to epigenetic mechanisms that explain the persistence of the effect of the mother's environment on our bodies across the life course. This may inform better ways to predict individuals at risk of adverse outcomes at birth and also over their lifetime; it could also help in devising pregnancy interventions (e.g., pharmaceutical, gene or nutritional therapies, diet and lifestyle advice) aimed at providing the best possible start to life.

The response by the fetus to maternal environmental cues is affected by the environment experienced earlier in pregnancy, even preconception. Improved preconception health care is considered to be a core part of public health solutions to setting up individuals for better health across the life course.[58] The solutions may be targeted to couples planning a family around the obvious potential benefits of specific and informed advice on exercise, diet, and weight management before and during pregnancy (for both father and mother).[182] But international programs that engage with a much younger public,[183] optimizing their healthy behaviors at ages when children and adolescents are not yet intending to become pregnant, will be very important in setting conditions for the best possible start of a future planned pregnancy and influencing the health of the next generation.

ACKNOWLEDGMENTS

Preparation of this chapter was supported by grants from the British Heart Foundation, the Biotechnology and Biological Sciences Research Council, and Gerald Kerkut Trust.

A complete reference list is available at www.ExpertConsult.com.

SELECT REFERENCES

3. Cardiovascular Diseases (CVDs). World Health Organization. 2017. https://www.who.int/news-room/fact-sheets/detail/cardiovascular-diseases-(cvds).
4. *Political Declaration of the High-Level Meeting of the General Assembly on the Prevention and Control of Non-Communicable Diseases*. 2012. https://www.who.int/nmh/events/un_ncd_summit2011/political_declaration_en.pdf.
5. WHO | What is the Global Strategy? *WHO*; 2017. Accessed December 13, 2019. https://www.who.int/life-course/partners/global-strategy/global-strategy-2016-2030/en/index1.html#.XfNPK7nWSlo.mendeley.
6. Barker DJ, Osmond C, Simmonds SJ, Wield GA. The relation of small head circumference and thinness at birth to death from cardiovascular disease in adult life. *BMJ*. 1993;306(6875):422–426. http://www.ncbi.nlm.nih.gov/pubmed/8461722.
12. Eriksson JG, Forsen T, Tuomilehto J, Osmond C, Barker DJ. Early growth and coronary heart disease in later life: longitudinal study. *BMJ*. 2001;322(7292):949–953. http://www.ncbi.nlm.nih.gov/pubmed/11312225.
14. Crozier SR, Inskip HM, Godfrey KM, et al. Weight gain in pregnancy and childhood body composition: findings from the Southampton Women's Survey. *Am J Clin Nutr*. 2010;91(6):1745–1751. https://doi.org/ajcn.2009.29128 [pii];10.3945/ajcn.2009.29128 ([doi]).
18. Ma RC, Chan JC, Tam WH, Hanson MA, Gluckman PD. Gestational diabetes, maternal obesity, and the NCD burden. *Clin Obstet Gynecol*. 2013;56(3):633–641. https://doi.org/10.1097/GRF.0b013e31829e5bb0.
21. Barker DJ, Shiell AW, Barker ME, Law CM. Growth in utero and blood pressure levels in the next generation. *J Hypertens*. 2000;18(7):843–846. http://www.ncbi.nlm.nih.gov/pubmed/10930180.
28. Burdge GC, Hanson MA, Slater-Jefferies JL, Lillycrop KA. Epigenetic regulation of transcription: a mechanism for inducing variations in phenotype (fetal programming) by differences in nutrition during early life? *Br J Nutr*. 2007;97(6):1036–1046. http://www.ncbi.nlm.nih.gov/pubmed/17381976.
31. Godfrey KM, Lillycrop KA, Burdge GC, Gluckman PD, Hanson MA. Epigenetic mechanisms and the mismatch concept of the developmental origins of health and disease. *Pediatr Res*. 2007;61(5 Pt 2):5R–10R. http://www.ncbi.nlm.nih.gov/pubmed/17413851.
33. Morgan HL, Paganopoulou P, Akhtar S, et al. Paternal diet impairs F1 and F2 offspring vascular function through sperm and seminal plasma specific mechanisms in mice. *J Physiol*. 2019;598:699–715. https://doi.org/10.1113/JP278270.
36. Painter RC, de Sr R, Bossuyt PM, et al. Early onset of coronary artery disease after prenatal exposure to the Dutch famine. *Am J Clin Nutr*. 2006;84(2):322–327. http://www.ncbi.nlm.nih.gov/pubmed/16895878.
41. Gopalakrishnan GS, Gardner DS, Rhind SM, et al. Programming of adult cardiovascular function after early maternal undernutrition in sheep. *Am J Physiol Regul Integr Comp Physiol*. 2004;287(1):R12–R20. http://www.ncbi.nlm.nih.gov/pubmed/14975924.
43. Cleal JK, Poore KR, Boullin JP, et al. Mismatched pre- and postnatal nutrition leads to cardiovascular dysfunction and altered renal function in adulthood. *Proc Natl Acad Sci USA*. 2007;104(22):9529–9533. http://www.ncbi.nlm.nih.gov/pubmed/17483483.
54. Watkins AJ, Platt D, Papenbrock T, et al. Mouse embryo culture induces changes in postnatal phenotype including raised systolic blood pressure. *Proc Natl Acad Sci USA*. 2007;104(13):5449–5454. http://www.ncbi.nlm.nih.gov/pubmed/17372207.
57. Torrens C, Noakes DE, Poston L, Hanson MA, Green LR. Impaired femoral resistance artery function in adult sheep offspring following pre- or peri-conceptional nutrient restriction. *Pediatr Res*. 2005;58(5):1131.
60. Torrens C, Brawley L, Anthony FW, et al. Folate supplementation during pregnancy improves offspring cardiovascular dysfunction induced by protein restriction. *Hypertension*. 2006;47(5):982–987. http://www.ncbi.nlm.nih.gov/pubmed/16585422.
67. Cleal JK, Hargreaves MR, Poore KR, et al. Reduced fetal vitamin D status by maternal undernutrition during discrete gestational windows in sheep. *J Dev Orig Health Dis*. 2017;8(3):370–381. https://doi.org/10.1017/S2040174417000149.
68. Cleal JK, Day PE, Simner CL, et al. Placental amino acid transport may be regulated by maternal vitamin D and vitamin D-binding protein: results from the Southampton Women's Survey. *Br J Nutr*. 2015;113(12):1903–1910. https://doi.org/10.1017/s0007114515001178.
71. Green LR. Programming of endocrine mechanisms of cardiovascular control and growth. *J Soc Gynecol Investig*. 2001;8(2):57–68. https://doi.org/S0143-4004(11)00575-3 [pii];10.1016/j.placenta.2011.12.003 ([doi]). https://doi.org/S1071557601000971.
82. Burrage D, Green LR, Moss TJM, et al. The carotid bodies influence growth responses to moderate maternal undernutrition in late-gestation fetal sheep. *BJOG An Int J Obstet Gynaecol*. 2008;115(2):261–268. https://doi.org/10.1111/j.1471-0528.2007.01607.x.
85. Haugen G, Hanson M, Kiserud T, Crozier S, Inskip H, Godfrey KM. Fetal liver-sparing cardiovascular adaptations linked to mother's slimness and diet. *Circ Res*. 2005;96(1):12–14. http://www.ncbi.nlm.nih.gov/pubmed/15576647.
87. Nishina H, Green LR, McGarrigle HHG, Noakes DE, Poston L, Hanson MA. Effect of nutritional restriction in early pregnancy on isolated femoral artery function in mid-gestation fetal sheep. *J Physiol*. 2003;553(2):637–647. https://doi.org/10.1113/jphysiol.2003.045278.
92. Torrens C, Ethirajan P, Bruce KD, et al. Interaction between maternal and offspring diet to impair vascular function and oxidative balance in high fat fed male mice. *PloS One*. 2012;7(12):e50671. https://doi.org/10.1371/journal.pone.0050671.

93. Samuelsson AM, Matthews PA, Jansen E, Taylor PD, Poston L. Sucrose feeding in mouse pregnancy leads to hypertension, and sex-linked obesity and insulin resistance in female offspring. *Front Physiol*. 2013;4:14. https://doi.org/10.3389/fphys.2013.00014.
96. Krause BJ, Herrera EA, Diaz-Lopez FA, Farias M, Uauy R, Casanello P. Pre-gestational overweight in Guinea pig sows induces fetal vascular dysfunction and increased rate of large and small fetuses. *J Dev Orig Heal Dis*. 2015:1-7. https://doi.org/10.1017/S2040174415007266.
102. Costello PM, Rowlerson A, Astaman NA, et al. Peri-implantation and late gestation maternal undernutrition differentially affect fetal sheep skeletal muscle development. *J Physiol*. 2008;586(9):2371-2380. http://www.ncbi.nlm.nih.gov/pubmed/18339691.
104. Burrage DM, Braddick L, Cleal JK, et al. The late gestation fetal cardiovascular response to hypoglycaemia is modified by prior peri-implantation undernutrition in sheep. *J Physiol*. 2009;587(3):611-624. https://doi.org/10.1113/jphysiol.2008.165944.
107. Cleal JK, Poore KR, Newman JP, Noakes DE, Hanson MA, Green LR. The effect of maternal undernutrition in early gestation on gestation length and fetal and postnatal growth in sheep. *Pediatr Res*. 2007;62(4):422-427. http://www.nature.com/pr/journal/v62/n4/pdf/pr2007248a.pdf.
108. Hanson MA, Gluckman PD. Early developmental conditioning of later health and disease: physiology or pathophysiology? *Physiol Rev*. 2014;94(4):1027-1076. https://doi.org/94/4/1027 [pii];10.1152/physrev.00029.2013 ([doi]).
109. King D. *Foresight Report-Tackling Obesities:Future Choices*. 2007. http://www.foresight.gov.uk/Obesity/obesity_final/17.pdf.
110. Vickers MH, Reddy S, Ikenasio BA, Breier BH. Dysregulation of the adipoinsular axis - a mechanism for the pathogenesis of hyperleptinemia and adipogenic diabetes induced by fetal programming. *J Endocrinol*. 2001;170(2):323-332. http://www.ncbi.nlm.nih.gov/pubmed/11479129.
114. Sellayah D, Anthony F, Hanson M, Cagampang F. Mismatched prenatal and post-weaning diet leads to sex-specific changes in expression of genes involved in the regulation of appetite and metabolism in the adult mouse offspring. *Early Hum Dev*. 2007;83:S131-S132.
124. Torrens C, Poston L, Hanson MA. Transmission of raised blood pressure and endothelial dysfunction to the F2 generation induced by maternal protein restriction in the F0, in the absence of dietary challenge in the F1 generation. *Br J Nutr*. 2008:1-7. http://www.ncbi.nlm.nih.gov/pubmed/18304387.
125. Fleming TP, Watkins AJ, Velazquez MA, et al. Origins of lifetime health around the time of conception: causes and consequences. *Lancet*. 2018;391(10132):1842-1852. https://doi.org/10.1016/S0140-6736(18)30312-X.
126. Lewis RM, Cleal JK, Hanson MA. Review: placenta, evolution and lifelong health. *Placenta*. 2012;33 Suppl:S28-S32. https://doi.org/S0143-4004(11)00575-3 [pii];10.1016/j.placenta.2011.12.003 ([doi]).
128. Sferruzzi-Perri AN, López-Tello J, Fowden AL, Constancia M. Maternal and fetal genomes interplay through phosphoinositol 3-kinase(PI3K)-p110α signaling to modify placental resource allocation. *Proc Natl Acad Sci*. 2016;113(40):11255-11260. https://doi.org/10.1073/pnas.1602012113.
141. Hawkins P, Steyn C, McGarrigle HH, et al. Effect of maternal nutrient restriction in early gestation on development of the hypothalamic-pituitary-adrenal axis in fetal sheep at 0.8-0.9 of gestation. *J Endocrinol*. 1999;163(3):553-561. http://www.ncbi.nlm.nih.gov/pubmed/0010588829.
155. Edwards LJ, McMillen IC. Periconceptional nutrition programs development of the cardiovascular system in the fetal sheep. *Am J Physiol Regul Integr Comp Physiol*. 2002;283(3):R669-R679. http://www.ncbi.nlm.nih.gov/pubmed/12185002.
156. Green LR, Hawkins P, McGarrigle HH, Steyn C, Noakes DE, Hanson MA. Effect of maternal nutrient restriction in early gestation on the plasma angiotensin II and arginine vasopressin responses during acute hypoxaemia in late gestation fetal sheep. *Pediatr Res*. 2001;50(1):24A.
157. Braddick LM, Burrage DM, Cleal JK, Noakes DE, Hanson MA, Green LR. The lack of impact of peri-implantation or late gestation nutrient restriction on ovine fetal renal development and function. *J Dev Orig Heal Dis*. 2011;2(4):236-249. https://doi.org/10.1017/s2040174411000237.
175. Sinclair KD, Allegrucci C, Singh R, et al. DNA methylation, insulin resistance, and blood pressure in offspring determined by maternal periconceptional B vitamin and methionine status. *Proc Natl Acad Sci USA*. 2007;104(49):19351-19356. http://www.ncbi.nlm.nih.gov/pubmed/18042717.
176. Stevens A, Begum G, Cook A, et al. Epigenetic changes in the hypothalamic proopiomelanocortin and glucocorticoid receptor genes in the ovine fetus after periconceptional undernutrition. *Endocrinology*. 2010;151(8):3652-3664. https://doi.org/en.2010-0094 [pii];10.1210/en.2010-0094 ([doi]).
178. Poore KR, Hollis LJ, Murray RJ, et al. Differential pathways to adult metabolic dysfunction following poor nutrition at two critical developmental periods in sheep. *PloS One*. 2014;9(3):e90994. https://doi.org/10.1371/journal.pone.0090994.
182. Barker M, Dombrowski SU, Colbourn T, et al. Intervention strategies to improve nutrition and health behaviours before conception. *Lancet*. 2018;391(10132):1853-1864. https://doi.org/10.1016/S0140-6736(18)30313-1.
183. Woods-Townsend K, Bagust L, Barker M, et al. Engaging teenagers in improving their health behaviours and increasing their interest in science (Evaluation of LifeLab Southampton): study protocol for a cluster randomized controlled trial. *Trials*. 2015;16(1):372. https://doi.org/10.1186/s13063-015-0890-z.

Mechanisms Regulating Closure of the Ductus Arteriosus

52

Ronald I. Clyman

INTRODUCTION[a]

The ductus arteriosus represents a persistence of the terminal portion of the sixth branchial arch. During fetal life, the ductus arteriosus serves to divert blood away from the fluid-filled lungs toward the descending aorta and placenta. After birth, constriction of the ductus arteriosus and obliteration of its lumen separates the pulmonary and systemic circulations. In full-term infants, obliteration of the ductus arteriosus takes place through a process of vasoconstriction and anatomic remodeling. In the preterm, the ductus arteriosus frequently fails to close. The clinical consequences of a patent ductus arteriosus (PDA) are related to the degree of left-to-right shunt through the PDA with its associated change in blood flow to the lungs, kidneys, and intestine.

[a]Portions of this chapter are reprinted from Chapter 54 in *Avery's Diseases of the Newborn,* 10th edition.

DIAGNOSIS

Phase contrast magnetic resonance imaging appears to offer the most accurate measurements of ductal shunt volume and the effects of a PDA on left ventricular and systemic blood flow volumes.[1] Unfortunately, these measurements are difficult to obtain in extremely immature, sick preterm infants. As a result, two-dimensional echocardiography and color Doppler flow mapping have been used as the standard for assessing the presence, magnitude, and direction of PDA shunting. Although pulsed Doppler echocardiographic assessments can consistently diagnose the presence of a PDA, determining its hemodynamic significance has been more challenging. Ductus diameter ≥1.5 mm (or >50% of the diameter of the left pulmonary artery), left atrial-to-aortic root (LA/Ao) ratio ≥1.5, reversal of forward blood flow in the descending aorta during diastole, and end diastolic flow velocity in the left pulmonary artery ≥0.20 m/s are signs consistent with a moderate-to-large PDA shunt.[1,2] Unfortunately,

Table 52.1 Incidence of Patent Ductus Arteriosus Among Infants <30 Weeks Gestation.

Presence of a PDA (%)

Gestation-Weeks	Day 4	Day 7	Day 20	Day 40	Day 60	Day 80
28–29 wk	55	33	20	10	8	
26–27 wk	84	68	48	38	27	27
24–25 wk	96	87	75	72	56	38

Presence of a Hemodynamically Significant PDA (Ductus Diameter ≥2 mm on Echocardiography *Plus* Need for Ventilator Support) (%)

Gestation-Weeks	Day 4	Day 7	Day 20	Day 40	Day 60	Day 80
27–28 wk		21	13	5	1	0
25–26 wk		64	50	22	3	0
23–24 wk		93	88	58	33	14

PDA, Patent ductus arteriosus.

the inter-observer repeatability of all echocardiographic parameters is relatively poor.[3]

Clinical signs of a PDA (systolic murmur, hyperdynamic precordial impulse, full pulses, widened pulse pressure, and/or worsening respiratory status) usually appear later than echocardiographic signs and are less sensitive in determining the degree of left-to-right shunt. Certain signs such as continuous murmur or hyperactive left ventricular impulse are relatively specific for a PDA but lack sensitivity; conversely, worsening respiratory status, while a sensitive indicator, is relatively nonspecific for a PDA. Tachycardia is not a useful or reliable indicator of a PDA in preterm infants. Infants with large left-to-right shunts may have evidence of cardiomegaly and increased pulmonary arterial markings on their chest x-rays; however, in general, the chest x-ray and electrocardiogram are not useful in diagnosing a PDA. Although elevated plasma concentrations of brain natriuretic peptide (BNP) and N-terminal pro-BNP (NTpBNP) have been found to correlate with the presence of a moderate sized left-to-right PDA shunt,[4] changes in BNP and NTpBNP concentrations have poor sensitivity and specificity in predicting increases or decreases in PDA shunt magnitude and cannot be used to replace echocardiography in the management of PDA shunts.[5]

Infants with persistent small PDA shunts appear to have similar neonatal outcomes as infants who close their ductus shortly after birth, whereas infants with moderate and large PDA shunt volumes appear to have increased neonatal morbidity.[6,7] While PDA shunt magnitude plays a significant role in creating its hemodynamic significance, equally important are the duration of exposure to the shunt[7] and the infant's ability to compensate for the shunt. Infants with poor ventricular diastolic function and a PDA are more likely to develop morbidities like bronchopulmonary dysplasia (BPD) than infants with normal diastolic function.[8] Similarly, adverse perinatal and neonatal events, lower gestational age, and the degree of respiratory support that an infant requires all contribute to exacerbating detrimental effects of a PDA shunt. At this time, a consistent definition of hemodynamically significant PDA, which includes both markers of shunt volume and clinical characteristics, has yet to be agreed upon.

INCIDENCE

Pulsed Doppler echocardiographic assessments of full-term infants indicate that functional closure of the ductus has occurred in almost 50% by 24 hours, in 90% by 48 hours, and in all by 72 hours. Ductus closure is delayed in preterm infants; however, essentially all healthy preterm infants (and 90% of those with respiratory distress syndrome) who are at least 30 weeks gestation will close their ductus by the fourth day after birth. Infants born at less than 30 weeks gestation have a 65% incidence of persistent ductus patency beyond day 4 (Table 52.1). Even among the most immature infants (≤27 weeks gestation), spontaneous closure can occur during the neonatal period. However, when it does occur, it usually occurs late during the neonatal course (average age 61 ± 37 days).[9-15] Eighty-six percent of preterm infants with a persistent PDA at the time of discharge from the hospital will close their PDA by 1 year of age. The remainder will require continued observation or transcatheter device closure.[9-15]

Several prenatal and postnatal factors also appear to alter the incidence of PDA in preterm infants. Chorioamnionitis increases the incidence of PDA; however, its effects may depend more on its ability to induce preterm birth than its effect on ductus pathobiology.[16] Surfactant administration can lead to early clinical presentation of the left-to-right shunt by altering pulmonary vascular resistance, even though it has no direct effect on ductus contractile behavior.[9,17-21] Infants who have late-onset septicemia[22] or receive excessive fluid administration during the first days of life also are more likely to develop a clinically symptomatic PDA.[23] Small-for-gestational age infants delivered between 23 and 24 weeks have a decreased risk of PDA, while those delivered at 26 to 29 weeks have an increased risk.[24] Non-Caucasian infants and infants who receive antenatal glucocorticoids have a reduced risk of PDA.[25-31]

REGULATION OF DUCTUS ARTERIOSUS PATENCY

In the full-term infant, closure of the ductus arteriosus occurs in phases: (1) "functional" closure of the lumen within the first hours after birth by smooth muscle constriction, and (2) "anatomic" occlusion of the lumen over the next several days due to extensive neointimal thickening and loss of smooth muscle cells from the inner muscle media.

FUNCTIONAL CLOSURE: BALANCE BETWEEN VASOCONSTRICTION AND VASORELAXATION

Ductus arteriosus patency is determined by the balance between dilating and constricting forces. The factors known to play a prominent role in ductus arteriosus regulation involve those that promote constriction (oxygen, endothelin, calcium channels, catecholamines, and Rho kinase) and those that oppose it (intraluminal pressure, prostaglandins [PGs], nitric oxide [NO], carbon monoxide, potassium channels, cyclic adenosine monophosphate [AMP], and cyclic guanosine monophosphate [GMP]). The relative importance of each of these factors depends on the intrauterine and extrauterine environment, the degree of ductus maturation, and the genetic background and species being studied.

VASOCONSTRICTION/VASORELAXATION: IN UTERO REGULATION

The fetal ductus normally has a high level of intrinsic tone caused by elevated levels of intracellular calcium, which activates myosin light chain kinase, producing myosin light chain phosphorylation and smooth muscle constriction.[32] Extracellular calcium enters the smooth muscle cytosol primarily through voltage–operated calcium channels (Ca_L and T-type channels) in the plasma membrane. Transient receptor potential (TRP) cation channels have also been detected in the ductus.[33,34] However, only a portion of fetal ductus tone is dependent on the influx of extracellular calcium.[35] Calcium is also released from intracellular stores in the sarcoplasmic and endoplasmic reticulum (SR and ER) through calcium–release channels, which consist of ryanodine receptors (RyRs) and inositol 1,4,5–trisphosphate receptors (IP3Rs).[34,36]

The contractile proteins of the fetal ductus (smooth-muscle myosin, calponin, and caldesmon) are more differentiated than they are in adjacent fetal arteries.[37-39] In addition, the fetal ductus arteriosus is more sensitive to the contractile effects of calcium than are the aorta and the pulmonary artery.[40] This may be due in part to increased Rho kinase activity in the ductus,[41] which increases smooth muscle sensitivity to calcium by inhibiting myosin light chain dephosphorylation. Endothelin-1 also appears to play a role in producing the elevated basal tone of the fetal ductus arteriosus.[42] The presence of catecholamine containing nerves varies with the species being studied.[43] Although catecholamines can constrict the ductus arteriosus[44] and are present in high circulating concentrations during the transition to extrauterine life,[45] there is little information about their role or the role of ductus innervation in regulating ductus tone. A role for serotonin in promoting fetal ductus tone has been suggested, since selective serotonin reuptake inhibitors appear to constrict the ductus in utero.[46]

The factors that oppose ductus arteriosus constriction in utero are better understood. The elevated vascular pressure within the ductus lumen (due to the constricted pulmonary vascular bed) plays an important role in opposing ductus constriction.[47]

K^+ channels, which regulate the smooth muscle cell's resting membrane potential, are the primary gatekeeper for extracellular calcium entry into the smooth muscle cells. When K^+ channels are open, K^+ exits the cell, turning the membrane potential more negative (i.e., hyperpolarizing the cell). Hyperpolarization inhibits ductus tone by inhibiting extracellular calcium influx through voltage-gated L-type calcium (CaL) channels. Several K^+ channels (voltage-gated [Kv], calcium-activated [K_{Ca}], and ATP-dependent [K_{ATP}]) are present in fetal ductus smooth muscle cells. Their relative contribution to resting membrane potential depends on the animal species and the stage of development.

The fetal ductus also produces several vasodilators that help to maintain ductus patency. Vasodilator PGs appear to be the dominant vasodilators that oppose ductus constriction in the later part of gestation.[48] Inhibitors of PG synthesis constrict the fetal ductus both in vitro and in vivo. PGE_2 is the most potent PG produced by the ductus[49,50] and appears to be the most important prostanoid to regulate ductus patency. The response of the ductus to PGE_2 is unique among blood vessels since it is extraordinarily sensitive to this vasodilating substance. PGE_2 produces ductus relaxation by interacting with several of the PGE receptors (EP2, EP3, and EP4).[35] In the ductus, all three of the EP receptors participate in vasodilation by activating adenylate cyclase and increasing ductus smooth muscle cyclic AMP and cAMP-dependent protein kinase (PKA).[35] Increased cyclic AMP production inhibits myosin light chain kinase and myosin light chain phosphorylation, thereby inhibiting the sensitivity of the contractile proteins to calcium.[40]

Inhibitors of phosphodiesterase (the enzyme that degrades cyclic AMP) relax the ductus in utero.[51] Low phosphodiesterase levels in the fetal ductus account for its increased sensitivity to PGE_2.[52] In addition, EP3 receptors in lamb and EP4 receptors in rabbit relax the ductus smooth muscle by opening potassium channels (K_{ATP} and Kv, respectively) and hyperpolarize the muscle cells.[35,53]

Both isoforms of the enzyme responsible for synthesizing PGs (cyclooxygenase [COX]-1 and COX-2) are expressed in the fetal ductus.[54] Depending on the species, both nonselective (e.g., indomethacin and ibuprofen) and selective COX inhibitors constrict the ductus. In the fetal mouse, COX-2 appears to be the COX isoform responsible for producing PGs that regulate the ductus[55]; whereas in the fetal sheep, both COX-1 and COX-2 play a role in ductus patency.[54]

In addition to the PGs that are made within the ductus, the fetal ductus is under the influence of circulating concentrations of PGE_2. Circulating PGE_2 appears to be of placental origin[56] and is particularly high (approximately 1 nmol/L) in the late gestation fetus because of low fetal pulmonary blood flow and reduced pulmonary clearance.[57] In the late-gestation fetal lamb circulating concentrations of PGE_2 are close to those that produce maximal relaxation of the ductus.[58]

NO, formed mainly by eNOS, is made by the fetal ductus arteriosus and appears to play an important role in maintaining ductus patency in rodent fetuses early in gestation.[48] NO activates soluble guanylyl cyclase and increases ductus smooth muscle cyclic GMP (cGMP) and cGMP-dependent PKG. In addition to decreasing intracellular calcium (by inhibiting calcium influx and stimulating calcium uptake and removal), cGMP and PKG also lead to decreased myosin light chain phosphorylation and decreased tone. PGE_2 and NO appear to be preferentially coupled for reciprocal compensation since COX inhibition upregulates NO.[59] Although NO is also made in the ductus of larger species, its importance in maintaining ductus patency under normal in utero conditions has not been conclusively demonstrated[60] (see below for the role of NO in fetuses exposed to indomethacin tocolysis and in premature newborns).

Carbon monoxide relaxes the ductus arteriosus and both heme oxygenase -1 and -2 (the enzymes that make carbon monoxide) are found within the endothelial and smooth muscle cells of the ductus. Under physiologic conditions the amount of carbon monoxide made by the ductus does not seem to affect ductus tone; however, in circumstances where its synthesis is upregulated, for example, endotoxinemia, it may exert a relaxing influence on the ductus.[61,62] Hydrogen sulfide (made by ductus endothelial and smooth muscle cells) also has been identified as another endogenous factor that inhibits fetal ductus tone.[63] Little evidence exists to suggest that either adenosine or β-adrenergic stimulation play a significant role in ductus patency.[64]

CHRONIC INHIBITION OF PROSTAGLANDIN SIGNALING IN UTERO

Although short-term pharmacologic inhibition of PG synthesis and signaling produces ductus constriction in utero,[65] chronic inhibition of PG synthesis[55,66] and signaling[67] in mice produces the opposite effect: a persistent patent ductus in utero and a persistent patent ductus after birth.[55,67] Although chronic inhibition of PG production in utero leads to increased NO production in the fetal ductus,[68,69] inhibition of NO production does not appear to increase the rate of ductus closure in newborn mice with a persistent PDA due to chronic PG synthesis inhibition in utero.[66] It is now clear that, in addition to its role in maintaining fetal ductus patency, PGE_2 is essential for vascular homeostasis[70] and for the induction of pathways necessary for postnatal closure.[71] Interruption of the PG receptor EP4 decreases the expression of several genes that control postnatal oxygen-induced ductus constriction (see below). Similarly, chronic inhibition of PG synthesis decreases Ca_L- and K^+-channel genes (Ca_Lalpha1c, Ca_Lbeta2, Kir6.1, and Kv1.5), which regulate calcium entry, without affecting genes that regulate calcium sensitization (Rho-kinase-associated genes). Conversely, the addition of PGE_2 increases the expression of the same Ca_L- and

K+-channel genes.[71] Chronic COX inhibition also decreases phosphodiesterase expression, which, in turn, increases the ductus' sensitivity to cAMP- or cGMP-dependent vasodilators.[71] Both ablation of the PG receptor EP4 gene and chronic EP4 blockade produce a marked reduction in α-SM actin, SM22α, and smooth muscle differentiation genes (myosin heavy chain and serum response factor)[70] by altering Wnt/β-catenin signaling.[72]

Inhibition of PG signaling may also contribute to delayed closure by inhibiting hyaluronic acid production and intimal cushion formation in the ductus.[73] Intimal cushions play an important role in permanent ductus closure after birth (see below). PGE2, acting through its EP4 receptor, has been shown to affect intimal thickening, elastogenesis, and contraction related genes through pathways that involve cyclic AMP, cAMP-protein kinase A, exchange protein activated by cAMP, phospholipase C, alpha1G T-type voltage dependent channels, and Wnt/β-catenin.[74,75]

Similar to its effects during rodent gestation, pharmacologic inhibition of PG synthesis during human pregnancy also is associated with an increased incidence of PDA after birth.[76] However, in the human newborn, the PDA that persists after antenatal indomethacin exposure appears to be due to indomethacin's ability to produce ductus constriction in utero. Constriction in utero produces ischemic hypoxia, increased NO production, and smooth muscle cell death within the ductus wall. These changes are similar to the events that occur postnatally (see "Relationship Between Vasoconstriction and Anatomic Closure"). These factors prevent the ductus from constricting after birth and make it resistant to the constrictive effects of postnatal indomethacin.[77,78]

VASOCONSTRICTION/VASORELAXATION: POSTNATAL REGULATION

There are several events that promote ductus constriction in the full-term newborn following delivery: (1) an increase in arterial PO_2, (2) a decrease in blood pressure within the ductus lumen (due to the postnatal decrease in pulmonary vascular resistance), (3) a decrease in circulating PGE_2 (due to loss of placental PG production, increased pulmonary blood flow, and increased pulmonary PG clearance), and (4) a decrease in the number of PGE_2 receptors in the ductus wall.[35] Although the newborn ductus continues to be sensitive to the vasodilating effects of NO, it loses its ability to respond to PGE_2.[79,80] All of these factors promote ductus constriction after birth. The ductus is also sensitive to the constrictive effects of angiotensin II, and angiotensin type 1 receptors are selectively induced at birth. However, studies have found no role for Ang II in the functional closure of the ductus at birth.[81,82]

The postnatal increase in arterial Pao_2 plays an important role in postnatal ductus constriction. Infants born in low oxygen environments, at higher elevations, have an increased incidence of PDA.[83] Oxygen-induced contraction can be demonstrated in the absence of the ductus endothelium,[84] and in the presence of inhibitors of PG, NO and endothelin signaling. This suggests that these vasoactive substances are not essential for normoxic constriction. In most species, oxygen appears to constrict the ductus arteriosus through mechanisms that involve smooth muscle depolarization as well as those that are independent of membrane depolarization.[33] Oxygen depolarizes the ductus smooth muscle cells by inhibiting K^+ channels.[85,86] Following the depolarization of the membrane, calcium enters the ductus smooth muscle through L-type[27,87] and T-type[75,88] voltage dependent, calcium channels. Several O_2 sensitive K^+ channels have been found in the fetal ductus (including Kv1.5 and Kv2.1). These vary with species and gestational age and may account for the differing sensitivity of the ductus to oxygen.[89,90] Rising oxygen tensions have also been found to inhibit ductus K_{ATP} channels by increasing mitochondrial oxidative phosphorylation and ATP production.[87] Conversely, diazoxide, a K_{ATP} channel opener, inhibits oxygen-induced constriction.[91] Oxygen also appears to have a direct effect on the calcium L-channels themselves,[92] as well as on the voltage-dependent T-type calcium channels,[75] and the store-operated calcium channels.[34,36] In addition, oxygen may increase smooth muscle sensitivity to calcium by activating Rho kinase mediated pathways that inhibit myosin light chain dephosphorylation resulting in persistent myosin light chain phosphorylation.[33,34,36,93]

Mitochondria in the ductus smooth muscle cells appear to be an important upstream oxygen sensor. Elevated PO_2 causes mitochondrial fission, mediated by dynamin-related protein-1, which increases electron transport chain complex I activity and production of reactive oxygen species (superoxide and H_2O_2).[85,94-98] Inhibition of mitochondrial fission selectively inhibits O_2-induced H_2O_2 production and ductus constriction, without altering constriction to other agonists.[94,95] In most species H_2O_2 appears to stimulate vasoconstriction by increasing calcium influx and calcium sensitization by regulating K^+ channels, calcium channels, and Rho kinase. However, in some species H_2O_2 acts only as a vasodilator,[99] or as both a vasodilator and a vasoconstrictor (depending on its concentration).[100]

In the chicken ductus, reactive oxygen species appear to activate their own amplification pathway by activating neutral sphingomyelinase and increasing ceramide production. Ceramide can activate NADPH oxidase, which increases the formation of reactive oxygen species by transferring electrons from NADPH to oxygen. Inhibitors of either neutral sphingomyelinase or NADPH oxidase blunt the formation of reactive oxygen species in the chicken ductus and block the effects of oxygen on contractile tone.[101]

Studies in animals suggest that a cytochrome P450 hemoprotein also appears to be involved with oxygen-induced constriction.[102-105] This mechanism may have parallels in preterm human ductus since cytochrome P450 inhibitors increase the incidence of PDA.[106,107] Oxygen also activates the epidermal growth factor receptor (EGFR) in ductus smooth muscle cells.[94] EGFR inhibition attenuates oxygen-induced constriction. The EGFR's effect on oxygen-induced constriction appears to be mediated by its effects on tyrosine kinase.[94]

During the transition from fetus to newborn oxygen increases the formation of isoprostanes. Isoprostanes are formed nonenzymatically by free radical-mediated peroxidation of phospholipid-bound arachidonatic acid. In mice, isoprostanes have both contractile and vasodilatory effects on the ductus by activating both thromboxane and EP4 receptors, respectively. With advancing gestation, the balance shifts in favor of the contractile effects of thromboxane stimulation.[108]

Oxygen also increases the formation of the potent vasoconstrictor, endothelin-1.[109] The role of endothelin-1 in postnatal ductus closure is still unclear[42,86,110-112] due to the marked species variation in its contribution to oxygen-induced ductus constriction.[86,112] Endothelin receptor stimulation accounts for 44% of the oxygen-induced constriction in the rat, but only 13% in the rabbit.[112] In the human ductus, inhibition of endothelin production does not inhibit oxygen-induced constriction.[86]

The postnatal increase in PaO_2 also has profound modulatory effects on other vasoactive systems.[113] Elevated oxygen tensions can increase the ductus' contractile response to neural mediators[114] and can decrease the formation of vasodilator PGs.[35]

Although the contractile effects of oxygen play an important role in postnatal ductus constriction, they may not be essential for postnatal ductus closure. For example, mice lacking the endothelin A receptor have diminished oxygen-induced ductus constriction; however, their ductus closes normally after birth.[42]

VASOCONSTRICTION/VASORELAXATION: DEVELOPMENTAL REGULATION

Gestational age has a marked effect on the rate of ductus closure after birth. In contrast with the full-term ductus, the premature ductus is less likely to constrict after birth. This is due to several mechanisms. The intrinsic tone of the extremely immature ductus (<70% of gestation) is decreased compared to the ductus at term.[32] This may be due to the presence of immature smooth muscle myosin isoforms, with a weaker contractile capacity,[37,39] and to decreased Rho kinase expression and activity.[41,93,96] Calcium entry through L-type calcium channels appears to be impaired in the immature ductus (especially under hypoxic conditions).[41,92,96] The potassium channels that promote ductus relaxation also change during gestation (switching from K_{Ca} channels (which are not regulated by oxygen tension) to Kv channels (which can be inhibited by increased oxygen concentrations).[89,115,116] Reduced expression and function of the putative oxygen-sensing Kv channels appear to contribute to ductus patency in the preterm rabbit, sheep, baboon, mouse, and chicken.[96,115,116] In contrast, a decrease in Kv channel expression occurs with advancing gestation in the rat, which suggests that in that species DA closure may occur by eliminating Kv channels.[89]

Although circulating catecholamine concentrations are elevated during the transition to extrauterine life,[45] immature animals are less responsive to circulating catecholamines than are animals near term.[45,117]

Premature infants have elevated circulating concentrations of PGE_2, which may play a significant role in maintaining ductus patency during the first days after birth. This is due to the decreased ability of the premature lung to clear circulating PGE_2.[57] In addition, during episodes of bacteremia and necrotizing enterocolitis, circulating concentrations of PGE_2 reach the pharmacologic range. These elevated concentrations (along with increased tumor necrosis factor α and inducible NO synthase production in the ductus[118]) are often associated with reopening of the ductus arteriosus.[22]

Probably the most important mechanism preventing the preterm ductus from constricting after birth is its increased sensitivity to the vasodilating effects of PGE_2. Inhibitors of PG production (e.g., indomethacin, ibuprofen, mefanamic acid, and acetaminophen) induce ductus closure in approximately 70% of premature infants. The increased sensitivity to PGE_2 is due to both increased cyclic AMP production (from enhanced receptor coupling with adenyl cyclase) and decreased cyclic AMP degradation by phosphodiesterase.[52,119]

Although inhibitors of PG production are very effective in closing the ductus when given on postnatal day 1, they become less effective by the end of the first postnatal week in preterm infants.[120-122] A number of factors conspire to make indomethacin and ibuprofen less effective by the end of the first week in preterm infants. Following delivery, COX-2 expression and PGE_2 production increase in the ductus wall.[123] However, in contrast with the full-term ductus, where all of the PGE_2 EP receptors are down-regulated after birth, in the preterm ductus, the dominant PGE_2 receptor, EP4, continues to be synthesized after birth and the ductus continues to relax with PG stimulation. In addition, despite the presence of persistent ductus luminal blood flow, there is a progressive decrease in ATP concentrations within the preterm newborn ductus smooth muscle cells. The decreased ATP concentrations limit the preterm newborn ductus' ability to constrict.[124] Similarly, the mild degrees of hypoxia that develop within the postnatal preterm ductus induce the production of other vasodilators within its wall that do not depend on PG signaling to affect contractility (e.g., NO, tumor necrosis factor [TNF]α, and interleukin [IL]-6).[125,126] These "other" vasodilators produce a change in the vasodilator-balance that maintains ductus patency. Ductus patency becomes less dependent on PG generation and more dependent on "other" vasodilators after the first postnatal week. These postnatal changes may explain why the effectiveness of indomethacin wanes with increasing postnatal age.[127,128] In premature animals and humans, the combined use of a NO synthase-inhibitor and indomethacin produces a much greater degree of ductus constriction than indomethacin alone.[129,130] It follows that drugs that interfere with NO synthesis could become a useful adjunct, especially in situations where indomethacin has been found to be ineffective.

PGs may also contribute to persistent ductus patency when it occurs in full-term infants. Indomethacin can produce a substantial degree of ductus constriction even in full-term infants[131] and term infants with congenital anomalies.[132]

Several other prenatal and postnatal factors also affect the rate of ductus constriction in preterm newborns. There appears to be a linear relationship between infant birth weight and the ductus' response to PDA treatment, since the failure rate of ibuprofen increases with increasing degrees of growth restriction[133]

Circulating concentrations of thyroid hormones and cortisol increase with advancing fetal gestation. Thyroid hormones may play a role in ductus arteriosus maturation since full-term infants with congenital hypothyroidism have an increased incidence of PDA that appears to respond to thyroid hormone replacement therapy.[134] Similarly, a lower occurrence of PDA has been found in thyroid hormone–treated preterm infants.[135,136]

Elevated fetal cortisol concentrations also foster ductus maturation by decreasing the sensitivity of the ductus to the vasodilating effects of PGE_2[137] and increasing its sensitivity to the contractile effects of oxygen.[31] Prenatal administration of glucocorticoids significantly reduces the incidence of PDA in premature humans and animals.[31,137-141] Postnatal glucocorticoid administration also reduces the incidence of PDA.[142,143] However, caution must be used when administering postnatal glucocorticoids since they increase the risk of spontaneous intestinal perforation when administered concurrently with indomethacin or ibuprofen.[143a,143b]

Prenatal administration of vitamin A has been shown to increase both the intracellular calcium response and the contractile response of the preterm ductus to oxygen.[144] However, two randomized controlled trials (RCTs) did not find an increased rate of spontaneous ductus closure in preterm infants treated with vitamin A.[145,146] Although vitamin A administration did not alter the rate of spontaneous constriction in these studies, a decreased need for ductus ligation among appropriate for gestational age infants treated with vitamin A was noted in a secondary analysis of the data.[146]

Preterm infants with a PDA have lower circulating concentrations of glutamate than infants with a closed ductus. Although glutamate can promote ductus constriction in rats through what appears to be glutamate receptor-mediated noradrenaline production,[147] parenteral glutamine supplementation has not been shown to alter the incidence of PDA in preterm infants.[148] Whether glutamate supplementation, by itself, might help to prevent PDA in extremely preterm infants has yet to be tested.

BNP is produced by the myocardium under conditions that produce myocardial deformation. Elevated circulating BNP concentrations have been used as a clinical biomarker for moderate sized left-to-right PDA shunts,[4] heart failure, and pulmonary hypertension. BNP has natriuretic and potent vasodilating properties mediated through the cGMP pathway. In rats, BNP has both vasodilating and anti-remodeling effects on the ductus and can prevent postnatal ductus closure.[149] It is interesting to note that the ductus' response to indomethacin-induced constriction is reported to be poor in preterm infants when circulating BNP concentrations are elevated.[150]

ANATOMIC CLOSURE-HISTOLOGIC CHANGES

Anatomic remodeling of the ductus arteriosus is essential for permanent luminal closure. In the full-term ductus arteriosus there is fragmentation of the internal elastic lamina and progressive intimal thickening that starts in the second half of gestation and accelerates rapidly once functional constriction occurs after birth. As the intima increases in size, it ultimately forms mounds that occlude the already constricted lumen. The increase in intimal thickening is due (1) to migration of smooth muscle cells from the muscle media into the neointima and (2) to proliferation of luminal endothelial cells. The process of intimal cushion formation starts with the accumulation of hyaluronic acid (hyaluronan or HA) below the luminal endothelial cells. This is accompanied by the loss of laminin and collagen IV from the basement membrane of the endothelial cells and their subsequent separation from the internal elastic lamina. Laminin and collagen IV ultimately reform under the detached endothelial cells but HA continues to accumulate in the subendothelial space. The hygroscopic properties of HA cause an influx of water and widening of the subendothelial space; this creates an environment well suited for cell migration.[151] The endothelial and smooth muscle cells of the ductus arteriosus differ from those of the adjacent vessels in their ability to form neointimal cushions. Isolated endothelial cells of the ductus arteriosus have an increased rate of HA accumulation compared with endothelial cells of the aorta or pulmonary artery; this increase appears to be due to transforming growth factor β (TGFβ),[152] which is markedly increased in the ductus after birth.

Hyaluronan makes ductus smooth muscle cells migrate faster than aortic smooth muscle cells. The potentiating effect of HA on ductus smooth muscle cells is mediated through a hyaluronan binding protein (RHAMM). Ductus smooth muscle cells synthesize more RHAMM than aortic smooth muscle cells and concentrate it at the leading edges of the cells. Antibodies against RHAMM will reduce the migration of ductus smooth muscle cells to the level found in aortic smooth muscle cells.[151]

PGs, acting through the EP4 receptor, also appear to play a stimulatory role in ductus HA production and neointimal thickening by increasing cAMP production and protein kinase A signaling.[73,153] PGE_2 also enhances rat ductus arteriosus smooth muscle migration and intimal thickening through Epac (exchange protein directly activated by cAMP), another downstream target of EP4-induced cAMP production.[154] On the other hand, PGE_2 promotes secretion of the cysteine-rich protein CCN3 from rat ductus smooth muscle cells that inhibits rat ductus intimal cushion formation. CCN3 appears to play a role in fine-tuning the stimulatory effects of PGE_2-EP4 on intimal cushion formation.[155]

Accompanying the increase in HA is an increase in fibronectin (FN) and chondroitin sulfate (CS) in the neointimal space.[156] Ductus smooth muscle cells secrete more FN and CS than those of the aorta or pulmonary artery.[157] This does not appear to be due to TGFβ. FN plays an important role in facilitating ductus smooth muscle cell migration.[151] When FN production in the ductus is inhibited, intimal cushion formation is blocked.[158] In contrast, FN has no effect on the migration of aortic smooth muscle cells.[151] CS appears to have no direct effect on either ductus or aortic smooth muscle cell migration.[151]

Ductus arteriosus smooth muscle cells use a family of cell surface receptors, called *integrins*, to interact with, adhere to, and migrate through the extracellular matrix that surrounds them. When smooth muscle cells of the ductus are in a quiescent, contractile state, they express the same integrins on their cell surface as smooth muscle cells of the aorta. However, when ductus smooth muscle cells of the inner muscle media begin to migrate into the subendothelial space, two new integrin complexes appear on their cell surface: the αvβ3 and the α5β1 receptors. The αvβ3 integrin is a promiscuous receptor that interacts with most extracellular matrix glycoproteins and is essential for migration of ductus smooth muscle cells in vitro. The α5β1 integrin binds exclusively to FN and mediates the potentiating effects of FN on ductus smooth muscle cell migration.

During the process of migration, ductus smooth muscle cells secrete laminin, which also has an important promigratory role. Laminin facilitates smooth muscle cell migration by destabilizing the interactions of the cell's integrin receptors with other matrix glycoproteins. Because strong adhesion between a cell and its surrounding matrix makes a cell ill-suited for migration, this anti-adhesive property of laminin allows the cell to make and break contacts with the surrounding matrix, thus promoting locomotion. Antibodies against laminin inhibit ductus smooth muscle cell migration.

Intimal cushion formation in the ductus is also associated with disruption of the internal elastic laminae underlying the ductus luminal endothelial cells. Compared with aortic endothelial cells, ductus endothelial cells have high levels of tissue-type plasminogen activator that activates the elastolytic enzyme matrix metalloproteinases two at sites of disruption of the internal elastic laminae.[159] In contrast with the aorta where well-developed elastic laminae surround smooth muscle cells in the muscle media and prevent the vascular wall from collapsing, smooth muscle cells in the ductus muscle media are surrounded by thin and fragmented elastin fibers that do not prevent it from collapsing and closing when the ductus vasoconstricts. In the ductus neointima, muscle cells are surrounded by even fewer elastin fibers.[160] The disruption of normal elastin fiber assembly in the ductus muscle media does not appear to be due to increased elastase activity or decreased tropoelastin production. Rather, it appears to be due to a developmental mechanism that reduces insolubilization of elastin and prevents formation of intact elastic laminae.

Vascular smooth muscle cells synthesize a 67-kD elastin binding protein (EBP) that is central to the assembly of soluble tropoelastin molecules into a mature matrix of insoluble elastic fibers.[161] It has three separate binding sites: one for the VGVAPG hydrophobic region of tropoelastin, one for the cell membrane, and one for galactosugars.[162] The 67-kD EBP binds the tropoelastin molecule, escorts it through the smooth muscle cell's secretory pathways, and attaches it to the cell's surface. When galactosugars come in contact with the lectin-binding site of the 67-kD EBP, the affinity for both tropoelastin and the cell binding site is lowered and tropoelastin is released. Coordinated presentation of galactosugars, contained within the growing elastin microfibrillar scaffold, regulate the orientation and proper alignment of tropoelastin for crosslinking during normal elastin fiber assembly. On the other hand, galactosugars from other matrix elements may compete with this process and lead to abnormal assembly (see CS below).[163] Ductus smooth muscle cells have less 67-kD EBP on their cell surface when compared with aortic smooth muscle cells.[164] As a result, ductus smooth muscle cells deposit little insoluble elastin when compared with aortic smooth muscle cells. They also secrete large amounts of a truncated form of tropoelastin due to proteolytic intracellular degradation caused by the 67-kD EBP deficiency.[165,166] As noted above, ductus smooth muscle cells secrete increased amounts of CS compared with aortic smooth muscle cells. CS, through its galactosugar side chains, removes the 67-kD EBP from smooth muscle cell surfaces, thereby interfering with elastin fiber assembly.[164]

The exact relationship between impaired elastin assembly and smooth muscle migration into the neointima is still open for speculation. Impaired assembly of thick elastic laminae might facilitate smooth muscle cell migration by removing a physical barrier to which they might attach. Ductus smooth muscle cells are able to migrate through elastin membranes that restrain aortic smooth muscle cell migration. Treatment of aortic smooth muscle cells with CS causes the release of the 67-kD EBP from the aortic cell's surface and enables them to migrate through elastin membranes at the same rate as ductus smooth muscle cells.[167] Finally, the accumulation of a relatively stable, soluble, truncated tropoelastin may act as a chemoattractant for smooth muscle cells.[168] Thus, there appear to be mechanisms that link elastin fragmentation with formation of ductus intimal cushions. Conversely, in some genetic forms of PDA the ductus' elastic laminae appear abnormally well developed and similar to those in the aorta; when this occurs, intimal cushions fail to develop.[160,169,170]

PGE_2 and its receptor EP4 appear to play a critical role (through an EP4-cSrc-PLCγ-signaling pathway) in inhibiting thick elastin fiber formation in the ductus. Lysyl oxidase, which catalyzes elastin crosslinking, is degraded when the EP4 receptor is stimulated.[170] Conversely, the ductus of the EP4 knockout mouse has an increased elastic phenotype that is similar to the aorta.[170] Decreased expression of the EP4 receptor can also be found in the ductus of the brown Norway rat, which has increased amounts of elastin in its internal elastic lamina and develops a PDA after birth.[169]

Antenatal betamethasone, which increases the sensitivity of the ductus to the contractile effects of oxygen,[31] also appears to promote neointimal thickening by increasing the expression of ADP-ribosyltransferase three, which stimulates ductus smooth muscle migration.[171] The postnatal increase in oxygen also activates the RhoA-ROCK-PTEN pathway, which plays a role in ductus smooth muscle proliferation and migration.[172]

RELATIONSHIP BETWEEN VASOCONSTRICTION AND ANATOMIC CLOSURE

In full-term animals, both the loss of vasodilator regulation and the anatomic events that lead to permanent closure appear to be controlled by the degree of ductus smooth muscle constriction. Constriction produces ischemic hypoxia of the vessel wall (Fig. 52.1).[173] Experimental models that alter the ability of the ductus to constrict at term also prevent the normal histologic changes that occur after birth.[47,55,67,158,174,175] Due to of the thickness of the full-term ductus, intramural vasa vasorum that originate from the ductus's adventitia are needed to provide oxygen and nutrients to the outer half of its wall. These thin-walled intramural vasa vasorum collapse during ductus constriction providing the ductus with a unique mechanism for controlling the maximal diffusion distance for oxygen and nutrients across its wall. Increased intramural pressure during ductus constriction obliterates vasa vasorum blood flow within its outer muscle media. This turns the entire thickness of the muscle media into a virtual avascular zone.[176] The profound ischemic hypoxia of the ductus muscle media that occurs following ductus constriction inhibits local smooth muscle production of PGE_2 and NO, induces local production of hypoxia-inducible factors like HIF1α and vascular endothelial growth factor (VEGF), and produces smooth muscle apoptosis in the ductus wall. VEGF plays a critical role in the migration of the ductus smooth muscle cells into the neointima and in the proliferation of intramural vasa vasorum.[126] After postnatal ductus constriction, several genes known to be essential for vascular remodeling (HIF1α, VCAM-1, E-selectin, IL-8, MCSF-1, CD154, IFNγ, IL-6, and TNFα) are increased in the ductus wall. In primates, circulating mononuclear cells are attracted to the ductus and, once adherent to the ductus wall, they become activated monocytes/macrophages and produce PDGF. PDGF stimulates smooth muscle migration and proliferation into the neointima.[125] The mononuclear cell adhesion to the ductus wall and inflammatory response that follows postnatal ductus constriction appears to be necessary for neointimal remodeling since the extent of remodeling is directly associated with the degree of mononuclear cell adhesion.[125]

Low platelet counts also have been associated with persistent ductus patency and failure of indomethacin/ibuprofen to close the PDA in preterm infants.[177] However, the role of platelets in human ductus remodeling is still in doubt. An RCT attempting to maintain a platelet count greater than 100,000 per μL by liberally transfusing platelets in preterm thrombocytopenic neonates did not hasten PDA closure.[178] In contrast with the human ductus, where large, occlusive neointimal mounds are needed to fill the residual lumen that remains following ductus constriction,[125] the mouse ductus has a much smaller lumen and thinner neointima following ductus constriction. In mice, platelets appear to play an essential role in luminal closure by forming a platelet plug that seals the small residual lumen.[179] Thromboxane, produced during platelet activation, may play an important role in rodent neointima formation.[180]

In preterm infants, the ductus frequently remains open for many days after birth. Even when it does constrict, the premature ductus frequently fails to develop profound hypoxia and anatomic remodeling. The preterm infant requires a greater degree of ductal constriction than the term infant to develop a comparable degree of hypoxia. In contrast with the full-term ductus, where vasa vasorum are needed to provide oxygen and nutrients to the outer two-thirds of the ductus wall, intramural vasa vasorum are absent from the ductus wall of infants born before 26 weeks gestation where luminal blood flow can provide all the oxygen and nutrients the thin-wall ductus requires. The absence of intramural vasa vasorum leaves the preterm ductus without a mechanism to rapidly increase the diffusion distance across its wall during postnatal constriction. As long as any degree of luminal patency exists, the thin-wall preterm

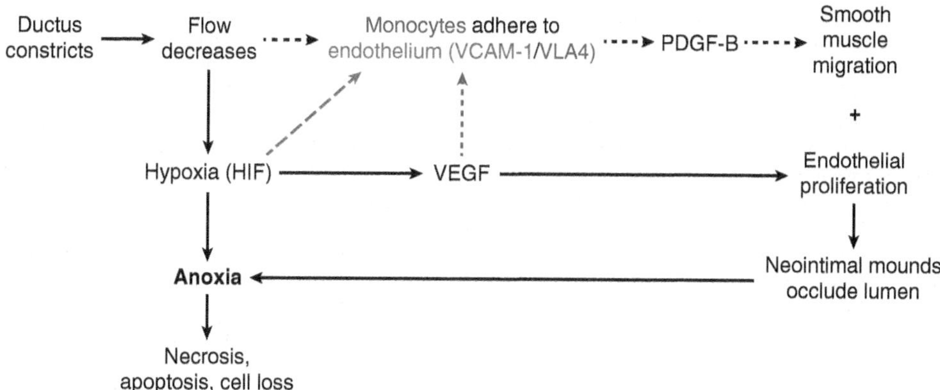

Fig. 52.1 Ductus arteriosus remodeling. Role of constriction, hypoxia, and mononuclear cell adhesion in neointima formation and smooth muscle cell death postnatal constriction produces hypoxia in the ductus arteriosus wall. The hypoxic smooth muscle and endothelial cells increase their expression of vascular endothelial growth factor *(VEGF)* and vascular cell adhesion molecule 1 *(VCAM-1)*, respectively. VEGF is required for endothelial cell proliferation. VEGF also attracts circulating mononuclear cells (expressing VLA4 [very late antigen-4]) to the endothelial cell surface. Under very low flow conditions, the weakly adherent VLA4+ mononuclear cells attach to VCAM-1 on the endothelial cell surface and release platelet-derived growth factor *(PDGF)* and matrix metalloproteinase 9 (which promote smooth muscle migration into the neointima). Therefore tight constriction and loss of luminal flow are essential for VEGF expression, mononuclear cell adhesion, neointimal formation, and luminal occlusion. *HIF,* Hypoxia-inducible factor.

ductus fails to become profoundly hypoxic and fails to undergo anatomic remodeling after birth. As a result, the preterm ductus requires complete cessation of luminal flow before it can develop the same degree of hypoxia as found at term. Once the preterm ductus develops the same degree of hypoxic ischemia as the term ductus, most of the anatomic changes seen at term will occur.[32,130] However, if the premature ductus does not develop the degree of ischemic hypoxia needed to induce cell death and anatomic remodeling, it will continue to be responsive to vasodilators and continue to be susceptible to vessel reopening.

GENETIC REGULATION

Studies have used genome-wide transcriptome analysis to examine differences in gene expression between the ductus and the aorta (as well as the effects of oxygen and preterm birth on ductus gene expression). In the ductus the expression of genes related to neural crest migration (TFAP2b), TGF-β signaling, matrix molecules (like FN and lysyl oxidase), actin-myosin interactions, potassium and calcium ion signaling, as well as PG, endothelin, and angiotensin II signaling, are increased compared with the aorta. Mutations in several of these ductus-dominant genes/pathways (examined in either mouse knock-out models or human genetic syndromes) are associated with persistent ductus patency in term neonates (Table 52.2).[42,55,72,179,181-220] Single nucleotide polymorphisms (SNPs) have also been associated with persistent ductus patency in term infants (e.g., in TGFBR2).[221]

However, both species and genetic background play a significant role in determining the relative importance of ductus regulatory pathways.[31,182,222-227] Although several pathways appear to be commonly involved among different species, the relative expression and importance of individual orthologous genes frequently differ between species.[181,182,227] For example, endothelin receptor stimulation may account for 44% of the oxygen-induced contraction in the rat, whereas it only contributes to 13% of the contraction in the rabbit,[112] and has a negligible role in the human ductus.[86] Oxygen depolarizes the ductus smooth muscle cells by inhibiting K^+ channels.[85,86] In the rabbit, an increase in the expression of Kv channels appears to be responsible for the developmental increase in the oxygen-induced contraction.[116] In contrast, in the rat, Kv channel expression decreases with advancing gestation.[89] Ductus patency is critically dependent on vasodilator PGs in most species; however, notable exceptions exist in the guinea pig, chicken, and emu ductus, where locally derived PGs do not appear to play a significant role in its patency.[117,228-230]

Genetic and familial factors may also play a role in persistent ductus patency in preterm infants.[231,232] SNPs in several genes have been associated with preterm PDA (ATR type 1,[233] IFNγ,[234] estrogen receptor-alpha PvuII,[235] TFAP2B, PGI synthase, TRAF1),[236] and its response to indomethacin treatment (CYP2C9).[237] There is a growing body of evidence to suggest that SNPs in TFAP2B may be responsible for some of the PDAs that occur in preterm infants. TFAP2B is uniquely expressed in ductus smooth muscle[238]; it regulates other genes that are important in ductus smooth muscle development[238]; mutations in TFAP2B produce PDA in mice and humans[211]; and TFAP2B polymorphisms are associated with preterm PDAs (especially those that are unresponsive to indomethacin).[236] However, race, ethnicity, and ancestral background appear to be important modifiers of these effects since not all populations have been similarly affected by the presence of these PDA-risk-inducing SNPs.[239]

HEMODYNAMIC AND PULMONARY ALTERATIONS

The pathophysiologic features of a PDA depend both on the magnitude of the left-to-right shunt and on the cardiac and pulmonary responses to the shunt. The PDA left-to-right shunt lowers systemic blood pressures (both systolic and diastolic)[240] and adds to the incidence of inotrope-dependent hypotension often observed among preterm infants (born before 28 weeks gestation) at the end of the first week.[241]

There are important differences between immature and mature infants in the heart's ability to handle the increased volume load from the PDA. Immature infants have less cardiac sympathetic innervation. The preterm myocardium has more water and less contractile mass. Therefore, the immature fetal ventricles are less distensible than at term and generate less force per gram of myocardium (even though they have the same ability to generate force per sarcomere).[242] The relative lack of left ventricular distensibility in immature infants is more a function of the ventricle's tissue constituents than of poor muscle function. As a result, left ventricular distension secondary to a large left-to-right PDA shunt may produce a higher left ventricular end-diastolic pressure at smaller ventricular volumes. The increase in left ventricular pressure increases pulmonary venous pressure and contributes to pulmonary congestion.

Studies in preterm animal and human newborns[240,243] have shown that despite these limitations, preterm newborns are able to increase left ventricular output, and maintain their "effective" systemic blood flow, even with left-to-right PDA shunts equal to 50% of left ventricular output. With shunts greater than 50% of left ventricular output, "effective" systemic blood flow falls, despite a continued increase in left ventricular output. The increase in left ventricular output associated with a PDA is accomplished not by an increase in heart rate, but by an increase in stroke volume.[240,243] The presence of a PDA does not appear to affect myocardial contractility.[244] Instead, stroke volume increases primarily as a result of a simultaneous decrease in afterload (due to the decrease in arterial pressure and elastance) and increase in left ventricular preload. Several weeks of PDA exposure causes the left heart to remodel to a larger, more spherical shape with an increase in wall thickness. This returns to normal values following PDA closure.[244]

Despite the ability of the left ventricle to increase its output in the face of a left-to-right ductus shunt, blood flow distribution is significantly rearranged. This redistribution of systemic blood flow occurs even with small shunts.[240] Blood flow to the skin, bone, and skeletal muscle is most likely to be affected by the left-to-right ductus shunt. The next most likely organs to be affected are the gastrointestinal tract and kidneys due to a combination of decreased perfusion pressure and localized vasoconstriction. Mesenteric blood flow is decreased in both fasting and fed states in the presence of a PDA,[245] as is mesenteric regional oxygen saturation.[246] Significant decreases in organ blood flow and oxygenation may occur before there are signs of left ventricular compromise[243,247] and may contribute to the decreased glomerular filtration rate that has been observed with ductus patency.[127,248,249]

Cerebral blood flow and oxygenation are also compromised in the presence of a moderate-to-large left-to-right PDA shunt due to the limited ability of the preterm newborn to autoregulate cerebral blood flow.[250] Small-for-gestational age infants are at even greater risk for having low cerebral oxygen saturations due to an increased incidence of impaired cerebrovascular autoregulation.[251,252] Evidence suggests that any negative impact of a PDA on neonatal brain growth may have more to do with its effects on cerebral oxygen saturation than on the magnitude of the shunt or the treatments used to close it.[253] In contrast with the effects of a PDA on mesenteric and renal oxygen saturations, cerebral oxygen saturations may be preserved in the presence of a moderate-to-large PDA if cerebral autoregulation remains intact.[254] Therefore, as long as continuous cerebral oxygen monitoring demonstrates that cerebral oxygenation is not compromised, it may be reasonable to delay treatments to close the PDA while awaiting spontaneous closure.[253]

Table 52.2 Partial List of Gene Mutations or Deletions Associated With a Persistent Patent Ductus Arteriosus in Animal and Human Full-Term Neonates.

Mouse Knockout Models			Human Genetic Syndromes		
Name	**Description**	**Function**	**Name**	**Description**	**Function**
Ptger4	Prostaglandin E receptor 4	Receptor (prostaglandin signaling)	TFAP2B (Char)	Transcription factor AP-2 β	Transcription factor (neural crest differentiation)
Ptgs1, Ptgs2	Prostaglandin-endoperoxide synthase 1 and 2	Enzyme (prostaglandin signaling)	TBX1 (DiGeorge)	T-box transcription factor 1	Transcription factor
Hpgd	Hydroxyprostaglandin dehydrogenase 15	Enzyme (prostaglandin signaling)	TBX5 (Holt-Oram)	T-box transcription factor 5	Transcription factor
Slco2a1	Prostaglandin transporter	Transporter (prostaglandin signaling)	ZIC3 (Visceral heterotaxy)	Zic family member 3	Transcription factor
Notch2 and 3	Notch receptor 2 and 3	Receptor (notch signaling)	CHD7 (CHARGE)	Chromodomain helicase DNA binding protein 7	Chromatin remodeling
Ednra	Endothelin receptor type A	Endothelin receptor	EP300 (Rubinstein-Taybi)	E1A binding protein p300	Chromatin remodeling, cAMP regulation, HIF1A co-activator
Jag1	Jagged canonical Notch ligand 1	Ligand for notch (notch signaling)	CREBBP (Rubinstein-Taybi)	CREB binding protein	Transcriptional co-activator
Lox	Lysyl oxidase	Enzyme (elastin crosslinking)	TGFBR1/2 (Loeys-Dietz)	TGF-β receptor ½	TGF-β receptor
Tfap2b	Transcription factor AP-2 β	Transcription factor (neural crest differentiation)	SMAD4 (Myhre)	SMAD family member 4	TGF-β signaling
Myocd	Myocardin	Transcription coactivator (modulates smooth muscle target genes)	ZEB2/SMADIP1 (Mowat-Wilson)	Zinc finger E-box binding homeobox 2	Transcriptional repressor that interacts with TGF-β/SMAD signaling
Myh11	Myosin heavy chain 11	Smooth muscle myosin	PTPN11 (Noonan)	Protein tyrosine phosphatase non-receptor type 11	Protein tyrosine phosphatase
Brg1	Brahma-related gene 1	Chromatin-remodeling complexes	MYH11	Myosin heavy chain 11	Smooth muscle myosin
Bmp9/Gdf2	Growth differentiation factor 2	Ligand for TGF-β receptor	ACTA2	Actin α 2, smooth muscle	Smooth muscle actin
Nfe2	Nuclear factor, erythroid derived 2	Transcription factor (platelet biogenesis)	ABCC9 (Cantu)	ATP binding cassette subfamily C member 9	ATP-sensitive potassium channel transporter
Itga2b	Integrin subunit α 2b	Integrin subunit α 2b (platelet adhesion)	KCNJ8 (Cantu)	Potassium voltage-gated channel subfamily J member 8	Inward-rectifier type potassium channel
Ilk	Integrin linked kinase	Integrin signaling	CACNA1C (Timothy)	Calcium voltage-gated channel subunit α1 C	Voltage-dependent calcium channel
Cx43	Connexin 43	Gap junction communication	PTEN (VACTERL)	Phosphatase and tensin homolog	Dephosphorylates phosphoinositide substrates
Prrx1	Paired related homeobox 1	Transcription co-activator	RAB23 (Carpenter)	RAB23, member RAS oncogene family	GTPase of the Ras superfamily
Foxc1	Forkhead box C1	Transcription factor	FLNA (Periventricular heterotopia)	Filamin A	Crosslinks actin filaments
Matr3	Matrin 3	Nuclear matrix protein expressed in neural crest	FLNB (Larsen)	Filamin B	Platelet glycoprotein Ib interaction
			SEMA3E (CHARGE)	Semaphorin 3E	Cell migration
			ERK2/MAPK1	Mitogen-activated protein kinase 1	RAF/MEK/ERK/serum response factor signaling pathway
			NKX2.5	NK2 homeobox 5	Homeobox-containing transcription factor
			UBR1 (Johanson-Blizzard)	Ubiquitin protein ligase E3 component n-recognin 1	Ubiquitin proteolytic pathway
			MATR3	Matrin 3	Nuclear matrix protein expressed in neural crest
			G6PC3 (Severe congenital neutropenia type 4)	Glucose-6-phosphatase catalytic subunit 3	Hydrolysis of glucose-6-phosphate
			PRDM6	PR/SET domain 6	Transcriptional repressor of vascular smooth muscle contractile proteins
			PDA1 (on chromosome 12q24)	Patent ductus arteriosus, susceptibility to	?
			Cri-du-chat (chromosome 5)		

PDA, Patent ductus arteriosus; *TGF,* transforming growth factor.

The decreased ability of the preterm infant to maintain active pulmonary vasoconstriction[255] may be responsible in part for early development of a "large" left-to-right PDA shunt.[256,257] RCTs have shown that the presence of a PDA increases the incidence of early hemorrhagic pulmonary edema/pulmonary hemorrhage.[258-260] Therapeutic maneuvers or prenatal conditions that lead to a rapid postnatal drop in pulmonary vascular resistance, such as surfactant replacement[21,261,262] or intrauterine growth retardation,[21,261,262] can exacerbate the amount of left-to-right shunt and lead to pulmonary hemorrhage. Although fluid restriction and elevated mean airway pressure may decrease the effects of edema on lung mechanics (see below), these maneuvers have little effect on the volume of the left-to-right ductus shunt.[263,264] Phototherapy has been associated with persistence of a PDA; however, RCTs have not found that chest shielding alters the incidence or severity of PDA.[265]

In premature animals, a wide-open PDA increases the hydraulic pressures in the pulmonary vasculature on both the arterial and venous sides of the capillary bed. In addition, the increased pulmonary blood flow and immature precapillary arterial tone cause the hydraulic pressure head to shift downstream toward the capillary fluid filtration sites[266] increasing the rate of fluid transudation into the pulmonary interstitium.[267] In premature infants with respiratory distress syndrome, low plasma oncotic pressures and increased capillary permeability increase the rate of fluid transudation with any increase in microvascular perfusion pressure. If plasma proteins enter the alveolar space, surfactant function is inhibited and surface tension is increased in the immature air sacs[268] already compromised by surfactant deficiency. The increased FiO_2 and mean airway pressures required to overcome these early changes in compliance may play a role in the development of chronic lung disease.[127,269,270] Depending on the gestational age and the species examined, changes in pulmonary mechanics may occur as early as 1 day after birth or not before several days of exposure to a PDA left-to-right shunt.[266,271]

Although preterm animals with a PDA have increased fluid and protein transudation into the lung interstitium, a simultaneous increase in lung lymph flow appears to eliminate the excess fluid and protein flux into the lung.[267] This compensatory increase in lung lymph acts as an "edema safety factor," inhibiting fluid accumulation in the lungs. As a result, during the first days after birth there is no net increase in water or protein accumulation in the lung and there is no change in pulmonary mechanics.[17,127,266,272,273] This delicate balance between the PDA-induced fluid filtration and lymphatic reabsorption is consistent with the observation, made in human infants, that closure of the ductus arteriosus, within the first 24 hours after birth, has no effect on the course of the newborn's hyaline membrane disease. However, after several days of mechanical ventilation, there is a decrease in pulmonary capillary surface area,[274] which increases both the pulmonary microvascular pressure and rate of hydraulic fluid filtration. If lung lymphatic drainage also is impaired, as it is in the presence of pulmonary interstitial emphysema or fibrosis, the likelihood of edema increases dramatically. As a result, it is not uncommon for infants with a persistent PDA to develop pulmonary edema and alterations in pulmonary mechanics at 6 to 10 days after birth. In these infants, improvement in lung compliance occurs following closure of the PDA.[127,275-279]

A baboon model of PDA, using preterm newborns (delivered at 67% term gestation—equivalent to 26 weeks human gestation) that are mechanically ventilated for 2 weeks, has been used to examine the factors responsible for alterations in pulmonary mechanics in the presence of a PDA.[271] Newborns were either treated with a COX inhibitor to close the ductus or allowed to have a moderate size persistent PDA. Exposure to a persistent PDA for 2 weeks did not appear to alter surfactant secretion, pulmonary epithelial protein permeability, or presence of surfactant inhibitory proteins, compared with animals with a closed ductus. Although numerous changes occur in the preterm newborn lung in the expression of genes that regulate inflammation and tissue remodeling, the presence of an open ductus did not appear to alter the expression of any of the pro-inflammatory or tissue remodeling genes that were examined. In contrast with full-term newborns, which mobilize lung fluid rapidly after birth, preterm newborns (including those with a closed ductus) mobilize lung fluid much more slowly.[271] Preterm baboons with an open ductus had an altered distribution and increased amount of water in their lungs compared with animals with a closed ductus. The persistent PDA led to a small but significant increase in lung water at 2 weeks after delivery. On the other hand, closure of the PDA with a COX inhibitor, like indomethacin or ibuprofen, produced increased expression of alveolar epithelial sodium channels, which facilitate fluid removal from the alveolar compartment. This finding may account for the decreased incidence of pulmonary edema and hemorrhage in infants treated with prophylactic indomethacin after birth.[258-260]

Pharmacologic closure of the PDA was associated with improved lung development in the preterm baboons. In contrast to the animals with an open ductus, where an arrest in alveolar development (the hallmark of the new BPD) was noticeable by 2 weeks after birth, pharmacologic closure of the PDA led to improved alveolarization.[271] Whether the improvement in alveolarization is due to the closure of the ductus or the pharmacologic agents (indomethacin/ibuprofen) used to close it is unknown at this time. Neutrophil counts are elevated in the tracheal fluid of human infants with a PDA[280] and indomethacin can decrease tracheal neutrophil accumulation. However, the decreased neutrophil accumulation occurs in both those who close and in those who fail to close their PDA after indomethacin.[281]

The same improvements in pulmonary mechanics and alveolar surface area have not been observed after surgical ligation of the PDA. Early surgical ligation increases the expression of genes involved with pulmonary inflammation and decreases the expression of pulmonary epithelial sodium channels (that are critical for alveolar water clearance).[282] These changes may contribute to the lack of improvement in pulmonary mechanics after PDA ligation. In addition, early surgical ligation impedes lung growth.[271,283,284] These findings raise the possibility that early ductus ligation, while eliminating the detrimental effects of a PDA on lung development, may create its own set of problems that counteract many of the benefits derived from ductus closure.[285,286]

Transcatheter PDA closure is becoming a feasible alternative to surgical ligation in infants less than 1000 g.[287] Early studies suggest that transcatheter PDA closure may improve an infant's respiratory status and decrease overall exposure to mechanical ventilation.[288] However, no controlled studies to date have compared the outcomes after transcatheter PDA closure with those of pharmacologic treatment or conservative-nontreatment of the PDA.

Not all of the changes associated with a PDA are necessarily detrimental to the immature infant with respiratory distress syndrome. Persistence of the left-to-right shunt maintains an elevated Pa_{O_2} in the presence of atelectasis. This phenomenon is due to recirculation of oxygenated arterial blood through lungs that are not fully expanded.[240,289] Decreases in systemic arterial O_2 content have been observed after PDA closure, despite the absence of any alterations in pulmonary mechanics.

CONCLUSION: PATENT DUCTUS ARTERIOSUS AND NEONATAL MORBIDITY

Although a prolonged, persistent left-to-right shunt through a PDA shortens the life span of animals and humans,[55,290-292] there has been a growing debate about whether or not the PDA needs to be closed during the neonatal period.[293-297] Published RCTs provide only limited information about the consequences of a persistent PDA since none of the trials were designed to address the question of whether to close the PDA or to leave it alone and just deal with its symptoms. These RTCs show that exposure to a moderate-to-large PDA during the first week increases the risk of severe early pulmonary hemorrhage during the first week as well as the incidence of dopamine-dependent hypotension and higher levels of ventilator support at the end of the first week.[128,258,259,298-300] However, little information exists about the consequences of exposure to a persistent moderate-to-large PDA shunt for greater than 1 week. Only two small RCTs, performed almost 40 years ago, specifically examined the role of a persistent untreated symptomatic PDA on neonatal morbidity.[270,301] Both studies found that a persistent PDA increased pulmonary morbidity and prolonged the need for respiratory support. Whether these findings are still applicable in the setting of modern neonatal respiratory care, with "gentle ventilation" and acceptance of elevated arterial Pco_2, needs to be reexamined in future RCTs. Even the authors of the original studies speculated that the increased respiratory morbidity might be due to the "extensive use of mechanical ventilation" used to control PDA-induced pulmonary edema rather than the PDA shunt itself.[270] In the absence of appropriate and current RCTs, several cohort controlled trials have examined whether exposure to moderate-to-large PDA shunts for greater than 8 days increases morbidity.[302,303] These studies found no increase in the incidence of NEC, ROP, or death but did find an increased incidence of BPD and BPD/death among infants that were exposed to a moderate-to-large PDA for greater than 2 weeks. In addition, the longer infants were exposed to a PDA before PDA treatment was initiated, the less likely PDA treatment was associated with a reduction in BPD and BPD/death.[302,303] Whether exposure to a moderate-to-large PDA shunt for more than 2 weeks actually contributes to the development of BPD and BPD/Death is a question that still needs to be tested in appropriately designed RCTs. At this time what we do know is that neither a delay of two-to-five days before starting PDA treatment, nor treatment that starts only after infants have been exposed to a moderate-to-large shunt for longer than 2 weeks appear to affect the incidence of BPD and BPD/death. Further investigations will be needed to determine which infants are likely to benefit from PDA treatment and which infants might best be left untreated.

 A complete reference list is available at www.ExpertConsult.com.

SELECT REFERENCES

1. Broadhouse KM, Finnemore AE, Price AN, et al. Cardiovascular magnetic resonance of cardiac function and myocardial mass in preterm infants: a preliminary study of the impact of patent ductus arteriosus. *J Cardiovasc Magn Reson*. 2014;16:54.
2. El Hajjar M, Vaksmann G, Rakza T, et al. Severity of the ductal shunt: a comparison of different markers. *Arch Dis Child Fetal Neonatal Ed*. 2005;90:F419–F422.
4. El-Khuffash A, Molloy EJ. Are B-type natriuretic peptide (BNP) and N-terminal-pro-BNP useful in neonates? *Arch Dis Child Fetal Neonatal Ed*. 2007;92:F320–F324.
7. Schena F, Francescato G, Cappelleri A, et al. Association between hemodynamically significant patent ductus arteriosus and bronchopulmonary dysplasia. *J Pediatr*. 2015;166:1488–1492.
14. Sung SI, Chang YS, Kim J, et al. Natural evolution of ductus arteriosus with noninterventional conservative management in extremely preterm infants born at 23-28 weeks of gestation. *PloS One*. 2019;14:e0212256.
15. Semberova J, Sirc J, Miletin J, et al. Spontaneous closure of patent ductus arteriosus in infants ≤1500 g. *Pediatrics*. 2017;140:e20164258.
22. Gonzalez A, Sosenko IR, Chandar J, et al. Influence of infection on patent ductus arteriosus and chronic lung disease in premature infants weighing 1000 grams or less. *J Pediatr*. 1996;128:470–478.
23. Bell EF, Acarregui MJ. Restricted versus liberal water intake for preventing morbidity and mortality in preterm infants (Cochrane Review). *Cochrane Database Syst Rev*. 2001;3.
30. Waleh N, Barrette AM, Dagle JM, et al. Effects of advancing gestation and non-Caucasian race on ductus arteriosus gene expression. *J Pediatr*. 2015;167:1033–1041.
31. Shelton EL, Waleh N, Plosa EJ, et al. Effects of antenatal betamethasone on preterm human and mouse ductus arteriosus. comparison with baboon data. *Pediatr Res*. 2018;84(3):458–465.
32. Kajino H, Chen YQ, Seidner SR, et al. Factors that increase the contractile tone of the Ductus Arteriosus also regulate its anatomic remodeling. *Am J Physiol Regul Integr Comp Physiol*. 2001;281:R291–R301.
34. Hong Z, Hong F, Olschewski A, et al. Role of store-operated calcium channels and calcium sensitization in normoxic contraction of the ductus arteriosus. *Circulation*. 2006;114:1372–1379.
35. Bouayad A, Kajino H, Waleh N, et al. Characterization of PGE2 receptors in fetal and newborn lamb ductus arteriosus. *Am J Physiol Heart Circ Physiol*. 2001;280:H2342–H2349.
36. Keck M, Resnik E, Linden B, et al. Oxygen increases ductus arteriosus smooth muscle cytosolic calcium via release of calcium from inositol triphosphate-sensitive stores. *Am J Physiol Lung Cell Mol Physiol*. 2005;288:L917–L923.
40. Crichton CA, Smith GC, Smith GL. a-Toxin-permeabilised rabbit fetal ductus arteriosus is more sensitive to Ca^{2+} than aorta or main pulmonary artery. *Cardiovasc Res*. 1997;33:223–229.
41. Clyman RI, Waleh NS, Kajino H, et al. Calcium-dependent and calcium-sensitizing pathways in the mature and immature ductus arteriosus. *Am J Physiol Regul Integr Comp Physiol*. 2007;293:R1650–R1656.
42. Coceani F, Liu Y, Seidlitz E, et al. Endothelin A receptor is necessary for O_2 constriction but not closure of ductus arteriosus. *Am J Physiol*. 1999;277:H1521–H1531.
52. Liu H, Manganiello VC, Clyman RI. Expression, activity and function of cAMP and cGMP phosphodiesterases in the mature and immature ductus arteriosus. *Pediatr Res*. 2008;64:477–481.
55. Loftin CD, Trivedi DB, Tiano HF, et al. Failure of ductus arteriosus closure and remodeling in neonatal mice deficient in cyclooxygenase-1 and cyclooxygenase-2. *Proc Natl Acad Sci U S A*. 2001;98:1059–1064.
61. Coceani F, Kelsey L, Seidlitz E, et al. Carbon monoxide formation in the ductus arteriosus in the lamb: implications for the regulation of muscle tone. *Br J Pharmacol*. 1997;120:599–608.
66. Reese J, Anderson JD, Brown N, et al. Inhibition of cyclooxygenase isoforms in late- but not midgestation decreases contractility of the ductus arteriosus and prevents postnatal closure in mice. *Am J Physiol Regul Integr Comp Physiol*. 2006;291:R1717–R1723.
68. Baragatti B, Brizzi F, Ackerley C, et al. Cyclooxygenase-1 and cyclooxygenase-2 in the mouse ductus arteriosus: individual activity and functional coupling with nitric oxide synthase. *Br J Pharmacol*. 2003;139:1505–1515.
71. Reese J, Waleh N, Poole SD, et al. Chronic in utero cyclooxygenase inhibition alters PGE_2-regulated ductus arteriosus contractile pathways and prevents postnatal closure. *Pediatr Res*. 2009;66:155–161.
74. Yokoyama U. Prostaglandin E-mediated molecular mechanisms driving remodeling of the ductus arteriosus. *Pediatr Int*. 2015;57:820–827.
76. Norton ME, Merrill J, Cooper BAB, et al. Neonatal complications after the administration of indomethacin for preterm labor. *N Engl J Med*. 1993;329:1602–1607.
78. Clyman RI, Chen YQ, Chemtob S, et al. In utero remodeling of the fetal lamb ductus arteriosus: the role of antenatal indomethacin and avascular zone thickness on vasa vasorum proliferation, neointima formation, and cell death. *Circulation*. 2001;103:1806–1812.
85. Reeve HL, Tolarova S, Nelson DP, et al. Redox control of oxygen sensing in the rabbit ductus arteriosus. *J Physiol*. 2001;533:253–261.
86. Michelakis E, Rebeyka I, Bateson J, et al. Voltage-gated potassium channels in human ductus arteriosus. *Lancet*. 2000;356:134–137.
92. Thebaud B, Wu XC, Kajimoto H, et al. Developmental absence of the O_2 sensitivity of L-type calcium channels in preterm ductus arteriosus smooth muscle cells impairs O_2 constriction contributing to patent ductus arteriosus. *Pediatr Res*. 2008;63:176–181.
93. Kajimoto H, Hashimoto K, Bonnet SN, et al. Oxygen activates the Rho/Rho-kinase pathway and induces RhoB and ROCK-1 expression in human and rabbit ductus arteriosus by increasing mitochondria-derived reactive oxygen species: a newly recognized mechanism for sustaining ductal constriction. *Circulation*. 2007;115:1777–1788.
95. Hong Z, Kutty S, Toth PT, et al. Role of dynamin-related protein 1 (Drp1)-mediated mitochondrial fission in oxygen sensing and constriction of the ductus arteriosus. *Circ Res*. 2013;112:802–815.
104. Baragatti B, Ciofini E, Scebba F, et al. Cytochrome P-450 3A13 and endothelin jointly mediate ductus arteriosus constriction to oxygen in mice. *Am J Physiol Heart Circ Physiol*. 2011;300:H892–H901.
107. Cotton RB, Shah LP, Poole SD, et al. Cimetidine-associated patent ductus arteriosus is mediated via a cytochrome P450 mechanism independent of H2 receptor antagonism. *J Mol Cell Cardiol*. 2013;59:86–94.
109. Coceani F, Armstrong C, Kelsey L. Endothelin is a potent constrictor of the lamb ductus arteriosus. *Can J Physiol Pharmacol*. 1989;67:902–904.
110. Fineman JR, Takahashi Y, Roman C, et al. Endothelin-receptor blockade does not alter closure of the ductus arteriosus. *Am J Physiol*. 1998;275:H1620–1626.
116. Thebaud B, Michelakis ED, Wu XC, et al. Oxygen-sensitive Kv channel gene transfer confers oxygen responsiveness to preterm rabbit and remodeled human ductus arteriosus: implications for infants with patent ductus arteriosus. *Circulation*. 2004;110:1372–1379.
118. Kajimura I, Akaike T, Minamisawa S. Lipopolysaccharide delays closure of the rat ductus arteriosus by induction of inducible nitric oxide synthase but not prostaglandin E2. *Circ J*. 2016;80:703–711.

120. Ohlsson A, Shah SS. Ibuprofen for the prevention of patent ductus arteriosus in preterm and/or low birth weight infants. *Cochrane Database Syst Rev.* 2011:CD004213.
121. Fowlie PW, Davis PG. Prophylactic intravenous indomethacin for preventing mortality and morbidity in preterm infants. *Cochrane Database Syst Rev.* 2010:CD000174.
125. Waleh N, Seidner S, McCurnin D, et al. The role of monocyte-derived cells and inflammation in baboon ductus arteriosus remodeling. *Pediatr Res.* 2005;57:254-262.
126. Clyman RI, Seidner SR, Kajino H, et al. VEGF regulates remodeling during permanent anatomic closure of the ductus arteriosus. *Am J Physiol.* 2002;282:R199-R206.
129. Keller RL, Tacy TA, Fields S, et al. Combined treatment with a non-selective nitric oxide synthase inhibitor (L-NMMA) and indomethacin increases ductus constriction in extremely premature newborns. *Pediatr Res.* 2005;58:1216-1221.
130. Seidner SR, Chen Y-Q, Oprysko PR, et al. Combined prostaglandin and nitric oxide inhibition produces anatomic remodeling and closure of the ductus arteriosus in the premature newborn baboon. *Pediatr Res.* 2001;50:365-373.
143. Shaffer ML, Baud O, Lacaze-Masmonteil T, et al. Effect of prophylaxis for early adrenal insufficiency using low-dose hydrocortisone in very preterm infants. an individual patient data meta-analysis. *J Pediatr.* 2019;207:136-142.
146. Londhe VA, Nolen TL, Das A, et al. Vitamin A supplementation in extremely low-birth-weight infants: subgroup analysis in small-for-gestational-age infants. *Am J Perinatol.* 2013;30:771-780.
147. Fujita S, Yokoyama U, Ishiwata R, et al. Glutamate promotes contraction of the rat ductus arteriosus. *Circ J.* 2016;80:2388-2396.
153. Yokoyama U, Minamisawa S, Katayama A, et al. Differential regulation of vascular tone and remodeling via stimulation of type 2 and type 6 adenylyl cyclases in the ductus arteriosus. *Circ Res.* 2010;106:1882-1892.
154. Yokoyama U, Minamisawa S, Quan H, et al. Prostaglandin E2-activated Epac promotes neointimal formation of the rat ductus arteriosus by a process distinct from that of cAMP-dependent protein kinase A. *J Biol Chem.* 2008;283:28702-28709.
156. de Reeder EG, Girard N, Poelmann RE, et al. Hyaluronic acid accumulation and endothelial cell detachment in intimal thickening of the vessel wall. The normal and genetically defective ductus arteriosus. *Am J Pathol.* 1988;132:574-585.
158. Mason CA, Bigras JL, O'Blenes SB, et al. Gene transfer in utero biologically engineers a patent ductus arteriosus in lambs by arresting fibronectin-dependent neointimal formation. *Nat Med.* 1999;5:176-182.
164. Hinek A, Mecham RP, Keeley F, et al. Impaired elastin fiber assembly related to reduced 67-kD elastin-binding protein in fetal lamb ductus arteriosus and in cultured aortic smooth muscle cells treated with chondroitin sulfate. *J Clin Invest.* 1991;88:2083-2094.
167. Hinek A, Boyle J, Rabinovitch M. Vascular smooth muscle cell detachment from elastin and migration through elastic laminae is promoted by chondroitin sulfate-induced "shedding" of the 67-kDa cell surface elastin binding protein. *Exp Cell Res.* 1992;203:344-353.
170. Yokoyama U, Minamisawa S, Shioda A, et al. Prostaglandin E2 inhibits elastogenesis in the ductus arteriosus via EP4 signaling. *Circulation.* 2014;129:487-496.
173. Clyman RI, Chan CY, Mauray F, et al. Permanent anatomic closure of the ductus arteriosus in newborn baboons: the roles of postnatal constriction, hypoxia, and gestation. *Pediatr Res.* 1999;45:19-29.
177. Mitra S, Chan AK, Paes BA. The association of platelets with failed patent ductus arteriosus closure after a primary course of indomethacin or ibuprofen: a systematic review and meta-analysis. *Matern Fetal Neonatal Med.* 2017;30:127-133.
179. Echtler K, Stark K, Lorenz M, et al. Platelets contribute to postnatal occlusion of the ductus arteriosus. *Nat Med.* 2010;16:75-82.
182. Yarboro MT, Durbin MD, Herington JL, et al. Transcriptional profiling of the ductus arteriosus: comparison of rodent microarrays and human RNA sequencing. *Semin Perinatol.* 2018;42:212-220.
238. Ivey KN, Sutcliffe D, Richardson J, et al. Transcriptional regulation during development of the ductus arteriosus. *Circ Res.* 2008;103:388-395.
240. Clyman RI, Mauray F, Heymann MA, et al. Cardiovascular effects of a patent ductus arteriosus in preterm lambs with respiratory distress. *J Pediatr.* 1987;111:579-587.
241. Liebowitz M, Koo J, Wickremasinghe A, et al. Effects of prophylactic indomethacin on vasopressor-dependent hypotension in extremely preterm infants. *J Pediatr.* 2017;182:21-27.e22.
243. Shimada S, Kasai T, Konishi M, et al. Effects of patent ductus arteriosus on left ventricular output and organ blood flows in preterm infants with respiratory distress syndrome treated with surfactant. *J Pediatr.* 1994;125:270-277.
245. McCurnin D, Clyman RI. Effects of a patent ductus arteriosus on postprandial mesenteric perfusion in premature baboons. *Pediatrics.* 2008;122:e1262-1267.
253. Lemmers PM, Benders MJ, D'Ascenzo R, et al. Patent ductus arteriosus and brain volume. *Pediatrics.* 2016;137:e20153090.
258. Al Faleh K, Smyth J, Roberts R, et al. Prevention and 18-month outcome of serious pulmonary hemorrhage in extremely low birth weight infants: results from the trial of indomethacin prophylaxis in preterms. *Pediatrics.* 2008;121:e233-e238.
264. De Buyst J, Rakza T, Pennaforte T, et al. Hemodynamic effects of fluid restriction in preterm infants with significant patent ductus arteriosus. *J Pediatr.* 2012;161:404-408.
266. Perez Fontan JJ, Clyman RI, Mauray F, et al. Respiratory effects of a patent ductus arteriosus in premature newborn lambs. *J Appl Physiol.* 1987;63:2315-2324.
267. Alpan G, Scheerer R, Bland RD, et al. Patent ductus arteriosus increases lung fluid filtration in preterm lambs. *Pediatr Res.* 1991;30:616-621.
271. McCurnin D, Seidner S, Chang LY, et al. Ibuprofen-induced patent ductus arteriosus closure: physiologic, histologic, and biochemical effects on the premature lung. *Pediatrics.* 2008;121:945-956.
282. Waleh N, McCurnin DC, Yoder BA, et al. Patent ductus arteriosus ligation alters pulmonary gene expression in preterm baboons. *Pediatr Res.* 2011;69:212-216.
284. Chang LY, McCurnin D, Yoder B, et al. Ductus arteriosus ligation and alveolar growth in preterm baboons with a patent ductus arteriosus. *Pediatr Res.* 2008;63:299-302.
285. Clyman R, Cassady G, Kirklin JK, et al. The role of patent ductus arteriosus ligation in bronchopulmonary dysplasia: reexamining a randomized controlled trial. *J Pediatr.* 2009;154:873-876.
296. Benitz WE, Committee on Fetus and Newborn. Patent ductus arteriosus in preterm infants. *Pediatrics.* 2016;137:e20153730.
302. Liebowitz M, Clyman RI. Prophylactic indomethacin compared with delayed conservative management of the patent ductus arteriosus in extremely preterm infants: effects on neonatal outcomes. *J Pediatr.* 2017;187:119-126.

53 Umbilical Circulation

Torvid Kiserud | Guttorm Haugen

INTRODUCTION

The fetoplacental circulation, also known as *umbilical circuit,* with its transport of nutrients, gases, and endocrine signaling, is critical for fetal development. A long tradition of animal experiments has given us indispensable insights into its physiology.[1-4] However, the introduction of ultrasound techniques enabled studies of the human version of this physiology free from the surgical trauma hampering the experimental procedures. This chapter prioritizes human data where possible, as animal and human physiology are different. For example, fetal lambs have a fundamentally different placenta; four vessels in the umbilical cord; different anatomy of the liver, portal veins, ductus venosus, and intrathoracic inferior vena cava; faster growth; shorter pregnancy; lower hemoglobin; and higher heart rate and temperature than the human fetus.

ANATOMY

Technically, the fetoplacental circuit starts in the heart as it ejects blood into the aorta and pulmonary artery, and ends with the

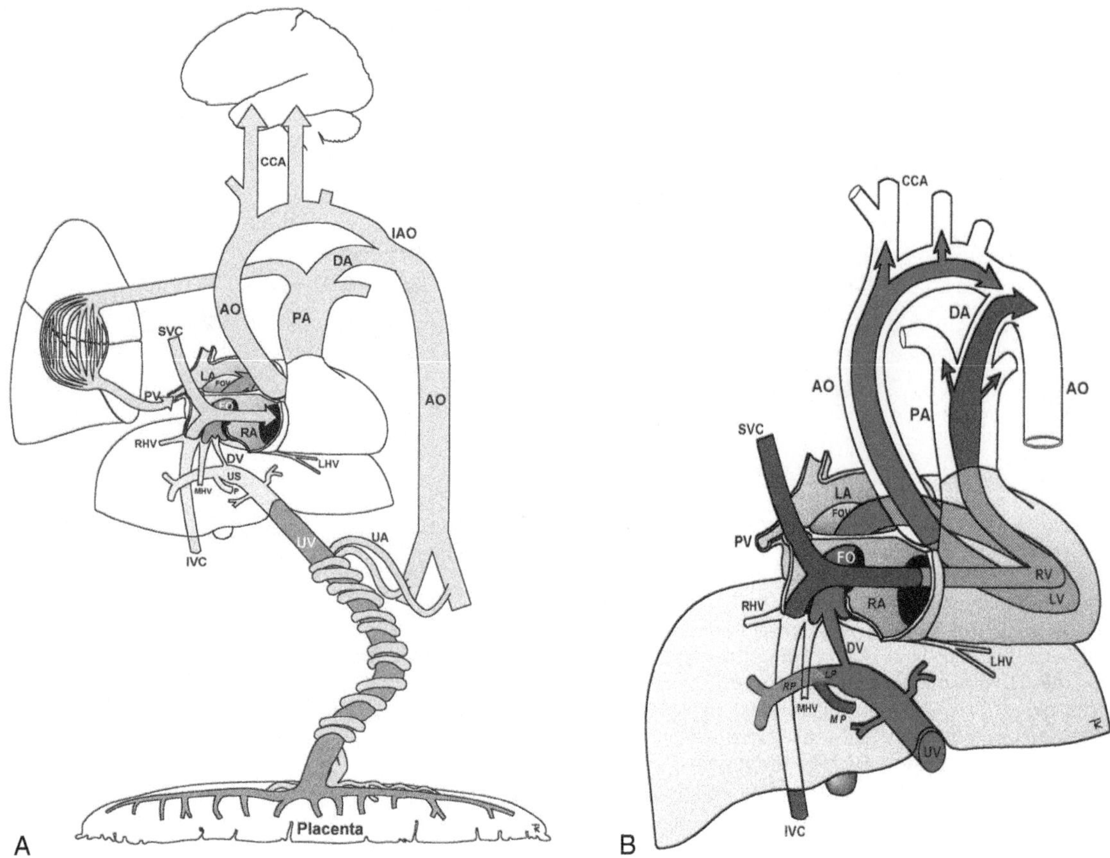

Fig. 53.1 Overview of the umbilical circulation as part of the entire fetal circulation (A) and the distribution of umbilical venous return with central pathways (B). While low-oxygenated blood follows the pathway of "via dextra" *(blue)*, well-oxygenated venous return is fed into the "via sinistra" *(red)* via the ductus venosus *(DV)*, foramen ovale *(FO)*, left atrium *(LA)*, left ventricle *(LV)*, and aorta *(Ao)*, to feed the coronary and cerebral arteries *(CCA)* before joining the via dextra in the descending Ao. *DA*, Ductus arteriosus; *FOV*, foramen ovale valve; *IAO*, isthmus of the aorta; *IVC*, inferior vena cava; *LHV*, left hepatic vein; *LP*, left portal branch; *MHV*, medial hepatic vein; *MP*, main portal vein; *PA*, pulmonary artery; *PV*, pulmonary vein; *RA*, right atrium; *RHV*, right hepatic vein; *RP*, right portal branch; *RV*, right ventricle; *SVC*, superior vena cava; *UA*, umbilical artery; *US*, umbilical sinus of the left portal branch; *UV*, umbilical vein. ([A] reproduced with permission from Hanson M, Kiserud T. Circulation. In: Harding R, Bocking A, eds. *Developmental Physiology*. Cambridge: Cambridge University Press; 2001; and [B] modified from Kiserud T, Rasmussen S, Skulstad S. Blood flow and the degree of shunting through the ductus venosus in the human fetus. *Am J Obstet Gynecol*. 2000;182:147–153.)

inferior vena cava entering the heart (Fig. 53.1A). However, the umbilical circulation starts as the umbilical arteries branch from the internal iliac arteries, passing the fetal urinary bladder on both sides to enter the umbilical cord through the umbilical ring. Here the two arteries are bundled with the umbilical vein to communicate with the placenta. The vessels are suspended in Wharton jelly, which prevents external compression of the vessels,[5] and covered with the amniotic membrane to form the free loop of the cord (the amniotic part of the umbilical circuit). At the insertion of the cord in the placenta, the arteries commonly communicate (Hyrtl's anastomosis) before branching on the amniotic surface of the placenta.[6] The anastomosis equalizes blood pressure and stabilizes the distribution into the smaller arteries in the depths to reach the capillary system of the villi.[7] In the villi, the capillaries communicate extensively with each other before fusing into venules and veins to finally form a single umbilical vein (two umbilical veins in early embryonic development; see Chapter 45) that joins the two arteries in the cord on its way to the fetal umbilicus. Here, it enters through the somehow constricting umbilical ring[8-10] to become the intra-abdominal umbilical vein, embedded in the inferior surface of the liver, and connects with the portal system (see Fig. 53.1B). During fetal life, the nutritious umbilical venous return feeds the left side of the liver through branches of the left portal system then feeds the shunt ductus venosus that directs blood into the inferior vena cava and foramen ovale. The remainder flows beyond the ductus venosus inlet to merge with blood from the main portal stem and circulate through the right liver lobe ultimately reaching the heart via the hepatic veins and inferior vena cava (Fig. 53.2).

After birth, as the umbilical arteries obliterate and cord is clamped (see "Umbilical Circulation at Birth and Timing of Cord Clamping"), the intra-abdominal umbilical vein obliterates distal to the first portal branches into the left liver lobe (see Fig. 53.2), and the entire portal system including the ductus venosus is now supplied from the main portal stem. As for the ductus venosus, 76% obliterate within a week in healthy term neonates,[11,12] while in premature neonates[13,14] or neonates with pulmonary hypertension, it may stay open for 2 to 3 weeks.[15]

In singleton pregnancies, 0.5% to 1.0% of the umbilical cords have a single artery.[16] These pregnancies have an increased risk of adverse perinatal outcome including small for gestational age neonates. While conventionally the umbilical cord has a central insertion into the placenta, 6% to 7% have a marginal insertion (<3 cm from the placental border) and 1% to 2% a velamentous insertion into the fetal membranes, both associated with an increased risk of adverse perinatal outcome including prematurity and low birth weight.[17]

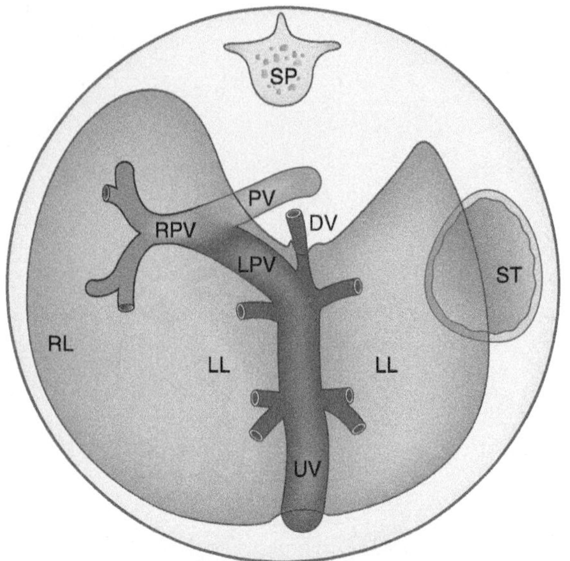

Fig. 53.2 In the fetus, oxygenated blood *(red)* in the umbilical vein *(UV)* is either shunted through the ductus venosus *(DV)*, 20% to 30%, or perfuses the liver, 70% to 80%, feeding the left liver lobe *(LL)* and then flowing through the transverse part of left portal vein *(LPV)* and the right portal vein *(RPV)* to circulate the right liver *(RL)* blended with low-oxygenated blood *(blue)* from the main portal vein *(PV)*. After birth, the UV obliterates and the PV is the sole venous supply to the entire liver. *SP*, Spine; *ST*, stomach. (Modified with permission from Kessler J, Rasmussen S, Kiserud T. The fetal portal vein: normal blood flow development during the second half of human pregnancy. *Ultrasound Obstet Gynecol.* 2007;30:52–60.)

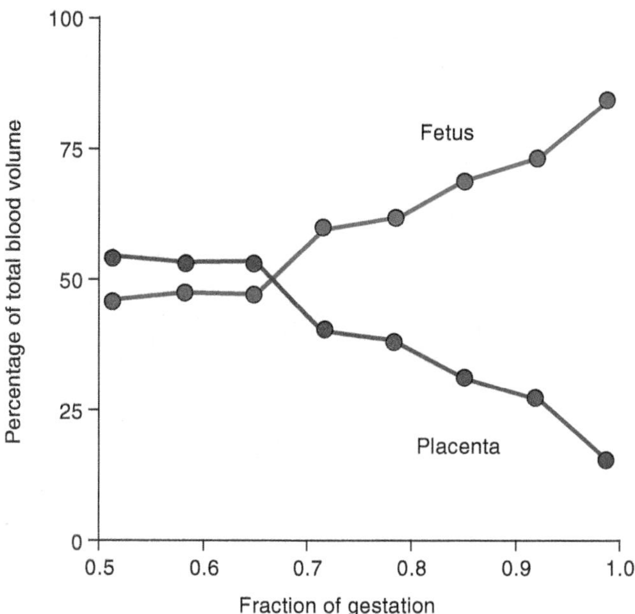

Fig. 53.3 Fraction of total blood volume contained within the placenta and fetus during the second half of pregnancy. (Based on sheep data from Barcroft J. *Researches on Pre-natal Life*. Oxford: Blackwell Scientific Publications; 1946.)

THE VOLUME OF BLOOD IN THE UMBILICAL CIRCUIT

The fetus circulates a blood volume corresponding to 11% to 12% of its weight, which is considerably higher than the 7% during adult life.[18-20] The reason is that at any time a large proportion of blood is contained within the placenta. This fraction, however, decreases from 50% at mid-gestation to below 25% near term, according to sheep data (Fig. 53.3).[2] Although the fetal liver and splanchnic circuit have a capacity to accumulate blood volume and act as a buffer within the circulation, the umbilical circuit with the huge placental volume represents a correspondingly larger volume buffer.

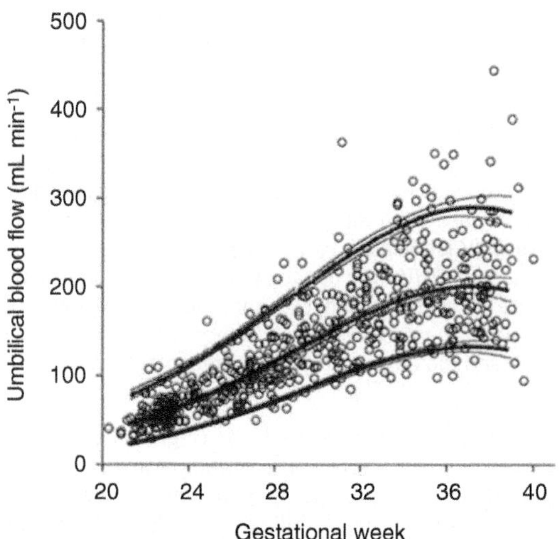

Fig. 53.4 During the second half of a human pregnancy the umbilical flow grows exponentially, but with a blunted pattern after 32 weeks. Lines = 5th, 50th, and 95th percentiles with 95% confidence intervals *(thin lines)*. (Reproduced with permission from Kessler J, Rasmussen S, Godfrey KM, et al. Longitudinal study of umbilical and portal venous blood flow to the liver: low pregnancy weight gain is associated with preferential supply to the fetal left liver lobe. *Pediatr Res.* 2008;63:315–320.)

UMBILICAL BLOOD FLOW

Umbilical blood flow (mL/min) is a key determinant for fetal growth, has attracted numerous experimental and clinical studies, and is still today of great physiologic interest but has not fully reached clinical applicability. With improved ultrasound techniques and study designs, a number of studies have confirmed and refined the pioneering studies by Gill and colleagues[21,22] showing that umbilical blood flow grows steadily during the second half of pregnancy, with some blunting toward term (Fig. 53.4).[23-30] However, fetuses developing birth weight exceeding the 90th percentile without hyperglycemia have less or no blunting.[31] Although small dimensions impose substantial measurement variation, umbilical flow has been described for gestational weeks 11 to 20.[32]

Before 20 weeks of gestation, umbilical blood flow normalized for fetal weight (mL/min/kg) increases steadily (Fig. 53.5).[32] This hemodynamic development is also reflected in the increasing distribution of fetal cardiac output to the umbilical circuit—that is, from 14% to 21% during 11 to 20 weeks of gestation (see Fig. 53.5).[32] These findings in early human pregnancies corroborate previous animal data.[33] These events coincide with establishment of intervillous circulation at the end of the first trimester, which is followed by rapid expansion of the vascular cross-section and a corresponding fall in resistance.[34,35]

After 20 weeks of gestation, however, the umbilical flow per kilogram of fetal weight declines from 105 to 65 mL/min at term (Fig. 53.6A).[26-29] During gestational weeks 20 to 30, a steady fraction (30%) of the total cardiac output is distributed to the placenta. Beyond 30 weeks, the fraction declines to reach 20% or less before term (see Fig. 53.6B).[36] In contrast, the fetus maintains a combined cardiac output of 400 mL/min/kg during

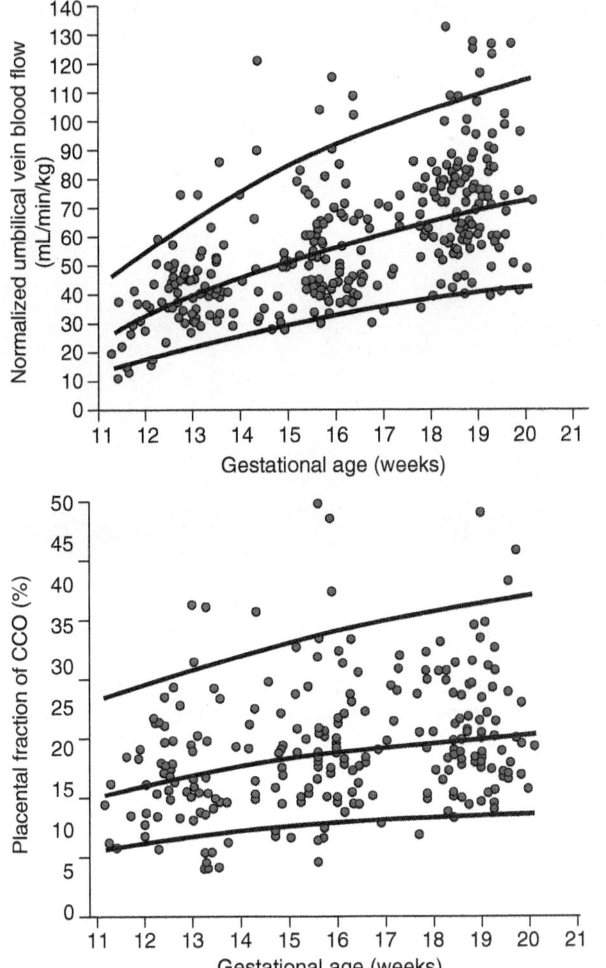

Fig. 53.5 Umbilical blood flow per kg increases during gestational weeks 12 to 19 *(upper panel)* and constitutes an increasing fraction of the combined cardiac output *(CCO)* in the human fetus *(lower panel)*. Lines = 5th, 50th, and 95th percentiles. (Reproduced with permission from Vimpeli T, Huhtala H, Wilsgaard T, et al. Fetal cardiac output and its distribution to the placenta at 11–20 weeks of gestation. *Ultrasound Obstet Gynecol.* 2009;33:265–271.)

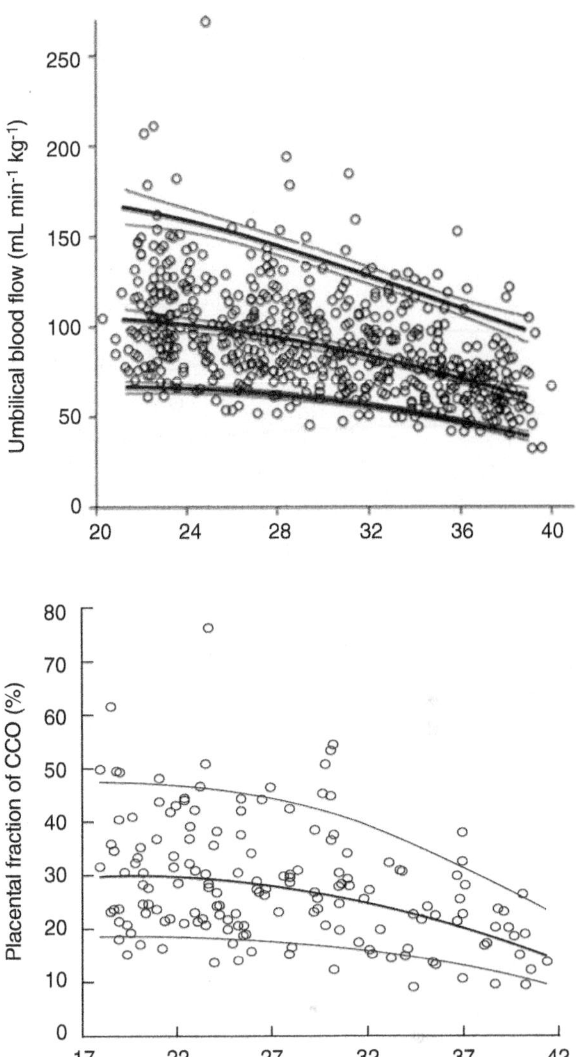

Fig. 53.6 Umbilical blood flow normalized for fetal weight declines during the second half of human pregnancies *(upper panel)*. That is also reflected in the decreased fraction of combined cardiac output *(CCO)* distributed to the umbilical circulation *(lower panel)*; 30% before 30 weeks and at average 20% after. Lines = 5th, 50th, and 95th percentiles with 95% confidence intervals *(thin lines)* in upper panel, and 10th, 50th, and 90th percentiles in lower panel. (Reproduced with permission from Kessler J, Rasmussen S, Godfrey KM, et al. Longitudinal study of umbilical and portal venous blood flow to the liver: low pregnancy weight gain is associated with preferential supply to the fetal left liver lobe. *Pediatr Res.* 2008;63:315–320; and Kiserud T, Ebbing C, Kessler J, et al. Fetal cardiac output, distribution to the placenta and impact of placental compromise. *Ultrasound Obstet Gynecol.* 2006;28:126–136.)

the entire second half of pregnancy.[36] Thus the fetus seems to have a tight regulation to maintain cardiac output per kilogram of body weight, and at mid-gestation it uses 70% of its cardiac output to perfuse its body as the rest (30%) is directed to the placenta. During the last trimester, 80% is circulating to the body, whereas only 20% is directed to the placenta.

Interestingly, normalized cardiac output is maintained equally well in growth-restricted fetuses, even with the most severe placental compromise (Fig. 53.7A),[36] while the fraction distributed to the placenta is significantly reduced and may reach 10% or less in the most severe cases (see Fig. 53.7, *B*). This implies that 90% or more of the blood is recycled within the fetal body without being rejuvenated in the placenta.

UMBILICAL ARTERY HEMODYNAMICS

UMBILICAL ARTERY PRESSURE

Typically, the mean arterial pressure in fetal lambs increases exponentially during the second half of pregnancy, reaching 40 to 60 mm Hg at term.[3,4] Less is known of the human fetus. During cordocentesis, Castle and MacKenzie determined mean umbilical artery pressure to be 15 mm Hg at gestational weeks 19 to 21,[37] and during the latter part of pregnancy, Weiner and coworkers measured systolic/diastolic pressures of 63/40, 31/26, and 39/19 mm Hg in three fetuses.[38] Intraventricular measurements suggest that systemic systolic pressure increases from 15 to 20 mm Hg at 16 weeks to 30 to 40 mm Hg at 28 weeks, with negligible difference between the left and the right side.[39] Using mathematical modeling of volume blood flow and diameter variation as measured by Doppler ultrasound, mean aortic blood pressure was estimated to increase from 21 to 45 mm Hg during gestational weeks 21 to 40.[40]

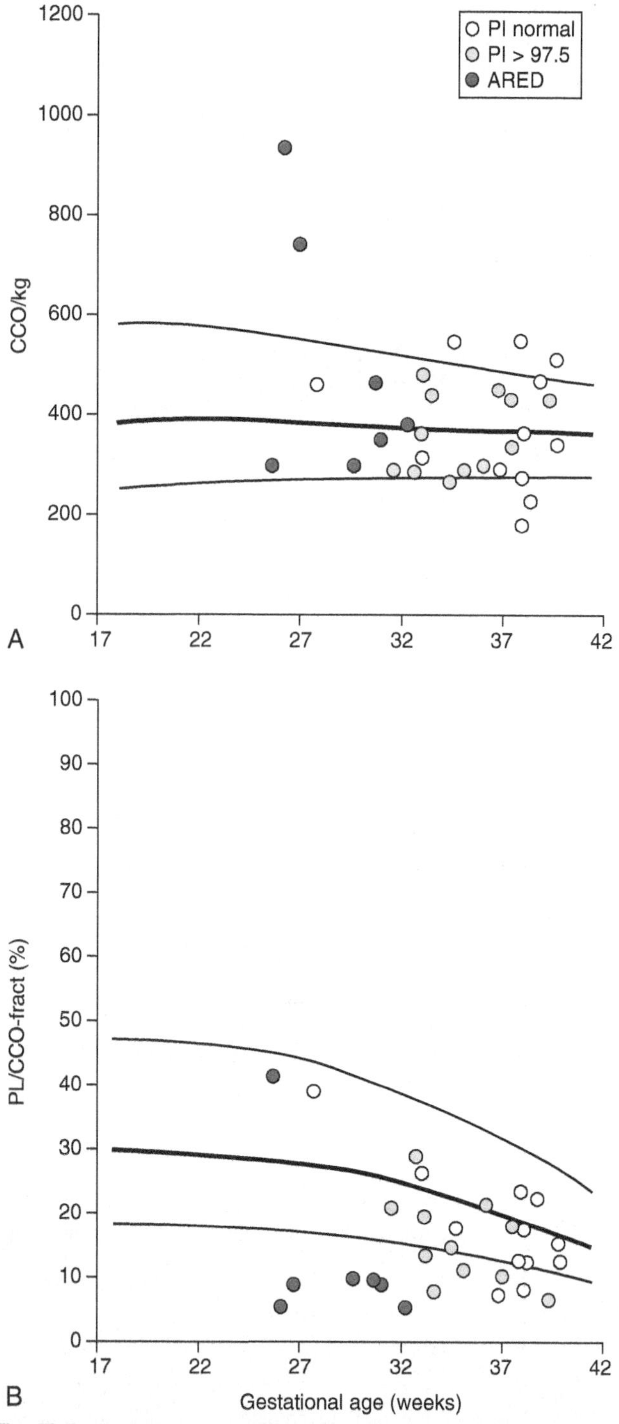

Fig. 53.7 Fetuses with intrauterine growth restriction maintain a normal combined cardiac output *(CCO)* (mL/kg/min) during the second half of pregnancy (A), but distribute a smaller fraction of the CCO to the placenta *(PL)* (B) graded according to umbilical artery impedance (≈ pulsatility index *[PI]*). The most extreme cases with absent or reversed end-diastolic flow *(ARED)* in the umbilical artery direct ≤10% of CCO to the placenta. Lines = 5th, 50th, and 95th percentiles. (Reproduced with permission from Kiserud T, Ebbing C, Kessler J, et al. Fetal cardiac output, distribution to the placenta and impact of placental compromise. *Ultrasound Obstet Gynecol.* 2006;28:126–136.)

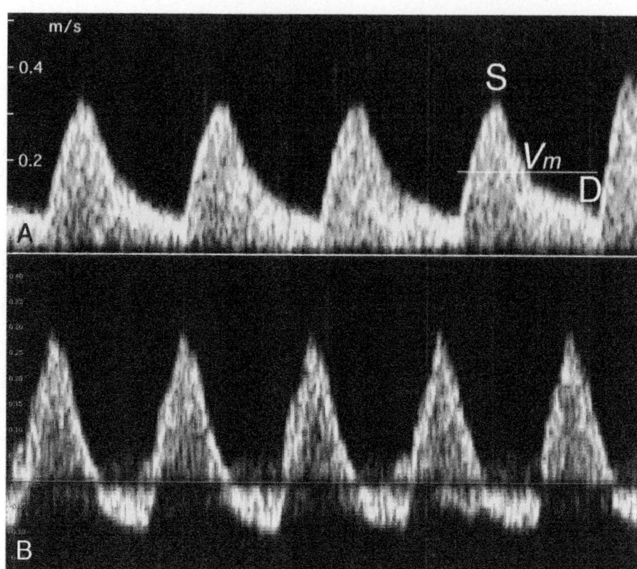

Fig. 53.8 Normal umbilical artery blood velocity pulse waves recorded with Doppler ultrasound during second trimester (A). Pulsatility index (PI = $[S - D] / V_m$) is a robust way of documenting the wave form. Increased impedance during placental compromise is visualized in a reduced end-diastolic velocity that in extreme cases may be absent or reversed as in the present recording during 24 weeks of gestation (B). *D,* End-diastolic velocity; *S,* systolic peak velocity; V_m, time-averaged maximum velocity *(white line).*

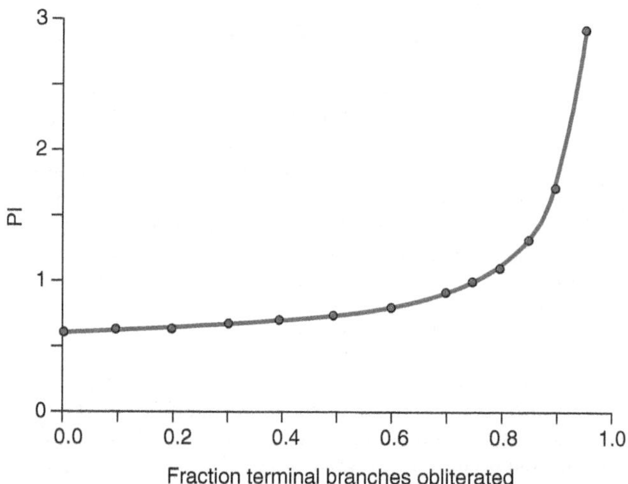

Fig. 53.9 Extensive obliteration (e.g., >60%) of the fetoplacental vascular bed is needed to create any discernable impact on the umbilical artery blood velocity waveform, expressed as pulsatility index *(PI)*, as demonstrated in a mathematical model. (Modified and reproduced with permission from Trudinger B. Doppler ultrasonography: applications in clinical practice. In: Hanson MA, Spencer JAD, Rodeck CH, eds. *Fetus and Neonate. Physiology and Clinical Application: The Circulation.* Cambridge: Cambridge University Press; 1993.)

ARTERIAL PULSATION

The pulsation of the umbilical artery blood flow velocity is extensively used in obstetrics because the waveform recorded using Doppler ultrasound indicates the downstream impedance. The waveform is quantified by various indices, the most robust being the pulsatility index (Fig. 53.8A).[41] An increased pulsatility index is associated with increased impedance in the umbilical circuit—that is, hemodynamic compromise (see Fig. 53.8B).[42,43] However, the relation between the waveform and resistance in the placental bed is not linear. Obliterating half of the fetoplacental vessels may hardly impact the pulsatile waveform, as shown in embolization experiments and mathematical modeling (Fig. 53.9).[44,45] Part of the explanation is that the resistance to pulsatile

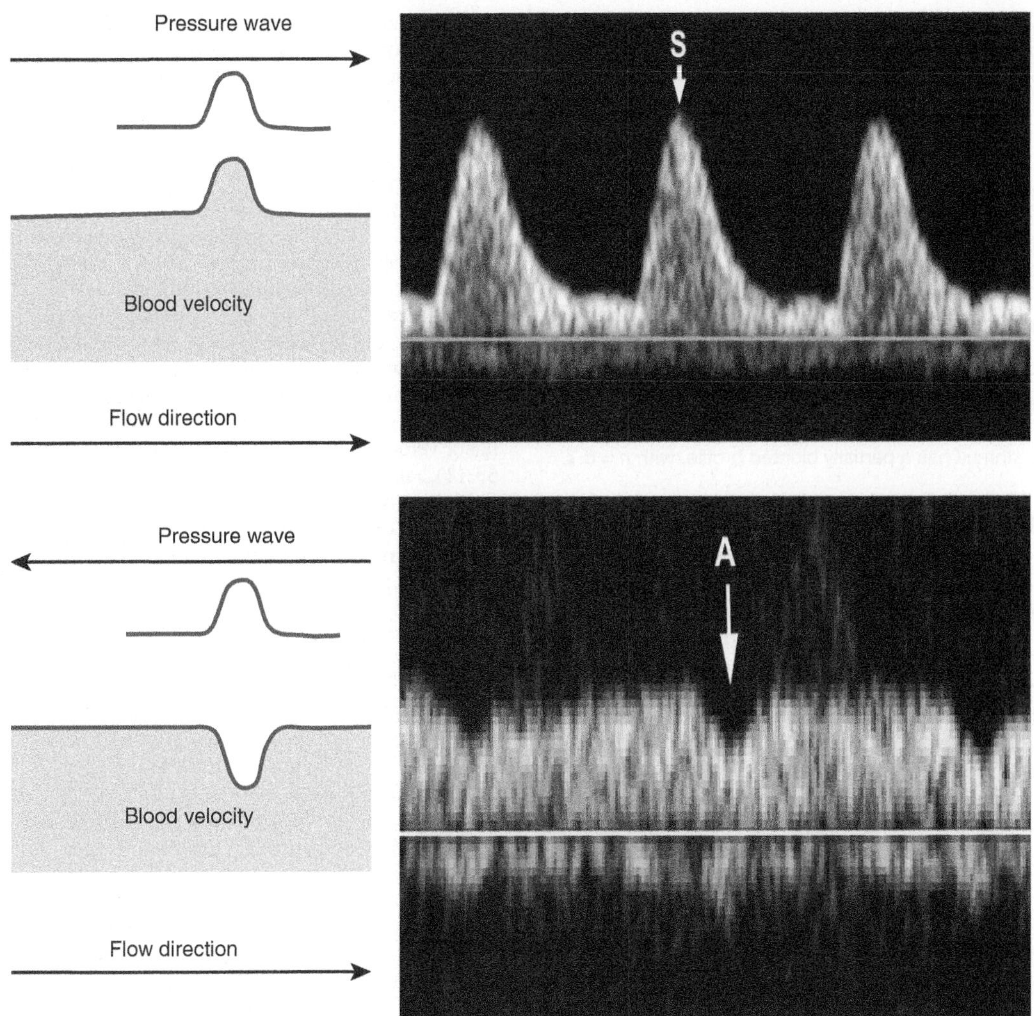

Fig. 53.10 Arterial blood flows in the direction away from the heart, and the pressure pulse generated in the ventricle runs in the same direction, resulting in a blood velocity increment during systole *(S) (upper panel)*. However, if the pressure wave runs in the direction opposite to flow, the result is a velocity deflection *(lower panel)*. That is the case with a reflected wave in arteries, or as here, the atrial contraction wave running away from the heart along the veins in the opposite direction of the venous flow causing a velocity deflection *(A)*.

flow—that is, impedance, in addition to vascular cross-section and length—is governed by the fluid dynamic determinants of pulsation that include frequency, pressure amplitude, and vessel compliance,[46-48] as well as viscosity when velocities are low.

The arterial pulse wave consists of three components: pressure, vessel diameter, and blood velocity wave. As the pulse wave travels downstream in the vascular tree, it moves considerably faster than the average blood velocity in the vessel.[49] The stiffer the vessel, the faster the pressure wave travels. In the fetus, it is estimated that the speed climbs from less than 2m/s to 10 m/s within the first 20 cm from the heart.[50] Thus the pressure wave reaches the periphery early and is reflected whenever there is a change of impedance (which is determined by local vessel geometry and distensibility and blood viscosity). The reflected pressure wave interferes with the downstream velocity wave,[49] which is the reason why velocity waves in the umbilical artery indicate details of the downstream vasculature. Conventionally, the reflected wave will hit the downstream wave with a phase shift and cause a velocity deflection because now it is running in the opposite direction of flow (Fig. 53.10).[51] This is particularly seen in the extreme cases of placental compromise, when the umbilical artery end-diastolic velocity is zero or reversed (see Fig. 53.8B). In the normally developing umbilical vasculature, this reflected pulse-wave interference is less marked, probably signifying the diffuse distribution of a large number of bifurcations causing the various reflected waves to cancel out each other.[47] The blood velocity waveform in the umbilical artery changes to a less pulsatile pattern with advancing gestation, reflecting continued vascular proliferation.[52]

VISCOSITY

At a high blood velocity, which is common in main arteries, the physical behavior of blood is "Newtonian"—that is, like water, with a low viscous resistance and a linear relation to vascular surface and flow velocity.[53] However, viscosity becomes an issue when blood velocities are low (near zero). The placental arterial tree branches up to a huge cross-sectional area where flow velocity is low. The large cross-section indicates low resistance, but the blood that runs with the very low velocity has become non-Newtonian with a correspondingly high viscous friction. If the blood in some of these sections comes to a standstill, there has to be an opening pressure (or closing pressure) to overcome before the blood starts moving (a phenomenon that is also seen in the fetal venous liver circulation).[53-55] Some anatomic studies of the capillary formation in compromised placentas suggest that there is a reduced branching and increased elongation of capillaries, which implies that the resistance increases also because of an increase in the length of the vessel,[55] a significant contribution to local vascular resistance.

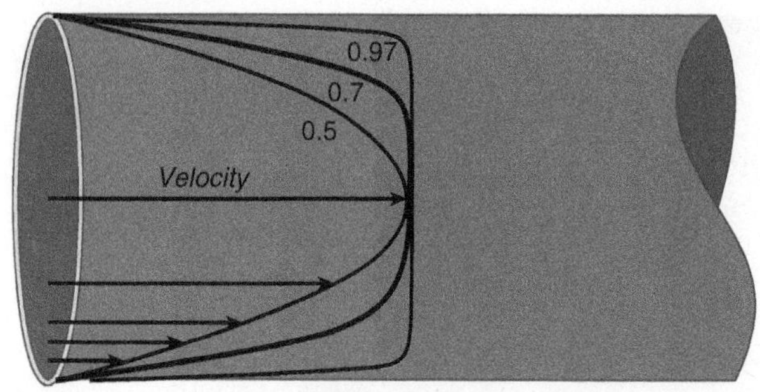

Fig. 53.11 The velocity profile is characterized by the quotient h = (spatial average velocity) / (peak velocity). A steady laminar flow has a parabolic velocity profile with $h = 0.5$. At the aortic valve, where blood velocity is high, the profile will be flat (blunted) with a typical $h = 0.97$. Blood that accelerates from the umbilical vein through the ductus venosus isthmus has a partially blunted profile, with $h = 0.7$.

VELOCITY PROFILE

Impedance is lowest when flow is laminar.[49] The higher the velocity, the greater is the risk of developing turbulent flow, which is characterized by a mixture of unpredictable velocity directions that forms a blunted (flat) velocity profile in the vessel cross-section (Fig. 53.11). Turbulent flow represents higher resistance to flow. The *Reynolds number* characterizes the vessel and indicates the level of velocity when turbulence may develop.[49] In addition to magnitude of velocity, the vessel cross-sectional area is important; the wider the vessel, the more likely turbulence develops. Steady flow has a greater risk of turbulence than flow with velocity variation (e.g., pulsation). Also, directional variation reduces the risk of turbulence formation. In the long umbilical arteries of the cord, velocities are kept high enough to have the low viscous friction of Newtonian fluids. Because the flow in the cord normally is distributed between two rather than a single artery, the vessel cross-section is low and reduces the risk of turbulence. The pulsatile velocity reduces turbulence formation and so does the continuously changing direction (coiling). These characteristics all optimize blood transportation at minimal energy expenditure. However, several studies have reported increased perinatal risk associated with reduced and increased coiling of the umbilical cord vessels[56] suggesting that this geometry matters and operates best within certain limits.

HEMODYNAMICS OF THE UMBILICAL VENOUS RETURN

VELOCITY AND VELOCITY PROFILE

The umbilical venous flow is governed by the same fluid-dynamic mechanisms as the arterial flow. However, the venous flow is slow (mean 16 to 22 cm/s from 19 to 41 weeks of gestation),[28] mostly not pulsatile, and thus laminar with a parabolic spatial distribution of velocities ($h = 0.5$) (see Fig. 53.11). At the junction between the placenta and the cord, there is a venous confluence feeding the single vein in the cord. The corresponding reduction in cross-section causes an acceleration in blood velocity and, thus, a slightly blunted velocity profile.[57]

At the fetal end, there is a similar phenomenon where the umbilical vein enters through the abdominal wall.[8] Here, a restrictive ring impacts the vein diameter (once the period of physiologic umbilical herniation is completed at 12 weeks of gestation), as reflected in a substantial increase in velocity and a more blunted velocity profile.[9] This constriction is maintained with some variation for the rest of pregnancy, and 20% to 30% of normally developing fetuses at some stage have a velocity increase of 300% corresponding to a diameter reduction by half.[10,58] The physiologic significance is not well understood, but it has been suggested that increased pressure in the placental venules caused by a venous constriction may contribute to proliferation of villous vasculature in the placenta. Because of the physiologic constriction at the umbilical ring, there is regularly a "poststenotic" dilation of the vein inside the abdominal wall signifying pressure regain—that is, the high velocity is taken down to expected ranges and the corresponding kinetic energy is transformed to pressure, producing the dilation. Since the constriction is short, the loss of energy is minimal. A constriction extending for many millimeters, however, may represent a considerable resistance (and loss of energy) and thus affect venous return and fetal development.

The next "rapid" for the umbilical venous flow comes as it enters the ductus venosus.[59,60] Flow acceleration starts before the narrow entrance to the ductus, similar to water in the river accelerating as it approaches the edge of the waterfall.[61] The peak velocity is reached at the narrowest cross-section where the blood has a velocity profile of $h = 0.7$ (i.e., partially blunted) (see Fig. 53.11), a finding that is predicted by mathematical modeling using fluid dynamic laws and physiologic boundaries, and validated in sheep experiments and in human ultrasound studies.[62–65] However, in early pregnancy when velocities are low (e.g., 11 to 14 weeks), the velocity profile is close to parabolic ($h = 0.53$).[66] At this stage of pregnancy, the precordial venous pulsations drive the velocity toward zero during the atrial contraction phase, and the profile distorts and may at times have simultaneous antegrade and retrograde velocities in the same vessel cross-section,[66] which may cause a problem when interpreting Doppler recordings.

UMBILICAL VENOUS PRESSURE

The venous pressure in the intra-abdominal umbilical vein is important for the further transportation and distribution of oxygenated blood through the fetal liver or ductus venosus. In 111 normal human pregnancies, Ville and colleagues found that mean umbilical venous pressure increases from 4.5 mm Hg at 18 weeks to 6 mm Hg near term,[67] which was similar to previous measurements.[38,68] However, it is difficult to assess the umbilical vein pressure because the amniotic pressure needs to be controlled for simultaneously, which is not always possible in the practical situation, and amniotic pressure tends to vary with time.

UMBILICOCAVAL (PORTOCAVAL) PRESSURE GRADIENT

Rather than the absolute umbilical venous pressure, it is the pressure gradient $\Delta P_{UV\text{-}IVC}$ between the umbilical vein and the inferior vena cava (which postnatally continues as portocaval pressure gradient) that drives the umbilical perfusion of the liver and the ductus venosus flow.[62,69,70] Because the ductus venosus blood velocity (55 to 90 cm/s)[71] is accelerated compared with the umbilical venous blood velocity, the velocity difference represents the pressure gradient. Using human Doppler recordings, the simplified Bernoulli equation

$$\Delta P_{UV-IVC} = 4(V_{DV})^2 \quad [53.1]$$

yields 0 to 3 mm Hg during the cardiac cycle in the second half of pregnancy (the ductus venosus blood velocity, V_{DV}, is entered in m/s and the output comes in mm Hg).[69] The values seem low but have been verified in sheep experiments and are fluid-dynamically validated in mathematical models.[61,62,72,73] The pressure gradient may increase when an increased volume load is imposed on the umbilical circuit, for example, hyperkinetic circulation during fetal anemia. An increase in the vascular resistance of the liver tissue (e.g., inflammation or infiltration) may also cause a raised pressure gradient. Particularly in the latter case, the ductus venosus blood velocity is overly increased.

VENOUS PULSATION

During the second half of pregnancy, umbilical venous velocity rarely pulsates, and if it does, it commonly represents waves generated in the heart transmitted along the transmission lines

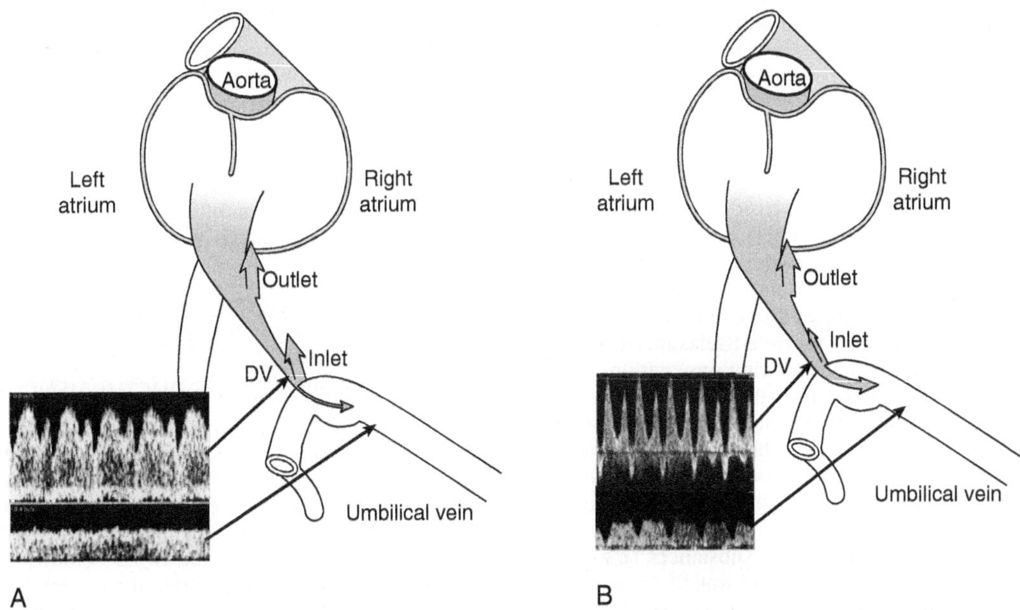

Fig. 53.12 (A) The pressure wave generated in the atria propagates *(broad gray arrows)* into the precordial veins and is partially reflected, partially transmitted at the junctions due to difference in impedance (mainly vessel area). When the difference is substantial, most is reflected and what is transmitted is hardly causing pulsation as shown in the Doppler recording at the umbilical vein, whereas above the junction pulsations are recorded in the ductus venosus *(DV)*. (B) During severe placental compromise the umbilical vein is slim and the DV distended, causing less difference in cross-section and impedance with corresponding less reflected wave and more transmitted. The result is that pulsations are also recorded in the umbilical vein. An augmented pressure wave further increases the probability of a visible pulse in the umbilical vein.

formed by the precordial veins. The transmission line inferior vena cava–ductus venosus–umbilical vein is clinically important (see Fig. 53.1B) and commonly used for recording and evaluating the hemodynamic status of the fetus.

Pulsations are regularly found in the ductus venosus down to the isthmic portion, whereas beyond the junction with the umbilical vein they are hardly observed. The fluid-dynamic reason for this is illustrated in Fig. 53.12. The wave generated in the atria represents the pressure variation during the cardiac cycle and is imposed on the local blood velocity and vessel cross-section as it travels along the vessels. On the arterial side the pressure wave travels in the same direction as the blood, and according to the concept of wave intensity,[51] the pressure wave causes a velocity and diameter increment (see Fig. 53.10). On the venous side, however, the pressure wave runs in the opposite direction of the venous flow, and the result is a velocity deflection (see Fig. 53.12) and diameter distension.[74] The configuration of the resulting local wave depends on the pressure amplitude imposed, and on the other side, the local properties of the vessel. The single most important mechanism modifying the transmission of the pressure wave in the fetal precordial veins is reflection of the pressure wave at the junction of two vessels with its reflection coefficient ($R_{dv\text{-}uv}$),[74-76] here exemplified by the ductus venosus–umbilical vein junction:

$$R_{dv-uv} = \frac{Z_{uv} - Z_{dv}}{Z_{uv} + Z_{dv}} \qquad [53.2]$$

where Z_{UV} represents the impedance distally of the junction (umbilical vein) and Z_{DV} the proximal impedance (ductus venosus). Analogous to light being reflected or transmitted according to the density difference between air and water, the pressure wave is reflected according to the difference in impedance between the two sections of vasculature. The most decisive factor in the impedance *(Z)* is the vessel cross-section *(A)*:

$$Z = \rho c / A \qquad [53.3]$$

where ρ is density and c is wave velocity. There is a substantial step in impedance between the ductus venosus and the umbilical vein (e.g., diameter 1.5 vs. 6 mm at 37 weeks of gestation),[26] which means that almost the entire pressure wave is reflected and very little arrives in the umbilical vein (see Fig. 53.12).

Because the umbilical vein is wide and compliant (the fluid-dynamic "reservoir function"), the residual pressure wave arriving there will essentially be absorbed in a hardly traceable distension and no blood velocity pulse will be traced.[74] Had the umbilical vein been smaller (e.g., early pregnancy or growth-restriction) and under increased adrenergic tone, the compliance would have been reduced, permitting less diameter distension and more velocity pulsation. Growth-restricted fetuses tend to distend the ductus venosus inlet leading to less impedance difference between the ductus venosus and the umbilical vein contributing to more wave transmission across the junction and less reflection (see Fig. 53.12B). Because these fetuses commonly are challenged by hypoxemia, they may increase the adrenergic stimulation of the heart to increase atrial contraction, thus increasing the pressure amplitude and making it more likely that the pulse energy will travel further.

REGULATION OF VASCULAR TONE IN UMBILICOPLACENTAL VESSELS

The human placenta and umbilical cord vessels lack innervation.[77] The local regulation of the vascular smooth muscle tension is dependent on vasoactive substances within the circulation or on locally produced substances within the vessel wall. The impact of different autacoids has been examined in different human preparations taken from placental or umbilical cord vessels following delivery. Their response varies depending on the local concentration, vessel segment, and experimental method used. In preparations from the umbilicoplacental circulation, some of these substances (e.g., bradykinin) induce responses that are opposite or diverse from those observed in other vascular beds. Bradykinin is generally considered to relax vascular smooth muscle preparations, but in isolated, perfused human placental cotyledon, bradykinin induces concentration-dependent constriction.[78] In strips from umbilical cord arteries and veins, bradykinin produces only a monophasic constriction.[79,80] In the same experimental setup, serotonin and prostaglandin (PG)$F_{2\alpha}$ induce potent vasoconstriction. However, in in vitro perfused segments taken from intact umbilical cord arteries, these agents induce a biphasic response, starting with a small endothelial-dependent vasodilation followed by a dominant vasoconstriction.[81] In the same experimental setup, autacoid responsiveness varies depending on vessel segment; for example, angiotensin II induces a larger monophasic vasoconstriction in chorionic than umbilical cord arteries.[82,83]

The response to acetylcholine is also dependent on vessel segment and experimental design. Acetylcholine induces a modest monophasic vasoconstriction during experiments with umbilical cord arterial and venous strips,[80,84] whereas a relaxant response is observed in human villous stem arterial ring preparations,[85] and no change is seen in the perfusion pressure of isolated perfused human placental cotyledons.[78] Acetylcholine is additionally an example of autacoid interaction. The substance induces further constriction in umbilical arteries preconstricted with potassium chloride, serotonin, or PGE_2.[79,80,84] Thus the interaction between the different autacoids is complex. Circulating autacoids may also induce the production of other vascular substances (e.g., prostanoids and nitric oxide [NO]) in the vessel wall.[86]

The mechanisms involved in keeping these vessels dilated during pregnancy are unclear. Large amounts of prostanoids are produced in the vasculature of the human placenta[86] and in the umbilical cord vessels.[87] In vitro perfused umbilical cord vessel preparations showed lower production in veins than arteries.[88] These are primarily assumed to constitute local hormones, which exert their biologic activity at or close to the site of their production. The major prostanoid produced in these vessels is prostacyclin.[87] Prostacyclin is generally assumed to relax vascular smooth muscle and is mainly produced by the endothelial layer. However, infusion of prostacyclin into human umbilical arteries in vitro did not induce any significant changes in perfusion pressure, but it did reduce vasoconstriction induced by other vasoactive substances.[82,83]

NO is produced in the endothelial layer by the enzyme endothelial NO synthase (eNOS). NO is an essential vasodilating substance and is assumed to be the main vasodilator in the umbilicoplacental vessels.[89] NO is thought to be more significant than prostacyclin in maintenance of the low vascular resistance of the placenta.[90] Inhibition of the NO pathway increases the perfusion pressure of in vitro perfused human placentas,[91] and vascular smooth muscle preparations from human umbilical vessels relax following stimulation of NO synthesis.[92] In vitro studies of umbilical vessel preparations sampled after delivery is probably inadequate to give a comprehensive understanding of the mechanisms involved in the regulation of vascular smooth muscle tonus in the umbilicoplacental circulation. However, umbilical blood flow was reduced by inhibition of the NO pathway and increased by its stimulation in the in vivo chronically catheterized fetal sheep model, confirming the importance of NO in maintaining the low vascular tonus in the umbilicoplacental vessels.[93] The action of NO differs between arteries and veins,[92] and intrauterine growth restriction and preeclampsia are assumed to be associated with altered NO-induced relaxation of umbilical vessels.[94]

The final effects of different vasoactive substances on the umbilical circulation result from their systemic and local effects, as well as their interrelated and orchestrated effect with other substances. For example, adrenergic substances have a significant systemic effect on blood pressure and heart rate; whereas their effects on the vascular wall tension in the umbilical vessels are modest.[80] This contrasts with the dilating substances prostacyclin and NO, which have a short half-life and act locally where they are produced.[86,89]

The umbilical cord vessels constrict within a few minutes following delivery.[19,95] This is apparently an important response observed in different mammalian species to avoid exsanguination of the newborn. Mechanical traction on the cord, temperature changes, and changes in oxygen tension are thought to provoke this vasoconstriction. Most probably vasoactive substances are involved in this major response. However, human umbilical cord preparations used in in vitro experiments (such as the aforementioned studies on autacoid responsiveness) are necessarily sampled after birth, when the constriction is initiated. These preparations do not necessarily represent the in utero situation in which the umbilicoplacental vessels are believed to be nearly maximally dilated.

DISTRIBUTION OF UMBILICAL VENOUS RETURN

THE FETAL LIVER AND THE DUCTUS VENOSUS SHUNT

Oxygenated venous blood returning from the placenta enters the fetus to be distributed either to the liver or to the ductus venosus, which shunts the blood to the inferior vena cava as part of the via sinistra (see Fig. 53.1B). Animal experiments suggested that approximately 50% of the umbilical blood is shunted this way,[96-98] but ultrasound studies in humans have repeatedly shown that only 30% of the umbilical return enters the ductus venosus at 20 weeks and only 20% after 30 weeks (see Fig. 53.13).[26,31,99] Variation in reported measurements[100,101] is probably attributable to different measurement techniques, with the small diameter of the ductus venosus isthmus (0.5 to 2 mm) being the main challenge in controlling measurement errors.[102,103] Although the disparity between invasive experimental studies and the human results may be due to differences in techniques (e.g., microsphere distribution or implanted flow meters in the animal experiments versus ultrasound Doppler studies in humans), or to genuine variation between species, the most prominent reason may be that surgical trauma during preparation of animal experiments alters a very sensitive liver circulation. The fact that the liver is the first organ to receive rejuvenated umbilical blood and that the liver's share is 70% to 80% of the total umbilical flow underscores the developmental and physiologic importance of the fetal liver.

During experimental acute hypoxic challenges, the fraction of umbilical blood shunted through the ductus venosus increases substantially to prioritize blood flow to the heart and brain,[96,104] and a similar shift in shunting occurs during reduced umbilical flow.[104,105] During chronic placental compromise in humans, the ductus venosus volume flow is kept normal or near normal, but since umbilical flow is low in these fetuses,[23,25,27,106,107] the remaining fraction entering the liver is markedly reduced, thus the fraction shunted is relatively high (see Fig. 53.13).[100,108-110] In such cases, the blood from the spleen and bowel fed to the liver through the main portal vein constitutes a relatively larger venous source for the liver, although low on oxygen and nutritional content (Fig. 53.14).[29,99,110,111]

In diabetic mothers, the development of umbilical venous flow and its distribution between fetal liver and ductus venosus shunting are distorted; that is, the umbilical liver perfusion is prioritized at the expense of the ductus venosus shunting, leaving the fetus with less capacity to buffer acute hypoxic challenges in late pregnancy (Fig. 53.15).[112,113]

REGULATION OF UMBILICAL VENOUS DISTRIBUTION TO LIVER AND DUCTUS VENOSUS

The two competing circulatory sections, the liver parenchyma and the ductus venosus shunt, are very different both in terms of endocrine regulation and fluid dynamic properties: a huge hepatic vascular cross-section of portal venules and capillaries with a correspondingly low blood flow velocity versus a slim trumpet-like single vessel with a high blood velocity.

First, they are governed by "passive regulation" (i.e., fluid dynamic forces).[54,97,114] Blood pressure of the intra-abdominal umbilical vein, or rather the portocaval pressure gradient

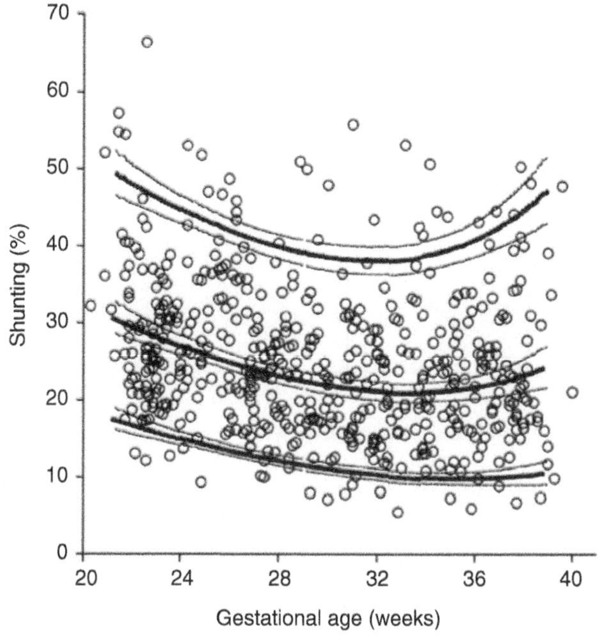

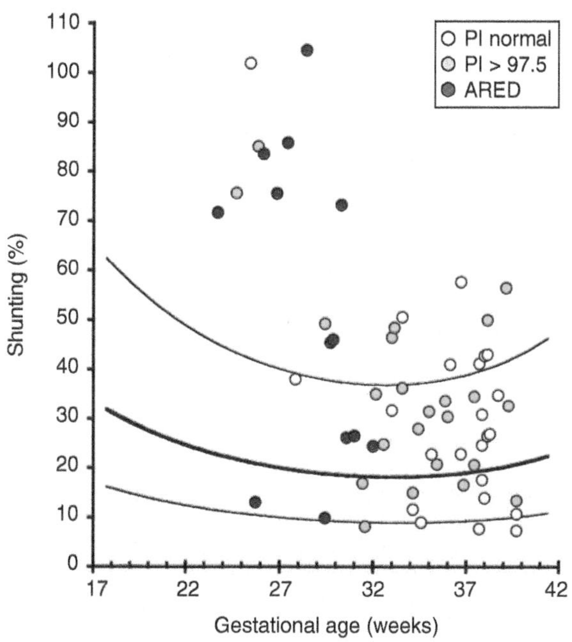

Fig. 53.13 *Upper panel:* Longitudinal study showing how the fraction of umbilical venous return shunted through the ductus venosus declines from one third to one fifth during normal pregnancy (5th, 50th, and 95th percentiles with 95% confidence intervals *[thin lines]*). *Lower panel:* In growth-restricted fetuses the fraction is increased particularly during the second trimester (10th, 50th, and 90th percentiles). *ARED,* Absent or reversed end-diastolic flow; *PI,* normal umbilical artery pulsatility index. (Reproduced from Kessler J, Rasmussen S, Godfrey KM, et al. Longitudinal study of umbilical and portal venous blood flow to the fetal liver: low pregnancy weight gain is associated with preferential supply to the fetal left liver lobe. *Pediatr Res.* 2008;63:315–320; and Kiserud T, Kessler J, Ebbing C, et al. Ductus venosus shunting in growth-restricted fetuses and the effect of umbilical circulatory compromise. *Ultrasound Obstet Gynecol.* 2006;28:143–149.)

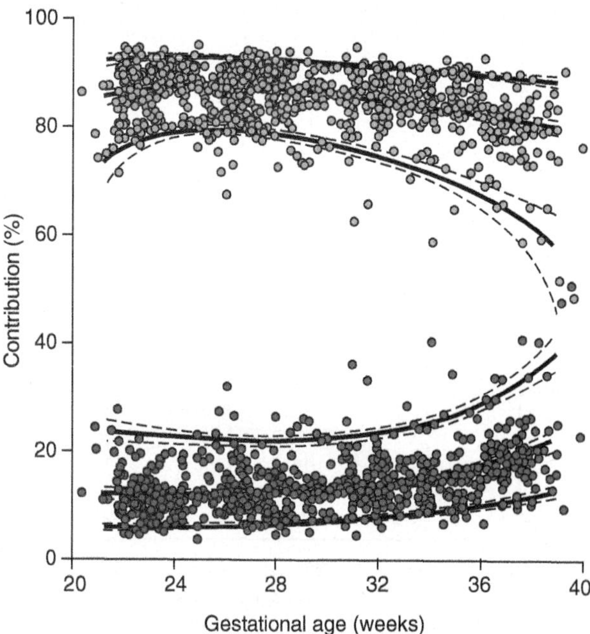

Fig. 53.14 Development of the umbilical *(gold circles)* and portal *(blue circles)* contribution to the venous perfusion of the fetal liver in the second half of pregnancy, presented with 5th, 50th, and 95th percentiles and 95% confidence intervals *(dashed lines).* Although small, the portal contribution increases from an average of 14% to 20% during this period. (Reproduced with permission from Kessler J, Rasmussen S, Godfrey KM, et al. Longitudinal study of umbilical and portal venous blood flow to the fetal liver: low pregnancy weight gain is associated with preferential supply to the fetal left liver lobe. *Pediatr Res.* 2008;63:315–320.)

($\Delta P_{UV\text{-}IVC}$), accelerates the blood in the ductus venosus to a velocity three times that of the umbilical vein. Thus, the oxygenated blood is ejected from the shunt with a higher kinetic energy than the surrounding bloodstreams and in the most favorable direction to press open the foramen ovale valve and reach the left atrium (see Fig. 53.1B).[59,115,116] In the ductus venosus, $\Delta P_{UV\text{-}IVC}$ (0.5 to 3.5 mm Hg) causes high systolic blood flow velocity of 60 to 90 cm/s—that is, kinetic energy—because little energy is consumed to overcome vascular resistance.

However, in the liver tissue, this energy is to a larger extent used to surmount vascular resistance where viscosity is decisive. At low velocities, blood turns non-Newtonian with a nonlinear relationship between velocity and resistance. Here a certain pressure has to build up before the blood even starts to move (the opening or closing pressure). The viscosity of blood is directly related to hematocrit, and a high hematocrit therefore requires an increased $\Delta P_{UV\text{-}IVC}$ to start the circulation and perfuse the liver tissue.[54] As can be seen from Fig. 53.16, these factors alone have a substantial influence on blood distribution between the liver and the ductus venosus shunt. A reduction in umbilical venous pressure or an increase in hematocrit shifts blood flow from the liver to the ductus venosus.

Second, active neuronal and endocrine regulation is also important.[117-121] Adrenergic nerve fibers have been identified at the ductus venosus in human fetuses at 20 to 24 weeks of gestation, and contractile responses to norepinephrine, acetylcholine, and 5-hydroxtryptamine have been demonstrated.[122,123] Later studies in fetal lambs confirmed α-adrenergic constriction and β-adrenergic relaxation, but responses to acetylcholine were inconsistent.[124] The ductus venosus dilates in response to NO and PGE_1.[124-126] During experimental work, the most efficient distension of the inlet of the ductus venosus is orchestrated by hypoxemia, which causes a 60% increase in its diameter.[126] This effect extends to the entire length of the ductus venosus,[126,127] making it a powerful mechanism for reducing resistance.

On the other hand, the venules of the portal system in the liver parenchyma are six times more sensitive to catecholamines (epinephrine and norepinephrine) than the ductus venosus, which is partly explained by the more distinctive presence of

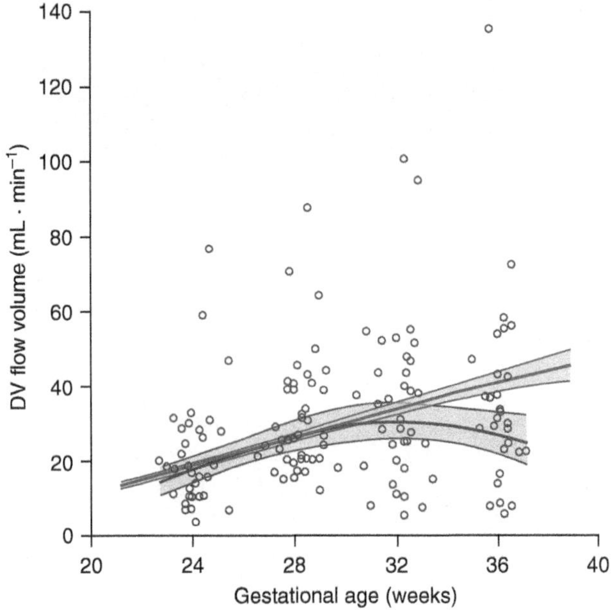

Fig. 53.15 Umbilical venous blood flow (mL/min) distributed to the fetal ductus venosus *(DV)* in 49 pregnancies with pregestational diabetes *(red)* shows a stunted development in the third trimester compared with reference population *(blue)*. In such pregnancies, umbilical liver perfusion is prioritized at the expense of the DV even when umbilical venous return is faltering. *Open circles*, individual observations; *solid lines*, mean and 95% confidence interval of the mean. (Reproduced with permission from Lund A, Ebbing C, Rasmussen S, Kiserud T, Kessler J. Maternal diabetes alters the development of ductus venosus shunting in the fetus. *Acta Obstet Gynecol Scand.* 2018;97:1032–1040.)

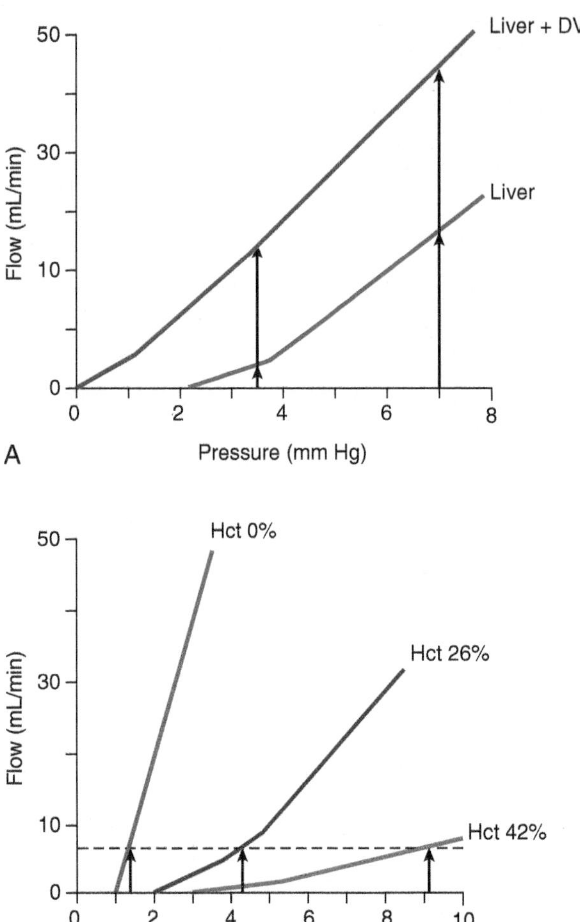

Fig. 53.16 Perfusion pressure (A) and viscosity (B) affect venous flow in the liver and ductus venosus *(DV)* differently in an in vitro fetal sheep preparation. At umbilical venous pressures of 2, 3.5, or 7 mm Hg, the proportion of shunting through the DV was 100%, 85%, and 50%, respectively. Perfusing the liver with saline solution or blood with *Hct* 26% or 42% demonstrates the profound effect of viscosity on opening (closing) pressure, being 1, 2, and 4 mm Hg, respectively. Achieve a flow of 7 mL/min required pressures of 1.4, 4.2, and 9 mm Hg, respectively. (Reproduced and modified with permission from Kiserud T, Stratford L, Hanson MA. Umbilical flow distribution to the liver and the ductus venosus: an in vitro investigation of the fluid dynamic mechanisms in the fetal sheep. *Am J Obstet Gynecol.* 1997;177:86–90.)

α-adrenergic receptors in the portal venules.[128] Such endocrine regulation augments the redistribution from the liver to the ductus venosus during stress. The magnitude of umbilical flow in the liver is also shown to induce fetal liver growth, suggesting mediation via sheer force and endothelial NO production in the portal vasculature.[129,130]

UMBILICAL BLOOD FLOW TO THE LIVER AND METABOLIC FUNCTION

It is well accepted that placental function is essential to fetal development and growth, but information is accumulating that the fetal liver is a key organ for translating transplacental information into differential growth and adaptive development.[129-132] By occluding or stenting the ductus venosus, Tchirikov, Schröder, and colleagues showed that increasing umbilical blood flow into the fetal lamb liver induced liver cell proliferation and increased production of insulin-like growth factor-1 and -2, resulting in fetal organ growth.[129] Applying this insight to human observations, it could be demonstrated that the fetal liver had an autoregulation in the sense that in slim mothers the fetal liver tended to take a larger share of the umbilical flow, an effect that was further augmented if the mother's diet was of poor quality.[131] These studies could also demonstrate that umbilical liver flow was a separate strong determinant for fetal fat accretion, across all maternal body compositions.[132,133] High umbilical flow to the fetal liver resulted in high fat content in the newborn and at 4 years of age. Development of fetal macrosomia in the absence of maternal hyperglycemia was associated with increased umbilical flow, particularly during the third trimester.[31] All parts of the liver received more umbilical blood and, thus, the right lobe had a lower fraction of splanchnic blood. A differential involvement of the fetal liver in metabolic adaptation was demonstrated when large fetuses responded with increased umbilical liver blood flow to a glucose tolerance test, while medium-sized or small fetuses did not.[134]

In growth-restricted fetuses, the liver has a lower priority and more umbilical blood bypasses the liver to reach the heart and brain directly. This causes a downregulation of liver size[135] and enzyme production[136] and reduces fat accretion, probably an important postnatal nutritional buffer. In addition, the right liver lobe is increasingly deprived of umbilical blood and relies more on low-oxygenated blood from the spleen and gut.[110] Thus, the fetal liver, with its umbilical perfusion, plays a key role in fetal development, metabolic responses, and adaptation.

UMBILICAL CIRCULATION AT BIRTH AND TIMING OF CORD CLAMPING

During the first minutes after delivery, there is a major reallocation of blood between the placenta and the newborn. Using ^{125}I-human-serum-albumin dilution technique the blood volume of the newborn increased from about 70 mL/kg birth weight following immediate cord clamping to more than 90 mL/kg birth weight if cord clamping was avoided for more than 3 minutes after birth.[95] Several randomized studies have examined the possible clinical benefits and disadvantages of late versus early umbilical cord clamping. A systematic review including 13 studies showed that late cord clamping increases birth weight, presumably reflecting larger placentofetal transfusion.[137] Newborn hemoglobin concentrations were increased 1 to 2 days after birth but not at later assessments. However, 3 to 6 months after birth, iron stores were significantly larger and the frequency of children with iron-deficiency anemia was reduced following late versus early cord clamping. Fewer neonates required phototherapy for jaundice in the early than in the late cord clamping group; the importance of this observation is disputed.[137] The included studies varied in their definition of early versus late cord clamping; overall, early clamping was performed less than 1 minute (mostly within 15 seconds) and late clamping more than 1 minute after birth. A Swedish study, using definitions of less than 10 seconds and more than 3 minutes to distinguish early versus late cord clamping, showed that infants in the late clamping group had higher birth weights (mean difference 96 g, 95% confidence interval [CI] 0.3 to 191 g) and hemoglobin levels at 2 days of age (mean difference 13.5 g/L, 95% CI 9.6 to 17.5).[138] At 4 months after birth, hemoglobin levels did not differ, but iron stores were 1.6 mg/kg (95% CI 0.9 to 2.3) greater in the late clamping group. The included studies varied in the use of uterotonic medication during the third stage of labor and in the level at which the newborn was placed relative to the placenta. In both intervention arms of the Swedish study, the newborn was placed 20 cm below the vulva for 30 seconds and then placed on the mother's abdomen.[138] Thus gravity plays a role in draining the blood from the placenta to the newborn infant. Additionally, the constriction of the umbilical cord vessels induced after birth is possibly important to avoid fetal exsanguination, and to squeeze blood from the larger vessels of the placenta and umbilical cord into the newborn.

Studies in preterm lambs demonstrated the importance of timing the clamping in relation to initiation of lung ventilation. Clamping of the low-resistance umbilical circulation leads to increased total systemic vascular resistance and thus an increase in blood pressure. Also, a reduction in venous return decreases cardiac output and reduces oxygen saturation. Beginning ventilation before cord clamping decreases pulmonary vascular resistance and increases pulmonary blood flow, the result being a smoother transition to neonatal circulation by avoiding the abrupt increase in impedance and blood pressure seen during early clamping.[139,140]

SUMMARY

The umbilical circulation receives 20% to 30% of the fetal combined cardiac output, loaded with a pulsatile energy that drives the blood through the placenta for rejuvenation and information exchange, and then brings it back to the fetus. At the receiver end, the fetal liver and the ductus venosus shunt determine the distribution between them. Under physiologic conditions it would be 75% versus 25%, respectively, but with wide variation according to gestational age and individual adaptation.

Classic passive fluid-dynamic regulation is important in the umbilical circuit with its long branchless vessels, large capillary bed of the placenta and the very differently acting receiving organs, the hepatic vasculature, and the slender ductus venosus. Intravascular pressure, vascular branching and cross-section, and viscosity are major determinants for how much blood can circulate through the placenta, and how it is distributed to the fetal liver and the ductus.

Active endocrine regulation is superimposed on this, using mechanisms similar to those acting elsewhere in the circulation but with a different response profile, keeping vessels rather extended and less sensitive to impulses than most other sections of circulation.

Although the distribution of umbilical venous return is prioritized into the low resistance of the liver vasculature, a reduced venous pressure, increased viscosity, and highly sensitive constriction in the portal venules constitute a powerful mechanism for redirecting blood to the ductus venosus, where the muscular layers are less sensitive to vasoconstrictive agents, making these redistribution mechanisms both an important response to challenges and a delicate adaptive mechanism.

The latter has gained interest as increasing observations suggest the liver is a key organ to sense available resources in the umbilical flow and translate this information into differential fetal organ growth, adapt to environmental conditions, and optimize the offspring's metabolic profile for postnatal life (or potentially to distort metabolic adaptation under the impact of perturbations such as maternal diabetes).

A complete reference list is available at www.ExpertConsult.com. 

SELECT REFERENCES

1. Barclay DM, Franklin KJ, Prichard MML. *The Foetal Circulation and Cardiovascular System, and the Changes that They Undergo at Birth*. Oxford: Blackwell Scientific Publications, Ltd.; 1944:275.
2. Barcroft J. *Researches on Pre-natal Life*. Vol 1. Oxford: Blackwell Scientific Publications; 1946:287.
4. Rudolph AM. Distribution and regulation of blood flow in the fetal and neonatal lamb. *Circ Res*. 1985;57:811-821.
7. Gordon Z, Eytan O, Jaffa AJ, et al. Hemodynamic analysis of Hyrtl anastomosis in human placenta. *Am J Physiol Regul Integr Comp Physiol*. 2007;292:R977-R982.
9. Skulstad SM, Rasmussen S, Iversen OE, et al. The development of high venous velocity at the fetal umbilical ring during gestational weeks 11-19. *Br J Obstet Gynaecol*. 2001;108:248-253.
11. Loberant N, Barak M, Gaitini D, et al. Closure of the ductus venosus in neonates: findings on real-time gray-scale, color-flow Doppler, and duplex Doppler sonography. *AJR Am J Roentgenol*. 1992;159:1083-1085.
12. Fugelseth D, Lindemann R, Liestol K, et al. Ultrasonographic study of ductus venosus in healthy neonates. *Arch Dis Child Fetal Neonatal Ed*. 1997;77:F131-F134.
13. Fugelseth D, Lindemann R, Liestol K, et al. Postnatal closure of ductus venosus in preterm infants or = 32 weeks. An ultrasonographic study. *Early Hum Dev*. 1998;53:163-169.
16. Ebbing C, Kessler J, Moster D, et al. Isolated single umbilical artery and the risk of adverse perinatal outcome and third stage of labor complications: a population-based study. *Acta Obstet Gynecol Scand*. 2020;99:374-380.
17. Ebbing C, Kiserud T, Johnsen SL, et al. Prevalence, risk factors and outcomes of velamentous and marginal cord insertions: a population-based study of 634,741 pregnancies. *PloS One*. 2013;8:e70380.
18. Brace RA. Blood volume and its measurement in the chronically catheterized sheep fetus. *Am J Physiol*. 1983;244:H487-H494.
19. Yao AC, Moinian M, Lind J. Distribution of blood between infant and placenta after birth. *Lancet*. 1969;2:871-873.
21. Gill RW. Pulsed Doppler with B-mode imaging for quantitative blood flow measurement. *Ultrasound Med Biol*. 1979;5:223-235.
23. Gill RW, Kossoff G, Warren PS, et al. Umbilical venous flow in normal and complicated pregnancies. *Ultrasound Med Biol*. 1984;10:349-363.
26. Kiserud T, Rasmussen S, Skulstad SM. Blood flow and degree of shunting through the ductus venosus in the human fetus. *Am J Obstet Gynecol*. 2000;182:147-153.
29. Kessler J, Rasmussen S, Godfrey K, et al. Longitudinal study of umbilical and portal venous blood flow to the fetal liver: low pregnancy weight gain is associated with preferential supply to the fetal left liver lobe. *Pediatr Res*. 2008;63:315-320.
30. Barbera A, Galan HL, Ferrazzi E, et al. Relationship of umbilical vein blood flow to growth parameters in the human fetus. *Am J Obstet Gynecol*. 1999;181:174-179.
32. Vimpeli T, Huhtala H, Wilsgaard T, et al. Fetal cardiac output and its distribution to the placenta at 11-20 weeks of gestation. *Ultrasound Obstet Gynecol*. 2009;33:265-271.
36. Kiserud T, Ebbing C, Kessler J, et al. Fetal cardiac output, distribution to the placenta and impact of placental compromise. *Ultrasound Obstet Gynecol*. 2006;28:126-136.
37. Castle B, Mackenzie IZ. *In vivo* observations on intravascular blood pressure in the fetus during mid-pregnancy. In: Rolfe P, ed. *Fetal Physiological Measurements*. London: Butterworths; 1986:65-69.

40. Struijk PC, Mathews VJ, Loupas T, et al. Blood pressure estimation in the human fetal descending aorta. *Ultrasound Obstet Gynecol*. 2008;32:673-681.
44. Thompson RS, Trudinger BJ. Doppler waveform pulsatility index and resistance, pressure and flow in the umbilical placental circulation: an investigation using a mathematical model. *Ultrasound Med Biol*. 1990;16:449-458.
45. Trudinger BJ, Stevens D, Connelly A, et al. Umbilical artery flow velocity waveforms and placental resistance: the effects of embolization of the umbilical circulation. *Am J Obstet Gynecol*. 1987;157:1443-1448.
47. Hanson M. The control of heart rate and blood pressure in the fetus: theoretical considerations. In: Hanson MA, Spencer JAD, Rodeck CH, eds. *The Circulation*. Cambridge: Cambridge University Press; 1993:438.
51. Parker KH, Jones CJH. Forward and backward running waves in the arteries: analysis using the method of characteristics. *ASME J Biomech Eng*. 1990;112:322-326.
54. Kiserud T, Stratford L, Hanson MA. Umbilical flow distribution to the liver and the ductus venosus: an *in vitro* investigation of the fluid dynamic mechanisms in the fetal sheep. *Am J Obstet Gynecol*. 1997;177:86-90.
56. Pergialiotis V, Kotrogianni P, Koutaki D, et al. Umbilical cord coiling index for the prediction of adverse pregnancy outcomes: a meta-analysis and sequential analysis. *J Matern Fetal Neonatal Med*. 2019:1-8.
57. Pennati G, Bellotti M, De Gasperi C, et al. Spatial velocity profile changes along the cord in normal human fetuses: can these affect Doppler measurements of venous umbilical blood flow? *Ultrasound Obstet Gynecol*. 2004;23: 131-137.
59. Kiserud T, Eik-Nes SH, Blaas HG, et al. Ultrasonographic velocimetry of the fetal ductus venosus. *Lancet*. 1991;338:1412-1414.
60. Huisman TWA, Stewart PA, Wladimiroff JW. Ductus venosus blood flow velocity waveforms in the human fetus - a Doppler study. *Ultrasound Med Biol*. 1992;18:33-37.
62. Hellevik LR, Kiserud T, Irgens F, et al. Simulation of pressure drop and energy dissipation for blood flow in a human fetal bifurcation. *ASME J Biomech Eng*. 1998;120:455-462.
67. Ville Y, Sideris I, Hecher K, et al. Umbilical venous pressure in normal, growth-retarded, and anemic fetuses. *Am J Obstet Gynecol*. 1994;170:487-494.
73. Schröder HJ, Tchirikov M, Rybakowski C. Pressure pulses and flow velocities in central veins of the anesthetized sheep fetus. *Am J Physiol Heart Circ Physiol*. 2003;284:H1205-H1211.
74. Hellevik LR, Stergiopulos N, Kiserud T, et al. A mathematical model of umbilical venous pulsation. *J Biomech*. 2000;33:1123-1130.
77. Reilly RD, Russell PT. Neurohistochemical evidence supporting an absence of adrenergic and cholinergic innervation in the human placenta and umbilical cord. *Anat Rec*. 1997;188:277-286.
80. Altura BM, Malaviya D, Reich CF, et al. Effects of vasoactive agents on isolated human umbilical arteries and veins. *Am J Physiol*. 1972;222:345-355.
81. Haugen G, Hovig T. Studies of autacoid responsiveness and endothelium dependency in human umbilical arteries. *Scand J Clin Lab Invest*. 1992;52: 141-149.
84. Chen N, Lv J, Bo L, et al. Muscarinic-mediated vasoconstriction in human, rat and sheep umbilical cords and related vasoconstriction mechanisms. *Br J Obstet Gynaecol*. 2015;122:1630-1639.
88. Bjøro K, Hovig T, Stokke KT, et al. Formation of prostanoids in human umbilical vessels perfused *in vitro*. *Prostaglandins*. 1986;31:683-698.
89. Krause BJ, Hanson MA, Casanello P. Role of nitric oxide in placental vascular development and function. *Placenta*. 2011;32:797-805.
90. Chaudhuri G, Cuevas J, Buga GM, et al. NO is more important than PGI_2 in maintaining low vascular tone in feto-placental vessels. *Am J Physiol*. 1993;265:H2036-H2043.
109. Kiserud T, Kessler J, Ebbing C, et al. Ductus venosus shunting in growth-restricted fetuses and the effect of umbilical circulatory compromise. *Ultrasound Obstet Gynecol*. 2006;28:143-149.
112. Lund A, Ebbing C, Rasmussen S, et al. Maternal diabetes alters the development of ductus venosus shunting in the fetus. *Acta Obstet Gynecol Scand*. 2018;97:1032-1040.
126. Kiserud T, Ozaki T, Nishina H, et al. Effect of NO, phenylephrine, and hypoxemia on ductus venosus diameter in fetal sheep. *Am J Physiol Heart Circ Physiol*. 2000;279:H1166-H1171.
128. Tchirikov M, Kertschanska S, Schroder HJ. Differential effects of catecholamines on vascular rings from ductus venosus and intrahepatic veins of fetal sheep. *J Physiol*. 2003;548:519-526.
130. Tchirikov M, Kertschanska S, Schroder HJ. Obstruction of ductus venosus stimulates cell proliferation in organs of fetal sheep. *Placenta*. 2001;22: 24-31.
132. Godfrey KM, Haugen G, Kiserud T, et al. Fetal liver blood flow distribution: role in human developmental strategy to prioritize fat deposition versus brain development. *PloS One*. 2012;7:e41759.
133. Ikenoue S, Waffarn F, Ohashi M, et al. Prospective association of fetal liver blood flow at 30 weeks gestation with newborn adiposity. *Am J Obstet Gynecol*. 2017;217:204.e201-204.e208.
139. Bhatt S, Alison BJ, Wallace EM, et al. Delaying cord clamping until ventilation onset improves cardiovascular function at birth in preterm lambs. *J Physiol*. 2013;591:2113-2126.
140. Polglase GR, Dawson JA, Kluckow M, et al. Ventilation onset prior to umbilical cord clamping (physiological-based cord clamping) improves systemic and cerebral oxygenation in preterm lambs. *PloS One*. 2015;10:e0117504.

54 Fetal and Placental Circulation During Labor

Karel Maršál

PHYSIOLOGIC BACKGROUND

A sufficient maternal blood supply to the placenta is of utmost importance to the fetus during pregnancy and labor. It has long been recognized that uterine contractions diminish uteroplacental blood flow. Contractions of myometrium compress the vessels traversing the uterine wall and increase intrauterine pressure, thus influencing the intervillous space pressure as well. The intrauterine pressure during labor usually ranges from 25 to 100 mm Hg. In contrast, the mean pressure in small arteries is 70 to 95 mm Hg and only 15 mm Hg at the venous end of the capillaries. Compression and even collapse of the myometrial vessels during labor are thus probable. Even a slight reduction in the diameter of an artery results in reduction of flow because resistance to flow is inversely proportional to the fourth power of the vessel radius, according to Poiseuille's law. Obviously, during a contraction the uterine veins are affected first, and the restricted venous outflow results in a reduction of the pressure gradient over the placenta. With use of the radioangiographic technique in pregnant women, it has been shown that the maternal blood flow to the placenta decreases markedly during contractions.[1] Similarly, in the rhesus monkey, diminished arteriolar jets have also been demonstrated.[2] However, flow to the intervillous space appears to remain constant.

The intermittent decrement in the blood flow during myometrial contractions has been found to be inversely related to the increase in intrauterine pressure.[3-6] During uterine relaxation after a contraction, an increase in blood flow—a reactive hyperemia—has been observed,[4,6] which compensates for the decreased oxygen delivery during the preceding contraction.

With the progress of labor, the peak intrauterine pressure during each contraction increases, and the time-averaged blood flow in the uterine artery diminishes (Fig. 54.1).[7] Woodbury and colleagues[8] described a "maternal effective placental arterial pressure," defined as the arterial pressure minus the pressure within the uterus (which opposes the inflow of maternal blood).

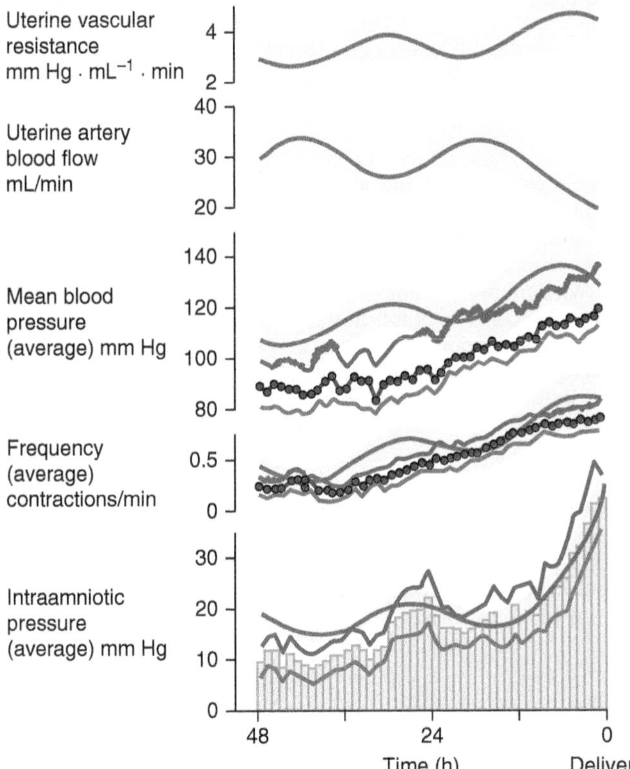

Fig. 54.1 Composite drawing showing the incorporation of the circadian changes of uterine dynamics into the process of labor and delivery. The *bars* depicting intraamniotic pressure and the *circles* depicting the frequency of contractions and mean blood pressure represent data obtained from five patients monitored continuously during the last 48 hours of pregnancy. Each *bar* and *circle* represents the mean of hourly average values. The *thin lines* delineate the 95% confidence intervals. The *thick lines* for intra-amniotic pressure, frequency of contraction, mean blood pressure, uterine artery blood flow, and uterine vascular resistance were calculated from continuous recordings made in 15 monkeys during the 48 hours terminating in spontaneous labor and delivery. The *shaded areas* represent the 95% confidence intervals determined for individual mean values. Uterine vascular resistance was calculated by the following formula: aortic blood pressure minus intraamniotic pressure divided by uterine artery blood flow. (From Harbert GM Jr. Circadian changes in uteroplacental blood flow. In: Rosenfeld CR, editor. *The Uterine Circulation. Reproductive and Perinatal Medicine.* Vol. X. Ithaca, NY: Perinatology Press; 1989:157.)

To ensure perfusion of the placenta, the maternal central blood circulation responds to contractions by increasing both blood pressure and cardiac output.[9,10]

The circulation of a healthy fetus in uncomplicated labor usually remains unaffected. The umbilical circulation is relatively unreactive and does not seem to respond to the changes in intrauterine pressure or to the short-term changes in the maternal placental blood flow during contractions. During normal labor, uterine contractions are not of sufficient magnitude to negatively affect gas exchange over the placenta, and therefore they do not endanger the fetus. In labor with a pathologic course, in which uteroplacental blood flow is diminished, fetal hypoxemia can develop. In that situation, the fetus reacts with changes in heart rate, blood pressure, and blood flow.[11] Uterine contractions can also cause a direct compression of the umbilical cord, with restriction of the umbilical blood flow, leading to changes in the fetal circulation.

METHODS OF RECORDING HUMAN FETAL AND UTEROPLACENTAL BLOOD FLOW

Previously, most of our knowledge of uteroplacental and fetal circulation was based on animal experiments, in which invasive methods were used. Approximately 40 years ago, a noninvasive method making use of Doppler ultrasonography was introduced in the field of perinatal medicine and has made it possible to obtain data on blood flow in human pregnancies.[12,13]

FLOW PROBE TECHNIQUES

Measurement of the uterine, uteroplacental, or fetal blood flow with a flow probe technique (measuring the flow in a single vessel by evaluating changes caused by the blood flow in either the electromagnetic field or the ultrasound passage time) requires an application of the probe on an exposed vessel. Only in exceptional circumstances has the electromagnetic method been used on a human uterine artery during laparotomy for hysterectomy in pregnancy.[14]

RADIOANGIOGRAPHY

The radioangiographic technique, with injection of contrast medium followed by serial x-ray exposures, has made it possible to establish the time of appearance and disappearance of contrast dye in various parts of the uteroplacental circulation.[1] However, absolute flow cannot be determined, and because of the high radiation hazard to the fetus, this method is not acceptable for use in humans.

PLACENTAL SCINTIGRAPHY

Radioactive isotopes (^{24}Na, ^{133}Xe) can be injected into either the myometrium or the intervillous space, and the rate of washout can then be determined by external measurement. This gives a semiquantitative measure of the maternal placental blood flow. To circumvent the disadvantage of the method's invasiveness, placental scintigraphy has been developed. This uses an intravenous injection of a radionuclide tracer (^{99m}Tc, ^{133}Xe, or ^{113m}In) and external measurement of accumulation or disappearance of radioactivity over the placenta.[15] Clinical application of this method is limited because it cannot be used for continuous measurement of the changes in placental blood flow over time, and only the anterior placenta can be examined. The most serious drawback of the method is exposure of the fetus to ionizing radiation.

THERMISTOR METHOD

One can evaluate the relative uterine blood flow by placing a preheated thermistor pearl into cervical tissue and then recording heat dispersal.[16] This method has the disadvantages of being invasive and of measuring flow in the cervix and lower segment of the uterus and not directly in the placenta.

LASER DOPPLER TECHNIQUE

Variability of fetal scalp blood flow during labor was measured using the continuous transcutaneous laser Doppler technique.[17] An overall reduction in the scalp blood flow during labor and a clear association with uterine contractions were found. Because of poor reproducibility, the method did not find any clinical application.

DOPPLER ULTRASOUND METHOD

PHYSICAL PRINCIPLE

The Doppler ultrasound method makes it possible to estimate blood velocity and blood flow in maternal and fetal vessels in a noninvasive way during pregnancy and labor. The first report on the detection of flow signals from the umbilical artery was in 1977 by FitzGerald and Drumm.[12] Doppler velocimetry has since

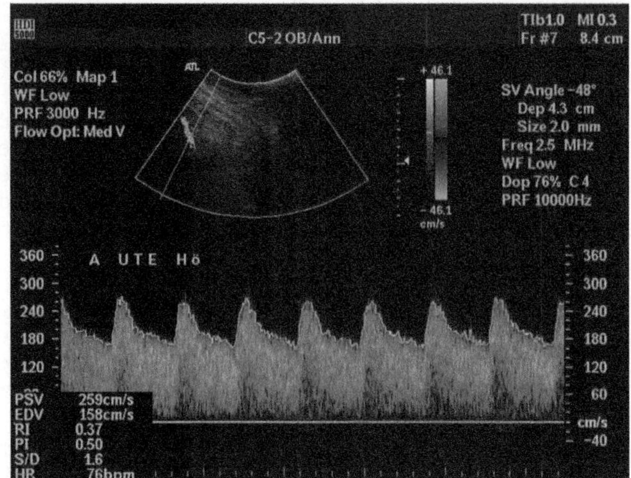

Fig. 54.2 Doppler shift spectrum recorded from the uterine artery in a term pregnancy. The high proportion of diastolic flow velocity indicates a very low resistance to flow in the uteroplacental circulation.

become a method of choice for evaluation of the uteroplacental and fetal circulation.

According to the Doppler principle, wave energy is reflected by a moving reflector with a wavelength (frequency) that is different from the emitted wavelength. The change in frequency (Doppler shift) is proportional to the velocity of the reflector. In the situation of blood flow measurement, ultrasound with a frequency of 1 to 10 MHz is transmitted to the tissue and reflected by the moving red cells within the vessel. The frequency of the received ultrasound is higher than the emitted frequency when the blood is moving towards the transducer, and it is lower when the blood is moving away from the transducer. The Doppler shift (f_d) is defined by the formula

$$f_d = 2 \cdot f_0 \cdot V \cdot \cos\theta / c \qquad [54.1]$$

where f_0 is the ultrasound frequency, V is the blood velocity, θ is the angle between the ultrasound beam and the bloodstream direction, and c is the velocity of ultrasound in tissue. The Doppler shift frequencies are within the range of audible sound. They can be analyzed, for example, by the fast Fourier transform and displayed as a Doppler shift spectrum (Fig. 54.2). From the spectrum, the mean and the maximum velocity can be estimated and further processed.

Doppler ultrasonography can be used in one of four modes: continuous-wave (CW) Doppler ultrasonography, pulsed-wave (PW) Doppler ultrasonography, color flow imaging, or power Doppler imaging. In the first mode, CW ultrasound is continuously transmitted by one piezoelectric crystal, and the reflected ultrasound is received by another crystal. Signals of blood flow are obtained from all vessels traversed by the ultrasound beam. The application of CW Doppler ultrasonography is limited because of the lack of range resolution.

In the PW mode, one single piezoelectric crystal is used for transmission and reception of the ultrasound bursts. By changing the time delay between the transmission and reception of signals, one can determine the range within the tissue from which the Doppler-shifted signals are received. In other words, it is possible to choose a specific vessel for recording blood velocity signals. PW ultrasonography is usually combined with imaging ultrasonography (linear array or sector real-time scanner) to locate and identify the vessel of interest.

The color flow imaging mode makes possible a color-coding of the received Doppler signals, usually red for the blood flow towards the transducer and blue for the flow in the opposite direction. The color signals are then superimposed on the two-dimensional real-time image. Color flow imaging facilitates detection of flow even in very small vessels (e.g., fetal cerebral vessels or maternal spiral arteries). It is often combined with PW Doppler ultrasonography for quantification of flow velocity (spectral Doppler imaging).

The amplitude of the received Doppler shift signals can be used to characterize the signal power, which is proportional to the number of blood cells moving within the investigated area, thus reflecting the perfusion of the organs examined. The power Doppler signals can also be color coded and displayed in the two-dimensional image. The power Doppler imaging mode allows detection of blood flow with low velocity; however, the information is nondirectional. In obstetric applications, this mode has been used for evaluation of perfusion of fetal organs (e.g., lungs[18]) or placenta.[19] The power Doppler signals can also be collected from a tissue volume and presented in three dimensions.

VOLUME FLOW ESTIMATION

The information on the time-averaged mean velocity (*V*) obtained from a specific vessel and corrected for cosθ can be used for calculation of the volume flow (*Q*) in milliliters per minute according to the formula

$$Q = V \cdot d^2 \cdot \pi / 4 \cos\theta \qquad [54.2]$$

This assumes that the diameter of the vessel (*d*) is known for the calculation of the cross-sectional area of the vessel. Originally, the method was applied for estimations of volume flow in large fetal vessels (i.e., abdominal aorta and umbilical vein).[13]

The measurement of vessel diameter using the two-dimensional ultrasound image is relatively inaccurate. The estimation of the volume blood flow also requires knowledge of the insonation angle and uniform insonation of the vessel for reliable estimation of the mean velocity. Because of all these possible sources of error, this method has not found wide application.[20] Nevertheless, it can be expected that further technical development will enable a more reliable estimation of flow. A certain revival of this method has occurred, and measurements of flow also in vessels of small caliber (e.g., maternal uterine arteries and umbilical arteries) have been reported.[21,22] Nevertheless, the reported variability in the resulting values was of similar magnitude as in the original reports 40 years ago and is, obviously, a combination of the physiologic variability and method errors.

VELOCITY WAVEFORM ANALYSIS

The maximum blood velocity (i.e., the envelope of the Doppler spectrum) recorded from an artery can be analyzed for its waveform and characterized by various indices (Fig. 54.3). These indices are angle independent. The diameter of the vessel needs not be known for waveform analysis, and the maximum velocity is easier to record than is the mean velocity. Thus many errors involved in the estimation of blood flow are eliminated. However, this method does not directly reflect flow, and the interpretation of results is not always obvious.

The diastolic part of the flow velocity waveform is mainly influenced by the peripheral vascular resistance; an increase in the resistance lowers the diastolic velocity and, consequently, increases the values of the waveform indices described in Fig. 54.3. However, cardiac performance, blood pressure, vessel wall properties, and viscosity of blood also influence the waveform and its indices.

A simple semiquantitative evaluation of the waveform recorded from the umbilical artery or fetal descending aorta with regard to the presence or lack of the end-diastolic flow (blood flow classes) has proven useful in the identification of fetuses with growth restriction and fetuses at risk of intrauterine asphyxia[23] (Fig. 54.4). In the cerebral vessels of hypoxic fetuses, an increase in diastolic velocity can be observed as an expression of decreased resistance in the cerebral vascular bed and redistribution of blood flow (brain-sparing phenomenon).

The resistance to flow in the uterine artery is reflected in the pulsatility index (PI) of the uterine artery waveform. With increasing resistance (e.g., in cases with intrauterine growth restriction and/or preeclampsia), the PI increases and a notch in the early diastole can occur. A bilateral notch in the uterine artery persisting after 26 weeks gestation has been shown to be associated with increased risk of development of preeclampsia and intrauterine growth restriction. For clinical use, a mean value of PI measured in the left and right uterine artery[24] or a scoring system (uterine artery score) can be used to characterize the resistance in both uterine arteries.[25]

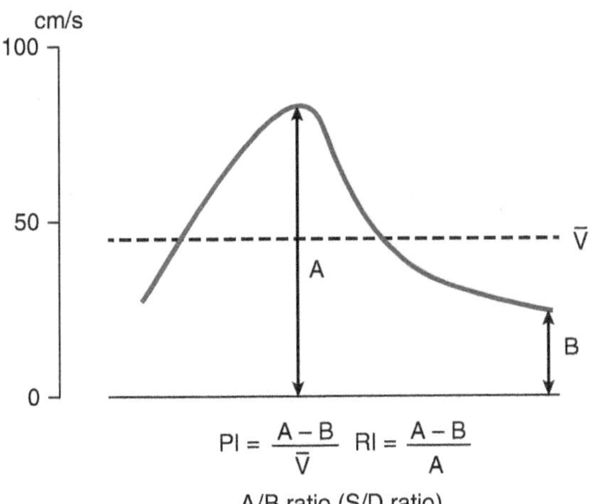

Fig. 54.3 Waveform analysis of the fetal arterial maximum blood velocity. *A/B* ratio according to Stuart and colleagues.[117] *A (S),* Peak maximum velocity; *B (D),* minimum diastolic velocity; *PI,* pulsatility index according to Gosling and King[118]; *RI,* resistance index according to Pourcelot[119]; $\bar{V}$, mean velocity over the cardiac cycle.

SAFETY ASPECTS OF USING DOPPLER ULTRASONOGRAPHY IN PREGNANCIES

Ultrasound with high intensity levels has known biologic effects (e.g., thermal effects and cavitation). Therefore it is necessary that users be constantly alert to the possibility of adverse effects of diagnostic ultrasound.[26] Hitherto, no harmful effects of ultrasound on human tissues have been found at the intensities used for diagnostic purposes, and epidemiologic follow-up studies have failed to elicit any evidence of adverse effects of exposure to diagnostic ultrasound in utero. Nevertheless, it is important that users of Doppler ultrasonography be aware of the output ultrasound energy of the equipment they are using for examining pregnancies. Some of the Doppler devices can produce output energy exceeding the upper limit for energy output to be used in pregnancy (720 mW/cm^2); it is the responsibility of the ultrasound operator to control the output on the basis of the output displays in the form of the mechanical index and thermal index.[27] The operator should always follow the ALARA principle (i.e., to use ultrasound energy "as low as reasonably achievable").

HUMAN UTEROPLACENTAL BLOOD FLOW DURING LABOR

PW Doppler ultrasonography has been used for recording flow velocity signals from the uteroplacental vessels in labor.[28,29] CW Doppler ultrasonography was also used for this purpose.[30,31] All Doppler studies on uteroplacental vessels in labor have shown that, during uterine contractions, both the systolic and the

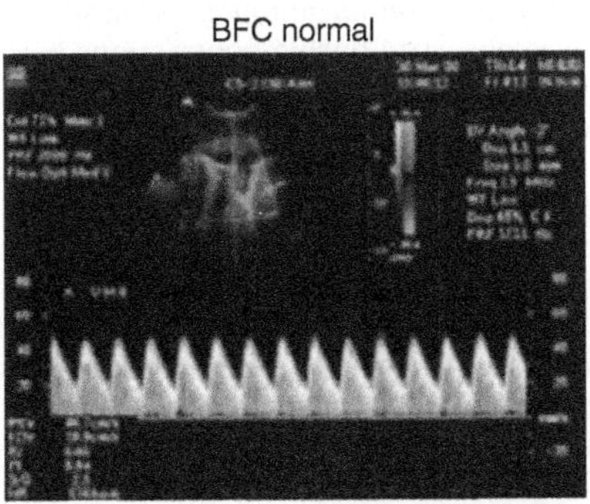

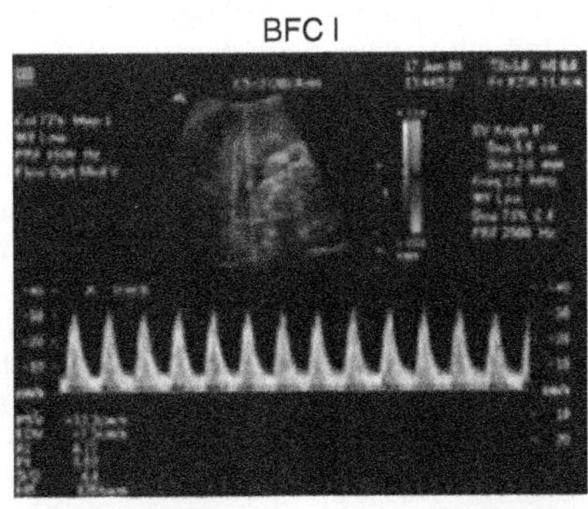

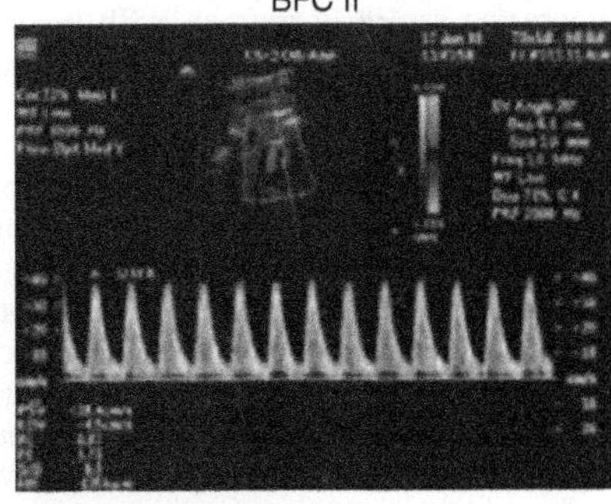

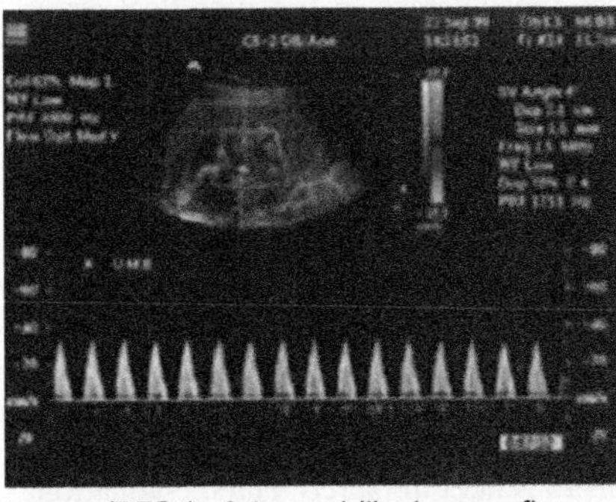

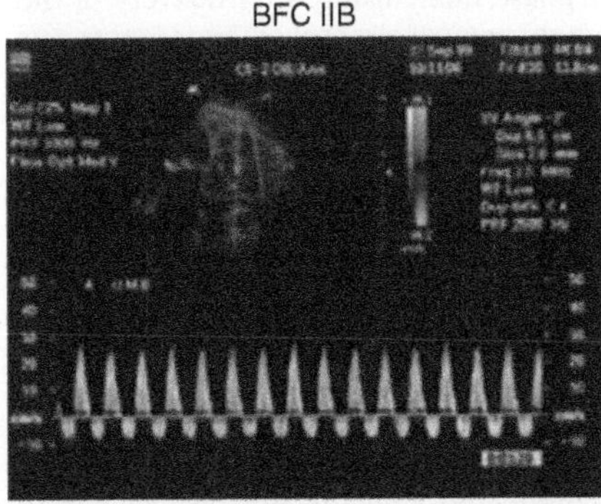

Fig. 54.4 Blood flow classes *(BFCs)* of the umbilical artery flow velocity waveforms. *BFC normal,* Positive diastolic flow, pulsatility index (PI) within normal limits; *BFC I,* positive diastolic flow, PI > mean + 2 standard deviations (SD) and ≤ mean + 3 SD of the reference curve; *BFC II,* positive diastolic flow, PI > mean + 3 SD of the reference curve; *BFC IIIA,* absent end-diastolic flow velocity; *BFC IIIB,* reverse end-diastolic velocity.

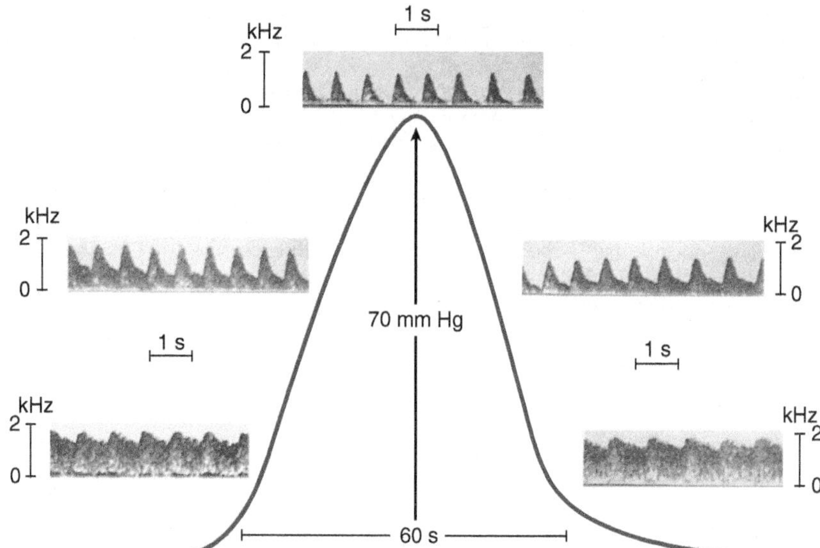

Fig. 54.5 Changes of the Doppler velocity waveforms recorded from the uterine artery before, during, and after uterine contraction. (From Fendel H, Fettweis P, Billet P, et al. Doppleruntersuchungen des arteriellen utero-feto-plazentaren Blutflusses vor und während der Geburt. *Z Geburtshilfe Perinatol* 1987;191:121–129.)

diastolic blood velocities diminish, suggesting a decrease in blood flow. At the acme of contraction, the diastolic velocities disappear completely. An inverse linear relationship has been found between the intensity of the contraction, measured as the intrauterine amniotic pressure, and the degree of the end-diastolic flow. When intraamniotic pressure exceeds 60 mm Hg, an elimination of end-diastolic flow velocity occurs in all cases (Fig. 54.5).[32]

A similar pattern of blood velocity changes as in spontaneous labor contractions was described for contractions induced by an oxytocin challenge test (OCT).[33] At the time of the acme of induced contractions, the diastolic flow velocities in the uterine artery diminished, were undetectable, or were even reversed. The reversal was significantly more often seen during induced contractions than during spontaneous contractions in a control group.[33]

The PI measured between contractions both in the left and right uterine artery in women with uncomplicated labor, was found to be lower in the second stage than in the first stage of labor, indicating a compensatory increase of placenta perfusion during uterus relaxation.[34]

During the third stage of labor, PW Doppler studies of uterine arteries showed that after a latent phase, during the contraction and detachment phase, a significant increase occurred in the resistance to flow, reflected by an increase in PI.[35] After placental separation, a slight uterine relaxation occurred, resulting in decreased resistance to flow in the uterine arteries. By use of color flow imaging, the changes of blood flow between myometrium and placenta can be followed.[36] In cases with normal placental separation, blood flow between myometrium and placenta ceases during the latent phase immediately after delivery of the neonate. In patients in whom manual removal of the placenta was necessary, the blood flow continued into the placenta beyond the latent phase. Thus color Doppler examination might be used to diagnose placenta accreta.

HUMAN FETAL BLOOD FLOW DURING LABOR

UMBILICAL ARTERY BLOOD FLOW

According to several reports, the waveform indices (see Fig. 54.3) of flow velocities recorded from the umbilical artery of healthy fetuses in uncomplicated labor do not change during contractions or with the progression of labor.[30,32,37,38] This suggests that normal uterine activity in labor does not increase the vascular resistance on the fetal side of the placenta, which helps the fetus to withstand the stress of labor. Fleischer and colleagues[39] found that the umbilical artery waveform did not change over a wide range of uterine pressures in labor. Conversely, Malcus and colleagues[40] examined 575 fetuses in early labor and found a significant increase in the PI during contraction, as compared with the recording taken before the onset of contraction. Nevertheless, the absolute difference in the PI was small and probably without importance for an undisturbed fetus. However, in fetuses with already compromised umbilical blood flow, such a slight increase in placental resistance might be of pathophysiologic and clinical importance. This is in agreement with the observation that fetuses that exhibit a lack of end-diastolic velocity during pregnancy often have signs of distress in labor and frequently require operative delivery.[23,41] In a study that recorded umbilical artery waveform changes continuously through different stages of labor, a significant increase in systolic-to-diastolic (S/D) ratio was observed during contractions in the second stage of labor.[42] The increase in S/D ratio correlated well with a decrease in umbilical artery pH. No significant changes in the umbilical artery velocity waveform were observed during the first stage of labor. In a more recent study,[34] an increase in the PI was found from the first to the second stage of normal labor.

During Braxton Hicks contractions the PI in the umbilical artery did not change, thus indicating that Braxton Hicks contractions have no effect on fetal hemodynamics and on fetal oxygenation in the healthy near-term fetus.[43]

In pregnant women with decelerations in the fetal heart rate (FHR) during contractions in labor, a concomitant increase in the PI,[37] or S/D ratio,[44] has been found. One study found that the increase in the umbilical artery resistance index (RI) was particularly pronounced at downward and bottom stages of variable decelerations.[45] During early decelerations or during contractions not associated with FHR decelerations, no changes were found in the resistance to flow. Tadmor and colleagues,[46] using computerized analysis of umbilical artery velocity waveforms, recorded an increase in S/D ratio and PI in approximately 50% of FHR variable decelerations. They showed that in one group of pregnancies the increase in the resistance to flow preceded the decrease in FHR. In other cases the deceleration was not preceded by a measurable increase in umbilical artery resistance. Tadmor and colleagues considered this to reflect impaired fetal oxygenation.

Operative delivery is significantly more frequent in patients with abnormal PI values. Brar and colleagues[47] compared the S/D ratio in a group of patients with late decelerations with the S/D ratio in matched controls. The mean S/D ratio in the former group was significantly higher than that in the latter group. Among women with late decelerations, a progressive increase was also seen in the incidence of adverse pregnancy outcome with increasing abnormality in the waveform. Patients with late decelerations and a normal umbilical S/D ratio had an incidence of adverse pregnancy outcome similar to that of controls. Feinkind and colleagues[48] performed a similar analysis of the relationships among FHR tracings and umbilical artery velocity waveforms during the first stage of labor and outcome of pregnancy in 273 unselected patients. Both the umbilical *A/B* ratio and the FHR had similar low positive predictive values (30% and 23%, respectively). When the two methods were combined, the predictive value increased to 56%. Somerset and colleagues[49] found the positive predictive values for prediction of cesarean delivery for fetal distress to be 31% for the umbilical artery S/D ratio and 15% for admission FHR recording. The positive predictive value of the umbilical artery PI in early labor was also examined by Malcus and colleagues[40] and was found to be 19% for fetal distress and 15% for intrauterine growth restriction. Similar results were subsequently reported by others.[50,51]

The rupture of membranes, or amniotomy, does not seem to have any influence on the umbilical velocity waveform.[38-40,52]

Li and colleagues[53] examined umbilical artery flow velocities during an OCT performed in a group of high-risk pregnancies. In cases of a positive OCT result, according to Freeman[54] the umbilical artery PI increased significantly both during and between contractions induced by oxytocin.[53]

Umbilical artery Doppler velocimetry has been shown to be a clinically useful test when applied for antenatal monitoring of fetal health in high-risk pregnancies.[55] However, clinical studies on umbilical artery velocimetry in labor reviewed by Farrell and colleagues[56] do not seem to provide similarly convincing results. Therefore this method has not found widespread clinical application in laboring patients.

FETAL AORTIC BLOOD FLOW

The fetal aortic blood flow, estimated on two occasions during the first stage of uncomplicated labor, increases with progression of labor.[57] These measurements were performed between contractions, and the finding of increased fetal flow might be a phenomenon similar to reactive hyperemia in the uteroplacental circulation described both in animal[9] and human[34] pregnancies. Lindblad and colleagues[57] found no change in the aortic PI with advancing labor, and no difference between patients with and patients without ruptured membranes. Fendel and colleagues[32] measured the mean fetal aortic velocity in labor and found a drop in the velocity during contractions. The aortic PI and RI remained unchanged.

FETAL CEREBRAL BLOOD FLOW

The flow velocity in cerebral arteries of fetuses during uncomplicated labor has been examined by use of the transcervical access without imaging with either CW[58] or PW[59] Doppler ultrasonography. Dougall and colleagues[58] did not find any change in the mean velocity or the RI of the anterior cerebral artery with advancing labor. During contractions, a fall occurred in the diastolic velocities, suggesting an increase in cerebral vascular resistance caused by head compression during contractions (assuming that the fetal cardiac output and blood pressure remain unchanged). The mean RI was between 0.69 between contractions and 0.81 during contractions ($P < .001$). However, this finding was not confirmed by Maesel and colleagues[59] in the fetal middle cerebral artery.

More recently, several research groups have examined the fetal cerebral circulation in labor using a combined two-dimensional real-time and PW Doppler ultrasonography. The waveforms of velocities recorded from the fetal internal carotid artery and middle cerebral artery were similar to those recorded before labor.[60,61] Furthermore, no significant difference was found in PI values of velocities recorded between and during uterine contractions.[61] In the late first and second stages of labor, lower PI values were found in the middle cerebral artery, suggesting a decrease in impedance to flow in fetal cerebral circulation with progress of labor.[62,63] Fetal cerebral oxygenation decreases in the second stage of labor,[64] which might lead to vasodilation of the cerebral vascular bed. This has been confirmed by Sütterlin and colleagues,[65] who measured fetal oxygen saturation simultaneously with Doppler waveforms of the fetal middle cerebral artery. They showed that in fetuses with abnormal heart rate patterns and oxygen saturation less than 30%, the PI and RI of the middle cerebral artery were significantly lower than in control fetuses. More recently, these findings were confirmed.[66]

During uterine contractions in late labor, transient increases in the PI were observed in the fetal internal carotid artery[67] and middle cerebral artery[68] as an expression of higher intrauterine pressure, compared with that in early labor. Braxton Hicks contractions did not change the resistance to flow in the fetal internal carotid artery.[43]

During the OCT of fetuses suspected of having intrauterine growth restriction, the PI of fetal middle cerebral and anterior cerebral arteries decreased significantly if the PI was primarily within normal limits.[69] No difference was seen between the two vessels in the PI response. No PI decrease occurred in cases where the PI was below the normal lower limit (i.e., if signs of so-called brain sparing were already seen before the OCT).

During the past decade, there was an increased interest in cerebroplacental ratio (CPR; i.e., the ratio between the fetal middle cerebral artery PI and umbilical artery PI), designed originally to enhance the detection of redistribution of fetal blood flow with preferential supply of fetal brain.[70] Dall'Asta and colleagues[71] measured the CPR in 562 low-risk pregnant women in early labor and found that fetal distress in labor was more than 3 times higher in women with low CPR. However, the positive predictive value of the CPR was low both for the intervention for imminent fetal asphyxia and for adverse neonatal outcome. Two studies investigated the potential of CPR to predict adverse perinatal outcome in women subsequently undergoing induction of labor.[72,73] In 1902 pregnancies with various indications for induction and in 210 pregnancies with small-for-gestational-age fetuses, respectively, the two studies found a significant association with the risk of emergency cesarean section and adverse neonatal outcome. However, Fiolna and colleagues[72] concluded that the CPR showed a poor predictive power to be used for screening before intended induction of labor.

FETAL VENOUS BLOOD FLOW

Murakami and colleagues[74] showed that the blood flow in the intraabdominal part of the umbilical vein decreased in association with late and variable FHR decelerations. The reduction of blood flow was more pronounced with variable decelerations than with late decelerations, and the blood flow change preceded the deceleration. The pattern of umbilical venous flow velocities during labor was evaluated by Ghosh and colleagues.[75] They found the occurrence of pulsatile flow to be predictive of fetal hypoxia and operative delivery for fetal distress.

Fetal ductus venosus blood flow velocity waveforms during the first stage of labor have been described by Krapp and colleagues.[76] In a group of normal term fetuses, they found that between contractions the mean values of the PI for veins and peak velocity index for veins were 0.48 (standard deviation 0.19) and 0.44 (standard deviation 0.18), respectively. During contractions, the mean values increased to 1.66 (standard deviation 0.85) and 1.46 (standard deviation 0.65), respectively. Krapp and colleagues proposed Doppler examinations of ductus venosus in labor to be possibly useful in fetuses at risk. Other researchers, who measured the ductus venosus PI between contractions, reported that in term pregnancies with premature rupture of membranes the PI was significantly increased.[77]

Li and colleagues[78] recorded blood flow patterns in fetal cerebral veins (vein of Galen, straight sinus, and transverse sinus) during the OCT. They found that the OCT increased blood velocities in uncompromised growth restricted fetuses, which they interpreted as a sign of an acute cerebral venous hyperperfusion in response to uterine contractions.

PHARMACOLOGIC EFFECTS ON UTEROPLACENTAL AND FETAL BLOOD FLOW IN LABOR

The possible effects on the fetal and uteroplacental circulation of drugs used in clinical obstetrics for treatment of preterm labor (tocolysis) or for obstetric analgesia in labor have been examined in a number of studies using various techniques. Ritodrine given to patients with preterm labor results in a significant decrease in the uterine and umbilical S/D ratio.[79] Similar effect on umbilical artery PI was observed after administration of fenoterol,[80] a finding interpreted by the authors as a decrease in vascular resistance and improved uteroplacental perfusion. However, the investigated tocolytic agents cause a concomitant increase in both the maternal heart rate and the FHR, suggesting that the response of waveform indices might be secondary to the changes in the heart rate. In a study comparing the effects of nifedipine and ritodrine in preterm labor, no significant effect on umbilical artery Doppler velocimetry findings was reported for either of the treatments.[81] In contrast, Gokay and colleagues[82] reported a decrease in the umbilical artery PI during ritodrine infusion. In addition, they found a selective increase of left cardiac output, indicating redistribution of fetal blood flow. Furthermore, an increase occurred in PI of the fetal middle cerebral artery. They commented that these changes might be of importance in preterm fetuses. Brar and colleagues[79] found that magnesium sulfate tocolysis was not associated with any significant changes in the S/D ratio, the maternal heart rate, or the FHR. Other authors observed a decrease in the uterine artery PI and an increase in the fetal middle cerebral artery PI during the administration of magnesium sulfate.[83] They interpreted these findings as a physiologic normalization process related to the stressed preterm fetus during labor.

Treatment of preterm labor with indomethacin[84] or sulindac[85] has been shown to cause a constriction of the fetal ductus arteriosus in approximately 50% of cases. In these cases, Doppler recordings showed very high ductal blood flow velocities. After discontinuation of the use of indomethacin, normal function of the ductus arteriosus usually returned. No increase in the ductal flow velocity was observed when a selective cyclooxygenase 2 inhibitor (celecoxib) was used in a comparative study by Stika and colleagues.[86]

Tocolysis with an oral dose of 30 mg nifedipine, followed by an additional oral dose of 20 mg after 4 hours, did not influence either fetal or uteroplacental circulation.[87] This is in agreement with other reports on sublingual administration of nifedipine[88] and with the observation from a study using orally administered nifedipine in women with pregnancy-induced hypertension.[89] Two days after nifedipine maintenance tocolysis (80 to 120 mg nifedipine daily), a decrease in the uterine artery PI and fetal middle cerebral artery PI was found.[90]

Nitric oxide donors administered for treatment of preterm labor sublingually or transdermally did not influence the RI or PI in the umbilical artery and fetal middle cerebral artery, respectively, but they decreased the resistance in the uteroplacental circulation.[91,92]

After epidural analgesia, a rapid uptake of local anesthetics in the maternal circulation and a rapid transport to the fetus occur. However, epidural analgesia for labor uncomplicated by hypotension is not associated with any alterations in placental blood flow as measured by placental scintigraphy.[93] Fetal aortic blood flow in women receiving epidural analgesia during labor increases with advancing labor in a fashion similar to that in women without any obstetric analgesia. Furthermore, no signs of negative effects on the fetal circulation are seen.[57] Several Doppler studies have examined umbilical and uterine artery S/D ratios or RI in term parturients before and after establishment of epidural block, and in none have any changes been found.[94-97] A similar observation was reported by Mires and colleagues[98] for women with normal pregnancy and uncomplicated labor. However, in women with pregnancy-induced hypertension, epidural analgesia led to a fall in maternal blood pressure and a concomitant decrease in umbilical artery S/D ratio.[98] Oláh[99] studied the effects of an epidural top-up in labor and did not find any change in the umbilical artery PI. However, a transient increase in the uterine artery PI was observed, with a maximum at 15 minutes after the top-up. This change in uteroplacental circulation was preceded by an increase in the maternal femoral artery flow, probably causing a loss of circulating volume in the uterine circulation.

Pethidine crosses the placenta rapidly, and maximum concentrations are found in fetal scalp blood and umbilical arterial blood between 1 and 5 hours after an intramuscular injection in the mother.[100] After intramuscular injection of 75 to 100 mg pethidine, fetal aortic blood flow decreases.[57]

Considerable maternal plasma and fetal scalp concentrations of local anesthetics have been found 20 to 30 minutes after paracervical block.[101] Reduced placental flow has been proposed as the cause of the fetal bradycardia that is sometimes observed after paracervical block.[102] However, no change in the intervillous blood flow[19] or in the uterine artery PI[103] has been observed after paracervical block. As long as no fetal bradycardia occurred, the umbilical artery PI remained unchanged.[103] In a study by Manninen and colleagues[104] paracervical block initiated a significant increase in uterine artery PI, suggesting a vasoconstrictive effect.

FETAL HEART RATE IN LABOR

Rhythmic contractions of the fetal heart are initiated by electric stimuli generated in the pacemaker, the sinus node. The rate of cardiac contractions is subject to autonomic central nervous influences, humoral factors, and the metabolic condition of the myocardium. The main determinants of FHR are the sympathetic and parasympathetic nervous systems, which are in continuous counteraction. This interplay causes changes in beat-to-beat intervals, expressed as heart rate variability. The variability also reflects the function of the fetal central nervous system and shows cyclic changes related to fetal behavioral states. The variability changes due to fetal behavior continue even during labor.[105]

During labor an increase in fetal blood pressure (e.g., caused by a compression of umbilical cord) leads to bradycardia by initiating a vagal nerve reflex. Fetal hypoxemia can have a direct depressing effect on the function of the central nervous system and fetal myocardium, which can result in a decrease in, or even loss of, FHR variability. The complex effects of hypoxemia and developing acidemia on chemoreceptors of the fetus result in an increase of blood pressure and bradycardia. During labor, signals of fetal heart action can be detected either transabdominally by use of a Doppler ultrasound transducer or, after rupture of membranes, transcervically with a fetal scalp electrode. From the measured beat-to-beat intervals, FHR is calculated and recorded simultaneously with the signals of uterine activity as a cardiotocogram. Uterine activity is recorded either with an external tocodynamometer or with an intrauterine pressure catheter. Cardiotocography is widely used today as the preferred method for monitoring fetal health in labor.[106,107]

FETAL ELECTROCARDIOGRAM IN LABOR

Fetal electrocardiogram (ECG) signals are easily obtained from the fetal scalp during labor. The early interest of researchers in revealing information on fetal myocardial function from the ECG was hampered by difficulties in obtaining signals of good quality and performing accurate waveform analysis.[108] Technologic developments have made it possible to design computerized techniques for improved isolation and analysis of fetal ECG signals.

In studies on animal fetuses, the ECG waveform is changed in a characteristic fashion with fetal hypoxia.[109,110] When the oxygen supply is insufficient to satisfy the energy needs of fetal myocardium, myocardial energy balance becomes negative, metabolism changes to anaerobic, and acidosis occurs. When the fetus compensates for hypoxia by additional glycogenolysis, an elevation occurs in the ST segment of the waveform and the height of the T wave increases. One can quantify this change by calculating the ratio between the amplitude of the QRS complex and that of the T wave, which in noncompromised fetuses does not exceed 0.25. In normal fetuses a direct correlation exists between the PR interval and FHR. This relationship is inverted, and the PR interval shortens[111] with fetal acidosis, which might enable a distinction to be made between FHR decelerations of various origins. The first studies in human fetuses during labor reported promising results, suggesting that changes in the fetal ECG waveform may be an early sign of fetal hypoxia.[112] The clinical usefulness of this new method of fetal surveillance during labor was tested in several large randomized controlled trials.[113-115] The latest meta-analysis demonstrated a significant reduction of metabolic acidosis rates by 36% and operative vaginal delivery rates by 8%, compared with cardiotocography alone.[116]

CONCLUSION

Uterine contractions during labor diminish the uteroplacental blood flow. The decrement in blood flow during contractions is inversely related to the increase in intrauterine pressure, and, at the contraction acme in late labor, the diastolic velocities in maternal uteroplacental vessels disappear. Doppler ultrasonography has made it possible to examine blood flow changes during labor in human pregnancies. Several studies confirmed that the fetal circulation during normal labor in uncomplicated pregnancy usually remains unaffected as the uncompromised fetus can cope with the intermittent decreases in the oxygen supply. Doppler velocimetry, performed between contractions, shows that the waveforms of blood velocities recorded from the umbilical artery and from the descending aorta, ductus venosus, and middle cerebral arteries of the fetus do not change during labor. A finding of increased PI values between contractions in the umbilical artery or ductus venosus is frequently associated with subsequent development of fetal asphyxia and operative delivery for fetal distress. However, the potential of Doppler examinations in labor as a clinical predictor of fetal asphyxia still awaits proof. Drugs clinically used in labor, such as tocolytics, opioids, or local anesthetics, can influence the fetal and uteroplacental blood flow.

 A complete reference list is available at www.ExpertConsult.com.

SELECT REFERENCES

1. Borell V, Fernstroem I, Ohlson L, et al. Influence of uterine contractions on the uteroplacental blood flow at term. *Am J Obstet Gynecol*. 1965;93:44-57.
2. Ramsey EM, Corner Jr GW, Donner MW. Serial and cineradioangiographic visualization of maternal circulation in the primate (hemochorial) placenta. *Am J Obstet Gynecol*. 1963;86:213-225.
6. Lees MH, Hill JD, Ochsner III AJ, et al. Maternal placental and myometrial blood flow of the rhesus monkey during uterine contractions. *Am J Obstet Gynecol*. 1971;110:68-81.
7. Harbert GM, Spisso KR. Biorhythms of the primate uterus (Macaca mulatta) during labor and delivery. *Am J Obstet Gynecol*. 1980;138:686-696.
11. Dawes GS. *Fetal and Neonatal Physiology*. Chicago: Year Book; 1968.
12. FitzGerald DE, Drumm JE. Non-invasive measurement of human fetal circulation using ultrasound. A new method. *BMJ*. 1977;2:1450-1451.
13. Eik-Nes SH, Marsal K, Brubakk AO, et al. Ultrasonic measurement of human fetal blood flow. *J Biomed Eng*. 1982;4:28-36.
15. Rekonen A, Luotola H, Pitkänen M, et al. Measurement of intervillous and myometrial blood flow by an intravenous 133Xe method. *Br J Obstet Gynaecol*. 1976;83:723-728.
17. Smits TM, Aarnoudse JG. Variability of fetal scalp blood flow during labour: continuous transcutaneous measurement by the laser Doppler technique. *Br J Obstet Gynaecol*. 1984;91:524-531.
18. Hernandez-Andrade E, Thuring-Jönsson A, Jansson T, et al. Lung fractional moving blood volume in normally grown and growth restricted fetuses. *Clin Physiol Funct Imaging*. 2004;24:69-74.
22. Bellotti M, Pennati G, De Gasperi C, et al. Simultaneous measurements of umbilical venous, fetal hepatic, and ductus venosus blood flow in growth-restricted human fetuses. *Am J Obstet Gynecol*. 2004;190:1347-1358.
24. Gómez O, Figueras F, Fernández S, et al. Reference ranges for uterine artery mean pulsatility index at 11-41 weeks of gestation. *Ultrasound Obstet Gynecol*. 2008;32:128-132.
25. Hernandez-Andrade E, Brodszki J, Lingman G, et al. Uterine artery score and perinatal outcome. *Ultrasound Obstet Gynecol*. 2002;19:438-442.
28. Fendel H, Fendel M, Pauen A, et al. Doppleruntersuchungen des arteriellen uterinen Flows während der Wehentätigkeit. *Z Geburtshilfe Perinatol*. 1984;188:64-67.
30. Brar HS, Platt LD, DeVore GR, et al. Qualitative assessment of maternal uterine and fetal umbilical artery blood flow and resistance in laboring patients by Doppler velocimetry. *Am J Obstet Gynecol*. 1988;158:952-956.
32. Fendel H, Fettweis P, Billet P, et al. Doppleruntersuchungen des arteriellen uterofeto-plazentaren Blutflusses vor und während der Geburt. *Z Geburtshilfe Perinatol*. 1987;191:121-129.
33. Li H, Gudmundsson S, Olofsson P. Uterine artery blood flow velocity waveforms during uterine contractions. *Ultrasound Obstet Gynecol*. 2003;22:578-585.
34. Baron J, Shwarzman P, Sheiner E, et al. Blood flow Doppler velocimetry measured during active labor. *Arch Gynecol Obstet*. 2015;291:837-840.
37. Fairlie FM, Lang GD, Sheldon CD. Umbilical artery flow velocity waveforms in labour. *Br J Obstet Gynaecol*. 1989;96:151-157.
39. Fleischer A, Anyaegbunam AA, Schulman H, et al. Uterine and umbilical artery velocimetry during normal labor. *Am J Obstet Gynecol*. 1987;157:40-43.
40. Malcus P, Gudmundsson S, Maršál K, et al. Umbilical artery Doppler velocimetry as a labor admission test. *Obstet Gynecol*. 1991;77:10-16.
42. Abitbol MM, Rochelson B, Castillo I, et al. Continuous monitoring of Doppler umbilical artery waveforms in labor. *J Matern Fetal Invest*. 1992;2:45-49.
43. Oosterhof H, Dijkstra K, Aarnoudse JG. Fetal Doppler velocimetry in the internal carotid and umbilical artery during Braxton Hicks' contractions. *Early Hum Dev*. 1992;30:33-40.
47. Brar HS, Platt LD, Paul RH. Fetal umbilical blood flow velocity waveforms using Doppler ultrasonography in patients with late decelerations. *Obstet Gynecol*. 1989;73:363-366.
48. Feinkind L, Abulafia O, Delke I, et al. Screening with Doppler velocimetry in labor. *Am J Obstet Gynecol*. 1989;161:765-770.
53. Li H, Gudmundsson S, Olofsson P. Acute increase of umbilical artery vascular flow resistance in compromised fetuses provoked by uterine contractions. *Early Hum Dev*. 2003;74:47-56.
55. Westergaard HB, Langhoff-Roos J, Lingman G, et al. A critical appraisal of the use of umbilical artery Doppler ultrasound in high risk pregnancies. use of meta-analyses in evidence-based obstetrics. *Ultrasound Obstet Gynecol*. 2001;17:466-476.
56. Farrell T, Chien PF, Gordon A. Intrapartum umbilical artery Doppler velocimetry as a predictor of adverse perinatal outcome: a systematic review. *Br J Obstet Gynaecol*. 1999;106:783-792.
57. Lindblad A, Bernow J, Maršál K. Obstetric analgesia and fetal aortic blood flow during labour. *Br J Obstet Gynaecol*. 1987;94:306-311.
59. Maesel A, Lingman G, Maršál K. Cerebral blood flow during labour in the human fetus. *Acta Obstet Gynecol Scand*. 1990;69:493-495.
63. Yagel S, Anteby E, Lavy Y, et al. Fetal middle cerebral artery blood flow during normal active labour and in labour with variable decelerations. *Br J Obstet Gynaecol*. 1992;99:483-485.
65. Sütterlin MW, Seelbach-Göbel B, Oehler MK, et al. Doppler ultrasonographic evidence of intrapartum brain-sparing effect in fetuses with low oxygen saturation according to pulse oximetry. *Am J Obstet Gynecol*. 1999;181:216-220.
66. Kassanos D, Siristatidis C, Vitoratos N, et al. The clinical significance of Doppler findings in fetal middle cerebral artery during labor. *Eur J Obstet Gynecol Reprod Biol*. 2003;109:45-50.

71. Dall'Asta A, Ghi T, Rizzo G, et al. Cerebroplacental ratio assessment in early labor in uncomplicated term pregnancy and prediction of adverse perinatal outcome: prospective multicenter study. *Ultrasound Obstet Gynecol.* 2019;53:481-487.
72. Fiolna M, Kostiv V, Anthoulakis C, et al. Prediction of adverse perinatal outcome by cerebroplacental ratio in women undergoing induction of labor. *Ultrasound Obstet Gynecol.* 2019;53:473-480.
74. Murakami M, Kanzaki T, Utsu M, et al. Changes in the umbilical venous blood flow of human fetus in labor. *Acta Obstet Gynaecol Jpn.* 1985;37:776-782.
75. Ghosh GS, Fu J, Olofsson P, et al. Pulsations in the umbilical vein during labor are associated with increased risk of operative delivery for fetal distress. *Ultrasound Obstet Gynecol.* 2009;34:177-181.
76. Krapp M, Denzel S, Katalinic A, et al. Normal values of fetal ductus venosus blood flow waveforms during the first stage of labor. *Ultrasound Obstet Gynecol.* 2002;19:556-561.
79. Brar HS, Medearis AL, DeVore GR, Platt LD. Maternal and fetal blood flow velocity waveforms in patients with preterm labor: effect of tocolytics. *Obstet Gynecol.* 1988;72:209-214.
84. Moise Jr KJ, Huhta JC, Sharif DS, et al. Indomethacin in the treatment of premature labor. Effects on the fetal ductus arteriosus. *N Engl J Med.* 1988;319:327-331.
88. Guclu S, Saygili U, Dogan E, et al. The short-term effect of nifedipine tocolysis on placental, fetal cerebral and atrioventricular Doppler waveforms. *Ultrasound Obstet Gynecol.* 2004;24:761-765.
94. Hughes AB, Devoe LD, Wakefield ML, et al. The effects of epidural anesthesia on the Doppler velocimetry of umbilical and uterine arteries in normal term labor. *Obstet Gynecol.* 1990;75:809-812.
104. Manninen T, Aantaa R, Salonen M, et al. A comparison of the hemodynamic effects of paracervical block and epidural anesthesia for labor analgesia. *Acta Anaesthesiol Scand.* 2000;44:441-445.
106. Macones GA, Hankins GD, Spong CY, et al. The 2008 National Institute of Child Health and Human Development workshop report on electronic fetal monitoring: update on definitions, interpretation, and research guidelines. *J Obstet Gynecol Neonatal Nurs.* 2008;37:510-515.
107. Ayres-de-Campos D, Spong CY, Chandraharan, et al. FIGO consensus guidelines on intrapartum fetal monitoring: cardiotocography. *Int J Gynecol Obstet.* 2015;131:13-24.
109. Greene KR, Dawes GS, Lilja H, et al. Changes in the ST waveform of the fetal lamb electrocardiogram with hypoxia. *Am J Obstet Gynecol.* 1982;144:950-958.
116. Amer-Wåhlin I, Ugwumadu A, Yli BM, et al. Fetal electrocardiography ST-segment analysis for intrapartum monitoring: a critical appraisal of conflicting evidence and a way forward. *Am J Obstet Gynecol.* 2019;221:577-601.e11.
117. Stuart B, Drumm J, FitzGerald DE, et al. Fetal blood velocity waveforms in normal pregnancy. *Br J Obstet Gynaecol.* 1980;87:780-785.
118. Gosling RG, King DH. Arterial assessment by Doppler-shift ultrasound. *Proc R Soc Med.* 1974;67:447-449.
119. Pourcelot L. Applications Clinique de l'Examen Doppler Transcutane. In: Peroneau P, ed. *Velocimetric Ultrasonor Doppler.* Paris: INSERM; 1974:213-240.

Normal and Abnormal Structural Development of the Lung

55

Xin Sun

INTRODUCTION

The respiratory system functions to provide oxygen from the external environment to the organism, while removing excess carbon dioxide from the blood. The respiratory system is divided into two parts, the upper and lower respiratory tracts. The upper respiratory tract is composed of the nasal cavity, sinuses, nasopharynx, and larynx (above the vocal fold), and it warms, moistens, and filters inspired air. The lower respiratory tract includes the larynx (below the vocal fold), trachea, bronchi, and bronchioles, and it distributes air throughout the alveolar region of the lung where exchange of oxygen and carbon dioxide occurs. Integral to respiration are the primary respiratory muscles, which include the intercostal muscles of the thoracic wall and the muscular thoracic diaphragm, which ventilate the lung, moving air in and out of the lung and across the respiratory surface. In addition, the blood vessels of the pulmonary circulation are an integral component of the lung, carrying deoxygenated blood from the heart to the lungs through the pulmonary arteries and returning oxygen-rich blood from the lung to the heart through the pulmonary veins. Appropriate specification of progenitors, patterning and alignment of tissues, differentiation and physiologic maturation of cell types, are all critical for efficient gas exchange and survival starting at birth. This chapter describes the development of the lung and its associated tissues, along with a review of the congenital malformations that arise from defects in pulmonary and vascular morphogenesis. Where known, chromosomal disorders and single-gene mutations associated with these malformations will be discussed.

OVERVIEW OF LUNG DEVELOPMENT

Human lung development can be divided into five overlapping chronologic stages of organogenesis, which describe the structural and histologic changes that occur during morphogenesis and maturation of the lung.[1] These stages are the embryonic, pseudoglandular, canalicular, saccular, and alveolar stages of lung development, which extend throughout gestation and into the postnatal period (Table 55.1). Lung development begins during the early embryonic period of gestation (at a gestational age [GA] of 3 to 7 weeks) as a small saccular outgrowth, or diverticulum, of the ventral wall of the foregut endoderm. This region is marked by expression of the transcription factor *NKX2-1*, which encodes thyroid transcription factor-1 (TTF1), a homeobox transcription factor critical for lung development.[2] During the subsequent pseudoglandular stage of lung development (5 to 17 weeks' GA), formation of the conducting airways, or tracheobronchial tree, occurs by a process called *branching morphogenesis*. This process involves rapid growth and repetitive and programmed branching of the epithelial-lined bronchial tubules until all of the branches of the tracheobronchial tree are formed. Outgrowth and branching of the bronchial tubules are dependent on interactions between the epithelium and the surrounding mesenchyme, which are facilitated by a number of pathways that signal across these tissue boundaries, including fibroblast growth factor (FGF), wingless-related integration site (WNT), transforming growth factor beta (TGFβ), bone morphogenetic protein (BMP), sonic hedgehog (SHH), and retinoic acid (RA) pathways.[2] Transcription factors regulating gene expression during this period include NKX2-1, FOXA2, GATA6, and SOX2, among many others (Fig. 55.1).[2] By the end of this stage, the terminal bronchioles have divided into two or more respiratory bronchioles, which will subdivide again into small clusters of short acinar tubules and buds at the periphery of the lung. These peripheral structures will become the adult pulmonary acinus, consisting of the alveolarized respiratory bronchiole, alveolar duct, and alveolus.

During the canalicular stage of lung development (16 to 26 weeks' GA), increased vascularization of the surrounding mesenchyme with formation of the peripheral intra-acinar capillary bed gives rise to the blood-air barrier, or alveolar-capillary membrane, of the gas-exchange region of the lung. Molecular pathways important for vascularization during this stage include the vascular endothelial growth factor (VEGF), platelet-derived growth factor (PDGF), epidermal growth factor (EGF), TGFα and TGFβ signaling pathways, as well as components of the extracellular matrix (ECM).[2] In addition, differentiation of type 1 and type 2 alveolar epithelial cells (AEC1s and AEC2s) initiated during this period of lung development. NKX2-1, FOXA2, and GATA6 continue to be important transcriptional regulators of target genes involved in AEC differentiation, as well as in surfactant synthesis and fluid and electrolyte transport at this stage (see Fig. 55.1).

Enlargement and expansion of the peripheral acinar tubules during the saccular stage of lung development (24 to 38 weeks' GA) result in formation of primitive sac-like alveoli with thick inter-alveolar septa. Thinning of these septa and remodeling of the alveolar-capillary membrane occur during the alveolar stage of lung development (36 weeks' GA to 8 years of age), giving rise to mature alveolar organization of the adult lung. This process of alveologenesis extends into the postnatal period, during which millions of additional alveoli are formed, greatly increasing the surface area of the lung available for gas exchange (Table 55.2). Molecular mechanisms that are important for alveolarization and differentiation of the alveolar epithelium during these last two stages include the PDGF, FGF, Hippo/yes-associated protein (YAP) signaling pathways, as well as steroid hormone pathways such as glucocorticoid and thyroid hormone receptors (see Fig. 55.1).[2]

Although definitive alveoli can be found in the human lung by 36 weeks' GA, greater than 85% to 90% of all alveoli are formed within the first 6 months of life.[3] After 6 months, alveolar formation continues at a slower pace until at least 8 years of age.[4-6]

Table 55.1 Human Lung Development.

Developmental Stage	Major Developmental Events
Embryonic 3–7 wk GA	Lung bud arises from ventral foregut endoderm Branching morphogenesis initiated Primary, secondary, and tertiary bronchi form Trachea and esophagus separate Pulmonary arteries bud off sixth pair of aortic arches Pulmonary veins develop as outgrowths of left atrium Autonomic innervation extends to trachea and bronchi
Pseudoglandular 5–17 wk GA	Branching morphogenesis continues and completes Formation of tracheobronchial tree complete by 17 wk Cartilage and mucus glands develop in trachea and bronchi Airway smooth muscle extends to respiratory bronchioles Ciliated, mucus, club, neuroendocrine, basal cells differentiate Respiratory bronchioles, acinar tubules/buds form in distal lung Pulmonary arterial development parallels airway branching Pulmonary lymphatics arise from veins/invest bronchi and vessels Pulmonary veins and lymphatics extend into interlobular septa Capillary blood vessels form in distal mesenchyme Autonomic innervation parallels airway branching Pleuroperitoneal cavity and diaphragm closes
Canalicular 16–26 wk GA	Acinar tubules/buds lengthen, subdivide, and widen Mesenchyme thins/condenses Primitive alveolar capillary network/blood-air barrier forms Type I/type II AECs differentiate Surfactant synthesized in lamellar bodies by type II AECs Fetal lung fluid production increases Fetal breathing-like movements initiated
Saccular 24–38 wk GA	Distal airspaces continue to branch and grow Acinar tubules/buds expand to form fluid-filled saccules Mesenchyme spreads to form alveolar septal walls Alveolar septa contain double capillary network Elastin deposited at sites of alveolar septal crest formation Type I AECs flatten and elongate Surfactant synthesized and secreted by type II AECs Ex utero breathing/gas exchange feasible
Alveolar 36 wk GA—8 yr	Alveolar surface area available for gas exchange increases Secondary alveolar septa subdivide saccules into true alveoli Alveolar septal walls thin with loss of connective tissue Microvasculature fuses into single capillary network Subset of interstitial fibroblasts differentiate into myofibroblasts Collagen, elastin, and fibronectin deposited Surfactant production increases in type II AEC Pulmonary vascular resistance decreases at birth

AECs, Alveolar epithelial cells; *GA*, gestational age.

A more recent study presented helium imaging data demonstrating that new alveoli may be added into the early 20-years-of-age period.[7] Overall, the number of alveoli increases from an average of 150 million alveoli (ranging from 110 to 174 million) in the term lung[8] to 480 million alveoli (ranging from 274 to 790 million) in the adult human lung.[4,6,8,9] Likewise, the conducting airways increase in length and diameter (see Table 55.2), whereas the diffusion capacity and surface area of the alveolar parenchyma increase linearly with body weight up to about 18 years of age.[6]

EMBRYONIC STAGE (3 TO 7 WEEKS' GESTATIONAL AGE)

The lung is a derivative of the definitive foregut endoderm and the adjacent mesoderm.[10,11] The respiratory primordium of the lung first appears at day 22 GA as an enlargement of the caudal end of the laryngotracheal sulcus, which is located in the medial pharyngeal groove, an outgrowth of the ventral wall of the definitive foregut endoderm.[12] The primitive respiratory diverticulum, or lung bud, appears at day 26 GA, when the embryo is only about 3 mm long, and grows ventrocaudally into the mesoderm surrounding the foregut in a position that is anterior and parallel to the primitive esophagus. Epithelial cells of the primitive respiratory diverticulum invade the surrounding mesoderm, or splanchnic mesenchyme. At day 28 GA, the respiratory diverticulum bifurcates into right, and left primary bronchial buds, which will become the main stem, or primary, right and left bronchi. The region proximal (or superior) to the first bifurcation becomes the trachea and larynx. Shortly thereafter, the trachea and the esophagus begin to separate into two distinct structures.

A second round of branching occurs during the fifth week of gestation (days 33 to 41 GA) to yield three secondary (or lobar) bronchial buds on the right and two on the left, which will become the primary lobes of the right and left lung. During the sixth week of gestation (days 41 to 44 GA), a third round of branching yields 10 tertiary (or segmental) bronchi on the right and 8 to 9 on the left. These will become the bronchopulmonary segments of the mature lung. During this period, there is extensive proliferation of both epithelial and mesenchymal cells, with focal apoptosis in the mesenchyme around bronchial branch points and in regions of new bronchial bud formation.[13]

At this stage of development, the mesenchyme is composed of a loose arrangement of primitive cells that will at a later stage give rise to the pulmonary vascular plexus, airway and vascular smooth muscle, cartilage, and other fibroblast-like cells. The ECM is composed primarily of hyaluronic acid, whereas the basement membrane underlying the epithelium contains type IV collagen, laminin, and fibronectin.[14] The trachea and bronchial tubules are lined by pseudostratified columnar epithelium, composed of relatively primitive and undifferentiated epithelial cells. At the end of this stage, the lung resembles a small tubuloacinar gland, and separation of the trachea and esophagus is complete.

Autonomic innervation of the lung is derived from the ectoderm, neural plate, and associated neural crest cells, which migrate through the mesoderm to take up positions in the walls of the trachea and lung buds before separation from the esophagus. Ganglion cells appear in the mesenchyme around the trachea by 7 weeks of gestation. As growth proceeds, these cells form segmental ganglia and nerve fibers that develop into primitive neural plexuses, encircling the trachea and extending as far as the main stem and lobar bronchi.[15]

Vascular connections with the right and left heart are established at the end of the embryonic stage (5 to 8 weeks' GA), creating the primitive pulmonary vascular circulation.[16,17] The pulmonary arteries arise from the sixth pair of aortic arches and grow into the surrounding mesoderm, where they accompany the developing airways, segmenting with each bronchial subdivision, and then anastomose with the vascular plexus developing in the pulmonary mesenchyme around the bronchial buds.[18] During fetal life, the pulmonary artery is connected to the aortic arch

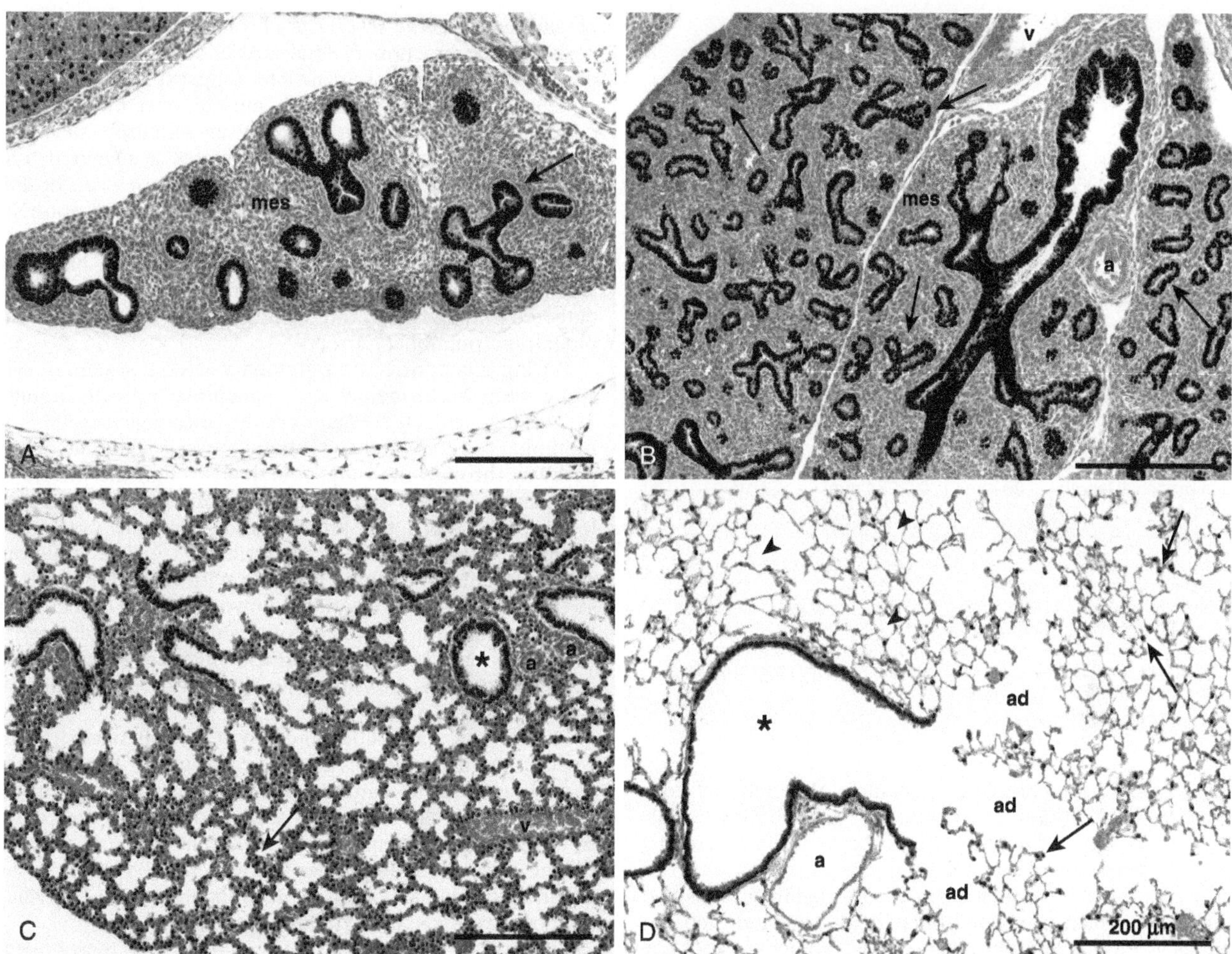

Fig. 55.1 The nuclear transcription factor, NKX2-1, is critical for the initiation of lung development, as well as differentiation of the alveolar epithelium during later stages of lung development in both human and mouse lungs. It is expressed throughout lung development, which is illustrated here during the embryonic (A), pseudoglandular (B), saccular (C), and alveolar (D) stages of mouse lung development. The canalicular stage is not shown. *NKX2-1* is detected by immunohistochemistry as a black precipitation product in the nuclei of epithelial cells lining the primitive bronchial tubules (A, *arrow*) and the acinar tubules and buds (B, *arrow*) during branching morphogenesis (A and B). In the saccular stage of lung development (C), *NKX2-1* is detected in the nuclei of epithelial cells lining the conducting airways *(asterisk)* and in the nuclei of differentiating type I and type II alveolar epithelial cells (AECs) *(arrow)* located in the expanding terminal saccules. In the alveolar stage mouse lung (D), *NKX2-1* is detected in the nuclei of epithelial cells lining the bronchioles *(asterisk)* and in type I and type II AECs *(arrow)* located in the alveolar septa *(ars)*. *a*, Pulmonary artery; *ad*, alveolar duct; *mes*, mesenchyme; *v*, pulmonary vein. Scale bars for all panels = 200 µm. Immunoperoxidase detection system, enhanced with TrisCobalt, and counterstained with nuclear fast red.

by the ductus arteriosus, which enables the right ventricular output from the heart to bypass the pulmonary vascular bed. The pulmonary veins originate from the left atrium and grow into the surrounding mesoderm, dividing several times before connecting to the pulmonary vascular bed.

Developmental abnormalities that arise during the embryonic stage of lung development are related to lung bud formation, separation of the trachea and esophagus, formation of the proximal conducting airways, and initial lobe formation. These abnormalities include laryngeal, esophageal, tracheal, and bronchial atresia; tracheal and bronchial stenosis; tracheo- and bronchoesophageal fistulas; pulmonary agenesis; bronchogenic cysts; ectopic lobes; and extralobar pulmonary sequestration.

PSEUDOGLANDULAR STAGE (5 TO 17 WEEKS' GESTATIONAL AGE)

The pseudoglandular stage of fetal lung development is marked by the formation of the bronchial portion of the lung. This occurs through a process during which the segmental tubules of the developing lung undergo a set program of branching morphogenesis to form the primitive bronchial tree.[19] Expansion of the bronchial tubules is due to rapid proliferation of their epithelial cells, particularly at the ends of the tubes, or bronchial buds. By the end of this stage, formation of the conducting airways, including the terminal bronchioles, is complete (17 weeks), with 12 to 17 generations of bronchial tubules in the upper lobes, 18 to 23 in the middle lobes, and 14 to 23 in the lower lobes.[15,20] Numerous acinar tubules and buds, which give rise to the adult pulmonary acinus, are formed in the periphery of the lung, arising as distal branches of the respiratory bronchioles.[21,22] By the end of this stage, the pseudoglandular lung is composed of millions of epithelial tubules surrounded by relatively extensive regions of mesenchyme, which gives it a distinct glandular appearance.

The bronchial tubules are lined initially by a pseudostratified columnar epithelium. These cells are morphologically undifferentiated and contain large pools of intracellular glycogen, deriving most of their energy needs from anaerobic glycolysis. A prominent basement membrane, rich in laminin and

Table 55.2 Postnatal Growth of the Human Lung and Conducting Airways.

	Term	Adult	Fold Change
Lung weight (mean)	50 g	800 g	~16
Lung volume (mean)	150–200 mL	4–6 × 10^3 mL	~25–30
Alveolar (Alv) surface area (SA)[a]	3–5 m^2	75–100 m^2	~20–25
SA/kg (mean)	0.4 m^2	1 m^2	~2.5
Alv number (mean)[a,b]	150 × 10^6	480 × 10^6	~3
Alv number (range)[a,b]	110–174 × 10^6	274–790 × 10^6	~2.5–4.5
Alv diameter (mean)	150 μm	300 μm	~2
Alv septal wall thickness (mean)	5 μm	2.5 μm	~2
Air-blood barrier (mean)	0.6 μm	0.6 μm	0
Tracheal length (mean)	26 mm	184 mm	~7
Main bronchial length (mean)	26 mm	254 mm	~10

[a]Hislop AA, Wigglesworth JS, Desai R. Alveolar development in the human fetus and infant. *Early Hum Dev*. 1986;13:1–11.
[b]Ochs M, Nyengaard JR, Jung A, et al. The number of alveoli in the human lung. *Am J Respir Crit Care Med*. 2004;169:120–124.
Adapted from Hodson WA. Normal and abnormal structural development of the lung. In: Polin RA, Fox WW, eds. *Fetal and Neonatal Physiology*. 2nd ed. Philadelphia: Saunders; 1998:1037.

collagen type IV, underlies the epithelium. Mesenchymal cells adjacent to these tubules differentiate into smooth muscle cells starting at 7 weeks' GA, aligning themselves in a circumferential orientation perpendicular to the long axis of the tubules. The ECM is composed of various types of glycosaminoglycans and proteoglycans, such as chondroitin, dermatan, and heparan sulfate, as well as laminin, fibronectin, tenascin, entactin, and type I and type III collagen.[14,23] These macromolecules are important for cell proliferation, migration, adhesion, and differentiation during lung development.

As branching progresses, the pseudostratified columnar epithelium is reduced to a tall columnar epithelium in the proximal airways and to a cuboidal epithelium in the distal acinar tubules and buds. Differentiation of the conducting airway epithelium occurs with ciliated, club (serous), goblet (mucus), neuroendocrine, and basal cells appearing first in the more proximal airways.[15,24,25] Isolated neuroendocrine cells, the first bronchial epithelial cells to differentiate, can be detected in the proximal airways by 8 to 9 weeks' GA.[25] Clusters of neuroendocrine cells, called *neuroepithelial bodies*, are detected by 9 to 10 weeks' GA. These are located at branch points along the bronchial tree and are innervated by parasympathetic, sympathetic, and sensory nerve fibers. Ciliated cells appear in the epithelium of the trachea by 10 weeks' GA, in the main stem bronchi by 12 weeks' GA, and in the segmental bronchi by 13 weeks' GA. Whereas mucus cells are present in the epithelium by 13 weeks' GA, submucosal glands appear in the trachea by 11 to 12 weeks' GA and in the bronchi by 13 weeks' GA, with active mucus production by 14 weeks' GA.[15,24] Epithelial cell differentiation is initiated in the distal acinar structures with the onset of surfactant protein B (SFTPB) and C (SFTPC) expression. These two hydrophobic lung-specific surfactant components are expressed selectively in the distal respiratory epithelium by 12 to 14 weeks of GA.[26]

Cartilage appears in the trachea and bronchi by 10 weeks' GA and in the segmental bronchi by 16 weeks.[20] By the end of this developmental stage, cartilaginous structures extend as far as the segmental bronchi, and airway smooth muscle extends as far as the respiratory bronchioles. Spontaneous and peristaltic contraction of fetal airway smooth muscle can be observed in cultured human fetal lung explants at this stage of development.[27] The smooth muscle layer enveloping the conducting airways is invested by an extensive network of neural ganglia and nerve bundles, which is detected by 7.5 to 8 weeks' GA.[28] Well-defined neural plexuses can be found between the cartilage and the tracheobronchial epithelium, with nerve fibers extending to the submucosal glands and trachealis muscle; ganglia are found at bronchial bifurcations and in the adventitia of smaller bronchi.[15] Elastic fibers are detected in the walls of the trachea and the main stem bronchi, pleura, and pulmonary artery.[14]

During this period, the pulmonary arterial system develops along with the bronchial and bronchiolar tubules, branching in parallel with these airways by *angiogenesis*.[8,16,29] The pulmonary veins and lymphatic vessels take a different pathway through the lung, coursing through the interlobular connective tissue septa that surround each pulmonary lobule.[30] Between the arteries and veins the preacinar, or capillary, blood vessels are formed.[16-18] The pulmonary arteries gradually become invested with smooth muscle cells, so that smooth muscle actin and myosin can be detected in all of the vasculature by the end of this developmental stage.[31,32] Intrapulmonary bronchial arteries, which are supplied by the descending aorta, extend along the airways in parallel with cartilage formation.[18,24]

Little is known about the ontogeny of the pulmonary lymphatic vessels, but these vessels appear to originate by budding, or sprouting, from the cardinal veins.[33] Progenitor cells in these sprouts then proliferate and migrate into the lung mesenchyme to form primitive lymphatic sacs adjacent to the hilar bronchi. During the pseudoglandular period, the lymphatic system expands, forming an extensive network around the bronchi and pulmonary vessels, and extends to the pleura.

A variety of congenital defects in branching morphogenesis may arise during the pseudoglandular stage of lung development, including tracheo- and bronchomalacia, intralobar bronchopulmonary sequestration, congenital pulmonary airway malformations, acinar aplasia or dysplasia, pulmonary hypoplasia, pulmonary lymphangiectasis, and other pulmonary vascular malformations. The pleuroperitoneal cavity also closes during the pseudoglandular period (6 weeks' GA), forming the diaphragm. Failure to close the pleural, or thoracic, cavity is often accompanied by herniation of the abdominal contents into the thorax (congenital diaphragmatic hernia), which limits the space available for further growth of the lung, causing pulmonary hypoplasia.

CANALICULAR STAGE (16 TO 26 WEEKS' GESTATIONAL AGE)

The *canalicular stage* is so named because of the appearance of vascular canals, or capillaries, that multiply in the interstitial compartment to form the blood-air barrier, or alveolar-capillary membrane, the future gas-exchange surface of the lung.[1] Development of the alveolar-capillary membrane, along with the synthesis and secretion of pulmonary surfactant, is critical for extrauterine survival of the immature fetus, if delivered prematurely near the end of this stage. Gas exchange cannot occur in the premature infant unless these capillaries are close enough to the adjacent alveolar epithelium for optimal gas diffusion to take place across their surfaces. Rapid expansion of the capillary bed, with condensation and thinning of the mesenchyme, is the first critical step in the formation of the gas-exchange regions of the lung. During this stage of lung development, the total surface area of the alveolar-capillary membrane increases exponentially with a concomitant decrease in the mean mesenchymal wall thickness, thereby increasing the potential for gas exchange in the immature lung.[1] Disturbances in this stage of lung development result in severe hypoxemia and are not compatible with life after birth.

At the beginning of the canalicular stage, branching morphogenesis and formation of the bronchial tree is complete, and the terminal bronchioles have divided into two or more respiratory bronchioles that have subdivided further into small clusters of short acinar tubules and buds lined by cuboidal epithelium. These structures undergo further differentiation to become the adult respiratory unit, or pulmonary acinus, consisting of two to four alveolarized respiratory bronchioles, each ending in six to seven generations of branched alveolar ducts and alveoli. Clusters of acinar tubules and buds grow by lengthening, subdividing, and widening at the expense of the surrounding mesenchyme. The proportion of epithelial and endothelial cells increases, and the proportion of interstitial fibroblasts decreases. Apoptosis of cells in the interstitial tissue contributes to mesenchymal involution and thinning of the alveolar septa at this stage.[13] Epithelial growth drops in the larger airways and cell proliferation occurs predominantly in the peripheral acinar tubules and buds. This peripheral growth is accompanied by the growth and development of inter-acinar capillaries, which align themselves around the air spaces, establishing contact with the adjacent epithelium to form the primitive alveolar-capillary membrane.

Epithelial cell differentiation becomes increasingly complex and is especially apparent in the distal regions of the lung parenchyma, where type I and type II AECs can be detected. Bronchiolar cells begin to express differentiated features and to synthesize cell-specific secretory proteins, such as secretoglobin 1A1.[34] Cuboidal type II AECs lining the distal acinar tubules express increasing amounts of surfactant proteins and phospholipids.[26,35-40] Nascent lamellar bodies, the storage form of pulmonary surfactant, are seen in association with rich glycogen stores in cuboidal pre-type II AECs lining the acinar tubules and buds.[41-44] Cells of the proximal acinar tubules become flattened and attenuated, acquiring features of typical squamous type I AECs. Type I AEC differentiation occurs in conjunction with formation of the alveolar-capillary membrane—that is, wherever endothelial cells of the developing capillary system come into contact with adjacent acinar epithelial cells. Where this occurs, the intercellular junctional complexes, originally localized around the epithelial cell apex, shift to the basolateral aspect of the intercellular cleft. The cells develop thin cytoplasmic attenuations, differentiating into squamous type I AECs and losing features previously associated with pre-type II AECs.

By the end of the canalicular stage of lung development, fully differentiated mucus and ciliated cells are found in the conducting airways, and cartilage, submucosal glands, and smooth muscle extend as far down the airway as they do in the adult lung. The epithelial cells are capable of producing fetal lung fluid, and the primitive alveolar-capillary membrane is thin enough to support gas exchange, although pulmonary surfactant production is low. Disturbances in this stage of lung development often result in severe hypoxemia and are incompatible with life after birth. Abnormalities of lung development associated with the canalicular stage include diverse causes of congenital alveolar dysplasia and pulmonary hypoplasia, which usually lead to severe respiratory insufficiency shortly after birth. In addition to genetic causes, acquired forms of pulmonary hypoplasia include (1) congenital diaphragmatic hernia, (2) compression from thoracic or abdominal masses, (3) decreased fetal breathing movements, (4) renal agenesis (such as with Potter syndrome) or obstruction of the urinary tract, in which amniotic fluid production is impaired, and (5) prolonged rupture of membranes in which amniotic fluid is lost.

Although postnatal gas exchange can be supported late in the canalicular stage, premature infants born during this period generally suffer severe complications related to low levels of pulmonary surfactant (surfactant deficiency of prematurity) with injury to the alveolar epithelium, which causes hyaline membrane disease (HMD) and respiratory distress syndrome (RDS).[45] The administration of exogenous surfactants improves survival in these infants,[46] but bronchopulmonary dysplasia (BPD), a complication secondary to antenatal or postnatal injuries that can include hyperoxia and ventilatory therapy for RDS, frequently develops as a consequence.[47-50] Surfactant synthesis and mesenchymal thinning can be accelerated by glucocorticoids,[51,52] which are administered to mothers to prevent RDS and HMD when a premature birth is anticipated.[53,54]

SACCULAR STAGE (24 TO 38 WEEKS' GESTATIONAL AGE)

During the saccular stage of lung development, the terminal clusters of acinar tubules and buds dilate and expand into thin smooth-walled transitory alveolar ducts and saccules, and there is a marked reduction, or condensation, of the surrounding mesenchymal tissue. The lung continues to grow peripherally by branching and growth of the transitory ducts, so that by the end of this period, three additional generations of transitory alveolar ducts ending in terminal, or primary, saccules have formed. The peripheral regions of the lung also increase in size as a result of lengthening and widening of all segments distal to the terminal bronchioles (respiratory bronchioles, transitory alveolar ducts, and terminal saccules). Intersaccular and interductal septa develop, which include myofibroblasts at the tip and contain delicate collagen fibers and a double capillary network.[1] Overall, cell proliferation slows as a result of a sharp drop in division of the epithelial cell population.

With the reduction in epithelial cell proliferation comes ultrastructural evidence of cell differentiation. Maturation of type II AECs continues and is associated with increased synthesis of surfactant phospholipids,[37,55] the surfactant-associated proteins A, B, C, and D,[26,35,36,38-40,56] and ABCA3, a phospholipid transporter important for lamellar body formation.[57] Glycogen content is reduced, and mitochondrial enzyme activity increases, indicating a shift to aerobic oxidative pathways. Lamellar bodies increase in number and size, and increasing amounts of tubular myelin, the secretory form of pulmonary surfactant, are seen in the terminal air spaces.[41] The concentration of pulmonary surfactant is still low, however, and its phospholipid composition differs significantly from that at term.[37]

Squamous type I AECs continue to differentiate from type II AECs and line an increasing proportion of the surface area of the distal lung. Enlargement of the potential gas exchange surface is dependent on the development of type I AECs with their flattened and squamous cell shape. Capillaries become more closely associated with squamous type I AECs, decreasing the diffusion distance between the air spaces and the capillary bed. The basal lamina of the epithelium and endothelium fuse to form the thin-walled alveolar-capillary membrane. In the newborn and adult lung, the mean thickness of the alveolar-capillary membrane is 0.6 μm, which permits passive diffusion of oxygen and carbon dioxide between the alveolar lumen and the capillary bed.[1] Near the end of this stage, the interstitial tissue, or stroma, contains increasing amounts of ECM, and elastin is deposited in areas where future interalveolar septa will form, subdividing the terminal alveolar saccules into true alveoli. At this time, the immature lung contains relatively few elastin and collagen fibers, has little elastic recoil, and can be easily ruptured by mechanical ventilation.[14] Abnormalities associated with the saccular stage of lung development are similar to those associated with the canalicular stage of lung development, including pulmonary hypoplasia, alveolar capillary dysplasia with or without misaligned pulmonary veins, and respiratory insufficiency, resulting in RDS, HMD, and BPD in the premature infant (Table 55.3).

ALVEOLAR STAGE (36 WEEKS' GESTATIONAL AGE TO 8 YEARS POSTNATAL)

The alveolar stage is the last stage of lung development and is marked by the formation of secondary alveolar septa, which partition the transitory ducts and terminal saccules into true alveolar ducts and alveoli, as well as by the maturation of the alveolar-capillary membrane. This process, known as *alveologenesis*, greatly increases the surface area of the lung available for gas exchange. A key cell type that drives the formation of new secondary septa is the myofibroblast; these cells differentiate from progenitors in the lung mesenchyme. At the beginning of this stage, the alveolar septa are relatively thick and contain a capillary network on each side of a central core of connective tissue, often referred to as a *double capillary network*.[1] With the appearance of myofibroblasts at organized positions, their contractile property leads to lengthening and thinning of the secondary septa.[58,59] This is accompanied by the reduction of septal interstitial tissue, and remodeling of the capillary bed by fusion of the two septal capillary networks into one.[1] Pulmonary vascular resistance decreases just before birth, allowing increased blood flow and commencement of gas exchange.

This stage is accompanied by a phase of rapid cellular proliferation in both the epithelial and mesenchymal cell populations. Interstitial fibroblasts actively proliferate early in this stage, but then slow down as increased synthesis and deposition of collagen, elastin, and fibronectin occur. Endothelial growth is brisk throughout this stage, and dividing endothelial cells are located primarily in the developing secondary alveolar septal crests. Both type II and type I AECs increase in number during this stage, but only type II AECs are proliferating actively, while type I AECs are derived from type II AECs. Type I AECs are thought to be terminally differentiated and to lack the capacity for mitosis. Although type II AECs account for two thirds of the total number of AECs in the adult human lung, the larger squamous type I AECs actually occupy 93% of the total alveolar surface. Although type I AECs form a tight epithelial barrier that is impervious to extracellular fluid and ions, they are easily injured by oxidants, barotrauma, and infection, readily detaching from the alveolar wall when injured. Injury to the lung during this stage of development can result in abnormal remodeling of the lung with a reduction in the number of alveoli and the development of chronic interstitial lung disease. Additional factors that may cause disturbances in alveolarization include administration of glucocorticoids, which inhibit cellular proliferation and reduce septation and formation of alveoli. Conversely, glucocorticoid administration enhances thinning of the alveolar septa, increases maturation of type II AECs, and enhances the production of surfactant in the premature lung.[51-54]

Disorders associated with disturbances in the alveolar stage of lung development, which present at birth, include persistent fetal circulation and pulmonary hypertension of the newborn, BPD, congenital lobar emphysema, alveolar capillary dysplasia with or without misaligned pulmonary veins (often due to a FOXF-1 gene mutation), pulmonary hypoplasia, and RDS caused by surfactant deficiency due to mutations in the *SFTPB*, *SFTPC*, and *ABCA3* genes.[60-64]

EMBRYOLOGY OF THE PULMONARY CIRCULATION

Formation of the pulmonary circulation is linked directly to cardiovascular development, which begins on day 19 GA with formation of the lateral endocardial tubes.[12] Subsequent embryonic folding on day 20 GA brings the endocardial tubes together in the midline, where they fuse to form a single primitive heart tube, or truncus arteriosus. Simultaneously, both the outflow (dorsal aortae) and inflow (venous) tracts of the heart form in the dorsal mesenchyme and connect with the endocardial tubes before they fuse. During additional embryonic folding (days 23 to 28 GA), the cranial ends of the dorsal aortae are pulled ventrally until they form a dorsoventral loop, or the first aortic arch, connecting the upper end of the truncus arteriosus to the paired dorsal aortae. Four additional pairs of aortic arches develop over the next week from the aortic sac, an expansion of the cranial end of the truncus arteriosus, and connect to the dorsal aortae. These arches will form the major arteries of the head, neck, upper thorax, upper extremities, lungs, and dorsal aorta. Along with remodeling of the atrial and ventricular chambers (5 to 8 weeks' GA), the truncus arteriosus eventually splits vertically to form the ascending aorta and the main pulmonary artery, which is complete by week 8 of GA. During this period, the right and left pulmonary arteries arise from the paired sixth aortic arches and grow towards the lung, where their distal ends anastomose with

Table 55.3 Human Lung Malformations and Associated Disorders.

Developmental Stage	Malformations/Disorders
Embryonic 3–7 wk GA	Laryngeal, esophageal, tracheal agenesis/atresia Tracheo- and bronchoesophageal fistula Tracheal and bronchial stenosis Bronchogenic cysts Extralobar bronchopulmonary sequestration Pulmonary agenesis/aplasia Pulmonary vascular malformations/cardiac defects
Pseudoglandular 5–17 wk GA	Tracheo- and bronchomalacia Intralobar bronchopulmonary sequestration Cystic pulmonary airway malformation Congenital acinar aplasia/dysplasia Pulmonary hypoplasia/renal agenesis with oligohydramnios Pulmonary hypoplasia/congenital diaphragmatic hernia Congenital pulmonary lymphangiectasis Pulmonary vascular malformations/cardiovascular defects
Canalicular 16–26 wk GA	Pulmonary hypoplasia/oligohydramnios Congenital alveolar dysplasia Pulmonary arteriovenous malformations Pulmonary immaturity/surfactant deficiency Respiratory insufficiency/RDS
Saccular 24–38 wk GA	Pulmonary hypoplasia/oligohydramnios Alveolar capillary dysplasia with misaligned pulmonary veins Pulmonary immaturity/surfactant deficiency Respiratory insufficiency/RDS Hyaline membrane disease Bronchopulmonary dysplasia
Alveolar 36 wk GA–2 yr	Congenital lobar overinflation Pulmonary hypoplasia/oligohydramnios Alveolar capillary dysplasia with misaligned pulmonary veins Persistent fetal circulation/pulmonary hypertension Genetic surfactant deficiency/dysfunction Alveolar simplification/lung growth disorders

GA, Gestational age; *RDS*, respiratory distress syndrome.

the vascular plexus developing in the mesenchyme surrounding the bronchial buds. Subsequent growth and development of the pulmonary arteries follow branching of the bronchial tree (5 to 17 weeks' GA). The bronchial arteries, which develop later (between 20 and 32 weeks' GA), arise from the descending aorta and also supply blood to the lung.[65] Along with the esophageal arteries, the bronchial arteries are remnants of the original, segmental, arterial supply from the aorta to the foregut vascular plexus, which include vessels to the esophagus, trachea, and lung buds.

ABNORMAL DEVELOPMENT OF THE LUNG AND CONDUCTING AIRWAYS

As can be seen from Table 55.3, most pulmonary malformations arise during the embryonic and pseudoglandular stages of lung development. These malformations represent a spectrum of closely related abnormalities associated with lung bud formation, branching morphogenesis, separation of the trachea from the esophagus, and failure of the pleuroperitoneal cavity to close properly. Abnormalities in other organ systems, such as renal agenesis, dysplastic growth of the kidney, or congenital diaphragmatic hernia, may also affect branching morphogenesis of the lung during these early developmental stages. Later during the canalicular and saccular stages of lung development, abnormalities related to growth and maturation of the respiratory parenchyma and its vasculature predominate, leading to abnormalities in acinar development, alveolar capillary dysplasia, pulmonary hypoplasia, and respiratory insufficiency. Infants born prematurely during the saccular and early alveolar stages of development are also subject to acute lung injury following ventilation and supplemental oxygen treatment in the neonatal period, resulting in BPD or chronic interstitial lung disease. Postnatally, mutations in the surfactant-related genes *SFTPB*, *SFTPC*, and *ABCA3*, have been associated with pulmonary surfactant deficiency and/or dysfunction, causing respiratory distress and failure in term infants,[66,67] as well as chronic interstitial lung disease in older infants, children, adolescents, and adults.[63,68–75]

MALFORMATIONS OF THE TRACHEOBRONCHIAL TREE

These are a group of rare malformations caused by defective budding, branching, or separation of the primitive lung from the foregut during early lung development. Often these lesions result in obstruction of the airway, which subsequently causes secondary cystic or dysplastic changes in the lung.[76–78] There are several categories, including those that impact formation of (1) the tracheobronchial tree, such as tracheoesophageal fistulas (TEFs), tracheal and bronchial agenesis, stenosis, or malacia, bronchogenic cysts, and bronchopulmonary sequestration; (2) the distal lung parenchyma, such as pulmonary agenesis, acinar dysplasia, alveolar capillary dysplasia, and pulmonary hypoplasia; and (3) the pulmonary vasculature, including pulmonary artery agenesis, aberrant pulmonary arteries, anomalous pulmonary venous drainage, and pulmonary arteriovenous malformations (PAVMs).

Multiple congenital malformations in other organ systems are often found in conjunction with these early pulmonary lesions, including musculoskeletal, cardiovascular, gastrointestinal (GI), and genitourinary (GU) abnormalities. Either large-scale chromosomal disorders or single-gene mutations have been found to be associated with these malformations; they are known to impact developmental processes important for organogenesis, such as the maintenance of self-renewing progenitor/stem cells, cell proliferation and differentiation, or migration and adhesion.

TRACHEOESOPHAGEAL FISTULAS

Most congenital malformations of the tracheobronchial tree arise during early formation of the respiratory diverticulum and branching morphogenesis of the lung. One of the most critical events in the formation of the respiratory system is the initial separation of the common definitive foregut into the respiratory and digestive tracts. This process begins during the third week of gestation and is complete by the sixth week. Failure of this process to proceed normally results in the formation of a TEF, one of the most commonly encountered abnormalities of the trachea. TEFs have an incidence of 1 in 3500 live births and are usually found in combination with various forms of esophageal atresia (EA).[79–82] The most common combination, accounting for 80% to 90% of all TEF cases, is EA with a lower, or distal, fistula where the upper segment of the esophagus ends in a blind pouch and the lower segment originates from the trachea just above the bifurcation into right and left main stem bronchi.[83] Other combinations are (1) an isolated EA without a fistula (8%); (2) an isolated, or common, fistula without EA (4%); (3) EA with a proximal fistula connecting the upper esophagus to the trachea, whereas the lower esophagus ends in a blind pouch (1%); and (4) EA with a double fistula, where both upper and lower portions of the esophagus join the trachea at separate points along its length (1%). In cases where both the trachea and esophagus are present and just defectively connected, the anomalies do not interfere with cellular differentiation, so that the tracheal segments contain pseudostratified ciliated epithelium and cartilaginous rings, whereas the esophageal segments contain stratified squamous epithelium and muscle.[65]

Survival from isolated TEF is almost 100% in term infants, but in low-birth-weight infants TEF is often associated with a variety of other organ malformations and carries a high risk of a poor outcome. Overall, 50% of all TEFs are associated with multiple organ abnormalities, the most common being cardiac malformations (13%), followed by skeletal defects (11%), anal atresia (10%), and renal malformations (17%).[84] For example, TEF with EA is found in 50% to 80% of patients with VATER/VACTERL syndrome (OMIM #192350), in association with multiple developmental malformations, including vertebral anomalies, anal atresia, cardiac defects, renal anomalies, and limb abnormalities.[85–87] Although the majority of EA/TEF cases (90%) arise as sporadic events with a low risk of recurrence,[84] a familial form of EA/TEF has been described in 30% to 40% of those with Feingold syndrome (OMIM #164280), which is also characterized by duodenal atresia, digital abnormalities, and microcephaly.[84]

Multiple congenital abnormalities and/or syndromes involving chromosomal disorders or single gene mutations have been associated with EA/TEF. For instance, chromosomal anomalies have been reported in 6% to 10% of EA/TEF patients with trisomy 18 (Edwards syndrome) and trisomy 21 (Down syndrome, OMIM #190685),[84,84,88] whereas single-gene mutations have been reported in Feingold, VATER/VACTERL, and Pallister-Hall (OMIM #146510) syndromes. Feingold syndrome is caused by heterozygous mutations in the oncogene *MYCN* (OMIM *164840), which is downstream of SHH signaling and regulates cell proliferation. VATER/VACTERL syndrome is caused by heterozygous mutations in the transcription factor, HOXD13 (OMIM *142989), a gene important for cell adhesion, which is also downstream of the SHH signaling pathway. TEF, tracheal stenosis, and pulmonary agenesis have been observed in some patients with Pallister-Hall syndrome (OMIM #146510), which is caused by mutations in the *GLI3* gene (OMIM *165240), a downstream transducer of the SHH signaling pathway that is active in mesenchymal cells.[89–91] Patients with *GLI3* mutations also exhibit malformations in the central nervous system (hypothalamic hamartoblastoma, pituitary aplasia/dysplasia), craniofacial features, limbs (postaxial polydactyly), kidneys (renal dysplasia), adrenals (adrenal hypoplasia), and heart.[85]

The incidence of EA is 100% in AEG syndrome (anophthalmia, esophageal, genital; OMIM #206900), which is caused by heterozygous mutations in *SOX2* (OMIM *184429), a transcription factor essential for maintenance of self-renewing progenitor/stem cells. EA/TEF occurs in 10% of patients with CHARGE syndrome (coloboma of the eye, heart defects, choanal atresia, retarded growth, genital hypoplasia, and ear anomalies, OMIM #214800), which is caused by heterozygous mutations in the transcriptional regulator, CHD7 (OMIM *608892), an important nuclear cofactor for *SOX2* activity.

TRACHEAL AGENESIS

Tracheal agenesis is a rare but fatal malformation with a prevalence of 1 in 50,000,[92] involving complete (8%) or partial absence of the trachea below the larynx. Approximately 53% of cases are associated with premature delivery. Classification of anatomic variations in this malformation is based on the length of the agenetic segment and the presence or absence of EA.[65,93,94] The most common variation is complete absence of the trachea below the larynx with the right and left main stem bronchi forming a common airway that is connected to the esophagus (56%). Other variations include (1) tracheal agenesis with fistulas connecting each main stem bronchi to the esophagus (10%); (2) agenesis of the proximal trachea with the main stem bronchi fused to form the distal trachea with (5%) or without (5%) a TEF; (3) a short segment of proximal trachea connected to the esophagus; (4) proximal and distal segments of the trachea, linked by a short atretic, or cordlike, fibrous band of tissue (5%); and (5) tracheal agenesis with an atretic strand joining the larynx to a distal tracheal segment with a fistula joining it to the esophagus (10%). As for EA/TEF, other congenital abnormalities are present in most cases, including additional lower respiratory tract malformations, such as abnormal lobe formation, and complex cardiac defects with a high incidence of abnormal vessels.[94]

TRACHEAL STENOSIS

Tracheal stenosis is also a rare malformation in which the trachea is narrowed, because of either intrinsic abnormalities in cartilage formation or extrinsic compression by abnormal vessel formation, such as vascular rings.[81,95] Narrowing of the trachea by compression results in local obstruction to the passage of air, whereas cartilage deformities may cause more widespread obstruction of the airway on both inspiration and expiration. The major underlying causes of intrinsic tracheal stenosis are abnormalities in cartilaginous ring formation, either due to posterior fusion of the normally C-shaped rings or to formation of a complete cartilaginous sleeve.[65] Generalized or complete stenosis is found in 30% of all cases, whereas segmental tracheal stenosis with local narrowing of the trachea, is seen in 50% of all cases and may occur anywhere along the tracheobronchial tree.[96] Segmental tracheal stenosis has been reported in children with craniosynostosis syndrome, including Apert (OMIM #101200), Pfeiffer (OMIM #101600), and Crouzon (OMIM #123500) syndromes.[85,97-102] These syndromes involve abnormal fusion of skeletal or osseous structures and are associated with heterozygous mutations in the fibroblast growth factor receptors, *FGFR2* (OMIM *176943) and *FGFR1* (OMIM *136350).[85,103-106] Craniosynostosis, cleft palate, and tracheal stenosis, with thickened, cartilaginous tracheal sleeves and atelectasis of the distal lung, have also been observed in transgenic mice wherein *Fgfr2* has been mutated or partially deleted.[107,108] These malformations represent mesenchymal defects in which the cells do not respond normally to FGF signaling, affecting both chondrogenesis and osteogenesis. As for TEF and tracheal agenesis, patients with congenital tracheal stenosis have other malformations, including additional airway and lung abnormalities, esophageal and diaphragmatic abnormalities, and cardiovascular, skeletal, GU, and GI tract anomalies.[65,109,110]

Tracheal abnormalities consistent with intrinsic tracheal stenosis have been reported in young children with cystic fibrosis (CF) (OMIM #219700), as well as in genetic animal models of CF caused by mutations or deletion of the *CFTR* gene (OMIM *602421). Neonatal CF pigs demonstrated luminal narrowing of both the trachea and main stem bronchi, as well as irregularly shaped cartilage rings, hypoplastic submucosal glands, and abnormal airway smooth muscle.[111] Likewise, previously published morphometric data and chest computed tomography scans from neonates with CF (<2 weeks old) showed alterations in the circular shape of the trachea and narrowing of the tracheal lumen.[111] Subsequent functional studies demonstrated air trapping and airflow obstruction in young children with CF,[112] as well as in the neonatal CF pig.[113] Previous studies in *Cftr* knockout and/or mutated mice also revealed disrupted or incomplete tracheal rings with tracheal stenosis in the upper trachea, as well as altered breathing patterns in both newborn and adult mutant mice.[114,115]

Extrinsic tracheal stenosis is caused by external compression of the trachea, usually associated with abnormally situated blood vessels, which are termed *vascular rings*.[93,110] These can include a double aortic arch, a right aortic arch with a left ligamentum arteriosum, an aberrant (retroesophageal) right subclavian artery, a right aortic arch with aberrant left subclavian artery, an anomalous left innominate or carotid artery, or a pulmonary artery sling (retrotracheal), which is found in 20% of tracheal stenosis cases.[96,110] In the case of pulmonary artery sling, the left pulmonary artery originates from the right pulmonary artery, encircling and compressing the right main stem bronchus and distal trachea.

TRACHEOMALACIA

Congenital, or primary, tracheomalacia occurs when there is an absence or abnormality of the cartilaginous rings with hypotonia of the muscular or membranous posterior wall (the trachealis muscle), which causes the trachea to collapse on expiration, obstructing the airway.[81,95] It is the most common congenital abnormality of the trachea with an estimated incidence of 1 per 1445 infants.[116] Primary tracheomalacia is caused by congenital immaturity of the tracheal cartilage but is often associated with marked redundancy of tissue growth in the posterior wall. In the normal trachea, the cartilage-to-soft tissue ratio is 4.5:1, a ratio that remains constant throughout childhood. In primary tracheomalacia, this ratio is reduced, in some instances as low as 2:1.[93,95,116] Most affected infants improve by 6 to 12 months of age, as the structural integrity of the trachea is gradually restored by further cartilage development and growth of the trachea.[65] Tracheomalacia may be associated with other lung/foregut defects, such as TEF, EA, and BPD.[116] It is often seen in connective tissue disorders, resulting in the formation of abnormal cartilaginous structures.[116] Tracheo- and bronchomalacia have been associated with Costello, or faciocutaneoskeletal, syndrome (OMIM #218040), which is caused by sporadic, autosomal dominant, heterozygous mutations in the *HRAS* gene (OMIM *190020), a member of the RAS family of small GTPases, which regulates cell division in response to growth factors. This is a rare syndrome with multiple congenital anomalies, most likely caused by abnormal cell division and cell overgrowth.

BRONCHIAL ATRESIA, STENOSIS, AND MALACIA

Bronchial atresia is a rare anomaly and is often identified as an incidental finding on chest x-ray. The most commonly affected lobe is the left upper lobe, but bronchial atresia of the right upper and lower lobes has also been reported. The segmental bronchus is the more common site of atresia, but subsegmental and lobar bronchi can also be affected.[81,95] The lung distal to the obstruction may be hypoplastic, emphysematous, or hyperinflated. Air may enter the affected lobe via collateral airways, causing mild overinflation or air trapping, whereas mucus may accumulate in the distal bronchial segments, causing a mucus plug or a mucus-filled cyst. Often there is loss of bronchi and vessels in the affected lobe, as well as absence of segmentation and interlobular septa.

Like tracheal stenosis, bronchial stenosis may be intrinsic or extrinsic, the latter due to external compression.[117] Intrinsic bronchial stenosis is rare and is usually associated with anomalous cartilage segmentation. Extrinsic bronchial stenosis due to external compression is usually associated with congenital heart disease. Compression occurs when the pulmonary arteries enlarge in response to pulmonary hypertension, compressing the left upper lobe bronchus. An enlarged left atrium, a bronchogenic cyst, or a teratoma may also compress the left main bronchus.

Bronchomalacia, or dynamic narrowing of the bronchi, is caused by congenital abnormalities in the bronchial cartilage, which leads to collapse, or bronchiectasis, of the affected airway during respiration. Primary bronchomalacia is a relatively common abnormality of the lower airways and is often associated with tracheomalacia. A variation of this is seen in Williams-Campbell syndrome (OMIM 211450), a familial disorder characterized by absent, diminished, or immature bronchial cartilage distal to the main segmental bronchi, resulting in bronchiectasis. Primary bronchomalacia may be associated with other anomalies, such as skeletal dysplasia, or diffuse congenital cartilage deficiency.[95] Secondary bronchomalacia may be caused by extrinsic compression, either from an enlarged vessel, a vascular ring, or a bronchogenic cyst.

Additional malformations of the bronchi include abnormal branching patterns that give rise to both minor and major anomalies.[82] Minor anomalies (or variations) include displaced lobar and apical bronchi, supernumerary lobar and apical bronchi, aberrant lobar bronchi, trifurcation of the left upper lobe bronchus, and double-stem superior segments of the lower lobe bronchi. Major anomalies include tracheal origin of the right upper lobe bronchus, which is associated with recurrent episodes of pneumonia.[82]

BRONCHOGENIC CYSTS

Abnormal budding of the ventral foregut during the embryonic stage of lung development causes bronchogenic cysts, also known as foregut duplications. Bronchogenic cysts are commonly found in the mediastinum, close to the trachea or main stem bronchi, and rarely communicate with the tracheobronchial tree. Bronchogenic cysts may also be found in the peripheral lung, most commonly in the lower lobes, and arise from abnormal branching of the tracheobronchial tree at a later time.[78,81,117-121] Approximately two-thirds are located in the mediastinum and one-third in the parenchyma. Although bronchogenic cysts are rare, with an incidence of 1 per 68,000,[121] they are the most common primary cyst of the mediastinum.[78,122]

Bronchogenic cysts located in the mediastinum may arise at any point along the tracheobronchial tree, commonly in paraesophageal, paratracheal, carinal, or hilar locations with the carinal location being the most frequent.[81,121] Although bronchogenic cysts do not communicate with the conducting airway, they may be attached to the trachea or bronchus by a strand of tissue. Bronchogenic cysts found in the lungs as peripheral cysts (usually in the medial third of the lung) may or may not communicate with the tracheobronchial tree.[81] Bronchogenic cysts are typically solitary, unilocular, thin-walled, cystic cavities that are filled with fluid or mucus. They are lined with bronchial epithelium composed of pseudostratified, ciliated, columnar or cuboidal, epithelial cells, and their walls contain cartilage, smooth muscle, and mucus glands.

BRONCHOPULMONARY SEQUESTRATION

This malformation develops as a mass of abnormal pulmonary tissue, which is not connected to the tracheobronchial tree and receives its blood supply from one or more anomalous systemic arteries arising from the aorta.[95,117,123,124] There are two forms of bronchopulmonary sequestration, intralobar and extralobar. Intralobar sequestrations (ILSs) are contiguous with the lung, sharing a common visceral pleura and venous drainage into the pulmonary veins. Extralobar sequestrations (ELSs) are anatomically separate from the lung, with a distinct pleural covering and venous drainage to systemic veins. ILSs are more common than ELSs, accounting for 75% to 80% of all cases of bronchopulmonary sequestration.[78,125,126] Both types of sequestration occur more frequently on the left side, sometimes in association with diaphragmatic defects. Rarely, a sequestration may be connected to the esophagus or to the stomach. Bronchopulmonary sequestration is most likely caused by formation of a supernumerary, or accessory, lung bud ventral to the primitive foregut. ILS results if the accessory lung bud develops before formation of the pleura, whereas ELS develops after formation of the pleura, and it becomes invested with its own pleural covering.[126]

ILSs are found most frequently in the posterior basal segment of the left lower lobe. The blood supply is derived from either the thoracic or abdominal aorta, whereas the venous drainage is to the pulmonary vein of the affected lobe. The affected tissue is often cystic, lined with either columnar or cuboidal epithelium, and filled with mucus. Although many cases of ILS occur in children, at least half of affected patients are over 20 years old when the diagnosis is made.[124,127]

ELSs develop as a separate but complete segment of pulmonary tissue (or accessory lobe), enclosed within its own pleural sac. ELS usually occurs on the lower left side of the thorax, often between the left lower lobe and the diaphragm. Other extrapulmonary sites of sequestration include paraesophageal, mediastinal, or paracardiac regions, as well as within the muscle of the diaphragm or below the diaphragm in the retroperitoneum. The arterial supply is from the abdominal aorta or one of its branches, whereas the venous drainage is into the azygous system or inferior vena cava, creating a left-to-right shunt. Histologically, the lesion may be composed of normal lung or immature or dysplastic pulmonary parenchyma, with absent or reduced cartilaginous bronchi and an irregular pattern of bronchiolar-like structures resembling congenital pulmonary airway malformations (discussed later). Most ELSs are found in children younger than 6 months of age, but the lesion occurs in older children and adults as well. This malformation is frequently associated with other congenital anomalies, especially congenital diaphragmatic hernia, which occurs in ~16% of cases.[78,124,127,128] Additional congenital lung abnormalities are present in 25% of ELSs, including pulmonary hypoplasia, congenital pulmonary adenomatous malformation (CPAM), congenital lobar overinflation, congenital pulmonary lymphangiectasia, and bronchogenic cysts. Cardiac abnormalities, foregut duplication cysts, chest wall and vertebral deformities, hindgut duplications, and accessory spleen can also be seen. Interestingly, bronchial atresia is often associated with both ILS and ELS,[129] whereas CPAM is present in 91% of both types of bronchopulmonary sequestration, suggesting that these malformations have a common etiology that may vary depending on timing, duration, or extent of the lesion.

MALFORMATIONS OF THE LUNG PARENCHYMA

PULMONARY AGENESIS AND APLASIA

Pulmonary agenesis (or atresia) and aplasia represent two different forms of arrested lung development that result in absence of the distal lung parenchyma.[81,95] Pulmonary agenesis is the complete absence of one or both lungs, including bronchi, bronchioles, vasculature, and respiratory parenchyma. In pulmonary aplasia, only rudimentary bronchi are present, each of which ends in a blind pouch, with no pulmonary vessels or respiratory parenchyma. Bronchial hypoplasia with variable reduction in lung tissue (hypoplasia) has also been reported.[95] The incidence of these anomalies is rare (1 in 100,000 births) and represents failure of the primitive foregut branches, or lung buds, to develop during the early, embryonic stage of lung development. Developmental arrest at a later stage may result in lobar agenesis or pulmonary dysplasia; some bronchial elements are present, but there are no alveoli. Pulmonary agenesis is frequently associated with other congenital anomalies of the lung, such as tracheal stenosis, EA, TEF, and bronchogenic cysts, as well as cardiac defects including patent ductus arteriosus, tetralogy of Fallot, and anomalies of the great vessels.

Bilateral agenesis of the lung is very rare, and only a small number of cases have been reported.[65] In one case, a trachea with 10 cartilaginous rings remained connected to the esophagus throughout its length. There were no lung buds or pleural cavities. In another case, the trachea was separated from the esophagus, but ended blindly with only two cartilaginous rings. In several other cases, branching morphogenesis was arrested at the bronchial bud stage.

Unilateral pulmonary agenesis is more common than bilateral pulmonary agenesis and may affect either lung, although the right side is more commonly affected. Patients with isolated unilateral pulmonary agenesis (25% of all cases) have a better prognosis than those with additional congenital abnormalities.[130] There are usually no serious clinical consequences owing to compensatory growth, or hyperplasia, of the contralateral lung, and often individuals with isolated unilateral pulmonary agenesis can live without limitations. Despite concerns related to diminished lung capacity and susceptibility to recurrent pulmonary infections, isolated unilateral pulmonary agenesis has been diagnosed incidentally in adults, providing further evidence that unilateral pulmonary agenesis can be associated with adequate respiratory function.[131,132]

These defects arise in early lung development, when the respiratory primordium bifurcates into the right and left primitive lung (bronchial) buds at the end of the fourth week of gestation. This is coincident with development of the first and second pharyngeal aortic arches and outgrowth of the forelimb bud. Each of these tissues is supplied by blood flow from specific regions of the aortic arch. It has been suggested that anomalous formation of the sixth aortic arch, which supplies the developing lung bud, causes primary agenesis of the pulmonary arteries, resulting in pulmonary agenesis.[133,134] Likewise, malformation of the first and second aortic arch segments would disrupt blood flow to the face, whereas malformation of the fourth aortic arch would disrupt blood flow to the developing limbs. This would explain the striking association of pulmonary agenesis with facial and limb defects,[133] as well as with DiGeorge-velocardiofacial syndrome (multiple OMIM entries involving regional disruption of chromosome 22q11.2), which exhibits cardiac defects, including interrupted aortic arch.[135] Alternative hypotheses include disruption of the inductive mechanisms responsible for early lung specification, including FGF, WNT, SHH and TGFβ/BMP signaling pathways and lung-specific transcription factors, such as *NKX2-1,* a homeobox gene critical for lung development.

Identification of *NKX2-1* (OMIM *600635) mutations in patients with brain-lung-thyroid syndrome (OMIM #610878) and corresponding phenotypes in *NKX2-1*-deficient mice (null and phosphorylation mutants), established *NKX2-1* as a critical gene driving lung development. *NKX2-1* encodes the protein TTF1. Expression of TTF1 is restricted to the developing lung, thyroid, and ventral forebrain, sites of expression that correspond with a defined group of syndromes, including respiratory distress, congenital hypothyroidism, and benign hereditary chorea, exhibited by patients with heterozygous *NKX2-1* mutations, as well as whole-gene deletions.[136-139] Although the pulmonary histopathology is heterogeneous, there are often clear growth abnormalities with alveolar simplification, lobular remodeling, and cyst formation in the lungs of these patients.[138] Related phenotypes in *NKX2-1*-deficient mice provide evidence for TTF1 loss or disruption as a cause for the human syndrome. Heterozygous *NKX2-1* loss in mice results in neurologic and thyroid dysfunctions, whereas homozygous deletion results in complete absence of the thyroid, as well as severe brain defects and lung hypoplasia.[136,140] The lungs in *NKX2-1*-null mice consist of bilateral saclike structures that originate from a common tracheoesophageal tube.[141]

Pulmonary agenesis is associated with malformations in other organ systems, including cardiovascular, GI, skeletal, GU, and the upper respiratory tract, as well as with limb and facial defects.[130,133] In fact, multiple congenital anomalies are detected in ~75% of cases with unilateral pulmonary agenesis. Pulmonary agenesis has been reported in several syndromes, including Mardini-Nyhan syndrome (OMIM %601612),[142] Goldenhar syndrome,[143] trisomy 21,[144] VATER/VACTERL syndrome (OMIM #192350), and DiGeorge syndrome with sporadic microdeletions in 22q11.2.[130]

PULMONARY DYSPLASIA

These are a group of fatal lung disorders that include congenital acinar dysplasia, congenital alveolar dysplasia, and alveolar capillary dysplasia with or without misalignment of the pulmonary veins (MPV).[145-150] Infants with these disorders have persistent pulmonary hypertension and unexplained severe respiratory distress requiring ventilation and/or ECMO; they deteriorate quickly when support is withdrawn.

These disorders represent a rare form of diffuse interstitial lung disease characterized by uniform developmental impairment of the distal pulmonary airspaces, or pulmonary acini, resulting in severe pulmonary hypoplasia. Although there is considerable overlap between the clinical and histologic features of these disorders, acinar dysplasia is the most severe phenotype, exhibiting an almost complete lack of mature alveoli, with little to no development of the pulmonary acini distal to the bronchioles. The lung lobules are composed of bronchioles lined by ciliated columnar epithelia surrounded by smooth muscle fibers, which terminate directly at the pleura and interlobular septa. Although acinar dysplasia is thought to represent arrest in the early pseudoglandular stage of lung development (8 to 16 weeks), the bronchiolar epithelium is well differentiated and representative of the term lung.[151] In some cases, a few immature canalicular or saccular structures may be found, but this is rare.[149] In comparison, congenital alveolar dysplasia represents arrest of acinar development in the late canalicular or early saccular stage of lung development (17 to 24 weeks) with the formation of primitive, somewhat simplified canalicular and/or saccular structures.[146,149] The airspaces have elongated primary septa, but secondary septation is incomplete. The interstitial regions are expanded and composed of loose, primitive mesenchyme with little collagen. Although the capillary bed is extensive, only a few of the capillaries are located adjacent to the epithelial surface of the distal airspaces. Thus, development of the alveolar-capillary membrane is impaired and gas exchange is severely compromised.

Alveolar capillary dysplasia (ACD) is similar to congenital alveolar dysplasia but exhibits reduced alveolar capillary formation, as well as ACD/MPV. In general, the capillaries are located in the interior of thickened alveolar septa instead of in close proximity to the alveolar epithelia.[145,147,148] Although the largest pulmonary veins may be located in the interlobular septa, the smaller pulmonary veins are displaced, or "misaligned," in that they are located adjacent to the pulmonary arteries in the peribronchiolar connective tissue.[148] Both the pulmonary veins and the lymphatic vessels are thin-walled and dilated, whereas there is increased medial hypertrophy and hyperplasia of the pulmonary arteries and muscularization of the smaller, peripheral arterioles. One third of the patients have lymphangiectasis. In addition, there is significant underdevelopment of the pulmonary lobules with reduction and simplification of the distal acinar structures with some alveolar type II AEC hyperplasia.[145] Three-dimensional reconstruction of lung tissue from patients with ACD/MPV demonstrated that there is a right-to-left vascular shunt linking the pulmonary and systemic circulation, which bypasses the alveolar capillary bed and causes respiratory insufficiency and persistent hypertension.[152] Patients with ACD/MPV often have additional organ abnormalities, including GI, GU, musculoskeletal, and cardiovascular malformations, as well as disruption of the normal left-right asymmetry of intrathoracic or intra-abdominal organs.[147,153-155] At least 60 distinct mutations and/or genomic deletions in *FOXF1* (OMIM *601089), a transcription factor important for vascular and alveolar development, have been identified in patients with ACD/MPV.[156] Most are sporadic, autosomal dominant mutations, although several have been inherited as autosomal recessive disorders with maternal inheritance, consistent with paternal imprinting.[157]

PULMONARY HYPOPLASIA AND CONGENITAL DIAPHRAGMATIC HERNIA

Pulmonary hypoplasia is defined as incomplete development of the lungs, resulting in a reduction in the number or size of the bronchopulmonary segments or pulmonary acini. It usually occurs as a result of other fetal abnormalities, such as congenital diaphragmatic hernia or renal agenesis, which interfere with normal lung development. It is a common cause of neonatal death[158] and is frequently associated with stillbirths. Incidence ranges from 9 to 14 per 10,000 births.[159] Lung weight, lung weight:body weight ratios, radial alveolar counts, and lung volume measurements are often used to determine the presence of pulmonary hypoplasia.[82] For example, the normal lung-to-body weight ratio for term infants is ~1.79%, for congenital diaphragmatic hernia, it is 0.98%, and for severe renal anomalies, 1.4%.[160] At autopsy, the lungs may be uniformly reduced in size or markedly asymmetric in the case of congenital diaphragmatic hernia. Histologically, the alveoli are small for GA, but alveolar and capillary development is normal.

Primary pulmonary hypoplasia is rare and occurs in the absence of any other identifiable cause or association. It is thought to result from alterations in transcription factor and/or growth factor signaling.[161] For example, retinoic acid signaling deficiencies in animal models result in severe respiratory phenotypes, including lung hypoplasia and agenesis.[162,163] Retinoic acid also influences perinatal alveolus formation, which has led to its clinical use for the prevention of BPD.[164,165]

Pulmonary hypoplasia can be seen in association with chromosomal abnormalities, including trisomy 13, 18, and 20, and as a component of multiple syndromes including Scimitar (OMIM #608281), Down (OMIM #190685), Eagle-Barret, and Pena-Ahokeir syndromes.[82] Developmental lung abnormalities, including pulmonary hypoplasia, abnormal pulmonary lobation, and anomalies of laryngeal and tracheal development, are also relatively common in Smith-Lemli-Opitz syndrome (OMIM #270400), an autosomal recessive malformation syndrome caused by mutations in the *DHCR7* gene (OMIM *602858), which encodes the enzyme 7-dehydrocholesterol reductase that catalyzes the final step in cholesterol biosynthesis.[166] *Dhcr7*-null mice, a model for the human disease, die within 24 hours of birth with lung saccular hypoplasia characterized by failure to terminally differentiate alveolar sacs, delayed differentiation of type I AECs and an immature vascular network.[167] Approximately one quarter of Smith-Lemli-Opitz syndrome patients also have renal anomalies, including renal hypoplasia or agenesis, which may contribute to the lung hypoplasia.[166]

Secondary pulmonary hypoplasia, which accounts for more than 85% of all cases, occurs in association with other abnormalities in the developing fetus,[82,168] the most frequent being congenital diaphragmatic hernia and renal defects, such as renal agenesis or dysplasia, polycystic renal disease, and urinary outlet obstruction (obstructive uropathy). Many of these abnormalities cause a reduction in the volume of the thoracic cavity, which physically restricts the growth of the peripheral lung. Thoracic space-occupying lesions include CPAM, bronchopulmonary sequestration, mediastinal masses, and lymphatic malformations. Disturbances in the production of fetal lung fluid, fetal breathing, loss of amniotic fluid (as in prolonged rupture of membranes), pleural effusion, or external compression of the thoracic cavity can all cause defects in the growth and/or expansion of the distal respiratory parenchyma, resulting in a reduced number of alveoli.

In congenital diaphragmatic hernia, which is the most common cause of pulmonary hypoplasia, the diaphragm fails to close.[95] This allows the developing abdominal viscera to bulge into the thoracic cavity and stunts the growth of the lung. Usually, the left side of the diaphragm is involved more often than the right, probably because the left pericardioperitoneal canal is larger and closes later than the right. The severity of the resulting pulmonary hypoplasia varies depending on the timing of the onset of compression. With early, severe compression of the lung, there is marked hypoplasia, resulting in the affected lung being less than half the weight of the contralateral lung. This is accompanied by a decrease in alveolar number and size, decreased gas-exchange surface area, and a proportional decrease in the pulmonary vasculature. Often there is evidence of severe pulmonary hypertension, most likely due to an increased proportion of muscular arteries in the periphery of the lung, which results in increased pulmonary vascular resistance.

CONGENITAL LOBAR OVERINFLATION

Congenital lobar overinflation (also known as *congenital* or *infantile lobar emphysema*) is overdistension or hyperplasia of an individual pulmonary lobe or segment, in response to partial or complete bronchial obstruction.[81,117] It is a rare condition with a prevalence of 1 per 20,000 to 30,000 deliveries.[128] The upper lobes are involved in over 95% of cases,[82] whereas multiple lobe involvement is seen in ~5% of cases.[82] Compression of the remaining, uninvolved, ipsilateral lung or lobes often occurs. Most cases are caused by partial bronchial obstruction due to intrinsic bronchial abnormalities, such as bronchial atresia, bronchial stenosis, and bronchial cartilaginous dysplasia with absent or incomplete cartilage rings. These abnormal bronchi collapse during expiration, leading to distal air trapping and overinflation of the affected lobe.[82,169] In regional or segmental pulmonary overinflation, only a small segment of the lung is hyperinflated, usually due to bronchial atresia. Extrinsic bronchial obstruction may be caused by vascular abnormalities such as pulmonary artery sling, anomalous pulmonary venous return, or a left-to-right shunt (patent ductus arteriosus) with increased blood flow through the pulmonary arteries. Intrathoracic masses, such as bronchogenic cysts, ELSs, and enlarged lymph nodes, also cause bronchial compression. Intrinsic bronchial obstruction is most often related to defects in the bronchial cartilage with absent or incomplete rings. Additional causes of intrinsic bronchial obstruction include mucus plugs, bronchial mucosal folds, or torsion of the bronchus. Abnormalities in other organ systems are seen ~40% of patients with lobar overinflation, most commonly (70%) in the cardiovascular system.[82,169] Less commonly, congenital lobar overinflation is associated with renal, GI, musculoskeletal, and cutaneous malformations.[128]

There are two different patterns of congenital lobar overinflation.[82] Most (70%) exhibit normal numbers of well-developed alveoli that are uniformly overdistended, and 3 to 10 times larger than normal. The remaining cases (30%) appear to have a more complex polyalveolar pattern of acinar formation with a larger number of alveoli than would be expected for the age of the child[82]; the lung is hyperplastic with little overdistension of the alveoli. It has been suggested that this is caused by severe or complete bronchial obstruction during early lung development, leading to accelerated lung growth similar to that seen in tracheal atresia or tracheal occlusion. Postnatally, the partially obstructed lobe becomes progressively hyperinflated due to gas-trapping distal to the obstruction and can require lobectomy as a surgical emergency. In these cases, the lung tissue itself can appear histologically normal except for the hyperinflation, suggesting an important postnatal role for the stenotic airway lesion.

CONGENITAL PULMONARY AIRWAY MALFORMATIONS

CPAMs (formerly termed *congenital cystic adenomatoid malformations*) are a heterogeneous group of cystic and noncystic lung lesions caused by abnormal fetal lung development. Although rare, CPAMs account for 30% to 40% of all congenital lung disease and ~95% of all congenital cystic lung diseases.[170-172] CPAMs are most often found in the lungs of infants and have features of malformation and/or immaturity of the small airways and distal lung parenchyma.[81,95,117,123] There are five types of CPAM, which are classified on the basis of size and histologic features. Type 0 lesions are rare and composed of 0.5-cm, bronchial-like, cystic structures with abundant cartilage in their wall, as well as glands and smooth muscle. Type 1 lesions are the most common, accounting for 65% of all cases,[83] and are composed of one or more large cysts ranging in size from 3 to 10 cm in diameter. These lesions resemble bronchi and/or proximal bronchioles and contain fibrous septa lined by pseudostratified, ciliated columnar or cuboidal cells, with clusters of mucus-filled cells resembling goblet cells. Cartilaginous foci are also present in 5% to 10% of these lesions. Type 2 lesions are the second most common, accounting for 10% to 15% of cases, and are characterized by evenly spaced, small, uniform cysts that are usually less than 2 cm in diameter. These bronchiolar-like structures are lined by cuboidal and/or ciliated columnar cells.[82] Type 3 lesions (5% of cases) are composed of large, solid air-containing masses of tissue with multiple, microscopic cysts of less than 0.2 cm that produce a mediastinal shift, often resulting in hypoplasia of the uninvolved lung. Histologically, the lesions are comprised of immature-appearing lung that is devoid of bronchi, consisting of bronchiolar-like structures surrounded by alveolar ducts and saccules lined by cuboidal or low columnar epithelial cells. Type 4 lesions are found in the peripheral lung and are characterized by large (up to 7 cm in diameter), thin-walled cysts that are lined by type I and/or type II AECs.[173] This variant typically presents in the newborn to 4 years of age range and accounts for 10% to 15% of cases. The morphology, cellular phenotypes, radiologic findings, and clinical presentation of type 4 CPAM are indistinguishable from cystic pleuropulmonary blastoma and likely represent the same lesion.[76,172,174,175] Cystic pleuropulmonary blastoma is a neoplastic process with the potential to progress to an overt sarcoma.

Immunohistochemical analysis of cell differentiation markers for specific pulmonary epithelial cells revealed that CPAM types 1, 2, and 3 contained clusters of gastrin-releasing peptide (GRP)-positive neuroendocrine cells and SCGB1A1-positive club cells, demonstrating a bronchiolar origin for these cysts.[173] The epithelial linings of CPAM type 4 cysts were immunopositive for a type I AEC-associated surface antigen and the type II AEC surfactant-associated proteins, SFTPA, SFTPB, and SFTPC.[173] These findings suggest that CPAM types 1, 2, and 3 arise during the embryonic and pseudoglandular stage of branching morphogenesis, whereas CPAM type 4 arises during the canalicular and/or saccular stage of acinar development.

CPAMs usually present as sporadic, nonhereditary lung abnormalities that are associated with other anomalies in 15% to 20% of cases, particularly in the cases of type 2 lesions.[82,170,174] The pathogenesis of CPAM remains unknown. These lesions are thought to result from abnormal branching morphogenesis during lung development. It has been proposed that airway obstruction is the basis for CPAM.[82,129,168,176] CPAMs usually communicate with the tracheobronchial tree and receive blood supply from pulmonary vessels, which differentiates CPAM from bronchopulmonary sequestration that has a systemic blood supply.[78,172] Hypothesized mechanisms for CPAM development are (1) failure of appropriate endoderm-mesoderm signaling, (2) imbalance between increased cell proliferation and decreased programmed apoptotic cell death, (3) altered gene expression, and (4) aberrant growth factor signaling during lung morphogenesis.[128,168] Experimental studies including genetic modifications in mouse models identify Ras, PI3K-AKT-mTOR, FGF-7, FGF-9, FGF-10, FRIZZLED2, HOXB-5, and SOX-2 as potential molecular mediators of CPAM.[128,168,177-184] A genetic basis for CPAM type 0 is supported by a tendency for the lesions to recur in families in up to 40% of cases, suggesting an autosomal dominant inheritance pattern.[185]

MALFORMATIONS OF THE PULMONARY VESSELS

Although congenital anomalies of the pulmonary circulation are rare, these anomalies range from total obstructive anomalous pulmonary venous return (TAPVR), which causes acute life-threatening respiratory distress, to agenesis of the right or left pulmonary artery, which may be asymptomatic. Usually, the more severe pulmonary vascular anomalies are associated with complex cardiac defects that disrupt cardiovascular function and/or normal blood supply and drainage of the lung.

The inflow, or venous flow, to the heart is initially supplied by six vessels, three on each side of the embryo: (1) the posterior cardinal veins draining the trunk, (2) the anterior cardinal veins, draining the head, and (3) the vitelline veins draining the yolk sac, all of which drain into the inferior aspect of the primitive heart tube, or the right and left horns of the primitive left atrium, or sinus venosus. Oxygenated blood from the placenta is delivered to the heart by the umbilical veins. Initially, the primitive lung bud is drained by the cardinal and vitelline veins, but this connection eventually regresses. The cardinal veins differentiate into the superior vena cava, whereas the vitelline and umbilical veins develop into the inferior vena cava. At the beginning of 4 week's GA, the common pulmonary vein arises from the cranial portion of the sinus venosus and immediately branches into right and left pulmonary veins, which bifurcate again to produce a total of four pulmonary veins. Like the pulmonary arteries, these veins grow toward the lung where they anastomose with the vascular plexus developing in the mesenchyme around the bronchial buds. During 5 weeks' GA, the first two branches of the pulmonary vein are incorporated into the posterior wall of the left side of the primitive atrium, where they form the definitive left atrium.

Formation of the pulmonary valve by 9 weeks' GA marks the beginning of the pulmonary arterial circulation, which originates from the right ventricular outflow tract. The ductus arteriosus, a remnant of sixth aortic arch on the left, connects the pulmonary artery to the aorta, shunting the fetal circulation of the immature lung from the right ventricle into the systemic circulation, whereas the patent foramen ovale allows blood to enter the left atrium from the right atrium, bypassing the right ventricle and pulmonary vein. Failure of the ductus arteriosus and/or foramen ovale to close at birth allows this shunting to persist and may require intervention.

PULMONARY ARTERY MALFORMATIONS

Events that disrupt development of the pulmonary arteries are rare and most commonly affect the proximal or extrapulmonary vessels. Most originate during embryonic development of the heart (5 to 9 weeks, GA) and are frequently associated with other cardiovascular abnormalities. For example, normal development of the main pulmonary artery and pulmonary valve is affected by cardiac anomalies that disrupt division of the truncus arteriosus into the ascending aorta and the pulmonary artery, such as tetralogy of Fallot (ventricular septal defect, pulmonary valve stenosis, displacement of the aorta, and right ventricular hypertrophy) or persistent truncus arteriosus (ventricular septal defect with incomplete separation of the aortic and pulmonary outflow tracts). These abnormalities create a right-to-to left shunt, bypassing the lungs and causing hypoxemia and cyanosis in the affected neonate.

Aberrant pulmonary arteries may originate from the descending or ascending aorta, from the brachiocephalic or subclavian arteries, or from a persistent ductus arteriosus, causing compression of the trachea and/or esophagus. Accessory arteries may also arise from the descending aorta in conjunction with accessory pulmonary lobes or pulmonary sequestration. Agenesis of the right or left pulmonary artery may be partial or complete and affects growth of the ipsilateral lung, which may be hypoplastic. Blood supply to the affected lung is from enlarged collateral vessels, including the bronchial arteries, intercostal arteries, coronary arteries, and/or a patent ductus arteriosus. Often patients are asymptomatic, unless additional cardiac abnormalities, such as a patent ductus arteriosus, coarctation, or tetralogy of Fallot, are present, creating a large left-to-right shunt.

Pulmonary artery sling is a rare malformation in which the left pulmonary artery originates from the posterior aspect of the right pulmonary artery. To get to the left lung, the artery passes anteriorly to the right main stem bronchus and then posteriorly between the trachea and esophagus, forming a partial sling around the trachea. This causes compression of the adjacent bronchus and/or trachea with air trapping and hyperinflation of the right lung, as well as recurrent respiratory infections. There are two distinct types of pulmonary artery slings: (1) type I, which is less common and is associated with secondary tracheobronchomalacia and right-sided air-trapping, and (2) type II, which is more common and is associated with congenital tracheal stenosis with complete cartilaginous rings, often affecting a long segment of the trachea.[186] Additional right lung abnormalities may be present, including abnormal bronchial branching, hypoplasia, agenesis, absent right pulmonary artery, and pulmonary sequestration. Pulmonary slings are usually associated with other organ abnormalities, including those found in VATER/VACTERL syndrome, as well as numerous cardiovascular and GI anomalies. Additional vascular abnormalities that cause compression of the tracheobronchial tree and/or esophagus include double aortic arch, right aortic arch with aberrant left subclavian artery, anomalous innominate artery, circumflex aorta, and cervical aortic arch.[120]

PULMONARY VEIN MALFORMATIONS

As for the pulmonary arteries, events that disrupt development of the pulmonary veins are rare but most commonly involve abnormal connection of the proximal veins to the right atrium or the systemic veins instead of to the left atrium, creating an extracardiac left-to-right shunt. Aberrant venous return may be total, involving all four pulmonary veins, or partial, involving only some of the veins, with either direct or indirect venous drainage into the left brachiocephalic vein, the right atrium, the superior or inferior vena cava, or the portal vein.[65] Partial anomalous pulmonary venous return (PAPVR) may be asymptomatic, unless there are associated cardiac anomalies, such as sinus venosus-atrial septal defects. Symptoms depend on hemodynamic changes that are secondary to the left-to-right shunt, to the magnitude of the shunt, and to the presence of cardiac defects. These include dyspnea, shortness of breath, fatigue, chest pain, palpitations, tachycardia, and peripheral edema.[187]

Scimitar syndrome, also known as *congenital venolobar syndrome* or *hypogenetic lung syndrome,* is a form of PAPVR in which an anomalous pulmonary vein drains into the inferior vena cava, portal or hepatic veins, coronary sinus, or right atrium, establishing a left-to-right shunt that can lead to pulmonary hypertension. On chest x-ray, the anomalous vein resembles a curved Turkish sword or "scimitar"—that is, a crescent-shaped tubular shadow or curvilinear density, located over the right lower lobe and coursing toward the right hemidiaphragm. Commonly, the defect affects the right pulmonary vein, which drains into the inferior vena cava, and is associated with right lung hypoplasia and dextroposition of the heart. The right bronchial tree may be abnormal, exhibiting a left-sided branching pattern with a reduction in lobes from three to two on the right side. Often, an anomalous systemic blood supply, with or without sequestered lung tissue, bronchogenic cysts, horseshoe lung, or diaphragmatic defects, may be found, as well as hypoplasia or absence of the right pulmonary artery. Associated cardiovascular defects include hypoplastic left heart, aortic coarctation, atrial septal defects, patent ductus arteriosus, tetralogy of Fallot, and a left pulmonary artery sling.[120]

TAPVR is a rare abnormality in which all of the pulmonary veins drain into the systemic veins, the right atrium, the coronary sinus, or the inferior vena cava. To be compatible with life, TAPVR requires a right-to-left shunt via a cardiac septal defect or a patent ductus arteriosus. There are four major types based on location of the drainage: supracardiac, cardiac, infracardiac, or mixed.[187] Supracardiac drainage is the most common, with venous connections to the left brachiocephalic vein, the superior vena cava, or azygos vein. Cardiac drainage is the second most common, with venous connections to the coronary sinus or the posterior wall of the right atrium. Infracardiac drainage usually involves some form of venous obstruction. In this type of TAPVR, the left and right pulmonary veins fuse behind the left atrium to form a common vertical descending vein, which is located anteriorly to the esophagus and passes through the diaphragm at the esophageal hiatus to join the portal vein. Infrequently, this vertical vein may join the ductus venosus, hepatic vein, or inferior vena cava. Obstruction may occur at any point along its path. In the mixed pattern, the pulmonary veins drain into more than one location, including the brachiocephalic vein, superior vena cava, azygos vein, coronary sinus, right atrium, or a vein below the diaphragm. This pattern is usually associated with other major cardiac defects.

PULMONARY ARTERIOVENOUS MALFORMATIONS

PAVMs (also known as *pulmonary arteriovenous fistulas, pulmonary arteriovenous aneurysms,* or *pulmonary telangiectasia*) are abnormal, or dysplastic, connections between the pulmonary arteries and veins. These malformations allow blood to bypass the pulmonary capillaries, which creates an extracardiac, or intrapulmonary, right-to-left shunt, leading to hypoxemia, dyspnea, cyanosis, clubbing, and polycythemia.[188] Respiratory symptoms may also be complicated by rupture of the PAVM, leading to hemoptysis and hemithorax. Age at presentation ranges from birth to the seventh or eighth decade of life, although most are diagnosed in the second or third decades. Although PAVM is rare in newborns, at least 34 cases have been reported in children.[189] In addition, 50% of patients with PAVM have clinical manifestations of this disorder during early childhood, but go undiagnosed. PAVM presents in infancy with mild cyanosis that progresses with age.

Most patients with PAVM have underlying hereditary hemorrhagic telangiectasia (HHT), also known as *Osler-Rendu-Weber disease* (OMIM #187300). This congenital vascular disorder is inherited as an autosomal dominant defect involving multiple AVMs in several organs, including skin, mucus membranes, retina, conjunctiva, thyroid, intestine, kidney, adrenal, brain, and lung. The most frequent form, HHT1, is caused by a heterozygous mutation in endoglin, or *ENG* (OMIM *131195), a transmembrane glycoprotein found on the surface of endothelial cells that is a component of the TGF-β receptor complex, binding TGFB1 with high affinity. HHT2 (OMIM #600376) is caused by mutations in an activin receptor–like kinase, or *ACVRL1* (also known as *ALK1*, OMIM #601284), which is another cell surface receptor for TGFB1. There is also a juvenile form of HTT (OMIM #175050) caused by mutations in *SMAD4* (OMIM *600993), a downstream component of the TGF-β signaling pathway that mediates transcriptional activation of target genes. The TGF-β signaling pathway is important for angiogenesis in the lung, regulating proliferation, differentiation, adhesion, and migration of angioblasts and endothelial cells.

PAVMs are dysplastic terminal capillary loops or connections between the arterial blood supply and venous drainage in the lung. PAVMs present as (1) large, thin-walled, single, or multiple vascular sacs; (2) distended plexiform-like masses of vascular channels; or (3) tortuous anastomoses between arteries and veins. PAVMs vary in number, size, and distribution; they may be single or multiple, unilateral, or bilateral. Typically, PAVMs are 1 to 5 cm in diameter, but diffuse, microvascular PAVMs may also be present. PAVMs smaller than 2 cm are often asymptomatic. PAVMs may increase in size over time, but rarely regress spontaneously. Most multiple PAVMs are found in the lower lobes, with the incidence of bilateral PAVMs being about 20%.[65] The majority of single PAVMS are also found in the lower lobes, with the left lower lobe being the most common location, followed by the right lower lobe.[190] Most PAVMs are simple and supplied by a single subsegmental pulmonary artery, whereas complex PAVMs are supplied by more than one subsegmental artery.

CONGENITAL PULMONARY LYMPHANGIECTASIS

Congenital pulmonary lymphangiectasis (also known as *congenital pulmonary lymphangiectasia*) is an extremely rare condition characterized by markedly distended or dilated pulmonary lymphatic vessels, which are located in the subpleural regions of the lung and extend into the interlobular septa and the bronchovascular connective tissue.[117] The dilated lymphatic vessels are thin-walled, lined by endothelial cells, and form a network of communicating channels. Pulmonary lymphangiectasis can be divided into three main categories: primary, secondary, and generalized.[117,191] Primary lymphangiectasis is a fatal developmental defect in which the pulmonary lymphatic vessels fail to communicate with the systemic lymphatic vessels. Affected infants present with respiratory distress and pleural effusions and die shortly after birth. Secondary pulmonary lymphangiectasis is associated with cardiovascular malformations, including anomalous pulmonary venous return, atrioventricular valve defects, ostium secundum, pulmonary stenosis, ventricular septal defect, mitral atresia, hypoplastic left heart, cor triatium, and atresia of the common pulmonary veins.[95] Generalized pulmonary lymphangiectasis is characterized by proliferation of the lymphatic spaces and occurs in the lung as part of a systemic abnormality in which multiple lymphangiomas are also found in the bones, viscera, and soft tissues. Cardiovascular anomalies are seen in 60% of these patients, whereas renal malformations, generalized lymphangiectasis, and other congenital anomalies are present in 20% of cases. Most cases of pulmonary lymphangiectasis are sporadic, with males more frequently affected than females (>2.5:1).[82,192]

Pulmonary lymphangiectasis has been described in association with multiple chromosomal abnormalities, including Turner (OMIM #309590, #309585), Down (OMIM #190685), Noonan (numerous OMIM entries), and Phelan McDermid (OMIM #606232) syndromes. Pulmonary lymphangiectasis can also be a component of other syndromes characterized by lymphedema or generalized lymphatic dysplasia, such as Hennekam syndrome (OMIM #235510, #616006). Pulmonary lymphangiectasis may be inherited as a dominant, recessive, or X-linked inheritance pattern. Mutations in genes associated with specific syndromes that have been identified in pulmonary lymphangiectasis patients include *PTPN11* (OMIM *176876) and *SOS1* (OMIM *182530), both components of the RAS signaling pathway that regulates cell growth and differentiation. Mutations in *FOXC2* (OMIM *602402) have also been described in families with lymphedema with venous reflux, suggesting that this gene may be important for normal development and maintenance of venous and lymphatic valves.[193-195] *VEGFR3* (*FLT4*, OMIM *136352) mutations have also been described in pulmonary lymphangiectasis, in association with Nonne-Milroy lymphedema syndrome (OMIM #153100). Interestingly, perinatal overexpression of the ligand for this receptor, VEGFC, was shown to induce pulmonary lymphangiectasis in a mouse model that phenotypically and histologically resembles the human condition.[196]

SUMMARY

Development of the lung and its conducting airways begins during early gestation as an outgrowth of the ventral foregut endoderm, which forms the primitive trachea and bronchial tubules. Thereafter, lung development proceeds in a stereotypical pattern, involving branching morphogenesis of the tracheobronchial tree followed by outgrowth, expansion, and maturation of the alveolar parenchyma, or gas-exchange regions of the lung. This process can be divided into five chronologic stages of morphogenesis, which extend throughout gestation and into childhood. These are the embryonic, pseudoglandular, canalicular, saccular, and alveolar periods of lung development, terms describing the anatomic, microscopic, biochemical, and physiologic changes that determine normal development and growth of the lung.

Pulmonary malformations that arise during the early embryonic and pseudoglandular stages of lung development are a heterogeneous group of closely related abnormalities associated with defective lung bud formation, separation of the trachea from the esophagus, branching morphogenesis, and formation of the conducting airways. These lesions often lead to obstruction of the airway, resulting in secondary cystic or dysplastic changes in the distal lung. Pulmonary vascular abnormalities that arise during this period of lung development also cause obstructive malformations of the lung and conducting airways. Multiple congenital malformations, including musculoskeletal, cardiovascular, GI, and GU abnormalities, are found in conjunction with these early lung malformations. In many cases, chromosomal disorders and single-gene mutations known to impact developmental processes important for organogenesis are associated with these malformations, including mutations in components of the SHH, FGF, TGF-β, WNT, BMP, and VEGF signaling pathways.

Pulmonary abnormalities related to growth and maturation of the respiratory parenchyma and its vasculature arise during the canalicular and saccular stages of lung development and generally result in abnormalities in alveolar and/or capillary development, as well as in pulmonary hypoplasia and respiratory insufficiency. Infants born prematurely during the late saccular or early alveolar stages of lung development exhibit biochemical immaturity of the lung, leading to surfactant deficiency, growth disorders of the parenchyma, or chronic interstitial lung disease. Mutations in genes important for lung and vascular development, such as

NKX2-1, *FOXF1*, and *DHCR7*, are associated with abnormal lung development and growth, whereas mutations in the surfactant-associated genes *ABCA3*, *SFTPC*, and *SFTPB* result in surfactant dysfunction, respiratory insufficiency, neonatal death, and/or chronic lung disease.

Chromosomal and genetic analyses of patients with hereditary lung malformations have been important for identifying molecular mechanisms underlying abnormal lung development. Integration of genomic studies in human patients with functional studies utilizing a variety of animal models will continue to be important for elucidating additional developmental and molecular pathways critical for both normal and abnormal lung development.

ACKNOWLEDGMENTS

The author thanks Dr. Susan E.Wert for her writing of this chapter for the fifth edition, which is the foundation for this updated chapter.The author would also like to thank Dr. Jamie Verheyden for assistance with this manuscript.

 A complete reference list is available at www.ExpertConsult.com.

SELECT REFERENCES

1. Burri PH. Structural aspects of prenatal and postnatal development and growth of the lung. In: McDonald JA, ed. *Lung Growth and Development*. New York: Taylor & Francis; 1997:1-36.
2. Morrisey EE, Hogan BL. Preparing for the first breath: genetic and cellular mechanisms in lung development. *Dev Cell*. 2010;18:8-23.
3. Langston C, Kida K, Reed M, et al. Human lung growth in late gestation and in the neonate. *Am Rev Respir Dis*. 1984;129:607-613.
5. Thurlbeck WM. Postnatal growth and development of the lung. *Am Rev Respir Dis*. 1975;111:803-844.
6. Zeltner TB, Caduff JH, Gehr P, et al. The postnatal development and growth of the human lung. *I. Morphometry. Respir Physiol.* 1987;67:247-267.
8. Hislop AA, Wigglesworth JS, Desai R. Alveolar development in the human fetus and infant. *Early Hum Dev*. 1986;13:1-11.
9. Ochs M, Nyengaard JR, Jung A, et al. The number of alveoli in the human lung. *Am J Respir Crit Care Med*. 2004;169:120-124.
12. Larsen W. *Human Embryology*. Philadelphia: Churchill Livingstone; 2001.
15. Jeffrey PK. The development of large and small airways. *Am J Respir Crit Care Med*. 1998;157:S174-S180.
16. deMello DE, Reid LM. Embryonic and early fetal development of human lung vasculature and its functional implications. *Pediatr Dev Pathol*. 2000;3:439-449.
17. Hislop A. Developmental biology of the pulmonary circulation. *Paediatr Respir Rev*. 2005;6:35-43.
24. Jeffery PK, Gaillard D, Moret S. Human airway secretory cells during development and in mature airway epithelium. *Eur Respir J*. 1992;5:93-104.
28. Sparrow MP, Weichselbaum M, McCray PB. Development of the innervation and airway smooth muscle in human fetal lung. *Am J Respir Cell Mol Biol*. 1999;20:550-560.
30. Hall SM, Hislop AA, Haworth SG. Origin, differentiation, and maturation of human pulmonary veins. *Am J Respir Cell Mol Biol*. 2002;26:333-340.
31. Hall SM, Hislop AA, Pierce CM, et al. Prenatal origins of human intrapulmonary arteries: formation and smooth muscle maturation. *Am J Respir Cell Mol Biol*. 2000;23:194-203.
32. Leslie KO, Mitchell JJ, Woodcock-Mitchell JL, et al. Alpha smooth muscle actin expression in developing and adult human lung. *Differentiation*. 1990;44:143-149.
33. Oliver G, Alitalo K. The lymphatic vasculature: recent progress and paradigms. *Annu Rev Cell Dev Biol*. 2005;21:457-483.
64. Whitsett JA, Wert SE, Weaver TE. Diseases of pulmonary surfactant homeostasis. *Annu Rev Pathol*. 2015;10:371-393.
72. Nogee LM. Genetic basis of children's interstitial lung disease. *Pediatr Allergy Immunol Pulmonol*. 2010;23:15-24.
78. Biyyam DR, Chapman T, Ferguson MR, et al. Congenital lung abnormalities: embryologic features, prenatal diagnosis, and postnatal radiologic-pathologic correlation. *Radiographics*. 2010;30:1721-1738.
81. Berrocal T, Madrid C, Novo S, et al. Congenital anomalies of the tracheobronchial tree, lung, and mediastinum: embryology, radiology, and pathology. *Radiographics*. 2004;24:e17.
84. Shaw-Smith C. Oesophageal atresia, tracheo-oesophageal fistula, and the VACTERL association: review of genetics and epidemiology. *J Med Genet*. 2006;43:545-554.
88. Felix JF, Tibboel D, de Klein A. Chromosomal anomalies in the aetiology of oesophageal atresia and tracheo-oesophageal fistula. *Eur J Med Genet*. 2007;50:163-175.
91. Spilde T, Bhatia A, Ostlie D, et al. A role for sonic hedgehog signaling in the pathogenesis of human tracheoesophageal fistula. *J Pediatr Surg*. 2003;38: 465-468.
93. Munzon GB, Martinez-Ferro M. Pediatric tracheal stenosis and vascular rings. *Bull Thorac Surg*. 2012;5:207-219.
94. de Groot-van der Mooren MD, Haak MC, Lakeman P, et al. Tracheal agenesis: approach towards this severe diagnosis. Case report and review of the literature. *Eur J Pediatr*. 2012;171:425-431.
102. Lertsburapa K, Schroeder Jr JW, Sullivan C. Tracheal cartilaginous sleeve in patients with craniosynostosis syndromes: a meta-analysis. *J Pediatr Surg*. 2010;45:1438-1444.
105. Gonzales M, Heuertz S, Martinovic J, et al. Vertebral anomalies and cartilaginous tracheal sleeve in three patients with Pfeiffer syndrome carrying the S351C FGFR2 mutation. *Clin Genet*. 2005;68:179-181.
111. Meyerholz DK, Stoltz DA, Namati E, et al. Loss of cystic fibrosis transmembrane conductance regulator function produces abnormalities in tracheal development in neonatal pigs and young children. *Am J Respir Crit Care Med*. 2010;182:1251-1261.
116. Carden KA, Boiselle PM, Waltz DA, et al. Tracheomalacia and tracheobronchomalacia in children and adults: an in-depth review. *Chest*. 2005;127:984-1005.
118. Aktogu S, Yuncu G, Halilcolar H, et al. Bronchogenic cysts: clinicopathological presentation and treatment. *Eur Respir J*. 1996;9:2017-2021.
120. Garcia-Pena P, Coma A, Enriquez G. Congenital lung malformations: radiological findings and clues for differential diagnosis. *Acta Radiol*. 2013;54:1086-1095.
124. Corbett HJ, Humphrey GM. Pulmonary sequestration. *Paediatr Respir Rev*. 2004;5:59-68.
126. Walker CM, Wu CC, Gilman MD, et al. The imaging spectrum of bronchopulmonary sequestration. *Curr Probl Diagn Radiol*. 2014;43:100-114.
128. Correia-Pinto J, Gonzaga S, Huang Y, et al. Congenital lung lesions–underlying molecular mechanisms. *Semin Pediatr Surg*. 2010;19:171-179.
129. Riedlinger WF, Vargas SO, Jennings RW, et al. Bronchial atresia is common to extralobar sequestration, intralobar sequestration, congenital cystic adenomatoid malformation, and lobar emphysema. *Pediatr Dev Pathol*. 2006;9:361-373.
134. Conway K, Gibson R, Perkins J, et al. Pulmonary agenesis: expansion of the VCFS phenotype. *Am J Med Genet*. 2002;113:89-92.
147. Bishop NB, Stankiewicz P, Steinhorn RH. Alveolar capillary dysplasia. *Am J Respir Crit Care Med*. 2011;184:172-179.
149. Chow CW, Massie J, Ng J, et al. Acinar dysplasia of the lungs: variation in the extent of involvement and clinical features. *Pathology*. 2013;45:38-43.
150. Langenstroer M, Carlan SJ, Fanaian N, et al. Congenital acinar dysplasia: report of a case and review of literature. *AJP Rep*. 2013;3:9-12.
152. Galambos C, Sims-Lucas S, Ali N, et al. Intrapulmonary vascular shunt pathways in alveolar capillary dysplasia with misalignment of pulmonary veins. *Thorax*. 2015;70:84-85.
153. Stankiewicz P, Sen P, Bhatt SS, et al. Genomic and genic deletions of the FOX gene cluster on 16q24.1 and inactivating mutations of FOXF1 cause alveolar capillary dysplasia and other malformations. *Am J Hum Genet*. 2009;84: 780-791.
138. Hamvas A, Deterding RR, Wert SE, et al. Heterogeneous pulmonary phenotypes associated with mutations in the thyroid transcription factor gene NKX2-1. *Chest*. 2013;144:794-804.
168. Gupta K, Das A, Menon P, et al. Revisiting the histopathologic spectrum of congenital pulmonary developmental disorders. *Fetal Pediatr Pathol*. 2012;31:74-86.
169. Ozcelik U, Gocmen A, Kiper N, et al. Congenital lobar emphysema: evaluation and long-term follow-up of thirty cases at a single center. *Pediatr Pulmonol*. 2003;35:384-3891.
170. Cloutier MM, Schaeffer DA, Hight D. Congenital cystic adenomatoid malformation. *Chest*. 1993;103:761-764.
186. Newman B, Cho Y. Left pulmonary artery sling—anatomy and imaging. *Semin Ultrasound CT MR*. 2010;31:158-170.
187. Katre R, Burns SK, Murillo H, et al. Anomalous pulmonary venous connections. *Semin Ultrasound CT MR*. 2012;33:485-499.
190. Cartin-Ceba R, Swanson KL, Krowka MJ. Pulmonary arteriovenous malformations. *Chest*. 2013;144:1033-1044.
192. Reiterer F, Grossauer K, Morris N, et al. Congenital pulmonary lymphangiectasis. *Paediatr Respir Rev*. 2014;15:275-280.
193. de Bruyn G, Casaer A, Devolder K, et al. Hydrops fetalis and pulmonary lymphangiectasia due to FOXC2 mutation: an autosomal dominant hereditary lymphedema syndrome with variable expression. *Eur J Pediatr*. 2012;171: 447-450.

56 Regulation of Alveolarization

Christophe Delacourt | Alice Hadchouel

INTRODUCTION

Lung development is a continuous process, starting very early in embryonic life with the differentiation of the tracheal bud from the ventral side of the primitive gut and ending in postnatal life with the multiplication of alveoli and the maturation of the pulmonary microvasculature. Alveoli represent the functional unit of the lung, the site at which oxygen and carbon dioxide are exchanged between inspired air and the blood. Alveolarization is controlled by many factors, whose expression is tightly regulated temporally and spatially. In humans, the most illustrative pathology of impaired alveolar multiplication is bronchopulmonary dysplasia (BPD), the most common chronic respiratory disease in premature infants, and a source of significant respiratory morbidity. Moderate and severe forms of this disease are characterized by prolonged respiratory insufficiency, with persistent requirement for supplemental oxygen beyond 36 weeks of postmenstrual age. Impaired alveolarization, with alveolar hypoplasia and altered microvascular maturation, are characteristic pathophysiologic features of BPD.[1]

TIMING OF ALVEOLAR MULTIPLICATION DURING LUNG DEVELOPMENT

The first distal air spaces are represented by primitive saccules during the saccular stage. The alveolar stage succeeds the saccular stage and is characterized by a dramatic increase in the gas exchange surface due to the subdivision of the primitive saccules by new interair-space walls resulting in new alveoli. Formation of alveoli may be pre- or postnatal, depending on the species. It is almost entirely prenatal in species such as guinea pigs[2] or lambs.[3] In contrast, in rodents and humans, the formation of alveoli is essentially postnatal.[4-6] Therefore, rodents are most often used as a model of human alveolar development. The duration of alveolar multiplication during postnatal life has been the subject of many studies. Most recent studies confirm that new septa are formed until young adulthood. Using a direct and unbiased assessment of the number of alveoli in the rat model, Tschanz and associates demonstrated a biphasic behavior of alveolarization.[7] In this model, the early phase of alveolarization corresponds to a very high production rate of alveoli, frequently described as *bulk alveolarization*. During this initial phase, the number of alveoli increased in rats from less than 1 million at postnatal day 4, to approximately 3.5 million at day 10, and to over 14 million at day 21.[7] This represents an impressive rate of 800,000 new alveoli per day. During this initial period, the volumetric expansion of the alveolar air space does not follow, and therefore the alveoli are becoming much smaller. This first phase is followed by a second phase from day 21 to day 60, corresponding to young adulthood, with a slower rate of alveolar multiplication, and the formation of an additional 5 million alveoli. During this second phase, the formation of new alveoli is less important than the growth of the alveoli, leading to an increase in the mean airspace volume.[7] Recent stereologic-based longitudinal study reported dynamic changes in structural changes during postnatal mouse lung development.[8] Alveologenesis was clearly evident over the early postnatal phase. The saccular or alveolar density was multiplied threefold between the 5th and 7th postnatal day, and fivefold between the 5th and 10th postnatal day. Alveolar density peaked at the 39th postnatal day and remained unchanged at 9 months but was reduced by 22 months. Stereologic analysis revealed a progressive decrease in the mean saccular or alveolar volume of the lung over the first 10 days of life. Mean septal wall thickness dramatically decreased over the first 10 days of postnatal life, with a twofold reduction between the 5th and 10th postnatal day, and continued to decrease to the 28th postnatal day.[8] These experimental data were confirmed in humans. Based on human lung tissues obtained by autopsy, Herring and associates demonstrated that the number of alveoli in the human lung increased exponentially during the first 2 years of life but continued to increase, albeit at a reduced rate, through adolescence.[9] The estimated number of alveoli for the whole human lung is around 100×10^6 alveoli by 1 month of postnatal age, and reaches over 500×10^6 alveoli by 15 years of age.[9]

STRUCTURAL CHANGES DURING THE ALVEOLAR STAGE

Primitive saccules are delineated by thick intersaccular walls, or *primary septa*. The alveolar stage is characterized by the formation of numerous small ridges from the saccular wall, called *secondary septa,* which grow in a centripetal manner into the saccules to subdivide them into alveoli.[10] Among the variety of factors that participate in the control of budding of secondary septa, spatial and temporal changes in extracellular elastin and laminin distribution appeared as critical.[11] Elastin deposition in the thickness of primary septa appears to have a spatially instructive role, as sites of elastic fiber formation correspond precisely to the location of future buds. However, 3-D analysis recently showed that the isolated patches in the tips of the "finger-like" protrusions were not actually isolated but were parts of continuous elastin fibers that rim the alveolar opening.[11] The growth of secondary septa into the lumen of the terminal saccule is accompanied by migration and proliferation of fibroblasts. Lipofibroblasts (LFs) and myofibroblasts (MFs) are two lineages of mesenchymal cells with fibroblast characteristics that are identified during alveolarization.[12] LFs contain lipid vacuoles and are located at the base of newly formed septa, in close proximity to the alveolar type II cells (AECII) and endothelial cells.[13] In the rat, the quantity of LFs doubles between P4 and P7, with an accompanying increase in cellular lipid content.[14] LFs may constitute a stem-cell niche for AECII stem cells.[15] MFs are nonlipid-containing, α-smooth muscle actin–positive interstitial cells and are located adjacent to collagen and elastic fibers.[13] MFs may be derived from platelet-derived growth factor receptor-α (PDGFRA)–positive cells[16] and play a key role in elastogenesis. Elastin fibers are arranged in an orderly and predictable manner within the alveolar septa.[17] Crosslinking of elastin monomers is a critical process in alveolarization, and inhibition of this process impairs secondary septation (see below). Elastin fibers are in close proximity with collagen fibers, suggesting that both fibers are mechanically interconnected.[17] Increased deposition of elastin and collagen fibers does not drive maturational changes in lung tissue mechanics. Indeed, changes in tissue viscoelastic properties with maturation are determined mainly by other components of extracellular matrix, such as glycosaminoglycans and proteoglycans,[18] which are dynamically controlled during postnatal stages of pulmonary development.[19] At the beginning of the alveolar stage, both primary and secondary septa show a double capillary layer, as one capillary is associated with each surface of the forming alveolar septa. In a recent study that imaged newborn mouse lung with serial block-face scanning electron microscopy, new 3D information was provided on the structure of the alveolar capillary network in the newborn lung. In particular, the so-called double-layered capillary network of developing lungs was identified more as a single network extending in all three dimensions rather than two (nearly separated) networks within one septum.[20]

Along with the emergence of secondary septa, a progressive thinning of interstitial tissue is observed.[21] It is likely that this decrease in interstitial volume allows both capillary networks to come into close contact and to potentially fuse, so that a single capillary system forms in the alveolar wall. It was postulated that the formation of secondary septa can continue as long as a double capillary network is present and that the end of alveolarization occurs in parallel with capillary fusion.[21] At the end of the bulk alveolarization in rats, a 20% to 25% fraction of the capillary network is still immature, thus potentially explaining the continued alveolarization beyond this period.[9,21] At 60 days in rodents, 5% to 10% of the capillary network remains immature[21] and might contribute to alveolar regeneration in adults. Furthermore, local reduplication of the capillary network was also described as the basis of newly forming septa in adult rodents.[22]

The period of alveolization is accompanied by the differentiation of alveolar epithelial cells, which is covered in another chapter of this book.

REGULATORS OF THE NORMAL ALVEOLAR MULTIPLICATION

ELASTOGENESIS

Elastogenesis is a complex multistep process in which elastin is incorporated into microfibril bundles to generate elastic fibers.[23] Elastic fibers are elaborated by crosslinking of a soluble precursor, known as *tropoelastin,* under the action of lysyl oxidase.[24] Tropoelastin is synthesized by MFs. Elastin fiber deposition also involves the coordinated expression of microfibril proteins such as fibrillins, fibulins, microfibril-associated glycoproteins (MAGPs), emilin, and latent transforming growth factor-beta (TGFβ) binding proteins (LTBPs) that act as a scaffold for elastin assembly.[25,26] Alveolar septation defects are observed in *Ltbp4*$^{-/-}$ lungs, due to several interacting mechanisms, including an absence of an intact elastic fiber network and reduced angiogenesis.[27]

Normal elastin synthesis and deposition requires tightly spatially regulated processes, including differentiation and migration of MFs, formation of elastic fibers from tropoelastin molecules and scaffold proteins, and specific deposition sites in the thickness of primary septa. The essential role of elastin for distal lung development has been elucidated by various experimental approaches that disrupt these processes. Mice with inactivation of the elastin gene display fewer and more dilated distal air sacs with attenuated tissue septa[28]; however, this is not a good model for studying alveolar growth, because mouse pups die early after birth, before the period of alveolar multiplication. The role of elastin deposition in alveolarization has been demonstrated indirectly in models characterized by loss of the genes for platelet-derived growth factor A (PDGFA, a chemoattractant for MFs[6]) or lysyl oxidase.[24] In these models, a profound reduction in elastin deposition occurs, resulting in the absence of secondary septa and definitive alveoli. Moreover, early and transient inhibition of the PDGF receptor by a specific antagonist leads to a long-term impairment of secondary septation characterized by abnormal elastic fibers deposition along with an increase in lung content of fibulin-5.[29] Finally, retinoic acid (RA) and fibroblast growth factor (FGF) 18 are key regulators of elastogenesis. RA enhances the expression of PDGFA/PDGFR α[30] and tropoelastin,[31] whereas vitamin A deficiency leads to delayed alveolar development[32] (see below). FGF18 is up-regulated in the postnatal rat lung and increases the expression of tropoelastin and lysyl oxidase in MFs.[33] In animal models with impaired alveolarization, elastogenesis and elastic fibers deposition are markedly altered. Exposure of rat pups to 95% FiO_2 from postnatal day 4 to day 14 led to a delay in peak tropoelastin mRNA, the level of which remained abnormally elevated until day 23, with a greater total length of elastic fibers in oxygen-exposed animals than controls.[34] Mechanical ventilation of newborn mice in room air or with 40% FiO_2 led to an increase in tropoelastin and lysyl oxidase mRNA relative to controls, with abnormal elastic fiber deposition throughout the walls of distal respiratory units.[35] In humans, most of the studies rely on autopsy specimen analyses from infants with "old" BPD, that is, before the prophylactic use of exogenous surfactant. These studies found that the volume, density, and absolute quantity of elastic tissue in BPD lungs are significantly higher than normal.[36] Alveolar elastic fibers have been described as thickened, tortuous, and irregularly distributed.[37] Nevertheless, altered elastogenesis was also observed in infants with "new" BPD, where lysyl oxidase expression and activity were found to be up-regulated.[38]

Recently, other factors controlling myofibroblastic differentiation have been identified, with possible involvement in the control of alveolarization. Sonic hedgehog (SHH) signaling, which regulates mesenchymal proliferation and differentiation during embryonic lung development, was also expressed in the postnatal lung with a peak expression during alveolarization. SHH signaling is required for MF differentiation during growth of the secondary alveolar septa, and early inhibition of SHH signaling reduces the number of new septa formed.[39] Hox5 genes *(Hoxa5, Hoxb5, Hoxc5)* were also demonstrated to peak during the first 2 weeks after birth and to direct elastin network formation during alveologenesis by regulating MF adhesion.[40]

MATRIX METALLOPROTEINASES

Extracellular matrix remodeling is an important element of harmonious pulmonary development. Up to 40% of the newly synthesized collagen is degraded within hours during alveolarization in the newborn rat.[41] This remodeling particularly involves the matrix metalloproteinases (MMPs) family of enzymes. Two proteases of this family play a crucial role in lung development, namely *MMP2* and *MMP14,* which progressively increase in activity and expression during rat lung alveolarization.[41,42] Moreover, alveolar multiplication in MMP2-null mice is initially delayed, but recovers over time, suggesting possible compensatory mechanisms.[43] Activation of MMP2 from proMMP2 requires the proteolytic action of MMP14.[44] MMP14-insufficient mice display disrupted alveolarization with fewer and enlarged alveolar spaces that persist into adulthood,[43] suggesting that the role of MMP14 in alveolar septation is partly independent of the activation of proMMP2.[45] The expression of MMP14 is modulated by the epidermal growth factor (EGF) signaling pathway: EGF receptor knockout mice have low expression of MMP14 and poor alveolarization, and administration of an EGF ligand in wild-type mouse fibroblasts' culture medium induces a 10-fold increase in MMP14 mRNA levels.[46] The activity of MMP is modulated by specific tissue inhibitors of metalloproteinases (TIMPs), whose expression also affects alveolar development.[47] In consistency with MMPs having a major role in alveolarization, low MMP2 levels in tracheal effluents and plasma were linked to an increased risk of BPD in infants.[48,49] In those studies, the level of another MMP, namely *MMP9,* which is the main MMP released by inflammatory cells, was significantly increased in infants who developed BPD.[48,49]

Phospholipid derivatives such as lysophosphatidic acid (LPA) can act as a signaling molecule contributing to extracellular matrix production, MMP and TIMP expression, and finally to alveologenesis. Alveolarization was demonstrated to be impaired in LPA1 knockout mice, with impaired alveolar septal elastogenesis, and reduced expression of MMP-2, MMP-7, and MMP-9 mRNA.[50]

FIBROBLAST GROWTH FACTOR SIGNALING

In addition to FGF18, other FGFs contribute to the control of alveolar growth, and/or to lung repair after neonatal injury. FGF receptors (FGFRs) 1 through 4 are expressed in the developing lung with specific spatial and temporal profiles, and alveolar formation coincides with increased expression of FGFR3 and 4.[51] Mice devoid of both FGFR3 and 4 manifest a failure of secondary septation not observed in either single mutant.[52] Although FGFR3 and FGFR4 are expressed throughout the epithelium and mesenchyme of the developing mammalian lung, reports demonstrate that FGFR3 and FGFR4 expression is required in the lung mesenchyme, but not the epithelium, for alveologenesis.[53] Three genes with increased transcript levels in the FGFR3;4 mutant lung are thought to contribute to the mechanisms underlying the elastin disorganization phenotype in this model: insulin-like growth factor-1 (IGF-1), fibrillin 2 (Fbn2), and microfibrillar-associated protein 5.[53]

Reduced expression of FGFR3 and 4 has been described in the lungs of neonatal rats exposed to hyperoxia.[54] Although FGF18 is a ligand for these receptors, it is probably not the factor responsible for these results. Indeed, elastin is deposited in primary septa in FGFR3/4-null mice and deposition even failed to cease with aging; this is inconsistent with the known role of FGF18 in elastogenesis. Therefore, other FGF-driven mechanisms must operate both to condition the septal surge associated with elastin deposition and to stop elastogenesis. FGF2 is a candidate for the latter process, because it has negative effects on tropoelastin production.[55,56] FGF2 is elevated in tracheal aspirates from preterm neonates who died or developed BPD.[56] However, no lung abnormality has been found in FGF2-null mice.

FGF signaling may also be involved in the migration of alveolar MFs that populate the lung during postnatal alveolarization.[57] In particular, it was shown experimentally that FGF signaling is required for the induction of α-SMA in the PDGFR α-positive MF progenitor.[58] It was further demonstrated that FGFR2B ligands were required for alveolar MFs formation during alveolar regeneration after pneumonectomy.[59] After birth, FGF10 transcripts are detected at considerable levels in the lung during the alveolar stage and during adulthood, suggesting that the role of this growth factor is not limited to embryonic life but rather extends to postnatal life.[60] In particular, FGF10 may significantly contribute to maintaining distal epithelial progenitors.[60] FGF10 deficiency was demonstrated as causative for lethality in a mouse model of hyperoxia-induced impaired alveolarization.[61] In this model, FGF10 deficiency was also shown to affect quantitatively and qualitatively the formation of AECII cells.[61] Recently, pulmonary vasculature formation was decreased in FGF10-deficient mice pups exposed to hyperoxia.[62] Nevertheless, the direct contribution of the FGF10-FGFR2 signaling pathway in normal alveologenesis remains debated. Blockade of the FGFR2 pathway during the alveolar stage does not result in any structural alterations.[63] Further, FGF10 deficiency is associated with impaired alveolarization only in models of neonatal injuries, and not in healthy neonates,[61,62] suggesting rather a protective and/or repair role of FGF10 against injury-driven alterations to lung development.

TRANSFORMING GROWTH FACTOR–β

The extracellular matrix is not simply structural, but functions as a dynamic modulator through the selective sequestration and subsequent release of growth factors and cytokines. A striking example of the importance of this function for alveologenesis is given by the simultaneous observation of impaired alveolar septation and enhanced proportion of active TGF-β through greater local activation, in mice deficient in fibrillin-1.[64] TGF-β signaling is dynamically regulated during alveolar development.[65] TGF-β1 overexpression in neonatal mouse lung induced pulmonary morphologic changes consistent with those seen in human BPD lung, including enlarged alveolar sacs, poor secondary septation, thick and hypercellular septa, and abnormal capillary development.[66] Neutralization of the abnormal TGF-β activity improves alveologenesis and microvascular development in the injured developing lung.[67] Canonical TGF-β signaling involves Smad2/3 phosphorylation, but accumulating evidence indicates that TGF-β can also cross-stimulate bone morphogenetic protein (BMP)–Smad1/5 signaling pathways. TGF-β–stimulated Smad1/5 activation was recently evidenced in the developing mouse lung.[68] TGF-β signaling also plays an important role in hypoxia-induced inhibition of lung development.[69] Hypoxia-induced inhibition of alveolar development was associated with increased TGF-β activation and signaling, and was prevented by inhibition of TGF-β signaling using a mouse model with an inducible dominant-negative TGF-β receptor.[69] Improved alveolarization in the oxygen-exposed newborn mouse lung was also recently observed after intraperitoneal injection of TGF-β-neutralizing antibodies.[70] Hypoxia-induced loss of Thy-1, a glycophosphatidylinositol-linked outer membrane leaflet glycoprotein, was demonstrated to contribute to these results, as newborn mice deficient in Thy-1 had impaired alveolarization and increased TGF-β signaling when exposed to hypoxia.[71] Thy-1 limits the ability of fibroblasts to activate latent TGF-β.[72] TGF-β expression was similarly found to be increased in various models of neonatal injury associated with impaired alveolar growth, including mechanical ventilation,[73] hyperoxia,[67] and antenatal inflammation.[74] In preterm-born human infants, dysregulated production of this cytokine appears to be a significant mechanism in the pathogenesis of BPD. Abnormally high levels of TGF-β have been detected in airway secretions from infants with BPD.[75]

VASCULAR ENDOTHELIAL GROWTH FACTOR AND ANGIOGENIC FACTORS

Normal angiogenesis is required for alveologenesis, as demonstrated by experiments in the developing rat involving angiogenesis inhibitors, including vascular endothelial growth factor (VEGF) receptor inhibitors and adrenomedullin antagonists.[76,77] These inhibitors not only impair pulmonary vascular growth, but also reduce septation and final alveolar number. This emphasizes close interactions between the growth of pulmonary capillaries and the formation of alveoli in the postnatal lung. VEGF and its receptors are expressed in the developing lung in a coordinated fashion that peaks during the bulk alveolarization.[78] VEGF signaling, through isoforms 164 and 188, is essential for correct microvascular lung development.[79] The absence of these heparin-binding VEGF isoforms is associated with rarefied and dilated peripheral vessels and with fewer air-blood barriers and a decreased air space-parenchyma ratio. The expression of VEGF is in part regulated by O_2 tension through the actions of hypoxia-inducible factors (HIFs). In vivo postnatal HIF inhibition using dominant-negative HIF-1α, or a pharmacologic inhibitor, disrupts normal alveolar development and angiogenesis.[80] VEGF-induced angiogenesis is at least partly mediated by nitric oxide (NO). NO synthase activity is considerably reduced by treatment with VEGF receptor inhibitor, and inhaled NO can correct the alveolar disorders in this model.[81] Interestingly, treatment of hyperoxia-exposed neonatal rats with an NO donor increased both VEGF mRNA and protein levels, and also restored the expression level of key controllers of alveolarization, particularly FGF18 and FGFR4, and enhanced elastin expression.[54] Close interactions between angiogenic factors and matrix remodeling controllers have been further highlighted by the demonstration that adrenomedullin is a major target of FGF18.[82] Strict control of VEGF expression is necessary during alveolar development, however, because marked VEGF overexpression in neonatal mouse lung causes increased mortality, pulmonary hemorrhage, hemosiderosis, alveolar remodeling, and inflammation.[83] Neonatal lung injuries in animal models with impaired alveolarization are associated with reduced pulmonary microvascular growth and decreased VEGF expression,[84] which are also found in several human studies. Infants with BPD have fewer air-blood barriers, less capillary density, and capillaries more distant from the air surface than controls.[36,85] VEGF mRNA and protein expressions are low in BPD infants.[85] In a therapeutic perspective, postnatal intratracheal adenovirus-mediated VEGF gene therapy improved survival, promoted lung capillary formation, and preserved alveolar development in neonatal rats exposed to hyperoxia.[86] Similarly, in vivo airway delivery of HIF-1α via adenovirus-mediated gene transfer increases lung expression of angiogenic growth factors, including VEGF, and preserves alveolar and vascular development in hyperoxia-induced impaired alveolarization in newborn rats.[80] Interestingly, this protective signaling pathway, that is, HIF-1/2α and its downstream genes, is induced by sildenafil in lungs of newborn rats exposed to hyperoxia.[87] This may largely contribute to the significant recovery of alveolarization in sildenafil-treated rats.[87] Early inhaled high-dose NO was shown to enhance rat lung development after birth.[88] In humans, however, providing inhaled NO to premature infants does not significantly improve survival without BPD.[89]

NFκB signaling play also a significant role in promoting pulmonary angiogenesis during alveolarization. In particular, silencing the NFκB activating kinase IKKβ in neonatal mouse lungs was associated with severe angiogenic defects and decreased vascular cell adhesion molecule expression.[90]

Intratracheal transplantation of human umbilical cord blood–derived mesenchymal stem cells (MSCs) was demonstrated to protect against neonatal hyperoxic lung injury.[91] Intranasal delivery of human umbilical cord Wharton's jelly MSCs was also demonstrated to restore lung alveolarization and vascularization in newborn rats exposed to hyperoxia.[92] The mechanisms by which MSCs exert their restorative effect are probably multiple. VEGF secreted by transplanted MSCs was proposed as one of the critical paracrine factors that play seminal roles in attenuating hyperoxic lung injuries in neonatal rats.[93] MSC treatment was shown to increase VEGF mRNA expression in lung homogenates compared to room air rats, but without difference from the hyperoxic animals.[92] MSCs were found to significantly increase the expression profile of two genes: *Anxa5*, implicated in cell signaling, vesicle trafficking, cell division/migration, and apoptosis, and *NPPB*, a neovascular factor that stimulates endothelial regeneration.[92]

Stem cell factor (SCF), or c-kit ligand, is commonly known to be a mobilizer of stem cells, and is particularly expressed on bronchial epithelial cells and pulmonary microvascular endothelial cells. Its receptor, c-kit, is expressed on endothelial progenitor cells, hematopoietic stem cells, mast cells, fetal lung stromal cells, and putative lung stem cells.[94] Binding of SCF to c-kit was demonstrated to promote angiogenesis. In neonatal rats with hyperoxia-induced lung injury, exogenous SCF was demonstrated to restore alveolar and vascular structure by promoting neoangiogenesis.[95] FOXF1 signaling in c-KIT+ endothelial progenitor cells was demonstrated to regulate postnatal alveologenesis.[96] In particular, neonatal hyperoxia decreases pulmonary c-KIT$^+$ endothelial progenitors in mice, and FOXF1 was demonstrated as critical for maintenance of c-KIT$^+$ endothelial cells.[96] Inactivation of either *Foxf1* or *c-Kit* caused alveolar simplification. Expression of FOXF1 and c-KIT was decreased in the lungs of infants with BPD.[96]

In a phase I study, intratracheal transplantation of allogeneic hUCB-derived MSCs was shown to be feasible and safe in preterm infants, with an apparent lower severity of BPD in the transplant recipients.[97] More recently, the off-label administration of repeated intravenous doses of MSCs in two human babies with severe and advanced BPD did not prevent the children's deaths.[98]

HORMONAL REGULATORS

Glucocorticoids (GCs) have a deleterious effect on alveologenesis, under physiologic conditions, in contrast with their well-recognized beneficial effect on the prevention of respiratory distress syndrome in preterm infants.[99] Indeed, GCs accelerate alveolar wall thinning and fusion of the two capillary layers, leading to early termination of the septation process and resulting in fewer and larger alveoli in the mature lung.[100,101] The GC effects on lung structure appear to be permanent in the rat.[102] GC-induced inhibition of septation in mice is associated with down-regulation of VEGFR2 and impaired angiogenesis.[103] Deleterious effects of GC are prevented by RA treatment.[103,104] However, interactions between GCs and RA are complex and depend on the conditions in which they are being investigated. Thus in a situation of hyperoxic injury, simultaneous treatment with RA and dexamethasone was shown to improve survival in oxygen-exposed newborn rats.[105] In such models, RA may compensate the accelerating effects of GCs on septal maturation while keeping the benefit of GC treatment for lung epithelial maturation and for lowering inflammation.[106] In A549 cell culture, it was also shown that GCs regulate vitamin A signaling via inhibition of β-carotene 15,15′-oxygenase (BCO1) gene expression in a PPARα-dependent manner.[107]

Thyroid hormone is known to accelerate lung maturation[108,109] but is also involved in alveolarization. Maternal hypothyroidism affects postnatal alveolar septation even before the functioning of fetal thyroid.[110] Newborn rats born to iodine-deficient mothers have larger and irregularly shaped alveoli.[109] Mechanisms by which thyroid hormone influence secondary septation are not known. Decreased MMP-9 mRNA levels were found in iodine-deficient pups, suggesting impairment in the process of basement membrane disruption required during lung development.[109]

RETINOIC ACID

RA and its receptors RARs/RXRs play a complex and critical role in alveolarization during the neonatal period of the lung, including both stimulatory and inhibitory influences.[106] During late gestation, the lungs of rats contain retinyl esters,[111] which are precursors of RA. The RA-synthesizing enzymes aldehyde dehydrogenase 1 (Aldh-1) and retinaldehyde dehydrogenase 2 (Raldh-2) are up-regulated during the period of maximal alveolar-wall cell proliferation.[112] RA enhances tropoelastin gene expression,[31] and use of inhibitors of retinoid metabolism to reduce the flux of retinyl esters to RA was linked to a decrease in the steady-state level of tropoelastin transcripts in rat lung fibroblasts and fetal lung explants.[111] RA also up-regulates the mRNA expression of PDGF-A and PDGFR-α and -β,[30] and of FGF18.[33] Postnatal treatment with RA increases the number of pulmonary alveoli in neonatal rat pups,[113] whereas vitamin A deficiency led to delayed alveolar development.[32] Simultaneous deletion of two RA receptors, RARγ and RXRα,[114] or overexpression of dominant negative RARα,[115] reduced alveolar number, whereas RARβ knockout mice exhibited higher alveolar number.[116] In newborn rats exposed to hyperoxia and studied at day 14 of life, RA treatment improved survival and increased lung collagen but did not improve alveolar development.[105] By contrast, at day 45, lungs were no longer different from those in controls, indicating complete recovery, whereas deficient alveologenesis remained obvious in hyperoxia-exposed rats that were not RA-treated.[117] In humans, blood retinol concentration was shown to be lower in prematurely born than in term infants, and lower in those who develop BPD than in those who do not.[118] In randomized controlled trials, vitamin A appeared to be beneficial in reducing death or oxygen requirement at 1 month of age, and oxygen requirement at 36 weeks' postmenstrual age.[119]

NUTRITION

Maternal food restriction causes intrauterine growth restriction (IUGR), which is a known risk for BPD in preterm infants. In a rat model of IUGR, maternal protein deprivation was associated with alveolarization arrest.[120] Expression of known growth factors involved in lung development were not altered in lungs of pups born from deprived mothers, raising the question of the possibility of programming of altered alveolarization.[120] In a more recent study, the same authors identified 13 miRNAs with more than twofold differential expression between control lungs and low protein diet–induced IUGR lungs.[121] Deregulation of several target genes of differentially expressed miRNAs could be predicted. Especially, E2F3, a transcription factor involved in cell cycle control, was expressed in developing alveoli, and its mRNA and protein levels were significantly increased after IUGR. Hence, IUGR affects the expression of selected miRNAs during lung alveolarization. These results provide a basis for deciphering the mechanistic contributions of IUGR to impaired alveolarization.[121] Maternal high fat diet–induced obesity was also demonstrated to alter lung development in mice pups, in part due to disruption of normal pulmonary angiogenesis in the developing lung.[122]

CONCLUSION

Alveolar multiplication is a phenomenon that takes place mainly postnatally in humans and in many animal species. Development of transgenic mouse models has led to substantial progress in understanding the regulation of alveolarization. However, the interactions between the multiple involved factors are still poorly understood. Rearrangement of the extracellular matrix and control of microvascular maturation are two critical phenomena for harmonious alveolarization. In humans, BPD, which represents the main respiratory sequela of prematurity, is characterized by impaired alveolarization. Better understanding of the mechanisms controlling the alveolarization may result in innovative treatments for this disease, whether preventive or curative.

 A complete reference list is available at www.ExpertConsult.com.

SELECT REFERENCES

1. Hadchouel A, Franco-Montoya ML, Delacourt C. Altered lung development in bronchopulmonary dysplasia. *Birth Defects Res A Clin Mol Teratol.* 2014;100:158-167.
5. Burri PH, Dbaly J, Weibel ER. The postnatal growth of the rat lung. I. Morphometry. *Anat Rec.* 1974;178:711-730.
8. Pozarska A, Rodriguez-Castillo JA, Surate Solaligue DE, et al. Stereological monitoring of mouse lung alveolarization from the early postnatal period to adulthood. *Am J Physiol Lung Cell Mol Physiol.* 2017;312:L882-L895.
9. Herring MJ, Putney LF, Wyatt G, et al. Growth of alveoli during postnatal development in humans based on stereological estimation. *Am J Physiol Lung Cell Mol Physiol.* 2014;307:L338-L344.
16. Lindahl P, Karlsson L, Hellstrom M, et al. Alveogenesis failure in PDGF-A-deficient mice is coupled to lack of distal spreading of alveolar smooth muscle cell progenitors during lung development. *Development.* 1997;124:3943-3953.
20. Buchacker T, Muhlfeld C, Wrede C, et al. Assessment of the alveolar capillary network in the postnatal mouse lung in 3D using serial block-face scanning electron microscopy. *Front Physiol.* 2019;10:1357.
27. Bultmann-Mellin I, Dinger K, Debuschewitz C, et al. Role of LTBP4 in alveolarization, angiogenesis, and fibrosis in lungs. *Am J Physiol Lung Cell Mol Physiol.* 2017;313:L687-L698.
37. Margraf LR, Tomashefski Jr JF, Bruce MC, et al. Morphometric analysis of the lung in bronchopulmonary dysplasia. *Am Rev Respir Dis.* 1991;143:391-400.
39. Kugler MC, Loomis CA, Zhao Z, et al. Sonic hedgehog signaling regulates myofibroblast function during alveolar septum formation in murine postnatal lung. *Am J Respir Cell Mol Biol.* 2017;57:280-293.
40. Hrycaj SM, Marty-Santos L, Cebrian C, et al. Hox5 genes direct elastin network formation during alveologenesis by regulating myofibroblast adhesion. *Proc Natl Acad Sci U S A.* 2018;115:E10605-E10614.
43. Atkinson JJ, Holmbeck K, Yamada S, et al. Membrane-type 1 matrix metalloproteinase is required for normal alveolar development. *Dev Dyn.* 2005;232:1079-1090.
52. Weinstein M, Xu X, Ohyama K, et al. FGFR-3 and FGFR-4 function cooperatively to direct alveogenesis in the murine lung. *Development.* 1998;125:3615-3623.
53. Li R, Herriges JC, Chen L, et al. FGF receptors control alveolar elastogenesis. *Development.* 2017;144:4563-4572.
60. El Agha E, Bellusci S. Walking along the fibroblast growth factor 10 route: a key pathway to understand the control and regulation of epithelial and mesenchymal cell-lineage formation during lung development and repair after injury. *Scientifica (Cairo).* 2014;2014:538379.
61. Chao CM, Yahya F, Moiseenko A, et al. Fgf10 deficiency is causative for lethality in a mouse model of bronchopulmonary dysplasia. *J Pathol.* 2017;241:91-103.
62. Chao CM, Moiseenko A, Kosanovic D, et al. Impact of Fgf10 deficiency on pulmonary vasculature formation in a mouse model of bronchopulmonary dysplasia. *Hum Mol Genet.* 2019;28:1429-1444.
63. Hokuto I, Perl AK, Whitsett JA. Prenatal, but not postnatal, inhibition of fibroblast growth factor receptor signaling causes emphysema. *J Biol Chem.* 2003;278:415-421.
68. Zhang H, Du L, Zhong Y, et al. Transforming growth factor-beta stimulates Smad1/5 signaling in pulmonary artery smooth muscle cells and fibroblasts of the newborn mouse through ALK1. *Am J Physiol Lung Cell Mol Physiol.* 2017;313:L615-L627.
70. Deng S, Zhang H, Han W, et al. Transforming growth factor-beta-neutralizing antibodies improve alveolarization in the oxygen-exposed newborn mouse lung. *J Interferon Cytokine Res.* 2019;39:106-116.
76. Jakkula M, Le Cras TD, Gebb S, et al. Inhibition of angiogenesis decreases alveolarization in the developing rat lung. *Am J Physiol Lung Cell Mol Physiol.* 2000;279:L600-L607.
79. Galambos C, Ng YS, Ali A, et al. Defective pulmonary development in the absence of heparin-binding vascular endothelial growth factor isoforms. *Am J Respir Cell Mol Biol.* 2002;27:194-203.
80. Vadivel A, Alphonse RS, Etches N, et al. Hypoxia-inducible factors promote alveolar development and regeneration. *Am J Respir Cell Mol Biol.* 2014;50:96-105.
82. Franco-Montoya ML, Boucherat O, Thibault C, et al. Profiling target genes of FGF18 in the postnatal mouse lung: possible relevance for alveolar development. *Physiol Genomics.* 2011;43:1226-1240.
85. Bhatt AJ, Pryhuber GS, Huyck H, et al. Disrupted pulmonary vasculature and decreased vascular endothelial growth factor, Flt-1, and TIE-2 in human infants dying with bronchopulmonary dysplasia. *Am J Respir Crit Care Med.* 2001;164:1971-1980.
86. Thebaud B, Ladha F, Michelakis ED, et al. Vascular endothelial growth factor gene therapy increases survival, promotes lung angiogenesis, and prevents alveolar damage in hyperoxia-induced lung injury: evidence that angiogenesis participates in alveolarization. *Circulation.* 2005;112:2477-2486.
90. Iosef C, Liu M, Ying L, et al. Distinct roles for IkappaB kinases alpha and beta in regulating pulmonary endothelial angiogenic function during late lung development. *J Cell Mol Med.* 2018;22:4410-4422.
92. Moreira A, Winter C, Joy J, et al. Intranasal delivery of human umbilical cord Wharton's jelly mesenchymal stromal cells restores lung alveolarization and vascularization in experimental bronchopulmonary dysplasia. *Stem Cells Transl Med.* 2020;9:221-234.
96. Ren X, Ustiyan V, Guo M, et al. Postnatal alveologenesis depends on FOXF1 signaling in c-KIT(+) endothelial progenitor cells. *Am J Respir Crit Care Med.* 2019;200:1164-1176.
107. Gong X, Marisiddaiah R, Rubin LP. Inhibition of pulmonary beta-carotene 15, 15'-oxygenase expression by glucocorticoid involves PPARalpha. *PLoS One.* 2017;12:e0181466.
120. Zana-Taieb E, Butruille L, Franco-Montoya ML, et al. Effect of two models of intrauterine growth restriction on alveolarization in rat lungs: morphometric and gene expression analysis. *PLoS One.* 2013;8. e78326.
121. Dravet-Gounot P, Morin C, Jacques S, et al. Lung microRNA deregulation associated with impaired alveolarization in rats after intrauterine growth restriction. *PLoS One.* 2017;12:e0190445.
122. Heyob KM, Mieth S, Sugar SS, et al. Maternal high-fat diet alters lung development and function in the offspring. *Am J Physiol Lung Cell Mol Physiol.* 2019;317:L167-L174.

Physiologic Mechanisms of Normal and Altered Lung Growth Before and After Birth

57

Megan J. Wallace | Stuart B. Hooper | Richard Harding

INTRODUCTION

Growth and development of the lung occurs both before and after birth and is a major determinant of respiratory health throughout postnatal life. Adequate lung growth before birth is necessary for the successful transition from fetal to postnatal life. Normal lung growth after birth is necessary to enable the lung to meet increasing metabolic demands during infancy and childhood and into adulthood. During its development, the lung must acquire an intricate system of airways allowing low-resistance airflow to and from the respiratory zone; the internal surface area of the respiratory zone must be large with a dense vascular network allowing a high level of blood flow. The distance between the distal airspaces and the surrounding vascular network must also be thin enough to enable efficient gas exchange. In terms of its mechanical properties, lung tissue must be easily expanded during inspiration but retain sufficient recoil to drive expiration, and surfactant is required to prevent collapse at the end of expiration. It is now apparent that the physiologic processes controlling lung growth before and after birth are quite different, although the molecular mechanisms are likely to be similar. This chapter presents an overview of the physiologic control of lung growth before and after birth, as well as pathophysiologic processes that perturb normal lung growth.

FETAL LUNG GROWTH

During fetal life, the future air spaces of the lungs are filled with a unique liquid that is produced by the lung as a result of net transepithelial ion movement into the lung that creates an osmotic gradient favoring movement of water into the lung. This osmotic gradient is primarily due to active secretion of chloride into the lung.[1] This fetal lung liquid (FLL) plays a critical role in lung development by maintaining the future air spaces in a distended state; it also limits entry of amniotic fluid into the lungs, which can have damaging effects. The volume of FLL within the future air spaces and its flux to and from the lower airways are influenced by fetal muscular activity, as well as by fetal posture and other factors that influence fetal transpulmonary pressure.[2] By maintaining this distended state, FLL serves as an internal "splint," which maintains a high degree of expansion of the distal air spaces.[1-3] Without this underlying expansion, the fetal lung is unable to grow and structurally mature.[2] Experimental manipulations have clearly demonstrated that sustained reductions in FLL volume reduce fetal lung growth and structural maturation, whereas sustained increases in FLL volume accelerate fetal lung growth and structural maturation.[1,2] Most clinical conditions that result in altered lung growth can also be explained by underlying alterations in FLL volume. Consequently, much attention has focused on understanding how the volume of FLL is controlled and the mechanisms by which it influences the growth and remodeling of fetal lung tissue. It is apparent that the fetal metabolic and endocrine environments also play important roles in lung development, especially in lung maturation, and studies in transgenic mice, genomics, transcriptomics, proteomics, and epigenetics are now elucidating the cellular and molecular mechanisms. The physical factors that are critical for normal lung development underlie many common disorders of fetal lung growth and are the major focus of this chapter.

CONTROL OF FETAL LUNG EXPANSION

Identification of the factors that control fetal lung expansion and its fundamental role in lung growth are derived primarily from studies of chronically catheterized fetal sheep.[1,2,4] During the latter half of ovine gestation, the volume of FLL within the fetal lungs progressively increases, reaching 35 to 45 mL/kg during the last weeks of gestation[2]; this is considerably greater than the functional residual capacity of the air-filled lung after birth (25 to 30 mL/kg) (Fig. 57.1).[5] The high level of fetal lung expansion is largely maintained by fetal muscular activity, involving fetal breathing movements (FBMs)[6,7] and laryngeal adductor muscles[2] (Fig. 57.2), but also depends on FLL secretion, resulting in the development of a transpulmonary pressure gradient. The degree to which the lungs can expand is ultimately dependent on the available intrathoracic and intrauterine space (see later). Values of lung expansion obtained from dead, anesthetized, exteriorized, or paralyzed fetuses will necessarily be underestimates, because FLL is lost under these conditions[2,7] (see Fig. 57.2). Similarly, measurements of FLL volume are questionable unless they were made in the absence of fetal hypoxemia or labor, and in the presence of normal amniotic fluid volumes.[8,9] Both labor and reduced amniotic fluid volume reduce FLL volume by increasing fetal transpulmonary pressure owing to increased flexion of the fetal trunk.[8,9]

In the absence of labor, the volume of FLL in healthy fetuses is largely determined by fetal muscular activity and the transpulmonary pressure gradient. Although continued FLL secretion must contribute to FLL volume, the rate of secretion is relatively unimportant as alterations in the FLL secretion rate have little or no effect on the resulting volume.[10] The rate of FLL efflux from the fetal lung via the trachea is dependent on the pressure gradient between the lung lumen and the amniotic sac (transpulmonary pressure), as well as the resistance to efflux in the upper respiratory tract.[11,12] In the absence of FBMs (i.e., during fetal apnea), the pulmonary intraluminal pressure is 1 to 2 mm Hg above amniotic sac pressure,[13] due to the inherent recoil of lung tissue and the resistance of the upper airway.[12] The resistance to liquid flow through the upper airway is high during apnea because laryngeal muscles are adducted. As a result, the rate of efflux of FLL through the trachea during apnea is, on average, lower than the rate of FLL production, and liquid accumulates within the lungs (Fig. 57.3).[4] During episodes of FBM, the resistance to efflux is reduced by phasic dilation of the glottis,[11,12] which together with the pressure gradient between the lungs and amniotic sac favors FLL efflux from the lungs (see Fig. 57.3).[4] Thus, despite rhythmic contractions of the diaphragm, the average net flow of liquid from the lungs during FBM episodes is two to three times greater than the rate of efflux during intervening nonbreathing (apneic) periods.[11] Although amniotic fluid can enter the fetal lungs during periods of accentuated FBM, the net flow is out of the lungs.[11] This essentially unidirectional flux of FLL helps maintain a constant chemical environment within the future air spaces, limiting

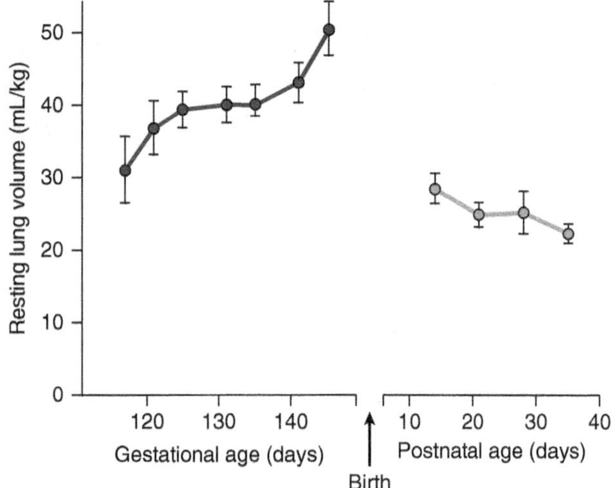

Fig. 57.1 Basal lung luminal volumes in fetal and postnatal sheep. The fetal data *(red circles)* are derived from measurements of fetal lung liquid volume made with a dye-dilution technique (*n* = 9 to 47 at each age). The postnatal data *(gold circles)* are derived from measurements of end-expiratory volume (functional residual capacity), made with a helium-dilution technique (*n* = 13 to 14 at each age). (From Harding R, Hooper SB. Regulation of lung expansion and lung growth before birth. *J Appl Physiol*. 1996;81:209–224.)

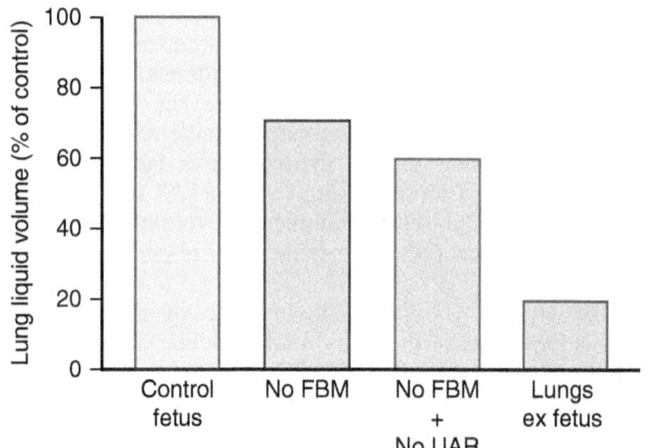

Fig. 57.2 The influence of fetal muscular activity on the volume of fetal lung liquid (FLL) retained within the future airways. The inhibition of fetal breathing movements *(FBMs)*, by fetal spinal cord transection[6] or selective blockade of the phrenic nerves,[7] causes an approximately 25% decrease in FLL volume from that in control fetuses, demonstrating the importance of FBMs in maintaining the FLL volume. If the fetal upper airway is bypassed, eliminating upper airway resistance *(UAR)* in addition to the abolition of FBMs, the FLL volume is reduced further, demonstrating the independent effect of the fetal upper airway on maintaining FLL volumes. The further reduction in FLL volume after the removal of the lungs from the fetus demonstrates the contribution of the fetal chest wall to maintaining FLL volumes. (From Harding R, Hooper SB. Regulation of lung expansion and lung growth before birth. *J Appl Physiol*. 1996;81:209–224.)

the entry of potentially harmful substances such as meconium. However, the occurrence of meconium aspiration syndrome in newborn infants[14] suggests that there are some circumstances in which substances dissolved or suspended in amniotic fluid can enter the fetal lungs, which most likely occurs during episodes of augmented fetal breathing[15] (or gasping) induced by fetal stress. Experimental studies injecting substances into the amniotic sac[16] suggest that brownian motion could potentially cause some

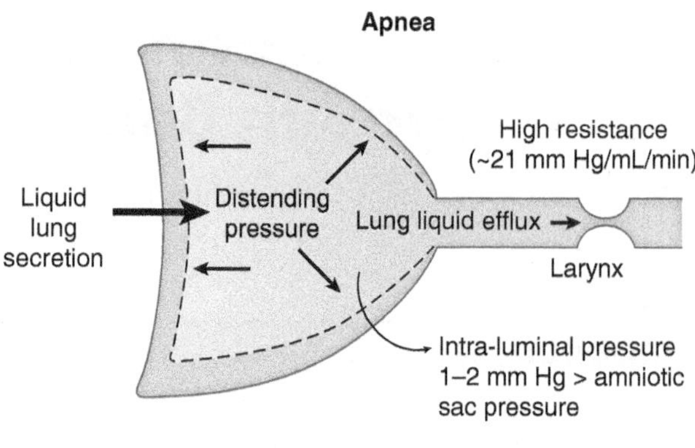

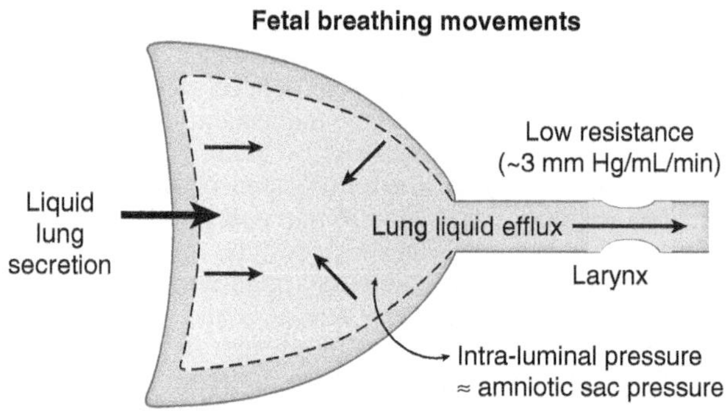

Fig. 57.3 The role of the fetal upper airway in regulating the efflux of fetal lung liquid (FLL) during periods of apnea *(upper panel)* and of fetal breathing movements (FBMs) *(lower panel)*. During periods of apnea, the resistance to FLL efflux through the upper airway is high (owing to a lack of laryngeal abductor activity and the presence of tonic adductor activity); as a result, FLL tends to accumulate within the future airways, causing the lungs to expand. This liquid accumulation is responsible for generating a transpulmonary pressure gradient of 1 to 2 mm Hg (intra-airway pressure greater than amniotic sac pressure). During periods of FBM, the resistance to FLL efflux through the upper airway decreases (owing to phasic dilator activity of glottic abductor muscles and lack of sustained activity in adductor muscles); therefore, FLL leaves the lungs at an increased rate.

exchange of substances between lung liquid and the amniotic sac. However, the differences in ionic and protein composition between lung liquid and amniotic fluid[17] support the notion that in healthy fetuses, the movement of lung liquid is essentially unidirectional from the lungs towards the amniotic fluid.

The transpulmonary pressure gradient, and hence the efflux of FLL, is also influenced by factors external to the lungs, such as fetal abdominal pressure.[8] Changes in fetal posture (e.g., trunk flexion) that increase abdominal pressure can increase the transpulmonary pressure gradient, leading to a reduction in FLL volume.[8] Such changes in transpulmonary pressure can be caused by uterine contractions or may develop when intrauterine space is limited as a result of oligohydramnios[8] or by the presence of multiple fetuses. Lack of amniotic fluid forces the fetus into a more flexed posture.[8] Increased flexion increases fetal abdominal pressure and thus transpulmonary pressure, leading to increased FLL efflux and a reduction in lung volume (Fig. 57.4).[8] This is the likely cause of lung hypoplasia associated with prolonged oligohydramnios.[8] Because the fetal lungs and chest wall are highly compliant, even small changes in transpulmonary pressure will have marked effects on the rate of FLL efflux and consequently, on the degree of lung expansion.

EFFECTS OF REDUCED LUNG EXPANSION ON FETAL LUNG GROWTH AND MATURATION

Sustained reductions in fetal lung expansion are a common cause of fetal lung hypoplasia and retarded lung development,

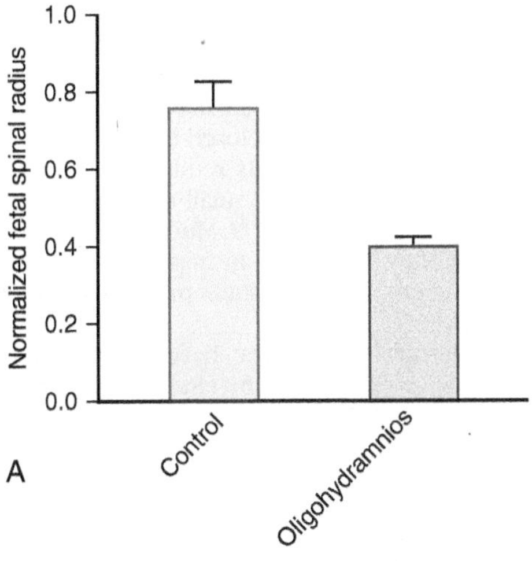

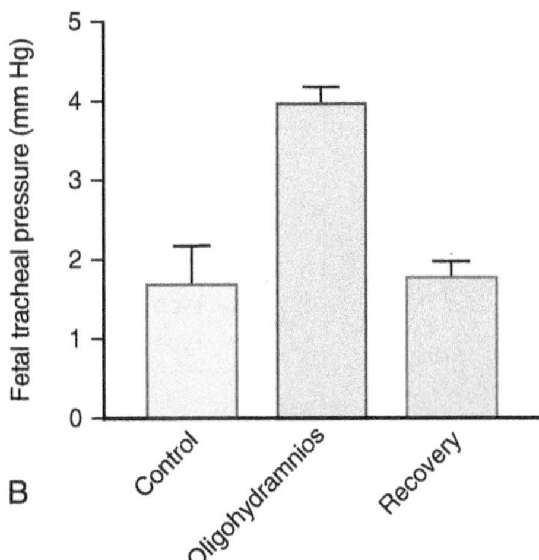

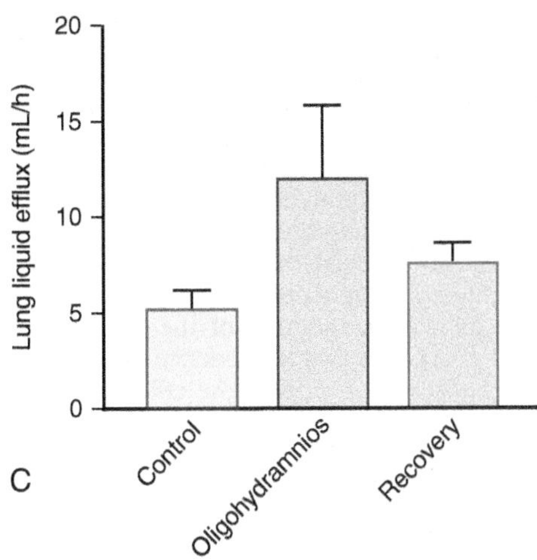

Fig. 57.4 The effect of oligohydramnios on spinal flexion, fetal tracheal pressure, and fetal lung liquid efflux. (A) Oligohydramnios induced by amniotic fluid drainage in fetal sheep increases spinal flexion (a smaller normalized spinal radius is indicative of greater curvature of the spine). Fetal tracheal pressure (B) and lung liquid efflux along the trachea (C) during a control period, a 48-hour period of oligohydramnios (induced by draining amniotic fluid) and after replacement of amniotic fluid (recovery) in fetal sheep. (From Harding R, Hooper SB, Dickson KA. A mechanism leading to reduced lung expansion and lung hypoplasia in fetal sheep during oligohydramnios. *Am J Obstet Gynecol* 1990;163:1904–1913.)

including effects on cell proliferation, extracellular matrix (ECM) deposition, alveolarization, vascular development, and alveolar epithelial cell (AEC) differentiation. The hypoplastic effects appear to depend on the degree to which lung expansion is decreased. For example, a 25% reduction in lung expansion causes lung growth to be reduced by approximately 25%,[6] whereas total lung deflation causes lung tissue growth to effectively cease.[3,18,19] The remodeling of lung parenchyma that characterizes normal lung maturation is also retarded by reduced lung expansion.[3] In particular, perialveolar tissue volume is increased,[3] leading to thicker septa and a reduced diffusing capacity for respiratory gases. Furthermore, alveolarization is attenuated,[3] which is probably related to impaired elastogenesis,[20] and there is a reduction in the growth and maturation of the pulmonary vascular bed, resulting in elevated pulmonary vascular resistance after birth.[21] These findings indicate that lung expansion is an essential and normal stimulus for fetal lung growth. It is likely that the high degree of lung expansion during fetal life provides a direct mechanical stimulus to cells that is required to activate or suppress key regulatory gene pathways (as discussed further below).[22-26]

The alveolar epithelium of the fetal lung is also affected by the degree of fetal lung expansion.[3,27] Prolonged reductions in expansion promote differentiation of type I AECs into type II AECs,[27] whereas prolonged overexpansion reduces the proportion of type II AECs to less than 2% and increases the proportion of type I AECs to greater than 90%.[28] These findings support in vitro evidence that type I AECs are not terminally differentiated and can transdifferentiate into type II AECs.[29] Indeed, the high degree of lung expansion during fetal life is associated with a predominance of type I AECs (60% to 70% of all AECs) relative to type II AECs (25% to 35% of all AECs).[28] After birth, when lung expansion decreases, there is an increase in the proportion of type II AECs (to approximately 53% of all AECs) and a reduction in the type I AEC phenotype (to approximately 45% of all AECs) (Fig. 57.5).[28]

EFFECTS OF INCREASED LUNG EXPANSION ON FETAL LUNG GROWTH AND MATURATION

Prolonged overexpansion of the fetal lungs is a very potent stimulus for fetal lung growth and tissue remodeling.[3,30] Experimentally, this can be induced by ligation or obstruction of the bronchus or trachea.[18,23,31-33] The increase in lung cell proliferation and cell hypertrophy in response to tracheal obstruction is time dependent[31] and is restricted to the expanded lung tissue.[18] This indicates that local factors, not circulating factors, must mediate the effect of lung expansion on lung development,[18] although basal levels of growth hormone are required.[22,31,34] The growth response to tracheal obstruction also differs according to the stage of fetal lung development. During the alveolar stage in fetal sheep, the acceleration in lung growth is completed within 7 days of tracheal obstruction, with proliferation of most cell types in the distal lung (fibroblasts, type II AECs, and endothelial cells)[30] resulting in an almost doubling of lung DNA content.[22,31] The eventual cessation of accelerated growth is probably due to the physical restraint imposed by the chest wall, which prevents further lung expansion. Structural maturation is also accelerated, with a reduced proportion of tissue space[3] and increased collagen and elastin deposition,[20] capillary formation,[33,35]

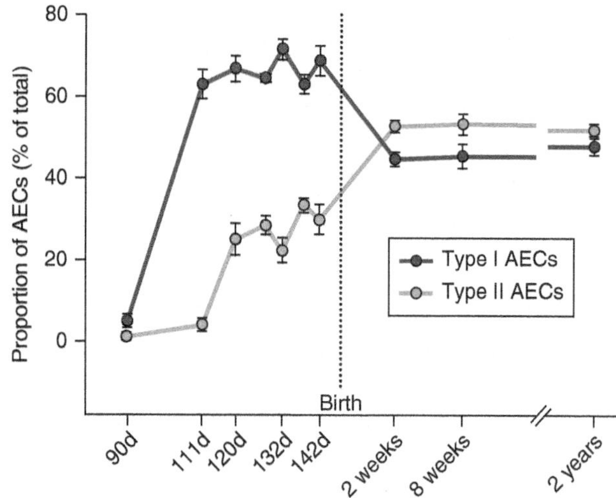

Fig. 57.5 Changes in alveolar epithelial cell proportions before and after birth. In fetal sheep, undifferentiated epithelial cells differentiate into type I *(red circles)* and type II *(gold circles)* alveolar epithelial cells *(AECs)* during the canalicular stage of lung development, between 90 and 120 days of gestational age (term is approximately 145 days). The type I AECs appear first, then remain stable until birth, accounting for 60% to 70% of all AECs. Type II AECs differentiate later, then remain stable until birth, accounting for approximately 30% of all AECs. After birth, the relative proportions of each AEC type reverse; the proportion of type I AECs decreases to approximately 45%, and the proportion of type II AECs increases to approximately 55% of all AECs. The change in AECs at birth is likely associated with the reduction in lung expansion, due to the loss of the distending influence of lung liquid and the development of an air-liquid interface. *d*, Days. (From Flecknoe SJ, Wallace MJ, Cock ML, et al. Changes in alveolar epithelial cell proportions during fetal and neonatal development in sheep. *Am J Physiol Lung Cell Mol Physiol*. 2003;285:L664–L670.)

alveolar number, and luminal surface area.[30] By contrast, during the late pseudoglandular to early canalicular stage, acceleration in lung growth in response to tracheal obstruction is slower[36] but eventually results in a greater (~200%) increase in lung DNA content,[36,37] primarily due to mesenchymal cell proliferation[36,37] with a large increase in perisaccular tissue volume.[36,37] Similar results have been obtained in fetal rabbits.[38] The lower rate of accelerated lung growth in younger fetuses may be due to lower lung compliance and thus less lung expansion at the initial stages of tracheal obstruction until more significant structural remodeling has commenced.[36,37] The eventual greater increase in lung DNA content in younger fetuses is probably due to greater compliance of the chest wall, allowing the lungs to expand to a greater degree than in older fetuses.[36,37]

The mechanisms by which lung expansion affects the rate of lung growth and structural maturation are under active investigation and are discussed below. However, it must be recognized that the mechanical stresses imposed on lung tissue by sustained alterations in lung expansion are likely to be very different depending on the location of cells within the tissue. For example, in response to increased lung expansion, some cells will experience a stretch-like stimulus, whereas others may experience compression.

THE ROLE OF FETAL BREATHING MOVEMENTS IN LUNG EXPANSION AND LUNG GROWTH

FBMs begin early in fetal life and progressively become organized into discrete episodes that are largely associated with a fetal behavioral state resembling rapid eye movement sleep.[39] During the latter half of gestation the incidence of FBMs is 40% to 50%.[4,12,39] The major muscle used in FBMs is the diaphragm; respiratory activity of the intercostal muscles is largely absent, as in postnatal rapid eye movement sleep. During FBM episodes the laryngeal abductor (dilator) muscles contract in phase with the diaphragm, whereas during fetal apnea this dilator activity is absent and the glottis is closed by sustained adductor activity.[4,12] Typically, individual FBMs reduce intrathoracic pressure by up to 5 mm Hg[39] and cause small oscillations of liquid flow within the fetal upper airway.[40,41] Much interest has focused on FBMs because they constitute an important determinant of fetal lung development, although their precise role in vivo took time to unravel.[1,2]

Numerous techniques have been used to explore the functional role of FBMs, by eliminating or blunting their effects, including fetal paralysis, phrenic nerve sectioning,[42,43] or reversible blockade,[7] sectioning of the fetal spinal cord above the outflow of the phrenic motoneurons,[6,44,45] or replacing sections of the thoracic wall with a compliant membrane.[46] However, the findings must be interpreted with caution owing to confounding factors associated with those procedures. For example, phrenic nerve section causes the diaphragm muscle to atrophy, whereas thoracoplasty may allow lung compression, and fetal paralysis abolishes laryngeal adductor activity and may alter fetal posture. To identify the specific role of FBMs in lung development, it is necessary to alter only FBM and then to measure FLL volume. With this investigative approach, it is apparent that the reduction in lung growth induced by the abolition of FBM can be explained by the associated decrease in the basal level of fetal lung expansion[6,7]; indeed, the percentage decrease in lung expansion is similar to the reduction in lung growth.[6] The decrease in lung expansion after abolition of the thoracic component of FBM can be explained by persistence of laryngeal dilator activity.[6] As a result of this activity, the efflux of FLL is increased during centrally generated FBMs over that observed in intact fetuses.[6,7] Thus in intact fetuses, rhythmic activation of the diaphragm in FBM apparently plays a key role in restricting the loss of FLL when the resistance to FLL efflux is lowered by glottic dilation.[1,2] Collectively, these data show that fetal muscular activity, whether it is active glottic adduction during apnea or activation of the diaphragm during FBM episodes, helps to defend FLL volume and hence the degree of lung expansion (see Figs. 57.2 and 57.3). At present, no in vivo evidence has emerged to show that phasic stretch, per se, of the lung during FBMs is an important determinant of fetal lung growth, although in vitro evidence suggests this is possible.

Numerous in vitro studies have used phasic stretch of fetal lung cells in culture in an attempt to simulate FBMs in vivo. Such studies usually expose isolated fetal lung cells to 5% phasic distension, either constantly at approximately 60 cycles/minute, or intermittently (e.g., for 15 minutes in each hour), in either two-dimensional or three-dimensional cultures.[47-49] Other studies use much higher levels of distension in culture (20% phasic stretch), but those studies are designed to mimic overdistension injury in ventilated patients, which leads to abnormal, not normal lung development, and are not therefore, included as part of this discussion.

The 5% distension regimen causes an increase in fetal lung cell proliferation[47-51] and differentiation of distal lung epithelial cells,[52-54] implying that phasic distension as a result of FBM may be important for lung development in a manner similar to basal distension. However, the stimulus used (approximately 5% stretch) probably exceeds that induced by FBMs in vivo. In vivo, individual FBMs are essentially isovolumic, so the percent length change experienced by a lung cell with each FBM will be negligible. This is because the fetal chest wall is very compliant, and FLL is very viscous compared with air and, owing to its mass, has a large inertia. Thus although activation of the diaphragm causes a reduction in intrathoracic pressure, very little liquid is inhaled with each inspiratory effort, because other sections of the chest wall are simultaneously drawn in[55] and free liquid must be present within the pharynx before any liquid can be inhaled.[12] As a result, the tidal volume in the fetus is very small. In late-gestation fetal sheep, the tidal volume is usually less than 0.5 mL[39] at FBM rates of up to 3/second. In human fetuses during the last trimester, the mean FBM frequency is approximately 1/second,[40] although respiratory cycle times of up to 1.5 to 2.0 seconds have been reported. Color Doppler ultrasound imaging has been used to measure liquid flow velocity waveforms in the trachea and nasopharynx of human fetuses, although the contribution of this liquid movement to lung volume changes is unclear.[41] Thus, at least in sheep, fetal tidal volume is less than 1% of resting lung luminal volume but markedly increases immediately after birth to approximately 20% of resting lung volume (functional residual capacity). Nevertheless, in vitro studies investigating the effects of phasic distension on lung cells have provided important information about the cellular mechanisms by which the fetal lung responds to physical forces. These experiments are described in more detail in the next section.

MECHANOTRANSDUCTION MECHANISMS AFFECTING LUNG GROWTH AND CELL DIFFERENTIATION

All cells, tissues, and even whole organs are subjected to physical forces in vivo, including shear stress, stretch, and compression. These forces can result from gravity, osmotic pressures, fluid flow, intracellular tensile forces, body movements, and changes in the internal volume of hollow organs such as the lung. It has been proposed that cells exist in a state of isometric tension that is generated by the intracellular contractile filaments of the cell.[56] In cultured AECs this tension is 0.1 to 0.2 kPa.[57] Thus, externally applied forces are imposed on a preexisting equilibrium of force, causing changes in cell shape and intracellular structural fiber alignment until the force equilibrium is reestablished.[56,58]

Physical forces play an important role in cell growth and differentiation, are critical regulators of three-dimensional tissue structure,[58] particularly in the lung,[1,59] and constitute an important means by which cells interact with and adapt to changes in their environment.[56] The transduction pathways by which physical forces are translated into chemical stimuli, and lead to changes in cell function, are still being explored. Transmembrane cell surface receptors, such as integrins, are ideally placed to detect and respond to alterations in the physical environment. Integrins bind to ECM proteins via their extracellular domain, whereas their intracellular domains are bound to fibrillar-actin bundles of the cell cytoskeleton via cytoskeleton-associated proteins (e.g., talin, vinculin, paxillin), and are associated with other signaling proteins, including phosphatidylinositol 3-kinase, pp60src, growth-factor-receptor-bound protein 2, and p130Cas.[60] The cell cytoskeleton is in turn coupled to the nuclear skeleton via the LINC complex composed of nesprins, SUN proteins, and lamins. Nesprin on the outer nuclear membrane binds intermediate and microfilaments of the cell cytoskeleton and connects with SUN proteins on the inner nuclear membrane. SUN proteins bind to the internal nuclear scaffold and to nuclear proteins via A-type lamins. Together these complexes form a structural continuum from the ECM to the nucleus. It is through these physical couplings that mechanical forces can be detected and translated into intracellular chemical signals.[58,61,62] The chemical signaling pathways are less well defined, but they are likely to include stretch-activated ion channels, activation of intracellular second messenger systems, direct activation of RNA polymerases and DNA-synthesis enzymes, and recruitment of messenger RNA and protein translation machinery, as well as alteration of chromatin structure allowing access of transcription factors to gene promoters.[56,63,64] Together, these pathways likely result in the synthesis or release of ECM proteins, growth factors, cytokines, and other factors that can act in an autocrine or paracrine manner to induce cell proliferation, differentiation, migration, or other alterations in cell function (Fig. 57.6) that lead to marked changes in the size, structure, and function of the lung.

The importance of signaling through mechanotransduction pathways has been highlighted by transgenic mice and isolated fetal lung cells exposed to cyclic stretch. Integrin α3-null mice have abnormal branching morphogenesis,[65] whereas double α3/α6 integrin null-mice have left lung agenesis and severe right lung hypoplasia.[66] The lungs of integrin α8-null mice have defective alveolarization and abnormal elastin deposition.[67] Epithelial cell differentiation also appears to require integrin signaling, as blocking antibodies against integrins β1, α3, and α6 reduce the increases in SP-C mRNA levels induced by 5% phasic stretch of cultured fetal lung epithelial cells.[68] Exposing fetal lung cells to cyclic stretch also increases pp60src activity and its translocation to the cytoskeleton,[69] which activates phospholipase Cγ1, leading to increases in diacylglycerol and inositol 1,4,5-trisphosphate (InsP3) content.[47] InsP3 releases calcium from intracellular stores via the InsP3 receptor (InsP3R), which, via diacylglycerol, activates protein kinase C and its downstream mitogenic effects. Activation of phospholipase Cγ1 and protein kinase C is required for cyclic stretch-induced proliferation of fetal lung cells in culture (see Fig. 57.6).[69]

Mechanical forces can also be converted into biochemical signals by activation of stretch-activated ion channels, which alter intracellular ion concentrations. Calcium, in particular, is an important cofactor for the activation of many signaling pathways. Blocking strain-induced calcium channels or chelating intracellular calcium stores abolishes the proliferation of lung cells in culture,[49] suggesting that calcium entry into cells, via stretch-activated ion channels, is vital for fetal lung growth. Blockade of voltage-dependent calcium channels also causes hypoplasia in lung explants.[70] Inhibiting calmodulin, a major calcium-signaling molecule, in type II AECs of transgenic mice disrupts lung development,[71] and postnatal rats treated with a calmodulin antagonist have impaired lung growth.[72] This is consistent with the finding that calmodulin mRNA levels are increased in response to an increase in fetal lung expansion,[73] when lung cells are proliferating at rates approximately 800% above that in control fetuses. Hemi-pneumonectomy in young rats induces compensatory lung growth in the remaining lung, which like fetal lung growth, is thought to be expansion mediated.[74,75] The time course for the increase in lung growth after postnatal hemi-pneumonectomy in rats is very similar to that induced by tracheal obstruction in fetal sheep,[30] with a maximal increase in both cell proliferation and calmodulin expression within 2 days.[72,73,75] The calmodulin inhibitor trifluoperazine reduces both calmodulin activity and the increase in lung growth induced by hemi-pneumonectomy.[75] These findings indicate that calcium signaling is critical for enabling expansion-induced lung growth both before and after birth.

Calcium may also mediate the effects of lung stretch on AEC differentiation. As noted above, 5% phasic stretch of cultured fetal lung epithelial cells increases SP-C mRNA levels; this effect is increased in the presence of an agonist for the calcium-permeable cation channel TRPV4, while a TRPV4 antagonist completely abolishes the effect of phasic stretch on SP-C expression.[76]

It is also possible that increased expansion of the fetal lung stimulates growth factors and/or an increase in their receptors that act locally, in an autocrine or paracrine manner, to stimulate cellular proliferation. The fetal lung produces a number of growth factors and their receptors, including platelet-derived growth factor,[77,78] vascular endothelial growth factor,[79] insulin-like growth factors 1 and 2,[80] fibroblast growth factors,[81] and transforming growth factor β,[82] which have been shown to be critical for fetal lung development. Furthermore, phasic distension of cells in culture induces the expression of many of

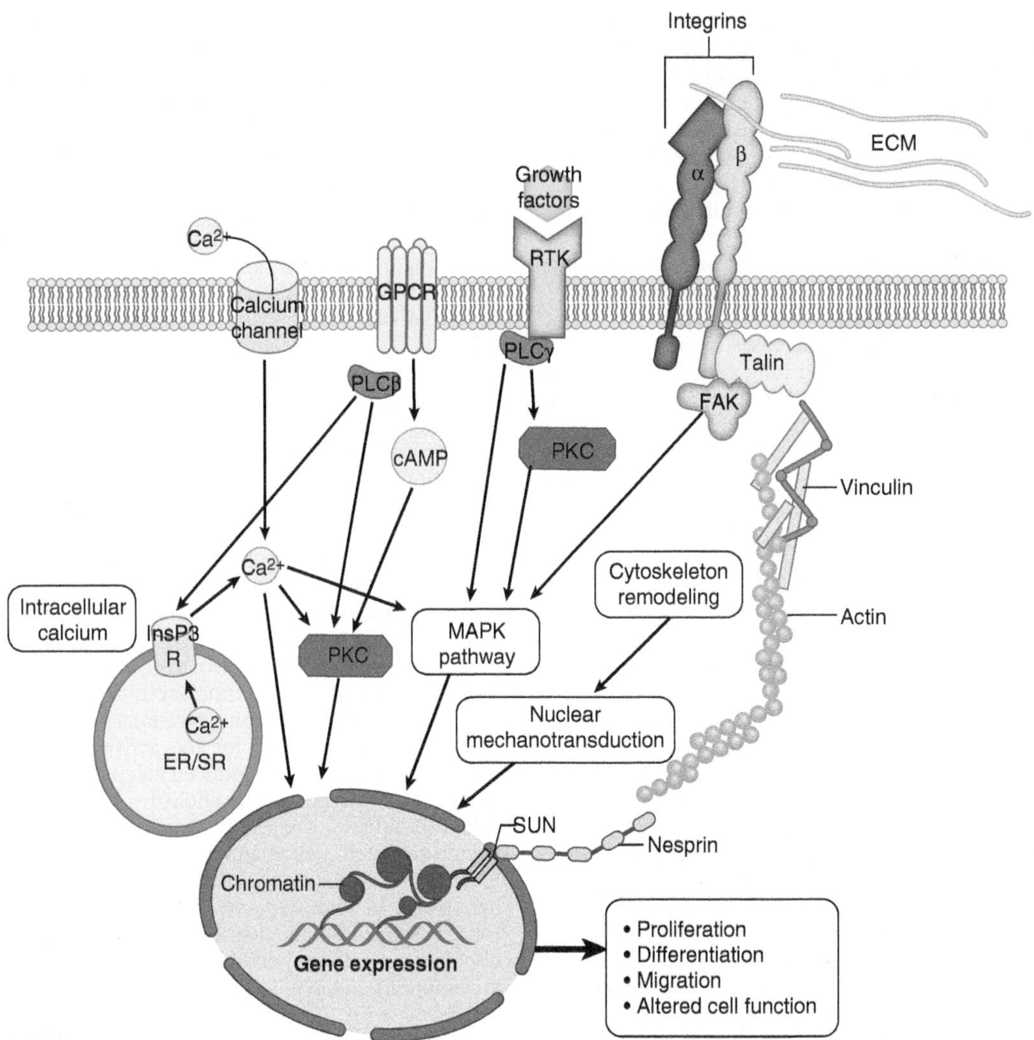

Fig. 57.6 Potential growth and mechanotransduction pathways in the developing lung. These pathways include increases in intracellular calcium concentration,[59] signaling through G protein–coupled receptors *(GPCRs)*,[242] growth factors binding to their receptor tyrosine kinases *(RTK)*,[50,83,86] and integrin signaling.[60] Calcium can enter the cell via stretch-activated calcium channels and can be released from intracellular stores when inositol 1,4,5-trisphosphate (InsP3) binds to its receptor *(InsP3R)*. Calcium can activate calcium-associated signaling. GPCRs are activated by factors known to influence lung development, including cytokines, parathyroid hormone–related protein, and prostaglandins. G proteins can activate or inhibit cyclic adenosine monophosphate *(cAMP)* signaling and activate phospholipase Cβ *(PLCβ)*, catalyzing the hydrolysis of phosphatidylinositol 4,5-bisphosphate to InsP3, activating calcium signaling pathways and diacylglycerol, which activates the protein kinase C *(PKC)* pathway. Growth factors bound to their RTKs activate phospholipase Cγ *(PLCγ)* and/or the mitogen-activated protein kinase *(MAPK)* pathway. Calcium, cAMP, PLCβ, and PLCγ can all activate the PKC pathway, which activates the MAPK pathway regulating transcription. Force changes in the extracellular matrix *(ECM)* can be transmitted through integrins to focal adhesions, which connect the ECM to actin and other connecting proteins, including talin, focal adhesion kinase *(FAK)*, and vinculin. Actin is connected to the nucleoskeleton via nesprin and SUN proteins to lamin, which in turn connects to chromatin, altering access to gene promoter regions. Force can therefore be transmitted from the ECM to the chromatin to alter gene transcription. Alteration of gene transcription via any of these pathways can lead to alterations in cell proliferation, differentiation, migration, and other cell functions, which coordinate to promote lung growth and development. *ER*, Endoplasmic reticulum; *SR*, sarcoplasmic reticulum. (From Wallace MJ, Hooper SB, McDougall ARA. Physical, endocrine and growth factors in lung development. In: Harding R, Pinkerton KE, eds. *The Lung: Development, Aging and the Environment*. 2nd ed. Waltham, MA: Academic Press; 2015:165.)

these growth factors,[50,54,83,84] suggesting that they may mediate the effects of lung expansion on lung development.

Insulin-like growth factor-2 expression is decreased by reductions and enhanced by sustained increases in lung expansion,[22,85] but the increase in insulin-like growth factor-2 expression occurs only after the maximal increase in expansion-induced DNA synthesis rates has already occurred.[86] Similarly, expression of platelet-derived growth factor subunit B is reduced in response to tracheal obstruction, when DNA synthesis rates are elevated, suggesting that expansion-induced lung growth is unlikely to be mediated by those growth factors.[86] Surprisingly, increased fetal lung expansion does not activate extracellular signal–regulated kinase 1 or extracellular signal–regulated kinase 2 of the mitogen-activated protein kinase pathway,[86] suggesting that growth factor receptor activation, at least via the extracellular signal–regulated kinase pathway, is unlikely to be a major mediator of expansion-induced fetal lung growth. However, basal levels of genes in the ERK pathway are critical for lung growth, as transgenic manipulations of these genes in a variety of lung cell types cause either lung agenesis or lung hypoplasia.[87] However, vascular endothelial growth factor expression is reduced in lung hypoplasia and transiently increased after tracheal obstruction, indicating that vascular endothelial growth factor may mediate impaired vascular development in lung hypoplasia and may regulate endothelial cell proliferation in growth-accelerated lungs,[33,86,88] potentially via activation of c-Jun N-terminal kinase instead of extracellular signal–regulated kinase 1.

Several studies have used transcriptomic or proteomic approaches to identify larger-scale changes in gene expression and protein levels in response to decreases or increases in lung fetal lung expansion.[23,25,89-95] Numerous genes likely to be involved in expansion-induced lung growth, epithelial cell differentiation, or alveolarization were identified by Sozo and colleagues, using subtraction hybridization in fetal sheep,[23] and by Seaborn and colleagues, using serial analysis of gene expression in fetal mice.[94] In the fetal rabbit model of surgically induced congenital diaphragmatic hernia (which induces lung hypoplasia) and restoration of growth using tracheal obstruction, targeted gene screening and mRNA sequencing has been used to identify candidate genes associated with expansion-induced alveolarization and angiogenesis.[25,95-97] More recently, Peiro and colleagues, used a proteomic approach to identify proteins in tracheal liquid from fetal sheep with congenital diaphragmatic hernia (CDH)-induced lung hypoplasia and tracheal obstruction.[26] Many of the genes and proteins identified in the above studies have strong correlations with cell proliferation or differentiation in vivo, and cell culture or transgenic mouse studies often support the likelihood of those factors being involved.[23,25,26,89-92,95-97] However, proving the involvement of the identified genes and proteins in mechano-transduction-mediated lung development is much more challenging. This is due to the difficulty of performing transgenic manipulations and the cost of performing siRNA and CRISPR technologies in the large animals commonly used to manipulate lung expansion and the difficulties of altering lung expansion in small animals used for transgenic studies.

However, where specific inhibitors are available, these studies are possible. For example, studies in fetal mice with reduced fetal lung expansion induced by oligohydramnios, and increased fetal lung expansion induced by tracheal occlusion, have demonstrated that the Rho/Rho-associated kinase (ROCK) pathway, which regulates actin cytoskeleton assembly, is a likely mechanosensory pathway critical for mediating the effects of lung expansion on the generation of distal airways.[24]

Recent studies have focused on identifying the molecular mechanisms that regulate lung development more broadly (not specifically in relation to effect of physical forces on the lung).[98-102] The rapidly evolving fields of genomics, transcriptomics, proteomics, metabolomics, lipidomics, and epigenomics techniques are identifying novel genes and proteins and regulatory mechanisms, in addition to the molecules already known to have roles in cell growth, cell survival, cell migration, cell differentiation, and remodeling of the ECM. These studies are generating information regarding entire protein pathways and interactions between pathways, that likely play important roles in stimulating and coordinating normal and abnormal fetal lung growth and maturation.[102,103]

Those studies are dramatically enhancing our understanding of the molecular mechanisms that regulate lung development and publicly available databases like LungMAP (the Molecular Atlas of Lung Development Program; https://lungmap.net/)[102,104,105] and Jackson Laboratory lung development database (http://lungdevelopment.jax.org/),[106] enable data sharing and interrogation by other investigators. Many of the genes, proteins and pathways identified in such studies are discussed in more detail in Chapters 55, 56, and 58 and have been the subject of numerous reviews.[101,107] Studies in transgenic mice, particularly those that use inducible, cell-specific transgenic techniques, are also rapidly improving our understanding of how individual genes regulate lung development, and improved imaging and molecular techniques in mice and cell culture are improving our knowledge of the cell types, structural context, stages of lung development, and species in which these genes are expressed. However, the exact roles of these genes in mediating the effect of lung expansion on lung development are less well understood.

Another exciting area of investigation is the role that extracellular vesicles (EV) are likely to play in cell-to-cell communication in the lung. EV are small membrane vesicles that are released from many cell types and can carry microRNA (miRNA), proteins, and lipids from one cell to another.[108,109] Numerous studies have identified miRNAs that may regulate the expression of genes that are critical for lung development.[110-113] A recent study by Najrana and colleagues demonstrated the presence of EV in lung liquid from late gestion and newborn mouse lungs and in cultured lung cells exposed to stretch.[109] Cells exposed to 10% cyclic stretch for 24 hours produced twice as many EVs as unstretched controls, and nine of the miRNAs isolated from the EVs were differentially expressed. In contrast, cells exposed to 5% continuous stretch had a similar number of EVs to unstretched controls, but contained nearly four times as many differentially expressed miRNAs, including several miRNA species known to regulate T1α.[109] T1α is a marker of type-I epithelial cells in mice and sustained increases in lung expansion promote the differentiation of alveolar type II cells into alveolar type-I cells.[27,28] EVs and associated miRNA molecules may mediate the effect of expansion by cell-cell transmission and also offer an exciting potential route for the targeted delivery of new therapeutics to the lungs.

PHYSICAL CAUSES OF FETAL LUNG HYPOPLASIA

Fetal lung hypoplasia, defined at autopsy as a reduction in lung DNA content or lung tissue weight relative to body weight or by fetal imaging as reduced fetal lung-to-head ratio, is associated with disorders in pregnancy. Such disorders include oligohydramnios secondary to premature rupture of membranes or fetal anuria, CDH, thoracic space–occupying lesions such as pulmonary cysts, tumors, and pleural effusions, and fetal musculoskeletal deformities. The common mechanism for inducing fetal lung hypoplasia in these situations is likely to be a prolonged reduction in the degree of fetal lung expansion.[2,8]

OLIGOHYDRAMNIOS

Oligohydramnios occurs in approximately 10% of pregnancies and is usually caused by premature rupture of the fetal membranes or by inadequate fetal urine production due to fetal urinary tract disorders, including renal agenesis or dysplasia, agenesis or stenosis of the ureters, urethra, or urethral valve.[114] The severity of the lung growth deficit depends on the gestational age at onset and the duration and severity of oligohydramnios.[115] The likely cause of fetal lung hypoplasia in oligohydramnios is a prolonged reduction in lung expansion.[8] In the absence of amniotic fluid, the intrauterine space is reduced, so the fetal trunk is increasingly flexed.[8,114] This positioning leads to an increase in abdominal pressure, elevation of the diaphragm, compression of the lungs, and loss of lung liquid[8] (see Fig. 57.4); the efflux of FLL is increased during nonlabor uterine contractions, which further increase the degree of fetal spinal flexion.

CONGENITAL DIAPHRAGMATIC HERNIA

CDH is less common than oligohydramnios (1 in 2000 infants to 1 in 5000 infants) but results in severe, often fatal, lung hypoplasia. CDH occurs when the diaphragm fails to close during embryonic development, allowing abdominal contents to enter the thorax.[116-118] The hernia is usually unilateral, with 85% to 90% occurring on the left side, approximately 10% on the right side, and occasionally it is bilateral (2%). The entry of abdominal contents into the chest causes chronic lung collapse on the affected side(s) and reduces the space available for lung growth. The distending influence of diaphragmatic contractions during FBMs is also lost. As a result, the ipsilateral lung is unable to expand, and lung growth ceases. The contralateral lung may also be affected as the abdominal contents can induce a lateral shift in the mediastinal ligament. Because the defect occurs early, it usually results in severe lung hypoplasia, with major impairments in lung structure and function. Defective retinoid signaling has been implicated both in the diaphragmatic defect and directly in the lung hypoplasia,[119] as described in more detail below.

MUSCULOSKELETAL DISORDERS

A variety of fetal musculoskeletal disorders can lead to severe lung hypoplasia.[114] Although the precise mechanisms depend on the type of disorder, they probably all involve a prolonged reduction in lung expansion. Because the activity of the diaphragm and that of glottic adductor muscles play a crucial role in maintaining fetal lung expansion,[2] interference with such activity would be expected to impact fetal lung growth. Experimentally induced perturbations of the fetal musculoskeletal system such as spinal cord transection,[6,44] removing ribs,[120] or replacing sections of the thoracic wall with a compliant membrane[46] all lead to lung hypoplasia, which has been attributed to a reduction in lung expansion. Similarly, knockout mice, which lack skeletal muscle[121] or have rib-cage defects,[122] also develop lung hypoplasia, which is likely due—at least in part—to reductions in the degree of lung expansion.

EFFECTS OF CORTICOSTEROIDS ON GROWTH AND MATURATION OF THE FETAL LUNG

During development, the fetal lung is exposed to corticosteroids of maternal and fetal origin, particularly during late gestation and fetal distress. Much attention has been devoted to corticosteroids owing to their therapeutic value in enhancing lung maturity, although the cellular mechanisms by which they enhance lung development in vivo are still unclear. In the fetal lung, elevated circulating corticosteroid levels have important effects on structural development, the surfactant system, and the reabsorption of FLL at birth. Other potential effects of corticosteroids include reduced lung tissue growth and stimulation of type II AEC differentiation. Here we focus on the role of cortisol in fetal lung growth and structural maturation.

It is often assumed that corticosteroids induce fetal lung maturation at the expense of lung growth but the in vivo data are contradictory, probably reflecting species differences, as well as differences in dose, number of doses, and route of administration. Most studies have used synthetic glucocorticoids (betamethasone or dexamethasone), with a 30- to 40-fold greater bioactivity than endogenous corticosteroids. When administered to the mother, betamethasone[123] causes a decrease in both fetal body and lung growth, effects that become greater with increasing number of doses.[124,125] However, when administered directly to the fetus, betamethasone does not affect fetal body or lung growth.[126] Similarly, physiologic doses of cortisol, infused directly into the fetus to simulate the preparturition increase in fetal plasma cortisol level, induce structural maturation of the lung without affecting either fetal lung or body growth.[127-129] These data suggest that the effects of maternally administered betamethasone on fetal body and lung growth are dose dependent, mediated through an effect on the placenta, or related to the duration of exposure (i.e., half-life).

Removing the sources of corticosteroids or preventing their actions has led to conflicting effects on lung growth. Adrenalectomy[130] and hypophysectomy[131] in fetal sheep reduce lung protein rather than DNA content,[130] indicating that endogenous cortisol contributes to lung protein accumulation. By contrast, glucocorticoid receptor (GR) knockout increases lung hypercellularity (DNA content) within the mesenchyme, indicating that endogenous corticosteroids suppress lung mesenchymal cell proliferation.[132]

One of the principal effects of corticosteroids is enhanced structural maturation of the fetal lung, which improves lung mechanics after birth.[133] Both natural and synthetic corticosteroids markedly reduce perialveolar tissue volume, leading to a reduction in cellularity (cell density within the tissue) and a marked increase in potential air space volume; these changes thin the blood-gas barrier and increase lung compliance. By contrast, adrenalectomized or hypophysectomized fetal sheep and fetal pigs[130,131,134] and GR-knockout mice[135,136] all have increased perialveolar tissue volumes, decreased air space volumes, and increased cellularity, resulting in respiratory failure at birth, presumably because of reduced lung compliance and increased thickness of the air/blood gas barrier. Thus, although it has often been assumed that the primary effect of corticosteroids is to induce differentiation of type II AECs, the reduction of perialveolar tissue volume is becoming increasingly recognized as one of the major benefits of corticosteroid therapy. Indeed, studies in GR-knockout mice have demonstrated that the proportion of type II and undifferentiated AECs increases in the absence of GR signaling, whereas the proportion of type I AECs decreases.[136] These changes in AEC phenotypes may be driven by the reduction in lung compliance and associated reduction in lung expansion in GR-knockout mice.[136] The administration of cortisol to fetal sheep with and without a reduction in lung expansion demonstrated that the degree of lung expansion was a more potent regulator of AEC differentiation than physiologic levels of corticosteroids.[137]

Corticosteroids can also affect alveolarization, although this effect is likely to be dose and species dependent. Dexamethasone causes an arrest of alveolarization in prenatal and postnatal rats.[138,139] This effect may be mediated by the retinoic acid system, as retinoic acid administration can partially rescue the glucocorticoid-induced deficit.[140] In contrast, physiologic doses of cortisol administered to fetal sheep increase alveolar number.[127] This effect may be mediated by an increase in fetal lung compliance, allowing increased lung expansion and resulting in expansion-induced lung growth and alveolarization.[128]

Antenatal corticosteroids also mature the pulmonary vascular bed in both normal and hypoplastic fetal sheep lungs.[141,142] In addition, antenatal corticosteroids enhance pulmonary vasodilator responsiveness and increase the fall in pulmonary vascular resistance and rise in pulmonary blood flow before birth, although the increase in pulmonary blood flow after birth was unaffected.[143] These effects may be mediated by acceleration of vascular and parenchymal maturity but are unlikely to involve changes in vascular density or wall structure.[142]

More recently, cell-specific GR-knock outs in endothelial cells, mesenchymal cells, or epithelial cells of the lung have revealed that loss of GR signaling in the lung's mesenchymal cells is responsible for the lethal phenotype of GR-knockout in mice.[132,135,144] In total GR knockout mice and mesenchymal GR knockout mice, the mesenchyme fails to thin during late gestation, consistent with the finding of increased mesenchymal cell proliferation in GR-knockout mice, and these mice do not survive after birth. In contrast, lung epithelial cell-specific GR knockout mice do survive postnatally, likely because the mesenchyme in those mice does decrease in thickness prior to birth (albeit not to the same degree as wild-type mice),[132,135,144] producing a relatively thin air-blood gas barrier. Those studies provide strong evidence that the primary maturational effect of the pre-parturient increase in corticosteroids is to thin the mesenchyme.

The effect of corticosteroids on lung structure is arguably the major beneficial effect of corticosteroids on the developing lung. The exact mechanisms by which activation of the GR achieves remodeling of the pulmonary mesenchyme, cell differentiation, alveolar development, and vascular development are now the subject of active investigation.[145-147] Studies using cell type-specific GR-knockout mice will make enormous contributions to elucidation of these pathways.[135,145,147-150]

EFFECTS OF METABOLIC FACTORS ON FETAL LUNG GROWTH AND MATURATION

Impaired nutrient and oxygen delivery during fetal life can affect the developing lung. Studies of respiratory function in infants,[151] children,[152] and adults[153] suggest that lung development may be affected by intrauterine conditions that inhibit fetal growth and lead to low birth weight. A common cause of fetal growth restriction (FGR) is chronic placental insufficiency, which reduces the delivery of nutrients and oxygen to the fetus. The effects of fetal hypoxemia differ from those of nutrient restriction. Prolonged hypoxemia in the absence of hypoglycemia leads to reduced DNA synthesis rates in ovine fetal lungs[154] and lung hypoplasia in fetal rats.[155] Nutrient restriction impairs alveolus formation. For example, in rats, in which alveolus formation occurs postnatally,[138] intermittent starvation soon after birth was associated with enlarged alveoli with thicker septa and reduced elastin deposition.[156] In sheep, hypoxemia, and nutrient restriction during late gestation (coinciding with saccular and alveolar formation), also reduces alveolarization.[157] Similar findings have been documented in guinea pigs exposed to antenatal undernourishment.[158] In rats, FGR induced by bilateral uterine artery ligation during the canalicular and saccular period of lung development caused a temporary delay in alveolarization that recovered after birth.[159] This delay was apparent only in females and was likely mediated by an increase in the amount of retinoic acid receptor β, a known inhibitor of alveolarization.[159] This is an interesting finding given that male FGR infants are more likely than females to have adverse respiratory outcomes.[160,161] It also suggests that there are likely to be complex interactions between sex and the timing and duration of FGR relative to the time of birth in regard to lung development. Impaired alveolarization secondary to FGR could result from fetal hypoxemia, hypoglycemia, elevated corticosteroid levels, or disrupted retinoic acid signaling.

The alveolar blood-gas barrier can also be affected by FGR. In sheep, severe FGR during late gestation increases the blood-air barrier thickness, an effect that persists for at least 2 years after birth.[162] In guinea pigs born after maternal undernutrition during pregnancy, the alveolar surface area was reduced, which reduced diffusing capacity.[158] A smaller surface area and alterations in airway development were still apparent at 18 weeks, despite a catch-up in body weight and lung volume, potentially impairing lung function later in life.[163,164]

Structural elements of the lung, such as elastic fibers, collagens, proteoglycans, and basement membrane proteins, are laid down during early development, and these processes may also be affected by nutritional status. Elastin is necessary for airway and alveolar development and affects lung compliance.[165] Owing to the long half-life of elastin,[166] alterations in elastin deposition during development may exert persistent effects on the mechanical properties of the lung, and it is now apparent that nutritional factors may affect elastin deposition. For example, in female FGR rats, reduced tropoelastin expression is coincident with an impairment in alveolarization,[159] and in growing rats, protein restriction caused a loss of lung desmosine and an increase in alveolar dimensions.[167] In humans, most elastin accumulates in the lungs between 25 weeks of gestation and 15 weeks after birth, and this accumulation is not significantly affected by FGR.[168] Similarly, pulmonary tropoelastin expression and elastin content are not altered in fetal sheep subjected to FGR during late gestation.[169]

During fetal life, both hypoxia and fetal undernutrition may increase corticosteroids,[170] which may affect elastin synthesis as exogenous corticosteroids can both increase[171] and decrease[172] elastin formation in the fetal lungs. Elastin deposition in the lung may also be affected by hypoxia, as it down-regulates tropoelastin in pulmonary fibroblasts[173] and in pulmonary artery smooth muscle cells.[174] Paradoxically, hypoxia increases the activity of pulmonary lysyl oxidase, the enzyme responsible for cross-linking elastin and collagen. However, an inhibitory effect of hypoxia on elastin synthesis was not observed in growing rats.[175]

Collagen provides the lung and airways with mechanical strength.[176] In contrast to elastin, collagen is synthesized and degraded throughout life.[176] It is well established that collagen metabolism is affected by nutritional status[177] and lung collagen content is reduced in postnatal rats fed a low-protein diet.[167]

The effects of undernutrition and hypoxia on type II AECs are likely to differ according to gestational timing and alterations in cortisol levels. Fetal lung extracts from undernourished pregnant rats have impaired surface tension–lowering properties.[178] The maturation of type II AECs in the offspring is also delayed, as evidenced by increased cellular glycogen content and fewer lamellar bodies.[179] In contrast, prolonged periods of fetal hypoxemia in sheep, induced by placental restriction, increase expression of surfactant proteins A and B at 0.88 of gestation[180] but not near term.[181] This observation suggests that FGR or nutrient restriction may advance aspects of lung maturity in preterm infants, but not in those born at term.

Maternal obesity also impairs lung development. Babies of obese mothers are at increased risk of respiratory complications at birth, and experimental models of maternal overnutrition impair fetal and postnatal lung development.[182] For example, 10-day glucose infusion in fetal sheep impaired surfactant protein mRNA levels and reduced levels of the GR,[183] but did not alter the density of type II cells. Mice fed high-fat diets before, during, and after pregnancy produce offspring that have fewer and larger alveoli with reduced markers of pulmonary vascular development and increased markers of inflammation.[184]

Certain micronutrients are essential for normal lung development[185]; vitamin A (retinol) and retinoic acid play important roles.[186] Retinoic acid induces heterodimerization of the retinoic acid receptors (RARs) and retinoid X receptors (RXRs). Both types of receptors have three subtypes (α, β, and γ). RAR-RXR heterodimers bind to retinoic acid response elements in the promoter region of DNA of target genes to alter gene expression.[186] Retinoic acid affects early airway branching, mesenchymal cell differentiation, regulation of the ECM (including elastin and collagen), formation of the basement membrane, alveolarization, the synthesis of surfactant and surfactant proteins,[187] and development of the diaphragm. The section below focuses on the role of retinoic acid in lung hypoplasia; several recent reviews include a broader overview of the role of RA in development of the respiratory system.[186,187] Nitrofen, the teratogen that induces CDH and lung hypoplasia, is now considered to exert its effects, at least in part, by interfering with retinoic acid synthesis.[119,188] Fetuses and infants with CDH have alterations in the retinoic acid pathway in lung tissue, suggesting that retinoids may directly contribute to lung hypoplasia in addition to the diaphragm defect.[119] RARα and RARγ promote alveolarization, whereas RARβ inhibits alveolarization,[189-191] suggesting a complex interplay between the different receptor subtypes. Retinoic acid reverses a glucocorticoid-induced impairment of septation in neonatal mice[140] and fetal lung hypoplasia in a rat model of nitrofen-induced CDH.[192,193] However, retinoic acid treatment did not reverse lung hypoplasia in a rabbit model of surgically induced CDH,[194] or in fetal rats with oligohydramnios,[195] and did not accelerate lung maturation in preterm fetal sheep.[196] Further studies are therefore required to determine the complex role of retinoic acid in fetal lung development and alveolarization.

Vitamin D can advance maturation of type II AECs by reducing glycogen content and increasing surfactant synthesis.[197] A vitamin D–responsive gene (*TXNIP*, also known as *VDUP1*), a known regulator of cell differentiation, is down-regulated after an increase in lung expansion[23,89] and may mediate the effects of lung expansion on type II AEC differentiation and surfactant protein expression.[27,89]

EFFECTS OF MATERNAL ASTHMA ON FETAL LUNG DEVELOPMENT

Maternal asthma also impacts lung development, although the mechanisms are not yet understood. Asthma during pregnancy increases the risk of respiratory distress syndrome and transient tachypnea of the newborn and increases the risk of hospitalization even in babies born at term.[198-200] Children from mothers with asthma have ~10% lower lung function through childhood and an increased risk of developing asthma.[201] Good asthma control decreases the risk of adverse outcomes, indicating that genetics alone do not explain these outcomes.[202] A sheep model of maternal asthma indicates that the increased risk of respiratory distress syndrome at birth may, at least in part, be due to reduced fetal lung type II AECs and reduced surfactant protein expression.[203,204]

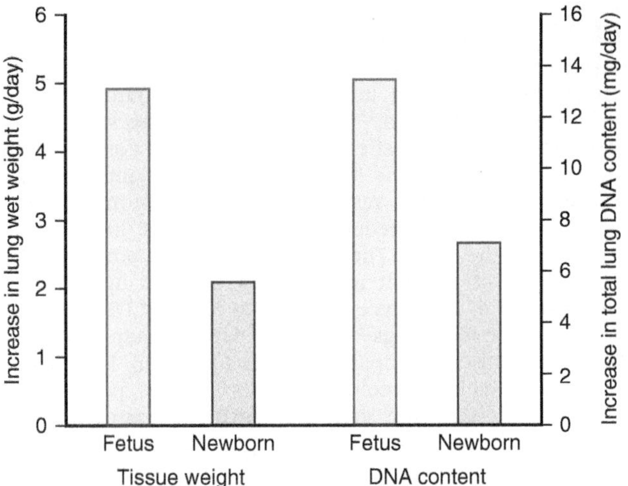

Fig. 57.7 Lung growth rates measured in fetal sheep during late gestation and in postnatal lambs. Lung growth rates were calculated as the increase in wet tissue weight (g/day) *(left)* and total DNA content (mg/day) *(right)* in fetal sheep killed at 114 and 138 days (term is approximately 147 days) and postnatal lambs killed at 1 day and 46 days after birth (n = 5 for each age-group). Note that lung growth rates in postnatal lambs are considerably lower than in the fetuses. (From Hooper SB, Wallace M. Role of the physicochemical environment in lung development. *Clin Exp Pharmacol Physiol*. 2006;33:273–279.)

POSTNATAL LUNG GROWTH

Until recently it was thought that alveolarization in humans ceases at 1.5 to 3 years after birth.[205] However, it has been demonstrated that the formation of new alveoli increases exponentially during the first 2 years of life and that alveoli continue to form at least until adolescence.[206] Alveolar development in mice and rats also continues until adulthood.[207,208] Lung growth per se also continues for 15 to 18 years after birth in humans, until the chest stops growing in late adolescence, and until adulthood in rodents.[208] This indicates that much more lung tissue growth occurs after birth than during fetal life. In sheep, for example, the weight of the lung tissue increases from approximately 100 g at birth to around 220 g at 6 weeks, and then to approximately 600 g in the mature animal. However, paradoxically, less is known about the physiologic control of lung growth after birth than before birth. Much of what is currently known about the control of postnatal lung growth has been derived from experimental and clinical studies observing lung growth after lung resection (i.e., postpneumonectomy lung growth) and in disorders affecting chest wall development (e.g., kyphoscoliosis).[209]

An understanding of lung growth after birth is of particular interest in the clinical approach to preterm infants, infants with hypoplastic lungs (e.g., after preterm premature rupture of membranes or CDH), infants affected by FGR (who then experience postnatal catch-up in body growth), and infants and children with feeding problems or nutritional deficiencies. Lung growth increases the surface area for gas exchange and is also necessary for normal development of the pulmonary vascular bed. Children with problems arising from impaired lung growth before or after birth may benefit from treatments that accelerate lung parenchymal growth and development, some of which are discussed later in this chapter.

THE ROLE OF THE PHYSICAL ENVIRONMENT

It is generally assumed that as the thoracic cavity enlarges with skeletal growth, lung growth follows passively to fill the chest; put simply, if the chest wall does not grow, then the lung is unlikely to grow. Indeed, alveolar growth remains fixed around the rate of lung volume expansion in postnatal rats, rhesus monkeys, and humans,[206] indicating that postnatal lung growth, like fetal lung growth, is sensitive to lung expansion, which is likely secondary to chest enlargement. Thus, a full understanding of postnatal lung growth will ultimately require knowledge of how chest wall growth and its stiffness are regulated. Because of their inherent recoil properties, the lungs exert a chronic traction on the chest wall, so an intimate relationship must exist between lung growth and thoracic wall growth, with each affecting the other. However, it is likely that the lung, which ultimately fills the space available, will stop growing once the chest is no longer enlarging. Immediately after birth, the chest wall is very compliant and can influence lung growth to a significant extent only after the ribs and sternum have become ossified; the rate at which this ossification proceeds will therefore affect lung growth. Ossification of the chest wall in preterm infants may be delayed, particularly if they receive a continuous positive airway pressure or a positive end-expiratory pressure, as the luminal distending pressure will greatly reduce the traction imposed by lung recoil on the chest wall.

Lung resection experiments have shown that the postnatal lung will grow to fill the space available, which may be dependent on the presence of a subatmospheric intrapleural pressure. This pressure differential in turn creates a transpulmonary pressure that effectively expands the lung by exerting chronic traction on the lung pleura.[210] The mechanical stress and strain imposed on the lung are presumed to activate intracellular processes that precipitate events that increase cell replication and tissue remodeling. The stimulated lung growth has the effect of reducing stress and strain in the alveolar septa, which limits the stimulus for further growth.[210]

Evidence suggests that the basal level of lung expansion is an important determinant of lung growth and structural development after birth, as it is in the fetus, although the mechanical forces exerted on the air-filled lung are considerably more complex. Indeed, in the fetus it is apparent that lung growth may drive chest wall growth, whereas the reverse seems to be true after birth. The relationship between the basal level of lung expansion and lung development is graphically demonstrated by the marked reduction in the rates of lung tissue growth[211] (Fig. 57.7), alveolarization[205,212] (Fig. 57.8), and reversal in AEC phenotypes[28] (see Fig. 57.5), which occurs after birth when the degree of lung expansion is chronically reduced,[2] as shown in Fig. 57.1.

Chronic, localized distension of a region of the lung with perfluorocarbon accelerates lung growth and alveolarization in the distended region, an effect seen in neonatal lambs but

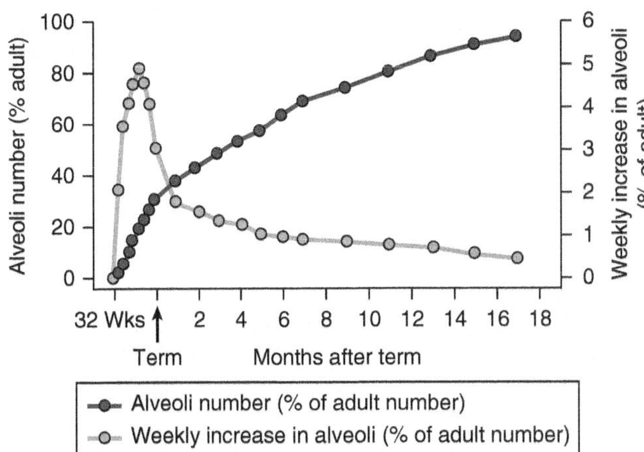

Fig. 57.8 Changes in alveolar number and weekly rate of alveoli accumulation of alveoli in humans. The gold circles show the weekly rate of alveolus formation expressed as a percentage of the final adult number of alveoli; the *red circles* show the percentage of the adult number of alveoli that have been formed at each time point. The rate of alveolus formation is markedly reduced after birth. *Wks*, Weeks. (Modified from Jobe A. Lung development and maturation. In: Martin RJ, Fanaroff AA, Walsh MC, eds. *Neonatal-Perinatal Medicine*. 8th ed. St Louis: Mosby; 2006:1069–1086. Idealized curves data from Langston C, Kida K, Reed M, et al. Human lung growth in late gestation and in the neonate. *Am Rev Respir Dis*. 1984;129:607–613; and Hislop AA, Wigglesworth JS, Desai R. Alveolar development in the human fetus and infant. *Early Hum Dev*. 1986;13:1–11.)

not adult sheep.[213] The use of continuous positive airway pressure and positive end-expiratory pressure (both of which increase the basal degree of lung expansion by increasing end-expiratory lung volume [i.e., functional residual capacity]) has been shown to enhance lung growth in growing ferrets[214] and lambs.[215] Similarly, the compensatory lung growth induced by partial resection of the air-filled lung after birth is thought to be expansion dependent.[74,210] Although it has been suggested that phasic lung expansion can stimulate postnatal lung growth, experimentally increasing the phasic component of postnatal breathing does not affect lung growth or lung structure.[216] These findings indicate that lung growth after birth is regulated primarily by the basal degree of lung expansion, as it is in the fetus. Indeed, a comparison of gene expression changes in prenatal[23] and postnatal[209,217] models of accelerated lung growth identifies some similar changes in gene expression, indicating that the cellular mechanisms may be similar.

EFFECTS OF METABOLIC AND ENDOCRINE FACTORS

Although it is now apparent that mechanical tissue strain is the major signaling mechanism underlying postnatal lung growth, nonmechanical factors are likely to play a role in modifying the growth response.[210] These include metabolic factors such as the availability of nutrients, micronutrients, and oxygen and endocrine factors such as corticosteroids, growth hormone, sex hormones, insulin-like growth factors, and thyroid hormones.

NUTRITION

Numerous studies have shown that, as in the fetus, postnatal nutrition can have a profound effect on lung development.[185] In children, severe malnutrition adversely affects lung function, but such effects could be related in part to altered musculoskeletal development.[218] Animal studies have shown that postnatal under nutrition impairs lung structure, including alveolarization,[156,185] with the adverse effects persisting into maturity. For example, a study has shown that sheep that grow slowly after birth have a smaller lung volume and a smaller pulmonary surface area relative to lung and body size than those measured in normally growing sheep.[219] Maternal high-fat diets before and after birth also impair alveolar development, with impairments extending into adulthood and worsened if the offspring continues on a high-fat diet.[184] The combination of maternal high-fat diet and high-environmental stress also impairs pulmonary capillary and alveolar development.[220] If the same is true in humans, the worldwide epidemic of obesity may lead to an increase in the burden of respiratory diseases in future generations.

CORTICOSTEROID EXPOSURE

Corticosteroids may be administered to preterm infants to accelerate lung maturity and to reduce the time spent on a mechanical ventilator. Although data on the structural effects of postnatal exposure to exogenous corticosteroids are very limited for human infants, such exposures have been shown to affect lung growth and alveolarization. In postnatal rats, dexamethasone accelerates thinning of interalveolar septa via remodeling of the ECM and suppression of cell proliferation.[145,146,221,222] However, it also inhibits alveolarization and pulmonary vascular growth[138,221,223,224], effects which may be mediated by down-regulation[145] of VEGFR (KDR), TGM2, and CRISPLD2.

POTENTIAL TREATMENTS FOR FETAL LUNG GROWTH DISORDERS

FETAL TREATMENTS

It is now clear that lung growth and structural development are a consequence of a complex interaction between mechanical, endocrine, and metabolic factors. The challenge is to translate this knowledge into therapeutic treatments that will improve outcomes for preterm infants and infants with hypoplastic lungs. Because increased fetal lung expansion is a potent stimulus for fetal lung growth and structural maturation, it has been trialed as an in utero treatment for severe lung hypoplasia. Experimental studies have shown that increases in fetal lung expansion induced by tracheal obstruction can rapidly reverse fetal lung growth deficits in utero[19,225,226] and can reverse postnatal respiratory dysfunction that would otherwise be fatal.[227] Clinical trials in fetuses with severe pulmonary hypoplasia resulting from CDH had mixed success, although more recent trials with less invasive approaches and more selective patient criteria, have improved outcomes.[116,228] The major problems relate to preterm labor, failure to adequately stimulate fetal lung growth, tracheal complications, and postnatal respiratory insufficiency despite induced lung growth. Some of the discrepancies between the results of animal experiments and the early clinical trials likely relate to the stage of lung development at which the treatment was applied, the duration and mode of the tracheal obstruction, and the severity of the fetal lung hypoplasia. For example, many tracheal obstruction procedures in humans have been performed before 28 weeks of gestation, during the early to mid-canalicular stage of development.[229,230] When tracheal obstruction is performed at this stage in fetal sheep, it is associated with increased perisaccular tissue volume.[37] Similarly, sustained increases in fetal lung expansion can severely reduce the numbers of type II AECs and surfactant protein gene expression,[231-234] and the obstruction must be released before birth for normalization to occur.[235] Thus inappropriate growth and reduced type II AEC numbers may explain why infants subjected to prolonged tracheal obstruction in utero can have respiratory insufficiency after birth, despite having normal-sized or larger-than-normal lungs.

The failure to stimulate lung growth by tracheal obstruction in some human fetuses with CDH may also be explained by the inability of secreted FLL to expand relatively noncompliant severely hypoplastic fetal lungs. If the internal distending pressure required to expand the lung is greater than the osmotic pressure driving FLL secretion (a hydrostatic pressure of 5 to 6 mm Hg),[31] the lung will not expand, despite the trachea being occluded. Ongoing FLL secretion and increased lung expansion are requirements for accelerated fetal lung growth,[31,128] because without continued secretion the lung growth response will not be activated.[229]

Another complication associated with tracheal obstruction for the correction of CDH-induced lung hypoplasia in human fetuses is fetal hydrops,[229] which has also been observed in fetal sheep[37] but only when tracheal obstruction was in the pseudoglandular-canalicular stages of lung development, not during the alveolar stage. The hydrops is thought to result from the more compliant immature chest at mid-gestation, which allows the lungs to expand to a much greater degree,[37] likely restricting venous return or mechanically constraining the heart. More recent trials in human fetuses with CDH have adopted a less invasive fetoscopic approach for obstructing the trachea, followed by a second fetoscopic procedure to release the tracheal obstruction before delivery to allow time for type II AEC transdifferentiation and surfactant production to occur.[228] Along with more specific patient selection criteria and improved neonatal management, at least some of these trials are reporting improved outcomes.[228,236]

POSTNATAL TREATMENTS

The stimulation of lung growth in the early postnatal period is of interest in the management of infants born with hypoplastic lungs, such as in CDH. Positive end-expiratory pressure is often used with preterm neonates to enhance oxygenation and to prevent lung collapse and injury. Because positive end-expiratory pressure causes a sustained increase in the basal degree of lung expansion (i.e., functional residual capacity), it may have the added effect of enhancing postnatal lung growth. This effect has not been demonstrated in human infants, but has been observed in normal postnatal ferrets[214] and lambs.[215] A potential complication of increasing end-expiratory lung volumes in ventilated preterm infants is a reduction in the number of type II AECs, but a study in normal lambs failed to detect an adverse effect of 48 hours of positive end-expiratory pressure on AECs.[215] Vitamin A administration has also received significant attention given its ability to reverse deficits in alveolar development[140,237] and the finding that preterm infants are often vitamin A deficient.[238] As a result, vitamin A is often administered to preterm and low-birth-weight babies to reduce the incidence of bronchopulmonary dysplasia, although initial findings vary.[239] Reduced vitamin D and E levels have also been associated with the development of bronchopulmonary dysplasia and supplementation of these vitamins are potential therapeutic options to reduce the severity of bronchopulmonary dysplasia.[240,241]

CONCLUSION

Growth and structural maturation of the lung both before and after birth result from a complex interaction among physical, endocrine, and metabolic factors. Sustained expansion of the developing lung appears to be crucial for normal lung development both before and after birth. In the fetus, a high degree of lung expansion is actively maintained and is dependent on diaphragmatic and laryngeal muscle activity. Factors that inhibit these muscles or alter the transpulmonary pressure gradient result in a reduction in fetal lung expansion, which is now recognized as the common underlying mechanism by which a variety of disorders result in pulmonary hypoplasia. After birth the major stimulus for lung growth is also likely to be physical lung expansion, which is provided by growth of the rib cage. The molecular mechanisms by which alterations in lung expansion accelerate or retard the growth and development of the lung are largely unknown but are vital areas of research that may yield substantial clinical benefits.

A complete reference list is available at www.ExpertConsult.com. 

SELECT REFERENCES

1. Hooper SB, Harding R. Fetal lung liquid: a major determinant of the growth and functional development of the fetal lung. *Clin Exp Pharmacol Physiol.* 1995;22(4):235–247.
2. Harding R, Hooper SB. Regulation of lung expansion and lung growth before birth. *J Appl Physiol.* 1996;81(1):209–224.
3. Alcorn D, Adamson TM, Lambert TF, Maloney JE, Ritchie BC, Robinson PM. Morphological effects of chronic tracheal ligation and drainage in the fetal lamb lung. *J Anat.* 1977;123(Pt 3):649–660.
5. Davey MG, Johns DP, Harding R. Postnatal development of respiratory function in lambs studied serially between birth and 8 weeks. *Respir physiol.* 1998; 113(1):83–93.
7. Miller AA, Hooper SB, Harding R. Role of fetal breathing movements in control of fetal lung distension. *J Appl Physiol.* 1993;75(6):2711–2717.
8. Harding R, Hooper SB, Dickson KA. A mechanism leading to reduced lung expansion and lung hypoplasia in fetal sheep during oligohydramnios. *Am J Obstet Gynecol.* 1990;163(6 Pt 1):1904–1913.
11. Harding R, Bocking AD, Sigger JN. Influence of upper respiratory tract on liquid flow to and from fetal lungs. *J Appl Physiol.* 1986;61(1):68–74.
12. Harding R, Bocking AD, Sigger JN. Upper airway resistances in fetal sheep: the influence of breathing activity. *J Appl Physiol.* 1986;60(1):160–165.
18. Moessinger AC, Harding R, Adamson TM, Singh M, Kiu GT. Role of lung fluid volume in growth and maturation of the fetal sheep lung. *J Clin Invest.* 1990;86(4):1270–1277.
23. Sozo F, Wallace MJ, Zahra VA, Filby CE, Hooper SB. Gene expression profiling during increased fetal lung expansion identifies genes likely to regulate development of the distal airways. *Physiol Genomics.* 2006;24(2):105–113.
24. Cloutier M, Tremblay M, Piedboeuf B. ROCK2 is involved in accelerated fetal lung development induced by *in vivo* lung distension. *Pediatr Pulmonol.* 2010;45(10):966–976.
25. Vuckovic A, Herber-Jonat S, Flemmer AW, Roubliova XI, Jani JC. Alveolarization genes modulated by fetal tracheal occlusion in the rabbit model for congenital diaphragmatic hernia: a randomized study. *PLoS One.* 2013;8(7):e69210.
26. Peiro JL, Oria M, Aydin E, Joshi R, Cabanas N, Schmidt R, et al. Proteomic profiling of tracheal fluid in an ovine model of congenital diaphragmatic hernia and fetal tracheal occlusion. *Am J Physiol Lung Cell Mol Physiol.* 2018;315(6):L1028–L1041.
27. Flecknoe SJ, Wallace MJ, Harding R, Hooper SB. Determination of alveolar epithelial cell phenotypes in fetal sheep: evidence for the involvement of basal lung expansion. *J Physiol.* 2002;542(Pt 1):245–253.
28. Flecknoe SJ, Wallace MJ, Cock ML, Harding R, Hooper SB. Changes in alveolar epithelial cell proportions during fetal and postnatal development in sheep. *Am J Physiol Lung Cell Mol Physiol.* 2003;285(3):L664–L670.
30. Nardo L, Maritz G, Harding R, Hooper SB. Changes in lung structure and cellular division induced by tracheal obstruction in fetal sheep. *Exp Lung Res.* 2000;26(2):105–119.
31. Nardo L, Hooper SB, Harding R. Stimulation of lung growth by tracheal obstruction in fetal sheep: relation to luminal pressure and lung liquid volume. *Pediatr Res.* 1998;43(2):184–190.
33. Cloutier M, Maltais F, Piedboeuf B. Increased distension stimulates distal capillary growth as well as expression of specific angiogenesis genes in fetal mouse lungs. *Exp Lung Res.* 2008;34(3):101–113.
37. Probyn ME, Wallace MJ, Hooper SB. Effect of increased lung expansion on lung growth and development near midgestation in fetal sheep. *Pediatr Res.* 2000;47(6):806–812.
55. Harding R, Liggins GC. Changes in thoracic dimensions induced by breathing movements in fetal sheep. *Reprod Fertil Dev.* 1996;8(1):117–124.
78. Lindahl P, Karlsson L, Hellstrom M, et al. Alveogenesis failure in PDGF-A-deficient mice is coupled to lack of distal spreading of alveolar smooth muscle cell progenitors during lung development. *Development.* 1997;124(20):3943–3953.
81. Wallace MJ, Hooper SB, McDougall ARA. Physical, endocrine, and growth factors in lung development. In: Harding R, Pinkerton KE, eds. *The Lung: Development, Aging and the Environment.* 2nd ed. Elsevier Academic Press; 2015:157–181.
86. Wallace MJ, Thiel AM, Lines AM, Polglase GR, Sozo F, Hooper SB. Role of platelet-derived growth factor-B, vascular endothelial growth factor, insulin-like growth factor-II, mitogen-activated protein kinase and transforming growth factor-beta1 in expansion-induced lung growth in fetal sheep. *Reprod Fertil Dev.* 2006;18(6):655–665.
89. Filby CE, Hooper SB, Sozo F, Zahra VA, Flecknoe SJ, Wallace MJ. VDUP1: a potential mediator of expansion-induced lung growth and epithelial cell

differentiation in the ovine fetus. *Am J Physiol Lung Cell Mol Physiol.* 2006;290(2):L250-L258.
90. McDougall AR, Hooper SB, Zahra VA, et al. Trop2 regulates motility and lamellipodia formation in cultured fetal lung fibroblasts. *Am J Physiol Lung Cell Mol Physiol.* 2013;305(7):L508-L521.
91. McDougall AR, Hooper SB, Zahra VA, et al. The oncogene Trop2 regulates fetal lung cell proliferation. *Am J Physiol Lung Cell Mol Physiol.* 2011;301(4):L478-L489.
94. Seaborn T, St-Amand J, Cloutier M, et al. Identification of cellular processes that are rapidly modulated in response to tracheal occlusion within mice lungs. *Pediatr Res.* 2008;63(2):124-130.
97. Engels AC, Brady PD, Kammoun M, et al. Pulmonary transcriptome analysis in the surgically induced rabbit model of diaphragmatic hernia treated with fetal tracheal occlusion. *Dis Model Mech.* 2016;9(2):221-228.
101. Surate Solaligue DE, Rodriguez-Castillo JA, Ahlbrecht K, Morty RE. Recent advances in our understanding of the mechanisms of late lung development and bronchopulmonary dysplasia. *Am J Physiol Lung Cell Mol Physiol.* 2017;313(6):L1101-L1153.
102. Moghieb A, Clair G, Mitchell HD, et al. Time-resolved proteome profiling of normal lung development. *Am J Physiol Lung Cell Mol Physiol.* 2018;315(1):L11-L24.
103. Ding J, Ahangari F, Espinoza CR, et al. Integrating multiomics longitudinal data to reconstruct networks underlying lung development. *Am J Physiol Lung Cell Mol Physiol.* 2019;317(5):L556-L568.
105. Ardini-Poleske ME, Clark RF, Ansong C, et al. LungMAP: the molecular atlas of lung development program. *Am J Physiol Lung Cell Mol Physiol.* 2017;313(5):L733-L740.
106. Beauchemin KJ, Wells JM, Kho AT, et al. Temporal dynamics of the developing lung transcriptome in three common inbred strains of laboratory mice reveals multiple stages of postnatal alveolar development. *PeerJ.* 2016;4:e2318.
129. Wallace MJ, Hooper SB, Harding R. Effects of elevated fetal cortisol concentrations on the volume, secretion, and reabsorption of lung liquid. *Am J Physiol.* 1995;269(4 Pt 2):R881-R887.
130. Wallace MJ, Hooper SB, Harding R. Role of the adrenal glands in the maturation of lung liquid secretory mechanisms in fetal sheep. *Am J Physiol.* 1996;270(1 Pt 2):R33-R40.
132. Bird AD, McDougall AR, Seow B, Hooper SB, Cole TJ. Minireview: glucocorticoid regulation of lung development: lessons learned from conditional GR knockout mice. *Mol Endocrinol.* 2015;29(2):158-171.
136. Cole TJ, Solomon NM, Van Driel R, et al. Altered epithelial cell proportions in the fetal lung of glucocorticoid receptor null mice. *Am J Respir Cell Mol Biol.* 2004;30(5):613-619.
140. Massaro GD, Massaro D. Retinoic acid treatment partially rescues failed septation in rats and in mice. *Am J Physiol Lung Cell Mol Physiol.* 2000;278(5):L955-L960.
145. Seow BKL, McDougall ARA, Short KL, Wallace MJ, Hooper SB, Cole TJ. Identification of betamethasone-regulated target genes and cell pathways in fetal rat lung mesenchymal fibroblasts. *Endocrinology.* 2019;160(8):1868-1884.
146. Short KL, Bird AD, Seow BKL, et al. Glucocorticoid signalling drives reduced versican levels in the fetal mouse lung. *J Mol Endocrinol.* 2020;64(3):155-164.
147. Bridges JP, Sudha P, Lipps D, et al. Glucocorticoid regulates mesenchymal cell differentiation required for perinatal lung morphogenesis and function. *Am J Physiol Lung Cell Mol Physiol.* 2020;319(2):L239-L255.
182. McGillick EV, Lock MC, Orgeig S, Morrison JL. Maternal obesity mediated predisposition to respiratory complications at birth and in later life: understanding the implications of the obesogenic intrauterine environment. *Paediatr Respir Rev.* 2017;21:11-18.
203. Clifton VL, Moss TJ, Wooldridge AL, et al. Development of an experimental model of maternal allergic asthma during pregnancy. *J Physiol.* 2016;594(5):1311-1325.
204. Wooldridge AL, Clifton VL, Moss TJM, et al. Maternal allergic asthma during pregnancy alters fetal lung and immune development in sheep: potential mechanisms for programming asthma and allergy. *J Physiol.* 2019;597(16):4251-4262.
211. Hooper SB, Wallace MJ. Role of the physicochemical environment in lung development. *Clin Exp Pharmacol Physiol.* 2006;33(3):273-279.
215. Flecknoe SJ, Crossley KJ, Zuccala GM, et al. Increased lung expansion alters lung growth but not alveolar epithelial cell differentiation in newborn lambs. *Am J Physiol Lung Cell Mol Physiol.* 2007;292(2):L454-L461.
227. Davey MG, Hooper SB, Tester ML, Johns DP, Harding R. Respiratory function in lambs after in utero treatment of lung hypoplasia by tracheal obstruction. *J Appl Physiol.* 1999;87(6):2296-2304.
228. Deprest J. Prenatal treatment of severe congenital diaphragmatic hernia: there is still medical equipoise. *Ultrasound Obstet Gynecol.* 2020;56(4):493-497.
236. Jani J, Nicolaides KH, Keller RL, et al. Observed to expected lung area to head circumference ratio in the prediction of survival in fetuses with isolated diaphragmatic hernia. *Ultrasound Obstet Gynecol.* 2007;30(1):67-71.

Molecular Mechanisms of Lung Development and Lung Branching Morphogenesis

58

Sandra L. Leibel | Martin Post

The need to extract and utilize sufficient amounts of oxygen from the environment to sustain life has had an incredible impact on the evolution of the respiratory systems. In particular, breathing amphibians and mammals with their high metabolic rates have been forced to evolve a sophisticated organ to meet their oxygen requirements and get rid of carbon dioxide, the cellular waste of aerobic metabolism. We explore this process of lung development and examine a variety of important molecular regulators mediating lung formation.

Lung development can be subdivided into six distinct stages (Table 58.1).[1,2] The embryonic and fetal stages of lung formation comprise the embryonic, pseudoglandular, canalicular, and saccular stages. The embryonic stage encompasses organogenesis of the lung and formation of the major airways and pleura. During the pseudoglandular stage, the bronchial tree and respiratory parenchyma begin to form and the primitive airway epithelium starts to differentiate. Neuroendocrine, ciliated, and goblet cells appear, whereas mesenchymal cells begin to form cartilage and smooth muscle cells. In the subsequent canalicular period, the airway branching pattern is completed and the prospective gas exchange region starts to develop. During this period, respiratory bronchioles appear, interstitial tissue volume decreases, vascularization within the peripheral mesenchyme increases, distal cuboidal epithelium differentiates into type I and type II cells, and surfactant begins to appear. In the saccular period, growth of the pulmonary parenchyma, thinning of the connective tissue between the air spaces, and maturation of the surfactant system occur in preparation for life ex utero. Although capable of functional gas exchange, the lung is structurally immature. The distal airspaces at this time consist of smooth-walled transitory ducts and saccules with thick primitive septa containing a double capillary network.

The final two stages of lung development include alveolarization and microvascular maturation. Depending on the species, alveolarization starts before or after birth. Secondary septa are formed and fusion of the dual-layer capillaries into a single-layer network occurs. The microvascular maturation period ensues concurrently with alveolarization with the remodeling and maturation of the alveolar septa and transformation of the capillary network into a single layer. One of the important hallmarks of lung development is the signaling crosstalk between the epithelial and mesenchymal tissue layers. The combination, concentration, and

Table 58.1 Stages of Lung Development.

Stage	Gestational Age: Human	Gestational Age: Mouse	Main Events	Epithelial Differentiation
Embryonic	3.5–8 wk	9.5–14.5 days	Formation of lung bud, trachea, left and right primary bronchi, and major airways	Undifferentiated columnar epithelium
Pseudoglandular	5–17 wk	14.5–16.5 days	Establishment of the bronchial tree; all preacinar bronchi are formed	Proximal: columnar epithelium; ciliated, nonciliated, basal, neuroendocrine cells Distal: cuboidal epithelium; precursor type II cells
Canalicular	16–26 wk	16.5–17.5 days	Formation of the prospective pulmonary acinus by narrowing of terminal buds and increase of capillary bed	Proximal: columnar epithelium; ciliated, nonciliated, basal, neuroendocrine cells Distal: differentiation of cuboid type II cells to squamous type I cells
Saccular	24–38 wk	17.5 days to 5 dpn	Formation of alveoli precursors: saccules, alveolar ducts, and alveolar air sacs	Proximal: ciliated, nonciliated club, basal, neuroendocrine cells Distal: type I cells flatten and type II cells mature
Alveolar	36 wk to 2 ypn	5–30 dpn	Formation of alveoli by septation of alveolar air sacs, thinning of interalveolar septa	Proximal: columnar epithelium; ciliated, nonciliated, basal, neuroendocrine cells Distal: type I cells and type II cells mature
Microvascular maturation	Birth to 3 ypn	14–21 dpn	Fusion of the capillary bed to a single layered network	

dpn, Days postnatally; *ypn*, years postnatally.

spatiotemporal localization of a multitude of molecular signaling factors working in harmony determines the fate of branching, proliferation, and cellular differentiation of the developing lung. This chapter summarizes studies on lung development from the past two decades and explore the current dogma on the molecular mechanisms that determine lung pattern formation.

EARLY LUNG DEVELOPMENT

Lung development starts as an endodermal outgrowth of the ventral foregut around the fourth week of human development. This foregut mass rapidly elongates into a single tube dividing into a dorsal esophagus and a ventral trachea.The buds of the right and left lungs appear as two independent outpouchings around the tracheal bud. In a similar process, the mouse respiratory system develops from a pair of endodermal buds in the ventral half of the primitive foregut, just anterior to the developing stomach at 9.5 days of gestation.The two buds elongate in a posteroventral direction, whereas starting from the primary branch point, the gut tube begins to pinch into two, creating the dorsal esophagus and ventral trachea.

In humans, the left lung bud gives rise to two main stem bronchi and the right lung bud gives rise to three main stem bronchi. In the mouse, the right lung bud forms four stem bronchi, whereas the left lung consists of one stem bronchus.The secondary bronchi will then branch and rebranch in a process termed *branching morphogenesis.* Endoderm-derived epithelial cells line the airways, whereas the surrounding mesenchyme provides the elastic tissue, smooth muscles, cartilage, vascular system, and other connective tissues. The visceral pleura forms from splanchnic mesoderm, whereas the parietal pleura forms from the somatic mesoderm layer. The first pulmonary vessels form as a plexus surrounding the lung buds by vasculogenesis.The formation of the bronchial tree is finished at 16 days of gestation in the mouse and at 16 weeks of gestation in the human. At this stage of development, the tracheobronchial tree from the trachea to the terminal bronchioles resembles a system of branching tubules that terminate in exocrine gland-like structures.

MOLECULAR BASIS OF LUNG BUD AND LOBE FORMATION

The outgrowth of the ventral foregut, formation of the trachea, and outgrowth of the main pulmonary bronchi occur during the embryonic period of lung development.The crucial event at this stage is the initiation of lung formation at the right place along the anteroposterior axis of the foregut. Genetic studies have implicated several transcription factors (TCFs), morphogens, peptide growth factors, and their cognate receptors in specifying the morphogenetic progenitor field of the lung along the foregut axis (Fig. 58.1). One important TCF in this process is forkhead box (Fox) A2 (FOXA2).[3,4] *Foxa2* is expressed in the ventral foregut endoderm before and immediately at the start of lung bud formation.[5-7] Targeted ablation of *Foxa2* in mice led to embryonic death between embryonic day 6.5 and embryonic day 9.5 before the onset of lung formation[8,9]; however, chimeras rescued for the embryonic-extraembryonic constriction showed that *Foxa2* was essential for foregut and lung formation.[10]

Fibroblast growth factor (FGF) 10 is a member of the large family of FGFs essential to many processes during embryonic development.[11,12] In the murine lung, *Fgf10* messenger RNA (mRNA) is dynamically expressed in the distal mesenchyme adjacent to the primitive lung buds.[13] The importance of FGF10 for lung development was shown in *Fgf10*-deficient mice that die at birth because of respiratory failure.[14,15] The *Fgf10*-deficient mice had complete lung agenesis; that is, lung development had stopped after the formation of the trachea.[14,15] FGF10 overexpression did not affect proper epithelial branching, which remained highly preserved. Instead, mesenchymal FGF10 maintained distal Sox-9 expressing epithelial progenitors in an undifferentiated state

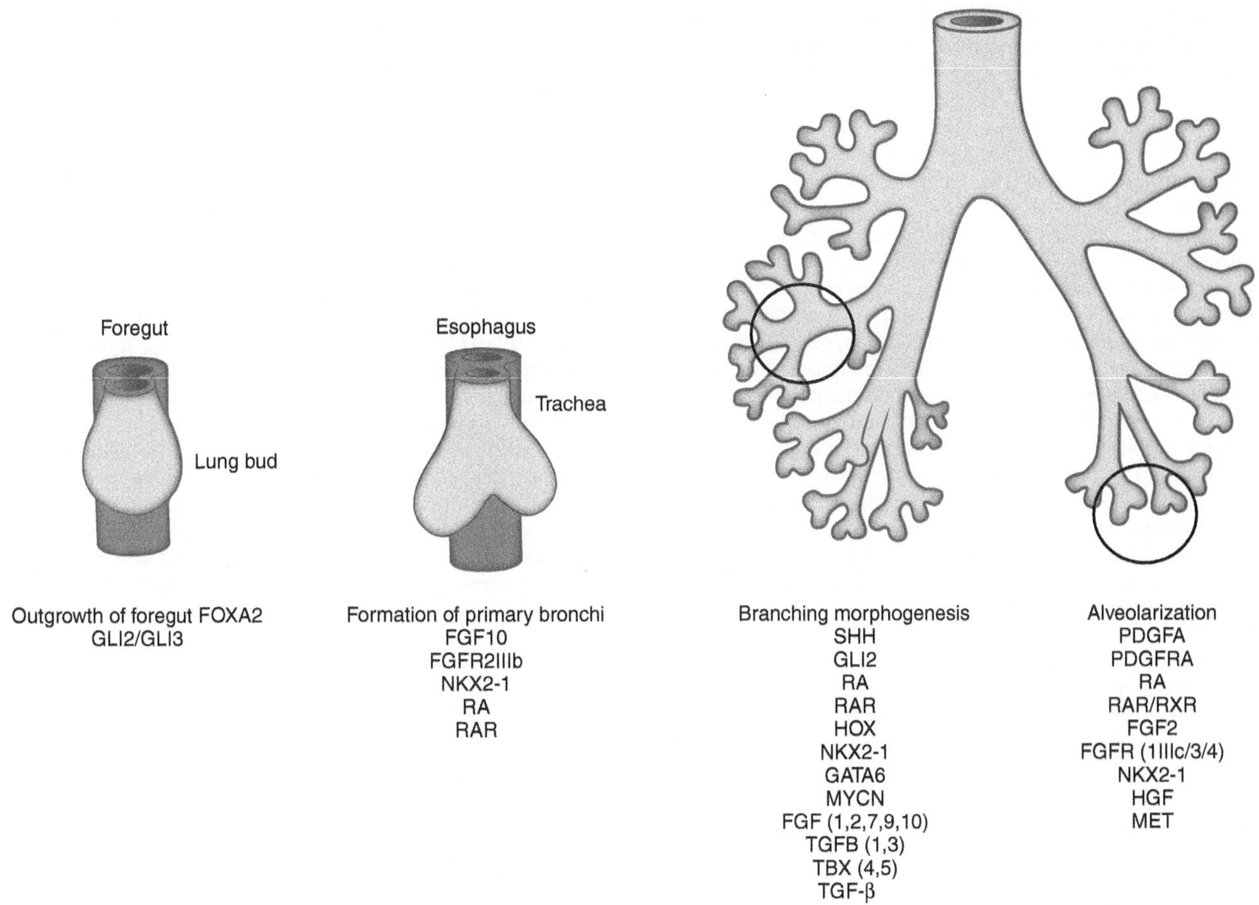

Fig. 58.1 Transcription and growth factors known to regulate lung development. *FGF,* Fibroblast growth factor; *HGF,* hepatocyte growth factor; *MET,* hepatocyte growth factor receptor; *RA,* retinoic acid; *RAR,* retinoic acid receptor; *SHH,* sonic hedgehog gene; *TGF,* transforming growth factor.

through the activation of β-catenin signaling.[16] FGFs bind to and signal via FGF tyrosine kinase receptors (FGFRs).[11,17] The FGF10 receptor (FGFR2IIIb), an FGFR2 splice variant, is expressed in lung bud epithelium.[18] FGFR2IIIb is also capable of binding FGF1 and FGF7, which have also been implicated in lung development.[11,13] Because targeted mutation of FGFR2 resulted in an early lethal phenotype caused by placental insufficiency,[19,20] *Fgfr2*$^{-/-}$ chimeras were created to overcome this early lethality and allow lung development to be analyzed.[21] Similarly to what occurred in the *Fgf10*-deficient mice, only the trachea formed, without further pulmonary branching.[21] Transgenic mice overexpressing a dominant negative FGFR2IIIb splice variant in distal lung epithelium show a severe pulmonary defect, forming only a trachea and two main bronchi, without any lateral branches.[22] Moreover, Cre recombinase-mediated excision to generate mice lacking the IIIb form of FGFR2 while retaining expression of the IIIc splice form resulted in mice that had no lungs and thus died at birth.[23] Taken together, these data indicate that FGF10 signaling via FGFR2IIIb plays a crucial role in the initiation of lung bud formation (see Fig. 58.1). The "no lung" phenotype as a result of inhibited FGF10 signaling shows a striking similarity to a phenotype resulting from the loss of function of either *branchless (bnl)* or *breathless (btl)* in *Drosophila*. The *bnl* gene encodes an FGF homologue that functions as a ligand for breathless, a *Drosophila* homologue of FGFR. Loss of function of either *bnl* or *btl* prevented tracheal branching in the fly.[24,25]

Sonic hedgehog (SHH) is a secreted signaling molecule and a mammalian homologue of *Drosophila* hedgehog (HH) that is known to be involved in many fundamental processes during *Drosophila* embryonic development.[26] *Shh* is expressed as early as ventral foregut endodermal development. It is induced by retinoic acid (RA) produced in the mesoderm and then signals back to activate the GLI2/3 TCFs, stimulating WNT2/2b and bone morphogenetic proteins (BMPs), which induce NKX2-1 expression.[27] SHH functions via paracrine signaling. It is produced by the epithelial cells and is handled by the mesenchymal-located Patched (PTC) receptor, suggesting that the SHH pathway is an important regulator of epithelial-mesenchymal signaling during lung development.[27] Its importance for lung development was shown when the *Shh* gene was genetically ablated, which resulted in a simplistic-looking lung consisting of only one lobe on each side of the trachea (pulmonary left isomerism).[28,29] In contrast to the FGF10-null mutant, the initiation of lung formation does occur in *Shh*-null mutants; however, there is an incorrect number of lobes and a subsequent failure of branching morphogenesis.[28,29] This was confirmed with generation of a lung-specific *Shh*-null mouse.[30] In this mouse, when *Shh* expression was removed before embryonic day 13.5, tracheal, bronchial, and peripheral lung defects were seen similar to those of the *Shh*-null mouse. The mesenchyme appears to be the primary target of SHH deficiency, showing decreased cell proliferation and increased cell death.[28] The effect of SHH on pulmonary mesenchyme was also demonstrated when *Shh* was overexpressed in distal lung epithelium with use of the surfactant protein C *(Sftpc)* promoter.[31] Overexpression of SHH resulted in smaller lungs at birth that lacked functional alveoli, most likely due to hypercellularity of the mesenchyme. Together, these results reveal the important function of SHH in epithelial-mesenchymal signaling during early lung formation.

Cubitus interruptus (CI) has been identified as a downstream target in HH signaling in *Drosophila*.[26] Mammalian Gli genes are the putative homologues of *Drosophila ci* and have also been implicated in mammalian SHH signaling.[26] Three Gli genes have been described in mice: *Gli1*, *Gli2*, and *Gli3*, all of which are expressed in the early pulmonary mesenchyme.[32] These TCFs are posttranslationally converted into their activator or repressor forms to regulate the expression of SHH target genes. *Gli3*-null mice show a mild lung defect with a slight reduction in size. However, *Gli2*-null mice have respiratory failure at birth, with defective airway branching, left pulmonary isomerism, and severe hypoplasia.[33] Concurrent deletion of both *Gli2* and *Gli3* revealed a more dramatic phenotype. These *Gli2/Gli3*$^{-/-}$ double-mutant mice have no lung, trachea, or esophagus and die early in gestation. Other foregut derivatives such as the pancreas, thymus, and stomach do develop in *Gli2/Gli3*$^{-/-}$ mutant mice, although they are hypoplastic. These findings indicate that GLI2 and GLI3 have distinct, overlapping, and vital functions during initiation of lung bud formation. The complete absence of trachea and lung formation was ameliorated by the presence of one *Gli3* gene, as the *Gli2*$^{-/-}$/*Gli3*$^{+/-}$ mutant had a lung consisting of one hypoplastic lobe.[33] Because the ablation of both *Gli2* and *Gli3* resulted in a far worse lung phenotype than *Shh* deficiency alone, SHH is likely not the only regulator of Gli genes during lung development. The complete absence of a lung in *Gli2/Gli3*$^{-/-}$ mutant mice is similar to the "no lung" phenotype seen in *Fgf10*-deficient mice. The difference is that the trachea and esophagus are present in *Fgf10*-deficient mice but absent in *Gli2/Gli3*-deficient mice, implicating different signaling pathways. Other single or compound mutants for the three Gli genes show a variable degree of lung hypoplasia with an aberrant number of lung lobes and decreased branching morphogenesis.[33,34] However, another compound mutant recently analyzed revealed an interesting relationship between SHH and GLI3 during lung development. The *Shh/Gli3*$^{-/-}$ mouse shows a phenotype that is less severe than the *Shh*-null lung alone, with enhanced vasculogenesis and growth potential.[35] For a complete review of the SHH-GLI pathway interactions and effect of mutations on lung development, see Rutter and Post.[36]

RA plays a crucial role during gestation and is involved in the developmental processes of almost every organ.[37,38] Both a deficiency and an excess of RA cause congenital defects during human development in a variety of organs.[37,38] RA exerts its effects via retinoic acid receptors (RARs) and retinoid X receptors (RXRs), tyrosine kinase receptors, which function as transcriptional regulators of RA target genes. The RAR family is composed of three genes producing several isoforms: $RARA_{1,2}$, $RARB_{1-4}$, and $RARG_{1,2}$, all activated by both all-*trans*-RA and 9-*cis*-RA, whereas the three isoforms from the RXR family, RXRA, RXRB, and RXRG, are activated only by 9-*cis*-RA.[38] RARs require heterodimerization with RXRs for DNA binding to RA response elements (RAREs). Mice deficient for only one of the isoforms show a milder phenotype than expected on the basis of their expression patterns, indicating a high degree of redundancy among the RARs.[38] In contrast, compound mutant mice had similar congenital defects as seen with fetal vitamin A deficiency.[37,38] *Rara2/Rarb2*$^{-/-}$ double-mutant mice die soon after birth with agenesis of the left lung and hypoplasia of the right lung.[39] Lung hypoplasia was also reported in *Rara1/Rarb*$^{-/-}$ and *Rxra/Rara*$^{-/-}$ double mutants.[40,41] RA has profound influences on lung development during branching morphogenesis and alveolarization. The localized expression of FGF10 in the mesenchyme requires RA signaling and may regulate the Hox genes.[42-45] Hox genes form a large family of homeobox-containing TCFs that are implicated in the specification of cells that form morphologic structures along an anteroposterior axis. Hox genes are arranged in four chromosomal clusters, and the 3′ to 5′ position of each gene within a cluster corresponds to their expression pattern along the anteroposterior axis of the developing body.[46] Genes of the 3′ regions of Hox clusters A and B are expressed in the developing lung, with the Hoxb cluster predominantly expressed in the early pulmonary mesenchyme.[42-45,47-52] Within the mesenchyme, Hoxb genes express in a proximal-distal expression gradient, suggesting a role for Hoxb genes in specifying proximal from distal pulmonary mesenchyme.[48] Several mutant models have been created that illustrate the importance of Hox genes during lung development. Single-mutant mice for Hox genes are generally normal, most likely because of redundancy. However, compound *Hoxa1/Hoxb1*$^{-/-}$ mutants have severe lung hypoplasia with phenotypes ranging from five hypoplastic lung lobes to a lung with only two lobes.[53] In the *Hox5* paralog group, *Hoxb5*$^{-/-}$ mice have lung phenotypes that are less severe than those in *Hoxa5* mutants. *Hoxa5*$^{-/-}$ mice die in the perinatal period and have laryngotracheal malformations, a reduced tracheal lumen, and lung hypoplasia. *Hoxa5* also plays specific roles in lung microvascular development and diaphragm innervation.[54]

Another homeodomain TCF expressed at the onset of lung morphogenesis is NKX2-1 (also known as *TTF1*).[55-57] Expression of *Nkx2-1* mRNA is localized to epithelial cells of the developing pulmonary tubules.[7,58,59] NKX2-1 continues to be expressed in adult bronchiolar and alveolar epithelial type II cells, where it plays an important role in the regulation of secretoglobin protein, SCGB1A1 (also known as *club cell secretory protein*), and surfactant protein synthesis.[60] Targeted disruption of NKX2-1 results in severe hypoplasia of the lung lacking separation of the trachea from the esophagus, arrest of branching morphogenesis, and epithelial cell differentiation at the pseudoglandular stage.[57,61]

SEPARATION OF ESOPHAGUS AND TRACHEA

The formation of a tracheoesophageal septum divides the ventral trachea from the dorsal esophagus. Failure of the trachea and esophagus to separate results in a congenital defect in humans called *tracheoesophageal fistula*. Deficiency of the growth and TCFs implicated in lung agenesis or hypoplasia also results in tracheoesophageal fistula with different gradations of severity (Table 58.2). *Gli2/Gli3*$^{-/-}$ mutant mice have no trachea, nor do they form an esophagus, and *Gli2*$^{-/-}$/*Gli3*$^{+/-}$ mutants have a single tracheoesophageal tube connected to the stomach.[33] In *Shh*$^{-/-}$ mutant mice, the trachea and esophagus fail to separate, resulting in tracheoesophageal fistula.[28,29] Mice haploinsufficient for the TCF *Foxf1* exhibit foregut abnormalities including narrowing and, sometimes, atresia of the esophagus, as well as frequent fusion of the trachea and esophagus.[62] *Foxf1* expression was absent in foregut derivates (trachea, esophagus, oral cavity, lungs) of *Shh*$^{-/-}$ mutants, indicating that SHH signaling is required for activation of FOXF1 in these tissues.[62] Surprisingly, separation of the trachea and esophagus occurs normally in *Fgf10*-deficient mice,[14,15] whereas *Nkx2-1*-deficient mice have a complete tracheoesophageal defect.[57] *Rara/Rarb2*$^{-/-}$, *Rara1/Rarb*$^{-/-}$, and *Rxra/Rara*$^{-/-}$ mutant mice all exhibit a tracheoesophageal septal defect and other tracheal malformations such as disorganized cartilaginous rings and shortening of the trachea.[39-41] The end result of RA signaling in relation to lung development appears to be mediated through FGF10. This became evident in studies using the pan-RAR antagonist BMS493 in foregut explant cultures, which resulted in failure of initial lung bud outgrowth in the prospective lung field due to inhibition of *Fgf10* expression in the foregut mesenchyme.[62]

Table 58.2 Separating Trachea and Esophagus.

Condition	Trachea	Esophagus	Remarks
Fgf10$^{-/-}$	+	+	Trachea-esophagus separation; trachea ends blind
Shh$^{-/-}$	+	+	Trachea-esophagus septal defect
Gli2$^{-/-}$	+	+	Trachea-esophagus separation with stenosis
Gli2$^{-/-}$/Gli3$^{-/+}$	+	–	Single (tracheal) tube connecting to the stomach, esophageal atresia
Gli2$^{-/-}$/Gli3$^{-/-}$	–	–	No esophagus, trachea, or lung
Rara$^{-/-}$/Rarb2$^{-/-}$ Rara1$^{-/-}$/Rarb$^{-/-}$	+	+	Trachea-esophagus septal defect, tracheal cartilage malformations
Nkx2-1$^{-/-}$	+	+	Trachea-esophagus septal defect

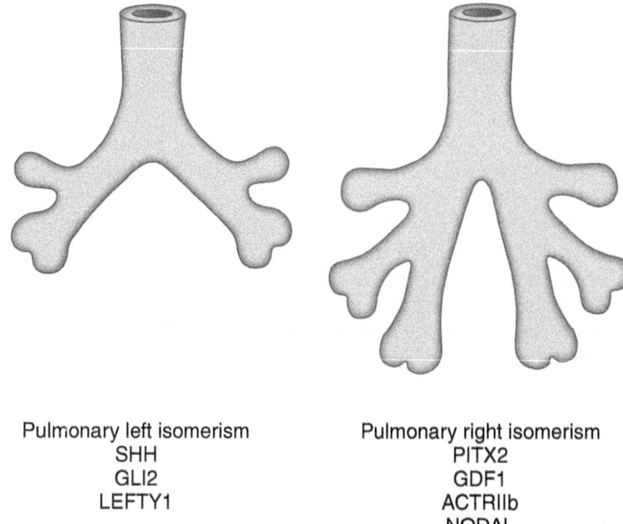

Fig. 58.2 Transcription and growth factors involved in left-right determination of the developing mouse lung. The drawings represent a human lung, which in the normal situation consists of two lobes on the left and three lobes on the right. *SHH*, Sonic hedgehog gene.

LEFT-RIGHT ASYMMETRY

At day 26 postconception in humans, the right and left lung buds appear at the sides of the tracheal bud and begin elongating and branching.[63] Around 5 weeks of gestation, five separate lobes can be identified in the human lung, two on the left and three on the right. In the mouse, the right side has four major lobes, whereas the left consists of one. Such left-right asymmetries during development are an integral part of the establishment of a body plan, and several highly conserved mechanisms have been found to initiate the vertebrate left-right axis, including the SHH signaling pathway.[64] Molecules such as SHH,[65,66] FGF8,[65] N-cadherin,[67] activin B, activin receptor IIb,[68] and FOXJ1[69] have all been shown to influence left-right asymmetry during development (Fig. 58.2). However, it appears that these pathways converge to influence the expression patterns of genes in the transforming growth factor β (TGF-β) family of cell-cell signaling, *NODAL*, *LEFTY1*, and *LEFTY2*.[69-72] Nodal acts as a left-side determinant whereas Lefty acts as a feedback inhibitor of Nodal. *Shh* and *Lefty1* mutants have left pulmonary isomerisms with only one lobe on each side of the lung.[27,28,66,71] Both SHH and FOXA2 are thought to act upstream of LEFTY1 and are normally expressed in *Lefty1*$^{-/-}$ mice.[71] Although no data are available regarding the expression of *Lefty1* in the *Shh*$^{-/-}$ mutant lung, LEFTY1 is absent in *Shh*$^{-/-}$ mutant lateral plate mesoderm (LPM).[66] *Lefty1*$^{-/-}$ mice show bilateral expression of *Nodal* and *Lefty2* in LPM, which results in ectopic expression of the homeobox transcription regulator paired-like homeodomain transcription factor 2 (PITX2) on the right side of the foregut region.[71] PITX2 is clearly a powerful determinant of left-right asymmetry as ectopic expression of *Pitx2* in the right LPM alters looping of the heart and gut and reverses body rotation in *Xenopus* embryos.[73] In contrast, the phenotype of *Pitx2*$^{-/-}$ mice demonstrates right pulmonary isomerism and altered cardiac position.[74-76] Growth differentiation factor 1 (GDF1) encodes another member of the TGF-β superfamily, and it is proposed to act upstream of *NODAL*, *LEFTY1*/*LEFTY2*, and *PITX2*. It increases Nodal activity by forming a Gdf1-Nodal heterodimer.[77] Mice deficient for this factor, as well as mutants hypomorphic for *Nodal*, exhibit right pulmonary isomerism.[70,77] Cerberus-like 2 (Cerl2) is an antagonist of Nodal and does not depend on SHH signaling.[78] *Cerl-2*$^{-/-}$ mice show bilateral or right-sided expression of Nodal in the LPM.[79] It has not been possible to investigate the role of FOXA2 in left-right asymmetry formation of the lung, because *Foxa2*-null mutant mice die before the onset of lung formation. However, in rescued *Foxa2* mutant mice, SHH was not detected in the foregut region.[10] Another FOX family member, FOXJ1, has been shown to have a critical role in left-right axis determination as the *Foxj1*-null mutant shows left-right asymmetry of the visceral organs (lung included) resulting from defective ciliary development.[69,80]

BRANCHING MORPHOGENESIS

Early branching of the primary bronchi is monopodal, and starting at the level of the secondary bronchus, each bronchus subsequently undergoes dichotomous branching where each branch bifurcates repeatedly into two branches. Careful morphometric analysis of mouse lung development has revealed a branching pattern that is highly stereotyped.[81] Each pattern is one of three modes that have been described as *domain branching*, *planar*, and *orthogonal bifurcation*, and the overall branching process is the repetition of these modes in different combinations. In humans, the enlarging bronchial tree expands through 23 generations of branching into the surrounding mesenchyme, eventually furrowing into the characteristic lobes of the lung.

Early studies have indicated that branching of the lung buds is controlled by epithelial-mesenchymal tissue interactions,[82,83] where a soluble factor from the mesenchymal compartment dictates the branching pattern of the epithelium.[84] The strong inductive capacity of pulmonary mesenchyme is prevalent by its ability to induce a lung epithelial phenotype in epithelial ureter buds[85] and early endoderm cultures.[18] Branching also appears to be regulated by positional information along the anteroposterior axis of the lung as proximal (trachea and main bronchi) and distal (lung bud) mesenchyme differ in their ability to support epithelial branching.[86-88] Some progress has been made in elucidating the complex mixture of TCFs and morphogens that guide this process (see Fig. 58.1). Alterations in cell adhesion and matrix remodeling at the epithelial-mesenchymal interface also contribute to lung branching morphogenesis (for a review of this topic, see Keijzer and Post).[89]

Several growth factors, including FGFs and different forms of TGF-β, have been shown to regulate lung branching morphogenesis.[89,90] FGFR2 is highly expressed during early lung development along the proximal-distal axis of lung epithelium, whereas different FGFs are present in the pulmonary mesenchyme.[91,92] This strongly suggests that the temporospatial control of branching is established through signaling crosstalk between these two compartments. FGF10 is expressed in the mesenchyme at sites of bud formation and exerts a chemotactic effect on the underlying lung epithelium. It binds to FGFR2IIIb, and both *Fgfr2IIIb*-null mutants and *Fgf10*-null mutants show complete lung agenesis.[14,15,23] Transcripts for *Fgf7* are also expressed at sites of active branching in the mesenchyme.[93,94] In vitro, FGF10 elicits endodermal expansion and bud formation, whereas FGF7 induces expansion of the endoderm but never progresses to bud formation.[15] Exogenous FGF7 inhibits rat lung branching morphogenesis in vitro[95] but stimulates proliferation of adult type II pneumocytes both in vitro[96] and in vivo.[97,98] This suggests that FGF7 and FGF10 signals are transduced in different physiologic responses and may explain why FGF7 cannot compensate for loss of FGF10. Surprisingly, mice bearing a null mutation of *Fgf7* had no obvious lung abnormalities,[99] suggesting that the function of FGF7 can be replaced by other factors such as FGF1 and/or FGF10. FGF1 binds to both FGFR2 splice variants, FGFR2IIIb and FGFR2IIIc, and is crucial for branching of embryonic mouse epithelium in mesenchyme-free culture.[100] FGF2, which binds to FGFR2IIIc, but not to FGFR2IIIb, did not affect epithelial branching in these cultures, suggesting that the effects of FGF1 on epithelial branching are mediated via FGFR2IIIb.[101]

Another member of the FGF family, FGF9, is expressed in pulmonary mesothelium and epithelium in early development and later only in the mesothelium.[21,102] However, more recent data indicate that FGF9 is expressed at significant levels in the lung epithelium at embryonic day 14.5.[103] This expression pattern is different from that of FGF1, FGF7, and FGF10, which are expressed only in the lung mesenchyme. Targeted deletion of *Fgf9* resulted in severe lung hypoplasia and immediate postnatal death.[102] Analysis of the lungs revealed decreased branching morphogenesis and a lack of alveoli; however, the number of lung lobes and primary bronchi were normal.[102] Studies using recombinant FGF9 on lung explant cultures showed potent effects on growth, differentiation, and branching morphogenesis, and furthermore FGF9 exerts its influence on both the epithelium and mesenchyme separately.[103] It also appears that the impact of FGF9 on lung development is effected through changes in expression of FGF10 and FGF7. Additional studies using an inducible system spatially regulated by the *Sftpc* promoter to express FGF9 during lung development also demonstrate that FGF9 has the ability to induce *Shh*, *Ptc*, *Spry2*, and *Bmp4* expression, indicating that FGF9 may be a crucial regulator of epithelial-mesenchymal signaling.[104] Interestingly, antisense oligonucleotides directed towards the T-box 4 gene (*Tbx4*) or the T-box 5 gene (*Tbx5*) to attenuate transcript levels reduced branching morphogenesis in mouse lung explant cultures.[105] Concurrent knockdown of both *Tbx4* and *Tbx5* resulted in complete loss of lung branching in culture. On closer examination it was found that *Fgf10* transcript levels were completely attenuated in the double-knockdown lung cultures and reduced by individual *Tbx4* or *Tbx5* targeting. Several FGF ligands and receptors were studied in human lung development using native human fetal lung explants. FGF7 was found to be expressed in both epithelium and mesenchyme while FGF9 was localized in the distal epithelium. FGF10 was diffusely expressed throughout the parenchyma. FGF7 and FGF9 had similar effects on human and mouse fetal lungs, but FGF10 caused human explants to form cysts instead of epithelial branching like in the mouse. All 3 FGFs decreased double-positive SOX2/SOX9 progenitor cells in the human fetal lung.[106]

TGF-β belongs to a superfamily that includes activin, BMP, and TGF-β_1, TGF-β_2, and TGF-β_3. These peptides can exert a variety of biologic effects, including regulation of cell growth and differentiation and expression of a variety of proteins. In the lung, *Tgfβ1* mRNA and protein are found in the mesenchyme and epithelium, respectively.[107-109] Addition of exogenous TGF-β_1 to cultured embryonic mouse lung explants and in vivo overexpression of *Tgfβ1* in distal lung epithelial cells resulted in decreased branching morphogenesis, inhibited distal epithelial cell differentiation, and inhibited formation of the pulmonary vasculature, indicating an inhibitory role for TGF-β_1 during branching morphogenesis.[110-114] Most or all biologic activities of TGF-β are transmitted via transmembrane Ser/Thr kinase receptors, known as type I and type II receptors.[115] Signal transduction requires the formation of a heteromeric complex of type I (TGFβR1) and type II (TGFβR2) receptors. Inhibition of TGFβR2 signaling stimulated lung morphogenesis in whole-lung explant cultures, underlining again the negative effects of TGF-β signaling on branching morphogenesis.[116] In vivo studies show that *Tgfβ1*-null mutants have no gross developmental abnormalities; however, 50% of the null mutants die before embryonic day 11.5 as a result of defects in yolk sac vascularization.[117,118] *Tgfβ3*-null mutants die after birth with defective lungs showing alveolar hypoplasia and mesenchymal thickening and *Tgfβ2*-deficient mice die after birth and display a lung phenotype with postnatal collapse of alveoli and terminal airways.[119] SMAD proteins are downstream effecter proteins in the TGF-β signaling pathway.[120] SMAD1, SMAD2, and SMAD3 are expressed in distal lung epithelium, and SMAD4 is expressed in both distal lung epithelium and mesenchyme.[121,122] TGFβR-I phosphorylates SMAD2 and SMAD3, which then interact with SMAD4 and translocate to the nucleus where they bind to SMAD-binding elements on TGF-β responsive genes. Down-regulation of *Smad2/Smad3* and *Smad4* expression increased branching morphogenesis in cultured lung explants. Exogenous TGF-β_1 did not reverse this inhibitory effect, which is consistent with TGF-β_1 being upstream of SMAD proteins.[122]

Although the previously mentioned TCFs belonging to the Gli, Hox, and FOX families are likely involved in branching morphogenesis, additional TCFs that have been implicated in lung branching morphogenesis include GATA-binding protein 6 (GATA6) and MYCN. GATA6 belongs to the GATA family of zinc finger–containing TCFs and is expressed in epithelial and mesenchymal cells of the developing lung bud.[123,124] GATA6 is essential for endoderm formation as its targeted deletion resulted in embryonic death due to failure of visceral endoderm formation.[125,126] In the lung, GATA6 appears to be important for branching morphogenesis as inhibition of expression in the lungs results in decreased branching.[123,126] Expression of a GATA6-Engrailed dominant negative fusion protein in the distal lung epithelium resulted in a lack of alveolar type I cells and a perturbation in alveolar type II cells together with a reduction in the number of proximal airway tubules.[127] On the other hand, overexpression of *Gata6* with use of the *Sftpc* promoter resulted in disrupted branching morphogenesis and a lack of distal epithelial cell differentiation.[128] This suggests that a balanced *Gata6* expression level is important for branching during the pseudoglandular period of lung development and also during later stages of lung development in alveolar type I and type II cell differentiation. MYCN is a member of the Myc family of protooncogenes, which includes MYCN, MYC, and MYCL, all belonging to the basic helix-loop-helix class of TCFs. In the lung, MYCN is expressed in pulmonary epithelium,[129,130] and mice homozygous for the *Mycn*-null mutation die at mid-gestation.[130,131] Leaky null mutants for *Mycn* survive until the onset of lung

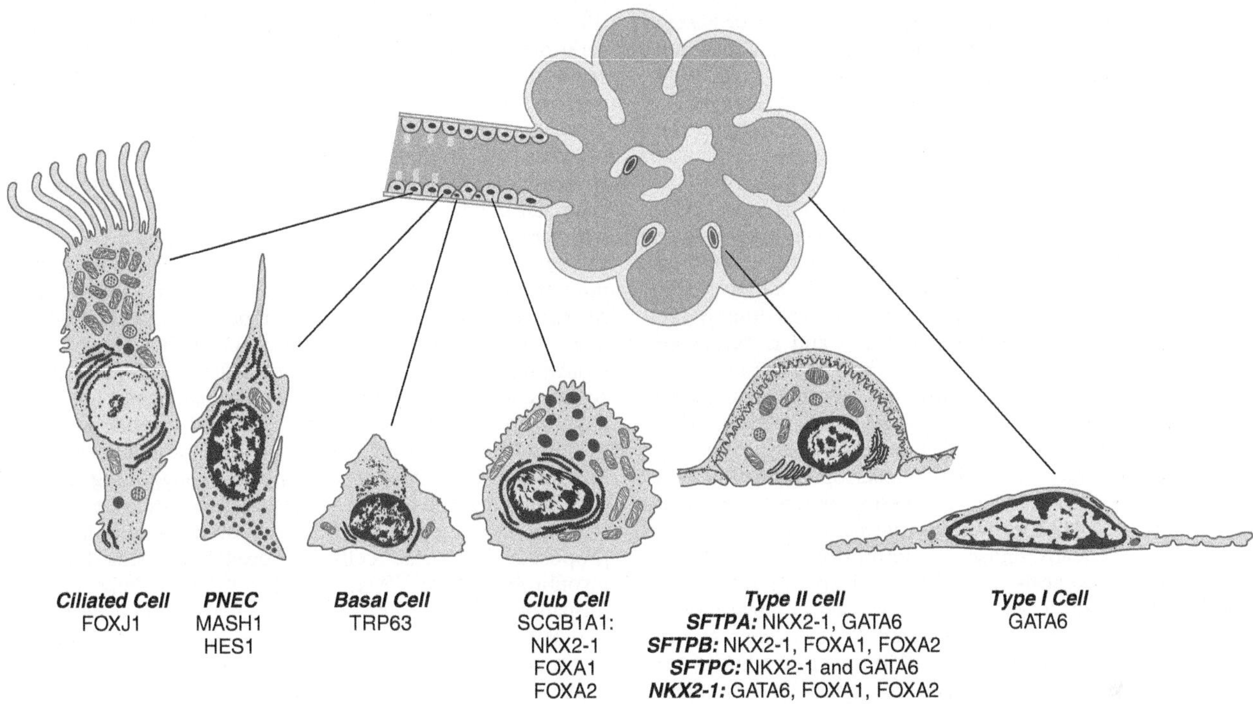

Fig. 58.3 Molecular control of airway and alveolar epithelial cell differentiation during lung development.

development; however, branching morphogenesis is dramatically reduced, resulting in severe lung hypoplasia.[129,132] More recently, mice containing a lung-specific *Mycn*-null mutation showed its critical role during lung development as these mice had abnormal lungs with a loss of proliferation, increased apoptosis, and reduced branching.[133]

EPITHELIAL DIFFERENTIATION

As branching proceeds, numerous different cell phenotypes emerge along the proximal-distal axis of the developing epithelial tubules and associated mesenchymal components, each with different morphologies and patterns of gene expression. Epithelial cell types of the proximal lung in the bronchi and bronchioles are pseudostratified and comprise mainly secretory and multiciliated cells. Pulmonary neuroendocrine cells (PNECs), unspecialized basal cells, and goblet cells within submucosal glands are also found in the upper airways. The distal part of the lung is composed of squamous alveolar type I cells that provide the gas exchange surface and cuboidal surfactant-producing type II cells. Recent studies have discovered bipotent alveolar progenitors that express markers of AT1 (HOPX) and AT2 (SFTPC) cells. These bipotent cells are, however, rareand barely contribute toward alveolar epithelial cell differentiation. Most alveolar lineages arise from uni-lineage-primed progenitor cells during the proximal-distal specification of the lung.[134] Over the last decade, some regulatory molecules involved in epithelial morphogenic patterning of the lung have been identified (Fig. 58.3).

PNECs are the first recognizable differentiated cells in humans and animals.[135,136] MASH1 is a basic helix-loop-helix TCF implicated in neural differentiation.[133] In the lung, *Mash1* is expressed in clusters or single-progenitor PNECs.[137] Mice deficient for *Mash1* do not develop PNECs, indicating an essential role for this TCF in their differentiation.[137] *Hes1* encodes a basic helix-loop-helix protein that is upregulated in response to Notch activation and represses downstream targets such as MASH1, thereby preventing neural differentiation.[134] This finding was supported with the use of approaches to both knock down and upregulate Notch1 expression to show effects on HES1 regulation and PNEC differentiation.[138] Indeed, HES1-deficient embryos have increased *Mash1* mRNA expression and PNECs in their lungs.[139] Whether the Notch signaling pathway plays a further role in distal epithelial specification remains to be elucidated. TCF21 is another basic helix-loop-helix protein that acts as a transcriptional regulatory protein that governs cell fate determination and differentiation in a variety of tissues. The *Tcf21*-null mutant dies at birth with severely hypoplastic lungs that have a reduced number of tertiary branches and a lack of acinar tubules, terminal air sacs, and alveoli.[140] Marker analysis revealed a disturbance in proximal-distal patterning of the lung epithelium with increased *Scgb1a1* and decreased *Sftpc* expression.

Epithelial TCFs such as FOXA2, GATA6, and NKX2-1 have been shown to influence lung epithelial specification. In both fetal mouse and human lung, the spatial-temporal distribution of NKX2-1 follows the pattern of expression of surfactant proteins.[7,58] It has been shown that NKX2-1 regulates the transcription of SFTPA, SFTPB, SFTPC, and SCGB1A1.[141-146] Consequently *Nkx2-1*-null mutants lack distal epithelial cell differentiation, whereas the ciliated cell marker FOXJ1 was unaffected.[147] Taken together, these data underline the importance of NKX2-1 for the establishment of the distal epithelial cell phenotype. Also, GATA6 transactivates SFTPA and NKX2-1,[148,149] and it has been shown that GATA6 acts synergistically with NKX2-1 to influence the activity of the *Sftpc* promoter.[150] In some respiratory epithelial cells, NKX2-1 is coexpressed with members of the FOX family of TCFs. Similarly to NKX2-1, FOXA1 and FOXA2 appear to modulate the expression of SFTPB and SCGB1A1.[141,151,152] It has been proposed that FOXA1 and FOXA2 are upstream regulators of NKX2-1[153] and that both members of the FOX family confer lung-specific gene expression in the primitive foregut through NKX2-1 as the intermediate. FOXJ1 is a TCF of the winged helix-forkhead family, expressed in various tissues during development. In the developing and adult lung, FOXJ1 expression is restricted to ciliated cells of the bronchial and bronchiolar epithelium.[147,154] The role of FOXJ1 in ciliated cell differentiation was clearly demonstrated when it was overexpressed in distal pulmonary epithelial cells. High levels of *Foxj1* expression inhibited branching morphogenesis and development of distal epithelial cells, while enhancing the development of ciliated cells.[155] In contrast, *Foxj1*-null mutant mice completely lack respiratory ciliated cells.[70,156]

The secreted morphogen SHH does not appear to be involved in regulating proximal-distal epithelial specification because SFTPC and SCGB1A1 are expressed in *Shh*-deficient mice.[29] In *Drosophila*, *Hh* may regulate the expression of decapentaplegic, the *Drosophila* counterpart of BMPs.[26] In the murine lung, BMP4 is implicated in lung epithelial specification and is expressed in early distal lung tips and at lower levels in the mesenchyme adjacent to the distal lung buds.[157,158] Overexpression of BMP4 in the distal epithelium in vivo resulted in hypoplastic lungs with grossly dilated terminal lung buds separated by abundant mesenchyme.[157] Distal epithelial differentiation was abnormal with decreased SFTPC expression, whereas proximal differentiation (SCGB1A1 expression) was normal.[157] In vitro, exogenous BMP4 clearly enhanced peripheral lung epithelial branching morphogenesis and SFTPC expression.[159] The secreted BMP antagonist Xnoggin is expressed in distal mouse lung mesenchyme early in development.[158] Its overexpression or that of the dominant-negative BMP receptor dnAlk6 in distal pulmonary epithelium resulted in a proximal pulmonary epithelial phenotype.[158] Similar results were obtained when Gremlin, another BMP antagonist, was overexpressed in the distal lung epithelium.[160] These studies clearly indicate a role for BMP4 in proximal-distal epithelial differentiation during lung development.

One of the current models of murine lung epithelial lineage specification depicts a multipotential progenitor population present during the pseudoglandular stage (up to embryonic day 13.5 in the mouse), located at the distal tips of the growing lung buds. This population expresses the TCFs *Id2* and *Sox9*[161-163] and can give rise to both the proximal and the distal lineage cells. The progeny left behind in the stalk of the outgrowth lose *Id2* and *Sox9* expression and begin to express *Sox2*. SOX2-positive cells continue to proliferate and differentiate to epithelial cells typically found in the bronchi and bronchioles: club cells, ciliated cells, goblet cells, and neuroendocrine cells.[164,165] At the canalicular stage, the multipotential ability of these distal tip cells is restricted to the alveolar lineage and gives rise to type I and type II alveolar cells. Recently a *Nkx2-1mcherry* reporter mouse line was used to identify a proximal progenitor population isolated from embryonic day 12.5 to embryonic day 14.5 mouse lungs. These cells were capable of self-renewal and expansion in vitro, and differentiation into polarized epithelium of multiple proximal lineages including basal and secretory cells.[166] Many questions remain regarding the fate of these progenitor cells and whether they represent a single progenitor population or a mixture of subpopulations with restricted differentiation potential. In the human, distal epithelial progenitors at the tips coexpress SOX2 and SOX9 and are critical to proximal-distal patterning and lung branching. They are no longer present at the canalicular stage.[167]

ALVEOLAR DEVELOPMENT

Alveolarization is the last step of lung development that induces physical changes to the internal surface area of the lung. Alveoli are formed by septation of the pulmonary saccules that form the immature lung. In both humans and mice, alveolarization occurs predominately after birth. One of the key players in the alveolarization process (see Fig. 58.1) appears to be one of the three isoforms of platelet-derived growth factor (PDGF)—namely, PDGF-A.[168] PDGF-A is normally expressed in early pulmonary epithelium and becomes undetectable at later stages of gestation.[169] Its receptor (PDGF receptor α, PDGFR-α) is expressed in the mesenchyme adjacent to the epithelium that expresses PDGF-A, signifying a paracrine signaling mechanism between the epithelium and the mesenchyme.[169-171] In mice, absence of PDGF-A results in prenatal and postnatal death. Postnatal deaths were characterized by emphysematous lungs with areas of atelectasis, without any formation of septa or alveoli; instead, dilated prealveolar saccules were found.[170,171] In normal mice, alveolar septa contain myofibroblasts positive for smooth muscle cell alpha actin. The postnatal *Pdgfa*-null mutant lungs lack alveolar staining for smooth muscle cell α actin, indicating a lack of alveolar myofibroblasts. In addition, they were almost completely devoid of parenchymal elastin fibers, which most likely contributed to the lack of alveolarization.[170,171] Myofibroblasts surrounding vessels and bronchioles appeared normal and were tropoelastin positive, suggesting a different developmental lineage.[171] Moreover, PDGFR-α were specifically missing from lungs of *Pdgfa*-null mutants, and it has been proposed that these cells are progenitor cells for alveolar myofibroblasts.[170,171] Taken together, PDGF-A is important for the formation of alveolar myofibroblasts that produce elastin, which in turn is important for alveolar formation. *Pdgfra*-deficient mice die in utero with severe skeletal malformations and incomplete cephalic closure. *Pdgfra*-deficient lungs were hypoplastic; however, primary branching and the histologic features were not affected.[172,173] Both FGFR3 and FGFR4 are expressed in postnatal pulmonary mesenchyme, whereas their ligands are expressed in pulmonary epithelial cells.[174] Although a null mutation of either *Fgfr3* or *Fgfr4* caused no obvious lung defects, concurrent silencing of both receptors resulted in severe overall body growth retardation and a failure of postnatal alveolar formation. Despite the lack of alveolar septation, differentiation (including myofibroblasts positive for smooth muscle cell alpha actin) and proliferation proceeded normally.[174] A study examining postnatal alveolar formation in the rat has found a new connection between FGF signaling in postnatal lung development.[175] When signaling of FGF2 (most likely through FGFR2IIIc) was blocked, it inhibited normal postnatal lung development. Histologically, these lungs exhibited a reduction in secondary septation and a decrease in apoptosis, resulting in an increased tissue-to-air ratio. Culture of stem cell-derived endoderm with embryonic mesenchyme resulted in differentiation of endodermal cells to an NKX2$^+$/SOX9$^+$/proSFTPC$^+$ lung lineage, whereas this differentiation was completely inhibited in the presence of truncated soluble FGFR2IIIc, but not by FGFR2IIIb. This suggests that FGFR2 signaling via FGFR2IIIc may be necessary for early lung specification.[18]

Besides its role in prenatal lung development, NKX2-1 also regulates postnatal lung development and homeostasis. After birth, *Nkx2-1* expression decreases dramatically; however, its expression remains detectable in adult alveolar type II cells. Overexpression of NKX2-1 in distal lung epithelial cells, with use of the *Sftpc* promoter, does not affect prenatal lung development but perturbs postnatal alveolarization, leading to emphysema, severe inflammation, and fibrosis.[174]

RA has been shown to increase the number of alveoli in postnatal rats and abrogates the decreased alveolarization seen after the experimental use of dexamethasone or elastase, which reduces alveolar formation. This indicates that RA is a potential controlling factor in "neoalveogenesis" in prematurity or after lung injury.[176-179] Similarly, compound mice homozygous for *Rarg* and heterozygous for *Rxra* deletion have a reduced number of alveoli and fewer elastic fibers in their alveolar walls.[180] RARB, however, appears to be an endogenous inhibitor of septation, and as a result, the *Rarb*-null mutant shows early-onset septation, resulting in twice as many alveoli in the null mutant lungs when compared with wild-type lungs.[181] Hepatocyte growth factor (HGF) is a heparin-binding glycoprotein with mitogenic and morphogenic effects on a variety of tissues. It has recently been shown that HGF-neutralizing antibodies injected intraperitoneally into rat pups caused a reduction in the number of alveoli.[182] This was also true when a truncated soluble form of HGF receptor was injected intraperitoneally. Combined, these findings clearly indicate an important and previously unknown role for HGF signaling in the lung during postnatal alveolarization.

VASCULAR DEVELOPMENT

The lung is composed of a complex network of airways and vessels, and, although a great deal has been discovered regarding the mechanisms controlling lung bud formation and airway branching, the elements guiding vascular formation remain obscure. The lung is unique among most organs in that it possesses a dual vascular system: the pulmonary system, which transports the blood to be oxygenated from and back to the heart, and the bronchial system, which provides oxygenated blood to the nonrespiratory parts of the lung. Three processes are believed to control pulmonary vascular development: (1) angiogenesis, which is defined as sprouting of new vessels from preexisting ones and gives rise to the central vessels; (2) vasculogenesis, which is de novo synthesis of blood vessels from blood lakes in the periphery of the lung; and (3) the fusion of proximal and peripheral vessels to form the pulmonary circulation.[183] More recently it was shown that vascular connections are well established even in the early stages of lung development and that pulmonary vascular formation occurs at all developmental stages, with completion of a single capillary network during the period of microvascular maturation.[184] A third mechanism of pulmonary vascular formation that relies heavily on vascular remodeling has been proposed and contradicts the other two. This theory uses a distal angiogenesis-driven model in which the vasculature is formed very early on in lung development and surrounds the epithelial bud tips as they grow out into the splanchnic mesenchyme.[185] As the epithelial buds branch and rebranch, growing outward, the developing vasculature rapidly expands and remodels with the bud tips. These epithelial-endothelial interactions between the capillary plexus and the epithelial bud tip coordinate growth between the developing airways and vasculature.

Members of the vascular endothelial growth factor (VEGF),[186,187] angiopoietin,[188,189] and ephrin families[190] have all been implicated in controlling vascularization of the pulmonary system. VEGF is a potent mitogen for endothelial cells, influencing angiogenesis and vasculogenesis.[191] It is essential for embryonic development, and even haploinsufficiency of VEGF results in embryonic lethality.[192,193] In both the embryonic and the adult lung, *Vegf* mRNA is detected in the lung epithelium[194-196] and signals via two high-affinity receptors: FLT1 and KDR (formerly FLK-1), which in the embryonic lung are localized to the mesenchyme.[194,195] The complementary expression patterns of VEGF in lung epithelium and the two VEGF receptors in the mesenchyme suggest an epithelial-mesenchymal signaling mechanism and an impact on lung development and branching morphogenesis.[197] Overexpression of the VEGF164 isoform in distal airway epithelium results in perinatal death.[198] The lungs appear abnormal, with dilated respiratory tubules and saccules and a decreased number of terminal buds. KDR expression in the mesenchyme was increased, indicative of a regulatory role of VEGF between pulmonary epithelium and mesenchyme. Mice that lack the VEGF isoforms 164 and 188 and express only the 120 isoform have decreased peripheral vascular development with fewer air-blood barriers and a general delay in lung development.[199] Another factor implicated in pulmonary vascular development is FOXF1. *Foxf1*-null mutant mice die in utero of defects in mesodermal differentiation and cell adhesion.[200] In the lung, FOXF1 is expressed in smooth muscle cells surrounding bronchioles and alveolar endothelial cells.[201,202] Heterozygous mutant mice carrying a disruption of the *Foxf1* gene, in which FOXF1 levels are reduced by 80%, displayed a 55% postnatal mortality with lung hemorrhaging. Analysis of the lungs revealed abnormalities in alveolar formation and pulmonary vasculature.[201] FOXA2 has also been demonstrated to have effects on vascular development of the lung. Experiments using the *Sftpc* promoter to express FOXA2 in the distal lung epithelium showed disrupted airway branching, vasculogenesis, and arrested differentiation of epithelial cells.[203] However, this finding was complicated by a more recent study using mice containing a conditional knockout for *Foxa2*, which showed defects only in alveolarization and differentiation.[204]

From these studies, one can reason that a disruption in pulmonary vascular development goes hand in hand with impaired branching morphogenesis and lung hypoplasia. Indeed, evidence suggests that development of the vascular system exerts a strong influence over lung morphogenesis. Blocking VEGF signaling by use of a pharmacologic inhibitor has been shown to impair not only vascular growth but also alveolarization.[205] This was confirmed in other experiments using antisense oligonucleotides targeted toward VEGF that caused a reduction in both airway branching and vascular development.[206] In vivo delivery of VEGF by means of intratracheal administration of an adenovirus carrying the *Vegf* expression construct not only results in increased vessel formation, but also restores alveolar growth in an experimental rat model of bronchopulmonary dysplasia.[207] Finally, both loss-of-function and gain-of-function experiments were used in mouse lung cultures to confirm the effect of VEGF on both the lung epithelium and the lung endothelium in terms of proliferation, differentiation, and branching morphogenesis.[208] However, the question still remains whether the airway branching phenotype is the direct result of physical disruption of blood vessel formation or whether it is the molecular signaling factors of vascular development alone that affect airway branching morphogenesis.

CONCLUSION

Molecular studies of lung development have started to unravel the complex series of events that control formation of the lung. One of the major complications with preterm birth is immaturity of the lung. Despite modern management, many infants exhibit lung dysfunction characterized by arrested lung development and interrupted alveolarization. A better understanding of the molecular basis of pulmonary development may guide clinicians in the design of strategies for promoting normal lung maturation in a premature infant. Identification of factors implicated in foregut specification and lung lineage morphogenesis is therefore important for understanding the cause of developmental and adult-onset lung morbidities and the generation of novel therapeutic options.

A complete reference list is available at www.ExpertConsult.com. 

SELECT REFERENCES

1. Schittny JC. Development of the lung. *Cell Tissue Res*. 2017;367:427–444.
2. Perl AK, Whitsett JA. Molecular mechanisms controlling lung morphogenesis. *Clin Genet*. 1999;56:14–27.
3. Ang SL, Wierda A, Wong D, et al. The formation and maintenance of the definitive endoderm lineage in the mouse: involvement of HNF3/*forkhead* proteins. *Development*. 1993;119:1301–1315.
4. Kaestner KH, Knochel W. Unified nomenclature for the winged helix/forkhead transcription factors. *Genes Dev*. 2000;14:142–146.

5. Monaghan AP, Kaestner KH, Grau E, Schütz G. Postimplantation expression patterns indicate a role for the mouse forkhead/HNF-3 alpha, beta and gamma genes in determination of the definitive endoderm, chordamesoderm and neuroectoderm. *Development*. 1993;119:567–578.
6. Stahlman MT. Temporal-spatial distribution of hepatocyte nuclear factor-3beta in developing human lung and other foregut derivatives. *J Histochem Cytochem*. 1998;46:955–962.
7. Zhou L, Lim L, Costa RH, Whitsett JA. Thyroid transcription factor-1, hepatocyte nuclear factor-3beta, surfactant protein B, C, and Clara cell secretory protein in developing mouse lung. *J Histochem Cytochem*. 1996;44:1183–1196.
8. Ang SL, Rossant J. HNF-3beta is essential for node and notochord formation in mouse development. *Cell*. 1994;78:561–574.
9. Weinstein DC, Altaba ARI, Chen WS, et al. The winged-helix transcription factor *HNF-3B* is required for notochord development in the mouse embryo. *Cell*. 1994;78:575–588.
10. Dufort D, Schwartz L, Harpal K, Rossant J. The transcription factor HNF3beta is required in visceral endoderm for normal primitive streak morphogenesis. *Development*. 1998;125:3015–3025.
11. Goldfarb M. Functions of fibroblast growth factors in vertebrate development. *Cytokine Growth Factor Rev*. 1996;7:311–325.
12. Ornitz DM, Itoh N. Fibroblast growth factors. *Genome Biol*. 2001;2:3005.1–3005.12.
13. Bellusci S, Grindley J, Emoto H, et al. Fibroblast growth factor 10 (FGF10) and branching morphogenesis in the embryonic mouse lung. *Development*. 1997;124:4867–4878.
14. Min H, Danilenko DM, Scully SA, et al. Fgf-10 is required for both limb and lung development and exhibits striking functional similarity to *Drosophila* branchless. *Genes Dev*. 1998;12:3156–3161.
15. Sekine K, Ohuchi H, Fujiwara M, et al. Fgf10 is essential for limb and lung formation. *Nat Genet*. 1999;21:138–141.
16. Volckaert T, De Langhe S. Lung epithelial stem cells and their niches. Fgf10 takes center stage. *Fibrogenesis Tissue Repair*. 2014;7:8.
17. Ornitz DM, Xu J, Colvin JS, et al. Receptor specificity of the fibroblast growth factor family. *J Biol Chem*. 1996;271:15292–15297.
18. Fox E, Shojaie S, Wang J, et al. Three-dimensional culture and FGF signaling drive differentiation of murine pluripotent cells to distal lung epithelial cells. *Stem Cells Dev*. 2015;24:21–35.
19. Arman E, Haffner-Krausz R, Chen Y, et al. Targeted disruption of fibroblast growth factor (FGF) receptor 2 suggests a role for FGF signaling in pregastrulation mammalian development. *Proc Natl Acad Sci U S A*. 1998;95:5082–5087.
20. Xu X, Weinstein M, Li C, et al. Fibroblast growth factor receptor 2 (FGFR2)-mediated reciprocal regulation loop between FGF8 and FGF10 is essential for limb induction. *Development*. 1998;125:753–765.
21. Arman E, Haffner-Krausz R, Gorivodsky M, Lonai P. Fgfr2 is required for limb outgrowth and lung-branching morphogenesis. *Proc Natl Acad Sci U S A*. 1999;96:11895–11899.
22. Peters K, Werner S, Liao X, et al. Targeted expression of a dominant negative FGF receptor blocks branching morphogenesis and epithelial differentiation of the mouse lung. *EMBO J*. 1994;13:3296–3301.
23. De Moerlooze L, Spencer-Dene B, Revest JM, et al. An important role for the IIIb isoform of fibroblast growth factor receptor 2 (FGFR2) in mesenchymal-epithelial signalling during mouse organogenesis. *Development*. 2000;127:483–492.
24. Klambt C, Glazer L, Shilo B-Z. *Breathless*, a *Drosophila* FGF receptor homolog, is essential for migration of tracheal and specific midline glial cells. *Genes Dev*. 1992;6:1668–1678.
25. Sutherland D, Samakovlis C, Krasnow MA. *Branchless* encodes a *Drosophila* FGF homolog that controls tracheal cell migration and the pattern of branching. *Cell*. 1996;87:1091–1101.
26. Ingham PW, McMahon AP. Hedgehog signaling in animal development: paradigms and principles. *Genes Dev*. 2001;15:3059–3087.
27. Rankin SA, Han L, McCracken KW. A retinoic acid-hedgehog cascade coordinates mesoderm-inducing signals and endoderm competence during lung specification. *Cell Rep*. 2016;28(1):66–78. 16.
28. Litingtung Y, Lei L, Westphal H, Chiang C. Sonic hedgehog is essential to foregut development. *Nat Genet*. 1998;20:58–61.
29. Pepicelli CV, Lewis PM, Mcmahon AP. Sonic hedgehog regulates branching morphogenesis in the mammalian lung. *Curr Biol*. 1998;8:1083–1086.
30. Miller LA, Wert SE, Clark JC, et al. Role of Sonic hedgehog in patterning of tracheal-bronchial cartilage and the peripheral lung. *Dev Dyn*. 2004;231:57–71.
31. Bellusci S, Furuta Y, Rush MG, et al. Involvement of Sonic hedgehog (Shh) in mouse embryonic lung growth and morphogenesis. *Development*. 1997;124:53–63.
32. Grindley JC, Bellusci S, Perkins D, Hogan BLM. Evidence for the involvement of the *Gli* gene family in embryonic mouse lung development. *Dev Biol*. 1997;188:337–348.
33. Motoyama J, Liu J, Mo R, et al. Essential function of *Gli2* and *Gli3* in the formation of lung, trachea and oesophagus. *Nat Genet*. 1998;20:54–57.
34. Bai CB, Joyner AL. *Gli1* can rescue the *in vivo* function of *Gli2*. *Development*. 2001;128:5161–5172.
35. Li Y, Zhang H, Choi SC, et al. Sonic hedgehog signaling regulates Gli3 processing, mesenchymal proliferation, and differentiation during mouse lung organogenesis. *Dev Biol*. 2004;270:214–231.
36. Rutter M, Post M. Shh/gli signalling during murine lung development. In: Howie S, Fisher CE, eds. *Shh and Gli Signaling and Development*. Georgetown, TX: Landes Bioscience; 2006:137.
37. Zile MH. Function of vitamin A in vertebrate embryonic development. *J Nutr*. 2001;131:705–708.
38. Ross SA, McCaffery PJ, Drager UC, De Luca LM. Retinoids in embryonal development. *Physiol Rev*. 2000;80:1021–1054.
39. Mendelsohn C, Lohnes D, Decimo D, et al. Function of the retinoic acid receptors (RARs) during development. (II) Multiple abnormalities at various stages of organogenesis in RAR double mutants. *Development*. 1994;120:2749–2771.
40. Kastner P, Messaddeq N, Mark M, et al. Vitamin A deficiency and mutations of RXRalpha, RXRbeta, RARalpha lead to early differentiation of embryonic ventricular cardiomyocytes. *Development*. 1997;124:4749–4758.
41. Luo J, Sucov HM, Bader JA, et al. Compound mutants for retinoic acid receptor (RAR) beta and RAR alpha 1 reveal developmental functions for multiple RAR-beta isoforms. *Mech Dev*. 1996;55:33–44.
42. Cardoso WV, Mitsialis SA, Brody JS, Williams MC. Retinoic acid alters the expression of pattern-related genes in the developing rat lung. *Dev Dyn*. 1996;207:47–59.
43. Packer AI, Mailutha KG, Ambrozewicz LA, Wolgemuth DJ. Regulation of the *Hoxa4* and *Hoxa5* genes in the embryonic mouse lung by retinoic acid and TGFbeta1. Implications for lung development and patterning. *Dev Dyn*. 2000;217:62–74.
44. Volpe MV, Martin A, Vosatka RJ, et al. Hoxb-5 expression in the developing mouse lung suggests a role in branching morphogenesis and epithelial cell fate. *Histochem Cell Biol*. 1997;108:495–504.
45. Cardoso WV. Transcription factors and pattern formation in the developing lung. *Am J Physiol*. 1995;269:L429–L442.
46. Krumlauf R. *Hox* genes in vertebrate development. *Cell*. 1994;78:191–201.
47. Bogue CW, Gross I, Vasavada H, et al. Identification of *Hex* genes in newborn lung and effects of gestational age and retinoic acid on their expression. *Am J Physiol*. 1994;266:L448–L454.
48. Bogue CW, Lou LJ, Vasavada H, et al. Expression Hoxb genes in the developing mouse foregut and lung. *Am J Respir Cell Mol Biol*. 1996;15:163–171.
49. Kappen C. Hox genes in the lung. *Am J Respir Cell Mol Biol*. 1996;15:156–162.
50. Krumlauf R, Holland PWH, McVey JH, Hogan BLM. Developmental and spatial patterns of expression of the mouse homeobox gene. *Hox2.1*. *Development*. 1987;99:603–617.

59 Regulation of Liquid Secretion and Absorption by the Fetal and Neonatal Lung

David P. Carlton

INTRODUCTION

Before birth, the lung is filled with liquid secreted by the epithelia lining the potential air spaces of the fetal lung. The amount of liquid retained in the fetal lung is similar to the functional residual capacity of the postnatal lung, and maintenance of this dynamic template is an important factor in fetal lung growth. Under normal circumstances, secretion of liquid into the potential airspaces slows as birth approaches, ultimately switching to frank liquid absorption during labor and after birth. Liquid is removed from the lung lumen by a combination of mechanical drainage and liquid absorption across the lung epithelium (Fig. 59.1). The

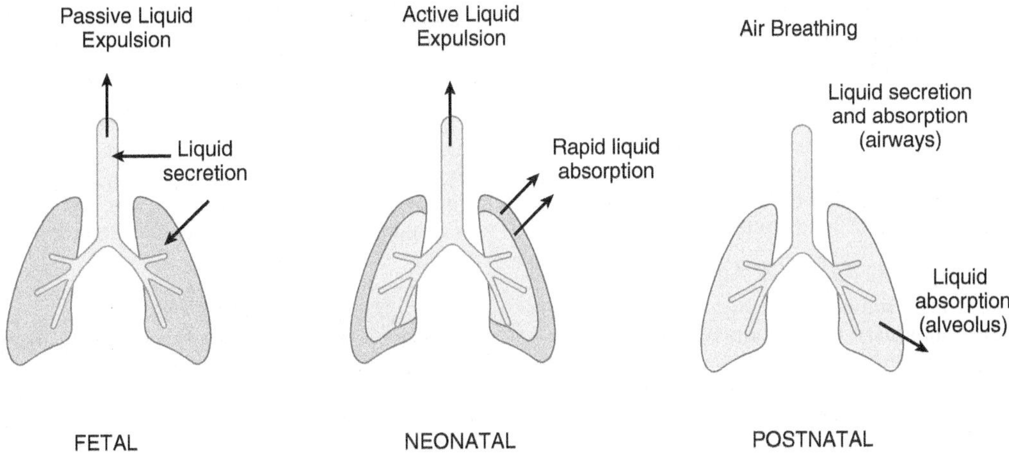

Fig. 59.1 Fetal, neonatal, and postnatal phases of liquid flow across lung epithelia.

liquid absorption mechanism is augmented by an increase in epinephrine associated with labor and delivery. This epinephrine responsiveness is absent in the very immature fetal lung and is triggered in the last half of gestation by thyroid and steroid hormones. The increase in oxygen tension associated with the onset of air breathing also contributes to the absorptive response of the epithelium. Because the absorptive mechanism of the fetal lung is maturationally regulated, premature infants and term infants who are "immature for gestational age" may not clear fluid from their airspaces in an effective manner.

DYNAMICS OF LUNG LIQUID FLOW BEFORE AND AFTER BIRTH

LUNG LIQUID FORMATION AND FLOW DURING FETAL LIFE

Initial observations about the nature of fetal lung liquid centered around the intuitive assumption that the liquid was amniotic fluid aspirated into the lung.[1] However, the observation that tracheal ligation allowed progressive lung distention made this proposal moot.[2] Later, experiments in fetal sheep showed not only that the electrolyte composition of the lung liquid and amniotic fluid were distinct, but also that the chloride (Cl) concentration of fetal lung liquid was higher than that in plasma, suggesting that there might be an active secretory component to the formation of fetal lung liquid.[3,4]

LIQUID SECRETION

Fetal lung liquid is generated by active secretion across the lung epithelium.[5] The rate of liquid secretion has been measured in fetuses of several mammalian species, but most confidently in the fetal lamb.[5-10] The secretion rate increases in fetal sheep from approximately 1.5 mL/kg/h at around midgestation to 5 mL/kg/h later in gestation.[11,12] After its secretion, the liquid exits the lung into the pharynx where it either contributes to the amniotic fluid or is swallowed and contributes to normal fetal gastrointestinal contents. The lung liquid generates a pressure of approximately 2 mm Hg relative to that measured in amniotic fluid, largely due to restriction to flow through the larnyx.[13-15] In the more mature fetal lamb, the lung volume has been found to be similar to that of the functional residual capacity of the postnatal lung, approximately 30 mL/kg body weight.[16] This filling of the lung with liquid results in a sort of "dynamic template," around which the lung architecture develops. If the expected fetal lung volume is diminished experimentally, the lung becomes hypoplastic, and if the volume is made to increase, the lung becomes, by some measures, hyperplastic.[17-19]

FETAL BREATHING MOVEMENTS

Fetal breathing results in small and irregular movements of liquid (~0.5 mL) in the fetal airways.[20-22] If fetal breathing is altered neurologically, the lung becomes hypoplastic, presumably as a result of alterations in fetal lung volume.[23-25]

AIRWAY WALL CONTRACTIONS

Peristaltic contractions of the developing airways cause changes in local lung liquid flow and pressure that may also be important in lung development. Striking contractions of embryonic airways were first observed in chick embryos in the 1920s.[26] Studies on various animal models demonstrate that these contractions cause peristalsis of the airway similar to that seen in the gut. These peristaltic waves propagate distal movement of intraluminal liquid and cause expansion of the endbuds.[27] Smooth muscle contractions were inhibited by the calcium (Ca^{2+}) channel blocker nifedipine.[28] However, it is not clear whether the observed lung hypoplasia after nifedipine administration was a result of the inhibition of peristalsis or whether liquid secretion was influenced by this intervention.

SURGICAL INTERVENTION

Given that ligation of fetal airways promotes lung growth distal to that point, surgical obstruction of the fetal airway has evolved as a technique for prevention or correction of potential lung hypoplasia, particularly with lung anomalies associated with congenital diaphragmatic hernia. However, early enthusiasm for fetal surgery has been tempered by poor results.[29] The traditional hypothesis that lung hypoplasia results from compression by herniating abdominal viscera has been challenged because pulmonary anomalies have been observed before herniation of abdominal contents into the chest.[30,31] The role of ion transport in the pathogenesis lung hypoplasia is not known.

CHANGES IN LUNG LIQUID AROUND BIRTH

At the time of birth, at least in the term newborn, approximately 100 mL of lung liquid must be removed. This is achieved as a result of a series of mechanical and ion transport events.

DECREASE IN LUNG LIQUID VOLUME BEFORE LABOR

Experiments in fetal animals demonstrate that both lung liquid volume and secretion decrease near delivery.[6,8,12,32] The decrease in lung liquid volume is likely a result not only of a decrease in transepithelial fluid movement, but also from the exit of fluid from the lung.[33]

ROLE OF LABOR

Several lines of evidence suggest that delivery by cesarean section (CS) slows lung liquid clearance, particularly when it occurs before the beginning of labor.[34,35] Rabbits that are born at term, either vaginally or by CS after the onset of labor, have less water in their lungs than do rabbits that are delivered by CS without prior labor (Fig. 59.2). This observation is one of several that challenge the intuitive appeal of the "thoracic compression" during vaginal birth as critical for lung liquid removal.

FATE OF LUNG LIQUID DURING LABOR AND DELIVERY

Once labor begins, at least some portion of lung liquid begins to move across the pulmonary epithelium in a direction the reverse of that before labor.[12] Active transcellular Na^+ absorption is the mechanism that drives liquid out of the lumen into the interstitial space.[36] The excess interstitial liquid then moves into the pulmonary circulation and lung lymphatics for return to the central circulation.[37]

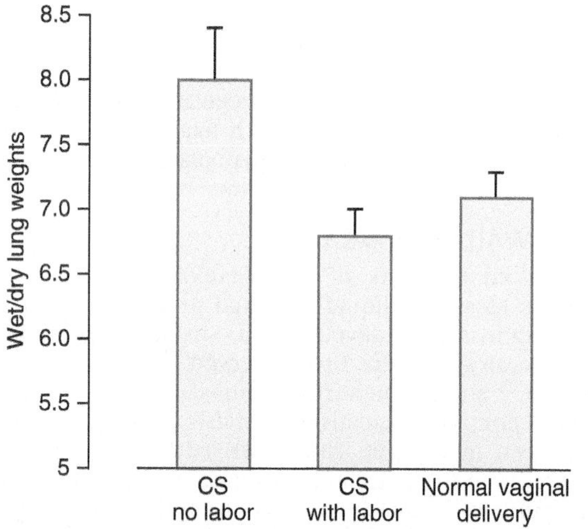

Fig. 59.2 Effect of labor on lung water content (wet/dry weight) of newborn rabbit pups born after normal vaginal delivery or by cesarean section *(CS)*. (From Bland RD, Bressack MA, McMillan DD. Labor decreases the lung water content of newborn rabbits. *Am J Obstet Gynecol.* 1979;135:364–337.)

LIQUID MOVEMENT AFTER BIRTH

After delivery, active liquid absorption continues, and most of the liquid is cleared from the term newborn lung within 2 hours after birth.[12,38] With the onset of breathing, solute permeability of the distal lung epithelium increases, and this increase in flux potential likely contributes in part to liquid removal.[39]

BASIC MECHANISMS OF TRANSEPITHELIAL ION TRANSPORT

Ion transport pathways common to other epithelia permit the secretion and absorption of liquid across the epithelium of the fetal and newborn lung. Our understanding of perinatal lung liquid flow is a result of the interrogation of these channels and transporters.

The initial studies of fetal lung liquid demonstrated that the fetal lung epithelium was highly restrictive to macromolecules compared with the endothelium. This characteristic accounts for the near absence of protein in the fetal lung lumen, in contrast to the significant protein concentration of the interstitium and circulation. Despite this oncotic gradient across the lung epithelium, lung liquid is secreted actively before birth by transcellular Cl^- transport. In a still incompletely understood sequence, clearance is then driven after birth by an active ion transport process, namely, Na^+ absorption.[5,11,36,40]

The basic configuration of ion transporters and channels is similar to that found in other mammalian ion-transporting epithelia. The electrochemical gradient for entry and exit of ions to and from the lung epithelial cells is established by Na^+,K^+-adenosine triphosphatase (ATPase) at the basolateral membrane. Activity of this transporter results in a low intracellular $[Na^+]$ that creates a gradient for Na^+ to enter the cell through either the basolateral membrane or through apical membrane. The main identified transporters and channels that result in liquid secretion and absorption are shown in Fig. 59.3.

The molecular identities of the important transporters and pumps located on the interstitial or basolateral membrane (Na^+

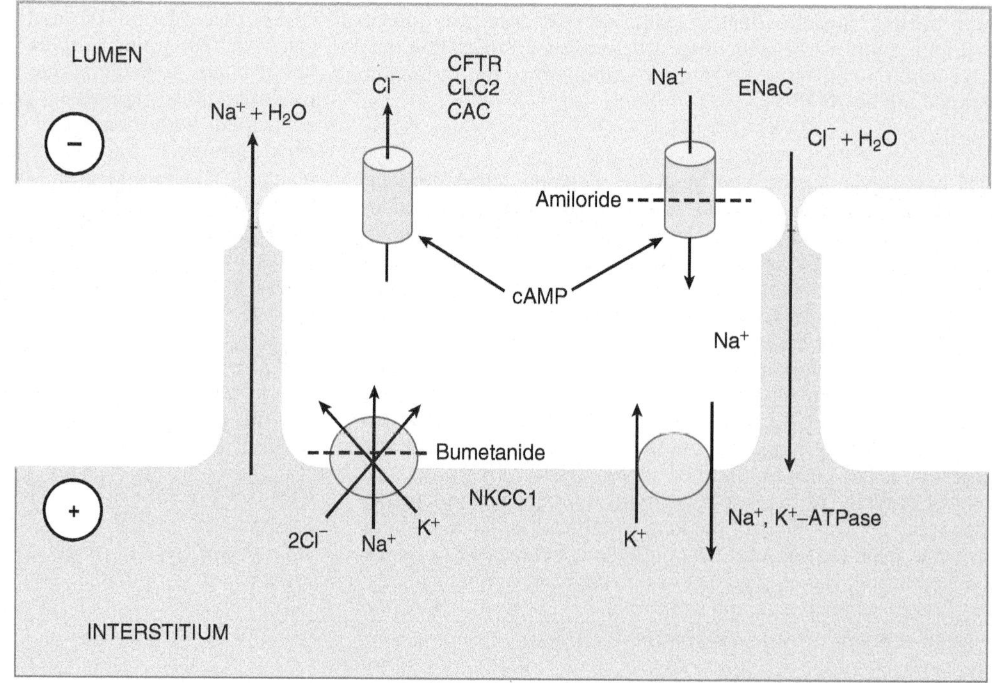

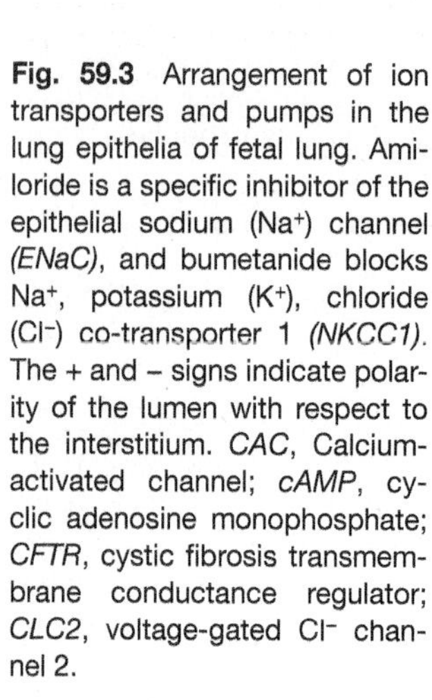

Fig. 59.3 Arrangement of ion transporters and pumps in the lung epithelia of fetal lung. Amiloride is a specific inhibitor of the epithelial sodium (Na^+) channel *(ENaC)*, and bumetanide blocks Na^+, potassium (K^+), chloride (Cl^-) co-transporter 1 *(NKCC1)*. The + and – signs indicate polarity of the lumen with respect to the interstitium. *CAC*, Calcium-activated channel; *cAMP*, cyclic adenosine monophosphate; *CFTR*, cystic fibrosis transmembrane conductance regulator; *CLC2*, voltage-gated Cl^- channel 2.

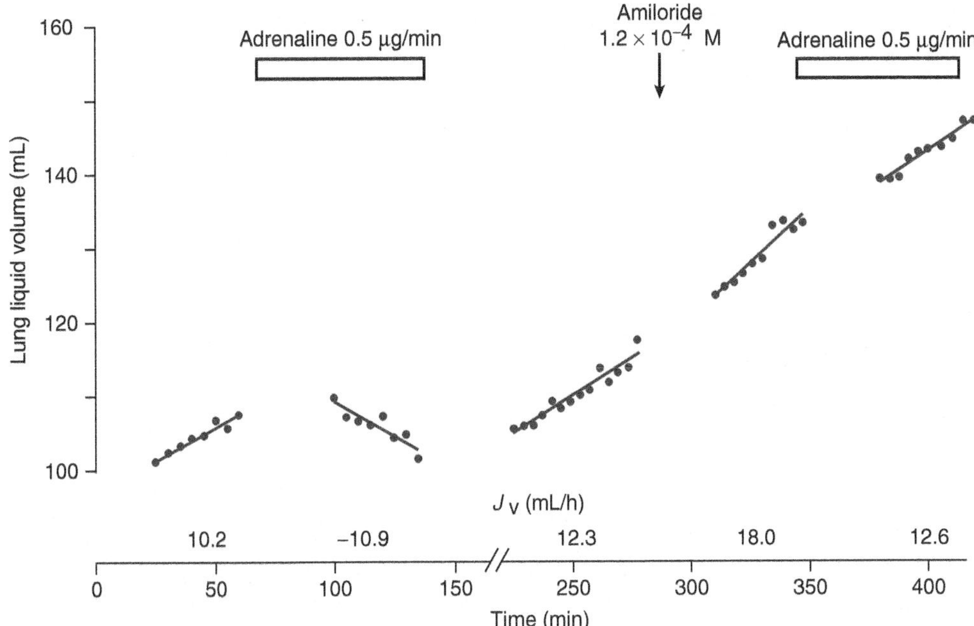

Fig. 59.4 Effect of epinephrine (adrenaline) infusion and topical amiloride on cumulative lung volume across the lung epithelium of a near-term fetal sheep. At the start of the study, volume increases because of liquid secretion (J_v 10.2 mL/h). Epinephrine infusion abruptly causes a decrease in lung volume, reversing the direction of flow (J_v −10.9 mL/h) from secretion to absorption. Secretion is restored when the epinephrine infusion is discontinued. Addition of the sodium channel blocker amiloride to lung liquid prevents liquid absorption when the epinephrine infusion is restarted. (From Olver RE, Ramsden CA, Strang LB, et al. The role of amiloride-blockable sodium transport in adrenaline-induced lung liquid reabsorption in the fetal lamb. *J Physiol* 1986;376:321–340.)

pump, Na^+,K^+-ATPase, and $Na^+,K^+,2Cl^-$ co-transporter [NKCC1]) are known (see Fig. 59.3). Likewise, the principal Na^+ channel on the luminal membrane (epithelial Na^+ channel [ENaC]) is well-characterized molecularly.[41] However, the identity of the principal mechanism responsible for fetal Cl^- secretion across the lumen membrane is not completely clear. Some of the candidates include the cystic fibrosis transmembrane conductance regulator (CFTR) and the voltage-gated Cl^- channels 2 and 3 (CLC2, CLC3), all of which are expressed in the fetal lung.[42-45] There is also evidence for a purinoceptor-Ca^{2+}-activated Cl^- channel in fetal lung epithelia.[46,47]

CHLORIDE SECRETION

The movement of Cl^- from the interstitium to the lung lumen is the driving force for fetal lung liquid secretion. From studies of other Cl^--secreting mammalian epithelia, NaK2Cl co-transporter (NKCC) family members are likely candidates for the Cl^- entry mechanism through the basolateral membrane. On the apical membrane, it is assumed that Cl^- channels, exchangers, or co-transporters are responsible for exit of Cl^- into the lumen.

SODIUM, POTASSIUM, CHLORIDE CO-TRANSPORTER

In the fetal lung, instillation of the loop diuretics bumetanide or furosemide (specific NKCC inhibitors) to lung liquid results in slowing of lung liquid secretion or frank liquid absorption.[48,49] Loop diuretics also inhibit liquid secretion in vitro by distal lung explants from fetal lung, and they decrease basal short-circuit current, at least in the fetal trachea.[50-53] Of the two NKCC isoforms that have been described, messenger RNA (mRNA) of NKCC1 but not NKCC2 is abundantly expressed in epithelia from all regions of the late-gestation fetal mouse lung.[54] Postnatally, there is a significant decrease in NKCC1 expression by mouse tracheal epithelia.[55] Because bumetanide only minimally inhibits basal and cyclic adenosine monophosphate (cAMP)-induced Cl^- secretion across fetal human and mouse distal lung epithelium, there are likely non-NKCC pathways for Cl secretion. This notion is supported by the observation that mice that lack the NKCC transporter ($NKCC^{-/-}$) have apparently normal lung function and development.[46,54-57] Studies of fetal NKCC1-null mice show that maximal, but not basal, Cl^- secretion is impaired.[55] The molecular interrogation of other potential Cl^- entry mechanisms in fetal lung epithelia are incomplete.

CYSTIC FIBROSIS TRANSMEMBRANE CONDUCTANCE REGULATOR

The CFTR provides a critical apical membrane conduit for Cl^- secretion and is an important regulator of Na^+ transport in lung epithelia after birth.[58,59] However, non-CFTR mechanisms are also capable of participating in liquid secretion by fetal lung epithelia because the lungs of fetuses with cystic fibrosis (CF) are normally developed and CF-affected human fetal lung explants are inflated with liquid.[60-63]

OTHER FETAL CHLORIDE CHANNELS

The identity of non-CFTR anion secretory pathways in fetal lung epithelia is uncertain. Purinoceptor-activated Cl^- secretion has been observed in CFTR-null mice fetal lung and in wild-type fetal rat and fetal human lung epithelia.[46,47,64] The developmental expression pattern of CLC2 and CLC3 indicates a possible role for these channels in fetal lung liquid secretion.[45]

ROLE OF SODIUM ABSORPTION IN PERINATAL LUNG LIQUID CLEARANCE

Spontaneous and epinephrine-induced absorption of fetal lung liquid is associated with a large increase in net Na^+ transport out of the lumen and is inhibited by amiloride, a Na^+ channel blocker (Fig. 59.4).[36] Na^+ and cation channels have been identified by electrophysiologic means on the apical membrane of fetal cells harvested from the distal lung.[65] In addition the observation that all activated and spontaneous liquid absorption could be inhibited by mixing the Na^+ channel blocker amiloride into fetal lung liquid demonstrates an essential role for amiloride-sensitive Na^+ transport in lung liquid clearance around the time of birth. The importance of amiloride-sensitive pathways is highlighted by the observation that amiloride instilled into the trachea of the newborn guinea pig impairs lung water clearance in a dose-dependent manner, and related studies later confirmed the importance of a specific channel, ENaC.[66,67] The roles of the high-energy Na^+,K^+-ATPase pump on the basolateral membrane and ENaC on the apical membrane have been well studied.[41,68]

Na^+,K^+-ADENOSINE TRIPHOSPHATASE

Processes associated with labor are important for activation of the lung epithelial Na^+,K^+-ATPase pump. Labor is associated with a several-fold increase in pump activity in fetal alveolar type II

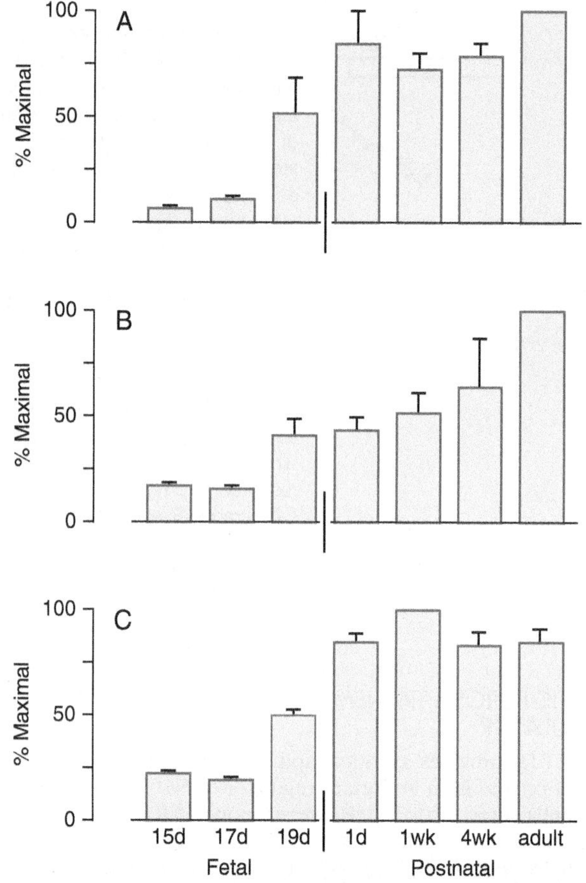

Fig. 59.5 α (A), β (B), and γ (C) epithelial sodium channel subunit mRNA expression in fetal (term = 19 days) and postnatal whole mouse lung. (From Talbot CL, Bosworth DG, Briley EL, et al. Quantitation and localization of ENaC subunit expression in fetal, newborn, and adult mouse lung. *Am J Respir Cell Mol Biol.* 1999;20:398–406.)

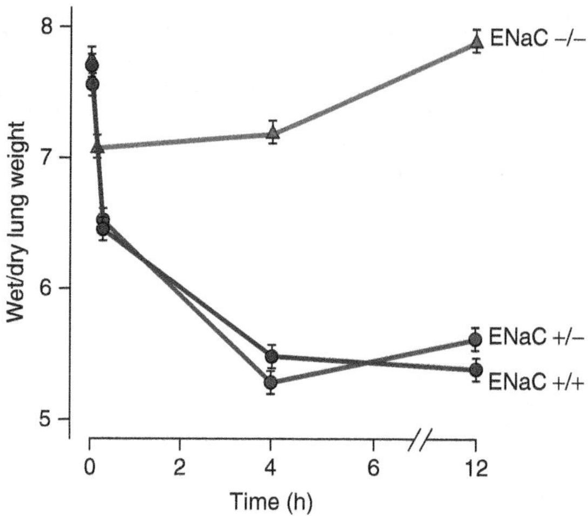

Fig. 59.6 Lung water content (wet/dry lung weight) before (0 hour) and after birth (15 minutes, 4 hours, 12 hours) in α-epithelial sodium channel (αENaC), knockout mice (αENaC –/–), and littermate controls (αENaC +/– and +/+). (From Hummler E, Barker P, Gatzy J, et al: Early death due to defective neonatal lung liquid clearance in α-ENaC-deficient mice. *Nat Genet.* 1996;12:325–328.)

cells.[69,70] Expression of the α1 and β1 subunits of this enzyme increase from low levels in early fetal life and peak around the time of birth.[71,72] During the first several days after birth, epithelial expression of α1 and β1 subunit mRNA is found in small airways and the basolateral surface of alveolar type II.[72,73]

EPITHELIAL SODIUM CHANNEL

ENaC subunit mRNA expression has been studied in human and rodent lung epithelia and demonstrate that αENaC mRNA expression in the lung shortly after birth is similar to levels seen in the adult lung.[74,75] There is a similar increase in expression of γENaC and a more gradual increase in βENaC that peaks in adult lung (Fig. 59.5). Expression of γENaC parallels that of αENaC, with intense expression of subunit mRNA in all regions of the fetal lung, whereas βENaC expression in fetal and early postnatal lung is restricted to the airway epithelium.[74] Both αENaC mRNA expression and the sensitivity of lung liquid clearance to amiloride and to β-adrenergic blockade are maximal soon after birth, and they decline in parallel with endogenous plasma epinephrine concentration. Immunocytochemical studies of human fetal lung show significant αENaC protein expression in early midtrimester fetal lung, at a time when the fetal lung is not thought to be capable of significant Na^+ transport.[76,77]

ALTERNATIVE SODIUM CHANNELS

Alternative amiloride-sensitive Na^+-permeable channels in fetal lung that may contribute to the driving force for lung liquid clearance have been described. These include certain amiloride-sensitive, poorly nonselective cation channels: G-protein-regulated, β-adrenergic agonist/Ca^{2+}-activated, and cyclic nucleotide-gated channels.[78-80] According to at least one school of thought, the β-adrenergic-responsive, nonselective channel may be a multimer of αENaC subunits, and the role of β and γ subunits may be to confer selectivity on the channel.[81] An additional pathway for Na^+ absorption is Na^+-glucose co-transport, which has been reported in fetal sheep lung epithelia.[82]

KNOCKOUT MODELS OF SODIUM TRANSPORT

Certain knockout and other transgenic mouse models have been used to explore the role of ion transport in the perinatal lung. Knockout mice for all three ENaC subunits have been studied.[67,83-86] Newborn mice that lack the αENaC gene are unable to clear liquid from the alveolar spaces after birth (Fig. 59.6). These mice show an increased work of breathing, they fail to eat, and move less than expected. Mice with γENaC- or βENaC-null mutations have delayed liquid clearance, but near-normal lung water content within the first day after birth. All subunit mutations resulted in severe hyperkalemia. αENaC-null mice demonstrate an improvement in fluid clearance following rescue with an αENaC transgene, with approximately 50% Na^+ channel activity.[86] These studies indicate that ENaC function is a critical requirement for clearance of neonatal lung liquid in the newborn period and suggest that the αENaC subunit is the core rate-limiting part of the Na^+ channel in lung epithelia.

HORMONAL REGULATION OF ION AND LIQUID TRANSPORT

CYCLIC ADENOSINE MONOPHOSPHATE-MEDIATED LIQUID TRANSPORT

Near the time of birth, cAMP stimulates the induction of liquid absorption, although early in gestation, cAMP stimulates liquid secretion.[46,61] Birth is known to be associated with a surge in fetal catecholamine secretion, and epinephrine causes lung liquid absorption, an effect that is inhibitable by propranolol.[12,87,88] In addition to effects on liquid secretion and lung water, β-adrenergic agonists cause release of surfactant and improve both early lung mechanics and gas exchange.[89-92] β-Adrenergic agonists act via the cAMP signaling pathway, and, as predicted, the addition of a

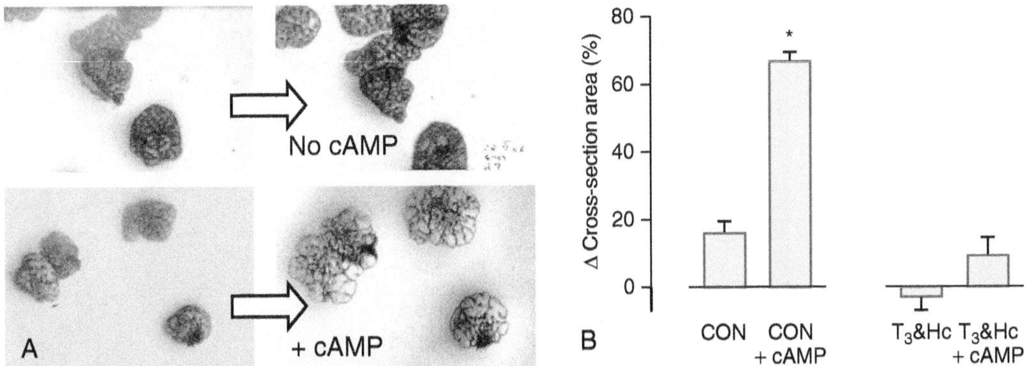

Fig. 59.7 (A) These 20-week human fetal lung explants expanded with liquid when they were exposed for 24 hours to 10^{-4} mol cyclic adenosine monophosphate *(cAMP)*. (B) This increase in diameter was attenuated in explants preincubated for 48 hours with 10^{-9} mol triiodothyronine (T_3) and 10^{-6} mol hydrocortisone (Hc). *CON,* Control.

lipid-soluble analogue of cAMP, dibutyryl cAMP (db-cAMP), can mimic the effect of epinephrine.[93]

Because cAMP mediates both liquid secretion and liquid absorption in the fetal lung, the potential exists for an epinephrine to cause inappropriate lung liquid secretion in neonates born very prematurely. In explants of human fetal lung, cAMP causes an increase in liquid volume (Fig. 59.7A). This effect is attenuated by pretreatment of explants with thyroid and steroid hormones (see Fig. 59.7B).

Arginine vasopressin, another hormone that increases cellular cAMP, increases during labor. Although it can be shown to inhibit lung liquid secretion, its effect is weaker than that of epinephrine, and its role is uncertain.[94-96] It has been suggested that arginine vasopressin may provide a redundant mechanism to the β-adrenergic-dependent pathway and may explain why β-adrenergic blockade fails to prevent lung liquid absorption during labor.[97]

THYROID AND STEROID HORMONES

Thyroid and glucocorticoid hormones are important in the maturation of the absorptive response of the lung to epinephrine.[98,99] In the absence of thyroid hormone, the lung liquid response to epinephrine (and db-cAMP) is blunted, but such a response is reinstated by infusion of triiodothyronine (T_3). Neither T_3 nor hydrocortisone is capable of advancing maturation of the epinephrine response in normal fetuses with intact thyroid glands when they were given separately, but they are synergistic when given concurrently (Fig. 59.8).[100] In fetal lambs that have had the thyroid gland removed, the response to epinephrine is detectable within 2 hours of the start of infusion of the hormone combination. This induction of epinephrine-sensitive liquid absorption is lost within 24 hours after stopping hormone administration.[101] These observations highlight the degree of coordination of hormonal development for efficient lung liquid clearance around the time of birth.[102]

The rise in αENaC expression parallels plasma cortisol concentration in late gestation and can be blocked by metyrapone after delivery by CS.[103] Prenatal steroids, but not thyroid hormones, advance the timing of the increase in αENaC mRNA in fetal rat lung, but neither hormone affects expression of βENaC or γENaC subunit mRNA.[75] Thyroid hormones have no effect on ENaC mRNA expression, but they do potentiate the effect of steroids on Na^+ transport, effects that are consistent with our understanding of molecular binding.[104,105]

A similar pattern of regulation has been reported for the subunits of the Na^+,K^+-ATPase. Steroid hormones increase α1 and β1 mRNA expression and enzyme activity.[106] In addition, the activity of Na^+,K^+-ATPase can be up-regulated by intracellular cAMP.[107,108] The similarity of hormonal regulation of ENaC and

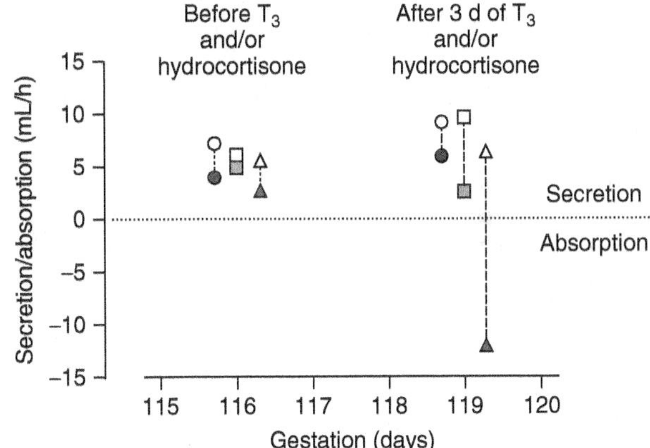

Fig. 59.8 Effect of thyroid and steroid hormone on basal secretion *(open symbols)* and the ability of immature fetal sheep (term = 145 days) to respond to epinephrine infusion *(closed symbols)*. Thyroid (triiodothyronine [T_3]) and steroid hormone exposure did not affect basal secretion rates. Only fetuses that had been treated with thyroid *and* steroid hormone for 3 days were able to absorb lung liquid during epinephrine infusion. *Dashed line,* Effect of IV epinephrine; *gold square,* hydrocortisone; *red circle,* T_3; *green triangle,* T_3 and hydrocortisone. (From Barker PM, Markiewicz M, Parker KA, et al. Synergistic action of triiodothyronine and hydrocortisone on epinephrine-induced reabsorption of fetal lung liquid. *Pediatr Res.* 1990;27:588–591.)

Na^+,K^+-ATPase demonstrates the linkage present between the two principal mechanisms that drive lung liquid absorption.

REGULATION OF ION TRANSPORT BY OXYGEN

Oxygen appears to be an important factor in maintaining liquid removal after birth.[109] The onset of breathing results in an increase in alveolar P_{O_2} from the fetal level of approximately 25 mm Hg to about approximately 100 mm Hg after birth. A shift from fetal P_{O_2} (~25 mm Hg) to room air (~150 mm Hg) inhibits liquid secretion by fetal lung explants in late gestation, whereas there is no inhibition of liquid secretion by elevated oxygen exposure at very early gestations (Fig. 59.9). By contrast, liquid secretion is not triggered in postnatal lung explants with exposure to fetal gas concentrations, suggesting that the switch to liquid absorption may be irreversible shortly after birth. The effect of O_2 on liquid secretion is induced in immature explants by treatment with thyroid and steroid hormones. These observations demonstrate

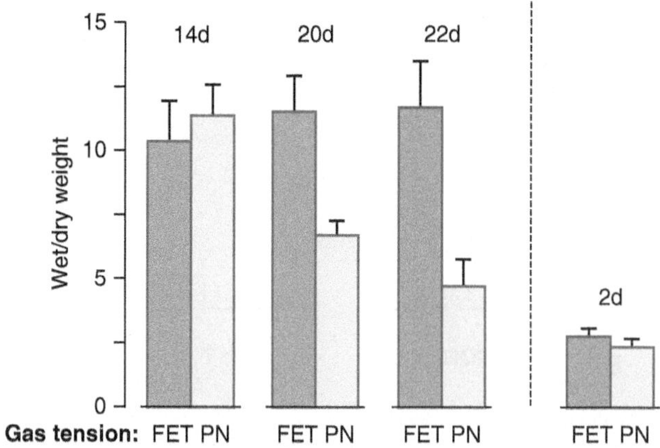

Fig. 59.9 Effect of fetal *(FET)* ambient O_2 of 3% or postnatal *(PN)* ambient O_2 of 21% conditions on liquid volume of distal lung explants derived from fetal mouse lung. (From Barker PM, Gatzy JT. Effect of gas composition on liquid secretion by explants of distal lung of fetal rat in submersion culture. *Am J Physiol.* 1993;265:L512–L517.)

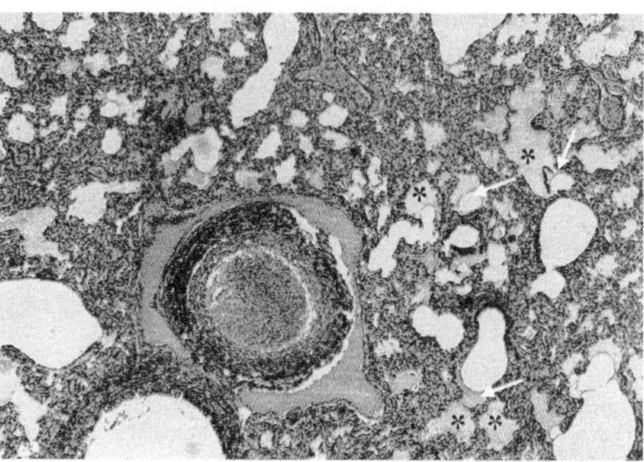

Fig. 59.10 Photomicrograph of a lung from a 1300-g infant who died of respiratory distress syndrome at 8 hours without mechanical ventilation. The *arrows* show meniscus of liquid *(asterisks)* contained inside the alveoli. (From DeSa DJ. Pulmonary fluid content in infants with respiratory distress. *J Pathol.* 1969;97:469–478.)

a critical role of thyroid and steroid hormones in priming the lung epithelium to respond to physiologic stimuli that promote transepithelial liquid flow from secretion to absorption at birth.

Studies with fetal lung cells show that the increase in Na^+ transport induced by raising Po_2 from 30 to 150 mm Hg is paralleled by an increase in ENaC mRNA expression.[110] This shift in Po_2 is accompanied by a temporary fall in epithelial resistance lasting several hours, consistent with the increase in solute permeability at the onset of breathing in vivo that may assist liquid absorption.[39] Hypoxia in adult animals decreases alveolar liquid clearance, an effect that is independent of ENaC and Na^+,K^+-ATPase subunit expression.[111] These studies indicate that the mechanisms of O_2-induced neonatal alveolar Na^+ and liquid transport include regulation of ENaC and may be reversible.

Glucocorticoid and thyroid hormones up-regulate Na^+ transport and β-agonist-induced apical Na^+ conductance (G_{Na}) independent of ambient Po_2, but a shift to neonatal Po_2 is a prerequisite for hormonal up-regulation of Na^+,K^+-ATPase.[112] This observation is contrasted with the effects of thyroid hormones and steroids on immature fetal sheep lung, which are restricted to induction of β-agonist-responsive liquid absorption, with no effect on basal secretion rates.[100] Postnatally, steroids and Po_2 also have an additive effect in up-regulating expression of ENaC-like Na^+ channels in type II alveolar cells.[113]

The promoter region of α-rENaC contains a consensus nuclear factor-κB (NF-κB) binding element. Further experiments in rat lung cells show that an increase in Po_2 induces this redox-sensitive transcription factor, and blocking NF-κB activation reduced the O_2-mediated increase in sodium conductance.[114,115] These findings could be interpreted as indicating that Po_2 activation of NF-κB up-regulated the expression of ENaC, thus increasing Na^+ transport at the onset of breathing. However, subsequent experiments demonstrate that a shift from fetal to postnatal Po_2 concentration results in an immediate increase in NF-κB expression and a detectable increase in Na^+ pump capacity within 6 hours. In contrast, activation of the αENaC promoter is not seen until after 24 hours, reaching a maximum (together with sodium conductance) at 48 hours.[116,117]

Therefore it appears that the early increase in fluid absorptive capacity in response to the rise in alveolar Po_2 at birth is primarily the result of an increase in Na^+,K^+-ATPase pump capacity, and the increase in sodium conductance may be secondary to this increase in Na^+ transport, not its cause. Both components of the response are enhanced by glucocorticoid and thyroid hormones, which are also required for β-adrenergic-mediated control of sodium movement.

LUNG LIQUID AND ION TRANSPORT IN NEONATAL RESPIRATORY DISEASE

This section reviews the evidence that lung water clearance is important in understanding neonatal lung disease and examines the contribution of abnormal airway ion transport.

LUNG LIQUID

Animal studies show a clear correlation between intraluminal liquid volume and respiratory function at birth. Residual lung liquid at birth influences gas exchange in lambs delivered by CS near term.[118] Animals that have approximately 50% of their lung liquid removed just before delivery have significantly better respiratory function than those delivered without liquid removal. The first clinical evidence that lung liquid may play a role in neonatal respiratory disease came from an analysis of postmortem lung findings.[119] Infants who died of idiopathic respiratory distress syndrome (RDS) had significantly higher lung liquid content compared with infants who died of nonrespiratory causes.[120] These findings were supported by other evidence of lung liquid excess on histologic examination after RDS (Fig. 59.10).[119]

Certain factors may predispose the newborn preterm infant to pulmonary edema[121]:

1. Persistent pulmonary hypertension is more common in this group of infants, particularly if they experience hypoxia or patent ductus arteriosus.
2. A large transpulmonary pressure that drives fluid into the alveolar compartment may develop in areas of the lung with surfactant deficiency. The advent of artificial surfactant therapy has significantly decreased the incidence of RDS, and some of its effect may result from decreased surface tension and improved gas exchange in areas of the preterm lung that are not completely emptied of alveolar liquid at birth.[122]
3. Mechanical ventilation likely disrupts the epithelial barrier and allows entry to the alveolar space of proteins that, in turn, may increase intra-alveolar fluid.
4. High inspired O_2 releases toxic metabolites that may interfere with essential cellular functions, including ion transport.

In addition to these factors that promote pulmonary edema, ion transport is almost certainly incompletely developed in infants born very prematurely.[123]

The correlation between preterm delivery and respiratory distress is clear; however, some clinical studies, both prospective and retrospective, also demonstrate a link between mode of delivery and respiratory condition in the neonate.[124-126] Elective CS without labor is associated with a small but significant increased risk of RDS. This risk is exacerbated by delivery even a couple of weeks before term.[127]

Transient tachypnea of the newborn (TTN) is probably the best-described consequence of inadequate neonatal lung liquid clearance. This self-limiting disease, characterized by an increase in respiratory rate or other clinical indications of respiratory malfunction, occurs more frequently in infants delivered by elective CS and is thought to result from delayed activation of liquid clearance in infants not subjected to the stress of labor.[128,129] These clinical data are consistent with animal studies demonstrating the importance of gestation and labor in perinatal lung water clearance and successful adaptation to air breathing.

AIRWAY ION TRANSPORT STUDIES

Some investigators have used nasal electrical potential difference (PD) to measure ion transport directly across the upper airway in vivo. Nasal PD measures the electrical potential generated by active transport of charged ions (Cl^- and Na^+) across the nasal membrane. The use of nasal PD to infer patterns of ion transport in the lower airways and alveoli has been validated by measurement of similar ion transport patterns in nasal and lower bronchial epithelia.[130,131] In addition, nasal PD can predict who will be susceptible to high-altitude pulmonary edema.[132] Nasal PD has been used to distinguish newborn infants with CF from healthy neonates and those with non-CF respiratory disease.[133] This test can also detect ion transport differences that reflected the mode of delivery. Nasal PD is significantly higher in infants born by elective CS than in those born normally or by CS after labor. Infants with TTN have the highest nasal PD, but they also have less amiloride-sensitive Na^+ transport compared with babies who do not have TTN.[134] These studies support the notion that TTN may result in persistence of a fetal ion transport phenotype after birth.

There are also nasal PD abnormalities in premature infants. Premature infants who have respiratory distress have significantly lower maximal PDs and less inhibition after amiloride perfusion (Fig. 59.11), a finding suggesting reduced ENaC-mediated Na^+ absorption.[135] However, because of a close correlation between maximal PD and birth weight, the lower birth weight of the RDS group could represent a significant confounding variable. Although more studies are needed in this area, the available evidence supports an etiologic role for immature ion transport processes in the evolution of acute and possibly chronic lung disease (CLD) in preterm infants.

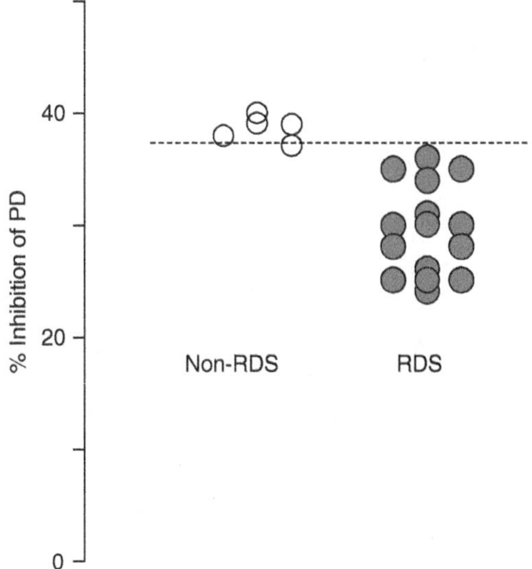

Fig. 59.11 The percentage of inhibition of nasal potential difference *(PD)* by the sodium channel blocker amiloride discriminates between infants who subsequently developed respiratory distress syndrome *(RDS) (green circles)* and those who did not *(white circles)*. (From Barker PM, Markiewicz M, Parker KA, et al. Synergistic action of triiodothyronine and hydrocortisone on epinephrine-induced reabsorption of fetal lung liquid. *Pediatr Res.* 1990;27:588–591.)

THERAPEUTIC CONSIDERATIONS

The role of labor in clearing fetal liquid from the perinatal lung is supported by clinical studies that show a protective effect of labor on subsequent respiratory outcome. Drugs that augment the switch from liquid secretion to liquid absorption at birth are candidates for novel therapies to treat lung disease associated with premature birth. Possible strategies include inhibiting Cl^- secretion and augmenting Na^+ transport across respiratory epithelia.

EFFECT OF LABOR

Respiratory morbidity of both term and preterm infants is related to mode of delivery. In term infants born to mothers undergoing repeat CS, there is a higher incidence of TTN after birth without a trial of labor (6%) compared with those born after a trial of labor (3%). The TTN rate in infants who had a trial of labor is similar to that of those born during routine vaginal births.[136] In both preterm and term infants, the rates of all respiratory problems are significantly higher in infants born by CS without labor compared with those born by either route with labor.[137]

β-ADRENERGIC STIMULATION

In term infants undergoing CS without labor, there is significant improvement in dynamic lung compliance and a decrease in respiratory rate for those whose mothers receive a β-adrenergic agonist during the last 2 hours of labor compared with infants who are not exposed to these drugs.[138] These studies confirm the important role of labor in clearing lung liquid in preparation for air breathing and thus supports the hypothesis that β-adrenergic stimulation induced by labor plays a key role in triggering the absorptive process. This beneficial effect of prenatal β-adrenergic stimulation on respiratory morbidity is also observed in preterm infants.[139]

SODIUM TRANSPORT

Steroid and thyroid hormones exert a major maturational effect on Na^+ transport in the developing fetal lung. Both hormones have been tested for prevention and treatment of neonatal lung disease. Multiple randomized trials suggest that prenatal glucocorticoids reduce the risk of RDS. But even combined with surfactant therapy, antenatal steroid therapy has not decreased CLD in preterm infants.[140,141] Some clinical trials examining the addition of thyrotropin-releasing hormone to antenatal steroids have been reported. Early trials suggested some reduction in respiratory morbidity in infants of mothers given the hormone; however, subsequent larger studies have not confirmed these findings and have suggested potentially negative outcomes, both short term and long term, after treatment with thyrotropin-releasing hormone.[142-146] Postnatal steroid administration has been used extensively to treat ventilator-dependent lung disease in preterm infants, and studies showed that short courses of dexamethasone given early (in the first 2 weeks of life) may prevent bronchopulmonary dysplasia.[147-150] However, enthusiasm for steroid therapy has been tempered by reports of negative effects of both prenatal and postnatal glucocorticoids on lung development and pathologic findings in multiple organs.[151] These concerns have generated interest in the possibility that lower doses of steroids may be effective and may generate fewer side effects. Pilot studies in very preterm infants suggest that adrenal insufficiency can be reversed and CLD can be prevented

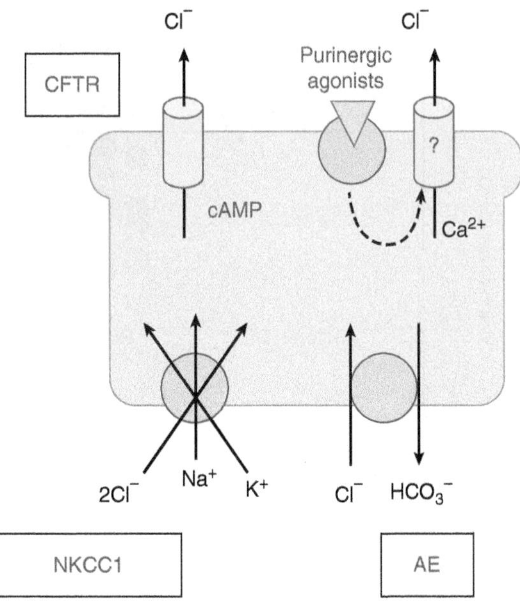

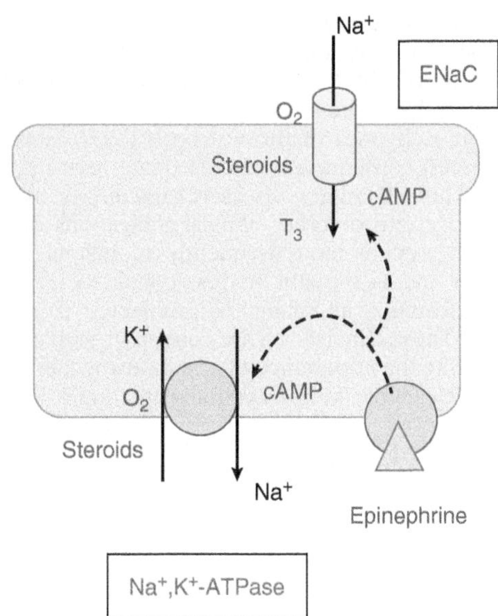

Fig. 59.12 Summary of ion transport components and regulations. *AE,* Anion exchanger; *cAMP,* cyclic adenosine monophosphate; *CFTR,* cystic fibrosis transmembrane conductance regulator; *ENaC,* epithelial sodium channel; *HCO_3^-,* bicarbonate; *NKCC1,* sodium-potassium-chloride co-transporter 1; *T_3,* triiodothyronine.

with low doses of glucocorticoids.[152-154] The mechanism of low-dose steroid benefit for CLD is not known, but it is possible that ion transport is favorably affected, resulting in more effective lung water clearance in these preterm infants.

CHLORIDE SECRETION

Furosemide, a drug that inhibits Cl^- secretion by blocking the basolateral NKCC, has been investigated for the treatment of CLD after preterm delivery. Two systematic Cochrane Database reviews examined the use of furosemide for CLD after preterm studies. Studies of aerosolized furosemide suggest a short-term benefit in lung mechanics after a single administration; however, no data are available on clinical outcome and repeated administration.[155] The effect of oral or intravenous administration is similar, although long-term administration by these routes was associated with a more consistent improvement in lung compliance and oxygenation.[156]

CONCLUSION

Ion transport has an important role in the switch from liquid-filled to air-filled lungs at birth. Although this physiologic process occurs over hours, the adaptive processes that prepare the fetal lung for birth are initiated as the end of gestation nears. There is clear evidence that active Cl^- secretion is linked to fetal lung liquid secretion and that this process is critical for normal lung growth in utero. Although there has been progress on elucidating mechanisms for Cl^- entry into the airway cells, the molecular identity of the channel or channels involved in transporting Cl^- into the lung lumen remains unknown. The functional and molecular basis of liquid absorption has been well characterized with detailed animal studies and molecular identification of the key components (ENaC and Na^+,K^+-ATPase) of this process (Fig. 59.12). Both Cl^- secretion and Na^+ absorption are triggered by an increase in cellular cAMP, and an alternative path for Cl^- secretion is activated by an increase in intracellular Ca^{2+}. At least some of the events that switch liquid secretion to liquid absorption are known. In late gestation, a rise in fetal glucocorticoids and active thyroid hormones plays a permissive role, but does not activate, the Na^+ absorptive mechanism. In the last few days of gestation, there is some decrease in lung liquid production and luminal liquid content. Labor has an important role in initiating lung liquid clearance in preparation for air breathing. During labor, some liquid is actively extruded, but the main mechanism for clearing liquid is the activation of Na^+ transport by the induction of ENaC and Na^+,K^+-ATPase. A rise in fetal epinephrine levels in response to the stress of contractions and birth can trigger the switch from liquid secretion to liquid absorption. After birth, a rise in ambient O_2 augments Na^+ absorption, which completes the transition to the postnatal state. There is circumstantial evidence that dysfunctional ion transport activity contributes to respiratory disease in very preterm infants, but determining the extent and magnitude across neonatal RDSs requires additional study.

ACKNOWLEDGMENT

The editors wish to thank David P. Carlton for his excellent work on this chapter in the fifth edition. It has been republished here essentially unchanged.

A complete reference list is available at www.ExpertConsult.com. 

SELECT REFERENCES

1. Preyer W. *Specielle Physiologiedes Embryo*. Leipzig: Greeben Verlag (L. Fernau); 1885:149.
2. Jost A, Policard A. Contribution expérimentale a l'etude du developpment prenatal du poumon chez le lapin. *Arch Anat Micr*. 1948;37:323–332.
3. Adamson TM, Boyd RDH, Platt HS, Strang LB. Composition of alveolar liquid in the foetal lamb. *J Physiol (Lond)*. 1969;204:159–168.
4. Adams FH. The tracheal fluid in the fetal lamb. *Biol Neonate*. 1963;5:151–158.
5. Olver RE, Strang LB. Ion fluxes across the pulmonary epithelium and the secretion of lung liquid in the foetal lamb. *J Physiol (Lond)*. 1974;241:327–357.
6. Kitterman JA, Ballard PL, Clements JS, et al. Tracheal fluid in fetal lambs: spontaneous decrease prior to birth. *J Appl Physiol*. 1979;47:985–989.
7. Mescher EJ, Platzker AC, Ballard PL, et al. Ontogeny of tracheal fluid, pulmonary surfactant, and plasma corticoids in the fetal lamb. *J Appl Physiol*. 1975;39:1017–1021.

8. Dickson KA, Maloney JE, Berger PJ, et al. Decline in lung liquid volume before labor in fetal lambs. *J Appl Physiol*. 1986;61:2266-2272.
9. Perks AM, Cassin S. The rate of production of lung liquid in fetal goats, and the effect of expansion of the lungs. *J Dev Physiol*. 1985;7:149-160.
10. Perks AM, Dore JJ, Dyer R, et al. Fluid production by *in vitro* lungs from fetal Guinea pigs. *Can J Physiol Pharmacol*. 1990;68:505-513.
11. Olver RE, Scheenberger EE, Walter DV. Epithelial solute permeability, ion transport and tight junction morphology in the developing lung of the fetal lamb. *J Physiol (Lond)*. 1981;315:395-412.
12. Brown MJ, Olver RE, Ramsden CA, et al. Effects of adrenaline and of spontaneous labour on the secretion and absorption of lung liquid in the fetal lamb. *J Physiol (Lond)*. 1983;344:137-152.
13. Vilos GA, Liggins GC. Intrathoracic pressures in fetal sheep. *J Dev Physiol*. 1982;4:247-256.
14. Adams F, Desilets DT, Towers B. Physiology of the fetal larynx and lung. *Ann Otol Rhinol Laryngol*. 1967;76:735-743.
15. Harding R, Bocking AD, Sigger JN. Influence of upper respiratory tract on liquid flow to and from fetal lungs. *J Appl Physiol*. 1986;61:68-74.
16. Klaus M, Tooley WH, Weaver KH, Clements JA. Lung volume in the newborn infant. *Pediatrics*. 1962;30:111-116.
17. Carmel JA, Friedman F, Adams FH. Tracheal ligation and lung development. *Am J Dis Child*. 1965;109:452-456.
18. Alcorn D, Adamson TM, Lambert TF. Morphological effects of chronic tracheal ligation and drainage in the fetal lamb lung. *J Anat*. 1977;123:649-660.
19. Moessinger AC, Collins MH, Blanc WA. Oligohydramnios-induced lung hypoplasia: the influence of timing and duration in gestation. *Pediatr Res*. 1986;20:951-954.
20. Maloney JE, Adamson TM, Brodecky AV, et al. Diaphragmatic activity and lung liquid flow in the unanesthetized fetal sheep. *J Appl Physiol*. 1975;39:423-428.
21. Harding R, Sigger JN, Poore ER, Johnson P. Ingestion in fetal sheep and its relation to sleep states and breathing movements. *Q J Exp Physiol*. 1984;69:477-486.
22. Dickson KA, Maloney JE, Berger PJ. State-related changes in lung liquid secretion and tracheal flow rate in fetal lambs. *J Appl Physiol*. 1987;62:34-38.
23. Goldstein JD, Reid LM. Pulmonary hypoplasia resulting from phrenic nerve agenesis and diaphragmatic amyoplasia. *J Pediatr*. 1980;97:282-287.
24. Wigglesworth JS, Desai R. Effect on lung growth of cervical cord section in the rabbit fetus. *Early Hum Dev*. 1979;3:51-65.
25. Hooper SB, Harding R. Fetal lung liquid: a major determinant of the growth and functional development of the fetal lung. *Clin Exp Pharmacol Physiol*. 1995;22:235-247.
26. Lewis M. Spontaneous rhythmical contraction of the muscles of the bronchial tubes and air sacs of the chick embryo. *Am J Physiol*. 1924;68:385-388.
27. Schittny JC, Miserocchi G, Sparrow MP. Spontaneous peristaltic airway contractions propel lung liquid through the bronchial tree of intact and fetal lung explants. *Am J Respir Cell Mol Biol*. 2000;23:11-18.
28. McCray Jr PB. Spontaneous contractility of human fetal airway smooth muscle. *Am J Respir Cell Mol Biol*. 1993;8:573-580.
29. Porter HJ. Pulmonary hypoplasia. *Arch Dis Child*. 1999;81:F81-F83.
30. Jesudason EC, Losty PD, Lloyd DA. Pulmonary hypoplasia: alternative pathogenesis and antenatal therapy in diaphragmatic hernia. *Arch Dis Child*. 2000;82:F172.
31. Kluth D, Tenbrinck R, von Ekesparre M, et al. The natural history of congenital diaphragmatic hernia and pulmonary hypoplasia in the embryo. *J Pediatr Surg*. 1993;28:452-462.
32. Bland RD. Edema formation in the lungs and its relationship to neonatal respiratory distress. *Acta Paediatr Scand Suppl*. 1983;305:92-99.
33. Pfister RE, Ramsden CA, Neil HL, et al. Volume and secretion rate of lung liquid in the final days of gestation and labour in the fetal sheep. *J Physiol*. 2001;535:889-899.
34. Adams FH, Yanagisawa M, Kuzela D, Martinek H. The disappearance of fetal lung fluid following birth. *J Pediatr*. 1971;78:837-843.
35. Bland RD, Bressack MA, McMillan DD. Labor decreases the lung water content of newborn rabbits. *Am J Obstet Gynecol*. 1979;135:364-367.
36. Olver RE, Ramsden CA, Strang LB, Walters DV. The role of amiloride-blockable sodium transport in adrenaline-induced lung liquid reabsorption in the fetal lamb. *J Physiol (Lond)*. 1986;376:321-340.
37. Bland RD, Hansen TA, Hazinski TA, et al. Studies of lung fluid balance in newborn lambs. *Ann N Y Acad Sci*. 1982;384:126-145.
38. Aherne W, Dawkins MJR. The removal of fluid from the pulmonary airways after birth in the rabbit, and the effect on this of prematurity and pre-natal hypoxia. *Biol Neonate*. 1964;7:214.
39. Egan EA, Olver RE, Strang LB. Changes in non-electrolyte permeability of alveoli and the absorption of lung liquid at the start of breathing in the lamb. *J Physiol (Lond)*. 1975;244:161-179.
40. Normand IC, Reynolds EOR, Strang LB. Passage of macromolecules between alveolar and interstitial spaces in foetal and newly ventilated lungs of the lamb. *J Physiol (Lond)*. 1970;210:151-164.
41. Canessa CM, Schild L, Buell G, et al. Amiloride-sensitive epithelial Na+ channel is made of three homologous subunits. *Nature*. 1994;367:463-467.
42. Kerem B, Rommens JM, Buchanan JA, et al. Identification of the cystic fibrosis gene: genetic analysis. *Science*. 1989;245:1073-1080.
43. Lengeling A, Gronemeier M, Ronsiek M, et al. Chloride channel 2 gene (Clc2) maps to chromosome 16 of the mouse, extending a region of conserved synteny with human chromosome 3q. *Genet Res*. 1995;66:175-178.
44. McGrath SA, Basu A, Zeitlin PL. Cystic fibrosis gene and protein expression during fetal lung development. *Am J Respir Cell Mol Biol*. 1993;8:201-208.
45. Murray CB, Morales MM, Flotte TR, et al. ClC-2: a developmentally dependent chloride channel expressed in the fetal lung and downregulated after birth. *Am J Respir Cell Mol Biol*. 1995;12:597-604.
46. Barker PM, Boucher RC, Yankaskas JR. Bioelectric properties of cultured monolayers from epithelium of distal human fetal lung. *Am J Physiol*. 1995;268:L270-L277.
47. Barker PM, Gatzy JT. Effects of adenosine, ATP, and UTP on chloride secretion by epithelia explanted from fetal rat lung. *Pediatr Res*. 1998;43:652-659.
48. Cassin S, Gause G, Perks AM. The effects of bumetanide and furosemide on lung liquid secretion in fetal sheep. *Proc Soc Exp Biol Med*. 1986;181:427-431.
49. Carlton DP, Cummings JJ, Chapman DL, et al. Ion transport regulation of lung liquid secretion in foetal lambs. *J Dev Physiol*. 1992;17:99-107.
50. Krochmal EM, Ballard ST, Yankaskas JR, et al. Volume and ion transport by fetal rat alveolar and tracheal epithelia in submersion culture. *Am J Physiol*. 1989;256:F397-F407.

Upper Airway Structure: Function, Regulation, and Development 60

Thomas H. Shaffer | Raymond B. Penn | Marla R. Wolfson

INTRODUCTION

Although the conducting airways are formed well in advance of fetal viability, they undergo significant maturational changes in late gestation. Conducting airways are susceptible to damage until they acquire the characteristics of more mature airways. Controversy exists concerning the pathogenesis of bronchopulmonary dysplasia (BPD) in the neonate[1-3]; in any case, prolonged mechanical ventilation and oxygen toxicity appear to be major contributing factors. Serial evaluations of pulmonary function in infants surviving hyaline membrane disease in whom BPD develops subsequently have demonstrated conclusively that the duration and pressure magnitude of mechanical ventilation, rather than increased inspired oxygen tension, damage the airways and lead to interference with their growth.[4,5] Within this context, the greater mechanical ventilation requirements of the very premature infant relative to the older infant precipitate an age-related predisposition to airway damage.

This chapter summarizes the function-structure characteristics and regulation of the developing upper airway and the impact of mechanical ventilation on airway function and reviews the clinical assessment of airway function.

STRUCTURE-FUNCTION CHARACTERISTICS

AIRWAY EMBRYOLOGY

Airway development in humans begins during the fourth week of gestation when the respiratory diverticulum, or lung bud, branches from the embryonic foregut.[6] The esophagotracheal septum forms and separates the foregut into the esophagus dorsally and the trachea ventrally; thus, the developing airway is of foregut endodermal origin. Elongation of the respiratory diverticulum forms the trachea, whereas the main bronchi are formed by branching. Growth and elongation continue in the caudal direction under the influence of airway secretions and physical forces.

Maturation of the airway occurs first in the trachea and proceeds distally. Tracheal cartilage formation begins during the seventh week of gestation, but full maturation of the distal airway cartilage is not completed until after birth. Epithelial differentiation begins in the trachea during week 10 of gestation. Together with the phasic contractions of the fetal airway smooth muscle, which are present after gestational week 23, lung fluid secreted from the epithelial cells promotes the growth and development of the respiratory system.[7]

AIRWAY STRUCTURE

The airway tree is a branched conducting system whose major functions include the delivery, distribution, and conditioning of gas to the gas exchange units of the lung. The lower airway has three primary components: epithelium, cartilage, and smooth muscle. The epithelium lines the entire length of the airway. From the trachea to the large bronchioles, it is composed of a pseudostratified ciliated columnar epithelium called the *respiratory epithelium.* The designation *pseudostratified* applies because the respiratory epithelium is one cell layer thick and all cells attach to the basement membrane but not all cells extend out to the airway lumen, giving the histologic appearance of multiple cell layers. Beyond the large bronchioles, the airway epithelium undergoes a gradual transition to a simple ciliated columnar epithelium and, finally, a cuboidal epithelium. The airway epithelium is composed of approximately eight different cell types. The primary cell type in the epithelium is the columnar epithelial cell, which contains a layer of cilia on its apical surface. Other cell types present include mucus-secreting cells, brush cells, small granule cells, and basal cells.

Cartilage is present from the trachea to the bronchioles. In the trachea, cartilage exists as C-shaped rings that are open posteriorly. In the bronchi, the cartilage forms plates that encompass the entire airway circumference. At more distal airway generations, the cartilage plates become smaller and more discontinuous, gradually disappearing before the bronchioles. As with the airway cartilage, the architectural disposition of airway smooth muscle also varies with different configurations along progressive airway generations. In the trachea, the airway smooth muscle is confined to the trachealis muscle. The trachealis, along with fibroelastic tissue, bridges the gap between the tips of the C-shaped cartilage rings and forms the posterior wall of the trachea. By contrast, bronchial airway smooth muscle forms a complete circumferential layer that gradually diminishes and becomes discontinuous at lower generations.

A mucosal layer covers the inner surface of the trachea. The mucosa consists of an epithelial layer supported by a basement membrane. This basement membrane is part of a loose connective tissue layer called the *lamina propria.* The lamina propria is very cellular and contains lymphocytes and lymphatic tissue, plasma and mast cells, eosinophils, and fibroblasts. Also included within the mucosal layer are glands that send ducts to the epithelial surface.

Below the mucosa lies the submucosa. The submucosa is a connective tissue layer containing the distributing blood vessels, lymphatics, and mucus-secreting glands. The submucosa ends when it blends into the perichondrium of the cartilage rings. The outer layer of the trachea consists of adventitia, which binds the trachea to adjacent structures such as the esophagus, neck musculature, and mediastinal structures. The adventitia contains the large blood vessels and nerves supplying the components of the tracheal wall.

The primary innervation of the trachea is cholinergic from the vagus nerve.[8] Vagal stimulation results in the contraction of airway smooth muscle. In addition, nonadrenergic, noncholinergic innervation controls both bronchoconstrictive and bronchodilatory actions through mediators such as nitric oxide, vasoactive intestinal peptide, neurokinins, and substance P. Little if any direct sympathetic innervation of the airway is present. Sympathetic control is provided primarily through circulating catecholamines.

More recent studies on structural maturation of airway smooth muscle at the cellular, ultrastructural, and protein expression levels have elucidated structural mechanisms for developmental changes in function.[9–11] Although the individual lengths of isolated tracheal smooth muscle cells increased from prematurity to adulthood, a linear increase in cell length was not demonstrated during the neonatal period, precluding cell length changes as a mechanism for functional development.[9] Similarly, developmental alterations in the electron-microscopic ultrastructure of the tracheal smooth muscle could not be identified as potential mechanisms. At the protein expression level, the expression of smooth muscle myosin SM1 and SM2 heavy chain isoforms increased across development. This increase correlates with the developmental increase in tracheal smooth muscle force development, providing a likely mechanism for the functional maturation of this airway smooth muscle.

In the developing rabbit trachea, clear patterns of expression or activation of matrix metalloproteinase (MMP)-2 and MMP-9, as well as their (tissue) inhibitors tissue inhibitor of metallinoproteinase (TIMP)-1 and TIMP-2, have been demonstrated during the progression of airway development.[12] In the lung, differences in MMP activity have been associated with BPD[13] and other chronic fibrotic lung diseases.[14] Thus, it is implied that the progression of lung disease involves the alteration in MMP activity. As noted by Miller and colleagues,[12] total MMP-2 quantity decreased steadily with increasing age in both the pregestational period and the postgestational period, whereas the active-to-latent ratio decreased only in the postgestational period. This change in the proteolytic potential of MMP-2 was compounded in the postgestational period by an age-dependent rise in TIMP-2 quantity. In that these arbitrary units of protein quantity are relative to a constant total protein load, the rise in TIMP-2 quantity affirms that the significant fall in MMP-2 levels is not likely to be the result of an increase in the quantity of inert, structural protein diluting the quantity of functional mediators of structural development. Of interest in this study is the lack of MMP-7 activity in the developing trachea, in contrast with the developing lung, where MMP-7 activity is present. These data support the assessment by other researchers that MMP-7 serves as a regulator for passage across the alveolar epithelium[15,16] and thus is not a mediator in the development of conducting airways. In this regard, MMP-7 may play a role in the differentiation between airway and lung development.

MECHANICS AND REGULATION OF THE DEVELOPING AIRWAY

It is well accepted that infant airways are more compliant than adult airways. Early studies in necropsied human tracheobronchial segments indicated that airway pressure-volume relationships could be correlated with maturity.[17,18] Accordingly, a reduction

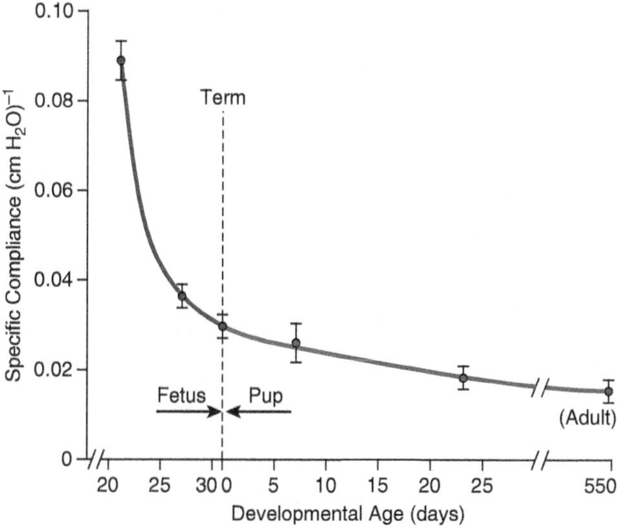

Fig. 60.1 Developmental change in specific tracheal compliance in the rabbit (term is 31 days). (From Bhutani VK, Rubenstein SD, Shaffer TH. Pressure-volume relationships of tracheae in fetal newborn and adult rabbits. *Respir Physiol.* 1981;43:221–231.)

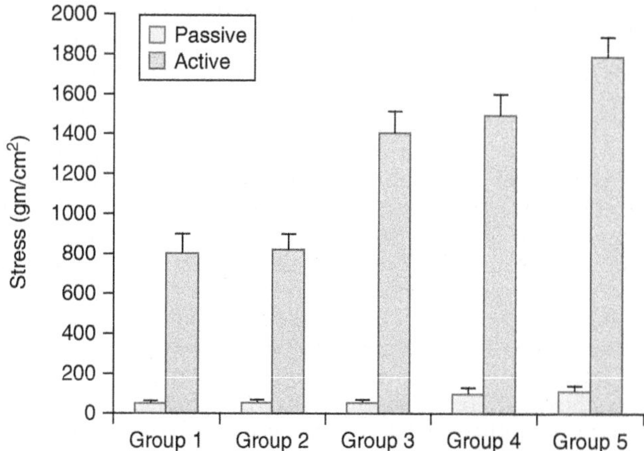

Fig. 60.2 Active and passive stress values from muscle bath studies in isolated trachealis muscle strips from preterm, newborn, and adult sheep (term is 147 ± 3 days of gestation). Data are normalized for the cross-sectional area and for the percentage of muscle fibers within the strip. *Group 1,* Preterm sheep at 110 days of gestation (n = 8); *group 2,* preterm sheep at 110 to 124 days of gestation (n = 25); *group 3,* preterm sheep at 125 to 140 days of gestation (n = 5); *group 4:* term newborn sheep (n = 10); *group 5,* adult sheep (n = 16). A significant increase in both active and passive stress as a function of age was noted (P < .001). Post hoc analysis revealed significant differences in active stress between group 1 and groups 3, 4, and 5, and between group 2 and groups 4 and 5. Similarly, passive stress increased between groups 1 to 3 and group 5. The values are the mean ± the standard error of the mean. (From Panitch HB, Deoras KS, Wolfson MR, et al. Maturational changes in airway smooth muscle structure-function relationships. *Pediatr Res.* 1992;31:151–156.)

in airway compliance with maturity results in decreased collapsibility and increased resistance to deformation during positive-pressure ventilation. Therefore, the immature airway is more likely to sustain deformational changes resulting from barotrauma than the less compliant airway of the older infant or adult.

Animal tracheae have been used extensively as models to study mechanisms that determine maturational changes in airway function. A study of in vitro rabbit tracheal segments,[19] as shown in Fig. 60.1, documented an age-related decrease in compliance in the developing rabbit airway that parallels that seen in neonates.[17] An in vivo study of the innervated and perfused trachea of the lamb demonstrated similar developmental changes in airway compliance and a decrease in the tracheal relaxation time constant.[20] It is noteworthy that in comparison with the results of in vitro studies, the absolute values of specific tracheal compliance in vivo were lower. Contribution of forces of surrounding connective tissue, or neurohumoral influences on airway smooth muscle tone, may affect the elastic properties of the developing airway and account for these observed differences. In addition, the decrease in the relaxation time constant with maturation is also suggestive of age-related differences in smooth muscle tone in vivo. Alterations of smooth muscle tone modulate mechanical properties and pressure-flow relationships of the trachea in preterm and newborn lambs.[21-23] In general, tracheae stimulated with acetylcholine become stiffer and are less compressible, as reflected by decreased resistance to airflow when they are subjected to compressive forces.[23-25] Specifically, however, the comparison of data suggests that the effect of pharmacologic stimulation on airway mechanics is age dependent and that the ability of airway smooth muscle to decrease airway compliance and increase flow may be limited in the preterm trachea.

The inability of fetal/premature airway smooth muscle to generate as much force as that produced by its adult counterpart probably contributes to this limitation. The effect of postnatal aging on airway smooth muscle maximal force production and sensitivity to various agonists remains controversial.[26] Some studies show that contractility and sensitivity increase with age,[8,27,28] whereas others suggest that contractility and sensitivity reach their peak early in postnatal life, declining thereafter.[29,30] When the extremes of the developmental spectrum are compared, however, a clear pattern emerges (Fig. 60.2). Several investigators have shown that the maximal contractility of airway smooth muscle increases between twofold and fourfold from preterm age or newborn to adult.[8,23,24,27] Furthermore, maximal active stress has been shown to increase significantly during late gestation in both the lamb[27] and the pig.[10] This change is not the result of an increase in smooth muscle mass because normalization for cross-sectional area eliminates that factor.

Developmental changes in force generation of airway and nonairway smooth muscle in various species have been related to an increase in the amount of contractile proteins (actin and myosin) per unit area and to age-related differences in the amount and type of myosin isoforms.[9,29,31,32] Age-related increases in contractile responses of vessels have also been related to alterations in the orientation of vascular smooth muscle cells, changing from circular to oblique relative to the long axis of the vessel wall.[33] Furthermore, age-related shifts in the synthetic activity of vascular smooth muscle cells have been identified in neonatal rats. Initially, synthetic activity is primarily secretory, producing extracellular proteins, collagen, and elastin; after the age of 4 weeks, synthetic activity is primarily contractile, producing the intracellular protein actomyosin.[34] Driska and colleagues[35] further identified age-related differences in morphometry and similar shortening responses in airway smooth muscle cells isolated from preterm and adult sheep. In size and appearance, adult cells were similar to adult arterial smooth muscle cells, but the velocity of shortening (0.54/s) was approximately three times faster. Isolated preterm airway smooth muscle cells were approximately half as long and thick as adult cells, but shortening velocities were similar.

Airway epithelium plays an important role in the modulation of smooth muscle function. Studies of adult airways have shown that airway epithelium generates relaxant and contractile factors that modulate the tone of the underlying smooth muscle.[36-40] The barrier function of airway epithelium, more commonly recognized for its protective role in inflammatory airway disease, undoubtedly also influences airway smooth muscle contractility throughout development. Epithelial damage has been associated with bronchial hyperreactivity.[41] In a study of deepithelialized preterm lamb trachea, force generation in response to acetylcholine stimulation was increased over that measured for the intact tracheal smooth muscle strip.[42] These data demonstrate that preterm airway epithelium can modulate the responsiveness of smooth muscle. Additionally, the magnitude of the effect was unchanged with maturation (from preterm to adult). Thus, even during late gestation, epithelial integrity may be an important determinant of smooth muscle function, bronchial hyper reactivity, and bronchodilator responsiveness. Whether regional differences in airway epithelium exert differential contractile or relaxant influences on airway smooth muscle in the developing airway is not completely understood.

The fact that the structural arrangement of muscle and cartilage in the adult trachea is different from that in the bronchi suggests that the functional effects of muscle contraction may also be different in these tissues in the adult, and presumably during development as well.[40] Studies of the adult trachea suggest that the elasticity of the passive trachealis muscle and connective tissue is greater than that of the bronchial wall.[43] Moreover, these studies demonstrated that tracheal smooth muscle can generate larger circumferential tensions than bronchial muscle, presumably because of the circumferential alignment and relatively greater proportion of the smooth muscle cells in the trachealis muscle, compared with the helical orientation and fewer smooth muscle cells in the bronchial wall. Regional differences in force generation have been noted in the airway of premature sheep as well.[42] Passive, active, and total stress development decreased significantly as a function of airway generation from the trachea (generation 0) to the subsegmental bronchi (generation 4). The receptor-mediated response to acetylcholine was significantly less in generations 0, 1, and 2 than in generations 3 and 4. In addition, the ratio of the internal radius to the wall thickness decreased from the trachea to the fourth-generation airway. The law of Laplace predicts that because of this decline in the ratio of the internal radius to the wall thickness, the trachea would be exposed to the greatest degree of wall stress during positive-pressure ventilation.[42] Taken together, these data help to explain the structural changes and physiologic changes in airway reactivity seen in the premature infant after mechanical ventilation.

Although the intact trachea serves as a suitable preparation for studying the mechanical function of the muscle and cartilage, it is important to consider the individual differences in airway smooth muscle function and the contribution of cartilage. Along these lines, several investigators have suggested that airway cartilage plays an important role in determining airway compressibility and inflatibility.[44-46] Moreno and colleagues[45] softened rabbit tracheae with papain and demonstrated alterations in unstressed tracheal volume and compliance. In a related study using papain-treated rabbits, McCormack and colleagues[47] observed changes in pulmonary function indicative of increased airway collapsibility. The maturational effects of cartilage contribution to airway function were demonstrated by Penn and colleagues,[46] who showed that tracheal cartilage in preterm lambs is extremely compliant relative to that in the adult sheep. In addition, it was suggested that these age-related changes in cartilage paralleled developmental differences in tracheal smooth muscle and tracheal mechanics.[22,27,48] Therefore, age-related differences in airway mechanical function may reflect an increase in stiffness that occurs in both airway muscle and cartilage.

EFFECTS OF MECHANICAL VENTILATION ON AIRWAY FUNCTION AND STRUCTURE

Although mechanical ventilation undoubtedly increases the survival of patients in respiratory compromise, it is also associated with increased morbidity.[49] The volumes, pressures, and oxygen concentrations that are incumbent in mechanical ventilation provide a mechanism of injury to a respiratory system that is not suited to such exposure.[50] This dilemma is most obvious in the premature and neonatal patient population.[51,52] Owing to the low compliance of the premature or surfactant-deficient lung, the inspired oxygen concentrations and ventilatory pressure requirements are often extreme.

Even though mechanical ventilation can be associated with systemic morbidity from specific nonpulmonary entities such as intraventricular hemorrhage, the primary pathologic changes consequent to mechanical ventilation involve the respiratory system. Mechanical ventilation is known to result in ventilator-induced lung injury and concomitant respiratory dysfunction. The signs of ventilator-induced lung injury include atelectasis, progressive respiratory failure, and pulmonary edema with hyaline membrane formation.

The current thinking regarding the minimization of lung injury includes limiting ventilatory pressures. Reduction of these pressures, however, comes with a paradox. Although elevated mean airway pressures are implicated in the pathogenesis of lung injury, maintaining adequate positive end-expiratory pressure may attenuate this damage. Including a level of positive end-expiratory pressure in the ventilation strategy sufficient to ensure that tidal ventilation occurs at pressures greater than the lower inflection point is thought to minimize lung damage. When end-expiratory pressures fall below the inflection point, some alveoli close. These closed alveoli must then reopen during subsequent inspiratory cycles. This alveolar opening-closing action is thought to be involved in the lung injury and inflammatory process.[53] Additionally, in the absence of positive end-expiratory pressure, the closing and reopening of the alveoli have been shown to disrupt the surfactant layer and thereby exacerbate already impaired lung function.

Under most circumstances, mechanical ventilation has little effect on adult airways but has been shown to alter the dimensions[53-56] and mechanical properties of preterm and newborn airways.[57,58] The extent of ventilation-induced deformation appears to be directly related to the compliance of the airway and inversely related to age. Our own observations in a preterm lamb model of the effects of mechanical ventilation included an increase in tracheal diameter, thinning of cartilage and muscle, disruption of the muscle-cartilage junction, and focal abrasions of the epithelium.[54] As shown in Fig. 60.3, in comparison with the unventilated trachea, decreased inflation and increased collapsing compliance of the trachea after ventilation produce a structure analogous to that of a fire hose, which is difficult to expand but easier to collapse.[58] In addition, ventilated tracheae showed greater resistance to airflow. The clinical implications of these studies include increased dead space, flow limitation, elevated airway resistance and work of breathing, and gas trapping.[59]

The mechanisms that mediate the alterations in mechanical properties of the ventilated trachea, and of the more distal airways, are unclear. One probable mechanism involves the altered architecture of extracellular matrix proteins, in which excessive strain promotes mechanical failure in elastin and collagen fibers, which in turn affects the mechanical properties of the more complex tissue. Collagen architecture has been shown to be altered in BPD infants with thick, disorganized fibers.[60,61] The findings are mixed with respect to whether the short-term effects of ventilation alter expression levels of extracellular matrix proteins; assessing the distal airways, Brew and colleagues[60] found that 24 hours after brief mechanical ventilation of lambs at

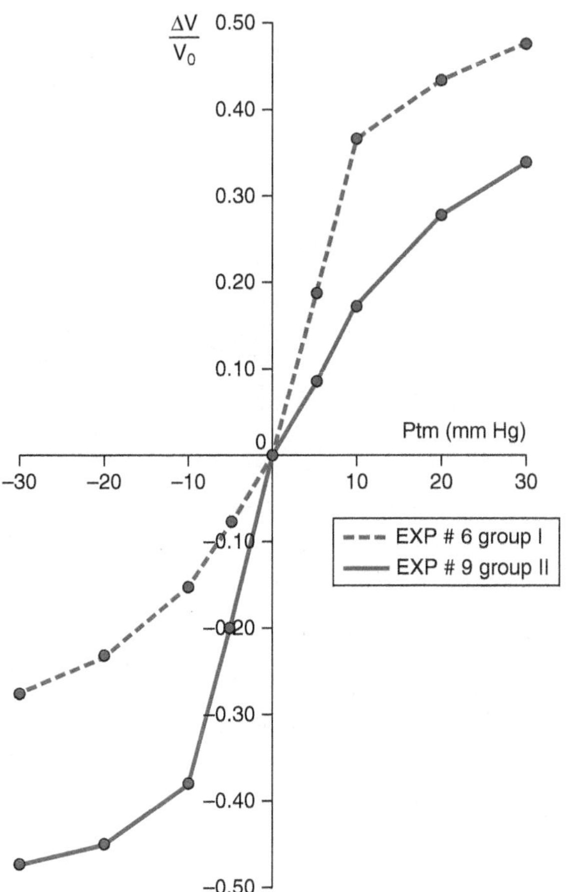

Fig. 60.3 Transmural airway pressure *(Ptm)* as a function of normalized volume change ($\Delta V/V_0$) in a typical unventilated *(group I)* and ventilated *(group II)* trachea segment. (From Penn RB, Wolfson MR, Shaffer TH. Effect of ventilation on mechanical properties and pressure-flow relationships of immature airways. *Pediatr Res.* 1988;23:519–524.)

75% of gestation, collagen and elastin fibers were deformed but the expression levels were unchanged. Increased muscle tone can decrease the compliance of the trachea in the term newborn lamb.[19] This finding suggests a mechanism whereby ventilation-induced alterations of the airway can be ameliorated. The ability of airway smooth muscle contraction to decrease pressure-induced deformation may help protect against the mechanical failure of elastin/collagen fibers and altered tissue mechanics. However, such a protective mechanism may be compromised by disruption of the muscle-cartilage junction, as noted for the trachea, or by pressure-induced alterations in the orientation of airway smooth muscle fibers in more distal airways that impair the ability of smooth muscle contraction to stiffen the airway and resist deformation. It also is possible that pressure-induced alterations in the alignment of cartilage components (i.e., proteoglycan-collagen configuration) may attenuate the contribution of cartilage as a structural support for the trachea and bronchi.

In addition to pressure-induced tracheomegaly, histologic studies of ventilated neonatal human and animal lungs describe the widening of the peripheral airways.[62,63] Recently, Hysinger et al. have shown that ultrashort echo-time magnetic resonance imaging (MRI), a noninvasive assessment approach, is effective at diagnosing tracheomegaly and have reported that tracheomegaly is associated with increased morbidity (longer and more complicated hospitalizations) in BPD.[64,65] Apart from the qualitative assessment of dimensions, the effects of ventilation on the peripheral airways are not known. Presumably, age-related and regional differences in the amount of cartilage and the orientation, force-generating capabilities, and contractility of airway smooth muscle may exacerbate the effect of ventilation on the relatively more compliant distal (as compared with proximal) airways. This effect would be further potentiated by a ventilatory scheme wherein an inspiratory hold is produced by long inspiratory times. Long inspiratory times favor equilibration of pressures throughout the tracheobronchial tree, thereby increasing the length of time over which the highly compliant distal airways are subjected to barotrauma. However, high-frequency jet ventilation evaluated in preterm rabbit airways was associated with significant dimensional and mechanical deformation of tracheal segments, as well as an increased propensity for collapsibility after cessation of the ventilation.[66] Therefore, ventilation techniques that attempt to minimize pulmonary barotrauma may potentially still have some deleterious effect on immature proximal airways.

Several in vitro, ex vivo, and in vivo studies strongly suggest that mechanical ventilation per se is sufficient to induce many of the pathologic features of BPD. However, infants with BPD experience both mechanical ventilation and hyperoxia; thus, pathogenic mechanisms mediated by mechanical ventilation are difficult to dissociate from those mediated by hyperoxia and oxidative stress and merit discussion here. Both mechanical ventilation and hyperoxia cause epithelia loss and inflammation and directly or indirectly affect airway cell biochemistry to promote airway injury and remodeling. Oxidative stress caused by hyperoxia has numerous effects on multiple cell types to promote tissue damage and remodeling evidenced in BPD. Such effects are mediated by altered cellular biochemistry consequent to the generation of intracellular reactive oxygen species or cell membrane damage caused by extracellular reactive oxygen species. Direct effects on inflammatory cells and induction of cytokine synthesis and radical and protease release from multiple cell types all exacerbate lung inflammation and promote necrotic and apoptic cell death, as well as damage/repair mechanisms that alter lung morphology, architecture, and mechanics (reviewed by Perrone and colleagues[67]). Similarly, mechanical ventilation can affect cell death and injury by strain effects: mechanical disruption of cell membranes, loss of compartmentalization due to epithelial barrier disruption (Fig. 60.4), alterations in cell and tissue morphology and architecture. Interestingly, in models of asthma, mechanical forces in the airway, imposed by bronchospasm alone in the absence of inflammation, acting on both airway epithelia and airway smooth muscle are sufficient to cause pathologic airway remodeling (Grainge et al.[68]). Potential mechanisms involve the induction of growth factors (Tschumperlin et al.[69], Ressler et al. [70]), as well as enhanced epithelial cell migration caused by "unjamming" likely associated with augmented epithelial-mesenchymal transition (Park et al.[71,72]). Such effects are likely experienced in the premature airway subject to mechanical ventilation, in addition to the more destructive effects imposed by high ventilatory pressures resulting in tissue mechanical failure/disruption.

Importantly, mechanical ventilation also impacts inflammation that is promoted by cell/tissue death, injury, and *mechanotransduction.*[73] In a recent translational cellular model, the impact of high-frequency oscillatory ventilation (HFOV) on human epithelial cell function was demonstrated by Mowes and associates.[74] Although HFOV has been proposed as a gentle ventilation strategy to prevent lung injury, this study demonstrated that hyperoxia and pressure (HFOV) independently resulted in significant cell dysfunction and inflammation, while in combination had a synergistic effect resulting in greater cell death. Although mechanotransduction-mediated inflammation is initiated (e.g., via ion channels, integrin receptors, and focal adhesion kinase complexes) in a manner distinct from that of hyperoxia-induced inflammation,

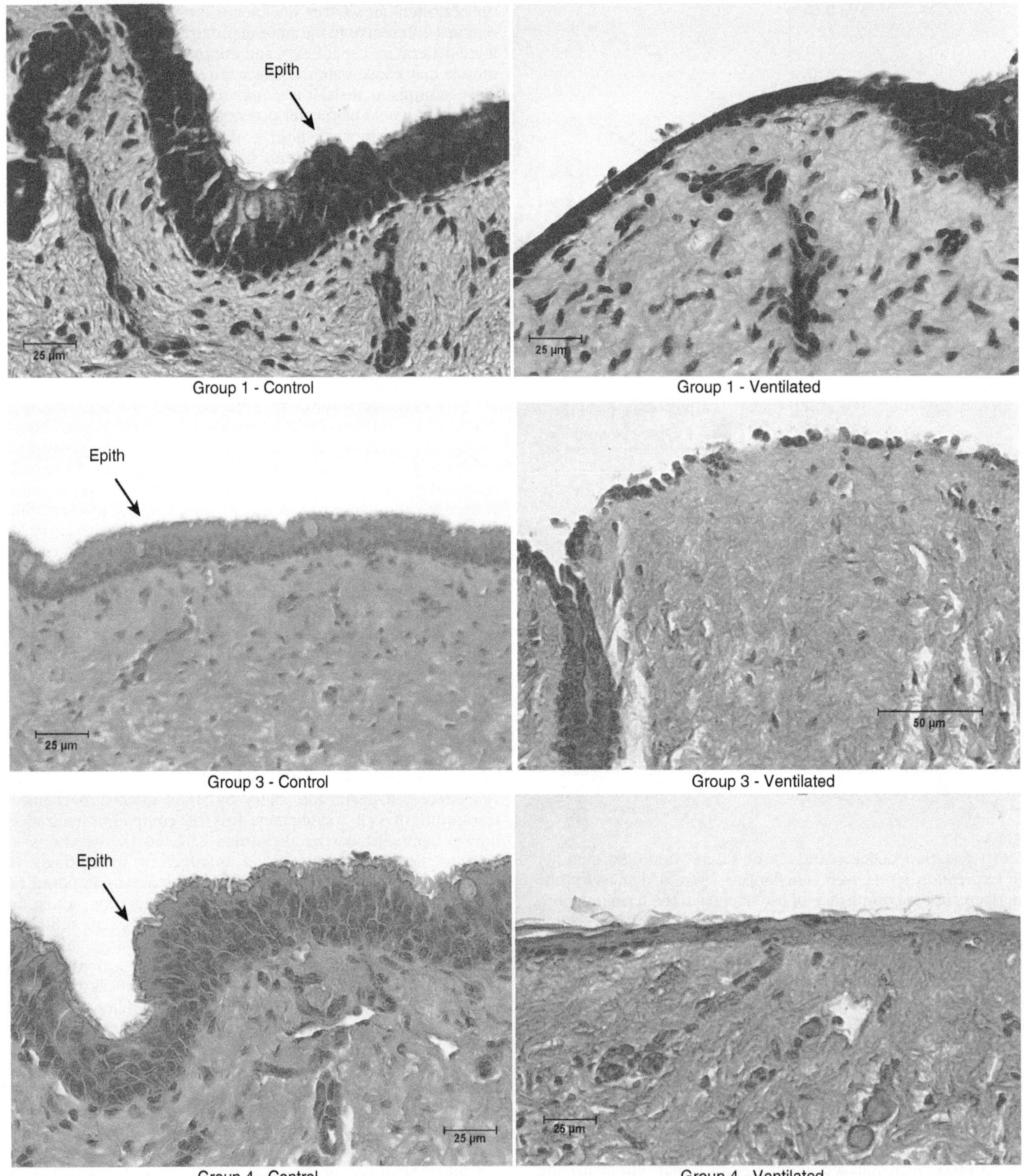

Fig. 60.4 Effect of mechanical ventilation on the epithelial lining (Epith) of neonatal lamb trachea in four different age-groups. *Group 1,* preterm lamb at 110 to 116 days; *group 3,* preterm lamb at 129 to 132 days; *group 4,* term lamb at 149 to 157 days. (Term is 147 ± 3 days of gestation.) *Left panels:* Nonventilated control lambs. *Right panels:* Lambs subjected to mechanical ventilation (mean airway pressure of 15 cm H_2O, duration 2.8 h). (From Cullen AB, Cooke PH, Driska SP, et al. The impact of mechanical ventilation on immature airway smooth muscle: functional, structural, histological and molecular correlates. *Biol Neonate.* 2006;90:17–27.)

many of the downstream signaling intermediates (mitogen-activated protein kinases and nuclear factor κB) are the same, as are the inflammatory cytokines (TNF-α, interleukins), proteases, and growth factors produced.[73-76] Thus, although numerous studies have shown that either reducing oxygen concentration or increasing antioxidant capabilities can ameliorate the BPD phenotype (reviewed by Perrone and colleagues[67]), the capacity of mechanical ventilation to promote damage through different mechanisms may limit the effectiveness of strategies that solely address oxidative stress. Consistent with this notion are the results obtained by Davis and colleagues,[77] who noted that premature infants treated with exogenous surfactant at birth for respiratory distress syndrome when treated for 1 month after birth with the antioxidant CuZn superoxide dismutase had improved pulmonary outcomes after 1 year but that the incidence of death or development of BPD was not reduced. The development of increasingly sophisticated imaging techniques should enable a better understanding of the relationship among developmental and ventilation-induced alterations in airway tissue morphology, biochemistry, and mechanical properties. It has been demonstrated that ultrasound imaging can provide insight into the basis of altered mechanical properties of the developing airway.[78] Ultrasound imaging of the isolated tracheal segment allows real-time assessment, with the following specific advantages: (1) airway dimensions can be assessed with the adhesions to surrounding tissue and blood supply and innervations intact; (2) static pressure-volume relationship data can be corrected with a more accurate resting volume calculation and without sacrifice of the preparation; and (3) stress-strain relationships can be recorded and analyzed during dynamic pressure pulses, which account for tissue kinetics and the trachea's elastic modulus. More importantly, an application of this method demonstrated that mechanical ventilation has a significant effect on both static and dynamic mechanical properties of the sheep neonatal trachea.[79] Furthermore, mechanical ventilation resulted in the breakdown and thinning of the trachealis muscle boundary, as well as increased segment volume and thus anatomic dead space. These data serve as a standard for comparison to evaluate various "protective" alternatives to conventional mechanical ventilation with respect to preservation of airway function. Moreover, future studies assessing morphologic and biochemical changes associated with altered airway dimensions and mechanical properties of the mechanically ventilated immature airway provide new insight into the pathogenesis of tracheomalacia and airway remodeling in BPD and further refine the analysis of ventilation strategies. Of note, Kim and colleagues[80] demonstrated that acute mechanical ventilation of neonatal lamb tracheae resulted in increased tracheal dimensions, an increase in bulk modulus and elastic modulus, and increased cartilage extracellular matrix content, including collagen and proteoglycan content.[80]

CLINICAL ASSESSMENT OF AIRWAY FUNCTION

Recently, Shepard et al. reported the importance of infant pulmonary function testing and phenotypes in severe BPD, as well as the need for the development of bedside tests to define phenotypes.[81] Modalities for evaluating airway function in the pediatric population include measurement of lung function during tidal breathing or forced exhalation, radiography, fluoroscopy, and airway endoscopy. In combination, these assessment modalities can be used to identify and quantitate the predicted functional abnormalities found in preterm airways exposed to positive-pressure ventilation, including elevated resistance, decreased forced expiratory flow, airway hyperreactivity, and excessive central airway collapsibility. In addition, these diagnostic procedures have provided important insight into the effects of early injury on future airway growth and function and can be used to test the effectiveness of newer therapies. Evaluation of airway function is especially useful and should be considered in infants whose clinical course is not one of gradual improvement or is marked by frequent severe pulmonary exacerbations and in infants who demonstrate stridor, chronic wheezing, or focal areas of chronic atelectasis or hyperinflation.

PULMONARY FUNCTION PROFILE

With the simultaneous measurement of respiratory pressures, volumes, and airflow, pulmonary mechanics can be monitored relatively noninvasively.[82] Pulmonary function profiles can be determined to assess initial disease cause, response to therapy, and disease sequelae during follow-up.[83] For example, the pressure-volume relationship for a premature infant can identify the degree of respiratory function and monitor the response after surfactant administration. In addition, the evaluation of tidal breath pressure-volume relationships serves as a tool to optimize the parameters of mechanical ventilation. Over time, sequential assessments of pulmonary mechanics can be used to monitor the progression of, or improvement in, both lung and airway abnormalities.

MEASUREMENTS OF AIRWAY FUNCTION DURING TIDAL BREATHING

Dynamic pulmonary compliance as measured by the esophageal balloon and pneumotachometry technique is significantly lower in infants in whom chronic lung disease develops subsequently than in normal infants or those who recover uneventfully from neonatal respiratory distress.[83-85] Although such measurements reflect the elastic properties of the lung to some degree, they also are influenced by the maldistribution of ventilation associated with regions having differing time constants (frequency dependence of compliance).[84] Thus, dynamic compliance measurements in infants with chronic lung disease probably also reflect some degree of airway obstruction. Quasi-static methods of measuring respiratory system compliance in infants with BPD have verified that alterations in the elastic properties of the lung contribute significantly to the observed decrease in compliance.[86] Studies comparing static and dynamic compliance measurements in this group of infants, however, have not been performed. Thus, it is not clear whether the improvement in dynamic compliance seen in infants with moderate to severe BPD studied longitudinally[83,85] represents a change in the characteristics of the lung parenchyma or if it is reflective of a coexistent decrease in respiratory rate or improvement in airway obstruction. Of interest, both static and dynamic measurements of compliance have been shown to have predictive value regarding the development of BPD in mechanically ventilated preterm infants.[87,88]

Resistance measurements, including airway resistance as determined by plethysmography, pulmonary resistance measured by the esophageal balloon and pneumotachometry technique, and respiratory system resistance determined by the airway occlusion technique, are significantly elevated in infants with BPD.[83,85,89-91] When measurements of resistance or its reciprocal, conductance, have been made serially, values have approached normal levels in the first 2 to 3 years of life.[83,85] Longitudinal changes in resistance can reflect either the resolution of airway obstruction or merely an increase in airway diameter related to growth. To eliminate the influence of growth or changes in lung volume on these measurements, investigators have also reported size-corrected values for resistance or conductance—namely, *specific conductance,* defined as the conductance divided by lung volume at functional residual capacity. Data reported in this way confirm the presence of airway obstruction in infants with BPD.[83,85] In the relevant study, although pulmonary resistance decreased to only one-fourth of the original measurement in the first 3 years of life, specific conductance rose only minimally and remained below the normal level at the end of the study period. Arad and colleagues[92] found that specific conductance rose from 57% ± 7% of that predicted in infancy to 90% ± 8% of that predicted by the age of 5 to 7 years, although the children who required mechanical ventilation in infancy demonstrated air trapping and small airway obstruction at the time of the study.

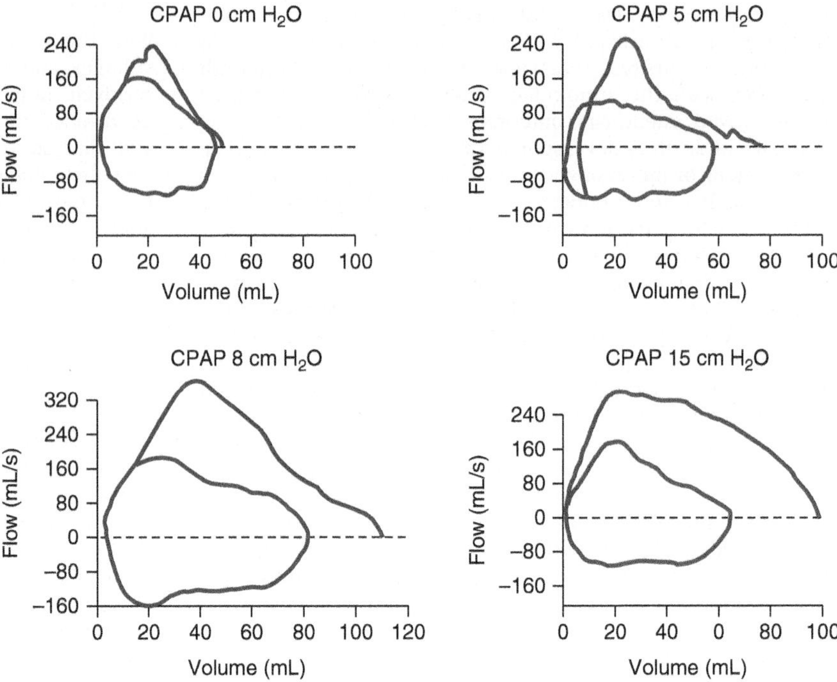

Fig. 60.5 Series of partial expiratory flow versus volume curves from an infant with bronchopulmonary dysplasia and bronchoscopically documented tracheobronchomalacia, showing the effect of increasing levels of continuous positive airway pressure *(CPAP)*. With no CPAP, the curve shape becomes straight, and at higher levels of CPAP, it becomes convex. At each level of CPAP, expiratory flow reserve increases as well. The values for maximal flow at functional residual capacity at each level of CPAP are 26 mL/s at 0 cm H_2O, 53 mL/s at 5 cm H_2O, 120 mL/s at 8 cm H_2O, and 204 mL/s at 15 cm H_2O. (From Panitch HB, Allen JL, Alpert BE, et al. Effects of CPAP on lung mechanics in infants with acquired tracheobronchomalacia. *Am J Respir Crit Care Med* 1994;150:1341–1346.)

FORCED EXPIRATORY FLOW MEASUREMENTS

Measurements of tidal mechanics include significant contributions of the nasopharynx, pharynx, and central airways. In a number of studies, either the rapid thoracic compression technique[89,93,94] or the rapid deflation technique[95,96] has been applied in infants with BPD to obtain information more reflective of small airway status and to compare data obtained in infancy more easily with spirometric measurements made in routine testing performed later in childhood. Such studies also demonstrate significant airway obstruction in infancy, with evidence of incomplete recovery with growth. When maximal expiratory flow versus volume curves were generated by the rapid deflation technique in a group of preterm infants during the acute phase of BPD, severe small airway obstruction as determined by a marked reduction in the maximal expiratory flow at 25% of functional residual capacity ($Vmax_{25}$) was noted, and the shape of the maximal expiratory flow versus volume curve was concave to the volume axis.[95] When patients with moderate BPD who were weaned from mechanical ventilation before 5 months of age were studied longitudinally with the same technique, there was a gradual increase in $Vmax_{25}$ to approximately 40% of that predicted by the age of 3 years.[96] By contrast, those patients who required extended periods of mechanical ventilation (>10 months) showed no increase in $Vmax_{25}$ over the same time period.

Similar evidence of airway obstruction has been demonstrated with the use of the rapid compression technique.[89,93] Partial expiratory flow versus volume curves were generated over the tidal range of breathing and quantitated by measurement of the maximal expiratory flow at functional residual capacity (VmaxFRC) in young infants with BPD. Furthermore, the separation between tidal flow and forced flow curves was interpreted as a measure of expiratory flow reserve.[93] The shape of the partial expiratory flow versus volume curve was typically concave to the volume axis, and the expiratory flow reserve was smaller than in infants with normal lungs. Size-corrected forced expiratory flows were only half those of normal controls and did not increase by the age of 14.5 to 22 months.[93] Furthermore, the slope of the regression equation for VmaxFRC versus age was lower in the BPD group than in normal infants. These data suggest that early exposure to positive-pressure ventilation and high concentrations of oxygen not only caused early airway damage but also interfered with subsequent normal airway growth.

Values of VmaxFRC have usually been considered to be representative of small airway function. More recently, however, studies have shown that central airway collapsibility (i.e., tracheomalacia or bronchomalacia) can cause a marked reduction in the values of VmaxFRC and appears graphically similar to small airway obstruction.[94,97] Panitch and colleagues[94] studied five infants with BPD who had bronchoscopic evidence of tracheobronchomalacia using the rapid compression technique. As shown in Fig. 60.5, when continuous positive airway pressure was applied to the airway opening, an incremental increase in VmaxFRC was observed. Additionally, in several subjects, the shape of the partial expiratory flow versus volume curve changed from concave to convex, suggesting that continuous positive airway pressure acted as an intraairway stent to prevent collapse. Furthermore, the ratio of forced-to-tidal flows at midexpiration, a reflection of expiratory flow reserve, increased with application of continuous positive airway pressure. Thus, reductions in VmaxFRC previously ascribed to small airway damage in infants with BPD may also represent a component of central airway injury.

ASSESSMENT OF AIRWAY REACTIVITY

Airway reactivity, as determined by bronchodilator responsiveness, has been well documented in infants with BPD through assessments of both tidal mechanics and forced expiratory flows. Acute decreases in pulmonary, respiratory system, and airway resistance ranging from 23% to 48% have been reported in response to several β-agonist and anticholinergic drugs.[90,91,98-102] The magnitude of this response was even more dramatic when forced flows were tested. Kao and colleagues[90] reported an increase of 86% over baseline values of VmaxFRC in 15 infants with BPD at a mean age of 15.8 weeks after treatment with metaproterenol and an increase of 45% over baseline values after treatment with atropine. Similarly, Motoyama and colleagues[95] found an increase of 214% over baseline values of $Vmax_{25}$ after isoetharine inhalation in 32 intubated and mechanically ventilated infants. Bronchodilator responsiveness could be demonstrated in infants as young as 26 weeks of postmenstrual age and as early as 12 days of postnatal age.

Other investigators have also demonstrated early evidence of bronchodilator responsiveness. Gomez-Del Rio and colleagues[100] found significant improvement in pulmonary resistance in 30 mechanically ventilated preterm infants younger than 20 days of age after isoetharine inhalation. The youngest was only 3 days of age, and gestational ages ranged from 27 to 34 weeks. Denjean and colleagues[98] measured significant decreases in respiratory system resistance after salbutamol inhalation in ventilator-dependent preterm infants at 13.3 ± 4.9 days of postnatal age.

That bronchodilator airway responses appear relatively high in BPD infants is intriguing and begs the question of "why?" In obstructive lung diseases such as asthma, increased airway smooth muscle tone occurs primarily as a result of inflammation, which serves to increase airway concentrations of procontractile agonists, increase parasympathetic cholinergic activation of airway smooth muscle, damage airway epithelium, and promote contractile (calcium) sensitization in airway smooth muscle.[103] Although a similar effect of inflammation could occur in the BPD lung, additional mechanisms consequent to ventilator-induced (or hypoxia-induced) injury are possible. Of note, mechanical ventilation alone is sufficient to denude the epithelial lining of preterm lamb tracheae (see Fig. 60.4). Regardless of the mechanism, the result of increased airway smooth muscle tone is an interesting adaptive (or possibly maladaptive) response. Although a detriment to inspiratory airflow, as noted above, it holds the benefit of reducing airway compliance to limit stress-induced strain/barotrauma and the inhibition of expiratory flow by compressive forces.

RADIOGRAPHIC EVALUATION OF AIRWAY INJURY

Acquired tracheomalacia has been evaluated fluoroscopically and by computed tomography. Sotomayor and colleagues[104] used fluoroscopy in anteroposterior, oblique, or lateral views to document central airway collapse in infants with BPD who required mechanical ventilation for 3 weeks to 4 months. These investigators also used fluoroscopy to determine the amount of distending pressure required to maintain airway patency in those infants. McCubbin and colleagues[105] studied central airway collapse in 10 infants (3.3 to 20.5 months of age) with BPD using cine computed tomography. A group of seven children of similar age with glottic or supraglottic obstruction but no evidence of lower airway disease was used as a control group. The median percent decrease in airway cross-sectional area during exhalation in the BPD group was 63.5% (range, 23% to 100%), whereas that of the control group was only 9% (range, 5% to 13%). This significant difference in collapsibility was present in a short segment of the airway in six children and was diffuse in the other four children. Because narrowing was not always diffuse, these authors speculated that the underlying cause of collapse must include local sites of injury as well as transmural pressure changes.

Bhutani and colleagues[56] described roentgenographic evidence of acquired tracheomegaly in very preterm neonates (i.e., with birth weight less than 1000 g) who had received mechanical ventilatory support. Increases in tracheal width at the level of the thoracic inlet and carina were present in the very preterm neonates when compared with individually weight-matched nonventilated control infants. These authors speculated that the persistent airway dimensional deformation seen in those infants resulted in increased anatomic dead space and contributed to carbon dioxide retention after extubation.

The ability to evaluate small airway abnormalities with conventional bronchographic agents has been limited by poor resolution of the bronchioles at the secondary lobule level.[97] Because of the high density, low surface tension, and radiopacity of the perfluorochemical liquid perflubron, it has been used as a bronchographic contrast agent for high-resolution computed tomography direct visualization of the airways through the centrilobar bronchioles and their first-order branches, with definition within a millimeter of the lung surface.[106,107]

Radiographic studies of the perflubron-filled lungs of animals and humans with congenital diaphragmatic hernia have proved informative in qualitatively delineating the degree of pulmonary hypoplasia and in identifying the distribution and elimination pattern of the perfluorocarbon liquid.[108,109] Regional differences in perfluorocarbon clearing, detected on x-ray studies, were related to localized bronchial obstruction.[108]

ENDOSCOPIC EVALUATION OF AIRWAY INJURY

Airway endoscopy allows both diagnosis and treatment of anatomic lesions of supraglottic, glottic, and subglottic regions, as well as of the trachea and bronchi down to the segmental level.[110-116] Two prospective studies of infants who required intubation in the newborn period found that the incidence of moderate to severe subglottic stenosis was 9.8% and 12.8%, respectively,[111,112] but the incidence of other fixed anatomic lesions is unknown. Endoscopy of the airway was selected when infants presented with acquired lobar emphysema, persistent lobar atelectasis, or unexplained medical failure.[114,115,117-121] Typically, with lobar emphysema, the right lower lobe and right middle lobes were more commonly affected.[114,115,117-119]

Direct visualization of the airways during spontaneous breathing is the most direct method of identifying central airway collapse. Although both rigid and flexible fiberoptic bronchoscopic techniques are available for the study of pediatric airways, rigid bronchoscopy must be performed while the patient is under general anesthesia. Often, the child receives assisted ventilation during the procedure. Consequently, the patient's effort of breathing is decreased, and exhalation may be completely passive. Thus, many cases of central airway collapse would be underdiagnosed with the use of this approach.

By contrast, flexible bronchoscopy is usually performed with conscious sedation. The patient breathes spontaneously but must breathe around the bronchoscope as well. Variation in the expiratory effort can influence the degree of intrathoracic airway collapse. Because of these technical considerations and the lack of universally agreed-on criteria, the frequency of diagnosis of central airway collapse varies from center to center. To circumvent these inconsistencies, some researchers have based the diagnosis on the extent of airway narrowing observed during exhalation.[94,116,122] Mair and Parsons[122] have recommended a grading system based on the percentage of airway narrowing present at the end of expiration during spontaneous respiration, together with an increase in the membrane-to-cartilage ratio. Other investigators have defined tracheobronchomalacia as collapse resulting in either less than 50%[94,123] or less than 75%[102] obstruction during spontaneous breathing, with no mention of changes in the proportion of membrane relative to cartilage. Acquired extrathoracic tracheomalacia has also been described in patients with BPD.[112]

To date, most quantitative studies of the inherent characteristics of the developing airway wall have required excision of an airway segment or surgical creation of an isolated segment. A laboratory study demonstrated that airway wall characteristics at various collapsing pressures and attendant changes in stiffness after smooth muscle stimulation could be quantitated bronchoscopically from airway pressure-area relationships.[124] Neonatal lamb tracheal segments were suspended over hollow mounts in a buffer-filled chamber and then subjected to a range (0 to −4.0 kPa) of pressures to determine wall stiffness under collapsing forces before and after stimulation of the trachealis with methacholine. Luminal images were recorded through a 3.6-mm flexible bronchoscope under the same conditions, and the cross-sectional area was calculated from the data thus obtained. Both pressure-volume and pressure-area relationships detected significant changes in airway wall stiffness after methacholine administration ($P < .002$), with similar magnitudes of change for both quantities. In a subsequent study, this same method was used to quantitate airway stiffness in vivo.[125] The speculation is that this technique may be clinically useful to quantitate airway collapsibility and can differentiate whether deformation is secondary to effort or to intrinsic abnormalities of the airway wall.

CONCLUSION AND FUTURE DIRECTIONS

Considerable progress has been made in characterizing developmental (preterm, newborn, and adult) differences in airway physiology with respect to pressure-volume and pressure-flow relationships, the effects of mechanical ventilation, and pharmacologic stimulation. In this regard, studies conducted using in vivo, in vitro, and muscle bath preparations have provided valuable insight into how the very premature infant may differ from the later-term and term neonate with respect to airway function. Nevertheless, little is known about how positive-pressure ventilation alters the cellular, biochemical, and molecular constituents of the components of the immature airway, and why mechanical ventilation is associated with the development of severe airway dysfunction in some premature infants but not in others. More sophisticated imaging analyses that enable visualization of airway morphology with greater sensitivity coupled with biochemical and molecular analyses assessing the effects of ventilator parameters and experimental/therapeutic interventions on morphology, architecture, and mechanics should improve current understanding of the pathogenesis of pressure- or stretch-related injury and facilitate continual advancement of neonatal and pediatric clinical respiratory management.

A complete reference list is available at www.ExpertConsult.com.

SELECT REFERENCES

1. Northway Jr WA, Rosan RC, Porter DY. Pulmonary disease following respiratory therapy of hyaline membrane disease. Bronchopulmonary dysplasia. *N Engl J Med*. 1967;276:357-368.
5. Stocks J, Godfrey S, Reynolds EO. Airway resistance in infants after various treatments for hyaline membrane disease: special emphasis on prolonged high levels of inspired oxygen. *Pediatrics*. 1978;61:178-183.
8. Haxhiu-Poskurica B, Ernsberger P, Haxhiu MA, et al. Development of cholinergic innervation and muscarinic receptor subtypes in piglet trachea. *Am J Physiol*. 1993;264:L606-L614.
9. Cullen AB, Cooke PH, Driska SP, et al. Correlation of airway smooth muscle function with structure during early development. *Pediatr Pulmonol*. 2007;42:421-432.
10. Booth RJ, Sparrow MP, Mitchell HW. Early maturation of force production in pig tracheal smooth muscle during fetal development. *Am J Respir Cell Mol Biol*. 1992;7:590-597.
12. Miller TL, Touch SM, Singhaus CJ, et al. Expression of matrix metalloproteinases 2, 7 and 9, and their tissue inhibitors 1 and 2 in developing rabbit tracheae. *Biol Neonate*. 2006;89:236-243.
13. Danan C, Jarreau PH, Franco ML, et al. Gelatinase activities in the airways of premature infants and development of bronchopulmonary dysplasia. *Am J Physiol*. 2002;283:L1086-L1093.
15. Dunsmore SE, Saarialho-Kere UK, Roby JD, et al. Matrilysin expression and function in airway epithelium. *J Clin Invest*. 1998;102:1321-1331.
17. Burnard ED, Grattan-Smith P, Picton-Warlow CG, Grauaug A. Pulmonary insufficiency in prematurity. *Aust Paediatr J*. 1965;1:12-38.
19. Bhutani VK, Rubenstein SD, Shaffer TH. Pressure-volume relationships of tracheae in fetal newborn and adult rabbits. *Respir Physiol*. 1981;43:221-231.
23. Penn RB, Wolfson MR, Shaffer TH. Effect of tracheal smooth muscle tone on collapsibility of immature airways. *J Appl Physiol*. 1988;65:863-869.
27. Panitch HB, Deoras KS, Wolfson MR, Shaffer TH. Maturational changes in airway smooth muscle structure-function relationships. *Pediatr Res*. 1992;31:151-156.
30. Murphy TM, Mitchell RW, Blake JS, et al. Expression of airway contractile properties and acetylcholinesterase activity in swine. *J Appl Physiol*. 1989;67:174-180.
35. Driska SP, Laudadio RE, Wolfson MR, Shaffer TH. A method for isolating adult and neonatal airway smooth muscle cells and measuring shortening velocity. *J Appl Physiol*. 1999;86:427-435.
42. Gauthier SP, Wolfson MR, Deoras KS, Shaffer TH. Structure-function of airway generations 0 to 4 in the preterm lamb. *Pediatr Res*. 1992;31:157-162.
44. Gunst SJ, Lai-Fook SJ. Effect of inflation on trachealis muscle tone in canine tracheal segments in vitro. *J Appl Physiol*. 1983;54:906-913.
46. Penn RB, Wolfson MR, Shaffer TH. Developmental differences in tracheal cartilage mechanics. *Pediatr Res*. 1989;26:429-433.
48. Panitch HB, Allen JL, Ryan JP, et al. A comparison of preterm and adult airway smooth muscle mechanics. *J Appl Physiol*. 1989;66:1760-1765.
49. The Acute Respiratory Distress Syndrome Network. Ventilation with lower tidal volumes as compared with traditional tidal volumes for acute lung injury and the acute respiratory distress syndrome. *N Engl J Med*. 2000;342:1301-1308.
51. Coalson JJ, Winter VT, Gerstmann DR, et al. Pathophysiologic, morphometric, and biochemical studies of the premature baboon with bronchopulmonary dysplasia. *Am Rev Respir Dis*. 1992;145:872-881.
55. Bhutani VK, Rubenstein D, Shaffer TH. Pressure-induced deformation in immature airways. *Pediatr Res*. 1981;15:829-832.
59. Cullen AB, Cooke PH, Driska SP, et al. The impact of mechanical ventilation on immature airway smooth muscle: functional, structural, histological and molecular correlates. *Biol Neonate*. 2006;90:17-27.
60. Brew BN, Hooper SB, Zahra V, et al. Mechanical ventilation injury and repair in extremely and very preterm lungs. *PLoS ONE*. 2013;8(5):e63905. 2013.
61. Thibeault DW, Mabry SM, Ekekezie II, et al. Collagen scaffolding during development and its deformation with chronic lung disease. *Pediatrics*. 2003;111:766-776.
64. Hysinger EB, Bates AJ, Higano NS, et al. Ultrashort echo-time MRI for the assessment of tracheomalacia in neonates. *Chest*. 2019;3692(19):34403-34404.
65. Hysinger EB, Friedman NL, Padula MA, et al. Children's Neonatal Consortium: tracheobronchomalacia is associated with increased morbidity in bronchopulmonary dysplasia. *Ann Am Thorac Soc*. 2017;14:1428.
67. Perrone S, Tataqranno ML, Buoncore G. Oxidative stress and bronchopulmonary dysplasia. *J Clin Neonatol*. 2012:1109-1114.
68. Grainge CL, LauL CK, Ward JA, et al. Effect of bronchoconstriction on airway remodeling in asthma. *N Engl J Med*. 2011;364:2006-2015.
69. Tschumperlin DJ, Dai G, Maly IV, et al. Mechanotransduction through growth-factor shedding into the extracellular space. *Nature*. 2004;429:83-86.
70. Ressler B, Lee RT, Randell SH, Drazen JM, Kamm RD. Molecular responses of rat tracheal epithelial cells to transmembrane pressure. *Am J Physiol Lung Cell Mol Physiol*. 2000;278:L1264-L1272.
71. Park JA, Kim JH, Bi D, et al. Unjamming and cell shape in the asthmatic airway epithelium. *Nat Mater*. 2015b;14:1040-1048.
73. Uhlig S. Ventilation-induced lung injury and mechanotransduction: stretching it too far? *Am J Physiol Lung Cell Mol Physiol*. 2002;282:L892-L896.
74. Mowes AK, de Jongh BE, Cox T, Zhu Y, Shaffer TH. A translational cellular model to study the impact of high frequency oscillatory ventilation (HFOV) on human epithelial cell function. *J Appl Physiol (1985)*. 2017;122(1):198-205.
77. Davis JM, Parad RN, Michele T, et al. Pulmonary outcome at 1 year corrected age in premature infants treated at birth with recombinant human CuZn superoxide dismutase. *Pediatrics*. 2003;111:469-476.
79. Miller TL, Zhu Y, Altman AR, et al. Sequential alterations in tracheal mechanical properties in the neonatal lamb: effects of mechanical ventilation. *Pediatr Pulmonol*. 2007;42:141-149.
80. Kim M, Pugarelli J, Miller TL, et al. Brief mechanical ventilation impacts airway cartilage properties in neonatal lambs. *Pediatr Pulmonol*. 2012;47:7630770.
81. Shepherd EG, Clouse BG, Hasenstab KA, et al. Infant pulmonary function testing and phenotypes in severe bronchopulmonary dysplasia. *Pediatrics*. 2018;141:e20173350.
83. Gerhardt T, Hehre D, Feller R, et al. Serial determination of pulmonary function in infants with chronic lung disease. *J Pediatr*. 1987;110:448-456.
88. Bhutani VK, Abbasi S. Relative likelihood of bronchopulmonary dysplasia based on pulmonary mechanics measured in preterm neonates during the first week of life. *J Pediatr*. 1993;120:605-613.
90. Kao LC, Durand DJ, Nickerson BG. Effects of inhaled metaproterenol and atropine on the pulmonary mechanics of infants with bronchopulmonary dysplasia. *Pediatr Pulmonol*. 1989;6:74-80.
93. Tepper RS, Morgan WJ, Cota K, Taussig LM. Expiratory flow limitation in infants with bronchopulmonary dysplasia. *J Pediatr*. 1986;109:1040-1046.
94. Panitch HB, Allen JL, Alpert BE, Schidlow DV. Effects of CPAP on lung mechanics in infants with acquired tracheobronchomalacia. *Am J Respir Crit Care Med*. 1994;150:1341-1346.
96. Mallory Jr GB, Chaney H, Mutich RL, Motoyama EK. Longitudinal changes in lung function during the first three years of premature infants with moderate to severe bronchopulmonary dysplasia. *Pediatr Pulmonol*. 1991;11:8-14.
97. Panitch HB, Keklikian EN, Motley RA, et al. Effect of altering smooth muscle tone on maximal expiratory flows in patients with tracheomalacia. *Pediatr Pulmonol*. 1990;9:170-176.
103. Deshpande DA, Penn RB. Targeting G protein-coupled receptor signaling in asthma. *Cell Signal*. 2006;2:2105-2120.

106. Stern RG, Wolfson MR, McGuckin JF, et al. High-resolution computed tomographic bronchiolography using perfluoroctylbromide (PFOB): an experimental model. *J Thorac Imaging*. 1993;8:300–304.
112. Downing GJ, Kilbride HW. Evaluation of airway complications in high-risk preterm infants: application of flexible fiberoptic airway endoscopy. *Pediatrics*. 1995;95:567–572.
122. Mair EA, Parsons DS. Pediatric tracheobronchomalacia and major airway collapse. *Ann Otol Rhinol Laryngol*. 1992;101:300–309.
124. Panitch HB, Talmaciu I, Heckman J, et al. Quantitative bronchoscopic assessment of airway collapsibility. *Pediatr Res*. 1998;43:832–839.
125. Panitch HB, Talmaciu I, Wolfson MR, Shaffer TH. In vivo quantitation of airway stiffness. *Am J Resp Crit Care Med*. 1998;157:A470.

Regulation of Lower Airway Function 61

Abhrajit Ganguly | Richard J. Martin | Peter M. MacFarlane | Y.S. Prakash | Thomas M. Raffay

INTRODUCTION

Significant progress has been made in elucidating the fetal and neonatal development of lower airway structures and regulation of their function. During early development, airway smooth muscle differentiates from the mesenchyme of the primordial lung and envelops the emerging bronchial tree. Airway smooth muscle at this early stage provides phasic rhythmic contractility that is thought to propel lung fluid distally and enhance lung development. Neural structures emerge in parallel to airway muscle, and their functional roles are rapidly integrated such that during postnatal life, tonic, rather than phasic, contractile, and relaxant functions dominate.

Although it is well accepted that the potential effect of the lower airway on prenatal and postnatal lung function is considerable, our understanding of the link between neurotransmitter-specific networks involved in the regulation of airway function is incomplete. Furthermore, compared with healthy and diseased adult airways, little attention has been paid to the diverse neural mechanisms that regulate airway caliber in the perinatal period. This subject has gained considerable interest because of the injurious effects of increased inspired oxygen and positive pressure ventilation on neonatal airway function. It is therefore important to gain a greater understanding of the normal maturational changes exhibited by airway smooth muscle contractile and relaxant mechanisms superimposed on the immature structural elements that compose the airways.

NEURAL REGULATION OF THE LOWER AIRWAYS

CHOLINERGIC EFFERENT CONTROL OF LOWER AIRWAYS

Most studies on neural control of the airways during development have focused on the regulation of smooth muscle, even though many of the same principles apply to control of mucus production and blood flow in the airways. In general, at any given age, neural control of airway functions (Fig. 61.1) involves integrated networks along the neural axis that funnel information to tracheobronchopulmonary effector units via airway-related vagal preganglionic neurons (AVPNs) in the medulla oblongata. The AVPNs are the final common pathway from the brain to the airways and transmit excitatory signals to the intrinsic tracheobronchial ganglia that are part of the network for feedback control.

The AVPNs, innervating airways from the extrathoracic trachea to the most distal bronchiole, arise mainly within the brain stem from the rostral nucleus ambiguus and to a lesser degree from the rostral portion of the dorsal motor nucleus of the vagus nerve. These cholinergic cells (see Fig. 61.1), which express vasoactive intestinal peptide and brain-derived neurotrophic factor (BDNF),[1] transmit cholinergic signals to intrinsic tracheobronchial ganglia. The individual innervation of postganglionic neurons from the vagus nerve gives rise to postganglionic fibers that regulate the functions of specific effector targets. In the postnatal period, neuronal innervation is already well developed, and choline acetyltransferase, a specific marker for cholinergic traits that synthesizes acetylcholine, appears in vagal preganglionic neurons, postganglionic neurons, and postganglionic fibers.

Signals transmitted through preganglionic nerves are relayed, filtered, integrated, and modulated by intrinsic ganglionic neurons before reaching their airway neuroeffector sites through postganglionic axons. This structural organization could explain the strong effects of a relatively small number of vagal efferent fibers on coordinated reflex changes in airway smooth muscle tone, submucosal gland secretion, and blood flow along the tracheobronchial tree. Postnatally, cholinergic innervation is the principal tonic input to airway smooth muscle bundles and may serve to protect the compliant immature airways from collapsing during expiration-induced compressive narrowing (Fig. 61.2).

Muscarinic receptors mediate the responsiveness of airway smooth muscle to acetylcholine during early development and adult life. Studies in the developing airways and porcine lung from birth to adulthood reveal maturational changes in muscarinic receptor subtypes (M_1, M_2, M_3) that may explain pharmacologic changes during development.[2] These muscarinic receptor subtypes, coupled to the family of G proteins, mediate airway contractile responses and their modulation. M_1 receptors are largely present on neuronal tissue and ganglia, and the selective M_1 receptor antagonist pirenzepine reduces the contractile response to vagal stimulation in newborn animals.[3,4]

M_2 receptors are located on prejunctional postganglionic cholinergic fibers in airway smooth muscle in some species and exhibit an autoinhibitory action whereby the quantal release of acetylcholine in response to nerve stimulation is reduced by feedback inhibition. Sinus node M_2 receptors also mediate the bradycardia seen with vagal stimulation. Selective blockade or down-regulation of M_2 receptors may enhance vagally-mediated bronchoconstrictor responses and cause a reduction in the bradycardia response. M_2 autoinhibitory actions may be reduced or absent in the newborn because blockade of M_2 receptors does not enhance bronchoconstrictor responses to vagal stimulation.[4] The potential role of lung injury and infection in modulating physiologic responses coupled to M_2 receptors in the newborn remains to be explored.

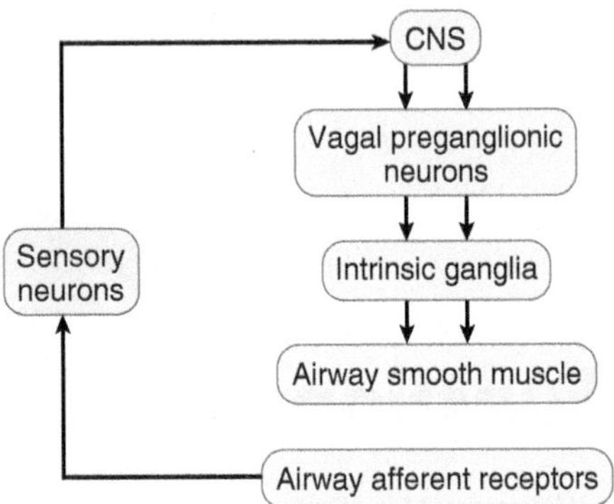

Fig. 61.1 The organization of autonomic parasympathetic control of airway functions. Central nervous system *(CNS)* cell groups regulate the activity of airway-related vagal preganglionic neurons (AVPNs) that present the final common pathway to the airways. Projections from the AVPNs synapse on intrinsic ganglionic neurons within the airway walls. These ganglia give rise to postganglionic fibers that control the function of specific effector targets (i.e., airway smooth muscle, mucus glands, and blood vessels). Sensory feedback for these systems occurs via sensory fibers originating from sensory ganglia (nodose and jugular ganglionic neurons). These fibers innervate sensory receptors and transmit information from the airways to the CNS. They modulate the activity of the AVPNs through the central multisynaptic pathways and may affect the function of effector organs via two ill-defined local networks that include axon reflex responses and sensory innervation of intrinsic airway ganglia.

M_3 receptors are present on smooth muscle and mucous glands and airway epithelial cells where they initiate the events leading to smooth muscle contraction, airway narrowing, and mucus secretion. In the newborn, the density of M_3 receptors has been reported to be similar to that in the adult; however, they do not appear to be tightly coupled to G-protein signal transduction mechanisms that lead to smooth muscle contraction.[3] In vivo studies show that M_3 receptor antagonism decreases bronchoconstrictor responses to vagal stimulation in the newborn that at low doses does not affect the bradycardic response.[4] Among the many unanswered questions in the newborn are the extent of receptor subtype differentiation in human neonates, investigation of G-protein signal transduction, the role of M_2 autoinhibitory receptors in modulating airway tone, and the possible effect of inflammatory lung disease on muscarinic receptor regulation and its pharmacologic manipulation.

VAGAL AFFERENT SENSORY FIBERS DERIVED FROM LOWER AIRWAYS

The bronchopulmonary sensory receptors are specialized units for detecting changes in chemical, mechanical, or thermal stimuli. They originate from the bipolar airway vagal afferent neurons that are located in the nodose and jugular ganglia and participate in reflex events. Sensory fibers affect the function of lower airway effector units via a local network that includes axon reflex responses. Endogenous substance P released from sensory nerve endings (i.e., C fibers that are mainly nonmyelinated nerve terminals) facilitates synaptic transmission in airway postganglionic neurons, suggesting the presence of control mechanisms within the tracheobronchial system, which also reflexly influence activity of AVPNs.

Sensory neural fibers from the airways also enter the brain stem through the solitary tract and make synapses with the

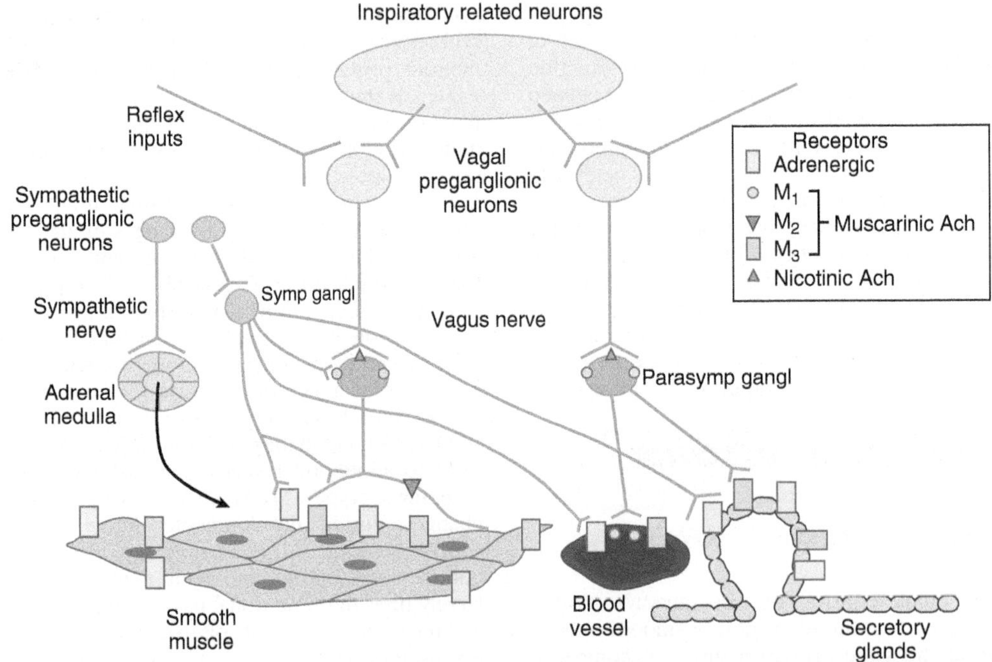

Fig. 61.2 The major parasympathetic, or cholinergic (contractile), and sympathetic, or adrenal adrenergic (relaxant), pathways that innervate (or regulate) airway smooth muscle. The efferent output from vagal preganglionic neurons to airways is influenced by various afferent reflex inputs and inspiratory-related neurons in the brain stem. Excitation of parasympathetic efferents also increases the output of submucosal secretory glands and results in the relaxation of adjacent vascular structures. See the text for the functional roles of the various muscarinic receptor subtypes. The role of nicotinic cholinergic receptors on parasympathetic ganglia regulating the lower airways is unclear. *Ach*, Acetylcholine; *parasymp gangl*, parasympathetic ganglion; *symp gangl*, parasympathetic ganglion.

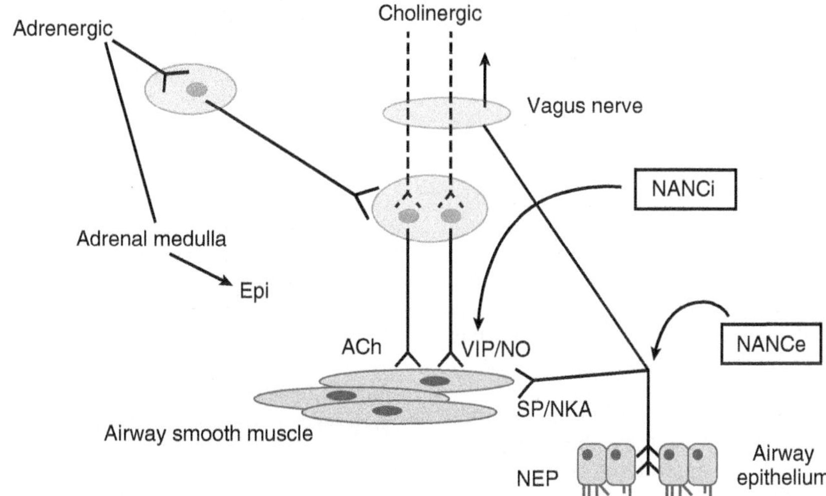

Fig. 61.3 The nonadrenergic noncholinergic *(NANC)* innervation of airway smooth muscle and related epithelium that complements traditional cholinergic and adrenergic pathways. The inhibitory component of this system *(NANCi)* appears to be mediated primarily by the release of nitric oxide *(NO)* and vasoactive intestinal peptide *(VIP)*. NANC excitatory mechanisms *(NANCe)* are initiated by the release of neuropeptides such as substance P *(SP)* and neurokinin A *(NKA)* from the C-fiber afferent nerve endings, and this is modulated by the neuropeptide degrading enzyme neutral endopeptidase *(NEP)* in epithelial cells. Epithelium-derived prostaglandin-mediated pathways *(Epi)* may be both inhibitory or excitatory of airway smooth muscle. *Ach,* Acetylcholine.

second-order nucleus tractus solitarius neurons that project to the AVPNs. Excitatory signals arise from bronchopulmonary rapidly adapting lightly myelinated receptor afferents or nonmyelinated C-fiber terminals via release of glutamate, which activates α-amino-3-hydroxy-5-methyl-4-isoxazolepropionic acid (AMPA) receptors expressed by these nucleus tractus solitarius neurons.[5] The processed information is then transmitted to AVPNs via the glutamate-AMPA signaling pathway and from the AVPNs to the bronchopulmonary effector system through acetylcholine release. Maturational data in ferrets indicate a decrease in the number of efferent AVPNs during the second postnatal week. It is possible that early postnatal injury may modify this normal remodeling.[6]

SYMPATHETIC CONTROL OF LOWER AIRWAYS

Extrinsic sympathetic innervation of airway smooth muscle is highly species-specific, and in airway smooth muscle in humans, direct sympathetic innervation appears to be lacking (Fig. 61.3). Nevertheless, circulating catecholamines activate airway adrenoreceptors to exert specific actions that affect smooth muscle contractile function. β-Adrenergic responses in airway smooth muscle are composed of two inhibitory actions. First, relaxation of airway smooth muscle mediated by airway β_2-receptors that are coupled to the stimulatory G protein and adenylate cyclase; and second, inhibition of acetylcholine release from postganglionic vagal axons through prejunctional α_2-adrenergic and β_1 receptors in some species. Activation of β-adrenergic receptors is the pharmacologic basis for neonatal bronchodilator therapy. The airway relaxant response to β-adrenoreceptor stimulation actually appears to decrease with advancing maturation, and several mechanisms, including greater muscarinic antagonism of β-receptor responses and attenuated expression of M_2 muscarinic receptors, have been proposed.[7]

The second category of adrenergic responses is attributed to α-adrenoceptors of which both α_1 and α_2 subtypes play a role. Data indicate that in adult humans, α-adrenergic contractile responses of airway smooth muscle are weak or absent, although this may not hold true for the newborn. A potential role for α-adrenergic receptors in the control of airway smooth muscle in newborn infants with bronchopulmonary dysplasia (BPD) is supported by observations in preterm infants with chronic lung disease in whom ophthalmic application of the α_1-adrenergic agonist phenylephrine resulted in an increase in total pulmonary resistance and a decrease in compliance.[8] The deterioration in lung mechanics was attributed to α_1-receptor-mediated contraction of airway smooth muscle.

NONADRENERGIC, NONCHOLINERGIC CONTROL OF THE LOWER AIRWAYS

Rather than representing a separate pathway for modulation of airway caliber, the nonadrenergic noncholinergic (NANC) system comprises both inhibitory and excitatory mechanisms modulated by several neurotransmitters located in intrinsic ganglia and their fibers (see Fig. 61.3). Vasoactive intestinal peptide was initially proposed as the primary neurotransmitter of the NANC system. Mice lacking the vasoactive intestinal peptide gene show airway hyperresponsiveness and airway inflammation, which is partially reversible by the administration of vasoactive intestinal peptide. Subsequently, nitric oxide (NO) was also shown to act as a NANC neurotransmitter, suggesting the involvement of multiple substances and molecules in airway smooth muscle relaxation, with considerable interspecies variation.[9]

Limited information is available about the ontogeny of this system in the airways. Activation of vagal preganglionic axons results in a NANC-mediated bronchodilation in newborn feline airways, a response that is eliminated by ganglionic blockade with hexamethonium, confirming the efferent nature of the response.[10] NANC inhibitory innervation also appears to be functional in young guinea pigs and rat pups. In some species, NANC inhibitory responses undergo significant developmental changes; for example, NANC relaxation responses are not present in rabbits until 2 weeks of age.[11] Allergen sensitization significantly reduced the NANC response at 2, 4, and 12 weeks of age,[11] suggesting that host or environmental factors may alter the maturation of the inhibitory NANC system and predispose to airway reactivity. The NANC inhibitory system has not been explored in human neonatal airways; data on other airway neurotransmitters suggest that it might be expected to be present.

NO has received considerable attention for its ability to reverse persistent pulmonary hypertension of the newborn, and this has largely overshadowed investigation of its role in the control of airway smooth muscle. Nevertheless, some evidence indicates that expression of neuronal NO synthase is developmentally regulated, declining during late gestation, but subsequently increasing postnatally in the rat. In developing sheep lungs, all three isoforms of NO synthase are expressed in airway epithelium and so might be expected to modulate underlying contractile responses.[12] Release of endogenous NO from airway epithelium opposes cholinergically mediated contraction of piglet tracheal smooth muscle. Furthermore, NO signaling in the form of protein S-nitrosylation may also play an important role in airway constriction and relaxation in newborn murine models.[13,14] Thus, the NANC inhibitory system and NO play a significant role in modulating airway and lung function in neonatal animal models. It is unclear whether this is important in human neonates and disturbed in response to inflammatory airway disease.

NANC excitatory mechanisms also play a role in modulating airway smooth muscle. Within this system, the tachykinin peptides, such as substance P and neurokinin A, have been studied during early postnatal development. Tachykinin released from C-fiber nerve endings may directly or reflexly elicit smooth muscle contraction, modulate cholinergic responses through muscarinic receptors, and induce histamine release from mast cells. In young rabbits, substance P–induced modulation of acetylcholine release increases with advancing postnatal age,[15] and in newborn piglets compared with older animals, exogenously administered substance P elicits weak contractile responses of tracheal smooth muscle.[16]

There is some debate about whether increased expression of substance P or other neuropeptides contributes to lung or airway pathophysiology. In mature animal models, long-term exposure to irritant gas increases substance P content; however, it is controversial whether this serves to aggravate airway hyperreactivity or serves a protective role for airway and lung structures. Furthermore, in addition to eliciting airway smooth muscle constriction, substance P may induce relaxation of preconstricted neonatal tracheal tissue by the release of NO and relaxant prostaglandins.[17] Newborn and 3-week-old rats exposed to hyperoxia exhibit increased tachykinin precursor expression, increased substance P content in the lung, and increased cholinergic responsiveness, although the relationship of the latter to the increased substance P content is not clear.[18] Ongoing developmental studies should focus on the signaling pathways that modulate airway smooth muscle relaxant responses through NO- and prostaglandin-mediated mechanisms in health and disease.

INTRACELLULAR CA^{2+} CONCENTRATION REGULATION IN DEVELOPING AIRWAY SMOOTH MUSCLE

Airway smooth muscle contraction is elicited when phosphorylation of the 20-kDa regulatory light chain of myosin allows cross-bridge formation of actin and myosin. This process of phosphorylation is regulated by Ca^{2+}/calmodulin-dependent myosin light chain kinase isoforms. Conversely, dephosphorylation of the 20-kDa regulatory light chain of myosin by myosin phosphatase leads to relaxation. Studies in rat pups have demonstrated that hyperoxic exposure inhibited myosin phosphatase and the resultant prolongation of phosphorylation of the 20-kDa regulatory light chain of myosin may have contributed to hyperoxia-induced enhanced airway contractility,[19] as discussed later. Both plasma membrane Ca^{2+} influx mechanisms and intracellular Ca^{2+} release and reuptake are involved in the intracellular Ca^{2+} concentration ($[Ca^{2+}]_i$) responses of airway smooth muscle to an agonist. Even in the first trimester, immature airway smooth muscle contains many of the $[Ca^{2+}]_i$-regulating mechanisms that are present in adult tissue, contributing to spontaneous and acetylcholine-induced $[Ca^{2+}]_i$ oscillations.[20] However, there is currently limited information on which of the $[Ca^{2+}]_i$ regulatory mechanisms are involved in mediating bronchoconstriction in the normal and injured developing airway.[21] In this regard, in human fetal airway smooth muscle (fASM), many calcium influx pathways appear to be present, as are intracellular calcium release pathways. However, compared with adult airway smooth muscle, in developing airway smooth muscle cells, $[Ca^{2+}]_i$ responses to an agonist appear to be smaller and slower, likely reflecting differences in the kinetics of regulatory mechanisms. Importantly, exposure of fASM cells to even moderate levels of hyperoxia causes enhanced $[Ca^{2+}]_i$ responses to an agonist,[22] and this may underlie the increased airway reactivity observed in vivo after hyperoxia.

MATURATIONAL CHANGES IN AIRWAY PHYSIOLOGIC RESPONSES

Elegant immunohistochemical studies of developing human and porcine fetal airways have been performed from as early as the first trimester. These have revealed the development of an airway smooth muscle layer by the end of the human embryonic period, extending from the trachea to terminal lung sacs, as well as an extensive nerve plexus comprising nerve trunks and ganglia, investing the airways and innervating the smooth muscle. This layer of airway smooth muscle is functional in the first trimester as evidenced by phasic spontaneous narrowing and relaxation of airways with back-and-forth movement of lung fluid. Phasic or tonic activity in airway smooth muscle might stimulate lung growth by providing positive intraluminal pressure. These data are consistent with human autopsy findings that airway smooth muscle is present at 23 weeks gestation at all levels of the conducting airways and is increased in amount during the earliest signs of developing chronic lung disease, as early as 10 days after birth.[23]

Despite clear evidence of an intact airway smooth muscle layer early in gestation, the effect of postnatal maturation on airway contractile responses is somewhat controversial. Physiologic studies using isolated tracheal smooth muscle strips from several species have demonstrated decreased cholinergic responsiveness in early postnatal life.[3,24] These in vitro studies are complicated by the need to carefully normalize the airway contractile response for smooth muscle mass and myosin content.[25] Maturational changes in airway reactivity may also be influenced by immature lung parenchymal structures and increased airway compliance, which may contribute to altered airway narrowing in more immature animal models,[26] as discussed later. Nonetheless, the weight of evidence appears to point to an anatomically intact airway smooth muscle layer superimposed on highly compliant airway structures in early postnatal life.

CONTRIBUTORS TO ABNORMAL AIRWAY FUNCTION

Wheezing disorders and asthma characterized by airway hyperreactivity are major and unintended longer-term respiratory morbidities seen in former preterm infants.[27] It is therefore important to characterize the biologic mechanisms that affect airway function and reactivity of the developing airway.[28,29] Airway function may be modulated by the structural integrity of the airways, changes in the lung parenchyma, and changes in the airway smooth muscle structure or function (Fig. 61.4).

INJURY TO THE LUNG PARENCHYMA

There has been considerable interest in investigating the effects of BPD and chronic lung injury on aberrant alveolar development.[30] Intrapulmonary vascular structures, vascular endothelial growth factor (VEGF), and its downstream signaling mechanism play an

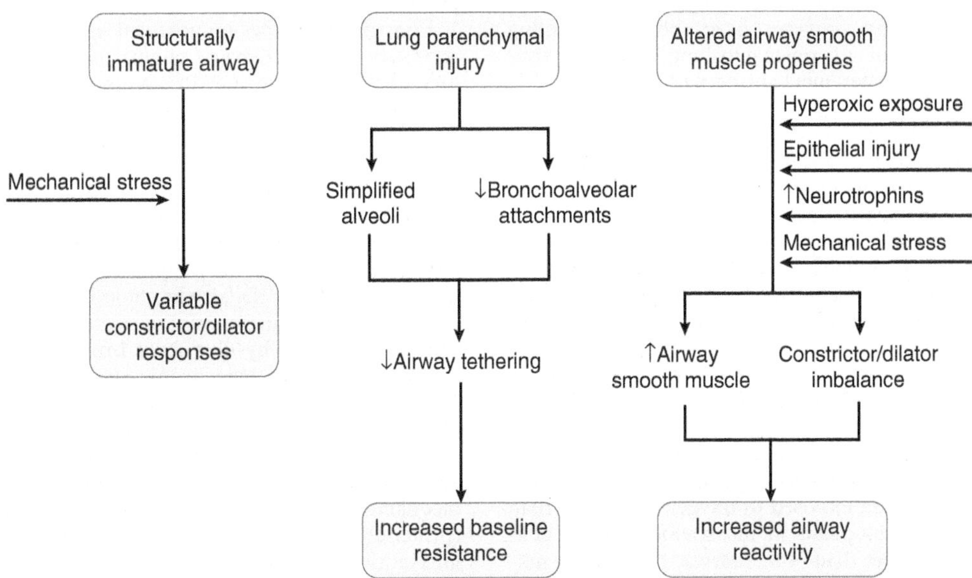

Fig. 61.4 Interacting contributors from the airways and lung parenchyma that are proposed to modulate airway activity in the face of neonatal lung injury.

important role in parenchymal development, and this VEGF effect may be disrupted when the lungs are exposed to hyperoxia.[31] Another important component of lung development is the close relation of the lung parenchyma and the intrapulmonary airways.[32] Disruption of this airway-parenchymal coupling is associated with decreased tethering between the airway and the lung parenchyma, compromising airway caliber.[33] This may eventually increase airway resistance causing future airway hyperresponsiveness. This concept is supported by hyperoxic exposure contributing to the long-term disruption of the airway-parenchymal coupling in neonatal mouse lungs.[34] While there are limited data regarding the effects of the parenchymal injury on altered airway function, these studies point toward an increased predisposition to airway hyperreactivity in the face of alveolar simplification.

NEURO-EPITHELIAL CONTRIBUTION

Airway epithelium plays an important role in modulating airway smooth muscle response. Epithelial damage secondary to mechanical ventilation and/or oxidative stress may lead to airway hyperreactivity seen in former preterm infants. Injury to the epithelial layer may augment the cholinergic pathway and at the same time result in a loss of airway relaxant factors, thus leading to exaggerated airway constriction response. This is supported by studies on tracheal strips from preterm sheep that show increased responsiveness to methacholine after the epithelial layer is removed[24] and diminished NO mediated relaxation in murine intrapulmonary airways after epithelial debridement.[14] Epithelial damage may also result in the release of important mediators that affect airway reactivity. This has been demonstrated in murine models of hyperoxic lung injury by nonspecific blockade of NO synthase. Under normoxic conditions, vagal stimulation-induced increases in airway resistance were further augmented with the blockade of NO synthase.[35] However, this augmentation effect appears to be lost after hyperoxic exposure. These findings indicate that NO released from vagal postganglionic fibers plays an important role in modulating airway constriction responses to endogenously released acetylcholine. In this regard, the prostaglandin/cyclic adenosine monophosphate (c-AMP) signaling pathway may be important in the airway constrictor/dilator imbalance. Hyperoxic injury to the airway seems to attenuate c-AMP mediated airway relaxation in rat pups when compared with animals under normoxic conditions.[36] This impairment in relaxation may be related to the impairment of dephosphorylation of airway smooth muscle myosin phosphatase as discussed earlier.[19]

The c-AMP pathway may also play a role in modulating the effects of neurotrophin in the developing airway smooth muscle.[37] Neurotrophins are a family of proteins that play an important role in neuronal plasticity of the vertebrate nervous system and are increasingly being isolated in non-neuronal tissues.[38,39] The neurotrophin family is principally composed of BDNF, nerve growth factor [NGF], neurotrophin 3, and neurotrophin 4. They share a common structural feature and act downstream through their corresponding tyrosine kinase receptor complex. Increased BDNF secretion following hyperoxia exposure has been associated with increased airway smooth muscle contractility and proliferation.[37,40] Consistent with these findings, neurotrophins are overexpressed in the lower airways of human infants infected with the respiratory syncytial virus that is well-known for increasing the risk of future airway hyperreactivity.[41]

ROLE OF INFLAMMATION

Factors affecting airway structure and function may begin in the prenatal period. Prematurity, intrauterine growth restriction (IUGR), and chorioamnionitis have all been associated with future airway hyperreactivity.[42] Among all the factors, chorioamnionitis was most strongly associated with airway hyperreactivity. This is supported by animal studies with prenatal administration of lipopolysaccharide (LPS) and subsequent finding of arrested alveolar and microvascular development, increased inflammation, and diminished lung compliance.[43,44] It is interesting to note that infants who are exposed to chorioamnionitis or other intrauterine infections rarely have organisms isolated from cultures. Data suggest that the response of the fetus to the infection rather than the actual infection may be more important in this regard.[45] Presence in the amniotic fluid of increased amounts of pro-inflammatory cytokines such as interleukin-6 (IL-6), interleukin-8 (IL-8), interleukin-1-beta (IL-1β), tumor necrosis factor-alpha (TNFα) has been associated with later pulmonary morbidity in preterm infants.[46] Prenatal inflammation caused by nicotine has also been shown to disrupt bronchopulmonary development in rat lungs.[47] Some studies with prenatal inflammation, however, have shown conflicting results with improvement of postnatal lung function, thus pointing toward a complicated mechanistic pathway.[48]

EFFECT OF HYPEROXIA ON DEVELOPING AIRWAYS

Postnatal interventions such as the use of oxygen and ventilation are important factors that affect airway remodeling in preterm infants.[18,49-51] Reactive oxygen species and free radical damage secondary to hyperoxic exposure have long been postulated as a cause of airway remodeling and altered airway function. Recent studies in murine models have explored different levels of hyperoxia on methacholine induced airway reactivity.[52] Mouse pups exposed to mild hyperoxia (40% FiO_2) demonstrated worse airway hyperreactivity and lung compliance when compared to the severe hyperoxia group (70% FiO_2).The airway reactivity and lung compliance in the severe hyperoxia group were similar to mice in the normoxia group.This interesting finding was supported by an in vitro study performed with human fASM cells that demonstrated increased proliferation when exposed to oxygen levels less than 60% FiO_2 and increased apoptosis in the smooth muscle cells when exposed to FiO_2 more than 60%.[22] Airway remodeling may also involve increased extracellular matrix (ECM) or proteoglycan deposition in the lung. Hyperoxia during the first 10 postnatal days was associated with increased hyaluronan (HA) deposition in the perivascular spaces and alveolar walls in rat pups.[53] These changes in the ECM interfere with normal airway development while increasing the risk for future airway reactivity.[54] A similar study done with fASM cells found that moderate hyperoxia-induced airway remodeling was associated with alteration in the ECM.[55] The changes in the ECM included increased collagen deposition along with an imbalance of several important ECM components, such as matrix metalloproteinase-9 (MMP-9), tissue inhibitor of metalloproteinase-1 (TIMP-1), and caveolin-1 (CAV-1), all of which have been associated with reactive airway diseases such as asthma.[56-59]

EFFECT OF INTERMITTENT HYPOXIA ON DEVELOPING AIRWAYS

Translational animal studies have incorporated moderate oxygen exposure with intermingled hypoxic episodes (i.e., intermittent hypoxia, IH).[60] In a recent study, mouse pups were exposed to various combinations of 50% oxygen with IH episodes (10% FiO_2) every 10 minutes for 7 days.[61] When compared with room-air controls, the mouse pups exposed only to IH did not exhibit increased airway reactivity. However, if hypoxic episodes were followed by hyperoxic recovery, airway resistance increased in response to methacholine and decreased compliance. Interestingly, the alveolarization and the airway smooth muscle mass were comparable between groups. Observational studies in extremely premature infants have shown associations between increased IH episodes in the first weeks of life and incidence of subsequent BPD diagnosis at 36 weeks corrected gestational age[62] and increased use of asthma medications and parental reported wheezing in childhood follow-up.[63]

EFFECT OF POSITIVE PRESSURE ON DEVELOPING AIRWAYS

Decreased airway smooth muscle contractility and inadequate cartilaginous support result in the high deformability or compliance of the airways in premature infants. The obvious result is that tracheas, and possibly lower airways, are vulnerable to deformation during positive pressure ventilation. This may result in the partial collapse of airways and impaired gas exchange. Bronchodilator therapy may aggravate this problem.[64] Avoidance of excessive volu- and baro-trauma has lessened this problem, especially with the recent shift toward noninvasive modes of ventilation (i.e., continuous positive airway pressure or CPAP).

Unfortunately, the longer-term issues of increased airway reactivity remain a major clinical issue, despite the increased use of noninvasive CPAP.[65] A murine model of normoxic CPAP exposure resulted in long-term (3 weeks of age) airway hyperreactivity.[66] Additionally, the effects of CPAP were more profoundly seen in smaller airways compared to larger airways. As described, the airway smooth muscle layer is present around the developing preterm airways at an early gestational age.[23] The larger airways are eventually stabilized with the cartilaginous layer. The lack of this cartilaginous support around the smaller airways means that the airway smooth muscle layer is potentially subjected to a higher amount of stretch secondary to ventilation. This is supported by data from bronchial segments of rabbits that demonstrated that chronic strain had a more detrimental effect on smaller airways.[67] This would explain the differential effects of CPAP seen on smaller versus larger airways.[66] Airway remodeling through disruption of ECM may also play a role in ventilator-induced lung injury.[68] Overdistension and mechanical stretch can cause fragmentation of ECM components (proteoglycans and glycosaminoglycans) of the airway setting into motion an inflammatory cascade downstream. Inflammatory cells (neutrophils and macrophages) accumulate, producing cytokines and further changes in the ECM components such as HA, collagen, and elastin.[69] HA, in particular, seems to be a major player in the inflammatory pathway signaling in lung injury.[70] The pro-inflammatory low-molecular-weight HA and hyaluronan synthase-3 (the enzyme that synthesizes low-molecular-weight HA) have been found at increased amounts in the lungs of various neonatal respiratory morbidities as well as juvenile airway diseases.[71,72] Interestingly, CPAP and positive end expiratory pressure have been shown to have a protective effect against airway hyperreactivity in an adult rat model.[73] Positive airway pressure may affect developing immature airways differently than it affects matured adult airways.

LONGER-TERM RESPIRATORY OUTCOMES AFTER PREMATURE BIRTH

The complex milieu of exposures and genetic susceptibilities associated with premature birth likely contributes to an observed increased risk for longer-term respiratory morbidities, particularly in regard to airway dysfunction and wheezing disorders (Fig. 61.5). In the United States, 1 in 12 children will receive a diagnosis of asthma (Centers for Disease Control and Prevention; 2017 National Health Interview Survey); in premature infants, the rate may be as high as one in three. Large international birth cohorts have similarly revealed elevated asthma risk in premature infants compared with their term peers. These studies have found

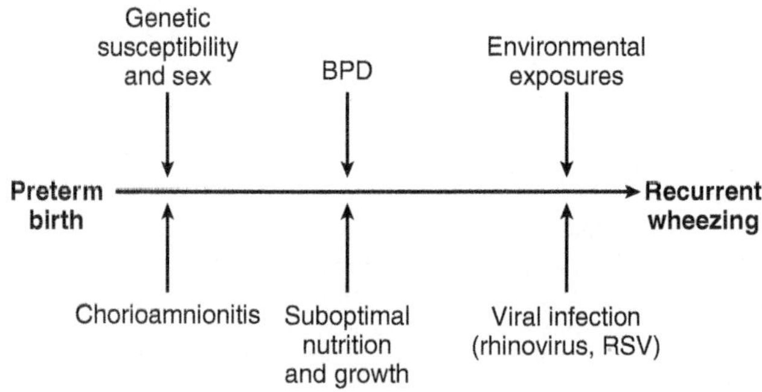

Fig. 61.5 Risk factors for recurrent wheezing in former preterm infants. *BPD,* Bronchopulmonary dysplasia; *RSV,* respiratory syncytial virus.

that the most premature infants have the most risk, but even moderately premature infants have a significantly increased risk for asthma.[74,75]

The asthma phenotype in preterm infants may differ from allergic asthma seen in their term peers. The airway hyperreactivity observed in former preterm neonates is strongly associated with a history of prolonged supplemental oxygen exposure and BPD compared with the airway hyperreactivity observed in term controls, which, instead, is associated with a history of genetic inheritance, allergy, airway inflammation, and cigarette exposure. Wheezing preterm infants, with and without BPD, display diminished airway reversibility, atopy, inflammation, and exhaled NO in comparison with their term counterparts with asthma.

Regarding longitudinal data, Hack and colleagues[76] have reported that extremely low-birth-weight children at 8 years of age were more likely than their normal-birth-weight controls to require medication for asthma (23% vs. 8%, respectively). The rates of asthma medication use did not change between the ages of 8 and 14 years among the extremely low-birth-weight cohort (23% at both ages) but did increase among controls (17%). As such, differences were no longer significant between groups, suggesting stability in wheezing prevalence among extremely low-birth-weight children as they age, with an increased incidence of allergic asthma among their teenage peers. Still, in follow-up studies of children and young adults born prematurely, there continues to be evidence of impaired pulmonary function, manifesting signs of obstructive pulmonary disease with decreased predicted forced expiratory volume in 1 second,[75] small airway impairments with decreased predicted forced expiratory flow at 25% to 75% of the pulmonary volume,[75] and reduced exercise capacity.

Treatment of wheezing disorders in former preterm infants can be challenging. Environmental triggers of wheezing are less likely to be allergen driven. Traditional asthma medications such as corticosteroids and bronchodilators[75] show variable responses, and leukotriene inhibitors have yet to be studied in this population. Furthermore, β-agonist bronchodilators may paradoxically increase airway resistance in some preterm infants, and regular use has further increased airway reactivity in hyperoxia-exposed neonatal rodents.[77]

CONCLUSION

In summary, recognition of prematurity as an independent risk factor for childhood wheezing, even among the late preterm infant and those infants who do not have BPD should prompt the clinician to diligently assess the patient for signs and symptoms of airway disease in the neonatal intensive care unit. Future investigation of the pathophysiology and clinical indicators of airway disease among former preterm infants will, hopefully, lead to targeted interventions and long-term management strategies in this high-risk population.

ACKNOWLEDGMENT

This chapter was prepared through the financial support of grant HL 56470 (R.J. Martin and Y.S. Prakash), HL138402 (P.M. MacFarlane), and HL 133459 (T.M. Raffay) from the National Institutes of Health.

 A complete reference list is available at www.ExpertConsult.com.

REFERENCES

1. Zaidi SI, Jafri A, Doggett T, et al. Airway-related vagal preganglionic neurons express brain-derived neurotrophic factor and TrkB receptors. Implications for neuronal plasticity. *Brain Res*. 2005;1044:133–143.
2. Hislop AA, Mak JC, Reader JA, et al. Muscarinic receptor subtypes in the porcine lung during postnatal development. *Eur J Pharmacol*. 1998;359:211–221.
3. Haxhiu-Poskurica B, Ernsberger P, Haxhiu MA, et al. Development of cholinergic innervation and muscarinic receptor subtypes in piglet trachea. *Am J Physiol*. 1993;264:L606–L614.
4. Fisher JT, Brundage KL, Anderson JW. Cardiopulmonary actions of muscarinic receptor subtypes in the newborn dog. *Can J Physiol Pharmacol*. 1996;74:603–613.
5. Haxhiu MA, Kc P, Moore CT, et al. Brain stem excitatory and inhibitory signaling pathways regulating bronchoconstrictive responses. *J Appl Physiol*. 2005;98:1961–1982.
8. Mirmanesh SJ, Abbasi S, Bhutani VK. Alpha-adrenergic bronchoprovocation in neonates with bronchopulmonary dysplasia. *J Pediatr*. 1992;121:622–625.
11. Colasurdo GN, Loader JE, Graves JP, et al. Maturation of nonadrenergic noncholinergic inhibitory system in normal and allergen-sensitized rabbits. *Am J Physiol*. 1994;267:L739–744.
13. Raffay TM, Dylag AM, Di Fiore JM, et al. S-nitrosoglutathione attenuates airway hyperresponsiveness in murine bronchopulmonary dysplasia. *Mol Pharmacol*. 2016;90:418–426.
16. Haxhiu-Poskurica B, Haxhiu MA, Kumar GK, et al. Tracheal smooth muscle responses to substance P and neurokinin A in the piglet. *J Appl Physiol*. 1992;72:1090–1095.
17. Mhanna MJ, Dreshaj IA, Haxhiu MA, et al. Mechanism for substance P-induced relaxation of precontracted airway smooth muscle during development. *Am J Physiol*. 1999;276:L51–L56.
18. Agani FH, Kuo NT, Chang CH, et al. Effect of hyperoxia on substance P expression and airway reactivity in the developing lung. *Am J Physiol*. 1997;273:L40–L45.
19. Smith PG, Dreshaj A, Chaudhuri S, et al. Hyperoxic conditions inhibit airway smooth muscle myosin phosphatase in rat pups. *Am J Physiol Lung Cell Mol Physiol*. 2007;292:L68–L73.
21. Prakash YS, Martin RJ. Brain-derived neurotrophic factor in the airways. *Pharmacol Ther*. 2014;143:74–86.
23. SwardComunelli SL, Mabry SM, Truog WE, et al. Airway muscle in preterm infants. Changes during development. *J Pediatr*. 1997;130:570–576.
24. Panitch HB, Allen JL, Ryan JP, et al. A comparison of preterm and adult airway smooth muscle mechanics. *J Appl Physiol*. 1989;66:1760–1765.
27. Reyburn B, Martin RJ, Prakash YS, et al. Mechanisms of injury to the preterm lung and airway: implications for long-term pulmonary outcome. *Neonatology*. 2012;101:345–352.
28. Ganguly A, Martin RJ. Vulnerability of the developing airway. *Respir Physiol Neurobiol*. 2019;270:103263.
29. Kistemaker LEM, Prakash YS. Airway innervation and plasticity in asthma. *Physiology*. 2019;34:283–298.
32. Mansell AL, McAteer AL, Oldmixon EH. Mechanical dissociation of bronchi from parenchyma in the immature piglet lung. *J Appl Physiol*. 2005;89:228–234.
34. O'Reilly M, Harding R, Sozo F. Altered small airways in aged mice following neonatal exposure to hyperoxic gas. *Neonatology*. 2014;105:39–45.
35. Iben SC, Dreshaj IA, Farver CF, et al. Role of endogenous nitric oxide in hyperoxia-induced airway hyperreactivity in maturing rats. *J Appl Physiol*. 2000;89:1205–1212.
36. Mhanna MJ, Haxhiu MA, Jaber MA, et al. Hyperoxia impairs airway relaxation in immature rats via a cAMP-mediated mechanism. *J Appl Physiol*. 2004;96:1854–1860.
40. Yao Q, Haxhiu MA, Zaidi SI, et al. Hyperoxia enhances brain-derived neurotrophic factor and tyrosine kinase B receptor expression in peribronchial smooth muscle of neonatal rats. *Am J Physiol Lung Cell Mol Physiol*. 2005;289:L307–L314.
44. Faksh A, Britt Jr RD, Vogel ER, et al. Effects of antenatal lipopolysaccharide and postnatal hyperoxia on airway reactivity and remodeling in a neonatal mouse model. *Pediatr Res*. 2016;79:391–400.
49. Uyehara CF, Pichoff BE, Sim HH, et al. Hyperoxic exposure enhances airway reactivity of newborn guinea pigs. *J Appl Physiol*. 1993;74:2649–2654.
51. Iben SC, Haxhiu MA, Farver CF, et al. Short-term mechanical ventilation increases airway reactivity in rat pups. *Pediatr Res*. 2006;60:136–140.
52. Wang H, Jafri A, Martin RJ, et al. Severity of neonatal hyperoxia determines structural and functional changes in developing mouse airway. *Am J Physiol Lung Cell Mol Physiol*. 2014;307:L295–L301.
53. Juul SE, Krueger Jr RC, Scofield L, et al. Hyperoxia alone causes changes in lung proteoglycans and hyaluronan in neonatal rat pups. *Am J Respir Cell Mol Biol*. 1995;13:629–638.
55. Vogel ER, Britt Jr RD, Faksh A, et al. Moderate hyperoxia induces extracellular matrix remodeling by human fetal airway smooth muscle cells. *Pediatr Res*. 2017;81:376–383.
59. Vogel ER, Manlove LJ, Kuipers I, et al. Caveolin-1 scaffolding domain peptide prevents hyperoxia-induced airway remodeling in a neonatal mouse model. *Am J Physiol Lung Cell Mol Physiol*. 2019;317:L99–L108.
61. Dylag AM, Mayer CA, Raffay TM, et al. Long-term effects of recurrent intermittent hypoxia and hyperoxia on respiratory system mechanics in neonatal mice. *Pediatr Res*. 2017;81:565–571.
62. Raffay TM, Dylag AM, Sattar A, et al. Neonatal intermittent hypoxemia events are associated with diagnosis of bronchopulmonary dysplasia at 36 weeks postmenstrual age. *Pediatr Res*. 2019;85:318–323.
63. Di Fiore JM, Dylag AM, Honomichl RD, et al. Early inspired oxygen and intermittent hypoxemic events in extremely premature infants are associated with asthma medication use at 2 years of age. *J Perinatol*. 2019;39:203–211.

65. Doyle LW, Carse E, Adams AM, et al. Ventilation in extremely preterm infants and respiratory function at 8 years. *N Engl J Me.d.* 2017;377:329-337.
66. Mayer CA, Martin RJ, MacFarlane PM. Increased airway reactivity in a neonatal mouse model of continuous positive airway pressure. *Pediatr Res.* 2015;78:145-151.
71. Savani RC. Modulators of inflammation in bronchopulmonary dysplasia. *Semin Perinatol.* 2018;42:459-470.
76. Hack M, Schluchter M, Andreias L, et al. Change in prevalence of chronic conditions between childhood and adolescence among extremely low-birth-weight children. *JAMA.* 2011;306:394-401.
77. Raffay T, Kc P, Reynolds J, et al. Repeated beta2-adrenergic receptor agonist therapy attenuates the response to rescue bronchodilation in a hyperoxic newborn mouse model. *Neonatology.* 2014;106:126-132.

62 Functional Development of Respiratory Muscles

Carlos B. Mantilla | Joline E. Brandenburg | Matthew J. Fogarty | Gary C. Sieck

INTRODUCTION

This chapter provides a snapshot of fetal and neonatal development of the diaphragm muscle (DIAm), the major inspiratory muscle in mammals, and partition between the thoracic and abdominal cavities. The DIAm appears rather late in evolution, being present only in mammals, while other vertebrates use different means of ventilation.[1] The embryologic origin of the DIAm has been elucidated by studies using molecular markers of muscle development, reflecting a common origin to the DIAm in the pleuroperitoneal fold. The traditional view of DIAm development called for multiple sites of origin reflecting a complex derivation, consistent with its multiple anatomic origin and insertion sites. The mechanical actions of the DIAm reflect its functions during ventilatory (inspiration) and several nonventilatory motor behaviors. These nonventilatory behaviors include expulsive maneuvers such as coughing, defecation, emesis, micturition, parturition, and sneezing; postural activations while performing lifting activities; and emotional behaviors such as vocalization and musicianship.[2]

Neural control of the DIAm is similar to other skeletal muscles and is based on recruitment and frequency coding of motor units.[3] Motor units in the adult DIAm, each comprising a motor neuron and the muscle fibers it innervates, vary considerably in their mechanical, histochemical, and biochemical properties,[4-6] and this heterogeneity provides the range of control of muscle force generation that occurs during different motor behaviors. It is the cumulative contractile and fatigue properties of the motor unit pool that determine the constraints under which the DIAm responds to the various mechanical demands placed upon it during different ventilatory and nonventilatory behaviors. Clearly, these motor demands can change during development, and the DIAm must adapt or remodel to accommodate these changing demands.

The DIAm becomes rhythmically active during late fetal development (fetal respiratory movements), and at birth, it must be ready to sustain ventilation. Postnatally, the DIAm is one of the most active skeletal muscles, with a duty cycle (time active versus relaxed) of ~30% to 40%, compared to limb muscles (duty cycles ranging from 2% to 15%).[7] It is not surprising, therefore, that the fetal and neonatal pathology of the DIAm often lead to ventilatory failure and premature death. Despite the vital importance of the DIAm, previous studies have provided mostly descriptive information about its development and growth. However, there is accumulating information about myogenesis and neural development that derives from in vitro model systems, which may be applicable to the mechanisms regulating DIAm development in vivo. Yet, the applicability of these in vitro results regarding the basis of myogenesis and neural development remains to be established, especially in the context of maturation of other systems, for example, the central nervous system (CNS), lung, and thoracic and abdominal walls. Unfortunately, such integrative information is lacking.

Rodent models are increasingly being used to explore the genetic basis for developmental plasticity in neuromotor control. Accordingly, in this chapter, we focus on recent results obtained in rats and mice. Benchmarks for the development of the mouse DIAm are summarized in Fig. 62.1. The fetal and neonatal developmental benchmarks in rats are generally comparable to those in mice (offset by ~2 days). In mice, developmental benchmarks for the DIAm begin at approximately embryonic day 11 or 12 (E11, E12) when the phrenic nerve makes initial contact with the primordial DIAm. In both rats and mice, the final pattern of adult motor units and muscle fiber types is not achieved until postnatal day 28 (D28). During this 5 to 6 week span, dramatic changes in DIAm innervation, contractile protein expression, and function occur. Obviously, the timeline for such developmental benchmarks in humans is far more protracted, but it is likely that similar convergence of neural and myogenic events also occurs. Therefore, much can be learned by studying the integrated aspects of myogenesis and neural development of the DIAm in rodent models.

EMBRYOLOGIC DERIVATION AND INNERVATION OF THE DIAPHRAGM MUSCLE

MYOGENESIS

Skeletal muscle fibers, including those in the DIAm, are formed in two stages: (1) commitment (also known as *determination*), when mesodermal progenitor cells are transformed to myoblasts; and (2) terminal differentiation, when myoblasts fuse to form myotubes and myofibers (Fig. 62.2). Myogenesis may proceed via an intrinsic genetic program, or it may require either the presence of positive extrinsic signals or the removal of inhibitory signals.[8] None of these potential mechanisms can be presently excluded. However, there is converging evidence that myogenesis is induced in a variety of nonmuscle cells by the expression of proteins belonging to the basic helix-loop-helix (bHLH) superfamily.[9,10] Collectively, these are known as *muscle regulatory factors (MRFs)* and include MyoD,[11] myogenin,[12] Myf-5,[13] and MRF4/Myf-6.[14] In addition to providing a molecular

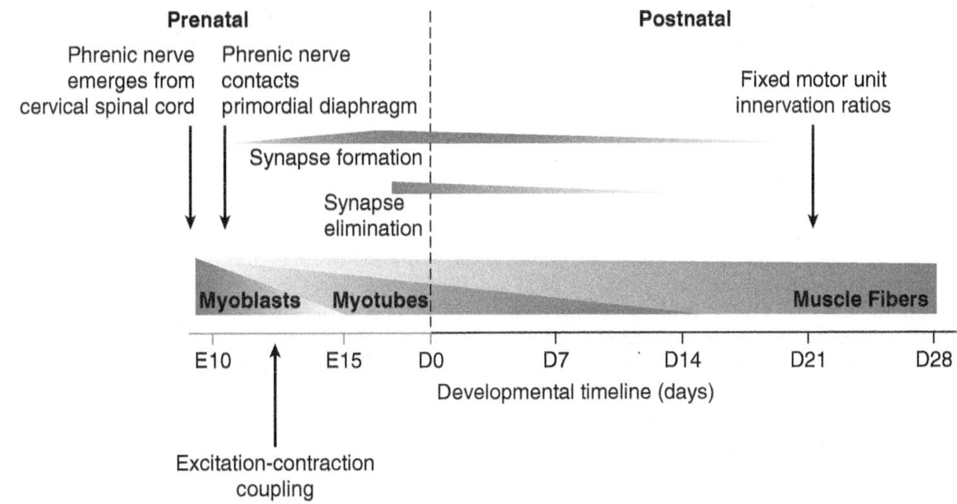

Fig. 62.1 Schematic showing the timeline for major events in the development of the mouse diaphragm muscle (DIAm). Similar seminal events occur in the embryonic and early postnatal development of the DIAm in other mammals including humans, although temporal characteristics and inter-relationships may vary.

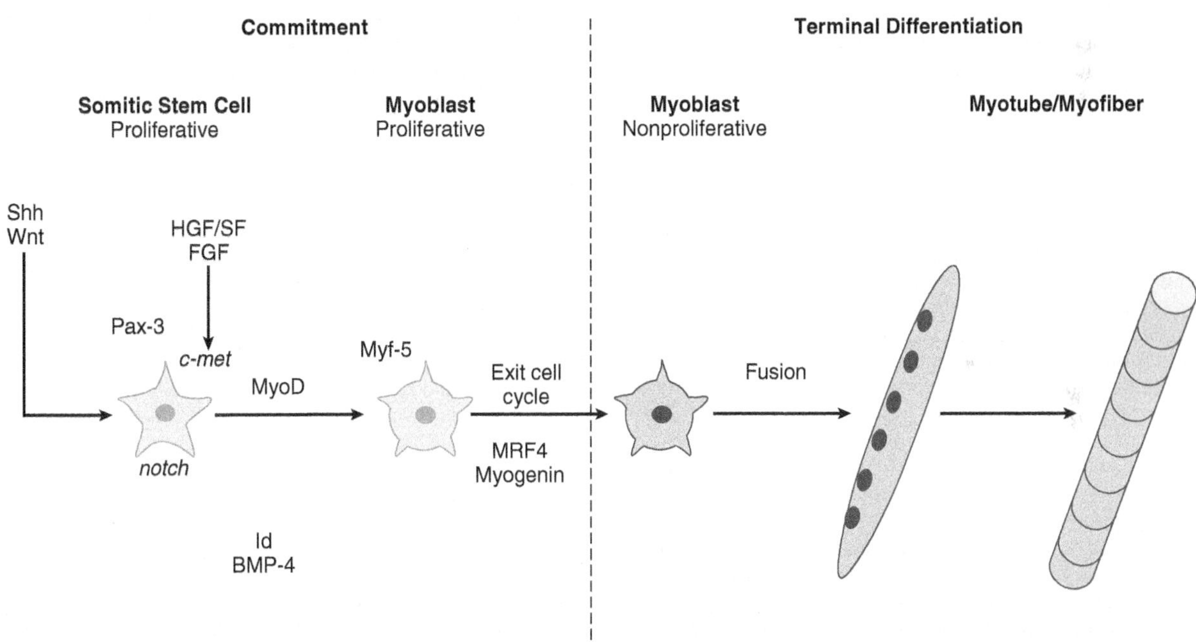

Fig. 62.2 Schematic demonstrating the two major stages of myogenesis—commitment and terminal differentiation. During commitment, somitic stem cells proliferate and are committed to myoblasts, a process marked by MyoD and Myf-5 expression. This process ends when proliferating myoblasts exit the cell cycle, influenced by the expression of MRF4 and myogenin. The exit of myoblasts from the cell cycle marks the beginning of the differentiation stage. Thereafter, nonproliferative myoblasts fuse to form myotubes and with the formation of distinct sarcomeres, myofibers. The differentiation process continues until adult fiber types are established. *Bmp,* Bone morphogenetic protein; *FGF,* fibroblast growth factor; *HGF/SF,* hepatocellular growth factor/scatter factor; *MyoD,* myoblast determination protein 1.

mechanism for the regulation of myogenesis in fetal and neonatal muscle, MRFs are also involved in determining the expression of myosin heavy chain (MyHC) isoforms in adult muscle.[15]

Genetic determinants of myoblast commitment have been most extensively studied in *Drosophila*, but this information is likely to be directly applicable to myoblast commitment in the mammalian DIAm as well. In *Drosophila*, it has been shown that neural-derived proteins (e.g., sonic hedgehog, Wnt 1, 3, and 4) promote commitment to myoblasts within a myotome.[8,16] Expression of sonic hedgehog and/or other signals commit mesodermal cells to form myoblasts possibly by releasing suppression of the expression of specific MRFs.[17] The process of myoblast commitment is marked by the expression of the paired-box protein *Pax-3*, which appears to positively regulate MRF expression, and in turn is regulated by Six1and Six4.[18] For example, the ectopic expression of *Pax-3* induces both MyoD and Myf-5 in embryonic tissue.[19] The consequent increase in MRFs then initiates a cascade of signals that continues through differentiation, thus sustaining myogenesis. Indeed, transplantation of *Pax-3*-expressing embryonic stem cells into dystrophic mice resulted in engraftment of stem cell precursors with adult myofibers and enhanced contractile function.[20]

MRFs function as molecular switches, initiating myogenesis by inducing expression of muscle-specific genes through binding of the bHLH motif to *cis*-acting DNA control elements of muscle-specific genes, known as *E-boxes*.[21] The E-box is a CANNTG sequence-containing motif present in the promoter regions of many skeletal muscle-specific genes.[22] Transcriptional regulation mediated by MRFs may also involve interactions of MRFs with the family of MADS-box proteins termed *myocyte enhancer factor 2 (MEF2A-D)*, which may determine muscle-specificity for genes lacking MRF binding domains. Binding sites for MEF2 factors are located in the promoter regions of many muscle-specific genes, including myogenin. However, MEF2 binding alone is not sufficient to induce myogenesis.

It is also possible that myoblast commitment is determined by release from inhibition by signals that actively suppress MRF expression. For example, a class of HLH proteins termed *Id factors* (Id1-Id4) inhibit MRF activity by forming heterodimers with E2 products (ubiquitously expressed HLH-containing proteins encoded for by E2 genes). These products prevent dimerization with MRFs and thus block subsequent activation of skeletal muscle-specific genes.[23] The Id proteins lack the basic DNA binding domain; therefore, the heterodimerization of bHLH proteins with Id proteins prevents the strong binding to DNA by either E-proteins or MRFs.[24] Twist is another protein in mice that sequesters E-proteins that inhibit MRF activity by preventing the formation of MRF-E protein heterodimers.[25] Yet another inhibitory factor is Mist1, which binds MyoD to form an inactive heterodimer.[26] The balance between inhibitory and pro-myogenic signals likely determines the timing and location of muscle precursor development. Calcineurin was shown to activate MyoD indirectly by decreasing the expression of the Id inhibitory proteins.[27] Others have shown that Nfix may also play a key role in the transition of embryonic to fetal skeletal muscle gene expression through binding with MEF2A.[28,29] A knockout mouse for Nfix (E16.5) shows disorganized sarcomeres, downregulation of β-enolase, and muscle creatine kinase (MCK) though myogenin expression remains intact.[29] Myogenic inhibitory signals may be critical to prevent the ectopic formation of skeletal muscle because mesodermal somite cells can follow both myogenic and nonmyogenic programs.

In hypaxial muscles (e.g., limb muscles, chest, and abdominal wall muscles and DIAm) MyoD is the first MRF to be expressed. MyoD expression then initiates a cascade resulting in subsequent expression of Myf-5, MRF4, and myogenin.[30] The sequence of MRF expression appears to be critical for the development of normal muscle. MyoD and Myf-5 are highly expressed in proliferating myoblasts, suggesting a primary role for these MRFs during this stage of myogenesis.[11] In mutant mice lacking MyoD or MRF4,[31,32] there is no apparent effect on normal skeletal muscle development, but Myf-5 and myogenin are upregulated, respectively. Therefore redundant MRF expression may rescue the normal skeletal muscle phenotype in these animals. Similarly, Myf-5 deficient mice appear to have normal skeletal muscle, but they succumb to asphyxiation soon after birth due to rib cage abnormalities.[33] In contrast, myogenin deficient mice have only myoblasts without the development of myotubes/myofibers,[34,35] suggesting that myogenin is indispensable for differentiation of myotubes/myofibers. In mice lacking both Myf-5 and MyoD, no myoblasts are present, suggesting that the expression of both of these MRFs is required for myoblast commitment.[36] Mice lacking both Myf-5 and MRF4 resemble Myf-5 knockouts, suggesting that MRF4 regulates later aspects of myogenesis.

With terminal differentiation, committed mononucleated myoblasts are nonreversibly transformed into multinucleated myotubes/myofibers with the expression of contractile proteins (see Fig. 62.2). Thus terminal differentiation represents the irreversible exit of proliferating myoblasts from the cell cycle. Yet, not all myoblasts lose their ability to proliferate because a pool of myoblasts (satellite cells) persists into adulthood, and their proliferative capacity is important in processes of injury and repair as well as other conditions of muscle remodeling. Throughout life, proliferating myoblasts are susceptible to apoptosis, that is, programmed cell death, until they are terminally differentiated and exit the cell cycle. The balance between proliferation and apoptosis may play an important role in controlling the total number of muscle fibers of a given type.[37] Terminal differentiation of myoblasts in hypaxial muscles does not occur in vivo until they have migrated from the myotome to their final location (e.g., thoracic or abdominal walls or to the limbs). As myoblasts migrate from the lateral dermomyotome, they express Myf-5 and *c-met* (a tyrosine kinase receptor for hepatocyte growth factor/scatter factor), which thus are used as markers for this process. In hypaxial muscle precursors (including DIAm), expression of Myf-5 and *c-met* begins at ~E10 and continues through E12.[38] The expression of MyoD is also important in the process of terminal differentiation and can be inhibited in vitro by bone morphogenic protein-4 or fibroblast growth factor-5,[17] both of which have been implicated in the maintenance of the myoblast proliferative capacity and inhibition of differentiation.

Following terminal differentiation, myoblasts fuse forming multinucleated myotubes/myofibers. Although the formation of myotubes/myofibers is coincident with the initial appearance of innervation in hypaxial muscles, converging evidence from in vitro and in vivo models indicates that terminal differentiation can be initiated in the absence of neural influence. Myotubes/myofibers can form in vitro in the absence of innervation, but at a much slower pace compared to that observed in vivo. This suggests that neural influence may facilitate the normal process of terminal differentiation and formation of myotubes/myofibers. This potential facilitating influence of innervation needs to be further explored. There is evidence, based on in vitro model systems, that terminal differentiation and myotube/myofiber formation depend on the expression of several non-neural proteins, including those present in the extracellular matrix (e.g., fibronectins and laminins), basal lamina (e.g., muscle cell adhesion molecule [M-CAM], neural cell adhesion molecule [N-CAM] and M-cadherin), cell membrane (e.g., β1-integrin), and cytoskeleton (e.g., actin and desmin).[39,40] Obviously, terminal differentiation and myotube/myofiber formation involve very complex interactions between differentiating cells and their surrounding environment. Current research is only starting to unravel these complex interactions. It should be noted that even though the process of myoblast fusion into myotubes/myofibers is called *terminal differentiation*, there is subsequent differentiation of these nascent muscle fibers into adult muscle fiber types (see below).

Other factors may also influence myogenesis. For example, in vitro passive mechanical strain results in both myotube hyperplasia and hypertrophy.[41,42] Thus, both myoblast proliferation and differentiation are affected by passive strain. Passive stretching can also prevent the atrophy of myotubes, which normally occurs in culture media lacking growth factors. The mechanisms responsible for the transduction of passive strain into a proliferative and/or trophic influence is unclear but may involve mediators such as prostaglandin (PG)$F_{2\alpha}$, insulin-like growth factor-1 (IGF-1), or other cytokines.[42] Although these in vitro studies employed passive strain, these results suggest that early mechanical activation of the fetal DIAm (e.g., via fetal respiratory movements) may be important in promoting further myogenesis.

MYOSIN HEAVY CHAIN

Myosin is a hexameric protein (MW = 480 kDa) comprising two heavy chains and four light chains. At the rod-shaped COOH-terminus end of the myosin molecule, the two heavy chains (MW = 200 kDa) dimerize into a 200-nm α-helical tail. At the NH_3-terminus, the heavy chains separate and form two distinct heads (S-1), which contain both actin and nucleotide-binding domains. The S-1 converts chemical energy into mechanical work through a process that involves stereo-specific docking of S-1 with actin, thereby reversing the intra-molecular conformational changes induced by ATP hydrolysis.[43,44] A number of MyHC isoforms exist, and all of which are encoded by a highly conserved multi-gene family located on chromosome 17 (human) or 11 (mouse).[45] The rate of ATP hydrolysis at the S-1 varies among the different MyHC isoforms, thereby providing the molecular basis for fiber type differences in mechanical properties.[6,46-48] The essential (MLC_{20}) and regulatory myosin light chains (MLC_{17}) provide structural support and possibly modulate the mechanical performance of the MyHC.[49] Different MLC isoforms may differentially modulate the kinetic properties of MyHC.[50] There is also evidence that both Ca^{2+} binding to MLC_{17} and phosphorylation of MLC_{17} modulate S-1 ATPase activity.[51-53]

Adult skeletal muscle fibers are classified histochemically as type I, IIa, and IIb based on the pH lability of myofibrillar ATPase staining.[54] Muscle fiber type classification in the adult corresponds with the expression of different MyHC isoforms; fibers classified as type I express $MyHC_{Slow}$, type IIa fibers express $MyHC_{2A}$, and type IIb fibers express $MyHC_{2B}$ and/or $MyHC_{2X}$.[45,55-57] Such histochemical classification of muscle fiber types is not possible during fetal and neonatal development. During this period, there are dramatic transitions in MyHC isoform expression, with a high incidence of co-expression of MyHC isoforms that precludes ready distinction of different muscle fiber types.[58-61] In the fetal mouse and rat DIAm, an embryonic MyHC isoform ($MyHC_{Emb}$) is predominantly expressed together with $MyHC_{Slow}$ and $MyHC_{2A}$. At or close to birth, the predominant isoform expression switches from an embryonic MyHC isoform ($MyHC_{Emb}$) to a neonatal ($MyHC_{Neo}$) isoform, together with $MyHC_{Slow}$ and $MyHC_{2A}$. Thereafter, $MyHC_{Neo}$ expression gradually disappears and is totally absent in the mouse and rat DIAm by D28. Expression of $MyHC_{2X}$ and $MyHC_{2B}$ isoforms emerges only after D14 in the mouse and rat DIAm, and the proportion of fibers expressing these isoforms increases until about D28, when the adult pattern of MyHC isoform expression is fully established.[62] This dramatic postnatal transition in MyHC isoform expression in the DIAm represents an important stage of muscle fiber differentiation, especially with respect to the development of mature contractile properties (see below). Beyond D28, the relative contribution of each MyHC isoform changes due to the disproportionate growth of DIAm fibers; for example, the growth of fibers expressing $MyHC_{2X}$ and $MyHC_{2B}$ is approximately two- to threefold greater than that of fibers expressing $MyHC_{Slow}$ and $MyHC_{2A}$ isoforms.[63,64] Based on the temporal associations between innervation and the major developmental events in myogenesis (see the following section), it would seem reasonable that the nervous system can either directly (e.g., activity, nerve traffic) or indirectly (e.g., secretion of trophic factors) influence DIAm development.[65] However, the precise mechanisms by which activation history and/or trophic factors influence DIAm development remain largely unknown.

The time course for developmental transitions in MyHC isoform expression in the DIAm is also influenced by the hormonal milieu (e.g., thyroid hormones, growth hormone, and IGF) surrounding the fibers. For example, MyHC expression is sensitive to thyroid hormone levels.[66,67] Nutritional status can also affect myogenesis and MyHC isoform expression.[63]

The determination of skeletal muscle fiber type has received considerable attention. Expression of class II histone de-acetylases (HDACs) may determine muscle fiber type by inhibiting the transcription factor MEF2.[68] MEF2 factors are required for the transcription of oxidative genes found in slow-twitch fibers.[69] HDAC activity is also regulated posttranslationally via ubiquitination and proteasome degradation.[70] Whether these mechanisms play a role in the developmental determination of muscle fiber type is still to be explored. We have examined MyHC mRNA expression during postnatal development of DIAm and found postnatal changes in mRNA and protein expression were not concordant for adult MyHC isoforms, suggesting that changes in MyHC expression in the developing rat DIAm are not driven solely by changes in mRNA expression.[62] Furthermore, myonuclear domain size (reflecting the volume of myoplasm under transcriptional control by a single myonucleus) increased postnatally as fibers increased in cross-sectional area, indicating that changes in transcriptional activity (although present) do not exclusively determine the postnatal growth of the DIAm.[71]

EMBRYOLOGIC ORIGIN

The DIAm derives from the pleuroperitoneal fold.[72] The pleuroperitoneal fold forms a partition separating the coelomic cavity into thoracic (superior; containing the developing heart and pericardium) and abdominal (inferior; containing the future peritoneal cavity) portions.[1] Growth of the embryonic axis causes a progressive caudal displacement of the pleuroperitoneal fold, with its anterior edge eventually becoming attached at the midthoracic level while its dorsal edge becomes attached at the lowest thoracic level. Committed myoblasts migrate within the pleuroperitoneal fold and eventually differentiate to form DIAm myotubes/myofibers. Coincident with myoblast migration, the phrenic nerves exit the cervical spinal cord following the septum transversum and migrating myoblasts. The exact target of phrenic nerve terminals is not clear, but the site of phrenic nerve contact seems to be consistent (located medially within the pleuroperitoneal fold) with nerve axons being surrounded by migrating myoblasts.[73,74] Phrenic motor axons start branching within the pleuroperitoneal fold as myoblasts radiate into the dorsocostal, sternocostal, and crural regions of the DIAm.[72] The mechanisms by which phrenic nerve axons are guided toward the primordial DIAm remain unclear. However, netrin-1 signaling via the Unc5c receptor has been implicated in motor axon guidance to the DIAm.[75]

INNERVATION

All regions of the DIAm are innervated by cervical spinal cord segments.[76-78] Innervation of the DIAm displays a somatotopic pattern, with the sternal and more ventral aspects of both costal and crural regions being innervated by phrenic motor neurons (~220 to 250 per side)[77,79,80] located in more rostral segments of the cervical spinal cord.[81] It remains unclear whether the somatotopic pattern of DIAm innervation develops before or after initial synapse formation (i.e., it could reflect either the pattern of phrenic nerve outgrowth or the location of myotubes/myofibers).

In the mouse, the phrenic nerve arrives at the developing DIAm by E11 (see Figs. 62.1 and 62.3), 2 days sooner than in the rat.[74] After arrival at the primordial DIAm, phrenic motor axons branch extensively, in close proximity with Schwann cells (see Figs. 62.3 and 62.4). Both Schwann cells and nerve terminals at this early stage display coated vesicles suggesting vesicular release (Fig. 62.5). A number of regulatory processes may be involved in guiding Schwann cell and phrenic axon terminal outgrowth, both with respect to the initial targeting to the pleuroperitoneal fold and the subsequent contact with myotubes/myofibers. These regulatory processes may involve components of the extracellular matrix, and/or the release of trophic factors and/or chemotactic substances. Schwann cell migration and branching may be essential to the outgrowth and branching of phrenic nerve terminals. Unfortunately, most of the available literature in this important area is limited by the fact that it is based on measurements of axonal outgrowth and branching using in vitro preparations. Some studies, however, suggest that perineurial sheaths may serve as a scaffold for Schwann cell growth and alignment, thus targeting motor axons toward muscle fibers.[82,83] Clearly, this is a complex integrated system where in vitro measurements may not accurately reflect in vivo conditions.

Trophic factors derived from motor axons may be important in determining DIAm development.[84] For instance, nerve-derived agrin is important not only for neuromuscular junction (NMJ) development but also for the development of

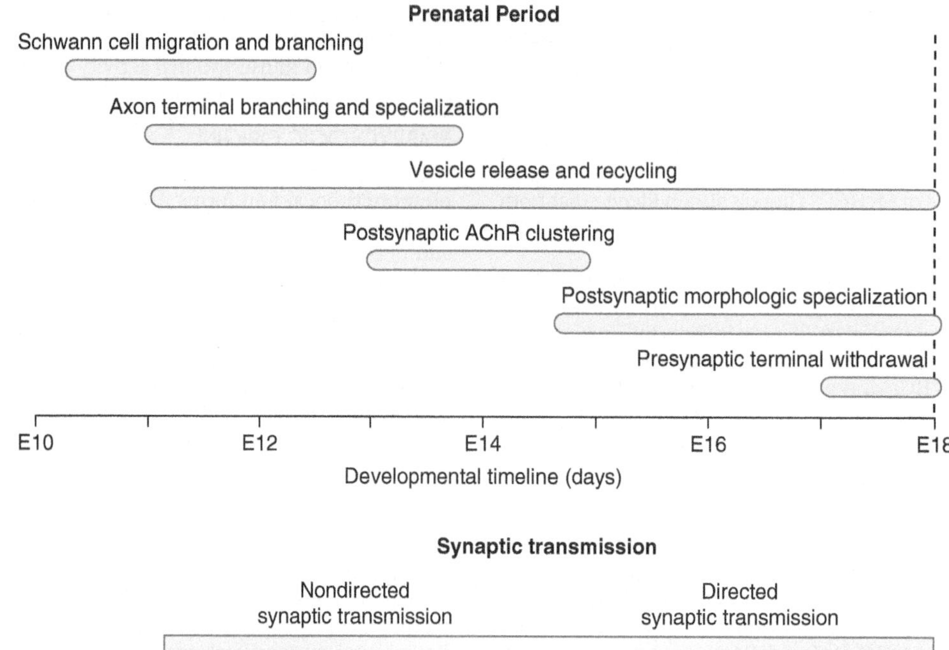

Fig. 62.3 Schematic demonstrating the timeline for major events in synapse formation in the mouse diaphragm muscle including differentiation of presynaptic and postsynaptic elements of neuromuscular junctions. Experimental evidence suggests that synaptic transmission is initially "non-directed" toward specific postsynaptic targets (i.e., cholinergic receptor clusters that define motor endplates). With cholinergic receptor clustering and differentiation of postsynaptic specializations, synaptic transmission becomes "directed" toward these targets.

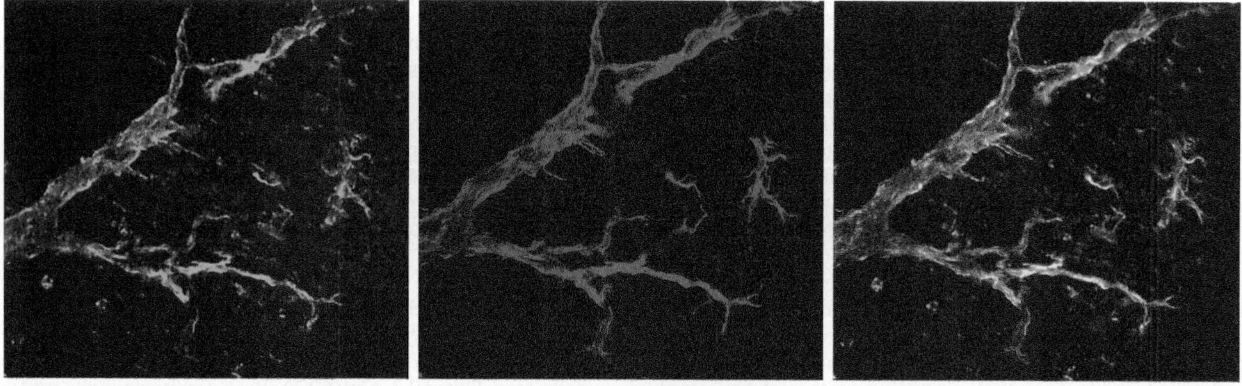

Fig. 62.4 Confocal photomicrographs displaying immunoreactivity for neurofilamin (NF - to mark branching nerve fibers) and S-100 (to mark Schwann cells) in the mouse diaphragm muscle at E12.5. Note the extensive branching and overlap of both nerve fibers and Schwann cells at this early age.

excitation-contraction coupling mechanisms in cultured human myotubes. Maturation of cultured myotubes including expression of ryanodine receptors and voltage-gated L-type Ca^{2+} channels is promoted by spinal cord explants as well as exogenous administration of neural agrin,[85,86] suggesting that soluble factors (rather than electrical activity) may be responsible for the effects of nerves on muscle development. Neuregulin (a member of the larger epidermal growth factor family)[87-90] is also expressed by motor neurons during embryonic and early postnatal development and may activate receptor tyrosine kinases of the ErbB family present in mature skeletal muscles,[91] including rat DIAm.[92] Neuregulin is known to induce acetylcholine receptor expression at embryonic via its effects on Schwann cells.[93] The relative importance of different trophic factor signaling pathways (e.g., agrin vs. neuregulin) remains to be determined.

Concurrent with the outgrowth of phrenic motor axons, there is also a progression of events on the postsynaptic side, with the expression and aggregation of cholinergic receptors. In the mouse DIAm, aggregation and clustering of cholinergic receptors is apparent ~E13 (see Figs. 62.3 and 62.6). The process of aggregation of cholinergic receptors has received considerable attention, and it is known that this process involves agrin secretion by the nerve terminal and incorporation into the basal lamina, with subsequent activation of MuSK receptors at the postsynaptic membrane and finally rapsyn-mediated cholinergic receptor clustering.[94-96] MuSK phosphorylation seems critical to cholinergic receptor clustering, as they are absent in MuSK double mutants and mice treated with inhibitory RNA designed to block MuSK transcription.[97] MuSK receptors show a gradient of expression in muscle fibers, being most abundant in their central regions where MuSK can undergo autoactivation,[98] leading to cholinergic receptor clustering in the absence of neural influence. In neighboring sections of the muscle fiber where MuSK is not as richly expressed, agrin released by motor axons can also lead to cholinergic receptor clustering.[99] This model for the formation of postsynaptic components of a NMJ can account for the apparent "targeting" of motor axons to "pre-formed" cholinergic clusters,[100,101] as well

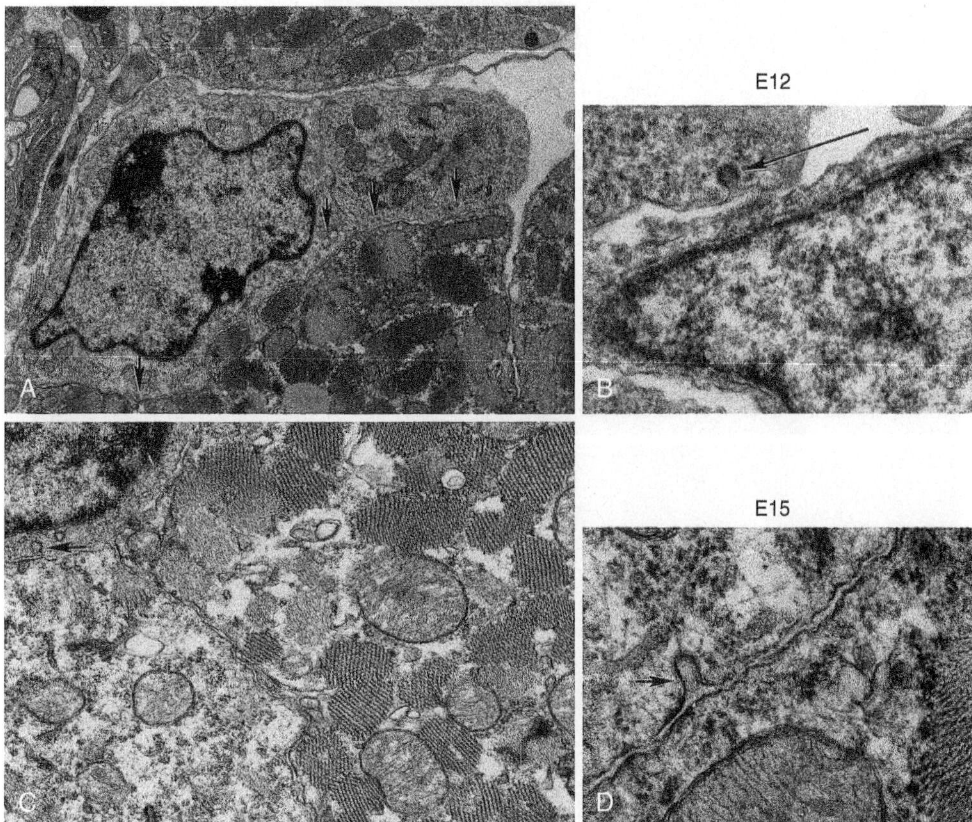

Fig. 62.5 Electron photomicrographs showing (A) the presence of coated vesicles *(arrows)* in both a nerve terminal and Schwann cell (noted by the presence of a distinct nucleus) and (B) an exocytotic vesicle at a nerve terminal in a mouse diaphragm muscle at E12. Evidence for nondirected vesicular release from both nerve terminals (C) and Schwann cells (D) continues through E15.

as the induction of new clusters by nerve-derived influences.[93] Following the aggregation of cholinergic receptors, there is a further specialization of the postsynaptic membrane with the formation of synaptic folds and differentiation of the complex NMJ structure characteristic of adult DIAm (see Figs. 62.3 and 62.7). Previously, we demonstrated that in the adult rat DIAm, NMJ morphology varies across different fiber types (Fig. 62.8), being far more complex in fibers expressing $MyHC_{2X}$ and MHX_{2B} isoforms as compared to fibers expressing $MyHC_{Slow}$ and $MyHC_{2A}$ isoforms.[102,103] NMJs are much smaller and morphologically far less complex in the fetal and neonatal DIAm compared to the adult (Fig. 62.9), but there is currently very little information regarding the mechanisms responsible for the development of fiber type-specific differences in NMJ structure.[104]

Initially, a single myotube/myofiber can be contacted by multiple motor neurons (polyneuronal innervation). Next, polyneuronal innervation disappears through the process of synapse elimination, which in the mouse and rat DIAm is complete by about D14 (see Figs. 62.1 and 62.10).[105-110] The process of synapse elimination is not fully understood. It has been suggested that there may be competition among motor neurons for target cell innervation depending on activity (Hebbian competition).[109,111,112] Accordingly, terminal synapses of more active motor neurons would persist at the expense of less active motor neurons. This theory is confounded by the fact that in adult muscle, motor units with the largest innervation ratio (i.e., number of muscle fibers innervated by a single motor neuron) are those that are least active (e.g., fast-fatigable motor units).[113-115] Thus, either the activity patterns of these motor neurons must change dramatically during development (transitioning from most to least active), or these motor neurons must initially innervate a greater number of muscle fibers to account for the subsequent greater loss of synaptic contacts (see Fig. 62.10). The pattern of activity (not total activity) and the secretion of so-called synaptotrophins or synaptotoxins may also contribute to the maintenance or elimination of synapses.[110] Another possibility is that muscle fibers use intracellular signals called *synaptomedins* to maintain contact with selected nerve terminals—this may or may not be dependent on differential activity.[116] Lastly, in *Drosophila*, a group of transmembrane proteins, Tenuerins (specifically Ten-a and Ten-m), interact pre- (Ten-A) and post-synaptically (Ten-m) impacting effective synaptic transmission.[117] Genetic knockout of Ten-A expression results in larger presynaptic boutons but a reduced number of boutons.[117] In contrast, knockout of Ten-m appears to primarily disrupt the postsynaptic spectrin cytoskeleton resulting in up to 70% disruption of the membranous subsynaptic reticulum, and an increased frequency of "ghost" boutons.[117] It is likely that a combination of mechanisms, some yet to be identified, is responsible for the final pattern of motor unit innervation. However, since differences in the innervation ratio exist across motor unit types, it is likely that the mechanisms underlying synapse elimination are linked to muscle fiber lineage and/or MyHC isoform expression. Ultimately, the motor unit composition may also be affected by on-going postnatal myogenesis and formation of new myotubes/myofibers that occurs until the third postnatal week in the rat and mouse DIAm.[63] The final innervation ratio of motor units is not established in the mouse and rat DIAm until about D21.

Fetal respiratory movements indicating intact inspiratory drive and functional synapses have been observed in a number of species, including humans. In the rat, fetal respiratory movements begin at about E17.[118] However, the onset of fetal respiratory movements does not necessarily denote the presence

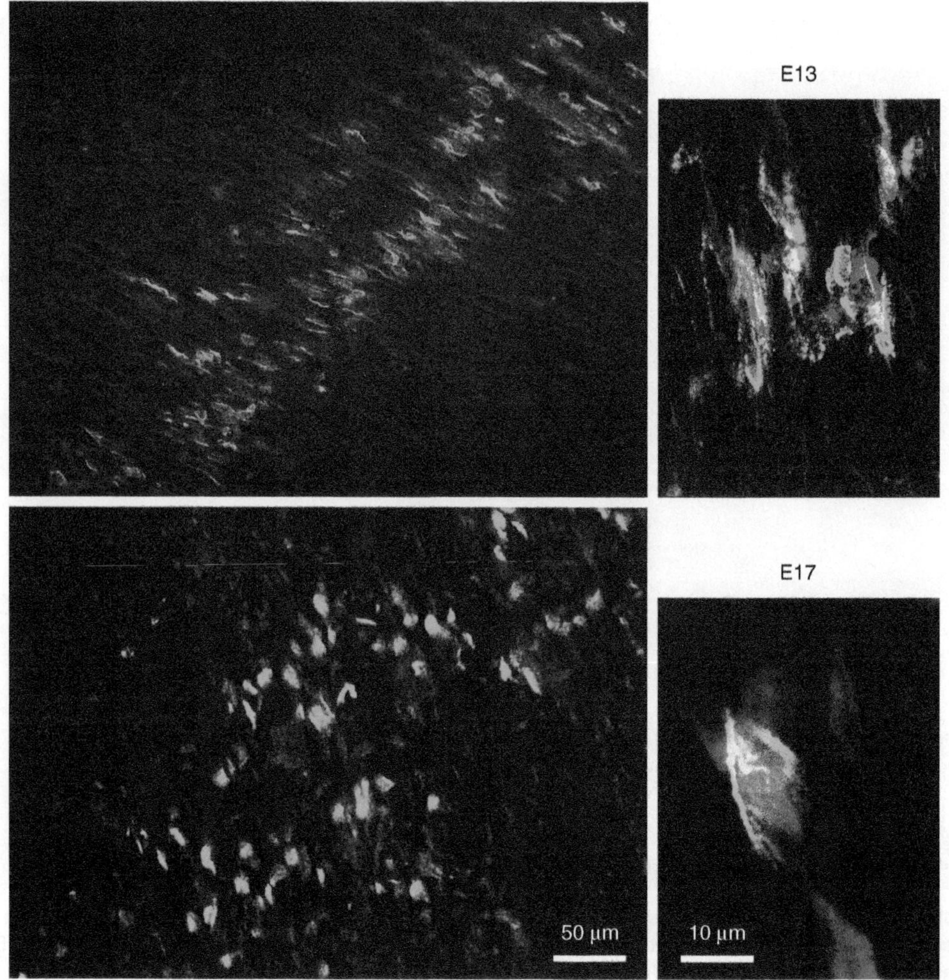

Fig. 62.6 Confocal photomicrographs displaying α-bungarotoxin (BTX) labeling (in green) of cholinergic receptors and neurofilamin (NF) labeling (in red) of phrenic nerve axons and nerve terminals in the mouse diaphragm muscle at E13 and E17. Note the more diffuse pattern of BTX staining at E13 compared to E17, indicating a progression toward the clustering of cholinergic receptors. Also note the greater overlap between nerve terminals (NF staining) and cholinergic receptors (BTX staining) at E17.

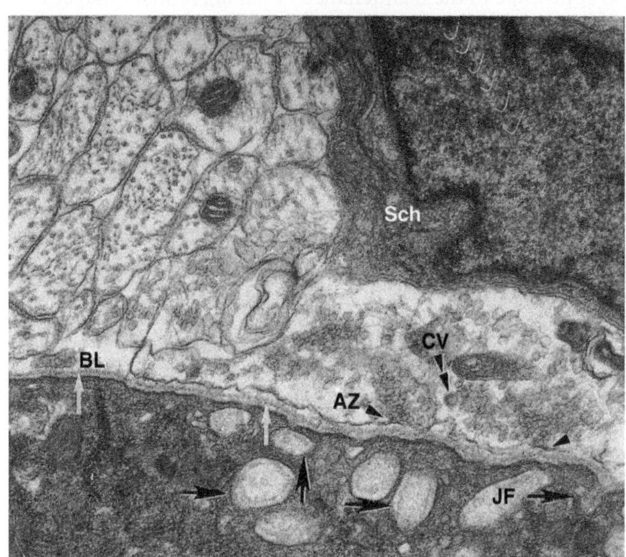

Fig. 62.7 Electron photomicrograph illustrating the presence of postsynaptic specializations (e.g., basal lamina—BL, white arrows, and junctional folds—JF, indicated by black *arrows*) at a neuromuscular junction in the mouse diaphragm muscle at E16. The electron micrograph also displays nerve terminals containing coated synaptic vesicles *(CV)* aggregating around active zones *(AZ)* and a Schwann cell *(Sch)*.

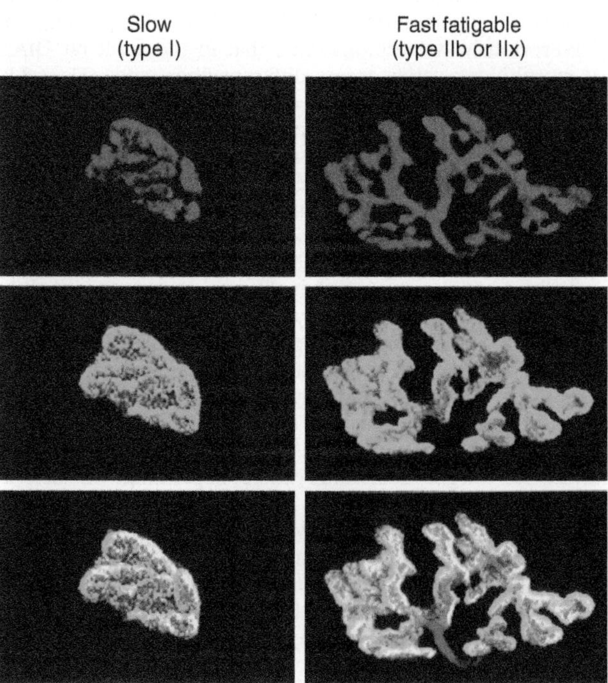

Fig. 62.8 Confocal photomicrographs of pre- *(red)* and postsynaptic *(green)* elements of neuromuscular junctions (NMJs) in the adult rat diaphragm muscle. Note differences in complexity and size of NMJs that depend on motor unit (muscle fiber) type.

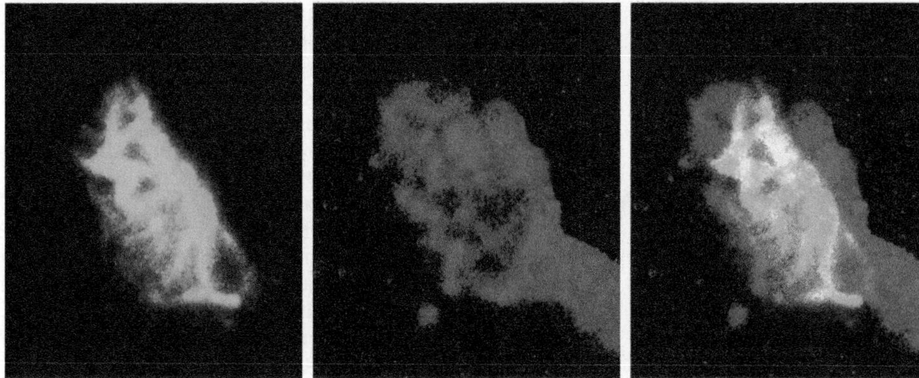

Fig. 62.9 Confocal photomicrograph showing the morphology of neuromuscular junctions (NMJs) in the mouse diaphragm muscle (DIAm) at E17. Note that in comparison to NMJs in the adult DIAm (see Fig. 62.8), NMJs at this age are substantially smaller and far less complex.

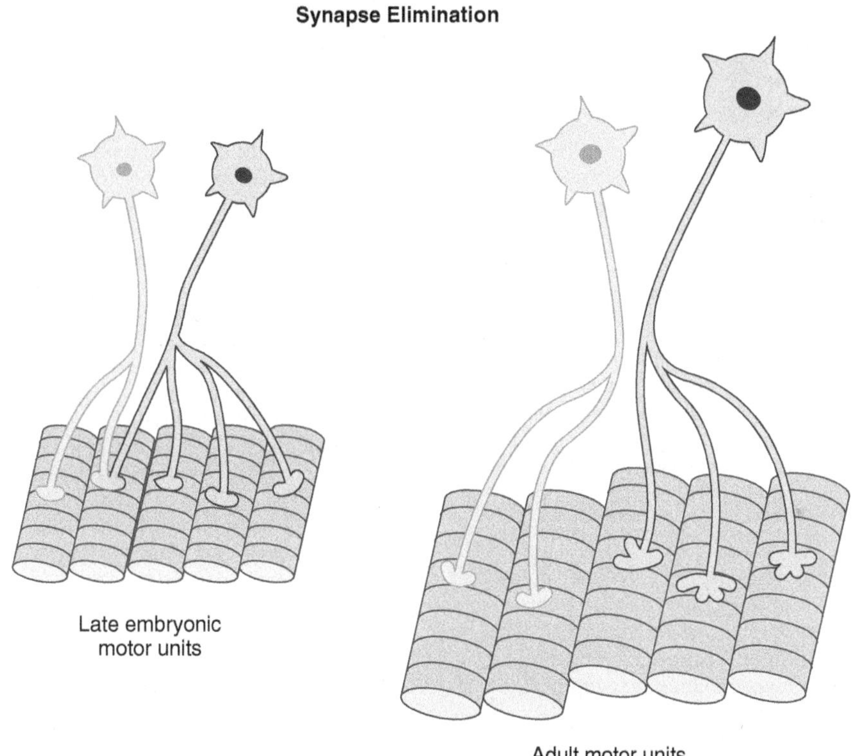

Fig. 62.10 Schematic illustrating the process of synapse elimination. It is thought that differential patterns of motor neuron activity lead to the selective withdrawal of motor axon terminals, which may be regulated by the secretion of synaptotrophins or synaptotoxins by the nerve terminal and/or production of synaptomedins within myofibers.

of functional synapses and excitation-contraction coupling in DIAm fibers. We found that intracellular Ca^{2+} and contractile responses could be elicited in the mouse DIAm by indirect nerve stimulation as early as E12.5 (Fig. 62.11). These intracellular Ca^{2+} and contractile responses were blocked by d-tubocurarine and α-bungarotoxin, indicating dependence on acetylcholine release and activation of cholinergic receptors. Yet, at this early age, synapses are only primordial at best, with no postsynaptic specialization and limited clustering of cholinergic receptors. These observations are consistent with the presence of coated vesicles and other indications of vesicular release (see Fig. 62.5). Myotubes/myofibers that are forming in the DIAm at this time also display the onset of sarcomeric organization necessary for a mechanical response (Figs. 62.12 and 62.13). Thus the nervous system appears to induce mechanical responses before well-defined synapses are present. Such mechanical responses may be important in the subsequent development of myofibers in the DIAm (e.g., sarcomeric organization and alignment).

Clearly, neuromuscular transmission in the fetal and neonatal DIAm is quite different from that of the adult muscle. In previous studies, it was shown that the neonatal rat DIAm is far more susceptible to neuromuscular transmission failure during repetitive activation than the adult.[119-122] Certainly, the increased susceptibility of the fetal and neonatal DIAm to neuromuscular transmission failure can be attributed, at least in part, to the more extensive branching of phrenic axons (due to polyneuronal innervation) and thus the greater likelihood of failure of action potential propagation at axonal branch points.[120,122-124] It is also likely that differences in the number of synaptic vesicles, presynaptic neurotransmitter release and/or consequent activation of cholinergic receptors all could account for the developmental differences in neuromuscular transmission failure.

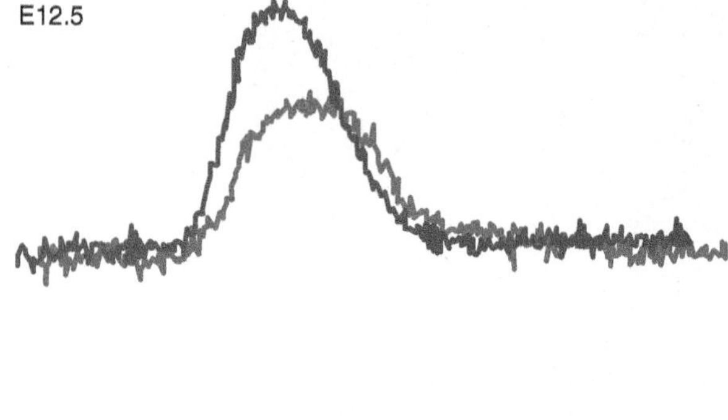

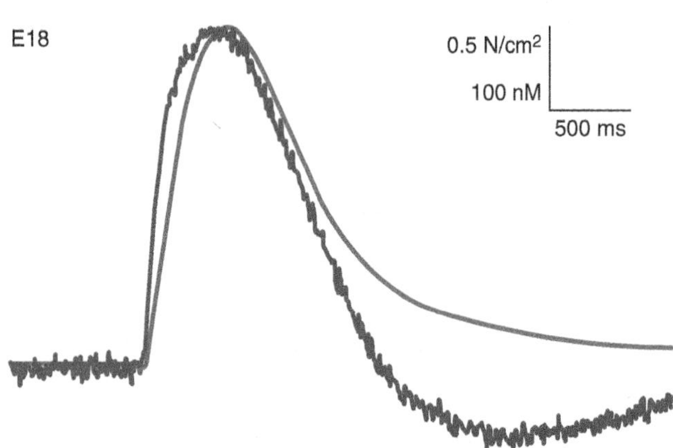

Fig. 62.11 Simultaneous measurement of force and intracellular Ca^{2+} responses to phrenic nerve stimulation in the mouse diaphragm muscle at E12.5 and E18. Myofibers mounted between force and length transducers in a flow-through chamber were loaded with Fluo-3AM. Phrenic nerve terminals were stimulated using low current short duration (0.1 ms) square wave pulses. Responses were blocked using d-tubocurarine (10 μM).

In the early postnatal DIAm, reduced spontaneous miniature endplate potential frequency and amplitude as well as evoked endplate potential amplitude compared to the adult are consistent with reduced neurotransmitter release and/or disproportionately smaller endplate regions (i.e., fewer cholinergic receptors).[119-121]

ACTIVITY-DEPENDENT DEVELOPMENTAL MOTOR NEURON DEATH

Developmental motor neuron death is influenced not only by descending input from the brain, but ascending input from target muscles, such as DIAm. This complex interplay shapes the final motor neuron number, and thus motor unit innervation ratio (i.e. number of muscle fibers innervated by a motor neuron), which may also influence motor neuron excitability (Henneman size principle). Early in embryonic development, a large pool of motor neurons exists.[125] Survival of these motor neurons is influenced by both the activity of the motor neuron and target muscle as well as a variety of trophic factors.[84,104,126] In turn, motor neuron and target muscle activity are influenced by the release of the neurotransmitters both at the periphery (acetylcholine) and in the CNS (excitatory and inhibitory). Important to note, key CNS neurotransmitters, glycine and gamma aminobutyric acid (GABA), are excitatory (depolarizing) during the embryonic stage rather than the inhibitory (hyperpolarizing) role they play in adults. This switch appears to be mediated by a transition in the expression of chloride co-transporters Na^+-K^+-Cl^- (NKCC1) and simultaneous up-regulation of the neuron-specific K^+-Cl^- co-transporter (KCC2).[127-130] The timing of this transition varies depending on location in the CNS, ranging from E16 to D15 in mice and rats with the transition for a respiratory system likely occurring around 2 weeks postnatal age in rats.[130-134]

Evidence for the excitatory to inhibitory switch in the effects of GABA and glycine on activity-dependent developmental motor neuron death is provided through work with mutant mice—specifically mice with GABA and/or glycine deficiencies. In the last trimester, E15.5 and E18 in mice, there is a profound developmental loss of motor neurons.[135] In mice lacking effective glycinergic (gephyrin mutant), GABAergic (GAD67) or both GABA and glycinergic neurotransmission (VGAT), increased developmental phrenic motor neuron death (decreased motor neuron survival)[136-138] is associated with increased motor neuron[139,140] and respiratory muscle[141] activity. In the gephyrin, GAD67 and VGAT mutants, the marked reduction in phrenic and hypoglossal motor neurons is contrasted with increased motor neuron survival in more rostral motor pools.[138,141,142] The marked difference between forelimb muscles and the diaphragm may reflect a rostral-caudal developmental progression in the "switch" of GABAergic and glycinergic receptors at motor neurons.

Clearly, any incidence of abnormal developmental motor neuron death has a profound impact on function later in life. Indeed, many animal models of motor neuron disease display abnormal motor neuron excitability prior to death of motor neurons.[143-145] In developmental conditions, such as individuals with cerebral palsy secondary to birth prematurity, birth occurs at a time critical to motor neuron development.[146] Interestingly, the hallmark definition of cerebral palsy includes a "nonprogressive disturbance of the developing fetal or infant brain,"[147] yet brain imaging alone is not predictive or diagnostic of cerebral palsy nor is brain imaging necessarily predictive of the severity of the spasticity or movement difficulty.[148-150] Therefore, it is plausible that at this critical time of development, abnormalities in motor neuron development may be occurring and contributing to the development of spasticity (hyperexcitability) and motor impairment seen later in infancy. Though not as well studied, there also appears to be impairment in the respiratory function that impacts the health and survival of individuals with cerebral palsy.[151-154] We are currently exploring this concept of abnormal developmental motor neuron death in spastic cerebral palsy and observe excessive loss of lumbar motor neurons in an animal model of hypertonia, the *spastic (spa)* mouse,[155] which has mutated glycine receptors. We have preliminary evidence suggesting that a similar reduction in phrenic motor neuron numbers also occur in *spa* mice. In both phrenic and lumbar motor neurons, these losses are disproportionately in the larger motor neurons,[155] likely to comprise FInt and FF motor units that innervate type IIx and or IIb muscle fibers.[1] The relative vulnerability of type FInt and FF motor neurons to loss in early onset hypertonia is strikingly similar to the vulnerability of these same motor neurons in aging[79] and motor neuron disease.[143,156-158] We theorize that individuals who have early onset hypertonia, including those with spastic cerebral palsy, have increased developmental motor neuron death and an increased innervation ratio. Smaller sizes of remaining motor neurons will result in increased motor neuron excitability, as described by the Henneman size principle. Both increased excitability and altered innervation ratio would contribute to spasticity and movement disorder.[159] Similar to observations in aging[160-162] and motor neuron disease,[163,164] we observe neuromuscular transmission failure and reduced DIAm specific force in *spa* mice, consistent with a selective loss of FInt and FF units. We are currently investigating whether the timing of these abnormalities coincides with the switch of GABA and glycine from excitatory to inhibitory.

MUSCLE FIBER CONTRACTILE PROPERTIES

EXCITATION-CONTRACTION COUPLING

As mentioned, fetal respiratory movements are present in the rat at about E17; but this does not necessarily reflect the

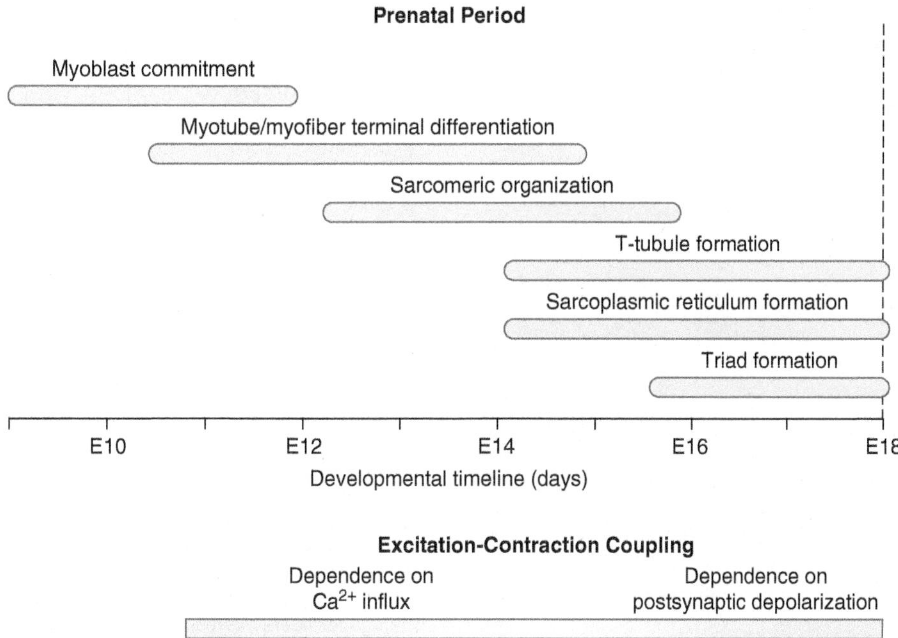

Fig. 62.12 Schematic demonstrating the timeline for major embryologic events in the formation of myotubes/myofibers in the mouse diaphragm muscle. It is likely that before the differentiation of distinct T-tubules, triads, and sarcoplasmic reticulum, excitation-contraction coupling is mediated primarily via Ca^{2+} influx, whereas in later embryonic stages, mechanisms underlying excitation-contraction coupling resemble those in the adult.

onset of excitation-contraction coupling. In fact, intracellular Ca^{2+} and contractile responses are elicited in the mouse DIAm by indirect nerve stimulation as early as E12.5 (see Fig. 62.11), indicating excitation-contraction coupling. These early mechanical responses are coincident with the earliest formation of myotubes/myofibers, expression of contractile proteins, and presence of rudimentary sarcomeres (see Figs. 62.12 and 62.13). However, the coordination of these events with the emergence of other structures important in excitation-contraction coupling (e.g., functional synapses, T-tubules, triads, and sarcoplasmic reticulum) remains obscure. A number of studies have focused on the embryologic development of the sarcoplasmic reticulum, T-tubules, and triads and their association with myofibrillar organization.[165-175] In ultrastructural studies, we observed the presence of T-tubules, triads, and sarcoplasmic reticulum in the mouse DIAm at E14 (Fig. 62.14). Takekura and colleagues also presented ultrastructural and confocal evidence for the presence of T-tubules, triads, and sarcoplasmic reticulum in the embryologic mouse DIAm but only as early as E17.[176] These investigators reported the consistent presence of ryanodine receptor clustering at E15 in the mouse DIAm, suggesting the presence of sarcoplasmic reticulum at this early developmental time point. Interestingly, knockout studies indicate that the apposition of sarcoplasmic reticulum to either plasmalemma or T-tubules occurs in the absence of ryanodine receptors and/or L-type Ca^{2+} channels (dihydropyridine receptors), despite the lack of functional activation in these mutants.[174,177,178] However, functional Ca^{2+} release is necessary for normal muscle development. Clearly, further studies are needed to elucidate the maturation of the excitation-contraction apparatus and its function during development.

ASSOCIATION OF CONTRACTILE PROPERTIES WITH FIBER TYPE AND/OR MYHC ISOFORM EXPRESSION

It is now well established that mechanical properties of skeletal muscle fibers correlate with fiber type and MyHC isoform composition.[45,48,179-185] In the rat and mouse DIAm, fibers that express $MyHC_{2X}$ and/or $MyHC_{2B}$ display faster maximum unloaded shortening velocities (V_o) (Fig. 62.15) and greater specific forces (i.e., force generated per muscle cross-sectional area) (Fig. 62.16) than fibers expressing $MyHC_{Slow}$ and $MyHC_{2A}$. In the adult rat DIAm, the greater maximum specific force of fibers expressing $MyHC_{2X}$ and/or $MyHC_{2B}$ is at least partially explained by differences in MyHC protein content per half-sarcomere (i.e., greater number of cross bridges in parallel) as well as the force per cross bridge (see Fig. 62.16).[184-187] Similarly, the faster V_o of adult rat DIAm fibers expressing $MyHC_{2X}$ and/or $MyHC_{2B}$ is partially explained by faster cross bridge cycling kinetics and a correspondingly higher rate of ATP consumption.[48,188]

During fetal and early postnatal development, DIAm fiber contractile properties change dramatically, corresponding with the transitions in MyHC isoform composition that occur. For example, from E15 to ~D28, the specific force generated by the rat DIAm increases almost 20-fold (Fig. 62.17),[61,63,64,67,189-192] together with an increase in the relative expression of fast MyHC isoforms and MyHC content per half-sarcomere.[61,64,185,189] The lower specific force of fetal and neonatal DIAm is due both to a lower MyHC content per half-sarcomere as well as reduced force per cross bridge.[185] During the same developmental period, V_o of the DIAm increases by over 6-fold (Fig. 62.18),[64,67,190,192] again corresponding with the increase in the relative expression of fast MyHC isoforms.[64] The slower V_o of fetal and neonatal DIAm reflects the slower rate of ATP consumption of these fibers, which predominantly express $MyHC_{Emb}$ and $MyHC_{Neo}$ isoforms (Fig. 62.19).[61] With an increase in both force and velocity, there is an accompanying increase in maximum power output and work performance of the rat DIAm from birth to D28.[192] However, as power output and work performance of the DIAm increase postnatally, fatigue resistance to repeated activation declines.[191,192]

While it is clear that the contractile properties of DIAm undergo profound shifts during early development that correspond to the transitions in MyHC isoform expression, the signals driving these changes are not yet known. Changes in contractile properties induced by pathophysiologic conditions may not always be reflected by changes in MyHC isoform

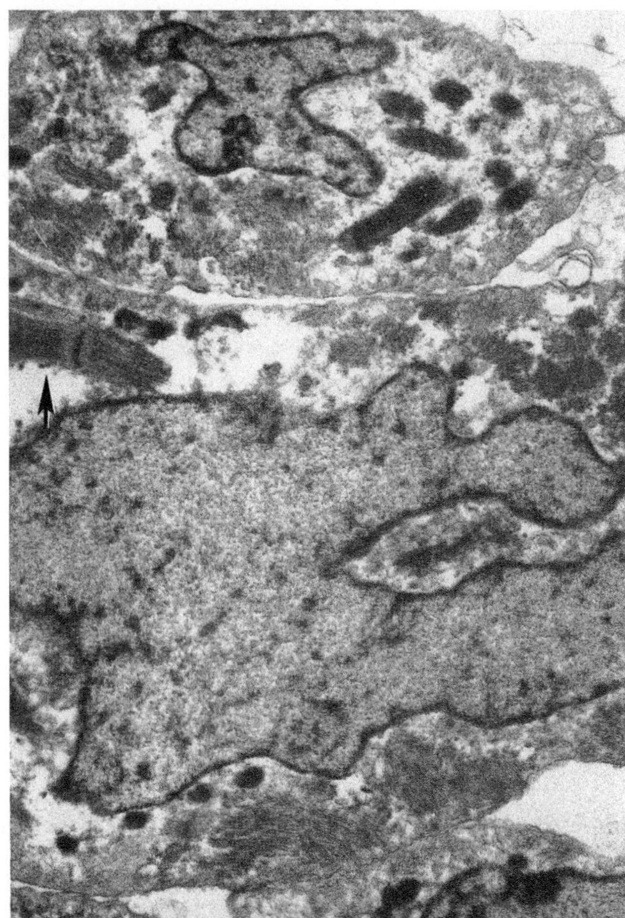

Fig. 62.13 Electron photomicrograph displaying rudimentary sarcomeric organization (indicated by an *arrow*) in the mouse diaphragm muscle at E12.5.

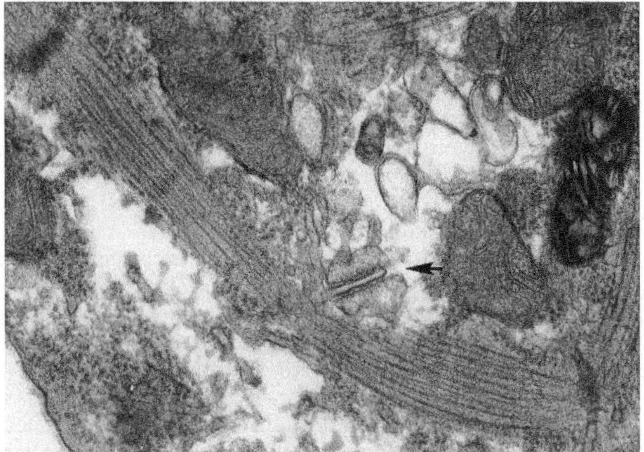

Fig. 62.14 Electron photomicrograph showing the presence of a triad (indicated by an *arrow*) in the mouse diaphragm muscle at E14.

composition alone. For example, with perinatal hypothyroidism there is a dramatic reduction in maximum specific force and a slowing of V_o in the rat DIAm that cannot be fully attributed to the moderate changes in MyHC isoform composition.[67] Similarly, following unilateral denervation of the DIAm at D7, there is a marked reduction in maximum specific force and a slowing of V_o that are not predicted from the slight changes in MyHC isoform composition. As mentioned above, the changes in specific force

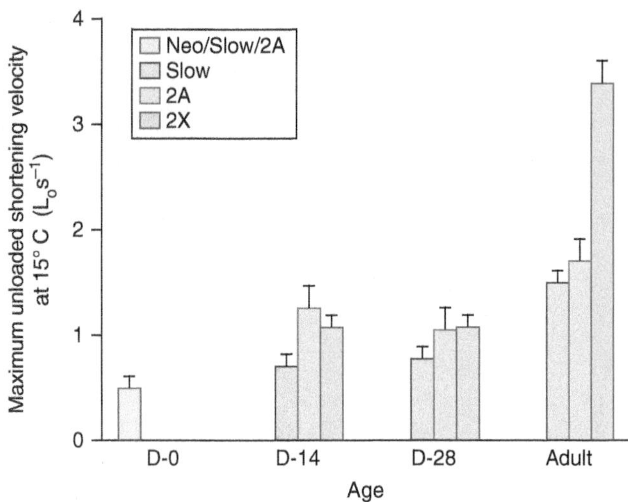

Fig. 62.15 Maximum unloaded shortening velocity of single triton-X permeabilized rat diaphragm muscle fibers expressing different myosin heavy chain (MyHC) isoforms. Maximum unloaded shortening velocity was not solely dependent on MyHC isoform expression but increased with age for fibers expressing the same MyHC isoform.

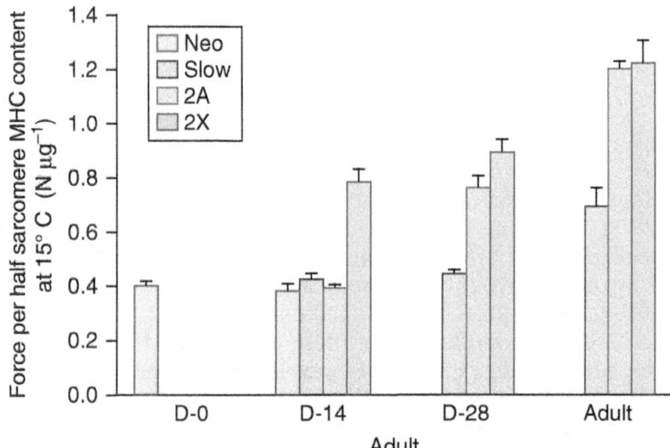

Fig. 62.16 Maximum force of single triton-X permeabilized rat diaphragm muscle fibers expressing different myosin heavy chain (MyHC) isoforms was normalized for MyHC content per half-sarcomere. Maximum force per half-sarcomere MyHC content (equivalent to force per cross bridge) varied with MyHC isoform as well as across age groups for a given isoform.

may reflect the total MyHC content per half-sarcomere (i.e., number of cross bridges in parallel) of DIAm fibers rather than MyHC isoform expression per se.[184] The slowing of V_o is more difficult to explain. Clearly, these results indicate that cross bridge cycling kinetics can be slowed independent of the MyHC isoform expressed. It is possible that these pathophysiologic conditions affect actomyosin ATPase activity of the myosin S-1 fragment or that there is an increased internal resistance to shortening. In support, we observed that following unilateral denervation of the adult rat DIAm maximum isometric ATP consumption rate was reduced independent of MyHC isoform expression.[193]

MYHC ISOFORM EXPRESSION AND CROSS BRIDGE CYCLING KINETICS IN SINGLE MUSCLE FIBERS

In the original model of muscle contraction proposed by Huxley,[194,195] cross bridges cycle between two functional states: a force-generating state, in which cross bridges are strongly attached to actin, and a nonforce-generating state, in which cross bridges are detached from actin. The transitions between the two

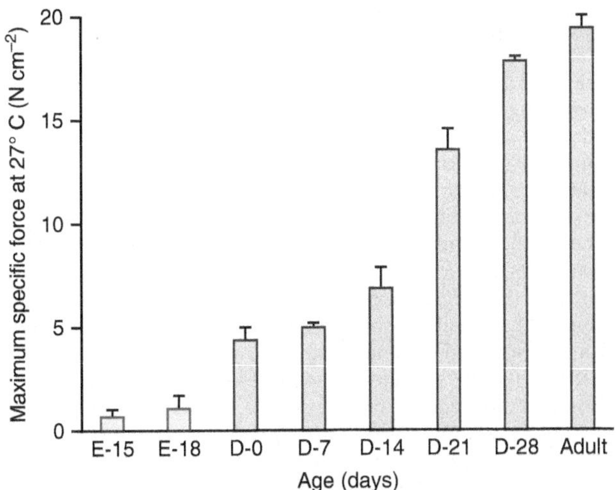

Fig. 62.17 Developmental changes in maximum specific force (force per cross-sectional area) of rat diaphragm muscle. Maximum specific force increases almost 20-fold from E15 to adulthood.

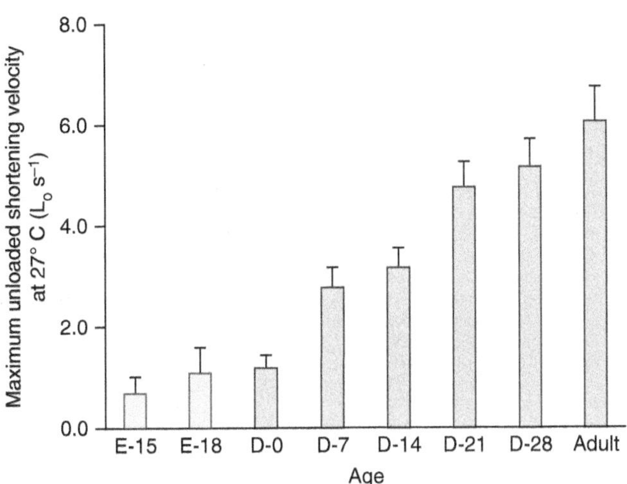

Fig. 62.18 Developmental changes in maximum unloaded shortening velocity (expressed as L_o s^{-1}) of the rat diaphragm muscle. Maximum unloaded shortening velocity increases more than 6-fold from E15 to adulthood.

primary functional states of cross bridges are described by two apparent rate constants: one for cross bridge attachment (f_{app}) and the second for cross bridge detachment (g_{app}). An increase in isometric force with increasing myoplasmic Ca^{2+} is explained by the recruitment of cross bridges into the force-generating state (described by f_{app}). The transition of cross bridges from force-generating to nonforce-generating states (described by g_{app}) requires the hydrolysis of ATP (actomyosin ATPase). Thus, in the Huxley model, the transduction of chemical to mechanical energy is implicit. Brenner proposed an analytical framework based on Huxley's two-state model of cross bridge cycling in which this transduction of chemical to mechanical energy is more explicitly described.[196-198] In the Brenner analytical framework, the steady-state fraction of strongly-bound cross bridges in the force generating state (α_{fs}) is given by:

$$\alpha_{fs} = f_{app}/(f_{app} + g_{app})$$

The isometric force generated by a muscle fiber is then described by the following relationship:

$$\text{Isometric force} = n \cdot F\,\alpha_{fs}$$

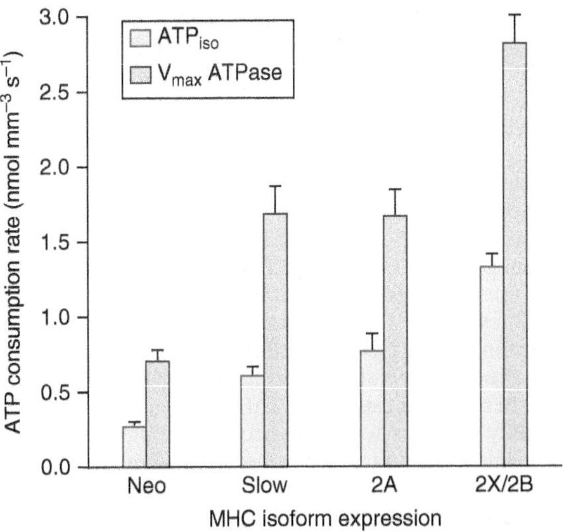

Fig. 62.19 Maximum velocity of the actomyosin ATPase reaction (Vmax ATPase) and maximum isometric ATP consumption rate (ATPiso) of the rat diaphragm muscle fibers expressing different MyHC isoforms. For each fiber type, Vmax ATPase was greater than ATPiso indicating substantial reserve capacity for ATP consumption. Although Vmax ATPase and ATPiso varied across MyHC isoforms and with age, the reserve capacity for ATP consumption remained relatively constant.

where n is the number of cross bridges in parallel per half-sarcomere, and F is the mean force per cross bridge in the force-generating state. Assuming the hydrolysis of one ATP molecule during each cross bridge cycle, isometric ATP consumption rate (actomyosin ATPase activity) is described by the following relationship:

$$\text{ATPase} = n \cdot b \cdot g_{app} \cdot \alpha_{fs}$$

where b is the number of half sarcomeres within the fiber. At maximal Ca^{2+} activation, where α_{fs} remains constant, actomyosin ATPase activity is directly proportional to g_{app}.

Previously, we employed a quantitative histochemical procedure to determine the maximum velocity of the actomyosin ATPase reaction (V_{max} ATPase) in DIAm fibers expressing different MyHC isoforms.[48,188,199] Fibers expressing $MyHC_{2X}$ and $MyHC_{2B}$ have higher V_{max} ATPase compared to fibers expressing $MyHC_{Slow}$ and $MyHC_{2A}$. To determine the ATP consumption rate of single permeabilized rat DIAm fibers during maximum isometric activation (ATP_{iso}), we used an NADH-linked fluorometric procedure.[48,188,193] ATP_{iso} was 30% to 45% lower than V_{max} ATPase, but the dependence on MyHC isoform expression was still present, being highest in fibers expressing $MyHC_{2X}$ and $MyHC_{2B}$ and lowest in fibers expressing $MyHC_{Slow}$ and $MyHC_{2A}$. This reflects a reserve capacity for ATP consumption in DIAm fibers, which is consistent with the well-known fact that ATP consumption rate increases in proportion to work.[200,201] Differences in a reserve capacity for ATP consumption may account, at least in part, for differences in fatigability among DIAm fibers.[48,188] We have shown that the postnatal transition from $MyHC_{Neo}$ to adult fast MyHC isoform expression in rat DIAm fibers is accompanied by an increase in V_{max} ATPase and ATP_{iso} (see Fig. 62.19).

MyHC ISOFORM EXPRESSION AND Ca^{2+} SENSITIVITY OF MUSCLE FIBERS

In skeletal muscle fibers, force generation depends on myoplasmic [Ca^{2+}]. The dependency of force generation of myoplasmic [Ca^{2+}] is usually expressed as the force/pCa (-log [Ca^{2+}]) relationship.

The force/pCa relationship of rat DIAm fibers expressing $MyHC_{Slow}$ is shifted leftward compared to fibers expressing adult fast MyHC isoforms,[183] consistent with greater Ca^{2+} sensitivity of $MyHC_{Slow}$-expressing DIAm fibers.[202-205]

It is widely recognized that in skeletal muscle, Ca^{2+} binding to the regulatory protein troponin C (TnC) underlies the dependency of force on myoplasmic [Ca^{2+}]. Ca^{2+} binding to TnC may simply act to increase the availability of myosin binding sites on actin and thus increase the probability of cross bridge formation. Different isoforms of TnC from fast (TnC-f) and slow (TnC-s) muscle fibers have different numbers of regulatory binding sites for Ca^{2+} (2 for TnC-f vs. 1 for TnC-s) and different binding affinities for Ca^{2+}. These differences in TnC isoforms may underlie the fiber type differences in force/pCa relationships. The role of other troponin subunits (TnI or TnT) in regulating muscle contractility is not as well understood, although both slow and fast isoforms exist and in agreement with TnC findings, fibers containing slow TnI and TnT have higher Ca^{2+} sensitivity than fast Tn-containing fibers.[206]

FUNCTIONAL IMPLICATIONS OF DEVELOPMENTAL CHANGES IN MECHANICAL PERFORMANCE OF THE DIAM

From the first neonatal breath onward, the DIAm sustains ventilation for the duration of the life span. However, DIAm mechanical performance changes during postnatal development of diaphragm motor units and the concurrent maturation of other structures. For example, following the maturation of limb muscles and the advent of locomotor behaviors the ventilatory demand on DIAm increases dramatically. In addition, DIAm must be capable of meeting the increased range of functional demands that coincide with postnatal development.[104] In addition, compliance of the lung and chest wall changes markedly during early development. The neonatal lung is stiffer due to greater alveolar recoil, which is offset by expression of surfactant, while the chest and abdominal walls are more compliant. As a result, the DIAm must generate greater relative intrathoracic pressures to produce a given level of inspiratory airflow and tidal volume. Yet, the neonatal DIAm generates much lower maximum tetanic force (Fig. 62.17) and has a much slower maximum unloaded shortening velocity (Fig. 62.18) compared to the adult. Thus, the functional reserve capacity of the neonatal DIAm is greatly reduced, and a far greater fraction of maximum power output must be recruited to accomplish ventilation. Polyneuronal innervation of DIAm fibers may be particularly important as a safeguard strategy to accomplish greater fractional recruitment of DIAm motor units. As synapse elimination proceeds, more selective recruitment of DIAm motor units becomes possible, coinciding with the increased range of functions required of the DIAm. In addition, during early postnatal expression of $MyHC_{2X}$ and $MyHC_{2B}$ isoforms in DIAm fibers increases overall functional range, but at the expense of lower energy-efficiency and greater susceptibility to fatigue.[4,6] It is likely that DIAm fibers expressing $MyHC_{2X}$ and $MyHC_{2B}$ isoforms are recruited only during expulsive maneuvers that require high force output and are of short duration. These maneuvers may be less necessary in the neonates, with common responses to tracheal obstruction being swallowing, apnea, gagging, or laryngeal closure rather than coughing, which is extremely rare.[207] The absence of such functional reserve and inadequate airway defense maneuvers may underlie increased neonatal susceptibility to aspiration, asphyxiation, and sudden infant death syndrome. Clearly, greater attention should be focused on the integrative aspects of DIAm development, and it will be important to place the genetic regulation of myogenesis and changing innervation patterns of the DIAm in this more physiologic context.

CONCLUSION

- The DIAm is the major inspiratory muscle in mammals, appearing rather late in evolution. Other vertebrates use different means of ventilation.
- The DIAm has a common embryologic origin in the pleuroperitoneal fold, contrasting traditional views of DIAm development that called for multiple sites of origin.
- The multiple anatomic origin and insertion sites of the DIAm reflect its major function in inspiration. The DIAm is also involved in several nonventilatory motor behaviors such as coughing, defecation, emesis, micturition, parturition, sneezing, vocalization, and weight lifting.
- MRFs function as molecular switches initiating myogenesis.
- Terminal differentiation of myoblasts results in multinucleated myotubes and myofibers that express the contractile protein machinery necessary for force generation.
- Motor unit properties are established postnatally in a relatively short period. Synapse elimination, loss of polyneuronal innervation, and motor neuron pruning contribute to the establishment of a motor unit innervation ratio.
- The diversity of muscle fiber types (e.g., slow-twitch fatigue-resistant to fast-twitch fatigable) appears postnatally at a time of rapid muscle fiber growth.

A complete reference list is available at www.ExpertConsult.com. 

SELECT REFERENCES

4. Sieck GC. Neural control of the inspiratory pump. *NIPS (News Physiol Sci)*. 1991;6:260-264.
48. Sieck GC, Han YS, Prakash YS, et al. Cross-bridge cycling kinetics, actomyosin ATPase activity and myosin heavy chain isoforms in skeletal and smooth respiratory muscles. *Comp Biochem Physiol*. 1998;119:435-450.
61. Watchko JF, Daood MJ, Sieck GC. Myosin heavy chain transitions during development. Functional implications for the respiratory musculature. *Comp Biochem Physiol*. 1998;119:459-470.
62. Geiger PC, Bailey JP, Mantilla CB, et al. Mechanisms underlying myosin heavy chain expression during development of the rat diaphragm muscle. *J Appl Physiol*. 2006;101:1546-1555.
64. Johnson BD, Wilson LE, Zhan WZ, et al. Contractile properties of the developing diaphragm correlate with myosin heavy chain phenotype. *J Appl Physiol*. 1994;77:481-487.
65. Sieck GC, Zhan WZ. Denervation alters myosin heavy chain expression and contractility of developing rat diaphragm muscle. *J Appl Physiol*. 2000;89:1106-1113.
67. Sieck GC, Wilson LE, Johnson BD, et al. Hypothyroidism alters diaphragm muscle development. *J Appl Physiol*. 1996;81:1965-1972.
71. Mantilla CB, Sill RV, Aravamudan B, et al. Developmental effects on myonuclear domain size of rat diaphragm fibers. *J Appl Physiol*. 2008;104:787-794.
74. Greer JJ, Allan DW, Martin-Caraballo M, et al. An overview of phrenic nerve and diaphragm muscle development in the perinatal rat. *J Appl Physiol*. 1999;86:779-786.
79. Fogarty MJ, Omar TS, Zhan WZ, et al. Phrenic motor neuron loss in aged rats. *J Neurophysiol*. 2018;119:1852-1862.
80. Prakash YS, Mantilla CB, Zhan WZ, et al. Phrenic motoneuron morphology during rapid diaphragm muscle growth. *J Appl Physiol*. 2000;89:563-572.
84. Mantilla CB, Sieck GC. Trophic factor expression in phrenic motor neurons. *Respir Physiol Neurobiol*. 2008;164:252-262.
96. Sanes JR, Lichtman JW. Induction, assembly, maturation and maintenance of a postsynaptic apparatus. *Nat Rev Neurosci*. 2001;2:791-805.
102. Prakash YS, Miller SM, Huang M, et al. Morphology of diaphragm neuromuscular junctions on different fibre types. *J Neurocytol*. 1996;25:88-100.
103. Mantilla CB, Rowley KL, Fahim MA, et al. Synaptic vesicle cycling at type-identified diaphragm neuromuscular junctions. *Muscle Nerve*. 2004;30:774-783.
104. Mantilla CB, Sieck GC. Key aspects of phrenic motoneuron and diaphragm muscle development during the perinatal period. *J Appl Physiol*. 2008;104:1818-1827.
105. Bennett MR, Pettigrew AG. The formation of synapses in striated muscle during development. *J Physiol*. 1974;241:515-545.
107. Brown MC, Jansen JKS, Van Essen D. Polyneuronal innervation of skeletal muscle in new-born rats and its elimination during maturation. *J Physiol*. 1976;261:387-422.
108. Redfern P. Neuromuscular transmission in new-born rats. *J Physiol*. 1970;209:701-709.
114. Fournier M, Sieck GC. Mechanical properties of muscle units in the cat diaphragm. *J Neurophysiol*. 1988;59:1055-1066.

116. Balice-Gordon RJ, Lichtman JW. In vivo observations of pre- and postsynaptic changes during the transition from multiple to single innervation at developing neuromuscular junctions. *J Neurosci*. 1993;13:834–855.
120. Fournier M, Alula M, Sieck GC. Neuromuscular transmission failure during postnatal development. *Neurosci Lett*. 1991;125:34–36.
122. Sieck GC, Prakash YS. Fatigue at the neuromuscular junction. Branch point vs. presynaptic vs. postsynaptic mechanisms. *Adv Exp Med Biol*. 1995;384: 83–100.
123. Krnjevic K, Miledi R. Failure of neuromuscular propagation in rats. *J Physiol*. 1958;140:440–461.
124. Krnjevic K, Miledi R. Presynaptic failure of neuromuscular propagation in rats. *J Physiol*. 1959;149:1–22.
135. Lance-Jones C. Motoneuron cell death in the developing lumbar spinal cord of the mouse. *Dev Brain Res*. 1982;4:473–479.
137. Fogarty MJ, Smallcombe KL, Yanagawa Y, et al. Genetic deficiency of GABA differentially
139. Fogarty MJ, Kanjhan R, Bellingham MC, et al. Glycinergic neurotransmission: a potent regulator of embryonic motor neuron dendritic morphology and synaptic plasticity. *J Neurosci*. 2016;36:80–87.
146. Brandenburg JE, Fogarty MJ, Sieck GC. A critical evaluation of current concepts in cerebral palsy. *Physiology*. 2019;34:216–229.
155. Brandenburg JE, Gransee HM, Fogarty MJ, et al. Differences in lumbar motor neuron pruning in an animal model of early onset spasticity. *J Neurophysiol*. 2018;120:601–609.
160. Greising SM, Mantilla CB, Gorman BA, et al. Diaphragm muscle sarcopenia in aging mice. *Exp Gerontol*. 2013;48:881–887.
161. Fogarty MJ, Gonzalez Porras MA, Mantilla CB, et al. Diaphragm neuromuscular transmission failure in aged rats. *J Neurophysiol*. 2019;122:93–104.
162. Khurram OU, Fogarty MJ, Sarrafian TL, et al. Impact of aging on diaphragm muscle function in male and female Fischer 344 rats. *Physiol Rep*. 2018;6:e13786.
172. Franzini-Armstrong C, Jorgensen AO. Structure and development of E-C coupling units in skeletal muscle. *Annu Rev Physiol*. 1994;56:509–534.
182. Sieck GC, Prakash YS. Cross bridge kinetics in respiratory muscles. *Eur Respir J*. 1997;10:2147–2158.
183. Geiger PC, Cody MJ, Sieck GC. Force-calcium relationship depends on myosin heavy chain and troponin isoforms in rat diaphragm muscle fibers. *J Appl Physiol*. 1999;87:1894–1900.
184. Geiger PC, Cody MJ, Macken RL, et al. Maximum specific force depends on myosin heavy chain content in rat diaphragm muscle fibers. *J Appl Physiol*. 2000;89:695–703.
185. Geiger PC, Cody MJ, Macken RL, et al. Mechanisms underlying increased force generation by rat diaphragm muscle fibers during development. *J Appl Physiol*. 2001;90:380–388.
186. Geiger PC, Cody MJ, Macken RL, et al. Effect of unilateral denervation on maximum specific force in rat diaphragm muscle fibers. *J Appl Physiol*. 2001;90:1196–1204.
187. Geiger PC, Cody MJ, Han YS, et al. Effects of hypothyroidism on maximum specific force in rat diaphragm muscle fibers. *J Appl Physiol*. 2002;92:1506–1514.
190. Sieck GC, Zhan WZ. Denervation alters myosin heavy chain expression and contractility of developing rat diaphragm muscle. *J Appl Physiol*. 2000;89: 1106–1113.
191. Watchko JF, Sieck GC. Respiratory muscle fatigue resistance relates to myosin phenotype and SDH activity during development. *J Appl Physiol*. 1993;75:1341–1347.
192. Zhan WZ, Watchko JF, Prakash YS, et al. Isotonic contractile and fatigue properties of developing rat diaphragm muscle. *J Appl Physiol*. 1998;84:1260–1268.
193. Sieck GC, Zhan WZ, Han YS, et al. Effect of denervation on ATP consumption rate of diaphragm muscle fibers. *J Appl Physiol*. 2007;103:858–866.
194. Huxley AF, Simmons RM. Proposed mechanism of force generation in striated muscle. *Nature*. 1971;233:533–538.
196. Brenner B. Kinetics of the crossbridge cycle derived from measurements of force, rate of force development and isometric ATPase. *J Muscle Res Cell Motil*. 1986;7:75–76.
198. Brenner B, Eisenberg E. Rate of force generation in muscle: correlation with actomyosin ATPase activity in solution. *Proc Natl Acad Sci USA*. 1986;83:3542–3546.

Mechanics of Breathing 63

Jacopo P. Mortola

INTRODUCTION

The human infant has at least two important advantages over the adult in the evaluation of respiratory mechanical function. First, the infant, like newborn mammals of many species, is often asleep and does not immediately react to gently performed maneuvers. Hence, a maneuver consisting of a very brief occlusion of the airways during spontaneous breathing is often used in the evaluation of the mechanical properties of the respiratory system in infants. Second, infants have a chest wall compliance (C_w) some five times higher than lung compliance (C_L).[1] Therefore because the reciprocal of respiratory system compliance $1/C_{rs}$ equals $1/C_L + 1/C_w$, C_{rs} is about 83% of C_L. This means that C_{rs} essentially reflects C_L in infants, which is an important practical advantage because C_{rs} can be measured much more easily than C_L. This chapter reviews some basic concepts and focuses on simple techniques that permit measurements of respiratory mechanics in newborn infants.

GENERAL CONCEPTS AND TERMINOLOGY

In the chain of events that contribute to the translation of the output of the respiratory rhythm generator into pulmonary ventilation, the mechanical properties of the respiratory system are a critical aspect (Fig. 63.1). After activation of the inspiratory muscles, the magnitude of the force generated depends on the force-length and force-velocity characteristics of the muscles. The physical translation of force into inspiratory pressure depends on the configuration of the muscle and the mechanical properties of the structure to which the force is applied. Finally, of the total muscle pressure generated, a part overcomes the elastic properties of the respiratory system to change lung volume (V) and a part is dissipated to overcome the resistive characteristics of the respiratory system to generate flow ($\dot{V}$). An additional pressure component for the acceleration of the gas depends on the inertia of the respiratory system; it is usually very small and can be disregarded. Hence, the total pressure P produced equals the sum of elastic (P_{el}) and resistive (P_{res}) components; the former is proportional to V and $1/C$, while the latter is proportional to $\dot{V}$ and R:

$$P = P_{el} + P_{res} = (V \cdot 1/C) + (\dot{V} \cdot R) \quad [63.1]$$

where C (compliance) and R (resistance) are proportionality factors determined by, respectively, the elastic and resistive characteristics of the system.

During *spontaneous breathing*, the total P for inflation is generated by the respiratory muscles. Hence, muscle pressure (P_{mus})

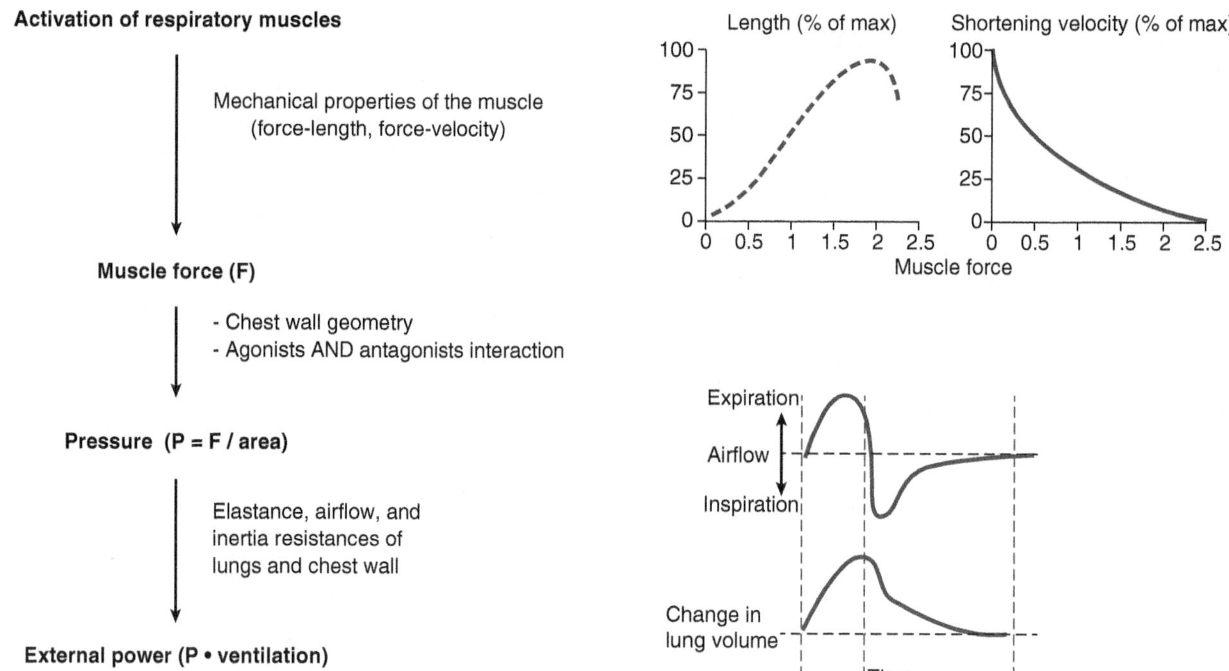

Fig. 63.1 *Left,* Summary of the processes involved in the translation of muscle activation into ventilation. *Right top,* Typical muscle force-length and force-velocity relationships. *Right bottom,* The pneumotachographic (time-airflow) and spirometric (time-volume) recordings.

equals P, and inflow occurs whenever $P_{mus} - P_{el}$ is greater than 0. During resting breathing, because the tidal volume is entirely above the resting volume of the respiratory system (V_r), the inspiratory muscles generate P_{mus} and expiration is passive. However, in some conditions, such as certain cases of hyperventilation or during breathing against a positive airway pressure, the expiratory muscles may become active and breathing occurs both above and below V_r. In these cases, inspiration originates from the recoil of the respiratory system after expiratory muscle relaxation plus the active contraction of the inspiratory muscles.

During *external (mechanical) ventilation,* P_{mus} = 0, and the driving pressure is generated by the ventilator, which opposes P_{el} and P_{res}. Whenever P_{mus} = 0, the system is in *passive* mode; this is the case during lung expansion by a ventilator or in the last portion of expiration during resting breathing. During this phase, the elastic pressure stored during inspiration (P_{el}) is the sole driving pressure generating expiratory flow—that is, $P_{el} = P_{res} = \dot{V} \cdot R_{rs}$.

Whenever P_{mus} differs from 0, the system is in an *active* mode; of course, this is the case during spontaneous inspiration or when $\dot{V} = 0$ during voluntary breath holding (in which case $P_{mus} = P_{el}$).

Whenever $\dot{V} = 0$, Equation 63.1 simplifies to

$$P = P_{el} = V \cdot 1/C \qquad [63.2]$$

This condition is defined as *static,* irrespective of whether P_{el} is offset by muscle activity (e.g., during breath holding) or by external means with P_{mus} = 0 (e.g., relaxation against an artificial occlusion of the airways). In contrast, whenever $\dot{V}$ differs from 0, the system is in a *dynamic* condition again, irrespective of whether the respiratory muscles are active (e.g., inflation during spontaneous inspiration) or not (e.g., inflation by a ventilator). In conclusion, the operating modes of the respiratory system can be summarized into four combinations, *static* or *dynamic,* depending on the absence or presence of $\dot{V}$, each either *active* or *passive,* depending on the presence or absence of muscle activity (Table 63.1).

A dynamic condition with changes in V so small that the component $V \cdot 1/C$ in Equation 63.1 is negligible is approached whenever $\dot{V}$ is very high and V is very small, such as with thermal panting or high-frequency ventilation. During an inspiratory effort against closed airways, because the change in lung volume equals 0 (and therefore $\dot{V} = 0$), no external work is performed and the energy of isometric contraction is dissipated entirely as heat.

PASSIVE MECHANICAL PROPERTIES OF THE RESPIRATORY SYSTEM

As defined already, the respiratory system is in a passive mode when P_{mus} = 0. This is the case during paralysis, with the lungs ventilated by external means (e.g., during positive pressure ventilation) or without paralysis after a period of hyperventilation. Hyperventilation lowers the arterial partial pressure of carbon dioxide below the threshold for muscle activation, which is just a few millimeters of mercury below the resting arterial partial pressure of carbon dioxide. During spontaneous breathing, the passive mode occurs when the subject relaxes at lung volumes above the resting position of the respiratory system; in infants, this is the case after an occlusion of the airways at the end of inspiration. The sustained lung inflation activates the airway slowly adapting stretch receptors, which trigger the vagally mediated Hering-Breuer inflation reflex and cause relaxation of the inspiratory muscles. This brief period of artificially provoked muscle relaxation is important in the context of pulmonary function testing in human neonates and is sufficient to evaluate the passive mechanical properties of the respiratory system (C_{rs}, R_{rs}) during spontaneous breathing.

RESPIRATORY SYSTEM COMPLIANCE AND RESPIRATORY SYSTEM RESISTANCE DURING MECHANICAL VENTILATION

Measurements of passive mechanics of the respiratory system are easier to perform during artificial ventilation than during spontaneous breathing because P_{mus} = 0 and the passive conditions are guaranteed. In addition, because it is customary to ventilate the lungs through an endotracheal tube, the infant's

Table 63.1 Terms, Units, and Common Terminology.

BTPS	Body temperature, ambient pressure, saturated with water vapor
C (C_L, C_{rs}, C_w)	Compliance (of lungs, respiratory system, chest wall), mL/cm H_2O
FRC	Functional residual capacity (end-expiratory volume), mL
P	Pressure, cm H_2O
P_{ao}	Pressure at the airway opening, cm H_2O
P_{el}	Elastic pressure (proportional to lung volume), cm H_2O
P_{es}	Esophageal pressure (proportional to pleural pressure), cm H_2O
P_{mus}	Pressure generated by the respiratory muscles, cm H_2O
P_{res}	Resistive pressure (proportional to airflow), cm H_2O
R (R_L, R_{rs}, R_w)	Resistance (of the lungs, respiratory system, chest wall), cm H_2O/mL/s
τ_{rs}	Passive time constant of the respiratory system, s
$\tau_{rs(exp)}$	Expiratory time constant of the respiratory system, s
V	Volume, mL_{BTPS}
V_r	Static relaxation volume of the respiratory system, mL
V_T	Tidal volume, mLBTPS
$\dot{V}$	Flow, mL_{BTPS}/s
Active mode	$P_{mus} > 0$, respiratory muscles are active
Passive mode	$P_{mus} = 0$, respiratory muscles are relaxed
Static condition	$\dot{V} = 0$. *Active:* breath holding by muscle contraction above or below V_r. *Passive:* relaxation against closed airways above V_r ($P_{ao} > 0$), below V_r ($P_{ao} < 0$), or at V_r ($P_{ao} = 0$)
Dynamic condition	$\dot{V} > 0$. *Active:* activation of the respiratory muscles, as during spontaneous breathing. *Passive*: respiration driven by external means, with respiratory muscles relaxed, as during mechanical ventilation or in the late portion of expiration during resting breathing

FRC, Functional residual capacity.

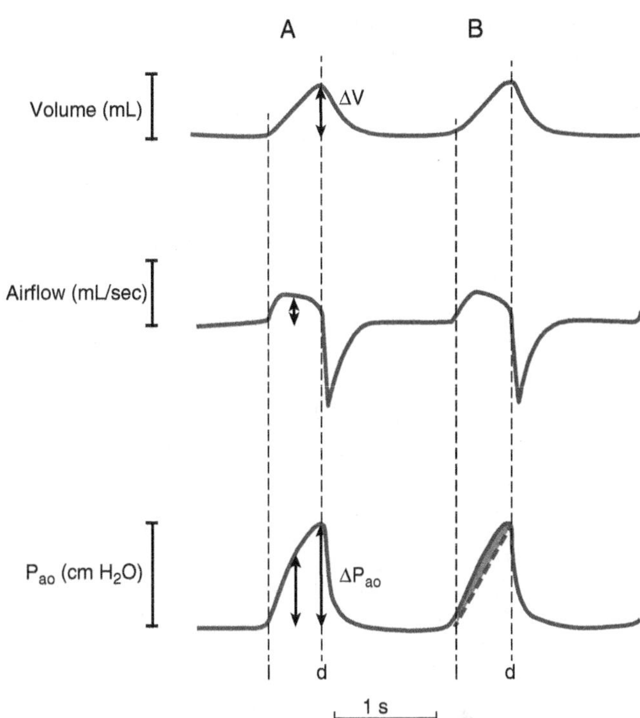

Fig. 63.2 The changes in lung volume, airflow, and pressure at the airway opening (P_{ao}), with the most common recording units, that can be observed in an intubated infant during mechanical ventilation. The dashed lines labeled *I* and *d* indicate the onset of, respectively, inflation and deflation. P_{ao} at the end of deflation is usually a few centimeters of water higher than zero. The compliance of the respiratory system is measured "dynamically," at the end of inflation, as $\Delta V/\Delta P_{ao}$. The resistance of the respiratory system can be measured by various analytical procedures—for example, at mid lung volume, when airflow is high *(A)*, or as average inflation by planimetry *(B)*. For further details, see the text.

upper airways are bypassed, eliminating an important source of nonlinear mechanical behavior. Therefore the respiratory system will likely perform as a first-order mechanical system, which simplifies the conceptual approach and the analysis of the measurements.

In intubated infants undergoing mechanical ventilation, the pneumotachograph, placed in series between the endotracheal tube and the ventilator, measures $\dot{V}$. The $\dot{V}$ signal is amplified and electronically integrated to obtain the changes in lung volume (V). The total P needed to inflate the whole respiratory system (P in Equation 63.1) is conveniently measured at the airway opening (P_{ao})—for example, at the mouth or at the inlet of the endotracheal tube. From these measurements, C_{rs} and R_{rs} are either separately computed or derived from the equation of motion of the respiratory system (Equation 63.1). Because three ($\dot{V}$, V, P_{ao}) of the five variables are measured, it is possible to derive mathematically the two unknown constants, C_{rs} and R_{rs}. Measurements of C_{rs} and R_{rs} during mechanical ventilation are often plagued by air leaks around the endotracheal tube; a cuffed tube would eliminate the problem, but it is rarely used in routine clinical management. Air leaks can introduce enormous errors in the computation of the volume of air delivered to the lungs and of the parameters related to it. Alternative methods for measurements of changes in lung volume in artificially ventilated infants, such as head-out body plethysmography and respiratory inductance plethysmography,[2] are cumbersome and of little value in the clinical setting. Measurements of R_{rs} as commonly performed (see later) need to take into account that the endotracheal tube resistance is often quite high in comparison with R_{rs},[3] and its computation can be difficult because the fluid dynamics of small tubes is prone to substantial errors.[4] The monitoring of the inflation pressure at the distal end of the tube, rather than at its proximal end, could eliminate this potential analytical problem.

COMPLIANCE

At the end of inflation, the compliance of the respiratory system, C_{rs}, equals $\Delta V/\Delta P_{ao}$, where ΔV and ΔP_{ao} represent the difference in V and P_{ao} between the onset of inflation and the zero-flow point at the end of inflation (Fig. 63.2). It is important to consider that at the onset of inflation P_{ao} is not necessarily zero. P_{ao} is above zero whenever the infant is ventilated with some positive end-expiratory pressure, which is the most frequent condition. Thus, if one computes C_{rs} simply as the ratio of V and P_{ao} instead of $\Delta V/\Delta P_{ao}$, C_{rs} will be incorrectly low. Lung compliance (C_L) is measured as the ratio between the change in V (ΔV) and the change in transpulmonary pressure (ΔP), defined as the difference between P_{ao} and pleural pressure; then, from C_{rs} and C_L, chest wall compliance (C_w) is computed as $C_w = 1/(1/C_{rs} - 1/C_L)$. As in adults, in newborns, pleural pressure is usually measured as esophageal pressure (P_{es}) with an esophageal liquid-filled catheter. To what extent P_{es} is a faithful representation of the mean change in pleural pressure is debatable.[5-7] Problems originate from the technical aspects of the measurements (including the frequency response of the esophageal catheter) and from the distortion of the chest, a phenomenon more pronounced in infants than in adults. In spontaneously breathing infants, the accuracy of the P_{es} recording is evaluated from the changes in P_{es} and P_{ao} during an inspiratory effort against occluded airways.[6,8,9] During the effort, because neither lung volume nor transpulmonary pressure changes, the $P_{ao} - P_{es}$ difference should remain zero. Even so, the possibility exists that the P_{es} signal, albeit adequate during the effort, may not be equally reliable during normal breathing because of differences in chest distortion.

Compliance measured as described above is often labeled *dynamic compliance,* a term that may be confusing because it seems to contradict the requirement for *static* conditions. The word *dynamic* is used to stress the fact that the measurement is performed during the dynamic state of continuous ventilation by taking advantage of the end-of-inflation condition when, in fact, $\dot{V} = 0$. One can achieve truly static conditions by stopping the ventilator and recording *P* while the lungs are kept inflated at a constant level. In healthy adults, the values of dynamic and static compliance are similar. In infants, dynamic compliance is consistently lower than static compliance,[10,11] mainly because of the lung stress relaxation.[12] Stress relaxation is a phenomenon originating from the viscous properties of biologic tissue and is substantially more marked in newborns than in adults.[13,14] The asynchronous behavior of peripheral lung units characteristic of the newborn lung contributes to the dynamic-static difference of compliance, especially in conditions of marked chest distortion.[1,15]

RESISTANCE

At any given time during lung *inflation*, the total resistance of the respiratory system (R_{rs}) corresponds to $P_{res}/\dot{V}$, where P_{res} is the difference between the total *P* of the respiratory system and its elastic components (see Equation 63.1).[16] The measurement of R_{rs} is more accurate at the time of peak flow, which is usually in the middle third of inflation (see Fig. 63.2A). Alternative analytic approaches are based on the computation of P_{res} by planimetry (see Fig. 63.2B) or on various solutions of Equation 63.1.[1] The planimetric method gives a time-averaged inflation resistance. By this method, the two P_{ao} points at the onset and at the end of inflation are joined, and the area enveloped between this line and the actual P_{ao} curve divided by the inflation time corresponds to the average resistive pressure during inflation. The ratio of this value and the mean inspiratory flow (tidal volume divided by inflation time) is the time-averaged inflation resistance.

The total pulmonary resistance (R_L) is computed in very similar ways; in this case, P_{res} is the difference between the total inflating transpulmonary pressure ($P_{ao} - P_{es}$) and its elastic component. Finally, chest wall resistance (R_w) is the difference $R_{rs} - R_L$.

During lung *deflation,* to the extent that the respiratory apparatus behaves mechanically as a first-order system, the decrease in volume and flow follow exponential trajectories. Therefore, during deflation, the logarithmic representation of either $\dot{V}$ or *V* yields a linear relation and the reciprocal of the slope represents the time constant (τ_{rs}).[17] By this approach, because the time constant of a first-order mechanical system is the product of *C* and *R*, R_{rs} is computed simply as τ_{rs}/C_{rs}. R_{rs} measured in this way during passive expiration is lower than R_{rs} measured during lung inflation because the lung volume history differs between the two conditions, the airways being more expanded (and therefore with lower *R*) after lung inflation.

RESPIRATORY SYSTEM COMPLIANCE AND RESPIRATORY SYSTEM RESISTANCE DURING SPONTANEOUS BREATHING

For these measurements, the infant breathes through a facemask connected to a $\dot{V}$-recording device, the pneumotachograph. The $\dot{V}$ signal is electronically integrated to obtain the changes in lung volume (*V*), and intra-airway pressure is measured at the airway opening (P_{ao}). The modification of the breathing pattern caused by the facemask because of the stimulation of the trigeminal area[18] and of the added dead space has no important effect on respiratory mechanics. In its simplest approach, the investigator covers the infant's mouth and nostrils with the facemask and performs a brief (approximately 1 to 2 second) occlusion of the pneumotachograph outlet, either manually or through a solenoid valve attached to the pneumotachograph. This brief airway occlusion aims to maintain lung volume elevated above the end-expiratory volume, which is the starting point for the measurements of compliance and resistance during spontaneous breathing.

COMPLIANCE

During the occlusion of the airways at the end of inspiration or at any time during expiration, P_{ao} rises to the recoil pressure of the respiratory system at that volume (Fig. 63.3). The time required for P_{ao} to reach its new equilibrium depends on the time needed by the inspiratory muscles to achieve relaxation. This relaxation is triggered by the activation of the airway slowly adapting stretch receptors that respond to transpulmonary pressure. Therefore the larger the lung volume at which the occlusion is performed, the greater the likelihood of complete muscle relaxation. The passive condition required for the measurement lasts less than a couple of seconds and is sufficient for the measurements; after this time, the same vagal reflex inhibiting the inspiratory muscles eventually activates the expiratory muscles. Because C_{rs} is the slope of the ΔP_{ao} versus ΔV relationship (*x*-axis and *y*-axis, respectively), the accuracy of the C_{rs} computation improves when many ΔP_{ao} and ΔV data points are collected over a wide range of *V*.[10,19-21]

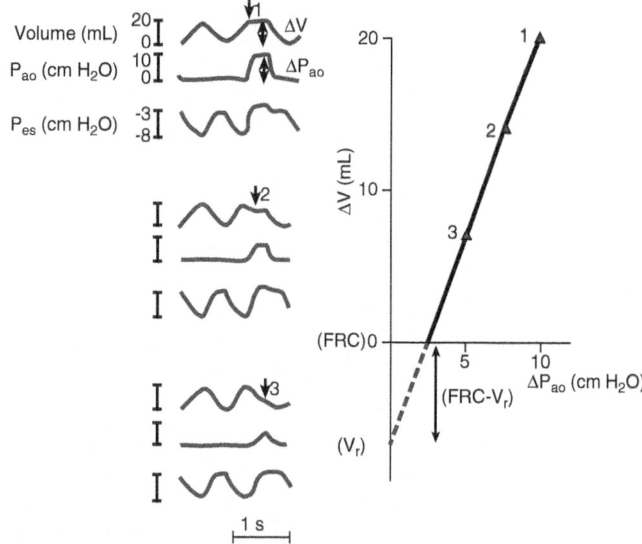

Fig. 63.3 The changes in lung volume (ΔV_T), pressure measured at the mouth (P_{ao}), and esophageal pressure (P_{es}) in a spontaneously breathing infant. In each of the three examples indicated, from top to bottom, the recordings start with a breathing cycle followed by an occlusion of the airways made by the investigator. At *1*, the occlusion is at the end of inspiration; at *2*, it is in the first third of expiration; at *3*, it is in the second half of expiration. The corresponding P_{ao}-*V* points are plotted in the diagram on the *right*; the slope of the linear regression represents the compliance of the respiratory system (C_{rs}), and the intercept on the *y*-axis represents the difference between the end-expiratory level and the resting volume (*FRC-V_r* difference). Although only three data points are represented, many more data points through the whole V_T range are desirable to improve the accuracy of the linear regression. *FRC,* Functional residual capacity.

Several other approaches have been proposed to compute C_{rs}, with small variations from the method just described[22-24]; each has advantages and limitations, as discussed in the original publications. Irrespective of the method used, if P_{es} is simultaneously monitored, as schematically indicated in Fig. 63.3, it is possible to partition C_{rs} into its lung and chest wall components (C_L and C_w, respectively).

TIME CONSTANT AND RESISTANCE

Both C_{rs} and R_{rs} vary with large changes in lung volume,[25] but within the V_T range, their values remain approximately constant. Therefore, during passive expiration, after the brief end-inspiratory airway occlusion discussed in the previous sections, the trajectories of the drop in V and $\dot{V}$ follow exponential functions. The semilog representations of such trajectories give a linear function, and the reciprocal of its slope is the passive time constant of the respiratory system (τ_{rs}).[26] This corresponds to the slope of the linear portion of the $\dot{V}$(*x*-axis) – *V*(*y*-axis) loop during passive expiration (Fig. 63.4).[19,22] Once τ_{rs} is known, R_{rs} is calculated as τ_{rs}/C_{rs}. This simple and very practical approach is not readily applicable whenever the expiratory trajectories of $\dot{V}$ and V deviate from the exponential pattern because of respiratory muscle activation, nonlinear mechanical behavior of the upper airways, or other reasons. In these cases, τ_{rs} and R_{rs} depend on the value of $\dot{V}$ at which they are measured.

In infants, during resting breathing, the extrapolation of the linear segment of the $\dot{V} - V$ expiratory curve to $\dot{V}=0$ hits the *V*-axis not quite at the functional residual capacity (FRC) but below it; this difference represents the dynamic elevation of the end-expiratory level (or FRC—V_r difference) (see Fig. 63.4), as it was derived from the measurements of C_{rs} (see Fig. 63.3).[19,20] In infants, the FRC – V_r difference, or *dynamic elevation of FRC*, originates from the fact that expiration is short with respect to τ_{rs}, so inspiration begins at a lung volume higher than V_r. In infants a few days old, FRC is about 7 to 15 mL higher than V_r, or at about 20% to 30% of tidal volume.

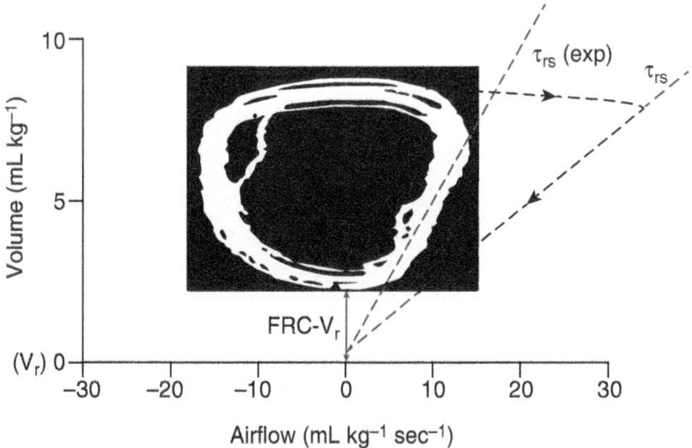

Fig. 63.4 Infant, spontaneously breathing. Respiratory airflow and volume are continuously recorded on the *x*-axis and the *y*-axis; inspirations are on the left with negative flows and expirations are on the right with positive flows *(superimposed white oscilloscope tracings on the black background)*. Eventually, at the end of inspiration, the airways are briefly occluded by the investigator (end-inspiratory occlusion); after the release of the occlusion *(arrowed dashed line)*, the slope of the deflation flow versus volume curve represents the passive time constant of the respiratory system (τ_{rs}). Usually, during resting breathing, the expiratory flow versus volume curve is at the left of the passive curve, indicating that the expiratory time constant $\tau_{rs(exp)}$ exceeds τ_{rs}. The extrapolation to zero flow of the linear portion of the expiratory flow versus volume relationships permits one to compute the volume difference between the end-expiratory volume (functional residual capacity, *FRC*) and the resting volume of the respiratory system (V_r).

Several reviews have discussed the technical details of the measurements of C_{rs} and R_{rs} in infants[21,27-29]; a common ongoing effort is to standardize the methods to facilitate comparisons among studies and identification of pathologic situations.

ACTIVE MECHANICAL BEHAVIOR OF THE RESPIRATORY SYSTEM

An important question is whether or not during spontaneous breathing the mechanical properties of the respiratory system are the same as those measured during passive conditions. The answer is that the system does not behave as expected based on passive measurements either in inspiration or in expiration. One reason is the difference between *dynamic* and *static* compliance, as mentioned earlier. Additional issues are the uneven distribution of forces applied to the chest wall during muscle contraction and, during expiration, the residual activities of the inspiratory muscles and the laryngeal control of expiratory flow.[1]

MECHANICS OF CHEST WALL DISTORTION

During passive inflation of the respiratory system (as during mechanical ventilation), the abdominal and pleural pressures increase. In the absence of diaphragmatic tension, the transdiaphragmatic pressure is zero; hence, the changes in pleural and abdominal pressures are the same, and the two main chest wall compartments, the rib cage and the abdomen, are driven by the same pressure applied uniformly to all regions (Fig. 63.5A).

Quite different is the situation in active (spontaneous breathing) conditions ($P_{mus} > 0$) when the diaphragm contracts and transdiaphragmatic pressure increases (see Fig. 63.5B). In this case, while the abdominal pressure increases and expands the abdomen (as it does with passive inflation), the motion of the rib cage depends on the interplay of several factors.[1] First, the subatmospheric pleural pressure tends to collapse both the upper and lower regions of the rib cage. One can appreciate this mechanical effect of diaphragmatic contraction on the rib cage by observing its motion in quadriplegic patients who have lost the use of all extradiaphragmatic muscles.[30] In the lower rib cage regions, the tendency to collapse is partly offset by the expanding action of the abdominal pressure (or "abdomen-rib cage interdependence") and by the direct outward pulling of the diaphragmatic fibers. In normal infants, the inspiratory collapse of the upper rib cage is common because of their high C_w and poor mechanical coupling between the upper and the lower rib cage. It follows that in infants the expansion of the rib cage, especially its upper regions, during spontaneous inspiration can occur only through the intervention of the intercostals and the other extradiaphragmatic muscles; indeed, these muscles are recruited to compensate for the otherwise inevitable distortion.[31] The motion of the rib cage during spontaneous breathing, because of recruitment of extradiaphragmatic muscles (*compensated* distortion), is an expansion similar to that during passive inflation (*absence* of distortion); however, the two situations are very different when examined in the light of the energetics of breathing.

Functional evaluation of the net effect of chest distortion can be done by comparison of lung volumes between active and passive conditions at the same abdominal pressure (or for the same abdominal expansion, because changes in abdominal pressure and abdominal displacement are closely related).[31] A schematic example is presented in Fig. 63.6, which refers to a newborn infant during sleep. Airflow ($\dot{V}$), changes in lung volume (*V*), pressure at the airway opening (P_{ao}), and the motion of the abdominal wall are recorded simultaneously. At the end of inspiration, the experimenter briefly occludes the infant's airways; the plateau in P_{ao} during the short time of the occlusion suggests relaxation of the respiratory muscles. Hence, at

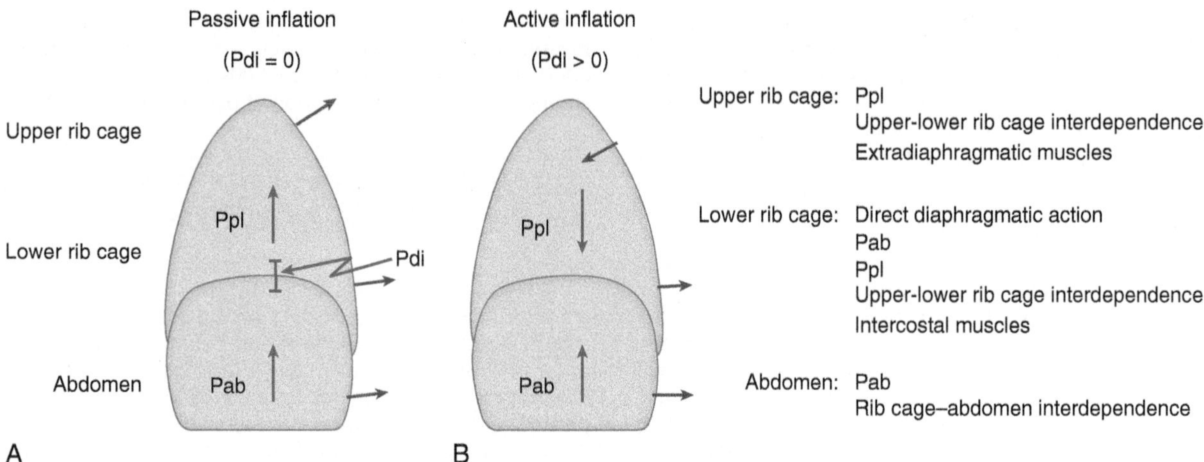

Fig. 63.5 The pressures applied to the chest wall and its components of the rib cage and the abdomen during passive inflation (A) and spontaneous (active) inspiration (B) in a normal newborn infant. *Blue arrows* indicate the changes in pleural *(Ppl)* and abdominal *(Pab)* pressures. Pdi is the transdiaphragmatic pressure, equal to Pab − Ppl. *Red arrows* indicate the expected direction of motion in passive and active conditions when Pdi is, respectively, zero or positive. At the extreme right, the pressures and forces responsible for the motion of upper rib cage, lower rib cage, and abdomen during spontaneous inspiration are summarized; the resulting motion is the net effect of all these factors.

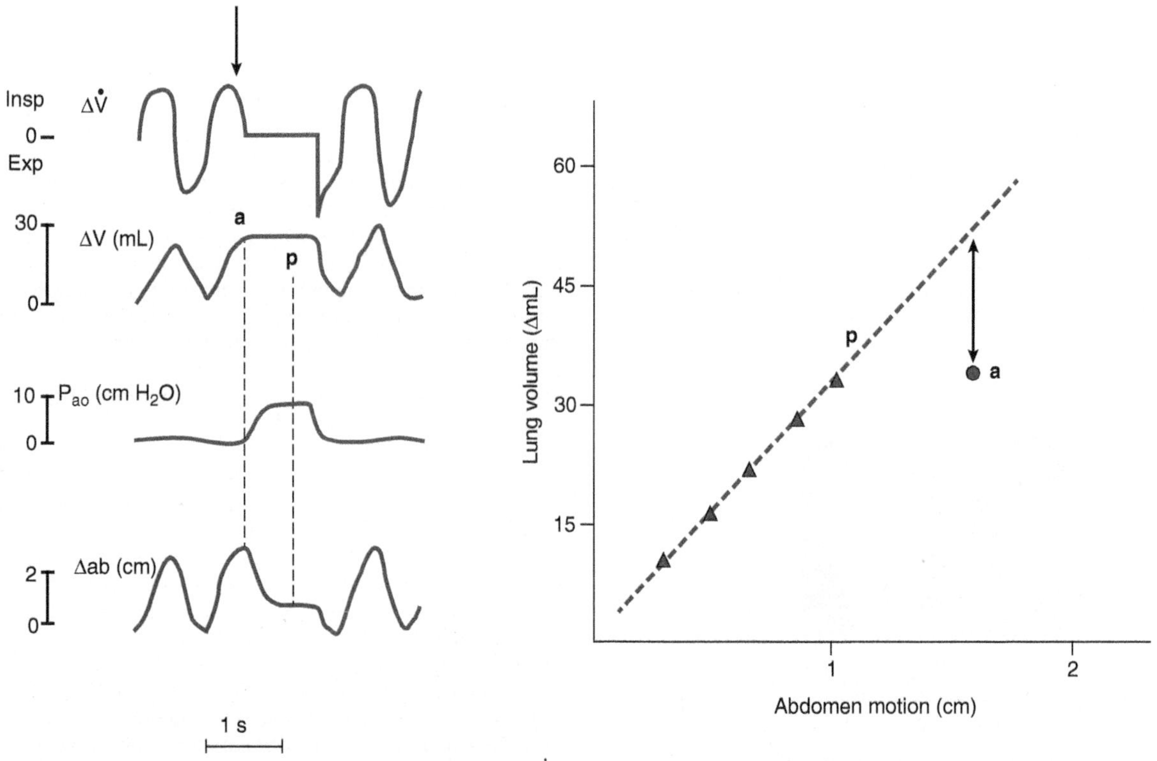

Fig. 63.6 From top to bottom, the changes in respiratory airflow ($\dot{V}$), lung volume *(V)*, pressure at the airway opening (P_{ao}), and motion of the abdominal wall *(ab)* in a spontaneously breathing infant. At the time indicated by the *arrow* (end of inspiration, *first dotted line*), the investigator briefly occludes the infant's airways; the occurrence of muscle relaxation is shown by the plateau of P_{ao} *(p, second dashed line).* The active *(a, solid circle)* and passive *(p)* ab-*V* data points are plotted on the right. The passive relationship *(open triangles)* is obtained by multiple occlusions at different lung volumes during expiration. The vertical distance between *a* and the passive curve *(blue double-ended arrow)* indicates the volume loss because of distortion. *Exp,* Expiration; *Insp,* inspiration.

the same lung volume (end of inspiration), two situations follow one another, the *active* condition at the end of the spontaneous inspiration and the *passive* condition during the occlusion. By performing many such maneuvers at different lung volumes during expiration (in a way similar to that described earlier for the measurement of C_{rs} during spontaneous breathing; see Fig. 63.3), one can construct the passive relationship between abdomen motion and *V* (see Fig. 63.6, right panel). The difference on the *y*-axis between the active points (at the end of inspiration) and the passive relationship represents the *V* difference between active and passive conditions. In normal infants, while resting breathing at any given abdominal pressure, tidal volume is less than the passive *V* by as much as 50%. This means that breathing in infants functionally involves a substantial loss of air volume.[31] The volume "loss" is likely to increase in REM sleep, when the intercostal muscles are less active and the inspiratory distortion of the rib cage is maximal. Equally, volume loss probably increases in the supine posture, compared with the prone position,[32] because abdominal compliance is higher in the former case. A very large volume loss could occur in conditions of high C_w/C_L ratio, as in premature infants; in diseases lowering C_L, such as bronchopulmonary dysplasia; or in conditions of increased airway resistance. Conversely, a very small volume loss, or eventually, a tidal volume in excess of the passive V, could occur in hypoxia or in other situations of increased ventilatory "drive" and elevated output to the extradiaphragmatic muscles.

EXPIRATORY TIME CONSTANT

Because in resting conditions expiration is a passive process, one may expect the expiratory $\dot{V}$ and V to follow exponential profiles; hence, the time constant measurable during tidal expiration, $\tau_{rs(exp)}$, should coincide with the passive time constant of the respiratory system, τ_{rs}. However, this is often not the case, as one can appreciate by comparing the tidal expiratory flow versus volume loop with the flow-volume curve obtained after the release of an end-inspiratory airway occlusion (see Fig. 63.4).[19,20] The fact that the expiratory curve is positioned at the left of the passive curve indicates that $\tau_{rs(exp)}$ is longer than τ_{rs} at all volumes during expiration.[19,20,33] There are two main reasons for this difference. First, the inspiratory activity does not cease abruptly at the end of inspiration but proceeds during part of the expiratory phase, effectively reducing the elastic recoil pressure of the respiratory system. Second, the adduction of the vocal folds during expiration increases airway resistance and prolongs $\tau_{rs(exp)}$.

The prolongation of $\tau_{rs(exp)}$ causes the mean lung volume to remain higher throughout the expiratory phase of the breathing cycle, and the next inspiration begins at a volume (FRC) higher than V_r. Indeed, almost half a century ago, Olinsky and colleagues[34] showed that during a short period of apnea, FRC decreases in infants; hence, they deduced that during resting breathing, the infant's FRC was maintained actively above V_r. Later, it was possible to compute the FRC – V_r difference from the static pressure versus volume curve (see Fig. 63.3) or from the expiratory flow versus volume curve (see Fig. 63.4).[19,20,33,35] The elevation of FRC above V_r results from the combined effects of the rather short expiratory time (because the breathing rate is higher in infants than in adults) and the expiratory action of inspiratory and laryngeal (vocal folds) muscles and is an important mechanism to counteract the infant's predisposition to a low V_r caused by the high C_w/C_L ratio.[1] These mechanisms to control FRC cannot be operative in infants artificially ventilated through an endotracheal tube because breathing frequency is controlled by the ventilator and the laryngeal region is bypassed. In these cases, therefore, an end-expiratory pressure of a few centimeters of water[36,37] must be added to the expiratory line of the ventilator to avoid the deflation of the lungs to V_r.

ASPECTS OF THE ENERGETICS OF BREATHING

Once C_{rs} and R_{rs} are known, the total pressure required to inflate the lung to a given volume in a given time is obtained from the equation of motion of the respiratory system (see Equation 63.1). Then, the total work can be calculated based on the assumption of a sinusoidal flow pattern, which is based on the formula originally proposed by Otis and colleagues.[38] These computations have indicated that in newborns, as in adults, breathing frequency at rest falls within the optimal range of minimal external work, although the mechanisms that regulate this optimality are still unknown.[19] The respiratory work calculated in this way represents the *passive* work of breathing because it is based on values of C_{rs} and R_{rs} obtained in passive conditions. During spontaneous breathing, the *active* work of breathing exceeds the passive value because the respiratory muscles cannot apply a force to the chest wall as uniformly as occurs in passive conditions. For example, as mentioned earlier (see Fig. 63.5), the diaphragm acts like a piston that expands the abdomen while simultaneously collapsing the upper rib cage. The result of this uneven distribution is that some muscle force is lost in the distortion of the chest wall instead of being translated into pressure driving the respiratory system. Furthermore, during contraction, muscles lose force according to their length and velocity of shortening (see Fig. 63.1). Therefore from the point of view of the dynamics and energetics of breathing, one can state that during active breathing the respiratory system behaves as if its impedance is higher than in passive conditions because of a lower C_{rs}, higher R_{rs}, or both.

Estimates of the active pressure required to expand the respiratory system have been obtained by measurement of the pressure in the airways (P_{ao}) generated during an inspiratory effort against an occlusion. In this condition, the change in lung volume is negligible and, supposedly, the inspiratory muscles are contracting isometrically. The main assumption underlying this approach is that P_{ao} generated by the muscles is the same pressure required to generate V and $\dot{V}$ during normal (open airways) breathing. Measurements of P_{ao} are made at known time intervals from the onset of the occluded inspiratory effort, and measurements of flow and volume are made at the corresponding times of the preceding open airway breath (Fig. 63.7A).[39] From these data, it is possible to construct the P_{ao}/V(*y*-axis) – $\dot{V}/V$(*x*-axis) relationship; the slope and intercept represent, respectively, the *active* R_{rs} and $1/C_{rs}$ (see Fig. 63.7B). From several studies that have applied this or similar approaches, it was concluded that the newborn infant's C_{rs} during spontaneous breathing is about 65% of the passive value, whereas R_{rs} is approximately the same as in passive conditions. This means that the elastic work (and cost) of breathing in a spontaneously breathing infant is approximately 50% (1/0.65) higher than expected from values of respiratory mechanics obtained in passive conditions. Notwithstanding the technical and analytic difficulties, estimates of the active work are useful because they provide a more realistic evaluation of the work imposed on the respiratory muscles than passive measurements would. In addition, the knowledge of the active values of C_{rs} and R_{rs} yields more accurate predictions of the ability to maintain ventilation in the face of external elastic or resistive loads.[40]

CONCLUSIONS

In addition to the techniques described, several other techniques are available to explore in more detail the mechanical conditions of the infant's respiratory pump; for example, methods oriented at measuring thoracic gas volume, the mechanical properties of the airways, and their interaction with those of the lung. Absolute lung volumes are usually measured by body plethysmography, and the mechanical properties of the airways are usually measured by forced expiratory maneuvers. These measurements, performed commonly in adults, have some practical difficulties when applied to the infant mainly because infants cannot cooperate.[41–43] As an example, in infants, forced expiratory maneuvers can be done only either by forced suction of air from the airways[41] or by forced squeezing on the thorax[44,45]; either approach yields results that depend greatly on how the pressure is applied.[46,47] Thus, these methods are usually confined to specific situations or to the research setting.[48,49] Differently, the measurements of C_{rs} and R_{rs} described in the previous sections are simple techniques readily applicable to a wide range of healthy and sick infants. Because in infants C_w is very high by comparison with C_L, C_{rs} can

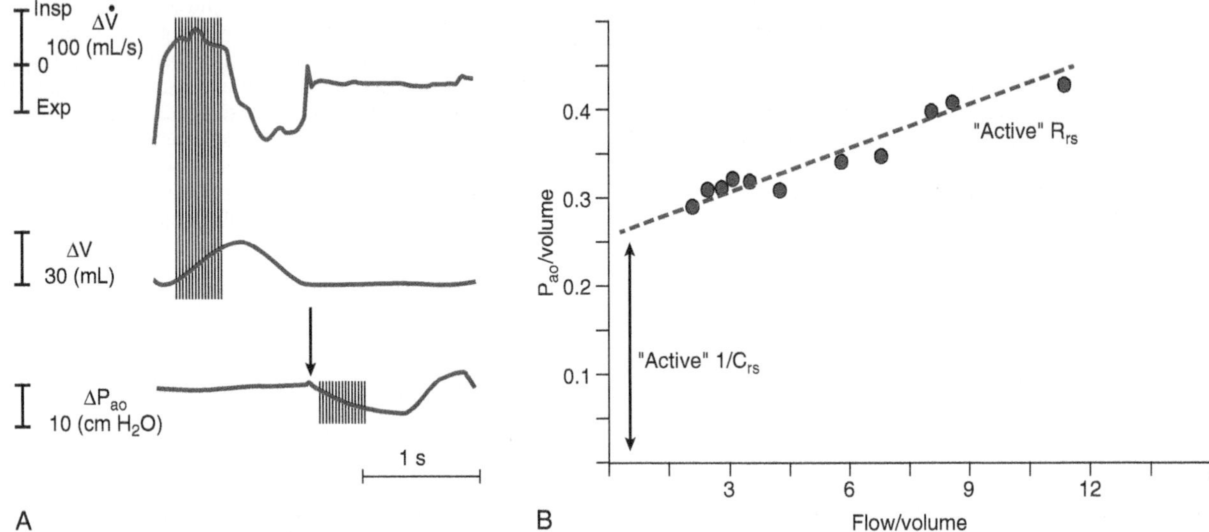

Fig. 63.7 (A) Newborn infant, spontaneously breathing. From top to bottom, records of respiratory airflow ($\dot{V}$), tidal volume (V), and mouth pressure (P_{ao}). At the time indicated by the *arrow,* the investigator occludes the infant's airways; then, the infant makes an inspiratory effort, as shown by the drop in P_{ao} with no changes in V. The *vertical parallel lines* indicate iso-time measurements of P_{ao} (from the onset of the effort), and $\dot{V}$ and V (from the onset of the preceding breath). (B) The iso-time $P_{ao}/V - \dot{V}/V$ points are plotted; from the linear regression through the data points, the slope and the reciprocal of the intercept represent, respectively, the active resistance (R_{rs}) and active compliance (C_{rs}) of the respiratory system. *Exp,* Expiration; *Insp,* inspiration.

reflect pathologic changes in C_L more readily than is the case in adults. Hence, measurements of C_{rs} have been found useful in predicting the course and outcome of neonatal respiratory problems, as well as in classifying the severity of some respiratory diseases.

REFERENCES

1. Mortola JP. *Respiratory Physiology of Newborn Mammals. A Comparative Perspective*. Baltimore: The Johns Hopkins University Press; 2001:344.
2. Brown K, Aun C, Jackson E, et al. Validation of respiratory inductive plethysmography using the qualitative diagnostic calibration method in anaesthetized infants. *Eur Respir J*. 1998;12:935.
3. Manczur T, Greenough A, Nicholson GP, Rafferty GF. Resistance of pediatric and neonatal endotracheal tubes: influence of flow rate, size, and shape. *Crit Care Med*. 2000;28:1595.
4. Chang HK, Mortola JP. Fluid dynamic factors in tracheal pressure measurement. *J Appl Physiol*. 1981;51:218.
5. LeSouef PN, Lopes JM, England SJ, et al. Influence of chest wall distortion on esophageal pressure. *J Appl Physiol*. 1983;55:353.
6. Asher MI, Coates AL, Collinge JM, Milic-Emili J. Measurement of pleural pressure in neonates. *J Appl Physiol*. 1982;52:491.
7. Dinwiddie R, Russell G. Relationship of intraesophageal pressure to intrapleural pressure in the newborn. *J Appl Physiol*. 1972;33:415.
8. Baydur A, Behrakis PK, Zin WA, et al. A simple method for assessing the validity of the esophageal balloon technique. *Am Rev Respir Dis*. 1982;126:788.
9. Coates AL, Davis GM, Vallinis P, Outerbridge EW. Liquid filled esophageal catheter for measuring pleural pressure in preterm neonates. *J Appl Physiol*. 1989;67:889.
10. Olinsky A, Bryan AC, Bryan MH. A simple method of measuring total respiratory system compliance in newborn infants. *S Afr Med J*. 1976;50:128.
11. Kano S, Lanteri CJ, Pemberton PJ, et al. Fast versus slow ventilation for neonates. *Am Rev Respir Dis*. 1993;148:578.
12. Sullivan KJ, Mortola JP. Dynamic lung compliance in newborn and adult cats. *J Appl Physiol*. 1986;60:743.
13. Sullivan KJ, Mortola JP. Age related changes in the rate of stress relaxation within the rat respiratory system. *Respir Physiol*. 1987;67:295.
14. Pérez Fontán JJ, Ray AO, Oxland TR. Stress relaxation of the respiratory system in developing piglets. *J Appl Physiol*. 1992;52:1297.
15. Sullivan KJ, Mortola JP. Effect of distortion on the mechanical properties of newborn piglet lung. *J Appl Physiol*. 1985;59:434.
16. Mead J, Whittenberger JL. Physical properties of human lung measured during spontaneous respiration. *J Appl Physiol*. 1953;5:779.
17. McIlroy MB, Tierney DF, Nadel JA. A new method for measurement of compliance and resistance of lungs and thorax. *J Appl Physiol*. 1963;18:424.
18. Dolfin T, Dufty P, Wilkes D, et al. Effects of a face mask and pneumotachograph on breathing in sleeping infants. *Am Rev Respir Dis*. 1983;128:977.
19. Mortola JP, Fisher JT, Smith B, et al. Dynamics of breathing in infants. *J Appl Physiol*. 1982;52:1209.
20. Mortola JP, Milic-Emili J, Noworaj A, et al. Muscle pressure and flow during expiration in infants. *Am Rev Respir Dis*. 1984;129:49.
21. Gappa M, Colin AA, Goetz I, et al. Passive respiratory mechanics: the occlusion technique. *Eur Respir J*. 2001;17:141.
22. LeSouef PN, England SJ, Bryan AC. Passive respiratory mechanics in newborns and children. *Am Rev Respir Dis*. 1984;129:552.
23. Mortola JP, Hemmings G, Matsuoka T, et al. Referencing lung volume for measurements of respiratory system compliance in infants. *Pediatr Pulmonol*. 1993;16:248.
24. Grunstein MM, Springer C, Godfrey S, et al. Expiratory volume clamping: a new method to assess respiratory mechanics in sedated infants. *J Appl Physiol*. 1987;62:2107.
25. Miller MJ, DiFiore JM, Strohl KP, Martin RJ. Effects of nasal CPAP on supraglottic and total pulmonary resistance in preterm infants. *J Appl Physiol*. 1990;68:141.
26. Brody AW. Mechanical compliance and resistance of the lung-thorax calculated from the flow recorded during passive expiration. *Am J Physiol*. 1954;178:189.
27. Frey U, Stocks J, Coates A, et al. Specifications for equipment used for infant pulmonary function testing. *Eur Respir J*. 2000;16:731.
28. Katier N, Uiterwaal CS, de Jong BM, et al. Feasibility and variability of neonatal lung function measurement using the single occlusion technique. *Chest*. 2005;128:1822.
29. Reiterer F, Müller W. Assessment of single-occlusion technique for measurements of respiratory mechanics and respiratory drive in healthy term neonates using a commercially available computerized pulmonary function testing system. *Biol Neonate*. 2003;83:117.
30. Mortola JP, Sant'Ambrogio G. Motion of the rib cage and the abdomen in tetraplegic patients. *Clin Sci Mol Med*. 1978;54:25.
31. Mortola JP, Saetta M, Fox G, et al. Mechanical aspects of chest wall distortion. *J Appl Physiol*. 1985;59:295.
32. Wolfson MR, Greenspan JS, Deoras KS, et al. Effect of position on the mechanical interaction between rib cage and abdomen in preterm infants. *J Appl Physiol*. 1992;72:1032.
33. Kosch PC, Stark AR. Dynamic maintenance of end-expiratory lung volume in full-term infants. *J Appl Physiol*. 1984;57:1126.
34. Olinsky A, Bryan MH, Bryan AC. Influence of lung inflation on respiratory control in neonates. *J Appl Physiol*. 1974;36:426.
35. Stark AR, Cohlan BA, Waggener TB, et al. Regulation of end-expiratory lung volume during sleep in premature infants. *J Appl Physiol*. 1987;62:1117.
36. Berman LS, Fox WW, Raphaely RC, Downes Jr JJ. Optimum levels of CPAP for tracheal extubation of newborn infants. *J Pediatr*. 1976;89:109.
37. Gregory GA, Kitterman JA, Phibbs RH, et al. Treatment of the idiopathic respiratory-distress syndrome with continuous positive airway pressure. *N Engl J Med*. 1971;284:1333.
38. Otis AB, Fenn WO, Rahn H. Mechanics of breathing in man. *J Appl Physiol*. 1950;2:592.
39. Mortola JP, Saetta M. Measurements of respiratory mechanics in the newborn: a simple approach. *Pediatr Pulmonol*. 1987;3:123.

40. Milic-Emili J, Zin WA. Breathing responses to imposed mechanical loads. In: Fishman AP, ed. *Handbook of Physiology; Section 3. The Respiratory System, Vol II, Part 2*. Bethesda, Maryland: American Physiological Society; 1986:751-769.
41. Beardsmore CS, Stocks J, Silverman M. Problems in measurement of thoracic gas volume in infancy. *J Appl Physiol*. 1982;52:995.
42. Helms P. Problems with plethysmographic estimation of lung volume in infants and young children. *J Appl Physiol*. 1982;53:698.
43. Stocks J, Thomson A, Silverman M. Pressure-flow curves in infancy. *Pediatr Pulmonol*. 1985;1:33.
44. Adler SM, Wohl MEB. Flow-volume relationship at low lung volumes in healthy term newborn infants. *Pediatrics*. 1978;61:636.
45. Taussig LM, Laundau LI, Godfrey S, Arad I. Determinants of forced expiratory flows in newborn infants. *J Appl Physiol*. 1982;53:1220.
46. Silverman M, Prendiville A, Green S. Partial expiratory flow-volume curves in infancy: technical aspects. *Bull Eur Physiopathol Respir*. 1986;22:257.
47. Hughes DM, Lesouëf PN, Landau LI. Effect of compression pressure on forced expiratory flow in infants. *J Appl Physiol*. 1986;61:1639.
48. Sly PD, Tepper R, Henschen M, et al. Tidal forced expirations. *Eur Respir J*. 2000;16:741.
49. Frey U. Clinical applications of infant lung function testing: does it contribute to clinical decision making? *Paediatr Respir Rev*. 2001;2:126.

Pulmonary Gas Exchange in the Developing Lung 64

Leif D. Nelin | John P. Kinsella | William E. Truog

INTRODUCTION

Integral to the system of pulmonary gas exchange are mechanisms to maintain matching of pulmonary perfusion and alveolar ventilation, known as *ventilation/perfusion matching*. The goal is that alveolar oxygen and pulmonary capillary blood have intimate contact to optimize diffusion of O_2 and CO_2. Requisite features of the efficient gas-exchange apparatus include sustained effective ventilation to replenish the oxygen stores in alveolar gas, free diffusion of both oxygen and carbon dioxide across the alveolar-capillary barrier, and sustained blood flow through the capillaries. Evolution has produced a situation in which gas exchange must switch sites from the placenta to the lung rapidly after birth. Strictly in terms of O_2 exchange, this switch represents a substantial improvement in the efficiency of the gas-exchange apparatus, from the circulatory countercurrent pattern of the human placenta to the alveolar-capillary interface in the lungs. Placental gas exchange is associated with a gradient from maternal uterine artery partial pressure of oxygen (PO_2) of approximately 85 mm Hg at sea level to a fetal umbilical venous PO_2 of approximately 40 mm Hg, a gradient of approximately 45 mm Hg. In normal adult lungs the gradient from alveolar oxygen tension (approximately 110 mm Hg in room air) to arterial blood oxygen tension (approximately 100 mm Hg) is approximately 10 mm Hg; this gradient is referred to as the alveolar-arterial difference in O_2 ($AaDO_2$). The mechanisms for maintaining the matching of alveolar ventilation ($\dot{V}_A$), usually referred to as $\dot{V}$, and pulmonary perfusion ($\dot{Q}_P$), usually referred to as $\dot{Q}$, and the factors that influence changes in the intrapulmonary distribution of $\dot{V}$ and $\dot{Q}$ and thereby the matching of $\dot{V}$ to $\dot{Q}$ ($\dot{V}/\dot{Q}$ matching) in neonates are the topics of this chapter.

A distinct feature of postnatal gas exchange to which the lung must accommodate is the different frequency at which $\dot{V}$ and $\dot{Q}$ occur. The pulmonary circulation maintains exclusively unidirectional flow, although at varying velocity, through the pulmonary microvasculature. By contrast, the inhalation of gases is periodic, occurring normally at a rate in neonates that is 20% to 50% of the cardiac rate during health and may be closer to 75% with pulmonary disorders. These different rates of ventilation and perfusion must be accommodated in achieving and maintaining optimal pulmonary gas exchange a continuous process. To help sustain sufficient O_2 and CO_2 flux between gas and blood, an adequate alveolar gas volume or functional residual capacity (FRC) must be established shortly after birth and sustained thereafter. Development of the FRC occurs in the process of transition from fetal to neonatal life as the fluid-filled fetal lung empties of liquid and refills with gas. Once established, this gas volume serves as an intrapulmonary reservoir for oxygen allowing for the continuous process of pulmonary gas exchange.

The newborn infant is particularly vulnerable to the development of arterial hypoxemia for several reasons. At the time of birth there is a rapid switch from the fetal circulatory pattern to the adult pattern, i.e., a rapid increase in pulmonary blood flow coupled with the onset of alveolar ventilation. If this does not occur, then the infant will maintain extra-pulmonary shunting of blood away from the lung across the patent ductus arteriosus (PDA) and/or foramen ovale leading to arterial hypoxemia. There are also postnatal characteristics of the neonatal lung that lead to this vulnerability to arterial hypoxemia. First, the partial pressure of oxygen in arterial blood (Pao_2) of normal newborns is low compared with that of adults.[1,2] Second, the FRC is relatively low given the compliant chest wall, resulting in less intravascular oxygen reserve during periods of no oxygen movement into the lungs (i.e., during apnea). Third, the FRC in the neonatal lung is close to the airway closing volume. Atelectasis, or airway closure, is more likely to develop, especially considering the relative paucity of channels of collateral ventilation in the newborn. Finally, the metabolic demand for oxygen in infants is greater on a per-kilogram basis than in adults. Therefore, the infant more quickly depletes oxygen stores in the blood and in resident alveolar gas in attempting to maintain aerobic metabolism. These factors are accentuated in premature infants, who are more susceptible to apnea because of their immature respiratory drive and because of lung segment collapse at the end of expiration due to extremely compliant chest walls.

ASSESSMENT OF VENTILATION-PERFUSION RELATIONSHIPS

OXYGEN GRADIENT

The measurement of P_aO_2 provides an excellent approximation of the efficiency of the lung as a gas-exchanging organ. One can use the P_aO_2 and some assumptions to calculate the idealized alveolar (A) to arterial (a) oxygen gradient (or $AaDO_2$) by first calculating the P_AO_2 by solving the alveolar air equation:

$$P_AO_2 = P_IO_2 - \frac{P_aCO_2}{R} + \left[F_IO_2 \times P_ACO_2 \times \frac{1-R}{R}\right],$$

where R is the respiratory exchange ratio. P_ACO_2 is assumed to be approximately equal to P_aCO_2 and P_IO_2 is calculated from measured barometric pressure and body temperature, and assumes that inspired gas is 100% saturated with water vapor ($PH_2O = 47$ mm Hg) on reaching the acinar space ($P_IO_2 = F_IO_2 \times [PB - PH_2O]$). Thus, at sea level, breathing ambient air, the $P_IO_2 = 150$ mm Hg. As an example, the P_AO_2 for a normal adult breathing ambient air at sea level and assuming a P_ACO_2 of 40 mm Hg and an R of 0.8 would be $P_AO_2 = 150 - 35/0.8 + [0.21 \times 40 \times (1 - 0.8)/0.8] = 108$ mm Hg. Thus, if the P_aO_2 is 100 mm Hg, then the $AaDO_2 = 108$ mm Hg − 100 mm Hg = 8 mm Hg. Neonates have larger $AaDO_2$ values than do adults during ambient air breathing, and the $AaDO_2$ can be as high as 40 to 50 mm Hg shortly after birth, even allowing for R values close to 1.0 in neonates (presumably based on relatively high utilization of carbohydrates). $AaDO_2$ may remain in the 20 to 40 mm Hg range for days after birth in term nondistressed infants[3,4] even with SpO_2 values greater than 90% (remember that the oxygen-hemoglobin dissociation curve for fetal hemoglobin is shifted to the left compared to adult hemoglobin).

$AaDO_2$ quantifies the degree of venous admixture plus alveolar-capillary membrane diffusion disequilibrium. However, neither $AaDO_2$ nor the calculated ratio of arterial-to-alveolar oxygen tension (P_aO_2/P_AO_2) discriminates between these components, and both are insensitive to situations with both intrapulmonary (or extrapulmonary) shunt and pulmonary parenchymal diseases. Venous admixture includes both intrapulmonary shunt (perfusion of pulmonary capillary blood past non-ventilated lung regions before joining the stream of pulmonary venous blood, see Fig. 64.1A and $\dot{Q}P_3$ in Fig. 64.2) and perfusion of low $\dot{V}/\dot{Q}$ areas (see Fig. 64.1B and $\dot{Q}P_2$ Fig. 64.2), in which alveolar ventilation is insufficient to restore P_AO_2 to the value predicted from the "idealized" P_AO_2 calculated earlier. Pulmonary end-capillary to alveolar space equilibrium can be predicted to occur for oxygen and carbon dioxide in low $\dot{V}/\dot{Q}$ areas because P_AO_2 is low and only a small rise in pulmonary P_aO_2 occurs as blood traverses the pulmonary microcirculation (Fig. 64.1B).[5] Depressed pulmonary end-capillary PO_2 is associated with disproportionately depressed oxygen content because of the shape of the oxygen-hemoglobin curve, leading to an exaggerated depression of the mixed arterial PO_2 as measured in the left atrium or systemic arteries (assuming no extrapulmonary right-to-left shunts). Therefore, overall pulmonary gas exchange is the flow-weighted and alveolar ventilation-weighted sum of gas exchange occurring across all of the lungs' $\dot{V}/\dot{Q}$ regions (see Fig. 64.2). Note that the rise in P_aO_2 in the high $\dot{V}/\dot{Q}$ region (see Fig. 64.1D) and the decrease in P_aCO_2 do not equal levels of alveolar gas partial pressures that would be found if no regional perfusion existed. Lung units with both low $\dot{V}/\dot{Q}$ and normal $\dot{V}/\dot{Q}$ relationships are depicted in Figs. 64.1 and 64.2. Also shown is a pulmonary arterial to pulmonary venous connection bypassing any aerated area (see Fig. 64.1A and $\dot{Q}P_3$ in Fig. 64.2), which in the neonate could represent shunt through the ductus arteriosus, the foramen ovale, connections between pulmonary and bronchial arteries, or through the Thebesian circulation (venous drainage from the myocardium directly to the left ventricle). In the preterm infant with surfactant deficiency, this could also represent blood flowing past atelectatic alveoli, which have collapsed due to increased surface tension. Indeed, one reason that preterm infants with surfactant deficiency respond to exogenous surfactant therapy with an increase in P_aO_2 (or SpO_2) is that $\dot{V}/\dot{Q}$ matching is improved as atelectatic alveoli are reinflated and ventilated.

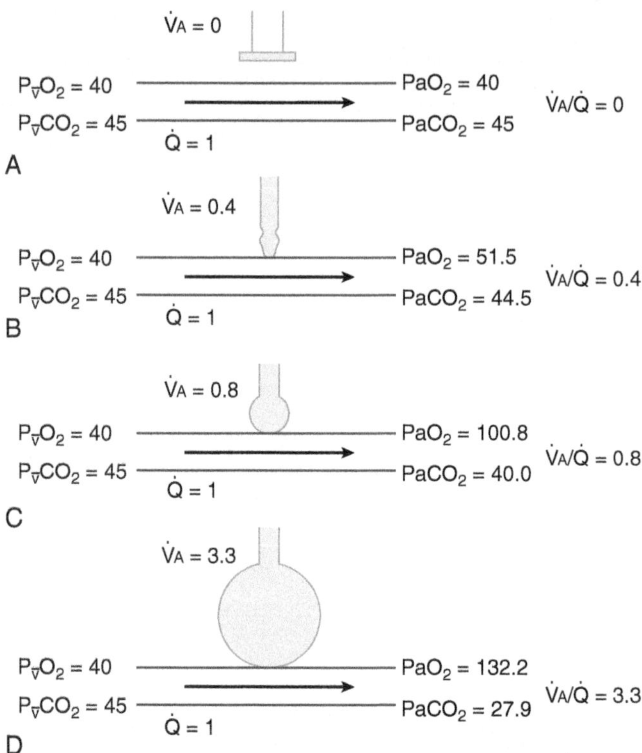

Fig. 64.1 Effects of $\dot{V}/\dot{Q}$ ratios on blood gas tensions expressed in millimeters of mercury. (A) Intrapulmonary shunt leaves mixed venous blood gas tensions unaltered. (B) Alveolus with low $\dot{V}/\dot{Q}$ ratio: only partial oxygenation occurs. (C) Relatively normal $\dot{V}/\dot{Q}$ ratio with satisfactory oxygenation of pulmonary capillary blood. (D) Underperfused alveolus with high $\dot{V}/\dot{Q}$ ratio. (From Thibeault DW, Gregory GA, eds. *Neonatal Pulmonary Care*. 2nd ed. Norwalk, CT: Appleton & Lang; 1986.)

Although the $AaDO_2$ measured in ambient air provides an overall summary of pulmonary oxygen exchange efficiency, it provides little information about pulmonary reserves or about the cause of an increased $AaDO_2$. A surrogate measure of pulmonary gas exchange that is related to the $AaDO_2$, the oxygenation index (OI) combines P_aO_2, F_IO_2, and lung distending pressure as measured by the mean airway pressure (MAP), where $OI = (MAP \times F_IO_2 \times 100)/P_aO_2$. The OI is commonly used in the neonatal intensive care unit (NICU), in particular in term infants, to help guide decisions related to need for advanced therapies. Although the OI is helpful in estimating $AaDO_2$ or the degree of $\dot{V}/\dot{Q}$ mismatch, it also does not discriminate between intrapulmonary and extrapulmonary causes of hypoxemia.

The effect of low $\dot{V}/\dot{Q}$ areas on $AaDO_2$ can be eliminated by breathing 100% oxygen to remove nitrogen from any open but underventilated lung regions (Fig. 64.3). However, breathing 100% oxygen is not sustainable as a method to improve $\dot{V}/\dot{Q}$ matching, since absorption atelectasis tends to develop, which would paradoxically increase the contribution of the intrapulmonary shunt and thereby result in an increase in $\dot{V}/\dot{Q}$

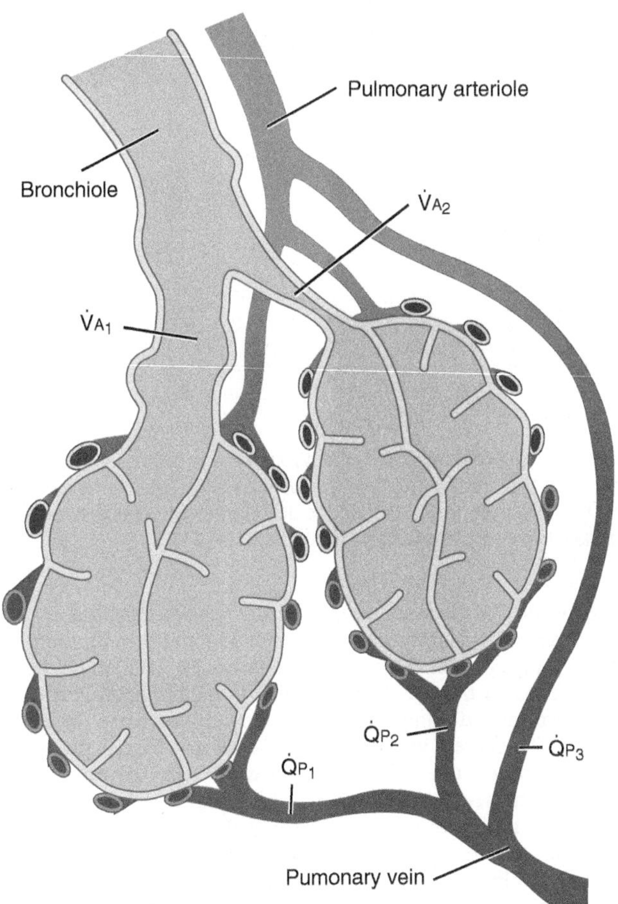

Fig. 64.2 Airway and vascular relationships. The acinar unit, containing many alveolar sacs, is shown with multiple pulmonary capillaries enveloping the saccules, providing the maximal gas-exchanging surface area. $\dot{V}_{A1}/\dot{Q}_{P1}$ corresponds to an acinar region (containing multiple alveoli) with normal $\dot{V}_A/\dot{Q}_P$; $\dot{V}_{A2}/\dot{Q}_{P2}$ represents an acinar region with a low $\dot{V}_A/\dot{Q}_P$ and poor gas exchange. The pulmonary arteriole to pulmonary venous connection $\dot{Q}P_3$, which bypasses any air-containing spaces, could represent intrapulmonary as well as extrapulmonary shunts.

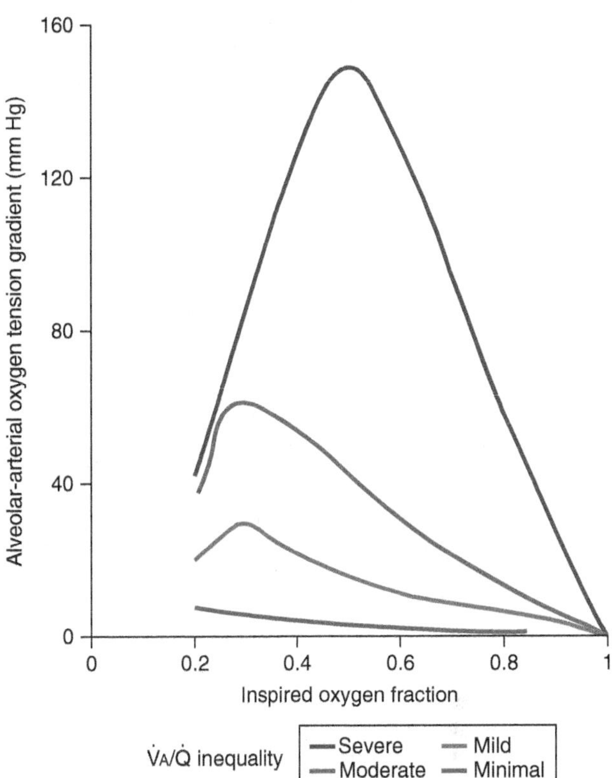

Fig. 64.3 The effects of changes in inspired oxygen fraction, shown on the abscissa, on the calculated alveolar-arterial oxygen gradient are plotted for various degrees of $\dot{V}/\dot{Q}$ inequality without any coexisting shunt. (From Dantzker DR. Physiology and pathophysiology of pulmonary gas exchange. *Hosp Pract (Off Ed)*. 1986;15:135.)

mismatch and a decrease in P_aO_2. Furthermore, prolonged exposure to 100% oxygen causes severe central nervous system and pulmonary toxicities. Interestingly, as shown in Fig. 64.3, the $AaDO_2$ tends to increase as the F_IO_2 is increased from 0.21, and then as the F_IO_2 continues to increase, slowly decreases until with an F_IO_2 of 1.00 there is no $AaDO_2$ (see Fig. 64.3).[6] The greater the degree of $\dot{V}/\dot{Q}$ mismatch, the larger the increase in $AaDO_2$ with increasing F_IO_2. There is evidence that increased shunt with oxygen breathing occurs in premature infants[7] and neonatal lambs but not in adult dogs.[8] These differences have been attributed to different degrees of development of pathways of collateral ventilation. Hence, neither P_aO_2 nor the ratio of arterial-to-alveolar PO_2 alone provides detailed knowledge of the state of the $\dot{V}/\dot{Q}$ relationships in the lung. The unique shape of the oxygen and carbon dioxide hemoglobin dissociation curves make precise quantification of exact patterns of $\dot{V}/\dot{Q}$ heterogeneity difficult to determine. Use of multiple inert gas techniques to directly measure $\dot{V}/\dot{Q}$ have not completely eliminated the uncertainty in $\dot{V}/\dot{Q}$ distribution. Furthermore, there is no clinically useful way of measuring $\dot{V}/\dot{Q}$ distribution in the neonatal lungs due to the size of infants, although some experimental techniques have been reported. There has been an attempt to model various $\dot{V}/\dot{Q}$ distributions using readily available bedside measurements such as Spo_2, arterial blood gases, and other means. However, all of these models have their own limitations and therefore there is no particular method that has come into widespread clinical use. Thus, Spo_2 and/or P_aO_2 are used in the NICU as surrogate measures of $\dot{V}/\dot{Q}$ matching, despite all of the weaknesses described above.

In an effort to separate the effects of intrapulmonary shunt from regions of low $\dot{V}/\dot{Q}$, Roe and Jones[9] and Smith and Jones[10] have created algorithms in which simultaneous measurements of Spo_2 were plotted against the calculated P_IO_2 value. Using these graphs, one can differentiate shunt from low $\dot{V}/\dot{Q}$ areas. The method assumes that changes in the shape of P_IO_2 versus Spo_2 curves, or changes in the position of the curves, are reflective of changes in shunt or in low $\dot{V}/\dot{Q}$ areas, or both. (Fig. 64.4). Thus, the degree of right shift of the curves away from the oxyhemoglobin dissociation curve is an index of reduced $\dot{V}/\dot{Q}$ matching. This technique may translate into individualization of approaches to improving gas exchange in the two different circumstances or in the circumstance in which both significant shunt and significant low $\dot{V}/\dot{Q}$ areas contribute to arterial hypoxemia. One limitation of the technique is the need to measure Spo_2 and P_IO_2 data points quickly. The measurement of Spo_2 in the NICU has its own limitations. Another limitation of the technique proposed[9,10] is that the low $\dot{V}/\dot{Q}$ area is not further quantifiable. The importance of the low $\dot{V}/\dot{Q}$ area, which is treated as a single value, may not be differentiated among different regions with variably low $\dot{V}/\dot{Q}$ areas (<0.8). As with other techniques, this assessment assumes standard hemoglobin concentration and pH. The model uses a three-compartment gas-exchange model: namely, shunt, a normal $\dot{V}/\dot{Q}$ region, and a low $\dot{V}/\dot{Q}$ region, as shown in Fig. 64.5. Differentiation of shunt from low $\dot{V}Q$ at the bedside

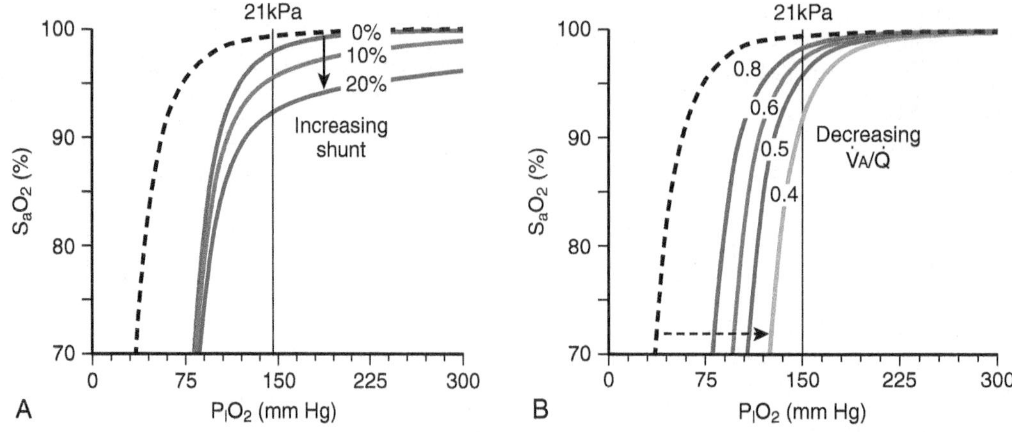

Fig. 64.4 The effects of arterial oxygen saturation *(S_aO_2)* with changing inspired oxygen pressure P_IO_2 *(heavy lines)*, with either (A) increasing shunt from 0% to 20% *(downward arrow)* or (B) reducing ventilation–perfusion ratio ($\dot{V}/\dot{Q}$ from 0.8 to 0.4 *[rightward arrow]*). The oxyhemoglobin dissociation curve is the *long dashed line,* which plots blood S_aO_2 versus P_aO_2. (Data from Smith HL, Jones JG. Non-invasive assessment of shunt and ventilation/perfusion ratio in neonates with pulmonary failure. *Arch Dis Child Fetal Neonatal Ed.* 2001;85:F127–132.)

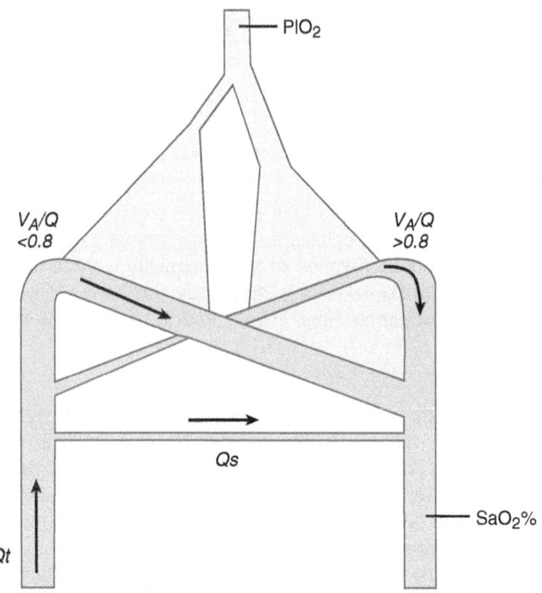

Fig. 64.5 Three-compartment gas-exchange model showing shunt *($\dot{Q}s$)* compartment, and two ventilation–perfusion ratio ($\dot{V}/\dot{Q}$) compartments. With use of a physiologic model,[8] the first step was to vary the shunt while keeping $\dot{V}/\dot{Q}$ of the two other compartments normal (0.8). The second step was to reduce $\dot{V}/\dot{Q}$ of the well-perfused compartment with the shunt set at zero.[8] P_IO_2, Inspired oxygen tension; S_aO_2, arterial oxygen saturation. (From Jones JG, Jones SE. Discriminating between the effect of shunt and reduced V˙A/Q˙ on arterial oxygen saturation is particularly useful in clinical practice. *J Clin Monit Comput* 2000;16:337–350.)

could contribute to both improved understanding of the cause of hypoxemia and consequently to more specific therapy.

NITROGEN GRADIENT

When P_AO_2 is low because of diminished alveolar ventilation (i.e., insufficient replacement of alveolar oxygen from inspiratory gas relative to the rate of removal by pulmonary capillary blood), the alveolar partial pressure of nitrogen (P_AN_2) rises because during "no flow" states (end-expiration and end-inspiration) the sum of gas partial pressures in the alveolar spaces will equal atmospheric pressure. P_AH_2O and P_ACO_2 are relatively constant; therefore, when P_AO_2 is diminished, P_AN_2 must be increased. If the elevated P_AN_2 is sustained, there will be increased absorption of nitrogen into pulmonary capillary blood and development of an arterial-to-alveolar nitrogen gradient ($aADN_2$), which has been used to identify the presence of low $\dot{V}/\dot{Q}$ lung regions. Perfusion of non-ventilated lung units produces no increase in P_AN_2, because the mixed venous and end-capillary partial pressures are the same for O_2, CO_2, and N_2, as well as for any other inert gas solution (see Fig. 64.1A). An $aADN_2$ gradient can develop because of the presence of either a small area of very low $\dot{V}/\dot{Q}$ or a larger region of low $\dot{V}/\dot{Q}$, as long as $\dot{V}/\dot{Q}$ is less than 1.0. Use of $aADN_2$ to indirectly estimate shunt ($\dot{V}/\dot{Q} = 0$) may result in an overestimation of shunt, because of the sigmoidal shape of the oxygen-hemoglobin dissociation curve (i.e., small reductions in P_AO_2 can disproportionately depress the arterial oxygen content on the steep part of the curve).

On the basis of measurements of $AaDo_2$ and $aADN_2$ in healthy newborn infants Krauss and colleagues[11,12] inferred that a relatively small low $\dot{V}/\dot{Q}$ region occurred after 1 to 2 days of postnatal life. Furthermore, the calculated $aADN_2$ in infants with respiratory distress syndrome (RDS) showed little contribution from low $\dot{V}/\dot{Q}$ areas.[13] This observation suggests that the large venous admixture occurring with RDS results from intrapulmonary and/or perhaps extrapulmonary shunt.

CARBON DIOXIDE GRADIENT

Arterial-to-alveolar differences for carbon dioxide ($aADCO_2$) reflect areas of the lungs that are poorly perfused but have a large dead space because they receive a substantial fraction of minute ventilation ($\dot{V}_E$). Dead space in the lung is defined as areas that are ventilated but do not participate in gas exchange. There is normally a part of the tidal volume that fills the parts of the respiratory apparatus not involved in gas exchange, but involved in getting air from the atmosphere to the alveoli, including the upper airways, trachea, and conducting airways, and this is referred to as the anatomic dead space. Physiologic dead space includes the anatomic dead space plus those areas of the lung that are ventilated but not perfused, or ventilated and very poorly perfused (high $\dot{V}/\dot{Q}$ areas). Mismatching of $\dot{V}/\dot{Q}$ as a cause of CO_2 retention has been emphasized to explain the development of respiratory acidosis when minute ventilation is elevated above normal levels.[14] A small $aADCO_2$ exists in some newborn infants,[4] but when a normal FRC has been established, the small magnitude of the gradient implies only a modest presence of high $\dot{V}/\dot{Q}$ areas, except in premature infants where the $aADCO_2$ gradient remains somewhat larger, suggesting the presence of relatively more high $\dot{V}/\dot{Q}$ areas.[4] Deficiencies in CO_2

exchange during respiratory disorders probably persist after the minute ventilation has been normalized (i.e., with mechanical ventilation) due to excess physiologic dead space ventilation.[15]

TRACE INERT GASES GRADIENT

Trace quantities of inert gases can be used to quantitate the continuous distribution of $\dot{V}/\dot{Q}$ from shunt to dead space ($\dot{V}/\dot{Q}$ of 0 to $\dot{V}/\dot{Q}$ of infinity).[16] Wagner and colleagues[17,18] described a technique that uses six inert gases (which encompass a wide range of solubility in blood, see Fig. 64.6A) and in which retention of each gas in blood perfusing the lung can be expressed by the simple relationship

$$\frac{P_a}{P_v} = \frac{P_{alv}}{P_v} = \frac{\lambda}{\left(\lambda + \frac{\dot{V}_A}{\dot{Q}_F}\right)}$$

where λ is the Ostwald blood-gas solubility coefficient (unique for each gas) and P_a, P_v, and P_{alv} are the partial pressures of the gas measured in arterial blood, mixed venous blood, and alveolar gas (in reality measured in mixed expired gas and corrected for dead space ventilation), respectively. The equation assumes that each gas demonstrates a linear dissociation between blood or plasma and air, behavior unlike that demonstrated by the respiratory gases O_2 and CO_2. Under conditions of presumed steady-state gas exchange, which is always an approximation of in vivo situations, the multiple inert gas elimination technique (MIGET) allows quantification of shunt, dead space, and low and high $\dot{V}/\dot{Q}$ lung regions during both normal and experimental conditions (see Fig. 64.6B). A major advantage of the technique is the quantification of shunt, separate from low $\dot{V}/\dot{Q}$ areas, without the need to resort to 100% oxygen breathing. The experimental data consist of the measured ratios of the mixed arterial to mixed venous and mixed expired to mixed venous partial pressure for each of the gases used (usually sulfur hexafluoride, ethane, cyclopropane, halothane, diethyl ether, and acetone) and the measured solubility of each gas (Fig. 64.7). Limitations of the inert gas technique include the lack of online analysis capacity for assessment of $\dot{V}/\dot{Q}$ relations and the necessity of the assumption of steady-state gas exchange.[19]

PULSE OXIMETRY

The substitution of pulse oximetry saturation (Spo_2) for P_aO_2 is seductive in the NICU setting but can be misleading. Spo_2 is precise, reproducible, harmless, and painless to obtain. However, change in Spo_2 may not reflect concomitant change in P_aO_2 but, rather, may reflect shifting position of the oxyhemoglobin dissociation curve. Sharp increases in pH and decreases in P_aCO_2 can produce a leftward shift of the curve, raising Spo_2 without changing P_aO_2. Transfusion of adult hemoglobin into term and especially preterm infants will alter P_{50}, producing a rightward shift and a lower Spo_2 with no change in P_aO_2. Lack of awareness of this potential discrepancy may result in inappropriate undertreatment or overtreatment in an effort to maintain Spo_2 in a narrow window. This limitation of Spo_2 for predicting P_aO_2 also is a limitation in the interpretation of the "physiologic" diagnosis of bronchopulmonary dysplasia (BPD).[20]

ASSUMPTIONS ABOUT ASSESSMENT OF VENTILATION AND PERFUSION

One important assumption is uniformity of the inspired gas composition. Inspired gas that is altered in composition by rebreathing of expired gas from more slowly emptying adjacent lung areas in the nonhomogeneously ventilated lung will produce series inequality of ventilation, which is difficult to differentiate from the more familiar parallel inequality.[21] This situation may be encountered in the NICU in patients with severe BPD on mechanical ventilation.

Although the composition of pulmonary arterial blood is relatively uniform, intraregional differences in hematocrit may affect gas exchange.[22] Gas exchange is impaired when lung units with low $\dot{V}/\dot{Q}$ are perfused by blood with high hematocrit. If high neonatal hematocrits predispose to greater pulmonary interregional variability, this effect could theoretically contribute to depressed oxygen exchange, but the effect even if present is likely minor.

Alveolar end-pulmonary capillary partial pressure disequilibrium, as may occur during a shortened transit time across the pulmonary capillary bed, may limit transport of oxygen. Alveolar end-capillary disequilibrium for inert gases, with their rapid equilibrium time, is less than for respiratory gases.[23]

All the techniques used for gas exchange analysis have limits because of invasiveness, inaccuracy, or irreproducibility. They depend on assumptions about steady-state conditions, which in periods of rapid transient changes in pulmonary blood flow or alveolar ventilation, or in the presence of pulmonary disease, may not be true. During rapidly evolving disease states, the techniques may not reflect rapidly changing contributions to overall gas exchange inefficiency of the lung.[24]

Even with all of these assumptions and issues discussed in the section above, $\dot{V}/\dot{Q}$ can be measured directly in adults. For example, $\dot{V}/\dot{Q}$ scans have been used for a long time in adult medicine and involve 2 nuclear scans, one to measure ventilation to the lungs and a second to measure perfusion. A radioactive tracer is used in both scans: for the first scan it is given via nebulization and for the second a different radioactive tracer is given intravenously. These scans entail minimal risk and are excellent for detecting areas of large $\dot{V}/\dot{Q}$ mismatch, as seen with pulmonary emboli or chronic obstructive pulmonary disease (COPD). Another method that is used in adults is the MIGET, as discussed above under "Trace Inert

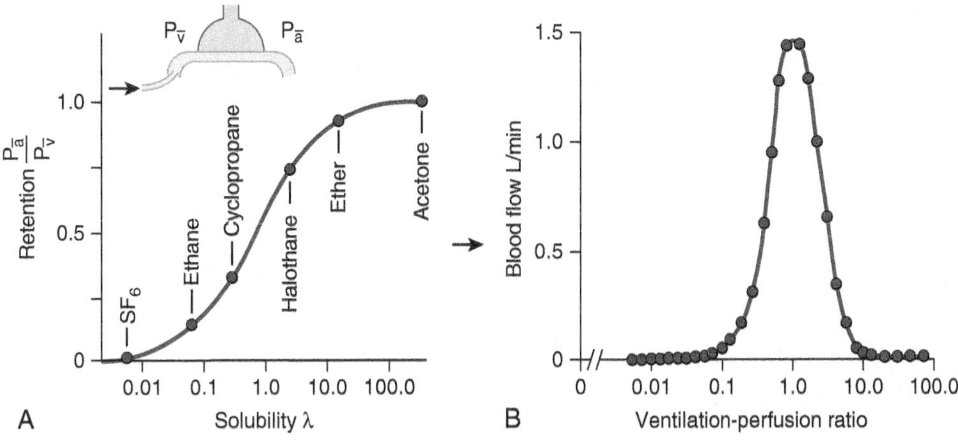

Fig. 64.6 (A) Retention–solubility curve created by the experimental techniques referred to in the text for six gases. (B) The retention–solubility curve can be used to derive a distribution of fractional perfusion to each of 50 theoretical lung compartments. P_a, Partial pressure of each inert gas in arterial blood; P_v, partial pressure in mixed venous blood. (From West JB. State of the art: ventilation–perfusion relationships. *Am Rev Respir Dis.* 1977;116:919.)

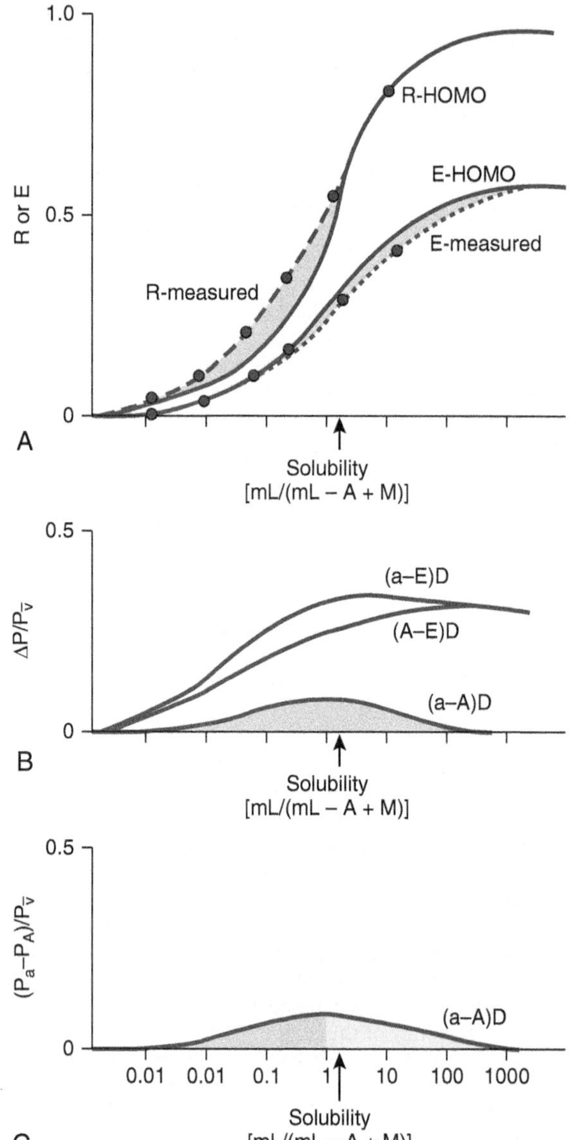

Fig. 64.7 (A) Measured and homogeneous *(HOMO)* retention *(R)* and excretion *(E)* versus solubility, with retention and excretion values shown as *circles*. The homogeneous curves would occur if there were no $\dot{V}/\dot{Q}$ heterogeneity in the lung (i.e., an idealized lung). *Pink areas* between measured and homogeneous retention and excretion curves occur because of $\dot{V}/\dot{Q}$ heterogeneity. (B) The sum of the areas under the aAD curve is shown. The area under the (a–A)D curve is calculated by subtraction of the (A–E)(D) curve from the (a–E)D curve. The *arrow* on the abscissa indicates solubility that is numerically equal to mean $\dot{V}/\dot{Q}$ in the lung. (C) The area under the curve to the left of the mean $\dot{V}/\dot{Q}$ represented by the *pink area* is an index of low $\dot{V}/\dot{Q}$ lung areas. (From Truog WE, Hlastala MP, Standaert TA, et al. Oxygen-induced alteration of ventilation–perfusion relationships in rats. *J Appl Physiol.* 1979;47:1112.)

Gas Gradients." Single photon emission computed tomography (SPECT) has been used, but mostly for research purposes. Recently, magnetic resonance (MR) techniques have been developed using pulse sequences and/or hyperpolarized gas lung MR imaging (MRI) to directly measure $\dot{V}/\dot{Q}$ matching in adults, particularly those with COPD.[25-27] Currently, in neonatology $\dot{V}/\dot{Q}$ matching is not directly measured clinically in our patients, due in large part to challenges with the size of the patient and relatively small tidal volumes and perfusion compared to adults. However, the

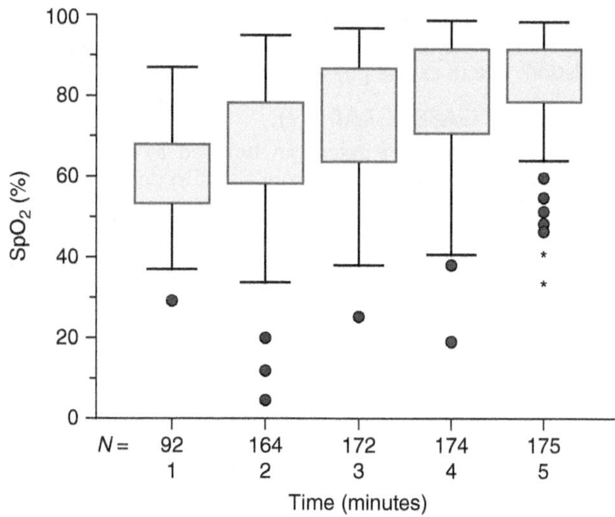

Fig. 64.8 Box plots showing the median, quartiles, range (1.5 times the quartile on that side), outliers, and extreme values for Spo_2 at each minute after birth for the first 5 minutes. *N* is the number of patients in whom Spo_2 was obtained. A number less than 175 indicates that Spo_2 was not obtained in all cases. (From Kamlin CO, O'Donnell CP, Davis PG, Morley CJ. Oxygen saturation in healthy infants immediately after birth. *J Pediatr.* 2006;148:585.)

field is moving rapidly, and these advanced imaging techniques may soon be available to assess $\dot{V}/\dot{Q}$ matching, at least for larger infants with bronchopulmonary dysplasia in our NICUs, within the assumptions and limitations outlined above.[28]

PERINATAL TRANSITION AND GAS EXCHANGE

The decline of pulmonary arterial pressure (*P*pa) and pulmonary vascular resistance (PVR) after birth occurs in conjunction with elimination of some of the intraparenchymal pulmonary fluid. Factors modulating the decline in *P*pa include the endogenously produced arachidonate metabolite and vasodilator prostacyclin[29] and endogenously produced nitric oxide.[30] Mean *P*pa does not approach adult values until days after birth. Wagner[31] has suggested that moderate elevation in *P*pa may help maintain $\dot{V}/\dot{Q}$ matching, given the relatively unstable lung volume of the neonate. However, elevations in PVR also favor passage of vascular fluid into the extravascular alveolar lung spaces, especially if the anatomic site of increased pressure is venular. Such fluid extravasation can have secondary deleterious effects on $\dot{V}/\dot{Q}$ matching by altering bronchiolar dimensions (see Fig. 64.2).[32]

The rate of change in SpO_2 in the minutes after delivery of healthy term infants has been assessed.[33,34] Combining a large number of observations in term infants, Kamlin and colleagues[33] demonstrated a rise in Spo_2 from 60% at 1 minute after clamping of the umbilical cord (range 38% to 82%) to a median of 84% by 5 minutes of age (Fig. 64.8).[33] They noted that saturation of greater than 80% was achieved at less than 4 minutes (median time of 2.5 minutes) and saturation of greater than 90% was achieved in less than 7 minutes in term infants born either vaginally or by cesarean delivery. This is consistent with a rapid and significant improvement in $\dot{V}/\dot{Q}$ matching within the lung occurring within minutes of birth. The previously noted limitations with the use of Spo_2 and their correlation with arterial oxygen tension in these infants breathing ambient air also apply to these studies.

FACTORS REGULATING VENTILATION–PERFUSION MATCHING IN THE NEONATAL LUNG

EFFECTS OF INCREASED PULMONARY ARTERIAL PRESSURE

In fetal life *P*pa equals or exceeds systemic arterial pressure (*P*sa), and *P*pa declines normally in the hours surrounding birth to a level approximately 50% of *P*sa. The further decline to adult levels occurs more slowly. Marked (suprasystemic) levels of *P*pa can cause hypoxemia due to extrapulmonary shunting, as seen in persistent pulmonary hypertension of the newborn (PPHN). It is unknown, however, to what extent increased *P*pa or persistent elevation of *P*pa undermines or contributes to the stability of $\dot{V}/\dot{Q}$ matching in the neonatal lung during the normal transition to extrauterine life or during pulmonary diseases. Neonatal pulmonary diseases are commonly characterized by marked vasoreactivity, leading to elevated PVR and *P*pa. The diseased neonatal lung may also demonstrate collapsed segments or lobes, which can interfere with $\dot{V}/\dot{Q}$ matching. An elevation in *P*pa may change the intrapulmonary distribution of blood flow. Elevations in *P*pa can occur either because of constriction of smooth muscle lining the vessels that constitute the pulmonary microvasculature (vasoreactivity) or because of an increase in left atrial pressure. Different vasoactive substances may mediate vasoconstriction at different sites within the microvasculature.[35] Changes in *P*pa are relevant to gas exchange in both the adult and the newborn. However, in establishing and maintaining $\dot{V}/\dot{Q}$ matching, neonates appear to respond differently from adults to certain stimuli affecting *P*pa, PVR, and at least theoretically, bronchial and bronchiolar smooth muscle constriction. For instance, lambs have a more vigorous hypoxic pulmonary vasoconstrictive response than do adult sheep, and the onset of the response can be detected at a higher P_{aO_2}.[36] If this phenomenon is also true in humans, it has implications in neonates regarding the effects of even brief apneic episodes on $\dot{V}/\dot{Q}$ matching. Inferences about effects of the changes in *P*pa in neonates with both regional and generalized lung injury cannot be easily extrapolated from results in adults.

HYPOXIC PULMONARY VASOCONSTRICTION AND $\dot{V}/\dot{Q}$ MATCHING

Hypoxic pulmonary vasoconstriction (HPV) prevents localized $\dot{V}/\dot{Q}$ mismatching by diminishing blood flow locally to those areas of the lungs that are underventilated or not ventilated at all. As regional alveolar and acinar PO_2 decline, due to reduced localized ventilation, blood flow through the local pulmonary microvasculature is decreased by an increase in resistance in muscular small arteries. Blood flow is then redirected into well-ventilated nonhypoxic lung regions. The mechanisms by which a decrease in local P_AO_2 induces constriction of vascular smooth muscle remain incompletely understood. Many modulators, including vasoconstrictive leukotrienes, have been described.[37] Mediation of this response, as opposed to modulation, may depend on the status of calcium- and potassium-selective membrane channels in the pulmonary vascular smooth muscle cells.[38]

When regional alveolar hypoxia is created by lobar or segmental atelectasis induced by endobronchial balloon obstruction, a relationship exists between the increase in local PVR in the atelectatic region and the increase in overall intrapulmonary shunt. This is shown in Fig. 64.9 by the greater than expected P_aO_2 suggesting that the local increase in PVR in the atelectatic region limited blood flow to the atelectatic region while increasing blood flow to the well ventilated parts of the lung and thereby maintaining better than expected $\dot{V}/\dot{Q}$ matching and P_aO_2. Marshall[39] showed that with progressively larger areas of pulmonary parenchymal collapse, up to unilateral atelectasis, the diversion away from atelectatic lung areas and the capacity to maintain satisfactory $\dot{V}/\dot{Q}$ matching becomes less effective (see Fig. 64.9). These studies are particularly relevant to neonatal respiratory conditions, in which both lobar and multiregional atelectasis can develop.

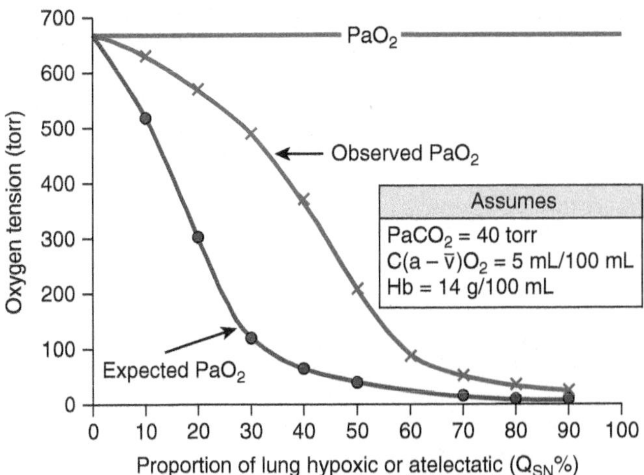

Fig. 64.9 The effect of progressively increasing size of the atelectatic lung region on arterial oxygen tension is demonstrated by the *red line*, which would occur if no redistribution of blood flow away from atelectatic area occurred. The *blue line* indicates effects of presumed hypoxic pulmonary vasoconstriction. Note the conversion of the two lines when more than 40% of the lung develops atelectasis. The assumptions regarding O_2 content (C_aO_2) are shown in the *inset*. (From Marshall BE. Importance of hypoxic pulmonary vasoconstriction with atelectasis. *Adv Shock Res* 1982;8:1.)

In addition to the size of the collapsed and nonventilated segment as a modifier of HPV and $\dot{V}/\dot{Q}$ matching, the presence of inflammatory cells and their products in the affected region have been found to modify HPV. Secretions containing bacteria and inflammatory cell products can become trapped in atelectatic regions, these products contain vasoactive substances. These vasoactive substances can then potentially inhibit local HPV. By inhibiting HPV, the regional blood flow to the atelectatic region is not decreased, maintaining $\dot{V}/\dot{Q}$ mismatch leading to decreased P_aO_2.

Global, or total, lung exposure to alveolar hypoxia produces a different challenge for control of pulmonary gas exchange. Global alveolar hypoxia has the potential to increase regional blood flow to preexisting shunt or low $\dot{V}/\dot{Q}$ regions, and thereby worsening $\dot{V}/\dot{Q}$ matching. However, in lambs exposed to acute alveolar hypoxia (F_{IO_2} = 0.12), there is no evidence of an alteration in $\dot{V}/\dot{Q}$ matching in spite of a doubling (beyond room air baseline values) of *P*pa and PVR. Hansen and colleagues[40] demonstrated redistribution of blood flow in neonatal lambs during acute alveolar hypoxia, providing indirect evidence of heterogeneity of local vascular resistance during conditions associated with elevated PVR.

An important effect of increasing *P*pa in the normal lung is the recruitment of previously underperfused or nonperfused pulmonary capillaries, particularly in the upper lobes. This recruitment serves the important physiologic mechanism of increasing the gas-exchange surface area and acts as a type of "reserve" mechanism to help sustain pulmonary gas exchange during various conditions, including exercise and assent to high altitude. However, evidence suggests that neonatal lambs have a fully recruited pulmonary microvasculature at rest, at least as assessed by direct vital microscopy during hypoxia[41] or measurement of carbon monoxide diffusing capacity (D_{LCO}) in conditions of altered pulmonary blood flow due to opening of an aorticopulmonary shunt.[42] Indirect evidence for full capillary recruitment present under baseline conditions has also been inferred from work in piglets.[43] If these findings can be generalized to newborn humans, they represent another instance of the decreased reserves available to sustain gas exchange in neonates and also point to a relative lack of vascular compliance in the neonatal lung.

The role of acute HPV in the maintenance of $\dot{V}/\dot{Q}$ matching has been tested in neonatal lambs subjected to 3 days of breathing more than 90% inspired oxygen,[44] a clinically important situation in the NICU given the propensity of neonates to desaturate despite being given supplemental oxygen. This was done to determine if hyperoxia caused blunting of the vascular response to acute alveolar hypoxia (F_IO_2 = 0.12) and if this would be associated with worsened $\dot{V}/\dot{Q}$ matching. Hyperoxia-treated animals demonstrated diminished acute HPV and resultant increase in $\dot{V}/\dot{Q}$ mismatching during exposure to acute vasoconstrictive stimuli, including alveolar hypoxia, compared with the normoxia-treated control animals.

Possible genetic contributions to postnatal regulation of gas exchange in a relatively hypoxic environment due to high altitude have been examined in Tibetan infants.[45] Comparisons of Spo_2 were made in healthy infants born at 3300 m (approximately 11,800 feet) and normalized for activity state. The infants of the Tibetan (multigenerational) dwellers at altitude demonstrated consistently higher Spo_2 than infants of the Han ethnic group (recent dwellers) during all relevant activity states (Fig. 64.10). Comparisons of Spo_2 were made from values obtained during active sleep, the behavioral state associated with irregular breathing effort and reduced FRC because of changes in intercostal muscle tone. Multiple factors contribute to maintenance of Spo_2 and the relevant ones that contributed to these findings could not be evaluated. However, the findings suggest that there are likely genetic determinants of the hypoxic response and its role in regulating $\dot{V}/\dot{Q}$ matching in the lung, even in very young infants.

VASOACTIVE MEDIATORS INFLUENCING PULMONARY VASCULAR RESISTANCE AND $\dot{V}/\dot{Q}$ MATCHING

Stimuli that produce an elevation in *P*pa may impair $\dot{V}/\dot{Q}$ matching in neonates by maintaining blood flow, particularly to areas of low or absent ventilation. Vasoactive peptides and phospholipid substances are two classes of such agents, which are synthesized and released into the circulation in response to stimuli including bacterial infusion or endotoxin infusion. Their effect on PVR and pulmonary gas exchange varies with the species and with postnatal age. Intravenous infusion of *Escherichia coli* endotoxin into adult goats produced a 200% to 250% rise in *P*pa and PVR, yet was associated with only a small decrease (of 8 to 9 mm Hg) in P_aO_2.[46] Infant or neonatal lambs demonstrate a response different from that of adults. In piglets, despite a similar rise in *P*pa as seen in adult animals, infusion of either group B *Streptococcus* (GBS) or other bacteria resulted in a 30 to 40 mm Hg decline in P_aO_2.[47–49] This decline was associated with a generalized mismatching of $\dot{V}/\dot{Q}$, with the development of low $\dot{V}/\dot{Q}$ areas, but was not associated with an increase in intrapulmonary shunt. The elevation in *P*pa induced by bacterial products correlated with increased plasma levels of the vasoconstrictor arachidonic acid metabolite thromboxane,[47] implying that arachidonate products can alter distribution of perfusion and ventilation and thereby affect $\dot{V}/\dot{Q}$ matching in the lung.

The young piglet has served as a useful model for examining the effects on pulmonary gas exchange of potential antiinflammatory or antiinfective therapies, including anti-vasoactive agents. After pretreatment with a thromboxane synthase inhibitor, the infusion of GBS into piglets led to no immediate increase in *P*pa, decrease in P_aO_2, or development of $\dot{V}/\dot{Q}$ mismatching due to an increase in the low $\dot{V}/\dot{Q}$ compartment.[50] When administered after 2 hours of bacterial infusion, inhibitors of thromboxane synthase decreased *P*pa and PVR but did not improve P_aO_2 or the low $\dot{V}/\dot{Q}$ compartment.[51] These findings are interesting in that they imply that regulation of hemodynamics (*P*pa and PVR) and the regulation of $\dot{V}/\dot{Q}$ matching may become increasingly independent phenomena under conditions of ongoing bacterial product stimulation, suggesting that there are conditions where increases in PVR have little effect on $\dot{V}/\dot{Q}$ matching. Gibson and colleagues[52] demonstrated that multiple vasoactive agents participate in the persistence of elevated PVR in experimental piglets during controlled bacteremia and that catecholamines are another class of substances that can alter $\dot{V}/\dot{Q}$ matching in the neonate by increasing *P*pa. Truog and Standaert[53] demonstrated that when dopamine was administered to neonatal lambs in which *P*pa and PVR were increased due to breathing of hypoxic gas (F_IO_2 = 0.12), a further rise is observed in *P*pa, coupled with a deterioration in gas exchange associated with an increase in both intrapulmonary shunt and $\dot{V}/\dot{Q}$ mismatching.

The effect of elevated *P*pa on gas exchange can be difficult to predict in neonates. Elevation of *P*pa may result from a diminished cross-sectional microvascular area secondary to either a primary developmental failure or delayed growth (or inappropriate regression) of the microvasculature. The diminished cross-sectional area increases vascular resistance and can result in an extrapulmonary shunt or failure to redistribute intrapulmonary blood flow. Presumably, a spectrum of regional resistances exists across the pulmonary microvasculature shortly after birth, as long as lung fluid is being removed from potential gas-exchange areas. Sudden vasoactive stimulation may result in a redistribution of pulmonary blood flow, leading to $\dot{V}/\dot{Q}$ mismatching and arterial hypoxemia, producing a vicious cycle with diminished pulmonary P_vO_2 and further decline in P_aO_2. Low mixed venous PO_2 is a secondary stimulus, inducing pulmonary arterial hypertension.[54] In situations characterized by low cardiac output and $\dot{V}/\dot{Q}$ mismatching, the low P_vO_2 increases *P*pa and PVR and may lead to intrapulmonary shunt or extrapulmonary shunt through the foramen ovale or ductus arteriosus. Measurement of simultaneously obtained pulmonary venous and preductal and postductal arterial PO_2 would be necessary to differentiate among the anatomic sites for the

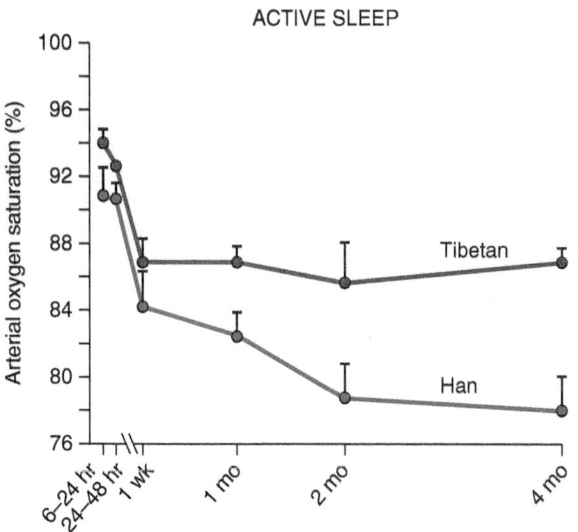

Fig. 64.10 Arterial oxygen saturation recorded in multigenerational dwellers' infants at high altitude (Tibetan) versus single-generation dwellers' infants (Han). Data were obtained during active sleep in apparently healthy term infants. (From Niermeyer S, Yang P, Shanmina, et al. Arterial oxygen saturation in Tibetan and Han infants born in Lhasa, Tibet. *N Engl J Med.* 1995;333:1248.)

shunt. Obviously, mixed venous sampling is not routinely clinically possible in sick neonates.

DISTRIBUTION OF VENTILATION AND $\dot{V}/\dot{Q}$ MATCHING

Although many studies have examined postnatal changes in lung mechanics, less information is available describing the distribution of ventilation within the lungs.[55] Analysis of the distribution of alveolar ventilation using nitrogen or xenon washout during 100% oxygen breathing is difficult to perform in neonates because of the need for multiple breath analysis and exposure to radioactivity. However, analysis of the distribution of alveolar ventilation in clinical studies suggested two types of acinar spaces that empty at different rates.[55] The pulmonary function measurement, pulmonary clearance delay, quantifies the presence of these two acinar compartments. It is difficult to draw conclusions about $\dot{V}/\dot{Q}$ matching from this index because it relates only to ventilation irrespective of the relative distribution of pulmonary perfusion. Engel[56] has reviewed the theoretical and experimental evidence for incomplete alveolar gas mixing with inspiration that develops because of the interaction between diffusion and convection at airway branch points subtending branches of unequal length. It is unknown if this problem is diminished or magnified in the much smaller neonatal lung or to what extent the resulting inhomogeneous alveolar gas mixtures contribute to overall $\dot{V}/\dot{Q}$ heterogeneity in the neonate. The immature lung, with its delayed and variable distal airway and acinar development, has not been well studied with regard to the contribution of "regional" $\dot{V}/\dot{Q}$ inequality to overall gas exchange abnormalities. Factors that influence bronchial and bronchiolar constriction can alter the distribution of each inhaled breath, and Box 64.1 lists some of the factors relevant to bronchial and bronchiolar constriction in young infants.

CARDIAC FUNCTION AND PULMONARY VASCULAR RESISTANCE

An additional factor influencing PVR is the diminished cardiac reserve of neonates, especially premature neonates, who depend largely on chronotropy for raising cardiac output. Older children or adults, by contrast, have effective inotropic mechanisms for increasing cardiac output. The newborn has difficulty doubling the resting cardiac output either by pharmacologic stimulation or by increased sympathetic nervous system activity. Thus, efforts to increase P_aO_2 (assuming constant tissue oxygen extraction and an unchanging degree of $\dot{V}/\dot{Q}$ mismatching) by increasing cardiac output (and thereby $P_{\bar{v}}O_2$) are not usually successful in the newborn.

Box 64.1 Some Factors Capable of Producing Bronchoconstriction or Bronchiolar Narrowing in the Newborn

- Airway inflammation
- Mucosal edema
- Excess mucous secretion
- Sloughing of damaged epithelial cells
- Hyperreactive bronchial smooth musculature
- Inspiration of cold, dry gas
- Increase in parasympathetic nervous system stimulation
- Congenital airway stenosis or deficient cartilage development
- Bronchiolar narrowing secondary to vascular engorgement
- Presence of any foreign body, including partially occluded endotracheal tubes
- Trauma from suction catheters
- Aspiration of stomach contents into upper airway
- Hypoosmolar or hyperosmolar solution in the airway

INHALED NITRIC OXIDE AND $\dot{V}/\dot{Q}$ MATCHING

The ability of inhaled nitric oxide therapy to selectively lower PVR and decrease extrapulmonary shunt accounts for the improvement in oxygenation observed in persistent PPHN.[57] However, oxygenation can also improve during inhaled nitric oxide therapy in critically ill patients who do not have extrapulmonary right-to-left shunting.[58,59] Hypoxemia in these cases is primarily due to intrapulmonary shunting caused by continued perfusion of lung units that lack ventilation (e.g., atelectasis), with variable contributions from $\dot{V}/\dot{Q}$ inequality. Distinct from its ability to decrease extrapulmonary right-to-left shunting by reducing PVR, inhaled nitric oxide therapy can in some circumstances also improve oxygenation by redirecting blood from nonventilated lung regions to ventilated distal air spaces (the so-called *microselective effect*).[60]

DIFFUSION AND PULMONARY GAS EXCHANGE

Respiratory gas exchange depends on prompt diffusion of respiratory gases between the tissue and plasma, erythrocyte and plasma, plasma and resident alveolar gas, and alveolar gas and gas in the conducting airways. Of these, alveolar-capillary membrane diffusion has been considered the likeliest barrier to gas exchange. Gas movement between alveolar space and pulmonary capillary blood is a passive process, summarized by Fick's law, which asserts that the amount of gas transferred is governed by the partial pressure of that gas in the two compartments, the inverse of the square root of the molecular weight of the gas, and the specific characteristics of the diffusion barrier (thickness and surface area). Thus, the movement of gas ($\dot{V}$) is expressed by $\dot{V} \propto D_m(P_A - P_b)$, where D_m is alveolar-capillary membrane diffusion conductance and $(P_A - P_b)$ represents the partial pressure difference across the membrane. To simplify the analysis, it is useful to study a single gas that binds firmly to hemoglobin. Because carbon monoxide (CO) combines avidly with hemoglobin, *PCO* in pulmonary capillary plasma is virtually zero when small quantities of carbon monoxide are inspired, simplifying the analysis of diffusing capacity. In clinical practice, the diffusing capacity of the lung for CO (D_{LCO}) is expressed by the following equation:

$$D_{LCO} = \frac{\dot{V}_{AC}}{P_{AC}}$$

The D_{LCO} is expressed as the volume of CO transferred in milliliters of CO per minute per mm Hg of alveolar partial pressure of CO. Both a single-breath technique (which is difficult to perform in a neonate) and a steady-state technique can be used for assessment of P_ACO.

Use of CO as the marker gas does not eliminate other variables in the interpretation. Ventilation-perfusion heterogeneity, reduced pulmonary capillary transit time, lung volume, and pulmonary capillary blood volume can affect the interpretation of diffusing capacity, as well as intrinsic properties of the alveolar capillary membrane itself, which is the actual subject of the measurement. Detailed analysis of the effects of these factors on diffusion measurement is available elsewhere.[61] Comparing serial measurements of D_{LCO} assumes that effective pulmonary blood flow (or total − shunt) is unchanged. This may be an unsupportable assumption in many neonatal pulmonary diseases. Rapid postnatal lung growth and alveolarization, with change in lung volumes, complicates interpretation of serial measurement of DLCO in the neonatal lung. However, Escourrou and colleagues[62] inferred from cross-sectional studies using the MIGET in neonatal and infant piglets that diffusion limitation may contribute to early postnatal hypoxemia in animals breathing room air. Either a reduction in surface area or an increase in thickness of the alveolar capillary membrane can reduce DLCO. Although these conditions may occur in neonatal pulmonary diseases, they probably have little practical significance for transport of oxygen because virtually every pulmonary disease is treated with increased F_IO_2, increasing P_AO_2. Hence, the driving pressure (partial pressure gradient) across the membrane becomes large for oxygen. Even in these circumstances, there may be lung regions in which diffusion disequilibrium may occur because neonatal pulmonary conditions rarely affect the lung uniformly.

Diffusing capacity for carbon monoxide has been measured in premature infants with and without RDS, and no significant differences were found.[63] However, DLCO was notably lower than the values measured in earlier studies conducted in term healthy infants.[64] The different results may relate to the smaller quantity of both intrapulmonary gas and blood found in the premature newborn. The differences highlight the problems in interpretation of cross-sectional studies of DLCO in the newborn. Perhaps the most important diffusing capacity measurements are made after recovery and growth. Hakulinen and colleagues[65] observed that children born very prematurely and studied at age 7 to 11 years demonstrated a modest but significant reduction in DLCO (single breath) compared to children born at term. This was true for premature infants with or without BPD. Some "normal" values for DLCO may have overestimated DLCO in some of these children because airflow obstruction, which was common in the preterm infants, may have produced an overestimation of the true DLCO.

IMPAIRED GAS EXCHANGE IN BRONCHOPULMONARY DYSPLASIA

The principles of pulmonary gas exchange discussed in the previous sections are supplemented here with a brief review of gas-exchange abnormalities arising from the important clinical disorder BPD. Pathologically, BPD is characterized by multifocal radiographic evidence of lung injury or by postmortem findings of airway and alveolar/acinar simplification with disordered development of the pulmonary microvasculature. Current definitions of BPD rely on assessment of need for respiratory support and/or supplemental oxygen at 36 weeks of postmenstrual age (PMA). Although the focus is on impairment in O_2 exchange, alveolar ventilation as assessed indirectly by serum bicarbonate measured at the same PMA is also impaired. Minute ventilation is normal or increased,[66] so the finding of elevated PCO_2 or serum bicarbonate level indicates alveolar hypoventilation and increased high $\dot{V}/\dot{Q}$ areas. The reasons for impairment in both O_2 and CO_2 exchange include the development of intrapulmonary shunt, the development of both high and low $\dot{V}/\dot{Q}$ areas, and possibly diffusion disequilibrium, depending on other circumstances as listed in Table 64.1. Infants requiring $F_IO_2 \geq 0.3$ at near-term equivalent age are at increased risk for recurrent hospitalization for pneumonia and for reactive airway disease, and the long-term consequences of their pulmonary insufficiency as measured at 36 weeks of PMA remain to be well defined. The very profound changes in small airway function documented in children years after their "recovering" from BPD provide a warning to work to reduce the gas-exchange inefficiencies accompanying profoundly preterm births.[67]

Alterations in $\dot{V}/\dot{Q}$ matching have been described in a few clinical studies of patients with BPD in the NICU. For example, using SPECT, Kjellberg and colleagues[68] found that in infants with BPD studied at a median PMA of 37 weeks that 60% patients with severe BPD had less than 50% of their lung volume with $\dot{V}/\dot{Q}$ between 0.6 and 1.4, which they termed satisfactory $\dot{V}/\dot{Q}$.[68] Furthermore, they[68] reported that in 30 patients with mild, moderate, or severe BPD that the percent of the lung with $\dot{V}/\dot{Q}$ between 0.6 and 1.4 was negatively correlated with days on mechanical ventilation (i.e., the less the percent of lung with satisfactory $\dot{V}/\dot{Q}$ the longer the duration of mechanical ventilation). Svedenkrans and colleagues[69] altered P_IO_2 to generate SpO_2/P_IO_2 curves (as discussed and similar to that shown in Fig. 64.4) to estimate $\dot{V}/\dot{Q}$ in preterm patients with and without BPD at a median PMA of 35 weeks. They found that infants with severe BPD had the lowest $\dot{V}/\dot{Q}$ and the greatest shunt fraction compared to infants without BPD, mild BPD, and moderate BPD.

The lungs in patients with BPD demonstrate marked heterogeneity of disease. There are lung regions that are essentially normal in terms of resistance and compliance, lung regions with elevated resistance and normal compliance, lung regions with elevated resistance and elevated compliance, and lung regions with normal resistance and elevated compliance. In general, most patients with BPD have some component of obstructive lung disease.[70] Thus the ventilation of the various lung compartments can be very different and may contribute to $\dot{V}/\dot{Q}$ mismatching and resultant hypoxemia. In particular this can be seen in the ventilator-dependent patient with severe BPD in the NICU, if one is using a strategy similar to that used early in neonatal life for lung diseases like RDS. In RDS it is important to utilize a lung-protective strategy characterized by a low tidal volume and fast rate, with short inspiratory times. However, if this lung-protective strategy is utilized in patients with severe BPD this will lead to areas of underventilation, particularly in those lung compartments with high airway resistance. Since the compartments with high airway resistance will have relatively long time constants, the fast rate, short inspiratory time strategy will not ventilate, or will poorly ventilate, the high resistance compartments, which will lead to $\dot{V}/\dot{Q}$ mismatch and hypoxemia requiring high levels of F_IO_2. Furthermore, the $\dot{V}/\dot{Q}$ mismatch may result in local areas of HPV, and if this affects a large enough portion of the pulmonary blood flow, it could contribute to an elevation of *Ppa* and potentially further worsen $\dot{V}/\dot{Q}$ matching by increasing local perfusion to the underventilated lung compartment. Thus in the patient with severe BPD, switching from a low tidal volume, fast rate strategy to one with high tidal volumes, low rates, and relatively long inspiratory times improves ventilation, particularly in the high resistance lung compartment, by allowing more time for inspiration in those long time constant compartments. This strategy thereby improves $\dot{V}/\dot{Q}$ matching

Table 64.1 Bronchopulmonary Dysplasia and Impaired Gas Exchange.

Abnormality	Effect
Distal airway simplification	Increase in high $\dot{V}/\dot{Q}$ areas and increase in dead space
Bronchial lining thickening	Maldistribution of $\dot{V}_E$
Decrease in capillary network	Increase in high $\dot{V}/\dot{Q}$ areas
Mesenchymal location of pulmonary capillary bed	Decrease in diffusing capacity
Pulmonary to bronchial venous connections	Increased intrapulmonary shunt
Anemia, decreased systemic venous O_2 saturation, decreased PvO_2	Increased risk for end capillary-alveolar disequilibrium
Altered metabolic function in the lung	Increased *Ppa* and PVR

Ppa, Pulmonary arterial pressure; *PVR*, pulmonary vascular resistance; $\dot{Q}_P$, pulmonary perfusion; $\dot{V}_A$, alveolar ventilation; $\dot{V}_E$, minute ventilation.

and hypoxemia, as evidenced by a decrease in the F_IO_2 needed to maintain the Spo_2 within the desired range.

It is also becoming increasingly clear that BPD is a lifelong disease with persistent elevations in airway resistance and the potential for alterations in cardiac function into adulthood. In fact, BPD is beginning to be referred to as a pre-COPD condition, given that patients with BPD are at high risk for developing COPD as young adults.[25] Thus, patients with BPD, and particularly severe BPD, are at risk for chronic or acute $\dot{V}/\dot{Q}$ mismatching leading to hypoxemia. Kjellberg and colleagues[71] measured $\dot{V}/\dot{Q}$ matching using SPECT in subjects with BPD at 10 years of age and found that they had reduced $\dot{V}/\dot{Q}$ matching. Um-Bergström[72] reported that young adults with BPD had increased ventilation inhomogeneity and lower DLCO compared to age matched healthy controls. Polverino and colleagues[25] demonstrated in a case of a young adult with BPD $\dot{V}/\dot{Q}$ abnormalities by ^{129}Xe MRI. These findings are consistent with persistent $\dot{V}/\dot{Q}$ abnormalities in patients with BPD as they age, even into young adulthood.

 A complete reference list is available at www.ExpertConsult.com.

SELECT REFERENCES

1. Nelson NM, Prod'hom LS, Cherry RB, et al. Pulmonary function in the newborn infant: the alveolar-arterial oxygen gradient. *J Appl Physiol*. 1963;18:534.
2. Oliver Jr TK, Demis JA, Bates GD. Serial blood gas tensions and acid-base balance during the first hour of life in human infants. *Acta Paediatr*. 1961;50:346.
3. Koch G. Alveolar ventilation, diffusing capacity, and the A-a PO_2 difference in the newborn infant. *Resp Physiol*. 1968;4:I68.
4. Thibeault DW, Poblete E, Auld PA. Alveolar-arterial oxygen O_2 and CO_2 differences and their relation to lung volume in the newborn. *Pediatrics*. 1968;41:574.
5. Krauss AN. Ventilation-perfusion relationships in neonates. In: Thibeault DW, Gregory GA, eds. *Neonatal Pulmonary Care*. Vol 2. East Norwalk, CT: Appleton & Lange; 1986.
6. Dantzker DR. Physiology and pathophysiology of pulmonary gas exchange. *Hosp Pract*. 1986;15:135.
7. Parks CR, Alden ER, Woodrum DE, et al. Gas exchange in the immature lung. II: method of estimation and maturity. *J Appl Physiol*. 1974;36:108.
8. Parks CR, Woodrum DE, Alden ER, et al. Gas exchange in the immature lung. I: anatomical shunt in the premature infant. *J Appl Physiol*. 1974;36:103.
9. Roe PG, Jones JG. Analysis of factors which affect the relationship between inspired oxygen partial pressure and arterial oxygen saturation. *Br J Anaesth*. 1993;71:488-494.
10. Smith HL, Jones JG. Non-invasive assessment of shunt and ventilation/perfusion ratio in neonates with pulmonary failure. *Arch Dis Child Fetal Neonatal Ed*. 2001;85:F127-F132.
11. Krauss AN, Auld PA. Ventilation-perfusion abnormalities in the premature infant: triple gradient. *Pediatr Res*. 1969;3:255.
12. Krauss AN, Soodalter JA, Auld PA. Adjustment of ventilation and perfusion in the full-term normal and distressed neonate as determined by urinary alveolar nitrogen gradients. *Pediatrics*. 1971;47:865.
13. Corbet AJ, Ross JA, Beaudry PH, Stern L. Ventilation-perfusion relationships as assessed by a-ADN_2 in hyaline membrane disease. *J Appl Physiol*. 1974;36:74.
14. West JB. State of the art: ventilation-perfusion relationships. *Am Rev Respir Dis*. 1977;116:919.
15. West JB. Causes of carbon dioxide retention in lung disease. *N Engl J Med*. 1971;284:1232.
16. Farhi LE. Elimination of inert gas by the lung. *Respir Physiol*. 1967;3:1.
17. Wagner PD, Naumann PF, Laravuso RB. Simultaneous measurement of eight foreign gases in blood by gas chromatography. *J Appl Physiol*. 1974;36:600.
18. Wagner PO, Saltzman HA, West JB. Measurement of continuous distributions of ventilation-perfusion ratios: theory. *J Appl Physiol*. 1974;36:588.
19. Hlastala MP. Multiple inert gas elimination technique. *J Appl Physiol*. 1984;56:1.
20. Walsh MC, Yao Q, Gettner P, et al. Impact of physiologic definition on bronchopulmonary dysplasia rates. *Pediatrics*. 2004;114:1305.
21. Hlastala MP, Robertson HT. Inert gas elimination characteristics of the normal and abnormal lung. *J Appl Physiol*. 1978;44:258.
22. Young IH, Wagner PD. Effect of intrapulmonary hematocrit maldistribution on O_2, CO_2, and inert gas exchange. *J Appl Physiol*. 1979;46:240.
23. Farhi LE. Ventilation-perfusion relationships. In: Farhi LE, ed. *Handbook of Physiology, Section 3: The Respiratory System*. Baltimore: Williams & Wilkins; 1987:199-215.
24. West JB, Wagner PD. Pulmonary gas exchange. *Am J Respir Crit Care Med*. 1998;157:S82.
29. Leffler CW, Hessler JR, Green RS. Onset of breathing at birth stimulates pulmonary vascular prostacyclin synthesis. *Pediatr Res*. 1984;18(10):932.
30. Fineman JR, Heymann MA, Soifer SJ. N omega-nitro-L-arginine attenuates endothelium dependent pulmonary vasodilation in lambs. *Am J Physiol*. 1991;260:H1299.
31. Wagner Jr WW. Control of the pulmonary circulation. *Sem Respir Med*. 1985;7:124.
32. Stenmark KR, James SL, Voelkel NF, et al. Leukotriene C_4 and D_4 in neonates with hypoxemia and pulmonary hypertension. *N Engl J Med*. 1983;309:77.
33. Kamlin CO, O'Donnell CP, Davis PG, Morley CJ. Oxygen saturation in healthy infants immediately after birth. *J Pediatr*. 2006;148:585.
34. Rabi Y, Yee W, Chen SY, Singhal N. Oxygen saturation trends immediate after birth. *J Pediatr*. 2006;148:590.
35. Dawson CA. Role of pulmonary vasomotion in physiology of the lung. *Physiol Rev*. 1984;64:544.
36. Custer JC, Hales C. Influence of alveolar oxygen on pulmonary vasoconstriction in newborn lambs vs. sheep. *Am Rev Respir Dis*. 1985;132:326.
37. Goldberg R, Suguihara C, Ahmed T, et al. Influence of an antagonist of slow reacting substance of anaphylaxis on the cardiovascular manifestations of hypoxia in piglets. *Pediatr Res*. 1985;19:1201.
38. Weir EK, Archer SL. The mechanism of acute hypoxic pulmonary vasoconstriction: the tale of two channels. *FASEB J*. 1995;9:183.
39. Marshall BE. Importance of hypoxic pulmonary vasoconstriction with atelectasis. *Adv Shock Res*. 1982;8:1.
40. Hansen TN, Le Blanc AL, Gest AL. Hypoxia and angiotensin II infusion redistribute lung blood flow in lambs. *J Appl Physiol*. 1985;58:812.
41. Means IJ, Hanson WL, Mounts KO, Wagner Jr WW. Pulmonary capillary recruitment in neonatal lambs. *Pediatr Res*. 1993;31:596.
43. Gibson RL, Truog WE, Redding GJ. Hypoxic pulmonary vasoconstriction during and after infusion of group B *Streptococcus* in neonatal piglets: vascular pressure-flow analysis. *Am Rev Respir Dis*. 1988;137:774.
44. Truog WE, Redding J, Standaert TA. Effects of hyperoxia on vasoconstriction and VA/Q matching in the neonatal lung. *J Appl Physiol*. 1987;63:2536.
45. Niermeyer S, Yang P, Shanmina, et al. Arterial oxygen saturation and Tibetan and Han infants born in Lhasa, Tibet. *N Engl J Med*. 1995;333:1248.
46. Rojas J, Green RS, Hellerqvist CG, et al. Studies on group B β-hemolytic *Streptococcus*. II: effects on pulmonary hemodynamics and vascular permeability in unanesthetized sheep. *Pediatr Res*. 1981;15:899.
47. Rojas J, Larsson LE, Hellerqvist CG, et al. Pulmonary hemodynamics and ultrastructural changes associated with group H streptococcal toxemia in adult sheep and newborn lambs. *Pediatr Res*. 1983;17:1002.
48. Runkle B, Goldberg RN, Streitfeld MM, et al. Cardiovascular changes in group B streptococcal sepsis in the piglet: response to indomethacin and relationship to prostacyclin and thromboxane A_2. *Pediatr Res*. 1984;18:874.
49. Sorenson GK, Redding GJ, Truog WE. Mechanisms of pulmonary gas exchange abnormalities during experimental group B streptococcal infusion. *Pediatr Res*. 1985;19:922.
50. Truog WE, Sorensen GK, Standaert TA, Redding GJ. Effects of the thromboxane synthetase inhibitor, dazmegrel (UK 38,485) on pulmonary gas exchange and hemodynamics in neonatal sepsis. *Pediatr Res*. 1986;20:481.
51. Truog WE, Gibson RL, Juul SE, et al. Neonatal group B streptococcal sepsis: effects of late treatment with dazmegrel. *Pediatr Res*. 1988;23:352.
52. Gibson RL, Truog WE, Henderson Jr WR, Redding GJ. Group B streptococcal sepsis: effect of combined pentoxifylline indomethacin pretreatment. *Pediatr Res*. 1992;31:222.
53. Truog WE, Standaert TA. Effect of dopamine infusion on pulmonary gas exchange in lambs. *Biol Neonate*. 1984;46:220.
54. Benumof J, Pirlo AF, Johanson I, Trousdale FR. Interaction of PVO2 with PaO2 on hypoxic pulmonary vasoconstriction. *J Appl Physiol*. 1981;51:871.
55. McCann EM, Goldman SL, Brady JP. Pulmonary function in the sick newborn infant. *Pediatr Res*. 1987;21:313.
56. Engel LA. Gas mixing within the acinus of the lung. *Appl Physiol*. 1983;54:609.
57. Kinsella JP, Neish SR, Ivy DD, et al. Clinical responses to prolonged treatment of persistent pulmonary hypertension of the newborn with low doses of inhaled nitric oxide. *J Pediatr*. 1993;123:103-108.
58. Abman SH, Griebel JL, Parker DK, et al. Acute effects of inhaled nitric oxide in severe hypoxemic respiratory failure in pediatrics. *J Pediatr*. 1994;124:881-888.
59. Gerlach H, Rossaint R, Pappert D, Falke KJ. Time-course and dose-response of nitric oxide inhalation for systemic oxygenation and pulmonary hypertension in patients with adult respiratory distress syndrome. *Eur J Clin Invest*. 1993;23:499-502.
60. Rossaint R, Falke KJ, Lopez F, et al. Inhaled nitric oxide for the adult respiratory distress syndrome. *N Engl J Med*. 1993;328:399-405.
61. Hlastala MP. Diffusing-capacity heterogeneity. In: Farhi LE, ed. *Handbook on Physiology, Section 3: The Respiratory System*. Baltimore: Williams & Wilkins; 1987.
62. Escourrou PJ, Teisscire DP, Herigault RA, et al. Mechanism of improvement in pulmonary gas exchange during growth in awake piglets. *J Appl Physiol*. 1988;65:1055.
63. Krauss AN, Klain DB, Auld PA. Carbon monoxide diffusing capacity in newborn infants. *Pediatr Res*. 1976;10:771.
64. Stahlman MT. Pulmonary ventilation and diffusion in the human newborn infant. *J Clin Invest*. 1957;36:1081.
65. Hakulinen AL, Järvenpää AL, Turpeinen M, Sovijärvi A. Diffusing capacity of the lung in school-aged children born very preterm, with and without bronchopulmonary dysplasia. *Pediatr Pulmonol*. 1996;21:353.
66. Hjalmarson O, Sandberg KL. Lung function at term reflects severity of bronchopulmonary dysplasia. *J Pediatr*. 2005;146:86.
67. Kilbride HW, Gelatt MC, Sabath RJ. Pulmonary function and exercise capacity for ELBW survivors in preadolescence: effect of neonatal chronic lung disease. *J Pediatr*. 2003;143:488.

65 Oxygen Transport and Delivery

Danielle R. Rios | Afif F. El-Khuffash | Patrick J. McNamara

INTRODUCTION

Because aerobic metabolism is critically dependent on a consistent and adequate supply of oxygen, oxygen is an essential fuel source for normal cellular metabolic function. Hence, control of oxygen uptake, transport, and release are essential functions. Although molecular oxygen participates in numerous oxidative reactions necessary for cellular metabolism (e.g., production of prostaglandins mediated by cyclooxygenase), its primary role is as the final electron acceptor in the mitochondrial respiratory chain—the process by which energy produced by the citric acid cycle is stored in high-energy phosphate bonds as adenosine triphosphate. Oxygen transport depends on many interrelated factors, including the fractional concentration or partial pressure of oxygen in inspired air, the adequacy of alveolar ventilation, the relation of ventilation to perfusion within the lungs, arterial blood pH and temperature, cardiac output, blood volume, hemoglobin concentration, and the affinity of hemoglobin for oxygen. The ability of this complex system to respond varies according to metabolic needs and maturation, and it may be confounded by coexisting disease processes, yet humans in good health have a reasonable reserve capacity and can respond rapidly to changes in oxygen needs. Birth and the immediate postnatal period represent situations that make special demands upon the oxygen transport system. In this chapter, we review the principal determinants of oxygen transport, with emphasis on the modulator role of the cardiovascular system.

OXYGEN DELIVERY: OVERVIEW OF BIOLOGIC CONTRIBUTORS

Oxygen delivery (DO_2), defined as the quantity of oxygen entering a tissue, organ, or the entire body in arterial blood each minute, is the product of the concentration (or content) of oxygen in arterial blood (C_aO_2) and the rate of blood flow to the region of interest. For the whole body, oxygen delivery is determined by the equation:

$$DO_2 = C_aO_2 \times CO/100 \qquad [65.1]$$

where C_aO_2 is the oxygen content of arterial blood (in mL/dL) and CO is the cardiac output (in L/min); the 100 is a unit reconciliation factor (100 mL/L). The oxygen content of arterial blood includes both oxygen carried by hemoglobin and oxygen in solution. Oxygen delivery therefore is determined by function of the lungs, heart, and hemoglobin.

This term may be somewhat of a misnomer, since not all the oxygen "delivered" to tissues in arterial blood remains there. It is important to distinguish DO_2 as so defined from oxygen uptake or utilization ($\dot{V}O_2$), which for the entire body is:

$$\dot{V}O_2 = (C_aO_2 - C_{\bar{v}}O_2) \times CO/100 \qquad [65.2]$$

where $C_{\bar{v}}O_2$ is the oxygen content of mixed venous blood. At the tissue or organ level, oxygen utilization is often expressed in terms of fractional tissue oxygen extraction (FTOE, often referred to simply as oxygen extraction):

$$FTOE = (C_aO_2 - C_{\bar{v}}O_2) / C_aO_2 \qquad [65.3]$$

CARDIOPULMONARY FACTORS

Under basal conditions, the lungs of a newborn infant load approximately 6 to 8 mL/kg/min onto hemoglobin (compared to 3 to 4 mL/kg/min typically for adults). This can be increased up to 15-fold in response to input from the carotid and aortic bodies (which sense arterial oxygen content) and brain stem chemoreceptors. The effectiveness of oxygen uptake from the lungs may be compromised by parenchymal lung disease, pulmonary vasoconstriction, or diseases leading to ventilation-perfusion mismatch. Arterial blood flow transports oxygen from the pulmonary capillaries to systemic tissues. The oxygen content of the arterial blood usually is high enough to readily meet cellular oxygen demands. When the oxygen content is decreased, however, local perfusion or hemoglobin oxygen affinity may change to compensate for the lower oxygen content.

The cardiovascular system regulates oxygen supply through variation in cardiac output and distribution of blood flow. Alterations in the metabolic rate of peripheral tissues activate local regulatory mechanisms that modulate arterial blood flow and venous return and, consequently, cardiac output. Accordingly, different controls exist in different tissues.[1] Coronary blood flow, for example, reflects the metabolic activity of heart muscle; because the oxygen extraction of cardiac muscle is normally high, changes in cardiac work must be matched closely by concomitant changes in coronary blood flow. In moderate or severe hypoxic-ischemic brain injury, cerebral oxygen extraction may be markedly reduced because of decreased oxygen utilization by injured brain cells.[2] When oxygen supply is limited, flow is reduced to tissues with low oxygen extraction (such as kidney and gut) in favor of tissues with high extraction (such as heart and brain). The high flow–low extraction areas of the circulation constitute an oxygen reserve capacity that may be deployed in times of oxygen deprivation. By contrast, total cardiac output does not appear to be directly responsive to moderate changes in either arterial partial pressure of oxygen or blood oxygen content (presumably because other mechanisms provide an adequate adjustment) and is virtually unaffected by increased arterial partial pressure of carbon dioxide up to 50 mm Hg. Blood viscosity and volume are additional determinants of cardiac output.

HEMOGLOBIN

Hemoglobin concentration is regulated by a renal sensing mechanism that operates to maintain a balance between oxygen supply and oxygen requirement of renal tissues. A decrease in concentration or arterial oxygen saturation of hemoglobin or any increase in hemoglobin affinity for oxygen causes increased erythropoietin production through increased expression of hypoxia-inducible factor.[3] The effect of erythropoietin on bone marrow is usually limited by available iron, so red blood cell production can only be stimulated to approximately double its basal value of 1% of the total red blood cell mass per day. Consequently, red blood cell mass increases slowly in response to hypoxia.[4] Because it increases blood viscosity, a higher hemoglobin concentration at the same total blood volume reduces blood flow, offsetting the increase in oxygen delivery. Normal cardiac output is reestablished by a proportionate increase in plasma volume (i.e., by an increase in total blood volume).[5] The affinity of hemoglobin for oxygen, in association with blood flow distribution, translates blood flow into oxygen availability. This characteristic of hemoglobin is classically depicted in the oxyhemoglobin dissociation curve (oxygen equilibrium curve). Because of its remarkable ability to combine reversibly with large quantities of oxygen, hemoglobin increases the oxygen transport capacity of blood approximately 70-fold over that of oxygen transported dissolved in plasma.

CELLULAR FACTORS

Diffusion of oxygen from capillaries to mitochondria within cells, the last step in oxygen transport, depends on several factors, including the oxygen pressure gradient between the capillary and the cell, the distance between the closest perfusing capillary and the cell, and impedance to diffusion within the tissue. The pressure gradient, which directly affects mitochondrial oxygen uptake, varies with regional oxygen delivery, tissue oxygen consumption, and the hemoglobin-oxygen affinity. In vitro, mitochondrial function remains at maximal levels at oxygen partial pressures (Po_2) as low as 0.5 mm Hg. In vivo, however, it is likely that mitochondrial respiration is compromised at oxygen tensions below a higher "critical" Po_2.[6]

DETERMINANTS OF CARDIAC OUTPUT

FETAL AND TRANSITIONAL CARDIOVASCULAR PHYSIOLOGY

The integrity of oxygen transport in the newborn period is dependent on adequacy of the cardiac output, which must be maintained through the transition from fetal to neonatal life. Therefore, a thorough understanding of the fetal, transitional, and neonatal circulations is essential. Similarly, an understanding of the terms used when one is defining the components determining cardiac output is necessary. Cardiac output is determined by *heart rate* (chronotropy), *preload* (amount of blood present in the ventricle at the end of diastole, which is dependent on hydration status, pulmonary and systemic venous return, and diastolic compliance of the ventricle [lusitropy]), *myocardial performance* (the intrinsic ability of the myocardium to contract [inotropy]), and *afterload* (force generation necessary to overcome the resistance against which the ventricle muscle must contract, which depends on vascular resistance and compliance, blood viscosity, ventricular muscle wall thickness, and ventricular outflow tract obstructions).[7] Intrauterine, transitional, and postnatal changes in each of these determinants of cardiac output have significant impacts on oxygen delivery before, during, and after birth.

CHARACTERISTICS OF FETAL AND EARLY NEONATAL MYOCARDIUM

Adult myocardium is more efficient at contraction than its neonatal and fetal counterparts. In adults, surface L-type calcium channels allow a small amount of extracellular calcium to enter the myocytes after depolarization. These in turn lead to further intracellular calcium release from intrinsic stores called the *sarcoplasmic reticulum,* leading to effective myofibril shortening and muscle contraction. The process is facilitated by the proximity of the sarcoplasmic reticulum to the L-type calcium channels and the presence of transverse tubules. Conversely, the immature fetal heart muscle relies on L-type calcium channels as a source of calcium to facilitate contraction, because of the lack of transverse tubules and the physical separation of the sarcoplasmic reticulum from the L-type calcium channels.[8] Furthermore, the immature myocytes have a higher surface area-to-volume ratio to compensate for the lack of the T-tubule system necessary for effective calcium entry into the cell. The arrangement of the myofibrils within the myocardium is also less organized during fetal life, with only 30% consisting of contractile tissue, compared with 60% in the adult myocardium. The ability of the fetal myocardium to relax (accommodate preload) is compromised with less compliant elastic tissue present. These developmental differences drastically reduce the functional reserve of the fetal heart in the face of postnatal stresses. In the early neonatal period, failure of a normal postnatal transition may place the infant in a vulnerable hemodynamic situation, which may lead to compromised cardiac output and tissue oxygenation.[9] This problem may be further compounded by any potential stressors, such as hypoxia, anemia, asphyxia, and mechanical ventilation, all of which can alter cardiac loading conditions and affect contractility.[10]

FETAL PHYSIOLOGY OF THE CARDIOVASCULAR SYSTEM

Fetal cardiac output rises from 50 mL/min at 18 weeks' gestation to 1200 mL/min at term, reflecting the growing demand placed on the myocardium to supply vital organs in the developing fetus. In utero, the left ventricle (LV) is subject to low afterload owing to sustained exposure to a low-resistance circuit that includes the highly compliant placental circulation; therefore, the LV, in particular, is subjected to less wall stress during the fetal period. This low-pressure system is suitable for the immature myocardium to ensure effective transplacental perfusion but also makes it vulnerable in the face of additional stresses. The major source of preload to the LV during fetal life is derived from the placenta through the umbilical circulation. Oxygenated blood returning from the placenta into the right atrium is directed through the foramen ovale into the left atrium, thus determining LV preload and LV output (LVO). Because of the low afterload to which the LV is subjected by the systemic circulation, most of the LVO, constituted of oxygenated blood, is directed to vital organs such as the brain. The right ventricle (RV) receives most of the blood draining from the superior vena cava, and a proportionately lower amount of oxygenated blood from the umbilical venous system. Ninety percent of the RV output flows from the pulmonary artery to the descending aorta across the ductus arteriosus (DA). This is a consequence of the high pulmonary vascular resistance (PVR) during fetal life. Pulmonary venous return into the left atrium is low, and as mentioned above, LV preload depends primarily on umbilical venous supply through the foramen ovale. Because the DA diverts the RV output to the low resistance systemic and placental circulation, the RV also is subjected to a low afterload in utero.

TRANSITIONAL CIRCULATION AFTER BIRTH

The cardiovascular system undergoes significant changes after birth. Important changes in both preload and afterload occur in quick succession after the loss of the uteroplacental circulation and the onset of reliance on the lungs as the organ of gas exchange. After birth, the loss of the low-resistance circulation of the placenta results in a sudden increase in systemic vascular resistance (SVR). This in turn leads to an increase in LV afterload. Another important transition faced by the neonate after birth is enhanced aeration of the lungs, the fall in PVR, and the increase in pulmonary blood flow, with commencement of gas exchange. During fetal life, the lungs are fluid filled. This liquid is necessary for fetal lung development. After birth a combination of mechanisms, including pressure gradients generated during inspiration and through sodium exchange channels, result in lung fluid clearance and enhanced lung compliance. The subsequent fall in PVR is promoted by increased alveolar oxygen content and lung recruitment. However, recent data demonstrate that oxygen is not the only contributor to the increase in pulmonary blood flow. Other active substances such as prostaglandins, bradykinins, and histamine may play a role in inducing pulmonary vasodilation after birth. This is supported by rabbit experimental models, where an increase in pulmonary blood flow independent of lung aeration was noted in nonventilated lungs.[10] The fall in PVR results in preferential flow of RV output through the pulmonary vascular bed, and not through the DA. The changes described above lead to a change in the circulation from a circuit in series to one in parallel. LV preload now becomes solely dependent on pulmonary venous return. Adequate LV preload is essential to maintain the necessary LVO in the face of increasing LV afterload. Therefore, the changes occurring in the lungs are essential for maintaining postnatal life. RV preload is now dependent on adequate systemic venous return from the upper and lower body. The fall in PVR occurring soon after birth ensures that the RV continues to be exposed to low afterload. Recent data shows a relative difference between the RV and LV performance immediately after birth. The RV improved in both systolic and diastolic function, whereas the LV showed no change in systolic performance and a small improvement in diastolic performance during the transitional period.[11] The authors demonstrated an increase in RVO and no change in LVO during the first day after birth.

REGULATION OF VASCULAR TONE DURING TRANSITION

The sudden increase in SVR immediately after birth can compromise organ blood flow by reducing cardiac output. After the transitional period, vascular tone is regulated by a balance between vasoconstrictors and vasodilators. Nitric oxide (NO), vasopressin, and prostaglandins all play vital roles. Immaturity of the autonomic nervous system may also have an impact on transitional vascular changes.[12] NO is produced by actions of NO synthase, present in abundance in smooth muscle tissue. NO acts via cyclic guanosine monophosphate on calcium-sensitive potassium channels and myosin light chain phosphatases to cause smooth muscle relaxation. Endotoxins and cytokines, such as tumor necrosis factor (TNF)α and a variety of interleukins, can induce NO synthase synthesis of NO, leading to profound dilatation and a reduced systemic blood flow in the presence of sepsis. In addition, excess NO leads to formation of free oxygen radicals, leading to vascular wall damage. Vasopressin plays an important role in regulating vascular tone during the postnatal period. Vasopressin increases vascular tone via specific vasopressin receptors that increase calcium release from the sarcoplasmic reticulum, up-regulate adrenergic receptors on smooth muscle walls, and reduce NO synthesis.[12] In adults, augmentation of vasopressin levels occurs in the early phase of shock to maintain vascular tone. As the degree of shock and hemodynamic compromise progresses, however, vasopressin stores are depleted and vascular tone is therefore compromised.[13] Vasopressin is a useful adjunctive pressor that spares epinephrine and norepinephrine requirements in patients with shock, but its use is not without risk, particularly when it is combined with sustained moderate to high infusions of norepinephrine.[14,15] Prostaglandins are eicosanoids derived from cell membrane arachidonic acid by the actions of cyclooxygenases and play an important role in regulation of vascular tone. An imbalance between prostaglandin I_2, a potent vasodilator, and thromboxane A_2, a vasoconstrictor, is implicated in the early regulation of vascular tone and may have a role in the pathogenesis of hypovolemia associated with shock.[8]

CONSEQUENCES OF EARLY UMBILICAL CORD CLAMPING

Umbilical cord clamping is commonly done immediately after the delivery of infants and should therefore be considered an important component of a normal transition. Early umbilical cord clamping at birth has a major impact on neonatal hemodynamics during transition. As the placental circulation acts as an organ with low vascular resistance, it may hold 30% to 50% of the fetus's blood volume at any given time. Experimental studies demonstrate that early umbilical cord clamping results in a rapid increase in SVR and arterial blood pressure.[16] This leads to a transient increase in cerebral blood flow because of the passive nature of the cerebral circulation in the early neonatal period. Early clamping may, however, also promote a reduction in LVO caused by early cessation of blood returning from the placenta to the heart. This may lead to significant fluctuations in cerebral perfusion in the early neonatal period, which may modify brain injury in certain situations. Cardiac output may remain low until pulmonary blood flow is established and LV preload is restored by pulmonary venous return.[17] Recent data suggest that allowing infants to breathe *and* establish pulmonary blood flow before cord umbilical cord clamping may allow a smoother transition with less fluctuation in blood pressure and cardiac output. Deferring umbilical cord clamping for up to 1 minute after birth may enhance the establishment of pulmonary blood flow. Augmentation of LV preload helps maintain LVO during the immediate postnatal period. Some of the clinical benefits of this approach on the hemodynamic status of neonates (preterm and term) include improved early oxygenation,[18,19] cardiac output,[18,20] and circulating blood volume[18,21] in addition to reduced hospital mortality in preterm infants.[22]

ROLE OF SHUNTS IN DETERMINING CARDIAC OUTPUT

Flow across the foramen ovale ceases soon after birth as the increase in left atrial pressure (becoming higher than right atrial pressure) leads to a change in the direction of flow across the foramen ovale (from a right-to-left direction to a left-to-right direction). This causes the displacement of the atrial septal flap over the fossa, thus abolishing flow. Flow across the DA also changes soon after birth. As PVR falls and SVR increases, the directionality of the shunt changes from right-to-left to bidirectional, and eventually from left-to-right before subsequent closure. Recent normative data from term human cohorts suggest that the transductal shunt is exclusively left-to-right by 24 hours.[23] DA patency and closure are influenced by a multitude of factors. In utero, low systemic oxygen tension and elevated circulating levels of prostaglandins are important to maintain ductal patency. Functional closure of the DA begins within a few hours after birth and is usually complete by 1 week of age in preterm infants. This is partly because of the increase in oxygen tension and the falling prostaglandin levels postnatally. Anatomic closure is achieved after ductal tissue is exposed to sustained hypoxia-ischemia, resulting in cell apoptosis, leading to the transformation of ductal tissue to a noncontractile element.[24]

SPECIAL CONSIDERATIONS FOR PRETERM INFANTS

The problem of low systemic blood flow in the early transitional period is further compounded by several factors in preterm neonates, and these need to be considered to optimize the management of low blood flow states and select the best therapy, preventing impaired tissue oxygenation:

1. *The neonatal myocardium is poorly tolerant of increased afterload compared with that of older children.*[8,25] Immaturity of myocyte calcium storage (t-tubules and sarcoplasmic reticulum) and myofibrillar organization drastically reduce the functional reserve of the premature heart in the face of postnatal stresses and increased afterload. The net effect is impaired myocardial systolic performance and consequential poor systemic blood flow because of low cardiac output, often despite a normal systemic blood pressure.
2. *The preterm myocardium has impaired diastolic function, resulting in abnormal relaxation and reduced ventricular filling during diastole.* The preterm heart spends a lower

percentage of the cardiac cycle in diastole, reducing the time available for ventricular filling and compromising preload.[26] This may be compounded by other factors, such as mechanical ventilation, which may reduce venous return.[8] In addition, these effects are often accentuated in patients with ventricular hypertrophy, which is increasingly seen in extremely low-birth-weight infants after prolonged courses of steroid treatment.[27,28]

3. *Resting peripheral vascular tone is high in preterm infants.* This may be due to the higher number of peripheral vasoconstrictor (α-adrenergic) receptors and a reduced number of peripheral vasodilator (β-adrenergic) receptors.
4. *The myocardium may have less adrenergic innervation and fewer adrenergic receptors,* thereby reducing the net inotropic effect of inotropes. As a result, most of the agents used in the early period may have more of a vasopressor than an inotropic effect, thereby potentially compromising cardiac output and systemic blood flow.
5. *Low-birth-weight infants have an immature hypothalamic-pituitary-adrenal axis.* Corticosteroids regulate vascular tone by up-regulating adrenergic receptors on vascular smooth muscle wall. Sick preterm neonates do not increase glucocorticoid production in response to stress; this may be due to the lack or immaturity of enzymes necessary for synthesis.[29,30] Inotrope-resistant preterm neonates have low cortisol levels.[31] This may contribute to the poor cardiopulmonary status in sick newborns.
6. *Left-to-right shunting across a patent DA (PDA) and patent foramen ovale (PFO) may compromise systemic blood flow by short-circuiting blood back to the lungs.* Patency of the DA may persist in more than 70% of infants less than 28 weeks' gestation. As PVR falls after birth (sometimes very dramatically in the first 24 hours), the magnitude of left-to-right transductal flow may increase to the extent that systemic blood flow is compromised, as a large percentage of LVO is redirected to the lungs. Consequently, increased pulmonary blood flow can reduce lung compliance as pulmonary edema ensues. Similarly, a PFO can remain open during the early preterm period. Left-to-right flow across the PFO can increase pulmonary blood flow, especially in the setting of a PDA, which causes pulmonary edema and further worsens lung compliance and gas exchange. In addition, rapid reduction in PVR that leads to dramatic increases in pre-ductal output may impact the rate of intraventricular hemorrhage.[32]

ROLE OF HEMOGLOBIN IN OXYGEN UPTAKE, TRANSPORT, AND DELIVERY

STRUCTURE OF HEMOGLOBIN

The hemoglobin molecule contains four heme groups bound to the protein globin. The heme groups, located in crevices near the exterior of the molecule, consist of an organic moiety, protoporphyrin, and an iron atom. The iron in heme binds to the four nitrogens in the center of the protoporphyrin ring (Fig. 65.1). The four oxygen-binding sites of hemoglobin are relatively far apart, the distance between the two closest sites being 2.5 nm. The primary structure of the hemoglobin molecule is genetically determined by the amino acid sequence of the globin chains. The three basic chain structures most important in humans are the α-chain (with 141 amino acids), the β-chain (with 146 amino acids), and the γ-chain (with 146 amino acids), which together form hemoglobin A, with a makeup of $\alpha_2\beta_2$, and hemoglobin F, which is $\alpha_2\gamma_2$. The β-chain and the γ-chain differ from each other by only a few amino acid residues. The quaternary structure of deoxyhemoglobin is termed the *T* or *tense form,* whereas that of oxyhemoglobin is the *R* or *relaxed form.* X-ray crystallographic studies have

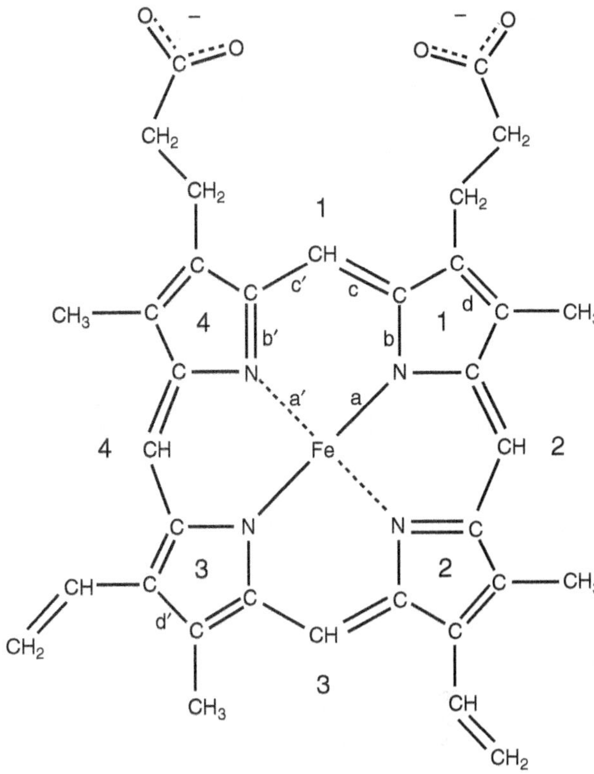

Fig. 65.1 The heme group is an essential component of hemoglobins, cytochromes, and enzymes such as catalase and peroxidase. The central porphyrin ring has various side chains: methyl, $-CH_3$; vinyl, $-CH-CH_2$; and propionic acid, $-CH-CH_2-COOH$.

confirmed that oxygenated and deoxygenated hemoglobin differ in their conformation, with the oxygenated form being more compact.[33] In the T form (deoxyhemoglobin), the iron atom is pushed out approximately 0.6 nm from the heme plane because of steric repulsion between the proximal histidine and nitrogen atoms of the porphyrin. On oxygenation, the iron atom moves into the plane of the protoporphyrin ring, forming a strong bond with oxygen. Because each hemoglobin molecule (tetramer) contains four iron atoms, it can combine with four oxygen molecules. Each mole of hemoglobin can thus combine with four moles of oxygen, for a normal blood oxygen capacity of 9.30 mmol/L (i.e., 2.32 mmol of hemoglobin per liter × 4 = 9.30, assuming a hemoglobin concentration of 15 g/dL). Expressed alternatively, 1 g of hemoglobin ideally can combine with up to 1.39 mL of oxygen. Measured values are typically slightly lower (1.31 to 1.37 ml O_2/g Hgb, and 1.34 is commonly used), likely reflecting inactivity of methemoglobin and other dyshemoglobins. The oxygen-carrying capacity of blood is therefore approximately 20 mL/dL at a hemoglobin concentration of 15 g/dL.[34]

The oxygen content of blood consists of both the component carried on hemoglobin and that in aqueous solution. The latter is directly proportional to the partial pressure of oxygen. The solubility of oxygen in water at 37°C is modest, however, at 0.0031 mL/dL/mm Hg. Accordingly, the oxygen content of blood (CO_2; mL/dL) can be calculated from hemoglobin concentration ([Hgb]; g/dL), oxygen saturation (SO_2; %), and oxygen partial pressure (PO_2; mm Hg):

$$CO_2 = [Hgb] \times 1.34 \times SO_2/100 + 0.003 \times PO_2 \quad [65.4]$$

Along with Eq. (65.1), this implies that oxygen delivery can be impaired by insufficient blood flow, anemia, or low oxygen saturation (and PO_2).

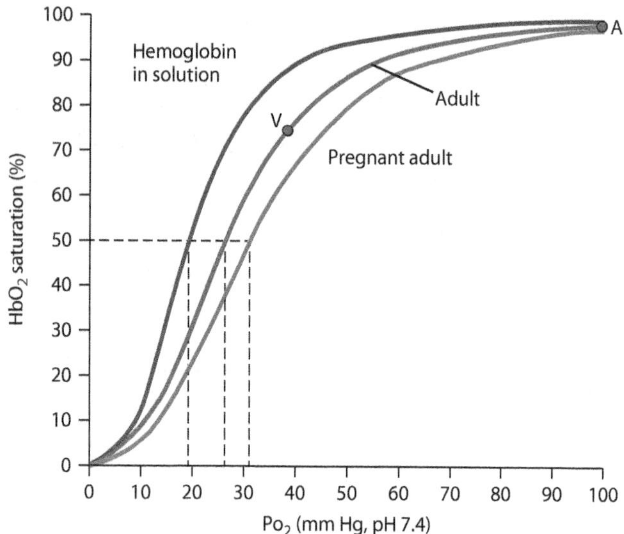

Fig. 65.2 Oxyhemoglobin *(HbO_2)* saturation curve under standard conditions for normal blood of pregnant and nonpregnant women. Also shown is the dissociation curve for hemoglobin in solution.

INTERACTIONS: AFFINITY/RELEASE

Hemoglobin oxygen affinity is the continuous relationship between hemoglobin oxygen saturation and oxygen tension. It is customarily plotted as the sigmoidal oxygen equilibrium curve, and it can be summarily expressed as P_{50}—that is, the oxygen tension at which 50% of hemoglobin is saturated with oxygen at standard temperature and pH (Fig. 65.2). The sigmoidal shape of the oxygen-hemoglobin equilibrium curve relates to the fact that the heme groups react with oxygen in sequence, and oxygenation and deoxygenation of one heme group profoundly affects the oxygenation and deoxygenation of the other heme groups. This phenomenon has been termed *heme-heme interaction*. As each heme group accepts oxygen, it becomes progressively easier for the next heme group of the molecule to pick up oxygen. This concept is implicit in the Hill equation for percent saturation:

$$\text{Hemoglobin saturation} = \Theta = (PO_2)^n / \left[(P_{50})^n + (PO_2)^n\right] \quad \textbf{[65.5]}$$

where Θ is percent saturation with oxygen, Po_2 is oxygen partial pressure, P_{50} is oxygen partial pressure at 50% hemoglobin saturation, and the exponent n is an interaction coefficient related to the cooperativity and number of oxygen-binding sites per hemoglobin tetramer. For normal hemoglobin, n is approximately 2.9.

As blood circulates through the normal lung, Po_2 increases from approximately 40 mm Hg to 110 mm Hg, a pressure sufficient to ensure at least 95% saturation of hemoglobin with oxygen. The oxygen-hemoglobin equilibrium relationship is such that any further increase of oxygen tension in the lung results in only a small increase in saturation. In the normal adult, when oxygen tension has fallen to approximately 27 mm Hg, at a pH of 7.40 and a temperature of 37°C, 50% of hemoglobin is saturated with oxygen (i.e., P_{50} for whole blood is 27 mm Hg).

The steep and flat parts of the curve reflect definitive processes in oxygen unloading. As oxygen diffuses from capillary to tissue, at first a rapid fall in Po_2 (represented by the flat part of the curve) occurs until the steep part is reached, after which capillary Po_2 decreases little even though large amounts of oxygen are released. Because oxygen tension at the mitochondrial surface, the point of oxygen utilization, is always approximately 0.5 to 1.0 mm Hg,[6] the driving pressure for, and consequently the rate of, oxygen delivery is determined solely by the mean Po_2 in capillary blood. This is in turn set by the position of the dissociation curve on the Po_2 axis and by its steepness, such that relatively little change in driving pressure occurs as the red blood cell moves through the capillary. As the partial pressure of oxygen decreases, tissue oxygenation may become impaired. The term *critical* Po_2 was introduced to indicate the oxygen tension of blood below which diffusion is impaired and organ function is disturbed.[35] A critical Po_2 cannot be a well-defined value, as cellular needs likely vary between organs and are influenced by metabolic activity. For example, in the brain, an organ in which an adequate oxygen supply is essential for maintaining energy metabolism, the critical Po_2 appears to be approximately 20 mm Hg.

When hemoglobin oxygen affinity is increased (i.e., with lower P_{50}), the curve is shifted to the left, and oxygen (which is bound more tightly to hemoglobin) is released only at lower partial pressures. For example, whereas a Po_2 of 40 mm Hg results in an oxygen saturation of 75% at 37°C and pH 7.40, a leftward shift of the curve results in a higher saturation at the same Po_2. The resulting change in oxygen unloading ultimately could result in impaired diffusion. When affinity is decreased (i.e., with higher P_{50}), the curve is shifted to the right. Consequently, oxygen is bound less tightly to hemoglobin and is released at higher partial pressures, thereby enhancing oxygen unloading at the tissue level. Therefore, the release of oxygen from the blood at the tissue level depends on the position of the oxygen equilibrium curve, which in turn is modified by intraerythrocytic pH, Pco_2, temperature, and other factors, including electrolyte concentration, organic phosphate levels, and hemoglobin type.

The effect of temperature on the oxygen equilibrium curve was first noted by Barcroft and King[36] in 1909. Increased temperature shifts the curve toward the right, thereby facilitating the release of oxygen. In addition, changes in temperature alter both the Bohr factor and the 2,3-diphosphoglycerate (2,3-DPG) effect.[37] The *Bohr effect* is the shift to the right of the oxygen equilibrium curve of both adult and fetal blood in response to an increase in PCO_2 or a decrease in pH, or both. Oxygen unloading is determined by the PO_2 gradient between blood and tissues. The shift of the oxyhemoglobin dissociation curve to the right as carbon dioxide enters the blood from the tissues tends to raise the oxygen tension, increasing the gradient for any given oxyhemoglobin saturation and facilitating transfer of oxygen to the tissues. The change in log P_{50} per unit change in pH (i.e., $\Delta\log(P_{50})/\Delta pH$) is known as the Bohr factor. Its value for adult human blood is -0.48, and for the newborn infant it is -0.44. The effective pH is the intracellular pH of the red blood cell, which is usually 0.2 unit less than plasma pH at physiologic levels, although the pH gradient across the red blood membrane cell may vary in disease states. Thus, an acute change in pH of 0.1 unit changes P_{50} by approximately 3 mm Hg. The Bohr effect is more pronounced, at least experimentally, as oxygen saturation decreases, and is diminished in 2,3-DPG-depleted blood.[38]

The Bohr effect produced by varying Pco_2 at constant fixed acid is larger (−0.48) than that induced by alterations in metabolic acids at constant Pco_2 (−0.40).[38] The molecular basis of the carbon dioxide effect is two-fold: It follows both carbon dioxide–induced changes in pH and the action of carbon dioxide as a ligand, binding reversibly to uncharged amino groups in the hemoglobin molecule to form carbamates.[39,40] Bound carbamates form salt bridges, stabilizing the T (deoxy) conformation of hemoglobin and decreasing hemoglobin oxygen affinity. In addition, the affinity of other sites on the hemoglobin molecule for the hydrogen ion (H^+) is enhanced by transition from oxyhemoglobin to deoxyhemoglobin, allowing deoxyhemoglobin to take up much of the H^+ generated from spontaneous dissociation of carbonic acid. By modifying hemoglobin oxygen affinity, carbon dioxide also facilitates respiratory gas exchange in the lungs. At the lungs, carbon dioxide is given up by red blood cells into the alveoli. Carbon dioxide concentration falls, thereby shifting the oxygen equilibrium curve to the left; the increase in hemoglobin oxygen affinity enhances uptake of oxygen from the alveoli.[41] The combined effects of pH, PCO_2, and temperature on the oxygen equilibrium curve can be viewed, in theory, as advantageous for species survival. An increase in tissue metabolism causes increases in local temperature, H^+ concentration, and PCO_2, all of which raise P_{50}. The result is a higher gradient of oxygen tension between the capillary and the mitochondrion at the site (tissue) where oxygen consumption is highest. For example, the in vivo oxygen equilibrium curve has been shown to shift markedly rightward during acute exercise because of the combined Bohr and temperature effects.[42] On the other hand, in therapeutic hypothermia, the curve shifts leftward because of temperature effects, resulting in the potential for a relative underestimation of P_aO_2 compared to pulse oximetry.[43]

It has long been recognized that the oxygen affinity of hemoglobin A in free solution is considerably greater than that of the intact fresh erythrocyte. In 1967, it was demonstrated that interaction with a number of organic phosphates decreased the affinity of a hemoglobin solution for oxygen, with 2,3-DPG being the most effective.[44,45] Of the organic phosphates normally found in the human erythrocyte, 2,3-DPG is present in the largest concentrations and thus is both qualitatively and quantitatively the most important phosphate with respect to modulation of hemoglobin oxygen affinity. Hemoglobin oxygen affinity as indicated by P_{50} is linear with respect to 2,3-DPG concentration over a wide range; a change of 0.43 mmol of 2,3-DPG/mL of red blood cells results in a 1 mm Hg change in P_{50}.[46] The highly negatively charged 2,3-DPG anion binds preferentially to deoxyhemoglobin in a 1:1 molar ratio under physiologic conditions of solute concentration and pH. On a molecular basis, 2,3-DPG decreases oxygen affinity by stabilizing the quaternary structure of deoxyhemoglobin through cross-linking of β-chains. A second mechanism by which 2,3-DPG reduces oxygen affinity is by altering the intraerythrocytic pH relative to plasma pH. The reduction in pH consequently decreases oxygen affinity by the Bohr effect.

FETAL OXYGEN TRANSPORT/DELIVERY

Compared with adult blood, fetal blood has a higher affinity for oxygen and lower P_{50}—an observation first made in 1930. Fig. 65.3 shows this relationship for the human fetus near term, when P_{50} is approximately 20 mm Hg under standard conditions. Barcroft and colleagues[47,48] and Hall[49] reported a gradual decrease in the blood oxygen affinity (increase in P_{50}) as gestation advances, such that the fetal curve progressively approximates the maternal curve. In the placenta, because of the low Po_2 at which transfer of oxygen is achieved, the high affinity of fetal hemoglobin favors oxygen uptake in the fetus. The highest Po_2 in the fetus is in umbilical venous blood, in which Po_2 usually does not go much above 30 mm Hg. At that oxygen tension, the saturation of human fetal blood is 6% to 8% higher than the saturation of maternal blood.[50]

These findings raised questions about the mechanism or mechanisms responsible for the increased oxygen affinity of fetal blood. In 1930, Haurowitz[51] demonstrated a difference in alkaline denaturation that resides in the globin chains of hemoglobin and proposed the presence of two hemoglobins in newborn blood: an alkali-susceptible adult fraction and a more resistant fetal fraction. In 1963, the human fetal α-chain was shown to have the same amino acid sequence as the α-chain of human adult hemoglobin.[52] In addition to the two α-chains, fetal hemoglobin was found to contain two non–α-chains (labeled γ-chains), which resemble the β-chain and contain the same number of amino acids (146) but differ in sequence by 39 amino acids. Each γ-chain contains four isoleucine residues not found in either the α-chain or the β-chain. In addition, three proline residues present in the β-chain have been substituted by other amino acids.

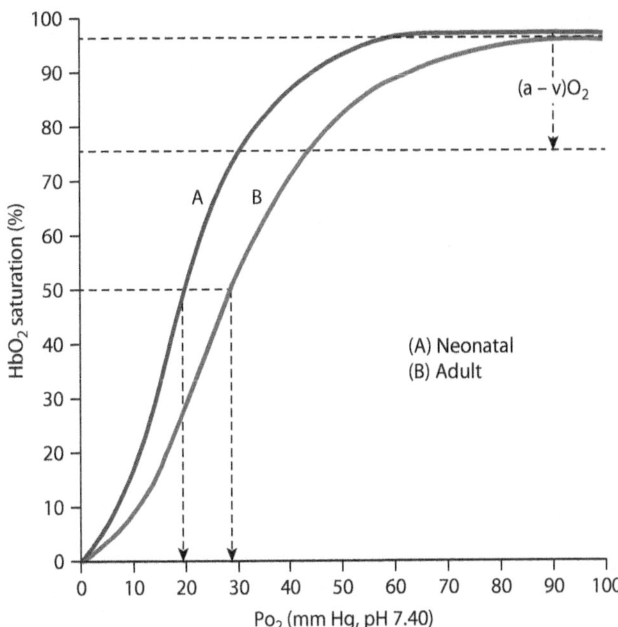

Fig. 65.3 Oxyhemoglobin *(HbO₂)* equilibrium curves for blood from term infants at birth and from adults.

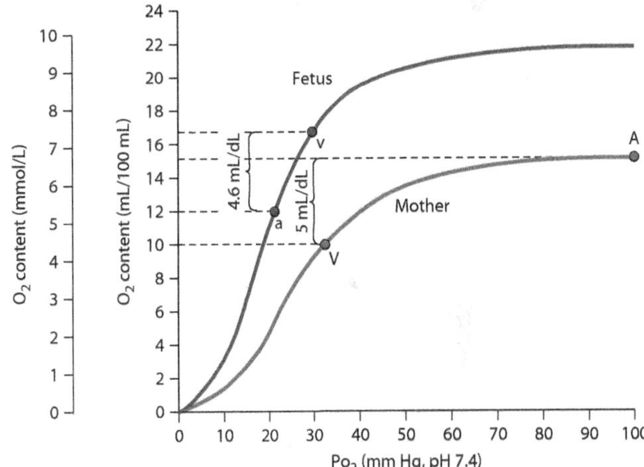

Fig. 65.4 Blood oxygen content as a function of oxygen tension in human maternal and near-term fetal blood.

A linear correlation between the proportional composition of fetal hemoglobin and P_{50} at the time of delivery has been noted in humans. At term, hemoglobin A accounts for approximately 25% of total hemoglobin, and the fetal P_{50} is approximately 19 mm Hg.[53,54] Birth, intrauterine hypoxia,[55] or hemolytic disease of the newborn do not cause a change in the proportions of hemoglobin A and hemoglobin F at any given gestational age. Despite an oxygen tension in fetal blood that is only one-fifth to one-fourth that of the adult, fetal arterial blood oxygen content and oxyhemoglobin saturation at term are not much lower than those in the adult (Fig. 65.4). This similarity, of course, results from a combination of the high oxygen-carrying capacity and increased oxygen affinity of fetal blood. The greater oxygen affinity of fetal blood is generally considered an advantage, in that it allows incorporation of oxygen to nearly saturate fetal hemoglobin at relatively low oxygen tensions. The possible disadvantage in oxygen delivery to fetal tissues is offset by the fact that the fetal oxyhemoglobin saturation curve is rather steep, so a small decrease in oxygen tension results in a major decrement in oxyhemoglobin saturation and

Table 65.1 Oxygen Transport in Term Infants: Selected Clinical Series.

No. of Infants	Age	Total Hb (g/dL blood)	Hct (%)	MCHC (%)	O_2 Capacity (mL/dL blood)	P_{50}[a] (mm Hg)	2,3-DPG (nmol/mL RBCs)	Fetal Hb (% of Total)	FFDPG (nmol/mL RBCs)	Reticulocyte Count (%)
19	1 day	17.8 ± 2.0	52.7 ± 7.1	34.2 ± 1.9	24.7 ± 2.8	19.4 ± 1.8	5433 ± 1041	77.0 ± 7.3	1246 ± 570	4.70 ± 1.74
18	5 days	16.2 ± 1.2	46.9 ± 6.0	34.1 ± 0.8	22.6 ± 2.2	20.6 ± 1.7	6580 ± 996	76.8 ± 5.8	1516 ± 495	2.15 ± 1.64
14	3 wk	12.0 ± 1.3	33.5 ± 4.3	35.9 ± 1.2	16.7 ± 1.9	22.7 ± 1.0	5378 ± 732	70.0 ± 7.33	1614 ± 252	0.88 ± 0.71
10	6–9 wk	10.5 ± 1.2	30.2 ± 3.9	34.9 ± 0.6	14.7 ± 1.6	24.4 ± 1.4	5560 ± 747	52.1 ± 11.0	2670 ± 550	1.63 ± 0.65
14	3–4 mo	10.2 ± 0.8	30.3 ± 2.4	33.8 ± 1.7	14.3 ± 1.2	26.5 ± 2.0	5819 ± 1240	23.2 ± 16.0	4470 ± 1380	1.36 ± 0.45
8	6 mo	11.3 ± 0.9	34.0 ± 3.6	33.4 ± 0.7	14.7 ± 0.6	27.8 ± 1.0	5086 ± 1570	4.7 ± 2.2	4840 ± 1500	1.42 ± 1.15
8	8–11 mo	11.4 ± 0.6	34.8 ± 1.9	32.8 ± 0.9	15.9 ± 0.8	30.3 ± 0.7	7381 ± 485	1.6 ± 1.0	7260 ± 544	0.82 ± 0.27

[a]At pH 7.40.

2,3-DPG, 2,3-Diphosphoglycerate; *FFDPG*, functioning fraction of 2,3-diphosphoglycerate; *Hb*, hemoglobin; *Hct*, hematocrit; *MCHC*, mean corpuscular hemoglobin concentration; *RBCs*, red blood cells.

Data from Delivoria-Papadopoulos M, Oski FA, Miller LD, Forster RE. The pathophysiology of exchange transfusion of the newborn infant with regard to oxygen transport. In: Chaplin H Jr, Jaffe ER, Lenfant C, et al., eds. *Preservation of Red Blood Cells*. Washington, DC: National Academy of Sciences; 1973:137–147.

unloading of oxygen to the tissues. The actual oxyhemoglobin saturation curve in vivo as blood flows through the placental exchange capillaries is an additional important consideration. Compared with standard conditions, maternal arterial blood is slightly hypocarbic (Pco_2 of 32 mm Hg) and alkalotic (pH 7.42), whereas fetal blood is slightly hypercarbic (Pco_2 of 45 mm Hg) and acidotic (pH of 7.34). As fetal blood courses through the exchange vessels, it gives up H^+ and carbon dioxide, leading to a rise in pH and a fall in Pco_2. The opposite changes occur in the maternal exchange vessels. Thus, in vivo, the maternal and fetal oxyhemoglobin saturation curves may be almost superimposed (see Fig. 65.4). Although the double Bohr effect in the placenta has been credited with significantly augmenting oxygen exchange, theoretical studies suggest that this accounts for only 2% of the total oxygen transferred. Below pH 7.2, however, the Bohr effect is greater for fetal blood than for maternal blood. An additional factor tending to shift the in vivo fetal dissociation curve to the right is the temperature of the fetus, which exceeds that of the mother by 0.5°C to 1.0°C. In human neonates the dissociation curve also shifts toward that of the mother as the proportion of hemoglobin F decreases.[50,56]

In 1971, investigation of the deoxygenation kinetics of isolated fetal and adult hemoglobin revealed significant functional differences.[57] Although 2,3-DPG bound to fetal hemoglobin, the binding constant was lower than for adult hemoglobin.[54] Other experiments performed on whole blood demonstrated a significant fall in P_{50} when erythrocytes were depleted of 2,3-DPG, even in samples of blood with a high percentage of fetal hemoglobin.[58] With the use of pure solutions of fetal and adult hemoglobin, it was subsequently shown that the effect of 2,3-DPG on P_{50} of fetal hemoglobin is approximately 40% of its effect on P_{50} of adult hemoglobin.[59] On the basis of these findings, P_{50} of neonatal whole blood can be expected to be related to both the 2,3-DPG level and the relative concentrations of adult and fetal hemoglobin. The correlation of P_{50} with gestational age is even closer than that with the functioning fraction of 2,3-DPG, suggesting that other factors contribute to the rise of P_{50} during gestation. No satisfactory explanation has emerged for the rise in 2,3-DPG levels during gestation. It has been speculated, however, that the increase is the result of increased synthesis of adult hemoglobin, because in vitro studies have shown that the reduced hemoglobin of adults is more effective than the reduced hemoglobin of fetuses in stimulating 2,3-DPG synthesis. This hypothesis is also supported by the significant correlation between the percentage of adult hemoglobin and 2,3-DPG content in the neonatal period (Table 65.1).

POSTNATAL CHANGES IN OXYGEN AFFINITY

The high oxygen affinity of fetal blood, which is well adapted to oxygen uptake in the placenta, has disadvantages in postnatal life. With adequate postnatal lung function, the pulmonary circulation is exposed to an oxygen tension of 80 mm Hg or more, so high affinity at low oxygen tensions has no advantage for oxygen uptake during the newborn period. At the tissue level, the low P_{50} decreases the driving potential for oxygen diffusion, limiting the rate at which oxygen can be unloaded. The newborn infant needs more oxygen than the fetus, for even in a neutral thermal environment and at minimal activity the oxygen consumption of most species increases by 100% to 150% in the first few days of life.[60] Colder environments and muscle activity further increase the metabolic demand for oxygen. Hence a P_{50} adequate for tissue supply in the fetus may not provide a sufficient rate of net oxygen diffusion in the neonate.

To meet the increased oxygen demands after birth, oxygen-carrying parameters of blood change drastically. In most species, postnatal changes occur in both oxygen affinity and oxygen-carrying capacity, but at different rates and by different amounts. Beginning at birth, the infant's blood oxygen affinity decreases rapidly.[53] On the first day of life, P_{50} in normal infants is 19.4 ± 1.8 mm Hg, in contrast with a value of 27.0 ± 1.1 mm Hg for the normal adult (all values are the mean ± standard deviation). In the term infant, P_{50} increases gradually and reaches normal adult values by 4 to 6 months of age (Fig. 65.5), corresponding to the time course of the replacement of fetal hemoglobin by adult hemoglobin. The red blood cell 2,3-DPG concentration on day 1 averages 5.43 ± 1.04 μmol/mL of red blood cells and thus does not differ significantly from the adult value of 5.11 ± 0.42 μmol/mL. By the fifth day, the 2,3-DPG concentration increases to 6.58 ± 1.00 μmol/mL of red blood cells.[52] Although this increment has only a modest direct effect on fetal hemoglobin oxygen affinity, it lowers the intracellular pH, thereby decreasing blood oxygen affinity. Therefore, the postnatal change in P_{50} correlates neither

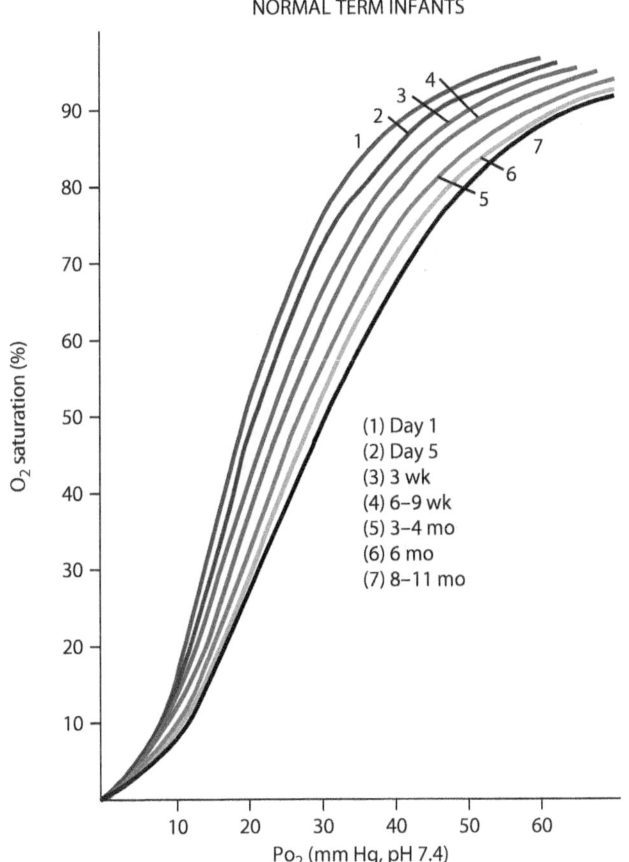

Fig. 65.5 Oxygen equilibrium curve for blood from term infants at different postnatal ages.

with the change in red blood cell 2,3-DPG content alone nor with the decline in fetal hemoglobin concentration alone. The changes in oxygen affinity during postnatal life should be considered when the oxygen saturation or content of arterial blood in the neonate is derived from measurements of arterial partial pressure of oxygen and pH. In the absence of other measurements, gestational age can be used for a reasonably accurate estimation of the oxygen affinity.

In general, compared with their larger term counterparts, preterm, low-birth-weight infants have a lower erythrocyte 2,3-DPG content, lower P_{50}, and higher fetal hemoglobin concentration. During the first several weeks after birth, these small infants have 2,3-DPG concentrations significantly lower than those in term infants. Premature infants have a smaller oxygen-unloading capacity initially than that measured in term infants and do not catch up during the first 3 months of life (Fig. 65.6).

CLINICAL ASSESSMENT OF THE ADEQUACY OF CARDIAC OUTPUT/ TISSUE OXYGENATION

An adequate cardiovascular system maintains sufficient oxygen transport to meet the metabolic demands of organs and cells (Fig. 65.7). The determination of an adequate circulation is based on a composite appraisal of clinical indices such as arterial pressure, heart rate, and capillary refill; end-organ well-being, including urinary output, muscle tone, and level of consciousness; and laboratory parameters such as arterial pH, lactate concentration, urea concentration, and creatinine concentration, which reflect adequacy of tissue perfusion. The value of these parameters is likely greatest when they are used in combination and longitudinally to document trends or responses to therapeutic interventions. Therapeutic decisions should not be based on any single parameter in isolation. In addition, decisions to intervene will likely depend on the underlying disease process; this in turn enables a more targeted approach to treatment.

HEART RATE

The conventional concept of heart rate being the main determinant of cardiac output in neonates and preterm infants has recently been challenged. Stroke volume may play a more important role in maintaining cardiac output. Recent data suggest that the increase in LVO seen soon after birth after an increase in pulmonary blood flow is a consequence of increasing stroke volume rather than heart rate.[61] Nonetheless, a heart rate greater than 160 beats per minute may be a physiologic response to hypovolemia. Extremes of tachycardia may have a negative impact on the force-frequency relationship. In patients with severe heart dysfunction, where increased heart rate caused by cardiotropic agents is not associated with positive inotropy, further deteriorations in heart function may occur due to rate-related compromised diastolic perfusion. Other causes of tachycardia in the neonate include pain, sepsis and fever, hyperthyroidism, catecholamine excess, drugs (caffeine), hypoglycemia, anemia, and neonatal arrhythmias.

ARTERIAL PRESSURE MEASUREMENT

Blood pressure is relatively easy to measure, so it is commonly and incorrectly used as a surrogate of cardiac output and systemic blood flow, for which it does poorly.[62] Ease of access does not confer accuracy of measurement, so invasive arterial monitoring is preferred to noninvasive (cuff) blood pressure measurements, which must be interpreted with caution, especially in very small infants. A normal mean arterial pressure does not ensure adequacy of cardiac output, as the blood pressure may be maintained by a high SVR in the face of reduced systemic blood flow. Similarly, low blood pressure may result from low peripheral vascular resistance despite normal or high cardiac output and systemic blood flow. There are no set criteria to define true hypotension in neonates. The most commonly used definition for hypotension—mean blood pressure in mm Hg less than gestational age in weeks—lacks scientific validation.[7] Little attention is paid to blood pressure components such as the systolic and diastolic arterial pressures in the adjudication of circulatory stability or selection of a cardiovascular intervention. Normative population-based data for systolic arterial pressures are available[63,64] and may be more useful than examination of mean blood pressure in isolation. Systolic arterial pressure is a useful surrogate of the adequacy of cardiac output and diastolic arterial pressure reflects SVR (Fig. 65.8).

CAPILLARY REFILL TIME

A capillary refill time of more than 5 seconds correlates weakly with low flow states.[65] In addition, cool extremities, acrocyanosis, and pallor are all early signs of peripheral vasoconstriction and redirecting of blood to vital organs. However, evaluations comparing a prolonged capillary refill time and echocardiography measurements of cardiac output show variable correlations.[66]

URINE OUTPUT

In the absence of parenchymal renal disease or obstructive uropathies, a low urinary output may suggest compromised renal perfusion secondary to low systemic blood flow. In preterm infants with renal tubular immaturity, urine output can remain normal despite reduced renal perfusion.

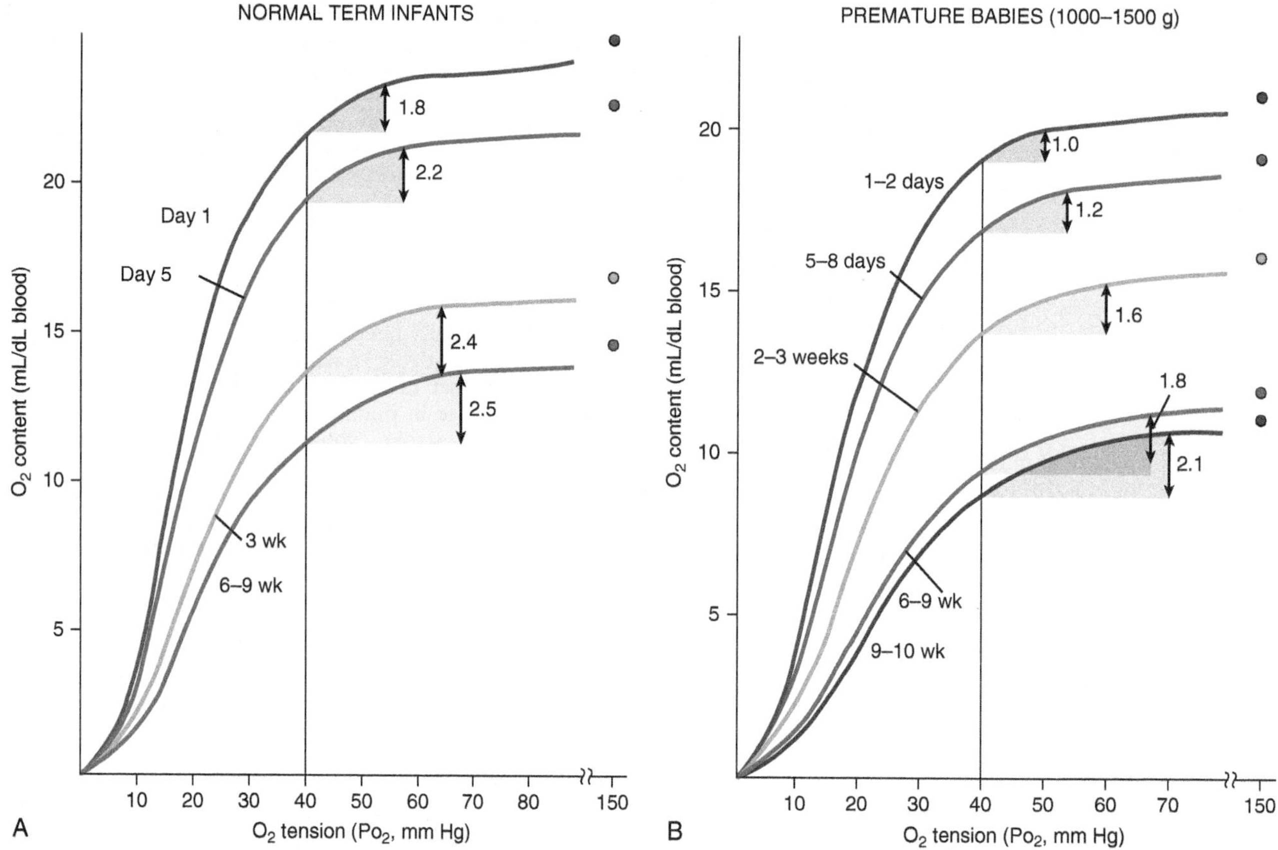

Fig. 65.6 Oxygen equilibrium curves for blood from term infants (A) and from preterm infants of birth weight 1000 to 1500 g (B) at different postnatal ages. *Double arrows* represent the oxygen-unloading capacity between given arterial and venous P_{O_2} values. *Points* corresponding to 150 mm Hg on the abscissa are the O_2 capacities; each *curve* represents the mean value for the infants studied in each age-group.

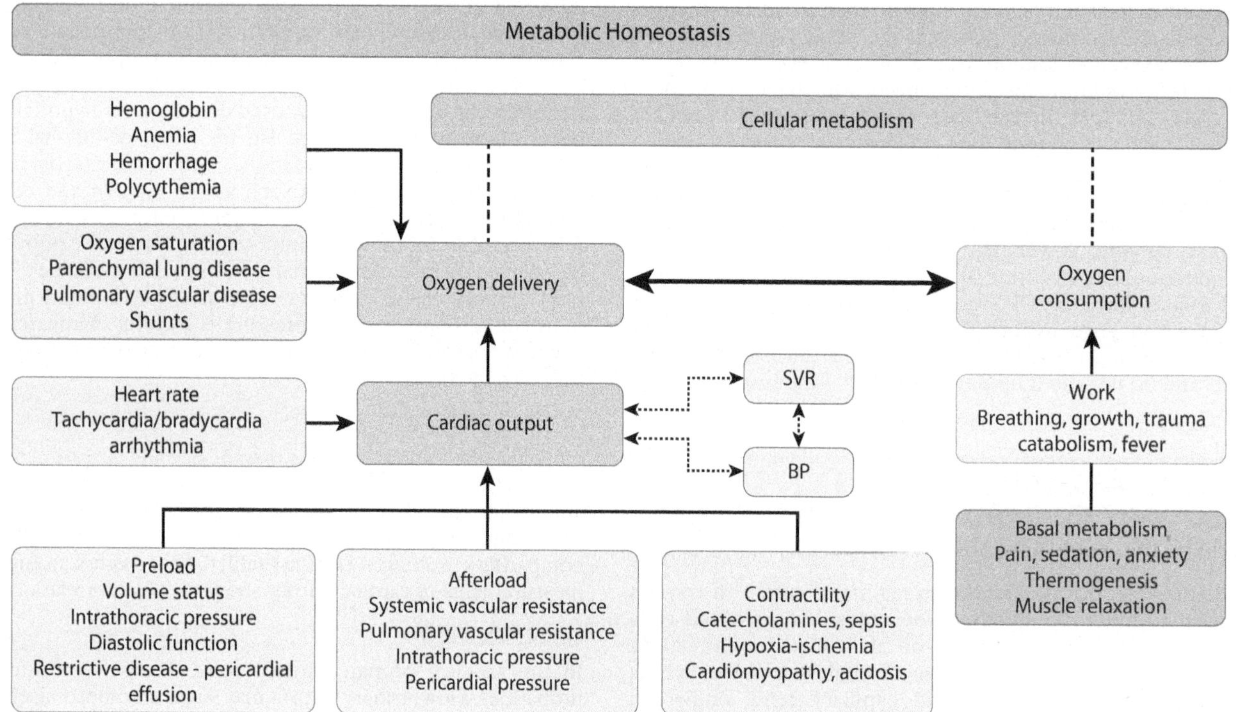

Fig. 65.7 Contributions to cellular metabolism required for maintenance of metabolic homeostasis. *BP*, Blood pressure; *SVR*, systemic vascular resistance. (Adapted from Giesinger RE, McNamara PJ. Hemodynamic instability in the critically ill neonate: an approach to cardiovascular support based on disease pathophysiology. *Semin Perinatol.* 2016;40:174–188. Fig. 1.)

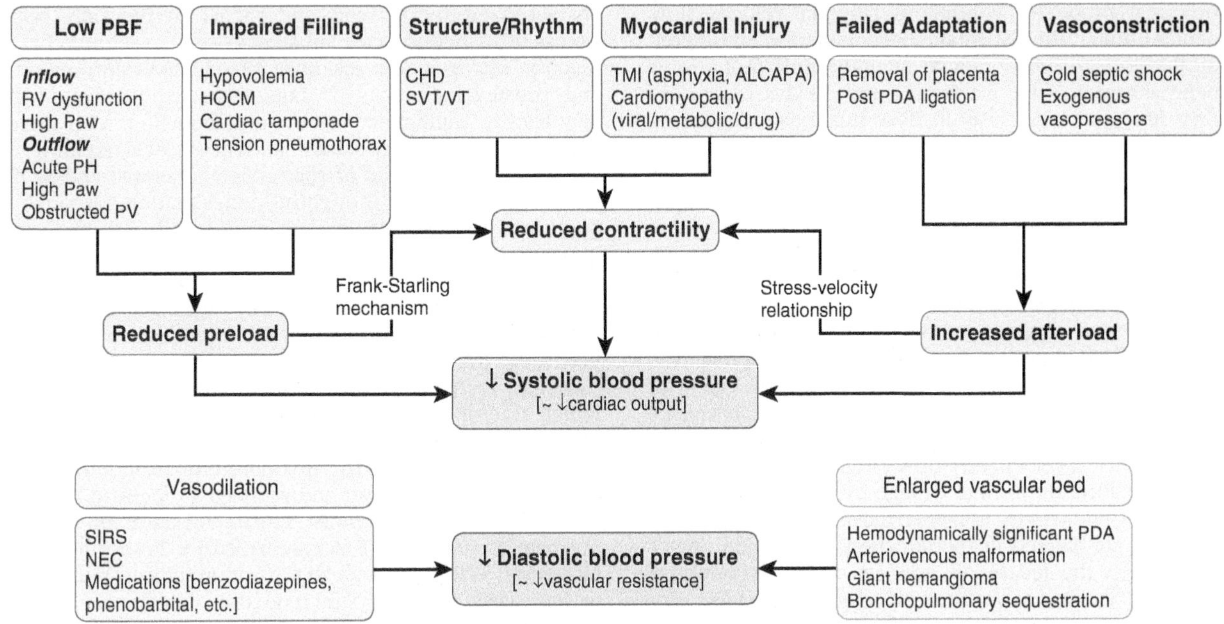

Fig. 65.8 Importance of investigating causes of low systolic and diastolic blood pressures. *ALCAPA*, Anomalous left coronary from the pulmonary artery; *CHD*, congenital heart disease; *HOCM*, hypertrophic cardiomyopathy; *NEC*, necrotizing enterocolitis; *Paw*, mean airway pressure; *PBF*, pulmonary blood flow; *PDA*, patent ductus arteriosus; *PH*, pulmonary hypertension; *PV*, pulmonary vein; RV, right ventricle; *SIRS*, systemic inflammatory response syndrome; *TMI*, transmural myocardial infarction; *SVT*, supraventricular tachycardia; *VT*, ventricular tachycardia. (Adapted from McNamara PJ, Giesinger RE, Fisk A, et al. *Anderson's Pediatric Cardiology.* 4th ed. Elsevier; 2020. Fig. 15.10.)

LABORATORY MARKERS

Anaerobic metabolism occurs when oxygen transport and tissue oxygenation are compromised. The resulting rise in serum lactate levels can be a marker for low cardiac output, albeit a late indicator of severe metabolic compromise. Elevated lactate levels in isolation can be a consequence of increased glycogenolysis or other inborn errors of metabolism. Conversely, lactate produced in poorly perfused tissue undergoing anaerobic metabolism may not be mobilized into the bloodstream until perfusion improves, with the rise of lactate level occurring only after restoration of an adequate systemic blood flow.[67]

Blood urea nitrogen levels gradually increase in response to renal hypoperfusion, without corresponding elevation in creatinine levels until glomerular filtration is impaired by severe underperfusion. These are late markers of compromised cardiac output.

TARGETED NEONATAL ECHOCARDIOGRAPHY

The overreliance on blood pressure in isolation as a surrogate marker of the adequacy of systemic blood flow and tissue oxygenation is problematic for several reasons. *First,* the arbitrary threshold of mean arterial pressure approximating the gestational age proposed in 1992 is a physiologic oversimplification that lacks scientific validation. *Second,* end-organ perfusion is dependent on systemic blood flow and vascular resistance; therefore reliance on blood pressure measurements alone provides limited information regarding the adequacy of organ blood flow.[68] There is poor correlation between blood pressure and LVO[62] and a weak relationship between blood pressure and superior vena cava flow[69] in the first few days after birth. Both blood pressure and systemic flow are important determinants of oxygen transport and tissue oxygenation; neither should be monitored nor treated in isolation, without consideration of the influence of the other. The lack of positive impact of treatment of hypotension has been interpreted as the lack of importance of BP thresholds. While normative data are lacking, an imprecise and non-judicious approach to selection of cardiovascular agents may provide an alternate explanation for the lack of positive effect. Serial targeted neonatal echocardiography (TnECHO) offers the potential for novel insights regarding real-time cardiovascular physiology; specifically, whether the apparent impairment of cardiac output relates to preload, afterload, or myocardial function (see Fig. 65.8). Furthermore, TnECHO can aid in examining the role of the various shunts (PDA and PFO) in hemodynamic instability, if present. It may provide longitudinal physiologic information that may enable more focused management and monitor the response to treatment. The use of TnECHO to manage cardiovascular health has become standard care in many institutions, but the training of hemodynamic experts/consultants needs to be extensive.[70-73] Recent expert opinion provides endorsement for the need for competency-based training, which considers not only imaging competencies but an advanced knowledge of imaging physics, cardiopulmonary physiology, and pharmacotherapeutic knowledge.[74] There is also mounting evidence that the regular use of TnECHO may improve outcomes[75] and limit unnecessary therapy.[76] Direct measurement of LV and RV output using TnECHO methods is feasible, with acceptable validity and reliability, but it provides only discrete intermittent readings and is dependent on the availability of personnel with expertise.[78,79] Additionally, caution is needed in certain scenarios. For example, LVO is not an accurate measure of true systemic blood flow in the presence of a high-volume left-to-right shunt, where LV preload and stroke volume are increased, but at the expense of postductal systemic blood flow. RV output measurements are confounded by interatrial shunt. Typically, atrial shunts are much smaller than ductal shunts, so RV output may be used as an estimation of systemic blood flow.[62,77]

NOVEL NONINVASIVE TECHNIQUES OF CONTINUOUS CARDIAC OUTPUT ASSESSMENT

Continuous assessment of cardiac output would be a valuable tool in the management of a wide range of neonatal illnesses. In pediatric and adult populations, this can be achieved by invasive methods such as continuous thermodilution with a pulmonary artery catheter, an arterial catheter for pulse contour analysis, an intratracheal tube for partial CO_2 rebreathing, or an intraesophageal probe for continuous Doppler velocity flow assessment. Although the thermodilution method is considered the clinical gold standard of central hemodynamic monitoring, it has been shown to have many risks and disadvantages. Size constraints have precluded use of those methods in neonates. Two relatively new approaches to continuous noninvasive measurement of cardiac output are based on the theory of bioimpedance. Noninvasive continuous cardiac output monitoring (NICOM) based on transthoracic bioreactance uses analysis of relative phase shifts of oscillating currents traversing the thoracic cavity (rather than a change of amplitude in bioimpedance). The degree of phase shift of the ingoing current compared with the outgoing current is proportional to the stroke volume of blood ejected from the aorta. Validation studies in infants show close correlation with invasive measurement of aortic blood flow in small animals but systematic differences when compared to echocardiographic measurements in infants.[80-82] Electrical velocimetry uses variation of conductivity of blood in the aorta during the cardiac cycle to derive aortic stroke volume. Conductivity is higher during systole, when all red blood cells are aligned in the direction of flow, and lower in diastole, when the red blood cells are randomly oriented. Cardiac output estimates obtained by electrical velocimetry correlated well with echocardiography.[83] Both methods remain investigative and their applicability in routine neonatal care is yet to be determined.

ASSESSMENT OF CEREBRAL PERFUSION

Continuous real-time monitoring of cerebral perfusion may provide important information about adequacy of oxygen delivery.[84] The relatively high degree of transparency of myocardial and brain tissue to near-infrared light enables real-time noninvasive detection of tissue oxygen saturation by transillumination spectroscopy.[85] Near-infrared spectroscopy (NIRS) is an important predictor of brain damage and long-term outcome during hypothermic cardiac arrest in animal studies[86,87] and may serve as a reliable diagnostic modality for monitoring cerebral metabolism during therapeutic hypothermia for cardiac surgery.[88] Studies of neonatal cerebral metabolism during cardiac surgery using NIRS provide a prototype for similar applications in other clinical contexts. NIRS-measured hemoglobin oxygenation parameters may reflect functional changes in cerebral hemodynamics and brain tissue oxygenation during neonatal cardiopulmonary bypass and deep hypothermic circulatory arrest.[89] In neonates undergoing an arterial switch procedure with deep hypothermia-induced circulatory arrest, NIRS-measured regional cerebral oxygen saturation (rSO_2) did not correlate with cerebral electrographic activity or arterial oxygen content and took longer than both of them to normalize.[90] Patients with a lower preoperative rSO_2, despite having no preexisting brain damage, had worse developmental outcomes at 30 to 36 months. This indicates that NIRS measurement of rSO_2 could be a superior measure of cerebral tissue oxygenation and may be a useful predictor of long-term neurologic outcome.

OXYGEN TRANSPORT/DELIVERY IN SPECIFIC CONDITIONS

ACUTE PULMONARY HYPERTENSION OF THE NEWBORN

Acute pulmonary hypertension (aPH) of the newborn is a relatively common condition, occurring in 0.5 to 7 per 1000 live births, with mortality rates ranging from 4% to 33%.[91,92] The hallmark clinical feature is hypoxemia secondary to failure of the normal postnatal fall in PVR. The consequences may include impaired right ventricular systolic function and low cardiac output. On a cellular level, the condition is characterized by marked endothelial dysfunction, with an excess of vasoconstrictor substances such as endothelin 1 and reactive nitrogen species over vasodilator compounds (NO and prostaglandin I_2).[93,94] Long-term exposure to hypoxia may lead to pulmonary arteriolar remodeling, with increased connective tissue deposition and neomuscularization.[95] The role of the persistence of right-to-left foraminal and/or ductal fetal channels needs thoughtful consideration. Although their continued patency may permit right-to-left flow and ongoing hypoxemia, they may have the advantages of protecting the RV from failing and augmentation of cardiac output, but at the expense of blood oxygenation. The right-to-left shunts across the PFO and PDA enhance preductal cardiac output, cerebral perfusion, and postductal cardiac output. This represents a paradigm shift in consideration of the role of these shunts, which traditionally were considered purely harmful through reducing effective pulmonary blood flow.

RV and LV function may be compromised in aPH as a result of increased RV afterload and reduced LV preload (because of reduced pulmonary venous return).[96] Failure of the normal postnatal decline in PVR accompanied by the normal postnatal increase in SVR after placental separation subjects both ventricles to increased afterload. The reduction in effective pulmonary blood flow secondary to vasoconstriction leads to suboptimal pulmonary venous return, LV preload, and cardiac output. The effects of a pressure-loaded, dilated right side of the heart include a shift in the interventricular septum and compression of the left atrium and ventricle, both resulting in decreased LV filling, further compromising LVO. The low cardiac output state resulting from reduced LV preload can lead to a fall in mean arterial pressure, prompting use of vasoactive inotropes such as dopamine and epinephrine. Animal experimental data have demonstrated that these inotropes raise both SVR and PVR and may further contribute to RV compromise in the setting of aPH.[97,98] Several studies have demonstrated the association of a low cardiac output in the setting of aPH with morbidity and mortality.[99-101] The choice of cardiovascular agents with inodilator effects (e.g., milrinone) that have beneficial effects on PVR and cardiac output would appear prudent. Early identification of low systolic arterial pressure may enhance the identification process and inform therapeutic choices.

CHRONIC PULMONARY HYPERTENSION

Chronic pulmonary hypertension (cPH) usually manifests in infants after 4 to 6 weeks of life and results from neonatal lung disease, congenital heart disease, or structural and genetic malformations of the airway, pulmonary vasculature, or lung parenchyma.[102] It is more commonly seen in extremely premature infants with bronchopulmonary dysplasia (BPD). Though the true prevalence of cPH is difficult to establish, a meta-analysis found a prevalence in extremely premature infants of 2% in the absence of BPD, 6% for mild BPD, 12% for moderate BPD, and 39% for severe BPD.[103] Infants with BPD have alveolar and vascular simplification and remodeling resulting in abnormal gas exchange, hypercapnia, and hypoxemia. Interventions to improve gas exchange, such as mechanical ventilation and oxygen supplementation, may further contribute to lung pathology. The result is a muscularized pulmonary vascular system with marked increase in PVR and decreased pulmonary blood flow. Over time, the increase in PVR leads to limited right ventricular adaptation, resulting in hypertrophy and/or dilation. When the RV is unable to sustain this response, right heart failure begins, and the RV uncouples from its afterload. Ventriculo-ventricular interaction at that time may lead to LV dysfunction as well. Notable comorbidities that may significantly affect the clinical course in the BPD patient with cPH include intra- and extra-cardiac shunts and pulmonary vein stenosis.[104] Cardiac shunts as a source of increased pulmonary circulation in the BPD patient may promote further vascular remodeling.[105] Pulmonary vein stenosis, congenital or acquired, may result in pulmonary venous congestion, interstitial edema, and an increase in upstream pulmonary artery pressure. Clinical detection is challenging in these patients with varying degrees of BPD and confounding illnesses. In addition, many infants with cPH present with nonspecific symptoms. Many of these symptoms, such as frequent desaturations, tachypnea, and persistent oxygen requirement, may be attributed to the patients' underlying prematurity or BPD, which can lead to a delay in diagnosis. These limitations suggest the need for monitoring with serial TnECHO. Recent evidence, however, highlights the poor reliability of subjective interpretation of echocardiography indices of cPH, prompting the need for standardized imaging protocols based on validated quantitative techniques.[106]

HEMODYNAMICALLY SIGNIFICANT DUCTUS ARTERIOSUS

The DA connects the main pulmonary artery to the descending aorta and is necessary for fetal survival. After birth the lungs expand and become the organ of oxygen exchange; the increase in arterial PO_2 promotes DA closure. In premature infants, because of immaturity of the ductal architecture, the DA may remain patent, allowing shunting of high blood volumes with potentially pathologic consequences. It is the most common cardiovascular abnormality of prematurity, occurring in about one-third of infants born before 30 weeks' gestation and in up to 60% of infants born at less than 28 weeks' gestation.[107] As PVR drops in the first few days of life, the PDA acts as a shunt, allowing blood flow from the systemic circulation to the pulmonary circulation. The consequences of high-volume left-to-right shunts include reduced systemic blood flow (systemic hypoperfusion) and increased pulmonary blood flow (pulmonary overcirculation). Persistent patency of the DA is associated with numerous morbidities potentially attributable to systemic hypoperfusion (e.g., necrotizing enterocolitis, intraventricular hemorrhage, metabolic acidosis, prerenal failure) or to pulmonary overcirculation (e.g., pulmonary hemorrhage, impairment of gas exchange, hypoxemia, increased ventilator dependence, BPD).[108-110] The odds of death are 4 to 8 times greater in infants whose DA remains patent despite attempted medical closure.[111,112] The causal role of hemodynamic consequences of PDA remains uncertain because numerous randomized controlled trials have failed to demonstrate that medical or surgical closure of the PDA leads to a reduction in morbidity or mortality. Most trials are, however, limited by the lack of standardized assessment of hemodynamic significance and variable physician equipoise such that patients with the most problematic shunts may not be enrolled.

OTHER CAUSES OF IMPAIRED TISSUE OXYGENATION

SEPSIS

Bacterial sepsis also affects tissue oxygen transport and utilization. Sepsis caused by group B streptococci, for example, is associated with a higher critical venous oxygen saturation (the levels below which tissue acidosis develops) than that typical for hypoxemia.[113] This higher critical point seems to be a specific effect of sepsis rather than a result of the alterations in circulatory status (e.g., increased catecholamine levels) that occur in response to infection. Oxygen consumption is increased during sepsis, while at the same time oxygen delivery may be decreased as a result of impairment of myocardial function by endotoxin.[114] Additional evidence suggests that sepsis may decrease oxygen extraction at the tissue level, further reducing tissue oxygen delivery.

ANEMIA

In otherwise normal infants with no evidence of cardiac disease, pulmonary disease, or increased metabolic needs, a decrease in the oxygen-carrying capacity is a source of concern only if oxygen delivery to the tissues approaches the limit of oxygen stores.

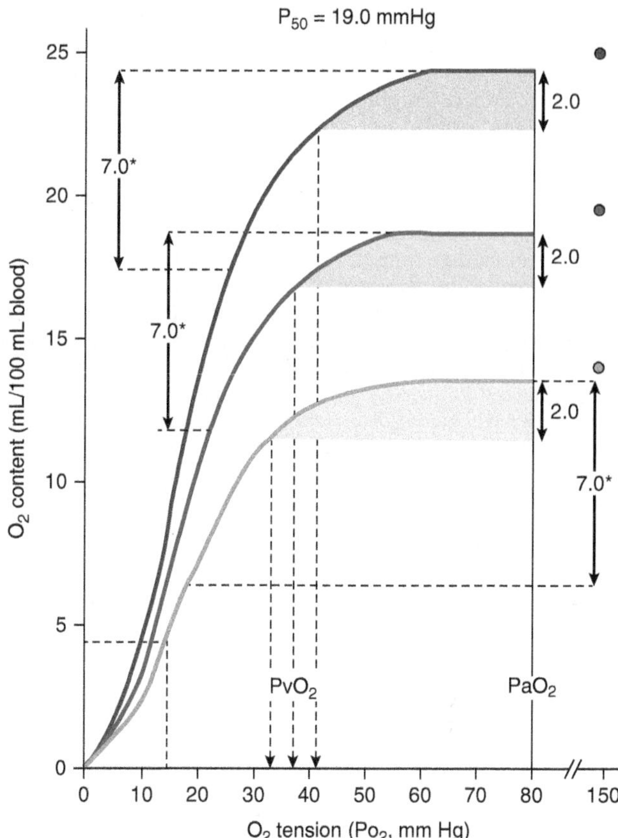

Fig. 65.9 The effect of altered hemoglobin concentrations (10, 14, and 18 g/dL in *yellow*, *blue*, and *red*, respectively) on tissue oxygen extraction, at a constant P_{50} of 19.0 mm Hg, fixed oxygen consumption and blood flow, for tissues with oxygen extractions of 2 or 7 mL/dL. Equivalent arteriovenous content differences are associated with lower venous oxygen saturations at lower hemoglobin concentrations.

As seen in Fig. 65.9, infants who exhibit significant differences in total oxygen-carrying capacity at birth, but similar oxygen affinities, will exhibit the same arteriovenous oxygen content differences. The effect of a decrease in Sa_{O_2} on oxygen delivery is significantly less than the effect of anemia.[115,116] For example, Sa_{O_2} would have to decrease from 95% to approximately 80% to have an effect on oxygen content comparable to a 2-g decrease in hemoglobin concentration. Thus, in situations of marginal oxygen delivery, maintenance of hemoglobin concentrations high enough to optimize oxygen-carrying capacity is essential.

POLYCYTHEMIA

Polycythemia, defined as a venous hematocrit of greater than 65%, can result from fetal transfusions, as a compensatory mechanism for intrauterine hypoxia, or secondary to fetal causes (e.g., trisomy 13/18/21, hypothyroidism, congenital adrenal hyperplasia).[117] The pathologic concern of polycythemic states relates to hyperviscosity of the blood leading to impaired tissue perfusion and oxygenation. Previous investigations have shown a linear relationship between blood viscosity and hematocrit up to 65%; thereafter, progressively disproportionate increases in viscosity are seen.[118]

CONCLUSION

Oxygen is an essential fuel for cellular metabolism and homeostasis; hence, effective uptake and delivery of oxygen are essential determinants of human existence. The latter is dependent on lung maturation and physiology, hemoglobin characteristics, myocardial performance, and vascular integrity. Differences in hemoglobin subtype in the fetus and intrauterine cardiovascular physiology allow effective control of tissue oxygenation in the fetus as organs mature and the fetus develops. After birth, oxygen transport is influenced by the partial pressure of oxygen in inspired air, the adequacy of alveolar ventilation, hemoglobin concentration, the affinity of hemoglobin for oxygen, and cardiac output. The clinical approach to impaired tissue oxygenation warrants thoughtful consideration of all potential physiologic contributors and how they influence each other, enabling a more precise and relevant approach to decision-making. The use of echocardiography by neonatology specialists with enhanced knowledge of cardiopulmonary physiology and therapeutics will guide advancements in the field and potentially facilitate improvements in patient care and neonatal outcomes.

ACKNOWLEDGMENT

This chapter is based on a previous contribution by Maria Delivoria-Papadopoulos and Jane E. McGowan.

 A complete reference list is available at www.ExpertConsult.com.

SELECT REFERENCES

5. Schruefer JJ, Heller CJ, Battaglia FC, Hellegers AE. Independence of whole blood and haemoglobin solution oxygen dissociation curves from haemoglobin type. *Nature*. 1962;196:550-553.
9. Fanaroff JM, Fanaroff AA. Blood pressure disorders in the neonate: hypotension and hypertension. *Semin Fetal Neonatal Med*. 2006;11(3):174-181.
11. Jain A, Mohamed A, Kavanagh B, et al. Cardiopulmonary adaptation during first day of life in human neonates. *J Pediatr*. 2018;200:50-57. e52.
12. Liedel JL, Meadow W, Nachman J, Koogler T, Kahana MD. Use of vasopressin in refractory hypotension in children with vasodilatory shock: five cases and a review of the literature. *Pediatr Crit Care Med*. 2002;3(1):15-18.
13. Landry DW, Oliver JA. The pathogenesis of vasodilatory shock. *N Engl J Med*. 2001;345(8):588-595.
15. Dries DJ. Vasoactive drug support in septic shock. *Shock*. 2006;26(5):529-530.
16. Hooper SB, Polglase GR, te Pas AB. A physiological approach to the timing of umbilical cord clamping at birth. *Arch Dis Child Fetal Neonatal Ed*. 2015;100(4):F355-F360.
17. van Vonderen JJ, Roest AA, Siew ML, et al. Measuring physiological changes during the transition to life after birth. *Neonatology*. 2014;105(3):230-242.
18. Yigit B, Tutsak E, Yıldırım C, Hutchon D, Pekkan K. Transitional fetal hemodynamics and gas exchange in premature postpartum adaptation: immediate vs. delayed cord clamping. *Matern Health Neonatol Perinatol*. 2019;5(1):5.
23. Jain A, Mohamed A, El-Khuffash A, et al. A comprehensive echocardiographic protocol for assessing neonatal right ventricular dimensions and function in the transitional period: normative data and z scores. *J Am Soc Echocardiogr*. 2014;27(12):1293-1304.
25. Rowland DG, Gutgesell HP. Noninvasive assessment of myocardial contractility, preload, and afterload in healthy newborn infants. *Am J Cardiol*. 1995;75(12):818-821.
26. Cox DJ, Groves AM. Inotropes in preterm infants–evidence for and against. *Acta Paediatr Suppl*. 2012;101(464):17-23.
27. Choudhry S, Salter A, Cunningham TW, et al. Risk factors and prognostic significance of altered left ventricular geometry in preterm infants. *J Perinatol*. 2018;38(5):543-549.
29. Ng PC, Lee CH, Lam CW, et al. Transient adrenocortical insufficiency of prematurity and systemic hypotension in very low birthweight infants. *Arch Dis Child Fetal Neonatal Ed*. 2004;89(2):F119-F126.
31. Noori S, Friedlich P, Wong P, et al. Hemodynamic changes after low-dosage hydrocortisone administration in vasopressor-treated preterm and term neonates. *Pediatrics*. 2006;118(4):1456-1466.
32. Noori S, McCoy M, Anderson MP, Ramji F, Seri I. Changes in cardiac function and cerebral blood flow in relation to peri/intraventricular hemorrhage in extremely preterm infants. *J Pediatr*. 2014;164(2):264-270. e263.
34. Scherrer M, Bachofen H. The oxygen combining capacity of hemoglobin. *Anesthesiology*. 1972;36:190.
42. Shappell SD, Murray JA, Bellingham AJ, et al. Adaptation to exercise: role of hemoglobin affinity for oxygen and 2,3-diphosphoglycerate. *J Appl Physiol*. 1971;30(6):827-832.
46. Oski FA, Gottlieb AJ, Miller WW, Delivoria-Papadopoulos M. The effects of deoxygenation of adult and fetal hemoglobin on the synthesis of red cell 2,3-diphosphoglycerate and its *in vivo* consequences. *J Clin Invest*. 1970;49(2):400-407.
53. Delivoria-Papadopoulos M, Oski FA, Gottlieb AJ. Oxygen-hemoglobulin dissociation curves: effect of inherited enzyme defects of the red cell. *Science*. 1969;165(3893):601-602.
54. Delivoria-Papadopoulos M, Morrow 3rd G, Oski FA. Exchange transfusion in the newborn infant with fresh and "old" blood: the role of storage on 2,3-diphosphoglycerate, hemoglobin-oxygen affinity, and oxygen release. *J Pediatr*. 1971;79(6):898-903.
57. Salhany JM, Mizukami H, Eliot RS. The deoxygenation kinetic properties of human fetal hemoglobin: effect of 2,3-diphosphoglycerate. *Biochem Biophys Res Commun*. 1971;45(5):1350-1356.
58. Brewer GJ, Eaton JW. Erythrocyte metabolism: interaction with oxygen transport. *Science*. 1971;171(3977):1205-1211.
61. van Vonderen JJ, Roest AA, Siew ML, et al. Noninvasive measurements of hemodynamic transition directly after birth. *Pediatr Res*. 2014;75(3):448-452.
62. Kluckow M, Evans N. Relationship between blood pressure and cardiac output in preterm infants requiring mechanical ventilation. *J Pediatr*. 1996;129(4):506-512.
63. Hegyi T, Carbone MT, Anwar M, et al. Blood pressure ranges in premature infants. I. The first hours of life. *J Pediatr*. 1994;124(4):627-633.
64. Hegyi T, Anwar M, Carbone MT, et al. Blood pressure ranges in premature infants: II. The first week of life. *Pediatrics*. 1996;97(3):336-342.
65. Osborn D, Evans N, Kluckow M. Randomized trial of dobutamine versus dopamine in preterm infants with low systemic blood flow. *J Pediatr*. 2002;140(2):183-191.
67. de Boode WP. Clinical monitoring of systemic hemodynamics in critically ill newborns. *Early Hum Dev*. 2010;86(3):137-141.
68. Evans JR, Lou Short B, Van Meurs K, Cheryl Sachs H. Cardiovascular support in preterm infants. *Clin Ther*. 2006;28(9):1366-1384.
69. Kluckow M, Evans N. Low superior vena cava flow and intraventricular haemorrhage in preterm infants. *Arch Dis Child Fetal Neonatal Ed*. 2000;82(3):F188-F194.
71. El-Khuffash AF, Jain A, Weisz D, Mertens L, McNamara PJ. Assessment and treatment of post patent ductus arteriosus ligation syndrome. *J Pediatr*. 2014;165(1):46-52. e41.
72. El-Khuffash AF, Jain A, McNamara PJ. Ligation of the patent ductus arteriosus in preterm infants: understanding the physiology. *J Pediatr*. 2013;162(6):1100-1106.
75. Jain A, Sahni M, El-Khuffash A, et al. Use of targeted neonatal echocardiography to prevent postoperative cardiorespiratory instability after patent ductus arteriosus ligation. *J Pediatr*. 2012;160(4):584-589. e581.
76. Carmo KB, Evans N, Paradisis M. Duration of indomethacin treatment of the preterm patent ductus arteriosus as directed by echocardiography. *J Pediatr*. 2009;155(6):819-822. e811.
77. Evans N, Kluckow M. Early determinants of right and left ventricular output in ventilated preterm infants. *Arch Dis Child Fetal Neonatal Ed*. 1996;74(2):F88-F94.
78. Mertens L, Seri I, Marek J, et al. Targeted neonatal echocardiography in the neonatal intensive care unit: practice guidelines and recommendations for training. Writing group of the American Society of Echocardiography (ASE) in collaboration with the European Association of Echocardiography (EAE) and the Association for European Pediatric Cardiologists (AEPC). *J Am Soc Echocardiogr*. 2011;24(10):1057-1078.
79. El-Khuffash AF, McNamara PJ. Neonatologist-performed functional echocardiography in the neonatal intensive care unit. *Semin Fetal Neonatal Med*. 2011;16(1):50-60.
80. Heerdt PM, Wagner CL, DeMais M, Savarese JJ. Noninvasive cardiac output monitoring with bioreactance as an alternative to invasive instrumentation for preclinical drug evaluation in beagles. *J Pharmacol Toxicol Methods*. 2011;64(2):111-118.
84. Murkin JM, Arango M. Near-infrared spectroscopy as an index of brain and tissue oxygenation. *Br J Anaesth*. 2009;103(suppl 1):i3-13.
87. Abdul-Khaliq H, Schubert S, Troitzsch D, et al. Dynamic changes in cerebral oxygenation related to deep hypothermia and circulatory arrest evaluated by near-infrared spectroscopy. *Acta Anaesthesiol Scand*. 2001;45(6):696-701.
90. Toet MC, Lemmers PM, van Schelven LJ, van Bel F. Cerebral oxygenation and electrical activity after birth asphyxia: their relation to outcome. *Pediatrics*. 2006;117(2):333-339.
93. Gao Y, Raj JU. Regulation of the pulmonary circulation in the fetus and newborn. *Physiol Rev*. 2010;90(4):1291-1335.
94. Hoeper MM, Galie N, Simonneau G, Rubin LJ. New treatments for pulmonary arterial hypertension. *Am J Respir Crit Care Med*. 2002;165(9):1209-1216.
98. Cheung PY, Barrington KJ. The effects of dopamine and epinephrine on hemodynamics and oxygen metabolism in hypoxic anesthetized piglets. *Crit Care*. 2001;5(3):158-166.
99. Evans N, Kluckow M, Currie A. Range of echocardiographic findings in term neonates with high oxygen requirements. *Arch Dis Child Fetal Neonatal Ed*. 1998;78(2):F105-F111.
108. McNamara PJ, Sehgal A. Towards rational management of the patent ductus arteriosus: the need for disease staging. *Arch Dis Child Fetal Neonatal Ed*. 2007;92(6):F424-F427.
112. Noori S, McCoy M, Friedlich P, et al. Failure of ductus arteriosus closure is associated with increased mortality in preterm infants. *Pediatrics*. 2009;123(1):e138-144.
113. Hammerman C. Influence of disease state on oxygen transport in newborn piglets. *Biol Neonate*. 1994;66(2-3):128-136.
116. van der Hoeven MA, Maertzdorf WJ, Blanco CE. Relationship between mixed venous oxygen saturation and markers of tissue oxygenation in progressive hypoxic hypoxia and in isovolemic anemic hypoxia in 8- to 12-day-old piglets. *Crit Care Med*. 1999;27(9):1885-1892.

Control of Breathing in Fetal Life and Onset and Control of Breathing in the Neonate

66

Ruben E. Alvaro

INTRODUCTION

There are at least three important considerations regarding the study of the control of breathing during the fetal and neonatal periods. First, the fetus sleeps all the time and the neonate most of the time.[1-4] This means that their control of breathing must be studied during sleep and compared with the control of breathing in adult subjects during sleep and not during wakefulness.[5-8] This has not been the norm in the past and accounts for some important misconceptions. Second, the fetus and the neonate are noncooperative subjects. This means that we must study their respiratory control without their being aware and try to compare the measurements with those of the adult under similar conditions. This is difficult to do. Third, measurements in the neonate are usually made, by necessity, in the decubitus position, whereas those in the adult subject are usually made in the sitting or standing position.[6,9] The implications of different positions on the control of breathing have also not been dealt with in the past. Unless there is some consistency in the methodology, it is difficult to define what is actually distinct or unique about the control of breathing in the neonate.

In this chapter, we review some of the concepts and the progress made in the area of control of breathing in the fetus and newborn. We also highlight major developments and critically analyze the scientific foundations of our knowledge in this area.

CONCEPTUAL AND HISTORICAL PERSPECTIVES

Although the major advances in our understanding of the control of breathing generally apply to the fetus and newborn, two major aspects make breathing during this period unique. One is the presence and purpose of fetal breathing, and the other is the physiologic mechanism responsible for the establishment of continuous breathing at birth.

In 1970, Dawes and co-workers presented evidence that the fetal sheep makes regular breathing movements during rapid eye movement (REM) sleep.[10] In their work, tracheal pressure changes were measured as an index of fetal breathing. Simultaneously, Merlet and colleagues, using changes in intraesophageal pressure as an index of fetal breathing, demonstrated respiratory activity in fetal sheep.[11] Subsequent work confirmed and expanded these findings by recording the electrical activity of the diaphragm and clearly showing the central origin of the respiratory output in utero.[2,12-16] It is now universally accepted that the fetus makes breathing exercises in utero beginning with early pregnancy that are a critical component of normal lung growth and in the development of respiratory muscles and neural regulation.[14,15,17-23] Failure of the fetus to generate breathing movements results in lung hypoplasia.

The discovery of fetal breathing brought a new dimension to the events occurring at birth. What had traditionally been called *the initiation of breathing at birth* must now be called *the establishment of continuous breathing at birth*. Breathing begins long before birth. The question now is not what determines the appearance of breathing at birth but what makes it continuous. Or from another perspective, we may ask what makes fetal breathing episodic, present only during low-voltage electrocortical activity. The answers to these questions remain essentially unknown.

THE FETUS

BREATHING PATTERN AT REST

Fetal breathing occurs primarily during periods of low-voltage electrocortical activity, which accounts for 40% of fetal life during the last trimester of gestation in sheep.[2,10,24-26] In the human fetus, this percentage is similar.[17,21,22] During the high-voltage electrocortical activity, there is no established breathing present, but occasional breaths may surface after episodic, generalized, tonic muscular discharges associated with body movements (Fig. 66.1).[2] During low-voltage electrocortical activity, breathing is irregular, the diaphragmatic electromyogram (EMG) being characterized by abrupt onset and ending. Less frequently, there is a progressive increase in envelope amplitude, comparable to the inspiratory slope observed in the anesthetized newborn lamb (Fig. 66.2). A gradual decrease in diaphragmatic EMG at the end of a breath, reflecting postinspiratory activity (as observed in the newborn infant), is rarely seen in the fetus.[2,19,23,27,28] This irregular diaphragmatic activity generates a negative tracheal pressure of about 2 to 5 mm Hg. The corresponding changes in tracheal flow are less than seen postnatally, likely owing to the higher viscosity of lung fluid in the system. The irregular breathing activity observed during this period probably reflects the influence of the reticular formation on breathing so characteristic of REM sleep. The average breath has an inspiratory time of 0.45 seconds, expiratory time of 0.74 seconds, and a total duration of 1.12 seconds.[27,29] The physiologic mechanism responsible for the occurrence of fetal breathing only during low-voltage electrocortical activity is unknown.

FETAL STATE

The occurrence of fetal breathing during low-voltage electrocortical activity has led some investigators to believe that the fetus might be awake during part of this period.[30-32] In fact, using electrophysiologic criteria, it was postulated that during the last part of gestation in sheep, the fetus was awake about 5% of the time.[12,13,32,33]

It was further postulated that a number of chemical and pharmacologic agents could alter fetal breathing by arousing the fetus.[12,32,33] In the late 1970s, our lab became interested in determining whether the fetus was at times awake in utero and whether arousal could be induced by chemical or pharmacologic agents. By implanting a window on the left flank of the ewe we were able to directly observe the fetus in utero (Fig. 66.3).[2,34] The technique proved to be powerful and has generated substantial information. Wakefulness, defined by open eyes and purposeful movement of the head, was never observed in the fetus under resting conditions. Analysis of videotapes, amounting to more than 5000 hours of observation over 8 years, has shown clearly that the fetus alternates between two basic behavioral states, REM (mostly low-voltage electrocorticographic activity [LVECoG]) and quiet (mostly high-voltage electrocorticographic activitym[HVECoG]) sleep.[2,3] Activities such as movement, swallowing, licking, and breathing occur during REM sleep (Fig. 66.4). During quiet sleep, the fetus is still and occasionally shows generalized movements associated with tonic discharges. Generalized tonic discharges and rotation of the body and head were observed during the transition from low- to high-voltage ECoG but were not associated with wakefulness.

Besides the normal irregularity of the respiratory pattern seen in REM sleep, licking and swallowing clearly disturb breathing activity[2,19,28]; breathing becomes slower and irregular, and diaphragmatic activity becomes interspersed with clusters of esophageal electromyographic activity. This digestive tract activity occurs primarily during REM sleep and is translated behaviorally and electrophysiologically as a general increase in EMG activity, blood pressure, and heart rate.

MODULATION OF FETAL BREATHING BY CARBON DIOXIDE, OXYGEN, PULMONARY REFLEXES, AND PHARMACOLOGIC AGENTS

Initially, fetal breathing was thought by some investigators to depend on behavioral influences because it was observed only during REM sleep and seemed somewhat refractory to chemical stimuli.[35] Subsequent studies, however, clearly showed that the fetal breathing apparatus is capable of responding well to chemical stimuli and other agents known to modify breathing postnatally. Thus it became clear that the fetus responds to an increase in Pa_{CO_2} with an increase in breathing.[17,18,27,29,33-36] This increase is associated with increases in tracheal pressure, integrated diaphragmatic activity, and frequency (Fig. 66.5). Both inspiratory and expiratory times decrease as would be expected from postnatal studies.[29] The increased breathing activity is prolonged into the transitional HVECoG but does not continue into the established HVECoG.[29] The increased fetal breathing in response to increased Pa_{CO_2} during rebreathing or during direct

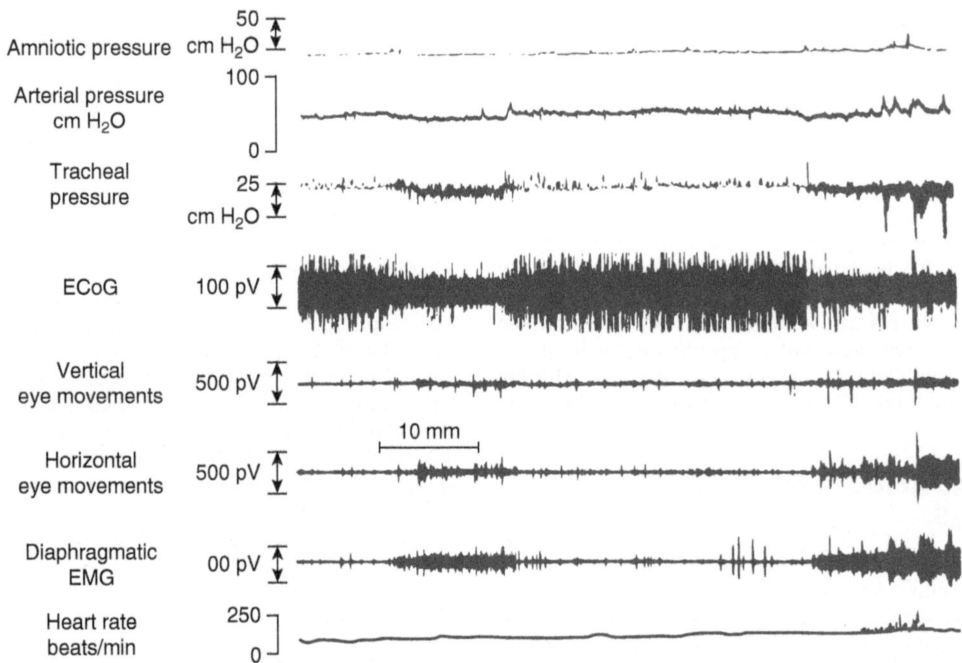

Fig. 66.1 Fetal breathing in a fetal lamb at 134 days' gestation. Note that the deflections in tracheal pressure and diaphragmatic activity occur during periods of rapid eye movement sleep in low-voltage electrocortical activity *(ECoG)* only. In high-voltage electrocortical activity (quiet sleep), breathing is absent. *EMG,* Electromyogram.

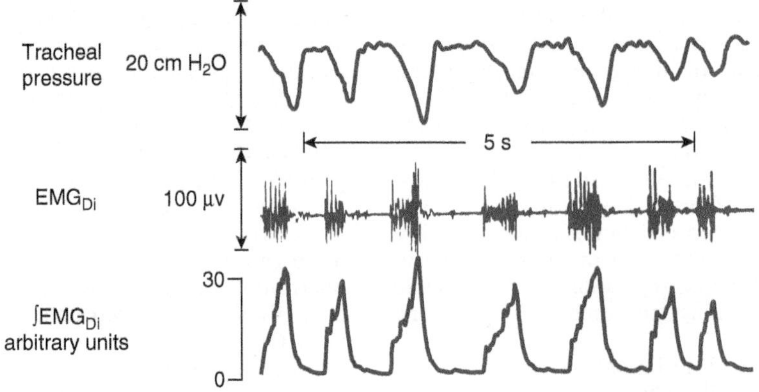

Fig. 66.2 Tracheal pressure and diaphragmatic activity *(EMG_{Di})* in a fetal lamb at 129 days' gestation. Note the abrupt beginning and ending of diaphragmatic activity in some of the breaths and the progressive increase in activity in others. A gradual decrease in diaphragmatic activity, reflecting postinspiratory activity, as seen in the newborn infant, is rarely seen in the fetus. *EMG,* Electromyogram.

administration of carbon dioxide to the fetus via an endotracheal tube[29] was always abolished in established HVECoG. Only when Pa_{CO_2} was unphysiologically high (>100 mm Hg) and pH low (<7.0) could breathing be initiated in HVECoG. At this level of acidosis, low pH could have been the primary stimulus to initiate breathing, as acidosis has been shown to induce continuous breathing.[37] This increased breathing activity was not associated with wakefulness.[29] Conversely, reducing Pa_{CO_2} below the "apneic threshold level" abolishes breathing activity,[38] as has been shown in postnatal life.[39,40–45]

Fetal breathing movements are abolished shortly after induction of hypoxia secondary to administration of low oxygen to the ewe, anemia, reduced uterine blood flow, or umbilical cord occlusion.[17,46] This is associated with a decrease in body movements.[18,47] Hypoxia does not alter amplitude or cycle time, indicating that the depression results from a reduction in the behavioral state.[48] This respiratory inhibition results mainly from direct effects of low O_2 tensions on the fetal brain through the activation of adenosine A_{2A} receptors.[49–51] Koos et al. have found that neuronal lesions of the diencephalon that included the posteromedial group of thalamic nucli abolished the depressant effects of hypoxia.[52] More recently, the same group of authors observed that neurons within, proximate, or connected to the thalamic parafascicular nuclei were crucially involved in the hypoxic arrest of fetal breathing.[53]

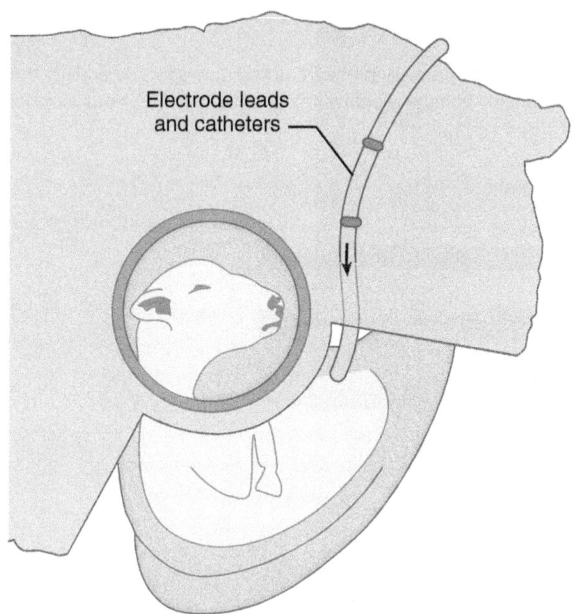

Fig. 66.3 View of the head of the fetus as it appears after surgery is completed. Note that the bundle with catheters and electrical leads crosses the abdominal and uterine walls at some distance from the window.

Conversely, an increase in arterial PO_2 to levels above 200 mm Hg through the administration of 100% oxygen via an endotracheal tube induced continuous fetal breathing in some experiments in sheep.[54]

Of the pulmonary reflexes, the inflation reflex of Hering-Breuer is present in fetal life. Lung distension with saline infusion produced decreased frequency of breathing.[14,15] However, fetoplacental gas exchange and the incidence of fetal breathing and sleep states were not affected by bilateral vagotomy during fetal life.[23,30] Although bilateral vagotomy did not prevent the establishment of continuous breathing at birth, vagal innervation was necessary to establish adequate alveolar ventilation in newborn lambs.[55]

A comprehensive review of the effects of various neurochemicals agents on fetal breathing has been published.[56] In general, fetal breathing is inhibited by the gamma-aminobutyric acid (GABA) agonist muscimol,[57] pentobarbitone,[58] and diazepam[59] acting at the $GABA_A$ receptor complex.[60] Other endogenous inhibitors include adenosine, PGE_2 (see later), and endorphins, which may be present at high levels in the fetal circulation. Agents that stimulate fetal breathing movements include prostaglandin inhibitors (such as indomethacin or meclofenamate), morphine, caffeine, pilocarpine, and 5-HTP. Fetal breathing is inhibited by maternal hypoglycemia, alcohol consumption, and intra-amniotic infection, whereas it is stimulated after maternal meals and hyperglycemia.

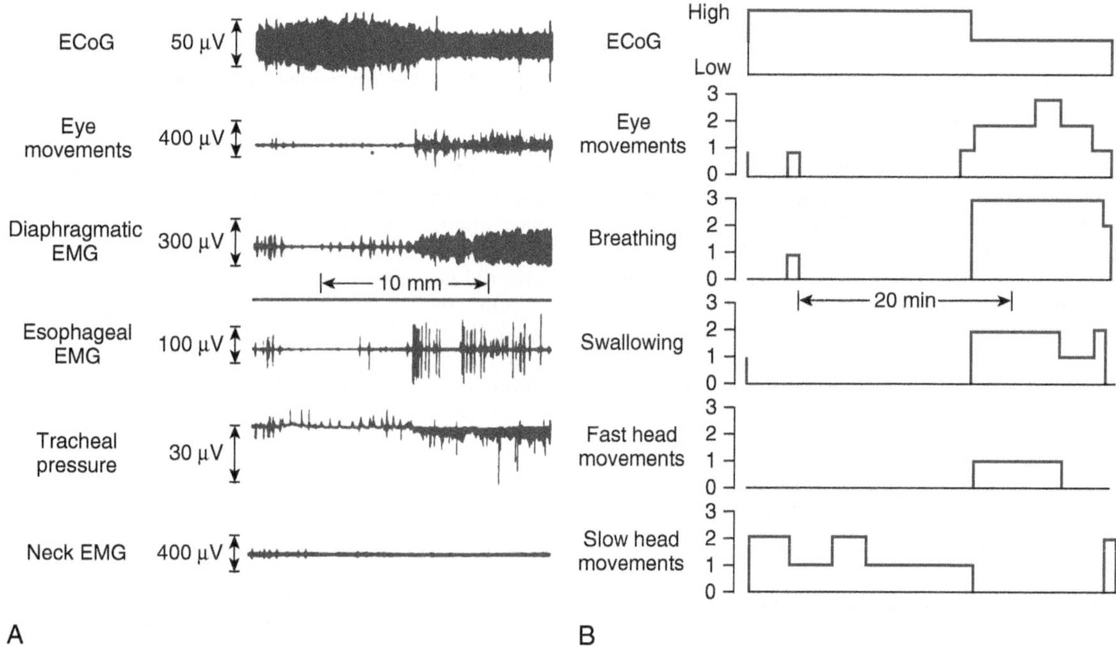

Fig. 66.4 A comparative representation of observations made (A) on a polygraph and (B) through a double-wall Plexiglas window. Fetal breathing, eye movements, and swallowing are predominantly present in low-voltage electrocortical activity *(ECoG)* (*0* = absent; *1* = low activity; *2* = medium; *3* = high). *EMG,* Electromyogram.

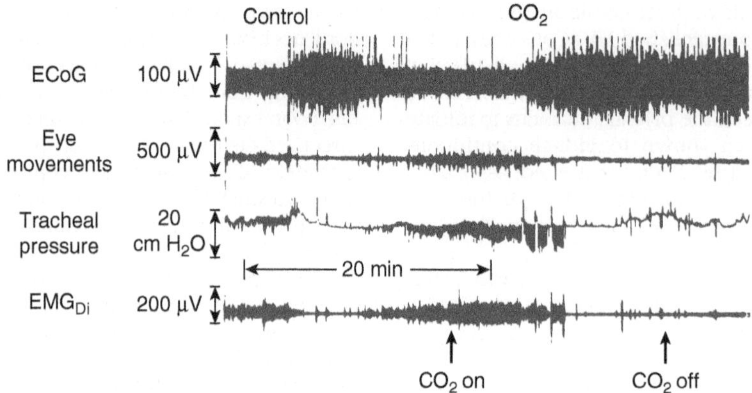

Fig. 66.5 Fetal breathing during control and during CO_2 rebreathing. Note the increase in tracheal pressure and diaphragmatic activity during CO_2 rebreathing. Fetal breathing was prolonged into the transitional low-voltage to high-voltage electrocortical activity *(ECoG)* but stopped in established high-voltage ECoG. *EMG,* Electromyogram.

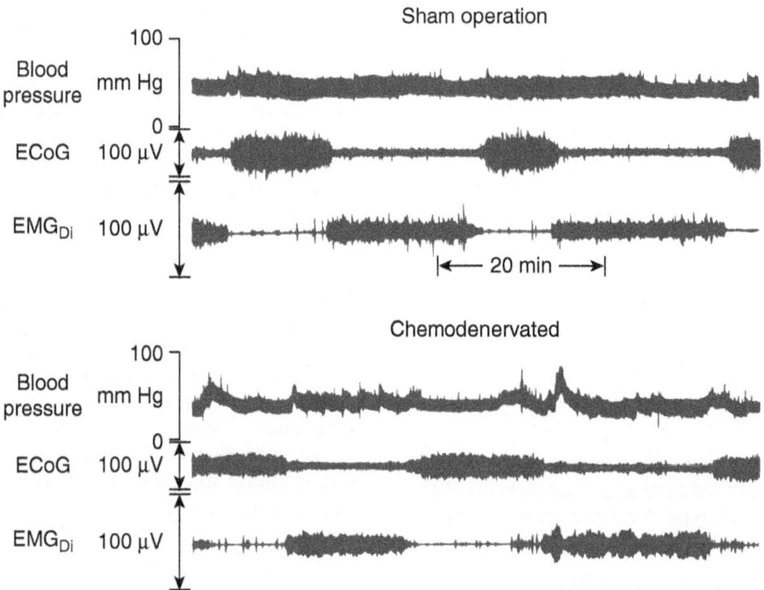

Fig. 66.6 Breathing activity in a sham-operated (132 days' gestation) and in a chemodenervated fetal sheep (130 days' gestation). Note that breathing activity remains intact in the chemodenervated fetus. Blood gases were comparable in the two fetuses. *ECoG,* Electrocortical activity; *EMG,* electromyogram.

There is much evidence suggesting that the actions of carbon dioxide and those of the pharmacologic agents are central. The effect of hypoxia is poorly understood, but it also seems to act centrally. The peripheral chemoreceptors were originally thought to be inactive in utero; however, the idea that they are completely silent was probably derived from incorrect experimental evidence.[61] Blanco and co-workers have clearly documented the activity of the peripheral chemoreceptors in the fetal lamb, showing that they are reset at the time of delivery.[62] Johnston and associates have found that the response to hypoxia in the fetal lamb with a pontine lesion is mediated through peripheral chemoreceptors.[63] Resection of the carotid bodies does not alter fetal breathing or fetal state substantially and apparently does not alter the establishment of breathing at birth.[64,65] The exact relevance of peripheral chemoreceptors to intrauterine breathing remains undetermined.

ESTABLISHMENT OF CONTINUOUS BREATHING AT BIRTH

The traditional view about the onset of continuous breathing at birth is that labor and delivery produce transient fetal asphyxia that stimulates the peripheral chemoreceptors to induce the first extrauterine breath. Breathing is then maintained through the input of other stimuli such as cold, touch, and other sensory stimuli.[10,66-69] This overall view was generated through experiments done many years ago in the acute exteriorized fetal preparation at a time when the general consensus was that the fetus did not breathe in utero.

More recent observations have made this general view open to question. First, denervation of the carotid and aortic chemoreceptors does not alter fetal breathing or the initiation of continuous breathing at birth (Figs. 66.6 and 66.7).[64,65] Second, continuous breathing can be initiated in utero, with manifestations of arousal, by raising arterial PO_2 with an administration of 100% oxygen to the fetus through an endotracheal tube (Fig. 66.8).[54] Continuous breathing does not occur if the arterial PO_2 does not rise. In fetuses in which Pao_2 does not rise, however, continuous breathing subsequently initiates on cord occlusion.[54] This continuous breathing in response to high arterial PO_2 or cord occlusion is independent of an increase in arterial Pco_2 because it remains when Pco_2 is kept constant by ventilating the fetus with high-frequency oscillation. These observations during the administration of 100% oxygen and cord occlusion suggest that the fetus can resemble a newborn in utero. Breathing can occur in the fetus in the absence of transient hypoxemia to stimulate the peripheral chemoreceptors and without any of the sensory stimuli, such as cold, once thought to be important for the establishment of continuous breathing at birth.

Thus the physiologic mechanism responsible for the inhibition of fetal breathing and the establishment of continuous breathing at birth remain unknown. It has been debated whether the key factors in inducing these changes are intrinsic to the fetal brain or are in the placenta. Because placental separation at birth is associated with the onset of continuous breathing, we together with others have hypothesized that the placenta is the main player responsible for the inhibition of fetal breathing.[70-74] This line of thinking is based on the assumption that the release of factors by the placenta into the fetal circulation prevents fetal breathing from being continuous, with inhibition during high-voltage ECoG, and present only during periods of reticular activation as it occurs during low-voltage ECoG.[75] In the absence of these factors from the placenta at birth, after cord clamping, the state-related inhibition observed during high-voltage ECoG is insufficient to disrupt continuous breathing. Teleologically, it is interesting that nature may have delegated to the placenta the important role of providing the fetus with gas exchange and nutrients, and it is conceivable that it may also have endowed the placenta with some form of chemoreceptor activity regulating fetal breathing and behavior by the secretion of chemical substances into the fetal circulation.

More direct evidence for a placental role has been present since Dawes and Harned and Ferreiro showed that only after clamping the umbilical cord does the newborn lamb start breathing and behaving like a neonate.[67,69] Subsequently, Adamson et al. induced breathing in the fetus with umbilical cord occlusion and supply of O_2 via an endotracheal catheter.[72] Upon release of the cord, breathing ceased immediately, before any change in blood gases or pH, suggesting that factors from the placenta might be involved. In our laboratory, we were able to induce continuous breathing and wakefulness in fetal sheep by occluding the umbilical cord, as long as we provided a gas exchange area for the fetus via an endotracheal tube.[71,76-78] These experiments suggest the origin is in the placenta of compounds that inhibit fetal breathing and fetal activity.

In trying to prove the hypothesis that factors released by the placenta were responsible for the inhibition of fetal breathing, we injected the fetal sheep with a placental extract (juice of cotyledons acutely dissected, sliced, and immersed in Krebs solution) after continuous breathing was induced by cord occlusion.[71] In all experiments, the placental extract decreased or abolished breathing. The infusion of the placental extract into the fetal circulation also inhibited spontaneous fetal breathing present during low-voltage electrocortical activity without inducing significant changes in blood gas tensions, pH, heart rate, and blood pressure.[79] This effect appeared specific to the placenta because the breathing response was absent with extracts from other tissues. We have then demonstrated that these factors in the placental extract are likely prostaglandins because treatment of the extract with indomethacin/aminosalicylic acid (ASA), which significantly reduced the concentration of prostaglandins, eliminated the activity of the extract (Fig. 66.9).[80]

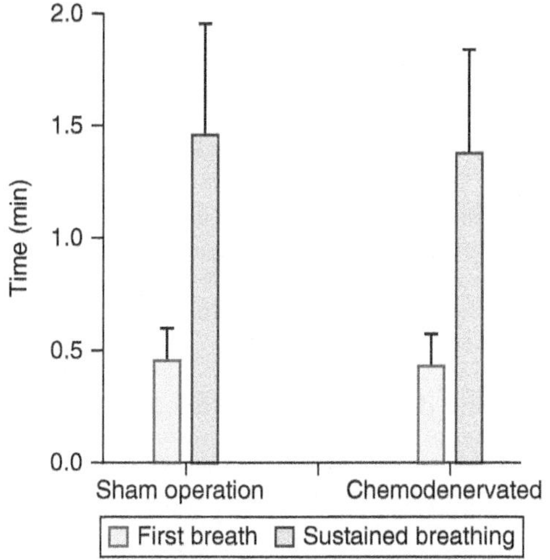

Fig. 66.7 Delay in minutes from the opening of the window to the appearance of the first breath and to sustained breathing. There were no significant differences between the two groups.

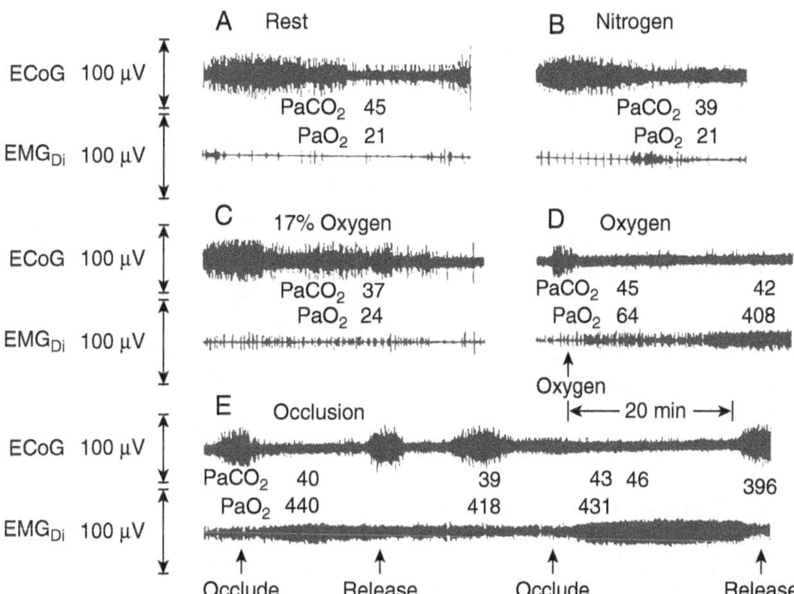

Fig. 66.8 Representative tracing showing the effect of various concentrations of O_2 on fetal breathing and electrocortical activity. (A) Control cycle showing little breathing in fetuses in early labor at 143 days of gestation. (B) Lung distension (mean airway pressure 30 cm H_2O) and inspired N_2 does not affect baseline tracing. (C) 17% O_2 also does not alter breathing. (D) 100% O_2 induces continuous breathing. (E) Occlusion on two occasions induces more forceful breathing than that observed with O_2 alone. Note that continuous breathing was elicited despite preventing the rise of Pa_{CO_2} by ventilating the fetus with high-frequency ventilation (15 Hz, stroke = 7 cm H_2O). *ECoG,* Electrocortical activity; *EMG,* electromyogram.

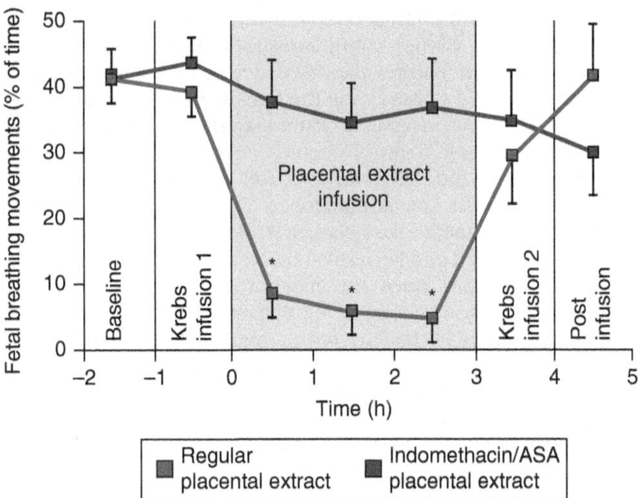

Fig. 66.9 Illustration of the effect of eliminating the prostaglandins from the placental extract on fetal breathing. Please note that fetal breathing remains essentially unchanged with the infusion of a regular placental extract (not treated with indomethacin/ASA), whereas it decreased significantly with the infusion of an indomethacin/ASA treated extract.

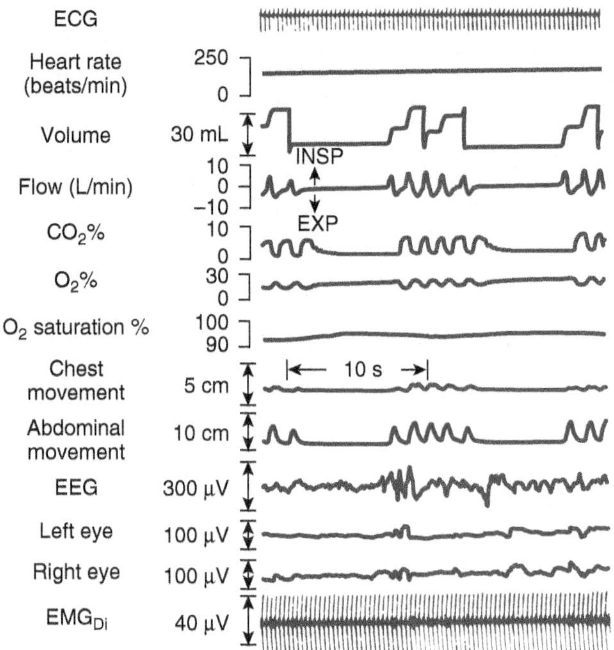

Fig. 66.10 Periodic breathing during quiet sleep in an 8-day-old preterm infant born at 32 weeks. Note the regular periodicity of breathing, with both apneic and breathing intervals keeping a constant length. Note also the classic tracé alternans pattern on the electroencephalogram *(EEG)*. *EMG,* Electromyogram.

Indirect evidence that placental prostaglandins, especially PGE_2, are the mediators responsible for the inhibition of breathing in fetal life has been demonstrated by Kitterman et al.[81] and Wallen et al.[82] who have shown that infusion of PGE_2 into the circulation of the fetal sheep induced a prompt and complete cessation of breathing movements. In addition, the incidence of fetal breathing movements was inversely correlated with both the PGE_2 dose and the mean PGE_2 concentration. Conversely, intravenous infusion of prostaglandin synthetase inhibitors, such as indomethacin or meclofenamate, induce continuous breathing for many hours in the fetus.[81-84] Thus the rate of placental prostaglandin production plays a significant role in setting the level of fetal breathing activity by producing a sleep-related inhibition in the fetal brainstem.

It is unlikely, however, that prostaglandins are involved in the inhibition of fetal breathing observed during hypoxia, because this inhibition persists after the administration of prostaglandin inhibitors. As mentioned earlier, several studies have shown that adenosine is the likely mediator of the respiratory depression observed during hypoxia because intravascular administration of adenosine inhibits fetal breathing and eye movements and the infusion of adenosine receptor antagonists blunts this inhibition.[85,86] Also, brain disruptions that eliminate hypoxic inhibition of breathing also abolish the depressant effects of adenosine.[87]

THE NEONATE

BREATHING PATTERN AT REST

It has been well described that the first postnatal breath tends to be the deepest and the slowest of the early pattern of breathing primarily due to a short deep inspiration followed by a prolonged expiratory time that helps to overcome the forces produced by the liquid-filled lungs and airways.[88] These initial breaths are actively exhaled by the high negative transpulmonary pressures. These expiratory breaths are also associated with interruptions in the expiratory flow (braking of the expiration) that help maintaining functional residual capacity (FRC). There are two mechanisms for stopping or slowing expiratory flow. The first one is the diaphragmatic postinspiratory activity that slows the rate of lung deflation by counteracting its passive recoil. The second one is the closure or narrowing of the pharyngeal/laryngeal region, as indicated by the radiographic studies of Bosma et al.[89] TePas et al. have recently found that this expiratory braking is achieved most commonly by crying.[90]

After these initial postnatal breaths, the neonate, and particularly the premature infant, breathes irregularly. There is great breath-to-breath variability, and there are long stretches of periodic breathing in which breathing and apnea alternate.[9,91-95] The resting breathing pattern of the neonate is not sleep-state dependent, although sleep greatly modulates it.[3,96] Sleep has traditionally been divided into quiet, REM, transitional, and indeterminate states. Twenty-nine percent of sleep time in neonates is spent in quiet sleep, 33% in REM, 7% in transitional sleep, and 31% in indeterminate sleep. The proportion of quiet sleep increases with age, while the amount of REM decreases with age. The proportion of wakefulness decreases with decreasing gestational age, and in very immature infants, it becomes difficult to define wakefulness or arousal.[97-99] We have shown that periodic breathing, a common breathing pattern in premature infants in which they alternate between breathing intervals and apneas lasting 5 to 10 seconds, occurs in the three states, wakefulness, REM, and quiet, but its prevalence is increased in REM sleep.[3] It is frequently stated in textbooks that in quiet sleep, in analogy with criteria used for adult subjects, breathing is regular. Prechtl and we, however, have clearly shown that periodic breathing is common in quiet sleep.[9,100,101] The difference is that periodic breathing in quiet sleep is regular—that is, the breathing and apneic intervals are of similar duration—and very irregular in REM sleep. The most well-defined periodic breathing observable in small babies is in quiet sleep during tracé alternant (Fig. 66.10). Therefore there are two major differences between neonates and adults regarding the staging of the sleep state. One difference relates to the patterns of breathing observed in quiet and REM sleep states, and the other relates to the presence of the tracé alternant electroencephalogram (EEG) during quiet sleep in the neonate. As this pattern subsides after 44 weeks'

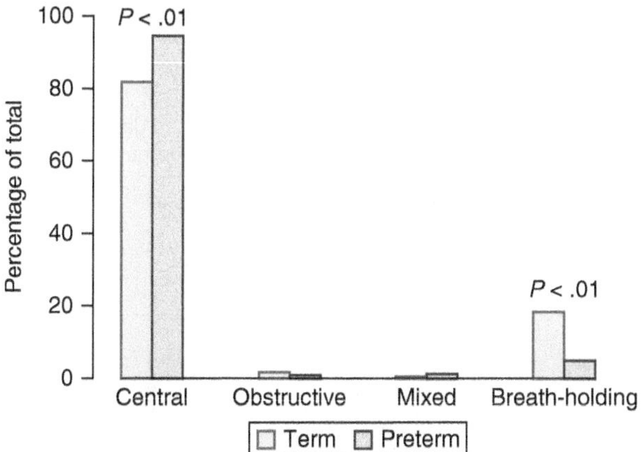

Fig. 66.11 Frequency distribution of the various types of apneas in healthy preterm and term infants. Central apneas are predominant. The frequency of breath-holding apneas is greater in term than in preterm infants. Obstructive and mixed types of apneas are rare.

postconceptional age, it is not used in adults to characterize quiet sleep. Finally, the overall minute ventilation is increased in REM sleep as compared with quiet sleep, and this is due to a primary increase in respiratory frequency with little change in tidal volume.[3,6,9]

PERIODIC BREATHING AND APNEA

Periodic breathing, defined as pauses in respiratory movements that last for up to 20 seconds alternating with breathing, is common in preterm infants. When the respiratory pause is longer than 20 seconds, it is called *apnea*.[102] Although the duration used to distinguish periodic breathing and apnea is arbitrary, it has proved useful and has been widely adopted. Periodic breathing is not as harmful as apnea since the respiratory pause is short and the decrease in heart rate is minor. In contrast, apnea is a more serious condition, the respiratory pause being longer and frequently associated with decreases in heart rate below 80 beats/min.[91,102] In very small preterm infants, significant bradycardia can occur with very short apneic pauses. In this instance, therefore, the length of the respiratory pause is not a very useful indicator of the severity of the disruption in breathing. For this reason, many centers, including ours, have decided to rely on heart rate and oxygen desaturation as the primary indicators of severity.

Apneic episodes in the neonate are classified according to the absence or presence of breathing efforts during the period of no airflow.[103] Central apneas are those with no flow and no observable breathing efforts. Obstructive apneas are those with no flow despite breathing efforts. Mixed apneas begin as central and end as obstructive apnea. Breath-holding apneas are those in which flow stops at mid-expiration, and the remaining expiration occurs just before breathing starts again. A new method of classifying apneas based on a magnified cardiac-induced pulse observed on the respiratory flow tracing has been described by us. This method can detect the presence and timing of airway obstructions with great precision. Using this method, it is obvious that some apneas, previously classified as central because of the absence of respiratory efforts, are indeed obstructive.[104]

In preterm infants with underlying disease followed longitudinally over a period of 3 months, central apneas predominate and purely obstructive apneas are rare (Fig. 66.11).[103] Obstructive apneas are more commonly noted as part of a mixed apneic event. In preterm infants recovering from respiratory support, with some degree of residual lung disease (bronchopulmonary dysplasia), the prevalence of obstructive apneas appears to be increased, comprising up to 48% of the apneas in some studies. There is no clear explanation for the obstruction, but it seems to be at the level of the larynx.[105] Our initial observations suggest that borderline hypoxemia of these infants may be a predisposing factor. One report has described obstruction in 80% of the pauses in preterm infants with periodic breathing.[106]

Periodic breathing and apnea are clearly a consequence of a disturbance of the respiratory control system, but the precise mechanisms are unclear. Investigators in this area tend to believe that the negative feedback loop controlling respiration is affected by multiple factors related primarily to anatomic and physiologic immaturity. Oscillation in arterial gas tensions, changes in circulation time, incoordination of the respiratory pump owing to a compliant chest wall, and changes in sleep state may all contribute to this instability of the respiratory control system.[102]

There has been controversy in the literature on whether periodic breathing and apnea are mechanistically different or whether long apneas are just a step further in the basic respiratory disturbance that induces the short apneas of periodic breathing. In a study carried out in our laboratory, we were able to show (1) a prolonged apnea almost never occurred in the absence of preceding short apneas and that (2) the risk of a prolonged apnea occurring increased significantly when the preceding period contained an increased number of apneic episodes, increased duration of the longest apneic interval, or increased duration of the apneic time.[107] More recently, we have shown that the periodic breathing cycles in REM but not in quiet sleep were associated with the progressive decrease in minute ventilation and oxygenation likely related to the mechanical and chemoreceptor limitations known to be present in this sleep state.[108] We believe that periodic breathing, especially during REM sleep, is a marker for apnea since apneas almost never occur abruptly in infants breathing regularly, but only in infants whose respiratory pattern is characterized by significant periodicity.

Compared with infants who breathe continuously, neonates breathing periodically have lower PO_2 values, and their peripheral chemoreceptors are more hyperactive, as reflected by the longer apneic period and more pronounced immediate decrease in ventilation in response to the inhalation of high oxygen mixtures.[91,92,109] Thus the basic reason for background instability appears to be the major contribution of the peripheral chemoreceptor drive to normal breathing at this age. Indeed, the arterial PO_2 tension of these infants sits on the steep portion of the minute ventilation-arterial PO_2 regression curve for human adults. This means that small changes in baseline arterial PO_2 produce large changes in baseline ventilation. Hypoxia may be a contributing factor because inhalation of a low-oxygen mixture easily induces periodic breathing and apnea in these infants.

We found that the average CO_2 apneic threshold in preterm infants is only 1.5 Torr lower than the eupneic P_{CO_2}, whereas in adults it is ~5 Torr lower.[43] The closeness of eupneic and threshold Pa_{CO_2} likely confers a great vulnerability to respiratory stability in these infants. It is not surprising, therefore, that brief startles, movements, or changes in sleep state could allow eupneic P_{CO_2} to dive below the P_{CO_2} apneic threshold, inducing periodic breathing and apnea in these infants (Fig. 66.12). We believe that the key element responsible for this narrow difference is the well-known hypoxemic status of these infants. Xie et al. have recently shown in adults that the time course of the occurrence of apnea after transient hyperpnea was consistent with a peripheral chemoreceptor mechanism. In this study, hypoxia shortened the apnea latency and narrowed the eupneic-apneic Pa_{CO_2} threshold, while hyperoxia delayed the onset of apnea and widened the eupneic-apneic Pa_{CO_2} threshold.[45] The same group had previously shown that the smaller difference between eupneic and apneic Pa_{CO_2} during hypoxia was due to a disproportionate reduction in the eupneic Pa_{CO_2} rather than a higher apneic threshold. The low arterial PO_2

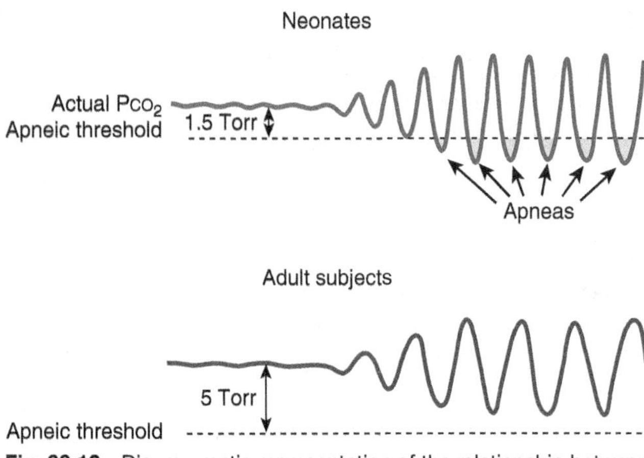

Fig. 66.12 Diagrammatic representation of the relationship between the CO_2 apneic threshold and the baseline or actual P_{CO_2} levels in neonates and adults. Because of the proximity of these two levels in neonates, P_{CO_2} is much more likely to dive below the apneic threshold than in the adult.

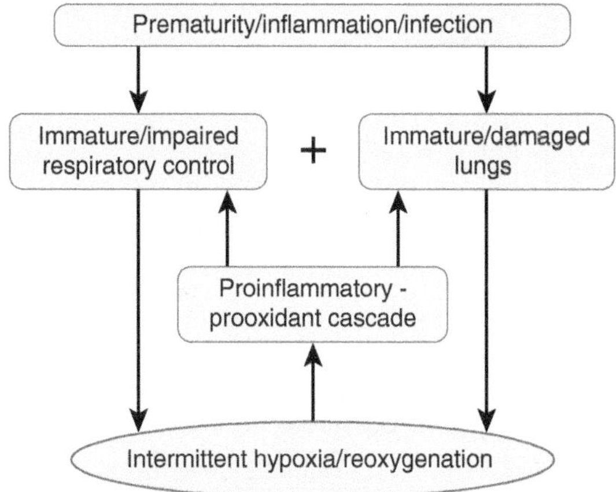

Fig. 66.13 A proposed vicious cycle triggered by prematurity, inflammation, and infection on lung development and respiratory control leading to intermittent hypoxia. (Adapted from Di Fiore J, Martin RJ, Gauda EB. Apnea of prematurity—perfect storm. Figure 2. *Respir Physiol Neurobiol.* 2013;189:213–222.)

in newborn infants may keep the eupneic P_{CO_2} relatively low, not by hyperventilation as in adult subjects but by a decrease in metabolism that parallels the decrease in arterial PO2.

The sleep state appears also to be a contributing factor because periodic breathing and apnea are more frequent in REM sleep than in quiet sleep. The neonate sleeps almost uninterruptedly, continuously alternating between REM sleep and quiet sleep. This pattern increases instability in the respiratory control system. Indeed, minor alterations during sleep, such as a startle or a sigh, produce apnea in these infants.

Although sleep modulates breathing, it does not cause apnea; apnea also occurs during wakefulness. The high prevalence of apnea during REM sleep may be related to muscle activity in this stage. During REM sleep, the tone of the intercostal muscles is abolished in conjunction with a decrease in diaphragmatic activity and in the tone of the adductor muscles of the upper airway—a combination of factors likely to induce chest distortion, impairment of the braking mechanism during expiration, pulmonary collapse, and apnea.[102] When chest distortion occurs, diaphragmatic work increases by about 40%, adding to the mechanical impairment. This observation is compatible with the finding that the application of continuous negative pressure around the chest tends to abolish apnea.[110]

THE EFFECT OF INFECTION AND INFLAMMATION ON THE CONTROL OF BREATHING

It is well known that perinatal infection and inflammation could impair both the pulmonary function and the control of breathing in preterm infants.[111-115] The progressive inflammation observed in the lungs of preterm infants secondary to intrauterine and extrauterine infection and the oxidative stress due to oxygen exposure and mechanical ventilation leads to respiratory morbidity. This negative effect on lung development would contribute to a worsening apnea of prematurity by altering FRC, the pulmonary vascular resistance, and the hypoxic pulmonary vasoconstriction. It is also well known that inflammatory mediators affect both peripheral and central structures that control breathing.[111,116] In preterm infants, environmental stimuli such as intermittent hypoxia and hyperoxia, inflammation, and infection could inhibit central respiratory output and may also adversely affect the structure and function of the carotid chemoreceptors that could contribute to intractable apnea.[112,113,117,118]

Although the mechanisms by which inflammation impairs the respiratory circuit are not fully understood, the release of peripheral proinflammatory cytokines, mainly i interleukin (IL)-1β, IL-6, and tumor necrosis factor, during the acute phase of immune response could affect carotid body function. These cytokines synthesized in the periphery may also alter the structure and function of the central chemoreceptors by crossing the blood-brain barrier, by induction of PGE_2 synthesis, and by afferent neuronal pathways such the vagus and the carotid body.[114,115]

INTERMITTENT CHRONIC HYPOXIC EPISODES

The respiratory pauses observed during periodic breathing and apnea are frequently associated with intermittent hypoxemic episodes, especially in infants with significant lung disease. These hypoxic events are secondary to the loss in lung volume and hypoventilation that occur during the respiratory pauses producing intrapulmonary shunting with a rapid fall in Sp_{O_2}. Di Fiore et al. have shown that in extremely low-birth-weight infants, these episodes progressively increase over the first 4 weeks of postnatal life, with a subsequent plateau followed by a slow decline beginning at 6 to 8 weeks.[119] The low incidence of hypoxemic events in the first 2 weeks of life may be related to the decreased activity of peripheral chemoreceptors, high concentration of fetal hemoglobin, and unharmed lungs. The progressive increase in their incidence at weeks 2 to 6 may be related to the increased periodic breathing and apneas due to the increased peripheral chemoreceptor activity, switch to adult hemoglobin, and development of lung injury. The slow decrease observed after week 6 may presumably be related to improvement in lung function and decrease apnea frequency.

There is mounting evidence mainly from animal studies and adults with sleep apnea syndrome that these intermittent episodes of hypoxemia and reoxygenation may also predispose to a selective activation of proinflammatory pathways. The reactive oxygen species generated during reoxygenation superimposed to the release of proinflammatory cytokines could further impair the respiratory control and lung development creating a vicious cycle (Fig. 66.13).[120-122]

Although still controversial, there is increasing evidence that these episodes of intermittent hypoxemia may have short- and long-term negative effects in preterm infants. Several studies have shown a strong association between hypoxemia episodes and neurodevelopmental impairment at 18 months of age,[123] the development of retinopathy of prematurity,[124] lung development and function with increased airway and vasculature reactivity,[125-127] growth, and cardiovascular control.[128-130]

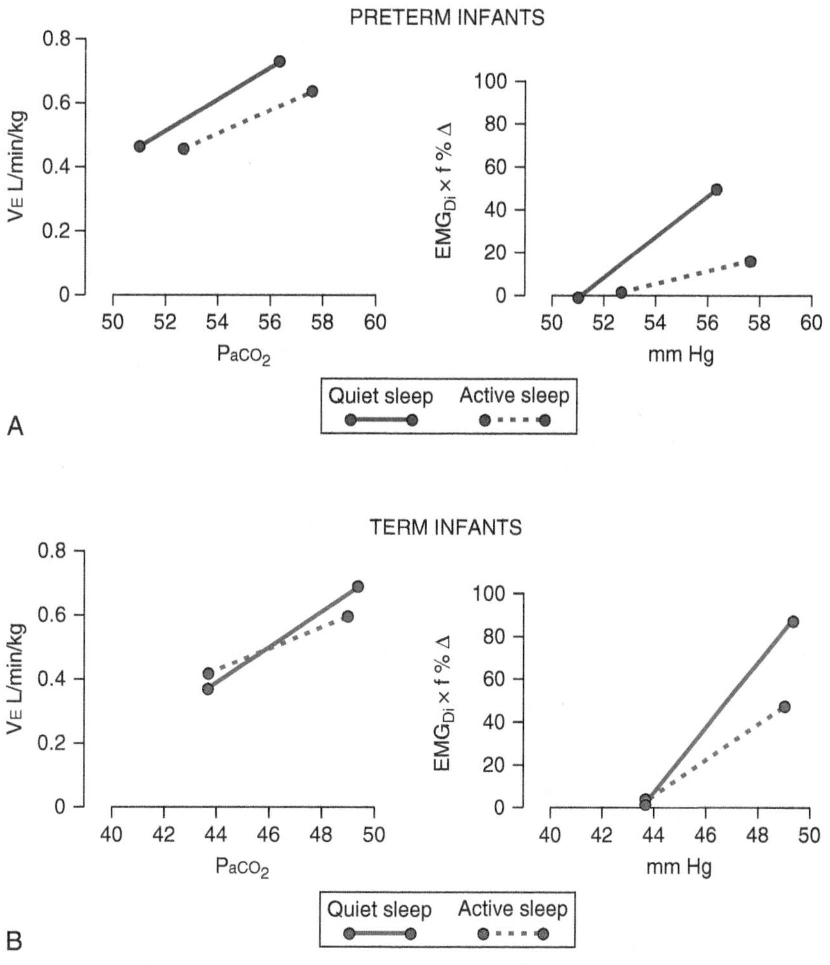

Fig. 66.14 The ventilatory response to CO_2 rebreathing in neonates. Note that (A) preterm and (B) term infants showed a decreased response to CO_2 in phasic rapid eye movement sleep, as compared with quiet sleep. *EMG,* Electromyogram.

CHEMICAL REGULATION

Inhalation of carbon dioxide increases ventilation during REM and quiet sleep in newborn infants. The response to steady-state inhalation of carbon dioxide is the same in these two sleep states, but the response during the rebreathing of carbon dioxide is less in REM than in quiet sleep (Fig. 66.14).[3,6,8,100] We postulated that the differences in response with these two techniques relate to the fact that when using rebreathing, it is possible to measure the response in phasic REM only, whereas when using the steady-state technique, the response always covers both phasic and tonic REM sleep.[100] As the carbon dioxide response in tonic REM is the same as that during quiet sleep, the results using the steady-state method tend to resemble those in quiet sleep.[7,131]

The pattern of breathing observed with inhalation of carbon dioxide varies with the percentage of carbon dioxide inhaled. If the percentage of inhaled carbon dioxide is low (<2%) during steady-state inhalation, the response consists primarily of an increase in tidal volume.[9] If the percentage of inhaled carbon dioxide is high (>2%), the response in both sleep states consists of an increase in respiratory frequency and in tidal volume.[92,100] Periodic breathing is abolished with a small increase in inhaled carbon dioxide of about 1% to 2%.[9,93] This response has been attributed to the increased central drive and increased stores of carbon dioxide, with better buffering capacity for the oscillations in $Paco_2$.

Inhalation of low oxygen produces an immediate increase in ventilation (1 minute) followed by a later decrease (5 minutes).[91,94,132,133] The response is similar in wakefulness, REM, and quiet sleep, although hyperventilation seems slightly more sustained during late hypoxia in quiet sleep.[3] The more sustained hyperventilation in these infants during quiet sleep reflects more autonomic control during this sleep state, the system being more responsive to chemical stimuli.[7,131] The immediate increase in ventilation reflects peripheral chemoreceptor stimulation and is associated with an increase in frequency and in tidal volume. The late response is primarily manifested by a decrease in frequency.[92,94] The mechanism responsible for this response is still unclear and may vary according to species. In humans, it is likely related to the central release of inhibitory neuromodulators.[134] However, experiments in kittens and in newborn monkeys suggest that the late decrease in ventilation may be a mechanical effect rather than a depression of the central respiratory neurons.[135,136] In these experiments, diaphragmatic activity and frequency remained elevated during hypoxia, but tidal volume decreased below control values during late hypoxia. These experiments were carried out during quiet sleep. The peculiar response of the neonate to low inhaled oxygen is of great clinical significance. Infants who are borderline hypoxic tend to breathe periodically or develop apneic spells. Hypoxia can induce periodic breathing in these infants, as shown previously.[69] The relief of these apneic spells, which are frequently associated with bradycardias, can be obtained by increasing the inspired oxygen concentration.[92,93]

Administration of high concentrations of oxygen, on the other hand, produces an immediate decrease in ventilation followed by hyperventilation, a response that is similar during wakefulness, REM, and quiet sleep. These findings suggest a lack of major differences in the activity of the peripheral chemoreceptors during these sleep states.[102,137] The immediate decrease in ventilation following the administration of 100% oxygen is related to a decrease in frequency (apnea being common in preterm infants) and a decrease in tidal volume. The late increase in ventilation with oxygen is likely related to cerebral vasoconstriction with increase H^+ concentration at the chemoreceptor site.[138]

PULMONARY REFLEXES

The inflation reflex of Hering-Breuer is much more active in the newborn period than in adult life.[139,140] Small increases in lung volume cause apnea. This response is so powerful in the newborn that many have used this inflation to produce apnea and then study the mechanical properties of the respiratory system during the passive expiratory phase following apnea. The action of the stretch receptors is much influenced by sleep, being abolished during REM sleep. The irritant receptors are also poorly developed in preterm infants, and the mediated reflexes are also abolished during REM sleep.[141] Therefore airway mechanisms responsible for clearing, such as cough, are impaired during REM sleep. The paradoxical reflex of the head is commonly observed in the neonate in the form of a sigh.[142] Many attribute the high prevalence of sighs to the greater need for lung recruitment at this age.[143] Sighs are more frequent in REM than in quiet sleep and are also more frequent during periodic than regular breathing. During periodic breathing, a sigh usually appears during the first or second breath after apnea. When it occurs during regular breathing, it tends to be followed by short apneas.[144] Efforts to discover the mechanisms triggering sighs have been fruitless. Thach and Tauesch showed that asphyxia does not seem to be a stimulus.[143] Alvarez and colleagues, however, have observed that airway occlusion in the presence of hypoxia predisposes to sighs.[145]

Studying the morphology of sighs in infants and adult subjects, we have found that the sighs in infants are relatively larger than those in adults and that while post-sigh ventilation is usually increased in adults, it is decreased in infants.[146] Because the drive to breathe early in life is dependent on increased peripheral chemoreceptor activity, it is conceivable that the sudden increase in arterial PO_2 with sighs could produce a rapid decline in the carotid body afferent discharge, leading to hypoventilation and apnea. The other almost instantaneous change that occurs with a sigh includes a decrease in Pco_2. Because the CO_2 apneic threshold is much closer to the baseline CO_2 in neonates compared with adults, the decline in CO_2 below the threshold during a sigh could trigger an apnea or initiate an epoch of periodic breathing in infants with an immature respiratory feedback loop.[43,147] These findings suggest that although the ability to sigh may be an important mechanism to restore lung volume, sighs have the potential to destabilize breathing and cause hypoventilation and apnea in infants at risk for inadequate control of breathing.[146]

RESPIRATORY MUSCLES

The activity of the respiratory muscles is much altered by sleep state. Tonic activity of most respiratory muscles is abolished during REM sleep.[19,27,148,149] The disappearance of tone in the intercostal muscles has been suggested as a major factor responsible for the increased chest distortion seen during REM sleep in infants with this condition. Lack of tone leads to chest wall collapse during inspiration, and caudal displacement of the diaphragm has to be twice as long to produce the same lung volume displacement.[148,149] Because of chest wall collapse, functional residual capacity is decreased in these infants during REM sleep.[148]

Postinspiratory activity of the diaphragm is also affected by sleep. This activity controls, in part, the duration of expiratory time.[150,151] In neonates, this activity is more pronounced in the lateral than in the crural part of the diaphragm, longer in quiet than in REM sleep, and more prolonged in preterm than in term infants.[152] The length and variability of this activity in preterm infants suggest that because of their highly compliant chest wall, these infants use the postinspiratory diaphragmatic activity as a braking mechanism whose role in maintaining lung volume and controlling expiratory time is much more important than in older children and adult subjects. Similarly, the sleep state profoundly affects the muscular control of upper airway resistance. Studies in fetal and neonatal lambs suggest that the abductor muscles of the larynx—the posterior cricoarytenoid and cricothyroid—have inspiratory activities in parallel with that of the diaphragm during both quiet and REM sleep. In contrast, the adductor muscles of the larynx—the thyroarytenoid, lateral cricoarytenoid, and intra-arytenoid—have a phasic expiratory activity during quiet sleep. This activity is lost during REM sleep in the fetus and in the newborn lamb.[19,27] A reduction in adductor activity of the larynx, in conjunction with decreased intercostal and decreased postinspiratory diaphragmatic activity during REM sleep, may cause the decrease in lung volume observed during this sleep state.

CONCLUSIONS

In summary, although the basic mechanisms involved in the control of breathing during fetal and neonatal life are similar to those investigated more extensively in adult subjects, some aspects make this control unique at this age. First, sleep seems to have a very profound effect during this period of life, particularly in the fetus, in which breathing is allowed to surface only during REM sleep. Second, breathing activity is present in utero since early gestation and without apparent reason because it is not responsible for gas exchange. The placenta is responsible for gas exchange, being the lung of the fetus. We must therefore discover the purpose of fetal breathing. Third, the discovery of fetal breathing is probably the most exciting contribution made in this area during the past 60 years. To explain why this episodic breathing in utero becomes continuous after birth is the major challenge of the moment. Trying to understand this change at birth may result in the discovery of key mediators that are at the heart of the mechanism controlling breathing in general.

ACKNOWLEDGMENT

The late Dr. Henrique Rigatto was the original author of this chapter, which still contains parts of those original contributions.

A complete reference list is available at www.ExpertConsult.com. 

SELECT REFERENCES

1. Parmelee AH, Wenner WH, Akiyama Y, Schultz M, Stern E. Sleep states in premature infants. *Dev Med Child Neurol*. 1967;9:70.
2. Rigatto H, Moore M, Cates D. Fetal breathing and behavior measured through a double-wall Plexiglas window in sheep. *J Appl Physiol*. 1986;61:160.
3. Rigatto H, Kalapesi, Leahy FN, Durand M, MacCallum M, Cates D. Ventilatory response to 100% and 15% O_2 during wakefulness and sleep in preterm infants. *Early Hum Dev*. 1982;7:1.
4. Stern E, Parmelee AH, Akiyama Y, Schultz MA, Wenner WH. Sleep cycle characteristics in infants. *Pediatrics*. 1969;43:65.
5. Bülow K. Respiration and wakefulness in man. *Acta Physiol Scand*. 1963;59(suppl 209):1.
6. Davi M, Sankaran K, Maccallum M, Cates D, Rigatto H. Effect of sleep state on chest distortion and on the ventilatory response to CO_2 in neonates. *Pediatr Res*. 1979;13:982.
7. Phillipson EA. Control of breathing during sleep. *Am Rev Respir Dis*. 1978;118:909.
8. Reed DJ, Kellogg RH. Changes in respiratory response to CO_2 during natural sleep at sea level and at altitude. *J Appl Physiol*. 1958;13:325.
9. Kalapesi Z, Durand M, Leahy FN, Cates DB, MacCallum M, Rigatto H. Effect of periodic or regular respiratory pattern on the ventilatory response to low inhaled CO_2 in preterm infants during sleep. *Am Rev Respir Dis*. 1981;123:8.

10. Dawes GS, Fox HE, Leduc BM, Liggins GC, Richards RT. Respiratory movements and paradoxical sleep in the fetal lamb. *J Physiol (Lond)*. 1970;210:47P.
11. Merlet C, Hoerter J, Devilleneuve C, Tchobroutsky C. Mise en evidence de mouvements respiratoires chez le foetus d'agneau. *CR Acad Sci Ser D*. 1970;270:2462.
12. Ioffe S, Jansen AH, Russell BJ, Chernick V. Respiratory response to somatic stimulation in fetal lambs during sleep and wakefulness. *Pfluegers Arch*. 1980;388:143.
13. Ioffe S, Jansen AH, Russell BJ, Chernick V. Sleep, wakefulness and the monosynaptic reflex in fetal and newborn lambs. *Pfluegers Arch*. 1980;388:149.
14. Maloney JE, Adamson TM, Brodecky V, Dowling MH, Ritchie BC. Modification of respiratory center output in the unanesthetized fetal sheep *in utero*. *J Appl Physiol*. 1975;39:552.
15. Maloney JE, Bowes G, Wilkinson M. Fetal breathing" and the development of patterns of respiration before birth. *Sleep*. 1980;3:299.
16. Rigatto H, Blanco CE, Walker DW. The response to stimulation of hindlimb nerves in fetal sheep, *in utero*, during the different phases of electrocortical activity. *J Dev Physiol (Lond)*. 1982;4:175.
17. Boddy K, Dawes GS, Fisher R, Pinter S, Robinson JS. Foetal respiratory movements, electrocortical and cardiovascular responses to hypoxaemia and hypercapnia in sheep. *J Physiol*. 1974;243:599–618.
18. Boddy K, Dawes GS, Fisher R, Pinter S, Robinson JS. Foetal respiratory movements, electrocortical and cardiovascular responses to hypoxaemia and hypercapnia in sheep. *J Physiol (Lond)*. 1974;243:599.
19. Harding R, Johnson P, McClelland ME, McLeod CN, Whyte PL. Laryngeal function during breathing and swallowing in foetal and newborn lambs. *J Physiol (Lond)*. 1977;272:14P.
20. Maloney JE, Adamson TM, Brodecky AV, et al. Diaphragmatic activity and lung liquid flow in the unanesthetized fetal sheep. *J Appl Physiol*. 1975;39:423.
21. Patrick J, Campbell K, Carmichael L, Natale R, Richardson B. A definition of human fetal apnea and the distribution of apneic intervals during the last ten weeks of pregnancy. *Am J Obstet Gynecol*. 1980;136:471.
22. Patrick J, Campbell K, Carmichael L, Natale R, Richardson B. Patterns of human fetal breathing during the last 10 weeks of pregnancy. *Obstet Gynecol*. 1980;56:24.
23. Hagan RAC, Bryan CA, Bryan MH, et al. The effect of sleep state on intercostal muscle activity and rib cage motion. *Physiologist*. 1976;19:214.
24. Dawes GS. Breathing before birth in animals and man. An Essay in Developmental Medicine. *N Engl J Med*. 1974;290:557.
25. Dawes GS, Fox HE, Leduc BM, Liggins GC, Richards RT. Respiratory movements and rapid eye movement sleep in the fetal lamb. *J Physiol (Lond)*. 1972;220:119.
26. Kitterman JA, Liggins GC, Clements JA, Tooley WH. Stimulation of breathing movements in fetal sheep by inhibitors of prostaglandin synthesis. *J Dev Physiol*. 1979;1:453.
27. Dawes GS, Gardner WN, Johnston BM, Walker DW. Effects of hypercapnia on tracheal pressure, diaphragm and intercostal electromyograms in unanesthetized fetal lambs. *J Physiol (Lond)*. 1982;326:461.
28. Harding R, Johnson P, McClelland ME. Respiratory function of the larynx in developing sheep and the influence of sleep state. *Respir Physiol*. 1980;40:165.
29. Rigatto H, Lee D, Davi M, Moore M, Rigatto E, Cates D. Effect of increased arterial CO_2 on fetal breathing and behavior in sheep. *J Appl Physiol*. 1988;64:982.
30. Condorelli S, Scarpelli EM. Somatic-respiratory reflex and onset of regular breathing movements in the lamb fetus *in utero*. *Pediatr Res*. 1975;9:879.
31. Condorelli S, Scarpelli EM. Fetal breathing. Induction *in utero* and effects of vagotomy and barbiturates. *J Pediatr*. 1976;88:94.
32. Ruckebusch Y. Development of sleep and wakefulness in the foetal lamb. *Electroencephalogr Clin Neurophysiol*. 1972;32:119.
33. Moss IR, Scarpelli EM. Generation and regulation of breathing *in utero*: fetal CO_2 response test. *J Appl Physiol. Respir Environ Exercise Physiol.* 1979;47:527.
34. Rigatto HA. New window on the chronic fetal sheep model. In: Nathanielsz PW, ed. *Animal Models in Fetal Medicine III*. Ithaca, NY: Perinatology Press; 1984:57–67.
35. Chernick V. Fetal breathing movements and the onset of breathing at birth. *Clin Perinatol*. 1978;5:257.
36. Jansen AH, Ioffe S, Russell BJ, Chernick V. Influence of sleep state on the response to hypercapnia in fetal lambs. *Respir Physiol*. 1982;48:125.
37. Molteni RA, Melmed MH, Sheldon RE, Jones MD, Meschia G. Induction of fetal breathing by metabolic acidemia and its effect on blood flow to the respiratory muscles. *Am J Obstet Gynecol*. 1980;136:609.
38. Kuipers IM, Maertzdorf WJ, DeJong DS, et al. Effect of mild hypocapnia on fetal breathing and behavior in unanesthetized normoxic fetal lambs. *J Appl Physiol*. 1994;76:1476–1480.
39. Phillipson E, Duffin J, Cooper JD. Critical dependence of respiratory rhythmicity on metabolic CO_2 load. *J Appl Physiol*. 1981;50:45–54.
40. Phillipson EA, Bowes G. Control of Breathing During Sleep. In: Fishman AP, Cherniack NS, Widdicombe JG, eds. *Geiger SR. Handbook of Physiology, vol II, pt 2*. Bethesda, MD: Am Physiol Soc; 1986:649–689.
41. Kolobow T, Gattinoni L, Tomlinson TA, et al. Control of breathing using an extracorporeal membrane lung. *Anesthesiology*. 1977;46:138–141.
42. Canet E, Praud JP, Laberge JM, et al. Apnea threshold and breathing rhythmicity in newborn lambs. *J Appl Physiol*. 1993;74:3013–3019.
43. Khan A, Qurashi M, Kwiatkowski K, et al. Measurement of the CO_2 apneic threshold in newborn infants: possible relevance for periodic breathing and apnea. *J Appl Physiol*. 2005;98:1171–1176.
44. Dempsey JA, Smith CA, Przybylowski T, et al. The ventilatory responsiveness to CO_2 below eupnoea as a determinant of ventilatory stability in sleep. *J Physiol*. 2004;560:1–11.
45. Xie A, Skatrud JB, Puleo DS, et al. Influence of arterial O_2 on the susceptibility to posthyperventilation apnea during sleep. *J Appl Physiol*. 2006;100:171–177.
46. Koos BJ, Sameshima H, Power GG. Fetal breathing, sleep state, and cardiovascular responses to graded hypoxia in sheep. *J Appl Physiol*. 1987;62:1033–1039.
47. Clewlow F, Dawes GS, Johnston BM, Walker DW. Changes in breathing, electrocortical and muscle activity in unanaesthetized fetal lambs with age. *J Physiol (Lond)*. 1983;341:463.
48. Koos BJ, Rajaee A. Fetal breathing movements and changes at birth. *Adv Exp Med Biol*. 2014;814:89–101.
49. Dawes GS. The central control of fetal breathing and skeletal muscle movements. *J Physiol*. 1984;346:1–18.
50. Koos BJ, Sameshima HJ. Effects of hypoxaemia and hypercapnia on breathing movements and sleep state in sinoaortic-denervated fetal sheep. *Dev Physiol*. 1988;10:131–144.

Basic Mechanisms of Oxygen Sensing and Adaptation to Hypoxia

67

Dan Zhou | Gabriel G. Haddad

INTRODUCTION

A large body of experimental work has been performed on oxygen sensing and on the cellular events that result from oxygen deprivation in a variety of cell types and organisms. Such comparative studies have contributed to our understanding of O_2 sensing and adaptation to hypoxia. As a result, a number of new concepts and mechanisms regarding O_2 sensing and hypoxia adaptation have emerged. It has been shown that neurons, renal and respiratory epithelial cells, hepatocytes, myocardial cells, vascular smooth muscle, or endothelial cells—virtually every cell type studied—can sense O_2, one way or another. This type of investigation has also been done at various ages, and age has been very important in determining sensing, responsiveness, and the ability to adapt to lack of O_2. Because in the past we have generally focused our study on nerve and glial cells during O_2 deprivation, this chapter summarizes mostly the studies on excitable tissues. However, an extensive body of new knowledge has demonstrated that much of what is known about the heart's sensing mechanisms can be applied to the central nervous system, for example, and much of what we know about the renal epithelium can be applied to the respiratory cells. It should be recognized that although there are similarities among tissues, there are often major differences. These differences reflect either differing environments or the function of that particular cell type of tissue. In certain instances, when the duration and severity of the stimulus are not too overwhelming, nerve cells may adapt and possibly survive hypoxia. Often, however, when the stress is too severe, the response time of the cells, from sensing to actual injury, is considerably shortened, and it is often difficult to tease apart the processes that control the various stages of response.

The aim of this chapter is to highlight observations that will demonstrate that a number of potential O_2 sensors exist in nerve cells. We detail results and data regarding ionic flux and controlling ionic flux mechanisms. We also detail some newer observations regarding expressional regulation of genes and adaptation to O_2 deprivation that occurs over much longer periods of time.

OXYGEN SENSING VIA MEMBRANE PROTEINS: IONIC ALTERATIONS

POTASSIUM IONIC FLUX AND ITS REGULATION: SHORT VERSUS LONG EXPOSURES

Potassium ion (K^+) channel modulation has been shown to be an integral and important cellular response to O_2 deprivation in nerve and cardiac cells. It is not clear, however, what signals precede the modulation of K^+ channels. This modulation could be direct or indirect.[1,2] Part of this modulation occurs as a result of changes in the concentrations of cytosolic factors (e.g., adenosine triphosphate and calcium ion [Ca^{2+}]) that are altered during O_2 deprivation. For example, a number of cytosolic factors change during hypoxia. Ca^{2+}, pH, sodium ion (Na^+), adenosine triphosphate-adenosine diphosphate-adenosine monophosphate ratios, and redox.[3-8] These, in turn, modulate a number of ion channels, including K^+ channels.

If K^+ channels can be modulated by cytosolic changes during hypoxia, one should question whether there are mechanisms originating from changes other than in the cytosol. For example, does the partial pressure of O_2 itself affect plasma membrane channels? To test the hypothesis that membrane-delimited mechanisms participate in the O_2-sensing process and are involved in the modulation of K^+ channel activity in central neurons, experiments were performed with use of patch-clamp techniques and dissociated cells from the rat neocortex and substantia nigra.[1,2] Oxygen deprivation produced a biphasic response in current amplitude. An initial transient increase was followed by a pronounced decrease in outward K^+ currents. The reduction in outward currents was a reversible process because perfusion with a normoxic medium with a Po_2 greater than 100 mm Hg (13.3 kPa) resulted in complete recovery. In cell-free excised membrane patches, we have demonstrated that a specific K^+ current (large conductance, inhibited by micromolar concentrations of adenosine triphosphate and activated by Ca^{2+}) was reversibly inhibited by lack of O_2. This was characterized by a marked decrease in channel open-state probability and a slight reduction in unitary conductance. The magnitude of channel inhibition by O_2 deprivation was closely dependent on O_2 tension. These studies demonstrated the selective nature of the hypoxia-induced inhibition of some K^+ channels[1,2,8] (Figs. 67.1 and 67.2) and also provided the first evidence for the regulation of K^+ channel activity by O_2 deprivation in cell-free excised patches of central neurons.[9,10]

It is not well understood how this inhibition occurs. With the use of specific agents that chelate metal, including heme and nonheme iron and copper, our laboratory has demonstrated that iron-center blockers inhibited the channel in excised patches in a fashion similar to that of low Po_2. These results suggested that K^+ channel activity is modulated during hypoxia by iron-containing proteins, thus providing evidence for an O_2-sensing mechanism in neuronal membranes.

Although most ionic fluxes that have been studied during hypoxia are plasma-membrane related, a number of reports on ion channels in mitochondrial membranes have been published.[11,12] However, it is unclear how these are involved in O_2 sensing or in hypoxic injury. We have obtained evidence that the maxi-K channels can be found in mitochondrial membranes and that they play a role in apoptotic cell death induced by serum deprivation. Furthermore, data demonstrate that mitochondrial channels (adenosine triphosphate-dependent K^+ channels) are present in myocardial cells and may be important for hypoxic injury.[13]

The observation of the relative "insensitivity" or the lack of response of the immature cells or tissues to low O_2 tensions compared with the more mature response of differentiated cells is of particular interest. On the basis of a large number of studies investigating ion fluxes and activities, release of neurotransmitters, or changes in membrane electrophysiologic properties, it is clear that the newborn exhibits a blunted response to hypoxia.[3,4,14-17] Although there is a paucity of cellular and molecular work on this subject in the fetus, it is clear from whole-body studies in the fetus exposed to hypoxia that its response is very blunted, if not totally eliminated. In other types of studies, however, investigating the response of the neonatal lung to hypoxia (compared with that of the adult), the response in terms of septation and alveolar formation was more severe in the neonate than in the adult.[18] For example, hypoxia in the first couple of weeks of life will inhibit septation, whereas in the adult there is very little effect on alveolar size.[18] Therefore, depending on the measured variable, the newborn infant may or may not be as responsive as the adult. Because most systems exhibit plasticity at an early stage in life, strong stimuli may affect function and structure much more in the neonate, especially when these stimuli occur over prolonged periods of time. Acute short stresses, however, especially those in the central nervous system, may not be so significant for the newborn infant.

SODIUM IONIC FLUX AND ITS REGULATION: SHORT VERSUS LONG EXPOSURES

The concentrations of Na^+ and chloride ion (Cl^-) change markedly during hypoxia. Anoxia induces a drop in extracellular Na^+ in brain slice, and removal of extracellular Na^+ prevents the anoxia-induced morphologic changes in dissociated hippocampal neurons.[6,19,20] For an understanding of the mechanisms that sense O_2 and lead to acute neuronal swelling during anoxia, the ionic movements of Cl^- and Na^+ during O_2 deprivation in the hypoglossal (XII) neurons of rat brain slices have been studied. Baseline extracellular Cl^- and Na^+ activities ($[Cl^-]_o$ and $[Na^+]_o$) were measured in both adult and neonatal brain slices.[6,19,20] During a period of anoxia (4 minutes), $[Na^+]_o$ decreased markedly in adult slices, whereas $[Na^+]_o$ did not show any significant change in the neonatal slice. Anoxia induced a significant decrease of $[Cl^-]_o$ in both the adult and neonate; however, $[Cl^-]_o$ dropped seven times more in the adult than in the neonate. Intracellular Cl^- activity ($[Cl^-]_i$) has been studied in adult hypoglossal cells. It is not surprising that an increase in $[Cl^-]_i$ with O_2 deprivation was seen. To also study intracellular Na^+ ($[Na^+]_i$) in isolated neurons, we used the fluorophore Sodium Green in freshly dissociated rat neurons, and sodium-binding benzofuran isophthalate (SBFI), a fluorescent indicator for sodium, in cultured cortical neurons. Ten minutes of anoxia caused an increase in Na^+_i with a latency of approximately 2 minutes. In these neurons, fluorescence increased by an average of approximately 20%. We conclude that during anoxia (1) intracellular $[Cl^-]$ and $[Na^+]$ increase in the adult, most likely because of entry of extracellular ions into the cytosol, and (2) a major maturational difference exists in mechanisms regulating Cl^- and Na^+ homeostasis between neonate and adult brain tissue.

Although it is well known that Na^+_i increases during hypoxia, the sensors for this ionic alteration are not well documented. It is possible that exchangers or transporters and channels are somehow located within the cascade of events that lead to this increase. The regulation of the voltage-sensitive Na^+ channels during hypoxia has been investigated with the use of isolated

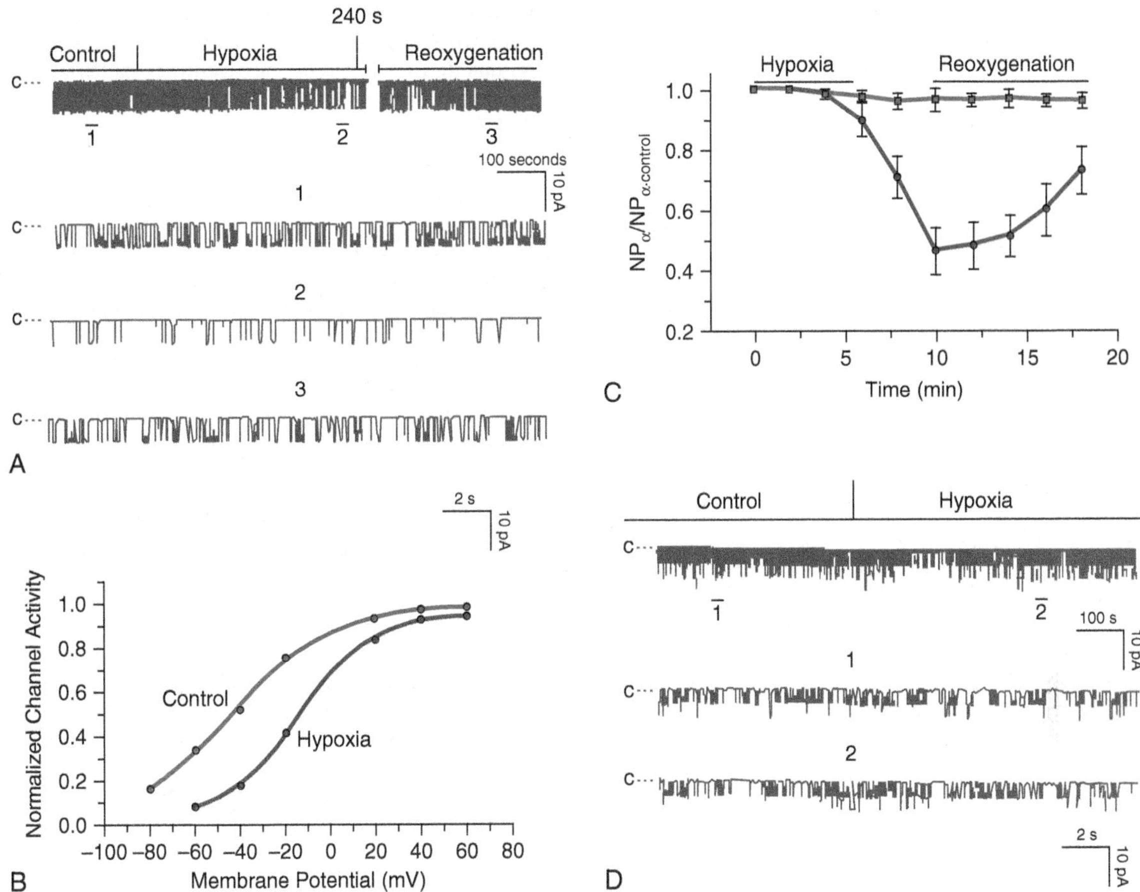

Fig. 67.1 Effect of hypoxia on single-channel BK_{Ca} current. (A) Effect of hypoxia on single BK_{Ca} channel in a cell-attached patch from a neocortical neuron. Current was recorded with high-KCl (140 mmol/L) solution in the pipette and physiologic solution in the bath at a V_m of −30 mV. The channel closed level is indicated by *C*. Three parts of the compressed trace are shown, as indicated by numbers *1* through *3* (fast-time resolution). (B) Effect of hypoxia on the voltage activation of BK_{Ca} channel under the ionic condition just described. The line is fitted to a Boltzmann distribution. $V_{0.5}$ shifted from −42.4 ± 4.8 mV to −18.6 ± 3.5 mV after exposure of hypoxia for 10 min. (C) Time course of the hypoxia-induced effect on NP_o. In cell-attached recordings *(filled squares)*, channel inhibition started about 5 min after the onset of hypoxia, and a maximum inhibition was reached in approximately 10 min. After that time, NP_o was markedly reduced to approximately 43% of control level. Reoxygenation led to partial recovery. In inside-out recordings *(filled circles)*, NP_o was not significantly affected during hypoxia. (D) Continuous recording of a single BK_{Ca} channel current from an inside-out patch of a neocortical neuron during hypoxia, with the use of a symmetric 140-mmol/L KCl on both sides of the membrane, with a V_m of −30 mV. The channel closed level is indicated by *C*. Two parts of the compressed trace (indicated by the numbers *1* and *2*) are shown at fast-time resolution. *BKCa*, Large-conductance calcium channel; *NPo*, product of number of channels open multiplied by the open probability. (From Liu H, Moczydlowski E, Haddad GG. O_2 deprivation inhibits Ca^{2+}-activated K^+ channels via cytosolic factors in mice neocortical neurons. *J Clin Invest.* 1999;104:577.)

hippocampal neurons.[5,20] Given the prior data demonstrating an increase in intracellular Na^+, it is somewhat surprising that hippocampal neurons respond to acute oxygen deprivation with inhibition of whole-cell Na^+ current (I_{Na}).[10,21] Because kinases can modulate I_{Na} and are activated during hypoxia, we hypothesized that kinase activation may play a role in the hypoxia-induced inhibition of I_{Na}. I_{Na} was recorded at baseline, during exposure to kinase activators (with and without kinase inhibitors), and during acute hypoxia (with and without kinase inhibitors). Hypoxia reduced I_{Na} to approximately 40% of initial values and shifted the steady-state inactivation in the negative direction.[22] Hypoxia produced no effect on activation or fast inactivation. Protein kinase A (PKA) activation with 3′,5′-cyclic adenosine monophosphate, N^6,O_2-dibutyryl, sodium salt (db-cAMP) resulted in a reduction of I_{Na} to 63% without an effect on activation or steady-state inactivation. I_{Na} was also reduced by activation of protein kinase C (PKC) with phorbol 12-myristate 13-acetate (PMA) to 40% or with 1-oleoyl-2-acetyl-*sn*-glycerol (OAG) to 46%. In addition, steady-state inactivation was shifted in the negative direction by PKC activation.

Neither the activation curve nor the kinetics of fast inactivation was altered by PKC activation. The response to PKA activation was blocked by the PKA inhibitor (H-89) and by PKA inhibitory peptide $PKA_{5\text{-}24}$ (PKA_i). PKC activation was blocked by the kinase inhibitor (H-7), by the PKC inhibitor calphostin C, and by the inhibitory peptide $PKC_{19\text{-}31}$ (PKC_i). The hypoxia-induced inhibition of I_{Na} and shift in steady-state inactivation were greatly attenuated by H-7, calphostin C, or PKC_i but not by H-89 or PKA_i. We conclude that hypoxia activates PKC in rat CA1 neurons and that PKC activation leads to the hypoxia-induced inhibition of I_{Na}. These data indicate that kinases can inhibit whole-cell Na^+ current very much like that observed during hypoxia. However, it is unclear how kinases are activated during hypoxia and what events occur upstream.

From this analysis, we should highlight a few issues pertaining to O_2 sensing. (1) Sensing can be very rapid; whatever the sensor is, the reactions that lead to the electrophysiologic responses observed by using our techniques and approaches must be very quick, on the order of seconds. (2) Most of the alterations are not genetically mediated, and no gene expression is presumably altered in this short period of time.

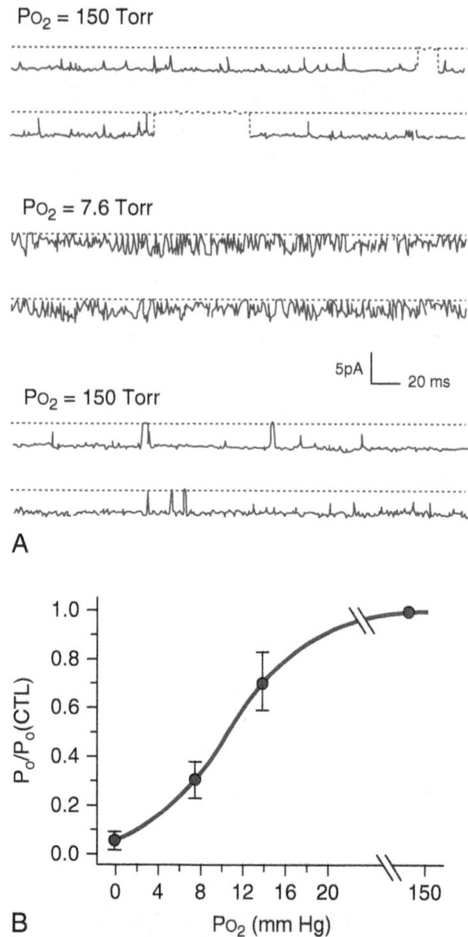

Fig. 67.2 A large conductance K^+ current is inhibited during O_2 deprivation. (A) Continuous recordings of a single K^+ current from an inside-out patch with the same solution (150 mmol/L K^+) in both internal and external sides, when the membrane potential was held at 20 mV. During baseline *(top two traces)*, this channel had a P_{open} of 0.92 and a unitary conductance of 188 picosiemens. *Straight lines* indicate the channel closed level. Hypoxia ($Po_2 \approx 8$ mm Hg) induced a decrease in P_{open} to 0.24 *(middle two traces)*. Recovery of P_{open} (0.96) is seen after reperfusion *(lower two traces)*. (B) Dose-dependent inhibition of P_{open} by graded hypoxia. Note that the P_{open} was normalized to its control level. Data presented as means ± SEM (n = 3) are fitted with an equation of $y = 1/\{1 + \exp[(K_d - x)/h]\}$, where $y = P_{open}/P_{open}$ (control), $x = Po_2$, $K_d = 11$, a Po_2 level for 50% inhibition of y, and $h = 4$. P_{open}, Probability of having a channel in the open state. (From Jiang C, Haddad GG. A direct mechanism for sensing low oxygen levels by central neurons. *Proc Natl Acad Sci U S A.* 1994;91:7198.)

Chronic hypoxia has also been studied in our laboratory, as well as in others.[23-25] With respect to Na^+ flux, it seems that Na^+ influx increases when neurons are subjected to hypoxia for days.[23,26] It is very important to note that Na^+ influx through voltage-sensitive Na^+ channels can lead to cell death, and this form of cell death is most likely a result of the activation of cell death genes.[25]

OXYGEN SENSING VIA GENE REGULATION

Neurons vary widely in their capacity to adapt to a limited oxygen supply to the brain, reflecting the diversity of neuronal function and their adaptive mechanisms to oxygen deprivation. The hypoxia-tolerant neurons can be found in every order of vertebrates, such as crucian carp,[27] tadpoles,[28] turtle,[29] and the naked Kenyan mole rat. Neurons from oxygen-sensitive species such as *Rattus norvegicus* are hypoxia tolerant during the embryonic and neonatal periods.[30,31] The discovery of the hypoxia-tolerant property of an invertebrate species, *Drosophila melanogaster*, provided researchers with a new model system to study the mechanism of hypoxia tolerance in the neuronal systems.[32,33] Those studies have prompted a number of questions. How do neurons "sense" the lack of microenvironmental O_2? How do they respond? How does sensing O_2 deprivation affect the cascade that follows the initial steps?

Multiple O_2 sensing systems most likely exist, and although much remains to be learned about how cells sense and adapt to conditions of oxygen scarcity, it is clear that O_2 sensing (and the cascade of events that follow O_2 deprivation) largely depends on the regulation of gene transcription. Such mechanisms are fairly quick, and targets can be multiple. Several transcription factors, such as the hypoxia-inducible factor (HIF), activator protein 1 (AP-1), early growth response protein-1 (EGR-1),[34] nuclear factor κB (NF-κB),[35]and CCAAT enhancer-binding protein beta (C/EBPβ/NF-IL-6),[36] were found to be involved in the modulation of gene expression by oxygen. Among these O_2-sensitive transcriptional systems, perhaps the best-described O_2-sensing pathway is the oxygen-sensitive transcription factor HIF, which activates the gene transcription machinery in an oxygen deprivation-dependent manner.[37]

HIFs are heterodimeric transcription factors containing an α- and a β-subunit that belong to the basic-helix-loop-helix (bHLH)-PAS protein superfamily. HIF-1α was first cloned from the human Hep3B cell line[38] and is a member of the PAS superfamily 1 (MOP1). The mouse and rat isoforms also have been cloned.[39,40] In addition, two other α-subunits were cloned, from humans and rats and mice (HIF-2α and HIF-3α). HIF-2α is known as *endothelial PAS domain protein 1 (EPAS1), HIF-1α-like factor (HLF),* or *HIF-related factor (HRF)*, and is a member of the PAS superfamily 2 (MOP2).[41] HIF-3α is also referred to as MOP7.[41] The β-subunits of HIF, HIF-1β, HIF-2β, and HIF-3β, are members of the arylhydrocarbon receptor nuclear translocator, ARNT family, also named as ARNT1, ARNT2, or ARNT3.[42] HIF-1α and β homologs also exist in *Drosophila* tissues, and studies in this species have provided new data on the cellular adaptive responses to chronic hypoxic stress.[15,43] HIF-1 has been the most extensively studied (Fig. 67.3).

Previous investigations have shown that HIF-1 messenger RNA (mRNA) was expressed in the mouse, rat, and human brain.[44] Because the brain is extremely sensitive to hypoxia and ischemia, the regulation of HIF-1 expression is highly relevant. Two of its target gene products in the brain are erythropoietin (EPO) and vascular endothelial growth factor (VEGF).[45,46] In the adult rat brain, HIF-1 mRNA was found in neuronal cells.[47] In hypoxia-treated rats or mice, an increase of HIF-1 mRNA was found in the brain, kidney, and lung. The HIF-1-regulated gene VEGF increased accordingly with a similar expression pattern as HIF-1. This provides evidence for a neuroprotective role of HIF-1 in the central nervous system. HIF-1 has been shown to mediate adaptive responses to reduced O_2 availability, including angiogenesis, glycolysis, and ischemia tolerance in the brain.

Control of angiogenesis through HIF-1 and HIF-2 is regulated by growth factors, including VEGF.[48] Numerous studies have demonstrated that chronic hypoxia induces angiogenesis in the adult brain with an increase in VEGF. A time-course study, however, has shown that, after exposure to 10% O_2, HIF-1 rapidly accumulated, remained at high levels for only 14 days, and then decreased by 21 days, despite continuous low arterial

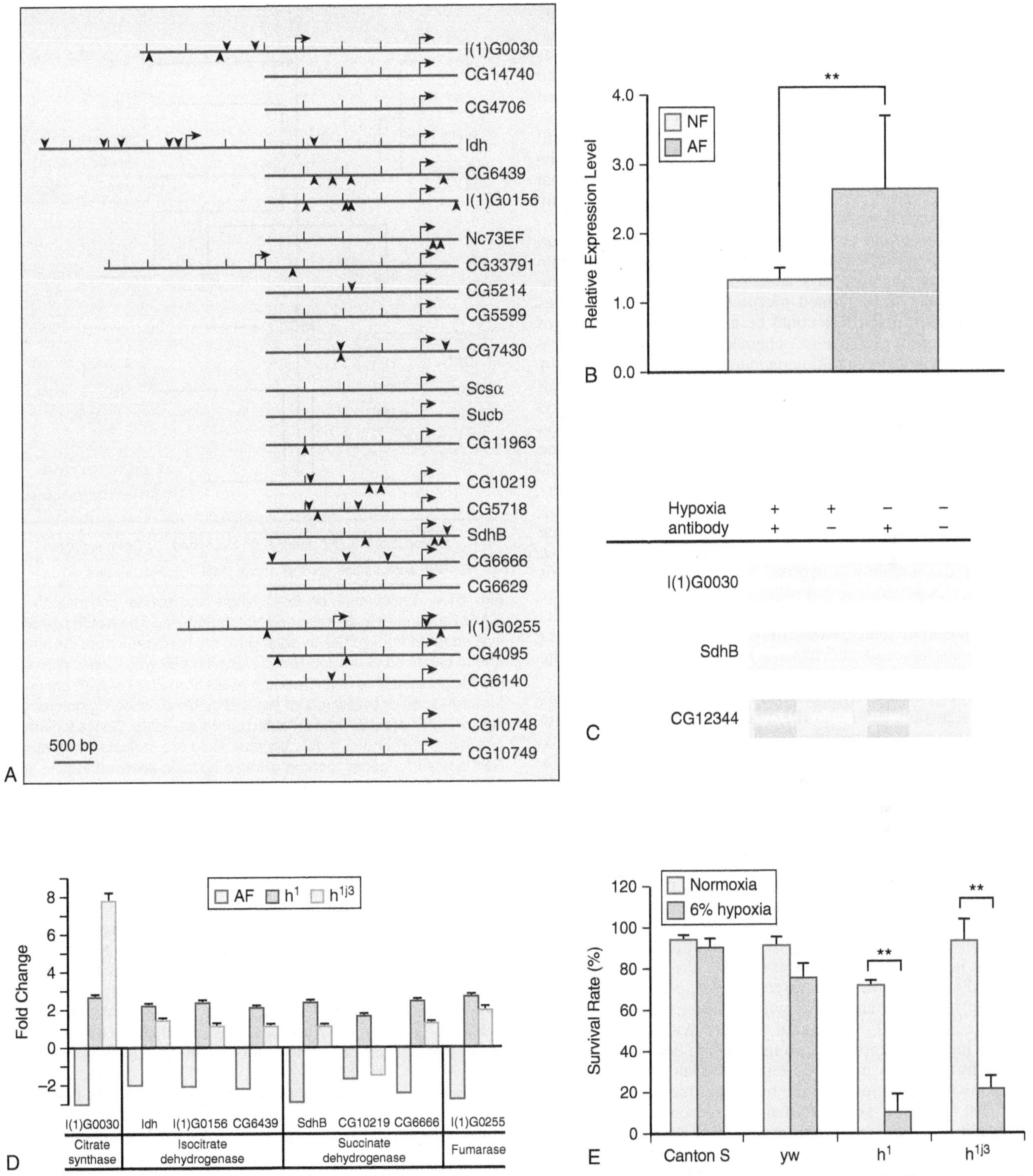

l(1)G0030
CG14740
CG4706
Idh
CG6439
l(1)G0156
Nc73EF
CG33791
CG5214
CG5599
CG7430
Scsα
Sucb
CG11963
CG10219
CG5718
SdhB
CG6666
CG6629
l(1)G0255
CG4095
CG6140
CG10748
CG10749
500 bp
A
**
NF
AF
Relative Expression Level
4.0
3.0
2.0
1.0
0.0
B
Hypoxia + + − −
antibody + − + −
l(1)G0030
SdhB
CG12344
C
AF h1 h1j3
Fold Change
8
6
4
2
0
−2
l(1)G0030
Idh
l(1)G0156
CG6439
SdhB
CG10219
CG6666
l(1)G0255
Citrate synthase
Isocitrate dehydrogenase
Succinate dehydrogenase
Fumarase
D
Normoxia
6% hypoxia
Survival Rate (%)
120
100
80
60
40
20
0
Canton S
yw
h1
h1j3
**
**
E

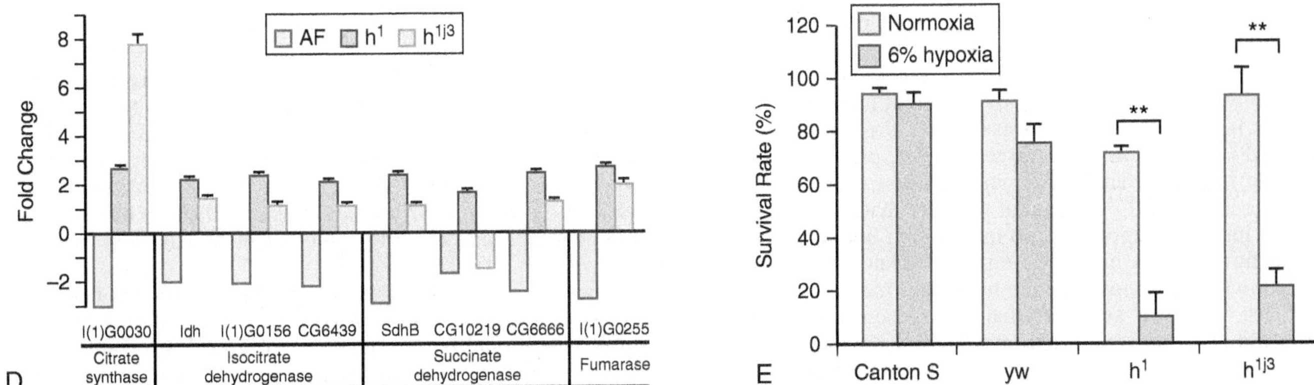

Fig. 67.3 Transcriptional suppressor hairy regulates TCA cycle gene expression and hypoxia tolerance. (A) Genomic localization of hairy binding elements in the *cis*-regulatory region of genes encoding TCA cycle enzymes. Arrowheads indicate consensus hairy binding sites, and arrows indicate transcriptional start sites. (B) Significant up-regulation of hairy expression in hypoxia-selected AF populations ($P < .01$). (C) Chromatin immunoprecipitation assay of gene *l(1)G0030, SdhB,* and CG12344 under normoxia or hypoxia. (D) Abolished suppression of genes encoding TCA cycle enzymes in *hairy* loss-of-function mutants. (E) Significant reduction in hypoxia survival in hairy loss-of-function mutants. Embryos from loss-of-function hairy mutants (h^1 and h^{1j3}) and controls (Canton-S and yw) were cultured at normoxic or 6% O_2 hypoxic condition. The ratio of adult flies to pupae was determined as survival rate of each stock. The loss-of-function hairy mutants exhibited a significantly reduced rate of hypoxia survival. Data are presented as means ± SD. $^{**}P < .01$. *AF,* Hypoxia-adapted flies; *TCA,* tricarboxylic acid. (Modified from Zhou D, Xue J, Lai JC, Schork NJ, et al. Mechanisms underlying hypoxia tolerance in *Drosophila melanogaster.* hairy as a metabolic switch. *PLoS Genet.* 2008;4(10):e1000221.)

oxygen tension. This would indicate either that HIF has a long-lasting effect on target genes or that other HIF targets or long-lasting hypoxia can maintain the induction of genes such as VEGF, because angiogenesis does not regress at a time when HIF has gone back to normal levels.[49] When 21-day adapted rats were exposed to a more severe hypoxic challenge (8% O_2), HIF-1 increased again indicating that the level of HIF-1 can still be upregulated with more severe stresses.[49] Thus HIF-1 and its regulated genes appear to have a role in vascular remodeling and metabolic changes that contribute to the adaptation of the chronic hypoxia condition.

It has been found that a non-injurious hypoxic stimulation can protect cells from an otherwise lethal hypoxic-ischemic attack several hours or days later. This non-injurious hypoxic stimulation has been termed *preconditioning*. Several studies have suggested that HIF-1 could be an important mediator of hypoxia-induced tolerance to ischemia by preconditioning.[50-52] Indeed, hypoxic preconditioning-induced expression of HIF-1 and its target genes has been found in the neonatal and adult brain. With the use of DNA microarray methods combined with real-time reverse transcriptase-polymerase chain reaction technologies, a set of HIF-1- but not HIF-2-mediated gene expression has been identified in the neonatal rat brain.[53] In this study, 12 genes were reported to be induced; they are *VEGF, EPO, GLUT-1, adrenomedullin, propyl 4-hydroxylase, MT-1, MKP-1, CELF, 12-lipoxygenase, t-PA, CAR-1*, and an expressed sequence tag. Some of these genes, such as *GLUT-1, MT-1, CELF, MKP-1*, and *t-PA*, did not show a hypoxic regulation in either neurons or astrocytes, suggesting that other cells are responsible for the upregulation of these genes in the hypoxic brain. These results also demonstrate that, besides HIF-1 pathway, a number of other endogenous molecular mechanisms might also be involved in the hypoxic preconditioning-induced tolerance.

If the responses to hypoxia over a longer term, such as hours and days, involve HIF-1 and HIF-2 and their target downstream genes, how about hypoxia over even longer periods of time, such as over generations? These types of studies have been relatively scarce. We have generated a hypoxia-tolerant *Drosophila* strain to study the genetic and molecular basis of adaptation to long-term (i.e., over generations) hypoxic environments.[54] Transcriptome and whole-genome analyses have shown that the survival of both larvae and adult flies was accompanied by alterations in a number of major signaling pathways, including Notch, EGF, Insulin, and Toll/Imd pathways. Furthermore, we also found that many genes encoding glycolytic enzymes were downregulated in the hypoxia-tolerant flies.[55] And, no significant lactate accumulation was found in the hypoxia-adapted flies (AF).[56] For more than three decades, physiologists have debated the importance of down-regulation of metabolism in hypoxia tolerance.[57,58] Although this idea, based on metabolic data, is intuitively appealing, no information has been obtained about how various metabolic enzymes could be coordinated to survive severe long-lasting hypoxia. Our work provided the first evidence showing that such coordination can be achieved at a transcriptional level by a seemingly metabolic switch (i.e., *hairy*, a transcriptional suppressor). This notion is supported by a number of observations: (1) expression of *hairy* was up-regulated in hypoxia-tolerant flies; (2) the *hairy*-binding region was present in the *cis*-regulatory regions of the down-regulated genes but not others; (3) functional chromatin immunoprecipitation analysis demonstrated that the down-regulation of these metabolic genes is based on the changes of *hairy* (it is noteworthy that its binding was not increased for other, nonmetabolic target genes—for example, CG12344); and (4) *hairy* loss-of-function mutations abolished the suppression on the expression of tricarboxylic acid (TCA) cycle genes and significantly reduced hypoxia survival in *Drosophila*[55] (see Fig. 67.3). Furthermore, whole genome sequence analysis revealed that the signaling mechanism regulating *hairy* (i.e., the Notch signaling pathway) was under hypoxia selection in the hypoxia-tolerant flies, suggesting that Notch signaling is a critical cellular mechanism regulating hypoxia adaptation during development. Indeed, genetic manipulation of Notch signaling altered hypoxia tolerance (Fig. 67.4; i.e., Notch activation enhanced hypoxia tolerance).[59] We also found that the adaptive mechanisms identified in this hypoxia-tolerant *Drosophila* model are evolutionarily conserved in highlander humans and may play a crucial role in protecting mammals from hypoxic injury.[60]

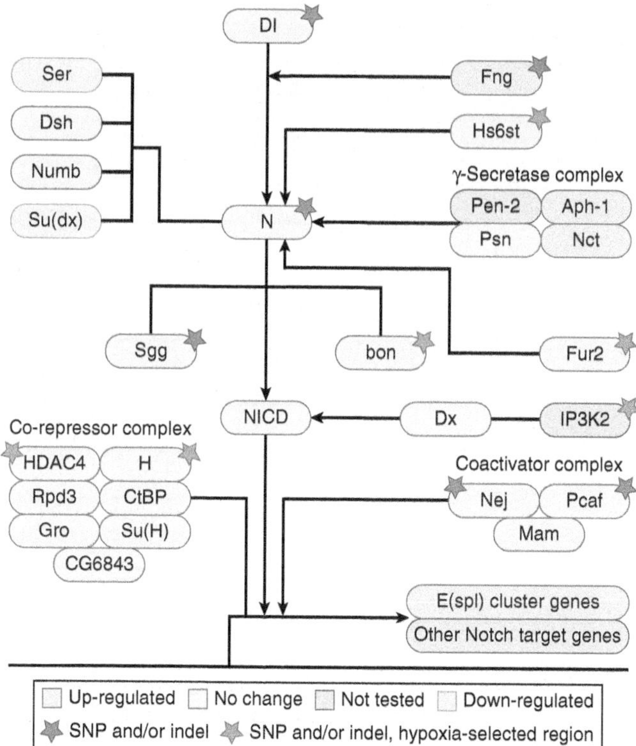

Fig. 67.4 Enrichment of fixed single nucleotide polymorphisms *(SNPs)* and Indels in an extended Notch pathway. The Notch pathway was adapted from KEGG by adding Notch interactors from the literature to create an expanded Notch signaling pathway. Genes differentially expressed in larva (expression levels from Zhou et al.)[55] are cyan (up-regulated) or yellow (down-regulated), genes showing no change in expression are gray, and untested genes are white. Genes for which one more SNP and/or indels became fixed are indicated with stars. Red is used for genes located within a hypoxia-selected region, and blue is used for all others. (From Zhou D, Udpa N, Gersten M, Visk DW, et al. Experimental selection of hypoxia-tolerant Drosophila melanogaster. *Proc Natl Acad Sci U S A*. 2011;108(6):2349–2354.)

A new important focus in the past few years has been the importance of epigenetics on gene expression during hypoxic stress. This should be considered as a sensing mechanism that plays an important role in hypoxia. A number of studies have shown that many genes are regulated by epigenetic mechanisms in CNS under hypoxic/ischemic conditions.[61-63]

Human adaptation to high altitude hypoxia is based on O_2 sensing and responses of a variety of tissues as well. It is possible that a number of sensors lead to such adaptation over generations over thousands of years.[64,65] To date, genome-wide studies have yielded a wealth of valuable information that increased our appreciation of the complexity of the molecular and genetic mechanisms underlying adaptation to long-lasting hypoxic stress. Indeed, a survey of the literature has suggested that greater than 1000 genes are potentially involved in adaptation to high-altitude hypoxia in different human populations across the world.[66-68] Interestingly, we found that

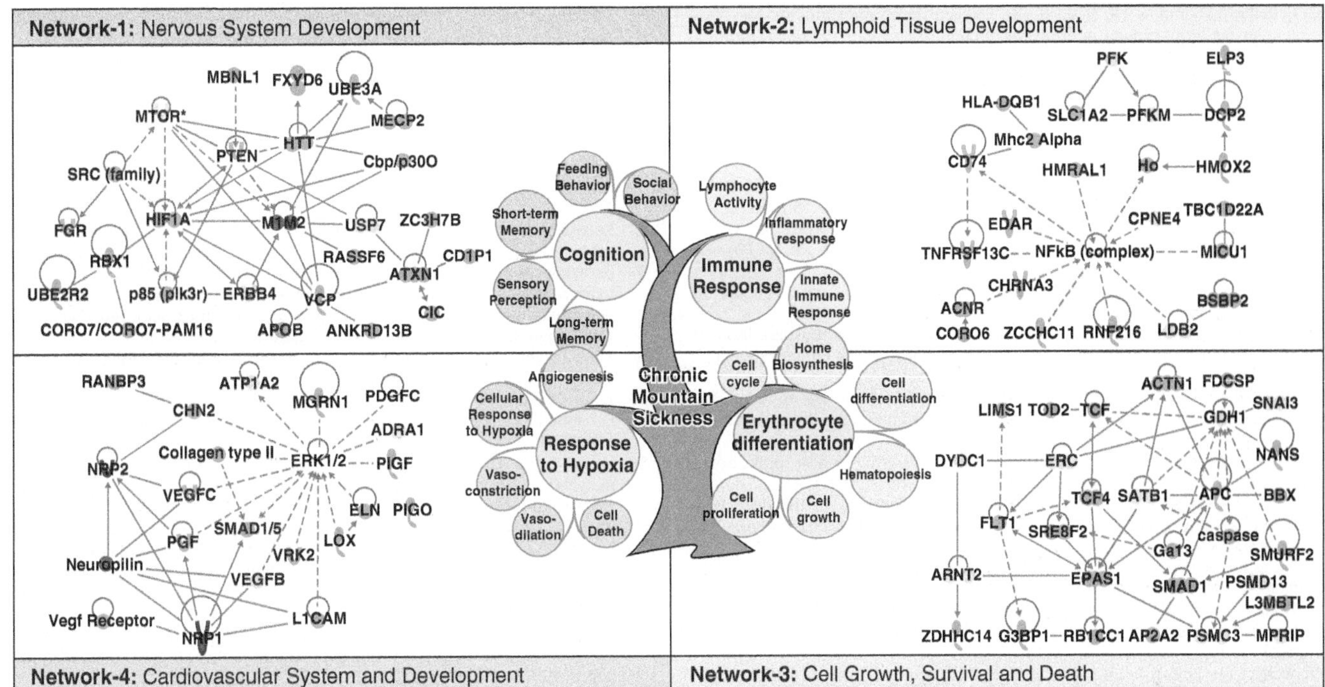

Fig. 67.5 Representative genetic interactions regulating biologic processes and physiologic functions involved in human adaption to high altitude. The central figure shows the complexity of the pathology linked to chronic mountain sickness. It involves various physiologic responses such as erythrocyte differentiation, immune response, response to hypoxia. Network 1 shows the gene interactions regulating posttranslational modification, cell-to-cell signaling and interaction, nervous system development and function. Network 2 shows the genetic network regulating hematologic system development and function, immunologic disease, lymphoid tissue structure, and development. Network 3 depicts the genetic interactions regulating cell death and survival, gene expression, and cell cycle, particularly during hematopoiesis. Network 4 shows the genetic network regulating cardiovascular system development and function, tissue development and organismal development. Color code: Yellow—genes identified in the Andean population, Blue—genes identified in the Ethiopian population, Green—genes identified in the Tibetan population, and Red—genes identified in both Andean and Tibetan populations. (Reprinted by permission from Springer Nature: Azad P, Stobdan T, Zhou D, et al. High-altitude adaptation in humans: from genomics to integrative physiology. *J Mol Med*. 2017;95(12): Fig. 1.)

many cellular signaling pathways were enriched in this set of genes, suggesting that adaptation to high altitude requires coordinated cellular signaling. For example, interactions between the candidate genes that were obtained by analyzing Andean, Ethiopian, and Tibetan highlander populations suggested that there is a coordination of functions and developmental processes in various organs/tissues, such as the function and development of the neuronal, hematologic, and cardiovascular systems, as well as the gene-gene interactions regulating cell death and survival (Fig. 67.5). Therefore, it is interesting to note that although different genetic networks involved genes that were identified in different human populations, these genes may nonetheless regulate similar biologic processes and physiologic functions.

Although a great deal of work has been done to understand the biologic role of hypoxia-induced gene expression in the brain, many important questions remain largely unanswered. For example, which genes are expressed and which are inactivated during hypoxia in different brain regions and cell types are still unknown. Further research is needed to describe the diversity of oxygen sensors and the mechanisms by which these sensors regulate the gene transcription machinery.

A complete reference list is available at www.ExpertConsult.com.

SELECT REFERENCES

1. Jiang C, Haddad GG. A direct mechanism for sensing low oxygen levels by central neurons. *Proc Natl Acad Sci U S A*. 199491:7198–7201.
2. Jiang C, Sigworth FJ, Haddad GG. O_2 deprivation activates an ATP-inhibitable K^+ channels in substantia nigra neurons. *J Neurosci*. 1994;14:5590–5602.
3. Xia Y, Haddad GG. Major difference in the expression of μ- and δ-opioid receptors between turtle and rat brain. *J Comp Neurol*. 2001;436:202–210.
4. Gu XQ, Yao H, Haddad GG. Effect of extracellular HCO_3^- on Na^+ channel characteristics in hippocampal CA1 neurons. *J Neurophysiol*. 2000;84:2477–2483.
5. Friedman JF, Haddad GG. Anoxia induces an increase in intracellular sodium in rat central neurons. *Brain Res*. 1994;663:329–334.
6. Chidekel AS, Friedman JE, Haddad GG. Anoxia-induced neuronal injury: role of Na^+ entry and Na^+-dependent transport. *Exp Neurol*. 1997;146:403–413.
7. Yao H, Ma E, Gu XQ, Haddad GG. Intracellular pH regulation of CA1 neurons in Na^+/H^+ isoform 1 mutant mice. *J Clin Invest*. 1999;104:637–645.
8. Liu H, Moczydlowski E, Haddad GG. O_2 deprivation inhibits Ca2+-activated K^+ channels via cytosolic factors in mice neocortical neurons. *J Clin Invest*. 1999;104:577–588.
9. Marks JD, Donnelly DF, Haddad GG. Adenosine-induced inhibition of vagal motoneuron excitability: receptor subtype and mechanisms. *Am J Physiol*. 1993;264:L124–L132.
10. Cummins TR, Jiang C, Haddad GG. Human neocortical excitability is decreased during anoxia via sodium channel modulation. *J Clin Invest*. 1993;91:608–615.
12. Douglas RM, Lai JC, Bian S. The calcium-sensitive large-conductance potassium channel (BK/MAXI K) is present in the inner mitochondrial membrane of rat brain. *Neuroscience*. 2006;139:1249–1261.
14. Ma E, Haddad GG. A Drosophila Cdk5α-like molecule and its possible role in response to O_2 deprivation. *BiochemBiophys Res Comm*. 1999;261:459–463.
15. Xia Y, Haddad GG. Effect of prolonged O_2 deprivation on Na^+ channels: differential regulation in adult versus fetal rat brain. *Neuroscience*. 1999;94:1231–1243.
16. Schmitt BM, Berger UV, Douglas RM, et al. Na/HCO_3 cotransporters in rat brain: expression in glia, neurons and choroid plexus. *J Neurosci*. 2000;20:6839–6848.
17. Jiang C, Haddad GG. Short periods of hypoxia activate a K^+ current in central neurons. *Brain Res*. 1993;64:352–356.
19. Xia Y, Haddad GG. Voltage-sensitive Na^+ channels increase in number in newborn rat brain after *in utero* hypoxia. *Brain Res*. 1994;635:339–344.
20. Friedman JE, Haddad GG. Removal of extracellular sodium prevents anoxia-induced injury in freshly dissociated rat CA1 hippocampal neurons. *Brain Res*. 1994;641:57–64.
21. Cummins TR, Donnelly DF, Haddad GG. Effect of metabolic inhibition on the excitability of isolated hippocampal CA1 neurons: developmental aspects. *J Neurophysiol*. 1991;66:1471–1482.

22. O'Reilly J, Cummins TR, Haddad GG. Oxygen deprivation inhibits Na+ current in rat hippocampal neurons via protein kinase C. *J Physiol (London)*. 1997;503:479-488.
24. Banasiak KJ, Xia Y, Haddad GG. Mechanism underlying hypoxia-induced neuronal apoptosis. *Prog Neurobiol*. 2000;62:215-249.
25. Banasiak KJ, Burenkova O, Haddad GG. Activation of voltage-sensitive sodium channels induces caspase-3-mediated neuronal apoptosis. *Soc Neurosc*. 2001;27:501.
26. Cummins TR, Xia Y, Haddad GG. Comparison of the functional properties of human and rat neocortical sodium currents. *Soc Neurosc*. 1992;18:1136.
28. West NH, Burggren WW. Gill and lung ventilation responses to steady-state aquatic hypoxia and hyperoxia in the bullfrog tadpole. *Respir Physiol*. 1982;47:165-176.
29. Belkin DA. Anaerobic brain function: effects of stagnant and anoxic anoxia on persistence of breathing in reptiles. *Science*. 1968;162:1017-1018.
30. Haddad GG, Donnelly DF. O_2 deprivation induces a major depolarization in brain stem neurons in the adult but not in the neonatal rat. *J Physiol*. 1990;429:411-428.
31. Haddad GG, Jiang C. O_2 deprivation in the central nervous system: on mechanisms of neuronal response, differential sensitivity and injury. *Prog Neurobiol*. 1993;40:277-318.
32. Haddad GG, Ma E. Neuronal tolerance to O_2 deprivation in drosophila: novel approaches using genetic models. *Neuroscientist*. 2001;7:538-550.
33. Zhou D, Visk DW, Haddad GG. *Drosophila*, a golden bug, for the dissection of the genetic basis of tolerance and susceptibility to hypoxia. *Pediatr Res*. 2009;66:239-247.
37. Wang GL, Semenza GL. Purification and characterization of hypoxia-inducible factor 1. *J Biol Chem*. 1995;270:1230-1237.
38. Wang GL, Jiang BH, Rue EA, Semenza GL. Hypoxia-inducible factor 1 is a basic-helix-loop-helix-PAS heterodimer regulated by cellular O_2 tension. *Proc Natl Acad Sci U S A*. 1995;92:5510-5514.
39. Wenger RH, Rolfs A, Marti HH, et al. Nucleotide sequence, chromosomal assignment and mRNA expression of mouse hypoxia-inducible factor-1 alpha. *Biochem Biophys Res Commun*. 1996;223:54-59.
42. Semenza GL. Regulation of mammalian O_2 homeostasis by hypoxia-inducible factor 1. *Annu Rev Cell Dev Biol*. 1999;15:551-578.
43. Lavista-Llanos S, Centanin L, Irisarri M, et al. Control of the hypoxic response in Drosophila melanogaster by the basic helix-loop-helix PAS protein similar. *Mol Cell Biol*. 2002;22:6842-6853.
44. Weiner CM, Booth G, Sementza GL. *In vivo* expression of mRNAs encoding hypoxia-inducible factor 1. *Biochem Biophys Res Commun*. 1996;225:485-488.
45. Sakanaga M, Wen TC, Matsuda S, et al. *In vivo* evidence that erythropoietin protects neurons from ischemic damage. *Proc Natl Acad Sci U S A*. 1998;95:4635-4640.
48. Carmeliet P. Mechanisms of angiogenesis and arteriogenesis. *Nat Med*. 2000;6:389-395.
49. Chavez JC, Agani F, Pichiule P, LaManna JC. Expression of hypoxia-inducible factor-1alpha in the brain of rats during chronic hypoxia. *J Appl Physiol*. 2000;89:1937-1942.
50. Bergeron M, Gidday JM, Yu AY, et al. Role of hypoxia-inducible factor-1 in hypoxia-induced ischemic tolerance in neonatal rat brain. *Ann Neurol*. 2000;48:285-296.
51. Jones NM, Bergeron M. Hypoxic preconditioning induces changes in HIF-1 target genes in neonatal rat brain. *J Cereb Blood Flow Metab*. 2001;21:1105-1114.
52. Bernaudin M, Nedelec AS, Divoux D, et al. Normobaric hypoxia induces tolerance to focal permanent cerebral ischemia in association with an increased expression of hypoxia-inducible factor-1 and its target genes, erythropoietin and VEGF, in the adult mouse brain. *J Cereb Blood Flow Metab*. 2002;22:393-403.
54. Zhou D, Xue J, Chen J, et al. Experimental selection for Drosophila survival in extremely low O_2 environment. *PloS One*. 2007;2:e490.
55. Zhou D, Xue J, Lai JC, et al. Mechanisms underlying hypoxia tolerance in Drosophila melanogaster: hairy as a metabolic switch. *PLoS Genet*. 2008;4:e1000221.
58. Hochachka PW, Clark CM, Brown WD, et al. The brain at high altitude: hypometabolism as a defense against chronic hypoxia? *J Cereb Blood Flow Metab*. 1994;14:671-679.
59. Zhou D, Udpa N, Gersten M, et al. Experimental selection of hypoxia-tolerant *Drosophila melanogaster*. *Proc Natl Acad Sci U S A*. 2011;108:2349-2354.
60. Jha AR, Zhou D, Brown CD, et al. Shared genetic signals of hypoxia adaptation in drosophila and in high-altitude human populations. *Mol Biol Evol*. 2016;33:501-517.
61. Hartley I, Elkhoury FF, Heon Shin J, et al. Long-lasting changes in DNA methylation following short-term hypoxic exposure in primary hippocampal neuronal cultures. *PloS One*. 2013;8:e77859.
64. Udpa N, Ronen R, Zhou D, et al. Whole genome sequencing of Ethiopian highlanders reveals conserved hypoxia tolerance genes. *Genome Biol*. 2014;15(2):R36.
65. Zhou D, Udpa N, Ronen R, et al. Whole-genome sequencing uncovers the genetic basis of chronic mountain sickness in Andean highlanders. *Am J Hum Genet*. 2013;93:452-462.
66. Zhou D, Haddad GG. Genetic analysis of hypoxia tolerance and susceptibility in Drosophila and humans. *Annu Rev Genomics Hum Genet*. 2013;14:25-43.
68. Azad P, Stobdan T, Zhou D, et al. High-altitude adaptation in humans. from genomics to integrative physiology. *J Mol Med (Berl)*. 2017;95:1269-1282.

68 Evaluation of Pulmonary Function in the Neonate

Emidio Sivieri | Kevin Dysart | Soraya Abbasi | Eric C. Eichenwald

INTRODUCTION

The ability to measure lung function is essential for understanding lung growth and developmental physiology, diagnosing pathologic conditions, and assessing therapeutic interventions and management. Neonatal pulmonary function evaluation in the 21st century has achieved a remarkable level of sophistication, making use of new and emerging technologic innovations; these advances stand in stark contrast to very early lung function evaluation efforts that occurred in the 19th century with the invention of a simple spirometer to measure vital capacity.[1,2] Modern pulmonary function testing in adults and children has been used effectively as a research and clinical tool since the 1950s.[3,4] Although testing of infant pulmonary function was introduced around the same time, its practical use lagged behind, owing to technical limitations, lack of patient cooperation, difficulty with the long duration of testing in this age group, and time-consuming manual analysis methods.[5-7] In the 1980s, improvements in technology, including sensor miniaturization and computerization, led to mobile equipment systems enabling the clinician to perform routine pulmonary function testing at the bedside. In the 1990s, a new generation of infant ventilators incorporating continuous display of pulmonary function data, as well as online graphic display of respiratory waveforms, became available. Infant pulmonary function testing has thus moved from the research laboratory to the patient bedside, while efforts to reduce invasiveness and improve accuracy continue. This chapter will give an overview of the basic principles and methods for evaluation of pulmonary function in the neonate from both a physiologic and technical perspective.

PHYSIOLOGIC BACKGROUND

Each respiratory cycle is governed by a driving pressure that moves a volume of air into and out of the respiratory tract, resulting in measurable airflow and volume changes. During unaided breathing, the driving force required for initiation of inspiratory airflow is generated by contraction of the respiratory muscles, causing a downward movement of the diaphragm and outward movement of the rib cage, resulting in a transient decrease in alveolar pressure from atmospheric pressure at end-expiration to a sub-atmospheric level and peak airflow at mid-inspiration (Fig. 68.1). During expiration, relaxation of the

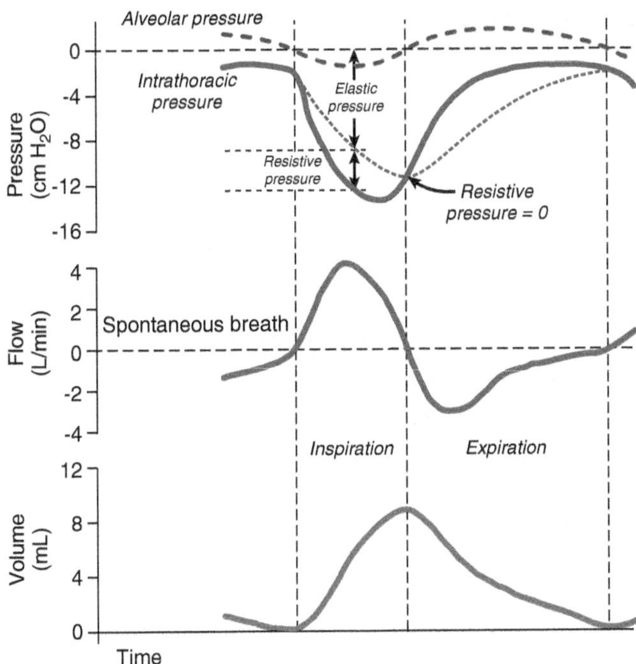

Fig. 68.1 Pressure, flow, and volume signals for a respiratory cycle during spontaneous breathing.

respiratory muscles and inward recoil of the lungs result in an increase in alveolar pressure, causing an expiratory airflow that reaches a peak near mid-expiration. At the end of expiration, alveolar pressure returns to atmospheric level, airflow returns to zero, and another respiratory cycle commences. Intrapleural pressure, however, remains sub-atmospheric throughout the breathing cycle owing to a balance of the opposing forces of lung elastic recoil and chest wall outward recoil.

During tidal spontaneous breathing in normal healthy lungs, pleural pressure decreases and increases with inspiration and expiration, respectively. The magnitude of these changes is determined by airflow and tissue resistances and by elastic forces in the lungs and chest wall, reaching a maximum at inspiratory and expiratory midpoints, as do the inspiratory and expiratory airflows.

Evaluation of pulmonary function is based on measurements of the interaction of driving pressure (*P*), volume (*V*), and airflow ($\dot{V}$). Early investigators developed an equation of motion relating the movement of gas, chest wall, and lungs in a force balance equating the total driving force for breathing to the sum of elastic, resistive, and inertial forces[8,9]:

$$P = EV + R\dot{V} + I\ddot{V} \qquad [68.1]$$

where E = elastance of the respiratory tract, or its tendency to recoil upon application of an expanding or compressing force; equivalent to the reciprocal of compliance, or $1/C$, R = frictional resistance of respiratory tract comprising both airflow and tissue resistances, and I = inertance of the respiratory tract, due to gas and tissue acceleration, usually considered negligible except at higher breathing frequencies and flow rates, V = volume, $\dot{V}$ = flow (rate of change in volume, dV/dt), and $\ddot{V}$ = acceleration (rate of change in flow = d^2V/dt^2).[10,11]

This equation describes a one-compartment linear model relating driving pressure to volume and flow and has been considered an ideal elemental equation as well as a basic principle of respiratory physiology.[12] However, it is well appreciated that the respiratory system is not a linear system and that resistance, compliance, and inertance are not constants, being dependent on lung volume, volume history, flow characteristics, and breathing frequency. The respiratory system is a complex system consisting of multiple components with differing mechanical properties. Despite its inexactness, however, and because of the complexities of dealing with nonlinear modeling, this simple linear model provides a useful framework for examining the dynamic behavior of the normal respiratory system.

INSTRUMENTATION

Instrumentation to measure the pressures, gas flows, and volumes in neonatal pulmonary function testing must meet basic physical capabilities for accuracy, precision, range, frequency response, and calibration integrity.[13,14] Computerized data collection systems also need to conform to signal processing standards, such as sufficient digitization resolution and adequate sampling rates to minimize aliasing in digitized signals and to permit the use of appropriate automated breath detection algorithms.[15,16] In addition, devices to be used in line with infant breathing circuitry also must meet minimum standards for safety, hygiene, dead space, and resistive load. Equipment specifications and methodologies have been studied extensively in an effort to achieve uniformity among research laboratories and also among the various commercially available infant pulmonary function assessment systems. To this end, comprehensive testing and measurement standards have been established and published.[17,18]

FLOW MEASUREMENT

Decades of pulmonary function research have advanced several flow measurement technologies for use in both term and preterm neonates.[19] In spontaneously breathing, nonintubated infants, airflow is measured using a flow sensor attached to a face mask, whereas in intubated infants, the flow sensor is placed in line with the endotracheal tube at the ventilator connection. A consistent objective has been to produce a smaller and lighter flow sensor having minimal dead space and airflow resistance. Some of the most commonly used flow measurement devices are described below.

PNEUMOTACHOMETERS

Pneumotachometers are flow-resistive type devices in which gas flows through a tube containing a fixed laminar flow-resistive element. The resistive element can be either a fine-mesh screen or a bundle of small capillaries (Fleish type),[20] both of which produce a pressure drop that is linearly proportional to flow so long as it is within a specified laminar flow range; higher flows give rise to turbulence and a nonlinear response.[21,22] Accordingly, pneumotachometers that have linear flow ranges appropriate to the maximum expected flow for a given subject should be selected. Condensation of water vapor on the resistive element can easily alter its resistive properties, so most pneumotachometers incorporate a heating element to prevent accumulation of moisture. The flow characteristics may also be altered by accumulation of secretions, varying gas viscosity, gas composition, and temperature.[23,24] Pressure drop across the resistive element is measured with a sensitive differential pressure transducer, which must have a linear response over the appropriate pressure range and with sufficient frequency response and phase characteristics to capture any rapid transients contained in the flow signal.[25,26] The pneumotachometer, as well as most other types of flow sensors, should be calibrated using the same connectors, adapters, and gas composition as will be used during actual measurements at the bedside.[27]

HOT WIRE ANEMOMETERS

Hot wire anemometers are flow sensors that operate on the principle that the electrical resistance of a metal is temperature dependent. In one application of this principle, the amount of electrical current needed to maintain a constant temperature in a fine heated wire suspended across an air stream is measured and related to the magnitude of the airflow; the added current increases as the airflow increases and more heat is dissipated. The response of the anemometer is inherently nonlinear, requiring linearization either in the signal conditioning circuitry or through computer signal processing. Another disadvantage is directional insensitivity, usually circumvented by the use of multiple sensor elements. Advantages are small size, good frequency response, and wide dynamic range. Furthermore, hot wire anemometers are relatively pressure-independent devices and thus are not subject to artifacts from sudden pressure transients, as are pressure-dependent devices.[28,29]

OTHER FLOW-RESISTIVE TYPE FLOW SENSORS

These include the fixed and variable orifice types and various pitot tube configurations.[30] These flow sensors also require a pressure measurement, but, unlike the laminar flow pneumotachometer, the flow-pressure relationship for these devices is nonlinear and requires hardware or software linearization. Like the anemometer, these sensors typically are smaller and lighter and thus have less dead space than the pneumotachometer. These factors, in addition to being less susceptible to moisture condensation errors, allow these devices to be more appropriate for long-term monitoring, especially as integral components of mechanical ventilators for flow control and tidal volume monitoring, as well as for breath detection and triggering.

ULTRASONIC-BEAM FLOW SENSORS

The theory behind operation of the ultrasonic-beam flow sensor is based on the fact that sound waves traveling through a medium in flux are either accelerated or slowed in accordance with the velocity of the medium. By measuring the transit time of a sound wave pulsed through a gas stream in a rigid conduit, the flow rate of the gas can be calculated. The main advantage of the ultrasonic-beam flow meter is a much lower sensitivity to changes in gas properties than is associated with a traditional pneumotachometer, but a major disadvantage of this flow meter is a larger dead-space volume.[31,32]

EMERGING TECHNOLOGIES

Two notable new classes of flow sensors are electro-optical and micro-machined sensors, both with various implementations of their basic operating principles. One variation of an electro-optical-type sensor is based on measurement of the deflection of a light beam emitted from a short length of optical fiber suspended in an air stream.[33] Micro-electro-mechanical systems-type sensors integrate micro-machining technology with micro-electronics and are based on measurements of mechanical deflection, thermal effects, or a combination of both. An example of a mechanical-type sensor utilizes a micro-cantilever machined on a silicon chip. Bending or vibration of the cantilever in a flow stream causes a change in a piezo-resistive element, which is transduced into an electrical output.[34] In addition to the low cost of manufacturing, advantages of these newer sensors are small size, low dead-space volume, fast response, wide dynamic range, and negligible resistive loading.

VOLUME MEASUREMENT AS DERIVED FROM A FLOW SIGNAL

When respiratory airflow is measured directly at the airway opening using a flow sensor, volume change in the lungs may be derived by integration of the flow signal over time, which is simply the area under the scalar flow waveform. With computerized signal processing, electronic integration of the flow signal has been largely replaced by digital integration. Sign reversals in the flow signal are used to detect inspiratory and expiratory endpoints, which are then used to identify individual breaths. Typically, the resultant tidal volume waveform will have slightly unequal inspiratory and expiratory portions owing to differences in inspired versus expired conditions in gas composition, water vapor, temperature, and viscosity. For these and other reasons, most volume signal conditioning routines correct for any baseline drift by incorporating an automatic return to zero at end-expiration. Differences in inspiratory and expiratory tidal volumes larger than 10%, however, may be indicative of airflow leakage around the endotracheal tube or face mask. Large baseline drifts may also indicate faulty flow sensor readings, which may be due to factors such as water vapor condensation or buildup of secretions.

INDIRECT VOLUME MEASUREMENTS

Indirect methods for measuring volume change, without connection to the airway opening, have also been implemented. These are useful, for example, when an infant is receiving non-invasive forms of respiratory support such as nasal continuous positive airway pressure (nCPAP) or heated and humidified high flow nasal cannula (HFNC). In these instances, the requirement of a nasal interface to apply the therapy precludes use of a traditional direct airflow sensor connected to a face mask. As a workaround, alternative techniques using measurements at the body surface instead of at the airway opening may be used to derive not only tidal volume but also various other indices of respiratory function. Advantages include elimination of face mask and flow sensor dead space and airflow resistance, which affect the actual parameters being measured.[35] These indirect measurement devices also have the advantage of allowing noninvasive continuous monitoring without alterations in the breathing pattern that occur with use of face masks or inline flow sensors, and are therefore especially useful for undisturbed measurements in spontaneously breathing and sleeping infants.[36,37] Some of these technologies are described below.

RESPIRATORY INDUCTANCE PLETHYSMOGRAPHY

Respiratory inductance plethysmography (RIP) was first developed in the early 1980s and has been commonly used for chest wall motion analysis and for monitoring breathing in sleep apnea studies, as well as for non-invasive spirometry.[38] The basic RIP apparatus consists of sinusoidally arranged thin wires embedded in two soft elastic bands, which are placed around the rib cage and abdomen as shown in Fig. 68.2. As a patient breathes and the bands expand and retract, changes in the magnetic field created by a low-level high-frequency current in the coils cause changes in their self-inductance. It follows that these inductance changes are proportional to changes in the cross-sectional areas circumscribed by the bands. The resulting small changes in frequency are transduced into electrical signals, which may then be recorded.[39] Rib cage (RC) and abdominal (ABD) excursions are measured separately and the summation of these two signals (SUM) is approximately proportional to the net pulmonary tidal volume change.

Calibration of the SUM signal to true tidal volume can be accomplished using one of several techniques that have been developed for this purpose by various investigators.[40,41] In general, all such calibration schemes require a period of restful breathing to generate separate RC and ABD weighting factors to account for their different contributions to the SUM. A period of breathing through a calibrated face mask-attached flow sensor, such as a pneumotachometer, is then used to convert the final corrected SUM signal to known volume changes and that can then be converted to flow through mathematic differentiation. Once calibrated, maintaining consistent accuracy is highly dependent on maintaining both body position and prevention of band slippage.

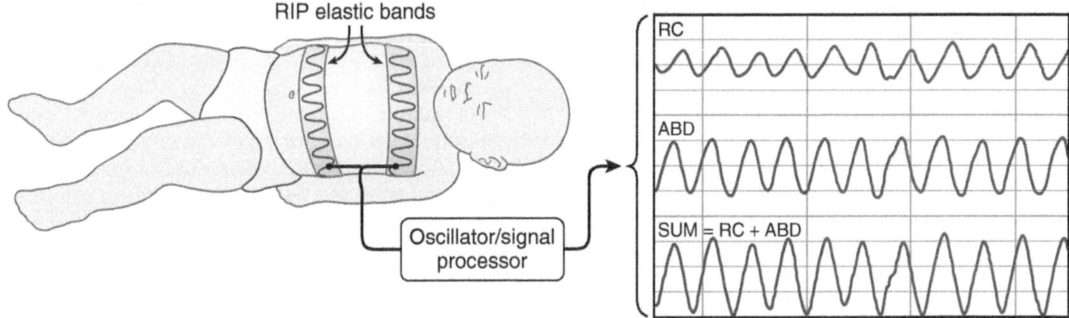

Fig. 68.2 Typical respiratory inductance plethysmography *(RIP)* setup showing the rib cage *(RC)* and abdominal *(ABD)* bands. Scalar display showing the summated signal *(SUM)* tracing.

Nonetheless, the RIP technique, when accurately calibrated and used in place of a mask-attached flow sensor, has been used to measure undisturbed tidal volume in respiratory assessment studies for bronchopulmonary dysplasia in VLBW premature infants[42] and in infants receiving non-invasive respiratory support.[43] Moreover, calibrated RIP has also been shown to yield clinically acceptable pulmonary mechanics measurements in infants on nCPAP or HFNC.[44–46] RIP technology has gone through several iterations in the last decades, the most recent being a wireless system (PneuRIP) that displays and records real-time measurements of several work of breathing and breathing efficiency indices (as described later in this chapter) on a small hand-held display.[47,48]

ELECTROMAGNETIC INDUCTANCE PLETHYSMOGRAPHY

Electromagnetic inductance plethysmography (EIP) is a novel technology that measures changes in an electromagnetic field induced in coils carrying a weak high-frequency current and embedded in an elastic vest encircling the infant's thorax and abdomen. An antenna positioned above the infant detects magnetic field changes that are proportional to cross-sectional respiratory volume changes from the chest and abdomen.[49,50] Advantages are subject-independent calibration and continuous undisturbed display of separate rib cage and abdominal volume excursions without the need for a face mask and flow sensor. Accuracy is dependent on proper fit of the elastic vest and the requirement for the patient to remain in a supine position with minimal hip flexion. In addition, the EIP system must be positioned to avoid nearby electromagnetic interference. EIP has been used successfully for infant spirometry as well as for measuring tidal breathing parameters with adequate clinical accuracy in term and preterm infants.[51]

OPTOELECTRONIC PLETHYSMOGRAPHY

Optoelectronic plethysmography (OEP) is a technically sophisticated technology that requires powerful computer software to process multi-camera video images from a grid-array of reflective markers strategically placed on an infant's thoracoabdominal surface. Markers are placed on both anterior and lateral surfaces. The number of markers can vary from 24 for neonates up to 89 markers for adults; accuracy increases as a function of the number of markers used. Respiratory volume is estimated by measuring the three-dimensional position of each marker using 4, 6, or 8 special video cameras and processing the signals through a motion analyzer.[52,53] The system measures volumes for three thoracoabdominal compartments, where the rib cage compartment is partitioned into pulmonary rib cage (RC_p) and abdominal (RC_{abd}) volumes in addition to the abdominal volume (ABD). These are further partitioned into left- and right-side measurements, or hemithoraxes. Synchrony and timing parameters between the various compartments can then be further analyzed separately. Studies with term and preterm infants have demonstrated accurate measurements of tidal volume as validated against pneumotachometry and showing good agreement.

Advantages of the OEP technique include its non-invasiveness and the ability for continuous uninterrupted monitoring and not requiring pre-calibration. In contrast to other indirect technologies, OEP is able to estimate not only tidal volume but also the total absolute thoracoabdominal as well as the various separate component volumes. The main disadvantages are the complex and cumbersome bedside instrumentation and the need for a large number of markers on an exposed skin surface, which also need to be precisely positioned in order to ensure accuracy. Nonetheless, OEP is a promising new technology for both research and clinical application enabling sophisticated and highly detailed measurements of a three-compartment model and their interaction.

STRUCTURED LIGHT PLETHYSMOGRAPHY

Structured light plethysmography (SLP) is a more recently developed three-dimensional optical, non-contact, technology. As with OEP, computer vision and processing is used to generate a three-dimensional reconstruction of the thoracoabdominal surfaces. But instead of tracking markers placed on the body surface, SLP uses a checkerboard grid light pattern that is projected onto the patient's frontal thoracoabdominal surface.[54] As the patient breathes, movement of distinct points in the light pattern are tracked by two cameras and image processing algorithms are used to display a three dimensional spatial image of the thoracoabdominal surface displacement. The system can differentiate rib cage and abdominal volume changes as well as left and right side hemithoraxes over time. The current state of SLP technology is not yet configured to output absolute volume measurements and thus the system does not require calibration prior to use. As with most non-invasive methodologies, accuracy is motion- and position-sensitive, requiring some patient cooperation. Therefore SLP has been used chiefly for measurements of tidal breathing timing indices in children and adults, but recent studies using SLP for measurements on neonates have also demonstrated promising results.[55] Integration of the light projector, cameras, and computer into a stand-alone unit has allowed a commercially available version of this device to be suitable for cordless bedside measurements.[56]

ELECTRICAL IMPEDANCE TOMOGRAPHY

Electrical impedance tomography (EIT) is an advanced imaging technology that measures the bioelectrical impedance within the thorax. Electrical conductivity varies for different materials such as air, blood, and tissues, with air having much less conductivity than the surrounding fluids and tissues. It follows that measurement of the impedance in a transthoracic cross-sectional slice using a series of surface electrodes can provide a two-dimensional image of the impedance distribution in the cross-section. Implementing this principle, EIT is used to image the pulmonary ventilation distribution over time by measuring impedance across sequentially alternating pairs of electrodes placed circumferentially across a given transthoracic cross-section.[57,58] This process may be performed both statically and dynamically to monitor the breath-by-breath ventilation distribution and regional lung perfusion as a function of time. An electrode belt of as many as 16 electrodes must be placed completely around the thorax for these measurements.

EECTRICAL IMPEDANCE SEGMENTOGRAPHY

A closely related technology developed into a commercially available device is electrical impedance segmentography (EIS).[59] EIS measures impedance changes in the four thoracic quadrants encompassing the upper left, upper right, lower left, and lower right pulmonary regions (Fig. 68.3). Four ventral and four dorsal current collection electrodes are placed in opposition across each of the four thoracic quadrants and a fifth ventral and dorsal current injection electrode is placed centrally along the sternum. A real-time computer display of the relative percent ventilation distribution in each quadrant is provided along with a scalar display of the tidal impedance changes for each breath.An animal study has demonstrated accurate calibration of tidal impedance to known pneumotachometer tidal volumes in milliliters, but this ability has not been repeated in infants. EIT and EIS have demonstrated usefulness in evaluating efficacy of respiratory support strategies, detection of pneumothoraxes, pulmonary recruitment maneuvers, and the study of ventilation inhomogeneity.[60–63] Limitations of this technology include low spatial resolution and effects of electrode placement difficulty on accuracy.

LUNG VOLUMES

DEFINITIONS

The components of lung volumes and capacities are illustrated in Fig. 68.4. The classical definitions of relevance for lung function testing in neonates are as follows:

Tidal volume (V_T): Tidal volume is defined as the volume of gas entering and leaving the respiratory tract with each breath. This is a dynamic measurement and varies with the activity of the baby. For infants, tidal volume is usually expressed in units of mL.

Minute volume: The total volume of gas expired over a period of 1 minute. Accurate measurement of V_T (no leak around endotracheal tube or face mask) and respiratory frequency (f_R) allows estimation of minute ventilation as the product: $V_T f_R$, and is usually expressed in units of L/min, or normalized for body weight as (L/min)/kg.

Functional residual capacity (FRC): Volume of air in the lungs at the end of expiration of a normal, resting tidal volume. Lung volume at FRC is maintained by the opposing forces of lung elastic recoil and chest wall outward recoil.

Residual volume: Volume of air remaining in the respiratory system at the end of a maximum possible expiration.

Thoracic gas volume (TGV): The total amount of gas in the lung at end expiration, irrespective of whether or not the gas is in communication with the airways. In healthy infants without air trapping, FRC is equivalent to TGV.

Expiratory reserve volume: Volume of air that is the difference between FRC and residual volume.

Total lung capacity: Volume of air that is in the respiratory system at the end of a maximum possible inspiration.

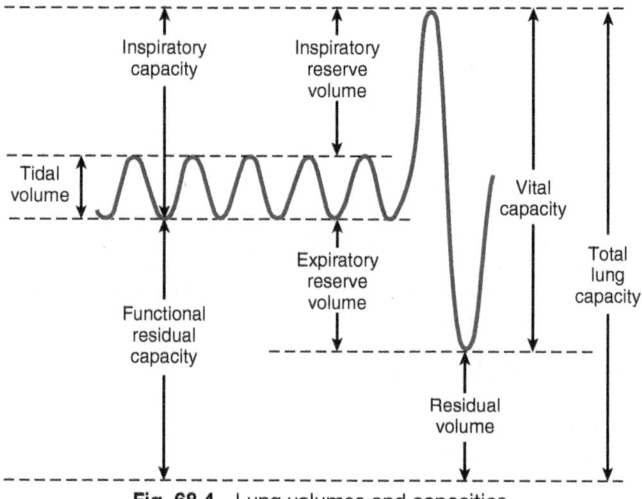

Fig. 68.4 Lung volumes and capacities.

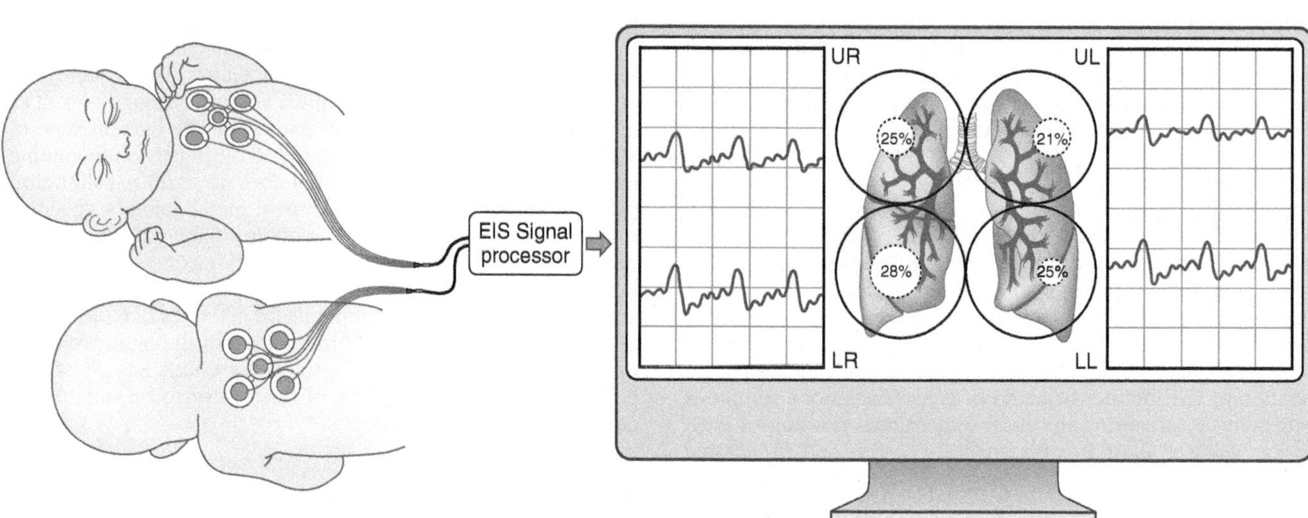

Fig. 68.3 Electrical impedance segmentography *(EIS)* system showing ventral and dorsal electrode placement and a simplified computer display showing breath-by-breath impedance changes as both scalar traces and as percentage ventilation relative to a baseline starting value in the four pulmonary quadrants of the thorax. (Angelie EIS system, EMS Biomedical, Korneuburg, Austria.)

FUNCTIONAL RESIDUAL CAPACITY MEASUREMENT BY PLETHYSMOGRAPHY

Whole-body plethysmography, first described by DuBois and colleagues in 1956, has been a standard modality for measurement of thoracic lung volume for many years.[64-66] From Boyle's law, it is known that under isothermal conditions, the gas pressure in a closed rigid chamber is inversely proportional to the gas volume, such that for initial and final conditions 1 and 2, respectively,

$$P_1 V_1 = P_2 V_2 \qquad [68.2]$$

For an infant placed in a rigid-body plethysmograph and breathing against a momentarily occluded airway,

$$P_1 V_1 = (P_1 + \Delta P)(V_1 + \Delta V) \qquad [68.3]$$

where P_1 is the pre-occlusion mouth pressure (which is the barometric pressure), V_1 is the initial lung volume, and ΔP and ΔV are the resultant changes in pressure and volume from respiratory efforts against the occlusion. For this measurement, the infant breathes through a face mask incorporating a remotely controlled shutter, a pneumotachometer to record flow, and a port for recording mouth pressure. When the occlusion is triggered at the end of a resting expiration, lung volume is at FRC (represented by V_1), and because no airflow is present, alveolar pressure equals barometric pressure. As the infant breathes against the closed shutter, alveolar pressure changes owing to alternating gas compression and decompression are recorded, as are the concomitant changes in plethysmograph pressure, which are directly proportional to changes in alveolar volume. With appropriate corrections for temperature drift and apparatus dead space, as well as water vapor and body temperature and pressure, saturated (BPTS), Boyle's law can be applied to solve for FRC as given by V_1.

In contrast to tracer gas techniques, which measure only those volumes in communication with airways undergoing tidal ventilation, plethysmography measures total TGV, including trapped air spaces in occluded airways. For this reason, FRC by plethysmography is usually denoted as FRC_{pleth}.

Although several commercial infant body-box systems are now available, whole-body plethysmography is not a practical technique for routine measurements in newborn infants in the intensive care nursery, particularly in infants receiving assisted ventilation. However, despite the complexities involved, the plethysmographic method has the advantage of allowing rapid repeat measurements within a period of only a few minutes.

FUNCTIONAL RESIDUAL CAPACITY BY CLOSED-CIRCUIT HELIUM DILUTION METHOD

For measurement of FRC by helium dilution, the infant's airway is connected to a closed breathing circuit containing a small amount of helium at a known concentration. After connection at end-expiration, as the infant breathes from the closed system, the helium concentration gradually equilibrates to a lower value due to addition of the infant's FRC.[67] Equilibration usually is complete within 45 to 60 seconds. By knowing the initial breathing circuit volume (V_i) and the initial and final helium concentrations from before and after equilibration (C_i and C_f), FRC may be calculated from a mass balance on helium,

$$V_i C_i = (V_a + \mathrm{FRC})\, C_f \qquad [68.4]$$

$$FRC_{He} = V_i C_i / C_f - V_a \qquad [68.5]$$

where V_a includes the initial system volume (V_i) plus volume changes resulting from the patient's oxygen consumption, carbon dioxide production, and the known dead space in the patient connection. The infant's oxygen consumption may be compensated for by either continuous monitoring of the breathing circuit volume and gradually adding oxygen to maintain a constant level during rebreathing, or by adding the infant's estimated oxygen consumption to the final system volume. Exhaled carbon dioxide is continuously scrubbed from the circuit through an absorbent. In variations of the technique, the final system volume of the breathing circuit is measured directly in a large collection reservoir.[68] Modifications of this technique have been used to measure FRC in mechanically ventilated infants using a "bag-in-box" system.[69-71]

TECHNICAL LIMITATIONS

Sick infants with airway disease and poor distribution of ventilation have prolonged equilibration time and require long periods of rebreathing, which may lead to hypoxia and hypercapnia. Leaks around the endotracheal tube or face mask also are a frequent source of error, and methods have been developed that attempt to correct for this error.[72] To achieve maximum helium measurement accuracy and to maximize the dilution effect, the total volume of the breathing circuit should be close to the approximate infant FRC; this may be impractical, however, owing to the small lung volumes in premature and small infants. In addition, helium analyzers are not insensitive to other ventilatory gases, thereby potentially affecting measurement accuracy.

FUNCTIONAL RESIDUAL CAPACITY MEASUREMENT BY NITROGEN WASHOUT

FRC also can be determined by measurement of the total expired nitrogen "washed out" of the lungs while the infant breathes either 100% oxygen or an oxygen-helium mixture (heliox). The basic principle is described by the mass balance equation,

$$FRC_{N_2} = V_{N_2} / (C_{iN_2} - C_{fN_2}) \qquad [68.6]$$

where V_{N_2} is the total volume of nitrogen washed out of the lungs and C_{iN_2} and C_{fN_2} are the pre-washout and post-washout alveolar nitrogen fractional concentrations assumed to be 0.79 and 0.0, respectively. The value V_{N_2} must be obtained by measuring the nitrogen concentration of the entire expired volume, making this method impractical because the entire expired washout volume must be collected and measured. Alternatively, in a technique known as the ***multiple-breath nitrogen washout method,*** V_{N_2} may be theoretically calculated from the integration of the product of instantaneous flow ($\dot{V}$) and the instantaneous nitrogen concentration (C_{N_2}) signals over time,

$$V_{N_2} = \int \dot{V}(t) C_{N_2}(t)\, dt \qquad [68.7]$$

This may be accomplished by passing the expired gas stream through a pneumotachometer and a rapid-response nitrogen analyzer. However, care must be taken to correct the flow for varying viscosity, temperature, and gas composition; most importantly, any phase lag between the flow and nitrogen concentration signals must be carefully synchronized.[73] Alternatively, to circumvent these complexities, V_{N_2} may instead be measured using a much-simplified method in which the infant breathes from a constant bias flow of 100% oxygen (or heliox mixture).[74] The expired gas is added to the bias flow, which is passed through a mixing chamber to produce an averaged nitrogen washout curve wherein the increase in flow during expiration is assumed to be equal to the decrease in flow during inspiration.[75] Thus the integrated nitrogen concentration signal is simply multiplied by the averaged bias flow ($\dot{V}$), which is treated as a constant in the equation,

$$V_{N_2} = \dot{V} \int C_{N_2}(t)\, dt \qquad [68.8]$$

The nitrogen washout technique has been widely implemented. When compared with the helium dilution technique, it was found to produce comparable estimates of FRC in infants and very young children.[76,77] When compared with FRC determined by whole-body plethysmography in paired measurements, nitrogen washout FRC was consistently lower, the difference being larger for infants with BPD than for healthy infants.[78,79] This difference, previously attributed mainly to trapped gases in obstructed airways, recently has been reevaluated as possibly also attributable to methodologic factors.[80] The nitrogen washout technique also has been adapted for application in mechanically ventilated infants through use of a secondary washout ventilator.[81,82]

TECHNICAL LIMITATIONS

Breathing oxygen at a high concentration may result in hyperoxia or absorption atelectasis in areas of lung with low ventilation. To circumvent this problem, heliox has been used in place of 100% oxygen with favorable results.[83] Lastly, as with the helium dilution method, the nitrogen washout technique is prone to gas leakage errors.

FUNCTIONAL RESIDUAL CAPACITY BY SULFUR HEXAFLUORIDE WASHOUT

An alternative washout technique that uses SF_6 as the tracer gas can be used with either spontaneously breathing or ventilated infants on high oxygen concentrations.[84,85] For this technique, an SF_6 dispenser is connected to the inspiratory portion of the breathing circuit, and a small amount of the inert gas SF_6 is washed into the lungs until a fixed alveolar level (usually <5%) is reached. The SF_6 dispenser is then switched off to initiate a washout period. A rapid-response SF_6 sensor in series with a flow sensor enables near-simultaneous recording of both signals for calculation of the cumulative expired volume of SF_6. In a manner similar to the multiple-breath nitrogen washout method, FRC is determined from the breath-by-breath integration of the product of flow and SF_6 concentration. In contrast to the nitrogen washout method, however, ventilator and FiO_2 settings need not be altered, no mixing chamber is needed, and flow sensor accuracy is not compromised by significant changes in gas composition during the testing procedure. Moreover, unlike with the bias-flow nitrogen washout method, infants on very high FiO_2 levels may be studied because oxygen levels up to 100%, as well as other ventilatory gases, have been shown to have negligible effect on SF_6 analyzer accuracy.[86] In commercially available systems, the SF_6 analyzer–flow sensor combination has been replaced by an ultrasonic flow meter capable of providing simultaneous measurements of airflow and SF_6 concentration in a single unit.[87,88] The SF_6 washout method, as well as the nitrogen multiple-breath washout method, may also be used for determination of ventilation distribution[89] and for estimation of trapped gas.[90]

RESPIRATORY MECHANICS

DEFINITIONS

COMPLIANCE

Lungs, airways, and thorax are elastic; these tissues stretch due to changes in pressure during inspiration. When the pressure change ceases, the tissues return or recoil to their resting positions. The compliance of a closed elastic structure is defined as the change in volume resulting from a unit change in pressure, or $\Delta V/\Delta P$, and usually expressed in units of mL/kPa or mL/cm H_2O.

Static compliance: Static compliance is an accurate determinant of lung elastic properties only. It measures the change in volume for a given pressure during static, non-flow conditions. Measurement of the systematic step changes in both pressure and volume during inflation and deflation allows a static pressure-volume curve of the lungs to be plotted. A sufficient equilibration period is required to ensure that the actual static pressure change is recorded. The curves that the lungs follow during inflation and deflation are different and are also influenced by surface tension and viscoelastic tissue resistances. This physical property of the lungs is known as *hysteresis.*

Pulmonary compliance (C_L): Compliance of the lung only, as determined from measurement of transpulmonary pressure (P_{tp}), that is, the difference between pleural and alveolar pressures. Under static conditions alveolar pressure is equivalent to airway pressure. Pleural pressure may be estimated from measurement of esophageal pressure.

Dynamic lung compliance ($C_{L,dyn}$): Dynamic compliance is the determination of the change in volume and pressure during the respiratory cycle while there is airflow, during either spontaneous breathing or mechanical ventilation, and is predominantly influenced by breathing frequency. During rapid breathing, there may not be sufficient equilibration time to determine the actual change in pressure accurately.

Respiratory system compliance (C_{rs}): Volume change of the entire respiratory system as related to the total driving pressure across the lungs and chest wall. During mechanical ventilation, the driving pressure is measured at the airway opening.

Chest wall compliance (C_{cw}): Volume change related to the pressure across the chest wall, or transthoracic pressure. Transthoracic pressure may be measured as the difference between airway opening and pleural pressure. Alternatively, if the total compliance and lung compliance are known, the following relationship may be used to calculate chest wall compliance: total respiratory system elastance = elastance of the lungs + elastance of the chest wall, or in terms of compliances: $1/C_{rs} = 1/C_L + 1/C_{cw}$.

Specific compliance (sC): Compliance normalized to lung volume, usually at FRC, or C/FRC expressed as (mL/kPa)/L or (mL/cm H_2O)/L. Alternatively, if FRC is unknown, compliance may also be expressed relative to body weight with units of (mL/kPa)/kg or (mL/cm H_2O)/kg.

RESISTANCE

Resistance is a frictional phenomenon that is due to the motion of both respiratory gases and tissues; thus resistance is absent during static respiratory conditions. Tissue resistance is due to the viscoelastic properties of biologic tissues during respiratory movements. Airflow resistance is defined as the pressure differential associated with a unit of flow of a gas through a conduit (i.e., resistance = $P/\dot{V}$), and is dependent on the length and diameter of the conduit and the density and viscosity of the gas. The magnitude of airflow resistance is also dependent on the fluid dynamics of the air stream—for example, turbulent airflow will produce a greater resistance than laminar airflow. Respiratory airflow requires a driving pressure generated by changes in alveolar pressure relative to the pressure at the airway opening or mouth. When alveolar pressure is less than or greater than atmospheric pressure, air flows into or out of the lungs accordingly, and the magnitude of this airflow is influenced by resistance. Resistance is usually expressed in units of kPa/(L/s) or cm H_2O/(L/s).

Total resistance (R_{rs}): The combined airway, lung tissue, and chest wall resistance of the respiratory system.

Pulmonary resistance (R_L): Resistance calculated using the pressure difference across the lung only, that is, transpulmonary pressure divided by the resultant airflow.

Airway resistance (R_{aw}): Resistance of the airway alone, equal to the pressure gradient between alveolar and atmospheric pressure divided by the resulting airflow. Airway resistance may be responsible for as much as 80% of the total pulmonary resistance in a normal lung and is influenced by the velocity and pattern of airflow, geometry of the airways, and the density or viscosity of the gas itself. Airway resistance may be measured by plethysmography, typically in conjunction with FRC_{pleth} measurements using similar instrumentation.[66]

Tissue frictional resistance normally accounts for approximately 20% of the pulmonary resistance and is influenced by the configuration of the chest wall and the lung, as well as by the fluid content of the pulmonary tissue. Inertial resistance, or inertance, which is less than 1% of pulmonary resistance, usually is more dependent on the breathing frequency and the density of the gas and typically is ignored within the normal range of breathing frequencies and flow rates.[10,11]

MEASUREMENT OF RESPIRATORY MECHANICS

DYNAMIC PULMONARY MECHANICS

Pulmonary mechanics are calculated from measurements of transpulmonary pressure, flow, and volume changes throughout the respiratory cycle. These are dynamic measurements obtained during either spontaneous breathing or mechanical ventilation. Airflow and volume are measured by pneumotachometry or other flow sensor technology, as described previously. Pleural pressure can be estimated from esophageal pressure[91] measured by a pressure transducer connected to either an air-filled balloon[92] or a fluid-filled catheter,[93] or by a microtransducer-tipped catheter.[94] The accuracy of the esophageal pressure measurement must be assessed by an occlusion test.[95] This is a brief, two- or three-breath airway occlusion performed either manually, or by an occlusion valve, preferably at end-inspiration. In the absence of airflow during the occlusion, pleural pressure changes produce equal changes in alveolar pressure, which can be measured directly at the airway opening (ΔP_{ao}) and compared to the simultaneously measured esophageal pressure changes (ΔP_{esoph}). Ideally, esophageal pressure will be an accurate measure of pleural pressure if the ratio $\Delta P_{esoph}/\Delta P_{ao}$ is equal to 1.0; acceptable values are 1.00 ± 0.05. In addition, it is essential that the P_{esoph} transducer be perfectly matched in phase and frequency response with the flow sensor transducer, as even small differences in timing can have a significant effect on accuracy of the calculated pulmonary mechanics variables.

The calculations of dynamic compliance and resistance are based on the assumption of the simplified, single-compartment linear model in which the transpulmonary pressure is equal to the sum of the elastic and resistive pressures and in which the inertance term is assumed negligible,

$$P_{tp} = P_{elastic} + P_{resistive} + k \quad [68.9]$$

$$P_{tp} = V/C + R\dot{V} + k \quad [68.10]$$

where the constants C and R may be evaluated manually or by any of several computerized techniques. The constant term, k, must be included to account for any residual end-expiratory transpulmonary pressure.

The Mead-Whittenberger Method

Before computer-aided analysis, the Mead-Whittenberger analysis method was a commonly used graphical procedure for calculating pulmonary mechanics from scalar tracings of pressure, flow, and volume signals as shown in Fig. 68.5.[3] Because there is no airflow at the end-inspiratory and end-expiratory points of the breathing cycle, there are no flow-resistive losses at these points, and the pleural pressure is dependent solely on elastic forces. Hence, between the zero-flow points we can obtain the following,

$$\Delta P_{tp} = \Delta P_{elastic} = V_T/C \quad [68.11]$$

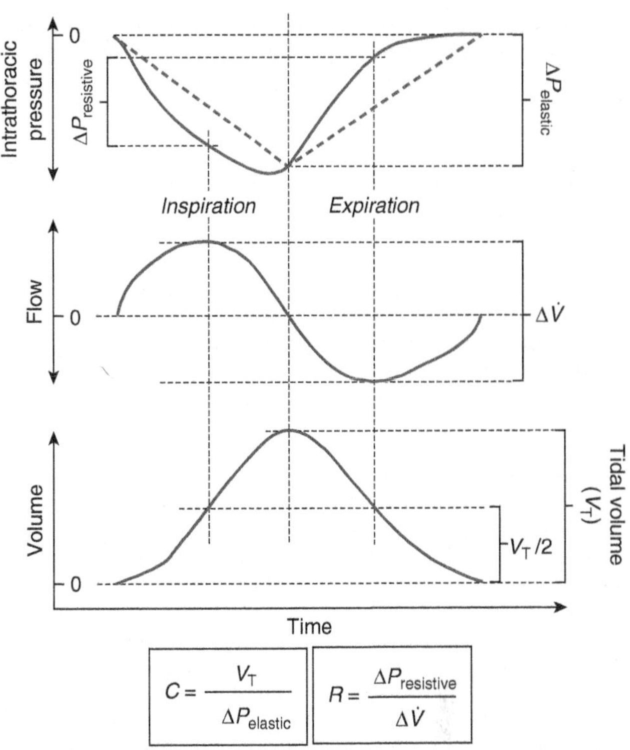

Fig. 68.5 Determination of pulmonary mechanics by analysis of intrathoracic pressure *(P)*, flow *($\dot{V}$)*, and volume *(V)* signals using the Mead-Whittenberger method. Measurements made during spontaneous respiration.

$$C = V_T/\Delta P_{elastic} \quad [68.12]$$

Similarly, R_L is calculated from the resistive pressure change ($\Delta P_{resistive}$) and difference in flow ($\Delta \dot{V}$) taken between the inspiratory and expiratory mid-isovolume flow points ($V_T/2$), where the inspiratory elastic recoil pressure is assumed to equal expiratory recoil pressure. Therefore the difference between mid-inspiratory and mix-expiratory flows is attributable only to the difference between mid-inspiratory and mix-expiratory pressures, or net resistive pressure difference. Then the ratio of these differences is

$$R_L = \Delta P_{resistive}/\Delta \dot{V} \quad [68.13]$$

Linear Regression Methods

In contrast to the traditional manual methods, in which calculations are based on a few discrete points in the respiratory cycle and for only a few breaths (at best), high-speed and high-resolution computerized data recording allows use of linear regression techniques that make use of all of the sampled data points in each breath, as well as for many breaths at once. Using multiple linear regression analysis, the equation $P_{tp} = V/C + R\dot{V}$ is solved for unique values of the coefficients C and R, which minimizes the mean squared error between the measured pressure and calculated pressure, resulting in the best fit of the linear model to the measured variables of pressure, flow, and volume.[96] A multiple correlation coefficient is also generated to provide an index of the goodness of fit to the model. Breaths with a poor correlation ($r^2 < 0.95$) are discarded from the final analysis. Because all breath data points are used, this method may also be applied to selected segments of a breath to allow separate calculation of inspiratory, expiratory, or whole-breath values of C and R.

The assumption of a simple linear lung model with constant coefficients is often not applicable, especially in very premature infants with a highly compliant chest wall, infants with severe lung disease, or infants on ventilatory support whose tidal breaths reside on nonlinear portions of the sigmoidal volume-pressure curve. Methods have been developed that attempt to analyze more accurately nonlinear pulmonary mechanics, for example by including a volume-dependent compliance term in the equation of motion[97,98] or by separately calculating compliance over the final 20% of inspired volume (C_{20}), where lung overdistension is most likely to occur. The C_{20} value is normalized to the total inspiratory compliance and expressed as the ratio C_{20}/C.[99]

Technical Considerations. Reliable esophageal pressure measurement by esophageal balloon catheter depends on proper size, positioning, and inflation of the balloon. Water-filled catheters need to be free of gas bubbles and have no accumulation of secretions at the tip. Placement of catheters may generate peristalsis, resulting in an initial pressure drift. Because measured esophageal pressure reflects pleural pressure only at a specific location, its accuracy depends on assuming that the pressure change at the site represents mean pleural pressure changes.[100] Altered patterns of inspiratory muscle contraction or esophageal muscle tone and distortion of the chest wall may potentially result in uneven pleural pressure distribution.[101]

Accuracy of measurements is also dependent on body position. Measurements should be done with the patient in supine neutral head position and preferably during quiet sleep with a regular breathing pattern. Flexion or extension of the neck in small infants can affect the airflow resistance.[102] Feeding volume also may affect the measurements and should be standardized in repeated studies[103] In mechanically ventilated infants, the ventilatory support should be maintained during sequential studies to prevent shifting of the tidal volume to a different portion of the volume-pressure curve.

Commercially available equipment should be tested with a calibrated lung simulator before clinical use to ensure accuracy at the expected infant tidal volumes and frequencies.[17] Furthermore, voluminous results of computerized analysis should be interpreted with caution, avoiding over-reliance on machine scoring of breaths. High correlation coefficients can be misleading, and visual inspection is still vital in identifying breaths with obvious anomalies and other signal artifacts. Experience in assessing test results, taking into account measurement conditions and the state of the infant during testing, is important.

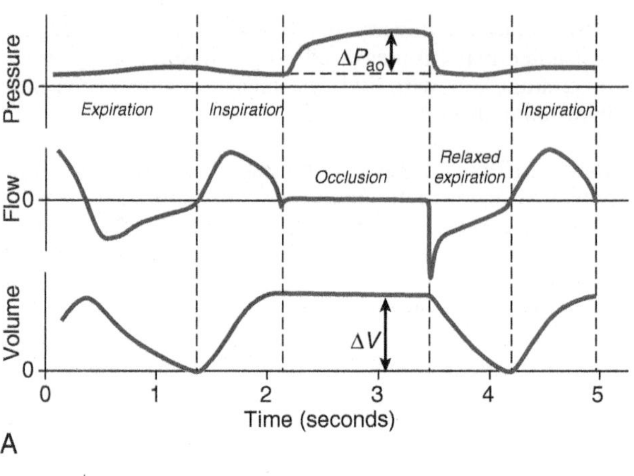

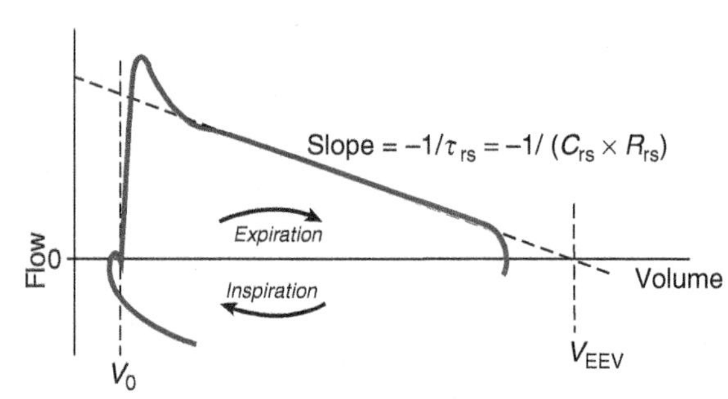

Fig. 68.6 Passive respiratory mechanics determined using the single occlusion technique (SOT). (A) Scalar tracing showing an end-inspiratory occlusion maneuver. ΔP_{ao}, Elastic recoil pressure plateau measured at the airway opening; ΔV, occluded volume difference. (B) Flow-volume curve demonstrating determination of respiratory system time constant (τ_{rs}) from the slope of relaxed expiration portion. V_{EEV}, Elastic equilibrium volume; V_0, volume at start of occlusion.

PASSIVE RESPIRATORY MECHANICS: THE OCCLUSION TECHNIQUES

Passive occlusion techniques constitute a relatively noninvasive method for determining total respiratory system compliance (C_{rs}), resistance (R_{rs}), and time constant (τ_{rs}) and therefore do not require measurement of esophageal pressure. These passive techniques rely on the Hering-Breuer inflation reflex[104] to relax both the inspiratory and expiratory respiratory muscles during an expiratory occlusion. Under the resultant condition of complete expiratory relaxation, driving pressure is zero, and the airway opening pressure comes into equilibrium with alveolar pressure.[105]

SINGLE-BREATH OCCLUSION TECHNIQUE

A single end-inspiratory occlusion (Fig. 68.6A) is performed to invoke the Hering-Breuer inflation reflex to induce relaxation of the respiratory muscles during both the occlusion and the post-occlusion passive expiration. Elastic recoil pressure is measured during the occlusion, and a passive flow-volume loop is recorded during the post-occlusion relaxed expiration (see Fig. 68.6B). The negative reciprocal of the slope of the linear portion of the expiratory flow-volume relationship gives the passive expiratory time constant ($\tau_{rs} = C_{rs}R_{rs}$). Extrapolation of this line to the zero flow point, that is, the elastic equilibrium volume (V_{EEV}), and to the volume at start of occlusion (V_0), allows estimation of the occluded volume above the V_{EEV}. Knowing the relaxed plateau pressure, P_{ao}, during zero flow allows estimation of compliance as $C_{rs} = (V_0 - V_{EEV})/P_{ao}$ and thus resistance as $R_{rs} = \tau_{rs}/C_{rs}$.

MULTIPLE OCCLUSION TECHNIQUE

A series of brief expiratory airway occlusions are performed on multiple spontaneous breaths. During each occlusion, the elastic recoil pressure measured at the airway opening (P_{ao}) reaches a plateau as it equilibrates with alveolar pressure (Fig. 68.7). An occlusion is repeated at each of several different volume points on separate breaths and over the first two thirds of expiration. A volume-versus-pressure plot is constructed from each of the resulting occluded ΔV and ΔP_{ao} measurement pairs. The slope of the linear regression line through these points is used to calculate $C_{rs} = \Delta V/\Delta P_{ao}$.

AIRWAY RESISTANCE BY WHOLE-BODY PLETHYSMOGRAPHY

The plethysmographic technique, described above for measuring FRC_{pleth}, may also be used for simultaneous measurements of R_{aw} with proper BPTS conditioning of the respired gas. The method was first described by DuBois and colleagues in 1955 for use in adults,[106] was soon after adapted to infants by Polgar in 1961,[107] and a more detailed methodology of the refined

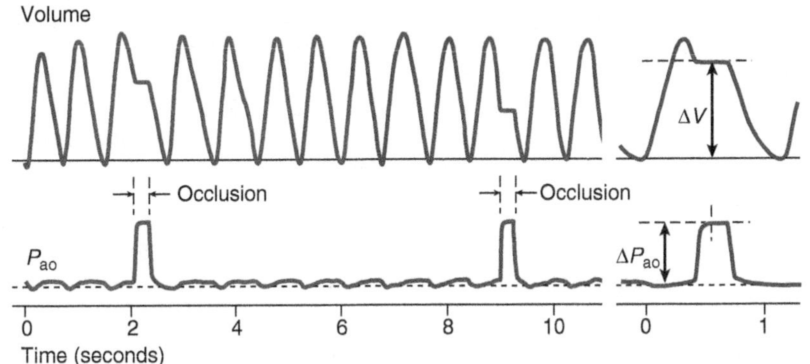

Fig. 68.7 Passive respiratory mechanics using the multiple occlusion technique (MOT). ΔP_{ao}, Airway opening pressure equilibrated with alveolar pressure during an occlusion; ΔV, plateaued volume difference during the occlusion.

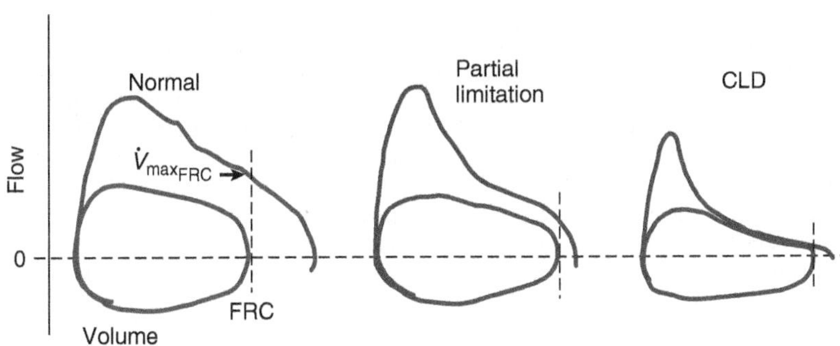

Fig. 68.8 Schematics of partial forced expiratory flow-volume relationship: infants with normal expiratory flow, moderate flow restriction (partial limitation), and severe chronic lung disease *(CLD)*. *FRC*, Functional residual capacity.

technique for infants was described by Stocks and colleagues in 2001.[66]

FORCED EXPIRATORY FLOW MEASUREMENTS

The tone of tracheobronchial smooth muscle provides a mechanism to stabilize the airways and prevent airway collapse.[108] Plugging of the airways, edema, or weakening of the airway walls and the resulting tracheobronchomalacia all may alter airflow.[109,110] In addition, the increased driving pressure secondary to the high elastic and resistive loads during tidal breathing in infants with bronchopulmonary dysplasia often leads to self-induced expiratory flow limitation. Forced expiration commonly is used to detect obstructive lung disease by determining the lung volume at which small airways begin to close. During expiration, flow is limited by airway compression, which in turn is determined by the elastic recoil of the lung, the resistance of the airway, and airway wall mechanics. In infants, forced expiratory flow may be generated by rapid thoracic compression (RTC) or by negative-pressure forced deflation. The RTC technique is preferred because it is noninvasive and does not require intubation, paralysis, or deep sedation. The RTC maneuver achieves forced expiratory flow using an inflatable jacket wrapped around the infant's thorax. At the end of a normal inspiration the jacket is rapidly pressurized to generate a partial forced expiratory flow-volume (PEFV) loop. Parameters used to characterize PEFV include peak expiratory flow, forced expiratory flow at FRC ($\dot{V}_{maxFRC}$), and the shape of the expiratory flow curve.[111] Fig. 68.8 illustrates typical PEFV loops representing normal, moderate, and severe flow limitation.

TECHNICAL LIMITATIONS

This technique generates only partial rather than complete forced flow-volume loops, which limits the evaluation of true flow limitation in response to the appropriate compression pressure for a particular infant. The main limitation is the variability of FRC in young infants because inspiration may start before the completion of a full expiration.

FORCED OSCILLATION TECHNIQUE

One last technique to include in this discussion of pulmonary function measurements is the forced oscillation technique first described in 1956 by Dubois and colleagues.[112] The key to this technique is the application of a pressure sine wave of a given frequency to the respiratory system while measuring the resultant flow. The amplitude of the sine wave is typically small enough to cause a reaction of the respiratory system without disrupting the behavior of the system itself. The reaction should be linear in response, while the flow generated should be at the same frequency as the pressure sine wave applied. Under these conditions, the respiratory impedance describes the response of the respiratory system and can be mathematically written as the ratio between the pressure applied and the resultant flow.[113] This respiratory impedance (Z_{rs}) is a complex number consisting of a real component representing the respiratory system resistance (R_{rs}), which includes airway, lung tissue, and chest wall frictional resistances; and an imaginary component, termed *reactance* (X_{rs}), which opposes elastic (compliance) and inertial forces. Both of these terms are a function of the frequency of oscillation.[114] While there are several testing apparatuses that can be conceived for applying the small frequency oscillations and measure airflow and airway pressure, the basic concepts are similar amongst these devices.

Frequency ranges that are applied to the respiratory system include low, medium, and high frequencies, where the low range includes spontaneous breathing rates, the most commonly used medium frequencies are typically between 2 to 4 and 20 Hz, and the high frequencies can be up to several hundred hertz. Across

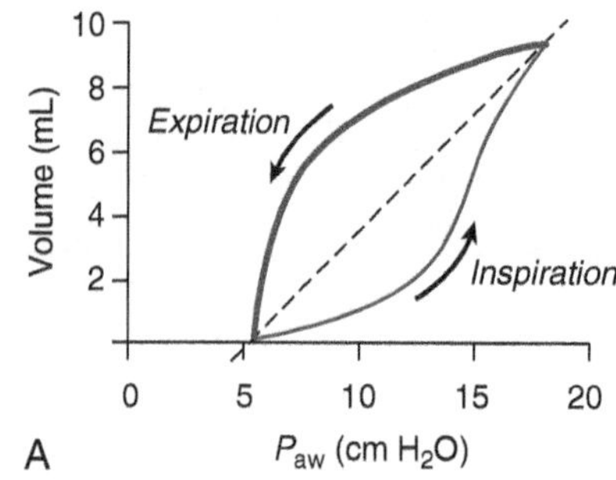

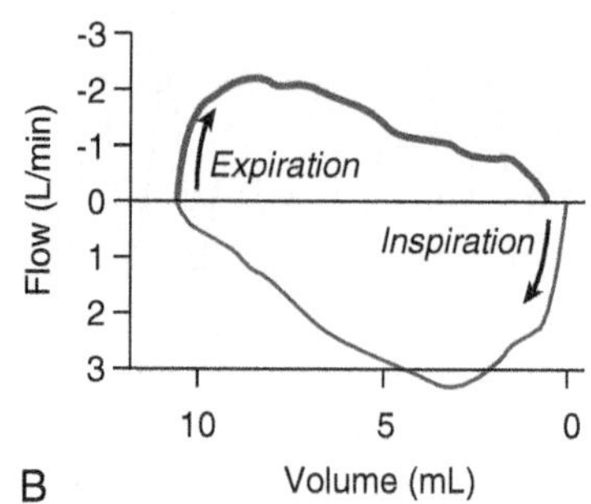

Fig. 68.9 Representation of a typical infant ventilator graphics display for a single breath. (A) Volume-pressure loop. (B) Flow-volume loop.

the frequency ranges, different properties of the respiratory system can be measured. At very low frequencies properties of the lung parenchyma dominate. Using the medium frequencies allows for the measurement of the real part of the impedance, R_{rs}. In some research studies the impedance between 4 and 6 Hz is used as a measure of simple airway resistance as is measured through the more classical methods described above. At higher frequencies, the inertive properties of the lung become dominant, revealing more information about airway wall mechanics. One of the central concepts of the forced oscillation technique is that there is a frequency applied to the respiratory system at which the elastic and inertive forces are equal and opposite in magnitude. This frequency is referred to as the *resonant frequency*. This frequency often falls in the medium frequencies where airway resistance dominates and explains why the range of 4 to 6 Hz is used as a surrogate, as mentioned previously.[113,114]

The forced oscillation technique holds the promise of providing better understanding of evolving lung injury and pulmonary outcomes, both in the intensive care nursery and throughout early childhood.[115,116] Potentially the greatest advantage is that there is no need for patient cooperation and also that the instrumentation is such that this technique may be performed rapidly at the bedside. Patients may be spontaneously breathing throughout or may be receiving conventional mechanical support via either an endotracheal tube or tracheostomy. Another important advantage is the fact that forced oscillation is a non-invasive technique that does not require placement of an esophageal pressure catheter as with more traditional PFT methods.

Although the forced oscillation technique provides a more complete characterization of the respiratory system, it continues to have the following limitations: lack of familiarity amongst clinicians caring for these patients, understanding of what the values reported would mean from a diagnostic testing standpoint, and the lack of established normative values in preterm infants and newborns. There have been only limited investigative uses in small cohorts of infants, specifically with chronic lung disease, utilizing this technique to evaluate long-term outcomes into childhood.[117-119]

REAL-TIME PULMONARY GRAPHICS MONITORING

The addition of pneumotachometers and waveform graphics to the latest generation of infant ventilators provides clinicians with respiratory function information that previously was available only with specialized instrumentation requiring specifically trained operators and frequent calibration. These dedicated bedside instruments at best sampled only a few minutes of data, as opposed to continuous monitoring; serial repeat measurements were therefore needed to observe the effect on pulmonary function resulting from changes in ventilator settings or other therapies. The newer graphics-based ventilators, as well as stand-alone respiratory monitors, make use of improved sensor and micro-processing technology to provide continuous real-time display of the fundamental measurable parameters of respiration, namely, the pressure, flow, and volume signals. These signals may be displayed as waveforms along a time axis or as plots of *x-y* relationships such as volume-versus-pressure and flow-versus-volume loops. In addition to graphic display, measurements from the three signals are used to calculate a limited set of respiratory function data useful in pulmonary focused research studies.[120]

VOLUME-PRESSURE LOOPS

A volume-pressure loop is an *x-y* plot of tidal volume as a function of airway pressure. Fig. 68.9A illustrates a volume-pressure loop from a mechanically ventilated neonate. The loop represents a single breath and is plotted in a counterclockwise direction as the breath progresses from inspiration to expiration. The slope of the dotted line, connecting the zero flow points at end-expiration and end-inspiration, is a good estimate of the overall elasticity or dynamic respiratory system compliance, defined as the ratio of tidal volume to driving pressure, i.e. the difference between peak inspiratory pressure (PIP) and positive end-expiratory pressure (PEEP), or V_T/(PIP − PEEP). Tilting of the loop toward the horizontal or toward the vertical is indicative of either decreased or increased compliance, respectively, as shown in Fig. 68.10A. Of note, the volume-pressure relationship follows a different course during expiration than during inspiration. The resulting hysteresis, depicted as the area within the loop, is due to resistive pressures. Increased inspiratory or expiratory resistive work expands the hysteresis to the right or left, respectively (see Fig. 68.10B).

Volume-pressure loops are useful in clinical practice for detection of ventilatory overdistension, evidenced by the "beaking" effect as illustrated in Fig. 68.10C. In this breath, the compliance in the flattened area within the final 20% of the inspiratory limb (C_{20}) is less than the dynamic compliance for the entire breath (C_{dyn}). It has been suggested that a C_{20}/C_{dyn} ratio less than 0.8 may be an indicator of lung overdistension.[99] Any further pressure increase in the flattened portion of the volume-pressure loop produces negligible volume change, and a small decrease in PIP may be used to reduce overdistension while maintaining the same tidal volume (see Fig. 68.10D).

Another abnormality easily detected from observation of the volume-pressure loop is lung atelectasis (see Fig. 68.10E), evidenced by a prolonged period of negligible volume

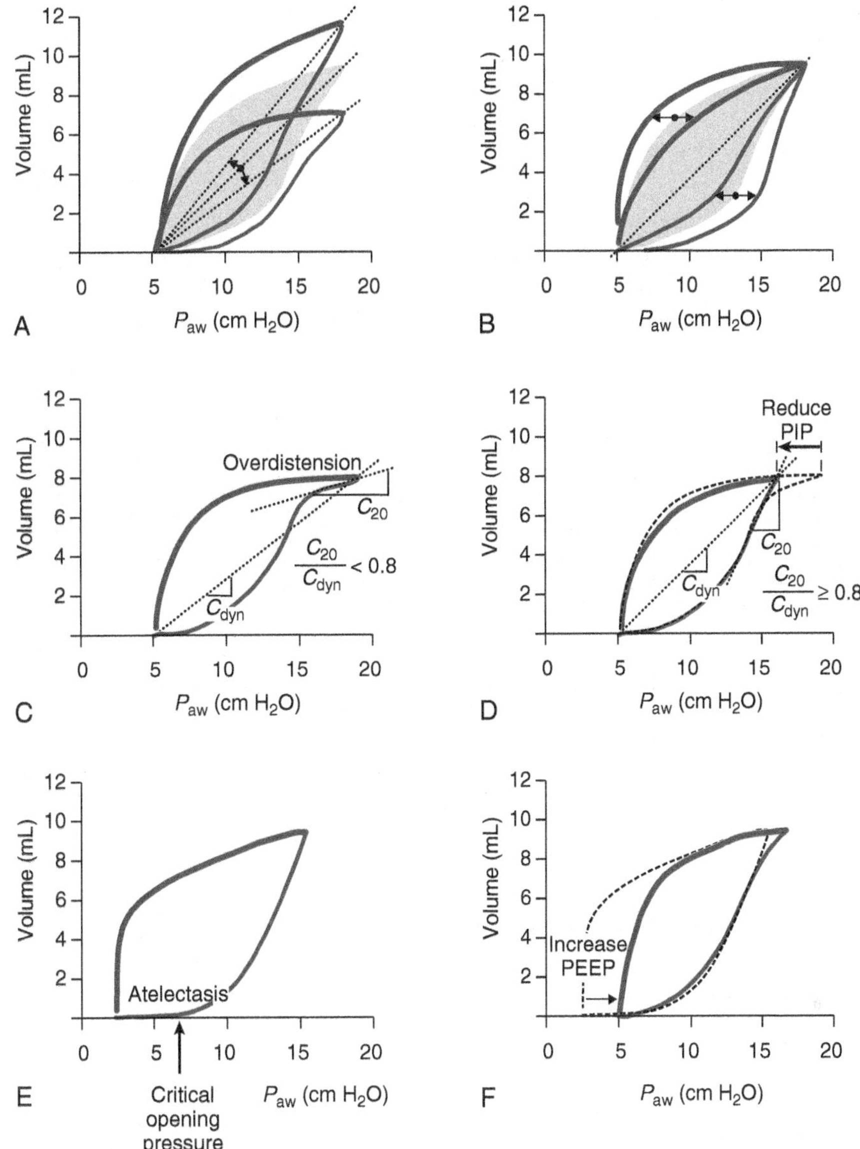

Fig. 68.10 Volume-pressure loop characteristics. (A) Compliance change with fixed peak inspiratory pressure *(PIP)* and fixed positive end-expiratory pressure *(PEEP)*. (B) Inspiratory and expiratory resistance changes. (C) "Beaking" effect seen with overdistension. (D) Effect of reducing PIP on overdistension. (E) Atelectasis due to insufficient functional residual capacity (FRC); *arrow* indicates critical opening pressure. (F) Increasing PEEP to reduce atelectasis.

recruitment at the start of inspiration. Fig. 68.10F illustrates how an increase in PEEP may be used to shift the FRC upward along the lung's sigmoidal volume-pressure characteristic to a point above the critical opening pressure, thereby preventing alveolar collapse at end-expiration.[71,121,122] The volume-pressure loop also is useful for detecting other ventilatory abnormalities such as endotracheal tube leaks and air trapping, both of which result in incomplete closure of the graphical volume-pressure loop during end of expiration.

FLOW-VOLUME LOOPS

A flow-volume loop is a plot of airflow versus tidal volume, as illustrated in Fig. 68.9B, which also shows the corresponding volume-pressure loop from the same mechanically ventilated breath. The loop represents one breath as it progresses downward with inspiration to an upward expiration in a clockwise direction (of note, the direction and orientation may vary among ventilators and monitors from different manufacturers). The tidal flow-volume loop is useful for evaluating changes in inspiratory and expiratory airflow-to-volume response during tidal breathing. In addition to determination of the peak flow values, the patterns of airflow and tidal volumes indicative of turbulence or obstructive flow limitation also may be evaluated.[123-125] A typical flow-volume loop for a healthy newborn infant is shown in Fig. 68.11A. Preterm neonates with high chest wall compliance and greater expiratory airway collapsibility, as well as infants with chronic lung disease, typically will show an early peak expiratory flow followed by a concave profile (see Fig. 68.11B).[126-128] Other loop shapes that are characteristic of intrathoracic and extrathoracic flow limitation are shown in Figs. 68.11C–F.

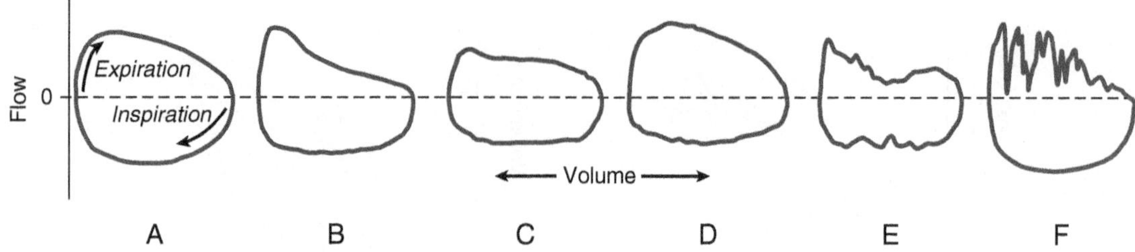

Fig. 68.11 Tidal flow-volume loops illustrating various types of flow limitation. (A) Healthy newborn. (B) Obstructive airway disease—expiratory airway collapse. (C) Fixed upper airway obstruction—inspiratory and expiratory flow limitation. (D) Extrathoracic inspiratory flow limitation. (E) Bronchomalacia—severe flow limitation. (F) Airflow turbulence possibly due to secretions in the airway from crying.

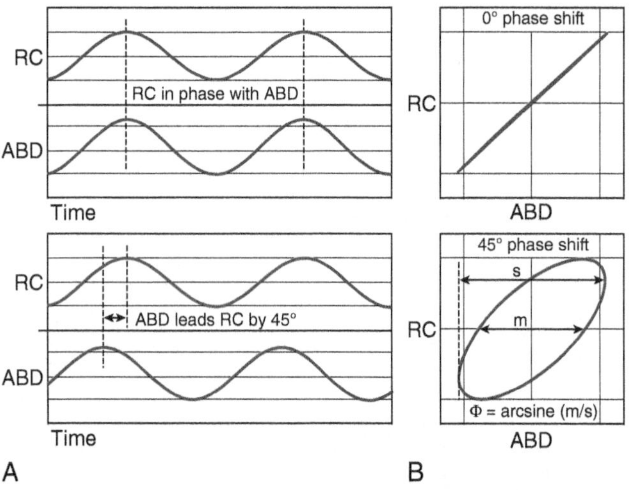

Fig. 68.12 (A) Idealized, scalar tracings of rib cage *(RC)* and abdominal *(ABD)* relative volume changes illustrating fully synchronized *(top panel)* and unsynchronized breathing having a 45-degree phase angle *(bottom panel)*. (B) The respective Konno-Mead Lissajous plots of RC versus ABD and calculation of the phase angle Φ.

OTHER NON-INVASIVE RESPIRATORY MEASURES

THORACOABDOMINAL MECHANICS

Analysis of chest wall dynamics, specifically, rib cage and abdominal movements, as recorded using several of the previously described thoracoabdominal body surface movement analysis technologies such as RIP, EIP, OEP, and SLP, allows evaluation of the following work of breathing and breathing efficiency indices:

THORACOABDOMINAL ASYNCHRONY

This is a measure of the degree of asynchrony between RC and ABD excursions as defined by the phase delay, either lagging or leading, between the sinusoidally varying movements of these two thoracic compartments. More precisely, this parameter is termed the *phase angle phi (Φ)* and may be visualized simply as the average "shift" between the peaks of the sinusoidal scalar tracings of RC and ABD as illustrated in Fig. 68.12A. An *x-y* plot of RC vs. ABD, also known as a *Konno-Mead plot*,[129] allows a practical method for calculation of the phase angle where, referring to Fig. 68.12B, Φ = arcsine(m/s), where m is measured as the width of the horizontal line intercepting the loop at one-half of the maximal RC excursion, and s is the maximal ABD excursion. A phase angle of zero degrees corresponds to complete synchrony between RC and ABD, whereas a phase angle of 180 degrees indicates complete asynchrony, or paradoxical movement. Fig. 68.13 illustrates several other idealized loop shapes and their associated phase angles in progression from full synchrony to full asynchrony. Because infants have a relatively compliant rib cage, ABD excursions tend to lead the RC excursions resulting in some asynchrony that is increased in the presence of any airway obstruction and leading to increased work of breathing. Thus, the phase angle is considered an index of thoracoabdominal asynchrony and work of breathing and is useful in quantifying obstructive airway disease.[42,130–132]

LABORED BREATHING INDEX

The Labored Breathing Index is defined as the ratio of the sum of the absolute values of maximal RC and ABD amplitudes to the actual resulting tidal volume as given by:

$$LBI = (|\Delta RC_{max}| + |\Delta ABD_{max}|)/V_T \quad [68.14]$$

In perfect synchrony the sum of changes in RC and ABD exactly equal tidal volume giving a ratio of 1.0. As breathing becomes more asynchronous volume increases in one compartment are counteracted by simultaneous decreases in the other compartment having a net effect of reducing tidal volume if left uncompensated.[133–135] To maintain tidal volume at a sufficient level an increase in either the RC or ABD excursions is needed. This, of course, requires more effort by the patient and the sum of RC and ABD excursions becomes greater than actual tidal volume resulting in LBI ratios greater than 1.0. The LBI is a work of breathing parameter and may be particularly useful in assessing breathing effort during non-invasive respiratory support. It is notable that the LBI, as defined above, requires measurement of volume-calibrated RIP signals. Although methodology for RIP calibration is well established,[40,41] the procedure may be disruptive and impractical at the infant's bedside. As a workaround to this complication, a study was performed comparing LBI calculated using uncalibrated vs. calibrated RIP signals and demonstrated clinically acceptable accurate evaluations of the LBI using only uncalibrated RIP signals.[136]

THE PHASE RELATION TOTAL BREATH

Phase relation total breath is defined as the percentage of time during a breath cycle in which the RC and ABD are nonsynchronous as illustrated in Fig. 68.14. With increasing time in asynchrony PhRTB increases and approaches 100% at complete paradoxical breathing.[135]

PERCENT RIB CAGE

This index quantitates the percentage of rib cage contribution to the tidal volume excursions and is simply: RC/(RC +ABD).[42,137]

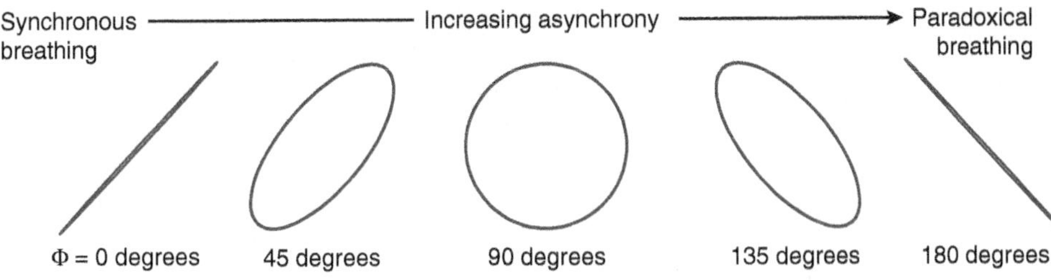

Fig. 68.13 Idealized Konno-Mead plots for phase angles representing full synchrony, at the far left, and increasing to complete asynchrony or paradoxical breathing at the far right.

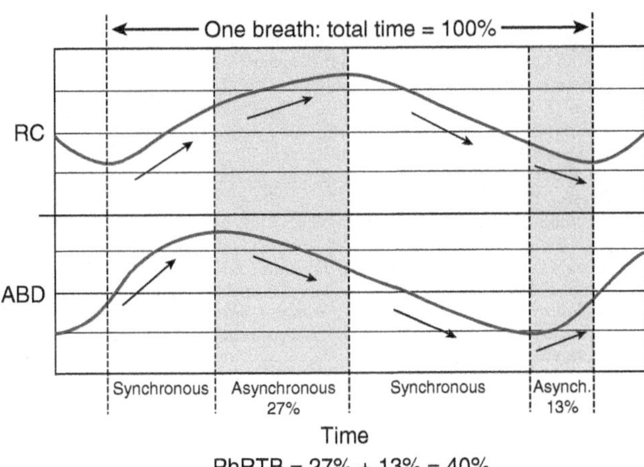

Fig. 68.14 Phase Relation Total Breath *(PhRTB)*. The grayed areas in the figure show where the rib cage *(RC)* and abdominal *(ABD)* excursions are moving in opposing directions resulting, in this example, in a PhRTB which totals 40% asynchrony.

CONCLUSION

The clinical usefulness of neonatal pulmonary function testing lies in the fact that the functional parameters define the magnitude and pattern of respiratory compromise. Individual disease processes are not differentiated by pulmonary function data. Infants with hyaline membrane disease, pulmonary edema, or pneumonia have low lung compliance, whereas infants with increased airway resistance may have an obstructive disease process such as meconium aspiration syndrome or bronchopulmonary dysplasia. However, pulmonary function data can be used to determine the severity of the pathologic condition, its resolution, and the effects of respiratory support.

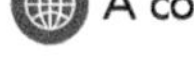 A complete reference list is available at www.ExpertConsult.com.

SELECT REFERENCES

1. Hutchinson J. On the capacity of the lungs, and on the respiratory functions, with a view of establishing a precise and easy method of detecting disease by the spirometer. *Med Chir Trans*. 1846;29:137-252.
4. Comroe Jr JH, Nisell OI, Nims RG. A simple method for concurrent measurement of compliance and resistance to breathing in anesthetized animals and man. *J Appl Physiol*. 1954;7:225-228.
7. Bancalari E. Pulmonary function testing and other diagnostic laboratory procedures in neonatal pulmonary care. In: Thibeault DW, Gary GA, eds. *Neonatal Pulmonary Care*. 2nd ed. East Norwalk, CT: Appleton-Century Crofts; 1986:195-234.
12. Rodarte JR, Rehder K. Dynamics of respiration. In: Fishman A, Macklem P, Mead J, Geiger SR, eds. *Handbook of Physiology. Section 3: The Respiratory System. Mechanics of Breathing, Part I*. Vol 3. Bethesda, MD: American Physiological Society; 1986:131-144.
14. Sly D, Davis M. Equipment requirements for infant respiratory function testing. In: Stocks J, Sly PD, Tepper RS, Morgan WJ, eds. *Infant Respiratory Function Testing*. New York: John Wiley & Sons; 1996:45-117.
17. Frey U, Stocks J, Coates A, et al. Specifications for equipment used for infant pulmonary function testing. ERS/ATS task force on standards for infant respiratory function testing. European Respiratory Society/American Thoracic Society. *Eur Respir J*. 2000;16:731-740.
21. Sullivan WJ, Peters GM, Enright PL. Pneumotachometers: theory and application. *Respir Care*. 1984;29:736-749.
27. Turner MJ, MacLeod IM, Rothberg AD. Calibration of Fleisch and screen pneumotachographs for use with various oxygen concentrations. *Med Biol Eng Comput*. 1990;28:200-204.
29. Zimova-Herknerova M, Plavka R. Expired tidal volumes measured by hot-wire anemometer during high-frequency oscillation in preterm infants. *Pediatr Pulmonol*. 2006;41:428-433.
32. Scalfaro P, Cotting J, Sly PD. In vitro assessment of an ultrasonic flowmeter for use in ventilated infants. *Eur Respir J*. 2000;15:566-569.
37. Dolfin T, Duffty P, Wilkes D, et al. Effects of a face mask and pneumotachograph on breathing in sleeping infants. *Am Rev Respir Dis*. 1983;128:977-979.
38. Sackner JD, Nixon AJ, Davis B, et al. Non-invasive measurement of ventilation during exercise using a respiratory inductive plethysmograph. I. *Am Rev Respir Dis*. 1980;122(6):867-871.
40. Sackner MA, Watson H, Belsito AS, et al. Calibration of respiratory inductive plethysmograph during natural breathing. *J Appl Physiol*. 1989;66:410-420.
42. Ren CL, Feng R, SD, Davis SD, et al. Tidal breathing measurements at discharge and clinical outcomes in extremely low gestational age neonates. *Ann Am Thorac Soc*. 2018;15:1311-1319.
44. Courtney SE, Aghai ZH, Saslow JG, et al. Changes in lung volume and work of breathing: a comparison of two variable-flow nasal continuous positive airway pressure devices in very low birth weight infants. *Pediatr Pulmonol*. 2003;36:248-252.
45. Sivieri EM, Wolfson MR, Abbasi S. Pulmonary mechanics measurements by respiratory inductive plethysmography and esophageal manometry: methodology for infants on non-invasive respiratory support. *J Neonatal Perinatal Med*. 2019;12:149-159.
47. Rahman T, Page R, Page C, et al. PneuRIP™: a novel respiratory inductance plethysmography monitor. *J Med Device*. 2017;11:0110101-0110106.
50. Pickerd N, Williams EM, Kotecha S. Electromagnetic inductance plethysmography to measure tidal breathing in preterm and term infants. *Pediatric Pulmonol*. 2013;48:160-167.
53. Reinaux M, Aliverti A, da Silva LG, et al. Tidal volume measurements in infants: Opto-electronic plethysmography versus pneumotachograph. *Pediatr Pulmonol*. 2016;51:850-857.
54. De Boer W, Lasenby J, Cameron J, et al. SLP: a zero-contact non-invasive method for pulmonary function testing. In: Labrosse F, Zwiggelaar R, Liu Y, Tiddeman B, eds. *Proceedings of the British Machine Vision Conference. 2010*. BMVA Press; 2010:85.1-85.12.
58. Van der Burg PS, Miedema M, de Jong FH, et al. Cross sectional changes in lung volume measured by electrical impedance tomography are representative for the whole lung in ventilated preterm infants. *Crit Care Med*. 2014;42:1524-1530.
59. Reiterer F, Vallant J, Urlesberger B. Electrical impedance segmentography: a promising tool for respiratory monitoring? *J Neonatal Perinatal Med*. 2020;13:489-494.
64. Dubois AB, Botelho SY, Bedell GN, et al. A rapid plethysmographic method for measuring TGV: a comparison with a nitrogen washout method for measuring functional residual capacity in normal subjects. *J Clin Invest*. 1956;35:322-326.
66. Stocks J, Godfrey S, Beardsmore C, et al. Plethysmographic measurements of lung volume and airway resistance. ERS/ATS task force on standards for infant respiratory function testing. European Respiratory Society /American Thoracic Society. *Eur Respir J*. 2001;17:302-312.
68. Krauss AN, Auld PA. Measurement of functional residual capacity in distressed neonates by helium rebreathing. *J Pediatr*. 1970;77:228-232.
70. Schwartz JG, Fox WW, Shaffer TH. A method for measuring functional residual capacity in neonates with endotracheal tubes. *IEEE Trans Biomed Eng*. 1978;25:304-307.

71. Da Silva WJ, Abbasi S, Pereira G, Bhutani VK. Role of positive end-expiratory pressure changes on functional residual capacity in surfactant treated preterm infants. *Pediatr Pulmonol*. 1994;18:89-92.
75. Morris MG, Gustafsson P, Tepper R, et al. The bias flow nitrogen washout technique for measuring the functional residual capacity in infants. ERS/ATS Task Force on Standards for Infant Respiratory Function Testing. *Eur Respir J*. 2001;17:529-536.
85. Schulze A, Schaller P, Töpper A, Kirpalani H. Measurement of functional residual capacity by sulfur hexafluoride in small-volume lungs during spontaneous breathing and mechanical ventilation. *Pediatr Res*. 1994;35:494-499.
88. Pillow JJ, Ljungberg H, Hulskamp G, Stocks J. Functional residual capacity measurements in healthy infants: ultrasonic flow meter versus a mass spectrometer. *Eur Respir J*. 2004;23:763-768.
91. Coates AL, Stocks J, Gerhardt T. Esophageal manometry. In: Stocks J, Sly PD, Tepper RS, Morgan WJ, eds. *Infant Respiratory Function Testing*. New York: John Wiley & Sons; 1996:241-258.
95. Beardsmore CS, Helms P, Stocks J, et al. Improved esophageal balloon technique for use in infants. *J Appl Physiol*. 1980;49:735-742.
96. Bhutani VK, Sivieri EM, Abbasi S, Shaffer TH. Evaluation of neonatal pulmonary mechanics and energetics: a two factor least mean square analysis. *Pediatr Pulmonol*. 1988;4:150-158.
98. Nikischin W, Gerhardt T, Everett T, Bancalari E. A new method to analyze lung compliance when pressure-volume relationship is nonlinear. *Am J Respir Crit Care Med*. 1998;158:1052-1060.
99. Fisher JB, Mammel MC, Coleman JM, et al. Identifying lung overdistention during mechanical ventilation by using volume-pressure loops. *Pediatr Pulmonol*. 1988;5:10-14.
104. Chan V, Greenough A. Lung function and the Hering Breuer reflex in the neonatal period. *Early Hum Dev*. 1992;28:111-118.
105. Gappa M, Colin AA, Goetz I, Stocks J. ERS/ATS task force on standards for infant respiratory function testing. European Respiratory Society/American Thoracic Society. Passive respiratory mechanics: the occlusion techniques. *Eur Respir J*. 2001;17:141-148.
106. Dubois AB, Botelho SY, Comroe JH. A new method for measuring airway resistance in man using a body plethysmograph: values in normal subjects and in patients with respiratory disease. *J Clin Invest*. 1956;35:327-335.
110. Bhutani VK, Deoras K, Shaffer TH, Sivieri EM. Determination of alterations in tracheobronchial airflow mechanics in preterm infants following mechanical ventilation. In: Gennser G, Marsal K, Svenningsen N, Lindström K, eds. *Fetal and Neonatal Physiological Measurements*. Vol 3. Malmo, Sweden: Flenhags Tryckeri; 1989:419-423.
111. Sly PD, Tepper R, Henschen M, et al. ERS/ATS task force on standards for infant respiratory function testing. European Respiratory Society/American Thoracic Society. Tidal forced expirations. *Eur Respir J*. 2000;16:741-748.
112. Dubois AB, Brody AW, Lewis DH, Burgess BF. Oscillation mechanics of lungs and chest in man. *J Appl Physiol*. 1956;8:587-594.
113. Frey U. Forced oscillation technique in infants and young children. *Paediatr Respir Rev*. 2005;6:246-254.
118. Hantos Z, Czövek D, Gyurkovits Z, et al. Assessment of respiratory mechanics with forced oscillations in healthy newborns. *Pediatr Pulmonol*. 2015;50:344-352.
120. Di Fiore JM, Hibbs AM, Zadell AE, et al. The effect of inhaled nitric oxide on pulmonary function in preterm infants. *J Perinatol*. 2007;27:766-771.
123. Schmalisch G, Wauer RR, Foitzik B, Patzak A. Influence of preterm onset of inspiration on tidal breathing parameters in infants with and without CLD. *Respir Physiol Neurobiol*. 2003;135:39-46.
129. Konno K, Mead J. Measurement of the separate volume changes of rib cage and abdomen during breathing. *J Appl Physiol*. 1967;22:407-422.
130. Allen JL, Wolfson MR, McDowell K, et al. Thoracoabdominal asynchrony in infants with airflow obstruction. *Am Rev Respir Dis*. 1990;141:337-342.
132. Wolfson MR, Greenspan JS, Deoras KS, et al. Effect of position on the mechanical interaction between the rib cage and abdomen in preterm infants. *J Appl Physiol*. 1992;72:1032-1038.
133. De Jongh BE, Locke R, Mackley A, et al. Work of breathing indices in infants with respiratory insufficiency receiving high-flow nasal cannula and nasal continuous positive airway pressure. *J Perinatol*. 2014;34:27-32.
136. Sivieri EM, Shaffer TH, Abbasi S. *Labored Breathing Index. Calculation Using Uncalibrated vs. Calibrated Respiratory Inductance Plethysmography in Premature Infants*. San Francisco, CA: Proceedings of the Pediatric Academic Society Annual Meeting; 2017.

69 Mechanisms of Neonatal Lung Injury

Anastasiya Mankouski | Richard Lambert Auten, Jr.

INTRODUCTION

At birth, the term newborn lung is at the alveolar phase of lung development, with a smaller number of alveoli normalized to body weight than an adult has. The lung must make the rapid transition from a fluid-filled structure with low stretch frequency and low strain, to an air-filled structure subjected to high strain at variable frequency to support gas exchange. Spontaneous breathing efforts just after delivery at 40 weeks gestation can generate high transpleural or transpulmonic pressures during the first few breaths. Failure to reabsorb amniotic fluid can lead to uneven gas distribution during spontaneous breathing or positive pressure ventilation, generating stress points that contribute to strain, injury, alveolar rupture, and *pneumothorax* (Fig. 69.1). The prevalence of spontaneous pneumothorax is undoubtedly higher than recognized because many are clinically insignificant. Pneumothorax is associated with meconium-stained amniotic fluid and elective repeat cesarean deliveries. In babies born very prematurely, at less than 26 weeks, the fetal lung is completing the transition from the canalicular stage to the saccular stage of development. Air sacs are relatively thick walled, and pulmonary capillaries are incompletely branched and do not extend to the ends of the alveolar septa. Surfactant synthesis and secretion are decreased. Enzymatic antioxidants, superoxide dismutase, catalase, and glutathione peroxidase are relatively low and less inducible than at term. Nutritional antioxidants such as vitamin E and retinoids are also relatively low.[1] To support ventilation, the extremely premature newborn lung with these liabilities is often subjected to supplemental oxygen, endotracheal intubation, and positive pressure ventilation, all of which can injure a developing lung, leading to impaired alveolar development and chronic lung disease of prematurity, or bronchopulmonary dysplasia (BPD) (Fig. 69.2). Neonatal lung injury likely impairs normal progenitor cell function during development and diminishes the capacity for repair following later insults.

Newer analyses of clinical approaches that avoid intubation, allowing for more gradual recruitment, appear to decrease the risk for BPD.

MECHANICAL MECHANISMS OF LUNG INJURY

Vulnerability to mechanical lung injury is significant immediately after birth.[2] Present methods of mechanical ventilation unavoidably deliver nonuniform distending forces, which worsen ventilation-perfusion matching and induce cellular injury. Animal studies have shown that structural damage and inflammatory response can be generated after only a few overdistending breaths. Significant lung injury can take place after brief periods of mechanical ventilation of the incompletely recruited lung. Forced "recruitment" maneuvers may be harmful. Despite the promise suggested by prolonged sigh maneuvers in some animal models, preterm newborns requiring intubation at birth did not benefit. In preterm, surfactant-treated lambs, initial recruitment maneuvers with tidal volumes varying from 8 to 30 mL/kg had no benefit, and caused "dose-dependent" histologic damage with increasing tidal volumes.[3] Lung volumes at less than optimal functional residual capacity (FRC) require higher than optimal peak pressures in later breaths to fully re-recruit alveoli.To minimize lung injury, strategies are aimed at identifying adaptive and proper goals of gas exchange which can decrease excessive administration of mechanical support to minimize harm and maximize benefit. These strategies include avoiding atelectrauma by promoting alveolar stability and minimizing de-recruitment, and the use of a broader range of acceptable target pulse oximetry (SpO_2) in the delivery room to minimize the need for positive-pressure ventilation during stabilization after delivery. Maneuvers designed to avoid de-recruitment, such as use of continuous positive airway pressure (CPAP),[4] have decreased injury markers in experimental models of prematurity and respiratory distress syndrome (RDS).To minimize volutrauma during the delivery room resuscitation, some recommend that the positive inspiratory pressure should be adjusted to deliver a tidal volume of 4 to 5 mL/kg.[5] Choosing and delivering the appropriate tidal volume during delivery room resuscitation remain important, but as yet unrealized, goals in the quest to minimize lung injury, particularly in the extremely premature newborn at high risk for developing BPD.

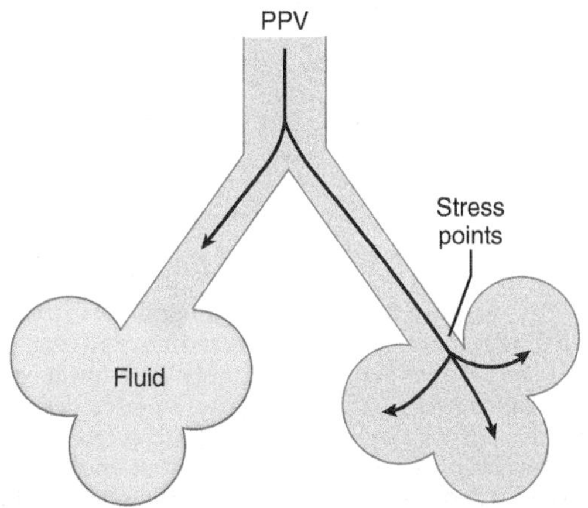

Fig. 69.1 During inspiration, fluid-filled atelectatic alveoli *(gray)* allow gas to be shunted to more compliant alveoli, leading to overdistension and alveolar wall stress. *PPV,* Positive pressure ventilation.

LUNG DE-RECRUITMENT

Trauma to delicate airways can easily result if the lung is de-recruited to volumes at less than FRC (Fig. 69.3), resulting in alveolar collapse (atelectasis). Higher airway pressures are then required during subsequent mechanical breaths to re-recruit alveoli, leading to stretch injuries in terminal airways.[6] The spontaneously breathing patient must generate greater negative pressures to achieve the same goal, also leading to the same stretch injury, higher work of breathing, and fatigued muscles of respiration. Considerations for mechanical ventilation strategies designed to avoid lung injury due to de-recruitment and atelectasis are discussed in Chapter 159.

LUNG OVEREXPANSION

As the mechanical breath volume increases to approach the total lung capacity, increased airway pressure and mechanical shear force are applied to the airways and alveoli without a proportional

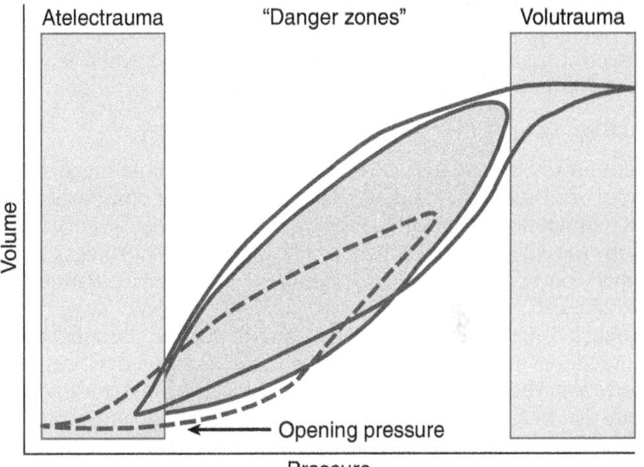

Fig. 69.3 Static pressure-volume loop after recruitment *(solid line, gray fill)* of lung volume above functional residual capacity. After derecruitment, the P-V loop demonstrates decreased hysteresis *(dashed line)*, decreased slope, and loss of lung volume at end-deflation, predisposing to "atelectotrauma." Overinflation *(dark solid line)* of the lung leads to increased luminal pressure without increased accumulation of lung volume, increasing shear stress to airways, and predisposing to "volutrauma."

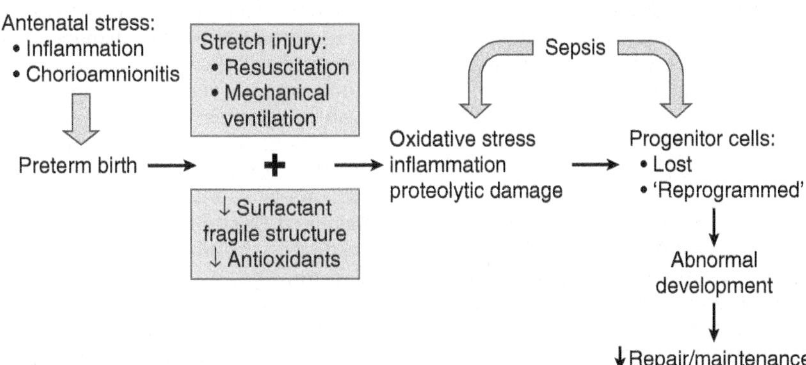

Fig. 69.2 Developmental lung vulnerabilities superimposed with mechanical injury and maladaptive inflammation, leading to disrupted lung development. Neonatal lung injury impairs the capacity of progenitor cells—both in situ and recruited—to conduct maintenance and repair.

increase in lung volume at the upper inflection point (see Fig. 69.3). The widespread use of in-line flow or pressure sensors capable of displaying the pressure-volume relationship can detect overinflation, demonstrating the flattened inspiration and expiration limbs and decreased pressure-volume loop hysteresis at the end of inspiration. Overinflation is more likely to occur when patients are receiving time-cycled, pressure-limited ventilation at a time when compliance rapidly improves, for example, immediately after surfactant therapy, or on achieving full alveolar recruitment.

Balancing the risks of lung injury due to de-recruitment or atelectotrauma against the risks of overinflation can be complex, particularly when the pathophysiology that affects the lung microenvironment is non-uniform, and produces underinflated and overinflated regions. Volume-targeted mechanical ventilation appears to achieve this balance, and meta-analysis of studies evaluating its effects suggests lower duration of mechanical ventilation and a lower risk to develop BPD.[7]

SQUARING THE CIRCLE: THE RIGHT KIND OF MECHANICAL SUPPORT

Neurally adjusted ventilatory assist (NAVA) takes advantage of physiologic signals to regulate the amount of positive pressure support. The number of assisted breaths is determined by the patient, since all breaths are assisted, but the magnitude of the delivered volume (flow × inspiratory time) is determined by the patient's diaphragmatic neural signaling. Since tidal volumes normally fluctuate, NAVA cooperates with the patient's effort. Risks and benefits of NAVA compared to other forms of ventilation for neonates are uncertain. Multicenter, randomized, adequately powered trials are needed to determine whether NAVA is more effective than other modes of ventilation.

SURFACTANT DEFICIENCY AND LUNG INJURY

Nonuniform compliance and resistance can promote mechanical strain, so it follows that achieving more uniform compliance by correcting surfactant deficiency common in those prematurely born should prevent mechanical injury. For short-term lung injury outcomes such as pneumothorax, and duration of mechanical ventilation, and for survival in some subgroups, surfactant treatment has been shown to be beneficial in multicenter randomized trials. Early use of selective, empiric surfactant therapy on very premature newborns, typically less than 26 weeks estimated gestational age, has been shown to reduce the risk of pneumothorax and BPD.[8] However, uneven surfactant distribution may contribute to the heterogeneous clinical response and may further contribute to lung injury by directing positive airway pressure preferentially to the compliant parts of the lung. This may injure compliant lung regions and spare (for a while) the noncompliant lung regions. In an effort to avoid mechanical ventilation, some have used immediate surfactant treatment followed by CPAP, but there is no clear evidence that this prevents BPD, as typically defined,[9,10] with its multifactorial etiology (see Chapter 159), even though this approach and similar approaches using intubation with small catheters to deliver surfactant are gaining wider usage. Some developed approaches to delivery of surfactant by aerosol may avoid intubation and laryngoscopy altogether.[11]

LUNG WATER, PATENT DUCTUS ARTERIOSUS CONTRIBUTE TO MECHANICAL LUNG INJURY

Patent ductus arteriosus (PDA) in the setting of low pulmonary vascular resistance contributes to pulmonary edema by allowing pulmonary overcirculation, which results in elevated left atrial pressures. PDA has been associated in numerous clinical studies with the development of chronic lung disease of prematurity and is discussed in detail in Chapters 52 and 159. Persistence or recurrence of a PDA is highly correlated with the development of BPD, probably because of uneven effects on lung compliance. Alternatively, recurrence of the PDA is often associated with sepsis, which itself may contribute to inflammatory lung injury.[12] Chorioamnionitis and fetal inflammation may also contribute to the production of prostaglandins that promote ductal patency by the same mechanisms, and may contribute to lung injury via inflammation, making it difficult to separate the physiologic contribution of the PDA to lung injury in the premature newborn.

Intravenous fluid management using rates exceeding 200 mL/kg/day in the first days of life for extremely premature newborns, has been linked to later development of BPD,[13] but the precise role in lung injury remains unclear because pulmonary lymphatic drainage appears to compensate for increased pulmonary blood flow in experimental animals given similarly high rates of intravenous fluids.[14] High fluid rates have been linked to arterial ductus patency in clinical trials and observational studies, and may contribute to lung injury through this mechanism. On the other hand, the impact of fluid restriction and/or routine use of diuretics on lung injury after the first 2 weeks of life have not been adequately evaluated.

HUMORAL LUNG INJURY: OXIDATIVE STRESS, INFECTION, AND INFLAMMATION

CONGENITAL, PERINATAL, AND POSTNATAL SEPSIS

Premature newborns are likely to have been exposed to infection in utero because preterm labor is often precipitated by infection.[15] Epidemiologic evidence correlates fetal exposure to chorioamnionitis with development of BPD.[16] Infection and inflammation damage lung cells as a result of the maladaptive inflammatory response that amplifies the cycle of mechanical or oxidative injury, which leads to inflammation and additional injury. Fetal exposure to inflammatory or immunologic challenge can directly injure lung cells without the additional burdens of oxygen therapy and mechanical ventilation.[17]

Postnatal sepsis may provoke a systemic inflammatory response, accompanied by significant pulmonary neutrophil influx, alveolar-capillary leak, and, in some cases, necrotizing tracheobronchitis. Premature newborns are more likely to develop BPD if they develop postnatal sepsis.[18] Death or dysregulation of lung progenitor cells, ordinarily destined to complete repair and development, may interrupt normal alveolar and capillary development. Exposure to proinflammatory cytokines or endotoxin components without actual infection can disrupt alveolar development (see Chapter 121). Late-onset sepsis in prematures has been strongly predictive of later development of BPD. In the premature newborn lung subjected to oxidative and mechanical stress, infection may represent another instance of the "second hit" that further amplifies inflammation and contributes to dysregulated lung development and repair.

Ureaplasma infection has been implicated in the pathogenesis of BPD and may impair lung development through its provocation of inflammation. Autopsy studies of premature newborns with pneumonia have linked the presence of *U. urealyticum* in the lung to fibrotic histologic changes often found in advanced BPD. These studies linked *Ureaplasma* infection with a "pro-fibrotic" phenotype in alveolar macrophages that strongly expressed transforming growth factor β, a cytokine linked to fibroblast proliferation. Experimental infection with *Ureaplasma* in premature baboons caused lung injury and abnormal alveolar development.[19] Whether it does so in humans remains to be determined. The role of *U. urealyticum* in apparent exacerbations of respiratory failure in very low-birth-weight prematures may be underestimated.

MECONIUM ASPIRATION

Passage of meconium is associated with compromised uteroplacental blood flow at or near full-term gestation, and under certain circumstances meconium may be aspirated in utero or at delivery. Animal models using human meconium routinely demonstrate lung injury but lack the in utero pulmonary vascular remodeling that may accompany clinical meconium aspiration syndrome (MAS). Mechanical obstruction of small airways with particulate meconium can lead to air trapping and pneumothorax. Meconium present at birth is associated with pneumothorax, as noted previously.

Meconium components are toxic to the lung. Meconium contains fatty acids, and oleic acid in particular can be directly toxic to epithelial membranes. In vivo aspiration models demonstrate elevated interleukin (IL)-8 levels in tracheal aspirates.[20] In addition, oleic acid, hemoglobin, and other components in meconium may inactivate lung surfactant, leading to alveolar instability that contributes to shear stress and cellular injury. Experimental and clinical treatment with exogenous surfactant restores minimum surface tension, improves oxygenation,[21] and reduces the need for extracorporeal membrane oxygen (ECMO) in patients with MAS.[22]

AMNIOTIC FLUID ASPIRATION

At first glance, it may seem paradoxical that amniotic fluid, which is produced in part by the fetal lung, would be toxic to pulmonary epithelium. However, the aspiration of cellular debris and the components of dead cells are likely to provoke an inflammatory response by the same mechanisms attributed to meconium aspiration: direct cellular toxicity, release of humoral mediators, and surfactant inactivation. Although the net flux of pulmonary fluid in fetal life is toward the mouth and away from the lung, mixing occurs during labor, particularly if the fetus gasps in response to hypoxia. Infected amniotic contents have been reported frequently in postmortem examinations. In addition, experiments in fetal lambs have demonstrated the exposure of the fetal lung to proinflammatory cytokines derived from inflamed fetal membranes.[17]

NEONATAL PULMONARY RESPONSES TO INFLAMMATION

Inflammation—regardless of its initiating cause—exacerbates newborn lung injury. Different injuries or exposures can alter the timing and sequence of inflammatory cell influx. In neonatal surfactant deficiency and in experimental oxygen toxicity in newborn rats, resident alveolar macrophages[23] both precede and succeed the influx of neutrophils[24] that are isolated from bronchoalveolar lavage fluid of newborns with RDS. Cellular inflammatory responses to mechanical or oxidative injury in the lung are prompted by release of prostanoids, or by the binding of pathogens to signal molecules that activate proinflammatory cytokines, such as IL-1β or tumor necrosis factor-alpha (TNFα). These stimulate expression of monocyte chemokines, such as monocyte chemoattractant protein-1 (now termed *CCL2*), known to be expressed in alveolar epithelium, which in turn recruits macrophages into the lung.[25] The recruitment of leukocytes, particularly neutrophils, into the lung hinges on the complex interplay of cytokines, chemokines, and cellular adhesion molecules summarized in Fig. 69.4.

Large animal models designed to mimic clinical BPD (use of appropriate oxygen therapy, moderate ventilation, and surfactant treatment after premature delivery) have shown a similar sequence of the development of injury and inflammation even though they lack antecedent labor.[26] Premature newborns that later develop BPD are likely to have elevations of proinflammatory cytokines and chemokines in tracheal aspirate samples.[27] These elevations may be present at birth, suggesting that the inflammatory response was begun antenatally, or shortly after delivery—perhaps during the initial resuscitation.

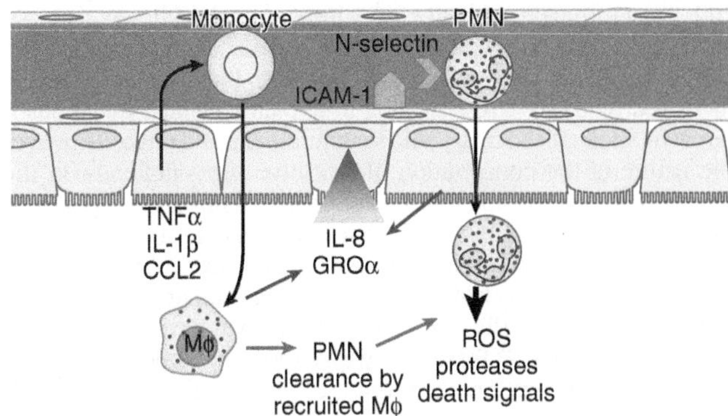

Fig. 69.4 Damaged cells release proinflammatory cytokines that up-regulate adhesion molecules—for example, N-selectin, *ICAM-1*—on circulating leukocytes (monocytes, polymorphonuclear cells, *PMNs*) and endothelium. Both epithelium and macrophages produce PMN chemokines, for example, GROα and interleukin 8 *(IL-8)*, that further up-regulate PMN adhesion and regulate chemotaxis, chemokinesis, and the reactive oxygen species *(ROS)* producing respiratory burst. On activation, the neutrophil requires continuous chemokine signal transduction, without which, the neutrophil undergoes apoptosis and is cleared by alveolar macrophages *(green arrows)*. Activated neutrophils release reactive oxygen species, proteases, and other toxic materials that can damage adjacent cells.

INFLAMMATORY PROCESSES INTERRUPT LUNG DEVELOPMENT

Damage to the developing lung may be sustained during a critical period, leading to death of particular progenitor cells necessary to orderly transition from the canalicular to the alveolar stage of lung development. Indirect effects of reactive oxygen species produced by leukocytes following oxidative stress in newborns[28] may damage lung cell deoxyribonucleic acid (DNA) in certain proliferating cell types,[29] necessitating DNA repair and thereby delaying orderly mitosis and tissue development.[30] This may occur by disrupting the normal order of cell proliferation or by accelerating pathologic lung cell apoptosis.[31] Therapies aimed at selective modification or prevention of maladaptive inflammatory responses may attenuate lung injury and permit orderly postnatal lung development.[32]

DEFICIENCY OF ANTIOXIDANT DEFENSES IN PREMATURITY

Numerous oxygen radicals including superoxide, hydrogen peroxide, peroxyl radical, singlet oxygen, and hydroxyl radical can develop in particular compartments (in vitro) within the lung and inside lung cells. These compounds can damage lipid, protein, carbohydrate, and nucleic acid cell components. What is presently unknown is whether they *do* occur in sufficient measure to cause enough lung cell injury to lead to BPD. The strength of the evidence implicating each reactive species in the pathology of newborn lung injury is variable and has been reviewed elsewhere.[33] Effects of reactive oxygen and nitrogen species on cell viability, function, and their ultimate effects on lung injury and development depend on the microenvironment in which they are formed and metabolized.

Premature newborns have relatively low chemical and enzymatic or inducible antioxidant systems compared with term and adult animals and are subjected to relatively high oxidative stress. The transition from the fetal milieu, wherein the oxygen delivery at relatively low arterial Po_2 is adequate to meet the metabolic demands, to the extrauterine existence with its significantly higher metabolic demands of thermogenesis and work of breathing, is typically accompanied by supplemental oxygen treatment.

Studies in premature animals have shown that gene expression and the enzymatic activities of superoxide dismutases, catalase, and glutathione peroxidase are decreased.[1] This suggests the circumstance of antioxidant deficiency in the face of relatively increased oxidative stress, leading to impaired cellular metabolism, direct biomolecular damage, and structural cellular damage. However, the nature of the contribution of oxidative stress depends on the relevant biologic compartments and relationships among potential molecular substrates.[34] Serum glutathione stores are diminished (relative to adults) in premature newborns at risk to develop BPD. Oxidation of proteins isolated from tracheal aspirates of newborns destined to develop BPD provides indirect evidence of inadequate antioxidant defense.[35] Treatment with exogenous antioxidants such as vitamin A[36] or superoxide dismutase[37] has been shown to reduce BPD or its sequelae.

MITIGATING OXYGEN TOXICITY EFFECTS ON LUNG INJURY

Despite this potential for harm, supplemental oxygen is a mainstay of therapy for many newborns during the adaptation to extra-uterine life, and afterwards. The goal of oxygen therapy is to deliver sufficient oxygen to the tissues while minimizing oxygen toxicity, but direct measurements of oxygen demand and delivery are seldom used in the newborn. Tissue bed near infrared spectroscopy is becoming increasingly used to monitor trends in tissue oxygenation, but its effectiveness in optimizing oxygen use has yet to be demonstrated in newborns with lung diseases. Clinical trials seeking to address this by stratifying oxygen delivery targets, mainly using different Spo_2 targets, have yielded mixed results, in part due to population differences and medical center treatment approach differences. This does not mean that the contribution of oxygen toxicity to lung injury is in doubt, but that the magnitude of the contributions of each component of injury can vary.

LUNG INJURY: LOSS OF REPAIR CAPACITY

Lung strain and stress, which may take place very soon after birth in very premature newborns or in full-term newborns with aspiration injuries, may affect progenitor cell phenotypes, thus influencing repair/differentiation capacity. For example, this may contribute to the vulnerability of patients with BPD for the later development of emphysematous pulmonary changes[38,39] and limitations of lung function[40] later in life. Our understanding of the contribution of these or other proposed underlying mechanisms to adult lung function is hampered by the scarcity of longitudinal assessments of respiratory outcomes in patients born extremely prematurely or with BPD.[41]

In the adult lung, the cellular turnover is relatively slow compared with the gastrointestinal tract or the hematopoietic system. However, during the perinatal period, and particularly after injury, turnover in the lung is relatively high. Understanding the regenerative capacity of the lung and the role of stem and progenitor cells and the paracrine factors that regulate their function will be important to future therapeutic development.

Over the past few years there have been significant advances in defining the cell lineages that contribute toward mammalian lung repair and regeneration.[42] Murine models of oxidative stress experienced during the saccular to alveolar phases of lung development demonstrate deranged alveolar type II cell proliferation and increased susceptibility to lung inflammation and injury when exposed to later insults, suggesting loss of normal repair capacity and/or ability to regulate inflammation.[43] Some type II alveolar epithelial cells appear to serve as progenitors for alveolar epithelium following injury, at least in mice.[44] Club cells in the bronchoalveolar duct junction have also been implicated as possible progenitors. Lineage tracing studies in mice exposed to hyperoxia as newborns did not demonstrate contribution of these cells to alveolar epithelium, whereas bleomycin treatment in adult mice did.[45] The plasticity of progenitor cells may vary with the injury and developmental stage.

Recent approaches using cell-based approaches to promote repair confirm that alveolar and pulmonary vascular development can be protected by treatment with bone marrow or cord blood derived mesenchymal stromal cells (MSCs), or umbilical cord derived perivascular cells, likely through paracrine effects, since engraftment is always quite low, and conditioned medium from the donor cells has some of the same effects.[46] Future lung regenerative therapies may achieve enhanced specificity with improved understanding of the paracrine mechanisms that program progenitor cell function in response to injury.[47] Evidence suggests that such cell-cell communication takes place through paracrine effects. These paracrine effects seem to be mediated through the release of nanosized extracellular vesicles important for cell-cell communication.[48] The community of alveolar and recruited cells that take part in repair is depicted in Fig. 69.5.

Although there have been great advances in our understanding of the mechanisms of lung injury and repair throughout the life span, it must be emphasized that most of these studies have relied on cell-fate or lineage tracing in murine models. It is likely that most of these general mechanisms are conserved across mammalian species, but the relative contributions to ultimate lung function in humans is limited by distinct species differences in lung anatomy, and in the ethologically distinct roles for innate immune and inflammatory responses that contribute to injury and repair.[49]

CONCLUSION

Lung injury with lifelong consequences for pulmonary function and cognitive development may occur during fetal life. Mechanical injury and resulting inflammation that may lead to nonuniform lung mechanics invite repetitive stretch injury in mechanically ventilated

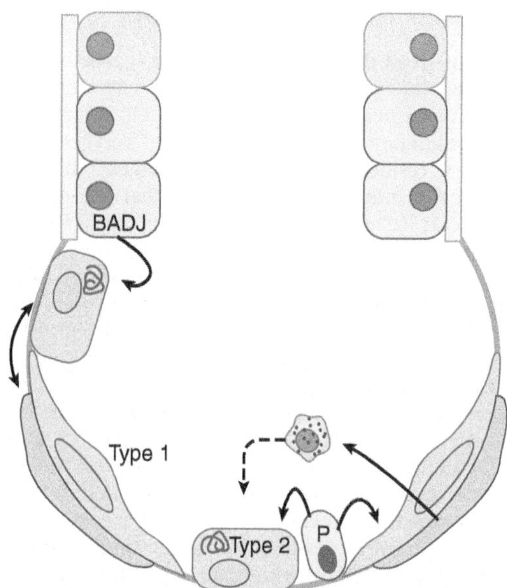

Fig. 69.5 Neonatal lung injury targets progenitor cells in the alveoli. Under some cases, bronchoalveolar duct junction cells *(BADJ)* may contribute to alveolar epithelium. A subset of progenitor cells (P) gives rise to both type 1 and type 2 alveolar epithelial cells. Bone-marrow-derived cells recruited from the circulation have paracrine effects *(dotted arrow)* that program differentiation of progenitor cells. Disrupted cross-talk between epithelial cells and vascular cells *(two-headed arrow)* impairs alveolar development.

patients, and may begin at birth during initial resuscitation. Individual differences in host antioxidant defenses, and in inflammatory responses and their regulation, very likely contribute substantially to variability of resistance to initial injury, and to the variability of successful repair in the vulnerable newborn lung (see Chapter 159). Direct cytotoxic injuries—oxygen, aspiration, sepsis—provoke inflammation, which is often maladaptive and contributes to further injury. Preventing, overcoming, and treating these inevitable early lung injuries will require improved understanding of the contributions of perinatal injury mechanisms to lifelong lung development, repair, and function. Given that variations in care approaches are among the largest predictors for the development of BPD,[50,51] future multicenter clinical trials aimed at BPD prevention will require much more uniformity in the clinical approach, and will require prospective stratification of study subjects according to likely contributory disease mechanisms. For example, the pathways in premature newborns born to mothers with pregnancy-induced hypertension are at increased risk to develop BPD, but this may be due to impaired fetal and postnatal growth. In contrast, the inflammatory burden in preterm newborns born to mothers with chorioamnionitis is likely higher. One might expect that a trial of antiinflammatory pharmacotherapy would have differing effects in these two patient categories, particularly non specific agents like corticosteroids that also affect growth and development.

REFERENCES

1. Frank L, Sosenko IR. Oxidants and antioxidants: what role do they play in chronic lung disease? In: Bland RD, Coalson J, eds. *Chronic Lung Disease in Early Infancy*. New York: Marcel Dekker; 2000:257-284.
2. Mosca F, Colnaghi M. Respiratory management of the premature infant in the delivery room. *J Matern Fetal Neonatal Med*. 2004;16(suppl 2):17-19.
3. Bjorklund LJ, Ingimarsson J, Curstedt T, et al. Lung recruitment at birth does not improve lung function in immature lambs receiving surfactant. *Acta Anaesthesiol Scand*. 2001;45:986-993.
4. Jobe AH, Kramer BW, Moss TJ, et al. Decreased indicators of lung injury with continuous positive expiratory pressure in preterm lambs. *Pediatr Res*. 2002;52:387-392.
5. Schmolzer GM, Te Pas AB, Davis PG, et al. Reducing lung injury during neonatal resuscitation of preterm infants. *J Pediatr*. 2008;153:741-745.
6. Auten RL, Vozzelli M, Clark RH. Volutrauma. What is it, and how do we avoid it? *Clin Perinatol*. 2001;28:505-515.
7. Peng W, Zhu H, Shi H, et al. Volume-targeted ventilation is more suitable than pressure-limited ventilation for preterm infants: a systematic review and meta-analysis. *Arch Dis Child Fetal Neonatal Ed*. 2014;99:F158-F165.
8. Kendig JW, Ryan RM, Sinkin RA, et al. Comparison of two strategies for surfactant prophylaxis in very premature infants: a multicenter randomized trial. *Pediatrics*. 1998;101:1006-1012.
9. Stevens TP, Blennow M, Soll RF. Early surfactant administration with brief ventilation vs selective surfactant and continued mechanical ventilation for preterm infants with or at risk for respiratory distress syndrome. *Cochrane Database Syst Rev*. 2004:CD003063.
10. Finer NN, Merritt TA, Bernstein G, et al. An open label, pilot study of Aerosurf(R) combined with nCPAP to prevent RDS in preterm neonates. *J Aerosol Med Pulm Drug Deliv*. 2010;23:303-309.
11. Gupta S, Donn SM. Novel approaches to surfactant administration. *Crit Care Res Pract*. 2012;2012:278483.
12. Stoll BJ, Hansen N. Infections in VLBW infants: studies from the NICHD Neonatal Research Network. *Semin Perinatol*. 2003;27:293-301.
13. Tammela OK, Koivisto ME. Fluid restriction for preventing bronchopulmonary dysplasia? Reduced fluid intake during the first weeks of life improves the outcome of low-birth-weight infants. *Acta Paediatr*. 1992;81:207-212.
14. Alpan G, Scheerer R, Bland R, et al. Patent ductus arteriosus increases lung fluid filtration in preterm lambs. *Pediatr Res*. 1991;30:616-621.
15. Maxwell NC, Davies PL, Kotecha S. Antenatal infection and inflammation: what's new? *Curr Opin Infect Dis*. 2006;19:253-258.
16. Watterberg KL, Demers LM, Scott SM, et al. Chorioamnionitis and early lung inflammation in infants in whom bronchopulmonary dysplasia develops. *Pediatrics*. 1996;97:210-215.
17. Kramer BW, Kramer S, Ikegami M, et al. Injury, inflammation, and remodeling in fetal sheep lung after intra-amniotic endotoxin. *Am J Physiol Lung Cell Mol Physiol*. 2002;283:L452-L459.
18. Bancalari E. Changes in the pathogenesis and prevention of chronic lung disease of prematurity. *Am J Perinatol*. 2001;18:1-9.
19. Viscardi RM, Atamas SP, Luzina IG, et al. Antenatal *Ureaplasma urealyticum* respiratory tract infection stimulates proinflammatory, profibrotic responses in the preterm baboon lung. *Pediatr Res*. 2006;60:141-146.
20. Lindenskov PH, Castellheim A, Aamodt G, et al. Meconium induced IL-8 production and intratracheal albumin alleviated lung injury in newborn pigs. *Pediatr Res*. 2005;57:371-377.
21. Auten RL, Notter RH, Kendig JW, et al. Surfactant treatment of full-term newborns with respiratory failure. *Pediatrics*. 1991;87:101-107.
22. Al Tawil K, Abu-Ekteish FM, Tamimi O, et al. Symptomatic spontaneous pneumothorax in term newborn infants. *Pediatr Pulmonol*. 2004;37:443-446.
23. Sherman MP, Truog WE. The role of pulmonary macrophages in chronic lung disease of early infancy. In: Bland RD, Coalson J, eds. *Chronic Lung Disease in Early Infancy*. New York: Marcel Dekker; 2000:813-839.
24. Jackson JC, Chi EY, Wilson CB, et al. Sequence of inflammatory cell migration into lung during recovery from hyaline membrane disease in premature newborn monkeys. *Am Rev Respir Dis*. 1987;135:937-940.
25. Vozzelli MA, Mason SN, Whorton MH, et al. Antimacrophage chemokine treatment prevents neutrophil and macrophage influx in hyperoxia-exposed newborn rat lung. *Am J Physiol Lung Cell Mol Physiol*. 2004;286:L488-L493.
26. Coalson J. Animal models of chronic lung injury. In: Bland RD, Coalson J, eds. *Chronic Lung Disease in Early Infancy*. New York: Marcel Dekker; 2000:927-956.
27. Kotecha S, Wilson L, Wangoo A, et al. Increase in interleukin (IL)-1 beta and IL-6 in bronchoalveolar lavage fluid obtained from infants with chronic lung disease of prematurity. *Pediatr Res*. 1996;40:250-256.
28. Liao L, Ning Q, Li Y, et al. CXCR2 blockade reduces radical formation in hyperoxia-exposed newborn rat lung. *Pediatr Res*. 2006;60:299-303.
29. Auten RL, Whorton MH, Nicholas Mason S. Blocking neutrophil influx reduces DNA damage in hyperoxia-exposed newborn rat lung. *Am J Respir Cell Mol Biol*. 2002;26:391-397.
30. Auten RL, O'Reilly MA, Oury TD, et al. Transgenic extracellular superoxide dismutase protects postnatal alveolar epithelial proliferation and development during hyperoxia. *Am J Physiol Lung Cell Mol Physiol*. 2006;290:L32-L40.
31. Dieperink HI, Blackwell TS, Prince LS. Hyperoxia and apoptosis in developing mouse lung mesenchyme. *Pediatr Res*. 2006;59:185-190.
32. Auten RL, Ekekezie II. Blocking leukocyte influx and function to prevent chronic lung disease of prematurity. *Pediatr Pulmonol*. 2003;35:335-341.
33. Asikainen TM, White CW. Pulmonary antioxidant defenses in the preterm newborn with respiratory distress and bronchopulmonary dysplasia in evolution: implications for antioxidant therapy. *Antioxid Redox Signal*. 2004;6:155-167.
34. Smith CV, Welty SE. Mechanisms of oxygen induced lung injury. In: Bland RD, Coalson J, eds. *Chronic Lung Disease in Early Infancy*. New York: Marcel Dekker; 2000:730-777.
35. Varsila E, Pesonen E, Andersson S. Early protein oxidation in the neonatal lung is related to development of chronic lung disease. *Acta Paediatr*. 1995;84:1296-1299.
36. Tyson JE, Wright LL, Oh W, et al. Vitamin A supplementation for extremely-low-birth-weight infants. National Institute of Child Health and Human Development Neonatal Research Network. *N Engl J Med*. 1999;340:1962-1968.
37. Davis JM, Richter SE, Biswas S, et al. Long-term follow-up of premature infants treated with prophylactic, intratracheal recombinant human CuZn superoxide dismutase. *J Perinatol*. 2000;20:213-216.
38. Wong PM, Lees AN, Louw J, et al. Emphysema in young adult survivors of moderate-to-severe bronchopulmonary dysplasia. *Eur Respir J*. 2008;32:321-328.
39. Wong P, Murray C, Louw J, et al. Adult bronchopulmonary dysplasia: computed tomography pulmonary findings. *J Med Imaging Radiat Oncol*. 2011;55:373-378.
40. Vom Hove M, Prenzel F, Uhlig HH, et al. Pulmonary outcome in former preterm, very low birth weight children with bronchopulmonary dysplasia: a case-control follow-up at school age. *J Pediatr*. 2014;164:40-45 e44.
41. Shetty S, Greenough A. Neonatal ventilation strategies and long-term respiratory outcomes. *Early Hum Dev*. 2014.
42. Hogan BL, Barkauskas CE, Chapman HA, et al. Repair and regeneration of the respiratory system: complexity, plasticity, and mechanisms of lung stem cell function. *Cell Stem Cell*. 2014;15:123-138.
43. Buczynski BW, Yee M, Martin KC, et al. Neonatal hyperoxia alters the host response to influenza A virus infection in adult mice through multiple pathways. *Am J Physiol Lung Cell Mol Physiol*. 2013;305:L282-L290.
44. Rock JR, Barkauskas CE, Cronce MJ, et al. Multiple stromal populations contribute to pulmonary fibrosis without evidence for epithelial to mesenchymal transition. *Proc Natl Acad Sci U S A*. 2011;108:E1475-E1483.
45. Rawlins EL, Okubo T, Xue Y, et al. The role of Scgb1a1+ Clara cells in the long-term maintenance and repair of lung airway, but not alveolar, epithelium. *Cell Stem Cell*. 2009;4:525-534.
46. Collins JJ, Thebaud B. Lung mesenchymal stromal cells in development and disease: to serve and protect? *Antioxid Redox Signal*. 2014;21:1849-1862.
47. Alphonse RS, Vadivel A, Fung M, et al. Existence, functional impairment, and lung repair potential of endothelial colony-forming cells in oxygen-induced arrested alveolar growth. *Circulation*. 2014;129:2144-2157.
48. Sdrimas K, Kourembanas S. MSC microvesicles for the treatment of lung disease: a new paradigm for cell-free therapy. *Antioxid Redox Signal*. 2014;21:1905-1915.
49. Wenzel S, Holgate ST. The mouse trap: it still yields few answers in asthma. *Am J Respir Crit Care Med*. 2006;174:1173-1176.
50. Ambalavanan N, Walsh M, Bobashev G, et al. Intercenter differences in bronchopulmonary dysplasia or death among very low birth weight infants. *Pediatrics*. 2011;127:e106-e116.
51. Lapcharoensap W, Gage SC, Kan P, et al. Hospital variation and risk factors for bronchopulmonary dysplasia in a population-based cohort. *JAMA Pediatr*. 2015;169:e143676.

70 Impaired Lung Growth After Injury in Preterm Lung

Kurt H. Albertine | Theodore J. Pysher | Bradley A. Yoder

INTRODUCTION

Infants born as early as 22 weeks estimated gestational age may survive if supported by neonatal intensive care, which includes the routine use of antenatal steroids, postnatal surfactant-replacement therapy, and respiratory support. These and other therapies are required because the gas-exchange regions of the lungs of prematurely born infants are structurally and functionally immature, with limited capacity to support extrauterine life. However, some approaches used for respiratory support are known to adversely affect ongoing lung development and contribute to lung injury, both acute and chronic. The goal of this chapter is to describe the impact of preterm birth and respiratory support on lung growth and development, with emphasis on impairment of alveolar formation.

ARCHITECTURAL ORGANIZATION OF THE MATURE LUNG

Before birth, fetal respiratory gas exchange is subserved by the placenta, the interface between the maternal and fetal circulations. At earlier gestational ages with more extreme fetal immaturity, the morphology of the human fetal lung is too immature to provide efficient exchange of oxygen (O_2) and carbon dioxide (CO_2). To emphasize the structural immaturity of the lung, this section provides context regarding architectural organization of the mature lung related to its respiratory gas-exchange function.

Exchange of O_2 and CO_2 in the mature lung occurs in relatively large units that are referred to as *terminal respiratory units* (TRUs). TRUs are defined anatomically as a terminal respiratory bronchiole and all its alveolar ducts, together with their accompanying alveoli.[1] In the adult human lung, each TRU contains approximately 100 alveolar ducts and 2000 anatomic alveoli. At functional residual capacity, TRUs are approximately 5 mm in diameter and have a volume of roughly 0.02 mL.[2] Together, the two lungs of the adult human contain approximately 150,000 TRUs.[3] Physiologically, diffusion of O_2 and CO_2 in the gas phase is so rapid that the partial pressures of each gas are uniform throughout a TRU. Because O_2 from incoming air has a higher O_2 partial pressure than the alveolar gas, O_2 diffuses across the gradient into all associated alveoli of the TRU. Subsequently, O_2 diffuses across the alveolar-capillary membrane and into the red blood cells, where O_2 combines with hemoglobin for transport and delivery to body tissues. CO_2 diffuses in the opposite direction.

In the normal adult human lung, the alveolar-capillary membrane is exceedingly thin, which facilitates gas diffusion through the barrier. The average width of the alveolar-capillary membrane is approximately 1.5 μm.[3,4] In the context of O_2 diffusion, the alveolar-capillary membrane's structural components are, in order, alveolar epithelium and its subjacent basal lamina, alveolar wall interstitium, basal lamina of the capillary endothelium and the capillary endothelium, plasma, the membrane of red blood cells, and, finally, hemoglobin molecules. For CO_2 transfer, the obstacles to diffusion are encountered in the opposite sequence.

ARCHITECTURAL ORGANIZATION OF THE PRETERM LUNG

TRUs of the prematurely born human infant are incompletely developed, and the gas-exchange membrane barrier is thicker, both of which impair efficient gas exchange postnatally. The structural barriers are greater with earlier preterm birth because development of the TRUs occurs during the second half of gestation and the thickness of the developing gas-exchange membrane barrier is inversely related to gestational age. A brief review of the stages of lung development in humans illustrates these points (Fig. 70.1).[5]

Before 16 weeks of gestation in humans, the future bronchi and bronchioles extend into a core of relatively undifferentiated mesenchyme that contains few blood vessels (see Fig. 70.1A). This period of lung development is called the *pseudoglandular stage*. From weeks 16 to approximately 28 of gestation, the human fetal lung is at the canalicular stage. Lung architecture at this stage is characterized by more elongated profiles of the distal-most airways and proliferation of capillaries. Although capillary proliferation is robust during the canalicular stage, the developing capillaries are distant from the air space canals (see Fig. 70.1B). The columnar epithelial cells that line the air space canals progressively become cuboidal (shorter) and show ultrastructural evidence of differentiation towards alveolar type II epithelial cells. These epithelial cells gradually develop lamellar bodies that are histologically recognizable at the transition from the canalicular to the saccular stages of lung development. Arising from alveolar type II cells are alveolar type I (squamous) epithelial cells. Although fewer in number than their alveolar type II counterparts, alveolar type I epithelial cells differentiate over time into an extremely thin cellular barrier that eventually covers approximately 90% to 95% of the alveolar surface area of the peripheral lung in the adult.[6] Thus the structural attributes of alveolar type I epithelial cells are particularly specialized for efficient movement of respiratory gases (O_2 and CO_2).

From approximately 28 to 36 weeks of gestation, lung development is at the saccular stage (see Fig. 70.1C). During this stage, the initially cylindrical air space canals become divided by primary septa, leading to formation of air space saccules. Capillaries extend into the primary septa; however, owing to a persistently thickened mesenchyme, the capillaries remain relatively distant from the epithelial cells that line the saccules. Continual saccular development is accompanied by an apoptotic-related gradual thinning of the interstitial mesenchyme that separates the air space epithelium from the capillaries.[7]

From the saccular stage to the end of term gestation, the concentrations of dipalmitoyl phosphatidylcholine and other surfactant phospholipids increase in lung tissue, lung lavage liquid, and amniotic liquid. In the developing human lung, surfactant components can be identified within type II alveolar epithelial cells as early as approximately 20 weeks' gestation,[8] although evidence for surfactant in the amniotic fluid is not typically noted until approximately 26 weeks or later.[9] Human SP-B and SP-C messenger RNAs (mRNAs) are detectable in lung tissue at very low levels, earlier than SP-A, during the transition from the canalicular to the saccular stage (approximately 24

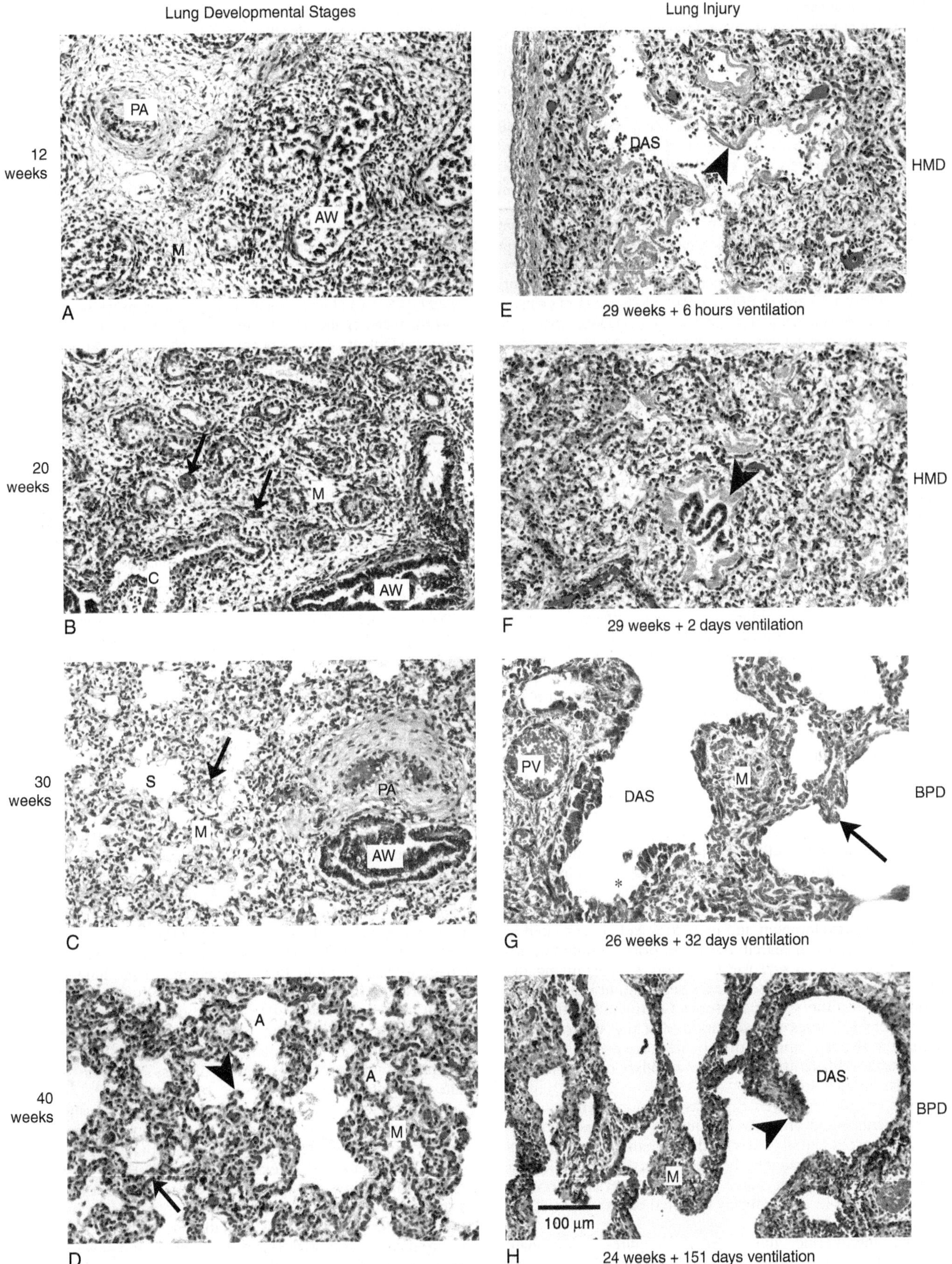

Fig. 70.1 See the following page for the explanation of the figure.

Fig. 70.1 Comparison of normal lung histology during development in humans to lung histopathology associated with hyaline membrane disease *(HMD)* or bronchopulmonary dysplasia *(BPD)*. The panels are shown at the same magnification (scale bar is 100 μm in length). (A to D) Ontogeny (H & E stain). All the lungs were fixed at low lung volume at autopsy. (A) Infant stillborn at 12 to 14 weeks of gestation. Although considerable autolysis (postmortem degeneration) is evident, airways *(AW)* are lined by columnar epithelium that is largely desquamated. The mesenchyme *(M)* is devoid of capillaries in this tissue section. (B) Infant stillborn at approximately 20 weeks of gestation. Canaliculi are lined by cuboidal epithelium. A larger AW is visible in this tissue section. The M remains thick and cellular, and contains capillaries deep within the mesenchyme, but not at the air-blood interface *(arrows)*. (C) Infant stillborn at approximately 30 weeks of gestation. Saccules *(S)* are separated from capillaries *(arrow)* by M that is thinner than during the canalicular stage but nonetheless remains relatively thick and cellular. An AW and pulmonary artery *(PA)* are visible in this tissue section. (D) Infant stillborn at approximately 40 weeks of gestation (term). Alveolar development has progressed to where the primary septa are thinner and secondary septa *(crests; arrowhead)* protrude into the developing alveoli. The alveolar walls have numerous capillaries *(arrow)*. (E to H) Histopathology of lung injury in preterm human infants who died. (E and F) HMD (H & E stain). (E) Birth at approximately 25 weeks of gestation followed by 6 hours of mechanical ventilation. At 6 hours of respiratory support, the preterm, mechanically ventilated lung shows uneven expansion of the distal air spaces *(DASs)*, vascular congestion, and interstitial edema. Hyaline membranes *(arrowhead)* are present. Some patchy hemorrhage also may be present. (F) HMD, birth at 29 weeks of gestation followed by 2 days of mechanical ventilation. Hyaline membranes *(arrowhead)* are present. The distribution of ventilation is uneven, with centriacinar expansion and peripheral collapse. (G and H) BPD. (G) Birth at 26 weeks of gestation followed by 32 days of mechanical ventilation (approximately 30 weeks' postconceptual age) (Masson trichrome stain). The DASs appear to have desquamated epithelial cells *(asterisk)*. Thick, cellular mesenchyme *(M)* separates the adjacent air spaces. *Arrow* indicates stunted secondary septa. (H) Birth at 24 weeks of gestation followed by 151 days of mechanical ventilation (approximately 46 weeks' postconceptual age) (H & E stain). Simplification and overdistension of the DASs is clearly evident. Primary septa have thick and cellular M. Secondary septa *(crests; arrowhead)* are infrequently visible; those that are visible are short, thick, and devoid of capillaries near their tip. *PV*, Pulmonary vein.

weeks of gestation).[10] Detection of SP-B and SP-C proteins, however, occurs later in development, during the saccular stage (approximately 30 weeks of gestation).[8] To our knowledge, human SP-D protein has been detected in amniotic liquid only during the transition from the canalicular to the saccular stage of lung development (approximately 24 weeks of gestation).[11,12] Thus the biochemical machinery to reduce surface tension at air-liquid interfaces in the future air spaces develops during the third trimester in humans. Many preterm human infants who are born before the third trimester are at risk for respiratory failure because their lungs are deficient in surfactant. An approach to assess lung development before birth is to measure these secretory products in amniotic liquid.[13,14]

Beginning at approximately 36 weeks of gestation and continuing through the first 18 to 24 months of postnatal life, alveoli are formed by progressive subdivision of the air space saccules by secondary septa (see Fig. 70.1D). At term, alveolar formation is less complete in humans, baboons, and mice[5,15-19] compared to sheep and other ruminants.[20-22] The interspecies developmental differences are important to keep in mind when comparing results within and among species (Table 70.1: Control interventions and Genetic background), and drawing analogies to human lung development and pathology. References cited in Table 70.1 are through March 2020. The primary outcome for Table 70.1 is impaired alveolar formation. Accompanying the subdivision of saccules by secondary septa is outward growth of capillaries into the secondary septa. Continuous thinning of the mesenchymal cores also occurs during the alveolar stage, such that the alveolar-capillary membrane barrier attains its adult thinness, with intimate juxtaposition of capillary endothelium to the alveolar lining epithelium.

Another impediment to efficient gas diffusion in the lungs of preterm infants is the presence of liquid in the interstitium and potential air spaces. Liquid (water) in the interstitium and potential air spaces is an impediment because diffusion of molecular oxygen is slower through water than gas phase. Therefore O_2 diffusion is slower in the relatively hydrated environment of the preterm lung.

Normal intrauterine lung growth requires appropriate distension by lung luminal liquid.[23] Fetal lung liquid moves into the fetal potential air space via an osmotic gradient that is generated by the active transport of chloride secreted across the fetal lung epithelium into the potential air spaces.[24] Under normal conditions, the liquid pressure within the lung's air space is higher than that within the amniotic cavity; thus lung luminal liquid is propelled centrally along the conducting airways to the oropharynx, where the liquid is either swallowed or expelled into the amniotic sac. Balance between production and drainage of lung luminal liquid is required for normal intrauterine lung growth.[23]

Near or at the time of term birth, the secretory activity of the lung epithelium switches from a predominantly chloride-secreting membrane to a predominantly sodium-absorbing membrane.[25-28] This molecular switch reverses water movement, thereby drying the potential air spaces for gaseous diffusion.

ACUTE LUNG INJURY OF PREMATURITY (RESPIRATORY DISTRESS SYNDROME)

When an infant is born prematurely, the structurally immature lungs are deficient in surfactant. Therefore surface tension forces are high, and the distal air spaces are unstable.[29] Air space instability results in air space collapse (atelectasis), which contributes to ventilation-perfusion mismatch. Such mismatch leads to intrapulmonary shunting that also contributes to poor oxygenation and ventilation.[30] Opening the collapsed air spaces requires high ventilatory pressures and/or volumes, which are transmitted to the immature parenchyma of the lung. In effect, the extreme effort required to expand the lungs with the first breath must be repeated with each subsequent breath because surfactant is not present to prevent collapse of the distal air spaces. Prematurely born infants who have these characteristics tire quickly and develop respiratory distress syndrome (RDS; also called *acute lung injury*).

RDS affects approximately 50,000 infants annually in the United States, with incidence inversely related to gestational age.[31-34] For example, RDS occurs in more than 50% of preterm infants born before 30 weeks of gestation.[35] However, the total number of late-preterm infants exceeds those born at earlier gestations. Therefore about half of all infants diagnosed with RDS are older than 33 weeks' gestation at birth.[36,37] For reasons that remain unclear, RDS is more prevalent and severe in male compared with female preterm infants. This sex difference is considered in Table 70.1 (sex as a biologic variable).

RDS is characterized by hypoxemia, tachypnea, and chest retractions shortly after birth. Chest radiographs reveal low

Table 70.1 Processes and Molecular Players in Impaired Alveolarization in Animal Models of Bronchopulmonary Dysplasia.

Process	Species	Molecular Players	Injury Model and Alveolarization Outcome	References
Control interventions	Mouse pups		Various control interventions	204
Genetic background	Mouse pups		Hyperoxia	205-209
Sex as Biologic Variable				
	Mouse pups		Hyperoxia	210, 211
	Mouse pups	TLR4-NF-κB signaling (innate immune response)	Administration with or without lipopolysaccharide (LPS) no impact on alveolar simplification—*no sex-specific effects*	212
	Mouse pups	Cytochrome P450 family 1 subfamily A member 2 (*Cyp1a2* gene)	Global knockout (*Nqo1* signaling) during hyperoxia: better alveolarization—*in females*	213
	Mouse pups	β-Naphthoflavone (Cyp1a2/NADPH quinone oxidoreductase, NQO1)	Administration during hyperoxia: better alveolarization and vascular growth—*in females*	213
	Mouse pups	Dihydrotestosterone	Administration during hyperoxia: worsened alveolar simplification—*in both sexes*	214
	Mouse pups	Androgens (Flutamide, competitive inhibitor for binding to androgen receptor; dihydrotestosterone)	Excess exogenous androgens during hyperoxia: worsened alveolar simplification—*in both sexes*	214
	Mouse pups	miR-146	Administration of mimic during hyperoxia: better alveolarization—*in males* Administration of inhibitor during LPS with hyperoxia: worsened alveolar simplification—*in females*	206
Respiratory Management				
	Mouse pups		Mechanical ventilation: alveolar simplification	215
	Mouse pups	Elafin (elastase inhibitor; targets epidermal growth factor receptor and Krüppel-like factor 4, EGFR-Klf4)	Mechanical ventilation: better alveolarization	216-218
	Rat pups		Mechanical ventilation: imbalance between fibulin-5 and elastin expression	53
	Preterm rabbit kits		Preterm birth with hyperoxia (not ventilated): alveolar simplification Preterm birth with hyperoxia and continuous positive airway pressure (CPAP): better alveolarization	147
	Fetal lambs		Mechanical ventilation (1 h) with umbilical cord blood: did not prevent alveolar simplification 24 h later	219
	Preterm lambs	Erythropoietin (EPO; targets inflammation)	Mechanical ventilation with EPO: EPO dose-dependent exacerbation of lung injury	220
	Preterm lambs		Mechanical ventilation 21 days: alveolar simplification with excess elastin accumulation	138, 139
	Preterm lambs	Vitamin A (targets vascular growth)	Administration during 21 days of mechanical ventilation: better alveolarization	173
	Preterm lambs	Parathyroid hormone-related protein-peroxisome proliferator-activated receptor gamma (PTHrP-PPARγ) signaling	Mechanical ventilation 21 days: lower level Noninvasive respiratory support 21 days: higher level	221
	Preterm lambs	Restricted nutrition (targets growth)	Enteral nutrition restriction during 21 days of noninvasive respiratory support: alveolar simplification and poor growth	184
	Preterm lambs	Noninvasive respiratory support (targets gentler respiratory management)	Compared to mechanical ventilation 3 days or 21 days: better alveolarization	7, 78
	Preterm baboons	Noninvasive respiratory support (targets gentler respiratory management)	Compared to mechanical ventilation 28 days: better alveolarization	76
	Preterm baboons	Proteases and protease inhibitors	Mechanical ventilation 14 days: imbalance between cysteine proteases and inhibitors	222
	Former preterm lambs	Long-term outcomes	Mechanical ventilation ~7 days, with follow-up at 5 months corrected postnatal age: persistent alveolar simplification	141
	Former preterm baboons	Long-term outcomes	Mechanical ventilation 14 days and hyperoxia, with follow-up at 8 months corrected postnatal age: persistent alveolar simplification	223

Continued

Table 70.1 Processes and Molecular Players in Impaired Alveolarization in Animal Models of Bronchopulmonary Dysplasia.—cont'd

Process	Species	Molecular Players	Injury Model and Alveolarization Outcome	References
Inflammation				
	Mouse pups	Nuclear factor kappa-light-chain-enhancer of activated B cells (NFκB) kinase subunit β (IKBKB; targets elastin)	Transactivation: alveolar simplification	224
	Mouse pups		LPS: alveolar simplification	225
	Mouse pups	NF-κB pathway inhibitor (BAY 11-7082)	Administration during LPS: worsened alveolar simplification	226
	Mouse pups	NF-κB signaling or C-X-C motif chemokine ligand 2 (CXCL2; targets macrophage inflammatory protein-2)	Blocking during LPS: worsened alveolar simplification	226
	Mouse pups	Cytoplasmic polyadenylation element-binding protein 2 (CPEB2)-activated PDGFRα	Administration during hyperoxia: better alveolarization	227
	Mouse pups	Interleukin 1 (IL-1) receptor	Agonists during hyperoxia: better alveolarization	228, 229
	Mouse pups	Nucleotide-binding oligomerization domain-like receptor pyrin domain-containing-3 (NLRP3; targets inflammasome)	Administration during hyperoxia: better alveolarization	230
	Mouse pups	Selective and irreversible inhibitor of the cysteine protease caspase-1 (Ac-YVAD-CMK; also known as *interleukin-1-converting enzyme*, ICE; targets inflammasome)	Administration during hyperoxia: better alveolarization	231
	Mouse pups	Ac-YVAD-CMK	Administration during hyperoxia: less inflammation and better alveolarization (and more proliferation in the brain)	231
	Mouse pups	*Adenovirus* transfected β-defensin-2 (AdhBD2; targets inflammation)	Administration during hyperoxia: better alveolarization	232
	Mouse pups	CD11b⁺ mononuclear cells	Depletion during hyperoxia: worsened alveolar simplification	233
	Mouse pups	Resident alveolar macrophages	Depletion during hyperoxia: better alveolarization	234
	Mouse pups	Anti-IL-33 antibody	Administration during hyperoxia: less inflammation and better alveolarization	235
	Rat pups	Human β-defensin-2 (hBD2; targets neutrophil extracellular traps)	Administration during hyperoxia: better alveolarization	232
	Rat pups	Adenovirus overexpressing tumor necrosis factor-stimulated protein 6 (AdTSG-6)	Administration during hyperoxia: better alveolarization	236
	Rat pups	Rac1 (member of subfamily of the Rho family of GTPases; affects structural changes to the actin cytoskeleton; targets inflammasome)	Administration of specific Rac1 inhibitor: better alveolarization	237
	Rat pups	Celecoxib (NSAID; targets NF-κB and aquaporin1)	Administration during hyperoxia; better alveolarization	238
	Rat pups	Lipoxin A4 (targets PTEN-induced putative kinase 1, PINK1)	Administration during hyperoxia: better alveolarization	239
	Rat pups	Leukocyte recruitment	Blocked during hyperoxia: better alveolarization	240, 241
	Rat pups	Low-dose heparin (targets neutrophil extracellular traps and histones)	Administration during hyperoxia: better alveolarization	242

Table 70.1 Processes and Molecular Players in Impaired Alveolarization in Animal Models of Bronchopulmonary Dysplasia.—cont'd

Process	Species	Molecular Players	Injury Model and Alveolarization Outcome	References
Oxidative Stress				
	Guinea pigs	Glutathione (GSSG)	Administration: improved alveolarization	243
	Mouse pups	Nuclear factor erythroid 2 p45-related factor, *Nrf2* gene (antioxidant response gene)	Knockout during hyperoxia: worsened alveolar simplification	244
	Mouse pups	*Nrf2* gene	Induction during hyperoxia: no impact on alveolar simplification	245
	Mouse pups	NAD(P)H quinone oxidoreductase (*Nqo1* gene expression in *Cyp1a1* knockout model)	Induction during hyperoxia: better alveolarization	246
	Mouse pups	Superoxide dismutase 2 (*Sod2* gene)	Knockout during hyperoxia: no impact on alveolar simplification	247
	Mouse pups	*Sod3*	Knockout during bleomycin: worsened alveolar simplification	248
	Mouse pups	BTB domain and CNC homolog 1 (*Bach1* gene; target transcriptional repressor of heme oxygenase)	Knockout during hyperoxia: better alveolarization	249
	Rat pups	Edaravone (free radical scavenger)	Administration during hyperbaric hyperoxia: better alveolarization	250
Oxidative Stress				
	Rat pups	Resveratrol (polyphenol; antioxidant)	Administration during hyperoxia: better alveolarization	251
	Rat pups	Rapamycin (autophagy agonist; targets are p62, Keap1, Nrf2, NQO1, GGLC, HO-1)	Administration during hyperoxia: better alveolarization	252
	Mouse pups	Aurothioglucose (thioredoxin reductase-1 inhibitor)	Administration during hyperoxia: no impact on vascular density	253
Extracellular Matrix Involvement				
	Mouse pups	Elastin	Normal lung development Haploinsufficiency during mechanical ventilation: no impact on alveolar simplification	155, 215, 254
	Mouse pups	Elafin	Mechanical ventilation: better alveolarization	217, 218
	Mouse pups	Elafin	Administration during hyperoxia: better alveolarization	255
	Mouse pups	β-Aminopropionitrile (lysyl oxidase inhibitor)	Administration during hyperoxia: no impact on alveolar simplification	53, 256
	Mouse pups	Transglutaminase 2 (*Tgm2*; targets ECM structure)	Knockout before hyperoxia: no impact on alveolar simplification	257
	Mouse pups	Cysteamine (transglutaminase inhibitor)	Administration during hyperoxia: better alveolarization	257
	Mouse pups	TSG-6 (hyaladherins; targets extracellular matrix stability and cell migration)	Administration during hyperoxia: worsened alveolar simplification	258
	Mouse pups	Cathepsin K	Over-expression and hyperoxia: airspace enlargement	259
	Mouse pups	Proteases, using human BPD exosomes (target neutrophil elastase)	Administration: alveolar simplification	260
	Preterm baboons	Proteases and protease inhibitors	Mechanical ventilation 14 days: imbalance between cysteine proteases and inhibitors	222
Corticosteroids				
		Use in BPD		261, 262
	Rat pups	Repeated doses of postnatal dexamethasone	Daily administration during postnatal days 3–14: decreased saccular subdivision into alveoli, with accelerated alveolar wall thinning and decreased replication of fibroblasts	263, 264

Continued

Table 70.1 Processes and Molecular Players in Impaired Alveolarization in Animal Models of Bronchopulmonary Dysplasia.—cont'd

Process	Species	Molecular Players	Injury Model and Alveolarization Outcome	References
Morphogenesis				
	Mouse pups	Transforming growth factor β (TGFβ) receptor and downstream signaling molecules	Hyperoxia: Upregulated and worsened alveolar simplification	265
	Mouse pups	TGFβ-induced protein (TGFBI)	Knockout: alveolar simplification	266
	Mouse pups	Latent TGFβ-binding protein 4 (LTBP4)	Hypomorphic: alveolar simplification	267
	Mouse pups	Caffeine (TGFβ signaling)	Administration during hyperoxia: better vascular growth Administration during hyperoxia: no impact on alveolar simplification	268, 269
	Mouse pups	Wingless-related integration site (Wnt) 5a	Conditional loss-of-function postnatally: alveolar simplification	270
	Mouse pups	Wnt5a	Inhibition of NF-κB (BAY-11-708) to reduce Wnt5a expression during hyperoxia: better alveolarization	271
	Mouse pups	Platelet-derived growth factor receptor alpha (*Pdgfrα* gene)	Haploinsufficiency during hyperoxia without PDGF-A treatment: worsened alveolar simplification Haploinsufficiency during hyperoxia with PDGF-A treatment: better alveolarization	272
	Rat pups	TGFβ receptor and downstream signaling molecules	Hyperoxia: upregulated and worsened alveolar simplification	273, 274
	Rat pups	Anti-placental growth factor (PGF) antibody (targets NF-κB signaling pathway suppression)	Administration during hyperoxia: better alveolarization and vascular growth	275
	Preterm rabbit kits		Preterm birth (not ventilated): alveolar simplification	142
Morphogenesis				
	Preterm rabbit kits	Simvastatin (targets vascular growth and inflammation)	Preterm birth with hyperoxia (not ventilated): no impact on alveolar simplification	276
Vascular Growth				
	Rat pups	Angiogenesis	Thalidomide, fumagillin, or SU-5416 (inhibitor of vascular endothelial growth factor receptor, kinase domain-containing receptor/fetal liver kinase 1 [KDR/flk-1]): alveolar simplification	171
	Mouse pups	Caffeine	Administration during hyperoxia: better vascular growth Administration during hyperoxia: no impact on alveolar simplification	268, 269
	Mouse pups	Iloprost (synthetic analog of prostacyclin, PGI_2)	Administration during hyperoxia: better alveolarization and vascular growth	277
	Mouse pups	Sildenafil (phosphodiesterase 5, PDE5, inhibitor)	Administration during hyperoxia: no impact on alveolar simplification	278
	Mouse pups	Glutaredoxin 1 (thiol esterase; targets vascular growth)	Knockout during hyperoxia: better alveolarization	279
	Mouse pups	Non-integrating expression plasmids with forkhead box m1 or f1, Foxm1, Foxf1; targets proangiogenic transcription factors)	Administration during hyperoxia: better alveolarization	280
	Mouse pups	Aurothioglucose (thioredoxin reductase-1 inhibitor; targets vascular growth)	Administration during hyperoxia: better alveolarization	253
	Mouse pups	Adrenomedullin (targets vascular growth)	Haplosufficiency during hyperoxia: worsened alveolar simplification	281

Table 70.1 Processes and Molecular Players in Impaired Alveolarization in Animal Models of Bronchopulmonary Dysplasia.—cont'd

Process	Species	Molecular Players	Injury Model and Alveolarization Outcome	References
	Rat pups	Cellular communication network factor 1 (CCN1; targets vascular growth and inflammation)	Administration during hyperoxia: better vascular growth and reduced inflammation	282
	Rat pups	Insulin-like growth factor 1/binding protein 3 (IGF-1/BP-3; targets vascular growth and inflammation)	Intraamniotic endotoxin or soluble fetal liver kinase1 followed by postnatal administration during hyperoxia: better alveolarization	283
Nutrition				
	Mouse pups	Quercetin (flavonoid; targets inflammation and oxidant injury)	Administration during hyperoxia: better alveolarization and vascular growth	284
	Mouse pups	All-*trans*-retinoic acid	Coincident daily (10 days) injection of retinoic acid and dexamethasone (the latter to inhibit alveolar): better alveolarization	285, 286
	Rat pups	Omega-3 fatty acids	Administration during hyperoxia: no impact on alveola simplification	287
	Rat pups	Vitamin D	Administration during LPS: better alveolarization	288
	Preterm lambs	Vitamin A (targets vascular growth)	Administration during 21 days of mechanical ventilation: better alveolarization	173
	Preterm lambs	Restricted nutrition (targets growth)	Enteral nutrition restriction during 21 days of noninvasive respiratory support: alveolar simplification and poor growth	184
Stem Cells/Extracellular Vesicles (Target Regeneration)				
	Mouse pups	Mesenchymal stem/stromal cell (MSC)-derived exosomes	Administration during hyperoxia: better alveolarization	289
	Mouse pups	MSC-derived exosomes (target tumor necrosis factor alpha-stimulated gene-6, TSG-6)	Administration during hyperoxia: better alveolarization	258
	Mouse pups	Erythropoietin and MSCs (target inflammation)	Administration during hyperoxia: better alveolarization	290, 291
	Mouse pups	Human aortic endothelial cells (target inflammation)	Administration during hyperoxia: better alveolarization	291
	Mouse pups	Human induced pluripotential stem cell-derived lung progenitor cells (target alveolar epithelial cells)	Administration during hyperoxia: better alveolarization	292
	Mouse pups	Human umbilical cord blood-derived MSCs (target formyl peptide receptor 1, FPR1)	Administration during hyperoxia: better alveolarization	293
Stem Cells/Extracellular Vesicles				
	Mouse pups	MSC-expressing anti-stromal derived factor-1 short hairpin RNA (target *Sdf-1* pathway)	Administration during hyperoxia: better alveolarization	294
	Mouse pups	Human umbilical cord Wharton's jelly-derived MSCs (target TGF-β1)	Administration during hyperoxia: better alveolarization	295
	Mouse pups	Human induced pluripotent stem cells (iPSCs; target inflammation)	Administration during hyperoxia: better alveolarization than exosomes or alveolar-like iPSCs	296
	Mouse pups	Proteases, using human BPD exosomes (target neutrophil elastase)	Administration: alveolar simplification	260
	Mouse pups	α1,3-Fucosyltransferase-IX (enzyme of pulmonary endogenous lung stem cell marker stage-specific embryonic antigen 1, SSEA-1; target inflammation)	Administration during hyperoxia: no impact on alveolar simplification	297
	Rat pups	Human MSCs (targets renin-angiotensin system)	Administration during hyperoxia: better alveolarization	298

Continued

Table 70.1 Processes and Molecular Players in Impaired Alveolarization in Animal Models of Bronchopulmonary Dysplasia.—cont'd

Process	Species	Molecular Players	Injury Model and Alveolarization Outcome	References
	Rat pups	Naked plasmid expressing stromal derived factor-1 (SDF-1; target inflammation and vascular growth)	Administration during hyperoxia: better alveolarization and vascular growth	299
	Rat pups	Decorin secreted by human umbilical cord-derived MSCs (target macrophage polarization)	Reduced secretion during hyperoxia: alveolar simplification Increased secretion during hyperoxia: better alveolarization	300
	Rat pups	Extracellular vesicles (target immunomodulation)	Administration during hyperoxia: better alveolarization	301
	Rat pups	MSC-derived extracellular vesicles (target inflammation and vascular growth)	Administration during hyperoxia: better alveolarization	302
	Rat pups	7ND truncated version of CC chemokine ligand 2 (CCL2)-transfected MSCs (target macrophage activation)	Administration during hyperoxia: better alveolarization than MSCs alone	303
	Rat pups	Human umbilical cord Wharton's jelly MSCs (target inflammation and vascular growth)	Administration during hyperoxia: better alveolarization	304
	Rat pups	Human umbilical cord Wharton's jelly-derived MSCs (target inflammation and vascular growth)	Late rescue with repeated administration after early hyperoxia: long-term outcome of better alveolar structure and vessel density	305
	Rabbit kits	Human amniotic fluid stem cells with upregulated VEGF expression (target VEGF)	Administration during hyperoxia: no effects	306
	Fetal lambs	Ovine umbilical cord blood	Mechanical ventilation for 1h in utero: did not prevent alveolar simplification 24 hours later	219
Epigenetics				
		microRNA pathways	Lung development	202, 203, 307, 308
	Mouse pups	microRNA (miR)-17/92 cluster (targets DNA methyltransferases, DNMT1, 3A and 3B)	Hyperoxia and LPS: lower levels	309
	Mouse pups	miR-29a (targets growth factor receptor-bound protein 2 (GRB2)-associated-binding protein 1)	Inhibition during hyperoxia: better alveolarization	310
	Mouse pups	miR-29b	Hyperoxia and LPS: lower levels Adeno-associated 9 (AAV9)-mediated restoration of miR-29 during hyperoxia and LPS: better alveolarization	309, 311
	Mouse pups	miR-34a (targets angiopoietin-1)	Hyperoxia: higher levels Inhibition during hyperoxia: better alveolarization Global knockout during hyperoxia: better alveolarization and vessel growth	312
	Mouse pups	miR-34a/*Pdgfra* interactions (targets PDGFRα+ myofibroblast abundance)	Administration of inhibitor during hyperoxia: better alveolarization	313
	Mouse pups	miR-146	Administration of mimic to males during hyperoxia: better alveolarization Administration of inhibitor to females during LPS with hyperoxia: worsened alveolar simplification	206
	Mouse pups	miR-150 (targets glycoprotein nonmetastatic melanoma protein B, GPNMB)	Hyperoxia: lower levels	314

Table 70.1 Processes and Molecular Players in Impaired Alveolarization in Animal Models of Bronchopulmonary Dysplasia.—cont'd

Process	Species	Molecular Players	Injury Model and Alveolarization Outcome	References
Epigenetics				
	Mouse pups	miR-199a-5p mimic	Administration of mimic during hyperoxia: worsened alveolar simplification Administration of inhibitor during hyperoxia: better alveolarization	315
	Mouse pups	miR-421 (targets Fgf10)	Administration of inhibitor during hyperoxia: better alveolarization	316
	Mouse pups	miR-489 (targets *Igf2* and *Tnc* mRNAs)	Hyperoxia: lower levels	317
	Mouse pups	miR-876-3	Administration of mimic during hyperoxia and LPS: better alveolarization	318
	Rat pups	Circular RNAs	Hyperoxia versus normoxia: profiles are different	319
Potpourri				
	Mouse pups	Carnitine palmitoyl transferase 1A (*Cpt1A* gene; targets carnitine shuttling)	Endothelial knockout during hyperoxia: better alveolarization	320
	Mouse pups	Cytochrome P450 family 1 subfamily A member 1 (*Cyp1a1* gene; targets NADP(H) quinone reductase)	Increase during hyperoxia: better alveolarization Global knockout during hyperoxia: better alveolarization	246, 321
	Mouse pups	Cytochrome P450 family 1 subfamily A member 2 (*Cyp1a2* gene; targets NQO1 signaling)	Global knockout during hyperoxia: better alveolarization—in females	213
	Mouse pups	Germ-free mice (target no microbiome)	Hyperoxia: better alveolarization	322
	Mouse pups	Extracellular signal-regulated kinases (ERK) 1/2 (targets mitogenesis)	Knockdown during hyperoxia: worsened alveolar simplification	323
	Rat pups	Necrostatin-1 (Nec-1; targets inhibition of kinase activity of receptor-interacting serine/threonine-protein 1 (RIP1) kinase, a mediator of necroptosis)	Administration during hyperoxia: better alveolarization	250
	Rat pups	*NSC23766* (inhibitor of Rac1, a Rho-family GTPase critical for guanine nucleotide exchange factor interaction)	Administration during hyperoxia: better alveolarization and vascular growth	237
	Rat pups	Riociguat (targets cGMP production)	Administration during hyperoxia: better alveolarization	324
	Rabbit kits		Delivered preterm and managed 7 days: alveolar simplification	142

lung volumes, air bronchograms, and diffuse opacification. Lung function studies reveal increased airway resistance and decreased pulmonary compliance.[37,38] Pulmonary vascular studies show increased pulmonary artery pressure and pulmonary vascular resistance in preterm infants with severe RDS.[39]

The pathologic findings in RDS are similar to those found in adults with acute RDS,[40] superimposed on the immature lung.[41] Histopathologic lesions in the immature lungs reflect both the disease and its treatment with mechanical ventilation and supplemental O_2 (see Fig. 70.1E and F). Within the first 3 to 4 hours, the lungs may show only uneven ventilation of distal air spaces, interstitial edema, and congestion of capillaries. By 12 to 24 hours, necrosis of alveolar and bronchiolar epithelial cells develops, and the denuded walls become coated by characteristic hyaline membranes.[42] Increased-permeability pulmonary edema is accompanied by accumulation of neutrophils in the vascular, interstitial, and airspace compartments of the lung.[43-45] A harbinger of impending accumulation of mature neutrophils in the lung and progression to acute injury is early decrease in the number of circulating neutrophils during the first 30 to 90 minutes after birth, demonstrated in preterm lambs that were ventilated with 100% O_2 for 8 hours.[44] The early decrease of neutrophils from the circulation correlated with accumulation of neutrophils in the airway and distal lung, as well as formation of pulmonary edema and hyaline membranes. The correlation in preterm lambs is consistent with a retrospective chart review for premature human infants,[46] which showed that a low number of mature neutrophils in the systemic circulation within 24 hours of birth is associated with more severe respiratory distress during the first week of postnatal life and increased need for mechanical ventilation with supplemental O_2.

Mode of respiratory support contributes to the pathogenesis of RDS (see Table 70.1: Respiratory management).[47-49] Mechanical ventilation stretches the lung, initiating responses from cells in the lung, even following repeated doses of exogenous surfactant. Primary among the responses are inflammatory responses (see

Table 70.1: Inflammation) that are initiated by the effects of expansion of air space volume, termed *ventilator-induced lung injury*.[50-53] The injurious effects of mechanical ventilation depend on a number of factors, among which are the magnitudes of stretch related to airway pressure (barotrauma) and lung volume (volutrauma),[54,55] the concentration of inspired O_2,[56,57] infection/inflammation (biotrauma),[58-61] and the duration of ventilation support. Several experimental studies compared indices of ventilator-induced lung injury between conditions that raised airway pressure and increased lung volume. Results of studies that strapped the thorax and abdomen of rats,[62] rabbit kits,[63] or lambs[64] demonstrated that large lung volume, rather than high peak airway pressure *per se*, is important in the pathogenesis of ventilator-induced lung injury, including increased-permeability pulmonary edema. Permeability in this context may be increased directly or indirectly through release of inflammatory mediators from sequestered neutrophils in the lung. Accumulation of edema liquid, particularly air-space edema liquid, is associated with inactivation of surfactant, which contributes to atelectasis and reduces lung compliance. If these events are not arrested, lung injury continues, necessitating larger tidal volume, higher airway pressure, and more supplemental O_2, all contributing to respiratory failure.

A problem with mechanical ventilation of immature lungs that are surfactant deficient is inhomogeneous distribution of ventilation, which leads to regional overinflation of ventilated units of the lung. Clinical studies suggest maturation-related effects of early nasal continuous positive airway pressure (CPAP), as reflected by high treatment failure rates in the extremely preterm newborns at many centers. Nonetheless, early use of noninvasive respiratory support, including nasal CPAP, is associated with better pulmonary outcomes.[65] For example, nasal CPAP is associated with less use and fewer days of mechanical ventilation, lower levels of inspired O_2-rich gas,[33,66-69] and lower incidence of bronchopulmonary dysplasia (BPD) or BPD with death.[70-72] Encouraging results from a randomized clinical trial show that use of extended CPAP led to significantly increased functional residual capacity through hospital discharge, which may lead to improved respiratory outcomes later in life.[73]

Animal studies demonstrate that 2 hours of bubble nasal CPAP support of preterm lambs is associated with less mRNA expression and protein abundance of inflammatory markers compared with 2 hours of mechanical ventilation.[74,75] Other animal studies reveal that early use of nasal CPAP or nasal pulsatile-flow ventilation improve respiratory gas exchange and alveolar formation.[7,76-78] An explanation for the beneficial outcomes is that much lower mean airway pressure reaches the lung parenchyma during noninvasive modes of respiratory support (approximately 10-fold lower than during mechanical ventilation),[7,78] which minimizes overstretch of the developing lung.[79,80]

Because RDS is a predictable consequence of lung immaturity, strategies have been developed to accelerate lung development before preterm delivery. One strategy is antenatal administration of corticosteroids, such as betamethasone (see Table 70.1: Corticosteroids).[81-84] The seminal studies of Liggins demonstrated that glucocorticoids accelerate lung maturation of fetal sheep and decrease the incidence of RDS in human infants after antenatal corticosteroid therapy.[85,86] Corticosteroids (betamethasone or dexamethasone) accelerate maturation of alveolar type II epithelial cells, which are the source of surfactant. For these reasons, most mothers likely to deliver a preterm birth are routinely treated with antenatal corticosteroids.[87]

A postnatal treatment strategy to reduce lung stiffness (increase lung compliance) after preterm birth is to instill surfactant into the airways.[88] Surfactant-replacement therapy is beneficial because once it becomes widely and thinly distributed in the lung, the exogenous surfactant reduces surface tension at air-liquid interfaces, thereby stabilizing distal air spaces when they deflate. After surfactant replacement, oxygenation improves swiftly, followed for several hours by progressive improvement in gas exchange and lung mechanics.[89-91] Other improvements, at least in preterm lambs, are reduced vascular injury and edema.[92] Thus surfactant-replacement therapy reduces the severity of RDS following preterm birth. Although instilled surfactant is not recycled as efficiently as native surfactant, this therapy improves the opportunity for the preterm lung to repair and grow by reducing the lung injury associated with RDS.[65]

Oxygen exposure, even room air exposure,[93] is toxic to the cells of the immature lung (see Table 70.1: Oxidative stress).[55,94-97] Related to oxygen toxicity is overwhelming of endogenous antioxidants in the immature lung. Evidence of oxidant stress in preterm human infants is detected as shifts in plasma concentrations of reduced glutathione and glutathione disulfide.[98] Sources of oxidant stress are endogenously released toxic metabolites of O_2, such as superoxide anion and hydroxyl radical from activated neutrophils and macrophages that accumulate in the lung.[44,45,99,100] Overwhelmed endogenous antioxidant enzymes (e.g., catalase, copper-zinc superoxide dismutase, or manganese superoxide dismutase) also may contribute to the evolution of RDS and subsequent BPD.

Oxygen exposure also is associated with increased levels of proteases, such as elastases and collagenases, and imbalance between proteases and protease inhibitors (see Table 70.1: Extracellular matrix involvement). Increased levels of elastase and collagenase may result in destruction of elastin and collagen, two prominent extracellular matrix molecules in the lung that are necessary for alveolar formation.[101-103] Oxygen exposure also inactivates proteinase inhibitors, such as α_1-antiproteinase, a consequence that may contribute further to acute lung injury.[104]

CHRONIC LUNG DISEASE OF PREMATURITY (BRONCHOPULMONARY DYSPLASIA)

Preterm human infants who develop BPD today are more immature (22 to 26 weeks' gestation compared with 31 to 34 weeks' gestation), are smaller (<1000 g vs. >2000 g at birth), and have radiologic and pathologic lung disease features that appear less severe and more peripheral[33,91,105-107] compared with the original description of BPD.[94,108,109] Radiologic features include lung hyperinflation, emphysema, and interstitial densities. Pathologic features, at autopsy, are distended and simplified air canals and air saccules.[105,106] As described earlier, survival rates at some centers are greater than 90% for preterm human infants weighing 500 to 1500 g at birth.[110-113] Nonetheless, more than 40% of preterm human infants, or 10,000 to 15,000 per year in the United States, develop BPD, despite high rates of usage of antenatal glucocorticoids and postnatal surfactant-replacement therapy.

Other epidemiologic studies identify a number of other risk factors for the development of BPD, including male sex, white race, and severity of RDS. Multifactorial modeling suggests that the major risk factors for development of BPD are birth weight, gestational age, infection, and need for continuous mechanical ventilation.[114,115] A recently published report on diagnosis of BPD in very preterm infants concluded that mode of respiratory support, specifically mechanical ventilation, at 36 weeks postmenstrual age, best predicted early childhood morbidity, regardless of use of supplemental O_2.[116]

ANTENATAL STRESS AND SUSCEPTIBILITY FOR POSTNATAL LUNG INJURY

Clinical and pre-clinical studies suggest that antenatal stress may set the table for postnatal lung injury in preterm neonates.[117]

Epidemiologic studies identify that antenatal factors, such as fetal growth restriction,[118-123] chorioamnionitis,[124-126] pre-eclampsia,[127] placental pathology,[128] or pre-existing hypertension, gestational diabetes, maternal obesity, or maternal smoking,[129,130] are associated with increased risk for BPD. Table 70.1 includes molecular players in impaired alveolarization in the context of pre-clinical studies of antenatal stress.

ALVEOLAR SIMPLIFICATION ASSOCIATED WITH BRONCHOPULMONARY DYSPLASIA

Simplification of distal airspaces is characteristic of the histopathology of BPD in the lungs of preterm infants today. Alveolar simplification is evident as distended distal airspaces, alveolar walls that are thick and cellular, and capillaries that are separated from the air spaces (see Fig. 70.1G and H). Simplification is related to failure (dysmorphogenesis) of primary septa to subdivide air space canals into saccules, and/or failure of secondary septa (crests) to subdivide air space saccules into alveoli (see Table 70.1: Morphogenesis), along with failure of alveolar capillary growth (see Table 70.1: Vascular growth). Failed secondary septation reduces air space surface area for respiratory gas exchange. These features are recapitulated in chronically ventilated preterm baboons[131-137] and preterm lambs,[7,78,138-141] as well as preterm rabbit kits that are not ventilated.[142] The molecular mechanisms that participate in normal or abnormal septation of air space canals and/or saccules are not known and are a topic of intense investigation today (see Table 70.1).

Because BPD in human infants occurs almost exclusively after preterm birth and weeks of mechanical ventilation with supplemental O_2, reproducing the clinical setting and prolonged neonatal intensive care in animal models of evolving neonatal chronic lung disease (CLD) requires intensive and expensive large-animal models. Coalson and colleagues developed the baboon (non-human primate) model that has the pathologic features of BPD, including alveolar simplification.[131-133,143] Those investigators showed that early application of high-frequency ventilation may reduce the severity of the histopathologic chan ges[136,144,145] and speculated that tidal ventilation and hyperoxia lead to lung overstretch and release of inflammatory mediators that cause loss of alveoli and alveolar capillary surface area.[133,143] Our model of BPD, using preterm lambs, is being used to identify mechanisms underlying mechanical ventilation for up to 4 weeks, using large tidal volume (13 to 15 mL/kg body weight), low tidal volume (5 to 7 mL/kg body weight), or noninvasive respiratory support (high-frequency nasal support).[7,78,138-140] Our results show that mechanical ventilation inhibits alveolar formation and alveolar capillary growth, diminishes microvessel number, disrupts respiratory gas exchange, and leads to persistent muscularization of resistance arterioles, increases pulmonary vascular resistance, and decreases expression of endothelial nitric oxide synthase protein.[139,140,146] Another model uses preterm rabbit kits to assess the impact of prematurity alone on alveolar formation[142] or the impact of intermittent continuous positive airway pressure on alveolar formation.[147] This model shows that prematurity alone leads to alveolar simplification.

A consequence of failed primary and/or secondary septation is reduced surface area for gas exchange, including the capillary surface area.[134,140,148] However, the latter observation in experimental animals with evolving neonatal CLD has not been confirmed in autopsy tissue from human preterm infants who died with established BPD.[149] One explanation for this discordance may be the time frame for disease development. Experimental animal models that include weeks of respiratory support and neonatal intensive care are relatively short (up to 4 weeks for evolving neonatal CLD), whereas preterm human infants with established BPD may be in the neonatal intensive care setting for months, suggesting that capillary proliferation may be a slow adaptive response to impaired primary and/or secondary septation related to established BPD.[141] Current studies suggest that even preterm infants not diagnosed with BPD have reduced lung growth and impaired lung function relative to infants born at term.[150-152] Given that lung function normally begins to decline around the end of the third decade of life, minimizing the interruption of alveolarization associated with very preterm birth and exacerbated through processes leading to BPD should be a top research priority.[153,154]

Studies using chronically ventilated preterm lambs with evolving neonatal CLD also indicate that the elastin gene is excessively and continuously upregulated.[138] Detectable upregulation occurs by the third day of continuous mechanical ventilation and remains up-regulated for the 3- to 4-week studies. Although results from studies of preterm lambs with evolving CLD and elastin knockout mice[155] seem contradictory, their results suggest that elastin gene expression must be tightly regulated in terms of quantity and site-specific expression for normal alveolar formation. Too little elastin gene expression (elastin knockout mice) or too much elastin gene expression (preterm lambs with evolving CLD) is detrimental to normal alveolar formation.

Knockout and transgenic mouse models identify molecular players that are important in postnatal alveolar formation. Numerous examples are provided in Table 70.1. One such molecular player is platelet-derived growth factor-A (PDGF-A).[156] Some PDGF-$A^{-/-}$ mice survive through the postnatal period; however, the surviving mice lack both alveolar myofibroblasts and alveolar elastin, and their lungs have simplified distal air spaces. Narrower focus on the important role of elastin was provided by elastin null mice.[155] $Elastin^{-/-}$ mice survive through the first several days of postnatal life, but the pups are cyanotic. Their lungs have distal air spaces that are arrested at the saccular stage. In addition, their lungs have reduced airway and vascular generations.

Appropriate stretch of the developing lung appears to be of key importance for formation of normal alveoli. Overstretch leads to distortion of cells and extracellular matrix in the developing lung. The distortion may lead to the local synthesis and release of regulatory molecules that affect cellular division, phenotype, and metabolic activity.[157] High lung inflation (overstretch), for example, increases mRNA levels for transforming growth factor (TGF)-β_1 fourfold and basic fibroblast growth factor (bFGF; or FGF2) by 60% compared with low lung inflation in adult rabbits.[158] In this regard, PDGF is involved in stretch-mediated signaling, and elastin is also a stretch-responsive gene. These data emphasize the importance of mechanical stretch in alveolar formation.

Among the mediators proposed to link overstretch and arrested alveolar formation are growth factors, cytokines, and matrix-degrading proteinases released by epithelial and mesenchymal cells, as well as resident and infiltrating inflammatory cells. For example, the developing lung has the ability to synthesize and release vascular endothelial growth factor (VEGF),[159] FGFs,[160] PDGFs,[156,161-163] TGFs,[164,165] insulin-like growth factors,[166,167] and epidermal growth factor (EGF),[168,169] as well as their receptors. Of these growth factors, VEGF[170-173] and related vascular growth signaling molecules[174,175] and FGF signaling[176,177] are implicated in alveolar formation.

VEGF expression is regulated by other growth factors, such as TGF-β[178] and PDGF,[179] and can be suppressed by dexamethasone.[159] The biologic function of VEGF in disease states may rely on altered amounts of VEGF protein, as well as altered VEGF receptor (VEGF-R) number and affinity. For example, hypoxia induces pulmonary production of VEGF and its receptor 2, VEGF-R2.[159,180] Hyperoxia, in comparison, inhibits pulmonary production of VEGF and VEGF-R2,[181] which is a risk factor for failed alveolar formation.[181,182] In this regard, disruption of pulmonary blood vessel formation in rats, by blocking binding of VEGF to its receptor, results in lung histopathologic changes that look like CLD.[170,171] Recovery of neonatal and adult rabbits from hyperoxia is associated with VEGF message expression by alveolar epithelial cells.[181,183] These findings suggest a role for VEGF in regulating alveolar capillary proliferation normally and after oxidant injury; the latter plays a central role in the pathogenesis of BPD.

Deficiencies in nutrition contribute to the development of BPD (see Table 70.1: Nutrition). For example, restricted nutrition was shown to lead to alveolar simplification in preterm lambs.[184] The preterm lambs were managed by noninvasive respiratory support for 21 days, because that mode and duration are associated with appropriate alveolar formation in preterm lambs.[7,78] The experiment compared restricted daily enteral nutrition (mL/kg/day; kcal/kg/day) to that tolerated by other preterm lambs that were managed by mechanical ventilation for 21 days. The results showed that restricted nutrition led to alveolar simplification, with biochemical and molecular indices of inappropriate formation of alveoli and alveolar capillaries.

Deficiencies in retinol or retinol-binding protein after preterm birth also are related to the development of BPD.[185-188] Clinical trials of retinol replacement of preterm human infants at risk for BPD, however, provide conflicting results. A randomized, double-blind, controlled trial[189] showed that preterm human infants who received vitamin A had significantly lower incidence of BPD and reduced need for supplemental O_2, mechanical ventilation, and intensive care. In a subsequent study, retinol supplementation had no effect on the incidence of BPD in preterm human infants.[190] In contrast, large multi-center studies of retinol versus placebo treatment of tiny preterm human infants showed significant reduction in the incidence of BPD among the retinol-treated infants.[191] However, the relative protection after vitamin A treatment was small, and no differences in respiratory morbidities were noted during cohort follow-up studies. Experimental animal studies provide supportive results in this regard. One study showed that retinoid signaling is required for alveolar formation.[192] Another study used pregnant rats treated with dexamethasone repeatedly to inhibit lung development in utero before treating with retinol.[193] The newborn pups, treated with all-*trans* retinoic acid postnatally, had greater alveolar formation than the untreated control rat pups. A third study showed that retinoids reversed steroid-induced suppression of lung growth and epithelial cell proliferation in cultured fetal rat lung.[194] A fourth study showed that retinoic acid treatment of adult rats with elastase-induced pulmonary emphysema was associated with reversal of emphysematous lesions.[195] Our studies using preterm lambs with evolving neonatal CLD showed that daily treatment with vitamin A (Aquasol A) is associated with greater formation of alveoli and alveolar capillaries, and increased expression of VEGF and VEGF-R2.[173] The molecular mechanisms by which vitamin A up-regulates expression of VEGF and VEGF-R2 are being investigated by our group.

POTENTIAL OF MESENCHYMAL STEM CELLS AND EXOSOMES (EXTRACELLULAR VESICLES)

Mesenchymal stem cell (MSC) therapies, or their extracellular vesicles, may represent a new opportunity to treat preterm human infants.[196,197] A phase 1 dose-escalation study used allogenic umbilical cord blood-derived MSCs in nine extremely preterm neonates at risk of BPD.[198] This study provides feasibility for the procedure and 2-year follow-up shows no adverse effects on growth or outcomes for the respiratory system and neurodevelopment. Determining how and where exogenously administered MSCs, or their isolated and purified exosomes, are beneficial is a hot topic in experimental studies of the pathogenesis of and potential treatment for alveolar simplification (see Table 70.1: Stem Cells/Extracellular Vesicles). An insightful study revealed that even room air is toxic to MSCs that should be developing at much lower levels of oxygen in utero.[93] Numerous proof-of-concepts provide biologic basis for utility of MSCs or their exosomes in human preterm infants at risk of developing BPD. Effects of MSCs or their exosomes include antiinflammatory, anti-fibrotic, anti-apoptotic, anti-oxidative, as well as pro-angiogenic and pro-growth. Another effect of MSCs or their exosomes is epigenetic.[199] Epigenetic contribution is through direction or redirection of gene expression by orchestrating the interactions among transcription machinery, transcription factors, and specific regions of DNA. Epigenetic mechanisms include DNA methylation,[200] histone protein covalent modifications,[201] and noncoding RNAs.[202,203] These beneficial effects are manifest structurally as better alveolar formation in the lungs of experimental animal pups (see Table 70.1: Epigenetics).

SUMMARY

Preterm human infants, especially those born less than 30 weeks gestational age, have marked structural and functional immaturity of the lung. Improvement in survival has occurred with aggressive perinatal and neonatal interventions, including antenatal steroids, perinatal surfactant-replacement therapy, noninvasive approaches to respiratory support, and other measures such as aggressive nutritional support. Acute lung injury as a result of lung immaturity is often exacerbated by supportive therapy (i.e., mechanical ventilation and supplemental O_2) that are necessary for survival. All very preterm infants have altered lung development, and a large proportion continue to progress to BPD. Although BPD continues to be one of the most serious of pediatric public health issues, important progress has been made. For example, BPD occurs in tinier infants than the population that Northway and colleagues described in the original paper on BPD.[94] Moreover, more severe fibroproliferative forms of BPD are less common today than 50 years ago. These encouraging changes reflect better understanding of lung developmental biology and improvements in clinical management of prematurely born infants, such as use of noninvasive modes of respiratory support. Nonetheless, challenges remain because rates of preterm birth remain high, the gestational age and size of preterm human infants who are supported are decreasing, and the incidence of BPD and mortality among the smallest preterm infants remain very high. The long-term pulmonary effects associated with very preterm birth and BPD are not yet completely clear,[141] but the most recent data suggest potential for earlier, and possibly more rapid, progression of the normal decline in adult lung function associated with aging. Identification of factors/processes critical to maintaining or restoring normal lung growth and development in preterm infants with or without BPD remain key challenges for the future. Another challenge is developing translational models that link early-life treatments to long-term outcomes, especially long-term neurodevelopmental outcomes.

ACKNOWLEDGMENTS

Portions of this work were supported by NIH grants HL110002 (KHA), HL62875 (KHA), HL56401 (KHA; PL Ballard, P.I.), and AHA Grant-in-Aid 96014370 (KHA).

A complete reference list is available at www.ExpertConsult.com. 

SELECT REFERENCES

1. Hayek H. *The Human Lung*. New York: Hafner; 1960.
2. Albertine KH. Anatomy of the lungs. In: Broaddus VC, ed. *Murray & Nadel's Textbook of Respiratory Medicine*. 6th ed. Philadelphia: Elsevier; 2016:3–21.
3. Weibel ER. *Morphometry of the Lung*. New York: Academic Press; 1963.
4. Crapo JD, Young SL, Fram EK, Pinkerton KE, Barry BE, Crapo RO. Morphometric characteristics of cells in the alveolar region of mammalian lungs. *Am Rev Respir Dis*. 1983;128:S42–S46.
5. Burri PH. Structural aspects of prenatal and postnatal development and growth of the lung. In: McDonald JA, ed. *Lung Growth and Development*. Vol 100. New York: Marcel Dekker, Inc; 1997:1–35.
6. Crapo JD, Barry BE, Gehr P, Bachofen M, Weibel ER. Cell number and cell characteristics of the normal human lung. *Am Rev Respir Dis*. 1982;126:332–337.
7. Reyburn B, Li M, Metcalfe DB, et al. Nasal ventilation alters mesenchymal cell turnover and improves alveolarization in preterm lambs. *Am J Respir Crit Care Med*. 2008;178(4):407–418.
8. Pryhuber GS, Hull WM, Fink I, McMahan MJ, Whitsett JA. Ontogeny of surfactant proteins A and B in human amniotic fluid as indices of fetal lung maturity. *Pediatr Res*. 1991;30(6):597–605.
13. Clements JA, Platzker AC, Tierney DF, et al. Assessment of the risk of the respiratory-distress syndrome by a rapid test for surfactant in amniotic fluid. *New Eng J Med*. 1972;286(20):1077–1081.
15. Boyden EA. The mode of origin of pulmonary acini and respiratory bronchioles in the fetal lung. *Am J Anat*. 1974;141(3):317–328.
16. Davies G, Reid L. Growth of the alveoli and pulmonary arteries in childhood. *Thorax*. 1970;25(6):669–681.
17. Langston C, Kida K, Reed M, Thurlbeck WM. Human lung growth in late gestation and in the neonate. *Am Rev Respir Dis*. 1984;129(4):607–613.
18. Emery JL, Wilcock PF. The post-natal development of the lung. *Acta Anat*. 1966;65(1):10–29.
23. Harding R, Hooper SB. Regulation of lung expansion and lung growth before birth. *J Appl Physiol*. 1996;81(1):209–224.
27. Olver RE, Robinson EJ. Sodium and chloride transport by the tracheal epithelium of fetal, new-born and adult sheep. *J Physiol*. 1986;375:377–390.
29. Avery ME, Mead J. Surface properties in relation to atelectasis and hyaline membrane disease. *Am J Dis Child*. 1959;97(5, Part 1):517–523.
36. Hibbard JU, Wilkins I, Sun L, et al. Respiratory morbidity in late preterm births. *JAMA*. 2010;304(4):419–425.
67. Colaizy TT, Younis UM, Bell EF, Klein JM. Nasal high-frequency ventilation for premature infants. *Acta Paediatr*. 2008;97(11):1518–1522.
69. Dumas De La Roque E, Bertrand C, Tandonnet O, et al. Nasal high frequency percussive ventilation versus nasal continuous positive airway pressure in transient tachypnea of the newborn: a pilot randomized controlled trial (NCT00556738). *Pediatr Pulmonol*. 2011;46(3):218–223.
73. Lam R, Schilling D, Scottoline B, et al. The effect of extended continuous positive airway pressure on changes in lung volumes in stable premature infants: a randomized controlled trial. *J Pediatr*. 2020;217:66–72 e61.
78. Null DM, Alvord J, Leavitt W, et al. High-frequency nasal ventilation for 21 d maintains gas exchange with lower respiratory pressures and promotes alveolarization in preterm lambs. *Pediatr Res*. 2014;75(4):507–516.
86. Liggins GC, Howie RN. A controlled trial of antepartum glucocorticoid treatment for prevention of the respiratory distress syndrome in premature infants. *Pediatrics*. 1972;50(4):515–520.
93. Mobius MA, Freund D, Vadivel A, et al. Oxygen disrupts human fetal lung mesenchymal cells. Implications for bronchopulmonary dysplasia. *Am J Respir Cell Mol Biol*. 2019;60(5):592–600.
94. Northway Jr WH, Rosan RC, Porter DY. Pulmonary disease following respirator therapy of hyaline-membrane disease. Bronchopulmonary dysplasia. *New Eng J Med*. 1967;276(7):357–368.
106. Margraf LR, Tomashefski Jr JF, Bruce MC, Dahms BB. Morphometric analysis of the lung in bronchopulmonary dysplasia. *Am Rev Respir Dis*. 1991;143(2):391–400.
107. Kirpalani H, Millar D, Lemyre B, et al. A trial comparing noninvasive ventilation strategies in preterm infants. *New Eng J Med*. 2013;369(7):611–620.
112. Alleman BW, Bell EF, Li L, et al. Individual and center-level factors affecting mortality among extremely low birth weight infants. *Pediatrics*. 2013;132(1):e175–e184.
113. Rysavy MA, Li L, Bell EF, et al. Between-hospital variation in treatment and outcomes in extremely preterm infants. *New Eng J Med*. 2015;372(19):1801–1811.
115. Klinger G, Sokolover N, Boyko V, et al. Perinatal risk factors for bronchopulmonary dysplasia in a national cohort of very-low-birthweight infants. *Am J Obstet Gynecol*. 2013;208(2):115–119.
116. Jensen EA, Dysart K, Gantz MG, et al. The diagnosis of bronchopulmonary dysplasia in very preterm infants. An evidence-based approach. *Am J Respir Crit Care Med*. 2019;200(6):751–759.
117. Taglauer E, Abman SH, Keller RL. Recent advances in antenatal factors predisposing to bronchopulmonary dysplasia. *Semin Perinatol*. 2018;42(7):413–424.
129. Keller RL, Feng R, DeMauro SB, et al. Bronchopulmonary dysplasia and perinatal characteristics predict 1-year respiratory outcomes in newborns born at extremely low gestational age: a prospective cohort study. *J Pediatr*. 2017;187:89–97.e83.
130. Morrow LA, Wagner BD, Ingram DA, et al. Antenatal determinants of bronchopulmonary dysplasia and late respiratory disease in preterm infants. *Am J Respir Crit Care Med*. 2017;196(3):364–374.
133. Coalson JJ, Winter VT, Gerstmann DR, Idell S, King RJ, Delemos RA. Pathophysiologic, morphometric, and biochemical studies of the premature baboon with bronchopulmonary dysplasia. *Am Rev Respir Dis*. 1992;145(4 Pt 1):872–881.
141. Dahl MJ, Bowen S, Aoki T, et al. Former-preterm lambs have persistent alveolar simplification at 2 and 5 months corrected postnatal age. *Am J Physiol Lung Cell Mol Physiol*. 2018;315(5):L816–L833.
142. Salaets T, Aertgeerts M, Gie A, et al. Preterm birth impairs postnatal lung development in the neonatal rabbit model. *Respir Res*. 2020;21(1):59.
147. Gie AG, Salaets T, Vignero J, et al. Intermittent CPAP limits hyperoxia induced lung damage in a rabbit model of bronchopulmonary dysplasia. *Am J Physiol Lung Cell Mol Physiol*. 2020.
152. Ronkainen E, Dunder T, Peltoniemi O, Kaukola T, Marttila R, Hallman M. New BPD predicts lung function at school age: follow-up study and meta-analysis. *Pediatr Pulmonol*. 2015;50(11):1090–1098.
154. Greenough A, Peacock J, Zivanovic S, et al. United Kingdom Oscillation Study: long-term outcomes of a randomised trial of two modes of neonatal ventilation. *Health Technol Assess*. 2014;18(41):1–95, v–xx.
155. Wendel DP, Taylor DG, Albertine KH, Keating MT, Li DY. Impaired distal airway development in mice lacking elastin. *Am J Respir Cell Mol Biol*. 2000;23(3):320–326.
156. Lindahl P, Karlsson L, Hellstrom M, et al. Alveogenesis failure in PDGF-A-deficient mice is coupled to lack of distal spreading of alveolar smooth muscle cell progenitors during lung development. *Development*. 1997;124(20):3943–3953.
157. Han B, Bai XH, Lodyga M, et al. Conversion of mechanical force into biochemical signaling. *J Biol Chem*. 2004;279(52):54793–54801.
158. Berg JT, Fu Z, Breen EC, Tran HC, Mathieu-Costello O, West JB. High lung inflation increases mRNA levels of ECM components and growth factors in lung parenchyma. *J Appl Physiol*. 1997;83(1):120–128.
159. Klekamp JG, Jarzecka K, Hoover RL, Summar ML, Redmond N, Perkett EA. Vascular endothelial growth factor is expressed in ovine pulmonary vascular smooth muscle cells in vitro and regulated by hypoxia and dexamethasone. *Pediatr Res*. 1997;42(6):744–749.
160. Han RN, Liu J, Tanswell AK, Post M. Expression of basic fibroblast growth factor and receptor: immunolocalization studies in developing rat fetal lung. *Pediatr Res*. 1992;31(5):435–440.
171. Jakkula M, Le Cras TD, Gebb S, et al. Inhibition of angiogenesis decreases alveolarization in the developing rat lung. *Am J Physiol Lung Cell Mol Physiol*. 2000;279(3):L600–L607.
184. Joss-Moore LA, Hagen-Lillevik SJ, Yost C, et al. Alveolar formation is dysregulated by restricted nutrition but not excess sedation in preterm lambs managed by non-invasive support. *Pediatr Res*. 2016:719–728.
197. Simones AA, Beisang DJ, Panoskaltsis-Mortari A, Roberts KD. Mesenchymal stem cells in the pathogenesis and treatment of bronchopulmonary dysplasia: a clinical review. *Pediatr Res*. 2018;83(1-2):308–317.
198. Chang YS, Ahn SY, Yoo HS, et al. Mesenchymal stem cells for bronchopulmonary dysplasia: phase 1 dose-escalation clinical trial. *J Pediatr*. 2014;164(5):966–972.e966.
203. Ameis D, Khoshgoo N, Iwasiow BM, Snarr P, Keijzer R. MicroRNAs in lung development and disease. *Paediatr Respir Rev*. 2017;22:38–43.

71 Antenatal Factors That Influence Postnatal Lung Development and Injury

Suhas G. Kallapur | Alan H. Jobe

SPECTRUM OF LUNG DISEASE IN PRETERM INFANTS

The normal fetal lung at 26 weeks gestation is in a late canalicular or early saccular stage of development and surfactant deficient. Surfactant treatment and the use of more gentle modes of assisted ventilation have resulted in populations of very preterm infants with a wide range of lung diseases not easily classifiable into the traditional categories of respiratory distress syndrome (RDS), lung hypoplasia, transient tachypnea, and normal. In one large series of 1340 preterm infants born between 23 and 27 weeks gestation, the mortality rate for infants weighing 501 to 1500 g at birth was 17% (excluding deaths <12 hours of age), and bronchopulmonary dysplasia (BPD), defined as the need for supplemental oxygen at 36 weeks, occurred in 42% of surviving infants.[1] Of the infants surviving for at least 14 days, 17% had very low supplemental oxygen needs in the first 2 weeks of postnatal life, yet these infants developed BPD.[2] Thus, in these infants, the clinical course was not characteristic of the usual progression from RDS to BPD associated with assisted ventilation in the neonate.

A complex interplay of antenatal and postnatal factors is now recognized to affect postnatal lung development after premature birth and, ultimately, the incidence of BPD (Fig. 71.1). This chapter explores some of the antenatal factors that may modulate lung development and thereby alter the postnatal clinical course of lung disease in preterm infants. Antenatal factors that influence postnatal lung development and injury are discussed below.

CHORIOAMNIONITIS—DEFINITION

Inflammation of the chorioamnion, termed *chorioamnionitis,* can be confirmed only by histopathologic examination to diagnose "histologic chorioamnionitis." In practice, clinical chorioamnionitis is diagnosed using a combination of indicators such as elevated maternal temperature, uterine tenderness, malodorous vaginal discharge, maternal leukocytosis, and fetal tachycardia.[3] In some centers, amniocentesis is performed to diagnose chorioamnionitis. Increases in leukocytes, low glucose, elevated interleukin (IL)-6 levels, and the presence of microorganisms in the amniotic fluid constitute amniotic fluid inflammation and/or amniotic fluid infection. In a report of women with preterm labor, the presence of amniotic fluid infection or IL-6 levels greater than 11.3 ng/mL were associated with shorter time from amniocentesis to delivery when compared with cases in which amniotic fluid IL-6 levels were between 2.6 and 11.2 ng/mL.[4] Interestingly, the majority of these women with amniotic fluid IL-6 levels greater than 11.3 ng/mL did not have microbes demonstrated in the amniotic fluid, even with the use of sophisticated sensitive molecular methods to detect microorganisms.[4] Due to the imprecise nature of the definition and heterogeneity of clinical manifestations a National Institutes of Health (NIH) expert panel proposed to replace the term *chorioamnionitis* with a more general, descriptive term, *Intrauterine Inflammation and/or Infection*, abbreviated as *Triple I*.[5] In this scheme, fever alone during labor is classified separately, while fever with one or more of the following: leukocytosis, fetal tachycardia, or purulent cervical discharge is classified as "suspected Triple I." To be confirmed, suspected Triple I should be accompanied by objective laboratory findings of infection in amniotic fluid (AF) (e.g., positive gram stain for bacteria, low AF glucose, high white blood cell (WBC) count in the absence of a bloody tap, and/or positive AF culture results) or histopathologic evidence of infection/inflammation in the placenta, fetal membranes, or the umbilical cord vessels (funisitis). How is it possible to explain severe amniotic fluid inflammation without the detection of microorganisms? An explanation is that the organisms may be localized deep in the fetal membranes, and the resultant inflammation in the fetal membranes may induce IL-6 in the amniotic fluid.[6] The most common microorganisms detected in the amniotic fluid with chorioamnionitis are the *Ureaplasma* species.[7] The presence of low-virulence organisms such as the *Ureaplasma* species may not cause much inflammation in the amniotic fluid. Thus, the diagnosis of chorioamnionitis can be problematic because the clinical, histologic, microbiologic, and amniotic fluid inflammation definitions of chorioamnionitis will lead to overlapping but distinct subsets of patients. As an illustration, in a cohort of very low-birth-weight infants weighing less than 1500 g at birth, the incidence of "clinical chorioamnionitis" was 18%, but the incidence of "histologic chorioamnionitis" was 48%.[1]

Growing evidence suggests that the endometrium is not normally sterile. In a clinical study using care to prevent contamination, Agostinis and colleagues[8] demonstrated that at least one organism was isolated from endometrial cultures in 85% of nonpregnant women.[9] Amniotic fluid sampled before 20 weeks gestation for genetic diagnostic indications can contain elevated proinflammatory mediators and be culture-positive for low-virulence pathogenic organisms.[10] Often the infants born to mothers with such amniotic fluid markers have no overt signs of infection at delivery. Thus, a majority of fetuses may be exposed to bacterial products for a long time in utero without clinically apparent complications. Nevertheless, the most common cause of fetal death or death soon after birth for very low-birth-weight infants was sepsis or pneumonia in an autopsy series.[11] Evidently, the effects of chorioamnionitis on the preterm fetus may range widely, from severe infection or death to normal fetal development with histologic chorioamnionitis as an incidental finding. Attempts to secure a definitive diagnosis of chorioamnionitis typically are limited by a lack of information about its duration, intensity, or extent or the organisms responsible for the clinical or histopathologic findings. In the face of exposure to commonly encountered infectious agents, down-regulation of inflammatory responses in utero may be a key coping mechanism of the fetus.

CHORIOAMNIONITIS—PATHWAY TO FETAL LUNG INFLAMMATION

The fetal lungs are protected from the traditional mechanisms of lung injury, but infection and inflammation can reach the fetal lung. Infective organisms from the lower genital flora can ascend through the cervix, with subsequent spread of infection between the chorioamnion and the uterus; this mode of transmission is commonly associated with early preterm

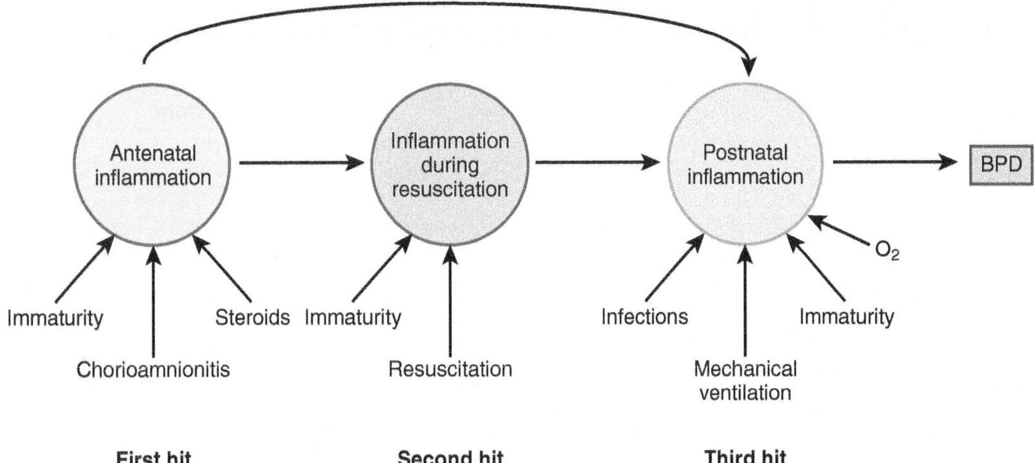

Fig. 71.1 A model for the interplay of fetal exposures on early postnatal events that may contribute to altered lung development and injury. *BPD,* Bronchopulmonary dysplasia.

labor.[12] Normal fetal swallowing will result in aspiration of any inflammatory products and organisms in the amniotic fluid. With pathogens such as group B streptococci (GBS), a pneumonia-sepsis syndrome is likely. More frequently, the fetus may mount a lung and systemic inflammatory response to signals from the inflamed fetal placenta and chorioamnion without obvious infection. The fetal inflammatory response to chorioamnionitis has been defined clinically as an elevation of IL-6 in fetal cord blood sampled by cordocentesis or in cord blood at delivery.[13] *Funisitis,* or histologic inflammation of the cord, correlates with elevated cord blood IL-6 levels and signs of generalized fetal inflammation.

The rapidly progressive chorioamnionitis or bloodstream infection caused by organisms such as *Escherichia coli, Listeria monocytogenes,* or GBS is relatively infrequent in the preterm population. By contrast, clinically asymptomatic histologic chorioamnionitis caused by low-virulence or commensal organisms increase in frequency as gestational age at delivery decreases. In one series, approximately 70% of infants (born before 30 weeks gestation) delivered by cesarean section with intact membranes had histologic chorioamnionitis.[14] This clinically inapparent chorioamnionitis is associated with recurrent preterm deliveries, and indicators of inflammation may be present before mid-gestation. The low frequency of blood culture–proven sepsis (approximately 2%) is remarkable because of the greater than 50% prevalence of histologic chorioamnionitis for very low-birth-weight deliveries.

CHORIOAMNIONITIS AND ADVERSE PULMONARY OUTCOMES

The associations of respiratory diseases including BPD with chorioamnionitis are complex. Although a systematic review showed an association between chorioamnionitis and the development of BPD, the authors concluded that there was "strong evidence of publication bias, which suggests potential overestimation of the measure of association between chorioamnionitis and BPD."[15] Been and colleagues reported that the severity of RDS may be greater with chorioamnionitis and a fetal inflammatory response (funisitis) than with chorioamnionitis and no funisitis.[16] Furthermore, clinical responses to surfactant may be less striking after exposure to chorioamnionitis with fetal inflammation.[17] It is thus very likely that respiratory outcomes may depend on a number of factors associated with exposure to chorioamnionitis, including timing, fetal involvement, and the underlying cause of the infective process. A new meta-analysis study associates BPD with chorioamnionitis.[18]

Chorioamnionitis in preterm infants may also be associated with adverse longer-term respiratory outcomes. Jones and colleagues classified 95 preterm infants according to histologic examination of the placenta.[19] They observed lower maximal expiratory flows at 40 weeks postconceptional age but interestingly noted that this outcome was mainly due to females being affected.[19] In the Boston prospective study of 1096 preterm subjects, those born at less than 33 weeks gestation with chorioamnionitis had the greatest risk for wheezing and physician-diagnosed asthma, up to the follow-up age of 2.2 years.[20] We reported that compared to non-exposed infants, late preterm infants exposed to chorioamnionitis had increased diagnosis of childhood asthma or wheezing disorders without an increase in neonatal morbidity.[21,22] Although the mechanisms are not well understood, chorioamnionitis decreased the activity of anti-inflammatory Tregs and increased cord blood IL-6 levels correlating with childhood wheezing.[22,23] Although chorioamnionitis certainly affects lung development, further work is required to identify the specific cell populations and associated inflammatory pathways that drive long-term high-risk respiratory compromise.

CLINICAL LUNG MATURATION

Although chorioamnionitis is generally considered to have adverse effects on the fetus, some reports indicate a clinical benefit. Watterberg and colleagues[24] reported that histologic chorioamnionitis and high IL-1β levels in airway samples determined on the first postnatal day predicted a decreased incidence of RDS but an increased incidence of BPD. Infants in whom blood cultures were positive for *Ureaplasma urealyticum* also had a lower incidence of RDS but a higher incidence of BPD than infants with negative blood cultures.[25] Higher cord plasma levels of IL-6 predicted a lower incidence of RDS in another report.[26] Although these small clinical series may reflect a reporting bias, chorioamnionitis was associated with improved survival for 881 infants born at less than 26 weeks gestation in the United Kingdom and Ireland in 1995.[27] Histologic chorioamnionitis also was associated with less RDS in 446 consecutive singleton births before 32 weeks gestation (Table 71.1).[28]

The associations of chorioamnionitis with outcomes such as RDS and BPD are quite complex. In a large epidemiologic report, histologic chorioamnionitis predicted a decreased incidence of BPD unless the infant received mechanical ventilation

Table 71.1 Associations Between Histologic Chorioamnionitis and Outcomes for 446 Consecutive Singleton Deliveries Before 32 Weeks Gestation.

	Neutrophils in Membranes		Neutrophils in Cord		
Clinical Outcome	**Yes (%)**	**No (%)**	**Yes (%)**	**No (%)**	**Statistically Significant**
Ureaplasma + Mycoplasma	81	32	49	21	•
RDS	61	73	57	72	•
BPD (need for O_2 at 36 weeks)	7	9	7	8	
IVH (grade 3 or 4)	10	8	11	9	
NEC	18	14	22	14	•
SIRS	44	18	55	20	
Death	10	9	11	10	•

BPD, Bronchopulmonary dysplasia; *IVH*, intravascular hemorrhage; *NEC*, necrotizing enterocolitis; *RDS*, respiratory distress syndrome; *SIRS*, systemic inflammatory response syndrome.
From Andrews WW, Goldenberg RL, Faye-Petersen O, et al. The Alabama Preterm Birth study: polymorphonuclear and mononuclear cell placental infiltrations, other markers of inflammation, and outcomes in 23- to 32-week preterm newborn infants. *Am J Obstet Gynecol*. 2006;195:803–808.

or developed postnatal sepsis, which in combination with histologic chorioamnionitis increased the risk for BPD.[29] This study suggests that fetal exposure to inflammation can induce clinically apparent maturation of the lung, but that subsequent injury (as from ventilation or sepsis) may increase the injury response, thereby resulting in BPD.

ANIMAL MODELS OF CHORIOAMNIONITIS

Bry and colleagues[30] reported that intraamniotic injections of recombinant IL-1α induced messenger RNA (mRNA) for surfactant proteins SP-A and SP-B and improved the pressure-volume curves in preterm rabbits. IL-1α also increased mRNA for SP-A, -B, and -C in early gestation explants of rabbit lung.[31] To further explore the relationships between inflammation and maturation, *E. coli* lipopolysaccharide (LPS, a component of cell wall of gram-negative bacteria) was given by intraamniotic injection in sheep.[32] The fetal sheep lung responded to intraamniotic LPS with improved gas exchange, a large increase in compliance, and a large increase in lung gas volume within 5 to 7 days. These improvements in lung function after preterm birth were accompanied by persistent increases in the mRNA for SP-A, -B, -C, and -D, and by large increases in the surfactant lipids and surfactant proteins in the air spaces.[33] The quantity of SP-B increased, as did the processed mature form of SP-B in the airways.

In the preterm lamb model, "clinical maturation" was a late response of the lung to inflammation (Fig. 71.2). Within hours of the intraamniotic injection of LPS, white cells producing the mRNA for the proinflammatory cytokines IL-1β, IL-6, and IL-8 infiltrated the chorioamnion and subsequently appeared in the amniotic fluid.[34] The cells in amniotic fluid expressed the mRNA for IL-1β and IL-8 for at least 1 week after the LPS exposure. Within 5 hours of intraamniotic LPS administration, the fetal lung contained activated granulocytes, and the airways expressed heat shock protein 70 (HSP70).[35] The amount of H_2O_2 in cells lavaged from the lungs was maximal at 24 hours, and both the lung tissue and lavage cells expressed proinflammatory cytokines.[36] Apoptosis increased at 24 hours, and cell replication increased by 72 hours. The fetal lung had an acute but modest generalized inflammatory response that resolved to "clinical maturation" in that lung function was strikingly improved after preterm delivery and ventilation.

The lung maturational response in the preterm lamb model required direct contact of the inflammatory products in the amniotic fluid.[37] Conversely, when the amniotic fluid containing inflammatory products was surgically separated from the lungs, no lung maturation was seen. The inflammation in the chorioamnion and lung did not result in increased plasma cortisol or a large systemic inflammatory response.[32] Therefore the inflammation-mediated mechanisms for inducing lung maturation were independent of the adrenal axis. When inflammatory cell recruitment to the lung was blocked with an anti-CD18 antibody, the lung maturational changes also did not occur.[38] The fetal sheep responded to intraamniotic administration of recombinant ovine IL-1α or IL-1β with chorioamnionitis and lung maturation.[39] Blocking IL-1 signaling using IL-1 receptor antagonist almost completely prevented intraamniotic LPS-induced lung maturation.[40] Similarly, LPS from periodontal organisms and chronic fetal colonization with live *Ureaplasma* organisms caused lung inflammation with improved lung function.[41,42] These findings clearly show that LPS and other inflammatory mediators, particularly IL-1, can induce lung maturation by direct contact with the fetal lung, indicating that lung maturation seems to be a consistent response of the fetal lung to inflammation.

MEDIATORS OF CHORIOAMNIONITIS INDUCE ALTERED LUNG DEVELOPMENT

Preterm infants in whom proinflammatory cytokines are increased in bronchoalveolar lavage fluid are at increased risk for the development of BPD.[43] Intraamniotic injection of IL-1 greatly increased the expression of IL-1β, IL-8, granulocyte-macrophage colony-stimulating factor (GM-CSF), monocyte chemoattractant protein-1, and the acute-phase reactant serum amyloid A3 in the lungs of fetal sheep and fetal monkeys. Interestingly, the Th1 cytokines IFNγ and IL-12, type I interferon inducible genes CXCL9 (MIG) and CXCL10 (IP-10), and the Th2 cytokines IL-4 and IL-13 were not induced. Intraamniotic LPS increased expression of additional genes inducible by the type I interferon signaling, including CXCL9 (MIG) and CXCL10 (IP-10). In the fetal sheep, intraamniotic LPS increased lung expression of TLR4 and TLR2 mRNA expression but decreased TLR4 expression in the gut, demonstrating organ-specific responses. Neither intraamniotic IL-1 nor LPS significantly increased expression of tumor necrosis factor (TNF)- α in the lung, and intraamniotic TNF did not induce chorioamnionitis or fetal lung inflammation.[44] The counter regulatory cytokines IL-10 and IL-1ra are only modestly increased in the fetal lung exposed to IL-1 or LPS.

The expression of multiple other genes is also associated with lung injury in model systems, and some of these have been assessed in the fetus. Caveolins (Cavs) are implicated as major modulators of lung injury and remodeling by virtue of their

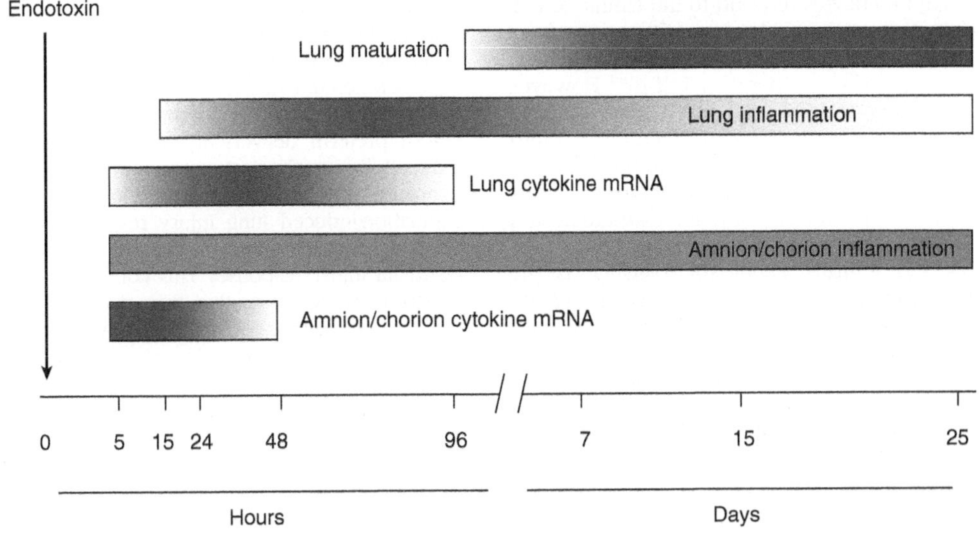

Fig. 71.2 The time course of lung inflammation and maturation after intraamniotic endotoxin in preterm lambs. The shading within each box is proportional to the intensity and magnitude of the responses. (Data from Kramer BW, Moss TJ, Willet KE, et al. Dose and time response after intra-amniotic endotoxin in preterm lambs. *Am J Respir Crit Care Med.* 2001;164:982–988; Kramer BW, Kramer S, Ikegami M, et al. Injury, inflammation, and remodeling in fetal sheep lung after intra-amniotic endotoxin. *Am J Physiol Lung Cell Mol Physiol.* 2002;283:L452–L459; and Kallapur SG, Willet KE, Jobe AH, et al. Intra-amniotic endotoxin: chorioamnionitis precedes lung maturation in preterm lambs. *Am J Physiol Lung Cell Mol Physiol.* 2001;280:L527–L536.)

strategic positioning in the lipid rafts of plasma membranes. Intraamniotic LPS decreased the expression of Cav-1 in the preterm fetal lung.[45] The decreased expression of Cav-1 was associated with the activation of the Smad2/3, Stat 3, and a-SMase/ceramide pathways and increased expression[45] of HO-1. Consistent with activation of Smads, intraamniotic LPS increased lung transforming growth factor (TGF)-β1 mRNA and protein expression.[46] However the lung expression of connective tissue growth factor, a key profibrotic protein induced by TGF-β, decreased upon lung exposure to LPS.[46]

Metalloproteinases regulate the breakdown of extracellular matrix in the lung. Lung expression of matrix metalloproteinase-9 was increased in sheep after intraamniotic LPS treatment[47] and in transgenic mice that overexpress IL-1β in the lung.[48] Sonic Hedgehog (Shh) signaling is a major pathway directing lung development. Intraamniotic LPS also decreased Shh mRNA levels and Gli1 protein expression in the fetal sheep.[49] In fetal mouse lung explants, LPS mediated abnormal saccular lung development due to NFκB activation in macrophages with enhanced IL-1β secretion.[50] Fibroblast growth factor (FGF)-10 linked inflammation and abnormal lung development in this mouse lung explant system, a finding that is consistent with reduced FGF-10 in the tracheal aspirates of preterm infants developing chronic lung disease.[51] In a study in rats, vitamin D administration prenatally and postnatally reversed intraamniotic LPS-induced aberrant alveolar and pulmonary vascular development.[52] Clearly, chorioamnionitis directly and indirectly changes multiple pathways that are linked to lung growth and development.

ANTENATAL INFECTION AND VASCULAR INJURY

Infants with BPD have decreased and disorganized lung microvasculature with decreased expression of angiogenic growth factors such as vascular endothelial growth factor (VEGF) and its receptors.[53,54] This decreased microvascular development also occurred in preterm lamb and baboon models of BPD caused by mechanical ventilation.[55,56] Alveolar development was also disrupted in transgenic mice that overexpressed VEGF or in mice lacking the higher-molecular-weight heparin-binding VEGF isoforms.[57,58] Hypoxia and hypoxia-inducible factor (HIF)-1 are well-known regulators of VEGF expression.[59] Pulmonary expression of HIF-1α, HIF-2α, and the downstream target of their regulation, VEGF mRNA, is impaired following RDS in neonatal lambs.[60]

There is crosstalk between the mediators of vascular and alveolar development in the lung.[61] In neonatal rat pups, inhibitors of the Flk-1/KDR receptor disrupted VEGF signaling and impaired alveolarization.[62] Intraamniotic LPS impairs alveolarization in lambs (Fig. 71.3).[63,64] The lung inflammatory response in these preterm lambs also decreased the expression of endothelial proteins in the lung important for blood vessel formation (e.g., VEGF receptor-2, endothelial nitric oxide synthase).[65] The lungs of preterm fetal lambs exposed to intraamniotic LPS developed smooth muscle hypertrophy in resistance arterioles and adventitial fibrosis in large blood vessels, as described in human infants with BPD.[66] Neonatal hyperoxia impairs vascular and alveolar growth in mice and decreases endothelial progenitor cells. Injection of bone marrow–derived angiogenic precursor cells restored lung alveolar and vascular structure after neonatal hyperoxia.[67] These experimental and clinical data demonstrate the tight linkage between alveolar and vascular growth in the developing lung.

IMMUNOLOGIC RESPONSES AFTER FETAL LUNG INFLAMMATION

The inflammatory responses of the fetal lung differ from adult responses in that multiple components of a mature inflammatory response to injury are deficient in the developing lung. The preterm fetal lung does not respond to bioactive TNF-α in the amniotic fluid or to TNF-α given intravenously.[38] The preterm fetal lung contains almost no macrophages or granulocytes, and normal host defense proteins such as SP-A and SP-D are present in very low amounts.[68] Although multiple components of innate immune response are deficient, preterm fetal sheep at 50% gestation can recruit inflammatory cells in the airway and mount an inflammatory response to intraamniotic LPS.[64]

Immature fetal lung monocytes respond to intraamniotic LPS in functionally distinct ways. Immature lung monocytes from preterm sheep have a minimal IL-6 secretory response to in vitro challenge with LPS and do not respond to TNF-α.[69] However, intraamniotic LPS induces GM-CSF and PU.1 expression to mature the lung monocytes. These monocytes then migrate into the fetal alveolar spaces and respond vigorously to both LPS and TNF-α in vitro.[69] Thus exposure to a proinflammatory agonist in the amniotic fluid is a potent stimulus for maturation and responsiveness of monocytes in the fetal lung.

In adult animals and humans, endotoxin tolerance is the suppression of LPS signaling caused by a complex reprogramming of inflammatory responses. As part of endotoxin tolerance, proinflammatory cytokine expression is down-regulated, while there is no change or an increase in the expression of antiinflammatory genes, antimicrobial genes, and genes mediating phagocytosis. Intraamniotic LPS can cause an innate immune tolerance in the fetus. Exposure of preterm fetal sheep to intraamniotic LPS 2 days before delivery induces a robust expression of multiple cytokines in the fetal lung. However, if the fetus is exposed to two intraamniotic LPS injections 7 days before delivery, a second exposure 2 days before delivery causes no secondary inflammatory responses.[70] Interestingly, both lung and blood monocytes that have been exposed to the two doses of LPS are refractory to in vitro challenge with LPS. The lung and blood monocytes from fetal sheep exposed to two injections of intraamniotic LPS are also refractory to stimulation by a host of other TLR agonists including PamCysK4 (TLR2), flagellin (TLR5), and CpG-DNA (TLR9),[71] implying a cross-tolerance to TLP receptors.

The phenomenon of innate immune tolerance in the fetus is not restricted to exposure to LPS. Exposure to intraamniotic live *Ureaplasma parvum* almost completely abolished responsiveness of the fetal lung to LPS, implying a profound immune paralysis in the fetal lung induced by *Ureaplasma* exposure.[72] Other interactive phenomena between antenatal LPS and postnatal inflammatory insults have also been reported. As in sheep, intraamniotic LPS in rats induced aberrant lung development and pulmonary hypertension. However, when these LPS-exposed fetal mice were exposed to postnatal moderate hyperoxia, the lung abnormalities were no longer evident. In contrast, exposure to postnatal severe hyperoxia further enhanced the pulmonary abnormalities caused by antenatal LPS.[73] Thus interactions between different inflammatory insults can be complex and either exacerbate or reduce lung injury. Because the innate immune tolerance is time-dependent, it is not clear how these experimental phenomena translate into clinical scenarios, where the timing of exposure to different inflammatory insults generally are not known. The complex effects of chronic exposure of the fetal lung to antenatal inflammation probably will alter postnatal lung and systemic inflammatory responses. Chronic exposure to inflammation may be quite common in infants born before 30 weeks gestation.

ANTENATAL INFLAMMATION AND POSTNATAL INFLAMMATION

BPD in preterm infants is multifactorial in etiology and results from the interaction of antenatal and postnatal risk factors (see Fig. 71.1).[74] In epidemiologic and clinical studies, chorioamnionitis was associated with BPD in some studies[24] but not in others.[75] Multiple reasons for this discrepancy of the association between chorioamnionitis and BPD are recognized: (1) definitions of chorioamnionitis vary (clinical chorioamnionitis versus histologic chorioamnionitis); (2) different consequences may result from chorioamnionitis with different organisms (*Ureaplasma* versus gram-negative organisms); and (3) there will be differing degrees of antenatal and postnatal inflammation in different populations. A way to interpret the interaction between antenatal and postnatal inflammation is by a "multiple-hit hypothesis" (see Fig. 71.1). Antenatal inflammation may "prime" the inflammation, leading to exacerbation or suppression of injury from postnatal inflammation.

Experimental evidence from the fetal sheep model supports a "multiple-hit" mechanism. Exposure to intraamniotic LPS 30 days before preterm delivery increased postnatal lung inflammation induced by mechanical ventilation in preterm lambs, whereas exposure to LPS 4 days before delivery did not amplify the ventilation-induced lung injury response.[76,77] The timing of the onset of antenatal inflammation may be important for modulating postnatal injury responses. This concept is best illustrated by the experiments demonstrating that exposure to antenatal infection may cause either innate immune paralysis or augmentation of innate immune responses, depending on the timing of the insult.[69,70]

Another variable that may contribute to lung injury is the fate of inflammatory mediators in the lungs of the infant at delivery. The epithelium of the uninjured fetal lung is quite impermeable to proteins and large-molecular-weight substances such as LPS. However, in two different studies, gentle mechanical ventilation of the preterm lamb lung following the addition of LPS or IL-1 to fetal lung fluid resulted in the transfer of the proinflammatory mediators to the systemic circulation and a systemic inflammatory response.[78,79] In an epidemiologic study, the risk for BPD did not increase on exposure to chorioamnionitis but was increased after exposure to chorioamnionitis and mechanical ventilation after birth.[29]

GLUCOCORTICOID EFFECTS ON THE FETAL LUNG

Although antenatal glucocorticoids decrease the incidence of RDS, they do not decrease the incidence of BPD in survivors.[80] This lack of clear benefit for prevention of BPD has been attributed to the increased survival of antenatal corticosteroid–exposed very preterm infants, who are most at risk for BPD. An alternative possibility, however, is the diminished alveolar septation observed after antenatal glucocorticoid treatment. Exposure of fetal monkeys or sheep to glucocorticoids decreased the lung mesenchyme, thinned the alveolus-capillary barrier, and increased potential lung gas volume, but inhibited alveolar septation (see Fig. 71.3).[63,81] Monkeys exposed to a relatively high dose of antenatal glucocorticoids had functionally more mature lungs that held more gas after preterm birth. However, when delivery was at term, the lungs were smaller, with fewer and larger alveoli.[82] Alveolar septation also was decreased in the fetal sheep lung by maternal betamethasone.[83] The magnitude of the arrest in alveolar septation was similar for both antenatal intraamniotic LPS and maternal betamethasone in sheep.[63] Although the mechanisms resulting in altered alveolar septation are not known, it is provocative that both proinflammatory and anti-inflammatory stimuli that induce clinical lung maturation also have as an adverse effect the inhibition of alveolar septation. As with LPS, antenatal glucocorticoids may alter the fetal lung responses to injury and initiate the anatomic changes characteristic of BPD.

INTERACTIONS OF ANTENATAL GLUCOCORTICOIDS AND INFLAMMATION

Most women at risk for very preterm delivery from chronic histologic chorioamnionitis and low-grade infection will be asymptomatic. On the basis of current recommendations, such women will receive antenatal glucocorticoids without an amniocentesis to evaluate for infection or inflammation. This clinical practice is based on clinical data and a meta-analysis indicating that antenatal glucocorticoids improved neonatal outcomes despite the presence of histologic chorioamnionitis or preterm rupture of membranes.[84] Studies in fetal sheep have evaluated the pulmonary effects of fetal exposure to chorioamnionitis and maternal

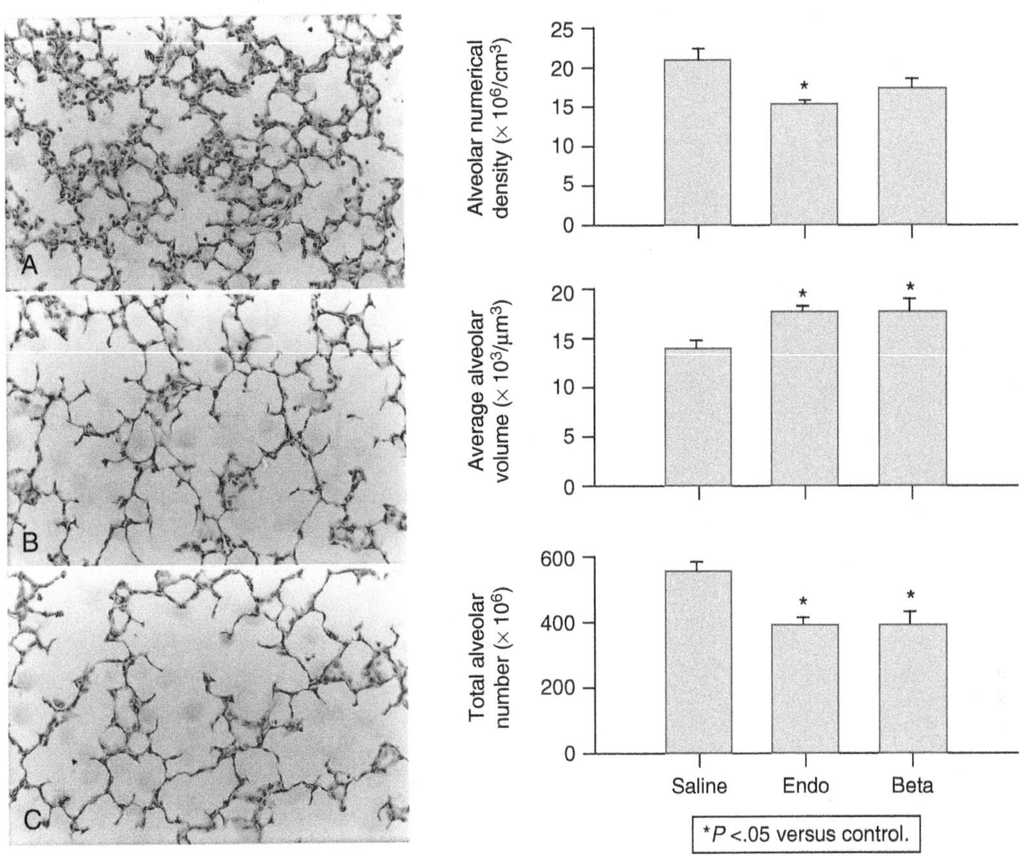

Fig. 71.3 Preterm lamb lungs at 125 days gestation, 7 days after administration of control intraamniotic saline (A), intraamniotic endotoxin *(Endo)* (B), or maternal betamethasone *(Beta)* (C). Bar graphs give indices of alveolar development in treated versus control groups of preterm lambs. Note that both endotoxin and maternal betamethasone impaired alveolar development. (From Willet KE, Jobe AH, Ikegami M, et al. Antenatal endotoxin and glucocorticoid effects on lung morphometry in preterm lambs. *Pediatr Res.* 2000;48:782–788.)

betamethasone. If intraamniotic LPS and maternal betamethasone were given simultaneously to pregnant ewes, there was an initial suppression of fetal lung inflammation induced by LPS. Curiously, there was amplification of pulmonary inflammation at later time points. Thus, maternal betamethasone had an initial innate immune suppressive effect as expected, but the unanticipated later amplification of innate immune response may result from maturational effects of betamethasone on inflammatory cells.[85] Despite the modulation of inflammatory response, the physiologic effects of the combined exposure were increased airway surfactant and improved lung mechanics compared with either exposure alone. When maternal betamethasone was administered before intraamniotic LPS in the ewes, lung inflammation was suppressed.[86] Interestingly, betamethasone treatment after LPS did not counteract inflammation but enhanced lung maturation (Fig. 71.4). Thus, the order of exposures of intraamniotic LPS or maternal betamethasone had large effects on fetal lung inflammation and maturation. Extrapolation of these experimental results supports the clinical practice of giving maternal betamethasone to women with suspected chorioamnionitis because the net physiologic effect of the combined exposure is for the fetal lung to be more clinically mature.

MATERNAL HYPERTENSIVE DISORDERS, FETAL GROWTH RESTRICTION, AND LUNG DEVELOPMENT

Fetal growth restriction is a common abnormality of pregnancy with a number of associations that include maternal hypertensive disorders, maternal smoking, severe nutritional deficiency, infections, and chromosome abnormalities. Fetal growth is decreased for infants born very prematurely in association with preeclampsia and as yet poorly defined placental vascular developmental abnormalities that also alter vascular development of the fetal lung.[87] From a physiologic perspective, decreased fetal growth results from decreased fetal perfusion due to increased placental resistance or abnormal fetal somatic growth. Decreased tissue perfusion causes hypoxemia, decreased delivery of nutrients, and increased cortisol concentrations, all of which may affect lung development. Fetal growth restriction is independently associated with an increased risk for neonatal death and chronic lung disease in preterm infants.[88,89] Infant mortality and the risk for BPD increase strikingly as the percentile Z-scores decrease relative to gestational age (Fig. 71.5). In a post-hoc analysis of the SUPPORT trial of comparison of lower vs. higher oxygen saturation targeting in preterm infants, higher mortality in the lower oxygen saturation targeting group was almost entirely attributable to small for gestation infants.[90] Thus, fetal growth compromise may increase vulnerability to hypoxemia in neonates. In animal models, calorie or protein restriction or placental blood restriction to the fetus causes fetal growth restriction. Intrauterine growth restriction (IUGR) decreases lung weight and total DNA content in proportion to body weight, decreases maturation of type II cells and subsequent surfactant maturation, decreases alveoli numbers, and thickens airway walls in animal models. The mechanisms by which growth restriction alters lung development are complex and model dependent. An example of a mechanism by which IUGR may interfere with lung development is via peroxisome proliferator-activated receptor (PPAR) γ, a transcription factor

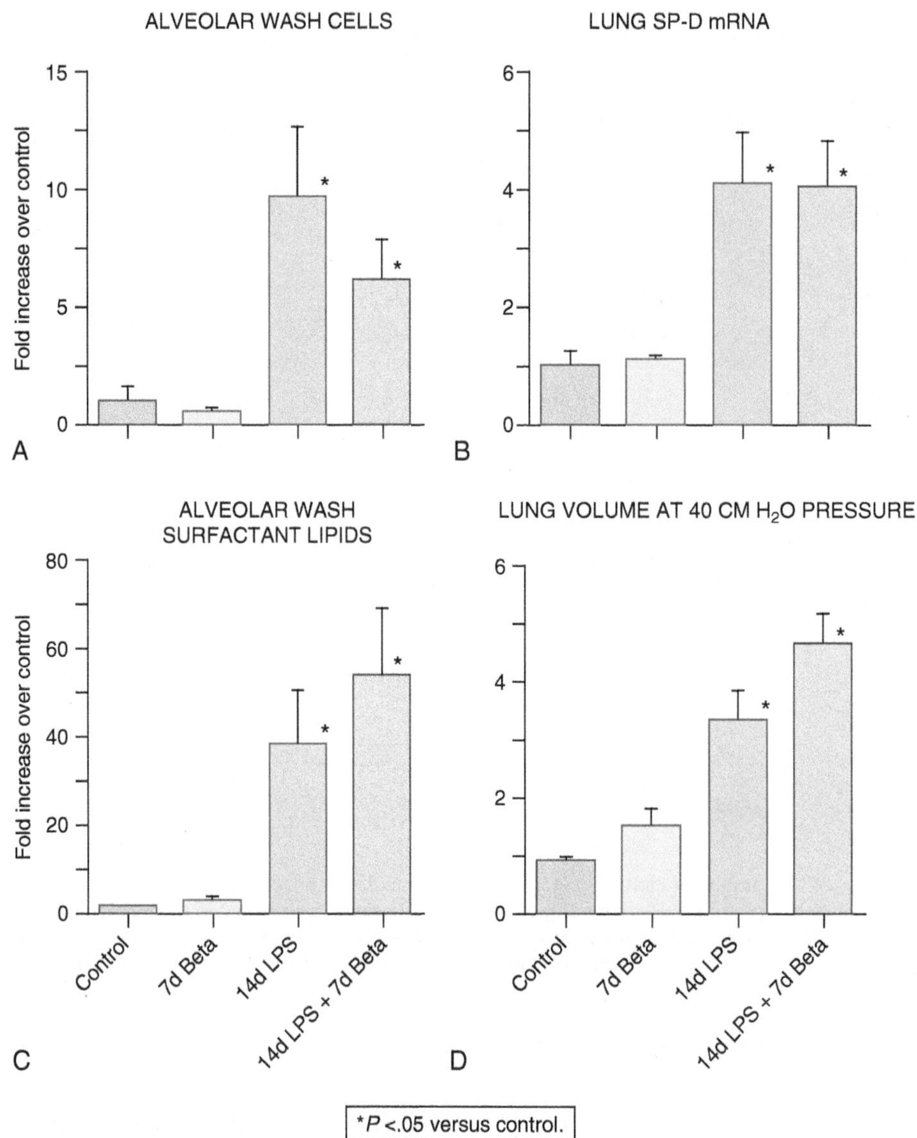

Fig. 71.4 Interplay between fetal exposures to intraamniotic lipopolysaccharide *(LPS)* and maternal betamethasone. Fetal sheep were delivered at approximately 125 days gestation (term = 150 days) after exposures to intraamniotic saline (control), maternal betamethasone 7 days before delivery (7d Beta), intraamniotic LPS 14 days before delivery (14d LPS), or a combination of 14d LPS+7d Beta. (A) Alveolar wash inflammatory cells (neutrophils + monocytes). (B) SP-D mRNA from whole lung homogenates. (C) Alveolar wash surfactant lipids (saturated phosphatidyl choline). (D) Lung volumes at 40 cm H_2O pressure. All measurements were normalized to controls (value designated as 1). Beta administration 7 days after LPS did not significantly attenuate lung inflammation, but the combined effect was more clinical lung maturation. (Data from Kuypers E, Collins JJ, Kramer BW, et al. Intra-amniotic LPS and antenatal betamethasone: inflammation and maturation in preterm lamb lungs. *Am J Physiol Lung Cell Mol Physiol.* 2012;302:L380–L389.)

that regulates epigenetic changes, particularly chromatin-modifying enzymes. In a rat model of growth restriction, maternal supplementation of docosahexaenoic acid increased PPAR γ levels and restored aberrant fetal lung development.[91] Effects of fetal growth abnormalities on lung function are of great interest. Epidemiologic studies from the United Kingdom reported increased cardiovascular disease in adults who had fetal growth restriction and decreased growth during the first year of life.[92] The hypothesis of fetal origins of disease in adulthood has expanded to include adverse cardiovascular, endocrine, and respiratory outcomes.[93] There is increasing evidence that growth restriction is associated with decreased lung function in childhood and beyond. In a meta-analysis of eight studies of lung function in adults, Lawlor and colleagues showed that birth weight was associated with an approximately 48 mL (95% CI, 26 to 70) increase in forced expiratory volume in 1 second (FEV_1) for each kg increase in birth weight.[94] Catch-up growth during childhood may improve the outlook,[95] but caution is required as increased weight gain during infancy may possibly worsen lung function.[96]

MATERNAL NUTRITION AND LUNG DEVELOPMENT

Both macro- and micronutrient deficiencies in the mother can cause abnormal lung development in the fetus. A striking example is increased incidence of airway obstruction even at 50 years in individuals whose mothers were exposed to the Dutch famine during midgestation during World War II. One mechanism causing aberrant fetal lung development during growth restriction is via retinoic acid signaling. The retinoids act on

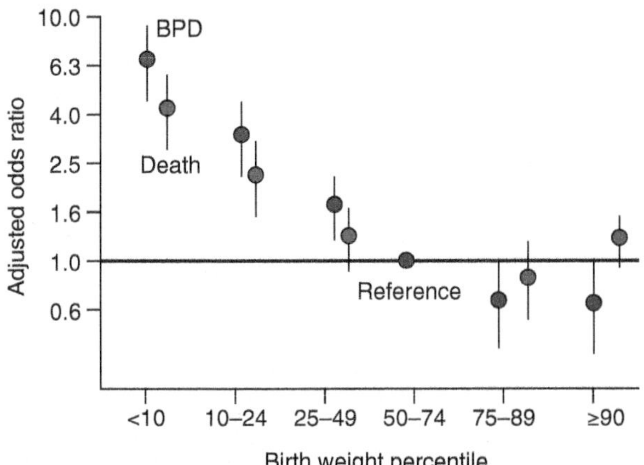

Fig. 71.5 Intrauterine growth restriction is associated with an increased risk for neonatal death and bronchopulmonary dysplasia *(BPD)*. The risk for infant mortality *(blue circle)* and BPD *(red circle)* in a cohort of 4525 preterm infants born between 24 and 31 weeks gestation are plotted against birth weight percentiles. The reference group is preterm infants born at 50th to 74th percentile weight, and the risks for BPD or death for other groups are expressed relative to the reference group. (Data from Zeitlin J, El Ayoubi M, Jarreau PH, et al. Impact of fetal growth restriction on mortality and morbidity in a very preterm birth cohort. *J Pediatr.* 2010;157:733–739.)

retinoic acid receptors (RARs) and retinoid X receptors (RXRs) and modulate alveolar formation, branching morphogenesis, and surfactant protein synthesis.[97] In a rat model of fetal growth restriction by caloric limitation during pregnancy, the resulting alveolar hypoplasia was reversible with postnatal vitamin A supplementation.[98] Administration of vitamin A also can reduce lung injury and BPD in sheep and humans.[99,100] In a randomized controlled trial in Nepali women with a high incidence of vitamin A deficiency, maternal supplementation of vitamin A during pregnancy resulted in improved lung volumes in their offspring at 9 to 13 years of age.[101] Maternal vitamin D deficiency has been correlated with increased risk for asthma and impaired lung function during childhood.[102] Thus, maternal nutrition is an important modulator of fetal lung development.

MATERNAL EXPOSURES AND FETAL LUNG DEVELOPMENT

Maternal cigarette smoking is a prevalent fetal exposure. Although the rate of smoking during pregnancy has decreased in the past decade in the United States, about 7% of all pregnant mothers reported smoking cigarettes in the United States with significant regional and socioeconomic disparities.[103] Nicotine has multiple direct effects on both the conducting airways and the parenchyma but also appears to alter the epigenome resulting in life-long pulmonary consequences. Maternal cigarette smoke exposure in rats results in fewer numbers of alveoli in exposed pups.[104] In fetal monkeys, prenatal exposure to nicotine also causes lung hypoplasia and increases collagen deposition around large airways and vessels.[105] Prenatal nicotine exposure of lambs and monkeys causes proximal airway obstruction.[106,107] However, not all nicotine exposure effects have detrimental fetal outcomes. Nicotine stimulated branching morphogenesis and increased expression of surfactant proteins in embryonic mouse lungs cultured in vitro and increased surfactant producing alveolar type II cells in monkeys.[105,108] In a human study, compared to healthy term infants, lung function of infants born to smokers was decreased at birth and these infants also had increased wheezing reports at 1 year of age.[109] This effect was particularly pronounced in mothers with homozygous mutant alleles in the $\alpha5$ nicotinic acetylcholine receptor. Remarkably, daily vitamin C supplementation (500 mg) of smoking mothers starting in the second trimester rescued decreased lung function at birth and the incidence of wheezing at 1 year of age.[109]

The fetal lung may also be affected by exposure to drugs. In a meta-analysis, the use of antidepressants, particularly selective serotonin reuptake inhibitor (SSRI) during pregnancy was associated with an increased risk for persistent pulmonary hypertension of the newborn if the drug was used in the third trimester (odds ratio 2.50; 95% confidence interval 1.32 to 4.73; P = .005) but not the first trimester (odds ratio 1.23; 95% confidence interval 0.58 to 2.60; P = .58).[110] Since the disease is not very common, the overall risk for neonatal pulmonary hypertension with maternal SSRI use is small when considered against the potential benefits.

Another area receiving increasing scrutiny is the exposure to environmental pollutions such as carbon particles and gases such as nitrous oxide and sulfur oxide particularly from automobile exhaust or charcoal and kerosene used for cooking and heating in the developing countries. Multiple studies have shown a clear association between prenatal exposure to environmental pollution and adverse pulmonary outcomes in the offspring.[111] Although the mechanisms are not completely understood, ambient black carbon particles have been shown to be deposited on the fetal side of human placenta.[112,113]

FETAL BREATHING, FETAL LUNG FLUID, AMNIOTIC FLUID, AND LUNG DEVELOPMENT

For optimal lung growth and development, adequate intra- and extrathoracic fluid, adequate intrathoracic space, pulmonary blood flow, and fetal breathing are required. Abnormalities of the thoracic cage or muscle disorders may also affect lung growth and development. The elegant experiments by Desai and Wigglesworth showed that transection of the phrenic nerve results in hypoplastic lungs, suggesting that breathing movements are essential to lung development.[114]

The importance of adequate fetal lung fluid volume was shown by Moessinger and colleagues, who observed that when one lobe in fetal lambs was allowed to drain freely, marked lung hypoplasia occurred.[115] In contrast, ligation of the contralateral lobe resulted in lung hyperplasia. Decreased amniotic fluid or oligohydramnios complicates about 10% of pregnancies.[116] Severe pulmonary hypoplasia associated with renal agenesis (Potter's syndrome) and prolonged oligohydramnios is characterized by a decrease in lung size and cell number along with narrow airways, delayed epithelial differentiation, and surfactant deficiency.[117] The importance of oligohydramnios was shown in a study of 5228 women with oligohydramnios during the third trimester.[118] When compared to 20,912 unaffected pregnancies, the offspring of the oligohydramnios group had increased rates of respiratory failure and increased rate of hospitalization. Even relatively short-term oligohydramnios caused by ruptured membranes in the 16th to 28th week of gestation can also result in pulmonary hypoplasia, the severity in general correlates with the length of the oligohydramnios.[119] There are several ongoing studies evaluating the efficacy of fetoscopic occlusion of trachea to reverse pulmonary hypoplasia resulting from severe forms of congenital diaphragmatic hernia.

CONCLUSION

There are clearly multiple antenatal associations of fetal exposures to long-term outcomes.[120,121] The most basic observation and consistent observation is that lung function trajectory from newborn to adulthood tracks across the life span of the individual. Is that because of unidentified exposures in a normal population of infants or simply biologic variability? This chapter reviews how complex some of the associations are. Fetal inflammation can injure the lung or induce early lung maturation as well as induce tolerance phenomena,[70,122] which may program the developing immune system for later adverse effects. The multiple variables and complexity tend to confound the clinical epidemiologic associations so that clinical studies do not reveal clear associations. For example, a presumed injury marker, chorioamnionitis, may induce lung maturation and also interact with postnatal exposure—oxygen or mechanical ventilation—to injure the lung. These interactive variables interfere with simple clinical and epidemiologic correlations.

A complete reference list is available at www.ExpertConsult.com.

SELECT REFERENCES

2. Laughon M, Allred EN, Bose C, et al. Patterns of respiratory disease during the first 2 postnatal weeks in extremely premature infants. *Pediatrics*. 2009;123(4):1124-1131.
3. Romero R, Espinoza J, Goncalves LF, Kusanovic JP, Friel LA, Nien JK. Inflammation in preterm and term labour and delivery. *Semin Fetal Neonatal Med*. 2006;11(5):317-326.
4. Combs CA, Gravett M, Garite TJ, et al. Amniotic fluid infection, inflammation, and colonization in preterm labor with intact membranes. *Am J Obstet Gynecol*. 2014;210(2):125.e1-e15.
5. Higgins RD, Saade G, Polin RA, et al. Evaluation and management of women and newborns with a maternal diagnosis of chorioamnionitis: summary of a workshop. *Obstet Gynecol*. 2016;127(3):426-436.
7. DiGiulio DB. Diversity of microbes in amniotic fluid. *Semin Fetal Neonatal Med*. 2012;17(1):2-11.
12. Goldenberg RL, Culhane JF, Iams JD, Romero R. Epidemiology and causes of preterm birth. *Lancet*. 2008;371(9606):75-84.
13. Gomez R, Romero R, Ghezzi F, Yoon BH, Mazor M, Berry SM. The fetal inflammatory response syndrome. *Am J Obstet Gynecol*. 1998;179(1):194-202.
14. Goldenberg RL, Hauth JC, Andrews WW. Intrauterine infection and preterm delivery. *N Engl J Med*. 2000;342(20):1500-1507.
18. Villamor-Martinez E, Alvarez-Fuente M, Ghazi AMT, et al. Association of chorioamnionitis with bronchopulmonary dysplasia among preterm infants: a systematic review, meta-analysis, and metaregression. *JAMA Netw Open*. 2019;2(11):e1914611.
20. Kumar R, Yu Y, Story RE, et al. Prematurity, chorioamnionitis, and the development of recurrent wheezing: a prospective birth cohort study. *J Allergy Clin Immunol*. 2008;121(4):878-884.e6.
22. McDowell KM, Jobe AH, Fenchel M, et al. Pulmonary morbidity in infancy after exposure to chorioamnionitis in late preterm infants. *Ann Am Thorac Soc*. 2016;13(6):867-876.
24. Watterberg KL, Demers LM, Scott SM, Murphy S. Chorioamnionitis and early lung inflammation in infants in whom bronchopulmonary dysplasia develops. *Pediatrics*. 1996;97(2):210-215.
28. Andrews WW, Goldenberg RL, Faye-Petersen O, Cliver S, Goepfert AR, Hauth JC. The Alabama Preterm Birth study: polymorphonuclear and mononuclear cell placental infiltrations, other markers of inflammation, and outcomes in 23- to 32-week preterm newborn infants. *Am J Obstet Gynecol*. 2006;195(3):803-808.
32. Jobe AH, Newnham JP, Willet KE, et al. Endotoxin-induced lung maturation in preterm lambs is not mediated by cortisol. *Am J Respir Crit Care Med*. 2000;162(5):1656-1661.
34. Kramer BW, Moss TJ, Willet KE, et al. Dose and time response after intraamniotic endotoxin in preterm lambs. *Am J Respir Crit Care Med*. 2001;164(6):982-988.
37. Kemp MW, Kannan PS, Saito M, et al. Selective exposure of the fetal lung and skin/amnion (but not gastro-intestinal tract) to LPS elicits acute systemic inflammation in fetal sheep. *PloS One*. 2013;8(5):e63355.
38. Kallapur SG, Moss TJ, Ikegami M, Jasman RL, Newnham JP, Jobe AH. Recruited inflammatory cells mediate endotoxin-induced lung maturation in preterm fetal lambs. *Am J Respir Crit Care Med*. 2005;172(10):1315-1321.
40. Kallapur SG, Nitsos I, Moss TJ, et al. IL-1 mediates pulmonary and systemic inflammatory responses to chorioamnionitis induced by lipopolysaccharide. *Am J Respir Crit Care Med*. 2009;179(10):955-961.
42. Moss TJ, Nitsos I, Ikegami M, Jobe AH, Newnham JP. Experimental intrauterine Ureaplasma infection in sheep. *Am J Obstet Gynecol*. 2005;192(4):1179-1186.
51. Benjamin JT, Smith RJ, Halloran BA, Day TJ, Kelly DR, Prince LS. FGF-10 is decreased in bronchopulmonary dysplasia and suppressed by Toll-like receptor activation. *Am J Physiol Lung Cell Mol Physiol*. 2007;292(2):L550-L558.
56. Albertine KH, Jones GP, Starcher BC, et al. Chronic lung injury in preterm lambs. Disordered respiratory tract development. *Am J Respir Crit Care Med*. 1999;159(3):945-958.
61. Le Cras TD, Kim DH, Gebb S, et al. Abnormal lung growth and the development of pulmonary hypertension in the Fawn-Hooded rat. *Am J Physiol*. 1999;277(4):L709-L718.
65. Kallapur SG, Bachurski CJ, Le Cras TD, Joshi SN, Ikegami M, Jobe AH. Vascular changes after intra-amniotic endotoxin in preterm lamb lungs. *Am J Physiol Lung Cell Mol Physiol*. 2004;287(6):L1178-L1185.
70. Kallapur SG, Jobe AH, Ball MK, et al. Pulmonary and systemic endotoxin tolerance in preterm fetal sheep exposed to chorioamnionitis. *J Immunol*. 2007;179(12):8491-8499.
72. Kallapur SG, Kramer BW, Knox CL, et al. Chronic fetal exposure to Ureaplasma parvum suppresses innate immune responses in sheep. *J Immunol*. 2011;187(5):2688-2695.
74. Kallapur SG, Jobe AH. Contribution of inflammation to lung injury and development. *Arch Dis Child Fetal Neonatal Ed*. 2006;91(2):F132-F135.
78. Kramer BW, Ikegami M, Jobe AH. Intratracheal endotoxin causes systemic inflammation in ventilated preterm lambs. *Am J Respir Crit Care Med*. 2002;165(4):463-469.
81. Bunton TE, Plopper CG. Triamcinolone-induced structural alterations in the development of the lung of the fetal rhesus macaque. *Am J Obstet Gynecol*. 1984;148(2):203-215.
84. Harding JE, Pang J, Knight DB, Liggins GC. Do antenatal corticosteroids help in the setting of preterm rupture of membranes? *Am J Obstet Gynecol*. 2001;184(2):131-139.
85. Kallapur SG, Kramer BW, Moss TJ, et al. Maternal glucocorticoids increase endotoxin-induced lung inflammation in preterm lambs. *Am J Physiol Lung Cell Mol Physiol*. 2003;284(4):L633-L642.
86. Kuypers E, Collins JJ, Kramer BW, et al. Intra-amniotic LPS and antenatal betamethasone: inflammation and maturation in preterm lamb lungs. *Am J Physiol Lung Cell Mol Physiol*. 2012;302(4):L380-L389.
87. Hansen AR, Barnes CM, Folkman J, McElrath TF. Maternal preeclampsia predicts the development of bronchopulmonary dysplasia. *J Pediatr*. 2010;156(4):532-536.
88. Zeitlin J, El Ayoubi M, Jarreau PH, et al. Impact of fetal growth restriction on mortality and morbidity in a very preterm birth cohort. *J Pediatr*. 2010;157(5):733-739.e1.
93. Barker DJ, Godfrey KM, Fall C, Osmond C, Winter PD, Shaheen SO. Relation of birth weight and childhood respiratory infection to adult lung function and death from chronic obstructive airways disease. *BMJ*. 1991;303(6804):671-675.
94. Lawlor DA, Ebrahim S, Davey Smith G. Association of birth weight with adult lung function: findings from the British Women's Heart and Health Study and a meta-analysis. *Thorax*. 2005;60(10):851-858.
95. Kotecha SJ, Watkins WJ, Heron J, Henderson J, Dunstan FD, Kotecha S. Spirometric lung function in school-age children: effect of intrauterine growth retardation and catch-up growth. *Am J Respir Crit Care Med*. 2010;181(9):969-974.
101. Checkley W, West Jr KP, Wise RA, et al. Maternal vitamin A supplementation and lung function in offspring. *N Engl J Med*. 2010;362(19):1784-1794.
104. Collins MH, Moessinger AC, Kleinerman J, et al. Fetal lung hypoplasia associated with maternal smoking: a morphometric analysis. *Pediatr Res*. 1985;19(4):408-412.
105. Sekhon HS, Jia Y, Raab R, et al. Prenatal nicotine increases pulmonary alpha7 nicotinic receptor expression and alters fetal lung development in monkeys. *J Clin Invest*. 1999;103(5):637-647.
109. McEvoy CT, Schilling D, Clay N, et al. Vitamin C supplementation for pregnant smoking women and pulmonary function in their newborn infants: a randomized clinical trial. *JAm Med Assoc*. 2014;311(20):2074-2082.
110. Grigoriadis S, Vonderporten EH, Mamisashvili L, et al. Prenatal exposure to antidepressants and persistent pulmonary hypertension of the newborn: systematic review and meta-analysis. *BMJ*. 2014;348:f6932.
111. Korten I, Ramsey K, Latzin P. Air pollution during pregnancy and lung development in the child. *Paediatr Respir Rev*. 2017;21:38-46.
114. Wigglesworth JS, Desai R. Effect on lung growth of cervical cord section in the rabbit fetus. *Early Hum Dev*. 1979;3(1):51-65.
115. Moessinger AC, Harding R, Adamson TM, Singh M, Kiu GT. Role of lung fluid volume in growth and maturation of the fetal sheep lung. *J Clin Invest*. 1990;86(4):1270-1277.
118. Chien LN, Chiou HY, Wang CW, Yeh TF, Chen CM. Oligohydramnios increases the risk of respiratory hospitalization in childhood: a population-based study. *Pediatr Res*. 2014;75(4):576-581.
119. Thibeault DW, Beatty Jr EC, Hall RT, Bowen SK, O'Neill DH. Neonatal pulmonary hypoplasia with premature rupture of fetal membranes and oligohydramnios. *J Pediatr*. 1985;107(2):273-277.
120. Agusti A, Hogg JC. Update on the pathogenesis of chronic obstructive pulmonary disease. *N Engl J Med*. 2019;381(13):1248-1256.
121. Postma DS, Bush A, van den Berge M. Risk factors and early origins of chronic obstructive pulmonary disease. *Lancet*. 2015;385(9971):899-909.

Regulation of Pulmonary Circulation

72

Yuansheng Gao | J. Usha Raj

INTRODUCTION

Throughout fetal life, the pulmonary circulation forms and establishes a hierarchical system that is essential for postnatal gas exchange. In humans, a continuity of the circulation between the heart and the capillary plexus of the lung appears at approximately 34 days of gestation.[1,2] There is no appreciable reactivity of pulmonary vessels at midterm gestation, but reactivity increases with advancing gestation thereafter, with increased pulmonary vascular resistance (PVR) and low pulmonary blood flow (PBF).[3,4] At birth, with the onset of breathing, PVR dramatically decreases and PBF increases to allow the entire right ventricular output to go into the lungs.[5,6] After birth, the pulmonary vasculature continues to grow in parallel with the growth of the airways to increase gas exchange capacity, making it compatible with somatic growth.[7,8] During the fetal and neonatal period, regulation of the pulmonary circulation—in comparison with that of adults—is more dynamic, complicated, and vulnerable to injury.[9-11] In this chapter, regulation of pulmonary circulation of the fetus in utero, at birth, and in the neonatal period is discussed, with a focus on the role of endothelium-derived nitric oxide (NO) and endothelin-1 (ET-1), two key regulators during these periods.[10,12,13] In addition, perinatal mechanisms underlying vascular remodeling and exaggerated vasocontractility, the hallmarks of pulmonary arterial hypertension (PAH), are also discussed.

DEVELOPMENT OF THE PULMONARY VASCULATURE

Lung development is divided into five distinct histologic stages: embryonic, pseudoglandular, canalicular, saccular, and alveolar. These overlap due to the nonsynchronous development of the lung.[14-16] During the embryonic stage (4 to 7 postconception weeks [pcw] in humans), the lung bud lined by epithelium first appears as a ventral diverticulum of the foregut at 4 pcw. A continuity of the circulation between the heart and the capillary plexus of the lung exists from at least 5 pcw, with the artery extending from the outflow tract of the heart and the veins connecting to the prospective left atrium. A capillary plexus in the mesenchyme forms between these arteries and veins.[1,2,17] During the pseudoglandular stage (5 to 17 pcw in humans), preacinar airway and vascular structures are formed and all preacinar pulmonary and bronchial arteries are in place, corresponding with the bronchial branching pattern. The canalicular stage (16 to 26 pcw in humans) marks a great increase in the number of lung capillaries in close apposition to the epithelium to form the first air-blood barrier, which is sufficient to sustain life in extremely premature infants. During the saccular stage (24 to 38 pcw in humans), the last generations of airways are formed, which end in clusters of thin-walled saccules. Capillaries form a bilayer within the cellular intersaccular septa. In the alveolar stage, starting at 36 pcw, the interalveolar septa are thinned, the double capillary layer matures into a single-layer adult form, and the microvasculature undergoes marked growth and development. At birth, about one-third to one-half of the adult number of alveoli are present. After birth there is further multiplication of alveoli and the adult number is reached by 3 years of age. The size and surface area of the alveoli increase until the end of adolescence.[8,14,15,18-21]

REGULATION OF THE PULMONARY CIRCULATION IN THE PERINATAL PERIOD

FETAL PERIOD

Fetal blood is oxygenated in the placenta and circulates through the inferior vena cava, right atrium, foramen ovale, left atrium, and left ventricle to the aorta. Blood received by the right ventricle is mainly from the superior and inferior venae cavae and has a relatively low oxygen content. A large portion of the blood pumped out by the right ventricle enters the aorta via the ductus arteriosus, and, owing to the high PVR, only a small portion enters the lungs (Fig. 72.1).[3,10,22] In human fetuses, blood flow to the lung increases from 13% to 25% of the combined ventricular output (CVO) from 20 to 30 weeks of gestation because of the growth of the pulmonary vascular bed. At this gestational age, the pulmonary vasculature in the fetus shows minimal vasodilation to acute maternal hyperoxygenation. From 30 to 38 pcw, blood flow of the lungs decreases from 25% to 21% of CVO, while the weight-indexed PVR significantly increases, mainly owing to increased vasomotor tone. This is evident from the decrease in PVR and increase in PBF that occurs in response to maternal hyperoxygenation.[3,4] In ovine fetal lungs, PBF represents only 3.7% and 7.0% of CVO at 40% and 100% gestational ages, respectively, which is accompanied by a progressive decrease in PVR, but PVRI (PVR indexed for growth) increases with gestation.[9,10,23] Similar phenomena have been reported in other species including rabbits, pigs, and primates.[24-26]

High PVR and low PBF are hallmarks of the fetal pulmonary circulation,[9,10,23,27,28] in part owing to the thick-walled fetal pulmonary vessels[18,19] but also because of a high myogenic tone that resists the actions of vasodilators in the low-oxygen-tension milieu of the fetus, in particular during late gestation.[29-32] In chronically catheterized late gestational fetal lambs, the myogenic response of pulmonary vessels is suppressed by brief intrapulmonary infusions of Y-27632 or HA-1077, inhibitors of Rho kinase (ROCK), leading to a sustained decrease in PVR and an increase in PBF without lowering the systemic arterial pressure. ROCK inhibits the dephosphorylation of myosin light chain (MLC), leading to vasoconstriction, and suggesting that high ROCK activity is involved in the maintenance of fetal pulmonary vasomotor tone.[31,32] ROCK is activated by RhoA, a member of the Rho family of small GTPase-binding proteins, which is stimulated by hypoxia and various vasoconstrictors; this indicates that RhoA/ROCK signaling is important in the maintenance of high PVR in the fetus.[33-36] RhoA/ROCK activity is also present in pulmonary arterial endothelial cells (PAECs), and ROCK has been shown to inhibit the synthesis of NO through the phosphorylation of endothelial nitric oxide synthase (eNOS) at threonine 495.[37] ROCK inhibition increases the production of NO by the PAECs of fetal lambs under normoxic but not hypoxic conditions. This could be because eNOS activity is already low in the fetal environment, so that ROCK cannot further reduce NO production.[38]

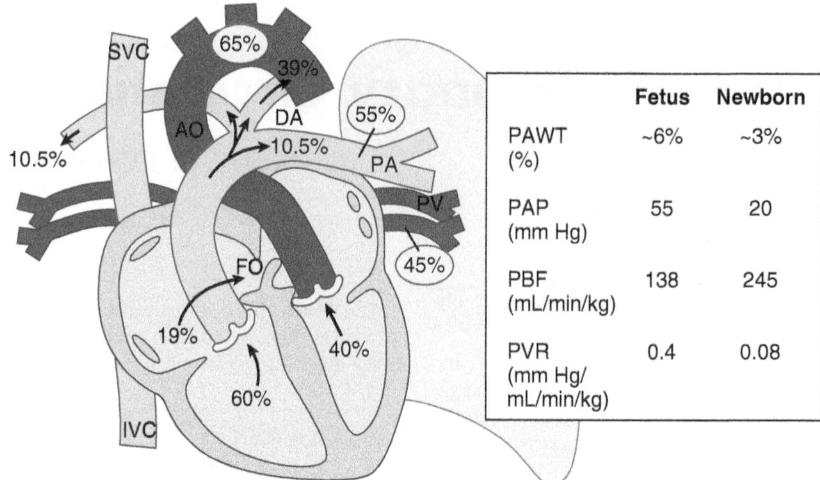

	Fetus	Newborn
PAWT (%)	~6%	~3%
PAP (mm Hg)	55	20
PBF (mL/min/kg)	138	245
PVR (mm Hg/ mL/min/kg)	0.4	0.08

Fig. 72.1 Pulmonary hemodynamic parameters of the term fetal human pulmonary circulation compared with that of the 2- to 3-day-old newborn. Fetal pulmonary circulation is characterized by high pulmonary arterial pressure *(PAP)*, high pulmonary vascular resistance *(PVR)*, and low pulmonary blood flow *(PBF)*. The wall thickness of the pulmonary arteries *(PAWT)* (expressed as a percentage of twice the wall thickness/ external diameter) with an external diameter of 200 μm is about twice as much in the term fetus as in the newborn. Owing to the high PVR, the major portion of the fetus's cardiac output is diverted to other organs instead of the lungs via the foramen ovale *(FO)* and the ductus arteriosus *(DA)*. The fetal blood is relatively hypoxic, with oxygen saturation (numbers in green circles) of 65%, 55%, and 45% for blood in the aorta *(AO)*, pulmonary artery *(PA)*, and pulmonary vein *(PV)*, respectively. At birth, PVR is markedly reduced by increased vasodilator activity evoked by ventilation, oxygenation, and increased shear stress. A rapid increase in the vessel diameter of resistance pulmonary arteries, resulting from reorganization of smooth muscle cells, also occurs. The numbers in vessel lumina and cardiac chambers represent the percent of the combined cardiac output of the left and right ventricles that flows through the PA, FO, and DA. *IVC*, Inferior vena cava; *SVC*, superior vena cava. (Modified with permission from Gao Y, Raj JU. Regulation of the pulmonary circulation in the fetus and newborn. *Physiol Rev.* 2010;90:1291–1335.)

NO plays a key role in the regulation of the pulmonary circulation in the fetus and newborn. NO is synthesized by eNOS during the conversion of L-arginine to L-citrulline and readily diffuses into the underlying smooth muscle cells to exert its vasodilatory effect.[10,39] In the human fetal lung, immunohistochemical examination shows that eNOS is highly expressed during the canalicular and saccular stages; expression falls sharply in the alveolar stage and decreases further after birth.[40] Lung NOS activity also rises and peaks at 118 days of gestation in the sheep fetus (term = 150 days) before falling in late gestation; it remains low in the newborn and adult.[41] In near-term and term fetal lambs, nitro-L-arginine, an inhibitor of eNOS, reduces pulmonary artery blood flow and increases pulmonary artery pressure, suggesting that NO is functional and exerts an inhibitory effect on fetal pulmonary vasomotor tone.[5] Since the fetal pulmonary vasculature exists in an environment of low oxygen tension (17 to 19 mm Hg), the formation of NO is relatively modest[42] but nevertheless significant, as inhibition of endogenous NO production in fetal lambs increases PVR.[5,43] In near-term lambs, the increase in fetal arterial oxygen tension from 25 to 55 mm Hg results in an increase of more than sevenfold in the proportion of right ventricular output distributed to the fetal lung. In contrast, an increase in oxygen tension from 27 to 174 mm Hg has no effect on PBF in early-term (approximately 65% of gestational period) lambs, indicating a minor role for NO at an early stage of gestation.[44] However, inhibition of endogenous NO production does increase PVR at this stage.[45]

NO stimulates soluble guanylyl cyclase (sGC), resulting in elevated levels of cGMP and the activation of cGMP-dependent protein kinase (PKG), followed by a Ca^{2+}-dependent and Ca^{2+}-independent decrease in MLC phosphorylation and vasodilation.[10,46–49] In pulmonary arterial smooth muscle cells (PASMCs), the protein level and enzyme activity of sGC are greater in normoxia than in hypoxia.[50,51] In vivo infusion of 8-Br-cGMP a cell-permeable cGMP analog, induces relaxation of the pulmonary circulation in fetal lambs.[52] Relaxation of isolated pulmonary arteries induced by 8-Br-cGMP is less in fetal than in newborn and adult sheep,[53] indicating a developmental increase in the responses to cGMP. In pulmonary arteries and veins of term fetal lambs, relaxation to 8-Br-cGMP is greater after exposure for 4 hours to normoxia (Po_2, 140 mm Hg) compared with hypoxia (Po_2, 30 mm Hg) in part because hypoxia reduces the expression of PKG protein and mRNA and also leads to posttranscriptional modification of PKG by peroxynitrite and other reactive oxygen species (ROS).[54–56] cGMP is degraded by phosphodiesterases (PDEs), in particular the type 5 PDE (PDE5).[57] The rates of degradation of cGMP in ovine pulmonary vessels are greater in the fetus than in the newborn lamb contributing to the greater vasomotor tone and contractility of fetal pulmonary vessels, particularly the veins.[58]

ET-1, a potent peptide vasoconstrictor, is mainly synthesized in endothelial cells (ECs), first as a 212-amino acid preproET-1 peptide; it is then transformed to pro-ET-1 by a signal peptidase, to big ET-1 by a furin convertase, and finally to the vasoactive ET-1 by ET-converting enzyme (ECE). Various stimuli such as shear stress, hypoxia, or ischemia, rapidly increase ET-1 synthesis, which is secreted within minutes, predominantly toward to the subluminal side.[59] Upon release, ET-1 exerts its effect by binding to its receptors ET_A and ET_B, with the former predominantly located in vascular smooth muscle cells (VSMCs) and the latter mainly in ECs. The activation of ET_A receptors on VSMCs leads to a potent and long-lasting vasoconstriction, primarily by increasing intracellular Ca^{2+} levels ($[Ca^{2+}]_i$) and increasing the sensitivity of myofilaments to $[Ca^{2+}]_i$ via Rho/ROCK and protein kinase (PKC).[60–62] The activation on ET_B receptors stimulates ECs to synthesize and release NO and PGI_2, leading to reduced pulmonary vascular tone.[10,62] In human fetuses, the expression of ET-1 in the lung is greater during the saccular and alveolar stages than in canalicular stages. ET_A expression is strong throughout gestation, whereas ET_B receptor expression is weak in the canalicular stage but increases markedly during the saccular and alveolar stages.[40] In late-gestation fetal lambs, intrapulmonary infusion of ET_A antagonist causes a sustained fetal pulmonary vasodilation, whereas infusion of an ET_B

receptor agonist has no effect on basal blood flow, suggesting that the endogenous ET-1 released in the fetal lungs may mainly activate ET_A receptors, leading to an increased high PVR.[63] In fetal lambs, intrapulmonary infusion of ET-1 increases the basal PBF in a manner sensitive to the inhibition of eNOS, indicating that the effect of exogenous ET-1 primarily results from ET_B-mediated NO.[64-67] However, infusion of big ET-1, which is converted to ET-1 inside ECs by ECE and released predominantly locally, exclusively causes fetal pulmonary vasoconstriction in utero.[59] Although the exact mechanism underlying the different effects between the infusion of ET-1 and big-ET-1 remain to be clarified, it is possible that the effect of big ET-1 is more closely related to the true in vivo role of endogenous ET-1.[63,68] Such a point of view is in line with the observations obtained with ET antagonists.[63]

AT BIRTH

At birth, with the onset of breathing, PVR dramatically decreases from 0.4 to 0.08 mm Hg/mL/min/kg (body weight); PBF increases from 21% CVO to nearly the entire cardiac output, pulmonary arterial pressure (PAP) gradually decreases while systemic pressure increases. The mean PAP approaches 50% of mean systemic pressure within the first day and reduces further to the adult level within 2 weeks after birth. The foramen ovale closes as soon as systemic vascular resistance exceeds PVR. The ductus arteriosus begins to close within the first few hours after birth and flow of blood through the ductus arteriosus becomes insignificant within 15 hours of birth.[3,10,11,69-71] The dramatic fall in PVR at birth results from many birth-related events, including an increase in oxygen tension, increase in shear stress from increased blood flow, changes in the activities of various vasoactive agents (e.g., NO, ET-1),[9,10,23,72,73] and mechanical causes such as expansion of vessels from changes in lung volume, creation of an air-liquid interface, and changes in surface tension.[74-76] In late gestation, the volume of fetal lung liquid in lambs (approximately 45 mL/kg) is much greater than the functional residual capacity (FRC; approximately 25 mL/kg) in newborns, which results in greater extraluminal pressures surrounding the pulmonary vasculature and compression of the vessels in the fetal lung. Following clearance of lung liquid after birth, there is a marked reduction in extraluminal pressures, which contributes to vascular expansion and increased PBF.[77-79] With onset of breathing, an air-liquid interface is established in the alveolus, with increased alveolar recoil, capillary distension, and a decrease in PVR.[76]

Oxygenation and increased shear stress are the most important factors in the fall in PVR at birth.[10] In fetal lambs near term, an increase in oxygen tension alone can increase PBF.[6,44,80] The increase in PBF causes further reduction of PVR via shear stress–induced vasodilation of pulmonary vessels.[81-83] These changes are largely abolished by nitro-L-arginine (a selective endothelium-derived NO antagonist), indicating a key role for NO as a signaling molecule.[43,81,84] Vasodilation induced by NO is suppressed by the inhibition of sGC and PKG; therefore the NO-cGMP-PKG signaling pathway plays a pivotal role in mediating the effects of oxygenation and shear stress.[85-88] As discussed earlier, the RhoA-ROCK signaling pathway contributes to the high fetal PVR.[29-31] In fetal lambs, inhibition of ROCK increases the production of NO of pulmonary arteries under normoxic but not hypoxic conditions. Moreover, even in the presence of NO inhibition the inhibition of ROCK inhibition caused pulmonary vasodilation of the fetal circulation. At birth, therefore, RhoA/ROCK signaling may exert counteractive actions both at the endothelial and smooth muscle levels.[38] However, under oxygenated conditions after birth, NO-cGMP-PKG exhibits potent inhibitory actions on RhoA/ROCK pathway.[33,89-91]

The plasma levels of ET-1 rise immediately after birth in humans.[92,93] In newborn lambs, circulating ET-1 level is high 8 hours after delivery.[94] Bosentan, a nonselective ET receptor blocker, does not affect the increase in PBF or decrease in PVR of term fetal lambs caused by oxygen ventilation.[95] However, selective blockade of ET_B receptors with BQ-788 attenuates the reduction in PVR induced by ventilation and oxygenation.[96] These data suggest that the net influence of ET-1 at birth may be minor. In primary cultures of ovine PAECs of newborn lambs, ET-1 secretion is inhibited by an NO donor, activator of sGC, and cGMP analog, together with a decrease in preproET-1 mRNA, indicating that the increased production of NO at birth may inhibit ET-1 production via cGMP pathway[97] (Fig. 72.2). Other vasoactive agonists are also involved in the changes in pulmonary circulation at birth, among them is PGI_2 (prostacyclin), a potent vasodilator, which is synthesized in the endothelium and released by both oxygenation and shear stress.[80,98-100] In fetal lambs, the increase in PBF induced by increasing oxygen tension from 20 to 54 torr is not significantly attenuated by indomethacin, an inhibitor of prostaglandin synthesis, indicating that PGI_2 may not play a major role in the birth-related change in PBF.[101] At birth, the plasma levels of PAF, a potent vasoconstrictor of pulmonary vasculature, is decreased by approximately 80% in fetal lambs, and the activity of PAF acetylhydrolase (PAF-Ah), which converts PAF into biologically inactive lyso-PAF, is increased in an oxygen tension-dependent manner, suggesting that the increased catabolism of PAF by PAF-Ah levels caused by oxygenation is involved in the birth-related reduction in PVR.[102-104] Exogenous PAF infusion in fetal lambs results in vasodilation[105] but infusion of PAF after birth, when vasomotor tone is low, results in vasoconstriction.[106] These data once again highlight the fact that the physiologic effects of various vasoactive agents depend on many factors such as basal vasomotor tone when an individual is exposed to the agent, the oxygen tension surrounding the blood vessels, and other interacting vasoactive agents.

NEONATAL PERIOD

Immediately after birth, there is reorganization of the cytoskeleton of both endothelial and smooth muscle cells in the pulmonary arterial wall, so that the cells become thinner and spread around a larger lumen, resulting in reduced medial thickness and increased luminal diameter. These changes are most pronounced in the first 19 days and continue for the first 3 months of life.[7,107-109] The number of pulmonary arteries increases rapidly in the first 2 months of life. Thereafter, arteries multiply at a rate similar to that of alveoli. The size of the arteries increases most rapidly during the first 2 months, but growth rate remains high during the first 4 years. Pulmonary veins also grow at a rate corresponding to the growth of the arteries, although the veins are thin-walled compared with arteries of the same order.[18,19,107] The growth of the pulmonary vasculature is closely linked to that of the airways throughout lung development.[110] After birth, the pulmonary capillary network continues to expand, leading to a 35-fold increase by adulthood, thus providing the necessary surface area for gas exchange to match the increasing cardiac output during somatic growth.[8,111,112]

In term neonates, after a 5- to 10-fold drop in PVR at birth, PVR continues to fall over the next 4 to 6 weeks to approach adult levels.[9,113] This continued fall in PVR results from morphologic changes in the vasculature and from continued upregulation of active mechanisms for maintaining low vasomotor tone. Ovine pulmonary arteries of term fetal, 1- to 2-week-old newborn, and adult sheep show an age-dependent increase in relaxation responses to NO, exogenous NO donors, and a cell membrane–permeable analog of cGMP, implying a maturational change in the NO-cGMP-PKG pathway.[53] In the porcine lung, eNOS protein increases after birth to a maximum at 3 days of age, associated with increased enzyme activity.[114] In porcine pulmonary arteries, coimmunoprecipitation

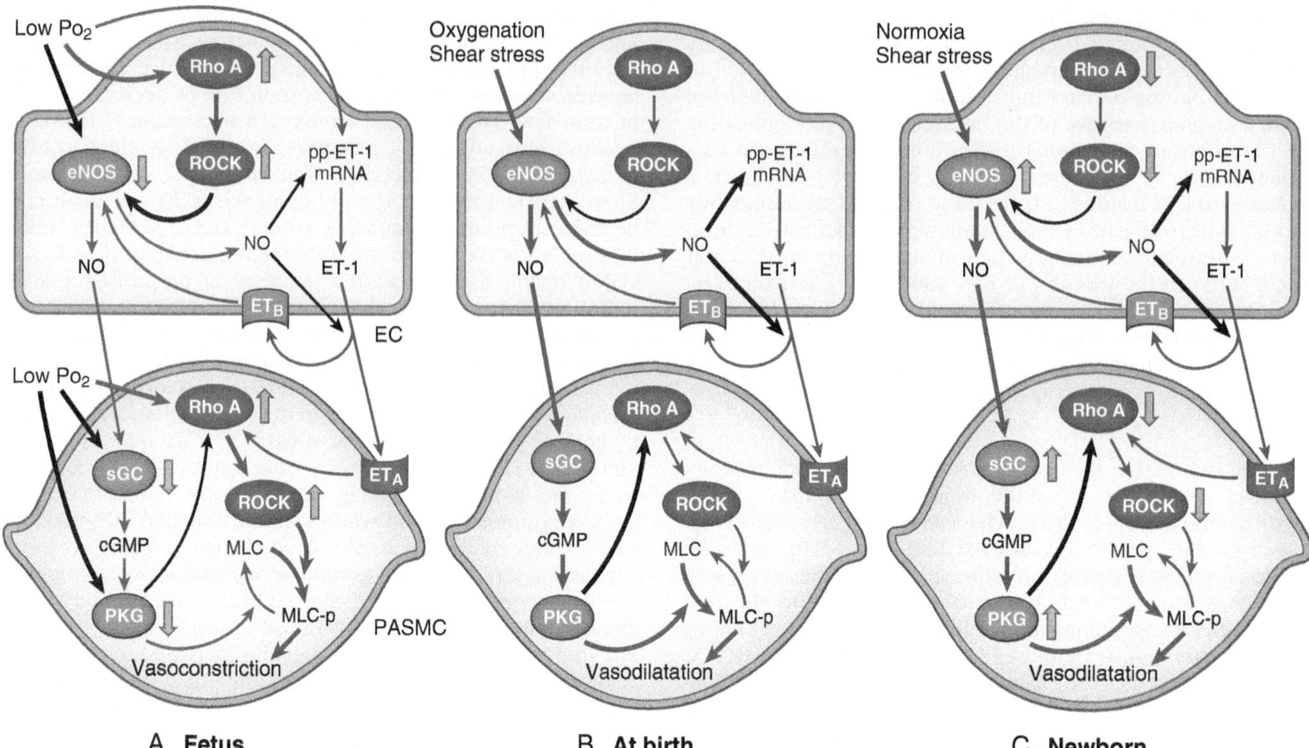

Fig. 72.2 Possible mechanism for the regulation of contractility of pulmonary arterial smooth muscle cells *(PASMCs)* by nitric oxide *(NO)* and endothelin-1 *(ET-1)* released from the endothelial cells *(ECs)* of the fetus (A), at birth (B), and in the newborn (C). (A) In fetal lungs the signaling of NO-cGMP-cGMP–dependent protein kinase *(PKG)* is suppressed owing to inhibition of the expression and activity of endothelial NO synthase *(eNOS)*, soluble guanylyl cyclase *(sGC)*, and PKG by low oxygen tension *(Po_2)*. By contrast, the expression and activity of RhoA-Rho kinase *(ROCK)* is upregulated, leading to high myogenic tone due to reduced dephosphorylation of myosin light chain *(MLC→MLCp)* and thus increased vasoconstriction and high pulmonary vascular resistance *(PVR)*. ET-1 is synthesized in the ECs from preproendothelin *(pp-ET-1)* and released to the extracellular space in response to various stimuli including hypoxia. ET-1 exerts its actions on PASMCs via the endothelin A receptor *(ET_A)* to cause vasoconstriction via the RhoA/ROCK pathway. ET-1 may also stimulate eNOS via the endothelin B receptor *(ET_B)*. Under low Po_2, however, the ET_B is oxidized and its effect on eNOS is rather limited. (B) With the onset of breathing, NO-cGMP-PKG is stimulated by oxygenation, resulting in increased dephosphorylation of myosin light chain (MLCp→MLC) promoted by cGMP-PKG activity and hence vasodilation, reduction in PVR, and increase in pulmonary blood flow *(PBF)*. The increased PBF further stimulates NO-cGMP-PKG activity via increased shear stress. NO signaling also exerts an inhibitory effect on the synthesis and release of ET-1 and on RhoA/ROCK activity. (C) After birth and during the neonatal period, continuous normoxia and shear stress upregulate the expression of eNOS, sGC, and PKG and downregulate the expression and activity of RhoA and ROCK, resulting in a prevailing role of NO signaling over that of ET_A. *Red* and *green arrows* represent stimulatory and inhibitory action, respectively. Thick and thin *arrows* represent enhanced and suppressed activity, respectively. Upward- and downward-pointing *orange thick arrows* represent increased and decreased expression, respectively, of the enzyme.

study has revealed that the interactions between Hsp90 and eNOS mature over the first weeks of life, which promotes eNOS synthetic activity and coincides with increased NO-induced pulmonary vasodilatation.[115] The expression of sGC[116] also increases in an age-dependent manner in the pulmonary arteries of newborn and 2-week-old piglets, which correlates with increased vasorelaxant responses to NO and the exogenous sGC activator YC-1.[117] The rate of hydrolysis of cGMP is faster in ovine fetal pulmonary arteries and veins than in the vessels of 3- to 7-day-old newborns, resulting in a greater accumulation of cGMP in newborn vessels and a greater vasodilator response to NO and other sGC stimulators.[58] Expression of eNOS mRNA and protein increases in ovine fetal PAECs exposed to 95% O_2 for 24 hours and/or fluid shear stress for 8 hours[118] or 24-hour exposure to oxygenation with Po_2 at 150 mm Hg.[119] Shear stress–induced upregulation of eNOS may result from increased transcriptional activity of AP-1 protein c-Jun in fetal PAECs[120] and inhibition of STAT3 effects on the eNOS promoter through the inhibition of PKC-δ.[121] In addition to eNOS, shear stress also stimulates inducible NO synthase in the pulmonary VSMCs of fetal lambs.[122] In the perinatal pulmonary vasculature, the activities of sGC and PKG increase with increased oxygen tension and decrease with reduced oxygen tension.[54-56,123,124] Low oxygen tension may inhibit sGC expression via Sp1, a hypoxia-sensitive transcription factor,[51] or suppress the activity of sGC by redox modification of the dimerization of the enzyme.[125] Changes in oxygen affect PKG activity by altering the abundance of PKG,[54,124] the nitration of PKG,[55,56] and the interaction of PKG with its downstream target myosin light chain phosphatase (MLCP) target subunit 1 (MYPT1).[126]

In the neonatal period, a balance in the activity of the NO-cGMP-PKG and ET-1-ET_A-Ca^{2+}/RhoA-ROCK pathways is essential to the maintenance of normal pulmonary vasomotor tone. In healthy human neonates the high plasma ET-1 level at birth falls by 5 days of life and stays stable at 30 days of life.[127] Similar changes have been described in piglet[128] but not in ovine lungs.[129] In porcine pulmonary arteries and veins, the dominant receptor is ET_A in the immediate newborn period (5 minutes after birth), and in neonatal and adult pigs, and the density is comparable among the different age groups. ET_B receptor density is also similar in these age groups with the exception of 2- to 3-day-olds, where it is higher.[130-132] In the rabbit there is also an age-related decrease in ET_A-mediated contraction and an increase in ET_B-mediated NO-dependent relaxation (see Fig. 72.2).[133]

ABNORMAL VASOCONTRACTILITY AND VASCULAR REMODELING IN THE FETAL AND NEONATAL PERIOD

After the immediate neonatal transitional period, pulmonary artery pressure reaches the low adult levels of the first few days of life and definitely reaches levels similar to those of the adult by 2 to 3 months of age.[134] Pediatric PAH is defined as a mean PAP (mPAP) equal to or greater than 25 mm Hg at rest after 3 months of age, with a normal pulmonary artery wedge pressure equal to or greater than 15 mm Hg and an increased PVR indexed to body surface area (PVRI) equal to or greater than 3 WU·m^2.[134,135] In the neonatal period there may be many causes of pulmonary hypertension, including the persistent pulmonary hypertension syndrome (group 1) and developmental lung diseases (group 3), as well as congenital heart defects (CHD) and idiopathic PAH (IPAH).[134,136-138]

VASCULAR REMODELING

Pediatric PAH is intrinsically linked with vascular remodeling, leading to medial hypertrophy of muscular arteries and muscularization of muscle-free peripheral arteries from a variety of causes.[17,139,140] The remodeling of pulmonary vasculature in PPHN is often triggered by the dysfunction of the endothelium and consequently altered mediator activities, including increased proproliferation and antiapoptosis signaling such as elevated levels of ET-1 and augmented RhoA/ROCK activity. Meanwhile, mediators that inhibit vascular remodeling—such as NO/cGMP signaling—are suppressed.[135,139,141-145] NO-cGMP-PKG activity is often compromised in PAH.[56,124,126,145,146] In eNOS-deficient fetal and neonatal mice, pulmonary arterial muscularity was greater.[147] In ovine fetal PASMCs, exogenous NO attenuates serum-induced proliferation, with arrest of cells in G0/G1 cycle in part owing to peroxynitrite-mediated protein nitration.[120] NO may also inhibit cell proliferation and differentiation by interfering with MAPK signaling in a cGMP-dependent and -independent manner.[148] In ovine fetal pulmonary venous smooth muscle cells, the hypoxia-induced phenotype change from contractile to synthetic is closely related to reduced PKG protein levels. Overexpression of PKG in SMC reverses the effect of hypoxia.[149] Myocardin and E-26-like protein 1 (Elk-1) are downstream effectors of PKG. Hypoxia or inhibition of PKG decreases the expression of myocardin but increases the expression of Elk-1. It is postulated that PKG induces displacement of myocardin from serum response factor and up-regulates myocardin expression, thus activating transcription of SMC contractile genes.[150]

The plasma ET-1 level is elevated in infants with PPHN.[151] An increased production of ET-1 and activation of ET$_A$ receptors is associated with aberrant vascular development in models of PPHN in mice, rats, and piglets.[152-154] Platelet-derived growth factor (PDGF), a potent smooth muscle cell mitogen, is a downstream mediator of vascular remodeling induced by ET-1 in neonatal lungs.[155] In an ovine PPHN model created by ligation of the ductus arteriosus, the expression of PDGF α- and β-receptor proteins was increased. Blocking PDGF action with NX1975, a high-affinity DNA-based aptamer to the PDGF-B chain, reduces muscular thickening of small pulmonary arteries and reduces right ventricular hypertrophy.[156] PDGF may promote PAH via the activation of c-Jun NH2-terminal kinase1/2 (JNK1/2)[157] or p38 mitogen-activated protein kinase (p38-MAPK),[158] and phosphatidylinositol 3-kinase.[159] The transforming growth factor β (TGF-β)/Smad3 pathway is also activated by ET-1, via ET$_A$ receptors in the lung.[160] In newborn mice, chronic hypoxia leads to PASMC proliferation and vascular remodeling and these effects are abrogated by dominant-negative mutation of the TGF-β type II receptor, indicating that in hypoxia ET-1 may promote PASMC proliferation via TGF-β and Smad2.[161,162] Vascular remodeling results from either increased proliferation and/or decreased apoptosis. In PASMCs of a neonatal PAH model the Bcl-2-associated X protein (Bax), a key proapoptotic factor, is downregulated while B-cell lymphoma–extra large (Bcl-xL), an antiapoptotic factor, is upregulated. These effects are blocked by ET receptor antagonism, suggesting that ET-1 may mediate remodeling of neonatal pulmonary arteries by inhibiting smooth muscle cell apoptosis.[155,163] In a juvenile rat model of PAH induced by chronic hypoxia, treatment with Y-27632 reverses arterial wall remodeling accompanied by increased apoptosis, attenuates right ventricular hypertrophy, and completely normalized right ventricular systolic function.[164] ROCK promotes PASMCs proliferation by promoting cytoplasmic-to-nuclear translocation of extracellular signal-regulated kinase (ERK) 1/ERK2[165] and by a permissive action for the ERK1/2-dependent production of tenascin-C (TN-C), an extracellular matrix (ECM) protein.[166]

Increased elastase activity is thought to be involved in pathogenesis of PPHN. Newborn mice with chronic hypoxia-induced pulmonary hypertension exhibit decreased MMP-2 and increased TIMP-2.[167] In extremely preterm newborns (born at 23 to 26 weeks' gestational age), there is an increased incidence of PAH associated with bronchopulmonary dysplasia (BPD), characterized by reduced alveolar and microvascular density in addition to an increase in the distal arteries' percentage of medial thickness; an extension of arterial smooth muscle into peripheral arteries has also been documented in BPD.[139,168,169]

ABNORMAL VASOCONTRACTILITY

Pulmonary hypertension in neonates is accompanied by increased vascular tone and vasoreactivity. Under pathologic conditions, the action of vasoconstrictors may prevail over that of vasodilators.[a] Decreased eNOS activity, reduced release of NO, and impaired pulmonary vasodilatation are reported in PPHN in human infants and in a number of animal models.[b] NO synthesis is suppressed by asymmetric dimethylarginine (ADMA), an endogenous inhibitor of eNOS generated in protein methylation.[173] In PPHN infants, urinary ADMA levels are markedly higher at day 1 and 3 postbirth than in control subjects.[174,175] ADMA is metabolized by dimethyl-arginine dimethylaminohydrolase (DDAH).[173] In the newborn pig model with PH, decreased type 2 DDAH is associated with elevated ADMA levels.[176] In pulmonary arteries from human neonates and animal models of PPHN, the elevated levels of ROS may oxidize tetrahydrobiopterin (BH$_4$), an essential eNOS cofactor, to dihydrobiopterin, which causes eNOS uncoupling. The uncoupled eNOS synthesizes less NO and generates more superoxide, which can rapidly scavenge NO, leading to the formation of peroxynitrite and decreased NO bioavailability.[177] In fetal lambs with PPHN associated with a surgically induced left diaphragmatic hernia, relaxation of pulmonary arteries in response to the NO donor sodium nitroprusside is impaired, suggesting that the signaling pathway downstream from NO may be impaired.[178] Indeed, substantial evidence indicates that reduced activity and expression of sGC and PKG contribute to the development of pediatric PAH.[33,54-56,124,126,146] In fetal lambs exposed to chronic high-altitude hypoxia, relaxation of pulmonary arteries induced by 8-Br-cGMP is diminished, in part due to decreased PKG specific activity,[33] in part due to increased nitration of PKG by ROS.[55,56] The interaction of the N-terminal leucine zipper (LZ) domain of PKG-Iα and the LZ and/or coiled coil (CC) domain of the regulatory subunit MYPT1 of MLCP is critical for cGMP-induced vascular relaxation. In fetal ovine

[a]References 10, 12, 13, 46, 139, 170.

[b]References 10, 12, 13, 46, 139, 141, 170–172.

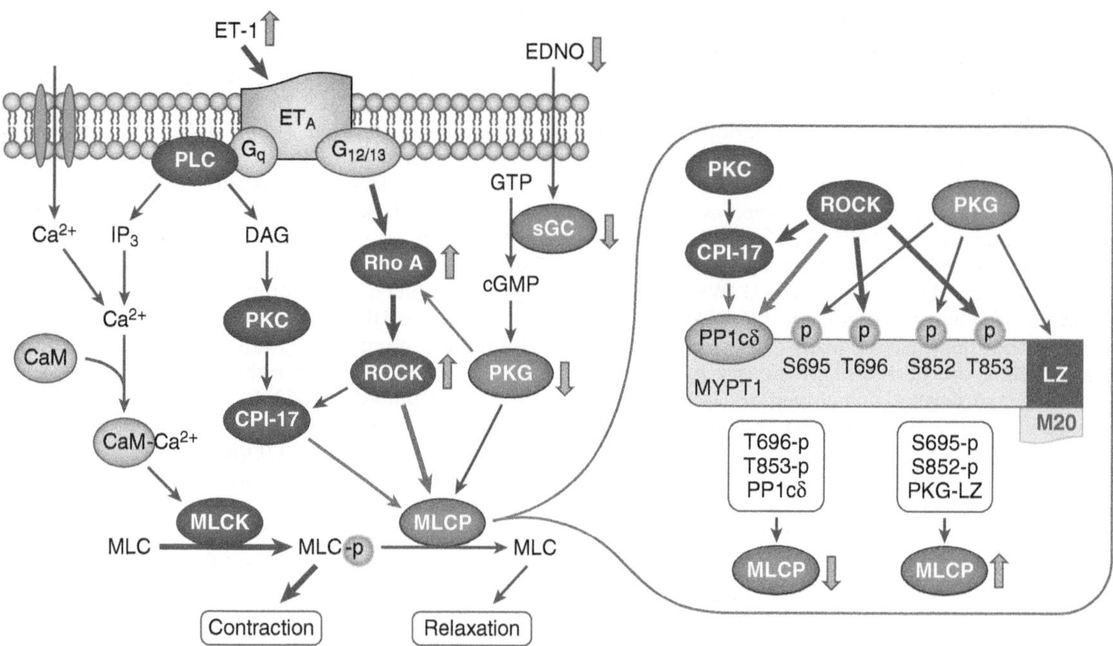

Fig. 72.3 Possible mechanism related to myosin light chain phosphatase *(MLCP)* for exaggerated vasoconstriction resulted from the augmented endothelin-1 *(ET-1)*-RhoA-rho kinase *(ROCK)* signaling and diminished endothelium-derived nitric oxide *(NO)*-cGMP-cGMP–dependent protein kinase *(PKG)* signaling in the pathogenesis of pulmonary arterial hypertension *(PAH)* in the neonate. In PAH, release of ET-1 from the endothelial cells is increased while that of NO is decreased. Moreover, the expression and activity of RhoA and ROCK are upregulated, whereas those of soluble guanylyl cyclase (*sGC*, which synthesizes cGMP from GTP when stimulated by NO) and PKG are downregulated. ET-1 stimulates RhoA-ROCK signaling through binding to ET$_A$ receptors and activating G$_{12/13}$ G-protein. ROCK and PKG may regulate vasocontractility through opposing actions on the regulatory subunit of MLCP *(MYPT1)*. ROCK causes phosphorylation of MYPT1 at threonine 696 *(T696)* and threonine (T853, human sequence), which leads to reduced MLCP activity, increased phosphorylation of myosin light chain (*MLC*→*MLC*-p), increased Ca^{2+} sensitivity of myofilaments, and thus augmented vasoconstriction. By contrast, after being activated by cGMP, PKG can phosphorylates MYPT1 at Serine 695 *(S695)* and Serine 852 *(S852)*, resulting in increased MLCP activity, increased dephosphorylation of myosin light chain (MLC-p→MLC), decreased Ca^{2+} sensitivity of myofilaments, and thus weakened vasoconstriction. ET-1 can also activate protein kinase C *(PKC)* via ET$_A$ receptors and G$_q$ G protein, followed by activated phospholipase C *(PLC)*, elevated diacyl glycerol *(DAG)* levels. PKC can enhance vasocontractility through inhibiting the δ isoform of catalytic unit of MLCP (PP1cδ) via PKC-potentiated phosphatase inhibitor protein-17 *(CPI-17)*. MLCP can also be inhibited by ROCK directly and via CPI-17, whereas MLCP is also stimulated by the binding of PKG to the leucine zipper *(LZ)* of MYPT1. MLCP consists of three subunits, MYPT1, PP1cδ, and a 20-kDa subunit of unknown function *(M20)*. The scheme in the box depicts the more detailed MLCP mechanism of ROCK and PKG. In addition, ET-1 can cause vasoconstriction through elevating the intracellular concentrations of Ca^{2+} via enhanced extracellular Ca^{2+} entry and inositol 1,4,5-trisphosphate *(IP$_3$)*-induced Ca^{2+} release from sarcoplasmic reticulum. Together with those entered from the membrane channels, these Ca^{2+} ions bind to calmodulin *(CaM)* and activate myosin light chain kinase *(MLCK)*, which promotes the phosphorylation of MLC *(MLC→MLCp)*, leading to an increased contractile response. *Red and green arrows* represent stimulatory and inhibitory action, respectively. Thick and *thin arrows* represent enhanced and suppressed activity, respectively. Upward- and downward-pointing *orange thick arrows* represent increased and decreased expression, respectively, of the enzyme.

PASMCs the interaction of LZ of MYPT1 with PKG is inhibited by hypoxia.[126] In mice, a selective mutation in the LZ domain of PKG-Iα leads to a progressive increase in right ventricular systolic pressure, indicating an increasing PVR.[146] In ovine fetal and newborn PASMCs hypoxia increases ubiquitination of PKG1, resulting in decreased binding of cGMP to PKG.[126]

In patients with PPHN, plasma levels of ET-1 are elevated and this may contribute to increased vasomotor tone.[151,179,180] Binding of ET$_A$ receptors sensitizes myofilaments to Ca^{2+} by inhibiting the activity of the catalytic subunit of MLCP , PP1cδ, via PKC- and PKC-potentiated phosphatase inhibitor protein-17 (CPI-17) and through RhoA/ROCK-dependent inhibition of MLCP.[60,180-182] Under pathologic conditions, ET$_B$ receptors can be inactivated by oxidative modification of cysteinyl thiols in the eNOS-activating region of ET$_B$ receptors, resulting in decreased NO production and thus the vasoconstrictive effect of ET-1 prevails.[183,184] In PAH binding to ET$_B$ receptors on VSMCs of intrapulmonary conduit and resistance arteries may induce vasoconstriction, so that dual blockade is necessary to maximize the inhibition of ET-1-induced pulmonary vasoconstriction.[185,186] In fetal lambs, chronic blockade of ET$_A$ receptors attenuates the development of PAH while chronic blockade of ET$_B$ receptors promotes PAH, suggesting a critical role for ET$_A$ receptors in the pathogenesis of PAH and a protective role for ET$_B$ receptors.[187,188]

Increased expression and activity of RhoA and ROCK have been documented in both adult and newborn PAH.[189-193] In pulmonary arteries from term ovine fetuses exposed in utero to chronic high-altitude hypoxia, the expression of type II ROCK and activity of type I and II ROCK I are increased. ET-1 induces phosphorylation of the regulatory subunit MYPT1 at threonine (Thr)-696 and Thr-853, which results in decreased activity of MLCP and consequently reduced dephosphorylation of the regulatory MLC and augmented vasoconstriction. The inhibitory action of ROCK on MLCP can be counteracted by PKG via phosphorylation of MYPT1 at serine (Ser)-695 and Ser-852.[48,89] In pulmonary arteries from fetal lambs exposed to chronic high-altitude hypoxia, phosphorylation of MYPT1 at Ser-695 and Ser-852 induced by 8-Br-cGMP, an activator of PKG, is attenuated, suggesting that increased ROCK activity following chronic hypoxia may suppress the vasodilatation mediated by PKG at MLCP level (Fig. 72.3).[33] In rat models of severe PAH that are refractory to NO treatment, ROCK inhibitors completely normalize PVR.[179] A number of studies demonstrate that ROCK activity is preferentially increased in PAH, indicating that inhibition of ROCK may be a promising therapy.[48,193]

ROLE OF MICRORNAS AND EPIGENETIC MODIFICATIONS

MicroRNAs (miRNAs) represent an evolutionarily conserved family of small noncoding RNAs consisting of 17 to 25 nucleotides,[194,195] which play important roles in lung development and pulmonary circulation via posttranscriptional regulation of gene expression. Altered expression and activity of miRNA are associated with aberrant development of pulmonary circulation and the pathogenesis of pediatric PAH.[196,197] A study of illumina HiSeq next-generation deep sequencing (NGS) shows that miRNA-210 (miR-210) of ovine pulmonary artery of term fetuses is greater than that of 5-day-old neonatal lambs.[197] miR-210 is augmented in hypoxic lungs and in PASMCs and other cell types exposed to hypoxic conditions. miR-210 increases resistance to apoptosis, resulting in hyperplasia of PASMCs.[7,194,198] In a murine model of hyperoxia-induced BPD, miR-34a levels in the lung are significantly increased. Deletion or inhibition of miR-34a improves the pulmonary phenotype and BPD-associated PAH, which, conversely, is worsened by miR-34a overexpression. miR34a may impair alveolarization through angiopoietin-1 and Akt (protein kinase B) pathway and through cyclin D1 and cyclin-dependent kinase 4 (CDK4). miR34a may also cause dysregulated vascularization via delta-like protein 1(DLL1)-Notch 1/2 pathway. In addition, miR34a enhances transcription of pro-inflammatory mediators by inhibiting the class III histone deacetylator sirtuin 1 (SIRT1).[199]

Endothelial-to-mesenchymal transition (EndMT) is an important contributor to vascular remodeling in the pathogenesis of PAH.[200,201] In pulmonary microvascular ECs from a rat model of PH induced by chronic hypoxia, the expression of platelet/EC adhesion molecule-1 (Pecam1) is decreased whereas that of α-smooth muscle actin (α-SMA) is increased, suggestive of EndMT. These changes are accompanied by an elevated expression of miR-126a-5p. Interestingly, the EndMT of pulmonary microvascular ECs is prevented by miR-126a-5p knockdown, implying a casual role for this miRNA. Further study suggests that miR-126a-5p may act through the p85-β/p-AKT pathway.[202]

Epigenetic regulation of gene expression through mechanisms other than miRs are also involved in the pathogenesis of PAH, including pediatric PAH.[203-206] In PASMCs of ovine fetal lungs, inhibition of G9a, a key enzyme for histone H3 dimethylation at position lysine-9, reduces cell proliferation, induces cell cycle arrest in G1 phase, inhibits contractility of fetal PASMCs, and decreases the expression of calponin and ROCK-II proteins, demonstrating that histone lysine methylation is involved in the cell proliferation and contractility of fetal PASMCs.[207] In newborn ovine PASMCs, the inhibition of class I histone deacetylase (HDAC-I), which removes acetyl groups from an ε-N-acetyl lysine amino acid on a histone, suppresses cell proliferation, and induces cell-cycle arrest in G1 phase. Contractility and global DNA methylation levels in newborn PASMCs are also markedly modulated, suggesting that HDAC-I is involved in phenotypic alteration of newborn pulmonary arterial SMCs.[208] Pulmonary arterial SMCs from fetal lambs exposed to high altitude chronic hypoxia in utero show reduced levels of global histone 4 acetylation and DNA methylation accompanied by diminished CDK inhibitor p21, a key regulator in hypoxia-induced cell progression. The inhibition of histone deacetylase (HDAC) reduces PASMC proliferation, in part due to altered expression of p21. HDAC inhibition also decreases PDGF-induced cell migration and ERK1/2 activation and increases global DNA methylation suggesting that reduced histone acetylation and DNA methylation caused by chronic hypoxia promotes fetal PASMC proliferation (Fig. 72.4).[209] In the PAECs of fetal lambs with PPHN induced by

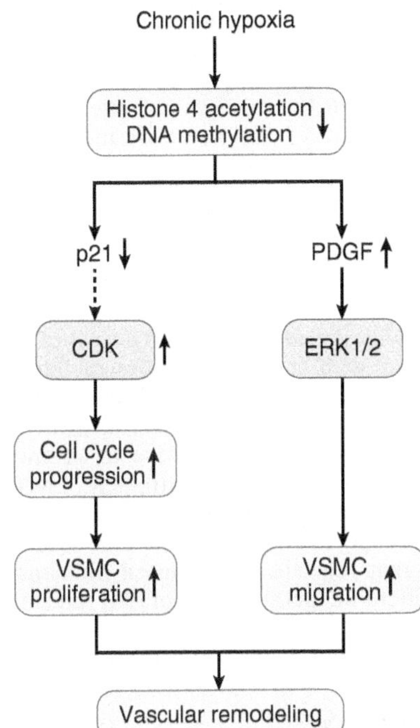

Fig. 72.4 Possible mechanism for epigenetic regulation of vascular remodeling of fetal pulmonary arteries in chronic hypoxia through the downregulation of histone 4 acetylation and DNA methylation. These epigenetic modifications lead to the downregulation of p21, an endogenous inhibitor of cyclin-dependent kinase *(CDK)*, increased CDK activity, increased cell cycle progression, and augmented vascular smooth muscle cell *(VSMC)* proliferation. The altered epigenetic activity also leads to enhanced VSMC migration by increasing activation of platelet-derived growth factor *(PDGF)*–extracellular signal–regulated kinases 1 and 2 *(ERK1/2)* signaling pathways.

ductus arteriosus constriction, the reduced expression and activity of eNOS are closely related to increased DNA CpG methylation in eNOS proximal promoter, altered modifications of histone H4K12ac in eNOS promoter, and histone H3K9me3 around Sp1 binding sites in PAECs.[210] Altered DNA methylation is also linked to predisposition to PAH in the newborn offspring of mice given a restrictive diet during pregnancy (RDP), as manifested by impaired endothelium-dependent pulmonary artery vasodilatation, an exaggerated increase in PAP, and right ventricular hypertrophy, in part due to increased oxygen stress. Administration of histone deacetylase inhibitors to the offspring normalizes pulmonary DNA methylation and vascular function.[211,212]

CONCLUSION

The fetal pulmonary circulation is characterized by a high PVR and low blood flow, which is largely ascribed to the morphologically thick vessel wall and high vascular tone. The fetal pulmonary vasculature possesses high myogenic tone, accompanied by low activity of intrinsic vasodilators mainly due to the low oxygen environment in the lung. With the onset of breathing at birth, PVR is dramatically and rapidly reduced, while PBF is markedly increased to accommodate the whole cardiac output. These hemodynamic changes predominantly result from increased vasodilator activity and decreased vasoconstrictor activity, in particular because of the increased production and action of NO in response to birth-related stimuli—particularly oxygenation and increased shear stress. Afterward, the up-regulation of eNOS and its downstream signaling enzymes, including sGC and PKG, contribute importantly to the maintenance of low PVR.[9,23,10,11]

Immediately after birth and during the neonatal period, the pulmonary vessel walls undergo structural reorganization resulting in thinner vessel wall and rapid growth of the pulmonary tree, with growth of the microvasculature in parallel with the growth of the airways and alveolarization. These processes occur at a high rate in early postnatal life but can extend beyond adolescence to match the increase in cardiac output and somatic growth.[7,8] Under pathologic conditions, there is persistence of elevated vasomotor tone as well abnormal and increased vasoreactivity and vascular remodeling, all of which result in increased PVR.

Compared with the adult, the pathogenesis of PAH of children is more related with the abnormalities of lung development. For instance, perinatal stresses—including chorioamnionitis, placental vascular lesions, and intrauterine growth restriction—are associated with PPHN. Also, owing to advances in medical interventions, the survival of extremely low-gestational-age newborns has markedly increased. This, however, leads to an increased incidence of BPD and PAH with BPD.[139,213,214] Mechanisms that regulate the perinatal pulmonary circulation and contribute to the pathogenesis of PAH remain under study.

 A complete reference list is available at www.ExpertConsult.com.

SELECT REFERENCES

1. Hall SM, Hislop AA, Pierce CM, Haworth SG. Prenatal origins of human intrapulmonary arteries. Formation and smooth muscle maturation. *Am J Respir Cell Mol Biol*. 2000;23:194-203.
2. Hall SM, Hislop AA, Pierce CM, Haworth SG. Origin, differentiation, and maturation of human pulmonary veins. *Am J Respir Cell Mol Biol*. 2002;26:333-340.
3. Rasanen J, Wood DC, Weiner S, et al. Role of the pulmonary circulation in the distribution of human fetal cardiac output during the second half of pregnancy. *Circulation*. 1996;94:1068-1073.
4. Rasanen J, Wood DC, Debbs RH, et al. Reactivity of the human fetal pulmonary circulation to maternal hyperoxygenation increases during the second half of pregnancy. A randomized study. *Circulation*. 1998;97:257-262.
5. Abman SH, Chatfield BA, Hall SL, McMurtry IF. Role of endothelium-derived relaxing factor during transition of pulmonary circulation at birth. *Am J Physiol Heart Circ Physiol*. 1990;259:H1921-H1927.
6. Morin 3rd FC, Egan EA. Pulmonary hemodynamics in fetal lambs during development at normal and increased oxygen tension. *J Appl Physiol*. 1992;73:213-218.
10. Gao Y, Raj JU. Regulation of the pulmonary circulation in the fetus and newborn. *Physiol Rev*. 2010;90:1291-1335.
12. Gao Y, Chen T, Raj JU. Endothelial and smooth muscle cell interactions in the pathobiology of pulmonary hypertension. *Am J Respir Cell Mol Biol*. 2016;54:451-460.
31. Parker TA, Roe G, Grover TR, Abman SH. Rho kinase activation maintains high pulmonary vascular resistance in the ovine fetal lung. *Am J Physiol Lung Cell Mol Physiol*. 2006;291:L976-L982.
33. Gao Y, Portugal AD, Negash S, et al. Role of Rho kinases in PKG-mediated relaxation of pulmonary arteries of fetal lambs exposed to chronic high altitude hypoxia. *Am J Physiol Lung Cell Mol Physiol*. 2007;292:L678-L684.
36. Herrera EA, Ebensperger G, Hernández I, et al. The role of nitric oxide signaling in pulmonary circulation of high- and low-altitude newborn sheep under basal and acute hypoxic conditions. *Nitric Oxide*. 2019;89:71-80.
52. Abman SH, Accurso FJ. Sustained fetal pulmonary vasodilation with prolonged atrial natriuretic factor and GMP infusions. *Am J Physiol Heart Circ Physiol*. 1991;260:H183-H192.
55. Negash S, Gao Y, Zhou W, et al. Regulation of cGMP-dependent protein kinase-mediated vasodilation by hypoxia-induced reactive species in ovine fetal pulmonary veins. *Am J Physiol Lung Cell Mol Physiol*. 2007;293:L1012-L1020.
63. Ivy DD, Kinsella JP, Abman SH. Physiologic characterization of endothelin A and B receptor activity in the ovine fetal pulmonary circulation. *J Clin Invest*. 1994;93:2141-2148.
73. Vali P, Lakshminrusimha S. The fetus can teach us. Oxygen and the pulmonary vasculature. *Children (Basel)*. 2017;4:pii. E67.
81. Wedgwood S, Bekker JM, Black SM. Shear stress regulation of endothelial NOS in fetal pulmonary arterial endothelial cells involves PKC. *Am J Physiol Lung Cell Mol Physiol*. 2001;281:L490-L498.
87. Gao Y, Dhanakoti S, Tolsa J-F, Raj JU. Role of protein kinase G in nitric oxide and cGMP-induced relaxation of newborn ovine pulmonary veins. *J Appl Physiol*. 1999;87:993-998.
96. Ivy DD, Lee DS, Rairigh RL, et al. Endothelin B receptor blockade attenuates pulmonary vasodilation in oxygen ventilated fetal lambs. *Biol Neonate*. 2004;86:155-159.
97. Kelly LK, Wedgwood S, Steinhorn RH, Black SM. Nitric oxide decreases endothelin-1 secretion through the activation of soluble guanylate cyclase. *Am J Physiol Lung Cell Mol Physiol*. 2004;286:L984-L991.
110. Hislop AA. Airway and blood vessel interaction during lung development. *J Anat*. 2002;201:325-334.
120. Wedgwood S, Black SM. Molecular mechanisms of nitric oxide-induced growth arrest and apoptosis in fetal pulmonary arterial smooth muscle cells. *Nitric Oxide*. 2003;9:201-210.
124. Ramchandran R, Pilipenko E, Bach L, et al. Hypoxic regulation of pulmonary vascular smooth muscle cyclic guanosine monophosphate-dependent kinase by the ubiquitin conjugating system. *Am J Respir Cell Mol Biol*. 2012;46:323-330.
134. Rosenzweig EB, Abman SH, Adatia I, et al. Paediatric pulmonary arterial hypertension: updates on definition, classification, diagnostics and management. *Eur Respir J*. 2019;53(1):1801916.
139. Abman SH, Baker C, Gien J, et al. The Robyn Barst Memorial Lecture. Differences between the fetal, newborn, and adult pulmonary circulations. Relevance for age-specific therapies (2013 Grover Conference series). *Pulm Circ*. 2014;4:424-440.
140. Stenmark KR, Frid MG, Graham BB, Tuder RM. Dynamic and diverse changes in the functional properties of vascular smooth muscle cells in pulmonary hypertension. *Cardiovasc Res*. 2018;114:551-564.
145. Beghetti M, Gorenflo M, Ivy DD, et al. Treatment of pediatric pulmonary arterial hypertension. A focus on the NO-sGC-cGMP pathway. *Pediatr Pulmonol*. 2019;54:1516-1526.
146. Ramchandran R, Raghavan A, Geenen D, et al. PKG-1α leucine zipper domain defect increases pulmonary vascular tone. Implications in hypoxic pulmonary hypertension. *Am J Physiol Lung Cell Mol Physiol*. 2014;307:L537-L544.
150. Zhou W, Negash S, Liu J, Raj JU. Modulation of pulmonary vascular smooth muscle cell phenotype in hypoxia. Role of cGMP-dependent protein kinase and myocardin. *Am J Physiol Lung Cell Mol Physiol*. 2009;296:L780-L789.
164. Xu EZ, Kantores C, Ivanovska J, et al. Rescue treatment with a Rho-kinase inhibitor normalizes right ventricular function and reverses remodeling in juvenile rats with chronic pulmonary hypertension. *Am J Physiol Heart Circ Physiol*. 2010;299:H1854-L1864.
170. Fuloria M, Aschner JL. Persistent pulmonary hypertension of the newborn. *Semin Fetal Neonatal Med*. 2017;22:220-226.
181. Chester AH, Yacoub MH. The role of endothelin-1 in pulmonary arterial hypertension. *Glob Cardiol Sci Pract*. 2014;2014:62-78.
188. Ivy DD, Parker TA, Abman SH. Prolonged endothelin B receptor blockade causes pulmonary hypertension in the ovine fetus. *Am J Physiol Lung Cell Mol Physiol*. 2000;279:L758-L765.
194. Zhou G, Chen T, Raj JU. MicroRNAs in pulmonary arterial hypertension. *Am J Respir Cell Mol Biol*. 2015;52:139-151.
203. Saco TV, Parthasarathy PT, Cho Y, et al. Role of epigenetics in pulmonary hypertension. *Am J Physiol Cell Physiol*. 2014;306:C1101-C1105.
209. Yang Q, Lu Z, Ramchandran R, et al. Pulmonary artery smooth muscle cell proliferation and migration in fetal lambs acclimatized to high-altitude long-term hypoxia. Role of histone acetylation. *Am J Physiol Lung Cell Mol Physiol*. 2012;303:L1001-L1010.
210. Ke X, Johnson H, Jing X, et al. Persistent pulmonary hypertension alters the epigenetic characteristics of endothelial nitric oxide synthase gene in pulmonary artery endothelial cells in a fetal lamb model. *Physiol Genomics*. 2018;50(10):828-836.

Historical Perspective

73

John A. Clements

As a first-time contributor to *Fetal and Neonatal Physiology,* I have wondered what motivation prompted the editors of this scholarly and compendious tome to invite me to prepare a historical and personal perspective for the section on pulmonary surfactant. Did they hope to lighten the intellectual load imposed on its readers? Were they fostering gender neutrality? (Mary Ellen Avery wrote the previous account.) Maybe they wished to avoid age discrimination by including an author in his tenth decade of life! Whatever the editors' reasons, my principal credential for this task is an interest in the subject that goes back more than six decades and has required continuing education in the mysteries and delights of surface phenomena. I hope that this brief essay will convey a little of the pleasure and excitement of contemplating, investigating, and applying the concepts, materials, and techniques of physics and chemistry to pulmonary biology and therapeutics.

The ideas and observations necessary to understand pulmonary surfactant were developing long before it was recognized as an important component of lung structure. These included the existence of surface tension or surface free energy of liquids and the properties of insoluble films at water surfaces. Other aspects, such as surfactant functions, morphology, chemical composition, metabolism, regulation, development in the fetus, and therapeutic use, have been elucidated much more recently and make up a large part of the relevant current literature. Many of these aspects are addressed in other chapters of this section.

The idea of surface tension and its connection with the rise of liquids in capillary tubes predated correct explanations by many years (summarized by Hardy[1]). For instance, the members of the Accademia del Cimento in Florence were interested in such phenomena. Their 1667 report was largely devoted to experiments in vacuo and included a demonstration that fluid rose in a capillary held in a vacuum. Boyle (of the gas laws) also showed the rise of liquids in capillary tubes (1682) but did not succeed with the vacuum experiment. In 1709 Hauksbee, Demonstrator of the Royal Society, London, showed that the height of liquid rise was the same in two tubes of the same internal diameter, but one had a wall 10 times as thick as the other. He reasoned, brilliantly, from this result that the attraction of the solid for the liquid is limited to the surface of the solid and is in a direction perpendicular to the sides of the cylindrical glass. This statement was remarkable because students of capillary attraction intuitively felt that a force parallel to the glass causes the liquid to rise (or fall). Jurin, Secretary of the Royal Society, showed in a lovely experiment (1718) that if water was drawn up into an inverted funnel whose stem had been pulled out to a capillary, the funnel remained full, even in a vacuum. He concluded that cohesion in the water suspended the lower part in the funnel from that in the capillary. He also surmised that the water particles were more strongly attracted by glass than by each other, and vice versa for mercury, explaining why water is raised and mercury is depressed in a glass tube.

Meanwhile, scientists in France were studying such phenomena, but they tended to describe them mathematically, though incorrectly, because they failed to take into account the double curvature of many of the liquid surfaces. It fell to Young (1805) and Laplace (1806) to correct this mistake and derive the equations necessary to relate the tension and the complex curvature to the pressure difference across various liquid surfaces. (We still use these formulas to calculate the mechanical effects of surface tension on the lungs.) Many leading scientists throughout the nineteenth century (Poisson, Dupré, van der Waals, Boltzmann, Maxwell, Kelvin, Raleigh, Gibbs) and in the twentieth century (Bakker, Guggenheim, Onsager, Kirkwood and Buff, Born, Ono and Kondo, and Defay and Prigogine) studied capillarity and greatly refined theories of intermolecular forces in relation to the origin of surface tension. Application of thermodynamic analysis led to the result that mechanical surface free energy is equal to surface tension times surface area—a relationship that became useful much later in the measurement of alveolar surface area.

The liquids at the surfaces of the pulmonary airspaces, however, are not simple like those considered in the classical systems, and one has to take into account other components that modify the surface tension. Many materials dissolved or suspended in water spontaneously accumulate in the interface, and these are commonly called *surfactants*. If such materials are freely soluble in water, their partition between interface and aqueous phase at equilibrium is described by the Gibbs-Duhem equation, and it turns out that changes in surface area do not change the surface tension significantly. If these substances have minute solubility in water so that they are in effect locked into the interface after adsorption, changes in the area of the surface cause large changes in surface tension. Lung surfactant acts in this way, and such behavior is critical to its ability to reduce surface tension and stabilize alveolar structure at low transpulmonary pressures and volumes.[2]

Just as the understanding of surface tension and its origin in intermolecular attractive forces evolved over several centuries, so too the investigation and theory of "insoluble" surface films required many years. For example, pouring oil on troubled waters to calm the waves was apparently known in ancient times. The earliest record of such surface films that I know of was from Pliny the Elder. He was a *self-taught* man of insatiable curiosity, who read voraciously and corresponded with prominent Roman scholars. He made notes on zoology, botany, agriculture, geology, mining, navigation, astronomy, and land warfare that are said to have occupied 160 volumes, which he boiled down to 37 books by the year 77 CE. Interestingly, Pliny included oil films on water in his writings.[3]

About 16 centuries later, another *self-taught* man, Benjamin Franklin, then living in London, became curious about films on water. He performed the famous experiment of pouring oil onto the surface of the pond at Clapham Common, in a town southwest of London. The day was windy and the water was rough. In a paper he read to the Royal Society in 1774, he wrote "the oil, though not more than a teaspoonful ... spread amazingly and extended itself gradually till it reached the lee side, making all that quarter of the pond, perhaps half an acre, as smooth as a looking glass."[3] His data would have allowed him to calculate the thickness of the film, approximately one 10-millionth of an inch, or about the length of an oil molecule, but he did not report doing that.

Moving along a century later, we find another *self-taught* person, Agnes Pockels, who kept house for her invalid parents in Braunschweig, Germany. Her natural curiosity was boundless. Denied entrance to university because she was a woman, she read the literature of physics and chemistry avidly and thoughtfully. The greasy films on cooking dishes annoyed others, but she found them captivating. She set up clean dishes filled to the brim with clean water, laid metal strips across the surface, applied known amounts of oils to the water between the strips, and measured the surface tension as she moved the barriers to decrease the area available to the oil film. This was a new method, and it gave her important results. She tried to publish them but had no success. Frustrated, she sent a letter describing her findings to Lord Raleigh in England, whose papers on surface phenomena she had read. Her letter was written in German, which Raleigh didn't understand. Fortunately, his wife was fluent in German and translated the letter for him. He saw the importance of Pockels's results and sent the letter to *Nature* with a request that it be published. It was, in 1891.[4] Pockels's apparatus was the precursor of a device we now call the *surface balance*, an instrument often used in physical chemistry laboratories. With various improvements, it has made possible the characterization of hundreds of insoluble interfacial films since Pockels invented it (Fig. 73.1).

The first time I saw a surface balance was in 1950 in the laboratory of Hans Trurnit. Hans worked in the Medical Laboratories of the Army Chemical Center in Maryland, where I was doing my national service in the Army Medical Corps. He was an expert on surface films of proteins. Quite by accident, we became friends. Hans burned with a gem-like flame, and nothing seemed to please him more than telling me about his work. Although my main assignment was to improve the treatment of nerve gas casualties, I enjoyed learning about surface effects and adding to what Hans told me by studying relevant textbooks. My formal education had not included any mention of surface properties, and so, without knowing it at the time, I became another in a long line of *self-taught* students of surface films.

The Medical Laboratories had a research contract with the Harvard School of Public Health to study lung edema caused by the war gas phosgene. The work was directed by Jere Mead, a brilliant pulmonary physiologist, and the results led him to wonder what effects the surface tension of the edema fluid and its foam bubbles had on the mechanical properties of the lungs. As a US Army officer, I was assigned an additional duty in 1951 to evaluate progress under the contract, and that meant visiting Jere's laboratory and discussing his ideas and results. Again, without my invitation, surface phenomena invaded my life. This time I was better prepared to understand and analyze them.

In 1952, Ted Radford, a member of Jere's group, began another project that involved surface effects. Ted wanted to estimate the area of the alveolar surface by a physicochemical method to check histologic estimates. His idea was to calculate the surface free energy of the alveoli from air and saline pressure-volume measurements and divide it by an assumed surface tension to compute alveolar area (Fig. 73.2). This method gave an area only one-tenth of morphometric estimates, and Ted concluded that the morphologists were wrong.[5] When I asked him to explain the discrepancy, he told me I would not understand it. That annoyed me, and I decided to analyze his results in detail. I made a calculation of the diffusion capacity of the lungs using his area value, and it came out far lower than measured diffusion values. His pressure-volume data seemed solid, but his assumption of a particular surface tension bothered me. So I turned the calculation backward and used the pressure-volume data and morphologic information to compute surface tension. A trial calculation assuming a surface tension of 50 dynes/cm at maximum lung volume and a relative alveolar radius proportional to the cube root of volume gave this astonishing result: on deflation of the lung, computed surface tension fell from 50 dynes/cm to very

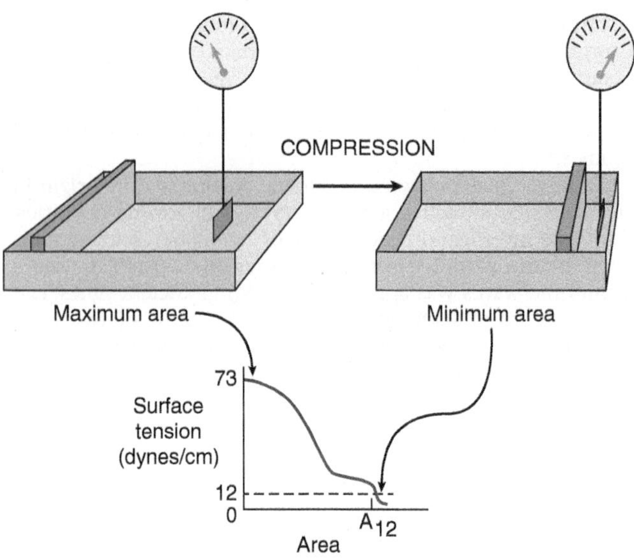

Fig. 73.1 Schematic diagram of a surface balance consisting of a trough containing water, a barrier to change the area available to a surface film at the air-water interface, a Wilhelmy plate dipping into the water surface, and a strain gauge to register the pull of surface tension on the plate. When an insoluble film occupies the water surface, reducing the area causes the surface tension to decrease as shown in the surface tension-area diagram.

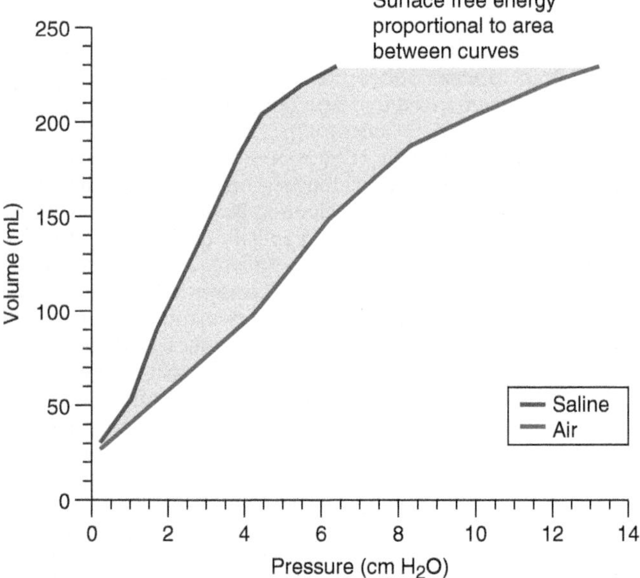

Fig. 73.2 Relationships of transpulmonary pressure and volume when cat lungs are filled with air or with normal saline. The area between the air and saline curves during emptying is proportional to the mechanical surface free energy of the alveoli. (Data from Radford EP. Method for estimating respiratory surface area of mammalian lungs from their physical characteristics. *Proc Soc Exp Biol Med.* 1954;87:58–61.)

low values, implying the presence of a unique surfactant in the alveoli.

Then, in 1955, Pattle reported that bubbles in pulmonary edema foam or squeezed from the cut surface of normal lungs contained "an insoluble protein layer which can abolish the tension of the alveolar surface."[6] I thought this conclusion was dubious because the pressure-volume data of Radford[5] and von Neergaard[7] suggested higher surface tension values for the airspaces.

Clearly, the next step was to demonstrate the surface tension-area behavior of the hypothetical surfactant directly. That meant extracting it from the lungs and observing it in a surface balance. I knew how to do that, from discussions with Trurnit, from papers I had read, and from my previous biochemical research. After some technical problems were solved, it turned out (Fig. 73.3) that the surface tension versus area relationships measured in the surface balance and calculated from pressure-volume and morphologic information agreed unbelievably well…EUREKA!

I presented my results at a 1956 meeting of the American Physiological Society, showing that lung extracts could lower surface tension to less than 10 dynes/cm when surface area was decreased, and theorized that this effect could stabilize alveoli against collapse.[2] The talk drew little attention and less interest. Despite that cold reception, I was sure that the ideas and data were important and wrote a short paper for *Science,* which was rejected. After a few months of misery, I asked a friend to introduce it to the *Proceedings of the Society for Experimental Biology and Medicine*, an unreviewed journal, where it appeared in May 1957.[8] (Years later, the Institute for Scientific Information announced that it had become a citation classic.)

In December 1957, Mary Ellen Avery visited my laboratory. She had gone to Harvard for a fellowship in pediatrics with Clement Smith and in lung physiology with Jere Mead, because of her strong interest in respiratory diseases in infants, especially hyaline membrane disease. I showed her my methods and told her all I knew about lung surfactant and lung physiology. Back in Boston, she and Jere Mead set up the methods, applied them to infant lungs, and showed that surfactant could not be found in infants with respiratory distress syndrome (RDS) who had died. Figure 73.4 shows data from the famous graph in their January 1959 paper,[9] demonstrating that fact, which launched a flood of research on lung surfactant and RDS. The relevant literature now contains more than 15,000 publications, of which more than 500 were added in the last year. Such a mountain of research cannot be properly summarized in this brief historical perspective. It does seem worthwhile, though, to mention a few milestones in the development of surfactant treatment for RDS.

It had been obvious from the start that if lack or dysfunction of lung surfactant caused pulmonary failure, this might be ameliorated by replacement therapy. Attempts in the 1960s failed[10,11] for various reasons: the necessary composition and physical properties of substitutes were not fully known; doses and delivery methods were inadequate; and nursery personnel lacked knowledge and methods of assessing the physiologic status of newborns, especially premature infants. Most of these problems were addressed in the ensuing decades, and surfactant treatment finally became feasible for RDS.

In 1972, Enhorning and Robertson[12] showed that instilling surfactant extracted from adult rabbits into the trachea of prematurely delivered rabbit fetuses enabled suitable expansion of the lung. Then, in 1980, Fujiwara and colleagues[13] reported that in a series of 10 infants with RDS, tracheal instillation of cow lung surfactant enriched in its main component (dipalmitoyl phosphatidylcholine) expanded the lungs and

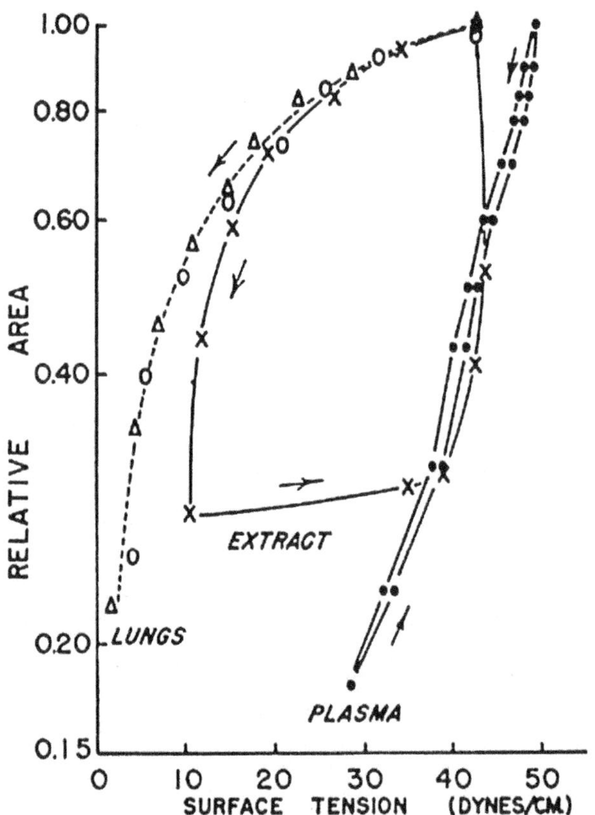

Fig. 73.3 Comparison of surface tension-area relationship of lung extract measured in a surface balance with that of alveolar surfaces computed from pressure-volume data. When area is decreased, both surfaces show surface tension falling to very low values. Blood plasma in the surface balance shows relatively high surface tensions and little hysteresis, unlike the lung extract. (With permission from Clements JA. Surface tension of lung extracts. *Proc Soc Exp Biol Med.* 1957;95:170–172.)

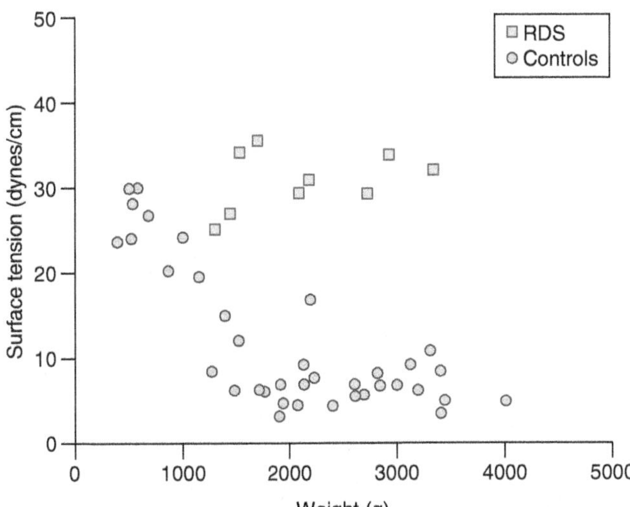

Fig. 73.4 Avery and Mead measured the surface tension-area relationships of lung extracts from newborn infants who died with or without respiratory distress syndrome *(RDS)*. They were not able to demonstrate surfactant in those with RDS and those with normal lungs who weighed about <1200 g. (Data from Avery ME, Mead J. Surface properties in relation to atelectasis and hyaline membrane disease. *Am J Dis Child.* 1959;97:517–523.)

improved oxygenation. This paper stimulated many randomized controlled trials over the next 10 years of a variety of surfactant preparations derived from animal lungs. The results have shown benefit for the most part and have led to the widespread use of surfactant substitution in infants with RDS, as well as to the evaluation of synthetic preparations containing surfactant protein B or peptides of similar structure.

The current state of the art is well summarized in the report and recommendations of the American Academy of Pediatrics 2012–2013 Committee on the Fetus and Newborn: *Surfactant Replacement Therapy for Preterm and Term Neonates with Respiratory Distress*.[14] In essence, the Committee endorses surfactant therapy for preterm infants with severe RDS after they are stabilized but also suggests that, in appropriate cases, one should consider immediate continuous positive airway pressure with subsequent surfactant administration if needed, rather than routine tracheal intubation and early surfactant dosing. Although the Committee's recommendations illustrate that surfactant therapy now has an established place in the management of the newborn with RDS, they also imply that there is room for further improvement. The incidence of chronic lung disease (bronchopulmonary dysplasia) remains distressingly high among RDS survivors, and the causes of premature birth need continuing study.[15]

Clearly, we still have much to learn, and if past history is a reliable guide, we can expect the application of fundamental concepts and methods of physics and chemistry to lead the way toward better understanding and care of the fetus and neonate.

REFERENCES

1. Hardy WB. Historical notes upon surface energy and forces of short range. *Nature*. 1922;109:375-378.
2. Clements JA. Dependence of pressure-volume characteristics of lungs on intrinsic surface-active material. *Am J Physiol*. 1956;187:592.
3. Gaines GL. Historical introduction. In: *Insoluble Monolayers at Liquid-Gas Interfaces*. New York: Interscience Publishers; 1966.
4. Pockels A. Surface tension. *Nature*. 1891;43:437-439.
5. Radford EP. Method for estimating respiratory surface area of mammalian lungs from their physical characteristics. *Proc Soc Exp Biol Med*. 1954;87:58-61.
6. Pattle RE. Properties, function and origin of the alveolar lining layer. *Nature*. 1955;175:1125-1126.
7. Neergaard KV. Neue auffassungenübereinengrundbegriff der atemmechanik. Die retraktionkraft der lunge, abhängig von der oberflächenspannung in den alveolen. *Z Gesamte Med*. 1929;66:1-22.
8. Clements JA. Surface tension of lung extracts. *Proc Soc Exp Biol Med*. 1957;95:170-172.
9. Avery ME, Mead J. Surface properties in relation to atelectasis and hyaline membrane disease. *Am J Dis Child*. 1959;97:517-523.
10. Robillard E, Alarie Y, DagenaisPerusse P, et al. Microaerosol administration of synthetic beta-gamma-dipalmitoyl-L-alpha-lecithin in the respiratory distress syndrome. A preliminary report. *Can Med Assoc J*. 1964;90:55-57.
11. Chu J, Clements JA, Cotton EK, et al. Neonatal pulmonary ischemia. Part I: clinical and physiological studies. *Pediatrics*. 1967;40:709-782.
12. Enhorning G, Robertson B. Lung expansion in the premature rabbit fetus after tracheal deposition of surfactant. *Pediatrics*. 1972;50:58-66.
13. Fujiwara T, Maeta H, Chida S, et al. Artificial surfactant therapy in hyaline membrane disease. *Lancet*. 1980;1:55-59.
14. Polin RA, Carlo WA, Committee on Fetus and Newborn. Surfactant replacement therapy for preterm and term neonates with respiratory distress. *Pediatrics*. 2014;133:156-163.
15. Behrman RE, Adashi EY, Allen MC. *Committee on Understanding Premature Birth and Assuring Healthy Outcomes: Preterm Birth: Causes, Consequences, and Prevention, Report Brief July 2006*. Washington, DC: Institute of Medicine, National Academies of Science USA, National Academies Press; 2006.

74 Developmental Biology of Lung Stem Cells

Ivana Mižíková | Chanèle Cyr-Depauw | Bernard Thébaud

INTRODUCTION

Abbreviations

Abbreviation	Meaning	Abbreviation	Meaning
αSMA	α-Smooth muscle actin	CCR2b	C-C motif chemokine receptor 2
ABCA3	ATP binding cassette subfamily A member 3	CD11b (ITGAM)	Integrin subunit α M
AcLDL	Acetylated low-density lipoprotein	CD13 (ANPEP)	Alanyl aminopeptidase membrane
ACTA2	Actin α 2, smooth muscle	CD14	Cluster of differentiation 14
AECI	Alveolar epithelial type 1 cell	CD19	Cluster of differentiation 19
AECII	Alveolar epithelial type 2 cell	CD24	Cluster of differentiation 24
AQP5	Aquaporin 5	CD31 (PECAM1)	Platelet and endothelial cell adhesion molecule 1
Axin2	Axis inhibition protein 2		
BADJ	Bronchoalveolar duct junction	CD34	Cluster of differentiation 34
BAL	Bronchoalveolar lavage	CD41 (ITGA2B)	Integrin subunit α 2b
BASC	Bronchial alveolar stem cell	CD45 (PTPRC)	Protein tyrosine phosphatase, receptor type, C
BM	Bone marrow	CD49 (ITGA4)	Integrin subunit α 4
BPD	Bronchopulmonary dysplasia	CD73 (NT5E)	5'-nucleotidase ecto
BST1 (CD157)	Bone marrow stromal cell antigen 1	CD79	Cluster of differentiation 79

Abbreviations—cont'd

Abbreviation	Meaning
CD90 (THY-1)	Thy-1 cell surface antigen
CD104 (ITGB4)	Integrin subunit β4
CD105	Endoglin
CD106 (VCAM)	Vascular cell adhesion molecule-1
CD117 (c-KIT)	KIT proto-oncogene receptor tyrosine kinase
CD133 (PROM1)	Prominin1
CD144 (CDH5)	Cadherin5, VE-cadherin
CD146 (MCAM)	Melanoma cell adhesion molecule
CD166	Cluster of differentiation 166
CD309 (KDR)	Kinase insert domain receptor
c-KIT (CD117)	KIT proto-oncogene receptor tyrosine kinase
COL1A1	Collagen 1a1
COL1A2	Collagen 1a2
DASC	Distal alveolar stem cell
Dermo1 (Twist2)	Twist basic helix-loop-helix transcription factor 2
DES	Desmin
ECFC	Endothelial colony-forming cells
EGFR	Epidermal growth factor receptor
ELN	Elastin
eNOS	Endothelial nitric oxide synthase
EpCAM	Epithelial cell adhesion molecule
EPCs	Endothelial progenitor cell
FGF10	Fibroblast growth factor 10
FN1	Fibronectin 1
FOXF1	Forkhead box F1
FOXI1	Forkhead box J1
FOXJ1	Forkhead box J1
HGF	Hepatocyte growth factor
HLA-A	Major histocompatibility complex, class I, A
HLA-DR	Major histocompatibility complex, class II, DR β 1
HOPX	HOP homeobox
IGFBP-2	Insulin-like growth factor-binding protein 2
KRAS	KRAS proto-oncogene
KRT14	Keratin 14
KRT5	Keratin 5
KRT8	Keratin 8
LNEP	Lineage-negative epithelial stem/progenitor cells
LR-MSC	Lung resident-MSC
Lyve1	Lymphatic vessel endothelial hyaluronan receptor 1
MAC	Myeloid angiogenic cell
MMT	Mesenchymal-myofibroblast transition
MS	Mesenchymal stromal cell
MYB	Myeloblastosis
MYH11	Myosin heavy chain 11
NFκB	Nuclear factor kappa B subunit 1
NKX2-1 (Tift1)	NK2 homeobox 1
OCT4 (POU5F1)	POU class 5 homeobox 1
PAEC	Pulmonary artery endothelial cells
PDGFRα	Platelet-derived growth factor receptor α
PDPN	Podoplanin
PMVEC	Pulmonary microvascular endothelial cells
PROCR	Protein C receptor
pro-SPC	Pro-surfactant protein C
Prox1	Prospero homeobox 1
RFX	Regulatory factor X
RMEPC	Resident microvascular endothelial progenitor cells
Sca1 (Ly6a)	Lymphocyte antigen 6 complex
SCGB1A1	Secretoglobin family 1A member 1
SP-A	Surfactant protein A1
SFTPC	Surfactant protein C
SP-D	Surfactant protein D
SM22 (TAGLN)	Transgelin
SOX2	SRY-box transcription factor 2
SP	Side population
TAGLN (SM22)	Transgelin
TBX2	T-box transcription factor 2
TGF-β	Transcription growth factor β
Tie2(Tek)	TEK receptor tyrosine kinase
TNF-α	Tumor necrosis factor α
TP65 (p65)	Tumor protein 65
TRP63 (p63)	Tumor protein 63
UC	Umbilical cord
VEGFR2	Vascular endothelial growth factor receptor 2
Vegfr3	Vascular endothelial growth factor receptor 3
vWF	von Willebrand factor
WNT	Wingless-related integration site
WNT7a	Wnt family member 7A

Insights into the biology and function of stem cells have revealed their therapeutic potential in the treatment of numerous diseases, including diseases of the lung.[1,2] Multiple studies to date have shown protective effects of mesenchymal stromal cells (MSCs) or endothelial progenitor cells (EPCs) derived from bone marrow (BM) or umbilical cord (UC) in animal models of neonatal lung diseases.[3-5] The discovery of resident stem/progenitor cells in adult tissues led to the development of a new field of investigation into the role of resident stem/progenitor cells in lung development, injury, and repair.[1,6,7]

Stem cells are identified by (1) their ability to self-renew (remain in an undifferentiated state) and (2) their potency (ability to produce differentiated cells). According to their ability to produce differentiated somatic cells, stem cells are characterized in four categories: (1) totipotent cells of zygote and morula, which can give rise to all embryonic and extraembryonic tissues; (2) pluripotent cells of the blastula capable of forming any cell type in the developing embryo; (3) multipotent cells, which are often found in adult organisms (e.g., hematopoietic stem cells) and can give rise to several cell types; and (4) unipotent cells, which can only differentiate into one cell type (e.g., alveolar epithelial type 2 cell [AECII] differentiating into type 1 cell [AECI]).[8] Somatic stem cells (also called *adult stem cells*) are typically multipotent or unipotent. While progenitor cells can also give rise to one specific type of cells, they are thought to lack the capacity to self-renew. Therefore they are typically distinguished from the population termed *stem cells*.[1]

Due to their low turnover, the lungs are relatively quiescent organs. This is particularly true in more distal alveolar regions, as cellular turnover time decreases along the proximal-distal axis.[9] Lung somatic stem cells are therefore activated through their microenvironment, especially following tissue damage, and participate in tissue repair and remodeling.[10-12] Injurious stimuli, however, can also cause substantial damage to resident stem cells. Such impacted cells may then undergo an unusual differentiation process, followed by the proliferation of abnormal cell populations and even tumorigenesis. In fact, the hypothesis that the proliferation of stem cells can drive carcinogenesis (so-called cancer stem cell hypothesis) has been widely accepted as one of the underlying principles of cancer research and therapy.[13] Alternatively, alterations to stem cells can result in increased or decreased production of a particular differentiated cell population leading to changes in tissue composition. Such mechanisms contribute, for example, to lung fibrosis in bronchiolitis obliterans syndrome following lung transplantation[14] or loss of tissue in chronic obstructive pulmonary disease,[15] respectively. Thus, impairment of somatic lung stem cells and progenitors and disturbance in their environmental niche may contribute to several pathologies in the developing lung.[2]

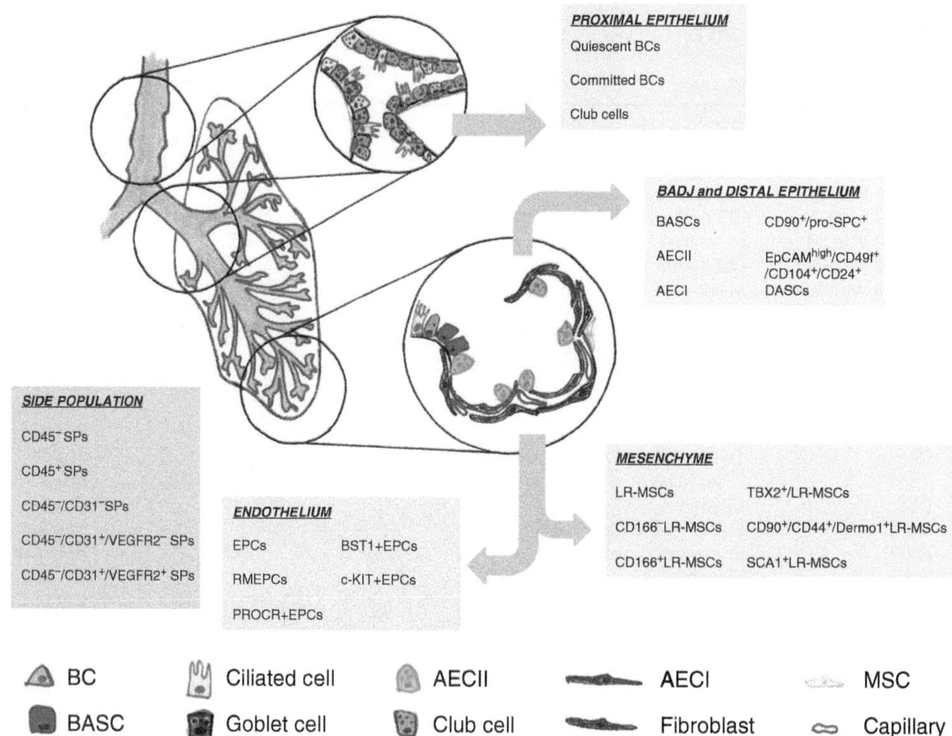

Fig. 74.1 Overview of distinct types of lung resident epithelial, endothelial, and mesenchymal stem cells.

To date, multiple populations of stem cells within the pulmonary endothelium, epithelium, and mesenchyme have been described. Putative epithelial stem or progenitor cells, such as basal cells of proximal airways, secretory cells of conducting airways, and bronchial alveolar stem cells (BASCs) have been extensively studied.[16-18] However, relatively little is known by comparison about mesenchymal and endothelial stem cells of distal alveolar regions (Fig. 74.1).[19]

ENDOTHELIAL PROGENITOR CELLS

The pulmonary vascular tree is formed by two processes of vessel formation: vasculogenesis (de novo vessel formation) and angiogenesis (formation of new vessels from pre-existing vessels).[7,20] The relative contribution and timing of the two processes during individual stages of lung development remain unclear, and two main hypotheses are currently considered: (1) proximal/distal angiogenesis model[21-23] and (2) proximal angiogenesis/distal vasculogenesis model.[24] The formation of the vascular tree during the pseudoglandular and canalicular stages is followed by the process of microvascular maturation. During the saccular stage, capillaries are organized in bilayers within the relatively thick intersaccular space. Progressive thinning of intersaccular (interalveolar) walls during the alveolar stage then leads to the remodeling of the double capillary layer and the formation of the single capillary layer.[25]

In a broader sense, EPCs represent a very heterogeneous and rare population of cells in peripheral and cord blood.[2] Typically, EPCs have been described as cells able to differentiate into endothelial cells and form new blood vessels. Expression of CD31 and vascular endothelial growth factor receptor 2 (VEGFR), as well as acetylated low-density lipoprotein (AcLDL) uptake and lectin binding, are often used as means to identify circulating EPCs in vitro. A proposed nomenclature differentiates between myeloid angiogenic cells (MACs) and endothelial colony-forming cells (ECFCs), representing two separate cell types promoting vascular repair by two distinct mechanisms of action. MACs are characterized as CD45+/CD14+/CD31+ and CD146−/CD133−/Tie2− cultured cells derived from peripheral blood mononuclear cells. While MACs do not have the capacity to become endothelial cells, they promote angiogenesis through paracrine mechanisms.[26] ECFCs, also known as late outgrowth endothelial cells, possess potent intrinsic angiogenic capacity and act as a source of angiogenic paracrine factors.[26] They are characterized by (1) their high proliferative potential, (2) the ability to form secondary and tertiary colonies in vitro, and (3) the de novo blood vessels in vivo.[27] The presence of resident EPCs has been demonstrated in rodent and human lungs.[28-32]

An ever-increasing number of studies reinforce the notion that blood vessel formation actively drives pulmonary growth and constitutes a critical aspect of alveolarization.[33] The hypothesis that angiogenesis drives alveolarization is for the most part founded on two experimental and clinical observations: (1) defects of vascular organization and production of angiogenic factors in patients with underdeveloped lungs suffering from bronchopulmonary dysplasia (BPD), as well as in animal models of BPD,[20,34-38] and (2) studies of angiogenesis inhibition in animal models of lung development.[38-41] This was best demonstrated by studies where the crucial angiogenic factor, vascular endothelial growth factor (VEGF), was pharmacologically or genetically inhibited.[38,39] Disruption of VEGF resulted in arrested alveolarization in the lungs of developing rats and in emphysema-like enlargement of airspaces in adult rats,[42,43] indicating its importance in development and maintenance of the alveolar architecture. Conversely, enhancing angiogenesis during the critical developmental period had partially rescued stunted alveolar formation in experimental models of BPD.[38,44-46] These observations suggest the existence of EPC populations in the distal pulmonary region.

EPCs in the developing lung are poorly understood (Table 74.1; see Fig. 74.1). Multiple reports of resident EPCs in developing mouse, rat, and human lung have been published over the past decade; however, these studies are often limited to in vitro characterization of the cells, and little is known about their location and active role in the developing lung.

In general, pulmonary EPCs population comprises populations of (1) lung resident (LR) and (2) circulating vascular progenitors expressing characteristic cell-surface markers, able

Table 74.1 Overview of Known Markers and Differential Potentials in Distinct Types of Lung Resident Epithelial, Endothelial, and Mesenchymal Stem Cells.

Lung Compartment	Cell Type	Cell Markers	Differentiation Potential
Endothelium	EPCs	CD31$^+$/CD34$^+$/CD144$^+$/CD45$^-$	
	RMEPCs$^+$		
	BST1$^+$		
	c-KIT$^+$		
	RMEPCs	CD31$^+$/CD34$^+$/CD144$^+$/CD309$^+$/CD105$^+$/ VEGFR2$^+$/vWF$^+$/CD45$^-$	
Proximal epithelium	BCs	TRP63$^+$/KRT5$^+$	→ Committed BCs
	Quiescent BCs		→ Goblet cells
	Committed BCs	TP63$^+$/KRT5$^+$/KRT8$^+$	→ Ciliated cells
	Club cells		→ Club cells → Ciliated cells
BADJ and distal epithelium	BASCs	SCGB1a1$^+$/SFTPC$^+$	→ AECIIs
	AECI	AQP5$^+$/PDPN$^+$/HOPX$^+$	→ AECIIs
	AECII	SFTPC$^+$	→ AECIs
	CD90$^+$/pro-SPC$^+$		→ AECIIs
	EpCAM^{high}/CD49f$^+$/CD104$^+$/CD24$^+$		→ Airway and alveolar epithelium
	DASCs	TRP63$^+$/KRT5$^+$	→ AECIs → AECIIs
Mesenchyme	LR-MSCs	CD73$^+$/CD90$^+$/CD105$^+$/CD34$^-$/CD45$^-$/ CD14$^-$/CD11b$^-$/CD19$^-$/CD79α/HLA-DR$^-$	
	CD166$^-$ LR-MSCs		→ Lipofibroblasts/ myofibroblasts
	CD166$^+$ LR-MSCs		→ Myofibroblasts
	TBX2$^+$ LR-MSCs		→ Fibroblasts → Endothelial cells → SMCs
	CD90$^+$/CD44$^+$/Dermo1$^+$ LR-MSCs		→ Club cells → Ciliated cells → Goblet cells
	SCA1$^+$ LR-MSCs		→ Myofibroblasts
Side population	SPs	CD44$^+$/CD90$^+$/CD105$^+$/CD106$^+$/CD73$^+$/ SCA1$^+$/c-KIT$^-$/CD11b$^-$/CD34$^-$/CD14$^-$	
	CD45$^+$ SPs		
	CD45$^-$ SPs		
	CD45$^-$/CD31$^-$ SPs		
	C45$^-$/CD31$^+$/VEGFR2$^-$ SPs		→ CD45$^-$/CD31$^+$/VEGFR2$^+$ SPs
	CD45$^-$/CD31$^+$/VEGFR2$^+$ SPs		

DASCs, Distal airway stem cells; *EPC*, endothelial progenitor cell; *SP*, side population; *VEGFR*, vascular endothelial growth factor receptor.

to proliferate and form colonies in vitro and to form de novo vessels in vitro and in vivo.[10,29] Unfortunately, no cell surface markers have yet been established to distinguish between the resident and circulating population, making it particularly challenging to determine their individual functions in tissue development and repair.[10,47]

Most authors identify EPCs as CD31$^+$, CD34$^+$, CD144$^+$, and CD45$^-$ cells.[28-31,48] Initial isolation of the cells, however, often relies on a single surface marker, CD31, with subsequent selection for EPCs during the in vitro culture. This practice is rooted in the notion that only cells with "stem-cell-like" characteristics will survive, proliferate, and form colonies in culture. One study characterized such cells isolated from human fetal lungs (17 to 20 weeks of gestation) and developing rat lungs (postnatal day [P]14). In addition to CD31, cells surviving in culture expressed CD105 (endoglin), CD144 (VE-cadherin), von Willebrand factor (vWF), and VEGFR2 and formed colonies and tube formations in vitro. Furthermore, when transplanted subcutaneously to mice in form of cell/matrix plugs, these cells formed de novo vessels, demonstrating their progenitor capacity.[30]

To better understand the nature of EPCs in their study, Alvarez and colleagues performed separate assessments of pulmonary artery endothelial cells (PAECs) and pulmonary microvascular endothelial cells (PMVECs)[29] in adult rats. While PAECs were isolated directly by manually scraping the intima of pulmonary arteries, PMVECs were isolated by bulk digestions of distal pulmonary regions. Interestingly, while the majority of PAECs were fully differentiated, three-fourths of PMVECs proliferated in culture, with 50% giving rise to large colonies. These cells, dubbed by authors as resident microvascular endothelial progenitor cells (RMEPCs), expressed CD31, CD34, CD144, CD309, CD105, VEGFR2, vWF, and endothelial nitric oxide synthase (eNOS), while lacking the expression of CD45. Similarly to other studies, these cells formed de novo vessels following transplantation in vivo.[29]

In addition to vascular endothelial progenitors, in their study, Schniederman and colleagues identified a subpopulation of progenitors of lymphatic endothelium.[28] Murine lung CD31$^+$ microvascular endothelial cells were cultured and assessed for colony formation and expression of endothelial and progenitor-specific cell antigens. All cells were CD31, CD34, CD105, VEGFR2, and CD144 positive and CD45, CD41, and CD117 negative. However, in addition, a considerable portion of cells also expressed *Lyve1*, *Prox1*, and *Vegfr3*, indicating their commitment to lymphatic endothelium. In fact, when these cells were transplanted in Matrigel plugs to recipient mice, de novo formation of both blood and lymphatic vessels was observed.[28]

The pivotal role of EPCs during lung development is further supported by studies of arrested lung development, particularly BPD, where both alveolar and vascular development are halted. A decrease in the number of both circulating and resident EPCs, likely MACs, was observed in a murine model of BPD.[32] Furthermore, ECFCs isolated from lungs of diseased rats exhibited reduced cell growth, formed less colonies, and had less complex tubular networks in vitro.[30]

More recently, several novel EPC-specific markers were proposed. BST1(CD157) was described as an endothelial stem cell marker in multiple mouse organs, including the lung.[49] BST1$^+$/CD31$^+$/CD45$^-$ cells constituted approximately 5.5% of all lung cells in mice and were localized within large vessels. However, these cells were absent from capillaries. Another proposed population of vascular endothelial stem cells, PROCR$^+$ cells, was identified in multiple organs, including the mammary gland—the only other organ that undergoes the process of alveolarization. PROCR$^+$ cells showed bipotent character and gave rise de novo to both endothelial cells and pericytes.[50] However, no further studies on the nature of these cells in the developing lung exist to date. Additional markers of pulmonary EPCs, c-KIT, and FOXF1 were proposed by Ren and colleagues.[51] A population of c-KIT$^+$ cells could be detected as early as E16.5 and represented approximately 50% of lung endothelial cells until birth (P1). By 2 weeks of life (P14), the number of c-KIT$^+$ endothelial cells decreased by 20%; this decrease was more severe in animals with hyperoxia-induced arrest in alveolarization. Furthermore, the numbers of both c-KIT$^+$ and FOXF1$^+$ cells were lower in the lungs of BPD patients.[51] Room-air housed transgenic mice with endothelial cells-specific deletion of c-Kit or Foxf1 displayed alveolar simplification. Similarly, FOXF1 haplo insufficient (Foxf1$^{+/-}$) developed spontaneous alveolar hypoplasia and exhibited worse alveolar structure after exposure to hyperoxia, when compared with wild-type mice. Alveolar simplification in both wild-type and Foxf1$^{+/-}$hyperoxia-exposed animals could be reversed by treatment with lung-derived c-KIT$^+$ endothelial cells.[51] These findings are in agreement with previous work by the same authors, demonstrating that FOXF1 is required for the formation of embryonic vasculature, endothelial proliferation, and VEGF signaling.[52]

A growing body of evidence points to the existence of resident pulmonary EPCs and their contribution to normal lung development and repair. New technologies will enable a better characterization of these cells to improve our understanding of normal lung development and disease. This, in turn, may lead to novel therapies to either protect resident EPCs from injury or provide exogeneous EPC for lung regeneration.

LUNG EPITHELIAL STEM CELLS

The pulmonary epithelium is initially formed by progenitor cells, progressively differentiating during embryonic and fetal development toward more restricted progenitor cells.[53] Among the key pathways associated with these processes are hedgehog, retinoic acid, WNT, and NOTCH signaling.[53] During the early stages of fetal development, endoderm-derived epithelial cells serve as early progenitors. It is believed that most, if not all, lung epithelium cells originate from endoderm NKX2-1$^+$ (or *Titf1*$^+$) progenitor cells.[54,55] The composition of the postnatal pulmonary epithelium differs greatly along the proximal-to-distal axis of the lung. Different regions of the lung are thus populated by distinct types of specialized epithelial cells (see Fig. 74.1 and Table 74.1)

PROXIMAL LUNG: TRACHEA AND PROXIMAL BRONCHI

The airways (from the trachea to the bronchioles) are lined by a pseudostratified mucociliary epithelium. This part of the lung acts as a first line of defense for pathogens and is made up of three types of luminal cells: ciliated cells, club cells, and neuroendocrine cells. Luminal airway cells are maintained by a population of basal cells characterized by the expression of TP63 and KRT5. In addition, a smaller population of basal cells also expresses KRT14. These cells are present as a single continuous layer along the airways.[16]

Lineage-tracing studies in mouse lungs revealed the existence of heterogeneity within basal cells. In fact, two equally distributed basal cell populations with diverse gene expression profiles exist: (1) the quiescent basal cells (basal stem cells) and (2) the committed progenitor basal cells, sometimes called *committed luminal progenitors*. Unlike quiescent basal cells, committed basal cells express the luminal cytokeratin KRT8 and rapidly differentiate into secretory and ciliated cells.[56] Furthermore, when cultured on an air-liquid interface, immortalized basal cells are able to form tight junctions and differentiate into ciliated, club, mucous, neuroendocrine, FOXI1$^+$ pulmonary ionocytes, and surfactant positive cells.[57]

Multiple studies to date have shown the importance of NOTCH signaling in the fate of basal cells.[58-60] In absence of NOTCH signaling, committed progenitor basal cells differentiate toward ciliated cells following ciliogenesis—a process characterized by the expression of Forkhead box J1 (FOXJ1), regulatory factor X (RFX), and myeloblastosis (MYB) proto-oncogene transcription factors.[61] The activation of NOTCH signaling induces distinct differentiation programs, depending on the intensity of NOTCH signal. Low levels of NOTCH expression promote secretory cell (club cell) differentiation, characterized by SCGB1A1 expression, while high levels of NOTCH expression promote differentiation into goblet cells.[60]

While ciliated and goblet cells are considered terminally differentiated cells, club cells are known to self-renew and even to produce new ciliated cells following tracheal injury.[62] Similarly, in bleomycin-induced fibrosis, a subset of club cells expressing Uroplakin 3a actively contributed to alveolar repair by differentiating into ciliated and AECII. This sort of unexpected plasticity has been seen in different injury models and will be further discussed herein.[63]

BRONCHOALVEOLAR DUCT JUNCTION

The transition sites between the bronchioles and alveoli are colonized by a small population of endogenous epithelial stem cells titled BASCs. Murine BASCs, which express the club cell marker, SCGB1A1, and the AECII marker, SFTPC, have the ability to self-renew and differentiate in culture, and proliferate in response to bronchiolar and alveolar lung damage in vivo.[17] However, the existence of SCGB1A1$^+$/SFTPC$^+$ cells in humans remains controversial.

BASCS from adult mice exhibited self-renewing and multipotent capacity in culture.[17] Furthermore, BASCs and club cells contribute to alveolar repair following bleomycin injury in adult mice.[64,65] However, in a contradicting study by *Rawlins* and colleagues, lineage-tracing and hyperoxic lung injury experiments showed no apparent contribution of BASCs to postnatal growth, adult homeostasis, or alveolar repair after lung injury.[62] Further studies are necessary to better elucidate the function of BASCs in normal lung development and in disease.

DISTAL LUNG

The alveolar wall is principally formed by a continuous layer of thin elongated AECIs. Markers of AECI include aquaporin 5 (AQP5) and podoplanin (PDPN). AECIs cover a large surface area necessary for proper gas exchange in the alveoli. AECIIs, which are fundamental to lung development, are interspersed between AECIs. AECIIs play pivotal roles in the formation and function of the alveoli, as they (1) produce surfactant proteins, (2) can self-renew, and (3) serve as precursors for AECI. Initial work by Evans and colleagues from the early 1970s showed that AECIIs contribute to alveolar repair by proliferating and differentiating into AECIs.[66] More recently, AECIIs were found to retain the repair capacity in the adult lung for as long as one year.[67] In addition, CD90+/pro-surfactant protein C (pro-SPC)+, potential epithelial progenitors isolated from adult human lungs, showed the ability to self-renew and differentiate into AECIIs in vitro.[68]

Disease models of neonatal lung injury contributed to our understanding of stem cell mechanisms and their contribution to alveolar growth. AECII proliferation and repair were investigated in developing mice, in which the arrest in alveolarization was induced by exposure to hyperoxia. Exposure to hyperoxia for the first 4 days of life led to a reduction in AECII proliferation, which persisted for up to 8 weeks. In addition, lung compliance was significantly increased, indicating that the timing of AECII proliferation and differentiation is essential for postnatal lung development and function.[69] Studies using other lung disease models, such as bleomycin injury and AECII ablation, further confirmed the ability of AECII to differentiate into AECI.[64,67,70]

It is apparent that severe damage or loss of AECII can induce major impairment to the lung alveolus. Conversely, as a response to the destruction of AECI, AECII have been shown to hyperproliferate. For example, hyperproliferation of AECII was observed in premature baboon ventilated with up to 50% oxygen for 6, 14, or 21 days.[71] Furthermore, multiple studies suggest a role for AECII in the development of pulmonary fibrosis by inducing the production of profibrotic factors.[72,73] In addition, AECII hyperplasia is a known marker of genetic neonatal pulmonary diseases, including surfactant protein deficiencies due to mutations in the genes encoding for ABCA3,[74] or in SP-A and SP-D double deficient mice.[75]

Among the signaling pathways believed to be involved in the AECII self-renewal and differentiation capacity is the WNT signaling pathway. Using a novel WNT signaling reporter mouse line ($Axin2^{CreERT2\text{-}Td\text{-}Tom}$), Frank and coworkers showed that a wave of WNT signaling is responsible for the increase of a subpopulation of WNT-responsive AXIN2+ AECII during late lung development.[76] Activation of WNT signaling promotes AECII self-renewal and increases organoid formation and proliferation and clonal expansion during alveologenesis. WNT7a was identified as a critical regulator of differentiation of AECII into AECI.[77] Other signaling pathways identified in regulating AECII progenitor activity include epidermal growth factor receptor (EGFR) and members of KRAS signaling pathways.[70] Further studies suggested that a subpopulation of AECII expressing high levels of laminin receptor $\alpha6\beta4$ but low levels of pro-SPC has progenitor cell maintenance capacity during lung repair.[78] Conclusively, the role of AECIIs in alveolar repair and their ability to differentiate into AECIs are well established. However, the mechanism of action remains to be better understood.

Finally, a minor population of $EpCAM^{high}/CD49f^{+}/CD104^{+}/CD24^{+}$distal epithelial stem cells in adult mouse lung was able to generate colonies comprising airway, alveolar, or mixed lung epithelial cells when co-cultured with $EpCAM^{-}/Sca1^{+}$ lung mesenchymal cells. This cross-talk was mediated via fibroblast growth factor-10 (FGF10) and hepatocyte growth factor (HGF) signaling.[79]

A study investigating the regeneration of mice lungs after H1N1 infection showed that a population of epithelial stem cells located in the small airways, called *distal airway stem cells (DASCs)*, proliferated in response to influenza-induced lung damage.[80] Moreover, ablation of DASCs halted lung regeneration following N1H1 infection in mice and resulted in lung fibrosis.[80] Activated DASCs, sometimes also called *lineage-negative epithelial stem/progenitor cells (LNEPs)*, express Trp63 (p63) and Keratin 5 (KRT5), and proliferate and migrate from the airways to the alveolar region, where they differentiate to pods of KRT5+ epithelial cells at sites of injury.[81] NOTCH signaling is required for the activation of DASCs, whereas in the absence of NOTCH, DASCs differentiate toward alveolar epithelial cells. Furthermore, DASCs were recently shown to improve lung function and increase survival in a bleomycin-induced mouse model of pulmonary fibrosis by promoting lung regeneration and inhibition of fibrogenesis.[82]

Interestingly, multiple studies have hinted at the potential plasticity of AECI. AECI, previously recognized as terminally differentiated, were shown to proliferate and exhibit phenotypic plasticity in vitro.[83] Moreover, Jain and colleagues showed that during lung development in mice, a small population of HOPX+AECI proliferates and differentiates into AECII, which was also observed in adult lungs following partial pneumonectomy.[84] Additional investigation revealed that HOPX+AECI can further be divided into two subpopulations: (1) the insulin-like growth factor-binding protein 2 (IGFBP2)+subpopulation and (2) the IGFBP2− subpopulation. Interestingly, only the HOPX+/IGFBP2− cells were able to differentiate into AECII.[85] Nevertheless, self-renewing and progenitor properties of AECI in other injury models remain controversial.

Given the importance of both AECI and AECII in lung development, a deeper understanding of stem-cell-like subpopulations among these cells will be crucial to identifying superior candidates for future cell therapies.

MESENCHYMAL STROMAL CELLS

Among all somatic stem cells, MSCs have undoubtedly attracted the most attention to date. This is primarily due to the relatively easy access to UC and BM MSCs, easy isolation, and cell culture conditions. The existence of MSCs was first described in BM in early 1970s, bringing excitement in the field of regenerative research.[86] Consecutive research revealed their therapeutic potential in numerous diseases, including those affecting the developing or adult lung. Further discoveries of MSCs in other organs, including the lung, opened a new field of research focused on their contribution to organ development and repair. While minimal criteria for MSCs characterization have been defined, this definition remains relatively rudimentary, resulting in sometimes imprecise or controversial reports in the literature.[1,87] Present research will likely improve the current definition and requirements for MSCs as we begin to study these cells using more sophisticated methods, such as lineage tracing or single-cell RNA sequencing.

MSCs constitute a heterogeneous population derived from the mesodermal or ectodermal germ layer.[2,88,89] They are generally described as fibroblast-shaped cells with characteristic expression pattern of cell surface markers: CD73+, CD90+, CD105+/CD34−, CD45−, CD14/CD11b−, CD79α/CD19−, HLA-DR−. In addition, minimal criteria for human BM-derived MSCs, as stated by *The International Society for Cellular Therapy*, include adherence to the culture-treated plastic surfaces and an ability to form colonies and differentiate along chondrogenic, adipogenic, and osteogenic lineages.[90]

Therapeutic effects of BM, UC, or adipose tissue-derived MSCs were investigated in numerous animal models of adult and developmental pulmonary diseases. Selected therapies are currently subjects to early phase clinical trials.[2,91] In developing rodent lungs, exogenous BM- or UC-derived MSCs were shown to restore lung architecture and function, attenuate inflammation, oxidative stress, fibrosis, and pulmonary hypertension. Multiple avenues by which MSCs exert their therapeutic effects are currently under investigation.[92]

While the clinical translation of exogenous MSCs has begun, insights into the role MSCs residing in the adult and developing lung[30,89,93-95] may yield a better understanding of the biology and function of these still ill-defined cells (see Fig. 74.1 and Table 74.1). LR MSCs comprise a diverse population of mesenchymal cells. Their direct descendants, lipofibroblasts and myofibroblasts, actively contribute to postnatal lung development. While myofibroblasts drive the process of alveolarization and formation of secondary septa, lipofibroblasts stimulate the production of retinoic acid and pulmonary surfactant.[2,96,97] The current state of research also indicates that MSCs further regulate the developing lung by coordinating the behavior and differentiation of other cells. Relatively little is known about the hierarchy and location of mesenchymal progenitors in the postnatally developing or adult lung. Furthermore, new lung-specific markers need to be defined in order to better understand the heterogeneous MSC population and to distinguish resident MSCs from other lung mesenchymal populations, which often express commonly used MSC cell surface markers.

McQualter and colleagues investigated the heterogeneous nature of LR-MSCs in adult mice. They identified two separate populations of MSCs based on their expression of CD166. Interestingly, CD166⁻ cells had higher proliferative potential and differentiated into both lipofibroblasts and myofibroblasts, while CD166⁺ were only able to produce myofibroblasts.[79] Furthermore, CD166⁻ MSCs were able to support lung epithelial colonies in vitro, which was dependent on transcription growth factor-β (TGF-β) expression. In addition, LR-MSCs could support the growth of epithelial progenitors, including AEC-II and club cells.[98]

In fact, several studies suggested that at least some LR-MSCs have multiple functions beyond their role of mesenchymal progenitors. It was proposed that LR-MSCs act as controllers of cellular fate for mesenchyme, mesothelium, endothelium, and epithelium.[79,99] Lung MSCs were shown to modulate the immune response by regulating T-cell proliferation.[100] When accordingly stimulated in vitro, LR-MSCs generated epithelial, endothelial, and even nerve cells.[100-105] In a recent publication, Wojahn and co-workers identified TBX2⁺ resident MSCs as a source of fibroblasts, endothelial, and smooth muscle cells in fetal lungs. In addition, approximately 50% of fetal mesothelial population was also generated by TBX2⁺ MSCs.[106] Furthermore, lineage-tracing studies in mice showed that following club cells injury, CD90/CD44/Dermo1⁺ LR-MSCs can differentiate into club, ciliated, and goblet cells.[107]

Studies of early (embryonic) lung development have shown that lung mesenchymal progenitors do not represent a homogeneous cell pool, but progenitors of different cell types display distinct spatial and temporal characteristics and are recruited in different ways.[99] Furthermore, the same progenitor population can generate diverse cell populations according to the developmental period or location.[108] For example, lineage-tracing studies showed that FGF10⁺ mesenchymal progenitors differentiate into smooth muscle cells and lipofibroblasts during the embryonic period, while during the later alveolar period they generate only lipofibroblasts. In adult lungs, FGF10⁺ show characteristics of LR-MSCs and exhibit an MSC-like cell markers pattern: CD45⁻/CD31⁻/SCA1.[108]

LR-MSCs from human or animal sources are often identified by the previously mentioned minimal criteria, including the presence of surface markers CD90 and CD73, and the absence of hematopoietic, epithelial, and endothelial markers CD45, CD31, and CD34.[95,109-113] Inconsistencies in isolation procedures and further characterization in vitro, however, complicate direct comparisons between individual studies. While in some studies cells are sorted based on their expression profile immediately after tissue dissociation and prior to culture,[94,113,114] many researchers choose to characterize cells only following culture.[95,109-111,115]

Resident MSCs have been characterized in human fetal lungs (embryonic week 15 to 17). Following the organ digest, cells were plated and surface markers were assessed in cultured cells. Cells were identified based on their MSC-specific expression profile (CD73⁺/CD90⁺/CD105⁺/CD146⁺, CD19⁻/CD14⁻/CD45⁻/CD34⁻/HLA-A⁻), as well as expression of progenitor markers SOX2 and OCT4. Furthermore, these cells differentiated along adipogenic, osteogenic, and chondrogenic lineages. MSCs, which were cultured in hypoxic conditions (5% O_2), formed large colonies; however, when cells were exposed to relative hyperoxia mimicking birth (21% O_2) or intense oxygen therapy (60% O_2) following premature birth, this ability was dramatically reduced.[109] The concept of lung MSCs playing a role in postnatal lung development is further supported by studies in rodent models of BPD—the most common disease of prematurity. CD31⁻/CD45⁻/Epcam⁻/CD146⁺ extracted from both healthy and hyperoxia-exposed developing rat pups differentiated along all three designated lineages and form colonies to the same extent. However, LR-MSCs from hyperoxia-exposed developing rat pups showed decreased angiogenic supportive capacity. This was also accompanied by decreased expression of the stem-cell marker CD73 and altered expression profile.[113]

The notion that disturbance to LR-MSCs may affect postnatal alveolar development stems from studies of MSCs in the tracheal aspirates of mechanically ventilated neonates. The presence of MSCs in bronchoalveolar lavage (BAL) from prematurely born infants was first detected in 2007.[110] Following isolation, cells were cultured up to the third passage prior to surface markers assessment. Cultured cells were positive for multiple MSC markers such as CD73, CD90, CD105, and CD166, as well as CCR2b, CD13, prolyl 4-hydroxylase, and α-smooth muscle actin (αSMA), while negative for the hematopoietic and endothelial cell markers CD11b, CD31, CD34, and CD45. Moreover, cells formed colonies in vitro and were able to differentiate into adipocytes, osteocytes, and myofibroblasts. Differentiation along the chondrogenic lineage was not demonstrated. Interestingly, more MSCs were present in the BAL of infants who went on to develop BPD than in those who did not.[110] Since this original report, several studies have built upon this initial finding. In four subsequent studies, Popova and colleagues identified the presence of MSCs in tracheal aspirates as an indicator of BPD morbidity and severity.[111] Poor outcome was particularly associated with low expression levels of PDGFRα. This observation was further supported by an analysis of the lungs of BPD patients and hyperoxia-exposed neonatal mice, which exhibited decreased populations of PDGFRα⁺ cells compared to healthy controls.[116] Cells from BPD patients also showed higher content of phosphor-GSK3, β-catenin, and α-actin.[117] Similar changes could be reproduced in lung MSCs in vitro following stimulation by TGF-β.[117] Treatment with TGF-β further induced the gene expression of contractile (ACTA2, MYH11, TAGLN, DES) and extracellular matrix proteins (FN1, ELN, COL1A1, COL1A2), and protein expression of α-SMA, myosin heavy chain, and SM22, promoting the myofibroblastic differentiation of neonatal lung MSCs.[118] This correlates with multiple studies demonstrating TGF-β–induced inhibition of PDGFRα in lung fibroblast populations.[119-121] MSCs from patients who were ventilated for longer periods also showed higher proliferative capacity and increased levels of NFκB/p65 and α-SMA, often associated with BPD.[115] While the presence of MSCs in tracheal aspirates clearly correlates with increased morbidity, the origin of these cells and their relationship to LR-MSCs remain unknown.

It is notable that studies of the role of LR-MSCs in the context of adult pulmonary diseases revealed deregulation of some of the same signaling pathways. Both WNT/TGF-β and TNF-α/NFκB signaling pathways induce mesenchymal-myofibroblast transition (MMT) in SCA1⁺ LR-MSCs from adult mice. Interestingly, WNT and TGF-β signaling, as well as MMT, were increased in murine models of pulmonary fibrosis, and WNT and TNF-α signaling were increased in patients with pulmonary fibrosis. These studies suggest that injury to resident MSCs can drive fibrosis, potentially via TGF-β and TNF-α signaling.[114,122,123]

It seems apparent that deleterious stimuli and tissue injury might alter the nature of LR-MSCs. Aberrant MSCs, in turn, may activate default differentiation pathways to contain the injury, leading to a profibrotic expression profile, further aggravating the disease process. A better characterization of MSC, in general, will be required to improve our understanding of the function of LR stem cells in normal and impaired pulmonary development, and this may lead to superior pharmacologic or cell-based therapies.

LUNG SIDE POPULATION

An additional, distinct population of lung progenitor cells that attracts researchers' attention is represented by the so-called lung side cells, or lung side population (SP; see Fig. 74.1 and Table 74.1). SP cells constitute a very small population found in multiple tissues, including adult and developing lung. They lack the expression of differentiated lineage markers and are distinctive by their ability to efflux the Hoescht 33342 DNA dye.[124,125] Lung SP represents a primitive multipotent population, with the ability to differentiate into epithelial, endothelial, mesenchymal, and hematopoietic cells. SP cells of two origins can be found in the lung. While $CD45^+$ SP cells are of hematopoietic origin, the origin of the $CD45^-$ population remains unknown.[125,126] $CD45^-$ SP cells further express well-known mesenchymal markers CD44, CD90, CD105, CD106, CD73, and SCA1, and lack the expression of hematopoietic markers c-KIT, CD11b, CD34, and CD14.

While similar to MSCs, SP cells represent a more heterogeneous cell population. Similarly to MSC populations, lung SP cells isolated from adult mice lungs form colonies in vitro and can differentiate along adipogenic, chondrogenic, and osteogenic lineages.[127] Lung SP cells isolated from developing mice pups showed the ability to form tubular networks in culture, indicating their endothelial potential. Furthermore, both $CD45^+$ and $CD45^-$ SPs were depleted in developing mice where arrest in alveolarization was induced by exposure to hyperoxia.[125] In their recent publication, Xu and colleagues further show that $CD45^-$ SPs can be subdivided into $CD31^+$ and $CD31^-$ subpopulations, and the $CD31^+$ fraction can be additionally classified based on the expression of endothelial marker VEGFR2. $CD45^-$/CD 31^+/$VEGFR2^-$ cells showed characteristics of smooth muscle and endothelial progenitors and differentiated into smooth muscle cells and endothelial cells in vitro. Authors further proposed that $CD45^-$/$CD31^+$/$VEGFR2^-$ cells differentiate into the $VEGFR2^+$ SP cells, possibly suggesting an existing hierarchy inside the population.[124]

Further in-depth studies are necessary to understand the full potential of various subtypes of lung SP cells and the specific roles they play in the postnatally developing lung.

CONCLUSION

Endogenous stem and progenitor cells play a pivotal role in early lung embryonic and fetal development. However, smaller populations of various multipotent progenitors remain in the early postnatal period and adulthood. Populations of lung endogenous stem cells consist of endothelial, epithelial, and mesenchymal populations, each comprising several specific subsets of cells with distinct phenotypes and functions. These resident stem/progenitor cells are instrumental for normal development, organ homeostasis, and repair. These functions are carried out either via direct differentiation into newly required cells or indirectly by influencing the fate of neighboring cell populations. An increasing number of studies suggest the involvement of endogenous stem cells in developmental and adult lung diseases. Exhaustion and/or dysfunction of these cells may impede the ability to contribute to tissue repair. Moreover, malfunctioning stem cells may proliferate and differentiate into undesirable cell types, causing dysplastic growth or fibrosis and ultimately contributing to BPD pathogenesis, accompanying pulmonary hypertension and early tissue aging. Treatments with exogenous MSCs have shown promise in experimental studies, and early phase clinical trials are underway. A better characterization of somatic stem cell populations is necessary to improve our understanding of their role during normal and impaired lung development. Improved knowledge of their function will conceivably open doors to pharmacologic or cell-based therapies protecting endogenous lung stem cell populations.

ACKNOWLEDGMENTS

This work was supported by the Canadian Institutes of Health Research (CIHR), the German Research Foundation (Deutsche Forschungsgemeinschaft), the Ontario Institute for Regenerative Medicine (OIRM), the Stem Cell Network, the Heart and Stroke Foundation Canada, the Ontario Graduate Scholarship, and the Canadian Lung Association—Breathing as One Studentship.

A complete reference list is available at www.ExpertConsult.com. 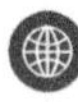

SELECT REFERENCES

1. Wagner DE, et al. An Official American Thoracic Society Workshop report 2015. Stem cells and cell therapies in lung biology and diseases. *Annals ATS*. 2016;13:S259–S278.
2. Möbius MA, Thébaud B. Bronchopulmonary dysplasia: where have all the stem cells gone? *Chest*. 2017;152:1043–1052.
3. O'Reilly M, et al. Late rescue therapy with cord-derived mesenchymal stromal cells for established lung injury in experimental bronchopulmonary dysplasia. *Stem Cells Dev*. 2020;29:364–371. https://doi.org/10.1089/scd.2019.0116.
6. Bertoncello I. Properties of adult lung stem and progenitor cells: lung epithelial stem and progenitor cells. *J Cell Physiol*. 2016;231:2582–2589.
7. Kotton DN, Morrisey EE. Lung regeneration: mechanisms, applications and emerging stem cell populations. *Nat Med*. 2014;20:822–832.
8. Barkauskas CE, et al. Type 2 alveolar cells are stem cells in adult lung. *J Clin Invest*. 2013;123:3025–3036.
10. Ciechanowicz A. Stem cells in lungs. In: Ratajczak MZ, ed. *Stem Cells*. Springer International Publishing; 2019:261–274. *Advances in Experimental Medicine and Biology*; vol 1201.
16. Morrisey EE. Basal cells in lung development and repair. *Dev Cell*. 2018;44:653–654.
17. Kim CFB, et al. Identification of bronchioalveolar stem cells in normal lung and lung cancer. *Cell*. 2005;121:823–835.
18. Rawlins EL. Lung epithelial progenitor cells: lessons from development. *Proc Am Thorac Soc*. 2008;5:675–681.
26. Medina RJ, et al. Endothelial progenitors: a consensus statement on nomenclature: endothelial progenitors nomenclature. *Stem Cells Transl Med*. 2017;6:1316–1320.
27. Yoder MC, et al. Redefining endothelial progenitor cells via clonal analysis and hematopoietic stem/progenitor cell principals. *Blood*. 2007;109:1801–1809.
29. Alvarez DF, et al. Lung microvascular endothelium is enriched with progenitor cells that exhibit vasculogenic capacity. *Am J Physiol Lung Cell Mol Physiol*. 2008;294:L419–L430.
30. Alphonse RS, et al. Existence, functional impairment, and lung repair potential of endothelial colony-forming cells in oxygen-induced arrested alveolar growth. *Circulation*. 2014;129:2144–2157.
38. Thébaud B, et al. Vascular endothelial growth factor gene therapy increases survival, promotes lung angiogenesis, and prevents alveolar damage in hyperoxia-induced lung injury: evidence that angiogenesis participates in alveolarization. *Circulation*. 2005;112:2477–2486.
51. Ren X, et al. Postnatal alveologenesis Depends on FOXF1 signaling in c-KIT^+ endothelial progenitor cells. *Am J Respir Crit Care Med*. 2019;200:1164–1176. https://doi.org/10.1164/rccm.201812-2312OC.
67. Barkauskas CE, et al. Type 2 alveolar cells are stem cells in adult lung. *J Clin Invest*. 2013;123:3025–3036.
68. Fujino N, et al. Isolation of alveolar epithelial type II progenitor cells from adult human lungs. *Lab Invest*. 2011;91:363–378.
70. Desai TJ, Brownfield DG, Krasnow MA. Alveolar progenitor and stem cells in lung development, renewal and cancer. *Nature*. 2014;507:190–194.
90. Dominici M, et al. Minimal criteria for defining multipotent mesenchymal stromal cells. The International Society for Cellular Therapy position statement. *Cytotherapy*. 2006;8:315–317.
91. Chang YS, et al. Human umbilical cord blood-derived mesenchymal stem cells attenuate hyperoxia-induced lung injury in neonatal rats. *Cell Transplant*. 2009;18:869–886.

94. McQualter JL, et al. Endogenous fibroblastic progenitor cells in the adult mouse lung are highly enriched in the sca-1 positive cell fraction. *Stem Cell*. 2009;27:623–633.
95. Khatri M, O'Brien TD, Chattha KS, Saif LJ. Porcine lung mesenchymal stromal cells possess differentiation and immunoregulatory properties. *Stem Cell Res Ther*. 2015;6:222.
96. McGowan SE, McCoy DM. Platelet-derived growth factor-A and sonic hedgehog signaling direct lung fibroblast precursors during alveolar septal formation. *Am J Physiol Lung Cell Mol Physiol*. 2013;305:L229–L239.
98. Möbius MA, Rüdiger M. Mesenchymal stromal cells in the development and therapy of bronchopulmonary dysplasia. *Mol Cell Pediatr*. 2016;3:18.
99. Kumar ME, et al. Mesenchymal cells. Defining a mesenchymal progenitor niche at single-cell resolution. *Science*. 2014;346:1258810.
100. Jarvinen L, et al. Lung resident mesenchymal stem cells isolated from human lung allografts inhibit T cell proliferation via a soluble mediator. *J Immunol*. 2008;181:4389–4396.
101. Yamamoto Y, Baldwin HS, Prince LS. Endothelial differentiation by multipotent fetal mouse lung mesenchymal cells. *Stem Cell Dev*. 2012;21:1455–1465.
108. El Agha E, et al. Fgf10-positive cells represent a progenitor cell population during lung development and postnatally. *Development*. 2014;141:296–306.
110. Hennrick KT, et al. Lung cells from neonates show a mesenchymal stem cell phenotype. *Am J Respir Crit Care Med*. 2007;175:1158–1164.
111. Popova AP, et al. Isolation of tracheal aspirate mesenchymal stromal cells predicts bronchopulmonary dysplasia. *Pediatrics*. 2010;126:e1127–e1133.
122. Cao H, et al. Inhibition of Wnt/β-catenin signaling suppresses myofibroblast differentiation of lung resident mesenchymal stem cells and pulmonary fibrosis. *Sci Rep*. 2018;8:13644.
124. Xu Y, et al. Differentiation of CD45-/CD31+ lung side population cells into endothelial and smooth muscle cells in vitro. *Int J Mol Med*. 2019:1128–1138. https://doi.org/10.3892/ijmm.2019.4053.
125. Irwin D, et al. Neonatal lung side population cells demonstrate endothelial potential and are altered in response to hyperoxia-induced lung simplification. *Am J Physiol Lung Cell Mol Physiol*. 2007;293:L941–L951.
127. Martin J, et al. Adult lung side population cells have mesenchymal stem cell potential. *Cytotherapy*. 2008;10:140–151.

75 Surfactant Homeostasis: Composition and Function of Pulmonary Surfactant Lipids and Proteins

Jeffrey A. Whitsett | Paul S. Kingma

INTRODUCTION

In vertebrates, adaptation to a nonaqueous respiratory environment was achieved by the development of lungs, which provide an extensive surface area for gas exchange. The unique physicochemical boundary between respiratory gases and the alveolar epithelium creates a region of high surface tension, generated by the unequal distribution of molecular forces on water molecules at the air-liquid interface. Unopposed, this surface tension creates collapsing forces that cause atelectasis and respiratory failure. Pulmonary surfactant creates lipid layers separating alveolar gas from the aqueous phase, decreasing these surface forces. It is not surprising that pulmonary surfactant is found in all air-breathing vertebrates studied, including animals as phylogenetically divergent as the lungfish and humans.[1]

Synthesis and secretion of an abundance of phospholipid-rich material accompany the maturation of the lung before birth. The lack of pulmonary surfactant in premature infants results in respiratory distress syndrome (RDS) after birth. Likewise, loss of surfactant function related to lung injury causes acute respiratory failure postnatally. Hereditary disorders of surfactant homeostasis cause respiratory failure in newborn infants and children. The specifics of structure and function of the surfactant complex have important implications for diagnosis and treatment of RDS and other pulmonary diseases. This chapter considers the maturation and function of the pulmonary surfactant system that is required for adaptation to air breathing after birth.

FORMING THE GAS-EXCHANGE REGION OF THE LUNG PARENCHYMA

The vertebrate lung is derived from epithelial progenitor cells from the anterior foregut endoderm that proliferate and branch within the splanchnic mesenchyme early in gestation. Complex paracrine signaling among diverse pulmonary cells directs stereotypic branching of conducting airways that end in acinar tubules that dilate in late gestation, forming the peripheral saccules that will create the alveolar gas-exchange region after birth.[2] Prior to birth, the stromal-mesenchymal components of the lung thin, and pulmonary capillaries expand as the pulmonary circulatory system comes in close apposition to the epithelial cells lining the peripheral saccules. Two distinct, differentiated epithelial cells, alveolar type 2 cells (AT2), and type 1 cells (AT1) line the peripheral lung saccules. AT1 cells are highly squamous that, together with endothelial cells, create the efficient gas-exchange structure in the alveoli; cuboidal AT2 cells cover much less of the alveolar surface but are critical for the synthesis and secretion of surfactant lipids and proteins needed to reduce surface tension, thereby enabling ventilation (Fig. 75.1). The signaling and transcriptional processes directing branching morphogenesis and lung maturation near the time of birth are increasingly understood.[3-6] The structural and biochemical maturation of the lung prior to birth include the interactions of multiple cell types, including diverse fibroblasts, myofibroblasts, pericytes, and endothelial cells that interact with epithelial progenitors in a precisely orchestrated temporal-spatial pattern to create the gas-exchange region critical for survival after birth.[7] Recent single cell RNA studies identify more than two dozen major cell types comprising the peripheral lung at the time of birth.[7,8] In humans, the perinatal lung is considered to be primarily in the late "saccular" stage of development. Further septation and elongation of the saccules during the "alveolar" stage occur after birth, resulting in the formation of the mature alveoli. Many of the nuclear transcription factors and signaling processes involved in early branching morphogenesis also play critical roles in the differentiation of the respiratory epithelium prior to birth. For example, FOXA1, FOXA2, FOXP1/P2, NKX2-1, SOX9, Wnt/β-catenin, GATA6, and CEBPα all play critical roles in the growth and differentiation of epithelial cells in peripheral lung, and therefore influence both lung architecture and pulmonary

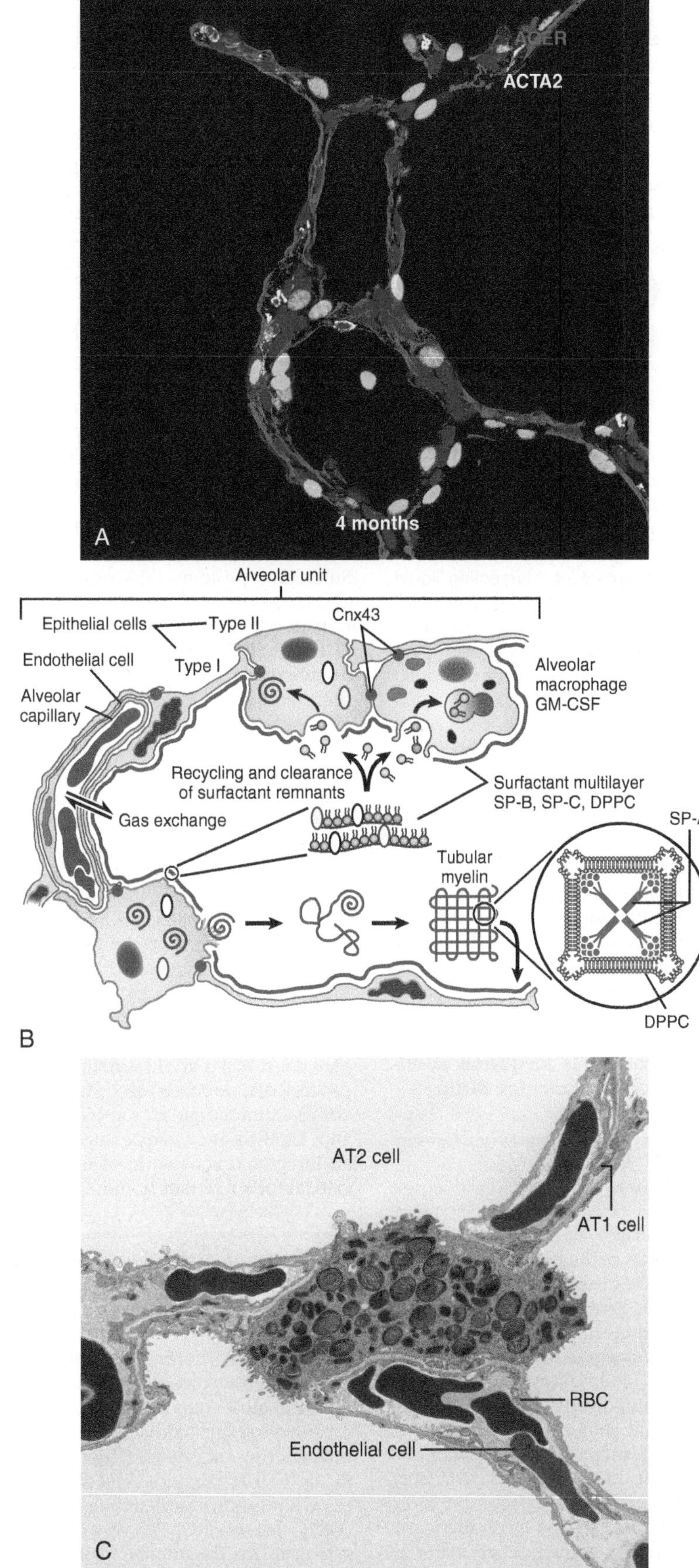

Fig. 75.1 Structure of the pulmonary alveolus. (A) Confocal image shows the human alveolar septae stained with NKX2-1 *(green)* identifying AT2 cells, advanced glycosylation end product specific receptor (AGER) *(red)* AT1 cells, and ACTA2 *(white)* smooth muscle actin. (B) A schematic of the alveoli identifies AT1 and AT2 and alveolar macrophages. Lamellar bodies are secreted into the alveoli and from tubular myelin from which surfactant multilayers form to reduce surface tension at the air-liquid interface. Alveolar macrophages clear the surfactant remnants. AT2 cells recycle surfactant components. (C) An electron micrograph of an AT2 cell with lamellar bodies in the corner of the alveolus is shown. *DPPC,* Desaturated palmitoyl-phosphatidylcholine; *GM-CSF*, granulocyte macrophage colony–stimulating factor; *SP*, surfactant proteins. (Adapted from Whitsett JA, Kalin TV, Xu Y, et al. Building and regenerating the lung cell by cell. *Physiol Rev*. 2019;99:513–554.)

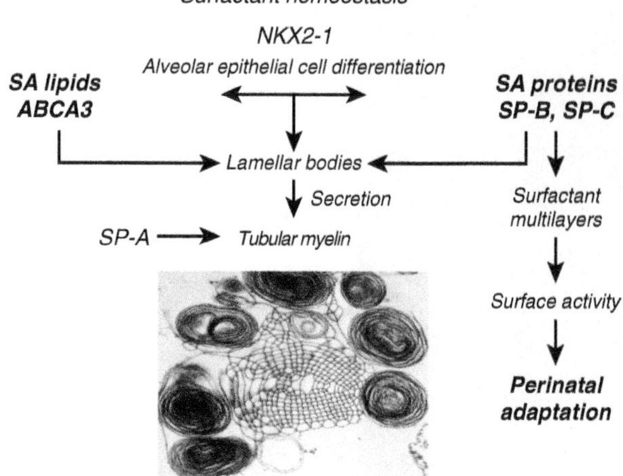

Fig. 75.2 Surfactant synthesis and trafficking. Lamellar bodies, the intracellular form of surfactant, are secreted into the alveolar lumen as concentrically arranged layers of tightly packed, phospholipid-rich membranes shown in the electron micrograph. They are converted into tubular myelin, a lattice-like arrangement of intersecting liquid tubules. Image is a transmission electron micrograph of glutaraldehyde-tannic acid–osmium tetroxide fixed lung. *NKX2-1* (thyroid transcription factor 1 [TTF-1]) regulates differentiation of AT2 cells, synthesis of surfactant proteins, *ABCA3*, and lipids, which are packaged with lipids in lamellar bodies and secreted in the alveolus. SP-B and SP-C interact with Ca^{2+} and SP-A to form tubular myelin, from which surface active multilayers are formed to reduce surface tension. (Magnification ×124,200.). *RBC,* Red blood cells; *SP,* surfactant proteins.

surfactant homeostasis.[2,6,9] Likewise, glucocorticoid signaling in mesenchymal cells of the lung plays an important role in the maturation of the respiratory epithelium, a process underlying the successful clinical use of antenatal maternal glucocorticoid therapy to enhance fetal lung maturation prior to preterm birth.[10,11] Since the processes of lung maturation are regulated in precisely timed sequences and occur relatively late in gestation, preterm infants are often born at a time in which neither lung structure nor surfactant homeostasis is adequately developed to support normal ventilation after premature birth.

SURFACTANT DEFICIENCY AND RESPIRATORY DISTRESS SYNDROME

Seminal studies by Avery and Mead[12] defined the critical role of pulmonary surfactant in the pathogenesis of RDS in preterm infants that led to the elucidation of the biochemical and physiologic requirements for the synthesis and function of pulmonary surfactant. Lungs from preterm infants dying from RDS lacked the lipid rich material needed to reduce surface tension at an air-liquid interface. Pulmonary surfactant is composed primarily of lipids present in distinct macromolecular aggregates whose structural forms are conferred by the relative abundance of surfactant associated proteins and phospholipids, as well as by the impact of mechanical forces on the surfactant material accompanying the compression and decompression during the respiratory cycle. Tubular myelin, the most abundant structural form of surfactant, is a highly surface-active material that sediments at relatively low gravitational forces and consists primarily of phospholipids and proteins; it is lacking in infants with RDS (Fig. 75.2). Tubular myelin serves as a reservoir from which multilayered lipid films that spread over the alveolar surface are formed. Differentiation of type II epithelial cells and associated production of both surfactant lipids and proteins are incomplete in many preterm infants.

SYNTHESIS, SECRETION, AND CATABOLISM OF SURFACTANT

Surfactant lipids are synthesized, stored, secreted, and recycled by type II epithelial cells (Fig. 75.3) (see also detailed reviews by Agassandian and Mallampalli,[13] Goss and colleagues,[14] and Whitsett and colleagues[15]). Metabolic substrates for lipid synthesis are derived from precursors taken up from the circulation, by de novo synthesis, by reuptake of lipids by type II epithelial cells, and from products of lipid degradation by alveolar macrophages. Within type II epithelial cells, lipids are synthesized in the endoplasmic reticulum (ER) and transferred to Golgi bodies. Alternatively, transport may be mediated by lipid transfer proteins or by direct contact of lamellar bodies (LBs) with the ER, for review see work by Brandsma and Postle.[16] Phosphatidylcholine (PC) transfer to LBs requires an adenosine triphosphate (ATP)-binding cassette transporter A3 (ABCA3), located on the limiting membrane of the LBs.[17] Surfactant proteins (SP) proSP-B and proSP-C are synthesized and transported via the ER and proteolytically processed during transport to LBs.The small, hydrophobic active peptides, mature SP-B and SP-C, are assembled with surfactant phospholipids into membranes that are stored in LBs. In contrast, SP-A and SP-D are secreted independently and are assembled into surfactant lipids after secretion. LBs are secreted into the airway via a process stimulated by catecholamines, purinoreceptor agonists, and stretch. Secretory processes are inhibited by GPR116, an orphan G protein–coupled receptor located on respiratory epithelial cells.[18,19] After secretion, LBs unwind and interact with SP-A and SP-D to produce tubular myelin and multilayered surface films that spread over the alveolus to reduce surface tension (see Fig. 75.3). SP-A and SP-B are required for formation of tubular myelin.[15,20] The pulmonary collectins, SP-A and SP-D, have important roles in innate host defense in the lung.[21,22] SP-D regulates extracellular forms of surfactant and has an important role in controlling the size of the surfactant lipid pool.[15,23] Pulmonary surfactant is recycled, catabolized, or reutilized actively by alveolar type II epithelial cells in a process influenced by SP.Alveolar macrophages play a critical part in surfactant uptake and degradation in a process that depends upon signaling by granulocyte-macrophage colony-stimulating factor (GM-CSF) and its receptors (CF2RA and CF2RB) in alveolar macrophages.[24,25] Fig. 75.3 provides an integrated schematic of important aspects of the processes critical for surfactant homeostasis in the alveolus.

METABOLIC PATHWAYS REGULATING SURFACTANT PRODUCTION AND HOMEOSTASIS

Major pathways controlling surfactant lipid synthesis are relatively well established, as recently reviewed in Brandsma and Postle.[16] PC is the most abundant lipid component of pulmonary surfactant, representing approximately 70% of the total lipid content.As the lung matures, the content of PC increases with increasing enrichment of PC 16.0/16.1 (palmitic acid at the C-1 position and palmitoleic acid at the C-2 position). Measurement of disaturated phosphatidylcholine (DSPC) (disaturated PC) by osmium tetroxide has been used as a surrogate for desaturated palmitoyl-phosphatidylcholine (DPPC), the most abundant species in surfactant. DPPC is synthesized de novo by the cytodine diphosphate choline (CDP) choline pathway and by reacylation of PC species in the Land cycle. Fatty acid chains are generated by the enzyme fatty acid synthase, controlled transcriptionally by sterol regulatory element binding

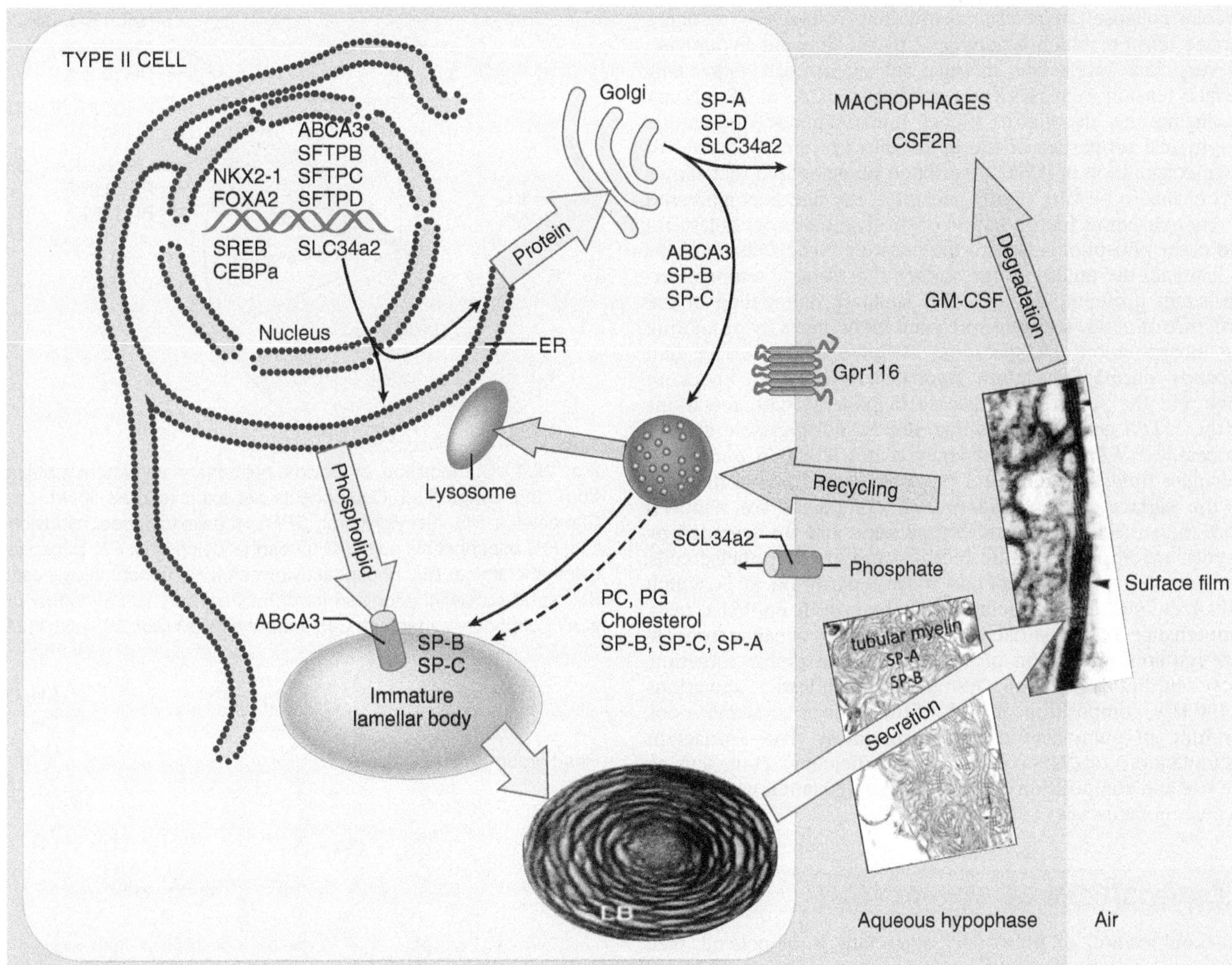

Fig. 75.3 Biosynthesis of surfactant involves distinct pathways for surfactant proteins and lipids. SP-B and SP-C are trafficked from the endoplasmic reticulum to lamellar bodies via the Golgi complex and MVB; in contrast, surfactant phospholipids are likely directly transported from the endoplasmic reticulum to specific lipid importers (ABCA3) in the lamellar body–limiting membrane. Surfactant proteins and lipids are assembled into bilayer membranes that are secreted into the alveolar airspace, where they form a surface film at the air–liquid interface. Cyclical expansion and compression of the bioactive film results in the incorporation *(large green arrow)* and loss *(red arrows)* of lipids and proteins from the multilayered surface film. Surfactant components removed from the film are degraded in alveolar macrophages or are taken up by type II epithelial cells for recycling or degradation in the lysosome *(red arrows)*. The MVB plays a key part in the integration of pathways for surfactant synthesis, recycling, and degradation. NKX2-1, FOXA2, SREBP, and CEBPα are transcription factors regulating surfactant protein and lipid synthesis. SLC34a2 is a phosphate transporter. GPR116 is a membrane receptor regulating surfactant secretion. *ABCA3*, ATP-binding cassette transporter A3; *ER*, endoplasmic reticulum; *GM-CSF*, granulocyte-macrophage colony–stimulating factor; *MVB*, multivesicular body; *PC*, phosphatidylcholine; *PG*, phosphatidylglycerol; *SP*, surfactant proteins.

proteins (SREBP),[26] that control lipid substrate supply in AT2 cells. The CDP-choline pathway is controlled by choline kinase (CK), phosphocholine cytidylyltransferase (CTP): choline phosphatidyl transferase (CCT), and choline phosphotransferase (CPT), and is activated by peroxisome proliferator-activated receptor (PPAR) γ, stretch, vasoactive intestinal peptide (VIP), and fibroblast growth factor 7. The ABCA3 transporter moves lipids into the lamellar body from the ER, selectively enriching for DPPC. Steady state cellular PC content is further maintained by the basolateral secretion of lipid into the systemic circulation and lymphatics in a process mediated by the transport protein ABCA1, which removes excess cholesterol ester and PC,[27] further enriching unsaturated species to enhance DPPC content in the AT2 cell and surfactant. Enrichment of PC with palmitate is maintained by acyl remodeling via phospholipase A2, peroxiredoxins 6 (Prdx6), and selective removal of unsaturated species by ABCA1 and LPCAT (lysophosphatidylcholine acyltransferase), which selectively incorporates palmitoyl CoA into DSPC.[28]

BIOPHYSICS OF PULMONARY SURFACTANT

The close apposition of alveolar type I epithelial cells to pulmonary endothelial cells lining the capillaries forms a highly diffusible air-blood barrier across which gas exchange occurs. The stabilization of alveolar structure during breathing-induced expansion and contraction is achieved by the formation and maintenance of a phospholipid-rich film that spreads over the thin liquid layer (the aqueous hypophase) that covers the alveolar epithelial cell surface (recently reviewed by Autilio and Perez-Gil[29]). The unique biophysical properties of surfactant prevent alveolar collapse (atelectasis) at low lung volumes by reducing surface tension, which is generated by the aqueous hypophase, to very low levels (<2 mN/m). During alveolar expansion, surface tension increases (to a maximum of 20 to 25 mN/m), stabilizing the alveolus at higher lung volumes. The unique biophysical properties of the lipid films are directly related to the incorporation of DPPC, a saturated phospholipid that allows acyl chains to be very tightly packed as the film is compressed during exhalation. Incorporation of small amounts of cholesterol and other phospholipids with the unsaturated acyl chains helps to maintain the fluidity of the surface film at body temperature. Surfactant proteins SP-B and SP-C facilitate remodeling of the structure of newly secreted surfactant membranes by promoting the incorporation and spreading of lipids as the surface film expands during inhalation. Neonatal lethality in knockout mice and the severe lung disease in patients with mutations in the *SFTPB* gene indicates that SP-B is indispensable for this process.[15,30] While SP-C deficiency is not lethal, in mice, SP-C enhances lipid spreading and is required for optimal function of the surface film.[31] Lipid–protein complexes are removed from the surface film during compression and are degraded by alveolar macrophages or are recycled in type II epithelial cells; the recycling process depends at least partly on SP-D, which enhances uptake of surfactant lipids by type II epithelial cells. Maintenance of the surface film is a highly dynamic process that requires integration of synthesis and assembly, secretion, recycling, and degradation. Dysregulation can lead to alterations in the size, composition, or both of the alveolar surfactant pool, resulting in pulmonary alveolar proteinosis (PAP—surfactant accumulation) or (RDS—surfactant insufficiency). Thus, sensing the size and composition of the alveolar surfactant is essential for alveolar homeostasis.

COMPOSITION OF SURFACTANT

The composition of pulmonary surfactant is, in general, well conserved among diverse species. The general composition of mammalian surfactant[32,33] is represented in Fig. 75.4. Surfactant is composed primarily of phospholipid (predominantly PCs), which represents approximately 80% to 90% of its mass; proteins generally contribute less than 10% of its mass. Lesser amounts of glycolipids and neutral lipids are detected in approximately equal amounts. Phospholipid is the primary surface tension–lowering component of pulmonary surfactant. The phospholipids form multilayered sheets that are derived from tubular myelin or other aggregate forms present in the alveolus. PC is uniquely enriched in disaturated forms of dipalmitoylphosphatidylcholine (Fig. 75.5). In human surfactant isolated from lung minces, PC represents 80% of the total phospholipid, of which 70% is present as the palmitoylphosphatidylcholine; 55% of this lipid species is in the form of disaturated palmitic acid acyl groups or DSPC. Phosphatidylglycerol is also uniquely enriched in pulmonary surfactant, generally representing 5% to 10% of surfactant phospholipids. Phosphatidylglycerol also is capable of reducing surface tension at an air-liquid interface; however, its precise role in surfactant function remains unclear. Other phospholipids, including phosphatidylinositol, phosphatidylserine, phosphatidylethanolamine, lysophosphatidylcholine, and sphingomyelin, are present in relatively low amounts in pulmonary surfactant. Glycolipids also are present in pulmonary surfactant and have been partially characterized in rabbit surfactant. Neutral lipids are present primarily as cholesterol esters and acylglycerol fatty acids. The biologic functions of these components, present in relatively low amounts, have not been determined with certainty.[13,14,32,33]

The molecular structures of PC and phosphatidylglycerol are represented in Fig. 75.5. Several aspects of their structures are critical for surface tension reduction at the alveolar-air interface. Each molecule consists of a three-carbon glycerol backbone. The C_1 carbon is modified by the addition of polar head groups (relatively more hydrophilic residues). In the case of pulmonary surfactant, the most abundant head groups are

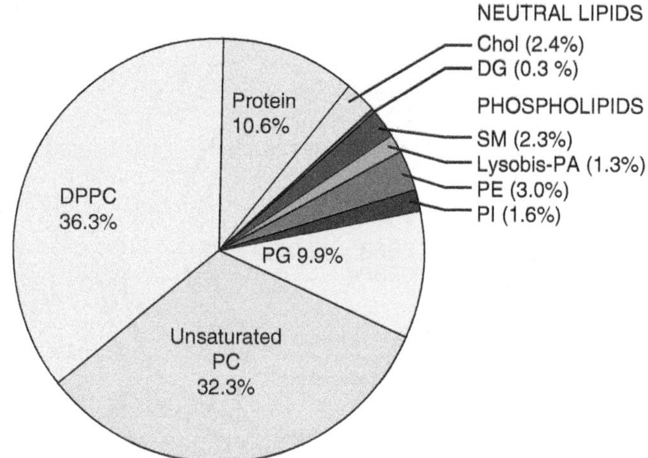

Fig. 75.4 Composition of bovine pulmonary surfactant obtained from lung lavage fluid. Components are expressed as % wt. *Chol,* Cholesterol; *DG,* diacylglycerol; *DPPC,* dipalmitoylphosphatidylcholine; *PA,* phosphatidic acid; *PC,* phosphatidylcholine; *PE,* phosphatidylethanolamine; *PG,* phosphatidylglycerol; *PI,* phosphatidylinositol; *SM,* sphingomyelin. (Modified from Possmayer F, Yu SH, Weber JM, et al. Pulmonary surfactant. *Can J Biochem Cell Biol.* 1984;62:1121.)

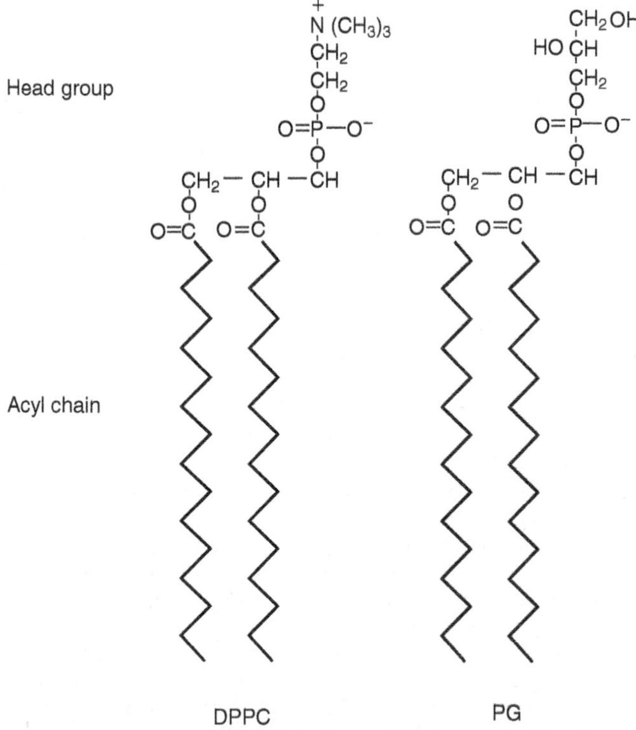

Fig. 75.5 Molecular structures of dipalmitoylphosphatidylcholine *(DPPC)* and phosphatidylglycerol *(PG)*. Phospholipid molecules pack densely, forming membrane monolayers, bilayers, and vesicles and other aggregate forms. Strong molecular interactions occur between polar head groups. Distinct interactions occur between atoms composing the more hydrophobic acyl chains. These lipids interact closely with surfactant proteins (SP)-B and SP-C, pack tightly, and spread at the alveolar surface to reduce surface tension.

choline and glycerol. The C_2 and C_3 carbons of the glycerol backbone contain acyl groups of long-chain fatty acids, which are highly hydrophobic and lacking in significant charge. The polar head groups—choline, glycerol, and inositol—of the phospholipids produce charge-dependent interactions among neighboring phospholipid molecules and with water. By contrast, the acyl groups are energetically more stable in a nonaqueous environment and are tightly associated with neighboring phospholipid molecules by interactions between carbon and hydrogen atoms of the acyl chains. Hence these molecules are inherently insoluble in aqueous environments and form a variety of complex structures that include membrane monolayers, bilayers, multilayers, micelles, inverted micelles, and vesicles.

The surface properties of surfactant phospholipids (spreading, stability, and surface tension reduction) are influenced by a number of factors, including the SP SP-B and SP-C, and the degree of saturation of the acyl chains, which alter the tightness of packing of phospholipid molecules in membranes. The surface activity of surfactant is readily inhibited by serum proteins, blood, edema fluid, or non-SP derived from lung injury, so maintenance of alveolar-capillary stability is critical for maintaining surfactant function. The fatty acid composition of the phospholipids in pulmonary surfactants has been determined for various species.[14] The structure of the acyl chains and the composition of the major phospholipids are important determinants of the organization of the membranes. PC isolated from pulmonary surfactant is uniquely enriched in forms with disaturated palmitic acid (C16) acyl chains. Enrichment of these phospholipid species at the surface results in densely packed lipid sheets, creating an interface with extremely low surface tension. Saturated acyl chains contain no methylene (C = C) bonds, and the carbon atoms are fully hydrogenated. Membranes containing such lipids pack densely through the hydrophobic interactions of the acyl chains. The ordering of phospholipid molecules in the surfactant membrane also is highly dependent on temperature. Surfactant lipids are present in a gel or crystalline state at the physiologic temperatures of homeothermic organisms because the transition temperature (temperature of melt) of DPPC is approximately 41°C. Therefore, DPPC would be present in a relatively rigid state at 37°C. However, the presence of minor lipids, proteins, and unique phospholipid acyl chains alters the packing characteristics of the phospholipids. The relative abundance of the major lipid classes and their acyl chain length and specific composition, including the proportion of molecular species with unsaturated acyl chains, therefore result in a unique pulmonary surfactant mixture that may alter the surface properties of the surfactant film. The characteristics of rapid adsorption and stability during compression of pulmonary surfactant are not properties inherent in the phospholipids alone, but require the presence of the SP SP-B and SP-C. The hydrophobic SP SP-B and SP-C are required for full surface-active properties of the lipids in surfactant and are active components of surfactant replacement preparations used to prevent or treat RDS in preterm infants.[34]

COMPOSITION OF LAMELLAR BODIES

Surface-active material can also be isolated from its primary intracellular storage site in LBs of alveolar type II cells. LBs are lysosomal-like organelles highly enriched in phospholipids, generally containing approximately 10 to 12 mg of phospholipid per mg of protein. A diversity of proteins are present in the LBs as identified by mass spectroscopy.[35] The limiting membrane of the lamellar body contains at least one ABC transporter, ABCA3, which plays an important role in importing phospholipids into the lamellar body. Mutations in the ABCA3 transporter block the formation of LBs and cause severe lung disease in newborn infants.[15,17] Lipid composition of LBs is similar to that for surfactant isolated from lung lavage fluid. The active, fully processed SP-B and SP-C peptides are highly enriched in LBs and are co-secreted with phospholipids into the air space. Like ABCA3, mutations in the genes encoding SP-B and SP-C (*SFTPB* and *SFTPC*) cause severe lung disease in neonates and infants.[15]

DEVELOPMENTAL CHANGES IN PHOSPHOLIPID COMPOSITION

The phospholipid composition of alveolar lavage material changes during perinatal development. Increased phospholipid synthesis and secretion occur with advancing gestation and are influenced by a variety of hormonal and cellular factors. Because pulmonary secretions contribute a significant volume to amniotic fluid, increased phospholipid in amniotic fluid accompanying advancing gestation has been used for determining the relative maturity of the fetal lung and thus predicting the risk of RDS in premature infants. The PC content of amniotic fluid increases during the last third of human gestation. The ratio of lecithin (PC) to sphingomyelin, otherwise known as the *L/S ratio*, has been useful in the clinical assessment of risk for RDS.[36] Surfactant content in amniotic fluid can be determined by a number of procedures that predict pulmonary maturity. Various amniotic fluid assays are useful in predicting surfactant function or lack of respiratory distress in preterm infants, including the L/S ratio; lamellar body counts; quantitation of phosphatidylglycerol, DSPC, or PC; and fluorescence anisotropy. Changes in total phospholipid content and in the relative abundance of phospholipid species also accompany respiratory failure in infants and adults.

ISOLATION OF PULMONARY SURFACTANT

Surface-active material usually is isolated by differential sedimentation of material collected by washing the lung with isotonic saline solutions. Centrifugation at low forces is used to remove mononuclear cells, which in the normal lung are primarily alveolar macrophages. Some surface-active material—specifically, large tubular myelin forms—generally sediments at low gravitational forces. Higher-speed centrifugation or buoyant density separation is then used to isolate subfractions of surfactant containing various physical forms. The dense, tubular myelin-rich material (large aggregate surfactant) is enriched in surfactant-associated proteins SP-A, SP-B, and SP-C and is highly active as a pulmonary surfactant. Less surface-active fractions containing primarily smaller or less dense vesicular forms (small aggregate forms) are relatively depleted of protein and are less surface-active than tubular myelin. SP-D is relatively enriched in the small lipid aggregate fraction that represents catabolic products generated during the respiratory cycle and therefore destined for uptake and catabolism by alveolar macrophages or reutilization by type II epithelial cells.

SURFACTANT PROTEINS

Four distinct surfactant-associated proteins have been purified from surfactant and their primary structures discerned. These proteins have been termed *surfactant proteins SP-A, SP-B, SP-C,* and *SP-D* (Table 75.1). Complementary DNAs and genes encoding each surfactant protein have been isolated and characterized. The human genes are termed *SFTPA, SFTPB, SFTPC,* and *SFTPD.* The roles of each of the proteins in surfactant function and pulmonary homeostasis have been clarified in gene-targeted mice and in clinical observations in children and adults (as reviewed

Table 75.1 Mutations in Genes Causing Surfactant Dysfunction.

	SFTPA	*SFTPB*	*SFTPC*	*SFTPD*	*ABCA3*	*CSF2RA* and *CSF2RB*	*NKX2-1*
Chromosome	10	2p11	8p21	10	16p13	Xp22 and 22p12	14q14.3
Protein	SP-A (30-30 KDa)	SP-B (8KDa)	SP-C (38KDa)	SP-D (43 KDa)	ABCA3	CSF2RA and CSF2RB	TTF-1
Primary Functions	Host defense/ tubular myelin	Surface activity	Surface activity	Host defense, surfactant pool size, inflammation	Lipid transport to lamellar body	Alveolar macro-phage function	Transcription factor
Human Mutation Phenotype	Emphysema-adenocarci-noma (adult)	Neonatal RDS, ILD	ILD, RDS	Influenza sus-ceptibility Emphysema; COPD, BPD	Neonatal RDS	Alveolar proteino-sis (PAP)	Brain-lung-thyroid
Pathogenesis	Abnormal SP-A folding	Lack of SP-B and surface activity	Misfolded protein with ER stress	Allele suscepti-bility	Defective phospholip-id transport into LBs	Defective surfac-tant catabo-lism	Abnormal mor-phogenesis and surfactant dysfunction
Usual Histopa-thology	Emphysema	PAP, DIP	Age-related ILD	NA	Age-related ILD	PAP	Diffuse lung disease

BPD, Bronchopulmonary dysplasia; *COPD*, chronic obstructive pulmonary disease; *DIP*, desquamative interstitial pneumonitis; *ER*, endoplasmic reticulum; *ILD*, interstitial lung disease; *LBs*, lamellar bodies; *NA*, not applicable; *PAP*, pulmonary alveolar proteinosis; *RDS*, respiratory distress syndromes; *SP*, surfactant proteins; *TTF*, thyroid transcription factor.

by Whitsett and colleagues[15,37]).The precise abundance of each of the proteins in pulmonary surfactant or surfactant subfractions has not been determined with certainty. Nevertheless, SP-A, SP-B, SP-C, and SP-D account for most of the nonserum proteins present in the lipid-associated fraction isolated from lung lavage.

SURFACTANT PROTEIN A

SP-A is an abundant nonserum lipid-associated protein in pulmonary surfactant. SP-A is a member of a related family of polypeptides termed the *collectins*,[38,39] that includes SP-D, mannose-binding lectin, conglutinin, and collectin-43 (CL-43).[21,22,39] These proteins share collagenous and lectin-containing domains that bind complex carbohydrates (Fig. 75.6). SP-A is a glycoprotein of 26,000 to 35,000 Da that undergoes sulfhydryl-dependent oligomerization and other posttranslational modifications, accounting for the significant molecular heterogeneity of its isoforms in pulmonary surfactant. Two human *SFTPA* genes have been identified, each consisting of five exons contained within approximately 4.5 kilobases (kb) of DNA.The *SFTPA* locus consists of two coding sequences and a noncoding sequence on human chromosome 10. SP-A is expressed primarily in respiratory epithelial cells but has been detected in other organs, including kidney, gastrointestinal tract, and reproductive tract.[40] Mutations in the *SFTPA* gene have been associated with late onset pulmonary fibrosis and adenocarcinoma, related in part to the toxicity of misfolding of the mutant gene product within type II cells.[41] SP-A is first synthesized as a 248 amino-acid precursor peptide from which a small signal sequence is cleaved.The remaining amino-terminal (N-terminal) domain of the mature SP-A peptide contains an extensive collagen-like region of approximately 10,000 Da. A discrete carboxyl-terminal (C-terminal) globular domain is homologous to other mammalian lectins (carbohydrate-binding proteins) and is structurally related to those in SP-D, mannose-binding lectin, and other members of the collectin family of polypeptides.[4] SP-A binds carbohydrates, phospholipids, and glycolipids that are surface components of numerous pathogens, including bacteria, viruses, and fungi.[21,42]

FUNCTIONS OF SURFACTANT PROTEIN A

In vitro and in vivo studies demonstrated a wide variety of biologic activities intrinsic to SP-A (reviewed by Nathan and colleagues[38]). SP-A binds carbohydrates and aggregates phospholipids in a calcium-dependent manner, forms tubular myelin-like structures in vitro, and enhances the biophysical activity of surfactant phospholipid-rich extracts.[43,44] In vitro, SP-A binds type II epithelial cells and macrophages and is internalized by receptor-mediated endocytosis.[45,46] After uptake, SP-A is detected in multivesicular bodies and vesicles within the cell cytoplasm. Receptor binding and internalization support the concept that SP-A is reutilized or is involved in cell signaling. Although in vitro findings support a role for SP-A in surfactant homeostasis, gene targeting experiments in transgenic mice do not support its critical importance in surfactant metabolism in vivo.[20] By contrast, a number of studies support an important role for SP-A in innate host defense of the lung. SP-A is a member of the Ca^{2+}-dependent lectins or "collectins" that serve as opsonins, enhancing binding, phagocytosis, and killing of a variety of bacterial, fungal, and viral pathogens. SP-A enhances binding or uptake of group B streptococci, subtypes of *Haemophilus influenzae, Staphylococcus aureus,* and *Pseudomonas aeruginosa* by alveolar macrophages and is therefore an important defense molecule in the both neonatal and mature lung.[21,47] SP-A activates alveolar macrophages in vitro and enhances their opsonin-type functions, oxidant production, and killing of pathogens.[48]

Transgenic SP-A-deficient mice, *Sftpa* gene-targeted mice, in which the SP-A gene was disrupted by homologous recombination, survive postnatally.[20] Although SP-A deficient mice do not form tubular myelin, intracellular and extracellular surfactant phospholipid content, uptake of PL by lung tissue, PL secretion, as well as surfactant function are not substantially altered by the absence of SP-A.

CONTROL OF SURFACTANT PROTEIN A EXPRESSION

Like other SP, SP-A is synthesized by respiratory epithelial cells in the developing fetal lung, and its expression increases in late gestation. SP-A is detected in nonciliated cells in tracheal bronchial glands, as well as in bronchiolar and alveolar epithelial cells of the lung. In the human, expression of SP-A increases with advancing gestational age in association with the maturation of type 2 epithelial cells occurring in the latter part of gestation. SP-A appears in increasing concentrations in amniotic fluid during advancing gestation and, like the L/S ratio, is a useful marker of

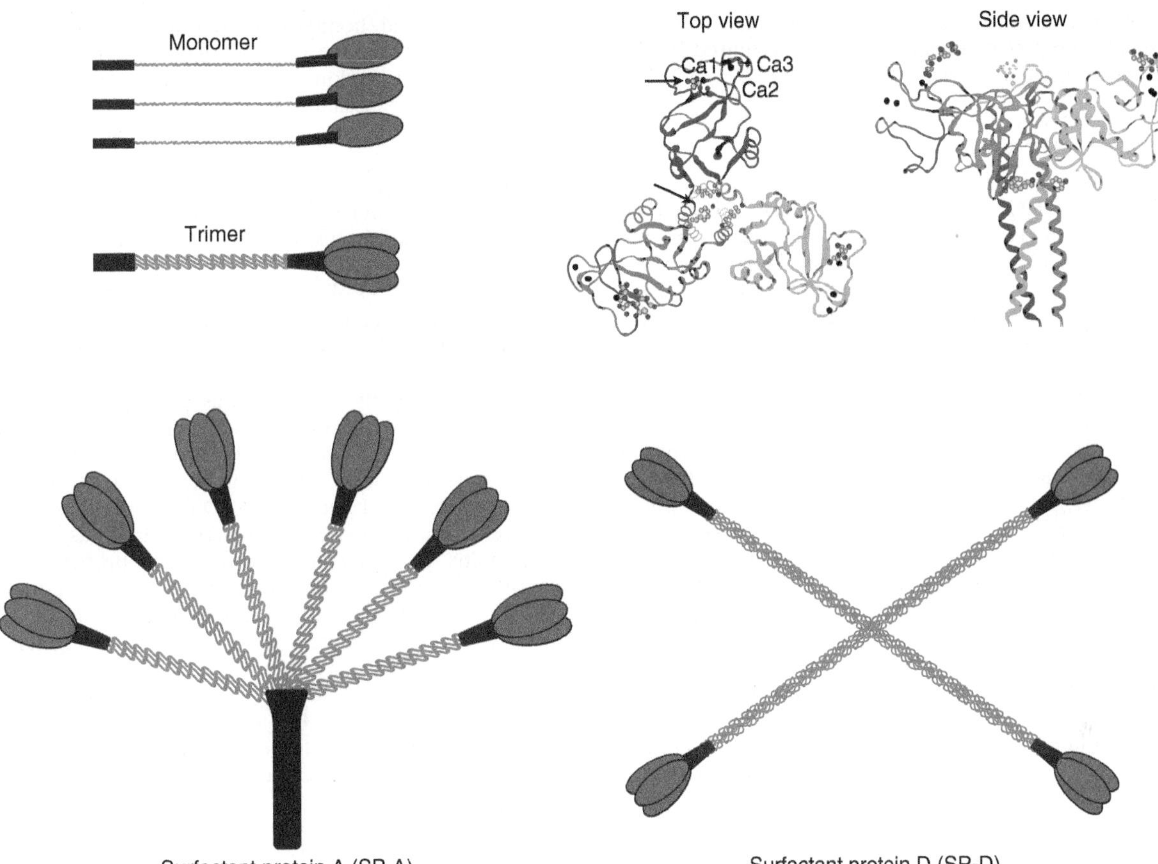

Fig. 75.6 Structure of surfactant proteins (SP)-A and SP-D. Translation of the mRNA from two *SFTPA* genes on chromosome 10 produces an SP-A monomer that forms trimers. Further, oligomerization through the amino-terminal (N-terminal) collagen-like domain *(hatched area)* results in larger assembled forms such as octadecamers found in association with tubular myelin in the alveolus. SP-D is formed by a similar process from a single human *SFTPD* gene locus, also located on chromosome 10; SP-D monomers form trimers that are organized into larger oligomers. Both proteins influence surfactant structure, innate host defense and inflammatory processes in the lung. (Adapted from Watson A, Phipps MJS, Clark HW, et al: Surfactant proteins A and D: trimerized innate immunity proteins with an affinity for viral fusion proteins. *J Innate Immun.* 2019;11:13–28.)

fetal lung maturity in humans.[49] SP-A synthesis in human fetal lung cultures is enhanced by a number of hormonal factors, including epidermal growth factor, interferon-γ, interleukin-1β, and cyclic adenosine monophosphate (cAMP),[50,51] and is inhibited by tumor necrosis factor (TNF)-α and transforming growth factor-β. Glucocorticoids both stimulate and inhibit human SP-A synthesis by distinct mechanisms, which include transcriptional enhancement and decreased messenger RNA (mRNA) stability in vitro.[52] Transcription of the *SFTPA* gene encoding SP-A is regulated by elements located in the 5′ region of the gene that bind to thyroid transcription factor-1 (TTF-1), a homeodomain-containing member of the NKX family of proteins that is inhibited by miR-199a/miR214.[53] Binding of TTF-1 confers lung epithelial specificity to *SFTPA* gene transcription.TTF-1 also regulates the transcription of a number of genes expressed selectively in the respiratory epithelium including *SFTPA, SFTPB*, and *SFTPC* and *SCGB1a1,* the latter encoding the club cell secretory protein (CCSP).[54] Mouse studies support the concept that increased fetal lung *SFTPA* prior to birth influences the timing of parturition.[55]

In summary, SP-A, encoded by two human genes (*SFTPA1* and *SFTPA2*), is an abundant pulmonary host defense protein that is strongly associated with surfactant phospholipids and is required for formation of tubular myelin. SP-A plays important roles in innate defense against bacterial, fungal, or viral pathogens, enhancing opsonization and killing of respiratory pathogens by alveolar macrophages.[56]

SURFACTANT PROTEIN D

SP-D is another member of the collectin family of polypeptides, sharing structural motifs with SP-A and other family members.[21,47] A single human SP-D gene *(SFTPD)* is located in close proximity to the SP-A genes on chromosome 10. *SFTPD* allelic variants resulting in decreased SP-D have been associated with severity of emphysema in patients with chronic obstructive lung disease and a number of alleles of *SFTPD* are associated with severity of neonatal lung disease.[57,58] SP-D is slightly larger than SP-A, being composed of 43-kDa monomers containing an approximate 15,000-kDa collagenous region that forms trimers and higher-ordered complexes that are found in the alveoli (see Fig. 75.6).[59] Like SP-A, SP-D expressed primarily in respiratory epithelial cells but is also expressed in many tissues. For example, SP-D mRNA and protein have been detected in various organs, including the gastrointestinal tract, pancreas, bile duct, cervical glands, and other sites.[40,60] In the lung, SP-D is highly expressed by type II epithelial cells in the alveoli, but it is also expressed in nonciliated bronchiolar and tracheal-bronchial epithelial cells, including cells lining tracheal-bronchial glands. SP-D is associated with small lipid vesicles (small aggregate surfactant) and is not required for the formation of tubular myelin or LBs.

ROLE OF SURFACTANT PROTEIN D IN INNATE HOST DEFENSE OF THE LUNG AND REGULATION OF SURFACTANT HOMEOSTASIS

The C terminus of SP-D consists of a globular carbohydrate recognition domain (CRD) that binds molecules on the surface of bacterial, viral, and fungal pathogens. SP-D has high affinity for various bacterial lipopolysaccharides (LPSs), complex carbohydrates, and phosphoinositol.[21] SP-D binds and agglutinates various bacteria (including *Escherichia coli*, *Salmonella*, and *Pseudomonas*), fungal, as well as viral pathogens (influenza virus A, adenovirus, and respiratory syncytial virus), enhancing their uptake and killing by alveolar macrophages.[21,47] Thus SP-D serves an important role in pathogen recognition critical to innate defense of the lung against infection. In vivo, SP-D–deficient (*Sftpd* gene-targeted) mice are susceptible to various bacterial and viral pathogens. SP-D enhances the clearance and suppresses inflammatory responses following viral and bacterial infection of the lung. SP-D also plays important roles in the regulation of surfactant phospholipid pool size and in the suppression of oxidant production by alveolar macrophages in the lung; deletion of SP-D in transgenic mice causing spontaneous emphysema, macrophage activation, accumulation of oxygen reactive species, and a pulmonary lipidosis.[61] Alveolar and tissue surfactant lipid pool sizes were markedly increased in the absence of SP-D. Thus SP-D plays a critical role in the regulation of surfactant lipid homeostasis, the inflammatory responses, and innate host defense of the lung. Because SP-D regulates inflammation and cytokine responses after exposure to various pulmonary pathogens, it also is highly likely that SP-D influences subsequent acquired immune responses after infection or exposure to inhaled antigens. Serum and bronchoalveolar lavage fluid (BALF) SP-D concentrations are used as biomarkers for a number of acute and chronic lung disease, including chronic obstructive pulmonary disease (COPD) and pulmonary fibrosis.[62]

REGULATION OF SURFACTANT PROTEIN D

SP-D is expressed at high levels in the lung, where it is regulated by C/EBPα (*C*CAAT/*e*nhancer-*b*inding *p*rotein-α), nuclear factor of activated T cells (NFAT), and TTF-1.[63] SP-D also is expressed in many other organs and in various cell types.[60] SP-D content in fetal lung and amniotic fluid increases with advancing gestational age, and its content is enhanced by glucocorticoids in experimental models. SP-D content is enhanced by allergens and interleukin (IL)-4 and IL-13. SP-D concentrations in alveolar fluid are decreased in various clinical conditions associated with pneumonitis, including cystic fibrosis and bronchopulmonary dysplasia in preterm infants. Like other surfactant components, SP-D accumulates in the lungs from patients with autoimmune and hereditary PAP associated with GM-CSF signaling defects and silicosis.

SURFACTANT PROTEIN B

SP-B is a small hydrophobic polypeptide comprising 79 amino acids (Fig. 75.7). SP-B structure and function were reviewed in

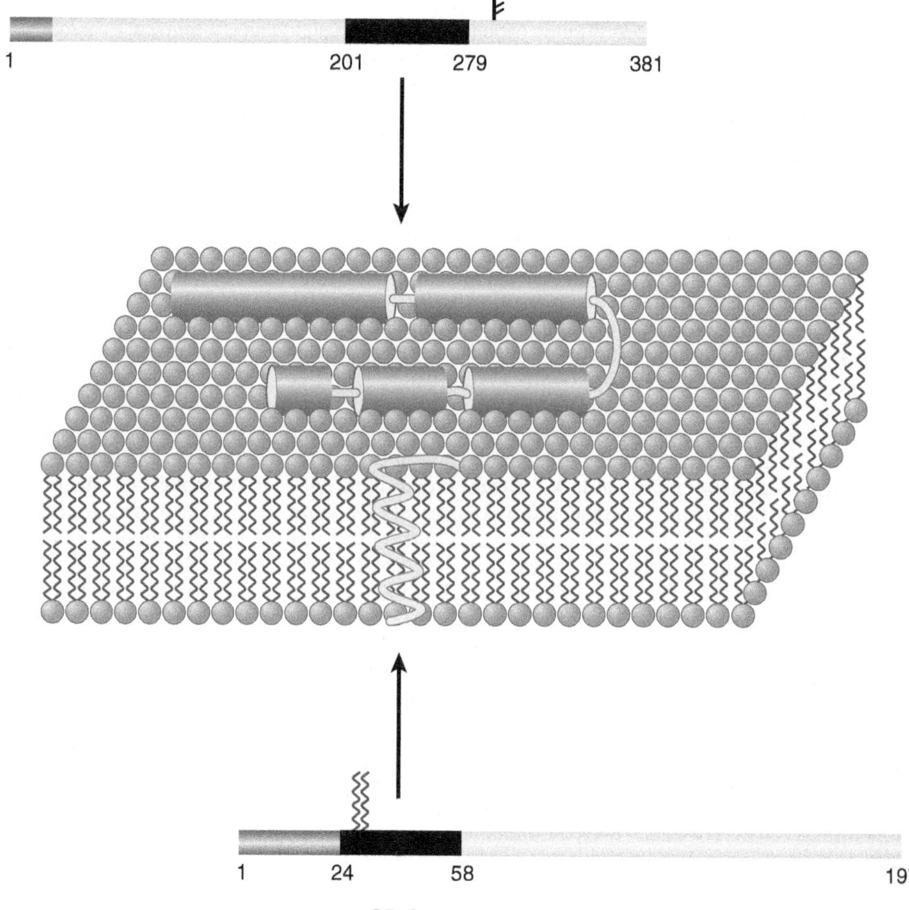

Fig. 75.7 cDNA and processing human surfactant proteins *(SP)*-B and SP-C. The *SFTB* gene comprises approximately 9.5 kb of genomic DNA located on human chromosome 2, which encodes the SP-B pre-proprotein that is proteolytically processed to produce the active SP-B peptide of 79 amino acids. The messenger RNA (mRNA) is approximately 2.0 kb in length and is translated to a preproprotein of approximately 39,000 Da that is proteolytically processed and glycosylated during transport to lamellar bodies. The active peptide is generated from proSP-B during proteolytic processing to form the 79–amino acid peptide (M_r of 8000), which forms oligomers that are tightly associated with phospholipids in the airway. Human SP-C is encoded by the *SFTPC* gene located on chromosome 8 that comprises approximately 3.5 kb of genomic DNA. The active peptide, of 35 or 36 amino acids, is encoded by a single exon and is palmitoylated. The mRNA is approximately 0.9 kb long and is translated to proSP-C (M_r of approximately 22,000), which is proteolytically processed to an M_r = 3800 monomer, and its oligomers found in the airway. SP-B and SP-C are tightly associated with phospholipid membranes in the alveolus and enhance spreading and stability of the surfactant at the alveolar surfaces. M_r, Molecular weight.

detail by Weaver and Conkright.[64] A single human SP-B gene *(SFTPB)* is composed of 10 exons, spanning approximately 10 kb of DNA located on chromosome 2.[65] Analysis of cDNAs encoding SP-B demonstrate that the SP-B polypeptide is produced by proteolytic processing of an approximately 40,000- to 46,000-Da glycosylated precursor comprising 381 amino acids. The active peptide found in the airway forms sulfhydryl-dependent oligomers that include dimers and tetramers. Proteolytic processing of the precursor proSP-B occurs in type II epithelial cells, during routing of the proSP-B from ER to multivesicular bodies and during transport from multivesicular body (MVB) and LBs before secretion. ProSP-B is expressed in both conducting airway and alveolar epithelial cells but is fully processed to the active SP-B peptide only in alveolar type II cells. Both SP-B and proSP-B are saposin-like proteins that have innate host defense functions against lung pathogens.[66] Immunostaining with antibodies generated against SP-B co-localize with apical intracellular inclusions in type II cells and stain material in the lumen of alveolar and airway structures. Although the biophysical mechanisms underlying the functions of SP-B have not been elucidated with certainty, SP-B is tightly associated with surfactant phospholipids and is required for formation of tubular myelin in the presence of SP-A, phospholipids, and calcium.[44] SP-B is highly fusogenic, generating phospholipid membranes from vesicular lipid forms and enhancing spreading and stability of surfactant. A model by which SP-B oligomers interact with phospholipid membranes to enhance lipid fusion and surface activity was recently proposed.[67] SP-B is required for conversion of vesicular lipids in the lumen of multivesicular bodies to the tightly packed membrane sheets observed in the LBs. Although SP-B enhances the uptake of phospholipid vesicles by type II epithelial cells in vitro, when present with SP-A, SP-B enhances formation of tubular myelin, a form of surfactant that remains in the alveolus. SP-B is critical for the enhancement of surface properties of surfactant phospholipids and is an important component of surfactant replacement mixtures made by organic solvent extraction of pulmonary surfactant or lung minces. Synthetic peptides with amphipathic structures based or that of SP-B are being developed for surfactant replacement preparations for clinical use in treatments of RDS.[68]

SURFACTANT PROTEIN B IS REQUIRED FOR LUNG FUNCTION AT BIRTH: HEREDITARY SP-B DEFICIENCY

Studies in SP-B gene *(Sftpb)*-targeted mice, and in full-term infants bearing mutations in *SFTPB*, demonstrated that SP-B is required for pulmonary function at birth.[15,30,69,70] Although pulmonary structure is normal, mice lacking SP-B die in respiratory distress immediately after birth. Decreased lung volumes, lack of hysteresis, and atelectasis were associated with the lack of LBs and accumulation of aberrant multivesicular bodies with type II cells. Decreased surfactant activity, lack of tubular myelin, and the synthesis of an abnormal proSP-C precursor demonstrated that SP-B is required for both intracellular and extracellular routing of surfactant lipids and proteins. Full-term human infants with mutations in *SFTPB* generally develop respiratory distress within hours after birth, with clinical and radiologic features typical of RDS in preterm infants. Respiratory failure is progressive and is not responsive to exogenous surfactant replacement therapy, affected infants dying of respiratory failure despite intensive ventilatory support. In SP-B–deficient infants, alveolar spaces are filled with proteinaceous material that consists primarily of SP and abnormally processed proSP-C. SP-B deficiency is inherited as an autosomal recessive disorder and is usually fatal in the first months of life but has been treated by lung transplantation. The diagnosis can be made prenatally or postnatally by sequencing the *SFTPB* gene. In summary, SP-B is required for packaging and processing of surfactant lipids and proteins intracellularly and for organization, function, and homeostasis of surfactant lipids and proteins in the alveolar space.

REGULATION OF EXPRESSION OF SURFACTANT PROTEIN B

The abundance of SP-B mRNA increases with advancing gestation in the human fetal lung, being expressed in both type II alveolar cells and nonciliated respiratory epithelial cells lining distal portions of the respiratory tract. In fetal lung, SP-B synthesis is stimulated by cAMP, IL-1β, glucocorticoids, and LPS.[50,51] The concentration of SP-B in human amniotic fluid increases with advancing gestation in association with increased L/S ratio and phosphatidylglycerol.[71] As with other SP, SP-B expression is regulated by a complex transcriptional network in which the homeodomain-containing nuclear protein TTF-1 plays a critical role.[5,6,54,63]

SURFACTANT PROTEIN C

SP-C is the most hydrophobic protein isolated from pulmonary surfactant (see Fig. 75.7). Like SP-A and SP-B, SP-C is relatively abundant in the dense surfactant fractions obtained by lung lavage. SP-C consists of only 34 to 35 amino acids, most of which are hydrophobic residues valine, leucine, and isoleucine, creating an α-helical domain that interacts within surfactant acyl chains in phospholipids (reviewed by Weaver and Conkright[64]). In humans, the *SFTPC* gene comprises approximately 3 kb of contiguous DNA and consists of six exons located on chromosome 8.[72] The precursor, proSP-C, contains neither an N-terminal signal sequence nor amino acid sequences predicting the addition of asparagine-linked carbohydrate. SP-C is palmitoylated and is transported as a pre-protein through the ER to multivesicular bodies with proSP-B; its folding and routing being dependent upon the C-terminal brichos domain.[15,64] Both proSP-C and proSP-B are proteolytically processed during transport to LBs, SP-B being required for normal proteolytic processing of proSP-C. The active 35-amino acid SP-C peptide is stored in LBs and is associated with surfactant lipid secreted into the alveolus. In the lung, synthesis of SP-C is restricted to type II alveolar cells.

SP-C or mixtures of SP-B and SP-C enhance the rate of absorption of surfactant phospholipids and confer important surfactant-like properties to the lipids.[73] Evidence from studies in *Sftpc* gene-targeted mice demonstrates that SP-C is not required for formation of LBs or tubular myelin but is required for optimal surface activity.[31] SP-C is taken up by alveolar epithelial cells; addition of SP-C peptides enhances uptake of phospholipid vesicles by type II epithelial cells in vitro.[74] SP-C is highly enriched in organic solvent extracts of surfactant and, like SP-B, is present in the surfactant extracts used for replacement therapy of RDS in infants.

ROLE OF SURFACTANT PROTEIN C IN SURFACTANT FUNCTION AND HOMEOSTASIS

Studies in SP-C gene–targeted mice and in humans bearing mutations in the SP-C gene demonstrate the important role of SP-C in surfactant function and pulmonary homeostasis.[73] Although SP-C gene–targeted mice survive perinatally, abnormalities in the stability of surfactant film formed from SP-C–deficient mice demonstrate the role of SP-C in recruiting phospholipids to monolayers/multilayers, as SP-C is required for the stability of phospholipid films during dynamic compression.[31] Formation of LBs and tubular myelin are not perturbed in SP-C deficient mice; however, SP-C–deficient mice develop strain-dependent interstitial lung disease associated with emphysema, epithelial cell dysplasia, and inflammation.[73] In vitro and in vivo studies also support a role for SP-C in innate host defense against both viral and bacterial pathogens.[75] Humans bearing mutations in the SP-C gene *(SFTPC)* develop various forms of acute and chronic pulmonary disease including acute respiratory distress syndrome

(ARDS) and diffuse lung disease.[76,77] *SFTPC* mutations generally are inherited as an autosomal dominant trait with variable penetrance and have been associated with the histopathologic diagnoses of usual interstitial pneumonitis, nonspecific interstitial pneumonitis, and desquamating interstitial pneumonitis.[15,70] Most *SFTPC* mutations occur in the brichos domain of the proprotein that disrupt normal preprotein folding and processing, the abnormal SP-C protein accumulating in type II cells causing cell injury. The diagnosis of SP-C related lung disease is made by identification of the gene mutation by genetic testing.

REGULATION OF SURFACTANT PROTEIN C SYNTHESIS

SP-C synthesis and mRNA content increase in association with type II cell maturation in fetal lung, and its expression is restricted to type II cells in the postnatal lung.[50,51] SP-C mRNA is detected early in embryonic lung development. SP-C mRNA are increased by glucocorticoids and cAMP.[50,51] Like the other SP, the transcription of the *Sftpc* gene in the lung requires TTF-1[54] and is influenced by a number of transcription factors that function together to regulate surfactant production.[5,6]

ROLE OF SURFACTANT PROTEINS IN SURFACTANT REPLACEMENT PREPARATIONS

The structures of each of the major SP are quite distinct, supporting the concept that each plays a unique role in the structure and function of surfactant. Surfactant phospholipids themselves, although providing the molecules critical for the reduction of surface tension in the alveolus, do not have the properties inherent in pulmonary surfactant. At physiologic temperatures, surfactant lipid is in a highly organized gel-crystalline state that is not capable of rapidly forming a surface film. Phospholipid molecules alone fail to rapidly spread and respread during compression and decompression. Their adsorption rates to surfaces are slow and do not generate stable surface tension–lowering film necessary to maintain surface forces during the respiratory cycle. SP-B and SP-C interact with surfactant phospholipids to produce surfactant with unique physicochemical properties, allowing formation and stability of the surfactant film during the respiratory cycle.

Both SP-B and SP-C confer important surfactant-like activity to phospholipids and are included in preparations used for treatment of surfactant-deficient states.[78-80] Preparations containing SP-A have not been used widely for clinical studies. Surfactant extracts based on organic solvent extracts of lung or surfactant preparations contain SP-B and SP-C (but not SP-A).[80] Survanta, Curosurf, BLES, and Infasurf are examples of such preparations. SP-B and SP-C, when mixed with phospholipids, appear to be sufficient to generate the surface-active properties of pulmonary surfactant. Synthetic peptides with structures similar to the SP are being studied for surfactant replacement.[68] Protein-free (Exosurf) surfactant preparations were developed but were less active than those containing SP-C and SP-B and are no longer used clinically.

GENETIC DISORDERS OF SURFACTANT HOMEOSTASIS

Mutations in genes encoding the SP SP-B and SP-C (*SFTPB* and *SFTPC*) and the lamellar body-associated lipid transporter protein (ABCA3) are causes of rare, but severe pulmonary disease in newborn infants and children (Table 75.1).[15,70,81] Although each protein has distinct structures and functions, these mutations generally cause acute respiratory failure in newborn infants or chronic interstitial lung disease in children. Pulmonary disease caused by mutations in *SFTPB* or *ABCA3* are inherited as autosomal recessive genes. These infants are generally born at term and present in the immediate neonatal period with progressive respiratory failure. Clinical and radiologic abnormalities are consistent with respiratory distress, and the infants typically fail to respond to surfactant replacement therapy and supportive care. Inheritance of a single *ABCA3* mutation allele is associated with increased risk for RDS in late preterm infants.[82]

While adults with single mutant alleles do not have a higher incidence of lung disease, histopathologic analysis of lung tissue from patients with mutations in *SFTPB*, *SFTPC*, or *ABCA3* reveals interstitial lung disease, consistent with chronic pneumonitis of infancy, nonspecific interstitial pulmonary disease, or desquamating interstitial pneumonitis. Abnormalities in surfactant lipid content associated with these disorders include decreased PC and phosphatidylglycerol content. Most patients with mutations in *SFTPC* present with the respiratory signs and symptoms later in infancy, but some have been symptomatic at birth. These mutations cause the synthesis of a misfolded or misrouted protein that in turn causes alveolar type II cell injury, disrupting the production of the active SP-C peptide. Although *SFTPC* mutations may be associated with disease manifestations in the newborn period, most affected patients present in infancy or childhood with chronic respiratory disease, often exacerbated by respiratory infection. Clinical, histopathologic, and immunohistochemical criteria are useful for identifying patients with disorders of surfactant homeostasis. Definitive diagnosis of mutations disrupting surfactant homeostasis requires their identification by gene sequencing.

The association of mutations in genes critical for surfactant homeostasis with acute and chronic interstitial or diffuse lung disease has enabled definitive clinical diagnoses and genetic counseling for infants and families. The heightened clinical awareness of the importance of genetic causes of pulmonary disorders previously considered idiopathic has led to the identification of a number of gene mutations associated with lung disease in infants. Mutations in *NXX2-1* (*TTF1*), a transcription factor regulating transcription of *ABCA3* and the surfactant protein genes, causes "brain-lung-thyroid" syndrome associated with severe diffuse lung disease. Other gene mutations causing lung disease in newborn infants include *FOXF1* (causing alveolar capillary dysplasia or ACD), *FGFR2* and *TBX4* (causing acinar-alveolar hypoplasia), and *filamin A* (causing emphysema).[83]

OTHER ALVEOLAR PROTEINS

Two-dimensional gel electrophoresis, sensitive silver staining, and mass spectroscopy reveal thousands of serum and nonserum proteins in BALF from normal individuals and are being used to develop biomarkers of lung diseases. The alveolar fluid contains a number of proteins and lipids that may play a role in host defense: fibronectin, lysozyme, antiproteases, immunoglobulins (particularly immunoglobulin A), defensins, mucins, and club cell proteins. Functional annotations in BALF proteins indicate their role in epithelial injury and repair, inflammation, innate immunity, coagulation, and acquired immune responses.[84] Products from type I and type II epithelial cells, alveolar macrophages, and lymphocytes are likely to contribute to the heterogeneity of proteins found in alveolar lavage fluid from the normal lung; however, the identity and functions of these proteins have not been clarified. It also is increasingly apparent that surfactant homeostasis may be disrupted by the presence of blood or serum proteins, including albumin and fibrin.[85] Thus, homeostatic mechanisms that exclude nonsurfactant proteins from the alveolus are likely to be highly critical for the function of surfactant and thus for gas exchange after birth.

CONCLUSION

Research efforts seeking to understand the pathogenesis of RDS in premature infants led to the elucidation of the structure and function of pulmonary surfactant. The lipids, proteins, and cellular processes mediating the synthesis, packaging, secretion, and function of surfactant were identified, providing new insights into alveolar function and innate defense of the lung. Mechanisms controlling surfactant homeostasis were identified that enabled the prevention and treatment of RDS with antenatal glucocorticosteroids and surfactant replacement therapy that together have enhanced the lives of countless preterm infants.

A complete reference list is available at www.ExpertConsult.com.

SELECT REFERENCES

1. Bernhard W. Lung surfactant. Function and composition in the context of development and respiratory physiology. *Ann Anat*. 2016;208:146-150.
2. Whitsett JA, Kalin TV, Xu Y, et al. Building and regenerating the lung cell by cell. *Physiol Rev*. 2019;99:513-554.
8. Guo M, Du Y, Gokey JJ, et al. Single cell RNA analysis identifies cellular heterogeneity and adaptive responses of the lung at birth. *Nat Commun*. 2019;10:37.
9. Hogan BL, Barkauskas CE, Chapman HA, et al. Repair and regeneration of the respiratory system. Complexity, plasticity, and mechanisms of lung stem cell function. *Cell Stem Cell*. 2014;15:123-138.
11. Dixon CL, Too G, Saade GR, et al. Past and present. A review of antenatal corticosteroids and recommendations for late preterm birth steroids. *Am J Perinatol*. 2018;35:1241-1250.
12. Avery ME, Mead J. Surface properties in relation to atelectasis and hyaline membrane disease. *AMA J Dis Child*. 1959;97:517-523.
13. Agassandian M, Mallampalli RK. Surfactant phospholipid metabolism. *Biochim Biophys Acta*. 2013;1831:612-625.
14. Goss V, Hunt AN, Postle AD. Regulation of lung surfactant phospholipid synthesis and metabolism. *Biochim Biophys Acta*. 2013;1831:448-458.
15. Whitsett JA, Wert SE, Weaver TE. Diseases of pulmonary surfactant homeostasis. *Annu Rev Pathol*. 2015;10:371-393.
17. Beers MF, Mulugeta S. The biology of the ABCA3 lipid transporter in lung health and disease. *Cell Tissue Res*. 2017;367:481-493.
20. Korfhagen TR, Bruno MD, Ross GF, et al. Altered surfactant function and structure in SP-A gene targeted mice. *Proc Natl Acad Sci U S A*. 1996;93:9594-9599.
23. Korfhagen TR, Sheftelyevich V, Burhans MS, et al. Surfactant protein-D regulates surfactant phospholipid homeostasis *in vivo*. *J Biol Chem*. 1998;273:28438-28443.
25. Trapnell BC, Nakata K, Bonella F, et al. Pulmonary alveolar proteinosis. *Nat Rev Dis Primers*. 2019;5:16.
29. Autilio C, Perez-Gil J. Understanding the principle biophysics concepts of pulmonary surfactant in health and disease. *Arch Dis Child Fetal Neonatal Ed*. 2019;104:F443-F451.
30. Clark JC, Wert SE, Bachurski CJ, et al. Targeted disruption of the surfactant protein B gene disrupts surfactant homeostasis, causing respiratory failure in newborn mice. *Proc Natl Acad Sci U S A*. 1995;92:7794-7798.
31. Glasser SW, Burhans MS, Korfhagen TR, et al. Altered stability of pulmonary surfactant in SP-C-deficient mice. *Proc Natl Acad Sci U S A*. 2001;98:6366-6371.
33. Possmayer F, Yu SH, Weber JM, et al. Pulmonary surfactant. *Can J Biochem Cell Biol*. 1984;62:1121-1133.
34. Curstedt T, Halliday HL, Hallman M, et al. 30 years of surfactant research - from basic science to new clinical treatments for the preterm infant. *Neonatology*. 2015;107:314-316.
37. Whitsett JA, Wert SE, Weaver TE. Alveolar surfactant homeostasis and the pathogenesis of pulmonary disease. *Annu Rev Med*. 2010;61:105-119.
50. Ballard PL. Hormonal regulation of pulmonary surfactant. *Endocr Rev*. 1989;10:165-181.
54. Bohinski RJ, Di Lauro R, Whitsett JA. The lung-specific surfactant protein B gene promoter is a target for thyroid transcription factor 1 and hepatocyte nuclear factor 3, indicating common factors for organ-specific gene expression along the foregut axis. *Mol Cell Biol*. 1994;14:5671-5681.
56. Whitsett JA, Alenghat T. Respiratory epithelial cells orchestrate pulmonary innate immunity. *Nat Immunol*. 2015;16:27-35.
61. Wert SE, Yoshida M, LeVine AM, et al. Increased metalloproteinase activity, oxidant production, and emphysema in surfactant protein D gene-inactivated mice. *Proc Natl Acad Sci U S A*. 2000;97:5972-59772000.
64. Weaver TE, Conkright JJ. Function of surfactant proteins B and C. *Annu Rev Physiol*. 2001;63:555-578.
67. Olmeda B, Garcia-Alvarez B, Gomez MJ, et al. A model for the structure and mechanism of action of pulmonary surfactant protein B. *FASEB J*. 2015;29:4236-4247.
69. Nogee LM, Garnier G, Dietz HC, et al. A mutation in the surfactant protein B gene responsible for fatal neonatal respiratory disease in multiple kindreds. *J Clin Invest*. 1994;93:1860-1863.
76. Nogee LM, Dunbar 3rd AE, Wert SE, et al. A mutation in the surfactant protein C gene associated with familial interstitial lung disease. *N Engl J Med*. 2001;344:573-579.
77. Thomas AQ, Lane K, Phillips 3rd J, et al. Heterozygosity for a surfactant protein C gene mutation associated with usual interstitial pneumonitis and cellular nonspecific interstitial pneumonitis in one kindred. *Am J Respir Crit Care Med*. 2002;165:1322-1328.
81. Griese M. Chronic interstitial lung disease in children. *Eur Respir Rev*. 2018;27:170100.
83. Nogee LM. Interstitial lung disease in newborns. *Semin Fetal Neonatal Med*. 2017;22:227-233.
85. Ikegami M, Jobe A, Jacobs H, et al. A protein from airways of premature lambs that inhibits surfactant function. *J Appl Physiol Respir Environ Exerc Physiol*. 1984;57:1134-1142.

Structure and Development of Alveolar Epithelial Cells 76

Henry J. Rozycki | Karen D. Hendricks-Muñoz

INTRODUCTION

The ultimate temporal and morphologic stage of lung development is the formation of millions of gas exchange units, the alveoli.[1] Life is possible without the alveolus; there are few in very premature infants. However, without expansion and maturation of the alveolar population, respiratory function and even survival are likely to be compromised.

In this chapter, the development and unique features of AT1 and AT2 cells are reviewed. The structure of the alveolus is fairly simple. In general, there are type I (AT1) and type II (AT2) alveolar epithelial cells, alveolar macrophages, endothelial cells, and pericytes. The last two are part of the vascular system. Macrophages act to intercept and process foreign material and to initiate and control local inflammatory responses.[2] The AT2, a cuboidal cell located in the alveolar corners, has critical roles in surfactant formation, secretion, and recirculation as well as in innate immunity and alveolar repair.[3] It constitutes 10% to 15% of lung cells and 60% of the cells within the alveolus but covers only some 4% of the alveolar surface. The AT1, which only constitutes about 10% of the total alveolar cells, covers more than 95% of the surface area. It is very large but very flat, resembling a snake after a recent large meal where the nucleus bulges out of the otherwise very thin cell profile. Based on its location, appearance, components, and the changes that occur when it is absent or damaged, the AT1 is believed to be essential for gas exchange as well as for the water and ion homeostasis that helps create the air–liquid interface within the alveolus. The AT1 cell may also have innate immune function.[4]

A cautionary note is warranted regarding the extrapolation of what is observed in the pulmonary development of animals to human lung development, because there are a variety of maturational and perhaps functional differences between species.[5] For instance, in sheep and rabbits, alveolarization is complete at birth. In contrast, marsupials such as the quokka wallaby are born with lungs equivalent to the canalicular stage. Lung development at birth coincides with the saccular stage of development in mice and rats. During human lung development, alveolarization starts 4 weeks before term (40 weeks postmenstrual age) and continues for as long as 2 years after birth, with the ultimate development of 300 to 480 million alveolar subunits.[1]

Whatever the species, the theme of alveolar development is one of thinning of the basement membrane and approximation of the epithelial and endothelial cell layers, with exponential growth of the surface area. This process optimizes gas diffusion and the movement of solutes and water within the air–liquid interface. This structural alveolar interface, in turn, provides the necessary environment for the function of AT2 cell surfactant. It therefore follows that if alveoli are underdeveloped because an individual is born before sufficient thinning and expansion of the surface area has occurred or if subsequent normal development is interrupted by injury from mechanical ventilation and high oxygen levels, significant compromise of normal pulmonary function may occur.

BASEMENT MEMBRANE

Juxtaposed between the airspace and the capillary lumen are the very thin AT1 cells, the endothelial cells, and the basement membrane. Within the alveolus is a thicker basement membrane made up primarily of capillary and alveolar basement membranes and a thinner portion where the membranes essentially fuse into one. Each type covers about 50% of the alveolar walls.[6] Morphologists have also noted interruption of the continuous basement membrane beneath the AT2 cells, permitting direct contact with the endothelium. It is speculated that this structural morphology facilitates the synthetic function and development AT2 cells.[7]

The basement membrane is made up of collagen, heparan sulfate proteoglycans, and laminins. This is not uniform throughout the alveolus. The basement membrane associated with AT2 cells is quantitatively less sulfated than the membrane associated with AT1 cells.[7] Histologically, the basement membrane progressively thins during lung development. It is unclear when the final fused endothelial/epithelial membrane becomes well established. The membrane components also change in the course of development. For example, laminin α-3, -4, and -5 are absent early in gestation, appearing only later, as distal and alveolar structures begin to form.[8]

These modifications may play a role in alveolar epithelial cell differentiation. For instance, in mice lacking laminin α-5, AT2 cells were diminished and AT1 cells absent,[8] whereas loss of type IV collagen had the opposite effect.[9] The addition of heparin (to mimic sulfated proteoglycans) to human AT2 cells in culture increased the expression of FoxA1 and Wnt7A, components of developmental pathways involved in the transdifferentiation of the AT2-to-AT1 cell phenotype, implying that these proteoglycans may have a regulatory role in the process of epithelial differentiation.[10]

THE TYPE I CELL

Before Frank Low's first detailed description of the AT1 cell, histologists generally felt that the capillary endothelium was "naked," separated from the air space only by a noncellular basement extracellular matrix and by noncellular "plaques."[11] Low demonstrated by electron microscopy that these plaques were, in fact, the thin cytoplasm of a large epithelial cell, subsequently called the type I alveolar epithelial cell.[10] Along with its size and shape, it was easily distinguishable from other nearby cell types because of the relative paucity of cytoplasmic organelles away from the nuclear bulge.[12]

Based on its appearance by light microscopy, the recognizable flat AT1 cell is not seen with any consistency before the second half of the canalicular phase, when the cuboidal airway cells at the distal tip of the lung branches begin to flatten and take on the appearance of AT1 cells. This occurs as the extracellular matrix thins, corresponding to the gestational age of clinical viability, which is around 22 to 24 weeks in humans.

In most descriptions of this temporal histologic progression, AT2 cells appear just before the point at which AT1cells can reliably be identified. This was one piece of evidence in support of the model in which AT1 cells are derived from AT2 cells.[13] Another was that in assessments of normal cell proliferation or turnover, it was difficult to see such activity in AT1 cells in contrast to AT2 cells. In 1989, Cheek and colleagues described how freshly isolated adult rat AT2 cells transdifferentiated into AT1 cells[14]; this model has produced significant insights into the molecular mechanisms needed for this differentiation. Perhaps the strongest evidence for the AT2-to-AT1 cell paradigm was the repeated observation that, after lung injury affecting AT1 cells, as by NO_2 or hyperoxia,[15,16] only AT2 cells demonstrate proliferation, and AT2 lineage markers are seen in the reconstituted AT1 cells.

The discovery of cell-specific markers greatly improved our understanding of AT1 biology. Using these cellular markers, cells with AT1 characteristics have been shown to appear in the lung earlier in gestation than previously thought. More recently, techniques such as single-cell RNA sequence analysis and lineage mapping have produced corroborating evidence to refute the concept that the AT1 cell is terminally differentiated, with functions limited to gas and water/solute exchange and that the sole source of the AT1 cell is the AT2 cell.

SOURCES OF AT1-CELL MARKERS

Desai and colleagues demonstrated that before birth there is a bipotent progenitor that expresses AT1 proteins such as T1α and RAGE as well as AT2 markers (SFTPC, MUC1, or CTSH).[17] Subsequently, AT1 cells progressively lose the AT2 markers and start expressing AQP5, whereas the cells leading to the AT2 phenotype stop expressing RAGE and T1α and start expressing proteins like SFTPB and ABCA3. These bipotent progenitors may be similar to the cells described in electron microscopic evaluations of fetal sheep, where cells that had both AT1 and AT2 characteristics were seen during development (Fig. 76.1).[18]

SOURCES OF AT1-CELL LINEAGE ANALYSIS

Using HOPX-promoter lineage mapping, Frank and colleagues showed that in cells labeled at E15.5, equivalent to the pseudoglandular stage, the label stayed within cells expressing AT1 markers through alveolarization.[19] Labeling with an Nkx2-1 promoter, which is expressed earlier in development, these researchers showed that at least half these cells are already committed to one or the other AT cell type. These studies imply that AT1 cell specification starts during branching morphogenesis. In another study, activating a rat podoplanin promoter in embryonic lungs at E12 marked cells carrying T1 markers exclusively at postnatal day 7. The authors speculate that the real earliest day might be as early as E10, based on the time needed for maternal doxycycline administration to activate gene transcription in the fetus.[20]

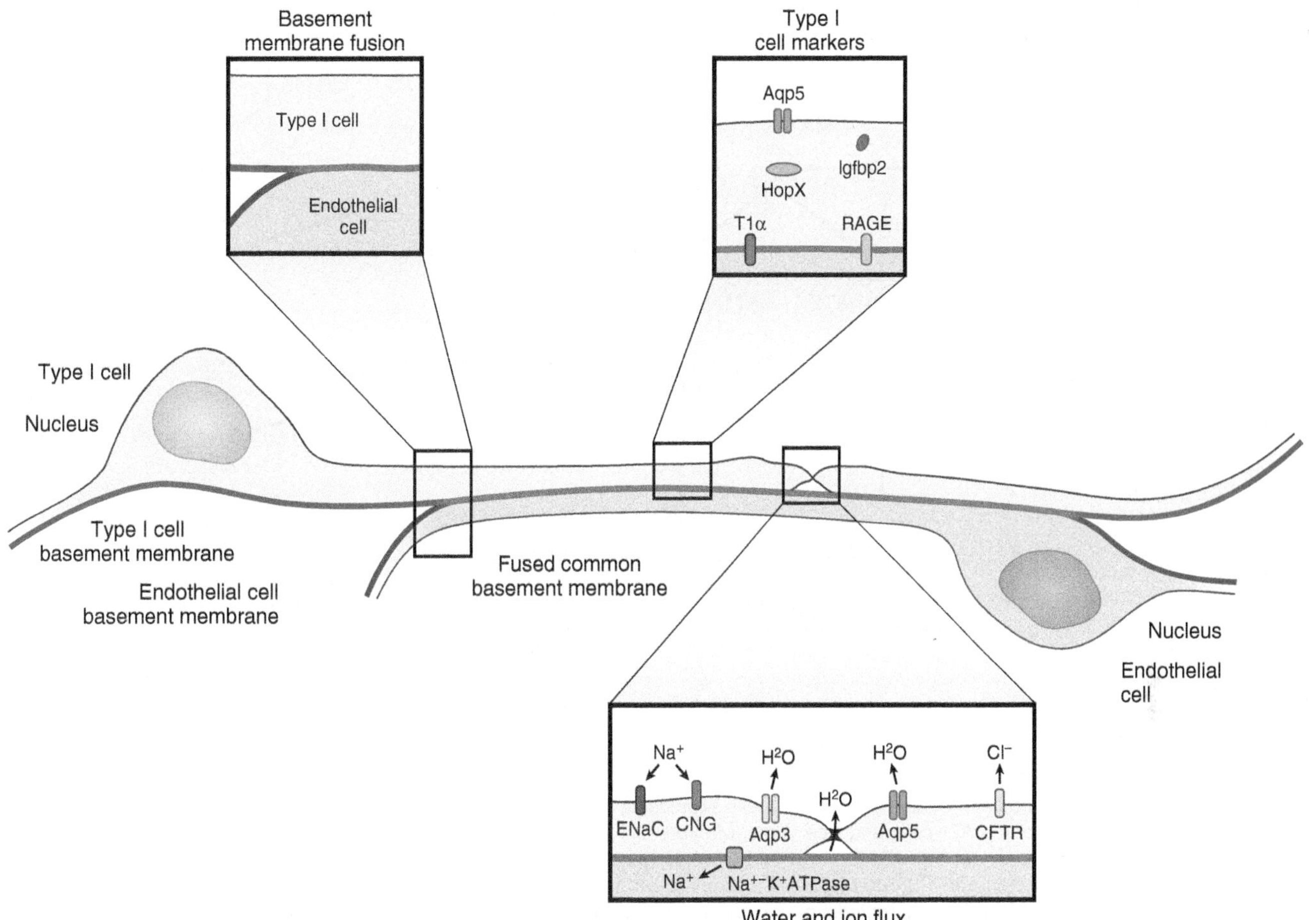

Fig. 76.1 Illustration of the contact between endothelial cells *(pink)* and the type I epithelial cell *(blue)* at the level of the alveolus. Boxes show the fusion of the basement membranes of the two cell types, localization of type 1 cell markers, and type I cell channels for water and ions.

SOURCES OF AT1 SINGLE-CELL RNA SEQUENCING AND MULTIOMICS

Single-cell RNA sequencing, which permits expression analysis of multiple genes from individual cells at various time points, has confirmed the presence of bipotent epithelial progenitors at E16.5, which then begins differentiating into AT1 and AT2 by E18.[21] Investigators from the LungMAP consortium are using multiple techniques—including single-cell RNA sequencing, DNA methylation, miRNA and proteomic analyses, immunofluorescence microscopy, and sophisticated software—to produce perhaps the most comprehensive dataset describing what happens during development. This is available to the public at www.lungmap.net.[22] The conclusions and implications of this massive effort are still being developed but are very likely to provide definitive information in the next few years.

SOURCES OF TYPE I CELLS

Before birth, multi- and bipotent progenitors are the primary sources of AT1 (Fig. 76.2). This progenitor system is not active after birth. AT2 cells are a self-renewing population and have been the presumed source of new AT1 cells, especially after injury. In addition, the bronchiolar epithelial club cell may replenish AT1 and AT2 cells after injury.[23] Additionally, some investigators have found cells that express both club- and AT2-cell characteristics. These cells, termed *bronchial alveolar stem cells (BASCs)*, may give rise to new AT1 and AT2 populations,[24] although this is not consistently observed.[25] Whether these postnatal repair processes are active in the premature infant with acquired lung injury is not yet established.

CONTROL OF DIFFERENTIATION AND DEVELOPMENT

Alveolar epithelial cell proliferation during lung development is an orchestrated event under precise regulatory signal control to generate the needed cell positional identity required for the final airway-alveolar exchange units.[26] For AT1 cells, a large number of molecular chaperone and control systems for both normal development and the postinjury repair of alveolar cells have been identified from whole lung and from the in vitro transdifferentiation of AT2 to AT1 cell phenotype.

A number of studies have found roles for the Wnt/β-catenin system in both the earliest stages of lung development, when the anterior foregut begins to branch, and later when the bipotent progenitor cells appear in the canalicular stage. Bmp-4 is also involved in the pre-AT cell stage, and in in vitro differentiation systems it delays the transition of AT2 to AT1 cells. Control of Bmp-4 signaling is done via Gremlin and Noggin. Members of the Forkhead box (Fox) family have been implicated in epithelial cell differentiation, most prominently FoxA2 but also FoxA1 (see earlier), and the loss of both leads to loss of epithelial cell differentiation. These in vitro studies have identified roles for transforming growth factor-β (promotes differentiation), insulin-like growth factor-1 (stimulates differentiation of AT2 cells to AT1-like cells through activation of Wnt5A),[27] and keratinocyte growth factor (which inhibits transdifferentiation).[28] Increasing attention is also being given to microRNA (miRNA) species in lung development. For example, miRNA375 is implicated in AT2 cell formation; its downregulation in vitro occurs during AT1 differentiation. Increases and decreases in miRNA-142 in

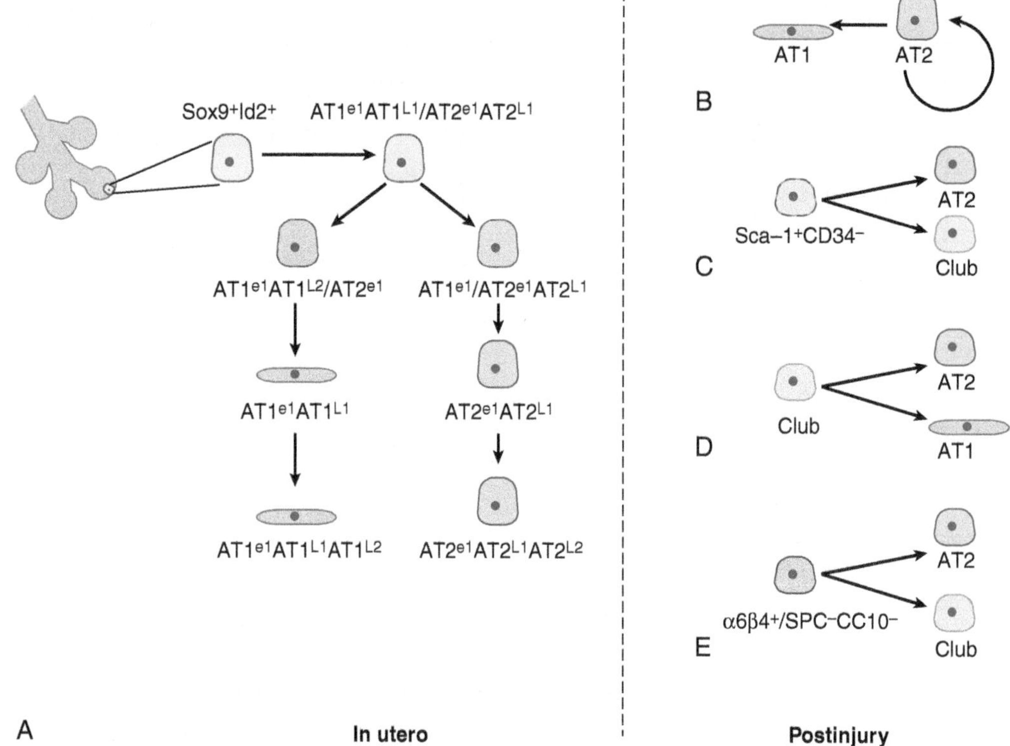

Fig. 76.2 Alveolar cell origins. (A) In utero. Progenitor cells within the budding endoderm after embryonic day (E) 12.5 in mice, which are positive for Sox9 and Id2, give rise to alveolar epithelial cells. By E17, cells expressing both AT1 and AT2 markers are present. The cells that progressively lose AT2 marker expression become AT1 cells and vice versa. Markers are as follows: AT1 e1 (RAGE, LEL [Lycopersicon esculentum lectin], RCA1 [Ricinus communis agglutinin I lectin]); AT1 L1 (T1α); AT1 L2 (AQP5); AT2 e1 (SftpC, Muc1, Ctsh); AT2 L1 (Nkx2.1, SftpB, SftpD); and AT2 L2 (Lyz2, ABCA3, Lamp-1, Lamp-2).[17,32,34] (B) After injury. AT2 cells are self-renewing and give rise to new AT1 cells. (C) Bronchoalveolar stem cells, which have both club- and AT2-cell characteristics, can give rise to both of these cell types after bleomycin injury.[25] (D) Club cells can replenish AT1 and AT2 populations after loss due to bleomycin or influenza.[24] (E) In adult mouse lungs, cells that express neither AT2 nor club cell markers (SPC− CC10−) but do express the integrin receptor α6β4 produce both AT2 and club cells when they are placed into embryonic organ culture and after bleomycin injury.[46]

alveolar progenitor cells increased and decreased the ratio of AT1 to AT1 cells, respectively.[29] More recently, evidence has been presented that most of the signaling systems involved in AT1 development may be under the control of Nkx2-1.[30]

Further knowledge of the similarities and differences in lung alveolar development before birth and epithelial cell response after injury is likely to continue to be important in understanding how premature birth and clinical risk factors for bronchopulmonary dysplasia lead to alveolar maldevelopment.

INNATE IMMUNE FUNCTION

Access to relatively pure populations of AT1 cells in vitro has revealed functions beyond the known ones involving gas exchange and ion and fluid homeostasis. For example, when exposed to endotoxin, AT1 cells produced several hundred-fold higher levels of tumor necrosis factor (TNF)-α, interleukin (IL)-6, and IL-1β than AT2 cells. In this model system, AT2 immune function was restored when macrophages were added to the AT2 cells in culture.[4]

THE TYPE II CELL

Uniquely situated within the alveolar epithelium, the AT2 pneumocyte is poised to contribute to airway stability, oxygen exchange, and immune defense.[3] Morphologically distinct from the AT1 pneumocyte, the cuboidal AT2 cells occupy less than 5% of the alveolar epithelial surface monolayer. Located in the septal corners of the alveolus, AT2 cells are best known for the synthesis, secretion, and recycling of surfactant as well as serving as progenitors to AT1 cells after injury (see earlier). AT2 cells have interfacing properties with the AT1 that are important for lung gas exchange, and they possess proliferative potential important for airway health and repair. Impairment of surfactant production or surfactant insufficiency as occurs during preterm birth or injury leads to severe alveolar compromise and pulmonary dysfunction.

BASIC ORIGINS

The understanding of the basic origins, development, and responses of AT2 cells has improved through studies in mouse cell and molecular biology. It is well recognized that the AT2 cell appears during what is described as the canalicular phase of lung development, which is approximately 16 to 26 weeks in humans and embryonic stages 16.5 to 17.5 days in mice.[3] During the subsequent saccular phase, 24 to 36 weeks (or the second half) of human gestation and embryonic day 17.5 to postnatal day 5 in the mouse, there is further differentiation and maturity of the AT2 cell associated with the ability to produce surfactant. In humans, because the period of alveolar growth continues through 2 years after birth, there is a sensitive period where injury or environmental factors may affect AT2 cells and overall lung development.[1] Although there is limited certainty regarding the exact origins of the AT2 cell, speculations suggest that these cells are derived from a pool of pulmonary progenitor cells that rely on fibroblast growth factor-10 (FGF10) and Wnt signaling factors.[31] These progenitors also give rise to nonciliated precursors of bronchiolar club cells.[32]

DEVELOPMENT

Similar to other differentiated cell types in lung structure development, control of AT2 cell differentiation and maturity is dependent on and responsive to a variety of signaling molecules and their associated receptors. The FGF family of soluble factors (especially FGF10) that often signal epithelial cell tyrosine kinase receptors plays a crucial regulatory role in lung bud development as well as further epithelial cell differentiation. Indeed, knockout deletion of FGF results in agenesis of the lung.[33,34] To achieve alveolar development, sequential interactions with core cell signaling networks, Wnt, Notch, and retinoic acid are crucial to distal lung generation.[31,35,36] Multiple signal antagonists provide feedback that result in pruning and refinement of alveolus. Notably during this developmental period, vascular endothelial growth factor (VEGF), commonly necessary for vascular development, becomes vital for lung airway morphogenesis and long-term maintenance.[37] In a variety of animal and human in vitro studies, AT2 cell growth and differentiation are dependent on VEGF, implicating the precise endothelial and epithelial cell coordination needed during this stage of lung development.[38]

FUNCTIONAL ROLES

Alveolar type II cells perform many critical functions that include production of pulmonary surfactant, stabilization of the airway epithelial barrier, immune defense, and airway regeneration in response to injury.

SURFACTANT

AT2 cells are critical for airway stabilization through the production and release of surfactant, discussed in detail elsewhere. The AT2 is the only pulmonary cell that synthesizes, stores, and secretes all components of pulmonary surfactant, including all four surfactant proteins, important to regulate surface tension, preventing atelectasis and maintaining alveolar fluid balance within the alveolus.[39] AT2 surfactant—produced by cellular classic mechanisms involving the rough endoplasmic reticulum, Golgi apparatus, and multivesicular bodies—is stored within the AT2 cell in specialized storage granules and lamellar bodies whose biochemical composition is reflected in bronchiolar lavage fluid.[40]

HOST DEFENSE

The AT2 cell resides at the air and pulmonary vascular interface and functions in the first line of host defense to protect the airway through a variety of mechanisms.[41] AT2 cells secrete antimicrobial lysozyme, iron-chelating lipocalin, β-defensins, and complement components that assist in pathogen elimination. As components of surfactant produced by the AT2 cell, SP-A and SP-D proteins act as host defense agents, binding to various surface pathogens to promote host pathogen clearance. SP-B protein boosts alveolar macrophage phagocyte function,[42] whereas SP-C is involved in regulating lung inflammation and repair. Additionally, AT2 cells express major histocompatibility complex class II molecules typically found in antigen-presenting cells.[43] Studies further delineate a unique adaptive immune role that AT2 cells play in response to pathogens through the induction of T-cell tolerance. Through antigen presentation, AT2 cells can dampen local pulmonary reactive inflammatory immune responses to inhaled antigens.[44] Finally, AT2 cell sensing of osmotic stress from bacterial pore-forming toxins enables early signals that activate inflammatory host responses to protect the airway.[45]

PROLIFERATIVE POTENTIAL

Postinjury regeneration of AT1 and AT2 epithelial cells within the alveolus has long been thought to originate from AT2 cell replication and proliferation.[13] Evidence now points to a population of bronchiolar alveolar stem cells as an additional source to replenish type I and AT1 cells after injury.[24] Current information implicates the bronchiolar club cell as an additional progenitor of type II and type I cells in response to injury.[23] Finally, a subset of lung cells that are positive for β4 integrin account for up to 10% of the normal total alveolar epithelial population. Residing at the bronchoalveolar junction, they can also proliferate to become AT2 cells.[46]

Proliferation of AT2 cells during development may present directly from a progenitor line, whereas injury that occurs after birth involves other sources and signals. Some studies point to epidermal growth factor receptor signal transduction as an important mediator for postinjury AT2 clonal cell expansion.[46]

CONCLUSION

The final phase of lung development, alveolarization, involves the complex orchestration of the development and proliferation of specialized cells. The large flat type I cells, along with the thin and partially fused basement membrane, create the surface area for gas exchange and alveolar lining fluid. They express unique markers that can be used to isolate and investigate new functions, including the production of proinflammatory mediators. The cuboidal type II cell produces functional surfactant and also supports lung defense through innate immune function. Before birth, both cell types are derived from bipotent progenitors. Several repair and replenishment mechanisms have been described to appear after birth and especially after lung injury, primarily in mice. Because bronchopulmonary dysplasia is due to injury to a lung that would be developing in utero and results in alveolar simplification and diminished numbers of alveolar epithelial cells, some or all of the described development, repair, and regeneration mechanisms likely have roles in the pathophysiology of the disease and the journey to lung recovery.

REFERENCES

1. Burri PH. Fetal and postnatal development of the lung. *Annu Rev Physiol.* 1984;46:617–628.
2. Hussell T, Bell TJ. Alveolar macrophages. Plasticity in a tissue-specific context. *Nat Rev Immunol.* 2014;14:81–93.
3. Fehrenbach H. Alveolar epithelial type II cell. Defender of the alveolus revisited. *Respir Res.* 2001;2:33–46.
4. Wong MH, Johnson MD. Differential response of primary alveolar type I and type II cells to LPS stimulation. *PloS One.* 2013;8. e55545.
5. Zoetis T, Hurtt ME. Species comparison of lung development. *Birth Defects Res (Part B).* 2003;68:121–124.
6. Vaccaro CA, Brody JS. Structural features of alveolar wall basement membrane in the adult rat lung. *J Cell Biol.* 1981;91:427–437.
7. Grant MM, Cutts NR, Brody JS. Alterations in lung basement membrane during fetal growth and type 2 cell development. *Dev Biol.* 1983;97:173–183.
8. Nguyen NM, Kelley DG, Schlueter JA, et al. Epithelial laminin alpha5 is necessary for distal epithelial cell maturation, VEGF production, and alveolization in the developing murine lung. *Dev Biol.* 2006;282:111–125.
9. Loscertales M, Nicolaou F, Jeanne M, et al. Type IV collagen drives alveolar epithelial-endothelial association and the morphogenetic movements of septation. *BMC Biol.* 2016;14:59–79.
10. Apparao KB, Newman DR, Zhang H, et al. Temporal changes in expression of FoxA1 and Wnt7A in isolated adult human alveolar epithelial cells enhanced by heparin. *Anat Rec.* 2010;293:938–946.
11. Low FN. Electron microscopy of the rat lung. *Anat Rec.* 1952;113:437–449.
12. Penney DP. The ultrastructure of epithelial cells of the distal lung. *Int Rev Cytol.* 1988;111:231–269.
13. Uhal BD. Cell cycle kinetics in the alveolar epithelium. *Am J Physiol Lung Cell Molec Physiol.* 1997;272:L1031–L1045.
14. Cheek JM, Evans ME, Crandall ED. Type I cell-like morphology in tight alveolar epithelial monolayers. *Exp Cell Res.* 1989;184:375–387.
15. Evans MJ, Cabral LJ, Stephens RJ, et al. Renewal of alveolar epithelium in the rat following exposure to NO. *Am J Pathol.* 1973;70:175–198.
16. Kapanci Y, Weibel ER, Kaplan HP, Robinson FR. Pathogenesis and reversibility of the pulmonary lesions of oxygen toxicity in monkeys. II. Ultrastructural and morphometric studies. *Lab Invest.* 1969;20:101–118.

17. Desai TJ, Brownfield DG, Krasnow MA. Alveolar progenitor and stem cells in lung development, renewal and cancer. *Nature*. 2014;507:190–194.
18. Flecknoe S, Harding R, Maritz G, Hooper SB. Increased lung expansion alters the proportions of type I and type II alveolar epithelial cells in fetal sheep. *Am J Physiol Lung Cell Mol Physiol*. 2000;278:L1180–L1185.
19. Frank DB, Penkala IJ, Zepp JA, et al. Early lineage specification defines alveolar epithelial ontogeny in the murine lung. *Proc Natl Acad Sci U S A*. 2019;116:4362–4371.
20. Gonzalez R, Leaffer D, Chapin C, et al. Cell fate analysis in fetal mouse lung reveals distinct pathways for TI and TII cell development. *Am J Physiol Lung Cell Mol Physiol*. 2019;317:L653–L666.
21. Pan H, Deutsch GH, Wert SE, et al. Comprehensive anatomic ontologies for lung development. A comparison of alveolar formation and maturation within mouse and human lung. *J Biomed Semantics*. 2019;10:18.
22. Ding J, Ahangari F, Espinoza CR, et al. Integrating multiomics longitudinal data to reconstruct networks underlying lung development. *Am J Physiol Lung Cell Mol Physiol*. 2019;317:L556–L568.
23. Zheng D, Limmon GV, Yin L, et al. Regeneration of alveolar type I and II cells from Scgb1a1-expressing cells following severe pulmonary damage induced by bleomycin and influenza. *PloS One*. 2012;7:e48451.
24. Kim CF, Jackson EL, Woolfenden AE, et al. Identification of bronchioalveolar stem cells in normal lung and lung cancer. *Cell*. 2005;121:823–835.
25. Rawlins EL, Okubo T, Xue Y, et al. The role of Scgb1a1+ Clara cells in the long-term maintenance and repair of lung airway, but not alveolar, epithelium. *Cell Stem Cell*. 2009;4:525–534.
26. Morrisey EE, Hogan BL. Preparing for the first breath: genetic and cellular mechanisms in lung development. *Dev Cell*. 2010;18:8–23.
27. Ghosh MC, Gorantla V, Makena PS, et al. Insulin-like growth factor-I stimulates differentiation of ATII cells to ATI-like cells through activation of Wnt5a. *Am J Physiol Lung Cell Mol Physiol*. 2013;305:L222–L228.
28. Qiao R, Yan W, Clavijo C, et al. Effects of KGF on alveolar epithelial cell transdifferentiation are mediated by JNK signaling. *Am J Respir Cell Mol Biol*. 2008;38:239–246.
29. Shrestha A, Carraro G, Nottet N, et al. A critical role for miR-142 in alveolar epithelial lineage formation in mouse lung development. *Cell Mol Life Sci*. 2019;76:2817–2832.
30. Little DR, Gerner-Mauro KN, Flodby P, et al. Transcriptional control of lung alveolar type 1 cell development and maintenance by NK homeobox 2-1. *Proc Natl Acad Sci U S A*. 2019;116:20545–20555.
31. Liu AR, Liu L, Chen S, et al. Activation of canonical wnt pathway promotes differentiation of mouse bone marrow-derived MSCs into type II alveolar epithelial cells, confers resistance to oxidative stress, and promotes their migration to injured lung tissue *in vitro*. *J Cell Physiol*. 2013;228:1270–1283.
32. Rawlins EL, Clark CP, Xue Y, Hogan BL. The Id2+ distal tip lung epithelium contains individual multipotent embryonic progenitor cells. *Development*. 2009;136:3741–3745.
33. Kotton DN, Morrisey EE. Lung regeneration. Mechanisms, applications and emerging stem cell populations. *Nat Med*. 2014;20:822–832.
34. Herriges M, Morrisey EE. Lung development. Orchestrating the generation and regeneration of a complex organ. *Development*. 2014;141:502–513.
35. Cardoso WV, Lu J. Regulation of early lung morphogenesis. Questions, facts and controversies. *Development*. 2006;133:1611–1624.
36. Tsao PN, Chen F, Izvolsky KI, et al. Gamma-secretase activation of notch signaling regulates the balance of proximal and distal fates in progenitor cells of the developing lung. *J Biol Chem*. 2008;283:29532–29544.
37. Yamamoto H, Yun EJ, Gerber HP, et al. Epithelial-vascular cross talk mediated by VEGF-A and HGF signaling directs primary septae formation during distal lung morphogenesis. *Dev Biol*. 2007;308:44–53.
38. Brown KR, England KM, Goss KL, et al. VEGF induces airway epithelial cell proliferation in human fetal lung *in vitro*. *Am J Physiol Lung Cell Mol Physiol*. 2001;281:L1001–L1010.
39. Hills BA. An alternative view of the role(s) of surfactant and the alveolar model. *J Appl Physiol*. 1999;87:1567–1583.
40. Chevalier G, Collet AJ. *In vivo* incorporation of choline-3 H, leucine-3 H and galactose- 3 H in alveolar type II pneumocytes in relation to surfactant synthesis. A quantitative radioautographic study in mouse by electron microscopy. *Anat Rec*. 1972;174:289–310.
41. Eisele NA, Anderson DM. Host defense and the airway epithelium. Frontline responses that protect against bacterial invasion and pneumonia. *J Pathogens*. 2011;2011:249802.
42. Yang L, Johansson J, Ridsdale R, et al. Surfactant protein B propeptide contains a saposin-like protein domain with antimicrobial activity at low pH. *J Immunol*. 2010;184:975–983.
43. Corbiere V, Dirix V, Norrenberg S, et al. Phenotypic characteristics of human type II alveolar epithelial cells suitable for antigen presentation to T lymphocytes. *Resp Res*. 2011;12:15.
44. Lo B, Hansen S, Evans K, et al. Alveolar epithelial type II cells induce T cell tolerance to specific antigen. *J Immunol*. 2008;180:881–888.
45. Ratner AJ, Hippe KR, Aguilar JL, et al. Epithelial cells are sensitive detectors of bacterial pore-forming toxins. *J Biol Chem*. 2006;281:12994–12998.
46. Chapman HA, Li X, Alexander JP, et al. Integrin alpha6beta4 identifies an adult distal lung epithelial population with regenerative potential in mice. *J Clin Invest*. 2011;121:2855–2862.

77 Regulation of Surfactant-Associated Phospholipid Synthesis and Secretion

Wolfgang Bernhard

INTRODUCTORY REMARKS ON MAMMALIAN SURFACTANT PHOSPHOLIPID ANALYSIS AND FUNCTIONS

Application of the Young-Laplace Equation (1805) by van Neergard in 1929 substantially promoted the understanding of lung physiology, showing that pulmonary retraction is primarily based on surface tension.[1] It took three decades to emphasize its clinical relevance and start the exploration of pulmonary *surface active agent* ("surfactant").[2,3] 1,2-Dipalmitoyl-glycero-3-phosphocholine, also named *1,2-dipalmitoyl-phosphatidylcholine*, DPPC, or PC16:0/16:0 (the term used in this chapter), was found critical to lower surface tension. PC16:0/16:0 is a zwitterionic glycerophospholipid with two straight saturated fatty acids, and a phase transition temperature of 41.5°C, optimal to achieve near-zero minimal surface tension upon lateral compression of air-liquid interfaces. Since then, our knowledge about surfactant function, structure, molecular composition, and metabolism has greatly increased. Advancements in phospholipid analysis significantly contributed to this progress.

Initially, phospholipid classes of lung tissue and lung lavage fluid (LLF) extracts were separated by column or thin layer

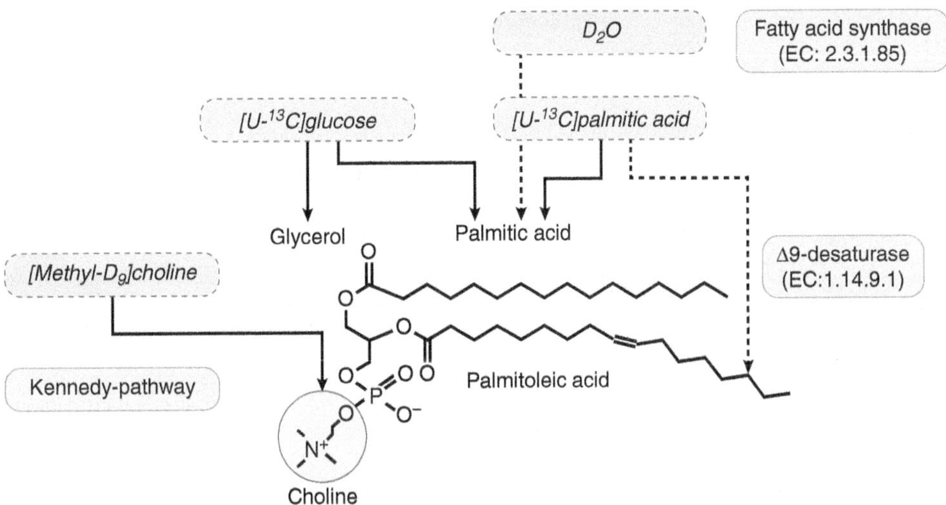

Fig. 77.1 Labeling strategies to address surfactant PC metabolism in human patients. Labeling with deuterated choline ([Methyl-D_9]choline) will address the CDP-choline (Kennedy) pathway of PC synthesis de novo and can be used for pulse-chase labeling approaches. Due to a mass shift of 9 mass units, tandem mass spectrometric analysis is specific for newly synthesized PC species.[13,62] Using labeled fatty acids is less specific because it can be incorporated into many glycerolipids, but allows for the investigation of fatty acid incorporation, desaturation, and elongation.[16,345,348,349] Labeling with deuterated water *(D_2O)* allows assessment of fatty acid synthesis, whereas using ^{13}C-labeled glucose may require sophisticated processing of surfactant PC samples because glucose can be used for the glycerol backbone as well as for fatty acid synthesis. *CDP-choline,* Cytidine-diphosphocholine; *EC,* Enzyme Commission number, *PC,* phosphatidylcholine.

chromatography, followed by gas-chromatographic fatty acid analysis. Techniques of lung tissue explants and culture of type II pneumocytes (also known as *alveolar epithelial type 2 cells [AECII]*) were developed. An approximative technique for quantification of PC16:0/16:0, named *disaturated PC (DSPC)*, was introduced, based on the removal of unsaturated phospholipids with osmium tetroxide (OsO_4).[4] However, Holm and colleagues[5] showed in 1996 that this OsO_4 technique does not reliably remove monounsaturated PC from samples. Moreover, monounsaturated palmitoyl-palmitoleoyl-PC (PC16:0/16:1) was found to be specific for mammalian surfactant.[6,7] Irrespective of such lack of validity, DSPC quantification is still in use.[8,9] However, techniques to quantify intact PC molecular species were developed, using high-performance liquid chromatography.[10,11] Finally, introduction of tandem mass spectrometry and stable isotope labeled precursors allowed for detailed insight into surfactant phospholipid metabolism in patients (Fig. 77.1).[12-16]

SURFACTANT COMPOSITION IN RELATION TO FUNCTION

Glycerophospholipids account for approximately 80% of surfactant. Cholesterol comprises approximately 10% in mammals, but its concentration can rapidly change in hibernating mammals to adapt surfactant function to body temperature.[17] Its origin from lipoproteins suggests that cholesterol may be essential to the developing lung.[18] Glycerophospholipids comprise a charged polar head group and a hydrophobic "tail" of two fatty acyl residues, ideal to form monolayers or multilayers at air-liquid interfaces, thereby reducing surface tension.

The need of low surface tension in terminal pulmonary air spaces is given by the Young-Laplace equation

$$p = \gamma\,(1/r_1 + 1/r_2) \qquad [77.1]$$

for any geometry,[19] where p is pressure, γ is surface tension, and r_1 and r_2 are the radii of curvature. When $r_1 = r_2$ (alveolus), $p = 2\gamma/r$. Consequently, when the alveolar radius decreases at end-expiration, high surface tension would increase the pressure forces required to resist effects of surface tension and cause alveolar collapse. In a tubule (bronchiole), r_2 approximates ∞, resulting in $p = \gamma/r$. Low surface tension is therefore essential to stabilize air-liquid interfaces of alveoli and bronchioles and of tubules and saccules of immature lungs of preterm infants as well (Fig. 77.2).[20-23] Notably, alveolarization and AECII differentiation are not synchronized: mammals and birds are born with a functioning surfactant system, whereas alveolarization proceeds from fetal age to childhood in humans, is completed in utero in Guinea pigs, starts 3 to 4 days after birth in small rodents, and does not occur in birds possessing air capillaries.[24-27]

Due to their rapid spreading on surfaces, surfactant phospholipids cover the air-liquid interface throughout the lung. Airways surfactant, from alveolar overspill, accounts for maximally 7% of surfactant turnover, which is ample with respect to small airway compared with alveolar surface.[6,28,29]

PHOSPHOLIPIDS AND PHOSPHATIDYLCHOLINE SPECIES IN SURFACTANT

PC comprises 80% of surfactant phospholipid, with a molecular composition different from that of other phospholipid-containing secretions.[30,31] In humans, it is mostly diacyl-PC, whereas alkyl-acyl-PCs are abundant in shrews, bats, and marsupials.[17] Anionic phospholipids, mostly phosphatidylglycerol (PG) and some phosphatidylinositol (PI), represent 10% of surfactant, with reciprocal relationship of their fractions. PG is a marker of human lung maturity, whereas in some mammals the switch from PI to PG occurs after term.[32] However, contrary to lung tissue, surfactant comprises little sphingomyelin—a sphingolipid containing a phosphocholine head group like PC—and phosphatidylethanolamine (PE), two major plasma membrane phospholipids (approximately 10% and ~25%, respectively).[6]

Surfactant PC composition changes during development.[33] Surfactant assembly is characterized by sorting processes according to fatty acyl chain length, with specific enrichment of PC16:0/16:0, palmitoyl-myristoyl-PC (PC16:0/14:0), myristoyl-palmitoyl-PC

High surface tension

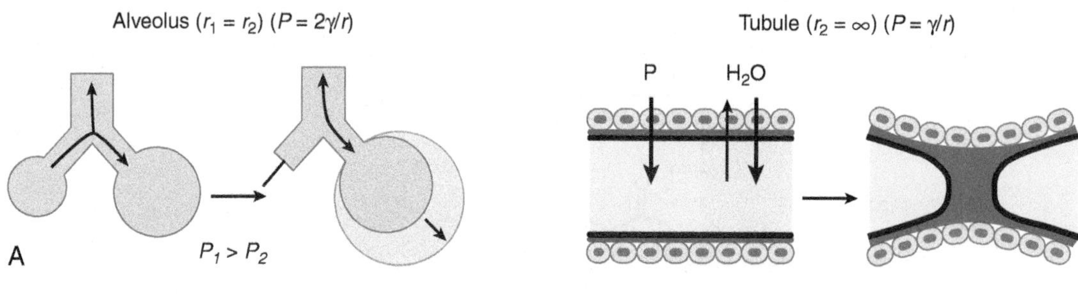

Low surface tension

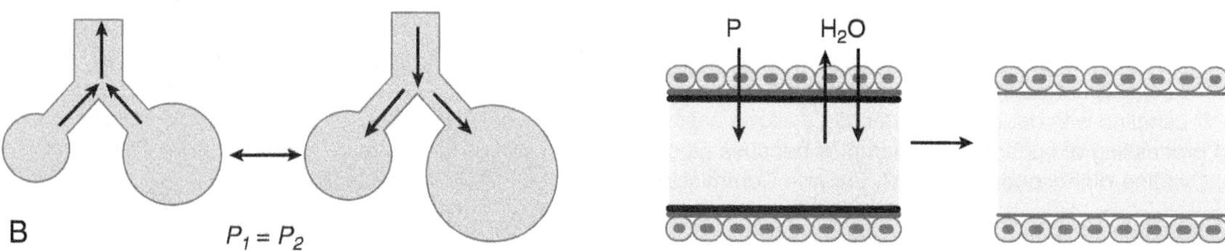

Fig. 77.2 Surfactant function at pulmonary air: liquid interfaces. The figure shows the consequences of high (A) versus low (B) surface tension for spherical structures ("alveolus") compared with a tubular structure (bronchioles, tubules, and saccules in immature mammalian lungs, air capillaries in bird lungs). When surface tension (γ) in the alveolus is high (A, *left*), low radius at end-expiration results in a higher pressure (*P*). Subsequent collapse results in the release of its gas content into the larger alveolus, with no reopening. When γ is near zero (B, *left*), *P* is nearly identically low under all conditions, with coexistence of larger and smaller alveoli and no collapse at end-expiration. Similarly, when surface tension in a tubule is high (A, *right*), transmural pressure will be high and induce collapse and/or water influx. Fluid influx will cause the generation of obstructing liquid drops, because surface tension of the fluid is high. This is prevented by low surface tension (B, *right*), decreasing fluid influx and formation of droplets, guaranteeing small airway patency while improving lung compliance.

(PC14:0/16:0), and palmitoyl-palmitoleoyl-PC (PC16:0/16:1). Together they comprise approximately 80% of the surfactant PC, and PC16:0/16:0 is inversely related to the fraction of these others.[17] PC16:0/16:0 maximally comprises 50% of surfactant PC (e.g., one third of surfactant). Only in birds, with no lung surface area changes during respiration, PC16:0/16:0 is higher (approximately 75%). In several mammals, particularly those with a high resting respiratory rate, PC16:0/16:0, including its alkyl-acyl-analogue, comprises only 20% of PC, providing good surface tension function (Fig. 77.3). This corrupts the paradigm that PC16:0/16:0 must predominate in mammalian surfactant.[8,17,27,34]

During alveolarization, PC16:0/14:0 increases at the expense of PC16:0/16:0 and is a better predictor of human fetal lung maturity than PC16:0/16:0. Aside from the contribution of these components to surface tension function under dynamic conditions, PC16:0/14:0 modulates macrophage functions, possibly relevant to alveolar protection.[35] In essence, mature human surfactant comprises 33% PC16:0/16:0, 15% of the other specific PC species, and 10% to 15% anionic phospholipids. The rest are other fluidic lipids and surfactant proteins (SPs; Fig. 77.4).

PC16:0/16:0 and PG are present in other organs such as the brain.[36-38] On the other hand, AECII and lung explants switch from PC16:0/16:0 synthesis to that of PC16:0/14:0 and PC16:0/16:1. In spite of using hormone and second messenger analogues in AECII cultures, lipid profiles remain different from in vivo conditions.[39-41] Hence only in vivo conditions reflect physiologic surfactant PC metabolism, in a defined species and at a defined developmental stage.

PATHWAYS OF PULMONARY PHOSPHOLIPID SYNTHESIS

Fig. 77.5 illustrates the pathways of PC, PG, and PI biosynthesis. Synthesis starts with the formation of phosphatidic acid (PA) from dihydroxyacetone phosphate (DHAP), which is derived from glycolysis. Two sequential acylations, using activated fatty acids (acyl-coenzyme A [CoA]), are required. DHAP can be 1-acylated followed by reduction or 1-acylated after reduction to glycerol 3-phosphate.[42,43] Acylation in position 2 then ends up in PA, the precursor of all other glycerophospholipids (and triglycerides).

Numerous precursors are used for PA synthesis, allowing for their stable isotope labeling to investigate surfactant phospholipid metabolism in patients (see Fig. 77.1): glucose, from blood or pulmonary glycogen stores, is used for the glycerol backbone and for fatty acid synthesis. Glycerol is incorporated after phosphorylation to glycerol-3-phosphate. Fatty acids originate from extrapulmonary and intrapulmonary lipids, fatty acid synthesis, and their desaturation or elongation. There is a wide range of experimental options, from deuterated water to fatty acids to address fatty acid synthesis, elongation, and desaturation in AECII.[44,45]

For PC biosynthesis, PA is dephosphorylated to 1,2-diacylglycerol (DAG; see Fig. 77.5). To transfer choline phosphate to DAG, choline is phosphorylated and then activated to cytidine-diphosphocholine (CDP-choline). For this, cytidine monophosphate is transferred from cytidine triphosphate (CTP) to phosphocholine by choline-phosphate cytidylyltransferase (CCT). The highly energetic diphosphoanhydride bond of

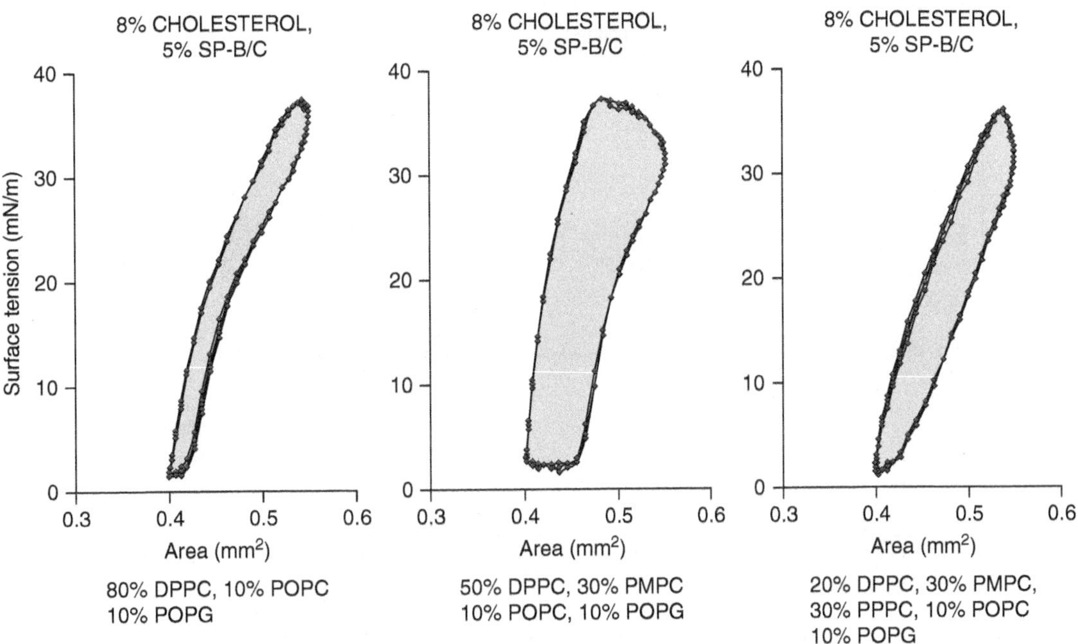

Fig. 77.3 Surface area versus surface tension of surfactant constructs in a captive bubble surfactometer (unpublished data of author). Surfactants were constructed as indicated elsewhere.[17] *DPPC*, 1,2-dipalmitoyl-PC; *PC*, phosphatidylcholine; *PMPC*, 1-palmitoyl-2-myristoyl-PC; *POPC*, 1-palmitoyl-2-oleoyl-PC; *POPG*, 1-palmitoyl-2-oleoyl-phosphatidylglycerol; *PPPC*, 1-palmitoyl-2-palmitoleoyl-PC; *SP-B/C*, mixture of surfactant proteins B and C from porcine lung lavage fluid. Figure shows that minimal surface tension upon lateral area compression is achieved with surfactant comprising only 20% DPPC relative to total phospholipid, while best hysteresis is achieved with 50% DPPC.

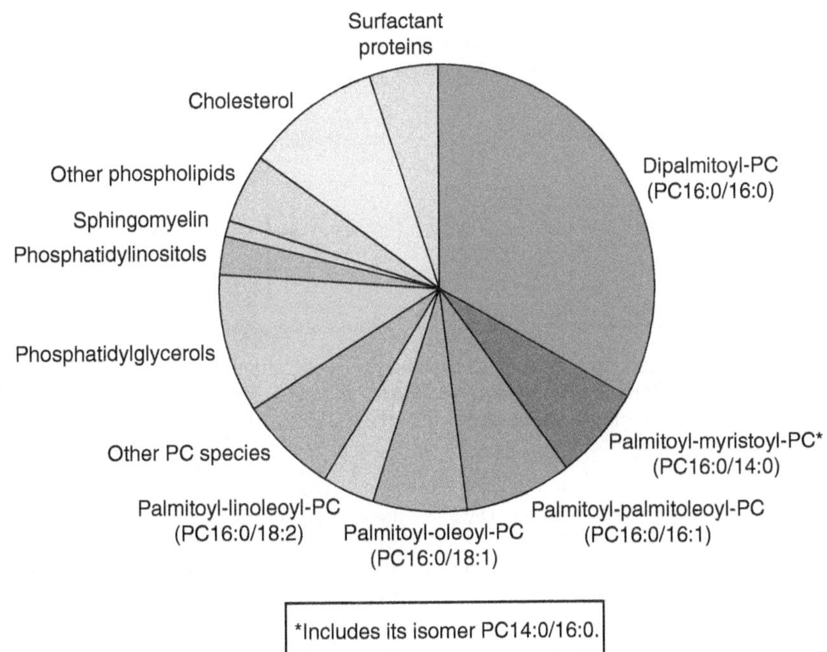

Fig. 77.4 Composition of regular adult mammalian surfactant. The green-colored components define those phospholipids being enriched in secreted surfactant over lung tissue, while those in grey color are increased in lung tissue over secreted surfactant. Nomenclature of fatty acids in PC species: the slash separates the fatty acids in positions sn-1 and sn-2 of PC; the number before the colon defines the number of carbon units of a fatty acid, whereas the figure after the colon defines the number of double bonds in it. Consequently, 18:2 means a fatty acid with 18 carbon units and two double bonds, that is, linoleic acid. *PC*, Phosphatidylcholine.

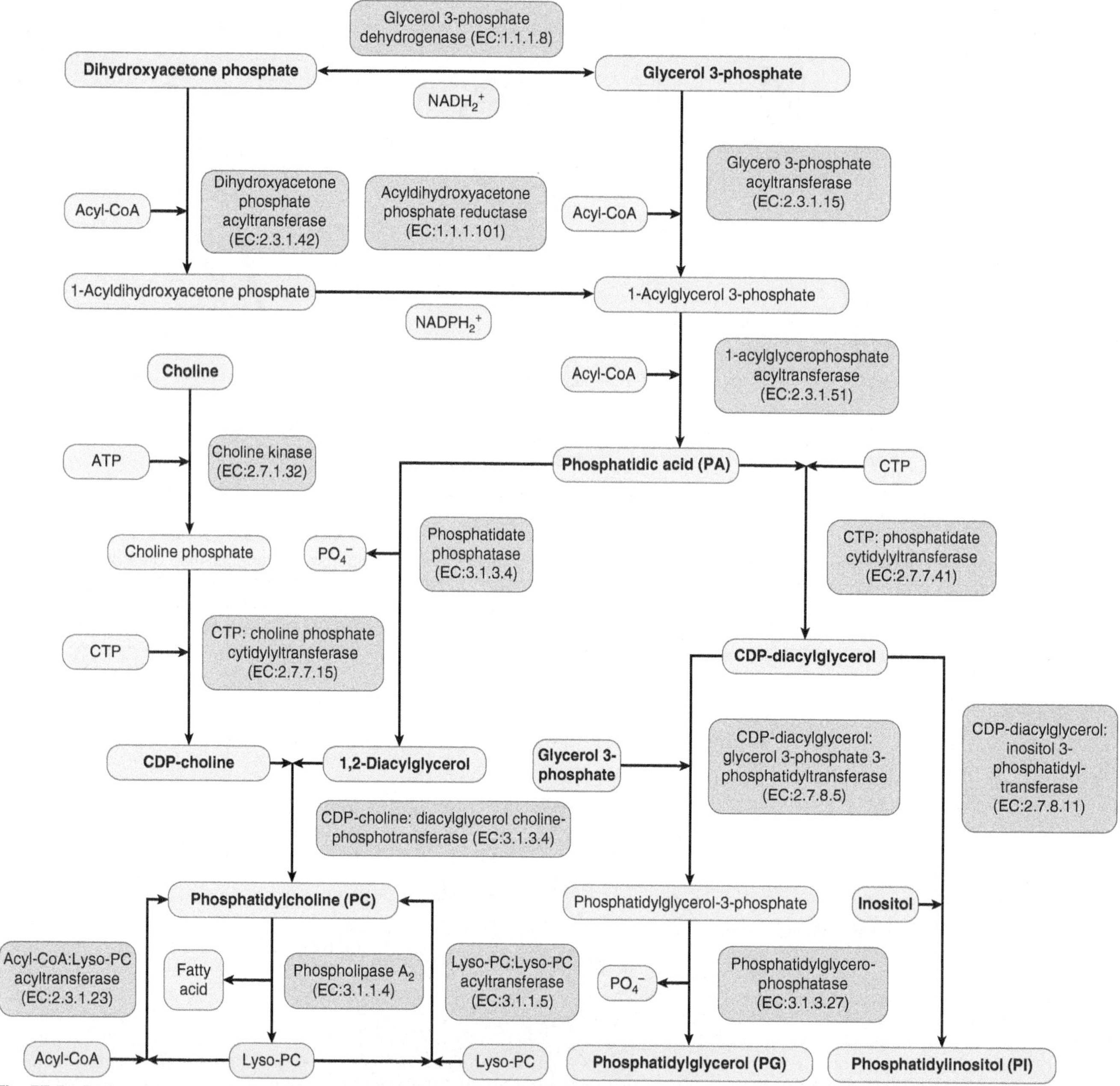

Fig. 77.5 Pathways in the biosynthesis of phosphatidylcholine, phosphatidylglycerol, and phosphatidylinositol. *CDP*, Cytidine-diphosphocholine; *CTP*, cytidine triphosphate; *EC*, Enzyme Commission number; *NAD(P)H2+*, reduced nicotinamide adenine dinucleotide (phosphate). (Modified from Rooney SA. The surfactant system and lung phospholipid biochemistry. *Am Rev Respir Dis*. 1985;131:439–460.)

CDP-choline drives the transfer of phosphocholine to DAG towards PC synthesis.

Although PC is primarily synthesized de novo, acyl remodeling contributes to approximately 50% of surfactant-specific PC species (see Fig. 77.5): deacylation of 1-palmitoyl-2-unsaturated-PC by phospholipase A_2 results in 1-palmitoyl-2-lyso-PC. Lyso-PC: acyl-CoA acyltransferase 1 (LPCAT-1) then reacylates lyso-PC to PC, mainly PC16:0/16:0 and PC16:0/14:0.[38,46,47] Consequently, absence of the remodeling pathway increases oleated and polyunsaturated PC in surfactant.[9,38]

Sorting mechanisms with a preference for PC containing two fatty acids of 14 or 16 carbon units assure the enrichment of these components in surfactant[39,44] but are not absolutely specific. In infants and newborn rats, surfactant comprises approximately 5% to 10% PC containing an arachidonic or docosahexaenoic acid residue. Notably, high contents of polyunsaturated fatty acids in surfactant correlates inversely with development of bronchopulmonary dysplasia (BPD) in preterm infants.[48,49] The responsible adenosine triphosphate (ATP)-binding cassette transporter A3 (ABCA3), located at the outer membrane of lamellar bodies (LBs), is regulated by glucocorticoids and triggers surfactant-PC and PG enrichment in LB of AECII. Consequently, several, but not all, ABCA3 mutations result in the absence of normal LB and acute neonatal respiratory failure of term infants.[50,51] In addition, ABCA3 knockout decreases the expression of proteins involved in lipid synthesis and trafficking, including LPCAT1, ABCA1, and steroidogenic acute regulatory domain protein 2 (stard2), highlighting the complexity of factors contributing to pulmonary PC metabolism.[52,53]

In contrast to PC, for PG and PI synthesis the phosphate group of PA is activated by CTP, resulting in CDP-DAG (see Fig. 77.5). Transfer of inositol or glycerol-3-phosphate to this intermediate yields PI, or PG-3-phosphate, which is immediately dephosphorylated to PG. PG and PI are enriched in unsaturated species and do not contain myristic acid, with the exception of rodent surfactant comprising 20% to 30% PG16:0/16:0. Differences in molecular species composition suggest different DAG/PA pools or different selection principles in trafficking.[17,54]

NORMAL DEVELOPMENT OF THE SURFACTANT SYSTEM

During fetal development, PC and PG increase at the expense of other glycerophospholipids and sphingomyelin.[55,56] PC16:0/14:0 and PC16:0/16:1 continuously increase, whereas the fraction of PC16:0/16:0 decreases from 34 weeks postmenstrual age onwards (i.e., when lung alveolarization has started). As the fetal lung secretes water, surfactant is carried out from the lung into amniotic fluid. Gastric and upper airway samples of newborns are similarly useful to characterize surfactant composition and function, as predictors of neonatal respiratory distress development. Increases in PG, in the ratio between PC ("lecithin") and sphingomyelin (L/S ratio), in PC16:0/14:0, PC16:0/16:1, and the PC16:0/14:0 to PC16:0/16:0 ratio are specific predictors of human lung maturity.[57-59] D9-choline labeling showed that airway samples reflect alveolar PC composition and metabolism,[60-62] whereas inhibition after meconium aspiration is not necessarily reflected by altered metabolism.[63,64] However, none of these functional or biochemical analyses was tested in randomized trials against clinical practice, of prophylactic surfactant application in very low-birth-weight preterm infants, or according to clinical status with measurement of oxygen saturation of hemoglobin, pressures required for adequate ventilation, and X-ray diagnostics.[65]

Prenatal increase of surfactant goes hand in hand with increased PC synthesis,[66] due to lung parenchymal growth and AECII proliferation. However, lung PC has a rapid turnover, and a major fraction is secreted into the circulation via basolateral ABCA1 transporters rather than into the airspaces,[67,68] thereby contributing to lipoprotein homeostasis and the choline/PC shuttle between liver and lung. Consequently, PC synthesis of the lungs and AECII does not simply represent surfactant metabolism but must be regarded in a systemic context.[50,51,69] Moreover, while incorporation of labeled precursors has been used to assess surfactant PC synthesis and secretion in humans,[13,15,16] isotope enrichment of precursors at the moment of synthesis and analysis of individual molecular species with their different turnover is necessary to assess synthesis rates.

REGULATION OF FETAL LUNG PHOSPHATIDYLCHOLINE BIOSYNTHESIS BY ENZYME ACTIVITY AND SUBSTRATE AVAILABILITY

The critical enzymes for PC synthesis de novo are choline kinase (CK) and CCT (see Fig. 77.5). CCT catalyzes the synthesis of CDP-choline. All CCT isoforms (α, β_1, and β_2) are expressed in fetal lung. The β isoforms are splice variants of the same gene. CCTα, the only isoform relevant to surfactant development and expressed in adult lung, is encoded by a different gene (*Pcyt1a*) and is found in association with cytosol and endoplasmic reticulum in the lung.[70-73] Increased CCT expression during development has become paradigmatic to explain for surfactant-PC enrichment.[73-78] However, this is questionable because mice overexpressing lung CCT four-fold have only modest or no increases in DSPC synthesis.[79] CCT activity increases during developmental lung growth and cell proliferation, whereas choline incorporation into PC remains unchanged relative to tissue weight. Moreover, accumulation of PC16:0/16:0 and PC16:0/14:0 at late gestation is due to decreased turnover and sequestration into LB rather than increased synthesis.[80,81]

Sphingosine and fibroblast growth factor 7 (FGF-7) enhance gene expression and/or activation of existing enzyme, whereas expression is inhibited by transforming growth factor-β1 (TGF-β1) and Zn deficiency.[77,78,82,83] However, CCT activity is disconnected from gene expression because the lipid-free cytosolic form is inactive, whereas translocation to the endoplasmic reticulum or other surrounding lipid (e.g., from fatty acid synthesis) activates the enzyme. Curvature and physical properties of lipids are critical to CCT activation. Notably, CCT stimulation by glucocorticoids, estrogens, progesterone, and thyroid hormones does not result from translocation but from increased fatty acid synthesis and presence. This alone results in maximal activation, so that hormones do not cause additional stimulation, whereas lipid removal abolishes any stimulatory effect.[84-97]

However, factors beyond CCT may be similarly important. CK (K_m = 13 μmol/L) for de novo PC synthesis is regulatory in other organs.[98] Lung tissue depends on exogenous choline supply, as choline synthesis by PE-*N*-methyltransferase (PEMT) is virtually absent from lung tissue and hepatic activity is low in the fetus and preterm infant.[99-102] The ubiquitous choline transporters have K_m values of greater than 30 μmol/L. Consequently, plasma choline concentration affects PC synthesis via cellular uptake, which may apply to the lungs as well. Notably, fetal plasma choline is approximately 40 μmol/L, which is three- to four-fold over adult values. Plasma PC concentration rapidly and untimely decreases to 20 μmol/L or less after preterm delivery.[103,104] Moreover, in choline deficiency PC is recruited from the lungs to supply the liver, possibly impacting on pulmonary PC and surfactant homeostasis.[105]

Fatty acid availability is similarly essential to lung tissue and surfactant PC synthesis as that of choline. Three sources of fatty acids are available: synthesis from carbohydrates via fatty acid synthase (FAS) within AECII, supply from pulmonary neutral lipid stores, and uptake from plasma, namely free fatty acids and lipoprotein lipids.[106] FAS expression is induced by glucocorticoids in fetal lungs but is down-regulated in the absence of ABCA3.[52] Notably, although retinoic acid (RA) is essential to lung maturation, it antagonizes FAS expression by glucocorticoids.[107-109] Increased surfactant PC pools in neonatal lungs after FGF-7 treatment go in line with increased pulmonary adipose triglyceride lipase (ATGL) rather than FAS expression.[110] ATGL is a ubiquitous lipase primarily acting on triglycerides, expressed in lungs together with hormone-sensitive lipase (HSL) and monoacylglycerol lipase (MGL).[111] Incorporation of fatty acids into surfactant-PC, derived from pulmonary lipofibroblasts, plasma lipoproteins, and free fatty acids, as well as from intrapulmonary fatty acid elongation or desaturation, suggests that lung tissue and surfactant PC synthesis depends on both intrapulmonary synthesis and the specific use of other fatty acid sources.[44,45,106] In this context, myristic acid (C14:0) is enriched in the lungs, whereas lauric acid (C12:0) is elongated to C14:0 for PC16:0/14:0 synthesis.[112,113] These complex, timely adjusted mechanisms may be corrupted, for example, by lipofibroblast to myofibroblast transdifferentiation by hyperoxia.[78,97,114-119]

FATTY ACID HOMEOSTASIS IN THE LUNG

Incorporation of tritiated or deuterated water into the fatty acids of lung PC and depletion of glycogen stores at

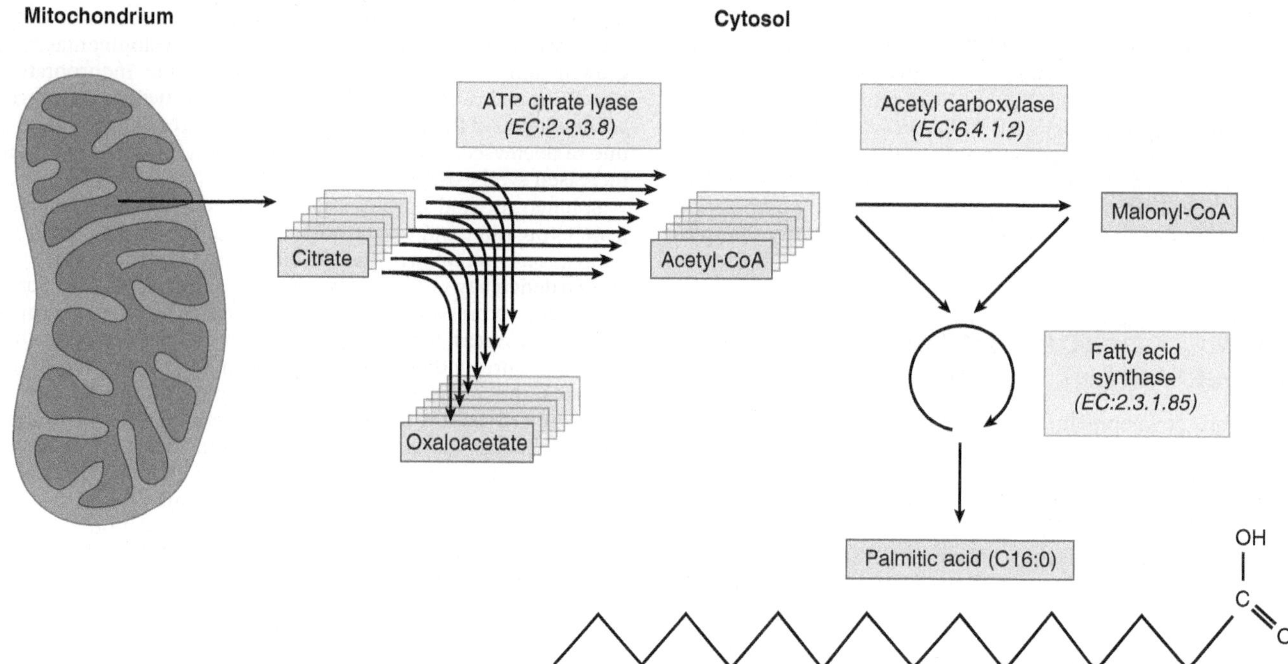

Fig. 77.6 Enzymes involved in fatty acid (primarily palmitic acid) biosynthesis. *ATP*, Adenosine triphosphate; *CoA*, coenzyme A; *EC*, enzyme Commission number.

end-gestation suggest intrapulmonary fatty acid synthesis from carbohydrates. It is accompanied by increased *FAS* gene expression and activity and by changes in the enzymes controlling glycogen synthesis and degradation, which in rats is followed by a decrease after birth.[120-125] In mammals, the seven FAS reactions are carried out by a single multifunctional protein complex. This addition reaction of 2-carbon units results in even-numbered fatty acids, mostly palmitic acid comprising[16] carbon units and no double bonds (C16:0). Initially, citrate is shuttled from the mitochondria to the cytosol (Fig. 77.6), where ATP-citrate lyase cleaves it to oxalacetate and acetyl-CoA. Acetyl-CoA is then carboxylated to malonyl-CoA, requiring carboxy-biotin. Starting with its transfer to the central sulfhydryl group of FAS, acetate from acetyl-CoA is transferred to malonyl-CoA, resulting in elongation to acetoacetate (C4-unit). Its reduction in several steps requires reduced niacin adenine dinucleotide phosphate ($NADPH_2^+$) and flavine mononucleotide ($FMNH_2$). Sequential repetition of this cycle ends up in C16:0-formation.[126,127] In essence, fatty acid synthesis for surfactant PC formation is highly substrate and energy consuming and is vitamin dependent.

Formation of surfactant PC in fetal lungs is connected to endogenous and exogenous neutral lipids as well as fatty acid modification.[128] In spite of molecular selection mechanisms, exogenous linoleic (C18:2*n*-6) and long-chain polyunsaturated fatty acids like arachidonic (C20:4*n*-6) and docosahexaenoic acid (C22:6*n*-3) are incorporated. C18:2 content of PC is increased by nutrition, and in neonatal organisms, requiring high amounts of C20:4 and C22:6 for the development of the brain and other organs, these fatty acids are increased. Moreover, myristic acid (C14:0), a saturated fatty acid like C16:0, is specifically enriched in mammalian surfactant. In Guinea pigs and humans, such enrichment starts in utero from alveolarization onwards. In rats, this occurs during postnatal alveolarization via exogenous supply, and under appropriate conditions PC16:0/14:0 is synthesized and enriched in AECII cultures without exogenous supply.[14,44,45] However, lauric acid (C12:0) is elongated to C14:0 prior to use for surfactant PC synthesis, and thereafter is used for PC16:0/14:0 synthesis in vivo.[35,39,44] Another fatty acid enriched in surfactant PC is palmitoleic acid (C16:1*n*-7), generated from C16:0 by stearoyl-CoA desaturase 1 (SCD-1) (EC:1.14.19.1).[129] Desaturase activity increases during lung maturation, differentially expressed in mammalian lungs, and is further up-regulated ex vivo. In vivo this process results in variable PC16:0/16:1 concentrations of surfactant that correlate with resting respiratory rate and are higher than PC16:0/16:0 in some species.[39] However, it cannot be replaced by palmitoyl-oleoyl-PC (PC16:0/18:1), which causes impaired surface tension function.[52] Enrichment of both PC16:0/14:0 and PC16:0/16:1 depends on LPCAT1 expression.[38] Whether C16:1 as a specific component of surfactant PC contributes to immune-regulating or antiinflammatory processes in the developing lung like C14:0 is unclear.[35,45,130]

ENDODERM-MESENCHYME INTERACTIONS IN PULMONARY FATTY ACID HOMEOSTASIS

Pulmonary fatty acid and surfactant PC homeostasis depend on endoderm-mesenchyme interactions, particularly between triglyceride-containing lipid interstitial cells (LICs, lipofibroblasts), located close to AECII.[131-133] LICs and exogenous fatty acid supply become increasingly important to PC formation when pulmonary glycogen stores are exhausted.[134,135] The contribution of LIC to surfactant homeostasis is underlined by experiments on sterol-responsive element-binding proteins (SREBPs). Down-regulation decreases expression of genes involved in fatty acid and cholesterol metabolism and decreases lung tissue PC and PG, while increasing triglycerides and cholesterol in LIC. Stretch acting on AECII induces parathyroid-hormone-related protein (PTHrP) and prostaglandin E2 (PGE2) acting on LIC, where mesenchymal peroxisomal proliferator-activated receptor-gamma (PPARγ) is up-regulated via protein kinase A. Adipocyte differentiation-related protein (ADRP) in LICs, triglyceride uptake by both LICs and AECII, and the action of LIC-derived leptin on AECII stimulate phospholipid synthesis in AECII. Down-regulation of PTHrP by traumata causes transdifferentiation of LICs to myofibroblasts, which has been suggested to perturb lung development and surfactant homeostasis.[133]

GLUCOCORTICOID ACTIONS ON SURFACTANT MATURATION IN ITS SYSTEMIC CONTEXT

In 1969, Liggins[136] reported that prenatal dexamethasone administration resulted in delivery of live preterm fetal lambs with partly expanded lungs. Subsequently, glucocorticoid treatment showed increased surfactant amounts in animal models and was successfully used in pregnant women to prevent respiratory distress in preterm infants. This finding dominates neonatal surfactant research and has resulted in the paradigm that glucocorticoids accelerate lung maturation.[137-140] However, glucocorticoids accelerate AECII differentiation, inhibit their proliferation, and antagonize anabolism.[141] Anticatabolic factors increasing surfactant in line with pulmonary and systemic anabolism may become increasingly important. It has long been known that direct or maternal injection of glucocorticoids increases the amounts of phospholipid, PC, the L/S ratio in fetal lungs in vivo. In lung explants and isolated AECII, glucocorticoids increase the pools of PC, DSPC, fatty acid biosynthesis, and CCT activity[142-153] and act on several levels of regulation in combination with other hormones.[154-156] However, in vitro data refer to increased parameters relative to protein or DNA. By contrast, in vivo glucocorticoids increase secreted surfactant at the expense of lung tissue phospholipids, AECII proliferation, and anabolism.[141]

INDIRECT GLUCOCORTICOID ACTIONS ON PHOSPHATIDYLCHOLINE METABOLISM IN ALVEOLAR TYPE 2 CELLS

Glucocorticoid act in a concentration-dependent manner on the lung, via receptors, *FAS* gene promoter, gene expression, and increased messenger RNA (mRNA) stability. In humans, increased mRNA stability predominates.[117,157] Glucocorticoid-deficient fetal mice show decreased FAS mRNA.[158-161] PC synthesis increases approximately 12 hours after treatment, and maxima are achieved in 20 to 36 hours.[162]

Glucocorticoids directly increase β-adrenoceptor–stimulated surfactant secretion by AECII.[163-166] However, effects on PC synthesis in adult or fetal AECII are indirect and require fibroblast-conditioned medium.[107,167,168] Components of such "fibroblast-pneumocyte factor" are FGFs like FGF-2, -3, -7, and -10, hepatocyte growth factor, neuregulin, PPAR, and ADRP.[133,169-173] However, their principle difference from glucocorticoids is that they are anabolic, maintaining or accelerating proliferation and growth.[141,174]

FIBROBLAST GROWTH FACTORS-7 AND ITS RELATION TO GLUCOCORTICOID EFFECTS

A brief communication by Danan and colleagues that FGF-7 concentrations in preterm infant airways relate inversely to BPD development, pointed to the role of FGFs in lung development and the deleterious effect of artificial ventilation.[175,176] FGF-7 is expressed in mesenchymal cells throughout the body,[177] and its receptor (KGFR), a splice variant of the FGF family receptors (FGFR2-IIIb), is exclusively expressed on epithelial cells.[178] FGF-7 knockout allows for viable animals, whereas absence of KGFR precludes lung development because FGF-10 stimulates pulmonary branching and differentiation via these receptors.[179-182] Glucocorticoids increase FGF-7 expression in fetal lungs, and anti-KGF antibodies block the glucocorticoid-augmented PC synthesis of fetal AECII in fibroblast-conditioned medium. Hence glucocorticoid effects on phospholipid synthesis in vitro are partly mediated by FGF-7.[183] FGF-7 increases DSPC and SP synthesis in fetal AECII, and pulmonary fluid secretion via chloride channels in utero.[184,185] However, during the perinatal switch, FGF-7 increases fluid absorption due to epithelial sodium/amiloride sensitive channel (ENaC) expression.[186,187] During alveolar formation, physiologic AECII proliferation is maintained by FGF-7, rather than blunted as with glucocorticoids,[141,188,189] and increases surfactant in neonatal hyperoxia, even after initiation of injury.[187] Both substances increase secreted surfactant in newborn rats, whereas later on only their combination is effective. Stimulation of fatty acid accretion by glucocorticoids is achieved by FAS expression, whereas FGF-7 increases accretion of ATGL.[110,141,190,191] Hence FGF-7 is a mediator of glucocorticoid actions, but direct actions on AECII underlie different mechanisms.

THYROID HORMONES AND THYROTROPIN-RELEASING HORMONE

Iodine deficiency is frequent among humans, with triiodothyronine (T_3) and thyroxine (T_4) affecting pulmonary structural and surfactant maturation. The impact of iodine deficiency and supplementation on fetal development is controversially discussed and regarded in the context of other nutrients.[192,193] Nevertheless, thyroid dysfunction is associated with respiratory failure in human neonates but is effectively treated by T_4 substitution.[194-196] Thyroid hormone receptors are present in fetal AECII, and fetal lungs of hypothyroid mice are less mature and contain less surfactant.[197-199] T_4 does not easily cross the placenta, whereas T_3 does and accelerates structural maturation and increases total and DSPC, CCT activity, secreted surfactant, and the L/S ratio in fetal lungs.[200-202]

In fetal lung explants, T_3 concentrations identical to the dissociation constant of its nuclear receptor exert half-maximal stimulation of PC synthesis via gene expression, as effects are abolished by actinomycin D and cycloheximide.[148,203] T_3/T_4 increase PC synthesis and CCT but not FAS activity.[148,149,203] Glucocorticoid effects on FAS activity are diminished by T_3/T_4.[204-206] In terms of organ development and epithelial-mesenchymal interaction, T_3/T_4 and glucocorticoid effects are additive,[207,208] suggesting complementary mechanisms.

In preterm infants, immaturity of the pituitary-thyroid axis and inflammation contribute to impaired lung development, as neonatal sepsis causes low plasma T_3 levels.[209] AECII homeostasis critically depends on T_3, because alterations in surfactant phospholipids and increased pulmonary surface tension are prevented by increasing plasma T_3 levels.[210,211] Clinically, pulmonary surfactant pools and function are improved by T_3, although PC synthesis and CCT activity are unchanged,[210,212] suggesting decreased turnover rather than increased synthesis.

Thyrotropin-releasing hormone (TRH) readily crosses the placenta and increases surfactant phospholipids in fetal LLF.[213-215] TRH receptors are present in fetal lung tissue, and ex vivo it stimulates CCT expression and PC synthesis.[216] Combination with cortisol is more effective than either hormone alone, with effects that depend on gestational age. Similar to FGF-7, TRH increases both tissue and secreted surfactant phospholipid. For respiratory distress syndrome (RDS) prevention, systemic administration of TRH to the mother is as effective as glucocorticoids, with both agonists increasing secreted surfactant to the same extent.[217-220]

ESTROGENS

Estrogens and progesterone are important for fetal development, alveolar formation, and surfactant formation, increasing thymidine incorporation, CCT activity, PC synthesis, and secreted surfactant PC, indicating lung growth together with surfactant maturation. Their decrease during late gestation dramatically impairs alveolar formation in pigs.[221-225] Low estrogen levels in maternal and cord blood correlate with increased RDS incidence, while estrogen administration to pregnant women resulted in an increased amniotic L/S ratio. According to ex vivo experiments, estrogen effects on the lungs are not direct, whereas estrogen administration in vivo accelerates development of the surfactant system equivalent to dexamethasone but without catabolic side effects.[226-231] However, there is no evidence that estrogen administration to preterm infants improves outcome.[232,233]

VITAMIN D

Human studies show that low plasma 25-hydroxy-cholecalciferol (25-OH-D_3), indicating severe vitamin D_3 (cholecalciferol) deficiency, is associated with preterm delivery, lung immaturity, and respiratory distress and is frequent in preterm infants. However, success of cholecalciferol supplementation depends on many factors, including the severity of deficiency.[234-236] Notably, the finally active calcitriol (1,25-$[OH]_2$-D_3) antagonizes placental inflammation via tumor necrosis factor (TNF)-α suppression, whereas the latter increases calcitriol catabolism.[237] 25-OH-D_3 does not cross the placenta; low plasma levels are frequent in mothers and fetuses and are associated with small-for-gestational-age (SGA) delivery.[238,239]

AECII, but not lung fibroblasts, convert 25-OH-D_3 to calcitriol. Its nuclear vitamin D receptor (VDR) is mostly restricted to AECII and lipofibroblasts. Perinatally, calcitriol increases the numbers of VDR on AECII and lipofibroblasts.[240,241] Acting via gene expression, calcitriol in vitro increases PC accumulation, and in vivo it increases secreted surfactant more than glucocorticoids.[242-245]

RETINOIC ACID, PROLACTIN, AND OTHER HORMONES

RA promotes fetal alveolar epithelial AECII proliferation, maturation, and differentiation to type I pneumocytes.[246,247] It increases choline incorporation and DSPC in fetal rat lungs, while vitamin A deficiency reduces surfactant pools.[248] This holds, although RA increases ABC-A1 expression and PC efflux to support systemic lipoprotein homeostasis (see later). RA antagonizes the stimulation of FAS expression by glucocorticoids but stimulates maturation of the surfactant system together with glucocorticoids in an orchestrated fashion in vivo.[107,169] Prolactin enhances the glucocorticoid effects on human lung explants, whereas prolactin alone does not increase surfactant.[249-251] Infants with RDS have decreased prolactin levels.[252-255] Hence the roles of RA and prolactin for human surfactant maturation lie in the systemic fetomaternal hormone milieu.

Other hormones and growth factors that may stimulate fetal surfactant maturation include corticotropin, corticotropin-releasing hormone, epidermal growth factor, parathyroid hormone, leptin, insulin-like growth factor, gastrin-releasing peptide, and other factors that increase cyclic adenosine monophosphate (cAMP) within the cells.[158,169,256-261] In essence, many hormones accelerate maturation of the surfactant system, but they generally do so without exhibiting catabolic side effects like glucocorticoids.

INHIBITION OF SURFACTANT ENRICHMENT IN THE LUNGS

Male preterm infants are more prone to develop RDS than female ones, due to a delay of 1 to 2.5 weeks in the development of the surfactant system.[262,263] This results from the inhibition of surfactant enrichment in males by dihydrotestosterone and its antagonism to glucocorticoids and triglyceride uptake and release by lipofibroblasts.[128,264] Androgen levels correlate inversely with epidermal growth factor (EGF) and directly with TGFβ1 receptor levels.

TGFβ1, important to inflammation in preterm infant lungs, tissue repair, and fibrotic remodeling, inhibits choline incorporation by glucocorticoids, FAS expression, and ultrastructural differentiation of AECII in human fetal lung explants.[265-268]

Gestational diabetes mellitus impairs surfactant maturation,[269] whereas glucose alone decreases lung tissue differentiation and surfactant production ex vivo only at 50 to 100 mM.[270] Streptozotocin- and alloxan-induced diabetes models show normal total PC but decreased CCT activity and DSPC at end-gestation.[271] Ex vivo, insulin does not decrease PC synthesis, but it diminishes the stimulatory effect of glucocorticoids.[272]

SECRETION AND HOMEOSTASIS OF SURFACTANT PHOSPHOLIPIDS

Surfactant secretion has been measured in vivo, in perfused lungs, and in isolated AECII from adult, neonatal, and fetal lungs.[165,273-275] Most studies were performed at a time before it was known that PC synthesis by AECII serves both apical surfactant secretion and basolateral PC secretion via ABCA1 transporters (see earlier).[67,152] In AECII, secretion was assessed by labeling PC synthesis with [3H]choline overnight and then measuring triggered compared with basal [3H]-PC/DSPC release. However, homeostatic distribution of precursor incorporation requires up to 48 hours so that surfactant may not be in equilibrium with cell membrane PC.[7,13,54] Moreover, only a few studies measured PC species characteristic of surfactant,[13,39,54] studied membrane fusion kinetics, assessed surfactant secretion in single AECII with fluorescence techniques, or measured PC molecular species rather than DSPC.[41,276-279]

Each AECII contains approximately 150 LBs storing surfactant, much less than the number of vesicles of other secreting cells. Up to 40% of this pool can be secreted per hour upon mechanical, hormonal, or paracrine stimulation.[280,281] Fig. 77.7 shows a scheme of processes of synthesis, storage, secretion, interface attachment, and turnover. At birth, secretion of surfactant increases in response to labor and ventilation, resulting in higher PC amounts in the air spaces.[131] Exercise-induced hyperventilation increases surfactant secretion up to 14-fold,[282] where inspiratory stretch rather than respiratory rate is the major trigger.[280,283,284] Neither vagotomy nor oxygen, CO_2, or pH affect this process.[280,285] Stretch of type I pneumocytes (alveolar epithelial cells type 1 [AECI]) and mechanotransduction and inositol-1,4,5-trisphosphate (IP_3) penetration from AECI to AECII via gap junctions may contribute.[280] Notably, with continued stretch events, surfactant increase reaches a plateau and returns to basal values within 4 hours after exercise, because secretion and recycling are tightly regulated to maintain surfactant homeostasis and to avoid AECII depletion.[280,282]

Surfactant secretion starts with rapid LB fusion with the plasma membrane, followed by a much slower release of LB contents depending on the size of fusion pores.[280,282] Not all LB of a AECII fuse upon stimulation, and not all AECII react simultaneously on a secretory stimulus.[286] Fusion events and surfactant secretion are connected to the cytoskeleton: depolymerization of F-actin via gelsolin in the presence of calcium (Ca^{2+}) increases secretion, whereas F-actin stabilization decreases it.[280,287,288] LB docking and membrane fusion requires t-SNAREs (target soluble N-ethylmaleimide-sensitive fusion protein-attachment protein receptors) and uses SNAP23, VAMP2, annexin A7, syntaxin 2, and others.[289-292] Because SNAREs are organized by lipid rafts, cholesterol deficiency inhibits surfactant secretion.[293]

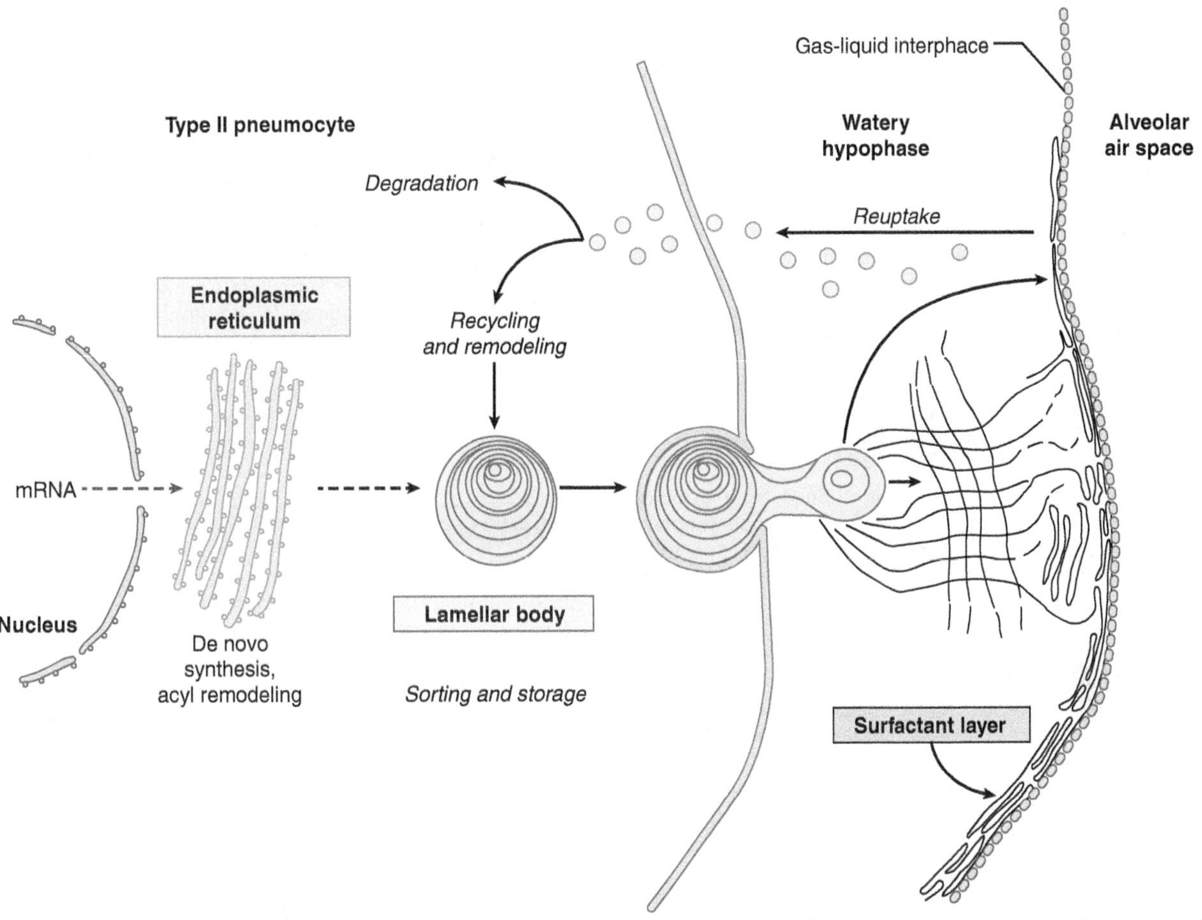

Fig. 77.7 Processes involved in lung surfactant homeostasis. After the expression of genes involved in surfactant metabolism and trafficking in the nucleus, proteins involved and phospholipids are synthesized. Surfactant components are transported to and stored in lamellar bodies. After a rapid constitutional or stimulated fusion of a lamellar body with the plasma membrane, its content is released and unfolds to form tubular myelin in the presence of surfactant proteins surfactant protein (SP)-A and SP-B, although direct surface-adsorption is possible.[52] Tubular myelin further develops towards the surface, forming and replenishing the surface associated reservoir in the presence of surfactant proteins SP-B and SP-C. "Used" surfactant material depleted of SPs will be reabsorbed and either degraded or recycled. During the recycling process surfactant undergoes a refinement of the composition of phosphatidylcholine molecular species requiring up to 48 hours in the healthy adult human.[13,54]

Cytoplasmic Ca^{2+} concentration is the central trigger of surfactant secretion, and Ca^{2+} removal blunts the action of secretagogues and protein kinase C activation. For short-term stimulation, Ca^{2+} ions originate from intracellular stores, and for long-term stimulation from the extracellular space.[294,286] IP_3, produced by cleavage of phosphatidylinositol 4, 5-bisphosphate (PIP_2) by phospholipase C-β_3 (PLC-β_3), promotes Ca^{2+} mobilization from intracellular stores,[295] which activates a Ca^{2+}/calmodulin-dependent protein kinase (CaCM-PK). It may also act synergistically with DAG. Protein phosphorylation by protein kinase A (PKA) or C (PKC) and/or CaCM-PK, together with Ca^{2+} mobilization, then leads to membrane fusion and surfactant secretion.[296] cAMP generation via adenylyl cyclase (AC), followed by activation of cAMP-dependent PKA works via β-adrenoceptor and adenosine A_{2B} receptor agonists. Both receptors belong to the seven-transmembrane domain receptors and activate AC through G_s proteins. Of the mammalian AC expressed in lung tissue, AC-II and AC-IV are present in AECII.[297-299] Other signaling mechanisms coupled to PKC, possibly contributing to surfactant secretion, include phospholipase A_2 and high- and low-density serum lipoproteins.[300,301]

There are many subtypes and isomers of receptors and signaling proteins in AECII. Pharmacologic data suggest that β_2-receptors, beyond stretch, are most important.[302-306] Of the adenosine receptors, A_{2B} stimulates surfactant secretion, due to its link to cAMP formation by AC.[296,307] Of the purinergic receptors, P_2Y_2 is expressed in AECII, with ATP and uridine triphosphate (UTP) being equally potent ligands.[308-311] P_2Y_2 receptors are coupled to PLC-β3,[312-314] followed by protein kinase D_1 (PKD_1) activation.[315]

Cholera toxin can pass the cell membrane and permanently activate G_s, whereas forskolin directly activates AC. Increased ATP and UTP release can transduce stretch to secretion in an autocrine or paracrine manner.[316-318] Their binding to P_2Y_2 receptors activates PLC-β_3, resulting in the cleavage of PIP_2 to DAG and IP_3. DAG then activates PKC, which in turn activates a phospholipase D_1 and D_2 to hydrolyze PC[319,320] to PA. Subsequent generation of DAG from PA by phosphatidate phosphatase (see Fig. 77.5) further activates PKC. Together with Ca^{2+}, this PLD loop may contribute to sustained surfactant secretion.[286,321] In addition, ATP stimulates surfactant secretion by the cAMP/PKA pathway.[311,322] Experimental tools like tetradecanoylphorbol-13-acetate (TPA), cell-permeable DAGs, and DAG "caged" in AECII, and then released by flash-photolysis, can directly activate PKC.[286]

These mechanisms of signal transduction are overlapping and interactive, linked to both plasma membrane receptors and mechanical stress.[286,323] All signal-transduction pathways result in phosphorylation of proteins after activation of the specific protein kinases. However, mitogen-activated protein (MAP) kinase activation is not involved in surfactant secretion or its feedback inhibition.[288,333,324-327] Agonist-induced surfactant secretion depends on lung development, as responses to them are low in fetal and newborn AECII.[298,299] Dexamethasone, and possibly calcitriol, significantly increase the response of AECII to other agonists, resulting in stronger effects.[166,242,328] Effects of mechanical forces are linked to receptor-stimulated secretion, because indomethacin, β-antagonists, and A_{2B} receptor blockade inhibit the effects of ventilation and labor. The m-cholinoceptor antagonist atropine blocks the effect of ventilation in vivo by decreasing catecholamine release from the adrenal medulla. This points to the close interaction of mechanical, paracrine, and systemic mechanisms, and of signal transduction systems, to ensure adequate secreted surfactant pools in vivo.[329-337]

SURFACTANT TURNOVER, RECYCLING, AND REFINEMENT

The pool size of secreted surfactant is defined by a dynamic equilibrium between secretion, bronchiolar clearance, reuptake into AECII, and removal by alveolar macrophages. Spreading to the air-liquid interface and ventilation provide the airways with conductive airways surfactant, accounting for up to 7% of turnover, ensuring small airway stability and contributing to lung compliance (see Fig. 77.2) and to the mucociliary clearance of inhaled particles.[20-22,338,339] Significant amounts of surfactant are metabolized by alveolar macrophages under control of granulocyte-macrophage colony-stimulating factor (GM-CSF). Lack of, or antibodies against, GM-CSF results in alveolar proteinosis.[340] Surfactant-PC species differentially influence macrophage function, with PC16:0/14:0 decreasing macrophage-induced T-lymphocyte proliferation.[35,45]

Finally, secreted surfactant is recycled by AECII.[52,341] Whereas secretion of surfactant phospholipids, SP-B and SP-C is simultaneous, and stimulated by the same agonists,[342-344] PC turnover is slower than that of PG and SP-B, and that of DSPC lower than unsaturated PC.[345-349] Recycling into AECII occurs through multivesicular bodies and is stimulated by SP-A to -D.[350,351] SP-D knockout decelerates alveolar PC turnover.[352,353] Phospholipids are directly recycled to LB or degraded and used for resynthesis.[354] The efficiency of surfactant recycling is much higher in newborn compared to adults and is impaired in lung injury because of changes in F-actin and β-tubulin homeostasis.[355-358]

Recycling is important for the refinement of surfactant PC, because the molecular composition of newly synthesized PC in the alveolar space comprises less PC16:0/16:0 than surfactant at equilibrium. This process was shown with labeled choline in mice, rats, and humans and takes 24 to 48 hours until newly synthesized surfactant PC in lung secretions reaches the composition of mature surfactant.[13,54,62,359] Whether different storage pools are responsible here is not clear,[282] but these data contradict the concept of primary storage of mature surfactant, and secretion of such finalized material.

SYSTEMIC CONTEXT OF PULMONARY AND SURFACTANT PHOSPHATIDYLCHOLINE METABOLISM

Total pulmonary PC synthesis is an order of magnitude higher than required for surfactant storage and its apical secretion. In the fetus this is due to both accelerated lung growth and AECII proliferation during the third and its dominating use for basolateral PC secretion throughout life.[68,141] AECII express ABCA3 for LB assembly but also ABCA1 for basolateral PC and cholesterol secretion and transfer to apo-lipoprotein A_1, connecting surfactant PC with systemic high-density lipoprotein metabolism.[52,360-362] Pulmonary ABCA1 expression is under control of 9-cis-RA and 22-hydroxycholesterol, stimulating pulmonary PC efflux manifold, whereas glucocorticoids and FGF-7 possibly decrease such efflux.[68] ABCA1 defects result in the absence of high density lipoproteins (HDL) including its PC moiety in plasma, pulmonary accumulation of total PC, DSPC, cholesterol, impaired function, and structural lung defects.[362-364]

Surfactant phospholipid metabolism is linked to that of systemic lipoprotein metabolism: a major fraction of lung PC synthesis is released into the circulation, due to ABCA1 expression on AECII, rather than for surfactant formation. Defective ABCA1 transporters cause pulmonary PC accumulation, whereas hepatic choline deficiency causes a PC redistribution at the expense of the lung. Notably, glucocorticoids may partly act by decreasing PC export rather than increasing synthesis.[365-369] The impact of choline deficiency in preterm infants on pulmonary phospholipid homeostasis requires further investigation.[370]

CONCLUSION

Mammalian surfactant is formed by AECII and comprises 80% phospholipids, 10% cholesterol, and less than 10% SP-A to -D. Its phospholipid molecular species composition is characteristic to assure function under respiratory air-liquid interface changes. Surfactant phospholipids spread to all pulmonary surfaces, stabilizing alveoli and small airways. Of total phospholipid content, 80% is PC and 10% to 15% is anionic phospholipids, mostly PG.

Four PC species are enriched in mammalian surfactant; they are dipalmitoyl-PC (PC16:0/16:0), palmitoyl-myristoyl-PC (PC16:0/14:0), myristoyl-palmitoyl-PC (PC14:0/16:0) and palmitoyl-palmitoleoyl-PC (PC16:0/16:1), comprising approximately 80% of PC. PC16:0/16:0 accounts for one third of human surfactant, is a minor surfactant component in some mammals, and during alveolarization decreases in favor of PC16:0/14:0 and PC16:0/16:1. These components possess different biophysical and immunomodulatory properties and seem adapted to alveolarization and respiration.

Fetal lung and surfactant maturation in vivo is regulated by many hormones, in a concerted or potentiating way. Glucocorticoids accelerate AECII differentiation, however at the expense of AECII proliferation and anabolism, but other mediators do so without catabolic effects, like RA, estrogens, calcitriol, thyroid hormones, FGF7, and other factors derived from fibroblasts. De novo PC synthesis increases with fetal lung growth. However, formation of specific surfactant PCs, like PC16:0/16:0 and PC16:0/14:0, is enhanced via acyl remodeling by LPCAT1. During AECII differentiation, they accumulate in LB by sequestration under control of ABCA3 rather than by increased synthesis.

PC synthesis by AECII is 10-fold higher than required for surfactant production and must be regarded in context with basolateral PC secretion via ABCA1 transporters, thereby contributing to HDL metabolism. ABCA1 transporter defects result in decreased plasma HDL-PC, increased pulmonary PC storage, and respiratory failure, underlining the role of pulmonary PC metabolism for systemic lipoprotein metabolism.

Surfactant secretion starts with rapid LB fusion with the plasma membrane and subsequent release of its contents. This occurs under control of cytoplasmic Ca^{2+} increase and actin, involving cAMP/protein kinase A and phospholipase C/protein kinase C pathways. AECII stretch is the main trigger of surfactant secretion in vivo, in interaction with β-adrenergic, purinergic, and cholinergic stimulation. Glucocorticoids improve the secretagogue insensibility of immature lungs.

Adjustment of the secreted pool size depends on respiratory requirements and is embedded into a system of factors determining turnover. These are clearance into the airways for airway stability, metabolism by alveolar macrophages under control of GM-CSF, modulating macrophage functions, and recycling into AECII. Recycling is more efficient in newborns than in adults and sick individuals, contributing to the molecular refinement of newly synthesized surfactant.

 A complete reference list is available at www.ExpertConsult.com.

SELECT REFERENCES

1. Neergard K. Neue Auffassungen über einen Grundbegriff der Atemmechanik. Die Retraktionskraft der Lunge, abhängig von der Oberflächenspannung in den Alveolen. *Z. gms.exptl. Med.* 1929;66:373-394.
2. Avery MEMead J. Surface properties in relation to atelectasis and hyaline membrane disease. *AMA J Dis Child.* 1959;97:517-523.
3. Klaus MH, Clements JA, Havel RJ. Composition of surface-active material isolated from beef lung. *Proc Natl Acad Sci U S A.* 1961;47:1858-1859.
4. Mason RJ, Nellenbogen J, Clements JA. Isolation of disaturated phosphatidylcholine with osmium tetroxide. *J Lipid Res.* 1976;17:281-284.
5. Holm BA, Wang Z, Egan EA, Notter RH. Content of dipalmitoyl phosphatidylcholine in lung surfactant: ramifications for surface activity. *Pediatr Res.* 1996;39:805-811.
6. Bernhard W, Haagsman HP, Tschernig T, et al. Conductive airway surfactant: surface-tension function, biochemical composition, and possible alveolar origin. *Am J Respir Cell Mol Biol.* 1997;17:41-50.
7. Bernhard W, Bertling A, Dombrowsky H, et al. Metabolism of surfactant phosphatidylcholine molecular species in cftr(tm1HGU/tm1HGU) mice compared to MF-1 mice. *Exp Lung Res.* 2001;27(4):349-366.
8. Veldhuizen R, Nag K, Sandra O, Possmayer F. The role of lipids in pulmonary surfactant. *Biochim Biophys Acta.* 1998;1408:90-108.
9. Bridges JP, Ikegami M, Brilli LL, Chen X, Mason RJ, Shannon JM. LPCAT1 regulates surfactant phospholipid synthesis and is required for transitioning to air breathing in mice. *J Clin Invest.* 2010;120:1736-1748.
10. Postle AD. Method for the sensitive analysis of individual molecular species of phosphatidylcholine by high-performance liquid chromatography using post-column fluorescence detection. *J Chromatogr.* 1987;415:241-251.
11. Caesar PA, Wilson SJ, Normand CS, Postle AD. A comparison of the specificity of phosphatidylcholine synthesis by human fetal lung maintained in either organ or organotypic culture. *Biochem J.* 1988;253:451-457.
12. Heeley EL, Hohlfeld JM, Krug N, Postle AD. Phospholipid molecular species of bronchoalveolar lavage fluid after local allergen challenge in asthma. *Am J Physiol Lung Cell Mol Physiol.* 2000;278:L305-L311.
13. Bernhard W, Pynn CJ, Jaworski A, et al. Mass spectrometric analysis of surfactant metabolism in human volunteers using deuteriated choline. *Am J Respir Crit Care Med.* 2004;170:54-58.
14. Ridsdale R, Roth-Kleiner M, D'Ovidio F, et al. Surfactant palmitoylmyristoylphosphatidylcholine is a marker for alveolar size during disease. *Am J Respir Crit Care Med.* 2005;172:225-232.
15. Postle AD, Hunt AN. Dynamic lipidomics with stable isotope labelling. *J Chromatogr B Analyt Technol Biomed Life Sci.* 2009;877:2716-2721.
16. Torresin M, Zimmermann LJ, Cogo PE, et al. Exogenous surfactant kinetics in infant respiratory distress syndrome: a novel method with stable isotopes. *Am J Respir Crit Care Med.* 2000;161:1584-1589.
17. Lang CJ, Postle AD, Orgeig S, et al. Dipalmitoylphosphatidylcholine is not the major surfactant phospholipid species in all mammals. *Am J Physiol Regul Integr Comp Physiol.* 2005;289:R1426-R1439.
18. Hass MA, Longmore WJ. Surfactant cholesterol metabolism of the isolated perfused rat lung. *Biochim Biophys Acta.* 1979;573:166-174.
19. Goldman S. Generalizations of the Young-Laplace equation for the pressure of a mechanically stable gas bubble in a soft elastic material. *J Chem Phys.* 2009;131(18):184502.
20. Enhorning G, Duffy LC, Welliver RC. Pulmonary surfactant maintains patency of conducting airways in the rat. *Am J Respir Crit Care Med.* 1995;151:554-556.
21. Enhorning G. Pulmonary surfactant function in alveoli and conducting airways. *Can Respir J.* 1996;3:21-27.
22. Hamm H, Fabel H, Bartsch W. The surfactant system of the adult lung: physiology and clinical perspectives. *Clin Investig.* 1992;70:637-657.
23. Im Hof V, Gehr P, Gerber V, Lee MM, Schürch S. *In vivo* determination of surface tension in the horse trachea and *in vitro* model studies. *Respir Physiol.* 1997;109:81-93.
24. Zeltner TB, Burri PH. The postnatal development and growth of the human lung. II. Morphology. *Respir Physiol.* 1987;67:269-282.
25. Massaro GD, Massaro D. Formation of alveoli in rats: postnatal effect of prenatal dexamethasone. *Am J Physiol.* 1992;263:L37-L41.
26. Sosenko IR, Frank L. Lung development in the fetal Guinea pig: surfactant, morphology, and premature viability. *Pediatr Res.* 1987;21:427-431.
27. Bernhard W, Gebert A, Vieten G, et al. Pulmonary surfactant in birds: coping with surface tension in a tubular lung. *Am J Physiol Regul Integr Comp Physiol.* 2001;281:R327-R337.
28. Pettenazzo A, Jobe A, Humme J, Seidner S, Ikegami M. Clearance of surfactant phosphatidylcholine via the upper airways in rabbits. *J Appl Physiol.* 1988;65(1985). 2151-2155.
29. Rau GA, Dombrowsky H, Gebert A, et al. Phosphatidylcholine metabolism of rat trachea in relation to lung parenchyma and surfactant. *J Appl Physiol.* 2003;95:1145-1152.
30. Bernhard W, Postle AD, Rau GA, Freihorst J. Pulmonary and gastric surfactants. A comparison of the effect of surface requirements on function and phospholipid composition. *Comp Biochem Physiol Mol Integr Physiol.* 2001;129:173-182.
31. Bernhard W, Postle AD, Linck M, Sewing KF. Composition of phospholipid classes and phosphatidylcholine molecular species of gastric mucosa and mucus. *Biochim Biophys Acta.* 1995;1255:99-104.
32. Rau GA, Vieten G, Haitsma JJ, et al. Surfactant in newborn compared with adolescent pigs: adaptation to neonatal respiration. *Am J Respir Cell Mol Biol.* 2004;30:694-701.
33. Bernhard W, Hoffmann S, Dombrowsky H, et al. Phosphatidylcholine molecular species in lung surfactant - composition in relation to respiratory rate and lung development. *Am J Respir Cell Mol Biol.* 2001;25:725-731.
34. Pynn CJ, Henderson NG, Clark H, Koster G, Bernhard W, Postle AD. Specificity and rate of human and mouse liver and plasma phosphatidylcholine synthesis analyzed *in vivo*. *J Lipid Res.* 2011;52:399-407.
35. Gille C, Spring B, Bernhard W, et al. Differential effect of surfactant and its saturated phosphatidylcholines on human blood macrophages. *J Lipid Res.* 2007;48:307-317.
36. Rooney SA. Phospholipid composition, biosynthesis, and secretion. In: Parent RA, ed. *Comparative Biology of the Normal Lung.* Boca Raton, FL: CRC Press; 1992:511.
37. Mason RJ. Disaturated lecithin concentration of rabbit tissues. *Am Rev Respir Dis.* 1973;107:678.
38. Harayama T, Eto M, Shindou H, et al. Lysophospholipid acyltransferases mediate phosphatidylcholine diversification to achieve the physical properties required *in vivo*. *Cell Metab.* 2014;20:295-305.
39. Longmuir KJ, Haynes S. Evidence that fatty acid chain length is a type II cell lipid-sorting signal. *Am J Physiol.* 1991;260:L44-L51.
40. Hunt AN, Clark GT, Neale JR, Postle AD. A comparison of the molecular specificities of whole cell and endonuclear phosphatidylcholine synthesis. *FEBS Lett.* 2002;530:89-93.
41. Postle AD, Gonzales LW, Bernhard W, et al. Lipidomics of cellular and secreted phospholipids from differentiated human fetal type II alveolar epithelial cells. *J Lipid Res.* 2006;47:1322-1331.
42. Rooney SA. The surfactant system and lung phospholipid biochemistry. *Am Rev Respir Dis.* 1985;131:439-460.
43. Rooney SA. Regulation of surfactant phospholipid biosynthesis. In: Rooney SA, ed. *Lung Surfactant: Cellular and Molecular Processing.* Landes: Austin, TX; 1998:29.
44. Pynn CJ, Picardi MV, Nicholson T, et al. Myristate is selectively incorporated into surfactant and decreases dipalmitoylphosphatidylcholine without functional impairment. *Am J Physiol Regul Integr Comp Physiol.* 2010;299:R1306-R1316.
45. Bernhard W, Raith M, Pynn CJ, et al. Increased palmitoyl-myristoyl-phosphatidylcholine in neonatal rat surfactant is lung specific and correlates with oral myristic acid supply. *J Appl Physiol.* 2011;111:449-457.
46. Batenburg JJ. Surfactant phospholipids: synthesis and storage. *Am J Physiol.* 1992;262:L367.
47. Shindou H, Shimizu T. Acyl-CoA: lysophospholipid acyltransferases. *J Biol Chem.* 2009;284:1-5.
48. Rüdiger M, von Baehr A, Haupt R, Wauer RR, Rüstow B. Preterm infants with high polyunsaturated fatty acid and plasmalogen content in tracheal aspirates develop bronchopulmonary dysplasia less often. *Crit Care Med.* 2000;28:1572.
49. Bernhard W, Schmiedl A, Koster G, et al. Developmental changes in rat surfactant lipidomics in the context of species variability. *Ped Pulmonol.* 2007;42:794-804.
50. Ban N, Matsumura Y, Sakai H, et al. ABCA3 as a lipid transporter in pulmonary surfactant biogenesis. *J Biol Chem.* 2007;282:9628-9634.

78 Antenatal Hormonal Therapy for Prevention of Respiratory Distress Syndrome

J.E. Harding | C.A. Crowther | C.J.D. McKinlay

INTRODUCTION

The use of antenatal hormone therapy to accelerate fetal maturation and decrease the incidence of respiratory distress syndrome (RDS) and other neonatal problems has been one of the great success stories of perinatal medicine. Here we describe the actions of glucocorticoids and other hormones on the lung and other tissues. We then review the evidence for the clinical use of antenatal glucocorticoids, including current recommendations and remaining uncertainties about this important treatment.

BIOLOGIC CONSIDERATIONS

PERIPARTUM ROLE OF GLUCOCORTICOIDS

Fetal glucocorticoids play a key role in late gestation in preparing the fetus for extra-uterine life and achieving synchrony between maturation and parturition. In virtually all mammalian species, fetal adrenal activity increases exponentially towards term, and the resulting increase in circulating glucocorticoid concentrations—cortisol in humans—induces a wide range of proteins and enzymes that produce morphologic and functional maturation in most fetal tissues. Concurrently, this late gestation fetal glucocorticoid surge contributes to several feed-forward loops that ultimately lead to myometrial prostaglandin synthesis and the onset of labor.

A key target for endogenous fetal glucocorticoids is the lung, as there is high expression of glucocorticoid receptors in fetal lung tissue from mid-gestation. At birth, survival depends on lung aeration and maintenance of functional residual capacity, increased pulmonary blood flow, and initiation of gas exchange across the alveolar wall. Antenatal glucocorticoids support this postnatal transition by (1) upregulating epithelial sodium channels and the sodium-potassium adenosine triphosphatase (ATPase) to promote clearance of fetal lung fluid, (2) increasing lung surfactant content to reduce the alveolar surface tension when the lung is aerated, (3) increasing alveolar airspace volume and thus the surface area for gas exchange, (4) reducing the thickness of the alveolar septae to increase diffusion capacity for gas exchange, and (5) maturation of pulmonary vasculature to reduce alveolo-capillary permeability to plasma proteins.

The effects of glucocorticoids in the fetal lung have been studied most extensively for surfactant synthesis. Glucocorticoids increase the synthesis of surfactant proteins (SP) A, B, C, and D in type II pneumocytes, with lung tissue content increasing about 48 hours after glucocorticoid exposure.[1] Glucocorticoids also increase the synthesis of phosphatidylcholine, but lung concentrations increase more slowly, as glucocorticoids act indirectly by inducing the lipogenic enzymes necessary for phospholipid synthesis (fatty acid synthetase, phosphatidyl acid phosphatase, lyso-phosphatidylcholine [PC]: acyl-coenzyme A [CoA] acyltransferase).[1] The duration of physiologic effect depends on the half-life of the induced proteins and enzymes. SP-A and SP-B levels remain elevated in lung tissue and alveolar fluid for up to 2 weeks but return to control levels by about 3 weeks in the absence of ongoing glucocorticoid exposure.[1,2] Phosphatidylcholine levels remain elevated for slightly longer, determined by the half-life of the induced lipogenic enzymes.

Glucocorticoids also produce multiple changes in fetal lung structure, including differentiation of alveolar type I and II epithelial cells, decreased interstitial tissue in the alveolar wall, increased deposition of supportive connective tissue matrix (elastin and collagen), enlargement of alveolar airspaces, and maturation of alveolar capillary vessels.[3] The net effect of these structural changes during postnatal transition is increased functional residual capacity, improved lung stability, reduced work of breathing, and enhanced gas exchange.

Glucocorticoids also promote maturation of several functional pathways in the fetal lung, the most important of which for birth transition is the clearance of fetal lung fluid. Glucocorticoids increase the synthesis of subunits of the epithelial sodium channel and basal sodium-potassium ATPase, which are critical for the movement of alveolar fluid from the alveolar airspace to the interstitium. Other pulmonary maturational effects of glucocorticoids include increased synthesis of antioxidant enzymes to reduce free radical injury (superoxide dismutase, catalase, glutathione peroxidase) and induction of glycogenolysis to provide substrates for phospholipid synthesis.

In addition to pulmonary maturation, glucocorticoids are responsible for a wide range of changes in other fetal tissues that support postnatal transition. In the liver, glucocorticoids increase the formation of bile canaliculi and induce multiple enzymes in metabolic pathways, including glycogenesis (glycogen synthetase) and gluconeogenesis (phospho-phenolpyruvate carboxykinase, glucose-6-phosphatase), fatty acid and protein synthesis (fatty acid synthetase, aminotransferases), and the conversion of thyroxine to triiodothyronine (5′-monodeiodinase). In the kidney, glucocorticoids increase renal blood flow and glomerular filtration rate and enhance tubular function. In the intestine, villus height and density are increased, as are brush border hydrolases, and secretion of gastric acid and pancreatic digestive enzymes is enhanced. Glucocorticoid-induced changes are also seen in the heart (myocyte differentiation), cerebral circulation (enhanced blood-brain barrier and maturation of microcirculation), endocrine pancreas (enhanced insulin response to glucose), skin (keratinization), bone marrow (hematopoiesis), and adrenal gland (enhanced catecholamine and cortisol secretion).

GLUCOCORTICOID MECHANISM OF ACTION IN THE FETUS

Glucocorticoid action is mediated primarily by activation of the cytosolic glucocorticoid receptor with subsequent effects on transcription, messenger RNA (mRNA) stability, and post-translational processing.[4] The activated glucocorticoid receptor induces a limited number of genes directly via nuclear response elements within the gene promoter, such as those encoding for SP-B, elastin, angiotensin, the β-1 subunit of the sodium-potassium ATPase, and the α subunit of the epithelial sodium channel. For these genes, maximal transcription rates are achieved within hours and are maintained with ongoing glucocorticoid exposure.[5] However, for most genes, transcription is induced indirectly through interactions with nuclear transcription factors that coordinate the expression of multiple genes.[5] Biphasic responses have been observed, such that with excessive glucocorticoid exposure, transcription of target genes may be suppressed.

Although molecular mechanisms have been well established for some glucocorticoid-induced effects, such as increased synthesis of surfactant components, mechanisms are less well established for others. For example, it is not entirely clear how glucocorticoids change lung architecture. This may result from effects on the cell cycle, induction of various growth factors, and antagonism of lung retinoids that promote alveolarization. Glucocorticoids also have a variety of non-genomic effects, including altered cell membrane permeability, mitochondrial function, and intracellular signaling, although the extent to which this occurs in the fetus is not known.

SYNTHETIC GLUCOCORTICOIDS FOR PRETERM BIRTH

Betamethasone and dexamethasone are the only parenterally administered glucocorticoids that reliably cross the placenta due to their limited affinity for 11-hydroxysteroid dehydrogenase (HSD)-2, a placental enzyme that metabolizes cortisol into inactive cortisone, thereby creating a functional barrier to the passage of maternal cortisol to the fetus. Hydrocortisone and prednisone do reach the fetus if given in sufficient amounts but are rapidly cleared from the fetal circulation and thus have limited effect on fetal maturation.

Betamethasone and dexamethasone are optical isomers of the same fluorinated synthetic steroid, differing in the orientation of a single methyl substituent at position C16. The pharmacokinetic properties of these drugs are similar, with fetal plasma concentrations being approximately one-third that of maternal. However, dexamethasone has a slightly greater affinity for the glucocorticoid receptor than betamethasone and a slightly longer duration of biologic activity with current antenatal dosing regimens.[6] Dexamethasone also appears to have greater potency for non-genomic effects.

The success of antenatal glucocorticoid therapy is due in large part to the fact that synthetic glucocorticoids accelerate a similar sequence of coordinated organ development in the preterm fetus as occurs typically with the increase in endogenous cortisol at term. Although the underlying developmental state of fetal tissues influences the maturation response, studies in preterm lambs and human lung explants have shown that glucocorticoids can induce marked increases in surfactant and changes to tissue architecture even during the early saccular phase of fetal lung development. While surfactant deficiency is central to the pathophysiology of RDS, immature lung structure underlies the acute respiratory distress seen in preterm infants. Thus, the clinical effect of synthetic glucocorticoids on the incidence and severity of RDS is due not only to increased lung surfactant but also wider maturational effects in the preterm fetus on lung structure and other functional pathways, which may occur more rapidly. This may explain why antenatal glucocorticoids are of benefit even with a short duration of exposure (<48 hours), before appreciable amounts of surfactant have been produced, and the synergism that has been observed between antenatal glucocorticoid and postnatal surfactant therapies.

In vitro studies have shown that the glucocorticoid receptor is saturated at low nanomolar concentrations of betamethasone and dexamethasone, and thus the fetal concentrations achieved with current clinical dosing regimens are likely in excess of that needed to induce gene transcription. Indeed, in sheep, a single maternal injection of the slowly absorbed betamethasone acetate was as effective as serial bolus dosing with betamethasone phosphate, despite considerably lower fetal plasma concentrations. However, with the commercial formulations available, current dosing regimens of dexamethasone and betamethasone are required to increase circulating fetal glucocorticoid concentrations for a sufficient duration (up to 60 to 72 hours).[7]

ROLE OF OTHER HORMONES IN RESPIRATORY DISTRESS SYNDROME

In addition to glucocorticoids, the fetal lung is also responsive to thyroid hormones and catecholamines. Triiodothyronine (T_3) directly stimulates phospholipid synthesis in type II epithelial cells, and in animal studies, T_3 and glucocorticoids were shown to act synergistically to increase the surfactant content of the fetal lung.[6] Indeed, glucocorticoids upregulate the deiodination of thyroxine in the fetal liver, and preterm babies with low cord blood T_3 concentrations have increased incidence and severity of RDS. Because T_3 does not readily cross the placenta, clinical trials have investigated co-administration of thyrotropin-releasing hormone (TRH) with betamethasone to women for prevention of RDS, but the addition of TRH did not offer any clinical advantage compared to betamethasone alone and maternal side effects were increased.[8]

Catecholamines stimulate surfactant release from type II epithelial cells and promote clearance of fetal lung fluid.[6] Catecholamine action is facilitated by glucocorticoids, which induce β-adrenergic receptors throughout the fetal lung. Although not given directly for prevention of RDS, use of β-agonists for tocolysis has not been associated with a reduced incidence of RDS.

LONG-TERM EFFECTS OF FETAL GLUCOCORTICOID EXPOSURE

In promoting tissue differentiation, antenatal glucocorticoids cause a shift in the cell cycle leading to decreased DNA synthesis and cell division. Although these genomic effects appear to be fully reversible, this has raised concern that excess fetal glucocorticoid exposure could permanently reduce the number of functional units in metabolic tissues, with effects on long-term health. For example, reduced nephrogenesis could contribute to later hypertension, and decreased alveolarization to emphysema in adulthood. Further, in some animal studies, fetal glucocorticoid exposure has been associated with altered homeostasis, including the hypothalamic-pituitary-adrenal and insulin-glucose axes, with long-term effects on stress responses and insulin sensitivity.

Consequently, fetal overexposure to glucocorticoids has been postulated as a potential mechanism to explain the known associations between fetal growth restriction and adult cardiometabolic diseases, such as diabetes, hypertension, stroke, and ischemic heart disease.[9] This is supported by experimental evidence showing that manipulations that inhibit placental 11-β-HSD-2 activity, and thereby increase the transfer of maternal cortisol to the fetus, are associated with both fetal growth restriction and components of the metabolic syndrome,[10] effects that can be prevented by blockade of maternal glucocorticoid synthesis.

CLINICAL EVIDENCE FOR EFFECTIVENESS OF ANTENATAL GLUCOCORTICOID THERAPY

IMPACT OF ANTENATAL GLUCOCORTICOID THERAPY ON RESPIRATORY DISTRESS SYNDROME

Liggins and Howie, working in Auckland, New Zealand, in the 1960s, showed in sheep that administration to the mother of a synthetic glucocorticoid that crossed the placenta (they used dexamethasone initially) resulted in preterm lambs surviving who would have been expected to die of lung immaturity.[11] They deduced that this approach could also be used to accelerate the maturation of the lungs in babies born preterm, and subsequently conducted the first randomized trial of giving antenatal glucocorticoids (betamethasone) to women at risk of preterm birth. Preliminary findings, reported in 1972, showed that this

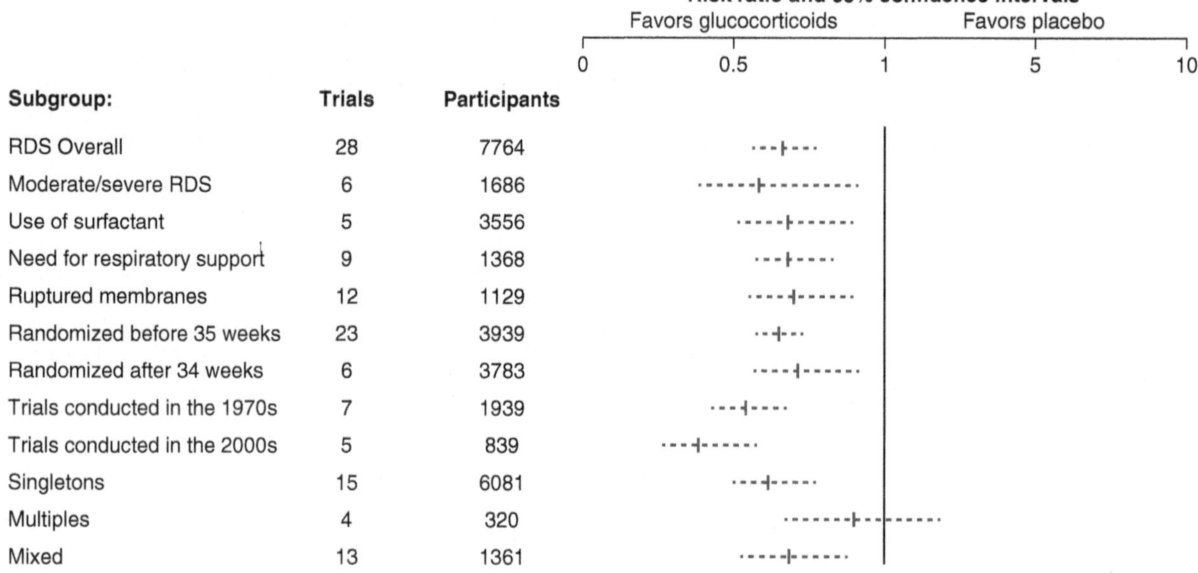

Fig. 78.1 Summary of meta-analysis of respiratory outcomes for those randomized to antenatal glucocorticoids compared with those randomized to placebo. (Data from Roberts D, Brown J, Medley N, Dalziel SR. Antenatal corticosteroids for accelerating fetal lung maturation for women at risk of preterm birth. *Cochrane Database Syst Rev.* 2017;3:CD004454.)

treatment significantly decreased neonatal mortality and the risk of RDS,[12] and in the final analysis, antenatal betamethasone was also associated with a reduction in the rate of intraventricular hemorrhage. Many other randomized trials followed, to date including more than 7000 mothers and 8000 babies, but the findings have changed little from those of the first trial.

The most recent Cochrane meta-analysis summarizes findings from 30 randomized trials, consistently showing that antenatal glucocorticoids reduce the incidence of RDS by approximately 45% (Fig. 78.1).[13] The need for mechanical respiratory support and for surfactant therapy are similarly reduced. These benefits are greatest if glucocorticoids are given 1 to 7 days before the birth but are also seen in babies born before or after this time. They are also greatest in babies randomized before 35 weeks but appear to be effective across the range of gestational ages. The beneficial effects on RDS are also seen in more recent trials conducted after the widespread adoption of artificial surfactant therapy. Indeed, these two treatments are synergistic in improving early lung function in babies at risk. This is likely to be because, in addition to surfactant production, glucocorticoids accelerate the development of lung structural components such as increased tissue elasticity, decreased mesenchymal volume and septal thickness, enlargement of alveolar airspaces, and maturation of alveolar capillaries. Studies in sheep suggest that these structural changes occur more rapidly than the effects on surfactant, the concentrations of which do not increase substantially for at least 48 hours after glucocorticoid exposure.[1]

EFFECT OF ANTENATAL GLUCOCORTICOID THERAPY ON MATERNAL AND OTHER NEONATAL MORBIDITIES

SHORT-TERM EFFECTS

Reduction in the incidence and severity of RDS was likely the major contributor to the significant reduction of neonatal mortality observed in the early randomized trials of antenatal glucocorticoids. This important benefit persists in the modern era, despite the decrease in overall mortality in preterm babies.[13] However, since glucocorticoids have widespread effects on maturation of different fetal tissues and organ systems, all of which may contribute to a more benign clinical course in babies exposed to antenatal glucocorticoids, it is perhaps not surprising that antenatal glucocorticoid therapy also reduces the risk of many of the other common complications of preterm birth (Fig. 78.2), including serious diseases of the intestines (necrotizing enterocolitis) and brain (intraventricular hemorrhage).

The extra-pulmonary benefits of antenatal glucocorticoids in preterm infants likely result from the combined maturational effects on multiple organ systems and pathways. For example, the risk of intraventricular hemorrhage is reduced by increased circulatory stability, maturation of cerebral microvasculature, improved lung function with reduced need for mechanical ventilation, and cerebral vasoconstriction at the time of birth.[14] Similarly, the incidence of necrotizing enterocolitis may be reduced due to increased maturation of the intestinal epithelium, increased secretion of gastric acid and digestive enzymes, improved humoral immunity, and better postnatal perfusion and oxygenation of the intestinal tissues.

The widespread effects of glucocorticoids also have the potential to result in adverse effects in clinical use. Glucocorticoids inhibit many aspects of immune defenses, including suppression of inflammatory mediators, attenuation of macrophage activation and leukocyte extravasation, and increasing lymphocyte apoptosis.[15] Thus, there have been concerns that antenatal glucocorticoids may increase the risk of infection in the mother and baby, particularly when that risk is already increased as a result of preterm prelabor rupture of the fetal membranes (PPROM). However, a meta-analysis of randomized trials shows that antenatal glucocorticoids reduce the rate of early-onset sepsis in newborns and maternal infection does not appear to be a significant problem in clinical practice, at least in high-income countries where most trials have been undertaken. In fact, in high-income countries, antenatal glucocorticoids may actually decrease the incidence of chorioamnionitis.[13]

In accelerating lung maturation, antenatal glucocorticoids may decrease alveolarization due to a decrease in secondary septal division, potentially resulting in impaired later lung function. For example, rats exposed to antenatal glucocorticoids

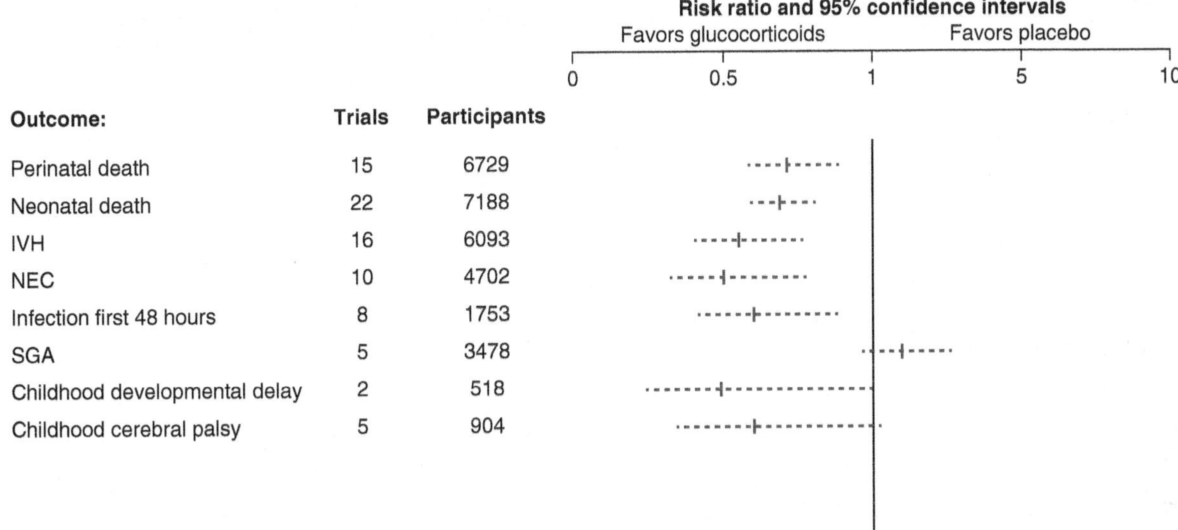

Fig. 78.2 Summary of meta-analysis of key neonatal and childhood outcomes for those randomized to antenatal glucocorticoids compared with those randomized to placebo. *IVH,* Intraventricular hemorrhage; *NEC,* necrotizing enterocolitis; *SGA,* small for gestational age. (Data from Roberts D, Brown J, Medley N, Dalziel SR. Antenatal corticosteroids for accelerating fetal lung maturation for women at risk of preterm birth. *Cochrane Database Syst Rev.* 2017;3:CD004454.)

had larger and fewer alveolar air spaces in adulthood.[16] However, there was no difference in lung function in childhood between those exposed to antenatal glucocorticoids and those in the placebo group for the two trials that have reported these outcomes.[13] Nor was there any difference in lung function between study groups in adult survivors of the original Liggins and Howie trial.[17] Further, children exposed to repeat doses of antenatal betamethasone had similar lung function at 6 to 7 years of age compared to those exposed to a single course of antenatal glucocorticoids.[18] This suggests that in humans, any effect on alveolarization is brief and reversible, as has also been demonstrated in fetal lambs.[3]

LONG-TERM EFFECTS

In animal studies, glucocorticoids inhibit brain growth, reducing the number of brain cells, particularly those undergoing rapid mitosis at the time of administration. Most of those studies used much larger doses of glucocorticoids and for proportionately a much longer period of gestation than in clinical use.[14] Nevertheless, these findings led to concern that the development of babies exposed to antenatal glucocorticoid therapy may be adversely affected. Evidence from randomized trials is once again reassuring, with a reduced incidence of developmental delay, and no effect on cerebral palsy, visual impairment, hearing impairment, or behavioral or learning difficulties in childhood.[13] Long-term follow-up of 534 participants in the original Liggins and Howie trial at 30 years of age also showed no adverse effects of antenatal glucocorticoid exposure on adult intelligence, memory, attention, psychiatric problems, handedness, education, employment, socioeconomic status, or health-related quality of life.[19]

Glucocorticoids also inhibit growth, alter body composition, and impair bone mineralization. In the fetus, glucocorticoids shift the cell cycle from proliferation to differentiation, with a decrease in DNA synthesis leading to reduced tissue accretion. Fetal growth may also be affected by slowing of placental growth and altered nutrient transfer, especially of amino acids.[20] In skeletal tissues, glucocorticoids may decrease fetal bone turnover, calcium uptake, and collagen turnover.[21] These changes are mediated, at least in part, by reduced fetal expression of the insulin-like growth factors (insulin-like growth factor [IGF]-1 and IGF-2).[22]

In animal studies, this can result in reduced size at birth, and in increased fat mass and relative obesity with aging, together with reduced bone density. Preterm birth in human cohorts is also associated with increased fat mass and increased risk of obesity with aging,[23] so data from randomized trials are important to separate any effects of antenatal glucocorticoid exposure from those of preterm birth itself. To date, data from the randomized trials have shown no change in birth size after antenatal glucocorticoid therapy.[13] Weight, height, and head circumference in childhood and into adulthood are also unchanged,[13] as are bone density, body mass index (BMI), waist–hip ratio, and skinfold thicknesses in adulthood.[24,25]

Similarly, given the substantial evidence from the experimental literature on the very widespread effects of early glucocorticoid exposure on later cardio-metabolic risk factors such as blood pressure and insulin sensitivity, there has been concern about these potential long-term adverse effects after clinical use. Limited data suggest that there are no effects on blood pressure or plasma concentrations of lipids, glucose, insulin, or cortisol.[25] However, consistent with the findings from animal experiments, 30-year-olds exposed to antenatal glucocorticoids in the Liggins and Howie trial did have evidence of possible insulin resistance.[25] This was of no clinical significance at that age, but longer-term follow-up is required to determine if this small physiologic effect results in any change in clinical outcomes as these adults age.

REPEAT COURSES OF ANTENATAL GLUCOCORTICOID THERAPY

The effects of glucocorticoids on many aspects of lung maturation are time-dependent, requiring gene transcription and protein synthesis. They also require repeated exposure for maximal effects, including on lung compliance and surfactant synthesis. In preterm lambs, maximal lung surfactant content and structural maturation were achieved with three to four maternal doses of antenatal glucocorticoids at weekly intervals.[3,26] Similarly, in mice, a multidose regimen of antenatal betamethasone promoted greater alveolar development in pups than a single dose.[27]

However, repeated exposure to glucocorticoids also increases the likelihood of all other effects, including potential adverse effects

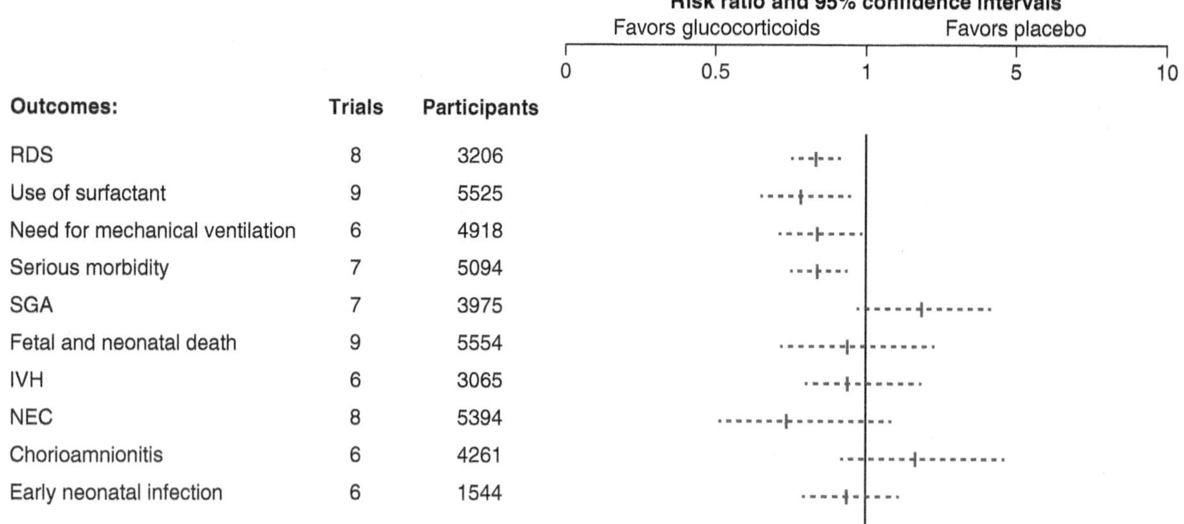

Fig. 78.3 Summary of meta-analysis of outcomes for mothers and babies randomized to repeat antenatal glucocorticoids compared with those randomized to placebo who therefore received only a single course. *RDS*, Respiratory distress syndrome. (Data from Crowther CA, McKinlay CJD, Middleton P, Harding JE. Repeat doses of prenatal corticosteroids for women at risk of preterm birth for improving neonatal health outcomes. *Cochrane Database Sys Rev.* 2015;7:CD003935.)

such as suppression of immune function and impaired growth, including brain growth. Studies in pregnant sheep particularly highlighted the potential benefits of repeat antenatal glucocorticoid exposure for lung development, balanced against adverse effects on overall short-term growth and brain development.[28] These effects varied with the specific drug and dose administered.

In clinical practice, approximately 25% of women thought to be at risk of preterm birth and thus eligible for the first course of antenatal glucocorticoids do not give birth within 7 days. In the original Liggins and Howie randomized trial, the benefits of antenatal glucocorticoid therapy were noted to be maximal for babies born 1 to 7 days later, and the authors raised the possibility of the need for repeat doses after this time if preterm birth still threatened but had not yet occurred. This led to the increasing use of repeat courses of antenatal glucocorticoids in clinical practice and, as concerns grew, to calls for randomized trials of repeat glucocorticoid therapy.

There have now been 10 randomized trials involving 4733 mothers and 5700 babies. As for a single course of antenatal glucocorticoids, the Cochrane meta-analysis of results to date shows repeat courses further reduce the risk of RDS by 17%, with similar reductions in the need for mechanical ventilation and use of surfactant.[29] Babies exposed to repeat courses also have a reduced risk of other serious neonatal morbidities, including intraventricular hemorrhage and necrotizing enterocolitis (Fig. 78.3). Indeed, the numbers of women who need to be treated with repeat courses of antenatal glucocorticoids to prevent one case of RDS (17; 95% confidence intervals [CI] 11 to 32) is only a little higher than the number for a single course (12; 95% CI 7 to 14).[29]

However, the risk of adverse effects may also be increased after repeat courses. In contrast to the effects of a single course of antenatal glucocorticoids, exposure to repeat courses results in reduced size at birth.[29] These effects are small (0.1 of a standard deviation) and of uncertain clinical significance, especially as they are no longer present by the time of discharge from hospital, and the proportion of babies born small for gestational age is not affected.[29] Importantly, subsequent growth appears unaffected, with no changes seen in weight, height, head circumference, or BMI in early childhood or at school age.[18,30]

Concerns about the effects on brain growth, in particular, make it important to carefully examine developmental outcomes after repeated antenatal glucocorticoids. An early non-randomized cohort study suggested that children exposed to repeat courses of antenatal glucocorticoids exhibited later behavioral difficulties. However, women for whom preterm birth is repeatedly threatened but does not occur, and who are therefore eligible to receive repeat courses of antenatal glucocorticoids, are inevitably different in many ways from those women where only a single course is administered, making data from cohort studies difficult to interpret. In contrast, limited data from four randomized trials show no differences between preschool children exposed to a single course and those exposed to repeat courses of antenatal glucocorticoids for developmental delay, blindness, deafness, cerebral palsy, or behavior problems.[29] Findings from the later follow-up of 1728 children at 5 years from one trial,[30] and 963 children at 6 to 8 years from another trial,[18] also showed no differences between study groups for these outcomes. Further, subgroup analysis has suggested that in the growth-restricted fetus, repeat antenatal glucocorticoids may even have a beneficial effect on attention and impulse control.[31]

Data from animal studies suggested that the possible adverse cardio-metabolic consequences of antenatal glucocorticoid exposure may also be greater after repeat doses.[32] Again, limited data from randomized trials are reassuring. In 258 children examined at 6 to 8 years of age, there was no evidence of any effects of exposure to repeat antenatal glucocorticoids compared to a single course on body composition, blood pressure, insulin sensitivity, kidney function, or cortisol secretion.[33]

RECOMMENDATIONS FOR ANTENATAL GLUCOCORTICOID THERAPY

It is clear that antenatal glucocorticoid therapy for women at risk of preterm birth substantially reduces the risk of mortality and serious morbidity including RDS in their offspring, with few short- or long-term adverse effects. Thus, the use of antenatal glucocorticoid therapy is recommended by all major international clinical practice guidelines for women at risk of preterm birth (Table 78.1).

While most guidelines recommend the use of a single course, there is less consistency in recommendations about

Table 78.1 Clinical Practice Guideline Recommendations Regarding Antenatal Glucocorticoid Therapy.

	World Health Organisation[43]	American College of Obstetrics and Gynecology[44]	International Federation of Gynecology and Obstetrics[45]	National Institute for Health and Care Excellence (UK)[46]	Australia and New Zealand Antenatal Corticosteroid Clinical Practice Guidelines Panel[47]
Publication date	2015	2017	2019	2015, updated 2019	2015
Eligible women	At risk of preterm birth	At risk of preterm delivery within 7 days. Glucocorticoids should not be administered unless there is substantial clinical concern for imminent preterm birth.	At risk of preterm birth within 7 days	Suspected, diagnosed, or established preterm labor, having a planned preterm birth, or have preterm prolonged rupture of the membranes.	At risk of early preterm, imminent birth, regardless of the reason
Gestation	24–34 weeks	24–33 weeks. May be considered at 23 weeks based on family's decision about resuscitation, and at 34–36 weeks in women who have not received a previous course.	24–34 weeks. Administration at less than 24 weeks is linked to a family's decision regarding resuscitation.	24–33 weeks, consider at 34–35 weeks.	34 weeks and 6 days or less
Dose and drug	Dexamethasone or betamethasone 24 mg intramuscularly in divided doses	Betamethasone 12 mg × 2 doses 24 h apart OR dexamethasone 6 mg × 4 doses 12 h apart	Betamethasone 12 mg × 2 doses 24 h apart OR dexamethasone 6 mg × 4 doses 12 h apart	NR	Betamethasone 24 mg in divided doses, completed between 12 and 36 h OR dexamethasone 24 mg in divided doses completed between 24 and 40 h
Timing	When preterm birth is considered imminent within 7 days of starting treatment, including within the first 24 h.	A first dose should be administered even if the ability to give the second dose is unlikely.	NR	NR	When preterm birth is planned or expected within the next 7 days, even if birth is likely within 24 h
Repeat	Single repeat course if preterm birth does not occur within 7 days after the initial dose, and high risk of preterm birth in the next 7 days.	A single repeat course if less than 34 weeks gestation, at risk of preterm delivery within 7 days, and prior course of antenatal glucocorticoids was more than 14 days previously. Rescue course could be provided as early as 7 days from the prior dose, if indicated by the clinical scenario. Regularly scheduled repeat courses or serial courses (more than two) are not recommended.	A single repeat course should be considered in women at less than 34 weeks gestation who have an imminent risk of preterm delivery within the next 7 days, and whose prior course was more than 7–14 days previously.	Do not routinely offer repeat courses, but take into account the interval since the end of last course, gestational age, the likelihood of birth within 48 h.	Use repeat antenatal glucocorticoids in women at risk for early preterm, imminent birth when gestation is 32 weeks and 6 days or less and preterm birth is planned or expected within the next 7 days, not less than 7 days following a single course. Use up to 3 single repeat doses (12 mg betamethasone) or 1 single repeat course (24 mg betamethasone in divided doses completed within 24 h).
Late preterm/ prior to cesarean section	Not recommended	Recommended between 34 0/7 weeks and 36 6/7 weeks if at risk of preterm birth within 7 days, and no previous course of antenatal glucocorticoids. No recommendations about cesarean section at term	Consider for women undergoing planned cesarean delivery at 37–38.6 weeks gestation.	NR	Use 48 h prior to cesarean birth planned beyond 34 weeks and 6 days if there is known fetal lung immaturity.

NR, No specific recommendation.

the use of repeat antenatal glucocorticoid treatment. Some authorities have recommended a single repeat "rescue" course for women who remain at risk of preterm birth at less than 34 weeks, 7 or more days after an initial course, but other repeat regimens are also advocated (see Table 78.1). An individual-participant data meta-analysis of data from 11 randomized trials found that to maximize clinical benefits for babies and minimize effects on fetal growth, repeat antenatal glucocorticoid therapy should be limited to a maximum of three repeat treatments and a total dose of betamethasone of between 24 and 48 mg.[34]

CHOICE OF SYNTHETIC GLUCOCORTICOID

There is considerable variation between countries as to which glucocorticoid is used, influenced by local availability, research findings, the influence of opinion leaders, and costs. For example, a course of betamethasone costs US\$60[35] compared with only about US\$5 for dexamethasone. Retrospective human studies comparing betamethasone and dexamethasone provide conflicting findings, with some studies reporting no differences between them in the risk of intraventricular hemorrhage, periventricular leukomalacia, or mortality,[36] while others suggest betamethasone results in a lower rate of periventricular leukomalacia[36] and neurosensory impairment.[37] The sulfite preservative previously used in some formulations for dexamethasone had been implicated in the effect on periventricular leukomalacia.

In the Cochrane meta-analysis of the randomized trials that have directly compared betamethasone with dexamethasone, neonatal findings were similar, although dexamethasone was associated with a lower risk of intraventricular hemorrhage than betamethasone.[38] The recent ASTEROID Trial randomized 1346 women at risk of preterm birth before 34 weeks gestation to receive dexamethasone or betamethasone.[39] The incidence of neonatal respiratory distress, intraventricular hemorrhage, periventricular leukomalacia, and maternal infections were similar for both drugs. However, fewer women given dexamethasone compared with betamethasone reported pain related to the injection or needed a cesarean birth, and their children at 2 years were less likely to be hypertensive. Both drugs showed a similar likelihood of survival free of neurosensory disability at 2 years.[39] These latest findings support the clinical practice guideline recommendations that either drug can be used. Choice of glucocorticoid will be influenced by availability, cost, and maternal and clinician preferences.

REMAINING UNCERTAINTIES ABOUT ANTENATAL GLUCOCORTICOID THERAPY

Many questions remain unanswered about the effects of antenatal glucocorticoids prior to preterm birth even though many thousands of women and babies have participated in randomized trials over the last 50 years. Recommendations for further research are provided within the latest clinical practice guidelines (Table 78.2).

VERY EARLY GESTATION

While randomized trials on the use of antenatal glucocorticoids recruited few women at risk of very early preterm birth before 26 weeks gestation,[13] cohort studies have consistently demonstrated benefit in survival and childhood neurodevelopment for babies exposed to antenatal glucocorticoids from 23 to 25 weeks gestation. The decision to use glucocorticoids at periviable gestational ages needs to be made with parental discussion and consideration of the clinical situation.

LATE GESTATION/TERM ELECTIVE CESAREAN SECTION

While there are strong recommendations to use antenatal glucocorticoids in women at risk of preterm birth at less than 35 weeks gestation, there is less certainty about use at later gestational ages, at or near term, when the risk of RDS may be increased (e.g., prior to cesarean birth or in women with diabetes). A systematic review that included six trials confirmed benefit at these later gestations for respiratory problems, and there was reduced need for admission to the neonatal nursery.[40] However, there is a paucity of information on use in late gestation and effects on childhood and later health. Importantly, the largest of these trials reported the unexpected finding of increased rates of low blood glucose concentrations (hypoglycemia) in infants exposed to antenatal glucocorticoids.[41] This may be because glucocorticoids increase maternal blood glucose concentrations via effects on glycolysis and gluconeogenesis, thus increasing fetal glucose and therefore insulin concentrations, which can persist after birth despite the cessation of glucose supply across the placenta. Hypoglycemia may be associated with later developmental impairment and lower educational achievement in childhood. Thus, further research is needed about the relative benefits and risks of antenatal glucocorticoid therapy after 35 weeks gestation before strong clinical recommendations can be made.

USE IN LOW- TO MIDDLE-INCOME COUNTRIES

Most randomized trials assessing the efficacy of antenatal glucocorticoids have been conducted in high-income countries where uptake has been high.[13] However, uptake in low- to middle-income countries has been varied. Given the known benefits, wider uptake has been strongly promoted. However, a population-based (99,742 women), cluster-randomized trial of a multifaceted intervention to implement the use of antenatal glucocorticoid treatment in six countries (Argentina, Guatemala, India, Kenya, Pakistan, and Zambia) unexpectedly showed increased neonatal mortality and increased risk of maternal infection after exposure to glucocorticoid treatment.[42] The reason for these findings is not clear, but some difficulties included a high rate of infection and growth restriction, uncertainty about gestational age, and limited access to medical care. Thus, the World Health Organization has recommended that antenatal glucocorticoid treatment should be used under circumstances when there is no evidence of maternal infection, gestational age is known, and mother and baby have access to adequate care.[43]

VERY LONG-TERM EFFECTS OF ANTENATAL GLUCOCORTICOID EXPOSURE

As concerns remain about the middle and old age effects of antenatal glucocorticoid exposure, follow-up of participants in the available trials is still required. Follow-up of the original Liggins and Howie randomized trial cohort into middle age is planned, as is adult follow-up of at least one of the repeat glucocorticoid trials.

CONCLUSION

Development of the fetal lung involves the coordinated action of many hormones, of which the glucocorticoids are arguably the most important. The increase in endogenous fetal glucocorticoids before birth coordinates structural and functional maturation of many fetal tissues, most notable the lung. This maturation can also be induced by exogenous glucocorticoids, an approach that is used clinically before preterm birth. There is robust evidence from large numbers of randomized trials that antenatal glucocorticoid administration before preterm birth has many beneficial effects and is safe in

Table 78.2 Clinical Practice Guideline Research Recommendations Regarding Antenatal Glucocorticoid Therapy.

	World Health Organization (2015)[43]	Australia and New Zealand Antenatal Corticosteroid Clinical Practice Guidelines Panel (2015)[47]
Use of a Single Course		
Understanding mechanisms		There is a need to better assess the impact, if any, of in utero exposure to a single course of antenatal glucocorticoids on: • the hypothalamic-pituitary adrenal axis of the infant, child, and adult; • the glucose-insulin axis in childhood; • the later risk of the infant developing diabetes in adulthood.
Use of a single course	What are the long-term outcomes of all infants exposed to antenatal glucocorticoids (including term infants)? What strategies can effectively and safely increase the use of glucocorticoids in low- and middle-income country settings to improve outcomes? What are the effects of antenatal glucocorticoids at different gestational ages at birth (using independent patient data analysis)? Assessment of coverage of antenatal glucocorticoids before and after guideline implementation (and associated reduction in neonatal mortality). Assessment of implementation strategies and monitoring of adverse events (in low- and middle-income settings). What are the effects of antenatal glucocorticoid administration in women undergoing prelabor cesarean section in late preterm? Are there differences in the pharmacokinetic properties of betamethasone acetate versus betamethasone phosphate? What is the impact of antenatal glucocorticoid administration among mothers with evidence of infection who also receive appropriate antibiotic therapy on both maternal and neonatal outcomes? What is the minimum effective dose of glucocorticoids to achieve fetal lung maturation and other improved outcomes?	Future research that investigates the use of a single course of antenatal glucocorticoids should include: • outcomes on maternal quality of life; • report on the risk factors for preterm birth of the included participants; • an assessment of the degree and health impact, if any, of changes in maternal blood glucose control.
Randomized trials needed to:	Antenatal glucocorticoid therapy in women undergoing planned cesarean section at late preterm gestations (34–36+ weeks). Assess differences in pharmacologic properties of dexamethasone and betamethasone dosage regimens. What is the most effective regimen and dose for antenatal glucocorticoids? In what contexts can antenatal glucocorticoids be used safely and effectively in low-income countries?	• compare betamethasone and dexamethasone to assess the effect on the short-term and long-term outcomes for the infant; • investigate the optimal timing for antenatal glucocorticoids where preterm birth is planned (e.g., maternal medical indications or fetal compromise) and women can be randomized to administration of antenatal glucocorticoids at different time intervals prior to birth; • investigate the neonatal benefits of antenatal glucocorticoids administered to women at less than 24 weeks gestation; • investigate if smaller doses are needed at lower gestational ages; • investigate the neonatal benefits of antenatal glucocorticoids administered late preterm (34 weeks and 6 days to <37 weeks gestation); • review the effect of a single course of antenatal glucocorticoids on women with systemic infection at risk of preterm birth.
To maximize benefit and minimize harm to the mother and infant there is a need to establish:		• the minimally effective dose per course of both betamethasone and dexamethasone; • the optimal timing interval per course between doses for both betamethasone and dexamethasone; • the optimal number of doses per course for betamethasone; • the optimal number of doses per course for dexamethasone; • the hemodynamic effects of antenatal glucocorticoids on the growth-restricted fetus; • the optimal timing of birth following administration of antenatal glucocorticoids to women with a fetus with intrauterine growth restriction.

Table 78.2 Clinical Practice Guideline Research Recommendations Regarding Antenatal Glucocorticoid Therapy.—cont'd

	World Health Organization (2015)[43]	Australia and New Zealand Antenatal Corticosteroid Clinical Practice Guidelines Panel (2015)[47]
Use of Repeat Antenatal Glucocorticoids		
Understanding mechanisms	What is the minimum effective dose required to achieve lung maturation or repeat courses of antenatal glucocorticoids?	There is a need to better assess the impact, if any, of in utero exposure to repeat antenatal glucocorticoids on: Physiologic outcomes: • the glucose-insulin axis in childhood, • hypothalamic-pituitary adrenal axis, • bone mass, • body size and body composition, • neurosensory impairments, • respiratory function. Health outcomes: • cardiovascular disease, • metabolic disease, • diabetes, • psychological health, • the later risk of developing diabetes in adulthood. Social outcomes: • educational attainment, • behavior, • cognitive ability.
Randomized trials needed to:		• evaluate dexamethasone as the repeat antenatal glucocorticoid; • compare the use of different timing of administration of repeat antenatal glucocorticoids prior to preterm birth where preterm birth is definitely expected or planned; • investigate the effects of repeat antenatal corticosteroids in women ≥32 weeks and 6 days gestation; • investigate if antenatal glucocorticoids should be repeated in women at risk of preterm birth who had antenatal glucocorticoids 7 days previously and then present with chorioamnionitis. Any future research to investigate the effects of treatment with repeat antenatal glucocorticoids should: • include outcomes for maternal quality of life, • report on the risk factors for preterm birth of the included participants, • assess the degree and health impact of changes in maternal blood glucose control.
Type of glucocorticoid to use		Further research is required to explore betamethasone and dexamethasone as the repeat antenatal glucocorticoid for: • the optimal dose, • the optimal number of dose(s) in a course, • the optimal interval between courses, • the effect of multiple repeat doses/courses.

usual clinical practice. Hence their routine use prior to preterm birth is strongly recommended, with widespread uptake. For the remaining uncertainties about their use, that lead to variation in clinical practice recommendations, further research is needed. The use of antenatal glucocorticoids to accelerate fetal lung maturation prior to preterm birth remains a significant success story in modern perinatal medicine.

REFERENCES

1. Ballard PL, Ning Y, Polk D, Ikegami M, Jobe A. Glucorticoid regulation of surfactant components in immature lambs. *Am J Physiol*. 1997;273(5 Pt 1):L1048-L1057.
2. Ikegami M, Polk DH, Jobe AH, et al. Effect of interval from fetal corticosteroid treatment to delivery on postnatal lung function of preterm lambs. *J Appl Physiol*. 1996;80(2):591-597.
3. Willet KE, Jobe AH, Ikegami M, Kovar J, Sly PD. Lung morphometry after repetitive antenatal glucocorticoid treatment in preterm sheep. *Am J Respir Crit Care Med*. 2001;163(6):1437-1443.
4. Venkatesh VC, Ballard PL. Glucocorticoids and gene expression. *Am J Respir Cell Mol Biol*. 1991;4(4):301-303.
5. Ballard PL, Ertsey R, Gonzales LW, Gonzales J. Transcriptional regulation of human pulmonary surfactant proteins SP-B and SP-C by glucocorticoids. *Am J Respir Cell Mol Biol*. 1996;14(6):599-607.
6. Ballard PL. *Hormones and Lung Maturation*. Berlin: Springer-Verlag; 1986.
7. Ballard PL, Gluckman PD, Liggins GC, Kaplan SL, Grumbach MM. Steroid and growth hormone levels in premature infants after prenatal betamethasone therapy to prevent respiratory distress syndrome. *Pediatr Res*. 1980;14(2):122-127.
8. Crowther CA, Alfirevic Z, Han S, Haslam RR. Thyrotropin-releasing hormone added to corticosteroids for women at risk of preterm birth for preventing neonatal respiratory disease. *Cochrane Database Syst Rev*. 2013;11:CD000019.
9. Barker DJP. The developmental origins of well-being. *Phil Trans R Soc Lond*. 2004;359(1449):1359-1366.
10. Langley-Evans SC, Phillips GJ, Benediktsson R, et al. Protein intake in pregnancy, placental glucocorticoid metabolism and the programming of hypertension in the rat. *Placenta*. 1996;17(2-3):169-172.
11. Liggins GC. Premature delivery of foetal lambs infused with glucocorticoids. *J Endocrinol*. 1969;45(4):515-523.

12. Liggins GC, Howie RN. A controlled trial of antepartum glucocorticoid treatment for prevention of the respiratory distress syndrome in premature infants. *Pediatrics*. 1972;50(4):515-525.
13. Roberts D, Brown J, Medley N, Dalziel SR. Antenatal corticosteroids for accelerating fetal lung maturation for women at risk of preterm birth. *Cochrane Database Syst Rev*. 2017;3:CD004454.
14. McKinlay CJ, Dalziel SR, Harding JE. Antenatal glucocorticoids: where are we after forty years? *J Dev Orig Health Dis*. 2015;6(2):127-142.
15. Cain DW, Cidlowski JA. Immune regulation by glucocorticoids. *Nat Rev Immunol*. 2017;17(4):233-247.
16. Blanco LN, Massaro GD, Massaro D. Alveolar dimensions and number: developmental and hormonal regulation. *Am J Physiol*. 1989;257(4 Pt 1):L240-L247.
17. Dalziel SR, Rea HH, Walker NK, et al. Long term effects of antenatal betamethasone on lung function: 30 year follow up of a randomised controlled trial. *Thorax*. 2006;61(8):678-683.
18. Crowther CA, Anderson PJ, McKinlay CJ, et al. Mid-childhood outcomes of repeat antenatal corticosteroids: a randomized controlled trial. *Pediatrics*. 2016;138(4):e20160947.
19. Dalziel SR, Lim VK, Lambert A, et al. Antenatal exposure to betamethasone: psychological functioning and health related quality of life 31 years after inclusion in randomised controlled trial. *BMJ*. 2005;331(7518):665.
20. Marconi AM, Mariotti V, Teng C, et al. Effect of antenatal betamethasone on maternal and fetal amino acid concentration. *Am J Obstet Gynecol*. 2010;202(2):166.e1-6.
21. Mosier Jr HD, Dearden LC, Roberts RC, Jansons RA, Biggs CS. Regional differences in the effects of glucocorticoids on maturation of the fetal skeleton of the rat. *Teratology*. 1981;23(1):15-24.
22. Ahmad I, Beharry KD, Valencia AM, et al. Influence of a single course of antenatal betamethasone on the maternal-fetal insulin-IGF-GH axis in singleton pregnancies. *Growth Horm IGF Res*. 2006;16(4):267-275.
23. Morrison KM, Ramsingh L, Gunn E, et al. Cardiometabolic health in adults born premature with extremely low birth weight. *Pediatrics*. 2016;138(4):e20160515.
24. Dalziel SR, Fenwick S, Cundy T, et al. Peak bone mass after exposure to antenatal betamethasone and prematurity: follow-up of a randomized controlled trial. *J Bone Miner Res*. 2006;21(8):1175-1186.
25. Dalziel SR, Walker NK, Parag V, et al. Cardiovascular risk factors after antenatal exposure to betamethasone: 30-year follow-up of a randomised controlled trial. *Lancet*. 2005;365(9474):1856-1862.
26. Ikegami M, Jobe A, Newnham J, Polk D, Willet K, Sly P. Repetitive prenatal glucocorticoids improve lung function and decrease growth in preterm lambs. *Am J Respir Crit Care Med*. 1997;156(1):178-184.
27. Stewart JD, Sienko AE, Gonzalez CL, Christensen HD, Rayburn WF. Placebo-controlled comparison between a single dose and a multidose of betamethasone in accelerating lung maturation of mice offspring. *Am J Obstet Gynecol*. 1998;179(5):1241-1247.
28. Jobe AH, Wada N, Berry LM, Ikegami M, Ervin MG. Single and repetitive maternal glucocorticoid exposures reduce fetal growth in sheep. *Am J Obstet Gynecol*. 1998;178(5):880-885.
29. Crowther CA, McKinlay CJD, Middleton P, Harding JE. Repeat doses of prenatal corticosteroids for women at risk of preterm birth for improving neonatal health outcomes. *Cochrane Database Sys Rev*. 2015;7:CD003935.
30. Asztalos EV, Murphy KE, Willan AR, et al. Multiple courses of antenatal corticosteroids for preterm birth study: outcomes in children at 5 years of age (MACS-5). *JAMA Pediatr*. 2013;167(12):1102-1110.
31. Cartwright RD, Crowther CA, Anderson PJ, Harding JE, Doyle LW, McKinlay CJD. Association of fetal growth restriction with neurocognitive function after repeated antenatal betamethasone treatment vs placebo: secondary analysis of the ACTORDS randomized clinical trial. *JAMA Netw Open*. 2019;2(2):e187636.
32. de Vries A, Holmes MC, Heijnis A, et al. Prenatal dexamethasone exposure induces changes in nonhuman primate offspring cardiometabolic and hypothalamic-pituitary-adrenal axis function. *J Clin Invest*. 2007;117(4):1058-1067.
33. McKinlay CJD, Cutfield WS, Battin MR, Dalziel SR, Crowther CA, Harding JE. Cardiovascular risk factors in children after repeat antenatal glucocorticoids: an RCT. *Pediatrics*. 2015;135(2):e405-e415.
34. Crowther CA, Middleton PF, Voysey M, et al. Effects of repeat prenatal corticosteroids given to women at risk of preterm birth: an individual participant data meta-analysis. *PLoS Med*. 2019;16(4):e1002771.
35. Gyamfi-Bannerman C, Zupancic JAF, Sandoval G, et al. Cost-effectiveness of antenatal corticosteroid therapy vs no therapy in women at risk of late preterm delivery: a secondary analysis of a randomized clinical trial. *JAMA Pediatr*. 2019;173(5):462-468.
36. Baud O, Foix-L'Helias L, Kaminski M, et al. Antenatal glucocorticoid treatment and cystic periventricular leukomalacia in very premature infants. *N Engl J Med*. 1999;341(16):1190-1196.
37. Lee BH, Stoll BJ, McDonald SA, Higgins RD. Neurodevelopmental outcomes of extremely low birth weight infants exposed prenatally to dexamethasone versus betamethasone. *Pediatrics*. 2008;121(2):289-296.
38. Brownfoot FC, Gagliardi DI, Bain E, Middleton P, Crowther CA. Different corticosteroids and regimens for accelerating fetal lung maturation for women at risk of preterm birth. *Cochrane Database Syst Rev*. 2013;8:CD006764.
39. Crowther CA, Ashwood P, Andersen CC, et al. Maternal intramuscular dexamethasone versus betamethasone before preterm birth (ASTEROID): a multicentre, double-blind, randomised controlled trial. *Lancet Child Adolesc Health*. 2019;3(11):769-780.
40. Saccone G, Berghella V. Antenatal corticosteroids for maturity of term or near term fetuses: systematic review and meta-analysis of randomized controlled trials. *BMJ*. 2016;355:i5044.
41. Gyamfi-Bannerman C, Thom EA, Blackwell SC, et al. Antenatal betamethasone for women at risk for late preterm delivery. *N Engl J Med*. 2016;374(14):1311-1320.
42. Althabe F, Belizan JM, McClure EM, et al. A population-based, multifaceted strategy to implement antenatal corticosteroid treatment versus standard care for the reduction of neonatal mortality due to preterm birth in low-income and middle-income countries: the ACT cluster-randomised trial. *Lancet*. 2015;385(9968):629-639.
43. World Health Organisation. *WHO Recommendations on Interventions to Improve Preterm Birth Outcomes: Evidence Base*. Geneva: WHO Press; 2015.
44. American College of Obstetricians and Gynecologists Committee on Obstetric Practice. Committee opinion No. 713: antenatal corticosteroid therapy for fetal maturation. *Obstet Gynecol*. 2017;130(2):e102-e109.
45. Good clinical practice advice: antenatal corticosteroids for fetal lung maturation. *Int J Gynaecol Obstet*. 2019;144(3):352-355.
46. Sarri G, Davies M, Gholitabar M, Norman JE. Preterm labour: summary of NICE guidance. *BMJ*. 2015;351:h6283.
47. Antenatal Corticosteroids Clinical Practice Guidelines Panel. *Antenatal Corticosteroids Given to Women Prior to Birth to Improve Fetal, Infant, Child and Adult Health. Clinical Practice Guidelines*. Auckland: Liggins Institute; 2015.

79 Surfactant Treatment

Alan H. Jobe | Suhas G. Kallapur

HISTORICAL BACKGROUND

A brief history of surfactant for the treatment of respiratory distress syndrome (RDS) provides perspective on this major therapeutic advance. In 1959, not long after surfactant had been identified as critical to maintaining lung inflation at low transpulmonary pressures,[1,2] Avery and Mead[3] reported that saline extracts from the lungs of preterm infants with RDS lacked the low surface tension characteristics of pulmonary surfactant. After unsuccessful attempts to treat infants with RDS with aerosolized phospholipids in the 1960s,[4] intratracheal administration of surfactant recovered by alveolar lavage from mature animal lungs was demonstrated to improve lung expansion and ventilation in preterm animals by Enhorning and Robertson in Sweden.[5,6] The clinical potential of surfactant treatment for RDS was shown by Fujiwara and colleagues[7] in a nonrandomized study in 1980, using a surfactant prepared from an organic solvent extract of bovine lung. Small, investigator-initiated, randomized controlled trials (RCTs) with surfactants prepared from bovine alveolar lavage or human amniotic fluid demonstrated significant decreases in pneumothorax and death by 1985.[8-10] Subsequent multicenter trials demonstrated decreased death rates and complications of RDS.[11] Surfactants were approved by the US Food and Drug Administration (FDA) for the treatment of RDS in 1990. They were a new class of drugs unique in the route of treatment—the airway—as an animal-sourced product developed specifically for preterm infants. Since 1990, surfactant treatments have been the standard of care for infants with RDS. Multiple studies have addressed questions about when to treat, how best to treat, and which infants respond.[12,13] New surfactants continue to be developed but need to be tested before general clinical use.[14]

CHARACTERISTICS OF SURFACTANTS FOR CLINICAL USE

Surfactants were developed empirically by testing the surface properties of mixtures of lipids and surfactant-specific proteins with the goal to emulate the properties of natural surfactant.[15] Although dipalmitoylphosphatidylcholine is the major and principal surface active component of surfactant, it is not an effective clinical surfactant because it is a solid at 37°C and does not rapidly spread or adsorb to a surface.[16] Surface adsorption of dipalmitoylphosphatidylcholine can be enhanced with the addition of other components, such as dioleoylphosphatidylcholine or phosphatidylglycerol. Simple mixtures of dipalmitoylphosphatidylcholine with other lipids can have surface properties similar to those of a natural surfactant.[17]

Two synthetic surfactants were extensively evaluated in clinical trials and were in clinical use until around the year 2000. A 7:3 weight ratio of dipalmitoylphosphatidylcholine and unsaturated phosphatidylglycerol was used in England.[18] The other synthetic surfactant used clinically was a mixture of dipalmitoylphosphatidylcholine, hexadecanol, and tyloxapol. These synthetic surfactants were not as effective as natural surfactants and are no longer used clinically.[18]

Highly surface-active surfactants purified from animal lungs were effective surfactant treatments for preterm surfactant-deficient lungs, demonstrating that formulations for clinical use could come from animal sources.[19] Surfactants from natural sources are of two general types: surfactants recovered from alveolar lavages or from saline extracts of minced lungs. Saline extracts then were extracted with organic solvents to yield phospholipids, neutral lipids, and small amounts of the hydrophobic surfactant protein (SP)-B and SP-C. The lipid extracts from lung contain the components of natural surfactant except SP-A and SP-D. However, they also have increased amounts of unsaturated phospholipids and neutral lipids that interfere with surface properties. Synthetic lipids can be added to improve surface properties,[15] or the neutral lipids can be removed by liquid-gel chromatography.[20] Another approach to making animal source surfactants is to prepare organic solvent extracts from alveolar lavages. The organic solvent extraction step removes nonessential proteins that might immune sensitize. Several commercial surfactants made from extracts from bovine or porcine lungs are in clinical use. These include beractant (Survanta), poractant (Curosurf), and calfactant (Infrasurf).

Surfactants that contain surfactant proteins or peptides that are completely synthetic are now being developed for clinical use.[21] A surfactant (lucinactant, Surfaxin) that contains synthetic lipids and small peptides that mimic the function of the native surfactant proteins is now FDA approved for the treatment of RDS.[21] Surfactants that contain minimally modified complete SP-C sequence and long sequences of SP-B have been tested in animal models and are in early phase clinical testing.[22] Synthetic surfactants have the theoretical benefit of not being derived from animal sources, although no adverse events have been attributed to the animal source surfactants in over 25 years of use. Surfactants that contain the innate host defense surfactant proteins SP-A and SP-D also have been tested in animal models but not in infants.[23] Surfactants are not difficult to make but should be tested in trials before widespread use. For example, a surfactant made from goat lungs in India was ineffective when recently tested in a RCT.[14]

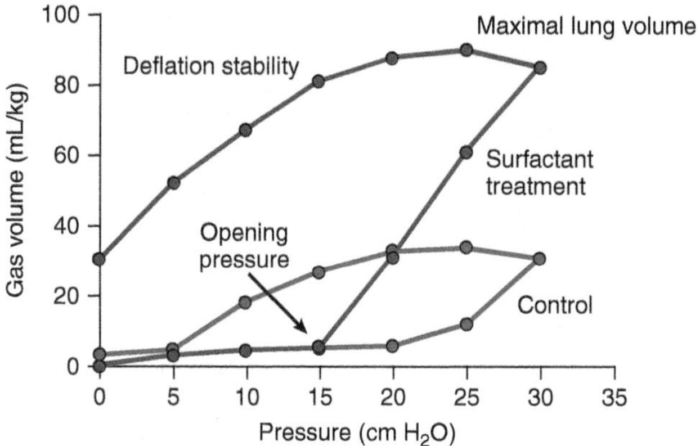

Fig. 79.1 Representative pressure-volume curves for 27-day preterm rabbit lungs treated with surfactant in comparison with control lungs. The curves were measured after a 30-minute period of ventilation. Surfactant had pronounced effects on opening pressure, maximal lung volume, and deflation stability relative to the control lungs. (Modified from Rider ED, Jobe AH, Ikegami M, et al. Different ventilation strategies alter surfactant responses in preterm rabbits. *J Appl Physiol.* 1992;73:2089.)

PHYSIOLOGIC EFFECTS OF SURFACTANT TREATMENT ON PRESSURE-VOLUME CURVES

The pressure-volume (P-V) curve defines the static effects of surfactant on the preterm lung (Fig. 79.1).[24] Surfactant treatment decreases the *opening pressure*, defined as the pressure at which the lung begins to fill above dead space volume, relative to lungs not treated with surfactant. The opening pressure of preterm surfactant-deficient rabbit lungs decreased from approximately 20 to 15 cm H_2O with surfactant treatment in this example. The explanation for this effect is that the surfactant-deficient immature lung resists inflation because of the high surface tensions at the interfaces of gas with fluid in small airways. Surfactant decreases the resistance to fluid movement in the airways and expansion of lung units is facilitated. The major clinically important effect of surfactant treatment is the large increase in lung volume at 30 cm H_2O. Because airway dead space volume will not change with surfactant treatment, this increase in volume represents the recruitment of the more distal lung surface area for gas exchange. In the mature lung maximal lung volume, V_{max} is defined by a flattening of the P-V curve at high pressure caused by the limits of expansion of the lung matrix and chest wall. The V_{max} for the surfactant-deficient preterm lung may not be achieved because inflation pressures needed to recruit that volume will exceed the rupture pressure.[25] Surfactant also stabilizes the lung during deflation to maintain a lung volume, functional residual volume (FRV), at 5 cm H_2O pressure in excess of the V_{max} achieved in control lungs.

Evaluation of degree and uniformity of inflation is another measure of surfactant effects on the lung. Based on the simplest model of two alveoli as interconnecting spheres, surfactant deficiency will cause alveolar (or small airway) instability characterized by collapse of units with small radii and dilation of units with larger radii. This instability results from Laplace's law: pressure at the surface of an alveolus = 2 × surface tension/radius. Because the alveolus is open to atmospheric pressure, the pressure outside must be balanced by the pressure on the inner surface or the alveolus will collapse. The forces acting on the alveolus are chest wall elasticity, lung tissue elasticity, and surface tensions at the alveolar surface and any continuous positive airway pressure

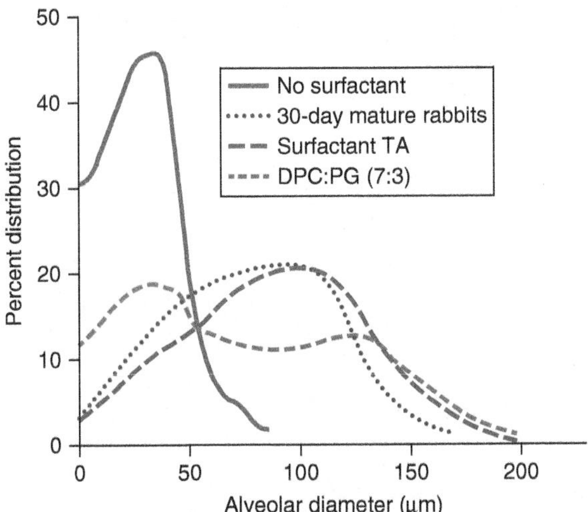

Fig. 79.2 Alveolar size distributions for 30-day-gestation mature rabbits, 27-day preterm rabbits receiving no surfactant, and preterm rabbits treated with a cow lung-derived surfactant or a dipalmitoylphosphatidylcholine:phosphatidylglycerol synthetic surfactant *(DPC:PG)* (lipid only synthetic surfactant). Surfactant treatment normalized alveolar diameters toward those measured for the mature newborn rabbits. (From Fujiwara T. Surfactant replacement in neonatal respiratory distress syndrome. In: Robertson B, van Golde LM, Battenberg JJ, eds. *Pulmonary Surfactant*. Amsterdam: Elsevier Science Publishers; 1984:480–503.)

(CPAP). All alveoli are not the same size. Therefore, Laplace's law predicts that the retractive force of surface tension will be greater on the small alveoli than on the large alveoli, with the result being collapse of the small alveoli with further filling of the large alveoli. However, surfactant has the unique property of variable surface tension, depending on the rate and amount of surface area compression. As alveolar radius decreases, surface tension falls, limiting the collapse of the small alveolus. This stabilizing influence is lost in the absence of surfactant.

The concept of alveolar interdependence results from the scaling up of the alveolar model. Each alveolus depends on the position and elasticity of the neighboring alveolar walls to maintain normal shape and volume. If adjacent alveoli collapse, an alveolus either tends to overexpand and distort or collapse. In surfactant-deficient states, the more normal alveoli tend to overexpand as other regional alveoli collapse, generating a nonhomogeneously inflated lung. Surfactant treatment improves uniformity of inflation, minimizes small airway dilation, and promotes alveolar inflation.[26] Surfactant treatment of 27-day preterm rabbits resulted in a distribution of alveolar sizes comparable to those of term rabbits (Fig. 79.2).[15] Surfactant treatment also resulted in more normal lung morphometry in preterm lambs receiving continuous mechanical ventilation 24 hours after delivery.[27] The alveoli of the lambs not treated with surfactant were shallow, and alveolar ducts were dilated. Most of these abnormalities were prevented with surfactant treatment (Fig. 79.3). This surfactant effect on uniformity of lung expansion may be the mechanism that decreases lung injury. There remains no sound consensus as to how to aerate the fluid-filled fetal lung to minimize injury. In new work by Tingay, the best approach may be a ramped increased in CPAP but not with a sigh.[28]

EFFECTS OF SURFACTANT TREATMENT ON DYNAMIC LUNG FUNCTION

If surfactant treatment were to normalize lung function completely, functional residual capacity (FRC) will increase, the time constant for inflation will decrease, and the time constant for expiration will increase. These effects occur to variable degrees, probably depending on factors related to the disease progression in each infant, the style of ventilatory management, and the surfactant used to treat the infant. The example in Fig. 79.4 demonstrates that the combination of surfactant and positive end-expiratory pressure (PEEP) increases FRC in ventilated surfactant-deficient preterm rabbit lungs more than either intervention alone following the initial 4 to 6 breaths. The effect of surfactant predominates for breaths 39 to 41.[26] FRC in infants with RDS increased by approximately 150% to approach a normal value after surfactant treatment in one report.[29] In another report, FRC increased from 7.6 mL/kg to 15.4 mL/kg 1 hour after surfactant treatment.[30] If PEEP is too high, FRC can be too high after surfactant treatment, resulting in CO_2 retention and a lower compliance.[31]

Compliance uniformly increases quickly in animal models of surfactant treatment.[32] As with FRC, compliance increased by breaths 4 to 6 in mechanically ventilated preterm rabbits treated with surfactant, and further increases with breaths 39 to 41 were not large (see Fig. 79.4). Consistent with this rapid increase in lung compliance, Miedema and colleagues[33] used electrical impedance tomography to measure 61% increases in lung gas volumes of infants treated with surfactant and high-frequency oscillation. However, compliance does not increase in infants soon after surfactant treatment in most clinical reports. For example, Davis and associates[34] reported no change in compliance for mechanical breaths with surfactant treatments, although spontaneous breaths after surfactant treatment had improved compliance. There are several explanations for this inconsistency. The animal models of RDS are ventilated in a standard fashion often with control of tidal volume. In the clinical evaluations of surfactant, tidal volumes were seldom measured. Large tidal volumes or high FRC may mask a "compliance effect" of surfactant treatment. Kelly and associates[35] found no improvement in dynamic compliance after treatment of infants with surfactant, whereas static compliance decreased as a result of lung volume recruitment. However, when the ventilator pressures were lowered, consistent improvements in both static and dynamic compliance occurred. The mix of PEEP, V_T targets, rates, and other ventilator-driven variables can change the surfactant responses that are measured. If peak inspiratory pressures and/or PEEPs are too high, compliance will decrease after surfactant treatment because the lung is overinflated.

Another variable in the compliance response is the type of surfactant used for treatment. A synthetic surfactant without surfactant proteins may not improve compliance in the first few hours after treatment. In contrast, treatment with animal-source surfactants can result in rapid improvements in compliance. These different responses between synthetic surfactants and surfactant from animal lungs were noted in preterm animal models[36] and in clinical practice.[37] Differences in acute physiologic responses between the surfactants from animal lungs that are now used clinically are not large. New surfactants will need to be tested for effects on lung mechanics as they become available.[14]

Surfactant treatments also will have effects on the time constants for lung inflation and deflation. The stiff, atelectatic lung of the infant with RDS does not inflate easily, and deflation to low lung volumes is rapid because the elastic recoil properties of the lungs are not counterbalanced by surfactant. With mechanical ventilation, inspiratory times and peak pressures are used empirically to adjust tidal volumes. The time constant for expiration (defined as the time required for the lung to empty two-thirds of its volume calculated from the peak tidal volume to FRC) is a passive property of the lung that is not controlled by the clinician. Although measurements of expiratory time constants have not been reported for surfactant-treated infants, the mean expiratory time constant increased from 25 ± 6 ms for

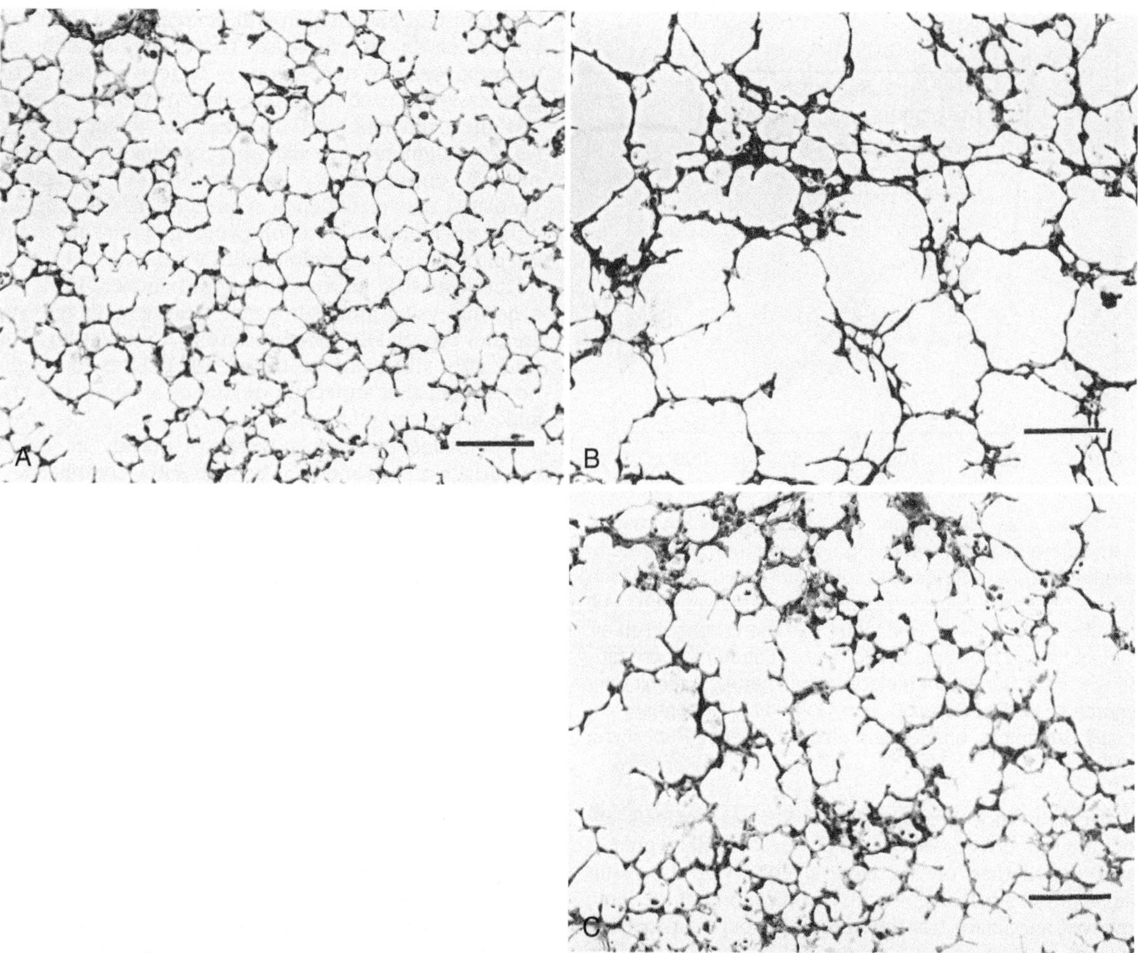

Fig. 79.3 Effect of surfactant on uniformity of alveolar expansion. (A) Light micrograph from a preterm fetal lamb lung fixed at delivery without mechanical ventilation demonstrates uniform alveolar sizes. (B) After ventilation for 24 hours without surfactant treatment, some alveoli are shallow and alveolar ducts are distended, and other alveoli are collapsed. (C) After surfactant treatment at birth and ventilation for 24 hours, alveolar sizes are more uniform. Bar is 100 μm in each figure. (From Pinkerton KE, Lewis JF, Rider ED, et al. Lung parenchyma and type II cell morphometrics: effect of surfactant treatment on preterm ventilated lamb lungs. *J Appl Physiol.* 1994;77:1953.)

controls to 50 ± 9 ms for surfactant-treated preterm rabbits.[38] The expiratory time constant increased as the SP-B content of the surfactant increased in preterm rabbits.[39] Increases in expiratory time constants in surfactant-treated infants ventilated at rapid rates could significantly increase expiratory lung volumes to the point of overdistention, resulting in decreased compliance and CO_2 retention. The combination of surfactant treatment and a ventilatory style that promotes air trapping may mask surfactant treatment effects. In contrast, lung that has not been "opened" may need long inspiratory times or higher pressure to recruit lung volume and avoid airway obstruction with surfactant treatment.[40]

OXYGENATION RESPONSE TO SURFACTANT

The most consistent response to surfactant treatment is an improvement in oxygenation,[11] which occurs within seconds to minutes after surfactant treatment of preterm animals (Fig. 79.5).[32] The rapid improvement in oxygenation results from the acute increase in lung volume and increases in the surface area for gas exchange with surfactant instillation. Fig. 79.6 demonstrates the relationship between surfactant, ventilatory pressures, and oxygenation in infants with RDS who are ventilated with high-frequency oscillators.[41] With initiation of ventilation, the mean airway pressures were increased until the oxygen need decreased to below 25%, and mean airway pressures of approximately 21 cm H_2O were needed to open the lungs. The pressures were decreased until oxygenation decreased, and an optimal mean airway pressure was then determined. These pressures were lower with surfactant treatment. These results parallel the pressures needed to recruit lung volume in surfactant-deficient rabbit lungs (see Fig. 79.1). Surfactant treatments also decrease pulmonary vascular resistance in infants with RDS.[42] Although the fall in pulmonary vascular resistance may reverse the ductal shunt (from right-to-left to left-to-right) and decrease hypoxic shunt,[43] this effect is probably delayed in most clinical situations until after the initial oxygenation response has occurred.[44] Surfactant treatments also can improve overall hemodynamics with an increase in systemic blood flow.[45] These changes in hemodynamics may acutely alter cerebral perfusion and the electroencephalogram.[46]

CLINICAL TRIALS OF SURFACTANT FOR RESPIRATORY DISTRESS SYNDROME

The use of surfactant in preterm infants is the most thoroughly studied therapy in neonatal care. The clinical trials comparing

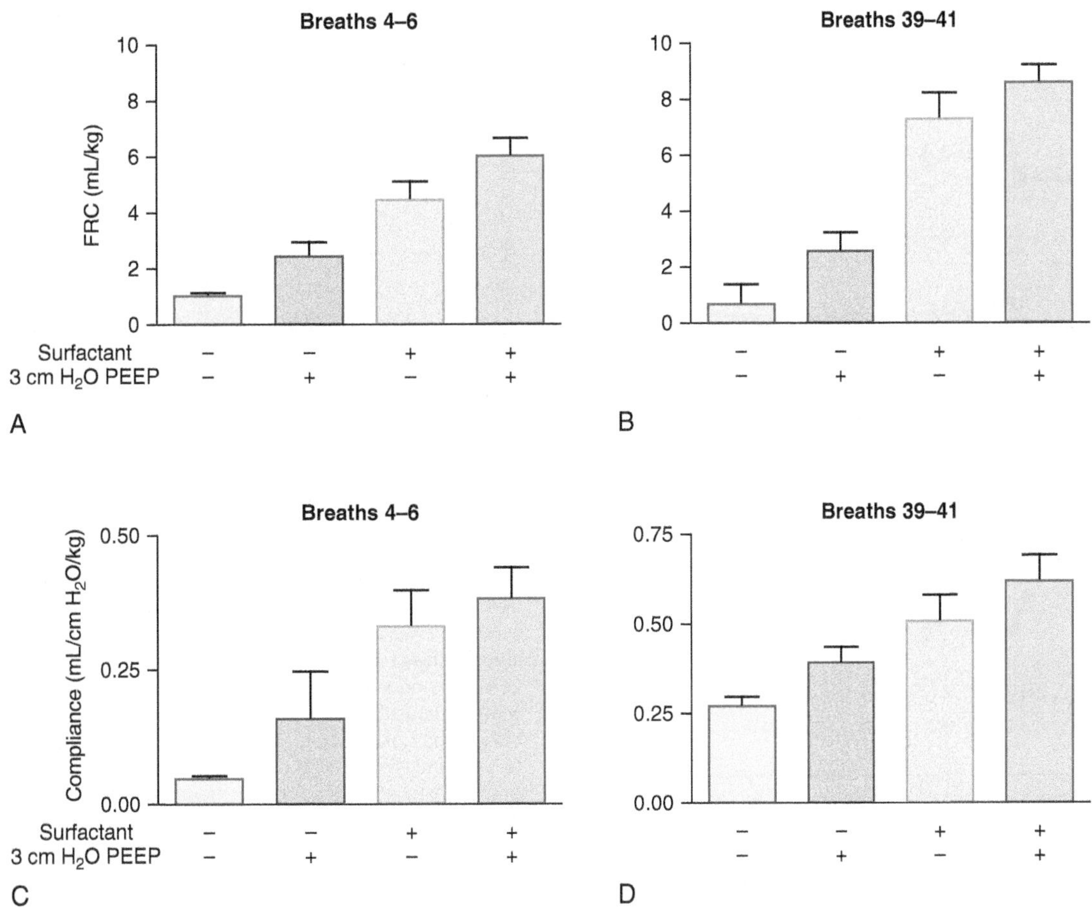

Fig. 79.4 Combined effects of positive end-expiratory pressure *(PEEP)* and surfactant treatment on functional residual capacity *(FRC)* and lung compliance with the initiation of ventilation in preterm rabbits. (A) Surfactant and PEEP have additive effects on FRC for the initial mechanical breaths 4 to 6. (B) By breaths 39 to 41, surfactant had the major effect on FRC. (C and D) Surfactant and PEEP also improved lung compliance for breaths 4 to 6, as well as for breaths 39 to 41. (Data from Siew M, TePas A, Wallace M, et al. Surfactant increases the uniformity of lung aeration at birth in ventilated premature rabbits. *Pediatr Res.* 2011;70:50.)

surfactant treatments with placebo were performed before 1990 and have been compiled by Seger and Soll[47,48] in a meta-analysis (Fig. 79.7). Two strategies for surfactant treatments were tested: the treatment of infants at high risk of RDS in the delivery room concurrently with the initiation of breathing and resuscitation or the treatment of infants at 2 to 24 hours of age after a diagnosis of RDS has been made. Treatment in the delivery room is referred to as *prevention* or *prophylactic treatment* because the goal is to prevent both RDS and any injury to the preterm surfactant-deficient lung that might result from oxygen exposure and mechanical ventilation associated with resuscitation and the subsequent need for ventilation.[49] The odds ratio for death by 28 days of age was approximately 0.6 for either treatment strategy.[11] With surfactant treatment, the absolute decrease in death from any cause was 30% to 40% in infants that were larger and more mature than those treated currently.

The major pulmonary complications of RDS are acute respiratory failure, air leaks (pneumothorax and pulmonary interstitial emphysema), and the chronic lung disease of infants called *bronchopulmonary dysplasia* (BPD).[50] Surfactant treatment improved lung function and greatly decreased pneumothorax and other air leaks. The incidence of BPD was not consistently lower, although it was reduced in individual studies. However, the severity of BPD was not quantified. Many tiny preterm infants have a supplemental oxygenation requirement and some radiographic abnormalities at 28 days of age, but they do not need oxygen or other treatments for lung disease at discharge.[51] The most frequently used definition for BPD is the use of oxygen at 36 weeks. Some infants who receive oxygen do not need oxygen when evaluated by objective oxygen saturation criteria.[52] Overall, the severity of BPD has decreased in the very low-birth-weight population, and surfactant treatments have contributed to this improved outcome.[53] Surfactant treatment increases survival, and these survivors may have the highest risk of BPD.[54]

An initial hope was that the improved cardiopulmonary stability and oxygenation resulting from surfactant treatment would protect preterm infants from the nonpulmonary complications of prematurity, such as patent ductus arteriosus, severe intraventricular hemorrhage, and necrotizing enterocolitis. Unfortunately, treatment has not consistently decreased the frequency of patent ductus arteriosus or severe intraventricular hemorrhage. Large decreases in intraventricular hemorrhage in association with surfactant treatment were reported in individual trials,[55] suggesting that other aspects of neonatal care may be interacting with surfactant therapy to influence the incidence of intraventricular hemorrhage. A thorough analysis of the available data on the possible association of intraventricular hemorrhage with surfactant treatment did not lead to any direct links.[56] Necrotizing enterocolitis and retinopathy of prematurity were not tabulated for the metanalyses, but no trends were reported in the individual trials. One study found a decrease in retinopathy of prematurity in the infants treated with surfactant.[57] Infants treated with surfactant generally perform as well as or better

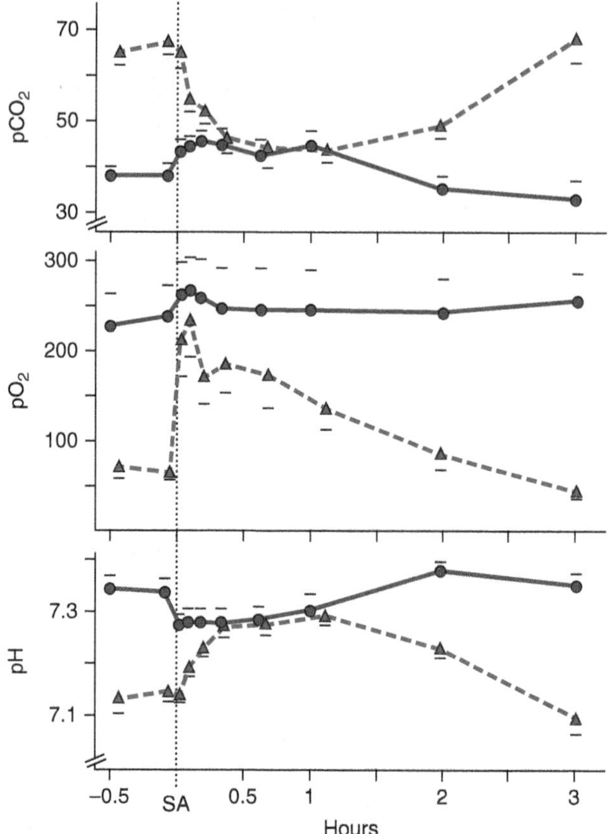

Fig. 79.5 Blood gas and pH responses of very preterm lambs to treatment with 100 mg/kg natural sheep surfactant from alveolar lavage. Preterm lambs were delivered at approximately 121 days of gestation (term is 150 days) and treated with surfactant either at birth *(red dot)* or after ventilation for approximately 30 minutes (SA) before surfactant treatment *(blue triangle)*. Oxygenation was good and P_{CO_2} values were normal with surfactant treatment at birth. Oxygenation improved very rapidly after surfactant treatment at 30 minutes of age, but the response did not persist because of lung injury from the initial period of ventilation before surfactant treatment. (From Jobe A, Ikegami M, Glatz T, et al. Duration and characteristics of treatment of premature lambs with natural surfactant. *J Clin Invest*. 1981;67:370, by copyright permission of The American Society for Clinical Investigation.)

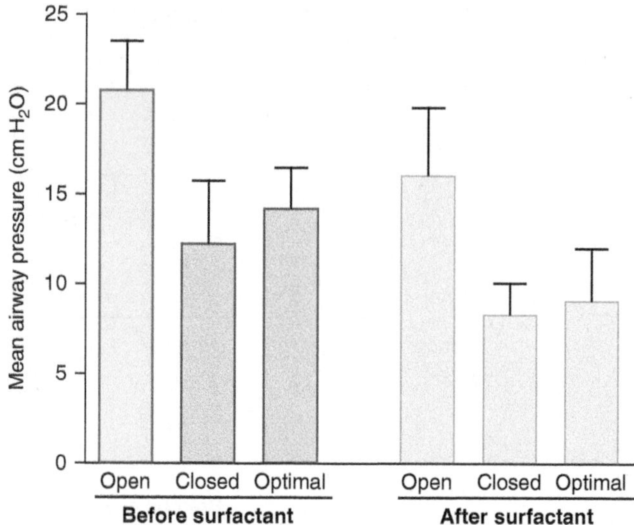

Fig. 79.6 Mean airway pressures and oxygenation in preterm infants ventilated with high-frequency oscillators before and after surfactant treatment. Infants who were intubated for severe respiratory distress syndrome were ventilated with oscillators with the mean airway pressures increased at brief intervals until the oxygen need was less than 25%. The goal was to open the lungs. Mean airway pressures then were decreased until the percentage of oxygen increased, defining the lung as closed. Optimum mean airway pressures were determined to be slightly higher than the closed values. Surfactant decreased the opening pressure, the closed pressure, and the optimal pressure. (Reprinted from data in the American Thoracic Society. Copyright © 2015 American Thoracic Society. De Jaegere A, van Veenendaal MB, Michiels A, van Kaam AH. Lung recruitment using oxygenation during open lung high-frequency ventilation in preterm infants. *Am J Resp Crit Care Med.* 2006;174:639, Figure 2. *The American Journal of Respiratory and Critical Care Medicine* is an official journal of the American Thoracic Society.)

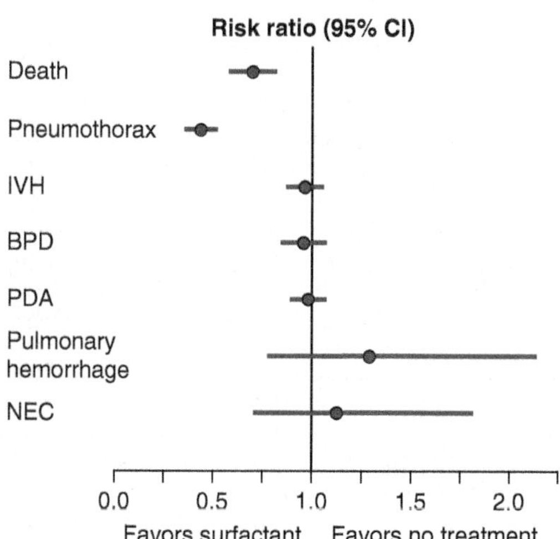

Fig. 79.7 Risk ratios and 95% confidence intervals (CIs) from meta-analysis of 13 clinical trials of natural surfactant treatments given for respiratory distress syndrome in comparison with untreated controls. No new trials have been published since 1990. *BPD,* Bronchopulmonary dysplasia; *IVH,* intraventricular hemorrhage; *NEC,* necrotizing enterocolitis; *PDA,* patent ductus arteriosus. (Data from Seger N, Soll RF. Animal derived surfactant extract for treatment of respiratory distress syndrome. *Cochrane Database Syst Rev.* 2009;CD0007836.)

than control infants when assessed at long-term follow-up.[58-60] Surfactant-treated infants needed less supplemental oxygen at 6 months and had less wheezing at 12 and 24 months of age relative to control infants.[61] In this study, less cerebral palsy also was diagnosed in surfactant-treated infants. It is important to remember that the more mature infants included in placebo-controlled trials of surfactant were cared for in an era with different ventilatory support strategies and minimal use of antenatal steroids.

TIMING OF SURFACTANT TREATMENT

In the initial trials, surfactant was administered 6 to 24 hours after birth when a diagnosis of severe RDS could be made more accurately. In contrast, delivery room treatment was considered to be optimal only if given before the infant breathed or received positive-pressure ventilation.[62] This delivery room strategy was based on information from surfactant treatment of preterm animals that demonstrated airway epithelial damage after very short-term periods of ventilation of the surfactant-deficient lung.[63] The two treatment strategies were compared in six trials using different surfactants.[64] Recognizing that only two studies reported on infants of less than 30 weeks gestation, delivery room treatment decreased death (risk ratio 0.84; 95% confidence interval [CI], 0.74 to 0.95), BPD (risk ratio 0.69; 95% CI, 0.55 to 0.86), and air leaks, versus delayed treatment. There were no differences in the incidences of intraventricular hemorrhage or patent ductus arteriosus. Treatment of infants at birth has two disadvantages: a number of the infants will be treated unnecessarily because they would not have developed RDS, and instillation of a large volume of surfactant soon after birth can interfere with normal efforts to stabilize the infant. Kendig and co-workers[62] demonstrated that surfactant treatment within the first 15 minutes after birth was equivalent and perhaps preferable to treatments before the infant was allowed to breathe.

Based on the metanalyses of the initial trials comparing delivery room treatment with later treatment of RDS, Horbar and colleagues[65] argued that the standard of care should be delivery room treatment for very low-birth-weight infants. However, in practice, the majority of infants were not treated in the delivery room. As a quality improvement initiative, they demonstrated that with education the age at treatment could be reduced from a mean of 78 minutes to 21 minutes, but the earlier surfactant treatment did not improve clinical outcomes.[66] A reasonable approach is to treat most infants as soon as clinical signs of RDS appear. Waiting for the disease to progress to establish the diagnosis more firmly before treatment will minimize the efficacy of the therapy and increase complications. Delivery room treatment is most appropriate for the smallest infants who are at the highest risk of RDS. However, delivery room treatment should be given by a person experienced in neonatal resuscitation.

SURFACTANT TREATMENTS INTEGRATED WITH NONINVASIVE STRATEGIES

The discussion of delivery room surfactant to prevent RDS or surfactant treatment early in the course of RDS has been superseded by strategies that integrate surfactant treatment with care strategies that avoid routine intubation of very low-birth-weight infants. CPAP is now used by many clinicians to help very low-birth-weight infants initiate breathing at birth.[67] The success rate for CPAP management increases as birth weight and gestational age increase, but even some infants at gestations of 25 weeks or less do not require surfactant treatment or mechanical ventilation following birth. A management strategy that emphasizes CPAP will decrease surfactant use in the delivery room, and many infants will not have RDS following stabilization.[68] This approach of CPAP and elective surfactant treatment or intubation and obligate surfactant treatment has been evaluated in large RCTs that demonstrate a marginal but significant benefit for CPAP plus elective surfactant treatment (Fig. 79.8).[69] The CPAP and elective surfactant treatment strategy has marginal benefits for decreased death and BPD as a combined outcome. This benefit is much less than would have been predicted for the protective effects of CPAP in lung injury animal studies. In practice, the benefits of avoiding mechanical ventilation for some infants may put other infants at risk of complications that result from delays in surfactant treatment. There are now a number of reports on using laryngeal mask or atomizer in the proximal airway.

Various approaches to give surfactant without intubation and ventilation are being actively investigated. The INSURE technique uses gentle intubation for infants on CPAP followed by a traditional surfactant treatment and extubation back to CPAP, with no or only short-term mechanical ventilation.[70] This approach has been modified for the use of fine feeding tubes or vascular catheters that are inserted into the trachea while attempting to maintain CPAP with high-flow nasal prongs.[71,72] The advantage of these approaches is that airway injury from intubation and any mechanical ventilation can be avoided. A disadvantage is not having control of the airway for surfactant treatment. These techniques require the infant to be spontaneously breathing, but the laryngoscopy procedure is viewed by some practitioners as requiring pain medications, whereas others will treat with surfactant without pain medications. The different management strategies depend on procedural skills, experience, and multiple aspects of the subsequent care, which may confound clear answers to when and how infants are best treated with surfactant.

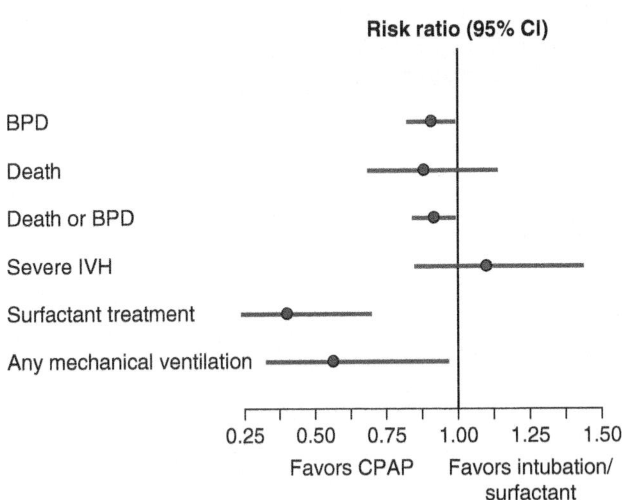

Fig. 79.8 Meta-analysis of outcomes of over 2700 infants randomized in four trials to receive continuous positive airway pressure *(CPAP)* or intubation and surfactant for respiratory support at birth. The outcomes of bronchopulmonary dysplasia *(BPD)* or death were not different, but the combined outcome just reached statistical significance. CPAP-treated infants received less mechanical ventilation and less surfactant and had similar rates of intraventricular hemorrhage *(IVH)*. *CI*, Confidence interval. (Modified from Schmolzer G, Kumar M, Pichler, G, et al. Non-invasive versus invasive respiratory support in preterm infants at birth: systematic review and meta-analysis. *BMJ*. 2013;347:f5980.)

European and American Academy of Pediatric guidelines for surfactant treatments have been published.[73,74] The European guidelines suggest that an early rescue treatment strategy is preferred over routine treatment at birth. Infants less than 26 weeks gestational age should receive surfactant for RDS for oxygen needs greater than 30%. For infants greater than 26 weeks, a reasonable oxygen need for surfactant treatment should be greater than 40%. Intubation or INSURE are reasonable approaches. The American Academy of Pediatrics guidelines are less specific but similar. Infants with RDS should be treated before disease progression, to decrease complications and to simplify clinical management. Other treatment approaches, using laryngeal masks,[75] atomizers in the large airways,[76] or aerosolized surfactant,[77] for example, are a very active area of investigation to minimize injury during surfactant treatment.

REPETITION OF TREATMENT

Multiple doses of surfactant were given in most trials because the response to an initial dose was often transient. In preterm animals, exogenously administered surfactant is not lost from the lungs,[78] but its function can be inhibited by soluble proteins and other factors. Surfactant function may be abnormal in the course of RDS secondary to inflammation, but late treatments

Table 79.1 Adverse Events Associated With Surfactant Treatment Among 17,641 Infants Treated.

Adverse Event	Rate of Occurrence (%)
Decreased O_2	16.6
Reflux	14.6
Bradycardia	4.2
Cyanosis	3.7
Increased O_2	3.3
Increased CO_2	0.5
Decreased CO_2	0.1
Others	2.7
At least 1 event	30.4

Data from Zola EM, Overbach AM, Gunkel JH, et al. Treatment investigational new drug experience with Survanta (beractant). *Pediatrics.* 1993;91:546.

with surfactant are of no benefit based on two RCTs but may have some benefits at 1 year of age.[79,80] Multiple doses of surfactant are thought to be useful because they can overcome this functional inactivation of surfactant. Multiple doses have been compared with single-dose treatments. In one trial, second and third doses given 12 and 24 hours after an initial treatment reduced the frequency of pneumothorax from 18% with a single dose to 9% with three doses of surfactant ($P < .01$), and the rate of deaths before 28 days decreased from 21% to 13% ($P < .05$).[81] In another study of 75 large infants with RDS (mean birth weight, 1900 g), those who received multiple doses had better oxygenation during the first several days of life.[82] All recent trials and treatment guidelines include retreatment as an option. Although most infants respond favorably to treatment, approximately 20% of infants thought to have RDS will have transient, modest, or no responses. These infants may have other diseases, such as pneumonia, pulmonary hypoplasia, or congenital heart disease.[68] Structural immaturity of the lungs and birth asphyxia with decreased cardiovascular performance can also blunt the response to surfactant. It is reasonable to re-treat with surfactant if the initial response to treatment was poor and other causes of respiratory failure have been excluded. In clinical practice, re-treatment should be individualized and considered for infants with enough residual lung disease to put them at risk of complications such as pneumothorax. The major reason for retreatment is to overcome inhibition of surfactant resulting from lung injury. If treatment is given early in the clinical course and a gentle approach to ventilation is used, significant lung injury can be avoided. The dose of 100 or 200 mg/kg surfactant, which is normally used, is large relative to the endogenous pool in a normal lung, and it is metabolized slowly.[78] Therefore, surfactant retreatment will not be for inadequate amounts of surfactant, but for inadequate surfactant function. On average, infants with RDS receive fewer than two doses of surfactant. Use of more than two doses of surfactant is excessive and is unlikely to improve outcomes.

COMPLICATIONS OF SURFACTANT TREATMENT

The documentation of treatment complications in Table 79.1 resulted from an extensive data collection required for the initial clinical approval of surfactant in 1990 and 1991.[83] Similar problems associated with surfactant treatments were reported by Horbar and colleagues.[84] The treatment procedures for each surfactant approved for clinical use differ in detail, but generally combine positioning of the infant and instillation of suspensions of surfactant in aliquots. The acute physiologic effects are related to the handling of the infant and the acute effects of the volume of vehicle in which surfactant is suspended in the lungs. Manipulation of the head, neck, and endotracheal tube can cause vagal responses resulting in bradycardia and cyanosis. The bolus of fluid can acutely obstruct airways leading to cyanosis, bradycardia, and CO_2 retention.[40] If surfactant is rapidly distributed to the distal lung, lung compliance can improve, the PO_2 will increase, and the PCO_2 will decrease. Reflux of some of the surfactant up the endotracheal tube is frequent. These acute effects of surfactant are easily dealt with by adjustments in the ventilator and probably have no long-term effect on outcome. Of more concern are the reports of transient changes in blood pressure, cerebral blood flow velocities, and electrocortical depression after surfactant treatments.[85-87] The mechanisms and importance of these effects are not known.

The only severe complication consistently associated with surfactant treatment is pulmonary hemorrhage. The overall relative risk of pulmonary hemorrhage after surfactant therapy was 1.47 (95% CI, 1.05 to 2.07) in the clinical trials.[88] Incidences ranged from approximately 1% to 5% of treated infants. A patent ductus arteriosus with a left-to-right shunt resulting in elevated pulmonary vascular pressures was linked to pulmonary hemorrhage in several trials. Although this association has not been identified in other trials, increased pulmonary vascular pressures leading to stress failure of alveolar capillaries is the likely explanation for the pulmonary hemorrhage.[89] Pulmonary hemorrhage after surfactant treatment does not often occur at the time of treatment. Hemorrhage can occur in the smallest infants a number of hours after surfactant treatment has improved lung function. Pulmonary hemorrhage is frequently found in autopsies of infants who have died of RDS. Surfactant treatment after pulmonary hemorrhage can improve subsequent lung function.[90] This result is consistent with the concept that pulmonary hemorrhage inactivates surfactant. Although not well documented, pulmonary hemorrhage seems to be less frequent in recent years. Perhaps changes in ventilation style toward the maintenance of better lung inflation, lower tidal volumes, and acceptance of higher CO_2 levels have contributed to the decrease in pulmonary hemorrhage.

ROUTINE CLINICAL USE OF SURFACTANT

Within the context of RCTs, surfactant treatment for RDS decreased deaths. However, did general clinical use have similar results? Incidences of death and other major neonatal complications were analyzed for the period before surfactant introduction (before 1989) and after general clinical availability. Horbar and colleagues[91] reported outcomes for 2870 infants weighing 601 to 1300 g before surfactant and 1413 infants after surfactant was available. Mortality decreased from 28% before surfactant to 20% after surfactant. This decrease in mortality was associated with an increase in the duration of ventilation and length of hospitalization and changes in secondary outcomes (Fig. 79.9).[91] Surfactant treatments were not associated with increased incidences of intraventricular hemorrhage, BPD, sepsis, or patent ductus arteriosus. Beneficial secondary effects were decreases in necrotizing enterocolitis, air leak, and severe retinopathy of prematurity. The increase in apnea probably resulted from the survival of more small infants. This favorable clinical experience was not replicated in a compilation of data for 5629 infants weighing 500 to 1500 g from 14 centers.[92] Although deaths decreased by 30% after the introduction of surfactant, intraventricular hemorrhage increased from 17% to 23% (adjusted risk ratio, 1.4; 95% CI, 1.2 to 1.6). Nevertheless, the effect of surfactant on death can explain 80% of the decline

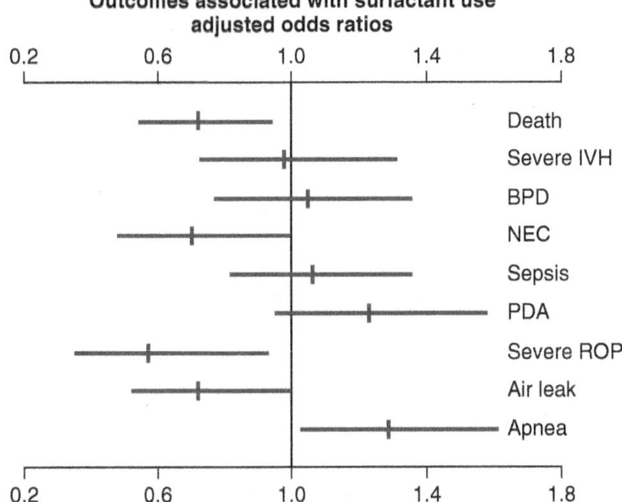

Fig. 79.9 Adjusted odds ratios for infants before and after the introduction of surfactant for the treatment of respiratory distress syndrome. The odds ratios and 95% confidence limits are from Horbar and colleagues. *BPD,* Bronchopulmonary dysplasia; *IVH,* intraventricular hemorrhage; *NEC,* necrotizing enterocolitis; *PDA,* patent ductus arteriosus; *ROP,* retinopathy of prematurity. (Data from Horbar JD, Wright EC, Onstad L, et al. Decreasing mortality associated with the introduction of surfactant therapy: an observed study of neonates weighing 601 to 1300 grams at birth. *Pediatrics.* 1993;92:191–196.)

in infant mortality between 1989 and 1990. The use of surfactant decreased overall costs for both survivors and infants who died. This epidemiology is important for understanding how the introduction of a new therapy affects overall outcomes.

ADMINISTRATION OF SURFACTANT

The instillation procedures used in the trials to treat RDS were selected empirically based on the techniques of treatment for preterm animal models of RDS. Surfactant has been given to infants at risk of developing RDS in the delivery room soon after delivery and intubation as a single bolus into the endotracheal tube followed by mechanical ventilation.[62] For infants with RDS, surfactant has been given by a variety of bolus injection schemes that include positioning the chest of the infant in an effort to optimize distribution. These treatment procedures were standardized for each clinical trial such that each surfactant in current use was given by a somewhat different technique. The essence of each treatment technique is the instillation of surfactant into the trachea with positioning of the chest. The only clinical trial comparing treatment techniques found that there were no differences in short-term efficacy when the surfactant dose was divided into two or four aliquots for administration or when two or four chest positioning maneuvers were used.[93]

The goal of the treatment technique is to get the surfactant into an infant's lungs with as little physiologic disturbance as possible. This clinical treatment goal may conflict with the goal of an optimal clinical outcome. At the level of the alveolus, the primary goal is to achieve as uniform a distribution of surfactant as possible. If distribution were perfectly uniform, expansion of the lung should be uniform. The physiologic result should be decreased oxygen and pressure needs and less lung injury. In contrast, if the distribution of surfactant were primarily to one lobe or one lung, that lung volume would expand if pressures were not decreased. The inflated lung would tend to over expand and potentially be injured.[94] If the pressures were decreased, the untreated lung would lose whatever gas volume it was receiving and become more atelectatic. At the alveolar level, alveoli are interdependent in that if a group of alveoli collapse, the adjacent alveoli may overinflate and distort (see Figs. 79.2 and 79.3).[27] The frequent occurrence of BPD after surfactant treatment may result in part from a nonhomogeneous distribution, contributing to focal lung injury.[28]

Experimental studies of surfactant distribution have used radiolabeled surfactant components or other easily measured substances mixed with surfactant.[95] van der Bleek and colleagues[96] reported that microaggregated technetium-albumin mixed with surfactant appeared to be uniformly distributed by external scanning of the lungs of saline-lavaged rabbits. However, the distribution was not homogeneous when the lungs were divided into 200 pieces and distribution per piece was measured. Analysis of lung pieces does not provide information about alveolar distribution. For example, if the preterm human lung at 32 weeks gestational age was cut into 200 pieces for a distribution measurement, each piece would contain approximately 200,000 saccules.[95] Therefore, even if distribution to lung pieces was homogeneous, significant inhomogeneity must exist at the saccular level.

VARIABLES THAT INFLUENCE SURFACTANT DISTRIBUTION

The biophysical properties of surfactant facilitate adsorption to an air-fluid interface and rapid spreading over a surface. Davis and associates[97] used external scanning to measure the kinetics of surfactant or saline distribution to the lungs of saline-lavaged piglets. They found that surfactant began to distribute within 5 seconds of dosing, with substantial distribution to the lung fields within 20 seconds. In contrast, saline did not distribute as rapidly, and multiple filling defects were noted on the scans. Surfactant given into single lobes in rabbits did not spread to other lobes even after 10 hours of spontaneous ventilation.[98] Therefore, surfactant treatments given into one lung or lobe will not treat other parts of the lung.

The surfactants used clinically are given as suspensions in volumes that range from 2.5 to 5 mL/kg. Intuitively, the larger the volume administered, the more likely multiple bronchi will be filled, and the better the distribution is likely to be. However, large volumes are more likely to cause airway obstruction, respiratory distress, cyanosis, and other undesirable side effects. New attempts for more gentle treatments have not been evaluated for effects of the treatment on surfactant distribution, effects on pulmonary blood flow or ventilation gas within the lung. A recent report identifies some of the distribution issues.[99] Gilliard and coworkers[100] found that instillation of 1.5-mL/kg surfactant into ventilated rabbits with normal lungs resulted in a nonuniform distribution. Increasing surfactant concentration did not improve the distribution. The same amount of surfactant suspended in 15 mL/kg resulted in a homogeneous distribution. The residual fetal lung fluid and alveolar edema associated with RDS may help distribute surfactant. Large treatment volumes are not realistic for clinical practice, and some nonhomogeneity of surfactant distribution is an inevitable consequence of present treatment techniques.

Given that surfactant distribution can be improved by increasing the treatment volume and that the administration of large volumes over short treatment intervals results in respiratory complications, it might seem logical to deliver surfactant to the lungs more slowly. This approach has been evaluated in two animal models of RDS. Segerer and associates[101] reported that 4 mL/kg of a surfactant suspension given as a bolus via the endotracheal tube in 10 seconds to saline-lavaged rabbits resulted in a reasonably uniform distribution. In contrast, infusion of the same volume of surfactant over 45 minutes through the pressure-monitoring channel in an endotracheal tube resulted in an extremely nonhomogeneous distribution. Ueda and associates[102] compared the four aliquot, four-position technique used clinically with a slow infusion in preterm lambs with RDS. The infusion-treated group received 2 mL/kg surfactant in the right lateral position in 15 minutes followed by 2 mL/kg in the left lateral position in 15 minutes. Both groups of lambs had improvements in Po_2 and lung mechanics, although the responses were not as large with the slow surfactant infusion. The bolus treatments delivered surfactant quite uniformly to the different lobes of the sheep lung, whereas infusion resulted primarily in upper lobe localization (Fig. 79.10). The animals received a second treatment 2 hours later, and the second treatment localized to the same lung pieces that received the majority of the surfactant with the initial treatment. Therefore, the first treatment determined primarily which lung volumes will open, and the second treatment tended to treat the same lung volumes. Pulmonary blood flow was relatively uniform across the lung pieces of the bolus-treated animals. In contrast, blood flow decreased to the lung pieces that received the most surfactant by infusion, probably because of over-inflation of those lung regions.

Surfactant distributes to the lungs by bulk movement of the suspension down the airways and by spreading. The style of ventilation immediately after treatment could affect the distribution. In clinical practice, conventional ventilation is routinely used after surfactant treatments. Walther and colleagues[103] reported that surfactant instilled into the airways of preterm lambs distributed similarly with conventional or high-frequency ventilation. In contrast, Heldt and coworkers[104] found that high-frequency ventilation seemed to delay surfactant delivery to distal airspaces of preterm rabbits. The efficacy of surfactant treatment techniques and distribution may be influenced by different ventilation strategies.

Surfactant distribution has not been evaluated for surfactant treatments given with fine catheters while the infants are breathing spontaneously.[71,72] The experimental information suggests that slow infusions without positioning the infant could cause very nonuniform distributions. Aerosolized or atomized surfactant could be a strategy to avoid the risks of intubation and the administration of large fluid volumes.[77] In models of RDS with ventilated animals, the aerosolized surfactant distributed to the ventilated lung and not the lung volumes that were not open.[105] However, atomized surfactant can achieve sustained physiologic responses in preterm ventilated lambs.[106] As reviewed by Abdel-Latif,[107] there are insufficient clinical data to evaluate aerosol strategies to deliver surfactant to infants with RDS.

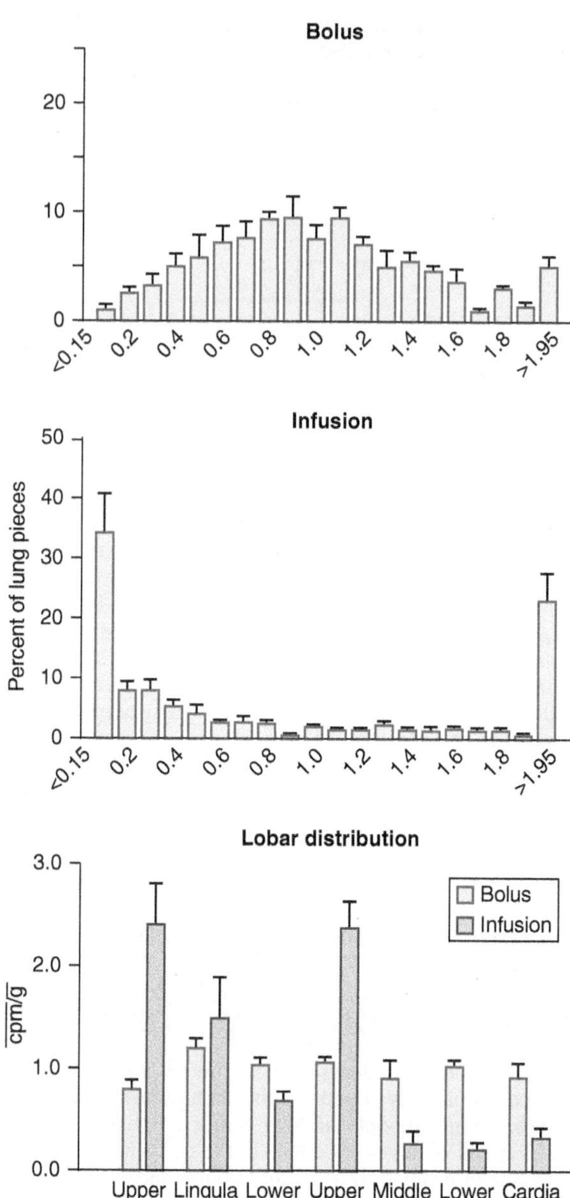

Fig. 79.10 Distribution of surfactant by bolus in comparison with a 30-minute infusion to preterm ventilated lamb lungs. The 100 mg/kg dose of surfactant was radiolabeled, and the amounts of surfactant recovered in lung pieces or by lobe were measured. Bolus treatment resulted in approximately 40% of the lung pieces containing within ±25% of the mean amount of surfactant. In contrast, infusion resulted in 7% of the pieces of lung receiving within ±25% of the mean. Most of the infused surfactant was found in the upper lobes. (Modified from Ueda T, Ikegami M, Rider ED, et al. Distribution of surfactant and ventilation in surfactant-treated preterm lambs. *J Appl Physiol.* 1994;76:45.)

VENTILATION EFFECTS ON SURFACTANT TREATMENT RESPONSES

Although mechanical ventilation and use of PEEP are routine in infants with RDS, multiple ventilatory techniques are in common use. The interaction between ventilatory management and surfactant treatment has not been studied extensively, although in experimental animals the ventilation technique is an important variable in the response of the preterm lung to surfactant treatment.[24] In clinical practice, surfactant does not have equivalent effects in different neonatal units, and the differences could be explained by ventilatory management.[108] Lung injury is induced by ventilation of the normal lung at volumes close to maximal lung volume.[109] With surfactant deficiency, ventilation at low lung volumes (below the normal FRC) also causes progressive injury and pulmonary edema.[110] If alveolar expansion is optimized in the saline-lavaged rabbit model of surfactant deficiency, the effectiveness of surfactant treatments is enhanced. The responses also depend on the type of surfactant used for treatment. Surfactants that contain only lipids are not as effective at improving compliances or pressure-volume curves of preterm rabbits.[111] Addition of the surfactant proteins SP-B and SP-C improves function, but enhanced function is evident only if PEEP is used to ventilate the animals.

The equipment used for the mechanical ventilation of preterm infants and the ventilatory goals have changed since surfactant was tested clinically in the 1980s. Most trials of respiratory management now focus on very low-birth-weight infants at highest risk of

BPD. These infants usually have RDS and have been treated with surfactant before trial enrollment. Examples are the trials comparing high-frequency oscillation with conventional ventilation.[112,113] The newer management approaches to keep the FRC relatively high (the open lung strategy) while ventilating with low tidal targets (4 to 6 mL/kg) to achieve CO_2 values higher than the normal range (>50 mm Hg) depend on good surfactant function. If surfactant is deficient, FRC cannot be maintained without excessive PEEP. Surfactant treatment before the initiation of high-frequency oscillation improves respiratory stabilization and allows oscillation at lower mean airway pressures.[41,114] CPAP is now used commonly as a primary therapy to decrease the need for mechanical ventilation and perhaps to decrease the incidence and severity of BPD. The biophysical properties of surfactant will optimally improve lung function in the preterm only when CPAP and ventilator support adequately maintains FRC and minimizes injury.[115]

SURFACTANT-MATERNAL CORTICOSTEROID INTERACTIONS

Prenatal corticosteroid therapy decreases the mortality rate and the incidence and severity of RDS and other complications of prematurity.[116] Prenatal corticosteroids and postnatal surfactant each decrease RDS or death by similar amounts. The question of clinical relevance is how these two effective therapies interact. The two therapies have additive effects on postnatal lung function in animal models (Fig. 79.11). After fetal cortisol exposure, preterm lambs treated with surfactant have improved lung compliance, increased lung volumes, and decreased alveolar edema relative to lambs receiving either treatment.[115] Prenatal corticosteroid treatment of preterm rabbits also resulted in an enhanced postnatal response to surfactant. Corticosteroid-exposed rabbits had larger compliance responses to lower doses of surfactant than did control animals.[117] Prenatal corticosteroid treatments also decreased vascular to alveolar protein leak in the preterm lung and changed the protein content of surfactant. The net effect was to decrease surfactant inhibition. If the only effects of prenatal corticosteroids on the developing lung were to increase surfactant, prenatal corticosteroids and postnatal surfactant treatments would be acting by the same mechanism. Experiments in developing animals indicate that the primary effects of prenatal corticosteroid treatments are on lung structure, causing increased lung gas volumes that resulted in improved ventilation and better responses to surfactant treatment.[118]

RCTs of the interactions between postnatal surfactant and prenatal corticosteroids are not available. It has not been ethical to randomize infants to receive either surfactant or prenatal corticosteroids as both are standard of care. Retrospective evaluations of the surfactant trial databases demonstrate a beneficial interaction between prenatal corticosteroids and postnatal surfactant. In one report, treatment with surfactant or prenatal corticosteroids decreased air leak and death similarly.[119] However, those infants who received both treatments had the best outcome, with fewer deaths, BPD, and air leaks. The combined use of antenatal corticosteroids and postnatal surfactant is a major contributor to improved outcomes of preterm infants.

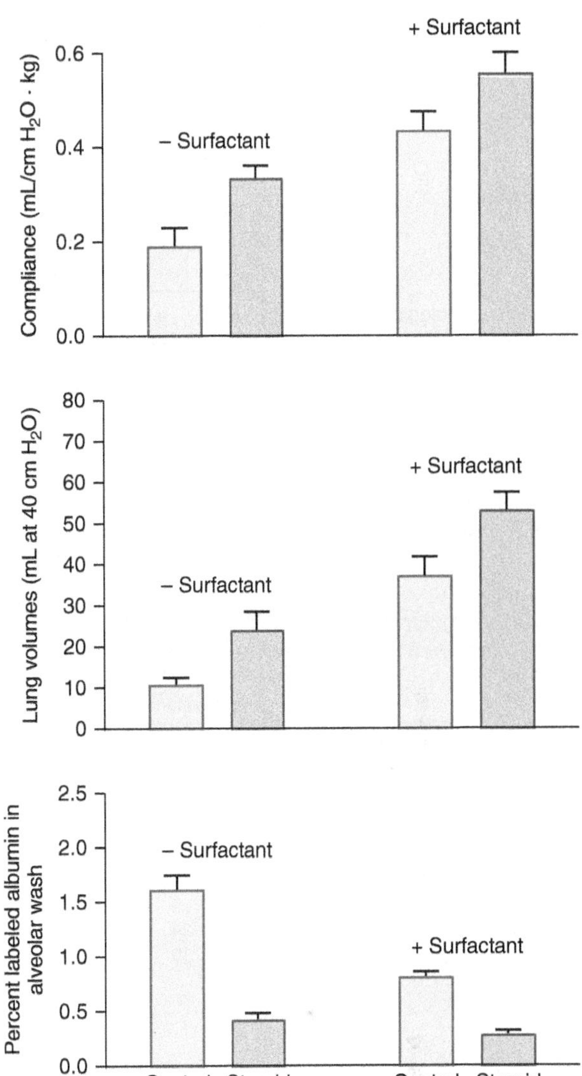

Fig. 79.11 Postnatal lung function in preterm lambs randomized to receive prenatal cortisol and postnatal surfactant treatments. Each treatment increased postnatal compliances, increased lung volumes, and decreased pulmonary edema as measured by the amount of intravascular125I-albumin that was recovered by alveolar wash. The lambs that received both treatments had responses that were approximately the sum of the surfactant and cortisol responses. (Data from Ikegami M, Polk D, Tabor B, et al. Corticosteroid and thyrotropin-releasing hormone effects on preterm sheep lung function. *J Appl Physiol.* 1991;70:2268.)

THE CHOICE OF SURFACTANTS FOR THE TREATMENT OF RESPIRATORY DISTRESS SYNDROME

The initial surfactants approved for clinical use by the FDA in 1990 were a synthetic surfactant that did not contain surfactant proteins and a surfactant made from bovine lungs. Subsequently, other animal lung-source surfactants and a synthetic surfactant containing surfactant protein-like peptides have been approved for clinical use. The clinician who selects a surfactant for clinical use for infants with RDS must sort through claims of product superiority. Surfactants have been directly compared in RCTs, and in general, the synthetic surfactants that do not contain surfactant proteins are less effective and are not used currently.[18,120] The animal-source surfactants have different characteristics: they are suspended in different volumes, different doses per kilogram are recommended, and treatment techniques vary somewhat. In general, surfactants that contain more of the surfactant proteins SP-B and SP-C have a more rapid onset of action in experimental models. However, in clinical practice, premature infants with RDS are much more diverse clinically than experimental animals. The reasons for the preterm delivery (e.g., antenatal infection, preeclampsia, multiple births) and prenatal corticosteroids will modulate the severity of RDS and clinical responses to surfactant. The example in Fig. 79.12 illustrates that oxygenation response

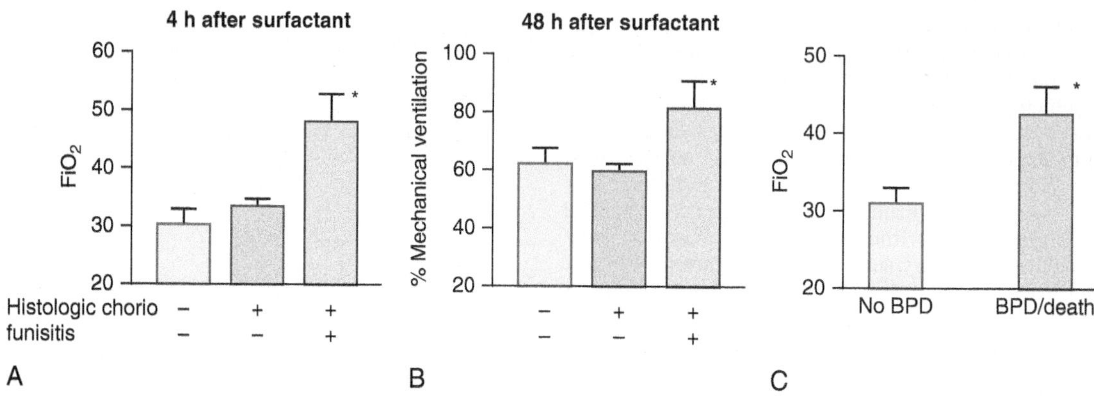

Fig. 79.12 Chorioamnionitis with funisitis decreased the oxygenation response to surfactant. (A) Preterm infants with respiratory distress syndrome and treated with surfactant had similar oxygenation responses at 4 hours unless they had both chorioamnionitis and funisitis. (B) More of the funisitis-exposed infants remained on mechanical ventilation at 48 hours. (C) Higher oxygen need resulted in more bronchopulmonary dysplasia *(BPD)*. (Modified from Been JV, Rours IG, Kornelisse RF, et al. Chorioamnionitis alters the response to surfactant in preterm infants. *J Pediatr.* 2010;156:10–15.)

Table 79.2 Comparison of Two Surfactants for Early Treatment of Respiratory Distress Syndrome.

	Surfactant 1	Surfactant 2
Characteristics of Populations		
Infants randomized *(n)*	375	374
Mean gestational age (weeks)	26.6	26.5
Age at treatment (minutes)	8	9
Median intubation (days)	3	4
Outcomes		
Died (%)	12	13
BPD; oxygen at 36 weeks (%)	34	33
Intraventricular hemorrhage; grades III or IV (%)	10	14
Pneumothorax	7	5

BPD, Bronchopulmonary dysplasia.
Data from Bloom BT, Clark RH. Comparison of Infasurf (calfactant) and Survanta (beractant) in the prevention and treatment of respiratory distress syndrome. *Pediatrics*. 2005;116:392.

to surfactant treatment is decreased and ventilation is prolonged if the infant was exposed to funisitis before delivery.[121] The decreased response is best explained by lung inflammation and surfactant inactivation. Furthermore, ventilation-induced lung injury will change surfactant responses and outcomes. With current management approaches, outcomes other than mild to moderate BPD are infrequent. In the example in Table 79.2, early treatment with two different surfactants resulted in similar low incidences of complications.[122] In an analysis of 51,282 surfactant treatments with three different surfactants, there were no differences in outcomes for air leak, BPD, or death.[123] New synthetic surfactants that contain the surfactant proteins or peptides that mimic surfactant protein function can be effective in animal models and clinically.[21] New surfactants will need to have cost, ease of use, and safety benefits to replace the very effective surfactants that are presently available.

CONCLUSION

Surfactant became the standard of care for the treatment of RDS shortly after its approval in the early 1990s. The trials used for approval are outdated for informing clinicians about surfactant use, because treatment strategies, modes of respiratory support, and the infant population at highest risk of complications and death from RDS are now different. The major differences are the frequent exposure to antenatal corticosteroids and the earlier gestational ages compared with infants in the efficacy trials. Present concerns are about when and how to most noninvasively treat infants with RDS with surfactant in an era when noninvasive respiratory support is favored over mechanical ventilation. Surfactant treatments are cornerstones for effective management of infants with RDS.

A complete reference list is available at www.ExpertConsult.com. 

SELECT REFERENCES

1. Clements JA. Surface tension of lung extracts. *Proc Soc Exp Biol Med.* 1957;95:170–172.
3. Avery ME, Mead J. Surface properties in relation to atelectasis and hyaline membrane disease. *AMA J Dis Child.* 1959;97:517–523.
7. Fujiwara T, Maeta H, Chida S, et al. Artificial surfactant therapy in hyaline-membrane disease. *Lancet.* 1980;1:55–59.
12. Sweet DG, Carnielli V, Greisen G, et al. European consensus guidelines on the management of respiratory distress syndrome - 2019 update. *Neonatology.* 2019;115:432–450.
13. Jobe AH. Why, when, and how to give surfactant. *Pediatr Res.* 2019;86:15–16.
14. Jain K, Nangia S, Ballambattu VB, et al. Goat lung surfactant for treatment of respiratory distress syndrome among preterm neonates: a multi-site randomized non-inferiority trial. *J Perinatol.* 2019;39:3–12.
26. Siew ML, Te Pas AB, Wallace MJ, et al. Surfactant increases the uniformity of lung aeration at birth in ventilated preterm rabbits. *Pediatr Res.* 2011;70:50–55.
27. Pinkerton KE, Lewis JF, Rider ED, et al. Lung parenchyma and type II cell morphometrics: effect of surfactant treatment on preterm ventilated lamb lungs. *J Appl Physiol.* 1994;77(1985):1953–1960.
28. Tingay DG, Pereira-Fantini PM, Oakley R, et al. Gradual aeration at birth is more lung protective than a sustained inflation in preterm lambs. *Am J Respir Crit Care Med.* 2019;200:608–616.
32. Jobe A, Ikegami M, Glatz T, et al. Duration and characteristics of treatment of premature lambs with natural surfactant. *J Clin Invest.* 1981;67:370–375.
33. Miedema M, de Jongh FH, Frerichs I, et al. Changes in lung volume and ventilation during surfactant treatment in ventilated preterm infants. *Am J Respir Crit Care Med.* 2011;184:100–105.
41. De Jaegere A, van Veenendaal MB, Michiels A, et al. Lung recruitment using oxygenation during open lung high-frequency ventilation in preterm infants. *Am J Respir Crit Care Med.* 2006;174:639–645.
45. Katheria AC, Leone TA. Changes in hemodynamics after rescue surfactant administration. *J Perinatol.* 2013;33:525–528.
47. Soll RF. Prophylactic natural surfactant extract for preventing morbidity and mortality in preterm infants. *Cochrane Database Syst Rev.* 2000;1997(2):CD000511.
48. Seger N, Soll R. Animal derived surfactant extract for treatment of respiratory distress syndrome. *Cochrane Database Syst Rev.* 2009;(2):CD007836.
49. Hillman NH, Moss TJ, Kallapur SG, et al. Brief, large tidal volume ventilation initiates lung injury and a systemic response in fetal sheep. *Am J Respir Crit Care Med.* 2007;176:575–581.

50. Thebaud B, Goss KN, Laughon M, et al. Bronchopulmonary dysplasia. *Nat Rev Dis Primers*. 2019;5:78.
58. Dunn MS, Shennan AT, Hoskins EM, et al. Two-year follow-up of infants enrolled in a randomized trial of surfactant replacement therapy for prevention of neonatal respiratory distress syndrome. *Pediatrics*. 1988;82:543-547.
59. Vaucher YE, Merritt TA, Hallman M, et al. Neurodevelopmental and respiratory outcome in early childhood after human surfactant treatment. *Am J Dis Child*. 1988;142:927-930.
65. Horbar JD, Carpenter JH, Buzas J, et al. Timing of initial surfactant treatment for infants 23 to 29 weeks' gestation: is routine practice evidence based? *Pediatrics*. 2004;113:1593-1602.
67. Ammari A, Suri M, Milisavljevic V, et al. Variables associated with the early failure of nasal CPAP in very low birth weight infants. *J Pediatr*. 2005;147:341-347.
68. Bancalari EH, Jobe AH. The respiratory course of extremely preterm infants: a dilemma for diagnosis and terminology. *J Pediatr*. 2012;161:585-588.
69. Schmolzer GM, Kumar M, Pichler G, et al. Non-invasive versus invasive respiratory support in preterm infants at birth: systematic review and meta-analysis. *BMJ*. 2013;347:f5980.
71. Gopel W, Kribs A, Ziegler A, et al. Avoidance of mechanical ventilation by surfactant treatment of spontaneously breathing preterm infants (AMV): an open-label, randomised, controlled trial. *Lancet*. 2011;378:1627-1634.
73. Sweet DG, Carnielli V, Greisen G, et al. European consensus guidelines on the management of neonatal respiratory distress syndrome in preterm infants–2013 update. *Neonatology*. 2013;103:353-368.
74. Polin RA, Carlo WA, Committee on Fetus and Newborn; American Academy of Pediatrics. Surfactant replacement therapy for preterm and term neonates with respiratory distress. *Pediatrics*. 2014;133:156-163.
77. Pillow JJ, Minocchieri S. Innovation in surfactant therapy II: surfactant administration by aerosolization. *Neonatology*. 2012;101:337-344.
79. Hascoet JM, Picaud JC, Ligi I, et al. Late surfactant administration in very preterm neonates with prolonged respiratory distress and pulmonary outcome at 1 year of age: a randomized clinical trial. *JAMA Pediatr*. 2016;170:365-372.
83. Zola EM, Overbach AM, Gunkel JH, et al. Treatment investigational new drug experience with Survanta (beractant). *Pediatrics*. 1993;91:546-551.
89. Costello ML, Mathieu-Costello O, West JB. Stress failure of alveolar epithelial cells studied by scanning electron microscopy. *Am Rev Respir Dis*. 1992;145:1446-1455.
93. Zola EM, Gunkel JH, Chan RK, et al. Comparison of three dosing procedures for administration of bovine surfactant to neonates with respiratory distress syndrome. *J Pediatr*. 1993;122:453-459.
101. Segerer H, van Gelder W, Angenent FW, et al. Pulmonary distribution and efficacy of exogenous surfactant in lung-lavaged rabbits are influenced by the instillation technique. *Pediatr Res*. 1993;34:490-494.
107. Abdel-Latif ME, Osborn DA. Nebulised surfactant in preterm infants with or at risk of respiratory distress syndrome. *Cochrane Database Syst Rev*. 2012;10:CD008310.
115. Ikegami M, Polk D, Tabor B, et al. Corticosteroid and thyrotropin-releasing hormone effects on preterm sheep lung function. *J Appl Physiol*. 1991;70(1985):2268-2278.
116. Roberts D, Dalziel S. Antenatal corticosteroids for accelerating fetal lung maturation for women at risk of preterm birth. *Cochrane Database Syst Rev*. 2006;(3):CD004454.
121. Been JV, Rours IG, Kornelisse RF, et al. Chorioamnionitis alters the response to surfactant in preterm infants. *J Pediatr*. 2010;156:10-15.

Genetics and Physiology of Surfactant Protein Deficiencies

80

Jennifer A. Wambach | Lawrence M. Nogee

INTRODUCTION

The principal cause of respiratory distress syndrome (RDS) in prematurely born infants is an inability to produce sufficient amounts of pulmonary surfactant because of immaturity. Surfactant phospholipids in combination with specific proteins help reduce alveolar surface tension at the air-liquid interface and prevent end-expiratory collapse. DNA sequence variants in the genes encoding proteins important for surfactant function and metabolism may result in diffuse lung disease in term neonates as well as older infants and children. Loss-of-function DNA sequence variants in the genes encoding surfactant protein B (SP-B) and adenosine triphosphate (ATP)-binding cassette member A3 (ABCA3) may cause neonatal respiratory failure inherited in an autosomal recessive fashion. Pathogenic variants in the gene encoding surfactant protein C (SP-C) cause lung disease of more variable onset and severity, either inherited in an autosomal dominant pattern or causing sporadic disease from de novo pathogenic variants.

Pathogenic variants in the gene *NKX2-1*, which encodes thyroid transcription factor 1 which is required for expression of surfactant-related and other genes, can also cause phenotypically similar lung disease. Pathogenic variants in *NKX2-1* may also cause disease in other organ systems including the brain and thyroid, whereas diseases due to pathogenic variants in the genes encoding SP-B, SP-C, or ABCA3 are restricted to the lung. These conditions are rare but cause significant morbidity and mortality, and it is important that they be recognized in a timely fashion to appropriately counsel families of affected infants and children. Treatments are limited and nonspecific, and lung transplantation, with substantial associated mortality and morbidities, remains the definitive treatment for progressive respiratory failure. Genetic surfactant dysfunction disorders also provide insights into the roles of these proteins in normal lung function and surfactant homeostasis and demonstrate how genetic mechanisms may contribute to the development of more common forms of lung disease.

PULMONARY SURFACTANT PROTEINS AND THEIR FUNCTION

SP-B and SP-C are extremely hydrophobic proteins that enhance the surface tension–lowering properties of surfactant phospholipids, and both are found in varying amounts in the mammalian-derived surfactant preparations used to treat premature infants with RDS.[1] SP-B and SP-C are encoded by single genes on chromosomes 2 and 8, respectively, with the genetic loci referred to as *SFTPB* and *SFTPC*. The mature forms of SP-B and SP-C are proteolytically processed from precursor proteins (pro-SP-B, pro-SP-C), routed in alveolar epithelial type II cells (AEC2s) to lysosomally derived intracellular organelles called *lamellar bodies,* and secreted by exocytosis along with surfactant phospholipids.[1] ABCA3 is a transmembrane protein located on the limiting membrane of lamellar bodies.[2] The ATP-binding cassette proteins are a large family of transporter proteins that use the energy from the hydrolysis of ATP to move substances across biologic membranes. ABCA3 transports phospholipids (e.g., phosphatidylcholine and phosphatidylglycerol) essential for surfactant function from the cytoplasm into lamellar bodies.

Pulmonary surfactant also contains two larger glycoproteins, surfactant protein A (SP-A) and surfactant protein D (SP-D). SP-A and SP-D are members of the collectin family, having both collagenous and carbohydrate-binding or lectin-like domains. SP-A and SP-D are important components of the innate immune system in the lung. They bind to a wide array of microorganisms, facilitate their uptake and/or killing by alveolar macrophages, and also have immunomodulatory functions.[3,4] Genetically engineered SP-A- and SP-D-deficient mice do not develop neonatal respiratory disease but do appear to have an increased susceptibility to infection with a variety of organisms that are relevant to human neonates, including group B streptococcus and respiratory syncytial virus.[5-9] With aging, SP-D-deficient mice develop emphysema and fibrosis, suggesting a role for SP-D and surfactant homeostasis in regulating chronic inflammation and lipoproteinosis.[10] Two genes (*SFTPA1*, *SFTPA2*) and a pseudogene for SP-A (*SFTPA3P*) and a single gene for SP-D (*SFTPD*) are located on chromosome 10. Variants in *SFTPA2* and rarely *SFTPA1* have been associated with adult-onset pulmonary fibrosis and lung cancer.[11,12] Variants in *SFTPD* have not yet been associated with human lung disease.[13]

SURFACTANT PROTEIN B DEFICIENCY

SP-B deficiency was the first recognized inborn error of surfactant metabolism.[14] Affected infants are usually term and present with clinical and radiographic features of RDS or hyaline membrane disease as observed in premature infants. Although some affected infants may have relatively milder initial respiratory symptoms, most have severe disease requiring positive pressure support. A need for support with high-frequency ventilation or even extracorporeal membrane oxygenation is not uncommon. Lung disease in SP-B deficiency is invariably progressive, with escalating need for respiratory support and persistent and worsening alveolar and interstitial infiltrates seen on chest radiographs. An initial positive response to surfactant replacement therapy may be observed but with diminished response to subsequent doses. Glucocorticoids may improve the lung disease in some affected infants, perhaps because they have variants that allow some SP-B production.[15] The disease is generally rapidly fatal, with the majority of affected infants dying within the first 3 to 4 months without lung transplantation.[16,17]

MOLECULAR GENETICS AND EPIDEMIOLOGY

The SP-B gene (*SFTPB*) contains 12 exons (initially thought to be 11), the first and last of which are untranslated, and is transcribed into a 2-kilobase messenger RNA, which directs the synthesis of a 393-amino acid pre-proprotein, with the signal peptide removed co-translationally. Mature SP-B corresponds to codons 213 (encoding phenylalanine) to 291 (encoding methionine) of the messenger RNA and is encoded in exons 7 and 8 of the gene. Pro-SP-B contains 3 tandem domains with structural homology to the saposins, lysosomal proteins that bind lipids and activate lysosomal hydrolases, with the 79-amino acid mature SP-B corresponding to the middle domain of the proprotein.[18]

The first and most frequently identified *SFTPB* pathogenic variant is a frameshift resulting from a substitution of three bases (GAA) for one base (C) located upstream of the sequence encoding mature SP-B.[19] This variant introduces a premature codon for the termination of translation, resulting in a transcript that is unstable owing to nonsense-mediated decay and a lack of detectable SP-B messenger RNA.[20] The frameshift upstream of the mature SP-B encoding sequence and premature termination codon would also preclude production of mature SP-B from the mutant sequence. This variant is thus a complete null allele, consistent with a loss-of-function mechanism. The variant was originally termed *121ins2* for the net 2-base insertion into codon 121 of the *SFTPB* transcript. On the basis of homology studies, the reference *SFTPB* transcript is now believed to contain an additional 12 upstream codons and the current nomenclature for this pathogenic variant is c.397delCinsGAA (or p.Pro133Gln*fs*Ter95 for the predicted change in the protein). Pathogenic variants on both *SFTPB* alleles in affected infants are consistent with an autosomal recessive inheritance pattern.

Multiple other pathogenic variants and a sizable deletion in *SFTPB* have been identified.[21-23] Some pathogenic variants allow production of pro-SP-B but processing of pro-SP-B to mature SP-B is impaired, resulting in the lack of mature SP-B in lung tissue and tracheal secretions of affected infants.[21] Pathogenic variants in the mature SP-B domain could theoretically result in the production of a SP-B with abnormal surface properties. However, a synthetic peptide containing one such variant (previously p.Arg236Cys, p.Arg248Cys in the current nomenclature) was able to augment surface tension lowering normally in an in vitro system, suggesting that the disease in infants with this variant also resulted from impaired processing of pro-SP-B containing the variant.[24] SP-B forms higher-order oligomers dependent on sulfhydryl-bond formation and ionic interactions. Variants that prevent oligomerization of SP-B could also in theory result in SP-B with decreased activity, and potentially act in a dominant negative fashion to interfere with SP-B from a normal allele, but such a mechanism for SP-B deficiency has not been reported.

The p.Pro133GlnfsTer95 variant has been identified mostly among individuals of European descent and likely results from a common ancestral origin (founder effect).[15] Two other *SFTPB* pathogenic variants have been identified within five nucleotides of the site of this variant, and a single nucleotide polymorphism is located within 30 base pairs of the site of the p.Pro133GlnfsTer95 variant, suggesting that this region of *SFTPB* could also be a "hot spot" for variation.[21] Other pathogenic variants have been observed in more than one unrelated individual from specific ethnic backgrounds. Rarely, children with biallelic *SFTPB* variants and relatively milder phenotypes have been identified.[16,23,25,26] The variants in these children may allow the production of some SP-B and thus result in partial deficiency. Whether the small amount of mature SP-B (approximately 8% to 10% of control levels) or some retained function of pro-SP-B accounts for the milder phenotype is unclear. These observations suggest that there is a critical level of SP-B needed for normal lung function. This hypothesis is supported by studies in which mice genetically engineered so that their production of SP-B could be experimentally reduced developed respiratory failure when their SP-B levels fell to 20% to 30% of those observed in control animals.[27]

An estimate of the incidence of SP-B deficiency may be derived from the frequencies of known or likely pathogenic variants in *SFTPB* in selected populations or from publicly available databases of genetic variants identified by whole-exome or whole-genome sequencing. The carrier frequency for the p.Pro133Gln*fs*Ter95 variant is approximately 1 in 2300 individuals in the gnomAD database of over 140,000 adults (https://gnomad.broadinstitute.org/)[28] with a greater carrier frequency among European-descent individuals (approximately 1 of 1200 individuals).[29,30] This variant has accounted for approximately two thirds of the variant *SFTPB* alleles identified among infants with progressive respiratory failure to date. SP-B deficiency is an autosomal recessive disorder with a 25% chance of an affected child when both parents carry a pathogenic variant. Using the frequencies of null (e.g., nonsense and frameshift) variants reported in gnomAD (97 null alleles identified in approximately 140,000 individuals) the predicted incidence of disease is approximately 1 in 5 to 10 million births, indicating that SP-B deficiency is a very rare disease. However, this is most certainly an underestimate as missense variants, whose effects on protein function are more difficult to predict, also contribute to disease incidence.

SP-B production increases with advancing gestational age and is down-regulated with inflammation. Lung disease could develop in individuals with loss-of-function variants on one *SFTPB* allele (haploinsufficiency) if other factors, such as prematurity[31] or infection, further delay or reduce SP-B expression below a critical level. Genetically engineered mice heterozygous for a null *Sftpb* allele have half normal levels of SP-B and were more

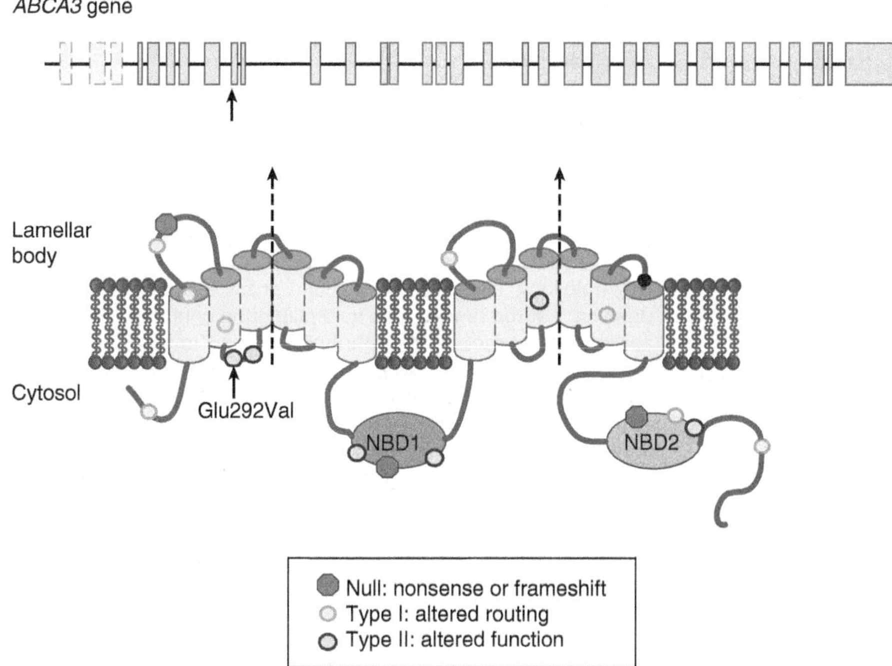

Fig. 80.1 Adenosine triphosphate (ATP)-binding cassette member A3 *(ABCA3)* gene and predicted protein structure and location of selected pathogenic variants. Translated exons are represented by *solid boxes*, and the introns are represented by *lines*. The locations of representative nonsense or frameshift variants predicted to result in no functional protein *(null)* are depicted, along with missense variants demonstrated in vitro to prevent proper trafficking of ABCA3 to lamellar bodies (type I) or to impair ATP binding, hydrolysis, or phospholipid transport into lamellar bodies (type II). The structure of ABCA3 is predicted by homology with other ATP-binding cassette subfamily A proteins, with 12 membrane-spanning domains *(cylinders)* and two nucleotide-binding domains *(NBD)* indicated by *ellipses*, with the exons in the gene encoding the nucleotide-binding domains *shaded*. The location of p.Glu292Val in both the protein and the gene *(arrow)* is indicated. *Dotted arrows* in the protein structure depict direction of phospholipid transport.

susceptible to pulmonary oxygen toxicity than their wild-type littermates but did not develop neonatal respiratory disease.[32,33] In a large study from Denmark, pulmonary function tests were performed in adult carriers of the *SFTPB* p.Pro133Gln*fs*Ter95 pathogenic variant. Abnormalities with reductions in the forced expiatory volume in the first second of expiration and the ratio of this to the forced vital capacity were observed in individuals who also smoked, suggesting that haploinsufficiency for SP-B in conjunction with an environmental insult could predispose to chronic obstructive lung disease.[29]

PATHOPHYSIOLOGY OF SURFACTANT PROTEIN B DEFICIENCY

Surfactant isolated from bronchoalveolar lavage fluid (BALF) of SP-B-deficient infants does not lower surface tension effectively, an unsurprising finding given the importance of SP-B in surfactant function.[34] Tubular myelin, the lattice-like extracellular form of surfactant, the formation of which requires SP-B (as well as SP-A and calcium), is also not found in lung tissue of affected infants.[35] However, additional disturbances in surfactant metabolism also contribute to the pathophysiology of the lung disease in SP-B-deficient infants. These include abnormal surfactant phospholipid composition, particularly a marked reduction in phosphatidylglycerol content, abnormal lamellar body formation, and an apparent block in posttranslational processing of pro-SP-C to mature SP-C.[20,21] Abnormal lamellar body formation and impaired pro-SP-C processing have also been observed in the lungs of genetically engineered mice unable to produce SP-B and that died within minutes of birth because of respiratory failure.[33] These observations indicate a fundamental intracellular role for SP-B (or pro-SP-B) in surfactant metabolism in addition to its extracellular role in lowering surface tension.

The block in the final processing steps of pro-SP-C would result in a relative deficiency of mature SP-C, further contributing to surfactant dysfunction. The abnormal pro-SP-C peptides found in BALF from affected infants contain relatively hydrophilic amino-terminal epitopes, are not very surface-active, and are likely to further inhibit surfactant function. The precise mechanisms underlying this block in pro-SP-C processing are unknown. Ultrastructural examination of the lungs of SP-B-deficient infants reveals a lack of normally formed lamellar bodies, and instead AEC2s have poorly organized lamellar bodies with abnormal-appearing lipid vesicles.[35,36] The final steps in processing of pro-SP-C to mature SP-C occur late in the secretory pathway, either in lamellar bodies or in their immediate precursors. Thus, the inability to form these organelles because of the lack of SP-B results in incompletely processed pro-SP-C, as well as inadequate packaging of surfactant components for secretion. SP-B facilitates membrane fusion, and an explanation for these observations is that without SP-B, transport vesicles containing incompletely processed pro-SP-C are unable to fuse with developing lamellar bodies, thus exposing the amino-terminal epitopes of pro-SP-C to the necessary processing enzymes.[37]

Treatments for infants with respiratory failure due to SP-B deficiency remain limited. However, recent applications of lentiviral-mediated gene correction and CRISPR-Cas9 gene editing to induced pluripotent stem cells (iPSC) from infants with SP-B deficiency have yielded promising results. Lentivirus carrying the wild-type *SFTPB* gene was used to restore SP-B protein production, lamellar body phenotype, and surfactant secretion in iPSC-derived lung organoids from an infant homozygous for p.Pro133Gln*fs*Ter95.[38] CRISPR-Cas9 gene editing resulted in in vitro correction of both mutant *SFTPB* alleles and restoration of SP-B and SP-C processing and lamellar body ultrastructure of AEC2s generated from iPSCs from an affected infant.[39] While significant challenges remain before these technologies can be applied clinically, these results offer hope for infants affected by this devastating disorder.

ADENOSINE TRIPHOSPHATE-BINDING CASSETTE MEMBER A3 DEFICIENCY

ABCA3 is a 1704-amino acid transmembrane protein that is highly expressed in AEC2s, where it is localized to the limiting membrane of lamellar bodies. The gene encoding ABCA3 *(ABCA3)* is large, spanning approximately 80,000 bases on the short arm of chromosome 16, and contains 33 exons. ABCA3 contains 12 membrane-spanning domains and two nucleotide-binding domains (Fig. 80.1). The localization of ABCA3 in AEC2s and the observations that other members of ATP-binding cassette subfamily A transport lipids suggested a role for ABCA3 in surfactant metabolism by importing lipids needed for surfactant function into lamellar bodies. This hypothesis was confirmed when *ABCA3* variants were found in 16 of 21 term newborns with severe lung disease who all had clinical and radiographic features of surfactant deficiency and no other cause for their lung disease identified.[2] Subsequent studies confirmed and extended these observations.[34,40,41]

Infants with biallelic *ABCA3* pathogenic variants often present with severe neonatal respiratory failure similar to that observed in SP-B-deficient infants, and many affected infants die or require lung transplantation within the first 3 to 4 months of life.[41] However, it has been increasingly recognized that infants with *ABCA3* variants may have no apparent neonatal lung disease or apparently transient, relatively mild disease.[42,43] Such infants may then present later in life with chronic interstitial lung disease,[44,45] and ABCA3 deficiency has been recognized as a cause of lung disease presenting in adulthood.[45-49]

MOLECULAR GENETICS AND EPIDEMIOLOGY

More than 250 different variants scattered throughout the *ABCA3* gene have been identified, as well as large deletions spanning one or more exons, indicating considerable allelic heterogeneity.[41,50,51] A predominant pathogenic variant has not been identified but an *ABCA3* variant consisting of a substitution of valine for glutamine in codon 292 (p.Glu292Val) has been observed in multiple unrelated individuals, often with interstitial lung disease.[41,46] Several studies have examined the frequency of the p.Glu292Val variant in selected populations, with carrier frequencies of approximately 1 of 215 individuals with a higher prevalence among individuals of European-descent (1 of 115 individuals, gnomAD).[28,30,52] The true disease incidence of ABCA3 deficiency is difficult to predict from large databases as the majority of pathogenic variants identified among symptomatic infants and children are private missense variants,[41,51] in silico algorithms used to predict their pathogenicity often give conflicting results,[53] and functional studies remain limited.

As with SP-B deficiency, the finding of patients with a milder phenotype implies that there is a critical level of ABCA3 expression needed for normal lung function, and *ABCA3* variants could thus contribute to the pathogenesis of other lung diseases, including RDS in premature infants.[31] Monoallelic *ABCA3* variants are overrepresented in late preterm infants with RDS compared with controls, which is consistent with the developmental expression of ABCA3.[42,43] A correlation of *ABCA3* genotype with age of presentation and outcome has been observed.[41,51] Infants with *ABCA3* variants likely to preclude any functional ABCA3 expression, such as nonsense or frameshift variants, presented at birth with respiratory failure and died or required lung transplantation within the first year of life.[41,51] In contrast, those infants who presented later with interstitial lung disease or survived into childhood had at least one allele with a sequence variant (missense variant, small in-frame insertion or deletion) that could potentially allow some ABCA3 expression.[41,51]

In contrast to the *SFTPB* p.Pro133Gln*fs*Ter95 variant, heterozygosity for *ABCA3* p.Glu292Val did not alter lung function in adults or increase the risk of chronic obstructive pulmonary disease in a large study.[52] However, the p.Glu292Val variant has been functionally characterized as a type 2 mutant (see following section) and not a complete loss-of-function mutant,[54] so these findings do not completely exclude this hypothesis. Experiments with mice heterozygous for a null *Abca3* allele indicated such mice had pulmonary abnormalities when exposed to hyperoxia, supporting the concept that haploinsufficiency for *ABCA3* could predispose to lung disease with exposure to environmental insults.[54a]

PATHOPHYSIOLOGY OF ADENOSINE TRIPHOSPHATE–BINDING CASSETTE MEMBER A3 DEFICIENCY

Ultrastructural examination of lung tissue from infants with biallelic *ABCA3* variants and severe neonatal respiratory failure have shown an absence of normal lamellar bodies in their AEC2s. Instead, small dense organelles with very tightly packed membranes and eccentrically placed electron-dense inclusions were observed, giving them a "fried egg" appearance, indicating a role for ABCA3 in lamellar body biogenesis.[2,35,36]

Whole-lung lavage fluid obtained from infants with ABCA3 deficiency at the time of lung transplantation contained decreased amounts of surfactant phospholipids and an impaired ability to lower surface tension.[34] Decreased amounts of SP-B and SP-C have also been demonstrated in BALF from some newborns with ABCA3 deficiency, which may have further contributed to impaired surfactant function.[40] In vitro studies in primary human AEC2s support a role for ABCA3 in surfactant lipid metabolism.[55] In vitro studies in pulmonary epithelial cell lines have demonstrated two classes of disease-associated, missense *ABCA3* variants: those that impair intracellular trafficking of ABCA3 (type 1) and those that impair ATP- mediated phospholipid transport (type 2).[54,56-65] Type 1 mutants do not traffic normally to the lysosomally derived vesicles and are retained in the endoplasmic reticulum (ER)[56-58,61,63] (see Fig. 80.1). Type 2 mutants traffic normally, but demonstrate reduced ATP binding, smaller lysosomally derived vesicles, or reduced lipid uptake into these vesicles compared with wild-type ABCA3.[54,57,58,64] This categorization is likely to be expanded into a schema similar to that of variants in the gene encoding cystic fibrosis transmembrane regulator *(CFTR)* as additional studies are performed.[66]

Genetically engineered mice homozygous for null *Abca3* alleles have a phenotype identical to that of human infants with loss-of-function *ABCA3* variants, with perinatal lethal respiratory failure, abnormal lamellar body formation, and abnormal lung phospholipid profiles.[67-69] Conditional deletion of the *Abca3* gene in mature mice resulted in surfactant deficiency (decreased phospholipids and increased surface tension), inflammation, alveolar capillary leak, and lethal respiratory failure.[70] While mice with near-total deletion of *Abca3* also demonstrated alveolar injury and inflammation, proliferation of diverse cell types was also observed, and resulted in restoration of ABCA3 expression, lung structure, and function.[70] Atypically activated (M2) macrophages were found in close proximity to proliferating AEC2 cells, however, it is unclear whether these macrophages, also identified in lung tissue from patients with ABCA3 deficiency, contribute to repair or injury mechanisms. Collectively, these observations indicate that loss-of-function *ABCA3* variants result in altered surfactant function and lipid metabolism, impaired lamellar body biogenesis, and alveolar injury and inflammation.

The pathophysiology of lung disease in older children with *ABCA3* variants is not well understood. Because many of these individuals present with lung disease beyond the neonatal period, presumably they were able to produce sufficient amounts of surfactant in the neonatal period to not develop RDS, despite the presence of biallelic *ABCA3* variants. Surfactant lipids in BALF from older children evaluated for diffuse lung disease had abnormal profiles similar to those of newborns with ABCA3 deficiency with decreased amounts of phosphatidylcholine, disaturated phosphatidylcholine, and phosphatidylglycerol.[71] Thus chronic surfactant deficiency could lead to recurrent alveolar collapse and regional atelectasis, resulting in hypoxemia and leading to alveolar injury and inflammation. Some *ABCA3* variants may cause ER stress and injury to AEC2s, leading to apoptosis.[59] Increased susceptibility to viral infections, specifically respiratory syncytial virus infection, has also been proposed on the basis of in vitro studies.[72] Surfactant is catabolized by alveolar macrophages, and accumulations of macrophages in distal air spaces are a prominent finding in the lungs of children with ABCA3 deficiency. Macrophage catabolism of the abnormal alveolar surfactant that results from *ABCA3* pathogenic variants may alter their metabolism, leading to release of cytokines contributing to lung injury. Finally, a role for ABCA3 in protecting cells from toxicity due to cholesterol accumulation has been proposed, providing another mechanism whereby ABCA3 deficiency could lead to chronic AEC2 injury and lung disease.[73] Elucidating the precise mechanisms whereby ABCA3 deficiency or dysfunction leads to chronic cellular injury and eventual fibrosis will be critical to developing therapeutic strategies to treat this lung disease.

SFTPC VARIANTS AND LUNG DISEASE

SP-C is a 35-amino acid extremely hydrophobic protein that also enhances the surface tension-lowering properties of surfactant phospholipids. SP-C is encoded by a small (<3.5 kilobases) gene *(SFTPC)* on human chromosome 8 containing six exons, the last of which is untranslated. The gene directs the synthesis of a proprotein (pro-SP-C) of either 191 or 197 amino acids, depending on alternative splicing at the beginning of the fifth exon. SP-C is extensively post-translationally modified, including the palmitoylation of cysteine residues at positions 5 and 6 of mature SP-C, such that it is a proteolipid.[37] Pro-SP-C is proteolytically processed at both the amino and carboxyl termini to yield the 35-amino acid mature SP-C that is secreted into the air spaces. Pro-SP-C does not contain a signal peptide, and the domain corresponding to mature SP-C is thought to anchor it in the membrane such that pro-SP-C is an integral membrane protein (Fig. 80.2).[37] The carboxy-terminal domain of pro-SP-C has homology with other proteins in what has been termed the *BRICHOS family*, membrane proteins in which abnormal aggregates have been implicated in the pathophysiology of familial dementia and neoplasia.[74] The BRICHOS domain of pro-SP-C may be important in binding to and stabilizing the mature SP-C domain in a conformation that is less prone to forming amyloid-like aggregates.[75,76] A disulfide bridge between cysteine residues at positions 121 and 189 is important in stabilizing the BRICHOS domain.[77]

Although SP-C enhances the surface activity of surfactant phospholipids, SP-C deficiency due to biallelic loss-of-function variants in *SFTPC* does not appear to be a cause of a neonatal RDS phenotype. Mice genetically engineered to lack SP-C do not develop neonatal lung disease (although depending on their genetic background they may develop emphysema with aging[78]), and humans with biallelic loss-of-function variants in *SFTPC* and lung disease have yet to be identified. Thus, SP-C does not appear to be essential for normal neonatal lung function.

However, pathogenic variants in *SFTPC* do cause human lung disease of variable severity and onset of symptoms, with some affected individuals remaining free of symptoms well into adulthood. Most individuals with pathogenic variants in *SFTPC* present later in life with chronic lung disease, and *SFTPC* variants are an unusual cause of neonatal respiratory failure.[16,79,80] Clinical symptoms in infants have included tachypnea, retractions, cough, hypoxemia in room air, failure to thrive, and digital clubbing.[81] The mechanisms responsible for the variability in disease severity remain largely unknown, although heterozygosity for an *ABCA3* variant may exacerbate the severity of the pulmonary symptoms.[82]

MOLECULAR GENETICS AND EPIDEMIOLOGY

As opposed to SP-B and ABCA3 deficiencies, where loss-of-function variants on both alleles result in loss of protein expression or function and lung disease is inherited in a recessive fashion, the lung disease caused by pathogenic *SFTPC* variants generally results from a variant on only one *SFTPC* allele. Lung disease is transmitted in an autosomal dominant pattern with a high degree of penetrance in familial cases, or sporadically caused by a de novo variant. More than 40 pathogenic variants scattered throughout the *SFTPC* gene have been reported.[16,76,79-83] One specific pathogenic *SFTPC* variant resulting in the substitution of threonine for isoleucine in codon 73 (p.Ile73Thr) has been identified in multiple unrelated families, is associated with both familial and sporadic lung disease, and has accounted for approximately 30% to 50% of reported cases.[79,82,83] Many of the known pathogenic variants in *SFTPC* are located in the BRICHOS domain in the carboxyl-terminal portion of pro-SP-C.[76,83] All reported pathogenic variants are predicted to result in an abnormal form of pro-SP-C, including missense variants, in-frame insertions or deletions, or distal frameshift variants that are likely associated with stable transcripts. Nonsense variants, early frameshifts that are likely to be associated with unstable *SFTPC* transcripts, or major deletions that would preclude SP-C production have not been reported, suggesting that haploinsufficiency is unlikely to be the mechanism for lung disease. Correlations of specific variants (genotype) with clinical features and the course (phenotype) have not been consistently observed.[83]

The incidence and prevalence of lung disease due to pathogenic variants in *SFTPC* have not been determined, although it is likely that the disease is quite rare. No individuals with the p.Ile73Thr variant are identified in the gnomAD database of ~120,000 adults.[28] Although many other *SFTPC* coding variants are listed in gnomAD[28] and other publicly available databases, it is uncertain how many represent pathogenic variants.

PATHOPHYSIOLOGY DUE TO *SFTPC* VARIANTS

Lung disease due to pathogenic variants in *SFTPC* results from multiple different mechanisms that may correlate with the nature and location of the variant in the proprotein.[84] The primary mechanism whereby *SFTPC* variants are thought to cause disease is due to a toxic gain-of-function mechanism from abnormal pro-SP-C expressed within AEC2s. *SFTPC* variants may induce misfolding of pro-SP-C with exposure of hydrophobic epitopes, resulting in accumulation of misfolded protein aggregates early in the secretory pathway.[76,84] Therefore, lung disease caused by pathogenic variants in *SFTPC* could represent a conformational disease. The presence of misfolded protein in the ER could result in stress, triggering the unfolded protein response, resulting in up-regulation of chaperone proteins and other downstream pathways, eventually leading to apoptosis and/or inflammation.[84-86] In support of such a toxic gain-of-function mechanism, robust rather than reduced or absent staining for pro-SP-C has been observed in the lung tissue of individuals with pathogenic variants in *SFTPC*, and aggregates of pro-SP-C, as well as amyloid-like deposits, have been observed both in vitro and in lung tissues from infants with *SFTPC* variants.[35,79,87] The potential toxicity of mutant SP-C towards lung epithelial cells has been demonstrated in vitro and by the observations that transgenic mice that overexpressed either mature SP-C without the flanking domains of the proprotein or the *SFTPC* exon 4 variant died of a marked disruption of lung development.[86,88] The impairment of normal lung development associated with high levels of SP-C expression in utero also suggests a potential mechanism whereby some pathogenic variants in *SFTPC* could result in severe neonatal lung disease.

A second mechanism whereby *SFTPC* variants could result in lung disease is through production of an unstable protein and a dominant negative mechanism. Pro-SP-C self-associates in the secretory pathway,[89] and mutant pro-SP-C that is targeted for degradation could interact with normal pro-SP-C, leading to its degradation as well, and thus SP-C deficiency. Pro-SP-C containing a variant identified in humans that

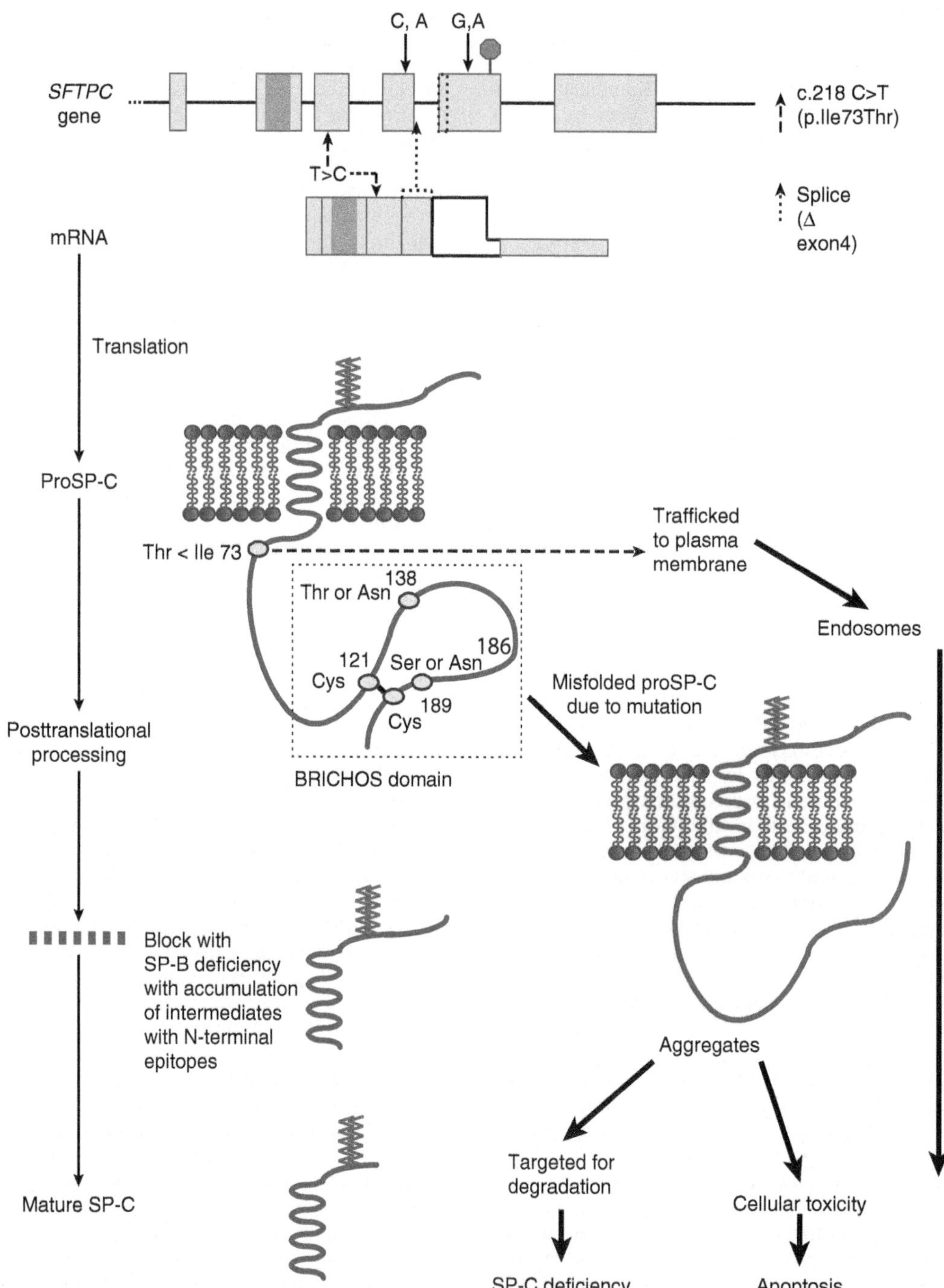

Fig. 80.2 Surfactant protein C gene *(SFTPC)*, surfactant protein C (SP-C), messenger RNA *(mRNA)*, proprotein, and effects of variants. The *SFTPC* gene is depicted at the top with the six exons represented by *blue boxes* and the introns represented by *lines.* Mature SP-C is encoded in exon 2 *(brown rectangle).* The locations of two frequent coding variants (p.Thr138Asn and p.Ser186Asn) in exons 4 and 5 are shown by *arrows,* along with the location of the termination codon *(octagon)* and the location of the pathogenic variant p.Ile73Thr *(dashed arrow).* The location of an intronic pathogenic variant that results in the skipping of exon 4 (Δ exon4) is indicated by a *dotted arrow,* and the skipped exon indicated in the mRNA. Pro-SP-C is depicted in the *middle* and is a transmembrane protein with the domain corresponding to the mature SP-C protein embedded in the membrane. The location of the most frequently observed *SFTPC* pathogenic variant (p. Ile73Thr) is shown, as are the locations of cysteine residues at positions 121 and 189 that form a disulfide bridge that stabilizes the *BRICHOS* domain *(dotted rectangle).* The p.Ile73Thr pathogenic variant results in altered trafficking and accumulation in endosomes. Misfolded pro-SP-C due to BRICHOS domain variants is depicted at *the right,* and results in an abnormal form of pro-SP-C that is rapidly degraded, leading to SP-C deficiency, or the misfolded protein may form aggregates that are toxic to the cell. The *thick dashed line* on the *left* depicts the block in processing of pro-SP-C to mature SP-C observed with surfactant protein B (SP-B) deficiency that results in the accumulation of partially processed intermediates.

resulted in the skipping of the fourth exon (Δexon4) is rapidly degraded in vitro in the absence of inhibitors of proteosome-mediated degradation.[90,91] Decreased expression of both pro-SP-C and mature SP-C were observed in patients with this variant, supporting such a mechanism.[80] Decreased amounts of mature SP-C have also been found in the BALF of patients with pathogenic variants in *SFTPC*. Precisely how deficiency of mature SP-C eventually results in interstitial lung disease is unknown.

A limited number of *SFTPC* variants have been studied in in vitro systems, and these studies support the pathophysiology of *SFTPC* variants, depending on the nature and location of the variants. Variants located in the BRICHOS domain (such as p.Cys121Gly or p.Leu188Gln) result in aggregation of misfolded protein in the ER, triggering of the unfolded protein response, and eventually apoptosis.[84,85,90-93] Variants in the domain bridging the mature peptide and the BRICHOS domain (such as p.Ile73Thr) are mis-trafficked to the plasma membrane rather than being trafficked to lamellar bodies and are subsequently internalized and trafficked to endosomes, where they may accumulate and inhibit recycling of surfactant components.[90,92,94] A block in macroautophagy has also been observed in association with the p.Ile73Thr mutant.[92] An important implication of these observations is that different treatment strategies may be needed depending on the nature of the variant.

Until recently, murine models that mimic human lung disease due to pathogenic variants in *SFTPC* have been limited. SP-C-null mice develop lung disease depending on their genetic background, but because SP-C deficiency due to biallelic loss-of-function variants has not been observed in humans, this is not an accurate model of the human disorder. Constitutive expression of mutant SP-C results in embryonic lethality during the saccular stage of lung development with impaired branching morphogenesis.[86,88,95,96] Transgenic mice expressing a human *SFTPC* BRICHOS domain variant, p.Leu188Gln, under the control of a regulatable promoter, demonstrated evidence of ER stress and the unfolded protein response on induction of the transgene expressing the mutant form or pro-SP-C; they were also more susceptible to lung injury.[97] However, these mice expressed the transgene in the context of two normal *Sftpc* alleles and thus were not completely representative of the human disease. Induced expression of another BRICHOS domain variant p.Cys121Gly in the endogenous *Sftpc* locus in adult mice resulted in ER-retained pro-SPC, AEC2 ER stress and activation of the unfolded protein response, AEC2 apoptosis, polycellular alveolitis, increased cytokine (CCL2, CCL7, CCL17) expression, macrophage recruitment, spontaneous fibrotic lung remodeling, and increased mortality.[95] BALF samples taken from children with interstitial lung disease due to BRICHOS domain variants similarly demonstrated increased cell count (including eosinophils) and increased cytokines, including CCL2, CCL7, and CCL17, which are associated with macrophage recruitment and subsequent fibrosis.[95,98,99] A knock-in mouse model capable of temporally regulated expression of SP-C^{I73T} within the endogenous *Sftpc* locus has also been developed.[96] Expression of the mutant SP-C^{I73T} allele after lung development resulted in spontaneous diffuse acute lung injury, polycellular alveolitis, fibrosis, restrictive lung physiology, and increased mortality in the homozygous mice and a similar but less severe phenotype in the heterozygous mice.[96] The lungs from affected mice demonstrated ultrastructural evidence of an acquired defect in macroautophagy and AEC2 cell hyperplasia with increased expression of CCL2 as well as transforming growth factor (TGF)-β1, which can induce production of collagen and other components of the extracellular matrix by mesenchymal cells.[96]

NKX2-1 HAPLOINSUFFICIENCY AND BRAIN-THYROID-LUNG SYNDROME

NKX2-1, located on the long arm of chromosome 14 (14q13.3), encodes thyroid transcription factor 1, a member of the homeodomain family. Two different protein isoforms have been reported depending on whether translation initiation sites in exon 1 or exon 2 are used, with the shorter isoform with the translation initiation site located in exon 2 predominating in the lung.[100] Thyroid transcription factor 1 plays an essential role in early development of the lung and thyroid gland and is important for the expression of numerous genes within the lung, including those in the surfactant system (*SP-A, SP-B, SP-C,* and *ABCA3* genes). The gene is also expressed in the basal ganglia. Pathogenic variants in or deletion of one *NKX2-1* allele results in a variable phenotype involving the three main organ systems in which the protein is expressed, "brain-thyroid-lung" syndrome, with all three organ systems involved in approximately 40% to 50% of identified cases (Fig. 80.3).[101]

Neurologic symptoms in older children and adults include movement disorders, and pathogenic variants in *NKX2-1* were first identified as a cause of benign familial chorea. Neonates and very young infants often exhibit hypotonia, but this may be perceived as secondary to the severe lung disease. In infants and older children, poor feeding and ataxia may be seen. The onset, nature, and severity of the lung disease is variable, ranging from RDS in newborn infants to diffuse lung disease or recurrent pulmonary infections in older children and adults. Pulmonary disease may be the sole manifestation of pathogenic variants in *NXK2-1*, although most affected individuals have thyroid or neurologic abnormalities as well.[102] Thyroid gland involvement ranges from agenesis of the gland to borderline chemical hypothyroidism with elevated serum thyroid-stimulating hormone (TSH) levels and low-normal levels of thyroxine; pathogenic variants in *NKX2-1* are a rare cause of isolated congenital hypothyroidism.[103]

MOLECULAR GENETICS AND EPIDEMIOLOGY

Chromosomal deletions encompassing the *NKX2-1* locus have been recognized and were the first reported genetic abnormality of *NKX2-1* in a newborn with a severe RDS phenotype and congenital hypothyroidism.[104] Because other genes were contained within the deleted regions, it was possible that deletion of contiguous genes contributed to the phenotype. Subsequently, DNA sequence variants were identified within *NKX2-1* as causes of benign hereditary chorea and individuals with combinations of neurologic and lung disease and hypothyroidism.[105,106] Multiple deletions incorporating *NKX2-1* and numerous pathogenic variants in exons 2 and 3 have been identified. Although some variants in unrelated individuals have been reported, most are private and no predominant pathogenic variant has been recognized. A long noncoding RNA immediately downstream of *NKX2-1* has been characterized that likely has a role in the regulation of *NKX2-1* expression. A child with the phenotype of brain-thyroid-lung syndrome, yet no sequence variant or deletion of the *NKX2-1* locus, was found to have a deletion in this region that would have disrupted a long noncoding RNA.[107] De novo variants in or deletions of *NKX2-1* may result in apparent sporadic disease. Familial cases are inherited in an autosomal dominant pattern with nearly complete penetrance, although the severity and patterns of disease of the three organ systems involved may vary even among family members with the same variant. Loss-of-function variants in *NKX2-1* are extremely rare (5 loss-of-function alleles identified in approximately 120,000 adults in gnomAD).[28] *NKX2-1* missense variants are more common in gnomAD; however, similar to variants in other surfactant genes, the majority of *NKX2-1* missense variants are rare or private, in silico algorithms use to predict pathogenicity often give conflicting results, and functional data remain limited thereby

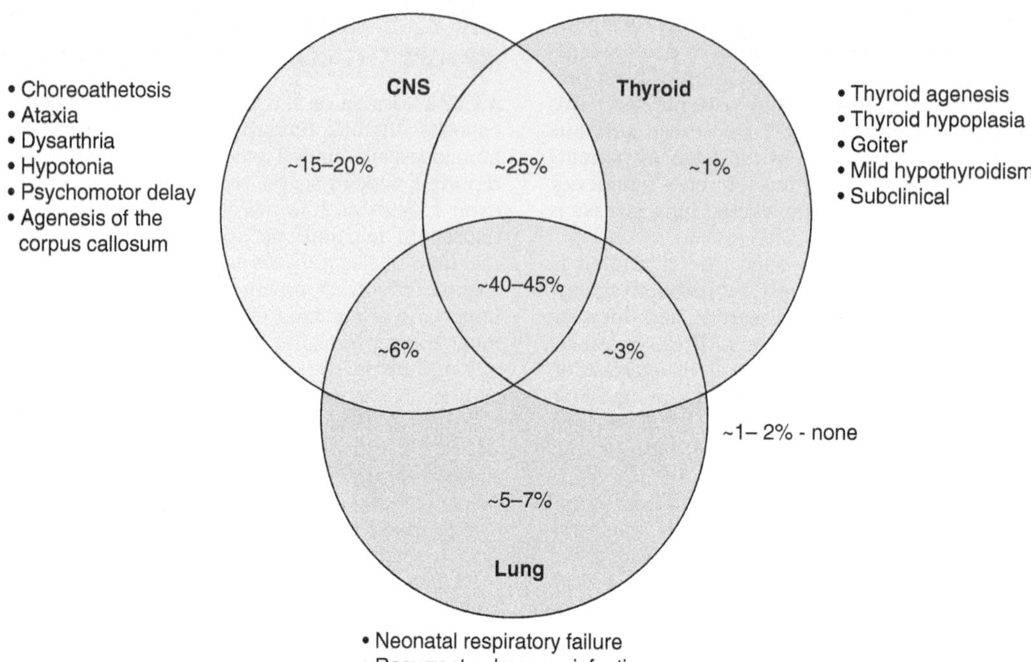

Fig. 80.3 Phenotypic spectrum associated with *NKX2-1* variants: diagram of findings in subjects with brain-thyroid-lung syndrome. The numbers are based on 284 published cases through 2019; the percentages are approximate, as complete organ system involvement was not reported in all individuals. *CNS,* Central nervous system.

complicating estimation of disease incidence. In addition, many de novo pathogenic variants may cause severe disease early in life and thus may be underestimated in large databases of adults.

PATHOPHYSIOLOGY OF *NKX2-1* VARIANTS

As complete deletions of the *NKX2-1* locus can result in lung disease, the primary mechanism by which pathogenic variants in *NKX2-1* cause disease is believed to be gene dose, where half the amount of the transcription factor (haploinsufficiency) results in inadequate production of downstream targets.[105,106] The findings of in vitro studies of some variants have generally been consistent with this mechanism, with decreased DNA binding of expressed *NKX2-1* mutants or reduced ability to express reporter constructs of target genes.[108–110] It is possible that some variants result in a gain of function, although it is less clear how this would result in lung disease.[108] Immunohistochemical staining of surfactant proteins in lung tissue of individuals with pathogenic variants in *NKX2-1* has demonstrated variable findings, with reduced expression of one or more surfactant proteins.[102] The most severe reductions in expression have correlated to some extent with the phenotype. For example, decreased staining for ABCA3 was observed in a child who presented with neonatal respiratory failure, and decreased staining for SP-D was observed in a child who presented with severe respiratory failure after a severe viral infection, with SP-D known to have role in innate immunity (Fig. 80.4).[111] A variant in *NKX2-1* also segregated with lung disease in a large kindred, where the pulmonary phenotype was more consistent with a different form of childhood interstitial lung disease—neuroendocrine cell hyperplasia of infancy—as opposed to surfactant dysfunction.[112] This observation suggests lung disease due to *NKX2-1* variants may result from altered expression of genes other than those in the surfactant system. *NKX2-1* is important for normal lung development, and abnormal lung development has also been observed in children with *NKX2-1* genomic deletions.[113]

LUNG PATHOLOGY FINDINGS WITH GENETIC SURFACTANT DYSFUNCTION DISORDERS

The histopathologic findings in the lungs of infants with pathogenic variants in *SFTPB*, *ABCA3*, *SFTPC,* or *NKX2-1* are similar and overlapping. Prominent findings include AEC2 cell hyperplasia, prominent collections of foamy macrophages in the air spaces, and interstitial thickening. Cholesterol clefts may be found in air spaces or within cells; nonspecific findings including diffuse alveolar damage and interstitial fibrosis may also be present.[35] Diagnostic terms that have been used to describe the lung pathology in these infants include *chronic pneumonitis of infancy, desquamative interstitial pneumonitis,* and *nonspecific interstitial pneumonia.* More recently, the term *surfactant dysfunction* has been used to encompass the pathologic findings related to all of these conditions, reflecting the nonspecific nature of the disease at the level of light microscopy.[114]

A prominent feature of the lung histopathology, particularly in newborn or young infants, is the presence of granular eosinophilic material in distal air spaces that stain positively with periodic acid–Schiff reagent and is diastase resistant. This finding resembles that seen in pulmonary alveolar proteinosis in adults, where there is marked accumulation of surfactant material in distal air spaces. Because of this similarity in appearance, the term *congenital alveolar proteinosis* was originally used to describe this clinical and histologic pattern.[14] However, the mechanism for pulmonary alveolar proteinosis in adults and some children is very different, being due to impaired catabolism of surfactant by alveolar macrophages as opposed to a disorder of surfactant production within AEC2s. This impairment in catabolism results from defective macrophage maturation due to lack of signaling by granulocyte-macrophage colony stimulating factor. Primary pulmonary alveolar proteinosis in adults is an autoimmune disorder resulting from neutralizing antibodies to

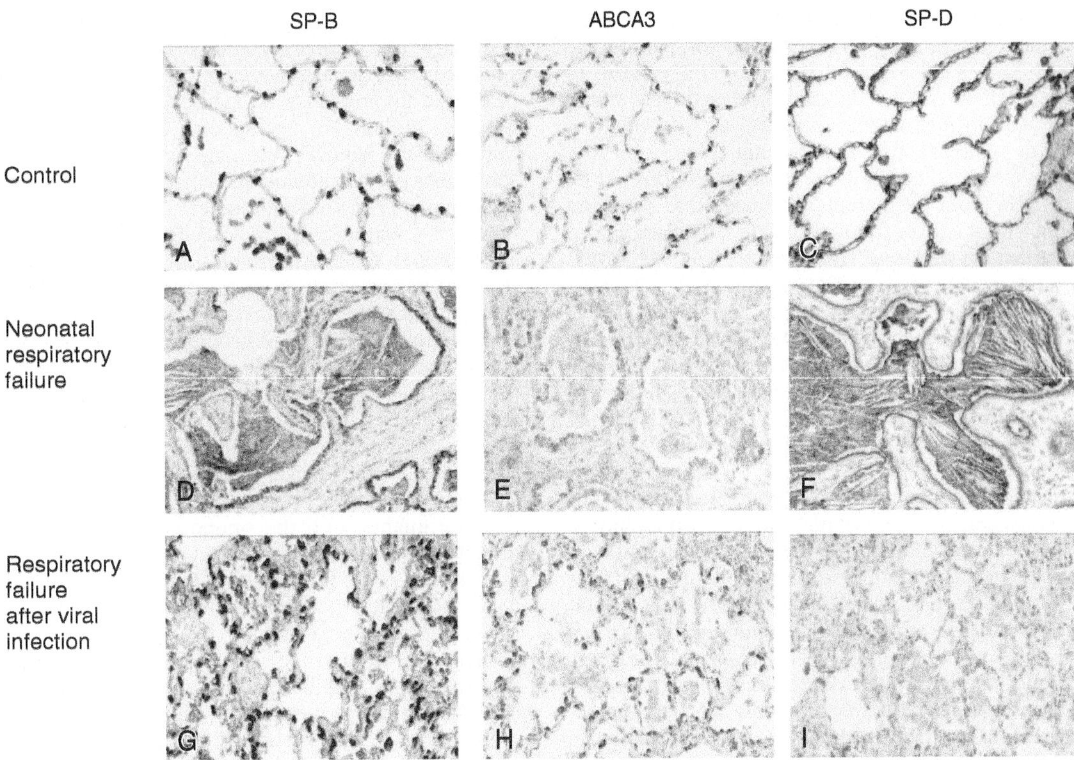

Fig. 80.4 Variable immunohistochemical staining for surfactant proteins associated with *NKX2-1* pathogenic variants. Lung tissue was immunostained for surfactant protein B (SP-B; *left*), adenosine triphosphate–binding cassette member A3 (ABCA3; *center*), and surfactant protein D (SP-D; *right*). Lung tissue from a control infant who died of chronic lung disease *(top)* demonstrates positive staining for mature SP-B (A), ABCA3 (B), and SP-D (C) observed in alveolar epithelial cells. In an infant who had severe neonatal respiratory failure and was heterozygous for a frameshift variant in *NKX2-1 (middle),* positive staining for mature SP-B (D) and SP-D (F) is observed in alveolar epithelium and air-space material, but staining is markedly reduced for ABCA3 (E). In contrast, in an infant who presented with respiratory failure after viral infection *(bottom),* positive staining in the alveolar epithelium is observed for SP-B (G) and ABCA3 (H) but is markedly reduced for SP-D (I). (Photographs courtesy Susan Wert, PhD, Children's Hospital Medical Center, Cincinnati, Ohio.)

granulocyte-macrophage colony-stimulating factor. Variants in the genes *(CSFR2A, CSFR2B)* encoding the components of the granulocyte-macrophage colony-stimulating factor receptor on alveolar macrophages have also been recognized as causes of pulmonary alveolar proteinosis in some children and adults.[115,116]

EVALUATION OF INFANTS WITH SUSPECTED GENETIC SURFACTANT DYSFUNCTION

The clinical features that distinguish SP-B or ABCA3 deficiency from reversible causes of neonatal respiratory failure have not been identified. Term infants with respiratory distress that is not explained by the clinical history and does not improve after the first week of life or infants who died of lung disease of unclear cause should be suspected of having one of these disorders. Although a family history of lung disease may prompt suspicion for a genetic disorder, a family history is often absent, given the autosomal recessive inheritance patterns for SP-B and ABCA3 deficiencies and that de novo pathogenic variants in *SFTPC* or *NKX2-1* may cause sporadic disease. Because the initial lung disease in some children with *ABCA3* variants may be very mild, these children may be discharged from the neonatal intensive care unit and be seen later with signs and symptoms of persistent diffuse lung disease without a clear cause. The differential diagnosis includes RDS, transient tachypnea of the newborn, pneumonia (both bacterial and viral), persistent pulmonary hypertension, pulmonary hypoplasia, unrecognized cardiac malformations, and developmental anomalies of the lung such as alveolar capillary dysplasia with misalignment of the pulmonary veins. This latter condition may result from pathogenic variants in or deletions of the gene encoding the transcription factor FOXF1, and these infants frequently have anomalies in other organ systems, particularly cardiac, gastrointestinal, or genitourinary malformations.[117] Patients with Niemann-Pick type C disease may have lung involvement and potentially present with a similar phenotype.[118]

Routine laboratory findings in children with genetic surfactant dysfunction are nonspecific. Tracheal aspirate samples for lecithin-to-sphingomyelin ratios have been reported as low and within the normal range from children with SP-B or ABCA3 deficiency but have not been systematically evaluated because such testing is not routinely done in term infants. Analysis of tracheal aspirate or BALF samples for surfactant protein levels is not available clinically and is also unlikely to provide a definitive diagnosis. Although SP-B levels are usually undetectable in SP-B-deficient infants, undetectable or very low levels may be present in children with other surfactant dysfunction disorders, particularly ABCA3 deficiency, as well as in children with diffuse alveolar injury and global surfactant deficiency not caused by genetic mechanisms.[40] Conversely, the presence of normal levels of SP-B in tracheal aspirate or BALF does not exclude the possibility of other surfactant dysfunction disorders due to pathogenic variants in *ABCA3, SFTPC,* or *NKX2-1*.[34]

Definitive diagnosis is established through genetic testing. Such testing is noninvasive, and sequenced-based analysis of all of the coding exons of *SFTPB, ABCA3, SFTPC,* and *NKX2-1* is available through certified diagnostic laboratories. A helpful resource listing laboratories providing testing for genetic disorders may be found on the National Center for Biotechnology website (www.ncbi.nlm.nih.gov/gtr). A finding of pathogenic variants on *both* alleles (biallelic) of either *SFTPB* or *ABCA3* is diagnostic for SP-B or ABCA3 deficiency, respectively. When two *SFTPB* or *ABCA3* pathogenic variants are identified, it is important to demonstrate that the variants are on opposite alleles (in *trans*), which is usually most easily accomplished by examination of DNA from the parents, because more than one variant has been identified on the same allele.[41] The finding of a pathogenic variant on only one allele (monoallelic) in *SFTPC* or *NKX2-1* is similarly diagnostic of SP-C dysfunction or NKX2-1 haploinsufficiency. Because genic or genomic deletions in *SFTPB*, *ABCA3*, and *NKX2-1* have been reported as causes of disease, specific approaches (e.g., chromosomal microarray or deletion/duplication studies) to detect such deletions should be part of clinical testing if there is a high index of suspicion for one of these disorders and pathogenic variants are not found through gene sequencing studies.[22,50,102]

Unfortunately, the interpretation of genetic testing is not always straightforward. It may be difficult or impossible to distinguish whether an identified DNA sequence variant will cause a functional change in the protein structure and thus potentially result in disease or represents a benign change. Such variants are referred to as *variants of unknown significance* and are usually missense variants or small in-frame insertions or deletions. Functional assays to determine the significance of such variants are generally not available or feasible for every such variant identified. Large-scale functional studies to evaluate the in vitro effects of all possible coding variants within specific genes ("saturational mutagenesis") are emerging to assist with interpretation of rare variants.[119,120] Knowledge of the frequency of a given variant in the general population may assist with interpretation, because variants that are not extremely rare are generally less likely to be pathogenic. For example, a variant in *SFTPC* resulting in an amino acid change in codon 167 (p.Arg167Gln) was originally reported as a cause of lung disease.[121] Newer data from population studies have demonstrated that this variant is present in approximately 1.5% of alleles among individuals of African descent, including several homozygous individuals (gnomAD).[28] Although not common, this frequency is inconsistent with the apparent rarity of lung disease due to *SFTPC* variants. Segregation studies within families may help in interpretation but may also be confounded by variable penetrance, such as seen with pathogenic variants in *SFTPC*, and may also lead to a diagnosis in a parent or extended family member who was previously unaware of his or her risk of lung disease.

Currently available clinical genetic testing for surfactant dysfunction disorders focuses on the coding regions (exon-targeted) and includes single gene, gene panels, or whole-exome sequencing (portion of genome that is translated into proteins). Genetic testing is not 100% sensitive, because functionally significant variants in the unexamined regions of the gene, including deep intronic variants, untranslated regions, or intergenic regions, will be missed with exon-targeted sequencing strategies. Children without identifiable *ABCA3* variants but with clinical and lung pathology phenotypic findings and genetic segregation findings consistent with ABCA3 deficiency have been reported, indicating that some *ABCA3* variants have gone undetected.[16,60,122,123] Genic or genomic copy number variants (deletions, duplications) or rearrangements may not be detected, depending on the method used. Chromosomal microarray may be useful for detecting large deletions or duplications but may miss smaller copy number variants or translocations. Whole-genome sequencing may address some of these limitations. Other limitations to genetic testing include the cost and the length of time needed for results to be reported, particularly for a child with rapidly progressive disease.

Tissue examination may be helpful if lung biopsy is deemed necessary for proper diagnosis or autopsy tissue when no suitable material is available for genetic studies. As discussed, histologic findings may be suggestive of surfactant dysfunction, but the findings are not specific for a given genetic disorder. Immunohistochemical staining for surfactant proteins can sometimes provide additional information. Staining of extracellular alveolar material with antibodies to the amino-terminal portion of pro-SP-C is indicative of SP-B deficiency (Fig. 80.5). Although antibodies to surfactant proteins are commercially available, such studies are not routinely performed by most clinical pathology laboratories, and the results must then be interpreted with caution. Because characteristic ultrastructural findings of abnormal lamellar bodies are associated with both ABCA3 and SP-B deficiency, lung tissue should be prepared for electron microscopy with proper fixatives if surfactant dysfunction is suspected.[35,124] Consideration should also be given to snap-freezing tissue in liquid nitrogen because such studies may facilitate future investigations including DNA and RNA studies.[124]

Some infants with the phenotype of surfactant dysfunction disorders may not have a known genetic cause identified.[2] With increased use of whole-exome and whole-genome sequencing, it is likely that other inherited disorders resulting in abnormal surfactant production will be discovered. Similar to the nonspecific appearance of a sepsis-like illness and metabolic disturbances in children with inborn errors of metabolism, children with inborn errors of lung cell metabolism may present with a nonspecific picture of neonatal respiratory distress and radiographically diffuse lung disease. Elucidation of these inborn errors should enhance our understanding of normal surfactant metabolism and may provide clues to the pathogenesis of lung diseases outside the neonatal period.

TREATMENT

There are no specific proven-effective therapies for surfactant dysfunction disorders. Medications that have been used in the treatment of affected infants have included systemic corticosteroids, hydroxychloroquine, and azithromycin.[51,125–128] Steroids might provide benefit to some patients by increasing expression of specific genes, particularly *ABCA3*. The mechanisms whereby hydroxychloroquine and azithromycin might improve lung function in surfactant dysfunction disorders are unclear, and these agents have been used on the basis of experiences in adults with various forms of interstitial lung disease or on the basis of studies in children with interstitial lung disease before the mechanisms for their lung disease were known.[129] Although there are single case reports or small series of patients demonstrating apparent improvement with these medications,[51] randomized trials demonstrating their efficacy have not been performed, and the design and conduct of such trials will be challenging, owing to the rarity of these conditions. The variability in the natural history of disease due to *SFTPC* and *ABCA3* variants also makes the interpretation of apparent responses to medical therapy difficult to determine.[130] Palliative care is an appropriate option for infants with SP-B deficiency or ABCA3 deficiency due to biallelic loss-of-function variants to preclude expression of any functional protein, given the associated very poor prognosis.[41,83]

Lung transplantation has been performed for surfactant dysfunction disorders with outcomes that are similar to those in infants with other pulmonary conditions.[17] Lung transplantation requires long-term immunosuppressive therapy and carries with it short-term and long-term risks for infection and rejection; long-term survival is often limited owing to the complication of bronchiolitis obliterans. The procedure is costly and available only at a limited number of medical centers, the availability of

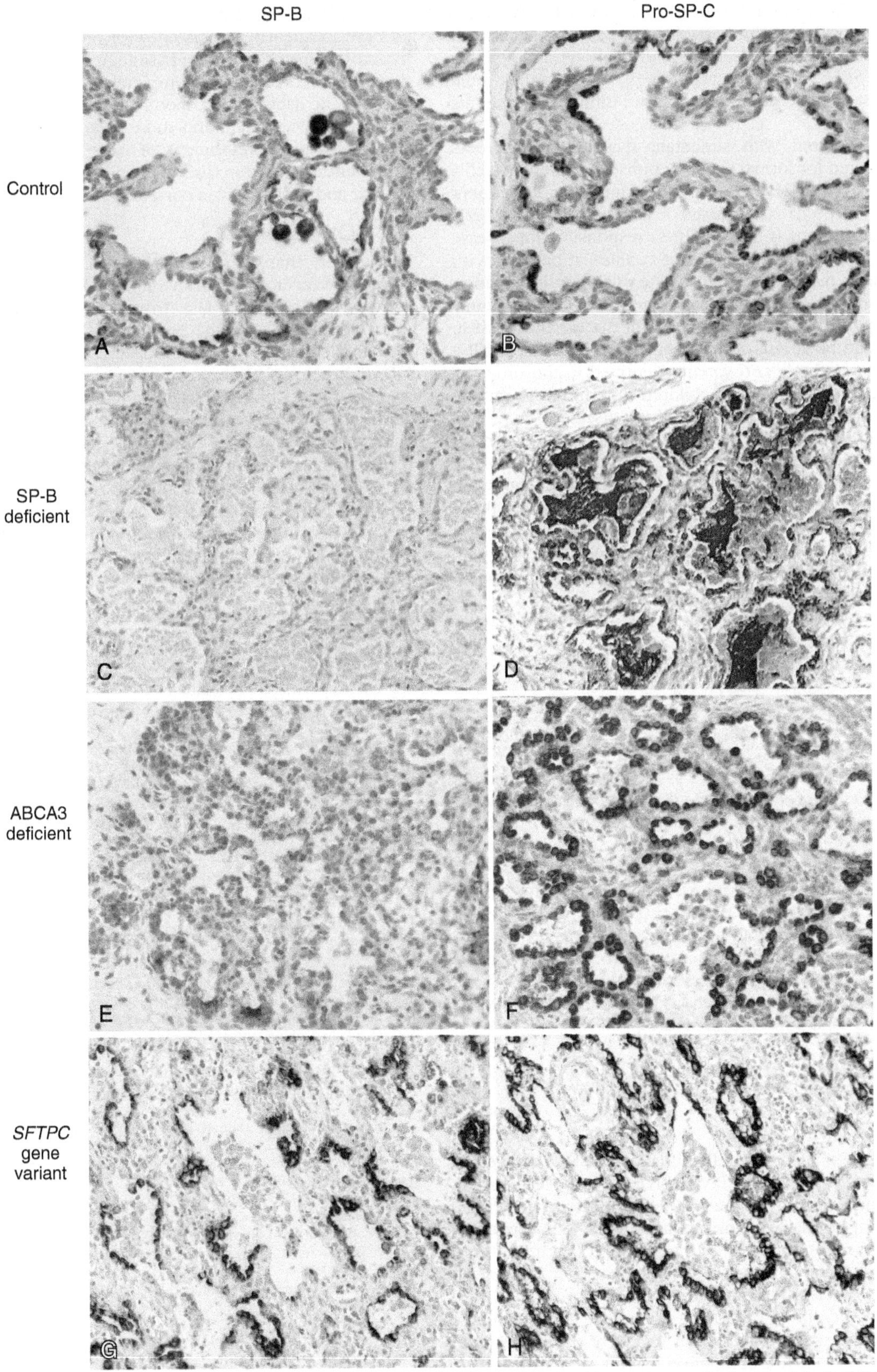

Fig. 80.5 Immunohistochemical staining of lung tissue. Lung tissue was immunostained for mature surfactant protein B (SP-B; *left)* and surfactant protein C precursor (pro-SP-C; *right)*. Lung tissue from a control infant who died of chronic lung disease demonstrates positive staining for both mature SP-B (A) and pro-SP-C (B) observed in alveolar epithelial cells *(top row)*. In contrast, absent staining for mature SP-B (C) but intense staining for pro-SP-C in the alveolar epithelium and extracellular proteinaceous material (D) is observed in lung tissue from an SP-B-deficient infant who was homozygous for the *SFTPB* pathogenic variant p.Pro133GlnfsTer95 *(second row)*. Staining for mature SP-B is also markedly reduced (E) in lung tissue from a patient who was a compound heterozygote for two *ABCA3* variants, with robust staining for pro-SP-C that is confined to the alveolar epithelium (F). Staining for mature SP-B (G) and for pro-SP-C (H) is robust in tissue from a patient with the most frequently found *SFTPC* pathogenic variant (p.Ile73Thr) on one allele *(bottom)*. (Photographs courtesy Susan Wert, PhD, Children's Hospital Medical Center, Cincinnati, Ohio.)

donor lungs is also limited, and death may occur before donor lungs become available. The variable courses associated with *ABCA3* missense, in-frame insertion and deletions, and splicing variants and *SFTPC* variants make decisions regarding lung transplantation or redirection of care more difficult for patients with these disorders.

Parents of children with surfactant dysfunction disorders should be referred for formal genetic counseling. There is a 25% recurrence risk with SP-B and ABCA3 deficiency for subsequent pregnancies, and prenatal diagnosis or preimplantation genetic testing may be options if the variant(s) responsible for disease in a family is identified. Counseling of families of patients with *SFTPC* variants is more difficult given the dominant inheritance, variable penetrance, and because parents or other family members may be asymptomatic carriers of the variant found in the proband and be at risk of development of lung disease. If a parent does carry the *SFTPC* variant identified in the proband, there is a 50% chance of future children inheriting the variant, but when those children will develop lung disease is unknown. Similarly, familial disease due to *NKX2-1* variants has also been reported, and the family history with particular emphasis on neurologic and thyroid disorders should be obtained from the family of an affected child. If neither parent of a child with an *SFTPC* or *NKX2-1* variant is found to carry the variant, then the risk for an affected child in subsequent pregnancies is very low, although not zero, owing to the potential of germ-line mosaicism or nonpaternity.

MODELS FOR STUDYING SURFACTANT DYSFUNCTION DISORDERS

Over the past decade, significant strides have been made in developing model systems by which to characterize encoded disruption of surfactant genes as well as the beginning of attempts at in vitro correction of these genetic disorders. A major limitation to identification of therapies for individuals with surfactant dysfunction disorders has been the need for suitable in vitro systems that accurately recapitulate the AEC2 and its cellular environment. Recent development of lung organoids, 3-dimensional organotypic culture, and generation of AEC2s from patient-derived iPSCs offer several advantages compared to pulmonary cell lines derived from cancerous or non-human cells, including improved disease modeling of pathogenic variants in a patient-specific context.[39,131,132] These models hold promise for identification of human-specific disease mechanisms and variant-specific therapies.

CONCLUSION

Genetic surfactant dysfunction disorders are rare but are associated with significant morbidity and mortality. SP-B deficiency is an extremely rare but almost invariably fatal cause of neonatal respiratory failure in term infants and demonstrates an essential role for SP-B in normal lung metabolism. ABCA3 deficiency is likely the most common of these disorders and may result in a clinical picture similar to that of SP-B deficiency or may result in interstitial lung disease presenting later in life; the specific *ABCA3* variants may be helpful in predicting prognosis. SP-B deficiency and ABCA3 deficiency are autosomal recessive disorders, with disease resulting from loss-of-function variants that result in a lack of functional protein. Variants in the gene encoding SP-C are associated with lung disease of variable severity and age of onset that may be sporadic or inherited in an autosomal dominant pattern. Lung disease due to pathogenic variants in *SFTPC* results from a gain of toxic function resulting in misfolded protein that is unstable, aggregates in the secretory pathway, or is abnormally routed in AEC2s. Deletions of or pathogenic variants in *NKX2-1* may result in lung disease of variable onset, severity, and nature and are frequently associated with neurologic findings and/or hypothyroidism. The pathophysiology of the lung diseases due to these disorders remains incompletely understood. Environmental and genetic factors that modify the course of these diseases need to be identified, and more effective treatments need to be developed. Development of new model systems to study surfactant dysfunction disorders and gene editing offer promise to treat and perhaps even correct these devastating disorders.

ACKNOWLEDGMENTS

The authors thank Jeffrey A. Whitsett, MD, Darrell Kotton, MD, Timothy Weaver, PhD, Aaron Hamvas, MD, F. Sessions Cole, MD, Frances V. White, MD, Lisa Young, MD, Robin Deterding, MD, Alicia Casey, MD, Martha Fishman, MD, Susan Guttentag, MD, Michael Beers, MD, Surafel Mulugeta, PhD, and Elizabeth Fiorino, MD, for their collaboration, along with Susan Wert, PhD, who also provided photographs of immunostained lung tissue. The authors also thank Dan Wegner, MS, Hillary B. Heins, BS, and Ping Yang, MS, at Washington University School of Medicine for their research contributions. This work was supported by grants from the National Institutes of Health, the American Thoracic Society/Children's Interstitial Lung Disease Foundation, the Children's Discovery Institute, and the Eudowood Foundation.

A complete reference list is available at www.ExpertConsult.com. 

SELECT REFERENCES

1. Whitsett JA, Weaver TE. Hydrophobic surfactant proteins in lung function and disease. *N Engl J Med*. 2002;347:2141-2148.
2. Shulenin S, Nogee LM, Annilo T, Wert SE, Whitsett JA, Dean M. ABCA3 gene mutations in newborns with fatal surfactant deficiency. *N Engl J Med*. 2004;350:1296-1303.
10. Wert SE, Yoshida M, LeVine AM, et al. Increased metalloproteinase activity, oxidant production, and emphysema in surfactant protein D gene-inactivated mice. *Proc Natl Acad Sci U S A*. 2000;97:5972-5977.
11. Maitra M, Wang Y, Gerard RD, Mendelson CR, Garcia CK. Surfactant protein A2 mutations associated with pulmonary fibrosis lead to protein instability and endoplasmic reticulum stress. *J Biol Chem*. 2010;285:22103-22113.
12. Nathan N, Giraud V, Picard C, et al. Germline SFTPA1 mutation in familial idiopathic interstitial pneumonia and lung cancer. *Hum Mol Genet*. 2016;25: 1457-1467.
14. Nogee LM, de Mello DE, Dehner LP, Colten HR. Brief report: deficiency of pulmonary surfactant protein B in congenital alveolar proteinosis. *N Engl J Med*. 1993;328:406-410.
19. Nogee LM, Garnier G, Dietz HC, et al. A mutation in the surfactant protein B gene responsible for fatal neonatal respiratory disease in multiple kindreds. *J Clin Invest*. 1994;93:1860-1863.
20. Beers MF, Hamvas A, Moxley MA, et al. Pulmonary surfactant metabolism in infants lacking surfactant protein B. *Am J Respir Cell Mol Biol*. 2000;22: 380-391.
21. Nogee LM, Wert SE, Proffit SA, Hull WM, Whitsett JA. Allelic heterogeneity in hereditary surfactant protein B (SP-B) deficiency. *Am J Respir Crit Care Med*. 2000;161:973-981.
29. Baekvad-Hansen M, Dahl M, Tybjaerg-Hansen A, Nordestgaard BG. Surfactant protein-B 121ins2 heterozygosity, reduced pulmonary function, and chronic obstructive pulmonary disease in smokers. *Am J Respir Crit Care Med*. 2010;181:17-20.
34. Garmany TH, Moxley MA, White FV, et al. Surfactant composition and function in patients with ABCA3 mutations. *Pediatr Res*. 2006;59:801-805.
39. Jacob A, Morley M, Hawkins F, et al. Differentiation of human pluripotent stem cells into functional lung alveolar epithelial cells. *Cell Stem Cell*. 2017;21: 472-488 e10.
40. Brasch F, Schimanski S, Muhlfeld C, et al. Alteration of the pulmonary surfactant system in full-term infants with hereditary ABCA3 deficiency. *Am J Respir Crit Care Med*. 2006;174:571-580.
41. Wambach JA, Casey AM, Fishman MP, et al. Genotype-phenotype correlations for infants and children with ABCA3 deficiency. *Am J Respir Crit Care Med*. 2014;189:1538-1543.
42. Wambach JA, Wegner DJ, Depass K, et al. Single ABCA3 mutations increase risk for neonatal respiratory distress syndrome. *Pediatrics*. 2012;130:e1575-e1582.
46. Bullard JE, Wert SE, Whitsett JA, Dean M, Nogee LM. ABCA3 mutations associated with pediatric interstitial lung disease. *Am J Respir Crit Care Med*. 2005;172:1026-1031.
51. Kroner C, Wittmann T, Reu S, et al. Lung disease caused by ABCA3 mutations. *Thorax*. 2017;72:213-220.

54. Matsumura Y, Ban N, Inagaki N. Aberrant catalytic cycle and impaired lipid transport into intracellular vesicles in ABCA3 mutants associated with non-fatal pediatric interstitial lung disease. *Am J Physiol Lung Cell Mol Physiol.* 2008;295:L698-L707.
55. Mulugeta S, Gray JM, Notarfrancesco KL, et al. Identification of LBM180, a lamellar body limiting membrane protein of alveolar type II cells, as the ABC transporter protein ABCA3. *J Biol Chem.* 2002;277:22147-22155.
56. Matsumura Y, Ban N, Ueda K, Inagaki N. Characterization and classification of ATP-binding cassette transporter ABCA3 mutants in fatal surfactant deficiency. *J Biol Chem.* 2006;281:34503-34514.
57. Wambach JA, Yang P, Wegner DJ, et al. Functional characterization of ATP-binding cassette transporter A3 mutations from infants with respiratory distress syndrome. *Am J Respir Cell Mol Biol.* 2016;55:716-721.
63. Kinting S, Hoppner S, Schindlbeck U, et al. Functional rescue of misfolding ABCA3 mutations by small molecular correctors. *Hum Mol Genet.* 2018;27:943-953.
64. Hoppner S, Kinting S, Torrano AA, et al. Quantification of volume and lipid filling of intracellular vesicles carrying the ABCA3 transporter. *Biochim Biophys Acta Mol Cell Res.* 2017;1864:2330-2335.
67. Ban N, Matsumura Y, Sakai H, et al. ABCA3 as a lipid transporter in pulmonary surfactant biogenesis. *J Biol Chem.* 2007;282:9628-9634.
68. Cheong N, Zhang H, Madesh M, et al. ABCA3 is critical for lamellar body biogenesis in vivo. *J Biol Chem.* 2007;282:23811-23817.
69. Fitzgerald ML, Xavier R, Haley KJ, et al. ABCA3 inactivation in mice causes respiratory failure, loss of pulmonary surfactant, and depletion of lung phosphatidylglycerol. *J Lipid Res.* 2007;48:621-632:e97381.
70. Rindler TN, Stockman CA, Filuta AL, et al. Alveolar injury and regeneration following deletion of ABCA3. *JCI Insight.* 2017;2:e97381.
71. Griese M, Kirmeier HG, Liebisch G, et al. Surfactant lipidomics in healthy children and childhood interstitial lung disease. *PloS One.* 2015;10:e0117985.
78. Glasser SW, Detmer EA, Ikegami M, Na CL, Stahlman MT, Whitsett JA. Pneumonitis and emphysema in sp-C gene targeted mice. *J Biol Chem.* 2003;278:14291-14298.
80. Nogee LM, Dunbar 3rd AE, Wert SE, Askin F, Hamvas A, Whitsett JA. A mutation in the surfactant protein C gene associated with familial interstitial lung disease. *N Engl J Med.* 2001;344:573-579.
82. Bullard JE, Nogee LM. Heterozygosity for ABCA3 mutations modifies the severity of lung disease associated with a surfactant protein C gene (SFTPC) mutation. *Pediatr Res.* 2007;62:176-179.
83. Kroner C, Reu S, Teusch V, et al. Genotype alone does not predict the clinical course of SFTPC deficiency in paediatric patients. *Eur Respir J.* 2015;46:197-206.
84. Mulugeta S, Nguyen V, Russo SJ, Muniswamy M, Beers MF. A surfactant protein C precursor protein BRICHOS domain mutation causes endoplasmic reticulum stress, proteasome dysfunction, and caspase 3 activation. *Am J Respir Cell Mol Biol.* 2005;32:521-530.
86. Bridges JP, Wert SE, Nogee LM, Weaver TE. Expression of a human surfactant protein C mutation associated with interstitial lung disease disrupts lung development in transgenic mice. *J Biol Chem.* 2003;278:52739-52746.
90. Stewart GA, Ridsdale R, Martin EP, et al. 4-Phenylbutyric acid treatment rescues trafficking and processing of a mutant surfactant protein-C. *Am J Respir Cell Mol Biol.* 2012;47:324-331.
91. Wang WJ, Mulugeta S, Russo SJ, Beers MF. Deletion of exon 4 from human surfactant protein C results in aggresome formation and generation of a dominant negative. *J Cell Sci.* 2003;116:683-692.
92. Hawkins A, Guttentag SH, Deterding R, et al. A non-BRICHOS SFTPC mutant (SP-CI73T) linked to interstitial lung disease promotes a late block in macroautophagy disrupting cellular proteostasis and mitophagy. *Am J Physiol Lung Cell Mol Physiol.* 2015;308:L33-L47.
94. Beers MF, Hawkins A, Maguire JA, et al. A nonaggregating surfactant protein C mutant is misdirected to early endosomes and disrupts phospholipid recycling. *Traffic.* 2011;12:1196-1210.
95. Katzen J, Wagner BD, Venosa A, et al. An SFTPC BRICHOS mutant links epithelial ER stress and spontaneous lung fibrosis. *JCI Insight.* 2019;4.
96. Nureki SI, Tomer Y, Venosa A, et al. Expression of mutant Sftpc in murine alveolar epithelia drives spontaneous lung fibrosis. *J Clin Invest.* 2018;128:4008-4024.
102. Hamvas A, Deterding RR, Wert SE, et al. Heterogeneous pulmonary phenotypes associated with mutations in the thyroid transcription factor gene NKX2-1. *Chest.* 2013;144:794-804.
105. Krude H, Schutz B, Biebermann H, et al. Choreoathetosis, hypothyroidism, and pulmonary alterations due to human NKX2-1 haploinsufficiency. *J Clin Invest.* 2002;109:475-480.
106. Pohlenz J, Dumitrescu A, Zundel D, et al. Partial deficiency of thyroid transcription factor 1 produces predominantly neurological defects in humans and mice. *J Clin Invest.* 2002;109:469-473.
112. Young LR, Deutsch GH, Bokulic RE, Brody AS, Nogee LM. A mutation in TTF1/NKX2.1 is associated with familial neuroendocrine cell hyperplasia of infancy. *Chest.* 2013;144:1199-1206.
114. Deutsch GH, Young LR, Deterding RR, et al. Diffuse lung disease in young children: application of a novel classification scheme. *Am J Respir Crit Care Med.* 2007;176:1120-1128.
116. Suzuki T, Sakagami T, Young LR, et al. Hereditary pulmonary alveolar proteinosis: pathogenesis, presentation, diagnosis, and therapy. *Am J Respir Crit Care Med.* 2010;182:1292-1304.
124. Langston C, Patterson K, Dishop MK, et al. A protocol for the handling of tissue obtained by operative lung biopsy: recommendations of the chILD pathology co-operative group. *Pediatr Dev Pathol.* 2006;9:173-180.
130. Liptzin DR, Patel T, Deterding RR. Chronic ventilation in infants with surfactant protein C mutations: an alternative to lung transplantation. *Am J Respir Crit Care Med.* 2015;191:1338-1340.
131. Wilkinson DC, Alva-Ornelas JA, Sucre JM, et al. Development of a three-dimensional bioengineering technology to generate lung tissue for personalized disease modeling. *Stem Cells Transl Med.* 2017;6:622-633.
132. Sucre JMS, Jetter CS, Loomans H, et al. Successful establishment of primary type II alveolar epithelium with 3D organotypic coculture. *Am J Respir Cell Mol Biol.* 2018;59:158-166.

81 Trophic Factors and Regulation of Gastrointestinal Tract and Liver Development

Douglas G. Burrin | Caitlin E. Vonderohe

FETAL AND NEONATAL GASTROINTESTINAL TRACT AND LIVER GROWTH

NATURE OF GROWTH

INTRODUCTION

To understand the role of trophic factors in fetal and neonatal gastrointestinal (GI) tract and liver growth, it is important to consider the elements of tissue growth. The fetal and neonatal period is the most dynamic period of postconceptual growth and includes critical developmental milestones, such as gastrulation, organogenesis, morphogenesis, cellular differentiation, and functional maturation, which are described in detail in other chapters. In the case of the intestine, key developmental steps include formation of the gut tube, the appearance of villi and digestive enzymes, and the development of swallowing and mature motility patterns.[1] Intestinal growth also encompasses different elements at the tissue and cellular level that are characterized by increased cellular numbers (hyperplasia) and size (hypertrophy). Intestinal growth involves expansion of the number and size of mucosal crypt and villus units,[2] as well as submucosal tissues, such as smooth muscle, neural, lymphoid, and immune cells. Moreover, the timing and characteristics of fetal and neonatal GI tract and liver growth are exquisitely coordinated with the events of birth and weaning to ensure survival of the organism. The regulation of the timing and nature of GI tract and liver growth is complex and involves multiple and often redundant factors. Among these factors are intrinsic cell programs or signals arising from gene expression, as well as extracellular signals, such as peptide growth factors, hormones, nutrients, and microbes, which originate from surrounding cells, the blood, and the gut lumen.

A fundamental aspect of growth in the gut is the continual proliferation, migration, and apoptotic loss of epithelial cells along the mucosal surface. In the small intestine this process involves four major cell lineages (absorptive enterocyte, goblet, Paneth, and endocrine cells) that differentiate from one pluripotent stem cell located in the crypt (Fig. 81.1). The application of molecular biologic techniques in model organisms such as the mouse, zebrafish, fruit fly, and nematode has revealed that genetic regulatory factors have a critical influence on early organogenesis and morphologic development of the gut, pancreas, and liver.[3,4] These studies have identified a group of key homeodomain transcription factor genes, *Pdx1* and *Cdx2*; GATA transcription factors, Gata4 and Gata6; signaling pathways, including Wnt/β-catenin, Hedgehog, and Notch; and new extracellular signals, including R-spondins.[5-7,8] Recent studies have identified several genes that play a key role in the determination of lineage cell commitment in the intestinal stem cell niche (Fig. 81.2), including *ATOH1*, *Notch1*, *Notch2*, *Hes1*, and *Neurog3*.[9-11] The homeodomain transcription factors are also involved in the anterior-posterior pattern formation of demarcations in muscular sphincters and regional epithelial morphology along the length of the gut.[1,4] Genetic regulation via homeodomain factors also influences functional maturation of the intestine that occurs during the late-gestation and neonatal period.

Development of in vitro models of fetal and neonatal GI physiology in the form of intestinal enteroids and organoids has further illuminated the role of crypt cells and growth factors in the proliferation and maintenance of the intestinal epithelium.[12] Intestinal organoids are specifically representative of fetal tissue and have been used to examine signaling pathways that determine the eventual developmental fate (endoderm, mesoderm, or ectoderm) of pluripotent stem cells, from gastrulation onward. Transforming growth factor β (TGFβ) initiates gastrulation, but Wnt, fibroblast growth factors (FGF), retinoic acid (RA), and bone morphogenic protein (BMP) pathways are essential for the development of the intestinal epithelium. Mesenchyme underlying intestinal epithelium produces laminins, which are also necessary for villus formation.[13] Conversely, enteroids are cultured from LGR5+ stem cells present in the base of intestinal crypts and represent the physiology of the tissue the LGR5+ cells were isolated from.[14] Paneth cells alternate with LGR5+ stem cells and produce Wnt3 (see Fig. 81.2), which maintains stemness of LGR5+ pluripotent stem cells. In enteroid culture, the Wnt3 signal is amplified by R-spondin to maximize enteroid proliferation and survivability, while epidermal growth factor (EGF) has a similar, profound mitogenic effect on stem cells. In intestinal tissue, BMP signaling is greatest at the villus tip, and lowest at the crypt base, driving terminal differentiation and repressing stemness; therefore Noggin is employed in enteroid culture to maintain the proliferative environment of the crypt compartment.[15]

ENVIRONMENTAL INFLUENCES

Normal GI tract growth and development during fetal life are critical to facilitate the successful adaptation from nutritional support via the umbilical circulation to that of oral ingestion of breast milk by the neonate. An increase in circulating fetal glucocorticoid concentration just before and during vaginal birth is an important trigger of gut functional development.[16] In the neonatal period, growth of the GI tract is influenced by multiple physiologic factors that serve to prepare the developing neonate for separation from maternal nutritional support (i.e., weaning). In addition, a number of important environmental cues signal adaptive changes in GI tract function to facilitate postweaning survival. The extent and diversity of microbial colonization of the gut serve to prime intestinal lymphoid cell development for normal innate immune function.[17-19] During these processes, extracellular signals, such as peptide growth factors, are often considered to be the major trophic factors that influence growth. However, the term *trophic* actually means "of or pertaining to

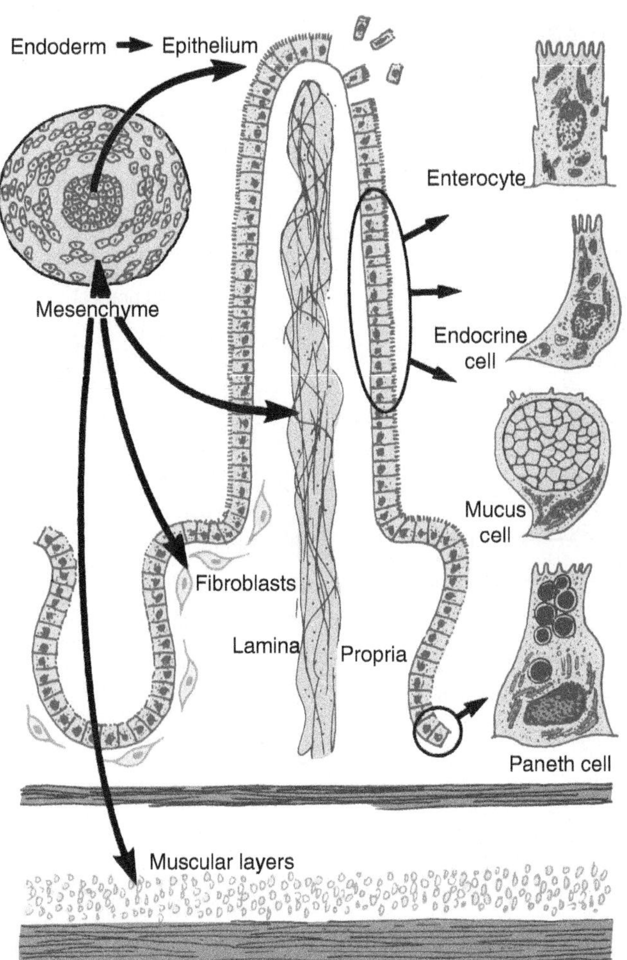

Fig. 81.1 Description and localization of the four intestinal epithelial cell lineages within the crypt-villus region. The stem cells located in the lower crypt area differentiate into absorptive enterocytes, mucin-secreting goblet cells, endocrine cells, and Paneth cells. (From Haffen K, Kedinger M, Simon-Assmann P. Cell contact dependent regulation of enterocytic differentiation. In: Lebenthal E, ed. *Human Gastrointestinal Development*. New York: Raven Press; 1989:20.)

nutrition," and in the case of the gut, nutrients present in amniotic fluid and breast milk are a major trophic influence. There are numerous extracellular trophic signals, including foods, nutrients, peptide growth factors, biliary and pancreatic secretions, gut peptide hormones, steroid and thyroid hormones, microbes, and neural inputs. The cells within the fetal and neonatal GI tract and liver are influenced by extracellular signals from multiple sources, including (1) blood-borne factors in the circulation such as hormones that act via endocrine mechanisms; (2) luminal factors derived from amniotic fluid, mammary secretions, or gut microbiota; and (3) local factors secreted via autocrine or paracrine mechanisms from surrounding cells (Fig. 81.3).

Recent studies have revealed novel insights into the role of mesenchymal cells, especially myofibroblasts,[20] and luminal microbes in intestinal epithelial growth and differentiation. Mesenchymal cell interactions are mediated via local secretion of tissue growth factors—for example, FGF, hepatocyte growth factor (HGF), keratinocyte growth factor (KGF), and insulin-like growth factor (IGF)—and basement membrane proteins (laminins, collagens, proteoglycans).[21] The extracellular matrix protein laminin may be particularly critical for expression of Cdx-2 and induction of epithelial differentiation genes, such as lactase. Interaction between the integrin receptors on the basal surface of epithelial cells with basement membrane proteins can also affect differentiation and cell death. Studies have shown that disruption of the integrin-receptor binding via protease degradation leads to detachment of epithelial cells from the basement membrane and activation of anoikis-mediated apoptotic signaling pathways.[22] Symbiotic relationships between commensal microorganisms and their mammalian host, such as ruminants, are well known. Yet in the past 10 years, molecular sequencing techniques and metagenomic analysis have markedly expanded our understanding of the microbiome and how it influences the health and disease of the human and mouse gut. Studies in conventional and germ-free animals demonstrated that the presence of intestinal microbes exerts a trophic effect on the gut, as evidenced by increased epithelial cell proliferation, mucosal thickness, and lymphoid cell density. Studies with germ-free mice monoassociated with specific bacterial species show that microbes can alter particular pathways of intestinal differentiation.[19] The emergence of molecular DNA analysis has led to the suggestion that the fetal gut contains a low abundance of microbes, but increased colonization and microbiome diversity during early postnatal life plays a critical role in development of mucosal immune function. Microbes also produce a wide range of bioactive molecules and substrates, including toxins and short-chain fatty acids (SCFAs) that influence the proliferation and function of mucosal epithelial and immune cells. The aim of this chapter is to provide a brief overview of some of the major trophic factors in these categories and discuss their relevance to the growth and development of the fetal and neonatal gut and liver. Most of the references cited in this chapter are review articles, and the number of original articles listed is limited owing to space restrictions.

MAJOR TROPHIC FACTORS

NUTRIENTS

ENTERAL VERSUS PARENTERAL NUTRITION

Nutrition is one of the most potent trophic stimuli of GI tract growth.[23-26] The diet supplies nutrients directly to mucosal epithelial cells for growth and oxidative metabolism, but it also acts indirectly by triggering the release of local growth factors and gut hormones and activating neural pathways. It has been shown that the trophic actions of several nutrients are mediated by specialized enteroendocrine cells within the mucosal epithelium that sense the amount and chemical composition of luminal nutrients and GI secretions, such as bile acids.[27-30] The molecular mechanisms for these responses are emerging; they show that membrane receptors and transport proteins act as chemical sensors that signal the presence of nutrients via enteric nerves to mediate local GI tract function and also peripheral responses via the extrinsic nervous system. Maternal malnutrition and neonatal starvation cause reduced gut tissue mass, shortened villi, and generalized increased catabolism and decreased protein synthesis.[31] However, the route of nutrient input, either enteral or parenteral, has a critical impact on the trophic response. In the late-gestation fetus, the onset of amniotic fluid swallowing coincides with increased intestinal growth and development. Studies in fetal sheep and pigs have shown that preventing this process by esophageal ligation suppresses intestinal growth.[16] In hospitalized premature neonates, early nutrition comes in the form of intravenous total parenteral nutrition (TPN), which leads to reduced growth and atrophy of the intestinal mucosa.[31] The TPN-induced intestinal atrophy is associated with reduced gut DNA and protein mass, cell proliferation, villus height, and protein synthesis, and increased apoptosis and proteolysis (see Fig. 81.3). Studies with neonatal pigs and human infants show that the lack of enteral nutrition is also associated with reduced secretion of many gut peptide hormones and growth factors.[31]

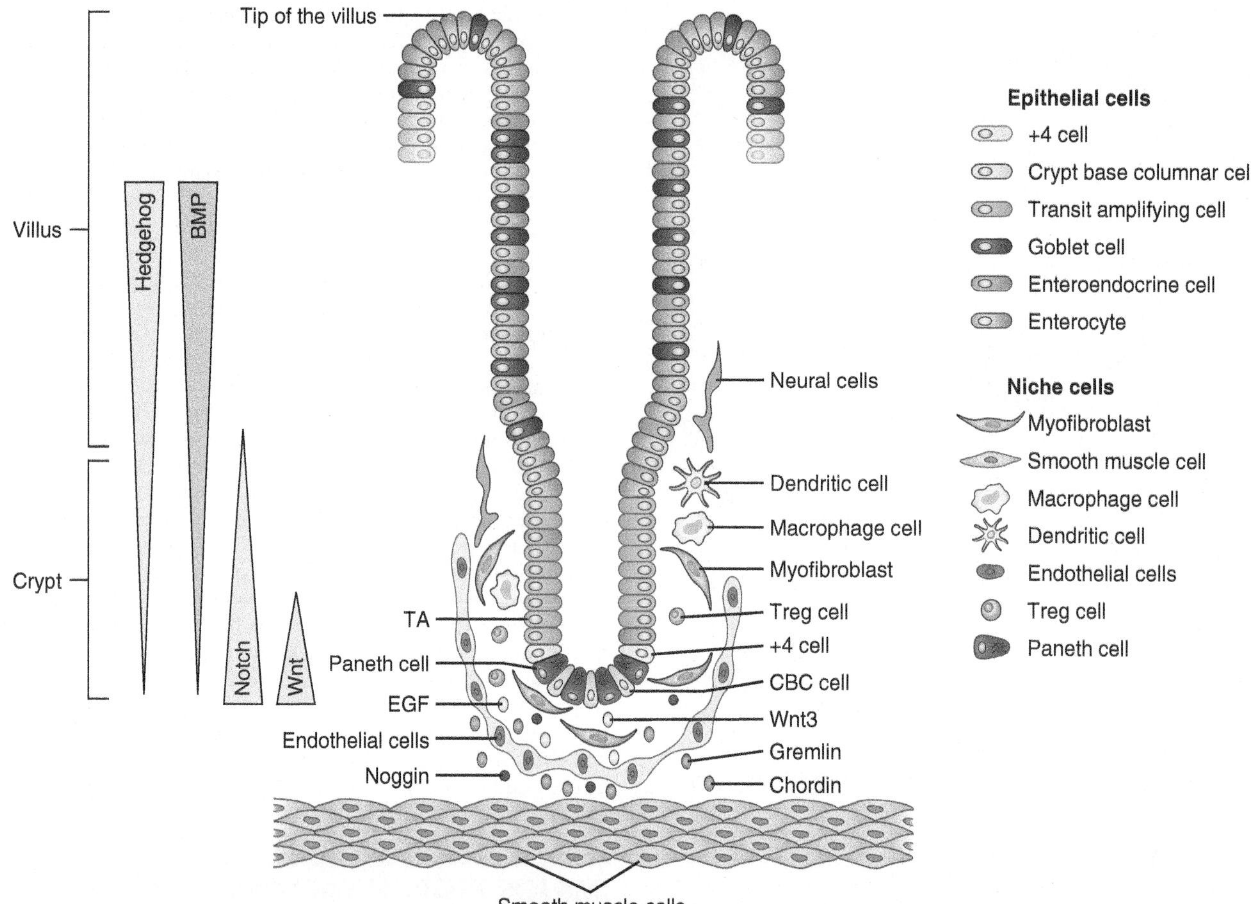

Fig. 81.2 The stem cell compartment resides at the base of the crypt consisting of crypt base columnar *(CBC)* and quiescent +4 stem cells. Rapidly dividing transit-amplifying *(TA)* cells arise from these stem cells and differentiate into absorptive lineages (enterocytes) or secretory lineages (enteroendocrine cells, goblet cells, tuft cells and Paneth cells). The niche consists of multiple components and cell types, including extracellular matrix, fibroblasts, myofibroblasts, smooth muscle cells, neural cells, endothelial cells, lymphocytes and macrophages along with secreted factors (Wnt3, epidermal growth factor *[EGF]*), and bone morphogenic protein *(BMP)* inhibitors (Noggin, Gremlin, and chordin) that support the regulation of stem cell activity. Wnt, BMP, Notch, Hh, and EGF signaling pathways are the regulators of stem cell activity. (This legend is adapted with permission from Sailaja BS, He XC, Li L. The regulatory niche of intestinal stem cells. *J Physiol.* 2016;594[17]:4827–4836.)

The practice of feeding small volumes of enteral nutrition, known as *minimal enteral feeding* or *trophic feeding,* has been shown to enhance GI tract motility and other functions.[32] The precise relationship between enteral feeding level and gut function has not been established, but studies in neonatal piglets suggest that an enteral intake of between 20% and 40% of the total nutrient intake is necessary to maintain normal growth.

BREAST MILK VERSUS FORMULA

The relative significance of milk-borne trophic factors is one of the most intensely studied areas of pediatric nutrition and gastroenterology.[17,33-36] Many of the trophic peptide growth factors discussed in this chapter are present in breast milk, but not infant formulas, and have been implicated in the beneficial outcomes of breast-fed infants. Studies have assessed the relative trophic effect of colostrum and mature milk compared with formula in neonatal rodent and pig studies. These studies have largely confirmed that idea that breast milk has a greater trophic effect on the GI tract than formula, as measured by typical indices of structural and cellular growth. However, the most significant advantage of breast milk on the neonatal intestine may be related not to growth but rather to mucosal barrier and immune function. There is considerable evidence suggesting that immunoprotective factors in breast milk (e.g., secretory IgA, lactoferrin, oligosaccharides) act to modulate mucosal immune function and bacterial colonization, thereby limiting the incidence of infection, sepsis, and necrotizing enterocolitis.[33,35,37] Many of the trophic factors in milk are polypeptides that survive digestion, retain their biologic activity, and interact with specific receptors present on the mucosal epithelium of neonates. A number of studies have shown that these milk-borne growth factors stimulate neonatal intestinal growth when given in purified and recombinant forms, either orally or systemically. Moreover, in preterm neonates the presence of increased intestinal permeability could facilitate the intestinal absorption of milk-borne peptide growth factors; however, there are few instances where this process has been found to be physiologically significant.

MACRONUTRIENTS

The chemical form and nutrient composition can also influence the impact of enteral nutrition on GI tract growth and function.[23] Some studies indicate that enteral nutrition in a complex, polymeric form is more trophic to the small intestine than enteral nutrition in a simpler, elemental form. The dietary restriction of protein and energy generally suppresses gut growth and mucosal immune function. The enteral infusion of individual nutrients, by themselves, can have a trophic stimulus on the gut if they are administered in a sufficient large amount. However, there are a number of

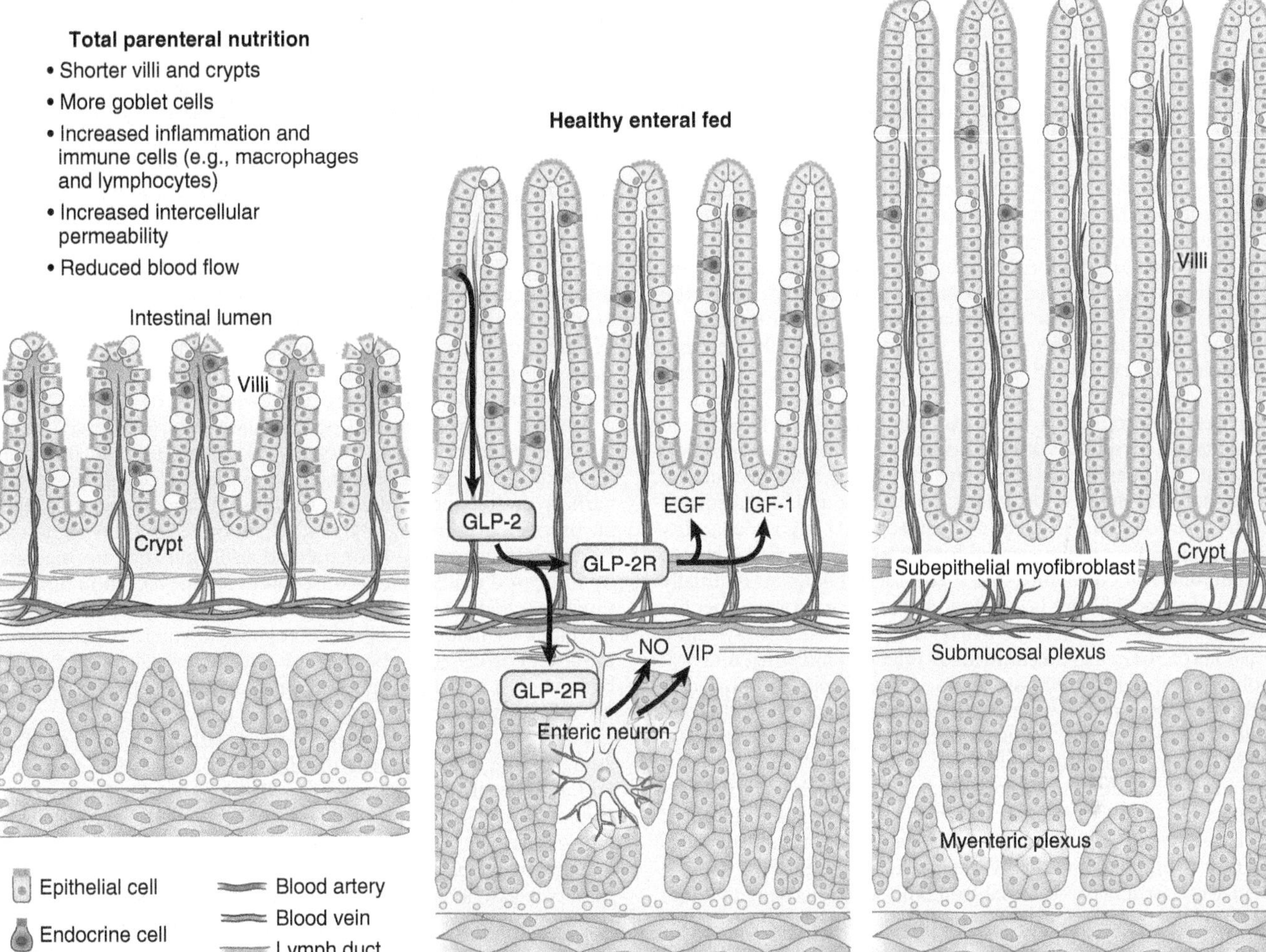

Fig. 81.3 Intestinal mucosal adaptation to TPN and intestinal resection. Illustrated is the influence of TPN, a common clinical practice in hospitalized preterm infants, which deprives the gut lumen of enteral nutrition and results in mucosal villus atrophy, deterioration of intestinal barrier function, and infiltration of immune cells. Also shown is the influence of surgical resection of intestine, which occurs due to congenital and acquired GI diseases, that results in activation of adaptive processes that promote mucosal growth, such as increased GLP-2 secretion, crypt cell proliferation, and blood flow. GLP-2 is a key gut hormone that functions to activate mucosal enteric neuron release of NO and VIP as well as subepithelial fibroblast release of EGF and IGF-1. *EGF*, Epidermal growth factor; *GI*, gastrointestinal; *GLP-2*, glucagon-like peptide 2; *GLP-2R*, glucagon-like peptide 2 receptor; *IGF-1*, insulin-like growth factor-1; *NO*, nitric oxide; *TPN*, total parenteral nutrition; *VIP*, vasoactive intestinal peptide. (This legend is adapted with permission from Burrin D, Sangild PT, Stoll B, et al. Translational advances in pediatric nutrition and gastroenterology: new insights from pig models. *Annu Rev Anim Biosci.* 2020;8:321–354.)

specific nutrients that have trophic actions when added to a complete diet, among which are glutamine, arginine, threonine, leucine, nucleotides, SCFAs, long-chain polyunsaturated fatty acids (LC-PUFAs), and RA.

Glutamine is a key intestinal oxidative fuel that is extensively metabolized and oxidized to CO_2 by intestinal tissues when fed either enterally or parenterally.[38] However, several studies have shown that enteral and parenteral glutamine also stimulates intestinal growth and enhances function in healthy and diseased conditions.[39] Studies in cultured intestinal epithelial cells indicate that glutamine, arginine, and leucine directly stimulate cell proliferation, activate mitogenic intracellular signaling pathways,[40] and may be critical precursors for glucosamine and arginine synthesis.[41] Arginine is an essential amino acid for neonates and may be an especially important substrate for maintenance of intestinal nitric oxide synthesis, blood flow, and immune function. Some studies have shown that enteral arginine supplementation can reduce the incidence of necrotizing enterocolitis in neonates.[42] Other nonessential amino acids, including glutamate, proline, and ornithine, have been shown to have stimulatory actions on the gut, perhaps because they are precursors for glutamine and arginine synthesis. Threonine is also a key nutrient for the intestine, because it is used for the synthesis of threonine-rich mucins by goblet cells; the intestinal threonine use by goblet cells appears to be dependent on the enteral rather than the parenteral route.[43,44]

Nucleotides are ubiquitous, low-molecular-weight, intracellular compounds that are integral to numerous biochemical processes, and are especially important as precursors for nucleic acid synthesis in rapidly dividing cells, such as epithelial and lymphoid cells in the mucosa.[45] Nucleotides consist of a purine or pyrimidine base, which can be synthesized within cells de novo from glutamine, aspartic acid, glycine, formate, and carbon dioxide as precursors, or these bases can be salvaged from the degradation of nucleic acids and nucleotides. Human milk is an excellent source of dietary nucleotides for infants during the first months of life, and its nucleotide content is markedly higher than that of cow's milk and most infant formulas, although several commercial formulas now include nucleotides. Numerous reports show that dietary supplementation with nucleosides, nucleotides, or nucleic acids supports small intestinal mucosal function, growth, and morphology.

SCFAs, largely in the form of acetate, propionate, and butyrate, are produced by microbial fermentation of carbohydrates in the large bowel.[46,47] Colonic epithelial cells derive most (60% to 70%) of their energy from SCFAs, and butyrate is the preferred oxidative fuel compared with glucose, glutamine, or ketone bodies. The diet of the human neonate is largely devoid of fiber, yet the production of SCFAs from large bowel microbial fermentation increases with the degree of microbial colonization and postnatal age. Normal substrates for colonic SCFA production in neonates include endogenous secretions and malabsorbed dietary carbohydrates, such as lactose and oligosaccharides. Oligosaccharides are the second most abundant carbohydrate in human milk, but cow's milk and infant formulas are substantially devoid of these.[48] There is considerable evidence for the specific intestinal trophic effects of SCFAs. Intraluminal and systemic infusions of SCFAs have a stimulatory effect on intestinal mucosal proliferation, gene expression, blood flow, and gut hormone secretion; yet studies with cultured colonic tumor cell lines indicate that butyrate induces differentiation and apoptosis, thereby suppressing neoplasia.[49]

There is considerable interest in dietary long-chain fatty acids because breast milk generally contains higher concentrations of *n*-3 LC-PUFAs than in formulas. As a result, many infant formulas are now formulated with these fatty acids. Interest in the *n*-3 LC-PUFAs, particularly docosahexaenoic acid, eicosapentaenoic acid, and arachidonic acid, has been heightened by recent studies showing that supplementing the diet with these fatty acids can lower the incidence and inflammatory effects of necrotizing enterocolitis in neonatal infants and rats.[50] There is limited information regarding the intestinal trophic effects of either *n*-3 LC-PUFAs or other long-chain fatty acids in developing animals. However, a series of studies have demonstrated that *n*-3 LC-PUFAs enhance intestinal adaptation after small bowel resection, and their effects were greater than those of less saturated oils; it was also found that medium-chain triglycerides are less trophic than long-chain triglycerides. In contrast, studies with neonatal piglets indicated that the long-chain fatty acid oleic acid can cause significant mucosal injury and increased permeability, and that this effect is more severe in newborn piglets than in 1-month-old piglets.[30]

BILE ACIDS

Historically, bile acids were solely considered to function as detergent molecules that emulsify lipids into absorbable micelles. In the past two decades, research has shown that bile acids play a much larger physiologic role in intestinal function and growth by acting as signaling molecules that can activate multiple cellular receptors, including the farnesoid x receptor (FXR), Takeda G protein-coupled receptor 5 (TGR5), and sphingosine-1-phosphate receptor 2.[30,51,52] Primary and secondary bile acids present in the small intestine and colon can directly stimulate epithelial proliferation by activating epithelial growth factor receptor pathways, which can lead to neoplasia.[53] Bile acids also activate intestinal TGR5 and FXR receptors and trigger the release of trophic gut hormone, glucagon-like peptide (GLP)-2, and the novel enterokine, fibroblast growth factor 19 (FGF19).[54] FGF19 has been shown to have trophic effects on liver tissue via activation of the receptors FGFR4 and βklotho, yet its trophic effects in the intestine have not been established.[55]

GASTROINTESTINAL HORMONES

The gut is one of the largest endocrine organs in the body and secretes numerous peptide hormones primarily in response to nutrient ingestion, but also according to the stage of development and disease. Many of the gut hormones discussed in this chapter have been implicated in the stimulation of gut and liver growth in response to enteral nutrition. Several of the gut hormones and local growth factors discussed in this section have been linked to intestinal adaptation after surgical resection of the intestine, a condition designated as *short bowel syndrome*.[56,57] Studies in rodent and pig models have shown beneficial effects of many of these hormones and growth factors, yet few have been developed for clinical practice in patients with short bowel syndrome, with the recent exception of GLP-2. GLP-2 is a product of the intestinal proglucagon gene expressed in the enteroendocrine L cells located predominantly in the distal intestine.[58,59] GLP-2 is secreted in response to feeding (especially carbohydrate), and studies in fetal and neonatal piglets suggest an ontogenic increase in GLP-2 secretion. GLP-2 has significant trophic effects on the neonatal and adult gut that are mediated by increased cell proliferation, protein synthesis, blood flow, and glucose transport (see Fig. 81.3). The trophic actions of GLP-2 are mediated by paracrine signals that are believed to originate from enteric neurons and subepithelial myofibroblasts. GLP-2 has also been shown to possess antiinflammatory effects in conditions of bowel injury resulting from colitis and chemotherapy.

Gastrin is secreted from the G cells within the antrum of the stomach and acts primarily to stimulate proliferation of parietal and enterochromaffin-like cells within the gastric mucosa.[60] Cholecystokinin is expressed in endocrine cells of the gut and in neurons within the gut and brain, and its primary target tissues are the pancreas and gallbladder. There is structural homology between gastrin and cholecystokinin with respect to both the peptide sequence and receptor function. Studies have shown that hypogastrinemia, produced by antrectomy and targeted disruption of the gastrin gene, leads to atrophy of the gastric mucosal cells. Cholecystokinin stimulates pancreatic growth and cell proliferation, and these trophic effects have been attributed exclusively to interaction via the cholecystokinin A receptor. The neonate exhibits hypergastrinemia and a comparatively high gastric pH, yet gastrin secretion is induced by feeding.[32] The development of pentagastrin-responsive gastric acid secretion occurs within 1 week in neonatal piglets and can be prematurely induced with glucocorticoids, consistent with up-regulation of gastrin receptor expression with age.[61] The trophic effects of gastrin are most evident in the stomach and are mediated by increased ornithine decarboxylase activity and cell proliferation.

Gastrin-releasing peptide is a 27-amino acid peptide with a carboxyl terminus region that is structurally related to bombesin, a 14-amino acid neuropeptide found in amphibian skin. Gastrin-releasing peptide is secreted from neurons located throughout the GI tract in response to vagal stimulation. Bombesin is also found in milk, and both oral and systemic administration to suckling animals stimulates intestinal growth.

Peptide YY is secreted from the same enteroendocrine cells as GLP-1 and GLP-2, and together these hormones have been implicated as factors in the "ileal-brake" phenomenon. Studies indicate that peptide YY stimulates gut growth in some but not all cases, and does not stimulate proliferation of cultured epithelial cells. Neurotensin is a 13-amino acid peptide secreted from the enteroendocrine N cells located exclusively in the gut within the distal small intestine.[62] Neurotensin expression is markedly increased during the neonatal period, and secretion is stimulated specifically by ingestion of fat. Administration of neurotensin stimulates gut growth in animals after small bowel resection, even in the absence of enteral nutrients.

TISSUE GROWTH FACTORS

Tissue growth factors can be generally categorized as polypeptides that are secreted locally and act via a paracrine or autocrine mechanism to affect cellular growth and function.[63] However, a number of the tissue growth factors are also present in the blood and GI secretions and thus may act via an endocrine mechanism—for example, IGF-1. Moreover, many of these growth factors are present in breast milk and are thought to influence neonatal gut growth.[64,65] Among the most well known of these is epidermal growth factor (EGF), a member of a family of peptides that includes transforming growth factor α (TGF-α), heparin-binding EGF, amphiregulin, epiregulin, betacellulin, neuregulin 1, and neuregulin 2. These factors act as ligands for membrane-bound EGF receptor and other EGF-related (ErbB family) receptors that become activated via phosphorylation on binding. EGF is widely distributed in most body fluids (notably mammary, salivary, biliary, and pancreatic secretions) but is not produced in the epithelial cells, in contrast to its homologue TGF-α. Most of the EGF family peptides are trophic to the gut, stimulating cell proliferation and suppressing apoptosis; however, they also modulate a number of other physiologic functions, including enhanced tooth eruption, decreased gastric acid secretion, increased mucus secretion and gastric blood flow, reduced gastric emptying, and increased sodium and glucose transport.[66] EGF has also been found to increase mucosal growth and functional adaptation after intestinal resection, diarrhea, and TPN, and to decrease the incidence of necrotizing enterocolitis.[67,68] Enteral nutrition stimulates GI secretion, resulting in the release of EGF into the gut lumen, where it is postulated to play a protective role, whereas TGF-α functions in the maintenance of epithelial cell proliferation and migration in the healthy gut. Stimulation of local EGF expression has also been shown to mediate some of the trophic actions of the gut hormone GLP-2. EGF appears to be more trophic to the gut when it is given intravenously than when it is given enterally, perhaps because the EGF receptor is localized to the basolateral membrane. However, many neonatal rodent and pig studies have shown that oral EGF administration does indeed augment gut growth and functional development. These findings combined with recent evidence from transgenic mice support the idea that both local expression and milk-borne ingestion of EGF and TGF-α play a physiologic role in neonatal gut growth and development.

The IGF family of peptides includes insulin, IGF-1, and IGF-2.[63,64,69,70] The biologic actions of insulin are mediated via the insulin receptor, whereas the actions of both IGF-1 and IGF-2 are largely mediated through the type 1 IGF receptor. The insulin and type 1 IGF receptors are present in epithelial cells; they are more abundant on the basolateral membrane than the apical membrane, and are more abundant in proliferating crypt cells than in differentiated enterocytes. Although insulin secretion is confined to the pancreas, both IGF-1 and IGF-2 are expressed throughout the body, including the gut. However, within the intestinal mucosa, expression of both IGF-1 and IGF-2 appears to be localized to mesenchymal cells in the lamina propria, although epithelial cells may also produce IGF-2. The expression of IGF-1 and IGF-2 in the gut is highest in the fetal and neonatal period and declines with age. In addition, insulin, IGF-1, and IGF-2 are present in milk, and IGF-1 is found in salivary, biliary, and pancreatic secretions and amniotic fluid. Numerous studies have shown that either administration of IGF systemically or increase of its expression locally (as in transgenic mice) stimulates intestinal growth and function in normal animals and under conditions of TPN, gut resection, dexamethasone treatment, sepsis, and radiation therapy.[71] The expression of IGF-binding proteins has been shown to inhibit IGF action in gut tissues. The effects of IGF-1 on intestinal development in fetal and neonatal animals given pharmacologic oral doses of insulin and IGF-1 have been variable. Some have demonstrated a stimulation of gut growth, disaccharidase activity, and glucose transport.[31] However, others have shown only limited effects of orally administered IGF on the neonatal gut, suggesting that the IGFs may not have a physiologic role in the neonate.

Growth hormone (GH) has a major influence on IGF-I expression during postnatal growth, and studies in postweaning rodents indicate that hypophysectomy results in gut atrophy, whereas transgenic overexpression of GH in mice increases gut growth.[31,70] However, the significance of GH in neonatal gut and liver growth may be limited by the abundance and responsiveness of the GH receptor. Studies with hypophysectomized neonatal rats suggest some degree of pituitary-dependent intestinal growth and development. Other studies in rats demonstrate that GH treatment does not prevent TPN-induced intestinal atrophy but may augment intestinal growth after massive small bowel resection. Like EGF, IGF-1 has been shown to mediate the local action of GLP-2.

Transforming growth factor β (TGF-β) is structurally unrelated to TGF-α and is found in three major forms (TGF-β_1, TGF-β_2, and TGF-β_3) in mammalian tissues.[63,72,73] TGF-β expression has been found throughout the small intestine in both lamina propria and epithelial cells; the levels are low in neonates and increase with age. In contrast, the levels of TGF-β_2 are high in early milk and decline as lactation progresses. At least five receptors (types I-V) have been found to bind one or more of the various TGF-β ligands, although the type I and type II receptors appear to mediate the effects on cell proliferation. TGF-β is a potent inhibitor of epithelial cell proliferation and may also induce differentiation. It has been implicated as an intermediate signal whereby butyrate suppresses proliferation and induces differentiation of colonic epithelial cells. It also stimulates epithelial cell migration and production of extracellular matrix proteins such as collagen via induction of connective tissue growth factor, thus making it a critical factor in the process of restitution of the epithelium after mucosal damage.[74] This latter function of TGF-β may play an important role in the intestinal inflammatory response, as evident by the fact that its expression is up-regulated in inflammatory bowel disease and that TGF-β-deficient transgenic mice develop inflammatory disease.

HGF, vascular endothelial growth factor (VEGF), FGF, and KGF are expressed in the gut tissues and may play a role in mucosal growth and repair.[31] HGF is expressed by mesenchymal but not epithelial cells, whereas the HGF receptor (c-Met) is found in epithelial cells; c-Met is localized on the basolateral membrane. Studies with cultured intestinal epithelial cells demonstrate that HGF stimulates cell proliferation and wound closure proliferation but decreases transepithelial resistance.[75] HGF is found in human milk mononuclear cells and partially accounts for the stimulatory effect of human milk on intestinal cell proliferation. Studies in rats have shown that HGF, given either systemically or orally, increased gut growth and nutrient transport after massive small bowel resection and colitis.

VEGF is expressed in the small intestine, predominantly in the lamina propria mast cells.[31,75] The receptor (Flt-1) for the VEGF 165-amino acid isoform is present in intestinal epithelial cells; however, VEGF does not stimulate proliferation of these cells. Studies in mice demonstrated that VEGF and FGF2 reduce the rate of crypt cell apoptosis after total body irradiation treatment. FGF and the FGF receptors have been found in intestinal tissues, yet their function remains poorly understood. Both VEGF and FGF2 have been implicated in angiogenesis during intestinal repair.[76] Increased local expression of KGF (FGF7) has been found in patients with inflammatory bowel disease, and administration of KGF enhanced mucosal healing in rats after induction of colitis.[77]

The trefoil factors are a family of peptides (TFF1, TFF2, TFF3) that play an important protective role in the gut.[68] TFF3 is expressed and secreted from goblet cells of the small and large intestine and interacts with mucins on the apical cell surface. Trefoil peptides have been shown to promote cell migration and suppress apoptosis via activation of intracellular signaling pathways linked to mitogen-activated kinase and the EGF receptor; however, trefoil factor receptors have not been identified.

Serotonin (5-HT) is a neurotransmitter primarily produced by enterochromaffin cells using the rate-limiting enzyme tryptophan hydroxylase (TPH2) in the small intestine with local and systemic effects. Epithelial cells present in the mucosal layer of the small intestine express serotonin reuptake transporter (SERT), which controls 5-HT levels by removing 5-HT molecules from the interstitium. Secreted 5-HT that diffuses into small intestine capillaries is taken up by platelets for later release. Dysregulation and dysfunction of SERT5-HT uptake has been associated with multiple GI pathologies, such as diverticulitis and celiac disease.[78] Development of SERT-knockout (SERTKO) andTPH2-knockout rodent models has also indicated the significance of 5-HT production and regulation in modulating and initiating intestinal motility, GI secretions, vasodilation, and activation of afferent nerves. 5-HT is also an factor to promote growth and survival of enterochromaffin cells and other enteric nerves.[78] Other investigators have implicated 5-HT and SERT as factors affecting mucosal wound healing in ulcerative colitis.[79] Additionally, SERKO mice have taller villi, deeper crypts, greater mucosal surface area, and increased nutrient absorption compared to WT mice, indicating that 5-HT may play a part in regulating mucosal proliferation and absorption.[79-81]

GLUCOCORTICOIDS

The role of glucocorticoids in neonatal intestinal development has been studied extensively, especially in rodents.[82,83] The impact of glucocorticoids, particularly dexamethasone, on human intestinal growth and development has received considerable attention in the past because of their use in treatment of pulmonary function in premature infants.[84] Studies in fetal rodents and pigs suggest that increased endogenous glucocorticoid levels are critical signals that stimulate GI tract development and growth.[28] The prenatal cortisol surge is an important signal for intestinal development of the neonate, and premature birth precludes exposure to this key maturational signal. This idea is supported by studies in infants and piglets showing that premature birth results in insufficient intestinal maturation of intestinal lactase and lactose digestive capacity.[16] Numerous studies demonstrate how glucocorticoids stimulate neonatal intestinal development and maturation, especially with regard to disaccharidase expression. However, their effects on neonatal mucosal growth, per se, as indicated by cell proliferation, cell cycle, protein turnover, and apoptosis are not completely understood. Studies in vivo and in vitro suggest that glucocorticoids inhibit intestinal mucosal growth by suppressing cell proliferation and increasing protein catabolism.[31] More recent studies have shown that glucocorticoids are synthesized in the intestinal mucosa, as well as the adrenals.[85] These studies show that the local production of corticosterone under the control of the nuclear receptor liver receptor homologue 1 has an important role in maintaining normal intestinal development and function.

CONCLUSION

The growth and development of the fetal and neonatal GI tract is more dynamic than any other time during the life cycle and is stimulated by a host of multiple factors, including intrinsic cellular and extracellular signaling pathways. Many of these signals, such as transcription factors, peptide growth factors, and hormones, are triggered by environmental cues, such as nutrients and microbes. Many of the cellular receptors that sense and transmit these extracellular growth signals, such as nutrients, are now emerging from nontargeted mining of the genome to reveal families of G protein–coupled receptors. Moreover, the use of metabolomic and metagenomic approaches is identifying new metabolites and small molecules derived from specific gut microbes that induce trophic and function effects on the GI tract. Growth of the organs and tissues involves changes in the number and size of cells, but also the phenotype and function of cells, with changes in maturation and ontogeny of the host. In the past 10 years, there has been rapid advancement in the tools and experimental approaches available to further elucidate the existing and new trophic factors that regulate GI tract growth, such as tissue organoids, stem cells, and the clustered regularly interspaced short palindromic repeat (CRISPR)/Cas system for gene editing of cells and animals. New growth factors continue to be discovered, and some of those, such as R-spondins, have potent effects on stem cell growth and function in the GI tract. These new approaches should provide important new advancements in the coming years in our understanding of the biology of GI tract growth during early development.

ACKNOWLEDGMENTS

This work is a publication of the U.S. Department of Agriculture/Agricultural Research Service, Children's Nutrition Research Center, Department of Pediatrics, Baylor College of Medicine and Texas Children's Hospital, Houston, Texas. The work was supported in part by federal funds from the U.S. Department of Agriculture/Agricultural Research Service, cooperative agreement no. 58-6258-6001, and by the National Institutes of Health (R01 HD33920 and DK094616). The contents of this publication do not necessarily reflect the views or policies of the U.S. Department of Agriculture, nor does the mention of trade names, commercial products, or organizations imply endorsement by the U.S. Government.

A complete reference list is available at www.ExpertConsult.com. 

SELECT REFERENCES

1. Montgomery RK, Mulberg AE, Grand RJ. Development of the human gastrointestinal tract: twenty years of progress. *Gastroenterology*. 1999;116(3):702-731.
2. Cheng H, Bjerknes M. Whole population cell kinetics and postnatal development of the mouse intestinal epithelium. *Anat Rec*. 1985;211(4):420-426.
3. Hooper LV, Midtvedt T, Gordon JI. How host-microbial interactions shape the nutrient environment of the mammalian intestine. *Annu Rev Nutr*. 2002;22:283-307.
6. Clevers H. Wnt/beta-catenin signaling in development and disease. *Cell*. 2006;127(3):469-480.
8. Bjerknes M, Cheng H. Gastrointestinal stem cells. II. Intestinal stem cells. *Am J Physiol Gastrointest Liver Physiol*. 2005;289(3):G381-G387.
10. Noah TK, Shroyer NF. Notch in the intestine: regulation of homeostasis and pathogenesis. *Annu Rev Physiol*. 2013;75:263-288.
15. Sato T, Clevers H. Growing self-organizing mini-guts from a single intestinal stem cell: mechanism and applications. *Science*. 2013;340(6137):1190-1194.
16. Sangild PT. Gut responses to enteral nutrition in preterm infants and animals. *Exp Biol Med*. 2006;231(11):1695-1711.
17. Calder PC, Krauss-Etschmann S, de Jong EC, et al. Early nutrition and immunity - progress and perspectives. *Br J Nutr*. 2006;96(4):774-790.
18. Macpherson AJ, de Aguero MG, Ganal-Vonarburg SC. How nutrition and the maternal microbiota shape the neonatal immune system. *Nat Rev Immunol*. 2017;17(8):508-517.
23. Jacobi SK, Odle J. Nutritional factors influencing intestinal health of the neonate. *Adv Nutr*. 2012;3(5):687-696.

24. Commare CE, Tappenden KA. Development of the infant intestine: implications for nutrition support. *Nutr Clin Pract*. 2007;22(2):159-173.
25. Tappenden KA. Mechanisms of enteral nutrient-enhanced intestinal adaptation. *Gastroenterology*. 2006;130(2 suppl 1):S93-S99.
26. Burrin D, Sanglid PT, Stoll B, et al. Translational advances in pediatric nutrition and gastroenterology: new insights from pig models. *Annu Rev Anim Biosci*. 2020;8:321-354.
27. Raybould HE. Visceral perception: sensory transduction in visceral afferents and nutrients. *Gut*. 2002;51(suppl 1):i11-i14.
29. Psichas A, Reimann F, Gribble FM. Gut chemosensing mechanisms. *J Clin Invest*. 2015;125(3):908-917.
30. Burrin D, Stoll B, Moore D. Digestive physiology of the pig symposium: intestinal bile acid sensing is linked to key endocrine and metabolic signaling pathways. *J Anim Sci*. 2013;91(5):1991-2000.
31. Burrin DG, Stoll B. Key nutrients and growth factors for the neonatal gastrointestinal tract. *Clin Perinatol*. 2002;29(1):65-96.
32. Berseth CL. Minimal enteral feedings. *Clin Perinatol*. 1995;22(1):195-205.
34. Jakaitis BM, Denning PW. Human breast milk and the gastrointestinal innate immune system. *Clin Perinatol*. 2014;41(2):423-435.
36. Martin CR, Ling PR, Blackburn GL. Review of infant feeding: key features of breast milk and infant formula. *Nutrients*. 2016;8(5):279.
38. Burrin DG, Davis TA. Proteins and amino acids in enteral nutrition. *Curr Opin Clin Nutr Metab Care*. 2004;7(1):79-87.
39. Huang Y, Shao XM, Neu J. Immunonutrients and neonates. *Eur J Pediatr*. 2003;162(3):122-128.
41. Naomoto Y, Yamatsuji T, Shigemitsu K, et al. Rational role of amino acids in intestinal epithelial cells (Review). *Int J Mol Med*. 2005;16(2):201-204.
44. Riedijk MA, van Goudoever JB. Splanchnic metabolism of ingested amino acids in neonates. *Curr Opin Clin Nutr Metab Care*. 2007;10(1):58-62.
47. Forchielli ML, Walker WA. The effect of protective nutrients on mucosal defense in the immature intestine. *Acta Paediatr Suppl*. 2005;94(449):74-83.
48. Smilowitz JT, Lebrilla CB, Mills DA, et al. Breast milk oligosaccharides: structure-function relationships in the neonate. *Annu Rev Nutr*. 2014;34:143-169.
50. Chapkin RS, Davidson LA, Ly L, et al. Immunomodulatory effects of (n-3) fatty acids: putative link to inflammation and colon cancer. *J Nutr*. 2007;137(suppl 1):200S-204S.
51. Hegyi P, Maléth J, Walters JR, et al. Guts and gall: bile acids in regulation of intestinal epithelial function in health and disease. *Physiol Rev*. 2018;98(4):1983-2023.
52. Thomas C, Gioiello A, Noriega L, et al. TGR5-mediated bile acid sensing controls glucose homeostasis. *Cell Metab*. 2009;10(3):167-177.
54. Jain AK, Stoll B, Burrin DG, Holst JJ, Moore DD. Enteral bile acid treatment improves parenteral nutrition-related liver disease and intestinal mucosal atrophy in neonatal pigs. *Am J Physiol Gastrointest Liver Physiol*. 2012; 302(2):G218-G224.
56. Sangild PT, Ney DM, Sigalet DL, Vegge A, Burrin D. Animal models of gastrointestinal and liver diseases. Animal models of infant short bowel syndrome: translational relevance and challenges. *Am J Physiol Gastrointest Liver Physiol*. 2014;307(12):G1147-G1168.
58. Burrin DG, Stoll B, Guan X. Glucagon-like peptide 2 function in domestic animals. *Domest Anim Endocrinol*. 2003;24(2):103-122.
59. Drucker DJ, Yusta B. Physiology and pharmacology of the enteroendocrine hormone glucagon-like peptide-2. *Annu Rev Physiol*. 2014;76:561-583.
60. Chao C, Hellmirch MR. Gastrointestinal peptides: gastrin, cholecystokinin, somatostatin, and ghrelin. In: FKG, Johnson LR, Kaunitz JD, Merchant JL, Said HM, Wood JD, eds. *Physiology of the Gastrointestinal Tract*. 5th ed. Waltham, MA: Elsevier Academic Press; 2012:115-154.
61. Trahair JF, Sangild PT. Systemic and luminal influences on the perinatal development of the gut. *Equine Vet J Suppl*. 1997;(24):40-50.
62. Gomez GA, Englander EW, Greeley Jr GH. Postpyloric gastrointestinal peptides. In: GFK, Johnson LR, Kaunitz JD, Merchant JL, Said HM, Wood JD, eds. *Physiology of the Gastrointestinal Tract*. 5th ed. Waltham, MA: Elsevier Academic Press; 2012:155-198.
63. Schumacher MA, Danopoulos S, Alam DA, Frey MR. Growth factors in the gastrointestinal tract. In: Said HM, Ghishan FK, Kaunitz JD, Merchant JL, Wood JD, eds. *Physiology of the Gastrointestinal Tract*. 6th ed. Waltham, MA: Elsevier Academic Press; 2018:71-101.
64. Donovan SM, Odle J. Growth factors in milk as mediators of infant development. *Annu Rev Nutr*. 1994;14:147-167.
65. Hamosh M. Bioactive factors in human milk. *Pediatr Clin North Am*. 2001;48(1):69-86.
66. Yang H, Teitelbaum DH. Novel agents in the treatment of intestinal failure: humoral factors. *Gastroenterology*. 2006;130(2 suppl 1):S117-S121.
67. Feng J, El Assal ON, Besner GE. Heparin-binding epidermal growth factor-like growth factor decreases the incidence of necrotizing enterocolitis in neonatal rats. *J Pediatr Surg*. 2006;41(1):144-149.
68. Warner BW, Erwin CR. Critical roles for EGF receptor signaling during resection-induced intestinal adaptation. *J Pediatr Gastroenterol Nutr*. 2006;43(suppl 1):S68-S73.
70. Bortvedt SF, Lund PK. Insulin-like growth factor 1: common mediator of multiple enterotrophic hormones and growth factors. *Curr Opin Gastroenterol*. 2012;28(2):89-98.
73. Biancheri P, Giuffrida P, Docena GH, et al. The role of transforming growth factor (TGF)-beta in modulating the immune response and fibrogenesis in the gut. *Cytokine Growth Factor Rev*. 2014;25(1):45-55.
78. Mawe GM, Hoffman JM. Serotonin signalling in the gut–functions, dysfunctions and therapeutic targets. *Nat Rev Gastroenterol Hepatol*. 2013;10(8):473-486.
81. Gross ER, Gershon MD, Margolis KG, et al. Neuronal serotonin regulates growth of the intestinal mucosa in mice. *Gastroenterology*. 2012;143(2):408-417 e2.
82. Xu H, Ghishan FK. Molecular physiology of gastrointestinal function during development. In: Said HM, Ghishan FK, Kaunitz JD, Merchant JL, Wood JD, eds. *Physiology of the Gastrointestinal Tract*. 6th ed. Waltham, MA: Elsevier Academic Press; 2018:235-269.
83. Drozdowski L. Intestinal hormones and growth factors: effects on the small intestine. *World J Gastroenterol*. 2009;15(4):385.
85. Bouguen G, Dubuquoy L, Desreumaux P, Brunner T, Bertin B. Intestinal steroidogenesis. *Steroids*. 2015;103:64-71.

Organogenesis of the Gastrointestinal Tract

82

Maxime M. Mahe | Michael A. Helmrath | Noah F. Shroyer

INTRODUCTION

Development of the gastrointestinal tract involves crucial processes, including endoderm formation and patterning along the anterior-to-posterior, dorsoventral, and left-right axis; gut tube morphogenesis into the foregut, midgut, and hindgut domains; assembly of mesenchyme, epithelial morphogenesis, and cytodifferentiation. The organogenesis of the gut tube and its derivatives starts around the third week of gestation from a primitive abdominal tube. From the initiation of gut tube formation until approximately the 12th week of gestation, the gut undergoes a series of events that will define the specific segments and organs of the digestive tract (Fig. 82.1). During the third trimester, organogenesis of the digestive tract is complete, but the intestines undergo rapid growth, resulting in a doubling of intestinal length that will continue over the first several years of life. In this chapter, we will detail the events occurring during the organogenesis of the digestive tract. We will emphasize the embryonic mechanisms, give a brief overview of the molecular pathways involved in the orchestration of the digestive tract organ formation, and describe the associated organogenesis defects.

FORMATION OF THE EMBRYONIC GUT

Around the second week of gestation, gastrulation starts in the epiblast with the formation of the primitive streak (Carnegie stage 6b). Two primitive germ layers arise by ingression and migration through the primitive streak to form endodermal and mesodermal layers below the epiblast; cells that do not migrate through the streak become the ectoderm, the third and last primitive germ layer.[1-3]

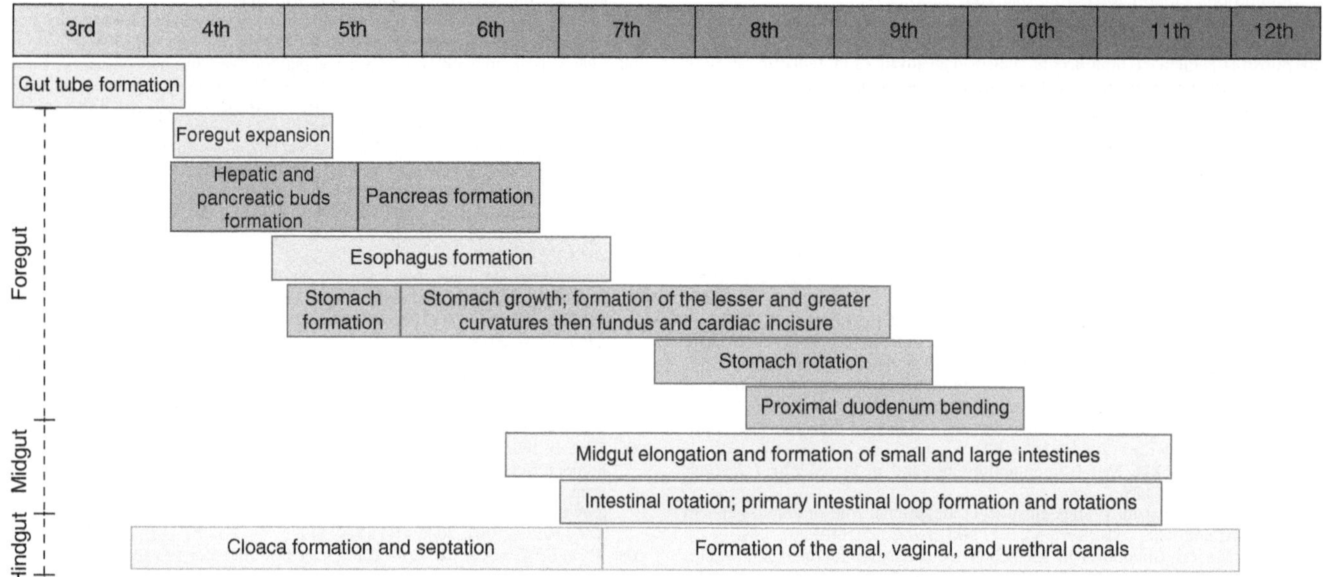

Fig. 82.1 Gastrointestinal tract organogenesis timeline. The organogenesis of the gut tube starts around the 3rd week of gestation to approximately the 12th week of gestation. The specific segments and organs of the digestive tract are derived from the endoderm and the primary gut tube. During the third trimester, organogenesis of the digestive tract is complete, but the intestines will continue to grow over the first several years of life.

During the third and fourth weeks, the three germ layers begin to fold into an elongated cylinder. The gut tube is first seen as pockets in the anterior (rostral) and posterior (caudal) aspect of the embryo, termed the *embryonic intestinal portals,* which are the primordial anlage of the foregut and hindgut. At this stage (Carnegie stage 9) the midgut has not yet formed a tube and is open to the yolk sac. As the embryo grows, the anterior and posterior intestinal portals deepen and extend toward the center of the embryo, and the lateral portions of the midgut fold toward the midline. This primitive gut consists of a blind-ending tube with the foregut terminating cranially in the buccopharyngeal membrane and the hindgut terminating caudally in the cloacal membrane.[1,4,5] The embryonic gut tube is lined by endoderm and surrounded by splanchnic mesoderm; the ectodermal contributions to the gut are derived from migrating neural crest cells that delaminate primarily from the vagal neural crest, with a smaller contribution from the sacral neural crest.[6]

By convention, the boundaries of the foregut, midgut, and hindgut correspond to the three arteries that supply the abdominal digestive tube: the celiac axis supplies the foregut, the superior mesenteric artery supplies the midgut, and the inferior mesenteric artery supplies the hindgut. The foregut gives rise to the anterior aspect of the digestive tube, including the pharynx and oral cavity, the esophagus, the stomach, and the upper duodenum. The foregut also gives rise to the endoderm-derived organs, including the thyroid, lungs, liver and biliary system, and pancreas. The midgut develops into the distal portion of the duodenum, jejunum, ileum, cecum, appendix, and proximal portion of the transverse colon. The hindgut gives rise to the distal portion of the transverse colon, descending colon, sigmoid colon, and rectum. The hindgut also gives rise to urogenital sinus derivatives, including the vaginal and urethral tracts. In addition, the gut tube regions are also defined by their specific structure, function, cell types, and gene expression. The establishment of the gastrointestinal territories is dependent on the rostrocaudal gradients of morphogen signals—Wnt, bone morphogenetic protein (BMP), and fibroblast growth factor (FGF)—provided by the mesoderm, as well as the expression of regional transcription factors (e.g., Hox-family and Caudal-family homeoproteins) in both the mesoderm and the endoderm.[7,8]

FOREGUT

During the fourth week of gestation the anterior intestinal portal of the primitive gut grows and forms an invagination that will constitute the foregut. The definitive endoderm is patterned along an anterior-posterior axis maintained by region-specific transcription factors—that is, the anterior portion of the foregut expresses hematopoietically expressed homeobox (HHEX), sex determining region Y (SRY)-box 2 (SOX2), and forkhead box A2 (FOXA2) proteins, whereas the posterior portion of the foregut expresses caudal-type homeobox 1, 2, and 4 (CDX1, CDX2, and CDX4), and pancreatic and duodenal homeobox 1 (PDX1) proteins.[7] From the foregut arise portions of the digestive tract: the pharynx, the esophagus, the stomach, the pylorus, and the anterior half of the duodenum. Also, the thyroid, the liver, the tracheal apparatus and lungs and the pancreas originate from the foregut. The precursors of both thyroid and lung buds are localized to the ventral midline of the foregut. Precursor cells of the liver and pancreas are localized at multiple sites in the foregut endoderm. Endodermal buds form the liver parenchyma and hepatic ducts, gallbladder and common bile ducts, and dorsal and ventral pancreatic buds.[3]

ESOPHAGUS

The esophagus connects, cranially, to the posterior end of the pharynx at the pharyngoesophageal junction and, caudally, to the stomach at the orifice of the cardia of the stomach. The average length of the esophagus ranges from 8 to 10 cm in the newborn, increasing to 18 to 26 cm in the adult. The esophagus lies ventrally to the vertebral column and dorsally to the trachea.[3,9]

ESOPHAGUS ORGANOGENESIS

Both the esophagus and the trachea are derived from the anterior portion of the foregut. At around 4 weeks (22 to 23 days of gestation), a median ventral diverticulum, the tracheal diverticulum, appears in the posterior region of the foregut. The tracheal diverticulum elongates with the proliferation of endodermal cells. Lateral ridges are formed, creating a separation between the trachea and the esophagus, the esophagotracheal septum, occurring at 34 to 36 days of gestation. The tracheal diverticulum ultimately becomes the primitive respiratory tract. As these tracheoesophageal folds continue to develop, the caudal part of the foregut forms a spindle-shaped dilation that becomes the stomach. The developing esophagus is localized between the caudal foregut dilation and the tracheal diverticulum. Elongation of the developing esophagus occurs first cranially and then caudally and reaches its final relative length by 7 weeks of gestation.[3]

MOLECULAR MECHANISMS REGULATING ESOPHAGUS DEVELOPMENT

The tracheoesophageal separation of the early foregut is controlled by signaling molecules and transcription factors that follow a specific dorsoventral patterning. Studies in the mouse reported several transcription factors involved in the anterior foregut separation. SOX2 is expressed within the epithelial cells of the dorsal foregut, whereas the NK2 homeobox 1 (NKX2-1, also known as *thyroid transcription factor [TTF1]*) is expressed in the ventral foregut, thus demarcating the separation between the presumptive ventral tracheal and esophageal diverticula.[10] Also, the separation of the esophagus from the early foregut is governed by several signaling pathways. The Sonic hedgehog (Shh) pathway induces foregut separation. In humans, *Shh* mutation leads to an abnormal foregut separation as seen in the VACTERL association.[11] The temporal Shh expression, from the ventral to the dorsal foregut endoderm, orchestrates the foregut separation.[12,13] Genetic deletion of Shh pathway effectors such as GLI family zinc finger 1-3 *(GLI1-GLI3)* or forkhead box F1 *(FOXF1)* causes abnormal foregut separation and esophageal atresia.[14,15] Whereas Shh is expressed by the epithelium, GLI1, GLI2, GLI3, and FOXF1 are expressed by the mesenchyme, highlighting an example of the continuous endoderm-mesoderm crosstalk that occurs during organogenesis of the digestive system. Wnt signaling is also essential to the generation of the esophagus. Several Wnt ligands have been identified both at the ventral side of the mesenchymal and at the endodermal foregut. For example, the ligands WNT2 and WNT2b are expressed in the mesenchyme and their simultaneous inhibition blocks the tracheoesophageal separation.[16] Importantly, epithelial inhibition of the Wnt pathway increased the expression of SOX2 at the ventral foregut despite NKX2-1 expression, resulting in an unseparated foregut.[16,17] Similarly to Wnt the BMP pathway forms a dorsoventral gradient where BMP4 and BMP7 are enriched at the ventral side of the foregut and the BMP inhibitor Noggin is enriched at the dorsal side. The disruption of this morphogenetic gradient leads to tracheoesophageal defects. BMP signaling also controls the expression of SOX2 within the foregut.[18,19] Retinoic acid signaling is also critical for the specification of both the trachea and the esophagus. Retinoic acid activity is seen in the anterior portion of the foregut both in mesenchyme and in epithelium and its alteration leads to foregut developmental anomalies. Moreover, a dorsoventral expression pattern exists for retinoic acid receptors.[20] For example, retinoic acid receptor β_2 in mice is localized to the dorsal epithelium and becomes more restricted during the tracheoesophageal separation.[21] Genetic deletion of retinoic acid receptors abrogates the tracheoesophageal separation.[22]

ESOPHAGUS ORGANOGENESIS DEFECT

TRACHEOESOPHAGEAL FISTULA AND ESOPHAGEAL ATRESIA

Esophageal atresia and tracheoesophageal fistula are commonly found in association and represent the most frequent congenital esophageal abnormalities. This defect results from the abnormal separation of the tracheal diverticulum from the foregut. The esophageal atresia is an interruption of the esophageal continuity resulting from a recanalization defect of the primitive gut during the eighth week. Esophageal atresia with tracheoesophageal fistula occurs in 1 in 3000 to 1 in 5000 live births. Five types of esophageal atresia with or without fistula have been classified. The most common is type C—esophageal atresia with distal tracheoesophageal fistula—with an incidence of 86.5% (Fig. 82.2).[23,24]

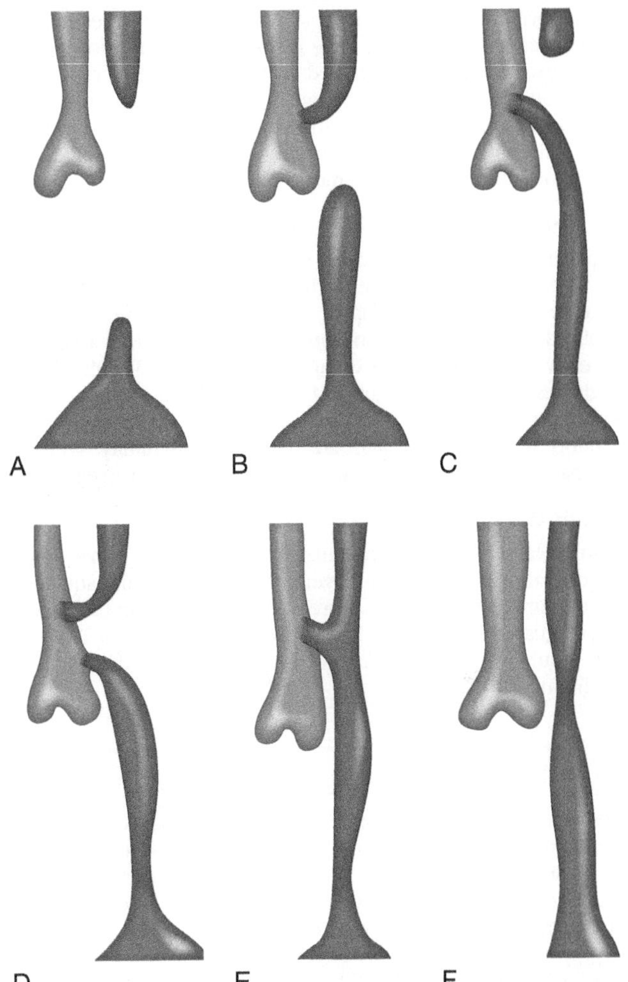

Fig. 82.2 Types of esophageal atresia and tracheoesophageal fistula. The tracheal pouch and the lower and upper esophageal pouches are represented in *blue* and *pink,* respectively. (A) Type A, isolated esophageal atresia. (B) Type B, blind-ending lower esophageal pouch with a fistula between the trachea and the upper esophageal pouch. (C) Type C, esophageal atresia with a blind proximal esophageal pouch and a distal tracheoesophageal fistula. This anomaly represents approximately 85% of all esophageal atresia. (D) Type D, esophageal atresia with two fistulas between the trachea and the lower and upper esophageal pouches. (E) Type E, fistula between the esophagus and the trachea. (F) Congenital esophageal stenosis.

ESOPHAGEAL STENOSIS AND RINGS

Esophageal stenosis is a narrowing of the esophagus that can be more frequently found in the middle to distal third of the esophagus and presents as a web (membranous diaphragm) or a long segment of narrowed esophagus (fibromuscular stenosis). This anomaly results from incomplete recanalization of the esophagus during the eighth week. It may also result from the absence of vascular ingrowth within the area or an incomplete tracheoesophageal separation as suggested by the presence of respiratory tissue.[24] The incidence of this congenital defect is 1 per 25,000 live births. This type of esophageal stenosis has been classified into three groups.[25] Another form of esophageal stenosis called *esophageal ring* is found within the lower third of the esophagus and is created by the presence of concentric extension of the normal esophageal tissue. These rings may result from an incomplete vacuolization of the columnar epithelium during the eighth week. Three types have been classified, with type B or Schatzki's ring the most common.[26]

ESOPHAGEAL DUPLICATION AND DUPLICATION CYST

Duplications can be found in direct communication with the esophagus or they may lie within the mediastinum completely separate from the esophagus. The origin of those intramural duplications within the esophagus could be caused by a failure of the early foregut to become completely vacuolated. The duplication originates from the foregut and thus could be attached to the esophagus or the tracheobronchial system. These duplications develop independently and are rarely in continuity with the esophagus but are contiguous with some gastrointestinal segments.[27]

ESOPHAGEAL WEB

Esophageal webs are thin transverse membrane consisting of a mucosal and submucosal layer covered by normal squamous epithelium. These webs are more frequently found in the cervical esophagus associated with heterotopic gastric mucosa. The webs may result from the incomplete vacuolization of the columnar epithelium.[26]

STOMACH

The stomach is cranially connected to the esophagus and caudally connected to the duodenum by the pylorus. The average volume of the stomach is about 30 mL in the newborn, increasing to 1.5 to 2 L in the adult. The stomach is divided into four regions: the cardia, the fundus, the body, and the antrum.

STOMACH ORGANOGENESIS

The stomach arises during the fourth week from the dilation of the posterior portion of the foregut. At 26 days of gestation, the foregut elongates to form a primitive stomach that expands in a spindle-shaped structure. During the fifth week the dorsal part of the stomach expands further than the ventral part, thus resulting in the formation of the greater and the lesser curvatures. By the end of the seventh week the expansion of the superior part of the greater curvature results in the formation of the fundus and the cardiac incisure. During the seventh and eighth weeks the stomach undergoes a 90-degree clockwise rotation (toward subject's left) around an anterior-posterior axis positioning the greater curvature to the left side and the lesser curvature to right side. The stomach also rotates slightly around a dorsoventral axis so the greater curvature is slightly upward and the lesser curvature downward. By approximately eight weeks of gestation, formation of the stomach is complete.[3]

MOLECULAR MECHANISMS REGULATING STOMACH DEVELOPMENT

During the formation of the stomach, anterior-posterior boundaries are maintained by specific transcriptional factors. SOX2 is expressed in the foregut epithelium and BarH-like homeobox 1 (BARX1) is expressed in the foregut mesenchyme. Both transcription factors block the intestinal program relying on Wnt signaling and the activation of the transcription factor CDX2.[28,29] Thus they establish the distinction between the stomach and the intestines. Also, other transcription factors are expressed along the anterior-posterior axis to delineate the forestomach and the posterior portion of the stomach. For example, the nuclear receptor COUP transcription factor 2 (NR2F2) is highly expressed in the proximal portion of the gastric mesenchyme and its deletion in the mouse induces a posteriorization of the forestomach.[30] In contrast, Bagpipe homeobox protein homologue 1 (BAPX1, also known as *NK3 Homeobox 2 [NKX3-2]*) is expressed in the distal mesenchyme and maintains a normal antrum to the duodenum by the pyloric boundaries.[31] BMP signaling is also established gradually along an anterior-posterior axis where it is posteriorly localized.[32,33] PDX1 is expressed in the distal portion of the foregut, demarcating the pancreatic, gastric antral, and proximal duodenal regions.[34] FGF10, produced by the mesenchyme, and its epithelial receptor fibroblast growth factor receptor 2 (FGFR2) act synergistically to control stomach morphogenesis and gland formation.[35,36] Crosstalk between the epithelium and the mesenchyme and these regional transcription factors creates and maintains the boundaries within the stomach. Studies in mice have also suggested that BARX1 enhances gastric smooth muscle development along with the expression of left-right transcription factors (ISL LIM homeobox 1 [ISL1], paired-like homeodomain 1 and 2 [PITX1 and PITX2] and Sine oculis homeobox homolog 2 [SIX2]), thus placing the stomach in its final position during the intestinal rotation.[37]

STOMACH ORGANOGENESIS DEFECT

GASTRIC ATRESIA

Gastric atresia is a rare condition located within the antral and pyloric regions, and infants present as newborns with complete gastric outlet obstruction. The prevalence of the disease is 1 in 100,000 live births.

GASTRIC VOLVULUS

Gastric volvulus is a rare condition that results in a 180-degree gastric rotation caused by the laxity or lack of the normal attachments of the stomach to the body. These attachments include the gastrophrenic ligaments, the gastrocolic ligament, the short gastric vessels, and the retroperitoneal fixation of the duodenum.[38]

CONGENITAL MICROGASTRIA

Microgastria is not uncommonly found and is the result of a developmental defect of the posterior portion of the foregut. Microgastria will occur as a result of an arrest in the early development of the foregut and an abnormal migration at the primitive streak stage. It is almost always associated with an enlarged esophagus and incomplete gastric rotation.[39,40]

GASTRIC DUPLICATION CYSTS

Gastric duplication cysts are rare and occur along the greater curvature or on the anteroposterior walls of the stomach. Communications to the stomach are not always present, and the mucosal lining is generally gastric. The prevalence of this disorder is 17 in 1,000,000 live births.[41,42]

PYLORUS

The stomach is separated from the duodenum by thick circular muscle rings: the sphincters. The pylorus is localized between the stomach and the proximal portion of the duodenum and acts as a sphincter to regulate chyme passage and avoid any backflow from the duodenum to the stomach.

PYLORUS ORGANOGENESIS AND MOLECULAR UNDERPINNINGS

The pylorus forms at the boundary between the stomach and the duodenum. This unique area is an important organ boundary but also a hub for the development of the digestive tract accessory organs.[43]

Several experiments in chick and mouse embryos unraveled the mechanisms that underlie pyloric sphincter formation. Studies in chicken have shown the importance of BMP4, expressed in the mesoderm of the small intestine, whereas BMP receptor 1 is expressed in the mesoderm of the posterior portion of the stomach.[44] The BMP signaling from the small intestine specifies the pyloric region by inducing the expression of NK2 homeobox 5 (NKX2-5) and SRY-box 9 (SOX9) in the posterior portion of the stomach.[44–46] Mouse studies have demonstrated that BMP4 is also expressed in the mesenchyme of the small intestine but also in the posterior portion of the stomach along with NKX2-5 in the mesoderm of the pyloric sphincter, suggesting a similar patterning mechanism.[47] The *SIX homeodomain family 6 (SIX6)* gene is also required to define the pyloric sphincter region.[48] Other transcription factors crucial in pyloric sphincter development have been identified. The GATA binding protein 3 (GATA3) and NKX2-5 are coexpressed along with SOX9 in the longitudinal muscle and the gastric ligament.[49,50] Also, the transcription factors identified in the foregut regionalization and stomach formation are required; *BARX1* or *BAPX1* deletion induces the loss of the pyloric constriction.[28,31] Similarly, an overexpression of WNT9b induces the same phenotype, suggesting an important role of Wnt signaling.[51]

PYLORUS ORGANOGENESIS DEFECTS

The infantile hypertrophic pyloric stenosis results from the hypertrophy of the circular muscle resulting in the narrowing and elongation of the pyloric channel. Concomitantly, the stomach gets obstructed with a compensatory gastric dilation, hypertrophy, and hyperperistalsis. The incidence of this disorder ranges from 0.5 to 5 per 1000 live births depending on ethnic demographics.[52,53] The ontogeny of the disease is rather complex, with possible causes combining genetic and environmental factors.[53] Duodenogastric reflux is a rare primary pyloric disorder. It results from the backflow of the duodenal content into the stomach. The cause is not known. This disorder is often observed secondary to surgery.[54]

DUODENUM

The average length of the small intestine is between 250 and 300 cm in the newborn, increasing to as much as 600 to 800 cm in the adult. The duodenum constitutes approximately the first 25 cm of the small intestine in adults; the remaining length is arbitrarily divided into the proximal two fifths, designated as the *jejunum,* and the distal three fifths, designated as the *ileum.* The transition from jejunum to ileum is arbitrary because there are no histologic or gross anatomic demarcations between these segments. The proximal portion of the duodenum is derived from the distal portion of the foregut, whereas the distal portion of the duodenum is derived from the midgut.

DUODENUM ORGANOGENESIS

At about 7 to 8 weeks, the rotations of the stomach bend the duodenum into a C shape and also place it to the right side until it lies against the dorsal body wall. The rotation of the stomach and the bending of the duodenum create an alcove dorsal to the stomach called the *lesser sac of the peritoneal cavity,* and the rest of the cavity constitutes the greater sac.

DUODENUM ORGANOGENESIS DEFECTS

ATRESIAS

Intestinal atresias are mostly duodenal atresia and occur in 1 in 10,000 live births.[55] Combined duodenal and jejunal atresias are very rare. Jejunal atresia occurs in 1 in 5000 to 1 in 14,000 live births. There are four different subtypes of duodenal atresias, ranging from a simple stenosis to an intestinal lumen gap with mesenteric defects (Fig. 82.3A and B).[56]

DIGESTIVE GLANDS

LIVER AND GALLBLADDER FORMATION

The liver, the gallbladder, and their associated ducts bud from the duodenal endoderm. Around day 22, the hepatic plate appears on the ventral side of the duodenum and will grow over the next few days to finally give rise to the liver (see Chapter 88). By day 26, a distinct endodermal thickening, on the ventral side of the duodenum, caudal to the base of the hepatic diverticulum, buds into the ventral mesentery. The hepatic diverticulum will form the gallbladder and the cystic duct. From the cystic duct and hepatic ducts, cells proliferate to form the common bile ducts.[3]

PANCREAS FORMATION

On day 26 of gestation, a duodenal bud begins to grow into the dorsal mesentery just opposite the hepatic diverticulum (see Chapter 86). This endodermal diverticulum is the dorsal pancreatic bud. Over the next few days, as the dorsal pancreatic bud grows into the dorsal mesentery, another endodermal diverticulum, the ventral pancreatic bud, sprouts into the ventral mesentery. By day 32, the main duct of the ventral pancreatic bud becomes connected to the proximal end of the common bile duct. During the fifth week the mouth of the common bile duct and the ventral pancreatic bud migrate posteriorly around the duodenum to the dorsal mesentery. By early in the sixth week the two pancreatic buds fuse to form the definitive pancreas. The dorsal pancreatic buds give rise to the head, body, and tail of the pancreas, whereas the ventral pancreatic bud gives rise to the uncinate process. The ductal systems become interconnected. The main pancreatic duct and the common bile duct meet at the major duodenal papilla or ampulla of Vater. A secondary pancreatic duct termed the *duct of Santorini* is also sometimes present.[3]

The annular pancreas is a common pancreatic anomaly. This defect is often a cause of duodenal obstruction. Defects in pancreatic duct formation are also common malformations in which the main pancreatic drainage occurs through the accessory duct.

MIDGUT

The embryonic midgut gives rise exclusively to intestinal segments: distal portion of the duodenum, jejunum, ileum, and proximal portions of the colon. There is no distinct demarcation between them, but progressive structural differences are present from the portions of the proximal jejunum to the distal portion of the ileum. The jejunal wall is thicker and more vascular than the ileum and diminishes in size with distal progression. The intestinal luminal diameter is also greatest in the jejunum, shrinking in diameter as it progresses distally.

ORGANOGENESIS

From the beginning of the sixth week the small and large intestines are formed by lengthening of the midgut and maturation of the mucosal, submucosal, and muscular layers.[57] This elongation of the midgut creates a dorsoventral hairpin fold called the *primary intestinal loop*. The cranial part of this loop gives rise to most of the ileum and the caudal part becomes the ascending colon and transverse colon. By early in the sixth week (Carnegie stage 15) the continuing elongation of the midgut, combined with the pressure due to the growth of other abdominal organs, forces the primary intestinal loop to herniate into the umbilicus. The herniated primary intestinal loop undergoes a 90-degree counterclockwise rotation (toward subject's left) around a dorsoventral axis. As the primary intestinal loop herniates into the umbilicus, it also rotates 90 degrees counterclockwise around the axis of the superior mesenteric artery. This rotation is complete by early in the eighth week. Meanwhile, the midgut continues to grow and mature. The lengthening jejunum and ileum form additional secondary and tertiary jejunal-ileal loops, and the expanding cecum sprouts a vermiform appendix.

During the 10th week the midgut retracts into the abdomen and rotates an additional 180 degrees. As the intestinal loop reenters the abdomen, it rotates 180 degrees counterclockwise

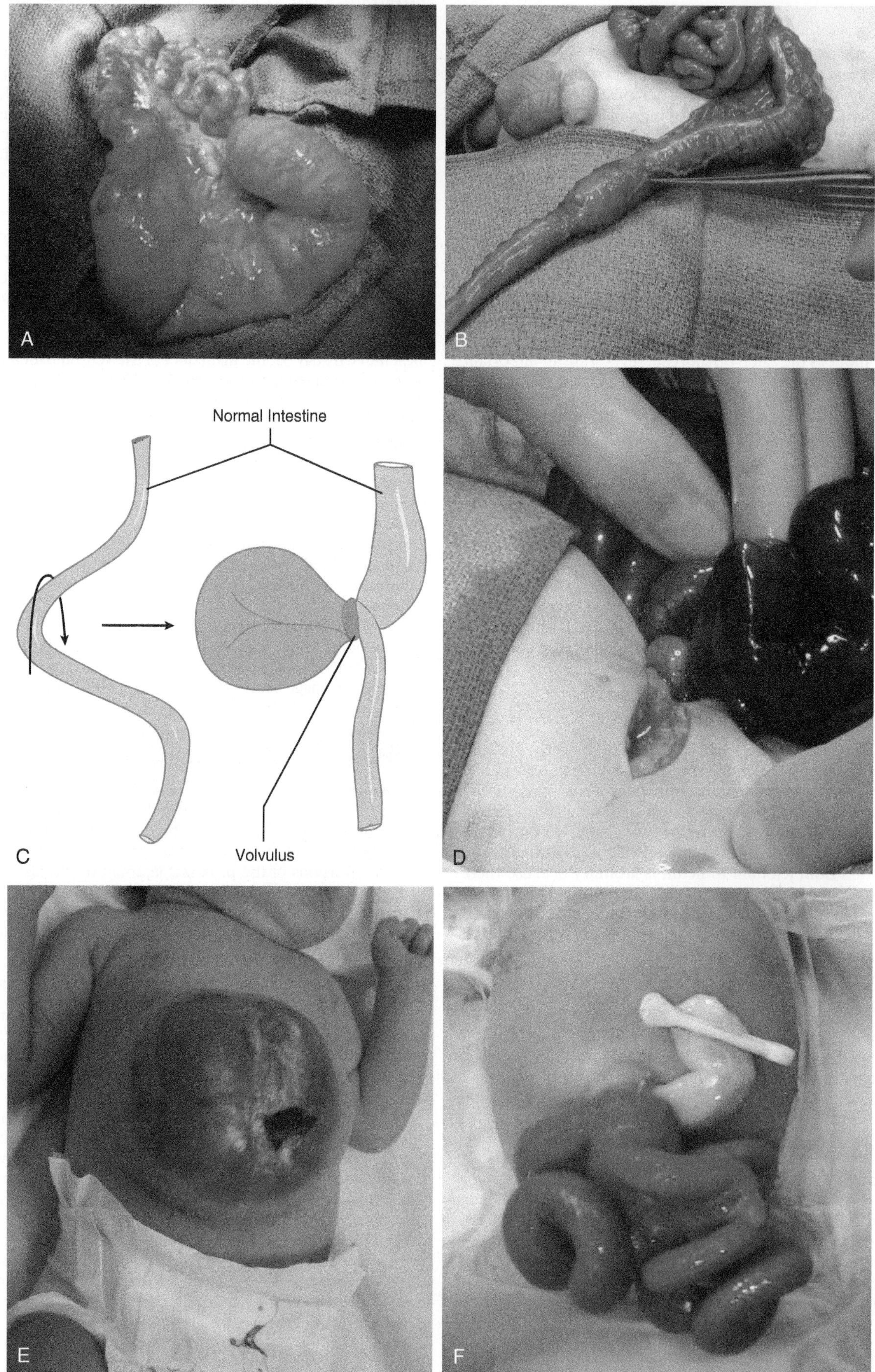

Fig. 82.3 Congenital midgut malformations and abdominal wall defects. (A) Duodenal atresia (type 3B) with dilation of the proximal bowel and, below the discontinuity, the atrophic distal bowel. (B) Jejunal atresia. (C) Small intestine malrotation inducing a volvulus. (D) Malrotated bowel with a volvulus. (E) Infant with a large omphalocele. The bowel and liver are seen outside the abdominal cavity in a sac. (F) Infant with gastroschisis. The bowel is seen outside the abdominal cavity.

(toward subject's left) around a dorsoventral axis, so that the retracting colon has rotated 270 degrees relative to the posterior wall of the abdominal cavity. The cecum consequently rotates to a position just inferior to the liver in the region of the right iliac crest. The intestines have completely returned to the abdominal cavity by the 11th week.[3]

MOLECULAR MECHANISMS REGULATING MIDGUT DEVELOPMENT

FGF4 plays an essential role in the midgut patterning as it inhibits the foregut development and promotes the midgut and hindgut identity. Thus FGF4 induces the intestinal fate, repressing anterior markers such as hematopoietically expressed homeobox 1 (HEX1) and enhancing midgut markers such as PDX1 and CDX2.[2] Also, Wnt signaling is essential to the midgut and hindgut development; high Wnt activity is required to repress foregut development and push toward an intestinal fate.[7] As an example, the aforementioned transcription factor BARX1, which is expressed during foregut embryogenesis, induces *SFRP1* and *SFRP2*, which in turn inhibit Wnt signaling, thus repressing midgut fate and favoring the foregut fate.[28] Another crucial transcription factor of intestinal specification is CDX2. CDX2 is expressed early during the anterior-posterior formation of the gut tube and is essential for specifying the intestinal endoderm. Wnt induces the expression of CDX2, thus reinforcing its predominant role in intestinal specification.[58]

An essential part of the midgut development is its lengthening. Studies in mice showed that hedgehog signaling plays an important role during that phase. Deletion of both *SHH* and *Indian hedgehog (IHH)* inhibits the expansion of the stomach and gut during development.[59] Crosstalk between the mesenchyme and the epithelial endoderm is also important. Soluble morphogens such as FGF9 or WNT5a participate in the intestinal expansion.[60,61] The rotation events occurring during the midgut expansion are also regulated by molecular cues received during development. The transcription factors PITX2 and ISL1 are asymmetrically expressed in the left side of the dorsal mesentery. Their expression induces the activation of downstream effectors to drive the aggregation of mesenchymal cells in an asymmetric manner, thus inducing looping.[62] Also, these loops happen in the presence of the mesentery, which is also driving the rotational forces.[63]

Boundaries between the small intestine and the large intestine are also defined by the regional expression of transcription factors. For example, the transcription factor GATA4 is restricted to the duodenum and jejunum and maintains their identity.[64] Also, the anterior-posterior axis of the intestine is determined by homeotic (Hox) genes that are expressed in a collinear manner along the digestive tract, thus defining the different intestinal segments.[65]

MIDGUT ORGANOGENESIS DEFECT

MALROTATION AND VOLVULUS

Malrotation is an anomaly of the intestinal positioning with an incidence of 1 per 2500 live births. Volvulus is a twisting of a portion of the bowel around the attached mesentery and often occurs on the mesentery where the base is narrow. Volvulus in the neonate is often due to a defect in intestinal rotation during the period of herniation of the intestinal loops through the anterior abdominal wall. The volvulus results in bowel obstruction and can cause abdominal distension, vomiting, and ischemia, leading to necrosis of the involved bowel (see Fig. 82.3C and D).[56]

ABDOMINAL WALL DEFECTS

Gastroschisis is an anterior abdominal wall defect in which abdominal organs protrude without any membrane or sac covering. The incidence is approximately 5 per 10,000 live births. The exact cause of gastroschisis is unknown, although it is believed to be due to occlusion of the omphalomesenteric artery, resulting in failure of the abdominal wall to develop normally.[66] Omphalocele is an outpouching of the peritoneum that protrudes through the umbilicus. In this condition, the intestines, liver, and other organs remain outside the abdomen contained within a sac. The incidence is approximately 4 per 10,000 births (see Fig. 82.3E and F).[66]

HINDGUT

ORGANOGENESIS

The hindgut gives rise to the distal third of the transverse colon, descending colon, sigmoid colon, and rectum, all of which receive blood from the inferior mesenteric artery.

The hindgut originates as the caudal intestinal portal grows both in length and circumference. By the fourth week the portion of the hindgut lying adjacent to the cloacal membrane forms a cavity lined by endoderm and is surrounded by mesenchyme called the *cloaca*. The cloaca is common to the anorectal and urogenital canals. Between the fourth week and the sixth week the anorectal and urogenital canals arise by septation of the cloaca; the cloaca is partitioned into a posterior rectum and an anterior primitive urogenital sinus by the growth of the urorectal septum. The distal edge of the urorectal septum fuses with the cloacal membrane, dividing the membrane into an anterior urogenital membrane and a posterior anal membrane. The zone of fusion between the urorectal septum and the cloacal membrane becomes the perineum. By the 12th week the anal, vaginal, and urethral canals have formed.[67-69]

After the large intestine returns to the abdominal cavity, the dorsal mesenteries of the ascending colon and descending colon shorten and fold, bringing these organs into contact with the dorsal body wall, where they adhere and become secondarily retroperitoneal. The cecum is suspended from the dorsal body wall by a shortened mesentery soon after it returns to the abdominal cavity. The transverse colon does not become fixed to the body wall but remains an intraperitoneal organ suspended by the mesentery. Pressure from this organ may help to fix the underlying duodenum to the body wall. The most inferior portion of the colon, the sigmoid colon, also remains suspended by the mesentery. The last part of the hindgut forms the rectum.[3]

MOLECULAR MECHANISMS REGULATING HINDGUT DEVELOPMENT

The Hox family is known to be expressed in the cecal primordium following a spatiotemporal collinearity, where each cluster (e.g., *HOXA*, *HOXB*, *HOXC*, *HOXD*) is expressed gradually along the tract and defines the cecal regions.[70,71] FGFs have also been shown to play a role in cecal development. For example, FGF10 acts downstream of the *HOXD* genes, where it is restricted to the cecal mesoderm and is required for epithelial budding. FGF9 is expressed within the epithelium and is essential to regulating cecal budding.[72] As the embryo develops, the posterior genes from the *HOXA* and *HOXD* clusters, *HOXA13* and *HOXD13*, are expressed in the hindgut and cloacal region.[73] It is thought that they play a crucial role in defining the hindgut territories. Also, CDX2 and CDX4 participate in hindgut patterning, where they act downstream of Wnt signaling.[74] The two Wnt ligands WNT3a and WNT5a play an important role in hindgut and anorectal development. WNT3a participates in the complete septation of the urogenital and anorectal tracts. WNT5a is expressed during hindgut formation and anorectal development but disappears once the anus has been formed.[75,76] The morphogen Shh is expressed by the endoderm of the cloaca and is important during septum formation. It has been shown that the deletion of key downstream effectors of Shh, GLI2 and GLI3, induces a persistent cloaca in mice.[77,78]

HINDGUT ORGANOGENESIS DEFECT

Hindgut developmental defect leads to various anorectal malformations. They are among the more frequent congenital anomalies encountered in the pediatric population, with an estimated incidence of 1 per 5000 live births.[79]

COLONIC ATRESIAS

Colonic atresias is a rare disorder with an estimated incidence of 1 per 10,000 to 1 per 66,000. The ascending colon is mostly affected associated with a mesenteric defect that separates the blind ends.[56]

CLOACAL ANOMALIES

The imperforate anus is the most common hindgut defect and results from the abnormal development of the urorectal septum; hence there is an incomplete separation of the cloaca into its urogenital and anorectal components. The incidence of this disorder is 1 per 10,000 to 1 per 40,000 live births. Anorectal malformations are categorized as either low or high, determined by whether the blind end of the rectum is above or below, respectively, the level of the levator musculature. The high type of lesion is more common than the low type (Fig. 82.4).[80]

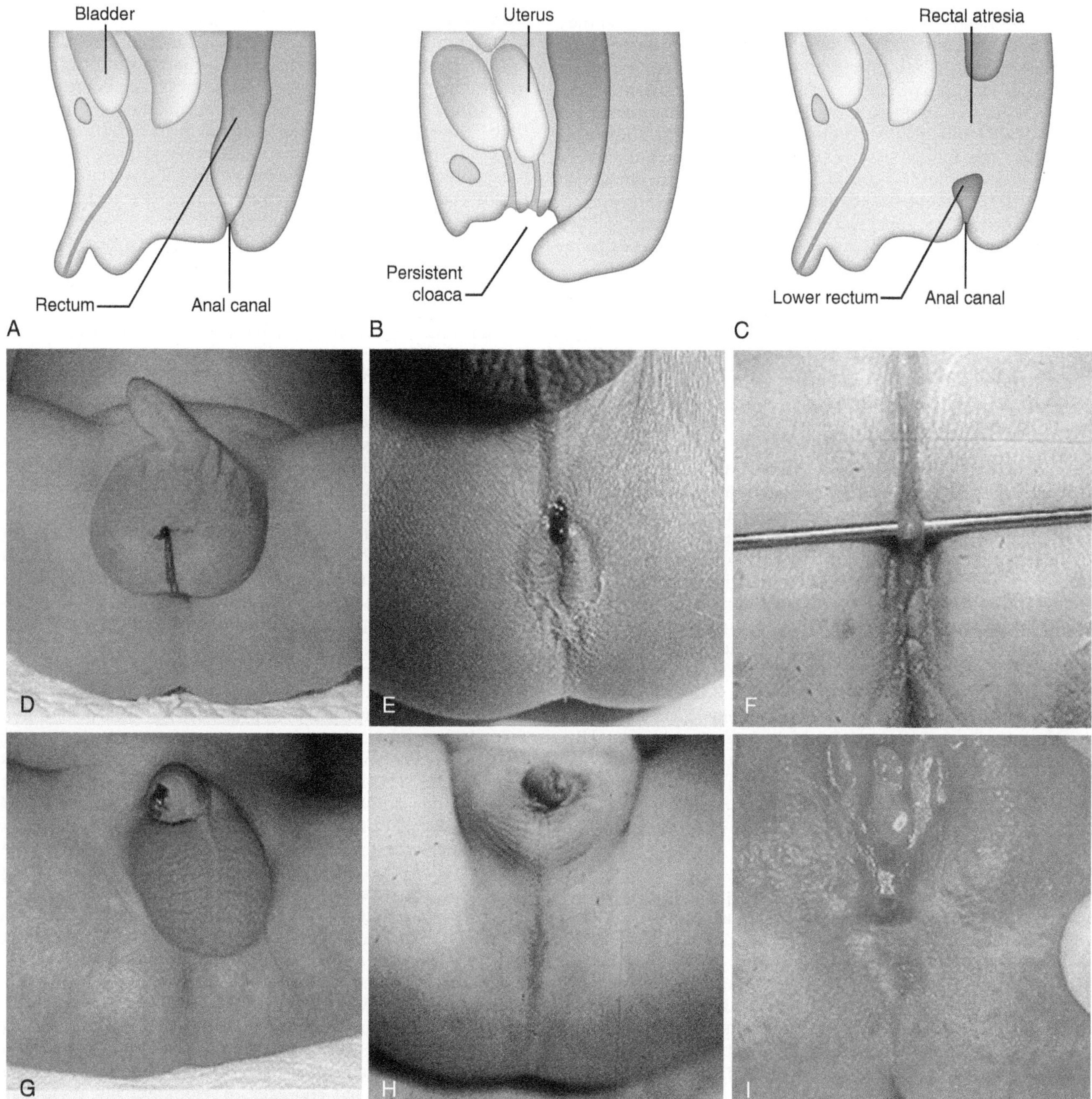

Fig. 82.4 Congenital anorectal anomalies. (A) A male with normal separated urogenital and intestinal tracts. (B) A female with a persistent cloaca resulting from a failure of urorectal septum formation. (C) A male with a rectal atresia. (D–F) Manifestations of low-type imperforate anus: (D) subepithelial fistula; (E) perineal fistula; (F) bucket-handle deformity. (G–I) Manifestations of high-type imperforate anus: (G) meatal meconium; (H) flat "rocker" bottom; (I) vestibular fistula.

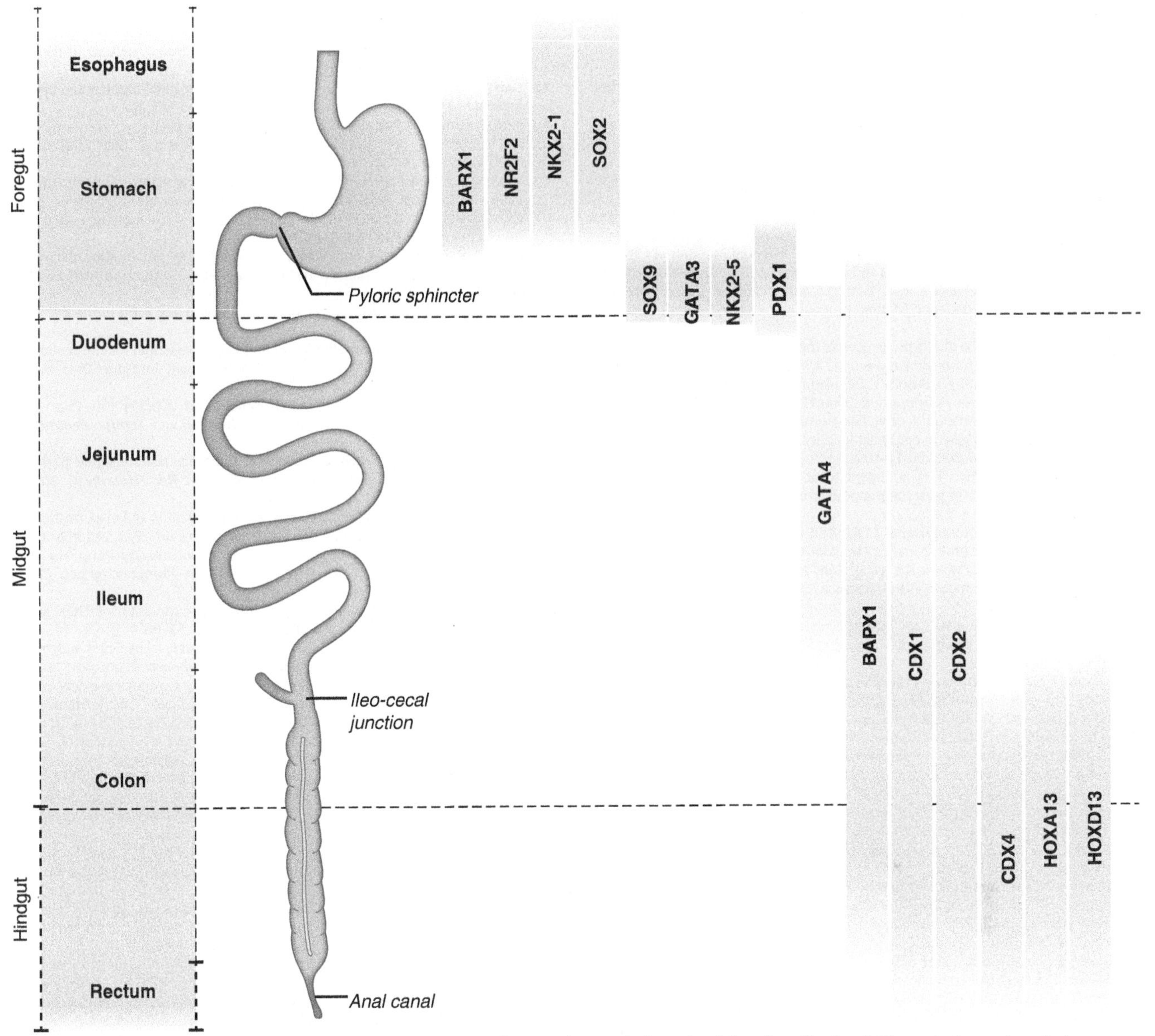

Fig. 82.5 Expression domains of transcription factors along the anterior-posterior axis of the digestive tract. The anterior and posterior expression limits on some of these factors establish organ identity and boundaries. *BAPX1,* Bagpipe homeobox protein homologue 1; *BARX1,* barH-like homeobox 1; *CDX1, 2, and 4,* caudal type homeobox 1, 2, and 4; *GATA3 and 4,* GATA binding protein 3 and 4; *HOXA13,* homeobox A13; *HOXD13,* homeobox D13; *NKX2-1,* NK2 homeobox 1; *NKX2-5,* NK2 homeobox 5; *NR2F2,* COUP transcription factor 2; *PDX1,*pancreatic and duodenal homeobox 1; *SOX2 and 9,* SRY (sex-determining region Y)-box 2 and 9. (From San Roman AK, Shivdasani RA. Boundaries, junctions and transitions in the gastrointestinal tract. *Exp Cell Res.* 2011;317:2711–2718.)

HIRSCHSPRUNG DISEASE

Hirschsprung disease is a congenital motility disorder characterized by the absence of ganglion cells, with an incidence of approximately 1 per 5000 live births.[81] The embryonic origin is a migratory defect of the vagal and sacral neural crest cells into the gut tube. The resulting aganglionosis is always observed in the more distal portions of the intestines. The most frequent region affected is the rectosigmoid location in 80% of cases. In the remaining 20% of cases, longer sections may be involved and can include the distal small bowel.

CONCLUSION

The gastrointestinal tract originates from the endodermal layer during the second and third weeks of gestation. At the fourth week, the primitive embryonic gut is formed, with the foregut developing anteriorly and the hindgut posteriorly. The different intestinal segments differentiate from the primary gut tube following a sequence of events tightly regulated by gradients of morphogens and regional expression of transcription factors (Fig. 82.5).

A complete reference list is available at www.ExpertConsult.com. 

SELECT REFERENCES

1. O'Rahilly R, Muller F. Developmental stages in human embryos: revised and new measurements. *Cells Tissues Organs.* 2010;192:73–84.
2. Wells JM, Melton DA. Vertebrate endoderm development. *Annu Rev Cell Dev Biol.* 1999;15:393–410.
3. Larsen WJ, Sherman LS, Potter SS, Scott WJ. *Human Embryology*. New York: Churchill Livingstone; 2001.

4. Grapin-Botton A. Antero-posterior patterning of the vertebrate digestive tract: 40 years after Nicole Le Douarin's PhD thesis. *Int J Dev Biol*. 2005;49:335-347.
5. Spence JR, Lauf R, Shroyer NF. Vertebrate intestinal endoderm development. *Dev Dyn*. 2011;240:501-520.
7. Zorn AM, Wells JM. Vertebrate endoderm development and organ formation. *Annu Rev Cell Dev Biol*. 2009;25:221-251.
8. San Roman AK, Shivdasani RA. Boundaries, junctions and transitions in the gastrointestinal tract. *Exp Cell Res*. 2011;317:2711-2718.
12. Ioannides AS, Henderson DJ, Spitz L, Copp AJ. Role of Sonic hedgehog in the development of the trachea and oesophagus. *J Pediatr Surg*. 2003;38:29-36, discussion 29-36.
13. Marti E, Takada R, Bumcrot DA, et al. Distribution of Sonic hedgehog peptides in the developing chick and mouse embryo. *Development*. 1995;121:2537-2547.
15. Motoyama J, Liu J, Mo R, Ding Q, Post M, Hui CC. Essential function of Gli2 and Gli3 in the formation of lung, trachea and oesophagus. *Nat Genet*. 1998;20:54-57.
16. Goss AM, Tian Y, Tsukiyama T, et al. Wnt2/2b and β-catenin signaling are necessary and sufficient to specify lung progenitors in the foregut. *Dev Cell*. 2009;17:290-298.
19. Que J, Choi M, Ziel JW, et al. Morphogenesis of the trachea and esophagus: current players and new roles for noggin and Bmps. *Differentiation*. 2006;74:422-437.
20. Malpel S, Mendelsohn C, Cardoso WV. Regulation of retinoic acid signaling during lung morphogenesis. *Development*. 2000;127:3057-3067.
28. Kim BM, Buchner G, Miletich I, et al. The stomach mesenchymal transcription factor Barx1 specifies gastric epithelial identity through inhibition of transient Wntsignaling. *Dev Cell*. 2005;8:611-622.
29. Kim BM, Miletich I, Mao J, et al. Independent functions and mechanisms for homeobox gene Barx1 in patterning mouse stomach and spleen. *Development*. 2007;134:3603-3613.
30. Takamoto N, You L-R, Moses K, et al. COUP-TFII is essential for radial and anteroposterior patterning of the stomach. *Development*. 2005;132:2179-2189.
31. Verzi MP, Stanfel MN, Moses KA, et al. Role of the homeodomain transcription factor Bapx1 in mouse distal stomach development. *Gastroenterology*. 2009;136:1701-1710.
33. McCracken KW, Cata EM, Crawford CM, et al. Modelling human development and disease in pluripotent stem-cell-derived gastric organoids. *Nature*. 2014;516:400-404.
34. Larsson LI, Madsen OD, Serup P, et al. Pancreatic-duodenal homeobox 1 -role in gastric endocrine patterning. *Mech Dev*. 1996;60:175-184.
35. Spencer-Dene B, Sala FG, Bellusci S, et al. Stomach development is dependent on fibroblast growth factor 10/fibroblast growth factor receptor 2b-mediated signaling. *Gastroenterology*. 2006;130:1233-1244.
36. Nyeng P, Norgaard GA, Kobberup S, Jensen J. FGF10 signaling controls stomach morphogenesis. *Dev Biol*. 2007;303:295-310.
37. Jayewickreme CD, Shivdasani RA. Control of stomach smooth muscle development and intestinal rotation by transcription factor BARX1. *Dev Biol*. 2015;405:21-32.
38. Cribbs RK, Gow KW, Wulkan ML. Gastric volvulus in infants and children. *Pediatrics*. 2008;122:e752-e762.
43. Udager A, Prakash A, Gumucio DL. Dividing the tubular gut: generation of organ boundaries at the pylorus. *Prog Mol Biol Transl Sci*. 2010;96:35-62.
44. Smith DM, Tabin CJ. BMP signalling specifies the pyloric sphincter. *Nature*. 1999;402:748-749.
45. Moniot B, Biau S, Faure S, et al. SOX9 specifies the pyloric sphincter epithelium through mesenchymal-epithelial signals. *Development*. 2004;131:3795-3804.
46. Theodosiou NA, Tabin CJ. Sox9 and Nkx2.5 determine the pyloric sphincter epithelium under the control of BMP signaling. *Dev Biol*. 2005;279:481-490.
56. Adams SD, Stanton MP. Malrotation and intestinal atresias. *Early Hum Dev*. 2014;90:921-925.
57. Soffers JH, Hikspoors JP, Mekonen HK, et al. The growth pattern of the human intestine and its mesentery. *BMC Dev Biol*. 2015;15:31.
58. Gao N, White P, Kaestner KH. Establishment of intestinal identity and epithelial-mesenchymal signaling by Cdx2. *Dev Cell*. 2009;16:588-599.
59. Mao J, Kim BM, Rajurkar M, et al. Hedgehog signaling controls mesenchymal growth in the developing mammalian digestive tract. *Development*. 2010;137:1721-1729.
60. Geske MJ, Zhang X, Patel KK, et al. Fgf9 signaling regulates small intestinal elongation and mesenchymal development. *Development*. 2008;135:2959-2968.
61. Cervantes S, Yamaguchi TP, Hebrok M. Wnt5a is essential for intestinal elongation in mice. *Dev Biol*. 2009;326:285-294.
62. Davis NM, Kurpios NA, Sun X, et al. The chirality of gut rotation derives from left-right asymmetric changes in the architecture of the dorsal mesentery. *Dev Cell*. 2008;15:134-145.
63. Savin T, Kurpios NA, Shyer AE, et al. On the growth and form of the gut. *Nature*. 2011;476:57-62.
64. Bosse T, Piaseckyj CM, Burghard E, et al. Gata4 is essential for the maintenance of jejunal-ileal identities in the adult mouse small intestine. *Mol Cell Biol*. 2006;26:9060-9070.
65. Beck F. Homeobox genes in gut development. *Gut*. 2002;51:450-454.
67. Kluth D. Embryology of anorectal malformations. *Semin Pediatr Surg*. 2010;19:201-208.
68. Fritsch H, Aigner F, Ludwikowski B, et al. Epithelial and muscular regionalization of the human developing anorectum. *Anat Rec (Hoboken)*. 2007;290:1449-1458.
69. Gupta A, Bischoff A, Pena A, et al. The great divide: septation and malformation of the cloaca, and its implications for surgeons. *Pediatr Surg Int*. 2014;30:1089-1095.
70. Duboule D, Dolle P. The structural and functional organization of the murine HOX gene family resembles that of Drosophila homeotic genes. *EMBO J*. 1989;8:1497-1505.
71. Illig R, Fritsch H, Schwarzer C. Spatio-temporal expression of HOX genes in human hindgut development. *Dev Dyn*. 2013;242:53-66.
72. Zhang X, Stappenbeck TS, White AC, et al. Reciprocal epithelial-mesenchymal FGF signaling is required for cecal development. *Development*. 2006;133:173-180.
73. Warot X, Fromental-Ramain C, Fraulob V, et al. Gene dosage-dependent effects of the Hoxa-13 and Hoxd-13 mutations on morphogenesis of the terminal parts of the digestive and urogenital tracts. *Development*. 1997;124:4781-4791.
74. van de Ven C, Bialecka M, Neijts R, et al. Concerted involvement of Cdx/Hox genes and Wntsignaling in morphogenesis of the caudal neural tube and cloacal derivatives from the posterior growth zone. *Development*. 2011;138:3451-3462.
75. Greco TL, Takada S, Newhouse MM, et al. Analysis of the vestigial tail mutation demonstrates that Wnt-3a gene dosage regulates mouse axial development. *Genes Dev*. 1996;10:313-324.
76. Li FF, Zhang T, Bai YZ, et al. Spatiotemporal expression of Wnt5a during the development of the hindgut and anorectum in human embryos. *Int J Colorectal Dis*. 2011;26:983-988.
77. Ramalho-Santos M, Melton DA, McMahon AP. Hedgehog signals regulate multiple aspects of gastrointestinal development. *Development*. 2000;127:2763-2772.
78. Mo R, Kim JH, Zhang J, et al. Anorectal malformations caused by defects in sonic hedgehog signaling. *Am J Pathol*. 2001;159:765-774.
81. Amiel J, Sproat-Emison E, Garcia-Barcelo M, et al. Hirschsprung disease, associated syndromes and genetics: a review. *J Med Genet*. 2008;45:1-14.

83 Development of Gastric Secretory Function

Joshua D. Prozialeck | Barry K. Wershil

INTRODUCTION

The stomach plays a number of roles in the digestive process and in host defense. Not only does the stomach serve as a reservoir for ingested foods and an important site of digestion; it is also exposed to a wide variety of swallowed bacteria, fungi, viruses, and parasites, and as such, it has a role in both innate and adaptive immunity. These functions are performed, in part, by a number of secretory processes, and the production of gastric acid is unique among them. The acidic environment created in the stomach also provides protective functions, such as gastric mucus and trefoil production, which require additional secretory activities.

The transition from the fetus to the newborn is accompanied by a rapid maturation of the secretory capacity of the stomach, but these processes develop in an asynchronous manner. In this chapter, we review the developmental biology and the developmental physiology of gastric secretory activity. Much of this information is derived from the experimental examination of either nonmammalian or lower mammalian species, so how this relates to human gastric development is still not entirely known.

ORGANOGENESIS

The stomach begins as an outpouching of the foregut at 4 weeks' gestation. It undergoes a 90-degree rotation at 8 weeks that establishes the left-sided greater curvature.[1] Stomach elongation occurs at variable rates, with the greater curvature forming from more rapid growth along the dorsum of the stomach. The combined effects of rotation and differential growth result in a transverse orientation from the upper-left quadrant to the midline. The fixation of the stomach is at two points, the gastroesophageal and gastroduodenal junctions, which provides considerable mobility. The final J-shaped appearance of the stomach can be seen at 22 weeks' gestation.[1] The innervation of the stomach by the vagus nerve reflects the rotational event, with the right vagus innervating the dorsal (right) wall and the left vagus innervating the anterior (left) wall.

The stomach can be divided into three anatomic regions or two functional zones. From an anatomic perspective, the proximal two-thirds of the stomach consists of the fundus and body, whereas the distal third is referred to as the *antrum*. The two functional zones refer to the oxyntic (acid) glands located primarily in the fundus and body (which constitute 80% of the glandular stomach) and pyloric glands, which make up the remaining 20% in the distal part of the stomach (antrum). The hallmark of the pyloric gland is the G or gastrin cell (Fig. 83.1). Glandular development is seen with the short gastric pits identifiable at 6 to 8 weeks' gestation. Definitive gastric glands are evident by the fourth month of gestation, with maturation continuing to the fifth and sixth months.[2]

The processes involved in stomach development are complex and still incompletely understood. There is exquisite spatial and temporal control of gene expression during development, and cell-to-cell contact (epithelial-to-mesenchymal transition) also plays a role in regionalization and elongation.[3,4] Many of the genes identified during development are shared between the stomach and the small intestine, with a small subset that is specific to the stomach.[5] Some of the more important signaling pathways involved in organ development and regionalization include sonic hedgehog, Indian hedgehog, bone morphogenetic protein, Wnt signaling, and fibroblast growth factor pathways.[4] This represents only a fraction of the genes and transcription factors that are expressed during organ development[5]; the relative importance of each remains to be defined. There does not appear to be transcription factors that function solely in stomach development, thus a "master" regulator has not been discovered.[6] The expression of genes is a critical factor in organogenesis, but what is also clear is that there is a precisely timed and orchestrated procession of gene expression and gene repression that has to occur for both the stomach and the intestinal tract to develop normally.

All gastric epithelial cells are thought to arise from a common progenitor cell located in the gastric gland,[7,8] which is supported by studies in murine species.[9,10] Originally, gastric progenitor cells were thought to be located only in the isthmus, but cell marker studies reveal that they may be located in different areas of the gland and that these cells can be mobile.[11] These studies also suggest that some progenitor cells may give rise to all the various types of gastric glandular cells, whereas others may be directed to more restricted lineages. The various mucosal cell types of the stomach express different transcription factors that control genes for cell type differentiation and function.[12-15]

GASTRIC CELL TYPE DEVELOPMENT

The gastric mucosa contains glands that are composed of secretory epithelial cells (see Fig. 83.1). The major cell types in the oxyntic mucosa are parietal cells, chief cells, and mucous neck cells. Parietal cells contain the machinery for acid secretion and are the most abundant secretory cell in the stomach. Mucous neck cells secrete a viscous glycoprotein to help maintain

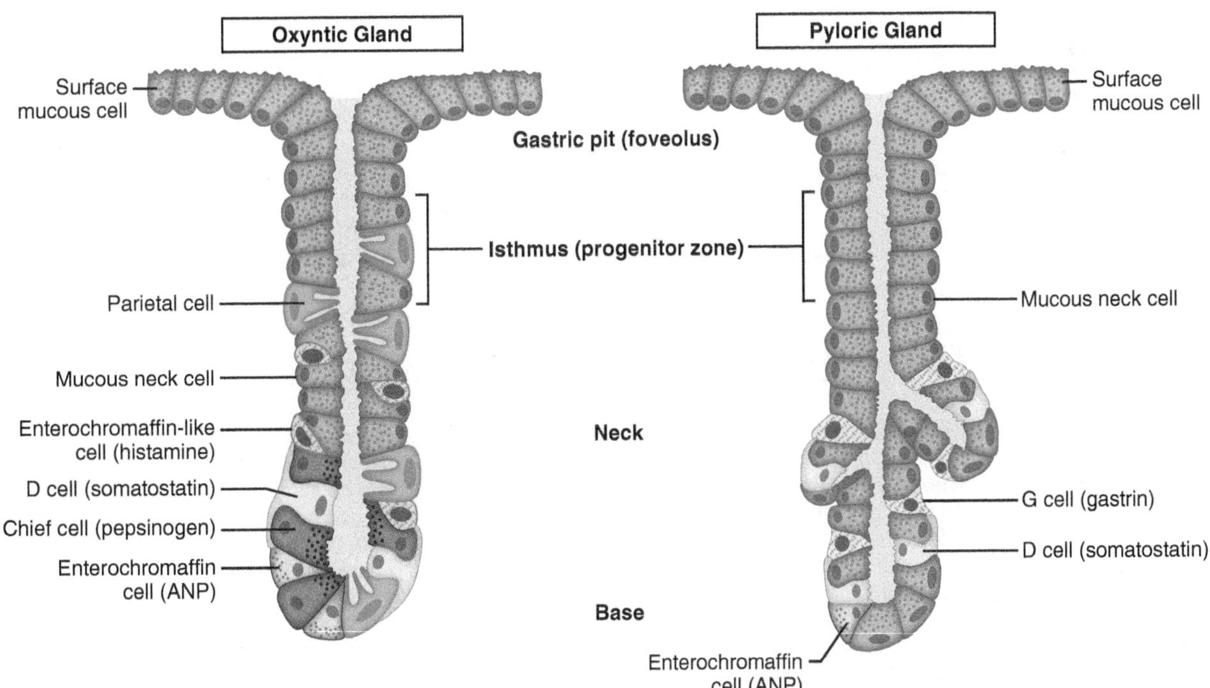

Fig. 83.1 Functional mucosal anatomy. Somatostatin-containing D cells contain cytoplasmic processes that terminate near acid-secreting parietal and histamine-secreting enterochromaffin-like cells in the oxyntic gland area (fundus and corpus) and gastrin-secreting G cells in the pyloric gland area (antrum). The functional correlate of this anatomic coupling is a tonic paracrine restraint exerted by somatostatin on acid secretion that is exerted directly on the parietal cell, as well as indirectly by inhibiting histamine and gastrin secretion. *ANP,* Atrial natriuretic peptide. (From Schubert ML, Peura DA. Control of gastric acid secretion in health and disease. *Gastroenterology.* 2008;134:1842–1860.)

the integrity of the gastric epithelium, whereas chief cells are responsible for the production of pepsinogen, which is the inactive form of pepsin. Additional secretory cells in the glands include histamine-producing enterochromaffin-like (ECL) cells, somatostatin-producing D cells, and enterochromaffin cells that produce a variety of regulatory peptides.

In fetal mice, gastric glands are present in the gastric epithelium at 18 days' gestation without evidence of the acid-producing pump, H^+, K^+-ATPase.[16] On day 19 of gestation, approximately 1 to 2 days before birth, parietal cells are observed along with α and β subunits of H^+,K^+-ATPase. In humans, parietal cells are present, marked with positive immunostaining of H^+,K^+-ATPase, as early as 13 weeks' gestation.[17] At this point in development, parietal cells are found throughout the entire stomach, but by the time of birth, parietal cells will disappear from the antrum, creating a transition zone from the body to the antrum.[18] However, in approximately 20% of adults, parietal cells can be found throughout the stomach extending to the pylorus.[19]

Gastrin-producing G cells in the pyloric mucosa are detected in the fetus as early as 12 weeks' gestation and are located only in the antrum,[18,20] and their numbers increase with gestational age. Neonates exhibit higher serum gastrin levels than what is considered normal in adults,[21] and this "physiologic hypergastrinemia" continues in the first 2 months of life.[22,23] This is thought to be due to the relative unresponsiveness of parietal cells to gastrin stimulation during this period of time (as discussed later).

In rats, histamine-producing mature ECL cells do not appear until after birth.[24] However, histamine immunoreactivity is observed in the oxyntic mucosa at day 18 of gestation.[25] On postnatal day 21, the number of histamine-immunoreactive ECL cells approaches adult levels. In humans, ECL cells are first observed at week 13 of gestation.[2] D cells first appear in humans at 10 weeks' gestation, although somatostatin-immunoreactive cells are noted as early as 8 weeks' gestation.[2,26]

REGULATION OF ACID SECRETION

The secretion of acid is a critical functional component of gastric physiology, with acid acting in the process of digestion by hydrolyzing proteins to more absorbable peptides and participating in host defense by preventing the growth of swallowed organisms. The regulation of acid secretion involves input from neuronal, hormonal, and endocrine circuits (Fig. 83.2) that all interplay to control acid secretion. It is widely accepted that the major pathway of gastric acid stimulation occurs along the gastrin-ECL cell-parietal cell axis (Fig. 83.3).

Gastrin, released by G cells in the antrum, stimulates acid secretion and promotes cell growth by binding to cholecystokinin B receptors on parietal cells and ECL cells.[27,28] Gastrin release is stimulated by food peptides in the stomach, an increase in gastric pH, and gastrin-releasing peptide from vagal activation; inhibition of gastrin secretion occurs secondary to acid secretion.[29] The mechanism of gastrin synthesis has been well studied and extensively reviewed.[27,29-31] Gastrin starts as a large precursor molecule, pre-progastrin, which is processed in the endoplasmic reticulum to progastrin. Sulfation and phosphorylation occur in the Golgi complex. In secretory granules, progastrin is

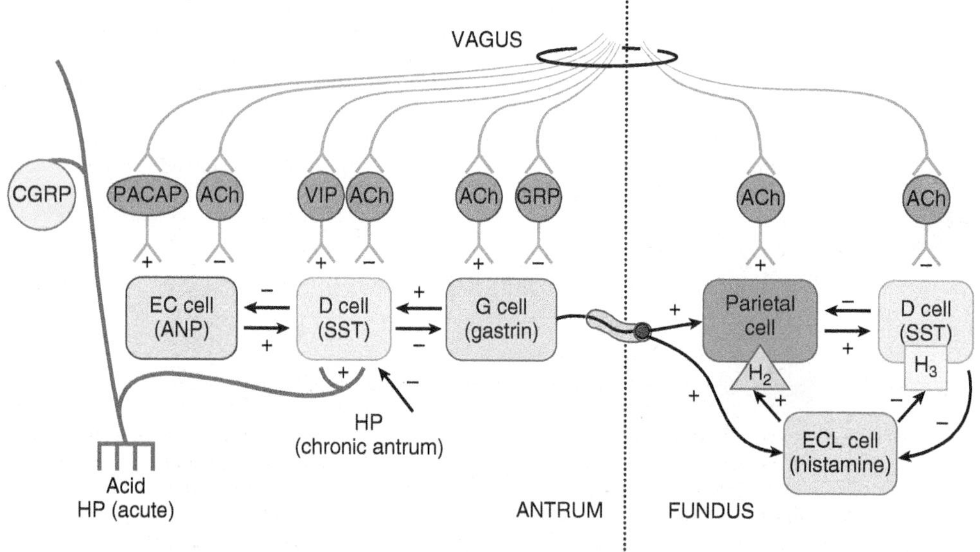

Fig. 83.2 Model illustrating the neural, paracrine, and hormonal regulation of gastric acid secretion. Efferent vagal fibers synapse with intramural gastric cholinergic (acetylcholine, *ACh*) and peptidergic (gastrin-releasing peptide, *GRP*; vasoactive intestinal peptide, *VIP*; and pituitary adenylate cyclase-activating peptide, *PACAP*) neurons. In the fundus (oxyntic mucosa), ACh neurons stimulate acid secretion directly via M_3 receptors on the parietal cell and indirectly by inhibiting somatostatin *(SST)* secretion, thus eliminating its restraint on parietal cells and histamine-containing enterochromaffin-like *(ECL)* cells. In the antrum (pyloric mucosa), ACh neurons stimulate gastrin secretion directly and indirectly by inhibiting SST secretion, the latter by a direct effect on the D cell and an indirect effect mediated by inhibition of atrial natriuretic peptide *(ANP)* secretion from enterochromaffin *(EC)* cells. GRP neurons, activated by intraluminal protein, also stimulate gastrin secretion. VIP neurons, activated by low-grade distension, stimulate SST and thus inhibit gastrin secretion. PACAP neurons stimulate SST, via the release of ANP, and thus also inhibit gastrin secretion. Dual paracrine pathways link SST-containing D cells to parietal cells and to ECL cells in the fundus. Histamine released from ECL cells acts via H_3 receptors to inhibit SST secretion. This serves to accentuate the decrease in SST secretion induced by cholinergic stimuli and thus augments acid secretion. In the antrum, dual paracrine pathways link SST-containing D cells to gastrin cells and to EC cells. Release of acid into the lumen of the stomach restores SST secretion in both the fundus and the antrum; the latter is mediated via release of calcitonin gene-related peptide *(CGRP)* from extrinsic sensory neurons. Acute infection with *Helicobacter pylori (HP)* also activates CGRP neurons to stimulate SST and thus inhibit gastrin secretion. In duodenal ulcer patients chronically infected with HP, the organism or cytokines released from the inflammatory infiltrate inhibit SST and thus stimulate gastrin (and acid) secretion. (From Schubert ML, Peura DA. Control of gastric acid secretion in health and disease. *Gastroenterology.* 2008;134:1842–1860.)

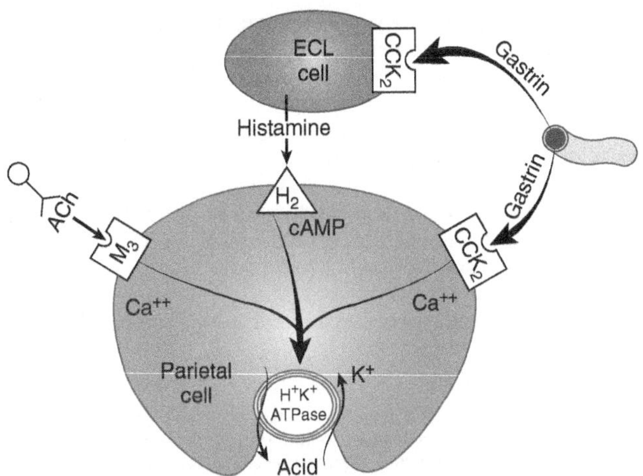

Fig. 83.3 Model illustrating parietal cell receptors and transduction pathways. The principal stimulants of acid secretion at the level of the parietal cell are histamine (paracrine), gastrin (hormonal), and acetylcholine (*ACh;* neurocrine). Histamine, released from enterochromaffin-like *(ECL)* cells, binds to H_2 receptors, which activate adenylate cyclase and generate cyclic adenosine monophosphate *(cAMP)*. Gastrin, released from G cells, binds to cholecystokinin B *(CCK_2)* receptors, which activate phospholipase C to induce the release of cytosolic calcium (Ca^{2+}). Gastrin stimulates the parietal cell directly and, more importantly, indirectly by releasing histamine from ECL cells. *ACh*, released from intramural neurons, binds to M_3 receptors, which are coupled to an increase in intracellular calcium concentration. The intracellular cAMP- and calcium-dependent signaling systems activate downstream protein kinases, ultimately leading to fusion and activation of H^+,K^+–ATPase, the proton pump. (From Schubert ML, Peura DA. Control of gastric acid secretion in health and disease. *Gastroenterology.* 2008;134:1842–1860.)

further processed by prohormone convertase enzymes and carboxypeptidase E to form glycine-extended gastrins and the carboxyl-terminal flanking peptides. Glycine-extended gastrin 34 is converted to its amidated form by peptidylglycine α-amidating monooxygenase, and bioactive gastrins, specifically gastrin 17 and gastrin 34, are produced after prohormone convertase 2 cleaves at lysine 53-lysine 54.

Histamine is an important stimulator of parietal cells. It is produced by ECL cells by the decarboxylation of l-histidine by the enzyme histidine decarboxylase. Histamine mediates acid secretion directly by activating H_2 receptors on parietal cells, which generates adenosine 3′,5′-cyclic monophosphate by the action of adenylate cyclase.[32] Histamine also activates H_3 receptors on somatostatin cells, which results in inhibition of somatostatin and thus indirectly promotes acid secretion.[33-35]

Acetylcholine is also an acid secretagogue. It is released from presynaptic enteric neurons and activates muscarinic M_3 receptors on parietal cells, whereas activation of muscarinic M_2 and M_4 receptors on D cells inhibits somatostatin, further promoting acid secretion. Other agents that can affect acid production include caffeine (stimulates), steroids (stimulates), and *Helicobacter pylori* (stimulates or inhibits depending on acute versus chronic infection).

The inhibition of gastric acid secretion is primarily mediated by somatostatin secreted by D cells located in both the oxyntic and the pyloric glands.[36,37] D cells communicate with parietal cells, ECL cells, and G cells through both paracrine and endocrine interactions.[38] Somatostatin receptors (somatostatin receptor 2, SSTR2) are found on parietal and ECL cells and facilitate a direct inhibitory effect on the parietal cell and the inhibition of gastrin-stimulated histamine release from the ECL cell.[39-44] There appears to be plasticity in this gastrin–ECL cell–parietal cell axis, as demonstrated in a murine model where SSTR2 had been genetically deleted (SSTR2-knockout mouse).[38,45] Zhao and colleagues found that gastrin and acid secretion remain unchanged in this SSTR2-deficient mouse, suggesting a shift from a paracrine pathway involving somatostatin to a neurocrine pathway that maintained the regulation of acid production.These results also suggest that there is a direct enhanced stimulatory effect of gastrin and vagal excitation on the parietal cell as a result of a shift from the gastrin–ECL pathway influencing parietal cell acid secretion.

PARIETAL CELL SECRETION IN THE NEONATE

Gastric secretions are relatively alkaline after birth in term infants, but within a few hours, the pH falls to less than 4.[46] Basal acid output, which is maintained predominantly by histamine and acetylcholine, exhibits no significant change between days 1 and 2 of life in term infants.[47] Basal acid output increases in preterm infants from the first week of life to the fourth week, when levels normalize to those seen in term infants.[48] When comparing preterm infants with term infants, Marino and colleagues did not find a significant difference in the volume of gastric secretion at 1 hour of life, when it was corrected for weight.[49] In the same study, term infants secreted significantly more acid and in a significantly higher concentration than preterm infants.

Acid secretion in newborns appears to be somewhat stimulus dependent. Betazole, a histamine analog, stimulated acid production in newborns in the first 12 to 24 hours of life.[50] By contrast, there was no difference between basal acid output and maximal acid output in healthy term infants after pentagastrin, a synthetic gastrin agonist, stimulation in the first 2 days of life.[47] This suggests that parietal cells are not responsive to pentagastrin during the first 2 days or that basal secretion is maximal in newborns. In rats, neither gastrin nor histamine stimulates acid secretion until day 20 of life.[51] Although the mechanism is unclear, gastric acid secretion can be stimulated by meals during the first 48 hours of life.[40] Thus it appears that the response of the newborn stomach to stimuli is different from that of older infants, children, and adults, but the significance of this difference remains unclear.

INTRINSIC FACTOR

Parietal cells also synthesize and secrete intrinsic factor, which binds to cobalamin (vitamin B_{12}) forms that are active in the body and facilitates absorption in the distal ileum. Intrinsic factor has been identified in both the pylorus and the body of human fetuses as early as 11 to 13 weeks' gestation,[52] but only small amounts of intrinsic factor can be measured at birth. There is no difference in basal intrinsic factor secretion between term and preterm infants.[49] After histamine stimulation, gastric secretions from birth to days 10 and 11 of life contain only small amounts of intrinsic factor, but thereafter the concentration rises to nearly adult levels by the third month of life.[50] Intrinsic factor receptor activity is detected throughout the entire small bowel in 10- to 19-week-old fetuses.[53] By 25 weeks' gestation, activity is noted only in the distal ileum, which is the site of absorption of intrinsic factor-bound vitamin B_{12} in adults.

GASTRIC LIPASE

Human gastric lipase is produced by chief cells and is collocated with pepsin.[54] Cells that have the appearance of chief cells appear at 12 to 13 weeks' gestation.[55] Gastric lipase appears in fetal stomachs as early as 10 to 11 weeks' gestation.[56,57] By 16 weeks' gestation, gastric lipase exhibits an adult-type distribution within the stomach—that is, a decreasing gradient from the fundus towards the pylorus.[57] Lipolytic activity is present in neonates with gestational ages ranging from 26 to 40 weeks.[58] Infants born at less than 26 weeks' gestation have low gastric lipase activity, and this increases to a peak activity level between 30 and 32 weeks' gestation.[59] Enzyme levels reach adult values by 3 months of life, and enzyme activity in older infants and children is similar to that of adults, indicating early maturation of this enzyme.[56,60] During the neonatal period, given the low concentrations of pancreatic lipase and bile salts, gastric and lingual lipases are an alternative and important pathway for fat digestion.[61,62]

PEPSINOGEN

Chief cells are also the cellular source of pepsinogen, the inactive precursor of pepsin. On secretion and exposure to stomach acid, inactive pepsinogen undergoes a conformational change, exposing its catalytically active site. This now-active form of pepsinogen generates pepsin from inactive pepsinogen by proteolysis. Pepsin plays an important role in protein digestion during the gastric phase of digestion.

Pepsinogen is identified by immunofluorescence in humans as early as 8 weeks' gestation.[63] By the sixteenth week of gestation, pepsin activity is seen in the stomach.[64] Pepsin secretion is lower in preterm infants than in term infants.[65] Basal pepsinogen secretion does not change significantly in the first few weeks of life in preterm infants, and before 31 weeks' gestation, meal stimulation does not significantly increase pepsinogen secretion.[66] Meal-stimulated pepsinogen secretion increases twofold by 36 weeks' gestation.

TREFOILS

Trefoil factors are peptides synthesized in and secreted by the mucin-producing cells of epithelial surfaces.[67] These peptides are thought to play an important role in the maintenance and protection of mucosal surfaces in the gastrointestinal tract through an interaction with mucins, enhancement of "restitution" (i.e., rapid mucosal repair by cell migration), modulation of mucosal regeneration by differentiation from stem cells, and modulation of the mucosal immune response.[68-72] Little is known about the developmental biology of trefoil proteins. There are at least three forms of the trefoil peptides (TFF1, TFF2, TFF3), and all are present in the stomach and duodenum of the developing fetus between 15 and 22 weeks' gestation.[67] The fetal distribution of these peptides (strong staining of all three trefoil peptides in the stomach) is different from the site-specific distribution seen in adults. (TFF1 is highly expressed in gastric surface epithelial cells; TFF2 is mostly detected in mucous neck cells of pyloric glands; and TFF3 is mostly expressed in the small and large intestines, with some expression in surface mucous cells of the cardia and antrum.) The fetal distribution is similar to the findings seen in inflammatory states, suggesting that increased numbers of trefoil peptides are seen in proliferating tissues.[71,73,74]

CONCLUSION

Our knowledge of human gastric secretory function remains somewhat rudimentary. We are still very reliant on studies from different species and on inferential speculation. There is much that remains to be learned about the course of gastric development, not just in structural terms but also from a developmental physiology perspective. This holds more than just academic interest because understanding the differences in maturation and the physiologic control of acid production in preterm and term infants compared with adults may have direct clinical applicability. For example, the use of acid-suppressing medication has become pervasive in the neonatal intensive care setting. It is not hard to envision how a greater understanding of the pathways regulating acid production in preterm infants may have a significant impact on the indications for and the class of an agent used to suppress acid production.

A complete reference list is available at www.ExpertConsult.com. 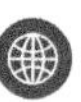

SELECT REFERENCES

1. Hawass NE, al-Badawi MG, Fatani JA, Meshari AA, Edrees YB. Morphology and growth of the fetal stomach. *Invest Radiol*. 1991;26(11):998-1004.
2. De Lemos C. The ultrastructure of endocrine cells in the corpus of the stomach of human fetuses. *Am J Anat*. 1977;148(3):359-383.
3. Fukuda K, Yasugi S. The molecular mechanisms of stomach development in vertebrates. *Dev Growth Differ*. 2005;47(6):375-382.
4. Khurana S, Mills JC. The gastric mucosa development and differentiation. *Prog Mol Biol Transl Sci*. 2010;96:93-115.
5. Choi MY, Romer AI, Hu M, et al. A dynamic expression survey identifies transcription factors relevant in mouse digestive tract development. *Development*. 2006;133(20):4119-4129.
6. Sherwood RI, Chen TY, Melton DA. Transcriptional dynamics of endodermal organ formation. *Dev Dyn*. 2009;238(1):29-42.
7. Brittan M, Wright NA. Gastrointestinal stem cells. *J Pathol*. 2002;197(4):492-509.
8. Han ME, Oh SO. Gastric stem cells and gastric cancer stem cells. *Anat Cell Biol*. 2013;46(1):8-18.
9. Canfield V, West AB, Goldenring JR, Levenson R. Genetic ablation of parietal cells in transgenic mice: a new model for analyzing cell lineage relationships in the gastric mucosa. *Proc Natl Acad Sci U S A*. 1996;93(6):2431-2435.
10. Bjerknes M, Cheng H. Multipotential stem cells in adult mouse gastric epithelium. *Am J Physiol Gastrointest Liver Physiol*. 2002;283(3):G767-777.
11. Qiao XT, Gumucio DL. Current molecular markers for gastric progenitor cells and gastric cancer stem cells. *J Gastroenterol*. 2011;46(7):855-865.
12. Verzi MP, Khan AH, Ito S, Shivdasani RA. Transcription factor foxq1 controls mucin gene expression and granule content in mouse stomach surface mucous cells. *Gastroenterology*. 2008;135(2):591-600.
13. Ramsey VG, Doherty JM, Chen CC, Stappenbeck TS, Konieczny SF, Mills JC. The maturation of mucus-secreting gastric epithelial progenitors into digestive-enzyme secreting zymogenic cells requires Mist1. *Development*. 2007;134(1):211-222.
14. Alaynick WA, Way JM, Wilson SA, et al. ERRgamma regulates cardiac, gastric, and renal potassium homeostasis. *Mol Endocrinol*. 2010;24(2):299-309.
15. Horst D, Gu X, Bhasin M, et al. Requirement of the epithelium-specific Ets transcription factor Spdef for mucous gland cell function in the gastric antrum. *J Biol Chem*. 2010;285(45):35047-35055.
16. Pettitt JM, Toh BH, Callaghan JM, Gleeson PA, Van Driel IR. Gastric parietal cell development: expression of the H+/K+ ATPase subunits coincides with the biogenesis of the secretory membranes. *Immunol Cell Biol*. 1993;71(Pt 3):191-200.
17. Kelly EJ, Brownlee KG. When is the fetus first capable of gastric acid, intrinsic factor and gastrin secretion? *Biol Neonate*. 1993;63(3):153-156.
18. Kelly EJ, Lagopoulos M, Primrose JN. Immunocytochemical localisation of parietal cells and G cells in the developing human stomach. *Gut*. 1993;34(8):1057-1059.
19. Naik KSLM, Primrose JN. Distribution of antral G-cells in relation to the parietal cells of the stomach and anatomical boundaries. *Clinical Anatomy*. 1990;3(1):17-24.
20. Grasso S, Buffa R, Martino E, Bartalena L, Curzio M, Salomone E. Gastrin (G) cells are the cellular site of the gastric thyrotropin-releasing hormone in human fetuses and newborns. A chromatographic, radioimmunological, and immunocytochemical study. *J Clin Endocrinol Metab*. 1992;74(6):1421-1426.
21. Euler AR, Byrne WJ, Cousins LM, Ament ME, Walsh JH. Increased serum gastrin concentrations and gastric acid hyposecretion in the immediate newborn period. *Gastroenterology*. 1977;72(6):1271-1273.
22. Treem W, Hu P, Sloan S. Normal and proton pump inhibitor-mediated gastrin levels in infants 1 to 11 months old. *J Pediatr Gastroenterol Nutr*. 2013;57(4):520-526.
23. Moazam F, Kirby WJ, Rodgers BM, McGuigan JE. Physiology of serum gastrin production in neonates and infants. *Ann Surg*. 1984;199(4):389-392.
24. Ekelund M, Hakanson R, Hedenbro J, Rehfeld JF, Sundler F. Endocrine cells and parietal cells in the stomach of the developing rat. *Acta Physiol Scand*. 1985;124(4):483-497.
25. Nissinen MJ, Hakanson R, Panula P. Ontogeny of histamine-immunoreactive cells in rat stomach. *Cell Tissue Res*. 1992;267(2):241-249.
26. Stein BA, Buchan AM, Morris J, Polak JM. The ontogeny of regulatory peptide-containing cells in the human fetal stomach: an immunocytochemical study. *J Histochem Cytochem*. 1983;31(9):1117-1125.

27. Chu S, Schubert ML. Gastric secretion. *CurrOpin Gastroenterol*. 2013;29(6):636-641.
28. Sandvik AK, Waldum HL. CCK-B (gastrin) receptor regulates gastric histamine release and acid secretion. *Am J Physiol*. 1991;260(6 Pt 1):G925-G928.
29. Chueca E, Lanas A, Piazuelo E. Role of gastrin-peptides in Barrett's and colorectal carcinogenesis. *World J Gastroenterol*. 2012;18(45):6560-6570.
30. Schubert ML, Peura DA. Control of gastric acid secretion in health and disease. *Gastroenterology*. 2008;134(7):1842-1860.
31. Dickinson CJ, Seva C, Yamada T. Gastrin processing: from biochemical obscurity to unique physiological actions. *News in Physiological Sciences*. 1997;12(9):9-15.
32. Soll AH, Wollin A. Histamine and cyclic AMP in isolated canine parietal cells. *Am J Physiol*. 1979;237(5):E444-E450.
33. Vuyyuru L, Schubert ML, Harrington L, Arimura A, Makhlouf GM. Dual inhibitory pathways link antral somatostatin and histamine secretion in human, dog, and rat stomach. *Gastroenterology*. 1995;109(5):1566-1574.
34. Vuyyuru L, Harrington L, Arimura A, Schubert ML. Reciprocal inhibitory paracrine pathways link histamine and somatostatin secretion in the fundus of the stomach. *Am J Physiol*. 1997;273(1 Pt 1):G106-G111.
35. Vuyyuru L, Schubert ML. Histamine, acting via H3 receptors, inhibits somatostatin and stimulates acid secretion in isolated mouse stomach. *Gastroenterology*. 1997;113(5):1545-1552.
36. Makhlouf GM, Schubert ML. Gastric somatostatin: a paracrine regulator of acid secretion. *Metabolism*. 1990;39(9 suppl 2):138-142.
37. Lloyd KC, Wang J, Aurang K, Gronhed P, Coy DH, Walsh JH. Activation of somatostatin receptor subtype 2 inhibits acid secretion in rats. *Am J Physiol*. 1995;268(1 Pt 1):G102-G106.
38. Corleto VD. Somatostatin and the gastrointestinal tract. *CurrOpin Endocrinol Diabetes Obes*. 2010;17(1):63-68.
39. Sandor A, Kidd M, Lawton GP, Miu K, Tang LH, Modlin IM. Neurohormonal modulation of rat enterochromaffin-like cell histamine secretion. *Gastroenterology*. 1996;110(4):1084-1092.
40. Prinz C, Kajimura M, Scott DR, Mercier F, Helander HF, Sachs G. Histamine secretion from rat enterochromaffinlike cells. *Gastroenterology*. 1993;105(2):449-461.
41. Prinz C, Sachs G, Walsh JH, Coy DH, Wu SV. The somatostatin receptor subtype on rat enterochromaffinlike cells. *Gastroenterology*. 1994;107(4):1067-1074.
42. Park J, Chiba T, Yamada T. Mechanisms for direct inhibition of canine gastric parietal cells by somatostatin. *J Biol Chem*. 1987;262(29):14190-14196.
43. Piqueras L, Tache Y, Martinez V. Somatostatin receptor type 2 mediates bombesin-induced inhibition of gastric acid secretion in mice. *J Physiol*. 2003;549(Pt 3):889-901.
44. Allen JP, Canty AJ, Schulz S, Humphrey PP, Emson PC, Young HM. Identification of cells expressing somatostatin receptor 2 in the gastrointestinal tract of Sstr2 knockout/lacZ knockin mice. *J Comp Neurol*. 2002;454(3):329-340.
45. Zhao CM, Martinez V, Piqueras L, Wang L, Tache Y, Chen D. Control of gastric acid secretion in somatostatin receptor 2 deficient mice: shift from endocrine/paracrine to neurocrine pathways. *Endocrinology*. 2008;149(2):498-505.
46. Avery GB, Randolph JG, Weaver T. Gastric acidity in the first day of life. *Pediatrics*. 1966;37(6):1005-1007.
47. Euler AR, Byrne WJ, Meis PJ, Leake RD, Ament ME. Basal and pentagastrin-stimulated acid secretion in newborn human infants. *Pediatr Res*. 1979;13(1):36-37.
48. Hyman PE, Clarke DD, Everett SL, et al. Gastric acid secretory function in preterm infants. *J Pediatr*. 1985;106(3):467-471.
49. Marino LR, Bacon BR, Hines JD, Halpin TC. Parietal cell function of full-term and premature infants: unstimulated gastric acid and intrinsic factor secretion. *J Pediatr Gastroenterol Nutr*. 1984;3(1):23-27.
50. Agunod M, Yamaguchi N, Lopez R, Luhby AL, Glass GB. Correlative study of hydrochloric acid, pepsin, and intrinsic factor secretion in newborns and infants. *Am J Dig Dis*. 1969;14(6):400-414.

Development of the Enteric Nervous System and Gastrointestinal Motility

84

Julie Khlevner | Andrew Del Colle | Kara Gross Margolis

INTRODUCTION

A critical modulator of gastrointestinal (GI) motility and secretion is the enteric nervous system (ENS). The ENS is a highly unique integrated neuronal circuitry, which, in contrast to other components of the peripheral nervous system, can and often does mediate reflex activity independent of the central nervous system (CNS). The ENS consists of two major plexuses (Fig. 84.1): the myenteric plexus (Auerbach plexus), located between the external circular and longitudinal muscle layers, and the submucosal plexus (Meissner plexus), which itself is divided even further in larger mammals.[1]

Although the ENS often acts independently, it also undergoes continuous, bidirectional communication with the CNS as well as other cell types, including immune, epithelial, and endocrine cells. All of these interactions play important roles in influencing the various physiologic roles within the intestine.

DEVELOPMENT OF THE ENTERIC NERVOUS SYSTEM

Enteric neurons and glial cells are derived from the migration of neural crest cells. Crest-derived cells from the vagal crest have been shown to colonize the entire bowel while those originating from the sacral crest contribute additional cells to the gut caudal to the umbilicus.[2,3] However, the vagal neural crest is the major source of ENS precursors.[2] Premigratory neural crest cells from either site are multipotent; these pre-enteric neural crest-derived cells (pre-ENCDCs) enter the foregut and begin to migrate through the bowel just prior to week 4 in utero.[4] As the ENCDCs migrate, they proliferate and differentiate into neurons, glia, and ganglia to form a network throughout the bowel (Fig. 84.2).[5] By week 7, this migration is complete.[6] Phenotypic expression of the neural crest cells is ultimately dictated by the enteric microenvironments they confront at their site of terminal differentiation.[7] After the initial gut colonization, ENCDCs undergo an inward radial migration, which results in the formation of the myenteric and submucosal plexuses.[8] Although beyond the scope of this chapter, it is important to note that each of these stages is highly regulated by an extensive matrix of receptors, ligands, morphogens, and signaling proteins, extensively reviewed elsewhere.[5,9] However, correct progression through all of these phases is critical for the functions discussed below.

SUCK AND SWALLOW

Ingestion of milk by the newborn infant depends on the ability to suck, in order to express milk from the breast or bottle into the oral cavity; to swallow, to propel milk from the oral cavity into the pharynx and then from the pharynx into the esophagus; and to coordinate sucking and swallowing with breathing.[10-12]

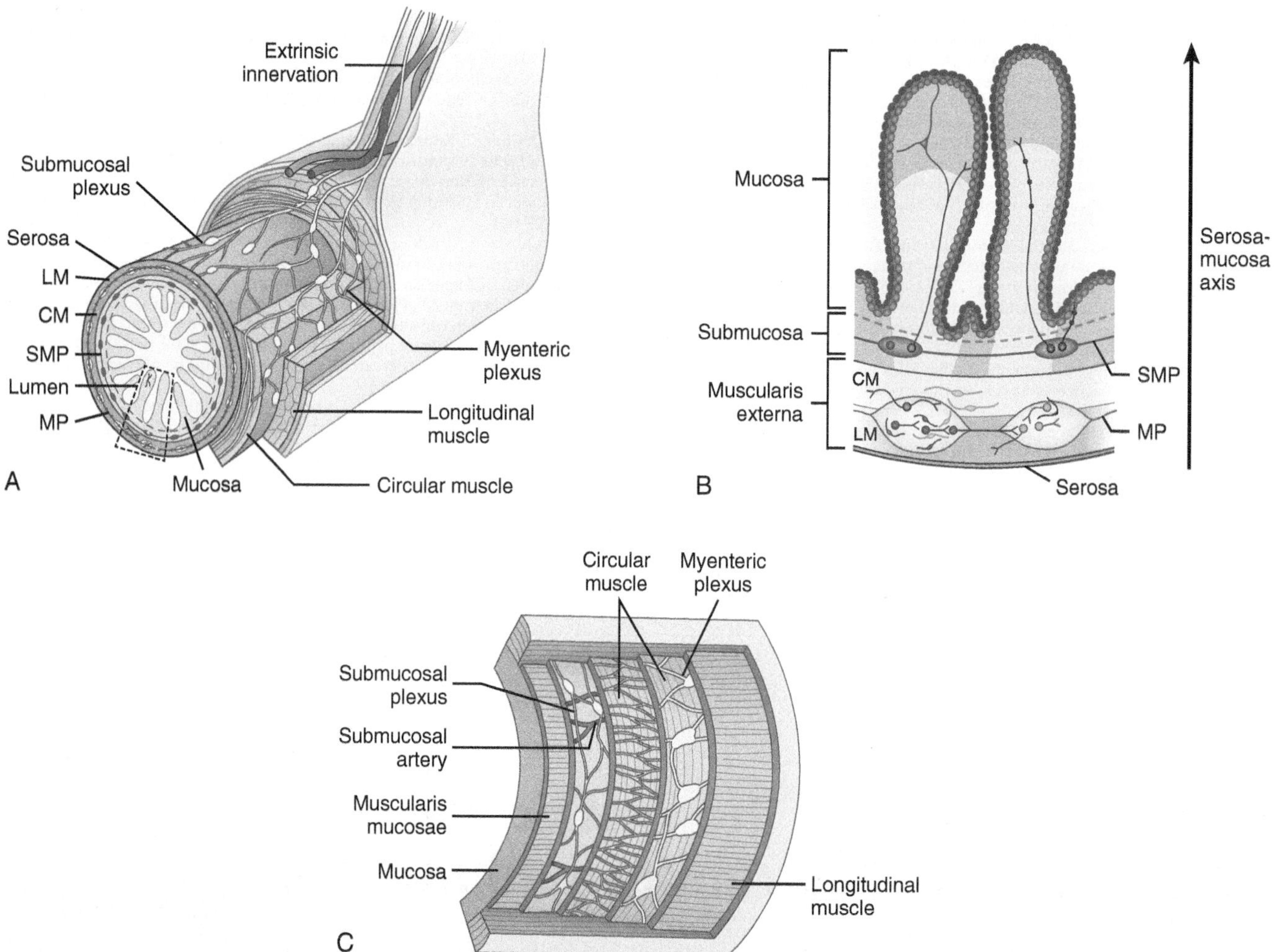

Fig. 84.1 (A) The organization of the ENS cross-sectional anatomy of intestinal and esophageal innervation: intestine (B) and esophagus (C). The boxed area (A) shows the neurons and glia of the mature ENS with the myenteric plexus *(MP)* located in the muscularis externa between the longitudinal *(LM)* and circular *(CM)* smooth muscle layers. The submucosal plexus *(SMP)* is located in the submucosal layer. *ENS*, Enteric nervous system. (Modified from Rao M, Gershon MD. Enteric nervous system development: what could possibly go wrong? *Nat Rev Neurosci.* 2018;19:552-565.)

This process can be divided into the four phases of deglutition. The first phase is the oral preparatory phase, during which milk is drawn into the mouth by negative suction, mixed with saliva forming a liquid bolus. The second phase is the oral phase, in which the tongue projects posteriorly while contacting the palate to propel the bolus into the pharynx and through the relaxed open upper esophageal sphincter (UES). The third phase is the pharyngeal phase, during which the pharyngeal constrictors contract sequentially, clearing the residue of the bolus through the UES and into the esophagus. During the final phase, the esophageal phase, esophageal peristalsis propels the bolus down the length of the esophagus through the relaxed lower esophageal sphincter (LES) into the stomach (Fig. 84.3).

The orientations of the neonatal tongue, gums, palate, larynx, epiglottis, and pharynx are specifically adapted to facilitate the entry of a liquid bolus into the esophagus. Sucking and swallowing is dependent on both the anatomic integrity of the feeding apparatus and the maturation of complex oropharyngeal neuromuscular control mechanisms. The primary mechanism of induction of bolus propagation progresses from swallow induced at a gestational age of approximately 26 weeks to esophageal distension at approximately 32 weeks. Most neonates are capable of a coordinated suck and swallow by 34 weeks.[11,12]

SUCKING (ORAL PREPARATORY PHASE)

Development of sucking begins in utero and continues well after birth. Mouthing and lingual movements begin as early as 15 weeks gestation and progress to coordinated sucks as early as 28 weeks.[10] Lingual movements begin with simple forward thrusting at approximately 21 weeks gestation and progress to cupping, which is a midline depression of the tongue, at approximately 28 weeks.[10] Anterior protrusion coordinated with posterior retraction of the tongue is consistently observed by 28 weeks gestation and can be triggered by oral-facial stimulation in utero.[10] The development of lingual movements coincides with myelination of the brain stem. In premature neonates, sucking patterns continue to mature through 36 weeks gestation.[11]

The oral cavity in the newborn infant is adapted to facilitate passage of a liquid bolus initiated by sucking (Fig. 84.4). The buccal fat pads and palate stabilize the lateral and superior walls of the cavity. The lips seal over the nipple, and the tongue presses against the soft palate to form a closed chamber in the oral cavity. The large tongue pulls inferiorly like a piston, creating a negative suction in the oral cavity, and the gums synchronously oppose this action to produce a positive expression pressure.[13] This sucking action is the same during bottle- and breast-feeding, with the exception of the tongue, which is projected farther forward during breast-feeding.[13]

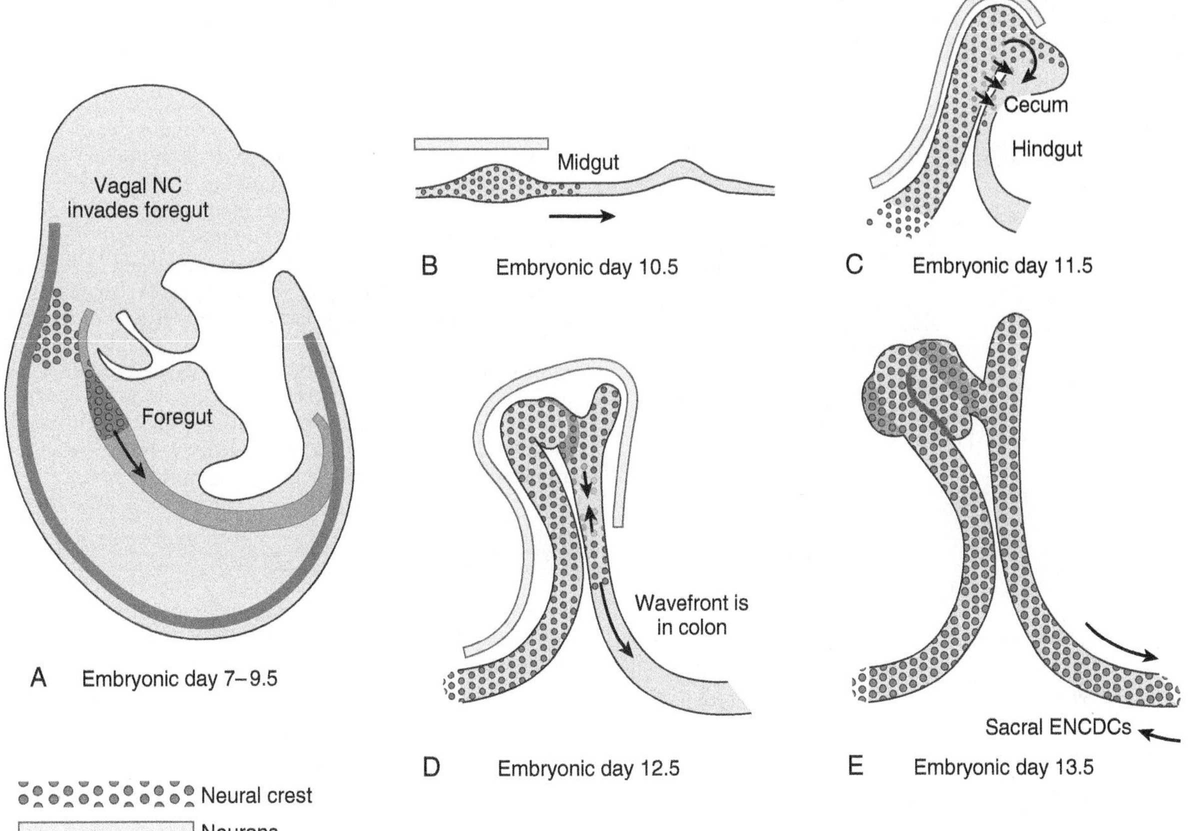

Fig. 84.2 Development of the murine enteric nervous system. (A) Vagal preenteric neural crest–derived cells enter the foregut and begin to migrate through the bowel. (B–E) Pre-enteric neural crest-derived cells migrate rostrocaudally and begin to differentiate into neurons and glial cells as the bowel lengthens and changes shape. (Modified from Lake JI, Heuckeroth RO. Enteric nervous system development: migration, differentiation, and disease. *Am J Physiol Gastrointest Liver Physiol.* 2013;305:G1-24.)

The development of oral motor skills starts with immature patterns of arrhythmic expression without suction (stage 1) and continues to a fully developed rhythmic expression-suction pattern (stage 5) (Fig. 84.5).[14] Both preterm and term infants exhibit maturation of sucking patterns postnatally, with preterm infants displaying the ability to attain full oral feeding at earlier post-gestational ages compared with those born at term.[13,15,16] As the infant matures, the oral cavity enlarges, allowing manipulation of pureed spoon feedings. At 3 to 4 months of age, tongue movements develop that move a food bolus from the front of the tongue back towards the pharynx. At 6 months, infants will occlude their lips to remove pureed foods from a spoon and will move the food towards the midline with their tongue for chewing. As alveolar ridges and teeth develop during the next year, the infant develops increased tongue mobility that allows lateralization of solid foods for mature mastication.[17]

SWALLOWING (ORAL AND PHARYNGEAL PHASES)

In the fetus and the neonate, the propagation of a liquid bolus through the pharynx and into the esophagus, known as *swallowing,* proceeds directly from the act of sucking. The distinction between bolus formation and swallowing matures as the mouth, the pharynx, the esophagus, and the neural networks that control the coordination of these structures develop.[18] Coordination of swallowing involves a complex interplay of neuromuscular fibers, cortical processing, and brain stem reflexes.[19]

As the milk bolus is sucked into the oral cavity, afferent sensory input to the brain stem triggers contraction of longitudinal and transverse intrinsic lingual muscles, distal elevation of the tongue, and a medial peristaltic wave that travels posteriorly along the tongue.[20] As the oral contents enter the pharynx, the soft palate and laryngeal musculature elevate, closing the nasopharynx and epiglottis while forming a conduit for passage of the milk bolus through the pharyngo-esophageal junction. Incoordination of this clearance from the oral cavity in premature infants may lead to residual overflow into the oropharynx, which may result in aspiration when the airway is not protected.[13]

The pattern of muscular contractions that coordinate the oropharyngeal and esophageal phases of swallowing is centrally integrated by two regionally distinct groups of medullary interneurons, the nucleus tractus solitarius and the nucleus ambiguus, which together form the "swallowing center."[21] The nucleus tractus solitarius acts as a pattern generator, whereas the nucleus ambiguus regulates the transmission of the signal, together coordinating the sequential activation of motor neurons responsible for pharyngeal and esophageal contraction and UES and LES relaxation.[18,21,22] Coordination becomes more efficient with maturity as sequential steps in the swallowing pathway occur in a more orderly manner.[12]

COORDINATION OF SWALLOWING WITH BREATHING

Respiration in the neonate depends on the normal development of the anatomic relationships of the pharynx, larynx, and esophagus, their respective protective reflexes, and the coordination of breathing patterns with swallowing. In utero, the pharynx is a conduit for fluid that facilitates the ingestion of up to 750 mL of amniotic fluid each day.[23] Swallowing contributes to amniotic fluid homeostasis, and the swallowed fluid appears to be trophic

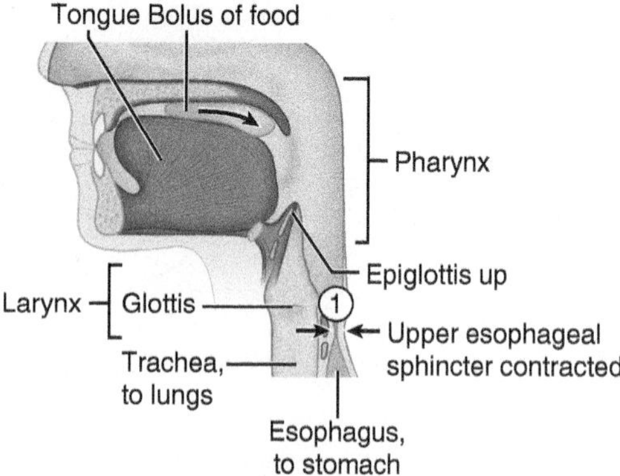

(1) At rest, when not swallowing, the upper esophageal sphincter muscle is contracted, the epiglottis is up, and the glottis is open, allowing air to flow through the trachea to the lungs.

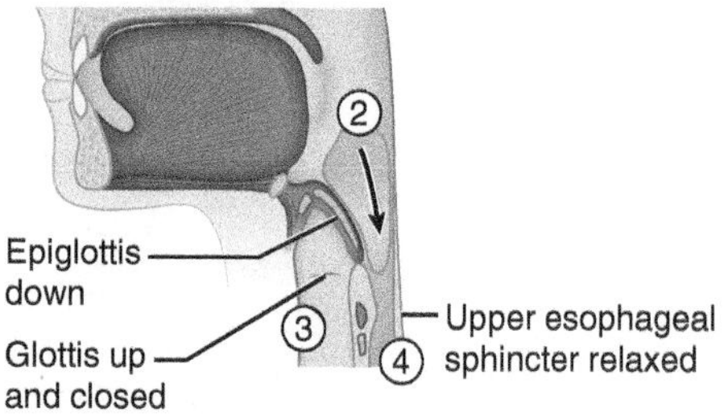

(2) The swallowing reflex is triggered when a bolus of food reaches the pharynx.

(3) The larynx, the upper part of the respiratory tract, moves upward and tips the epiglottis over the glottis, preventing food from entering the trachea.

(4) The esophageal sphincter relaxes, allowing the bolus to enter the esophagus.

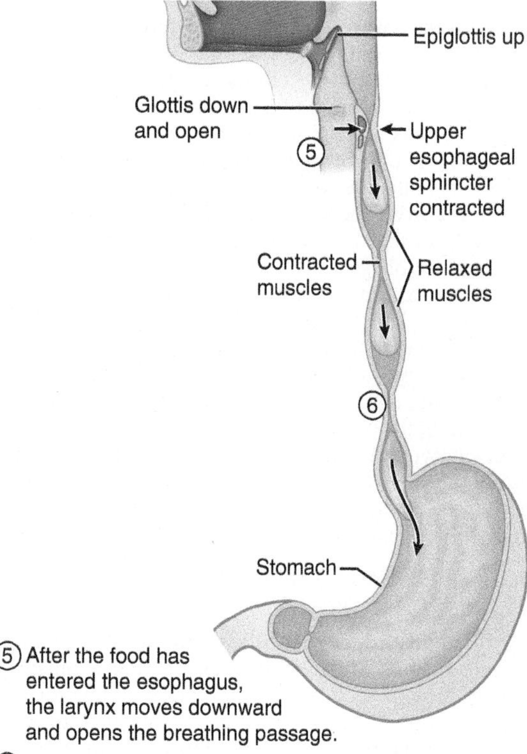

(5) After the food has entered the esophagus, the larynx moves downward and opens the breathing passage.

(6) Waves of muscular contraction (peristalsis) move the bolus down the esophagus to the stomach.

Fig. 84.3 Anatomy of swallow.

for mucosal development of the GI tract.[24,25] However, after birth, the pharynx performs a dual function, regulating the passage of food into the esophagus and air into the larynx.

Mature term infants possess an airway protection mechanism that is triggered before pharyngeal swallowing.[26] In contrast, recently born term infants and preterm infants rarely synchronize breathing and swallowing. Shortly after birth, term infants exhibit periods of rapid swallowing that are associated with unstable breathing, depressed respiratory rate, and reduced minute volume.[26,27] Premature infants alternate bursts of rapid swallowing with periods of rapid breathing.[13,28] When fluid enters the neonatal larynx, vagal afferents trigger a reflex of rapid swallowing, apnea, laryngeal constriction, hypertension, and bradycardia.[29,30] Although protective against aspiration, this reflex can threaten the infant and may exacerbate uncoordinated breathing and swallowing patterns. The coordination of breathing and swallowing depends on interneuronal pathways between the medullary swallow and respiratory centers; these pathways are poorly developed in premature infants.[31]

ESOPHAGEAL MOTILITY

The esophagus is a hollow muscular tube, closed proximally and distally by muscular sphincters.[32] The UES surrounds the upper part of the esophagus, and the LES surrounds the junction between the esophagus and the stomach. The main function of the esophagus is to propel swallowed food or fluid into the stomach, where digestion and absorption take place. This occurs through a series of peristaltic contractions of circular muscle in the esophageal body, in concert with appropriately timed relaxation of the UES and LES.

NEUROMUSCULAR COMPOSITION OF ESOPHAGUS

The UES and the proximal third of the esophageal body are composed of striated muscle. More distally, there is a transition zone where striated and smooth muscle intermix. The distal half to two thirds of the esophageal body and the LES are composed of smooth muscle.

The intrinsic innervation of the esophagus is made up of networks of nerves and ganglia that comprise the myenteric and submucosal plexuses (see Fig. 84.1). The myenteric plexus, located between the longitudinal and the circular layers of the tunica muscularis, regulates contraction of the outer muscle layers.[33] The submucosal plexus, located within the submucosa, regulates secretion and the peristaltic contractions of the muscularis mucosae.[33] Extrinsic innervation of the esophagus involves neurons located in the brain stem and spinal cord. Sympathetic and parasympathetic neurons originating in the nucleus ambiguus and vagus nerve supply the upper striated muscle and the UES.[34] Neurons from the dorsal motor nucleus and cervical and thoracic sympathetic trunks supply smooth muscle and the LES.[34]

UPPER ESOPHAGEAL SPHINCTER

The UES serves the dual role of accommodating boluses from the pharynx into the esophagus and maintaining a physical barrier to refluxed contents from the stomach entering the larynx.[35] UES function is controlled by a variety of reflexes that involve afferent inputs to the motor neurons innervating the UES.[36] These reflexes elicit either contraction or relaxation of the tonic activity of the UES.

UES pressure is generated predominantly by tonic contraction of the cricopharyngeus muscle. During the esophageal phase of swallowing, a propagated bolus exerts pressure to open the UES while the cricopharyngeus relaxes and the hyoid and larynx elevate.[37,38] Feeding difficulties may arise in premature infants who lack sufficient pharyngeal intrabolus pressure or lack coordination between oropharyngeal swallowing and UES

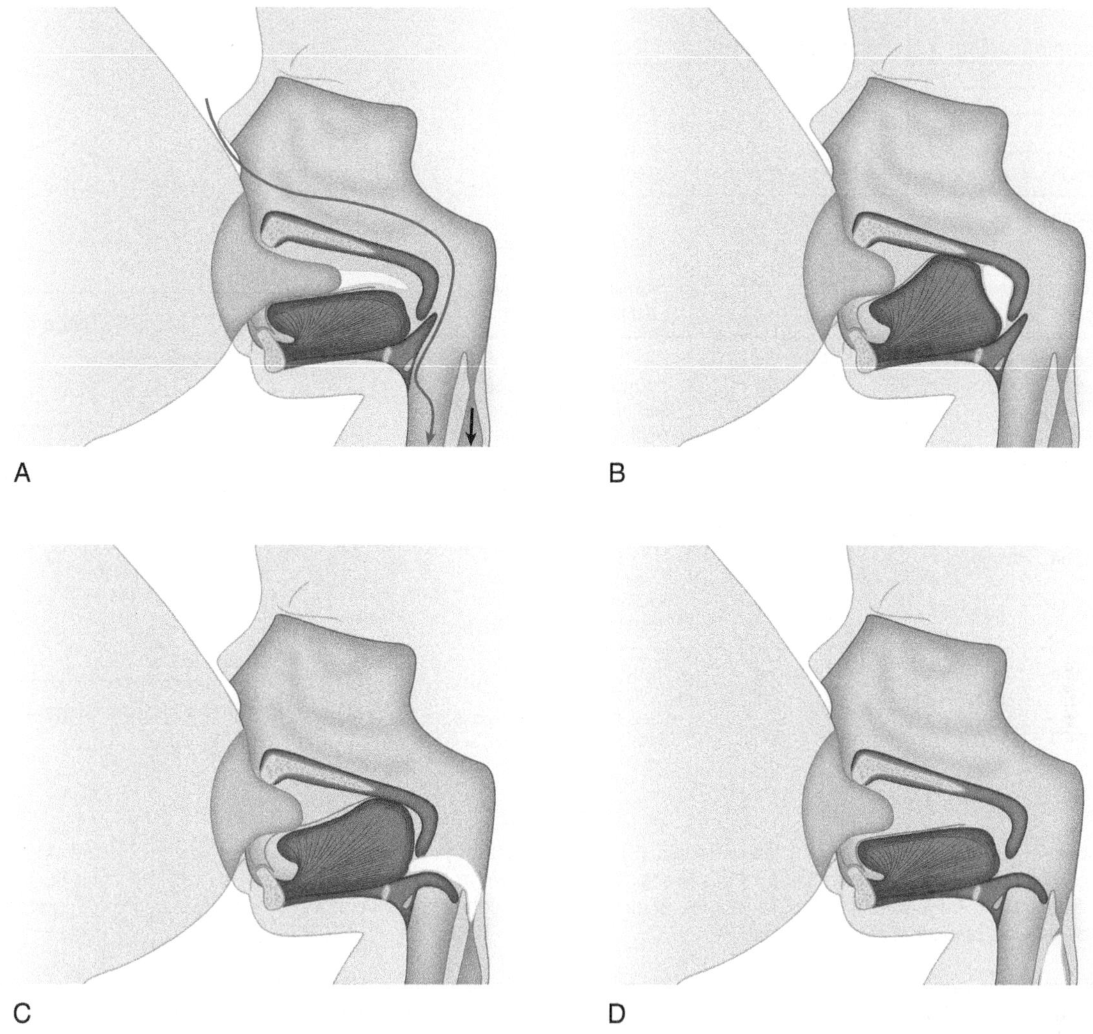

Fig. 84.4 Infant oropharyngeal anatomy: sucking and swallowing. (A) The tongue pulls inferiorly like a piston with the lips sealed over the nipple, creating a negative suction in the oral cavity to draw the nipple and expressed milk in. (B) The tongue presses against the soft palate to seal the milk into a bolus. (C) The bolus depresses the epiglottis and descends through the oropharynx into the upper esophageal sphincter. The tongue and soft palate remain sealed to create negative pressure for the subsequent suck. (D) The bolus proceeds into the upper esophagus as the oral cavity prepares for the next suck.

relaxation.[39,40] Reflex pathways of the vagus nerve and brain stem mature with age, and this maturation coincides with improved coordination of the timing of this sequence.[40,41] Esophageal distension, such as by refluxed gastric contents, causes UES relaxation in premature infants, which may lead to retrograde passage into the oropharynx. However, premature infants exhibit higher UES resting pressures during states of arousal or behavioral strain, which may serve as a protective mechanism.[42-44]

ESOPHAGEAL BODY PERISTALSIS

Esophageal peristalsis can be initiated by either sucking and swallowing or local distension. The sequential contraction of circular muscle of the esophageal body results in a peristaltic wave that pushes food towards the stomach.[45] The esophagus exhibits distinct peristaltic contractions by the second trimester.[46] Three different esophageal motility patterns have been described in utero: simultaneous opening of the esophageal lumen from the oropharynx to the LES, propulsive peristaltic contractions, and reflux from the stomach into the esophagus.[47] Although peristaltic movements are present in the second trimester, the propagation of peristalsis along the esophagus and LES is immature at birth, resulting in frequent regurgitation of food during the newborn period.[41,48]

LOWER ESOPHAGEAL SPHINCTER

The LES functions as a physical esophago-gastric anti-reflux barrier and is composed of two anatomic components, the intrinsic smooth muscle sphincter and the crural diaphragm, which provides extrinsic support and squeeze. Both components work together and contribute to LES pressure. To achieve LES relaxation, parasympathetic vagal nerve pathways, coordinated through the dorsal motor nucleus and nucleus tractus solitarius, are triggered by propagation of a food bolus through the esophageal body.[49] In addition, both swallowing and peristaltic activity trigger these reflex pathways to permit passage of food through the LES. Although not as mature as in term infants, preterm infants as young as 26 weeks gestational age exhibit well-developed swallow-related LES relaxation, as well as the ability to generate LES tonic pressures sufficient to maintain esophagogastric competence.[44,48,50]

CRICOPHARYNGEAL DYSFUNCTION AND ACHALASIA

Cricopharyngeal dysfunction (CPD; UES achalasia or cricopharyngeal achalasia) is a rare cause of dysphagia in infants that results from failure, incomplete, or uncoordinated relaxation of the UES, resulting in failed bolus propulsion and bolus stasis in the

Stage	Sample Tracing	Suction/Expression Amplitude (mm Hg)	Description
1A	Suction Expression	Absent +0.5 to +1.0	No suction Arrhythmic expression
1B	Suction Expression	−2.5 to −12.5 +0.5 to +1.0	Arrhythmic alternation Suction/expression
2A	Suction Expression	Absent +0.2 to +4.0	No suction Rhythmic expression
2B	Suction Expression	−7.5 to −150 +0.2	Arrhythmic alternation Suction/expression
3A	Suction Expression	Absent +0.8 to +1.0	No suction Rhythmic expression • Suction amplitude increase • Wide amplitude range • Prolonged sucking bursts
3B	Suction Expression	−15 to −75 +0.5 to +0.7	Rhythmic suction/expression
4	Suction Expression	−50 to −75 +0.4 to +1.0	Rhythmic suction/expression • Suction well defined • Decrease amplitude range
5	Suction Expression	−110 to −160 +0.6 to +0.75	Rhythmic/well defined suction/expression • Suction amplitude increase • Sucking pattern similar to that of full term infant

A

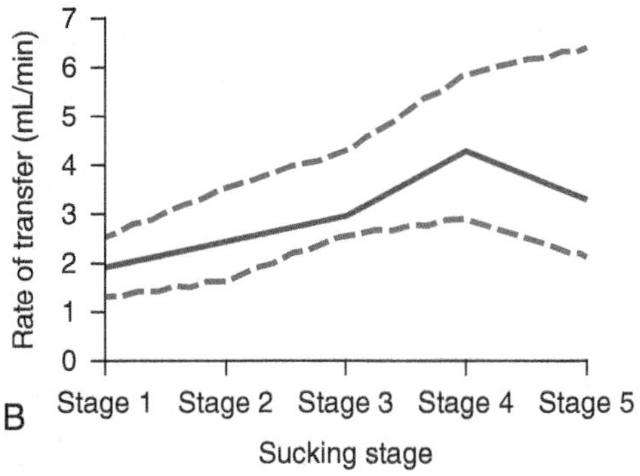

Fig. 84.5 (A) Stages of sucking characterized in preterm infants. (B) Rate of milk transfer during feeding in infants at the different stages of sucking. (C) Number of feedings per day at different stages of sucking. Data are shown as the median, with *dashed lines* indicating the interquartile range. (Modified from Lau C, Alagugurusamy R, Schanler RJ, et al. Characterization of the developmental stages of sucking in preterm infants during bottle feeding. *Acta Paediatr.* 2000;89: 846–552.)

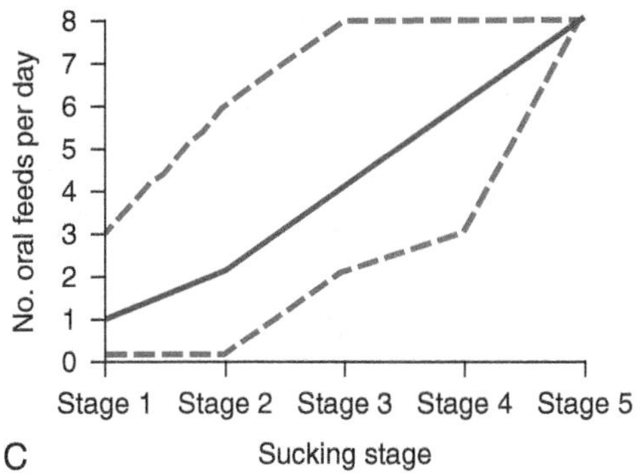

oropharynx. Infants often present with nonspecific symptoms such as feeding difficulties, wet voice, choking, regurgitation, cyanosis, growth failure, and recurrent respiratory infections and are at risk for aspiration. Although the exact mechanism is not well understood, CPD is thought to be caused by damage to the inhibitory oligosynaptic corticobulbar pathway to the motor neurons of the UES.[51]

Like CPD, achalasia is another rare neurodegenerative motor esophageal disorder that can occur in infants and can be associated with Trisomy 21, congenital hypoventilation syndrome, glucocorticoid insufficiency, familial dysautonomia, and Triple A syndrome (achalasia, alacrima, and ACTH insensitivity). It is characterized by the loss of the inhibitory myenteric plexus ganglia that innervate the LES and esophageal body.[52] The net result is an imbalance of inhibitory to excitatory neurons leading to failure of the LES to relax with swallowing, absence of peristalsis of the esophageal body, and increased LES resting pressures causing mid-esophageal body bolus stasis.[53] Similar to CPD, infants may present with feeding difficulties, regurgitation, emesis, and growth failure. Although the precise etiology of achalasia is not fully elucidated, depletion or absence of myenteric ganglion cells, destruction of myenteric nerves due to the presence of circulating antibodies to enteric neurons, variants in the HLA-DQ region, and/or chronic myenteric inflammation have all been proposed.[54]

SPHINCTERIC MECHANISMS AND GASTROESOPHAGEAL REFLUX

Gastroesophageal reflux (GER) results when gastric contents (liquid, gas, or a combination) are expelled into the esophageal lumen. GER is a normal physiologic phenomenon that often occurs during or after feeding.[55,56] Regurgitation—expulsion through the oropharynx—is also common and physiologic in infants. Abnormally frequent GER, poor clearance of refluxate from the esophageal lumen, or exposure of refluxate to airway structures may lead to the manifestation of GER disease (GERD), which has a number of clinical presentations, including feeding problems with or without weight loss, irritability, and obstructive apnea.[56,57] GER is more common in premature infants even though mechanisms of sphincter competence are well developed. The causes underlying GER are (1) swallow-related LES relaxation in association with failed peristalsis; (2) prolonged inhibition of LES tone and esophageal contraction induced by multiple swallows; and (3) transient LES relaxations, which are triggered in the absence of swallowing.[58]

Transient LES relaxation is the most common mechanism underlying GER and has been described in 26-week premature infants through adulthood.[59–61] The normal function of transient LES relaxations is to vent gases from the stomach during belching and to prevent GI bloating.[59,61] Compared with normal swallow-related LES relaxations, transient LES relaxations occur independently of pharyngeal swallowing, are prolonged in duration (>10 seconds), and result in greater relaxation. Gastric distension after a meal stimulates stretch-sensitive receptors in the smooth muscle of the stomach wall. A vagovagal reflex is triggered through the nucleus tractus solitarius, relayed down the dorsal motor nucleus of the vagus nerve, and propagated to the LES, esophagus, and crural diaphragm, enacting the transient LES relaxation.[62]

GASTRIC MOTILITY

The stomach serves to temporarily store ingested contents, mechanically and chemically break down food, and facilitate passage into the duodenum for further breakdown and absorption. To accomplish these roles, the stomach is divided into two functionally distinct regions. The proximal part of the stomach, comprising the fundus and proximal third of the corpus, provides gastric accommodation. The distal part of the stomach, comprising the remaining corpus, antrum, and pylorus, facilitates and regulates bolus passage into the duodenum.

GASTRIC ACCOMMODATION

Gastric accommodation is initiated by the swallowing of a food bolus and subsequent esophageal and gastric distension. Swallowing triggers a receptive relaxation of the gastric fundus that allows the stomach to prepare for acceptance of the bolus. Esophageal and gastric distension concomitantly trigger a vagally mediated inhibition of the gastric fundus, known as *adaptive relaxation,* with a simultaneous contraction of the antrum, allowing for substantial increases in gastric volume without compromising intragastric pressure.[63]

GASTRIC EMPTYING

As milk enters the antrum, the stomach is stimulated to contract, propelling the milk through the pylorus and into the duodenum by a process known as *gastric emptying.* During gastric filling, liquids separate from solids, partially through bulging of the greater curvature.[64] Tonic contraction of the proximal part of the stomach creates a pressure gradient downward into the duodenum, which regulates liquid emptying.[65] After initial liquid emptying, the greater curvature returns to its prior positioning and the antrum lines up with pylorus, positioning solids for passage into the duodenum.[64] Distally propagating antral contractions break up digestible solids and sweep particles towards the gastric opening. Particles greater than 1 mm in diameter are usually blocked by pyloric contractions, some of which can undergo retrograde flow from the duodenum, which returns particles to the antrum to be broken down further.[64]

The composition of gastric contents affects the rate of gastric emptying. Increased caloric density feeds slow gastric emptying, and long-chain triglycerides empty more slowly than medium-chain triglycerides.[66,67] Expressed breast milk empties at up to double the rate of formula at isocaloric levels, but the mechanism underlying this difference is unclear.[68]

DUODENAL FEEDBACK REGULATION

Gastric emptying is further regulated by mechanoreceptors and chemoreceptors of the duodenum. When food enters the duodenum, vagally mediated neural feedback decreases fundic tone, suppresses antral contraction, and stimulates the pylorus to contract, creating pyloric pressure waves.[69] Hormones also modulate gastric emptying; cholecystokinin, stimulated by protein and fat digestion, increases satiety, inhibits gastric motility, and stimulates duodenal contraction.[70] These regulatory actions are exhibited by infants as young as 32 weeks gestation.[71]

GASTROPARESIS

Gastroparesis, defined as delayed gastric emptying in the absence of mechanical obstruction, can be seen in premature infants (<34 weeks gestation), infants with pediatric intestinal pseudo-obstruction, or those who undergo surgeries resulting in vagal nerve injury.[72] Affected infants often present with feeding intolerance, emesis, nocturnal cough, aspiration, and growth failure.

Delayed gastric emptying in preterm infants is mostly due to immaturity of gastro-duodenal motor function and the absence of coordination between the antrum and the duodenum. During fasting, the stomach and small intestine exhibit cyclical groups of caudally migrating contractions known as *migrating motor complexes (MMCs).* The MMC is thought to sweep residual products of digestion toward the colon thus serving as a "housekeeper." MMCs are primarily controlled by the ENS but also modulated by hormones including motilin, somatostatin, and pancreatic polypeptides.[73] Motor patterns of the GI tract differ in preterm infants as compared to full term infants and older children. During fasting, most premature infants demonstrate episodes of motor quiescence that alternate with episodes of nonmigrating phasic activity instead of MMCs.[74] These differences in GI motor function in preterm infants result in less efficient gastric emptying and slower intestinal transit.

SMALL-INTESTINAL MOTILITY

The small intestine is a long tubular structure surrounded by layers of smooth muscle. The innermost smooth muscle layer, the muscularis mucosae, is surrounded by the circular muscle layer, which is arrayed circumferentially so that each contraction results in a narrowing of the lumen.[75] The outermost longitudinal layer contracts to foreshorten the intestine. The ENS of the small intestine, which integrates sensory input from the intestinal lumen and extrinsic input from the vagus nerve, is similar in composition to the esophagus, with myenteric and submucosal plexuses.[75]

As described earlier, the migration of the ENCDCs and their differentiation begins at approximately 4 weeks gestation, and completion takes approximately 3 weeks.[4,76,77] This coincides with the development of circular muscle layers, followed by longitudinal muscle development at approximately 10 weeks gestation.[78] The small intestine elongates, reaching a length of approximately four times the heel-to-crown length at birth (200 to 250 cm) and extends to approximately 6 meters by adulthood.[79,80]

SMALL-INTESTINAL CONTRACTION

Interstitial cells of Cajal function as the "pacemakers" of the intestine and play a critical role in small-intestinal contractile activity. Interstitial cells of Cajal form networks that are broadly distributed within the submucosal, intramuscular, and intermuscular layers throughout the GI tract. The interstitial cells of Cajal drive the electrical and mechanical activities of smooth muscle cells via "slow-wave" oscillations of membrane potential that are transmitted through the smooth muscle cells of the small intestine.[81] The slow wave is propagated rapidly around a localized ring of bowel, and when these slow-wave depolarizations reach a threshold potential, circumferential contraction occurs. This "spike" potential is then propagated longitudinally in concert with slow-wave depolarizations. Sequential, coordinated contractions along the longitudinal axis of the small intestine result in regions of high lumen pressure and low lumen pressure that move and mix the contents of the small intestine, respectively. Absent, poorly developed, or poorly distributed interstitial cells of Cajal have all been demonstrated to disrupt intestinal motility and can lead to chronic intestinal pseudoobstruction.[82]

COORDINATION OF SMALL-INTESTINAL CONTRACTION

The small intestine exhibits a characteristic pattern of contractions during fasting, known as the *MMC,* which travels from the antrum of the stomach to the cecum.[83] A cycle begins with no contractile activity (phase 1), followed by irregular activity (phase 2), and concluding with strong, regular contractions at a slow-wave frequency (phase 3). The migration velocity of the MMC along the small intestine decreases as it moves distally. The absence of this MMC pattern is associated with the development of bacterial overgrowth of the small intestine, which is likely attributable to the associated loss of strong phase 3 contractions that may sweep bacteria down the length of the bowel.[84]

Feeding replaces the fasting MMC pattern with a more irregular pattern of contractions that propel contents from the stomach to the cecum within 2 to 12 hours after feeding.[85] Meals containing primarily fat disrupt MMCs for longer periods of time than meals containing mainly protein or carbohydrate.[85] Vagal pathways modulate the conversion from a fasting to a fed pattern. After the meal has been propelled to the cecum, the fasting MMC pattern returns until the next feeding (Fig. 84.6).

DEVELOPMENT OF SMALL-INTESTINAL CONTRACTION

Contractile activity becomes more coordinated with increasing gestational age. At 25 to 30 weeks gestation, contractions are disorganized, of low amplitude, and irregular. By 30 to 33 weeks, rhythmic clusters of activity develop, with rare migration over long distances.[86,87] Between 33 and 36 weeks, migrating clusters display higher amplitudes, and by 36 weeks gestation, the mature MMC pattern is present.[86,87]

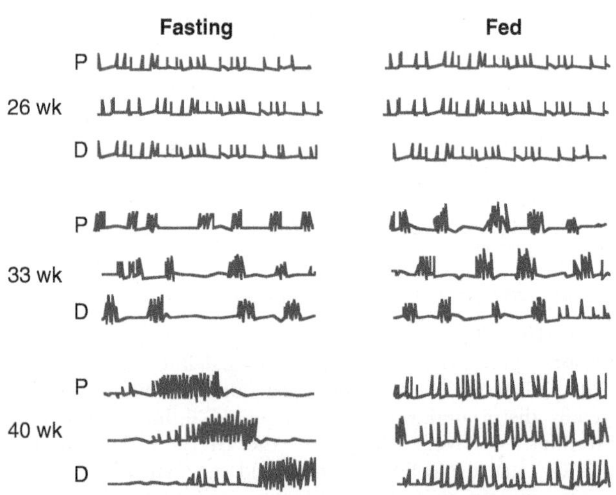

Fig. 84.6 Examples of fasted and fed intraluminal pressure recordings from the upper small intestine at increasing gestational age in human infants. At 26 weeks, a random disorganized pattern is present with low-amplitude contractile waves. No change in pattern occurs with feeding. At 33 weeks, clusters of contractions are prolonged with intervening quiescence. Cluster activity persists after feeding, with a decrease in the periods of quiescence. At 40 weeks gestation, an organized migrating motor complex exists. Feeding results in an irregular, disorganized contractile pattern. In normal newborn infants, cluster patterns can persist after feeding. *D*, Distal; *P*, proximal.

COLONIC AND ANORECTAL MOTILITY

COLON

The main functions of the colon are to move stool from the small intestine to the rectal vault, to serve as a storage space for fecal contents in the rectum until stooling is convenient, and to serve as a reservoir for fluid and gas absorption.

Fecal matter can be propelled down the colon by two types of movement. Small movements down the haustra occur regularly. High-amplitude propagated contractions are the larger and more effective mechanism for mass movement of intraluminal colonic contents and are thus likelier to be associated with defecation.[88,89] Colonic motility follows a circadian rhythm that begins after awakening and occurs cyclically throughout the day. Interstitial cells of Cajal, similarly to their role in the small intestine, serve as colonic pacemaker cells and act primarily in the transverse colon.[90] Both adults and children demonstrate an immediate postprandial colonic response that manifests itself as an increase in colonic motility in direct response to nutrient contact with the duodeno-jejunal mucosa. This response may also occur with gastric distension. The duration of this response increases with age, lasting 30 minutes in infants and 2 hours in adults.[91,92]

ANORECTUM

The rectum acts as a receptacle for fecal matter. Neonates usually defecate immediately on entry of stool into the rectum. As infants mature, they develop the ability to delay defecation until a socially appropriate time. This usually occurs in concert with toilet training. This bowel control requires coordination of the muscles of the sigmoid colon and rectum, the levator ani, the puborectalis, the internal anal sphincter, and the external anal sphincter (Fig. 84.7).[93,94] The external anal sphincter is under voluntary control via the pudendal nerve, and the internal anal sphincter is under both parasympathetic and sympathetic autonomic control.[93]

In the resting state, the puborectalis, internal anal sphincter, and the external anal sphincter remain in tonic contraction. During defecation, rectal contraction serves to position fecal material into the proximal part of the anal canal, where stretch receptors become stimulated. These receptors initiate recognition signals to the spinal cord neurons. In response, spinal reflexes are enacted through parasympathetic nerves that result in contraction of the sigmoid colon and rectum and relaxation of the internal anal sphincter (known as the *recto-anal inhibitory reflex*).[95] This relaxation of the internal anal sphincter is known as *the call to stool* and is the signal to the brain that defecation can occur. The ability of the external anal sphincter to develop adequate squeeze pressure is essential in the maintenance of fecal continence so it can override the effect of involuntary

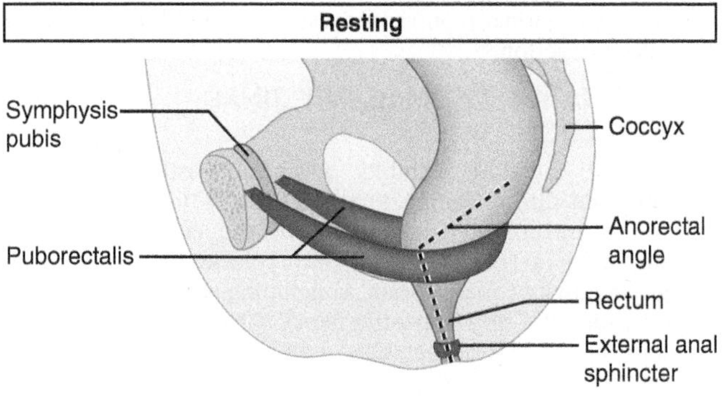

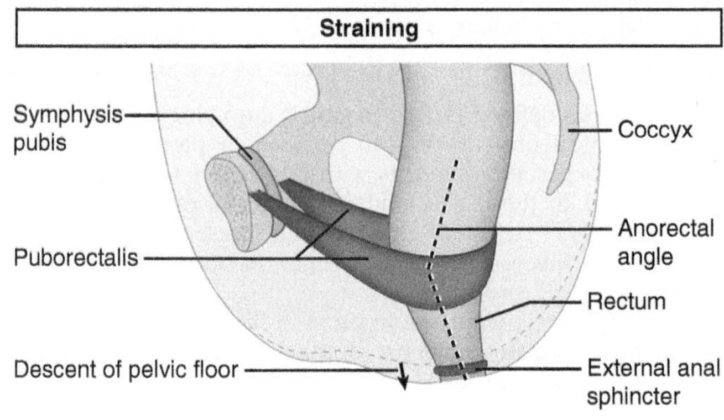

Fig. 84.7 Anorectal anatomy. (A) Resting. (B) Straining after recto-anal inhibitory reflex.

internal anal sphincter relaxation. Normal anorectal pressure and an intact recto-anal inhibitory reflex is present in infants as young as 26 weeks gestation.[96,97] The recto-anal inhibitory reflex is even normal in infants with delayed passage of meconium.[98,99]

Once the recto-anal inhibitory reflex has been initiated, the final extrusion of feces is under voluntary control and is achieved via relaxation of the puborectalis and contraction of the levator ani muscle. This allows the anorectal angle to straighten for easier stool passage.[100] Term infants pass their first meconium stool within 48 hours of birth, whereas premature infants may experience a delay of more than 1 week before their initial defecation.[101-103]

HIRSCHSPRUNG DISEASE

Hirschsprung disease is a GI disorder occurring in 1 in 5000 live births that results from the absence of neural crest–derived enteric ganglia in the terminal hindgut. Patients with Hirschsprung disease commonly present with partial or complete intestinal obstruction during the first year of life. Human genetic studies support the notion that a number of genetic mutations underlie the pathogenesis in Hirschsprung disease. Mouse models have been utilized to elucidate the underlying mechanisms of some of these mutations.

Pedigree studies in humans have shown that Hirschsprung disease is a heterogenous genetic disorder with autosomal dominant, autosomal recessive, and polygenic forms, as well as cases that result from environmental factors.[97] A well-studied autosomal dominant form of Hirschsprung disease has been mapped to human chromosome 10q11.1, in a region containing the *RET* protooncogene, a protein tyrosine kinase gene expressed in the cells derived from the neural crest.[99] Mutations in the *RET* gene of Hirschsprung disease have been identified in both sporadic and familial cases.[100,101] However, the existence of families with Hirschsprung disease without linkage to the *RET* gene suggests that there are additional genes affected in patients with Hirschsprung disease.[102]

Another susceptible chromosome in an inbred Mennonite kindred with Hirschsprung disease is chromosome 13q22.[103] Extensive molecular and genetic studies have implicated the endothelin-B (ET_B) receptor gene *(EDNRB)* as a gene candidate for Hirschsprung disease susceptibility within a subset of this kindred. Endothelins are a group of peptides that bind to two receptors, including ET_B. The ET_B receptor is expressed in the human colon, particularly in the myenteric plexus, mucosa, ganglia, and blood vessels of the submucosa,[104] areas that may be abnormal in Hirschsprung disease. Targeted disruption of the *EDNRB* gene in mice results in aganglionic megacolon, suggesting a direct relationship between this genetic abnormality and the development of Hirschsprung disease.[105]

Studies done in the lethal spotted *(ls/ls)* mouse, in which congenital aganglionosis is an autosomal recessive trait, have allowed investigators to elucidate possible mechanisms underlying the condition.[88] The aganglionosis in the *ls/ls* mouse develops as a result of the failure of precursors of enteric neurons and enteric glia to colonize the bowel wall.[89,90] Neurotrophins and laminin, in addition to other molecules, may play a role in the control of enteric neuron migration and differentiation.[91,92] After reaching the gut, neural crest cells express a 110 kDa cell-surface laminin-binding protein, which is not detected in ENS precursor cells.[92] It has been hypothesized that laminin interacts with the laminin-binding protein to cause neural crest cells to terminate migration. Neural crest cells from the *ls/ls* mouse can colonize the colonic walls of normal mice but not the distal colon of *ls/ls* mice.[93] Examination of the aganglionic segment of *ls/ls* bowel reveals that there is an overabundance of laminin and other components of the extracellular matrix in the gut wall.[94] It has been hypothesized that the accumulation of laminin could result in premature cessation of migration of crest-derived cells and therefore the absence of ganglionic cell bodies in the distal colonic segments of *ls/ls* mice.[92] The inhibition of cranial-to-caudal migration of vagal enteric neuroblasts to the large intestine of *ls/ls* mice suggests that a defect in the mesenchyme of the large intestine prevents colonization.[95] Similarly, a transgenic mouse model that expresses multiple copies of the *Hoxa-4* gene has crest-derived cells that can enter the terminal colon, but their development is abnormal, resulting in hypoganglionosis, suggesting that this gene may also be important in disease pathogenesis.[97]

ANORECTAL MALFORMATIONS

Anorectal malformations comprise a wide spectrum of anomalies of the anorectal system, urogenital system, sacral spine, and perineal musculature. They occur with a reported incidence of 1:3300 to 1:5000 live births.[106] The extent of the anomaly predicts the type of anorectal malformation (Table 84.1).[107] Most commonly, anorectal malformations present as an abnormally positioned anus. In the mild types of anal malformations, the bowel outlet opens in the perineal region outside the usually well-developed voluntary sphincter complex. In contrast, in the more severe anomalies the bowel outlet opens in an ectopic position in the urogenital tract in males or genital tract in females. Neonatal recognition of the type of the malformation is essential for the planning of the surgical management for correction.

The exact etiology of anorectal anomalies is not well defined. Embryologically, interference in the development of anorectal and genitourinary organs up to 7 to 8 weeks of gestation gives rise to a range of anomalies and severity that involve the musculoskeletal system of the hindgut.[108] There is evidence from animal models and the study of human fetuses with anorectal malformation that a deficiency in the dorsal component of the cloacal membrane and the adjacent dorsal cloaca may be causative. A subsequent malfunction of the primitive streak and tail bud in the early development phase around 3 to 4 weeks has been proposed—but is yet to be clearly defined—as the cause of associated anomalies of the pelvic floor.[109] Continued communication between the urogenital tract and rectal portions of the cloacal plate resulting in rectourethral fistulas or rectovestibular fistulas has also been proposed as a possible embryologic defect causing anorectal malformations.[110]

Table 84.1 Krickenbeck Classification of Anorectal Malformation Divided by Sex.

	Major Clinical Groups	Rare/Regional Variants
Males	Perineal (cutaneous) fistula Rectourethral fistula/atresia/stenosis Bulbar fistula Prostatic fistula Rectovesical fistula Imperforated anus with no fistula Anal stenosis	Pouch colon atresia/stenosis Rectal atresia/stenosis H-type fistula Others
Females	Vestibular fistula Cloaca with short common channel (<3 cm) Cloaca with long common channel (>3 cm) Imperforated anus with no fistula Anal stenosis	Rectal atresia/stenosis Rectovaginal fistula H-type fistula Others

Modified from Kluth D. Embryology of anorectal malformations. *Semin Pediatr Surg*. 2010;19:201–208.

Genetically determined syndromes with anorectal malformations are relatively uncommon. In contrast, anorectal anomalies are common in multi-anomaly sequences such as VACTERL (vertebral defects, anal atresia, cardiac defects, tracheoesophageal fistula, renal anomalies, and limb abnormalities) and CHARGE (coloboma, heart defects, choanal atresia, growth retardation, genital abnormalities, and ear abnormalities) associations. Anorectal malformations may develop in some syndromes that are caused by a mutation of a single gene. These include Currarino syndrome (sacral agenesis, anorectal malformation, and presacral mass), caused by a mutation in *HLXB9* gene in chromosome locus 7q39 and Townes-Brock syndrome (imperforate anus, abnormally shaped ears, and hand malformations), which has a mutated *SALL1* gene in chromosome locus 16q12.1.[106]

CONCLUSION

GI motility develops through a complex interplay of physiologic mechanisms that require proper anatomic and neural maturation. Sucking and swallowing is the fundamental mechanism by which ingested contents must enter the luminal tract efficiently without compromising respiration. Gastric accommodation and emptying are crucial for the receipt and mechanical breakdown of food and the timely passage into the absorptive sections of the GI tract. Small-intestinal contractions and peristalsis depend on the appropriate migration of ENCDCs and function of neuronal plexuses to effectively propagate luminal contents down the length of the small intestine. Colonic motor activity is essential for movement of fecal matter to the rectum. The final expulsion of fecal matter relies on proper recto-anal reflex networks and neuromuscular structures for effective defecation. Abnormalities in the development of any of these digestive and defecatory components can lead to long-lasting medical problems and disease states.

 A complete reference list is available at www.ExpertConsult.com.

SELECT REFERENCES

1. Gershon MD. Developmental determinants of the independence and complexity of the enteric nervous system. *Trends Neurosci*. 2010;33:446-456.
5. Lake JI, Heuckeroth RO. Enteric nervous system development: migration, differentiation, and disease. *Am J Physiol Gastrointest Liver Physiol*. 2013;305: G1-G24.
8. Jiang Y, Liu MT, Gershon MD. Netrins and DCC in the guidance of migrating neural crest-derived cells in the developing bowel and pancreas. *Dev Biol*. 2003;258:364-384.
9. Rao M, Gershon MD. Enteric nervous system development: what could possibly go wrong? *Nat Rev Neurosci*. 2018;19:552-565.
11. Mizuno K, Ueda A. The maturation and coordination of sucking, swallowing, and respiration in preterm infants. *J Pediatr*. 2003;142:36-40.
16. Qureshi MA, Vice FL, Taciak VL, et al. Changes in rhythmic suckle feeding patterns in term infants in the first month of life. *Dev Med Child Neurol*. 2002;44:34-39.
17. Stolovitz P, Gisel EG. Circumoral movements in response to three different food textures in children 6 months to 2 years of age. *Dysphagia*. 1991;6:17-25.
18. Miller AJ. The neurobiology of swallowing and dysphagia. *Dev Disabil Res Rev*. 2008;14:77-86.
29. Thach BT. Maturation and transformation of reflexes that protect the laryngeal airway from liquid aspiration from fetal to adult life. *Am J Med*. 2001;111(suppl 8A):69S-77S.
30. Rohof WO, Hirsch DP, Boeckxstaens GE. Pathophysiology and management of gastroesophageal reflux disease. *Minerva Gastroenterol Dietol*. 2009;55: 289-300.
33. Kumar D, Phillips SF. Human myenteric plexus: confirmation of unfamiliar structures in adults and neonates. *Gastroenterology*. 1989;96:1021-1028.
34. Cunningham Jr ET, Sawchenko PE. Central neural control of esophageal motility: a review. *Dysphagia*. 1990;5:35-51.
39. Singendonk MM, Rommel N, Omari TI, et al. Upper gastrointestinal motility: prenatal development and problems in infancy. *Nat Rev Gastroenterol Hepatol*. 2014;11:545-555.
46. Bowie JD, Clair MR. Fetal swallowing and regurgitation: observation of normal and abnormal activity. *Radiology*. 1982;144:877-878.
52. Franklin AL, Petrosyan M, Kane TD. Childhood achalasia: a comprehensive review of disease, diagnosis and therapeutic management. *World J Gastrointest Endosc*. 2014;6:105-111.
56. Vandenplas Y, Rudolph CD, Di Lorenzo C, et al. Pediatric gastroesophageal reflux clinical practice guidelines: joint recommendations of the North American Society for Pediatric Gastroenterology, Hepatology, and Nutrition (NASPGHAN) and the European Society for Pediatric Gastroenterology, Hepatology, and Nutrition (ESPGHAN). *J Pediatr Gastroenterol Nutr*. 2009;49:498-547.
62. Holloway RH. The anti-reflux barrier and mechanisms of gastro-oesophageal reflux. *Baillieres Best Pract Res Clin Gastroenterol*. 2000;14:681-699.
66. Siegel M, Lebenthal E, Krantz B. Effect of caloric density on gastric emptying in premature infants. *J Pediatr*. 1984;104:118-122.
70. Khoo J, Rayner CK, Feinle-Bisset C, et al. Gastrointestinal hormonal dysfunction in gastroparesis and functional dyspepsia. *Neuro Gastroenterol Motil*. 2010;22:1270-1278.
74. So AKW, Ng Pc, Fok TF. Gastrointestinal dysmotility in preterm infants HK. *J Paediatr*. 2003;8:101-106.
75. Furness JB, Bornstein JC, Smith TK. The normal structure of gastrointestinal innervation. *J Gastroenterol Hepatol*. 1990;5(suppl 1):1-9.
77. Obermayr F, Hotta R, Enomoto H, et al. Development and developmental disorders of the enteric nervous system. *Nat Rev Gastroenterol Hepatol*. 2013;10:43-57.
83. Sarna SK. Cyclic motor activity; migrating motor complex: 1985. *Gastroenterology*. 1985;89:894-913.
87. Berseth CL. Gestational evolution of small intestine motility in preterm and term infants. *J Pediatr*. 1989;115:646-651.
92. Di Lorenzo C, Flores AF, Reddy SN, et al. Use of colonic manometry to differentiate causes of intractable constipation in children. *J Pediatr*. 1992;120: 690-695.
94. Whitehead WE, Schuster MM. Anorectal physiology and pathophysiology. *Am J Gastroenterol*. 1987;82:487-497.
96. Benninga MA, Omari TI, Haslam RR, et al. Characterization of anorectal pressure and the anorectal inhibitory reflex in healthy preterm and term infants. *J Pediatr*. 2001;139:233-237.
95. Xu X, Pasricha PJ, Sallam HS, et al. Clinical significance of quantitative assessment of rectoanal inhibitory reflex (RAIR) in patients with constipation. *J Clin Gastroenterol*. 2008;42:692-698.
102. Clark DA. Times of first void and first stool in 500 newborns. *Pediatrics*. 1977;60:457-459.
106. Rintala RJ. Congenital anorectal malformations: anything new? *J Pediatr Gastroenterol Nutr*. 2009;48(suppl 2):S79-S82.
107. Levitt MA, Pena A. Anorectal malformations. *Orphanet J Rare Dis*. 2007;2:33.
108. Kluth D. Embryology of anorectal malformations. *Semin Pediatr Surg*. 2010;19:201-208.

85 Development of the Endocrine and Exocrine Pancreas

Lori Sussel

EMBRYOLOGY AND HISTOGENESIS OF THE HUMAN PANCREAS

The pancreas is a multifunctional organ consisting of three major tissues: exocrine tissue, endocrine islets, and epithelial ducts (Fig. 85.1). The exocrine compartment contains the largest proportion of cells within the adult pancreas and is composed of acinar cells, which synthesize and secrete digestive enzymes. The endocrine pancreas is composed of hormone-producing cells organized within the islets of Langerhans that are responsible for maintaining glucose homeostasis. These cells constitute approximately 1% to 2% of the adult pancreas. The epithelial

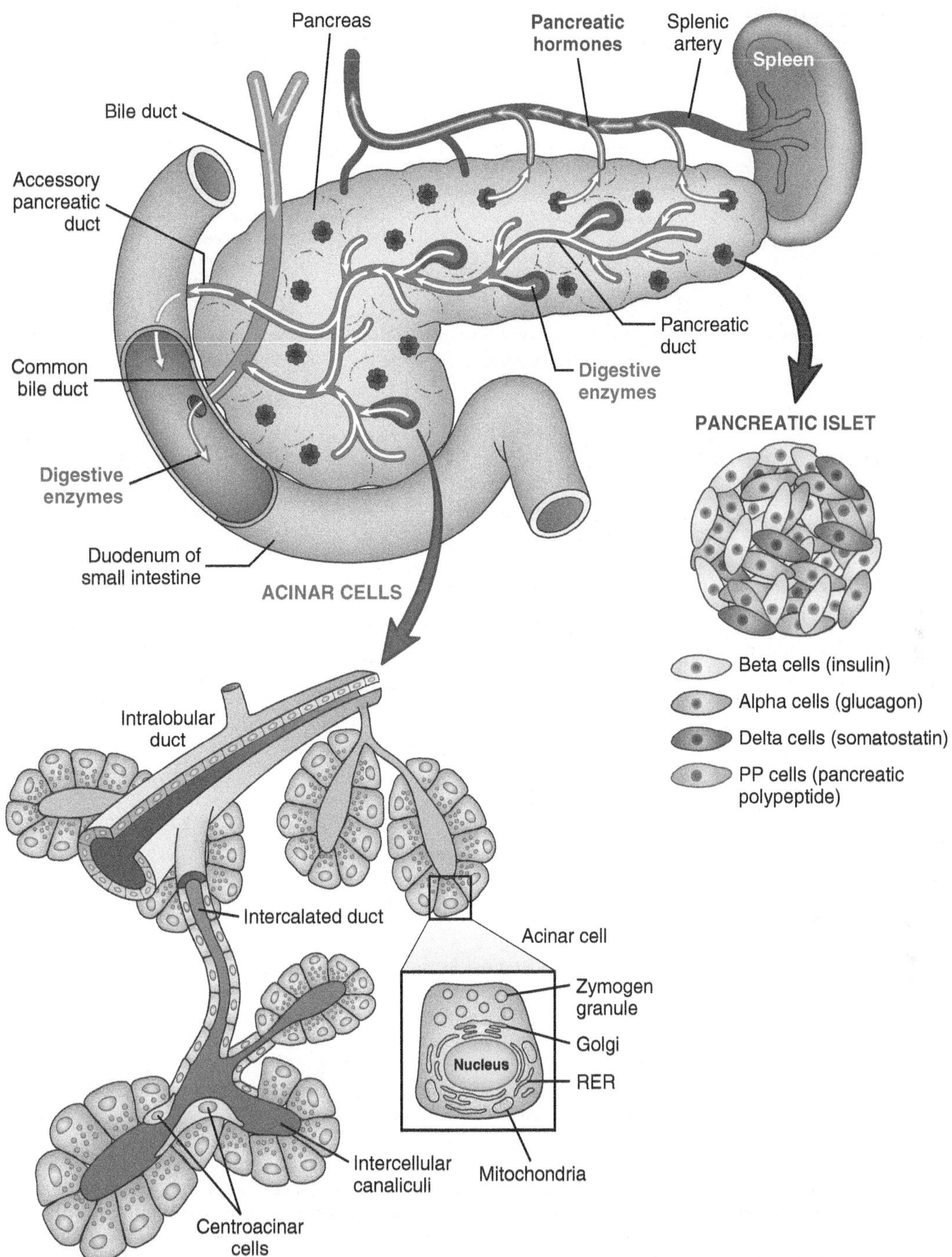

Fig. 85.1 The pancreas is a multifunctional, glandular organ nestled between the small intestine and spleen. It is comprised of the exocrine acinar cells that secrete digestive enzymes into the ductal system and endocrine cells that are located within the islets of Langerhans that secrete pancreatic hormones into the blood system.

ductal cells are also a small, but essential component of the pancreas, and act as a conduit for transporting the acinar enzymes into the intestinal lumen. Although each pancreatic tissue type performs diverse functions, they arise from a common progenitor pool in the foregut endoderm, and the respective developmental programs are closely associated. In this chapter, we will discuss what is known about the coordinated regulation of pancreas development and some of the diseases that are associated with defects in these developmental programs.

The pancreas is a unique organ in that it initially develops as two distinct anlagen. In most vertebrates, the dorsal and ventral pancreatic anlagen develop as evaginations of the primitive foregut endoderm (Fig. 85.2).[1-3] In humans, the larger dorsal anlage, which develops into the tail, body, and part of the head of the pancreas, grows directly from the duodenum and becomes visible by 26 days after conception.[3] The ventral anlage develops by 33 days after conception as two evaginations off the bile duct and eventually contributes to the head of the pancreas. The ventral anlagen are initially paired, with the left lobe ultimately disappearing over time.[4] At approximately 7 weeks gestation, the dorsal and ventral anlagen fuse as the buds develop and the gut rotates.[3] The ventral duct forms the proximal portion of the major pancreatic duct of Wirsung. The dorsal duct forms the distal portion of the duct of Wirsung and the accessory

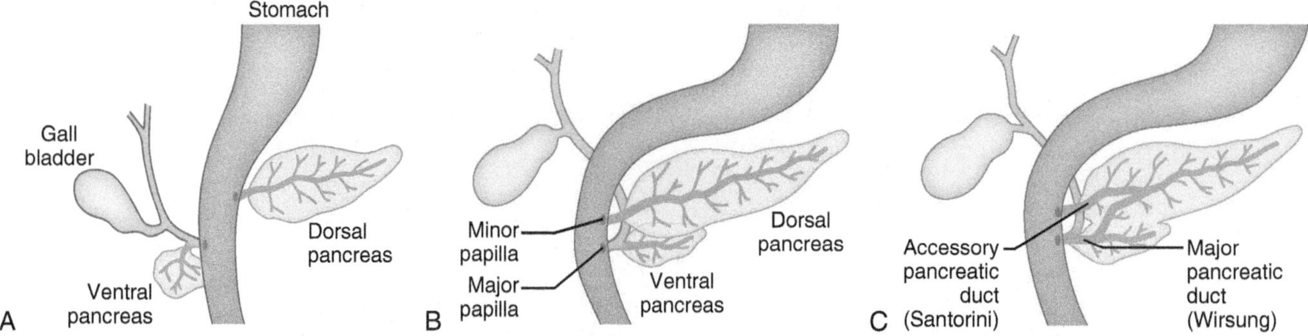

Fig. 85.2 Development of the human pancreas. (A) Gestational age 6 weeks. (B) Gestational age 7 to 8 weeks. The ventral pancreas has rotated but has not yet fused with the dorsal pancreas. (C) The ventral and dorsal pancreatic ductal systems have fused. (From Kelley VC, editor. *Practice of Pediatrics*. Vol V. Philadelphia: Harper & Row; 1987.)

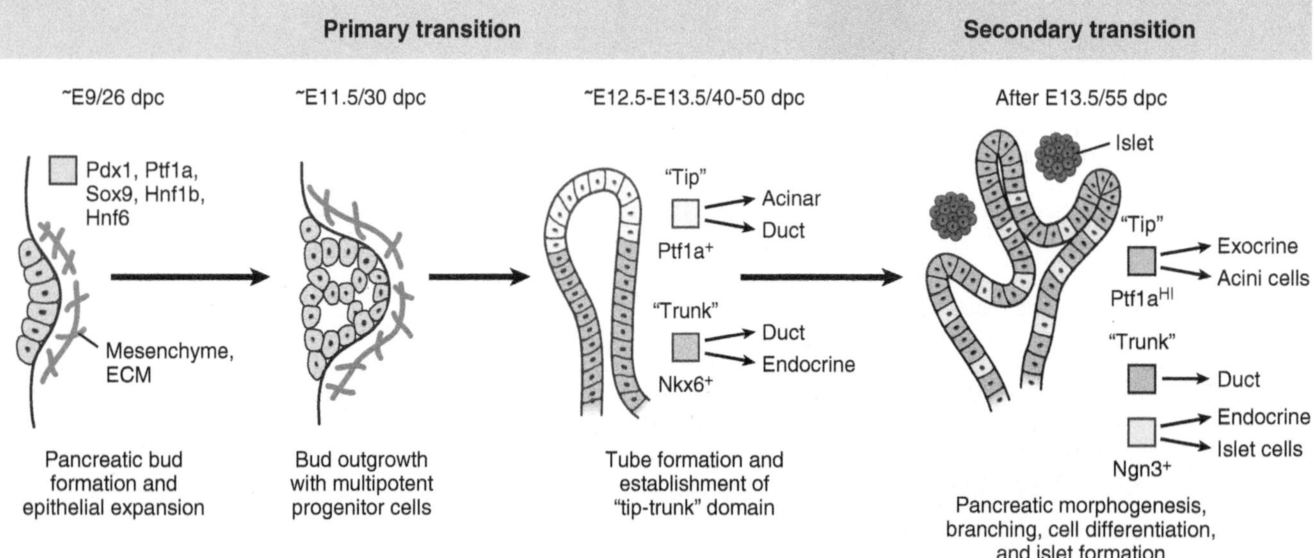

Fig. 85.3 Pancreatic morphogenesis in mouse and humans. During the stage referred to as the *primary transition*, the pancreas forms as an epithelial bud surrounded by mesenchymal tissue and extracellular matrix *(ECM)*. The epithelial bud continues to expand and forms a population of multipotent pancreatic progenitors that can give rise to all cell lineages within the pancreas. At the end of the primary transition, the pancreas undergoes a series of morphologic changes to form a tube-like structure that is divided into distinct domains. The "tip" domain gives rise predominantly to the acinar lineage, whereas the "trunk" domain predominantly gives rise to the ductal and endocrine lineages. During the "secondary transition" stage, pancreatic morphogenesis continues and cell lineage differentiation occurs to form the exocrine, ductal, and endocrine lineages. The endocrine cells begin to cluster into islets. (Adapted from Benitez CM, Goodyer WR, Kim SK. Deconstructing pancreas developmental biology. *Cold Spring Harb Perspect Biol*. 2012;4[6]:a012401. doi:10.1101/cshperspect.a012401. PMID: 22587935; PMCID: PMC3367550.)

duct of Santorini. Variations in fusion account for the variety of developmental abnormalities of the pancreas, such as anomalous pancreaticobiliary junction, annular pancreas, and pancreas divisum.[4] Pancreas divisum occurs in approximately 10% of the population, and although the majority of individuals are asymptomatic, some suffer from acute or chronic pancreatitis.[5]

Histologic examination of the emerging human pancreatic buds reveals predominantly undifferentiated epithelial cells that undergo active growth and branching morphogenesis to form a lobular-tubular pattern surrounded by loose mesenchymal stroma by 9 to 12 weeks after conception (Fig. 85.3).[6,7] The extracellular matrix present in the stromal compartment provides important signaling molecules that provide instructions for pancreatic differentiation into the different tissue cell types. During human development there is a significant amount of extracellular matrix fibers throughout the pancreas at 9 weeks after conception, and the extracellular matrix has intercalated between large numbers of epithelial cells by 14 to 20 weeks after conception.[8] Collagen I, collagen IV, fibronectin, and laminin are all expressed throughout the pancreas, especially within and around the endocrine cell clusters. In mice, laminin 1 has been shown to play a role in pancreatic duct formation, branching morphogenesis, induction of acinar cells, and enhancement of β cell differentiation.[9-11]

Several studies have indicated that signals from the vasculature are also required for morphogenesis, growth, and cytodifferentiation of the pancreas.[12-14] In humans, angiogenesis can be detected between 9 and 22 weeks after conception, at which time maturation is complete and the vasculature is able to provide a functional response.[15] Scanning electron microscopy analysis of the pancreatic vascular architecture between 18 and 25 gestational weeks demonstrated that the lobular structure of the pancreas influences the organization of the microvasculature. Similar to the adult organ, the vascular system of fetal human pancreas has many portal connections, including islet-lobule and islet-duct portal circulations.[3] In mice there is evidence that the vascular endothelial cells modulate both early and late pancreatic development and function to inhibit acinar cell differentiation.[16,17] Although there is currently no evidence that innervation influences developmental processes, significant innervation of the human pancreas can be detected shortly after vascularization at 13 weeks after conception; within the head of the pancreas there are two primary peaks of nerve growth at 14 and 22 weeks after conception, whereas in the body and tail of the pancreas a single growth peak can be observed at 20 weeks after conception.[18] That study also identified nerve fibers innervating distinct components of the vasculature. Furthermore, a study in mice demonstrated there is coordinated vascularization and innervation of the developing pancreas.[19]

PANCREATIC CELL LINEAGES

Pancreatic endocrine cells that make up the islets of Langerhans are the first lineage to form during vertebrate development. There are four hormone-producing endocrine lineages known to populate the adult islet: α cells (glucagon secreting), β cells (insulin secreting), δ cells (somatostatin secreting), and PP cells (pancreatic polypeptide secreting) (see Fig. 85.1). Two additional transient endocrine populations are present in prenatal mouse and human islets: ghrelin-producing epsilon cells and gastrin-producing cells.[20,21] With the increasing availability of human embryonic and fetal tissue, considerable insight has been gained regarding human endocrine cell development. In humans, rare insulin-positive cells are first apparent scattered throughout the epithelium at 52 days after conception, with isolated glucagon- and somatostatin-positive cells appearing approximately 1 week later at 8.5 weeks gestation.[3] The number of hormone-producing cells significantly increases by 10 weeks to constitute almost 1.5% of the total pancreatic cell population. Between 9 and 10 weeks after conception, PP and epsilon cells are also present. At this stage, insulin-positive cells are the most abundant cell type and begin to aggregate in progressively larger cell clusters.[3] Primitive islet clusters containing a mixture of endocrine hormone-expressing cells are first identifiable at 12 to 13 weeks after conception. Endocrine cells expressing almost all combinations of hormones, in addition to polyhormonal granules, are also frequently observed in the human fetal pancreas.[8,22] Between 11 and 13 weeks after conception, the highest ratio of insulin and glucagon co-expressing endocrine cell populations is present; however, this number significantly declines by 15 weeks after conception.[23] Ghrelin is the only hormone that does not colocalize with insulin or glucagon.[23] By 21 weeks after conception, single hormone expression has resolved into specific cell types, and the relative ratio of the distinct endocrine cell populations is comparable to that of the adult pancreas.[23] The histologic appearance of the pancreas in an infant born at term is similar to that in the adult.

Exocrine acinar cell differentiation is initiated between 8 and 9 weeks, although at this early-stage exocrine cells are rare and their secretory granules, referred to as *zymogen granules,* are not yet present.[4,8,24,25] Between 14 and 20 weeks, acinar cells rapidly mature and increase in number; and recognizable zymogen granules become visible by 14 to 16 weeks.[8,25] As the pancreas matures, the luminal volume decreases and acinar cell volume increases. The amount of connective tissue continues to decrease throughout gestation and in the postnatal period. By 20 weeks gestation, acinar cells contain mature-appearing proteolytic active zymogen granules, well-developed endoplasmic reticulum, and highly developed basolateral membranes. As development proceeds, the amount of stroma continues to decrease, and acinar cells gain a mature appearance. After birth the volume of the exocrine pancreas continues to grow and nearly triples in mass during the first year of life from 5.5 to 14.5 g.[26] The adult pancreas weighs approximately 85 g. During the first 4 months the ratio of acinar cells to connective tissue increases four-fold.

In rodents and humans, the acinar cell population is predominantly mononuclear at birth and acinus formation is due to proliferation of these mononuclear acinar cells and duct cells.[27] Postnatally, acinar cells become progressively binucleate. In the adult, the shape of the mature acinar cell is pyramidal with a basal nucleus. The most prominent organelles in the fasted state are large numbers of zymogen granules, located apically. Abundant rough endoplasmic reticulum and Golgi apparatus are present. Junctional complexes join adjacent acinar cells, and the apical membrane contains abundant microvilli projecting into the lumen. The final three-dimensional structure of the exocrine pancreas consists of a complex series of branching ducts surrounded by grapelike clusters of acinar cells. The ontogeny of cell surface glycoproteins is critical for normal cell-cell interactions and exocrine morphogenesis.[28,29] Stage-specific polylactosamine (carbohydrate) antigens are dynamically expressed during pancreas morphogenesis as they become preferentially localized to the differentiating cell lineages. These antigens are thought to be important for cell-to-cell communication and recognition.[30]

Duct and centroacinar cells are also found between 14 and 20 weeks after conception.[8] The ductal system constitutes less than 5% of the volume of the exocrine pancreas and only 0.5% of total pancreatic volume. The adult pancreatic ductal system is critical for secreting bicarbonate to dilute and neutralize the enzymes secreted by the acinar cells, in addition to acting as a conduit for these proteins into the intestinal lumen. Glycogen is highly expressed in human ductal cells at 8 weeks after conception, but by 20 weeks the glycogen expression domain shifts primarily into the acinar cell clusters.[8] In the adult pancreas there remains little detectable glycogen expression in ductal or islet cells; however, high glycogen expression can be detected in pancreatic microcystic adenomas.[31] The centroacinar cells lie at the nexus between the acinar cells and the terminal duct epithelium. The origin of the centroacinar cells has not been established; however, in humans, cytokeratin 19–labeled centroacinar cells can be located within amylase-expressing cell clusters between 14 and 20 weeks after conception. Emerging studies in mouse and zebrafish models suggest that centroacinar cells may represent a population of multipotent progenitor cells in the adult pancreas.[32]

LESSONS FROM THE NONHUMAN PANCREAS

Many of the concepts associated with human pancreatic development have historically been based on studies performed in model organisms. Although the relative time spans are different, comparative studies have demonstrated that the histologic, ultrastructural, and molecular developmental stages of rodent and human pancreas are very similar, although some important distinctions have also been identified.[3,8,23] Studies in mice have defined three distinct prenatal developmental periods.[33,34] Initially, a wave of pancreatic progenitor cell proliferation between embryonic day 9.5 and embryonic day 12.5 contributes to the development of a stratified epithelium that is referred to as the *primary transition* (see Fig. 85.3). This is followed by a major wave of cell type differentiation between embryonic day 13.5 and embryonic day 16.5, which is referred to as the *secondary transition* and describes the differentiation of the major pancreatic lineages. At this time acinar cells form from the extending tip epithelium and large numbers of acini differentiate and continue to proliferate past embryonic day 16.5. The third wave of development, or *tertiary transition,* occurs postnatally and refers to the adaptive regulation of hormone and enzyme secretion in response to dietary influences. In humans, similar waves of differentiation have been described, although the first phase of differentiation is less well defined.[3,6,8]

CONSERVED MOLECULAR REGULATION OF EARLY PANCREAS MORPHOGENESIS

Since the mid-1990s there has been progressive elucidation of the intrinsic and extrinsic molecular events that regulate mouse pancreas development (Fig. 85.4; reviewed by Jorgensen and

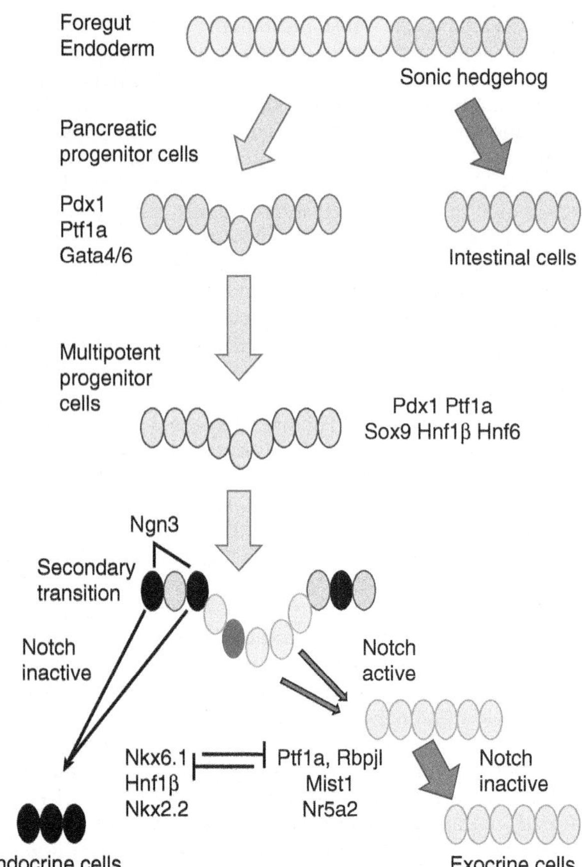

Fig. 85.4 Origin of the exocrine and endocrine cell lineages in the developing pancreas. This model is based on descriptions from various reports (e.g., see Hebrok and colleagues[42] and Jorgensen and colleagues[35]). *Arrows* indicate the sequential activities based on the appearance of specific cell markers in the developing mouse pancreas. (Modified from Edlund H. Pancreas: how to get there from the gut? *Curr Opin Cell Biol.* 1999;11:663–688; and Cleveland MH, Sawyer JM, Afelik S, et al. Exocrine ontogenies: on the development of pancreatic acinar, ductal and centroacinar cells. *Semin Cell Dev Biol.* 2012;23:711–719.)

colleagues[35]). More recently, access to human embryonic and fetal pancreas tissue, human-specific reagents and improved imaging technologies has resulted in demonstration of extensive conservation of many of the molecular pathways in normal human development, especially with regards to the intrinsic transcriptional regulatory programs (Fig. 85.5). It has been more difficult to gain insight into the signaling pathways given the challenges associated with culturing human pancreas.[6]

As described above, the parenchyma of both endocrine and exocrine glands originates from the endodermal epithelium of the primitive gut tube (see Fig. 85.4).[36] Genetic lineage tracing studies in mice have determined that all pancreatic cell types are derived from a common endodermal progenitor cell population.[37-39] Prior to the evagination of the pancreatic primordia from the primitive gut tube, the molecular programs specifying pancreatic fate have been initiated by the inductive influences of neighboring tissues. During gastrulation the endoderm is subdivided into anterior and posterior domains by signals from the adjacent mesectoderm. Retinoic acid,[40] bone morphogenetic proteins (BMPs), and fibroblast growth factors (FGFs)[41] play important roles during late gastrulation in localizing the prepancreatic domain, which will respond to subsequent instructive signals that induce pancreatic tissue and growth.

The ventral and dorsal aspects of the endoderm that will give rise to the pancreas are exposed to different local contacts and therefore rely on distinct signaling sources for their induction. The dorsal pancreas is induced by transient contact with the notochord, followed by interposition of the dorsal aorta. Contact with the notochord induces a localized exclusion of an important developmental signaling morphogen, sonic hedgehog (Shh), from the prepancreatic endoderm. This signaling event is necessary for dorsal pancreatic development; ectopic expression of *Shh* interferes with subsequent patterning events.[42] In humans there appears to be a similar exclusion of Shh from the dorsal epithelium.[6] In mice it has been shown that the dorsal aorta also provides essential signals to promote pancreatic fate,[43] among them vascular endothelial growth factor (VEGF).[44] The ventral pancreas emerges from a noncontiguous endodermal region that is in close association with the hepatic and bile duct endoderm, and is induced by sequential FGF and BMP signals derived from the adjacent cardiac and septum transversum mesoderm.[45]

These early events render the prepancreatic endoderm competent to form pancreatic tissue. The next step involves expression of transcription factors in the endoderm and in the surrounding mesenchyme to further specify a pancreatic fate. The pancreatic and duodenal homeobox 1 gene *(Pdx1)* is expressed in the prepancreatic endoderm at embryonic day 8.5 in the mouse,[46] and its ablation results in the arrest of pancreatic development shortly after formation of the pancreatic anlagen.[47] In humans PDX1 is expressed comparatively later in development, after the dorsal aortae have fused[6]; however, similarly to *Pdx1*-null mutations in mice, a mutation in the human *PDX1* gene was found to cause congenital pancreatic agenesis in an infant.[48]

Basic helix-loop-helix pancreas-specific transcription factor 1 α subunit *(Ptf1a)* is also expressed throughout the early pancreatic epithelium around embryonic day 9.5, shortly after *Pdx1* and in a domain more narrowly approximating the developing pancreas.[49] By embryonic day 12.5, *Ptf1a* expression becomes restricted to the epithelial tip domain and ultimately the acinar cells, where the gene product functions as part of a trimeric protein complex to regulate exocrine gene expression.[50] Genetic ablation of *Ptf1a* in mice also results in pancreas agenesis and has provided important insight into the early events of pancreatic specification.[51] By genetic tagging of the mutant cells that would otherwise express *Ptf1a*, cells lacking *Ptf1a* were incorporated into the developing duodenum as full-fledged intestinal epithelial cells. This illustrates the developmental plasticity of early pancreatic development and highlights the principle that multiple successive specification events are needed to guide cells from progenitor cells to a fully differentiated state. The expression domain of *PTF1A* in the developing human pancreas has not yet been determined; however, a recent study using RNA-based fluorescent probes has identified a pool of human multipotential progenitor cells located at the tips of the branching epithelium that co-express *SOX9* and *PTF1a*, similar to rodents.[52] Consistent with its expression within the earliest progenitor population, deletions of *PTF1a* and mutations in a distal enhancer of *PTF1A* in humans also cause pancreas agenesis.[53,54]

The genes encoding two members of the GATA family of transcription factors, GATA4 and GATA6, are also co-expressed with *Pdx1* and *Ptf1a* in early pancreatic endoderm of the mouse; *Gata4* subsequently becomes restricted to the exocrine compartment and *Gata6* becomes restricted to the ducts and the endocrine compartment.[55] Similarly in humans, GATA4 is expressed in the pancreatic buds and subsequently restricted to the acinar-fated tip cells (see Fig. 85.5); GATA6 expression has not been analyzed.[6] Heterozygous mutations in either *GATA4* or *GATA6* cause pancreas agenesis in humans, with disruption of GATA6 function causing most of the known pancreatic agenesis cases.[56] On the other hand, both *GATA4* and *GATA6* must be deleted from the pancreatic endoderm domain in mice to cause

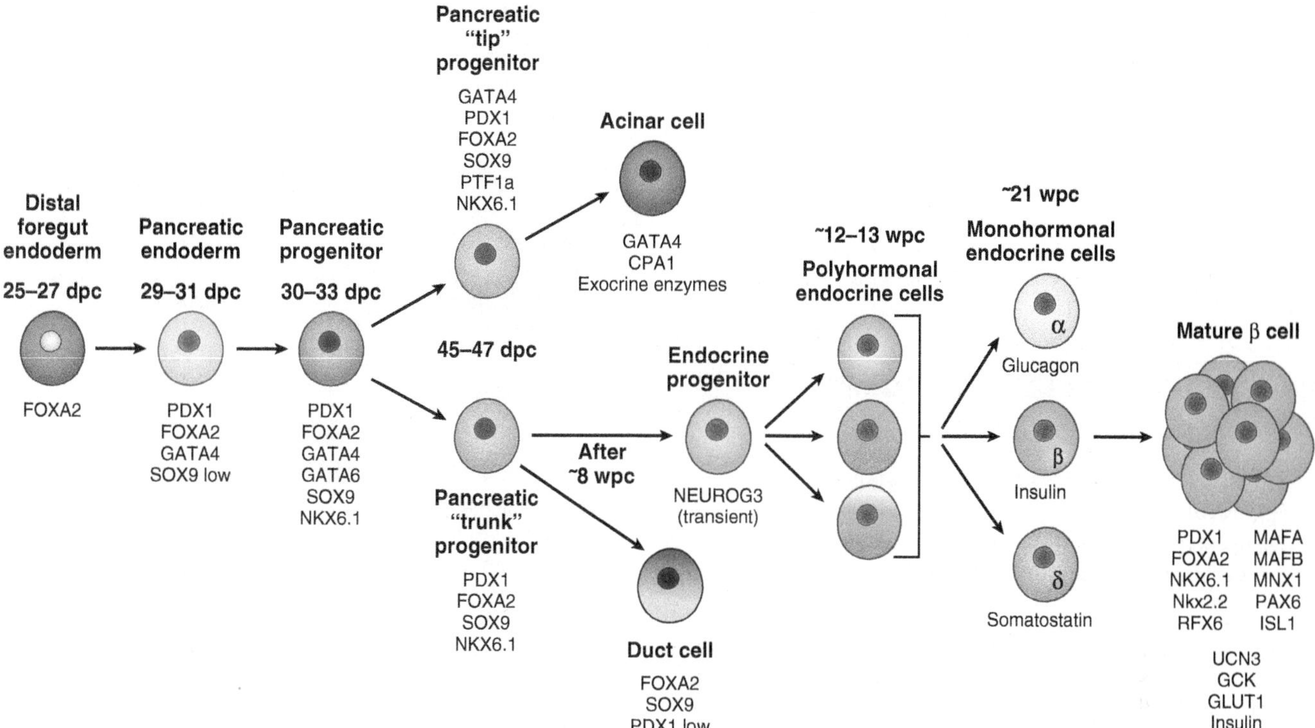

Fig. 85.5 Lineage specification of the human pancreas. The pancreas develops from a common progenitor population and progresses through sequential lineage decisions, similar to those observed in mice, but with some minor differences. The stages and known gene expression data are noted for each major lineage. (Modified from Jennings RE, Berry AA, Strutt JP, et al. Human pancreas development. *Development*. 2015;142:3126–3127.)

pancreas agenesis,[57,58] suggesting there has been a specialization of GATA functions during evolution.

Some of the earliest studies of exocrine pancreas development in rodents highlighted the influence of mesenchymal-epithelial interactions.[59,60] After initial budding of the pancreatic primordium in mice, FGF10 activates notch signaling to maintain the pool of pancreatic progenitors in an undifferentiated state and prevent their terminal differentiation.[61] Subsequently, mesenchymal signals were found to be critical for regulating pancreatic outgrowth and exocrine morphogenesis and cell differentiation, including FGF family members, epidermal growth factor, and members of the transforming growth factor (TGF) β/BMP superfamily (reviewed by Serup[62]). Currently, there is limited information on the endogenous mesenchymal signals required for human pancreas development; however, many of the mesenchymal signals identified in rodents are necessary for the stepwise differentiation of human embryonic stem cells into pancreatic lineages.[6,35,63–66]

Disruption of mesenchymal signaling pathways often results in reciprocal changes in the endocrine versus exocrine cell fates. Mouse studies have identified a population of multipotent progenitor cells that can give rise to all pancreatic lineages in response to secreted morphogens.[67] As pancreatic morphogenesis proceeds, the multipotent progenitor cells become allocated to specific tip and trunk domains within the pancreatic epithelium; cells within the trunk domain contribute to the duct and endocrine lineages, whereas the tip progenitors primarily give rise to the exocrine lineage (see Fig. 85.3). In humans, morphologic studies and limited marker analysis suggests that tip-trunk compartmentalization occurs in a similar manner between gestational weeks 7 and 14.[6]

Extensive molecular analyses in mice have identified many additional transcriptional regulators of pancreas development.[35] Shortly after bud evagination at embryonic day 9.5, *Sox9* becomes induced in the *Pdx1/Ptf1a*-expressing multipotent progenitor cell population. Between embryonic days 10.5 and 11.5, the multipotent progenitor cells acquire *Nkx2-2*, *Nkx6-1*, *Hes1*, *Hnf1b*, *Cpa1*, and *Nkx6-2* expression. Subsequently, at embryonic day 12.5, the pancreatic precursor cells become spatially and molecularly diversified into exocrine and endocrine lineages. In response to signaling events that are not well understood, epithelial stratification initiates a series of morphogenetic events, including tubulogenesis and epithelial tubule remodeling that shape the mature functional branching organ with distinct trunk and tip domains.[68] Concurrent with the morphologic changes, there is progressive restriction of transcription factor expression and corresponding lineage specification.[35] Cells within the trunk domains maintain expression of *Hnf1b*, *Nkx2.2*, *Nkx6-1*, and *Nkx6-2* to give rise to the ductal and endocrine lineages, whereas the tip domain maintains expression of *Ptf1a* and *Cpa1* to specify the exocrine lineage. *Pdx1* and *Sox9* continue to be expressed in all lineages. Reciprocal regulatory interactions between the Nkx6 factors and Ptf1α contribute to the delineation and maintenance of exocrine and endocrine lineages.[69] Several immunohistochemical studies of human fetal tissue have demonstrated that many of these morphologic and gene expression events are conserved in the human pancreas, with the exception of NKX2-2, which is not detected until after endocrine cell specification.[3,6,8,23]

In mice, Notch signaling is also a key participant in pancreatic cell fate decisions.[70,71] Notch signaling is active throughout the multipotent progenitor cells as indicated by the expression of *Hes1*, a major Notch target. Subsequent silencing of Notch signaling in the endocrine lineage leads to the down-regulation of *Hes1* and the induction of the basic helix-loop-helix transcription factor Neurogenin3 (Neurog3). *Neurog3* expression delineates the endocrine precursor population, and Neurog3 activity is required for all endocrine cell lineages.[72] Successive cell fate decisions further diversify the Neurog3-expressing precursor pool by induction of a combinatorial hierarchy of transcription factors that promote a lineage-specific program.[35] Whereas

Notch is required for activation of *Ptf1a* and early commitment to the exocrine lineage, continuous activation of Notch signaling eventually inhibits exocrine development.[70,71] Notch signaling remains active in the centroacinar and terminal duct cells, which co-express *Hes1* and *Sox9*. In humans, the relative *NOTCH1*, *NEUROG3*, and *HES1* expression domains are comparable to those in mice.[73,74] Furthermore, appropriate human endocrine cell development is dependent on functional NEUROG3 activity; human patients born with *NEUROG3* mutations have variable defects in pancreas development, and many of these *NEUROG3* alleles disrupt the differentiation of β cells from human pluripotent stem cells.[75,76]

PANCREATIC ISLET CELL DEVELOPMENT AND FUNCTION

MOLECULAR REGULATION OF ENDOCRINE DIFFERENTIATION

In rodents and humans, differentiation of the endocrine lineage precedes acinar cell differentiation. In mice, genetic lineage tracing analysis demonstrated that all endocrine cell populations arise from the Neurog3-expressing endocrine progenitor cells.[77] Unlike humans, the mouse endocrine cell populations emerge as single hormone-positive cells, with the glucagon-producing α cells arising first, followed by the insulin-producing β cells and somatostatin-producing δ cells, and finally the pancreatic peptide-producing PP cells.[35] Despite these differences, most of the transcriptional factors regulating α and β cell differentiation downstream of NEUROG3 are conserved, including PAX6, NKX2.2, NKX6.1, NEUROD1, RFX6, and ARX (see Fig. 85.5).[78,79] With only minor differences, these transcription factors are expressed in similar spatio-temporal patterns in human fetal pancreas compared to mice, suggesting there is conserved transcriptional regulator mechanisms between the two species. Furthermore, rare human mutations in NKX2.2, NEUROD1, and RFX6 have been shown to cause human neonatal diabetes, likely due to impaired β cell differentiation, and individuals with mutations in ARX lack α cells.[80,81] Compared to α and β cells, less is known about the determination of the other endocrine cell types in either mice or humans. Extensive summaries of transcription factor expression and function in the developing mouse and human pancreas is summarized in several comprehensive review articles, including a report that includes extensive three-dimensional imaging of the developing mouse pancreas (see Fig. 85.5).[35,82]

ISLET MORPHOGENESIS

In mice, beginning at the secondary transition, aggregated clusters of differentiated endocrine cells leave the ductal epithelium in what has been described as a "peninsular structure."[83] The e13.5 clusters are initially composed mostly of α cells, but over the following 2 days become populated with a progressively higher proportion of β cells. Concomitant with the increase in β cell numbers, the clusters begin to form cell aggregates in which the α and β cells become segregated. Shortly after birth, the islets become further organized into mature spherical structures with β cells located within the core of the islet and the non-β endocrine cells located at the mantle (Fig. 85.6). The signals that regulate the clustering process and islet assembly remain obscure, although they are believed to involve heterotypic and homotypic interactions between adhesion molecules, such as cadherins, integrins, and connexins (reviewed by Jain and lammert[84]). By 3 weeks postnatally, the full adult complement of islet cells has formed, with β cells representing the most abundant population (~70% to 75%), followed by α cells (~20%), δ cells (~5% to 10%), and PP cells (<5%) (see Fig. 85.6). The mature islets are also in close contact with endothelial cells and neurons, both of which are thought to influence islet architecture and function.

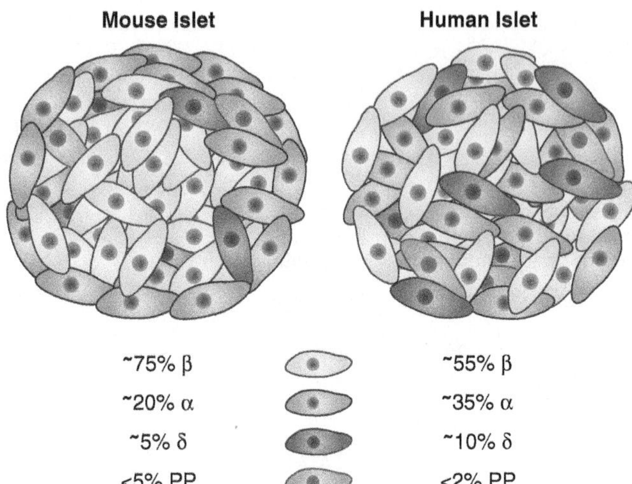

Fig. 85.6 Schematic of adult mouse and human islet morphology and endocrine cell composition. Mouse islets contain a higher proportion of β cells that are located in the core of the islet. The endocrine cell subtypes are intermingled throughout the islet.

It is currently not known whether clustered cell delamination also represents the mechanism through which human islets form. Although peninsular-like cap structures have been described in pseudo-islets derived from human embryonic stem cells,[83] this does not appear to be the primary method of human islet formation in vivo, especially since numerous single endocrine cells are found scattered throughout the epithelium shortly after endocrine cell differentiation.[7] Endocrine clusters do begin to appear at approximately 10 weeks post conception, and unlike mice, initially contain a higher ratio of β cells over α cells. By 14 to 16 weeks, α and β cells are present in relatively equal proportions.[23,85] Also unlike developing mouse islets, a large proportion of δ cells are present during the last trimester of gestation.[86] Interestingly, it has been discovered that the morphology of human fetal and neonatal islets is similar to that of mice, with β cells located within the islet core and surrounded by the other endocrine cell types.[85,87] Over time, however, the endocrine cell types become intermingled within the islet, a cellular organization that has postulated to be necessary for the human endocrine cells to achieve their mature functional state (see Fig. 85.6).[88] The cellular composition of the adult human islets is also different that the rodent islet, consisting of ~55% β cells, 35% α cells, 10% δ cells, and less than 2% PP cells.[89]

ISLET HORMONE SECRETION

Regulated secretion of islet endocrine hormones is critical for the control of metabolic homeostasis. The levels of insulin and glucagon vary reciprocally to regulate the balance of glucose in the circulation: insulin secreted from the islet β cells is required to promote the uptake and storage of circulating glucose following a meal, whereas glucagon produced from the α cells acts as a counter-regulatory hormone to stimulate glucose output from the liver during fasting conditions. The δ cells add an additional layer of regulation by secreting somatostatin, which functions to inhibit the release of insulin and glucagon. While extensive studies have elucidated the regulation of insulin secretion,[90] the regulation of glucagon secretion is less well understood, and few studies have investigated the regulation of somatostatin. The role and regulation of pancreatic polypeptide remains unknown.

Based on research from a large number of labs worldwide, a consensus model for glucose stimulated insulin secretion (GSIS) from β cells has been developed.[91] GSIS refers to the release of insulin from pancreatic β cells in response to circulating glucose. GSIS occurs in two phases, beginning with a transient spike in insulin release (first-phase GSIS), followed by a second longer phase response that can be sustained for hours in the presence of extracellular glucose. Both phases occur in rodents and humans, although with different kinetics. β Cells are able to sense elevated circulating glucose via the glucose transporter (Glut1 in humans, Glut2 in rodents) at the plasma membrane. Glucose uptake then triggers metabolism-dependent depolarization through the ATP-dependent closure of ATP-sensitive K+ (KATP) channels. This elicits action potential firing and allows calcium influx into cells through voltage-dependent calcium channels. The increased intracellular concentration of calcium then promotes insulin secretory granule biogenesis and trafficking of the granules to the cell periphery, where they are biochemically "primed" to for insulin release. Detailed description of the key aspects of secretory function can be found in several comprehensive reviews.[91,92]

MATURATION OF β CELL FUNCTION

At birth, β cells produce processed insulin, but have not yet undergone the physiologic maturation needed to optimally respond to glucose. Immature fetal and neonatal β cells are physiologic defined by their high basal insulin secretion and blunted insulin secretion response to glucose. Postnatally, β cells gradually mature to achieve the efficient GSIS response associated with adult functional β cells. In mice, β cell maturation is regulated by several transcription factors, including MafA and NeuroD1,[93,94] and is accompanied by the transition from anaerobic glycolysis to oxidative metabolism. In addition, there are changes in the expression of several molecules associated with β cell function, including and the upregulation of glucokinase (Gck), increased K_{ATP} channel activity, cell surface localization of glucose transporter 2 (GLUT2) and the expression of urocortin3 (Ucn3), and the downregulation of "disallowed genes," such as *Ldha* and *Npy* (see Fig. 85.5).[95,96] In addition to these molecular changes, formation of the three dimensional islet structure with the appropriate cell-cell interactions is also believed to be necessary to support optimal response to blood glucose levels.[97] Interestingly, even after β cells have become fully mature, maintained expression of several developmental transcription factors, including Pdx1, Pax6, Foxo1, and Nkx2.2, are required to preserve β cell identity in the adult islet.[98-101] Human β cells also do not become functionally mature until after birth and undergo a similar transition from glycolysis to oxidative metabolism to achieve optimal glucose responsiveness. Many of the molecular changes in humans are also conserved; however, GLUT1 is the predominant glucose transporter on human β cells and UCN3 is found in both mature α and β cells.[102,103]

Although, considerable information is becoming available about the intrinsic regulation of β cell maturation,[104] the environmental signals that regulate postnatal maturation are currently not known, despite extensive research efforts. This lack of information also represents the major barrier in generating fully functional β cells in vitro from human stem cell populations. Most of our current understanding of β cell maturation is derived from rodent studies. It has been demonstrated that exposure of immature β cells to glucose itself can enhance maturation.[105] Several studies in the early 1980s have also implicated adaptation to the neonatal diet as a factor in β cell maturation. More recently studies in rodent models and zebrafish have provided compelling evidence that exposure to thyroid hormone triiodothyronine (T3) regulates postnatal β cell maturation.[106,107] Notably, several groups have since demonstrated that addition of thyroid hormone T3 to the later stages of protocols differentiating human β cells from stem cell populations resulted in the induction of β cell maturation markers and enhanced β cell function, suggesting similar mechanisms may exist for postnatal human β cell maturation.[108,109]

β CELL PROLIFERATION

Coincident with postnatal β cell maturation is the predominant period of β cell expansion. In mice, β cell proliferation is highest in neonates and declines by 3 weeks after birth.[110] In humans, proliferation peaks between 4 and 6 months of age and becomes almost undetectable in adults. Studies in mice have identified several regulators required for neonatal β cell replication, including cyclin dependent kinases, D-type cyclins, and CDK (cyclin-dependent kinase) inhibitors (CKIs) (reviewed in[111]). Many of the same cell cycle proteins are present in human β cells but appear to be sequestered to the cytoplasm where they are not able to direct the essential cell cycle machinery.[111] Intensive efforts are underway to promote human β cell proliferation as a cell replacement therapy for diabetes; however, human β cells have proven to be extremely resistant to most proliferation-promoting strategies, and the ability to replicate often comes at the expense of β cell function.[112]

PANCREATIC EXOCRINE CELL DEVELOPMENT AND FUNCTION

MOLECULAR REGULATION OF EXOCRINE DEVELOPMENT

In rodents, a rapid increase in specific exocrine mRNA transcripts occurs late in gestation, shortly after endocrine cell differentiation, and is followed by a nonparallel increase in pancreas-specific proteins and zymogen granules.[113,114] Careful temporal characterization of exocrine transcript expression in rat showed that RNA synthesis peaks at embryonic day 18, followed by a peak in protein synthesis 1 day later. During this period, although total pancreatic protein synthesis increases by only 25%, synthesis of some exocrine pancreas-specific proteins (e.g., amylase and chymotrypsinogen) increases by more than 100%. Amylase-specific mRNA increases 600-fold at a gestational age between embryonic days 14 and 20, coincident with a 1000-fold increase in amylase-specific activity. During the final days of gestation and during early neonatal life, synthesis of secretory proteins accounts for more than 90% of all pancreatic protein synthesis.[115,116]

The first appearance of digestive enzymes in the human fetal pancreas has been variably described. Trypsin, chymotrypsin, phospholipase A, and lipase are present in the 14- to 16-week postconception fetus in low concentrations, and these steadily increase with gestation.[3,117,118] Chymotrypsin activity is low at birth, peaks at age 3 days, then declines slightly. Pancreatic secretory trypsin inhibitor is present in the fetal pancreas at 10 weeks gestation.[119] Pancreatic amylase is present in amniotic fluid at 14 weeks gestation.[120] A wide day-to-day variation of enzyme concentration is found; however, amylase, lipase, trypsinogen, and chymotrypsinogen are all present in the fetal pancreas by 16 weeks gestation, concurrent with the rapid development of zymogen granules. In rat, the presence of at least three different lipases, one of which may be identical to the zymogen granule membrane protein GP3, has been described.[121] Each lipase appears to be under different regulatory control, both before and after birth. In humans, Yang and colleagues[122] have also shown discoordinate expression of pancreatic lipase and two related proteins in the human fetal pancreas.

The initiation of individual exocrine enzyme synthesis appears to be distinct in different organisms, and the final levels are also dissimilar. However, the curves for the appearance of each protein are quite similar between humans and other organisms, and ultimately the final adult level of each enzyme is unrelated to the onset of synthesis or to the peak fetal level. Enzyme concentrations change considerably after birth,[114] and level of secretory protein in the mature pancreas represents the balance between synthesis and secretion.

Compared with the islet cells, considerably less is known about the molecular determinants of acinar cell differentiation. Currently, only a handful of factors are known to be specifically required for exocrine differentiation, including PFT1A, RBPJL, GATA4, LRH1/NR5A2, and MIST1. Pancreas-specific transcription factor 1 consists of a heterodimer comprising the ubiquitous transcriptional regulator E2A and a tissue-specific protein p48 (encoded by the *Ptf1a* gene).[50] This complex binds to the promoter regions of exocrine-specific genes and activates their transcription. Genetic ablation of *Ptf1a* in mice results in failure to form an exocrine pancreas, as well as morphologic deformities of the islets.[123] More recent studies using *Ptf1a*: Cre knock-in mice have broadened our understanding of the role of *Ptf1a* to include a much earlier function in specifying pancreatic identity from uncommitted endodermal precursors.[51]

RBPJL is a member of the pancreas-specific transcription factor 1 complex and functions with PTF1A to regulate acinar cell terminal differentiation and maintain acinar cell identity.[124] The nuclear receptor LRH1/NR5A2 has also been shown to physically interact with PTF1A and activate expression of acinar cell-specific genes.[125] Mice in which *Nr5a2* has been deleted are defective in several stages of exocrine development leading to a more than 90% loss of acini.[126]

MIST1 (encoded by the *Bhlha15* gene) is also a basic helix-loop-helix transcription factor expressed in the exocrine pancreas as well as in the salivary gland and stomach.[127] *Bhlha15*-null mice exhibit lesions in the exocrine pancreas, possibly resulting from defective cell-cell adhesion, but still retain exocrine-specific gene expression.[128] MIST1 has thus been proposed to function in cooperation with pancreas-specific transcription factor 1 to maintain a stable exocrine differentiated state. MIST1 is also required for granule organization in acinar and other exocrine cell types.[129]

SECRETION FROM THE EXOCRINE PANCREAS

Although a continuous slow basal secretion of pancreatic enzymes occurs, physiologically significant secretion occurs only after stimulation by a secretagogue. A large number of agents have been described that are effective secretagogues in the experimental animal, but only acetylcholine, secretin, and cholecystokinin (CCK) are of significance in humans. Acetylcholine is released locally in the pancreas after vagal stimulation. CCK and secretin are synthesized and stored in the intestinal amine precursor uptake and decarboxylation cells and are released after ingestion of a protein or fatty meal.

Each secretagogue then interacts with its specific receptor on the acinar cell membrane. Intracellular second and third messengers include Ca^{2+}, protein kinase C, diacylglycerol, and inositol phosphates.[130,131] This process eventually leads to fusion of zymogen granules and cell membranes and to exocytosis of pancreatic protein into the ductal system. Luminal factors, including the process of assembly and disassembly of a matrix (containing GP2 and proteoglycans), are thought to perform critical functions during storage and secretion of pancreatic secretory proteins.[132] Regulation by CCK and secretin is critical. Secretin acts directly on the pancreatic ducts. Human pancreatic acinar cells lack both CCK-A and CCK-B receptors. The primary target for CCK is now thought to be vagal receptors.[133] A portion of GP2 is cleaved by protein kinase C and released into the pancreatic duct during stimulated secretion.[134]

Fluid and electrolyte secretion from the centroacinar and ductal cells is controlled by secretin, which was the first hormone identified. The intracellular messengers in this system are cyclic adenosine monophosphate and protein kinase A. The concentrations of bicarbonate and chloride in pancreatic secretion depend on the flow rate. At lower flow rates, the concentration of bicarbonate is low and that of chloride is high.[135] As the flow rate increases, bicarbonate secretion increases and chloride secretion decreases, whereas sodium and potassium secretions remain constant.

The exocrine pancreas synthesizes more than 20 proteins specifically designed for export. After synthesis, it must segregate those proteins designated for export from those synthesized for internal use. Classic studies have demonstrated the synthetic pathway with use of the pulse-chase technique. Newly synthesized proteins travel from the endoplasmic reticulum to the Golgi apparatus, where they are "packaged" to the condensing vacuoles and then converted into mature zymogen granules in the apical portion of the cell. Little or no processing of individual proteins occurs from the time they leave the rough endoplasmic reticulum until the time they leave the cell. In rodents this entire process takes less than 1 hour. Molecular chaperones or chaperonins are involved in the transit process as they are in other cell types.[136]

ONTOGENY OF SECRETORY FUNCTION IN THE HUMAN

Because of both the technical difficulties and ethical concerns associated with performing invasive procedures in healthy infants, few studies of pancreatic secretory function in the human infant have been conducted. Because direct collection of pancreatic juice is not possible in the infant and young child, pancreatic secretions must be collected in the duodenum from the subject in the fasted or basal state, after indirect stimulation with a meal, or after direct stimulation with secretagogues such as secretin or CCK, or both. Pancreatic function may be determined indirectly by the measurement of fecal elastase and by fat balance studies.

Many of the early studies of exocrine pancreatic function in newborn infants are fraught with methodologic difficulties, including the qualitative nature of the collections and the lack of separation between the pancreatic and salivary amylase and lipase isoenzymes.[137-140] In a small group of children older than 9 months, Zoppi and colleagues[138] demonstrated that amylase secretion continues to increase with age (the oldest child studied was 13 years old), whereas output of lipase, proteinases, fluid, and bicarbonate was independent of age. A good correlation was found between protein secretion and enzyme activity. Norman and colleagues[141] measured pancreatic secretion in eight healthy term infants aged 3 to 15 days after a test meal of breast milk. Although the trypsin-to-chymotrypsin ratio was relatively constant, the levels of the individual enzymes varied considerably between infants. Salivary but not pancreatic amylase was present in low levels.

Basal and stimulated pancreatic secretion in groups of premature (32 to 36 weeks gestation) and term neonates, infants aged 1 month, and toddlers 2 years of age has been reported (Fig. 85.7).[142] The results obtained from term and premature infants were similar, and the data were pooled in the report. Although total protein content was similar in the pancreatic secretions collected from the duodenum of all three groups, each of the five individual secretory proteins studied had its own developmental profile. Trypsin level was low at 1 day, but at 1 month it was similar to the level seen at 2 years. Chymotrypsin level remained low at 1 month. The carboxypeptidase level was low both at 1 day and at 1 month when compared with the level found at 2 years. Amylase was not detected until age 2 years. Similarly, lipase was undetectable at 1 day and 1 month. Thus the ontogeny of the various enzymes is not parallel, a finding that has also been documented in rodents. Responses to secretin and CCK were poor in the newborn and the infant. Responses at 1 month were similar, whether the infants were fed a cow's milk-based formula or a soy formula.

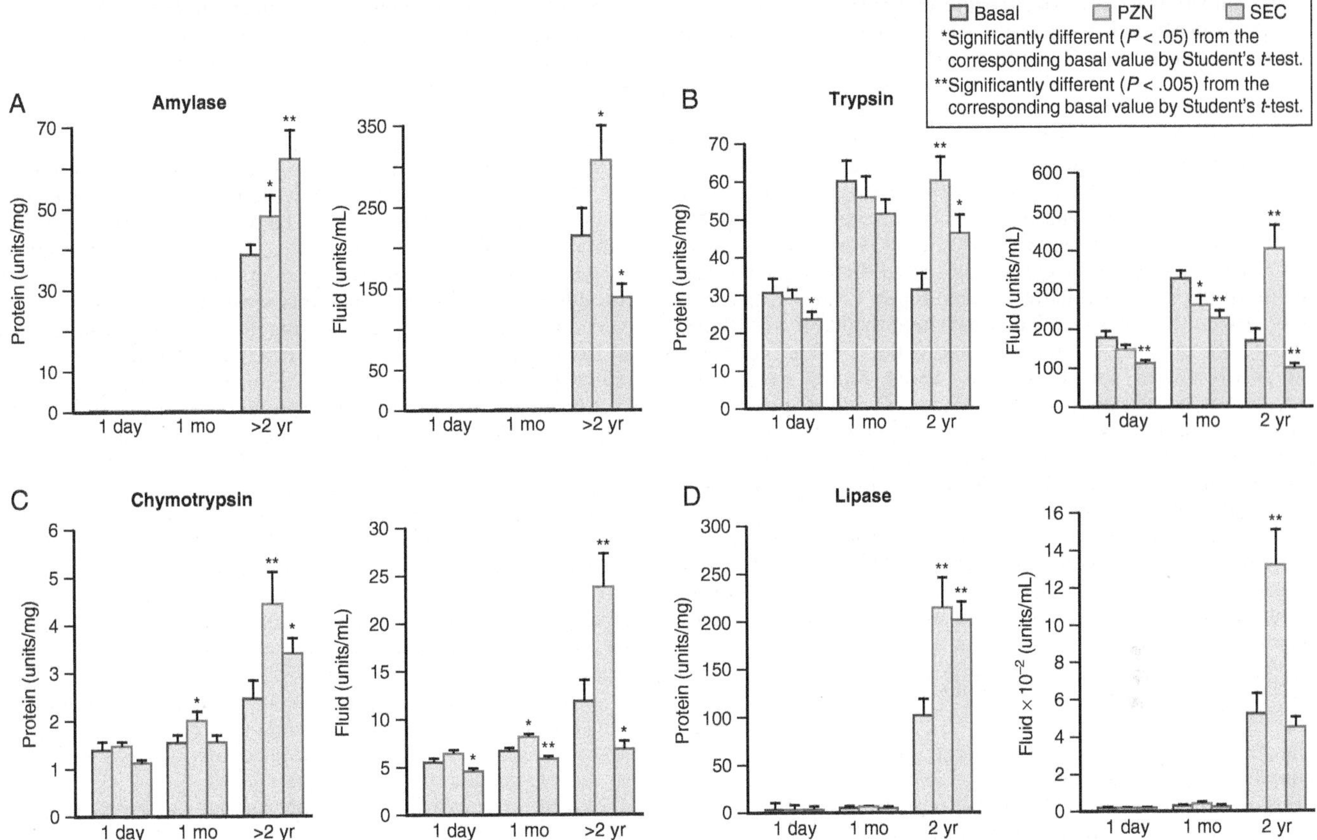

Fig. 85.7 Effect of cholecystokinin (CCK) and secretin on specific activities of pancreatic enzymes (amylase [A], trypsin [B], chymotrypsin [C], lipase [D]) in duodenal fluid in infants and children. *PZN,* Duodenal fluids collected after CCK-PZ (pancreozymin) administration (intravenously, 2 units/kg of body weight); *SEC,* duodenal fluids collected after secretin administration (intravenously, 2 units/kg of body weight).

These data confirm the findings of previous reports concerning proteinases but are contradictory with respect to amylase and lipase. It has clearly been shown that pancreatic amylase is present early in gestation. Similarly, salivary amylase is secreted in high concentration in the newborn. The serum levels of pancreatic isoamylase and isolipase are both low at birth and increase with age. These findings suggest that the newborn pancreas can synthesize but not secrete amylase. The failure to find a measurable amount of amylase may reflect the fasted state of the infants. A similar argument can be constructed to explain the extremely low levels of lipase.

Diet modulates pancreatic enzyme secretion in the human as it does in the animal models. Although these changes may occur at the level of synthesis, some changes reported to occur in animals clearly occur faster than can be explained by changes in synthesis. Premature infants fed a soy-based formula have greater stimulated secretion of lipase and trypsin compared with infants fed a cow's milk-based formula.[143] Total parenteral nutrition induces reversible pancreatic atrophy in animals and pancreatic hyposecretion in humans. Thus, as in the animal models described later in this chapter, some changes in pancreatic enzyme secretion are programmed, and others are inducible by diet.

ONTOGENY OF RODENT EXOCRINE PANCREATIC SECRETION

The pancreas of the newborn rat is both histologically and ultrastructurally fully developed; it is packed with secretory proteins. Although it appears poised to secrete proteins, it is functionally immature, and subsequent developmental steps correspond to the tertiary transition mentioned earlier. Immaturity has been documented at a number of steps along the stimulus-secretion chain. Responsiveness to cholinergic and peptidergic (e.g., CCK) secretagogues in a manner similar to, but not identical with, that of the adult gland does not occur until age 24 to 48 hours.[144-146] The newborn pancreas, although unresponsive to cholinergic agents and CCK, responded to the calcium ionophore A23187 with increased secretion of amylase in some studies but not in others.[146-148] Responsiveness suggests that the secretory mechanism distal to calcium mobilization is intact.

Muscarinic receptor density is low in the fetal and newborn periods and steadily increases with age, reaching maximal levels at age 1 month; it then decreases steadily until age 1 year.[149] A parallel increase occurs in secretory response and receptor density.

Binding of radiolabeled CCK to pancreatic acinar cells rises rapidly (from low levels at birth), reaching levels of the mature pancreas at age 3 weeks.[150,151] Others have found that the postnatal increase in secretory responsiveness was not associated with increased CCK binding.[148] These receptors are of the A or intestinal type that just after birth are already coupled to G proteins.[152] CCK-A glycoforms are different before birth. The results of these studies suggest that decreased receptor density cannot explain the lack of secretory responsiveness in the immature pancreas and that the immaturity is distal to calcium mobilization. The absence of the zymogen granule membrane protein GP2 in the fetus may contribute to secretory unresponsiveness.[153]

The ontogeny of the vasoactive intestinal polypeptide receptor has been described in rats and calves. In the rat, vasoactive intestinal polypeptide receptors are present at day 19 of gestation.[113,154] In the cow, a single class of receptors is present at birth; however, at 28 and 119 days after birth, two classes (high affinity and low affinity) of receptors are found.

Because protein phosphorylation appears to play an important role in the pancreatic response to secretagogues, the roles of protein kinases have been examined. Calcium-calmodulin–dependent protein kinase level increases in parallel with responsiveness to secretagogues from the late fetal to the newborn period.[155] Similarly, protein kinase C level was found to be low in the term fetus. The levels increased in the newborn period, reaching adult values by age 2 days.[156] The newborn rat pancreas was unresponsive to 12-*O*-tetradecanoylphorbol acetate, an activator of protein kinase C, but the 2-day-old pancreas responded to 12-*O*-tetradecanoylphorbol acetate with increased amylase secretion. These studies of protein kinases suggest immaturity of the secretory response to regulatory peptides at a number of levels.

Thus immaturity both of receptors to secretagogues and of protein kinases is found in the neonatal rat. At this time, the lack of responsiveness to secretagogues in the neonatal rat cannot be attributed to any one pharmacologic deficiency and may in fact be multifactorial.

EFFECTS OF DIET AND WEANING ON ACINAR CELL MATURATION

The pancreatic content of exportable proteins and zymogen granules falls dramatically after birth.[157] This fall is not preprogrammed but rather relates to feeding and stimulation of secretion.[158,159] Alterations in diet, time of weaning, and time of first feeding all affect the levels of secretory proteins in predictable ways.

Studies in which the diets of immature animals, including rats, pigs, and dogs, are altered have shown that the changes in the concentrations of various pancreatic enzymes are not all preprogrammed. The molecular basis for many of these effects has been reviewed.[160] Changing the diet from a high fat–low carbohydrate diet to a high carbohydrate–low fat diet by early weaning increases chymotrypsin and lipase and decreases amylase concentrations. Delaying weaning by prolonged nursing postpones these changes in enzyme concentration. Rats, pigs, or dogs weaned on a high-fat diet similar to mother's milk demonstrated changes in enzyme patterns similar to those found in animals prematurely weaned. The changes found with early weaning are similar to those induced with glucocorticoids. Premature weaning induces an increase in corticosteroid levels in the infant rat. Changes in diet after 21 days of age induce characteristic changes in pancreatic enzyme composition. Thus increasing the dietary intake of starch increases amylase concentration, increasing the intake of fat increases lipase concentration, and increasing the protein intake increases trypsin concentration. Glucocorticoids may modulate some effects of feeding; however, others seem to be preprogrammed.

ACINAR CELL REGULATORY FACTORS

Plasma CCK (CCK-8, CCK-33, and CCK-39) levels were measured before and after breast-feeding in 4-day-old infants.[161] A significant increase was seen immediately after a meal, followed by a decrease to basal levels at 10 minutes and a secondary increase at 30 and 60 minutes after feeding. This biphasic rise is not seen in older children or adults. Plasma gastrin 34 levels increased by 50% 5 and 10 minutes after the onset of suckling and immediately after breast-feeding in 3-day-old infants. Salmenperä and colleagues[162] measured postprandial levels of 11 regulatory hormones in 9-month-old infants who had been fed exclusively by either breast or bottle. The basal level of CCK and postprandial rise in CCK level were lower in breast-fed infants than in bottle-fed infants.

In the rat colon, CCK mRNA is found in low amounts in the fetus, is absent at birth, and then increases steadily until adulthood.[163] Immediately after birth, the rat small intestine contains CCK-like bioactivity. In the pig, CCK immunoreactivity is found in the small intestine at 6 to 8 weeks' gestation.[164] In the guinea pig, plasma CCK levels are low at birth but rise to near adult levels at day 15.[165] Thus CCK is present in the gut and is presumably available to participate in the regulation of pancreatic growth in the fetus.

Progastrin and gastrin are present in many species, including humans.[166] In the human fetal pancreas, the levels of gastrin and progastrin are low compared with those in other species. In the mouse, the gastrin gene is first expressed at 9.5 to 10 days gestation, whereas immunoreactivity does not develop until day 20. The gastrin gene is unique among those expressed by the pancreas in that it is active in the fetus but inactive in the adult, except when Zollinger-Ellison syndrome develops. Thus CCK and gastrin, both trophic agents for the pancreas, are present at birth when the rate of pancreatic growth is the greatest.

CCK controls gene expression at the translational level.[167] Long-term stimulation with CCK and cerulean (a CCK analogue) stimulates mRNA synthesis for genes coding for trypsinogen and chymotrypsinogen but not amylase.[168]

Pancreatic growth in the mature animal can be altered by a variety of agents, diets, and experimental procedures.[169] The trophic effects of CCK, gastrin, and CCK-like peptides have been well documented. In the adult rat the postprandial CCK level regulates ornithine decarboxylase and secretory protein gene expression at the translational level. Treatment of rats with the CCK antagonist L364718 not only prevents the trophic effects of exogenous CCK but also causes pancreatic atrophy, suggesting that CCK is necessary for both growth and maintenance of the gland.[170] When given to the immature rat, this agent does not alter normal growth but does block the trophic effects of exogenous CCK.[171] CCK-induced growth is mediated by a single-type variety of type A receptors with both high-affinity and low-affinity states.[172-175]

Although there are published studies concerning the roles of many of the previously discussed agents and treatments in the immature pancreas, interpretation and comparison of these studies present numerous difficulties in data analysis, including that (1) the various agents tested were given in different doses, at different ages, and for different lengths of time; and (2) the animals were evaluated for effects on growth in different ways. A major fact often overlooked is that the growth rate and the rates of synthesis of both DNA and protein vary considerably with developmental age.[176]

A great deal has been learned concerning the effects of many agents on the growth of the exocrine pancreas in the developing animal. CCK and CCK-like peptides have a variety of effects that seem to be age dependent. DNA synthesis is not increased by CCK before age 28 days, and variable effects on growth have been described depending on age, dosage, and CCK analogue studied.[177-179] The potent specific CCK antagonist L364718 blocks the effects of exogenous cerulean on the growth of the neonatal rat pancreas, but when given alone, it has no effect. This suggests that endogenous CCK is not a controlling factor in the growth of the neonatal rat pancreas.[180]

CCK action is mediated by CCK receptors. Of the two types of CCK receptors (A and B), the adult rat pancreas has only type A, which mediates pancreatic growth in adult rats. Although Otsuka Long-Evans Tokushima fatty rats lack the CCK-A receptor gene, pancreatic growth in the immediate postnatal life is normal although the pancreas is slightly smaller at 5 to 6 weeks of age.[181] However, in later growth at 24 to 25 weeks, Otsuka Long-Evans Tokushima fatty rats showed a significantly lower protein-DNA content than the wild-type strain, which suggests that the CCK-A receptor plays a small role in the early postnatal growth of the pancreas but is required for later cell growth. Thus CCK might not be important in regulating pancreatic growth in early postnatal life.

The role of gastrin is likewise questioned. Administration of a specific gastrin antagonist, CI-988, to neonates for 5 days reduced stomach growth but not pancreatic growth.[182] Thus although pharmacologic doses of gastrin and CCK are trophic for the neonatal exocrine pancreas, it is unclear whether they play a role in the early development of the exocrine pancreas.

Hydrocortisone decreases protein synthesis in the first week of life but has no effect on DNA synthesis in the immature animal.[177] Other studies have described hypertrophy and hyperplasia or hypertrophy alone,[178,183] depending on age. Cerulean and hydrocortisone potentiate each other's trophic effects. The lack of increase in DNA synthesis in the suckling animal after treatment with either CCK or hydrocortisone may be due to the finding that synthesis is already preceding at the maximum rate possible.

A temporal relationship exists between corticosterone levels, cytoplasmic corticosteroid receptors, and increases in pancreatic secretory products in the developing rat pancreas.[183,184] Corticosterone levels and dexamethasone binding increase from birth, reach a peak at approximately age 25 days, then decrease to adult levels. Increases in circulating levels of steroids precede increases in receptor density, which increases sharply after age 15 days. These increases parallel those of both amylase and hydrolase activities, which can be induced by exogenous steroids. The pancreatic glucocorticoid receptor is under autologous control of glucocorticoid. Early weaning, which augments corticosterone levels, causes similar changes in the content of exportable proteins in the pancreas. The highest density of steroid receptors occurs at age 21 to 28 days, the period of peak responsiveness of the pancreas to hydrocortisone. Thus glucocorticoids clearly modulate postnatal pancreatic development.[184]

Thyroxine induces precocious increases of amylase, lipase, chymotrypsin, and trypsin in neonatal rats, and chemical thyroidectomy retards pancreatic development.[185] The level of endogenous thyroxine peaks between days 10 and 16, the time point when amylase levels are also increasing. Thyroxine induces maturation of secretory function by modulating the maximum binding capacity of high-affinity CCK receptors. In the immature animal, thyroid hormone acts both directly on the pancreatic acinar cells and indirectly through the adrenal system.[185,186]

Pancreatic duct cells have high levels of epidermal growth factor.[187] Parenterally but not orally administered epidermal growth factor increases pancreatic amylase levels in suckling rabbits.[188] Inhibition of ornithine decarboxylase (and thus polyamine metabolism) inhibits stimulated pancreatic growth.[189,190] The role of polyamines in normal pancreatic growth and development has not been established. Secretin increases DNA, amylase, and chymotrypsin levels in 6-day-old rats.[191] The effects of peptide YY and somatostatin, which are antitrophic to the pancreas in mature animals, have not been studied in developing animals.

Other regulatory factors have also been implicated in rodent pancreatic exocrine development. Acting directly on the pancreas, bombesin induces hypertrophy and hyperplasia in newborn rats.[192] In adult animals bombesin regulates pancreatic gene expression at the level of mRNA.[193,194] This effect is not mediated by CCK.[194] TGF-α appears after birth and its level increases progressively with age in the exocrine pancreas.[195] Artificially mutated TGF-β receptor in mice leads to a pancreas with acinar hyperplasia and atypia.[196] Overexpression of TGF-β interferes with acinar differentiation.[197] TGF-β added to rat embryonic pancreatic rudiments resulted in differential gene activation.[198] FGFs and FGF receptors are important mediators of epithelial-mesenchymal interactions. FGFs are expressed throughout rat pancreatic development. In mesenchyme-free culture of embryonic pancreatic epithelium, addition of FGFs promotes growth, morphogenesis, and cytodifferentiation of exocrine pancreatic cells.[199] In the presence of mesenchyme, growth and development of pancreatic epithelium progresses without the addition of FGFs. Abrogation of FGF receptor 2 isoform IIIb in the system attenuates both growth and development.

FETAL ANTIGENS

Fetoacinar protein (FAP) is a specific acinar cell antigen found only in the exocrine pancreas. In the human fetus, FAP is present at 9 to 10 weeks gestation[200] and its level peaks at 15 to 25 weeks, when acinar cell proliferation is most intense. FAP synthesis then progressively decreases. The levels found in adults are lower than those in the fetus. FAP is found in high concentration in amniotic fluid. FAP can also be considered an oncodevelopmental antigen, because in pancreatic cancer and in some cases of chronic pancreatitis FAP level is elevated. FAP has been shown to be a variant of bile salt–dependent lipase, differing only by a decrease in *O*-glycosylation.[201]

A second fetal antigen, fetal antigen 1 (FA1), is found in both the exocrine and endocrine fetal pancreas and hepatocytes.[202] FA1 is found in high concentration in the fetal venous blood and amniotic fluid during the second and third trimesters. At 7 weeks gestation, FA1 is found in 94% of the ductal epithelial cells. By week 17, only 64% of the duct cells test positive for FA1 by immunoperoxidase staining, decreasing to only 11% in the 4-month-old infant. The role or roles and controls of FA1 in pancreatic development are not known.

SUMMARY

The pancreas is a relatively late-developing organ in the scheme of embryonic development. Its formation is contingent on the successive execution of multiple earlier steps, from specification of pancreatic cell fate in the endoderm, to fusion of two independent anlage, to cell lineage allocation, induction of outgrowth, and then completion of the differentiation program and maturation. In the last several years genetic technology and rodent models have helped to provide molecular annotation of these events, offering novel connections between genes and developmental mechanisms. More recently, access to human embryonic and fetal tissues has confirmed that many of the morphologic and molecular developmental events are conserved between rodents and humans. Furthermore, the knowledge of pancreas development that has been gained from model organisms has facilitated the successful differentiation of pancreatic lineages, and particularly islet β cells, from human stem cell populations.[108,109] Ironically, human pluripotent stem cell models of pancreas development have subsequently become important tools for characterizing human pancreas development and diseases.

ACKNOWLEDGMENT

Some content was based on a previous chapter by Steven L. Werlin, MD, and Alan N. Mayer, MD.

A complete reference list is available at www.ExpertConsult.com.

SELECT REFERENCES

1. Zorn AM, Wells JM. Vertebrate endoderm development and organ formation. *Annu Rev Cell Dev Biol*. 2009;25:221-251.
2. Bakhti M, Bottcher A, Lickert H. Modelling the endocrine pancreas in health and disease. *Nat Rev Endocrinol*. 2019;15(3):155-171.
3. Piper K, Brickwood S, Turnpenny LW, et al. Beta cell differentiation during early human pancreas development. *J Endocrinol*. 2004;181:11-23.
4. Tadokoro H, Takase M, Nobukawa B. Development and congenital anomalies of the pancreas. *Anat Res Int*. 2011;2001:351217.
6. Jennings RE, Berry AA, Kirkwood-Wilson R, et al. Development of the human pancreas from foregut to endocrine commitment. *Diabetes*. 2013;62:3514-3522.
7. Polak M, Bouchareb-Banaei L, Scharfmann R, Czernichow P. Early pattern of differentiation in the human pancreas. *Diabetes*. 2000;49(2):225-232.
8. Riopel M, Li J, Fellows GF, et al. Ultrastructural and immunohistochemical analysis of the 8-20 week old human fetal pancreas. *Islets*. 2014;6(4):e982949.
13. Reinert RB, Brissova M, Shostak A, et al. Vascular endothelial growth factor-a and islet vascularization are necessary in developing, but not adult, pancreatic islets. *Diabetes*. 2013;62:4154-4164.
16. Pierreux CE, Cordi S, Hick AC, et al. Epithelial: endothelial cross-talk regulates exocrine differentiation in developing pancreas. *Dev Biol*. 2010;347:216-227.
22. Lukinius A, Ericsson JL, Grimelius L, Korsgren O. Ultrastructural studies of the ontogeny of fetal human and porcine endocrine pancreas, with special reference to colocalization of the four major islet
23. Reidel MJ, Asadi A, Wang R, et al. Immunohistochemical characterization of cells co-producing insulin and glucagon in the developing human pancreas. *Diabetologia*. 2012;55:372-381.
24. Laitio M, Lev R, Orlic D. The developing human fetal pancreas: an ultrastructural and histochemical study with special reference to exocrine cells. *J Anat*. 1974;117(Pt 3):619.
25. Track NS, Creutzfeldt C, Bokermann M. Enzymatic, functional and ultrastructural development of the exocrine pancreas—II. The human pancreas. *Comp Biochem Physiol*. 1975;51(1A):95.
27. Oates PS, Morgan RGH. Cell proliferation in the exocrine pancreas during development. *J Anat*. 1989;167:235.
32. Cleveland MH, Sawyer JM, Afelik S, et al. Exocrine ontogenies: on the development of pancreatic acinar, ductal and centroacinar cells. *Semin Cell Dev Biol*. 2012;23:711-719.
33. Pictet R, Rutter WJ. Development of the embryonic endocrine pancreas. In: Steiner DF, Freinkel N, eds. *Handbook of Physiology, Section 7, Endocrinology*. Vol. 1. Washington, DC: American Physiological Society; 1972:25-66.
34. Gittes GK, Rutter WJ. Onset of cell-specific gene expression in the developing mouse pancreas. *Dev Biol*. 1992;89:1128.
35. Jorgensen MC, Ahnfelt-Ronne J, Hald J, et al. An illustrated review of early pancreas development in the mouse. *Endocr Rev*. 2007;28:685-705.
36. Slack JM. Developmental biology of the pancreas. *Development*. 1995;121:1569.
37. Percival AC, Slack JM. Analysis of pancreatic development using a cell lineage label. *Exp Cell Res*. 1999;247:123-132.
41. Wells JM, Melton DA. Early mouse endoderm is patterned by soluble factors from adjacent germ layers. *Development*. 2000;127:1563-1572.
52. Villani V, Thornton ME, Zook HN, et al. SOX9+/PTF1A+ cells define the tip progenitor cells of the human fetal pancreas of the second trimester. *Stem Cells Transl Med*. 2019;8(12):1249-1264.
59. Golosow N, Grobstein C. Epitheliomesenchymal interaction in pancreatic morphogenesis. *Dev Biol*. 1962;4:242-255.
60. Wessells NK, Cohen JH. Early pancreas organogenesis: morphogenesis, tissue interactions and mass effects. *Dev Biol*. 1967;15:237-270.
64. Irion S, Nostro MC, Kattman SJ, Keller GM. Directed differentiation of pluripotent stem cells: from developmental biology to therapeutic applications. *Cold Spring Harb Symp Quant Biol*. 2008;73:101-110.
65. Nostro MC, Keller G. Generation of beta cells from human pluripotent stem cells: potential for regenerative medicine. *Semin Cell Dev Biol*. 2012;23:701-710.
75. Zhang X, McGrath PS, Salomone J, et al. A comprehensive structure-function study of Neurogenin3 disease-causing alleles during human pancreas and intestinal organoid development. *Dev Cell*.
76. McGrath PS, Watson CL, Ingram C, Helmrath MA, Wells JM. The basic helix-loop-helix transcription factor NEUROG3 is required for development of the human endocrine pancreas. *Diabetes*.
78. Lyttle BM, Li J, Krishnamurthy M, et al. Transcription factor expression in the developing human fetal endocrine pancreas. *Diabetologia*. 2008;51(7):1169-1180.
79. Sarkar SA, Kobberup S, Wong R, et al. Global gene expression profiling and histochemical analysis of the developing human fetal pancreas. *Diabetologia*. 2008;51(2):285-297.
80. Folias AE, Hebrok M. Diabetes. Solving human beta-cell development–what does the mouse say? *Nat Rev Endocrinol*. 2014;10(5):253-255.
84. Jain R, Lammert E. Cell-cell interactions in the endocrine pancreas. *Diabetes Obes Metab*. 2009;11(suppl 4):159-167.
85. Jeon J, Correa-Medina M, Ricordi C, Edlund H, Diez JA. Endocrine cell clustering during human pancreas development. *J Histochem Cytochem*. 2009;57(9):811-824.
86. Gregg BE, Moore PC, Demozay D, et al. Formation of a human beta-cell population within pancreatic islets is set early in life. *J Clin Endocrinol Metab*. 2012;97(9):3197-3206.
87. Hart NJ, Powers AC. Use of human islets to understand islet biology and diabetes: progress, challenges and suggestions. *Diabetologia*. 2019;62(2):212-222.
88. Cabrera O, Berman DM, Kenyon NS, Ricordi C, Berggren PO, Caicedo A. The unique cytoarchitecture of human pancreatic islets has implications for islet cell function. *Proc Natl Acad Sci U S A*. 2006;103(7):2334-2339.
89. Brissova M, Fowler MJ, Nicholson WE, et al. Assessment of human pancreatic islet architecture and composition by laser scanning confocal microscopy. *J Histochem Cytochem*. 2005;53(9):1087-1097.
90. Rorsman P, Braun M. Regulation of insulin secretion in human pancreatic islets. *Annu Rev Physiol*. 2013;75:155-179.
91. Prentki M, Matschinsky FM, Madiraju SR. Metabolic signaling in fuel-induced insulin secretion. *Cell Metab*. 2013;18(2):162-185.
92. Thorn P, Zorec R, Rettig J, Keating DJ. Exocytosis in non-neuronal cells. *J Neurochem*. 2016;137(6):849-859.
105. Freinkel N, Lewis NJ, Johnson R, Swenne I, Bone A, Hellerstrom C. Differential effects of age versus glycemic stimulation on the maturation of insulin stimulus-secretion coupling during culture of fetal rat islets. *Diabetes*. 1984;33(11):1028-1038.
106. Aguayo-Mazzucato C, Zavacki AM, Marinelarena A, et al. Thyroid hormone promotes postnatal rat pancreatic beta-cell development and glucose-responsive insulin secretion through MAFA. *Diabetes*. 2013;62(5):1569-1580.
108. Rezania A, Bruin JE, Arora P, et al. Reversal of diabetes with insulin-producing cells derived in vitro from human pluripotent stem cells. *Nat Biotechnol*. 2014;32(11):1121-1133.
109. Pagliuca FW, Millman JR, Gurtler M, et al. Generation of functional human pancreatic beta cells in vitro. *Cell*. 2014;159(2):428-439.
110. Georgia S, Bhushan A. Beta cell replication is the primary mechanism for maintaining postnatal beta cell mass. *J Clin Invest*. 2004;114(7):963-968.
111. Wang P, Fiaschi-Taesch NM, Vasavada RC, Scott DK, Garcia-Ocana A, Stewart AF. Diabetes mellitus–advances and challenges in human beta-cell proliferation. *Nat Rev Endocrinol*. 2015;11(4):201-212.
112. Puri S, Roy N, Russ HA, et al. Replication confers beta cell immaturity. *Nat Commun*. 2018;9(1):485.
113. Przybyla AE, MacDonald RJ, Harding JD, et al. Accumulation of the predominant pancreatic mRNAs during embryonic development. *J Biol Chem*. 1979;254:2154.
115. Kemp JD, Walther BT, Rutter WJ. Protein synthesis during the secondary developmental transition of the embryonic rat pancreas. *J Biol Chem*. 1972;247:3941.
118. Carrère J, Figarella-Branger D, Senegas-Balas F, et al. Immunohistochemical study of secretory proteins in the developing human exocrine pancreas. *Differentiation*. 1992;51:55.
130. Grossman A. An overview of pancreatic exocrine secretion. *Comp Biochem Physiol*. 1984;78B:1.
134. Wagner AC, Williams JA. Pancreatic zymogen granule membrane proteins: molecular details begin to emerge. *Digestion*. 1994;55:191.
135. Scheele G, Kern H. Cellular compartmentation, protein processing and secretion in the exocrine pancreas. In: Go VLW, DiMagno EP, Gardner JD, et al., eds. *The Pancreas*. 2nd ed. New York: Raven; 1993.
140. Zoppi G, Andreotti G, Pajno-Ferrara F, et al. Exocrine pancreas function in premature and full term infants. *Pediatr Res*. 1972;6:880.
145. Doyle CM, Jamieson JD. Development of secretagogue response in rat pancreatic acinar cells. *Dev Biol*. 1978;65:11.
159. Merchant Z, Jiang LX, Lebenthal E, Lee PC. Pancreatic exocrine enzymes during the neonatal period in post mature rats. *Int J Pancreat*. 1987;2:325.
160. Le Huerou-Luron I, Lhoste E, Wicker-Planquart C, et al. Molecular aspects of enzyme synthesis in the exocrine pancreas with emphasis on development and nutritional regulation. *Proc Nutr Soc*. 1993;52:301.
164. Alumets J, Håkanson R, Sundler F. Ontogeny of endocrine cells in porcine gut and pancreas. *Gastroenterology*. 1983;85:1359.

Digestive-Absorptive Functions in Fetuses, Infants, and Children

86

Diomel de la Cruz | Josef Neu

INTRODUCTION

The developing gastrointestinal (GI) tract is the largest and most active immune organ of the body and supports important endocrine and exocrine roles in addition to its role for digestion. It encompasses a large mass of neural tissue that interacts closely with the developing central nervous system. In addition to intestinal tissue that is derived from the human sperm and egg, the intestinal microbiome is increasingly recognized as having a major role in development of the immune system, development of the brain, metabolism, and epigenetics. Fig. 86.1 depicts the myriad of integrated functions that transcend the digestive and absorptive role of the GI tract. The neonatal GI tract plays an important role in the pathogenesis of obesity, autoimmune diseases, allergy, and even neurodevelopmental disorders. In this chapter, we review the ontogeny and basic physiology of some of the major aspects of intestinal macronutrient (protein, carbohydrate, and lipid) digestion and absorption. The metabolic and immunologic aspects of the microbiome as related to digestion and absorption will be briefly discussed.

It is important to distinguish between the processes of digestion, absorption, and assimilation, with digestion primarily involving mechanisms that occur in the lumen of the intestine, absorption occurring at the intestinal mucosal surface, and assimilation occurring within and beyond the epithelial cells. A brief general overview of macronutrient digestion, absorption, and, where appropriate, assimilation is first provided and then the ontogeny of these processes will be presented during early fetal and postnatal life. Several of these descriptions of basic physiology will be augmented with clinically relevant correlations.

INTESTINAL GROWTH

Data accumulated by autopsy reports show the following small intestinal growth prenatally and postnatally: Mean length at 20 weeks gestation is 125 cm, at 30 weeks 200 cm, at term gestation 275 cm, at 1 year 380 cm, at 5 years 450 cm, at 10 years 500 cm, and at 20 years 575 cm.[1] Although this growth, especially during fetal life, appears to be large, it belies the fact that the surface area of the intestine is growing much faster during this time. When one accounts for the total surface provided by the villi and microvilli, this surface area becomes the largest in the body, which is also exposed to an external environment that includes a vast variety of antigens, microbes, and foods. The major component of the intestinal barrier between the external environment and the interior consists of a single layer of intestinal epithelium.

The intestine is subdivided into five functional areas along the proximal-to-distal gradient: the small intestine comprises the duodenum, jejunum, and ileum; the large intestine encompasses the cecum and colon. Specialized cell and tissue types originating from all three germ layers are found: endoderm-derived epithelium includes specialized intestinal stem cells,[2]

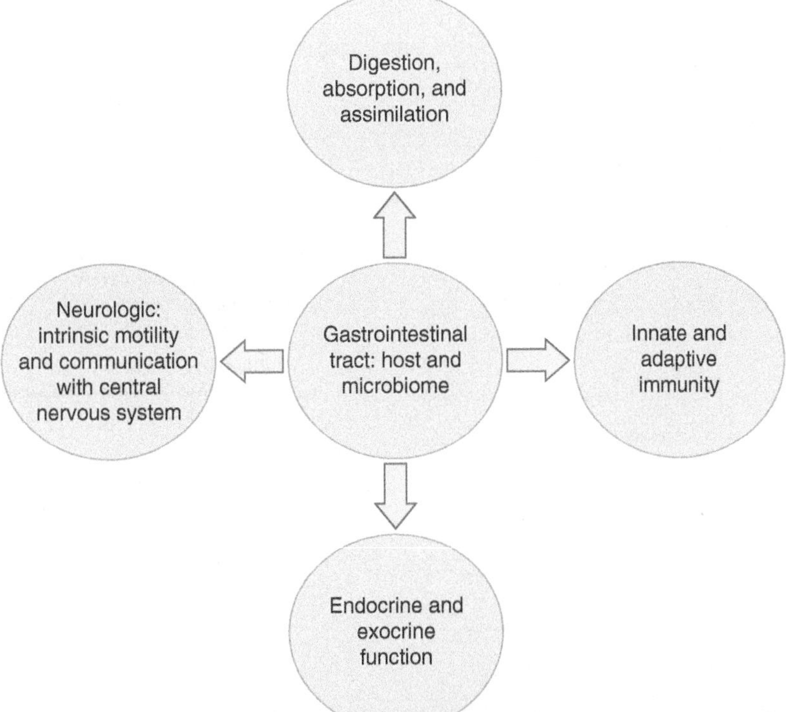

Fig. 86.1 Integrated functions of the intestinal tract and the intestinal microbiome.

smooth muscle, vascular, lymphatic and immune cells derived from mesoderm, and the enteric nervous system cells derived from ectoderm.

INTESTINAL EPITHELIAL CELLULAR DIVERSITY AND KINETICS

The intestinal epithelium is comprised of a diverse population of cells that differ depending on the aboral gradient region that spans the mouth to the rectum. These cells also differ in function depending on what region of the GI tract they are located. The intestinal epithelium functions as a selective barrier by restricting microbes and other antigens to the gut lumen.[3] The absorptive enterocyte along with cells of three secretory lineages comprise the epithelium. The epithelial cells of the intestine secrete digestive enzymes and mucus, absorb food particles, and produce hormones. The secretory cells involved in barrier function include goblet cells, which secrete mucin and Paneth cells, which release antimicrobial factors. The enteroendocrine cells secrete hormones involved in satiety, motility, secretion of digestive enzymes.[4]

A crypt to villus gradient of cells is present wherein epithelial cells undergo mitosis in the crypt region. Most of these cells migrate along the villus to the tip, where they are eventually extruded into the lumen of the intestine. The turnover and migration time from cell production in the crypt to extrusion from the villus tip ("anoikis") differs depending on age and region of the intestine, with younger animals showing longer migration times than adult animals.[5,6] Although most of the cells migrate to the villus tip, Paneth cells remain in the crypt region, where they perform the critical function of defending the mitotically active stem cells from pathogens using a myriad of defensive molecules.[7] The different regions across the crypt to villus axes serve different functions. Cells of the crypt are highly proliferative, whereas cells in the mid to the upper villus become increasingly differentiated as they migrate to the villus tip for absorptive as well as immunologic and neuroendocrine functions.

GENERAL ASPECTS OF DIGESTION, ABSORPTION, AND ASSIMILATION

An overview of major digestive absorptive processes is provided in Fig. 86.2. Food introduced into the mouth and stomach generally consists of large molecular aggregates that need to be further simplified by mechanical and biochemical means. However, milk presented to the newborn does not require chewing. Suck-swallow incoordination persists until 34 weeks gestational age,[8] necessitating tube feeding. With tube feeding, digestive processes in the oral cavity are bypassed, and thus digestion begins in the stomach. Enzymatic and other chemical processes include interactions between the food and gastric acid, proteases, lipases, salivary- and pancreatic-derived carbohydrases, and emulsifiers such as bile acids. In addition to the digestive processes provided by the human host, microbes residing in various parts of the GI tract metabolize various foods, and the metabolites produced from these microbes may be further digested and absorbed by the human host. These metabolites can be used for energy production purposes such as occurs with the short-chain fatty acids and for various other metabolic processes such as with certain vitamins (e.g., vitamins K and B12).

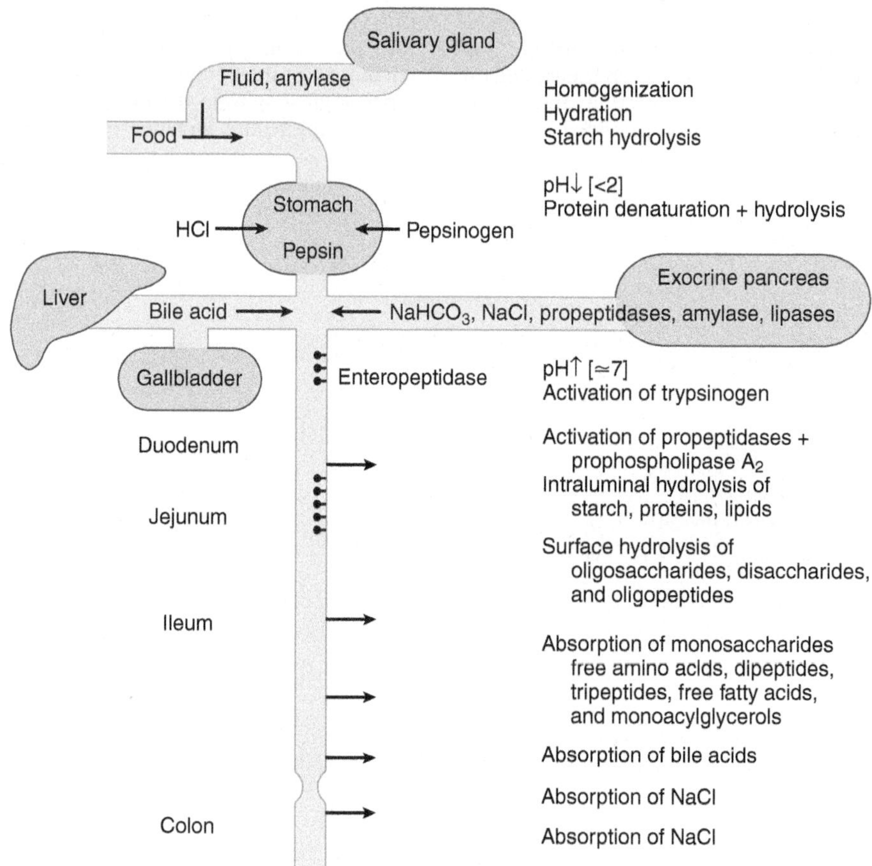

Fig. 86.2 Overview of digestion and absorption. (Modified from Johnson LR, ed. *Physiology of the Gastrointestinal Tract*. New York: Raven Press; 1994:1751–1772.)

PROTEIN

Human and cow's milk proteins comprise most of the proteins provided to the newborn infant, depending on whether the infant is breast- or formula-fed. Whey and casein synthesized in the mammary epithelial cells comprise the primary groups of milk proteins derived from these sources.[9] Other protein components include immunoglobulins and albumin, which are not synthesized by the epithelial cells but rather are absorbed from the maternal blood or from plasma cells, which reside in the mammary tissue. Caseins can be separated from the whey fraction of milk using precipitation with the acid. This precipitation separates the supernatant whey fraction from the precipitate, which is the casein fraction. Both fractions contain important essential amino acids that are required for normal metabolic functions, growth, and development.

The processes for protein digestion are summarized in Box 86.1 and Fig. 86.2. Digestion of proteins begins in the acidic environment of the stomach and continues in the small intestine under the influence of pancreatic proteases and peptidases. This process is accomplished by proteolytic cleavage of peptide bonds by enzymes that are secreted into the lumen of the upper digestive tract. In the stomach, pepsinogen is secreted and, in turn, is converted to the active protease pepsin by the action of acid. Secondly, the pancreas secretes proteases, such as trypsin, chymotrypsin, and carboxypeptidases, that require activation by the enzyme enterokinase; enterokinase is produced by the upper small intestinal epithelium, primarily in response to food. These proteases induce hydrolysis of the whole proteins within the lumen of the small intestine and result in the production of the medium to small amino acid chains called *oligopeptides*, *dipeptides*, or *single amino acids*.

Box 86.1 Protein Digestive Processes

Stomach

Proteolytic enzymes contained in gastric juice
Requires acid environment of stomach to hydrolyze protein
Synthesized in the gastric chief cells as inactive pre-proenzymes (pepsinogen)

Pancreas

Enterokinase: an intestinal brush border enzyme that activates pancreatic proteases. Stimulated by trypsinogen contained in pancreatic juice.

Pancreatic Endopeptidases

Trypsin: cleaves peptide bonds on the carboxyl side of basic amino acids (lysine and arginine)
Chymotrypsin: cleaves peptide bonds on the carboxyl side of aromatic amino acids (tyrosine, phenylalanine, and tryptophan)
Elastase: cleaves peptide bonds on the carboxyl side of aliphatic amino acids (alanine, leucin, glycine, valine, isoleucine)

Pancreatic Exopeptidases

Carboxypeptidases A and B: zinc-containing metalloenzymes that remove single amino acids from the carboxyl-terminal ends of proteins and peptides
Carboxypeptidase A: polypeptides with free carboxyl groups are cleaved to lower peptides and aromatic amino acids
Carboxypeptidase B: polypeptides with free carboxyl groups are cleaved to lower peptides and dibasic amino acids

Absorption of the products of digestion are depicted in Fig. 86.3. Oligopeptides are absorbed into the small intestinal epithelial cell primarily by co-transport with hydrogen ions.[10,11] These oligopeptides are further hydrolyzed within the epithelial cell into single amino acids by cytoplasmic peptidases and subsequently exported from the intestinal epithelial cell into the bloodstream. Only a very small number of these oligopeptides enter the blood intact.

Single amino acids can also be absorbed by the intestinal epithelial cell via several sodium-dependent amino acid transporters. These can be specific for acidic, basic, and neutral amino acids.[12] After binding sodium, these transporters bind the amino acids, which undergo a conformational change; this permits entry into the cytoplasm. Along with sodium, the amino acids are then reoriented to their original form. Absorption of amino acids is similar to those of the monosaccharides and contributes to osmotic gradients that drive water absorption. The basolateral membranes of the intestinal epithelial enterocytes contain additional transporters that are not dependent on sodium gradients, which export amino acids from the cell into the blood.

ONTOGENY OF PROTEIN DIGESTION AND ABSORPTION

GASTRIC ACID

The human fetus has the potential to produce gastric acid from the middle of the second trimester. By the 13th week, parietal cells that produce the acid are present in the pyloric regions of

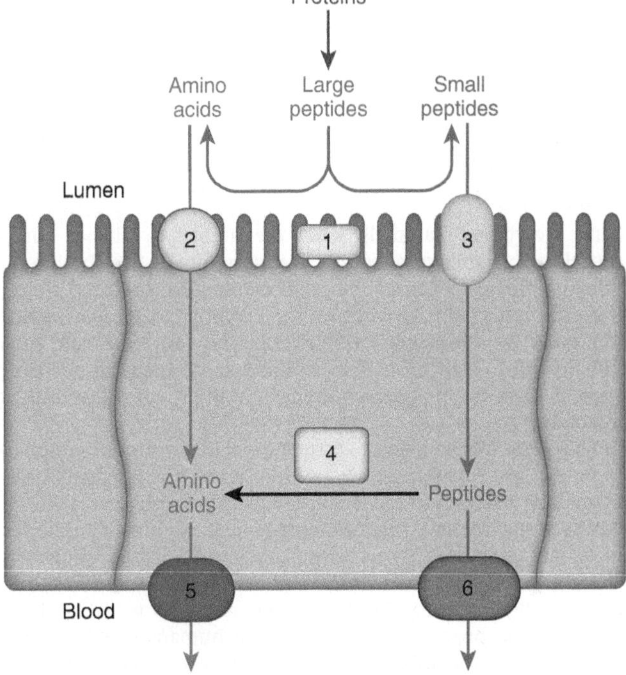

Fig. 86.3 Protein absorption. (Modified from Johnson LR, ed. *Physiology of the Gastrointestinal Tract*. New York: Raven Press; 1994:1751–1772.)

the fetal stomach.[13-15] Premature infants have considerably lower hydrochloric acid secretion in their stomach than do infants born at term.[16-18]

Although gastric acid secretion is limited in very low-birth-weight infants, it doubles from the first to the fourth week of postnatal life.[18] Food is a major stimulus to pH changes, where the entry of milk in the infant's stomach causes a sharp increase in the pH of the gastric contents and a slower return to lower pH values when compared with the older children and adults.[19,20]

UPPER GASTROINTESTINAL PROTEOLYTIC ENZYMES

The capability for proteolysis can be demonstrated as early as 16 weeks gestation.[21] The enzymes pepsinogen and cathepsin appear at approximately 17 to 18 weeks gestation.[22] The activity of the pepsin in the stomach of newborn infants is proportional to the degree of maturity.[23] Shortly after birth, in the fundus of the stomach it increases approximately four-fold after food intake in the first few days after birth.[24]

Pepsin production in the stomach of the newborn remains relatively low until the third postnatal month.[25] However, there were no differences in pepsin activity found via biopsy specimens of the gastric body in subjects aged 6 months to 15 years.[26]

Food stimulates secretion of enterokinase, which originates from the upper small intestinal epithelium. Enterokinase triggers a cascade of protease activity by catalyzing the activation of several inactive proteases into active forms, which perform their function in the intestinal lumen. Enterokinase is detectable at approximately 24 weeks of gestation, but its concentration is low and reaches only approximately 25% of adult activity at term.[27] This is potentially limiting to protein digestion.

Pancreatic enzymes are present at the later part of the first trimester, and secretion of these enzymes is initiated at approximately the fifth month of gestation.[21] Immunoreactive trypsin-1 and immunoreactive chymotrypsin A are detectable in amniotic fluid at 17 to 18 weeks of pregnancy.[28] Levels of trypsin are relatively low prior to 3 months, but chymotrypsin activity is also low in the newborn. These enzymes increase gradually, approaching the levels of older children at approximately 6 months of age.[29] Measurement of the fecal trypsin concentrations in preterm infants from 23 to 32 weeks gestational age during first 4 weeks of life demonstrates values that are similar to those found in term infants.[30]

ABSORPTION

Many newborn mammals have the ability to absorb intact proteins. This ability, called *closure*, is rapidly lost in the human when compared with several other mammalian species,[31-33] but it is important because it allows the newborn to acquire passive immunity by absorbing immunoglobulins and colostrum milk. This form of absorption is indispensable in shielding newborn animals from the possibility of succumbing to an opportunistic infection.

This same mechanism of absorption of intact proteins appears to be not as critical in newborn humans as it is for many other mammals. Preterm neonates, particularly those less than 33 weeks gestation, have higher serum concentrations of antibodies to β-lactoglobulin than term neonates given equivalent feeding.[33] This suggests that the ability of the GI tract to exclude antigenically intact food proteins increases with gestational age, and thus the process of gut closure in humans usually occurs before birth. Using nonabsorbable sugar markers such as lactulose and mannitol in preterm infants from 26 to 36 weeks gestation, intestinal permeability does not seem to be related to gestational age or birth weight but was found to be higher in the first 2 days after birth, than 3 to 6 days later. This relationship holds true in preterm infants when measured within 2 days after birth, suggesting the rapid postnatal adaptation of the small intestine in these preterm infants.[34]

A major component of absorption includes brush border enzymes that are found in the small intestine. In the jejunum, aminopeptidase activity does not change markedly between weeks 8 to 17, but a pronounced increase occurs in the ileum.[35] Another enzyme that displays the relatively high activity is dipeptyl peptidase IV (DPP IV). The activity of this peptidase is similar in the fetus and in older children and adults.[36] This finding suggests that the preterm infant should be able to efficiently absorb peptides as long as they are provided as oligopeptides or single amino acids.

With the presence of these enzymes in the fetal intestine, a question is raised whether there may be protein digestion and absorption in the fetus. Amniotic fluid contains a wide spectrum of proteins, which can be transferred to the fetus by the swallowing of amniotic fluid, and this in turn could play a role in fetal nutrition.[37] Approximately 50% of the amniotic fluid is swallowed by the fetus daily.[38] Thus the fetus can absorb a considerable amount of protein through the GI tract during fetal development.

Studies have indicated that there is increased small intestinal permeability for intact food during the neonatal period and that the serum of infants contains a higher percentage of antibodies to food antigens than the serum of adults.[33] This suggests that food proteins are absorbed in sufficient quantities for the immunologic response in these infants.

CLINICAL CORRELATIONS

Histamine blockers have been widely prescribed in the neonatal intensive care units. One of the major rationales for this is to prevent apnea and bradycardia that might be a result of gastroesophageal reflux. Of interest, the benefit of this intervention in the prevention of apnea and bradycardia has never been substantiated by well-controlled studies.[39] Concern for this practice stems from the fact that the ability of these preterm infants to secrete acid is limited, and this should be kept in mind when considering the use of H2 blockers.[18] There are currently several studies that show a relationship with an increased incidence of the nosocomial sepsis and necrotizing enterocolitis and even death in infants who received H2 blockers.[40-42] It is possible that with the already limited hydrogen production in the stomach of the preterm infant, additional inhibition of acid secretion further diminishes the acid barrier to microorganisms and allows for a higher load of bacteria to the more distal regions of the intestine. Importantly, certain types of microbes such as the Proteobacteria phylum have been found to survive very poorly in an acid environment.[43] Eliminating acid may promote the growth of Proteobacteria, which have been associated with the development of the intestinal inflammatory processes including necrotizing enterocolitis.[44-46] Proteobacteria are primarily gram-negative microorganisms that include the *Klebsiella, E. coli*, and other taxa containing high levels of lipopolysaccharide (LPS) in their cell wall, which promotes the production of proinflammatory mediators from both the intestinal epithelium and some of the underlying mucosal macrophages present in the intestine.[47] Of interest in this regard is a small study done approximately 2 decades ago that suggested that acidification of formula could potentially prevent necrotizing enterocolitis.[48] Using 16S sequencing, the effect of H2 blockers was shown to increase the relative abundance of Proteobacteria (primarily of the family Enterobacteriaceae),[49] blooms of which have previously been associated with development of necrotizing enterocolitis (NEC). An increase in the incidence of NEC was found in association with H2 blocker therapy in a study of 11,000 infants of 401 to 1500 g birth weight.[50] Thus use of H2 blockers may affect gastric acid production, which is important for initiation of protein digestive processes, and also affect the development of the microbiota and have additional deleterious consequences.

Overall, the mechanisms for brush border hydrolysis are present very early in the intestine; thus oligopeptides are readily absorbed. Furthermore, certain dipeptides and tripeptides are absorbed even faster than single amino acids.[51] Despite some potential limitations of digestive capability in the preterm infants compared with term infants related to lower gastric acid secretion and the limited conversion of pancreatic proenzymes by low levels of enterokinase in preterm infants, studies evaluating the potential benefits of hydrolyzed formulas compared with whole protein formulas appear to demonstrate only very small benefits in terms of lower length of hospitalization and time to reach full enteral feeding.[52]

CARBOHYDRATE DIGESTION AND ABSORPTION

GENERAL

The overall carbohydrate digestive-absorptive processes are described in Figs. 86.2 and 86.4 and Box 86.2. Complex carbohydrates and starches must first be hydrolyzed to oligosaccharides by digestive processes in the upper GI tract. This is accomplished via amylases derived from salivary and pancreatic sources. These oligosaccharides must then be hydrolyzed at the epithelial brush border to monosaccharides before absorption. The brush border hydrolases, which include maltase, lactase, and sucrase, are primarily involved in these processes. Maltase will cleave maltose into two molecules of glucose. Lactase cleaves lactose into glucose and galactose, and sucrase cleaves sucrose into glucose and fructose. The monosaccharides glucose and galactose are taken into the small intestinal epithelial cell by co-transport with sodium. Fructose enters the cell from the intestinal lumen by facilitated diffusion that does not require sodium co-transport. Lactase activity appears to be of major importance because lactose is the primary carbohydrate found in human milk. Other carbohydrates are present in human milk, the majority of which comprise the human milk oligosaccharides.[53] The microbiota of the GI tract have a major role in the breakdown of these nutrients, and these may play a significant role in the predominance of certain microorganisms that play a protective role in the developing GI tract.

DEVELOPMENTAL ASPECTS OF CARBOHYDRATE DIGESTION AND ABSORPTION

The functions of carbohydrate digestive enzymes such as amylase that are found in human milk are not clearly understood. α-Amylase is present in preterm colostrum. This enzyme activity slowly decreases during first 2 months after birth and is able to survive the relatively mild acidity and low activity of pepsin in the stomach of the newborn infant.[54-56]

Pancreatic amylase activity has been demonstrated in amniotic fluid and pancreatic tissue from 14- to 16-week-old fetuses.[57,58] Although salivary amylase activity increases after term birth, pancreatic amylase activity remains low for several months after birth and usually does not reach adult levels until approximately 2 years of age.[59] Thus the digestion of starch in the newborn infant appears to be limited. Providing an equal caloric amount of a glucose solution versus starch resulted in a much greater and earlier increase in blood glucose in infants receiving the glucose solution. This was accompanied by an earlier return to starting values within 120 minutes after the feeding with the glucose solution versus the starch solution.

The activities of sucrase and lactase are lower in young fetuses compared with the small intestine from adults. Sucrase activity is actually present in the fetal colon and disappears before birth. Lactase activity has also been described in the fetal intestine between 13 and 20 weeks of gestational age. Lactase activity at birth in term neonates is up to three times that of infants 2 to 11 months of age then slowly declines over time.

Despite the activities of lactase being low in the intestine of the fetus, it is of interest that the preterm infant appears

Box 86.2 Monosaccharide Transport

Glucose uptake is Na^+ dependent
Fructose is absorbed via facilitated diffusion
Galactose and glucose are actively transported
1. Sodium-glucose–linked transporter 1 (SGLT1) is the transport protein responsible for Na^+-dependent glucose transport
2. Glucose transporter 2 (GLUT-2) transports glucose out of the cell into the portal circulation

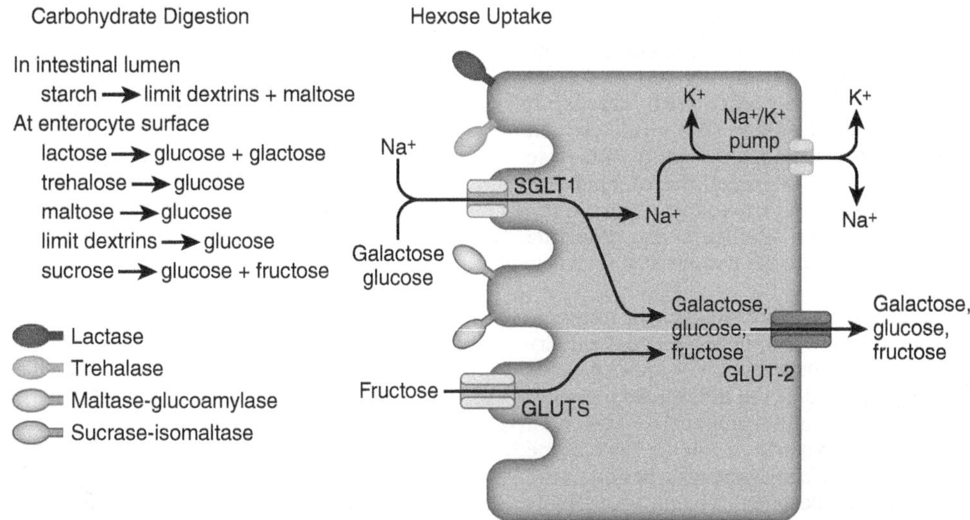

Fig. 86.4 Digestion and absorption of carbohydrates. *GLUT,* Glucose transporter; *SGLT1,* sodium-glucose–linked transporter 1.

to absorb lactose relatively well. Studies suggest that colonic fermentation of nonhydrolyzed lactose provides a colonic salvage pathway that results in efficient absorption of lactose breakdown products (short-chain fatty acids) in preterm infants.

As previously mentioned, monosaccharides are transported by sodium-dependent mechanisms and facilitated transport as with fructose. These transporters have been found to be present in abundant quantities and human fetal and adult intestine. Although the transporter GLUT-1 has been found to be higher in the fetal than adult small intestine, glucose absorption in infants is less efficient than in adults. The kinetics of glucose absorption is affected by gestational age, diet, and exposure to glucocorticoids.

CLINICAL CORRELATES

Many infant formulas, including those designed for preterm infants, contain partially hydrolyzed starches. The more extensively the starches are hydrolyzed the less reliance is placed on immature digestive capability. Because pancreatic secretion is poorly developed in the first several months after birth, pancreatic amylase hydrolysis is likely to be a limiting factor that leaves a substantial amount of undigested starch in the intestine. Whether there is any advantage of the hydrolyzed starch formulas or those containing the disaccharides maltose, sucrose, or lactose has not been established. Salivary amylase may play an important role when the pancreatic amylases are limited. Some data suggest that 18 to 29 glucose polymer units can be hydrolyzed by salivary amylases, but this still falls short of that accomplished by the usual concentrations of the pancreatic amylase.[60,61] In actual clinical practice, it is not clear whether these limitations of amylase play a significant role because the major carbohydrate in human milk or most cows' milk-based formulas is lactose. In addition, many preterm infants are fed by nasogastric or gastric tubes, which at least partially bypass the action of the salivary amylase.

As mentioned, a shortage of lactase activity in preterm infants[27] may result in unhydrolyzed lactose reaching the distal small intestine and colon, where it is fermented by microbes into short-chain fatty acids. The short-chain fatty acids can be absorbed and used for energy production purposes.[62,63] It is important to note that these short-chain fatty acids, especially butyrate, may play a major role in proliferation, differentiation, and apoptosis in the intestinal on colonic epithelium.[64] Butyrate also serves as a major fuel for the colonic epithelial cell. Propionate and butyrate have also been found to have important actions in terms of the immune modulation of the intestine.[65] Thus, in preterm infants, unhydrolyzed lactose may actually play a beneficial role when short-chain fatty acids are produced by microbes in the distal GI tract. Furthermore, very low-gestational-age infants are usually not provided large quantities of enteral feedings shortly after birth but rather receive minimal enteral (trophic) feedings. Thus it is likely that most of these babies do not receive a high quantity of lactose in their GI tracts and are unlikely to exceed the capability of the preterm infants' lactase hydrolytic capability at least in the first week of life. Thus the common practice of the providing non-lactose-containing carbohydrates in commercial formulas is of questionable value.

Studies examining the crypt to villous gradient of intestinal carbohydrase activities demonstrate that the most lactase activity is found at the mid to upper villous level.[66-68] Sucrase, maltase, and glucoamylase are concentrated at the mid-villous region. It is thought that this is pertinent to intestinal injury because, with injury, lactase would be the first enzyme lost and the last enzyme to be regenerated fully. Whether this necessitates a period of the lactose-free nutrition is debatable, despite this being a commonly used practice.

LIPID DIGESTION AND ABSORPTION

GENERAL

Most dietary lipid is in the form of triglyceride that is composed of a glycerol backbone with each carbon link to a fatty acid via ester bonds. Two main processes occur in the digestion of triglycerides. First, large aggregates of dietary triglyceride must be broken down physically and held in suspension, a process called *micellar emulsification*. These triglyceride molecules must then be enzymatically digested by triglyceride hydrolysis to yield a monoglyceride and free fatty acids, both of which can be transported into the enterocyte. These two processes are mediated by bile acids and lipases, respectively, and are depicted in Figs. 86.2, 86.5–86.7.

Bile acids promote lipid emulsification because they consist of hydrophobic and hydrophilic domains (see Fig. 86.5). On exposure to large aggregates of triglyceride, the hydrophobic portion of the bile acid intercalates into the lipid, with the hydrophilic domain remaining at the surface. This results in the breakdown of large aggregates into smaller droplets. The smaller the droplet size, the greater the surface area, and this in turn provides greater surface area for interaction with the lipase enzymes (see Fig. 86.6). These enzymes result in hydrolysis of triglycerides into monoglyceride and free fatty acids. This is accomplished primarily by pancreatic lipase, but there are several other lipases found in feedings and the GI tract (see Fig. 86.7). These include bile salt–stimulated lipases (BSSLs) found in human milk, lingual lipases found at the base of the tongue, gastric lipases, and intestinal epithelial brush border lipases.

By the process of simple diffusion, products of lipid digestion, such as fatty acids and monoglycerides, enter the intestinal epithelial cell by simple diffusion across the plasma membrane. There are also specific fatty acid transporter proteins present in the membrane of the intestinal epithelial cell. These lipids in turn are transported from the enterocyte into the blood by mechanism different from that of the monosaccharides and amino acids. This process also depends on the chain length of the fatty acids. Long-chain fatty acids and monoglycerides are transported in the endoplasmic reticulum of the intestinal epithelial cell, where they are used to resynthesize triglyceride. Continuing into the Golgi, the triglyceride is repackaged with cholesterol, lipoproteins, and other lipids into particles called

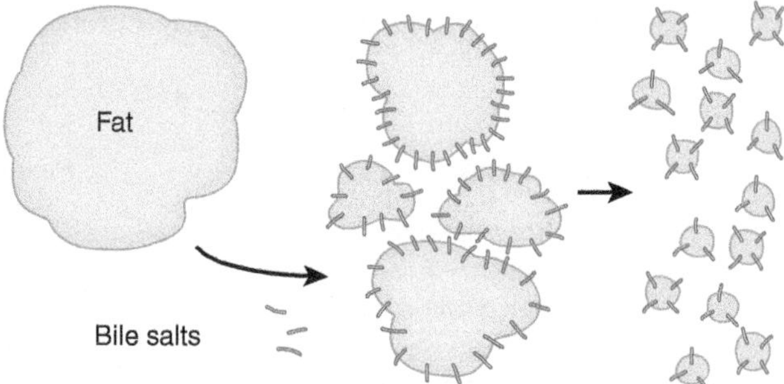

Fig. 86.5 Digestion of lipids: micellar emulsification.

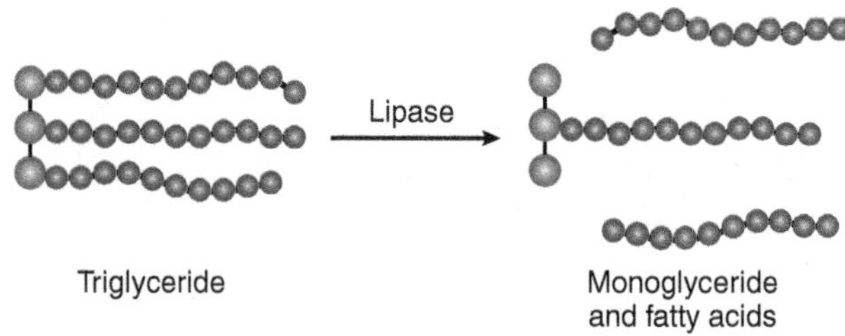

Fig. 86.6 Digestion of lipids—triglyceride hydrolysis. (From www.vivo.colostate.edu/hbooks/pathphys/digestion/smallgut/lipased.gif.)

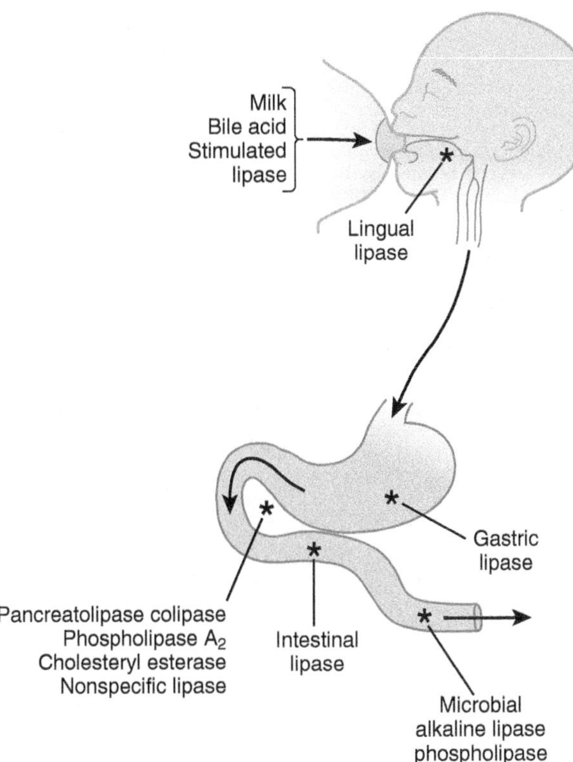

Fig. 86.7 Lipases from different sources.

chylomicrons. These are extruded from the Golgi into exocytic vesicles that are then transported through the basolateral aspect of the enterocyte. Chylomicrons are transported first into lymphatic vessels that penetrate into each villous, which in turn drain into the lymphatic system, before flowing into the blood. These lipids are rapidly disassembled, and their constituents are used throughout the body. Unlike the long-chain lipids, the medium-chain triglycerides require minimal emulsification by bile acids and undergo a relatively simple process of assimilation into the portal venous system, where they do not undergo reesterification and chylomicron formation. In conditions that involve obstruction of the lymphatics, using formulas containing primarily medium-chain triglycerides rather than long-chain triglycerides is recommended. Medium-chain triglycerides are fatty acids with 6 to 12 carbons versus long-chain triglycerides, which have more than 12 carbons.

DEVELOPMENTAL ASPECTS OF LIPID DIGESTION AND ABSORPTION

Although lipases are present in the stomachs of fetuses in early gestation,[69,70] their full functional capability at various gestational is not fully understood. Human milk contains lipase activity that is not detectable in cows' milk.[71] This enzyme is primarily functional in the presence of the bile salts and thus is classified as BSSL, which is present in human colostrum and in preterm and term milk.[72,73] Some of the properties of BSSL make it suitable to survive in the stomach with minimal loss of activity, and in the duodenum, BSSL is activated by bile acids such as cholate and chenodeoxycholate in concentrations close to those found in the infant duodenum.[74] Thus BSSL found in human milk may facilitate fat absorption by the hydrolysis of the long-chain triglycerides. BSSL hydrolyzes long-chain triglycerides with no positional specificity to glycerol and free fatty acids.

Pancreatic juice in adults contains two enzymes that are active in the hydrolysis of the neutral lipids. Pancreatic lipase is more active against insoluble, emulsified substrates than against soluble ones. The second lipase, also called *pancreatic carboxylase esterase*, is more active against micellar or soluble substrates than against the insoluble, emulsified substrates. Lipases show the lowest values after birth.[75] However, these increase toward adult values during the first 6 months after birth, which is faster than the amylase enzyme.

Pancreatic lipase is secreted in an active form, but its activity is enhanced by bile salts. Bile salts enhance the efficiency of lipolysis by increasing the surface area of oil-water interfaces at which water-soluble lipase is effective. Colipase is a small protein, synthesized in the pancreas, which allows pancreatic lipase to function in spite of micellar concentrations of conjugated bile salts. Bile salts by themselves hinder lipase adsorption onto triglycerides by covering the whole water-substrate interface. Colipase tends to prevent this and acts as an anchor for lipase adsorption, thus allowing lipase to hydrolyze substrate.

The presence of the serous glans located in the proximal dorsal side of the tongue was first described by Von Ebner in the late 1800s.[76] These glands appear to be the source of lingual lipase.[77] This lingual lipase activity is stimulated by feeding and is present in gastric aspirates as early as 6 months gestation and increases around 8 to 9 fetal months. Lingual lipase activity appears to be lower at birth in infants at 26 weeks, peaks at 30 to 32 weeks, and declines to lower levels at term.[78] Continuous enteral feeding appears to promote the development activity of this lipase.[79]

CLINICAL CORRELATIONS

As previously mentioned, medium-chain triglycerides do not require bile acid emulsification as do long-chain fats. The complexity of medium-chain triglyceride absorption and assimilation is also considerably less complex than the long-chain fats. Studies have shown that the medium-chain triglycerides appear to be just as readily absorbed as the long-chain triglycerides, and the mechanisms of this are speculated to reside in the greater gastric lipolytic activity of the longer-chain lipids. A Cochrane review supports this by showing no differences in growth, necrotizing enterocolitis, or other morbidities in infants fed primarily medium- versus long-chain triglycerides.[80]

The essential fatty acids linoleic and linolenic are converted into longer-chain fatty acids by desaturation and elongation. These long-chain polyunsaturated fatty acids are critical in the formation of eicosanoids and structural components of the central nervous system and retina. They are found in relatively high concentrations in human milk but are not provided in commonly used lipid solutions that are given intravenously to preterm infants. Because most preterm infants also do not take large quantities of food into their GI tract in the first week or two after birth, many of these babies are left with deficits of the long-chain fatty acids.[81]

The intravenous lipids that are provided to most preterm infants are very high in the omega-6 families. The clinical implications of this are just beginning to be appreciated, with amelioration of severe cholestatic jaundice with the use of the higher quantities of omega-3 fatty acid–containing intravenous lipids.[82] There is also an association with increased risk of chronic lung disease in preterm infants who received lower quantities of docosahexaenoic acid (DHA).[83] Whether it is necessary to provide these very-long-chain fatty acids by the intravenous route is not clear. Studies have shown that provision of a soybean-based lipid by the enteral route results in a fairly high absorption of the 18 carbon fatty acids, and it is thus likely that the longer-chain fatty acids could also be absorbed by the enteral route.[84] A meta-analysis has suggested that use of fish oil–containing lipid emulsions may reverse parenteral nutrition-associated cholestasis. This potential benefit deserves additional studies.

A complete reference list is available at www.ExpertConsult.com.

SELECT REFERENCES

1. Weaver LT, Austin S, Cole TJ. Small intestinal length: a factor essential for gut adaptation. *Gut*. 1991;32:1321-1323.
2. Sato T, Clevers H. Growing self-organizing mini-guts from a single intestinal stem cell: mechanism and applications. *Science*. 2013;340:1190-1194.
3. Turner JR. Intestinal mucosal barrier function in health and disease. *Nat Rev Immunol*. 2009;9:799-809.
4. Engelstoft MS, Egerod KL, Lund ML, Schwartz TW. Enteroendocrine cell types revisited. *Curr Opin Pharmacol*. 2013;13:912-921.
5. Koldovsky O, Sunshine P, Kretchmer N. Cellular migration of intestinal epithelia in suckling and weaned rats. *Nature*. 1966;212:1389-1390.
6. Holt PR, Kotler DP, Pascal RR. A simple method for determining epithelial cell turnover in small intestine. Studies in young and aging rat gut. *Gastroenterology*. 1983;84:69-74.
7. Clevers HC, Bevins CL. Paneth cells: maestros of the small intestinal crypts. *Annu Rev Physiol*. 2013;75:289-311.
8. Bertoncelli N, et al. Oral feeding competences of healthy preterm infants: a review. *Int J Pediatr*. 2012;2012:896257.
9. Berger HM, Scott PH, Kenward C, Scott P, Wharton BA. Curd and whey proteins in the nutrition of low birthweight babies. *Arch Dis Child*. 1979;54:98-104.
10. Fairclough PD, Silk DB, Clark ML, Dawson AM. Proceedings: new evidence for intact di- and tripeptide absorption. *Gut*. 1975;6:843.
11. Adibi SA, Morse EL, Masilamani SS, Amin PM. Evidence for two different modes of tripeptide disappearance in human intestine. Uptake by peptide carrier systems and hydrolysis by peptide hydrolases. *J Clin Invest*. 1975;56:1355-1363.
12. Mailliard ME, Steven SBR, Mann GE. Amino acid transport by small intestinal, hepatic, and pancreatic epithelia. *Gastroenterology*. 1995;108:888-910.
13. Kelly EJ, Brownlee KG, Newell SJ. Gastric secretory function in the developing human stomach. *Early Hum Dev*. 1992;31:163-166.
14. Kelly EJ, et al. The effect of intravenous ranitidine on the intragastric pH of preterm infants receiving dexamethasone. *Arch Dis Child*. 1993;69:37-39.
15. Kelly EJ, Lagopoulos M, Primrose JN. Immunocytochemical localisation of parietal cells and G cells in the developing human stomach. *Gut*. 1993;34:1057-1059.
16. Mignone F, Castello D. Research on gastric secretion of hydrochloric acid in the premature infant. *Minerva Pediatr*. 1961;13: 1098-1030.
17. Euler AR, Byrne WJ, Meis PJ, Leake RD, Ament ME. Basal and pentagastrin-stimulated acid secretion in newborn human infants. *Pediatr Res*. 1979;13:36-37.
18. Hyman PE, et al. Gastric acid secretory function in preterm infants. *J Pediatr*. 1985;106:467-471.
19. Harries JT, Fraser AJ. The acidity of the gastric contents of premature babies during the first fourteen days of life. *Biol Neonat*. 1968;12. 186-103.
20. Hyman PE, Feldman EJ, Ament ME, Byrne WJ, Euler AR. Effect of enteral feeding on the maintenance of gastric acid secretory function. *Gastroenterology*. 1983;84:341-345.
21. Keene MFL, Hewer EE. Digestive enzymes o fthe human foetus. *Lancet*. 1924;1:767.
22. Reid WA, et al. Immunolocalisation of aspartic proteinases in the developing human stomach. *J Dev Physiol*. 1989;11:299-303.
23. Werner B. Peptic and tryptic capacity of the digestive glands in newborns: a comparison between premature and full-term infants. *Acta Paediatr Jpn*. 1948;35n(suppl. 5):1.
24. Wagner H. The development to full functional maturity of the gastric mucosa and the kidneys in fetus and newborn. *Biol Neonat*. 1961;3:257-274.
25. Agunod M, Yamaguchi N, Lopez R, Luhby AL, Glas SGB. Correlative study of hydrochloric acid, pepsin, and intrinsic factor secretion in newborns and infants. *Am J Dig Dis*. 1969;14:400-414.
26. DiPalma J, et al. Lipase and pepsin activity in the gastric mucosa of infants, children, and adults. *Gastroenterology*. 1991;101:116-121.
27. Antonowicz I, Lebenthal E. Developmental pattern of small intestinal enterokinase and disaccharidase activities in the human fetus. *Gastroenterology*. 1977;72:1299-1303.
28. Carrère J, Figarella-Branger D, Senegas-Balas F, Figarella C, Guy-Crotte O. Immunohistochemical study of secretory proteins in the developing human exocrine pancreas. *Differentiation*. 1992;51:55-60.
29. Bujanover Y, et al. The development of the chymotryptic activity during postnatal life using the bentiromide test. *Int J Pancreatol*. 1988;3:53-58.
30. Kolacek S, Puntis JW, Lloyd DR, Brown GA, Booth IW. Ontogeny of pancreatic exocrine function. *Arch Dis Child*. 1990;65:178-181.
31. Lecce JG, Morgan DO. Effect of dietary regimen on cessation of intestinal absorption of large molecules (closure) in the neonatal pig and lamb. *J Nutr*. 1962;78:263-268.
32. Chastant-Maillard S, et al. Timing of the intestinal barrier closure in puppies. *Reprod Domest Anim*. 2012;47(suppl 6):190-193.
33. Roberton DM, et al. Milk antigen absorption in the preterm and term neonate. *Arch Dis Child*.(1082);57, 369-372.
34. van Elburg RM, Fetter WP, Bunkers CM, Heymans HS. Intestinal permeability in relation to birth weight and gestational and postnatal age. *Arch Dis Child Fetal Neonatal Ed*. 2003;88:F52-F55.
35. Heringová A, et al. Proteolytic and peptidase activities of the small intestine of human fetuses. *Gastroenterology*. 1966;51:1023-1027.
36. Auricchio S, Stellato A, De Vizia B. Development of brush border peptidases in human and rat small intestine during fetal and neonatal life. *Pediatr Res*. 1981;15:991-995.
37. Mulvihill SJ, Stone MM, Debas HT, Fonkalsrud EW. The role of amniotic fluid in fetal nutrition. *J Pediatr Surg*. 1985;20:668-672.
38. Gilbert WM, Brace RA. Amniotic fluid volume and normal flows to and from the amniotic cavity. *Semin Perinatol*. 1993;17:150-157.
39. Abu Jawdeh EG, Martin RJ. Neonatal apnea and gastroesophageal reflux (GER): is there a problem? *Early Hum Dev*. 2013;89(suppl 1):S14-S16.
40. Dalton J, Schumacher R. H2-blockers are associated with necrotizing enterocolitis in very low birthweight infants. *J Pediatr*. 2012;161:168-169.
41. Terrin G, et al. Ranitidine is associated with infections, necrotizing enterocolitis, and fatal outcome in newborns. *Pediatrics*. 2012;129:e40-e45.
42. Guillet R, et al. Association of H2-blocker therapy and higher incidence of necrotizing enterocolitis in very low birth weight infants. *Pediatrics*. 2006;117:e137-e142.
43. Duncan SH, Louis P, Thomson JM, Flint HJ. The role of pH in determining the species composition of the human colonic microbiota. *Environ Microbiol*. 2009;11:2112-2122.
44. Mai V, et al. Fecal microbiota in premature infants prior to necrotizing enterocolitis. *PloS One*. 2011;6:e20647.
45. Mai V, et al. Distortions in development of intestinal microbiota associated with late onset sepsis in preterm infants. *PloS One*. 2013;8:e52876.
46. Claud EC, et al. Bacterial community structure and functional contributions to emergence of health or necrotizing enterocolitis in preterm infants. *Microbiome*. 2013;1:20.
47. Yang Y, Jobin C. Microbial imbalance and intestinal pathologies: connections and contributions. *Dis Model Mech*. 2014;7:1131-1142.
48. Carrion V, Egan EA. Prevention of neonatal necrotizing enterocolitis. *J Pediatr Gastroenterol Nutr*. 1990;11:317-323.
49. Gupta RW, et al. Histamine-2 receptor blockers alter the fecal microbiota in premature infants. *J Pediatr Gastroenterol Nutr*. 2013;56:397-400.
50. Guillet R, et al. Association of H2-blocker therapy and higher incidence of necrotizing enterocolitis in very low birth weight infants. *Pediatrics*. 2006;117:e137-e142.

87 The Developing Microbiome of the Fetus and Neonate: A Multiomic Approach

Josef Neu | Neel Kamal Singh

INTRODUCTION

In the past two decades, DNA-based technologies have identified a myriad of difficult-to-culture microbes in the human body, including the gastrointestinal tract, skin, vaginal tract, urethra, and reproductive tract. In addition to the DNA-based technologies, newly developed bioinformatics are being developed that integrate microbial metagenomes, genomics, transcriptomes, proteomes, and metabolomes (or multi-omics) into system-based schema that more clearly illustrate the pathophysiology of diseases. Problems seen during pregnancy and the neonatal period beg for application of these newly developed techniques, which will enable better understanding of their pathophysiology in order to improve prevention, diagnosis, and treatment.

In this chapter, we will summarize some of the most recent studies pertaining to in utero microbial environment and how "omic" perturbations may result in preterm birth. The effects of mode of delivery on the developing microbiota-host-immune system interactions, and the effects of environmental factors such as antibiotic usage and diet will also be reviewed. In addition to the consequences of these early perturbations on health and disease in the individual, we will also speculate on transgenerational effects.

IS THE UTERUS "STERILE"?

Microbial exposure in utero can be at different levels. One involves direct exposure via live reproducing microbes that reside in niches such as the placenta, amniotic fluid, or fetal gastrointestinal tract. The other is indirect exposure to microbial components that are passed via the bloodstream to the placenta and fetus. A combination of these is also possible.

The widely held concept that the in utero environment under normal conditions is "sterile" continues to be a matter of controversy.[1–5] It is most commonly thought that the presence of microbes in the uterine cavity implies an infectious process, but there is considerable information that this may not be the case. In fact, a nonsterile environment is seen in numerous nonhuman animals[6] and may be quite beneficial in humans as well. When considered from the perspective of immunologic regulation and tolerance, exposure to certain microbes may play a vital role in the maintenance of pregnancy[7] and has implications for the early developmental processes that lead to the hosts' subsequent ability to counteract infections, experience normal brain development, or develop autoimmunity.[8]

Despite the presence of various barriers in the maternal-fetal interface, it is difficult to exclude the possibility of placental and/or fetal exposure to microbial components that originate from the maternal vagina, gastrointestinal tract, oral cavity, or skin. However, more recent data support that microbes likely harbor and colonize the placenta, amniotic fluid, and fetal gastrointestinal tract.[4,9,10,11–14] This may have major implications for the production of various metabolites with high physiologic activity. These include metabolites such as serotonin, very important in neurodevelopment, and short-chain fatty acids, which are very important in terms of immune development and epigenetic mechanisms.[15,3,8,16–19] Other studies suggest that the microbiology may be important for the development of the heart.[20]

The pregnant woman harbors microbes in her gastrointestinal tract, mouth, vaginal tract, skin, and other niches. Studies have shown that the vaginal tract harbors different sets of microbes depending on location in the vagina (upper vs. lower) and stage of gestation.[21,22] Previous studies have suggested that ascending microbes may translocate through the choriodecidual membrane into the amniotic fluid.[23] The extent to which this occurs under healthy conditions is unclear. However, studies evaluating amniotic fluid microbes using both culture- and nonculture-based studies support their presence, with the greatest quantity found in preterm versus term deliveries.[9] Studies of the placental microbiome have also suggested the presence of microbes that vary in their taxonomy depending on the stage of pregnancy.[4]

Even if one invokes the possibility of a sterile womb, microbes or microbial components transferred from maternal sites such as the intestine likely signal and interact with the fetal immune system. Studies have demonstrated that inoculation of germ-free pregnant mice with a single microbe results in major postnatal modifications of the innate immune system, with enhanced responses in mice whose mothers were exposed to the microbes during pregnancy.[24] Thus, the environment in which the mother resides may be very important in terms of her microbial composition, the interaction between her microbes, their components and/or metabolites, and the developing fetus. Maternal diet, and medications such as antibiotics, antacids, stress, and other environmental factors, likely play major roles in these microbial host interactions.

Although the most recent data suggest that the fetal environment is not sterile, challenges to this concept are being made because of the possibility that some studies had inadequate controls, where a "kitome" or environmental contaminant is detected.[1,25,26] In other words, microbes are present in the ambient environment or in the kits that are utilized to evaluate the microbiota in certain environments. Therefore, when low biomass samples are analyzed (as present in placenta and amniotic fluid), it is possible that the microbes detected in these niches may actually be a part of the background ("blank") environment rather than resident microbes in such an environment. Although it appears from a large number of recent studies that there actually is an in utero microbiome, future studies with better quality control techniques will be necessary.[2,3]

THE VAGINAL MICROBIOME: IMPLICATIONS FOR MODE OF DELIVERY

There is a body of literature supporting a lack of microbial diversity, with a predominance of *Lactobacillus crispatus*, in the healthy vaginal tract in mothers who deliver their babies at term.[27,28] This is reflected by a study of term and preterm infants' first gastric aspirate, wherein those born at term exhibited a preponderance of *L. crispatus,* and those born preterm had a wider variety of microbes with a relative scarcity of *L. crispatus.*[29] This may have implications in terms of the pathophysiology of some forms of spontaneous preterm birth.[30]

Could microbes acquired by the newborn during vaginal delivery differ from those acquired during cesarean section delivery, and what might be the implications of these differences? Since the beginning of the early 20th century, cesarean deliveries have become more common.[31] In several areas of the world, they are the most common form of delivery. Although there are certainly indications for many of these cesarean sections, the high variability between countries and hospitals suggests that some cesarean sections are not medically indicated.[1] With this in mind, the question has been raised about whether the high incidence of cesarean sections may be a trigger that increases the risk for obesity, autoimmune disease, infectious diseases, and allergic and atopic diseases. Epidemiologic studies support that cesarean section deliveries are associated with a greater risk for these problems.[32] Several studies support that differences in the acquisition of microbes do occur depending on the mode of delivery.[33,34] Whether this difference is directly secondary to the mode of delivery or whether other mitigating factors are involved—including high antibiotic use in cesarean-delivered babies, the longer duration of hospital stays for these babies, and longer time to enterally feed cesarean-delivered babies—has yet to be determined.[35,36] Whether major differences actually occur depending on mode of delivery is not supported by at least one study, where no significant differences were seen depending on mode of delivery at 6 weeks after birth (Fig. 87.1).[2,37] Sources of the neonatal microbiome likely originate from numerous sources.[38] Whether the difference in microbial colonization in cesarean section versus vaginally delivered infants has a role in health and disease is still not known, but it is potentially important from the perspective of therapeutics.[39]

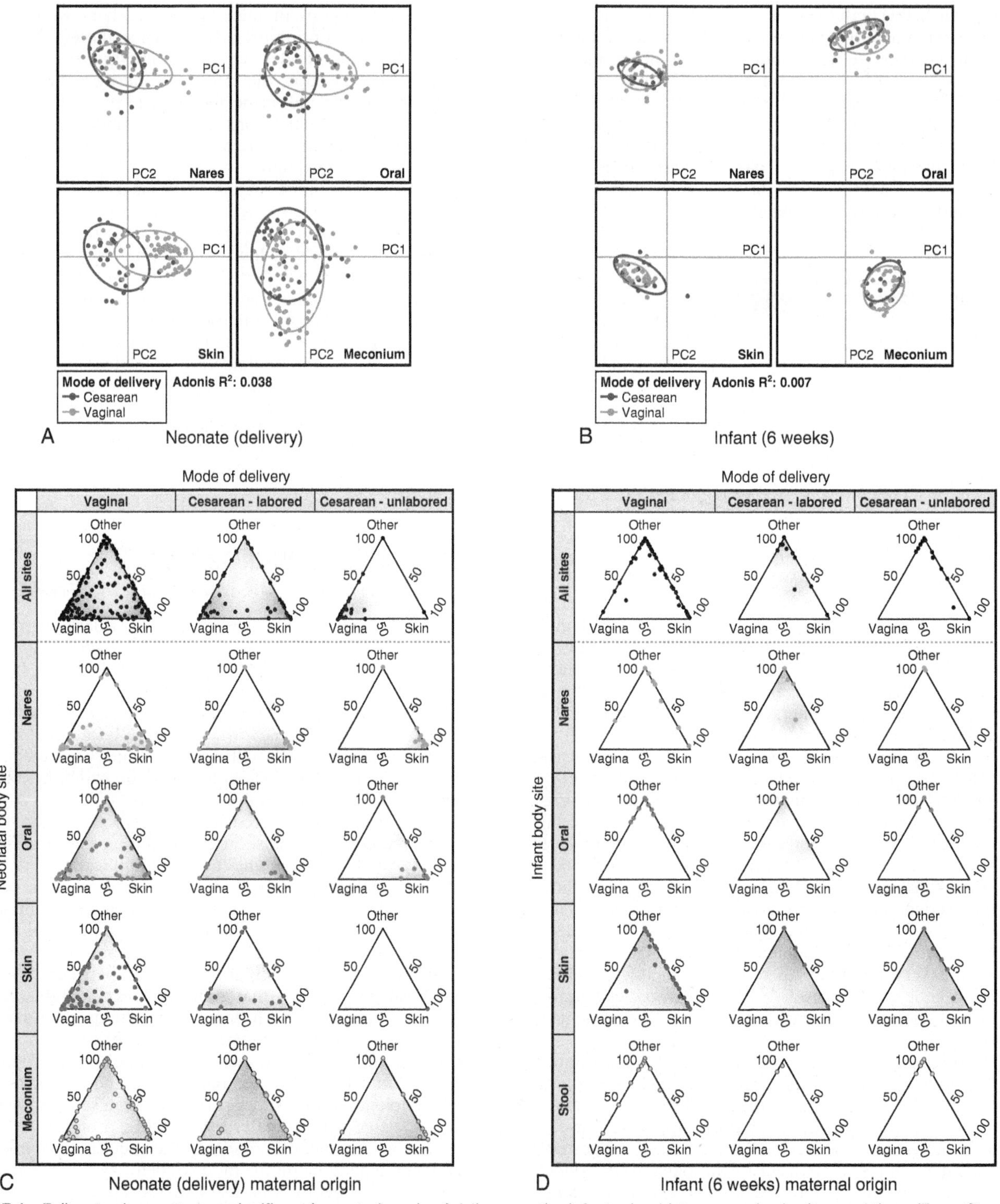

Fig. 87.1 Failure to demonstrate a significant impact of mode of delivery on the infant microbiota across body sites and time. (From Chu DM, Ma J, Prince AL, et al. Maturation of the infant microbiome community structure and function across multiple body sites and in relation to mode of delivery. *Nat Med.* 2017;23:314–326.)

The notion that the differences in acquisition of vaginal microbes during vaginal delivery may play a role in prevention of certain diseases has led to the practice of "seeding" of the vaginal microbes into the baby's mouth using a swabbing technique, whereby the vaginal microbes of the mother are put onto a gauze pad and then swapped into the cesarean section-delivered newborn's mouth. A small preliminary study supports that vaginal microbes can be transferred using this technique.[40] Whether this has implications in terms of health and disease remains speculative, and there are ongoing studies addressing this question. However, the safety of this procedure has been questioned, and recommendations against it have been made by obstetrical societies because of the possibility of seeding the newborn with potentially pathogenic microbes.[41]

MATERNAL-FETAL-MICROBIAL INTERACTIONS: METABOLIC, NUTRITIONAL, IMMUNOLOGIC, AND EPIGENETIC CONSIDERATIONS

Microbes in the pregnant woman's intestine may produce various metabolic products that get transferred to the fetus via the bloodstream. One would thus anticipate that maternal intestinal microbial changes that occur during pregnancy would result in a different pattern of metabolites being delivered to the fetus. Studies by Koren and colleagues[42] demonstrate that while the first-trimester maternal intestinal microbes do not differ from the nonpregnant state, by the third trimester the microbial pattern suggests a dysbiosis that resembles that seen in metabolic syndrome, with greater insulin resistance and obesity. In fact, the transfer of fecal microbiota from third-trimester mothers to germ-free wild-type mice resulted in greater insulin resistance, an increase in inflammatory markers, and a state that resembled metabolic syndrome. It remains unclear whether these microbial and metabolic alterations affect pregnancy in a negative or positive manner. However, it suggests that environmental alterations in the pregnant mother that change her normal intestinal microbiota may also have significant metabolic consequences, which in turn may have epigenetic consequences.[43] For example, the short-chain fatty acids acetate and propionic butyrate produced in the mother's distal small intestine and colon by microbial fermentation can be transferred to the fetus by the bloodstream. These can epigenetically affect the germ cell lines of the fetus via histone modifications, which can be very important to the fetus during critical developmental windows. Not only can these affect the fetus during the rest of its lifetime, but can also be transferred to subsequent generations.[3,4] Other metabolites that depend on intestinal microbial production, such as serotonin and dopamine, which have been implicated in the gut-brain axis and may be associated with long-term consequences,[44] need further investigation.

Dietary composition during pregnancy also is of major interest. A high-fat diet is associated with changes in the neonatal intestinal microbiome that persist through the first 4 to 6 weeks of age.[45] These effects are independent of the maternal body mass. Other studies[46] suggest that a high-fat diet prior to and during pregnancy also shifts the composition of the maternal intestinal microbiota, which impairs barrier integrity and exposes the fetus and placenta to proinflammatory mediators and ultimately to fetal intestinal inflammation. Placentas from obese mothers showed blood vessel immaturity, hypoxia, increased transcript levels of inflammation, autophagy, and altered levels of endoplasmic reticulum stress markers. The relative quantity of the type of fat also appears to be consequential. A preliminary investigation of n-3 PUFA intake during pregnancy demonstrated the potential to influence DNA methylation of several genes of the offspring, including those involved in innate immune responses, the onset of insulin resistance and adiposity, and several others.[47-49] This underlines the necessity of future studies that integrate several "omics" layers with environmental perturbations and the developing phenotype.

The in utero microbial environment is likely to play a major role in the pathogenesis of autoimmune and allergic diseases. The fetus is exposed to a myriad of metabolites that originate from the commensal microbiota of the mother that are passed on to the developing fetus. These metabolites may provide signals that contribute to immune development in the offspring, which include expansion of the innate immune populations in the intestine, mucus development, maturation of intestinal epithelial cells, and the secretion of antibodies into the intestinal lumen.[50] In this way, metabolites that originate either from the maternal diet or from her intestinal microbial metabolism (depending on the capabilities of the resident microbes) can be transferred to the offspring and alter its immunity.

THE NEONATE'S POSTNATAL MICROBIAL ENVIRONMENT

MECONIUM

As previously mentioned, the prenatal microbial environment of the fetus and mother can have marked effects on the newborn. The mode of delivery and attendant factors associated with operative versus vaginal delivery also appear to play a role in subsequent microbial colonization. Several studies show that the meconium of the newborn is not sterile[10,14,51] and may have altered composition due to maternal factors,[52] but also has a relatively low diversity, and may play a role in subsequent health and disease via microbe-host interactions.[53]

ANTIBIOTICS

Antibiotic use is extremely common during pregnancy and in the newborn period, especially when the infant is born preterm. In the very low-birth-weight (VLBW) preterm infant, the rationale for routine administration of antibiotics shortly after birth is speculative, based on immaturity of the neonatal immune system, the possibility that preterm delivery may be caused by an intra-amniotic infection, and that respiratory distress in these infants may be related to infection rather than lung immaturity. It has also been speculated that antibiotic use is safe in this population and the risks of pre-emptive antibiotic use are outweighed by the risk of possible morbidity or death due to sepsis. These assumptions may be incorrect because they are not based on solid evidence. The average length of treatment of this "standard of care" practice is between 5 and 7 days.[54,55] Yet, observational studies show an association between duration of early antibiotic use with increased odds of developing necrotizing enterocolitis (NEC),[54,56,57] a disease with high mortality and morbidity.[57,58]

It has been shown that microbial taxonomy is significantly affected by the early use of antibiotics (Fig. 87.2).[5,59] This effect may last well after discontinuation of the antibiotic. It is thus very concerning that infants who receive 5 to 7 days of antibiotics in their first week after delivery had increased relative abundance of *Enterobacteriaceae* and low diversity in the second and third weeks after birth.[60] Only 2 days of antibiotic use after birth has been associated with a "dysbiosis" well after these

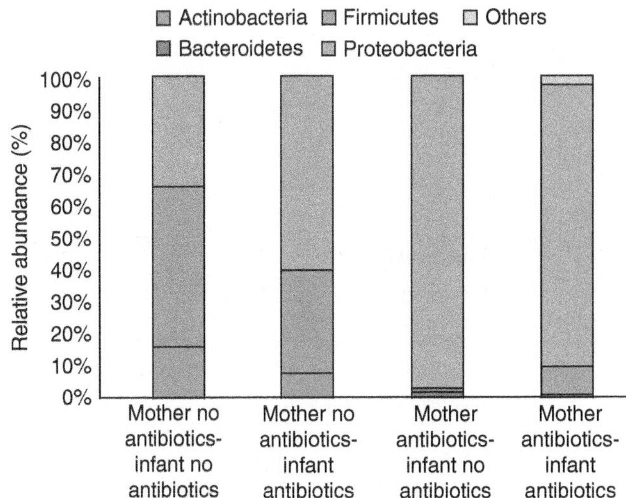

Fig. 87.2 Relative abundance (%) of phylum-level distributions of the fecal microbiota in the different antibiotic exposure groups classified into four classes, depending on mother and infant antibiotic exposure at 30 days of life. (From Arboleya S, Sánchez B, Solís G, et al. Impact of prematurity and perinatal antibiotics on the developing intestinal microbiota: a functional inference study. *Int J Mol Sci.* 2016;17:649.)

antibiotics have been discontinued.[61,62] These studies show long-term elevations of *Proteobacteria* and decreased *Firmicutes* in treated infants, which are microbial taxonomic changes found to be associated with the development of NEC.[63]

Studies have shown that NEC and late-onset sepsis (LOS) is preceded by an intestinal dysbiosis,[63-68] which may partially be due to antibiotic usage (Fig. 87.3).[63] Antibiotic use is also associated with an increase in a set of adverse outcomes.[69-72] Other retrospective observational data from the NIH Neonatal Research Network (NRN) suggests that prolonged early antibiotic use is not significantly associated with NEC or death, contrary to previous results. This same retrospective study shows a strong

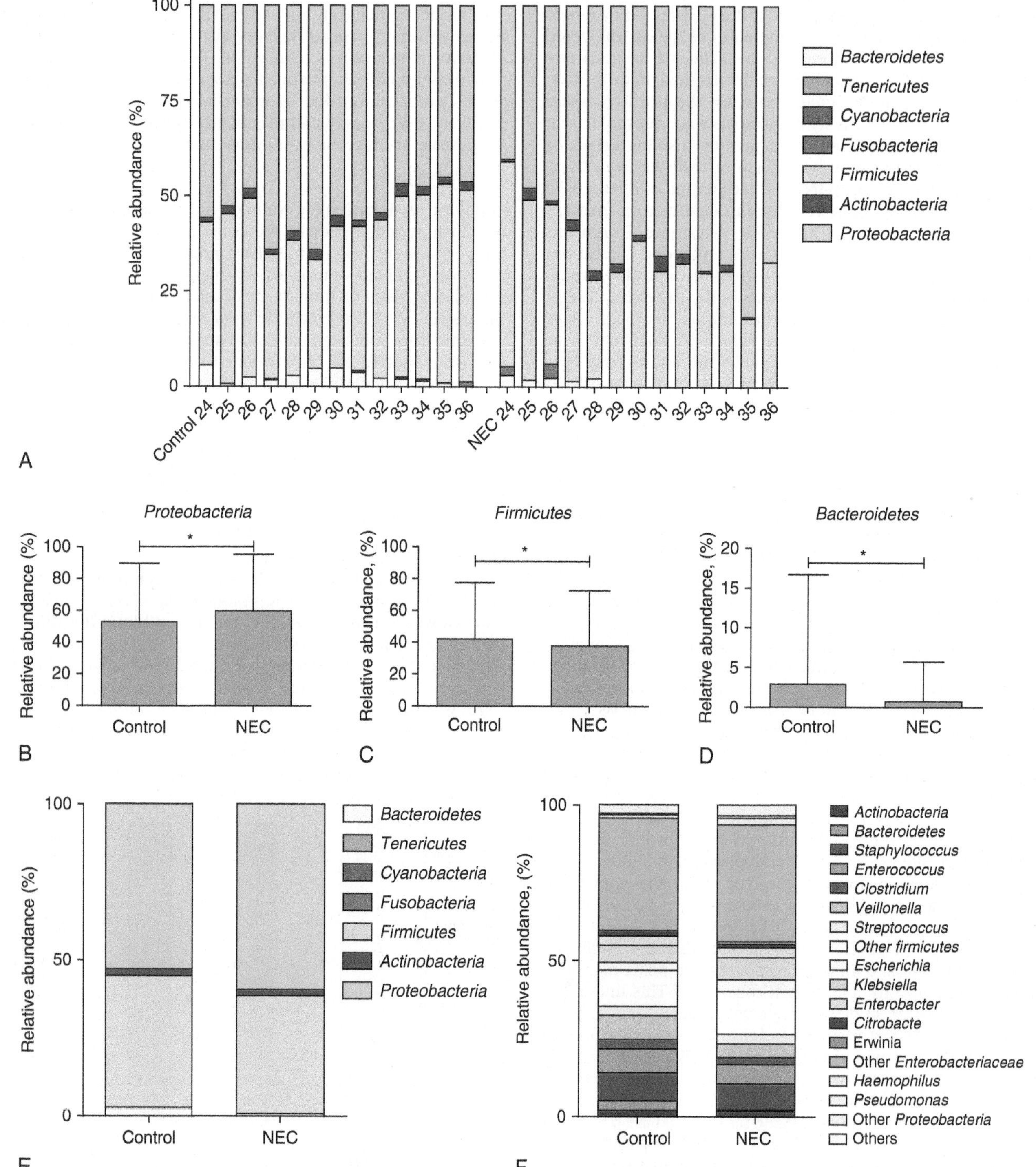

Fig. 87.3 Comparison of taxonomic profiles between infants with necrotizing enterocolitis *(NEC)* and controls. (A) NEC infants had trends of increased relative abundance in *Proteobacteria* from 24 to 36 weeks corrected gestational age (CGA) accompanied by decreased abundances in *Firmicutes* and *Bacteroidetes,* relative to controls. In control infants, the relative abundance of *Proteobacteria* decreased after 27 weeks and coincided with an increase in *Firmicutes* and *Bacteroidetes.* (B–D) Phylum-level differences between NEC cases and controls across CGA (data in means and SD) showed significant differences in *Proteobacteria, Firmicutes,* and *Bacteroidetes* (*$P < .05$). (E and F) Mean relative abundance distributions between NEC cases and controls at the phylum level (E) and genus level (F) when data from all CGAs are included. (From Pammi M, Cope J, Tarr PI, et al. Intestinal dysbiosis in preterm infants preceding necrotizing enterocolitis: a systematic review and meta-analysis. *Microbiome.* 2017;5:31.)

relationship between early antibiotics and late-onset fungal sepsis.[73] However, retrospective observational studies are fraught with the potential for confounding factors that are difficult to account for statistically. None of these studies were done in a randomized prospective manner and are thus prone to error due to confounding factors, such as greater initial degree of illness in the treated infants. In summary, the potential harm of antibiotics in preterm infants is concerning.[62,74-77] Prospective, randomized studies are clearly needed that obviate these confounding factors.

INFANT DIET: HUMAN MILK

The sterility of milk fed to human infants has long been a concern. Milk containing microbes has been considered to be a significant cause of disease and may be discarded when microbes have been found. Microbes in milk are killed using pasteurization, and almost all donor milk is pasteurized before use. Maternal breast milk is immediately frozen to decrease multiplication of bacteria. Certainly, milk can be contaminated with pathogens, but recently, it has become clear that human milk contains a wide variety of microbes that are likely to be of maternal origin, are not pathogenic, or are merely skin contaminants, and may provide a benefit to the infant.[78-82] A likely source of these microbes is from the mother's gastrointestinal tract, but studies tracking the source of these microbes are still in progress.[80,83] The exact mechanism of transfer of microbes to the mother's breast remains speculative, but there are reasonable data suggesting a maternal gastrointestinal tract origin.[84,85] The higher permeability of the intestinal tract during pregnancy may be more conducive to microbial translocation. The possibility that dendritic cells that underlie the intestinal mucosa can sample the bacteria in the intestinal lumen and ultimately transfer these cells to the mother's breast has also been proposed.[80]

Over time, the microbes from an individual mother's milk vary slightly, but the microbes from individual mothers differ markedly from other lactating mothers.[78] Whether this individual specificity represents an individualized microbiome that is the best for that particular mother's baby is speculative. However, the existence of the enteromammary system, which may offer dynamic immunologic responses from the mother to the newborn,[86,87] suggests there may be individual benefits. Donor milk, formula, or baby's own mother's milk that has been stored in a freezer for prolonged periods may not provide these potentially bioactive microbes to the infant.

Other components of breast milk that appear to be of major importance are milk oligosaccharides. There are numerous oligosaccharides in human milk, and several of these appear

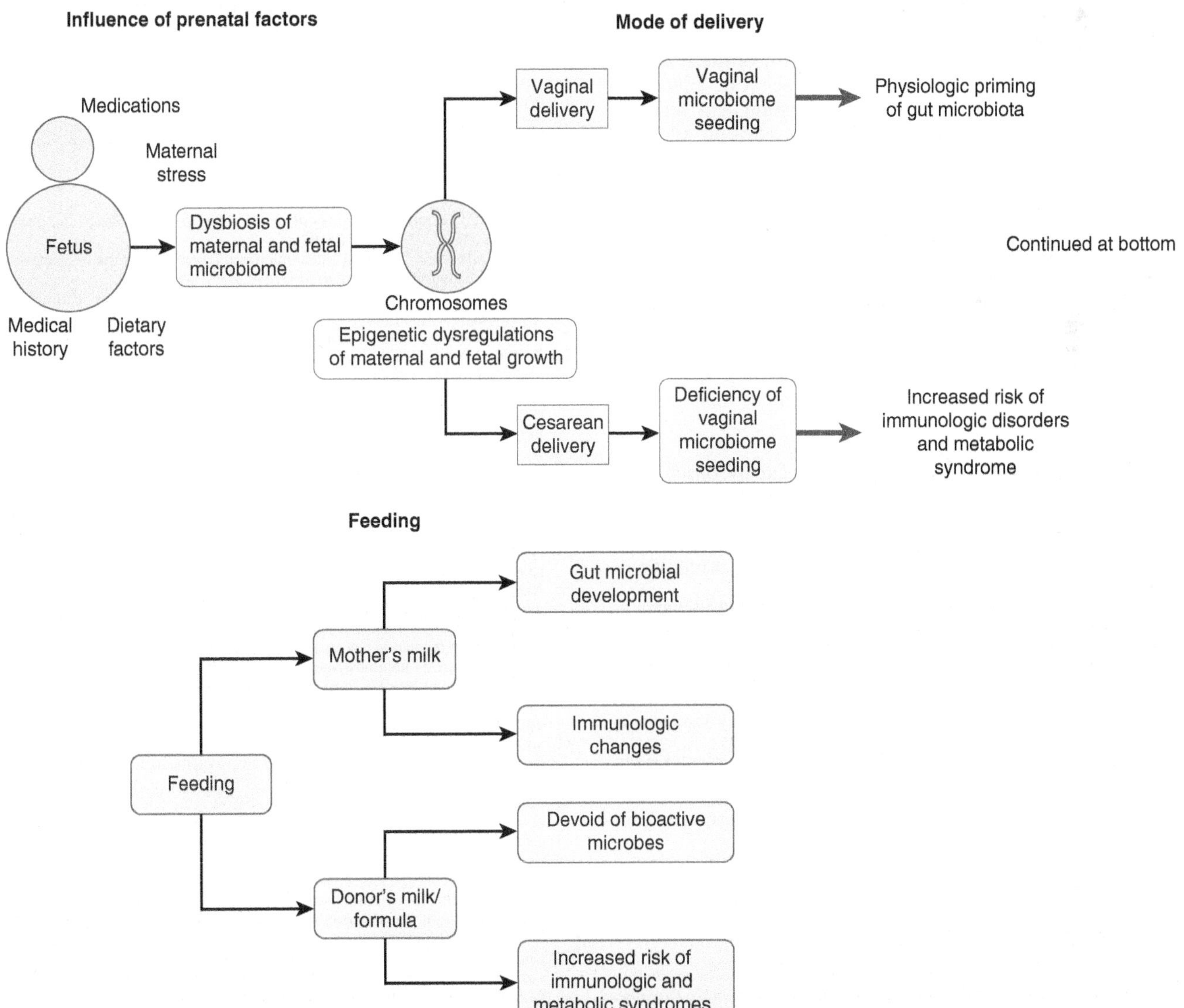

Fig. 87.4 Our algorithm summarizes various factors related to alterations in microbes related to pregnancy and early postnatal life.

to perform a prebiotic function that promotes the growth of certain taxa of bacteria that may play beneficial roles in the infant gastrointestinal tract.[88]

The American Academy of Pediatrics recommends that extremely preterm infants receive the mother's own milk when available or pasteurized donor breast milk (DBM) when mother's own milk is unavailable. Donor milk is devoid of live microbes and several other bioactive components that are destroyed during the pasteurization process. Many mothers may not be able to produce the quantities of milk required for the overall nutrition of their infants, and thus donor milk is thought to be a reasonable substitute. It has been hypothesized that small quantities of babies' own mothers' milk can be added to donor milk ("refaunation") to provide the personalized microbes that may benefit that infant. Preliminary studies to test this hypothesis have been done that support this technique is possible,[89] and further studies are underway to determine proof of principle, safety, and efficacy of this method.

CONCLUSION

New technologies that do not rely on culture-based methods have brought the sterility of the human womb into question. Whether one invokes in utero colonization or not, it remains true that the maternal microbiome is dynamic and influenced by factors such as diet, drug intake, and physiologic/pathologic state of the mother (Fig. 87.4). Alteration in any of these factors changes the microbiome composition, which can affect the mother's metabolic profile and gene expression, and serve as a trigger for future pathologic/disease processes. In addition, the altered microbiome can affect the developing fetus either by direct exposure to the microbes or indirectly through an altered maternal metabolomics/metabolic profile, which changes the epigenetic expression of the growing fetus. Furthermore, diversity or change in the maternal microbiome can also be used to predict the degree of prematurity, and the neonatal microbiome in the future. The neonatal microbiome is influenced by vaginal flora, meconium biome, neonatal antibiotic use, mother's milk, and the mode of delivery, which can further predict the risk for the development of complications ranging from NEC in the immediate neonatal period to later acquisition of immunologic disorders and metabolic syndrome.

A complete reference list is available at www.ExpertConsult.com.

SELECT REFERENCES

1. Willyard C. Could baby's first bacteria take root before birth? *Nature*. 2018;553:264-266.
2. Perez-Munoz ME, Arrieta MC, Ramer-Tait AE, Walter J. A critical assessment of the "sterile womb" and "in utero colonization" hypotheses: implications for research on the pioneer infant microbiome. *Microbiome*. 2017;5:48.
3. Stinson LF, Boyce MC, Payne MS, Keelan JA. The Not-so-Sterile Womb: evidence that the human fetus is exposed to bacteria prior to birth. *Front Microbiol*. 2019;10:1124.
4. Aagaard K, Ma J, Antony KM, Ganu R, Petrosino J, Versalovic J. The placenta harbors a unique microbiome. *Sci Tran Med*. 2014;6:237ra65.
5. Seferovic MD, Pace RM, Carroll M, et al. Visualization of microbes by 16S in situ hybridization in term and preterm placentas without intraamniotic infection. *Am J Obstet Gynecol*. 2019;221:146. e1-.e23.
6. Funkhouser LJ, Bordenstein SR. Mom knows best: the universality of maternal microbial transmission. *PLoS Biol*. 2013;11:e1001631.
7. Chu DM, Seferovic M, Pace RM, Aagaard KM. The microbiome in preterm birth. *Best Pract Res Clin Obstetr Gynaecol*. 2018;52:103-113.
8. Jasarevic E, Bale TL. Prenatal and postnatal contributions of the maternal microbiome on offspring programming. *Front Neuroendocrinol*. 2019;55:100797.
9. DiGiulio DB. Diversity of microbes in amniotic fluid. *Semin Fetal Neonatal Med*. 2012;17:2-11.
10. Ardissone AN, de la Cruz DM, Davis-Richardson AG, et al. Meconium microbiome analysis identifies bacteria correlated with premature birth. *PloS one*. 2014;9:e90784.
11. Borghi E, Massa V, Severgnini M, et al. Antenatal microbial colonization of mammalian gut. *Reproduct Sci (Thousand Oaks, Calif)*. 2019;26:1045-1053.
12. Walker RW, Clemente JC, Peter I, Loos RJF. The prenatal gut microbiome: are we colonized with bacteria in utero? *Pediatr Obes*. 2017;12(suppl 1):3-17.
13. Collado MC, Rautava S, Aakko J, Isolauri E, Salminen S. Human gut colonisation may be initiated in utero by distinct microbial communities in the placenta and amniotic fluid. *Sci Rep*. 2016;6:23129.
14. Younge N, McCann JR, Ballard J, et al. Fetal exposure to the maternal microbiota in humans and mice. *JCI Insight*. 2019;4:e127806.
15. Tamburini S, Shen N, Wu HC, Clemente JC. The microbiome in early life: implications for health outcomes. *Nat Med*. 2016;22:713-722.
16. Mei C, Yang W, Wei X, Wu K, Huang D. The unique microbiome and innate immunity during pregnancy. *Front Immunol*. 2019;10:2886.
17. Hsu CN, Chang-Chien GP, Lin S, Hou CY, Tain YL. Targeting on gut microbial metabolite Trimethylamine-N-Oxide and short-chain fatty acid to prevent maternal high-fructose-diet-induced developmental programming of hypertension in adult male offspring. *Mol Nut Food Res*. 2019;63:e1900073.
18. Cerdo T, Dieguez E, Campoy C. Early nutrition and gut microbiome: interrelationship between bacterial metabolism, immune system, brain structure, and neurodevelopment. *Am J Physiol Endocrinol Metab*. 2019;317:E617-e30.
19. Gur TL, Palkar AV, Rajasekera T, et al. Prenatal stress disrupts social behavior, cortical neurobiology and commensal microbes in adult male offspring. *Behav Brain Res*. 2019;359:886-894.
20. Guzzardi MA, Ait Ali L, D'Aurizio R, et al. Fetal cardiac growth is associated with in utero gut colonization. *Nut Metabol Cardiovas Dis: NMCD*. 2019;29:170-176.
21. Chen C, Song X, Wei W, et al. The microbiota continuum along the female reproductive tract and its relation to uterine-related diseases. *Nat Com*. 2017;8:875.
22. Li F, Chen C, Wei W, et al. The metagenome of the female upper reproductive tract. *GigaScience*. 2018;7:giy107.
23. Goldenberg RL, Hauth JC, Andrews WW. Intrauterine infection and preterm delivery. *N Engl J Med*. 2000;342:1500-1507.
24. Gomez de Aguero M, Ganal-Vonarburg SC, Fuhrer T, et al. The maternal microbiota drives early postnatal innate immune development. *Science (New York, NY)*. 2016;351:1296-1302.
25. Theis KR, Romero R, Winters AD, et al. Does the human placenta delivered at term have a microbiota? Results of cultivation, quantitative real-time PCR, 16S rRNA gene sequencing, and metagenomics. *Am J Obstet Gynecol*. 2019;220:267.e1-267.e39.
26. Leiby JS, McCormick K, Sherrill-Mix S, et al. Lack of detection of a human placenta microbiome in samples from preterm and term deliveries. *Microbiome*. 2018;6:196.
27. Lepargneur JP. Lactobacillus crispatus as biomarker of the healthy vaginal tract. *Annal De Biol Clin*. 2016;74:421-427.
28. Fettweis JM, Serrano MG, Brooks JP, et al. The vaginal microbiome and preterm birth. *Nat Med*. 2019;25:1012-1021.
29. Bajorek S, Parker L, Li N, et al. Initial microbial community of the neonatal stomach immediately after birth. *Gut Microbes*. 2019;10:289-297.
30. Staude B, Oehmke F, Lauer T, et al. The microbiome and preterm birth: a change in paradigm with profound implications for pathophysiologic concepts and novel therapeutic strategies. *BioMed Res Int*. 2018;2018:7218187.
32. Rushing J, Neu J. Probiotics for pregnant women and preterm neonates. *Am J Clin Nutr*. 2011;93:3-4.
33. Dominguez-Bello MG, Costello EK, Contreras M, et al. Delivery mode shapes the acquisition and structure of the initial microbiota across multiple body habitats in newborns. *Proc Natl Acad Sci U S A*. 2010;107:11971-11975.
34. Negele K, Heinrich J, Borte M, et al. Mode of delivery and development of atopic disease during the first 2 years of life. *Pediatr Allergy Immunol*. 2004;15:48-54.
35. Chu DM, Ma J, Prince AL, Antony KM, Seferovic MD, Aagaard KM. Maturation of the infant microbiome community structure and function across multiple body sites and in relation to mode of delivery. *Nat Med*. 2017;23:314-326.
36. Shao Y, Forster SC, Tsaliki E, et al. Stunted microbiota and opportunistic pathogen colonization in caesarean-section birth. *Nature*. 2019;574:117-121.
38. Aagaard KM. Mode of delivery and pondering potential sources of the neonatal microbiome. *EBioMedicine*. 2019;51:102554.
39. Montoya-Williams D, Lemas DJ, Spiryda L, et al. The neonatal microbiome and its partial role in mediating the association between birth by cesarean section and adverse pediatric outcomes. *Neonatology*. 2018;114:103-111.
40. Dominguez-Bello MG, De Jesus-Laboy KM, Shen N, et al. Partial restoration of the microbiota of cesarean-born infants via vaginal microbial transfer. *Nat Med*. 2016;22:250-253.
41. Stinson LF, Payne MS, Keelan JA. A critical review of the bacterial baptism hypothesis and the impact of cesarean delivery on the infant microbiome. *Front Med*. 2018;5:135.
42. Koren O, Goodrich JK, Cullender TC, et al. Host remodeling of the gut microbiome and metabolic changes during pregnancy. *Cell*. 2012;150:470-480.
43. Calatayud M, Koren O, Collado MC. Maternal microbiome and metabolic health program microbiome development and health of the offspring. *Trend Endocrinol Metabol:TEM*. 2019;30:735-744.
44. Jheeta S, Smith D. Seeing the wood for the trees: a new way to view the human intestinal microbiome and its connection with non-communicable disease. *Med Hypoth*. 2019;125:70-74.
45. Chu DM, Antony KM, Ma J, et al. The early infant gut microbiome varies in association with a maternal high-fat diet. *Genome Med*. 2016;8:77.
46. Gohir W, Kennedy KM, Wallace JG, et al. High-fat diet intake modulates maternal intestinal adaptations to pregnancy and results in placental hypoxia, as well as altered fetal gut barrier proteins and immune markers. *J Physiol*. 2019;597:3029-3051.

47. Bianchi M, Alisi A, Fabrizi M, et al. Maternal intake of n-3 polyunsaturated fatty acids during pregnancy is associated with differential methylation profiles in cord blood white cells. *Front Genet*. 2019;10:1050.
50. Macpherson AJ, de Aguero MG, Ganal-Vonarburg SC. How nutrition and the maternal microbiota shape the neonatal immune system. *Nat Rev Immunol*. 2017;17:508–517.
51. Moles L, Gomez M, Heilig H, et al. Bacterial diversity in meconium of preterm neonates and evolution of their fecal microbiota during the first month of life. *PloS one*. 2013;8:e66986.
52. Hu J, Ly J, Zhang W, et al. Microbiota of newborn meconium is associated with maternal anxiety experienced during pregnancy. *Dev Psychobiol*. 2019;61:640–649.
53. Wilczynska P, Skarzynska E, Lisowska-Myjak B. Meconium microbiome as a new source of information about long-term health and disease: questions and answers. *J Maternal-Fetal Neonatal Med*. 2019;32:681–686.
54. Cotten CM, Taylor S, Stoll B, et al. Prolonged duration of initial empirical antibiotic treatment is associated with increased rates of necrotizing enterocolitis and death for extremely low birth weight infants. *Pediatrics*. 2009;123:58–66.

Organogenesis and Histologic Development of the Liver

Steven Lobritto

INTRODUCTION

The liver is the largest internal organ of the body, compromising approximately 6% to 7% of the total weight of an adult. The organ is unique in that it receives dual supply, including venous inflow via the portal vein—predominantly from the intestines, pancreas, and spleen—and arterial inflow from the aorta via the hepatic artery. Together these sources provide the delivery of nutrients, hormones, toxins, and oxygen to hepatic tissues (Fig. 88.1).[1] The parenchyma of the liver is dominated by bipolar hepatocytes, organized into linear plates that are exposed to these blood elements on their basolateral surface that abuts a plexus of sinusoidal capillaries.[2-4] Although hepatocytes are the predominant cellular element of the liver, their function, structure, and differentiation are supported by interactions with other cellular components including cholangiocytes, stellate cells, Kupffer cells, Ito cells, endothelial cells, and hematopoietic elements. An intercellular matrix provides structural integrity and supports intracellular communications between these cellular elements.[5-7]

The hepatocytes perform various secretory and metabolic functions, including but not limited to detoxification of drugs and toxins, synthesis of key serum proteins (e.g., albumin, clotting factors, complement, apolipoproteins), synthesis and metabolism of dietary lipids, glucose homeostasis, and bile production.[8-12] Distortion of the normal architecture of the liver either by chronic disease states or congenital malformations can have significant impact on the ability of the liver to perform these complex functions. As expected, the developmental steps necessary to ensure proper hepatic organization and function involve multiple and complex communications between the cellular and matrix components of the organ during organogenesis of the liver.[13-16] Investigators continue to discover new intracellular signals (specific growth factors and transcription factors) that appear to combine to initiate and propagate the transformation of fetal endodermal tissue into differentiated hepatic cellular elements and a functioning organ. This chapter will attempt to summarize some of the experiments using molecular genetics, molecular biology techniques, and tissue explant culture techniques that have shed light on our understanding of early steps in hepatic development.

EARLY EMBRYOGENESIS: AN OVERVIEW

Extensive investigations have helped to clarify many of the steps involved with the early development of the liver and the specific messengers and tissue signals that orchestrate this process, as well as directing the maturation of the hepatocytes.[16,17] Specific signaling molecules, hormones, growth factors, transcriptional factors, and intracellular matrix interactions have been shown to contribute to the induction of pluripotential primitive tissues into cells committed to a hepatic fate. In addition, these molecules are critical to the maturation of the cells into specialized epithelium and contribute to the proper organization of these cells into the correct configuration constituting the fully functioning organ. Much of this work has been derived from observations in genetically altered mice, zebrafish, and tissue culture systems. During the third to fourth week of gestation, a bud of proliferating endodermal tissue is observed originating from the ventral foregut constituting the hepatic diverticulum. The progenitor cells of this region are derived from three domains that fuse to form a single prehepatic domain adjacent to the cardiogenic mesoderm.[18] Cells of this endodermal region become committed to hepatic fate by a process referred to as hepatic specification.[19] The primitive cells of this bud, referred to as hepatoblasts, appear to be bipotential, with the ability to differentiate into either mature hepatocytes or cholangiocytes.[20] These cells are in contact with embryonic cardiac mesoderm and abut the septum transversum mesenchyme.[16,17] Following inductive signaling from adjacent mesoderm, liver bud morphogenesis proceeds by conversion of cubital foregut epithelium to columnar hepatoblasts that subsequently change to pseudostratified epithelium mediated by transcription factor Hhex; they then migrate into adjacent mesenchyme.[21] The hepatoblasts migrate as cords into the septum transversum, closely associated with primitive sinusoidal endothelial cells. The migration process is mediated by a loss of contact between hepatoblasts as a result of downregulation of E-cadherin as well as concomitant extracellular matrix remodeling of the basal membrane, mediated in part by mesenchyme-derived Mmp2 and hepatocyte-expressed Mmp14.[22-24] As the process progresses, the sinusoidal structure is established, initially lacking the fenestrations observed at the latter stages of maturity. The undifferentiated hepatoblasts have few organelles at this stage, with a high nuclear to cytoplasmic ratio, scant rough endoplasmic reticulum, and few lysosomes.[9] Intercellular communication appears to be mediated via cell surface adhesions with other hepatoblasts and surrounding mesenchymal cells.[25] The anterior vitelline vessels of the yolk sac are the initial source of sinusoidal blood.[26] Early synthesis and secretion of α-fetoprotein, albumin, transthyretin, transferrin, and α-1-antitrypsin can be observed from these immature prehepatic cells.[27,28]

LATE EMBRYOGENESIS: AN OVERVIEW

Early in the second month of gestation, the hepatoblasts gradually begin to differentiate into mature hepatocytes with the necessary intercellular components (rough endoplasmic reticulum and Golgi apparatus) to conduct their multiple synthetic and metabolic functions.[9] These cells also acquire polarity with the increased production of specific membrane-associated proteins and transmembrane transporters.[29] This process creates a basolateral hepatocyte domain with clusters

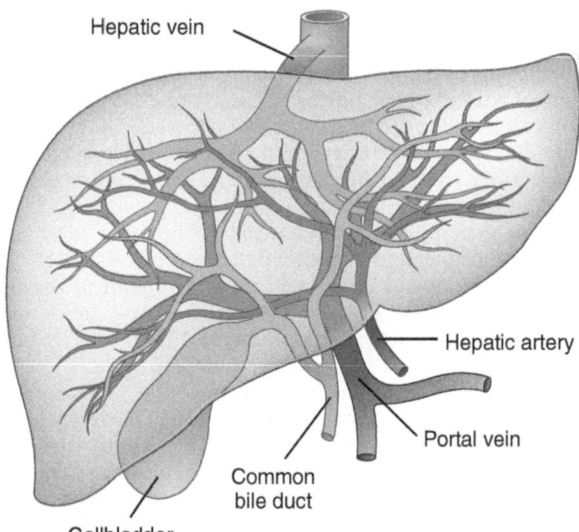

Fig. 88.1 Schematic depicting the unique vascular innervation of the liver. Unlike every organ in the body the liver has dual vascular inflow from the portal vein and from the hepatic artery. The blood traverses the liver parenchyma, coalescing into the hepatic veins that carry blood away from the organ. The intimate relationship between vessels and the biliary system is shown, with implications for the development of the biliary system, facilitating signaling between structures during development.

Table 88.1 Liver Cell Derivations.

	Tissue of Origin
Hepatocytes	Foregut endoderm bipotential hepatoblast
Endothelial cells	Septum transversum mesenchyme-angioblast
Biliary epithelial cells	Foregut endoderm-bipotential hepatoblast
Hematopoietic cells	Septum transversum mesenchyme
Kupffer cells	Yolk sac and bone marrow
Ito cells	Septum transversum mesenchyme

of membrane-associated receptors and transporters for protein secretion in association with sinusoidal vessels, and an apical hepatocyte domain constituting of the bile canaliculi with transporters related to bile secretion.[30] Both these surfaces develop microvillus architecture, presumably to optimize surface area for extracellular contact. Other hepatoblasts are thought to develop into cholangiocytes that organize into the hepatic biliary system.[31,32] The intrahepatic bile ducts are formed from periportal hepatoblasts forming the ductal plate. Differentiation and maturation of the intrahepatic ducts occurs via interactions with periportal connective tissue, glucocorticoid hormones, and basal laminar components.[20] Intrahepatic hematopoiesis increases at this stage and appears to progress with interactions between maturing hepatocytes and undifferentiated mesenchymal elements.[33-35] These hematopoietic precursors release interleukin 6, stimulating hepatocyte differentiation, which is also mediated by *Hnf4α*, an important transcriptional regulator of hepatocyte maturation.[36,37]

SPECIFIC INTERACTIONS PROMOTING HEPATOGENESIS

The initial induction of the ventral foregut to commit to a hepatic fate has been shown, in embryo tissue transplant studies in the chick, to be a function of interactions of this endodermal region with cardiac mesoderm (Table 88.1).[38] The growth factors found to mediate this process produced by cardiac mesoderm are fibroblast growth factors (FGFs) FGF-1 and FGF-2. Further studies using purified FGFs and FGF inhibitors confirmed this interaction.[28] The specificity of FGF for this region appears to be related to the fact that FGF migration is limited by high-affinity interactions with extracellular matrix.[39,40] In fact, further explanted embryonic tissue studies demonstrate that without this induction stimulus the fate of the ventral foregut that normally gives rise to the hepatic diverticulum will default to a pancreatic fate.[41] Specifically, FGF stimulation of the ventral foregut endoderm inhibits pancreatic genes and induces liver genes in this bipotential precursor cell population.

The induction stimulus provided by FGF is not sufficient to stimulate hepatocyte differentiation. Hepatocyte differentiation appears to be a function of a second induction stimulus from another mesoderm-derived tissue, the septum transversum mesenchyme. The signal proteins for this interaction appear to be bone morphogenetic proteins (BMPs).[42] Specifically, BMP-2, BMP-4, and BMP-7 are produced by the septum transversum mesenchyme cells. Further studies using a BMP signal inhibitor, Noggin, demonstrated that BMP as well as FGF were needed to achieve hepatoblast induction from ventral gut endoderm.[42] These mechanisms controlling the initiation of liver development are well conserved among various organisms, as demonstrated in studies in chick and zebrafish models.[12,14,43] The stimulatory effects of FGFs are focused to the prehepatic endodermal tissue by a network of transcription factors expressed in embryonic gut tissue. One such molecule is hepatocyte nuclear factor (HNF) 3B.[44] These transcription factors appear to be important mediators of hepatocyte differentiation that bind to specific hepatic gene enhancer regions promoting gene expression and cellular differentiation.[45]

The structure of the liver is organized into bipolar hepatocytes in linear plates interfacing with sinusoids on their basolateral surface and bile canaliculi at their apical pole. The molecular mechanisms responsible for hepatocyte polarity have been studied in vivo using HepG2, MDCK, and WIF-B cell lines as well as sandwich cultures of primary hepatocytes.[29,46,47] Despite these investigations, the mechanisms responsible for the establishment of hepatocyte polarity during development are as yet unknown.

The importance of the interaction between the septum transversum mesenchyme and the developing prehepatic endoderm cannot be overemphasized. The septum transversum mesenchyme is the source of BMP signaling, leading to induction of hepatoblast differentiation and propagation of the hepatocyte maturation process.[48] Extracellular matrix components of the septum transversum mesenchyme aid in the regulation of differentiation by binding and concentrating signaling molecules.[49,50] In addition, extracellular matrix components can directly mediate intracellular communication through interactions with integrins, focal adhesion kinase, and other signaling molecules.[7,51]

Membrane trafficking pathways and intracellular trafficking contribute to hepatocyte maturation and polarity regulated by liver kinase B1. This molecule mediates its effects through adenosine monophosphate (AMP) activated protein kinase.[46]

Hepatocyte growth factor (HGF) is a potent hepatocyte proliferation stimulant that affects cell migration as well as differentiation.[52,53] Retinoic acid is one additional factor that indirectly stimulates hepatoblast proliferation and stellate cell formation by inducing production of trophic factors by mesodermal cells, as demonstrated in chick embryo studies.[54] In addition, retinoic acid signaling has been characterized as an early regulator of liver asymmetry in zebrafish, leading to differential morphogenesis of the right and left liver lobes, but whether this contributes to liver symmetry in mammals is unknown.[55] These are but a few of the recognized components of the septum transversum mesenchyme and its extracellular matrix that are part of an integrated and diverse signaling process ensuring integrity of the hepatocyte maturation process and the overall hepatic structural organization.[56]

HEPATIC VASCULAR ANATOMY

During fetal development, highly oxygenated blood is delivered to the liver through the falciform ligament from the placenta via the umbilical vein.[1,57,58] The blood supply to the right lobe is derived from the right branch of the portal vein. The left branch of the portal vein connects via the portal sinus to the umbilical vein. The blood supply to the left lobe of the liver is derived from direct branches of the umbilical vein. This difference in blood oxygen saturation gives preferential dominance to the left lobe in utero. The umbilical vein continues past these branch points as the ductus venosus, delivering well-oxygenated blood to the inferior vena cava, which is then directed across the patent foramen ovale to the left heart.[26,58,59] After birth, the ductus venosus and umbilical veins obliterate and the normal adult hepatic vascular supply is established.

INTRAHEPATIC VASCULAR DEVELOPMENT

In the adult, the portal vein enters the liver and branches into smaller and smaller vessels that travel along with branches of the hepatic artery and the interlobular bile ducts within the portal tracts. The portal veins terminate in the sinusoids of the liver, which are characterized by fenestrated endothelial epithelium. Sinusoids are separated by single-cell-thick sheets of hepatocytes referred to as the *hepatic plates*. Therefore, the hepatocytes are directly exposed to portal blood, permitting transfer of macromolecules. The sinusoidal blood empties into the central vein branches of the hepatic veins, which terminate into the left, right, and middle hepatic veins, which return blood to the inferior vena cava and back to the heart. This important anatomic arrangement is critical for proper gland function and is under the control of a number of factors during hepatic development.[1,56]

Angioblasts, or primitive precursors to functional endothelial cells, have been found in an intermediate position between the prehepatic endoderm and the surrounding septum transversum mesenchyme (see Table 88.1).[16] These cells intermingle with hepatoblasts as the endoderm organizes into the hepatic bud. The development of this cell population is under the influence of vascular endothelial growth factor (VEGF) 2.[60,61] Observations in transgenic mice and explant systems of liver bud tissue suggest that angioblasts stimulate development of the hepatic bud in endodermal tissues before the local blood vessels are formed.[62] The exact origin of the angioblast cells remains unknown. Hepatocyte endothelial cells derive from the mesoderm and endoderm, but all sources have not yet been identified. The current thinking is that vessel anatomy does not follow a rigid predetermined pattern; rather, vasculogenesis appears to be guided both by local needs and flow dynamics. The vascular endothelium may well be equally important in providing signaling to the surrounding tissue affecting the differentiation of organ cell precursors and the ultimate structural integrity of the organ.[63,64] It remains unclear how the branching pattern is established during embryogenesis; it may be the result of either angiogenesis or vasculogenesis or both. Branching of the portal vein is the first to occur; it provides a framework for the development of the bile duct plate. Biliary cells in turn promote hepatic artery morphogenesis mediated through VEGF and angiopoietin.[65,66]

BILIARY DUCT DEVELOPMENT

In the adult liver, mature hepatocytes secrete bile into the canaliculi, small channels along their apical surface created by clusters of adjacent hepatocytes. These channels coalesce into a network of intrahepatic bile ducts and eventually into the main hepatic ducts lined by biliary epithelial cells or cholangiocytes. Bile is exported from the liver and stored and concentrated in the gallbladder for excretion during a meal.

The origin of biliary cells appears to be from bipotential hepatoblasts originating at the hepatic bud (see Table 88.1).[20] Bile duct development is initiated near the hilum of the liver and later propagates into the liver lobes. These cells under the influence of the transcription factor HNF-6 and its effect on HNF 1B undergo differentiation and proliferation.[67] Other key factors in the signaling of cholangiocyte differentiation include transforming growth factor (TGF)-β, Notch, Wnt, FGF, laminin, Hippo, and epimorphin.[19,68-70] These subsets of hepatoblasts strongly express biliary-specific cytokeratins.[31] Among the molecules produced by the biliary ductal cells is laminin α 5, which activates integrin β1, necessary throughout morphogenesis and differentiation.[71] These biliary precursor cells form the ductal plate that is characterized as a continuous single-layered ring around the portal mesenchyme. The ductal plate proliferates into a bilayer. Focal dilatations of the ductal plate along the bilayer give rise to the bile ducts. The newly formed ducts are incorporated into the hepatic mesenchyme. The above process is moderated by biliary precursor cell interactions with neighboring cells and with matrix proteins including laminin, fibronectin, and collagen types I and IV.[49,50,72,73] The process of bile duct formation also appears to be influenced by interactions with the nearby developing blood vessels as evidenced by abnormities in bile duct morphology observed with genetic deficiencies in the vascular Notch pathways.[74] Candidates for genetic modifiers of Notch signaling deficiencies affecting the phenotype have been described and include o-glycosyltransferase 1 *(POGLUT1)*, *Hnf6*, and the fringe family of glycosyltransferases.[75-77]

The extrahepatic biliary tree is derived from ventral endoderm and shares a common origin with the ventral pancreas.[78] *Sox17* originating from common progenitor cells mediates the lineage progression to hepatic ductal tissue as demonstrated by *Sox17* mouse knock-out models. Other genes shown to affect the development of the extrahepatic ductal system include *Hhex*, *Hnf1β*, *hnf6*, *leucine-rich repeat containing coupled receptor 4*, and *Fork-head box factor 1*.[67,79-82] Glypican 1 *(GCP1)* is a heparan sulfate proteoglycan that binds FGF19, resulting in gallbladder hypoplasia and intrahepatic bile duct paucity when knocked down in zebrafish.[83] Although the extrahepatic ducts are in the vicinity of the intrahepatic ducts in the hilum, how they anastomose remains unknown.[65]

HEPATIC HEMATOPOIESIS

The yolk sac contributes significantly to early fetal hemopoiesis.[33] The yolk sac delivers blood from the anterior vitelline vessels to the developing sinusoids of the liver. Around the sixth week of gestation the earliest hematopoietic elements appear to differentiate from the undifferentiated mesenchymal cells derived from the septum transversum (see Table 88.1).[84] These cells appear to interact with the developing hepatocytes and may derive trophic signals stimulating growth and development.[34] This stimulatory effect appears to change with time, diminishing as the hepatocyte matures.[35] Hematopoietic elements produced in the liver migrate through regulated temporary migration pores, not between the intact endothelial cell lining of the sinusoids, in a process termed *diapedesis*.[2,4] Interesting evidence suggests that hepatocytes themselves may be derived from multipotential bone marrow cells as well as arising from prehepatic endoderm.[85,86] As the hepatocyte matures and differentiates into the cells responsible for serum protein production near the end of gestation and in the early postnatal period, there appears to be a diminished role for intrahepatic hematopoiesis, which is then assumed by migration of hematopoietic precursor cells to the bone marrow.

SINUSOIDAL CELLS—KUPFFER AND ITO CELLS

Kupffer cells are manifested during the second month of gestation. These specialized cells residing on sinusoidal surface of the endothelium have macrophage-like activity.[2] These cells appear to originate from both the embryonic yolk sac and from the bone marrow at later stages of development (see Table 88.1).[87] The position of these cells permits regulation of migration across the endothelium of the sinusoid.

Ito cells are specialized cells that reside in the peri-sinusoidal space of Disse between the endothelial cells and the developing hepatocytes of the hepatic plate.[88] These cells appear to originate from the undifferentiated mesenchyme of the septum transversum (see Table 88.1).[88] These cells store fat and vitamin A. Along with endothelial cells these cells are involved with the production and secretion of basement membrane collagen and may therefore contribute to fibrosis in chronic liver injury.[88,89]

ACINAR ORGANIZATION

The functional unit of the liver is known as the *acinus*. This functional unit is defined by the hepatic blood flow from the portal vein branches within adjacent portal tracts, through the hepatic sinusoids separated by hepatocyte palates, and terminates in the central vein branches of the hepatic veins. (Fig. 88.2). These basic units of function are recognized in the second and third months of gestation, as the cell elements of the liver differentiate and as the matrix elements proliferate. In the mature liver, the hepatocytes within this functional unit perform differential functions depending on their position within the acinus. This concept, known as *metabolic zonation*, begins in the first weeks after birth.[10] The hepatocytes within the acinus can be divided into three zones. Zone one cells are closest to the portal tracts and therefore receive blood with the highest nutrient and oxygen content. These cells appear to be best suited to extract bile acids, perform gluconeogenesis, produce glycogen, produce and secrete protein, and metabolize lipids.[90-94] Zone three cells are located adjacent to the branches of the hepatic vein. Zone three hepatocytes appear to have a higher capacity to perform glycolysis, have higher cytochrome P450 expression, and perform various metabolic reactions including drug detoxification, glycosylation events, and ureagenesis.[10,95-97] Zone two cells are intermediate in position and the hepatocytes in this zone appear to express activities similar to the cells of the other two zones depending on their relative proximity. HNF-4α and Wnt signaling have been implicated in the regulation of metabolic zonation.[10]

Investigations as to the differences in the functions of the cells within these defined zones have led to two likely overlapping theories.[98] The first assumption is that differences in the oxygen and macromolecule content of the blood supply to these zones may influence the development and differentiation of hepatocytes. The second theory is that regional differences in cell signaling and matrix element interactions influence hepatocyte differentiation in local populations. Modulators of gene function and expression within the hepatocytes of a particular zone will ultimately define and refine their respective functions.[99] In addition, intercellular communications between adjacent hepatocyte populations will further affect hepatocyte differentiation and regional coordination of function. The likely conclusion to this process is that both these influences are responsible for the observed differences and similarities in hepatocyte function within the acinus.

REGULATION OF FETAL LIVER GROWTH AND MATURATION

As cell differentiation is proceeding, the fetal liver is undergoing growth and structural organization. The molecules stimulating these processes are poorly understood. The process seems to be under the influence of circulating hormones and various growth factors (Table 88.2). Specifically, growth hormone and its gestational homologue, placental lactogen, are believed to provide important stimuli to hepatocellular hyperplasia.[100,101] Insulin, cortisol, and thyroid hormone have been shown to alter

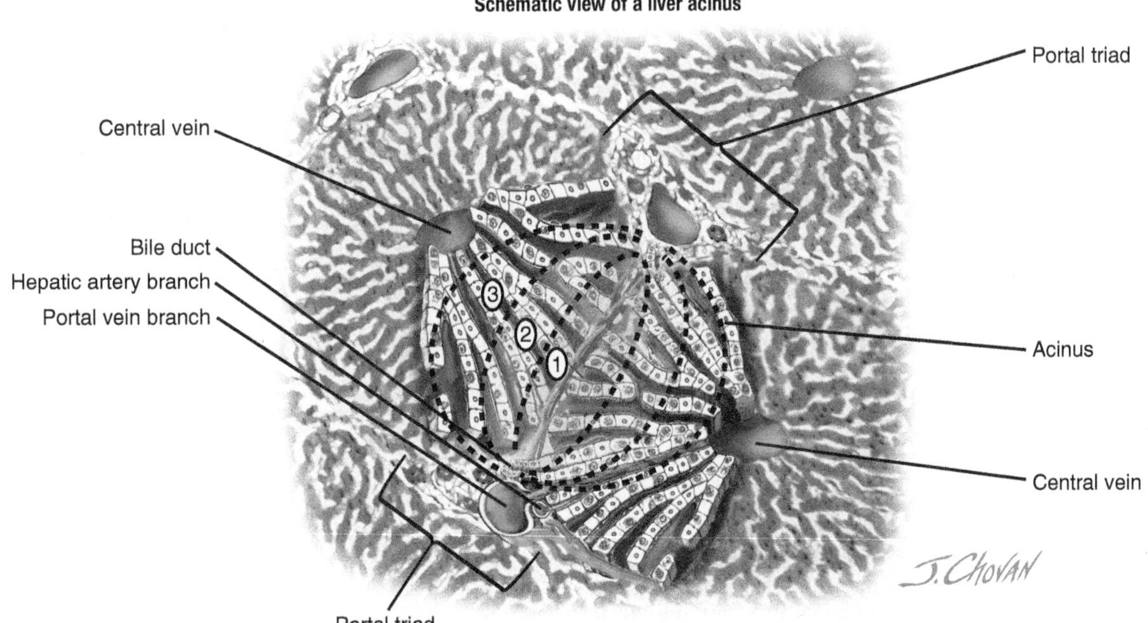

Fig. 88.2 Acinar organization. Schematic representing the microscopic infrastructure of the liver, which facilitates the absorption and excretion of macromolecules. The hepatic vascular inflow originates from branches of the portal vein and the hepatic artery. Blood from these two vessels intermixes in the hepatic sinusoids lined by cords of hepatocytes along their basolateral surface. Blood trickles across this space, ultimately emptying into branches of the hepatic vein for return to the heart. (Copyright 2021. Elsevier, NetterImages.com.)

Table 88.2 Stimuli of Hepatocellular Development.

Hormonal	Growth hormone, placental lactogen Thyroid hormone Cortisol Insulin
Growth Factors	Insulin-like growth factor-1 Insulin-like growth factor-2 Hepatocyte growth factor Epidermal growth factor

protein production and growth factor receptor expression in the developing liver and may be important mediators of growth and maturation of the organ both in utero and postpartum.[102-104] In part the effect of these hormones is a function of their effect on the production and binding of secondary messenger molecules, the insulin-like growth factors.[101-107] Differential production and binding of these messengers may contribute to cell growth and replication, cell migration, and tissue organization and maturation.

Other molecules considered to be contributors to cell hyperplasia, migration, and tissue organization are HGF and epidermal growth factor (see Table 88.2). HGF has emerged as an important tissue-specific signaling molecule between epithelial and mesenchyme tissues. This molecule is a ligand for the c-met protooncogene product of receptor tyrosine kinase and originates from mesenchymal tissues.[108] As such this paracrine molecule supports organogenesis, mature organ regeneration, and neoplastic processes.[108,109] HGF and the expression of its receptor in liver and other tissues have been demonstrated in association with tissue injury suggesting a focused tissue-specific regeneration response.[109] The diverse biologic functions of this multipotent polypeptide lead investigators to consider it a key molecule for tissue organization, organogenesis, and organ repair.

The factors influencing the integrity of the hepatic tissue architecture are believed to be a function of coordinated bidirectional cell interactions between adjacent differentiating hepatoblasts and sinusoidal endothelial cells. Studies in mutant zebrafish have shown that the regular spacing of hepatocytes between the sinusoidal plexus and the biliary system is regulated by cerebral cavernous malformation 2 (*ccm2*—expressed in endothelial cells) and EGF-like domain containing *gene heart of glass* (*heg1*).[43] Mouse studies have demonstrated that *Hnf4a* not only leads to the differentiation of polarized hepatic epithelium but also to the formation of a functional sinusoidal network.[37]

Epidermal growth factor has been identified as a key molecule involved with liver regeneration and may play a role in embryogenesis and fetal growth, since receptors have been found in fetal tissues.[54,110] The liver appears to modulate serum levels of this molecule, providing efficient clearance and degradation of the internalized protein.[111] There is also extensive data to indicate interactions between epidermal growth factor and other circulating hormones.[54] Growth hormone increases epidermal growth factor binding in the liver.[112] Thyroid and steroid hormones modulate both epidermal growth factor and its receptors in multiple tissues.[113] Epidermal growth factor itself stimulates hormone release from the pituitary, the placenta, and the adrenal gland but inhibits hormone production by the gonads and thyroid. The effect on fetal growth and development may be mediated by direct effects on gene activation or may be a function of other protein interactions.[114] The significance of this molecule for hepatic growth and maturation has yet to be proven.

CONCLUSION

In summary, the development of the liver from primitive endoderm and mesoderm is a complicated yet orchestrated process that mandates continued intercellular and matrix signaling. Our current knowledge of the multitude of contributing messengers to this process is likely just the tip of the proverbial organogenesis iceberg. Our expanding knowledge base of the steps ensuring proper hepatocyte differentiation, growth, and organization will permit us to apply learned techniques to promote regeneration and restoration of the damaged mature organ. In addition, by increasing our knowledge of the signaling pathways governing normal growth and development of the liver, we may expand our understanding and ability to manage the uncontrolled growth of hepatic malignancies. Our knowledge of the mechanisms regulating hepatic epithelial cell differentiation has been essential in the development of cell culture protocols for programmed differentiation of stem cell to hepatocytes, permitting the study of genetic inborn errors of the liver. The key to the evolution of this process in the short term is our expanding technical expertise with tissue culture systems and transgenic animal models.

A complete reference list is available at www.ExpertConsult.com. 

SELECT REFERENCES

1. Valette PJ, De Baere T. [Biliary and vascular anatomy of the liver]. *J Radiol.* 2002;83:221-234.
3. Enzan H, Hara H, Yamashita Y, et al. Fine structure of hepatic sinusoids and their development in human embryos and fetuses. *Acta Pathol Jpn.* 1983;33:447-466.
4. Zamboni L. Electron microscopic studies of blood embryogenesis in humans. II. The hemopoietic activity in the fetal liver. *J Ultrastruct Res.* 1965;12:525-541.
5. Chagraoui J, Lepage-Noll A, Anjo A, et al. Fetal liver stroma consists of cells in epithelial-to-mesenchymal transition. *Blood.* 2003;101:2973-2982.
7. Schwartz MA. Integrin signaling revisited. *Trends Cell Biol.* 2001;11:466-470.
10. Kietzmann T. Liver zonation in health and disease: hypoxia and hypoxia-inducible transcription factors as concert masters. *Int J Mol Sci.* 2019;20.
12. Quistorff B. Metabolic heterogeneity of liver parenchymal cells. *Essays Biochem.* 1990;25:83-136.
15. Zaret KS. Hepatocyte differentiation: from the endoderm and beyond. *Curr Opin Genet Dev.* 2001;11:568-574.
16. Zaret KS. Regulatory phases of early liver development: paradigms of organogenesis. *Nat Rev Genet.* 2002;3:499-512.
17. Duncan SA. Mechanisms controlling early development of the liver. *Mech Dev.* 2003;120:19-33.
18. Ober EA, Lemaigre FP. Development of the liver: Insights into organ and tissue morphogenesis. *J Hepatol.* 2018;68:1049-1062.
19. Zong Y, Stanger BZ. Molecular mechanisms of liver and bile duct development. *Wiley Interdiscip Rev Dev Biol.* 2012;1:643-655.
24. Yin C, Kikuchi K, Hochgreb T, et al. Hand2 regulates extracellular matrix remodeling essential for gut-looping morphogenesis in zebrafish. *Dev Cell.* 2010;18:973-984.
25. Cayuso J, Dzementsei A, Fischer JC, et al. EphrinB1/EphB3b coordinate bidirectional epithelial-mesenchymal interactions controlling liver morphogenesis and laterality. *Dev Cell.* 2016;39:316-328.
28. Jung J, Zheng M, Goldfarb M, et al. Initiation of mammalian liver development from endoderm by fibroblast growth factors. *Science.* 1999;284:1998-2003.
29. Treyer A, Musch A. Hepatocyte polarity. *Compr Physiol.* 2013;3:243-287.
31. Lemaigre FP. Development of the biliary tract. *Mech Dev.* 2003;120:81-87.
37. Parviz F, Matullo C, Garrison WD, et al. Hepatocyte nuclear factor 4alpha controls the development of a hepatic epithelium and liver morphogenesis. *Nat Genet.* 2003;34:292-296.
41. Deutsch G, Jung J, Zheng M, et al. A bipotential precursor population for pancreas and liver within the embryonic endoderm. *Development.* 2001;128:871-881.
42. Rossi JM, Dunn NR, Hogan BL, et al. Distinct mesodermal signals, including BMPs from the septum transversum mesenchyme, are required in combination for hepatogenesis from the endoderm. *Genes Dev.* 2001;15:1998-2009.
43. Antoniou A, Raynaud P, Cordi S, et al. Intrahepatic bile ducts develop according to a new mode of tubulogenesis regulated by the transcription factor SOX9. *Gastroenterology.* 2009;136:2325-2333.
45. Duncan SA. Transcriptional regulation of liver development. *Dev Dyn.* 2000;219:131-142.
48. Houssaint E. Differentiation of the mouse hepatic primordium. I. An analysis of tissue interactions in hepatocyte differentiation. *Cell Differ.* 1980;9:269-279.

54. Fisher DA, Lakshmanan J. Metabolism and effects of epidermal growth factor and related growth factors in mammals. *Endocr Rev*. 1990;11:418-442.
55. Garnaas MK, Cutting CC, Meyers A, et al. Rargb regulates organ laterality in a zebrafish model of right atrial isomerism. *Dev Biol*. 2012;372:178-189.
56. Sanchez-Romero N, Sainz-Arnal P, Pla-Palacin I, et al. The role of extracellular matrix on liver stem cell fate: a dynamic relationship in health and disease. *Differentiation*. 2019;106:49-56.
62. Matsumoto K, Yoshitomi H, Rossant J, et al. Liver organogenesis promoted by endothelial cells prior to vascular function. *Science*. 2001;294:559-563.
65. Fabris L, Cadamuro M, Libbrecht L, et al. Epithelial expression of angiogenic growth factors modulate arterial vasculogenesis in human liver development. *Hepatology*. 2008;47:719-728.
67. Clotman F, Lannoy VJ, Reber M, et al. The onecut transcription factor HNF6 is required for normal development of the biliary tract. *Development*. 2002;129:1819-1828.
68. Gerard C, Tys J, Lemaigre FP. Gene regulatory networks in differentiation and direct reprogramming of hepatic cells. *Semin Cell Dev Biol*. 2017;66:43-50.
71. Tanimizu N, Kikkawa Y, Mitaka T, et al. Alpha1- and alpha5-containing laminins regulate the development of bile ducts via beta1 integrin signals. *J Biol Chem*. 2012;287:28586-28597.
73. Terada T, Nakanuma Y. Expression of tenascin, type IV collagen and laminin during human intrahepatic bile duct development and in intrahepatic cholangiocarcinoma. *Histopathology*. 1994;25:143-150.
74. Li L, Krantz ID, Deng Y, et al. Alagille syndrome is caused by mutations in human Jagged1, which encodes a ligand for Notch1. *Nat Genet*. 1997;16:243-251.
76. Thakurdas SM, Lopez MF, Kakuda S, et al. Jagged1 heterozygosity in mice results in a congenital cholangiopathy which is reversed by concomitant deletion of one copy of Poglut1 (Rumi). *Hepatology*. 2016;63:550-565.
78. Spence JR, Lange AW, Lin SC, et al. Sox17 regulates organ lineage segregation of ventral foregut progenitor cells. *Dev Cell*. 2009;17:62-74.
80. Hunter MP, Wilson CM, Jiang X, et al. The homeobox gene Hhex is essential for proper hepatoblast differentiation and bile duct morphogenesis. *Dev Biol*. 2007;308:355-367.
82. Yamashita R, Takegawa Y, Sakumoto M, et al. Defective development of the gall bladder and cystic duct in Lgr4- hypomorphic mice. *Dev Dyn*. 2009;238:993-1000.
83. Cui S, Leyva-Vega M, Tsai EA, et al. Evidence from human and zebrafish that GPC1 is a biliary atresia susceptibility gene. *Gastroenterology*. 2013;144:1107-1115 e1103.
85. Austin TW, Lagasse E. Hepatic regeneration from hematopoietic stem cells. *Mech Dev*. 2003;120:131-135.
86. Oh SH, Witek RP, Bae SH, et al. Bone marrow-derived hepatic oval cells differentiate into hepatocytes in 2-acetylaminofluorene/partial hepatectomy-induced liver regeneration. *Gastroenterology*. 2007;132:1077-1087.
89. Fujita M, Spray DC, Choi H, et al. Extracellular matrix regulation of cell-cell communication and tissue-specific gene expression in primary liver cultures. *Prog Clin Biol Res*. 1986;226:333-360.
90. Aggarwal SR, Lindros KO, Palmer TN. Glucagon stimulates phosphorylation of different peptides in isolated periportal and perivenous hepatocytes. *FEBS Lett*. 1995;377:439-443.
93. Rempel A, Bannasch P, Mayer D. Differences in expression and intracellular distribution of hexokinase isoenzymes in rat liver cells of different transformation stages. *Biochim Biophys Acta*. 1994;1219:660-668.
99. Gumucio JJ, May M, Dvorak C, et al. The isolation of functionally heterogeneous hepatocytes of the proximal and distal half of the liver acinus in the rat. *Hepatology*. 1986;6:932-944.
101. Strain AJ, Hill DJ, Swenne I, et al. Regulation of DNA synthesis in human fetal hepatocytes by placental lactogen, growth hormone, and insulin-like growth factor I/somatomedin-C. *J Cell Physiol*. 1987;132:33-40.
103. Rajaratnam VS, Webb PJ, Fishman RB, et al. Maternal diabetes induces upregulation of hepatic insulin-like growth factor binding protein-1 MRNA expression, growth retardation and developmental delay at the same stage of rat fetal development. *J Endocrinol*. 1997;152:R1-R6.
107. Serna J, Gonzalez-Guerrero PR, Scanes CG, et al. Differential and tissue-specific regulation of (pro)insulin and insulin-like growth factor-I mRNAs and levels of thyroid hormones in growth-retarded embryos. *Growth Regul*. 1996;6:73-82.
108. Matsumoto K, Nakamura T. Emerging multipotent aspects of hepatocyte growth factor. *J Biochem*. 1996;119:591-600.
110. Marti U, Burwen SJ, Jones AL. Biological effects of epidermal growth factor, with emphasis on the gastrointestinal tract and liver: an update. *Hepatology*. 1989;9:126-138.
114. Murray MA, Dickson BA, Smith EP, et al. Epidermal growth factor stimulates insulin-like growth factor-binding protein-1 expression in the neonatal rat. *Endocrinology*. 1993;133:159-165.

Bile Acid Metabolism During Development 89

Linda X. Wang | Rohit Kohli

INTRODUCTION

Bile acids have long been understood to be physiologic detergent molecules synthesized from cholesterol and critical for the absorption of intestinal lipids. More recently we have come to comprehend their broader role as signaling molecules in a variety of metabolic processes such as glucose homeostasis, immune cell function, and regulation of cell growth and proliferation.[1] Thus, it is not surprising that bile acid physiology is a tightly regulated process of synthesis in the liver, transport and biotransformation in the intestines, followed by reabsorption in the ileum. Any alteration in this homeostasis has effects on hepatic metabolic processes, resulting in inflammation and development of diseases such as cholestatic liver diseases, dyslipidemia, diabetes, and even tumorigenesis.[1,2] This chapter provides an overview of bile acid synthesis and metabolism with a focus on disorders of bile acid metabolism that result in neonatal liver disease.

ANATOMY OF THE LIVER

DEVELOPMENT OF THE LIVER AND BILIARY TREE

The liver begins as an endodermal bud from the ventral foregut above the yolk sac that forms around the third week of gestation. This bud enlarges and differentiates into a semblance of the adult lobulated structure by the sixth week of gestation.[3,4] Concurrently, the intrahepatic biliary tree develops from the cranial bud while the caudal portion gives rise to the extrahepatic biliary tree (gallbladder, common bile duct, and cystic duct) via differentiation of ductal plates.[3,5] The vitelline veins, which pass between the yolk sac and the sinus venosus of the heart, eventually form the portal vein by the seventh week. The portal vein then joins with the umbilical vein to form the ductus venosus (Fig. 89.1). In contrast to adult circulation, in the fetus, the ductus venosus shunts blood from the left umbilical vein to the inferior vena cava directly. After birth, enteral feedings trigger the closure of this physiologic shunt, allowing systemic blood flow to instead reach the liver.[3,4,6] The hepatic artery forms at the eighth week, after the venous system and the establishment of ductal plates. Intrahepatic arterial branches extend into the liver parenchyma and portal tracts between the 10th and 15th weeks of gestation.[7] Therefore, the framework for the hepatic arterial circulation is dependent on the development of the intrahepatic portal and biliary system.

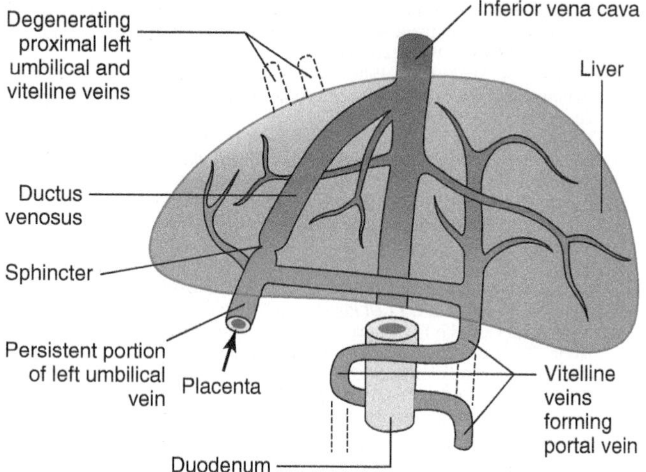

Fig. 89.1 Dorsal view of the liver demonstrating the venous circulation at 7 weeks gestation. Note the path from the umbilical vein through the ductus venosus to the inferior vena cava and the vitelline veins forming the portal vein. (From Moore KL. *The Developing Human: Clinically Oriented Embryology.* 3rd ed. Philadelphia: WB Saunders; 1982.)

Approximately 80% of the blood reaching the liver is poorly oxygenated blood from the portal vein, which is composed of blood from the intestines, pancreas, and spleen. The other 20% is well-oxygenated blood from the hepatic artery.[4] The two blood sources converge at the level of the hepatic sinusoids (Fig. 89.2), a vascular channel with a fenestrated endothelium that allows the exchange of nutrients, toxins, endobiotics, and xenobiotics between the blood and the adjacent hepatocytes. These sinusoids are lined by endothelial cells that lack a basement membrane and perform endocytotic and synthetic activity.[8,9] Other cells present in the lumen of sinusoids include hepatic stellate cells, which play a role in regulation of sinusoidal blood flow, storage of vitamin A, and liver fibrogenesis[10-12]; pit cells, which are immunoreactive natural killer (NK) cells[13]; and phagocytic Kupffer cells.[14] The sinusoids are separated from the hepatocytes by the perisinusoidal space, or the space of Disse, through which nerve fibers course on their way to the lobules. The sinusoids drain into the central veins, which join to form the hepatic veins. The hepatic veins comprise the outflow from the liver that eventually empties into the supra-hepatic inferior vena cava.[4,15]

HEPATIC LOBULE

The functional unit of the liver is the hepatic lobule, a polygonal structure with a central vein as its axis and radially arranged sheets of hepatocytes with portal triads (portal vein, hepatic artery, bile duct) at the vertices of the imaginary transverse

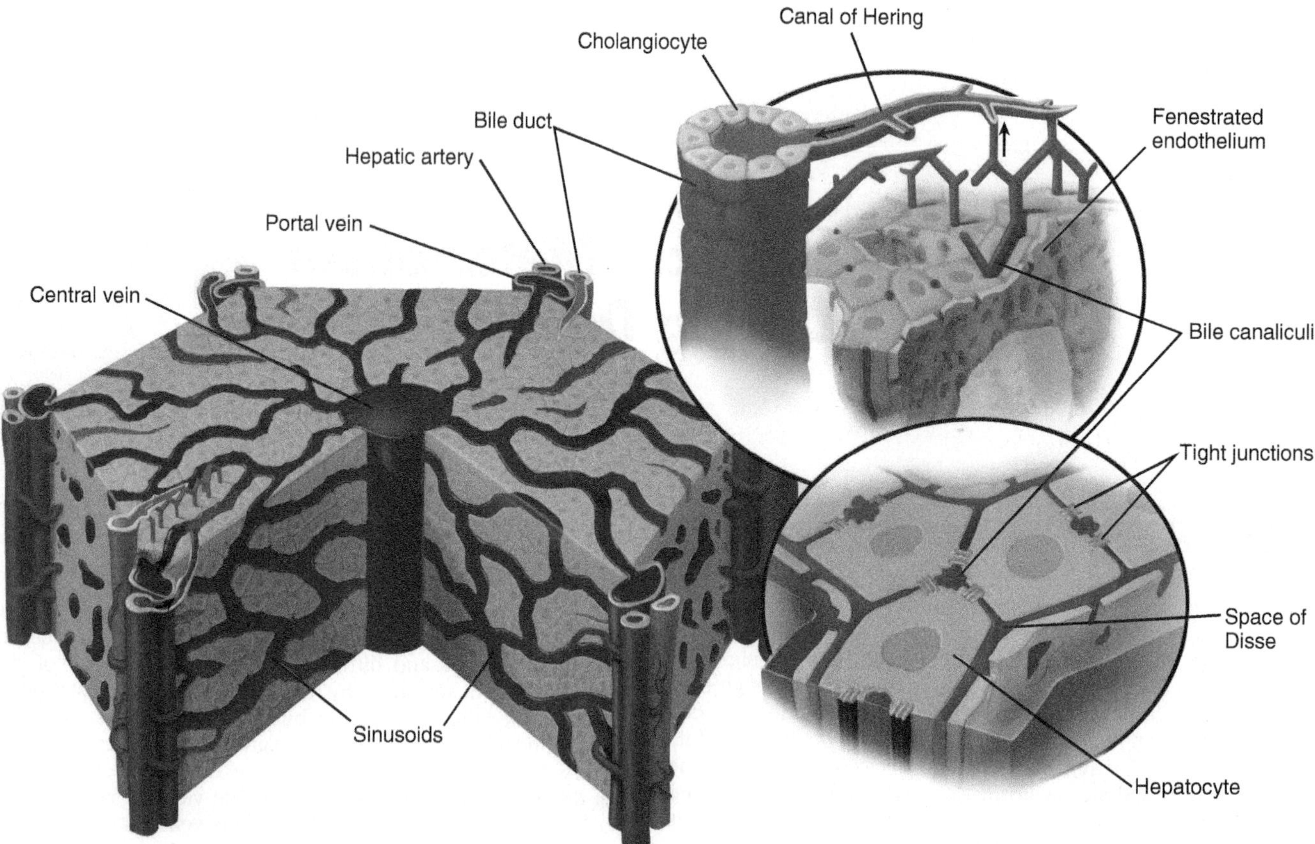

Fig. 89.2 Schematic view of the liver lobule. The central vein is shown in the center of the lobule, separated by cords of hepatocytes forming sinusoids from six portal areas at the periphery. The portal areas contain a portal vein, hepatic artery, and bile duct. Blood flows toward the center of the lobule, while bile flows toward the portal triads at the margins. Note the hepatic artery providing oxygenated blood to the hepatic sinusoids and the peribiliary plexus. The top inset provides a more detailed view of the fenestrated endothelium and the connections between intercellular canaliculi and the canals of Hering. The lower inset emphasizes the separate basolateral and canalicular membranes, as well as the junctional complexes.

polygon (see Fig. 89.2). The mixed venous and arterial blood from the portal tract flow through the sinusoids past the sheets of hepatocytes, creating a zonal gradient. The periportal region is the closest to the vascular inflow and therefore exposed to the highest concentration of nutrients and is richest in oxygen. The pericentral region is most distal and thus has the lowest oxygen content.[4] In addition, lobular heterogeneity in subcellular structure and gene expression creates a functional zonation with a distinct gradient in relation to fatty acid, glucose, toxin, and bile acid metabolism from periportal to the pericentral regions.[16-19]

HEPATOCYTES

The liver parenchyma is composed primarily of hepatocytes (>70%). Hepatocytes themselves are polarized cells with a basolateral surface that faces the sinusoids and apical surface facing a network of tiny passages that form the bile canaliculi. Both surfaces of the cells have microvilli that increase the surface area available for exchange of different substrates between the spaces.[3,4] The lateral surface lies between adjacent hepatocytes and is contiguous with the basal. The basolateral surface has a number of plasma membrane transporters dedicated to the exchange of organic and inorganic solutes. The lateral plasma membrane contains gap junctions that facilitate signaling between hepatocytes.[20] The apical surface also has transporters that allow for secretion of anions and solutes into bile.[21]

BILIARY TREE

The biliary tree begins at the canal of Hering, a transitional zone, wherein the bile canaliculi join the rest of the tree. The canals of Hering contain liver progenitor stem cells capable of regenerative activity when the liver sustains damage.[22] The canals drain into bile ductules that combine to form interlobular ducts, which combine with other interlobular ducts to form septal ducts. These septal ducts coalesce into progressively larger ducts to eventually form segmental and, finally, the right and left hepatic ducts. These two lobular ducts then converge to form the common hepatic duct, which joins the cystic duct to form the common bile duct. The common bile duct combines with the pancreatic duct that empties bile into the intestine.[23]

CHOLANGIOCYTES

Cholangiocytes are polarized epithelial cells that line the canals of Hering, bile ducts, and gallbladder (see Fig. 89.2).[4] They comprise approximately 5% of the cells of the liver. These cells modify bile composition by secreting electrolytes, organic solutes, and water in response to hormonal signals. As gastric contents enter the duodenum, gastric acid, fat, and protein stimulate the production of several hormones, including secretin. Secretin, in turn, binds to the secretin receptor on cholangiocytes, leading to stimulation of the cystic fibrosis transmembrane conductance regulator (CFTR) and transport of chloride out of the cell. The chloride gradient that is created drives the Cl^-/HCO_3^- anion exchanger with final excretion of bicarbonate into bile, thereby alkalinizing the bile.[2] Mutation of the gene encoding CFTR can lead to neonatal jaundice and liver disease in approximately 10% of patients with cystic fibrosis.[24]

Cholangiocytes also absorb glucose, amino acids, and other molecules, further modifying the bile. A small fraction of bile acids in bile are absorbed and returned to the hepatocytes in a pathway known as the *cholehepatic shunt*, which is hypothesized to promote bile flow.[1,4,25]

BILE ACID METABOLISM

BILE ACID SYNTHESIS

Bile acids are synthesized from cholesterol through a complex multi-enzyme series of reactions in the hepatocytes (Fig. 89.3). The enzymes for these reactions are found in the cytosol, peroxisomes, mitochondria, and endoplasmic reticulum.[26-29] There are two main pathways responsible for bile acid synthesis. In the neutral or classic bile acid pathway, the rate-limiting cytochrome P_{450} enzyme, cholesterol 7α-hydroxycholesterol (CYP7A1), initiates the conversion of cholesterol to the primary bile acid, cholic acid (CA). In the acidic or alternative pathway, cholesterol 27-hydroxylase (CYP27A1), a mitochondrial P_{450} enzyme, catalyzes the first reaction that leads to the final production of chenodeoxycholic acid (CDCA).[30] The acidic pathway contributes to less than 10% of the total bile acid production in humans.[31] Of note, the acidic pathway has been found to be more important in those with liver disease and in neonates.[32,33] Mutations of CYP7B1 in neonates have been reported to result in significant cholestatic liver injury, with accumulation of hepatotoxic monohydroxy bile acids.[34]

BILE ACID CONJUGATION

Typically, the primary bile acids, CA and CDCA, are conjugated to the amino acids glycine and taurine in a 3:1 ratio, depending on the availability of dietary taurine and species (e.g., in mice most bile acids are taurine-conjugated).[35,36] In contrast, in neonates, the majority (>80%) of bile acids are taurine-conjugated, due to an abundance of taurine stores in the liver.[37,38] Conjugation serves to increase the solubility of the bile acids and enables their transport via bile acid transporters on hepatocytes into the bile canalicular system and subsequently into the gallbladder. It also limits their passive reabsorption as they pass down the biliary system. After a meal, the secretion of cholecystokinin induces gallbladder contraction, which releases its contents into the gastrointestinal tract.[39] Greater than 70% of the stored bile is expelled into the proximal small intestine.

Intestinal bile acids act as detergents to emulsify dietary fats and form mixed micelles. Dietary fats and lipid-soluble vitamins are then absorbed by the intestine.[36]

ENTEROHEPATIC CIRCULATION

Some of the bile acids are passively absorbed in the proximal small intestine. The vast majority of bile acids secreted into the intestines each cycle are reabsorbed in the ileum by active transport back into the portal system and circulated back to the liver. Transporters on the apical membrane of ileal enterocytes (the apical sodium-dependent bile acid transporter or ASBT, SLC10A2) and on the sinusoidal membrane of the hepatocyte (the Na^+-taurocholate cotransporting polypeptide or NTCP, SLC10A1) are highly efficient in this process, with recovery of about 95% of secreted bile acids.[1,27,36] In adults, this bile acid pool of approximately 4 to 5 g is recycled 6 to 10 times per day, with only a small fraction (averaging 0.5 g) lost into the stool. The fecal losses are replenished by de novo bile acid synthesis in the liver.[40] Synthesis of bile acids is regulated by negative feedback by bile acids returning to the liver. (Please see the following discussion of feedback signals.)[41] A small fraction (0.5 mg/day) of circulating bile acid spills over into the systemic circulation and is excreted in urine.[1,42]

The enterohepatic circulation of bile acids serves to control bile acid synthesis through a negative feedback mechanism. Studies of rats fed with bile acids strongly reduced the activity of CYP7A1 and bile acid synthesis, whereas interruption of the enterohepatic circulation with use of bile acid binding resins (e.g., cholestyramine) increased the activity of CYP7A1.[43]

THE NEW ROLE OF BILE ACIDS

In addition to their historically defined role as emulsifiers, bile acids are now well understood to be ligands for nuclear receptors. These include the farnesoid X receptors (FXR), the vitamin D receptor (NR1I1), the pregnane X receptor (NR1I2), and the liver X receptor (NR1H3), as well as G protein coupled transmembrane receptor protein, TGR5. FXR has been implicated in the regulation of the enterohepatic circulation through downstream activation of fibroblast growth factor-19 (FGF19) and its receptor

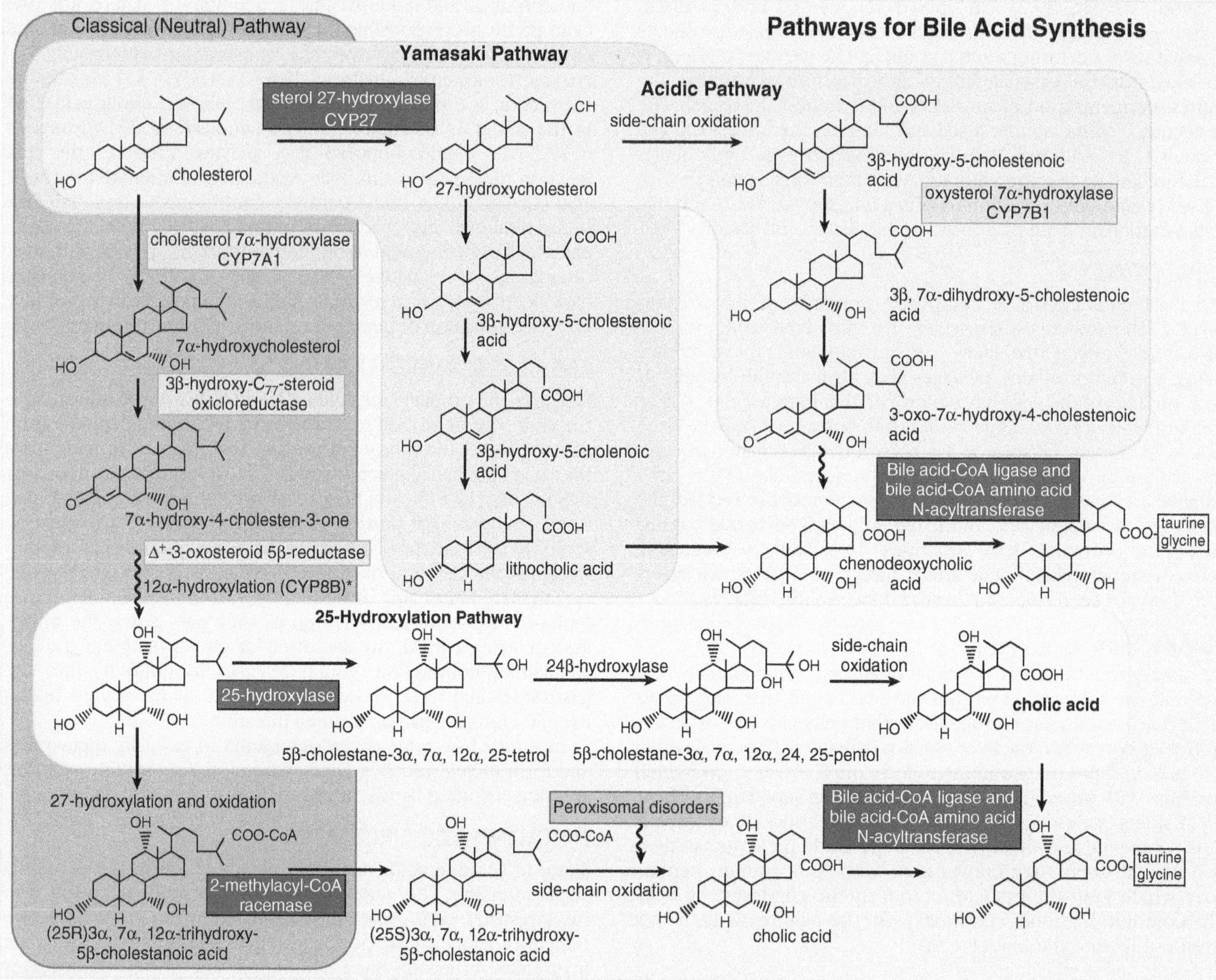

Fig. 89.3 The classic and alternative bile synthetic pathways. Known defects in sterol modification are highlighted in *yellow*. Known defects in side-chain modification are highlighted in *dark blue boxes*. (Adapted from Bove KE, Heubi JE, Balistreri WF, Setchell KDR. Bile acid synthetic defects and liver disease: a comprehensive review. *Pediatr Dev Pathol.* 2004;7:315–334.)

FGFR4 leading to inhibition of CYP7A1. FXR knockout mice have increased bile acid synthesis and CYP7A1 expression. FXR has also been shown to induce a bile salt export pump (BSEP) on the canalicular membrane of hepatocytes and inhibit a sinusoidal sodium-dependent taurocholate cotransporter (NTCP) that helps in the uptake of bile acids into hepatocytes.[39,41]

BILE ACID TRANSFORMATION

The small percentage of primary bile acids that reach the colon undergo significant structural modifications by intestinal bacteria, leading to the formation of secondary bile acids, deoxycholic acid (DCA), and lithocholic acid (LCA), respectively. DCA and LCA are both hydrophobic and known to be hepatotoxic but are mostly excreted into feces.[44]

Bacterial deconjugation creates unconjugated mono- or dihydroxy bile acids, which can be passively absorbed through colonic membrane and recycled to the liver. The enzymes that catalyze the transformations are found in bacterial organisms such as *Bacteroidetes*, *Clostridium* species, *Bifidobacteriaceae*, and *Enterococcus*.[31,44] Gut bacteria are thought to benefit from bile metabolism through acquisition of glycine and taurine, which can be utilized as an energy source in metabolism.[45,46] These alterations in intestinal microbiota can also have effects on bile acid pool size and composition, relevant to multiple chronic disease states.[47–49]

BILE POOL AND COMPOSITION

Bile is a complex aqueous secretion that consists of 95% water and organic and inorganic solutes, the most abundant being bile acids, which are found at concentrations of 20 to 30 mmol/L (Fig. 89.4). Adult human bile acids consist of approximately 40% CA, 40% CDCA, 20% DCA, and trace amounts of LCA.[39] Phosphatidylcholine is the major phospholipid in bile, whereas cholesterol, which makes up approximately 3% of biliary solute, is the predominant sterol.[50] The formation of micelles with phosphatidylcholine and bile acids/cholesterol (2:1 ratio) lowers the free bile acid concentration, thereby protecting the canalicular membranes from the detergent action of bile acids. This point is made clear through animal models wherein the absence of phosphatidylcholine is associated with rapid development of liver injury.[51] Imbalances in the bile acid/cholesterol to phospholipid ratio can result in the formation of sludge and gallstones.[52] Finally, waste products such as bilirubin (from heme degradation, which gives bile its characteristic yellow color) are also eliminated via bile secretion.[21]

Heavy metals such as iron, copper, manganese, and zinc are also excreted in bile. Retention of these substances and impairments in the processing of these potentially toxic components due to inherited mutations in genes involved in these pathways can contribute to liver disease, as seen in

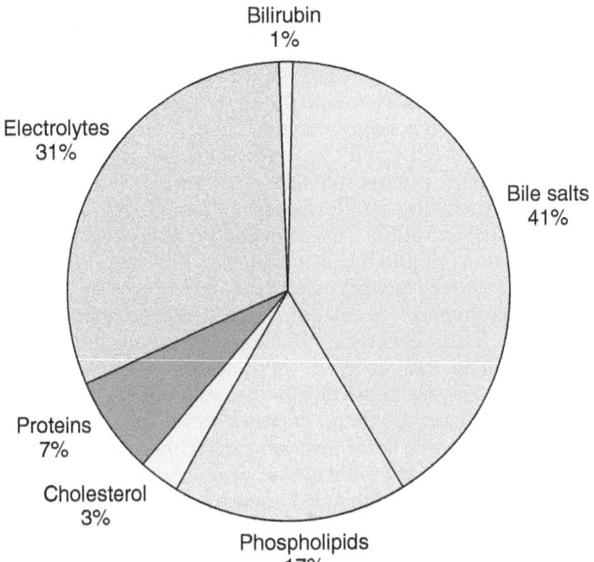

Fig. 89.4 Solute composition of human bile. Note that bile acids are the most prevalent solute, followed by phospholipids and cholesterol. Conjugated bilirubin makes up a small fraction of biliary solute loads. (From Vlahcevic et al. In: Zakim D, Boyer TD, eds. *Hepatology: A Textbook of Liver Disease.* Philadelphia: Saunders; 1996:381.)

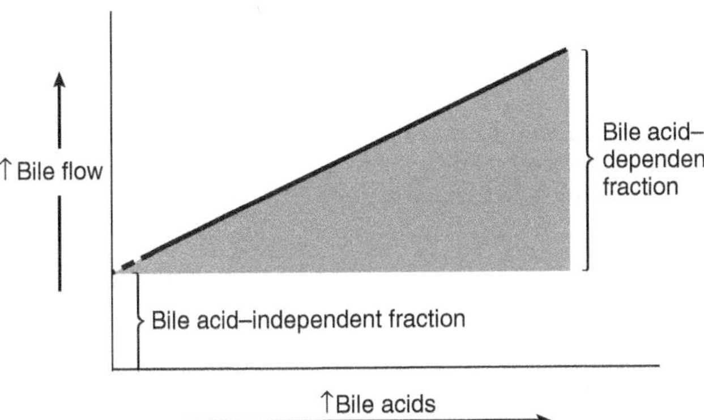

Fig. 89.5 Bile acid–dependent flow and bile acid–independent flow. Note the linear relationship between bile acid secretion and bile acid–dependent flow (BADF). The majority of bile flow is BADF that is reduced with smaller bile acid pool sizes, such as those of infants. The contribution made by bile acid–independent flow (BAIF) to total bile flow is approximately 25% and estimated by the extrapolation of the relationship between biliary flow and bile acid excretion to the y-axis, the imaginary point at which no bile acid secretes.

adult-onset hemochromatosis (iron) and Wilson disease (copper), but impairments in metal-handling processes are not clinically relevant in infants and young children.[53,54]

BILE FLOW

The average human adult liver produces up to 600 mL of bile per day. Bile flow into the canalicular system is divided into two components: bile acid-dependent bile flow and bile acid-independent flow (Fig. 89.5). The major driving force for bile secretion is the active transport of bile acids into the canalicular lumen. There is a linear relationship between the secretion of bile acids and bile flow.[21]

Bile acid-independent bile flow is largely dependent on the secretion of other solutes such as glutathione and glutathione conjugates, which are present in hepatocytes at relatively high concentrations of 5 to 10 mmol/L. Water, electrolytes, and other solutes follow passively in response to the osmotic gradient primarily by way of the paracellular route via tight junctions, although aquaporins are also present.[55] In patients with cholestasis, administration of bile acids such as ursodeoxycholic acid will increase bile acid pool size and promote increased bile flow through the biliary system.[56]

Canalicular bile is further modified by bicarbonate secretion from cholangiocytes in response to stimulation by hormones such as secretin. The binding of secretin to the bile duct cell results in phosphorylation of a chloride channel that increases chloride diffusion into the bile duct lumen. Chloride is then transported back to the cell via a chloride/bicarbonate antiporter at a ratio of $2Cl^-/3HCO_3^-$.[2,57]

CHOLESTASIS

Disruption of normal flow of bile at any level results in cholestasis, an abnormal retention of bile acids and bilirubin in the blood and liver. Cholestatic disorders can be separated into extrahepatic or biliary causes (e.g., structural abnormalities such as biliary atresia) and intrahepatic or hepatocellular causes (e.g., impairment in bile transport, genetic or metabolic disorders, infection).[58,59] Cholestasis in infants manifests as jaundice, acholic or hypopigmented stools, pruritus, and fat-soluble vitamin deficiencies. Long-standing cholestasis can result in injury to hepatocytes, leading to hepatocellular synthetic dysfunction and eventual liver failure.[60] In in vitro experiments, exposure of the basolateral membrane of hepatocytes and cholangiocytes to high bile acid concentrations caused disruption of cellular membranes, apoptosis, and necrosis. In reaction to chronic cholestasis, human hepatocytes undergo a number of adaptations mediated by FGF19 (Fgf15 in mice). In normal conditions, bile acids reaching the terminal ileum activate FXR and produce FGF19. During cholestasis, interruption of the enterohepatic cycle results in decreased bile acid absorption in the ileum. However, the serum level of FGF19 is actually elevated in cholestatic patients, due to ectopic production of FGF19 by the liver. FGF19 subsequently binds to its receptor FGFR4 causing downregulation of CYP7A1, thereby decreasing bile acid synthesis. In mice that have undergone bile duct ligation, adaptations of the canalicular system occur with increases in diameter of the canaliculi and length of spine-like protrusions into hepatocytes.[61] This is similar to morphologic changes that occur in the obstructive disease, biliary atresia.

Serum levels of bilirubin and bile acids are used as clinical markers of cholestasis, and tests are cost effective. To distinguish cholestasis from benign causes of jaundice, serum bilirubin should be separated into unconjugated and conjugated fractions. Unconjugated hyperbilirubinemia is commonly seen and may be due to physiologic jaundice, breastmilk or breastfeeding jaundice, Gilbert syndrome, Crigler-Najjar syndrome, and other systemic diseases.[62] Conjugated hyperbilirubinemia, however, is likely pathologic and is defined by a conjugated bilirubin level greater than 1 mg/dL (if total bilirubin is less than 5 mg/dL) or greater than 20% of the total bilirubin (if total bilirubin is greater than 5 mg/dL).[63] If conjugated hyperbilirubinemia is found, serum aspartate aminotransferase (AST), alanine aminotransferase (ALT), gamma-glutamyl transpeptidase (GGT), alkaline phosphatase (AP), prothrombin time (PT) and international normalized ratio (INR), and albumin levels should be checked. Elevations of AST and ALT indicate damage to hepatocytes. Elevated levels of GGT and AP suggest damage to cholangiocytes; however, some cholestatic disease (e.g., PFIC 1) may present with normal or low GGT.[64,65] Disturbances in PT, INR, and albumin levels are indicators of liver synthetic function.

Imaging studies can be obtained to assess liver and biliary structures, detect abnormalities in arterial or venous flow, or identify splenic malformations. A percutaneous liver biopsy remains integral to the diagnostic workup of infants with cholestasis. In addition to providing potential diagnostic data, a liver biopsy can also offer prognostic information to predict outcomes.[64]

FETAL BILE ACID METABOLISM

FETAL BILE ACID SYNTHESIS AND METABOLISM

In the fetus, the placenta is the primary site of bile acid metabolism and detoxification and elimination of lipophilic organic anions.[66] In fact, the fetal liver functions as the major site of hematopoiesis and does not play a major part in bile acid metabolism. At birth, there is an immediate transition wherein the role of metabolism and detoxification transfers from placenta to the liver.[67] However, the relative immaturity of the neonatal liver at birth is seen in studies demonstrating low bile acid synthesis and clearance. This hepatic immaturity is further compounded if the birth is premature.

Having said that, bile acids have been detected in the fetal liver and gallbladder as early as 14 to 16 weeks gestation,[68] and by 22 to 26 weeks gestation, the principal bile acids found in fetal gallbladder bile are taurine-conjugated dihydroxy bile acids.[69] After approximately 28 weeks' gestation, taurocholic acid (TCA), a trihydroxy bile acid, and glycocholic acid are also present.[37,68,70] In newborn infants, analysis of meconium and bile reveal a predominance of CDCA, which may indicate utilization of an alternative pathway favoring CDCA production. By 2 to 7 months of age, the proportion of glycine conjugates increases and reaches adult levels.[71-73]

Another distinction in bile acid composition in the fetus is the lack of secondary bile acid production. Secondary bile acids are unable to be produced in the fetus as this process requires enzymatic cleavage by colonic bacteria, which are not present in the relatively sterile fetal intestine. The presence of secondary bile acids in human fetal circulation implies transfer occurring from the maternal pool to the fetus. Specific transporters found on the brush-border and basolateral membranes of the placental syncytiotrophoblast may therefore provide bidirectional transport of bile acids between the fetal and maternal circulations (Fig. 89.6).[74]

Elimination of bile acids from the fetal liver occurs first with hydroxylation of bile acids into more hydrophilic forms by phase I enzymes CYP3A4 and CYP3A7 present in hepatocytes.[74-76] Export of these bile acids across the basolateral membrane occurs via transporters belonging to the organic anion-transporting polypeptide (OATP) family as well as adenosine triphosphate (ATP)-dependent pumps of the ATP-binding cassette (ABC) superfamily, including multidrug resistance protein (MRP)1 and isoforms, MRP3 and MRP4.[77] Next, carrier proteins such as albumin and lipoproteins shuttle bile acids through the fetal circulation to the basolateral (fetal-facing) membrane of the placenta.

The enterohepatic circulation is relatively immature in the developing fetus. Perfusion studies performed in near-term fetal dog using radiolabeled taurocholate suggest that bile reabsorption occurs passively in the jejunum, but active bile salt reabsorption in the ileum is poorly developed.[78] In fact, the ability to excrete bile acids into the canaliculus does not mature until the first year after birth. The poor reabsorptive capacity of the fetus coupled with the immaturity of hepatic synthetic mechanisms for bile acid production and efficient clearance through the maternal placenta leads to a small bile acid pool size in the fetus and neonate.[79,80] The term neonate has a reduced bile acid pool size that is approximately half of that of an adult. The premature neonate's bile acid pool size is even more reduced at one-third that of a term neonate.[80] It is of note that term neonates are capable of responding to increased fecal losses with the synthesis of new bile acids.[80] This may represent a step-up in bile acid synthesis in order to grow an effective bile acid pool.

Further, the adrenal axis appears to play a role in maturation of the synthesis and enterohepatic recirculation of bile acids in the fetus. This is likely through an increase in transporter expression and function as the fetus develops.[81] The administration of prenatal dexamethasone to healthy premature infants has been shown to increase the bile acid pool size in preterm neonates to levels equivalent to those for full-term infants and nearly

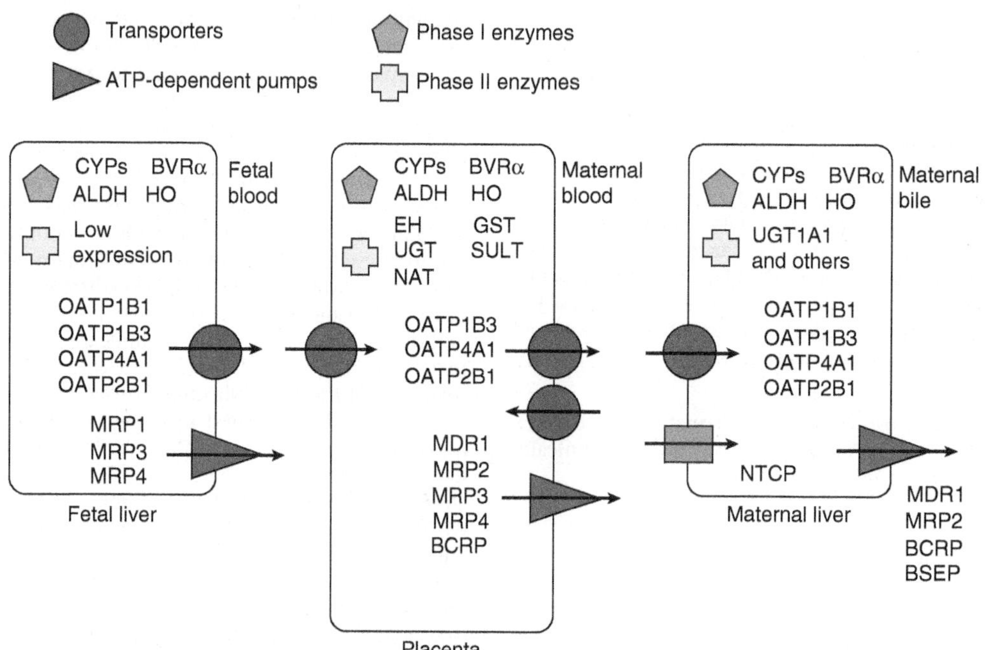

Fig. 89.6 The fetal-maternal hepatic excretory pathway: schematic representation of enzymes and transporters, adenosine triphosphate *(ATP)*-dependent pumps, and phase I and II enzymes involved in excretion of biliary compounds during intrauterine life. *ALDH,* Aldehyde dehydrogenase; *BCRP,* breast cancer resistance protein; *BSEP,* bile salt export pump; *BVR,* biliverdin reductase; *CYP,* cytochrome P450 enzyme; *EH,* epoxide hydrolase; *GST,* glutathione-S-transferase; *HO,* heme oxygenase; *MDR,* multidrug resistance protein; *MRP,* multidrug resistance–associated protein; *NAT,* N-acetyltransferase; *NTCP,* sodium-taurocholate cotransporting polypeptide; *OATP,* organic anion-transporting polypeptide; *SULT,* sulfotransferase; *UGT,* UDP-glucuronosyltransferase. (Adapted from Macias RIR, Marin JJG, Serrano MA. Excretion of biliary compounds during intrauterine life. *World J Gastroenterol*. 2009;15:817–828.)

four times those for untreated premature infants.[80] Additional animal studies demonstrate increase in bile acid synthesis after treatment with cortisone.[82]

The immaturity of the fetal liver and the reduced bile acid pool size may result in an intraluminal bile acid concentration too low to support normal lipid absorption efficiently.[83-85] Effects of this are manifest as fat malabsorption, poor growth, and deficiencies in fat-soluble vitamins, such as vitamin D.

Despite a lower bile acid synthesis rate and small bile acid pool size, serum bile acid levels are notably increased in term and preterm neonates, reaching values as high as those found in adults with cholestasis.[79] This degree of "physiologic cholestasis" improves over the first years of life with improvement in hepatic uptake of bile acids from the portal circulation.

FETAL BILE ACID TRANSPORT

Bile acids can easily pass through the placenta in a bidirectional process that is dependent on relative concentration gradients between the fetal and maternal circulation. As the bile acid concentration in the fetus is higher than in maternal serum because there is no significant excretion through the normal hepatobiliary systems,[86-88] transfer of bile acids typically occurs across the placenta toward the mother and is subsequently eliminated via the maternal liver. However, in cases of maternal cholestasis (e.g., intrahepatic cholestasis of pregnancy), the increased levels of maternal bile acids counterbalance or even reverse bile acid flux across the placenta.[89] However, accumulation of bile acids in the fetal compartment is potentially toxic and can result in fetal distress and even sudden intrauterine death.[90-92] Thus, the maintenance of a normal fetal-maternal bile acid steady state favoring bile acid flux from fetus to mother is crucial to normal fetal physiology.

PLACENTAL BILE ACID TRANSPORT

The placenta is composed of the endothelium of chorionic vessels, the stroma of chorionic villi, and the trophoblast layer, which contain phase I enzymes and phase II enzymes (Fig. 89.6) such as UDP-glucuronosyltransferases, sulfotransferases, and glutathione-S-transferases, which are involved in detoxification of xenobiotics as well as biotransformation of hepatobiliary compounds that can be readily exported across the apical pole.[74]

Fetal bile acids are imported across the basolateral plasma membrane of the placental trophoblast layer via a Na^+-independent bicarbonate anion transporting polypeptide, OATP.[93-96] OATP1A2, OATP1B1, OATP1B3, OATP2B1, and OATP4A1 expression in the human placenta has been detected using real-time quantitative polymerase chain reaction with varying expressions during gestation.[93,97,98] Subcellular localization of the OATPs in the placenta is poorly known. It has been postulated that OATP2B1 would be localized in the basal plasma membrane of the trophoblast[99] while OATP4A1 has been detected in the apical plasma membrane.[93]

Export of bile acids into the maternal circulation occurs primarily via ATP-dependent transporters of the ABC family—MRP1 *(ABCC1)*, MRP2 *(ABCC2)*, MRP3 *(ABCC3)*, and MRP4 *(ABCC4)*.[100] Although the cellular localization of these proteins remains controversial, they have been identified in the apical (maternal-facing) membrane of the syncytiotrophoblast.[101,102] These apical export pumps are noted to be upregulated during states of cholestasis or endotoxemia, which can contribute to the protection of the fetus.[103]

Another member of the ABC family of transporters that plays a major role in the export of placental substrates is the breast cancer resistance protein (BCRP, ABCG2). ABCG, found on both on the apical membrane of trophoblasts and in fetal vessels, has the ability to export sulfated and non-sulfated bile acids.[104]

A third ABC transporter, MDR1 *(ABCB1)* is highly expressed during early gestation in the syncytiotrophoblast. It is responsible for the export of organic and inorganic cations such as xenobiotics thus contributing to the protection of the fetus from a wide variety of toxic metabolites.[100]

From the placenta, the bile acids circulate through the maternal systemic bloodstream bound to carrier proteins such as albumin and lipoproteins[105,106] to arrive at the maternal liver where they are processed by previously described pathways.

REGULATION OF HEPATOBILIARY BILE FLOW

BASOLATERAL TRANSPORTERS

Bile acid clearance from circulating portal blood into the hepatocytes is a highly efficient process with about 75% to 90% of conjugated bile acids extracted from the first pass. Their clearance is largely accomplished by periportal hepatocytes (zone 1). Uptake of bile acids occurs by two processes: Na^+-dependent and Na^+-independent transport (Fig. 89.7).

Na^+-TAUROCHOLATE COTRANSPORTING POLYPEPTIDE

Approximately 75% of the uptake of conjugated bile acids and 50% of unconjugated bile acids occurs across the sodium-dependent transporter, Na^+-taurocholate cotransporting polypeptide (NTCP in humans, Ntcp in other species, SLC10A1), expressed on the basolateral (sinusoidal) membrane of hepatocytes.[107-109] This uptake process is driven by an inward Na^+ gradient that is maintained by a Na^+/K^+-ATPase.[57,107,110] NTCP has also been shown to be a transporter of steroidal hormones and a variety of drugs.[111,112] NTCP gene expression is post-transcriptionally regulated via activation of the nuclear receptor, FXR (NR1H4).[113] The binding of bile acids to FXR induces expression of short heterodimer partner (SHP), which inhibits the retinoic acid and retinoid X receptor RAR/RXR heterodimer on the NTCP promoter.[114] This in turn decreases expression of NTCP, which is essential for the protection of hepatocytes in times of excess bile acid loads (e.g., cholestasis) that can lead to cellular damage and apoptosis. Studies of $FXR^{+/+}$ mice fed a 1% CA diet showed a marked reduction of NTCP RNA levels. $FXR^{-/-}$ mice fed the same diet showed no change in NTCP and continued bile acid import.[115] In inflammatory states, endotoxin and proinflammatory interleukin IL1β also downregulate RAR/RXR to suppress NTCP expression.[116,117]

NTCP is thought to play an important role in infants with physiologic cholestasis, as studies in mice and rats demonstrate low Ntcp expression in newborns with a gradual increase in expression to adult levels with age.[118] Additionally, human hepatic NTCP mRNA levels in adults are noted to be 50-fold higher than in the fetus.[119] Polymorphisms in the NTCP gene in varying ethnic groups have previously been identified and are associated with decreased transport function.[120] There has been one reported case of hypercholanemia in a patient with NTCP deficiency.[121]

ORGANIC ANION-TRANSPORTING POLYPEPTIDE

The Na^+-independent bile acid transport is responsible for the majority of the uptake of unconjugated bile acids from the portal system.[110,122,123] It is mediated by organic anion transporting polypeptides (human OATP, Oatp in rodents) belonging to the SLC gene superfamily of transporters. These transporters consist of 12 transmembrane domains, typically function bidirectionally, and are expressed in a variety of tissues such as brain, liver, colon, and hepatocytes. They mediate the exchange of a wide spectrum of substrates, mostly amphipathic, including drug compounds, steroid conjugates, thyroid hormones, and bile acids, with intracellular HCO_3^- or glutathione.[124]

OATP transporters appeared to be regulated at the transcriptional level. Mice fed cholate showed a decrease in the expression of Oatp1a1 and Oatp1b2.[125] In patients with primary sclerosing cholangitis, expression of OATP1B1 is suppressed, while OATP1B3, a transporter whose substrates include peptides and xenobiotics, is induced by bile acids.[126,127]

This may represent differential regulation to reduce effects of cholestasis while maintaining sufficient ability to extract toxic drugs and xenobiotics. mRNA levels of Oatp1 and 2 are rapidly and profoundly suppressed in animal models of sepsis and cholestasis.[128,129] While the actual molecular mediators of these transporters are still under investigation, these studies suggest that both OATP and NTCP transporters are under coordinated suppression in sick, cholestatic infants.

BILE ACID EFFLUX

Bile acid influx is the predominant path of transport across the basolateral membrane under normal physiologic conditions. However, in cholestatic conditions, bile acid efflux becomes upregulated.

MULTIDRUG RESISTANCE PROTEIN 3/4

This process is mainly mediated by the multidrug resistance proteins, MRP3 (ABCC3) and MRP 4 (ABCC4), members of the ABC protein superfamily of transporters (see Fig. 89.7).[130] They are constitutively expressed at a low level on the basolateral membranes of cholangiocytes and perivenous hepatocytes and function as ATP-dependent pumps for substrates such as conjugated organic anions and retained bile acids. Their expression is induced under cholestatic conditions in both animal models and humans. However, other studies showed no changes in bile acid homeostasis in $Mrp^{-/-}$ mice.[131] Elevated levels of MRP3 expression are seen in patients with MRP2 dysfunction (e.g., Dubin-Johnson), which indicates a potential compensatory mechanism for bile acid elimination from the hepatocyte.[132]

OSTα-OSTβ

The heterodimeric organic solute transporter α and β (OSTα-OSTβ, SLC51) also mediate basolateral efflux of intracellular bile acids.[36,57,133] Both hypoxia and cholestasis have been shown to induce the expression of these transporters via transcription factor mediated pathways activated by FXR.[133-135]

INTRACELLULAR TRANSPORT

Transport of bile acids through the hepatocyte is not well understood. Two proposed methods are protein-mediated transport and vesicle-mediated transport. Members of the fatty acid binding protein family, FABP1 (also L-FABP), 3α-hydroxysteroid dehydrogenase (3α-HSD), and glutathione S-transferases are thought to be involved in the protein-mediated process.These are small, intracellular proteins that bind to bile acids.[110] Reclaimed unconjugated bile acids are reconjugated by bile acid coenzyme A:amino acid N-acyltransferase enzymes in peroxisomes prior to shuttle out of the cell.[136] In vivo studies with mice lacking FABP1 have disruption in bile acid metabolism and increased gallstone formation.[137]

Early studies indicated possible vesicle-mediated transport in hepatocytes from observations that demonstrated partitioning of bile acids into intracellular organelles such as the Golgi apparatus and endoplasmic reticulum;[138,139] however, later studies do not support the presence of this mechanism under physiologic conditions.[140]

CANALICULAR (APICAL) TRANSPORTERS

Canalicular bile acid transport is the rate-limiting step in hepatic excretion and bile formation. Excretion across the canalicular membrane occurs against a steep 1000-fold concentration gradient maintained by ATP-dependent transport.[110,141] The transporters responsible for this are the BSEP (ABCB11) and MRP 2 (see Fig. 89.7).

BILE SALT EXPORT PUMP

BSEP is the primary transporter of conjugated monovalent bile acids. Upon binding by bile acids, FXR forms a heterodimer with retinoid X receptor (RXR) to induce BSEP expression in a positive

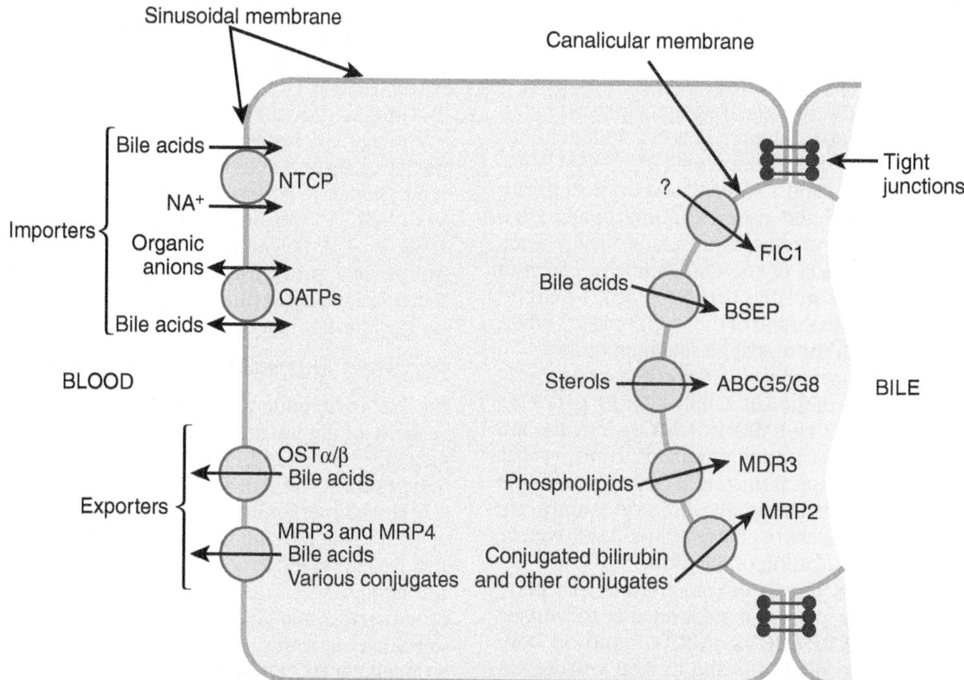

Fig. 89.7 Composite schematic of select hepatobiliary transporters involved in bile formation. The hepatocyte is oriented with sinusoidal (BLOOD) transporters on the left, canalicular (BILE) on the right. *Arrows* connote general directions that the listed solutes may be transported. *Arrows* denote distinct membranes and the tight junctions that help define these membrane domains. Note that the resident canalicular transporters are responsible for active secretion of nearly all components of bile. *BSEP,* Bile salt export pump; *MDR,* multidrug resistance protein; *MRP,* multidrug resistance-associated protein; *NTCP,* Na+/taurocholate cotransporting polypeptide; *OA,* organic anion; *OATP*, organic anion-transporting polypeptide; *OC,* organic cation; *OST,* organic solute transporters.

feed forward manner, leading to enhanced bile acid secretion. This mechanism has been demonstrated by the induction of BSEP mRNA and protein in mice fed a large dose of bile acid. FXR-deficient mice have low levels of BSEP expression that do not change after being fed a bile-acid enriched diet.[115] Therefore, FXR-mediated induction of BSEP is essential for the protection of hepatocytes against the toxic effects of accumulating intracellular bile acid levels.

Mutations in BSEP lead to development of the inherited cholestatic disorder, progressive familial intrahepatic cholestasis type 2 (PFIC2). This disease, which presents in infancy, is characterized by severe jaundice, hepatomegaly, and pruritus. Patient have elevated levels of serum bile acids and aminotransferases but low to normal serum GGT levels.[141,142] Extremely low canalicular BSEP expression leads to accumulation of bile acids within hepatocytes and a low concentration of biliary bile acids (nearly 1% of normal). Because efflux of bile acids is the driving force for bile flow, their intracellular retention leads to cholestasis and liver injury.[143]

MULTIDRUG RESISTANCE PROTEIN 2

MRP2 (ABCC2) is an ABC transporter localized to the canalicular membrane of hepatocytes as well as the apical membrane of enterocytes of the duodenum and jejunum and kidneys. MRP2 mediates the export of divalent bile acids and bilirubin conjugates. It also transports glutathione, sulfated and glucuronidated conjugates of drugs, toxins, and is responsible for bile acid–independent bile flow across the canaliculus.[144-146]

In animal models of sepsis and inflammation, levels of MRP2 are dramatically reduced leading to associated cholestasis.[147,148] Mutations in MRP2 result in Dubin-Johnson syndrome, a rare but benign disorder characterized by conjugated hyperbilirubinemia.[144]

MULTIDRUG RESISTANCE PROTEIN 3

The formation of micelles with phospholipids in bile is necessary for the protection of duct cells from hydrophobic bile acids. Multidrug resistance protein 3 (MDR3, ABCB4) is an ABC transporter "flippase" that transfers phosphatidylcholine from the outer leaflet of the canalicular membrane into bile.[149]

Mdr3 knockout mice do not secrete phospholipids into bile and subsequently incur severe biliary ductal damage.[150] Homozygous mutations of the ABCB4 gene in humans have been identified in persons with PFIC type 3; a cholestatic disease characterized by elevated serum bile acid levels and increased GGT levels.[151] Heterozygous mutations have been implicated in cases of intrahepatic cholestasis of pregnancy.[152]

ABCG5/ABCG8

Biliary secretion of cholesterol and phytosterols is dependent on the ABCG5/ABCG8 transporters. They are found in the canalicular membrane of hepatocytes and apical membrane of enterocytes. Mouse models deficient in ABCG5/ABCG8 show a 70% to 90% reduction in biliary cholesterol concentration.[153] In humans, mutations in ABCG5/ABCG8 result in sitosterolemia, a rare disease that is characterized by hypercholesterolemia, phytosterolemia, and coronary artery disease.[154,155] In inflammatory states (exposure to endotoxin or cytokines), mRNA levels of ABCG5 and ABCG8 are significantly decreased in the liver.[156]

INTESTINAL BILE ACID TRANSPORT

Once secreted in the lumen of the duodenum, bile acids mix and form micelles with dietary lipids, cholesterol, and fatty acids. Absorption of these lipids begins in the proximal to mid small intestine. Bile acids are recovered through passive absorption in the small and large intestine and active transport in the ileum (Fig. 89.8). Unconjugated bile acids or glycine-conjugated bile acids can be absorbed passively across the apical brush-border membrane.

The uptake of conjugated bile acids occurs in the terminal ileum via apical sodium-dependent bile acid transporter, ASBT (SLC10A2).[36,157] The driving force for bile acid uptake is provided by an inward Na^+ gradient maintained by the basolateral Na^+/K^+-ATPase. This transporter is highly efficient in recovering more than 95% of bile acids from the intestine.

Mutations in ASBT result in primary bile acid malabsorption (PBAM), an idiopathic congenital disorder associated with chronic diarrhea, interruption of the enterohepatic circulation of bile acids, and reduced plasma cholesterol levels. Diseases affecting the ileum such as Crohn disease and radiation enteritis are associated with ASBT dysfunction.[65]

Regulation of ASBT is extensive and can be mediated by sterols, bile acids, cytokines, glucocorticoids, and vitamins.[36,158]

INTRACELLULAR TRANSPORT

Bile acids are transported across the enterocyte bound to cytosolic intestinal bile acid binding protein, IBABP 6 (FABP6). IBABP is under tight regulation by different sterol sensors. IBABP gene expression is upregulated by bile acids through activation of nuclear FXR.[65] Dysregulation of IBABP has been suggested to be involved in necrotizing enterocolitis in rat models.[159]

BASOLATERAL MEMBRANE TRANSPORT

The heteromeric organic solute transporter OSTα-OSTβ has been proposed as the major exporter of bile acids across the intestinal basolateral membrane. Co-expression of both subunits is required for transport activity. OSTα-OSTβ not only transports bile acids but also steroids and prostaglandins.[158] Human ileal biopsies exposed to CDCA demonstrated elevated levels of OSTα-OSTβ.[160] $Ost\alpha^{-/-}$ mice exhibited reduced bile acid pool size and a decrease in hepatic bile acid synthesis. Loss of FXR in $Ost\alpha^{-/-}$ mice resulted in a reversal of decreases in hepatic bile acid synthesis and bile acid pool size.[161] This finding again emphasizes the complexities of the bile acid–FXR signaling.

CONGENITAL CHOLESTATIC DISORDERS

DISORDERS OF BILE ACID SYNTHESIS

Primary bile acids are synthesized from cholesterol through a complex series of enzymatic reactions. Defects in this process lead to overproduction and accumulation of hepatoxic intermediates proximal to the defective enzyme (Table 89.1).[162,163] These disorders are usually characterized by progressive cholestatic liver disease, fat malabsorption, and neurologic disease, except in cases of bile acid conjugation defects where elevated levels of unconjugated bile acids are able to maintain bile flow. Serum and urine studies may demonstrate marked alterations in bile acid levels, elevated serum aminotransferases, and normal GGT. Treatment with primary bile acids is a therapeutic option for many of these diseases.[164]

Disorders that can secondarily affect the synthesis of bile acids include ileal resection, bacterial overgrowth (bile acid malabsorption), and Smith-Lemli-Opitz syndrome (in which genetic defects in cholesterol synthesis subsequently reduce availability of cholesterol for bile acid synthesis).[165]

DISORDERS OF BILE ACID TRANSPORT

PROGRESSIVE INTRAHEPATIC CHOLESTASIS SYNDROMES

Progressive familial intrahepatic cholestasis (PFIC) is a group of autosomal recessive disorders in which defects occur in the transport or processing of bile acids.[166-168] These patients typically present in infancy or childhood with jaundice, pruritus, and progressive liver disease.

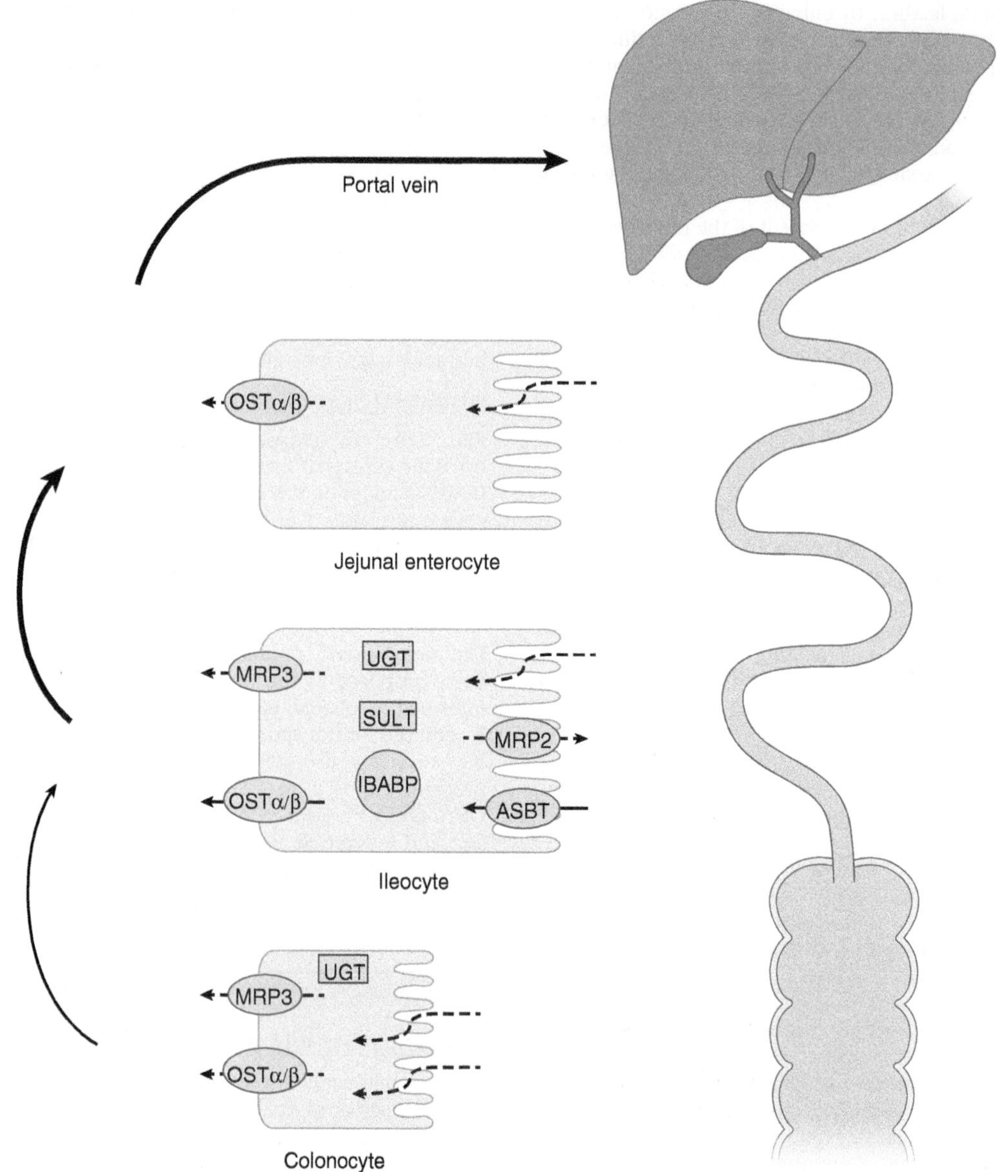

Fig. 89.8 Schematic of intestinal transport and metabolism of bile acids. *ASBT,* Apical sodium-dependent bile acid transporter; *IBABP,* ileal bile acid–binding protein; *MRP,* multidrug resistance–associated protein; *OST,* organic solute transporters; *SULT,* sulfotransferase; *UGT,* UDP-glucuronosyltransferase. (Adapted with permission from Dawson PA, Karpen SJ. Intestinal transport and metabolism of bile acids. *J Lipid Res.* 2015;56:1085–1099; and Walters JRF. Bile acid diarrhoea and FGF19: new views on diagnosis, pathogenesis and therapy. *Nat Rev Gastroenterol Hepatol.* 2014;11:426–434.)

PROGRESSIVE FAMILIAL INTRAHEPATIC CHOLESTASIS TYPE 1

PFIC1, previously known as *Byler disease*, is caused by a mutation in the FIC1 gene *(ATP8B1)*, a P-type ATPase gene located on chromosome 18q21-22.[169] FIC1 has been localized in the canalicular member of hepatocytes and cholangiocytes. It functions as an aminophospholipids transporter (flippase) in the movement of phosphatidylserine and phosphatidylethanolamine from the outer to inner canalicular leaflet, thus protecting the membrane from high bile acid concentrations in the lumen. The exact mechanism leading to cholestasis is still under investigation. The current proposed mechanism is that the defect of FIC1 results in downregulation of FXR, which in turn leads to downregulation of BSEP and upregulation of bile acid synthesis in hepatocytes. There is also a concurrent upregulation of ASBT in the small intestine, which increases absorption of bile acids.[170] Patients with PFIC1 have a low-GGT cholestasis that presents in the neonatal period with a wide range of phenotypes. Those with severe disease develop progressive cholestasis and portal hypertension. Others may experience extrahepatic symptoms of poor growth, pancreatic insufficiency, diarrhea, and sensorineural deafness. A milder form of FIC1 deficiency is termed *benign recurrent intrahepatic cholestasis (BRIC) 1* and characterized by recurrent episodes of cholestasis and pruritis.[151] Treatment with the hydrophilic bile acid, ursodeoxycholic acid, induces BSEP and MDR3 expression, which leads to improvement in cholestasis and pruritus.[170]

PROGRESSIVE FAMILIAL INTRAHEPATIC CHOLESTASIS TYPE 2

PFIC2 is the most commonly seen form of PFIC. Mutations in the ABCB11 gene encoding the BSEP protein lead to accumulation of bile acids within the hepatocytes. Patients typically present in infancy with elevated serum bile acids and aminotransferases, normal GGT levels and often progress to end-stage liver disease

Table 89.1 Bile Acid Synthetic Disorders.

Diagnosis	Genetics	Clinical Symptoms
CYP7A1 deficiency[a]	Chromosome 8q11-12	Hyperlipidemia, increased hepatic cholesterol, gallstones, premature cardiovascular disease
CYP7B1 deficiency	Chromosome 8q21.3	Severe neonatal cholestasis and cirrhosis, elevated transaminases but normal γ-GT
3β-Hydroxysteroid-Δ^5-C_{27}-steroid dehydrogenase deficiency[a]	Chromosome 16p11.2-12	Progressive neonatal cholestasis, hepatomegaly, fat malabsorption, fat-soluble vitamin deficiencies, rickets
Δ^4-3-Oxosteroid 5β-reductase deficiency (AKR1D1 or SRD5B1)[a]	Chromosome 7q32-33	Severe cholestasis, elevated transaminases but normal γ-GT, fat-soluble vitamin deficiencies
Cerebrotendinous xanthomatosis; sterol 27-hydroxylase (CYP27A1) deficiency[a]	Chromosome 2q33-qter	Elevated plasma concentrations of cholesterol and cholestanol, neurologic symptoms, including dementia, psychiatric disturbances, pyramidal or cerebellar signs, and seizures; diarrhea; tendon xanthomas; cataracts
2-Methyl coenzyme A racemase deficiency	Chromosome 5p11-13	Neuropathy (in adults), coagulopathy (in infants), vitamin D and E deficiency, mild liver impairment but no neurologic disease
Peroxisomal disorders		
1. D-bifunctional protein deficiency (HSD-17B4)	Chromosome 5q2	Neonatal seizures, hypotonia, hepatomegaly; usually fatal before 2 years of age
2. Trihydroxycholestanoic acid CoA oxidase deficiency	Chromosome 3p14.3	Ataxia with onset around 3 years of age, liver dysfunction
Amidation defects		
1. Bile acid CoA ligase	Chromosome 19q13.43	Cholestasis, elevated transaminases
2. Bile acid CoA amino acid N-acyl transferase	Chromosome 9q31.1	Neonatal cholestasis, fat-soluble vitamin deficiencies, growth failure

[a]Denotes disorders amenable to treatment with bile acid replacement.
Key features of known bile acid synthetic disorders.

within a few years. Liver histology shows intracellular cholestasis with positive BSEP antibody stain in over 90% of cases.[151,171,172] There are currently no effective drug therapies to treat this disorder. Up to 15% of patients with PFIC2 develop hepatocellular carcinoma by the age of 5.[173] Therefore, liver transplantation has become routinely performed as treatment. However, recurrence of the disease has been noted in some patients post transplantation, which is theorized to be secondary to allo-reactive antibodies to BSEP. This may require an increase in immunosuppression or more intensive management with B-cell depletion or allogenic hematopoietic stem cell transplant.[174,175]

Milder forms of BSEP deficiency include BRIC type 2, transient neonatal cholestasis, and intrahepatic cholestasis of pregnancy type 2 (ICP2).[174,176]

PROGRESSIVE FAMILIAL INTRAHEPATIC CHOLESTASIS TYPE 3

PFIC 3 is caused by a mutation in *ABCB4* gene that encodes the multidrug resistance 3 protein (MDR3). A defect in MDR3 results in impairment of phosphatidylcholine transport from the inner to the outer canalicular leaflet. In the absence of phosphatidylcholine, free bile acids cause damage to cholangiocytes and cholesterol crystallizes into stones that cause liver injury. Patients with MDR3 deficiency have a wide range of phenotypes but typically present in late adolescence or adulthood with elevated GGT levels.[169,177] Liver histology demonstrates portal fibrosis and bile duct proliferation with absent or decreased MDR3 antibody stain.[170] Cholangiocarcinoma and hepatocellular carcinoma have both been reported in patients with PFIC 4.[178] The use of ursodeoxycholic acid can improve biochemical markers in those with mild forms of the disease; however, there has been no data on long-term outcomes.

PROGRESSIVE FAMILIAL INTRAHEPATIC CHOLESTASIS TYPE 4

Biallelic mutations in tight junction protein 2 (TJP2) result in neonatal cholestasis with normal GGT levels.[179] TJP2 functions as an intracellular anchor for canalicular tight junctions preventing toxic bile acids from entering the paracellular space. Liver pathology demonstrates intracellular cholestasis with absence of TJP2 stain.[174] Most patients discovered to have TJP2 defect required liver transplantation in the first few years of life. Hepatocellular carcinoma has been described in these patients.[180]

OTHER CONGENITAL CHOLESTATIC DISORDERS

FARNESOID X RECEPTOR DEFICIENCY (NR1H4)

The *NR1H4* gene encodes FXR, which produces FGF19 to repress bile acid synthesis and also induces expression of BSEP to enhance bile acid secretion from hepatocytes. Patients with these defects have high serum bile acid levels and α-fetoprotein (AFP) levels, normal liver enzymes, and normal GGT. Liver pathology shows intralobular cholestasis, ductular reaction, giant cell transformation with hepatocyte ballooning. They progress very quickly to end-stage liver disease requiring liver transplantation.[181,182]

TIGHT JUNCTION PROTEIN DEFICIENCY

Tight junction proteins are cytoplasmic proteins that serve as anchors for proteins that form the tight junctions (e.g., claudins). Disruption of this junctional integrity allows toxic molecules to leak through the paracellular space. Biallelic mutations of these proteins result in cholestatic liver disease as well as extrahepatic manifestations of respiratory and neurologic disease. Liver pathology shows intracellular cholestasis with giant cell formation.[151,174] Hepatocellular carcinoma has been described in these patients.[183]

MYOSIN 5B DEFICIENCY

Precise intracellular trafficking of BSEP to the apical membrane is dependent on myosin 5B (MYO5B). Mutations in MYO5B have been seen in patients with microvillus inclusion disease and isolated cholestatic disease due to impaired bile acid secretion. Affected individuals present with low-GGT cholestasis, elevated serum bile acid levels, and normal aminotransferases within 2 years of life.[151,174,184]

INTRAHEPATIC CHOLESTASIS OF PREGNANCY

ICP affects approximately 0.1% to 2% of all pregnancies with higher prevalence in South American and Scandinavian countries. Familial clustering has been documented with higher incidences in mothers and sisters of patients with ICP.[185] Clinical manifestations include pruritus, hepatic dysfunction, and elevated serum bile acid levels. A high level of bile acids in the maternal circulation reverses the normal fetal to maternal bile flow and results in accumulation of bile acids in the fetus.[89] Elevation of serum bile acid levels greater than 100 μmol/L increases the risk for fetal loss.[186] A number of genes have been implicated in ICP including *ABCB4* (MDR3 transporter), *ABCB11* (BSEP), and *TJP2*.[152,187] Hormonal factors may also play a role in the pathogenesis of ICP. Administration of estrogen to rats resulted in decreased bile flow and bile acid uptake at the basolateral membrane of hepatocytes.[188] Pregnant women who received oral progesterone treatment for risk of premature delivery had higher rates of ICP.[189] This is further supported by the increase in severity of symptoms during the third trimester when hormones levels are the highest, followed by improvement after delivery. Preeclampsia and gestational diabetes have been associated with ICP during pregnancy as well as future development of immune-related diseases and hepatobiliary cancer.[190] Ursodeoxycholic acid (UDCA) has been used as treatment for ICP as it was thought to increase placental bile transporters; however, recent data does not show a significant reduction in fetal distress, preterm delivery, or fetal death after administration of UDCA.[191,192]

DUBIN-JOHNSON SYNDROME

Dubin-Johnson syndrome is a rare, benign disorder characterized by mildly elevated levels (typically 2 to 5 mg/dL) of conjugated bilirubin. It results from mutation of the ABCC gene encoding MRP2, important for the transport of bilirubin and other anions out of hepatocytes.[144] It typically manifests in adolescence or adulthood and rarely in infancy. Most patients are asymptomatic with no other laboratory abnormalities except elevated conjugated bilirubin levels. The liver will appear grossly black on histology with accumulation of dark granular pigment within hepatocytes.[192]

ACQUIRED CHOLESTATIC DISORDERS

DRUG-INDUCED CHOLESTASIS

Drug-induced liver injury can be separated into cholestatic, hepatocellular, and mixed cholestatic liver injury with cholestasis occurring in half of all cases.[193] Mechanisms for cholestatic injury include inhibition or reduced expression of transporters such as BSEP and MDR3, disruption of tight junctions, and alterations in bile canalicular dynamics (e.g., dilatation or constriction of canaliculi) resulting in accumulation of bile.[194] Recent studies also propose that toxic metabolites may also interact with nuclear receptors such as FXR or PXR or TGR5, a G-protein coupled bile acid receptor.[195]

Neonates are especially vulnerable to drug-induced liver injury due to the relative immaturity of liver in detoxification, impaired response to oxidative stress, and increased inflammatory response to injury.

SEPSIS-ASSOCIATED CHOLESTASIS

Sepsis or dysregulation of the systemic inflammatory response can occur with exposure to toxin, infections, or trauma. In animal models with induced sepsis, liver dysfunction often occurs early (<24 hours after onset). This is often due to an influx of inflammatory cells that flow through and adhere to sinusoidal endothelial cells causing cellular damage and formation of microthrombi. Persistent inflammation and hypoperfusion eventually leads to liver damage and failure.[196,197] Liver injury is associated with decreased ability to clear bacteria from the blood stream.

In response to endotoxin, Kupffer cells in the liver increase production of proinflammatory mediators, which act on receptors on the hepatocytes. This causes secretion of many factors (e.g., protease inhibitors, C-reactive peptide, compliment proteins) that work to restore homeostasis.[198,199] The liver also produces anti-inflammatory mediators such as IL-10 and glucocorticoids, which contribute to immunosuppression. An imbalance of pro-inflammatory and anti-inflammatory mediators increases mortality.[128,200]

Cholestasis in sepsis is attributed to several mechanisms. Circulating endotoxin and lipopolysaccharide have been seen to inhibit bile excretion.[201] In rat models of sepsis, pro-inflammatory cytokines suppress transcription factors that result in significant downregulation of NTCP and OATP at the basolateral membrane and BSEP and MRP2 at the canalicular membrane.[202] These alterations in the hepatobiliary transporters cause accumulation of bile acids. Basolateral export pumps MRP3 and MRP4 are upregulated facilitating the transport of bile acids back into the blood circulation. This suggests a possible compensatory reaction to cholestasis.[203]

Additionally, analysis of liver biopsies of critically ill patients with demonstrated elevated bile acid and bilirubin levels did not show a decrease in CYP7A1 protein expression when compared with controls. This indicates loss of feedback regulation of bile acid synthesis during critical illness.[204]

INTESTINAL FAILURE ASSOCIATED LIVER DISEASE

The development of parental nutrition has revolutionized the care of patients unable to receive enteral nutrition. However, this method of nutrition delivery has multiple complications including infections, metabolic disorders, and parenteral nutrition-associated liver disease (PNALD) or intestinal failure associated liver disease (IFALD).[205-208] The earliest case of IFALD was described in 1971 in a preterm neonate with cholestasis on autopsy.[209] It is estimated that 20% to 30% of infants or children who require long-term parenteral nutrition will develop IFALD.[210] Previously, the only treatment options for IFALD was organ transplantation whether isolated small bowel or combined liver-small bowel. However, clinical outcomes after transplantation were poor with high mortality and morbidity.

IFALD can be separated into two phases. Phase I is characterized by cholestasis and inflammation with other causes of cholestasis excluded. Phase II is generally associated with steatosis and fibrosis of the liver. Risk factors for IFALD include prematurity, low birth weight, duration of PN therapy, and type of intravenous lipid emulsion (ILE) (Fig. 89.9).[211,212]

The pathogenesis of IFALD is likely multifactorial with several proposed mechanisms. One is a lack of enteral stimulation of the gastrointestinal tract. This causes intestinal stasis, enterocyte hypoplasia, and impaired intestinal barrier function, which predisposes patients to bacterial growth.[210] Small intestinal bacterial overgrowth increases deconjugation of primary bile acids and disrupts ileal bile acid uptake, both of which leads to cholestasis. In a mouse model with intestinal injury on PN, treatment of the animals with enteral antibiotics prevented liver injury and cholestasis.[213] In addition, important gastrointestinal hormones involved in enterocyte proliferation and maturation are not produced and gallbladder emptying is disturbed. This leads to further bile stasis and a decrease in enterohepatic circulation. Decreased delivery of bile acids to the terminal ileum in cholestasis can cause further worsening through its effect on FXR. Under normal conditions, bile acids activate FXR leading to production of FGF19, which binds to FGFR4 to suppress CYP7A1, thus creating a negative feedback loop.[214] In patients dependent on PN, serum levels of FGF19 were found to be one-third of those in controls. Therefore, this could indicate a lack of negative feedback and continued synthesis of bile acids. In a piglet model of parenteral nutrition-associated cholestasis, administration of CDCA prevented cholestasis and liver disease.[215]

Another factor implicated in the pathogenesis of IFALD is the toxicity of PN components. High glucose, lipid, and amino acid concentrations have all been associated with hepatic dysfunction. The most widely known and important component is the amount and source of ILE.

The most commonly used ILE over the last decade is Intralipid, which is composed of 100% soybean oil. SO-ILE are abundant in ω–6 polyunsaturated fatty acids (PUFAs) and phytosterols. Phytosterols are sterol compounds found in plants that are minimally absorbed in enteral feeding and normally excreted into bile by canalicular ABCG5/ABCG8 transporter. One particular phytosterol, stigmasterol, has been found to cause downregulation of BSEP and MRP2 through modulation of FXR signaling leading to bile acid retention and hepatic injury. Further work in mouse models with IFALD showed that phytosterols also activated hepatic macrophages with subsequent cytokine release (primarily IL-1β), which also caused downregulation of FXR, BSEP, and MRP2.[216] A study of pediatric IFALD patients found that histologic hepatic inflammation and fibrosis and clinical cholestasis paralleled serum sterol concentrations.[217] ω–6 PUFAs are proinflammatory and produce mediators such as leukotrienes and tumor necrosis factor (TNF)–α that cause liver damage.

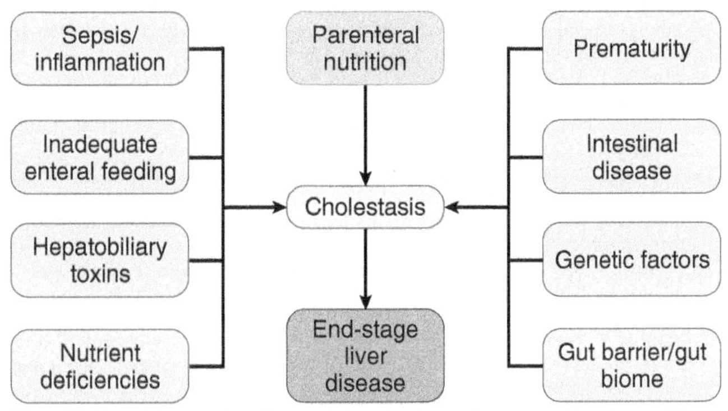

Fig. 89.9 Schematic of key risk factors for parenteral nutrition–associated liver disease.

ENTERAL FEEDINGS

Early enteral feeding has been associated with reversal of cholestasis in patients with IFALD. Enteral feedings stimulate intestinal motility, induce production of gastrointestinal hormones that promote intestinal adaptation, decrease small intestinal bacterial growth, and enhance bile flow.[218,219] Implementation of early feeding in infants post-intestinal surgery reduced the time to reach feeding goals, thereby significantly reducing the incidence of severity of IFALD.[220]

LIPID RESTRICTION

SO-ILE is traditionally dosed at 2 to 3 g/kg/day resulting in high levels of circulating phytosterols. Some evidence supports lipid restriction in an effort to decrease the risk of IFALD. In a study of postsurgical infants on PN, reductions in SO-ILE dose to 1 g/kg/day has been shown to reduce the incidence of IFALD by 21%.[221] However, other studies have reported no difference in incidence of cholestasis in neonates given a lower dose of SO-ILE.

Reductions in SO-ILE can increase the risk for deficiency of essential fatty acids important for brain growth and neurodevelopment. Newborn piglets given a half dose of SO-ILE showed decreased brain weight compared to those given the full dose.[222] Therefore, lipid reduction should be used cautiously and monitored closely.

ALTERNATIVE LIPID EMULSIONS

Due to the increased risk of IFALD with soy-based lipid emulsions, alternative lipid emulsions have been created (Table 89.2). One of the most widely used is Smoflipid (Fresenius Kabi, Bad Homburg, Germany), a mixture of soybean oil (30%), coconut oil (30%), olive oil (25%), and fish oil (15%). Medium-chain triglyceride (MCT) in coconut oil contain less ω–6 PUFAs than soybean-derived products. The metabolism of MCT is partially independent of the carnitine pathway, allowing for more rapid plasma clearance, metabolism, and energy utilization without accumulating in the liver. Olive oil is high in ω-9 PUFAs and α-tocopherol, a major

Table 89.2 Characteristics and Composition of Structurally Different Parenteral Lipid Emulsions.

Emulsion % Fat (g/100 mL) (Manufacturer)	Lipid Source (v/v %)	Linoleic Acid (% of Total FA)	Omega-6/Omega-3 Ratio	Phytosterols (mg/L)	α-Tocopherol (μmol/L)
Intralipid 20% (Fresenius Kabi, Bad Homburg, Germany)	SO, 100%	53	7:1	348 ± 33	87
Lipofundin 20% (B. Braun, Melsungen, Germany)	SO, 50%; MCT, 50%	29	7:1	No data	502
ClinOleic = Clinolipid 20% (Baxter, Maurepas, France)	SO, 20%; OO, 80%	19	9:1	327 ± 8	75
Lipoplus 20% (B. Braun)	SO, 40%; MCT, 50%; FO, 10%	24.5	2.7:1	No data	562
Smoflipid 20% (Fresenius Kabi)	SO, 30%; MCT, 30%; OO, 25%; FO, 15%	20	2.5:1	47.6	500
Omegaven 10% (Fresenius Kabi)	FO, 100%	4.5	1:8	0	505

FA, Fatty acid; *FO*, fish oil; *MCT*, medium-chain triglyceride oil; *OO*, olive oil; *SO*, soybean oil.
From Wanten GJA. Parenteral lipid tolerance and adverse effects: fat chance for trouble? *JPEN J Parenter Enteral Nutr*. 2015;39:33S–8S.

antioxidant from the vitamin E family capable of scavenging free radicals, which may be beneficial in patients at risk for oxidant damage or stress.

This formulation allows for reduction in phytosterol and ω–6 fatty acids delivery while providing essential fatty acids. Patients switched from SO-ILE to combination ILE (c-ILE) were noted to have improvement in liver function with decreased cholestasis and inflammation.[214,223,224] In a randomized study of children who received Smoflipid versus Intralipid for 1 month, those who received Intralipid had increased total bilirubin levels, while those who received Smoflipid demonstrated decreased bilirubin levels.[225]

Fish-oil based ILE (Omegaven, FreseniusKabi, Bad Homburg, Germany) are composed of mostly ω-3 PUFAs, such as docosahexaenoic acid (DHA) and eicosapentaenoic acid (EPA), with little ω-6 PUFAs. These fatty acids are anti-inflammatory and suppress macrophage production of cytokines.[226,227] Fish oil does not contain phytosterols and are enriched with α-tocopherol. In studies of infant switched from SO-ILE to FO-ILE, the FO-ILE group demonstrated significant improvement in biochemical markers and reversal of cholestasis.[228-230] Neonates who develop IFALD on Smoflipid also demonstrate reversal when switched to FO-ILE.[231] Utilization of FO-ILE has been associated with decreased need for small bowel and/or liver transplantation. Omegaven was approved for therapeutic use for reversal of IFALD in 2018 by the United States Food and Drug Administration.

Despite FO-ILE's effects on the reversal of cholestasis and inflammation, there have been no reported effects on hepatic fibrosis, which can persist for years even after switching to FO-ILE or after cessation of all parenteral nutrition.

As with lipid restriction, one area of concern with FO-ILE is the development of essential fatty acid deficiency given the lower ratio of ω-6 PUFAs. Thus far, no trials have demonstrated this.

Lastly, cycling PN, in which PN is delivered over a shorter period of time, allowing for time off, has also been shown to decrease cholestasis.[232,233] However, cycling needs to be closely monitored in the premature population due to increased risk for hypoglycemia.

INTESTINAL ADAPTATION

While no hormonal therapies have been shown to reverse IFALD, they have been effective in promoting intestinal adaptation with decrease in need for parenteral nutrition. Teduglutide (Gattex, Takeda, Tokyo, Japan) is a glucagon-like peptide (GLP)-2 analogue that has been shown to stimulate villus growth thus increasing intestinal absorptive capacity. In a clinical trial of pediatric patients with short bowel syndrome and PN dependence, administration of teduglutide helped reduce PN requirement and increase enteral intake. A small number of patients were successfully weaned off of PN.[234] Gattex has been approved for pediatric use as of 2019.

CONCLUSION

The liver, as the largest organ in the human body, consists of an extraordinarily complex system of biosynthetic and biotransformative pathways that serve to maintain metabolic and physiologic homeostasis. As the primary site of bile acid synthesis, regulatory mechanisms set in place allow for the effective synthesis and transport of bile acids and other organic solutes out of the hepatocyte. Subsequently, modification and transport of bile through the enterohepatic circulation back to the liver is a result of further tight regulation and signaling crosstalk. Extensive research over the last decade has also revealed bile acids to be important signaling molecules for nuclear receptors and cell surface receptors that can impact bile acid metabolism, gut microbiome, and other metabolic pathways.

Dysregulation at any step can result in cholestatic disease, especially in neonates who have an inherent immaturity of the hepatobiliary system. Further advances in the study of neonatal cholestasis have identified a number of causative genetic defects of transporters, synthetic enzymes, and nuclear receptors, which in turn has led to early diagnosis, evaluation, and life-saving treatment. Recent research in the interaction of bile acids and gut microbiota in health and disease states and the effect of bile acids on intestinal growth may advance our understanding of bile acids as potential therapeutic agents.

A complete reference list is available at www.ExpertConsult.com. 

SELECT REFERENCES

1. Chiang JYL, Ferrell JM. Bile acid metabolism in liver pathobiology. *Gene Expr*. 2018;18(2):71-87.
2. Copple BL, Li T. Pharmacology of bile acid receptors: evolution of bile acids from simple detergents to complex signaling molecules. *Pharmacol Res*. 2016;104:9-21.
3. McLin VA, Yazigi N. 67 - Developmental anatomy and physiology of the liver and bile ducts. In: Wyllie R, Hyams JS, eds. *Pediatric Gastrointestinal and Liver Disease*. 4th ed. Saint Louis: W.B. Saunders; 2011:718-727.e712.
4. Qin L, Crawford JM. 1 - Anatomy and cellular functions of the liver. In: Sanyal AJ, Boyer TD, Lindor KD, Terrault NA, eds. *Zakim and Boyer's Hepatology*. 7th ed. Philadelphia: Elsevier; 2018:2-19.e14.
5. Crawford JM. Development of the intrahepatic biliary tree. *Semin Liver Dis*. 2002;22(3):213-226.
6. Lautt WW, Greenway CV. Conceptual review of the hepatic vascular bed. *Hepatology*. 1987;7(5):952-963.
7. Collardeau-Frachon S, Scoazec JY. Vascular development and differentiation during human liver organogenesis. *Anat Rec*. 2008;291(6):614-627.
8. Rieder H, Meyer zum Buschenfelde KH, Ramadori G. Functional spectrum of sinusoidal endothelial liver cells. Filtration, endocytosis, synthetic capacities and intercellular communication. *J Hepatol*. 1992;15(1-2):237-250.
9. Smedsrod B, De Bleser PJ, Braet F, et al. Cell biology of liver endothelial and Kupffer cells. *Gut*. 1994;35(11):1509-1516.
10. Puche JE, Saiman Y, Friedman SL. Hepatic stellate cells and liver fibrosis. *Compr Physiol*. 2013;3(4):1473-1492.
11. Friedman SL. Hepatic stellate cells: protean, multifunctional, and enigmatic cells of the liver. *Physiol Rev*. 2008;88(1):125-172.
12. Mathew J, Geerts A, Burt AD. Pathobiology of hepatic stellate cells. *Hepatogastroenterology*. 1996;43(7):72-91.
13. Winnock M, Barcina MG, Lukomska B, Bioulac-Sage P, Balabaud C. Liver-associated lymphocytes: role in tumor defense. *Semin Liver Dis*. 1993;13(1):81-92.
14. Canbay A, Feldstein AE, Higuchi H, et al. Kupffer cell engulfment of apoptotic bodies stimulates death ligand and cytokine expression. *Hepatology*. 2003;38(5):1188-1198.
15. McCuskey RS. The hepatic microvascular system in health and its response to toxicants. *Anat Rec (Hoboken)*. 2008;291(6):661-671.
16. Schleicher J, Tokarski C, Marbach E, et al. Zonation of hepatic fatty acid metabolism - the diversity of its regulation and the benefit of modeling. *Biochim Biophys Acta*. 2015;1851(5):641-656.
17. Katz NR, Fischer W, Giffhorn S. Distribution of enzymes of fatty acid and ketone body metabolism in periportal and perivenous rat-liver tissue. *Eur J Biochem*. 1983;135(1):103-107.
18. Novikoff AB. Cell heterogeneity within the hepatic lobule of the rat: staining reactions. *J Histochem Cytochem*. 1959;7(4):240-244.
19. Evans JL, Quistorff B, Witters LA. Zonation of hepatic lipogenic enzymes identified by dual-digitonin-pulse perfusion. *Biochem J*. 1989;259(3):821-829.
20. Amaya MJ, Nathanson MH. Calcium signaling in the liver. *Compr Physiol*. 2013;3(1):515-539.
21. Boyer JL. Bile formation and secretion. *Compr Physiol*. 2013;3(3):1035-1078.
22. Theise ND, Saxena R, Portmann BC, et al. The canals of Hering and hepatic stem cells in humans. *Hepatology*. 1999;30(6):1425-1433.
23. Kanz MF. 9.04 - Anatomy and physiology of the biliary epithelium. In: McQueen CA, ed. *Comprehensive Toxicology*. 2nd ed. Oxford: Elsevier; 2010:43-108.
24. Feranchak AP, Sokol RJ. Cholangiocyte biology and cystic fibrosis liver disease. *Semin Liver Dis*. 2001;21(4):471-488.
25. Masyuk AI, Masyuk TV, LaRusso NF. Chapter 44 - physiology of cholangiocytes. In: Said HM, ed. *Physiology of the Gastrointestinal Tract*. 6th ed. Academic Press; 2018:1003-1023.
26. Axelson M, Sjovall J. Potential bile acid precursors in plasma–possible indicators of biosynthetic pathways to cholic and chenodeoxycholic acids in man. *J Steroid Biochem*. 1990;36(6):631-640.
27. Chiang JY. Bile acids: regulation of synthesis. *J Lipid Res*. 2009;50(10):1955-1966.
28. Russell DW. Fifty years of advances in bile acid synthesis and metabolism. *J Lipid Res*. 2009;50(suppl):S120-S125.

29. Russell DW, Setchell KD. Bile acid biosynthesis. *Biochemistry*. 1992;31(20):4737-4749.
30. Swell L, Gustafsson J, Schwartz CC, Halloran LG, Danielsson H, Vlahcevic ZR. An in vivo evaluation of the quantitative significance of several potential pathways to cholic and chenodeoxycholic acids from cholesterol in man. *J Lipid Res*. 1980;21(4):455-466.
31. Ridlon JM, Kang DJ, Hylemon PB, Bajaj JS. Bile acids and the gut microbiome. *Curr Opin Gastroenterol*. 2014;30(3):332-338.
32. Vlahcevic ZR, Schwartz CC, Gustafsson J, Halloran LG, Danielsson H, Swell L. Biosynthesis of bile acids in man. Multiple pathways to cholic acid and chenodeoxycholic acid. *J Biol Chem*. 1980;255(7):2925-2933.
33. McCormick 3rd WC, Bell Jr CC, Swell L, Vlahcevic ZR. Cholic acid synthesis as an index of the severity of liver disease in man. *Gut*. 1973;14(11):895-902.
34. Setchell KD, Schwarz M, O'Connell NC, et al. Identification of a new inborn error in bile acid synthesis: mutation of the oxysterol 7alpha-hydroxylase gene causes severe neonatal liver disease. *J Clin Invest*. 1998;102(9):1690-1703.
35. Haslewood GA. Bile salt evolution. *J Lipid Res*. 1967;8(6):535-550.
36. Dawson PA, Karpen SJ. Intestinal transport and metabolism of bile acids. *J Lipid Res*. 2015;56(6):1085-1099.
37. Poley JR, Dower JC, Owen Jr CA, Stickler GB. Bile acids in infants and children. *J Lab Clin Med*. 1964;63:838-846.
38. Jacobsen JG, Smith LH. Biochemistry and physiology of taurine and taurine derivatives. *Physiol Rev*. 1968;48(2):424-511.
39. Li T, Apte U. Bile acid metabolism and signaling in cholestasis, inflammation, and cancer. *Adv Pharmacol*. 2015;74:263-302.
40. Kullak-Ublick GA, Stieger B, Meier PJ. Enterohepatic bile salt transporters in normal physiology and liver disease. *Gastroenterology*. 2004;126(1):322-342.
41. Chiang JY. Bile acid metabolism and signaling. *Compr Physiol*. 2013;3(3):1191-1212.
42. Hofmann AF. The continuing importance of bile acids in liver and intestinal disease. *Arch Intern Med*. 1999;159(22):2647-2658.
43. Pandak WM, Vlahcevic ZR, Heuman DM, Redford KS, Chiang JY, Hylemon PB. Effects of different bile salts on steady-state mRNA levels and transcriptional activity of cholesterol 7 alpha-hydroxylase. *Hepatology*. 1994;19(4):941-947.
44. Ridlon JM, Kang DJ, Hylemon PB. Bile salt biotransformations by human intestinal bacteria. *J Lipid Res*. 2006;47(2):241-259.
45. Wang W, Wu Z, Dai Z, Yang Y, Wang J, Wu G. Glycine metabolism in animals and humans: implications for nutrition and health. *Amino Acids*. 2013;45(3):463-477.
46. Long SL, Gahan CGM, Joyce SA. Interactions between gut bacteria and bile in health and disease. *Mol Aspects Med*. 2017;56:54-65.
47. Staley C, Weingarden AR, Khoruts A, Sadowsky MJ. Interaction of gut microbiota with bile acid metabolism and its influence on disease states. *Appl Microbiol Biotechnol*. 2017;101(1):47-64.
48. Sayin SI, Wahlstrom A, Felin J, et al. Gut microbiota regulates bile acid metabolism by reducing the levels of tauro-beta-muricholic acid, a naturally occurring FXR antagonist. *Cell Metab*. 2013;17(2):225-235.
49. Duboc H, Rajca S, Rainteau D, et al. Connecting dysbiosis, bile-acid dysmetabolism and gut inflammation in inflammatory bowel diseases. *Gut*. 2013;62(4):531-539.
50. Hofmann AF. Biliary secretion and excretion in health and disease: current concepts. *Ann Hepatol*. 2007;6(1):15-27.

Fetal and Neonatal Bilirubin Metabolism

90

Ryoichi Fujiwara

INTRODUCTION

Bilirubin, a neurotoxic pigment, is the end product of heme catabolism in mammals. In adults, bilirubin is extensively metabolized by hepatic UDP-glucuronosyltransferase (UGT) 1A1 and thereby cleared from the body almost immediately. Expression and function of UGT1A1 is much less in the neonatal liver, allowing accumulation of unconjugated bilirubin in the body. Mild hyperbilirubinemia is commonly observed in human neonates. However, neonates who develop severe hyperbilirubinemia have a higher risk for kernicterus, an irreversible brain injury caused by invasion and accumulation of bilirubin into the brain. This chapter summarizes metabolism of bilirubin in the fetus and in neonates, which is important to the understanding and prevention of neonatal hyperbilirubinemia and kernicterus.

FORMATION OF BILIRUBIN

Heme proteins are a family of metalloprotein that contain a heme moiety, which consists of an Fe^{2+} ion in the center of porphyrin protoporphyrin–IX. Among a number of hemoproteins, hemoglobin, the main component of red blood cells and transporter of oxygen and carbon dioxide in the blood, is the largest contributor to the production of heme and its catabolite bilirubin. The first catabolic reaction is mediated by heme oxygenase–1 (HO-1), which metabolizes heme, producing α-hydroxyheme, α-verdoheme, ferric biliverdin, and then biliverdin.[1] While it is the end product of heme catabolism in some species such as birds, reptile, and amphibians, biliverdin is further metabolized to bilirubin by biliverdin reductase in mammals (Fig. 90.1).[2] Compared with healthy adults or older children, newborn infants have an increased rate of bilirubin production, and preterm infants generally have higher rates of bilirubin production than term newborns.[3,4] Catabolism of 1 mole of heme to 1 mole of bilirubin releases 1 mole of carbon monoxide (CO); thus the rate of bilirubin formation can be estimated from the rate of carboxyhemoglobin production or by trace gas analysis of CO in expired breath.[3-5] Approximately 80% of bilirubin is converted from the breakdown of hemoglobin in senescent red blood cells and prematurely destroyed erythroid cells in the bone marrow. The remainder originates from the turnover of various other hemoproteins found in other tissues, primarily the liver and muscles.[6,7]

GENERAL MECHANISM OF TRANSPORT, CONJUGATION, AND EXCRETION OF BILIRUBIN

Albumin delivers bilirubin to fenestrated sites in the hepatic sinusoids within the space of Disse,[8] by passage of the albumin-bilirubin complex through the fenestrae and dissociation of bilirubin from albumin at the hepatic cell surface. Bilirubin is not the sole substance that binds to albumin. Many other endogenous substances and xenobiotics such as drugs can competitively bind to albumin. Theoretically, if there is a substance that has a higher binding affinity to albumin than that of bilirubin, the substance can displace bilirubin from its albumin-binding sites, resulting in an increase of free bilirubin. It is not conclusive whether the passage of bilirubin across the basolateral portion of the hepatocyte membrane is carrier-mediated or by diffusion of free bilirubin.[8] However, due to its hydrophobic nature and high permeability, passive diffusion is more likely the main transport mechanism for unconjugated free bilirubin. Bilirubin is efficiently transported into hepatocytes in organic anion transporting polypeptide (OATP) knockout mice (which lacked *Slco1a/1b*

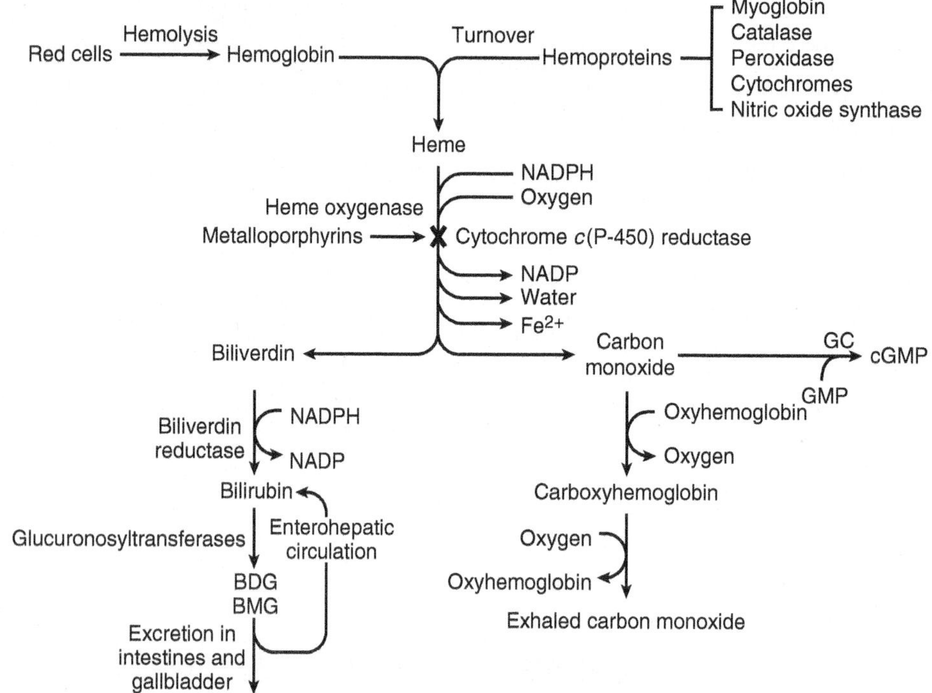

Fig. 90.1 Metabolic pathway for the degradation of heme and the formation of bilirubin. *BDG,* Bilirubin diglucuronide; *BMG,* bilirubin monoglucuronide; *cGMP,* cyclic guanosine monophosphate; GC, guanylyl cyclase; *GMP,* guanosine monophosphate; *NADP,* nicotinamide adenine dinucleotide; *NADPH,* nicotinamide adenine dinucleotide phosphate. (Modified from Vreman HJ, Wong RJ, Stevenson DK. Carbon monoxide in breath, blood, and other tissues. In: Penney DG, ed. *Carbon Monoxide Toxicity.* Boca Raton, FL: CRC Press; 2000:2-2.)

isoforms).[9] There are several methods to measure albumin-bound and free bilirubin in blood samples. The simplest method is the hematofluorometer that utilizes the fluorescent properties of bilirubin to measure albumin-bound bilirubin, reserve binding capacity, and total whole blood bilirubin.[10]

Bilirubin is transported within the hepatocyte to the smooth endoplasmic reticulum, where its carboxyl groups are conjugated with glucuronic acid. Conjugation of bilirubin is catalyzed by one of the isoforms of the UGT enzyme super family, UGT1A1,[11] which catalyzes glucuronidation of a number of endogenously produced or exogenously introduced small molecules, such as bilirubin, bile acids, and drugs.[12] UGTs utilize UDP-glucuronic acid as a co-substrate and mediate the transfer of glucuronic acid to their substrate.[13] Once conjugated, with the glucuronic acid moiety, bilirubin is highly water-soluble, facilitating its excretion. There are two types of conjugated bilirubin, bilirubin monoglucuronide and bilirubin diglucuronide; both are often called *direct bilirubin*, while unconjugated bilirubin is called *indirect bilirubin*. Although UGT1A1 expressed in the gastrointestinal tract can also metabolize bilirubin, its contribution to the overall metabolism in adults is minor.

In hepatocytes, conjugated bilirubin is subsequently excreted into bile through the ATP-dependent efflux transporter multidrug–resistance protein 2 (MRP2; encoded by ABCC2).[14] While the majority of conjugated bilirubin transported into the intestine is excreted in the feces, part of it undergoes hydrolysis by bacterial β-glucuronidase, converting it back into unconjugated bilirubin, which is reabsorbed into the body. This cycling between the liver and the small intestine is called *enterohepatic circulation of bilirubin*. The homeostasis of bilirubin is shown in Fig. 90.2.[15]

FETAL BILIRUBIN METABOLISM

Various enzymes are functional in the fetal body, contributing to detoxification of potentially toxic substances. However, the expression of bilirubin-glucuronidating UGT1A1 in the fetal liver is quite low.[16] Although UGT1A1 expression is high in intestinal tissue,[17] it appears that the fetal body is protected from accumulation of bilirubin by two independent mechanisms: (1) maternal bilirubin metabolism and (2) the placental barrier. Bilirubin is efficiently metabolized by UGT1A1 in heterozygous *Ugt1a1*$^{+/-}$ mice even during pregnancy.[18] The serum bilirubin level of a newborn mouse that is genetically deficient for UGT1A1 (*Ugt1a1*$^{-/-}$) is close to 0 mg/dL immediately upon birth,[18] which is likely because bilirubin is systematically metabolized and cleared by maternal UGT1A1. Interestingly, the serum bilirubin level of a newborn mouse with a *Ugt1a1*$^{-/-}$ genotype is still lower when it is born from a mouse that is genetically deficient for UGT1A1 (*Ugt1a1*$^{-/-}$).[18] This observation indicates the existence of an active transporting system of bilirubin that aids the passage of unconjugated bilirubin from fetal to maternal circulation, protecting against accumulation of neurotoxic bilirubin in the fetal body. Individuals with Crigler-Najjar type I, who develop severe unconjugated hyperbilirubinemia due to homozygous deficiency in *UGT1A1*, can be successfully pregnant as long as their newborns receive proper treatment to prevent kernicterus.[19]

NEONATAL BILIRUBIN METABOLISM AND HYPERBILIRUBINEMIA

After birth, exposure to increased amounts of oxygen accelerates hemolysis, resulting in overproduction of bilirubin. Because the bilirubin detoxification pathway is not yet fully developed, imbalance of bilirubin production and clearance results in mild hyperbilirubinemia in almost all human newborns. Preterm infants generally have even higher rates of bilirubin production than term newborns.[3,4] The biggest contribution to neonatal hyperbilirubinemia is the lack of UGT1A1 in the developing liver tissue.[20] Neonatal bilirubin glucuronidation, instead, is carried out in the gastrointestinal tract.[21] Compared to the liver,

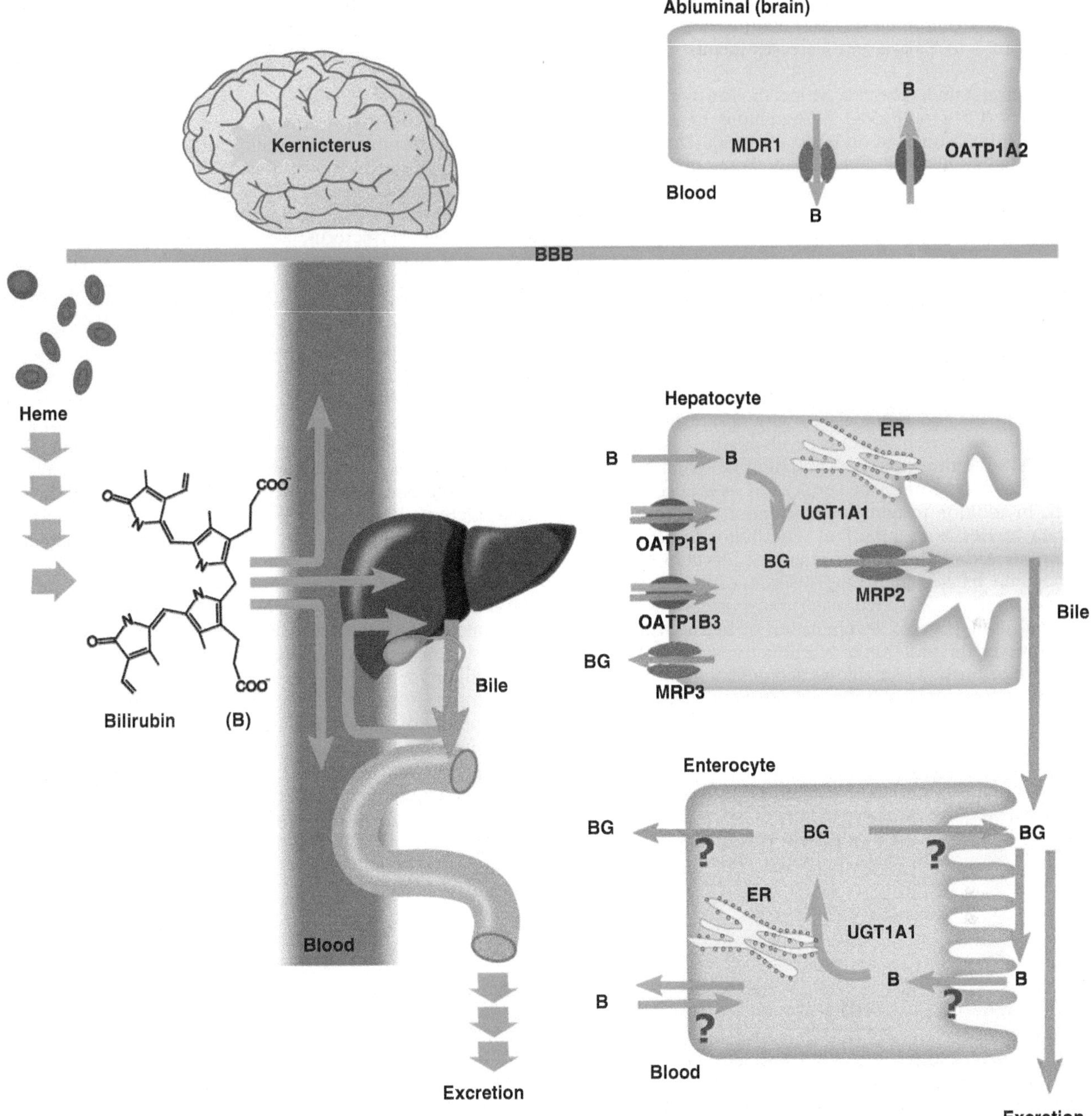

Fig. 90.2 Schematic representation of bilirubin homeostasis. Bilirubin, an end product of heme catabolism, is taken up into the hepatocyte, where it is glucuronidated by UGT1A1 and actively secreted into bile. Bilirubin glucuronide can be excreted or deconjugated and reabsorbed in the small intestine, where deconjugated bilirubin is glucuronidated again by UGT1A1. Significantly elevated serum bilirubin levels allow the entrance of bilirubin into the brain, causing irreversible brain damage, kernicterus. In contrast to the detailed knowledge on the transporters in the liver and blood-brain barrier, information on the transport of bilirubin and its glucuronide in the small intestine remains limited. *B,* Bilirubin *(blue arrows)*; *BBB,* blood-brain barrier; *BG,* bilirubin glucuronide *(orange arrows)*; *ER,* endoplasmic reticulum; *MDR,* multidrug resistance protein (P-glycoprotein); *MRP3,* multidrug resistance-associated protein 3. (From Fujiwara R, Haag M, Schaeffeler E, et al. Systemic regulation of bilirubin homeostasis: Potential benefits of hyperbilirubinemia. *Hepatology*. 2018;67(4):1609-1619. https://www.ncbi.nlm.nih.gov/pubmed/29059457 [Fig. 1].)

UGT1A1 is relatively highly expressed in the small intestine.[17] Intestinal UGT1A1 activity and serum bilirubin levels indeed correlate well.[17] The rate of metabolic clearance of bilirubin in formula-fed infants is faster than in breast-fed infants.[22] Serum bilirubin levels as well as the risk of developing kernicterus are therefore statistically higher in breast-fed infants compared to formula-fed infants.[23] This difference in bilirubin glucuronidation rate in formula-fed and breast-fed infants can be explained by a few mechanisms. Certain nutrients present in breast milk, such as fatty acids or 5β-pregnane-3α,20β-diol, can inhibit bilirubin glucuronidation catalyzed by UGT1A1.[24] Also, it seems that unidentified substances in breast milk suppress the expression of gastrointestinal UGT1A1, which results in reduced detoxification in the small intestine.[17] On the other hand, when formula-feeding replaces the UGT1A1-suppressing breast milk, it induces its expression, accelerating glucuronidation of bilirubin.[17] Additionally, breast-feeding might cause increased enterohepatic circulation of bilirubin, inhibition of binding of bilirubin to serum albumin, suboptimal fluid intake, weight loss, and intestinal colonization, all of which result in increased serum bilirubin levels. The system for hepatic uptake, enzymatic conjugation, and biliary excretion of bilirubin eventually matures, over an average time interval of 3 to 7 days, and increases infants' capacity to clear bilirubin.

Bilirubin can also undergo oxidative metabolism by cytochrome P450 enzymes (CYPs or P450s).[25] Continuous treatment with beta (β)–naphthoflavone, an inducer of P450s that mediate oxidative metabolism of bilirubin, delays onset of kernicterus in a Crigler-Najjar type I model,[18] indicating that P450-mediated oxidation could be an essential metabolic pathway of bilirubin if glucuronidation is genetically restricted.

KERNICTERUS AND ITS RISK FACTORS

When free unconjugated bilirubin invades and accumulates in the brain, it can cause irreversible brain damage—kernicterus—which has an incidence of about 1 in 50,000 to 100,000 live births and is associated with severe hyperbilirubinemia with total serum bilirubin levels higher than 30 mg/dL.[26] Therefore the threshold concentration of serum bilirubin level that leads to the onset of kernicterus is generally above 30 mg/dL. In addition to metabolic clearance of bilirubin, the blood-brain barrier is an important contributor to prevention of kernicterus. Although free unconjugated bilirubin can pass the blood-brain barrier, multidrug–resistance protein (MDR1; P-glycoprotein) and MRP1, two major transporters involved in efflux of bilirubin, prevent accumulation of bilirubin into the brain.[27] However, the function of bilirubin transporters has not fully matured at birth, which allows accumulation of bilirubin in the brain in preterm newborns and in the early life of full-term newborns; expression of bilirubin transporters gradually increases as newborns develop.[20] After acquiring the bilirubin efflux system, kernicterus is not observed even with hemolysis-induced elevation of serum bilirubin levels.[20] Crigler-Najjar type I neonates require extensive treatment to lower serum bilirubin levels and prevent kernicterus. However, bilirubin cannot pass the fully matured blood-brain barrier, which is developed in early childhood, and therefore they do not require extensive care, though serum bilirubin levels may exceed 30 mg/dL.[18]

Binding of bilirubin to albumin is another key factor affecting development of kernicterus. As mentioned above, a certain portion of bilirubin is bound to albumin in circulating blood, while the rest is present as free (unbound) bilirubin. Due to its complex and bulky structure, albumin- bound bilirubin cannot pass the blood-brain barrier. If bilirubin binding to albumin is impaired (e.g., by exposure to drugs that compete with bilirubin), newborn infants are prone to develop low-bilirubin kernicterus, which is a type of kernicterus induced at bilirubin levels much lower than presumed toxic threshold concentrations.[28] Hypoalbuminemia is a clinical condition in which the albumin level in blood is abnormally low due to inflammation, infection, or tissue diseases, or a combination of these. Increased free bilirubin in neonates with hypoalbuminemia increases the likelihood of accumulation of bilirubin in the brain. There are clinical cases of kernicterus in neonates who were administered with sulfamethoxazole and trimethoprim individually, as well as with their combination, known as *cotrimoxazole*, both of which strongly bind albumin, although the association between the medication and the onset of kernicterus is not entirely conclusive.[29] Compared to usual high bilirubin-induced kernicterus, low bilirubin kernicterus is rare and unpredictable.

Suppression of bilirubin production could be the ideal method to prevent high serum bilirubin levels and the onset of kernicterus. Untreated Crigler-Najjar type I models develop lethal kernicterus. However, continuous administration of an inhibitor for HO-1, the enzyme that metabolizes heme and produces a precursor of bilirubin, not only delays infants' development of kernicterus, but also completely protects them from bilirubin–induced neonatal lethality and permits normal development into adulthood, when the inhibitor treatment is no longer required.[18] Metalloporphyrins, which are derivatives of heme, are known as ***inhibitors of HO-1***. Among them, zinc protoporphyrin is a naturally occurring metalloporphyrin that has a potent inhibitory effect against HO–1 (Fig. 90.3). Zinc

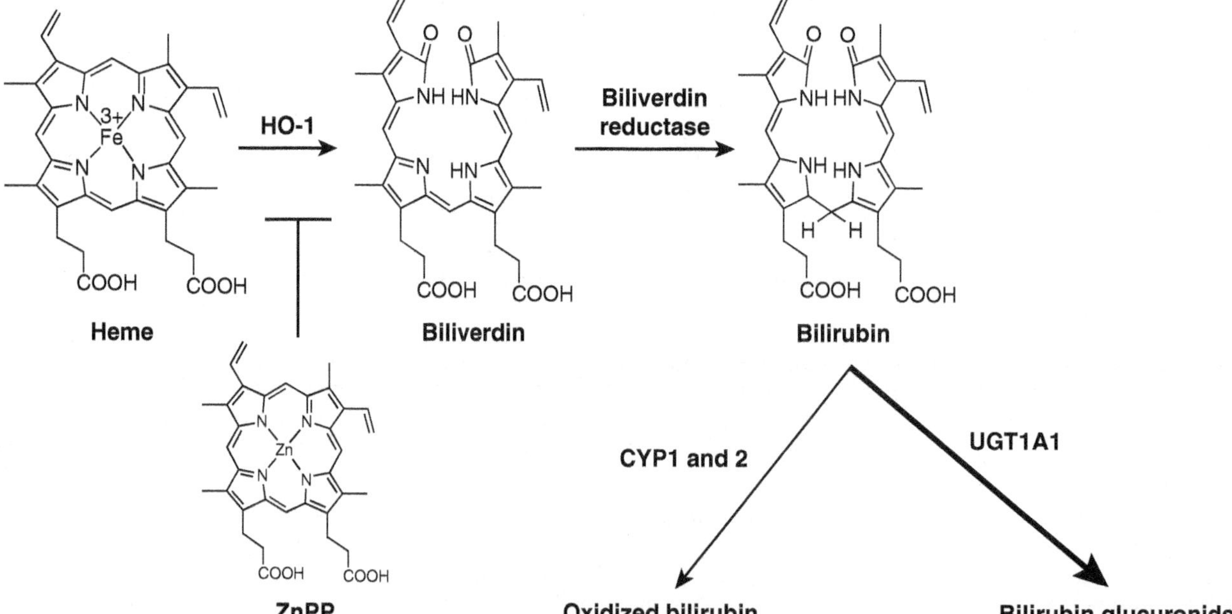

Fig. 90.3 Generation and metabolism of bilirubin. Heme oxygenase *(HO-1)* mainly contributes to the catabolism of heme, producing biliverdin. Biliverdin reductase converts biliverdin into bilirubin. Bilirubin is mainly metabolized by UGT1A1 but is partially metabolized by CYP enzymes. Genetic deficiency in UGT1A1 results in the onset of severe hyperbilirubinemia, which leads to the development of kernicterus. Zinc protoporphyrin (ZnPP) is a potent inhibitor of HO-1. (From Fujiwara R, Mitsugi R, Uemura A, et al. Severe neonatal hyperbilirubinemia in Crigler-Najjar syndrome model mice can be reversed with zinc protoporphyrin. *Hepatol Commun*. 2017;1(8):792-802. https://www.ncbi.nlm.nih.gov/pubmed/29399656 [Fig. 1].)

protoporphyrin even has the potential to become an anticancer drug. However, the biggest disadvantage of this therapy is that inhibition of HO-1 can cause massive oxidative stress in healthy tissue due to suppressed production of bilirubin, which is also a potent antioxidant.

CONCLUSION

Bilirubin homeostasis is systemically regulated. Human adults have a fully matured bilirubin detoxification system in the liver, in which UGT1A1 increases the solubility of bilirubin by transferring glucuronic acid to bilirubin. While the maternal liver plays the major role in metabolism of bilirubin in fetus, newborns have only limited metabolic function due to the extremely low expression of UGT1A1. Furthermore, onset of spontaneous breathing after birth increases the amount of oxygen in the body, accelerating hemolysis and production of bilirubin. Imbalance of bilirubin production and metabolism leads to development of hyperbilirubinemia in most neonates. Preterm birth and breast-feeding are two major factors that increase the risk of severe hyperbilirubinemia, which may cause kernicterus. Although neonatal hyperbilirubinemia has been a well-known physiologic condition for more than 70 years, its underlying mechanism had not been fully determined until recently because of the lack of animal models displaying the human-specific neonatal hyperbilirubinemia. Recent advances in biotechnology have enabled us to gain insights into the molecular mechanisms of neonatal jaundice and kernicterus. The next goal is the complete elimination of kernicterus, many cases of which are seen worldwide. In addition, potential benefits of bilirubin and neonatal hyperbilirubinemia need to be mechanistically determined.[15]

REFERENCES

1. Kikuchi G, Yoshida T, Noguchi M. Heme oxygenase and heme degradation. *Biochem Biophys Res Commun*. 2005;338:558-567.
2. Baranano DE, Rao M, Ferris CD, Snyder SH. Biliverdin reductase: a major physiologic cytoprotectant. *Proc Natl Acad Sci USA*. 2002;99:16093-16098.
3. Maisels MJ, Pathak A, Nelson NM, et al. Endogenous production of carbon monoxide in normal and erythroblastotic newborn infants. *J Clin Invest*. 1971;50:1-13.
4. Bartoletti AL, Stevenson DK, Ostrander CR, Johnson JD. Pulmonary excretion of carbon monoxide in the human infant as an index of bilirubin production. I. Effects of gestational age and postnatal age and some common neonatal abnormalities. *J Pediatr*. 1979;94:952-955.
5. Dennery PA, Seidman DS, Stevenson DK. Neonatal hyperbilirubinemia. *N Engl J Med*. 2001;344:581-590.
6. Kalakonda A, John S. *Physiology, Bilirubin*. Treasure Island (FL): StatPearls Publishing; 2019.
7. Ngashangva L, Bachu V, Goswami P. Development of new methods for determination of bilirubin. *J Pharm Biomed Anal*. 2019;162:272-285.
8. Sorrentino D, Berk PD. Mechanistic aspects of hepatic bilirubin uptake. *Semin Liver Dis*. 1998;8:119-136.
9. van de Steeg E, Wagenaar E, van der Kruijssen CM, et al. Organic anion transporting polypeptide 1a/1b-knockout mice provide insights into hepatic handling of bilirubin, bile acids, and drugs. *J Clin Invest*. 2010;120:2942-2952.
10. Spear ML, Baumgart S. The hematofluorometer: a rapid assay for bilirubin and bilirubin binding. *Med Instrum*. 1985;19:88-92.
11. Ritter JK, Chen F, Sheen YY, et al. A novel complex locus UGT1 encodes human bilirubin, phenol, and other UDP-glucuronosyltransferase isozymes with identical carboxyl termini. *J Biol Chem*. 1992;267:3257-3261.
12. Burchell B, Nebert DW, Nelson DR, et al. The UDP glucuronosyltransferase gene superfamily: suggested nomenclature based on evolutionary divergence. *DNA Cell Biol*. 1991;10:487-494.
13. Fujiwara R, Yokoi T, Nakajima M. Structure and protein-protein interactions of human UDP-glucuronosyltransferases. *Front Pharmacol*. 2016;7:388.
14. Nies AT, Schwab M, Keppler D. Interplay of conjugating enzymes with OATP uptake transporters and ABCC/MRP efflux pumps in the elimination of drugs. *Expert Opin Drug Metab Toxicol*. 2008;4:545-568.
15. Fujiwara R, Haag M, Schaeffeler E, Nies AT, Zanger UM, Schwab M. Systemic regulation of bilirubin homeostasis: potential benefits of hyperbilirubinemia. *Hepatology*. 2018;67:1609-1619.
16. Grimmer I, Moller R, Gmyrek D, Gross J. Bilirubin UDP-glucuronyltransferase activity in human fetal liver homogenates. *Acta Biol Med Ger*. 1978;37:131-135.
17. Fujiwara R, Chen S, Karin M, Tukey RH. Reduced expression of UGT1A1 in intestines of humanized UGT1 mice via inactivation of NF–κB leads to hyperbilirubinemia. *Gastroenterology*. 2012;142:109-118.
18. Fujiwara R, Mitsugi R, Uemura A, et al. Severe neonatal hyperbilirubinemia in crigler-najjar syndrome model mice can be reversed with zinc protoporphyrin. *HepatolCommun*. 2017;1:792-802.
19. Gajdos V, Petit F, Trioche P, et al. Successful pregnancy in a Crigler-Najjar type I patient treated by phototherapy and semimonthly albumin infusions. *Gastroenterology*. 2006;131:921-924.
20. Fujiwara R, Nguyen N, Chen S, Tukey RH. Developmental hyperbilirubinemia and CNS toxicity in mice humanized with the UDP glucuronosyltransferase 1 (UGT1) locus. *Proc Natl Acad Sci USA*. 2010;107:5024-5029.
21. Fujiwara R, Maruo Y, Chen S, Tukey RH. Role of extrahepatic UDP–glucuronosyltransferase 1A1: advances in understanding breast milk-induced neonatal hyperbilirubinemia. *Toxicol Appl Pharmacol*. 2015;289:124-132.
22. Wu TC, Huang IF, Chen YC, Chen PH, Yang LY. Differences in serum biochemistry between breast–fed and formula–fed infants. *J Chin Med Assoc*. 2011;74:511-515.
23. Gartner LM. Breastfeeding and jaundice. *J Perinatol*. 2001;21(suppl 1):S25-S29; discussion S35-S39.
24. Shibuya A, Itoh T, Tukey RH, Fujiwara R. Impact of fatty acids on human UDP–glucuronosyltransferase 1A1 activity and its expression in neonatal hyperbilirubinemia. *Sci Rep*. 2013;3:2903.
25. Abu–Bakar A, Moore MR, Lang MA. Evidence for induced microsomal bilirubin degradation by cytochrome P450 2A5. *Biochem Pharmacol*. 2005;70:1527-1535.
26. Bhutani VK, Johnson L. Kernicterus in the 21st century: frequently asked questions. *J Perinatol*. 2009;29(suppl 1):S20-S24.
27. Ostrow JD, Pascolo L, Brites D, Tiribelli C. Molecular basis of bilirubin-induced neurotoxicity. *Trends Mol Med*. 2004;10:65-70.
28. Watchko JF, Maisels MJ. The enigma of low bilirubin kernicterus in premature infants: why does it still occur, and is it preventable? *SeminPerinatol*. 2014;38:397-406.
29. Thyagarajan B, Deshpande SS. Cotrimoxazole and neonatal kernicterus: a review. *Drug Chem Toxicol*. 2014;37:121-129.

Hereditary Contributions to Neonatal Hyperbilirubinemia

91

Michael Kaplan | Cathy Hammerman

INTRODUCTION

Neonatal jaundice is a common phenomenon, noted in more than 80% of otherwise healthy, term newborns.[1,2] In the majority of cases, the jaundice is transient, usually resolving by the end of the first postnatal week, and serum total bilirubin (STB) concentrations are not harmful. In some infants, severe hyperbilirubinemia may develop with the potential for acute bilirubin encephalopathy.[3,4] Some of these cases may progress to the chronic athetoid form of cerebral palsy (kernicterus) or other

Box 91.1 Mutations and Polymorphisms of Genes Active in the Formation and Elimination of Bilirubin With the Potential for Modulating Neonatal Hyperbilirubinemia

A. Increased heme catabolism
 Heme oxygenase-1 (*HO-1*) promoter polymorphisms
B. Diminished bilirubin formation
 Bilirubin reductase polymorphisms
C. Diminished bilirubin hepatic uptake
 Solute carrier organic anion transporter (*SLCO1B1*) polymorphisms
D. Diminished bilirubin conjugation
 Uridine diphosphate-glucuronosyltransferase 1A1 (*UGT1A1*) promoter and coding area polymorphisms and mutations

forms of bilirubin neurotoxicity. These include deafness or mild neurologic sequelae attributed to high serum levels of bilirubin, called *bilirubin-induced neurologic dysfunction (BIND)*. Because of the wide range of clinical features resulting from bilirubin neurotoxicity, Le Pichon et al. suggested use of the term *kernicterus spectrum disorders* to include all above-mentioned forms of neurologic sequalae of bilirubin neurotoxicity.[5]

In recent years it has become apparent that much of the mediation of bilirubin metabolism and the determination of whether STB concentrations remain within the physiologic range or increase to potentially harmful concentrations lies within genetic control.[6-10] Indeed, one of the most important advances in our understanding of the genomics of bilirubin metabolism was the elucidation of the *UGT1A1* gene encoding the bilirubin-conjugating enzyme, uridine diphosphate-glucuronosyltransferase 1A1 (UGT1A1). It is now apparent that a number of genes control both the production and elimination of bilirubin and that polymorphisms or mutations of these genes, sometimes acting in combination or synergistically, have the potential to cause extreme hyperbilirubinemia. Additionally, genetically inherited diseases due to mutations of genes not normally involved in the physiology of bilirubin are associated with increased hemolysis, sometimes to a marked degree. Select hereditary conditions with the potential to moderate bilirubin metabolism are listed in Box 91.1. Furthermore, in addition to specific mutations and polymorphisms, there are racial and ethnic influences on bilirubin values and neonatal hyperbilirubinemia, as will be discussed. Finally, next-generation DNA sequencing, a modern diagnostic tool, has the potential to determine a specific genetic etiology in many newborns with extreme hyperbilirubinemia.

As reviewed in the ensuing chapter, hyperbilirubinemia is not dependent on increased bilirubin production or diminished elimination as individual processes. Rather, these forces may combine and even interact to increase the STB at any point in time.

THE SERUM TOTAL BILIRUBIN: WHAT DOES IT IMPLY?

The STB at any point in time represents two cardinal contributing processes: bilirubin production and bilirubin elimination, the latter primarily by conjugation but also including bilirubin uptake into the hepatocyte and excretion of the conjugated product. In neonates, bowel reabsorption of bilirubin via the enterohepatic circulation may further add to the bilirubin pool.

In healthy adults and older children and infants, bilirubin production and elimination are in equilibrium, and the STB remains within normal limits. During the first postnatal days, however, physiologically increased heme formation and its catabolism result in increased bilirubin production, while diminished activity of the bilirubin-conjugating enzyme, UGT1A1,[11] results in decreased bilirubin conjugation. Mild or moderate imbalance between these processes may pose little threat to an otherwise healthy, term infant. Almost all newborns have UGT1A1 enzyme immaturity; therefore, diminished bilirubin conjugation is universally present. In the immediate postnatal period, bilirubin production exceeds its elimination, resulting from a high intrauterine (and postnatal) hemoglobin concentration, a shortened red blood cell (RBC) life span, and elimination of transplacental clearance. Consequently, a physiologic increase in STB occurs during the first postnatal days.[12] Given universally diminished bilirubin conjugation in the newborn and the delicate balance between production and excretion, increased hemolysis will be the mediating factor in the pathophysiology of hyperbilirubinemia in most cases.[13]

IMBALANCE BETWEEN BILIRUBIN PRODUCTION AND ELIMINATION

Despite the significance of increased hemolysis, bilirubin accumulation in a hemolytic state should not always be assumed. Of prime importance is the concept of lack of equilibrium between bilirubin production and conjugation. Thus, in an infant who is hemolyzing but has efficient bilirubin-conjugating capacity, STB may not rise. On the other hand, in an infant with immature bilirubin-conjugating capacity, due, for example, to late prematurity or the presence of 7, rather than the wild-type 6, thymine adenine $(TA)_7$ repeats in the promoter region of the *UGT1A1* gene *(UGT1A1*28)*, associated with Gilbert syndrome, even minimally increased hemolysis may result in hyperbilirubinemia.

This lack of equilibrium between bilirubin production and conjugation in the pathophysiology of hyperbilirubinemia has been demonstrated mathematically. Kaplan and colleagues investigated the individual contributions of bilirubin production and conjugation to the STB concentration, and also the combined effects of these processes, in healthy, term neonates on the third postnatal day.[14] Blood carboxyhemoglobin determinations corrected for ambient carbon monoxide (COHbc) were used as an index of heme catabolism, whereas bilirubin conjugation was reflected by serum total conjugated bilirubin expressed as a percentage of STB (TCB[%]). As expected, over the range of STB concentrations observed, STB increased in positive correlation with COHbc, and in inverse correlation with TCB(%) (Fig. 91.1). An index or ratio, COHbc/TCB(%), termed the *production-conjugation index*, was constructed to reflect the combined forces of bilirubin production and conjugation. Correlation of this index with STB concentrations was higher than those for either COHbc or TCB(%) independently (Fig. 91.2), confirming the importance of imbalance between bilirubin production and conjugation, rather than the independence of these processes, in the physiologic rise of serum bilirubin. Although the relationship between the index and STB tended to plateau with increasing index values, at the lower end of the index scale, small increases in the index were associated with large increases in STB.

GENETICALLY DETERMINED METABOLIC STEPS ON THE PATHWAY FROM HEME TO CONJUGATED BILIRUBIN

HEME OXYGENASE-1

Heme oxygenase-1 (HO-1) is the rate-limiting enzyme in the heme degradation pathway. Biliverdin, which is formed as a result of this reaction, is subsequently converted to bilirubin.

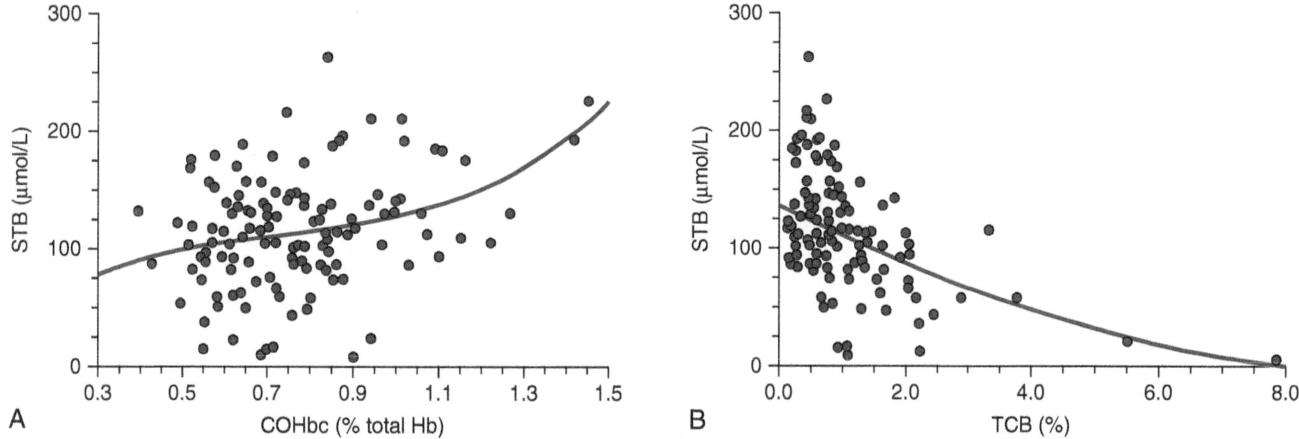

Fig. 91.1 (A) Regression analysis between total serum bilirubin *(STB)* and carboxyhemoglobin corrected for ambient carbon monoxide *(COHbc)* values. Increasing STB values correlated positively with COHbc (r = 0.38; s = 46.1; $y = 9.36 + 323.5x - 378.4x^2 + 172.5x^3$). (B) Regression analysis between STB values and total conjugated bilirubin *(TCB)*, expressed as a percentage of STB (TCB[%]). Increasing STB values were inversely proportional to TCB(%) ratio (r = 0.40; s = 45.8; $y = 136.5 - 27.0x + 1.3x^2$). (From Kaplan M, Muraca M, Hammerman C, et al. Imbalance between production and conjugation of bilirubin: a fundamental concept in the mechanism of neonatal jaundice. *Pediatrics.* 2002;110:e47, with permission.)

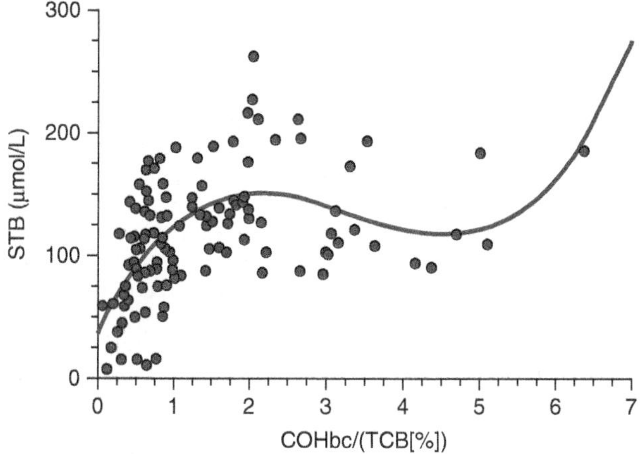

Fig. 91.2 Curvilinear regression analysis between total serum bilirubin *(STB)* values and the combined effect of bilirubin production and conjugation, reflected by the bilirubin production/conjugation index *COHbc/(TCB*[%]). Increasing values of STB correlated positively to this index (r = 0.61; s = 39.1; $y = 32.1 + 132.1x - 45.8x^2 + 4.6x^3$). (From Kaplan M, Muraca M, Hammerman C, et al. Imbalance between production and conjugation of bilirubin: a fundamental concept in the mechanism of neonatal jaundice. *Pediatrics.* 110:e47, 2002, with permission.)

It is logical, therefore, to expect that increased activity of HO-1 should lead to increased heme catabolism and thereby enhanced bilirubin production. The gene encoding HO-1, the inducible isoform of HO, has a polymorphic dinucleotide guanine thymine repeat $(GT)_n$ in the promoter region.[15,16] This regulatory region modulates gene transcription. Expression of *HO-1* is enhanced by a lower number of $(GT)_n$ repeats. Therefore, short *HO-1* promoter sequences should be associated with increased HO activity and lead to increased bilirubin production.

$(GT)_n$ promoter repeat lengths range from 12 to 40 repeats with a bimodal distribution at or around 23 and 30 repeats (Fig. 91.3).[16,17] This has allowed the identification of three subclasses according to the number of $(GT)_n$ repeats: fewer than 25 repeats (short); between 25 and 30 repeats (medium); and more than 30 repeats (long).[15] The impact of various $(GT)_n$ repeat lengths on the transcriptional activity of the *HO-1* promoter has been studied. Compared with constructs with greater than 25 repeats, those with fewer than 25 repeats showed increased *HO-1* promoter activity,[15,16,18] HO-1 messenger RNA (mRNA) expression, and enzyme activity.[19] *HO-1* $(GT)_n$ allele length combinations have been used to designate promoter genotypes including short/short, short/medium, short/long, medium/medium, medium/long, and long/long.

Variations in the distributions of the short, medium, and long promoter length sequences may be due to ethnicity or classification differences. Thus the distribution of short, medium, and long promoter alleles differed significantly in three separate studies.[15,17,20] However, the data are not entirely clear because the exact cutoff points defining short, medium, and long $(GT)_n$ alleles are somewhat arbitrary. This is a key issue because only the short allele is likely to affect heme catabolism. It is unlikely that variation in the cutoff point between the medium and long alleles would have a significant effect on the variation in bilirubin levels between studies.

In adults in the steady state, some studies have demonstrated increased STB values in carriers of the short *HO-1* allele, compared with those without any short allele. Differences in STB values between groups were often minor but did reach statistical significance; it is not clear, however, whether these variations had any clinical significance.[21,22]

Variations in STB values among varying *HO-1* $(GT)_n$ lengths are not necessarily consistent and may demonstrate ethnic distinction. Lin and colleagues studied three distinct Asian ethnic populations, finding an association between STB values and *HO-1* $(GT)_n$ polymorphisms in Uyghurs, but not in the Han or Kazak populations.[23] It is possible that during hemolysis the large amounts of heme released may induce HO-1 expression. This is consistent with a report of a boy with exceptionally elevated STB values during an episode of autoimmune hemolytic anemia, who was found to be homozygous for short *HO-1* $(GT)_n$ promoter alleles.[24]

HO-1 POLYMORPHISMS AND NEONATAL HYPERBILIRUBINEMIA

The case cited above and adult studies suggest the potential for *HO-1* $(GT)_n$ promoter polymorphisms to modulate the severity of neonatal hyperbilirubinemia. However, few studies have investigated the relationship of short promoter polymorphism and neonatal hyperbilirubinemia. Kanai and colleagues studied *HO-1* $(GT)_n$ promoter sequences in Japanese infants who had undergone phototherapy[25] and found no relationship between these polymorphisms and neonatal hyperbilirubinemia. Similarly, Bozkaya and colleagues did not detect significant differences

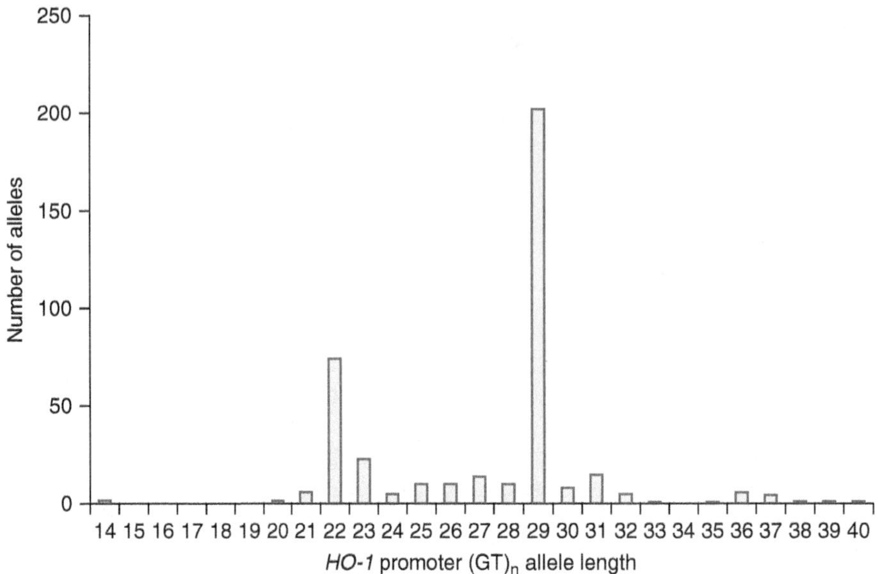

Fig. 91.3 Distribution of *HO-1* promoter $(GT)_n$ repeats according to allele length of 199 newborns. Note the bimodal distribution similar to other population groups (see text). (From Kaplan M, Renbaum P, Hammerman C, et al. Heme oxygenase-1 promoter polymorphisms and neonatal jaundice. *Neonatology.* 2014;106:323–329, with permission.)

in *HO-1* promoter allele lengths between newborns with STB values greater than 12.9 mg/dL and those in whom the STB value did not exceed this level.[20] They did, however, find a correlation between alleles with fewer than 24 $(GT)_n$ repeats and prolonged hyperbilirubinemia.

In a study by Kaplan and colleagues, in which both glucose 6-phosphate dehydrogenase (G6PD)-normal and -deficient newborns were analyzed, no significant correlation was found between the frequency of *HO-1* $(GT)_n$ promoter polymorphism genotypes, or the presence of any short *HO-1* promoter allele, and STB concentrations of 15.0 mg/dL or greater.[17] There was a trend, however, for the G6PD-normal, but not G6PD-deficient, newborns with COHbc values exceeding the 75th percentile to have a higher percentage of short *HO-1* promoter alleles, suggesting a possible role of short *HO-1* alleles in modulating heme catabolism. Absence of this pattern among the G6PD-deficient newborns excludes, at least in the steady state, any potential role of the short *HO-1* allele in modulating heme degradation in this subgroup. These findings do not, however, exclude a role for short *HO-1* promoter expression in exacerbating hyperbilirubinemia in acute hemolytic episodes associated with G6PD deficiency or other hemolytic conditions, in which the large amounts of heme released may induce HO-1 expression.

In contrast to the above studies, Tiwari and colleagues did find a significant association between homozygosity for the short $(GT)_n$ promoter genotype and STB levels exceeding the 95th percentile on the hour-specific bilirubin nomogram in North Indian newborns.[26] Also, in a report from Japan, a higher proportion of allele frequencies in class S (small alleles) was found in hyperbilirubinemic infants than in non-hyperbilirubinemic neonates, while homozygous or heterozygous S allele carrier individuals were encountered more frequently in hyperbilirubinemic neonates than in non-hyperbilirubinemic counterparts.[27]

BILIVERDIN REDUCTASE

Biliverdin reductase A reduces biliverdin to bilirubin, and the potential exists for polymorphisms of the gene encoding this enzyme to affect neonatal hyperbilirubinemia. However, the biliverdin reductase variant studied in adults is not associated with elevated STB levels, and there are no studies of these polymorphisms in neonates.

SOLUTE CARRIER ORGANIC ANION TRANSPORTER

Hepatic cellular uptake of bilirubin is mediated by the solute carrier organic anion transporter polypeptide 1 enzyme (OATP1B1). This enzyme and the gene encoding it, solute carrier organic anion transporter *(SLCO1B1)*,[28] therefore play an important role in modulating serum bilirubin levels. Variations in the *SLCO1B1* gene include 388 G>A, 521 T>C, and 463 C>A.[29] Laboratory expression studies have demonstrated that 388 G>A is associated with reduced transport activity of OATP1B1 and that transient hyperbilirubinemia may result from transporter inhibitors such as rifampin.[30,31] It is therefore logical to suspect that in populations with a high frequency of *SLCO1B1* 388 G>A, such as Asians, who also have a high incidence of neonatal hyperbilirubinemia,[32] this polymorphism may play a role in the pathogenesis of jaundice. In a meta-analysis of studies of neonatal hyperbilirubinemia, Liu and colleagues found no statistically significant differences in the overall incidence of hyperbilirubinemia in association with *SCLO1B1* 388 G>A.[29] When focusing on the specific ethnic subgroups included in this analysis, it did become apparent that this polymorphism was associated with the development of hyperbilirubinemia in Chinese neonates (odds ratio [OR], 1.39; 95% confidence interval [CI], 1.07 to 1.28), but not in other ethnic subgroups, which included whites, Asians, Thai, Brazilians, and Malaysians. Overall *SCLO1B1* 521 T>C was not associated with increased risk for hyperbilirubinemia and was actually associated with diminished risk in Chinese newborns (OR, 0.60; 95% CI, 0.40 to 0.92). The C>A substitution at nucleotide 463 was detected in only one study from the United States in which no statistical association was determined between this polymorphism and the development of neonatal hyperbilirubinemia.[8]

In a study that included 18 *SLCO1B1* variants, no significant differences were observed in the frequency of these variants between those with STB values exceeding the 95th percentile on the hour-specific bilirubin nomogram (hyperbilirubinemia) versus those with STB values not exceeding the 40th percentile.[7] There was, however, an effect of *SLCO1B1* variants when they occurred in combination with additional genetic factors (see below). Huang and colleagues found an association between the *SCLO1B1* 388 G>A variant and the development of neonatal hyperbilirubinemia (OR, 2.10; 95% CI, 1.02 to 4.30), but not for

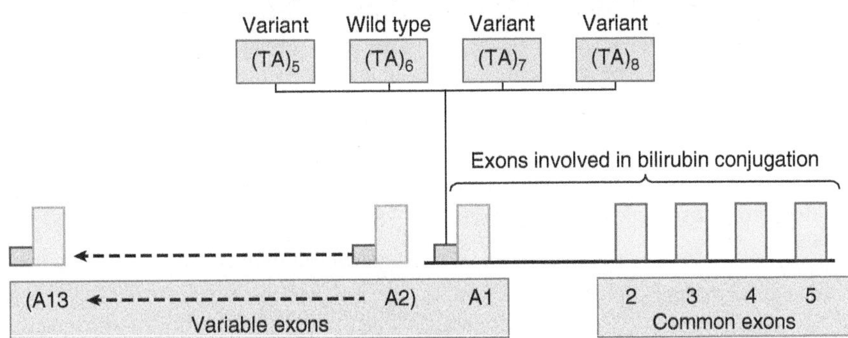

Fig. 91.4 Schematic representation of the genomic structure of the *UGT1* gene complex. Variable exon 1A1 and common exons 2 to 5 of the gene complex are the sites encoding the bilirubin-conjugating enzyme, uridine diphosphate-glucuronosyltransferase. Variable exons 1A2 to 1A13 do not participate in bilirubin metabolism. Genetic mutations associated with absent or decreased enzyme activity, which cause deficiencies of bilirubin conjugation, have been localized to this variable exon 1A1, its promoter, or the common exons 2 to 5. The upper section of the diagram demonstrates the 1A1 promoter TATAA box possibilities. Varying combinations of the promoter alleles derive promoter genotypes, the most common of which are the wild type $(TA)_6/(TA)_6$, heterozygote $(TA)_6/(TA)_7$, and the variant homozygote form $(TA)_7/(TA)_7$.

the other variants studied.[33] Coexpression of this polymorphism with additional risk factors, not necessarily genetic, such as breast-feeding, was instrumental in increasing the risk for hyperbilirubinemia.

GENETICS OF BILIRUBIN CONJUGATION

URIDINE DIPHOSPHATE-GLUCURONOSYLTRANSFERASE 1A1 AND THE *UGT1A1* GENE

THE *UGT* GENE

The *UGT* gene is a superfamily of genes whose function is to encode the conjugation of glucuronic acid to a variety of substrates and to facilitate their elimination from the body. The *UGT1A1* gene isoform, which belongs to the *UGT1* gene family, plays an important role in the conjugation and, therefore, elimination of bilirubin. The gene isoform has been mapped to chromosome 2q37 and was cloned by Ritter and colleagues in 1991.[34] *UGT1A1* is a major locus influencing bilirubin levels. Multiple genome-wide association studies have identified variants in *UGT1A1* to be associated with STB levels in European, East-Asian, and African American populations.[35]

As seen in Fig. 91.4, the gene-coding area comprises four common exons (exons 2, 3, 4, and 5) and 13 variable exons.[36] However, only one of the variable exons, A1, is of importance with regard to bilirubin conjugation. Variable exon A1 functions in conjunction with common exons 2 to 5 to splice mRNA from the variable exon to the common exons. This process provides a template for the synthesis of an individual enzyme isoform. Upstream of each variable exon is a regulatory noncoding promoter that contains a TATAA box sequence of nucleic acids. Coding-area mutations of variable exon A1 or the common exons 2 to 5 may result in deficiencies of bilirubin conjugation due to *structural* alterations in the UGT1A1 enzyme, such as in Crigler-Najjar syndrome. Polymorphisms of the noncoding promoter area affect bilirubin conjugation by diminishing *expression* of a normally structured enzyme. The wild-type promoter contains six sequences of TA nucleotides $(TA)_6$. Shorter TATAA box sequences $(TA)_5$, although rare, are associated with enhanced *UGT1A1* expression and, therefore, more effective bilirubin conjugation. Longer TATAA polymorphisms, such as the not infrequent $(TA)_7$ or the rare $(TA)_8$, are associated with diminished expression and, therefore, less effective bilirubin conjugation. Using a reporter gene, Beutler and colleagues demonstrated an inverse relationship between the number of (TA) repeats and the activity of the promoter through the range of five to eight (TA) repeats.[37] Allele frequency of the $(TA)_7$ promoter varies among populations (0.35 in Sephardic Jews in Israel,[7] 0.39 in Caucasians, 0.16 in Asians, and 0.43 in individuals of African descent[37]), while in Nigerian neonates the distribution of $(TA)_6$ and $(TA)_7$ was almost equal.[38] Homozygosity for $(TA)_7$, also known as *UGT1A1*28*, is associated with Gilbert syndrome in adults and with hyperbilirubinemia in neonates, primarily when in combination with additional icterogenic factors such as G6PD deficiency.[7] The high frequency of $(TA)_7$ in Nigerians and individuals of African descent may contribute to the high incidence of kernicterus associated with G6PD deficiency in these ethnic groups.[39,40]

HEREDITARY DISEASES RESULTING IN HYPERBILIRUBINEMIA

HEREDITARY CONDITIONS RESULTING IN INCREASED HEMOLYSIS

HEMOLYSIS: A POTENTIATOR OF BILIRUBIN NEUROTOXICITY

There are considerable data[13,41] to suggest that increased hemolysis may potentiate bilirubin neurotoxicity—that is, in the presence of hemolysis, neurotoxicity may develop at lower levels of STB than in newborns without obvious hemolysis. Furthermore, some hemolytic conditions with a hereditary basis are important in the pathophysiology of acute bilirubin encephalopathy and kernicterus (Box 91.2). Because of their clinical importance regarding bilirubin neurotoxicity and their relative frequency in some populations, G6PD deficiency, hereditary spherocytosis (HS), and pyruvate kinase (PK) deficiency will be discussed in some detail.

GLUCOSE-6-PHOSPHATE DEHYDROGENASE DEFICIENCY

G6PD deficiency is a common enzyme deficiency, estimated to affect hundreds of millions of people globally.[42-45] The condition is a well-documented hereditary cause of extreme hyperbilirubinemia and bilirubin encephalopathy and as such has major public health implications.[46-49] It is not surprising that in low- and middle-income countries, especially where G6PD deficiency is indigenous and occurs with a frequency of 10% or greater, the condition is frequently associated with neonatal mortality and/or neurodevelopmental disorders.[50] Moreover, it is remarkable that in series of neonates with extreme hyperbilirubinemia and/or kernicterus from Western countries, including the United States (Kernicterus Registry), Canada, the

Box 91.2 Some Hereditary Conditions Known to, or With the Potential to, Influence the Pathophysiology of Neonatal Hyperbilirubinemia

A. Hereditary conditions with the potential of increasing bilirubin production
 Glucose-6-phosphate dehydrogenase deficiency
 Hereditary spherocytosis
 Pyruvate kinase deficiency
 Red blood cell membrane abnormalities
 Hereditary spherocytosis
 Elliptocytosis, ovalocytosis, pyknocytosis
 Hemoglobinopathies
 Unstable hemoglobinopathies
B. Hereditary conditions with the potential of diminishing bilirubin conjugation
 Gilbert syndrome
 Crigler-Najjar syndrome types I and II

United Kingdom and Ireland, the Netherlands and Australia, G6PD deficiency featured prominently among identified etiologies for hyperbilirubinemia and was overrepresented relative to the low overall background frequency in these countries.[39,51-54] In a recent report from northern California, G6PD activity was deficient in 40% of infants tested for the condition who had STB levels of 30 mg/dL or greater.[55] Of 20 claims against the UK National Health Service alleging that kernicterus was preventable, G6PD deficiency was found in 6 (30%).[56] The high incidence of G6PD deficiency associated with severe neonatal hyperbilirubinemia in countries with a low overall frequency of the condition can be attributed to immigration patterns, slave trade, and modern-day ease of travel. These factors have changed the distribution of G6PD deficiency from one confined to the regions in which it is indigenous, including the Mediterranean basin, Central and West Africa, the Middle East, and Asia, to one that reaches many parts of the globe.

Physiology of Glucose-6-Phosphate Dehydrogenase

The primary function of G6PD is the stabilization of the RBC membrane and protection from oxidative damage, which may lead to hemolysis.[43-45] The enzyme catalyzes the first step in the hexose monophosphate pathway. Oxidation of glucose-6-phosphate to 6-phosphogluconolactone results in the reduction of nicotinamide adenine dinucleotide phosphate (NADP) to its reduced form, NADPH. The latter substance is cardinal to the glutathione antioxidative mechanism by which reduced glutathione is oxidized. For the system to function, reduced glutathione must be regenerated from the oxidized form. This process is dependent on hydrogen ion donation, which is contributed by NADPH produced by G6PD. In the G6PD deficiency state, NADPH will not be available, and reduced glutathione will not be regenerated. The pathway also contributes to catalase function, another important antioxidant. As complete absence of G6PD is probably incompatible with life, in the steady state, residual G6PD may be sufficient to prevent significant oxidative damage. However, in a situation of oxidative stress, an excess of oxygen free radicals may overwhelm the remaining protective mechanisms, and cell damage will occur. Unlike other body cells, in RBCs there is no substitute source of NADPH, explaining the predilection of the RBC membrane to G6PD deficiency-associated oxidative damage with resultant hemolysis.[45]

Extreme Hyperbilirubinemia in G6PD-Deficient Neonates

The most dreaded form of hemolysis associated with G6PD deficiency occurs in neonates. An exponential rise in STB to extreme levels may be sudden, severe, and unpredictable. Acute bilirubin encephalopathy may ensue with the potential for chronic manifestations of KSD or even death. Frequently no specific trigger can be identified, but because the episodes resemble those associated with exposure to known triggers, it is presumed that these attacks are trigger induced. Extreme hyperbilirubinemia with a sudden and unpredictable onset in G6PD-deficient newborns may limit the potential for complete elimination of kernicterus.

In spite of the severe hyperbilirubinemia, the typical hematologic findings that suggest hemolysis in adults and older children (e.g., decreasing hemoglobin/hematocrit, elevated reticulocyte count, and morphologic changes suggestive of hemolysis on the peripheral blood smear) may be absent in hemolyzing G6PD-deficient neonates. This has led some to conclude, erroneously, that these events are not the result of hemolysis.[33,57] Kaplan and colleagues, however, reported a 35-week gestation, G6PD-deficient neonate who was readmitted with sudden-onset jaundice and an STB value of 33 mg/dL.[58] The blood carboxyhemoglobin (COHb) level, reflective of hemolysis, was several-fold that of normal, clearly demonstrating the presence of a severe hemolytic process; however, the hemoglobin was slightly higher (15.1 g/dL) than it had been prior to discharge (14.8 g/dL), and the reticulocyte count was only 1.4%.

Additional evidence supporting the role of hemolysis in severely hyperbilirubinemic G6PD-deficient neonates was recently reviewed.[59] Slusher and colleagues demonstrated significantly higher levels of blood COHb in Nigerian hyperbilirubinemic G6PD-deficient neonates compared with those with a normal G6PD screen. In addition, G6PD deficiency was associated with a poorer prognosis with regard to jaundice-related death, kernicterus, and the need for exchange transfusion.[40] Similarly, Necheles and colleagues demonstrated high levels of COHb in Greek G6PD-deficient newborns with severe hyperbilirubinemia.[59]

Moderate Neonatal Hyperbilirubinemia

Many G6PD-deficient neonates manifest a moderate form of jaundice. STB levels are significantly higher than those of the G6PD-normal population.[60-62] The jaundice may either resolve spontaneously or require phototherapy; exchange transfusion may occasionally be necessary. Studies using COHbc and end-tidal carbon monoxide (ETCOc) have demonstrated that G6PD-deficient neonates had moderately increased rates of hemolysis compared with normal controls.[60-62] However, G6PD-deficient infants in whom moderate hyperbilirubinemia developed had similar levels of COHbc or ETCOc compared with those G6PD-deficient newborns who remained non-hyperbilirubinemic. Furthermore, increase COHbc concentrations did not correlate with the STB in the G6PD-deficient newborns as they did in controls. Increased hemolysis, therefore, could not be implicated as the primary icterogenic factor in this moderate form of jaundice. Decreased serum concentrations of diconjugated bilirubin, reflective of reduced UGT1A1 enzyme activity, were demonstrated in hyperbilirubinemic (STB >15 mg/dL) neonates with G6PD deficiency compared with healthy controls, demonstrating a predilection for diminished bilirubin conjugation in these neonates.[63,64] Diminished concentrations of total conjugated bilirubin as well as its mono- and diconjugated fractions were also reported in G6PD-deficient neonates who were non-hyperbilirubinemic at the time of sampling but who subsequently developed hyperbilirubinemia.[64] Consequently, the diminished bilirubin conjugation was found to be due to an

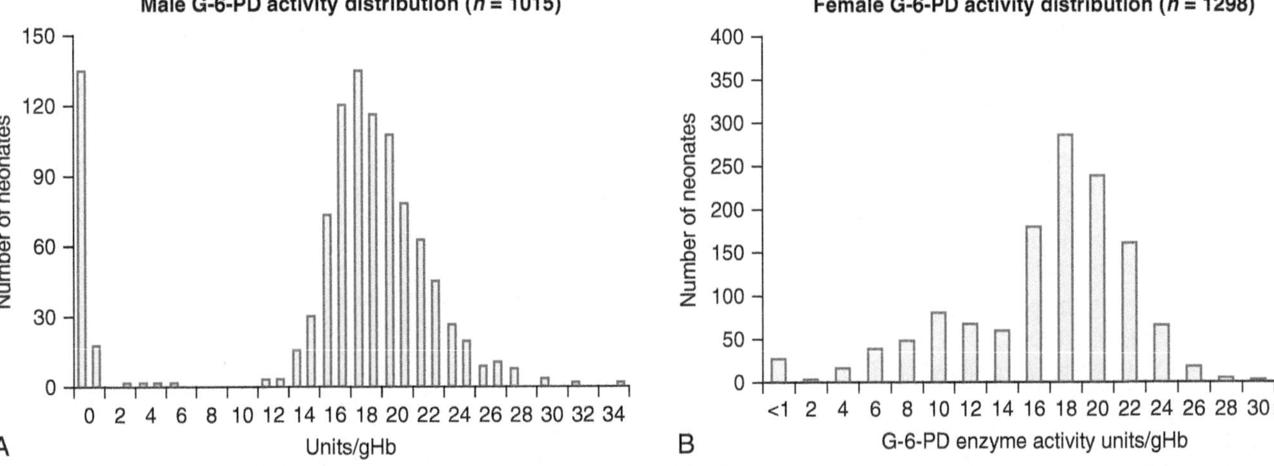

Fig. 91.5 (A) Distribution of glucose 6-phosphate dehydrogenase *(G6PD)* activity among the male neonates. Note separation into two subgroups, G6PD deficient and G6PD normal, with no overlap between the groups. (B) Distribution of G6PD activity among the female neonates. In contrast to the male distribution, there was no clear distinction among the three subgroups (G6PD–deficient homozygotes, normal homozygotes, and heterozygotes) based on phenotype. (From Algur N, Avraham I, Hammerman C, Kaplan M. Quantitative neonatal glucose-6-phosphate dehydrogenase screening: distribution, reference values, and classification by phenotype. *J Pediatr.* 2012;161:197–200, with permission.)

interaction between G6PD deficiency and the *UGT1A1* $(TA)_7$ promoter polymorphism.[7]

It is important to note that in many G6PD-deficient newborns, the bilirubin production-conjugation equilibrium is inherently imbalanced. Should an infant be exposed to additional oxidative stress or should the bilirubin-elimination system be further compromised, such as by late prematurity, the equilibrium may be placed in jeopardy with the potential for severe hyperbilirubinemia.[65] In contrast to the jaundice that follows the acute and unpredictably severe hemolysis, this milder form of jaundice can be predicted by predischarge serum bilirubin testing.[66]

Genetics of G6PD Deficiency: Genotype Versus Phenotype[43–45]

Because G6PD deficiency is an X-linked trait, males may be either normal hemizygotes or deficient hemizygotes depending on whether the maternally derived X chromosome is mutated. There should be no problem in differentiating between the two genotypes using biochemical enzyme assays. Females, on the other hand, because they have one maternally derived and one paternally derived X chromosome, may be normal homozygotes, deficient homozygotes, or heterozygotes depending on the possible combinations of normal or mutated chromosomes.[67] Heterozygotes may be difficult to categorize. Because of nonrandom X chromosome inactivation, up to 10% of heterozygotes may be phenotypically G6PD deficient, while another 10% may have normal enzyme activity. As shown in Fig. 91.5, males separate into two distinct groups (see Fig. 91.5A), but in females there is actually a continuum with no clear distinction among the three possible genotypes (see Fig. 91.5B).[68] In many heterozygotes, however, substantial numbers of G6PD–deficient RBCs may coexist with normal RBCs.[69] Should exposure to a hemolytic trigger occur, these G6PD-deficient cells may hemolyze with the release of heme and an increase in STB. Despite previous teaching that heterozygotes have sufficient enzyme activity to protect against the dangers of hemolysis,[44] extreme hyperbilirubinemia with encephalopathy and even death have been reported in heterozygotes.[70–72]

PYRUVATE KINASE DEFICIENCY

PK deficiency is a common glycolytic defect causing nonspherocytic hemolytic anemia.[73,74] In the United States, it is a common etiology for nonspherocytic, DAT-negative, hemolytic neonatal jaundice, second only to G6PD deficiency.[74,75] In the newborn the condition is associated with severe hemolytic crises and hyperbilirubinemia,[76–78] and kernicterus has been reported.[79]

PK is crucial to energy production as it catalyzes the conversion of phosphoenolpyruvate to pyruvate and the formation of adenosine triphosphate (ATP) from adenosine diphosphate in the Embden-Meyerhof pathway. Because RBCs lack mitochondria, it is responsible for the production of nearly 50% of their total ATP.

In humans, four PK isoenzymes (M1, M2, L, and R) are encoded by two separate genes (*PK-M* and *PK-LR*). Erythrocyte PK is synthesized under the control of the *PK-LR* gene located on chromosome 1 (1q21). Although there are both hepatic and RBC forms of the enzyme, in the deficiency state, only the RBC form is affected.[73] Ethnic and regional differences may modify the occurrence of some of the mutations. Inheritance is autosomal recessive.[80] Most people with the clinical form of the deficiency are compound heterozygotes, having inherited one paternal and one maternal mutant *PK* gene.[75]

Lack of ATP results in hemolysis and may lead to severe neonatal anemia and early hyperbilirubinemia.[81,82] In patients with homozygous null mutations, no functional enzyme is formed, and newborns may be born severely anemic or even die in utero.[73] In those born alive, anemia, reticulocytosis, and severe jaundice may be encountered.

HEREDITARY SPHEROCYTOSIS

HS occurs in one in 2500 to 5000 persons of Northern European descent[83,84] and is the most common hereditary RBC membrane defect that leads to acute hemolysis in the newborn.[85–87] The principal abnormality in HS erythrocytes is loss of membrane surface area relative to intracellular volume, which leads to spherical, rather than biconcave-shaped erythrocytes.[88] HS is characterized by a deficiency in one or more RBC membrane proteins, resulting in RBCs that have higher than usual metabolic requirements and are prematurely trapped and destroyed in the spleen.[89] Inheritance is autosomal dominant, but can also be recessive or due to de novo mutations.[88]

Mutations responsible for HS can lie in one of five genes that encode transmembrane proteins (i.e., band 3), membrane skeletal proteins (i.e., a- and b-spectrin), or proteins mediating the attachment of the latter to the former (i.e., protein 4.2 and ankyrin). The majority of mutations leading to HS are found in ankyrin and spectrin.[88-91]

HS may be associated with hyperbilirubinemia, and kernicterus has been described.[91] Of 178 affected Italian term, predominantly breast-fed newborns, 112 (63%) developed neonatal hyperbilirubinemia requiring phototherapy.[92] Variability in the clinical picture may be due to different molecular defects or to bone marrow compensation.[89] In its most severe form, HS may result in hydrops fetalis with intrauterine death.[93]

HEREDITARY CONDITIONS CAUSING DIMINISHED BILIRUBIN CONJUGATION

UGT1A1 POLYMORPHISMS AND MUTATIONS IN THE MANIFESTATION OF DISEASE

UGT1A1 (TA)$_7$ Promoter Polymorphism

Gilbert syndrome is a condition, manifest in adolescents and adults, in which the STB is modestly elevated in the absence of additional evidence of hepatic insufficiency. The genetic background to the condition has been identified in Caucasian populations as an additional TA repeat, (TA)$_7$, in the TATAA box of the *UGT1A1* gene promoter (*UGT1A1*28*).[94,95] In the absence of additional icterogenic factors, bilirubin values are only modestly elevated in association with the gene polymorphism, but overt hyperbilirubinemia does not usually occur.[7,96-100] Studies from Italy and Denmark examined the role of *UGT1A1*28* in the pathophysiology of severe hyperbilirubinemia. Neither study demonstrated an effect of the (TA)$_7$ polymorphism on severe neonatal hyperbilirubinemia. In combination with additional icterogenic factors, however, this gene's effect may be exacerbated (see below).

Gly71Arg Mutation

UGT1A1 promoter polymorphisms, while common in Caucasian populations, are rare in Asians.[36] The most common mutation associated with Gilbert syndrome in Asians is a coding area mutation, G>A at nucleotide 211, in which arginine replaces glycine at position 71 of the corresponding protein product. The variant gene, *G71R*, is known as *UGT1A1*6*. In a population of Japanese newborns, Maruo and colleagues[101] demonstrated that in those with hyperbilirubinemia, carriage of the *G71R* mutation was twice that of non-hyperbilirubinemic counterparts (allele frequency 0.34 versus 0.16). Several additional studies have confirmed the association of *G71R* with neonatal hyperbilirubinemia in Asian populations.[102] In contrast to *UGT1A1*28*, in which additional icterogenic factors appear to be necessary to cause neonatal hyperbilirubinemia, *UGT1A1*6* does not seem to require potentiating factors but functions independently in the pathogenesis of jaundice. In a recent meta-analysis comprising 18 studies from six countries,[103] the risk for neonatal hyperbilirubinemia was significantly increased in carriers of the 211 G>A allele than in those who were G/G allele carriers (OR, 2.37; 95% CI, 1.99 to 2.81). Studies using blood carboxyhemoglobin, corrected for ambient CO to reflect endogenous carbon monoxide production (COHbc), demonstrated a slightly although significantly increased hemolysis in Japanese newborns compared with Caucasians.[104] As hemolysis was only slightly increased, it stands to reason that diminished conjugation should be more contributory to neonatal hyperbilirubinemia in Asians.

GILBERT SYNDROME MARKERS AND PROLONGED BREAST MILK JAUNDICE

Genetic mutations may be important in the pathophysiology of prolonged breast milk jaundice. A genetic predisposition to develop prolonged neonatal hyperbilirubinemia in breast-fed infants was reported in association with the TATA box promoter polymorphism of the *UGT1A1* gene.[103] In this study, the incidence of homozygosity for *UGT1A1* promoter genotypes (TA)$_7$ and 5/7 heterozygosity was five times greater in cases of very prolonged jaundice (31%) than in cases of acute jaundice (6%). Žaja and colleagues reported a 42% frequency of homozygosity for *UGT1A1*28* in breast-fed newborns with prolonged jaundice, compared with 12% in controls.[105]

*UGT1A1*6* may also contribute to the pathophysiology of prolonged breast milk jaundice. Maruo and colleagues[106] documented at least one *UGT1A1* mutation in 16 of 17 Japanese breast-fed infants with prolonged hyperbilirubinemia, of whom 7 were homozygous for 211 G>A (*G71R*). This same group reported homozygosity for *UGT1A1*6* in 51.7% of 170 affected infants and heterozygosity for this mutation in 15.2%. These gene frequencies far exceed the background frequency in the Japanese population (estimated allele frequency 0.16, estimated homozygosity 2.56%).[107] In a study from Taiwan, Chang and colleagues reported that of 35 newborns with prolonged breast milk jaundice, 29 had at least one mutation of the *UGT1A1* gene, of which variation at nucleotide 211 was the most frequent.[108]

CRIGLER-NAJJAR SYNDROME[109,110]

Crigler-Najjar Syndrome Type I

Crigler-Najjar syndrome type I is a rare, autosomal recessive disease characterized by an almost complete absence of hepatic UGT activity. Because the coding area of the *UGT* gene is mutated, the enzyme produced is structurally abnormal, with no bilirubin-conjugating capacity. In the homozygous form, severe unconjugated hyperbilirubinemia develops during the first 3 days of life and progresses in an unremitting fashion. Stools are pale yellow, and bile bilirubin concentrations are less than 10 mg/dL (171 μmol/L) (normal being 50 to 100 mg/dL [855 to 1710 μmol/L]), with total absence of bilirubin glucuronide in bile. Bilirubin glucuronide formation measured in vitro with liver obtained by biopsy is absent. Formation of most non-bilirubin glucuronides is either severely reduced or absent.

With either direct hepatic enzymatic assay or indirect measurement of glucuronide formation, both parents are found to have partial defects (approximately 50% normal). Persistence of unconjugated hyperbilirubinemia at STB concentrations of greater than 20 mg/dL (342 μmol/L) beyond the first week of life, or repeated need for phototherapy in the absence of an obvious cause of hemolysis, should prompt investigation for this syndrome. Diagnosis is currently performed by *UGT1A1* gene analysis. An update of the genetic mutations known to date was recently published.[111]

Crigler-Najjar Syndrome Type II

Crigler-Najjar syndrome type II (also known as *Arias disease*) is more common than type I and is typically benign. STB levels generally do not exceed 20 mg/dL (342 μmol/L), and kernicterus is rare. Evidence of hemolytic disease is absent (although it may occur coincidentally), and neonates are otherwise healthy. A difference between Crigler-Najjar syndrome type I and type II is the response to phenobarbital among patients with type II disease.[112] Jaundiced neonates with type II disease respond readily to oral administration of phenobarbital with a sharp decline in STB concentrations, whereas individuals with type I disease demonstrate no such change. Crigler-Najjar syndrome type II occurs both as an autosomal recessive and dominant inheritance. As with Crigler-Najjar syndrome type I, current diagnostic methods for type II disease include *UGT1A1* gene sequencing.[113]

GENETIC INTERACTIONS IN THE PATHOPHYSIOLOGY OF NEONATAL HYPERBILIRUBINEMIA

Seldom is one single etiology responsible for the development of neonatal hyperbilirubinemia. Just as bilirubin production and elimination combine to result in a given STB, so may interaction between genes affecting the metabolism of bilirubin increase the STB to a degree greater than would be expected by a simple arithmetic addition. Kaplan and colleagues reported an intriguing interaction between G6PD deficiency and *UGT1A1* $(TA)_7$ promoter polymorphism.[7] In the absence of the variant promoter, the incidence of any STB value greater than 15 mg/dL was similar between G6PD-deficient and G6PD-normal newborns (9.7% and 9.9%, respectively). However, the combination of G6PD deficiency with $(TA)_7$ promoter polymorphism led to a dramatic increase in the incidence of hyperbilirubinemia. This additive effect was not seen in newborns with normal G6PD levels. Subsequently Huang and colleagues demonstrated a similar icterogenic effect in Taiwanese newborns who were both G6PD-deficient and homozygous for the 211 G>A variation.[114] Interactions between icteric risk factors (e.g., genetic mutations and polymorphisms) and environmental factors may exacerbate hyperbilirubinemia to an even greater degree. A paradigm of this concept may be the interaction of G6PD deficiency, *UGT1A1* $(TA)_n$ promoter polymorphism (*UGT1A1*28*), and the environment.[49]

Interactions between *UGT1A1* promoter polymorphism and hemolytic conditions in the pathophysiology of neonatal hyperbilirubinemia have been reported with HS[115,141] and ABO incompatibility,[116] although this latter finding was not confirmed in a recent study from Denmark.[117]

To estimate the risk for gene interactions in the development of neonatal hyperbilirubinemia in the United States, Lin and colleagues[119] studied allele frequencies of mutations and polymorphisms of *G6PD, UGT1A1*, and *SLCO1B1* in DNA samples obtained from the National Human Genome Research Institute and thought to be representative of the US population. A high rate of gene coinheritance in samples suggested a potentially important role for genetic polymorphism coexpression in neonatal hyperbilirubinemia. As stated earlier, Kaplan and colleagues studied possible interactions between *HO-1* promoter polymorphisms and G6PD deficiency, but did not demonstrate a cumulative interaction on serum bilirubin concentrations.[17]

The cumulative effect of genetic and nonhereditary risk factors, including breast-feeding, variant 211 in the *UGT1A1* gene, and variant 388 in the *OATP2* gene, on the development of neonatal hyperbilirubinemia was demonstrated by Huang and colleagues.[6] Presence of one, two, or three significant risk factors increased the OR for hyperbilirubinemia progressively to 8.46 (95% CI, 2.75 to 34.48; $P < .001$), 22.0 (95% CI, 5.50 to 88.0; $P < .001$), and 88.0 (95% CI, 12.50 to 642.50; $P < .001$), respectively.

GENOME WIDE ASSOCIATION GENETIC STUDIES

We are unaware of any genome wide association studies investigating the control of bilirubin metabolism in newborns. Adult studies have demonstrated that *UGT1A1* and *SLCO1B1* are important genes controlling serum bilirubin levels, reaching genome wide significance.[120,121] In Sardinia, three loci (*UGT1A1*, G6PD, and the *SLCO1B1* variant *SLCO1B3)* were associated with the modulation of STB levels, although *UGT1A1* had a predominant effect.[122] It would thus appear that three genes, *UGT1A1, SLCO1B1* or its B3 variant, and G6PD deficiency, are the important genes modulating serum bilirubin levels.[123]

HETEROZYGOSITY AND THE POTENTIAL FOR SEVERE HYPERBILIRUBINEMIA

Although previously thought not to play an important part in the pathogenesis of disease, heterozygosity is becoming more apparent as a factor with the potential to influence STB concentrations. The potential exists for several heterozygosities to combine, resulting in severe disease phenotypes, a phenomenon known as *synergistic heterozygosity*.[124] Combinations may be *compound*, in which two different mutations are present at a given locus, or *double*, in which mutated alleles are found in each of two separate gene loci. Extreme hyperbilirubinemia with kernicterus and death in a female newborn resulting from synergistic heterozygosity of a single G6PD gene and a single *UGT1A1*28* gene has been reported.[70] In a recent study by Skierka and colleagues, 7 of 11 infants younger than 3 months of age with hyperbilirubinemia were compound heterozygotes for coding or noncoding *UGT1A1* polymorphisms or mutations.[10]

RACIAL AND ETHNIC CONTRIBUTIONS TO NEONATAL HYPERBILIRUBINEMIA

The severity of jaundice and hyperbilirubinemia varies significantly among different ethnic groups. Some races or ethnicities, among which African American and Asian neonates are well-noted, have lower or higher incidences of hyperbilirubinemia than others. American Black race has long been considered protective against hyperbilirubinemia. In a Boston, MA-based epidemiologic study of 12,023 newborns, Black race was protective against any STB value of 10 mg/dL or greater (OR 0.49, 95% CI 0.40 to 0.60).[125] In that study, Black race was also protective against higher levels of hyperbilirubinemia: of the subgroup who did develop a STB of 10.0 mg/dL or greater, 6.9% of white but only 2.2% of Black infants developed an STB of 15.0 mg/dL or greater. In a study of 1370 neonates[126] from 9 multinational centers, 120 (8.8%) developed hyperbilirubinemia, defined as an STB greater than or equal to the 95th percentile on the hour-specific bilirubin nomogram.[127] Eleven percent of the white newborns developed hyperbilirubinemia, compared with only 4.9% of Black newborns. Black race is listed in the 2004 AAP Hyperbilirubinemia Guidelines as a factor decreasing the risk of significant jaundice.[128]

On the other hand, Kirkman reported a higher incidence of ABO incompatibility disease in Black neonates than in whites.[129] Kaplan et al. found a 12.8% frequency of G6PD deficiency among 500 African American neonates in Chicago.[129] Although no cases of kernicterus were encountered in this series, G6PD deficient newborns had a higher rate of hyperbilirubinemia (STB > 95th percentile) than controls (21.9% vs. 6.7%, relative risk 3.27, 95% CI 1.83 to 5.86). End tidal carbon monoxide values, reflecting hemolysis, were also higher in the G6PD deficient group than in controls. Black infants are also at increased risk of kernicterus. In the US-based Kernicterus Registry comprising a series of 125 cases of kernicterus, 32 (26%) were of Black race,[39] overrepresented among the 12% of individuals who are Black in the US population. In the United Kingdom and Ireland, Black race was found to be an independent risk factor for bilirubin encephalopathy.[52] Recently, in a Californian survey, Wickramasinghe et al. confirmed that black infants had a lower risk of developing total serum bilirubin levels greater than or equal to 20 mg/dL than white counterparts, but were at greater risk than white infants of developing extreme hyperbilirubinemia (levels ≥30 mg/dL) (relative risk 4.2, 95% CI 1.33 to 13.2).[131] Black newborns in Central and West Africa have a high incidence of severe neonatal hyperbilirubinemia and kernicterus.[40,50]

The increased risk of extreme hyperbilirubinemia and kernicterus in black newborns may be explained in part by the high incidence of G6PD deficiency in this population group[130] and a higher frequency of the $(TA)_7$ promoter polymorphism *UGT1A1*28* than Caucasian populations,[38] as described earlier in this chapter, which may be further exacerbated when coexpressed with G6PD deficiency.[7] Thus within the African or African American population there may be a subgroup of neonates at risk of developing hyperbilirubinemia or kernicterus.

Asian newborns, including Chinese, Japanese, and Koreans, have mean maximal STB concentrations higher than those of Caucasian and African American neonates. Autopsy proven kernicterus is also higher in Asians than in the latter groups.[132,133] Asian ethnicity is also associated with prolonged neonatal jaundice.[134]

RACIAL AND ETHNIC EFFECTS ON TRANSCUTANEOUS NOMOGRAMS

Both the 2004 AAP hyperbilirubinemia guidelines[128] and a subsequent 2009 update with clarifications[135] recommend that STB or transcutaneous bilirubin (TcB) values be plotted, for their interpretation and for prediction of subsequent hyperbilirubinemia, on a nomogram. The nomogram referred to in both statements is that of Bhutani et al., which is an hour-specific nomogram derived from serum bilirubin values from 2840 well term and late preterm newborns, 35 weeks gestational age or greater, in Philadelphia.[127] To our knowledge, no other serum bilirubin nomogram has been published, and the Bhutani et al. nomogram is used worldwide.[127] Because serum bilirubin testing involves painful blood drawing procedures for the neonate, it is unlikely that additional serum-based bilirubin nomograms will be constructed.

TcB values are frequently plotted on the serum-based nomogram. This nomogram should be reliable for interpreting TcB values less than 15 mg/dL, but because of potential discrepancies at higher bilirubin concentrations, use of the serum-based nomogram for higher TcB values may lead to inaccuracies. The advent of modern, painless, TcB devices has made construction of TcB nomograms for various population groups feasible. In a review of 12 TcB nomograms available in 2013, de Luca demonstrated differences between various population groups, primarily related to population demographics and the predictive value of TcB values greater than 75th percentile.[135] More recently, Kaplan and Bromiker analyzed the 95th and 75th percentiles of 19 published TcB nomograms constructed in 12 different countries (Fig. 91.6).[136] These percentiles were chosen for analysis as they are thought to be predictive of hyperbilirubinemia and are also included in all the published nomograms. A wide range of TcB readings was found through the first 5 postnatal days. For the 95th percentile analysis, highest readings at 48 hours were from Greece, Taiwan, Italy, and Mongolia, while at 96 hours the highest readings were from Greece, Taiwan, Italy, and India. On the other hand, the lowest readings at 48 hours were from Israel, China, the United States and Thailand, and at 96 hours from the United States, Israel, Brazil, and Thailand. As the wide range persisted in a subanalysis performed according to the two different TcB devices used, the authors speculated that the differences documented are likely of racial or ethnic origin, reflective of variations in bilirubin metabolism between various ethnic or racial groups. Differences in feeding practices and breastfeeding rates, however, may also have contributed to the contrasting results. The authors recommend that different population and ethnic groups should construct and use their own TcB nomograms, and that use of a nomogram constructed from a population different from that of the specific newborn being tested should be carried out with caution and clinical judgment.

NEXT-GENERATION DNA SEQUENCING: WHEN CONVENTIONAL DIAGNOSTIC METHODS FAIL

Next-generation sequencing is a method for sequencing genomes at high speed and low cost. The technology enables the sequencing of thousands to millions of molecules of DNA simultaneously and offers high throughput option with the capability of sequencing multiple individuals simultaneously. Multigene evaluation can not only facilitate the diagnosis but also explain the etiology of these multigene disorders. Correct diagnosis is critical in understanding the disease process and guiding the clinical management and appropriate genetic counseling for these patients and their families.[138] Christensen and colleagues recently reported that in neonates with STB values greater than 30 mg/dL, a specific diagnosis to explain the hyperbilirubinemia was not identified in 66%.[139] To pinpoint a diagnosis, next-generation DNA sequencing using a panel of 27 genes associated with

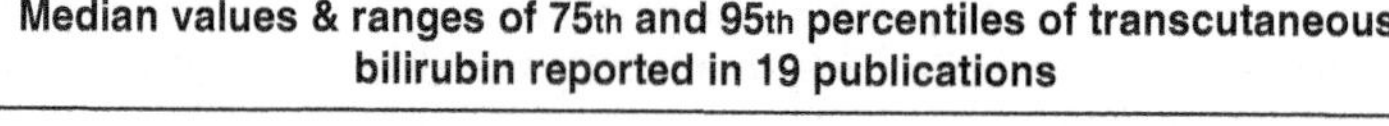

Median values & ranges of 75th and 95th percentiles of transcutaneous bilirubin reported in 19 publications

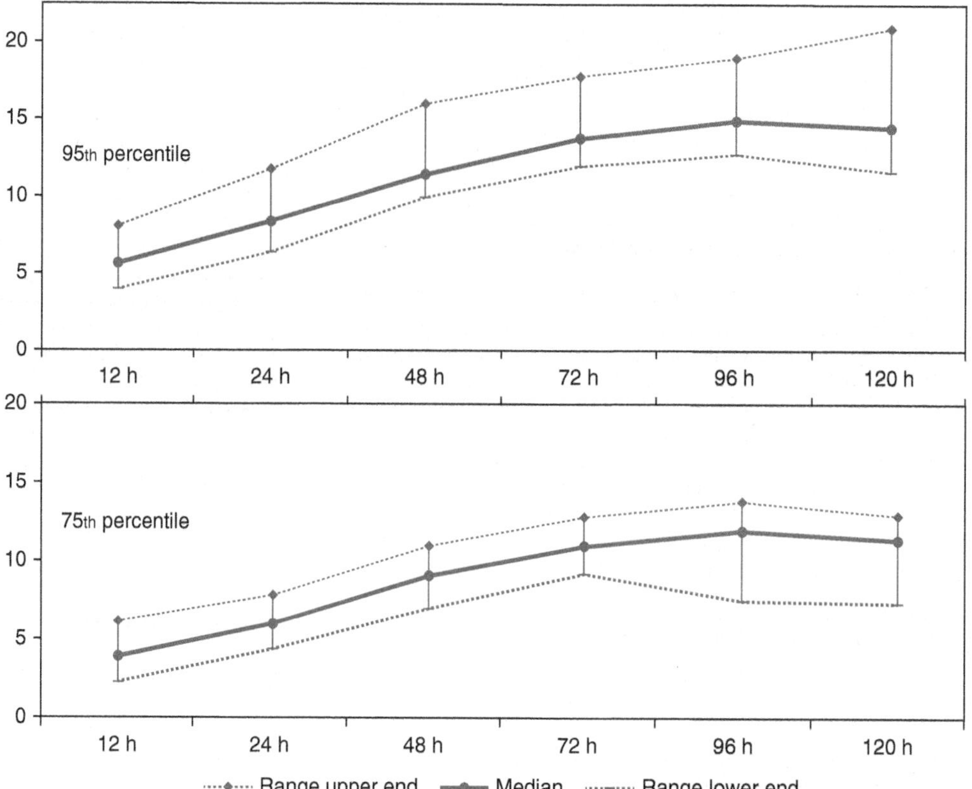

Fig. 91.6 Median transcutaneous bilirubin values, interquartile range, and upper and lower values for the range at each point studied, for 19 transcutaneous bilirubin nomogram studies analyzed. *Upper panel:* 95th percentile. *Lower panel:* 75th percentile. *IQR*, Interquartile range. (From Kaplan M, Bromiker R. variation in transcutaneous bilirubin nomograms across population groups. *J Pediatr.* 2019;208:273–279, with permission.)

neonatal hyperbilirubinemia was implemented in 10 neonates. An etiology for the hyperbilirubinemia was accomplished in every case including HS, some combined with ABO hemolytic disease, PK deficiency, severe G6PD deficiency, and ABO hemolytic disease. In a subsequent Utah registry of 7 cases of acute bilirubin encephalopathy, using a panel of 28 genes involved in increased bilirubin production or bilirubin uptake or bilirubin conjugation, Christensen et al. determined a genetic diagnosis for all.[140] These reports contrast with the high percentage of newborns labeled idiopathic in the Kernicterus registry[39] and in a report from Utah.[139] Bahr et al. proposed that using next-generation sequencing, most, if not all, cases of extreme hyperbilirubinemia will be found to have mutations or polymorphisms of genes encoding the bilirubin production or conjugation processes.[140] In an attempt to expand the above-mentioned database a study is underway in which next-generation sequencing will be used to determine the genetic etiology of 100 US cases of acute bilirubin encephalopathy.

CONCLUSION

Variations in bilirubin metabolism, the incidences of hyperbilirubinemia and bilirubin encephalopathy between racial and ethnic groups lend support to the concept of a hereditary setting in the control of extreme hyperbilirubinemia. More and more it is being determined that the metabolism of bilirubin is under genetic control. Extreme neonatal hyperbilirubinemia with feared bilirubin neurotoxicity and its devastating potential of kernicterus spectrum disorder are often the result of genetic polymorphisms and mutations. Whereas in the past the etiology of hyperbilirubinemia was frequently undetermined, it is foreseeable that in the not distant future genetic explanations will replace "idiopathic" in our designation of a diagnosis.

A complete reference list is available at www.ExpertConsult.com.

SELECT REFERENCES

4. Watchko JF, Tiribelli C. Bilirubin-induced neurologic damage-mechanisms and management approaches. *N Engl J Med*. 2013;369:2021–2030.
5. Le Pichon JB, Riordan SM, Watchko J, Shapiro SM. The neurological sequelae of neonatal hyperbilirubinemia: definitions, diagnosis and treatment of the kernicterus spectrum disorders (KSDs). *Curr Pediatr Rev*. 2017;13:199–209.
6. Huang MJ, Kua KE, Teng HC, et al. Risk factors for severe hyperbilirubinemia in neonates. *Pediatr Res*. 2004;56:682–689.
7. Kaplan M, Renbaum P, Levy-Lahad E, et al. Gilbert syndrome and glucose-6-phosphate dehydrogenase deficiency: a dose-dependent genetic interaction crucial to neonatal hyperbilirubinemia. *Proc Natl Acad Sci U S A*. 1997;94:12128–12132.
8. Watchko JF, Lin Z, Clark RH, et al. Complex multifactorial nature of significant hyperbilirubinemia in neonates. *Pediatrics*. 2009;124:e868–e877.
9. Watchko JF. Genetics and pediatric unconjugated hyperbilirubinemia. *J Pediatr*. 2013;162:1092–1094.
10. Skierka JM, Kotzer KE, Lagerstedt SA, et al. UGT1A1 genetic analysis as a diagnostic aid for individuals with unconjugated hyperbilirubinemia. *J Pediatr*. 2013;162:1146–1152.
11. Kawade N, Onishi S. The prenatal and postnatal development of UDP-glucuronyltransferase activity towards bilirubin and the effect of premature birth on this activity in the human liver. *Biochem J*. 1981;196:257–260.
12. Bhutani VK, Johnson L, Sivieri EM. Predictive ability of a predischarge hour-specific serum bilirubin for subsequent significant hyperbilirubinemia in healthy term and near-term newborns. *Pediatrics*. 1999;103:6–14.
14. Kaplan M, Muraca M, Hammerman C, et al. Imbalance between production and conjugation of bilirubin: a fundamental concept in the mechanism of neonatal jaundice. *Pediatrics*. 2002;110:e47.
15. Yamada N, Yamaya M, Okinaga S, et al. Microsatellite polymorphism in the heme oxygenase-1 gene promoter is associated with susceptibility to emphysema. *Am J Hum Genet*. 2000;66:187–195.
17. Kaplan M, Renbaum P, Hammerman C, et al. Heme oxygenase-1 promoter polymorphisms and neonatal jaundice. *Neonatology*. 2014;106:323–329.
23. Lin R, Wang X, Wang Y, et al. Association of polymorphisms in four bilirubin metabolism genes with serum bilirubin in three Asian populations. *Hum Mutat*. 2009;30:609–615.
29. Liu J, Long J, Zhang S, et al. The impact of SLCO1B1 genetic polymorphisms on neonatal hyperbilirubinemia: a systematic review with meta-analysis. *J Pediatr (Rio J)*. 2013;89:434–443.
30. Kameyama Y, Yamashita K, Kobayashi K, et al. Functional characterization of SLCO1B1 (OATP-C) variants, SLCO1B1*5, SLCO1B1*15 and SLCO1B1*15+C1007G, by using transient expression systems of HeLa and HEK293 cells. *Pharmacogenet Genomics*. 2005;15:513–522.
34. Ritter JK, Crawford JM, Owens IS. Cloning of two human liver bilirubin UDP-glucuronosyltransferase cDNAs with expression in COS-1 cells. *J Biol Chem*. 1991;266:1043–1047.
35. Chen G, Ramos E, Adeyemo A, et al. UGT1A1 is a major locus influencing bilirubin levels in African Americans. *Eur J Hum Genet*. 2012;20:463–488.
37. Beutler E, Gelbart T, Demina A. Racial variability in the UDP-glucuronosyltransferase 1 (UGT1A1) promoter: a balanced polymorphism for regulation of bilirubin metabolism? *Proc Natl Acad Sci U S A*. 1998;95:8170–8174.
38. Kaplan M, Slusher T, Renbaum P, et al. (TA)n UDP-glucuronosyltransferase 1A1 promoter polymorphism in Nigerian neonates. *Pediatr Res*. 2008;63:109–111.
39. Johnson L, Bhutani VK, Karp K, et al. Clinical report from the pilot USA Kernicterus Registry (1992 to 2004). *J Perinatol*. 2009;29:S25–S45.
43. Beutler E. G6PD deficiency. *Blood*. 1994;84:3613–3636.
44. Cappellini MD, Fiorelli G. Glucose-6-phosphate dehydrogenase deficiency. *Lancet*. 2008;371:64–74.
45. WHO Working Group. Glucose-6-phosphate dehydrogenase deficiency. *Bull World Health Organ*. 1989;67:601–611.
49. Kaplan M, Hammerman C. Glucose-6-phosphate dehydrogenase deficiency and severe neonatal hyperbilirubinemia: a complexity of interactions between genes and environment. *Semin Fetal Neonatal Med*. 2010;15:148–156.
51. Sgro M, Campbell D, Shah V. Incidence and causes of severe neonatal hyperbilirubinemia in Canada. *CMAJ*. 2006;175:587–590.
52. Manning D, Todd P, Maxwell M, Jane Platt M. Prospective surveillance study of severe hyperbilirubinaemia in the newborn in the UK and Ireland. *Arch Dis Child Fetal Neonatal Ed*. 2007;92:F342–F346.
53. Gotink MJ, Benders MJ, Lavrijsen SW, et al. Severe neonatal hyperbilirubinemia in the Netherlands. *Neonatology*. 2013;104:137–142.
54. McGillivray A, Polverino J, Badawi N, Evans N. Prospective surveillance of extreme neonatal hyperbilirubinemia in Australia. *J Pediatr*. 2016;168:82–87.e3.
58. Kaplan M, Hammerman C, Vreman HJ, et al. Severe hemolysis with normal blood count in a glucose-6-phosphate dehydrogenase deficient neonate. *J Perinatol*. 2008;28:306–309.
63. Kaplan M, Herschel M, Hammerman C, et al. Hyperbilirubinemia among African American, glucose-6-phosphate dehydrogenase-deficient neonates. *Pediatrics*. 2004;114:e213–e219.
64. Kaplan M, Rubaltelli FF, Hammerman C, et al. Conjugated bilirubin in neonates with glucose-6-phosphate dehydrogenase deficiency. *J Pediatr*. 1996;128:695–697.
65. Kaplan M, Muraca M, Vreman HJ, et al. Neonatal bilirubin production-conjugation imbalance: effect of glucose-6-phosphate dehydrogenase deficiency and borderline prematurity. *Arch Dis Child Fetal Neonatal Ed*. 2005;90:F123–F127.
68. Algur N, Avraham I, Hammerman C, Kaplan M. Quantitative neonatal glucose-6-phosphate dehydrogenase screening: distribution, reference values, and classification by phenotype. *J Pediatr*. 2012;161:197–200.
94. Bosma PJ, Chowdhury JR, Bakker C, et al. The genetic basis of the reduced expression of bilirubin UDP-glucuronosyltransferase 1 in Gilbert's syndrome. *N Engl J Med*. 1995;333:1171–1175.
95. Monaghan G, Ryan M, Seddon R, et al. Genetic variation in bilirubin UPD-glucuronosyltransferase gene promoter and Gilbert's syndrome. *Lancet*. 1996;347:578–581.
107. Maruo Y, Morioka Y, Fujito H, et al. Bilirubin uridine diphosphate-glucuronosyltransferase variation is a genetic basis of breast milk jaundice. *J Pediatr*. 2014;165:36–41.
118. Lin Z, Fontaine J, Watchko JF. Coexpression of gene polymorphisms involved in bilirubin production and metabolism. *Pediatrics*. 2008;122:e156–e162.
126. Bhutani VK, Johnson L, Sivieri EM. Predictive ability of a predischarge hour-specific serum bilirubin for subsequent significant hyperbilirubinemia in healthy term and near-term newborns. *Pediatrics*. 1999;103:6–14.
127. American Academy of Pediatrics Subcommittee on Hyperbilirubinemia. Management of hyperbilirubinemia in the newborn infant 35 or more weeks of gestation. *Pediatrics*. 2004;114:297–316.
129. Kaplan M, Herschel M, Hammerman C, et al. Hyperbilirubinemia among African American, glucose-6-phosphate dehydrogenase-deficient neonates. *Pediatrics*. 2004;114:e213–e219.
130. Wickremasinghe AC, Kuzniewicz MW, Newman TB. Black race is not protective against hazardous bilirubin levels. *J Pediatr*. 2013;162:1068–1069.
136. Kaplan M, Bromiker R. Variation in transcutaneous bilirubin nomograms across population groups. *J Pediatr*. 2019;208:273–278.e1.
137. Rets A, Clayton AL, Christensen RD, Agarwal AM. Molecular diagnostic update in hereditary hemolytic anemia and neonatal hyperbilirubinemia. *Int J Lab Hematol*. 2019;41(suppl 1):95–101.
138. Christensen RD, Lambert DK, Henry E, et al. Unexplained extreme hyperbilirubinemia among neonates in a multihospital healthcare system. *Blood Cells Mol Dis*. 2013;50:105–109.
139. Christensen RD, Agarwal AM, George TI, et al. Acute neonatal bilirubin encephalopathy in the State of Utah. *Blood Cells Mol Dis*. 2009-2018;72:10–13.
140. Bahr TM, Christensen RD, Agarwal AM, et al. The Neonatal Acute Bilirubin Encephalopathy Registry (NABER): background, aims, and protocol. *Neonatology*. 2019;115:242–246.

92 Mechanistic Aspects of Phototherapy for Neonatal Hyperbilirubinemia

Vinod K. Bhutani | Christina M. Konecny | Ronald J. Wong

INTRODUCTION

The pathways by which light reduces levels of circulating bilirubin and how these mechanisms decrease the levels of possible toxic byproducts of bilirubin have been subjects of intense inquiries and debates since the 1960s.[1] The first United States national symposium on neonatal hyperbilirubinemia and phototherapy convened in 1969 by the March of Dimes Foundation reported on the effect of light on bilirubin metabolism and delineated potential clinical implications for application of phototherapy to neonatal practice.[2] Key recommendations for the clinical use of phototherapy included a directive to "involve judgments similar to those made in deciding upon the clinical use of a new drug." A new standard of care was then established with consideration of the advantages and risks of phototherapy, the likelihood of injury from hyperbilirubinemia, and risks associated with alternative treatment strategies. Over the intervening years, the mechanism of action of phototherapy has been extensively studied, and sufficient evidence is available to guide its use in term and late-preterm neonates.[3-5] However, use of phototherapy in very or extremely preterm hyperbilirubinemic infants, although apparently effective, is confounded by preterm biology, state of maturation, concurrent disease, choice of light source, device design, and inconsistent clinical implementation.

The primary success of phototherapy has been attributed to its ability to reduce an infant's risk for bilirubin neurotoxicity (i.e., *kernicterus*) and the need for exchange transfusions.[6] When phototherapy is instituted as an emergency measure in infants presenting with extreme hyperbilirubinemia (total serum/plasma bilirubin [TB] levels > 20 or 25 mg/dL) or early neurologic signs, care is taken to maximize the intensity of phototherapy delivered and to concurrently reduce the enterohepatic circulation of bilirubin.[4,7,8] This approach, previously based only on hypothesis, has been validated by recent observations that 20% to 25% of circulating bilirubin can be converted to more water-soluble, and directly excretable, configurational photoisomers within 30 minutes of exposure to light of sufficient intensity.[9] Phototherapy also generates structural isomers of bilirubin, called *lumirubins*, which are produced less efficiently but excreted more rapidly. Both types of photoproducts are believed to be less likely than bilirubin to cross the blood-brain barrier (BBB), and some investigators have proposed that this may confer neuroprotection even without enhancing excretion.

Phototherapy for neonatal hyperbilirubinemia is relatively simple and efficacious if properly applied. Disciplined efforts are now aimed at standardizing prescribing practices. Furthermore, a much better definition of the phototherapy *action spectrum* has emerged, taking into account improvements in light sources, variables affecting efficacy (such as dosimetry and hematocrit levels), and potential undesirable effects (such as heating by absorption of light wavelengths that are relatively useless therapeutically).[10-13] The advent of blue light-emitting diodes (LEDs) with their narrow bandwidths has significantly contributed to development of affordable and optimized phototherapy devices.

In this chapter, we review bilirubin photochemistry, photobiology, and photomedicine to delineate how phototherapy should be viewed as a drug that interacts with bilirubin molecules (Table 92.1). A review of selected terms related to photobiology products can be found in Box 92.1. In the spirit of *primum non nocere*, there is an obligation for clinicians to optimize therapy and deliver the safest and most effective care.

BACKGROUND

ORIGIN AND MEDICAL INNOVATION[14]

Of the three naturally occurring biologic pigments (the red of hemoglobin, the yellow of bilirubin, and the green of chlorophyll), bilirubin (Fig. 92.1) is unique in that it retains its

Table 92.1 Indices for Optimal Administration of Phototherapy.

Checklist	Recommendation	Implementation
Light source (nm)	Emission spectrum in 460–490 nm blue-green light region	Know the spectral output of the light source
Light irradiance (μW/cm²/nm)	Irradiance: ≥30 μW/cm²/nm within the 460–490-nm wavelength band	Measure irradiance over entire light footprint area to ensure uniformity
Body surface area (cm²)	Expose maximal skin area (35%–80%)	Reduce blocking of light
Timeliness of implementation	Urgent or *crash-cart* intervention for excessive hyperbilirubinemia	May perform other procedures while infant is under phototherapy
Continuity of therapy	May briefly interrupt for feeding, parental bonding, and nursing care	After confirmation of adequate TB decrease
Efficacy of intervention	Periodically measure rate of response in bilirubin load reduction	Degree of TB concentration decrease
Duration of therapy	Discontinue at desired bilirubin threshold; be aware of possible rebound increase	Serial TB measurements based on rate of decrease

TB, Total serum/plasma bilirubin.
Republished with permission from Bhutani VK, Committee on Fetus and Newborn, American Academy of Pediatrics. Phototherapy to prevent severe neonatal hyperbilirubinemia in the newborn infant 35 or more weeks of gestation. *Pediatrics*. 2011;128:1046–1052.

Box 92.1 Selected Definitions of Photobiology Products

1. Biliprotein: This is a molecular complex containing stoichiometric proportions of bile pigment and protein. The term is limited to molecules in the bile pigment.
2. Bilirubin: This term refers specifically, by convention, to the naturally produced *4Z,15Z*-IXa isomer, unless indicated otherwise.
3. Chiral: A structure that is not superimposable on its mirror image is said to be chiral.
4. Configurational isomers: These are molecules that have the same sequence of atoms and bonds but different fixed three-dimensional arrangements of these atoms. They can only be interconverted by breaking and remaking chemical bonds between adjacent atoms.
5. Conformation isomers: These are molecules that can be interconverted by rotations about single bonds between atoms and without making or breaking covalent bonds between atoms. In general, conformational isomers interconvert very rapidly at room temperature and cannot be separated.
6. *E/Z* bilirubin: A nomenclature system for unambiguously designating the arrangement of atoms around double bonds in molecules is derived from the German words *entgegen* (opposite) and *zusammen* (together). Asymmetric substituted double bonds that are not contained within a ring system can have two possible configurations, which are designated as *E* and *Z*. Pairs of *E/Z* configurational isomers are also called *geometric isomers*.
7. Photo-bilirubins: A nonspecific term that has been used to designate several products obtained by irradiating bilirubin with light. Because the structures of most bilirubin photoproducts have been elucidated, the term is now redundant and may be abandoned except for use as a collective term to describe photoisomers derived from bilirubin.
8. Photoisomerization: This reflects conversion of a bilirubin molecule to an isomeric molecule by irradiation with light.

Data from McDonagh AF, Lightner DA. 'Like a shrivelled blood orange'—bilirubin, jaundice, and phototherapy. *Pediatrics* 1985;75:443–455.

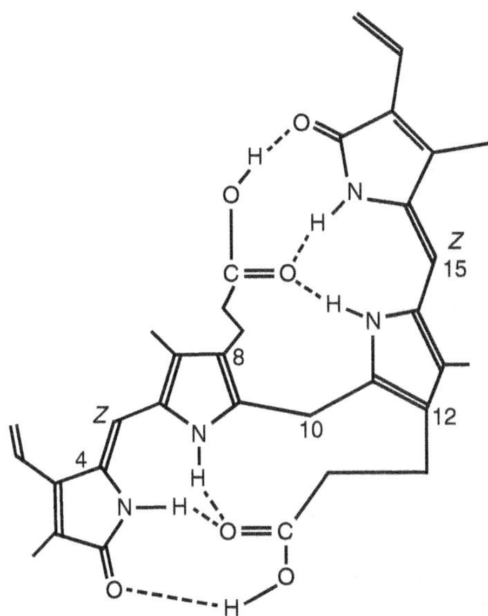

Fig. 92.1 A representation of the structure of naturally occurring bilirubin, the *Z,Z*-configurational isomer. This configuration allows all the polar groups in the molecule to be internally hydrogen bonded to other polar groups. The structure presents only a carbon-hydrogen hydrophobic surface and greatly reduced water solubility. (From McDonagh AF, Lightner DA. 'Like a shrivelled blood orange'—bilirubin, jaundice, and phototherapy. *Pediatrics.* 1985;75:443–455.)

photosensitivity.[1] Ancient and traditional knowledge of this yellow compound and social practices to use natural sunlight to reduce hyperbilirubinemia in newborns[14] intersected with scientific inquiry in 1956 to 1958 at the Rochford General Hospital, Essex, United Kingdom, where the photoreactivity of bilirubin was originally observed.[15] The scientific community was first introduced to this phenomenon at a meeting on June 1957. The "device-biodesign innovation team" included Dr. RJ Cremer (pediatrician in training), Dr. PW Perryman (biochemist), DH. Richards (laboratory technician), and B Holbrook (device engineer). They provided "evidence for the reduction of circulating bilirubin levels in some cases of neonatal jaundice by exposing these infants to sunlight." Details were published in their landmark paper in *The Lancet*, which described their "cradle illumination machine."[16] It consisted "of a hemi-cylindrical stainless-steel reflector suspended on a movable gantry and adjustable for height. Eight 24-inch 40W blue fluorescent tubes (General Electric Corporation) at 2-inch separation were arranged around the curve of the reflector." The equipment was designed for use with a bassinet that was wheeled beneath the lights, and a switch was provided to allow illumination to be halved, if desired. Light in the region of 420 to 480 nm, filtered of any dangerous ultraviolet (UV) or x-ray components, was delivered at a very high intensity. Although *The Lancet* recognized this as a contribution of importance to merit publication, it received only limited attention both in Europe and North America. The breakthrough scientific concepts, novel prototype device, and change in clinical practice, however, subsequently made their way to Italy, Brazil, and other Latin American nations.[17] A decade after the original scientific publication, Dr. JF Lucey opined "no adverse effects had been noted" with the use of phototherapy devices in Latin America.[18] However, his own studies led to serious debates about the effectiveness, timeliness, and safety of using phototherapy.[19-21] Dr. AK. Brown then conducted the pivotal National Institutes of Health (NIH)-sponsored clinical study of the effectiveness of phototherapy to prevent exchange transfusions in preterm infants.[22,23]

DEFINING BILIRUBIN LOAD: PRODUCTION AND ELIMINATION

Catabolism of heme from red blood cells (RBCs) occurs in the reticuloendothelial system, where heme oxygenase (HO) degrades heme to biliverdin, which is then rapidly reduced to the lipid-soluble unconjugated bilirubin.[24] Almost all of the bilirubin in blood is reversibly bound to its transport protein, albumin, in a form that can be distributed to a variety of tissues.[6] The bilirubin-binding capacity (BBC) of albumin controls a dynamic relationship between an infant's levels of bound and unbound ("free") bilirubin (UB) and his/her ability to *tolerate* increasing bilirubin loads.[25] The ability of albumin to bind bilirubin is influenced by a variety of molecular, biologic, and metabolic factors, including the rate of bilirubin production, an infant's gestational age (GA), and the presence of circulating competitive antagonists. UB, in dynamic equilibrium with albumin-bound

Table 92.2 Biomarkers Utilized to Assess Risk for Bilirubin Neurotoxicity and to Provide Thresholds for Phototherapy.

Biomarkers	Specifications	Clinical Use
Total serum/plasma bilirubin[6]	Consensus threshold values	Adjusted for maturity
Rate of bilirubin rise[40]	Increased; at any age	≥0.2 mg/dL/h
Bilirubin production rate[2]	Exhaled carbon monoxide (ETCOc)	>3.5 ppm
Bilirubin production rate	Carboxyhemoglobin (COHbc)	>2.5%
Unbound bilirubin[25]	≥10 nmol/L	Phototherapy threshold
Unbound bilirubin[25]	≥18 nmol/L	Crash-cart phototherapy threshold or exchange
Utilized bilirubin-binding capacity[25]	≥45%	Phototherapy threshold
Utilized bilirubin-binding capacity[25]	≥65%	Crash-cart phototherapy threshold or exchange

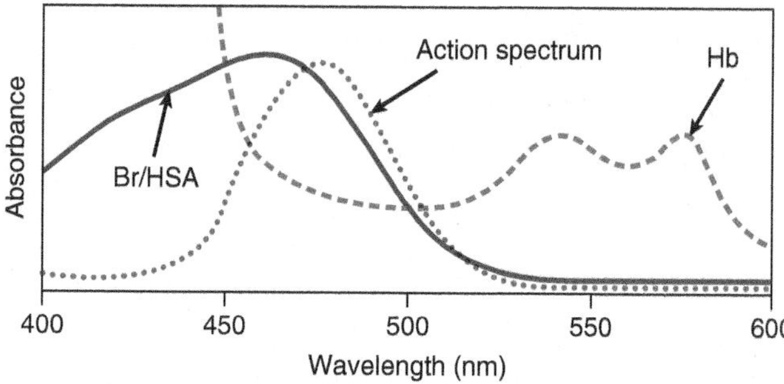

Fig. 92.2 The absorption spectrum of bilirubin: bound to albumin *(solid line)* and that of hemoglobin *(Hb)* (at 75% oxygenation, the average between venous and arterial blood in the skin) *(dashed line)*. The relative magnitudes of the two spectra represent that for total serum/plasma bilirubin at 15 mg/dL and blood *Hb* at 16.5 g/dL (hematocrit = 50%) except that the bilirubin spectrum is enhanced by a factor of four for easier visualization. It is easily seen that the Hb can effectively compete with bilirubin for light absorption. The *dotted line* is the relative fraction of light absorbed by the bilirubin and, as such, represents the first order *action spectrum* (relative efficacy as a function of *wavelength*) for bilirubin photochemistry in the blood. *Br/HSA*, Bilirubin bound to human serum albumin.

bilirubin, can cross membranes and enter cells. The cellular uptake of bilirubin is considered a reversible, passive diffusion process, such that bilirubin can be "pulled out of cells" by increasing the extracellular BBC.

The normal lipid- to water-soluble conversion of unconjugated bilirubin is mediated through a process of conjugation occurring in the liver. The uridine diphosphoglucuronosyltransferase (UGT) family of microsomal enzymes mediates active glucuronidation. Once conjugated, the now water-soluble bilirubin is excreted into urine or bile. Phototherapy-induced conversion of bilirubin to more water-soluble and colorless products bypasses this hepatobiliary excretion process.[1]

CURRENT MEASURES OF BILIRUBIN NEUROTOXICITY

Direct neurologic measures that quantify bilirubin toxicity have remained elusive. Precise assessment of neurotoxicity must address multiple domains of sensory processing. Table 92.2 lists current and prospective biomarkers for identifying infants most at risk for neurotoxicity. In clinical practice, the ability to use phototherapy more effectively and to reduce the need for exchange transfusion warrants development of an evidence-based risk assessment paradigm to replace the current consensus-based TB thresholds modulated by GA, clinical signs of hemolysis, and the bilirubin-albumin molar ratio (BAMR).[6,26]

PHOTONS, PHOTOCHEMISTRY, AND ABSORPTION SPECTRA: LIGHT AS A DRUG

Light absorption by bilirubin in the vasculature and extravascular space in the skin transforms the native toxic, nonpolar *Z,Z*-bilirubin into more readily excretable polar photoisomers: the configurational isomers *Z,E*- and *E,Z*-bilirubin and the structural isomers *Z*- and *E*-lumirubin.[5] The matching of the absorption spectrum of a bilirubin-albumin solution in vitro with a source of blue light with a peak emission of approximately 460 nm is now considered the global standard of treatment for hyperbilirubinemia.[6]

The perception of light as a continuous energy stream obscures the reality that it comprises discrete packets (quanta) of energy called *photons*. The energy *(E)* carried by a photon (quantum) is inversely proportional to the wavelength (λ) of the light as follows:

$$E = \hbar c/\lambda$$

where $\hbar$ is Planck's constant, and c is the velocity of light. From this equation, a photon at 400-nm wavelength (visibly blue) contains approximately 25% more energy than one at 500-nm wavelength (visibly green)—that is, the same light exposure measured in energy units (such as μW/cm^2) delivers approximately 25% more photons at 500 than would be the case for light at 400 nm. Photochemical reactions require absorption of single photons by individual molecules. The absorption spectrum is a plot of the probability of light absorption as a function of the wavelength of the light. Fig. 92.2 shows the absorption spectra of hemoglobin and bilirubin. Bilirubin appears yellow-orange in white light because it absorbs the blue light portion of the visual spectrum (as well as the UV portion that we cannot see). Fig. 92.2 also shows that hemoglobin strongly absorbs light throughout most of the region of the bilirubin spectrum. The spectrum in this illustration is actually that of bilirubin bound to albumin, which is the form of virtually all the bilirubin in blood.

Photons are analogous to the molecules of a drug. Therefore, the wavelength (color) of light (drug) designed to interact with the molecular target (bilirubin) can be predicted by determining its absorption by the molecular target. Additional specificity of the wavelength range may be dictated by the avoidance of untoward side effects. For example, bilirubin absorbs UV light, as do almost all biologic molecules, such as proteins and nucleic acids. UV light absorption by the latter can lead to photochemical alterations that can be deleterious. However, those without prosthetic groups do not absorb blue light; therefore, it is possible to have blue light absorbed by bilirubin without affecting proteins and nucleic acids. The number of therapeutic photons absorbed by the molecular target is analogous to the dose of a drug. The intensity or irradiance (photons per unit time) of the light is analogous to the drug dose. One way absorbed light generally differs from molecular drugs is in the deposition of heat. When a photon is absorbed by a molecule of bilirubin, the energy of the photon

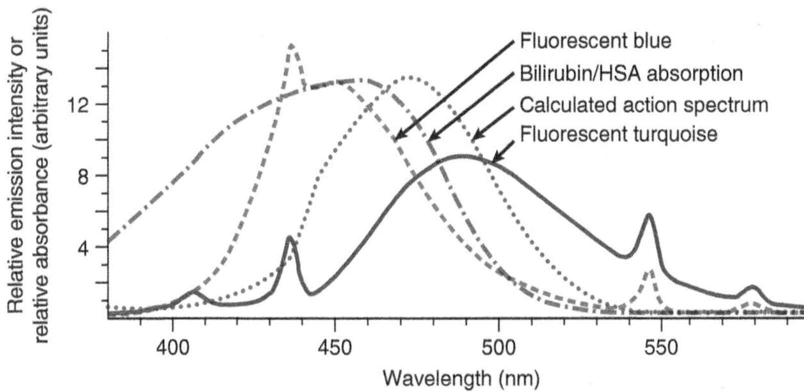

Fig. 92.3 The absorption spectrum of bilirubin bound to human serum albumin and the "action spectrum" for bilirubin photochemistry. Both are taken from Fig. 92.2, superimposed on the emission spectra of blue and turquoise fluorescent lamps. Although the blue lamp emission overlaps better with the bilirubin absorption, the turquoise lamp emission overlaps better with the action spectrum such that, for equal total irradiance, the turquoise may be more effective at driving the photochemistry of bilirubin in blood. *HSA,* Human serum albumin.

is transferred to the molecule and transformed into heat that is quickly transferred to the surrounding environment. These principles of molecular photochemistry are well described.[27]

THE ACTION SPECTRUM FOR BILIRUBIN PHOTOTHERAPY

The action spectrum of a light-driven process is a measure of its efficacy as a function of the wavelength of the light.[27] The measure of efficacy might be, for example, the rate of formation of a photochemical product for a given irradiance. For a sufficiently dilute solution of a photochemically reactive material, the action spectrum generally is identical to the absorption spectrum. This follows the basic law of photochemistry that states that light must be absorbed for a photochemical reaction to occur.[9] There are, however, many factors that can cause the action spectrum to differ, such as inhomogeneity of the material, as has been observed for a solution of bilirubin bound to albumin. In complex environments, such as in vivo, other materials present in tissues may compete for the light, acting as filters to block some wavelengths. Hemoglobin in the skin of adults and newborns is the main absorber of visible light, especially blue light, and is, in fact, an effective filter.[11] As shown in Fig. 92.3, the probability of blue light absorption by hemoglobin overwhelms the light absorption by bilirubin for the range of TB and hematocrit levels commonly found in infants. Lamola and colleagues proposed a semi-empirical model for the calculation of the action spectrum for bilirubin photochemistry in vivo using available data on skin optics.[11] The model is based upon one used to develop advanced transcutaneous bilirubinometers that can relate light reflected from the skin to assess the TB. In the model, key factors include the diffuse nature of light entering the skin, the wavelength dependence of back scatter of light from the skin, the absorbance due to melanin in the epidermis, the wavelength dependence of bilirubin photochemistry, the oxygenation level of the blood, the hemoglobin, and both intravascular and extravascular bilirubin. Calculations based on the model showed that the effect of competitive absorption of light by hemoglobin remains the predominant factor controlling the light that is absorbed by bilirubin. The result is that the probability of light-driven alterations of bilirubin in the skin of neonates as a function of wavelength (i.e., the action spectrum for phototherapy of neonatal jaundice) is predicted to be that shown in Fig. 92.2.[11] The spectrum peaks near 476 nm rather than at the maximum of the bilirubin-albumin absorption spectrum (460 nm). A corollary of the predominance of light absorption by hemoglobin in the range of light used in phototherapy is a predicted dependence of phototherapy efficacy upon the hemoglobin level of the infant; the higher the hemoglobin concentration, the lower the expected efficacy.[11,28]

PHOTOTHERAPY EFFICACY: LIGHT SOURCES, IRRADIANCE, AND DOSE

It is evident that the wavelength range of the light source must overlap the action spectrum for phototherapy to be effective. Near the beginning of the development of phototherapy, it was recognized that blue light should be effective because the visible absorption spectrum of bilirubin, presumed to reflect the action spectrum, is mainly in the blue region.[16] It is well known that UV light is deleterious and should be avoided. Therefore, the spectral region currently recommended is 400 to 520 nm, but more specifically 460 to 490 nm, to exclude potentially harmful UV light.

FLUORESCENT LAMP SOURCES

Because direct sunlight contains wavelengths of light that are (e.g., UV light), artificial light sources, which exclude harmful wavelengths, have been developed. Fig. 92.3 shows the emission spectrum of a lamp (Philips/52) that is typical of the "super" blue fluorescent lamps that have been used for phototherapy. This spectrum has very good overlap with the bilirubin-albumin absorption spectrum. Also shown is the emission spectrum of a turquoise colored fluorescent lamp (Osram Turquoise), which has less overlap with the bilirubin-albumin spectrum, yet several studies have shown that lamps utilizing green lights are equally or more effective than the blue lamps.[3,19-21] This observation is in quantitative agreement with the calculated expectation based upon the action spectrum of Figs. 92.2 and 92.3, but not the bilirubin-albumin absorption spectrum.[21,29]

LED LIGHT SOURCES

The observations discussed above strongly support the action spectrum of Fig. 92.3 and infer that a narrow-band source, such as LEDs with peak wavelength near 476 nm, would be most efficacious.[11,21,29] The use of an LED light source with peak emission near 460 nm is gaining in popularity; however, LEDs with a spectral output centered at 476 nm should be approximately 15% more efficacious than those centered at 460 nm at equal irradiance (Table 92.3). One can, however, increase the rate of TB reduction by simply increasing the irradiance (dose) by increasing lamp input power, adding more lamps, moving lamps closer to the infant, or increasing the light footprint. Therefore, if the irradiance of a 460-nm light source was increased by 15%, it should equalize the rate of bilirubin photo-alteration by a 476-nm light source. The risk-benefit ratio of that approach versus using longer-wavelength light (476 nm) would need to be ascertained to inform clinical decisions.

The use of a source that is the most effective at providing wavelengths of light that are maximally absorbed by bilirubin while reducing therapeutically useless and possibly harmful light absorption by other entities, a priori, should underscore clinical

Table 92.3 Summary of Relative Risks of Mortality Associated With Phototherapy in Extremely Low-Birth-Weight Infants Reported From NICHD Trials.

NICHD Trial	Study Cohort (g)	Deaths/Subjects (g)		RR (95% CI)
		Phototherapy	**No Phototherapy**	
Brown, 1985[22]	<1000	23/39	15/38	1.49 (0.93–2.4)
		Aggressive Phototherapy	**Conservative Phototherapy**	
Oh, 2005[41] (Post-hoc analysis of Morris et al)[42]	500–750	163/417	142/412	1.13 (0.96–1.34)
	500–650	106/214	80/212	1.27 (1.05–1.53)
	750–1000	67/529	76/532	0.93 (0.77–1.12)

NICHD, National Institute of Child Health and Human Development; *RR*, relative risk.
Data from Brown AK, Kim MH, Wu PY, et al. Efficacy of phototherapy in prevention and management of neonatal hyperbilirubinemia. *Pediatrics*. 1985;75: 393–400; Oh W, Tyson JE, Fanaroff AA, et al. Association between peak serum bilirubin and neurodevelopmental outcomes in extremely low birth weight infants. *Pediatrics*. 2003;112:773–779; Morris BH, Tyson JE, Stevenson DK, et al. Efficacy of phototherapy devices and outcomes among extremely low birth weight infants: multi-center observational study. *J Perinatol*. 2013;33:126–133.

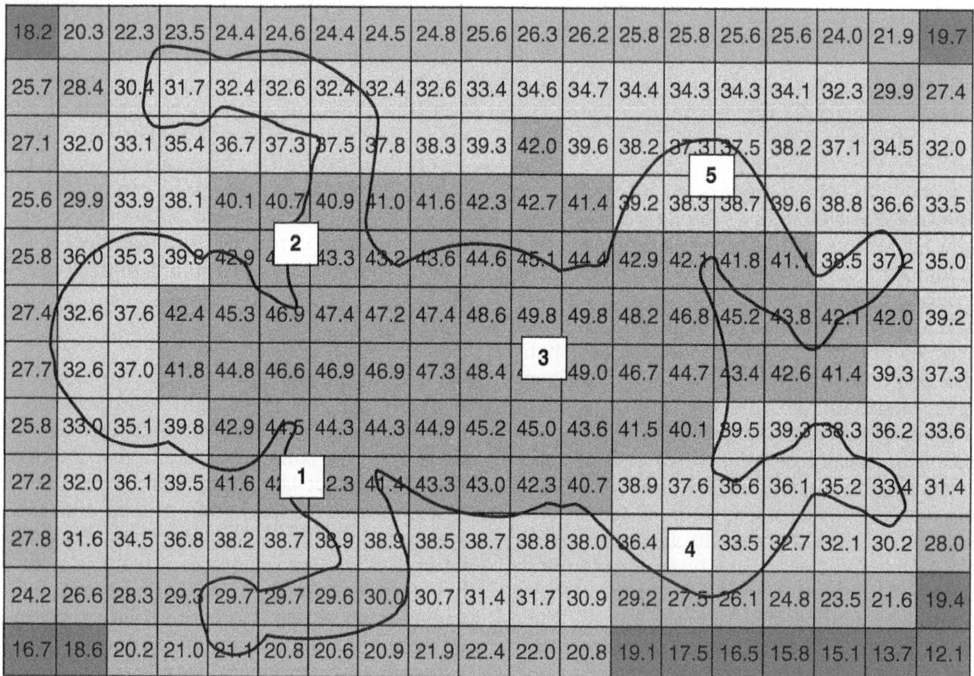

Fig. 92.4 Light footprint. An acceptable distribution of irradiance levels within the footprint of the phototherapy light, showing a pattern of homogenous exposure. Numbered sites indicate clinical sites at which irradiance measures (by dosimeter) should be similar: *1*, right shoulder; *2*, left shoulder; *3*, umbilicus; *4*, right knee; and *5*, left knee. (From Bhutani VK, Wong RJ. Neonatal phototherapy: a choice of device and outcome. *Acta Paediatr.* 2012;101:441–443.)

practice.[4] For example, it is calculated that for equal therapeutic efficacy, use of the typical blue fluorescent source *heats* the infant at a rate 1.5 times greater than a 476-nm LED source because of the absorption of *therapeutically useless* lower-wavelength blue light by hemoglobin.[11] The *heat* or energy transfer is not due to radiant heat from the device, and it may not translate to increased core temperature. The effect of the deposition of the absorbed light energy has not been clinically determined. However, this energy load has to be dissipated and could be potentially deleterious for a sick preterm infant.

LEDs have several other advantages over fluorescent lamps besides their narrow emission spectra and the ability to pick the desired peak emission wavelength (color). Although their initial cost may be higher than that of fluorescent lamps, LEDs use much less power, last much longer, and maintain a much more constant light output over time. The intensity of light emission from LEDs can be electronically controlled. Using such control and the employment of light management films or lenses may allow design of LED arrays that can provide a relatively uniform distribution of intensities over a variety of distances and angles.

REVIEW OF EFFICACY OF PHOTOTHERAPY DEVICES

Several commercial and indigenous device adaptations of current (or available devices) have been performed without rigor of scientific inquiry regarding the safety, efficacy, and actual performance of these devices prior to their clinical use. Of these, homogeneous exposure to a light source has been the most challenging (Fig. 92.4). In 1998, Vreman and colleagues pioneered the use of LEDs as phototherapy light sources.[13] Systematic analyses of the efficacy of both LED and non-LED sources were published independently by Kumar[10] and colleagues and by Tridente and De Luca.[30] Table 92.4 shows the similarities and the diverse perspectives of both systematic reviews. The Cochrane Library review[10] concluded that use of LEDs can decrease TB at rates similar to non-LED sources. They added that further randomized controlled trials are needed to determine the efficacy indices of phototherapy in neonates with severe hyperbilirubinemia associated with hemolysis.

Table 92.4 Recent Systematic Reviews of Phototherapy in Infants at Least 35 Weeks' Gestational Age.

Systematic Review	Cochrane Review	Meta-analysis
Publications identified	1215	103
Selected manuscripts	630	81
Comprehensive review	6	6
Studies of infants with gestational age ≥35 wk	4	4
Total number of infants	511	511
Randomized Controlled Trials: LED vs. non-LED Light Sources		
Weightage of single study	–	61.4%
Heterogeneity	NS	$\chi^2 = 3.44$; $p = 0.488$
Forrest plot test	NS	I^2 value = 0%
Funnel plot test	NS	NS; $p = 0.149$
TB decline	0.01 (95% CI, −0.02–0.04)	–
Duration of phototherapy	0.43 (95% CI, −1.91–1.05)	–
Treatment failure	1.83 (95% CI, 0.47–7.17)	

LED, Light-emitting diode; *TB*, total serum/plasma bilirubin.
Data from Kumar P, Chawla D, Deorari A. Light-emitting diode phototherapy for unconjugated hyperbilirubinaemia in neonates. *Cochrane Database Syst Rev*. 2011;12:CD007969; Tridente A, De Luca D. Efficacy of light-emitting diode versus other light sources for treatment of neonatal hyperbilirubinemia: a systematic review and meta-analysis. *Acta Paediatr*. 2012;101:458–465.

MEASURING EFFICACY

Many factors influence the efficacy of phototherapy. Clinical efficacy is associated with timely decrease of TB to an apparently safe level. Use of a change in TB as a marker for efficacy is complicated and depends upon various factors, such as the rates of bilirubin production and hepatic-mediated excretion, transport of bilirubin to or from the extravascular space, and phototherapy-mediated excretion. However, the TB level currently remains the only biomarker that can be tracked during phototherapy. The phototherapy-mediated excretion rate depends on the light intensity or irradiance at the exposed skin, the area of skin irradiated, the spectrum of the light, the action spectrum, the quantum efficiency of conversion of bilirubin to photoproducts, and the excretion rates of the photoproducts.[4,6,7] Thus the independent operational elements that control phototherapy are the emission spectrum of the light source, the irradiance at the skin surface, and the exposed body surface area (BSA).

MEASURING IRRADIANCE

Clinical guidelines recommend irradiating as much BSA as possible (roughly 1500 cm^2 or approximately 80% of the BSA).[7] Using a lamp or LED light source from above and below an infant can easily achieve an even larger exposed BSA. The irradiance at the distance from the light source to the skin surface should be measured with an appropriate spectroradiometer. The irradiance should be uniform over the footprint of the light-exposed BSA (see Fig. 92.4). The measure of intensity is usually given in energy units of $\mu W/cm^2$. Integrating over the wavelength range of the light source and then multiplying the result by the exposed BSA (assuming uniform intensity over the area) and the time in seconds gives the total dose in joules. If desired, the dose measured in joules can be converted to photons, remembering that the conversion factor depends on the wavelength such that for the same energy there are more photons at higher wavelengths. Although this may be of interest to researchers, in clinical practice commercial radiometers measure the average irradiance over a wavelength range determined by the bandwidth filters in the device. The units are usually expressed as $\mu W/cm^2/nm$. Unfortunately, the various available radiometers have different wavelength ranges and can give different readings for the same light source.[7] Thus, to predict the expected efficacy of a phototherapy device, one needs to consider concurrently manipulating three different spectral distributions: the sensitivity spectrum of the radiometer, the emission spectrum of the light source, and the bilirubin action spectrum. This has not generally been done in practice, so although intrastudy comparisons of efficacy can be made, comparisons of observations from one study to another may not be reliable.

ASSESSING EFFICACY OF LIGHT SOURCES

For the clinician, it is important to know with certainty that sufficient irradiance is delivered to an infant, that harmful wavelengths are excluded, and that light of ineffective wavelengths is minimized. It is also important to remember that radiometers from different suppliers can have different ranges of sensitivity that are specific to their device. Furthermore, lamps and LEDs have different emission spectra. Appropriate practice demands that the TB levels be monitored at a frequency determined by the clinical status of the infant to ensure that the TB is being reduced to a safe level at a rate commensurate with clinical needs. Thus, reliance on the irradiance level and dose (irradiance x time) alone may not be sufficient.

BILIRUBIN STRUCTURE, PHOTOCHEMISTRY, AND PHOTOTHERAPY MECHANISMS

An abridged description of the structure and photochemistry of bilirubin is presented here with the aim of addressing only salient features related to phototherapy. This brief description does not begin to honor the painstaking work required to uncover the complicated chemistry by many experts. Interested readers are directed to the recent, well-detailed historical and technical treatise by DA Lightner.[1] Although many investigators have made important contributions to the long saga, the current representation of the chemistry involved in phototherapy is based primarily on the works of AF McDonagh and DA Lightner and is reviewed by them.[5,31]

Upon absorption of light, bilirubin can undergo a variety of geometric and structural alterations with widely differing rates. Photooxidation to low-molecular-weight, colorless products is observed in vitro, and similar products have been observed in vivo.[5,31] However, this is a multistep process, and the rate (amount over time) at which it occurs is very low, by a factor one hundredth to one thousandth, compared to other alterations. These products are excretable. However, it has been concluded that this low efficiency photodegradation does not account for much of the therapeutic effect of phototherapy compared to more efficient isomerization processes.

As produced from the degradation of heme, bilirubin exists in a particular geometric form, *4Z,15Z*-bilirubin, in which the groups attached to the two key carbon-carbon double bonds are in the so-called *Z* configuration. This is denoted, without the positional numbers, as the *Z,Z* structure in Fig. 92.5. The most efficient photochemical processes involve isomerization between *Z* and *E* conformations, related by twists around the two key double bonds. The four possible configurational isomers are *Z,Z; Z,E; E,Z;* and *E,E* (see Fig. 92.5). These engender four distinct shapes of the bilirubin molecule. All three isomers that have an *E* component are more water soluble than the natural *Z,Z* isomer and are excretable without glucuronidation. Binding of bilirubin to human albumin restricts configurational photoisomerization, at least initially, to the *Z,E* isomer. All three *E* isomers have absorption spectra that are similar to that of the *Z,Z* isomer and can undergo the reverse photoisomerization to the

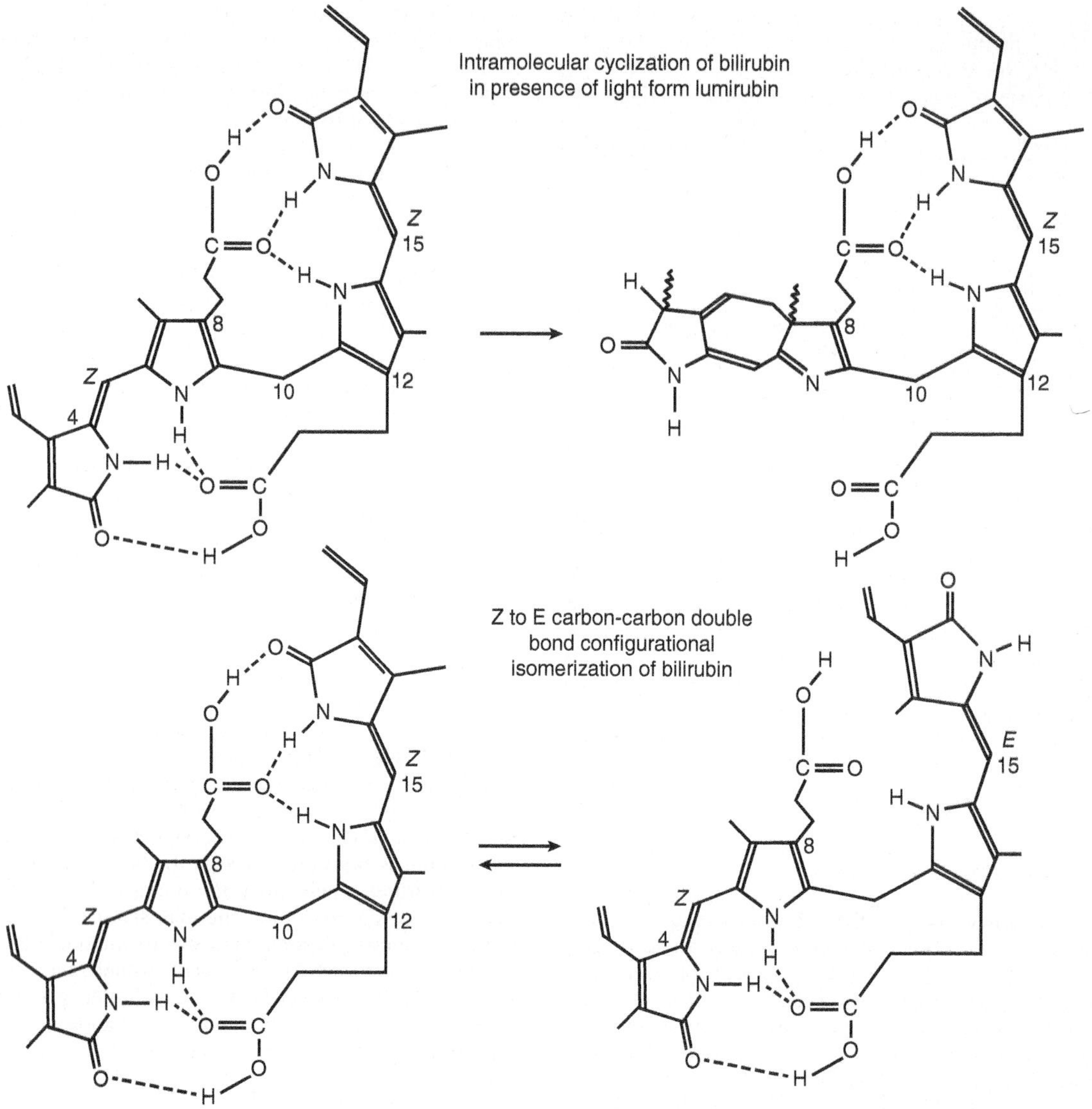

Intramolecular cyclization of bilirubin in presence of light form lumirubin

Z to E carbon-carbon double bond configurational isomerization of bilirubin

Fig. 92.5 The four configurational isomers of bilirubin: *Z,Z; Z,E; E,Z; and E,E*. They represent the four possible structures with respect to configuration around the two double bonds at positions *4* and *15* in the drawings. Absorption of light by bilirubin weakens the double bonds and allows the rotations to interconvert these configurational isomers. The *E* isomers cannot adopt the folded structure of the *Z,Z* isomer and consequently are more polar and more water soluble. (From McDonagh AF, Lightner DA. 'Like a shrivelled blood orange'—bilirubin, jaundice, and phototherapy. *Pediatrics.* 1985;75:443–455.)

respective *Z* isomer. *Z,Z* to *Z,E* isomerization is highly quantum efficient, with 10% to 20% of bilirubin molecules that absorb light converted to the *Z,E* isomer. Reverse photoisomerization from *Z,E* to *Z,Z* occurs with 40% to 80% quantum efficiency (quantum yield). The reversibility and high efficiencies of this interconversion lead to a rapid establishment of equilibrium at a mix of approximately 20% *Z,E*- and 80% *Z,Z*-bilirubin, which can be observed in vivo after less than an hour of therapy at the levels of irradiance commonly used. The *Z,E* isomer has a serum half-life of approximately 15 hours, indicating a relatively slow excretion rate. The *E* isomers are not thermally stable and can revert to *Z* isomers in the dark at rates dependent on their environment.

Structural isomerization, involving a cyclization with new bond formations within bilirubin, leads to a set of isomers collectively called *lumirubin*. This is less efficient than configurational isomerization. The photo-formation of lumirubin has quantum efficiency on the order of only 0.1%. Both structural considerations and experimental observations indicate that the lumirubins are formed from precursor *E* isomers. Their formation is irreversible. Lumirubin isomers are more water soluble than *Z,Z*-bilirubin and directly excretable at a relatively fast rate (serum half-life of approximately 2 hours). The relative contributions of the various photoproducts to the phototherapy-enabled excretion of bilirubin remain controversial. However, it is thought that, despite its low efficiency of production, the excretion pathway via lumirubin has greater importance. The difference in the photo-reversibility of lumirubin and the *Z,E* isomer has clinical implications. If formation of the *Z,E* isomer were essential to the light-induced excretion of bilirubin, the maximum fraction of *Z,E* isomer produced of approximately 20% to 25% (the photo-stationary fraction) would predict a limit to the useful light intensity. Once the stationary amount was reached, only enough light to maintain that amount against the excretion rate would be useful. Higher irradiance would not increase therapeutic efficacy and would only heat the infant. This suggests the possible benefit of using intermittent phototherapy, wherein sufficient irradiance to produce a photo-stationary mixture of *Z,Z* and *Z,E* isomers is employed, followed by a dark period, and then cycled again. However, if irreversible conversion to lumirubin substantially contributes to net bilirubin elimination, and given that lumirubin is formed from *E* isomers, then use of continuous, high-irradiance phototherapy would maximize the rate of reduction of TB. Greater doses of phototherapy are more effective in reducing the TB concentration, but it is uncertain whether there is a maximally effective dose.

OTHER EFFECTS OF PHOTOTHERAPY LIGHT

Despite the extensive use of phototherapy over the past 50 years, there have been limited long-term follow-up studies. Recent reports of presumed adverse effects are more likely associated with the use of early device designs that may not have effectively eliminated UV light. Unanticipated effects of phototherapy were an initial concern because of the potential for direct effect on structures at or near the body surface. UV light contamination was the most likely reason for cutaneous changes similar to sunburn. Other concerns, such as up-regulation of tyrosine kinase in melanocytes, alterations of vitamin D metabolism, disruption of circadian rhythms, effects on indole-O-methyltransferase (a pineal enzyme), and gonadal and retinal injury, have not been substantiated despite detailed inquiry.[6,7] It has been suggested that phototherapy may lead not only to alterations of various moieties that absorb blue light, such as riboflavin, but also to oxidative damage subsequent to free radical formation from photo-oxidation reactions.[32] Infants with thin, translucent skin with almost no subcutaneous tissue may be more vulnerable to the oxidants generated by light exposure. The lower wavelength portion of the blue light region is the more relevant in this regard, providing further impetus to confine the phototherapy wavelength range to the higher blue and blue-green regions.

EFFECT OF PHOTOTHERAPY ON DIRECT BILIRUBIN

Direct bilirubin is a mixture of mono and di-glucuronides, with both having multiple variants. Together with δ-bilirubin, the proportions of these three (or more) species probably differs among babies, with δ-bilirubin increasing with time in chronic cases of cholestasis because it is covalently linked to albumin and is not excreted.[33] Because of their inherent instability, none of these forms of direct diazo-reacting bilirubin are easy to study. Consequently, there is no secure literature on the photochemistry of conjugated forms of bilirubin. The bronze baby syndrome is an uncommon condition associated with phototherapy in infants with cholestatic jaundice.[34] It is manifest as dark grayish discoloration of the skin, urine, and serum that resolves with time. It has been conjectured that these abnormal pigments arise because of impaired biliary excretion of bilirubin photoproducts that undergo polymerization. Bronze skin has not been reported in adults with elevated direct hyperbilirubinemia. Currently, there is no evidence that the bronze baby-associated cutaneous pigment is neurotoxic.

Table 92.5 Calculated Relative Photon Absorption Rates by Bilirubin (15 mg/dL; Hct = 50%) in Neonate Skin at Equal Irradiance for Various Light Sources.[a]

Source	Peak Wavelength (nm)	Relative Photon Absorption Rate
LED[b]	450	0.62
LED	460	0.85
LED	470	0.96
LED	476	1.0[c]
LED	480	0.98
LED	490	0.79
Philips TL20W/52 Blue lamp	450	0.61
OSRAM L18W/860	490	0.72

[a]The photon absorption rate should predict the rate of bilirubin photochemistry.
[b]LED half-bandwidths ≈20 nm.
[c]LED source with 476-nm peak wavelength taken as reference = 1.0.
Hct, Hematocrit; *LED,* light-emitting diode.
Data from Lamola AA, Bhutani VK, Wong RJ, et al. The effect of hematocrit on the efficacy of phototherapy for neonatal jaundice. *Pediatr Res.* 2013;74:54–60.

TRANSLATION TO CLINICAL PRACTICE

Optimization and standardization of phototherapy for the management of neonatal hyperbilirubinemia have been the subjects of several literature reviews and guidelines (Table 92.5).[6,7,35] Blue LED light sources are preferred, followed by compact fluorescent tubes, tungsten-halogen lamps, and fiberoptic blankets that help BSA exposure to light. Devices that meet dose specifications include blue Philips TL20W/52 and turquoise Osram L18W/860 tubes. The key *device* characteristics that contribute to effectiveness include (1) emission of light in the blue-to-green range that overlaps with the in vivo plasma bilirubin absorption spectrum (460 to 490 nm); (2) irradiance of at least 30 μW/cm²/nm at a suitable distance (confirmed with an appropriate irradiance meter calibrated over the appropriate wavelength range); and (3) minimization of light outside the therapeutically efficient wavelength range. Irradiance of more than 65 μW/cm²/nm has not been adequately tested for safety. Due to reports of potentially increased mortality with phototherapy in infants weighing less than 1000 g, experts have recommended using less intensive levels of irradiance upon initiation of phototherapy, unless TB levels continue to rise.[36] Important *non-device* factors include (1) illumination of 35% to 80% of exposed BSA with multiple devices and (2) demonstration of a decrease in TB concentrations during the first 4 to 6 hours of exposure in the absence of excessive hemolysis. Standardization of irradiance meters, improvements in device design, and identification of lower and upper limits of light intensity for phototherapy devices merit further study. Comparing the clinical efficacy of phototherapy devices accurately is difficult with the present lack of an easily implemented standardized procedure.

BIOENGINEERING PERSPECTIVES

Barriers to effective phototherapy include use of unproven light sources, poor device maintenance, erratic or inconsistent power sources, and operational impediments.[37] To promote implementation of effective phototherapy at all birthing facilities, minimal technology criteria have been proposed to complement the safety and regulatory standards listed by the International Electrotechnical Commission.[38] Table 92.6 lists the minimum checklist to operationalize the use of phototherapy.

GUIDELINES FOR PHOTOTHERAPY

The initial provisional recommendation guidelines[2] have generally withstood the test of time. These are briefly listed here:

1. The cause of hyperbilirubinemia should always be investigated. Categorizing the cause as increased bilirubin production, decreased elimination, or increased enterohepatic circulation may allow for targeted intervention and/or follow up.
2. Phototherapy should be used for infants with unconjugated hyperbilirubinemia and not prior to onset of an elevated TB level. Phototherapy should be administered continuously but may be interrupted for breastfeeding. Use of cycled (intermittent) phototherapy is still being investigated.[39]

Table 92.6 Minimum Specifications for an Effective Phototherapy Device.

Technical Requirement	Clinical Specifications
Regulatory approval	FDA, 510 K, and/or CE mark
Emission spectrum	Blue or blue-green (range 430–490 nm); preferably narrow band and peaks at 470 ± 10 nm
Spectral irradiance	25 to <45 μW/cm²/nm at body surface
Light source	LED (preferred), 20,000 hours lifetime with irradiance ≥30 μW/cm²/nm
Light footprint	5-point measure; 30 by 50-cm area with minimum to maximum ratio >0.4
Device energy source(s)	Compatible with 90–240 V and 48–60-Hz power input, built-in circuit-breaker
Device structure (and stand)	UV protection; topple-resistant, portable (castors with brakes); height adjustable; base allows stand to fit under radiant warmers, bassinets, or isolettes

CE, Conformité Européenne; *FDA,* Food and Drug Administration; *LED,* light-emitting diode; *UV,* ultraviolet.
Data from Bhutani VK, Cline BK, Donaldson KM, et al. The need to implement effective phototherapy in resource-constrained settings. *Semin Perinatol.* 2011;35:192–197.

3. Phototherapy should be used for infants in whom adverse hyperbilirubinemia-related neurologic risks outweigh the therapy-related risks. Phototherapy should be used for infants with TB levels that do not yet meet the threshold for exchange transfusion when there is a reasonable chance of exceeding that threshold based on the rate of TB rise.
4. Even when infants meet thresholds for exchange transfusion, an immediate *crash-cart* approach should be implemented and may avert the need for the exchange procedure. In some infants, such as those with Rh hemolytic disease and rapidly increasing TB levels, the exchange transfusion should not be delayed.
5. Phototherapy is prescribed when an abnormal rate of bilirubin production has been demonstrated (>0.2 mg/dL/h).
6. Response to phototherapy, measured by TB (not transcutaneous bilirubin), is generally noted within 4 hours and continues to be observed in 24 to 36 hours. With 8 to 12 hours of effective phototherapy, there is an average decrease in TB of 3 to 4 mg/dL in infants who do not have active hemolysis.
7. Serial TB measurements should be obtained during the course of phototherapy. By eliminating visible jaundice, phototherapy may mask mild hemolysis due to ABO incompatibility, hereditary spherocytosis, or glucose 6-phosphate dehydrogenase (G6PD) deficiency.

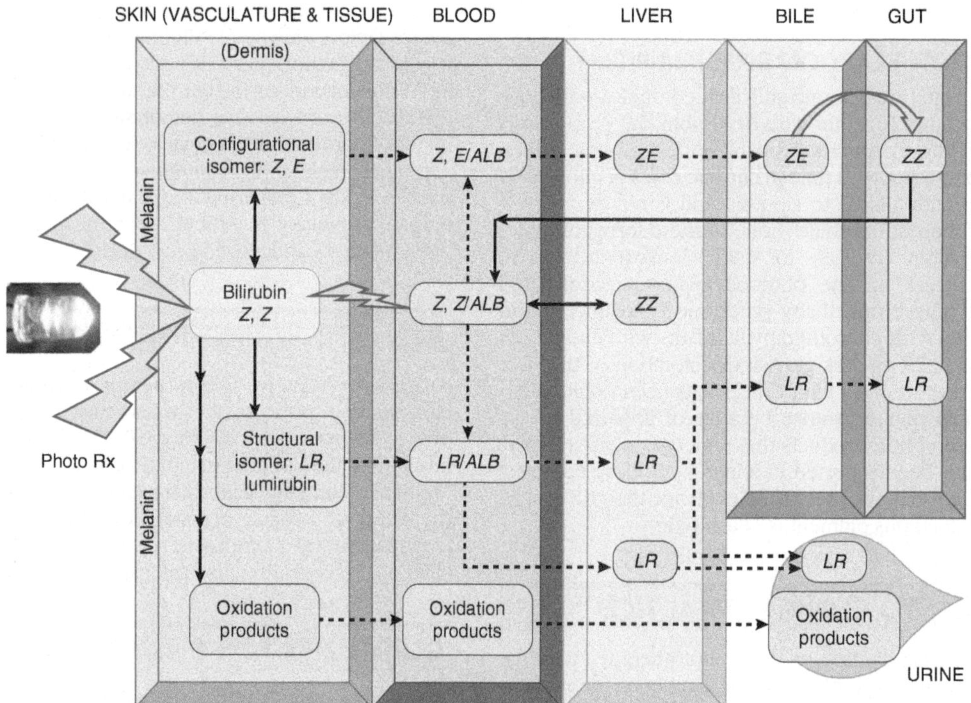

Fig. 92.6 Schematic of the salient features of phototherapy of unconjugated hyperbilirubinemia. The light must first pass through the epidermis, where it is weakly diminished by any melanin (does not affect the action spectrum). Entering the dermis, the light is quickly rendered diffuse and is absorbed by the hemoglobin and bilirubin present there. The competition for light absorption by hemoglobin essentially dictates the wavelength range where bilirubin most effectively absorbs the light. The bilirubin that absorbs light undergoes efficient conversion to the *Z,E* isomer until a steady-state level of approximately 20% of the bilirubin is reached. The bilirubin also undergoes a less efficient conversion to lumirubin in a process that is not photo-reversible. Much less efficient, requiring multiple chemical reactions, is the conversion of bilirubin to low-molecular-weight oxidation products. All of these products are transported (the *E* isomers and lumirubin are probably mostly bound to albumin) by the circulating blood to the liver and other sites and excreted. *E* isomers can be reverted to their *Z* counterparts by mechanisms not requiring light. (Adapted from McDonagh AF, Lightner DA. 'Like a shrivelled blood orange'—bilirubin, jaundice, and phototherapy. *Pediatrics.* 1985;75:443–455.)

8. The use of phototherapy in infants with concurrent conjugated hyperbilirubinemia remains controversial.
9. Infants who complete successful phototherapy do not require follow-up unless there is a need to determine the underlying cause of jaundice or the infant is at risk for the sequelae of extreme hyperbilirubinemia.
10. Currently, phototherapy has not been associated with either short- or long-term consequences. Eye patches are important for eye protection from bright lights; diapers serve as aids for comfort and hygiene.

INNOVATION AND FUTURE DIRECTIONS

TB levels remain an imprecise indicator of both bilirubin exposure and neurotoxicity. A specific threshold-based relationship between TB and subtle or moderate diverse-domain neurotoxicity (such as the syndrome of bilirubin-induced neurologic dysfunction [BIND]) has been elusive, indicating that additional critical factors contribute to a phenotype that could be either transient or irreversible. Novel and translational neonatal functional biomarkers of increased bilirubin load due to increased bilirubin production, disordered albumin binding, and ensuing reduced BBC are the subject of ongoing studies.[11,25] The ratios of UB to TB (which is inversely related to the reserve binding capacity) and TB to BBC (the extent of saturation of the BBC) present two different views of bilirubin-binding status. Considering them together, as a plot of UB/TB versus percent of saturation, may provide an improved assessment of risk. These extrapolations also suggest a potential role for individually measured BBC and TB.[25]

CONCLUSION

Neonatal phototherapy is the current standard of care for treatment of significant hyperbilirubinemia, which can result in bilirubin neurotoxicity including kernicterus. Much of the current knowledge of the mechanisms underlying this therapy is represented in Fig. 92.6. Drug effective absorbed dose of blue-green light (460 to 490 nm) depends on its wavelength-specific irradiance and an infant's skin tissue characteristics. The mechanism of action of phototherapy on the native unconjugated bilirubin proceeds via efficient photochemical reactions providing configurational and structural isomers that are more soluble than the native isomer. These polar isomers are eliminated through bile and urine and bypass the need for UGT conjugation. Because of their polarity, these isomers should be less able to cross the BBB, and therefore their formation could be beneficial. Though suggestive, this lowered neurotoxic potential of photoisomers has yet to be validated. Oxidants formed through photochemical reactions, perhaps especially at the lower wavelengths of blue light, could have adverse consequences for extremely low-birth-weight neonates and possibly those who are extremely small for GA. Further optimization of the therapy's benefits and risks based on the relative efficacy of continuous versus cycled light delivery[39] awaits further clinical investigation.

ACKNOWLEDGMENTS

This chapter was supported in part by the Ahlfors Center for Unbound Bilirubin Research & Development and the Kaplan-Goldstein Family Foundation. No commercial financial assistance was received in support of this chapter. We would also like to thank Angelo A. Lamola, PhD, for his contributions in the original chapter.

REFERENCES

1. Lightner DA. *Bilirubin: Jekyll and Hyde Pigment of Life: Pursuit of its Structure Through Two World Wars to the New Millenium*. Vienna: Springer-Verlag Wien; 2013.
2. Behrman RE, Hsia DY. Summary of a symposium on phototherapy for hyperbilirubinemia. *J Pediatr*. 1969;75:718–726.
3. Ennever JF, Sobel M, McDonagh AF, et al. Phototherapy for neonatal jaundice: *in vitro* comparison of light sources. *Pediatr Res*. 1984;18:667–670.
4. Maisels MJ, McDonagh AF. Phototherapy for neonatal jaundice. *N Engl J Med*. 2008;358:920–928.
5. McDonagh AF, Lightner DA. Phototherapy and the photobiology of bilirubin. *Semin Liver Dis*. 1988;8:272–283.
6. American Academy of Pediatrics Subcommittee on Hyperbilirubinemia. Management of hyperbilirubinemia in the newborn infant 35 or more weeks of gestation. *Pediatrics*. 2004;114:297–316.
7. Bhutani VK. Committee on Fetus and Newborn, American Academy of Pediatrics. Phototherapy to prevent severe neonatal hyperbilirubinemia in the newborn infant 35 or more weeks of gestation. *Pediatrics*. 2011;128:e1046–e1052.
8. Hansen TW, Nietsch L, Norman E, et al. Reversibility of acute intermediate phase bilirubin encephalopathy. *Acta Paediatr*. 2009;98:1689–1694.
9. Mreihil K, McDonagh AF, Nakstad B, et al. Early isomerization of bilirubin in phototherapy of neonatal jaundice. *Pediatr Res*. 2010;67:656–659.
10. Kumar P, Chawla D, Deorari A. Light-emitting diode phototherapy for unconjugated hyperbilirubinaemia in neonates. *Cochrane Database Syst Rev*. 2011;12:CD007969.
11. Lamola AA, Bhutani VK, Wong RJ, et al. The effect of hematocrit on the efficacy of phototherapy for neonatal jaundice. *Pediatr Res*. 2013;74:54–60.
12. Seidman DS, Moise J, Ergaz Z, et al. A prospective randomized controlled study of phototherapy using blue and blue-green light-emitting devices, and conventional halogen-quartz phototherapy. *J Perinatol*. 2003;23:123–127.
13. Vreman HJ, Wong RJ, Stevenson DK, et al. Light-emitting diodes: a novel light source for phototherapy. *Pediatr Res*. 1998;44:804–809.
14. Hansen TWR, Maisels MJ, Ebbesen F, et al. Sixty years of phototherapy for neonatal jaundice - From serendipitous observation to standardized treatment and rescue for millions. *J Perinatol*. 2020;40:180–193.
15. Cremer RJ, Perryman PW, Richards DH, et al. Photo-sensitivity of serum bilirubin. *Biochem J*. 1957;66:60.
16. Cremer RJ, Perryman PW, Richards DH. Influence of light on the hyperbilirubinaemia of infants. *Lancet*. 1958;1:1094–1097.
17. Lucey J, Ferriero M, Hewitt J. Prevention of hyperbilirubinemia of prematurity by phototherapy. *Pediatrics*. 1968;41:1047–1054.
18. Lucey J, Hewitt J, Brown A, et al. Recent observations on light and neonatal jaundice. In: Brown AK, Showacre J, eds. *Phototherapy for Neonatal Jaundice, DHEW Publication No (NIH) 76-1075*. Bethesda, MD: Department of Health, Education, and Welfare; 1977:170–179.
19. Ennever JF. Blue light, green light, white light, more light: treatment of neonatal jaundice. *Clin Perinatol*. 1990;17:467–481, 1990.
20. Ennever JF, McDonagh AF, Speck WT. Phototherapy for neonatal jaundice: optimal wavelengths of light. *J Pediatr*. 1983;103:295–299.
21. Mreihil K, Madsen P, Nakstad B, et al. Early formation of bilirubin isomers during phototherapy for neonatal jaundice: effects of single vs. double fluorescent lamps vs. photodiodes. *Pediatr Res*. 2015;78:56–62.
22. Brown AK, Kim MH, Wu PY, et al. Efficacy of phototherapy in prevention and management of neonatal hyperbilirubinemia. *Pediatrics*. 1985;75:393–400.
23. Brown AK, McDonagh AF. Phototherapy for neonatal hyperbilirubinemia: efficacy, mechanism and toxicity. *Adv Pediatr*. 1980;27:341–389.
24. Tenhunen R, Marver HS, Schmid R. The enzymatic conversion of heme to bilirubin by microsomal heme oxygenase. *Proc Natl Acad Sci USA*. 1968;61:748–755.
25. Lamola AA, Bhutani VK, Du L, et al. Neonatal bilirubin binding capacity discerns risk of neurological dysfunction. *Pediatr Res*. 2015;77:334–339.
26. Vreman HJ, Wong RJ, Stevenson DK. Phototherapy: current methods and future directions. *Semin Perinatol*. 2004;28:326–333.
27. Turro NJ, Ramamurthy V, Scaiano JC. *Principles of Molecular Photochemistry: an Introduction*. Sausalito, CA: University Science Books; 2009.
28. Linfield DT, Lamola AA, Mei E, et al. The effect of hematocrit on *in vitro* bilirubin photoalteration. *Pediatr Res*. 2016;79:387–390.
29. Ebbesen F, Madsen P, Stovring S, et al. Therapeutic effect of turquoise versus blue light with equal irradiance in preterm infants with jaundice. *Acta Paediatr*. 2007;96:837–841.
30. Tridente A, De Luca D. Efficacy of light-emitting diode versus other light sources for treatment of neonatal hyperbilirubinemia: a systematic review and meta-analysis. *Acta Paediatr*. 2012;101:458–465.
31. McDonagh AF, Lightner DA. 'Like a shrivelled blood orange'—bilirubin, jaundice, and phototherapy. *Pediatrics*. 1985;75:443–455.
32. Gathwala G, Sharma S. Oxidative stress, phototherapy and the neonate. *Indian J Pediatr*. 2000;67:805–808.
33. Kuenzle CC, Sommerhalder M, Ruttner JR, et al. Separation and quantitative estimation of four bilirubin fractions from serum and of three bilirubin fractions from bile. *J Lab Clin Med*. 1966;67:282–293.
34. Rubaltelli FF, Da Riol R, D'Amore ES, et al. The bronze baby syndrome: evidence of increased tissue concentration of copper porphyrins. *Acta Paediatr*. 1996;85:381–384.

35. Okwundu CI, Okoromah CA, Shah PS. Cochrane review: prophylactic phototherapy for preventing jaundice in preterm or low birth weight infants. *Evid Based Child Health*. 2013;8:204–249.
36. Maisels MJ, Watchko JF, Bhutani VK, et al. An approach to the management of hyperbilirubinemia in the preterm infant less than 35 weeks of gestation. *J Perinatol*. 2012;32:660–664.
37. Bhutani VK, Cline BK, Donaldson KM, et al. The need to implement effective phototherapy in resource-constrained settings. *Semin Perinatol*. 2011;35:192–197.
38. International Electrotechnical Commission. *Medical Electrical Equipment. Part 2-50: Particular Requirements for the Basic Safety and Essential Performance of Infant Phototherapy Equipment*; 2009. IEC 60601-2-50:2020 RLV. Available at: https://webstore.iec.ch/publication/67568.
39. Arnold CC, Tyson JE, Pedroza C, et al. Cycled phototherapy: dose-finding study for extremely low birth weight infants: a randomized clinical trial. *JAMA Pediatr*. 2020;174:649-656.
40. Slusher TM, Vreman HJ, Olusanya BO, et al. Safety and efficacy of filtered sunlight in treatment of jaundice in African neonates. *Pediatrics*. 2014;133:e1568–e1574.
41. Oh W, Tyson JE, Fanaroff AA, et al. Association between peak serum bilirubin and neurodevelopmental outcomes in extremely low birth weight infants. *Pediatrics*. 2003;112:773–779.
42. Morris BH, Tyson JE, Stevenson DK, et al. Efficacy of phototherapy devices and outcomes among extremely low birth weight infants: multi-center observational study. *J Perinatol*. 2013;33:126–133.

Index

Page numbers followed by *f* indicate figure, by *t* table, and by *b* box.

C

J

O

P

Q

R

Sixth Edition

Fetal and Neonatal Physiology

Richard A. Polin, MD
William T. Speck Professor of Pediatrics
College of Physicians and Surgeons
Columbia University
Executive Vice-Chair
Department of Pediatrics
Morgan Stanley Children's Hospital of New York–Presbyterian
Columbia University Irving Medical Center
New York, New York

Steven H. Abman, MD
Professor, Department of Pediatrics
Director, Pediatric Heart Lung Center
University of Colorado School of Medicine and Children's Hospital Colorado
Aurora, Colorado

David H. Rowitch, MD ScD FMedSci FRS
Professor and Head
Department of Paediatrics
Wellcome Trust—Medical Research Council Stem Cell Institute
University of Cambridge
Cambridge, United Kingdom
Adjunct Professor
Department of Pediatrics
University of California, San Francisco
San Francisco, California

William E. Benitz, MD
Philip Sunshine Professor in Neonatology Emeritus
Division of Neonatal and Developmental Medicine
Stanford University School of Medicine
Stanford, California

William W. Fox, MD
Editor Emeritus
Perelman School of Medicine,
The University of Pennsylvania

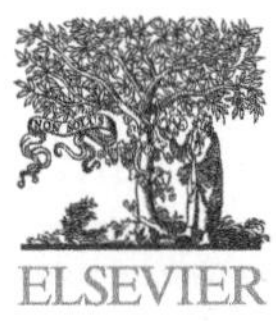

Elsevier
1600 John F. Kennedy Blvd.
Ste. 1800
Philadelphia, PA 19103-2899

FETAL AND NEONATAL PHYSIOLOGY: SIXTH EDITION

ISBN-13: 978-0-323-71284-2
Vol 1: 978-0-323-82555-9
Vol 2: 978-0-323-82556-6

Library of Congress Control Number: 2021940940

Publisher: Sarah Barth
Senior Content Development Specialist: Mary Hegeler
Publishing Services Manager: Catherine Albright Jackson
Senior Project Manager: Doug Turner
Designer: Brian Salisbury

Printed in the United States of America

Last digit is the print number: 9 8 7 6 5 4 3 2

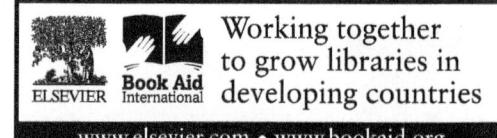

W

X

Y

Z

DEDICATED TO

Our spouses –
Helene Polin, Carolyn Abman, Risa Sorkin, and Andrea Benitz

Our children –
Allison Polin Steinbrenner, Mitchell Polin, Jessica Moseley, and Gregory Polin
Ryan Abman, Lauren Abman, Mark Abman, and Megan Abman
Sophie Rowitch
Lindsey Benitz, Maija Benitz, and Annika Benitz Chaloff

And our grandchildren –
Lindsey Steinbrenner, Eli Steinbrenner, Willa Polin, Jasper Polin, Elliot Polin, Lily Polin, Casey Moseley, Smith Moseley, Calla Moseley, Winslow Broderick, Mieke Broderick, Isla Abman, and Alina Abman

Contributors

Soraya Abbasi, MD
Professor
Department of Pediatrics
Perelman School of Medicine
University of Pennsylvania
Philadelphia, Pennsylvania
Evaluation of Pulmonary Function in the Neonate

Yalda Afshar, MD, PhD
Assistant Professor
Department of Obstetrics and Gynecology
Division of Maternal Fetal Medicine
David Geffen School of Medicine
University of California, Los Angeles
Los Angeles, California
Angiogenesis

Sun-Young Ahn, MD
Associate Professor
Pediatric Nephrology
Children's National Hospital
The George Washington University
Washington, District of Columbia
Organic Anion Transport in the Developing Kidney

Kurt H. Albertine, PhD
Professor
Edward B. Clark Endowed Chair IV in Pediatrics
Department of Pediatrics
University of Utah Health
Editor-in-Chief, *The Anatomical Record*
Salt Lake City, Utah
Impaired Lung Growth After Injury in Preterm Lung

Karel Allegaert, MD, PhD
Professor
Department of Development and Regeneration
Department of Pharmaceutical and Pharmacological Sciences
KU Leuven
Leuven, Belgium
Department of Clinical Pharmacy
Erasmus Medical Center
Rotterdam, The Netherlands
The Physiology of Placental Drug Disposition

Seth L. Alper, MD, PhD
Professor of Medicine
Harvard Medical School
Division of Nephrology and Vascular Biology Research Center
Beth Israel Deaconess Medical Center
Boston, Massachusetts
Urinary Acidification

Gabriel Altit, MDCM, MSc
Assistant Professor
Department of Pediatrics
McGill University
Neonatologist
Division of Neonatology
Montreal Children's Hospital
Montreal, Quebec, Canada
Basic Pharmacologic Principles

Ruben E. Alvaro, MD
Medical Director of Neonatology
St Boniface Hospital
Associate Professor
Department of Pediatrics
University of Manitoba
Winnipeg, Manitoba, Canada
Control of Breathing in Fetal Life and Onset and Control of Breathing in the Neonate

Cristina M. Alvira, MD
Associate Professor of Pediatrics
Division of Critical Care Medicine
Stanford University School of Medicine
Stanford, California
Developmental Biology of the Pulmonary Vasculature

Natália Carlos Maia Amorim, MS
Master in Nutrition
Postgraduate Program in Nutrition
Nutritionist of University Hospital Ana Bezerra-Federal University of Rio Grande do Norte
Santa Cruz, Brazil
Vitamin E Nutrition in Pregnancy and the Newborn Infant

Kelsey L. Anbuhl, PhD
Postdoctoral Fellow
Center for Neural Science
New York University
New York, New York
Early Development of the Human Auditory System

Claus Yding Andersen, MSc, DMSc
Professor
Laboratory of Reproductive Biology
University Hospital of Copenhagen
Copenhagen, Denmark
Differentiation of the Ovary

Richard A. Anderson, MD, PhD
Professor
MRC Centre for Reproductive Health
University of Edinburgh
Edinburgh, United Kingdom
Differentiation of the Ovary

Katrina A. Andrews, MB BChir
Department of Clinical Genetics
Cambridge University Hospitals NHS Foundation Trust
Department of Medical Genetics
University of Cambridge and NIHR Cambridge Biomedical Research Centre
Cancer Research UK Cambridge Centre
Cambridge Biomedical Campus
Cambridge, United Kingdom
Pathophysiology of Genetic Neonatal Disease

David J. Askenazi, MD, MSPH
Professor
Director, Pediatric and Infant Center for Acute Nephrology
Department of Pediatrics
Division of Nephrology
University of Alabama Birmingham
Birmingham, Alabama
Pathophysiology of Neonatal Acute Kidney Injury

Débora Gabriela Fernandes Assunção, MD
Nutritionist
Specialist in Neonate Intensive Care
Postgraduate Program in Nutrition
Federal University of Rio Grande do Norte
Natal, Brazil
Vitamin E Nutrition in Pregnancy and the Newborn Infant

Richard Lambert Auten Jr., MD
Professor
Department of Pediatrics (Neonatology)
Cone Health System
Greensboro, North Carolina
Mechanisms of Neonatal Lung Injury

Julie Autmizguine, MD, MHS
Associate Professor
Departments of Pharmacology and Pediatrics
University of Montreal
Infectious Disease Pediatrician
Department of Pediatrics
CHU Sainte-Justine
Montreal, Quebec, Canada
Basic Pharmacologic Principles

Timur Azhibekov, MD, MS CBTI
Assistant Professor
Department of Pediatrics
Case Western Reserve University School of Medicine
Department of Pediatrics
MetroHealth Medical Center
Cleveland, Ohio
Regulation of Acid-Base Balance in the Fetus and Neonate

Stephen A. Back, MD, PhD
Clyde and Elda Munson Professor of Pediatric Research
Department of Pediatrics
Oregon Health & Science University
Portland, Oregon
Pathophysiology of Neonatal White Matter Injury

Timothy M. Bahr, MD
Department of Pediatrics-Neonatology
University of Utah Health
Salt Lake City, Utah
Developmental Erythropoiesis

Peter Russell Baker II, MD
Associate Professor
Department of Pediatrics
Section of Clinical Genetics and Metabolism
University of Colorado School of Medicine
Aurora, Colorado
Fetal Origins of Adult Disease: A Classic Hypothesis With New Relevance

Eduardo H. Bancalari, MD
Professor
Department of Pediatrics—Neonatology
University of Miami Miller School of Medicine
Miami, Florida
Pathophysiology of Bronchopulmonary Dysplasia

Tatiana Barichello, PhD
Assistant Professor
Department of Psychiatric and Behavioral Sciences
The University of Texas Health Science Center at Houston
McGovern Medical School
Houston, Texas
Professor
Laboratory of Experimental Pathophysiology
Graduate Program in Health Sciences
University of Southern Santa Catarina
Criciúma, Brazil
Pathophysiology of Neonatal Acute Bacterial Meningitis

Frederick C. Battaglia, MD
Professor Emeritus
Department of Pediatrics
University of Colorado School of Medicine
Aurora, Colorado
Placental and Fetal Circulatory and Metabolic Changes Accompanying Fetal Growth Restriction

Andrew J. Bauer, MD
Director, The Thyroid Center
Division of Endocrinology and Diabetes
Children's Hospital of Philadelphia
Professor
Department of Pediatrics
Perelman School of Medicine
University of Pennsylvania
Philadelphia, Pennsylvania
Fetal and Neonatal Thyroid Physiology

Michel Baum, MD
Professor of Pediatrics and Internal Medicine
Sarah M. and Charles E. Seay Chair in Pediatric Research
UT Southwestern Medical Center
Dallas, Texas
Renal Transport of Sodium During Development

Ryan W. Bavis, PhD
Helen A. Papaioanou Professor of Biological Sciences
Department of Biology
Bates College
Lewiston, Maine
Pathophysiology of Apnea of Prematurity

Kathryn Beardsall, BSc, MBBS, MD
Lecturer
Department of Paediatrics
University of Cambridge
Physician
Department of Neonatology
Cambridge University Hospitals NHS Trust
Cambridge, United Kingdom
Role of Glucoregulatory Hormones in Hepatic Glucose Metabolism During the Perinatal Period

Simon Beggs, PhD
Associate Professor
UCL Great Ormond Street Institute of Child Health
London, United Kingdom
Developmental Aspects of Pain

Corinne Benchimol, DO
Assistant Professor
Department of Pediatrics
Mount Sinai Hospital
New York, New York
Potassium Homeostasis in the Fetus and Neonate

Manon J.N.L. Benders, MD, PhD
Professor
Department of Neonatology
University Medical Center Utrecht
Utrecht, The Netherlands
Cerebellar Development—The Impact of Preterm Birth and Comorbidities

Laura Bennet, PhD
Professor
Department of Physiology
The University of Auckland
Auckland, New Zealand
Neuroprotective Therapeutic Hypothermia

Phillip R. Bennett, MD, PhD
Clinical Professor
Faculty of Medicine
Department of Metabolism, Digestion, and Reproduction
Institute of Reproductive and Developmental Biology
Imperial College Parturition Research Group
Researcher
March of Dimes Prematurity Research Centre
Imperial College London
London, United Kingdom
Pathophysiology of Preterm Birth

Melvin Berger, MD, PhD
Adjunct Professor
Pediatrics and Pathology
Case Western Reserve University School of Medicine
Cleveland, Ohio
The Complement System of the Fetus and Newborn

Wolfgang Bernhard, MD
Professor
Department of Neonatology
Children's Hospital
Eberhard-Karls-University
Tübingen, Germany
Regulation of Surfactant-Associated Phospholipid Synthesis and Secretion

John F. Bertram, BSc, PhD, DSc
Head, Anatomy and Developmental Biology
Professor
Biomedicine Discovery Institute
Monash University
Melbourne, Victoria, Australia
Development of the Kidney: Morphology and Mechanisms

Shazia Bhombal, MD
Clinical Associate Professor of Pediatrics
Division of Neonatal and Developmental Medicine
Stanford University School of Medicine
Stanford, California
Developmental Biology of the Pulmonary Vasculature

Vinod K. Bhutani, MD
Professor
Department of Pediatrics
Lucile Packard Children's Hospital at Stanford
Stanford, California
Mechanistic Aspects of Phototherapy for Neonatal Hyperbilirubinemia

Mary Jane Black, BSc (Hons), PhD
Associate Professor
Deputy Head
Department of Anatomy and Developmental Biology
Biomedicine Discovery Institute
Monash University
Melbourne, Victoria, Australia
Development of the Kidney: Morphology and Mechanisms

Joseph M. Bliss, MD, PhD
Associate Professor
Department of Pediatrics
Women & Infants Hospital of Rhode Island
Warren Alpert Medical School of Brown University
Providence, Rhode Island
Normal and Abnormal Neutrophil Physiology in the Newborn

David L. Bolender, PhD
Professor
Cell Biology, Neurobiology, and Anatomy
Medical College of Wisconsin
Milwaukee, Wisconsin
Basic Embryology

Sarah C. Bowdin, MD
Department of Clinical Genetics
Cambridge University Hospitals NHS Foundation Trust
Cambridge, United Kingdom
Pathophysiology of Genetic Neonatal Disease

Scott D. Boyd, MD, PhD
Associate Professor
Department of Pathology
Stanford University School of Medicine
Stanford, California
B-Cell Development

Joline E. Brandenburg, MD
Assistant Professor
Physical Medicine and Rehabilitation
Pediatrics and Adolescent Medicine
Mayo Clinic
Rochester, Minnesota
Functional Development of Respiratory Muscles

Laura D. Brown, MD
Associate Professor
Department of Pediatrics
University of Colorado School of Medicine
Aurora, Colorado
Placental Transfer and Fetal Requirements of Amino Acids

Douglas G. Burrin, PhD
Research Physiologist and Professor
USDA-ARS Children's Nutrition Research Center
Department of Pediatrics
Baylor College of Medicine
Houston, Texas
Trophic Factors and Regulation of Gastrointestinal Tract and Liver Development

Barbara Cannon, BSc, PhD
Professor
Department of Molecular Biosciences
The Wenner-Gren Institute
Stockholm University
Stockholm, Sweden
Brown Adipose Tissue: Development and Function

Michael Caplan, MD
Chairman
Department of Pediatrics
NorthShore University HealthSystem
Evanston, Illinois
Clinical Professor
Department of Pediatrics
University of Chicago Pritzker School of Medicine
Chicago, Illinois
Pathophysiology and Prevention of Neonatal Necrotizing Enterocolitis

Susan E. Carlson, PhD
A. J. Rice Professor of Nutrition and University Distinguished Professor
Department of Dietetics and Nutrition
University of Kansas
Kansas City, Kansas
Long-Chain Polyunsaturated Fatty Acids in Neurodevelopment

David P. Carlton, MD
Marcus Professor and Chief
Division of Neonatology
Emory University
Atlanta, Georgia
Regulation of Liquid Secretion and Absorption by the Fetal and Neonatal Lung
Pathophysiology of Edema

Piya Chaemsaithong, MD, PhD
Division of Maternal Fetal Medicine
Department of Obstetrics and Gynecology
Faculty of Medicine
Ramathibodi Hospital
Mahidol University
Bangkok, Thailand
Intra-Amniotic Infection/Inflammation and the Fetal Inflammatory Response Syndrome

Jill Chang, MD
Assistant Professor
Department of Pediatrics
Division of Neonatology
Northwestern University Feinberg School of Medicine
Chicago, Illinois
Placental Function in Intrauterine Growth Restriction

Jennifer R. Charlton, MD
Associate Professor
Department of Pediatrics
Division of Nephrology
University of Virginia Children's Hospital
Charlottesville, Virginia
Response to Nephron Loss in Early Development
Pathophysiology of Neonatal Acute Kidney Injury

Sylvain Chemtob, MD, PhD
Professor
Departments of Pediatrics and Pharmacology
CHU Ste-Justine and University of Montreal
Professor
Department of Ophthalmology
Hospital Maisonneuve Rosemont and University of Montreal
Montreal, Quebec, Canada
Basic Pharmacologic Principles

Sadhana Chheda, MBBS, DTMH
Assistant Professor
Department of Pediatrics
Texas Tech University Health Sciences Center–El Paso
El Paso, Texas
Immunology of Human Milk

Andrew J. Childs, BSc (Hons), MSc, PhD
Lecturer
Institute of Reproductive and Developmental Biology
Imperial College London
London, United Kingdom
Differentiation of the Ovary

David H. Chu, MD, PhD
Staff Physician
Division of Dermatology and Cutaneous Surgery
Scripps Clinic Medical Group
La Jolla, California
Structure and Development of the Skin and Cutaneous Appendages

Wendy K. Chung, MD, PhD
Kennedy Family Professor of Pediatrics and Medicine
Department of Pediatrics
Division of Molecular Genetics
Columbia University Irving Medical Center
New York, New York
Basic Genetic Principles

Maria Roberta Cilio, MD, PhD
Professor
Department of Pediatrics
Saint-Luc University Hospital
Université Catholique de Louvain
Brussels, Belgium
Electroencephalography in the Preterm and Term Infant

David A. Clark, MD
Chairman and Professor
Department of Pediatrics
Albany Medical College
Albany, New York
Development of the Gastrointestinal Circulation in the Fetus and Newborn

Paul Clarke, MD, DCH DCCH
Professor
Neonatal Intensive Care Unit
Norfolk and Norwich University Hospitals NHS Foundation Trust
Professor
Norwich Medical School
University of East Anglia
Norwich, United Kingdom
Vitamin K Metabolism in the Fetus and Neonate

Jane K. Cleal, PhD
Lecturer in Epigenetics
School of Human Development and Health
Faculty of Medicine
University of Southampton
Southampton, United Kingdom
Mechanisms of Transfer Across the Human Placenta

Ethel G. Clemente, MD
Assistant Professor
Department of Pediatrics
Western Michigan University Homer Stryker MD School of Medicine
Kalamazoo, Michigan
Luteinizing Hormone and Follicle-Stimulating Hormone Secretion in the Fetus and Newborn Infant

John A. Clements, MD
Professor Emeritus
Department of Pediatrics
University of California, San Francisco
San Francisco, California
Historical Perspective

Ronald I. Clyman, MD
Professor Emeritus
Department of Pediatrics
University of California, San Francisco
San Francisco, California
Mechanisms Regulating Closure of the Ductus Arteriosus

Jennifer L. Cohen, MD
Assistant Professor
Department of Pediatrics
Division of Medical Genetics Pediatrics
Duke University School of Medicine
Durham, North Carolina
Genetic Variants and Neonatal Disease

Susan S. Cohen, MD
Associate Professor
Department of Pediatrics
Medical College of Wisconsin
Milwaukee, Wisconsin
Development of the Blood-Brain Barrier

Amélie Collins, MD, PhD
Assistant Professor
Department of Pediatrics
Columbia University Irving Medical Center
New York, New York
Developmental Biology of Hematopoietic Stem Cells

Allan Collodel, PhD
Laboratory of Experimental Pathophysiology
Graduate Program in Health Sciences
University of Southern Santa Catarina
Criciúma, Brazil
Pathophysiology of Neonatal Acute Bacterial Meningitis

John Colombo, PhD
Professor
Department of Psychology
University of Kansas
Lawrence, Kansas
Long-Chain Polyunsaturated Fatty Acids in Neurodevelopment

Alexander N. Combes, PhD
Senior Research Fellow
Monash Biomedicine Discovery Institute
Department of Anatomy and Developmental Biology
Biomedicine Discovery Institute
Monash University
Melbourne, Victoria, Australia
Development of the Kidney: Morphology and Mechanisms

Andrew J. Copp, MBBS, DPhil
Professor
GOS Institute of Child Health
University College London
London, United Kingdom
Pathophysiology of Neural Tube Defects

C. Michael Cotten, MD
Professor
Chief, Division of Pediatric Neonatology
Department of Pediatrics
Duke University School of Medicine
Durham, North Carolina
Genetic Variants and Neonatal Disease

Peter A. Crawford, MD, PhD
Professor
Vice Chair for Research
Department of Medicine
Director, Division of Molecular Medicine
University of Minnesota Medical School
Minneapolis, Minnesota
Ketone Body Metabolism in the Neonate

James E. Crowe, Jr., MD
Director
Vanderbilt Vaccine Center
Ann Scott Carell Chair
Pediatrics and Pathology, Microbiology and Immunology
Vanderbilt University Medical Center
Nashville, Tennessee
Host Defense Mechanisms Against Viruses

C.A. Crowther, MBChB, DCH, MD, CMFM
Professor
Liggins Institute
University of Auckland
Auckland, New Zealand
Antenatal Hormonal Therapy for Prevention of Respiratory Distress Syndrome

Luise A. Cullen-McEwen, BSc, PhD
Research Fellow
Department of Anatomy and Developmental Biology
Biomedicine Discovery Institute
Monash University
Melbourne, Victoria, Australia
Development of the Kidney: Morphology and Mechanisms

Wayne S. Cutfield, MD
Professor
Liggins Institute
University of Auckland
Auckland, New Zealand
Epigenetics

Chanèle Cyr-Depauw, MSc
PhD Candidate
Sinclair Centre for Regenerative Medicine
Ottawa Hospital Research Institute
Department of Cellular and Molecular Medicine
University of Ottawa
Ottawa, Ontario, Canada
Developmental Biology of Lung Stem Cells

Karla Danielly da S. Ribeiro, PhD
Nutritionist
Professor Adjunct
Department of Nutrition
Researcher
Postgraduate Program in Nutrition
Federal University of Rio Grande do Norte
Natal, Brazil
Vitamin E Nutrition in Pregnancy and the Newborn Infant

Nicolas Dauby, MD, PhD
Deputy Head of Clinic
Infectious Diseases
CHU Saint-Pierre
Post-Doctoral Researcher
Institute for Medical Immunology
Université Libre de Bruxelles
Brussels, Belgium
Host Defense Mechanisms Against Bacteria

Patricia Davenport, MD
Instructor of Pediatrics
Division of Newborn Medicine
Children's Hospital Boston and Harvard Medical School
Boston, Massachusetts
Developmental Megakaryopoiesis

Joanne O. Davidson, PhD
Senior Research Fellow
Department of Physiology
University of Auckland
Auckland, New Zealand
Neuroprotective Therapeutic Hypothermia

Diomel de la Cruz, MD
Assistant Professor
Department of Pediatrics
Division of Neonatology
University of Florida College of Medicine
Gainesville, Florida
Digestive-Absorptive Functions in Fetuses, Infants, and Children

Priscila Gomes de Oliveira, MD
Nutritionist
Specialist in Neonate Intensive Care
Postgraduate Program in Nutrition
Federal University of Rio Grande do Norte
Natal, Brazil
Vitamin E Nutrition in Pregnancy and the Newborn Infant

Barbra de Vrijer, MD
Associate Professor
Department of Obstetrics and Gynaecology
Western University
London, Ontario, Canada
Placental and Fetal Circulatory and Metabolic Changes Accompanying Fetal Growth Restriction

Andrew Del Colle, MS
Research Assistant
Department of Pediatrics
Columbia University Vagelos College of Physicians and Surgeons
New York, New York
Development of the Enteric Nervous System and Gastrointestinal Motility

Christophe Delacourt, MD, PhD
Physician
Department of Paediatric Pulmonology and Allergology
University Hospital Necker-Enfants Malades
Assistance Publique-Hôpitaux de Paris
Paris, France
Regulation of Alveolarization

Thomas G. Diacovo, MD
Professor
Department of Pediatrics
University of Pittsburgh School of Medicine
Chief, UMPC Division of Newborn Medicine
University of Pittsburgh Medical Center
Pittsburgh, Pennsylvania
Platelet–Vessel Wall Interactions

Clémence Disdier, PhD, PharmD
Postdoctoral Fellow
Department of Pediatrics
The Warren Alpert Medical School of Brown University
Providence, Rhode Island
Development of the Blood-Brain Barrier

John P. Dormans, MD
Chief, Pediatric Orthopedic Surgery
Riley Hospital for Children
Garceau Professor of Orthopedic Surgery
Indiana University School of Medicine
Indianapolis, Indiana
The Growth Plate: Embryologic Origin, Structure, and Function

François Duhamel, BPharm, MSc
PhD Candidate
Department of Pharmacology
University of Montreal
Montreal, Quebec, Canada
Basic Pharmacologic Principles

Minh Dien Duong, MD
Department of Pediatrics
Division of Nephrology
The Children's Hospital at Montefiore
Albert Einstein College of Medicine
Bronx, New York
Role of the Kidney in Calcium and Phosphorus Homeostasis

Kevin Dysart, MD
Associate Medical Director
Division of Neonatology
Children's Hospital of Philadelphia
Philadelphia, Pennsylvania
Evaluation of Pulmonary Function in the Neonate

Eric C. Eichenwald, MD
Professor of Pediatrics
Department of Pediatrics/Neonatology
Perelman School of Medicine
University of Pennsylvania
Chief, Division of Neonatology
Children's Hospital of Philadelphia
Philadelphia, Pennsylvania
Evaluation of Pulmonary Function in the Neonate

Afif F. El-Khuffash, MB, BCh, BAO, BA(Sci), MD, DCE
Consultant Neonatologist and Pediatrician
Department of Neonatology
The Rotunda Hospital
Clinical Professor
Department of Paediatrics
Royal College of Physicians in Ireland
Dublin, Ireland
Oxygen Transport and Delivery

Peter James Ivor Ellis, PhD
Senior Lecturer
School of Biosciences
University of Kent
Canterbury, United Kingdom
Genetics of Sex Determination and Differentiation

Kerry M. Empey, PharmD, PhD
Associate Professor
Department of Pharmacy and Therapeutics
Associate Professor (secondary appointment)
Clinical Translational Science Institute
Associate Professor (secondary appointment)
Department of Immunology
University of Pittsburgh
Pittsburgh, Pennsylvania
Neonatal Pulmonary Host Defense

Baris Ercal, MD, PhD
Instructor
Department of Psychiatry
Washington University School of Medicine
St. Louis, Missouri
Ketone Body Metabolism in the Neonate

Melinda Erdős, MD, PhD
Associate Professor
Primary Immunodeficiency Clinical Unit and Laboratory
Department of Dermatology, Venereology, and Dermatooncology
Faculty of Medicine
Semmelweis University
Budapest, Hungary
Host Defense Mechanisms Against Fungi
T-Cell Development

Mariella Errede, MD, PhD
Department of Basic Medical Sciences, Neurosciences, and Sensory Organs
Human Anatomy and Histology Unit
University of Bari School of Medicine
Bari, Italy
Development of the Blood-Brain Barrier

Brian J. Feldman, MD, PhD
Walter L. Miller Distinguished Professorship
Department of Pediatrics
University of California San Francisco
San Francisco, California
Development of the Hypothalamus-Pituitary-Adrenal Axis in the Fetus

Mario Fidanza, PhD
Postdoctoral Scientist
Systems Vaccinology
Telethon Kids Institute
Perth, Western Australia, Australia
Host Defense Mechanisms Against Bacteria

Matthew J. Fogarty, BVSc, PhD
Assistant Professor
Physiology and Biomedical Engineering
Mayo Clinic
Rochester, Minnesota
Functional Development of Respiratory Muscles

Philippe S. Friedlich, MD, MS Epi, MBA
Teresa and Byron Pollitt Family Chair in Fetal & Neonatal Medicine
Professor
Departments of Pediatrics and Surgery
Keck School of Medicine
University of Southern California
Co-Director, Fetal and Neonatal Institute
Children's Hospital Los Angeles
Chief, Division of Neonatology
Department of Pediatrics
Children's Hospital Los Angeles
Los Angeles, California
Regulation of Acid-Base Balance in the Fetus and Neonate
Pathophysiology of Shock in the Fetus and Neonate

Ryoichi Fujiwara, PhD
Assistant Professor
Department of Pharmaceutical Sciences
College of Pharmacy
University of Arkansas for Medical Sciences
Little Rock, Arkansas
Fetal and Neonatal Bilirubin Metabolism

Vittorio Gallo, PhD
Chief Research Officer
Center for Neuroscience Research
Children's National Research Institute and George Washington University School of Medicine and Health Sciences
Washington, District of Columbia
Cellular and Molecular Mechanisms of Neonatal Brain Injury and Neuroprotection

Abhrajit Ganguly, MD
Assistant Professor of Pediatrics
Section of Neonatal-Perinatal Medicine
Center for Pregnancy & Newborn Research
University of Oklahoma Health Science Center
Oklahoma City, Oklahoma
Regulation of Lower Airway Function

Yuansheng Gao, PhD
Professor
Department of Physiology and Pathophysiology
Peking University Health Science Center
Beijing, China
Regulation of Pulmonary Circulation

Marianne Garland, MB ChB
Associate Professor
Department of Pediatrics
Columbia University Vagelos College of Physicians and Surgeons
Attending Neonatologist
Department of Pediatrics
Children's Hospital of New York
New York, New York
Drug Distribution in Fetal Life

Donna Geddes, Post Grad Dip (Sci), PhD
Professor
School of Molecular Sciences
The University of Western Australia, Perth
Perth, Western Australia, Australia
Human Milk Composition and Function in the Infant

Michael K. Georgieff, MD
Professor
Department of Pediatrics
University of Minnesota Medical School
Minneapolis, Minnesota
Fetal and Neonatal Iron Metabolism

Jason Gien, MD
Associate Professor
Department of Pediatrics
Section of Neonatology
University of Colorado School of Medicine
Aurora, Colorado
Pathophysiology of Meconium Aspiration Syndrome

Dino A. Giussani, PhD, ScD
Professor
Department of Physiology Development and Neuroscience
Professorial Fellow
Gonville & Caius College
Cambridge, United Kingdom
Regulation of Cardiovascular Function During Fetal and Newborn Life

Armond S. Goldman, MD
Emeritus Professor
Department of Pediatrics
University of Texas Medical Branch
Galveston, Texas
Immunology of Human Milk

Nardhy Gomez-Lopez, PhD
Associate Professor
Division of Maternal-Fetal Medicine
Department of Obstetrics and Gynecology
Wayne State University School of Medicine
Detroit, Michigan
Intra-Amniotic Infection/Inflammation and the Fetal Inflammatory Response Syndrome

Misty Good, MD
Assistant Professor
Division of Newborn Medicine
Departments of Pediatrics, Pathology, and Immunology
Washington University School of Medicine
St. Louis, Missouri
Neonatal Pulmonary Host Defense
Pathophysiology and Prevention of Neonatal Necrotizing Enterocolitis

Pamela I. Good, MD
Instructor
Division of Neonatology-Perinatology
Department of Pediatrics
Columbia University Vagelos College of Physicians and Surgeons
New York, New York
Response to Nephron Loss in Early Development

Scott M. Gordon, MD, PhD
Attending Physician
Division of Neonatology
Children's Hospital of Philadelphia
Instructor
Perelman School of Medicine
University of Pennsylvania
Philadelphia, Pennsylvania
Cytokines and Inflammatory Response in the Fetus and Neonate

Lucy R. Green, BSc, PhD
Physician
Institute of Developmental Sciences
University of Southampton
Southampton, United Kingdom
Nutritional and Environmental Effects on the Fetal Circulation

Nicholas D.E. Greene, PhD
Professor
Great Ormond Street Institute of Child Health
University College London
London, United Kingdom
Pathophysiology of Neural Tube Defects

Zoya Gridneva, BSc, PhD
Research Associate
School of Molecular Sciences
The University of Western Australia, Crawley
Crawley, Western Australia, Australia
Human Milk Composition and Function in the Infant

Emmanouil Grigoriou, MD
Pediatric Orthopaedic Surgery
Texas Scottish Rite Hospital for Children
Dallas, Texas
The Growth Plate: Embryologic Origin, Structure, and Function

Adda Grimberg, MD
Professor
Department of Pediatrics
Perelman School of Medicine
University of Pennsylvania
Scientific Director
Diagnostic and Research Growth Center
Children's Hospital of Philadelphia
Philadelphia, Pennsylvania
Hypothalamus: Neuroendometabolic Center

Ruth E. Grunau, PhD
Professor
Department of Pediatrics
University of British Columbia
Vancouver, Canada
Developmental Aspects of Pain

Jean-Pierre Guignard, MD
Honorary Professor of Pediatric Nephrology
Lausanne University Medical School
Lausanne, Switzerland
Postnatal Development of Glomerular Filtration Rate in Neonates
Concentration and Dilution of Urine

Alistair J. Gunn, MBChB, PhD
Professor
Department of Physiology
University of Auckland
Auckland, New Zealand
Neuroprotective Therapeutic Hypothermia

Nursen Gurtunca, MD
Assistant Professor
Department of Pediatrics
Division of Endocrinology and Diabetes
Children's Hospital of Pittsburgh
Pittsburgh, Pennsylvania
Growth Hormone, Prolactin, and Placental Lactogen in the Fetus and Newborn

Kathleen M. Gustafson, PhD
Associate Professor
Department of Neurology
Hoglund Biomedical Imaging Center
University of Kansas Medical Center
Kansas City, Kansas
Long-Chain Polyunsaturated Fatty Acids in Neurodevelopment

Alice Hadchouel, MD, PhD
Physician
Department of Paediatric Pulmonology and Allergology
University Hospital Necker-Enfants Malades
Assistance Publique-Hôpitaux de Paris
Paris, France
Regulation of Alveolarization

Gabriel G. Haddad, MD
Professor
Department of Pediatrics
University of California, San Diego
La Jolla, California
Basic Mechanisms of Oxygen Sensing and Adaptation to Hypoxia

Thomas W. Hale, RPh, PhD
Professor
Associate Dean of Research
Texas Tech University Health Science Center
Department of Pediatrics
School of Medicine
Amarillo, Texas
Drug Transfer During Breastfeeding

K. Michael Hambidge, MD, ScD
Professor Emeritus
Department of Pediatrics
Section of Nutrition
University of Colorado School of Medicine
Aurora, Colorado
Zinc in the Fetus and Neonate

Cathy Hammerman, MD
Professor of Pediatrics
Faculty of Medicine
Hebrew University
Director, Newborn Nurseries Division
Neonatology
Shaare Zedek Medical Center
Jerusalem, Israel
Hereditary Contributions to Neonatal Hyperbilirubinemia

Thor Willy Ruud Hansen, MD, PhD, MHA
Professor Emeritus
Division of Pediatric and Adolescent Medicine
Oslo University Hospital and Institute of Clinical Medicine
Oslo, Norway
Pathophysiology of Kernicterus

Mark A. Hanson, MA, DPhil
Director
Institute of Developmental Sciences
University of Southampton
Southampton, United Kingdom
Nutritional and Environmental Effects on the Fetal Circulation

Danny Harbeson, PhD
Experimental Medicine
University of British Columbia
Vancouver, British Columbia, Canada
Host Defense Mechanisms Against Bacteria

J.E. Harding, MBChB, DPhil
Professor
Liggins Institute
University of Auckland
Auckland, New Zealand
Antenatal Hormonal Therapy for Prevention of Respiratory Distress Syndrome

Richard Harding, PhD, DSc
Emeritus Professor
Department of Anatomy and Developmental Biology
Monash University
Melbourne, Victoria, Australia
Physiologic Mechanisms of Normal and Altered Lung Growth Before and After Birth

Mary Catherine Harris, MD
Professor
Division of Neonatology
Department of Pediatrics
Children's Hospital of Philadelphia
Philadelphia, Pennsylvania
Cytokines and Inflammatory Response in the Fetus and Neonate

Peter Hartmann, BSc, PhD
Emeritus Professor
School of Molecular Sciences
The University of Western Australia, Perth
Perth, Western Australia, Australia
Human Milk Composition and Function in the Infant

M. Elizabeth Hartnett, MD
Distinguished Professor in Ophthalmology and Visual Sciences
Department of Ophthalmology
John A. Moran Eye Center
University of Utah Health
Salt Lake City, Utah
Pathophysiology of Retinopathy of Prematurity

Rodrigo Hasbun, MD, MPH
Professor
Division of Infectious Diseases
The University of Texas Health Science Center at Houston
McGovern Medical School
Houston, Texas
Pathophysiology of Neonatal Acute Bacterial Meningitis

Guttorm Haugen, MD
Consultant
Department of Fetal Medicine
Division of Obstetrics and Gynaecology
Oslo University Hospital
Professor
Institute of Clinical Medicine
Faculty of Medicine
University of Oslo
Oslo, Norway
Umbilical Circulation

Colin P. Hawkes, MD, PhD
Physician
Division of Endocrinology and Diabetes
Children's Hospital of Philadelphia
Adjunct Professor
Department of Pediatrics
Perelman School of Medicine
University of Pennsylvania
Philadelphia, Pennsylvania
Consultant Paediatric Endocrinologist
Department of Paediatrics and Child Health
University College Cork
Cork, Ireland
Growth Factor Regulation of Fetal Growth
Pathophysiology of Neonatal Hypoglycemia

William W. Hay, Jr., MD
Professor (Retired)
Department of Pediatrics
University of Colorado School of Medicine
Aurora, Colorado
Placental and Fetal Circulatory and Metabolic Changes Accompanying Fetal Growth Restriction
Placental Transfer and Fetal Requirements of Amino Acids

Vivi M. Heine, PhD
Assistant Professor
Pediatrics/Child Neurology
Vrije University Medical Center
Amsterdam, The Netherlands
Cerebellar Development—The Impact of Preterm Birth and Comorbidities

Michael A. Helmrath, MD
Professor
Division of Pediatric General and Thoracic Surgery
Cincinnati Children's Hospital Medical Center
Cincinnati, Ohio
Organogenesis of the Gastrointestinal Tract

Karen D. Hendricks-Muñoz, MD, MPH
William Tate Graham Professor
Chair, Neonatal Medicine
Department of Pediatrics
Virginia Commonwealth University School of Medicine
Richmond, Virginia
Structure and Development of Alveolar Epithelial Cells

Emilio Herrera, PhD
Emeritus Professor of Biochemistry and Molecular Biology
Department of Chemistry and Biochemistry
Faculties of Pharmacy and Medicine
University San Pablo-CEU
Madrid, Spain
Maternal-Fetal Transfer of Lipid Metabolites
Lipids as an Energy Source for the Premature and Term Neonate

Michael J. Hiatt, PhD
Senior Scientist Research and Development
Stemcell Technologies
Vancouver, British Columbia, Canada
Functional Development of the Kidney in Utero

Stuart B. Hooper, BSc (Hons), PhD
Professor
The Ritchie Centre
Hudson Institute for Medical Research
Professor
Department of Obstetrics and Gynaecology
Monash University
Melbourne, Victoria, Australia
Physiologic Mechanisms of Normal and Altered Lung Growth Before and After Birth
Physiology of Neonatal Resuscitation

Thomas A. Hooven, MD
Assistant Professor
Department of Pediatrics
University of Pittsburgh School of Medicine
Pittsburgh, Pennsylvania
Pathophysiology of Chorioamnionitis: Host Immunity and Microbial Virulence

Silvia Iacobelli, MD, PhD
Professor of Pediatrics
Réanimation Néonatale et Pédiatrique, Neonatologie
Centre Hospitalier Universitaire La Réunion
Saint Pierre, France
Centre d'Etudes Périnatales de l'Océan Indien
Université de la Réunion
Réunion, France
Postnatal Development of Glomerular Filtration Rate in Neonates
Concentration and Dilution of Urine

Terrie E. Inder, MBChB, MD
Chair
Pediatric Newborn Medicine
Brigham and Women's Hospital
Professor
Department of Pediatrics
Harvard Medical School
Boston, Massachusetts
Intraventricular Hemorrhage in the Neonate

M. Luisa Iruela-Arispe, PhD
Stephen Walter Ranson Professor and Chair
Department of Cell and Developmental Biology
Feinberg School of Medicine
Northwestern University
Chicago, Illinois
Angiogenesis

Sudarshan Rao Jadcherla, MD, DCH, AGAF
Professor
Department of Pediatrics
Sections of Neonatology and Pediatric Gastroenterology & Nutrition
The Ohio State University College of Medicine
Attending Neonatologist
Section of Neonatology
Director
Neonatal and Infant Feeding Disorders Program
Nationwide Children's Hospital
Principal Investigator
Center for Perinatal Research
Abigail Wexner Research Institute at Nationwide Children's Hospital
Columbus, Ohio
Pathophysiology of Gastroesophageal Reflux

Deepak Jain, MD
Associate Professor
Department of Pediatrics
Division of Neonatology
Rutgers Robert Wood Johnson Medical School
New Brunswick, New Jersey
Pathophysiology of Bronchopulmonary Dysplasia

Jennifer G. Jetton, MD
Medical Director, Pediatric Dialysis Unit
Clinical Associate Professor
Division of Nephrology
Stead Family Department of Pediatrics
University of Iowa Health Care
Iowa City, Iowa
Pathophysiology of Neonatal Acute Kidney Injury

Alan H. Jobe, MD, PhD
Professor
Department of Pediatrics
Director, Division of Perinatal Biology
Cincinnati Children's Hospital Medical Center
Cincinnati, Ohio
Antenatal Factors That Influence Postnatal Lung Development and Injury
Surfactant Treatment
Pathophysiology of Respiratory Distress Syndrome

Helen Jones, PhD
Associate Professor
Department of Physiology and Functional Genomics
Department of Obstetrics and Gynecology
University of Florida College of Medicine
Gainesville, Florida
Placental Development

Pedro A. Jose, MD, PhD
Professor
Departments of Medicine and Pharmacology-Physiology
The George Washington University School of Medicine & Health Sciences
Washington, District of Columbia
Development and Regulation of Renal Blood Flow in the Neonate

Eunjung Jung, MD
Assistant Professor
Division of Maternal-Fetal Medicine
Department of Obstetrics and Gynecology
Wayne State University School of Medicine
Detroit, Michigan
Intra-Amniotic Infection/Inflammation and the Fetal Inflammatory Response Syndrome

Suhas G. Kallapur, MD
Professor
Department of Pediatrics
Division of Neonatology
UCLA David Geffen School of Medicine
UCLA Mattel Children's Hospital
Los Angeles, California
Antenatal Factors That Influence Postnatal Lung Development and Injury
Surfactant Treatment

Michael Kaplan, MB ChB
Emeritus Director
Department of Neonatology
Shaare Zedek Medical Center
Professor of Pediatrics
Faculty of Medicine
Hebrew University
Jerusalem, Israel
Hereditary Contributions to Neonatal Hyperbilirubinemia

S. Ananth Karumanchi, MD
Professor
Department of Medicine
Harvard Medical School
Boston, Massachusetts
Staff Physician
Medallion Chair in Vascular Biology
Director, Nephrology
Cedars-Sinai Medical Center
Los Angeles, California
Pathophysiology of Preeclampsia

Frederick J. Kaskel, MD, PhD
Professor
Department of Pediatrics
Division of Nephrology
The Children's Hospital at Montefiore
Albert Einstein College of Medicine
Bronx, New York
Role of the Kidney in Calcium and Phosphorus Homeostasis

Lorraine E. Levitt Katz, MD
Physician
Division of Endocrinology and Diabetes
Children's Hospital of Philadelphia
Professor
Perelman School of Medicine
University of Pennsylvania
Philadelphia, Pennsylvania
Growth Factor Regulation of Fetal Growth

Haluk Kavus, MD
Medical Geneticist, Postdoctoral Research Scientist
Pediatrics, Division of Molecular Genetics
Columbia University Vagelos College of Physicians and Surgeons
New York, New York
Basic Genetic Principles

Susan E. Keeney, MD
Associate Professor
Department of Pediatrics
University of Texas Medical Branch
Galveston, Texas
Immunology of Human Milk

Steven E. Kern, PhD
Deputy Director, Quantitative Sciences
Global Health-Integrated Development
Bill & Melinda Gates Foundation
Seattle, Washington
Principles of Pharmacokinetics

Shirin Khanjani, MD, PhD
University College London Hospitals
London, United Kingdom
Pathophysiology of Preterm Birth

Julie Khlevner, MD
Associate Professor
Department of Pediatrics
Columbia University Vagelos College of Physicians and Surgeons
New York, New York
Development of the Enteric Nervous System and Gastrointestinal Motility

Laurie E. Kilpatrick, PhD
Professor
Department of Thoracic Medicine and Surgery
Lewis Katz School of Medicine
Temple University
Philadelphia, Pennsylvania
Cytokines and Inflammatory Response in the Fetus and Neonate

Chang-Ryul Kim, MD, PhD
Professor
Department of Pediatrics
Hanyang University College of Medicine
Seoul, South Korea
Director in NICU
Hanyang University Guri Hospital
Guri-si, South Korea
Fluid Distribution in the Fetus and Neonate

Paul S. Kingma, MD, PhD
Associate Professor of Pediatrics
Division of Neonatology
University of Cincinnati
Cincinnati Children's Hospital Medical Center
Cincinnati, Ohio
Surfactant Homeostasis: Composition and Function of Pulmonary Surfactant Lipids and Proteins

John P. Kinsella, MD
Professor
Department of Pediatrics
Section of Neonatology
University of Colorado School of Medicine
Aurora, Colorado
Pulmonary Gas Exchange in the Developing Lung
Pathophysiology of Meconium Aspiration Syndrome

Torvid Kiserud, MD, PhD
Professor
Department of Clinical Science
University of Bergen
Consultant
Fetal Medicine Unit
Department of Obstetrics and Gynecology
Haukeland University Hospital
Bergen, Norway
Umbilical Circulation

Joyce M. Koenig, MD
Professor
Division of Neonatal/Perinatal Medicine
Department of Pediatrics
Saint Louis University School of Medicine
St. Louis, Missouri
Normal and Abnormal Neutrophil Physiology in the Newborn

Rohit Kohli, MBBS, MS
Chief, Division of Gastroenterology
Children's Hospital Los Angeles
Professor of Pediatrics
Keck School of Medicine
University of Southern California
Los Angeles, California
Bile Acid Metabolism During Development

Tobias R. Kollmann, MD, PhD
Professor
Systems Biology and Pediatric Infectious Diseases
Telethon Kids Institute
Perth, Western Australia, Australia
Host Defense Mechanisms Against Bacteria

Jay K. Kolls, MD
Professor of Pediatrics
Medicine and Pediatrics
Tulane University School of Medicine
New Orleans, Louisiana
Neonatal Pulmonary Host Defense

Christina M. Konecny, MD
Postdoctoral Scholar
Department of Pediatrics
Stanford University School of Medicine
Stanford, California
Mechanistic Aspects of Phototherapy for Neonatal Hyperbilirubinemia

Panagiotis Kratimenos, MD, PhD
Assistant Professor
Center for Neuroscience Research
Children's National Research Institute and George Washington University School of Medicine and Health Sciences
Department of Pediatrics
Division of Neonatology
Children's National Hospital
Washington, District of Columbia
Cellular and Molecular Mechanisms of Neonatal Brain Injury and Neuroprotection

Nancy F. Krebs, MD
Professor
Department of Pediatrics
Section of Nutrition
University of Colorado School of Medicine
Aurora, Colorado
Zinc in the Fetus and Neonate

Kaytlin Krutsch, PharmD, MBA
Assistant Professor
Texas Tech University Health Sciences Center
Department of Obstetrics and Gynecology
School of Medicine
Amarillo, Texas
Drug Transfer During Breastfeeding

Kara Kuhn-Riordon, MD
Assistant Clinical Professor
Department of Pediatrics
Division of Neonatology
University of California Davis School of Medicine
Sacramento, California
Endocrine Factors Affecting Neonatal Growth

†Thomas J. Kulik, MD
Senior Associate in Cardiology
Department of Cardiology
Boston Children's Hospital
Associate Professor of Pediatrics
Harvard Medical School
Boston, Massachusetts
Physiology of Congenital Heart Disease in the Neonate

T. Rajendra Kumar, PhD
Professor and Edgar L. Patricia M. Makowski and Family Endowed Chair
Department of Obstetrics and Gynecology
University of Colorado School of Medicine
Aurora, Colorado
Luteinizing Hormone and Follicle-Stimulating Hormone Secretion in the Fetus and Newborn Infant

Jessica Katz Kutikov, MD
Pediatrics Specialist
Voorhees, New Jersey
Hypothalamus: Neuroendometabolic Center

Satyan Lakshminrusimha, MBBS, MD
Professor
Dennis and Nancy Marks Chair of Pediatrics
Pediatrician-in-Chief
UC Davis Children's Hospital
Sacramento, California
Pathophysiology of Persistent Pulmonary Hypertension of the Newborn

Miguel Angel Lasunción, PhD
Head, Servicio de Bioquímica-Investigación
Hospital Universitario Ramón y Cajal, IRyCIS, and CIBEROBN
Madrid, Spain
Maternal-Fetal Transfer of Lipid Metabolites

Pascal M. Lavoie, MDCM, PhD
Associate Professor
Department of Pediatrics
University of British Columbia
Clinician-Scientist
BC Children's Hospital Research Institute
Canada Staff Neonatologist
Children's & Women's Health Centre of British Columbia
Vancouver, British Columbia, Canada
Mononuclear Phagocyte System

Shelley M. Lawrence, MD
Associate Professor
Department of Pediatrics
Divisions of Neonatal-Perinatal Medicine and Host-Microbe Systems and Therapeutics
University of California, San Diego
La Jolla, California
Neutrophil Granulopoiesis and Homeostasis

Mark K. Lee, MD
Professor and Chief Physician
Nemours Children's Hospital
Wilmington, Delaware
Regulation of Embryogenesis

Mary M. Lee, MD
Professor
Department of Pediatrics
Sidney Kimmel Medical College
Jefferson University
Philadelphia, Pennsylvania
Physician-in-Chief
Nemours, AI duPont Hospital for Children
Chief Scientific Officer
Nemours Health Care System
Wilmington, Delaware
Testicular Development and Descent

†Deceased.

Yvonne K. Lee, MD
Pediatric Endocrinology
Department of Pediatrics
Kaiser Permanente
Oakland, California
Endocrine Factors Affecting Neonatal Growth

Sandra L. Leibel, MD
Assistant Professor
Department of Pediatrics
University of California, San Diego
La Jolla, California
The Extracellular Matrix in Development
Molecular Mechanisms of Lung Development and Lung Branching Morphogenesis

Ofer Levy, MD, PhD
Director, Precision Vaccines Program
Division of Infectious Diseases
Boston Children's Hospital
Professor
Department of Pediatrics
Harvard Medical School
Boston, Massachusetts
Associate Member
Broad Institute of MIT and Harvard
Cambridge, Massachusetts
Mononuclear Phagocyte System

Philip T. Levy, MD
Physician
Department of Neonatology
Division of Newborn Medicine
Boston Children's Hospital
Harvard Medical School
Boston, Massachusetts
Physiology of Congenital Heart Disease in the Neonate

Rohan M. Lewis, PhD
Professor
School of Human Development and Health
Faculty of Medicine
University of Southampton
Southampton, United Kingdom
Mechanisms of Transfer Across the Human Placenta
Placental Transfer and Fetal Requirements of Amino Acids

Changgong Li, PhD
Associate Professor
Department of Pediatrics
Keck School of Medicine
University of Southern California
Los Angeles County-University of Southern California Medical Center
Los Angeles, California
Regulation of Embryogenesis

Fangming Lin, MD, PhD
Director, Pediatric Nephrology
Department of Pediatrics
Columbia University Vagelos College of Physicians and Surgeons
New York, New York
Response to Nephron Loss in Early Development

Steven Lobritto, MD
Professor
Department of Pediatrics
NY Presbyterian–Columbia
New York, New York
Organogenesis and Histologic Development of the Liver

Cynthia A. Loomis, MD
Assistant Professor
Ronald O. Perelman Department of Dermatology
NYU Grossman School of Medicine
New York, New York
Structure and Development of the Skin and Cutaneous Appendages

Peter M. MacFarlane, PhD
Associate Professor
Department of Pediatrics
Division of Neonatology
Case Western Reserve University School of Medicine
Cleveland, Ohio
Regulation of Lower Airway Function
Pathophysiology of Apnea of Prematurity

David A. MacIntyre, PhD
Senior Lecturer
Faculty of Medicine
Department of Metabolism, Digestion, and Reproduction
Institute of Reproductive and Developmental Biology
Imperial College Parturition Research Group
Researcher
March of Dimes Prematurity Research Centre
Imperial College London
London, United Kingdom
Pathophysiology of Preterm Birth

Maxime M. Mahe, PhD
Assistant Professor
TENS, The Enteric Nervous System in Gut and Brain Diseases
INSERM
Université de Nantes
Nantes, France
Adjunct Assistant Professor
Department of Pediatric General and Thoracic Surgery
Cincinnati Children's Hospital Medical Center
Department of Pediatrics
University of Cincinnati
Cincinnati, Ohio
Organogenesis of the Gastrointestinal Tract

Linn Salto Mamsen, MSc, PhD
Researcher
Laboratory of Reproductive Biology
University Hospital of Copenhagen, Rigshospitalet
Copenhagen, Denmark
Differentiation of the Ovary

Anastasiya Mankouski, MD
Assistant Professor
Department of Pediatrics
Division of Neonatology
University of Utah Health
Salt Lake City, Utah
Mechanisms of Neonatal Lung Injury

Carlos B. Mantilla, MD, PhD
Professor and Chair
Anesthesiology and Perioperative Medicine
Professor
Physiology and Biomedical Engineering
Mayo Clinic
Rochester, Minnesota
Functional Development of Respiratory Muscles

Arnaud Marchant, MD, PhD
Director
Institute for Medical Immunology
Université Libre de Bruxelles
Brussels, Belgium
Host Defense Mechanisms Against Bacteria
Host Defense Mechanisms Against Viruses

Kara Gross Margolis, MD
Associate Professor
Department of Pediatrics
Columbia University Vagelos College of Physicians and Surgeons
New York, New York
Development of the Enteric Nervous System and Gastrointestinal Motility

László Maródi, MD, PhD
Professor
Primary Immunodeficiency Clinical Unit and Laboratory
Department of Dermatology, Venereology, and Dermatooncology
Faculty of Medicine
Semmelweis University
Budapest, Hungary
Host Defense Mechanisms Against Fungi
T-Cell Development

Karel Maršál, MD, PhD
Professor Emeritus
Department of Obstetrics and Gynecology
Lund University
Lund, Sweden
Fetal and Placental Circulation During Labor

Richard J. Martin, MBBS
Professor of Pediatrics, Reproductive Biology, and Physiology & Biophysics
Division of Neonatology
Case Western Reserve University School of Medicine
Drusinsky-Fanaroff Professor
Director, Neonatal Research
Department of Pediatrics/Neonatology
Rainbow Babies and Children's Hospital
Cleveland, Ohio
Regulation of Lower Airway Function

Jayne F. Martin Carli, PhD
Fellow
Department of Pediatrics
University of Colorado School of Medicine
Aurora, Colorado
Physiology of Lactation
Pathophysiology of Apnea of Prematurity

Hugo R. Martinez, MD
Assistant Professor
Department of Pediatrics
University of Tennessee Health Science Center
Cardiomyopathy and Transplant Cardiology
Cardio-Vascular Genetics Service
Le Bonheur Hospital
Cardio-Oncology Service
St. Jude Children's Research Hospital
Memphis, Tennessee
Pathophysiology of Cardiomyopathies

Douglas G. Matsell, MDCM
Head, Division of Nephrology
British Columbia Children's Hospital
University of British Columbia
Vancouver, British Columbia, Canada
Functional Development of the Kidney in Utero

Dwight E. Matthews, PhD
Professor Emeritus
Chemistry and Medicine
University of Vermont
Burlington, Vermont
General Concepts of Protein Metabolism

Harry J. McArdle, BSc (Hons), PhD
Professor
Rowett Institute of Nutrition and Health
University of Aberdeen
Aberdeen, United Kingdom
Fetal and Neonatal Iron Metabolism

C.J.D. McKinlay, MBChB, PhD
Senior Lecturer
Liggins Institute
University of Auckland
Auckland, New Zealand
Antenatal Hormonal Therapy for Prevention of Respiratory Distress Syndrome

James L. McManaman, PhD
Professor
Department of Obstetrics and Gynecology
University of Colorado School of Medicine
Aurora, Colorado
Physiology of Lactation

Patrick J. McNamara, MD, MRCPCH, MSc
Professor
Department of Pediatrics
Director, Division of Neonatology
University of Iowa Health Care
Iowa City, Iowa
Oxygen Transport and Delivery

Giacomo Meschia, MD
Emeritus Professor
Department of Physiology
University of Colorado School of Medicine
Aurora, Colorado
Placental and Fetal Circulatory and Metabolic Changes Accompanying Fetal Growth Restriction

Karen Mestan, MD
Associate Professor
Department of Pediatrics
Northwestern University Feinberg School of Medicine
Chicago, Illinois
Placental Function in Intrauterine Growth Restriction

Steven P. Miller, MDCM, MAS
Division Head, Neurology
Bloorview Children's Hospital
Chair, Paediatric Neuroscience
The Hospital for Sick Children
Professor
Department of Pediatrics
University of Toronto
Senior Scientist, Chair
Neuroscience and Mental Health
SickKids Research Institute
Toronto, Ontario, Canada
Pathophysiology of Neonatal White Matter Injury

Parviz Minoo, PhD
Professor
Department of Pediatrics
Keck School of Medicine
University of Southern California
Los Angeles County—University of Southern California Medical Center
Los Angeles, California
Regulation of Embryogenesis

Imran N. Mir, MD
Assistant Professor
Department of Pediatrics
University of Texas Southwestern Medical Center
Dallas, Texas
Regulation of the Placental Circulation

Lisa J. Mitchell, DO
Assistant Professor
Department of Pediatrics
F. Edward Hébert School of Medicine
Uniformed Services University of the Health Sciences
Bethesda, Maryland
Medical Director
Neonatal Intensive Care Unit
Carl R. Darnall Army Medical Center
Fort Hood, Texas
Pathophysiology of Apnea of Prematurity

Ivana Mižíková, PhD
Postdoctoral Fellow
Sinclair Centre for Regenerative Medicine
Ottawa Hospital Research Institute
Department of Cellular and Molecular Medicine
University of Ottawa
Ottawa, Ontario, Canada
Developmental Biology of Lung Stem Cells

Tomoyuki Mizuno, PhD
Assistant Professor
Division of Clinical Pharmacology
Cincinnati Children's Hospital Medical Center
Assistant Professor
Department of Pediatrics
University of Cincinnati College of Medicine
Cincinnati, Ohio
Pharmacogenomics

Jeremiah D. Momper, PharmD, PhD
Associate Professor
Skaggs School of Pharmacy and Pharmaceutical Sciences
University of California, San Diego
La Jolla, California
Organic Anion Transport in the Developing Kidney

Paul Monagle, MBBS, MD, MSC
Professor
Department Paediatrics
University of Melbourne
Haematologist
Department of Haematology
Royal Children's Hospital
Group Leader
Haematology Research
Murdoch Childrens Research Institute
Melbourne, Victoria, Australia
Staff Specialist
Kids Cancer Centre
Sydney Children's Hospital
Sydney, New South Wales, Australia
Developmental Hemostasis

Jenifer Monks, PhD
Assistant Professor
Department of Obstetrics and Gynecology
University of Colorado School of Medicine
Aurora, Colorado
Physiology of Lactation

Jacopo P. Mortola, MD
Professor
Department of Physiology
McGill University
Montreal, Quebec, Canada
Mechanics of Breathing

Louis J. Muglia, MD, PhD
Adjunct Professor
Department of Pediatrics
Cincinnati Children's Hospital Medical Center
Cincinnati, Ohio
President and CEO
Burroughs Wellcome Fund
Research Triangle Park, North Carolina
Fetal and Neonatal Adrenocortical Physiology

Upender K. Munshi, MBBS, MD
Associate Professor
Department of Pediatrics
Albany Medical Center
Albany, New York
Development of the Gastrointestinal Circulation in the Fetus and Newborn

Sumana Narasimhan, MD
Assistant Professor
Pediatric Endocrinology
Case Western Reserve University
Cleveland, Ohio
Luteinizing Hormone and Follicle-Stimulating Hormone Secretion in the Fetus and Newborn Infant

Vivek Narendran, MD, MRCP (UK), MBA
Professor of Pediatrics
Perinatal Institute
Cincinnati Children's Hospital and Medical Center
Director UCMC-NICU
University of Cincinnati Medical Center
Cincinnati Children's Hospital Medical Center
Cincinnati, Ohio
Physiologic Development of the Skin

Jan Nedergaard, PhD
Professor
Department of Molecular Biosciences
The Wenner-Gren Institute
Stockholm University
Stockholm, Sweden
Brown Adipose Tissue: Development and Function

Leif D. Nelin, MD
Dean W. Jeffers Chair in Neonatology
Nationwide Children's Hospital
Professor and Chief
Division of Neonatology
The Ohio State University
Columbus, Ohio
Pulmonary Gas Exchange in the Developing Lung

Josef Neu, MD
Professor
Department of Pediatrics
Division of Neonatology
University of Florida College of Medicine
Gainesville, Florida
Digestive-Absorptive Functions in Fetuses, Infants, and Children
The Developing Microbiome of the Fetus and Neonate: A Multiomic Approach

Sandra C.A. Nielsen, PhD
Scientist
Department of Pathology
Stanford University School of Medicine
Stanford, California
B-Cell Development

Sanjay K. Nigam, MD
Nancy Kaehr Chair in Research
Pediatrics and Medicine
University of California, San Diego
La Jolla, California
Organic Anion Transport in the Developing Kidney

Victor Nizet, MD
Distinguished Professor
Vice Chair for Basic Research
Department of Pediatrics
Distinguished Professor
Department of Pharmacy and Pharmaceutical Sciences
University of California, San Diego
La Jolla, California
Neutrophil Granulopoiesis and Homeostasis

Lawrence M. Nogee, MD
Professor
Eudowood Neonatal Pulmonary Division
Department of Pediatrics
Johns Hopkins University School of Medicine
Baltimore, Maryland
Genetics and Physiology of Surfactant Protein Deficiencies

Shahab Noori, MD, MS CBTI
Professor
Department of Pediatrics
Keck School of Medicine
University of Southern California
Administrative Director of Clinical Research
Division of Neonatology
Children's Hospital Los Angeles
Los Angeles, California
Pathophysiology of Shock in the Fetus and Neonate

Andrew W. Norris, MD, PhD
Professor
Department of Pediatrics
University of Iowa Health Care
Iowa City, Iowa
Glucose Metabolism in the Fetus and Newborn, and Methods for Its Investigation

Barbara M. O'Brien, MD
Beth Israel Deaconess Medical Center
Department of Obstetrics and Gynecology
Boston, Massachusetts
Prenatal Diagnosis

Lori L. O'Brien, PhD
Assistant Professor
Department of Cell Biology and Physiology
University of North Carolina at Chapel Hill
Chapel Hill, North Carolina
Development of the Kidney: Morphology and Mechanisms

Karen M. O'Callaghan, PhD
Research Fellow
Centre for Global Child Health
SickKids Research Institute
The Hospital for Sick Children
Toronto, Ontario, Canada
Fetal and Neonatal Calcium, Phosphorus, and Magnesium Homeostasis

Amanda Ogilvy-Stuart, BM, DM
Consultant Neonatologist
Department of Neonatology
Cambridge University Hospitals NHS Trust
Cambridge, United Kingdom
Role of Glucoregulatory Hormones in Hepatic Glucose Metabolism During the Perinatal Period

Robin K. Ohls, MD
Professor
Department of Pediatrics-Neonatology
University of Utah Health
Salt Lake City, Utah
Developmental Erythropoiesis

Henar Ortega-Senovilla, PhD
Adjunct Professor
Department of Chemistry and Biochemistry
Faculties of Pharmacy and Medicine
Universidad San Pablo-CEU
Madrid, Spain
Lipids as an Energy Source for the Premature and Term Neonate

Justin M. O'Sullivan, PhD
Professor
Deputy Director, Liggins Institute
University of Auckland
Auckland, New Zealand
Epigenetics

Howard B. Panitch, MD
Medical Director, Technology Dependence Program
Division of Pulmonary and Sleep Medicine
Children's Hospital of Philadelphia
Professor
Department of Pediatrics
Perelman School of Medicine
University of Pennsylvania
Philadelphia, Pennsylvania
Pathophysiology of Ventilator-Dependent Infants

Anna A. Penn, MD, PhD
Associate Professor
Department of Pediatrics
George Washington University School of Medicine
Attending Physician and Director
Translational Research for Hospital-Based Services
Co-Director, Cerebral Palsy Prevention Program
Fetal and Transitional Medicine, Neonatology
Investigator
Children's Research Institute Center for Neuroscience
Children's National Medical Center
Washington, District of Columbia
Endocrine and Paracrine Function of the Human Placenta

Raymond B. Penn, PhD
Robley Dunglison Professor of Pulmonary Research
Director, Center for Translational Medicine
Director, Pulmonary Research
Jefferson Jane and Leonard Korman Lung Institute
Vice Chair, Research
Department of Medicine
Division of Pulmonary, Allergy, and Critical Care Medicine
Thomas Jefferson University
Philadelphia, Pennsylvania
Upper Airway Structure: Function, Regulation, and Development

Margaret G. Petroff, PhD
Associate Professor
Pathobiology and Diagnostic Investigation
Michigan State University
East Lansing, Michigan
Placental Development

Anthony F. Philipps, AB, MD
Professor
Department of Pediatrics
University of California Davis School of Medicine
Sacramento, California
Oxygen Consumption and General Carbohydrate Metabolism of the Fetus

Francesco Pisani, MD, PhD
Professor
Child Neuropsychiatry Unit
Department of Medicine and Surgery
Neuroscience Section
University of Parma
Parma, Italy
Electroencephalography in the Preterm and Term Infant

David Pleasure, MD
Distinguished Professor
Department of Neurology and Pediatrics
University of California Davis School of Medicine
Sacramento, California
Trophic Factor, Nutritional, and Hormonal Regulation of Brain Development

Scott L. Pomeroy, MD, PhD
Bronson Crothers Professor
Department of Neurology
Harvard Medical School
Neurologist-in-Chief and Chairman
Department of Neurology
Boston Children's Hospital
Boston, Massachusetts
Development of the Nervous System

Martin Post, PhD
Senior Scientist
Translational Medicine
The Hospital for Sick Children
Professor
Department of Physiology
Laboratory Medicine and Pathobiology
University of Toronto
Toronto, Ontario, Canada
The Extracellular Matrix in Development
Molecular Mechanisms of Lung Development and Lung Branching Morphogenesis

Y.S. Prakash, MD, PhD
Professor
Anesthesiology and Physiology
Mayo Clinic
Rochester, Minnesota
Regulation of Lower Airway Function

Joshua D. Prozialeck, MD, MSA
Assistant Professor
Department of Pediatrics
Northwestern University Feinberg School of Medicine
Ann & Robert H. Lurie Children's Hospital of Chicago
Chicago, Illinois
Development of Gastric Secretory Function

Theodore J. Pysher, MD
Professor
Chief, Division of Pediatric Pathology
Department of Pathology
University of Utah Health
Salt Lake City, Utah
Impaired Lung Growth After Injury in Preterm Lung

Raymond Quigley, MD
Professor
Department of Pediatrics
UT Southwestern Medical Center
Dallas, Texas
Potassium Homeostasis in the Fetus and Neonate
Transport of Amino Acids in the Fetus and Neonate

Marlene Rabinovitch, MD
Professor of Pediatrics
Division of Cardiology
Stanford University School of Medicine
Stanford, California
Developmental Biology of the Pulmonary Vasculature

Thomas M. Raffay, MD
Assistant Professor of Pediatrics
Division of Neonatology
Case Western Reserve University
Rainbow Babies and Children's Hospital
Cleveland, Ohio
Regulation of Lower Airway Function

J. Usha Raj, MD, MHA
Anjuli S. Nayak Professor of Pediatrics
University of Illinois at Chicago
Chicago, Illinois
Regulation of Pulmonary Circulation

Laura B. Ramsey, PhD
Assistant Professor
Divisions of Clinical Pharmacology and Research in Patient Services
Cincinnati Children's Hospital Medical Center
Assistant Professor
Department of Pediatrics
University of Cincinnati College of Medicine
Co-Director, Genetic Pharmacology Service
Cincinnati Children's Hospital Medical Center
Cincinnati, Ohio
Pharmacogenomics

Sarosh Rana, MD, MPH
Professor
Division of Maternal Fetal Medicine
Department of Obstetrics and Gynecology
University of Chicago
Chicago, Illinois
Pathophysiology of Preeclampsia

Tara M. Randis, MD
Associate Professor
Department of Pediatrics and Molecular Medicine
USF Health Morsani College of Medicine
Tampa, Florida
Pathophysiology of Chorioamnionitis: Host Immunity and Microbial Virulence

Manon Ranger, PhD
Assistant Professor
School of Nursing
University of British Columbia
Vancouver, British Columbia, Canada
Developmental Aspects of Pain

Timothy R.H. Regnault, PhD
Associate Professor
Departments of Obstetrics/Gynaecology and Physiology/Pharmacology
Western University
London, Ontario, Canada
Placental and Fetal Circulatory and Metabolic Changes Accompanying Fetal Growth Restriction
Placental Transfer and Fetal Requirements of Amino Acids

Danielle R. Rios, MD
Associate Professor
Department of Pediatrics
Division of Neonatology
University of Iowa Health Care
Iowa City, Iowa
Oxygen Transport and Delivery

Roberto Romero, MD, DMedSci
Chief, Perinatology Research Branch
Eunice Kennedy Shriver National Institute for Child Health and Human Development
National Institutes of Health
U.S. Department of Health and Human Services
Detroit, Michigan
Intra-Amniotic Infection/Inflammation and the Fetal Inflammatory Response Syndrome

Charles R. Rosenfeld, MD
Professor Emeritus
Departments of Pediatrics, Obstetrics/Gynecology, Anesthesiology
University of Texas Southwestern Medical Center
Dallas, Texas
Regulation of the Placental Circulation

A. Catharine Ross, PhD
Professor of Nutrition and Physiology
Nutritional Sciences
Pennsylvania State University
University Park, Pennsylvania
Vitamin A Metabolism in the Fetus and Neonate

Daniel E. Roth, MD, PhD
Staff Pediatrician
Division of Pediatric Medicine
The Hospital for Sick Children
Associate Professor
Departments of Pediatrics and Nutritional Sciences
University of Toronto
Toronto, Ontario, Canada
Fetal and Neonatal Calcium, Phosphorus, and Magnesium Homeostasis

Henry J. Rozycki, MD
Professor and Vice Chair for Research
Department of Pediatrics
Children's Hospital of Richmond at VCU
Director, Children's Health Research Institute
Virginia Commonwealth University School of Medicine
Richmond, Virginia
Structure and Development of Alveolar Epithelial Cells

Thomas D. Ryan, MD, PhD
Associate Professor
Department of Pediatrics
University of Cincinnati College of Medicine
Director, Clinical Operations, Cardiomyopathy, and Heart Failure
Co-Director, Cardio-Oncology Program
The Heart Institute
Cincinnati Children's Hospital Medical Center
Cincinnati, Ohio
Pathophysiology of Cardiomyopathies

Rakesh Sahni, MBBS
Professor
Department of Pediatrics
Columbia University Vagelos College of Physicians and Surgeons
New York, New York
Temperature Control in Newborn Infants

Harvey B. Sarnat, MD
Professor
Departments of Paediatrics, Pathology (Neuropathology), and Clinical Neurosciences
University of Calgary Faculty of Medicine and Alberta Children's Hospital Research Institute
Calgary, Alberta, Canada
Development of Olfaction and Taste in the Human Fetus and Neonate
Ontogenesis of Striated Muscle

Lisa M. Satlin, MD
Professor and System Chair
Department of Pediatrics
Icahn School of Medicine at Mount Sinai
Pediatrician-in-Chief
Mount Sinai Kravis Children's Hospital
New York, New York
Potassium Homeostasis in the Fetus and Neonate

Joseph Scafidi, DO, MS
Associate Professor
Department of Neurology and Pediatrics
Kennedy Krieger Institute
Johns Hopkins School of Medicine
Baltimore, Maryland
Cellular and Molecular Mechanisms of Neonatal Brain Injury and Neuroprotection

Michael A. Schellpfeffer, MD
Professor
Departments of Cell Biology, Neurobiology, and Anatomy
Medical College of Wisconsin
Milwaukee, Wisconsin
Developmental Electrophysiology in the Fetus and Neonate

William Schierding, PhD
Senior Research Fellow
Liggins Institute
University of Auckland
Auckland, New Zealand
Epigenetics

George J. Schwartz, MD
Professor
Department of Pediatrics
Division of Nephrology
University of Rochester Medical Center and Golisano Children's Hospital
Rochester, New York
Urinary Acidification

Jeffrey L. Segar, MD
Physician
Department of Pediatrics
University of Iowa Children's Hospital
Iowa City, Iowa
Regulation of Cardiovascular Function During Fetal and Newborn Life

David T. Selewski, MD
Associate Professor
Department of Pediatrics
Division of Nephrology
Medical University of South Carolina
Charleston, South Carolina
Pathophysiology of Neonatal Acute Kidney Injury

Istvan Seri, MD, PhD, HonD
Professor
Pediatrics (Research)
First Department of Pediatrics
Semmelweis University
Budapest, Hungary, Professor of Pediatrics (Adjunct)
Pediatrics/Neonatology
Children's Hospital Los Angeles
Keck School of Medicine
University of Southern California
Los Angeles, California
Regulation of Acid-Base Balance in the Fetus and Neonate
Pathophysiology of Shock in the Fetus and Neonate

Thomas H. Shaffer, MSE, PhD
Professor Emeritus
Physiology, Pediatrics, and Medicine
Lewis Katz School of Medicine at Temple University
Professor of Pediatrics
Sidney Kimmel Medical College
Thomas Jefferson University
Philadelphia, Pennsylvania
Associate Director, Biomedical Research
Alfred I. duPont Hospital for Children
Wilmington, Delaware
Upper Airway Structure: Function, Regulation, and Development

Martin J. Shearer, BSc, PhD, FRCPath
Physician
Centre for Haemostasis and Thrombosis
St Thomas' Hospital
London, United Kingdom
Vitamin K Metabolism in the Fetus and Neonate

Noah F. Shroyer, PhD
Associate Professor
Department of Medicine
Section of Gastroenterology and Hepatology
Baylor College of Medicine
Houston, Texas
Organogenesis of the Gastrointestinal Tract

Gary C. Sieck, PhD
Professor
Physiology and Biomedical Engineering
Mayo Clinic
Rochester, Minnesota
Functional Development of Respiratory Muscles

Rebecca A. Simmons, MD
Hallam Hurt Professor Pediatrics
Department of Pediatrics
Children's Hospital of Philadelphia
Philadelphia, Pennsylvania
Cell Glucose Transport and Glucose Handling During Fetal and Neonatal Development

Neel Kamal Singh, MBBS, MD
NICU Fellow
Department of Pediatrics
Division of Neonatology
University of Florida College of Medicine
Gainesville, Florida
The Developing Microbiome of the Fetus and Neonate: A Multiomic Approach

Emidio Sivieri, MS, BE
Biomedical Engineer
Department of Neonatology
CHOP Newborn Care at Pennsylvania Hospital
Children's Hospital of Philadelphia
Philadelphia, Pennsylvania
Evaluation of Pulmonary Function in the Neonate

Laura Smith, MD
Beth Israel Deaconess Medical Center
Department of Obstetrics and Gynecology
Boston, Massachusetts
Prenatal Diagnosis

Ian M. Smyth, PhD
Group Leader
Department of Anatomy and Developmental Biology
Biomedicine Discovery Institute
Associate Professor of Pediatrics
Department of Biochemistry and Molecular Biology
Biomedicine Discovery Institute
Monash University
Melbourne, Victoria, Australia
Development of the Kidney: Morphology and Mechanisms

Martha C. Sola-Visner, MD
Associate Professor of Pediatrics
Department of Medicine
Division of Newborn Medicine
Children's Hospital Boston and Harvard Medical School
Boston, Massachusetts
Developmental Megakaryopoiesis

Michael J. Solhaug, MD
Professor of Pediatrics and Physiology
Physiological Sciences
Eastern Virginia Medical School
Norfolk, Virginia
Development and Regulation of Renal Blood Flow in the Neonate

Markus Sperandio, MD
Professor
Institute for Cardiovascular Physiology and Pathophysiology
Walter Brendel Center for Experimental Medicine
Ludwig-Maximilians-Universität
Munich, Germany
Normal and Abnormal Neutrophil Physiology in the Newborn

Mark A. Sperling, MBBS
Emeritus Professor and Chair
Department of Pediatrics
Children's Hospital University of Pittsburgh
Pittsburgh, Pennsylvania
Professorial Lecturer
Pediatric Endocrinology and Diabetes
Icahn School of Medicine at Mt. Sinai
New York, New York
Growth Hormone, Prolactin, and Placental Lactogen in the Fetus and Newborn

Lakshmi Srinivasan, MBBS
Assistant Professor
Department of Pediatrics
Children's Hospital of Philadelphia
Philadelphia, Pennsylvania
Cytokines and Inflammatory Response in the Fetus and Neonate

Diana E. Stanescu, MD
Assistant Professor
Department of Pediatrics
Perelman School of Medicine
University of Pennsylvania
Philadelphia, Pennsylvania
Pathophysiology of Neonatal Hypoglycemia

Charles A. Stanley, MD
Senior Endocrinologist
Division of Endocrinology and Diabetes
Children's Hospital of Philadelphia
Professor Emeritus
Department of Pediatrics
Perelman School of Medicine
University of Pennsylvania
Philadelphia, Pennsylvania
Pathophysiology of Neonatal Hypoglycemia

Robin H. Steinhorn, MD
Senior Vice President and Executive Director
Rady Children's Specialists of San Diego
Vice Dean, Children's Clinical Services
University of California, San Diego
La Jolla, California
Pathophysiology of Persistent Pulmonary Hypertension of the Newborn

Lisa Stinson, BSc, MMedSci, PhD
Research Fellow
School of Molecular Sciences
The University of Western Australia, Perth
Perth, Western Australia, Australia
Human Milk Composition and Function in the Infant

Barbara S. Stonestreet, MD
Professor
Department of Pediatrics
Women & Infants Hospital of Rhode Island
The Warren Alpert Medical School of Brown University
Providence, Rhode Island
Fluid Distribution in the Fetus and Neonate
Development of the Blood-Brain Barrier

Janette F. Strasburger, MD
Professor
Department of Pediatrics
Medical College of Wisconsin
Attending Cardiologist
Herma Heart Institute
Children's Hospital of Wisconsin
Milwaukee, Wisconsin
Developmental Electrophysiology in the Fetus and Neonate

Dennis M. Styne, MD
Yocha Dehe Chair of Pediatric Endocrinology
Professor
Department of Pediatrics
University of California Davis School of Medicine
Davis, California
Endocrine Factors Affecting Neonatal Growth

Xin Sun, PhD
Professor
Pediatrics and Biological Sciences
University of California, San Diego
La Jolla, California
Normal and Abnormal Structural Development of the Lung

Lori Sussel, PhD
Professor
Barbara Davis Center for Diabetes
University of Colorado School of Medicine
Aurora, Colorado
Development of the Endocrine and Exocrine Pancreas

Emily W.Y. Tam, MDCM, MAS
Associate Professor
Department of Paediatrics
University of Toronto
Toronto, Ontario, Canada
Cerebellar Development—The Impact of Preterm Birth and Comorbidities

Libo Tan, PhD
Assistant Professor
Human Nutrition and Hospitality Management
University of Alabama
Tuscaloosa, Alabama
Vitamin A Metabolism in the Fetus and Neonate

Arjan B. te Pas, MD, PhD
Professor
Department of Pediatrics
Leiden University Medical Center
Leiden, The Netherlands
Physiology of Neonatal Resuscitation

Vadim S. Ten, MD, PhD
Professor
Department of Pediatrics
Division of Neonatology
Columbia University Irving Medical Center
New York, New York
Pathophysiology of Neonatal Hypoxic-Ischemic Brain Injury

Bernard Thébaud, MD, PhD
Senior Scientist
Sinclair Centre for Regenerative Medicine
Ottawa Hospital Research Institute
Professor
Department of Pediatrics
Neonatologist
Children's Hospital of Eastern Ontario
University of Ottawa
Ottawa, Ontario, Canada
Developmental Biology of Lung Stem Cells

Claire Thornton, PhD
Senior Lecturer
Comparative Biomedical Sciences
Royal Veterinary College
London, United Kingdom
Mechanisms of Cell Death in the Developing Brain

Daniel J. Tollin, PhD
Professor
Department of Physiology and Biophysics
University of Colorado School of Medicine
Aurora, Colorado
Early Development of the Human Auditory System

Jeffrey A. Towbin, MD
Executive Co-Director
The Heart Institute
Le Bonheur Children's Hospital
Professor and Chief
Pediatric Cardiology
Medical Director, Cardiomyopathy, Heart Failure, and Transplant Services
University of Tennessee Health Science Center
Memphis, Tennessee
Pathophysiology of Cardiomyopathies

William E. Truog III, MD
Sosland Endowed Chair in Neonatal Research
Center for Infant Pulmonary Disorders
Children's Mercy Hospital
Professor
Department of Pediatrics
University of Missouri Kansas City School of Medicine
Kansas City, Missouri
Pulmonary Gas Exchange in the Developing Lung

Kristin M. Uhler, PhD
Audiologist/Associate Professor
Otolaryngology, Physical Medicine & Rehabilitation
University of Colorado School of Medicine
Chair
Audiology, Speech Pathology, and Learning
Children's Colorado Hospital
Aurora, Colorado
Early Development of the Human Auditory System

Chris H.P. van den Akker, MD, PhD
Pediatrician, Neonatologist
Amsterdam UMC—Emma Children's Hospital
Department of Pediatrics/Neonatology
University of Amsterdam and Vrije Universiteit Amsterdam
Amsterdam, The Netherlands
General Concepts of Protein Metabolism

John Nicolaas van den Anker, MD, PhD
Chief, Clinical Pharmacology
Department of Pediatrics
Children's National Health System
Washington, District of Columbia
Chair, Paediatric Pharmacology and Pharmacometrics
Department of Pediatrics
University Children's Hospital Basel
Basel, Switzerland
Faculty, Intensive Care
Pediatric Surgery
Erasmus Medical Center–Sophia Children's Hospital
Rotterdam, The Netherlands
The Physiology of Placental Drug Disposition

Maurice J.B. van den Hoff, PhD
Associate Professor
Department of Medical Biology
Amsterdam UMC
Amsterdam, The Netherlands
Cardiovascular Development

Johannes (Hans) B. van Goudoever, MD, PhD
Professor
Amsterdam UMC—Emma Children's Hospital
Department of Pediatrics
University of Amsterdam and Vrije Universiteit Amsterdam
Amsterdam, The Netherlands
General Concepts of Protein Metabolism

Mark H. Vickers, PhD
Professor
Liggins Institute
University of Auckland
Auckland, New Zealand
Epigenetics

Alexander A. Vinks, PhD, PharmD
Cincinnati Children's Research Foundation Endowed Chair
Professor of Pediatrics and Pharmacology
University of Cincinnati College of Medicine
Director, Division of Clinical Pharmacology
Director, Pediatric Clinical Pharmacology Fellowship Program
Scientific Director, Pharmacy Research in Patient Services
Cincinnati Children's Hospital Medical Center
Cincinnati, Ohio
Pharmacogenomics

Daniela Virgintino, MD
Professor
Department of Basic Medical Sciences, Neurosciences, and Sensory Organs
University of Bari School of Medicine
Bari, Italy
Development of the Blood-Brain Barrier

Marty O. Visscher, PhD
Professor
James L. Winkle College of Pharmacy
University of Cincinnati College of Medicine
Cincinnati, Ohio
Physiologic Development of the Skin

Caitlin E. Vonderohe, DVM, PhD
Postdoctoral Fellow
USDA-ARS Children's Nutrition Research Center
Department of Pediatrics
Baylor College of Medicine
Houston, Texas
Trophic Factors and Regulation of Gastrointestinal Tract and Liver Development

Neha V. Vyas, MD
Pediatric Endocrinology Fellow
Pediatric Endocrinology
Rainbow Babies and Children's Hospital
Cleveland, Ohio
Luteinizing Hormone and Follicle-Stimulating Hormone Secretion in the Fetus and Newborn Infant

Annette Wacker-Gussmann, MD
Department of Sport and Health Sciences
Institute of Preventive Pediatrics
Department of Pediatric Cardiology and Congenital Heart Defects
German Heart Center
Munich, Germany
Developmental Electrophysiology in the Fetus and Neonate

Abby Walch, MD
Clinical Fellow
Pediatric Endocrinology
University of California, San Francisco
San Francisco, California
Development of the Hypothalamus-Pituitary-Adrenal Axis in the Fetus

Megan J. Wallace, BSc, BSc (Hons), PhD
Associate Professor
Department of Obstetrics and Gynaecology
Director, Medical Student Research
School of Medicine
Monash University
Head, Lung Development Research Group
The Ritchie Centre
Hudson Institute of Medical Research
Clayton, Victoria, Australia
Physiologic Mechanisms of Normal and Altered Lung Growth Before and After Birth

Brian H. Walsh, MB, BCh, PhD
Physician
Department of Neonatology
Cork University Maternity Hospital
Cork, Ireland
Intraventricular Hemorrhage in the Neonate

Jennifer A. Wambach, MD
Associate Professor
Edward Mallinckrodt Department of Pediatrics
Washington University School of Medicine
St. Louis, Missouri
Genetics and Physiology of Surfactant Protein Deficiencies

Linda X. Wang, MD
Division of Gastroenterology
Children's Hospital Los Angeles
Clinical Instructor of Pediatrics
Keck School of Medicine
University of Southern California
Los Angeles, California
Bile Acid Metabolism During Development

David Warburton, DSc, MD
Professor
Developmental Biology and Regenerative Medicine Program
Saban Research Institute
Children's Hospital Los Angeles
Los Angeles, California
Regulation of Embryogenesis

Robert M. Ward, MD
Professor Emeritus
Department of Pediatrics
Division of Pediatric Clinical Pharmacology
Adjunct Professor
Department of Pharmacology/Toxicology
University of Utah Health
Salt Lake City, Utah
Principles of Pharmacokinetics

Kevin M. Watt, MD, PhD
Chief, Division of Clinical Pharmacology
Associate Professor
Department of Pediatrics
Division of Pediatric Critical Care Medicine
University of Utah Health
Salt Lake City, Utah
Principles of Pharmacokinetics

Kristi L. Watterberg, MD
Professor Emerita
Division of Neonatology
University of New Mexico
Albuquerque, New Mexico
Fetal and Neonatal Adrenocortical Physiology

Lynne A. Werner, PhD
Professor Emeritus
Department of Speech & Hearing Sciences
University of Washington
Seattle, Washington
Early Development of the Human Auditory System

Sarah A. Wernimont, MD, PhD
Assistant Professor
Department of Obstetrics, Gynecology, and Women's Health
University of Minnesota Medical School
Minneapolis, Minnesota
Glucose Metabolism in the Fetus and Newborn, and Methods for Its Investigation

Barry K. Wershil, MD
Professor
Department of Pediatrics
Feinberg School of Medicine at Northwestern
Chief, Division of Gastroenterology, Hepatology, and Nutrition
Department of Pediatrics
Ann & Robert H. Lurie Children's Hospital of Chicago
Chicago, Illinois
Development of Gastric Secretory Function

Andy Wessels, PhD
Professor
Regenerative Medicine and Cell Biology
Pediatric Cardiology
Medical University of South Carolina
Charleston, South Carolina
Cardiovascular Development

Jeffrey A. Whitsett, MD
Professor of Pediatrics
Divisions of Pulmonary Biology and Neonatology
Perinatal Institute
University of Cincinnati
Cincinnati Children's Hospital Medical Center
Cincinnati, Ohio
Surfactant Homeostasis: Composition and Function of Pulmonary Surfactant Lipids and Proteins

Fabienne Willems, PhD
Professor
Institute for Medical Immunology
Université Libre de Bruxelles
Brussels, Belgium
Host Defense Mechanisms Against Viruses

Myat Su Win, MBBS, MRCPCH
Physician
Department of Paediatrics
Cambridge University Hospitals NHS Trust
Cambridge, United Kingdom
Role of Glucoregulatory Hormones in Hepatic Glucose Metabolism During the Perinatal Period

Christoph Wohlmuth, MD, PhD
Department of Obstetrics and Gynecology
Paracelsus Medical University
Salzburg, Austria
The Pathophysiology of Twin-Twin Transfusion Syndrome, Twin-Anemia Polycythemia Sequence, and Twin-Reversed Arterial Perfusion

Matthias T. Wolf, MD
Associate Professor
Department of Pediatrics
UT Southwestern Medical Center
Dallas, Texas
Potassium Homeostasis in the Fetus and Neonate

Marla R. Wolfson, PhD
Professor
Departments of Physiology, Medicine, and Pediatrics
Center for Inflammation, Translational, and Clinical Lung Research
Associate Chair
Department of Physiology
Lead Researcher
CENTRe: Collaborative for Environmental and Neonatal Therapeutics Research
Lewis Katz School of Medicine
Temple University
Philadelphia, Pennsylvania
Upper Airway Structure: Function, Regulation, and Development

Ronald J. Wong, MD
Senior Research Scientist
Department of Pediatrics
Stanford University School of Medicine
Stanford, California
Mechanistic Aspects of Phototherapy for Neonatal Hyperbilirubinemia

James L. Wynn, MD
Professor
Departments of Pediatrics and Pathology, Immunology, and Laboratory Medicine
University of Florida College of Medicine
Gainesville, Florida
Pathophysiology of Neonatal Sepsis

Lami Yeo, MD
Professor
Division of Maternal-Fetal Medicine
Department of Obstetrics and Gynecology
Wayne State University School of Medicine
Director, Fetal Cardiology
Perinatology Research Branch, NICHD/NIH/DHHS
Detroit, Michigan
Intra-Amniotic Infection/Inflammation and the Fetal Inflammatory Response Syndrome

Bradley A. Yoder, MD
Professor
Department of Pediatrics
University of Utah Health
Salt Lake City, Utah
Impaired Lung Growth After Injury in Preterm Lung

Christopher J. Yuskaitis, MD, PhD
Assistant
Department of Neurology
Boston Children's Hospital
Instructor in Neurology
Harvard Medical School
Boston, Massachusetts
Development of the Nervous System

Jennifer Zabinsky, MD
Clinical Fellow
Pediatric Endocrinology
University of California, San Francisco
San Francisco, California
Development of the Hypothalamus-Pituitary-Adrenal Axis in the Fetus

Dan Zhou, PhD
Scientist
Department of Pediatrics
University of California San Diego
La Jolla, California
Basic Mechanisms of Oxygen Sensing and Adaptation to Hypoxia

Preface

The care of critically ill newborn infants has its foundations in neonatal physiology. Practitioners have traditionally used general physiologic principles in combination with clinical effectiveness studies to provide the most appropriate care. The sixth edition of *Fetal and Neonatal Physiology* marks the beginning of a new era in our specialty in which care providers will use genetic information, biomarkers, and big data to make clinical decisions. We are poised to rapidly diagnose and better understand the genetic basis of a variety of diseases affecting newborn infants, including chronic lung disease, necrotizing enterocolitis, retinopathy of prematurity, white matter injury, and sepsis. Whole genome sequencing (WGS) to identify the genetic basis for complex neonatal diseases (and to identify potentially treatable conditions) is becoming a bedside tool and will practically support pharmacogenomics to tailor treatments for neonatal conditions and limit side effects. Indeed, in the next 2 decades we expect WGS to augment newborn screening, providing information not only for NICU care but extending across the life span. In a critically ill infant, repeated RNA sequencing may be needed as a new parameter to monitor changes during the course of the illness. Well done randomized clinical trials will always be necessary to test the hypotheses that a new therapy is better or equivalent to a current therapy. However, success of any clinical trial begins with having a strong physiologic basis for any given intervention, and ensuring the enrollment of well-phenotyped and endotyped subjects will enhance the precision, success, and impact of such studies. Unfortunately, most randomized trials are based upon a best guess or power analysis of sample size and with limited insights into critical differences within the cohort that may affect outcomes. No matter how carefully patients are selected for a trial, underlying biases and physiologic differences will still exist and must be considered a priori. Data unable to demonstrate differences in two treatment arms does not mean an individual patient may not benefit. For precision medicine to be effective, genetic information must become available on a continuous and real-time basis and linked with ongoing assessment of organ function. This concept is not unique to neonatology and has been termed *personalized physiologic medicine* by Can Ince.[1] Dr. Ince has suggested four pillars of personalized physiology: fitness and frailty (to determine physiologic reserve), organ function response to therapy, hemodynamic coherence (assessment of the macro- and micro-circulations to determine appropriate resuscitation), and integration and feedback (which provides ongoing assessments and includes predictive models).

Our specialty is poised to apply these four pillars to neonatal intensive care, and we believe the sixth edition of *Fetal and Neonatal Physiology* will help support this. Most of the 174 chapters in the book have been extensively updated by nearly 400 authors. More than 1500 visual elements—photographs, illustrations, diagrams, charts, tables—are included, and we are pleased to offer over 100 brand new color illustrations and diagrams to illuminate the text. The genetics content has been expanded to include new chapters such as "Pathophysiology of Genetic Neonatal Disease" and "Genetic Variants and Neonatal Disease." Each of the chapters on disease pathophysiology has been extensively revised by leading experts in our specialty.

We want to thank many individuals who made this edition possible, including foremost the chapter authors who not only wrote superb chapters but who also adhered to the tight production schedule. We deeply appreciate the editorial help from two individuals at Elsevier. Mary Hegeler was our content development specialist, without whom we could never have done this revision. She was with us every step of the way and provided invaluable guidance as we moved through the stages of book development. We also wish to thank Sarah Barth at Elsevier who supported the decision to undertake the sixth edition.

Finally, we would like to thank the many readers of *Fetal and Neonatal Physiology,* who provided the stimulus and encouragement to revise the book.

RAP
SHA
WEB
DHR

[1]Ince C. Personalized physiological medicine. *Crit Care* 2017;21:308.

Contents

†Deceased.

SECTION XII THE LUNG

SECTION XIII SURFACTANT

SECTION XIV PHYSIOLOGY OF GASTROINTESTINAL TRACT IN THE FETUS AND NEONATE

SECTION XXIV ENDOCRINE FUNCTION

SECTION XXV OVARY AND TESTIS

SECTION XXVI PATHOPHYSIOLOGY OF NEONATAL DISEASES

Development of the Kidney: Morphology and Mechanisms

93

Ian M. Smyth | Luise A. Cullen-McEwen | Alexander N. Combes | Lori L. O'Brien | Mary Jane Black | John F. Bertram

INTRODUCTION

The development of the mammalian kidney has been extensively studied for the past 60 to 70 years, and our understanding of renal development and molecular regulation is perhaps better understood than that of any other organ. This chapter provides an overview of the development of the three mammalian excretory organs (pronephroi, mesonephroi, and metanephroi) but explores metanephric development in detail. The processes of ureteric budding, ureteric branching morphogenesis, and nephrogenesis are also described in detail, as is our current understanding of the nature and roles of renal progenitor cells. In addition, the roles of the renal stroma in kidney development are considered, and renal vascular development is described. Finally, the effects of preterm birth on kidney development are addressed.

DEVELOPMENT OF THE MAMMALIAN RENAL EXCRETORY SYSTEM

During mammalian embryogenesis, three pairs of excretory organs form from the intermediate mesoderm, which lies between the developing somites and the lateral plate on the flanks of the developing embryo.[1] These are the pronephroi, mesonephroi, and metanephroi, which develop in a cranial to caudal fashion, respectively (Fig. 93.1). The development of the permanent mammalian kidneys, or *metanephroi,* takes place after the successive formation and regression of the pronephroi and mesonephroi. All three pairs of kidneys are induced to develop from an epithelial tube, the nephric duct that migrates caudally through the nephrogenic cord along the anterior-posterior axis of the embryo and fuses with the cloaca.[2]

Bone morphogenetic protein (Bmp) signaling plays a critical role in the specification of the intermediate mesoderm, wherein a gradient of signaling orchestrates the differentiation of the lateral plate (high), intermediate mesoderm (intermediate), and paraxial mesoderm and somites (low levels).[3] Simultaneous deletion of the functionally redundant transcription factors *paired box 2* (*Pax2,* a Bmp target gene[4]) and *paired box 8* (*Pax8*) results in a failure of nephric duct formation, without induction of associated renal lineage genes such as *rearranged during transfection (Ret)* and *Lim1*.[5] These actions appear to be complemented by nodal-like signaling (mediated by Vg1/Nodal) in a manner that intersects with Bmp signaling.[6] Retinoic acid (RA), produced by paraxial mesoderm, is also required for initial specification of renal progenitor cells.[7-9]

The first indication of renal development in humans is evident at approximately embryonic day 22 (E22) with the appearance of the nephric or wolffian duct (WD). In mice, this occurs at E8. The nephric duct forms as a consequence of a mesenchymal to epithelial transition. Both the surface ectoderm and somites appear to play an inductive role in triggering the formation of the nephric duct. As the embryo ages, the nephric duct extends caudally through a process of migration and changes in cell shape that, depending on the species concerned, involve further contribution from cells derived from the uncommitted intermediate mesoderm. As the duct elongates and development progresses, the pronephros, mesonephros, and finally the metanephros are sequentially formed. The last of these structures ultimately develops into the functional or permanent mammalian kidney.

THE PRONEPHROS

The pronephros is the first of the excretory organs to form as the nephric duct differentiates. In humans, as with other amniotes, this is a transitory structure, which appears as 5 to 7 paired pronephroi that connect to the nephric duct around 3 weeks' gestation. In mice, elements of this structure appear in a highly rudimentary form at E8.5 to E9, but by E9 the mesonephros, the "second" excretory structure in developing amniotes, is established in the intermediate mesoderm field adjacent to the nephric duct. In humans, the pronephros begins to develop around E22 in the cervical region of the embryo. At this time, segmentally arranged sets of epithelial tubules appear within the nephrogenic cord. These structures are known as *nephrotomes,* and they connect to the anterior region of the nephric duct (pronephric duct). The pronephroi are nonfunctional in mammals; however, amphibians and fish have well-developed and functional pronephroi that persist throughout life to regulate water and solute balance and blood pH. The mammalian pronephric tubules regress around 5 weeks' gestation in humans, but the pronephric duct persists and becomes the mesonephric or WD.[2,10]

THE MESONEPHROS

The mesonephros is the second transient kidney and appears in humans at 3 to 4 weeks' gestation immediately caudal to the last pronephric tubules. The WD induces the adjacent mesenchyme within the nephrogenic cord to undergo a mesenchymal to epithelial transition to induce a renal vesicle. This differentiates into an S-shaped structure that elongates and eventually forms a proximal tubule connected to the WD. These structures develop a vascularized, glomerulus-like filtering component connected to proximal and distal tubules draining into the WD and are the first definitive functional unit or nephron in the renal excretory system. The mesonephric nephrons are transient structures, with up to 40 present at any one time in humans. As with the pronephros, the mesonephros degenerates in a craniocaudal direction from 5 to 12 weeks' gestation and ceases to function as an excretory organ.[2,11,12] Remnant structures of the mesonephros are involved in

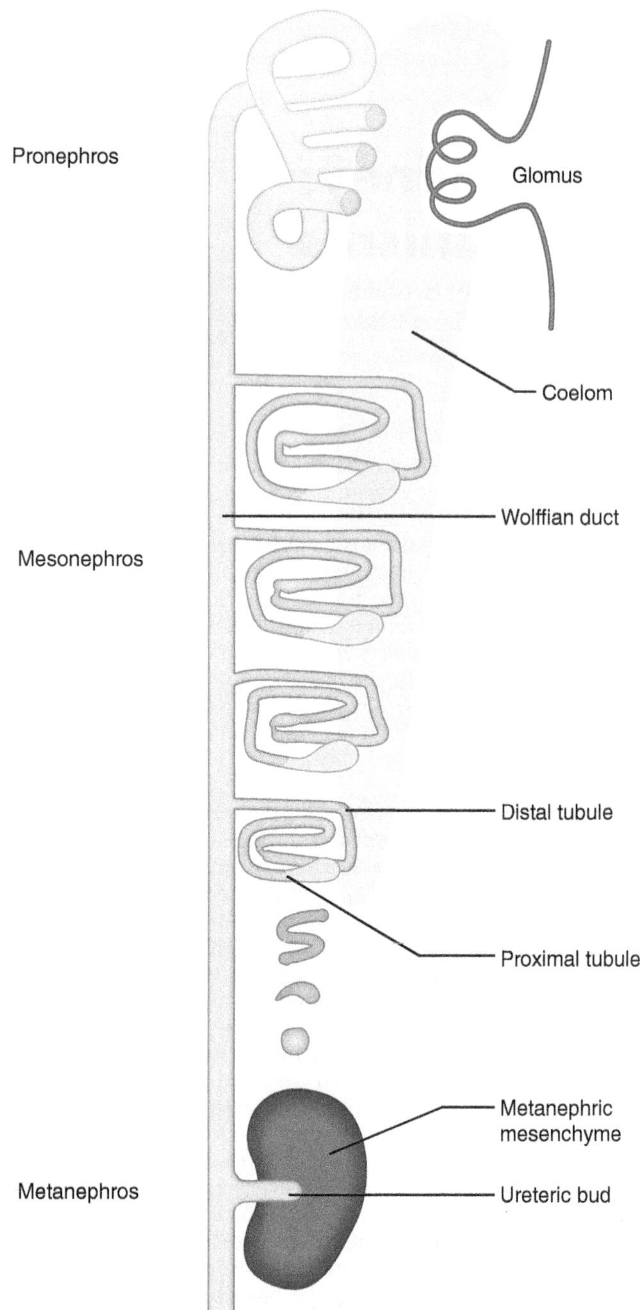

Fig. 93.1 Schematic representation showing development of the pronephros, mesonephros, and metanephros. The pronephros, composed of a single glomus, projects into the nephrocoel but filters directly into the coelom and is depicted as having already degenerated. The mesonephros consists of multiple nephrons that develop in a cranial to caudal fashion such that the most caudal structures are still in the process of developing into complete nephrons that will attach to the wolffian duct. The metanephros at this stage comprises the ureteric bud, which has entered the metanephric mesenchyme but has not yet branched. (Reprinted with permission from Moritz KM, Wintour EM, Black MJ, et al. Factors influencing mammalian kidney development: implications for health in adult life. *Adv Anat Embryol Cell Biol.* 2008;196:1–78.)

genitourinary development. In females, the mesonephric duct completely disappears during the third embryonic month, whereas some mesonephric tubules persist as the epoöphoron and paroöphoron, which have no known function in humans. In males, mesonephric tubules in the area of the gonad form the efferent ductules, whereas the mesonephric duct gives rise to the epididymis and the ductus deferens.[13]

THE METANEPHROS

The formation of the metanephros gives rise to the permanent kidney in humans, as well as in other mammals, reptiles, and birds. The development of the metanephros is initiated by the outgrowth of the ureteric bud (UB) from the caudal end of the WD at 4 to 5 weeks' gestation. The timing and site at which the UB emerges from the WD are well orchestrated such that it enters the adjacent metanephric mesenchyme. Reciprocal inductive signals occur between the UB and the metanephric mesenchyme (Fig. 93.2A).[1] The metanephric mesenchyme induces the UB to grow and repetitively bifurcate to form the ureteric tree via branching morphogenesis. The ureteric tree subsequently forms the collecting ducts, calyces, and renal pelvis. The region of the UB that does not enter the metanephric mesenchyme becomes the ureter. Simultaneously, the tips of the ureteric tree induce subpopulations of committed metanephric mesenchyme cells to condense and undergo a mesenchymal to epithelial transition to form a renal vesicle that further differentiates into the functional unit of the kidney, the *nephron* (see Fig. 93.2B). This process is known as *nephrogenesis*. Branching morphogenesis and nephrogenesis occur in the human embryo from 6 to 36 weeks' gestation.[14]

As the metanephros develops, it is drawn in a cranial direction. The upward movement of the metanephros from a pelvic position to its final lumbar position is complete by the eighth embryonic week. On emerging from the pelvis, the metanephros undergoes a 90-degree rotation so that the original ventral hilum takes its final medial position.

The principal feature presaging the development of the metanephros is the demarcation of the metanephric mesenchyme, which is marked by the expression of Wilms tumor-1 (Wt1) and *Pax2*.[15,16] This occurs at E10 of development in the mouse and approximately E30 in humans. Even at this early stage, the metanephric mesenchyme contains progenitor cell populations, which will ultimately form nephrons, stromal cells, and some of the vascular elements of the adult kidney. The positional specification of the metanephric kidney relies on molecules expressed in both the differentiating nephric duct and in the adjacent metanephric mesenchyme. The ultimate product of these interactions is the initiation of an outgrowth of a single structure from the nephric duct—the UB.[1] Unlike with the pronephros or mesonephros, it is critical that a single UB forms on each side of the metanephros and that it does so in a defined rostrocaudal position. Multiple or positionally inappropriate UBs contribute to the development of a number of diseases of the congenital abnormalities of the kidney and urinary tract (CAKUT) spectrum, including hypodysplasia, urinary outflow obstruction, and vesicoureteric reflux.[17] Notably, mouse and human kidneys have both conserved and divergent features of their structure and molecular and cellular features[18] although the contribution of these differences to development of pathology following gene mutation is poorly understood.

The poor structural outcomes due to inappropriate positional or numeric induction of UB formation are further reflected in altered communication between epithelial and mesenchymal cells, especially regarding signaling between the mesenchymally expressed *glial cell-derived neurotrophic factor (Gdnf)* and its co-receptors *Ret* and *glial cell line derived neurotrophic factor family receptor alpha 1 (Gfra1)* (see Fig. 93.2A).[19-21] These genes are all required for kidney development.[22-26] In the duct, *Pax2* and *Gata3* are required to establish the position of the UB (see Fig. 93.2A).[16,27,28] In parallel, the formation and position of the metanephric mesenchyme is dictated by expression of a collection of transcription factors that includes members of the *Hox11* gene

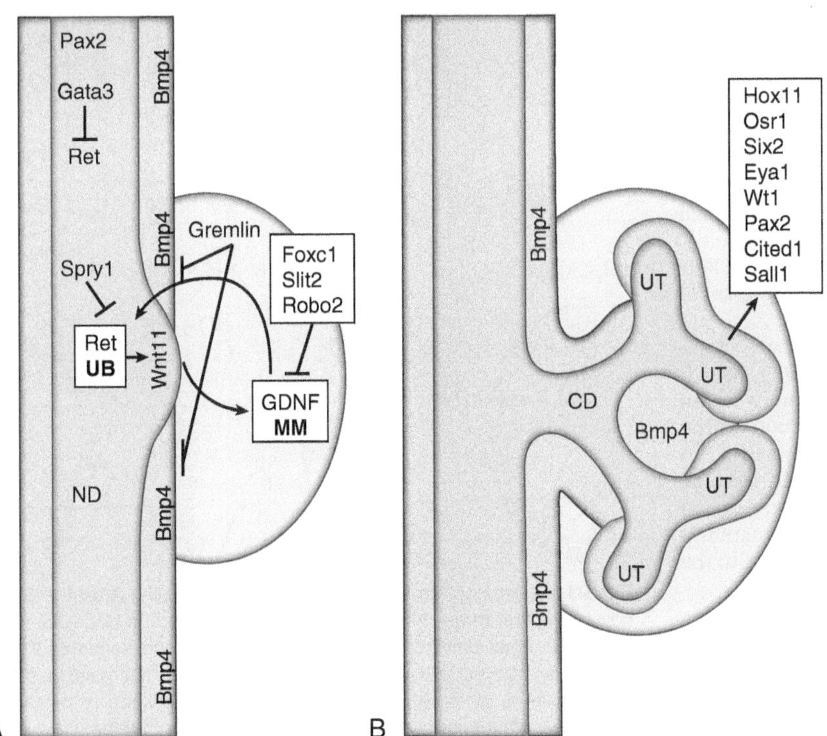

Fig. 93.2 (A) Schematic diagram illustrating key genes expressed in the nephric duct (ND, *blue*) and metanephric mesenchyme (MM, *green*) that regulate ureteric budding. Note that Bmp4 is expressed in a sleeve of tissue *(purple)* that surrounds the ND. (B) The earliest stages of ureteric branching morphogenesis. Note that the field of Bmp4 expression *(purple)* is now extended and prevents ectopic branching events. Genes expressed by the cap mesenchyme *(orange)* are shown. *CD,* Collecting duct; *GDNF,* glial cell–derived neurotrophic factor; *UT,* ureteric tree.

family (*Hoxa11, Hoxc11,* and *Hoxd11*[29]) and *odd-skipped related 1 (Osr1)*, a member of the odd-skipped family of zinc finger proteins.[30] Wt1 is also expressed in the neighboring intermediate mesoderm and is required to maintain the competency of the mesenchyme for metanephric kidney growth.[15] As the embryo develops, further cohorts of mesenchyme-expressed factors direct metanephric differentiation including Sall1, Eya1, Six1, Six4, and Gdf11,[31-35] which themselves reinforce positionally appropriate *Gdnf* expression next to the site of UB outgrowth. A complementary program of repression in the more rostral mesenchyme serves to suppress *Gdnf* and includes Foxc1,[36] Slit2, and Robo2[37] (see Fig. 93.2A). The capacity of the rostral part of the nephric duct to form the metanephric kidney is also repressed by the action of Bmp4 (expressed in the metanephric mesenchyme)[38] and Sprouty *(Spry1*; expressed in the nephric duct downstream of Wt1).[39] The actions of Bmp4 are overcome in the region of eventual metanephric growth by the expression of Gremlin *(Grem1)* (see Fig. 93.2A).[40] The relative importance of these different genes in metanephric specification is reflected in the findings of causative roles for *BMP4, SIX2,*[41] *PAX2,*[42] *EYA1,*[43] *SIX1,*[44] and *SIX5*[45] in renal hypodysplasia. The end result of these complex interactions is the emergence of the UB.

URETERIC BUD OUTGROWTH

Between E9.5 and E10.5 in mice the caudal end of the nephric duct undergoes a distinctive thickening that presages the emergence of the UB. This thickening is evidence of a pseudostratification of epithelial cells in this region, which is driven, at least in part, by signals from the metanephric mesenchyme.[1,46] It is from this thickened region that the UB is generated in a process mediated in large part by cell movements orchestrated by *Ret/Gdnf* signaling (see Fig. 93.2A). In a series of elegant experiments analyzing chimeric mice composed of a mixture of Ret^+ and Ret^- cells, it was found that the formed UBs were composed principally of Ret^+ cells, which assembled in the very tip of the emerging bud.[47] Further evidence supporting a role for Ret signaling in this process was provided by complementary experiments in which cells with heightened Ret signaling (by loss of a downstream regulator Sprouty) were added and which preferentially occupied the UB tip in competition with wild-type cells.[47] Even in wild-type nephric ducts there exists a considerable range in Ret activation, as assessed by surrogate markers of pathway activation, so it seems likely that a similar "sorting" mechanism is employed to generate the UB.

The downstream targets of Ret signaling are activated by a range of other receptor tyrosine kinases, raising the possibility that cell signaling pathways activated by growth factors other than GDNF might contribute to UB outgrowth. Evidence for such a pathway is provided by the observation that UB outgrowth and subsequent development in mice lacking *Ret* or *Gdnf* can be rescued by the deletion of *Spry1* (see Fig. 93.2A).[48] A prime candidate for such an alternate signaling molecule is fibroblast growth factor 10 (FGF10), which is normally expressed in the metanephric mesenchyme and plays a role in branching morphogenesis in the kidney and other organs.[49] Indeed, deletion of *Fgf10* in a *Spry1/Gdnf* null background blocks UB outgrowth, indicating that FGF signaling most likely acts to facilitate UB outgrowth by impacting on common cell signaling pathways downstream of a number of different receptor tyrosine kinases.[48] Whether there are further contributors to this process and which exact downstream signaling pathways are involved remain to be fully defined. Having initiated outgrowth, the UB then enters into a process of branching morphogenesis, largely driven by bifurcation events. Considerable evidence, particularly from live imaging in organ culture,[50] suggests that this process is mediated by increased cell division in the tips. Some cells are then maintained in this domain, whereas others remain in the "trunk," and the tip pushes into the surrounding metanephric mesenchyme. These choices in cell fate are reflected in heterogeneity in gene expression within the tip progenitor cell niches.[51] Although the evidence for lateral branching from established ureteric trunks in the mouse kidney is relatively scarce,[52] it is clear that, at least in culture, trunk cells do remain competent to initiate new branch formation in response to exogenous signals.[50]

A number of members of the *Wnt* gene family are also dynamically expressed during metanephric kidney development.

One of these in particular, *Wnt11*, seems to be intimately associated with UB outgrowth. Although it occurs in a number of other organ systems, *Wnt11* expression in the kidney is notable because it is restricted to UB tips (see Fig. 93.2A).[53] When exogenous sources of GDNF are focally added in cultured kidney, corresponding increases in *Wnt11* expression were detected,[54,55] suggesting that the gene is a downstream target of GDNF signaling. Engineered loss of *Wnt11* results in renal hypoplasia and concomitant decreases in *Gdnf* expression,[56] suggesting a positive, autoregulatory feedback loop between Ret/GDNF and Wnt11 that is required for maintaining the program of branching morphogenesis (see Fig. 93.2B).

Having "invaded" the neighboring metanephric mesenchyme, the UB begins to undergo a process of branching, which essentially establishes the future collecting duct network of the adult kidney. None of this epithelium will contribute to the nephrons. In the mouse, the UB undergoes approximately 12 to 13 branching events, although its extent is determined to some degree by the position of the tip in the organ (the anterior and posterior poles have greater depth).[52] In humans the situation is similar with a proposed 15 branch generations giving rise to the adult organ.[57]

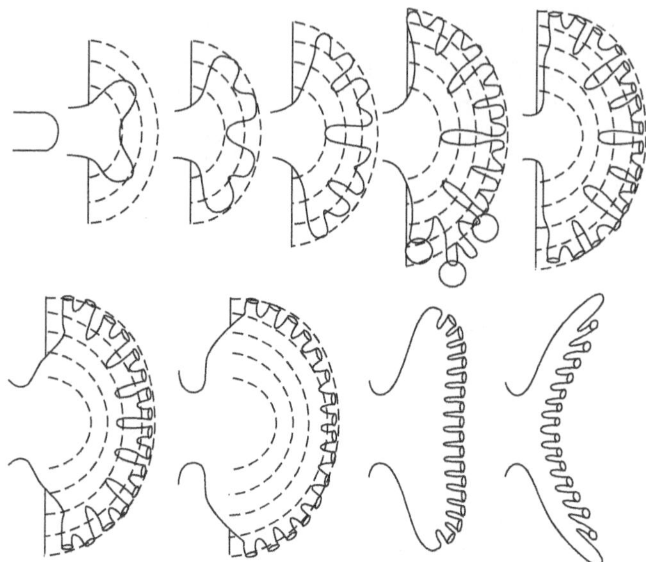

Fig. 93.3 Development of a minor calyx and papilla. After the dilation of the first three to five generations of the ureteric bud (UB) that forms the renal pelvis and major calyces, a second series of three to five generations of UB divisions occurs in rapid succession. This second series of rapidly formed short tubules expands to produce the cavity of the minor calyx, whereas the tubules of the next generations expand to become the cribriform plate that covers the papillary surface. It is thought that the definitive cup shape of the calyx and the conical form of the papilla are formed by the combination of intratubular pressure generated by urine formation and the extratubular pressure generated by enlargement and differentiation of nephrons distally. (From Potter EL. *Normal and Abnormal Development of the Kidney*. Chicago: Year Book Medical Publishers; 1972.)

COLLECTING DUCT ARCHITECTURE

Mammalian kidney function requires the coordinated development of specialized cell types within a precise architectural framework. The morphogenesis of the collecting system and the distinct zonal arborization of the developing kidney are a result of the patterned divisions of the nephron-inducing UB. The renal pelvis, calyces, and intrarenal collecting ducts arise from phases of rapid dichotomic branching of the UB, which alternate with phases of enlargement, branch resorption, or remodeling (Fig. 93.3). In humans this has been proposed to occur for the first five branching generations,[57] and in mice a similar "disappearance" of approximately the first three branching generations has been flagged.[52] Dilation of the early generations of UB branches and final structural modification of the pelvis, calyces, and papillae occur concomitantly with the formation of functional nephrons and probably result from accumulation of urine.

The pattern of UB branching determines the topographic distribution of nephrons and the elaborate "arcades" in which multiple nephrons connect in series to the cortical collecting ducts. The branching of the UB is highly structured, and dissection of early human embryonic kidneys revealed several types of repeating patterns of divisions.[18,58-60] The budding of the UB from the WD is a lateral branch that then divides, producing the first bifid branch point. The two daughter branches then divide again until a terminal set of branches is reached. The angle of bifurcation is variable but is as large as 180 degrees in the first bifurcation of the UB. The branching is often considered as being a bifid division. However, dissection of early embryonic kidneys revealed the presence of lateral branches and, although rare, trifid and carrefour (four-way) branches.[18,57-60] By birth, growth and differentiation has "corrected" them so all branches appear dichotomous. As each ureteric tip connects to a nephron, it is effectively removed from further branching events.[61]

The early patterns of renal branching morphogenesis had been previously inferred from static observations derived from microdissections and serial reconstruction of sectioned kidneys.[57-59] Dynamic observations of murine renal organ cultures,[56,60] in vivo time-lapse analysis of UB-branching mice expressing green fluorescent protein specifically in the UB epithelium have confirmed many of the hypothesized branching events.[62,63] More recently, three-dimensional imaging and analysis has provided new insights and quantification of this complex, highly regulated process during kidney development in mouse[64-66] (Fig. 93.4) and human.[18]

The structural development of the human kidney occurs in four periods[57]: period 1 (embryonic weeks 5 through 14), in which ampullae actively divide and induce formation of nephrons only when not carrying an attached nephron (Fig. 93.5); period 2 (embryonic weeks 14 to 15 through 20 to 22), when ampullae rarely divide but induce new nephrons while carrying an attached nephron, resulting in arcade formation (Fig. 93.6); period 3 (embryonic weeks 20 to 22 through 32 to 36), in which ampullae do not divide but induce new nephron formation (Fig. 93.7); and period 4 (embryonic weeks 32 to 36 through adult life), when ampullae are inactive and do not divide or induce formation of new nephrons. All renal growth in period 4 is a result of enlargement of existing structures and expansion of interstitial tissue.

The programmed stages of UB division and induction result in a predictable pattern of nephron arborization in the newborn kidney (Fig. 93.8). Because nephrons are successively attached to the UB within a zone of accelerated interstitial growth, they advance with the ampullae in a centrifugal fashion from generation to generation of UB branches. The connecting tubules of all nephrons in the mature kidney are therefore connected to the last two to three generations of collecting ducts (13th to 15th generations of UB branches).[58]

MOLECULAR REGULATION OF BRANCHING MORPHOGENESIS

The process of ureteric branching is regulated by a complex molecular interplay between progenitor cells in the UB tips and

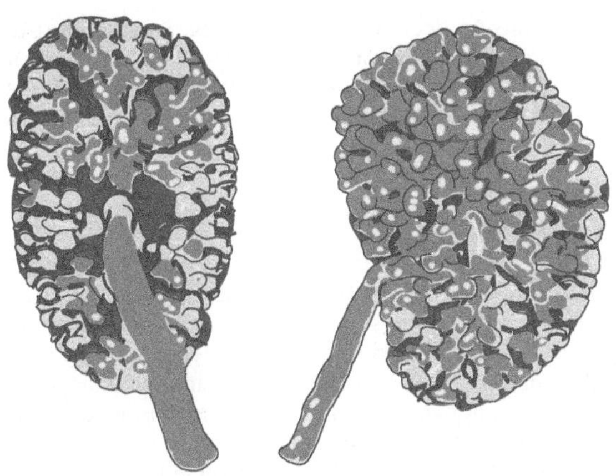

Fig. 93.4 Optical projection tomography images of ureteric branching in an E15.5 mouse kidney. Whole-mount kidneys were fluorescently immunostained for the ureteric epithelium, scanned by optical projection tomography (OPT) and three-dimensional OPT datasets rendered using Drishti software. (Courtesy Stacey Hokke, Monash University.)

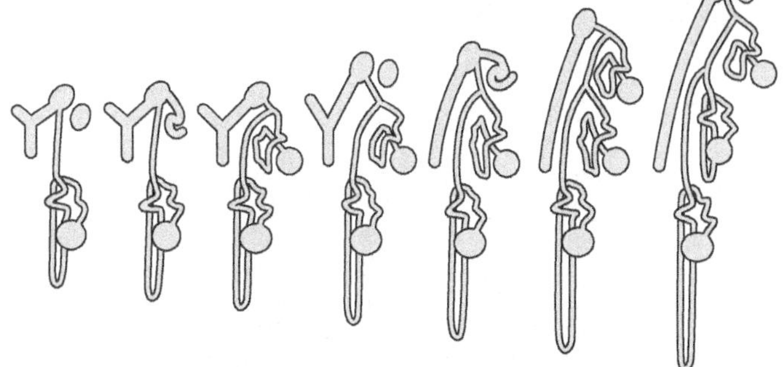

Fig. 93.6 Period 2 of nephron formation (embryonic weeks 14 to 15 through 20 to 22). Ampullae no longer actively divide and become capable of inducing new nephrons, even though they already carry an attached nephron. Although two nephrons may be attached to each terminal ampulla temporarily, the connecting piece of the more mature nephron shifts to communicate only with the connecting piece of the younger nephron. In this fashion, arcades of four to six nephrons become attached to each tubule. (From Potter EL. *Normal and Abnormal Development of the Kidney*. Chicago: Year Book Medical Publishers; 1972.)

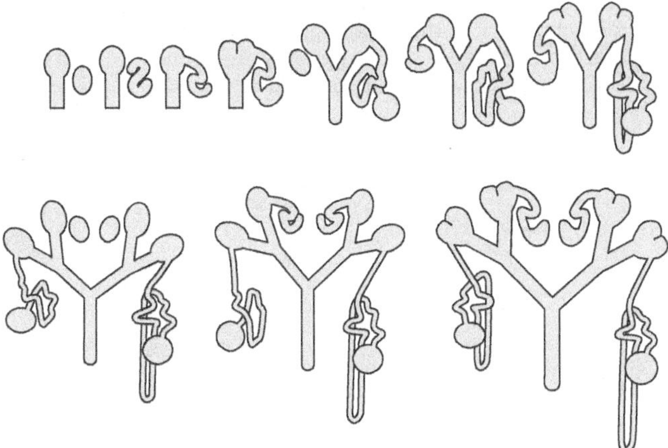

Fig. 93.5 Period 1 of nephron formation (embryonic weeks 5 to 14). Ampullae actively divide and induce formation of nephrons only when not carrying an attached nephron. (From Potter EL. *Normal and Abnormal Development of the Kidney.* Chicago: Year Book Medical Publishers; 1972.)

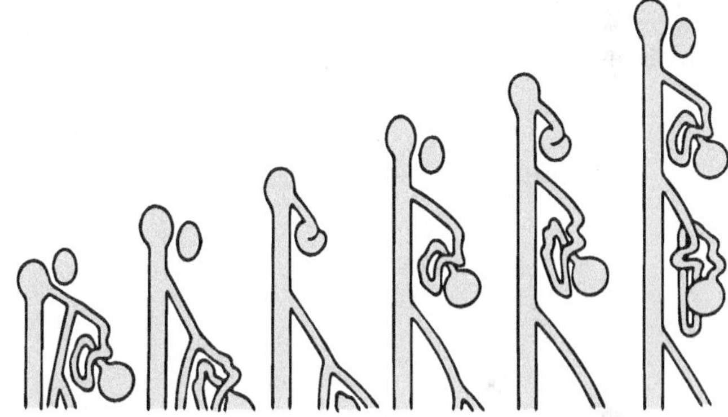

Fig. 93.7 Period 3 of nephron formation (embryonic weeks 20 to 22 through 32 to 36). During this period, ampullae branch rarely, induce formation of new nephrons when not already carrying nephrons, and permit attachment of new nephrons only behind the active growth zone at the junction of ampulla and collecting tubule. This results in direct attachment of nephrons to the terminal portion of each collecting tubule. (From Potter EL. *Normal and Abnormal Development of the Kidney*. Chicago: Year Book Medical Publishers; 1972.)

associated cell populations in the metanephric mesenchyme. Although UB branching can continue in culture conditions when supported by an extracellular matrix, doing so requires the provision of growth factors, either through the use of metanephric mesenchyme-conditioned media[67] or, to varying degrees, through specific supplementation with factors including GDNF and members of the FGF family.[67,68] Using either in vivo or "manipulated" ex vivo cultures, it appears that the mesenchymal cell population is important for directing the differentiation of the corresponding epithelial population.

A number of different cell-signaling pathways are integral to the ongoing branching of the UB (see Fig. 93.2B). As during early UB formation, Ret-GDNF signaling is central to ongoing branching morphogenesis. This signaling axis, in which GDNF is secreted by cells in the cap mesenchyme (CM) and received by Ret (and the co-receptor *Gfra1*), is central to the ongoing elaboration of the ureteric tree and is likely to be mediated by activation of the extracellular-signal-regulated kinase (ERK)/ mitogen-activated protein kinase (MAPK), phosphoinositide 3-kinase (PI3K), and phospholipase C (PLCg) pathways because inhibition or modulation of these pathways leads to reductions in the rate of branching.[50,69–71] Proteins like Hnf1β act upstream and downstream of Ret signaling by regulating the expression of *Gfra1* and *Etv5*[72] and others like MITF regulation of *Ret* itself.[73] The importance of the metanephric mesenchyme is highlighted by studies in which these cells were specifically ablated.[74] Even with a modest deletion of 40% of these cells, a reduced rate of branching was observed. In addition, the reduction in branching correlated with a period of "recovery" of the depleted cap cell niche. Maintenance of *Gdnf* expression is also regulated by the stroma. For example, targeted deletion of the Tcf21 protein results in attenuated branching as a consequence of attenuated GDNF signaling.[75]

A number of other secreted factors from the metanephric mesenchyme are required to maintain or modulate ureteric branching. FGF10 produced by the metanephric mesenchyme is necessary for the ongoing branching of the UB as deletion of this factor leads to abrogated elaboration.[48] The actions of FGF10 (and FGF7, produced principally in the stroma) are mediated by members of the FGF receptor (FGFR) family. Among these, FGFR2 appears to play a central role in regulating the actions of the stromal and mesenchymally produced FGF ligands as UB-specific

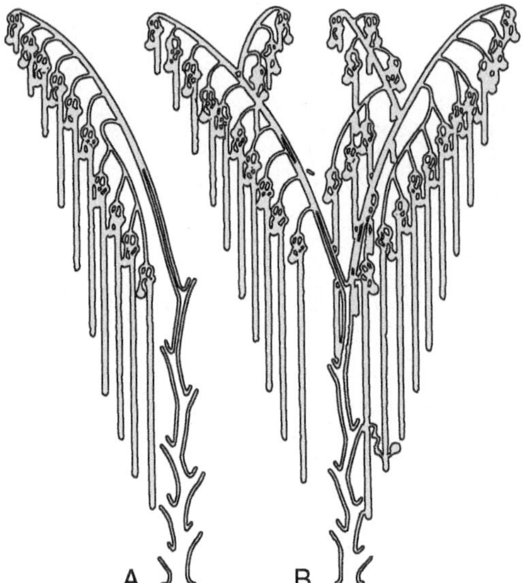

Fig. 93.8 Nephron arborization in the newborn kidney. The programmed periods of ureteric bud (UB) division and induction result in a predictable pattern of nephron arborization in the newborn kidney. (A) The most common arrangement. (B) Possible variations. (From Potter EL. *Normal and Abnormal Development of the Kidney.* Chicago: Year Book Medical Publishers; 1972.)

deletion results in decreases in branching.[76] Signaling through the canonical Wnt pathway, presumably in response to one of the several Wnt proteins expressed in the mesenchyme, is also important for UB elaboration as deletion of b-catenin specifically in the UB leads to reduced branching.[77,78]

NEPHROGENESIS

The formation of nephrons begins relatively early in embryonic development, during the second month of gestation in humans and at E12.5 in mice. Nephrons form when a subpopulation of CM cells come together to form pretubular aggregates that then undergo a mesenchymal to epithelial transition to form a renal vesicle, a structure that rapidly assumes polarity and undergoes its own process of tubulogenesis involving integration into the UB tip next to which it was generated. These events are part of a highly orchestrated process of tissue specification and differentiation and represent a fine balance between preservation of nephron progenitor cell populations over time and the commitment of these cells to enter the nephrogenic program.

Nephron development proceeds through a series of intermediate forms, beginning with condensation or aggregation of induced mesenchyme around the UB tips (Fig. 93.9). There are two distinct parts to these aggregates, the cap surrounding the tip and the pretubular aggregate lying just beneath the tips of the UB at the juncture of the ampulla and stalk. The pretubular

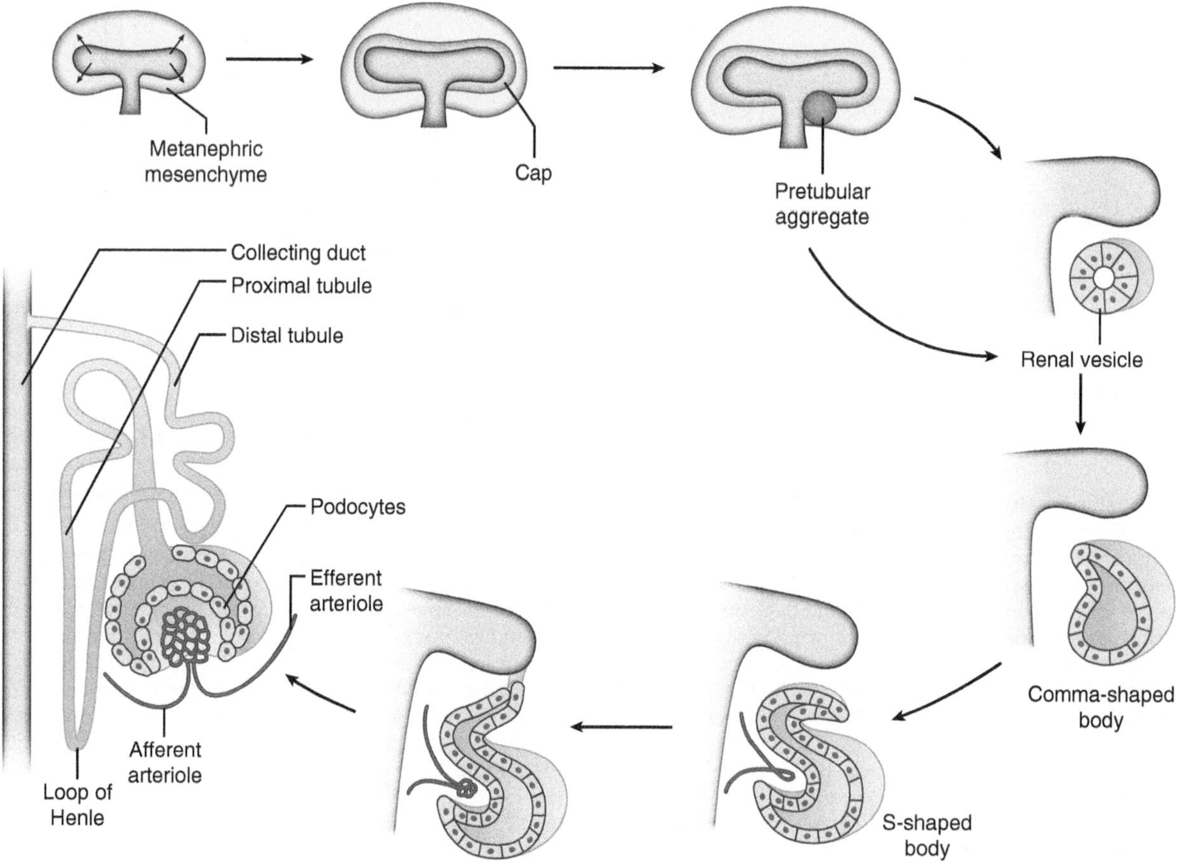

Fig. 93.9 The stages of normal nephron formation. Signals from the ureteric epithelial tip cells induce the adjacent metanephric mesenchyme to condense, forming a cap-like structure *(orange)*. A subset of these cells further aggregate to form the pretubular aggregates that undergo mesenchyme-to-epithelial transformation, forming the renal vesicle. The renal vesicle further differentiates into the comma- and S-shaped bodies. Endothelial cells migrate into the cleft of the S-shaped body, which will contribute to the formation of the renal corpuscle. The upper limb of the S-shaped body fuses to the tip of the ureteric duct (future collecting duct). The lower limb of the S-shaped body gives rise to the podocytes and Bowman capsule. The upper limb differentiates and elongates, forming the distal tubule, and the middle section forms the loop of Henle and proximal tubule. (Reprinted with permission from Moritz KM, Wintour EM, Black MJ, et al. Factors influencing mammalian kidney development: implications for health in adult life. *Adv Anat Embryol Cell Biol.* 2008;196:1–78; and modified by Justin Hewlett, Multimedia Services, Monash University.)

aggregate proliferates, undergoes a mesenchymal to epithelial transition, and ultimately forms the nephron. Expressed by the ureteric epithelium, Wnt9b is the initiating signal, inducing a mesenchymal to epithelial transition and the formation of nephrons.[79,80] Studies have shown that Wnt9b not only triggers differentiation of the pretubular aggregate but also activates proliferation and renewal of nephron progenitor cells, a process under the control of the transcriptional regulator Six2 (further described below).[81] Upon Wnt9b induction, committing nephron progenitor cells begin to express several growth factors such as *Fgf8* and *Wnt4* promoting nephrogenesis.[81,82]

Nephron development proceeds by segmentation and patterning of the renal vesicle into morphologically defined stages known as the comma- and S-shaped bodies before elongation and eventual fusion with the ureteric tip, forming a continuous uriniferous tubule. The comma-shaped body stage is defined by the development of a proximal-distal polarity axis in response to signals from the UB[83]; the proximal portion elongates, forming a cleft and establishing a distal and proximal segment. The S-shaped body is formed by elongation and folding of the comma-shaped body and is generally regarded as the precursor of two distinct processes, that is, glomerulogenesis and tubulogenesis, which are related to the spatial segmentation of the S-shaped body into three segments (proximal, medial, and distal). The proximal segment differentiates into two distinct epithelial layers of the glomerulus, the visceral (podocytes) and parietal (Bowman capsule) layers. The medial segment gives rise to the proximal tubule, and the distal segment forms the distal tubule, which ultimately fuses to the collecting tubule.[84] Further development of the S-shaped body sees the formation of glomerular capillary loops (through vasculogenesis and angiogenesis).[85] This is followed by the progressive development of specialized epithelial intercellular connections and basal lamina formation with consequent endothelial fenestration and differentiation of podocytes, including formation of foot processes and filtration slit diaphragms.[86-88] Continued branching of the UB and inductions of new nephrons occur in a radial fashion, such that the first nephrons that develop lie near the corticomedullary junction and the final nephrons form in the outer cortex close to the renal capsule.

MOLECULAR REGULATION OF NEPHROGENESIS

The use of mice with targeted genetic mutations has conclusively identified a number of key molecules that regulate the early events of nephron formation and epithelialization. In mice with homozygous mutations in *Wnt4*,[82] *Foxd1*,[89] or *Emx2*,[90] nephrogenesis halts at the condensation stage, resulting in the development of very few, if any, nephrons. The epithelialization of metanephric mesenchyme is delayed or reduced in mice lacking expression of cadherin-6 *(Cdh6)*, and the tubules that do form do not fuse to the UB.[91] Genetic deletion of *Wnt9b* leads to an arrest of epithelialization in the metanephric mesenchyme before occurrence of *Wnt4* positive pretubular aggregates. Epithelialization can be rescued in *Wnt9b*$^{-/-}$ mice by overexpressing Wnt1 in the UB, indicating that a Wnt signal is essential and permissive for epithelialization.[79]

The molecular specification of the proximo-distal axis of the nephron has been the subject of intense research. In vitro studies involving mouse and human tissue have shown that a gradient of Wnt activity is capable of programming proximal-distal nephron identity.[92,93] It is proposed that this Wnt gradient emanates from the UB with the forming distal nephron receiving the highest levels of exposure and the proximal nephron and podocytes receiving the lowest.[92] Notch signaling also plays an important role in nephron specification and patterning.[94,95] Asymmetric expression of *Brn1*,[96] *Cdh1* (E-cadherin), and *Cdh6*[97] provides the first known evidence of polarization of the proximo-distal axis. Although not identifiable histologically, gene-expression patterns suggest the proximo-distal axis exists at the renal vesicle stage,[83,84] with precursors of each segment of the nephron identifiable within the renal vesicle.[96,98,99] By the S-shaped-body stage, *Pax2* is highly expressed within the distal portion of the S-shaped body, including the region that fuses to the UB.[100] Podocyte precursors reside in the proximal limb of the S-shaped body and express high levels of Wt1.[15] Many genes such as *Brn1*, *Pax2*, and *Wt1* that display restricted expression patterns in the early nephron are also required for the formation of the nephron segment they are usually expressed within.[95]

EXPANSION AND SURVIVAL OF RENAL PROGENITOR CELLS

As described previously, a number of progenitor cell populations exist within the developing kidney, but arguably the three most important are those located in the tips of the branching UB, nephron progenitor cells, and the cortical stroma. Loss of any of these populations results in disruptions to kidney development. Nephron progenitor cells promote branching in the tips of the ureteric epithelium, which is necessary to generate sufficient niches for nephron formation. Nephron progenitors are also required to provide a pool of cells to facilitate the formation of nephrons themselves. Because nephrogenesis occurs throughout much of human gestation, a delicate balance between progenitor self-renewal and differentiation must be maintained. Perturbation of this balance, whether genetic or as a consequence of a suboptimal fetomaternal environment, can result in changes in the final number of nephrons (see below).

Several signaling pathways including Fgf, Wnt, Notch are known to regulate the commitment of nephron progenitor cells to the nephrogenic program. Wnt9b, produced by the ureteric epithelium, is a major regulator of nephron commitment. Loss-of-function studies show that Wnt9b is required for the earliest inductive response in the metanephric mesenchyme, in a mechanism that involves the related protein Wnt4.[79] One of the most critical mediators of the tip-cap inductive interactions is the transcription factor Six2. Deletion of this protein causes all of the cells within the specific mesenchyme to enter the nephrogenic program, leading to an eventual cessation of nephron formation (because progenitor cells are no longer present) and a breakdown in the process of branching morphogenesis (because the mesenchymal factors that normally potentiate this process are no longer produced). Indeed, lineage tracing of Six2-expressing cells indicates they are all fated to form nephrons.[81]

Further study on most of the signaling pathways has revealed that the roles of individual signaling pathways or ligands are not as clear cut as once thought. For example, low levels of Wnt9b have been shown to help maintain nephron progenitor self-renewal, whereas high levels induce commitment (Fig. 93.10). The prevailing view suggests that this is likely the result of gradients in the expression of the protein, shaped by the influence of other signaling molecules, including molecules that originate outside the cap-tip niche. In this respect, recent interest has focused on the role of the juxtaposed cortical stromal cells, which lie at the periphery of the metanephros. Evidence of a role for these cells in shaping progenitor cell behavior is provided by analysis of mice carrying mutations in the forkhead transcription factor family member Foxd1, which results in an expansion in the size of the Six2^{+} nephrogenic pool.[101] Foxd1 in turn acts by regulating a collagen-associated proteoglycan decorin, which is thought to bind to Bmp7 and to indirectly regulate Wnt signaling. Further influence of stromal cells on CM is mediated by the Hippo/Warts signaling pathway, which itself also affects b-catenin function—a downstream target of Wnt9b activity.[102] Perturbation in this pathway resulting from deletion of decorin

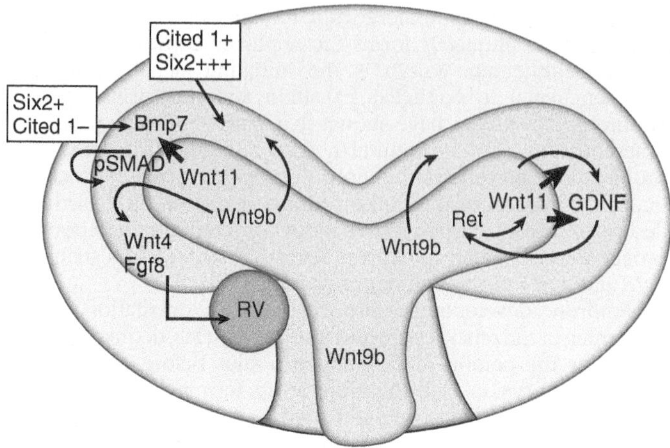

Fig. 93.10 Cap mesenchyme survival and nephron induction. Wnt9b produced by the ureteric epithelium *(blue)* is required for both commitment to the nephrogenic program and maintenance of the progenitor mesenchyme cell population. The cap mesenchyme cell population *(orange)* can be subdivided into uninduced highly Six2 positive (Six2+++) cells, which encompass a more restricted population of Cited1+ cells, providing a progenitor-like population. These Six2+++/Cited1+ cells are refractory to Wnt9b until they have undergone Bmp7-mediated SMAD activation. Six2+/Cited1– cells are able to respond to Wnt9b and are therefore able to differentiate and form a renal vesicle *(RV)*, which gives rise to a nephron. The GDNF-Ret-Wnt11 feedback loop regulates branching morphogenesis, metanephric mesenchyme, and Bmp4 expression. *Bmp,* Bone morphogenetic protein; *GDNF,* glial cell–derived neurotrophic factor.

(Dcn) and modulation of Hippo effectors, such as *Fat4* (stromal) or *Yap* and *Taz* (mesenchymal), alters the progenitor cell pool. Taken together, these studies propose a model in which the stroma acts on the CM in a process involving Fat4 activation of Hippo signaling that is affected through the actions of *Yap* and *Taz*. However, considerable work needs to be done to better understand these interactions and the occasionally conflicting reports of the effects of deletion of these genes.[103]

Given the influence of these different signaling pathways and tissue components on the cap niche and the presumably divergent choices in cell fate made by cap cells, one might speculate that cells within this population are in some way heterogeneous. Evidence supporting this view has come from a number of sources. First, the $Six2^+$ cap cell population encompasses a more restricted population of $Cited1^+$ cells, which has been mooted as a more progenitor-like cell niche.[104] These observations and others have led to a proposed model in which $Cited1^+$ cells are refractory to Wnt9b produced by the UB until they have undergone a Bmp7-mediated SMAD activation (see Fig. 93.10).[105] However, recent work has shown that commitment to nephron formation is not unidirectional. Cells can begin to express markers of nephron commitment such as *Wnt4*, then reintegrate back into the CM and remain there long term.[106] This phenomenon is facilitated by the random migration of CM cells out of the region of induction and back into an environment supporting self-renewal.[106,107] Thus, CM fate is much more plastic than previously appreciated. Heterogeneity of the CM is further evidenced by the observation that cells within this population display graded levels of Six2 expression that relate both to their position relative to the organ periphery and to their proliferation (see Fig. 93.10).[52] By modeling the incorporation of the nucleotide analogue EdU injected into pregnant mice, Short and colleagues[52] were able to model a system in which two distinct fast- and slow-cycling populations of $Six2^+$ cells exist and in which the slow-cycling cells come to predominate over the course of gestation.

The behavior of cap cells is also influenced in an autocrine manner.[108] CM progenitor cells produce both FGF9 and FGF20, and these factors, along with a second source of FGF9 from the UB, are required for maintenance of the nephrogenic progenitor cell populations. Deletion of *Fgf9* and *Fgf20* in mice halts UB branching shortly after outgrowth, either as a result of the high rates of apoptosis in the mesenchyme and/or a failure in the activation of downstream factors such as Etv4 and Etv5 that are necessary for epithelial proliferation. Although human and mouse kidneys are differentially sensitive to perturbation of these genes (*FGF20* acts alone in humans), this protein family is also important in human disease. For example, mutations in *FGF20* are associated with renal agenesis. Taken together, these findings suggest that the Fgfs are essential to maintaining a self-renewing progenitor population in the CM, upon which signals from the surrounding stroma and adjoining ureteric tree act to initiate the program of nephron differentiation. Global analysis of receptor-ligand interactions in the developing mouse kidney from single cell sequencing data has identified scores of known and new signaling interactions between cell types in the nephrogenic niche.[109] While the significance of these interactions is unclear until tested, this represents a valuable resource to use in optimizing media conditions to maintain isolated progenitors in culture.

DEVELOPMENT OF THE RENAL VASCULATURE

The mature kidneys are highly vascularized organs that contain a complex arterial and venous network that facilitate glomerular filtration and tubular reabsorption and secretion. The adult kidneys receive approximately 20% to 25% of cardiac output.[14,110] As the blood enters the kidneys via the renal arteries (direct branches from the abdominal aorta), the majority (90%) of renal blood flow is directed to the glomerular capillary beds, with the remaining 10% of blood flow directed to the medulla.[111] Blood vessel formation begins early in kidney development, and nephrogenesis and vascularization are highly synchronized.[112,113] As a result, glomerular filtration commences soon after formation of the first nephrons at approximately 9 weeks of human gestation.[110,114]

The exact mechanisms leading to the formation of the renal vasculature are not fully understood, with much of our knowledge to date derived from mouse studies. By E11.5 in the mouse, when the first UB branching occurs, a vascular plexus surrounds the UB stalk. Although the metanephric mesenchyme itself is relatively avascular at this time, it is enveloped by blood vessels. At E12.5, once the UB has undergone a few branchings, endothelial networks extend into the metanephric mesenchyme and it becomes vascularized. Endothelial plexuses, which form around each CM niche, are evident by E13.5 and connect to the internal vascular network.[115-119] Between E13 and E15 (equivalent to approximately 8 to 10 weeks' gestation in the human), the metanephric vasculature increases in complexity with the first glomerular capillary loops visible within the S-shaped bodies.[117] Around this time a single renal artery, running from the aorta to the metanephros, is visible.[120] This vessel branches into smaller arteries that terminate in afferent glomerular arterioles. The first renal arterioles are apparent in the mouse kidney by E15 to E16. By E18 to E19, a basic blueprint for arterial, arteriolar, and glomerular vascular development is apparent.[121]

It remains unclear whether the renal vasculature results from angiogenesis (sprouting from existing blood vessels) or vasculogenesis (de novo formation of blood vessels from endothelial cell precursors).[122] It is currently generally considered that both angiogenesis and vasculogenesis contribute to the formation of the renal vasculature.

Angiogenesis involves the sprouting, migration, and proliferation of already-differentiated endothelial cells and the recruitment of perivascular cells as the blood vessels form. Early studies supported the idea that development of the renal vasculature occurred via angiogenesis, which was initiated by a pair of vessels originating from the aorta.[2] Within the developing kidney, these vessels were thought to follow the branching ureteric tree and to invade the lower cleft of the S-shaped bodies, giving rise to the glomerular capillaries.[123] Evidence for this angiogenic theory of renal vascularization was provided by experiments in which undifferentiated avascular embryonic mouse kidneys were transplanted onto the quail chorioallantoic membrane.[124,125] In the following 7-day period, the transplanted kidneys were observed to develop chimeric glomerular-type structures containing quail endothelial cells. Similar findings of angiogenesis leading to the formation of glomerular capillaries were described in quail-chicken chimeras.[124,125] It has also been shown that the angiogenic response is dependent on the presence of factors within the differentiating tissue in the metanephric mesenchyme that stimulate an angiogenic response.[113]

However, the relevance of the findings from many of these early studies supporting angiogenesis as the process of renal vascular growth has been questioned.[117] In these early studies, the avascular kidneys were grown in a normoxic milieu, which is not reflective of the hypoxic environment of the developing fetus; therefore, it is possible that different mechanisms of vascular growth may have come into play. In support of this idea, several studies have since shown that low oxygen conditions lead to vasculogenesis in cultured metanephroi.[126,127] In relation to the chorioallantoic membrane studies, it has been suggested that the blood vessels of the chorioallantoic membrane may be intrinsically highly invasive and not representative of the vasculature in the developing kidney.[117]

An increasing amount of evidence suggests that vasculogenesis plays an important role in development of the renal vasculature.[122,128-131] Lineage tracing studies indicate an endogenous and likely heterogeneous population of endothelial progenitors exist in the developing kidney.[130,131] These cells contribute to endothelial structures such as the peritubular capillaries.[131] It has been proposed that local differentiation and assembly of endothelial precursors within the metanephric mesenchyme leads to glomerular capillary formation.[129,132] Expression of a number of endothelial markers including vascular endothelial growth factor receptor 1 (VEGFR1; Flt1), VEGFR2 (Flk1), angiopoietin 1 and 2 (Angpt1/2), and Tie2 in the avascular metanephric mesenchyme supports this concept.[115,122,126,133-135] In the case of larger vessels, it has been proposed that the formation of endothelial tubes is followed by recruitment of local mesenchymal cells that differentiate into smooth muscle cells to coat the growing endothelial tube.[136]

Early immunohistochemical studies by Kloth and colleagues[112] showed that capillary precursors were present in the developing kidney at a time when blood vessels were still absent. They also described a network of vessel-like structures in the differentiating glomerulus that subsequently connected with preexisting vessels. Since then, many studies have described the importance of vascular endothelial growth factor (VEGF) in the development of the renal vasculature. VEGF binds exclusively to VEGFR1 and VEGFR2, tyrosine kinase receptors that are expressed exclusively on endothelial cells and endothelial precursors.[137,138] All of these ligands and receptors have been detected in the metanephric mesenchyme and indicate the presence of endothelial precursors.[139] The importance of VEGF to glomerular capillary growth was demonstrated when injection of anti-VEGF antibodies into the cortex of developing mouse kidneys prevented the formation of glomerular capillaries, resulting in avascular glomeruli.[140]

Podocytes are rich sources of VEGF, which appears to attract endothelial precursors into the vascular clefts of the S-shaped bodies and thereby promote glomerular capillary formation.[134,140,141] VEGF and VEGFR expression is regulated by hypoxia-inducible factors that are activated by tissue hypoxia.[142] Within the cleft of the S-shaped body, the vascular precursors undergo homotypic aggregation and form into precapillary cords,[128] with the lumen of the cords subsequently formed through transforming growth factor β1 (Tgfβ1)-dependent apoptosis of a subset of endothelial cells.[143] The final stage of glomerular capillary formation involves flattening of remaining endothelial cells along the glomerular basement membrane and formation of fenestrae.[128]

A number of other receptor-ligand signaling systems are reported to play a role in glomerular capillary formation, including the Tie/angiopoietin and platelet-derived growth factor/receptor (PDGFR/PDGF) families.[144-149] In addition, CXCR4 (a chemokine) and its ligand CXCL12 are implicated in formation of glomerular capillaries.[150] Both mesangial cells and podocytes in the developing glomerulus express CXCL12, and its receptor CXCR4 is expressed by endothelial cells. Targeted deletion of *Cxcr4* or *Cxcl12* leads to impaired glomerular capillary formation, resulting in dilated single-looped capillaries.[151] The renin-angiotensin system also plays a role in kidney development,[152] with angiotensin II acting via the type 1 (AT1) receptor shown to be important in the development of the vasculature.[153-155] Blockade of the AT1 receptor has been shown to lead to fewer, thicker, and shorter afferent arterioles in newborn rats, together with alterations in kidney architecture.[155] There is evidence to suggest that angiotensin II effects on the renal vasculature are mediated by VEGF.[156]

To date, most of our understanding of renal vasculature development has been derived from animal studies. Given the differences in the spatial and temporal ontogeny of the human kidney, the challenge in the future will be to determine whether the same mechanisms of renal vascular growth occur in humans.

THE STROMA IN KIDNEY DEVELOPMENT

The metanephric mesenchyme gives rise to cell types other than those that contribute to nephrons, including vascular progenitor cells,[131] vascular smooth muscle cells, pericytes, mesangial cells,[157] and fibroblasts.[157,158] The renal stroma plays much more than a supportive role during metanephric development, regulating key processes such as formation of the renal capsule, nephrogenesis, ureteric branching, and smooth muscle formation.

The most important finding to date in identifying cells of the renal stroma was the discovery of *Foxd1*, with the production of *Foxd1*-mutant mice defining a role for stromal cells in metanephric development.[8,89,159] *Foxd1* is expressed by stromal progenitor cells and by stromal cells in the cortex and medulla. Loss of *Foxd1* expression results in an abnormal and thickened renal capsule.[89,159] In addition, ectopic Bmp4 expression in the capsule[159] disrupts branching morphogenesis and spatial patterning of the nephrogenic zone (ectopic condensates in medulla, hyperproliferation of condensates, and failure of differentiation), resulting in mice with only 7% of the normal nephron complement.[89,159,160] As described previously, studies have identified that stromal cells play a key role in the differentiation of nephron progenitor cells, highlighted by the abnormally maintained Cited1 expression in nephron progenitor cells of *Foxd1* mutants; that expression is normally lost when pretubular aggregates differentiate.[101]

Evidence also suggests that stromal cell–derived signaling regulates ureteric branching morphogenesis.[161,162] A signaling loop exists between UB cells and stromal cells, whereby RA receptors RARa and RARb2 induce stromal cells to secrete signals that control Ret expression in the UB and, therefore, branching morphogenesis. At the same time, adequate Ret expression regulates normal stromal cell patterning. Raldh2, expressed by cortical stromal cells surrounding developing nephrons, is the enzyme that converts retinaldehyde to RA.[163] Raldh2 in the cortical stroma restricts RA synthesis to the periphery, limiting signaling to the domain where Ret is localized (UB tips), thereby initiating and promoting branching.

By late gestation, the interstitium can be divided into cortical and medullary stroma. The medullary stroma expresses FGF7, which is critical for maintaining branching morphogenesis and thereby ensuring the formation of an appropriate number of nephrons.[164] Medullary stromal cells also express Bmp4, which inhibits ectopic budding along the duct.[162,165] By birth, many of the medullary stromal cells have undergone apoptosis to promote elongation of the loops of Henle and collecting ducts towards the papilla. The medullary interstitium gives rise to mature interstitial cells, vascular smooth muscle cells, and pericytes.[157] Once growth and differentiation of the kidney are complete, the primary interstitium differentiates into a diverse adult interstitium.

EXPLORING HUMAN KIDNEY DEVELOPMENT WITH SCRNA-SEQ AND STEM CELL MODELS

Technological advances in high throughput single cell RNA sequencing (scRNA-seq) and directed differentiation of human induced pluripotent cells have enabled new capabilities for investigating kidney development in human tissue. scRNA-seq and related technologies have facilitated rapid insight into the cellular composition of the human fetal kidney by revealing the transcriptional profile of thousands of component cells. Application of this approach to the human fetal kidney (reviewed by Little and Combes[95]) has identified a broad conservation of cell types characterized in the developing mouse kidney with a few notable differences such as human nephron progenitor cells expressing a more comprehensive array of stromal markers than seen in mouse. The resulting cell-type profiles from the human fetal kidney have served as a valuable reference for kidney organoids—miniature stem cell-derived models of the developing kidney. Containing patterned nephrons, stroma, and endothelial cells, kidney organoids self-organize after pluripotent cells are exposed to a series of signals that direct the formation of renal progenitors during embryogenesis. Kidney organoids represent a promising model for some aspects of human kidney disease but are currently limited in size, maturity, and by the absence of a functional blood supply and immune system.[95]

VARIABILITY IN NEPHRON NUMBER

Only a handful of studies have reported estimates of total nephron number in human kidneys. This is due to the painstaking histologic sectioning and morphometric/stereologic measurements typically required. Nevertheless, it is now well established that total nephron number varies widely in adult human kidneys. This was shown in studies of 37 Danish kidneys,[166] 28 French kidneys,[167] 20 German kidneys,[168] 47 Senegalese kidneys,[169,170] 19 Australian Aboriginal kidneys,[171] 24 kidneys from Australian non-Aborigines,[156] 132 kidneys from white Americans,[172] and 176 African American kidneys.[172] Interestingly, the mean nephron counts in kidneys from these seven racial groups was approximately 900,000, although Aboriginal Australian kidneys contained fewer nephrons than those from white Australians, and the nephron count in kidneys of the older Danish cohort was lower than that in all other groups.

The mean estimates of nephron number provided above fail to reveal the considerable variability in human nephron number. For example, in the French study, Merlet-Benichou and colleagues (1999)[167] reported a 2.4-fold range in nephron number, whereas the Senegalese study reported a 3.3-fold range[169,170] and the Danish study reported a 4.3-fold range.[166] In the large American cohorts, a 7.3-fold range was reported in white Americans and a 9.6-fold range was reported in African Americans, with counts ranging from 210,000 to 2.7 million, a 12.8-fold range.[172] The studies cited above reported nephron number in kidneys obtained at autopsy. However, in recent years a new approach involving a combination of computer tomographic (CT) estimation of renal cortical volume with morphometric estimation of glomerular density in biopsies has been used to estimate nephron number in living donors.[173-175] This represents a significant advance and is likely to be the first of several methods that will emerge in the next decade for estimating nephron number in donors, patients, and those at risk of developing kidney disease such as those born premature and/or with low birth weight.

The total nephron number in adult kidneys reflects the number of nephrons formed during development (nephron endowment) minus the number of nephrons subsequently lost.[176] This raises a question regarding the variability in nephron endowment in humans at birth. Few data are available to answer this question, but in one study of 15 children aged younger than 3 months, a 4.5-fold range in nephron number was reported.[177] One can speculate that with a larger sample size, a much larger range in nephron number would have been found.

Given the complex events involved in kidney development and nephrogenesis, and the numerous signaling molecules and pathways involved, it is perhaps not surprising that nephron number varies widely in the human population. In 2011, full or partial deletion of more than 25 genes in mice had been reported to result in kidney hypoplasia.[178] Polymorphisms in *Pax2,*[179] *RET,*[177] and *OSR1*[180] have also been shown to be linked to small kidney size in humans.

Perturbations to the fetomaternal environment have also been shown to influence nephron endowment. Most evidence has come from animal studies, in which global food restriction, maternal low-protein diet, placental insufficiency, vitamin A deficiency, and maternal exposure to natural and synthetic glucocorticoids, alcohol, and certain antibiotics have all resulted in reduced nephron endowment.[14,181,182] The size of the resulting nephron deficit is often influenced by dosage, timing and duration of the perturbation, and species. In humans, low vitamin A levels have been associated with small kidney size.[183]

PREMATURITY, BIRTH WEIGHT, AND NEPHRON NUMBER

Over recent decades it has become well recognized that body weight at birth has the potential to influence lifelong renal health.[184-187] Low birth weight (<2.5 kg at birth) imparts a 70% increase in the risk of developing chronic kidney disease.[187] Advances in the survival of low-birth-weight infants have contributed to an escalation in the incidence of chronic renal disease. In this regard, it is proposed that the high incidence of renal disease in the Australian Indigenous population is a legacy of the improved survival of low-birth-weight neonates over recent decades.[171,188,189] Low birth weight is linked to an increased risk of developing hypertension,[190-193] which is likely to be renal in origin,[182,194] and/or renal disease later in life.[187,195-197] Indeed, the associated long-term rise in blood pressure in subjects born of low birth weight renders vulnerability to both renal[187] and cardiovascular disease,[198] the both of which are inextricably linked. Hence the improved survival over recent decades of low-birth-weight infants is associated with a number of emerging long-term renal health costs, as the long-term renal sequelae begin to emerge. Notably, a systematic review in 2009 of 32 observational studies reported a 70% greater risk of developing chronic kidney disease later in life (as defined according to albuminuria, low estimated glomerular filtration rate [GFR], or end-stage renal disease) in individuals born of low birth weight.[187]

Low birth weight can be the result of intrauterine growth restriction (IUGR) and/or preterm birth (birth prior to 37 weeks' gestation).[197] IUGR occurs when there is poor growth of the fetus in utero and is defined as birth weight below the 10th percentile for gestational age.[199] IUGR is multifactorial in origin and generally occurs as a result of restricted blood flow, and thus inadequate delivery of oxygen and nutrients, to the developing fetus.[200,201] In developing countries the major cause of IUGR is maternal malnutrition and/or undernutrition, whereas in developed countries the major cause of IUGR is placental insufficiency,[202,203] which often occurs in the third trimester.

The etiology leading to the elevated risk of renal disease and/or elevated blood pressure in subjects born of low birth weight is not well understood. It is considered likely that early life adverse effects on nephrogenesis and on the number of nephrons formed within the kidneys may mediate, at least in part, the elevated risk in later life.[172,182,197,204] Notably, in the human kidney approximately 60% of nephrons are formed in the third trimester.[1,205] In the case of the many infants exposed to placental insufficiency, this is the critical time period in gestation when the infants are growth restricted. Likewise, it is during the third trimester when the majority of preterm infants are delivered. In this regard, there are many experimental studies linking IUGR with reduced nephron endowment at birth.[206-214] Preterm birth is also linked to impairment of nephrogenesis.[215-218] Therefore, both IUGR and preterm birth have the potential to adversely affect lifelong renal functional reserve. Indeed, given that it is the loss of functional nephrons throughout life (through lifestyle factors, aging, and disease) that ultimately leads to renal impairment, it is likely that subjects who commence life with a reduced nephron endowment will have an elevated risk.

As described previously, stereologic studies of more than 400 autopsied human kidneys from subjects with normal renal morphology have demonstrated a 13-fold range in nephron number, with values ranging from as low as 210,000 to 2.7 million nephrons in a single kidney.[166,169,176,219,220] Autopsied kidneys from 15 children also demonstrated a wide variability (4.5-fold range) in nephron number, supporting the concept that much of the variability in adult human nephron number is present at birth.[177] It appears that much of the variation in human nephron endowment observed at birth can be attributed to variations in birth weight. A direct linear relationship between human birth weight and nephron number has been reported, with the linear regression predicting an additional 250,000 nephrons for each 1-kg increase in birth weight.[220,221] However, it is important to point out that a high proportion of these kidneys were obtained from adults, so nephron numbers may not completely reflect nephron endowment at birth.

In a small autopsy study, a marked reduction in nephron number was reported in severely growth-restricted stillborn babies and in IUGR infants who had died during the first year of life, compared with infants who had been appropriately grown in utero.[222] In another autopsy study of 35 neonates, a significant linear correlation was observed between the number of glomeruli per area of cortex and birth weight.[223]

In addition to IUGR, low birth weight can result from preterm birth, and in many infants IUGR is a comorbidity of preterm birth.[224,225] During normal human pregnancies, nephrogenesis is complete prior to birth[1,58]; however, this is not the case for many preterm babies (born prior to 37 weeks of gestation). A high proportion of preterm infants are born at a time when their kidneys are very immature and nephrogenesis is still ongoing. Of particular concern are infants born very (28 to 32 weeks' gestation) or extremely (<28 weeks' gestation) preterm. There has been a marked increase in the survival of these infants in recent decades due to advances in neonatal care. In developed countries, babies born as early as 25 weeks' gestation now have approximately an 80% chance of survival.[226] Importantly, it has been shown in non-human primate studies and in human infants that nephrogenesis continues after preterm birth.[216,218,227] In studies of preterm baboon kidneys in which the timing of nephrogenesis is similar to that in humans,[228] the number of nephrons in extremely preterm offspring that survived for several weeks was significantly greater than in offspring born of the same gestational age but did not survive beyond birth, thus demonstrating that new nephrons were formed in the neonatal period.[215]

In human studies there is often evidence of a nephrogenic zone in the kidneys of preterm infants who have survived several days/weeks after birth. Furthermore, the number of glomerular generations formed within the kidneys has been shown to increase with postnatal age after birth, indicative of new nephrons forming in the extrauterine environment.[216,218] Of concern, however, as seen in the experimental baboon studies, preterm birth is associated with negative impacts on nephrogenesis with potential adverse impacts on nephron endowment and lifelong renal functional reserve. In autopsy studies of the kidneys of human babies, preterm birth has been shown to (1) accelerate renal maturation (with a significant reduction in the width of the nephrogenic zone and in the proportion of glomeruli in the most immature stage of development when compared to age-matched normally grown fetal kidneys)[218]; (2) result in gross glomerular abnormalities in the outer renal cortex in some preterm infants (these glomeruli with a cystic Bowman space are unlikely to ever be functional)[218]; and (3) lead to fewer generations of glomeruli formed within the kidneys (IUGR was a comorbidity in a number of babies in that study).[216]

The cause of the glomerular abnormalities associated with preterm birth is currently unknown. The fact that they are found only in the outer cortex suggests that only the most recently formed glomeruli are at risk. Indeed, the extrauterine environment must be considered an abnormal environment for nephrogenesis, and it may be that the changes in oxygen levels and/or hemodynamics that occur at the time of birth lead to these abnormalities. In contrast to the in utero environment (with low oxygen levels, high renal resistance, and low renal blood flow),[110,229-232] after birth the immature kidneys are exposed to a normoxic environment,[233,234] and there is a marked increase in blood pressure and renal blood flow.[235,236] It is also possible that the factors that led to preterm delivery and/or factors in the neonatal care have contributed to these glomerular abnormalities in preterm infants. Because these factors differ among babies, this would account for why the kidneys of some infants are adversely affected and others are not.[237-239] Several studies have shown that certain antibiotics (e.g., aminoglycosides) can be nephrotoxic in newborns,[238] and in experimental studies administration of antibiotics has been linked to impaired nephrogenesis.[240-243] In addition, animal studies report that in utero exposure to maternal glucocorticoids leads to reduced nephron endowment in offspring[244-246] and that exposure of immature kidneys to nonsteroidal antiinflammatory drugs leads to severe renal injury.[247] Notably, however, in morphologic studies in autopsied kidneys, no particular medication administered to preterm infants could be identified as the direct cause of the glomerular abnormalities observed,[218] and encouragingly studies in nonhuman primates have shown that prenatal exposure to betamethasone (which is administered to most women at risk of delivering preterm) does not lead to glomerular abnormalities.[215]

Renal function can also be adversely influenced by preterm birth.[238] Renal function in preterm neonates during the first month of life is significantly affected by gestational age at birth and by postnatal age; ethnicity can also be a contributing factor in this renal vulnerability.[248] Preterm infants experience a low GFR at birth, which increases with gestational and postnatal age.[249-251] Plasma creatinine is highest in the most preterm neonates and decreases gradually with increasing postnatal age.[252-254] Concomitantly, creatinine clearance increases with increasing gestational age at birth and increasing postnatal age.[251,253] The fractional excretion of sodium (a measure of tubular function) is inversely related to gestational age at birth and decreases with postnatal age.[251,253] A study of postnatal renal function in preterm infants showed that the fractional excretion of sodium was not different between term and preterm infants by 28 days after birth, whereas creatinine clearance remained significantly lower.[249] Both urinary protein and urinary neutrophil gelatinase-associated lipocalin (NGAL) levels (markers of renal injury and/or immaturity) were inversely associated with gestational age at birth.[249] Of concern, there is a high prevalence of acute kidney injury in preterm infants[255] with the causes often prerenal in origin, arising from conditions that affect renal perfusion such as hypotension, hypoxia, and sepsis.[256-258] In addition, many of the life-saving medications routinely used in contemporary neonatal care are known to adversely affect renal function[259]; both prenatal and postnatal medical interventions are also linked to acute kidney injury.[260]

Another common renal complication of preterm birth is nephrocalcinosis (deposition of calcium phosphate and/or calcium oxalate) within the tubulointerstitial regions of the kidney. The reported prevalence of nephrocalcinosis differs widely among populations (ranging from 7% to 41% or more[259,261]; differences in the study populations, ultrasound equipment, and study criteria contribute to the differences in the reported prevalence between studies. Factors such as a high intake of calcium, phosphorous, and ascorbic acid; a low urinary citrate/calcium ratio; a high urinary calcium/creatinine ratio; and medications to prevent or treat chronic lung disease (with hypercalciuric side effects) are associated with the high incidence of nephrocalcinosis in preterm neonates.[261]

With the improved survival of preterm infants over recent decades (especially those born very and extremely preterm), the long-term consequences on renal function are now becoming clinically apparent. Indeed, given the negative impact of preterm birth and IUGR (which is a common comorbidity of preterm birth) on nephron endowment and renal function it is not surprising that low birth weight is associated with an increased incidence of hypertension and renal disease later in life.

CONCLUSION

Kidney development is regulated by a host of gene products and signaling pathways and can be significantly and permanently affected by a suboptimal fetomaternal environment. Many gene factors and environmental agents can permanently reduce nephron endowment at birth, increasing the risk of adult cardiovascular and renal disease.

CHAPTER GLOSSARY

Angpt1: angiopoietin 1; vascular growth factor expressed by metanephric mesenchyme suggesting presence of endothelial precursors in the kidney

Angpt2: angiopoietin 2; vascular growth factor expressed by metanephric mesenchyme suggesting presence of endothelial precursors in the kidney

AT1 (Agtr1a): angiotensin II receptor, type 1a; receptor for angiotensin II, which supports development of kidney vasculature

Bmp4: bone morphogenetic protein 4; growth factor, which restricts ureteric bud outgrowth and supports ureteric bud branching

Bmp7: bone morphogenetic protein 7; growth factor, which supports nephron progenitor maintenance and responsiveness to Wnt9b induction

Brn1 (Pou3f3): brain-specific homeobox/POU domain protein 1; transcription factor; asymmetrically expressed during nephrogenesis establishing proximo-distal polarity; promotes distal tubule formation

Cdh1: cadherin-1 (E-cadherin); asymmetrically expressed during nephrogenesis establishing proximo-distal polarity

Cdh6: cadherin 6; promotes nephrogenesis and tubule fusion to the ureteric bud; asymmetrically expressed during nephrogenesis establishing proximo-distal polarity

Cited1: cbp/p300-interacting transactivator with Glu/Asp-rich carboxy-terminal domain 1; transcriptional regulator that marks the uninduced nephron progenitor pool

CXCR4: chemokine (C-X-C motif) receptor 4; endothelial receptor for CXCL12 important for glomerular capillary formation

CXCL12: chemokine (C-X-C motif) ligand 12; ligand for CXCR4 important for glomerular capillary formation

Dcn: decorin; antagonizes Bmp signaling to promote Wnt-induced nephron progenitor differentiation

Emx2: empty spiracles homeobox 2; transcription factor required for ureteric bud branching and nephrogenesis

ERK: extracellular-signal-regulated kinase; downstream signaling pathway involved in ureteric bud branching

Etv4: ets variant 4; transcription factor downstream of Ret that support ureteric bud branching

Etv5: ets variant 5; transcription factor downstream of Ret that support ureteric bud branching

Eya1: eyes absent homolog 1; transcriptional regulator that specifies the metanephric mesenchyme through interactions with Hox and *Pax* transcription factors; supports GDNF expression

Fat4: FAT atypical cadherin 4; receptor expressed by stroma that supports ureteric bud branching

FGF7: fibroblast growth factor 7; growth factor that promotes continued ureteric bud branching

FGF8: fibroblast growth factor 8; growth factor that marks induced nephron progenitors and supports nephrogenesis

FGF9: fibroblast growth factor 9; growth factor produced by ureteric bud and nephron progenitors to support nephron progenitor maintenance

FGF10: fibroblast growth factor 10; growth factor that promotes continued ureteric bud branching

FGF20: fibroblast growth factor 20; growth factor produced by nephron progenitors to support their maintenance

FGFR2: fibroblast growth factor receptor 2; receptor for FGF that promotes ureteric bud branching

Foxc1: forkhead box protein C1; transcription factor that suppresses GDNF expression and restricts ureteric bud outgrowth to a single site

Foxd1: forkhead box D1; transcription factor expressed by stromal progenitors required for nephrogenesis; modulates size of the nephron progenitor pool

Gata3: GATA binding protein 3; transcription factor, which helps establish ureteric bud position

Gdf11: growth differentiation factor 11; growth factor, which promotes GDNF expression and ureteric bud outgrowth

GDNF: glial cell-derived neurotrophic factor; ligand that promotes ureteric bud outgrowth and branching

Gfra1: glial cell line derived neurotrophic factor family receptor alpha 1; receptor for GDNF; promotes ureteric bud outgrowth and branching

Grem1: gremlin 1, DAN family Bmp antagonist; secreted factor, which inhibits Bmp4 to promote ureteric bud outgrowth and branching

Hnf1β: Hepatocyte nuclear factor 1β; transcription factor acting up and downstream of Ret to regulate ureteric bud branching

Hoxa/c/d11: homeobox A11/C11/D11; family of transcription factors, which support formation and positioning of the metanephric mesenchyme

Lim1: LIM homeobox 1; transcription factor, which promotes extension of nephric duct and ureteric bud branching

MAPK: mitogen-activated protein kinase; downstream signaling pathway involved in ureteric bud branching

MITF: Microphthalmia-associated transcription factor, also known as *melanogenesis-associated transcription factor*; transcription factor that modulates Ret to regulate ureteric bud branching

Notch: signaling pathway that promotes nephrogenesis

Osr1: odd-skipped related 1; transcription factor, which supports formation and positioning of the metanephric mesenchyme

Pax2: paired box 2; transcription factor, which promotes nephric duct formation and establishes ureteric bud position; expressed by metanephric mesenchyme to promote maintenance; expressed in developing nephrons and supports proper nephrogenesis

Pax8: paired box 8; transcription factor, which promotes nephric duct formation

PDGF: platelet derived growth factor; growth factor important for glomerular capillary formation

PDGFR: platelet derived growth factor receptor; receptor for PDGF important for glomerular capillary formation

PI3K: phosphoinositide 3-kinase; downstream signaling pathway involved in ureteric bud branching

PLCγ: phospholipase C; downstream signaling pathway involved in ureteric bud branching

RA: Retinoic acid; metabolite derived from retinol (vitamin A) that promotes specification of renal progenitors

Raldh2 (Aldh1a2): aldehyde dehydrogenase family 1, subfamily A2; enzyme that converts retinaldehyde to RA; restricts RA signaling to region of ureteric tips to promote branching

Rara: retinoic acid receptor, alpha (RARα); RA receptor, which induces the production of signals by stromal cells that modulate Ret expression and ureteric bud branching

Rarb: retinoic acid receptor, beta (RARβ); RA receptor induces the production of signals by stromal cells that modulate Ret expression and ureteric bud branching

Ret: rearranged during transfection; receptor for GDNF; promotes ureteric bud outgrowth and branching

Robo2: roundabout guidance receptor 2; receptor for Slit2 that suppresses GDNF expression and restricts ureteric bud outgrowth to a single site

Sall1: spalt like transcription factor 1; transcription factor that supports metanephric mesenchyme competency

Six1: sine oculis-related homeobox 1; transcription factor that promotes GDNF expression and metanephric mesenchyme competency

Six2: sine oculis-related homeobox 2; transcription factor required for nephron progenitor self-renewal and maintenance

Six4: sine oculis-related homeobox 4; transcription factor that promotes GDNF expression and metanephric mesenchyme competency

Slit2: slit guidance ligand 2; signaling ligand that suppresses GDNF expression and restricts ureteric bud outgrowth to a single site

SMAD: signaling pathway downstream of Tgfβ/Bmp

Spry1: sprouty RTK signaling antagonist 1; factor, which modulates signaling downstream of GDNF-Ret

Taz (Wwtr1): WW domain containing transcription regulator 1; effector of Hippo signaling that supports nephron progenitors and nephrogenesis

Tcf21: transcription factor 21; transcription factor that modulates GDNF and ureteric bud branching

Tgfb1: transforming growth factor β1; growth factor supporting lumenization of capillaries through apoptosis

Tie2 (Tek): Tyrosine-protein kinase receptor 2; receptor for Angpt1/2 and endothelial marker expressed by metanephric mesenchyme suggesting presence of endothelial precursors, regulates capillary formation

VEGF: vascular endothelial growth factor; endothelial growth factor expressed by the metanephric mesenchyme and podocytes, supports glomerular capillary formation

VEGFR1 (Flt1): vascular endothelial growth factor receptor 1; receptor for VEGF expressed by endothelium and metanephric mesenchyme, supports glomerular capillary formation

VEGFR2 (Flk-1): vascular endothelial growth factor receptor 2; receptor for VEGF expressed by endothelium and metanephric mesenchyme, supports glomerular capillary formation

Wnt4: wingless-type MMTV integration site family, member 4; signaling ligand that marks induced nephron progenitors and supports nephrogenesis

Wnt9b: wingless-type MMTV integration site family, member 9B; signaling ligand that induces nephron progenitor differentiation and helps promote their self-renewal

Wnt11: wingless-type MMTV integration site family, member 11; signaling ligand that promotes ureteric bud branching through GDNF-Ret

Wt1: Wilms tumor-1 (Wt1); transcription factor, which maintains competency of the metanephric mesenchyme

Yap (Yap1): yes-associated protein 1; effector of Hippo signaling that supports nephron progenitors and nephrogenesis

A complete reference list is available at www.ExpertConsult.com. 

SELECT REFERENCES

1. Saxen L, Sariola H. Early organogenesis of the kidney. *Pediatr Nephrol.* 1987;1(3):385-392.
14. Moritz KM, Wintour EM, Black MJ, Bertram JF, Caruana G. Factors influencing mammalian kidney development: implications for health in adult life. *Adv Anat Embryol Cell Biol.* 2008;196:1-78.
15. Kreidberg JA, Sariola H, Loring JM, et al. WT-1 is required for early kidney development. *Cell.* 1993;74(4):679-691.
18. Lindstrom NO, McMahon JA, Guo J, et al. Conserved and divergent features of human and mouse kidney organogenesis. *J Am Soc Nephrol.* 2018;29(3): 785-805.
27. Grote D, Souabni A, Busslinger M, Bouchard M. Pax 2/8-regulated Gata 3 expression is necessary for morphogenesis and guidance of the nephric duct in the developing kidney. *Development.* 2006;133(1):53-61.
29. Wellik DM, Hawkes PJ, Capecchi MR. Hox11 paralogous genes are essential for metanephric kidney induction. *Genes Dev.* 2002;16(11):1423-1432.
33. Kobayashi H, Kawakami K, Asashima M, Nishinakamura R. Six1 and Six4 are essential for Gdnf expression in the metanephric mesenchyme and ureteric bud formation, while Six1 deficiency alone causes mesonephric-tubule defects. *Mech Dev.* 2007;124(4):290-303.
38. Miyazaki Y, Oshima K, Fogo A, Hogan BL, Ichikawa I. Bone morphogenetic protein 4 regulates the budding site and elongation of the mouse ureter. *J Clin Invest.* 2000;105(7):863-873.
39. Gross I, Morrison DJ, Hyink DP, et al. The receptor tyrosine kinase regulator Sprouty1 is a target of the tumor suppressor WT1 and important for kidney development. *J Biol Chem.* 2003;278(42):41420-41430.
40. Michos O, Goncalves A, Lopez-Rios J, et al. Reduction of BMP4 activity by gremlin 1 enables ureteric bud outgrowth and GDNF/WNT11 feedback signalling during kidney branching morphogenesis. *Development.* 2007;134(13):2397-2405.
52. Short KM, Combes AN, Lefevre J, et al. Global quantification of tissue dynamics in the developing mouse kidney. *Dev Cell.* 2014;29(2):188-202.
58. Osathanondh V, Potter EL. Development of human kidney as shown by microdissection. III. Formation and interrelationship of collecting tubules and nephrons. *Arch Pathol.* 1963;76:290-302.
59. Osathanondh V, Potter EL. Development of human kidney as shown by microdissection. II. Renal pelvis, calyces, and papillae. *Arch Pathol.* 1963;76:277-289.
62. Short KM, Combes AN, Lisnyak V, et al. Branching morphogenesis in the developing kidney is not impacted by nephron formation or integration. *eLife.* 2018;7:e38992.
65. Short KM, Hodson MJ, Smyth IM. Tomographic quantification of branching morphogenesis and renal development. *Kidney Int.* 2010;77(12):1132-1139.
74. Cebrian C, Asai N, D'Agati V, Costantini F. The number of fetal nephron progenitor cells limits ureteric branching and adult nephron endowment. *Cell Rep.* 2014;7(1):127-137.
79. Carroll TJ, Park JS, Hayashi S, Majumdar A, McMahon AP. Wnt9b plays a central role in the regulation of mesenchymal to epithelial transitions underlying organogenesis of the mammalian urogenital system. *Dev Cell.* 2005;9(2): 283-292.
81. Kobayashi A, Valerius MT, Mugford JW, et al. Six2 defines and regulates a multipotent self-renewing nephron progenitor population throughout mammalian kidney development. *Cell Stem Cell.* 2008;3(2):169-181.

82. Stark K, Vainio S, Vassileva G, McMahon AP. Epithelial transformation of metanephric mesenchyme in the developing kidney regulated by Wnt-4. *Nature*. 1994;372(6507):679-683.
89. Hatini V, Huh SO, Herzlinger D, Soares VC, Lai E. Essential role of stromal mesenchyme in kidney morphogenesis revealed by targeted disruption of Winged Helix transcription factor BF-2. *Genes Dev*. 1996;10(12):1467-1478.
95. Little MH, Combes AN. Kidney organoids: accurate models or fortunate accidents. *Genes Dev*. 2019;33(19-20):1319-1345.
101. Fetting JL, Guay JA, Karolak MJ, et al. FOXD1 promotes nephron progenitor differentiation by repressing decorin in the embryonic kidney. *Development*. 2014;141(1):17-27.
102. Karner CM, Das A, Ma Z, et al. Canonical Wnt9b signaling balances progenitor cell expansion and differentiation during kidney development. *Development*. 2011;138(7):1247-1257.
104. Mugford JW, Yu J, Kobayashi A, McMahon AP. High-resolution gene expression analysis of the developing mouse kidney defines novel cellular compartments within the nephron progenitor population. *Dev Biol*. 2009;333(2):312-323.
106. Lawlor KT, Zappia L, Lefevre J, et al. Nephron progenitor commitment is a stochastic process influenced by cell migration. *eLife*. 2019;8:e41156.
109. Combes AN, Phipson B, Lawlor KT, et al. Single cell analysis of the developing mouse kidney provides deeper insight into marker gene expression and ligand-receptor crosstalk. *Development*. 2019;146(12).
112. Kloth S, Aigner J, Schmidbauer A, Minuth WW. Interrelationship of renal vascular development and nephrogenesis. *Cell Tissue Res*. 1994;277(2):247-257.
131. Sims-Lucas S, Schaefer C, Bushnell D, et al. Endothelial progenitors exist within the kidney and lung mesenchyme. *PloS One*. 2013;8(6):e65993.
136. Sequeira Lopez ML, Gomez RA. Development of the renal arterioles. *J Am Soc Nephrol*. 2011;22(12):2156-2165.
140. Kitamoto Y, Tokunaga H, Tomita K. Vascular endothelial growth factor is an essential molecule for mouse kidney development: glomerulogenesis and nephrogenesis. *J Clin Invest*. 1997;99(10):2351-2357.
150. Herzlinger D, Hurtado R. Patterning the renal vascular bed. *Semin Cell Dev Biol*. 2014;36:50-56.
164. Qiao J, Uzzo R, Obara-Ishihara T, Degenstein L, Fuchs E, Herzlinger D. FGF-7 modulates ureteric bud growth and nephron number in the developing kidney. *Development*. 1999;126(3):547-554.
165. Levinson R, Mendelsohn C. Stromal progenitors are important for patterning epithelial and mesenchymal cell types in the embryonic kidney. *Semin Cell Dev Biol*. 2003;14(4):225-231.
166. Nyengaard JR, Bendtsen TF. Glomerular number and size in relation to age, kidney weight, and body surface in normal man. *Anat Rec*. 1992;232(2):194-201.
172. Bertram JF, Douglas-Denton RN, Diouf B, Hughson MD, Hoy WE. Human nephron number: implications for health and disease. *Pediatr Nephrol*. 2011;26(9):1529-1533.
174. Sasaki T, Tsuboi N, Okabayashi Y, et al. Estimation of nephron number in living humans by combining unenhanced computed tomography with biopsy-based stereology. *Sci Rep*. 2019;9(1):14400.
175. Denic A, Elsherbiny H, Rule AD. In-vivo techniques for determining nephron number. *Curr Opin Nephrol Hypertens*. 2019;28(6):545-551.
176. Puelles VG, Hoy WE, Hughson MD, Diouf B, Douglas-Denton RN, Bertram JF. Glomerular number and size variability and risk for kidney disease. *Curr Opin Nephrol Hypertens*. 2011;20(1):7-15.
182. Luyckx VA, Bertram JF, Brenner BM, et al. Effect of fetal and child health on kidney development and long-term risk of hypertension and kidney disease. *Lancet*. 2013;382(9888):273-283.
187. White SL, Perkovic V, Cass A, et al. Is low birth weight an antecedent of CKD in later life? A systematic review of observational studies. *Am J Kidney Dis*. 2009;54(2):248-261.
188. Hoy WE, Nicol JL. The Barker hypothesis confirmed: association of low birth weight with all-cause natural deaths in young adult life in a remote Australian Aboriginal community. *J Dev Orig Health Dis*. 2019;10(1):55-62.
194. Luyckx VA, Brenner BM. *Clinical Consequences of Developmental Programming of Low Nephron Number*. Hoboken, NJ: Anat Rec; 2019.
196. Vikse BE, Irgens LM, Leivestad T, Hallan S, Iversen BM. Low birth weight increases risk for end-stage renal disease. *J Am Soc Nephrol*. 2008;19(1):151-157.
204. Luyckx VA, Brenner BM. Low birth weight, nephron number, and kidney disease. *Kidney Int Suppl*. 2005;(97):S68-S77.
205. Hinchliffe SA, Sargent PH, Howard CV, Chan YF, van Velzen D. Human intrauterine renal growth expressed in absolute number of glomeruli assessed by the disector method and Cavalieri principle. *Lab Invest*. 1991;64(6):777-784.
211. Woods LL, Weeks DA, Rasch R. Programming of adult blood pressure by maternal protein restriction: role of nephrogenesis. *Kidney Int*. 2004;65(4):1339-1348.
212. Zimanyi MA, Bertram JF, Black MJ. Does a nephron deficit in rats predispose to salt-sensitive hypertension? *Kidney Blood Press Res*. 2004;27(4):239-247.
221. Hughson M, Farris 3rd AB, Douglas-Denton R, Hoy WE, Bertram JF. Glomerular number and size in autopsy kidneys: the relationship to birth weight. *Kidney Int*. 2003;63(6):2113-2122.
238. Black MJ, Sutherland MR, Gubhaju L, Kent AL, Dahlstrom JE, Moore L. When birth comes early: effects on nephrogenesis. *Nephrology*. 2013;18(3):180-182.
239. Gubhaju L, Sutherland MR, Black MJ. Preterm birth and the kidney: implications for long-term renal health. *Reprod Sci*. 2011;18(4):322-333.
248. Sutherland MR, Chatfield MD, Davison B, et al. Renal dysfunction is already evident within the first month of life in Australian Indigenous infants born preterm. *Kidney Int*. 2019;96(5):1205-1216.
SECTION XVI — The Kidney

94 Functional Development of the Kidney in Utero

Douglas G. Matsell | Michael J. Hiatt

INTRODUCTION

The mature and differentiated mammalian kidney assumes a number of diverse, complex, and related functions in the postnatal environment. These functions include glomerular filtration, salt and water reabsorption, acid-base homeostasis, regulation of blood pressure, tubular secretion, and endocrine functions including vitamin D, calcium and phosphate metabolism, erythropoiesis, immune regulation, and circulating drug and toxin metabolism, among others. Most of these important postnatal physiologic functions that regulate normal body homeostasis have their origins in fetal life. Their ontogeny is directed by the development of kidney structure, which itself is under the tight control of precisely orchestrated spatial and temporal gene and protein expression.

The important events in fetal life that precede the acquisition of kidney function include the induction of embryonic kidney progenitor cell populations to differentiate into kidney-specific cells, the development and differentiation of glomeruli and associated vascularization, segment-specific differentiation of the kidney tubules, and terminal differentiation of the various cellular compartments of the kidney.

While much of our knowledge to date regarding fetal kidney physiology is based on large mammal experimental observation, and while there are a number of phylogenetic similarities in kidney embryogenesis (e.g., pro- and metanephric development of glomeruli and tubules), it should be noted that substantial variation exists in the periods of nephrogenesis that occur during fetal life and postnatally.

For example, in humans, nephrogenesis, as defined by the period of time during which new nephrons are formed, begins at approximately 8 weeks gestation and is complete by 36 weeks gestation. In other species (and in human infants born prematurely) nephron induction continues postnatally and is

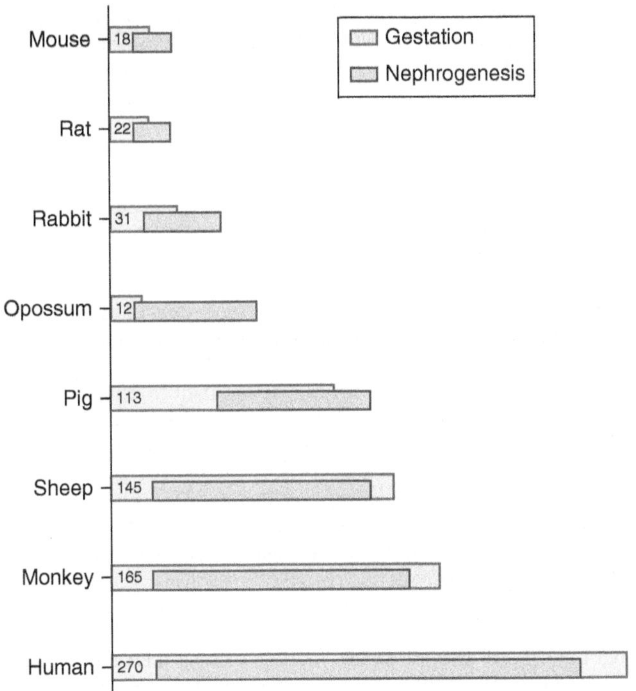

Fig. 94.1 Mammalian nephrogenesis. Schematic representation of the relative lengths of nephrogenesis in different mammalian species compared to the duration of their respective gestational period. In certain species, including the mouse, rat, rabbit, and pig, nephrogenesis continues into the postnatal period. Numbers in the green boxes indicate length of gestation in days. (Modified from Matsell DG, Tarantal AF. Experimental models of fetal obstructive nephropathy. *Pediatr Nephrol*. 2002;17:470–476.)

influenced by ex utero factors. The requirements for mature kidney function in the human fetus are supplanted by the interposition of the maternal placenta. Therefore, our knowledge of normal fetal kidney physiology is inferred from either observational data in preterm infants or from experimental data from animal models, whose period of gestational nephrogenesis may or may not correspond to the length of human gestation (Fig. 94.1).[1]

Why then is an understanding of normal fetal renal physiology important, particularly if growth and maturation of the fetus is dependent on the placenta and maternal circulation?

The development of normal kidney function originates in utero as soon as nephrogenesis begins and continues into the neonatal period. Fetal kidney function impacts normal fetal development and is linked to the normal development of other fetal organ systems such as the lung and genitourinary systems.

Alteration of normal kidney development and, therefore, normal kidney structure and kidney function by factors such as placental insufficiency, protein restriction, preterm birth, in utero exposure to toxins such as inhibitors of prostaglandin synthesis, corticosteroids, and inhibitors of the renin-angiotensin-aldosterone axis, impacts not only fetal development but also postnatal kidney function and long-term kidney health.[2] Abnormal fetal kidney development and fetal kidney function therefore portend long-term physiologic consequences.

In a more practical sense, in the developed world there is almost universal access to antenatal screening to evaluate fetal health. The most common abnormalities discovered during early second trimester ultrasound screening (16 to 20 weeks gestation) are anomalies associated with urinary tract and kidney structure. Information gained from early gestation fetal ultrasounds, particularly in the cases in which kidney abnormalities are found, is used to predict fetal outcome, to influence families' decisions regarding the future of their pregnancies, and to inform counseling around future pregnancies.

ANTENATAL ASSESSMENTS OF KIDNEY FUNCTION

A number of tests are used to estimate kidney health and to extrapolate postnatal kidney function during antenatal assessments of pregnancies complicated by fetal kidney anomalies. These include imaging studies of fetal kidney morphology, structure and differentiation, fetal blood and urine sample estimates of fetal glomerular filtration rate (GFR), amniotic fluid (AF) concentrations of analytes, AF volumes, fetal urine flow rates, and proteomic and metabolomic analysis of fetal urine and AF.

Antenatal imaging using second trimester screening ultrasound identifies most cases of severe developmental kidney anomalies including congenital urinary tract obstruction. Typically, the normal fetal bladder can be visualized from the onset of urine production at approximately 10 weeks gestation and in all pregnancies by 18 to 20 weeks. Increased echogenicity of the kidneys, a poorly defined cortico-medullary border, and parenchymal cystic changes are suggestive of abnormal kidney development.[3] When associated with severe oligohydramnios in early pregnancy, these changes carry a poor prognosis and are associated with a less than 90% perinatal mortality.[4]

Studies analyzing the value of screening antenatal ultrasounds in predicting postnatal kidney outcomes are conflicting. The predictive value of echogenic and/or cystic changes of fetal kidneys to detect either dysplasia histologically or chronic kidney disease on postnatal follow-up was only 59%. In contrast, the predictive value of normal parenchyma on prenatal ultrasound to detect no dysplasia or normal renal function was 56%.[5] Detailed ultrasound examination of the urinary tract, particularly when performed by an experienced operator, yields a higher accuracy of diagnosis of congenital kidney anomalies.[6] Fetal magnetic resonance imaging (MRI) can provide more detailed assessment of the fetal urinary tract,[7-9] and future applications of functional MRI, such as diffusion weighted imaging, may provide information regarding fetal GFR.[10] Predictive values of MRI for congenital urinary tract obstruction, however, are difficult to ascertain due to its selective use and small numbers of published cases.

Given the inherent drawbacks of antenatal imaging in affected fetuses with kidney disorders, antenatal evaluation strategies have included measures of fetal renal function. Measurement of fetal GFR would be an ideal determinant of renal function and likely a good surrogate for the severity of dysplasia; however, there are no normative data in uncomplicated pregnancies,[11] and GFR is somewhat challenging to determine accurately during prenatal life. β_2-microglobulin, the light chain of the class I major histocompatibility antigens, has been used as an indirect measure of fetal GFR. It is an attractive candidate for GFR estimation because of a constant production rate by the fetus, inability to cross the placenta, and free filtration at the level of the glomerulus. Thus, fetal blood levels reflect fetal GFR in the same manner that blood levels of creatinine reflect kidney function postnatally. Several groups of investigators have measured the levels of β_2-microglobulin in fetal blood obtained by cordocentesis at different stages of pregnancy.[12-16] Fetuses with congenital kidney anomalies affecting normal kidney function, such as urinary tract obstruction, had higher serum levels than those without obstruction, and β_2-microglobulin was shown to be a better predictor of postnatal kidney function in fetal uropathy than either α1-microglobulin or cystatin C (Fig. 94.2).[16]

A fetal serum β_2-microglobulin cutoff of 5.6 mg/L had a sensitivity of 80%, a specificity of 98.6%, a positive predictive value of 88.9%, and a negative predictive value of 97.1% for postnatal renal failure.[12] Filtered β_2-microglobulin normally undergoes 99.9%

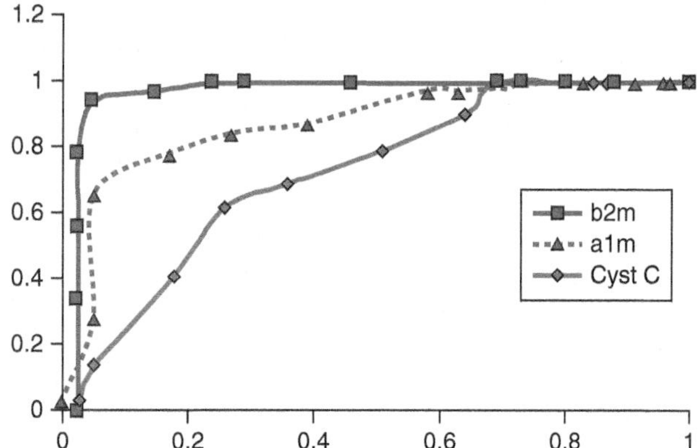

Fig. 94.2 Predictive value of fetal serum analytes. Receiver operating curves of the three fetal serum markers: α1-microglobulin *(a1m)*, β_2-microglobulin *(b2m)*, and cystatin C *(Cyst C)*. As a predictor of postnatal kidney function in cases with fetal uropathy, β_2-microglobulin had the best predictive value. (Reproduced with permission from Nguyen C, Dreux S, Heidet L, et al. Fetal serum alpha-1 microglobulin for renal function assessment: comparison with beta2-microglobulin and cystatin C. *Prenat Diagn*. 2013;33:775–781.)

degradation by proximal tubular cells. Urinary levels lower than 6 mg/L are considered "normal" in fetuses with congenital urinary tract obstruction,[17] while levels greater than 13 mg/L, which reflect tubular damage, were invariably associated with perinatal death.[18] The usefulness of serum β_2-microglobulin is, however, limited due to the lack of normative data based on the small numbers of patients, measurements at different stages of gestation, and variable measures of outcome. In addition, fetal blood sampling carries the risks of bleeding, AF leak, infection, and fetal death.

Fetal urine analyte analysis has also been used in the antenatal evaluation of kidney function. Similar to GFR, tubular function undergoes significant changes during fetal maturation. During early development, the urinary ultrafiltrate is minimally modified by passage through the nephron. With maturation, the tubules and collecting ducts become more efficient in water and electrolyte reabsorption. Based on these physiologic observations, normal fetal urinary thresholds have been correlated with autopsy and biopsy findings and clinical outcome in fetuses with bladder outlet obstruction.[19] Fetal urine sodium less than 100 mEq/L, chloride less than 90 mEq/L, and urine osmolality greater than 210 mEq/L at a mean gestational age of 23.8 weeks predicted a "good outcome," based on the presence of non-dysplastic kidneys at autopsy or biopsy, or normal renal and pulmonary function at birth. Values above or below these thresholds reflected poor tubular function of dysplastic kidneys with presumed altered reabsorption of filtered electrolytes and water. Since this report, multiple studies of the best predictors of poor outcome based on the composition of fetal urine, including sequential fetal urine sampling, have added little information, correlating only modestly with postnatal renal function.[20] A comprehensive systematic literature review on the accuracy of fetal urine analysis to predict postnatal renal function revealed that there is currently no individual analyte or threshold with significant clinical accuracy.[21] The thresholds of the most widely investigated analytes (e.g., sodium, chloride, calcium, osmolality, and β_2-microglobulin) varied widely among the studies, and not all studies correlated these thresholds with gestational age. The same analytes in fetal urine have also been used to select fetuses for prenatal intervention but, unfortunately, have not resulted in improved outcomes. More recently unbiased analyses of fetal urine peptidome and metabolome signatures have been used to more reliably predict postnatal kidney function outcomes in fetuses affected by bladder outlet obstruction.[22]

Serum cystatin C has also been used and promoted as a reliable measure of postnatal GFR.[23] It is a 13-kDa protein produced by all nucleated cells that is freely filtered in the glomerulus and almost completely reabsorbed in the proximal tubule. Serum cystatin C levels are higher in preterm infants than in newborn infants.[23] The metabolism of cystatin C by fetal kidneys has not been described, and the value of fetal urine, fetal blood, or AF cystatin C levels in assessing fetal kidney function is unknown. During normal pregnancy AF cystatin C levels decrease with increasing gestational age but are increased in pregnancies associated with fetal uropathy.[24]

AF volume can also be used as a surrogate marker of fetal GFR during the second half of pregnancy. In the early fetal period, most of the AF is produced by the amnion, placenta, and umbilical cord. AF volume increases from approximately 25 mL at 10 weeks gestation to approximately 400 mL at 20 weeks gestation when fetal kidneys become the main source, although the total volume of AF can vary substantially. By 28 weeks gestation, AF volume reaches a plateau of approximately 800 mL until term, with a slight decline post-term.[25] Any impairment of fetal kidney function, including urinary tract obstruction, will manifest as oligo/anhydramnios from mid-trimester onward.

Since fetal GFR increases with fetal weight and urine output increases with advancing gestation, fetal urinary flow rates have been used as a surrogate marker of fetal GFR and can be calculated from changes in fetal bladder volumes on repeat ultrasound examinations over time.[26,27]

DEVELOPMENT OF THE GLOMERULAR FILTRATION BARRIER

Development of glomeruli, the glomerular vasculature, and the glomerular filtration barrier occurs in a centrifugal fashion continuously between 8 and 36 weeks gestation in humans. Therefore juxtamedullary glomeruli form first and outer cortical glomeruli form last.

Following induction by the ureteric bud, pluripotent cells of the metanephric mesenchyme condense to form aggregates adjacent to the ureteric bud.[28-30] These aggregates subsequently undergo mesenchymal-epithelial transdifferentiation to form epithelialized structures called *renal vesicles*. Cell-to-cell adherence via the expression of adherens and tight junctional proteins allows cell polarization and the deposition of a provisional basement membrane and formation of a lumen. The immature epithelium of the renal vesicle will constitute all of the epithelial components of the nephron including the podocytes and parietal epithelium of the glomerulus. The differentiation of the simple renal vesicle to the complex structure of the final nephron proceeds through two recognizable intermediates: the comma shaped and S-shaped bodies.[28,29] The invasion of FLK1-positive angioblasts into the proximal cleft of the S-shaped body provides the precursors for the vascular bundles comprising the future glomerular capillary network. Mesangial precursors provide structural support for the growing capillary loops and serve an important role in the patterning and final development of the glomerular tuft.

The most proximal end of the S-shaped body, together with its vascularized cleft, differentiates into the glomerulus. The epithelium in this region specializes into precursors of the podocyte and parietal epithelium. Adjacent podocytes produce modified junctions that form the slit diaphragm, a crucial feature of the glomerular filtration barrier. The remaining epithelium of the proximal arm of the S-shaped body subsequently forms the parietal epithelial layer of the Bowman capsule and encloses the glomerular urinary space, or Bowman space. The glomerular filtration barrier then consists of the fenestrated glomerular capillary endothelium with its associated charged glycocalyx, the glomerular basement membrane whose components derive from both the developing endothelium and epithelium, and the developing podocyte or glomerular epithelial cell layer. Normal podocyte development is instrumental in determining normal glomerular filtration. Podocyte development and maintenance of glomerular integrity is under the control of numerous genes and the proteins they encode, and monogenic mutations have been defined in various childhood disorders associated with urinary protein losses and progressive decline in GFR.[31,32]

DEVELOPMENT OF GLOMERULAR FILTRATION

Fetal renal function is neither sufficient to balance all the metabolic requirements of the growing fetus, nor is it necessary, given the interposition of the placenta and maternal-fetal membranes. Nevertheless, the contribution of fetal kidneys to fluid and electrolyte homeostasis gradually increases as gestation progresses, eventually replacing the placenta at the time of birth.

In humans, glomerular filtration begins shortly after 8 weeks gestation, when the first glomeruli appear,[33] shows a slow linear increase reflecting new nephron development before 34 weeks gestation, and increases rapidly thereafter with completion of nephrogenesis,[34] renal blood redistribution, and engagement of younger cortical nephrons (Fig. 94.3).[35]

With the increase in cardiac output and growth of the renal vascular bed during gestation, renal blood flow also increases.[36] The kidneys of the human fetus at 10 to 20 weeks gestation receive about 5% of the cardiac output, compared to 9% in 1-week-old term infants and 25% in adults.[37] The intrarenal distribution of blood flow also changes during gestation as a result of a centrifugal pattern of new glomerular development. The hemodynamic evolution of the fetal kidney is thus characterized by a shift from a low-flow, high-resistance organ, with most of the blood supply to the inner cortex to a high-flow, low-resistance organ, with most of the blood flow supplying the outer cortex.[38]

Glomerular numbers are also proportional to fetal weight. The increase in GFR and fetal urine flow correlate closely with the increase in kidney mass, and thus it is reasonable to assume that a main contributing factor is the addition of new nephrons (Fig. 94.4).[39-41]

The attainment of the final nephron number and, therefore, the establishment of GFR are influenced by genetic and environmental factors. Conditional gene targeting in mice has implicated a number of individual genes and their protein products in determining nephron number.[42] These mutations include genes responsible for induction, specification, and maturation of glomerular cells. Similarly, in utero exposure to environmental factors, or developmental kidney injury, such as placental insufficiency, protein restriction, or urinary tract obstruction can impact normal nephrogenesis and result in a deficit of nephron endowment and associated decrease in renal function (Fig. 94.5).[43,44]

THE DETERMINANTS OF FETAL GLOMERULAR FILTRATION RATE

As in the postnatal kidney, glomerular filtration in the fetal kidney is the cumulative effect of single nephron GFR (SNGFR). The determinants of SNGFR in the fetal kidney, like the adult kidney, include the development of renal blood flow, the difference in trans capillary hydrostatic pressure across the filtration barrier, the difference in oncotic pressure between the capillary and urinary spaces, and the hydraulic permeability and surface area of the filtration membrane. The gestational changes in fetal GFR result from maturational changes in these variables, from changes in regulatory mechanisms with fetal maturation, and, ultimately, from an increase in number and size of glomeruli over the period of in utero nephrogenesis.

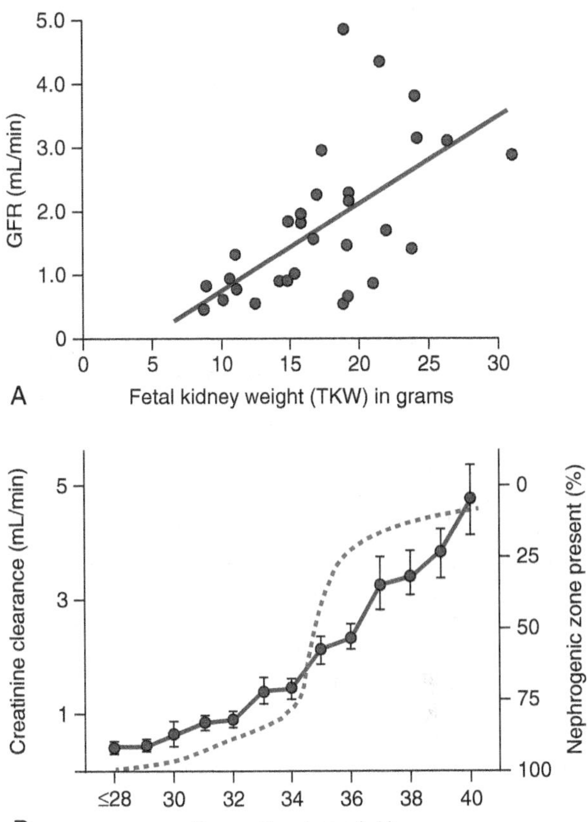

Fig. 94.3 Relationship between fetal glomerular filtration rate *(GFR)* and fetal kidney weight and gestational age. (A) Changes in GFR in fetal sheep in relation to total kidney weight during gestation. GFR increases in a linear fashion as fetal kidney weight increases. (B) Pattern of change in GFR *(solid line)* and persistence of the nephrogenic zone of the human fetal kidney cortex *(dashed line)*. As the gestational age increases, the nephrogenic zone decreases and disappears by 36 weeks gestation. This is associated with a corresponding increase in GFR as reflected by creatinine clearance. Data from 205 neonates, *N* ranging from 7 to 26 in each group at different gestational ages. (Reproduced with permission from Trnka P, Hiatt MJ, Tarantal AF, Matsell DG. Congenital urinary tract obstruction: defining markers of developmental kidney injury. *Pediatr Res*. 2012;72:446–454.)

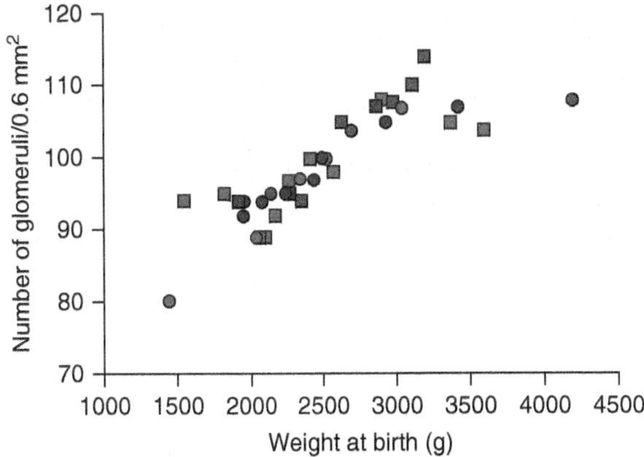

Fig. 94.4 Relationship between the number of glomeruli and birth weight. In humans, the number of glomeruli increases progressively until the birth weight reaches 3 kg; thereafter, it remains constant. Circles represent females, squares represent males. (Reproduced with permission from Manalich R, Reyes L, Herrera M, Melendi C, Fundora I. Relationship between weight at birth and the number and size of renal glomeruli in humans: a histomorphometric study. *Kidney Int*. 2000;58:770–773.)

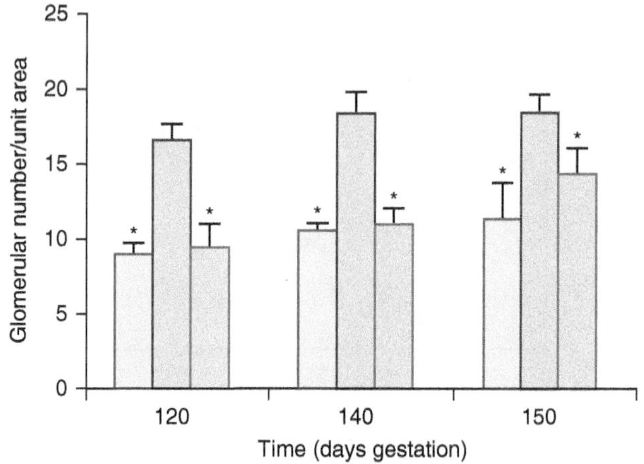

Fig. 94.5 Reduction of nephron number due to congenital urinary tract obstruction. In utero unilateral ureteric obstruction in fetal non-human primates results in a significant reduction in glomerular numbers at late gestation (120 and 140 days) and at term (150 days) in obstructed fetal kidneys *(green bars)* compared to control non-obstructed kidneys *(purple bars)* and to contralateral kidneys *(pink bars)*. *P <0.01 versus control kidneys. (Modified from Matsell DG, Mok A, Tarantal AF. Altered primate glomerular development due to in utero urinary tract obstruction. *Kidney Int*. 2002;61:1263–1269.)

CHANGES IN FETAL GLOMERULAR FILTRATION RATE

Using a combination of studies of fetal blood and urine sampling fetal GFR, as measured by creatinine clearance, has been estimated as early as 20 weeks gestation in humans.[33,45,46] While the absolute creatinine clearance for a fetus at 20 weeks gestation is estimated to be less than 1 mL/min, over the subsequent period of nephrogenesis and at term, the GFR increases approximately fivefold to 4 to 5 mL/min, with a further doubling of the GFR in the 2 weeks after birth (Fig. 94.6).[33]

FILTRATION COEFFICIENT

Hydraulic permeability and filtration membrane surface area constitute the filtration coefficient of the glomerular filtration membrane. Little is known about the changes that occur in hydraulic permeability in the developing fetal glomerulus; however, both indirect experimental evidence in late gestation fetal lambs[47] and direct measurement using antiglomerular basement membrane antibodies in newborn and growing rats[48] have demonstrated a significant increase in the glomerular filtration membrane surface area. Therefore, while an increase in the fetal filtration coefficient up to the end of nephrogenesis is accounted for by both the increase in the number of glomeruli and in the filtration surface area after nephrogenesis is complete, in later gestation this increase is due primarily to an increase in surface area.

HYDROSTATIC PRESSURE

The increase in GFR during fetal life is also attributable to an increase in fetal mean arterial pressure, which in turn increases the glomerular capillary hydrostatic pressure of the developing glomerular filtration barrier. These increases were first described using newborn guinea pigs, in which fetal kidney maturation is incomplete and superficial nephrons are accessible for micro puncture study. In the immediate neonatal period the effective hydrostatic filtration pressure increased 2.5-fold, which when combined with the increase in filtration barrier surface area, accounted for a 20-fold increase in GFR in this species (Fig. 94.7).[49,50]

RENAL PLASMA FLOW

Renal plasma flow has been defined in neonatal rats from 17 to 60 days after birth. As mentioned earlier, rat nephrogenesis is likely incomplete until approximately 4 weeks postnatally; therefore these studies include the changes in flow during the period of active nephrogenesis. With maturation during this period, renal blood flow increases, with a corresponding increase in SNGFR, slowly during the period of active nephrogenesis and rapidly thereafter (Fig. 94.8).[51,52]

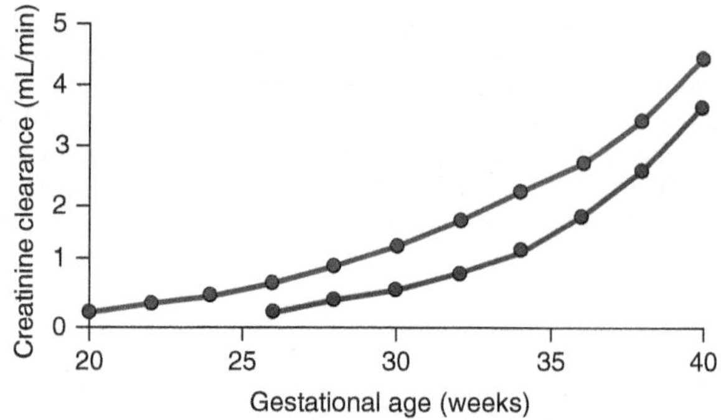

Fig. 94.6 Increase in fetal glomerular filtration rate (GFR) during gestation. Creatinine clearance was calculated from fetal urine and blood sample values during fetal life and in preterm infants, and used as a surrogate measure of fetal GFR. In both the fetus *(upper line)* and in the preterm infant *(lower line)* creatinine clearance increased with increasing gestational age. (Reproduced with permission from Haycock GB. Development of glomerular filtration and tubular sodium reabsorption in the human fetus and newborn. *Br J Urol*. 1998;81[suppl 2]:33–38.)

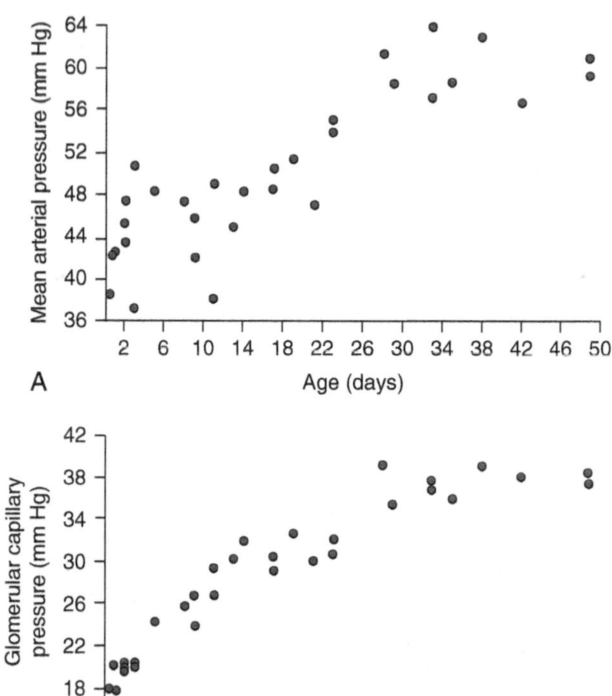

Fig. 94.7 Relationship of mean arterial pressure with glomerular capillary pressure in the developing kidney. (A) In guinea pigs in which nephrogenesis continues after birth, there is a linear increase in mean arterial pressure with increasing postnatal age. (B) With increasing postnatal age there is also a corresponding increase in glomerular capillary pressure, which plateaus at approximately 28 days. (Modified from Spitzer A, Edelmann CM Jr. Maturational changes in pressure gradients for glomerular filtration. *Am J Physiol*. 1971;221:1431–1435.)

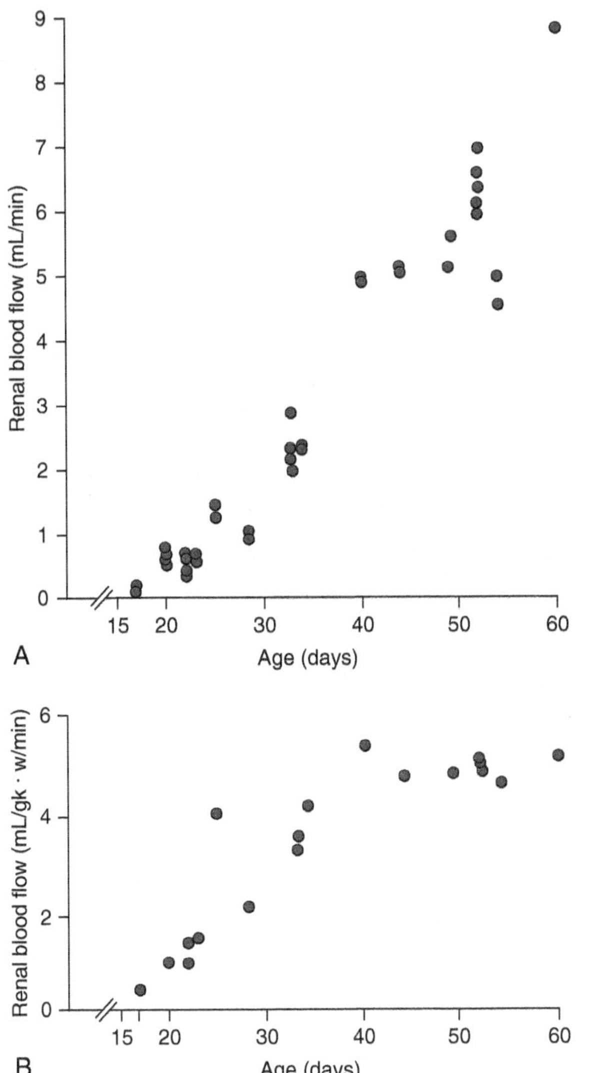

Fig. 94.8 Changes in renal blood flow in neonatal rat kidneys. (A) Total renal blood flow in young rats in which nephrogenesis continues after birth increases in a linear fashion as the postnatal age increases. (B) When corrected for absolute kidney weight, renal blood flow/kidney weight also increases as postnatal age increases. (Modified from Aperia A, Herin P. Development of glomerular perfusion rate and nephron filtration rate in rats 17–60 days old. *Am J Physiol.* 1975;228:1319–1325.)

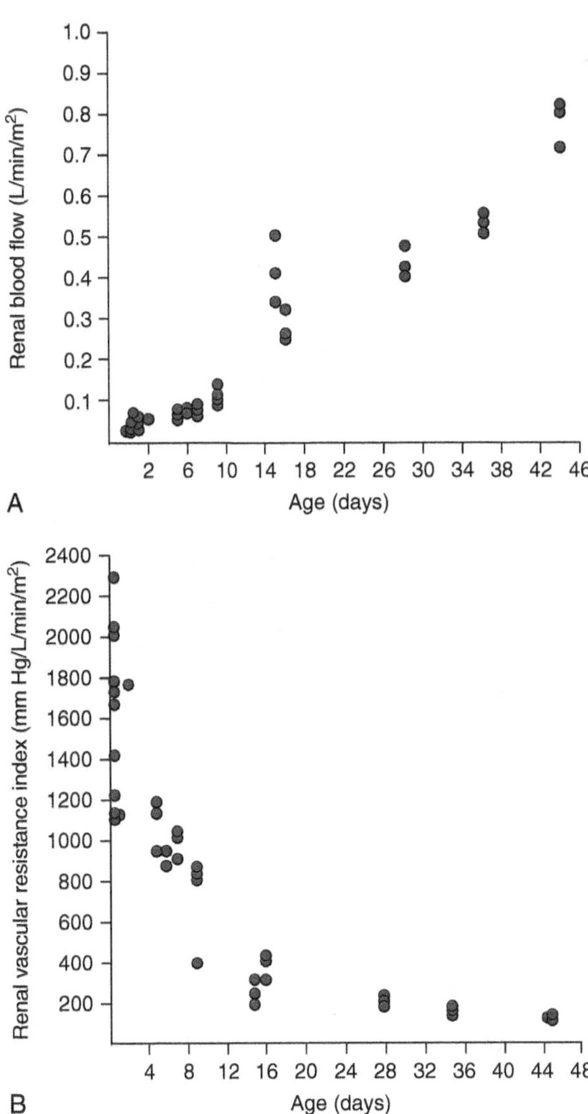

Fig. 94.9 Changes in renal vascular resistance in newborn piglet kidneys. (A) In newborn piglet kidneys, in which nephrogenesis continues after birth, increasing postnatal age is associated with a linear increase in renal blood flow. (B) With increasing postnatal age, particularly in the first 2 weeks, there is a corresponding decrease in renal vascular resistance. (Modified from Gruskin AB, Edelmann CM Jr, Yuan S. Maturational changes in renal blood flow in piglets. *Pediatr Res.* 1970;4:7–13.)

RENAL BLOOD FLOW AND RENAL VASCULAR RESISTANCE

Fetal renal blood flow is low due to the relatively high renal vascular resistance compared to the postnatal and adult kidney. With in utero kidney maturation, fetal renal blood flow increases as renal vascular resistance decreases. During the first 45 days of life of the piglet, during active nephrogenesis, renal blood flow increases 18 times its initial value, as a result of a 7.2-fold increase in cardiac index, a 2.5-fold increase in fractional flow to the kidney, and an 86% drop in actual renal vascular resistance index.[53] This is mostly due to the increase in vascular bed accompanying the increase in glomerular number (Fig. 94.9).[54]

REGULATION OF FETAL GLOMERULAR FILTRATION RATE

With maturation of the kidney, the increase in GFR parallels the increase in fetal size, kidney mass, increase in glomerular number, and expansion of the glomerular capillary bed. In addition, the changes in glomerular filtration are affected by a number of important proteins and peptides that regulate vascular muscle tone and undergo maturational changes during fetal kidney development. Interestingly a number of these factors, including members of the renin-angiotensin system (RAS) and of the prostaglandin compounds, not only regulate glomerular vascular tone but also are necessary for normal kidney development and differentiation.

RENIN ANGIOTENSIN SYSTEM

The RAS plays a major role in controlling systemic blood pressure in the developing fetus by maintaining systemic and renal vascular resistance. The RAS directly regulates GFR in the fetal kidney through its effects on vascular tone. Compared to the postnatal and mature adult kidney, the relative expressions of renin, angiotensin converting enzyme (ACE), and angiotensin II are higher in the fetal kidney.[55] In addition, angiotensinogen and ACE expression and activity increase during late gestation.[56]

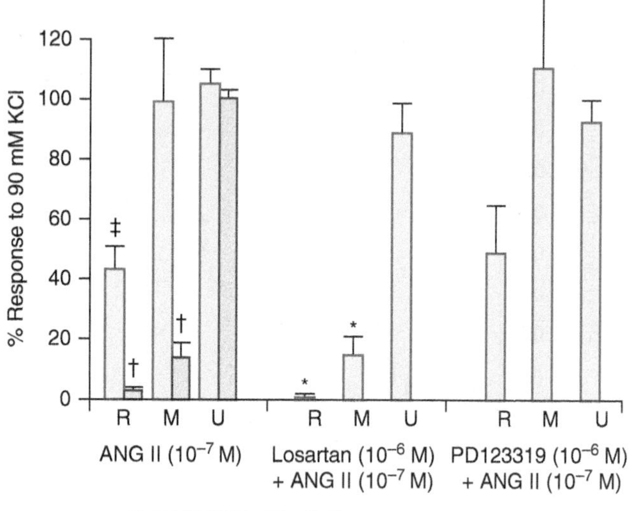

Fig. 94.10 Effects of angiotensin II *(ANG II)* on the contractile response in fetal lamb arteries. ANG II causes an increase in arterial vasoconstriction in the renal *(R)*, mesenteric *(M)*, and umbilical *(U)* arteries in the fetal lamb *(first panel)*. When pretreated with the AT1 receptor antagonist losartan, the contractile response is significantly attenuated in the renal artery *(middle panel)*, but not when pretreated with the AT2 antagonist PD 123319 *(last panel)*. $^{*}P < 0.5$ compared with ANG II alone for similar vessels. $^{\dagger}P < 0.05$ compared with maximal response for similar vessels. $^{\ddagger}P < 0.05$ compared with mesenteric and umbilical artery responses to ANG II alone. (Modified from Segar JL, Barna TJ, Acarregui MJ, Lamb FS. Responses of fetal ovine systemic and umbilical arteries to angiotensin II. *Pediatr Res*. 2001;49:826–833.)

Angiotensin II preferentially increases glomerular efferent arteriolar tone, resulting in an increase in glomerular capillary hydrostatic pressure and in SNGFR. The effects of angiotensin II on the renal vasculature are mediated through the type 1 angiotensin (AT1) receptor, which itself is upregulated in the renal vasculature during fetal kidney maturation.[57,58] In fetal lambs, the selective inhibitor of the AT1 receptor, losartan, completely attenuates the contractile effects of angiotensin II on renal arterioles; an effect not seen when the type 2 angiotensin (AT2) receptor is inhibited (Fig. 94.10).[59]

RENAL NERVES AND CATECHOLAMINES

The high renal vascular resistance seen in the fetus is also due, in part, to an increase in sympathetic nervous system (SNS) activity, an increase in α 1 receptor activity, and an increase in secreted catecholamines.[60] This preferentially increases the afferent arteriolar tone of the fetal glomerulus, with a consequent decrease in glomerular capillary hydraulic pressure and in SNGFR. Circulating catecholamine levels fall immediately after birth, with a corresponding increase in GFR.

The effects of the SNS on the renal vasculature and therefore on fetal GFR appear to be mediated, in part, through the stimulation of renin release.[61] In lambs with renal denervation there is an associated decrease in circulating plasma renin activity associated with the stress of birth (Fig. 94.11).[62]

ENDOTHELIN

Endothelin is another potent vasoconstrictor whose expression is upregulated in the fetal kidney. Endothelin production is stimulated by angiotensin II, bradykinin, epinephrine, and shear stress, and its sources include the vascular endothelium, glomerular mesangium, and distal tubular epithelial cells. Both endothelin and the endothelin receptor (ETR) are increased during fetal life but levels decrease after the first week of life.[63]

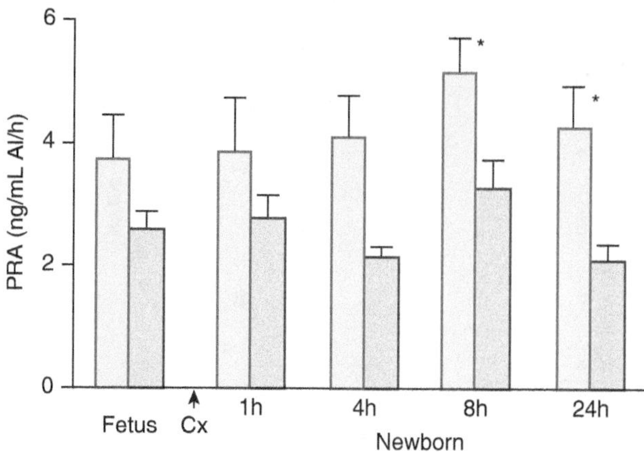

Fig. 94.11 Effects of renal denervation on plasma renin activity *(PRA)*. In fetal sheep in which the kidneys were denervated, the normal increase in renin response after birth was significantly attenuated. *Green bars* are intact animals, *purple bars* are denervated animals. *Cx*, Cesarean section delivery. $^{*}P < 0.05$ intact compared with denervated lambs. (Modified from Smith FG, Smith BA, Guillery EN, Robillard JE. Role of renal sympathetic nerves in lambs during the transition from fetal to newborn life. *J Clin Invest*. 1991;88:1988–1994.)

PROSTAGLANDINS

Like the RAS, members of the prostaglandin family, including PGE2, PGD2, and PGI2, are important during fetal life both in their role as renal vasoregulators and in determining normal kidney development. PGE2 in particular is a potent vasodilator that increases fetal GFR by decreasing afferent arteriolar tone and may be particularly important in maintaining GFR in states of intravascular volume depletion as a counterregulatory influence to the vasoconstrictor compounds such as AII.[64]

The importance of PG vasodilatation in the developing kidney is particularly evident in preterm infants exposed to indomethacin, an inhibitor of cyclooxygenase activity. Treatment causes a transient decrease in GFR and a predisposition to long-term kidney injury.[65] In experimental animal models, disruption of the cyclooxygenase gene results in significant developmental kidney anomalies including a decrease in glomerular number and hypoplasia.[66]

NITRIC OXIDE

Nitric oxide (NO) is an endothelium-derived relaxing factor, or vasodilator, which is synthesized in various tissues in the body under basal conditions. Endogenously produced NO is involved in the maintenance of blood flow and blood pressure through its effects on vascular smooth muscle relaxation. Under normal physiologic conditions the capacity of the fetal and newborn vasculature to release NO for a given stimulus is greater than later in life.[67] NO also appears to play a role in maintaining GFR in the developing kidney,[68] mediated, in part, by inhibiting the effects of angiotensin II (Fig. 94.12).[69]

In fetal kidneys, the enzyme most responsible for NO synthesis in the kidney, endothelial nitric oxide synthase (eNOS), is expressed early in embryonic life (embryonic day 14) in intrarenal capillaries, endothelial cells of renal vesicles, S-shaped bodies, and glomeruli. At later embryonic stages the eNOS expression is reduced. After birth, eNOS expression gradually increases in the vascular bundles and peritubular capillaries in the medulla. The strong expression of eNOS in the early stages of developing glomeruli and vasculature suggests that eNOS plays a role in regulating renal hemodynamics of the immature kidney.[70]

DEVELOPMENT OF TUBULAR FUNCTION

During nephrogenesis, the tubular portions of the nephron develop from the S-shaped body in a proximal-distal

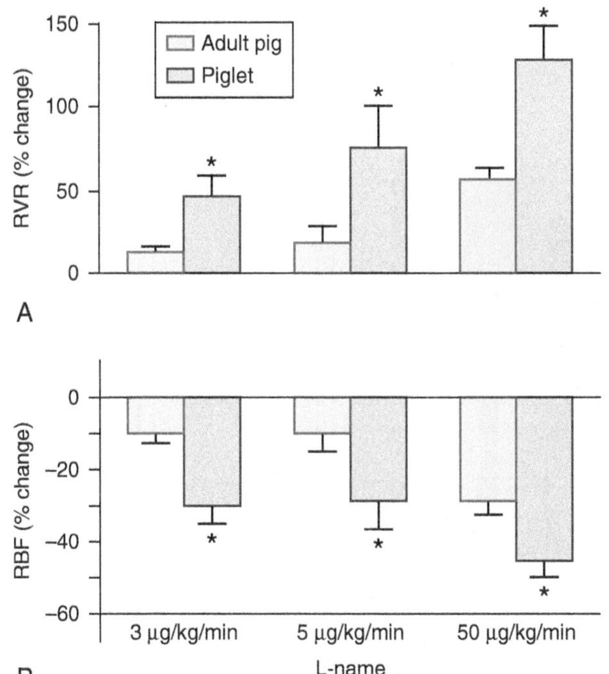

Fig. 94.12 Effects of nitric oxide (NO) on renal vascular resistance. Inhibition of NO production in newborn piglets by intrarenal infusion of the inhibitor L-NAME at increasing concentrations (3, 5, and 50 μg/kg/min) resulted in an increase in renal vascular resistance *(RVR)* (A) and a corresponding decrease in renal blood flow *(RBF)* (B). The newborn piglet *(purple bars)* demonstrated a significantly greater response to NO inhibition than the adult pig *(green bars)*. *$P < 0.05$ developing piglet vs. adult pig. (Modified from Solhaug MJ, Wallace MR, Granger JP. Nitric oxide and angiotensin II regulation of renal hemodynamics in the developing piglet. *Pediatr Res*. 1996;39:527–533.)

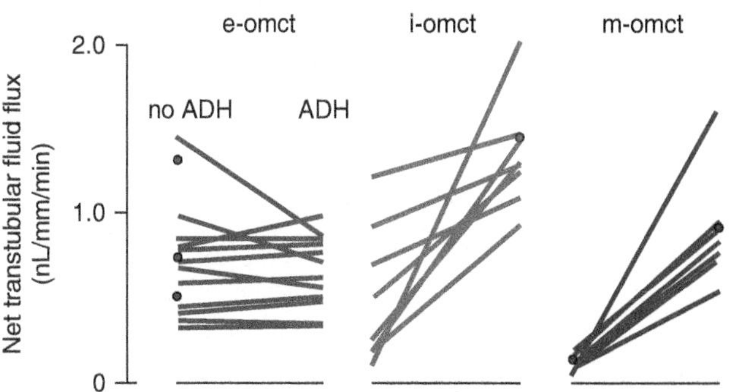

Fig. 94.13 Collecting duct responsiveness to antidiuretic hormone *(ADH)*. The outer medullary collecting tubule *(OMCT)* response to ADH was evaluated by measuring the transtubular fluid flux in rabbits of various postnatal ages: e-omct (<4 days old), i-omct (10 to 15 days old), and m-omct (30 to 35 days old). Collecting tubules from the early postnatal animals showed minimal responsiveness to ADH. (Modified from Horster MF, Zink H. Functional differentiation of the medullary collecting tubule: influence of vasopressin. *Kidney Int*. 1982;22:360–365.)

sequence.[28,29] The tubular region adjacent to the nascent glomerulus forms the proximal convoluted tubule, followed by the loop of Henle. The distal convoluted tubule forms from the most distal portion of the S-shaped body immediately adjacent to the ureteric bud tip. Throughout the epithelialization of the developing nephron precursor, signaling via the Notch pathway is central to the establishment of local proximal-distal patterning. Specifically, NOTCH2 expressed in the metanephric mesenchyme has been shown to control the differentiation of proximal epithelial types, but not of the distal convoluted tubule. The role of distal patterning may reside with other notch ligands yet to be identified. Following their formation, these tubular precursors undergo extensive proliferation to establish their mature structure. In particular, the long segments of the loop of Henle proliferate in conjunction with the convergent extension of the later branches of the ureteric bud, allowing the loop to maintain its position in the medullary region.

WATER TRANSPORT

Fetuses and preterm infants lack the ability to fully dilute and to fully concentrate their urine. Given their higher body water content and the evolutionary need to maintain adequate AF volumes, term infants can attain adequately dilute urines down to approximately 52 mOsm/kg after a hypotonic fluid challenge.[71,72] Urine concentrating ability increases with increasing gestational age reflecting the fetal kidney's increased responsiveness to antidiuretic hormone (ADH), water channel development, and renal medullary maturation.[73]

In the mature kidney, ADH exerts its effect on the principal cell of the collecting duct. Circulating ADH binds with the basolateral vasopressin (V2) receptor, which, through stimulation of the second messengers c-amp and protein kinase A, results in phosphorylation of the cytoplasmic water channel aquaporin-2 (AQP-2), resulting in its insertion into the principal cell apical membrane. Water passes from the tubule lumen through the principal cell apical AQP-2 channel, and then through the basolateral AQP-3 and AQP-4 channels, driven by the tonicity of the medullary interstitium.[74]

The inability of the fetal kidney to fully concentrate the urine is not due to low circulating ADH levels, which at birth for both term and preterm infants are higher than adult levels.[75] As demonstrated in dissected rabbit medullary collecting ducts, ADH-responsiveness, measured by transtubular fluid movement, increases with kidney maturation, with collecting ducts in the less than 4-day-old animal demonstrating minimal responsiveness (Fig. 94.13).[76]

In addition, the V2 receptor is expressed in the collecting duct cells of fetal rat kidneys as early as 16 to 17 days gestation.[77] Mechanisms therefore contributing to the blunted ADH- response in the immature collecting duct include inhibition of cAMP generation by endogenous prostaglandins,[78] rapid degradation of formed cAMP,[79] a deficit of AQP-2 channels, and relative medullary interstitial hypotonicity.

Aquaporin channels are expressed during fetal development, undergoing maturation during postnatal life.[80] In the mature kidney, AQP-1 is present in the proximal tubule, the descending limb of the LOH, and the fenestrated endothelium of the vasa recta.[81] However, the bulk of urine concentration occurs in the collecting duct, where AQP-2 is expressed on the apical membrane of principal cells, while AQP-3 and AQP-4 co-localize on the basolateral membrane. Expression is spatially and temporally regulated, with AQP-2 expression apparent as early as 18 weeks gestation in the developing human fetal collecting duct and as early as the S-shape phase of nephron development.[82] Similarly, AQP-2 expression has been detected as early as 18 days gestation in fetal rat kidneys,[83,84] and as early as 75 days gestation in fetal sheep kidneys,[85] while AQP-1 and AQP-3 are expressed as early as 16 to 18 days in the fetal rat kidney.[80,86,87] While the expression of AQP-2 is restricted to the collecting duct during kidney development, with branching morphogenesis and increase in renal mass, its abundance increases proportionately, associated with an increasing urine concentrating capacity.[88]

Another important contributing factor to the decreased responsiveness to ADH and the low concentrating ability of the fetal kidney is the relative hypotonicity of the fetal medullary

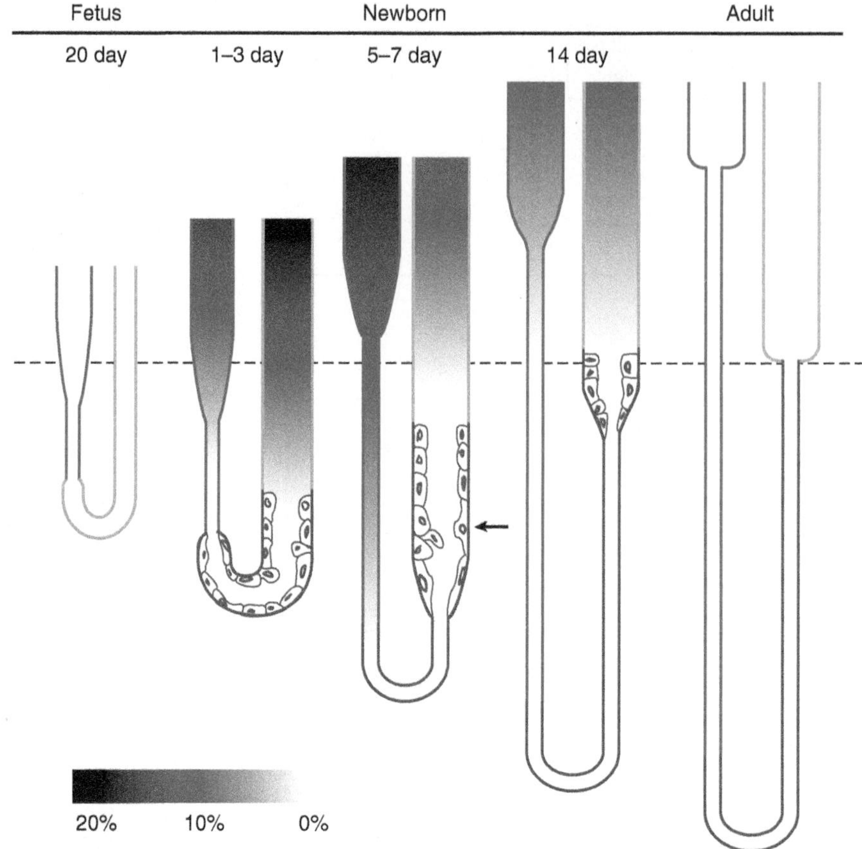

Fig. 94.14 Development of the loop of Henle. The loop of Henle develops by extension into the developing renal medulla through cell proliferation, differentiation, and apoptosis. The descending limb is shown in *blue*, the thick ascending limb in *yellow*. The *open arrow* indicates cells undergoing apoptosis and transformation into cells of of the thin ascending limb, shown in *red*. The *intensity of purple* indicates the presence of cells undergoing proliferation. (Reproduced from Cha JH, Kim YH, Jung JY, et al. Cell proliferation in the loop of Henle in the developing rat kidney. *J Am Soc Nephrol: JASN*. 2001;12:1410–1421.)

interstitium compared to the mature adult kidney. This is due to a number of developmental factors including lower protein intake, particularly in the preterm infant, decreased density of the Na-K-ATPase transporter with lower rates of sodium transport in the thick ascending limb (TAL) of the loop of Henle,[89] a lower expression of urea transporters,[90] and relatively shorter TAL segments in the developing renal medulla.[91]

The mature postnatal kidney contains both juxtamedullary and superficial nephrons.[91] Juxtamedullary nephrons have long loops of Henle that descend into the inner medulla and reach the tip of the papilla. They have a long descending thin limb and an ascending thin limb that continues into the TAL. Superficial nephrons have short loops of Henle, and they do not have an ascending thin limb.[91] During earlier kidney development, and at birth in rats, there is no distinct border between the outer and inner medulla, due to the immaturity of the loops of Henle. The immature nephrons have no ascending thin limbs, and therefore all nephrons have the same structural composition as the short-looped superficial nephrons of the adult kidney.[92] In the postnatal period, the kidney medulla matures with transformation of the epithelium of the TAL into the squamous epithelium of the thin ascending limb.[93] In addition, elongation of the loops of Henle and extension of the cortico-medullary axis occur through selective cell proliferation and apoptosis in the outer medulla.[91] In the postnatal rat, by 3 weeks of age, the medullary nephrons resemble those of the adult kidney. This elongation and remodeling of the loops of Henle is under genetic control,[94] and several genes have been implicated including the transcription factor gene *Irx* for intermediate tubule formation,[95] *Adamts-1* in the remodeling of the ECM facilitating elongation,[96] and the transcription factor *Brn1*, through the suppression of cell apoptosis (Fig. 94.14).[97]

SODIUM TRANSPORT

Considerable changes occur in sodium transport in the developing fetal kidney. Urinary sodium losses, as reflected by the fractional excretion of sodium (FENa), decrease with increasing gestational age and fetal kidney maturity. At birth, in term infants, the FENa is less than 1%, while in preterm and small for gestational age infants it approaches 2.4%—the more preterm the infant is, the higher the percentage.[98,99] After birth, in the preterm infant, there is a progressive decrease in the FENa, approaching the normal term infant values within 2 to 3 weeks of life (Fig. 94.15).

A number of maturational changes occur in sodium handling in the developing fetal kidney,[100] including tubule-segment-specific differentiation with increased abundance of sodium transporters and enhanced paracellular transport;[101] increased responsiveness to circulating hormones including angiotensin II,[102] catecholamines,[103] and glucocorticoids;[104] and a postnatal decrease in circulating atrial natriuretic peptide.[105]

Almost all sodium transport is driven by the effect of the energy-dependent Na-K-ATPase pump on the basolateral membrane of the cells of all segments of the nephron. When Na-K-ATPase activity is compared between dissected neonatal and mature rabbit kidney tubules, the activity overall is 40% to 80% less in the neonatal preparations, and all neonatal tubule segments have less activity than the corresponding adult segment, varying from being 2-fold less in the proximal tubule to as much as 5 to 10-fold less in the TAL (Fig. 94.16).[106]

The ontogeny of expression of the Na-K-ATPase pump is complex, since the transporter is a heterodimer of α and β subunits. The adult kidney consists of the $\alpha1\beta1$ subunits co-localized to the basolateral cell membrane. In humans the $\alpha1$ and $\beta2$ subunits can be detected as early as 12 weeks gestation in the apical epithelial plasma membranes of distal nephron segments of early stage nephrons, maturing loops of Henle, and

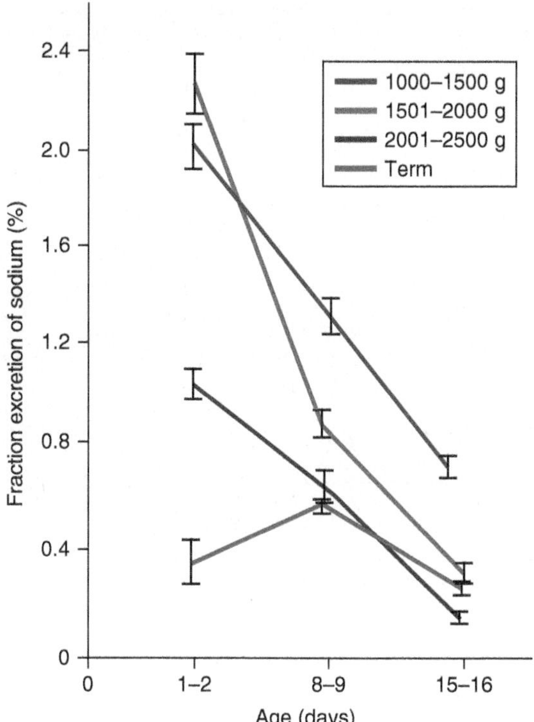

Fig. 94.15 Changes in sodium excretion in the developing kidney. At birth, urinary sodium losses, measured by the fractional excretion of sodium (FENa), decrease with increasing gestational age. For example, the FENa is significantly higher in the infant born between 1000 and 1500 g *(red line)* than in the term infant *(blue line)*. In the preterm and low-birth-weight infant, the FENa decreases after birth and approaches that of the term infant by 2 to 3 weeks. (Modified from Bueva A, Guignard JP. Renal function in preterm neonates. *Pediatr Res*. 1994;36:572–577.)

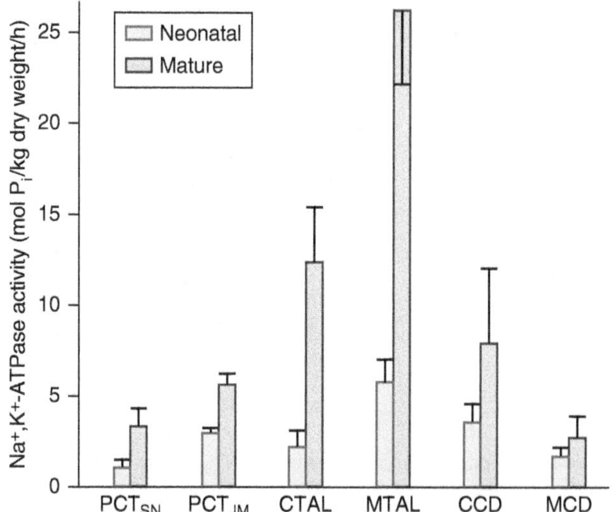

Fig. 94.16 Nephron segment-specific changes in Na-K-ATPase activity in the developing kidney. In the neonatal rabbit kidney, Na-K-ATPase activity is significantly higher in the medullary thick ascending limb *(MTAL)* than in other segments. With maturation there is a significant increase in all segments of the nephron, varying from a 2- to 10-fold increase. *CCD,* Cortical collecting duct; *CTAL,* cortical thick ascending limb; *MCD,* medullary collecting duct; *PCT_{JM},* proximal convoluted tubule (early segment from juxtamedullary nephron); *PCT_{SN},* proximal convoluted tubule (early segment from subcapsular nephron). (Modified from Schmidt U, Horster M. Na-K-activated ATPase: activity maturation in rabbit nephron segments dissected in vitro. *Am J Physiol*. 1977;233:F55–F60.)

collecting ducts. With maturation and into postnatal life the β2 expression is replaced by the β1 subunit.[107]

In the proximal tubule the NHE3 exchanger (or the Na-H antiporter) also effects sodium reabsorption, driven by the gradient created by the Na-K-ATPase pump, and is an important mechanism for proton excretion and thereby bicarbonate reabsorption in the proximal tubule. NHE3 expression and activity increase with advancing gestational age and in the transition from neonatal to adult life, as demonstrated in sheep and rats.[108] In the adult kidney NHE3 is found in apical vesicles and the apical plasma membrane of the proximal tubule, and in both the thin and thick limbs of the loop of Henle. When localized in the developing rat kidney, NHE3 is first detected in the late stages of the S-shaped body. In later stages of nephron development, the pattern of NHE3 staining is similar to that seen in the adult kidney.[109] There is also evidence for a fetal NHE8 transporter, as demonstrated in mice with a conditional NHE3 gene disruption.[110]

In the TAL of the loop of Henle, transcellular sodium reabsorption occurs via the Na-K-2Cl co-transporter (NKCC2). In the fetal rat kidney, the transporter mRNA is expressed as early as embryonic day 14.5 and is expressed in the immature loops of Henle but is absent from the ureteric bud, S-shaped bodies, and earlier nephrogenic structures.[111,112]

Sodium transport in the distal and connecting tubule cells occurs through the NaCl co-transporter (NCC).[113] The NCC is expressed in the developing kidney, exclusively in the cells of the nascent distal tubule, but not in the nephrogenic zone structures. It appears to be expressed before the NKCC2, and its abundance increases with kidney maturation.[112]

Fine-tuning of sodium reabsorption occurs through the epithelial sodium channel (ENaC) of the distal tubule and cortical collecting duct. Low levels of expression of ENaC subunits may limit distal Na absorption in more immature kidneys, such as those of very premature human infants.[114,115] In developing fetal rat kidneys, all three ENaC subunit mRNAs are detected in the distal convoluted tubule, connecting tubule, cortical collecting duct, and outer medullary collecting duct. Levels are low or undetectable on gestational day 16 and only slightly higher before birth. A sharp rise occurs soon after birth with levels at postnatal days 1 to 3 approaching those of adult kidneys (Fig. 94.17).

ACID-BASE REGULATION

Both the placenta and the fetal kidney maintain fetal acid-base balance; however, in the placenta, the rate of transfer of hydrogen ions and bicarbonate ions is slow. The fetal kidneys are able to reabsorb filtered bicarbonate and generate new bicarbonate by excreting titratable acid and ammonium.[116] The capacity to do so is less than in the adult kidney as reflected by lower serum bicarbonate levels in the preterm and term infant.[117,118] The capacity to generate bicarbonate increases with gestational age, mirroring the increase in fetal GFR. This adaptive capacity is limited, however, as demonstrated in fetal sheep rendered volume-depleted and in those in which maternal hypoxia is induced.[116,119,120]

As seen with sodium reabsorption, the fetal kidney's ability to generate bicarbonate and to excrete acid increases with gestational age. In the proximal tubule the expression of NHE3, Na-K-ATPase, and type IV carbonic anhydrase increases with kidney maturation, kidney growth, and proximal tubule elongation and differentiation; however, at birth, their expression is still less abundant than in adult kidneys.[121-123]

Similarly the fetal kidney has a reduced ability to secrete both organic and inorganic acids when compared to the adult kidney.[124] In the fetal cortical collecting duct of a number of

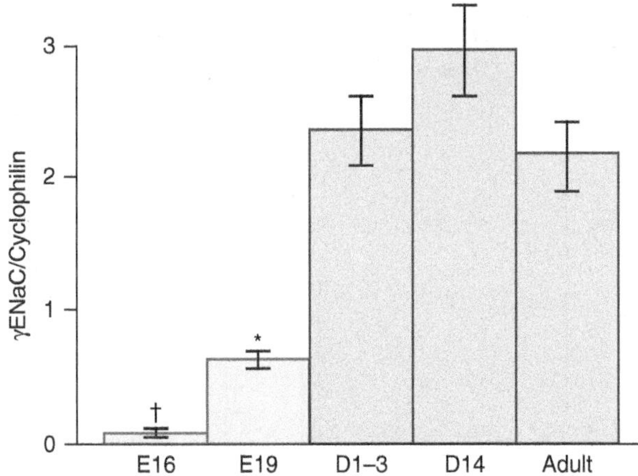

Fig. 94.17 Epithelial sodium channel *(ENaC)* expression in the developing kidney. ENaC mRNA expression, measured by quantitative polymerase chain reaction, increases during embryonic life in the developing rat kidney, with a sharp rise before birth and an incremental increase in expression to postnatal day 3. **P* <0.05; †*P* <0.01 vs. D1–3. (Modified from Vehaskari VM, Hempe JM, Manning J, Aviles DH, Carmichael MC. Developmental regulation of ENaC subunit mRNA levels in rat kidney. *Am J Physiol*. 1998;274:C1661–C1666.)

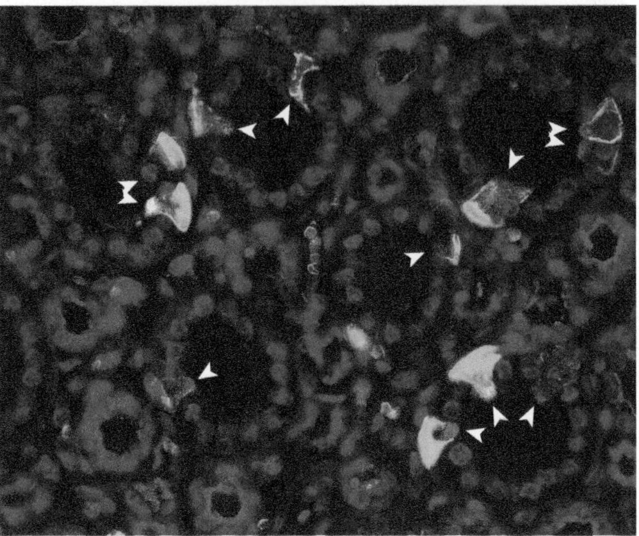

Fig. 94.18 Intercalated cells in the developing human kidney *(arrowheads)*. The fetal kidney's ability to secrete acid by the collecting duct results, in part, from the development and differentiation of Type A intercalated cells. Early in gestation intercalated cells are present but are undifferentiated. Type A intercalated cells are identified as early as 26 weeks gestation.

different species, the intercalated cell population is significantly less abundant than in the adult kidney, including the type A intercalated cell that is responsible for proton excretion.[125,126] In the human fetal kidney, intercalated cells originate in the medullary collecting duct at 8 weeks gestation and remain abundant in the inner medulla throughout gestation. In the cortex, intercalated cells are rare before 26 weeks gestation and are in low abundance by 36 weeks gestation. Early in gestation, intercalated cells exhibit an immature phenotype; however, by 36 weeks, type A intercalated cells predominate. The differentiated intercalated cells appear to arise from an undifferentiated pool of collecting duct epithelial cells and continue to differentiate into postnatal life (Fig. 94.18).[127]

POTASSIUM TRANSPORT

Somatic growth of the fetus requires a positive potassium balance.[128] Potassium excretion is almost entirely derived from its secretion by the principal cells of the distal tubule and collecting duct under the influence of aldosterone.[129,130] Potassium excretion is decreased in the preterm infant and neonate due primarily to an attenuated response of the immature collecting duct to this hormone.[130,131] However, in the TAL, there is postnatal functional maturation of transporters responsible for potassium transport, including the Na-K-ATPase pump, the NKCC2, and the apical ROMK channel.[73] In the collecting duct, potassium is handled through basal secretion via the ROMK channel in principal cells, and by maxi-K+ channels, which are flow-stimulated and expressed in principal and intercalated cells.[132,133] The ROMK channel is expressed in the developing human fetal kidney, as early as 21 weeks gestation. During fetal life its expression is restricted to the TAL; however, postnatally this extends to the CD.[134] As in the TAL, there is postnatal functional maturation of CD ROMK function.[135]

CALCIUM AND PHOSPHATE TRANSPORT

High-circulating calcium levels are required for normal fetal skeletal growth and are maintained through in utero placental transport.[136] The mature kidney plays an important role in the control of calcium homeostasis and secretion. Of the filtered calcium, only ~1% to 2% is excreted in the urine.[137] Although the majority is reabsorbed in the proximal tubule and TAL of the loop of Henle via paracellular pathways,[138] up to 7% of the filtered Ca^{2+} is reabsorbed in the distal convoluted tubule and collecting duct via the transient receptor potential-vanilloid-5 (TRPV5) channel.[139] TRPV5 in the apical plasma membrane provides a channel for calcium entry; its subsequent reabsorption across the basolateral membrane occurs via the Na/Ca exchanger NCX1 and Ca-ATPase (PMCA1b).[139,140] The fetal kidney expression of TRPV5 is not well described.

A positive phosphate balance is also essential for rapid fetal growth.[141] The ability to reabsorb phosphate is greater in immature and neonatal kidneys compared to adult kidneys,[142] a result of a physiologic adaptation to the demands of rapid growth rather than immaturity of transport systems for phosphate. In the developing proximal tubule, phosphate reabsorption occurs through the type IIc Na/Pi co-transporter.[143]

CONCLUSION

In humans, nephrogenesis occurs in utero during a lengthy gestation. In many species, kidney development begins in utero but is completed in the postnatal period. In either case, the development of kidney function follows the same well-orchestrated series of events that occur with the development of normal kidney structure and form. Kidney development begins at 8 weeks gestation, marking the beginning of kidney function. After vascularization of the glomerulus, regulated renal blood flow develops, followed by the establishment of the glomerular filtration barrier and the onset of glomerular filtration. Designated expression of transporter and channel genes and proteins that regulate tubular transport follow the spatial and temporal specification and segmentation of the tubules. These processes originate in fetal life and undergo significant maturation in utero, despite the interposition of placental function.

In this chapter we have focused on several of the well-studied functions of the fetal kidney, including the acquisition and development of glomerular filtration and its regulation, and the expression and maturation of tubular transporters involved in water, sodium, acid-base, potassium, and calcium and phosphate homoeostasis. Many of the other specialized functions, such as glucose and amino acid transport, are described in other chapters.

A complete reference list is available at www.ExpertConsult.com. 

SELECT REFERENCES

1. Matsell DG, Tarantal AF. Experimental models of fetal obstructive nephropathy. *Pediatr Nephrol*. 2002;17:470-476.
2. Carmody JB, Charlton JR. Short-term gestation, long-term risk: prematurity and chronic kidney disease. *Pediatrics*. 2013;131:1168-1179.
3. Winyard P, Chitty L. Dysplastic and polycystic kidneys: diagnosis, associations and management. *Prenatal Diag*. 2001;21:924-935.
6. Robyr R, Benachi A, Daikha-Dahmane F, Martinovich J, Dumez Y, Ville Y. Correlation between ultrasound and anatomical findings in fetuses with lower urinary tract obstruction in the first half of pregnancy. *Ultrasound Obstetr Gynecol*. 2005;25:478-482.
10. Chalouhi GE, Millischer AE, Mahallati H, et al. The use of fetal MRI for renal and urogenital tract anomalies. *Prenat Diagn*. 2020;40:100-109.
16. Nguyen C, Dreux S, Heidet L, et al. Fetal serum alpha-1 microglobulin for renal function assessment: comparison with beta2-microglobulin and cystatin C. *Prenat Diagn*. 2013;33:775-781.
21. Morris RK, Quinlan-Jones E, Kilby MD, Khan KS. Systematic review of accuracy of fetal urine analysis to predict poor postnatal renal function in cases of congenital urinary tract obstruction. *Prenata Diagn*. 2007;27:900-911.
22. Buffin-Meyer B, Tkaczyk M, Stanczyk M, et al. A single-center study to evaluate the efficacy of a fetal urine peptide signature predicting postnatal renal outcome in fetuses with posterior urethral valves. *Pediatr Nephrol*. 2020;35:469-475.
24. Mussap M, Fanos V, Pizzini C, Marcolongo A, Chiaffoni G, Plebani M. Predictive value of amniotic fluid cystatin C levels for the early identification of fetuses with obstructive uropathies. *BJOG*. 2002;109:778-783.
29. Dressler GR. Advances in early kidney specification, development and patterning. *Development*. 2009;136:3863-3874.
31. Grahammer F, Schell C, Huber TB. The podocyte slit diaphragm–from a thin grey line to a complex signalling hub. *Nat Rev Nephrol*. 2013;9:587-598.
33. Haycock GB. Development of glomerular filtration and tubular sodium reabsorption in the human fetus and newborn. *Brit J Urol*. 1998;81(suppl 2):33-38.
38. Satlin LMWC, Schwartz GJ. Development of function in the metanephric kidney. In: Vize PDWA, Bard JBL, eds. *The Kidney: From Normal Development to Congenital Disease*. London: Academic Press; 2003:267-325.
41. Hughson M, Farris 3rd AB, Douglas-Denton R, Hoy WE, Bertram JF. Glomerular number and size in autopsy kidneys: the relationship to birth weight. *Kidney Int*. 2003;63:2113-2122.
44. Matsell DG, Mok A, Tarantal AF. Altered primate glomerular development due to in utero urinary tract obstruction. *Kidney Int*. 2002;61:1263-1269.
47. Turner AJ, Brown RD, Carlstrom M, Gibson KJ, Persson AE. Mechanisms of neonatal increase in glomerular filtration rate. *Am J Physiol Regul Integr Comp Physiol*. 2008;295:R916-R921.
50. Ichikawa I, Maddox DA, Brenner BM. Maturational development of glomerular ultrafiltration in the rat. *Am J Physiol*. 1979;236:F465-F471.
51. Aperia A, Herin P. Development of glomerular perfusion rate and nephron filtration rate in rats 17-60 days old. *Am J Physiol*. 1975;228:1319-1325.
53. Gruskin AB, Edelmann Jr CM, Yuan S. Maturational changes in renal blood flow in piglets. *Pediatr Res*. 1970;4:7-13.
55. Wolf G. Angiotensin II and tubular development. *Nephrol Dial Transplant*. 2002;17(suppl 9):48-51.
60. DiBona GF, Kopp UC. Neural control of renal function. *Physiol Rev*. 1997;77:75-197.
65. Akima S, Kent A, Reynolds GJ, Gallagher M, Falk MC. Indomethacin and renal impairment in neonates. *Pediatr Nephrol*. 2004;19:490-493.
67. Sener A, Smith FG. Renal hemodynamic effects of L-NAME during postnatal maturation in conscious lambs. *Pediatr Nephrol*. 2001;16:868-873.
70. Han KH, Lim JM, Kim WY, Kim H, Madsen KM, Kim J. Expression of endothelial nitric oxide synthase in developing rat kidney. *Ame J Physiol Renal Physiol*. 2005;288:F694-F702.
71. Rodriguez-Soriano J, Vallo A, Castillo G, Oliveros R. Renal handling of water and sodium in infancy and childhood: a study using clearance methods during hypotonic saline diuresis. *Kidney Int*. 1981;20:700-704.
74. Bonilla-Felix M. Development of water transport in the collecting duct. *Am J Physiol Renal Physiol*. 2004;287:F1093-F1101.
76. Horster MF, Zink H. Functional differentiation of the medullary collecting tubule: influence of vasopressin. *Kidney Int*. 1982;22:360-365.
82. Baum M, Quigley R, Satlin L. Maturational changes in renal tubular transport. *CurrOpinNephrol Hypertension*. 2003;12:521-526.
83. Devuyst O, Burrow CR, Smith BL, Agre P, Knepper MA, Wilson PD. Expression of aquaporins-1 and -2 during nephrogenesis and in autosomal dominant polycystic kidney disease. *Am J Physiol*. 1996;271:F169-F183.
87. Yamamoto T, Sasaki S, Fushimi K, et al. Expression of AQP family in rat kidneys during development and maturation. *Am J Physiol*. 1997;272:F198-F204.
88. Bonilla-Felix M, Jiang W. Aquaporin-2 in the immature rat: expression, regulation, and trafficking. *J Am Soc Nephrol*. 1997;8:1502-1509.
91. Cha JH, Kim YH, Jung JY, Han KH, Madsen KM, Kim J. Cell proliferation in the loop of Henle in the developing rat kidney. *J Am Soc Nephrol*. 2001;12:1410-1421.
92. Madsen K, Tinning AR, Marcussen N, Jensen BL. Postnatal development of the renal medulla; role of the renin-angiotensin system. *Acta Physiologica*. 2013;208:41-49.
94. Song R, Yosypiv IV. Development of the kidney medulla. *Organogenesis*. 2012;8:10-17.
100. Baum M, Quigley R. Ontogeny of renal sodium transport. *Semin Perinatol*. 2004;28:91-96.
102. Chevalier RL, Thornhill BA, Belmonte DC, Baertschi AJ. Endogenous angiotensin II inhibits natriuresis after acute volume expansion in the neonatal rat. *Am J Physiol*. 1996;270:R393-R397.
104. Beck JC, Lipkowitz MS, Abramson RG. Ontogeny of Na/H antiporter activity in rabbit renal brush border membrane vesicles. *J Clin Investigat*. 1991;87:2067-2076.
107. Burrow CR, Devuyst O, Li X, Gatti L, Wilson PD. Expression of the beta2-subunit and apical localization of Na+-K+-ATPase in metanephric kidney. *Am J Physiol*. 1999;277:F391-F403.
108. Guillery EN, Karniski LP, Mathews MS, Robillard JE. Maturation of proximal tubule Na+/H+ antiporter activity in sheep during transition from fetus to newborn. *Am J Physiol*. 1994;267:F537-F545.
111. Igarashi P, Vanden Heuvel GB, Payne JA, Forbush 3rd B. Cloning, embryonic expression, and alternative splicing of a murine kidney-specific Na-K-Cl cotransporter. *Am J Physiol*. 1995;269:F405-F418.
112. Schmitt R, Ellison DH, Farman N, et al. Developmental expression of sodium entry pathways in rat nephron. *Am J Physiol*. 1999;276:F367-F381.
118. Edelmann CM, Soriano JR, Boichis H, Gruskin AB, Acosta MI. Renal bicarbonate reabsorption and hydrogen ion excretion in normal infants. *J Clin Investigat*. 1967;46:1309-1317.
119. Kesby GJ, Lumbers ER. Factors affecting renal handling of sodium, hydrogen ions, and bicarbonate by the fetus. *Am J Physiol*. 1986;251:F226-F231.
121. Schwartz GJ, Evan AP. Development of solute transport in rabbit proximal tubule. I. HCO-3 and glucose absorption. *Am J Physiol*. 1983;245:F382-F390.
127. Hiatt MJ, Ivanova L, Toran N, Tarantal AF, Matsell DG. Remodeling of the fetal collecting duct epithelium. *Am J Pathol*. 2010;176:630-637.
128. Satlin LM. Maturation of renal potassium transport. *Pediatr Nephrol*. 1991;5:260-269.
134. Nusing RM, Pantalone F, Grone HJ, Seyberth HW, Wegmann M. Expression of the potassium channel ROMK in adult and fetal human kidney. *Histochem Cell Biol*. 2005;123:553-559.
137. Hoenderop JG, Bindels RJ. Epithelial Ca2+ and Mg2+ channels in health and disease. *J Am Soc Nephrol*. 2005;16:15-26.
140. Dimke H, Hoenderop JG, Bindels RJ. Molecular basis of epithelial Ca2+ and Mg2+ transport: insights from the TRP channel family. *J Physiol*. 2011;589:1535-1542.
142. Kaskel FJ, Kumar AM, Feld LG, Spitzer A. Renal reabsorption of phosphate during development: tubular events. *Pediatr Nephrol*. 1988;2:129-134.

95 Development and Regulation of Renal Blood Flow in the Neonate

Michael J. Solhaug | Pedro A. Jose

INTRODUCTION

Newborn mammals, including humans, exhibit lower renal blood flow than their adult counterparts.[1-4] The low fetal and neonatal renal blood flows are maintained by a high renal vascular resistance and establish the newborn's unique renal functional state, which is characterized by a low glomerular filtration rate. The unique renal hemodynamic state at birth affects the clinical management of the newborn. The low renal blood flow and resultant low glomerular filtration rate contribute

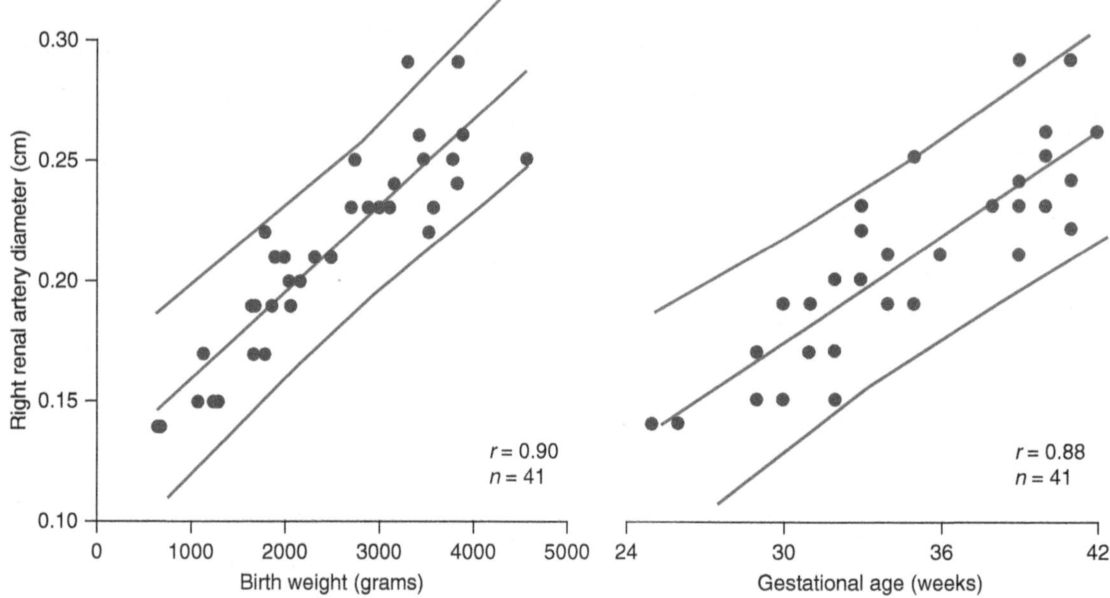

Fig. 95.1 Graph of correlation between right renal artery diameter versus birth weight and gestational age (regression line ±2 standard deviations). (From Visser MO, Leighton JO, van de Bor M, Walther FJ. Renal blood flow in neonates: quantification with color flow and pulsed Doppler US. *Radiology*. 1992;183[2]:441.)

to the newborn's altered pharmacokinetics of medications excreted by the kidney, as decreased tubular secretion.[5,6] The newborn's renal hemodynamic state modifies the development and severity of pathophysiologic conditions. These include acute renal failure resulting from hypoxic ischemic perinatal events and complications of respiratory distress syndrome.[1-4,7] Having an understanding of the regulation of renal blood flow in the newborn may provide insights into creating therapies directed at the prevention and treatment of renal injury in the neonate.

The postnatal maturation of renal hemodynamics involves a progressive increase in renal blood flow to reach adult capability (Fig. 95.1).[1-4,8-10] The major factor influencing the maturational increase in renal blood flow is the synchronous drop in renal vascular resistance, which occurs most notably in the immediate postnatal period.[1-4,8-11] Renal blood flow in the postnatal developing kidney is influenced by structural factors, such as the number of existing vascular channels, as well as functional factors, offered by the glomerular resistance vessels.[1-4,8] Several studies confirmed that in the developing kidney the functional maintenance of vascular tone (principally through a balance of vasoactive factors) is the paramount mechanism affecting renal hemodynamics.[1-4,10-13] The maturational changes in renal blood flow and renal vascular resistance must proceed normally to achieve adult capability for fully integrated renal-cardiovascular homeostasis. Disruption of the maturation of renal hemodynamics may lead to inadequate renal-cardiovascular function in the adult and may produce pathologic conditions, such as hypertension.

CHARACTERISTICS OF RENAL BLOOD FLOW IN THE IMMATURE KIDNEY

TOTAL RENAL BLOOD FLOW

In most mammalian species, with the horse as one exception,[14] renal blood flow in the neonate is lower than in the adult compared on the basis of body weight, kidney weight, or surface area.[1-4,8-11] In human newborns and infants, total renal blood flow has been determined by the clearance of *p*-aminohippurate (PAH), which measures effective renal plasma flow (ERPF)[8] and by Doppler ultrasonography.[10,11] Renal blood flow measured by Doppler and ERPF by clearance of PAH is lowest in newborns, and it correlates with gestational age. The increase in renal blood low, measured by pulsed Doppler ultrasonography, is related to an increase in vessel diameter and flow velocity.[10,11] After birth, following the short-term occlusion of the umbilical cord, renal blood flow does not change immediately, but there is redistribution of blood to the renal outer cortex (see below). There are also no significant changes in renal blood flow velocity or in renal vascular resistance during the transition from fetal to newborn life, rather renal blood flow increases after 24 hours of postnatal life.[12,13] After birth, the increase in renal blood flow is most likely related in part to an overall increase in blood pressure,[15] cardiac output,[10] as well as a decrease in renal vascular resistance.[16,17] In humans, the proportion of cardiac output distributed in the kidney in fetal life is 2% to 3%,[18,19] 4% to 6% in the first 12 hours of life, 10% at one day of age,[20] and 16% at 2 days of age,[10] which are less than the 20% to 25% observed in adults.[21,22] A decreased proportion of cardiac output to non-human fetuses has also been reported.[3,19] Using 3D-power Doppler ultrasonography, renal blood flow/index was reported to increase linearly from 23 to 40 weeks of gestational age.[23-25] By contrast, in fetuses with intrauterine growth retardation, the renal blood flow index plateaued at 34 weeks of gestational age. Renovascular reactivity index, which can detect changes in renal blood flow, can be monitored by reflectance near-infrared spectroscopy.[26,27] However, renal oxygen saturation may slightly increase, not change, or even decrease over the first few weeks of life of preterm infants instead of the expected increase in renal blood flow after birth.[28,29]

The increase in renal blood flow after birth in preterm infants is influenced by postconceptional rather than postnatal age. ERPF increases from 20 mL/min/1.73 m^2 at 30 weeks gestation to 50 mL/min/1.73 m^2 by 35 weeks gestation and 80 mL/min/1.73 m^2 at term gestation.[30] During the first 3 months of human postnatal life, ERPF increases rapidly to 300 mL/min/1.73 m^2. Thereafter, ERPF increases gradually, reaching values of 650 mL/min/1.73 m^2 by 12 to 24 months of age (Fig. 95.2).[8,31] However, the clearance of PAH underestimates ERPF in the neonatal period because the renal extraction of PAH is only 60% during the first 3 months of age compared with 94% by 5 months of age.[32] The low renal extraction of PAH in the neonate[15,32-34] has been attributed to shunting of blood to non-PAH-extracting tissues (e.g., relatively greater medullary blood flow and intracortical efferent arteriovenous shunting). PAH clearance also increases

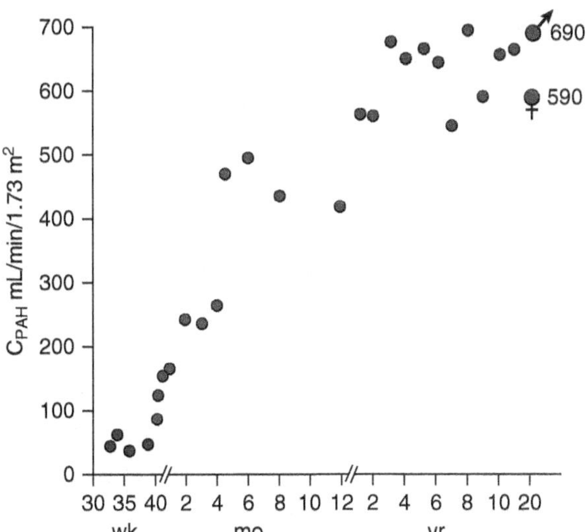

Fig. 95.2 The clearance of *p*-aminohippurate (C_{PAH}) with age. (From Rubin MI, Bruck E, Rapoport M, et al. Maturation of renal function in childhood: clearance studies. *J Clin Invest.* 1949;28:1144, by copyright permission of the American Society for Clinical Investigation.)

postnatally in the mouse.[35] However, PAH is also transported by OAT1 (SLC22a6) in renal proximal tubules and increases with maturation.[35] Thus, the PAH clearance, as an index of renal plasma flow, may be overestimated by renal proximal tubular secretion.[35,36] Increasing blood pH with use of bicarbonate or maternal use of antihypertensive drugs does not affect fetal renal oxygen saturation, which may be related to autoregulation of renal blood flow.[37,38]

Intrarenal Blood Flow

The renal vasculature is characterized by two capillary networks (the glomerular and peritubular capillary system) linked in series with each other. The major sites of renal vascular resistance are the glomerular arterioles. Blood enters the glomerulus via the afferent arteriole that arises from the interlobular artery, and it exits via the efferent arteriole. Vasoconstriction or vasodilation at these sites regulates blood flow to the glomerulus (hence, glomerular filtration rate) and the intrarenal distribution between the cortex, which contains all the glomeruli, and the medulla, which contains vasa recta and tubules but not glomeruli. In the mature kidney, the afferent arteriole of inner cortical nephrons accounts for the entire preglomerular resistance to blood flow, whereas in superficial cortical nephrons, the interlobular arteries offer the largest resistance to blood flow.[39] Blood flow to each region of the kidney (cortical, medullary, and papillary) increases with maturation.[15,21,34,40-42] The distribution of intrarenal blood flow in the young, however, is different from that reported in adults. The neonatal kidney has a greater percentage of blood flow to the inner cortical and medullary areas than the adult kidney.[43,44] In newborn lambs, clamping the umbilical cord increases renal outer cortical blood flow.[45] The low extraction ratio of PAH in infants younger than 3 months of age may be related to a relatively greater perfusion of juxtamedullary nephrons. As total renal blood flow reaches adult levels with maturation, a greater fraction of renal blood flow is received by the outer cortical nephrons. The duration of this maturational period varies from species to species.[9,34,41-46]

AUTOREGULATION OF RENAL BLOOD FLOW IN THE YOUNG

The mature kidney exhibits autoregulation; that is, renal blood flow remains constant even though renal perfusion pressure (determined by mean arterial pressure) varies throughout a range from low to high. Autoregulation depends on intrarenal mechanisms which is modulated by intrarenal factors.[47] The myogenic response and macula-densa-tubuloglomerular feedback mediate the autoregulation of renal blood flow.[48] In the newborn, the range of autoregulation is set at lower perfusion pressures than seen in the adult, and the renal pressure-flow relationship changes with renal growth.[26-29,42,49-51] Autoregulation of renal blood flow has been claimed to be negligible at birth[42] and less efficient in the young than in the adult. Furthermore, uninephrectomy impairs the autoregulatory response in young rats but does not affect this response in adult rats. This reduced autoregulatory efficiency in the neonate is apparently the result of prostaglandin-dependent renin release, which causes vasoconstriction at lower levels of perfusion pressure.[48] In pigs, the reduced autoregulatory efficiency in the neonate is not due to impaired myogenic responses.[51,52] The genetics and epigenetics of autoregulation have to be taken into consideration.[53] For example, TRPV4 channels[52] and γ-adducin[54] are involved in myogenic autoregulation. TRPV4 channels in preglomerular arteriolar smooth muscles contribute to renal myogenic autoregulation in neonatal pigs.[55] In the fetal lamb kidney, the sensitivity of the tubuloglomerular feedback is increased and decreases after birth; this is believed to be important in the postnatal increase in glomerular filtration rate.[18] In human infants, the frequency of a negative sodium balance is inversely proportional to gestational age and suggests immaturity of glomerulotubular feedback.[56]

Maturational relationships between tubular flow and glomerular filtration rate (tubuloglomerular feedback) occur with postnatal growth. The tubuloglomerular feedback mechanism is maximally sensitive at a tubular flow range that corresponds to the normal operating range. As the glomerular filtration rate increases with maturation, the maximal response and flow range also increase, so the relative sensitivity of the tubuloglomerular feedback mechanism is unaltered during growth.[57] However, gestational exposure to glucocorticoids increases the sensitivity of the tubuloglomerular feedback.[58] The relative roles of endothelial cell and smooth muscle in tubuloglomerular feedback have not been fully defined in the developing animal.

REGULATION OF POSTNATAL RENAL HEMODYNAMICS

The low renal blood flow of the preterm and full-term neonate and the increase that occurs with maturation are the result of a combination of effects, including alterations in cardiac output, perfusion pressure, and renal vascular resistance.[10,15-17] Lower cardiac output and perfusion pressure may partially account for the decreased renal blood flow noted in the newborn infant. In the dog, however, cardiac output corrected for body weight is highest in the youngest puppies, which also have the lowest renal blood flow per body weight.[34,59] As aforementioned, the proportion of cardiac output distributed in the kidney in fetal life is 2% to 3%.[10] The proportion of cardiac output distributed to the kidneys is 4% to 6% in the first 12 hours of life and increases to about 10% at one day of age,[20] 16% at two days of age.[10] These are in contrast to the 20% to 25% of cardiac output distributed to the kidneys in the normal adult.[21,22] As noted earlier, a decreased proportion of cardiac output to non-human fetuses has also been reported.[3,19] Systemic vascular resistance decreases markedly after birth. This may cause a redistribution of blood flow to organs other than the kidney and may immediately contribute to the low neonatal renal blood flow. Systemic vascular resistance gradually increases with maturation and therefore is not a factor in the increase in renal blood flow with age. However, in most species, renal vascular resistance is the most important component contributing to postnatal renal hemodynamics. Gruskin and colleagues[16] demonstrated that, in the developing

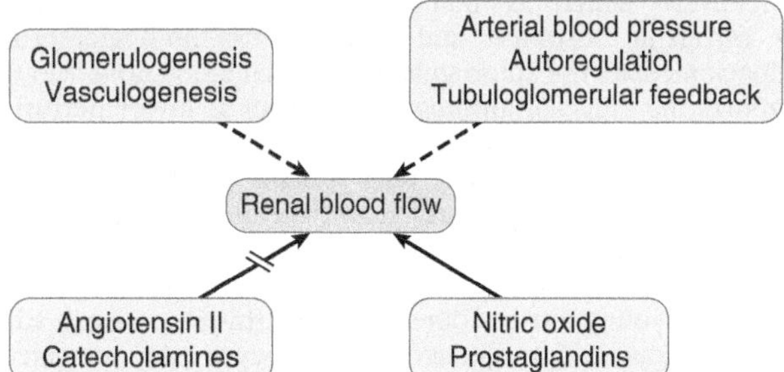

Fig. 95.3 Factors that influence the development of renal blood flow include anatomic factors (glomerulogenesis and vasculogenesis), physical factors (arterial blood pressure, myogenic autoregulatory response), and vasoactive factors (autoregulation, tubuloglomerular feedback, angiotensin II, catecholamines, renal nerves, nitric oxide, and prostaglandins). Other vasoactive agents can regulate renal blood flow; however, renal vascular resistance in the newborn regulated by vasoactive agents is probably the result of a balance between the vasoconstrictor influences of angiotensin II and catecholamines or renal nerves and the vasodilatory influences of nitric oxide and prostaglandins.

piglet, the major factor influencing the maturational increase in renal blood flow was an 86% decrease in renal vascular resistance. Renal vascular resistance in the developing kidney is influenced by *structural* factors, the number and size of vascular channels, as well as by *functional* vasoactive factors, the modulators of the resistance offered by the glomerular arterioles (Fig. 95.3).[9,60–62]

ROLE OF ANATOMIC DEVELOPMENT

The contribution of structural changes to the maturational changes of renal vascular resistance in the developing kidney is an important consideration.[63] Renal vascular resistance in the developing kidney is a function of the number of existing vascular channels, as well as the arteriolar resistance offered by each channel.[9,60–62] The two main progenitors from which renal arterioles are derived consist of the hemangioblast and Foxd1$^+$ cell. Endothelial cells originate from hemangioblasts, whereas vascular smooth muscle cells and mesangial cells originate from Foxd1$^+$ cells. The prorenin receptor, via Foxd1$^+$ cells, is important in nephron development, including the differentiation of the renal artery and arterioles.[64] In addition, the transcription factor *RBP-J* (via Foxd1$^+$ cells) is critical in the differentiation of vascular smooth muscle cells and pericytes of the renal arteries, arterioles, and glomerular mesangial cells.[65] The main structural development that could influence renal hemodynamics postnatally is the addition of vascular channels by nephrogenesis, resulting in a decrease in renal vascular resistance. The increase in renal blood flow after birth is caused by development and formation of new glomeruli and vascular remodeling. This increase may play a role in the postnatal renal hemodynamic development of several of the mammalian species in which nephrogenesis continues after birth, such as canines, swine, and rodents. Renal blood flow, however, continues to increase in these species long after glomerulogenesis is completed.[8,33,34,66] In addition, the increase in the diameter of resistance vessels during maturation is greater in the kidneys than in other organs.[67] In studies in canine puppies, Evan and colleagues[60] found substantial differences, both quantitative and qualitative, between neonatal and adult renal vasculature.[9] However, morphologic changes in renal resistance vessels cannot account for the rapid decreases in renal vascular resistance that occur in the period of renal hemodynamic maturation. Specifically, in humans, nephrogenesis is completed at 34 weeks gestation, yet renal blood flow continues to rise and renal vascular resistance continues to decrease with postnatal age, a finding indicating that the functional vasoactive characteristics of the immature renal vessels determine this fall in vascular resistance. Several studies confirmed the major contribution of the functional vasoactive attributes of the developing renal vasculature in altering renal blood flow.[a] Thus, although structural development may contribute to the changes in developing kidney by decreasing renal vascular resistance during nephrogenesis, the functional vasoactive changes of the resistance vessels are the main factors producing the maturational changes in renal hemodynamics.

ROLE OF VASOACTIVE FACTORS

High renal vascular resistance accounts for the low renal blood flow at birth, and the increase in renal blood flow with maturation mainly results from the progressive reduction in renal vascular resistance.[b] Vasoactive factors modulate renal blood flow through the alteration of renal vascular resistance by (1) the extent of participation of resistance vessels (interlobular artery and afferent and efferent arterioles), (2) the intrinsic properties of immature resistance renal vasculature, and (3) neurohormonal factors unique to the immature kidney. The site of high renal vascular resistance in the newborn guinea pig has been localized mainly to the preglomerular resistance vasculature, the interlobular artery, and the afferent arteriole.[70] The efferent arteriole may also participate, at least in the young rat.[71] The decrease in renal vascular resistance with age may be modulated by developmental changes in the intrinsic properties of the renal resistance vasculature. However, more information is needed on the myogenic internal vasoactive capabilities of these vessels or about any developmental differences in resistance vessel responsiveness to vasoactive factors. As aforementioned, in pigs, the reduced autoregulatory efficiency in the neonate is not due to impaired myogenic response.[52] Ultimately, the characteristics of postnatal renal hemodynamics are considered to be a balance of neurohormonal vasoactive factors. Both the vasoconstrictors and the vasodilators producing this immature renal condition have differing effects, intrarenal levels, and sites of action compared with the mature adult. Several vasoactive agents participate in the regulation of renal blood flow in the postnatal maturing kidney, including adenosine, arginine vasopressin (AVP), angiotensin II, atrial and other natriuretic peptides, bradykinin, endothelin, nitric oxide (NO), prostaglandins, renal nerves, urotensin, and the adrenergic nervous system.

Adenosine

The intrarenal vasodilator action of adenosine is as an important mediator of tubuloglomerular feedback in the adult.[47,48] Tubuloglomerular feedback is important in the renal autoregulation of glomerular filtration rate and blood flow. Adenosine, formed by the breakdown of adenosine triphosphate, can be a renal vasodilator or vasoconstrictor. Several adenosine receptor subtypes have been cloned: A_1R, $A_{2A}R$, $A_{2B}R$, and A_3R.[72] A_1R and $A_{2B}R$ are expressed to a greater extent than $A_{2A}R$ and A_3R in the mouse afferent arteriole.[73] Lower concentrations of adenosine cause vasoconstriction via A_1R, while higher concentrations cause vasodilation via A_2R, and A_3R only causes vasodilation, at least in afferent arterioles. The transient receptor potential cation channel, subfamily C, member 3 (TRPC3) in afferent arterioles increases with age in pigs and may be responsible for the vasoconstrictor effect of adenosine in the young because A_1R expression does not change with maturation.[74] In the adult, adenosine via A_1R decreases the glomerular filtration rate by constricting the afferent arteriole, apparently mainly in superficial nephrons. However, this can be counteracted by the vasodilatory effect of adenosine, via the $A_{2A}R$.[47,48] In one study,

[a] References 1–4, 8–11, 16, 17, 68, 69.
[b] References 1–4, 8–11, 16, 17, 34, 43, 68, 69.

intrarenal adenosine reduced cortical blood flow via adenosine A_1R and increased medullary blood flow via adenosine A_2R.[75] The stimulation of renal adenosine A_1R is associated with inhibition of renin release and constriction of afferent arterioles, whereas A_2R receptors promote renin release and dilate afferent and efferent arterioles.[47,48,76,77] Xanthines block all the adenosine receptor subtypes. In the adult, methylxanthines produce no consistent change in renal blood flow. Theophylline, however, via its adenosine receptor blocking property (independent of phosphodiesterase inhibition), increases renal vascular resistance in newborn rabbits.[78] This result is supported by the ability of a selective A_1R antagonist to decrease renal blood flow in these newborn rabbits.[79] However, in fetal sheep, the intravenous infusion of a selective A_1R agonist decreased renal blood flow without affecting blood pressure.[80] The adenosine analogue 2-chloroadenosine decreased renal blood flow in 3-day-old but not 3-week-old piglets.[81] Thus the role of adenosine receptors in the control of renal blood flow during development remains to be determined.

ARGININE VASOPRESSIN

AVP functions as an intrarenal vasoconstrictor. There are three major AVP receptor subtypes: $V_{1a}R$, $V_{1b}R$, and V_2R.[82,83] The V_2R, expressed in the principal cells of collecting ducts of the kidney, increases hydraulic conductivity via aquaporin 2, increases sodium reabsorption via the epithelial sodium channel ENaC, and increases urea transport. The V_2R is also expressed in the cells of the thick ascending limb of Henle, where it stimulates sodium transport by increasing Na-K-2Cl cotransporter activity. $V_{1a}R$ constricts the descending vasa recta and vascular smooth muscle cells while $V_{1a}R$ in renal medullary interstitial cells increases medullary blood flow by increasing the production of prostaglandins.[83,84] However, V_1R does not affect juxtamedullary afferent or afferent arterioles.[85] V_2R is vasodilatory, presumably by presence in vascular endothelial cells, that can stimulate NO production.[83-88] The role vasopressin plays in regulating basal renal hemodynamics in the young remains to be defined. In extremely low-birth-weight infants, the intravenous infusion of AVP has been reported to increase not only blood pressure but also renal blood flow.[89] In extremely low-birth-weight infants with patent ductus arteriosus, which is resistant to the vasoconstrictor effect of dopamine, an analogue of vasopressin, terlipressin has also been shown to increase both blood pressure and renal blood flow.[90] In fetal sheep (126 to 130 days), the intravenous infusion of AVP (6 hours) increased blood pressure that remained elevated after three days, although not as high as that seen acutely. Renal blood flow was also acutely increased by AVP but subsequently decreased after 1 day of infusion.[91] Similarly, in another study in fetal sheep (106 to 142 days), the intravenous administration of AVP (60 minutes) increased blood pressure, but renal blood flow was not altered (although there was a non-significant increase in renal vascular resistance).[92] The failure to observe a decrease in renal blood flow and an increase in renal vascular resistance in the latter study may be related to the duration of AVP infusion. Thus, in fetal life, AVP increases systemic vascular resistance; however, it initially decreases renal vascular resistance but subsequently increases it.

ANGIOTENSIN II AND THE RENIN-ANGIOTENSIN SYSTEM

The highly activated renin-angiotensin system, through the vasoconstriction properties of angiotensin II, contributes to the high renal vascular resistance in the immature kidney.[21,48-53,93-98] Renin cells and renin in the vasculature are important for nephron development, including the differentiation of the renal artery and arterioles.[63,97-100] The prorenin receptor is important in nephron and renal arterial development[64,101] and the angiotensin type 1 receptor, AT_1R, is apparently not involved in normal kidney development, at least in mice.[102] Circulating renin, angiotensin I, and angiotensin II levels are high in most neonatal mammals, including humans, and they decrease with age.[93-96,103] There are no data on angiotensin-(1 to 7), angiotensin III, angiotensin IV, angiotensin A, and alamandine levels in infants. Plasma prorenin and soluble prorenin receptor are higher in preterm than full-term neonates.[104] Plasma angiotensinogen is not different between preterm and full-term infants. However, the urinary angiotensinogen to creatinine ratio is higher in preterm than full-term infants and decreases with postnatal age.[105,106] The renin-angiotensin system is now classified into the classical pathway and the non-classical or counterregulatory pathway (Fig. 95.4).[107-111] The classical pathway starts with angiotensinogen, its conversion to angiotensin I by renin, and conversion of angiotensin 1 to angiotensin II by angiotensin converting enzyme. This pathway causes vasoconstriction and stimulation of renal sodium transport. In the non-classical or counterregulatory pathway angiotensin converting enzyme 2 converts angiotensin II from the classical pathway to angiotensin 1 to 7 or alamandine from angiotensin A and in general opposes the effects of the classical pathway. There are three angiotensin II receptors: AT_1R, AT_2R, and AT_4R, and two angiotensin 1 to 7 receptors, MrgD and Mas. AT_1R is a vasoconstrictor while AT_2R, AT_4R, MrgD, and Mas are vasodilators. In association with vascular endothelial growth factor, angiotensin II (via AT_1R, expressed in vasa recta pericytes) is important in the development of renal cortical and medullary capillaries and vasa recta in neonatal rats in the third postnatal week.[112,113] By contrast, AT_2R is the predominant angiotensin receptor in fetal and postnatal rats up to 3 days of life, after which their expression is negligible while AT_1R expression increases.[114-117] Human fetal kidneys only express the AT_2R.[118] The increased renal AT_2R expression in fetus and neonate is also seen in pigs and sheep.[119,120] AT_1R receptors, which mediate vasoconstriction, are expressed at later stages in the glomerulus, resistance arterioles, and medulla, including the period of hemodynamic development. Studies show that angiotensin via their receptors has a significant role in renal formation and postnatal function. Abnormalities in renal development are noted in human infants and neonatal rats treated with angiotensin-converting enzyme inhibitors. In neonatal rats, AT_1R but not AT_2R, antagonists produce renal defects similar to those noted with angiotensin-converting enzyme inhibitors, a finding further attesting to the importance of this receptor subtype in kidney development.[116,121-123] However, disruption of both AT_1R and AT_2R can lead to malformations of the kidney and urinary tract.[121] Specific blockade of the AT_1R in neonatal rats results in significant functional changes later in life; however, the degree and persistence of the functional changes is greater in males than females.[123] AT_1R inhibition for 2 weeks after birth in rats increases blood pressure and decreases nephron number in both males and females. However, only males exhibit decreased papillary volume, significant proteinuria, and reduced GFR at 3 months of age.[123] Unilateral ureteral obstruction in neonatal rats increases renal renin and angiotensin production and AT_1R expression.[124] Although nonspecific inhibition of angiotensin II has not revealed developmental differences in renal hemodynamics, the regulatory role of the renin-angiotensin system has been clarified with the use of non-peptide antagonists of angiotensin II receptors. Systemic infusion of an angiotensin-converting enzyme inhibitor in conscious newborn sheep decreases renal vascular resistance, but does not change renal blood flow.[125] Administration of the nonselective angiotensin receptor antagonist saralasin by Osborn and colleagues[126] in piglets and Jose and colleagues[50] in puppies did not significantly alter renal hemodynamics. However, the intrarenal infusion of a non-peptide-specific AT_1R antagonist produces greater increase in renal blood flow in 3-week-old piglets than the adult, suggesting that angiotensin II, via the AT_1R, is a more important renal vasoconstrictor in the immature kidney than

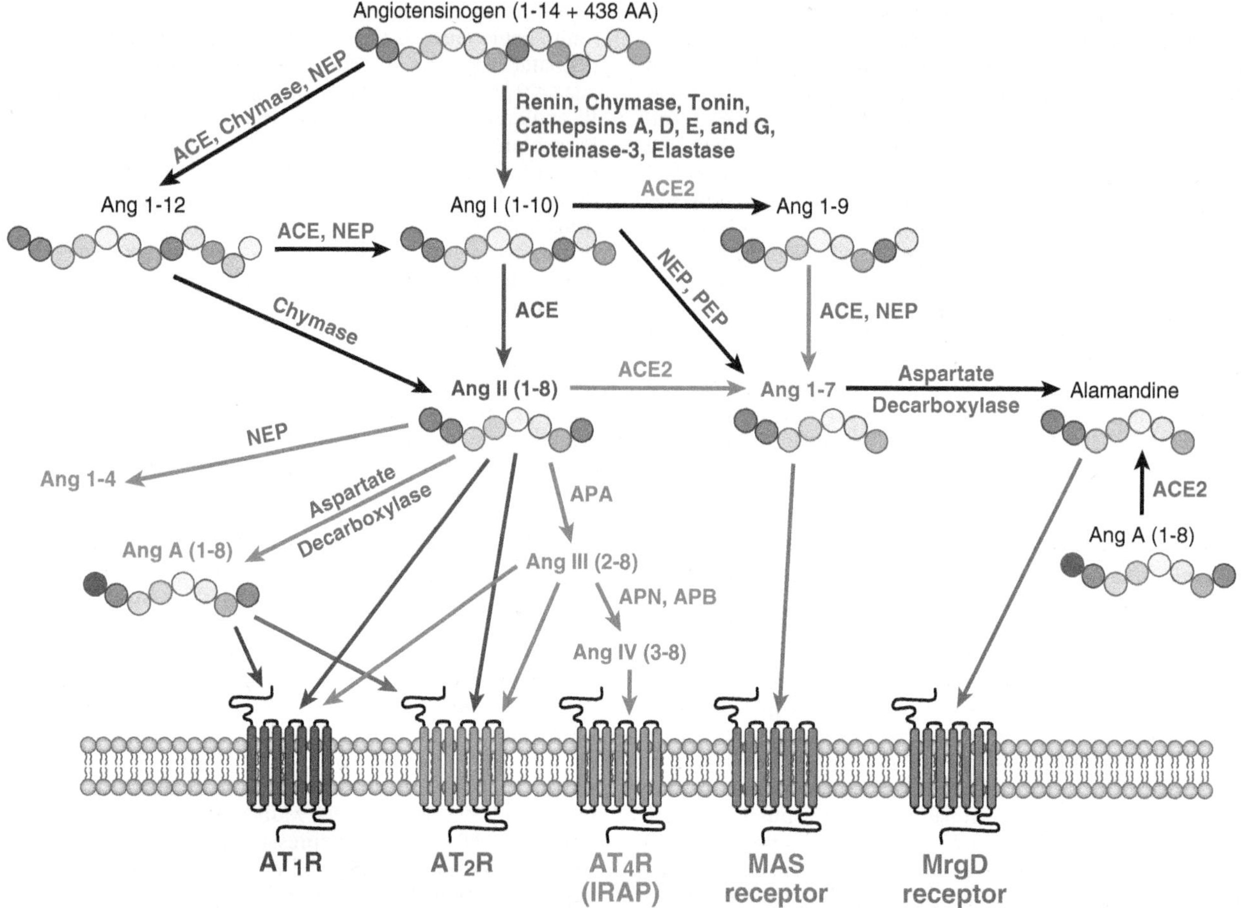

Fig. 95.4 The renin-angiotensin system (RAS) is currently divided into the classical RAS and the non-classical RAS pathways. Both the classical and non-classical pathways are initiated by renin cleaving angiotensinogen to angiotensin 1 *(Ang I)*. The classical pathway is initiated mainly by angiotensin converting enzyme *(ACE)* to angiotensin II ($D^1R^2V^3Y^4I^5H^6P^7F^8$). The non-classical pathway is comprised of two components: one pathway is initiated by *ACE2*, and the other component has three pathways, Ang A ($A^1R^2V^3Y^4I^5H^6P^7F^8$), Ang II, and Ang (1 to 7) ($D^1R^2V^3Y^4I^5H^6P^7F^8$). Shown as well is the conversion of Ang III to Ang IV ($V^3Y^4I^5H^6P^7F^8$) by aminopeptidase N. Ang IV binding to AT1R causes vasoconstriction[244] but causes vasodilation via the AT4R[245]. The corresponding receptors are indicated. *AA*, Amino acid; *APA*, amino peptidase A; *APB*, amino peptidase B; *IRAP*, insulin-regulated aminopeptidase; *NEP*, neprilysin.

the adult.[98] Chappallez and Smith[127] determined the individual roles of the AT_1R and AT_2R in renal hemodynamics of conscious 1- and 6-week-old lambs. In both age groups, AT_1R inhibition decreased renal vascular resistance and increased renal blood flow, while decreasing mean arterial pressure only at high doses. Furthermore, the pressor responses to angiotensin infusion were abolished by AT_1R inhibition. By contrast, AT_2R blockade did not change any of these parameters,[127] AT_2R, being vasodilatory.[107-111,128] Angiotensin-converting enzyme inhibition did affect renal blood flow in 4- to 5-days piglets.[129] However, in 5- to 8-day-old rabbits, angiotensin converting enzyme inhibition increased renal blood flow and decreased renal vascular resistance, indicating species-related differences.[130] In contrast to the apparently increased vasoconstrictor effect of angiotensin I via AT_1R a few weeks after birth, angiotensin II may actually be needed to maintain glomerular filtration rate in the neonatal rabbit. Pharmacologic inhibition of AT_1R in neonatal rabbits (~6 days) decreases glomerular filtration rate without affecting renal blood flow.[131] The above studies suggest that angiotensin II, via the AT_2R, plays an important role in the regulation of renal blood flow in the fetus and the immediate postnatal period, while AT_1R plays that role a few days after birth and during the postnatal period. However, the increased expression of AT_2R in fetal organs has been challenged; western blotting studies showed that AT_2R expression in kidney, liver, and whole brain homogenates is lowest in fetal rats and increases with age.[132-134] Real-time PCR also showed a greater AT_2R to AT_1R ratio in developing kidneys. Previous studies used autoradiography, ligand binding, and in situ hybridization techniques that can distinguish expression in glomeruli, tubules, and vessels.

ATRIAL AND OTHER NATRIURETIC PEPTIDES

There are several natriuretic peptides: atrial natriuretic peptide (ANP), brain natriuretic peptide (BNP), and C-type natriuretic peptide (CNP).[135] ANP and BNP (originally described in brain) are produced in the atria and ventricles, whereas CNP is found mainly in the brain, pituitary gland, vascular endothelium, kidney, and female genitourinary tract. ANP is present in both atria and ventricles of the fetus in several species, and plasma levels of this peptide are significantly elevated compared with those of the adult.[136-140] The fetal atrium may be the primary source of ANP synthesis.[136] Within the first few weeks of life, however, the plasma concentrations of ANP fall to adult levels. During the early developmental period, the release of ANP appears to be in response to various stimuli that are associated with volume overload. The most important vascular and renal effects of ANP in mature animals are (1) vasodilation and decrease in mean blood pressure; (2) increase in renal blood flow, glomerular filtration rate, and filtration fraction; (3) inhibition of sodium and water reabsorption in proximal and distal tubules; and (4) decrease in concentrating ability. Although ANP may play a role in sodium and volume homeostasis during the perinatal period, its role in the regulation of renal hemodynamics is uncertain. However, plasma ANP is increased by saline infusion in ovine fetuses, which already have high basal levels of ANP.[141] In rabbits, clear age differences in the renal response to intravenous infusions of α-human ANP have been noted. In newborn rabbits, ANP decreases renal blood flow, GFR, and urine flow without affecting sodium excretion, while in adult rabbits, ANP produces a marked diuresis and natriuresis with no effect on GFR and slight decrease in renal blood flow.[142] The infusion of recombinant ANP into fetal sheep results in minimal decline in mean arterial blood pressure. By contrast, significant decreases in blood pressure and increments in heart rate have been observed in newborn and adult sheep during continuous infusion of pharmacologic doses of ANP. ANP reduces renal blood flow in fetal and newborn sheep. This effect, however, decreases with maturation,[143] and its significance is not clear. Systemic clearance of ANP is increased in the newborn and decreases with development.[144] The decreased effects of ANP in the newborn period (in most but not all studies)[145] could be explained by increased clearance of ANP or decreased production of cyclic guanosine monophosphate but not by receptor number.[145-148] However, in fetal sheep ANP gene expression is increased by endothelin,[149] and the diuretic effects of low concentrations of ANP in fetal sheep is increased by ganglionic blocker hexamethonium, which blocks both sympathetic and parasympathetic pathways.[150]

BRADYKININ

Bradykinin is the major functional vasodilator produced by the kallikrein-kinin system. Bradykinin exerts its effects via B_1 and B_2 receptors.[151] Under physiologic conditions, most of the effects of bradykinin are mediated by the B_2 receptor. NO and prostaglandin E2, and suppression of renal nerve activity, may in part mediate the vasodilatory effect of bradykinin.[152-154] Kallikreins are proteinases that liberate vasoactive kinins from the protein precursor kininogen. The bradykinin-synthesizing enzyme, kininase II, is identical to angiotensin-converting enzyme, which produces angiotensin II. Although bradykinin may play a role in renal morphogenesis,[155-157] the role of this vasodilator in the renal hemodynamics is less certain. Several studies indirectly suggest that bradykinin may participate in the maturational increase in renal blood flow. Urinary kallikrein excretion corrected for either renal mass or glomerular filtration rate increases with maturation.[158,159] Kininase II mRNA and enzymatic activity are low in newborn rat kidney and peak at 2 to 3 weeks of age.[160]

Bradykinin B_2 receptor is overexpressed in several organs, including the kidney, in fetal and neonatal rats, relative to adult rats. However, there is no bradykinin B2 receptor expression in renal blood vessels.[161] Studies have also failed to demonstrate a significant role for bradykinin in immature renal hemodynamics. The intrarenal arterial injection of bradykinin increased renal blood flow that was greater in conscious 6-week-old than 1-week-old lambs.[162] However, acute intravenous injection of a selective kinin B_2 antagonist, icatibant, had no effect on renal plasma flow, although glomerular filtration rate was decreased.[162] Therefore, bradykinin, produced endogenously by the kidney, does not modulate the maturational increase in renal blood flow in the lamb. This conclusion is supported by studies in neonatal rats. Long-term administration of the same B_2 antagonist to neonatal rats from birth to 3 weeks did not alter the maturational increase in renal blood flow.[163] By contrast, in newborn rabbits, bradykinin B_2 antagonist given subcutaneously actually increased renal blood flow and decreased renal vascular resistance.[164] Thus, the increase in renal blood flow with maturation is probably not related to bradykinin.[163] Nevertheless, the possibility remains that bradykinin opposes the basal vasoconstriction of angiotensin II in the immature rat kidney.[163]

ENDOTHELIN

Endothelin, one of the vasoconstricting factors produced by the endothelium, is one of the most potent endogenous vasoconstrictors, second only to urotensin II.[125] I-Endothelin binding in renal cortex, medulla, and vessels is greater in fetal than adult humans.[165] There are three different endothelin peptides encoded by three distinct genes: endothelin-1 (ET-1), endothelin-2 (ET-2), and endothelin-3 (ET-3). Human endothelial cells synthesize ET-1 and ET-2 but not ET-3. All the endothelins can induce vasoconstriction. Two ET receptors, ET_AR and ET_BR,[166] mediate endothelin action. ET-1, ET-2, and ET-3 have the same affinity for the ET_BR, but ET-3 has a lower affinity to ET_AR, relative to ET-1 and ET-2. ET_AR is responsible for the ET-1 vasoconstrictor action; endothelins can also mediate vasodilation via ETB.[167-169] ET-1, produced by vascular endothelial cells, is the most abundant endothelin isoform in the cardiovascular system. In newborn mice, carotid arterial endothelial cells express high levels of ET-1.[170] The fetal pulmonary vascular endothelin converting enzyme-1 (ECE-1) increases after birth. There are no studies on ECE-1 or specifically the isoforms of ECE-1 (ECE-1a-d) in the developing kidney. ET-1 produces vasoconstriction in both the renal afferent and efferent arterioles and mesenteric arteries.[172-174] ET_AR is mainly expressed in vascular smooth muscles while ET_BR is mainly expressed in endothelial cells. ET_AR predominates in the afferent arteriole while ET_BR predominates in the efferent arteriole.[172] Vascular smooth muscles in brain and kidney express more ET_BR than other organs.[169] There are three splice variants of ET_AR, but their physiologic significance has not been demonstrated. The presence of two ET_BRs has not been confirmed.[169] There are splice variants of ET_BR but as with ET_AR, their physiologic significance has not been demonstrated. ET_BR expressed in endothelial cells (tunica intima) causes vasodilation because of linkage to NO, prostaglandins, and endothelium-derived hyperpolarizing factor. However, low concentrations of ET may cause vasoconstriction, via ETBR, expressed in vascular smooth muscle cells.[175] ET_BR is also negatively regulated by the dopamine D_2R.[176]

In term infants, the urinary excretion of ET-1 remains constant in the first month of life. In premature infants, ET-1 excretion increases with maturation such that, after the first week, postnatal values exceed those found in older children.[177] In newborn rabbits, ET-1 failed to change renal hemodynamics at doses that decreased renal blood flow in adults; however, at higher doses, exogenous endothelin induced a marked reduction in renal blood flow and glomerular filtration rate in the newborn as well.[178] Blockade of endogenous ET-1 activity in newborn rabbits by ET-1 antiserum increased renal vascular resistance and decreased renal blood flow.[179] These studies suggest that ET-1 may not be responsible for the increased renal vascular resistance in the newborn period. Rather, ET-1, via endothelial ETB, may function as a renal vasodilator to counteract the vasoconstrictor effects of other systems (e.g., angiotensin II and catecholamines). Dual ETAR and ETBR blockade in one study decreased the number of glomeruli, juxtamedullary filtration surface area, and glomerular filtration rate.[180] However, the finding that ETA and ETB blockade in the newborn increases renal blood flow indicates that endothelin is probably not an important factor in the increase of renal blood flow with age.[181]

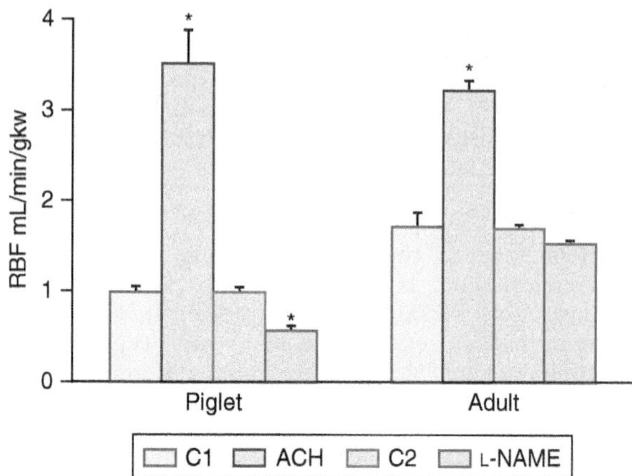

Fig. 95.5 Comparison of the renal blood flow *(RBF)* responses in immature and adult renal vasculature to vasoactive agents that act on the nitric oxide synthesizing enzyme, nitric oxide synthase (NOS). RBF responses were directly measured by electromagnetic flow probe in anesthetized 3-week-old piglets and adults ($n = 4$) during the sequential intrarenal infusions of NOS stimulation with acetylcholine, 0.05 μg/kg/min *(ACH)*, and NOS inhibition with L-NAME, 3 μg/kg/min (L-NAME) with interval control periods (C1 and C2). The immature kidney demonstrates lower baseline RBF in both control periods. RBF responses were greater in the immature kidney to NOS stimulation, ACH, and inhibition with L-NAME. *gkw,* Gram kidney weight. *$P < .05$ versus others within each group. (Modified from Solhaug MJ, Ballèvre LD, Guignard JP, et al. Nitric oxide in the developing kidney. *Pediatr Nephrol.* 1996;10:529.)

NITRIC OXIDE

NO synthesized by nitric oxide synthase (NOS) is an important endogenous regulator of renal hemodynamics in the immature kidney, functioning as a critical vasodilator to counterbalance highly activated vasoconstrictors, such as angiotensin II.[66] Angiotensin II, via AT_1R and AT_2R, increases nNOS expression in renal afferents of developing pigs.[182] Three NOS isoforms exist: endothelial (eNOS), inducible (iNOS), and neuronal (nNOS).[183] However, only eNOS and nNOS participate in regulating basal renal hemodynamics. The immature renal vasculature is highly responsive to alterations of the NO synthesizing enzyme, NOS. Fig. 95.5 shows the renal blood flow responses of the 3-week-old piglet to sequential intrarenal infusions of acetylcholine, a NOS stimulator, and L-NAME, an arginine analogue that non-selectively and competitively inhibits all NOS isoforms.[68] Several reports identify NO as a vital participant in postnatal developing renal hemodynamics under physiologic and pathophysiologic conditions.[66,68,184-186] The intrarenal infusion of the NOS inhibitor, L-NAME, in both whole animals (piglets, newborn lambs, and rabbits)[66,186,187] and isolated perfused kidneys (newborn rabbits)[188] produces greater renal hemodynamic responses than the adult. However, the intravenous administration of L-NAME had no effect on renal blood flow in 1- and 6-week-old lambs, suggesting that extra-renal effects could have confounding effects.[189] Indeed, renal NO production by NOS and resultant vasodilation is greater in the immature kidney compared with the adult. NOS enzymatic activity is significantly upregulated in microdissected resistance vessels (afferent interlobular and arcuate) immediately after birth but decreases to adult levels with maturation.[190,191] This increased NO production in the neonate is supported by the distinct developmental patterns in the postnatal maturing porcine kidney of two NOS isoforms: nNOS and eNOS. Both eNOS and nNOS demonstrate reciprocal developmental expression patterns during postnatal renal maturation. In whole kidney and corticomedullary sections in swine, eNOS concentration is least in the newborn and greatest in the adult, whereas nNOS is greatest in the newborn and least in the adult.[192,193] This reciprocal developmental pattern is also seen in discrete, microdissected resistance vessels (afferent, interlobular, and arcuate) from swine. nNOS levels are greatest in all vessels, decreasing with age to very low levels in the adult, whereas eNOS levels exhibit developmental changes in the afferent arteriole only; levels are relatively low in the immature afferent and significantly increase with age.[190,191]

The distinct expression patterns of the two NOS isoforms suggests nNOS may be the more important NOS isoform participating in immature renal hemodynamics. Indeed, studies using a combination of intrarenal infusions of a nNOS specific inhibitor and a global inhibitor of both nNOS and eNOS demonstrated that only nNOS, and not eNOS, was functionally significant in the immature kidney, compared with the major role of eNOS in the adult kidney,[194] consistent with previous studies in which eNOS is the functional isoform in adult kidneys.[195] Thus developmental patterns of NOS expression and functional activity suggest nNOS is the crucial enhanced isoform that provides counter-balancing NO vasodilation, which opposes augmented angiotensin II vasoconstriction characteristic of newborn renal hemodynamics. Sufficient evidence now exists to identify the major vasoactive factors regulating renal hemodynamics in the postnatal developing kidney. Angiotensin II functions as the predominant vasoconstrictor,[98] and NO, via the nNOS isoform, is the major vasodilator counter balancing highly activated angiotensin II.[98,182,194] Angiotensin II regulates NO function and NOS expression through the AT_1R and AT_2R. Inhibition of the AT_1R with the intrarenal infusion of a selective AT_1R antagonist abolishes renal functional responses to NO inhibition in the developing piglet.[115] Angiotensin II selectively regulates NOS enzymatic activity (via AT_1R and AT_2R) and nNOS and eNOS expression in afferent arterioles of the developing kidney. In microdissected afferent arterioles from immature and adult swine treated with angiotensin II and selective AT_1R or selective AT_2R inhibition, NOS enzymatic activity and nNOS expression were greater in the newborn afferents than in the adult, whereas eNOS expression was greater in the adult. Angiotensin II increased NOS activity and eNOS expression at all ages but increased nNOS expression only in developing afferents.[182] Both AT_1R and AT_2R blockade significantly attenuated NOS activity and eNOS expression at all ages but attenuated nNOS expression only in developing afferents.[182] The ability of NO to counteract the effects of vasoconstrictor agents, principally angiotensin II, under physiologic conditions suggests that NO may be even more important in pathologic conditions (e.g., perinatal hypoxemia).[185] In newborn rabbits, the renal blood flow responses to L-NAME were significantly greater during hypoxemia. These conditions induced an intense renal vasoconstriction, mediated by angiotensin II, often resulting in acute renal failure.[196] Thus, NO may serve to protect the immature kidney from the deleterious effects of adverse perinatal events that lead to vasoconstriction-induced acute renal failure.

PROSTAGLANDINS

Arachidonic acid is an essential fatty acid that is metabolized through different pathways: 5-lipoxygenase leads to formation of leukotrienes, 15-lipoxygenase leads to formation of lipoxins, cytochrome P450 leads to formation of epoxy-20:3, and cyclooxygenase (COX) leads to formation of prostaglandins and thromboxanes. In rats, arachidonic acid metabolism in the kidney shifts from a lipoxygenase-dependent to a cytochrome P450-dependent pathway during development.[197,198] Renal production of cytochrome P450-dependent metabolites of arachidonic, which is localized in the proximal tubule, is low in the fetus and newborn.[199] Two COX isoforms are present in the kidney: COX-1 and COX-2. COX-1 is found in glomerular mesangial cells, arteriolar endothelial cells, and cortical and medullary collecting duct across species.[198] However, COX-2 intrarenal localization is species-dependent. In rats, rabbits, and dogs, COX-2 is expressed in the macula densa, and thick ascending limb of the loop of Henle. In humans, COX-2 is also expressed in the loop of Henle and glomerular podocytes, but COX-2 expression in the macula densa is mainly evident in the elderly.[197,200] Several therapeutic agents such as nonsteroidal anti-inflammatory drugs, including aspirin, ibuprofen, and indomethacin, non-selectively inhibit both COX-1 and COX-2.[201] Celecoxib and rofecoxib are selective COX-2 inhibitors. Although COX-1 may not undergo postnatal regulation, COX-2 is highest after birth (between 1 and 2 weeks in rats) and declines with age.[197,200,202–204] COX-2 is constitutively active in the fetal kidney while there is minimal COX-2 expression in the adult kidney.[197,200,202–205] COX-2 inhibition during nephrogenesis may contribute to renal dysgenesis syndromes. In fetal kidneys, COX-2 strongly localizes to tubular structures, which differ from the adult.[200] Selective COX-2 inhibition leads to disruption of nephrogenesis in both mice and rats.[206] Genetic ablation of COX-2 results in severe morphologic abnormalities, including impaired glomerulogenesis, cortical dysplasia, and diffuse tubular cyst formation.[207] These studies confirm the teratogenic potential of prenatal use of nonsteroidal drugs. Administration of selective COX-2 inhibitors may also lead to acute renal failure and renal dysgenesis.[207–210] Apparently, AT_1R signaling is needed for COX-2-dependent effects.[211]

Despite the increasing information about the role of COX isoforms in nephrogenesis, the functional vasoactive role of the COX products (prostaglandins) in the immature kidney is uncertain. In fact, the relation of specific COX isoforms to renal function is not well understood. In general, thromboxanes and leukotrienes vasoconstrict the kidney, whereas prostaglandins and lipoxins vasodilate it. Cytochrome P450 metabolites of arachidonic acid can act as vasoconstrictors or vasodilators. Renal prostaglandin production is increased during the perinatal period. In preterm infants, the urinary excretion of prostaglandin E and a prostacyclin metabolite is five times that noted at term and is 20 times greater than that observed in physiologically normal children.[209] Glomerular prostaglandin synthesis and adenylate cyclase response to prostaglandin E_2 also decrease with maturation.[210,212] Moreover, when prostaglandin synthesis is inhibited by indomethacin in unstressed adults[213] or neonatal animals, renal blood flow is either decreased,[214–217] unchanged,[218–220] or redistributed to the outer cortex.[217] By contrast, indomethacin decreases renal blood flow in 2-day-old or 10-day-old premature human infants.[201,221] Therefore, if prostaglandin synthesis was deficient in the newborn infant, one could expect a pattern of blood flow converse to that normally found in the neonatal kidney. Likewise, the increased renal blood flow found in the uninephrectomized young rat is not maintained by increased prostaglandin or decreased thromboxane effects.[49] While neonatal rabbits may be more sensitive to the vasoconstrictor effects of acetylsalicylic acid,[222] prostaglandin inhibition does not alter basal renal blood flow in the immature piglet kidney.[68] Moreover, the COX inhibitor ibuprofen does not affect renal blood flow in preterm neonates.[223]

In young and adult rats, the major pathway of arachidonic acid metabolism in glomeruli occurs via the lipoxygenase pathway.[210,224] The conversion of arachidonic acid into 12-HETE does not vary with age in rats.[225] However, it is 20-HETE that has been shown to be important in the myogenic and tubuloglomerular feedback, via the afferent arteriole.[226] 20-HETE inhibits while epoxyeicosatrienoic acids activate renal microvascular smooth muscle cell large-conductance calcium-activated K^+ channels; 20-HETE is predominant in vascular smooth muscle cells.[227] The effects of this pathway on basal renal blood flow during development remains to be determined. Moreover, the renal development of the nine prostanoid receptors has not been determined.[228] As aforementioned, arachidonic acid can be metabolized by 5-lipoxygenase leeukotrienes.[227] The infusion of a lipoxygenase metabolite, leukotriene C4, does not affect renal blood flow although it decreases blood flow in the skeletal muscle and intestine.[229]

In neonates, as in adults, prostaglandins play little or no role in the control of renal blood flow in the normal animal at rest,[230] but prostaglandins may attenuate renal vasoconstriction in pathologic conditions. Indeed, in the fetus, prostaglandins may be important in the regulation of renal blood flow under both basal and stress conditions.[223] The role of other arachidonic acid metabolites on the maturation of renal blood flow needs more studies.

RENAL NERVES AND THE ADRENERGIC SYSTEM

The influence of renal innervation and the adrenergic nervous system is both maturation- and species-dependent.[231] The renal circulation of the pig is under tonic neural vasoconstrictor influence. Thus, low-frequency sciatic nerve stimulation in newborn pigs decreases renal blood flow but high-frequency stimulation increases renal blood flow.[231] Renal denervation increases the renal blood flow in piglets. By contrast, renal denervation does not alter basal renal blood flow in fetal lambs. However, in sheep, efferent renal nerve activity is present before birth and may influence renal hemodynamics in stressful conditions during renal maturation.[232]

Overall, the renal vascular bed of the newborn seems to be more sensitive, but less reactive, than that of the adult in response to renal nerve stimulation.[121,122] Low-level stimulation of the renal nerve of fetal sheep and 1- to 2-week-old piglets results in a greater increase in renal vascular resistance than in their adult counterparts. During higher levels of renal nerve stimulation, however, renal vascular resistance increases to a greater extent in older animals than in younger animals. In the presence of α-adrenergic blockade, renal nerve stimulation induces an increase in renal blood flow in fetal and newborn lambs, but not in adults. This effect is apparently the result of a greater density of α- (versus β-) adrenergic receptors in neonatal sheep. After the immediate newborn period, the neonatal renal circulation is more sensitive to α-adrenergic stimulation in several species (dogs, pigs, guinea pigs, sheep) compared with adults.[23,233–235] An age-dependent increase in renal blood flow and a concomitant decrease in renal vascular resistance with α-adrenergic blockade have been shown in piglets[236] and in canine puppies.[17,235] Isolated renal vessels of fetal lambs, studied in vitro, are also more sensitive and reactive to α-adrenergic agonists than are their newborn or adult counterparts. The rabbit seems to be an exception in that the renal vasculature in the adult is more sensitive to catecholamines compared with newborns. In sheep, renal nerve stimulation produces renal vasodilation in immature animals by activating β-adrenoceptors, providing evidence of an age-dependent neural renal vasodilator mechanism.[232] β-Adrenergic agonists increase renal blood flow to a greater extent in neonatal than in adult sheep, an opposite effect has been noted in piglets. The renal vasodilator effect of dopamine increases with maturation in several species (pigs, dogs, sheep).[234–236] The earlier reports of apparent absence of ontogenic differences in the renal catecholamine response in sheep can now be attributed to bolus versus constant intrarenal infusions. Fetal and newborn sheep are more responsive to the vasoconstrictor effects of α-adrenergic ligands and less responsive to the vasodilator effects of dopaminergic ligands.[232,233,236–239]

Low dose dopamine does not increase renal blood flow in preterm and term piglets.[240]

Gases such as carbon monoxide[241] and hydrogen sulfide[242] regulate renal blood flow in the adult, but there are no studies in the fetus, newborn, or developing kidney.

CONCLUSION

The low renal blood flow in the young is the result of several factors, including smaller vessel size, decreased number of glomeruli, and lower systemic pressure, but it is mainly caused by high renal vascular resistance. The increased renal vascular resistance in the newborn is predominately caused by increased activity of the renin-angiotensin system via angiotensin II, as well as increased sensitivity to vasoconstrictor catecholamines, as the result of receptor and postadrenergic receptor mechanisms. Critical vasodilators, such as NO, act to counterbalance these vasoconstrictor forces. NO function via the nNOS isoform is greater in the immature resistance vasculature compared with the adult and may undergo regulation via the AT_1R and AT_2R. The increase in renal blood flow with age presumably occurs as vasoconstrictor influences decline, accompanied by a concordant alteration in vasodilators, such as NO. New ligands and receptors continue to be discovered, but their roles, if any, in the development of renal blood flow remain to be determined. Moreover, the effect of circadian rhythm on the postnatal regulation of the development renal blood flow remains to be defined.[243]

 A complete reference list is available at www.ExpertConsult.com.

SELECT REFERENCES

1. McCrory WW. *Developmental Nephrology*. Cambridge: Harvard University Press; 1972.
2. Segar JL. Renal adaptive changes and sodium handling in the fetal-to-newborn transition. *Semin Fetal Neonatal Med*. 2017;22(2):76.
3. Sulemanji M, Vakili K. Neonatal renal physiology. *Semin Pediatr Surg*. 2013;22(4):195.
4. Saint-Faust M, Boubred F, Simeoni U. Renal development and neonatal adaptation. *Am J Perinatol*. 2014;31(9):773.
5. Ruggiero A, Ariano A, Triarico S, et al. Neonatal pharmacology and clinical implications. *Drugs Context*. 2019;8:21260.
6. Lim SY, Pettit RS. Pharmacokinetic considerations in pediatric pharmacotherapy. *Am J Health Syst Pharm*. 2019;76(19):1472.
7. Frazier KS. Species differences in renal development and associated developmental nephrotoxicity. *Birth Defects Res*. 2017;109(16):1243.
10. Visser MO, Leighton JO, van de Bor M, Walther FJ. Renal blood flow in neonates: quantification with color flow and pulsed Doppler US. *Radiology*. 1992;183(2):441.
12. Nakamura KT, Matherne GP, McWeeny OJ, et al. Renal hemodynamics and functional changes during the transition from fetal to newborn life in sheep. *Pediatr Res*. 1987;21:229.
15. Kleinman LI, Lubbe RJ. Factors affecting the maturation of glomerular filtration rate and renal plasma flow in the new-born dog. *J Physiol*. 1972;223(2):395.
16. Gruskin AB, Edelmann Jr CM, Yuan S. Maturational changes in renal blood flow in piglets. *Pediatr Res*. 1970;4:7.
27. Huber W, Zanner R, Schneider G, Schmid R, et al. Assessment of regional perfusion and organ function: less and non-invasive techniques. *Front Med*. 2019;6:50.
30. Fawer CL, Torrado A, Guignard JP. Maturation of renal function in full-term and premature neonates. *Helv Paediatr Acta*. 1979;34:11.
34. Jose PA, Logan AG, Slotkoff LM, et al. Intrarenal blood flow distribution in canine puppies. *Pediatr Res*. 1971;5:335.
40. Aperia A, Broberger O, Herin P. Maturational changes in glomerular perfusion rate and glomerular filtration rate in lambs. *Pediatr Res*. 1974;8:758.
42. Buckley NM, Brazeau P, Frasier ID. Renal blood flow autoregulation in developing swine. *Am J Physiol*. 1983;245:1.
46. Chevalier RL. Hemodynamic adaptation to reduced renal mass in early postnatal development. *Pediatr Res*. 1983;17(8):620.
50. Jose PA, Slotkoff LM, Montgomery S, et al. Autoregulation of renal blood flow in the puppy. *Am J Physiol*. 1975;229:983.
52. Soni H, Peixoto-Neves D, Matthews AT, Adebiyi A. TRPV4 channels contribute to renal myogenic autoregulation in neonatal pigs. *Am J Physiol Renal Physiol*. 2017;313(5):F1136.
57. Briggs JP, Schubert G, Schnermann J. Quantitative characterization of the tubuloglomerular feedback response: effect of growth. *Am J Physiol*. 1984;247:808.
62. Zhang J, Cong J, Yang J, et al. Morphologic and morphometric study on microvasculature of developing mouse kidneys. *Am J Physiol Renal Physiol*. 2018;315(4):F852.
66. Solhaug MJ, Wallace MR, Granger JP. Endothelium-derived nitric oxide regulates renal hemodynamics in the developing piglet. *Pediatr Res*. 1993;34:750.
68. Solhaug MJ, Ballèvre LD, Guignard JP, et al. Nitric oxide in the developing kidney. *Pediatr Nephrol*. 1996;10:529.
71. Ichikawa I, Maddox DA, Brenner BM. Maturational development of glomerular ultrafiltration in the rat. *Am J Physiol*. 1979;236:F465.
73. Lu Y, Zhang R, Ge Y, et al. Identification and function of adenosine A3 receptor in afferent arterioles. *Am J Physiol Renal Physiol*. 2015;308:F1020.
79. Prévot A, Mosig D, Rijtema M, Guignard JP. Renal effects of adenosine A1-receptor blockade with 8-cyclopentyl-1,3-dipropylxanthine in hypoxemic newborn rabbits. *Pediatr Res*. 2003;54(3):400.
85. Correia AG, Denton KM, Evans RG. Effects of activation of vasopressin-V1-receptors on regional kidney blood flow and glomerular arteriole diameters. *J Hypertens*. 2001;19(3 Pt 2):649.
92. Robillard JE, Weitzman RE. Developmental aspects of the fetal renal response to exogenous arginine vasopressin. *Am J Physiol*. 1980;238(5):F407.
94. Pelayo JC, Eisner GM, Jose PA. The ontogeny of the renin-angiotensin system. *Clin Perinatol*. 1981;8:347.
98. Solhaug MJ, Wallace MR, Granger JP. Nitric oxide and angiotensin II regulation of renal hemodynamics in the developing piglet. *Pediatr Res*. 1996;39:527.
108. Chappell MC. Biochemical evaluation of the renin-angiotensin system: the good, bad, and absolute? *Am J Physiol Heart Circ Physiol*. 2016;310(2):H137.
119. Bagby SP, LeBard LS, Luo Z, et al. ANG II AT1 and AT2 receptors in developing kidney of normal microswine. *Am J Physiol Renal Physiol*. 2002;283:755-764.
122. Friberg P, Sundelin B, Bohman SO, et al. Renin-angiotensin system in neonatal rats: induction of a renal abnormality in response to ACE inhibition or angiotensin II antagonism. *Kidney Int*. 1994;45:485.
124. Yoo KH, Norwood VF, el-Dahr SS, et al. Regulation of angiotensin II AT1 and AT2 receptors in neonatal ureteral obstruction. *Am J Physiol*. 1997;273:503.
126. Osborn JL, Hook JB, Bailie MD. Effect of saralasin and indomethacin on renal function in developing piglets. *Am J Physiol*. 1980;238:438.
134. García-Villalba P, Denkers ND, Wittwer CT, et al. Real-time PCR quantification of AT1 and AT2 angiotensin receptor mRNA expression in the developing rat kidney. *Nephron Exp Nephrol*. 2003;94(4):e154.
142. Semmekrot BA, Wiesel PH, Monnens LA, Guignard JP. Age differences in renal response to atrial natriuretic peptide in rabbits. *Life Sci*. 1990;46:849.
151. Coulson J, Couture R, Faussner A, et al. Bradykinin receptors (version 2019.4) in the IUPHAR/BPS guide to pharmacology database. *IUPHAR/BPS Guide to Pharmacology CITE*. 2019;2019(4).
163. el-Dahr SS, Yosipiv IV, Lewis L, Mitchell KD. Role of bradykinin B2 receptors in the developmental changes of renal hemodynamics in the neonatal rat. *Am J Physiol*. 1995;269:786.
179. Semama DS, Thonney M, Guignard JP. Role of endogenous endothelin in renal haemodynamics in newborn rabbits. *Pediatr Nephrol*. 1993;7:886.
181. Chin A, Radhakrishnan J, Fornell L, John E. Effects of tezosentan, a dual endothelin receptor antagonist, on the cardiovascular and renal systems of neonatal piglets. *J Pediatr Surg*. 2001;36:1824.
182. Ratliff BB, Sekulic M, Rodebaugh J, Solhaug MJ. Angiotensin II regulates NOS expression in afferent arterioles of the developing porcine kidney. *Pediatr Res*. 2010;68(1):29.
185. Ballèvre L, Thonney M, Guignard JP. Role of nitric oxide in the hypoxemia-induced renal dysfunction of the newborn rabbit. *Pediatr Res*. 1996;39:725.
190. Ratliff B, Rodebaugh J, Sekulic M, et al. Nitric oxide synthase and renin-angiotensin gene expression and NOS function in the postnatal renal resistance vasculature. *Pediatr Nephrol*. 2009;24:355-365.
191. Ratliff B, Sekulic M, Rodebaugh J, Solhaug MJ. Angiotensin II regulates NOS expression in afferent arterioles of the developing porcine kidney. *Pediatr Res*. 2010;68:29-34.
194. Rodebaugh J, Sekulic M, Davies W, et al. Neuronal nitric oxide synthase, nNOS, regulates renal hemodynamics in the postnatal developing piglet. *Pediatr Res*. 2012;71:144.
196. Tóth-Heyn P, Drukker A, Guignard JP. The stressed neonatal kidney: from pathophysiology to clinical management of neonatal vasomotor nephropathy. *Pediatr Nephrol*. 2000;14:227.
202. Ogawa T, Tomomasa T, Hikima A, et al. Developmental changes in cyclooxygenase mRNA expression in the kidney of rats. *Pediatr Nephrol*. 2001;16:618.
207. Norwood VF, Morham SG, Smithies O. Postnatal development and progression of renal dysplasia in cyclooxygenase-2 null mice. *Kidney Int*. 2000;58:2291.
223. Romagnoli C, De Carolis MP, Papacci P, et al. Effects of prophylactic ibuprofen on cerebral and renal hemodynamics in very preterm neonates. *Clin Pharmacol Ther*. 2000;67:676.
226. Ge Y, Murphy SR, Lu Y, et al. Endogenously produced 20-HETE modulates myogenic and TGF response in microperfused afferent arterioles. *Prostaglandins Other Lipid Mediat*. 2013;42:102-103.
232. Robillard JE, Nakamura KT. Neurohormonal regulation of renal function during development. *Am J Physiol*. 1988;254(6 Pt 2):F771.
235. Felder RA, Jose PA. Development of adrenergic and dopamine receptors in the kidney. In: Strauss J, ed. *Homeostasis, Nephrotoxicity, and Renal Anomalies in the Newborn*. The Hague: Martinus-Nijhoff; 1986:3-10.
240. Eiby YA, Shrimpton NY, Wright IM, et al. Inotropes do not increase cardiac output or cerebral blood flow in preterm piglets. *Pediatr Res*. 2016;80(6):870.

Postnatal Development of Glomerular Filtration Rate in Neonates

96

Jean-Pierre Guignard | Silvia Iacobelli

INTRODUCTION

The production of urine begins with the formation of an ultrafiltrate of plasma by the glomerulus. The function of the tubule is to modify this ultrafiltrate to allow an efficient excretion of waste products and the retention of those substances required to maintain constant body fluid volume and homeostasis. Glomerular filtration is also essential for the elimination of drugs. Alterations in glomerular filtration rate (GFR) have severe consequences for body fluid homeostasis. An estimate of GFR may be required to prescribe fluids, electrolytes, or drugs excreted by the kidney. This chapter reviews the factors that regulate GFR and the methods available to assess GFR in the newborn infant. It also briefly discusses the factors that may impair GFR during early development.

PHYSIOLOGY OF GLOMERULAR FILTRATION

Each kidney contains approximately 1 million nephrons (227,327 to 1,825,380) consisting of a glomerulus and a tubule. The number of nephrons correlates with birth weight (Fig. 96.1),[1,2] the count increasing by 25,743 for each 100 g of birth weight.[1] The glomerulus is a unique structure made out of a capillary network, the glomerular capillaries, supplied and drained by two resistance vessels, the afferent and the efferent arterioles.[3] This specialized bundle of capillaries is contained within the Bowman capsule. Urine formation starts with the production of an ultrafiltrate of plasma across the permselective glomerular capillary wall.[4,5] This wall consists of three layers: (1) the endothelial cell lining of the glomerular capillaries; (2) the glomerular basement membrane (GBM), composed of connective, noncellular tissues; and (3) the visceral epithelial cells of the Bowman capsule. The endothelial cells have numerous fenestrae with a diameter of 70 to 100 nm. The capillary endothelium acts as a screen to prevent blood cells and platelets from entering into contact with the GBM. The endothelial cells contain on their surface negatively charged sialoproteins and proteoglycans. The endothelial glycocalyx contributes to a primary glomerular anionic barrier, which diminishes the load of macromolecules being passed to the GBM and through the slit diaphragms.[6] Underneath the endothelium, the GBM forms a continuous layer that probably behaves as the filtration barrier for large molecules. It is an amorphous, 300- to 350-nm-thick extracellular structure formed of negatively charged glycoproteins, mainly triple-helical type IV collagen, proteoglycans, laminins, and fibronectins. The GBM-specific heparin sulfate proteoglycan 2 (perlecan) and agrin probably contribute to its charged selectivity because of the negatively charged heparan sulfate side chains they contain. The GBM is the main filtration barrier. The epithelium is formed by highly specialized visceral cells called *podocytes,* which are attached to the GBM by foot processes known as *pedicels.*[7] Membrane proteins such as nephrin and podocin are found in the foot processes and slit membranes. Mutations in these proteins result in massive proteinuria.[8] Adjacent pedicels are separated by filtration slits measuring approximately 25 nm by 60 nm in width, and a thin diaphragm bridges each gap. The diaphragms, in turn, contain rectangular "pores" with a dimension of 4 nm by 14 nm. Thus the filtration slits with their diaphragms could also constitute a size-selective filtration barrier. The podocytes may help in the phagocytosis of macromolecules. The size of the apertures in the glomerular filtration "barrier" is not the only factor that limits the passage of compounds through the glomerular capillary wall. The shape of the molecule, its flexibility and deformability, and its electric charge also play important roles. The molecular mass cutoff for the glomerular filter is approximately 70,000 Da. Thus albumin, with a molecular mass of 69,000 Da, passes through the filter in minute quantities. Smaller molecules pass through the filter more easily. Molecules with a molecular mass of less than 7000 Da pass through the filter freely. The glomerular ultrafiltrate thus initially contains small solutes and ions in the same concentration as present in the plasma.

The central part of the glomerular tuft is composed of irregularly shaped cells, the mesangial cells that hold the delicate glomerular structures. By contracting, the mesangial cells can modify the filtering surface area of the glomerular capillaries. The mesangial cells also act as phagocytes to prevent the accumulation of macromolecules in the GBM that have escaped from the capillaries.

The rate of ultrafiltration is governed by several factors: the balance of Starling forces across the capillary wall, the rate at which plasma flows into the glomerular capillaries, the permeability of the glomerular capillary wall to water and small solutes, and the total surface area of the capillaries.[4] The ultrafiltration coefficient (K_f) is defined as the product of the glomerular capillary permeability and the area of the capillary available for filtration. The permeability of the glomerular capillaries is approximately 100 times greater than the permeability of other capillaries elsewhere in the body. The hydrostatic pressure within the glomerulus favors filtration. It is opposed by the oncotic pressure within the lumen of the glomerular capillary. ΔP and $\Delta\pi$ represent the glomerular transcapillary hydrostatic and oncotic pressure, respectively. The net ultrafiltration pressure (P_{UF}) is defined as $\Delta P - \Delta\pi$. GFR is proportional to the sum of the Starling forces across the glomerular capillaries ($\Delta P - \Delta\pi$) times K_f.

$$GFR = K_f(\Delta P - \Delta\pi) \quad [96.1]$$

In normal conditions, P_{UF} and GFR are highly dependent on the arterial pressure within the glomerular capillaries, on renal blood flow (RBF), and on the glomerular plasma flow rate. The transcapillary hydrostatic pressure is also regulated by the balance between the afferent and efferent arteriolar resistance (Fig. 96.2). Pathologic conditions and drugs can affect GFR by modifying the pressure within the glomerular capillary (severe hypotension), K_f (drugs, diseases), or the oncotic pressure within the glomerular capillary (changes in the concentration of plasma proteins).

VASOACTIVE AGENTS

Several vasoactive agents modulate GFR and RBF during fetal and postnatal life.[9] Such agents include angiotensin II, the prostaglandins, atrial natriuretic peptide, endothelin, nitric oxide, bradykinin, and adenosine. Sympathetic nerves can also

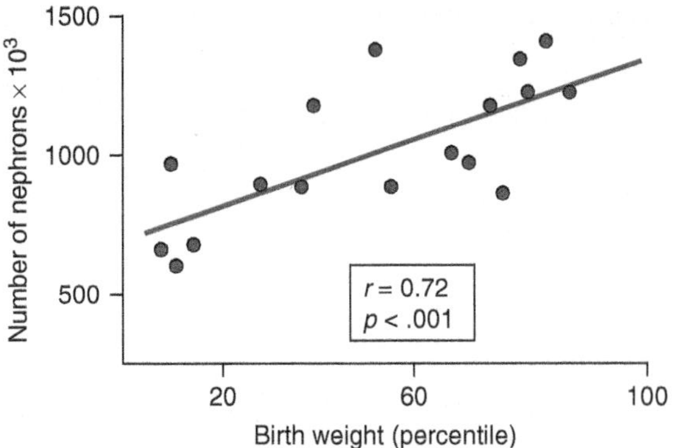

Fig. 96.1 In humans the number of nephrons correlates positively with birth weight, here expressed in percentiles. (Modified from Merlet-Bénichou C, Gilbert T, Vilar J, et al. Nephron number: variability is the rule—causes and consequences. *Lab Invest.* 1999;79:515.)

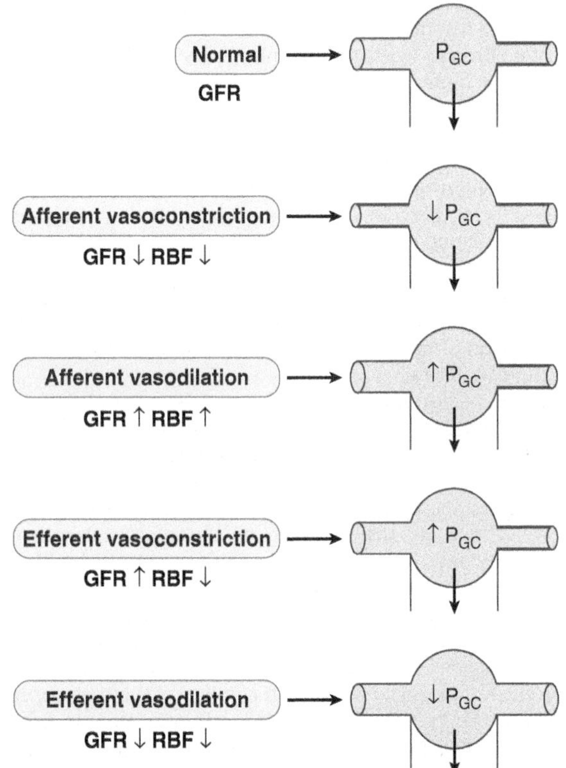

Fig. 96.2 Effects of changes in the afferent or efferent arteriolar tone on renal blood flow *(RBF)* and glomerular filtration rate *(GFR)*. P_{GC}, Glomerular capillary hydraulic pressure.

affect vascular tone. All these factors modulate GFR by affecting afferent or efferent vascular tone (see Fig. 96.2), as well as mesangial contractility. The main actions of the vasoactive agents are as follows:

- *Angiotensin II:* This peptide is a very potent constrictor of the afferent and efferent arterioles, acting on two types of receptors, the AT_1 and the AT_2 receptor subtypes. The AT_1 receptors are widely distributed and appear to mediate most of the biologic effects of angiotensin II. The exact role of the AT_2 receptors remains uncertain. Angiotensin II predominantly vasoconstricts the efferent arteriole, thereby increasing the intraglomerular pressure.[10] This mechanism serves to maintain GFR when the renal perfusion pressure decreases to low levels. Angiotensin also constricts the mesangial cells, with a consequent decrease in the ultrafiltration coefficient K_f. It also increases the sensitivity of the tubuloglomerular feedback mechanism.
- *Prostaglandins:* The prostaglandins are potent vasoactive metabolites of arachidonic acid.[11] In the kidney, prostaglandins are synthesized through the cyclooxygenase pathway by vascular smooth muscle cells, mesangial cells, and tubular and interstitial cells of the renal medulla. They are of major importance for maintaining constant the GFR of the newborn kidney perfused at low arterial pressures. They further protect the kidney when vasoconstrictor forces are activated (e.g., with hypotension, hypovolemia, sodium depletion states, and congestive heart failure).[9]
- *Atrial natriuretic peptide:* This 28-amino acid polypeptide is released by atrial myocytes in response to increased arterial pressure and effective circulating volume. It increases GFR by producing afferent vasodilation and relative efferent vasoconstriction, thus increasing GFR without significantly affecting RBF.[12] At high levels, atrial natriuretic peptide decreases systemic arterial pressure and increases the permeability of the glomerular capillaries. The kidney also produces a 32-amino acid natriuretic peptide, urodilatin, with the same local actions as atrial natriuretic peptide.
- *Nitric oxide:* Nitric oxide is a very potent vasodilator synthesized from L-arginine in endothelial cells throughout the body. In superficial nephrons, nitric oxide appears to decrease the preglomerular resistance but has much less effect on the postglomerular resistance.[13] In juxtamedullary nephrons, nitric oxide decreases the resistance in afferent and efferent arterioles. Nitric oxide appears essential to fine-tune the vasoconstrictor action of angiotensin II.[13,14]
- *Bradykinin:* This vasodilator and diuretic peptide is produced in the kidney by the effect of the enzyme kallikrein on kininogen. Bradykinin exerts its renal effects via β_2 receptors. The expression of β_2 receptors is higher in neonatal kidneys than in adult kidneys, a finding suggesting a role for this peptide during renal development. Bradykinin vasodilates the newborn kidney, as evidenced by the renal vasoconstriction that results from β_2-receptor blockade.[15] Therefore bradykinin decreases the ultrafiltration coefficient.
- *Adenosine:* Adenosine is an end product of adenosine triphosphate metabolism. Adenosine decreases GFR by vasodilating the efferent arteriole via A_2-receptor stimulation and by vasoconstricting the afferent arteriole via A_1-receptor stimulation.[16] By constricting the mesangial cells, adenosine further decreases the ultrafiltration coefficient.
- *Endothelin:* This peptide released from endothelial cells constricts the afferent and the efferent arterioles, thereby decreasing both GFR and RBF. However, there is circumstantial evidence that, at low endogenous concentrations, endothelin may actually vasodilate the glomerular vessels in fetuses and neonates.[17,18] Endothelin stimulates whole-kidney production of vasodilating prostaglandins that can partially balance its vasoconstrictive effects.
- *Sympathetic nervous system:* The sympathetic nerve endings are primarily of the α_1-adrenergic and β-adrenergic subtypes and secrete norepinephrine. Modest increases in renal nerve activity produce equivalent constrictions of both the afferent and the efferent arterioles, reducing RBF without significantly affecting GFR.[19] At elevated concentrations, as occurs in severe acute hemorrhage fetal distress and asphyxia, norepinephrine vasoconstricts the mesangial cells, thus decreasing GFR.

AUTOREGULATION OF GLOMERULAR FILTRATION RATE AND RENAL BLOOD FLOW

Autoregulation is necessary to prevent changes in GFR and RBF when blood pressure varies abruptly. Two systems are responsible for renal autoregulation: (1) a myogenic mechanism and (2) a tubuloglomerular feedback mechanism.

The *myogenic mechanism* refers to the intrinsic ability of arteries to constrict when blood pressure rises and to vasodilate when it decreases. This phenomenon modulates changes in RBF and GFR when blood pressure varies. The vascular constriction present in the myogenic response is effected by the opening of stretch-activated, nonselective cation channels in vascular smooth muscle.

The *tubuloglomerular feedback mechanism* involves the juxtaglomerular apparatus made of the macula densa and the juxtaglomerular cells. The macula densa cells sense the changes in sodium chloride delivery to the distal tubule that follow changes in blood pressure. When blood pressure increases, the macula densa cells actually sense the higher luminal concentrations of sodium or chloride that result from increased luminal flow. A drop in blood pressure and the consequent decrease in sodium chloride delivery stimulate angiotensin II formation by the juxtaglomerular cells. By constricting the efferent arteriole, angiotensin II increases the intraglomerular hydrostatic pressure and thus returns GFR toward normal levels.

CONCEPT OF CLEARANCE

The most common measurement of GFR is based on the concept of *clearance,* which relates the quantitative urinary excretion of a substance per unit time to the volume of plasma that, if "cleared" completely of the same contained substance, would yield a quantity equivalent to that excreted in the urine. The clearance (*C*) of a substance is expressed by the following formula:

$$C = U \cdot V / P, \quad [96.2]$$

where *U* represents the urinary concentration of the substance, *V* the urine flow rate, and *P* the plasma concentration of the substance. For its clearance to be equal to GFR, a substance must have the following properties: (1) it must be freely filterable through the glomerular capillary membranes—that is, not be bound to plasma proteins or sieved in the process of ultrafiltration; (2) it must be biologically inert and neither reabsorbed nor secreted by the renal tubules; and (3) it must be nontoxic and not alter renal function when infused in quantities that permit adequate quantification in plasma and urine.

Several substances, endogenous or exogenous, have been claimed to have the foregoing properties: inulin, creatinine, iohexol, diethylenetriaminepentaacetic acid, ethylenediaminetetraacetic acid, and sodium iothalamate. The experimental evidence that this is true has been produced only for inulin. The most commonly used markers in neonates are creatinine and inulin.

GLOMERULAR MARKERS

INULIN

Inulin, a fructose polysaccharide derived from dahlia roots and Jerusalem artichokes, has an Einstein-Stokes radius of 1.5 nm and a molecular mass of approximately 5200 Da. Inulin is inert, is not metabolized, and can be recovered quantitatively in the urine after parenteral administration.

The rate of excretion of inulin is directly proportional to and a linear function of the plasma concentration of inulin over a wide range. The clearance of inulin ($U \cdot V/P$) is consequently independent of its plasma concentration. Evidence that inulin is neither reabsorbed nor secreted by the renal tubules has been obtained in experimental micropuncture studies showing that (1) the concentration of inulin was identical in the Bowman space fluid and plasma, (2) 99.3% of inulin injected in the proximal tubule was collected in the distal tubule, and (3) the rate of recovery was the same when the peritubular plasma was loaded with inulin.[20]

Because the renal excretion of inulin thus occurs exclusively by glomerular filtration, its clearance is the most accurate index of GFR. Estimates of inulin clearance provide the basis for a standard reference against which the route or mechanisms of excretion of other substances can be ascertained. It should be stressed that inulin is a gold marker of GFR only when the $C = U \cdot V / P$, formula is used.

INULIN AS A MARKER OF GLOMERULAR FILTRATION RATE IN NEONATES

The same conclusion was reached from studies in preterm infants that showed that higher-molecular-mass inulin did not accumulate in the plasma of very immature babies into whom inulin was infused for several days, thus excluding any retention of the larger molecules.[21,22] In clinical practice, sinistrin, a readily soluble preparation of polyfructosan with side branching (extracted from bulbs of *Urginea maritima*), is more widely used. The clearance of sinistrin is identical to that of inulin. Because complicated analytic methods are required for its measurement, inulin and sinistrin cannot be used for routine clinical purposes. In neonates, only creatinine has been used broadly to assess GFR.

CREATININE

Creatinine is the anhydride of creatine, a compound that exists in skeletal muscle as creatine phosphate. It has a molecular mass of 113 Da. Conversion of creatine to creatinine is nonenzymatic and irreversible. The serum creatinine level reflects total body supplies of creatine and correlates with muscle mass. Creatinine is excreted through the kidneys in quantities proportional to the serum content. The renal excretion of endogenous creatinine is very similar to that of inulin in humans and several animal species. However, in addition to being filtered through the glomerulus, creatinine is secreted in part by the renal tubular cells. In spite of this, creatinine clearance correlates well with inulin clearance when the GFR is normal. This agreement results from the balance of two factors: (1) the excretion rate of creatinine is higher than the filtered rate because of the occurrence of tubular secretion of creatinine, and (2) the measured plasma creatinine concentration is higher than the true creatinine concentration because of the presence of non-creatinine chromogens that interfere with the colorimetric analysis of creatinine (*Jaffe reaction).*

Overestimation of GFR by creatinine clearance is usually more evident at low GFR. As GFR falls progressively during the course of renal disease, the renal tubular secretion of creatinine contributes an increasing fraction to urinary excretion, so creatinine clearance may substantially exceed the actual GFR.

The use of creatinine clearance to estimate GFR may be poorly reliable in uremic patients. Creatinine is uniformly distributed in the body water, and it diffuses into the gut. At a normal plasma concentration, the amount of creatinine entering the gut is negligible; it may become significant during renal failure, when the plasma creatinine concentration increases.[23] This phenomenon may also explain why creatinine clearance overestimates true GFR in patients with renal failure.

Although in use for decades, the methods available for the chemical determination of creatinine still present important drawbacks. As noted above, the traditional assay for measuring creatinine (the Jaffe reaction) substantially overestimates true serum creatinine levels because of the presence of interfering pseudochromogenic constituents in the blood. The major drawback for routine use in neonates is interference by bilirubin. Adaptations of the alkaline picrate assay have reduced the overestimation without totally eliminating the interference.[24] Although more specific than the Jaffe method, the enzymatic techniques are still biased by various interfering substances.[24] A new method coupling high-performance liquid chromatography

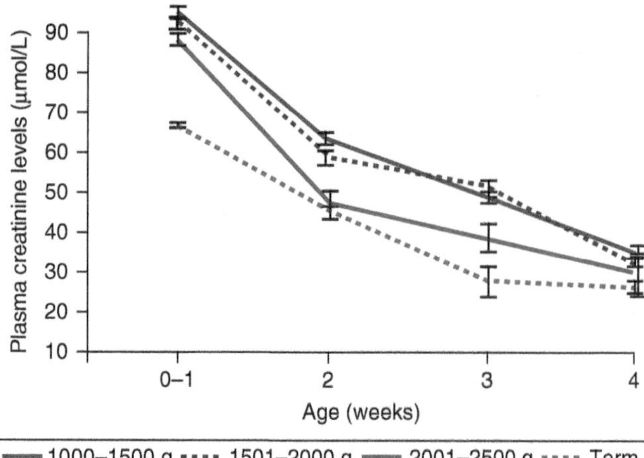

Fig. 96.3 Plasma creatinine concentrations (micromoles per liter) during the first weeks of life. (From Bueva A, Guignard JP. Renal function in preterm neonates. *Pediatr Res.* 1994;36:572.)

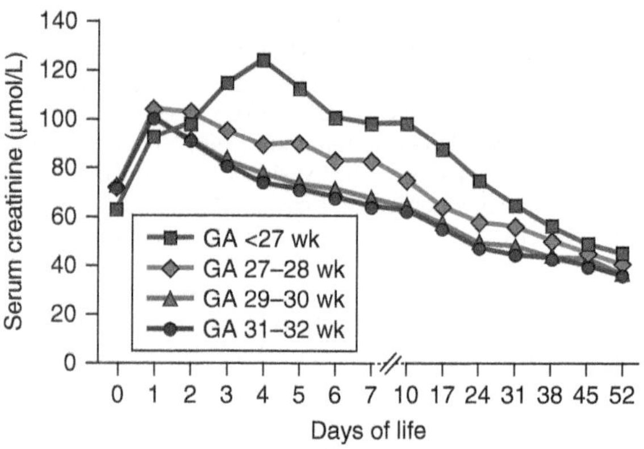

Fig. 96.4 Changes in serum creatinine in preterm neonates during the first 52 hours of postnatal life. Peak increases were noted on day 4 in the most premature infants. *GA*, Gestational age; *wk*, weeks. (Modified from Gallini F, Maggio L, Romagnoli C, et al. Progression of renal function in preterm neonates with gestational age ≤32 weeks. *Pediatr Nephrol.* 2000;15:119.)

and isotope dilution mass spectrometry appears to have an excellent specificity and low relative standard deviation.[25]

CREATININE AS A MARKER OF GLOMERULAR FILTRATION RATE IN NEONATES

The plasma creatinine concentration varies during the first postnatal weeks.[26,27] It is elevated at birth and decreases rapidly during the first week of life (Fig. 96.3); values stabilize at approximately 0.40 mg/dL (35 μmol/L; range, 0.14 to 0.70 mg/dL [12 to 61 μmol/L]) on the fifth postnatal day in term infants and somewhat later in very low-birth-weight infants.[27,28] A perfect equilibrium between fetal and maternal plasma creatinine concentrations has been observed throughout gestation.[29,30] So, the plasma creatinine concentration at the time of birth reflects maternal creatinine levels and maternal serum creatinine may affect neonatal levels for the first several days of life. In very premature neonates, the elevated plasma creatinine concentration at birth increases transiently; the highest levels are reached by the third day of life (Fig. 96.4 and Table 96.1).[31,32] The plasma urea level also rises significantly over time, but it does so in a more variable manner. Moreover, rising and high plasma urea levels can be expected in postnatal life in very low-birth-weight infants administered parenteral nutrition according to current recommendations.[33,34]

The transient postnatal increase in plasma creatinine concentration is probably the consequence of creatinine reabsorption (back diffusion) across leaky tubules,[35] as suggested by studies in piglets and newborn rabbits.[35,36] Plasma creatinine levels may take a month to reach *neonatal* levels in very low-birth-weight infants.[28,29]

IOHEXOL

Iohexol is a nonionic contrast agent with a molecular mass of 821 Da that appears to be eliminated exclusively by glomerular filtration. It exhibits minimal binding to proteins. In spite of a few reports showing a significant correlation between the urinary clearance of iohexol and the standard clearance of inulin,[37] the usefulness of iohexol in clinical pediatric practice remains unproven. It should not be used in the neonatal period.

IOTHALAMATE SODIUM

Iothalamate sodium is an ionic contrast agent with a molecular mass of 637 Da. It binds only minimally to plasma proteins,[38] and its clearance is independent of variations in plasma activity. The clearance of iothalamate was initially shown to correlate well with that of inulin; however, later studies unequivocally demonstrated that iothalamate is actively secreted by the renal tubules and perhaps also undergoes tubular reabsorption in humans and animal species. The agreement of iothalamate clearance with inulin clearance appears to be a fortuitous cancellation of errors between tubular reabsorption and secretion of iothalamate, and protein binding. In healthy adults, iothalamate clearance significantly overestimates inulin clearance, with a precision that is far from optimal.[39] Iothalamate has rarely been used in human neonates and in neonatal animal studies. Its use during the first month of life should be avoided.

AMINOGLYCOSIDES (GENTAMICIN, AMIKACIN)

Aminoglycoside antibiotics are potent antibacterial agents that are frequently used in high-risk neonates. After parenteral administration, they rapidly distribute in the extracellular space and are then eliminated, almost exclusively by glomerular filtration. They bind minimally to proteins and are excreted unchanged in the urine. Koren and colleagues[40] were the first to suggest that the clearance of gentamicin could be used to simply assess GFR in neonates receiving the drug. A significant correlation ($r = 0.77$; $P < .001$) was found between the urinary clearance of creatinine and the clearance of gentamicin calculated from its pharmacokinetic parameters.[40]

More recently, the clearance of amikacin, another aminoglycoside antibiotic, has been used to estimate GFR in sick neonates and predict the dosage regimens of other drugs eliminated by glomerular filtration.[41,42] The benefits of such an approach are obvious, and the hypothesis that the clearance

Table 96.1 Changes in Plasma Creatinine Over Time for Different Gestation Groups.

Group Gestational Age (wk)	Birth Plasma Creatinine (μmol/L)[a]	Peak Plasma Creatinine (μmol/L)[a]	Time to Peak Plasma Creatinine (h)[a]
23–26	67–92	195–247	40–78
27–29	65–89	158–200	28–51
30–32	60–69	120–158	25–40
33–45	67–79	99–140	8–23

[a]Ninety-five percent confidence intervals.

Modified from Miall LS, Henderson MJ, Turner AJ, et al. Plasma creatinine rises dramatically in the first 48 hours of life in preterm infants. *Pediatrics.* 1999;104:e76.

of amikacin or other aminoglycosides could provide valuable information on GFR in high-risk neonates under treatment should be validated.

RADIOISOTOPIC CLEARANCE STUDIES

Radioisotopic substances should not be used in the neonatal period and will not be discussed here.

CLINICAL ASSESSMENT OF GLOMERULAR FILTRATION RATE IN NEONATES

STANDARD CLEARANCES

INULIN URINARY CLEARANCE

Classic inulin clearance studies have been performed in premature and term neonates to provide data on (1) the reliability of inulin as a marker of GFR in human neonates, (2) the development of GFR in early postnatal life, and (3) the effect of disease states on GFR.

In the classic method, inulin is administered as a priming dose to achieve plasma concentrations close to 300 to 400 mg/L and is constantly infused to maintain constant levels. Accurate urine collection is performed by use of bladder catheterization, spontaneous voiding into plastic bags, or a collection tray. The clearance study is performed over a period of 3 to 4 hours. As in older children and adults, inulin is freely filtered even in the most immature human patients.[21,22] The standard inulin clearance must thus be considered the reference test in human neonates with which all other methods of estimating GFR should be compared.

CREATININE URINARY CLEARANCE

Creatinine is the most commonly used marker of GFR. Its clearance has been claimed to approximate true GFR in both term and preterm neonates. The validity of creatinine clearance has been assessed in low-birth-weight infants (mean birth weight, 1600 g; range, 1040 to 2275 g; postnatal age, 10 hours to 10 days). A significant correlation was found (r = 0.738) between inulin and creatinine clearance, but the scatter of values was substantial.[43] In infants with the lowest GFR (C_{in} < 12.5 mL/min/1.73 m^2), creatinine clearance overestimates true GFR, whereas it underestimates it in infants with higher filtration rates. Furthermore, a substantial underestimation of GFR by creatinine clearance has been demonstrated in both preterm and mature neonates.[44] Measurement of creatinine by a manual resin adsorption method, rather than by the automated method, improved the correlation.[44] Several factors can account for the variability of creatinine clearance determinations in very premature infants. These factors fall into two major categories: (1) those related to the transport of creatinine by the premature kidney and (2) those affecting the accuracy of plasma creatinine assays (noted earlier). Because of the low-normal levels of creatinine in the blood of neonates, small variations in laboratory measurements may spuriously alter the estimated concentration. Creatinine values obtained by the standard (Jaffe) method greatly overestimate the true creatinine concentration at values lower than 1.0 mg/dL.[45]

Other factors, such as hepatic injury, variations in muscle mass, abnormalities in protein catabolism, and/or patient fluid status, may further complicate the accuracy of GFR values determined using creatinine clearance.[46]

Inaccuracies in determining the true creatinine concentration in neonates, as well as uncertainties in renal tubular handling, point to a possible drawback in the use of creatinine as a glomerular marker, at least in very low-birth-weight infants. With these limitations in mind, the true creatinine clearance remains to date the best index of GFR for routine use.[47,48]

ESTIMATION OF GLOMERULAR FILTRATION RATE WITHOUT URINE COLLECTION

CONSTANT INFUSION OF INULIN WITHOUT URINE COLLECTION

The constant-infusion technique[49] assumes that the rate of intravenous infusion needed to maintain the plasma concentration of inulin at a constant level is equal to the rate of its excretion. At constant plasma levels, after inulin has equilibrated in its diffusion space, the clearance ($U \cdot V/P$) must be equal to the rate of infusion (I) divided by the plasma concentration: $C = U \cdot V/P = I/P$. To accelerate the achievement of a steady plasma concentration of inulin, a loading dose of inulin precedes the constant intravenous infusion. An estimate of the extracellular fluid volume (where inulin distributes) and of GFR is required to select the correct loading dose and infusion rate.

In studies in which inulin was constantly infused for only a few hours, significant overestimation of true GFR was observed.[50] As demonstrated by Coulthard and Ruddock,[21] reliable estimates of GFR can be obtained, provided inulin is constantly infused for 24 hours, with or without bolus injection at the start of the test. This method has the obvious advantage of eliminating the need for urine collection. Its main disadvantage is that it requires a constant infusion of long duration, as well as careful supervision of the test. Should the infusion stop for a moment, a long extra period of infusion will be necessary because the plasma inulin level falls exponentially but rises again only asymptomatically. The constant-infusion method also has the disadvantage of not reflecting acute changes in GFR.[49,51]

SINGLE-INJECTION (PLASMA DISAPPEARANCE CURVE) TECHNIQUE

The mathematical model for this technique is an open two-compartment system. The glomerular marker is injected in the first compartment, equilibrates with the second compartment, and is excreted from the first compartment by glomerular filtration. To obtain a well-defined plasma disappearance curve, and therefore an accurate calculation of the plasma clearance, numerous blood samples are required. Extension of the sampling period to 4 to 5 hours improves the precision of the results.

The single-injection method has been used in neonates, most often with inulin as a glomerular marker. Inulin is injected intravenously at a dose of 100 mg/kg, and the plasma concentration is measured at regular intervals over a few hours. Simplified techniques have been proposed that are based on a single-compartment model. They obviate the need for frequent blood sampling, but they are less accurate.

Results comparing data obtained by the single-injection technique with those obtained by the standard inulin clearance method are conflicting. Early studies using the plasma disappearance curve of inulin or polyfructosan claimed it to be a reliable index of GFR.[52] Later studies, however, questioned the validity of the single-injection technique in neonates. A large overestimation of 30% was demonstrated during the first week of life of neonates, when comparing the data of traditional urinary clearance of inulin with that observed with the plasma disappearance curve of inulin.[51,53] The overestimation in the younger neonates was ascribed to incomplete equilibration of inulin in its diffusion space during the duration of the test.[53]

SIMPLE CREATININE CLEARANCE METHOD IN NEONATES WITHOUT URINE COLLECTION

A formula often used to estimate GFR in children is as follows:

$$\text{GFR (mL/min)} \cdot 1.73\ \text{m}^2 = k \cdot L/P_{Cr}, \qquad [96.3]$$

where k is a constant, L (centimeters) represents body length, and P_{Cr} (milligrams per deciliter) is the plasma creatinine concentration. This formula is based on the assumption that creatinine excretion is proportional to body height and is inversely proportional to plasma creatinine concentration.[54] The value of factor k can be obtained from the formula k = GFR · L/P_{Cr}. Under steady-state conditions, k should be directly proportional to the muscle component of body weight, which correlates reasonably well with the daily urinary creatinine excretion rate. The mean value of k, calculated in 118 low-birth-weight infants with a corrected age of 25 to 105 weeks, was 0.33 ± 0.01. It rose to 0.45 in term infants up to 18 months.[54] When the plasma creatinine concentration was expressed in micromoles per liter, the corresponding values were 29 and 40, respectively. In both groups, a large scatter of values for k was observed, which the authors ascribed to the variability in body composition, differences in diet and creatinine excretion, errors in collection of urine, and inaccuracies in the measurement of creatinine. In spite of these limitations, the formula was claimed to be useful because it correlated well with the values obtained with the inulin single-injection technique.[55] However, it is unfortunate that the $k \cdot L/P_{Cr}$ formula has not been validated in neonates by comparison of its results with those given by the standard urinary $U \cdot V/P$ inulin clearance.

The accuracy of the $k = L/P_{Cr}$ formula as an estimate of GFR has been questioned.[50,56] In a study in infants younger than 1 year of age, k varied from 0.17 to 0.82, even though it was derived from the standard inulin clearance, and was found to vary markedly with the state of hydration. Moreover, the regression line relating the clearance estimated from the formula with the results obtained from the standard inulin clearance method differed significantly from the identity line.[50]

It is true that the $k \cdot L/P_{Cr}$ formula may be more informative clinically than the plasma creatinine value alone because the creatinine value is critically dependent on the percentage of muscle mass. Caution should be exercised, however, when one is using the formula as an estimate of GFR in studies aimed at defining pathophysiologic mechanisms in neonates.

DETECTION OF AN ABNORMAL GLOMERULAR FILTRATION RATE BY ALTERNATIVE ENDOGENOUS MARKERS

For a long time, some endogenous markers alternative to creatinine have been studied in adult and pediatric subjects, in order to detect an abnormal GFR.[57] These include cystatin C, β-trace protein (BTP), and β-2 microglobulin (B2M) to which studies on renal volumetry have been added. Among markers, cystatin C is an interesting contender in newborn life; however neonatal studies are limited.[58-62]

Cystatin C, a nonglycosated 13-kDa basic protein, is a proteinase inhibitor involved in the intracellular catabolism of proteins.[63] It is produced by all nucleated cells, freely filtered across the glomerular capillaries, almost completely reabsorbed, and catabolized in the renal proximal tubular cells. Its production rate is apparently constant and was initially claimed to be independent of inflammatory conditions, muscle mass, and sex. This claim has been questioned by a large study in 8058 adult inhabitants of Groningen.[64] In this study, male sex, older age, greater weight, higher serum C-reactive protein levels, and cigarette smoking were independently associated with higher cystatin C levels after adjustment for creatinine clearance. It thus appears that, in adults at least, cystatin C levels are influenced by factors other than renal function alone. Cystatin C concentrations are elevated in preeclamptic mothers toward term, and cystatin C m-RNA is highly expressed in their placenta.[65]

Initial studies suggested that cystatin C does not cross the placenta, and the same seems to apply to BTP,[66] but this has been questioned by a new report showing that small amounts of cystatin C cross the placenta.[67]

Cystatin C concentrations are highest at birth and then decrease, to stabilize after 12 months of age. It is uncertain whether cystatin C concentration is significantly higher in premature infants as compared with term infants.[60,68,69] Values of 1.63 ± 0.26 mg/L (mean ± standard deviation) were recorded during the first month of life, 0.95 ± 0.22 mg/L during months 1 to 12, and 0.72 ± 0.12 mg/L after the first year of life.[70] The concentration of cystatin C has been claimed to offer a greater sensitivity than creatinine concentration in detecting an abnormal GFR in newborn infants, as well as in children or adults. It is doubtful, however, whether this advantage is clinically significant. The use of cystatin C to predict GFR has important drawbacks. Because cystatin C is not excreted in the urine, the GFR predicted from its plasma concentration cannot be verified by its clearance. Cystatin C predicts only the presence of renal failure and does not measure the precise level of GFR. The extrarenal elimination of cystatin C at high serum levels, as well as higher intraindividual variation compared with the extrarenal elimination of creatinine, have been observed, in particular among transplant patients.[70] Estimates of GFR derived from equations based on serum levels of cystatin C, either alone or in combination with serum creatinine levels, have been published.[62] These equations have variable performance. Calibration of assays of serum cystatin C, as well as of creatinine, will require standardization before the routine use of these formulae. The complexity of some formulae is not a proof of accuracy. In a study of 75 neonates, cystatin C was not found to be more sensitive than creatinine as a marker of GFR.[71] In children, cystatin C has also been shown to be less reliable than the Schwartz formula in distinguishing impaired from normal GFR.[72] In addition, the assessment of GFR by the Schwartz formula has the obvious advantage of providing rational semiquantitative values of GFR related to the body surface area.

With regard to other markers, it is worthwhile to note that (1) increased serum B2M concentrations have been detected in newborns with respiratory distress syndrome, compared with healthy controls, thus questioning the feasibility of B2M to serve as a marker of estimated neonatal GFR[73]; (2) even if one review suggests that BTP may be a promising and more suitable marker, as it is unaffected by transplacental transport, its availability is even more limited than that of cystatin C.[74] Finally, a constructed cystatin C-based formula that includes kidney volume measures and body surface area has been proposed for estimating GFR in neonates.[75] However, this was not validated by the gold-standard inulin clearance.

DEVELOPMENT OF GLOMERULAR FILTRATION RATE

GLOMERULAR FILTRATION RATE AT BIRTH

GFR is low at birth. Standard inulin clearance studies performed by Guignard and colleagues[76-78] on the first 2 days of life indicated that GFR related to the body surface area increases rapidly from 28 to 35 weeks of gestation (Fig. 96.5). At 35 weeks of gestation, GFR reaches a plateau that is maintained up to the time of birth, a finding reflecting the parallel increase in kidney size and function. In these studies, GFR was approximately 20 mL/min/1.73 m² at birth in term infants and 12 to 13 mL/min/1.73 m² in preterm infants at 28 to 30 weeks of gestation. With use of the constant inulin infusion technique, low values for GFR (0.85 mL/kg/min) were also observed by van der Heijden and colleagues[79] in preterm

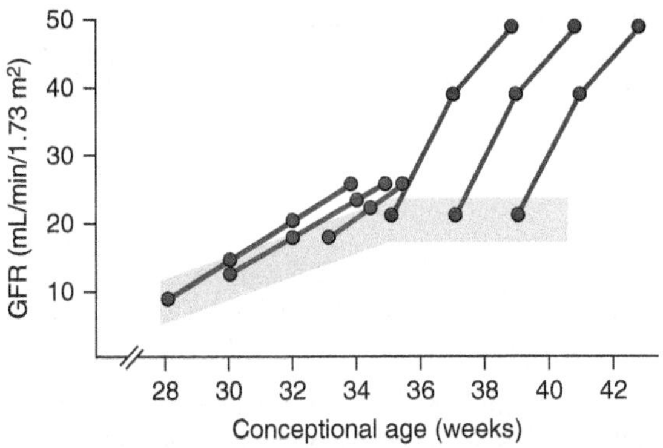

Fig. 96.5 Development of glomerular filtration rate *(GFR)* in relation to conceptional age during the last 3 months of gestation and the first month of life. The *shaded area* represents the range of normal values. The postnatal increase in GFR observed in neonates born before *(red dots)* or after *(purple dots)* 35 weeks of gestation is schematically represented. (Modified from Guignard JP. Renal function in the tiny, premature infant. *Clin Perinatol.* 1986;13:377.)

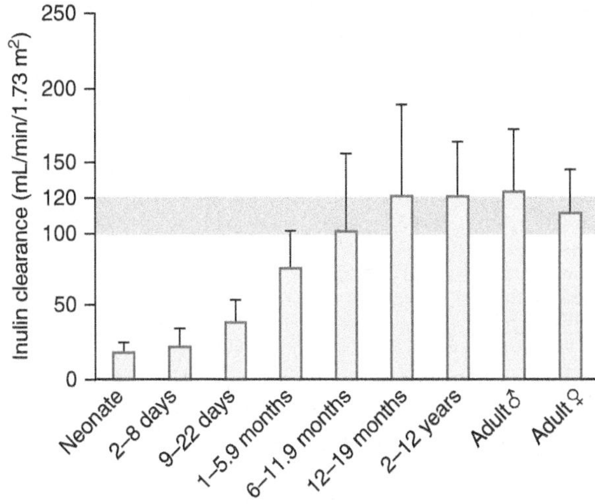

Fig. 96.6 Changes in glomerular filtration rate (inulin clearance) as a function of age.

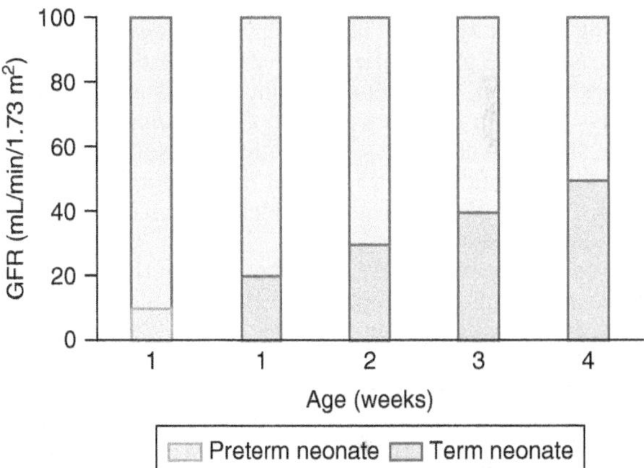

Fig. 96.7 Maturation of glomerular filtration rate during the first month of life of newborn infants. The *green area* of the columns represents normal adult values. (From Guignard JP, Drukker A. Clinical nephrology. In: Barratt TM, Avner ED, Harmon WE, eds. *Pediatric Nephrology*. Baltimore: Lippincott Williams & Wilkins; 1999.)

neonates on the second day of life. Siegel and Oh[48] and Gallini and colleagues[32] reported somewhat lower values of GFR in 2-day-old premature infants with a gestational age of less than 30 weeks using standard creatinine clearance techniques to assess GFR. This underestimation of GFR by the clearance of creatinine was also observed by Coulthard and colleagues.[80] Such an underestimation can be accounted for by the reabsorption of creatinine across leaky immature tubules.[29,35] In all these studies performed on the first few days of life, GFR correlated with gestational age.

MATURATION OF GLOMERULAR FILTRATION RATE IN THE FIRST MONTH OF LIFE

A rapid increase in GFR occurs in the first month of life. As shown in Fig. 96.6, inulin clearance doubles in the first 15 days of life.[76-79] The rate of increase in GFR is somewhat lower in the most premature infants. In spite of this impressive increase in GFR, as expressed in milliliters per minute per 1.73 m^2, the values achieved at 1 month of life are still only 50% of the adult values that are reached at the end of the first year of life (Fig. 96.7). This can be considered a state of "physiologic" renal insufficiency. Using the 24-hour constant infusion of inulin method in preterm infants, van der Heijden and colleagues[79] confirmed that GFR increases rapidly after birth; the postnatal increase is independent of body weight.

A similar pattern of maturation was observed in 66 physiologically stable term and premature infants undergoing creatinine clearance studies.[28] The lowest values of creatinine clearance were observed in the infants with the lowest birth weight (mean birth weight, 1332 ± 40 g; mean gestational age, 31.3 ± 0.5 weeks). This was true both for absolute values of creatinine clearance and for values expressed in relation to the body surface area. The progressive increase in creatinine clearance observed in the first 15 days of life also correlated significantly with postnatal age.[28,79,81,82] The study by Gallini and colleagues[32] confirmed the occurrence of a steady increase in creatinine clearance during the first 52 days of life, at which time values close to 42 and 27 mL/min/1.73 m^2 were recorded in 83 neonates born at gestational ages of 31 to 32 weeks and less than 27 weeks, respectively.

In a large, more recent study, Vieux and colleagues[81] described results for the urinary clearance of creatinine in 275 premature neonates (27 to 31 weeks of gestation) on days 7, 14, 21, and 28. These values should be used as reference values of GFR in the first month of life of neonates hospitalized in neonatal intensive care units. From their data, they propose simple formulae to calculate the expected median GFRs at different postnatal ages for a determined gestational age:

- Day 7: GFR = −63.57 + 2.85 × gestational age
- Day 14: GFR = −60.73 + 2.85 × gestational age
- Day 21: GFR = −53.97 + 2.85 × gestational age
- Day 28: GFR = −55.93 + 2.85 × gestational age

DETERMINANTS OF THE POSTNATAL INCREASE IN GLOMERULAR FILTRATION RATE

Several factors account for the striking postnatal maturation of GFR: (1) a decrease in renal vascular resistance and consequent increase in RBF, (2) an increase in systemic blood pressure and glomerular plasma flow rate, (3) an increase in the effective filtration pressure, and (4) an increase in K_f.

1. Renal vascular resistance is elevated at birth. It decreases rapidly in the first postnatal weeks. In rats, both afferent and efferent arteriolar resistances decrease by a factor of 3 during maturation.[83] The elevated renal vascular resistance is mainly the result of the high activity of vasoactive agents and hormones and the relative responsiveness of the newborn

Table 96.2 Normal Mean Arterial Blood Pressure in the Newborn Infant.

Age	<1.0 kg	1.0–1.5 kg	>2.5 kg
Birth	33 ± 15	39 ± 18	49 ± 19
1 wk	41 ± 15	47 ± 18	60 ± 19
2 wk	45 ± 15	50 ± 18	64 ± 19
4 wk	48 ± 15	53 ± 18	68 ± 19

From Ong WH, Guignard JP, Sharma A, Arandaet JV. Pharmacological approach to the management of neonatal hypertension. *Semin Neonatol.* 1998;3:149.

infant to these vasoconstrictor and vasodilator substances. The decrease is associated with a rise in RBF and an improvement in glomerular plasma flow rate. In human neonates the maturational increase in GFR parallels the increase in RBF.[76] Improved RBF and glomerular plasma flow rate probably explain the 30% immediate increase in inulin clearance associated with delayed clamping of the umbilical cord.[84]

2. The striking increase in systemic blood pressure occurring during the first weeks of life (Table 96.2) is associated with an increase in the glomerular capillary hydrostatic pressure. This favors filtration. Creatinine clearances measured on the first 2 days of life in neonates of 28 to 43 gestational weeks have been shown to correlate significantly with blood pressure.[28,76]
3. The low oncotic pressure present in newborn infants resulting from low plasma protein concentrations favors the ultrafiltration pressure. Furthermore, because the glomerular hydrostatic pressure increases more rapidly than the oncotic pressure during development, the effective filtration pressure rises. Because of the low systemic blood pressure, the glomerular capillary hydraulic pressure is extremely low in early life and increases in parallel with the rise in blood pressure. The glomerular transcapillary hydraulic pressure difference increases by 10 mm Hg from the third week of life to adulthood in rats.[85] In guinea pigs the effective filtration pressure increases 2.5 times in the first 50 days of life.[86] Increases in glomerular capillary hydraulic pressure and glomerular transcapillary hydraulic pressure difference could contribute to changes in GFR during early maturation.
4. K_f reflects both the surface and the permeability of the filtration barrier. Maturational changes in K_f also account for the postnatal rise in GFR. K_f is low in the newborn. It is significantly lower in 40- to 64-day-old rats than in adult animals.[87,88] The GBM surface area has been shown to increase 3.5-fold from birth to adulthood in rats,[89] whereas the glomerular capillary cross-sectional area increased 10-fold from 3 weeks to adulthood in dogs.[90] A 40% increase in glomerular corpuscular diameter has been observed in humans from birth to adulthood.[91] If this corresponds to increases in the glomerular filtering area, these changes should improve GFR. The increases in the area of the endothelial fenestrae observed in growing rats can also explain the postnatal rise in GFR. From studies in 1- and 6-week-old dogs, Goldsmith and colleagues[92] concluded that an increase in both the glomerular filtering area and the pore density accounted for the postnatal increase in GFR.

The increase in the number of negatively charged sites in the GBM[93] and the 2.5-fold increase in GBM thickness[88] observed in growing rats could account for the decreased permeability to large molecules (proteins) in the first postnatal weeks of human neonates. Clearance studies in human infants into whom inulin or polyfructosides with variable molecular masses were infused have clearly shown that the high-molecular-mass inulin did not accumulate in preterm infants (birth weight of 850 to 1250 g) into whom inulin was infused for 2 to 10 days.[21] The filterability of inulin (molecular mass 5200 Da) appears similar in neonates and older children. This does not, however, exclude subtle changes in glomerular capillary permeability during growth. Experimental studies on isolated rat glomeruli also failed to demonstrate an increase in glomerular hydraulic permeability during growth.[94]

FACTORS THAT CAN IMPAIR GLOMERULAR FILTRATION RATE IN THE PERINATAL PERIOD

The low GFR of the very low-birth-weight infant is maintained by a delicate balance of intrarenal vasoconstrictor and vasodilator forces. In immature animals, various conditions such as hypoxemia, hypercapnia, metabolic acidosis and alkalosis, hypothermia, and hyperthermia can dramatically increase renal vascular resistance.[95] Similarly, human neonates are prone to the development of vasomotor nephropathy and acute renal failure; the main causes include hypotension, hypovolemia, hypoxemia, and perinatal asphyxia.[95] Other causes of renal failure include the administration of angiotensin-converting enzyme inhibitors and nonsteroidal antiinflammatory drugs. Positive-pressure artificial ventilation at high mean airway pressure can also decrease RBF and impair GFR. In all these situations, the interaction between vasoconstricting and vasodilating forces is rather complex and their effects on the systemic and the intrarenal circulations can differ.

Perinatal hypoxemia and *asphyxia* are common causes of impaired GFR in neonates. The renal vasoconstriction is the consequence of increased activation of the renin-angiotensin system, changes in intrarenal adenosine levels, and increased levels of vasopressin, catecholamines, or other vasoconstrictor substances.[95] Contraction of blood volume (hypovolemia) with or without failure of the cardiac pump is often present in the neonates.[96] Experimental studies on the hypoxemia-induced decrease in GFR suggest a key role for intrarenal adenosine[97] in mediating the vasomotor nephropathy. By decreasing the postglomerular resistance, this agent induces a fall in the intraglomerular pressure and consequently GFR (Fig. 96.8). The hypothesis that adenosine plays a key role in the pathogenesis of the hypoxemic vasomotor nephropathy is supported by the fact that theophylline, an antagonist of adenosine cell surface receptors, protects the immature kidney from the deleterious hypoxemic stress.

Clinical studies using *theophylline* in high-risk asphyxiated term neonates,[98-100] in premature neonates with asphyxia,[101] and in very premature neonates with severe idiopathic respiratory distress syndrome[102] suggest a beneficial effect of theophylline in protecting GFR, and one recent systematic review concludes that a single dose of prophylactic theophylline helps in prevention of acute kidney injury/severe renal dysfunction in term neonates with severe birth asphyxia.[103] In the neonatal rabbit model, the specific adenosine A_1 receptor antagonist 8-cyclopentyl-1,3-dipropylxanthine does not offer the same protection as theophylline.[104]

In preterm neonates, administration of a single oral dose of *caffeine* (15 mg/kg) rapidly increased urine flow rate, the water output-input ratio, and creatinine clearance.[105] Like theophylline, at pharmacologic doses, caffeine acts by blocking the adenosine receptors A_1 and A_{2a}, by inhibiting phosphodiesterase and consequently increasing the cyclic 3,5-adenosine monophosphate concentration, and by translocating intracellular calcium.[106] The hypothesis that the various benefits of caffeine, which include the prevention of bronchopulmonary dysplasia, are in part related to a sustained improvement in GFR and diuresis remains to be demonstrated.

Ventilation of human neonates and newborn animals with high airway pressures has deleterious effects on renal function,

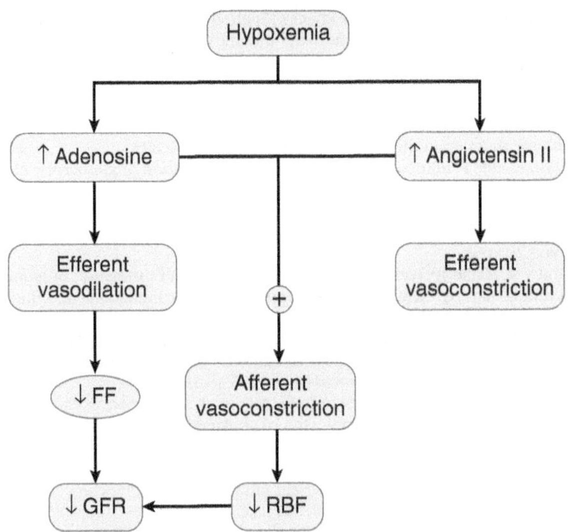

Fig. 96.8 Hypoxemia activates the release of intrarenal adenosine and angiotensin II. Whereas angiotensin II preferentially vasoconstricts the efferent arteriole, adenosine effectively vasodilates it. The decrease in the filtration fraction *(FF)* induced by hypoxemia reflects net efferent vasodilation. The combined net effect of angiotensin II and adenosine is thus afferent vasoconstriction and efferent vasodilatation. This results in a decrease in the intraglomerular pressure and consequently in glomerular filtration rate *(GFR)*. *RBF,* Renal blood flow.

resulting from decreased venous return and low cardiac output, increased renal sympathetic nervous activity, and high serum vasopressin levels.[107] Recent observations in preterm lambs suggest that mechanical ventilation may also impair nephrogenesis, as demonstrated by a long-lasting decrease in the glomerular capillary surface area.[108] Whether the same occurs in human neonates is not yet known.

Angiotensin-converting enzyme inhibitors can lead to a dramatic fall in mean arterial pressure, accompanied by persistent oliguria.[95] The oliguric renal insufficiency is similar to that observed in fetuses and neonates of women who are given angiotensin-converting enzyme inhibitors shortly before birth. Angiotensin-converting enzyme inhibitors interfere with the renin-angiotensin system, which is physiologically active during fetal and neonatal life.[95]

High prostaglandin activity is physiologically necessary to maintain sufficient perfusion of the newborn kidney. Serum prostaglandin levels are also high in infants with chronic cardiac failure, patent ductus arteriosus, hypotension, or hypovolemia.[109] Prostaglandin synthesis inhibitors, used before birth to prevent the premature onset of labor or after birth to promote the closure of a hemodynamically active patent ductus arteriosus, reduce GFR and RBF.[110-112] They do so by blunting the effect of vasodilator prostaglandins on the afferent arteriole. Decreases in GFR have been described in neonates exposed to indomethacin before birth, as well as in neonates given indomethacin for the closure of a patent ductus arteriosus. The deleterious effect is usually transient and results in water retention and hyponatemia.[110,111] Other nonselective (ibuprofen) or selective (nimesulide) cyclooxygenase inhibitors likely share the same adverse effects.[113,114] In a study by De Cock and colleagues[41] both ibuprofen and acetylsalicylic acid impaired the clearance of amikacin, and thus presumably reduced GFR. More recently, ibuprofen administered for closure of a patent ductus arteriosus in 74 very preterm infants (gestational age, 27 to 31 weeks) impaired GFR, as measured by the urinary clearance of creatinine (Fig. 96.9).[115] The decrease in GFR was sustained for 1 month. In experimental immature animals, cyclooxygenase-nonselective and cyclooxygenase 2-selective inhibitors similarly impair GFR and RBF.[116]

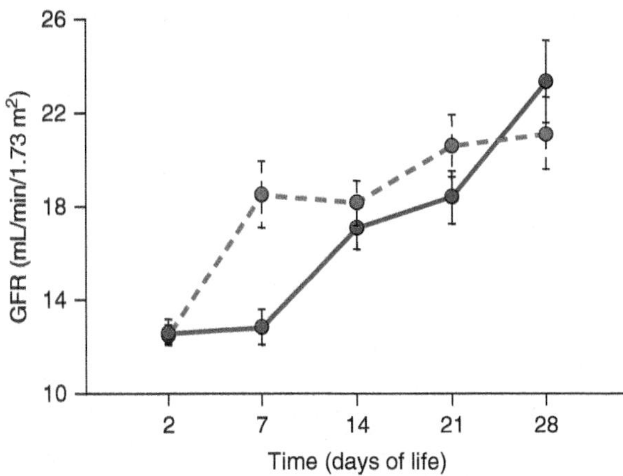

Fig. 96.9 Glomerular filtration rate *(GFR)* in infants receiving ibuprofen *(red dots and line)* and control infants *(green dots and line)* during the first month of life; 148 infants, 74 pairs on day 7. Values are the mean ± standard error of the mean. Overall adjusted difference $P = .003$. (From Vieux R, Desandes R, Boubred F, et al. Ibuprofen in very preterm infants impairs renal function for the first month of life. *Pediatr Nephrol*. 2010;25:267.)

CONCLUSION

Glomerular filtration is the first essential step in urine formation. Its maintenance within narrow limits is mandatory and requires subtle autoregulatory mechanisms that involve the action of autacoids, vasoactive substances, and intrinsic myogenic mechanisms. Physiologic changes in GFR during maturation may affect body fluid homeostasis and the excretion of drugs by the neonate; therefore an estimation of GFR will help the neonatologist to rationally prescribe fluids, electrolytes, and drugs.

A complete reference list is available at www.ExpertConsult.com. 

SELECT REFERENCES

1. Hughson M, Farris 3rd AB, Douglas-Denton R, et al. Glomerular number and size in autopsy kidneys: the relationship to birth weight. *Kidney Int*. 2003;63:2113.
2. Merlet-Bénichou C, Gilbert T, Vilar J, et al. Nephron number: variability is the rule. Causes and consequences. *Lab Invest*. 1999;79:515.
3. Pollak MR, Quaggin SE, Hoening MP, Dworkin LD. The glomerulus: the sphere of influence. *Clin J Am Soc Nephrol*. 2014;9:1461.
4. Deen WM, Lazzara MJ, Myers BD, et al. Structural determinants of glomerular permeability. *Am J Physiol*. 2001;281:F579.
5. Tryggvason K, Wartiovaara J. How does the kidney filter plasma? *Physiology*. 2005;20:96.
6. Haraldsson B, Sörensson J. Why do we not all have proteinuria? An update of our current understanding of the glomerular barrier. *News Physiol Sci*. 2004;19:7.
7. Pavenstädt H, Kriz W, Kretzler M. Cell biology of the glomerular podocyte. *Physiol Rev*. 2003;83:253.
8. Tryggvason K, Patrakka J, Wartiovaara J. Hereditary proteinuria syndromes and mechanisms of proteinuria. *N Engl J Med*. 2006;354:1387.
9. Guignard JP, Gouyon JB, John EG. Vasoactive factors in the immature kidney. *Pediatr Nephrol*. 1991;5:443.
10. Arendshorst WJ, Brännström K, Ruan X. Actions of angiotensin II on the renal microvasculature. *J Am Soc Nephrol*. 1999;10:S149.
11. Morris JL, Rosen DA, Rosen KR. Nonsteroidal anti-inflammatory agents in neonates. *Paediatr Drugs*. 2003;5:285.
12. Semmekrot BA, Wiesel PH, Monnens LA, Guignard JP. Age differences in renal response to atrial natriuretic peptide in rabbits. *Life Sci*. 1990;46:849.
13. Ballèvre L, Thonney M, Guignard JP. Role of nitric oxide in the hypoxemia-induced renal dysfunction of the newborn rabbit. *Pediatr Res*. 1996;39:725.
14. Krämer BK, Kammerl MC, Kömhoff M. Renal cyclooxygenase-2 (COX-2). Physiological, pathophysiological, and clinical implications. *Kidney Blood Press Res*. 2004;27:43.
15. Toth-Heyn P, Guignard JP. Bradykinin in the newborn kidney. *Nephron*. 2002;9:571.
16. Gouyon JB, Arnaud M, Guignard JP. Renal effects of low-dose aminophylline and enprofylline in newborn rabbits. *Life Sci*. 1988;42:1271.

17. Semama DS, Thonney M, Guignard JP. Role of endogenous endothelin in renal haemodynamics of newborn rabbits. *Pediatr Nephrol*. 1993;7:886.
18. Hunley TE, Kon V. Update on endothelins—biology and clinical implications. *Pediatr Nephrol*. 2001;16:1752.
19. Yuan BH, Robinette JB, Conger JD. Effect of angiotensin II and norepinephrine on isolated rat afferent and efferent arterioles. *Am J Physiol*. 1990;258:F741.
20. Marsh D, Frasier C. Reliability of inulin for determining volume flow in rat renal cortical tubules. *Am J Physiol*. 1965;209:283.
21. Coulthard MG, Ruddock V. Validation of inulin as a marker for glomerular filtration in preterm babies. *Kidney Int*. 1983;23:407.
22. Wilkins BH. The glomerular filterability of polyfructosan-S in immature infants. *Pediatr Nephrol*. 1992;6:319.
23. Jones JD, Burnett PD. Implication of creatinine and gut flora in the uremic syndrome: induction of "creatininase" in colon contents of the rat by dietary creatinine. *Clin Chem*. 1972;18:280.
24. Myers GL, Miller WG, Coresh J, et al. Recommendations for improving serum creatinine measurement: a report from the laboratory working group of the National Kidney Disease Education Program. *Clin Chem*. 2006;52:5.
25. Stokes P, O'Connor G. Development of a liquid chromatography-mass spectrometry method for high-accuracy determination of creatinine in serum. *J Chromatogr B Analyt Technol Biomed Life Sci*. 2003;25:125.
26. Feldman H, Guignard JP. Plasma creatinine in the first month of life. *Arch Dis Child*. 1982;57:123.
27. Stonestreet BS, Oh W. Plasma creatinine levels in low-birth-weight infants during the first three months of life. *Pediatrics*. 1978;61:788.
28. Bueva A, Guignard JP. Renal function in preterm neonates. *Pediatr Res*. 1994;36:572.
29. Guignard JP, Drukker A. Why do newborn infants have a high plasma creatinine? *Pediatrics*. 1999;103(4):e49.
30. Forestier F, Daffos F, Rainaut M, et al. Blood chemistry of normal human fetuses at mid-trimester of pregnancy. *Pediatr Res*. 1987;21:579.
31. Miall LS, Henderson MJ, Turner AJ, et al. Plasma creatinine rises dramatically in the first 48 hours of life in preterm infants. *Pediatrics*. 1999;104:e76.
32. Gallini F, Maggio L, Romagnoli C, et al. Progression of renal function in preterm neonates with gestational age ≤32 weeks. *Pediatr Nephrol*. 2000;15:119.
33. van Goudoever JB, Carnielli V, Darmaun D, Sainz de Pipaon M. ESPGHAN/ESPEN/ESPR/CSPEN working group on pediatric parenteral nutrition. ESPGHAN/ESPEN/ESPR/CSPEN guidelines on pediatric parenteral nutrition: amino acids. *Clin Nutr*. 2018;37(6 Pt B):2315–2323.
34. Yang S, Lee BS, Park HW, et al. Effect of high vs standard early parenteral amino acid supplementation on the growth outcomes in very low birth weight infants. *J Parenter Enteral Nutr*. 2013;37(3):327–334.
35. Matos P, Duarte-Silva M, Drukker A, Guignard JP. Creatinine reabsorption by the newborn rabbit kidney. *Pediatr Res*. 1998;44:639.
36. Alt JM, Colenbrander B, Forsling ML, Macdonald AA. Perinatal development of tubular function in the pig. *Q J Exp Physiol*. 1984;69:693.
37. Nilsson-Ehle P. Iohexol clearance for the determination of glomerular filtration rate: 15 years' experience in clinical practice. *eJIFCC*. 2002;13:1–5.
38. Anderson CF, Sawyer TK, Cutler RE. Iothalamate sodium I 125 vs cyanocobalamin Co 57 as a measure of glomerular filtration rate in man. *J Am Med Assoc*. 1968;204:653.
39. Botev R, Mallie JP, Wetzels JF, et al. The clinician and estimation of glomerular filtration rate by creatinine-based formulas: current limitations and quo vadis. *Clin J Am Soc Nephrol*. 2011;6:937.
40. Koren G, James A, Perlman M. A simple method for the estimation of glomerular filtration rate by gentamicin pharmacokinetics during routine drug monitoring in the newborn. *Clin Pharmacol Ther*. 1985;38:680.
41. De Cock RFW, Allegaert K, Schreuder MF, et al. Maturation of the glomerular filtration rate in neonates, as reflected by amikacin clearance. *Clin Pharmocokinet*. 2012;51:105.
42. Zhao W, Biran V, Jacqz-Aigrain E. Amikacin maturation model as a marker of renal maturation to predict glomerular filtration rate and vancomycin clearance in neonates. *Clin Pharmacokinet*. 2013;52:1127.
43. Stonestreet BS, Bell EF, Oh W. Validity of endogenous creatinine clearance in low birthweight infants. *Pediatr Res*. 1979;13:1012.
44. Wilkins BH. A reappraisal of the measurement of glomerular filtration rate in pre-term infants. *Pediatr Nephrol*. 1992;6:323.
45. Huang YC, Chiou WL. Creatinine XII: comparison of assays of low serum creatinine levels using high-performance liquid chromatography and two picrate methods. *J Pharmacol Sci*. 1983;72:836.
46. Kastl JT. Renal function in the fetus and neonate - the creatinine enigma. *Semin Fetal Neonatal Med*. 2017;22:83–89.
47. Ross B, Cowett RM, Oh W. Renal function of low birth weight infants during the first two months of life. *Pediatr Res*. 1977;11:1162.
48. Siegel SR, Oh W. Renal function as a marker of human fetal maturation. *Acta Paediatr Scand*. 1976;65:481.
49. Cole BR, Giangiacomo J, Ingelfinger JR, Robson AM. Measurement of renal function without urine collection. *N Engl J Med*. 1972;287:1109.

97 Renal Transport of Sodium During Development

Michel Baum

INTRODUCTION

The kidney is responsible for maintaining a constant composition and volume of the extracellular fluid. This steady state is achieved by the remarkable capacity of the kidney to maintain sodium balance between what is absorbed in the intestine and what is excreted in the urine. To achieve this, the adult kidney filters approximately 150 L of an ultrafiltrate of plasma from which the tubules reabsorb the vast majority of the filtered solutes and water. This leaves the urine with not only waste products but also the amount of sodium and water virtually equal to that consumed.

The glomerular filtration rate of the term neonatal kidney is approximately 2 mL/min.[1] When factored for an adult's surface area, the glomerular filtration rate is still only 25% of the adult's rate of 100 to 120 mL/min/1.73 m^2. The adult glomerular filtration rate, corrected for body surface area of 1.73 m^2, is reached at approximately 2 year of age.[2] Thus, during the course of postnatal renal development, there is a substantial increase in the glomerular filtration rate that must be matched by an increase in the capacity to reabsorb sodium, which is called *glomerular-tubular balance*. In other words, the developmental increase in sodium absorption matches the developmental increase in glomerular filtration rate. Postnatal renal development is not only characterized by an increase in the abundance of sodium transporters along the nephron but also by isoform changes in some key transporters, as well as maturational changes in the hormones that regulate sodium transport to match sodium intake and to protect the composition and volume of the extracellular fluid during times of stress such as volume depletion.

The very premature neonate has glomerular-tubular imbalance. Although the glomerular filtration rate in a premature infant may be only a fraction of that of the term infant,[1] it nonetheless filters an ultrafiltrate of plasma containing sodium at a rate greater than the immature tubule's capacity to reabsorb sodium.[1,3-6] Shown in Fig. 97.1 is the fractional excretion of sodium, the percentage of filtered sodium excreted in the urine, in premature compared with term infants. As can be seen, very premature infants excrete 5% to 10% of the filtered sodium, whereas the term infant has urine that has approximately 0.1% to 0.2% of the filtered sodium in the urine.[7] Thus there is substantive salt wasting by the premature neonate.[7] Glomerular-tubular imbalance is also found for glucose, in which neonates less than 30 weeks gestation often have significant glucosuria.[1,8] Neonates normally consume breast milk, which has a very low concentration of sodium. Thus very premature infants will develop hyponatremia and volume depletion if their milk is not supplemented with sodium. Fig. 97.2 depicts that premature neonates will be in negative sodium balance and will thus require sodium supplementation. Another important point shown in Fig. 97.2 is that term neonates are in slightly positive salt balance, which is essential for growth.

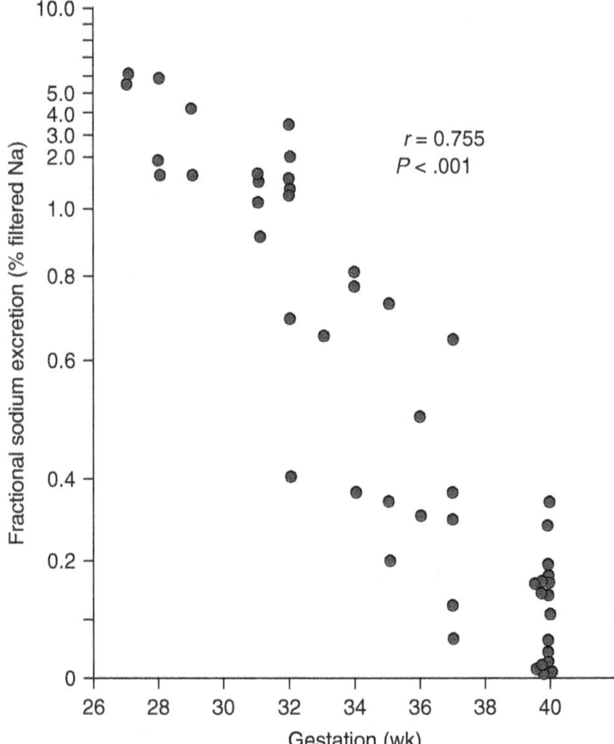

Fig. 97.1 Fractional excretion of sodium in infants of different gestational age. The percentage of filtered sodium excreted in the urine was higher in premature infants and decreased to very low levels as the infants approach term. (From Siegel SR, Oh W. Renal function as a marker of human fetal maturation. *Acta Paediatr Scand.* 1976;65:481.)

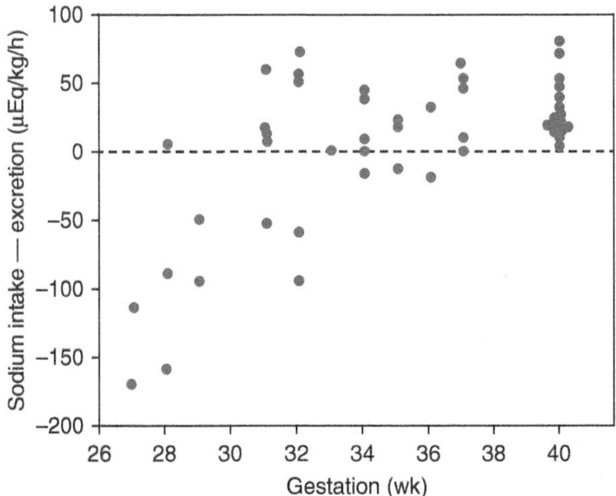

Fig. 97.2 Sodium balance in neonates as a factor of gestational age. Premature neonates are in negative salt balance due to immature tubular transport. Term neonates are in positive salt balance, which is essential for growth. (From Siegel SR, Oh W. Renal function as a marker of human fetal maturation. *Acta Paediatr Scand.* 1976;65:481.)

The term neonate is able to maintain a positive sodium balance over a wide range of sodium intake.[4,9] In addition, the neonate is less able to excrete a sodium load than an adult. This was exemplified by studies comparing the ability of neonatal and adult dogs to excrete a volume of saline equal to 10% of their weight.[10] Neonatal dogs had a blunted natriuretic response to saline loading compared with adults excreting only 10% of the sodium infused in 2 hours compared with 50% of the sodium infused in adult dogs. The ability to excrete a sodium load was not explained by the difference in glomerular filtration rate (GFR) with saline expansion in the two groups. The authors concluded that the difference was due to enhanced distal sodium absorption in the neonate.

PRINCIPLES OF MEMBRANE SODIUM TRANSPORT

The huge volume of isotonic fluid filtered each day by the glomerulus is delivered to the proximal tubule. The glomerular filtrate contains the same concentration of solutes as that in the blood, but it by and large is lacking the large molecular weight proteins in plasma. The proximal tubule reabsorbs approximately two thirds of the glomerular ultrafiltrate in an isotonic fashion. In other words, the glomerular ultrafiltrate has a sodium concentration of 140 mEq/L and osmolality of 290 mOsm/kg water. By the end of the proximal tubule the luminal fluid sodium concentration and osmolality are unchanged. However, the composition of the fluid changes substantively.

The proximal tubule predominantly reabsorbs organic solutes, sodium bicarbonate and sodium chloride. Reabsorption of solutes without water would result in a hypotonic luminal fluid if it were not for the fact that the proximal tubule has abundant expression of aquaporin 1, a water channel found on the apical and basolateral membranes of most cells.[11,12] Thus the high water permeability of the proximal tubular cell results in osmotic equilibration of the luminal fluid to that of the blood in the peritubular capillaries. The osmotic permeability of the neonatal proximal tubule is higher than that of the adult tubule.[13] A cartoon of the nephron is shown in Fig. 97.3.

Following the proximal tubule is the thin descending limb that also expresses aquaporin 1 and is thus highly permeable to water. The expression of aquaporins on the apical and basolateral membrane allows water to flow into the hypertonic medulla and concentrate the luminal fluid. At the bend of the thin limb the characteristics of the tubule changes significantly. The thin ascending limb is water impermeable, and it has a high sodium permeability. The high sodium permeability of the thin ascending limb results in the accumulation of NaCl into the interstitium of the medulla. Neither the thin descending limb nor the thin ascending limb actively transports solutes. This hairpin tubular structure is part of the countercurrent multiplication system that contributes to a hypertonic medullary interstitium.

As the tubular fluid ascends the loop of Henle, it flows into the thick ascending limb that is also water impermeable. The thick ascending limb reabsorbs salt without water. Approximately 25% of the filtered sodium is reabsorbed in the thick ascending limb via the electroneutral sodium-potassium-2 chloride co-transporter. The transepithelial potential difference is lumen positive due potassium recycling (secretion) into the lumen via the apical membrane potassium channel. The lumen positive potential difference provides a driving force for calcium and magnesium transport across the paracellular pathway. The fluid leaving the thick ascending limb has an osmolality of 50 mOsm/kg water regardless of the final urinary osmolality. This tubular fluid then flows into the distal convoluted tubule, where an additional 5% to 10% of the filtered sodium is reabsorbed via a sodium chloride co-transporter that is electroneutral. Finally, 1% to 3% of the filtered sodium is reabsorbed by the collecting tubule across the epithelial sodium channel, which is under the control of aldosterone. Whether the urine will be hypertonic or hypotonic will be dependent on whether vasopressin is present to cause the insertion of aquaporin 2, another water channel, into the apical membrane of the collecting duct.

In all of the nephron segments that actively transport sodium, the cells are poised for the vectorial transport of sodium from the lumen across the epithelium to the peritubular capillaries. The driving

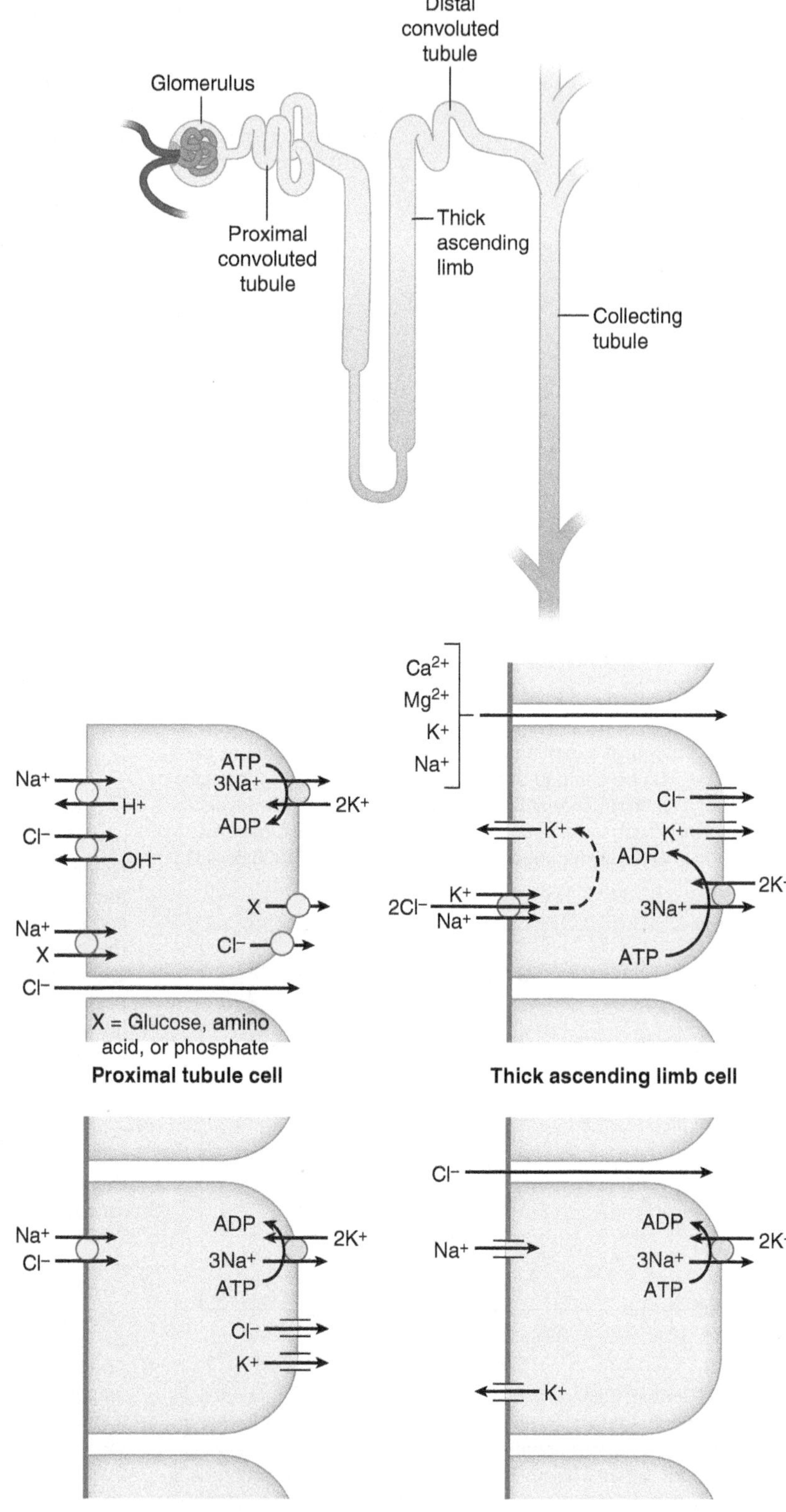

Fig. 97.3 Cartoon depicting the nephron and the cells that actively transport sodium. The glomerulus produces an ultrafiltrate of plasma, which is delivered to the proximal tubule. Sixty percent of the filtered sodium is reabsorbed in the proximal tubule with organic solutes (designated X), NaCl via parallel Na^+/H^+ and Cl^-/base exchangers and passively across the tight junction. The thick ascending limb has a NaK2Cl co-transporter that in parallel with the apical potassium channel results in a positive potential difference that is a driving force for paracellular cation transport. The distal convoluted tubule has NCC, which is electroneutral and thiazide sensitive. Finally, the final modulation of sodium transport occurs in the collecting tubule, where there is an apical sodium channel that generates a lumen negative potential difference that provides a driving force for potassium secretion via an apical potassium channel or paracellular chloride absorption. The driving force for apical sodium transport is generated by the basolateral Na^+/K^+-ATPase, which decreases intracellular sodium and generates a negative cellular potential difference.

force for all active transport of sodium is the Na^+/K^+-ATPase on the basolateral membrane. The Na^+/K^+-ATPase uses ATP to transport three sodium ions out of the cell and two potassium ions into the cell. The intracellular sodium concentration is approximately 10 mEq/L, and the intracellular potassium concentration is approximately 140 mEq/L. The low intracellular sodium concentration provides a driving force for the uptake of sodium across the apical membrane of cells along the nephron. In addition, the pump is electrogenic due to the stoichiometry of Na and K transport. With three sodium ions exiting the cell for two potassium ions entering the cell, the cellular potential difference is negative (−60 to −90 mV). This provides another driving force for sodium entry across the apical membrane.

The apical membrane of cells is a lipid bilayer that is impermeable to sodium. Thus, for sodium to enter the cell down its electrochemical gradient, there has to be a protein transporter in the membrane. There are three modes of sodium entry that are used along the nephron. The cartoon shown in Fig. 97.3 shows all three of these transporters. First, sodium can pass across an apical channel. This occurs in the collecting tubule principal cell where the epithelial sodium channel, designated ENaC, facilitates sodium entry down its electrochemical gradient. The abundance of ENaC on the apical membrane is regulated by aldosterone. Entry of the positive sodium ion leaves the lumen with a negative potential difference that serves as a driving force for potassium secretion, proton secretion, or chloride absorption. The second type of transport process is a sodium chloride co-transporter or sodium-other solute symporter. In this type of transporter, sodium enters the cell down its electrochemical gradient in the same direction as another solute. In the distal convoluted tubule, that transporter is the sodium chloride co-transporter, designated NCC. This is the transporter that is inhibited by thiazide diuretics and is electroneutral. Sodium can also enter cells along with another solute such as glucose, as occurs in the proximal tubule. In this case, there is a net positive charge entering the cell because glucose is electroneutral. This leaves the tubular lumen with a negative transepithelial potential difference. The lumen negative transepithelial potential can serve as a driving force for the passive transport of negative ions such as chloride that may be transported across the paracellular pathway. Finally, sodium may be transported in exchange for another ion. In the proximal tubule, there is a sodium hydrogen exchanger designated NHE. The NHE results in the reabsorption of sodium and secretion of a proton into the cell. NHE is electroneutral, and the secretion of a proton will titrate filtered bicarbonate and result in net bicarbonate reabsorption.

Cells are linked to the adjoining cells by a tight junction, which is the most apical structure of the paracellular pathway. The proteins that make up the tight junction are a rather ubiquitously expressed molecule designated occludin and a family of tight junction proteins called *claudins*. There are more than 20 claudins, and they all have four transmembrane domains, a short intracellular loop, and two extracellular loops that bind to the claudin expressed on the adjoining cell.[14] Claudins form the pore and barrier function of the paracellular pathway. Depending on the characteristics of the first loop, claudins will affect the ability of solutes to pass across the paracellular pathway.

Some claudins deserve discussion, such as claudin 16 and 19 in the thick ascending limb. Sodium enters the thick ascending limb via a sodium, potassium, two-chloride co-transporter designated NKCC. This is the transporter that is inhibited by furosemide. This transporter is electroneutral and is described in Fig. 97.3. Potassium recycles into the tubular lumen via a potassium channel designated ROMK, leaving the tubular lumen with a positive transepithelial potential difference. This positive potential provides a driving force for the passive paracellular absorption of magnesium and calcium. Mutations in either claudin 16 or 19 prevent the passive absorption of calcium and magnesium across the paracellular pathway, resulting in an autosomal recessive disorder called *familial hypomagnesemia with hypercalciuria and nephrocalcinosis (FHHNC)*.[15-17] In this disorder, large amounts of magnesium and calcium are excreted in the urine, causing hypomagnesemia, nephrocalcinosis, and renal stones.

The reabsorption of glucose and other neutral organic solutes with sodium leaves the lumen of the early proximal tubule with a negative potential difference.[18] This provides a driving force for passive paracellular chloride reabsorption in the proximal tubule. In addition, the composition of the luminal fluid changes along the proximal tubule.[18] The preferential reabsorption of bicarbonate over chloride ions in the early proximal tubule results in a higher chloride and lower bicarbonate concentration than that of the peritubular fluid. Thus chloride diffuses down its concentration gradient across the paracellular pathway and is reabsorbed.

There are developmental changes in the passive permeability properties of the proximal tubule.[19-23] These developmental changes in permeability are due to changes in the abundance of some claudins, such as claudin 2, which is more highly expressed in the neonate than the adult.[21] There are also claudins that are expressed in the neonate, such as claudin 6, 9, and 13, which are not expressed in the adult.[24] In the adult, approximately one third of chloride transport is passive and paracellular and is mediated by the electrochemical driving forces discussed earlier.[25,26] The chloride permeability of the adult proximal tubule is far greater than the neonate, which limits passive paracellular chloride transport by the neonatal segment to almost zero.[19,23,27] The lower chloride permeability in the neonate compared with the adult is likely due to the expression of claudin 6 and 9 by the neonatal proximal tubule and not by the corresponding adult segment.[24] Expression of either claudin 6 or 9 into Madin-Darby canine kidney (MDCK) cells in vitro results in a decrease in chloride permeability.[28] Thus not only are there maturational changes in active NaCl transport but also of passive paracellular transport.

DEVELOPMENTAL CHANGES IN THE Na^+/K^+-ATPASE

The Na^+/K^+-ATPase is composed of three subunits.[29] The α subunit is the enzymatic subunit that binds the sodium, potassium, and ATP. The α subunit also binds to ouabain, an inhibitor of the Na^+/K^+-ATPase. The β subunit is a regulatory subunit that is necessary for pump activity. The γ subunit is also a regulatory subunit that is induced by hypertonic conditions. Although the γ subunit it is not necessary for Na^+/K^+-ATPase activity, it plays a regulatory role in activity of the pump under conditions where there is a reduction in ATP such as in the medulla of the kidney.[30]

The Na^+/K^+-ATPase is necessary for active sodium transport in each nephron segment of the kidney. Na^+/K^+-ATPase activity is lower in neonatal kidneys compared with adults.[31-37] As will be discussed, sodium transport is lower in all the nephron segments in the neonate. As shown in Fig. 97.4, there is a developmental

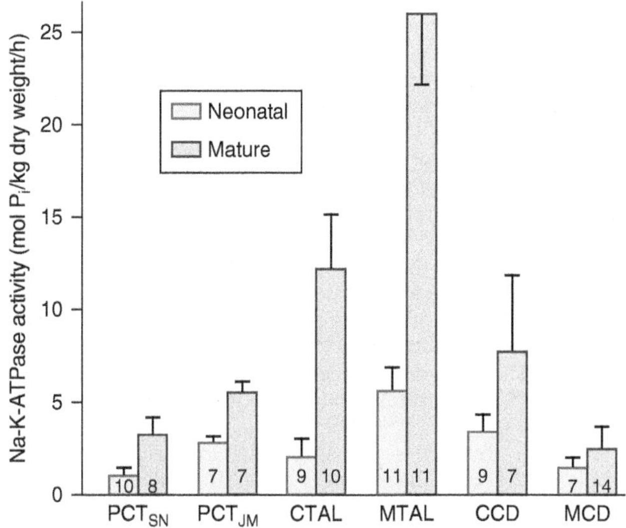

Fig. 97.4 Na^+/K^+-ATPase activity along the nephron. Na^+/K^+-ATPase activity was measured in isolated rabbit nephron segments in neonatal and adult tubules. Na^+/K^+-ATPase was significantly less in all neonatal nephron segments which transport sodium. *CCT,* Cortical collecting duct; *CTAL,* cortical thick ascending limb, *MCD,* medullary collecting duct; *MTAL,* medullary thick ascending limb; *PCT,* proximal convoluted tubule. (From Schmidt U, Horster M. Na-K activated ATPase activity maturation in rabbit nephron segments dissected in vitro. *Am J Physiol Renal Physiol.* 1977;233:F55.)

increase in Na^+/K^+-ATPase activity in all nephron segments involved in sodium transport along the nephron.[34]

There are a number of factors that have been shown to cause the postnatal increase in Na^+/K^+-ATPase activity. At the time of weaning in the rodent, there is an increase in both glucocorticoid and thyroid hormone levels.[38–41] The postnatal rise in glucocorticoid and thyroid levels parallel the developmental increase in Na^+/K^+-ATPase activity. In addition, administration of glucocorticoids and thyroid hormone before the postnatal increase in these hormones increases Na^+/K^+-ATPase activity.[32,35,42–45]

During postnatal development, there is an increase in a number of sodium transporters on the apical membrane that parallels the developmental increase in Na^+/K^+-ATPase.[37,46] This suggests that the increase in apical membrane transport and intracellular sodium could be a factor causing the induction of Na^+/K^+-ATPase. Indeed, in cell culture experiments an increase in intracellular sodium was shown to induce Na^+/K^+-ATPase activity.[47,48]

MATURATION OF PROXIMAL TUBULE SODIUM TRANSPORT

Active sodium transport in the proximal tubule is mediated by an apical Na^+/H^+ exchanger. For there to be net active sodium chloride transport, chloride must be also be transported across the apical membrane or passively diffuse across the paracellular pathway. As previously discussed, chloride permeability is very low in the neonate and there is very little passive chloride transport.[19,23,27] This is unlike the adult segment where approximately one third of chloride transport is passive and paracellular.[18,25,26] This section will discuss the developmental changes in active NaCl transport in the proximal tubule.

As shown in the cartoon in Fig. 97.3, net sodium chloride absorption can occur by the parallel operation of a Na^+/H^+ exchanger and a Cl^-/base exchanger. Both transporters are electroneutral, but it is not clear as to the nature of the base transported in exchange for chloride. There is evidence that the base is OH^-, so that for every Cl^- absorbed a OH^-would be secreted so that the parallel operation with the Na^+/H^+ exchanger would result in NaCl entering the cell and water being secreted.[49] However, there is also evidence for a Cl^-/formate exchanger with formic acid being recycled.[50–55] The rate of Cl^-/base exchange was five-fold less in the neonate than that in the adult, which results in a low rate of active NaCl transport.

The Na^+/H^+ exchanger is also responsible for two thirds of luminal proton secretion and for bicarbonate reclamation in the proximal tubule.[56,57] Neonatal Na^+/H^+ exchanger activity is significantly less than that in the adult.[58–62] This is in part responsible for the lower rate of both sodium chloride and sodium bicarbonate absorption in the neonate compared with the adult. In the adult, the Na^+/H^+ exchanger is due to NHE3 in rodents.[63] There is a developmental increase in NHE3 messenger RNA (mRNA) and protein abundance with postnatal proximal tubule development.[60–62,64,65]

Although there was a maturational increase in proximal tubule Na^+/H^+ exchanger activity and NHE3 mRNA and protein abundance, there was evidence that not all of the neonatal proximal tubule acidification was mediated by NHE3.[62] Indeed there was evidence that there must be other Na^+/H^+ exchangers mediating luminal acidification. NHE3-null mice were generated to better define the importance of NHE3 in proximal tubule acidification.[66] NHE3-null mice have metabolic acidosis and a lower rate or proximal tubule sodium and bicarbonate transport.[66] However, studies examining renal acidification showed that there was still significant Na^+/H^+ exchanger activity in NHE3-null mice.[67,68]

A number of Na^+/H^+ exchangers have been cloned, including NHE8, which was found to be present on the brush border membrane of the proximal tubule.[69,70] Studies in rodents looking at the ontogeny of NHE8 and NHE3 mRNA and protein abundance show that the neonate predominantly expresses NHE8 and there is an isoform switch from NHE8 to NHE3 during the course of postnatal maturation.[64,65] This isoform switch is depicted in Fig. 97.5, where the protein expression of NHE3 and NHE8 exchangers are shown during the course of postnatal development. NHE8 expression and activity is upregulated by metabolic acidosis,[71] and NHE8 expression is increased in NHE3 null mice.[68] Na^+/H^+ exchanger activity was essentially absent in NHE3/NHE8-double knockout mice, indicating that NHE8 was responsible for the residual activity in NHE3-null mice.

INDUCTION OF TUBULAR TRANSPORTER MATURATION

As noted, there are maturational changes in transporter abundance and isoform changes in transporters that occur during development. Thus there must be a factor or factors that are responsible for these changes. For a substance to be considered as a developmental inductive substance, it must fulfill four criteria.

1. The inducer must increase or decrease in concentration in concordance with the developmental change in transporter abundance.
2. Administration of the inducer before the developmental change will result in a premature change in the transporter abundance.
3. Prevention of the change in concentration of the inducer will result in a delay or total prevention of the developmental change in transporter abundance.
4. The inducing substance must be able to have its effect on transport in vitro.

During postnatal development, there is a rise in both glucocorticoid and thyroid hormone levels at the time of weaning in rodents.[40,41] The developmental changes in transporter abundance that occur coincide with the developmental changes in these hormones.

As an example of how developmental changes in thyroid hormone and glucocorticoids can cause induction of transport, we will use proximal tubule acidification mediated by the Na^+/H^+ exchanger. The increase in Na^+/H^+ exchanger activity occurs at the time of weaning in concordance with the increase in bicarbonate absorption and NHE3 mRNA and NHE3 protein abundance.[72,64,65] Administration of glucocorticoids before the developmental increase in transport prematurely increases the maturational increase in bicarbonate transport as well as NHE3 mRNA and protein abundance.[60,61,73–76] Adrenalectomy in neonates before the increase in glucocorticoid level attenuated the maturational increase in Na^+/H^+ exchanger activity and NHE3 protein abundance but did not affect NHE3 mRNA abundance.[61] However, glucocorticoid deficiency did not totally prevent the maturation of NHE3, indicating that there were other factors involved.

The effect of thyroid hormone on maturation of proximal tubule acidification has also been examined. Administration of thyroid hormone to neonates before the increase that occurs at the time of weaning results in an increase in proximal tubule bicarbonate transport, Na^+/H^+ exchanger activity, NHE3 mRNA, and protein abundance.[38,77,78] Prevention of the normal developmental increase in thyroid hormone levels delayed the maturational increase in proximal tubule acidification, Na^+/H^+ exchanger, and NHE3 and protein abundance.[38,77,78] However, as with glucocorticoids, thyroid hormone was not solely

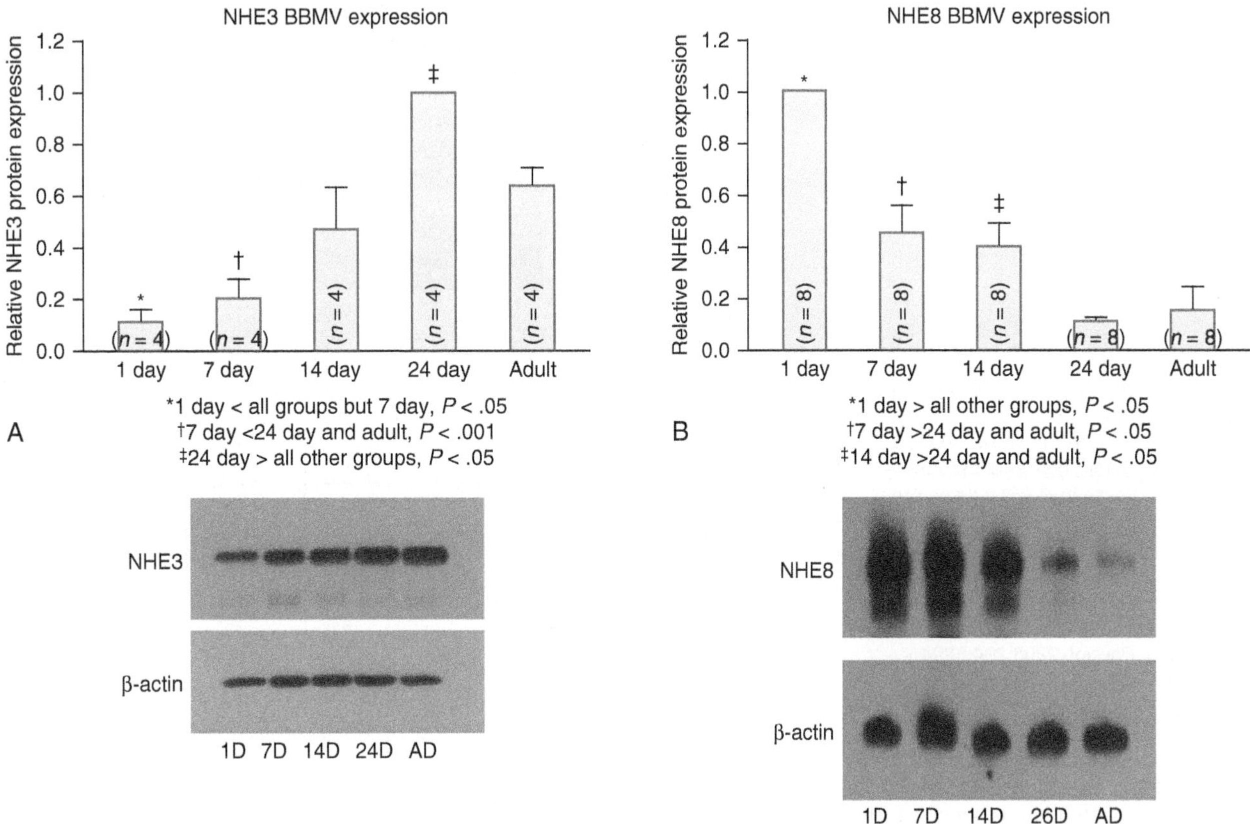

Fig. 97.5 Expression of NHE3 and NHE8 during postnatal maturation of the rat. The proximal tubule reabsorbs 60% of the filtered NaCl and 80% of the filtered $NaHCO_3$. The Na^+/H^+ exchanger is responsible for most of most of sodium transport in the proximal tubule. There is a developmental isoform switch from NHE8, which is highly expressed in the neonate, to NHE3, which is the predominant isoform in the adult. (From Becker A, Zhang J, Goyal S, et al. Maturation of NHE8 in the rat proximal tubule. *Am J Physiol Renal Physiol*. 2007;293:F255.)

responsible for the increase in proximal tubule maturation by itself and hypothyroidism did not affect NHE3 mRNA abundance. Thus it was likely that both hormones were necessary for the induction of proximal tubule acidification or that one hormone played a compensatory role in the absence of the other.

To examine whether both glucocorticoids and thyroid hormone were necessary for the maturational increase in NHE3 and proximal tubule acidification, a neonatal hypothyroid adrenalectomized rat was studied.[79] The hypothyroid adrenalectomized rat was allowed to develop to a young adult when the maturation of proximal tubule acidification would be complete. However, in the absence of both glucocorticoids and thyroid hormone, proximal tubule acidification and the increase in NHE3 mRNA and protein were totally prevented.

As noted earlier, it is possible for the effect of thyroid hormone and glucocorticoids to have an indirect effect in vivo. To demonstrate a direct effect of these hormones proximal tubule cells were studied in vitro. Both thyroid hormone and glucocorticoids had a direct epithelial action in increase Na^+/H^+ exchanger activity and NHE3 mRNA and protein abundance when added to proximal tubule cells in vitro.[74,77,80,80–82]

As noted earlier, although there is a developmental increase in NHE3, there is a concomitant decrease in NHE8. The maturational decrease in NHE8 coincides with the increase in NHE3. Administration of thyroid hormone to neonatal rats caused a premature isoform switch with a decrease in NHE8 protein abundance and an increase in NHE3 protein abundance.[77] Furthermore, prevention of the postnatal increase in thyroid hormone resulted in continued high expression of NHE8 and low expression of NHE3. Finally, thyroid hormone caused a reduction in NHE8 surface expression and NHE8 activity in proximal tubule cells in vitro that express NHE8 and not NHE3 (Fig. 97.6). Glucocorticoids have also been shown to result in a premature decrease in NHE8 protein expression when administered to neonatal rats.[83] In addition, glucocorticoids had a direct epithelial effect to decrease NHE8 protein expression in vitro as well as Na^+/H^+ exchanger activity in proximal tubule cells that express NHE8.[83]

MATURATION OF DISTAL TUBULE SODIUM TRANSPORT

The thick ascending limb reabsorbs approximately 30% of the filtered sodium. A thick ascending limb cell is shown in Fig. 97.3. Sodium transport in the thick ascending limb has been directly examined in vitro using in vitro microperfusion and shown to be five-fold lower in the neonate than in the adult.[84] There is a maturational increase in several of the transporters necessary for sodium transport in the thick ascending limb, including NKCC, ROMK, and Na^+/K^+-ATPase mRNA and protein abundance.[85] Administration of glucocorticoids to neonates results in a premature increase in these transporters. Bartter syndrome is due to a mutation in one of the transporters in the thick limb or stimulation of the calcium sensing receptor on the basolateral membrane that regulates transport in this segment. Neonatal Bartter syndrome that presents with polyhydramnios is usually due to a mutation in either NKCC or ROMK on the apical membrane or ClC-Kb on the basolateral membrane of the thick ascending limb. Patient's with Bartter syndrome have renal salt wasting and hypokalemia and usually develop nephrocalcinosis.

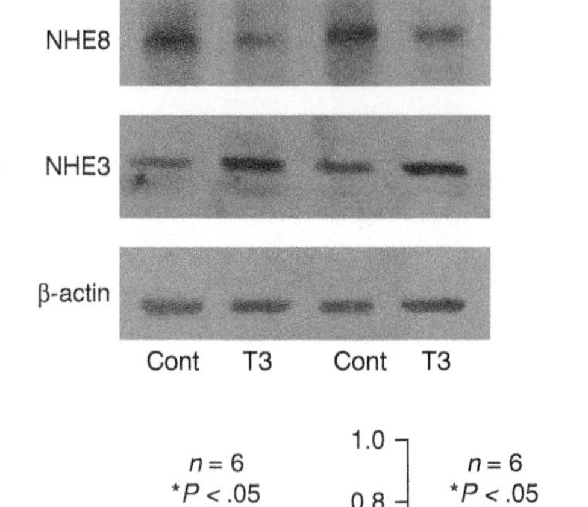

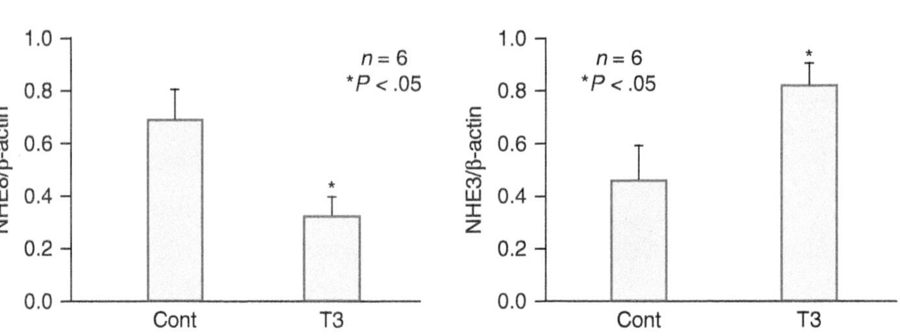

Fig. 97.6 Effect of thyroid hormone on the developmental isoform switch from NHE8 to NHE3. This study shows that administration of thyroid hormone before the maturational increase in NHE8 causes premature increase in NHE3 and a premature decrease in NHE8 brush border membrane protein abundance. (From Gattineni J, Sas D, Dagan A, et al. Effect of thyroid hormone on postnatal renal expression of NHE8. *Am J Physiol Renal Physiol*. 2008;294:F294.)

As noted, the neonate has a blunted ability to excrete a sodium load with volume expansion.[4,9,10] It is unclear how this occurs. The only study directly examining the location for this phenomenon was performed in volume depleted and volume expanded rats.[86] With volume depletion the fraction of sodium delivered to the early and late distal tubule was comparable in 24- and 40-day-old rats. With volume expansion the fraction of sodium delivered to the late distal tubule was lower in young rats compared with the older rats.[86] These data imply that the site of increased sodium absorption with volume expansion in young rats lies in the distal convoluted tubule. However, the mechanism of how this occurs is unclear because there are developmental changes in transporters in the distal convoluted tubule, including NCC, which suggest that sodium transport would be lower in the neonate than in the adult.[87] A distal convoluted tubule cell is depicted in Fig. 97.3. Mutation in NCC results in Gitelman syndrome. Gitelman syndrome is a salt wasting disorder with characteristics comparable with chronic administration of a thiazide diuretic, including hypomagnesemia, hypokalemia, and hypocalciuria. These patients have intense salt craving.

The cortical collecting tubule is the final segment that regulates sodium reabsorption in the nephron. As shown in Fig. 97.3, there is an electrogenic sodium channel designated ENaC, which is regulated by aldosterone. Satlin and colleagues used the isolated perfused tubule to examine the maturation of sodium absorption by the neonatal rabbit collecting duct.[88] There was no sodium channel activity in the newborn, but by 2 weeks of age, the sodium absorptive capacity was half that of the adult segment. Using patch clamp to measure the epithelial sodium channel, she found that the neonate had fewer sodium channels, which had a lower probability of being open to allow sodium entry into the cell than that of the adult. This is consistent with the lower sodium absorption seen in the isolated perfused tubule studies.[89] The maturational increase potassium secretion via an apical membrane potassium channel (ROMK) in this segment occurred after the developmental increase in sodium absorption.[88] There is a maturational increase in Na^+/K^+-ATPase activity in this segment as shown in Fig. 97.4.[34]

HORMONAL REGULATION OF TUBULAR TRANSPORT

There are a number of homeostatic mechanisms that protect the volume and composition of the extracellular fluid volume. If one thinks about our salt intake over the previous 24 hours, it is likely quite different than that of the previous day. We are often challenged by a loss of fluid from our extracellular volume such as occurs with vomiting and diarrhea. Faced with volume depletion, our kidneys act to conserve salt and water to maintain a constant composition of the extracellular milieu. If we did not have homeostatic mechanisms to protect us by conserving salt and water, we would not be able to survive these challenges.

There are a number of hormones as well as renal nerves that act on the kidney to conserve sodium and water to prevent volume depletion. In adults, volume depletion results in the activation of the renin-angiotensin system. The increase in angiotensin II causes vasoconstriction and a decrease in glomerular filtration rate; the latter is a protective means of limiting filtration of sodium and thus salt loss in the urine. Angiotensin II also acts on the proximal and distal tubule to increase sodium transport, and aldosterone acts on the collecting tubule in increase the apical expression of sodium channels.

Premature neonates that are fed regular formula are in negative salt balance as shown in Fig. 97.2. This negative salt balance can result in volume depletion. Fig. 97.7 depicts the difference in plasma renin activity, plasma aldosterone, and urinary aldosterone levels between salt supplemented and presumably euvolemic premature neonates and premature neonates that were not supplemented. As can be seen, there is an upregulation of the renin-angiotensin-aldosterone system in the neonates that are not salt supplemented and thus volume depleted.[90]

As previously described, neonates have limited ability to excrete a sodium load compared with adults. To examine if this was due to angiotensin II, losartan (an angiotensin II receptor blocker) or vehicle was administered for the first 2 weeks of life in rats, followed by a volume challenge.[91] The losartan-treated neonates had a 10-fold greater increase in urinary sodium excretion compared with vehicle-treated controls. Thus

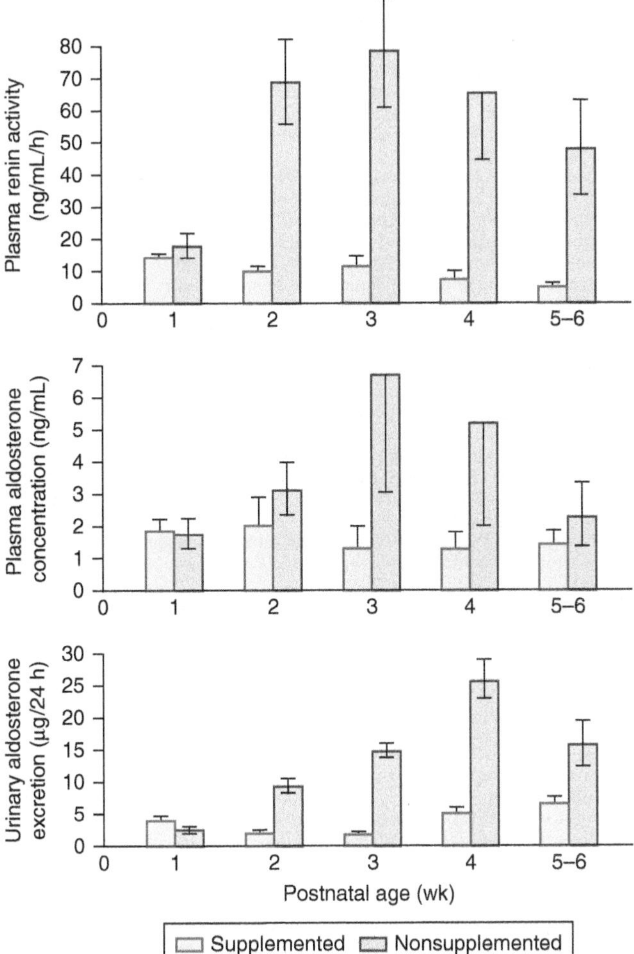

Fig. 97.7 Plasma renin activity, plasma aldosterone, and urinary aldosterone levels in preterm infants with and without salt supplementation. One- to 6-week-old preterm infants were either salt supplemented or given regular formula. As can be seen the salt-supplemented neonates had a lower plasma renin and aldosterone level and lower urinary aldosterone level compared with the nonsupplemented neonates. This indicates that, in volume-contracted premature infants that are not salt supplemented, the levels of aldosterone and renin are appropriately increased. The non–salt-supplemented data are shown in the *open bars.* (From Sulyok E, Németh M, Tényi I, et al. Relationship between the postnatal development of the renin angiotensin aldosterone system and electrolyte and acid-base status of the NaCl-supplemented premature infants. In: Spitzer A, editor. *The Kidney During Development*. New York:, Masson; 1982:273–281.)

neonates are able to respond to angiotensin II to increase tubular transport, which is a factor that explains the decreased ability to excrete a sodium load.

Aldosterone acts on the collecting tubule to increase sodium transport through the epithelial sodium channel, which secondarily results in increased potassium secretion as shown in Fig. 97.3. One can get an indication of aldosterone's tubular effect by examining the urinary sodium/potassium (U_{Na}/U_K) ratio. In adult rats, adrenalectomy resulted in a 40-fold increase in U_{Na}/U_K ratio, whereas there was no effect of adrenalectomy on U_{Na}/U_K in neonatal rats.[92] In addition, administration of aldosterone to adrenalectomized adult rats caused a decrease in the U_{Na}/U_K ratio but had no effect in neonatal adrenalectomized rats. Finally, aldosterone administration in vivo increased sodium transport in adult rabbit cortical collecting ducts perfused in vitro but had no effect in neonates.[93] Even though neonates have higher levels of plasma aldosterone than do adults,[94,95] the attenuated effect of aldosterone is not due to a paucity of mineralocorticoid receptors in the neonatal kidney[92] but rather is a postreceptor phenomenon.

The kidney is richly innervated, and sympathetic nerves act to increase vascular resistance, decrease the glomerular filtration rate, and increase sodium absorption in the proximal tubule, thick ascending limb, and distal convoluted tubule. Therefore renal sympathetic nerves play an important role in mediating sodium conservation in response to volume depletion. The sheep fetal kidney has a higher expression of α-adrenoreceptor abundance than the neonate, which is higher than the adult.[96] However, infusion of phenylephrine results in a greater decrease in urine flow and urine sodium excretion in the neonatal lamb than in the fetus and the adult.[97] Renal nerves also play a role in the transition from fetal to extrauterine life. Renal denervation of lamb fetuses results in a greater natriuresis and diuresis compared with control intact lambs.[98] Renal denervation also attenuated the rise in plasma renin activity with birth.[98] Thus renal sympathetic nerves likely play an important role in decreasing glomerular filtration rate and thus salt delivery to the proximal tubule, as well as increasing sodium transport during states of volume contraction.

We also must have a means to increase sodium excretion with volume expansion. Dopamine acts on the kidney to increase renal blood flow and glomerular filtration rate and inhibits sodium reabsorption in multiple nephron segments. L-dopa is filtered by the glomerulus and converted to dopamine in the lumen of the proximal tubule. Dopamine inhibits transport in a number of segments largely by inhibiting the Na^+/K^+-ATPase.[33,99] The intrarenal dopamine content is higher in neonates than in adult rats. Nonetheless, the effect of dopamine to inhibit the Na^+/K^+-ATPase and natriuretic effect of dopamine is blunted in the neonate.[33]

Atrial natriuretic peptide is a factor that is produced in the heart and causes an increase in glomerular filtration rate and a natriuresis. In the premature neonate administration of sodium supplements causes an increase in atrial natriuretic peptide levels.[100] Although there is an appropriate change in plasma atrial natriuretic peptide levels in the premature neonate, the effect of the peptide to cause a natriuresis is blunted in neonatal rats compared with adults.[101]

CONCLUSION

There are maturational changes in renal sodium handling in all nephron segments. The very premature infant has renal sodium wasting that can lead to volume depletion and hyponatremia. The term neonate must be in positive sodium balance for growth, which is reflected by the fact that the neonate has a decreased ability to excrete a sodium load compared with the adult. The maturation of sodium transport during renal development is due to changes in both paracellular and transcellular transport. There is a developmental increase in a number of transporters along the nephron during postnatal maturation as well as isoform changes of some important sodium transport proteins such as the Na^+/H^+ exchanger on the apical membrane of the proximal tubule. Finally, there are mechanisms to increase sodium reabsorption during volume depletion, as well as to promote sodium excretion with volume expansion. There are maturational changes that occur in these homeostatic mechanisms that are essential for survival.

A complete reference list is available at www.ExpertConsult.com. 

SELECT REFERENCES

1. Arant Jr BS. Developmental patterns of renal functional maturation compared in the human neonate. *J Pediatr*. 1978;92:705-712.
2. Rubin MI, Bruck E, Rapoport M. Maturation of renal function in childhood: clearance studies. *J Clin Invest*. 1949;28:1144-1162.
3. Aperia A, Broberger O, Elinder G, Herin P, Zetterstrom R. Postnatal development of renal function in pre-term and full-term infants. *Acta Paediatr Scand*. 1981;70(2):183-187.
4. Aperia A, Broberger O, Thodenius K, Zetterstrom R. Renal response to an oral sodium load in newborn full-term infants. *Acta Paediatr Scand*. 1972;61:670-676.
5. Al-Dahhan J, Haycock GB, Chantler C, Stimmler L. Sodium homeostasis in term and preterm neonates. *Arch Dis Child*. 1983;58:335-342.
6. Engelke SC, Shah GL, Vasan J, Raye JR. Sodium balance in very low-birth-weight infants. *J Pediatr*. 1978;93:837-841.
7. Siegel SR, Oh W. Renal function as a marker of human fetal maturation. *Acta Paediatr Scand*. 1976;65:481-485.
8. Tuvad F, Vesterdal J. The maximal tubular transfer of glucose and para-aminohippurate in premature infants. *Acta Paediatr Scand*. 1953;42:337-345.
9. Spitzer A. The role of the kidney in sodium homeostasis during maturation. *Kidney Int*. 1982;21(4):539-545.
10. Goldsmith DI, Drukker A, Blaufox MD, Edelmann Jr CM, Spitzer A. Hemodynamic and excretory response of the neonatal canine kidney to acute volume expansion. *Am J Physiol*. 1979;237(5):F392-F397.
18. Rector Jr FC. Sodium, bicarbonate, and chloride absorption by the proximal tubule. *Am J Physiol*. 1983;244(5):F461-F471.
20. Baum M. Developmental changes in proximal tubule NaCl transport. *Pediatr Nephrol*. 2008;23(2):185-194.
24. Abuazza G, Becker A, Williams SS, et al. Claudins 6, 9, and 13 are developmentally expressed renal tight junction proteins. *Am J Physiol Renal Physiol*. 2006;291(6):F1132-F1141.
27. Quigley R, Baum M. Developmental changes in rabbit proximal straight tubule paracellular permeability. *Am J Physiol Renal Physiol*. 2002;283(3):F525-F531.
31. Aperia A, Larrson L. Induced development of proximal tubular NaKATPase, basolateral cell membranes and fluid reabsorption. *Acta Physiol Scand*. 1984;121:133-141.
32. Aperia A, Larrson L, Zetterstrom R. Hormonal induction of Na-K-ATPase in developing proximal tubular cells. *Am J Physiol*. 1981;241:F356-F360.
33. Fukuda Y, Bertorello A, Aperia A. Ontogeny of the regulation of Na+,K(+)-ATPase activity in the renal proximal tubule cell. *Pediatr Res*. 1991;30(2):131-134.
34. Schmidt U, Horster M. Na-K-activated ATPase: activity maturation in rabbit nephron segments dissected in vitro. *Am J Physiol*. 1977;233(1):F55-F60.
35. Celsi G, Nishi A, Akusjarvi G, Aperia A. Abundance of Na(+)-K(+)-ATPase mRNA is regulated by glucocorticoid hormones in infant rat kidneys. *Am J Physiol*. 1991;260(2 Pt 2):F192-F197.
37. Schwartz GH, Evan AP. Development of solute transport in rabbit proximal tubule. III. Na-K-ATPase activity. *Am J Physiol*. 1984;246:F845-F852.
38. Baum M, Dwarakanath V, Alpern RJ, Moe OW. Effects of thyroid hormone on the neonatal renal cortical Na+/H+ antiporter. *Kidney Int*. 1998;53(5):1254-1258.
48. Larsson SH, Rane S, Fukuda Y, Aperia A, Lechene C. Changes in Na influx precede post-natal increase in Na, K-ATPase activity in rat renal proximal tubular cells. *Acta Physiol Scand*. 1990;138(1):99-100.
57. Baum M. Developmental changes in rabbit juxtamedullary proximal convoluted tubule acidification. *Pediatr Res*. 1992;31(4 Pt 1):411-414.
59. Beck JC, Lipkowitz MS, Abramson RG. Ontogeny of Na/H antiporter activity in rabbit renal brush border membrane vesicles. *J Clin Invest*. 1991;87(6):2067-2076.
60. Baum M, Biemesderfer D, Gentry D, Aronson PS. Ontogeny of rabbit renal cortical NHE3 and NHE1: effect of glucocorticoids. *Am J Physiol*. 1995;268(5 Pt 2):F815-F820.
61. Gupta N, Tarif SR, Seikaly M, Baum M. Role of glucocorticoids in the maturation of the rat renal Na+/H+ antiporterNHE3). *Kidney Int*. 2001;60(1):173-181.
62. Shah M, Gupta N, Dwarakanath V, Moe OW, Baum M. Ontogeny of Na+/H+ antiporter activity in rat proximal convoluted tubules. *Pediatr Res*. 2000;48(2):206-210.
64. Twombley K, Gattineni J, Bobulescu IA, Dwarakanath V, Baum M. Effect of metabolic acidosis on neonatal proximal tubule acidification. *Am J Physiol Regul Integr Comp Physiol*. 2010;299(5):R1360-R1368.
65. Becker AM, Zhang J, Goyal S, et al. Ontogeny of NHE8 in the rat proximal tubule. *Am J Physiol Renal Physiol*. 2007;293:F255-F261.
72. Schwartz GJ, Evan AP. Development of solute transport in rabbit proximal tubule. I. HCO-3 and glucose absorption. *Am J Physiol*. 1983;245(3):F382-F390.
73. Baum M, Quigley R. Prenatal glucocorticoids stimulate neonatal juxtamedullary proximal convoluted tubule acidification. *Am J Physiol*. 1991;261(5 Pt 2):F746-F752.
74. Baum M, Quigley R. Glucocorticoids stimulate rabbit proximal convoluted tubule acidification. *J Clin Invest*. 1993;91(1):110-114.
75. Baum M, Moe OW, Gentry DL, Alpern RJ. Effect of glucocorticoids on renal cortical NHE-3 and NHE-1 mRNA. *Am J Physiol*. 1994;267(3 Pt 2):F437-F442.
77. Gattineni J, Sas D, Dagan A, Dwarakanath V, Baum M. Effect of thyroid hormone on the postnatal renal expression of NHE8. *Am J Physiol Renal Physiol*. 2008;294(1):F198-F204.
78. Shah M, Quigley R, Baum M. Maturation of proximal straight tubule NaCl transport: role of thyroid hormone. *Am J Physiol Renal Physiol*. 2000;278(4):F596-F602.
79. Gupta N, Dwarakanath V, Baum M. Maturation of the Na/H antiporter (NHE3) in the proximal tubule of the hypothyroid adrenalectomized rat. *Am J Physiol Renal Physiol*. 2004;287:F521-F527.
86. Aperia A, Elinder G. Distal tubular sodium reabsorption in the developing rat kidney. *Am J Physiol*. 1981;240(6):F487-F491.
87. Schmitt R, Ellison DH, Farman N, et al. Developmental expression of sodium entry pathways in rat nephron. *Am J Physiol*. 1999;276(3 Pt 2):F367-F381.
88. Satlin LM. Postnatal maturation of potassium transport in rabbit cortical collecting duct. *Am J Physiol*. 1994;266(1 Pt 2):F57-F65.
89. Satlin LM, Palmer LG. Apical Na+ conductance in maturing rabbit principal cell. *Am J Physiol*. 1996;270(3 Pt 2):F391-F397.
90. Siegel SR, Fisher DA, Oh W. Serum aldosterone concentrations related to sodium balance in the newborn infant. *Pediatrics*. 1974;53(3):410-413.
91. Chevalier RL, Thornhill BA, Belmonte DC, Baertschi AJ. Endogenous angiotensin II inhibits natriuresis after acute volume expansion in the neonatal rat. *Am J Physiol*. 1996;270(2 Pt 2):R393-R397.
92. Stephenson G, Hammet M, Hadaway G, Funder JW. Ontogeny of renal mineralocorticoid receptors and urinary electrolyte responses in the rat. *Am J Physiol*. 1984;247(4 Pt 2):F665-F671.
93. Vehaskari VM. Ontogeny of cortical collecting duct sodium transport. *Am J Physiol*. 1994;267(1 Pt 2):F49-F54.
94. Sulyok E, Nemeth M, Tenyi I, et al. Postnatal development of renin-angiotensin-aldosterone system, RAAS, in relation to electrolyte balance in premature infants. *Pediatr Res*. 1979;13(7):817-820.
95. Sulyok E, Nemeth M, Tenyi I, et al. Relationship between maturity, electrolyte balance and the function of the renin-angiotensin-aldosterone system in newborn infants. *Biol Neonate*. 1979;35(1-2):60-65.
98. Smith FG, Smith BA, Guillery EN, Robillard JE. Role of renal sympathetic nerves in lambs during the transition from fetal to newborn life. *J Clin Invest*. 1991;88(6):1988-1994.
100. Tulassay T, Rascher W, Seyberth HW, Lang RE, Toth M, Sulyok E. Role of atrial natriuretic peptide in sodium homeostasis in premature infants. *J Pediatr*. 1986;109(6):1023-1027.

98 Potassium Homeostasis in the Fetus and Neonate

Matthias T. Wolf | Corinne Benchimol | Lisa M. Satlin | Raymond Quigley

INTRODUCTION

Potassium is the most abundant intracellular cation. Maintenance of a high intracellular potassium concentration (100 to 140 mEq/L) is essential for many basic cellular processes, including cell growth and division, DNA and protein synthesis, conservation of cell volume and pH, and optimal enzyme function. The steep gradient between potassium concentration in the cell and that in the extracellular fluid, maintained by the ubiquitous sodium-potassium adenosine triphosphatase (Na^+, K^+-ATPase) pump, is the major determinant of the resting membrane potential across the cell membrane; thus it affects neuromuscular excitability and contractility. Approximately 98% of the total body potassium content in the adult resides within cells (primarily muscle) (Fig. 98.1), whereas the remaining 2% is located within the extracellular fluid. The extracellular potassium concentration

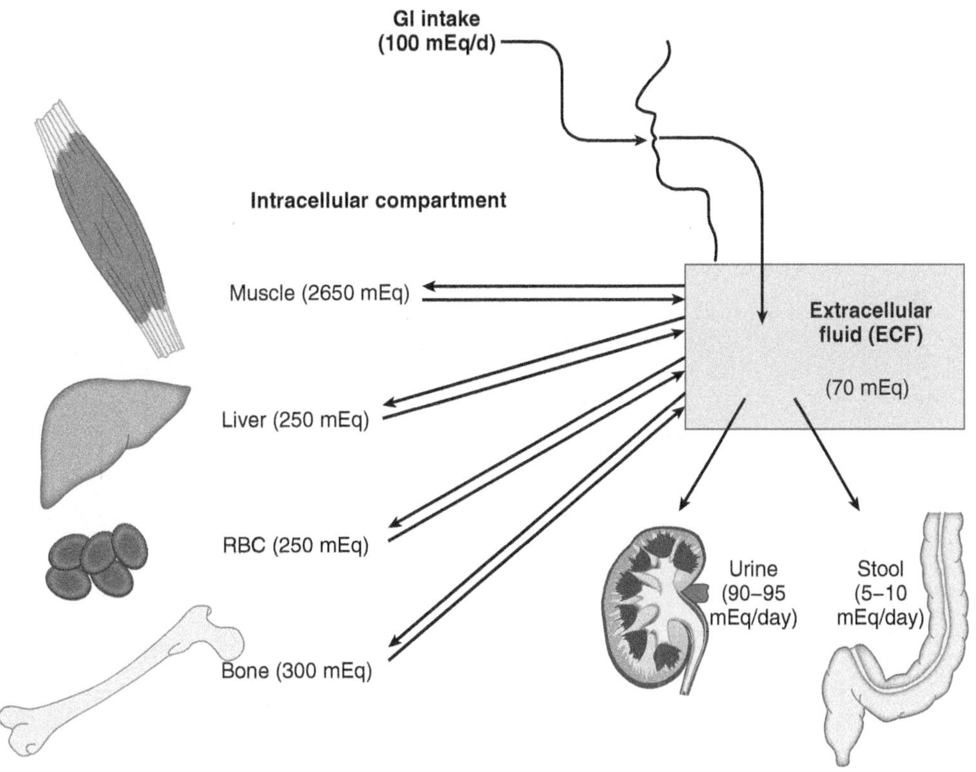

Fig. 98.1 Potassium homeostasis in the adult: *internal* and *external* balance. *External* potassium balance is maintained by the urinary (90% to 95%) and fecal (5% to 10%) excretion of the daily potassium intake of approximately 1 mEq/kg/day in the typical adult. *Internal* potassium balance depends on the distribution of potassium between the extracellular fluid *(ECF)* compartment and the vast intracellular storage reservoirs provided by muscle, liver, erythrocytes *(RBC)*, and bone. *GI*, Gastrointestinal.

(generally ranging from 3.5 to 5.0 mEq/L) is tightly regulated by mechanisms that govern the *internal* distribution between the intracellular and extracellular compartments and the *external* balance between intake and output.

POTASSIUM HOMEOSTASIS

The homeostatic goal of the adult is to remain in zero potassium balance. Thus, of the typical daily potassium intake of 1 mEq/kg body weight, approximately 90% to 95% is ultimately eliminated from the body in the urine; the residual 5% to 10% of the daily potassium load is lost through the stool (see Fig. 98.1). Normally, the amount of potassium lost through sweat is negligible.

In contrast to the situation in the adult, infants older than approximately 30 weeks' gestational age (GA) must conserve potassium for growth.[1,2] Postnatal growth is associated with an increase in total body potassium from approximately 8 mEq/cm body height at birth to more than 14 mEq/cm body height by 18 years of age.[3,4] The rate of accretion of body potassium per kilogram of body weight in the neonate is greater than that in later childhood (Fig. 98.2), a finding reflecting an increase in both cell number and potassium concentration (at least in skeletal muscle) with advancing age.[4-6] Given the requirement of the growing organism for potassium conservation, infants must maintain a state of positive potassium balance.[2,7] This tendency to retain potassium early in postnatal life is reflected in part in the higher plasma potassium values in infants, particularly in preterm neonates.[2,7] In fetal life, potassium is transported across the placenta from mother to fetus. Indeed, the fetal serum potassium concentration is maintained at levels exceeding 5 mEq/L even in the presence of maternal potassium deficiency.[8,9]

Urinary potassium excretion varies considerably, depending in large part on dietary intake. Children and adults ingesting an average American diet that contains sodium in excess of potassium excrete urine with a sodium-to-potassium ratio greater than 1.[2,10] Although breast milk and commercially available infant formulas generally provide a sodium-to-potassium ratio of approximately 0.5 to 0.6, the urinary sodium-to-potassium ratio in the newborn up to 4 months of age generally exceeds 1. This high ratio may reflect the greater requirement of potassium over sodium for growth. In fact, some premature (<34 weeks' GA) newborns may excrete urine with a sodium-to-potassium ratio greater than 2, a finding suggesting significant salt wasting and a relative hyporesponsiveness of the neonatal kidney to mineralocorticoid activity.[2] Because of the many vital processes that are dependent on potassium homeostasis, multiple complex and efficient mechanisms have developed to regulate total potassium balance and distribution.

REGULATION OF INTERNAL POTASSIUM BALANCE

The task of maintaining potassium homeostasis is complex, in large part because the daily dietary intake of potassium (approximately 100 mEq in the adult) typically approaches or exceeds the total potassium normally present within the extracellular fluid space (approximately 70 mEq in 17 L of extracellular fluid, with a potassium concentration averaging approximately 4 mEq/L) (see Fig. 98.1). To maintain zero balance in the adult, all the dietary intake of potassium must ultimately be eliminated, a task performed primarily by the kidney. However, renal excretion of potassium is rather sluggish, requiring several hours to be accomplished. Approximately 50% of an oral load of potassium is excreted during the first 4 to 6 hours after it is ingested, yet life-threatening hyperkalemia is not generally observed during this period because of the rapid (within minutes) hormonally mediated translocation of extracellular potassium into cells, particularly those of muscle and liver. The buffering capacity of the combined cellular storage reservoirs in the adult, capable of sequestering up to approximately 3500 mEq of potassium, is vast compared with that of the extracellular pool (see Fig. 98.1).

Cells must expend a significant amount of energy to maintain the steep potassium and sodium concentration gradients across their cell membranes. This is accomplished by the Na^+, K^+-ATPase pump, which catalyzes the hydrolysis of cytosolic adenosine triphosphate, thereby providing energy for the active extrusion of sodium from cells in exchange for the uptake of

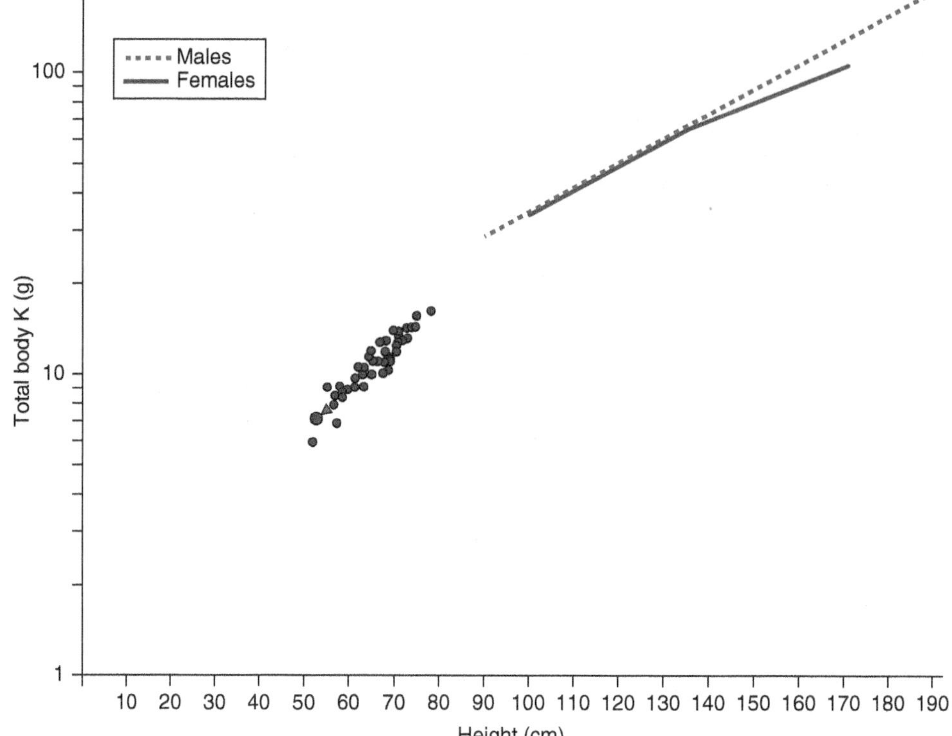

Fig. 98.2 Relationship between total body potassium (K^+) and height for infants and children. The rate of accretion of body potassium in the neonate is faster than in later childhood, likely reflecting an increase in both cell number and potassium concentration, at least in skeletal muscle, with advancing age. (From Flynn MA, Woodruff C, Clark J, et al. Total body potassium in normal children. *Pediatr Res.* 1972;6:239.)

potassium in a ratio of 3:2, respectively. A cell interior negative potential is created by the unequal cation exchange ratio and the subsequent leak of potassium out of the cells through potassium-selective channels in the plasma membrane. The Na^+, K^+-ATPase pump consists of a catalytic (α) and a regulatory (β) subunit.

Thirty percent to 50% of very-low-birth-weight and premature infants of less than 28 weeks' GA exhibit nonoliguric hyperkalemia (defined as a serum potassium concentration of >6.5 mEq/L) during the first 48 hours after birth despite the intake of negligible amounts of potassium.[11-15] This phenomenon is not observed in mature infants or very low-birth-weight infants after 72 hours.[13,14] This biochemical observation has been proposed to reflect a shift of potassium from the intracellular to the extracellular fluid space because of low Na^+-K^+ pump activity as well as a limited renal potassium secretory capacity.[13,14,16] Prenatal steroid treatment may prevent this nonoliguric hyperkalemia via induction of Na^+,K^+-ATPase pump activity in the fetus.[17,18]

Na^+,K^+-ATPase pump activity is regulated by numerous circulating hormones that exert short- and long-term control.[19] Whereas long-term stimulation of pump activity is generally mediated by changes in gene and protein expression, short-term regulation generally results from alterations in the phosphorylation status of the pump, changes in the subcellular or cell surface distribution of pumps (i.e., membrane trafficking), and/or interaction with regulatory proteins.[19] Regulation of internal potassium balance in the neonate may be influenced by developmental stage-specific expression of potassium transporters (such as the cation pump) and channels, receptors, and signal transduction pathways.

The chemical, physical, and hormonal factors that acutely influence the *internal* balance of potassium are listed in Table 98.1. Potassium uptake into cells is acutely stimulated by insulin, β_2-adrenergic agonists, and alkalosis and is impaired by α-adrenergic agonists, acidosis, and hyperosmolality. Generally, deviations in extracellular potassium concentration arising from fluctuations in internal distribution are self-limited as long as the endocrine regulation of *internal* balance and mechanisms responsible for regulation of *external* balance are intact.

PLASMA POTASSIUM CONCENTRATION

Active cellular potassium uptake in large part determines the intracellular pool of potassium. An increase in plasma potassium, either because of a dietary or parenteral potassium load or a chronic progressive loss of functional renal mass, decreases the concentration gradient (dependent on the ratio of intracellular to extracellular potassium concentration) against which the Na^+, K^+-ATPase pump must function. Thus an increase in cellular potassium uptake is favored. In those cells of the kidney and colon specifically responsible for potassium secretion, the resulting increase in intracellular potassium maximizes the concentration gradient between cell and lumen, thereby promoting potassium diffusion into the tubular lumen and thus potassium excretion.

HORMONES

Insulin, the most important hormonal regulator of *internal* potassium balance, stimulates Na^+, K^+-ATPase-mediated potassium uptake and sodium efflux in the kidney, skeletal muscle, adipocytes, and brain, a response that is independent of the hormonal effects on glucose metabolism.[20] The mechanism of insulin's action in these tissues differs, in part because of differences in the isoform complement of the catalytic α subunit of the pump. Insulin stimulates Na^+, K^+-ATPase activity by promoting the translocation of preformed pumps from intracellular stores to the cell surface (as in skeletal muscle),[21-24] and/or increasing cytoplasmic sodium content (as in adipocytes),[25-27] or by increasing the apparent affinity of the enzyme for sodium (as in kidney).[28] Basal insulin secretion is necessary to maintain the fasting plasma potassium concentration within the normal range. An increase in plasma potassium in excess of 1.0 mEq/L in the adult induces a significant increase in peripheral insulin levels to aid in the rapid disposal of the potassium load, yet a more modest elevation of approximately 0.5 mEq/L is without effect.[29]

Table 98.1 Factors Relevant to the Infant That Acutely Regulate the Internal Balance of Potassium.

Factor	Effect on Cell Uptake of Potassium
Physiologic Factors	
Plasma K Concentration	
Increase	Increase
Decrease	Decrease
Insulin	Increase
Catecholamines	
α-Agonists	Decrease
β-Agonists	Increase
Pathologic Factors	
Acid-Base Balance	
Acidosis	Decrease
Alkalosis	Increase
Hyperosmolality	Enhances cell efflux
Cell breakdown	Enhances cell efflux

The effect of epinephrine on potassium balance in the adult is biphasic and characterized by an initial increase, followed by a prolonged fall in plasma potassium concentration to a final value lower than baseline. The initial transient rise in plasma potassium results from stimulation of the α-adrenergic receptor, causing release of potassium from hepatocytes.[30,31] Stimulation of the β_2-receptor, via stimulation of adenylate cyclase leading to generation of the second messenger cyclic adenosine monophosphate, activates the Na^+, K^+-ATPase pump and thus promotes enhanced uptake of potassium by skeletal and cardiac muscle. These effects are inhibited by β_2 blockers.[30-35] Interestingly, similar effects are also seen with β_1-selective antagonist metoprolol and the nonselective β antagonist carvedilol, which has α-adrenergic effects.[36,37] β_2 blockers also contribute to hyperkalemia by a reduction of circulating angiotensin and possibly renin, thereby reducing the potassium secretory activity of the renin-angiotensin-aldosterone (RAAS) axis.[37,38] The observation that the potassium-lowering effects of insulin and epinephrine are additive suggests that their responses are mediated by different signaling pathways.

The effects of these hormones on the distribution of potassium between the intra- and extracellular compartments have been exploited to effectively treat disorders of homeostasis. For example, the β_2-adrenoreceptor agonist albuterol has been used to treat life-threatening hyperkalemia in premature and term neonates, children, and adults.[39-41] Administration of albuterol to treat hyperkalemia is associated with few side effects (mild, reversible tachycardia and tremors).[42] Administration of glucose, insulin, and furosemide may be associated with significant fluid, electrolyte, and glucose derangements in premature infants.[43-45] Administration of sodium bicarbonate has been associated with an increased incidence of intraventricular hemorrhage.[46] Oral or rectal administration of ion exchange resins can increase total body sodium and cause cecal perforation.[47] Furthermore, it may be ineffective in small infants.[43,48]

The side-effect profile of the newly approved calcium-based cation exchanger patiromer is not well studied in neonates, but it can be used to decant formula and reduce the potassium content.[49,50]

Aldosterone is best known for its effect on "transporting tissue"—that is, increasing potassium secretion in distal segments of the nephron and colon (discussed later). Thyroid hormone may also promote the cellular uptake of potassium as a result of its long-term stimulation of Na^+-K^+ pump activity.[19]

ACID-BASE BALANCE

It is well known that the transcellular distribution of potassium and acid-base balance are interrelated.[51] Whereas acidemia (increased extracellular hydrogen ion concentration) is associated with an increase in plasma potassium resulting from potassium release from the intracellular compartment, alkalemia (decrease in extracellular hydrogen ion concentration) results in a shift of potassium into cells and a consequent decrease in plasma potassium. However, the reciprocal changes in plasma potassium that accompany acute changes in blood pH differ widely among the four major acid-base disorders; metabolic disorders cause greater disturbances in plasma potassium than do those of respiratory origin, and acute changes in pH result in larger changes in plasma potassium than do chronic conditions.[51]

Acute metabolic acidosis after administration of a mineral acid including an anion that does not readily penetrate the cell membrane, such as the chloride of hydrochloric acid or ammonium chloride, consistently results in an increase in plasma potassium. As excess extracellular protons, unaccompanied by their nonpermanent anions, enter the cell where neutralization by intracellular buffers occurs, potassium (or sodium) is displaced from the cells, thus maintaining electroneutrality. However, comparable acidemia induced by acute organic anion acidosis (lactic acid in lactic acidosis, acetoacetic, and β-hydroxybutyric acids in uncontrolled diabetes mellitus) may not elicit a detectable change in plasma potassium.[51-53] In organic acidemia, the associated anion diffuses more freely into the cell and thus does not require a shift of potassium from the intracellular to the extracellular fluid.

In respiratory acid-base disturbances, in which carbon dioxide and carbonic acid readily permeate cell membranes, little transcellular shift of potassium occurs because protons are not transported in or out in association with potassium moving in the opposite direction.[51]

Changes in plasma bicarbonate concentration, independent of the effect on extracellular pH, can reciprocally affect plasma potassium concentration. Movement of bicarbonate (outward at a low extracellular bicarbonate concentration and inward at a high extracellular bicarbonate concentration) between the intra- and extracellular compartments may be causally related to a concomitant transfer of potassium. This may account for the less marked increase in plasma potassium observed during acute respiratory acidosis, a condition characterized by an acid plasma pH with an elevated serum bicarbonate (hence inward net bicarbonate and potassium movement) as compared with acute metabolic acidosis with a low serum bicarbonate concentration (hence outward net bicarbonate and potassium movement).

OTHER FACTORS

Many other pathologic perturbations alter the *internal* potassium balance. An increase in plasma osmolality resulting from severe dehydration causes water to shift out of cells. The consequent increase in intracellular potassium concentration exaggerates the transcellular concentration gradient and favors movement of this cation out of cells. The effect of hyperosmolality on potassium balance becomes especially troublesome in patients with hyperglycemia, as observed in those with diabetes, in whom the absence of insulin exacerbates the hyperkalemia.

REGULATION OF EXTERNAL POTASSIUM BALANCE

RENAL CONTRIBUTION

The kidney is the major excretory organ for potassium. In adults, urinary potassium excretion parallels dietary intake (see Fig. 98.1), and the speed of renal adaptation depends on the baseline potassium intake and the magnitude of the change in

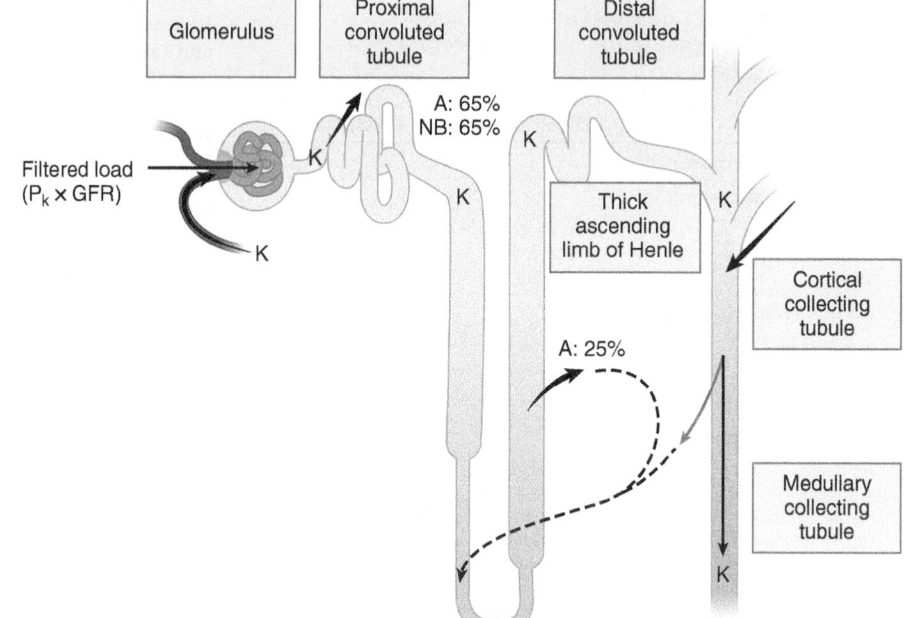

Fig. 98.3 Tubular sites of potassium (K^+) transport along the nephron. The percentages of filtered potassium reabsorbed along the proximal tubule and the thick ascending limb of the loop of Henle are indicated for the adult *(A)* and, when known, the newborn *(NB)*. *Arrows* identify the direction of net potassium transport as either out of (reabsorption) or into (secretion) the urinary fluid. *GFR*, Glomerular filtration rate.

dietary potassium intake. Extreme adjustments in the rate of renal potassium conservation cannot be achieved as rapidly as for sodium, and the adjustments are not as complete. In contrast, urinary sodium can be virtually eliminated within 3 to 4 days of sodium restriction, and a minimum urinary potassium loss of approximately 5 mEq/day occurs in the adult, even after several weeks of severe potassium restriction. An increase in dietary potassium intake is matched by a parallel increase in renal potassium excretion within hours, yet maximal rates of potassium excretion are not attained for several days after increasing potassium intake. In adults, renal potassium excretion follows a circadian rhythm, presumably determined by hypothalamic oscillators, and it is characterized by maximum output during times of peak activity.[54,55] Interestingly, in pinealocytes, calcium-activated potassium channels (BKCa, which are also localized in the kidney) are involved in melatonin secretion in a negative-feedback mechanism and thereby contribute to the regulation of the circadian rhythm.[56] It is unknown whether a circadian cycle of urinary potassium excretion exists in infancy.

The processes involved in renal potassium handling in the fully differentiated kidney include filtration, reabsorption, and secretion (Fig. 98.3).[57] Filtered potassium is reabsorbed almost entirely in proximal segments of the nephron, and urinary potassium is derived predominantly from distal secretion. Therefore renal secretion, rather than a balance of filtration and tubular reabsorption, maintains potassium homeostasis at least in the adult.

Renal potassium clearance is low in newborns, even when it is corrected for their low glomerular filtration rate.[2,7] Infants, like adults, when given a potassium load, can excrete potassium at a rate that exceeds its glomerular filtration—a finding indicating the capacity for net tubular secretion.[58] However, the rate of potassium excretion per unit of body weight or kidney weight in response to exogenous loading is less in newborns than in older animals.[59,60] Clearance studies in saline-expanded dogs also provide indirect evidence of a diminished secretory and enhanced reabsorptive capacity of the immature distal nephron to potassium.[61] A similar conclusion can be drawn from a longitudinal prospective study in premature neonates demonstrating a 50% reduction in the fractional excretion of potassium between 26 and 30 weeks' GA in the absence of significant change in absolute urinary potassium excretion.[1] To the extent that the filtered load of potassium increased almost threefold during this same time interval, the constancy of renal potassium excretion could be best explained by a developmental increase in the capacity of the kidney for potassium reabsorption.[1] In general, the limited potassium secretory capacity of the immature kidney becomes clinically relevant only under conditions of potassium excess. As stated earlier, under normal circumstances, potassium retention by the newborn kidney is appropriate and is required for somatic growth.

SITES OF POTASSIUM TRANSPORT ALONG THE NEPHRON

Potassium is freely filtered at the glomerulus. Approximately 65% of the filtered load of potassium is reabsorbed along the proximal tubule of the suckling rat, a fraction similar to that measured in the adult (see Fig. 98.3).[62-65] Reabsorption is passive in this segment, closely following water reabsorption, and is driven in part by the positive transepithelial voltage that prevails along part of the proximal tubule.

Approximately 10% of the filtered load of potassium reaches the early distal tubule of the adult, a finding reflecting significant further net reabsorption of this cation in the thick ascending limb of the loop of Henle (TALH) (see Fig. 98.3).[64] In contrast, up to 35% of the filtered load of potassium reaches the distal tubule of the very young (2-week-old) rat.[62] Observations in the maturing rodent—that the fractional reabsorption of potassium along the TALH, expressed as a percentage of delivered load, increases by 20% between the second and sixth weeks of postnatal life and that both the diluting capacity and TALH Na^+, K^+-ATPase pump activity increase after birth—are consistent with a developmental maturation of potassium absorptive pathways in this segment.[62,66,67] However, direct functional analysis of the potassium transport capacity of the TALH in the developing nephron has not been performed.

The avid potassium reabsorption characteristic of the fully differentiated TALH is mediated by a Na^+, K^+-$2Cl^-$ co-transporter, which translocates a single potassium ion into the cell accompanied by a sodium and two chloride (Cl^-) ions (Fig. 98.4A). This secondary active transport is ultimately driven by the basolateral Na^+, K^+-ATPase pump, which generates an

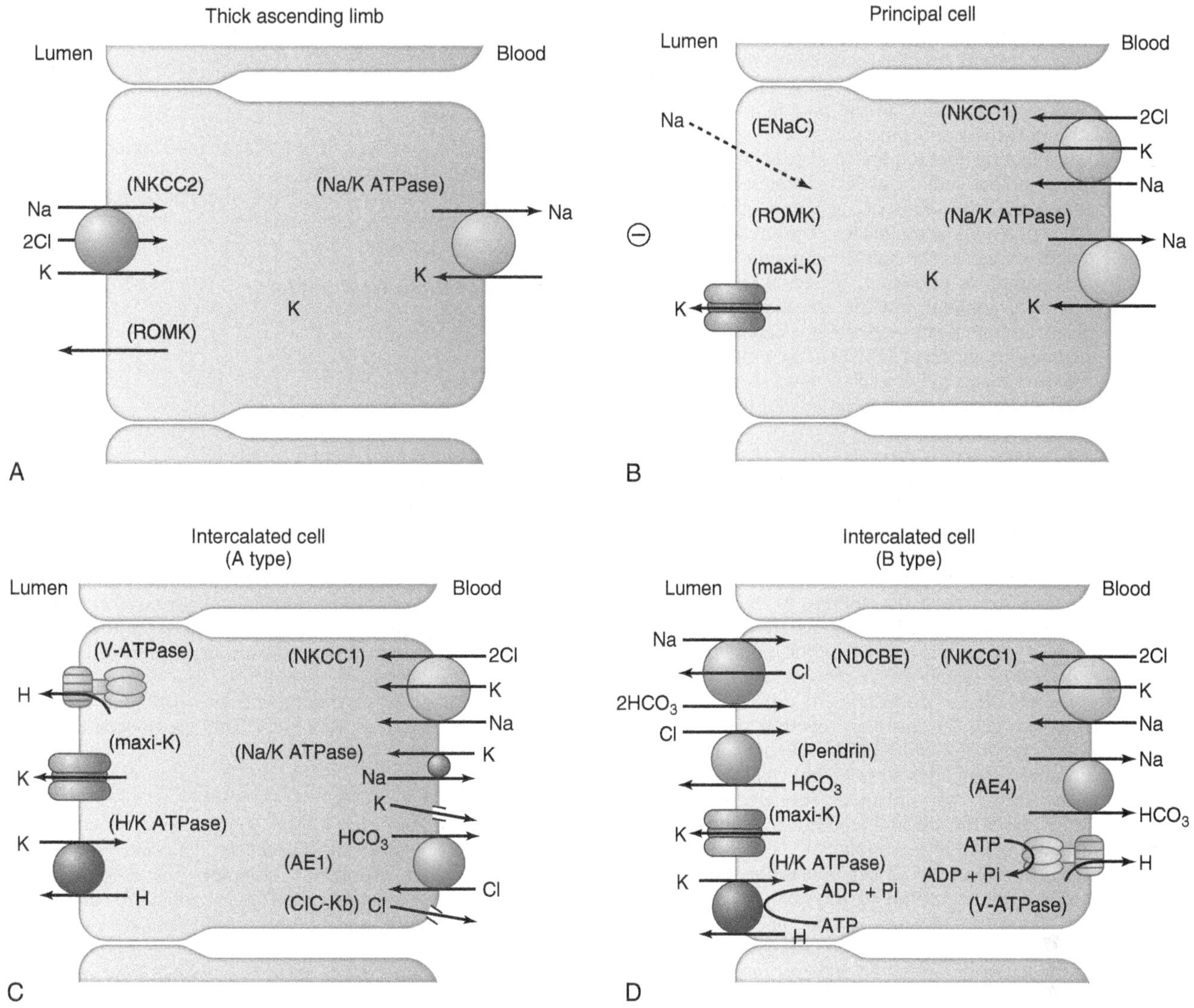

Fig. 98.4 Potassium (K^+) transport pathways in specific renal tubular cells. (A) In the thick ascending limb of the loop of Henle, potassium is avidly absorbed by specialized luminal Na^+-K^+-$2Cl^-$ *(NKCC2)* co-transport. A luminal secretory potassium channel, the renal outer medullary potassium channel *(ROMK)* in this cell, allows potassium to recycle back into the tubular fluid, thereby ensuring a continuous and abundant supply of potassium for the co-transporter. (B) In the cortical collecting duct, potassium is pumped into the cell in exchange for sodium by the basolateral Na^+, K^+-ATPase. Basolateral *NKCC1* also contributes to uptake of intracellular potassium. After entry into and accumulation in the cell, potassium is secreted preferentially across the apical membrane through the *ROMK* or BK channel, a process driven by a favorable electrochemical gradient. The electrochemical gradient is composed of two components: the cell-to-lumen concentration, or chemical gradient, and the cell-to-lumen electrical gradient. The latter is generated by apical sodium entry through amiloride-sensitive epithelial sodium channels *(ENaCs)* and its electrogenic basolateral extrusion. (C) Type A intercalated cells of the collecting duct mediate potassium absorption via apical H^+, K^+-ATPase, a pump that catalyzes the exchange of a single proton for potassium. BK channels secrete potassium in a flow-dependent manner. At the basolateral membrane, potassium absorption occurs by *NKCC1* and Na^+, K^+-ATPase. While the chloride channel ClC-Kb facilitates chloride movement outside the cell, the anion exchanger *(AE1)* exchanges intracellular bicarbonate *(HCO_3^-)* with extracellular chloride *(Cl)*. (D) Type B intercalated cells of the collecting duct mediate potassium absorption via apical H^+,K^+-ATPase, while BK channels secrete potassium. NDCBE and pendrin channels contribute to cellular uptake and secretion of HCO_3^-. At the basolateral membrane anion exchanger, AE4 moves bicarbonate out of the cell.

electrochemical gradient favoring sodium entry at the apical membrane. Diuretics such as furosemide and bumetanide, which inhibit the Na^+, K^+-$2Cl^-$ co-transporter, block potassium reabsorption at this site and promote potassium secretion, leading to profound urinary potassium losses.

Activity of the Na^+, K^+-$2Cl^-$ transporter requires the presence of a parallel potassium conductance in the urinary membrane. This luminal secretory potassium (SK) channel is encoded by the renal outer medullary K^+ channel *(ROMK)* gene.[68,69] Loss-of-function mutations in *ROMK* lead to antenatal Bartter syndrome, also known as the *hyperprostaglandin E syndrome,* which is characterized by severe renal salt and water losses, consistent with a pattern of impaired TALH function and similar to the clinical picture observed with the chronic administration of loop diuretics.[70] The typical presentation of antenatal Bartter syndrome includes polyhydramnios, premature delivery, and life-threatening episodes of dehydration during the first week of life. This group of patients also has severe growth failure, hypercalciuria with early-onset nephrocalcinosis, hyperreninism, and hyperaldosteronism but normal blood pressure.[71]

In the healthy adult, regulated potassium secretion by the distal tubule and the collecting duct contributes prominently to urinary potassium excretion, which can approach 20% of the filtered load (see Fig. 98.3).[57] Two major populations of cells compose the distal nephron. Principal cells reabsorb sodium and secrete potassium, whereas intercalated cells primarily function in acid-base homeostasis but can reabsorb potassium in response to dietary potassium restriction or metabolic acidosis. Potassium secretion by the collecting duct requires potassium to be actively transported into principal cells in exchange for sodium at the basolateral membrane by the action of the Na^+, K^+-ATPase pump (see Fig. 98.4B). Potassium accumulates within the cell and then passively diffuses across the apical membrane through SK channels. The magnitude of potassium secretion is determined by its electrochemical gradient and the apical permeability to this cation. The electrochemical gradient is established by the potassium concentration gradient between the cell and lumen and lumen-negative voltage, generated by apical sodium entry through epithelial sodium channels (ENaCs), and its basolateral electrogenic extrusion.

Two apical potassium-selective channels have been functionally identified in the distal nephron. The small-conductance SK channel, encoded by the *ROMK* gene, is considered to mediate baseline potassium secretion, whereas the high-conductance, stretch- and calcium-activated BK (maxi-K) channel mediates flow-stimulated potassium secretion.[72] Whereas BK channels in intercalated cells are now considered to mediate flow-stimulated potassium secretion, BK channels are also localized in the primary cilia of principal cells in the collecting duct, where they mediate flow signaling.[73] Surprisingly, in the primary cilia, the BK channels do not contribute to urinary potassium secretion but mediate cellular signaling together with calcium channels such as polycystin-2 and TRPV4.[74] Higher intracellular calcium concentration stimulates stretch- and calcium-activated BK channels. Any factor that enhances the electrochemical driving force or increases the apical membrane's permeability to potassium will favor potassium secretion.

The direction and magnitude of net potassium transport in the distal nephron vary according to physiologic need. Thus, in response to dietary potassium restriction or potassium depletion, the distal nephron may reabsorb potassium. Potassium reabsorption is mediated by an H^+, K^+-ATPase, an enzyme that exchanges a single potassium ion for a proton (see Fig. 98.4C), localized to the apical membrane of acid-base-transporting intercalated cells.

Potassium secretion in the distal nephron and specifically in the cortical collecting duct (CCD) is low early in life and cannot be stimulated by high urinary flow rates.[75] The limited capacity of the neonatal CCD for baseline potassium secretion appears not to be due to an unfavorable electrochemical gradient. Although Na^+, K^+-ATPase activity in neonatal collecting duct segments is only 50% of that measured in the mature nephron, cell potassium content of this segment is similar at both ages, presumably reflecting a relative paucity of membrane potassium channels early in life.[66,76,77] The rate of sodium absorption in the CCD at 2 weeks of age is approximately 60% of that measured in the adult and is not considered to be limiting for potassium secretion.[72] Electrophysiologic analysis has confirmed the absence of functional potassium secretory channels in the luminal membrane of the neonatal CCD.[78] Cumulative evidence now suggests that the postnatal increase in the potassium secretory capacity of the distal nephron is due to a developmental increase in number of SK/ROMK and BK channels, reflecting an increase in transcription and translation of functional channel proteins.[78-80] Molecular analyses demonstrate that *ROMK* messenger RNA and protein are first detectable in the second week of postnatal life in the rodent, immediately preceding the appearance of functional channels and potassium secretion in this segment.[75,78-80] Messenger RNA encoding the BK channel first becomes detectable after weaning in the rodent, as does functional BK channel activity.[81]

Box 98.1 Factors Regulating the External Balance of Potassium

Renal Factors

1. Distal sodium delivery and transepithelial voltage
2. Tubular (urinary) flow rate
3. Potassium intake–plasma potassium concentration
4. Hormones (mineralocorticoids, vasopressin)
5. Acid–base balance

Gastrointestinal Tract Factors

6. Stool volume
7. Hormones

Indirect evidence suggests that the neonatal distal nephron absorbs potassium. As indicated earlier, saline-expanded newborn dogs absorb 25% more of the distal potassium load than adult animals.[58] Functional analysis of the collecting duct in the rabbit has shown that the activity of apical H^+, K^+-ATPase in neonatal intercalated cells is equivalent to that in mature cells.[82] The latter data alone do not predict transepithelial potassium absorption under physiologic conditions. However, high distal tubular fluid potassium concentrations, as measured in vivo in the young rat, may facilitate lumen-to-cell potassium absorption mediated by the H^+, K^+-ATPase pump.[62]

The major factors that influence the *external* balance of potassium are listed in Box 98.1 and are discussed in the following sections.

DISTAL SODIUM DELIVERY AND TRANSEPITHELIAL VOLTAGE

As predicted from the principal cell model (see Fig. 98.4B), an increase in sodium absorption enhances the electrochemical driving force for potassium diffusion into the lumen. The magnitude of passive apical sodium entry and its electrogenic basolateral extrusion determine the apical membrane electrical potential and rate of basolateral Na^+-K^+ exchange. The dependence of potassium secretion on distal sodium delivery becomes evident at tubular fluid sodium concentrations less than 30 mEq/L, a value below which potassium secretion falls sharply.[83,84] In vivo measurements of the sodium concentration in distal tubular fluid generally exceed 35 mEq/L in both adult and suckling rats and thus should not restrict distal potassium secretion.[62,67,83,85]

Extracellular volume expansion or administration of many diuretics (osmotic diuretics, carbonic anhydrase inhibitors, loop and thiazide diuretics) is accompanied by an increase in excretion of both sodium and potassium. The kaliuresis is mediated not only by the increased delivery of sodium to the distal nephron but also by the increased tubular fluid flow rate, which activates the BK channel and maximizes the chemical driving forces, as described later, favoring potassium secretion. Other potassium-sparing diuretics, such as amiloride and triamterene, block distal sodium reabsorption, which reduces the electrical potential gradient favoring potassium secretion.

Sodium delivered to the distal nephron is generally accompanied by chloride. Chloride reabsorption across the paracellular pathway tends to reduce the lumen-negative potential that would otherwise drive potassium secretion. When sodium is accompanied by an anion less reabsorbable than chloride, such as bicarbonate (in proximal renal tubular acidosis), β-hydroxybutyrate (in diabetic ketoacidosis), or carbenicillin (during antibiotic therapy), luminal electronegativity is maintained, thereby eliciting more potassium secretion than occurs with a comparable sodium load delivered with chloride.

TUBULAR FLOW RATE

High rates of urinary flow in the mature but not neonatal or weanling rabbit distal nephron stimulate potassium secretion.[75] Thus volume expansion and diuretics, both of which increase distal tubular fluid flow rate, enhance potassium secretion in the fully differentiated kidney. A number of factors are responsible for the flow stimulation of potassium secretion. First, flow stimulates sodium reabsorption, which enhances the electrochemical gradient favoring potassium secretion.[86,87] Second, the higher the urinary flow rate in the distal nephron, the slower the rate of rise of tubular fluid potassium concentration because secreted potassium is rapidly diluted in urine of low potassium concentration. Maintenance of a low tubular fluid potassium concentration maximizes the potassium concentration gradient (and thus the chemical driving force) favoring net potassium secretion. Finally, increases in tubular fluid flow rate increase the intracellular calcium concentration, which activates the BK channel in the collecting duct to secrete potassium, thereby enhancing urinary potassium excretion.[72,81]

The capacity for flow-stimulated potassium secretion is developmentally regulated. Flow-stimulated potassium secretion, studied in single rabbit CCDs, does not appear until week 5 of postnatal life, approximately 2 weeks after baseline potassium secretion is first detected.[75,81] BK channel messenger RNA and protein are not consistently detected in the CCD until weeks 4 and 5 of life, respectively, suggesting that the postnatal appearance of flow-dependent potassium secretion is determined by the transcriptional and/or translational regulation of expression of BK channels in the distal nephron.[81]

POTASSIUM INTAKE AND CELLULAR POTASSIUM CONTENT

Ingestion of a potassium-rich meal is rapidly followed by enhanced urinary excretion of potassium. The increase in potassium entry into principal cells from the basolateral (blood) side maximizes the concentration gradient favoring apical potassium secretion into the urinary fluid (see Fig. 98.4B). Simultaneously, the increase in circulating levels of plasma aldosterone that accompanies potassium loading enhances the electrochemical driving force favoring potassium secretion in the distal nephron. It has also been suggested that a reflex increase in potassium excretion via vagal afferents follows activation of potassium-specific sensors in the gut or hepatic portal circulation, a control system that may be regulated in the absence of change in the plasma potassium concentration.[54,88]

Chronic potassium loading leads to potassium adaptation, an acquired tolerance to an otherwise lethal acute potassium load.[57] This adaptation occurs in the distal nephron and colon; the rate of potassium secretion in these segments varies directly with body stores of potassium. A similar adaptive response is seen in renal insufficiency, such that potassium balance is maintained during the course of many forms of progressive renal disease. The mechanisms underlying this adaptation in the principal cell include an increase not only in the density of apical membrane potassium channels but also in the number of conducting sodium channels and activity of the basolateral Na^+-K^+ pump. The latter two processes result in increases in transepithelial voltage and the intracellular potassium concentration, events that enhance the driving force favoring potassium diffusion from the cell into the urinary fluid.

When potassium intake is chronically reduced, potassium secretion by principal cells falls as reabsorption by intercalated cells increases. Stimulation of luminal H^+, K^+-ATPase activity in intercalated cells results not only in potassium retention but also in urinary acidification and metabolic alkalosis.

HORMONES

Mineralocorticoids stimulate sodium reabsorption and potassium secretion in principal cells of the distal nephron.[89,90] In the adult, the mineralocorticoid-induced stimulation of renal potassium secretion is considered to be due primarily to an increase in the electrochemical driving force favoring potassium exit across the apical membrane generated by stimulation of apical sodium entry and reabsorption. Aldosterone action requires its initial binding to the mineralocorticoid receptor, followed by translocation of the hormone-receptor complex to the nucleus in which specific genes are stimulated to code for physiologically active proteins (e.g., Na^+, K^+-ATPase). Cellular effects within the fully differentiated CCD include increases in the density of active ENaC channels, caused by recruitment of intracellular channels to the apical membrane, de novo synthesis of ENaC subunits, and activation of preexisting channels.[91,92] Aldosterone also stimulates Na^+, K^+-ATPase activity through both recruitment of preexisting pumps to the plasma membrane and increased total amounts of sodium pump subunits.[93] The sum effect of these actions is the stimulation of net sodium absorption, leading to an increase in lumen negative transepithelial voltage and thereby facilitating net potassium secretion. The effects of aldosterone on ENaC and, to some extent, the Na^+-K^+ pump appear to be indirect, mediated by aldosterone-induced proteins, including serum- and glucocorticoid-inducible kinase.[94]

Plasma aldosterone concentrations in the newborn are high compared with those in the adult.[2,95] Yet clearance studies in fetal and newborn animals demonstrate a relative insensitivity of the immature kidney to this hormone.[2,96-98] The density of aldosterone-binding sites, receptor affinity, and degree of nuclear binding of hormone receptor are thought to be similar in mature and immature rats.[98] Thus the early hyposensitivity to aldosterone is considered to represent a postreceptor phenomenon.[2,98]

Angiotensin II (ANGII) also modifies ROMK activity via angiotensin II type 1 (AT_1R) and type 2 (AT_2R) receptors. In animals during a dietary potassium restriction, ANGII stimulation of AT_1R inhibits ROMK, whereas in animals on a high-potassium diet, ANGII stimulation of AT_2R, increased potassium secretion via ROMK.[99] The transtubular potassium gradient (TTKG) provides an indirect, semiquantitative measure of the renal response to mineralocorticoid activity in the aldosterone-sensitive cortical distal nephron and is calculated by using the equation:

$$\text{TTKG} = \left[K^+\right]_{\text{urine}} / (U/P)_{\text{osmolality}} / \left[K^+\right]_{\text{plasma}} \qquad [98.1]$$

where $[K^+]$ equals the potassium concentration in either urine (U) or plasma (P), as indicated.[100-102] Measurements of TTKG have been reported to be lower in 27- than in 30-week GA preterm infants followed over the first 5 weeks of postnatal life.[103] The low TTKG has been attributed to a state of relative hypoaldosteronism but may also reflect the absence of potassium secretory transport pathways (i.e., channel proteins).[103]

ACID–BASE BALANCE

Disorders of acid–base homeostasis can induce changes in tubular potassium secretion. Acute metabolic acidosis decreases the urine pH and reduces potassium excretion, whereas both acute respiratory alkalosis and metabolic alkalosis result in increases in urine pH and potassium excretion. Chronic metabolic acidosis has variable effects on urinary potassium excretion.

The alkalosis-induced stimulation of potassium secretion reflects two direct effects on principal cells: (1) the stimulation of Na^+, K^+-ATPase activity and basolateral potassium uptake and (2) an increase in the permeability of the apical membrane to potassium, resulting from an increase in the length of time the potassium-selective channels remain open.[57] Alkalosis also decreases acid secretion in intercalated cells, thereby reducing H^+,K^+-ATPase-mediated countertransport.

Acute metabolic acidosis reduces cell potassium concentration and leads to a reduction in urine pH, which in turn inhibits apical potassium channel (SK/ROMK) activity.[57] The net effect is a fall in urinary potassium secretion. The effect of chronic metabolic acidosis on potassium secretion is more complex and may be influenced by modifications of the glomerular filtrate (e.g., chloride and bicarbonate concentrations), tubular fluid flow rate, and circulating aldosterone levels.[57] The latter two factors may lead to an increase rather than a decrease in potassium secretion and excretion.

CONTRIBUTION OF THE GASTROINTESTINAL TRACT

Under normal conditions in the adult, 5% to 10% of daily potassium intake is excreted in the stool (see Fig. 98.1).The colon is considered to be the main target for the regulation of intestinal potassium excretion.[104] Potassium transport in the colon represents the balance of secretion and absorption.[105] Under baseline conditions, net potassium secretion predominates over absorption in the adult, whereas the neonatal gut is poised for net potassium absorption.[104]

Potassium secretion requires potassium uptake by the Na^+, K^+-ATPase pump and Na^+,K^+-$2Cl^-$ co-transporter located in the basolateral membrane of colonocytes; potassium is then secreted across the apical membrane through potassium channels, including a calcium-activated BK channel similar to that found in the distal nephron.[106-109] Stool potassium content can be enhanced by any factor that increases colonic secretion, including aldosterone, epinephrine, and prostaglandins.[110-112] Indomethacin and dietary potassium restriction reduce potassium secretion by inhibiting the basolateral transporters and apical potassium channels. Diarrheal illnesses are typically associated with hypokalemia, presumably because of the presence of non-reabsorbed anions (which obligate K^+ secretion), an enhanced electrochemical gradient established by active chloride secretion, and secondary hyperaldosteronism resulting from volume contraction.

Potassium adaptation in the colon is demonstrated by increased fecal potassium secretion after potassium loading and increased excretion with renal insufficiency. Fecal potassium excretion may triple in patients with severe chronic renal insufficiency.[110,113-115] The enhanced colonic potassium secretion characteristic of chronic renal insufficiency requires induction and/or activation of apical BK channels in surface colonic epithelial cells.[116]

Net colonic potassium absorption is significantly higher in young versus adult rats.[104]The higher rate of potassium absorption during infancy is due to robust activity of potassium absorptive pumps located in apical membrane and limited activity of the basolateral transporters that mediate secretion.[117,118]

CONDITIONS OF ABNORMAL POTASSIUM LEVELS

HYPERKALEMIA

In preterm infants and neonates, reference ranges for serum potassium are usually higher than those in adults; this is consistent with the increased physiologic requirement for potassium due to accelerated growth and cell division in infancy. In addition, higher baseline serum potassium levels in preterm infants and neonates are partially due to a lower response of the distal nephron to aldosterone, owing to these subjects' immaturity. Frequently, hyperkalemia, defined as serum potassium levels above 6.5 mmol/L, is due to extrarenal etiologies (Table 98.2).[119] For example, hyperkalemia is observed with severe bruising, cephalohematoma, hemolysis, acidosis, thrombocytosis, hypoglycemia, and ischemia.[120] Renal causes of hyperkalemia may include poor renal perfusion due to a traumatic delivery and subsequent renal injury or medications such as indomethacin or angiotensin-converting enzyme (ACE) inhibitors (see Table 98.2). Hyperkalemia can be diagnosed by analysis of blood chemistry and confirmed by peaked T waves on an electrocardiogram. Hyperkalemia may cause fatal cardiac arrhythmia, brain hemorrhage, periventricular leukomalacia, and sudden death.[121]

Table 98.2 Etiology of Hyperkalemia in Preterm Infants and Neonates.

Extrarenal	Renal
Hemolysis	Renal failure (e.g., prerenal, intrinsic, or postrenal)
Bruising	Pseudohypoaldosteronism (PHA) type I
Cephalohematoma	PHA type II
Thrombocytosis	Transient PHA due to urinary tract infection, obstructive uropathy
Acidosis	Renal tubular dysplasia
Medication (angiotensin-converting enzyme inhibitors, indomethacin)	Renal outer medullary K^+ channel mutations in Bartter syndrome (transient hyperkalemia)
Nonoliguric hyperkalemia	
Congenital adrenal hyperplasia	

NONOLIGURIC HYPERKALEMIA

As discussed, up to 50% of all premature infants with very low or extremly low birth weight develop hyperkalemia within the first 72 hours of life with no obvious organ injury owing to a condition termed *nonoliguric hyperkalemia.*[122-124] Most infants with this condition are asymptomatic. Nonoliguric hyperkalemia is thought to be due to loss of intracellular potassium into the extracellular space caused by immature Na^+/K^+-ATPase activity.[125] Lower erythrocyte Na^+/K^+-ATPase activity has been described in hyperkalemic premature infants compared with infants with normal potassium levels.[16] No relationship between nonoliguric hyperkalemia and hemolysis, bruising, or intracranial hemorrhage has been found.[14] Prenatal steroid treatment could potentially prevent hyperkalemia by up-regulating Na^+/K^+-ATPase.[18] Early initiation of parenteral and enteral nutrition is believed to have reduced the incidence of this disorder.

PSEUDOHYPOALDOSTERONISM TYPE I

Pseudohypoaldosteronism type I (PHAI) is caused by mineralocorticoid resistance due to rare mutations in the genes encoding either the mineralocorticoid receptor (*NR3C2* for the renal form of PHAI) or one of the three subunits that form the apical epithelial Na^+ channel, called *ENaC* (*SCNN1A, SCNN1B, SCNN1G* for the generalized form of PHAI).[126] Classic features of PHAI include neonatal renal salt wasting, failure to thrive, and dehydration (Table 98.3). PHAI is characterized by inadequate potassium and hydrogen secretion resulting in hyperkalemia and metabolic acidosis; it is associated with hyponatremia and highly elevated renin and aldosterone levels. Patients have inappropriately high urine Na^+ excretion, reduced urinary K^+ secretion, and occasional hypercalciuria.[127] Two different forms of PHAI are differentiated; they vary significantly regarding disease severity (see Table 98.3).

RENAL PSEUDOHYPOALDOSTERONISM TYPE I

Renal PHAI is caused by heterozygous mutations of the mineralocorticoid receptor (encoded by the gene *NR3C2*) and is inherited in an autosomal-dominant fashion.[128,129] Due to the tissue distribution of *NR3C2*, mineralocorticoid resistance is restricted to the kidney. Mutations, including de novo mutations, have been identified throughout the entire *NR3C2* gene. Renal PHAI is typically milder and more common than the general form of PHAI.[128] Infants with renal PHAI exhibit renal salt wasting, hyponatremia, hyperkalemia, failure to thrive, vomiting, dehydration, metabolic acidosis, and elevated renin and aldosterone levels in early infancy. Symptoms usually improve

Table 98.3 Clinical and Laboratory Characteristics of Pseudohypoaldosteronism (PHA) Type I: Renal and Generalized Forms.

	Renal PHAI	Generalized PHAI
Gene	*NR3C2*	*SCNN1A, SCNN1B, SCNN1G*
Inheritance	Autosomal dominant	Autosomal recessive
Disease severity	Mild	Severe
Failure to thrive	+	+
Dehydration	Mild	Severe
Hyponatremia	+	+
Hyperkalemia	+	+
Renin	Elevated	Elevated
Aldosterone	Elevated	Elevated
Cardiac involvement	–	+
Respiratory involvement	–	+
Skin eczema	–	+
Sweat Na^+	Normal	Elevated

+, Present; –, absent.

in early infancy, between 18 and 24 months of age. It remains unclear which mechanism results in improvement of symptoms with increasing age, but it is suspected that maturation of tubular function, compensatory increase of proximal Na^+ reabsorption, and easier access to salt play a role. In an inducible nephron-specific mineralocorticoid receptor knockout mouse model, animals survived and presented with similar characteristics as the human phenotype. However, on a sodium-deficient diet, these animals die.[130]

GENERALIZED PSEUDOHYPOALDOSTERONISM TYPE I

The generalized form of PHAI is due to homozygous- or compound heterozygous-inactivating mutations of one of the three ENaC subunits—*SCNN1A, SCNN1B,* and *SCNN1G*—resulting in nonfunctional ENaC protein in kidney, colon, sweat, and salivary glands.[131] In contrast to the clinically more benign form of renal PHAI, generalized PHAI is characterized by severe renal salt wasting, hyponatremia, and dehydration due to systemic salt loss in early infancy.[126] Because of end-organ resistance, renin and aldosterone levels are elevated. In contrast to renal PHAI, patients with generalized PHAI can also develop cardiac, respiratory, or skin involvement.[132-134]

The clinical course can be complicated by arrhythmias, collapse, shock, and cardiac arrest. The Na^+ concentration in sweat and saliva is typically elevated, and this finding can be utilized as an additional diagnostic tool. Pulmonary involvement is characterized by cough, tachypnea, and wheezing and is due to impaired Na^+-dependent fluid absorption in the lung. Absence of the amiloride-sensitive Na^+ channel ENaC was found in a neonate with generalized PHAI.[133,135] Pulmonary involvement can be confused with cystic fibrosis. Generalized PHAI is a lifelong condition; it does not improve with age and remains life threatening due to the risk of dehydration and hyperkalemia. Animal studies for generalized PHAI have been complicated by the fact that constitutive inactivation of different ENaC subunits has been lethal in neonatal mice. The hyperkalemia seems to be the determinant factor for downregulation of sodium-chloride co-transporter (NCC) activity. Using an inducible, nephron-specific knockout mouse model for the α subunit of ENaC, characteristics mimicking the human PHAI phenotype were described and less expression and phosphorylation of NCC was found. Using a high-salt and low-potassium diet, NCC expression returned to normal levels in knockout mice.[136] These findings were also confirmed for nephron-specific knockout mouse models for the β and γ subunits of ENaC.[137,138]

TRANSIENT PSEUDOHYPOALDOSTERONISM

Considered to be a secondary form of PHAI, transient PHA is frequently caused by medications, urinary tract infections, urinary tract malformations, or tubulo-interstitial nephropathies.[139] Transient PHA is thought to be caused by tubular resistance to aldosterone.[139,140] The clinical presentation is very similar to PHAI with dehydration, hyperkalemia, hyponatremia, metabolic acidosis, hyperaldosteronism, and elevated renin levels. Medications causing transient PHA include amiloride, triamterene, trimethoprim, and pentamidine as ENaC blockers. In addition, spironolactone (a mineralocorticoid receptor antagonist) and cyclosporine can contribute to transient PHA.[141] Other medications contributing to transient PHA either interfere with the renin-angiotensin system (e.g., ACE inhibitors) or are nonsteroidal antiinflammatory substances or β blockers. The most common causes of transient PHA in neonates are urinary tract infections and obstructive uropathy.[142] Neonatal medullary necrosis and renal vein thrombosis can also result in transient PHA.[143]

PSEUDOHYPOALDOSTERONISM TYPE II

CLINICAL PRESENTATION

Both PHAI and PHAII share metabolic acidosis and hyperkalemia. In contrast to the volume depletion characteristic of PHAI patients, PHAII patients present with salt-sensitive hypertension, low plasma renin activity, and inadequately normal aldosterone levels (given the level of hyperkalemia), suggesting renal Na^+ retention and volume expansion.[143,144] PHAII patients respond well to thiazides, suggesting a role for thiazide-sensitive NCC in the enhanced Na^+ retention. Individuals with PHAII, which is also called *Gordon syndrome,* can present in preterm or in early infancy with hyperkalemia and metabolic acidosis in the presence of normal adrenal and renal function. Frequently, hyperkalemia presents first and hypertension may occur later.

GENETICS

Initially, heterozygous mutations causing PHAII were found in two genes called *WNK1* and *WNK4*, which encode With-no-lysine (K) kinases 1 and 4.[145] The name derives from the replacement of a highly conserved lysine residue by cysteine in the catalytic unit of these two proteins. Persons with PHAII were found to carry either intronic *WNK1* deletions, resulting in a higher *WNK1* abundance, or *WNK4* missense mutations.[145] In 2012, Boyden and colleagues identified mutations in two additional genes called cullin 3 *(CUL3)* and kelch-like 3 *(KLHL3)* causing PHAII in 52 families.[146,147] The two encoded proteins are components of an E3 ubiquitin ligase complex that degrades WNKs.[148,149] Interestingly, *KLHL3* mutations can be inherited in a dominant or recessive fashion, whereas *CUL3* mutations are solely inherited in a dominant fashion. Disease severity is dependent on the affected gene with *CUL3* mutations causing the most severe phenotype, presenting in early infancy with more severe hyperkalemia and acidosis. This has been confirmed by other reports of hyperkalemia and acidosis in young infants.[150,151] Carriers of recessive *KLHL3* mutations are more severely affected than patients with dominant *KLHL3, WNK4,* or *WNK1* mutations. All mutations causing PHA2 eventually result in accumulations of WNK proteins.

PHYSIOLOGY

By identifying the link between PHAII and *WNK1* or *WNK4* mutations, our understanding of Na^+ and K^+ homeostasis and blood pressure regulation has much improved. *WNK1* and

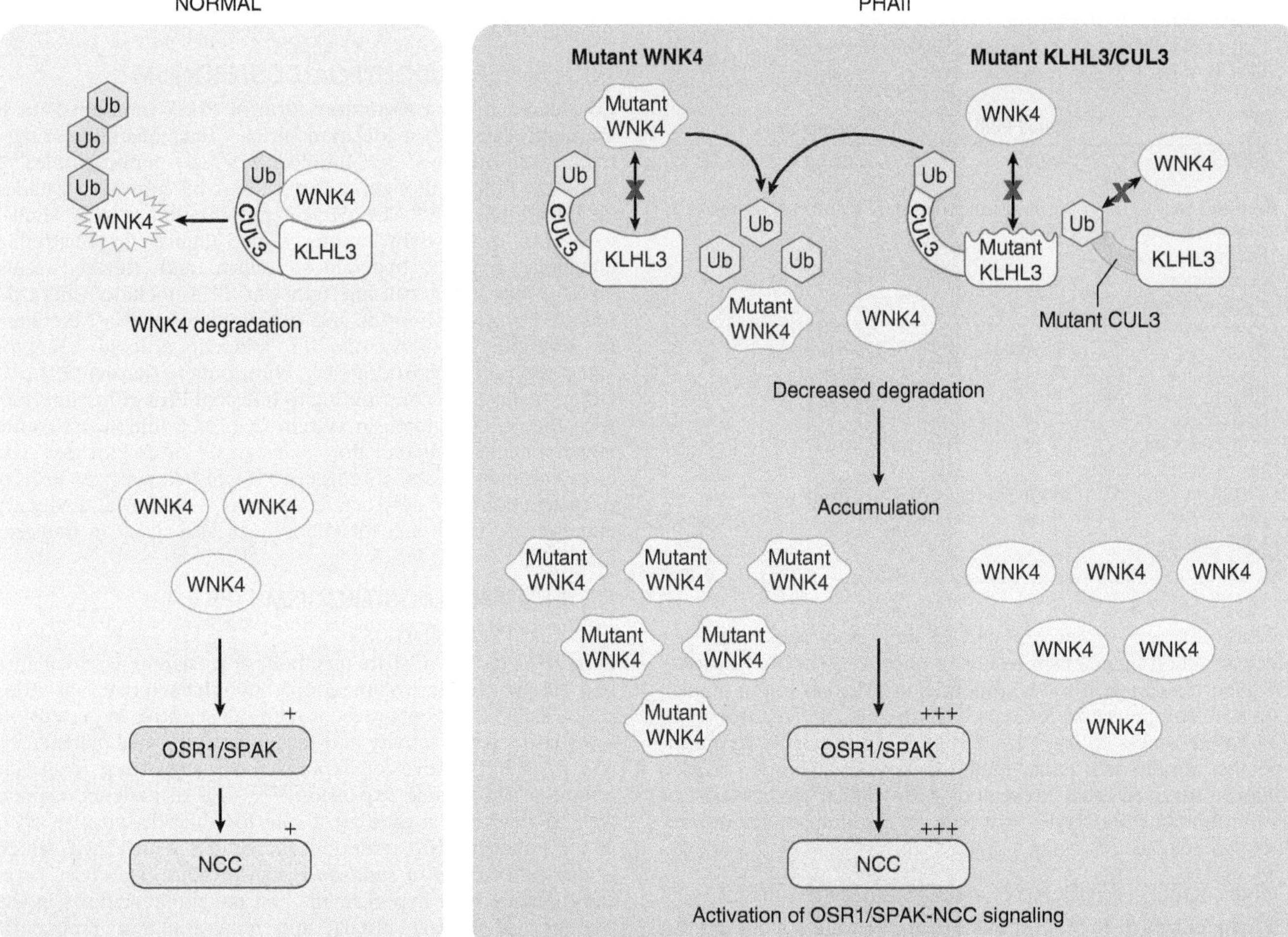

Fig. 98.5 Under physiologic conditions *WNK4* levels are maintained at a lower level due to ubiquitination. The *KLHL3-CUL3* E3 ligase complex binds and transfers WNK4 to ubiquitination. Pseudohypoaldosteronism type II (PHAII)-causing mutations in WNK4 or KLHL3 affect the binding of WNK4, which results in decreased WNK4 ubiquitination. CUL3 mutations result in decreased E3 ligase activity, which also increases WNK4 levels. Increased WNK4 levels were confirmed in a PHAII mouse model together with elevated *OSR1/SPAK* levels. Finally, along the WNK-OSR1/SPAK axis, NCC activity is enhanced. (With permission from Uchida S, Sohara E, Rai T, et al. Regulation of with-no-lysine kinase signaling by Kelch-like proteins. *Biol Cell.* 2014;106:45–56.)

WNK4 are expressed in the aldosterone-sensitive distal nephron. *WNKs* are thought to switch the aldosterone response in the kidney to be kaliuretic or antinatriuretic, depending on the physiologic requirement.[152] Because of the impressive response of PHAII patients to thiazides, a link between *WNK1* and *WNK4* was hypothesized to modulate NCC. *Wnk4* knockout mice displayed a phenotype similar to NCC loss-of-function mutations suggesting that *WNK4* is actually a positive regulator of NCC in vivo, thereby contributing to sodium and fluid absorption while also resulting in fluid retention and hypertension (Fig. 98.5).[153] Animal studies of transgenic and knockin mice carrying a *WNK4* mutation (Q562E or D561A) exhibit a phenotype similar to that in PHAII patients.[154,155] A chloride-binding site close to the conserved domain of WNK kinases is important for the inhibition of WNKs as the bound chloride stabilizes an inactive conformation.[156] The hyperkalemia in PHAII patients may be due to increased NCC activity in the DCT, which results in decreased distal Na^+ delivery, subsequently less lumen-negative potential difference, and thus less K^+ secretion in the connecting tubule, and protein inhibition of ENaC and ROMK.[157,158] An additional component in the hyperkalemia of PHAII patients is that *WNK1* and *WNK4* mutations result in even further decreased cell surface abundance of *ROMK* by increasing *ROMK* endocytosis.[159,160] Finally, increased distal chloride reabsorption was hypothesized to contribute to a less electronegative lumen, which subsequently decreases the electrochemical gradient for K^+ secretion.[161-163] Interestingly, patients with *WNK4* mutations exhibit hypercalciuria, and in vitro experiments demonstrated less activity of renal calcium channel TRPV5 due to increased endocytosis of TRPV5 by *WNK4* (see Fig. 98.5).[164]

WNK regulation of NCC, NKCC, and ROMK channels also involves two other kinases called *SPAK (Ste20p family protein kinases)* and *OSR1 (oxidative stress responsive kinase-1)* that are downstream of *WNK1* and *WNK4* (Figs. 98.5 and 98.6).[165,166] *WNK1* and *WNK4* associate with OSR1/SPAK and activate OSR1/SPAK by phosphorylation that in turn results in increased NKCC activity. *WNK1* is phosphorylated by hyperosmotic stress and releases OSR1 to interact with NKCC1. Interestingly, OSR1/SPAK signaling was increased in mice mimicking PHAII.[155] OSR/SPAK is also involved in the regulation of NCC, and the phenotype of PHAII does not develop in a *Wnk4* D561A-mutant mouse if OSR and SPAK are mutated.[167] Constitutively active SPAK in mice is characterized by hypertension and hyperkalemia and results in remodeling of the distal nephron with a lower connecting tubule mass, and less apical ENaC and ROMK expression.[168]

The physiologic significance of *WNKs* comes into play when the body has to regulate Na^+ and K^+ homeostasis in individuals with hypovolemia or hyperkalemia. In individuals with hypovolemia,

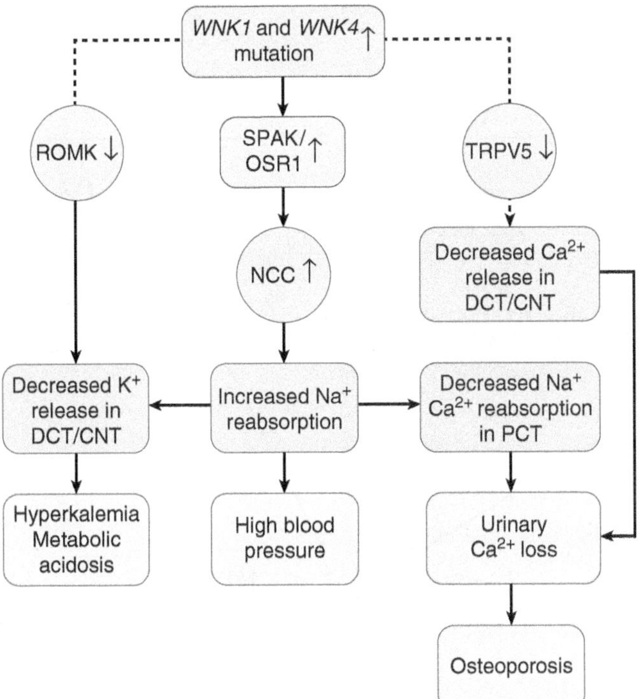

Fig. 98.6 Physiologic consequences of *WNK1* and *WNK4* mutations regarding Na^+, K^+, and Ca^{2+} channel regulation. Increased *NCC* activity due to *WNK1* and *WNK4* mutations increase tubular Na^+ and Cl^- absorption and contribute to hypertension. Hyperkalemia in pseudohypoaldosteronism type II is caused by stronger inhibition of renal outer medullary K^+ channel *(ROMK)* activity due to enhanced ROMK endocytosis. In addition, increased Na^+ reabsorption in distal convoluted tubule *(DCT)* results in decreased Na^+ delivery to the collecting duct, thus further aggravating hyperkalemia. Finally, increased paracellular Cl^- shunting may decrease the lumen negative charge and so also decrease a stimulus for K^+ secretion. TRPV5 (transient receptor potential vanilloid 5) activity is further inhibited by *WNK4* mutations, which result in hypercalciuria and subsequently osteoporosis. (With permission from Pathare G, Hoenderop JG, Bindels RJ, et al. A molecular update on pseudohypoaldosteronism type II. *Am J Physiol Renal Physiol.* 2013;305:F1513–1520.)

Na^+ reabsorption is increased without any effect on K^+ secretion, and in those with hyperkalemia, Na^+ reabsorption is decreased and K^+ secretion is increased (see Fig. 98.6). High versus low salt intake decreased or increased the phosphorylation of OSR1/SPAK and NCC in the kidney, thus adjusting urinary salt excretion dependent on dietary intake. *WNK1* also activates SPAK/OSR1 and increases NKCC activity. The WNK-OSR1/SPAK-NCC axis is also regulated by potassium with high K diet decreasing the signaling and low K diet increasing the signaling.[169] As distal sodium delivery increases distal potassium secretion, NCC activity depends on extracellular potassium concentration, thereby contributing to a lower urinary potassium excretion in the context of hypokalemia.[169-172]

In conclusion, the hypertension observed in PHAII patients may be caused by elevated Na^+ reabsorption via NCC, NKCC2, ENaC, and paracellular Cl^- pathways. A combination of events contributes to the laboratory constellation seen in PHAII: (1) increased NCC activity, contributing to hypervolemia and decreased distal sodium delivery, thus impairing distal K^+ secretion via ROMK, (2) directly depressed ROMK activity, and (3) increased paracellular Cl^- reabsorption causing a less electronegative lumen in the collecting duct and less ENaC activity, thus decreasing K^+ secretion via ROMK. The discovery of novel proteins, including WNKs, *CUL3,* and *KHLH3,* contributing to Na^+ and K^+ homeostasis has expanded our understanding of electrolytes and volume regulation significantly.

CONGENITAL ADRENAL HYPERPLASIA

Severe aldosterone deficiency is seen in neonates with salt-losing congenital adrenal hyperplasia (CAH) due to 21-hydroxylase activity or aldosterone synthase defects. Whereas the first group of children is glucocorticoid- and mineralocorticoid-deficient because of compromised hydrocortisone and aldosterone synthesis, the latter group has no genital or glucocorticoid abnormalities. Characteristic symptoms include hyponatremia, hyperkalemia, failure to thrive, hypotension, and dehydration. For more details regarding CAH, refer to Chapter 144. Alternatively, primary hypoaldosteronism may be caused by trauma, infections, hemorrhage, or thrombosis of the adrenal cortex.

RENAL TUBULAR DYSGENESIS

Homozygous- or compound heterozygous-inactivating mutations of different components of the renin-angiotensin system, including renin, angiotensinogen, ACE, and the ANGII receptor were found to cause inherited forms of renal tubular dysgenesis (RTD).[173] RTD is characterized by oligohydramnios, fetal anuria, perinatal death, and frequently wide fontanels. The clinical presentation can also be mimicked by the maternal intake of ACE inhibitors or angiotensin receptor blockers (Fig. 98.7).[174]

HYPOKALEMIA

Hypokalemia can be transient as a result of shifting of potassium from the extracellular fluid compartment into the intracellular fluid compartment, or it can be chronic as a result of excess potassium excretion or insufficient potassium intake. Conditions that cause a shifting of potassium from the extracellular fluid into the cells include acute metabolic alkalosis or administration of insulin or β-agonists (see Table 98.1). As discussed, TTKG can be helpful in determining if there is excess loss of potassium from the kidneys.[103] In conditions of hypokalemia with a normal renal response, one should expect a low value of TTKG. Thus, an inappropriately high value would indicate renal wasting of potassium in the face of hypokalemia.

Chronic hypokalemia is usually the result of a genetic disease that results in the wasting of potassium from the kidney. The most common cause of renal potassium wasting is Bartter syndrome.[71,175-177] This can be caused by a mutation of one of the transport proteins involved in ion transport in the TALH (listed in Box 98.2). Many of these patients will have polyhydramnios because of the polyuria in utero. It should be noted that patients with the *ROMK* defect will often present with hyperkalemia in the neonatal period because they have a limited ability to excrete potassium (previously discussed). As the infant matures, the BK channel expression will increase and they will then become hypokalemic.

Gitelman syndrome also causes renal wasting of potassium.[175,176] This is due to a defect in the thiazide-sensitive NCC in the distal convoluted tubule. These patients usually present as older children and in general have milder symptoms compared with patients with Bartter syndrome. Hypomagnesemia is more consistent with Gitelman syndrome than with Bartter syndrome.

Another cause of renal potassium wasting is the rare EAST syndrome,[178,179] which causes epilepsy, ataxia, sensorineural deafness, and renal tubulopathy. It stems from a defect in a potassium channel, KCNJ10. Children with renal tubular acidosis types 1 and 2 can present with hypokalemia due to renal wasting of potassium.

Potassium can also be lost through the stool in a condition known as *congenital chloride diarrhea*,[180] which is due to a mutation in the chloride hydroxyl exchanger in the gastrointestinal tract. Thus the TTKG would be low, indicating a nonrenal source of potassium loss.[103]

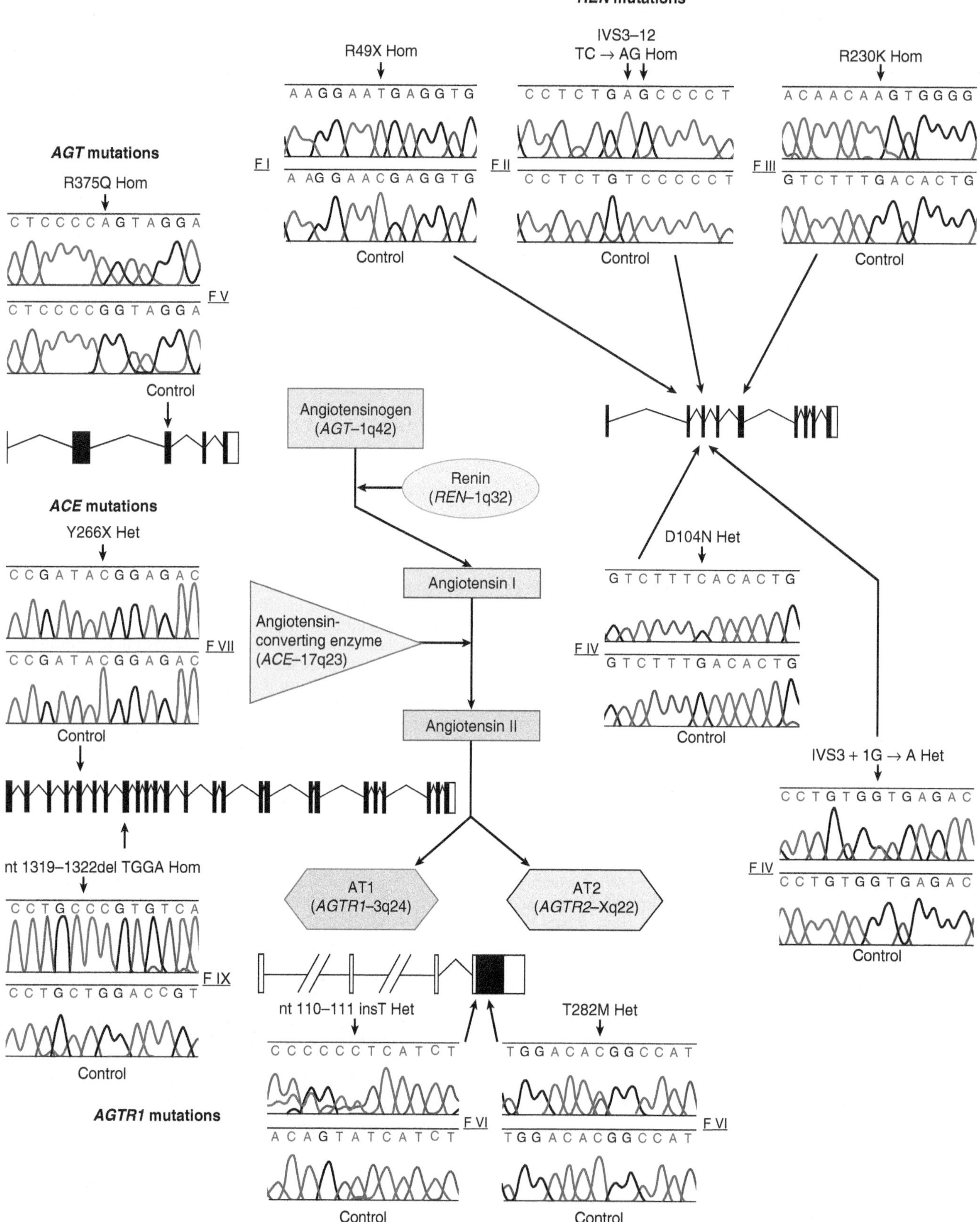

Fig. 98.7 Mutations in different components of the renin-angiotensin system *(RAS)* (e.g., angiotensinogen *[AGT]*, renin *[REN]*, angiotensin-converting enzyme *[ACE]*, and angiotensin II receptor type 1 *[AGTR1]*) result in the same phenotype of renal tubular dysplasia. Diagrams outline the intron-exon structure. Chromatograms of the different mutations are shown for each family. *F,* Family; *het,* heterozygous; *hom,* homozygous. (With permission from Gribouval O, Gonzales M, Neuhaus T, et al. Mutations in genes in the renin-angiotensin system are associated with autosomal recessive renal tubular dysgenesis. *Nat Genet.* 2005;37[9]:964–968.)

Box 98.2 Genetic Causes of Bartter Syndrome

1. Na-K-Cl-co-transporter 2 (NKCC2)
2. Chloride channel subunit B *(CLCNKB)*
3. Renal outer medullary K^+ channel *(ROMK)*
4. Barttin (with sensorineural deafness) *(BSND)*
5. Calcium-sensing receptor (*CaSR*)
6. MAGE-D2 (*MAGED2*)

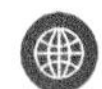
A complete reference list is available at www.ExpertConsult.com.

SELECT REFERENCES

1. Delgado MM, Rohatgi R, Khan S, et al. Sodium and potassium clearances by the maturing kidney: clinical-molecular correlates. *Pediatr Nephrol.* 2003;18(8):759-767.
2. Sulyok E, Nemeth M, Tenyi I, et al. Relationship between maturity, electrolyte balance and the function of the renin-angiotensin-aldosterone system in newborn infants. *Biol Neonate.* 1979;35(1-2):60-65.
3. Butte NF, Hopkinson JM, Wong WW, et al. Body composition during the first 2 years of life: an updated reference. *Pediatr Res.* 2000;47(5):578-585.
4. Flynn MA, Woodruff C, Clark J, Chase G. Total body potassium in normal children. *Pediatr Res.* 1972;6(4):239-245.
5. Dickerson JW, Widdowson EM. Chemical changes in skeletal muscle during development. *Biochem J.* 1960;74:247-257.
6. Rutledge MM, Clark J, Woodruff C, et al. A longitudinal study of total body potassium in normal breastfed and bottle-fed infants. *Pediatr Res.* 1976;10(2):114-117.
7. Satlin LM. Regulation of potassium transport in the maturing kidney. *Semin Nephrol.* 1999;19(2):155-165.
8. Serrano CV, Talbert LM, Welt LG. Potassium deficiency in the pregnant dog. *J Clin Invest.* 1964;43:27-31.
9. Dancis J, Springer D. Fetal homeostasis in maternal malnutrition: potassium and sodium deficiency in rats. *Pediatr Res.* 1970;4(4):345-351.
10. Rodriguez-Soriano J, Vallo A, Castillo G, Oliveros R. Renal handling of water and sodium in infancy and childhood: a study using clearance methods during hypotonic saline diuresis. *Kidney Int.* 1981;20(6):700-704.
11. Leslie GI, Carman G, Arnold JD. Early neonatal hyperkalaemia in the extremely premature newborn infant. *J Paediatr Child Health.* 1990;26(1):58-61.
12. Gruskay J, Costarino AT, Polin RA, Baumgart S. Nonoliguric hyperkalemia in the premature infant weighing less than 1000 grams. *J Pediatr.* 1988;113(2):381-386.
13. Lorenz JM, Kleinman LI, Markarian K. Potassium metabolism in extremely low birth weight infants in the first week of life. *J Pediatr.* 1997;131(1 Pt 1):81-86.
14. Sato K, Kondo T, Iwao H, et al. Internal potassium shift in premature infants: cause of nonoliguric hyperkalemia. *J Pediatr.* 1995;126(1):109-113.
15. Shaffer SG, Kilbride HW, Hayen LK, et al. Hyperkalemia in very low birth weight infants. *J Pediatr.* 1992;121(2):275-279.
16. Stefano JL, Norman ME, Morales MC, et al. Decreased erythrocyte Na+,K(+)-ATPase activity associated with cellular potassium loss in extremely low birth weight infants with nonoliguric hyperkalemia. *J Pediatr.* 1993;122(2):276-284.
17. Uga N, Nemoto Y, Ishii T, et al. Antenatal steroid treatment prevents severe hyperkalemia in very low-birthweight infants. *Pediatr Int.* 2003;45(6):656-660.
18. Omar SA, DeCristofaro JD, Agarwal BI, LaGamma EF. Effect of prenatal steroids on potassium balance in extremely low birth weight neonates. *Pediatrics.* 2000;106(3):561-567.
19. Therien AG, Blostein R. Mechanisms of sodium pump regulation. *Am J Physiol Cell Physiol.* 2000;279(3):C541-C566.
20. Zierler KL, Rabinowitz D. Effect of very small concentrations of insulin on forearm metabolism: persistence of its action on potassium and free fatty acids without its effect on glucose. *J Clin Invest.* 1964;43:950-962.
21. Hundal HS, Marette A, Mitsumoto Y, et al. Insulin induces translocation of the alpha 2 and beta 1 subunits of the Na+/K(+)-ATPase from intracellular compartments to the plasma membrane in mammalian skeletal muscle. *J Biol Chem.* 1992;267(8):5040-5043.
22. Omatsu-Kanbe M, Kitasato H. Insulin stimulates the translocation of Na+/K(+)-dependent ATPase molecules from intracellular stores to the plasma membrane in frog skeletal muscle. *Biochem J.* 1990;272(3):727-733.
23. Marette A, Krischer J, Lavoie L, et al. Insulin increases the Na(+)-K(+)-ATPase alpha 2-subunit in the surface of rat skeletal muscle: morphological evidence. *Am J Physiol.* 1993;265(6 Pt 1):C1716-C1722.
24. Kanbe MK, Kitasato H. Stimulation of Na,K-ATPase activity of frog skeletal muscle by insulin. *Biochem Biophys Res Commun.* 1986;134(2):609-616.
25. Lytton J. Insulin affects the sodium affinity of the rat adipocyte (Na+,K+)-ATPase. *J Biol Chem.* 1985;260(18):10075-10080.
26. Sargeant RJ, Liu Z, Klip A. Action of insulin on Na(+)-K(+)-ATPase and the Na(+)-K(+)-2Cl- cotransporter in 3T3-L1 adipocytes. *Am J Physiol.* 1995;269(1 Pt 1):C217-C225.
27. Sweeney GK, Klip A. Regulation of the Na+/K+-ATPase by insulin: why and how? *Mol Cell Biochem.* 1998;182(1-2):121-133.
28. Feraille E, Carranza ML, Rousselot M, Favre H. Insulin enhances sodium sensitivity of Na-K-ATPase in isolated rat proximal convoluted tubule. *Am J Physiol.* 1994;267(1 Pt 2):F55-F62.
29. Dluhy RG, Axelrod L, Williams GH. Serum immunoreactive insulin and growth hormone response to potassium infusion in normal man. *J Appl Physiol.* 1972;33(1):22-26.
30. DeFronzo RA, Bia M, Birkhead G. Epinephrine and potassium homeostasis. *Kidney Int.* 1981;20(1):83-91.
31. Williams ME, Gervino EV, Rosa RM, et al. Catecholamine modulation of rapid potassium shifts during exercise. *N Engl J Med.* 1985;312(13):823-827.
32. Rosa RM, Silva P, Young JB, et al. Adrenergic modulation of extrarenal potassium disposal. *N Engl J Med.* 1980;302(8):431-434.
33. Angelopoulous M, Leitz H, Lambert G, MacGilvray S. In vitro analysis of the Na(+)-K+ ATPase activity in neonatal and adult red blood cells. *Biol Neonate.* 1996;69(3):140-145.
34. Gillzan KM, Stewart AG. The role of potassium channels in the inhibitory effects of beta 2-adrenoceptor agonists on DNA synthesis in human cultured airway smooth muscle. *Pulm Pharmacol Ther.* 1997;110(2):71-79.
35. Clausen TF, Flatman JA. The effect of catecholamines on Na-K transport and membrane potential in rat soleus muscle. *J Physiol.* 1977;270(2):383-414.
36. Barold SS, Upton S. Hyperkalemia induced by the sequential administration of metoprolol and carvedilol. *Case Rep. Cardiol.* 2018;10:7686373.
37. Aggarwal A, Wong J, Campbell DJ. Carvedilol reduces aldosterone release in systolic heart failure. *Heart Lung Circ.* 2006;15(5):306-309.
38. Lindner A, Douglas SW, Adamson JW. Propranolol effects in long-term hemodialysis patients with renin-dependent hypertension. *Ann Intern Med.* 1978;88(4):457-462.
39. Mandelberg A, Krupnik Z, Houri S, et al. Salbutamol metered-dose inhaler with spacer for hyperkalemia: how fast? How safe? *Chest.* 1999;115(3):617-622.
40. Singh BS, Sadiq HF, Noguchi A, Keenan WJ. Efficacy of albuterol inhalation in treatment of hyperkalemia in premature neonates. *J Pediatr.* 2002;141(1):16-20.
41. Helfrich E, de Vries TW, van Roon EN. Salbutamol for hyperkalaemia in children. *Acta Paediatr.* 2001;90(11):1213-1216.
42. Semmekrot BA, Monnens LA. A warning for the treatment of hyperkalaemia with salbutamol. *Eur J Pediatr.* 1997;156(5):420.
43. Shortland D, Trounce JQ, Levene MI. Hyperkalaemia, cardiac arrhythmias, and cerebral lesions in high risk neonates. *Arch Dis Child.* 1987;62(11):1139-1143.
44. Yeh TF, Raval D, John E, Pildes RS. Renal response to frusemide in preterm infants with respiratory distress syndrome during the first three postnatal days. *Arch Dis Child.* 1985;60(7):621-626.
45. Lui K, Thungappa U, Nair A, John E. Treatment with hypertonic dextrose and insulin in severe hyperkalaemia of immature infants. *Acta Paediatr.* 1992;81(3):213-216.
46. Papile LA, Burstein J, Burstein R, et al. Relationship of intravenous sodium bicarbonate infusions and cerebral intraventricular hemorrhage. *J Pediatr.* 1978;93(5):834-836.
47. Bennett LN, Myers TF, Lambert GH. Cecal perforation associated with sodium polystyrene sulfonate-sorbitol enemas in a 650 gram infant with hyperkalemia. *Am J Perinatol.* 1996;13(3):167-170.
48. Malone TA. Glucose and insulin versus cation-exchange resin for the treatment of hyperkalemia in very low birth weight infants. *J Pediatr.* 1991;118(1):121-123.
49. Weir MR, Bakris GL, Bushinsky DA, et al. Patiromer in patients with kidney disease and hyperkalemiareceiving RAAS inhibitors. *New Engl J Med.* 2015;372(3):211-221.
50. Paloian NJ, Bowman B, Bartosh SM. Treatment of infant formula with patiromer dose dependently decreases potassium concentration. *Pediat Nephrol.* 2019;34(8):1395-1401.

99 Role of the Kidney in Calcium and Phosphorus Homeostasis

Minh Dien Duong | Frederick J. Kaskel

INTRODUCTION

Calcium and phosphate serve many complex and vital functions. They are key components of the cartilage and skeleton systems. Calcium is an important cofactor in many complex enzymatic reactions and a main messenger in signaling pathways in excitability of nerve and muscle, signal transduction, clotting of blood, and muscle contraction. Phosphate plays an important role in metabolic processes, including adenosine triphosphate (ATP) formation, and is a component of nucleosides, nucleotides, and phospholipids. Together with the bone and intestinal tract, the kidney plays a key role in maintaining serum calcium and phosphate levels as well as calcium and phosphate balance in the body.

CALCIUM

Calcium, which ranges from 1000 to 1200 g in adults, is the fifth most abundant element in the human body.[1-3] It plays both a structural role as a constituent of the bone and tooth matrices and a functional role in processes as diverse as blood coagulation, regulation of endocrine and exocrine secretory activities, complement system activation, neuromuscular activity, intracellular adhesion, and signal transduction. A total of 99% of calcium is stored in bone and teeth, approximately 1% is found in the intracellular fluid (ICF), and 0.1% is in the extracellular fluid (ECF).[1-4] Serum calcium concentration is normally maintained within very narrow ranges of 8.8 to 10.4 mg/dL.[4,5] Approximately 50% of the total calcium in plasma is ionized, 40% is bound to plasma proteins (albumin 80% to 90%, and globulins), and 10% is complexed to several anions including citrate, phosphate, bicarbonate, and sulfate.[1-6] The ionized calcium is available for transport and cellular metabolism. Protein binding of calcium is affected by pH, the serum sodium concentration, and serum albumin concentration. Acidemia increases the percentages of ionized calcium, and alkalemia decreases the ionized calcium. Both hydrogen ions and calcium are bound to serum albumin; in the presence of alkalemia, bound hydrogen ions dissociate from albumin, phosphate, bicarbonate, citrate, and sulfate, freeing up the albumin to bind with more calcium leading to the decrease in ionized calcium. The increase in hydrogen in metabolic acidosis causes more hydrogen to bind to plasma proteins, phosphate, citrate, and sulfate, thereby displacing calcium, resulting in the increase of the plasma ionized calcium.[2,4,5] For every 0.1 change in pH, ionized calcium changes by 0.12 mg/dL.[7] Similarly, an increase in serum albumin concentration of 1 g/dL increases protein-bound calcium by 0.8 mg/dL and decreases ionized calcium in plasma. Hyponatremia increases protein-bound calcium. Extracellular Ca^{2+} homeostasis is dependent on complex interactions among several hormones (parathyroid hormone [PTH], vitamin D, and calcitonin) and multiple organs (the gastrointestinal tract, bone, and kidney).

Within cells, calcium is mainly sequestered in the endoplasmic reticulum and mitochondria, or it is bound to cytoplasmic proteins including calmodulin and other calcium-binding proteins (CaBPs) and ionic ligands.[7] The fraction of ionized Ca^{2+} is four times lower in the intracellular than the extracellular compartment.[8,9] The large concentration gradient for calcium across the cell membrane is maintained by a calcium adenosine triphosphatase (ATPase) (PMCA1b) in all cells and by a 3Na-Ca exchanger (NCX)1 in some cells.[4] Furthermore, the fraction of free intracellular Ca^{2+} available for signaling and various cellular processes is approximately 10^{-4} fold lower than that present in the extracellular milieu.[10]

During certain physiologic states, calcium requirements are greatly increased, such as in children during skeletal growth and during pregnancy and lactation. During lactation, plasma Ca^{2+} levels can significantly drop because of Ca^{2+} excretion in the milk, and during pregnancy, Ca^{2+} transport from the mother to the fetus across the placenta affects the plasma Ca^{2+} concentration.[11,12]

Calcium homeostasis depends on two factors, the total amount of calcium in the body and the distribution of calcium between bone and ECF. The calcium balance is determined by the net difference between the amount of calcium absorbed by the intestinal tract and the amount of calcium excreted by the kidneys, intestines, and sweat glands. Regulation of calcium excretion by the kidneys is one of the major ways that the body regulates ECF calcium.[2-5]

The balance of calcium in bone depends on relative rates of bone formation and resorption. Children are in positive bone balance (formation > resorption), which ensures healthy skeletal growth. Healthy young adults are in neutral bone balance (formation = resorption) and have achieved peak bone mass. Elderly individuals are typically in negative bone balance (formation < resorption), which leads to age-related bone loss. Factors that promote positive bone balance in adults include exercise, anabolic and antiresorptive drugs, and conditions that promote bone formation over bone resorption (e.g., "hungry bone" syndrome, osteoblastic prostate cancer). On the other hand, immobilization, weightlessness, and sex steroid deficiency, among others, produce negative bone balance.[2]

An adult ingests the average amount of 1000 mg of calcium daily from which 200 mg is absorbed in the small intestine through an active, carrier-mediated transport mechanism stimulated by calcitriol, the active metabolite of vitamin D3, 1,25(OH)2, which is produced in the proximal tubule of the kidneys. When calcitriol levels rise, the intestine is able to absorb up to 600 mg of calcium a day. To maintain calcium balance, the kidney must excrete the same amount of calcium that the small intestine absorbs 200 mg a day (Fig. 99.1).[4] The kidneys do this by filtration of calcium across the glomeruli and reabsorption along the renal tubules. The identified epithelial Ca^{2+} channels, transient receptor potential vanilloid (TRPV) 5 and TRPV6, are the rate-limiting step in Ca^{2+}-transporting cells. TRPV5 acts primarily as a gatekeeper of epithelial Ca^{2+} transport in the kidney, whereas TRPV6 is the main Ca^{2+} influx pathway in the small intestine. They form the main target for action of hormones to control active Ca^{2+} movement from the intestinal lumen or urine space to the blood compartment. The second factor controlling calcium homeostasis is the distribution of calcium between bone and the ECF, which is regulated by PTH and calcitriol. Other factors including pH and extracellular Ca^{2+} have been shown to influence the calcium movement across epithelia.[2,4,5,13,14]

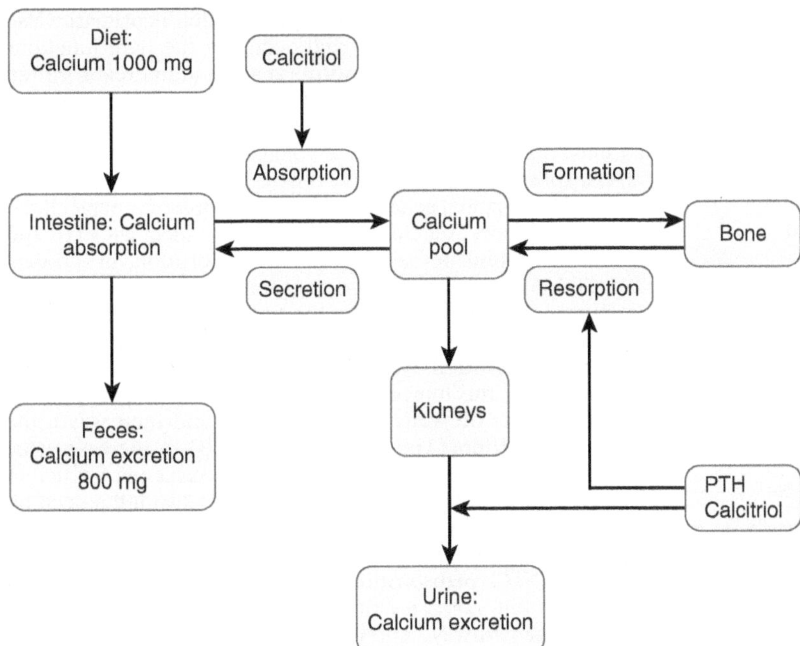

Fig. 99.1 Overview of calcium homeostasis. *PTH*, Parathyroid hormone. (Modified from Koeppen BM, Stanton BA. Regulation of calcium and phosphate homeostasis. In: Koeppen BM, Stanton BA, eds. *Renal Physiology*. 6th ed. Elsevier; 2019:138–150.)

RENAL HANDLING OF CALCIUM

The kidney contributes to the maintenance of Ca^{2+} homeostasis by regulating Ca^{2+} reabsorption (Figs. 99.2, 99.3, and 99.4).[15] Clearance studies in humans and animals have shown that, if the filtered load of Ca^{2+} is increased (by infusing Ca^{2+}), absolute calcium reabsorption increases, as does urinary Ca^{2+} excretion. Sodium (Na^+) and Ca^{2+} excretion often increases or decreases in parallel.[16] The relationship between Na^+ and Ca^{2+} reabsorption is maintained during various conditions that ultimately alter Ca^{2+} excretion, including the use of furosemide and thiazide diuretics, metabolic acidosis and metabolic alkalosis, phosphate depletion, PTH administration, and volume depletion or repletion.

The calcium available for glomerular filtration is approximately 60% of the plasma calcium, consisting of the ionized calcium fraction and the amount with anions. Normally, 99% of the filtered calcium is reabsorbed by the renal tubules. Filtered calcium is reabsorbed throughout the nephron by various active and passive processes. The proximal tubule reabsorbs approximately 50% to 60% of the filtered calcium. The loop of Henle, mainly the cortical portion of the thick ascending limb (TAL), reabsorbs 15%. The remaining 10% to 15% is reabsorbed by the distal segments of the nephron.[4,17,18] The distal cortical nephron plays an important role in maintaining calcium excretion based on physiologic needs. Approximately 1% of the filtered load of Ca^{2+} is excreted in the urine.

In the proximal tubules, Ca^{2+} is mainly reabsorbed via the passive paracellular pathway, which accounts for approximately 80% of calcium reabsorption in this segment of the nephron. This paracellular pathway is driven by solvent drag, the lumen positive transepithelial voltage across the second haft of the proximal tubule, and by a favorable concentration gradient of calcium. Both are established by transcellular sodium and water reabsorption in the first haft of the proximal tubule. The rate of transport depends on the magnitude of the electrochemical gradient, the Ca^{2+} permeability coefficient, the delivery of Ca^{2+} to the transport site, and the rate of Ca^{2+} extrusion from the interstitium. A small but significant component of active calcium transport is observed in the proximal tubules. The active transport of calcium proceeds in a two-step process, with calcium entry from the tubular fluid across the apical membrane

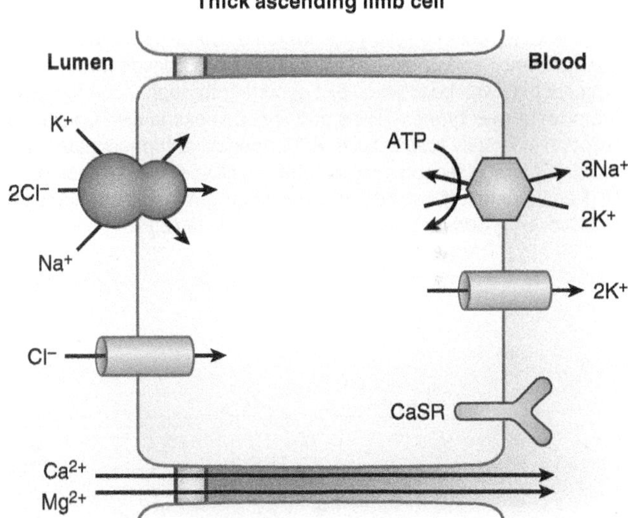

Fig. 99.2 Model of calcium absorption by the thick ascending limb of Henle. Calcium absorption is via both an active transcellular pathway and by a passive paracellular pathway. Only transport pathways relevant to calcium absorption are shown. Basal absorption is passive and is driven by the ambient electrochemical gradient for calcium. The apical Na^+-K^+-$2Cl^-$ co-transporter and the renal outer medullary potassium K^+ channel generate the "driving force" for paracellular cation transport. The apical Na^+-K^+-$2Cl^-$ co-transporter mediates apical absorption of Na, K, and Cl. The apical renal outer medullary K channel mediates apical recycling of K back to the tubular lumen and generates lumen-positive voltage. Cl channel Kb mediates Cl exit through the basolateral membrane. Here Na^+-K^+-ATPase also mediates Na exit through the basolateral membrane and generates the Na gradient for Na absorption. *ATP*, Adenosine triphosphate; *CaSR*, calcium-sensing receptor. (Modified from Blaine J, Chonchol M, Levi M. Renal control of calcium, phosphate, and magnesium homeostasis. *Clin J Am Soc Nephrol.* 2015;10[7]:1257–1272.)

and exit through the basolateral membrane. This active transport is generally considered to constitute 10% to 15% of total proximal tubule calcium reabsorption, and it is mainly regulated by PTH and calcitonin.[4,5,19,20]

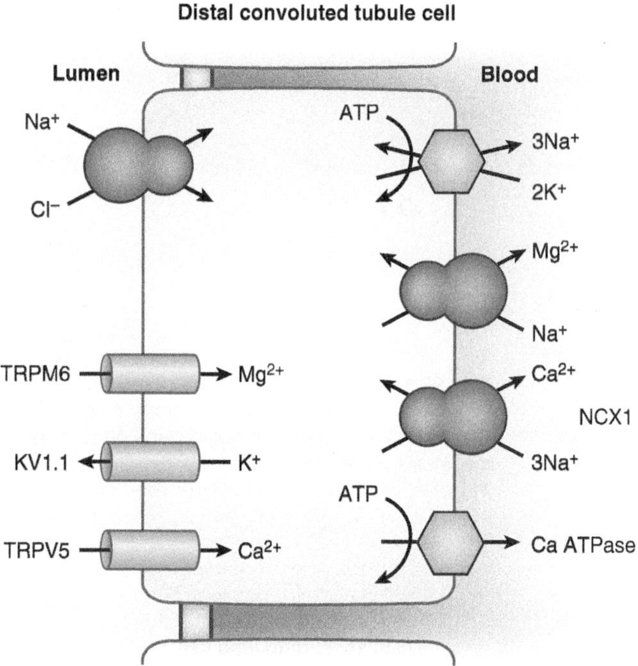

Fig. 99.3 Model of calcium absorption by distal convoluted tubules. Calcium entry across the plasma membrane proceeds through calcium channels with basolateral exit occurring through a combination of the plasma membrane ATPase and Na^+-Ca^+ exchanger. Calcium absorption is entirely transcellular. *ATP*, Adenosine triphosphate; *CaSR*, calcium-sensing receptor. (Modified from Blaine J, Chonchol M, Levi M. Renal control of calcium, phosphate, and magnesium homeostasis. *Clin J Am Soc Nephrol.* 2015;10[7]:1257–1272.)

In the TAL of Henle, calcium reabsorption is primarily also via the paracellular pathway and occurs at the tight junctions (see Fig. 99.2). Calcium reabsorption and sodium reabsorption parallel each other, along the proximal tubule. Calcium reabsorption is secondary to sodium reabsorption, generating a lumen-positive transepithelial voltage. The apical Na^+-K^+-$2Cl^-$ co-transporter (NKCC2) and the renal outer medullary potassium K1 (ROMK) channel generate the "driving force" for paracellular cation transport. Calciotropic hormones, such as PTH and calcitonin, stimulate active calcium absorption in cortical TALs. Inhibition of NKCC2 co-transporter by loop diuretics or in Bartter syndrome decreases the transepithelial voltage, thus diminishing passive calcium absorption. Loop diuretics inhibit sodium reabsorption by inhibiting NKCC2, which reduces the magnitude of the lumen positive transepithelial voltage. This action inhibits the calcium reabsorption and increases urine calcium excretion.[5] Loop diuretics are used to increase renal calcium excretion in patients with hypercalcemia.[4] Calcium transport in the TAL of the loop of Henle is also influenced by the calcium-sensing receptor (CaSR), which is localized in the basolateral membrane.[5] An acute inhibition of the CaSR does not alter NaCl reabsorption or the transepithelial potential difference but increases the permeability to calcium in the paracellular pathway.[5] The tight junction in the TAL expresses several claudins (claudin-14, claudin-16, and claudin-19). A normal expression of claudin-16 and claudin-19 is required for a normal absorption of divalent cations in this tubular segment. Claudin-16 (previously termed *paracellin-1*) is a claudin family tight junction protein that plays a critical role in calcium and magnesium reabsorption.[5] Loss-of-function mutations in claudin-16 result in the syndrome of familial hypomagnesemic hypercalciuria and nephrocalcinosis.[18] This disorder is characterized by enhanced excretion of calcium and magnesium due to a decrease in the passive reabsorption of these ions by the paracellular route. Treatment with cinacalcet (a calcimimetic that lowers the amount of PTH) increases the abundance of claudin-14 messenger RNA (mRNA), and in cell culture models, overexpression of claudin-14 decreases the paracellular permeability to calcium.[5]

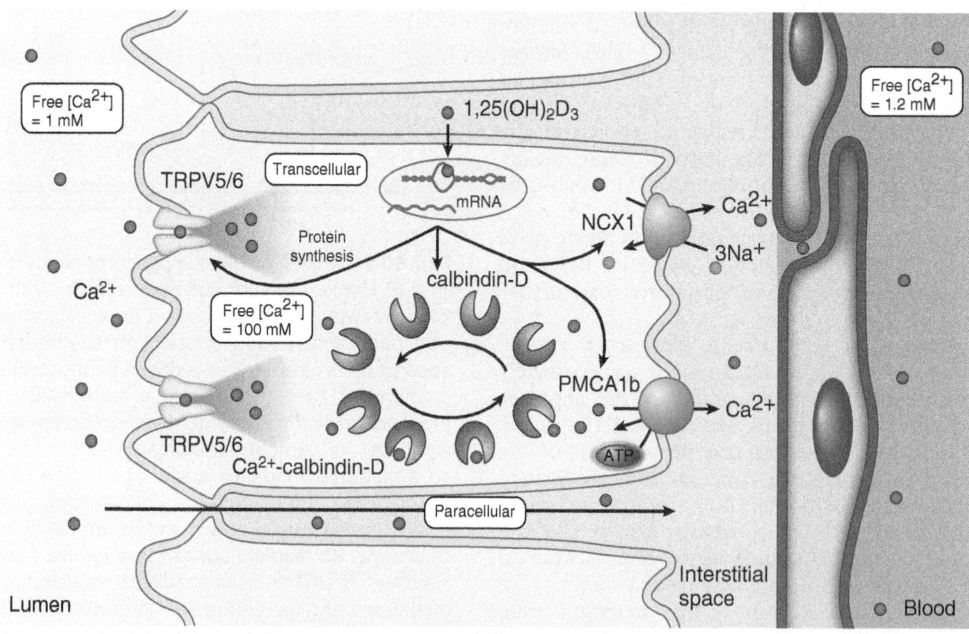

Fig. 99.4 Mechanism of epithelial calcium *(Ca^{2+})* transport. Entry of Ca^{2+} is facilitated by the apical Ca^{2+}channel *(transient receptor potential vanilloid [TRPV]5/6)*. In the cell, Ca^{2+} binds to calbindin-D and diffuses through the cytosol to the basolateral membrane. There Ca^{2+} is extruded via a Na^+-Ca^{2+} exchanger *(NCX1)* and a Ca^{2+}-ATPase *(PMCA1b)*. (Modified with permission from Hoenderop JG, Nilius B, Bindels RJ. Calcium absorption across epithelia. *Physiol Rev.* 2005;85:373–422.)

In the distal convoluted tubules (DCTs), where the voltage in the tubule lumen is electrically negative, calcium reabsorption is entirely active because calcium is reabsorbed against its electrochemical gradient (Figs. 99.3 and 99.4). The distal tubule reabsorbs calcium exclusively via the transcellular route. This active process can be divided into three steps. The first step requires calcium influx across the apical membrane by calcium permeable ion channels, the TRPV5. The second step is the diffusion of calcium through the cytosol. Inside the cell, calcium binds to calbindin-D28k and shuttles it through the cytosol towards the basolateral membrane, where calcium is extruded via the NCX1 and the plasma membrane calcium-ATPase (PMCA)1b, which is the final step in this process. The calcium and sodium excretions do not change in parallel because the reabsorption of Na^+ and Ca^{2+} in the distal tubule is independent and is differentially regulated.[4,5,21-29] Calciotropic hormones such as PTH and calcitonin stimulate calcium absorption. Calcitriol [1,25(OH)2D] stimulates calcium absorption through the activation of nuclear transcription factors. Inhibition of the apical NaCl co-transporter by thiazide diuretics or in Gitelman syndrome indirectly stimulates calcium absorption.[5] Thiazide diuresis inhibits Na reabsorption but stimulates calcium reabsorption in this renal segment. Thiazide inhibits the entry of NaCl into the cell and causes the membrane potential to hyperpolarize. This hyperpolarization in turn activates the TRPV5 channel to increase calcium flux into cells. Thiazide is given for patients with kidney stones to reduce urinary calcium excretion.[4,5]

TRANSIENT RECEPTOR POTENTIAL VANILLOID 5

Ca^{2+} movement across TRPV5 is controlled in multiple ways. TRPV5 gene expression is regulated by calciotropic hormones such as vitamin D3 and PTH.[30,31] Channel activity is modulated by intracellular Ca^{2+} by feedback inhibition. TRPV5 is also controlled by mobilization of the channel towards the plasma membrane. The hormone α-klotho expressed in the renal distal tubule enhances TRPV5 activity via a novel mechanism modifying its glycosylation status and entrapping the channel at the cell surface, resulting in a prolonged expression of TRPV5 at the plasma membrane.[32,33] The immunosuppressant tacrolimus is shown to decrease activity of TRPV5 and calbindin-28K, causing hypercalciuria.[34] Extracellular pH determines the cell surface expression of TRPV5 via a unique mechanism. Extracellular alkalinization causes a pool of TRPV5-containing vesicles to be rapidly recruited to the cell surface without collapsing into the plasma membrane, resulting in increased TRPV5 activity. In contrast, extracellular acidification causes the vesicles to be retrieved from the plasma membrane, resulting in decreased TRPV5 activity. This effect could explain the molecular basis of acidosis-induced calciuresis.[35] In the distal tubules, intracellular calcium concentration is increased by osmosensitive, nonselective ion channels such as TRPV4, especially under hypotonic stimulus.[36]

CALCIUM BUFFERING WITHIN THE CELL

The vitamin D–dependent CaBPs named *calbindins* are expressed in cells that are challenged by a high Ca^{2+} influx such as in brain, bone, teeth, inner ear, placenta, mammary gland, kidney, and intestine. In these tissues, CaBPs (i.e., CaBP9K and CaBP28K) are a key component in cellular Ca^{2+} handling (see Fig. 99.4). In the kidney, calbindin-D (CaBP28K) facilitates Ca^{2+} diffusion from the luminal Ca^{2+} entry side of the cell to the basolateral side, where Ca^{2+} is extruded into the extracellular compartment. CaBP28K provides protection against toxic high intracellular Ca^{2+} levels by buffering the cytosolic Ca^{2+} concentration during high Ca^{2+} influx.[37] Studies using protein-binding analysis, subcellular fractionation, and evanescent-field microscopy have shown that CaBP28K translocates towards the plasma membrane and directly associates with TRPV5 at a low Ca^{2+} concentration. CaBP28K tightly buffers the flux of Ca^{2+} entering the cell via TRPV5, facilitating high Ca^{2+} transport rates by preventing channel inactivation. Therefore CaBP28K acts in calcium-transporting epithelia as a dynamic Ca^{2+} buffer, regulating Ca^{2+} in close vicinity to the TRPV5 pore by direct association with the channel. Calbindins are regulated by calciotropic hormones including vitamin D, estrogens, PTH, and dietary calcium.[38]

CaBP28K was originally identified as a high-capacity Ca^{2+} buffer with Ca^{2+} affinities fitting the classic properties of a Ca^{2+} buffer. However, sequential Ca^{2+} binding and conformational changes suggested that CaBP28K can act as a Ca^{2+} sensor controlling downstream cellular processes.[39-42]

Inside the cell, calbindin directly interacts with a calmodulin-binding isoleucine-glutamine motif present in the C-tail of TRPV5 and TRPV6 channels. Deletion of the first eight amino acids of the isoleucine-glutamine motif in the carboxyl terminus tail of the Ca^{2+}-channel subunit a1C eliminates Ca^{2+}-dependent inactivation of voltage-gated, L-type Ca^{2+} channels.[43] Ca^{2+}-dependent interaction also occurs between calbindin and a novel site in the C-terminal domain of the 1A subunit of P/Q-type Ca^{2+} channels (calbindin-binding domain). In the presence of low concentrations of intracellular Ca^{2+} chelators, Ca^{2+} influx through P/Q-type channels enhances channel inactivation, increases recovery from inactivation, and produces a long-lasting facilitation of the Ca^{2+} current.[28] Ca^{2+} "shuttling" across the intracellular organelles such as mitochondria or endoplasmic reticulum depends on a Ca^{2+} electrochemical gradient, driven by internally negative membrane potential across the inner mitochondrial or endoplasmic reticular membrane.

CALCIUM TRANSPORT ACROSS THE BASOLATERAL MEMBRANE

The extrusion of Ca^{2+} across the basolateral membrane into the interstitium occurs against an electrochemical gradient and, as such, is an energy-dependent process. Transport is primarily mediated by two calcium transporters located at the basolateral membrane: NCX[44] and the Ca^{2+}-ATPase (PMCA).[45]

Na^+-Ca^{2+} Exchanger

Three genes for NCX, known as *NCX1, NCX2,* and *NCX3,* have been identified in mammals. In the kidney the expression of this transporter is restricted to the distal part of the nephron, where it predominantly localizes along the basolateral membrane.[46,47] *NCX1* is widely distributed in many different mammalian tissues, whereas *NCX2* and *NCX3* are expressed only in brain and skeletal muscle.[48,49] It has been demonstrated that *NCX1* is the primary extrusion mechanism, whereas only a minor amount of Ca^{2+} in the distal tubular cells is extruded by the plasma Ca^{2+} pump.[44] It has also been shown that targeted deletion of *NCX1* results in *NCX1*-null embryos that do not have a spontaneously beating heart and die in utero.[50,51] Studies in oocytes and mammalian cell systems show that NCX is regulated by several factors, including the membrane potential, protein kinase C (PKC) activation, protons, nucleotides, and calciotropic hormones.[52] PTH markedly stimulates Ca^{2+} reabsorption in the distal part of the nephron, primarily by augmenting *NCX1* activity via a cyclic adenosine monophosphate (cAMP)-mediated mechanism.

Plasma Membrane Ca^{2+}-Adenosine Triphosphatase

PMCA belongs to a class of P-type, ion-motive ATPase proteins with molecular weights ranging from 120,000 to 140,000 Da. PMCAs are high-affinity Ca^{2+} efflux pumps present in almost all cells and are responsible for the maintenance and resetting of the resting intracellular Ca^{2+} levels.[53] Four different isoforms—PMCA1 to A4—are encoded by separate genes. PMCAs are a universal system for the extrusion of Ca^{2+} in cells. In the kidney, PMCAs are present in all nephron segments, with highest expression in the basolateral membrane of cells lining the distal part of the nephron. The DCT possesses the highest Ca^{2+}-ATPase activity and exhibits the strongest immunocytochemical reactivity for PMCA protein expression.[54–56]

In humans, PMCAs are found along the DCT and, in contrast to other species, along the cortical collecting duct.[46] Studies suggest that PMCA1 and PMCA4 are the major isoforms expressed in the kidney, whereas PMCA2 and PMCA3 are more tissue specific. PMCA1 and PMCA4 are involved in the maintenance of cellular Ca^{2+} homeostasis.[57] PMCA4b plays a significant role in basolateral Ca^{2+} extrusion. PMCA1b is the predominant isoform and abundantly expressed in the small intestine, where *NCX1* is expressed at a low level. It is the major Ca^{2+} extrusion mechanism in intestinal Ca^{2+} absorption. PMCA also plays a role in cytosolic acidification, which in turn, acts a signal for activation of the sarcoplasmic reticulum Ca^{2+}-ATPase and other cellular functions in muscle. Limited data are available regarding the regulation of PMCA by hormones or signaling mechanisms. Several studies indicate that PMCA is positively regulated by 1,25-dihydroxyvitamin D3, [1,25(OH)2D3], in the intestine to increase Ca^{2+} absorption. In addition, several potassium (K^+)-dependent Na^+-Ca^{2+} exchangers (NCKXs) have been described.[53,58] Northern blot analysis demonstrated that some isoforms (i.e., NCKX4 and NCKX6) of this family are expressed in epithelia, including small intestine and kidney.[59,60]

These exchangers are found in various tissues, suggesting a key role in regulating intracellular Ca^{2+} homeostasis in mammalian cells. Ca^{2+} extrusion from the cell is a Na^+-Ca^{2+} countertransport driven by the Na^+ concentration gradient across the basolateral membrane maintained by Na^+-K^+-ATPase. Ca^{2+} removal by this exchanger is slowed when extracellular Na^+ concentration is diminished or when Na^+-K^+-ATPase is inhibited with ouabain.[61]

REGULATION OF CALCIUM TRANSPORT

The factors relating to calcium homeostasis are summarized in the Table 99.1.

PARATHYROID HORMONE

The parathyroid glands play an important role in maintaining the extracellular Ca^{2+} concentration by stimulating calcium absorption. PTH is a primary hormone responsible for maintaining Ca^{2+} hemostasis and the most powerful control on renal Ca^{2+} excretion. They have the capacity to sense changes in the level of blood Ca^{2+} from its normal level via the CaSR. In response to low blood Ca^{2+} levels, PTH is secreted into the circulation and then acts primarily on kidney and bone, where it activates the PTH-PTH-related peptide (PTHrP) receptor. PTH acts to increase the plasma calcium concentration by three ways: stimulated bone resorption, enhanced intestinal calcium and phosphate absorption by promoting the kidney 1,25(OH)2D3, and increased renal calcium absorption by the TAL of the Henle loop and the distal tubule. PTH secretion is regulated by a transcriptional and posttranscriptional level dependent on the extracellular level of calcium.[5] PTH gene transcription is increased by hypocalcemia, glucocorticoids, and estrogen. Hypercalcemia can increase the intracellular degradation of PTH.[5] Hypercalcemia leads to a reduction in PTH levels, which suppresses Ca^{2+} reabsorption by the distal tubule.[4]

In the kidney, PTH augments active renal absorption by stimulating transcellular Ca^{2+} reabsorption via a slow genomic pathway and a rapid nongenomic pathway. The rapid pathway is via activation of adenylyl cyclase, accumulation of cAMP, and stimulation of protein kinase A (PKA), resulting in an increase in the cytosolic concentration and transcellular Ca^{2+} transport. PKA inhibitors reduce the PTH-mediated rise of cytosolic Ca^{2+}, which suggests that cAMP-dependent phosphorylation is an essential step in short-term PTH stimulation. In addition to cAMP, PKC is also involved in the short-term PTH response. The slow pathway results in an elevated expression of the Ca^{2+} transport proteins TRPV5, calbindin-D28K, NCX1, and PMCA1b. The PTH receptor directly enhances the tubular Ca^{2+} reabsorption, and it stimulates the activity of 1α-hydroxylase, thereby increasing the 1,25(OH)2 D3-dependent absorption of Ca^{2+} from the intestine. PTH binds to two types of receptors: PTHR1, which also binds the PTH-PTHrP,[62] and PTHR2, which binds only PTH.[63] The PTHR1 receptor is the predominant receptor found in the kidney, and it is expressed in glomeruli and all tubule segments, except the TAL and collecting duct. The PTHR2 receptor is distributed primarily in brain, lung, pancreas, and vasculature (including the vascular pole of the glomerulus). Signal transduction for both PTH and PTHrP is via adenylate cyclase and phospholipase C.[64,65] PTH stimulates active Ca^{2+} reabsorption in the distal part of the nephron. PTH increases transepithelial Ca^{2+} transport via a dual signaling mechanism involving PKA- and PKC-dependent processes.[66,67] PTH has various actions such as membrane insertion of apical Ca^{2+} channels, opening of basolateral chloride channels resulting in cellular hyperpolarization, and modulation of PMCA activity.[68–70]

PTH activates dihydropyridine-sensitive channels responsible for Ca^{2+} entry. Once inserted or activated, these dihydropyridine-sensitive channels could mediate Ca^{2+} entry into Ca^{2+}-transporting epithelial cells. It is thought that dihydropyridine-sensitive Ca^{2+} channels play a role in signal transduction processes to maintain the cellular Ca^{2+} homeostasis. PTH affects renal Ca^{2+} handling through the regulation of the expression of the active renal Ca^{2+} transport proteins, including the epithelial Ca^{2+} channel TRPV5. PTH also stimulates the PMCA activity by increasing the affinity for Ca^{2+} in the distal tubule, unlike 1,25-(OH)2D3 that does not directly affect the basolateral membrane PMCA activity.[71]

In bone, PTH can induce a rapid release of Ca^{2+} from the bone matrix and can also mediate long-term changes in Ca^{2+} metabolism by acting directly on the bone-forming osteoblasts and indirectly on bone-resorbing osteoclasts by increasing their number and activity.

Table 99.1 Factors of Renal Regulation of Calcium.[4,5]

Increase Calcium Reabsorption	Decrease Calcium Reabsorption
Hyperparathyroidism	Hypoparathyroidism
Calcitriol	Low calcitriol
Hypocalcemia	Hypercalcemia
Volume contraction	Extracellular fluid excess
Metabolic alkalosis	Metabolic acidosis
Hyperphosphatemia	Hypophosphatemia
Thiazides	Loop diuretics: furosemide

Data from Koeppen BM, Stanton BA. Regulation of calcium and phosphate homeostasis. In; Koeppen BM, Stanton BA, eds. *Renal Physiology.* 6th ed. Philadelphia: Elsevier; 2019:138–150; Blaine J, Chonchol M, Levi M. Renal control of calcium, phosphate, and magnesium homeostasis. *Clin J Am Soc Nephrol.* 2015;10(7):1257–1272.

CALCIUM-SENSING RECEPTOR

CaSR was discovered in 1993. It is a plasma membrane-bound G protein-coupled receptor found in many tissues, including the parathyroid gland, thyroid, kidney, intestine, bone, bone marrow, brain, skin, pancreas, lung, and heart. CaSR plays a critical role in Ca^{2+} homeostasis by inducing changes in PTH secretion and renal Ca^{2+} reabsorption in response to variations in the extracellular concentration of Ca^{2+}. CaSR is not specific for calcium alone; it responds to other cations such as magnesium, aluminum, and gadolinium, but it has the highest affinity for calcium. The human CaSR is encoded by six exons of the CaSR gene located on chromosome 3q13.3-21.[72] The receptor is expressed abundantly in the parathyroid glands and, to less extent, along the length of the kidney tubule.[47] Activation of the CaSR on the parathyroid gland cells by elevated serum Ca^{2+} leads to activation of many secondary messengers, resulting in inhibition of PTH synthesis and the production of calcitriol by proximal tubule.[4] Moreover, the reduction of PTH secretion also contributes to calcitriol production because calcitriol is stimulated by PTH. A decrease in serum calcium has the opposite effect on PTH and calcitriol.[4] Activation of the CaSR in response to hypercalcemia produces several different effects in the renal tubules. In the TAL, an increase in serum calcium activates CaSR, which inhibits calcium absorption and thereby increases calcium excretion. This occurs due to a decrease in Na^+, K^+, and Cl^- reabsorption accompanied by a decrease in K^+ transfer across a specific potassium channel at the apical membrane. This causes a decrease in the lumen positive voltage in the tubular lumen, leading to decreased calcium and magnesium reabsorption and increased distal delivery. In the distal tubule, CaSR stimulation on the basolateral membrane results in inhibition of calcium transport. In the medullary collecting duct epithelium, CaSRs are found on the apical side. At that location, they reduce the insertion of aquaporin-2 water channels when the luminal calcium concentration is high, decreasing water reabsorption and thereby decreasing calcium concentration, and calcium crystal formation in the urine.[73-75] Inactivating mutations in the CaSR gene are associated with familial hypocalciuric hypercalcemia, neonatal severe hyperparathyroidism, and autosomal dominant hypocalcemia.[76-80] Hypocalciuria is caused by enhanced calcium reabsorption in the TAL and distal tubule due to elevated PTH levels and defective CaSR regulation of calcium transport in the kidneys. Autosomal dominant hypoparathyroidism results from an activating mutation in CaSR. Hypercalciuria is caused by decreased PTH levels and defective CaSR-regulated calcium transport in the kidneys.[4] In contrast, activating mutations of the CaSR result in a Bartter-like syndrome (Bartter syndrome type V) characterized by calcium, magnesium, sodium, potassium, chloride, and water wasting.[81]

VITAMIN D

The physiologic actions of vitamin D are mediated by its metabolite 1,25(OH)2D3 as the most active form of vitamin D, which is formed by 1-hydroxylation of 25(OH)D produced by the liver via 1α-hydroxylase (CYP24B1) in proximal tubules. There is 24α-hydroxylase, which forms 24,25-dihydroxyvitamin D as an inactive metabolite. Serum 25(OH)D, which is the precursor form of the biologically active vitamin D, is the best indicator of overall vitamin storage.[5] The 1,25(OH)2D3 enters the circulation and acts upon the target organ receptors to maintain calcium hemostasis and bone health. Both 25(OH)D and 1,25(OH)2D3 are carried in the circulation by vitamin D-binding protein (DBP).[33] In small intestine, 1,25(OH)2D3 enhances calcium absorption. An intact 1,25(OH)2D3 receptor system is important for PTH-induced osteoclastogenesis. Calcium and phosphate are released from mature osteoclasts to maintain the two minerals in serum.[5] Rickets due to gene defects in FGD23 decreases the conversion of 25(OH)D to 1,25(OH)2D.

In the kidney, the most important effect of 1,25(OH)2D3 is tight control of its own homeostasis through simultaneous suppression of 1α-hydroxylase and stimulation of 24α-hydroxylase.[5] The 1,25(OH)2D3 increases renal calcium absorption. Oral 1,25 (OH)2D3 is used to suppresses PTH in patients with chronic kidney disease (CKD) and end-stage kidney disease. The 25(OH)D inhibits PTH but requires higher levels.[33] In the kidneys, vitamin D receptor (VDR) is expressed in epithelia that play a role in Ca^{2+} reabsorption. Microarray analysis of 1,25(OH)2D3 has shown that TRPV6 is one of the most highly vitamin D-responsive genes.[82] In the cell, 1,25(OH)2D3 can be inactivated by mitochondrial 24-hydroxylase (CYP24A1) or bind to the VDR in the cytoplasm.[33] Once the VDR binds its ligand, the VDR translocates to the nucleus. The classic action of vitamin D is to stimulate transcription by binding to nuclear receptors. It binds with VDR in a ligand-dependent manner. Degradation of 1,25(OH)2D3 is believed to occur in the kidneys from side cleavage and oxidation by CYP24A1 to form 24,25(OH)2D. The CYP24B1 to produce 1,25(OH)2D synthesis is regulated by low calcium, low phosphate, increased PTH, estrogen, prolactin, growth hormones (GHs), fibroblast growth factor (FGF)23, and 1,25(OH)2 itself.[33]

CALCITONIN

Calcitonin is a 32-amino acid peptide secreted by the parafollicular cells of the thyroid gland. It is released in response to hypercalcemia and lowers serum calcium by various mechanisms. Its main action for lowering calcium is by inhibiting bone resorption. Calcitonin receptors are found on osteoclasts. The signal transduction pathways for calcitonin receptors are adenylate cyclase-PKA and phospholipase C-PKC via linking with G proteins. In the kidney, calcitonin increases the urinary excretion of calcium and phosphorus, independent of PTH.[83-86] Calcitonin has not been shown to affect intestinal calcium absorption, but it may decrease phosphorus absorption. Calcitonin is a major regulator of renal 1,25-hydroxylase gene expression.[87]

PLASMA CALCIUM CONCENTRATION

HYPERCALCEMIA

Hypercalcemia results in an increase in Ca^{2+} excretion caused by a net increase in the filtered load and a decrease in tubular reabsorption. Hypercalcemia, in the presence of intact parathyroid glands, decreases the glomerular ultrafiltration coefficient (Kf) and causes renal vasoconstriction, which tends to offset the increase in filtered load. Both together cause a decline in glomerular filtration rate (GFR).[88,89] Hypercalcemia also causes a decline in the tubule reabsorption of Ca^{2+} by PTH-independent and PTH-dependent mechanisms.[5,90] This effect is mediated by stimulation of the CaSR, which inhibits the apical K^+ channel and K^+ recycling, necessary for the activity of the Na^+-K^+-$2Cl^-$ transporter.[81,91] Decreased activity of the transporter decreases the lumen-positive potential difference and thus Na^+, Ca^{2+}, and Mg^{2+} reabsorption. In addition, a decrease in intestinal Ca^{2+} absorption is brought about by diminished synthesis of 1,25(OH)2D3.

HYPOCALCEMIA

In acute hypocalcemic conditions, PTH secretion increases, which results in the mobilization of Ca^{2+} from bone and soft tissues. This produces a gradual fall in PTH that, in turn, promotes a decrease in fractional excretion of Ca^{2+} and a decline in net Ca^{2+} excretion.[2,4,5] Hypocalcemia decreases renal calcium excretion by decreasing the filtered load and enhancing the tubular reabsorption of calcium. The CaSR is thought to play a significant role in the enhancement of Ca^{2+} reabsorption in the TAL.[81,92] A decreased Ca^{2+} concentration in the vasa recta contributes to enhanced extrusion of Ca^{2+} at the basolateral membrane. Hypocalcemia also stimulates the production of 1,25(OH)2D3, which increases the intestinal absorption of Ca^{2+}.[2,4,5]

PHOSPHATE AND MAGNESIUM

Hypophosphatemia produces a decrease in PTH resulting from an increase in plasma Ca^{2+} concentration. However, the ensuing hypercalciuria is only partially corrected by the administration of PTH, a finding suggesting a direct effect of phosphate (PO_4^{3-}) deprivation on renal Ca^{2+} transport.[93] Phosphate infusion enhances Ca^{2+} reabsorption in the distal nephron and reduces Ca^{2+} excretion, even in the setting of volume expansion. Mg^{2+}

infusion produces an increase in Ca^{2+} excretion that is not corrected by PTH infusion.[94]

VOLUME STATUS

Expansion of intravascular space produces natriuresis and increases Ca^{2+} excretion by inhibiting Na^+ (and therefore Ca^{2+}) reabsorption in the proximal tubule and Ca^{2+} reabsorption in the distal tubule.[5,95] This effect, which is independent of circulating PTH levels,[95] is used in treating patients with hypercalcemia. Contraction of the extracellular volume increases proximal tubular reabsorption of Na^+ (and Ca^{2+}) and results in decreased Ca^{2+} excretion.

ACID-BASE STATUS

Both acute and chronic metabolic acidosis has been shown to induce the release of Ca^{2+} from bone and to inhibit distal reabsorption of Ca^{2+}, resulting in hypercalciuria independent of PTH changes.[5,96] The calciuria may be due to the mobilization of calcium from bone, as the hydrogen ion is buffered in the skeleton; and direct effects of acidosis on tubular calcium resorption.[5] The effect of acidosis on tubular transport is mediated by a reduction in TRPV5 activity.[97] Metabolic alkalosis increases Ca^{2+} reabsorption in proximal tubule and decreases Ca^{2+} excretion.[98]

INSULIN, GLUCAGON, AND GLUCOSE

Ca^{2+} excretion is enhanced by glucose infusion. Insulin infusion and hyperinsulinemia are associated with reduced proximal reabsorption of Na^+, water, and Ca^{2+}, but only Ca^{2+} excretion is increased. Insulin induces a rise in near-membrane Ca^{2+} but not in free intracellular Ca^{2+} in muscle cells. The rise in near-membrane Ca^{2+} is the result of an increase in influx through L-type Ca^{2+} channels.[99,100] Glucagon has a natriuretic and calciuretic effect caused by increases in renal blood flow and GFR.[101]

MINERALOCORTICOIDS

Acute mineralocorticoid excess is associated with the retention of Na^+ but not Ca^{2+}. Chronic mineralocorticoid excess, conversely, results in an escape from Na^+ retention (after 3 to 5 days) and a concomitant rise in Ca^{2+} excretion.[102] This phenomenon occurs in patients with Bartter syndrome, which is characterized by high aldosterone levels, salt wasting, hypokalemic alkalosis, hypercalciuria, and normal plasma Mg^{2+} levels. These manifestations are consequent to genetic defects in the NKCCS transporter or the ATP-sensitive K^+ channel (ROMK) in the TAL and are similar to those consequent to the administration of loop diuretics.[103] Gitelman syndrome is also associated with salt wasting and hypokalemia, but, unlike in Bartter syndrome, the excretion of Ca^{2+} is reduced and plasma levels of Mg^{2+} are low. The genetic defect resides in the thiazide-sensitive Na^+-Cl^- co-transporter of the DCT encoded by the human thiazide-sensitive Na^+-Cl^- co-transporter *(SLC12A3)* gene. Reduced function of this co-transporter results in an increase in Ca^{2+} reabsorption because of stimulation of the basolateral extrusion of Ca^{2+} through the NCX transporter and a decrease in Mg^{2+} reabsorption because of inhibition of an apical Na^+-Mg^{2+} exchanger.[104]

DIURETICS

Loop diuretics (furosemide, ethacrynic acid, and bumetanide) inhibit the NKCC2 transporter present in the apical membrane of the TAL, resulting in a reduction in NaCl reabsorption and K^+ recycling across the apical membrane. This action diminishes the lumen-positive potential, which is the driving force for paracellular Ca^{2+} reabsorption in this particular nephron segment and explains the hypercalciuric effect of furosemide. The calciuric effect of furosemide enhances the delivery of Ca^{2+} to DCT and connecting tubule (CNT), which are the primary sites of active Ca^{2+} reabsorption. It is currently unknown whether these latter nephron segments partly compensate for the hypercalciuric effect of the loop diuretics.[105] Thiazide diuretics cause a decrease in urinary Ca^{2+} excretion. Two main mechanisms have been proposed to explain the effect of thiazides on calcium excretion: (1) increased proximal sodium and water reabsorption due to volume depletion and (2) increased distal calcium reabsorption at the thiazide-sensitive site in the DCT.[5] They increase renal Na^+ excretion by inhibiting the Na^+-Cl^- co-transporter present in the apical membrane of DCT cells. This inhibition of Na^+ reabsorption results in increased renal salt and water loss and a decreased extracellular volume.[106] The underlying mechanism is an enhancement of proximal Na^+ reabsorption secondary to volume contraction, which leads to an increase in the electrochemical driving force for passive Ca^{2+} reabsorption.[107-110] Thiazide diuretics can reduce Ca^{2+} excretion in the absence of PTH or volume contraction. They increase Ca^{2+} reabsorption and inhibit Na^+ reabsorption, thus revealing the dissociation in the transport of these ions in distal nephron.[111]

AUTOCRINE AND PARACRINE CALCITROPIC HORMONES

ARGININE VASOPRESSIN

Arginine vasopressin is the key regulator of water reabsorption in the distal nephron. In addition, it has a Ca^{2+}-sparing effect, mediated by an increase in the paracellular transport.[112]

PROSTAGLANDIN E_2

In the cortical collecting duct, prostaglandin E_2 has a dual effect on Ca^{2+} transport. By interacting with apical and basolateral prostaglandin EP2 or EP4 receptors, prostaglandin E_2 stimulates Ca^{2+} transport. In contrast, it inhibits the stimulatory action of other calciotropic hormones by interacting with basolateral EP3 receptors.[113] The G protein–coupled EP3 receptor modulates cAMP via G1 activation (inhibiting adenylyl cyclase) and via Gs activation (stimulating adenylyl cyclase activity).[114] The molecular mechanism by which EP2 or EP4 stimulates and EP3 inhibits the action of calcitropic hormones is unknown.

ADENOSINE

Acting via apical A1 receptors, adenosine increases transcellular Ca^{2+} transport to the same extent as PTH, arginine vasopressin, and prostaglandin E_2.[115]

ADENOSINE TRIPHOSPHATE

ATP inhibits the action of stimulatory calciotropic hormones. The effect is mediated via both apical and basolateral P2y receptors.[116]

NITRIC OXIDE

Nitric oxide activates Ca^{2+} reabsorption via cyclic guanosine monophosphate.[117]

THYROID HORMONE

Ca^{2+} uptake is increased in renal brush border membrane vesicles from hyperthyroid rats and is decreased in those from hypothyroid rats.[118] PTH regulates bone and mineralization through actions on osteoblasts, kidneys, and intestines by indirectly stimulating calcitriol production.[119]

FETAL AND NEONATAL ASPECTS OF RENAL TRANSPORT OF CALCIUM

Ca^{2+} is vital for adequate mineralization, growth, and development of the fetal skeleton. Approximately 30 g of Ca^{2+} is transferred via the human placenta from the mother to the fetus, mainly during the third trimester. The syncytiotrophoblasts actively transport 80% of Ca^{2+} from maternal to fetal circulation, where it is needed for fetal skeleton growth, especially during the third trimester of pregnancy.[119-121] Syncytiotrophoblasts of the placenta have mechanisms of calcium transport that are similar to those found in the distal renal tubules.[119,122] TRPV6 expression in the human placenta is much higher compared with its level in the kidney and small intestine. This higher TRPV6 placental expression is needed, given that transplacental Ca^{2+} transport is critical for normal fetal growth and development. This is also an indication that the transcellular, rather than the paracellular, pathway of the transepithelial Ca^{2+} transport, in which the TRP proteins do not participate, may be dominant in the placenta.[123]

Towards the end of gestation, the Ca^{2+} levels in fetal plasma (total and ionized) are 0.3 to 0.5 mmol/L higher than they are in the mother.[119,124] Hormones such as calcitonin, PTH, and PTHrP have been found in maternal and fetal circulations, and they originate from mother, fetus, and placenta.[119,125] The human fetal circulation is characterized by low PTH, calcitriol, and high levels of PTHrP and calcitonin.[119]

Fetal serum calcitriol is less than 50% of the maternal value.[119] Calcitriol synthesis is likely suppressed due to high serum calcium, high phosphate, and low PTH.[119] The available data show that human placentas likely metabolizes 25OH vitamin D to 24,25 dihydroxyvitamin D instead of calcitrilol.[119]

PTHrP has been found in the parathyroid glands of fetal sheep, in a 7-week-old human fetus, and in human placenta.[126] This protein is reported to stimulate placental Ca^{2+} transfer from mother to fetus in animals and in humans.[127] However, fetal PTH is not required for transplacental Ca^{2+} transfer.[128] It remains unclear whether the parathyroid glands, placenta, or both are a main source of PTHrP in the fetal circulation.[119] PTHrP plays several key roles in fetal bone and mineral metabolism that include the regulation of serum calcium and phosphate regulation, stimulation of placental calcium and magnesium transport, and control of endochondral development by delaying terminal differentiation of chrondrocytes.[119] The placenta has most of the G protein–coupled receptors that bind the calcitropic hormones. CaSR is expressed in both villous and extravillous regions of the human placenta and contributes to the local control of transplacental Ca^{2+} transport and to the regulation of placental development.[129] Polycystin-2, a ubiquitous transmembrane glycoprotein mutated in autosomal dominant polycystic kidney disease, is present in the term human syncytiotrophoblast, in which it behaves as a nonselective cation channel.

In humans, the parathyroid glands and thymus develop from the third pharyngeal pouch.[119] PTH is detected at 10 weeks gestation.[119] Fetal parathyroids produce low amounts of PTH.[119] Fetal PTH may play a greater role than PTHrP in determining serum calcium levels. PTH is a key regulator for fetal calcium, phosphate, and magnesium.[119] PTH increases after the first 12 hours of life and plays a role as dominant regulator of bone by acting in osteoblasts and kidneys.[119]

Fetal renal cortex adenylate cyclase activity increases in response to PTH, as evidenced by an increase in urinary cAMP excretion after PTH administration in fetal sheep preparations[130] and by adenylate cyclase responsiveness in fetal rabbit[131] and fetal rat kidney preparations.[132] PTH infusion into fetal lambs results in a rise in plasma Ca^{2+}, a decline in plasma phosphate, and increases in urinary flow rate and urinary Ca^{2+} excretion.[133] Several studies in young animals, as well as in premature and term human neonates, revealed an increase in PTH levels during hypocalcemia and a calcemic response to PTH.[126,134] Yet premature infants given exogenous PTH had minimal increases in urinary cAMP until day 6 of life, a finding suggesting a maturational delay in response to PTH by the nephron. Perfusion of isolated newborn guinea pig kidneys with a PTH-containing solution increased Ca^{2+} reabsorption and cAMP excretion, but it did not affect reabsorption of phosphate.[135] Similar effects have been observed in term human newborns.[136] Vitamin D-dependent CaBPs, thought to be involved in transepithelial Ca^{2+} transfer, have been found in human kidneys as early as 14 weeks gestation.[137] Yet the major function of the kidneys in fetal Ca^{2+} homeostasis appears to be the production of 1,25(OH)2D3, rather than renal regulation of Ca^{2+} excretion.[138] The urinary calcium-creatinine ratio (millimoles to millimoles) was reported to increase from 0.05 to 1.2 in term neonates and from 0.3 to 2.3 in preterm neonates during the first week of life. Children older than 1 year of age have a mean urinary calcium-creatinine ratio (millimoles to millimoles) of 0.40, and school-aged children have a ratio of less than 0.21.[139] These findings suggest that the fractional excretion of Ca^{2+} is high in newborns, especially in those born prematurely.[140] However, the high excretion rates observed in these infants may have been caused, at least in part, by a low phosphate intake because these children were largely breast-fed.[141] Urinary calcium excretion in preterm neonates has been also found to vary directly with urinary flow rate and with urinary Na^+ excretion. However, young animals given a saline load had an attenuated natriuretic response but a similar calciuretic response when compared with adult animals.[142] This finding suggests a linked proximal tubular Ca^{2+} and Na^+ reabsorptive mechanism and an unlinked distal mechanism in newborn animals.[143]

PHOSPHORUS

The importance of maintaining proper phosphate balance is illustrated by the wide variety of biologic processes that use phosphate, including ATP production, coenzymes, and signaling proteins, in addition to its role as a major constituent of bone, muscle, and even the cellular bilipid membrane. Although an acute decrease in circulating plasma phosphate produces symptoms consisting of myopathy (weakness, rhabdomyolysis, and myalgia), sinus bradycardia, and hematologic disturbances, chronic hypophosphatemia can contribute to development of congestive heart failure, as well as bone demineralization (leading to osteomalacia in adults and rickets in children).[4,144] Thus a positive phosphate balance in neonates and children is critical for proper growth and development. During the perinatal period, phosphate homeostasis, like that of calcium, involves the integrated action of several hormonal systems and certain key factors. The high metabolic demand of the neonate for phosphate is met through a relatively high intake of dietary phosphate, efficient intestinal phosphate absorption, and reduced urinary phosphate loss. The kidneys play a critical role in this process by limiting the urinary excretion of phosphate through enhanced tubular phosphate reabsorption.[145-151] The rate of renal phosphate uptake largely determines the level of extracellular phosphate and, ultimately, regulates phosphate homeostasis.

Of the total body phosphorus, approximately 85% is present in the skeleton and teeth, approximate 14% is in the ICF, and 1% is in the ECF.[4] Approximately two thirds of the circulating pool of phosphorus is in the form of organic phosphates (e.g., esters and phospholipids), and one third is as inorganic phosphate, essentially all in the form of orthophosphate. It is estimated that the latter fraction, which represents the plasma phosphate concentration, exists as free phosphate (ionized phosphate 45%), complexed with calcium or magnesium (30%), or protein bound (25%). The plasma phosphate concentration is highest in infants (4.5 to 9.3 mg/dL) and is higher in children (4.5 to 6.5 mg/dL) than in adults (3.0 to 4.5 mg/dL).[152]

Maintenance of serum phosphate within the normal range depends on the balance of intestinal phosphate absorption, exchange with bone stores, shifts between intracellular and intravascular compartments, and renal excretion. Phosphate absorption increases as dietary phosphate rises and is stimulated by calcitriol. Daily phosphate intake in adults is between 800 and 1500 mg a day, and the kidneys maintain the total body phosphate balance.[4,153-155]

PHOSPHATE REABSORPTION AND THE TRANSPORT MAXIMUM

In normal adults, between 3700 and 6100 mg a day of phosphorus is filtered by the glomerulus. Net renal excretion of phosphorus is between 600 and 1500 mg a day. Ninety percent of plasma phosphate is freely filterable across the glomerular capillary, and 10% is protein bound. Under normal conditions, the kidney reabsorbs 75% to 85% of the filtered phosphate load, with the remainder delivered to the collecting duct acting as a titratable acid and excreted in the urine. Approximately 85% of phosphate reabsorption occurs within the proximal tubule. The remainder of the nephrons plays a minor role in phosphate regulation.[5]

In the proximal tubule, phosphate is reabsorbed by a transcellular route that enhances phosphate uptake across the apical membrane via three Na-P co-transporters (Npt2a and 2c and PiT-2). These transporters use the energy derived from the transport of sodium down its gradient to move inorganic phosphate from the luminal filtrate into the cell (Fig. 99.5).[4,5] In humans, Npt2a and Npt2c are believed to play the most important role in phosphate reabsorption. Type 2a transports three Na with one divalent phosphate (HPO_4) and carries a positive charge into the cell. Type 2c transports two Na with one monovalent phosphate (H_2PO_4) and is electrically neutral. Phosphate exits across the basolateral membrane by a P-inorganic anion antiporter that has not been characterized.[5,156] The amount of phosphate reabsorption is determined by the abundance of the phosphate co-transporters in the apical membrane of proximal tubule cells and not by any alternations in phosphate transport by posttranscription modifications. Hormones or dietary factors alter phosphate reabsorption by changing the abundance of the phosphate co-transporters.

Npt2a is encoded by SLC34A1, whereas Npt2c is encoded by SLC34A3. PiT-2 is encoded by SLC20A2.[5] In humans, Npt2a and Npt2c may contribute equally to phosphate reabsorption. The importance of PiT-2 in the renal control of Pi in humans remains unclear. Knockout studies in mice have shown that approximately 70% of renal phosphate handling is mediated by Npt2a and the remaining (30%) by Npt2c. Double knockout Npt2a/Npt2c mice still exhibit some renal phosphate reabsorption, indicating a role for PiT-2 in this process.[156] There are a number of functional differences between the three co-transporters (Fig. 99.5, Table 99.2). Both Npt2a and Npt2c preferentially transport divalent phosphate. However, Npt2a is electrogenic, transporting three sodium ions into the cell for every one phosphate ion, whereas Npt2c is electroneutral, transporting two sodium ions for every one phosphate ion. In contrast, PiT-2, although electrogenic like NaPi2a, preferentially transports monovalent phosphate. Changes in pH also affect the transporters differently. Npt2a and Npt2c show a doubling of Pi transport between pH 6.5 and 8, whereas the transport rate of PiT-2 is constant over this range.[5]

The tubular reabsorption of phosphate is a saturable process characterized by a transport maximum (TmPi), although the TmPi is not a fixed value but rather influenced by the actions of hormones, dietary phosphate, and growth.[153,155] To facilitate comparison of TmPi values from individuals or animals of different sizes, values are normalized by kidney, body mass, or, more commonly, the GFR. On this basis, the TmPi GFR in infants[157,158] and neonates[136,157,159,160] is greater than in corresponding adults.

The bulk of filtered phosphate is reabsorbed in the proximal convoluted tubule. The rate of renal reabsorption can increase to 85% to 90% in states of phosphate retention such as hyperparathyroidism,[152-155] dietary phosphate deprivation, and respiratory alkalosis.[161-164] This increase in phosphate retention is facilitated by reabsorption in segments beyond the proximal

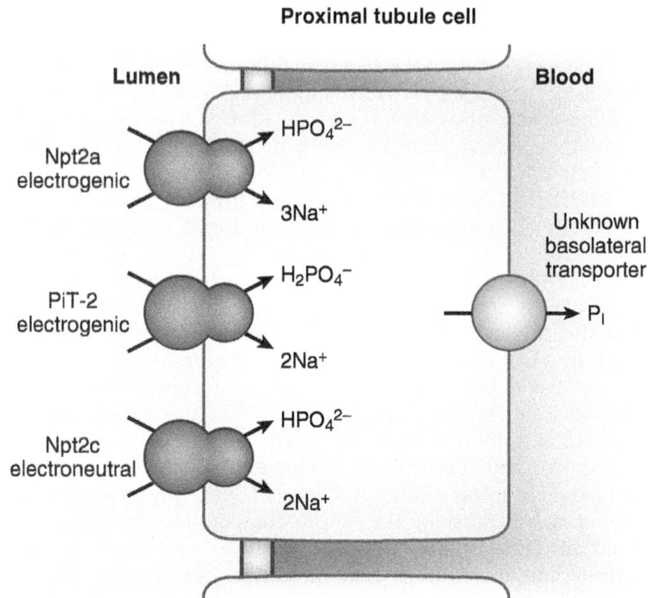

Fig. 99.5 Model of phosphate reabsorption in the renal proximal tubule. Phosphate is reabsorbed via three sodium phosphate co-transporters: Npt2a, Npt2c, and PiT-2. The sodium phosphate co-transporters, which are positioned in the apical membrane of renal proximal tubule cells, use energy derived from the movement of sodium down its gradient to move phosphate from the filtrate to the cell interior. The amount of phosphate reabsorbed is dependent on the abundance of the sodium phosphate co-transporters in the apical brush border membrane and hormones such as parathyroid hormone and fibroblast growth factor-23 decrease phosphate reabsorption by decreasing the abundance of the sodium phosphate co-transporters in the brush border. Movement of phosphate from the interior of renal proximal tubular cells to the peritubular capillaries occurs via an unknown transporter. (From Blaine J, Chonchol M, Levi M. Renal control of calcium, phosphate, and magnesium homeostasis. *Clin J Am Soc Nephrol.* 2015;10[7]:1257–1272.)

Table 99.2 Differences Between the Three Renal Sodium-Phosphate Co-transporters.

Npt2a	Npt2c	PiT-2
Electrogenic	Electroneutral	Electrogenic
Transports divalent Pi	Transports divalent Pi	Transports monovalent Pi
Found in S1, S2, and S3 segments of the proximal tubule	Only found in S1 and S2 segments of the proximal tubule	Found predominantly in S1 segments
Responds rapidly to changes in dietary Pi	Responds slowly to changes in dietary Pi	Responds slowly to changes in dietary Pi
Responds rapidly to PTH	Responds slowly to PTH	Responds rapidly to PTH
Higher activity at alkaline pH	Higher activity at alkaline pH	Higher activity at acidic pH

PTH, Parathyroid hormone.
From Blaine J, Weinman EJ, Cunningham. The regulation of renal phosphate transport. *Adv Chronic Kidney Dis.* 2011;18(2):77–84.

convoluted tubule, such as the proximal straight tubule (pars recta),[164-166] DCT,[162,167] and cortical collecting tubule,[168] particularly in states of phosphate conservation.[161,163,166,169] The postnatal period of rapid growth and development may represent a state of phosphate conservation that involves avid renal phosphate retention.

Studies using nuclear magnetic resonance techniques on isolated kidney cells have reported lower intracellular phosphate concentrations in kidneys of neonates compared with adults,[170,171] despite the known higher rate of phosphate entry into these tubular cells. This suggests that the rate of basolateral phosphate efflux must also be elevated in newborns and may contribute to their high reabsorptive capacity for phosphate. The concentration of intracellular phosphate has been directly correlated with postnatal age and dietary phosphate supply and inversely correlated with the TmPi. However, it is not significantly altered when TmPi is increased or decreased because of changes in the demand for phosphate that result from reductions in the rate of body growth or bone mineralization.[171] This suggests that variations in intracellular phosphate concentration do not contribute to those renal adaptations.

Both the descending and ascending limb of Henle probably do not contribute to the reabsorption of phosphate because the permeability of these segments to phosphate is extremely low.[152-155] Heterogeneity of phosphate reabsorption between superficial and juxtamedullary nephrons is another important element to consider in the tubular handling of phosphate by the newborn. The intrinsic capacity to transport phosphate in single nephron proximal tubules in vivo is greater in deep than superficial nephrons.[172] This observation could have significant implications for the developmental period, in view of the centrifugal pattern of nephron maturation. Because nephrogenesis begins in the juxtamedullary region and continues with the development of outer cortical nephrons,[173] the relative preponderance of deep nephrons (with a higher capacity for phosphate transport) in the immature kidney may contribute to the high capacity for phosphate reabsorption during development.[146]

REGULATION OF URINARY PHOSPHATE EXCRETION AND REABSORPTION

Estimates based on the differences between proximal tubular phosphate reabsorption and urinary phosphate excretion indicate that phosphate uptake in nephron sites beyond the superficial proximal tubule is enhanced in the newborn compared with the adult.[160] Phosphate excretion is low at birth and subsequently increases. Low PTH, low renal blood flow, and low GFR contribute to low phosphate excretion. An increase in phosphaturic response to PTH has been demonstrated in preterm and term infants. An increase of calcitriol after birth is due to up-regulation of the renal 1α-hydrolase by a PTH increase.[174]

Several hormones and factors regulate urinary phosphate excretion, but PTH is the most important hormone that controls phosphate excretion by inhibiting phosphate reabsorption in the proximal tubules and thereby increasing phosphate excretion (Table 99.3). PTH stimulates an endocytic removal of Na-P co-transporters from the brush border membrane of the proximal tubule. Dietary phosphate intake also regulates phosphate excretion. Phosphate loading increases excretion. Dietary or hormonal changes result in relatively rapid (minutes to hours) insertion or removal of Npt2a from the brush border membrane, whereas regulation of Npt2c and PiT-2 occurs more slowly (hours to days).[5]

EFFECTS OF DIETARY PHOSPHATE ON RENAL PHOSPHATE REABSORPTION

Dietary phosphate intake regulates P excretion by mechanisms unrelated to changes in PTH level. Changes in phosphate diet modulate phosphate transport by the transport rate of each Na-P co-transporters and the number of co-transporters in the apical membrane of the proximal tubule.[4,5] Ingestion of phosphorus-containing foods leads to removal of Npt2a, Npt2c, and PiT-2 from the proximal tubule brush border membrane, thereby decreasing phosphate reabsorption from the ultrafiltrate. By contrast, dietary Pi restriction leads to insertion of the sodium phosphate co-transporters in the proximal tubule brush border membrane, increasing phosphate reabsorption. In the adult, phosphate deprivation is associated with increased membrane fluidity and reduced membrane cholesterol content, which may facilitate the observed increase in Vmax.[169] Conversely, aging is associated with loss of membrane fluidity, increased cholesterol,[175] and reduced phosphate reabsorption.[176] The elevated TmPi in the phosphate-deprived newborn serves to maintain avid reabsorption of phosphate and facilitate the accelerated rate of growth that occurs on the restoration of phosphate to the diet.[147,150]

Table 99.3 Factors of Renal Regulation of Phosphate.

Change in Phosphate Absorption	Factors
Increase phosphate absorption	Low-phosphate diet 1,25-Vitamin D3 Thyroid hormone
Decrease phosphate absorption	Phosphatonins (FGF23) High-phosphate diet Metabolic acidosis Potassium deficiency Glucocorticoids Dopamine Hypertension Estrogen

FGF, Fibroblast growth factor.
Data from Koeppen BM, Stanton BA. Regulation of calcium and phosphate homeostasis. In: Koeppen BM, Stanton BA, eds. *Renal Physiology*. 6th ed. Philadelphia: Elsevier; 2019:138–150; Blaine J, Chonchol M, Levi M. Renal control of calcium, phosphate, and magnesium homeostasis. *Clin J Am Soc Nephrol*. 2015;10(7):1257–1272; Blaine J, Weinman EJ, Cunningham. The regulation of renal phosphate transport. *Adv Chronic Kidney Dis*. 2011;18(2):77–84.

Potassium deficiency leads to an increase in phosphate excretion in the urine despite a paradoxic increase in the abundance of Npt2a in the proximal tubule brush border membrane that should increase phosphate reabsorption. Potassium deficiency leads to changes in the brush border membrane lipid composition that are thought to inhibit Npt2a activity.[5]

EFFECTS OF PARATHYROID HORMONE ON RENAL PHOSPHATE REABSORPTION

PTH causes decreased renal reabsorption of phosphate and phosphaturia by decreasing the abundance of Npt2a, Npt2c, and PiT-2 in the renal proximal tubule brush border membrane. In response to PTH, Npt2a is removed rapidly (within minutes), whereas the decrease in apical membrane abundance of Npt2c and PiT-2 takes hours. The sodium phosphate co-transporter response to PTH involves several kinases, including protein kinases A and C and mitogen-activated protein kinase extracellular signal-regulated kinase 1/2, as well as a myosin motor (myosin VI).[5,177,178] It is interesting to note that juxtamedullary (deep) nephrons elicit a greater phosphaturic response to PTH than do superficial nephrons[179]; whether this effect is due to an increase in PTH receptors or increased maturation of the deep nephrons is not known.

PTH, the principal hormonal regulator of renal phosphate transport, is released from the parathyroid glands in response to hypocalcemia or hyperphosphatemia and acts on the kidney to increase calcium reabsorption while decreasing phosphate uptake. Of interest, evidence shows that exposure of the gut to a high Pi diet rapidly (within 10 minutes) can affect PTH secretion, independent of changes in serum calcium or phosphate.[180,181]

THYROID HORMONE

Thyroid hormone receptors are present in the fetus, with the hormone peaking at birth in humans and decreasing by 4 or 5 weeks after birth to levels maintained through adulthood. The kidney is a target organ for thyroid hormone and contains the iodothyronine deiodinase enzyme that converts the main circulating hormone T4 to the more potent T3.[182] Thyroid hormone increases phosphate absorption by increasing proximal tubule transcription and expression of Npt2a. The Npt2a gene contains a thyroid response element, and transcription of Npt2a mRNA is regulated by 3,5,3-triiodothyronine.[5]

FIBROBLAST GROWTH FACTOR 23

FGF23 is produced in osteoblasts and osteocytes in response to increases in serum phosphate and increased PTH and calcitriol.[4,5,119] FGF23 requires the presence of a cofactor, Klotho, which is produced in the kidney and activates FGF receptor 1. Klotho is a membrane-bound protein and a soluble protein.[4] Klotho promotes phosphate excretion by the kidney and reduces serum levels of 1,25OH vitamin D3.

FGF23 has decreased Na-dependent Pi transport[183] through down-regulation of NaPi IIa expression and activity in the proximal tubule.[184] FGF23 also decreases the activity of the intestinal sodium phosphate co-transporter.[5] FGF23 reduces serum levels of calcitriol by decreasing the renal expression of 1α-hydroxylase, which is the rate-limiting step in calcitriol synthesis, and increasing renal expression of 24-hydroxylase, which is required for calcitriol degradation.[5] In addition, FGF23 suppresses PTH synthesis, although the parathyroid glands are believed to become resistant to FGF23 as kidney disease progresses. Of clinical importance is the fact that patients with CKD have exceptionally high levels of circulating FGF23,[185-187] and the levels inversely correlate with the maximum tubular capacity of phosphate reabsorption.[186] Furthermore, hemodialysis plays no role in lowering the elevated FGF23 levels in these patients.[188] Increase in FGF23 levels in patients with CKD contributes to the suppression of 1,25-(OH)2D3 levels, which is involved in maintaining efficient intestinal calcium absorption. This also leads to secondary hyperparathyroidism, which has implications in producing bone mineralization abnormalities in these patients. Studies have shown that elevated FGF23 in CKD is likely associated with mortality, cardiovascular disease events, anemia, infection, and progression in CKD.[189] There have been clinical trials of new therapies and repurposing of existing drugs targeting on FGF23 in CKD, including calcimimetics that increase sensitivity of CaSR to serum calcium leading decrease in PTH, calcium, and 1,25(OH)2D and subsequently resulting in reduction of FGF23 production, and FGF23-blocking antibody (Burosumab).[189]

Of note, FGF23 may also be involved in the pathogenesis of McCune-Albright syndrome because circulating levels appear to correlate with the severity of hypophosphatemia and bone dysplasia in affected individuals.[190] Because binding of FGF23 to the FGF receptor elicits mitogen-activated protein kinase activation and tyrosine kinase signaling,[191] FGF23 inhibitors or blockers of the FGF receptor signaling cascade may have the potential to prevent the significant Pi losses and bone abnormalities seen in these patients. Activating mutations in the FGF23 gene lead to hypophosphatemia, low serum calcitriol, and rickets or osteomalacia. In terms of hypophosphatemic rickets with elevated FGF-23 levels, X-linked, autosomal dominant, and autosomal recessive forms are caused by pathogenic variants of the genes *PHEX, GGF23,* and *DMP1* (or *ENPP1*), respectively.[192] Conventional treatment with phosphate supplements and active vitamin D may require the addition of GH and calcimimetics. New biologic therapeutics, including FGF23 targeting monoclonal antibodies or recombinant receptor blockers, are being developed and becoming available.[192] Inactivating mutations cause hyperphosphatemia, high serum calcitriol, and calcification of soft tissue.[4] Hyperphosphatemic familial tumoral calcinosis (HFTC) is an autosomal recessive inherited hyperphosphatemic disease due to the mutations of GALNTs, FGF23, and Klotho leading FGF23 insufficiency that presents clinically with ectopic calcified masses, hyperphosphatemia, and elevated 1,25(OH)2D.[193]

1,25(OH)2 VITAMIN D

Calcitriol increases phosphate reabsorption in the proximal tubule, but the effects are confounded by the fact that changes in 1,25(OH)2D also alter plasma calcium and PTH levels.[4,5]

INSULIN-LIKE GROWTH FACTOR GROWTH HORMONE

GH is a key factor regulating renal phosphate reabsorption, particularly in the postnatal period. GH hypersecretion is associated with hyperphosphatemia and a reduction in urinary phosphate excretion.[194,195] Conversely, GH deficiency (dwarfism) is associated with an attenuated growth rate and increased excretion of phosphate.[195] When GH-deficient individuals are given GH injections, growth rate acutely increases and phosphate excretion diminishes.[195] In opossum kidney cells (a well-established model of the renal proximal tubule), insulin-like growth factor-1 (IGF-1) increases Pi uptake and increases NaPi-4 (the opossum kidney homologue of Npt2a) abundance by stabilization of the NaPi-4 protein within the brush border membrane and is independent of any increase in transcription of NaPi-4.[156]

GLUCOCORTICOIDS

Increased glucocorticoid levels lead to decreased proximal tubule synthesis and abundance of Npt2a as well as changes in brush border membrane lipid composition, which is thought to modulate sodium phosphate co-transporter activity.[5]

ESTROGEN

Estrogen causes phosphaturia by decreasing the abundance of Npt2a in the proximal tubule without altering Npt2c levels.[48] Estrogen also increases FGF23 synthesis.[5]

DOPAMINE

Dopamine leads to phosphaturia by inducing internalization of Npt2a from the proximal tubule brush border membrane. Dopamine-mediated internalization of Npt2a is dependent on a scaffolding protein (sodium-hydrogen exchanger regulatory factor 1) because dopamine does not induce phosphaturia in sodium-hydrogen exchanger regulatory factor 1 knockout mice.[5]

METABOLIC ACIDOSIS

Chronic metabolic acidosis increases phosphate excretion in urine, which helps to remove acid from the blood because phosphate serves as a titratable acid. Systemic acidosis causes glucocorticoid secretion, which inhibits phosphate reabsorption as well.[4] Acidosis also directly inhibits phosphate reabsorption in the proximal tubule. By contrast, metabolic alkalosis increases renal phosphate absorption.[4,5] In mice, acidosis increases proximal tubule brush border membrane abundance of Npt2a and Npt2c, suggesting that phosphaturia results from inhibition of sodium phosphate co-transporter activity rather than changes in the levels of these proteins.[196,197]

HYPERTENSION

An acute increase in BP leads to decreased renal phosphate reabsorption by inducing removal of Npt2a from the proximal tubule brush border membrane microvilli to subapical endosomes.[5]

EXTRACELLULAR FLUID VOLUME

Expansion of ECF enhances phosphate excretion by (1) increasing GFRs and thus the filtered amount of phosphate, (2) decreasing Na-P coupled reabsorption to reduce ECF volume expansion, and (3) reducing serum calcium, which increases PTH leading inhibition of phosphate reabsorption in proximal tubule.[4]

CIRCADIAN RHYTHM

Renal phosphate excretion is influenced by circadian rhythms.[156] A study by Bielesz and colleagues studied whether the diurnal changes in the renal excretion of Pi corresponded with changes in Npt2a protein abundance. These investigators concluded that the diurnal changes that have been known to occur in the urinary excretion of phosphate are most likely the result of changes in the serum phosphate concentration and the tubular threshold of phosphate and not because of changes in Npt2a expression within the brush border membrane. The role of Npt2c and PiT2 in the diurnal variation of renal phosphate excretion remains to be determined.[198]

FETAL AND NEONATAL ASPECTS OF RENAL TRANSPORT OF PHOSPHATE

The endochondral skeleton formation begins in the embryo, with substantial bone mineralization by the third trimester and afterward.[174] The placenta plays a main role in transporting minerals from the maternal circulation to fetus and returning waste products from fetus back to the mother. The normal fetal circulation displays higher levels of calcium, magnesium, and phosphate than maternal and normal adult values with serum phosphate ranging approximately 0.5 mmol/L higher. Despite a high calcium × phosphate product, there is no abnormal calcification development in normal fetus.[119,174] This is likely due to rapid uptake of mineral into developing skeleton. The fetal circulation presents with high levels of calcitonin and PTHrP but low concentrations of PTH, calcitriol, and sex steroids.[119,174] Low PTH, high phosphate, and calcium lead to suppression of 1α-hydroxylase expression, causing low calcitriol. FGF23 does not play a main role in fetal regulation of serum phosphate, placental phosphate transport, or skeleton development. Limited data indicate that fetal serum FGF23 level is at less than one third the normal adult. FGF23 begins to have significant roles within days after birth. Intact FGF23 levels increase fourfold at day 4 to 5 of life.[174] Phosphate excretion is low at birth and subsequently increases. Low PTH, low renal blood flow, and GFR over the first 12 to 24 hours after birth result low phosphate renal excretion.[174] Simultaneously there is a decrease in serum calcium concentration, and neonatal serum phosphate increases over the first 24 to 48 postnatal hours before decreasing to normal adult values. PTH increases significantly after 48 hours. Calcitriol slowly increases likely in response to PTH stimulating renal 1α-hydroxylase.[174]

CONCLUSION

The regulation of calcium and phosphate homeostasis requires a complex interplay between absorption from the intestine and exchange from bone, as well as the balance of renal excretion and absorption that occurs along different parts of the nephron. An intricate relationship between the many known factors influencing dietary, hormonal, environmental, and other variables results in the fine balance of calcium and phosphorous in health and disease.

ACKNOWLEDGMENTS

We acknowledge the coauthors of this chapter in the previous edition: Drs. Abhijeet Pal, Juhi Kumar, Craig B. Woda, Robert P. Woroniecki, and Susan E. Mulroney.

A complete reference list is available at www.ExpertConsult.com. 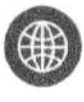

SELECT REFERENCES

2. Peacock M. Calcium metabolism in health and disease. *Clin J Am Soc Nephrol*. 2010;5(1):S23-30.
3. Weaver CM, Peacock M. Calcium. *Adv Nutr*. 2019;10(3):546-548.
4. Koeppen BM, Stanton BA. Regulation of calcium and phosphate homeostasis. In: Koeppen BM, Stanton BA. *Renal Physiology*. 6th ed. Philadelphia: Elsevier; 2019.
5. Blaine J, Chonchol M, Levi M. Renal control of calcium, phosphate, and magnesium homeostasis. *Clin J Am Soc Nephrol*. 2015;10(7):1257-1272.
11. Belkacemi L, Simoneau L, Lafond J. Calcium-binding proteins: distribution and implication in mammalian placenta. *Endocrine*. 2002;19:57-64.
15. Hoenderop JG, Nilius B, Bindels RJ. Calcium absorption across epithelia. *Physiol Rev*. 2005;85:373-422.
23. Hsu YJ, Hoenderop JG, Bindels RJ. TRP channels in kidney disease. *Biochim Biophys Acta*. 2007;1772:928-936.
25. Hoenderop JG, Nilius B, Bindels RJ. Epithelial calcium channels: from identification to function and regulation. *Pflügers Arch*. 2003;446:304-308.
26. Hoenderop JG, Vennekens R, Muller D, et al. Function and expression of the epithelial Ca2+ channel family: comparison of mammalian ECaC1 and 2. *J Physiol*. 2001;537:747-761.
29. Nijenhuis T, Hoenderop JG, van der Kemp AW, Bindels RJ. Localization and regulation of the epithelial Ca2+ channel TRPV6 in the kidney. *J Am Soc Nephrol*. 2003;14:2731-2740.
33. Moe SM. Calcium homeostasis in health and in kidney disease. *Compr Physiol*. 2016;(6):1781-1800.
35. Lambers TT, Oancea E, de Groot T, et al. Extracellular pH dynamically controls cell surface delivery of functional TRPV5 channels. *Mol Cell Biol*. 2007;27:1486-1494.
38. Lambers TT, Mahieu F, Oancea E, et al. Calbindin-D28K dynamically controls TRPV5-mediated calcium transport. *EMBO J*. 2006;25:2978-2988.
41. Venyaminov SY, Klimtchuk ES, Bajzer Z, Craig TA. Changes in structure and stability of calbindin-D (28K) upon calcium binding. *Anal Biochem*. 2004;334:97-105.
46. Biner HL, Arpin-Bott MP, Loffing J, et al. Human cortical distal nephron: distribution of electrolyte and water transport pathways. *J Am Soc Nephrol*. 2002;13:836-847.
47. Loffing J, Loffing-Cueni D, Valderrabano V, et al. Distribution of transcellular calcium and sodium transport pathways along mouse distal nephron. *Am J Physiol*. 2001;281:F1021-F1027.
54. Blaustein MP, Juhaszova M, Golovina VA, et al. Na/Ca exchanger and PMCA localization in neurons and astrocytes: functional implications. *Ann N Y Acad Sci*. 2002;976:356-366.
58. Philipson KD, Nicoll DA. Sodium-calcium exchange: a molecular perspective. *Annu Rev Physiol*. 2000;62:111-133.
59. Cai X, Lytton J. Molecular cloning of a sixth member of the K+-dependent Na+/Ca2+ exchanger gene family, NCKX6. *J Biol Chem*. 2004;279:5867-5876.
69. Friedman PA, Gesek FA. Hormone-responsive Ca2+ entry in distal convoluted tubules. *J Am Soc Nephrol*. 1994;4:1396-1404.
74. Blankenship KA, Williams JJ, Lawrence MS, et al. The calcium-sensing receptor regulates calcium absorption in MDCK cells by inhibition of PMCA. *Am J Physiol*. 2001;280:F815-F822.
81. Tyler Miller R. Control of renal calcium, phosphate, electrolytes, and water excretion by the calcium-sensing receptor. *Best Prac Res Clin Endocrinol Metab*. 2013;27(3):345-358.
106. Monroy A, Plata C, Hebert SC, Gamba G. Characterization of the thiazide-sensitive Na+-Cl- cotransporter: a new model for ions and diuretics interaction. *Am J Physiol Renal Physiol*. 2000;279:F161-F169.
115. Hoenderop JG, Müller D, Van Der Kemp AW, et al. Calcitriol controls the epithelial calcium channel in kidney. *J Am Soc Nephrol*. 2001;12:1342-1349.
116. Nilius B, Prenen J, Vennekens R, et al. Modulation of the epithelial calcium channel, ECaC, by intracellular Ca2+. *Cell Calcium*. 2001;29:417-428.
119. Kovacs CS. Bone development and mineral homeostasis in the fetus and neonate: role of the calciotrophic and phosphotropic hormones. *Physio Rev*. 2014;94:1143-1218.
128. Kovacs CS, Manley NR, Moseley JM, et al. Fetal parathyroids are not required to maintain placental calcium transport. *J Clin Invest*. 2001;107:1007-1015.
129. Bradbury RA, Cropley J, Kifor O, et al. Localization of the extracellular Ca2+-sensing receptor in the human placenta. *Placenta*. 2002;23:192-200.
149. Mulroney SE, Woda CB, Halaihel N, et al. Central control of renal sodium-phosphate (NaPi-2) transporters. *Am J Physiol Renal Physiol*. 2004;286(4):F647-F652.

153. Knochel JP, Jacobson HR. Renal handling of phosphorus, clinical hypophosphatemia, and phosphorus deficiency. In: Brenner BM, Rector FC, eds. *The Kidney*. 3rd ed. Philadelphia: Saunders; 1986.
154. Chesney RW, Dabbah S. Calcium, phosphorus, and magnesium. In: Holliday M, Barratt TM, Vernier RL, eds. *Pediatric Nephrology*. 2nd ed. Baltimore: Williams & Wilkins; 1987.
156. Blaine J, Weinman EJ, Cunningham. The regulation of renal phosphate transport. *Adv Chronic Kidney Dis*. 2011;18(2):77-84.
158. Brodehl J, Gellissen K, Weber HP. Postnatal development of tubular phosphate reabsorption. *Clin Nephrol*. 1982;17(4):163-171.
172. Haramati A. Tubular capacity for phosphate reabsorption in superficial and deep nephrons. *Am J Physiol*. 1985;248(5 Pt 2):F729-F733.
174. Calcium Kovacs. Calcium, phosphorus, and bone metabolism in the fetus and newborn. *Early Hum Dev*. 2015;91(11):623-628.
178. Bacic D, Schulz N, Biber J, et al. Involvement of the MAPK-kinase pathway in the PTH-mediated regulation of the proximal tubule type IIa Na+/Pi cotransporter in mouse kidney. *Flügers Arch*. 2003;446:52-60.
180. Martin DR, Ritter CS, Slatopolsky E, Brown AJ. Acute regulation of parathyroid hormone by dietary phosphate. *Am J Physiol Endocrinol Metab*. 2005;289:E729-E734.
187. Larsson T, Nisbeth U, Ljunggren O, et al. Circulating concentration of FGF-23 increases as renal function declines in patients with chronic kidney disease, but does not change in response to variation in phosphate intake in healthy volunteers. *Kidney Int*. 2003;64:2272-2279.
189. Musgove J, Wolf M. Regulation and effects of FGF23 in chronic kidney disease. *Annu Rev Physiol*. 2020;82:23.1-23.13.26.
191. Yamashita T, Konishi M, Miyake A, et al. Fibroblast growth factor (FGF)-23 inhibits renal phosphate reabsorption by activation of the mitogen-activated protein kinase pathway. *J Biol Chem*. 2002;277:28265-28270.
192. Bitzan M, Goodyer. Hypophosphatemic ricket. *Pediatr Clin North Am*. 2019;66(1):179-207.
193. Kinoshita Y, Fukumoto S. X-linked hypophosphatemia and FGF23-related hypophosphatemic diseases: prospect for new treatment. *Endocrine Review*. 2018;39:274-291.

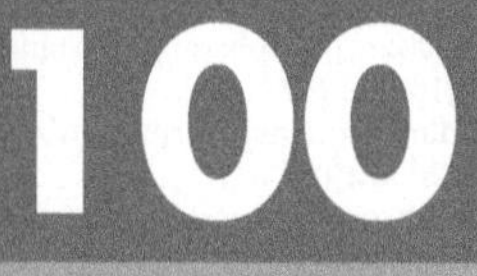

100 Transport of Amino Acids in the Fetus and Neonate

Raymond Quigley

INTRODUCTION

Amino acids are the building blocks for proteins and are critical for growth. In addition, they are involved in many metabolic processes within mammalian cells. Thus, regulating their circulating concentrations in the bloodstream is very important for many metabolic processes, including protein synthesis, which results in the growth and development of the fetus and neonate. This chapter reviews the regulation of amino acid transport in the fetus and the newborn. This will include a general description of epithelial transport systems for amino acids, including a more detailed description of the various classes of amino acid transporters that are known. The developmental expression of these transporters in the placenta and the developing kidney will also be discussed. In addition, the role these transporters play in the placenta of neonates with intrauterine growth restriction will be discussed.

EPITHELIAL TRANSPORT OF AMINO ACIDS

Amino acids are hydrophilic molecules and therefore do not easily diffuse through lipid bilayer membranes. There are a number of transport systems that facilitate the diffusion of amino acids through cell membranes. In addition, the epithelia of the proximal tubule of the kidney, the small intestine, and the syncytiotrophoblast of the placenta have active transport systems to move amino acids from one compartment to another against a concentration gradient. These active transport systems derive their energy from the inwardly directed sodium gradient that is generated from the sodium-potassium ATPase. This is depicted in a generic epithelial cell in Fig. 100.1. One side of the epithelial cell is the *lumen*, and the opposite membrane is the *basolateral membrane*. The sodium-potassium ATPase is located on the basolateral membrane and is responsible for maintaining a very low intracellular sodium concentration. Thus, the amino acid transporter located on the luminal membrane can harness the sodium gradient energy to transport amino acids from the lumen into the cell. The concentration of the amino acid in the cell then becomes much higher than that in the lumen and the bloodstream, and thus the amino acid can diffuse through the basolateral membrane by way of a facilitative transporter into the bloodstream.

Although this transport system seems very simple for many of the solutes reabsorbed in the proximal tubule, it is much more complicated for amino acid transport because amino acids have several different structural classes. Another feature that makes these systems complicated is that some amino acids can be transported by more than one system but with different affinities. There are five known systems of amino acid transporters responsible for the different classes of amino acids.[1] The nomenclature for these systems has also become very complex owing to the history of the discovery of these systems. A full discussion of all the known amino acid transporters is beyond the scope of this chapter (see Broer[1] for a more in-depth review). These systems will be reviewed briefly, and their development in the kidney and placenta will be discussed.

NEUTRAL AMINO ACIDS

The first system is designed to transport neutral amino acids and is depicted in Fig. 100.2.[1,2] As shown in the figure, the transporters found in the proximal convoluted tubule are very similar to those found in the small intestine. The proximal straight tubule, in general, has different amino acid transporters that have higher affinities for the amino acids because their concentrations in the lumen of the tubule will be much lower. The transporters on the basolateral membrane of the tubule have been much less characterized, so in Fig. 100.2 there are question marks on those transporters.

The main protein that has been identified in the system has been labeled *B^0AT1*, as shown in Fig. 100.2.[1,2] This transporter carries one sodium ion with the amino acid molecule, so it uses the sodium gradient as the energy source for active transport. The transporters on the basolateral membrane are less well characterized but serve to facilitate the diffusion of the amino acids out of the cell and into the bloodstream. The primary protein, TAT1, is a facilitative transporter that allows the amino acid to go down its concentration gradient from the intracellular compartment into the interstitial fluid. From the interstitial fluid compartment, the amino acid will diffuse into the bloodstream.

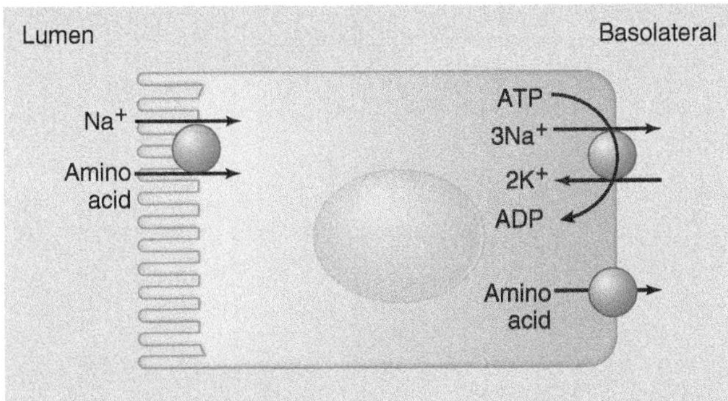

Fig. 100.1 A generic epithelial cell. The sodium-potassium ATPase is on the basolateral membrane. This active transporter is responsible for maintaining a very low intracellular sodium concentration. In addition, it is electrogenic and helps to maintain a negative intracellular potential difference. Thus there is a lumen-to-intracellular electrochemical gradient for sodium entry. The sodium-coupled amino acid transporter on the luminal membrane uses this gradient as its energy source to actively transport amino acids into the cell. In general, there is a facilitative transporter on the basolateral membrane for the diffusion of amino acids from the intracellular pool into the bloodstream.

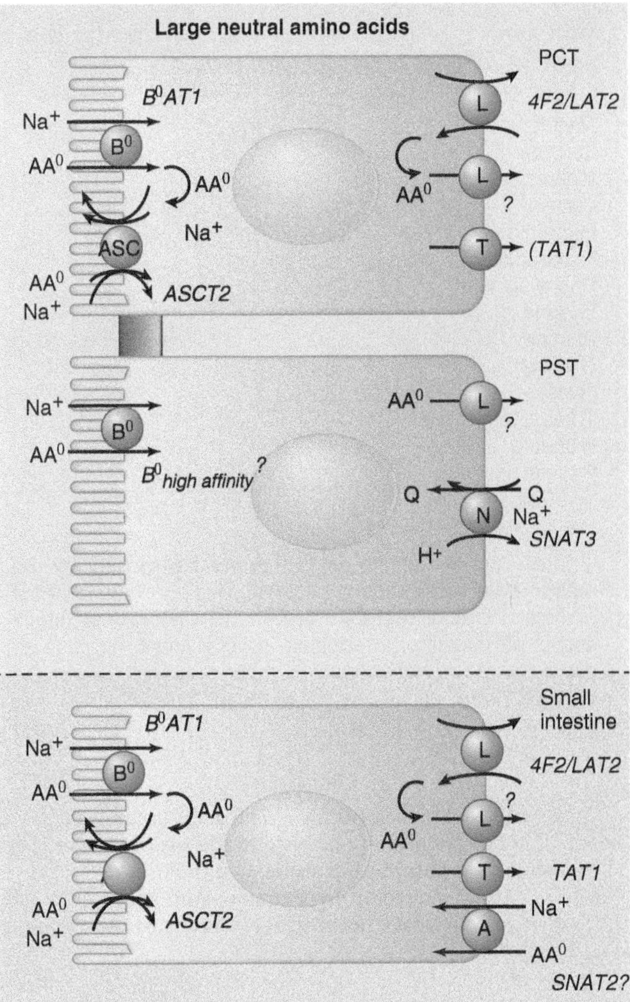

Fig. 100.2 This neutral amino acid transporter is responsible for the absorption of most of the amino acids, as listed in Box 100.1. Mutations in this transporter are responsible for several diseases, including Hartnup disorder and tryptophan malabsorption. *AA,* Amino acid; *PCT,* proximal convoluted tubule; *PST,* proximal straight tubule. (From Bröer S. Amino acid transport across mammalian intestinal and renal epithelia. *Physiol Rev.* 2008;88:249–286.)

Box 100.1 lists the various amino acids that are transported by this system in order of their affinities. As shown, a number of the amino acids that can be carried by the B^0AT1 transporter are also substrates for other transporters; for example, the cationic amino acid transporter also transports cystine actively.

Mutations in these neutral amino acid transporters result in several diseases. Hartnup disorder is caused by a mutation in B^0AT1 depicted in Fig. 100.2.[3,4] People with this disorder can develop a pellagra-like rash, as well as cerebellar ataxia, and exhibit aminoaciduria of neutral amino acids, including tryptophan. Tryptophan is a precursor of niacin. Thus, people with Hartnup disorder can easily become niacin deficient and often require supplementation. Another disorder resulting in tryptophan malabsorption is known as *blue diaper syndrome.*[5] This blue diaper syndrome is secondary to the increased amounts of tryptophan in the stool and urine, which are converted by bacteria into compounds known as *indoles.* These compounds can then be metabolized to indigo, which causes the blue coloration in the diapers. Although the transporter that is mutated in this syndrome has not been identified, a candidate protein is TAT1, which is located on the basolateral membrane (see Fig. 100.2). Recently, a patient with this syndrome was found to have a mutation in proprotein convertase subtilisin/kexin type 1 *(PCSK1).*[6] It remains unclear if this syndrome is the result of a defect in amino acid transport or possibly a defect in protein metabolism.

CATIONIC AMINO ACIDS AND CYSTINE

The cationic amino acids include lysine, arginine, ornithine, and cystine. The main transporter identified for these amino acids is referred to as *rBAT.*[1] However, transport of these amino acids is very complex and includes other proteins that may function as exchangers. In addition, it is unclear if these transporters require sodium. Because the cationic amino acid carries a charge, it can utilize the electric potential difference across the luminal membrane as its driving force. Although these transporters do not directly carry sodium, they are still dependent on the sodium-potassium ATPase to maintain the electrical gradient across the luminal membrane.

Evidence also indicates that the transport system functions as an exchanger for neutral amino acids.[7] Thus, instead of directly using the sodium gradient as its energy source, it uses the neutral amino acid gradient. This means that the neutral amino acids are shuttled back into the lumen of the tubule (or intestine) and then reabsorbed by means of the neutral amino acid transport system discussed above. As shown in Fig. 100.3, the transporters on the basolateral membrane are also very complex.

The most common disorder of this system is cystinuria.[8] People with cystinuria excrete excessive amounts of arginine, lysine, ornithine, and cystine. Because cystine is very insoluble, kidney stones develop that are almost 100% cystine. The excessive excretion of arginine, lysine, and ornithine does not seem to cause any problems because these amino acids are much more soluble and do not precipitate into stones. Most patients with cystinuria have a mutation in rBAT. A few patients have a mutation in $b^{0,+}AT$, which combines with rBAT to function as the transporter.[9] This probably explains some of the heterogeneity in the characteristics of the patients.

Another genetic defect in the system results in lysinuric protein intolerance.[10] In this disorder, there are very low

Box 100.1 Amino Acids Transported by the Neutral Amino Acid System B^{0}AT1

Methionine
Leucine
Isoleucine
Valine
Glutamine
Asparagine
Phenylalanine
Cystine
Alanine
Glycine
Tyrosine
Threonine
Histidine
Proline
Tryptophan
Lysine

These are the amino acids that are transported by the neutral amino acid transport system. This accounts for most of the amino acids that are transported in the proximal tubule and small intestine. In addition, several amino acids (e.g., cystine) that are transported by other systems can also be transported by this system but at much lower affinities.

concentrations of these cationic amino acids in serum. This can cause difficulty with the urea cycle in the liver because of the involvement of ornithine and arginine in the urea cycle. People with this disorder develop hyperammonemia when they have excessive protein intake because of an inadequate substrate for the urea cycle.

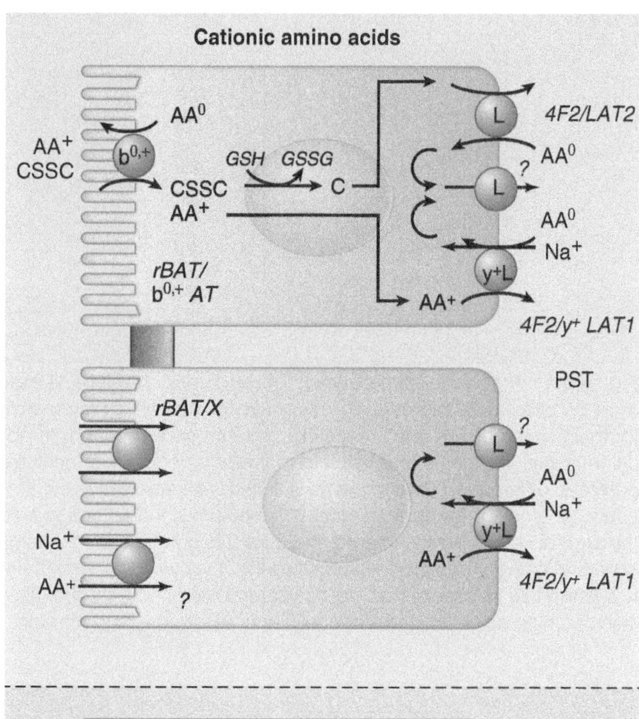

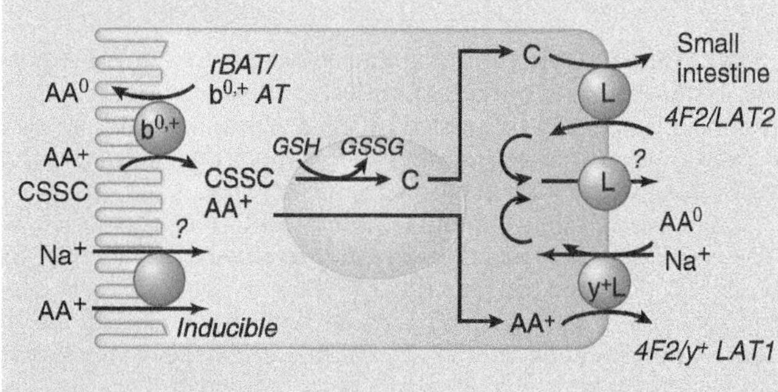

Fig. 100.3 The cationic amino acid transporter is responsible for the absorption of lysine, arginine, ornithine, and cystine. Mutations in this transporter result in cystinuria. *AA*, Amino acid; *C*, cysteine; *CSSC*, cystine; *GSH*, reduced glutathione; *GSSH*, oxidized glutathione; *PST*, proximal straight tubule. (From Bröer S. Amino acid transport across mammalian intestinal and renal epithelia. *Physiol Rev.* 2008;88:249–286.)

ANIONIC AMINO ACIDS

The transporter for these anionic amino acids is termed *EAAT3*.[1] It is primarily responsible for reabsorbing aspartate and glutamate. Inherited disorders of this transporter are extremely rare. People with this disorder, dicarboxylic aminoaciduria, can excrete these amino acids at a rate higher than the glomerular filtration rate.[11,12] This indicates that the basolateral uptake of these amino acids is mediated by a mutation in EAAT3 (the transporter for glutamate and aspartate), which is responsible for the secretion of these amino acids in the urine (Fig. 100.4).

PROLINE, HYDROXYPROLINE, AND GLYCINE

There are several transporters that are responsible for the reabsorption of these amino acids. These are depicted in Fig. 100.5.[1] The disorders that results from a mutation of one of these transporters are termed *iminoglycinuria* and *hyperglycinuria*.[13] People with this disorder have increased excretion of glycine, proline, and hydroxyproline. Patients that are heterozygotes for this disorder have hyperglycinuria while homozygotes have iminoglycinuria.[13]

These transporters undergo significant maturational changes during the first weeks of life.[14] This explains why many neonates and premature infants in particular can have significant amounts of glycine in their urine. This will be discussed in the section entitled "Developmental Changes in Neonatal Renal Function."

TAURINE AND OTHER β-AMINO ACIDS

There is a transporter in the proximal tubule responsible for transporting taurine, β-alanine, and gamma-aminobutyric acid (GABA). This is the high-affinity transporter that has been termed *TauT*.[1] It is dependent on sodium and chloride for its function. There is also a lower-affinity transporter (dependent on protons), similar to the transporter for proline, hydroxyproline, and glycine, which will transport these anionic amino acids (see Fig. 100.6).[1] In addition, there appears to be a low-affinity transporter in the proximal convoluted tubule. This transporter undergoes significant developmental changes. While almost 100% of the filtered taurine is reabsorbed in the adult rat proximal tubule, only approximately 50% is reabsorbed in the neonatal rat tubule. This appears to be due to lower uptake by the tubular cells as well as efflux from the tubule cells. The intracellular concentration of taurine was found to be higher in the neonatal tubule cells because of the slower efflux from the cells.

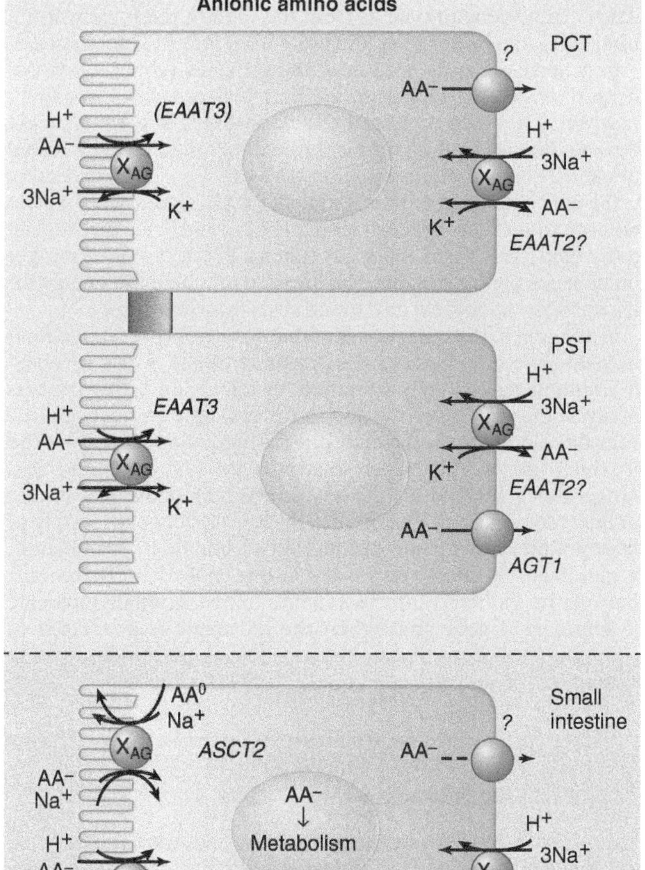

Fig. 100.4 The anionic amino acid transporter primarily reabsorbs aspartate and glutamate. As can be seen, there is also active transport on the basolateral membrane. Thus mutations in this system can result in excretion of these amino acids at a rate greater than the glomerular filtration rate. *AA*, Amino acid; *PCT*, proximal convoluted tubule; *PST*, proximal straight tubule. (From Bröer S. Amino acid transport across mammalian intestinal and renal epithelia. *Physiol Rev.* 2008;88:249–286.)

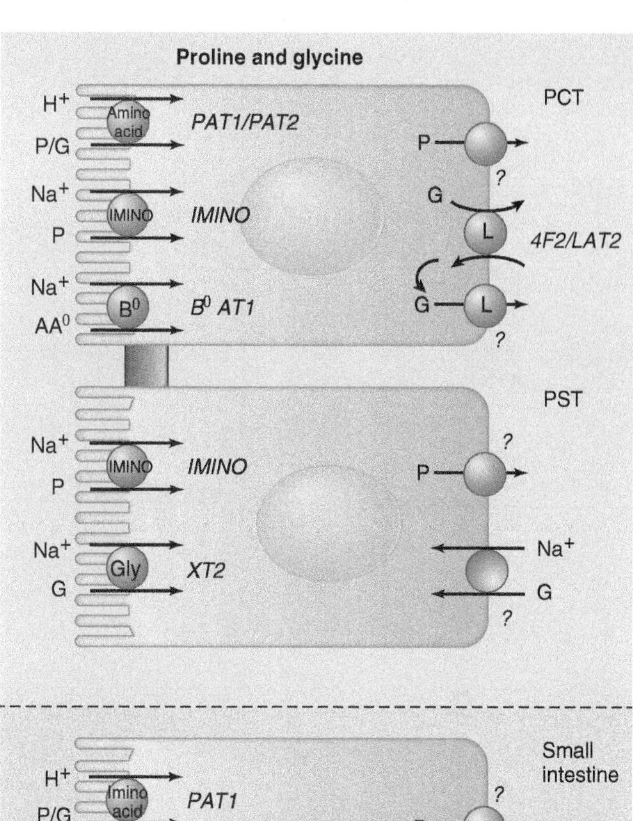

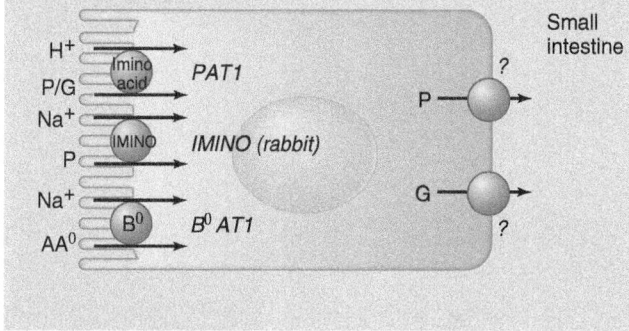

Fig. 100.5 The amino acid transporter depicted is responsible for transport of the imino group of amino acids, which includes proline (P), hydroxyproline, and glycine (G). *AA*, Amino acid; *PCT*, proximal convoluted tubule; *PST*, proximal straight tubule. (From Bröer S. Amino acid transport across mammalian intestinal and renal epithelia. *Physiol Rev.* 2008;88:249–286.)

PLACENTAL AMINO ACID TRANSPORT

During fetal development the placenta provides the regulation of solute concentrations in the blood. Although the fetal kidney starts to function in the 10th week of gestation, any solutes that are excreted into the amniotic fluid will be reabsorbed by the fetus. Thus, the fetus is dependent on the placenta for its nutrients, as well as for excretion of metabolic waste products.

In addition to the transport of amino acids by the placenta, there is significant metabolism of amino acids in the placenta and in the fetal liver.[15,16] Over the past 10 to 20 years our understanding of the transport of amino acids by the placenta has improved.[17,18] The complex interchange between the mother, placenta, and fetus in terms of the transport and metabolism of amino acids and other nutrients has shown how a systems approach will be necessary to understand how to care for these patients.[19]

It has been known for some time that the concentrations of amino acids in the fetus are higher than those in the mother's serum.[20] This is achieved by active transport of amino acids through the syncytiotrophoblast epithelial cells. A number of studies have examined the biochemical characteristics of these amino acid transporters using vesicles made from the microvilli of the syncytiotrophoblast. These characteristics are identical to those of the proximal tubule and small intestine transport systems.[21,22] More recently, many of these transporters have been identified genetically.

The transporter B^0AT1 is highly expressed and appears to be the main transporter for neutral amino acid uptake into the placenta.[22] As with the renal and intestinal neutral amino acid transporter, it transports a very wide range of amino acids. It was cloned from a placental choriocarcinoma cell line almost 25 years ago.[23] The concentration of taurine is very high within the placenta, indicating a high activity for the β-amino acid transporter. Biochemical studies have demonstrated the transport characteristics in placental tissue.[22] The transporter has also been cloned from placental tissue.[24]

In addition to the transport of amino acids, the placenta has a high rate of metabolism of amino acids. There is evidence that many of the nonessential amino acids are synthesized within the placenta.[15,25,26] In addition, many of the amino acids undergo extensive metabolism in the liver of the fetus.[25]

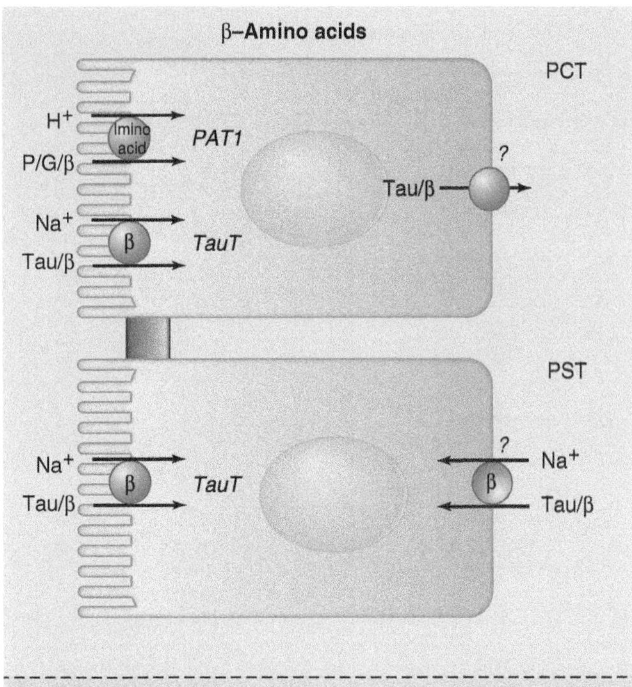

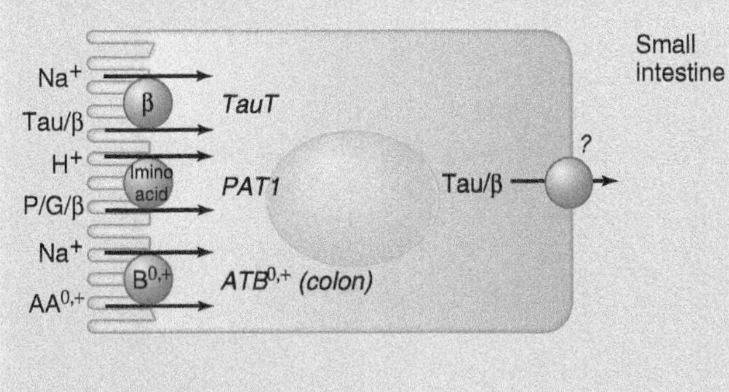

Fig. 100.6 Transporters involved in the absorption of taurine and β-amino acids. *AA*, Amino acid; *G*, glycine; *P*, proline; *PCT*, proximal convoluted tubule; *PST*, proximal straight tubule. (From Bröer S. Amino acid transport across mammalian intestinal and renal epithelia. *Physiol Rev.* 2008;88:249–286.)

The importance of the placenta in supplying the fetus with amino acids for substrates for protein synthesis is evident from the decreased transport of amino acids in the growth-restricted states of the fetus.[27-32] It is not clear if the cause of the growth restriction is due to the amino acid deficit or some other underlying factor that affects both the growth of the fetus and the function of the placenta. This has led to an understanding of the role that the placenta might play in chronic diseases of the fetus.[33] There are a number of reviews describing the changes that have occurred in the placental transport of amino acids in the setting of intrauterine growth retardation.[28,34,35] In addition, the growth of the neonate after birth has been shown to be critically linked to the administration of amino acids.[36,37]

RENAL HANDLING OF AMINO ACIDS

Amino acids are relatively small molecules that are freely filtered in the glomerulus. The mammalian kidney functions with a high glomerular filtration rate to excrete the nitrogenous waste products as urea. This results in a large amount of amino acids being filtered that could ultimately be excreted in the final urine. The proximal tubule is then responsible for reabsorbing almost the entire filtered load of amino acids to prevent losses. As discussed earlier, there are multiple active transport systems that reclaim the amino acids from the fluid in the lumen of the tubule and transport the amino acids back into the bloodstream.

In general, the early section of the proximal tubule, known as the *proximal convoluted tubule*, has high-capacity-low-affinity transport systems to reclaim the bulk of the filtered amino acids. Thus, as the tubular fluid travels through the proximal convoluted tubule, the concentrations of amino acids will decrease considerably. As the fluid enters the proximal straight tubule, more energy will be required to reclaim the small amounts of amino acids that remain in the fluid. Thus, these transport systems in the proximal straight tubule generally have higher affinities and require more energy for this transport to prevent any amino acids from being lost.

In addition to the transport of amino acids from the filtered fluid back into the bloodstream, the proximal tubule is also involved in ammoniagenesis (see reference 38 for review). This process involves the transport of glutamate and glutamine primarily from the bloodstream through the basolateral membrane of the proximal tubule. This is probably why the anionic amino acid transporter is located on the basolateral membrane and on the luminal membrane to ensure that there is an adequate supply of these amino acids for the production of ammonia. Deamination of glutamine to glutamate results in one molecule of ammonia that can be excreted into the tubule lumen. Another molecule of ammonia is generated when the glutamate is converted to α-ketoglutarate. Thus, it can be seen that there is considerable metabolism of amino acids within the proximal tubule.[38]

DEVELOPMENTAL CHANGES IN NEONATAL RENAL FUNCTION

The kidney in the fetus begins to function and make urine by the 10th week of gestation.[39] After the infant has been born, there are a number of developmental changes that occur during the first year of life. More importantly, if the neonate is born prematurely, many of these functions are not fully developed and result in excessive excretion of solutes such as glucose and some amino acids.

The glomerular filtration rate of the term normal newborn infant is approximately 30% of the normal adult rate, when factored for the body surface area.[39] During the first 12 to 18 months of life, this will increase to the adult rate. Because of the lower glomerular filtration rate, the quantity of amino acids that need be reabsorbed is actually much lower in the neonate than in the adult.

The proximal tubule also undergoes many developmental changes after the neonate is born. As outlined earlier, most of the transport in the proximal tubule is linked to the sodium-potassium ATPase. Several studies have shown that the activity of this enzyme is very low in the neonatal tubule and increases during the first month of life.[40,41] Furthermore, most of the other transport systems in the proximal tubule also undergo similar developmental changes. For example, the sodium-hydrogen exchanger has very low activity in the neonatal tubule, which explains the low rate of bicarbonate reabsorption. This is why most neonates and preterm neonates in particular have low serum bicarbonate concentrations. Glucose reabsorption is also low in preterm infants and can result in glucosuria in an otherwise healthy preterm infant.[42]

The primary function of the proximal tubule is to reabsorb approximately three fourths of the glomerular filtrate. The volume reabsorption rate of the proximal tubule undergoes a significant developmental increase during the first few months of life.[43] Thus, the ability to reabsorb amino acids will be affected by the rate of maturation of transport systems. The developmental change of specific amino acid transporters has been less well studied. We will now review the few specific amino acid transporters that have been studied.

It has been known for some time that neonates can have significant amounts of imino amino acids (proline and hydroxyproline) and glycine in their urine.[14] The specific amino acid transporters responsible for transport of these amino acids were first identified in patients who had mutations in these transporters; therefore these individuals lose those amino acids in their urine throughout their lifetime.[13] These are the transporters depicted in Fig. 100.5.

Developmental expression of these transporters was then examined in mice. As expected, the expression during the first 1 to 2 weeks of life was very low, leading to the excretion of proline, hydroxyproline, glycine, and leucine in the urine.[14] Thus this change in the delayed expression of these transporters explains the presence of these amino acids in the urine of many neonates.

Another system that has been studied extensively is the transporter for taurine. These studies examined the uptake of taurine in neonatal and adult rats and were primarily performed with brush-border vesicles that contain membranes from the lumen of the proximal tubule. Chesney and colleagues demonstrated a developmental increase in the ability to transport taurine.[44,45] This explained, to some degree, the finding of excess amounts of taurine in the urine of young rats. In addition, Friedman and colleagues identified both a high-affinity transport system and a low-affinity transport system.[46] Interestingly, they had to alter the diet of the mother that was feeding the young to bring out the different transport systems in the nursing offspring.[47]

In addition to the dependence of the taurine transporter on sodium and chloride, it has been demonstrated that there is an effect of the bilayer lipid membranes on the function of the transport process.[48] The fluidity of the lipid bilayer is highly dependent on the lipid composition of the membrane and can have multiple effects on the kinetics of membrane transporters. These studies showed that manipulation of the membrane fluidity by alteration of the sulfur content of the diet in experimental rats affected amino acid transport in the luminal membrane of the proximal tubule. Thus some of the changes in the transport rates might be intrinsic to the structure of the membrane and not just the expression of the specific transporters. This effect has also been seen in the water transport characteristics of the proximal tubule.[49]

CONCLUSION

The developing kidney in the fetus and neonate undergoes major change in the glomerular filtration rate as well as in the transport characteristics of the proximal tubule. These changes occur in concert with each other to help maintain appropriate concentrations of solute in the blood of the developing organism. There are changes in the expression of specific transporters and in basic membrane characteristics that regulate solute transport in the epithelia. The importance of these transporters is evident from the fact that mutations in many of these transporters result in significant disease processes. Understanding these changes can help explain many of the findings in neonates, in particular preterm neonates, which may be part of the physiologic developmental process.

SELECT REFERENCES

1. Broer S. Amino acid transport across mammalian intestinal and renal epithelia. *Physiol Rev*. 2008;88(1):249-286.
2. Broer S. Apical transporters for neutral amino acids: physiology and pathophysiology. *Physiology*. 2008;23:95-103.
3. Kleta R, Romeo E, Ristic Z, et al. Mutations in SLC6A19, encoding B0AT1, cause Hartnup disorder. *Nat Genet*. 2004;36(9):999-1002.
4. Seow HF, Bröer S, Bröer A, et al. Hartnup disorder is caused by mutations in the gene encoding the neutral amino acid transporter SLC6A19. *Nat Genet*. 2004;36(9):1003-1007.
5. Drummond KN, Michael AF, Ulstrom RA, Good RA. The blue diaper syndrome: familial hypercalcemia with nephrocalcinosis and indicanuria; a new familial disease, with definition of the metabolic abnormality. *Am J Med*. 1964;37:928-948.
6. Distelmaier F, Herebian D, Atasever C, et al. Blue diaper syndrome and PCSK1 mutations. *Pediatrics*. 2018;141(suppl 5):S501-S505.
7. Chillaron J, Estevez R, Mora C, et al. Obligatory amino acid exchange via systems bo,+-like and y+L-like. A tertiary active transport mechanism for renal reabsorption of cystine and dibasic amino acids. *J Biol Chem*. 1996;271(30):17761-17770.
8. Calonge MJ, Gasparini P, Chillarón J, et al. Cystinuria caused by mutations in rBAT, a gene involved in the transport of cystine. *Nat Genet*. 1994;6(4):420-425.
9. Dello Strologo L, Pras E, Pontesilli C, et al. Comparison between SLC3A1 and SLC7A9 cystinuria patients and carriers: a need for a new classification. *J Am Soc Nephrol*. 2002;13(10):2547-2553.
10. Perheentupa J, Visakorpi JK. Protein intolerance with deficient transport of basic amino acids. Another inborn error of metabolism. *Lancet*. 1965;2(7417):813-816.
11. Melancon SB, Dallaire L, Lemieux B, Robitaille P, Potier M. Dicarboxylic aminoaciduria: an inborn error of amino acid conservation. *J Pediatr*. 1977;91(3):422-427.
12. Swarna M, Rao DN, Reddy PP. Dicarboxylic aminoaciduria associated with mental retardation. *Hum Genet*. 1989;82(3):299-300.
13. Broer S, Bailey CG, Kowalczuk S, et al. Iminoglycinuria and hyperglycinuria are discrete human phenotypes resulting from complex mutations in proline and glycine transporters. *J Clin Invest*. 2008;118(12):3881-3892.
14. Vanslambrouck JM, Bröer A, Thavyogarajah T, et al. Renal imino acid and glycine transport system ontogeny and involvement in developmental iminoglycinuria. *Biochem J*. 2010;428(3):397-407.
15. Battaglia FC. In vivo characteristics of placental amino acid transport and metabolism in ovine pregnancy--a review. *Placenta*. 2002;23(Suppl):S3-8.
16. Regnault TR, de Vrijer B, Battaglia FC. Transport and metabolism of amino acids in placenta. *Endocrine*. 2002;19(1):23-41.
17. Cleal JK, Lewis RM. The mechanisms and regulation of placental amino acid transport to the human foetus. *J Neuroendocrinol*. 2008;20(4):419-426.
18. Grillo MA, Lanza A, Colombatto S. Transport of amino acids through the placenta and their role. *Amino Acids*. 2008;34(4):517-523.
19. Cleal JK, Lofthouse EM, Sengers BG, Lewis RM. A systems perspective on placental amino acid transport. *J Physiol*. 2018;596(23):5511-5522.
20. Philipps AF, Holzman IR, Teng C, Battaglia FC. Tissue concentrations of free amino acids in term human placentas. *Am J Obstet Gynecol*. 1978;131(8):881-887.
21. Moe AJ. Placental amino acid transport. *Am J Physiol*. 1995;268(6 Pt 1):C1321-C1331.
22. Jansson T. Amino acid transporters in the human placenta. *Pediatr Res*. 2001;49(2):141-147.
23. Kekuda R, Prasad PD, Fei YJ, et al. Cloning of the sodium-dependent, broad-scope, neutral amino acid transporter Bo from a human placental choriocarcinoma cell line. *J Biol Chem*. 1996;271(31):18657-18661.
24. Ramamoorthy S, Leibach FH, Mahesh VB, et al. Functional characterization and chromosomal localization of a cloned taurine transporter from human placenta. *Biochem J*. 1994;300(Pt 3):893-900.
25. Cetin I. Amino acid interconversions in the fetal-placental unit: the animal model and human studies in vivo. *Pediatr Res*. 2001;49(2):148-154.
26. Battaglia FC, Regnault TR. Placental transport and metabolism of amino acids. *Placenta*. 2001;22(2-3):145-161.
27. Cetin I. Placental transport of amino acids in normal and growth-restricted pregnancies. *Eur J Obstet Gynecol Reprod Biol*. 2003;110(suppl 1):S50-S54.
28. Avagliano L, Garo C, Marconi AM. Placental amino acids transport in intrauterine growth restriction. *J Pregnancy*. 2012;2012:972562.
29. Galan HL, Marconi AM, Paolini CL, Cheung A, Battaglia FC. The transplacental transport of essential amino acids in uncomplicated human pregnancies. *Am J Obstet Gynecol*. 2009;200(1):e1-7. 91.
30. Marconi AM, Paolini CL. Nutrient transport across the intrauterine growth-restricted placenta. *Semin Perinatol*. 2008;32(3):178-181.
31. Marconi AM, Paolini CL, Stramare L, et al. Steady state maternal-fetal leucine enrichments in normal and intrauterine growth-restricted pregnancies. *Pediatr Res*. 1999;46(1):114-119.
32. Paolini CL, Marconi AM, Ronzoni S, et al. Placental transport of leucine, phenylalanine, glycine, and proline in intrauterine growth-restricted pregnancies. *J Clin Endocrinol Metab*. 2001;86(11):5427-5432.
33. Burton GJ, Fowden AL, Thornburg KL. Placental origins of chronic disease. *Physiol Rev*. 2016;96(4):1509-1565.
34. Pardi G, Marconi AM, Cetin I. Placental-fetal interrelationship in IUGR fetuses--a review. *Placenta*. 2002;23(suppl A):S136-S141.
35. Regnault TR, Friedman JE, Wilkening RB, Anthony RV, Hay Jr WW. Fetoplacental transport and utilization of amino acids in IUGR--a review. *Placenta*. 2005;26(suppl A):S52-S62.
36. Hay Jr WW, Thureen PJ. Early postnatal administration of intravenous amino acids to preterm, extremely low birth weight infants. *J Pediatr*. 2006;148(3):291-294.
37. Poindexter BB, Langer JC, Dusick AM, et al. Early provision of parenteral amino acids in extremely low birth weight infants: relation to growth and neurodevelopmental outcome. *J Pediatr*. 2006;148(3):300-305.
38. Weiner ID, Mitch WE, Sands JM. Urea and ammonia metabolism and the control of renal nitrogen excretion. *Clin J Am Soc Nephrol*. 2015;10(8):1444-1458.
39. Quigley R. Developmental changes in renal function. *Curr Opin Pediatr*. 2012;24(2):184-190.
40. Fukuda Y, Bertorello A, Aperia A. Ontogeny of the regulation of Na+,K(+)-ATPase activity in the renal proximal tubule cell. *Pediatr Res*. 1991;30(2):131-134.
41. Schwartz GJ, Evan AP. Development of solute transport in rabbit proximal tubule. III. Na-K-ATPase activity. *Am J Physiol*. 1984;246(6 Pt 2):F845-F852.
42. Wilkins BH. Renal function in sick very low birthweight infants: 4. Glucose excretion. *Arch Dis Child*. 1992;67(spec no 10):1162-1165.

43. Gattineni J, Baum M. Developmental changes in renal tubular transport-an overview. *Pediatr Nephrol*. 2015;30(12):2085–2098.
44. Chesney RW, Jax DK. Developmental aspects of renal beta-amino acid transport I. Ontogeny of taurine reabsorption and accumulation in rat renal cortex. *Pediatr Res*. 1979;13(7):854–860.
45. Chesney RW, Zelikovic I, Friedman AL, et al. Renal taurine transport--recent developments. *Adv Exp Med Biol*. 1987;217:49–59.
46. Friedman AL, Jax DK, Chesney RW. Developmental aspects of renal beta-amino acid transport. III. Ontogeny of transport in isolated renal tubule segments. *Pediatr Res*. 1981;15(1):10–13.
47. Friedman AL, Albright PW, Gusowski N, Padilla M, Chesney RW. Renal adaptation to alteration in dietary amino acid intake. *Am J Physiol*. 1983;245(2):F159–F166.
48. Chesney RW, Gusowski N, Zelikovic I. Developmental aspects of renal beta-amino acid transport. VI. The role of membrane fluidity and phospholipid composition in the renal adaptive response in nursing animals. *Pediatr Res*. 1987;22(2):163–167.
49. Quigley R, Mulder J, Baum M. Ontogeny of water transport in the rabbit proximal tubule. *Pediatr Nephrol*. 2003;18(11):1089–1094.

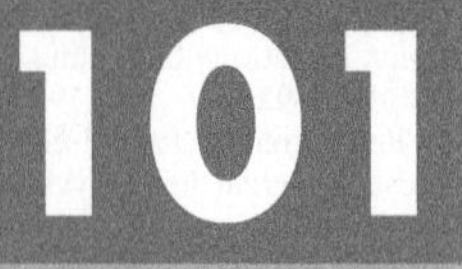

Organic Anion Transport in the Developing Kidney

Sun-Young Ahn | Jeremiah D. Momper | Sanjay K. Nigam

INTRODUCTION

Rapid and complex changes in physiology occur when the fetus transitions from an intrauterine to an extrauterine environment. From dependency on the maternal circulation via the placenta for nutrition, oxygen, and waste excretion, the infant shifts to reliance on its own organ systems for vital functions. These organ systems include the pulmonary system for oxygen and carbon dioxide exchange, the cardiovascular system for blood circulation, the gastrointestinal system for food absorption, and the renal system for waste excretion, fluid, and acid-base balance.[1]

The kidneys and the tubular transporters, in particular, play an important role in maintaining the chemical homeostasis within the body as the infant adapts to its rapidly changing environment. The transporters involved include the solute carrier (SLC) and ATP-binding cassette (ABC) family of transporters. A major subfamily of the SLC family of transporters is the organic anion transporters (OATs), multispecific transporters located in the proximal tubule that mediate the secretion and absorption of a wide array of endogenous solutes and drugs including diuretics, methotrexate, β-lactam and sulfonamide antibiotics, nonsteroidal antiinflammatory drugs (NSAIDs), angiotensin-converting enzyme (ACE) inhibitors, and antiviral drugs.[2–4] The OATs, especially OAT3, also transport glucuronides and sulfate esters, phase II reaction products, and therefore may play an essential role in elimination of toxic organic anions in the infant.[5] Members of the OAT family share structural similarities, including a putative 12 transmembrane helical domain, with an extracellular loop containing N-linked glycosylation sites between helices 1 and 2, and an intracellular loop containing protein kinase C (PKC) phosphorylation sites between helices 6 and 7.[6,7] Probably the most studied OATs are OAT1, the prototypical OAT originally identified as NKT,[8] and OAT3, which are located on the basolateral membrane of the proximal tubule where they function via a tertiary transport system.[2,9] This transport system begins with the Na^+ gradient generated by the Na^+/K^+-ATPase, which drives the sodium-dicarboxylate co-transporter (NaDC3) to transport Na^+ and dicarboxylates, including α-ketoglutarate, into the cell. The resulting high intracellular concentration of dicarboxylates then drives the outward movement of dicarboxylates and the inward movement of organic anions, an exchange mediated by the OATs (Fig. 101.1).[7]

Several studies have shown time-dependent expression patterns in the OATs and ABC transporters with kidney development, and these expression patterns appear to be affected by gender and transcriptional and posttranscriptional regulation.[9] The difference in expression patterns of OATs in the infant likely contributes to the differences in drug pharmacokinetics and therapeutic efficiency observed in children compared to adults, and emphasizes the importance of special consideration in drug dosing for pediatric patients. Furthermore, the immaturity of the transport system[10] can render the newborn more vulnerable to drug overdosing and to environmental stressors such as ischemia.

AGE-DEPENDENT EXPRESSION AND ACTIVITY OF RENAL OATS IN RODENT AND MAMMALIAN MODELS

Several studies have described the temporal expression patterns of the SLC and ABC transporter families in the mammalian kidney. Initial studies investigated the transport of p-aminohippurate (PAH), the prototypical substrate for OAT1, in mammalian models, and reported rapid increases in renal PAH transport activity within the first few weeks of life in rabbit kidney slices[11] and within the first few days after birth in newborn sheep.[12] Transcript analysis and live in vitro influx/efflux assays showed that OAT1 and OAT3 expression begins as early as embryonic(e) day 10.5 in the murine mesonephros.[13] These findings suggest that the mammalian mesonephros, a transient renal structure, can play an important role in the excretion of products in conjunction with the placenta in the developing embryo.[13] The expression of *Oat1* mRNA levels was detected on embryonic day 18 in the fetal rat kidney, with levels remaining low prenatally and dramatically increasing on the day of birth until postnatal day 2. The expression levels from postnatal days 1 and 2 were equivalent to adult rat expression levels.[14] Other studies have shown that *Oat1* mRNA levels increased gradually until 30 days of age, at which point they reached adult levels.[15]

Rat *Oat2* and *Oat3* mRNA levels were also shown to be low at birth. *Oat2* expression remained low until 30 days of age and increased from day 35 to 45 in only female rats and not male rats. An increase in *Oat3* expression occurred earlier compared to the other *Oats*, with mRNA levels increasing significantly during the first 10 days of life.[15] In the mouse, *Oat1* mRNA transcripts were first detected by in situ hybridization in the proximal tubules at e14, with expression levels increasing throughout the rest of gestation and into adulthood.[16] Organic cation transporter 1 (*Oct1*) expression was first detected in the mouse kidney between e15 and e16, and was found to increase postnatally until adult levels. *Oat2* mRNA levels were detected by in situ hybridization at e14 in the murine kidney, and these levels also increased postnatally.[16] Sweeney and colleagues performed time-series microarray experiments and found a

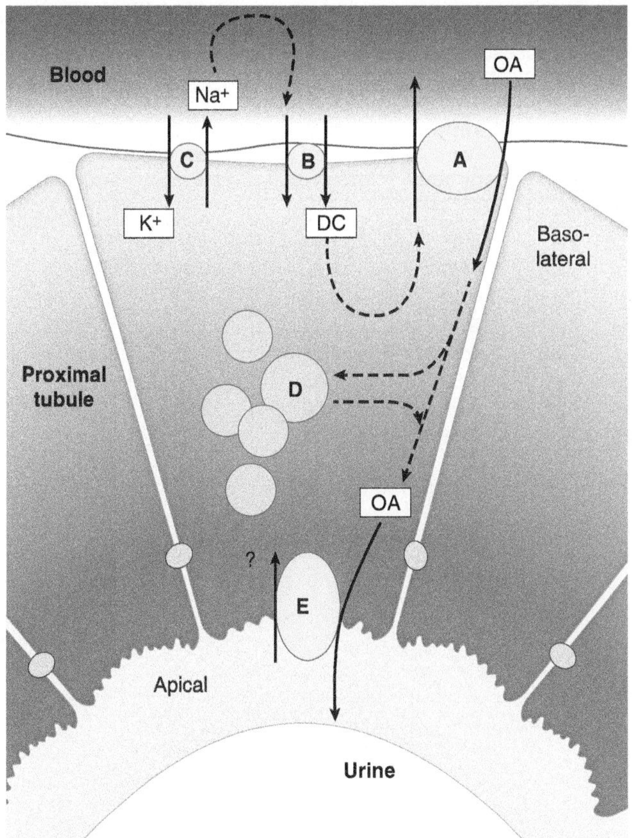

Fig. 101.1 Transport of organic anions in the renal proximal tubule. OAT1 and OAT3 *(A)* transport organic anions *(OA)* in exchange for dicarboxylates *(DC)* at the basolateral membrane. The Na^+/dicarboxylate co-transporter *(B)* accumulates dicarboxylates intracellularly through the Na^+ gradient generated by the Na^+/K^+ ATPase *(C)*. The organic anions may be concentrated in cytoplasmic vesicles *(D)*. The OA exits on the apical side *(E)* into the luminal urinary space. (From Eraly SA, Bush KT, Sampogna RV, et al. The molecular pharmacology of organic anion transporters: from DNA to FDA? *Mol Pharmacol.* 2004;65:479–487.)

twofold or greater increase in mRNA expression between two temporally consecutive stages of kidney development in Slc22 transporters, including *Oat1, 2, 3,* and *5*; *Oct1, 2*; *Octn1*; *Octn2*; and *Rst* (the murine URAT1 ortholog).[17] Interestingly, the largest increase in expression occurred between the postnatal stage (birth to week 1) and the mature stage (week 4 to adult) (Fig. 101.2). Furthermore, an increase in the expression of ABC transporters with renal development was also observed, again with the largest increase occurring between the postnatal and mature stage of kidney development (Fig. 101.3).[17] Using the GUDMAP consortium microarray datasets, the expression of six transporters including *Oat1*, *Oat3*, *Oct 1 Oct 2 Mate 1* and *Pept 2* were found to be increased at least twofold compared to other structures in the developing proximal tubules at e15.5.[17] These findings suggest that drug transport may occur as early as e15.5 and that the transporters already have a distinct localization in the nephron at this early stage.[17]

The up-regulation of the transporters studied correlated with an increase in PAH clearance observed in vivo during 1, 2, and 3 weeks of age and in the mature stages, supporting the finding that although the transporters are present and functional at an early age, they do not possess full activity until later in age.[17] Clearance of PAH was also investigated in *Oat1* and *Oat3* knockouts at 2 weeks of age, and confirmed that, as in the adult kidney, OAT1 is the main transporter of PAH in the postnatal kidney.[17]

Further localization of OAT1 and OAT3 expression was also described by immunohistochemical analysis of murine kidneys.[18] OAT1 immunoreactivity was noted at e15 in the proximal tubules of mice and in the outer cortex 7 days postnatally. OAT3 was found to be expressed in the distal tubule of e14 mice and in the S2 segment of the proximal tubule of e16 mice. At the time of birth, expression of OAT3 shifted to the S1 and S3 segments.

EXPRESSION AND ACTIVITY OF OATS IN THE DEVELOPING HUMAN KIDNEY AND COMPARISON WITH ANIMAL MODELS

Relatively sparse data are available on the ontogeny of OATs in humans. Cheung and colleagues evaluated the mRNA expression and protein abundance of OAT1 and OAT3 in 184 human postmortem kidney cortical samples ranging from newborns to adults.[19] Protein abundance levels of OAT1 and OAT3 were significantly lower in newborn and infants as compared with older age groups. Further, mRNA expression of these transporters as a function of age was highly correlated. The postnatal age at which half of the adult expression was reached (TM_{50}) was 19.71 weeks for OAT1 and 30.7 weeks for OAT3.[19]

As with rodents, an up-regulation of renal OAT expression with developmental time is accompanied by an increase in OAT functional activity. A recent reanalysis of data pooled from multiple older physiologic studies of PAH provides a quantitative description of OAT-mediated tubular secretion across the pediatric age continuum.[20] The maximum tubular secretory capacity of PAH (Tm_{PAH}) — representing the difference between the total rate of excretion and the quantity filtered by the glomeruli which is primarily attributable to OAT activity — increases markedly after birth reflective of increased OAT expression and/or function. Tm_{PAH} reaches 50% of the adult value (80 mg/min) at 8.3 years of age. In addition, during the first 2 years of life, Tm_{PAH} is lower than that of GFR when viewed as the fraction of the adult value, indicating that the acquisition of filtration and secretion do not occur at identical rates.

In addition to studies with PAH, the pharmacokinetics of OAT 1/3 drug substrates may be leveraged to evaluate developmental aspects of anionic transport function in humans. Tenofovir, an antiviral agent indicated for the treatment of HIV-1 infection and chronic hepatitis B, is a suitable surrogate for organic anion transport capacity. Tenofovir is not metabolized by hepatic CYP enzymes and is renally eliminated by glomerular filtration and tubular secretion with 70% to 80% of the administered dose recovered in urine. The renal clearance of tenofovir is two to three times the creatinine clearance, demonstrating tubular secretion. Tenofovir tubular secretion involves basolateral uptake by OAT1 and apical efflux out into urine by multidrug resistance protein 4 (MRP4).[21] In HIV-infected pediatric patients between 8 and 17 years of age, the BSA-normalized renal clearance of tenofovir is similar to that observed in adults.[22] These findings support the view that OAT1 expression and activity reaches adult levels by at least middle childhood.

Overall, the general pattern of renal OAT1 expression and activity (i.e., PAH clearance) is largely concordant between humans and rodents, particularly when rodent age and human age are related in terms of fraction of their respective adult ages. In both rodents and humans, an up-regulation of OAT1 expression with developmental time is accompanied by an increase in the clearance of PAH. In mice, when age is 30% and 40% of adult age (i.e., 3 and 4 weeks), renal Slc22a6 mRNA expression and PAH clearance are 73% and 42% of adult values, respectively.[17] Comparable values are seen in humans. For example, when human age is 30% of adult (i.e., 5.4 years), renal OAT1 protein expression and PAH clearance are 76% and 40% of adult values, respectively.[19,20] These similar results provide confidence that

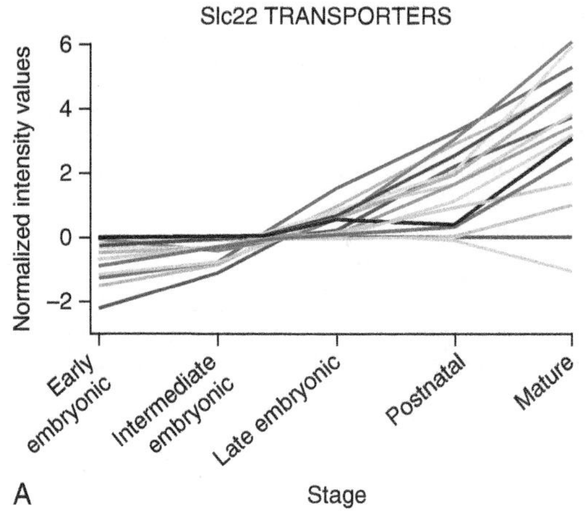

Gene Symbol	Title	Interm emb vs. Early emb	Late emb vs. Interm emb	Postnatal vs. Late emb	Mature vs. Postnatal
Slc22 transporters regulated at least two-fold in at least one pair between consecutive stages of kidney development					
		Fold change between consecutive stages			
Slc22a2	Oct2	1.00	2.20	2.41	14.33
Slc22a12	Rst	1.51	1.84	5.53	7.98
Slc22a9	Oat5	1.30	2.50	0.92	6.20
Slc22a1	Oct1	0.92	2.10	3.67	4.78
Slc22a6	Oat1	2.14	3.84	1.70	4.59
Slc22a7	Oat2	0.98	1.01	1.32	4.35
Slc22a8	Oat3	1.53	3.63	3.80	3.44
Slc22a4	Octn1	1.21	1.08	2.94	3.43
Slc22a5	Octn2	1.16	1.37	4.07	2.87

B

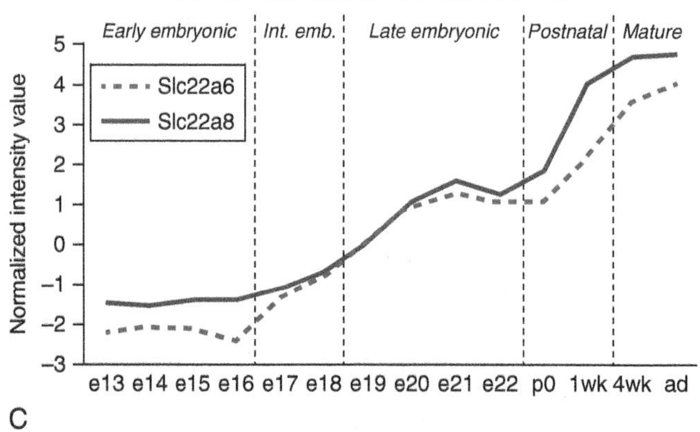

Fig. 101.2 Increase in mRNA expression of most SLC22 transporters during kidney development. (A) Large increase in expression of certain Slc22 (organic anion transporter [Oat]) transporters was observed in the postnatal to mature stage. (B) Fold change in expression of certain Slc22 genes between consecutive stages of kidney development. The shaded cells indicate the stage comparison that demonstrates the largest change in expression. *Early emb*, early embryonic stage; *interm emb*, intermediate embryonic stage; *late emb*, late embryonic stage. (C) Increase in expression of Slc22a6 *(broken line)* and Slc22a8 *(solid line)* from e13 to adulthood. (From Sweeney DE, Vallon V, Rieg T, et al. Functional maturation of drug transporters in the developing, neonatal, and postnatal kidney. *Mol Pharmacol.* 2011;80:147–154.)

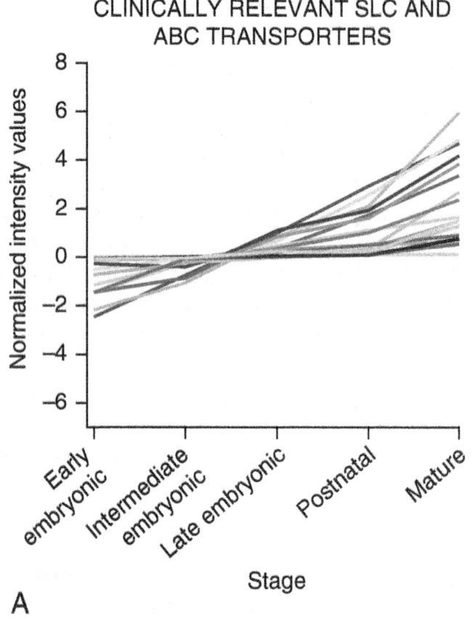

Gene Symbol	Title	Interm emb vs. Early emb	Late emb vs. Interm emb	Postnatal vs. Late emb	Mature vs. Postnatal
		Fold change between consecutive stages			
Slc22a2	Oct2	1.00	2.20	2.41	14.33
Slc15a2	Pept2	2.56	1.218	1.12	5.06
Slc47a1	MATE1	3.23	3.67	1.74	4.86
Slc22a1	Oct1	0.92	2.10	3.67	4.78
Slc22a6	Oat1	2.14	3.84	1.70	4.59
Slc22a8	Oat3	1.53	3.63	3.80	3.44
Abcg2	Bcrp	1.33	1.42	2.50	3.16
Abcb1a	Mdr1a/P-gp	1.00	1.06	1.08	2.59
Abcc4	Mrp4	1.89	1.57	1.54	2.53
Abcc2	Mrp2	1.03	1.06	1.29	2.21
Abcb1b	Mdr1/Pgy1	0.96	0.96	1.24	2.11

B

Fig. 101.3 Increase in expression of clinically relevant SLC and ABC transporters through kidney development. (A) The expression of clinically relevant SLC and ABC transporters[85] during kidney development was observed. (B) Fold change in expression of clinically relevant transporters between consecutive stages of kidney development. The shaded cells indicate the stage comparison with the largest change in expression. *ABC*, ATP-binding cassette; *early emb*, early embryonic stage; *interm emb*, intermediate embryonic stage; *late emb*, late embryonic stage. *SLC*, solute carrier. (From Sweeney DE, Vallon V, Rieg T, et al. Functional maturation of drug transporters in the developing, neonatal, and postnatal kidney. *Mol Pharmacol.* 2011;80:147–154.)

rodent studies aimed at characterizing the regulation of OAT1 expression and function during postnatal renal development can be useful for understanding these processes in humans.

REGULATION OF OAT EXPRESSION DURING KIDNEY DEVELOPMENT

The regulatory mechanisms controlling levels of OAT expression during kidney development remain unclear. Several factors, including hormones, transcriptional and posttranscriptional changes, and substrates may influence the expression of OATs, and these factors may come into play at different stages of kidney development to induce the upregulation or downregulation of OAT expression. Consistent with this is the upsurge in the levels of thyroid hormones, catecholamines, and glucocorticoids at birth, which may be responsible for the changes in OAT expression observed.[23,24] These factors will be briefly reviewed here.

HORMONAL REGULATION OF OAT EXPRESSION

OAT expression is under the regulation of various hormones, including thyroid hormones, sex steroid hormones, and catecholamines.[25] Renal excretion of PAH was found to be increased with triiodothyronine (T3) and tetraiodothyronine (T4) pretreatment[26] in rats starting on the second day after birth; furthermore, treatment with these thyroid hormones appeared to be more effective in increasing PAH accumulation in kidney cortical slices from young compared to adult rats.[27]

The effect of sex steroid hormones on OAT expression has been studied extensively,[28-30] and the gender-dependent expression of the OATs is well-established. Female rats were shown to have a longer elimination half-time for PAH than male rats, a difference that was overcome with testosterone treatment.[31] PAH transport was also found to be higher in intact male rat kidney cortical slices than in those of orchiectomized male rats, supporting the effect of androgens.[31] These differences appeared to be due to a lower number of functional transporters, rather than transporting capacity, in the orchiectomized rats compared to the intact rats. At the transcriptional level, *Oat1* mRNA expression in the kidney was found to be higher in murine males compared to females.[28] Differences in expression levels through development were also found between male and female mice. *Oat1* mRNA levels decreased slightly until 10 days of age, after which they reached a plateau, and began to rise between 25 and 30 days of age, until 40 days of age in male mice. Female levels of *Oat1* mRNA, on the other hand, remained relatively unchanged.[28]

Male *Oat2* mRNA levels also increased at higher rates compared to female mice by 40 days of age.[28] These findings, however, were seemingly contradictory to results of studies showing increased protein levels of OAT2 in female compared to male mice, which suggest possible gender-dependent posttranscriptional modifications in mice.[32] Estradiol and progesterone weakly stimulated OAT2 protein expression, while androgens inhibited expression. *Oat5* mRNA and protein expression were also found to be higher in postpubertal female compared to male rats.[33] In castrated males, mRNA expression was increased, an effect that was reduced by testosterone and increased by estradiol and progesterone treatment. These findings also correlated with findings in mice.[33] Progesterone was also found to suppress human OAT4 cell surface expression.[34]

The expression of OATPs is also under the regulation of sex hormones. *Oatp1* mRNA expression was found to be lower in female than in male rats, and castration of male rats resulted in decreased OATP1 expression.[35] In agreement with these observations, treatment of female rats with testosterone increased, while the treatment of male rats with estradiol decreased the level of kidney *Oatp1* mRNA.[35]

Glucocorticoids, such as prednisolone and dexamethasone, have been shown to increase PAH excretion and PAH accumulation in renal cortical slices from 5- and 10-day old rats with immature kidney function.[36] Dexamethasone increased the excretion of PAH in a dose-dependent manner in immature rats, whereas it did not increase PAH excretion in adult rats.[37] Furthermore, T3 acted synergistically with dexamethasone to increase the renal tubular transport of PAH.[38]

Catecholamines have also been shown to regulate the activity of organic anion transport. Jensen et al. have shown that epinephrine and norepinephrine, possibly via the modulation of Na^+-K^+-ATPase activity, stimulated the uptake of PAH in rat proximal tubular basolateral membrane vesicles, an effect that was inhibited by yohimbine (an alpha-2 adrenergic antagonist) and phentolamine.[39]

TRANSCRIPTIONAL AND POSTTRANSCRIPTIONAL REGULATION OF OAT EXPRESSION

The various hormonal, morphogenetic, and environmental factors discussed above most probably act through transcriptional, translational, and posttranslational mechanisms to affect OAT expression and function. This is partly supported by the observation that several conserved binding sites for transcription factors important in kidney development, such as Pbx, Tcf, Wt-1, Pax1, and hepatocyte nuclear factor (HNF-1), are present in the promoter regions of murine and human *OAT1* and *3* genes.[40-42] As discussed earlier, OAT1, 2, and 3 expression is first noted at e14 to e15 in mice, which is approximately similar to the time that proximal tubule differentiation occurs. It is therefore possible that the transcription factors that regulate kidney development may also simultaneously coordinate the activation of OAT expression. HNF1, for example, also regulates the transcription of type II sodium-glucose co-transporter (SGLT2)[43] and sodium/phosphate co-transporters,[44,45] which supports its potential role in proximal tubule function maturation. Motif analysis of enhancer elements in the rat kidney cortex identified HNF-4α and HNF-1α as the major transcriptional regulators of drug-metabolizing enzymes and transporters in the proximal tubule.[46]

Subsequent investigations have established the regulation of *Oat1, 2, 3, 5, 7* and *Urat1* promoter activities by HNF isoforms. Significant downregulation of *Oat1*, *Oat2*, and *Oat3* mRNA expression was found in kidneys of HNF-1α-null mice compared to wildtype,[47] and transactivation assays demonstrated that HNF-1α/β enhanced the activity of human and mouse *Oat1* promoters.[48] These findings were consistent with ensuing studies that showed human and mouse *Oat1* promoter activation with forced expression of HNF-1α alone or both HNF-1α and HNF-1β. In vitro studies further confirmed direct binding of the HNF-1α/HNF-1α homodimer and the HNF-1α/HNF-1β heterodimer to a HNF-1 motif in the human *OAT1* promoter.[48]

Similarly, the HNF-1α/HNF-1α homodimer and the HNF-1α/HNF-1β heterodimer stimulated *hOAT3* promoter activity in human embryonic kidney (HEK) 293 cells, while DNA methylation repressed the promoter activity.[49] This regulatory mechanism was also observed for the mouse/human URAT1 promoter, which was found to be activated by the HNF-1α/HNF-1β heterodimer and repressed by DNA methylation.[50] More recently, HNF-1α has also been shown to increase the promoter activities of human *OAT5* and *OAT7*, whereas knockdown of HNF-1α using short interfering RNAs decreased *OAT5* and *OAT7* mRNA expression.[51]

Another HNF isoform, HNF-4α has also been implicated in enhancing *hOAT1* promoter activity.[52] HNF-4α appears to interact with the *OAT1* promoter through regions encompassing -1191 to -700 base pairs and -140 to -79 base pairs. These areas contained a consensus sequence with a direct repeat separated by two nucleotides and a novel response element consisting of an inverted repeat of hexamers separated by eight nucleotides (IR-8).[52]

OAT expression is also under the control of proteins such as caveolins and PDZ proteins.[53] PDZ proteins bind to PDZ consensus binding sites at the carboxyl-terminus of transporters and target them to the plasma membrane, where they also are involved in their retention and regulation.[54] The PDZ domain-containing proteins, PDZK1 and NHERF1, have been shown to interact with hOAT4, increasing its expression at the apical membrane and also transport of estrone-3-sulfate in HEK293 cells.[55] PDZK1 was also demonstrated to interact with URAT1 through yeast two-hybrid assays; when transfected into HEK293 cells, PDZK1 increased the surface expression and transport activity of URAT1.[56]

Other proteins that have been implicated in the regulation of OAT expression include prostaglandin E_2 (PGE2), epidermal growth factor (EGF) and its receptor, the MAP kinase pathway, protein kinase A, serine/threonine phosphatases, PKC, phosphatidylinositol 3-kinase, tyrosine kinase, and the angiotensin-1 receptor.[25,57] Among these proteins, EGF was shown to increase basolateral PAH uptake in opossum kidney and rabbit proximal tubule cells through generation of PGE2 via arachidonic acid, MAP kinase, COX1, and phospholipase A2 (PLA_2).[58,59] PGE2 expression, in turn, has been shown to be stimulated by thyroid hormones in the late gestational fetal sheep kidney, which supports the possibility of hormonal regulation of OAT1 expression through a PGE2 mediated pathway during kidney development.[60]

SUBSTRATES AFFECTING OAT EXPRESSION

With the dramatic environmental changes that occur after birth, the kidney is suddenly exposed to a host of xenobiotics and endogenous factors that can account for the marked increase in OAT expression observed after birth. This is consistent with several studies that have shown that OAT expression can be induced by the substrates themselves, especially in the postnatal period. Endogenous substrates such as folic acid have been shown to stimulate PAH transport in the kidney.[61] Penicillin also stimulated the maturation of the renal organic acid transport system, resulting in increased PAH clearance, in newborn rabbits and dogs.[11,62,63] These findings were supported by a subsequent study that similarly showed an increase in PAH transport after penicillin pretreatment in immature rats.[64] Inulin clearance, on the other hand, did not increase in these rats, suggesting that the increase in PAH transport observed was not due to an increase in glomerular filtration, but to an increase in OAT expression or function. Further evidence for the increase in PAH clearance being due to increase in OAT expression was the observation that cycloheximide, an inhibitor of protein synthesis, blocked the increase in PAH uptake in renal cortical slices induced by penicillin.[65] Interestingly, pretreatment of 2-week-old rabbits with penicillin increased PAH transport, whereas it did not in 4-week-old rabbits, indicating an important role for drug modulation of OAT expression in the developing kidney.[63]

Other drugs that have been shown to upregulate the expression of OATs include diuretics. Previous in vivo and in vitro studies have demonstrated that both OAT1 and OAT3 contribute to the renal secretion of furosemide (loop diuretic) and bendroflumethiazide (thiazide diuretic)[66] in mice. In rats administered furosemide and hydrochlorothiazide for 7 days subcutaneously, the levels of OAT1 protein increased significantly in renal cortical homogenates. More importantly, no change in body weight and creatinine clearance was observed, indicating that chronic furosemide or hydrochlorothiazide infusion upregulated OAT1 expression.[67] These have significant implications for pharmacokinetics in the pediatric patient, and especially neonates in the neonatal intensive care unit, who are chronically exposed to diuretics. The increase in OAT1 expression resulting from diuretic administration may affect the clearance of and hence the response to other drugs that are being administered concomitantly, special factors that need to be taken into consideration.

STRUCTURAL AND ENVIRONMENTAL CHANGES AFFECTING OAT EXPRESSION

The significant increases in OAT expression and function that are generally observed postnatally in the rodent models could be explained by the growth of new nephrons and the maturation of the different segments of the proximal tubule. In the mouse, nephrogenesis continues until approximately postnatal days 7 to 10, while in humans, kidney development reaches completion at around 34 weeks' gestation.[17] In rabbits, the S1, S2, and S3 segments of the proximal tubule show a progressive increase in length, with all segments of the outer cortical tubules becoming fully developed at postnatal day 40.[68] The formation of new nephrons and the lengthening of the proximal tubules can contribute to the increase in OAT-mediated transport observed postnatally. A study done on rabbit proximal straight tubules showed, however, that the majority of the increase in absolute PAH transport observed with age was due to an increase in the intrinsic transport capacity, with 33% of the transport due to tubular elongation.[69,70]

The newborn or child can be exposed to numerous environmental stressors such as ischemic insults during delivery or sepsis. These stressors can result in altered levels of OAT expression in kidneys that can significantly change the patient's metabolism and response to drugs. In rat models of ischemia/reperfusion injury, a decreased transcriptional expression of *Oat1* and *Oat3*, together with a decrease in OAT1 and OAT3 protein levels, was reported. These changes corresponded with a reduction in PAH clearance.[71-73] Furthermore, lipopolysaccharide (endotoxin) induced a dose-dependent decrease in OAT1 and OAT3 expression in the renal cortex of rats.[74] This was also followed by reduced PAH clearance. Interestingly, increased cyclooxygenase-2 (COX-2) and PGE_2 expression was observed with the decrease in OAT1 and OAT3 expression, indicating that the downregulation in OAT expression may be mediated by prostaglandins generated from COX-2. Parecoxib, a COX-2 inhibitor, mitigated the downregulation of OAT1 and OAT3 induced by endotoxemia.[74] Similarly, indomethacin, a COX inhibitor, has been reported to prevent the downregulation of OAT1 and OAT3 expression seen during ischemic acute kidney injury.[75] These findings suggest a possible protective role for inhibitors of prostaglandin synthesis in ischemia or sepsis-induced downregulation of OATs, which may have important applications in the clinical setting for pediatric patients exposed to these environmental insults. Furthermore, consideration should be given to the possibility that different pathophysiologic states (e.g., diabetic ketoacidosis) can lead to changes in the body fluid pH, which in turn could lead to alterations in the charges of drugs and endogenous metabolites, such that although they do not bind OATs under normal physiologic conditions, they could interact with and modify the expression of OATs in diseased states.[76]

CONNECTIONS BETWEEN OATS AND EXTRA-RENAL METABOLIC ENZYMES: THE REMOTE SENSING AND SIGNALING THEORY

Proximal tubule transporters have overlapping substrate specificity with extra-renal drug metabolizing enzymes (DMEs)— which are particularly well-expressed in the liver and intestine—including several physiologically relevant metabolites and signaling molecules such as bile acids, uric acid, eicosanoids, fatty acids, uremic toxins, and gut microbiome products.[77,78] Hepatic and intestinal enzymes have unique patterns of expression during development with significant maturation occurring during the first few years of life, generally similar to what is known about renal OATs.[79-83] During the birth transition—a period during which multiple organs must communicate remotely to maintain homeostasis and respond to the requirements of tissue growth and maturation—OATs and DMEs may be involved in crosstalk via small molecule signaling and remote organ sensing (i.e., the mutual sensing of the transport capacity and types of substrates by the kidney, liver, intestine, and other organs).

How metabolism and transport in different organs is orchestrated to achieve homeostasis of small molecules during development is not well understood, yet must depend upon constant feedback during this particularly dynamic period of life. The Remote Sensing and Signaling Theory attempts to explain how this "remote interorgan and inter-organismal communication" might occur in the context of the need to optimize organ and systemic homeostasis of small molecules transported by OATs and other transporters with postnatal organ maturation being one important context.[2,9,84] Such a coordinated DME and transporter network—functioning to optimize metabolites (e.g., uric acid, carnitine) and signaling molecules (e.g., α-ketoglutarate, β-hydroxybutyrate, short chain fatty acids, bile acids) at the cellular, organ, and system levels—must be closely linked to classical homeostatic systems such as the neuroendocrine system, the growth factor-cytokine system, and autonomic nervous system.[77]

Coordination of DME and transporter activity would be especially important in the immediate postnatal period when defects could lead to disease or death. Different points during postnatal development (e.g., infancy vs. the late juvenile period) would also require the system to optimize for entirely different sets of small molecules. Furthermore, individual organs such as the liver and kidney may need to optimize for entirely different small molecules (compared to the whole system), depending on organ functional requirements at that point in development. Finally, the optimal degree of inter-organ communication (e.g., gut-liver-kidney) and, indeed, inter-organismal (e.g., gut microbiome) communication is likely to change during postnatal development (as will the microbiome itself).

CONCLUSION

Recent studies have provided some insight into the developmental changes in the expression and function of the OATs in the maturing kidney. OAT expression generally increases in an age-dependent manner, correlating with an increase in transport function. OAT expression and function have been shown to be under the control of many regulatory mechanisms; however, further investigations are required to elucidate the precise manner by which these regulatory mechanisms come into play during the different developmental stages of the kidney. Much remains unknown regarding drug metabolism and clearance by the kidneys in pediatric patients, especially in the newborn, underscoring the importance of further studies investigating OAT expression and regulation in the developing kidney.

ACKNOWLEDGMENTS

This work was partly supported by NIH grant U54 HD090259.

 A complete reference list is available at www.ExpertConsult.com.

SELECT REFERENCES

1. Behrman RE, Kliegman R, Jenson HB. *Nelson Textbook of Pediatrics*. 17th ed. Philadelphia: Saunders; 2004.
2. Nigam SK, Bush KT, Martovetsky G, et al. The organic anion transporter (OAT) family: a systems biology perspective. *Physiol Rev*. 2015;95:83–123.
3. Burckhardt BC, Burckhardt G. Transport of organic anions across the basolateral membrane of proximal tubule cells. *Rev Physiol Biochem Pharmacol*. 2003;146:95–158.
4. Ahn SY, Bhatnagar V. Update on the molecular physiology of organic anion transporters. *Curr Opin Nephrol Hypertens*. 2008;17:499–505.
5. De Gregori S, De Gregori M, Ranzani GN, Borghesi A, Regazzi M, Stronati M. Drug transporters and renal drug disposition in the newborn. *J Matern Fetal Neonatal Med*. 2009;22(suppl 3):31–37.
6. Burckhardt G, Wolff NA. Structure of renal organic anion and cation transporters. *Am J Physiol Renal Physiol*. 2000;278:F853–F866.
7. Eraly SA, Bush KT, Sampogna RV, Bhatnagar V, Nigam SK. The molecular pharmacology of organic anion transporters: from DNA to FDA? *Mol Pharmacol*. 2004;65:479–487.
8. Lopez-Nieto CE, You G, Bush KT, Barros EJ, Beier DR, Nigam SK. Molecular cloning and characterization of NKT, a gene product related to the organic cation transporter family that is almost exclusively expressed in the kidney. *J Biol Chem*. 1997;272:6471–6478.
9. Nigam SK. What do drug transporters really do? *Nat Rev Drug Discov*. 2015;14:29–44.
10. Jones DP, Chesney RW. Development of tubular function. *Clin Perinatol*. 1992;19:33–57.
11. Hirsch GH, Hook JB. Maturation of renal organic acid transport: substrate stimulation by penicillin and p-aminohippurate (PAH). *J Pharmacol Exp Ther*. 1970;171:103–108.
12. Alexander DP, Nixon DA. Plasma clearance of p-aminohippuric acid by the kidneys of foetal, neonatal and adult sheep. *Nature*. 1962;194:483–484.
13. Lawrence ML, Smith JR, Davies JA. Functional transport of organic anions and cations in the murine mesonephros. *Am J Physiol Renal Physiol*. 2018;315:F130–F137.
14. Nakajima N, Sekine T, Cha SH, et al. Developmental changes in multispecific organic anion transporter 1 expression in the rat kidney. *Kidney Int*. 2000;57:1608–1616.
15. Buist SC, Cherrington NJ, Choudhuri S, Hartley DP, Klaassen CD. Gender-specific and developmental influences on the expression of rat organic anion transporters. *J Pharmacol Exp Ther*. 2002;301:145–151.
16. Pavlova A, Sakurai H, Leclercq B, Beier DR, Yu AS, Nigam SK. Developmentally regulated expression of organic ion transporters NKT (OAT1), OCT1, NLT (OAT2), and Roct. *Am J Physiol Renal Physiol*. 2000;278:F635–F643.
17. Sweeney DE, Vallon V, Rieg T, Wu W, Gallegos TF, Nigam SK. Functional maturation of drug transporters in the developing, neonatal, and postnatal kidney. *Mol Pharmacol*. 2011;80:147–154.
18. Hwang JS, Park EY, Kim WY, Yang CW, Kim J. Expression of OAT1 and OAT3 in differentiating proximal tubules of the mouse kidney. *Histol Histopathol*. 2010;25:33–44.
19. Cheung KWK, van Groen BD, Spaans E, et al. A comprehensive analysis of ontogeny of renal drug transporters: mRNA analyses, quantitative proteomics, and localization. *Clin Pharmacol Ther*. 2019;106:1083–1092.
20. Momper JD, Yang J, Gockenbach M, Vaida F, Nigam SK. Dynamics of organic anion transporter-mediated tubular secretion during postnatal human kidney development and maturation. *Clin J Am Soc Nephrol*. 2019;14:540–548.
21. Imaoka T, Kusuhara H, Adachi M, Schuetz JD, Takeuchi K, Sugiyama Y. Functional involvement of multidrug resistance-associated protein 4 (MRP4/ABCC4) in the renal elimination of the antiviral drugs adefovir and tenofovir. *Mol Pharmacol*. 2007;71:619–627.
22. King JR, Yogev R, Jean-Philippe P, et al. Steady-state pharmacokinetics of tenofovir-based regimens in HIV-infected pediatric patients. *Antimicrob Agents Chemother*. 2011;55:4290–4294.
23. Brooks AN, Hagan DM, Howe DC. Neuroendocrine regulation of pituitary-adrenal function during fetal life. *Eur J Endocrinol*. 1996;135:153–165.
24. Freemark M. The fetal adrenal and the maturation of the growth hormone and prolactin axes. *Endocrinology*. 1999;140:1963–1965.
25. Terlouw SA, Masereeuw R, Russel FG. Modulatory effects of hormones, drugs, and toxic events on renal organic anion transport. *Biochem Pharmacol*. 2003;65:1393–1405.
26. Braunlich H. Postnatal development of kidney function in rats receiving thyroid hormones. *Exp Clin Endocrinol*. 1984;83:243–250.
27. Braunlich H. Transport of p-aminohippurate in renal cortical slices of rats of different ages following treatment with thyroid hormones. *Biomed Biochim Acta*. 1987;46:251–257.
28. Buist SC, Klaassen CD. Rat and mouse differences in gender-predominant expression of organic anion transporter (Oat1-3; Slc22a6-8) mRNA levels. *Drug Metab Dispos*. 2004;32:620–625.
29. Kobayashi Y, Hirokawa N, Ohshiro N, et al. Differential gene expression of organic anion transporters in male and female rats. *Biochem Biophys Res Commun*. 2002;290:482–487.
30. Kudo N, Katakura M, Sato Y, Kawashima Y. Sex hormone-regulated renal transport of perfluorooctanoic acid. *Chem Biol Interact*. 2002;139:301–316.

31. Reyes JL, Melendez E, Alegria A, Jaramillo-Juarez F. Influence of sex differences on the renal secretion of organic anions. *Endocrinology*. 1998;139:1581-1587.
32. Ljubojevic M, Balen D, Breljak D, et al. Renal expression of organic anion transporter OAT2 in rats and mice is regulated by sex hormones. *Am J Physiol Renal Physiol*. 2007;292:F361-F372.
33. Breljak D, Ljubojevic M, Balen D, et al. Renal expression of organic anion transporter Oat5 in rats and mice exhibits the female-dominant sex differences. *Histol Histopathol*. 2010;25:1385-1402.
34. Zhou F, Hong M, You G. Regulation of human organic anion transporter 4 by progesterone and protein kinase C in human placental BeWo cells. *Am J Physiol Endocrinol Metab*. 2007;293:E57-E61.
35. Lu R, Kanai N, Bao Y, Wolkoff AW, Schuster VL. Regulation of renal oatp mRNA expression by testosterone. *Am J Physiol*. 1996;270:F332-F337.
36. Braunlich H, Rassbach H, Vogelsang S. Stimulation of renal tubular transport of p-aminohippurate in rats of different ages by treatment with adrenocortical steroids. *Dev Pharmacol Ther*. 1992;19:1-5.
37. Braunlich H, Kohler A, Schmidt I. Acceleration of p-aminohippurate excretion in immature rats by dexamethasone treatment. *Med Biol*. 1986;64:267-270.
38. Braunlich H, Pils W. Synergistic effect of triiodothyronine and dexamethasone on renal tubular transport of p-aminohippurate in rats of different ages. *Dev Pharmacol Ther*. 1992;19:50-56.
39. Jensen RE, Berndt WO. Epinephrine and norepinephrine enhance p-aminohippurate transport into basolateral membrane vesicles. *J Pharmacol Exp Ther*. 1988;244:543-549.
40. Barasch J. Genes and proteins involved in mesenchymal to epithelial transition. *Curr Opin Nephrol Hypertens*. 2001;10:429-436.
41. Schnabel CA, Selleri L, Jacobs Y, Warnke R, Cleary ML. Expression of Pbx1b during mammalian organogenesis. *Mech Dev*. 2001;100:131-135.
42. Eraly SA, Hamilton BA, Nigam SK. Organic anion and cation transporters occur in pairs of similar and similarly expressed genes. *Biochem Biophys Res Commun*. 2003;300:333-342.
43. Pontoglio M, Prie D, Cheret C, et al. HNF1alpha controls renal glucose reabsorption in mouse and man. *EMBO Rep*. 2000;1:359-365.
44. Cheret C, Doyen A, Yaniv M, Pontoglio M. Hepatocyte nuclear factor 1 alpha controls renal expression of the Npt1-Npt4 anionic transporter locus. *J Mol Biol*. 2002;322:929-941.
45. Soumounou Y, Gauthier C, Tenenhouse HS. Murine and human type I Na-phosphate cotransporter genes: structure and promoter activity. *Am J Physiol Renal Physiol*. 2001;281:F1082-F1091.
46. Martovetsky G, Tee JB, Nigam SK. Hepatocyte nuclear factors 4alpha and 1alpha regulate kidney developmental expression of drug-metabolizing enzymes and drug transporters. *Mol Pharmacol*. 2013;84:808-823.
47. Maher JM, Slitt AL, Callaghan TN, et al. Alterations in transporter expression in liver, kidney, and duodenum after targeted disruption of the transcription factor HNF1alpha. *Biochem Pharmacol*. 2006;72:512-522.
48. Saji T, Kikuchi R, Kusuhara H, Kim I, Gonzalez FJ, Sugiyama Y. Transcriptional regulation of human and mouse organic anion transporter 1 by hepatocyte nuclear factor 1 alpha/beta. *J Pharmacol Exp Ther*. 2008;324:784-790.
49. Kikuchi R, Kusuhara H, Hattori N, et al. Regulation of the expression of human organic anion transporter 3 by hepatocyte nuclear factor 1alpha/beta and DNA methylation. *Mol Pharmacol*. 2006;70:887-896.
50. Kikuchi R, Kusuhara H, Hattori N, et al. Regulation of tissue-specific expression of the human and mouse urate transporter 1 gene by hepatocyte nuclear factor 1 alpha/beta and DNA methylation. *Mol Pharmacol*. 2007;72:1619-1625.

102 Concentration and Dilution of Urine

Silvia Iacobelli | Jean-Pierre Guignard

PHYSIOLOGY OF THE URINARY CONCENTRATING MECHANISM

The osmolality and volume of body fluids are maintained within narrow limits despite wide variations in water and solute intake. The kidneys play a key role in maintaining the constant homeostasis of body fluids by excreting or retaining water as needed, which keeps the osmolality of the extracellular fluids constant. Antidiuretic hormone (ADH or vasopressin) plays a central role in the defense of the osmolality of the extracellular compartment, while sodium, the main solute in the extracellular fluid, regulates its volume.[1,2] The excretion of sodium is mainly under the control of aldosterone.

RENAL MECHANISM FOR CONCENTRATION AND DILUTION OF URINE

The concentration and dilution of urine involve several transport mechanisms along the different segments of the nephrons (Fig. 102.1). The thick ascending limb of Henle loop, located in the outer medulla,[2-4] plays a key role in diluting and concentrating mechanisms. This segment of the nephron has a very low hydraulic conductivity and can reabsorb NaCl in the relative absence of water. The result is dilution of fluid remaining in the tubular lumen and an increase in the interstitial concentration of NaCl surrounding the thick limbs and collecting ducts. Isotonic fluid from the proximal tubule enters the descending loop of Henle at the level of the outer medulla and is exposed to increased interstitial osmolality. Descending loop segments have a high hydraulic conductivity, but a low sodium permeability. As a consequence, water in the descending limb moves osmotically into the interstitium, and fluid in the lumen of this segment becomes more concentrated.

Urine flowing through the thick ascending limb becomes progressively dilute by virtue of the relative impermeability of this segment to water. It then enters the distal convoluted tubule, a cortical segment in which water and salt reabsorption and equilibration with blood produce a largely isotonic urine entering the outer medullary collecting duct. In a hypertonic outer medulla, water is osmotically removed from the tubule lumen, and solutes in the collecting duct become increasingly concentrated. Urea movement in distal tubules is limited, but water reabsorption is substantial, so that cortical collecting tubules receive urine with a high urea concentration. This segment has low urea permeability in both the presence and absence of ADH, so that a high urea concentration is maintained in the urine entering the outer medullary collecting duct. This segment has also a low permeability to sodium and probably does not transport NaCl actively. Thus it does not contribute to the high interstitial salt content.

In contrast to the more proximal collecting duct, the inner medullary collecting duct is permeable to urea in the presence of ADH.[5,6] Urea diffuses down a chemical gradient to enter the medullary interstitium. Urea can also enter the descending limb, and its concentration actually rises in this segment. Accumulation of urea in the interstitium provides an osmotic driving force that further abstracts water from medullary portions of the descending loop. This increases the luminal concentration of NaCl and urea. The urine begins to become progressively less concentrated, and NaCl accumulates in the interstitium. The presence of this added interstitial NaCl abstracts more water from urine in the inner medullary collecting duct as this segment courses through the interstitium, a step that further concentrates the final urine. In addition, urea can reenter the lumen of the thin ascending limbs to recycle back to the collecting tubule.

ROLE OF SHORT-LOOP NEPHRONS AND UREA

Recycling of urea (to maintain a high medullary urea content) is critical for maximal efficiency of the concentrating process and

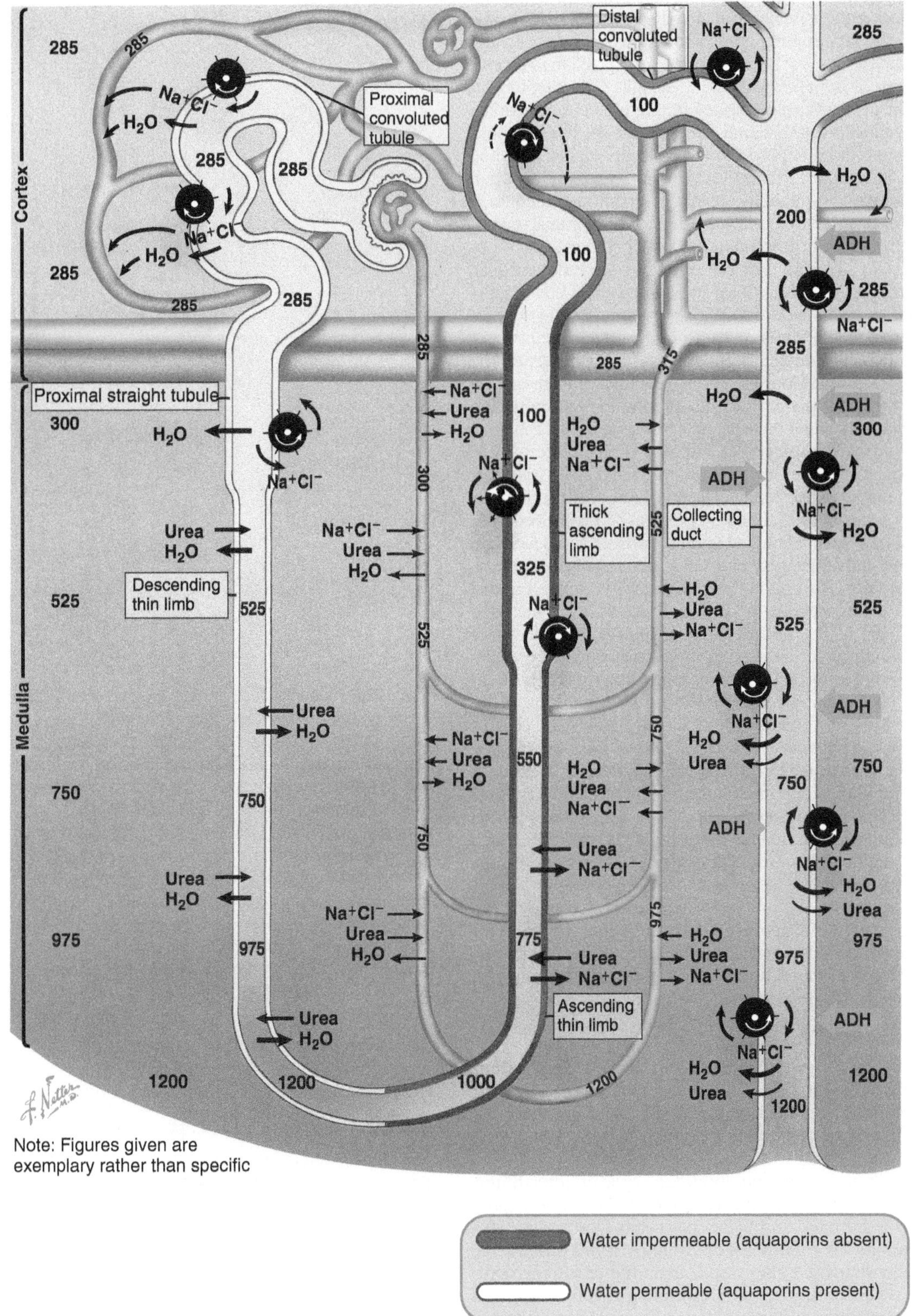

Fig. 102.1 The countercurrent movement of water and solutes between the loops of Henle and the collecting tubule. NaCl is actively reabsorbed from the thick limb, diluting urine and increasing osmolality of the outer medulla. Water reabsorption continues in the distal tubule and the cortical and outer medullary collecting duct, leading to increased urea concentration. Water and urea are reabsorbed from the inner medullary collecting duct. Urea accumulates in the interstitium, osmotically abstracts water from the descending limb and allows NaCl concentration in the descending limb fluid to increase and in the interstitium to decrease. The thin ascending limb is permeable to NaCl and receives fluid rich in NaCl. NaCl enters the interstitium down its concentration gradient, and urine becomes hypoosmotic to the surrounding interstitium. See text for details. (Reprinted with permission from Kelly CR, Landman J. *The Netter Collection of Medical Illustrations (vol 6), Urinary System*. Philadelphia: Elsevier; 2012.)

is facilitated by short-looped nephrons that do not descend deep into the inner medulla.[7,8] These nephrons reabsorb a large portion of filtrate, reducing the volume of fluid and solute that needs to be concentrated. Short-looped nephrons also exhibit permeability and anatomic characteristics that place them in a good position to receive urea and facilitate its recycling to the inner medulla.[9] The inter-tubular recycling of urea is likely accomplished through three major routes. First, urea in the ascending thin limb can remain in the tubule lumen, travel through the distal nephron to the collecting ducts, and then recycle to the interstitium. Second, urea in thin ascending limbs can reach the thick ascending limb, a segment that, in the outer medulla, is permeable to urea and is in close relationship to the proximal straight tubules (and therefore the descending limbs) of both long- and short-loop nephrons. At this site, urea can return to the inner medulla directly via proximal straight tubules and descending limbs of long-loop nephrons, or it can cycle through loops and collecting ducts of short nephrons to reenter the medulla. Third, urea can leave the inner medullary interstitium through ascending vasa recta and reenter the descending limbs of short-loop nephrons. This urea can similarly be carried back through superficial distal nephrons and transported to collecting ducts in the inner medulla.

The role of urea is complex. Urea had been thought to cross cell membranes solely by passive diffusion, but rapid urea transport rates in some tissues suggested a facilitating transport mechanism. As reviewed,[10] several urea transporter isoforms (UTs) derived from the *UT-A* gene have been identified in renal tissue that can facilitate transmembrane movement of urea and can help generate the hypertonic medulla. UT-A1 and UT-A3 are restricted to the terminal portion of the inner medullary collecting duct. UT-A2 is localized in the lower part of the thin descending limb of short-loops of Henle in the inner stripe of the outer medulla, and also in the thin descending limb of long-loop nephrons in the inner medulla under more prolonged antidiuretic conditions. The *UT-B* gene produces the UT-B1 transporter protein located in the endothelial cells of medullary descending vasa recta. UT-B1 allows urea leaving the ascending vasa recta to reenter the descending vasa recta, become trapped in the medulla, and maintain a high medullary urea concentration. This transporter protein is down-regulated by ADH and may serve different functions (favoring nitric oxide over urea synthesis and limiting urea production in endothelial cells when a very high inner medullary content of urea is already present).[11,12]

Finally, animal and human studies[13-15] suggest that urea is not an effective osmole when vasopressin acts in fed mammals (to allow for water conservation). Nevertheless, when the urine is electrolyte-poor, and in the context of water dehydration, urea becomes an effective osmole to ensure a safe minimum urine flow rate.

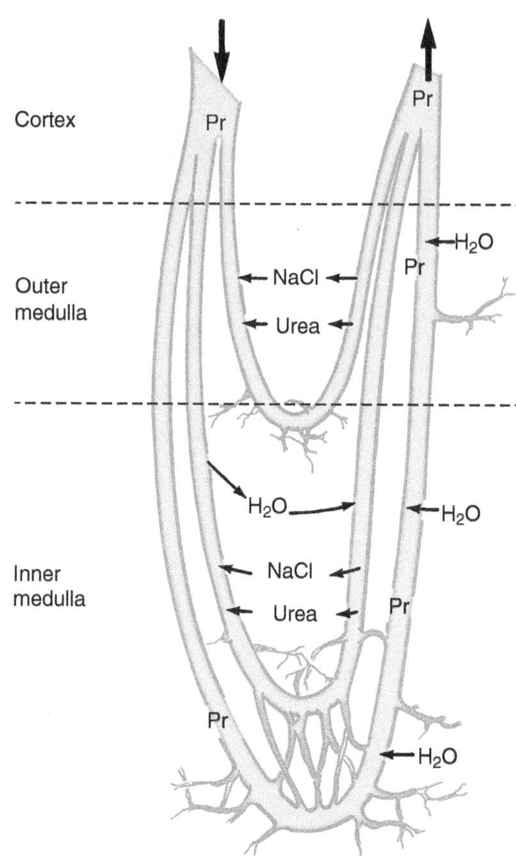

Fig. 102.2 Countercurrent exchange in vasa recta. Medullary circulation includes network of interconnecting vessels and main thoroughfares. Vessels are freely permeable to NaCl, urea, and water. Loops of Henle and collecting ducts are responsible for increasing concentration of interstitial NaCl and urea. Solutes can enter descending vasa recta and leave ascending vasa recta to remain trapped in medulla. As water leaves and descends the vasa recta, protein concentration increases. High osmotic and oncotic pressures in ascending vasa recta enhance capillary fluid uptake, returning water, reabsorbed from tubules, to general circulation. Therefore vasa recta trap solute and remove water, preserving hyperosmolality of the renal medulla. *Pr,* Plasma protein. (By permission of the *New England Journal of Medicine:* Jamison RL, Maffly RH. The urinary concentrating mechanism. *N Engl J Med.* 1976;295:1059.)

ROLE OF VASA RECTA

Vasa recta are blood vessels coursing through the interstitium. Vasa recta provide substrate for, and removal of end products of, metabolic reactions. In addition, due to their high permeability, they play an important role in salt and water balance. The vessels descend into the medulla to varying degrees, break up into small capillaries that course through localized areas of interstitium, and rejoin to ascend toward the cortex (Fig. 102.2). Ascending vasa recta are fenestrated and highly permeant. Descending vasa recta have continuous endothelial cells and pericytes (contractile smooth muscle remnants). They also contain the urea transporter UT-2 as well as aquaporin (AQP)-1. Descending vasa recta are well situated adjacently in vascular bundles and in deeper portions of the medulla to receive NaCl and urea from ascending vasa recta and to deliver water toward the ascending vessels down concentration gradients.[8,16] Accordingly, solutes such as NaCl and urea found in high concentration in ascending vasa recta can enter descending vasa recta that contain a fluid of lower solute concentration, whereas water can move in the opposite direction.

The ability of the vasa recta to maintain the medullary interstitial gradient is flow dependent. A substantial increase in vasa recta blood flow dissipates the medullary gradient. Alternatively, decreased blood flow reduces oxygen delivery to the nephron segments within the medulla.

ROLE OF THE RENAL PELVIS

The renal pelvis may contribute to urinary concentration.[17] Epithelium covering the inner medulla and papilla and facing the pelvic space is similar to that of papillary collecting ducts. During water diuresis, these cells are closely apposed and intercellular spaces are narrow. During antidiuresis, individual cells are more distinct, and intercellular spaces are widely dilated. This may reflect enhanced transepithelial movement of fluid.[18] Pelvic extensions in some species allow the urinary space to surround vascular bundles and much of the papillae and may reach the cortex.[7] Increased urine concentration has been related to an increase in contact surface area between papilla and pelvic urine.[18,19]

ROLE OF AQUAPORINS

AQPs are a family of highly selective transmembrane channels that mainly transport water across the cell and some facilitate low-molecular-weight solutes. To date, nine AQPs, including

Table 102.1 Characteristics of Aquaporins Found in Kidney Tissue.

Genetic Designation	Renal Localization	Proposed Physiologic Role
Aquaporin-1	Proximal tubule S1, S2, and S3 segments of short- and long-looped nephrons Descending thin limb of Henle in long-loop nephrons Nonfenestrated descending vasa recta Limited in vesicles and vacuoles Present in both apical and basolateral membranes (basal and lateral aspects)	Major transmembrane pathway for H_2O flow, including entry and exit sites Not under hormonal control
Aquaporin-2	Outer and inner medullary collecting duct Primarily apical membrane and intracellular vesicles	The vasopressin-regulated H_2O channel; ADH induces movement of an intracellular vesicle pool of H_2O channels to the apical membrane
Aquaporin-3	Collecting duct principal cells in cortex and medulla; strongest medullary label is at base, not tip, of papilla Mainly in lateral and basolateral infoldings, not in basal aspect, of basolateral plasma membrane Virtually absent from apical membrane; minimally found in intracellular vesicles	Major exit site for osmotically driven H_2O transport; not regulated through vesicular trafficking via ADH; may provide for small nonelectrolyte solute movement
	Inner medullary collecting duct principal cells, especially proximal two-thirds of segment; little in cortex and outer medulla Distributed roughly equally in basal and lateral domains of basolateral plasma membrane, and not in intracellular vesicles	Basolateral exit site of cellular H_2O transport of inner medullary collecting ducts

ADH, Antidiuretic hormone.

AQP1, AQP2, AQP3, AQP4, AQP5, AQP6, AQP7, AQP8, and AQP11, have been identified in different segments and various cells of the kidney to maintain normal urine concentration function.[20,21]

Some features of AQPs 1 to 3 are summarized in Table 102.1.

AQP-1 is found in renal proximal tubules, long-loop thin descending limbs of Henle, and non-fenestrated endothelium of descending vasa recta. AQP-1 imparts high osmotic water permeability. In nephron segments, this protein is identified in both apical and basolateral membranes, including both basal and lateral infoldings, but not to any substantial degree in cytoplasmic vesicle and vacuole membranes. Accordingly, AQP-1 is poised to facilitate transcellular water movement in segments responsible for reabsorbing a major portion of the glomerular filtrate, but it does not appear to require hormonal regulation and therefore is not the ADH-sensitive water channel.[22–24] This protein is also abundant in red blood cells, where it is thought to increase membrane permeability. Although individuals without functional AQP channel-forming integral protein (CHIP) water channels do not appear to have clinical abnormalities, such as polyuria,[25] rare individuals lacking AQP-1 have a urinary concentrating defect in response to ADH or to water deprivation.[26] The role of AQP-1 in maintaining urinary concentrating ability is appreciated from studies of transgenic knockout mice lacking AQP-1. These mice are polyuric and do not tolerate water deprivation.[27] Moreover, perfused proximal tubules[28] and descending thin limbs[29] from such mice have reduced osmotic water permeability. Thus AQP-1 is necessary for maximal concentrating ability. This is likely related to the need for rapid equilibration of water across the thin descending limb of Henle in helping to establish the countercurrent multiplication process.

AQP-2 is the most important ADH-regulated water channel and mediates the short-term renal response to the hormone. This conclusion is supported by the following cumulative observations. Vasopressin binds to a basolateral membrane receptor and initiates a cyclic adenosine monophosphate (cAMP)-mediated chain of signaling events leading to the insertion of water channels and increased osmotic water permeability of the collecting duct apical membrane.[30,31] AQP-2 protein is present primarily in cytoplasmic vesicles and in apical plasma membranes of collecting duct principal cells. Furthermore, some staining for AQP-2 occurs in basolateral plasma membranes of inner medullary collecting-duct principal cells.[21] After stimulation by ADH, apical membrane staining for AQP-2 intensifies, but it decreases in the subapical vesicles (i.e., AQP-2 redistributes from vesicles to membrane).[32,33] Therefore there is a reservoir of cellular AQP-2 protein capable of actually recycling between intracellular cytoplasmic vesicles and the plasma membrane.[34] Despite inhibition of protein synthesis in LLC-PK1 epithelial cells—cells that express many features of renal proximal tubule epithelia—AQP-2 staining was primarily localized to intracellular vesicles in nonstimulated cells and quickly redistributed (within 10 minutes) to the plasma membrane after exposure to ADH. The pattern was reversible on removal of ADH.

There is also evidence that AQP-2 plays a major role in the long-term adaptation to pathophysiologic stimuli known to alter urinary concentrating ability. For example, lithium, a drug used in affective disorders, induces an ADH-resistant concentrating defect characterized by the down-regulation of AQP-2 expression in rat inner medullary membranes that coincides with the development of polyuria.[35,36] The ADH-resistant urinary concentrating defect occurring after the release of bilaterally obstructed ureters is also associated with a marked down-regulation of inner medullary AQP-2 expression that correlates with polyuria. In addition, the slow recovery is marked by persistence of decreased AQP-2 expression.[37]

Chronic hypokalemia may lead to ADH-resistant nephrogenic diabetes insipidus. When hypokalemia was induced by potassium deprivation for 11 days, polyuria correlated with the down-regulation of AQP-2 in both the cortex and the inner medulla of rat kidneys. Polyuria expression of AQP-2 corrected within a week of potassium repletion.[37] Hypercalcemia is another electrolyte disorder in which a concentrating defect and polyuria have been associated with the down-regulation of AQP-2.[38,39] Thirsting increases expression of AQP-2 in rat collecting ducts, and in Brattleboro rats, a model of central diabetes insipidus, expression of AQP-2 in collecting ducts is reduced in the basal state and is significantly increased on exposure to ADH.[40,41] The decreased urinary-concentrating ability associated with protein-depleted or malnourished subjects is thought to relate to a decrease in the deep medullary urea content. However, rats kept on a low-protein diet for 2 weeks, without malnutrition, demonstrate decreased maximal urine osmolality after water deprivation, reduced ADH-stimulated osmotic water permeability, and decreased expression of AQP-2 protein in terminal portions of the inner medullary collecting ducts.[42]

In both acute and chronic renal failure, the contribution of dysregulation of several AQPs in defining a nephrogenic diabetes insipidus state has been described. In a renal artery clamp model of ischemic acute renal failure, decreased collecting ducts AQP-2, -3, and -4 have been documented, in association with impaired components of the countercurrent concentrating mechanism, which generates the hyperosmotic driving force for water transport through the AQPs water channels.[43] In a 5/6 nephrectomy rat model of chronic renal failure, several defects have been identified, including absence of the arginine vasopressin (V2) receptor mRNA as well as decreased AQP-2.[44] A rat model of nephrotic syndrome (using puromycin aminonucleoside) is also another example of nephrogenic diabetes insipidus associated with dysfunction of collecting duct AQPs and a significant decrease of both AQP-2 and -3 in the inner medulla. Finally, in the hypothyroid rat a significant diminution in renal concentrating capacity has been documented. This defect appeared multifactorial and in part due to a decrease in AQP-2 expression and trafficking to the apical membrane of the collecting duct.[45]

These examples of limitations in urinary concentrating ability associated with long-term alterations in AQP-2 are of particular interest considering the presence of AQPs in fetal and neonatal renal tissues (see later discussion). Moreover, AQP-2 appears to be necessary for ADH-dependent concentration of urine in humans, as evidenced by a patient with autosomal recessive nephrogenic diabetes insipidus who had two mutations in the gene encoding AQP-2. Expression of the defective proteins in *Xenopus* oocytes showed nonfunctional water channel proteins that failed to increase osmotic water permeability.[46] Such abnormalities may become definable by analyzing urine from such patients.[47,48]

Previous studies have also revealed a non–ADH-mediated regulation of AQP-2.

In animal models decreased prostaglandin E_2 (PGE_2) production, as induced by cyclooxygenase inhibition, results in reduced endocytosis of AQP-2 and therefore increased abundance of AQP-2 in the plasma membrane with associated water reabsorption.[49] Effective osmolality/tonicity has also been associated with increased expression of AQP-2.[50]

As proven by both animal and human studies, several drugs may modulate AQP-2 expression or regulation, and this effect may be different in infant versus adult kidney. In infant but not in adult rats, a single injection of betamethasone induces an increase in urine osmolality, renal medullary AQP-2 mRNA, and protein levels[51] in the 24 hours following treatment. This finding has been confirmed in human preterm neonates, as well.[52]

In patients with chronic heart failure, furosemide administration increased the vasopressin level and stimulated water reabsorption via the AQP-2 water channels.

In human healthy adults, ibuprofen administration increased urinary AQP-2 excretion without changes in ADH, urinary output, or urinary osmolality—this effect being mediated via the inhibition of renal prostaglandin synthesis.[53] These effects have not been proven during the first months of life in very preterm neonates treated by ibuprofen and presenting with oligo/anuria.[54]

AQP-3 is expressed along the connecting tubule and entire length of the collecting duct (in principal cells) from the cortex and the outer and inner medulla, especially the base, rather than the tip, of the inner medulla.[55,56] The protein is found primarily in the lateral and basal infoldings of the basolateral membrane and is regulated by thirst and aldosterone. Under long-term influence of ADH, AQP-3 is integrally involved in urinary concentration Transgenic knockout mice lacking AQP-3 have a concentrating defect and polyuria.[57] AQP-3 also appears to conduct small nonelectrolyte solutes, such as urea.[58]

AQP-4 expression is found primarily in inner medullary collecting duct principal cells. It is more prominent in the inner medullary base than in the papillary tip and is found in basolateral (both basal and lateral domains) rather than apical membranes. Little staining is found in intracellular vesicles. When rats were either water restricted for 48 hours or infused with ADH for 5 days, no increase in expression of AQP-4 over a baseline water-loaded state was observed.[56,59] These findings are consistent with a role for AQP-4 as a basolateral exit pathway for transcellular movement of water in the inner medulla, perhaps in response to osmotic gradients, and not in response to the secretion of ADH. The role of AQP-4 has been further assessed in transgenic knockout mice lacking AQP-4. Such mice had a mild urinary concentrating defect,[60] and their perfused inner medullary collecting ducts exhibit reduced ADH-stimulated osmotic water permeability.[61]

Four other AQPs have been identified in kidney tissue, but their physiologic roles are unclear.[20,21] Procino and colleagues[62] first reported that AQP5 is expressed in type-B intercalated cells in the collecting duct system of the rat, mouse, and human kidney, making the hypothesis that AQP5 may serve an osmosensor for the composition of the fluid coming from the thick ascending limb.

AQP-6, which has minimal water permeability, is expressed in collecting-duct intercalated cells from cortex to inner medulla. One study from Agre[63] suggests that this AQP could be implicated in the urine acidification process. The protein appears to be present in intracellular vesicles, not plasma membranes, and may represent an intracellular water and ion channel.[64] AQP-7 is present in the proximal tubular brush border, particularly in the S3 segment,[20,21] and effects metabolism by regulating the transportation of glycerol. AQP-8 is found in proximal tubule and collecting duct cells intracellular domains as well as other tissues.[65] AQP-11 has also been identified in mammalian kidney at low abundance by Northern blot and reverse transcriptase-polymerase chain reaction techniques, but its functional significance has not been clarified yet.[20,21] However, AQP-11 knockout mice have been shown to have polycystic kidneys and to develop uremia.

ROLE OF CHLORIDE CHANNELS

Rapid abstraction of NaCl down its concentration gradient occurs in medullary thin ascending limbs and is an integral part of the countercurrent multiplication process. This segment is particularly permeant to chloride. Chloride channels would be poised to facilitate transmembrane movement of solute and, in fact, such channels (e.g., ClC-K1) have been identified in the inner medullary thin ascending limbs of Henle in the rat kidney. The channel was localized to both apical and basolateral membranes in one study[66] and primarily on the basolateral membrane in another.[67] Although this channel is also found in other, more distal segments in both cortex and medulla, its location in the thin ascending limb underscores its role in concentrating and diluting urine. In this regard, dehydration was shown to increase expression of the ClC-K1 channel in cortical and medullary segments. Moreover, knockout mice without ClC-K1 showed clinical nephrogenic diabetes insipidus, a defect that was attributed to impaired generation of inner medullary hypertonicity rather than decreased collecting duct water permeability.[68,69] The role of chloride channels in urinary concentration as well as other ion channels along the nephron has been reviewed.[70,71]

To summarize, due to the countercurrent relationships of the loops of Henle, vasa recta, and proximal straight and collecting tubules, several cycles of solute transfer appear to take place more or less simultaneously. At all levels of the medulla (outer and inner stripes of the outer medulla as well as the inner medulla), but particularly in the inner stripe, in which the vessels located within the vascular bundle are separated only by a thin layer of interstitium, solute has the potential to leave the ascending vasa recta and enter the descending vasa recta. Some of this solute can be taken up by the descending loops of Henle from short-loop nephrons that are also within the bundle. This solute can ascend to the cortex and then move to the collecting tubules. When deep in the medulla, the solute can be transferred to the ascending vasa recta or to the ascending loops of Henle and can then reenter the descending loop of Henle to recycle in the medulla. In the outer stripe of the outer medulla, fluid in the ascending loop, as well as the ascending vasa recta, may also be able to enter the proximal straight tubules of the short- and long-looped nephrons. These relationships provide an ongoing transfer of solute between vessels and tubule segments to maintain sodium chloride and urea gradients in the medulla, allowing extraction of water from collecting ducts when there is need to concentrate urine. Urine leaving the renal papillary collecting ducts enters the renal pelvis and may be able to circulate in the pelvic spaces to bathe portions of the outer medulla. There is the potential for urea to recycle back to the medulla and contribute further to urinary concentration. Functional water channels appear to be amply present in both apical and basolateral membranes and are neatly poised to reclaim water by processes that are dependent on, as well as independent of, ADH.

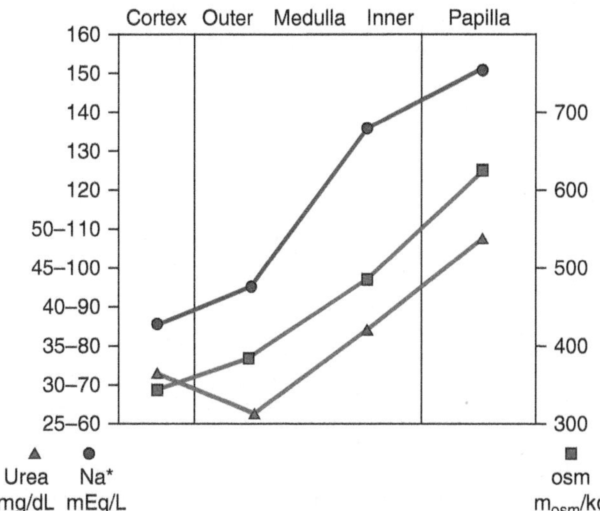

Fig. 102.3 Intrarenal solute gradients in fetal lambs at mid-gestation. (From Moore ES, Kaiser BA, Simpson EH, McMann BJ: Ontogeny of intrarenal solute gradients in fetal life. In: Spitzer A, ed. *The Kidney During Development: Morphology and Function.* New York: Masson; 1982:223–231.)

URINARY CONCENTRATION IN THE FETUS

The placenta, not the kidneys, maintains normal extracellular salt concentration in utero, and there is no practical need for the fetus to concentrate or dilute urine during pregnancy. Information on human fetal renal tubular reabsorption of water and response to ADH is limited. Most information comes from animals in which chronic catheters were inserted. Fetal metabolism, ontogeny, and ADH secretion are conveniently studied in the third trimester of sheep. This model is similar to humans because both placentas are impermeant to ADH, so that fetal blood ADH levels reflect fetal production.[72] To maximally concentrate urine, ADH must be synthesized, released into the circulation, and carried to collecting tubules, which must respond to the hormone. Loops of Henle, vasa recta, and tubules must have established the necessary anatomic relationship. Fetal urine, in a variety of species, is usually hypotonic to plasma.[73-79] This observation led to the conclusion that fetal kidneys could not concentrate urine, perhaps because ADH is either unavailable or the fetus is unresponsive to it. That this is not the case is evident from the following considerations.

MATURATION OF FETAL WATER REABSORPTION

A slight increase in urinary concentration occurs during fetal development.[78,80] At a time when plasma solute concentrations are stable, fetal sheep late in gestation (130 days of a normal 145-day gestation) have a urine osmolality significantly higher than that in younger fetuses of less than 130 days. Both urea and nonurea urinary solutes are seen to increase, whereas some investigators[81,82] found that intrarenal urea and salt gradients were present in fetal lamb medulla by mid-gestation (Fig. 102.3), the actual contribution of urea to total urinary osmolality was relatively small. During late gestation, urine flow rates decrease, but osmolar clearance remains unchanged. Therefore free water clearance, defined as urine flow rate minus osmolar clearance, is reduced, indicating that free water is more effectively separated (reabsorbed) from solute in the older fetal kidney.[80] Although the degree of urinary concentration in late gestation is unimpressive, the increase in water reabsorption is consistent with a heightened response to endogenous levels of ADH in the older fetus.

AVAILABILITY OF AND RESPONSIVENESS TO VASOPRESSIN

Although fetal pituitary content at term is much less than that of the adult, ADH has been identified in the human pituitary by week 12 of gestation, with a demonstrable increase over the ensuing weeks.[83-85] Neurosecretory granules and material are found in hypothalamic nuclei, the hypothalamohypophysial tract, and the infundibular process of the neurohypophysis by 16 weeks' gestation in the human fetus.[86] Clearly, ADH is produced at an early fetal age. Vasopressin mediates its tubular effect on water permeability by stimulating the generation of cAMP.[87-89] Compared with adults, fetal ADH causes a smaller increase in cAMP from renal medullary tissue obtained from the early fetus.[90-93] To achieve osmotic equilibrium (i.e., osmolality approximately 300 mOsm/kg H_2O), the fetal kidney needs higher plasma levels of ADH (approximately 5 μU/mL) than the adult, who requires only approximately 0.7 μU/mL. Moreover, maximal urine osmolality is achieved in both the fetus and adult at similar plasma levels of ADH, 4 to 6 μU/mL, but adult urine is much more concentrated.[80] Therefore the fetal nephron appears to be less sensitive than the adult to vasopressin.

EXOGENOUS VASOPRESSIN

The fetus responds to exogenous ADH by increasing urine osmolality,[94] a response linearly related to age over the third trimester of the fetal ewe (Fig. 102.4).[95-96] The human fetal nephron responds to ADH as shown in previous studies carried out in an isolated perfused human medullary collecting duct obtained from a 5.5-month male abortus with trisomy 13.[97] This tubule increased transmembrane water flow from 2.1 to 12.0 μL/cm²/Osm/min following exposure to peritubular ADH. Cells swelled with conspicuous dilation of intercellular spaces, indicating outward net flow of water through intercellular spaces and through cell membranes. Thus collecting duct receptors to ADH are well developed functionally in prenatal life.

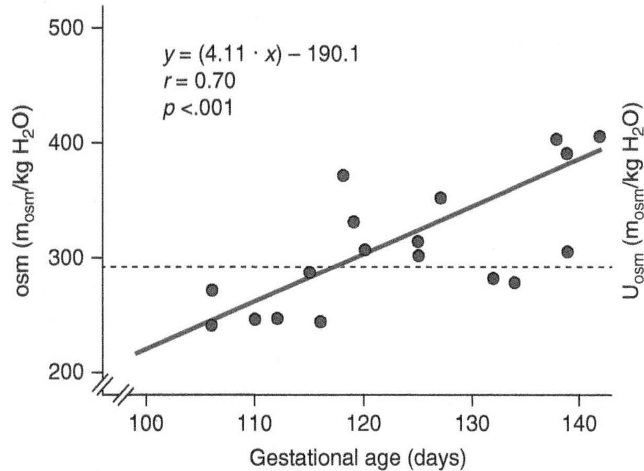

Fig. 102.4 The relationship between gestational age and urine osmolality in fetal lambs during an infusion of vasopressin (600 μU/min/kg). The *horizontal dashed line* represents mean plasma osmolality (291 mOsm/kg) during the infusion of vasopressin. (From Robillard JE, Weitzman RE. Developmental aspects of the fetal renal response to exogenous arginine vasopressin. *Am J Physiol.* 1980;238:F407.)

ENDOGENOUS VASOPRESSIN

In addition to the availability of ADH and tubular reactivity to the hormone, the fetus responds to osmotic, nonosmotic, and volume stimuli (hypertonic saline, hypoxia, hemorrhage, furosemide, and dehydration) by a prompt increase in endogenous plasma levels of ADH.[98-103] Infusing hypertonic saline into a fetus causes an increased level of plasma ADH that closely relates to plasma osmolality.[78,79,102] Fetal infusion of hypertonic saline increases fetal urine osmolality and decreases fetal urine flow rate. This response can be blocked by an ADH antagonist.[104] When water deprivation is imposed on a pregnant ewe, the older fetus, compared with the young fetus, has a higher plasma ADH level for a given plasma osmolality and, for a given plasma ADH level, the older fetus has a greater reduction in urinary water clearance.[98,100] When varying degrees of hemorrhage are induced in lamb fetuses during the third trimester of pregnancy, plasma ADH levels increase nearly 50-fold and correlate with the degree of blood removed.[105] In late gestation—more than 130 days—a hypoxic stimulus causes fetal plasma ADH levels to rise, which are accompanied by an increase in urine osmolality and a decrease in water clearance without a change in osmolar clearance. This response occurs in nearly all (9 out of 10) near-term fetuses of more than 130 days and approximately half (5 out of 9) of young fetuses of less than 120 days.[80,100,106] Therefore fetal hypoxemia induces antidiuresis, particularly in a near-term fetus. AVP levels are also elevated during labor, with higher levels observed in infants born by vaginal delivery (versus cesarean section without labor), which is consistent with an enhancement in AVP secretion by the fetus in response to increases in intracranial pressure or hypoxia.[107]

It appears then that in a fetus during the last trimester, volume, osmotic, and non-osmotic receptors for the production and release of ADH are functional, ADH is available, and tissue response to the hormone is intact. Animal data demonstrate that the V2 receptor is present very early in gestation. In rats, the number of receptors does not change during the first 2 weeks of postnatal life. There is a sharp increase after 20 days, reaching adult levels by the fifth week of life. Thus expression of the V2 receptor does not seem to be involved in the low response of the immature kidney to AVP.[108]

However, other steps of the AVP response are developmentally regulated; several investigations have demonstrated that AVP-stimulated cAMP generation is markedly lower during the neonatal period in different species, including rats, rabbits, and dogs.[109] Moreover, direct stimulation of adenylyl cyclase by forskolin (which does not require a functional G protein to stimulate the enzyme) failed to elicit maximal cAMP generation in the immature collecting duct.

Finally, tubular stimulation with 8-chlorophenylthiol cAMP, a cAMP analogue, failed to increase hydraulic permeability in the immature collecting duct.[110] These observations demonstrate that not only AVP-stimulated cAMP production is low in the immature kidney, but also that alteration in AVP response is localized, at least in part, at a segment distal to cAMP generation.

Other steps limiting the ADH activity in the immature cortical collecting duct are the elevated phosphodiesterase activity, as proven in neonatal kidney rat[111] and the inhibitory effect of PGE2 on AVP-stimulated cAMP generation. However, other factors may contribute more to limited concentrating ability. Loops of Henle are short,[112,113] and salt reabsorption in thick ascending limbs is limited in early life.[114] Total cortical flow exceeds that to the medulla, but blood flow/nephron is proportionately greater in the medulla than in the outer cortex in early development.[115-117] These factors tend to limit the efficiency with which a medullary osmotic gradient can be generated and maintained in fetal kidneys. Regardless of quantitative limitations on urinary concentration, a mature fetus or a premature infant is establishing means to tolerate stresses that may alter the osmolality or volume of its fluid environment.

Other Effects of Vasopressin

Vasopressin receptors are found in mesangial cells, aortic smooth muscle, liver, brain, and anterior pituitary. Thus ADH has several potential roles,[118] including (1) blood pressure control by effects on vasculature and baroreceptor reflexes, (2) platelet aggregation, (3) regulation of factor VIII and von Willebrand factor, (4) release of adrenocorticotropic hormone, (5) glomerular mesangial cell contraction with some control of filtration, (6) synthesis of prostaglandins, and (7) control of/effects on hepatic metabolism by stimulating gluconeogenesis and exerting a glycogenolytic effect on hepatocytes. Some of the responses require high ADH concentration and may be more of pharmacologic interest.

Vasopressin may influence fetal water and electrolyte balance in ways separate from its effect on the kidney. Vasopressin appears to exert some control over fetal osmolar homeostasis through an effect on the placenta.[83] An osmolar gradient, generated by infusing hypertonic saline or mannitol into the mother,[83,100,119] favors transfer of fluid from fetus to mother. In the presence of hypertonic saline, neither sodium nor ADH appears to cross the placenta, but fetal serum sodium and plasma ADH increase, and fetal ADH levels exceed those in the mother. Infusing hypertonic saline into the mother causes net water flux from the fetus to the maternal fluid compartment, inducing fetal water loss and increased fetal secretion of ADH. This effect is blunted if the fetus is given an ADH infusion. Similarly, mannitol infused into the mother does not cross the placenta, but induces sufficient fetal water flow to raise fetal serum osmolality. Infusing ADH into the fetus blunts this response and may even drop fetal, and slightly raise maternal, osmolality. Therefore fetal ADH can induce transplacental water flow and cause a net gain of fetal water by inhibiting fetal to maternal water flow despite a hyperosmolar stimulus sufficient to move water from the fetus to the mother.

Vasopressin may help regulate the volume of amniotic fluid by its direct effect on urine flow and its regulatory effect on lung fluid production.[120] Vasopressin also affects fetal cardiovascular homeostasis.[121,122] Vasopressin infusion into a sheep fetus slows the heart rate and raises the blood pressure within 4 to 5 minutes. Vasopressin also causes redistribution of blood flow so that the proportion of cardiac output to gastrointestinal and peripheral circulation drops, and the percentage of cardiac output to umbilical-placental, cerebral, and myocardial circulations increases. These changes are similar to those following hypoxia and suggest that ADH release helps support the fetal cardiovascular response to stress. Moreover, fetal hemorrhage induces a drop in blood pressure, but ADH provides some protection; the fall in pressure is less, and the time for fetal blood pressure recovery towards normal after hemorrhage is shorter in the presence of the hormone.

AQUAPORINS

AQP-1 expression has been shown to increase dramatically (approximately sevenfold) from 60 to 140 days of gestation in the ovine fetus, reaching adult levels by 6 weeks of postnatal age. This correlates with the maturational changes occurring in the kidney. Although nephrogenesis is complete by birth in the ovine fetus, there is a marked increase in postnatal glomerular filtration rate (GFR) and considerable tubular growth. This relates to the need for an increased capability for Na and water reabsorption and the need for functional and abundant water channels in portions of the nephron where a large amount of filtrate is absorbed.[123] Expression of AQP-2 is limited early in gestation in the ovine fetus. None was detected in 40-day-old or younger fetuses. It was present in low levels at 64 days; expression increased from 80 through 140 days' gestation, and much more occurred by adulthood. The increased expression of AQP-2 during gestation correlates with the heightened sensitivity of the older fetal kidney to ADH to form a concentrated urine. It is emphasized that this process is physiologic. The purpose of fetal urine is mainly to provide an adequate volume of amniotic fluid. Maximal concentrating ability is not needed. ADH and AQP-2 expressions are low enough to allow continued excretion of high volumes of dilute urine in the fetal kidney.[124]

In summary, fetal renal concentrating ability increases with gestation, but actual concentrating capacity is small, and the impact of ADH on urine concentration is relatively unimportant. Adult and immature subjects differ in tissue sensitivity to ADH, the generation of cAMP, and tubule permeability to salt and urea. However, ADH is present early in gestation, nephrons respond to the hormone, and volume and osmotic responses for ADH release appear to function in the last trimester of pregnancy in the fetal lamb. Therefore the absence of, or nonresponsiveness to, ADH does not explain the limited concentrating ability in the premature or term neonate. A more likely explanation is the inadequate generation and maintenance of a hypertonic medulla. ADH under adverse circumstances helps alter electrolyte and water transfer across the placenta, maintain adequate blood pressure, and redistribute circulating blood volume, all of which would help stabilize fetal circulation. The response to exogenous ADH and the release of ADH in response to adverse stimuli both mature with advancing age. Therefore, although kidneys are not needed to maintain electrolyte balance in utero, fetal kidneys respond to hypoxemia, asphyxia, and volume depletion and probably contribute to electrolyte, volume, osmolar, and blood pressure homeostasis. In late gestation, amniotic fluid volume is regulated by fetal urine and lung fluid production and fetal swallowing. Accordingly, fetal kidneys and ADH may be important for normal fetal and lung development.

URINARY CONCENTRATION IN THE NEONATE

In practical terms, low neonatal concentrating capacity is of little importance unless the infant is given insufficient water to compensate for dietary solute load and high rate of insensible water loss. A low concentrating ability makes the infant more vulnerable to extrarenal water depletion, as occurs in diarrhea, febrile states, and excessive insensible skin loss. The water needs of premature infants are even greater because of higher skin losses, but the higher water intake needed to offset these losses must be provided with care to prevent overhydration since the ability to excrete a water load is limited by a very low GFR until approximately 34 weeks of gestation.

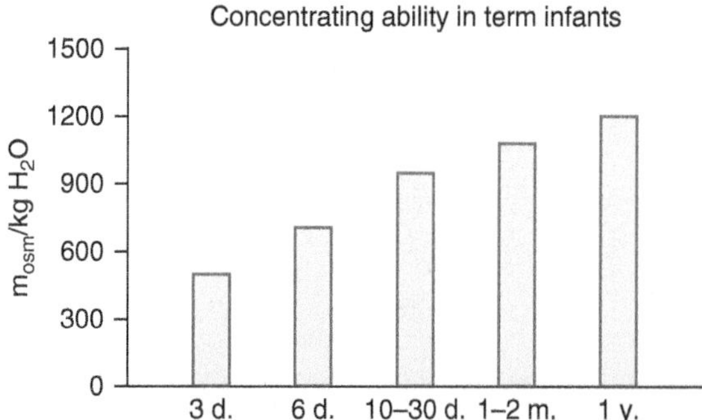

Fig. 102.5 The maximal concentrating ability in healthy infants and children up to 1 year of age. (From Polácek E, Vocel J, Neugebauerová L, et al. The osmotic concentrating ability in healthy infants and children. *Arch Dis Child.* 1965;40:291.)

NEONATAL URINARY CONCENTRATING CAPACITY

In the presence of ADH, human newborn infants produce a urine that is only modestly more concentrated than plasma and much less concentrated than that in the adult.[125-130] Svenningsen and Aronson[129] gave 10 μg of 1-deamino-(8-D-arginine)-vasopressin (DDAVP) to 20 healthy term and preterm infants (30 to 35 weeks' gestational age) and found that by 4 to 6 weeks of age, their mean maximal urinary concentrating capacity was only 565 and 524 mOsm/kg H_2O, respectively, although some infants concentrated urine to greater than 600 mOsm/kg H_2O.[129] Pratt and Snyderman[128] found that premature infants, 11 to 23 days of age, ingesting evaporated milk and small amounts of water, concentrated their urines to a maximal osmolality of 637 to 985 mOsm/kg H_2O.[128] Calcagno and colleagues[125] found that maximal urine osmolality ranged from 588 to 648 mOsm/kg H_2O in five premature infants 5 to 25 days of age after 12 to 18 hours of water restriction.

The striking maturation in concentrating ability has been appreciated from older studies in a larger group of children.[127] Urine osmolality exceeded 600 mOsm/kg within a week of life, was greater than 1000 mOsm/kg H_2O by 1 to 2 months, and was more than 1100 mOsm/kg H_2O by 1 year. Children reached the adult level of maximal urine concentrating ability, 1300 to 1400 mOsm/kg H_2O by 2 years of age (Fig. 102.5).[131] These values are comparable with the concentrating ability of a group of children 2 to 16 years of age reported by Edelmann and colleagues.[132] After nearly 20 hours of standardized water deprivation, these children concentrated urine to a mean osmolality of 1089 mOsm/kg H_2O (range, 873 to 1305 mOsm/kg H_2O), with little change occurring beyond 2 years of age. Clearly, with a urine osmolality of 1000 mOsm/kg H_2O, the 1- to 2-month-old infant is well protected from transient mild to moderate reductions in water intake. In fact, a non-highly concentrated urine of 600 to 700 mOsm/kg H_2O is adequate for the neonate's physiologic needs and would even be adequate for an adult under most clinical circumstances. Physiologic and anatomic factors contributing to a low neonatal renal concentrating capacity are summarized in the next section.

FACTORS LIMITING CONCENTRATING ABILITY IN THE NEONATE

Physiologic Considerations

Fluid Transport in Superficial Nephrons. Micropuncture studies on animal models reveal a maturation in water and solute transport in loops of Henle from superficial nephrons

Table 102.2 Effect of High Protein Intake on Maximal Urine Concentration.

	Protein Intake (g/kg)	Fluid Intake (mL/kg)	BUN (mg/dL)	Urine Osmolality (mOsm/kg H_2O)
Group 1	8.75	115	29	931
	2.3	215	9	571
Group 2	8.4	172	26	844
	2.4	164	9	657

Group 1 included four infants 13 to 38 days old, birth weight 1840 to 2800 g, first on high-protein, low-fluid intake, then on low-protein, high-fluid intake. Group 2 included five infants 7 to 32 days of age, birth weight 1980 to 3620 g, first on high-protein then low-protein diet without altering fluid intake.
BUN, Blood urea nitrogen.
Data from Edelmann CM, Jr, Barnett HL, Stark H, et al. A standardized test of renal concentrating capacity in children. *Am J Dis Child.* 1967;114:639.

Table 102.3 Concentrations of Vasopressin in Newborn Lambs.

	Plasma Vasopressin (μU/mL)	
Condition	**Baseline Values**	**Peak Values**
Hypertonic saline (10 mEq/kg; *N* = 11)	2.9 ± 0.7	22.2 ± 9
Phlebotomy (10 mL/kg; *N* = 10)	1.9 ± 0.4	72.0 ± 40
Dehydration (18 h; *N* = 9)	0.6 ± 0.1	4.8 ± 1.8
Water loading (100 mL/kg; *N* = 7)	3.4 ± 1.2	1.1 ± 0.3

Plasma vasopressin levels in newborn lambs (1 to 7 weeks) change appropriately with above stimuli. Values are mean ± standard error; $P < .05$ for all peak versus baseline values.
Data from Jamison RL, Maffly RH. The urinary concentrating mechanism. *N Engl J Med.* 1976;295:1059.

after birth.[114,133-135] with corresponding increases in osmolality and fractional reabsorption of sodium and chloride along the loop.

Ascending Thin Limb. The ascending thin limb of Henle is highly permeable to chloride, likely related to its chloride channel ClC-K1. By facilitating efflux of NaCl to the interstitium, salt can osmotically induce movement of collecting duct water to the interstitium and increase the osmolality of collecting duct fluid. Failure to express this channel causes diabetes insipidus in the mouse,[68] and the maturation of the channel and the thin ascending limb during development coincides with the increase in concentrating ability.[136] AQP-1 is present in inner medullary tubules by postnatal day 1, but its expression is weak. It increased to reach adult levels by day 14. AQP-2 is present in the premature kidney throughout the inner medullary collecting duct, and its pattern does not change with maturation. Therefore water channels are present to allow for urinary concentration by water abstraction, and chloride channels mature to facilitate solute movement from the medullary ascending thin limb to the interstitium to help establish and maintain a medullary gradient.

Fluid Transport in Collecting Tubules. Unlike the adult, the newborn collecting tubule is unable to maintain an adequate sodium (osmolar) gradient and, consequently, is unable to build a driving force to abstract water efficiently from more distal parts of the nephron.[137]

Urea. The importance of urea to mammalian urinary concentration was recognized nearly by Gamble and colleagues,[138] who noted that adult rats fed urea excreted a more concentrated urine than rats fed a nonurea diet made equimolar by adding inorganic solutes. High-protein diets and urea loads increase urine concentration in the human adult.[139] Urea, a protein metabolic waste product, normally represents approximately 50% of the solute in maximally concentrated urine, but this is not the case in the neonate. Infants and adults have a similar urinary content of nonurea (electrolyte) solute, but the urinary urea solute content of the infant is distinctly lower. Most of the increase in concentrating capacity occurs after birth and can be augmented by dietary alterations.[140,141]

Edelmann and colleagues[132] determined maximal urine concentrating ability in nine full-term and premature infants (7 to 39 days of age) who had been placed on protein-variable diets. Before a protein load, concentrating ability in infants was approximately half that of adults. When given a high-protein diet or a urea load, infants increased their maximal urine osmolality independent of fluid intake or urine output (Table 102.2). The low neonatal concentrating ability seemed to reflect the type of solute available to the renal medulla rather than an intrinsic problem related to the newborn kidney. It was postulated that because the infant is in a highly anabolic state, concentrating ability was limited by the efficient use of protein, which would tend to minimize the amount of urea available to build up a medullary gradient. However, despite the high-protein diet, urine osmolality still did not reach adult levels, and the levels actually reached required an extremely high protein intake (i.e., 8 g/kg) and a very high blood urea nitrogen concentration (up to 45 mg/dL).

It is also evident from other studies that urinary concentrating ability does not depend on diet alone.[142-145] Rane and colleagues[145] found that maximal concentrating ability increased during the third week both in rats who were normally weaned and in those who continued to nurse, indicating that the improvement in concentrating ability was independent of dietary composition or protein content.[145] Also no concomitant change occurred in the serum level of ADH. Therefore the maturational effect is intrarenal. Rather than simply due to an insufficient urea content, the low level of neonatal urinary concentration is more likely related to some difference in the manner in which urea is handled by the kidney. However, the gradual increase in urea synthetic function that occurs during the neonatal period might contribute in part to the progressive increase in concentrating ability.[146]

Response to Vasopressin. The newborn lamb responds to stimuli such as hypertonic saline, water loading, furosemide, dehydration, and blood loss (Table 102.3),[125,147] by appropriately elevating or suppressing ADH levels. The human newborn infant responds to hypertonic saline.[148] Human neonatal concentrating capacity remains limited even in the presence of elevated plasma ADH levels typical of the immediate newborn period in term and preterm infants.[83,107,149-151] Clearly, lack of ADH does not explain a gross reduction in neonatal concentrating ability. Nonetheless, investigators still consider that the neonatal ADH-renal axis may be inadequate because, in the immediate newborn period of the rat, urinary osmolality is lower than papillary tip osmolality, and hormone levels in young animals are further increased (to levels comparable with that of older animals) in response to dehydration. Rather than an insufficient circulating level of ADH, the limited newborn concentrating ability may reflect decreased responsiveness to the hormone or a decreased number of ADH receptors.

Supporting this hypothesis, Schlondorff and colleagues[92,93] found that, in the newborn rabbit, basal adenylate cyclase activity was considerably lower and stimulation of adenylate cyclase by ADH was much less than in the adult. The adult basal level of adenylate cyclase was 2.5 times that of the newborn rabbit. After stimulation with ADH, adult levels increased 10-fold in contrast to the 2.5-fold increase observed in newborn tubules.[92,93] In

Table 102.4 Postnatal Maturation of Vasopressin-Dependent Adenylate Cyclase in Rat Medullary Collecting Tubules.

Age (days)	ΔcAMP Formed in Collecting Tubule (fmol/mm/30 min)
3 (*N* = 4)	203 ± 50 (28%)
28 (*N* = 3)	536 ± 56 (75%)
60 (adult; *N* = 6)	719 ± 68

Values (stimulated minus basal adenylate cyclase activity) are mean ± standard error; response to 1 μM vasopressin in immature rat as percentage of the response of cyclic adenosine monophosphate (cAMP) formed in adult rat tubules given in parentheses. Note progressive sensitivity of tubule cAMP stimulation by vasopressin.

From Imbert-Teboul M, Chabardès D, Clique A, et al. Ontogenesis of hormone-dependent adenylate cyclase in isolated rat nephron segments. *Am J Physiol*. 1984;247:F316.

isolated rat collecting tubules, Imbert-Teboul and colleagues[90] reported a blunted ability of ADH to stimulate adenylate cyclase in the neonate[90] (Table 102.4) and adult levels were reached by day 35.[90] Moreover, several findings in animal models suggest that the cAMP system or the binding properties or response to ADH are immature in the neonate.[91,152,153]

In more recent studies, immature, isolated, perfused cortical collecting ducts were shown to have basal osmotic water permeability similar to mature tubules. However, the increase in water permeability after exposure to ADH was considerably less than that observed in adult tubules. The blunted response of immature tubules to ADH could not be abolished by exposing tubules to the stimulating effect of cAMP or to the inhibition of prostaglandin synthesis by indomethacin. The investigators concluded that, in addition to any impairment in ADH-stimulated cAMP generation or antagonism of cAMP by prostaglandins, there is likely a more distal pathway disruption, perhaps at the level of the basolateral membrane.[110]

Sulyok[154] suggested that the response of a premature infant kidney to ADH may be blunted by the presence of hyponatremia, a state that may occur in the first few weeks of life. Premature infants with "late hyponatremia" show an *increase* in ADH excretion with age, even though their serum sodium levels and osmolality fall and their urine osmolality diminishes as urine flow rate increases. Renal salt wasting and hyponatremia may hinder the establishment of an intrarenal salt gradient at a time when salt, rather than urea, would be the primary medullary solute. Although there might be a delay in maturation of concentrating ability, a blunted response to ADH could minimize the retention of excess water and may thereby serve to limit the severity of the hyponatremia. The late development of hyponatremia in premature infants can be prevented by the administration of supplemental NaCl. Such infants have increased sodium excretion; nevertheless, they are in positive sodium balance and their ADH secretion is increased. The salt supplement appears to enhance ADH secretion with resultant water retention, although this occurs in proportion to salt retention, because serum sodium concentration remains relatively constant.[155]

Aquaporins. AQP-1 is present in rat renal proximal tubules and thin descending limbs of Henle and is expressed in these tissues shortly before birth. However, the amount of renal AQP-1 messenger RNA (mRNA) is decreased in the kidney before and shortly after birth. Significant expression of AQP-1 does not occur until well after birth.[156] Peak levels appear around 3 weeks of postnatal age. AQP-1 is present in both apical and basolateral membranes in an equivalent staining intensity, suggesting that this protein appears simultaneously in both membranes.[157,158] Betamethasone stimulates a modest, yet significant, induction of AQP-1 in neonatal rat kidneys at 4 days of age. Adult rats did not show such a response.[159] By contrast, AQP-1 was detected by immunohistochemical staining techniques in the human fetus at 14 weeks of gestation in a newly developing proximal tubule, and, by 17 weeks, staining was evident in both developing proximal tubules and in newly forming thin limbs from the outer cortex. By 24 weeks, staining was noted in thin limbs of the medulla. At 1 month of postnatal age, AQP-1 immunostaining was prominent over apical and basolateral membranes of proximal tubules and thin descending limbs of Henle.[160] These findings correlate with differences in concentrating ability; the human kidney concentrates urine at birth, and the concentrating ability approaches that of the adult by 1 to 2 months (see earlier discussion); however, the rat concentrates urine primarily at the time of weaning.[145]

In other studies, AQP-1 was observed as early as 12 weeks of gestation in the human fetus, although not at 8 weeks, and was shown to increase steadily to reach 47% of adult levels at birth and 79% of adult levels by 15 months of postnatal age.[161] This coincides approximately to the age when urine concentrating ability reaches adult values. In this study, AQP-1 was initially localized to newly forming proximal tubular structures in the inner cortex. S-shaped bodies, glomeruli, and tubular structures of ureteric bud origin did not stain for AQP-1. By 15 to 20 weeks, proximal tubular structures in the cortex were better differentiated, and staining could be seen to localize mainly in the apical membrane of polarized epithelial cells to include proximal tubules and thin descending limbs of Henle. Basolateral staining, evident in proximal tubules and thin descending limbs in adult kidneys, was not clearly defined in the fetal kidneys, even at 24 weeks' gestation.[161]

Quigley and colleagues[162] reported that in rabbit proximal tubular basolateral membrane vesicles, both the expression of AQP-1 protein and osmotic water permeability were lower in neonates than in adults, although solute permeability (NaCl, $NaHCO_3$) was similar. They concluded that the higher neonatal transepithelial osmotic permeability in the neonate is not related to increased water movement across water channels.

AQP-1 is also present in descending vasa recta of adult kidneys. However, an interesting pattern of distribution of this protein is seen in the developing rat kidney.[163] AQP-1 was found throughout the arterial vascular tree of fetal and neonatal kidneys from 17 days of gestation to 7 days of postnatal age. During the next week, expression regressed and was limited to descending vasa recta. After approximately 3 weeks of age, AQP-1 also appeared in lymphatic vessels. This persisted in adults. The investigators suggest that the transient developmental expression may relate to fluid equilibrium in the developing kidney, or perhaps to a role in regulating fetal growth or branching of the vascular tree.

AQP-2 protein and AQP-2 mRNA have been reported to increase in rats during 10 to 40 days of life and particularly over the weaning period from 15 to 20 days of life, a period of time when urinary concentrating ability dramatically increases. As already mentioned, when rats were exposed to a single injection of betamethasone, which is known to accelerate maturation in other organs, an increase in renal medullary AQP-2 protein and mRNA, as well as in urine osmolality, occurred.[51] In studies of AQP expression during human nephrogenesis, AQP-2 was seen by week 12 of gestation, but not at 8 weeks. In contrast to AQP-1, AQP-2 was found only in structures derived from the ureteric bud. For example, in a 13-week fetal human kidney, AQP-2 stained in apical cell membranes in the collecting system and branching ureteric bud as it extended from the medulla towards the cortex. Comma- and S-shaped bodies, glomeruli, and proximal tubular structures did not stain for AQP-2, and this pattern continued throughout development. Therefore, it was evident from early in gestation that AQP-1 staining was limited to proximal segments and thin descending limbs, whereas AQP-2 was exclusively found in ureteric bud-derived cortical and medullary collecting duct segments.[161]

Bonilla-Felix and Jiang[164] found that AQP-2 expression was reduced in immature rats compared with adults. In addition, there was a close relationship between AQP-2 expression and urinary osmolality in rats receiving ad libitum fluid intake. However, while immature rats increased their AQP-2 content after stimulation by dehydration or exogenous ADH, concentrating ability was not concurrent or equal. Immature rats did show an ability to translocate AQP-2 from intracellular vesicles (during water loading) to plasma membranes (during dehydration or treatment with ADH). Thus, although AQP-2 expression and trafficking were present in immature kidneys, concentrating ability was still limited. It is noteworthy that in the human fetus the pattern of glycosylation of AQP-2 is altered when compared to that in adults. This could explain the ineffective action of AQP-2 in the immature kidney, despite a "normal" protein channel expression and excretion.[161]

Baum and colleagues[165] found expression of AQP-2 (apical membrane) and AQP-3 (basolateral membrane) in rat epithelial cells derived from ureteric bud and collecting ducts. Expression was detected as early as 16 to 18 days of gestation. They also found expression of both AQPs in comparable membranes of collecting ducts in human 3-day-old and adult kidneys. The rat kidneys showed little change in AQP expression over the first 3 days of life, but showed a dramatic (2.5-fold) increase in AQP-2 mRNA by 10 to 14 days of life. Given the presence of fetal and neonatal AQPs, the delay in maturation of maximal concentrating ability in neonates does not appear to be simply related to a lack of water channels. However, the importance of functional AQP-2 protein in neonates was illustrated in an AQP-2 knock-in mouse model of recessive diabetes insipidus. Gene replacement caused a mutant protein leading to death within approximately 6 days of life without supplemental fluid.[166]

In one study, AQP-3 and AQP-4 expression was demonstrated in rat kidney basolateral membrane collecting duct cells after birth, and staining intensity was stable throughout life. By contrast, AQP-2 staining increased with age.[167] In another study, AQP-4 was detected early in the postnatal period of mice and rats, and there was a gradual increase in immunostaining during development.[167] Although the correlation between AQP expression and increasing concentrating ability during maturation may not be unequivocal, a general increase in AQP expression that occurs as concentrating ability matures is clearly seen.[168]

Studies of AQP-2 activity in human developing kidney and during early postnatal life have yielded contrasting results regarding the correlation between urinary AQP-2 excretion and urinary osmolality, especially in preterm infants.[169-172] This is probably due to the heterogeneity of urine collection methods for AQP-2 (random, spot, or once-only measurements, which are considered a poor index of renal vasopressin action).[173]

Based on these studies, it appears that significant variations occur in AQP-2 expression and excretion levels during the first weeks of life in preterm infants. However, AQP-2 does not seem to be a limiting step in the development of urinary concentrating ability after birth.

Prostaglandins. Prostaglandins regulate medullary functions such as blood flow, sodium chloride transport, and water reabsorption. Accordingly, they could play a role in urinary concentration.[174,175] In experimental animals, PGE_2 was found to inhibit sodium chloride transport in the medullary thick ascending limb.[176] PGE_2 antagonizes ADH-mediated water flow across the collecting tubule and bladder,[4] inhibits urea flux across toad bladder epithelium, and decreases urea reabsorption in the rat collecting tubule.[177,178] PGE_2 also can induce renal vasodilation and increase medullary blood flow.[179] These effects tend to wash out a medullary osmolar gradient and decrease maximal concentrating ability. In fact, prostaglandins reduce the corticomedullary osmotic gradient and the medullary solute (salt and urea) content,[180] thereby reducing the driving force for water reabsorption. It has been suggested that increased prostaglandin synthesis in fetal and neonatal kidneys and blood vessels may interfere with neonatal concentrating ability.[181-183] However, the relationship between prostaglandin excretion and maturation of renal function is not firmly established,[184] and a role for prostaglandins becomes clouded when one recognizes that prostaglandin excretion increases with age. Surprisingly, Benzoni and colleagues[185] noted that urinary excretion of PGE increased during the first 24 months of life and correlated linearly with urine osmolality. The overall role of the prostaglandins during maturation of the concentrating mechanism is still debatable. So far at least three different receptors for PGE_2 have been identified. They activate different intracellular signaling mechanisms. For example, the EP3 receptor, which is coupled to an inhibitory guanine nucleotide-binding G protein, inhibits the generation of cAMP when stimulated by PGE_2. Immature collecting ducts have decreased the generation of cAMP when stimulated by ADH. This response is mediated by prostaglandin probably by activating the inhibitory G protein.[186] Receptor mRNA expression was found primarily in the distal nephron (i.e., in medullary thick ascending limbs) as well as cortical and inner medullary collecting ducts. During development, rabbit kidney expression for the EP3 receptor mRNA increased to a maximum at 2 weeks of postnatal age and then decreased to reach adult levels by 8 to 10 weeks of postnatal age.[187] This finding lends credence to the idea that part of the blunted concentrating ability in maturation relates to increased expression of an inhibitory receptor stimulated by PGE_2 that blunts the ability of ADH to stimulate cAMP in collecting ducts.

Renin-Angiotensin System. It has become clear that the renin-angiotensin axis must be intact during nephrogenesis for normal development of urinary concentration. Profound adverse effects on adult renal function occur when the angiotensin-converting enzyme inhibitor enalapril or the angiotensin II type 1 receptor antagonist losartan are given early in neonatal life during nephrogenesis. For example, use of these agents in neonatal rats and piglets causes irreversible histologic changes, including chronic interstitial inflammation and fibrosis, renal vascular changes involving interlobular arteries, and, particularly, profound papillary necrosis. Functionally, such animals present with polyuria and decreased urinary concentrating ability in adult life. The effect on other functions is variable. Proximal tubular fluid reabsorption is reduced, whereas glucose reabsorption, acidifying ability, glomerular filtration, and renal blood flow are largely unaffected.[188-192] The most critical period for renal vulnerability to adverse effects appears to be the first 13 days of life in the rat, coinciding with the duration of continued postnatal nephrogenesis.[189] Of interest, histologic and functional abnormalities were normalized in enalapril-treated rats when they were concomitantly treated with insulin-like growth factor-1, another renal growth-promoting factor.[193] In functional studies, decreased urine concentrating ability was associated with a decrease in negative free-water clearance (T_cH_2O), medullary tissue osmolality, Na, and urea concentration, and density of inner medullary AQP-2. Because density of AQP-2 is higher in the proximal one third than the more distal two thirds of the inner medullary collecting duct located mainly in the papilla, it would seem that the decreased concentrating ability is not wholly due to papillary atrophy.[191]

Anatomic Considerations

Loops of Henle of Deep Nephrons. Maximal concentrating ability directly correlates with the length of long loops of Henle as they descend into the medulla. Species able to develop highly concentrated urine tend to have both longer loops of Henle and a greater proportion of nephrons that send their loops deep into the medulla.[7] In the newborn infant, the length of loops and the renal papillae are relatively short, but they increase during maturation.[112] In the newborn rabbit, the inner medulla and papilla are underdeveloped, but during the first week of postnatal life the medulla becomes larger and the papillae become longer and the improved concentrating ability during development, might reflect the development of these anatomic changes.

Loops of Henle of Short Nephrons. Long loops of juxtamedullary nephrons help determine the degree to which urine can be concentrated, but the shorter loops of superficial nephrons also play a pivotal role in this process.[7,143] These nephrons allow accumulation of urea in the inner medulla by increasing the load and concentration of urea delivered to medullary collecting ducts and recycling urea to minimize its loss from the medulla. Were interstitial urea to enter long loops and vasa recta and leave the medulla, the medullary urea gradient would become depleted. By entering descending limbs of superficial nephrons, urea can recycle to the medulla and maintain the gradient. In fact, the descending limbs of short loops of superficial nephrons, not long loops of deep nephrons, are the ones that accompany vascular bundles of the inner stripe of the outer medulla.

Edwards and colleagues[143] clarified the role of short-loop nephrons in maturation of the concentrating mechanism (Fig. 102.6). In the rat, 40% to 50% of total solute in the adult papillary interstitium is urea. During nephrogenesis, superficial nephrons are the least mature and the last to develop. Their entrance or elongation into the deeper cortical and outer medullary portion of the kidney coincides with improvement in concentrating ability. During the first 16 days of life, the length of the corticopapillary gradient increased 3.4-fold and the superficial nephrons elongated markedly so that they came to cross more than 70% of the outer medulla. During this time, urinary osmolality increased following a period of water deprivation. After maximal penetration of superficial loops to the outer medulla had occurred, urinary concentrating ability increased even more sharply, coincident with a marked increase in papillary tip osmolality and an increase in the proportion of the papillary solute composed of urea. It should be reemphasized that the bulk of filtered fluid is reabsorbed in the cortex. This decreases the amount of fluid delivered to the collecting ducts. Therefore deeper tissues are not faced with the need to reabsorb so much water that the medullary solute gradient would be diluted and dissipated. The arcade segments in the renal cortex appear to play an important role in this regard.

The ability to use urea to enhance urinary concentration matures over the first 3 weeks of life in rabbits and rats.[194,195] For example, Trimble[195] found that an acute exogenous non-diuretic urea load given subcutaneously had no effect on urinary concentrating ability in rats 10 days of age, but it increased the medullary urea content and maximal concentrating ability in rats 20 days of age (Table 102.5). During this time, developmental changes occur in the length of the corticopapillary gradient and the length of superficial loops so that they penetrate well into the outer medulla. In addition, complex vascular bundles appear in the outer medulla, and the diluting capacity of superficial loops of Henle improves.

Renal Inner Medullary Tubule Organization. Liu and colleagues[196] analyzed organization and function of inner medullary tubules during development in isolated perfused tubules from rat kidneys. In thin descending limbs, hydraulic water conductivity was absent on day 1, appeared by day 4, but remained low until day 14 of life. This segment was impermeable to water early in life. Diffusional water permeability of thin ascending limbs was low from day 1 to adulthood, emphasizing low water permeability of this segment. Basal water permeability remained low in inner medullary collecting ducts until adulthood. Water permeability was mildly enhanced by vasopressin in this segment early in life but remained low and only reached adult levels by day 14. Therefore little water reabsorption occurred from these segments early in life.

Urea permeability was low in thin descending limbs throughout development and adulthood. In thin ascending limbs, urea permeability was low but reached two-thirds of adult value by day 14. In the inner medullary collecting duct, basal urea permeability was negligible until day 7 and remained low into adulthood. Vasopressin induced little increase in urea permeability in this segment until day 14, although this value was still less than one third that of the adult (Fig. 102.7). Expression of the urea transporter UT-A1 was not apparent until the late neonatal period. Therefore urea transport contributed little to neonatal urinary concentration. The chloride channel ClC-K1 was expressed in thin ascending limbs from day 1 through adulthood, but it was functionally absent early in life because chloride permeability via this channel was not appreciable. The Na-K-Cl2 co-transporter CCC2 was prominent in the thin ascending limb early in life, similar to that in the thick ascending limb, but it regressed in the thin limb by adulthood to be replaced functionally by the chloride channel. In addition, early in life, transepithelial voltages in the thin ascending limb were inhibited by bumetanide (inhibitor of the Na-K-Cl2 co-transporter in the thick ascending limb) and ouabain (inhibitor of the Na pump), and transepithelial voltages in the inner medullary collecting duct were inhibited by amiloride (inhibitor of Na channel and active electrogenic Na reabsorption). These results indicate capability for active NaCl reabsorption in the thin ascending limb early in life, in contrast to its passive reabsorption in this segment in adults. AQP-1 was observed by day 4 in thin descending limbs and persisted into adulthood, and AQP-2 was present throughout development. These findings, taken with others, indicate that water channels became poised to support water transfer once other medullary relationships are in place. The investigators concluded that there is a fundamentally different organization of the inner medulla between neonates and adults (Fig. 102.8). Early in life, the inner medulla is transiently characterized by active reabsorption and accumulation of NaCl. Compared with that of the adult, the thin descending limb is much less permeant to water. Because the thin ascending limb remains impermeant to water, the neonatal inner medulla is poised to reabsorb NaCl actively without water transfer, allowing urinary dilution early in life. At the same time, the inner medullary collecting duct is not geared to recycle urea. Subsequently, tubular transport properties appear that include increased thin descending limb water permeability, passive NaCl reabsorption in the thin ascending limb with functional maturation of a chloride channel, and increased urea permeability and responsiveness to vasopressin. Efficient urinary concentration requires that these properties be fully effective.

Renal Blood Flow. In the adult kidney, approximately 90% of blood flows through the cortex, 10% perfuses the outer medulla, and 1% to 2% reaches the inner medulla and papilla. This arrangement helps preserve the osmotic gradient established by the countercurrent mechanism. Rapid flow through the medulla tends to dissipate it. Neonatal renal blood flow is proportionately greater to deeper medullary regions of the kidney, and glomerular blood flow is greater in deep than in superficial nephrons.[115-117] After birth, renal vascular resistance drops more than resistance in systemic vessels, cardiac output and surface area increase briskly, and renal blood flow rises. Increases in single-nephron blood flow are proportionally greater in outer than in deep cortical nephrons. A relatively greater medullary flow in neonatal kidneys may delay establishing the corticomedullary gradient.

Renal Pelvis. The renal pelvis in the newborn animal is relatively narrow. As the animal matures, secondary fornices and outpouchings of the renal pelvis come to extend well towards the renal cortex so that urine in the pelvis will bathe a greater

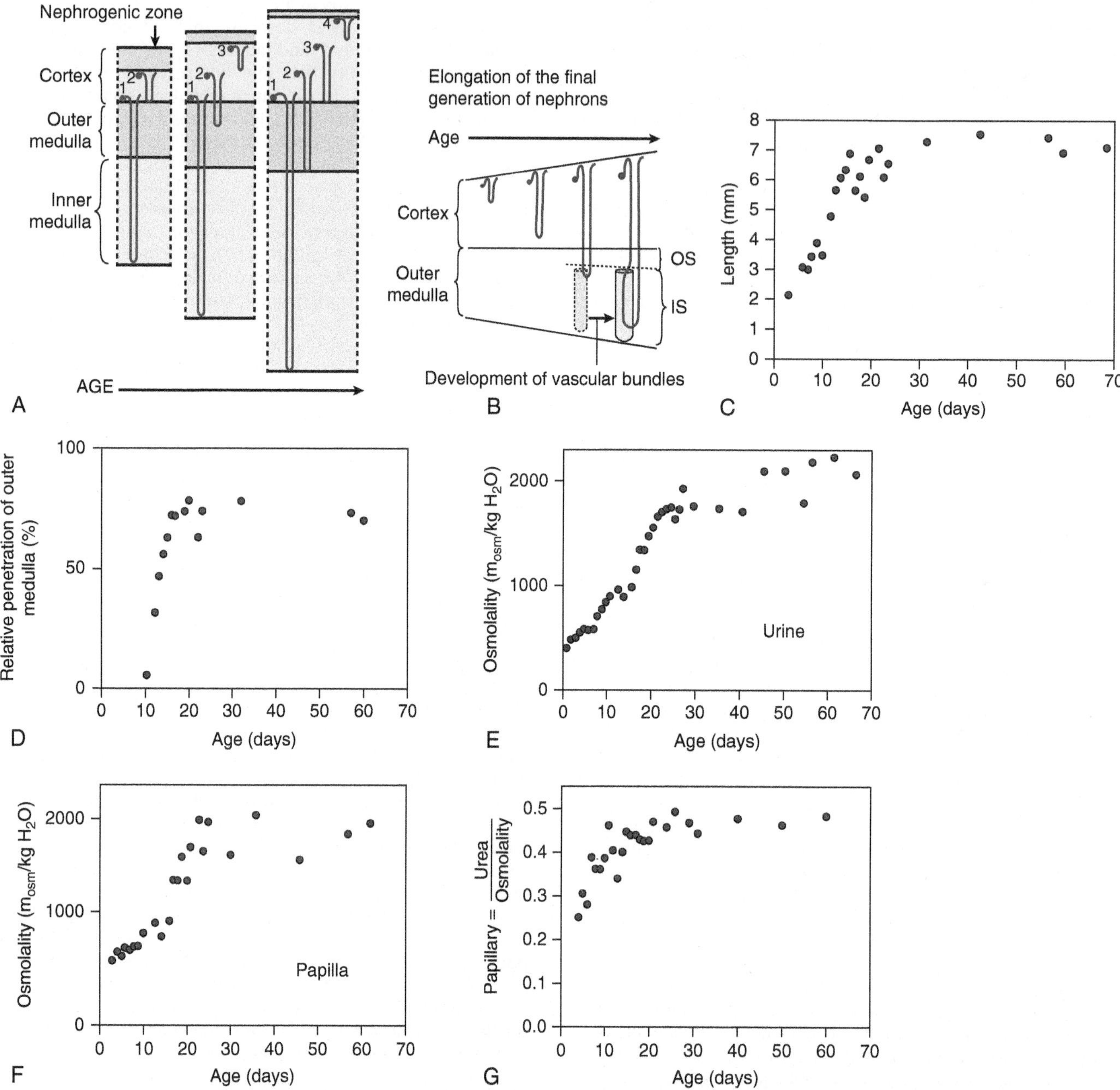

Fig. 102.6 Anatomic maturation of superficial and deep nephrons, penetration of short-looped nephrons toward outer medulla, and maturation of concentrating ability. (A) Simplified scheme of nephrogenesis in the rat. Numbers refer to successive generations of nephrons. (B) Diagrammatic representation of elongation of the loop of Henle belonging to a surface nephron. In the rat, the vascular bundles are recognizable at 20 days of age but not at 10 days. The descending limbs of superficial loops become incorporated with these structures. *IS,* Inner stripe; *OS,* outer stripe. (C) Length of the corticopapillary gradient as a function of age in the rat (*N* = 28). Each point represents a single animal except for days 13, 15, and 18 (2 rats each) and day 14 (3 rats), for which averages are shown. (D) Penetration of outer medulla by superficial loops of Henle. Each point represents a single animal except for day 13 (2 rats) and day 14 (3 rats). An average of three loops per rat was examined. (E) Urinary osmolality, after 8 hours of dehydration, as a function of age in the rat (*N* = 138). Each point represents the average value for one to eight rats (mean rats). (F) Osmolality of the papillary tip, after 8 hours of dehydration, as a function of age in the rat (*N* = 56). Each point represents the average value for one to five rats (mean = 2.3 rats). (G) Fraction of total papillary osmolality contributed by urea as a function of age in 67 rats dehydrated for 18 hours. Length of corticopapillary gradient increases with age, particularly in the first 16 days, corresponding to time of most marked elongation of superficial loops. Urine and papillary tip osmolality increase primarily in the first 3.5 weeks and most steeply after approximately day 16. The proportion of urea composing papillary osmolality increases until adult proportions are reached by approximately 15 to 20 days. (From Edwards BR. Postnatal development of urinary concentrating ability in rats: changes in renal anatomy and neurohypophysial hormones. In: Spitzer A, ed. *The Kidney During Development: Morphology and Function*. New York: Masson; 1982:223–240.)

Table 102.5 Urine Concentrating Capacity in Rats 10 to 20 Days of Age.

	Maximal Urinary Osmolality ($mOsm/kg\ H_2O$)		Urine (Urea) (mmol/L)		Urine/Plasma Osmolar Ratio	
	10 days	**20 days**	**10 days**	**20 days**	**10 days**	**20 days**
Control	938 ± 28	1449 ± 71	469 ± 23	774 ± 49	3.3 ± 0.1	4.8 ± 0.2
Urea load	907 ± 29	1716 ± 59	482 ± 27	1049 ± 70	3.1 ± 0.1	5.5 ± 0.3

Modified from Trimble ME. Renal response to solute loading in infant rats: relation to anatomical development. *Am J Physiol*. 1970;219:1089.

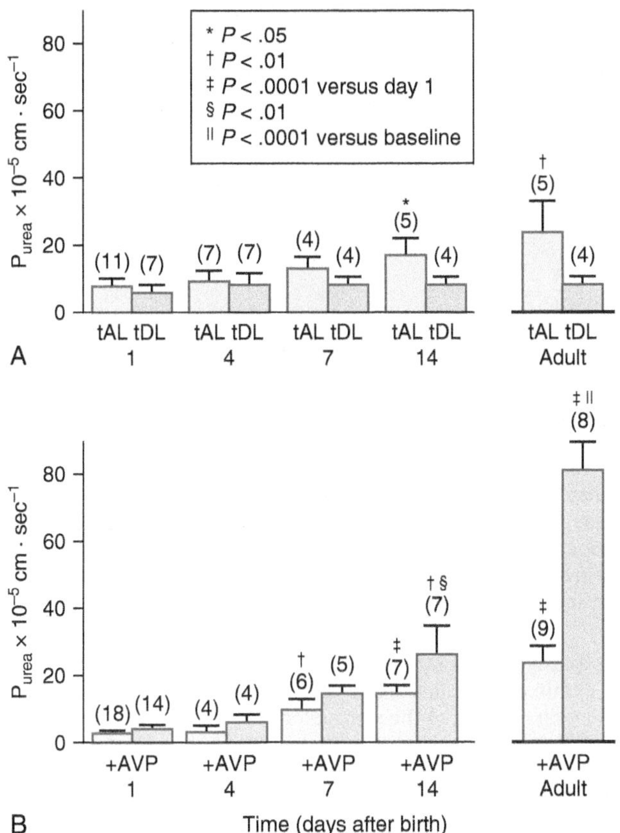

Fig. 102.7 Maturational changes in urea permeability. (A) Urea permeability (Purea) was low through adulthood in thin descending limb *(tDL)* and gradually increased in thin ascending limb *(tAL)*, approaching adult values only by day 14. (B) In the inner medullary collecting duct, basal urea permeability increased by day 7 and increased only mildly thereafter. Vasopressin *(AVP)* stimulated urea transport by day 14, but the value was considerably less than that of the adult. *Number in parentheses* indicates number of tubules examined. (From Liu W, Morimoto T, Kondo Y, et al. "Avian-type" renal medullary tubule organization causes immaturity of urine-concentrating ability in neonates. *Kidney Int*. 2001;60:680.)

part of the papilla.[131,195] As mentioned previously, this pelvic maturation may facilitate recycling of urea from pelvic urine back to medullary interstitium to further increase both interstitial solute concentration and final urine osmolality. ADH appears to have some impact on the growth of the renal medulla and renal pelvis. In young growing lambs, 13 weeks of treatment with DDAVP starting 2 weeks after birth induced an increase in the size of the renal medulla, especially the outer medulla, and the surface area of the renal pelvis. Ruminants have particularly well-developed renal pelvic fornices in their outer medulla. This is the area where dimensions were most impressively enlarged by vasopressin. Therefore the outer medulla may play an important role in the reabsorption and recycling of urea in these animals.[197]

In summary, the low urinary concentrating capacity of newborn mammals is related to a variety of anatomic and functional factors. The loops of Henle are relatively short, the transport properties of the thick ascending limb of Henle are immature, and the number of loops of Henle from more superficial nephrons that penetrate deeper into the cortex and outer medulla is low. Renal blood flow to deeper juxtamedullary nephrons is proportionally greater in the newborn than in the adult. Enhanced prostaglandin production has the potential to reduce salt, water, and urea transport at critical sites and to increase medullary blood flow. These factors may all contribute to the smaller medullary gradient and the lower medullary urea content found in the newborn. Neonatal collecting duct cells have decreased responsiveness to ADH and limited ability to maintain a transepithelial sodium (osmolar) gradient. Pelvic spaces surrounding papillae are narrower and more extensive in adults. This latter anatomic difference may contribute to a low concentrating ability during maturation because urine bathing the papillae may enhance urine and papillary osmolality. AQP-1 may also limit neonatal concentrating ability because the amount of this protein is decreased in the human kidney at birth and increases gradually to approach adult levels at a time when the young kidney concentrates urine nearly as well as the adult. Less likely to play a role is AQP-2 because this protein is not only present in utero at 20 weeks of gestation, but also must be functional as evidenced by the response of the isolated human fetal medullary collecting tubule of similar gestational age to vasopressin.

PHYSIOLOGY OF THE URINARY DILUTING MECHANISM

Urinary dilution is thought to have developed when our primitive ancestors left the briny seas for more freshwater habitats. In so doing, they were forced to develop mechanisms that could separate water from solute to preserve needed solute, eliminate imbibed excess water, and avoid fatal dilution of body fluids. It was considerably later in evolution when creatures had to develop a renal concentrating system to retain water as they traveled from one water environment to another.[198] Diluting capacity is considerable in the human adult, who can excrete 10% to 12% of the filtered load, or approximately 14 to 17 L of water/day if the GFR is 100 mL/min. More water can be excreted with higher rates of filtration. In terms of absolute volume, this capacity is considerably more limited in the infant, although the young subject can excrete 15%, and perhaps more, of the filtered load.

Our ability to dilute urine and remove excess water is more efficient than our ability to concentrate urine and retain needed water. For example, suppose a 70-kg subject has a

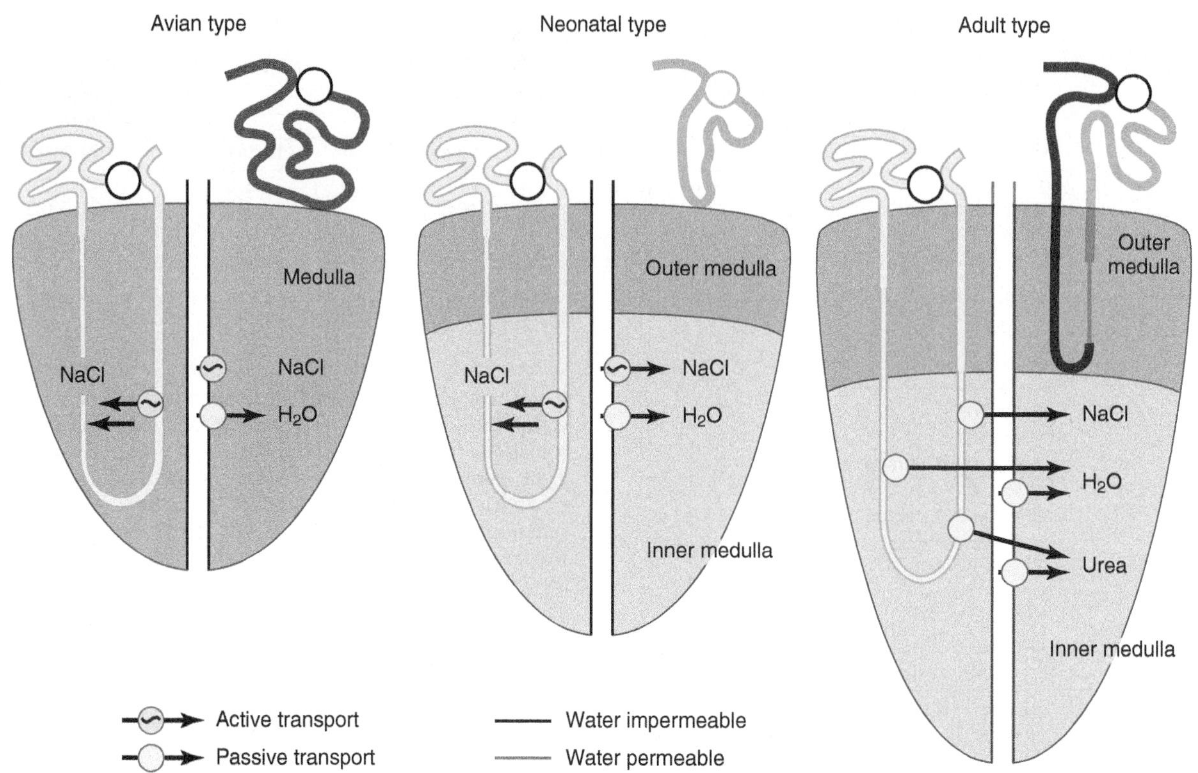

Fig. 102.8 Comparison of neonatal and adult renal medullary tubule organization. In the neonatal kidney, only long-looped nephrons penetrate the medulla, and the medulla has essentially no water movement in the loops of Henle. Medullary NaCl accumulates by active transport in the thin ascending limb, and there is amiloride-sensitive Na reabsorption in the inner medullary collecting duct. During maturation, cortical loops come to penetrate the outer medulla. In addition, NaCl reabsorption becomes passive in the thin ascending limb, collecting duct amiloride-sensitive Na reabsorption disappears, the thin descending limb becomes water permeant, and urea permeability in the inner medullary collecting duct becomes highly sensitive to vasopressin. Neonatal tubule organization is likened to the avian kidney. Delayed maturation of neonatal concentrating ability is related to a more "primitive" tubule organization early in life. (From Liu W, Morimoto T, Kondo Y, et al. "Avian-type" renal medullary tubule organization causes immaturity of urine-concentrating ability in neonates. *Kidney Int.* 2001;60:680.)

serum osmolality of 300 mOsm/kg H_2O and a daily renal solute excretory load of 600 mOsm. If urine osmolality is 300 mOsm/kg H_2O and the 600 mOsm solute load is excreted in 2 L of water, the subject is in water balance because urine is isotonic to plasma and the kidney has neither to concentrate nor to dilute urine to maintain a normal serum sodium level. If the subject is water deprived, urine osmolality can increase to a maximum of approximately 1200 mOsm/kg H_2O. At this urine concentration, 500 mL of water is needed to excrete the 600-mOsm solute load. Stated another way, of the 2 L of water/day needed to excrete this solute isotonically, a maximum of approximately 1500 mL of water/day can be retained to maintain normal serum osmolality; however, 600 mOsm cannot be concentrated in a volume of less than 500 mL. If the subject is water loaded, excess water can be excreted by reducing urine osmolality to a minimum of approximately 50 mOsm/kg H_2O. In this case, the kidney can excrete the 600 mOsm of solute in a urine volume of 12 L and remove 10 L of "pure" water in the process to maintain a normal serum sodium level.

In this example, renal diluting capacity (10 L water) is nearly sevenfold the concentrating capacity (1.5 L water) in terms of actual volume of water handled to maintain osmolar balance. This translates to a 24-fold increase in urine osmolality and urine volume when the urine changes from maximally dilute (osmolality, 50 mOsm/kg H_2O; volume, 12,000 mL) to maximally concentrated (osmolality, 1200 mOsm/kg H_2O; volume, 500 mL). Renal excretory solute loads in children usually range from 10 to 40 mOsm/100 calories expended. Urine volume required to excrete this solute varies with diet and availability of water.[199] Ingested water enters the total body water compartment where it is partly incorporated into new cells during growth. Extra water is eliminated by insensible losses and urine output, the latter allowing removal of the renal excretory solute load. A net excess or deficit of water leads to alterations in electrolyte balance.

When water intake is sufficient to lower serum osmolality by 1% (approximately 3 mOsm/kg H_2O), ADH secretion is suppressed. Solute reabsorption continues in the thick ascending limb, distal nephron, collecting tubule, and collecting duct. The latter segments become less permeable to water when ADH is absent. As a consequence, fluid traversing the distal nephron and entering the medulla becomes progressively dilute. Because water remains in the tubule lumen, urea concentration is reduced, and a major urea concentration difference between collecting duct fluid and interstitium will fail to develop. Because urea permeability in the medullary collecting duct is also decreased in the absence of ADH, urea entering this segment will be more easily excreted. The overall effect is that urea tends to be eliminated from, rather than recycled in, the medullary system. Interstitial as well as urinary urea concentrations decrease, whereas total urea excretion actually increases (but in a larger volume of water).

Reduced tubule permeability to water and continued reabsorption of solute in more distal parts of the nephron might be expected to increase interstitial solute concentrations. However, interstitial solute concentrations are actually reduced compared with the antidiuretic state. It is likely that the water gradient from lumen to interstitium at the medullary collecting duct is high enough to overcome the low water permeability induced by lack of ADH. As a result, reabsorption of water in medullary collecting ducts is actually greater, not less, during water diuresis. Perhaps as much as half the water delivered to collecting ducts back-diffuses into the interstitium, but NaCl is sufficiently reabsorbed along this segment so that the urine actually becomes more dilute.[4,200]

Another factor of potential importance to urinary dilution and water excretion is the reflux of urine around the renal papilla and medulla.[17] The renal pelvis has contractile properties and can induce reflux of urine. Full retrograde pelvic reflux is not typical of the antidiuretic state, but exposure of medullary structures to urine occurs much more often with the high flow rates associated with dilute urine. Urine refluxing into the fornices may actually reduce the amount of urea in the renal medulla. Accordingly, full pelvic reflux may help eliminate a fluid load. Investigators have noted a lack of clear correlation between concentrating ability and size and complexity of pelvic extensions, but a correlation exists between the size of pelvic extensions and the need to excrete a water load. Animals living in arid areas, with little water at their disposal, exhibit a high urinary concentrating ability, but have difficulty excreting a water load rapidly enough to avoid water intoxication and possible death. Such animals do not have large pelvic fornices. Animals that tolerate dehydration, but periodically need water, must be able to eliminate water reasonably rapidly and tend to have large pelvic extensions. Experimental evidence shows that during antidiuresis, water exchanges across the pelvic epithelium and hypotonic fluid can be added to pelvic urine from the medulla to enhance papillary osmolality.[201] It could well be that during water diuresis, water from dilute urine could enter the medulla from pelvic extensions and dilute the medullary interstitium, facilitating excretion of water.

Fluid along the proximal tubule is reabsorbed isotonically and does not directly add to urinary dilution. However, the amount of fluid reabsorbed at this site determines, to a major extent, the volume of dilute urine that can later be formed. A drop in filtration rate or an increase in proximal tubular reabsorption allows less fluid to arrive at the diluting site and therefore will limit the actual amount of water excretion. Some segment must be capable of reabsorbing solute in excess of water to allow luminal fluid to become dilute. This process occurs along the entire length of the ascending limb of Henle, especially along its thick portion. Any problem in solute reabsorption along this site will effectively prevent excretion of dilute urine. After urine passes into the distal nephron, in which solute reabsorption continues, water must remain largely in the lumen. Vasopressin determines the degree to which water will be reabsorbed because the water permeability of collecting duct epithelium depends on the presence of this hormone.

It becomes apparent, then, that to dilute urine, three fundamental conditions must be met. First, a sufficient amount of filtrate must escape reabsorption along the proximal tubule and reach the diluting segment (ascending loop of Henle) to deliver a sufficient amount of potential pure water. Second, this segment must be able to reclaim NaCl and separate reabsorbed solute from water so that urine becomes dilute (water stays in the lumen for excretion). Third, as solute continues to be reabsorbed from more distal sites, further diluting the urine, the ADH-sensitive nephron segments must not be exposed to ADH. Accordingly, urinary dilution results from the active reabsorption of NaCl along the thick ascending limb of Henle and the continued reabsorption of solute along more distal nephron segments in concert with a disproportionate reduction in reabsorption of water. Absence of any of these factors may lead to a defect in urinary dilution.

URINARY DILUTION IN THE FETUS

The human kidney can dilute urine early in fetal life.[131] Urine voided at birth (i.e., formed in utero) is hypotonic compared with the infant's serum. In contrast, maternal urine osmolality is fivefold more concentrated than that of the infant. Urine voided during the first 24 hours after birth becomes more concentrated than serum, but still has an osmolality less than half that of the mother's urine.[202] Amniotic fluid is hypotonic, particularly toward the end of pregnancy. A term fetus ingests substantial amounts of dilute amniotic fluid (approximately 5 mL/kg/h).[203] This value is similar to the estimated urine flow rate of 5 mL/kg/h in primates[75] and is close to the amount of breast milk ingested per day by a healthy newborn infant. A need to excrete this fluid load would account for dilution of fetal urine. Because infants often are not given oral fluid immediately after birth, subsequent concentration of urine represents another appropriate response.[131]

URINARY DILUTION IN THE NEONATE

Although the newborn infant is able to decrease urine osmolality to levels as low as 50 mOsm/kg H_2O,[204-206] the low GFR present at this stage limits the volume of free water that can be formed at the diluting site. This phenomenon is of limited importance beyond a few weeks of age. Although data were not strictly limited to neonates, Rodriquez-Soriano and colleagues[205] found that during periods of maximal free water clearance, urine osmolality in infants dropped to 52 mOsm/kg H_2O on average, and urine flow rates reached nearly 23 mL/dL of glomerular filtration. These infants and children effectively eliminated a water load with minimal impact on serum sodium and osmolality. In this study, fractional delivery of sodium to the distal nephron was high, indicating decreased proximal tubular salt reabsorption. However, reabsorption of salt along diluting segments of the distal nephron increased, indicating that enhanced distal reabsorption compensated for decreased proximal reabsorption. In general, the youngest infants tended to have high rates of delivery of sodium to the distal nephron, but they also had high rates of distal tubular sodium reabsorption. Clearly, at a young age, diluting segments have the potential to reabsorb solute avidly, and ADH-sensitive segments can be inhibited effectively from reabsorbing excess water. Therefore the primary limitation in neonatal water excretion falls largely on the low rates of filtration.

The rapid maturation of an infant's ability to excrete an acute water load was illustrated in a study by Ames.[207] Premature and term infants of different postnatal ages received 30 mL/kg of either an oral water load or an intravenous 2.5% dextrose solution load. Water excretion was initially low (Fig. 102.9). On average, infants in the first 24 hours of life excreted only 10% to 15% of the fluid load in 2 to 3 hours, with only a mild increase by 3 days of age. However, the ability to excrete the water load improved quickly. Infants 8 to 14 days of age excreted 60% of the load, and most infants older than 15 days (and all infants older than 30 days) excreted the total fluid load within 2 hours. One premature infant of birth weight 1.2 kg excreted 50% of an infused fluid load by the fourth day of life and excreted 100% by 12 days of age. Infants older than 7 days of age effectively reduced urine specific gravity to 1.002. The increasing ability to excrete water was associated with a higher GFR. This finding is consistent with the notion that low GFR limits the absolute amount of water that can be excreted.

Calcagno and colleagues[125] found that, 60 minutes after an acute water load, a 1.6-kg, 23-day-old premature infant was able to increase urine flow to 8.3 mL/min/1.73 m^2 (compared with 12 to 14 mL/min/1.73 m^2 in the adult) and to decrease urine osmolality to 50 mOsm/kg H_2O. Barnett and coworkers[204] gave 5 premature infants a 40-mL/kg oral water load. Urine osmolality decreased to 40 to 63 mOsm/kg H_2O. Although their urine flow rates after an hour were, in general, only approximately half that of adults, one 36-day-old premature infant not only diluted the urine maximally, but also had a urine flow rate fully comparable with that of the adult. Clearly, the postnatal maturation of this particular function is fairly rapid.

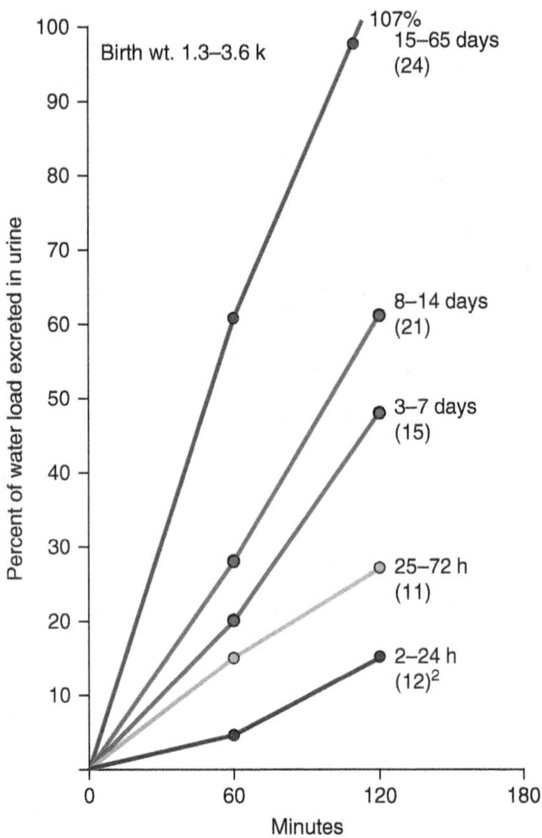

Fig. 102.9 Comparison of ability to excrete water load by infants of various ages after intravenous administration of 2.5% glucose, 30 mL/kg body weight given at −10 to 0 minutes. *Number in parentheses* is number of infants per group. (By permission of *Pediatrics:* Ames RG. Urinary water excretion and neurohypophysial function in full-term and premature infants shortly after birth. *Pediatrics.* 1953;12:272.)

It should be noted that although the ability to excrete an acute water load matures quickly, a sustained water load is more difficult to excrete in infants who have a low GFR and a limited ability to reabsorb solute along the distal nephron.[206] Fortunately, GFR matures relatively early in life and allows efficient elimination of a sustained water load.

In the acutely or chronically water-loaded state, ADH is suppressed. AQP-2 staining becomes more prominent in cytoplasmic vesicles and less so in the apical membrane of collecting ducts. Because AQP-2 is thought to be the actual ADH-sensitive water channel, excretion of a water load is likely made possible largely by acutely removing or more chronically down-regulating water channels from the membrane, thereby reducing apical membrane water reabsorption.[32,33,59] Recovery from the down-regulation of apical membrane water channels will take time because this protein up-regulates its production and membrane content in response to subsequent water restriction.

Torres and colleagues[207] provide a compelling example of potential clinical utility of such observations. In patients with autosomal dominant polycystic kidney disease, cAMP stimulates epithelial cell proliferation and fluid secretion into cysts, leading to cyst enlargement and renal dysfunction. Cyclic AMP is promoted by ADH acting through V2 receptors. Decreasing cyclic AMP may delay cyst/renal enlargement. Water loading can suppress ADH. These investigators suggest that, in patients with this disease and normal renal function, continuous water intake evenly throughout the day may mitigate the effect of cAMP and delay progression towards renal failure.

CONCLUSION

In summary, the dilution of urine depends on the ability to deliver adequate quantities of filtrate to nephron segments that can separate solute from water. More distal segments must be relatively water impermeant. Infants can maximally dilute their urine at an early age. Their ability to excrete an acute water load matures within a few weeks of birth. Limited excretion of large amounts of free water relates to the low GFR present at this age. Diluting capacity is quantitatively greater than concentrating capacity and tends to mature at an earlier age. The range of diluting and concentrating abilities in healthy newborn infants is such that even those of very low birth weight can tolerate a large range of fluid intake without major alterations to their fluid and electrolyte homeostasis.

ACKNOWLEDGMENTS

We acknowledge with great sadness the passing of Dr. Michael Linshaw, the renowned pediatric nephrologist who contributed the "Concentration and Dilution of Urine" chapter to this textbook for several editions. He was a beloved teacher and mentor who enjoyed solving the mysteries of the kidneys. His passion and tenacity for doing so improved the lives of many children and their families.

A complete reference list is available at www.ExpertConsult.com. 

SELECT REFERENCES

1. De Rouffignac C, Jamison RL. The urinary concentrating mechanism. *Kidney Int.* 1987;31:501.
2. Jamison RL, Maffly RH. The urinary concentrating mechanism. *N Engl J Med.* 1976;295:1059.
3. Kokko JP, Rector Jr F. Countercurrent multiplication system without active transport in inner medulla. *Kidney Int.* 1972;2:214.
4. Roy DR, Jamison RL. Countercurrent system and its regulation. In: Seldin D, Giebisch G, eds. *The Kidney: Physiology and Pathophysiology*. New York: Raven Press; 1985:903–932.
5. Knepper MA, Roch-Ramel F. Pathways of urea transport in the mammalian kidney. *Kidney Int.* 1987;31:629.
6. Kokko JP. The role of the collecting duct in urinary concentration. *Kidney Int.* 1987;31:606.
7. Jamison RL. Short and long loop nephrons. *Kidney Int.* 1987;31:597.
8. Lemley KV, Kriz W. Cycles and separations: the histotopography of the urinary concentrating process. *Kidney Int.* 1987;31:538.
9. Hebert SC, Reeves WB, Molony DA, Andreoli TE. The medullary thick limb: function and modulation of the single-effect multiplier. *Kidney Int.* 1987;31:580.
10. Fenton RA, Knepper MA. Urea and renal function in the 21st century: insights from knockout mice. *J Am Soc Nephrol.* 2007;18:679.
11. Timmer RT, Klein JD, Bagnasco SM, et al. Localization of the urea transporter UT-B protein in human and rat erythrocytes and tissues. *Am J Physiol Renal Physiol.* 2001;281:C1318.
12. Trinh-Treng-Tan MM, Lasbennes F, Gane P, et al. UT-B1 proteins in rat: tissue distribution and regulation by antidiuretic hormone in kidney. *Am J Physiol Renal Physiol.* 2002;283:F912.
13. Soroka SD, Chayaraks S, Cheema-Dhadli S. Minimum urine flow rate during water deprivation: importance of the nonurea versus total osmolality in the inner medulla. *J Am Soc Nephrol.* 1997;8:880.
14. Gowrishankar M, Lenga I, Cheung RY, et al. Minimum urine flow rate during water deprivation: importance of the permeability of urea in the inner medulla. *Kidney Int.* 1998;53:159.
15. Kamel KS, Cheema-Dhadli S, Shafiee MA, Halperin ML. Dogmas and controversies in the handling of nitrogenous wastes: excretion of nitrogenous wastes in human subjects. *J Exp Biol.* 2004;207:1985.
16. Zimmerhackl BL, Robertson CR, Jamison RL. The medullary microcirculation. *Kidney Int.* 1987;31:641.
17. Schmidt-Nielsen B. The renal pelvis. *Kidney Int.* 1987;31:621.
18. Bonventre JV. Renal papillary epithelial morphology in antidiuresis and water diuresis. *Am J Physiol.* 1978;235:F69.
19. Pfeiffer EW. Comparative anatomical observations of the mammalian renal pelvis and medulla. *J Anat.* 1968;102:321.
20. He J, Yang B. Aquaporins in renal diseases. *Int J Mol Sci.* 2019;20(2).
21. Nielsen S, Frøkiaer J, Marples D. Aquaporins in the kidney: from molecules to medicine. *Physiol Rev.* 2002;82:205.
22. Agre P, Preston GM, Smith BL. Aquaporin CHIP: the archetypal molecular water channel. *Am J Physiol.* 1993;265:F463.

23. Maeda Y, Smith BL, Agre P, Knepper MA. Quantification of aquaporin-CHIP water channel protein in microdissected renal tubules by fluorescence-based ELISA. *J Clin Invest*. 1995;95:422.
24. Nielsen S, Pallone T, Smith BL. Aquaporin-1 water channels in short and long loop descending thin limbs and in descending vasa recta in rat kidney. *Am J Physiol*. 1995;268:F1023.
25. Preston GM, Smith BL, Zeidel ML, et al. Mutations in aquaporin-1 in phenotypically normal humans without functional CHIP water channels. *Science*. 1994;265:1585.
26. King LS, Choi M, Fernandoz P, et al. Brief report: defective urinary concentrating ability due to a complete deficiency of aquaporin-1. *N Engl J Med*. 2001;345:175.
27. Ma T, Yang B, Gillespie A. Severely impaired urinary concentrating ability in transgenic mice lacking aquaporin-1 water channels. *J Biol Chem*. 1998;273:4296.
28. Schnermann J, Chou CL, Ma T. Defective proximal tubular fluid reabsorption in transgenic aquaporin-1 null mice. *Proc Natl Acad Sci U S A*. 1998;95:9660.
29. Chou CL, Knepper MA, Hoek AN. Reduced water permeability and altered ultrastructure in thin descending limb of Henle in aquaporin-1 null mice. *J Clin Invest*. 1999;103:491.
30. Brown D. Membrane recycling and epithelial cell function. *Am J Physiol*. 1989;256:F1.
31. Harris HWJ, Strange K, Zeidel ML. Current understanding of the cellular biology and molecular structure of the antidiuretic hormone-stimulated water transport pathway. *J Clin Invest*. 1991;88:1.
32. Marples D, Knepper MA, Christensen EI, Nielsen S. Redistribution of aquaporin-2 water channels induced by vasopressin in rat kidney inner medullary collecting duct. *Am J Physiol*. 1995;269:C655.
33. Nielsen S, Chou CL, Marples D. Vasopressin increases water permeability of kidney collecting duct by inducing translocation of aquaporin-CD water channels to plasma membrane. *Proc Natl Acad Sci U S A*. 1995;92:1013.
34. Katsura T, Ausiello DA, Brown D. Direct demonstration of aquaporin-2 water channel recycling in stably transfected LLC-PK1 epithelial cells. *Am J Physiol*. 1996;270:F548.
35. Marples D, Christensen S, Christensen EI, et al. Lithium-induced downregulation of aquaporin-2 water channel expression in rat kidney medulla. *J Clin Invest*. 1995;95:1838.
36. Frokiaer J, Marples D, Knepper MA, Nielsen S. Bilateral ureteral obstruction downregulates expression of vasopressin-sensitive AQP-2 water channel in rat kidney. *Am J Physiol*. 1996;270:F657.
37. Marples D, Frøkiger J, Dørup J, et al. Hypokalemia-induced downregulation of aquaporin-2 water channel expression in rat kidney medulla and cortex. *J Clin Invest*. 1996;97:1960.
38. Earm JH, Christensen BM, Frøkiaer J. Decreased aquaporin-2 expression and apical plasma membrane delivery in kidney collecting ducts of polyuric hypercalcemic rats. *J Am Soc Nephrol*. 1998;9:2181.
39. Sands JM, Flores FX, Kato A. Vasopressin-elicited water and urea permeabilities are altered in IMCD in hypercalcemic rats. *Am J Physiol Renal Physiol*. 1998;274:F978.
40. DiGiovanni SR, Nielsen S, Christensen EI, Knepper MA. Regulation of collecting duct water channel expression by vasopressin in Brattleboro rat. *Proc Natl Acad Sci U S A*. 1994;91:8984.
41. Nielsen S, Digiovanni SR, Christensen EI, et al. Cellular and subcellular immunolocalization of vasopressin-regulated water channel in rat kidney. *Proc Natl Acad Sci U S A*. 1993;90:11663.
42. Sands JM, Naruse M, Jacobs JD, et al. Changes in aquaporin-2 protein contribute to the urine concentrating defect in rats fed a low-protein diet. *J Clin Invest*. 1996;97:2807.
43. Fernández-Llama P, Andrews P, Turner R, et al. Decreased abundance of collecting duct aquaporins in post-ischemic renal failure in rats. *J Am Soc Nephrol*. 1999;10:1658.
44. Kwon TH, Frøkiaer J, Knepper MA, Nielsen S. Reduced AQP1, -2, and -3 levels in kidneys of rats with CRF induced by surgical reduction in renal mass. *Am J Physiol*. 1998;275:F724.
45. Cadnapaphornchai MA, Kim YW, Gurevich AK, et al. Urinary concentrating defect in hypothyroid rats: role of sodium, potassium, 2-chloride co-transporter, and aquaporins. *J Am Soc Nephrol*. 2003;14:566.
46. Deen PMT, Verdijk MA, Knoers NV. Requirement of human renal water channel aquaporin-2 for vasopressin-dependent concentration of urine. *Science*. 1994;264:92.
47. Deen PMT, Van Aubel RA, vab Lieburg AF, van Os CH. Urinary content of aquaporin 1 and 2 in nephrogenic diabetes insipidus. *J Am Soc Nephrol*. 1996;7:836.
48. Elliot S, Goldsmith P, Knepper M, et al. Urinary excretion of aquaporin-2 in humans: a potential marker of collecting duct responsiveness to vasopressin. *J Am Soc Nephrol*. 1996;7:403.
49. Zelenina M, Christensen BM, Palmér J, et al. Prostaglandin E(2) interaction with AVP: effects on AQP2 phosphorylation and distribution. *Am J Physiol Renal Physiol*. 2000;278:F388.
50. Kasono K, Saito T, Saito T, et al. Hypertonicity regulates the aquaporin-2 promoter independently of arginine vasopressin. *Nephrol Dial Transplant*. 2005;20:509.

Urinary Acidification 103

Seth L. Alper | George J. Schwartz

INTRODUCTION

The functions of the fetal kidney in utero remain little understood. Prior to delivery, the placenta regulates fetal homeostasis of salt and water, and fetal acid-base balance in the context of the acid load generated by intrauterine metabolism and growth. The fetal kidney in utero generates the amniotic fluid that contributes to fetal pulmonary development and provides mechanical protection to the enlarging fetus. Parturition marks the abrupt beginning of the fetal transition to extrauterine life, accompanied by transfer of the responsibility for organismal homeostatic regulation from the maternal placenta to the fetus' own regulatory mechanisms, including those of the kidney. This transition is accompanied by initiation of breathing and by rapid increases in blood pressure, cardiac output, and renal blood flow, as well as by the start of postnatal nephron maturation. Although human nephrogenesis is complete by 36 weeks gestation, the neonatal kidney continues to mature in many ways during the first 1 to 2 years of life before it achieves adult-level function as scaled to body mass. This chapter will review the neonatal kidney's handling of systemic acid-base balance, after briefly reviewing urinary acidification mechanisms of the adult kidney. Acid-base regulation by the neonatal and postnatal kidney has been the subject of several recent reviews.[1-6]

URINARY ACIDIFICATION MECHANISMS IN THE ADULT

Acid-base buffering in the body is accomplished by the volatile CO_2/HCO_3^- buffer system, with lesser contribution from fixed buffers, including phosphates, ammonium, citrate, and the proteins, proteoglycans, and numerous mobile buffers of cells and extracellular fluids. The 2 million glomeruli of the two human adult kidneys generate 150 to 180 L of glomerular filtrate each day. This filtrate contains 4000 mmoles of HCO_3^- that must be recovered to sustain systemic buffering and to provide one-carbon equivalents for biosynthetic pathways. Eighty percent of

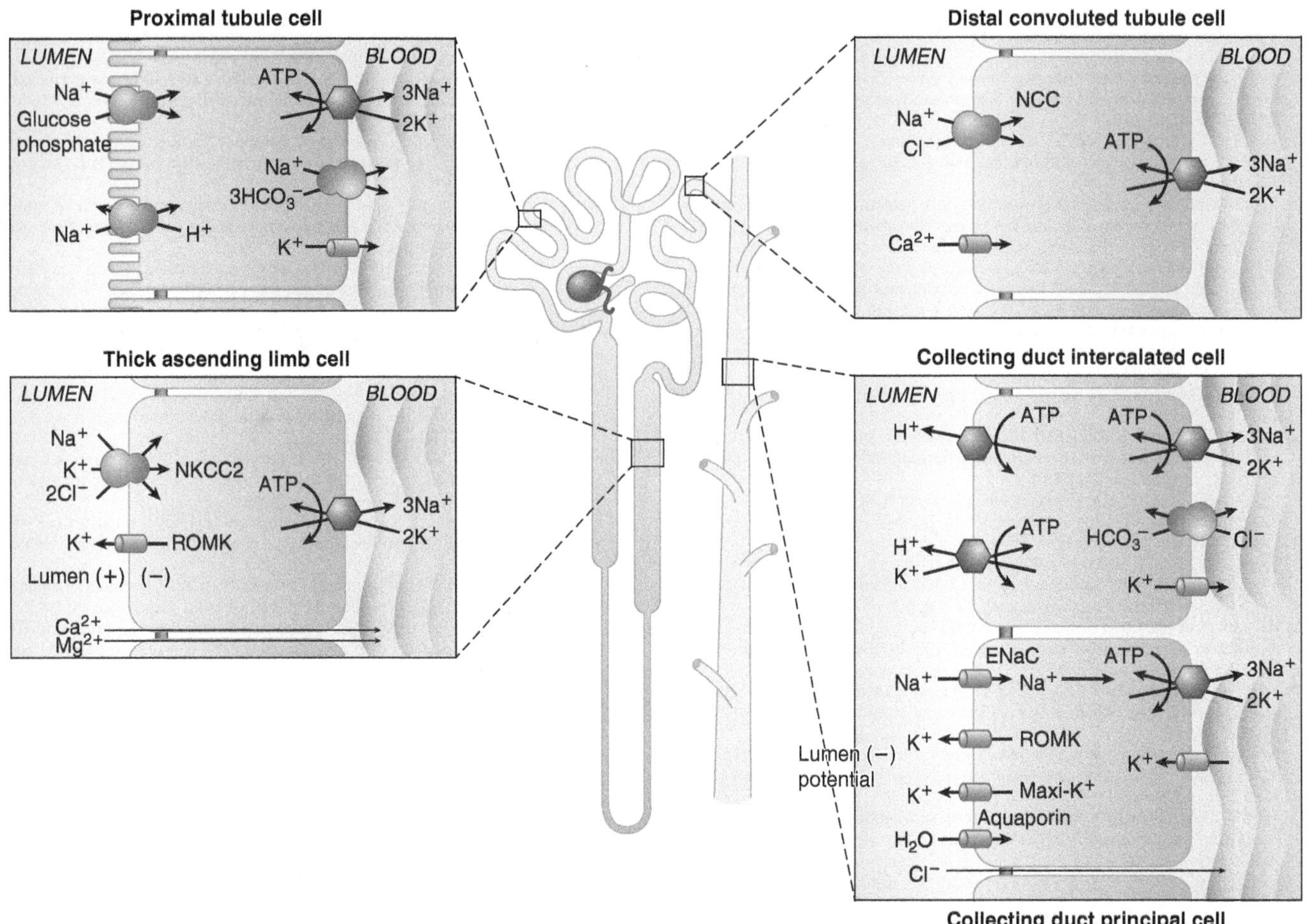

Fig. 103.1 Structure of adult nephron, without the surrounding renal vasculature. The glomerulus *(red)* provides glomerular filtrate to the proximal tubule. The tubular fluid then passes through descending and ascending thin limbs, the medullary and cortical thick limbs, the distal convoluted tubule and (not labeled) connecting segment, and the collecting duct, with cortical, outer medullary, and inner medullary segments. *ATP,* adenosine triphosphate; *NCC,* sodium chloride co-transporter. (Modified from Hoenig MP, Zeidel ML. Homeostasis, the milieu interieur, and the wisdom of the nephron. *Clin J Am Soc Nephrol.* 2014;9[7]:1272–1281.)

this HCO_3^- reclamation is accomplished by the proximal tubule, with the remainder reabsorbed by the thick ascending limb (TAL) and less quantity by downstream nephron segments (Fig. 103.1). The adult body on a regular Western diet also generates approximately 50 to 70 mmoles of protons from metabolism that must be excreted by the kidney to avoid uncompensated neutralization of HCO_3^-, with its resultant loss to the environment through pulmonary exhalation of CO_2. This process is mediated by secretion of H^+ into the urinary space by the type A intercalated cells of the collecting duct, which also reabsorb molar equivalent HCO_3^- newly generated in the process (see Fig. 103.1). The secreted proton equivalents are trapped by the major urinary buffer ammonium, with smaller buffering contributions from phosphate, citrate, and other organic ions.

ACID-BASE REGULATION IN THE MATURE PROXIMAL TUBULE

HCO_3^- reabsorption by the proximal tubule is carried out largely in the convoluted segments S1 and S2 (Fig. 103.2A), whereas the proximal straight tubule (S3 segment) preferentially reabsorbs chloride.[7] The proximal tubule reabsorbs 70% to 90% of filtered HCO_3^-, mostly via transcellular ion transport. Paracellular transport across tight junctional barriers via claudins 10a and 17 accounts for most of reabsorbed Cl^-, whereas claudin 17-assisted paracellular transport contributes up to 20% of reabsorbed HCO_3^- and to a portion of paracellular Cl^- transport.[8] As shown in Fig. 103.2A, the microvillar apical membrane of the proximal convoluted tubule secretes protons to acidify the urinary space. Proton secretion is mediated 65% by the sodium/proton exchanger NHE3/SLC9A3 and 35% by the complex multisubunit vacuolar H^+-ATPase. The glomerular filtration rate (GFR) likely helps to regulate this bicarbonate reabsorption through both mechanisms, because both are stimulated by axial fluid flow.[9] The secreted proton and the tubular fluid HCO_3^- are converted, with the catalytic assistance of the glyosylphosphatidylinositol-linked carbonic anhydrase IV of the apical membrane, to CO_2, which diffuses into the proximal tubular cell, and OH^-, which is instantaneously buffered in the tubular fluid.

The CO_2 in the proximal tubular cell cytoplasm encounters abundant cytosolic carbonic anhydrase II, which regenerates intracellular HCO_3^-. This newly regenerated HCO_3^- serves as substrate, along with cytosolic Na^+ imported from the tubular fluid by the action of NHE3 and other proximal tubular sodium/solute co-transporters, for the bicarbonate efflux transporter of the proximal tubular basolateral membrane, NBCe1A/SLC4A4. NBCe1 operates with a stoichiometry of 2 to 3 HCO_3^- per 1 Na^+. This stoichiometry, in the presence of proximal tubular cells' highly negative intracellular voltage and elevated intracellular concentrations of Na^+ and HCO_3^-, favors efflux of Na^+ and HCO_3^- from cytosol into basolateral interstitial fluid, and on

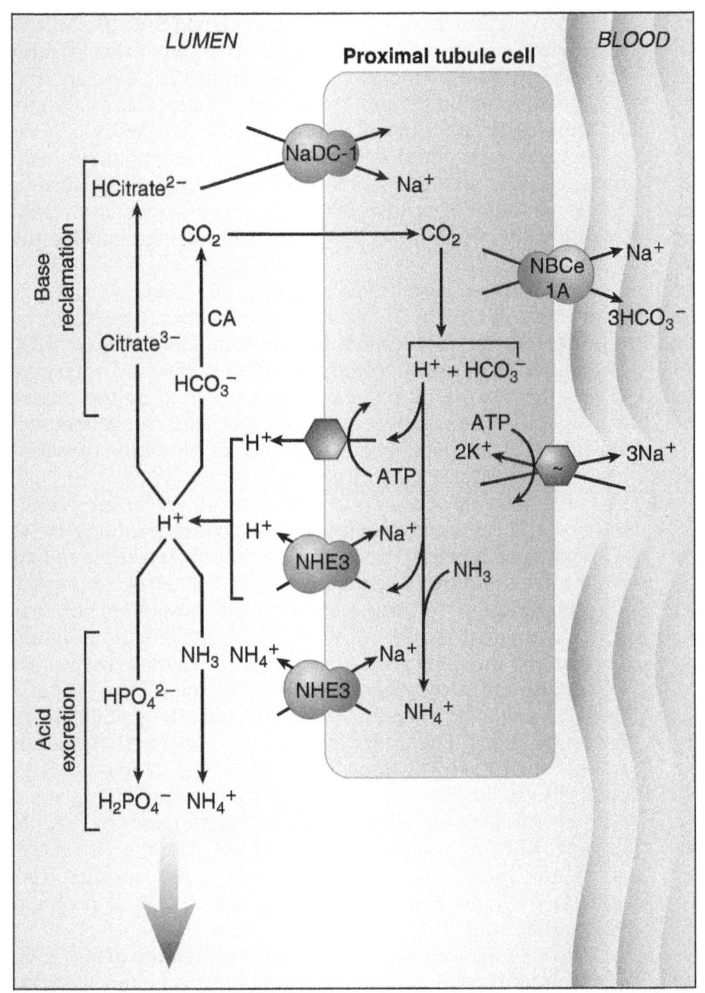

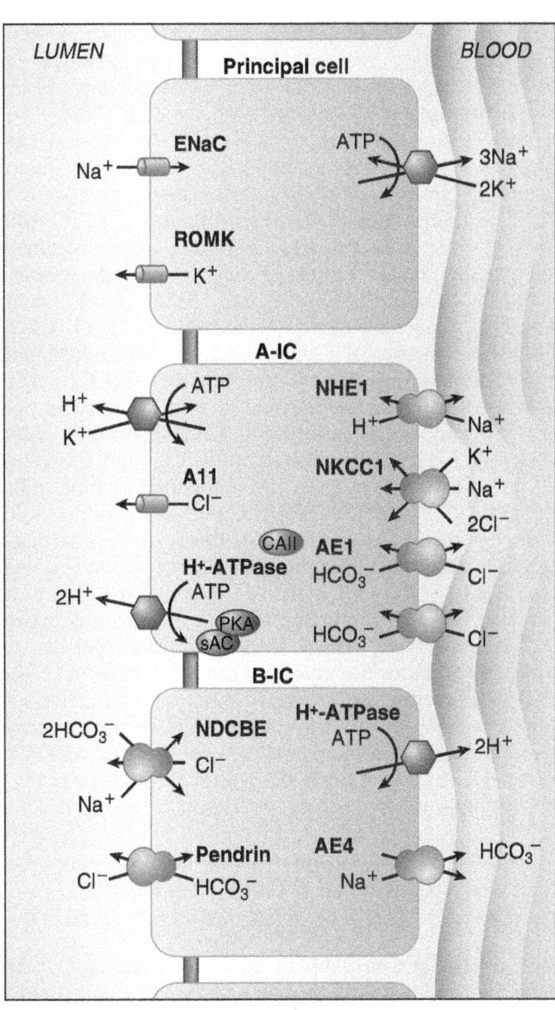

A B

Fig. 103.2 Nephron cell types regulating systemic acid-base balance. (A) Proximal tubule cell from the S1 or S2 convoluted segment. Apical membrane NHE3 and vH+-ATPase secrete protons into luminal fluid. Most protons serve to protonate bicarbonate with the catalytic help of carbonic anhydrase in the luminal membrane. Protons are also buffered by phosphate, ammonium, and citrate. Reclamation of tubular citrate is another source for regeneration of bicarbonate. Cytosolic bicarbonate exits the cell into the interstitium via the basolateral membrane NBCe1A. The entire process of bicarbonate regeneration and reabsorption is powered by the basolateral membrane Na^+,K^+-ATPase. Proximal tubular cells also take up and use glutamine as a source for ammonium biosynthesis and secretion. This ammonium is important for collecting duct acid secretion. (B) Cortical collecting duct cell types are arranged in a mosaic of principal cells (PCs) and intercalated cells (ICs) of A and B types. The A-IC secretes protons to acidify the urine via the apical vH^+-ATPase, and the intracellular bicarbonate so generated exits the basolateral membrane via chloride-bicarbonate exchanger AE1. The B-IC secretes bicarbonate under conditions of dietary base load via the B-IC–specific chloride-bicarbonate exchanger, pendrin. However, under usual conditions of acid load, the B-IC is dedicated to reabsorption of luminal chloride accompanied by Na^+, with apical recycling of bicarbonate. The basolateral $Na^+(K^+)$ HCO_3^-/Cl^- exchanger AE4/SLC4A9 may function in basolateral Na^+ egress from type B ICs, which express low levels of Na^+,K^+-ATPase. The PC reabsorbs tubular fluid Na^+ through the amiloride target, ENaC, secretes K^+ via the ROMK K^+ channel, and reabsorbs water through the vasopressin-regulated water channel, aquaporin 2. Although not itself secreting acid-base equivalents, the principal cell can regulate IC function directly and via paracrine mechanisms. (A, From Curthoys NP, Moe OW. Proximal tubule function and response to acidosis. *Clin J Am Soc Nephrol.* 2014;9:1627–1638. B, From Roy A, Al-Bataineh MM, Pastor-Soler NM. Collecting duct intercalated cell function and regulation. *Clin J Am Soc Nephrol.* 2015;10:305–324.)

across the fenestrated endothelial cells of peritubular capillaries back into the systemic circulation. Additional contributors to the electrochemical gradient favoring HCO_3^- reabsorption from lumen to blood include the basolateral membrane electrogenic Na^+,K^+-ATPase and basolateral membrane K^+ channels. By the end of the proximal tubule, luminal pH has decreased from the original glomerular filtrate value of 7.4 down to 6.8 to 6.9.[7]

Proximal tubular HCO_3^- reabsorption can be inhibited by the carbonic anhydrase inhibitor diuretic, acetazolamide. Potent and specific diuretics are not available clinically for NBCe1A or for the voltage-dependent (v)H^+-ATPase. Tenapanor, a potent and specific inhibitor of gut NHE3 engineered to be nonabsorbable, has entered clinical use for treatment of systemic fluid overload by reduction of intestinal Na^+ uptake.[10,11]

The proximal tubule also generates all the ammonium found in the final urine.[7] Proximal tubular cells take up glutamine and shuttle it to the mitochondria, where each glutamine undergoes two sequential deaminations by glutaminase and glutamate dehydrogenase. The two ammonium molecules generated exit the mitochondria as NH_3 via AQP8 into the cytosol. Two bicarbonates are also generated. The cytosolic pH (alkalinized by elevated HCO_3^- and NH_3) has been postulated to stimulate NHE3 to carry NH_4^+ from cytosol into luminal fluid. (However, NH_4^+ is excreted by alternate pathways in two models of NHE3 knockout mouse.[12,13])

Proximal tubular ammonium production and secretion are enhanced during metabolic acidosis by increased levels of glutaminase and glutamate dehydrogenase secondary to stabilization of the messenger RNAs (mRNAs) encoding these enzymes in response to the fall in intracellular pH.[7] The normal increase in proximal tubular NH_3 generation in response to hypokalemia requires expression of Na^+/HCO_3^- co-transporter NBCe1.[14]

The proximal tubule also reabsorbs nearly all the phosphate filtered by the glomerulus. Reabsorption at the proximal tubular luminal membrane occurs primarily via the electroneutral NaPi-2c/SLC34A3 (1 HPO_4^{2-} per $2Na^+$), with smaller contributions by electrogenic NaPi-2a/SLC34A1 (1 HPO_4^{2-} per $3Na^+$), electroneutral Pit-2/SLC20A2, and paracellular phosphate reabsorption. Inhibition of gut luminal NHE3 by the NHE3 inhibitor, tenapanor, can be used to control intestinal phosphate uptake during maintenance hemodialysis[11] through reduction of paracellular phosphate absorption.[15] Although the identities of the phosphate exporters of the basolateral membrane have not yet been confirmed,[7,16] XPR1/SLC53A1 is a strong candidate.[17]

In response to systemic acidosis, the proximal tubule increases uptake of glutamine (largely via basolateral membrane SNAT3/SLC38A3), with increased generation of ammonium by increased activity of glutaminase and glutamate dehydrogenase. Na^+/H^+ exchanger NHE3 is translocated from its vesicular storage sites under the apical membrane to fuse with the apical microvillar membrane, where it is subject to further activation. Citrate reabsorption by apical Na^+/citrate co-transporter NaDC-1/SLC13A2 is increased in response to acidosis, whereas phosphate reabsorption is decreased through direct inhibition and internalization of NaPi-2c and -2a.[7,16]

ACID-BASE REGULATION IN THICK ASCENDING LIMB AND DISTAL TUBULE

The TAL may reabsorb up to 20% of filtered HCO_3^-. As in the proximal tubule, apical activities of carbonic anhydrase IV and Na^+/H^+ exchanger NHE3 work together to mediate CO_2 entry into the epithelial cells. As in the proximal tubule, cytoplasmic carbonic anhydrase 2 can catalyze regeneration of HCO_3^- from the CO_2. Multiple basolateral efflux mechanisms for HCO_3^- in TAL cells include AE2/SLC4A2 Cl^-/HCO_3^- exchanger and a yet undefined K^+/HCO_3^- co-transport mechanism. The basolateral membrane also hosts Na^+-HCO_3^- co-transporters and Na^+/H^+ exchangers NHE1 and NHE4 to regulate HCO_3^- absorption. Metabolic acidosis increases TAL bicarbonate reabsorption, whereas metabolic alkalosis decreases it. Bicarbonate reabsorption is inhibited by medullary hypertonicity but stimulated by hypotonicity.[18]

The TAL also participates in urinary acidification through its role in uptake of the NH_4^+ generated in and secreted by the proximal tubule. This luminal NH_4^+ uptake is via multiple K^+ pathways such as the bumetanide-sensitive NKCC1/SLC12A2 Na^+-K^+-$2Cl^-$ co-transporter and the ROMK/KCNJ1 K^+ channel. NH_4^+ leaves the basolateral membrane to enter the medullary interstitium on Na^+/H^+ exchanger NHE4, SLC12 K-Cl co-transporters, and K+ channels. This interstitial NH_4^+ is then ready for secretion by the collecting duct.[18]

The distal convoluted tubule reabsorbs a small component of filtered bicarbonate through apical proton secretion via the Na^+/H^+ exchanger, NHE2.[19] This component can be enhanced in the setting of metabolic acidosis.

ACID-BASE REGULATION IN THE MATURE COLLECTING DUCT

The type A intercalated cells of the collecting duct (see Fig. 103.2B) are responsible for terminal urinary acidification.[20] Proton secretion is powered by the vH^+-ATPase of the apical membrane, a complex multisubunit H^+ pump[21] that harnesses the energy from adenosine triphosphate (ATP) cleavage by its V1 cytosolic subunit complex, through a molecular rotary motor that drives H^+ translocation along routes transiently generated by several proteolipid subunits of its V0 membrane-spanning complex. The vH^+-ATPase can generate a theoretical maximum proton gradient of nearly 1000-fold, to yield a maximum urinary acidification of pH 4.5 to 5.0 while maintaining cytosolic pH at 7.5 to 7.6.

The ability to sustain such a steep pH gradient is required to excrete the 50 to 70 mmol of mineral acid generated each day from dietary intake and metabolism. The cytosolic HCO_3^- remaining after apical proton secretion must be transported across the basolateral membrane to the blood by the action of the Cl^-/HCO_3^- exchanger, kAE1/SLC4A1, and the generation of H^+ and HCO_3^- at the needed rates requires the action of cytosolic carbonic anhydrase 2 (see Fig. 103.2B).

In the absence of urinary buffers, the minimal urine pH of 4.5 to 5 would be rapidly achieved, and proton pumping by vH^+-ATPase would reach steady state without secreting the total proton load required to achieve systemic acid-base homeostasis. This is the important role played by the ammonium generated in the proximal tubule, as well as any phosphate and sulfate that might have escaped the proximal tubular reabsorption mechanism: to allow continued net acid secretion without the need to generate a maximal transluminal pH gradient at high energetic cost. The proximal tubule-generated ammonium reabsorbed by the TAL (largely via apical NKCC1 and basolateral NHE4) into the medullary interstitium is taken up across the type A intercalated cell basolateral membrane by the NH_3 channel RhBG/SLC42A2. Intracellular NH_3 can then be released across the apical membrane by the related NH_3 channel RhCG/SLC42A3[22,23] into the urinary space, where NH_3 is protonated and trapped as NH_4^+.

Metabolic acidosis leads to increased expression of vH^+-ATPase, carbonic anhydrase 2, and AE1/SLC4A1 in type A intercalated cells. However, the immediate response of these intercalated cells to acute acidosis is massive exocytic insertion of apical membrane containing preformed vH-ATPase, emptying out the acidic vesicle contents and secreting continuously generated H^+ into the urinary space. This process is additionally controlled by cyclic adenine monophosphate (cAMP)-regulated protein kinase A and by cyclic guanosine monophosphate (cGMP) generated by Ca^{2+}-dependent soluble guanylate cyclase, among other regulatory pathways, including metabolic regulator AMPK and pH-sensitive kinase Pyk2. Acid secretion by type A intercalated cells is also regulated by angiotensin II, aldosterone, P2 purinergic receptors, the prorenin receptor (a vH^+-ATPase assembly factor), and the CaSR calcium-sensing receptor.[6,20,24]

Under conditions of dietary alkali load or metabolic alkalosis, type A intercalated cells down-regulate their acid-secretory mechanism, and the type B intercalated cells are activated to secrete bicarbonate via the apical Cl^-/HCO_3^- exchanger, pendrin/SLC26A4.[25,26] In response to chloride load, pendrin in type B cells coordinates its activity with other type B cell transporters to recycle bicarbonate while promoting transepithelial reabsorption of chloride.[27] Pendrin is regulated by acid-base status, chloride delivery, and angiotensin II. Pendrin is also regulated by an incompletely understood protein kinase C–mediated mechanism through activation of OXGR1, an apical receptor of the type B cell that binds α-ketoglutarate released by upstream proximal tubular cells.[28,29] Favorable electrochemical gradients for apical HCO_3^- secretion by type B cells are maintained by the basolateral vH^+-ATPase.[30]

The principal cells of the collecting duct are involved with Na^+ reabsorption and K^+ secretion. Principal cell ENaC Na^+ channel–mediated Na^+ reabsorption, by generating a lumen-negative electrical potential, can regulate vH^+-ATPase activity. ENaC also regulates pendrin activity by mechanisms less well understood. Systemic regulation of principal cell K^+ secretion requires coordination with flow-sensitive K^+ secretion by intercalated cells. In addition, principal cell K^+ secretion may influence type A intercalated cell H^+/K^+-ATPase activity, which can exploit K^+ reabsorption or recycling to drive additional H^+ secretion.[31] The several proposed mechanisms of acid-base sensing by intercalated cells[32] will undergo reevaluation in light of recent novel evidence that strongly supports a central sensing and intermediary signaling role for principal cells in the regulation of intercalated cell acid/base secretion.[33] Moreover, intercalated cells have recently been demonstrated to regulate principal cell water homeostasis.[34]

EARLY KIDNEY DEVELOPMENT

The nephrotome arises from *Osr1/Lhx1*-positive intermediate mesoderm of the urogenital ridge as early as 3 weeks gestation, differentiating first into *Pax2/Pax8*-positive pronephros/nephric duct, and then into transient mesonephric tubules after week 5. Starting at week 6, the metanephric duct gives rise to the metanephric mesenchyme and ureteric bud.[35] The ureteric bud differentiates into distal nephron segments, while ureteric bud induction of metanephric mesenchyme leads to differentiation of glomerular structures and proximal nephron structures. This differentiation process proceeds through a stereotypic process of complex nephron patterning precisely coordinated with lineage specification and restriction, and with maturation of specialized cell types that will later mediate specified subsets of the many functions of the mature nephron.[36,37]

These processes involve induction and repression of coordinate transcription of sets of genes under epigenetic controls that remain poorly understood.[38] Metanephric kidney structures first make urine and mediate a degree of tubular solute reabsorption by week 13 of gestation. Nephrogenesis is completed by week 34 to 36 of a normal gestation, with 60% of nephrons generated during the third trimester. However, nephron maturation continues through the early postnatal period and afterward.

GLOMERULOVASCULAR DEVELOPMENTAL CONTEXT OF URINARY ACIDIFICATION

Adult GFR is 100 to 120 mL/min. The GFR of 0.5 mL/min at 28 to 34 weeks gestation increases to 1 mL/min at 34 to 37 weeks, then to 2 mL/min by 40 weeks. Normalized to body surface area, this GFR is equivalent to approximately 30/mL min in an adult. The fetal kidney is perfused with only 2% of cardiac output (normalized to body surface area) between midgestation through preterm, with normalized neonatal renal perfusion 15% to 20% that of the adult kidney. Neonatal renal function is predominantly influenced by renal structural maturity,[39] governed by gestational age and additional exposure to injury and/or drug treatment.[40] During the first postnatal week, the proportion of cardiac output directed to the kidney reaches mature levels of 15% to 20%, but during the subsequent 1 to 2 years of postnatal life, GFR normalized to body surface area increases fourfold to finally achieve adult levels.[41] Renal perfusion increases in parallel, reflecting increased glomerular surface area without further increase in glomerular number, accompanied by redistribution of renal blood flow to the cortex from the medulla, reflecting decreased renocortical vascular resistance.[5]

Increasing tubular flow accompanying increased renal blood flow and GFR regulates mature tubular function and very likely is important in promoting its maturation. This maturation of tubular transport processes is clinically and developmentally apparent in most nephron segments, and is described segment-by-segment later in this chapter. Urinary acidification has not been extensively studied in human neonates. Human amniotic fluid is largely fetal urine, and its pH between 7.0 and 7.5 suggests that fetal urinary acidification is minimal if not absent during development. Term infants increase net acid excretion appropriately in response to an NH_4Cl acid load during the first month of life, whereas preterm infants born at gestational ages 29 to 36 weeks demonstrate reduced net acid excretion that normalizes by the third week of extrauterine life.[42-44] This acquisition of the ability to respond to an acid load is accompanied by the expression before or shortly after birth of renal ion transport proteins that contribute to renal acid-base regulation.

PROXIMAL BICARBONATE REABSORPTION IN THE NEONATE

Metabolic acidosis is common in premature or low-birth-weight infants, with serum bicarbonate values as low as 14.5 mM and with a median value of 19.5 mM.[42,45] Such low serum bicarbonate values contrast with those normally present in term infants (19 to 21 mM) and children (24 to 28 mM). These differences in serum bicarbonate reflect changes in the renal bicarbonate threshold (defined as that plasma $[HCO_3^-]$ at and beyond which HCO_3^- begins to appear in the urine) and are determined by maturation of the proximal tubular reabsorption of filtered bicarbonate. Another determinant may be changes in the proportion of birth weight contributed by extracellular fluid (typically 40% to 60%). Perinatal urine pH may be alkaline, reflecting some bicarbonate wasting and chloride retention. However, normal postnatal diuresis reduces extracellular fluid volume to less than 30% of body weight, accompanied by gradual acidification of the urine. In contrast, premature or low-birth-weight infants exhibit minimal urinary bicarbonate excretion, despite the low renal bicarbonate threshold, in association with extracellular volume contraction.

Nearly every element of proximal tubular ionic homeostasis must undergo postnatal maturation, as judged from studies in experimental animals. Neonatal ion transport rates tend to be low and are generally up-regulated at time of weaning, in parallel with the maturational increase in GFR.[46] This up-regulation is often dependent on the action of glucocorticoids and thyroid hormone, which increase at time of weaning.[5,47] For example, the basolateral membrane Na^+,K^+-ATPase that powers all active transport exhibits relatively low activity in newborn rabbits and newborn rodents and increases three- to fourfold in magnitude in the rabbit proximal tubule after weaning.[48] This process has been attributed to the action of weaning-associated elevations in glucocorticoids and thyroid hormone, leading to increased transcriptional activation of $\alpha1$ and $\beta1$ subunits of the Na^+,K^+-ATPase.

The isolated perfused proximal tubule from a juxtamedullary nephron of a rabbit 1 week of age displays a rate of bicarbonate reabsorption only one third that of the adult proximal tubule.[5,46] That low reabsorption rate is maintained until weaning at age 4 weeks. By age 6 weeks, bicarbonate reabsorption in rabbit proximal tubules is at the adult level. Although the adult proximal tubular apical membrane relies on both NHE3 and vH^+-ATPase for the luminal acidification needed to drive HCO_3^- reabsorption, the fetal and neonatal proximal tubules of rabbit express very low levels of vH^+-ATPase activity. A total of 95% of luminal acidification in neonatal proximal tubule can be attributed to Na^+/H^+ exchange, and all maturation through the time of weaning is accounted for by increased Na^+/H^+ exchange activity (threefold as measured in isolated perfused tubules, fourfold as measured in brush border membrane vesicles).[5,47] However, unlike the NHE3 of adult proximal tubule, neonatal proximal tubular Na^+/H^+ exchange activity is mediated largely or entirely by the neonatal isoform, NHE8. At the time of birth, NHE3 is active and localized to the proximal tubular brush border. During postnatal maturation under the influence of thyroid hormone, NHE8 is progressively internalized to intracellular compartments while NHE3 expression increases, with substantial increase in abundance and activity at time of weaning.[49] The maturational decrease in NHE8 is mediated by posttranscriptional regulation under the control of thyroid hormone. The coincident maturational and weaning-associated increase in NHE3 is stimulated by glucocorticoids, and prenatal delivery of glucocorticoids leads to early transcription and membrane insertion of NHE3, accompanied by accelerated development of adult levels of Na^+/H^+ exchange activity. Glucocorticoid administration just prior to delivery leads to a doubling of NHE3 abundance.[5,47]

The NHE8-NHE3 maturational transition has recently been studied in detail in neonatal knockout mice.[49] The abundance of NHE3 mRNA, total protein, and brush border membrane protein in NHE8 knockout mouse kidney was unchanged from control levels. Similarly, the abundance of NHE8 mRNA, total protein, and brush border membrane protein in NHE3 knockout mouse kidney was unchanged from control levels. However, both NHE3 and NHE8 knockout mice exhibited the same degree of reduction in proximal tubular NHE activity. Despite the reduced Na^+/H^+ exchange activity, NHE3 knockout mice at 7 days of age responded to subacute metabolic acidosis of 1 week's duration with increased NHE8 protein and Na^+/H^+ exchange activity, and comparably treated NHE8 knockout mice increased NHE3 protein and transport activity. Thus either transporter alone can partially fulfill the needs of proximal tubular bicarbonate reabsorption. Although NHE8 plays little or no role in the normal adult proximal tubule, NHE8 does undergo compensatory up-regulation in adult NHE3 knockout mice.[50]

Adult levels of proximal tubular carbonic anhydrase activity have been reported in human fetal kidney of 26 weeks gestation.[51,52] However, cytosolic carbonic anhydrase II in rabbit proximal tubule increases 10-fold between postnatal weeks 1 and 12 and in rat kidney increases 8-fold from the time of birth until achieving adult levels at age 7 weeks. Membrane-associated carbonic anhydrase IV also increases up to 10-fold after birth. In contrast to the substantial developmental changes in isoform expression and magnitude of activity of Na^+/H^+ exchangers and carbonic anhydrases, the proximal tubular basolateral membrane Na^+-bicarbonate co-transport activity in rabbit neonates was nearly as high as that in adults.

The developmental changes in transepithelial bicarbonate reabsorption are attributed almost entirely to changes in transcellular uptake because transepithelial resistance of the neonatal proximal tubule is higher than in the adult, with lower paracellular permeability. The low paracellular resistance of the adult proximal tubule is characterized by expression of claudins 1, 2, 10a, and 12.[53] In contrast, the neonatal proximal tubule expresses these as well as the additional claudins 6, 9, and 13. Claudins 6 and 9 have been shown to increase transepithelial resistance and to decrease paracellular anion permeability in heterologous expression experiments using confluent monolayers of MDCK dog kidney cells grown on filter supports. The elevated transepithelial resistance of neonatal proximal tubule has thus been attributed to expression of claudins 6 and 9.[5,54,55]

Phosphate plays an important role as a urinary buffer increasing net acid excretion in the urine. Human neonates have higher levels of serum phosphate than do adults, reflecting a proximal tubular reabsorption maximum for phosphate that is twofold higher than that in adults, as normalized to kidney mass. Neonatal fractional excretion of phosphate is only 0.2% for the first 36 hours of life, then increases to nearly 7% within 1 week after birth. The fractional excretion of phosphate in adult urine is 10% to 20%. A similar developmental phenomenon has been observed in rats, in which Na^+-phosphate co-transporter NaPi-2a is the major route of proximal phosphate reabsorption, rather than the Na^+-phosphate co-transporter NaPi-2c, as in humans.[7] Weaning of rats is accompanied by decreased NaPi-2a expression in proximal tubule and by increased urinary phosphate excretion. Tubular epithelial cell phosphate levels are lower than in adults during the first postnatal week, suggesting enhanced basolateral phosphate exit into the interstitium by still undefined pathways.[5,16,55]

Unlike the Na^+-dependent reabsorption of the fixed buffer phosphate, Na^+-dependent reabsorption of amino acids, glucose, urate, and oxalate all exhibit maturational increases that approximately parallel those of bicarbonate reabsorption. The maturational pattern of citrate reabsorption has not been reported, but in adult mice, Na^+-citrate co-transporter and urinary citrate excretion are regulated by expression of the proximal tubular sodium-bicarbonate co-transporter NBCe1-A.[56] Studies of maturation of bicarbonate reabsorption by neonatal TAL or distal convoluted tubule have not been reported.

DISTAL PROTON SECRETION IN THE NEONATE

In addition to reclamation of filtered bicarbonate, the neonate must excrete the acid equivalents generated by rapid growth and metabolism, as well as those released during active osteogenesis and calcification that accompanies postnatal growth. Thus the kidney in the postnatal period must excrete up to twice the number of acid equivalents per kg body weight as does the adult kidney. However, neonatal and postnatal net acid excretion (urinary ammonium + titratable acid/kg) is limited by delayed maturation of proximal tubular glutaminase and glutamine synthase activity. The need for acid excretion can be lowered in nursing infants by the lower contents of protein, phosphate, and acid in human milk than in infant formula, cow milk,[57] or goat milk.[58]

The excretion of mineral acid equivalents is the task of the A-type intercalated cells of the renal connecting segment, cortical collecting duct, and medullary collecting duct. Intercalated cells have been detected in the normal human fetal medullary collecting duct by 8 weeks gestation and were found throughout subsequent gestation, with highest abundance in the inner medulla.[59] Cortical intercalated cells were few at 18 and 25 weeks gestation and minimally increased by 36 weeks gestation. Intercalated cells had a poorly differentiated phenotype during early development. Type A intercalated cells constituted the majority of medullary intercalated cells at 26 and 36 weeks gestation. During the postnatal period, intercalated cells increased in abundance in the cortex but disappeared from the inner medulla.

In the postnatal mouse cortex, vH^+-ATPase subunits, AE1, and pendrin mRNA and protein increased in abundance from postnatal day 3 to days 18 and 24. Cortical collecting duct type A and non-type A cells both increased in number over this time, but the localization of vH^+-ATPase in these cells became progressively less apical, possibly reflecting development of additional regulatory pathways.[60]

Pendrin-positive intercalated cells first appear in mouse kidney in connecting segments at embryonic day 14, then in medullary collecting duct at embryonic day 17 to 18, where they are present at birth. Pendrin-positive intercalated cells appear in the mouse cortical collecting duct during the first week of postnatal life, in cortical collecting duct by day 4, and in medullary collecting duct by day 7. However, in medullary collecting duct, pendrin-positive intercalated cells undergo gradual apoptosis during the first 2 to 3 weeks of postnatal life, after which time they are absent from inner and outer medullary collecting duct.[60,61] Similar developmental patterns of intercalated cells were observed in embryonic and postnatal rat kidney.[62] In kidneys of postnatal age 18 weeks subjected to mild or moderate obstruction, intercalated cells increased further in abundance and apparent differentiation state. However, in the setting of severe obstruction and at later postnatal times, the number of intercalated cells was reduced.[59]

Expression of RhBG and RhCG polypeptides paralleled type A-intercalated cell development in the developing rat kidney.[22] The multiple subunits of the vH-ATPase show a more complicated developmental pattern. The ubiquitous subunits (present in all cell types) are detectable early in mouse nephrogenesis, at embryonic day 13.5, and expression remains stable throughout subsequent nephrogenesis. However, the intercalated cell-specific subunits were detected only after embryonic day 15.5, following induction of Foxi1,[63] a transcription factor with properties of a master regulator of intercalated cell differentiation.[64] Foxi1 is also involved in differentiation of mitochondria-rich acid-base regulatory cells in mouse epididymis[65] and in amphibian and fish skin ionocytes.[66]

The ancestral cell type(s) that give rise to mature intercalated cells during embryonic development have been the subject of intense debate. The immature collecting duct of Foxi1 knockout mice was characterized by a single hybrid cell type expressing both the principal cell marker AQP2 and intercalated cell marker carbonic anhydrase 2,[64] suggesting such a cell type as a possible physiologic precursor of mature intercalated cells. Indeed, genetic deficiency of carbonic anhydrase 2 also leads to reduced intercalated cell number.[67] More recent genetic lineage marker studies in mouse kidneys have shown that both intercalated cell types can arise from AQP2-expressing progenitor cells (and/or from mature principal cells),[68] a finding to be further tested in lineage-marked mice of still greater specificity.[69] The transcription factor TP63 is necessary but not sufficient for generation of intercalated cells from the ureteric bud tip.[70] The Notch signaling pathway also plays an important role in specifying coordinated development of principal and intercalated cells, as well as determining physiologically regulated proportions of intercalated cell subtypes in the cortical collecting duct.[71] Additional regulatory factors implicated in the regulated differentiation of intercalated cells include the transcription factor TFCP2L1,[72] the histone H3 K79 demethylase DOT1L,[73] the Notch regulator ADAM10,[73] the Notch signaling pathway components RBPJ and presenilins 1 and 2,[74] and the E3 ubiquitin ligase Mib1, required for initiation of Notch signaling.[75] It is likely that additional transcription factors and pathways determining intercalated cell differentiation and development remain to be elucidated, and these further studies will certainly be aided by the new analytic methods of single cell RNA sequencing[76] as validated by single tubule RNA sequencing.[77]

HEREDITARY DISORDERS OF ACID-BASE BALANCE

Mutations in eight genes have been reported to cosegregate with Mendelian forms of familial renal tubular acidosis (Table 103.1).[78-80] Autosomal recessive proximal tubular acidosis is caused by loss-of-function mutations in the proximal tubular basolateral Na^+/HCO_3^- co-transporter, NBCe1/SLC4A4. The syndrome is often accompanied by anterior ocular abnormalities, less frequently by poor dentition, and occasionally by pancreatic dysfunction.

Autosomal recessive and autosomal dominant forms of distal renal tubular acidosis are caused by loss-of-function mutations in the type A intercalated cell basolateral membrane Cl^-/HCO_3^- exchanger, kAE1/SLC4A1. The autosomal dominant forms are either dominant negative trafficking mutants that retain the wild-type gene product in the endoplasmic reticulum or the Golgi apparatus, or trafficking mutants that accumulate exclusively or nonexclusively in the apical membrane, where they function to partially neutralize apical H^+ secretion. Most recessive forms of mutant AE1 are nondominant trafficking mutants or protein-destabilizing mutants, but a minority of recessive mutants exhibit loss of transport function without polypeptide destabilization.[78]

Autosomal recessive distal renal tubular acidosis is also caused by loss-of-function mutations in ATP6V1B1 and perhaps also ATP6V1C2, the B1 and C2 cytosolic domain subunits of the vH^+-ATPase, as well as in ATP6V0A4, the a4 transmembrane domain subunit of the vH^+-ATPase. ATP6V1B1 mutations are usually accompanied by congenital or early-onset deafness, the latter by variable penetrance deafness of later onset.[78,79,81] Recessive mutations in the master transcriptional regulator of collecting duct cell differentiation, FOXI1, also cause distal renal tubular acidosis with deafness.[82] In addition, recessive mutations in the vH^+-ATPase binding protein, WDR72, have been found to cosegregate with distal renal tubular acidosis in patients with amelogenesis imperfecta.[81,83]

A syndrome of combined proximal and distal tubular acidosis is caused by autosomal recessive mutations in carbonic anhydrase II, which plays crucial roles in transport of acid-base equivalents across both proximal tubular cells and collecting duct intercalated cells. This syndrome is accompanied by osteopetrosis and cerebral calcifications with variable intellectual developmental disability[84] and can, as with other causes of renal tubular acidosis, increase propensity to urinary tract infection.[85] Type A intercalated cells are sources of antimicrobial peptides lipocalin-2 and RNAse 4,[86] as well as of peptide defensins.[87]

Several other hereditary disorders are often but not invariably accompanied by renal tubular acidosis (see Table 103.1). Proximal tubular acidosis contributes to the presentations of autosomal dominant generalized proximal tubular dysfunction (Fanconi syndrome) caused by a mistargeting mutation in the peroxisomal gene product enoyl-coA hydratase/3-hydroxyacyl-coA dehydrogenase (EHHADH) that misdirects the protein to mitochondria,[88] or caused by mutations in the mitochondrial gene product glycine amidinotransferase (GATM) leading to intramitochondrial precipitation of the mutant protein.[89] Autosomal dominant Fanconi syndrome accompanied by the atypical Fanconi phenotypes of hypercalciuria and nephrocalcinosis is caused by heterozygous mutations in the transcription factor hepatocyte nuclear factor 4A (HNF4A, in which distinct mutations cause type 1 maturity-onset diabetes of the young).[90]

Several additional hereditary syndromes variably present with or include metabolic acidosis (see Table 103.1). A recessive mutation in the proximal tubular Na^+-phosphate co-transporter NaPi-2A has been shown to cause an incomplete Fanconi syndrome with rickets[91] but without metabolic acidosis (and for this reason excluded from Table 103.1). Additional examples include the X-linked proximal tubular disorders of Dent disease (caused by mutations in the endo/lysosomal Cl^-/H^+ exchanger CLCN5), Dent-2 disease and Lowe syndrome (caused by mutations in the phosphatidylinositol phosphatase gene OCRL1), and the autosomal recessive Donnai-Barrow syndrome (caused by mutations in the broad-specificity receptor for endocytosis LRP2/megalin).[92]

Pseudohypoaldosteronism type 1 in its autosomal dominant renal form is caused by loss-of-function mutations in the mineralocorticoid receptor, and in its autosomal recessive multiorgan form is caused by loss-of-function mutations in any one of the three subunits of the ENaC sodium channel of collecting duct principal cells. Pseudohypoaldosteronism type 2 (PHA2, or hyperkalemic hypertension) is caused by autosomal dominant mutations in the with-no-lysine kinases WNK1 and WNK4, whose dysregulation in distal tubule and connecting segment epithelial cells ultimately serves to up-regulate

Table 103.1 Hereditary Syndromes of Renal Tubular Acidosis Attributed to Mutations in Defined Human Genes.

Syndrome	MIM	Chromosomal Localization	Locus Symbol	Gene Product
Primary Proximal RTA (Type 2)				
Autosomal recessive with ocular abnormalities	603345, 604278	4q21	SLC4A4	NBCe1
Autosomal dominant?	179830	?	?	?
Primary Distal RTA (Type 1)				
Autosomal dominant	179800, 109270	17q21-22	SLC4A1	AE1
Autosomal recessive	602272, 109270	17q21-22	SLC4A1	AE1
Autosomal recessive with deafness	192132, 267300	2p13 subunit	ATP6V1B1	vH^+-ATPase B1
Autosomal recessive with variable deafness	602272, 605239	7q33-34	ATP6V0A4	vH^+-ATPase a4 subunit
Autosomal recessive	618070	2p25.1	ATP5V1C2	vH^+-ATPase C2 subunit
Autosomal dominant with amelogenesis Imperfecta	613211	15q21.3	WDR72	WDR72
Autosomal recessive	601093	5q35.1	FOXI1	Forkhead Box I1
Combined Proximal and Distal RTA (Type 3)				
Autosomal recessive with osteopetrosis	259730	8q22	CA2	CAII
Fanconi syndrome with proximal RTA				
Autosomal dominant	615605, 607037	3q27.2	EHHADH	EHHADH
Autosomal dominant	612718, 602360	15q21.1	GATM	GATM
Autosomal dominant	616026, 600281	20q13.12	HNF4A	HNF4A
Dent disease	300009	Xp11.22	CLCN5	CLC-5
Dent-2 disease, Lowe syndrome	300555, 300535, 309300	Xq26.1	OCRL1	OCRL
Donnai-Barrow syndrome	222448, 600073	2q31.1	LRP2	Megalin
Secondary hyperkalemic distal RTA (type 4)				
Pseudohypoaldosteronism type 1				
Autosomal dominant renal form	4q31.1	MR	Mineralocorticoid receptor	
Autosomal recessive multiple-organ form	12p13.1	SCNN1A	ENaC α subunit	
	16p12-13.11	SCNN1B	ENaC β subunit	
	16p12-13.11	SCNN1G	ENaC γ subunit	
Pseudohypoaldosteronism type 2	145260, 605232	12p13.3	WNK1	WNK1 kinase
Hyperkalemic hypertension	145260, 601844	17p11-q21	WNK4	WNK4 kinase
Gordon syndrome	614495, 605775.5p31	KLHL3	Kelch-like 3	
	614496, 603136.2q36	CUL3	Cullin-3	

Italics denote familial syndromic conditions often but not always accompanied by distal renal tubular acidosis.
EHHADH, Enoyl-coA hydratase/3-hydroxyacyl-coA dehydrogenase; *GATM*, glycine amidinotransferase; *MIM*, Mendelian Inheritance in Man; *RTA*, renal tubular acidosis.

thiazide-sensitive NCC1 Na^+/Cl^- co-transporter activity. PHA2 is also caused by mutations in the *KLHL3* and *CUL3* genes encoding subunits of the ubiquitin ligase system that degrades the WNK1 and WNK4 kinases. A mouse PHA2 model engineered with the equivalent of the human WNK4 mutation Q562E revealed that pendrin up-regulation in type B intercalated cells was essential to the metabolic acidosis phenotype,[93] suggesting that distal HCO_3^- wasting might also contribute in some types of human distal renal tubular acidosis.

Many of the afore-described genetic loss-of-function diseases of human renal acid-base homeostasis have been reproduced with varying degrees of clinical fidelity in corresponding genetic knockout or knockin mouse models. (In the mouse, for example, knockout of ATP6V0A4 turns out to cause a mixed distal-proximal renal tubular acidosis,[94] unlike in humans with distal renal tubular acidosis). Moreover, many additional mouse models of renal tubular acidosis have been reported as genetic knockouts of genes expressed in mouse acid-base transporting cells but have not yet been reported as genes responsible for familial renal tubular acidosis in humans. These genes include two mouse proximal tubular acidosis genes encoding the proximal tubular basolateral membrane K^+ channels TASK2/KCNK5[95] and Kir4.2/KCNJ15.[96] Kir4.2 deficiency was notable for impairment of proximal ammoniagenesis without impairment of tubule lumen acidification.[95,96] Additional mouse distal tubular acidosis genes include the intercalated cell NH_3 channels RhBG and RhCG,[97] the intercalated cell basolateral K-Cl cotransporter KCC4,[98] the intercalated cell H^+,K^+-ATPases α1 and α2,[31] the proposed intercalated cell vH^+-ATPase binding proteins, NCOA7[99] and the prorenin receptor ATP6AP2,[100] the intercalated cell AE1-binding protein PRDX6,[101] the electrogenic Na^+/HCO_3^- co-transporter NBCe2,[102] the vasopressin receptor V1AR,[103] the SLC26A7 Cl^-/HCO_3^- exchanger and anion channel of the type A intercalated cell,[104] proton receptor GPR4,[105] and possibly, certain matrix components with trophic signaling properties.[106]

CONCLUSION

The fetal transition to extrauterine life at parturition challenges the kidney to assume the burden of maintaining systemic ionic and volume homeostasis. The neonatal kidney has the ability to respond to acid loading but further develops that ability during the early postnatal period, gradually increasing serum bicarbonate concentration and renal bicarbonate reabsorption threshold. Renal acid-base regulation does not achieve adult-level function as normalized to body mass until the age of 1 to 2 years. In rodents, maturation of the proximal tubule is accompanied by increased levels of NHE3 and CA2 and increased function of preexisting levels of NBCe1. Appearance of vH-ATPase in the proximal tubule occurs only after weaning. Collecting duct type A intercalated cells develop prenatally and postnatally in a gradual fashion, with increasing levels of transport proteins. Type B intercalated cells populate the entire collecting duct during embryonic development. Medullary type B cells then undergo apoptosis, leaving only the cortical collecting duct as a site for type B cells in the mature kidney. Similar morphologic changes may mark human nephron maturation. Mendelian forms of primary human renal tubular acidosis, most clinically apparent in infancy, have been attributed to mutations in eight genes. Genetically engineered knockout of these and additional genes in the mouse has generated numerous additional models of proximal and of distal renal tubular acidosis. Many of the ion transporters regulating renal acid-base regulation in the neonate have now been identified. However, the development and function of acid-base sensing and of communication between distinct cell types and nephron segments in the control of renal acid-base homeostasis and host defense during postnatal nephron maturation (as well as in the adult) remain among the most compelling problems in renal acid-base physiology requiring further investigation.

A complete reference list is available at www.ExpertConsult.com.

SELECT REFERENCES

1. Eladari D, Kumai Y. Renal acid-base regulation: new insights from animal models. *Pflugers Arch*. 2015;467(8):1623–1641.
2. Alexander RT, Law L, Gil-Pena H, Greenbaum LA, Santos F. Hereditary distal renal tubular acidosis. In: *GeneReviews 1993-2019*. Seattle, WA: University of Washington; 2019.
3. Alexander RT, Bitzan M. Renal tubular acidosis. *Pediatr Clin North Am*. 2019;66(1):135–157.
4. Iacobelli S, Guignard JP. Renal aspects of metabolic acid-base disorders in neonates. *Pediatr Nephrol*. 2020;35(2):221–228.
5. Gattineni J, Baum M. Developmental changes in renal tubular transport-an overview. *Pediatr Nephrol*. 2015;30(12):2085–2098.
6. Rao R, Bhalla V, Pastor-Soler NM. Intercalated cells of the kidney collecting duct in kidney physiology. *Semin Nephrol*. 2019;39(4):353–367.
7. Curthoys NP, Moe OW. Proximal tubule function and response to acidosis. *Clin J Am Soc Nephrol*. 2014;9(9):1627–1638.
8. Fromm M, Piontek J, Rosenthal R, Gunzel D, Krug SM. Tight junctions of the proximal tubule and their channel proteins. *Pflugers Arch*. 2017;469(7-8):877–887.
9. Du Z, Yan Q, Duan Y, Weinbaum S, Weinstein AM, Wang T. Axial flow modulates proximal tubule NHE3 and H-ATPase activities by changing microvillus bending moments. *Am J Physiol Ren Physiol*. 2006;290(2):F289–F296.
10. Spencer AG, Labonte ED, Rosenbaum DP, et al. Intestinal inhibition of the Na+/H+ exchanger 3 prevents cardiorenal damage in rats and inhibits Na+ uptake in humans. *Sci Transl Med*. 2014;6(227):227ra236.
11. Block GA, Rosenbaum DP, Yan A, Chertow GM. Efficacy and safety of tenapanor in patients with hyperphosphatemia receiving maintenance hemodialysis: a randomized phase 3 trial. *J Am Soc Nephrol*. 2019;30(4):641–652.
12. Li HC, Du Z, Barone S, et al. Proximal tubule specific knockout of the Na(+)/H(+) exchanger NHE3: effects on bicarbonate absorption and ammonium excretion. *J Molecul Med*. 2013;91(8):951–963.
13. Wang T, Yang CL, Abbiati T, et al. Mechanism of proximal tubule bicarbonate absorption in NHE3 null mice. *Am J Physiol*. 1999;277(2 Pt 2):F298–F302.
14. Lee HW, Harris AN, Romero MF, et al. NBCe1-A is required for the renal ammonia and potassium response to hypokalemia. *Am J Physiol Renal Physiol*. 2019;318(2):F402–F421.
15. King AJ, Siegel M, He Y, et al. Inhibition of sodium/hydrogen exchanger 3 in the gastrointestinal tract by tenapanor reduces paracellular phosphate permeability. *Sci Transl Med*. 2018;10(456).
16. Biber J, Murer H, Mohebbi N, Wagner CA. Renal handling of phosphate and sulfate. *Compreben Physiol*. 2014;4(2):771–792.
17. Ansermet C, Moor MB, Centeno G, et al. Renal Fanconi syndrome and hypophosphatemic rickets in the absence of xenotropic and polytropic retroviral receptor in the nephron. *J Am Soc Nephrol*. 2017;28(4):1073–1078.
18. Capasso G, Unwin R, Rizzo M, Pica A, Giebisch G. Bicarbonate transport along the loop of Henle: molecular mechanisms and regulation. *J Nephrol*. 2002;15(suppl 5):S88–S96.
19. Bailey MA, Giebisch G, Abbiati T, et al. NHE2-mediated bicarbonate reabsorption in the distal tubule of NHE3 null mice. *J Physiol*. 2004;561(Pt 3):765–775.
20. Roy A, Al-bataineh MM, Pastor-Soler NM. Collecting duct intercalated cell function and regulation. *Clin J Am Soc Nephrol*. 2015;10(2):305–324.
21. Vasanthakumar T, Bueler SA, Wu D, Beilsten-Edmands V, Robinson CV, Rubinstein JL. Structural comparison of the vacuolar and Golgi V-ATPases from Saccharomyces cerevisiae. *Proc Natl Acad Sci U S A*. 2019;116(15):7272–7277.
22. Han KH, Lee SY, Kim WY, Shin JA, Kim J, Weiner ID. Expression of ammonia transporter family members, Rh B glycoprotein and Rh C glycoprotein, in the developing rat kidney. *Am J Physiol Ren Physiol*. 2010;299(1):F187–F198.
23. Weiner ID, Mitch WE, Sands JM. Urea and ammonia metabolism and the control of renal Nitrogen excretion. *Clin J Am Soc Nephrol*. 2015;10(8):1444–1458.
24. Prieto MC, Gonzalez AA, Navar LG. Evolving concepts on regulation and function of renin in distal nephron. *Pflugers Arch*. 2013;465(1):121–132.
25. Wall SM, Lazo-Fernandez Y. The role of pendrin in renal physiology. *Annu Rev Physiol*. 2015;77:363–378.
26. Wagner CA, Devuyst O, Bourgeois S, Mohebbi N. Regulated acid-base transport in the collecting duct. *Pflugers Archiv*. 2009;458(1):137–156.
27. Quentin F, Chambrey R, Trinh-Trang-Tan MM, et al. The Cl-/HCO3- exchanger pendrin in the rat kidney is regulated in response to chronic alterations in chloride balance. *Am J Physiol Ren Physiol*. 2004;287(6):F1179–F1188.
28. Tokonami N, Morla L, Centeno G, et al. alpha-Ketoglutarate regulates acid-base balance through an intrarenal paracrine mechanism. *J Clin Invest*. 2013;123(7):3166–3171.
29. Lazo-Fernandez Y, Welling PA, Wall SM. Alpha-Ketoglutarate stimulates pendrin-dependent Cl(-) absorption in the mouse CCD through protein kinase C. *Am J Physiol Renal Physiol*. 2018;315(1):F7–F15.
30. Chambrey R, Kurth I, Peti-Peterdi J, et al. Renal intercalated cells are rather energized by a proton than a sodium pump. *Proc Natl Acad Sci U S A*. 2013;110(19):7928–7933.
31. Greenlee MM, Lynch IJ, Gumz ML, Cain BD, Wingo CS. The renal H,K-ATPases. *Curr Opin Nephrol Hypertens*. 2010;19(5):478–482.
32. Brown D, Wagner CA. Molecular mechanisms of acid-base sensing by the kidney. *J Am Soc Nephrol*. 2012;23(5):774–780.
33. Schwartz GJ, Gao X, Tsuruoka S, et al. Principal Cells sense acid and secrete SDF1 to regulate H+ and HCO3- secretion by kidney intercalated cells. *J Clin Invest*. 2015;125(12):4365–4374.
34. Nair AV, Yanhong W, Paunescu TG, Bouley R, Brown D. Sex-dependent differences in water homeostasis in wild-type and V-ATPase B1-subunit deficient mice. *PloS One*. 2019;14(8):e0219940.
35. Sulemanji M, Vakili K. Neonatal renal physiology. *Semin Pediatr Surg*. 2013;22(4):195–198.
36. McMahon AP. Development of the mammalian kidney. *Curr Top Dev Biol*. 2016;117:31–64.
37. Rosenblum S, Pal A, Reidy K. Renal development in the fetus and premature infant. *Semin Fetal Neonatal Med*. 2017;22(2):58–66.
38. Patel SR, Dressler GR. The genetics and epigenetics of kidney development. *Semin Nephrol*. 2013;33(4):314–326.
39. Gubhaju L, Sutherland MR, Horne RS, et al. Assessment of renal functional maturation and injury in preterm neonates during the first month of life. *Am J Physiol Ren Physiol*. 2014;307(2):F149–F158.
40. Kitterer D, Schwab M, Alscher MD, Braun N, Latus J. Drug-induced acid-base disorders. *Pediatr Nephrol*. 2015;30(9):1407–1423.
41. Abitbol CL, DeFreitas MJ, Strauss J. Assessment of kidney function in preterm infants: lifelong implications. *Pediatr Nephrol*. 2016;31(12):2213–2222.
42. Schwartz GJ, Haycock GB, Edelmann Jr CM, Spitzer A. Late metabolic acidosis: a reassessment of the definition. *J Pediatr*. 1979;95(1):102–107.
43. Edelmann CM, Soriano JR, Boichis H, Gruskin AB, Acosta MI. Renal bicarbonate reabsorption and hydrogen ion excretion in normal infants. *J Clin Invest*. 1967;46(8):1309–1317.
44. Svenningsen NW. Renal acid-base titration studies in infants with and without metabolic acidosis in the postneonatal period. *Pediatr Res*. 1974;8(6):659–672.
45. Arant Jr BS. Postnatal development of renal function during the first year of life. *Pediatr Nephrol*. 1987;1(3):308–313.
46. Schwartz GJ, Evan AP. Development of solute transport in rabbit proximal tubule. I. HCO-3 and glucose absorption. *Am J Physiol*. 1983;245(3):F382–F390.
47. Baum M, Gattineni J, Satlin LM. Postnatal renal development. In: Alper R, Caplan M, Moe O, eds. *Seldin and Geibisch's the Kidney*. 5th ed. Vol 1. Elsevier; 2013:911–931.
48. Schwartz GJ, Evan AP. Development of solute transport in rabbit proximal tubule. III. Na-K-ATPase activity. *Am J Physiol*. 1984;246(6 Pt 2):F845–F852.
49. Pirojsakul K, Gattineni J, Dwarakanath V, Baum M. Renal NHE expression and activity in neonatal NHE3- and NHE8-null mice. *Am J Physiol Ren Physiol*. 2015;308(1):F31–F38.
50. Baum M, Twombley K, Gattineni J, et al. Proximal tubule Na+/H+ exchanger activity in adult NHE8-/-, NHE3-/-, and NHE3-/-/NHE8-/- mice. *Am J Physiol Ren Physiol*. 2012;303(11):F1495–F1502.

104 Response to Nephron Loss in Early Development

Pamela I. Good | Fangming Lin | Jennifer R. Charlton

INTRODUCTION

Glomerular endowment is highly variable in humans. Although each kidney contains approximately 1 million nephrons, glomerular number ranges from 210,000 to 2,700,000 per kidney representing a 10-fold difference.[1,2] Both environmental and genetic factors influence nephrogenesis, a complex developmental program including renal cell fate determination, stem and progenitor renewal and differentiation, nephron patterning and lineage maturation, and the coordinated development of the kidney and urinary tract.[3-5] Human nephrogenesis is not complete until approximately 36 weeks of gestation,[6] and infants born preterm have decreased nephron number at birth. Some studies suggest that nephrogenesis ends at birth in both term and preterm humans;[7] however, conflicting data suggests that nephrogenesis continues for a limited time postnatally.[8] Importantly, studies suggesting that postnatal nephrogenesis occurs have shown that this process is abnormal and may result in nonfunctional glomeruli.[9]

Congenital anomalies of the kidney and urinary tract, which are usually associated with gene mutations, may also result in decreased nephron formation at birth and accelerated decline in nephron number over time. Furthermore, with age and insults such as sepsis and hypotension leading to acute kidney injury (AKI), there could be a further reduction in the number of functional nephron throughout life. When faced with a nephron deficit, the kidney undergoes adaptive responses that have both short- and long-term effects. This chapter reviews the causes and consequences of low nephron number, emphasizing the unique features of the vulnerable developing kidney.

KEY DETERMINANTS OF NEPHRON ENDOWMENT

While considerable variation exists with regard to the number of nephrons in humans, a relationship between glomerular number and birth weight has been reported. It has been estimated, from autopsy studies, that each kilogram in birth weight confers on average 260,000 more nephrons.[9] Additionally, 60% of nephrons are formed during the third trimester, making preterm birth a risk factor for low nephron endowment.[6] In an elegant human autopsy study, Sutherland and colleagues showed that during the first 40 days of life nephrogenesis continues. Yet the glomeruli formed were abnormal appearing, suggesting that nephrons formed after birth may not function normally.[8] This suggests that preterm birth may result in a functional nephron deficit. Since low nephron number can lead to chronic kidney disease (CKD)[10] preterm birth and low-birth-weight infants are expected to have an increased risk of CKD. Indeed, recent epidemiologic studies have identified preterm birth and low birth weight as risk factors for CKD.[11-14]

A broader understanding of normal nephrogenesis has identified genetic and environmental factors that play a key role in determining glomerular number. The kidneys develop through branching morphogenesis, whereby an outgrowth of the wolffian duct, the ureteric bud (UB), undergoes iterative branching events that are dependent on signaling with the surrounding metanephric mesenchyme (MM). The epithelial-mesenchymal interactions at the tips of the branching UB are essential for nephron formation. *Ret*, a receptor tyrosine kinase, is expressed in the UB, and its ligand, glial-cell derived neurotrophic growth factor, glial cell line-derived neurotrophic factor (GDNF), is secreted by surrounding mesenchyme. The interaction between Ret and GNDF results in UB branching that induces cells in the MM to condense around UB tips, transition to renal progenitor cells, and ultimately form the nephron.[3-5] Disruptions in genes and pathways that regulate the progenitor cell or mesenchymal population and those involved in the branching morphogenesis result in deficits in nephron number.[15] Fig. 104.1 highlights the major factors that contribute to the number of nephrons in the metanephric kidney.

GENETIC FACTORS

Advanced DNA sequencing and analysis has led to the discovery of hundreds of single genes that, if mutated, are responsible for isolated or syndromic kidney and urogenital malformations that can alter nephron endowment.[16] *Six2* is expressed in the cap mesenchyme surrounding the UB, and the progenitor cell population is reduced when it is inactivated.[17] Perturbations in the UB or its ability to branch also affect final nephron number. For example, infants with a common *Ret* variant (the RET[1476A] allele) have a kidney volume that is 10% smaller than controls.[18] The association between low kidney volume and low nephron number in *Ret* variants is supported by animal studies; homozygous *Ret* knockout mice do not develop kidneys, and heterozygotes have reduced nephron number.[19]

Although most mutations known to affect nephron number result in fewer nephrons, variants that may increase nephron number also exists. El Kares and associates found that newborns with a variant in ALDH1A had a 22% greater kidney volume.[20] *ALDH1A* encodes an enzyme, RALDH2, which converts nutritional vitamin A to active retinoic acid; retinoic acid is critical for UB branching. Manipulation of mechanistic target of rapamycin (Mtor), a regulator of cellular growth, metabolism, proliferation, and survival, can alter nephron number. Disinhibition of Mtor signaling through deletion of Hamartin, a negative regulator of Mtor, results in a 25% increase in nephron number.[20a] Altered heterochronic genes may also impact glomerular number by prolonging the duration of nephrogenesis. Yermalovich and colleagues discovered that the heterochronic genes *Lin28* and *Let7*, which code for highly conserved RNA binding proteins, have an important role in the cessation of nephrogenesis in mice.[21] *Lin28b* is expressed in MM during nephrogenesis and when present inhibits *Let7* expression. Over time *Lin28* expression decreases allowing for increased *Let7* activity, which includes inhibition of *Lin28.* Overexpression of *Lin28b* in the developing MM results in ectopic, nephron containing renal mass. Alternately, suppressing *Let7* miRNA during nephrogenesis results in prolonged nephron formation in the outer nephrogenic zone, effectively increasing nephron number. While manipulating heterochronic gene expression poses significant risk for oncogenesis, understanding what signals terminate nephrogenesis in humans could lead to therapeutic interventions to potentially increase nephron endowment.

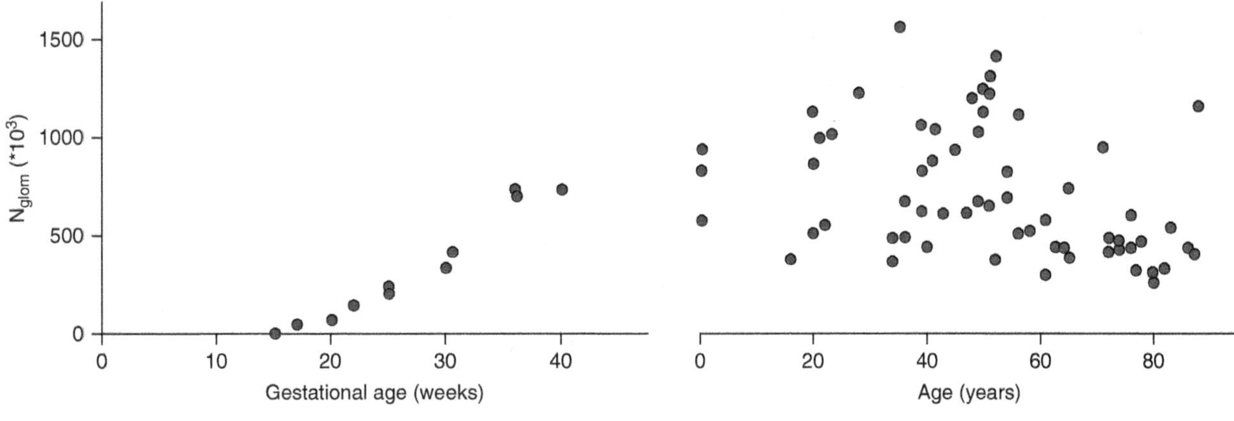

Genetic	Prenatal (prematurity)		Pediatric	Adult
RET	Nutrition	Tobacco	Nutrition	Diabetes
PAX2	IUGR	Medications:	AKI	Hypertension
ACE	Iron deficiency	-Cyclosporine	Medications	Acute kidney injury
OSR1	Vitamin A deficiency	-ACEI	Chronic illnesses	Autoimmune diseases
	Vitamin D status	-NSAIDs	Hypertension	UTIs
ALDH1A2	Hyperglycernia	-Aminoglycosides	UTIs	Urinary tract obstruction
	Ethanol		Urinary tract obstruction	Medications
	Obstruction			
	Potassium intake			
	Asphyxia			

Fig. 104.1 Factors affecting nephron number. A multitude of factors affect a human's final nephron number. With nephrogenesis complete in humans at the end of normal gestation, there are many etiologies that result in the variability in nephron number that occurs in adults. *ACE*, Angiotensin-converting enzyme; *ACEI*, angiotensin-converting enzyme inhibitor; *AKI*, acute kidney infection; *ALDH1A2*, retinaldehyde dehydrogenase 2; *IUGR*, intrauterine growth restriction; *NSAIDs*, nonsteroidal antiinflammatory drugs; *OSR1*, odd-skipped related 1; *PAX2*, paired box gene 2; *Ret*, receptor tyrosine kinase; *UTI*, urinary tract infection. (Modified from Charlton JR, Springsteen CH, Carmody JB. Nephron number and its determinants in early life: a primer. *Pediatr Nephrol.* 2014;29:2299–2308.)

Although genetic factors are important, other regulators such as epigenetic factors and microRNAs are likely to play a significant role in the determination of nephron number in humans.[22] Indeed, Nakagawa and colleagues showed that deleting an essential microRNA-activating enzyme, Dicer1, in developing renal stromal cells resulted in hypoplastic kidneys with abnormal tubules and vasculature.[23] Other groups have gone on to show that in mice, microRNAs regulate kidney development through inhibiting gene expression, particularly pro-apoptotic transcripts in nephron progenitors.[24,25]

ENVIRONMENTAL FACTORS

Infants with intrauterine growth restriction (IUGR) are born with low birth weight and fewer nephrons than those whose birth weight is appropriate for gestational age.[26] Data from experimental models of IUGR suggest that the timing of growth restriction determines nephron reduction, with perturbations that occur during periods of robust nephrogenesis associated with lower nephron endowment and higher blood pressure later in life.[27] Fetal rats of mothers whose uterine artery has been ligated, or rats with spontaneous IUGR, have reduced nephron number.[28,29] Reduced maternal calorie or protein intake leads to reduced nephron number in experimental animals and may program the individual for salt-sensitive adult hypertension.[27,28,31,32] Intrauterine malnutrition in Aborigine humans is associated with low birth weight and impaired renal function in adulthood, suggesting that optimizing fetal growth may reduce renal disease and hypertension.[33] In a provocative study, mild vitamin A deficiency was shown to lead to inborn nephron deficits in the rat, with a linear relationship between maternal plasma retinol levels and the number of glomeruli in the pups.[34] This study and many others suggest that small variations in maternal nutritional status may have significant implications for the ultimate complement of nephrons.

The connection between in utero nutritional deprivation and altered nephrogenesis is not fully understood. Animal data has implicated an adverse effect of increased renin-angiotensin signaling during nephrogenesis.[35] Studies have also shown altered DNA methylation patterns in human offspring exposed to in utero nutrient deprivation.[36] Recently Wanner and colleagues showed that deletion of a specific DNA methyltransferase in mice leads to impaired nephrogenesis that resembles models of growth restriction-induced nephron deficits,[37] supporting the role of epigenetic modification in nephron formation. In some cases nutrient deprivation can increase nephron number. In rats, vitamin D deficiency during pregnancy increased nephron number by roughly 20%, suggesting that vitamin D deficiency may stimulate nephrogenesis.[38]

Beyond nutrition, there are a wide range of fetal and early neonatal exposures that have been linked to altered nephron endowment. Fetal exposure to toxins, such as maternal smoking or alcohol consumption, can impair kidney development.[39–42] Exposure of the fetus to maternal angiotensin-converting enzyme (ACE) inhibitors or to prostaglandin synthesis inhibitors impairs nephrogenesis and renal maturation.[43,44] Maternal exposure to glucocorticoids, aminoglycosides, β-lactam antibiotics, or cyclosporine may also impair nephrogenesis and contribute to hypertension.[45–49]

Infants of diabetic mothers have an increased incidence of congenital malformations, and maternal hyperglycemia in rats leads to nephron deficits.[50] Early postnatal hyperglycemia may also alter nephrogenesis. In a study of preterm lambs, hyperglycemia was associated with accelerated nephron maturation. This altered nephrogenesis was thought to be due to increased reactive oxygen species found in hyperglycemic kidneys.[51] Perinatal factors such as asphyxia and severe circulatory disturbances can also cause irreversible nephron loss.[52]

Early human fetal urinary tract obstruction can result in abnormal kidney development and reduced number of nephrons, and the number of glomeruli can be related to the time of developmental arrest.[53] Similarly, animal models of ureteral obstruction also result in reduced glomerular number, and ureteral obstruction impairs nephrogenesis in direct proportion to the duration of obstruction.[54-57] These findings further support the interdependence of UB and MM for proper kidney development.

PRETERM BIRTH

Experimental data focused on the effect of prematurity on glomerular endowment is limited in part due to a lack of animal models. Baboons delivered prior to the completion of gestation are suitable models for studying the effects of prematurity on renal development as they have a long gestation and can survive in a primate intensive care unit after premature birth. When baboons are delivered at a gestational age equivalent to a 27-week human gestation, there is no difference in the number of nephrons at 3 weeks of life compared to gestational age matched controls, suggesting that baboons born preterm undergo postnatal nephrogenesis. However, nephrogenesis after early delivery does not appear to recapitulate normal kidney development in utero, as there are histologic abnormalities within the glomeruli.[58] Mice are commonly used laboratory animals to address many research questions. Unlike humans and primates, they complete nephrogenesis about 4 days after birth. The delivery of pups 1 to 2 days prior to term gestation results in low nephron endowment and evidence of CKD at 5 weeks with albuminuria, hypertension, and lower glomerular filtration rate (GFR).[20a]

There are few human studies that examine the effect of a premature birth on the development of the kidney.[60-62] Autopsy studies have provided insight into the postnatal adaptations that occur in infants born during a rapid phase of nephrogenesis. In a study of premature infants where the investigators matched to controls based on gestational age (n = 32), the kidneys were examined by stereologic and histologic methods to count and measure the glomeruli. The investigators found an accelerated termination of kidney development with a decreased nephrogenic zone and more abnormal glomeruli with a larger surface area.[60] In a similar study, 66 infant kidneys were examined from premature infants weighing less than 1000 g who were grouped based on gestational and postnatal age, in addition to exposure to AKI. The investigators provided evidence that glomerulogenesis ceased 40 days after birth. Additionally, there were smaller radial glomerular counts in the premature infants, particularly if there was exposure to AKI, implying fewer nephrons. The kidneys from the premature infants also had increased mesangial tufts and capsular areas when they lived for more than 40 days,[62] which may predispose them to vasomotor or nephrotoxic injury in the postnatal period or in later life. Taken together, these studies suggest that there may be a limited period of postnatal nephrogenesis but that if so, ex-utero nephrogenesis is likely abnormal.

The association between preterm birth and low nephron number in non-autopsy samples has been studied mostly through imaging modalities that use kidney size as surrogate for nephron endowment. A study following preterm children through 18 months found that children born prematurely had smaller kidneys than term children.[63] In a Dutch cohort of premature infants (less than 32 weeks) renal ultrasound performed at 20 years of age revealed smaller renal volumes compared with term controls; the average reduction was 47 mL.[64] These studies suggest that these children born preterm have lower nephron number; however, as explored in subsequent parts of this chapter, kidney size is not a precise surrogate for nephron number.

METHODS OF DETERMINING NEPHRON ENDOWMENT

Currently there are no direct, noninvasive methods to measure nephron number in living humans. The average observed number of nephrons in humans is estimated to be approximately 900,000, but considerable variability exists between individuals (210,000 to 2.7 million).[1] These data are derived from postmortem human kidneys using techniques whereby a small fraction of the total glomeruli within the kidney is counted. One of the unbiased methods for estimating nephron number is a stereologic technique using the physical dissector-fractionator combination[65]; this involves sectioning a kidney into progressively smaller pieces and systematically counting random samples of glomeruli. A second approach utilizes acid to digest the entire kidney and counting a fraction of the disassociated glomeruli.[66] An additional approach combines data extracted from a kidney biopsy and cortical volume derived from imaging to estimate glomerular number and size.[67,68] As kidney disease can be heterogeneous, sampling biases may limit the generalizability of these estimations to the whole kidney.

More recently, advanced imaging techniques have been used in experimental animals to estimate glomerular number. Cationized ferritin enhanced magnetic resonance imaging (CFE-MRI) is one such promising modality. Cationic ferritin is injected intravenously into animals and delivered through the vasculature to glomeruli, where it binds to anionic sites on the glomerular basement membrane. When animals are imaged via MRI, the glomerular basement membrane bound to this iron oxide core distorts the magnetic field, resulting in visible punctate spots on 3D reconstructions of kidneys. These studies have been performed on ex vivo kidneys from humans, mice, rats, and rabbits[69-71] and in vivo on mice and rats.[72-74] CFE-MRI can also be integrated with other imaging modalities to colocalize glomerular and vascular pathology as seen in a model of neonatal AKI in rabbits.[74]

Another promising method of determining nephron number is microcomputed tomography with barium sulfate contrast. Mice are perfused with a contrast agent, barium, and then kidneys are placed in a microcomputed tomography machine. Using image processing tools, authors are able to determine glomerular number.[75] Both MRI- and micro CT-based technologies require intravenous contrast agents that may be associated with risks in humans. However there have been several publications showing the safety of cationic ferritin when used as a contrast agent in CFE-MRI in animals.[76,77] At this time these emerging technologies have not been adopted for clinical use.

Although clinicians utilize various surrogates for nephron number, including renal volume and GFR, these are not ideal biomarkers. Renal sonography to estimate renal volume can serve as a surrogate for renal weight, which in some studies correlates with nephron number,[77] but is an inconsistent finding,[78] probably because tubular, not glomerular, hypertrophy accounts for the most renal growth. The exception to this principle may occur in the case of kidney loss during nephrogenesis, where the remaining contralateral kidney has the potential for increased nephron formation and a larger size may represent more nephrons. Conversely, renal volume is less likely to be helpful with nephron loss due to AKI or exposure to nephrotoxic medications, particularly in light of the significant variability in human nephron number. This finding is highlighted by a report of autopsies of middle-aged hypertensive subjects killed in motor vehicle accidents in whom the median number of glomeruli was 50% of that in matched normotensive subjects (hypertensive group:

702,379 vs. nonhypertensive controls: 1,429,200). Although there were fewer and larger glomeruli in the hypertensive group, there was no difference in the absolute weight of the kidneys, indicating that renal volume may not be an ideal surrogate for nephron number in adults.[79] Further work is necessary to determine if renal volume early in life can be a surrogate for CKD later in life.

Estimation of GFR, particularly with clearance of endogenous creatinine, provides information about the entire kidney, but is an insensitive surrogate unless a large loss of functioning nephrons occurs. Because of the lack of a direct, noninvasive method to quantify nephron number and the limitations surrounding surrogates for nephron number, most of the knowledge regarding the causes and consequences of nephron loss is derived from epidemiologic data and animal studies.

RESPONSE TO NEPHRON LOSS

COMPENSATORY RENAL ADAPTATION IN THE FETUS

Until recently, experimental evidence for compensatory renal growth in the fetus had not been clearly established. Peters and colleagues[80] induced unilateral ureteral occlusion in the fetal lamb at midtrimester and observed a significant increase in contralateral kidney weight within 2 weeks, which became maximal by 1 month (50% increase). The increase in renal mass in this study was not associated with a detectable increase in the total number of nephrons. More recent studies suggest that the timing and mechanism of nephron loss may affect compensatory nephrogenesis. In a study of ovine fetal uninephrectomy, animals were found to have a 45% increase in the number of nephrons in the remaining kidney when compared to a single kidney of a sham operated animal. Overall uninephrectomized lambs had 30% fewer nephrons than sham-operated animals, with a lower mean glomerular volume.[81] Over time, the glomerular volume of the uninephrectomized sheep increased and renal growth reached its limit by the age of 4 years.[82]

A study of 26-week-old pigs born with a solitary kidney also found that contralateral kidneys underwent compensatory growth and nephrogenesis. These remaining kidneys had weights that were increased by 84%, with a 50% increase in nephron number.[83] Rodent studies of congenital unilateral renal agenesis also report a similar increase in glomerular number.[84] Although removal of a kidney during fetal life can result in a greater number of nephrons in the remnant kidney, the individual's total number of nephrons is likely to be less than in those with two kidneys. The interpretation of these animal models of low nephron number must be made with caution when applied to humans; these scenarios do not recapitulate preterm or growth-restricted humans and the finding of compensatory increase in nephron number found with in utero renal loss has not been validated in humans. Moreover, in the case of humans born with a solitary kidney the etiology is often genetic; genetic defects resulting in renal agenesis can be associated with developmental abnormalities of the contralateral solitary kidney.[85]

MECHANISM OF POSTNATAL NEPHRON GROWTH

Renal size increases in response to a postnatal reduction in nephron mass, and this compensatory growth following nephron loss is proportionately greater in the newborn than in the adult.[7,8]

Despite a significant increase in glomerular volume, both normal and compensatory renal growth are primarily caused by an increase in proximal tubular growth.[86,87] Numerous studies indicate that experimental reduction in renal mass results in release of renotropic factors and/or suppression of inhibitors of renal growth.[88] Although blood-borne factors that stimulate renal growth are probably not released from the kidneys themselves, renal tissue factors may be necessary to activate humoral compounds.[89,90] The enhanced compensatory renal hypertrophy observed in the neonate may relate to differences in tissue factors. In this regard, kidneys of adult rats and mice have been found to contain a renal growth inhibitory factor; however, none was found in neonatal kidneys.[91] The initial phase of compensatory renal growth following unilateral nephrectomy in immature rats is independent of growth hormone secretion but is associated with an increase in insulin-like growth factor-1 (IGF-1) and IGF-1 receptor gene expression.[92,93]

Numerous compounds have also been shown to stimulate renal growth, including sodium, ammonium chloride, folic acid, thyroxine, growth hormone, and mineralocorticoids.[94-96] One stimulus to renal hypertrophy and hyperfiltration that has generated much interest is increased dietary protein intake.[97,98] The ribonucleic acid (RNA)-protein ratio and DNA content of the remaining kidney are increased as a result of uninephrectomy, but not with increased dietary protein.[99] Thus, the additive effect of dietary protein is probably caused by a separate mechanism rather than being an amplification of the normal hypertrophic response. Although angiotensin II has been shown to act as a renal growth factor, compensatory renal growth in neonatal mice subjected to unilateral ureteral obstruction is not impaired in animals lacking functional angiotensinogen genes.[100]

Perhaps as important as what stimulates compensatory renal growth is what limits compensatory renal growth. Mice lacking the gene for cyclin-dependent kinase inhibitor p21 do not develop progressive renal insufficiency after renal ablation.[101] A shift from renal cellular hypertrophy to proliferation in these mutants may underlie the protective effect.[102]

The inverse correlation between the number of nephrons at birth and blood pressure in adulthood suggests conservation of nephrons is particularly important in early life.[103,104] When a kidney is removed after nephrogenesis is complete, nephron enlargement occurs and is more significant when the insult occurs earlier in life. The degree of compensatory hypertrophy is indirectly related to age and directly related to the degree of nephron loss. Compared with glomeruli hypertrophy, tubules undergo a proportionately greater adaptive growth following uninephrectomy as the proximal and distal tubules increase in length substantially.[86,105]

Increased intraglomerular pressure and blood flow, and consequent hyperfiltration, may lead to progressive glomerular injury, a maladaptive response.[106,107] The mechanisms responsible for this process are not completely understood, but they include increased filtration of protein and other macromolecules that are taken up by mesangial cells, which are thereby damaged.[107,108] Proteinuria also leads to injury of the renal tubules and interstitium. Proteinuria can lead to apoptosis of tubular cells and the development of interstitial fibrosis.[109,110] Uninephrectomy in the neonatal rat has been shown to result in greater degrees of proteinuria and glomerular sclerosis of the remaining kidney than occurs following uninephrectomy in the adult.[111,112] Increased protein intake in the young rat can stimulate kidney growth by promoting cell proliferation and by increasing the GFR.[113] However, studies of young rats undergoing unilateral nephrectomy reveal that survival was significantly reduced in animals receiving a high-protein compared to a low-protein diet.[114] Moreover, this was preceded by an increase in urinary protein excretion.[115] These data have disturbing implications for neonates with nephron loss, as a more vigorous early adaptive response in remaining renal tissue may lead to progressive renal insufficiency during development. However, attempts to slow this progression by restricting protein in infancy carry the risks of protein malnutrition and impairment of normal somatic growth.

In cases of unilateral loss of nephrons (or more severe impairment of one kidney than the other), the contralateral kidney generally compensates accordingly. This phenomenon, first called *renal counterbalance* by Hinman,[116] appears to be exaggerated in early development.[117,118] The postnatal hypertrophic response of the less impaired kidney can be further compromised by the presence of vesicoureteral reflux or infection.[119,120] As in experimental studies, the hypertrophic response of the intact kidney is dependent on the proportion of nephron loss in the contralateral kidney.[121,122] Adaptation by remaining nephrons can also be influenced by iatrogenic factors such as radiation or chemotherapy, which may impair compensatory hypertrophy to a greater extent in patients younger than in those older than 2 years of age.[123]

CLINICAL CONSEQUENCES OF NEPHRON LOSS

ACUTE KIDNEY INJURY

Results from the international retrospective observational cohort study, Assessment of Worldwide AKI Epidemiology in Neonates (AWAKEN), indicate that the prevalence of neonatal AKI is high, and it is associated with poor outcomes.[124] In many cases the etiology of kidney injury is multifactorial. Neonates who are premature, septic, asphyxiated, or treated with extracorporeal membrane oxygenation (ECMO) are high-risk groups that have rates of AKI ranging from 12.5% to 71%.[125-131] While many studies have looked at AKI during an infant's entire hospitalization, the response to injury is likely different depending on the gestational age and chronologic age of the baby. A subgroup analysis from the AWAKEN study found that there is a high incidence of AKI in the first week of life and these infants are at increased risk of death or increased length of stay.[132] Because we currently lack experimental models of congenitally reduced nephron number and there are limited animal models of neonatal AKI, we know very little about the response to kidney injury during the first days of postnatal adaptation.

An additional concern of the premature population is the near universal prenatal and postnatal exposure to nephrotoxins, particularly aminoglycosides and nonsteroidal antiinflammatory drugs (NSAIDs).[133] There are significant limitations to studying the renal effects of these medications on neonates as there are few relevant and practical animal models. Existing data suggests that these exposures may perturb normal nephrogenesis and predispose individuals to CKD. Rodent studies reveal that prenatal exposure to gentamicin results in nearly 20% fewer nephrons. These animals have evidence of glomerulosclerosis as adults.[134] A similar study in rats highlights the differences in the long-term renal effects of NSAIDs on nephron number. In this study, indomethacin administration during early postnatal nephrogenesis (postnatal days 1 to 5), but not ibuprofen, reduced nephron number in adult rodents.[135] In rabbits, administration of indomethacin and gentamicin during postnatal nephrogenesis results in a circumferential ring of nephron injury and loss.[136] Although animal studies have shown the toxic potential of commonly utilized medications such as oxygen, aminoglycosides, and NSAIDs,[137-142] the studies have been performed in rodents that naturally complete nephrogenesis postnatally limiting their applicability to humans and highlighting the time-sensitive nature of these exposures.

In humans, exposure to AKI appears to either exacerbate or unmask the risk for CKD,[143,144] although there are few long-term studies of infants who have developed AKI during the neonatal period. In premature infants, a serum creatinine level of greater than 0.6 mg/dL, a urinary protein-creatinine ratio of greater than 0.6 at a year of life, and a body mass index higher than the 85th percentile have been proposed as predictors of poor renal outcomes.[145] More recently, the Follow-up of Acute kidney injury in Neonates during Childhood Years (FANCY) study found that neonatal AKI was associated with renal dysfunction. Investigators found that AKI was associated with a 4.5-fold higher risk of renal dysfunction (as defined by GFR <90) by 5 years of age. Of note the children in the AKI group had lower gestational age and birth weight, already putting them at increased risk of CKD given their likely lower glomerular endowment.[146] The IRENEO study, a prospective study of children born less than 33 weeks, compared kidney size and function in children with and without documented AKI in the neonatal period. While they found no difference in GFR or microalbuminuria, the children exposed to AKI did have smaller kidneys. This group defined AKI using gestational age specific creatinine values that they had previously determined were associated with increased mortality.[147] This approach may have identified a different population than studies using universal or standardized definitions for AKI.

PRETERM BIRTH AND LOW BIRTH WEIGHT

Infants with a lower nephron endowment may have decreased renal reserve putting them at high risk of CKD. Animal models of surgically reduced nephron mass suggest that animals with reduced glomerular number are more susceptible to injury and are at increased risk of developing CKD.[148] From an epidemiologic perspective, recent studies suggest that both low birth weight and prematurity, surrogate markers of low functional nephron endowment, are risk factors for CKD. Low-birth-weight infants have a 70% higher risk of developing CKD as adults,[149] and this risk can be identified during childhood.[150]

More recent studies have shown the association between preterm birth and CKD. A recent large cohort study from Sweden showed that those born preterm or extremely preterm (<28 weeks gestation) had a two- to threefold increased risk of developing CKD.[11] Interestingly, even early term infants (37 to 38 weeks) had increased odds of CKD, suggesting that there may be some renal benefit to continued gestation even after nephrogenesis is complete. Alternatively this suggests other mechanisms aside from nephron number that increase the risk for CKD. Multiple smaller cohorts have validated the finding that preterm birth is a risk factor for CKD.[151-153]

UNILATERAL MULTICYSTIC KIDNEY AND RENAL AGENESIS

The most obvious etiology for nephron loss in the neonate results from fetal renal maldevelopment, collectively named congenital abnormalities of the kidney and urinary tract (CAKUT). Unilateral multicystic renal dysplasia results in a nonfunctional kidney early in gestation and, similar to renal agenesis, provides an opportunity to study the adaptation that occurs in the remaining kidney. An autopsy study of 20 human fetuses with a unilateral kidney revealed a significant increase in the proportional weight of the single kidney.[154] These findings are corroborated by two clinical studies that show the human kidney appears to hypertrophy in utero. In 2000, Hill and associates published a study of 36 fetuses with a solitary kidney secondary to unilateral renal agenesis or multicystic dysplastic kidney.[155] They showed that 16 out of those 36 had a renal length greater than the 95th percentile, and this hypertrophy could be seen as early as 22 weeks' gestation. In a larger study of fetuses with a solitary kidney where 60 participants had unilateral multicystic dysplastic kidney and 7 had unilateral renal agenesis, 88% had compensatory renal hypertrophy at a mean gestational age of 29.7 weeks, but the hypertrophy could be visualized as early as 20 weeks' gestation.[156] In infants born with unilateral renal agenesis, renal volume increases to 188% of that of a single normal kidney during postnatal development.[157]

Sonography permits serial measurement of renal size in the fetus such that renal growth can be compared with normal ranges and followed beyond birth. Such tracking of renal size may be clinically useful in monitoring the function of an abnormal contralateral kidney in infants with two functioning kidneys. An exaggerated rate of increase in renal size has been correlated with contralateral renal function that contributes less than 15% of total function.[158] Consistent with the hypothesis that hypertrophy and prolonged hyperfiltration by remnant glomeruli lead to progressive renal injury, patients with unilateral renal agenesis may develop focal glomerular sclerosis and renal insufficiency in adulthood.[159-161] It is important to note that the remaining kidney may have development abnormalities,[162-164] which may contribute to the development of CKD. This is particularly relevant if genetic factors are responsible for the contralateral multicystic kidney or renal agenesis.

RENAL HYPOPLASIA

Because of the wide variation in functional nephron loss resulting from renal hypoplasia, it has been difficult to systematically examine the adaptation of remaining nephrons in these disorders. However, in oligomeganephronia, a rare form of congenital renal hypoplasia, infants are born with less than 25% of the normal nephron number.[165] Presumably, because of the severity of nephron loss, compensatory hypertrophy is pushed to its limits, resulting in glomerular volumes that are several-fold greater than normal.[166] This disorder is associated with the eventual development of focal glomerular sclerosis.[165,166]

CONGENITAL HYDRONEPHROSIS

Along with renal hypoplasia-dysplasia, congenital urinary tract obstruction accounts for most cases of nephron loss in the neonate. Complete ureteral obstruction (atresia) early in gestation results in multicystic dysplasia and a nonfunctional kidney.[167] However, most forms of hydronephrosis in the neonate result from incomplete obstruction of the urinary tract or vesicoureteral reflux. Severe bladder obstruction resulting from posterior urethral valves can cause renal maldevelopment in utero such that adaptive renal growth is impaired despite either prenatal or postnatal relief of obstruction.[168,169] Unilateral ureteropelvic junction obstruction, on the other hand, may be relatively mild in utero such that most renal damage occurs postnatally unless the obstruction is relieved.[170] Severe vesicoureteral reflux can eventually lead to glomerulosclerosis, proteinuria, and renal insufficiency if both kidneys are involved.[171]

Although compensatory growth of the contralateral kidney has been suggested as an index of functional impairment in children with unilateral ureteropelvic junction obstruction, biologic variability and limitations of clinical ultrasonographic imaging limit the early detection of compensatory renal growth.[172,173]

It is becoming increasingly clear that there is an insufficient follow-up period of children born with congenital anomalies of the kidney and urinary tract. In a study of 312 patients with CAKUT,[174] Sanna-Cherchi and associates demonstrated that by the age of 30, 18.5% of these patients started dialysis. Although it is not surprising that patients with posterior ureteral valves were at significant risk for requiring dialysis, the patients with a solitary kidney had a hazard ratio (HR) of 2.42 (95% CI [confidence interval]: 1.08, 5.40) for the development of end-stage renal disease, which was worse if vesicoureteral reflux was also present (HR 7.5, 95% CI: 2.72, 20.68).[174] This study challenges the previously accepted belief that unilateral renal agenesis represented a benign condition. A study of young adults with a solitary kidney demonstrated that 50% of this population had hypertension or microalbuminuria. Particularly worrisome were those born small for gestational age (SGA), another risk factor for nephron reduction, because they had smaller kidneys and lower estimated GFRs.[175] Additionally a meta-analysis of 2684 solitary kidney cases demonstrated that 16% were hypertensive, 21% had microalbuminuria, and 10% had a GFR of less than 60 mL/min.[176]

As shown in Fig. 104.2, maldevelopment of the kidneys or urinary tract, intrauterine or perinatal insults, or extreme prematurity can reduce renal function at birth. In general, the better the initial renal function, the better the outcome (trajectory A, see Fig. 104.2). Infants with compromised renal function at birth can subsequently develop a gradual decline in function (trajectory B), or a more rapid decline (trajectory C). The infant with a GFR of less than 50% of normal for age at the time of diagnosis is even more likely to experience progressive renal insufficiency.[177,178] Although infants with posterior urethral valves and a serum creatinine concentration less than 0.8 mg/dL during the first 12 months of life are likely to maintain adequate renal function for a number of years, acceleration of the rate of renal deterioration may increase at adolescence or during adulthood.[179] As discussed above, a number of conditions are associated with impairment of nephrogenesis (see Fig. 104.1), which may predispose patients to hypertension, proteinuria, and renal insufficiency in adulthood.[180]

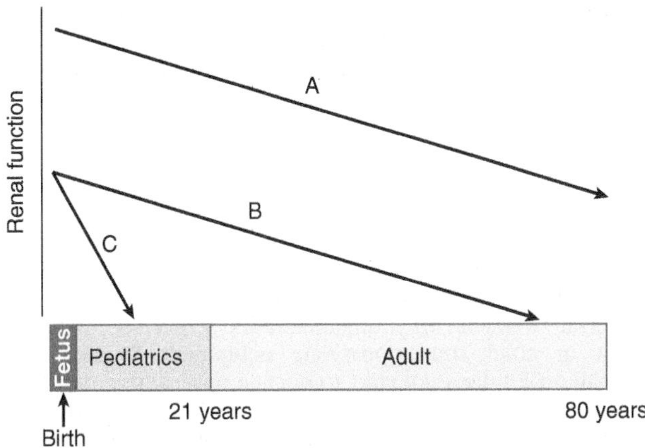

Fig. 104.2 Scheme showing long-term impact of congenital renal disorders. The urinary tract abnormality develops in embryonic and fetal life, but if mild *(A)*, the consequences of the condition may become apparent only later in adulthood, if at all. If moderate *(B)*, progression of renal insufficiency may develop earlier in adulthood. If severe *(C)*, renal failure develops in infancy or childhood. Long-term follow-up of blood pressure and urine protein excretion is desirable in virtually all patients discharged from a neonatal intensive care unit. (Modified from Chevalier RL. Obstructive uropathy: assessment of renal function in the fetus. In: Oh W, Guignard JP, Baumgart S, eds. *Nephrology and Fluid/Electrolyte Physiology: Neonatology Questions and Controversies*. Philadelphia: Elsevier; 2008: 226.)

LONG-TERM FOLLOW-UP

A major problem confronting the physician caring for the infant with reduced functioning renal mass is the lack of a reliable means of predicting which individuals will have compensatory renal adaptation and identifying those with greater risk of developing CKD. Will the infant require dialysis or renal transplantation, and if so, when? As described earlier, normal and compensatory renal development is interdependent and significantly influenced by the etiology of nephron loss, the proportion of intact nephrons remaining, and the presence of factors that impair adaptive processes. Because nephrogenesis is not complete until 36 weeks gestation, preterm infants with nephron loss may have a slower increase in postnatal renal mass and function than term infants. Moreover, because even an abnormal kidney undergoes accelerated growth at the time of the pubertal growth spurt, the patient with limited "renal reserve" may not manifest evidence of CKD until adolescence or later.[177,181] Identifying children with mild CKD in adolescence is essential for early lifestyle modifications to prevent further disease progression. This is particularly important in children born preterm or SGA who are at increased risk of metabolic and cardiovascular disease, both of which increase the risk for development of CKD.[182,183]

Until more comprehensive predictive data are available, the most prudent approach to follow-up of the neonate with possible nephron loss from any cause is periodic measurement of somatic and renal growth (by ultrasonography), blood pressure, GFR (by serum creatinine or cystatin C concentration), and urine protein excretion (by urine protein-creatinine ratio). Unfortunately, these monitoring modalities have a limited positive predictive value. Renal growth measured by ultrasonography may be difficult in large patients, is subject to interobserver variability, and changes in kidney size after the perinatal period represent largely tubular compensation. Accurate blood pressure assessment is not universally available for young infants and requires a cooperative infant or child and appropriate equipment. Whole kidney estimated GFR does not start to decline until a large number of nephrons are nonfunctional, and even clearance techniques will not reveal compensation by remaining nephrons. Orthostatic or transient proteinuria is common and must be ruled out in the evaluation where proteinuria is present.

We currently lack formal evidence-based guidelines to help practitioners identify which preterm neonates should be seen by a pediatric nephrologist and when follow-up should occur. A review article in Pediatrics in 2013 suggested that neonates could be risk stratified (low vs. high risk for CKD). Those with the lowest gestational ages, significant SGA, history of AKI, or any structural anomalies fall into the category of higher risk for CKD and should be followed by a pediatric nephrologist.[184] In addition, American Academy of Pediatrics recommends blood pressure monitoring before the age of 3 years for this "high risk" group.[185] As more information is obtained regarding the long-term outcomes of the preterm neonate, guidelines for follow up will become more evidence based.

It appears that the progression of renal disease may be slowed by the judicious inhibition of angiotensin II by using either an ACE inhibitor, an angiotensin receptor blocker,[186] or combined use of both. In addition to controlling hypertension, a number of experimental studies have shown a salutary effect of angiotensin inhibition on proteinuria and the development of interstitial fibrosis. As noted above, because angiotensin II is necessary for normal renal development and for maintaining renal hemodynamics perinatally, inhibition of angiotensin should be avoided if possible during the perinatal and neonatal periods. Studies in neonatal rats with partial ureteral obstruction show that ACE inhibitors or angiotensin receptor blockers can actually exacerbate renal lesions if administered too early.[187,188] However, if given after the period of nephron maturation (after weaning in the rat), the effects are salutary.[189,190] ACE inhibition in rodents with considerably low nephron endowment has also been shown to have a positive effect on renal and cardiac structure and function. Unfortunately, targeting the population of humans at risk that could benefit from angiotensin inhibitor is still unclear.

In view of their vasoconstrictor effects, patients with a reduced number of nephrons should also avoid the use of NSAIDs. The combination of improved perinatal/neonatal evaluation and management, as well as seamless longitudinal follow-up by the pediatrician and internist, should lead to optimal preservation of renal function in humans born with a reduction in renal mass.

CONCLUSION

Early adaption to reduced nephron number depends on when the nephron reduction occurs, pre- or postnephrogenesis, and whether there is ongoing renal injury. Evidence exists that nephron formation can be enhanced if the insult is early, but after the completion of nephrogenesis, the main compensatory mechanism is through glomerular and tubular hypertrophy. Given our lack of diagnostic testing to determine nephron number in humans, it is critical to monitor and educate high-risk children and their families about their risk for CKD due to low nephron number.

ACKNOWLEDGMENTS

The authors are supported by the following funding:

PG: NICHD, Pediatric Scientist Development Program (PSDP) and K12-HD000850.

FL: R01DK118140, R01DK107653.

JC: R01DK110622, R01DK111861, U34DK117128.

A complete reference list is available at www.ExpertConsult.com. 

SELECT REFERENCES

1. Bertram JF, Douglas-Denton RN, Diouf B, et al. Human nephron number: implications for health and disease. *Pediatr Nephrol.* 2011;26:1529–1533.
2. Douglas-Denton RN, McNamara BJ, Hoy WE, et al. Does nephron number matter in the development of kidney disease? *Ethn Dis.* 2006:16(2 suppl 2):S40–S45.
3. Lindström NO, McMahon JA, Guo J, et al. Conserved and divergent features of human and mouse kidney organogenesis. *J Am Soc Nephrol.* 2018;29(3):785–805.
4. Lindström NO, Tran T, Guo J, et al. Conserved and divergent molecular and anatomic features of human and mouse nephron patterning. *J Am Soc Nephrol.* 2018;29(3):825–840.
5. Lindström NO, De Sena Brandine G, Tran T, et al. Progressive recruitment of mesenchymal progenitors reveals a time-dependent process of cell fate acquisition in mouse and human nephrogenesis. *Dev Cell.* 2018;45(5):651–660.e4. https://doi.org/10.1016/j.devcel.2018.05.010.
6. Hinchliffe SA, Sargent PH, Howard CV, Chan YF, Van Velzen D. Human intrauterine renal growth expressed in absolute number of glomeruli assessed by the disector method and Cavalieri principle. *Lab Invest.* 1991;64(6):777–784.
7. Hughson M, Farris 3rd AB, Douglas-Denton R, Hoy WE, Bertram JF. Glomerular number and size in autopsy kidneys: the relationship to birth weight. *Kidney Int.* 2003;63(6):2113–2122.
8. Rodríguez MM, Gómez AH, Abitbol CL, Chandar JJ, Duara S, Zilleruelo GE. Histomorphometric analysis of postnatal glomerulogenesis in extremely preterm infants. *Pediatr Dev Pathol.* 2004;7(1):17–25. https://doi.org/10.1007/s10024-003-3029.
9. Sutherland L, Gubhaju L, Moore, et al. Accelerated maturation and abnormal morphology in the preterm neonatal kidney. *J Am Soc Nephrol.* 2011;22(7):1365–1374.
10. Hoy WE, Hughson MD, Bertram JF, Douglas-Denton R, Amann K. Nephron number, hypertension, renal disease, and renal failure. *J Am Soc Nephrol.* 2005;16(9):2557–2564. https://doi.org/10.1681/ASN.2005020172.
11. Crump C, Sundquist J, Winkleby MA, Sundquist K. Preterm birth and risk of chronic kidney disease from childhood into mid-adulthood: national cohort study. *BMJ.* 2019;365:l1346. https://doi.org/10.1136/bmj.l1346. Published 2019 May 1.
12. Horie A, Abe Y, Koike D, et al. Long-term renal follow up of preterm neonates born before 35 weeks of gestation. *Pediatr Int.* 2019;61(12):1244–1249. https://doi.org/10.1111/ped.14004.
13. White SL, Perkovic V, Cass A, et al. Is low birth weight an antecedent of CKD in later life? A systematic review of observational studies. *Am J Kidney Dis.* 2009;54(2):248–261. https://doi.org/10.1053/j.ajkd.2008.12.042.
14. Hsu CW, Yamamoto KT, Henry RK, De Roos AJ, Flynn JT. Prenatal risk factors for childhood CKD. *J Am Soc Nephrol.* 2014;25(9):2105–2111. https://doi.org/10.1681/ASN.2013060582.
15. Short KM, Smyth IM. The contribution of branching morphogenesis to kidney development and disease. *Nat Rev Nephrol.* 2016;12(12):754–767. https://doi.org/10.1038/nrneph.2016.157.
16. van der Ven AT, Vivante A, Hildebrandt F. Novel insights into the pathogenesis of monogenic congenital anomalies of the kidney and urinary tract. *J Am Soc Nephrol.* 2018;29(1):36–50. https://doi.org/10.1681/ASN.2017050561.
17. Self M, Lagutin OV, Bowling B, et al. Six2 is required for suppression of nephrogenesis and progenitor renewal in the developing kidney. *EMBO J.* 2006;25:5214–5228.
18. Zhang Z, Quinlan J, Hoy W, et al. A common RET variant is associated with reduced newborn kidney size and function. *J Am Soc Nephrol.* 2008;19:2027–2034.
19. Schuchardt A, D'Agati V, Pachnis V, Costantini F. Renal agenesis and hypodysplasia in ret-k- mutant mice result from defects in ureteric bud development. *Development.* 1996;122:1919–1929.
20. El Kares R, Manolescu DC, Lakhal-Chaieb L, et al. A human ALDH1A2 gene variant is associated with increased newborn kidney size and serum retinoic acid. *Kidney Int.* 2010;78:96–102.
21. Yermalovich AV, Osborne JK, Sousa P, et al. Lin28 and let-7 regulate the timing of cessation of murine nephrogenesis [published correction appears in Nat Commun. 2020 Mar 9;11(1):1327]. *Nat Commun.* 2019;10(1):168. https://doi.org/10.1038/s41467-018-08127-4. Published 2019 Jan 11.
22. Yu J. miRNAs in mammalian ureteric bud development. *Pediatr Nephrol.* 2014;29:745–749.
23. Nakagawa N, Xin C, Roach AM, et al. Dicer1 activity in the stromal compartment regulates nephron differentiation and vascular patterning during mammalian kidney organogenesis. *Kidney Int.* 2015;87(6):1125–1140. https://doi.org/10.1038/ki.2014.406.

24. Ho J, Pandey P, Schatton T, et al. The pro-apoptotic protein Bim is a microRNA target in kidney progenitors. *J Am Soc Nephrol*. 2011;22(6):1053–1063. https://doi.org/10.1681/ASN.2010080841.
25. Cerqueira DM, Bodnar AJ, Phua YL, et al. *Bim* gene dosage is critical in modulating nephron progenitor survival in the absence of microRNAs during kidney development. *FASEB J*. 2017;31(8):3540–3554. https://doi.org/10.1096/fj.201700010R.
26. Hinchliffe SA, Lynch MR, Sargent PH, et al. The effect of intrauterine growth retardation on the development of renal nephrons. *Br J Obstet Gynaecol*. 1992;99:296–301.
27. Woods LL, Weeks DA, Rasch R, Programming of adult blood pressure by maternal protein restriction: role of nephrogenesis. *Kidney Int*. 2004;65:1339–1348.
28. Merlet-Benichou C, Gilbert T, Muffat-Joly M, et al. Intrauterine growth retardation leads to a permanent nephron deficit in the rat. *Pediatr Nephrol*. 1994;8:175–180.
29. Schreuder MF, Nyengaard JR, Fodor M, et al. Glomerular number and function are influenced by spontaneous and induced low birth weight in rats. *J Am Soc Nephrol*. 2005;16:2913–2919.
31. Gopalakrishnan GS, Gardner DS, Dandrea J, et al. Influence of maternal pre-pregnancy body composition and diet during early-mid pregnancy on cardiovascular function and nephron number in juvenile sheep. *Br J Nutr*. 2005;94:938–947.
32. Gilbert JS, Lang AL, Grant AR, Nijland MJ. Maternal nutrient restriction in sheep: hypertension and decreased nephron number in offspring at 9 months of age. *J Physiol*. 2005;565:137–147.
33. Hoy WE, Rees M, Kile E, et al. A new dimension to the Barker hypothesis: low birthweight and susceptibility to renal disease. *Kidney Int*. 1999;56:1072–1077.
34. Lelievre-Pegorier M, Vilar J, Ferrier ML, et al. Mild vitamin A deficiency leads to inborn nephron deficit in the rat. *Kidney Int*. 1998;54:1455–1462.
35. Gilbert JS, Lang AL, Grant AR, Nijland MJ. Maternal nutrient restriction in sheep: hypertension and decreased nephron number in offspring at 9 months of age. *J Physiol*. 2005;565:137–147.
36. Lumey LH, Terry MB, Delgado-Cruzata L, et al. Adult global DNA methylation in relation to pre-natal nutrition. *Int J Epidemiol*. 2012;41(1):116–123. https://doi.org/10.1093/ije/dyr137.
37. Wanner N, Vornweg J, Combes A, et al. DNA methyltransferase 1 controls nephron progenitor cell renewal and differentiation. *J Am Soc Nephrol*. 2019;30(1):63–78. https://doi.org/10.1681/ASN.2018070736.
38. Maka N, Makrakis J, Parkington HC, et al. Vitamin D deficiency during pregnancy and lactation stimulates nephrogenesis in rat offspring. *Pediatr Nephrol*. 2008;23:55–61.
39. Hoy WE, Hughson MD, Bertram JF, et al. Nephron number, hypertension, renal disease, and renal failure. *J Am Soc Nephrol*. 2005;16:2557–2564.
40. Gray SP, Denton KM, Cullen-McEwen L, et al. Prenatal exposure to alcohol reduces nephron number and raises blood pressure in progeny. *J Am Soc Nephrol*. 2010;21:1891–1902.
41. Gray SP, Kenna K, Bertram JF, et al. Repeated ethanol exposure during late gestation decreases nephron endowment in fetal sheep. *Am J Physiol Regul Integr Comp Physiol*. 2008;295:568–574.
42. Taal HR, Geelhoed JJ, Steegers EA, et al. Maternal smoking during pregnancy and kidney volume in the offspring: the generation R study. *Pediatr Nephrol*. 2011;26:1275–1283.
43. Sedman AB, Kershaw DB, Bunchman TE. Recognition and management of angiotensin converting enzyme inhibitor fetopathy. *Pediatr Nephrol*. 1995;9:382–385.
44. Kaplan BS, Restaino I, Raval DS, et al. Renal failure in the neonate associated with in utero exposure to non-steroidal anti-inflammatory agents. *Pediatr Nephrol*. 1994;8:700–704.
45. Ortiz LA, Quan A, Weinberg A, Baum M. Effect of prenatal dexamethasone on rat renal development. *Kidney Int*. 2001;59:1663–1669.
46. Gilbert T, Lelievre-Pegorier M, Merlet-Benichou C. Long-term effects of mild oligonephronia induced in utero by gentamicin in the rat. *Pediatr Res*. 1991;30:450–456.
47. Nathanson S, Moreau E, Merlet-Benichou C, Gilbert T. In utero and in vitro exposure to beta-lactams impair kidney development in the rat. *J Am Soc Nephrol*. 2000;11:874–884.
48. Tendron A, Decramer S, Justrabo E, et al. Cyclosporin A administration during pregnancy induces a permanent nephron deficit in young rabbits. *J Am Soc Nephrol*. 2003;14:3188–3196.
49. Wintour EM, Moritz KM, Johnson K, et al. Reduced nephron number in adult sheep, hypertensive as a result of prenatal glucocorticoid treatment. *J Physiol*. 2003;549:929–935.
50. Amri K, Freund N, Vilar J, et al. Adverse effects of hyperglycemia on kidney development in rats: in vivo and in vitro studies. *Diabetes*. 1999;48:2240–2245.

105 Fluid Distribution in the Fetus and Neonate

Chang-Ryul Kim | Barbara S. Stonestreet

INTRODUCTION

The human body is composed of fluids and solids (proteins, fat, and minerals). Total body water (TBW) is inversely related to body fat content because fat has very low water content. Body water also contains an array of dissolved substances. Water is the largest single constituent of body composition. TBW is divided into two compartments: intracellular fluid (ICF) and extracellular fluid (ECF). ECF is further divided into the intravascular and interstitial compartments, lymphatics, and transcellular fluid. Intravascular compartment (blood volume, or BV), in turn, is subdivided into plasma volume (PV), as a part of the ECF, and red blood cell volume (RCV) as a part of the ICF, because white blood cells and platelets contribute negligibly to the total BV. Therefore, the ECF consists of plasma and interstitial fluid (ISF), so that TBW is distributed among the three major fluid spaces: ICF, plasma, and ISF (Fig. 105.1).

There is a constant flux of fluid among the compartments. Redistribution of fluid across the vascular endothelium under normal conditions allows overflow of excess volume from the intravascular compartment into the interstitial compartment. Consequently, volume overload of the cardiovascular system is prevented. The distribution of blood and plasma volumes is regulated by various hormones, which include the renin-angiotensin-aldosterone system, antidiuretic hormone, and atrial natriuretic factor. RCV is regulated by erythropoietin and growth factors.

ICF and ECF are governed by multiple forces that include active transport, osmotic pressure, epithelial permeability, crystalloid and colloid concentrations, intravascular and interstitial hydraulic pressures, hormones, and blood and lymph circulation.

The most abundant cation is Na^+, and the most abundant anion is Cl^- in the ECF. The most abundant cation is K^+, and the predominant anion is HPO_4^{2-} (phosphate) in ICF. There are more protein anions in ICF than in ECF so that ICF has a higher osmotic pressure than ISF. Normally, the higher intracellular osmotic pressure is balanced by forces that move water out of the cell, so the amount of water inside the cell does not change. When fluid imbalances between these two compartments occur, it is usually caused by a change in Na^+ or K^+ concentrations.

Plasma and ISF compositions are similar but differ from the composition of ICF. The main difference between plasma and ISF is that plasma contains quite a few protein anions and ISF has very little. Plasma contains more Na^+ but less Cl^- than ISF. The proteins stay within the plasma and do not move out of the blood into the ISF because normal capillary membranes are practically impermeable to proteins (Fig. 105.2).[1]

Fluid leaves the plasma and enters the interstitium because of the combined effects of hydrostatic and osmotic pressure gradients at the capillary membrane. The lymphatic system counterbalances this egress by pumping ISF through the lymphatic vessels back into the circulation. Thus, the distribution of fluid between plasma and ISF depends on the balance between capillary permeability and lymphatic function under steady-state conditions.

The most dramatic changes in body fluid compartments occur during intrauterine fetal growth and development and the postnatal adaptation of the neonate from the "aquatic" intrauterine to the "terrestrial" extrauterine environment.

The amount of TBW and its distribution into the body fluid compartments are markedly different in the fetus and newborn compared with the adult. The volume-regulatory mechanisms during the fetal and perinatal period are functioning at a level that is unique compared with those in later life. This chapter describes fetal, perinatal, and postnatal changes in body fluid compartments.

MEASUREMENT OF BODY WATER COMPARTMENTS

There are various techniques to measure body fluid volumes, such as whole-body desiccation, dynamic skinfold thickness measurement with a Harpenden caliper, bioelectrical impedance analysis, and indicator dilution techniques. The indicator dilution techniques are more valuable for clinical studies using Fick's law of diffusion. It is essentially the restatement of the law of conservation of mass, in which a known amount of the indicator is administered to the subject, and its concentration is then measured in samples of the body fluid space of interest. The ideal indicator is devoid of toxicity and is measurable in blood or other body fluids with sufficient accuracy and reproducibility with the use of small blood samples. It rapidly reaches equilibrium in its distribution and is neither metabolized nor excreted during the desired period of study. Table 105.1 lists the various methods used to determine the volume and distribution of body water in the fetus, neonate, child, and adult.

Accurate measurement of red cell mass, plasma, blood, and ISF volumes in the fetus and newborn as well as in the adult is difficult because the methods are technically complex and time consuming, and radioactive methods are no longer considered ethical in human subjects.

BLOOD VOLUME

When blood volume is calculated from measured plasma volume or red cell mass and hematocrit, the errors in plasma volume measurement produce major errors in blood volume determinations. Hematocrit determinations are also a potential source of error.

Large vessel (venous or arterial) hematocrits are higher than the total body hematocrit because of rheologic factors.[2] The total-body to venous hematocrit ratio (F-ratio)[3] is 0.87[4] or 0.91[5] in normal neonates. The ratio could be lower in severely sick neonates. Thus, both the use of an incorrectly high body to

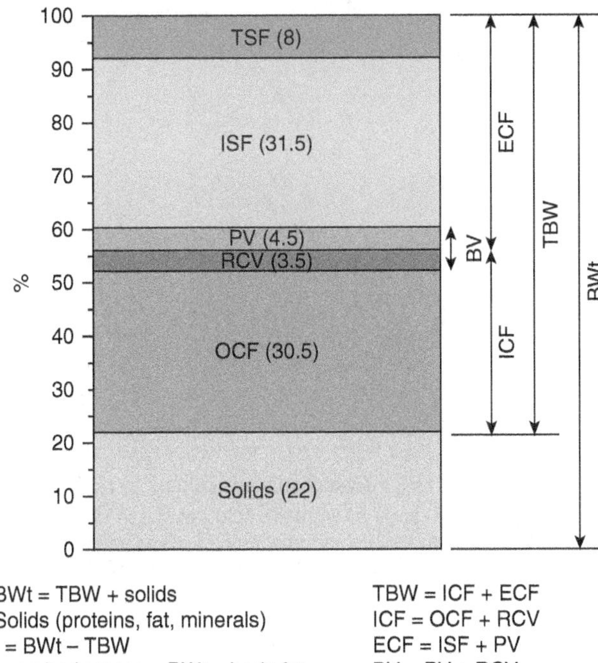

Fig. 105.1 Body water distribution in a term newborn infant. *BV*, Blood volume; *BWt*, body weight; *ECF*, extracellular fluid; *ICF*, intracellular fluid; *ISF*, interstitial fluid; *OCF*, organ cell fluid; *PV*, plasma volume; *RCV*, red cell volume; *TBW*, total body water; *TSF*, transcellular fluid.

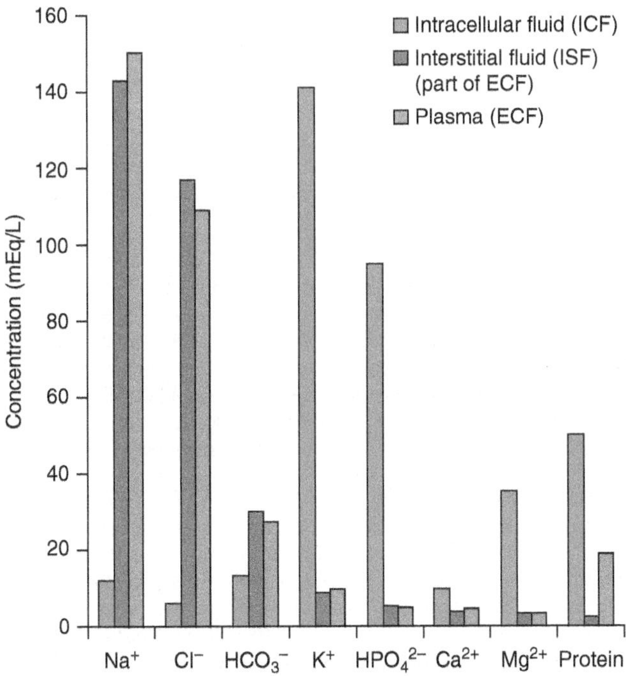

Fig. 105.2 The graph shows the composition of the intracellular fluid, interstitial fluid, and plasma in humans. *ECF*, extracellular fluid. (From ERservices. *Anatomy and Physiology II: Body Fluids and Fluid Compartments*. https://courses.lumenlearning.com/suny-ap2/chapter/body-fluids-and-fluid-compartments-no-content/. Accessed August 10, 2019.)

Table 105.1 Techniques for In Vivo Investigations of Human Body Water Volume and Distribution.

Body Water Compartment	Technique
Total body water (TBW)	Dilution (D_2O, $H_2{}^{18}O$, antipyrine), total body electrical conductivity
Extracellular water (ECW)	Dilution (bromide, sucrose, thiocyanate, thiosulfate, inulin, mannitol, ^{22}Na or ^{24}Na), bioelectrical reactance, dynamic skinfold thickness
Interstitial water (ISW)	ISW = ECW – PV, electrical conductivity, dynamic skinfold thickness
Intracellular water (ICW)	ICW = TBW – ECW, dilution (^{40}K)
Blood volume (BV)	BV = PV + RCV [a]BV = [PV/(100 – Hematocrit)] × 100 Automated blood volume analyzer (BVA, Volemetron)
Plasma volume (PV)	Dilution [Evans blue (T-1824), Indocyanine green, ^{131}I- or ^{125}I]
Red cell volume (RCV)	RCV = BV – PV, dilution (biotin, ^{51}Cr, ^{32}P, ^{99m}Tc)

Body solids = Body Weight – TBW.
[a]Blood volume = (PV x 100)/[100 - (Hct x F-cell ratio)][2,3]

venous hematocrit ratio and the delayed withdrawal of a blood sample after injection of a plasma label result in overestimation of blood volume. Therefore, an RBC label produces a more precise blood volume estimate in the fetus than double indicator dilution techniques that separately measure RBC and plasma volumes. The most accurate estimate of plasma volume is obtained by measuring blood volume with an RBC label and then multiplying by one minus the fractional large vessel hematocrit. Thus, labeled RBCs provide better estimates of plasma, RBC, and blood volume, provided that errors due to unbound labels are minimized.

PLASMA VOLUME

Plasma volume is measured as the dilution space of labeled high-molecular-weight substances, such as dyes (Evans Blue[6] or indocyanine green[7]) or radiolabeled (^{131}I or ^{125}I) human serum albumin or plasma proteins,[8] after injection into the circulation (indicator dilution technique). Plasma labels mix completely with the circulating plasma within 5 minutes.[4]

These measurements are frequently corrected for the loss of the label from the circulation by extrapolating the concentration-time curve backward to the original time of injection. Even with this correction, plasma volume measurements are subject to large errors for two major reasons: (1) All plasma labels are rapidly lost from the circulation through the capillary membranes of organs, such as the liver, even in normal neonates, which exhibit high permeability even to high-molecular-weight substances. Extrapolating back to the time of injection does not correct for this loss because it is too rapid to be detected. (2) Most labels such as radioisotopes or dyes are not completely bound to the plasma proteins when injected into the circulation. Unbound labels are rapidly lost from the circulation and again result in an overestimation of plasma volume.

RED BLOOD CELL MASS

Red cell mass is determined as the dilution space of a known quantity of labeled erythrocytes (indicator dilution technique; Biotin, ^{51}Cr, ^{32}P, ^{99m}Tc) or calculation from blood and plasma volumes. To measure red cell mass, blood is taken from the study subject, mixed with the erythrocyte label, and then retransfused into the subject. Labeled red blood cells (RBCs) do not leave the circulation for several hours, but the mixing time might be markedly prolonged compared with labeled plasma.[9] Biotin has been validated as a red cell label in neonates because there is a consensus that the use of radioactive materials was not ethical for research studies in human fetuses and neonates.[10,11]

EXTRACELLULAR FLUID AND INTERSTITIAL VOLUME

ISF volume can be calculated as the difference between ECF and plasma volume. However, measurement of each of these volumes is subject to error. ECF volume has been measured as the volume of distribution of a variety of labels injected into the circulation (indicator dilution technique: bromide, sucrose, thiocyanate, thiosulfate, inulin, mannitol, ^{22}Na, or ^{24}Na).

Each of these labels has a unique distribution space that does not exactly match the biologic ECF volume. Therefore, the comparison of ECF volumes measured with different methods is difficult. Bromide and sucrose are more widely used as ECF markers in the newborn.[12,13] Bromide may not be adequate in the fetus because of transplacental losses[12] and because it has an intracellular distribution in the fetus and neonate.[13] Sucrose is not metabolized, does not enter cells, and has been validated in neonates and children.[14,15]

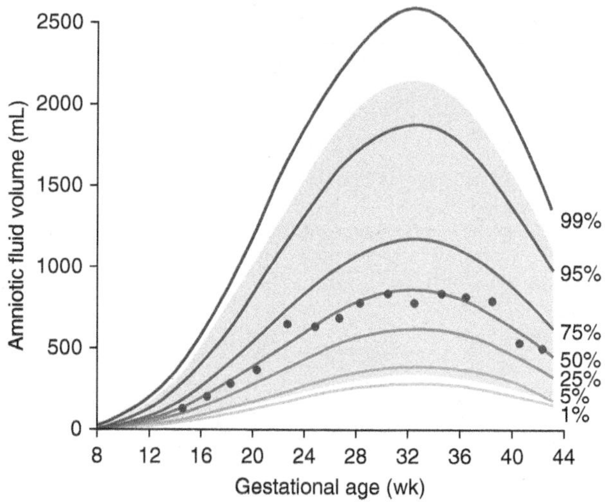

Fig. 105.3 Normal range of amniotic fluid volume in human gestation. (From Brace RA, Wolf EJ. Normal amniotic fluid volume changes throughout pregnancy. *Am J Obstet Gynecol.* 1989;161(2):382–388, used with permission.)

DEVELOPMENTAL CHANGES IN BODY FLUID VOLUMES IN FETUS AND NEONATE

AMNIOTIC FLUID VOLUME

Water is partitioned between the fetus, placenta, chorionic and amniotic membranes, and amniotic fluid (AF) during fetal life. The AF that surrounds the fetus is often considered to be an extension of the fetal extracellular space under unique volume regulatory mechanisms before birth. AF is formed from either a transudate of fetal plasma through nonkeratinized skin or from maternal plasma across the uterine decidua or placental surface.[16] AF most likely represents trophoblastic or fetal transudation early in gestation, which is isotonic with fetal and maternal plasma[17] but contains minimal protein. AF reflects the fetal ECF to around the 20th week of gestation because the fetal skin is permeable to free exchange of substances.

Approximately 4000 mL of water accumulates in the human uterus (2800 mL in the fetus, 800 mL in AF, and 400 mL in placenta) near term. The amniotic fluid volume (AFV) may vary from 500 mL to more than 1200 mL. Although AFV does not necessarily correlate with fetal weight, AF volume is lower in growth-restricted fetuses and higher in macrosomic fetuses.

AFV is 98% to 99% water and is regulated within a narrow range to maintain fetal fluid status throughout gestation.[18] Fetal organ function becomes more important for the regulation of AFV as gestation advances. AFV gradually increases during the first trimester, remaining relatively stable with an average volume of 700 to 800 mL between 22 and 39 weeks of gestation. There is also a peak at 33 weeks of gestation. Thereafter, AF decreases by 8%/week with a mean volume of approximately 500 mL at 40 to 42 weeks of gestation (Fig. 105.3).[19]

The two primary sources of AF influx during the latter half of gestation are fetal urine and lung liquid, with additional small contributions from fetal oral-nasal secretions. However, fetal urine is the main source of AF. The two primary routes of AF egress are fetal swallowing and the intramembranous absorption of water into fetal vasculature,[20,21] as schematically summarized in Fig. 105.4.[22]

The fetus produces hypotonic urine of 300 mL/kg/day after mid-gestation. This reduces AF osmolality and provides a large potential force for the outward flow of water across the intramembranous pathway (AF to fetal circulation). AF osmolality declines from 290 mOsm/kg in the first trimester to

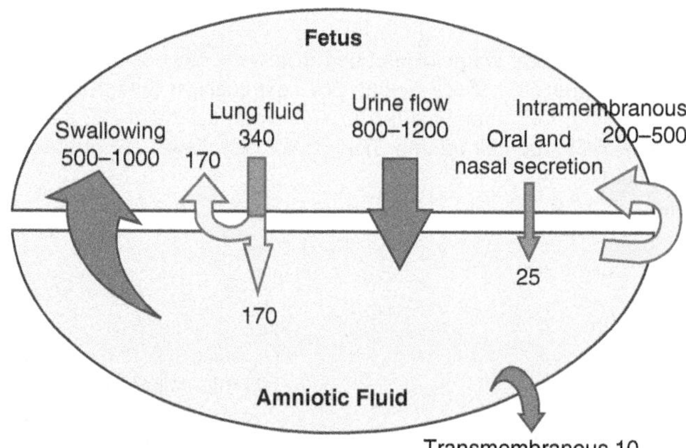

Fig. 105.4 Summary of water flows into and out of the amniotic space in late gestation (mL/day). Arrow size is proportional to flow rate. (Republished with permission from Gilbert WE, Brace, RA. Amniotic fluid volume and normal flows to and from amniotic cavity. *Semin Perinatol.* 1993;17:150–157.)

approximately 255 mOsm/kg near term, which favors water transfer from the amniotic cavity into the fetal blood across the fetal placental surface.[19-21,23] Maternal and fetal osmolality are very similar, which limits the quantity of water transfer to and from the fetus under normal conditions.[24] The chemical composition of AF also changes during gestation. AF urea, creatinine, and uric acid increase during the second half of pregnancy because of increased renal excretion.[25]

The volume of fetal lung fluid depends on the developmental stage of the lungs. Lung fluid volume is very low early in gestation and increases rapidly with the accelerated lung growth late in gestation. This large volume suggests that lung fluid could be a potential water source for the fetus. The fetus secretes isotonic lung fluid of 60 to 100 mL/kg/day at term, which serves to expand the airways and promote normal lung growth. This fluid is formed by active secretion of chloride ions into the alveolar spaces, resulting in a progressive accumulation of fluid in the lungs as gestation progresses. Pulmonary transepithelial chloride secretion appears to be the major driving force responsible for the production of liquid in the fetal lung lumen. Since the secretion of fetal lung fluid far exceeds that needed for lung volume expansion, the excess lung fluid exits via the trachea. The fluid appears to exit the trachea intermittently rather than making a gradual egress.[26] At least half of secreted lung fluid is immediately swallowed, and approximately half flows into the amniotic cavity.[24] Removal of AF occurs by fetal swallowing and the intramembranous absorption of AF into the fetal blood through the fetal surface of the placenta.

Fetal swallowing is the major mechanism by which fluid is removed from the amniotic cavity, comprising 500 to 1000 mL/day. Factors known to increase fetal swallowing include decreased amniotic osmolality, increased fetal plasma osmolality, and increased AFV.[24]

The total turnover of the AF (1170 mL/day, urine production plus lung fluid egress and minus volume swallowed of 750 mL/day) leaves a surplus influx of fluid into the amniotic cavity of at least 400 mL/day. This difference is compensated for by another pathway, termed the *intramembranous pathway*. The daily AF turnover of 1000 mL in the near-term fetus is actually higher than the absolute AFV of 700 to 800 mL. Therefore, AFV must be highly regulated to avoid oligohydramnios or polyhydramnios.

Regulatory mechanisms for AFV act at three levels:

1. Transfer of water between mother and fetus across the placenta. Transplacental transfer is dependent on the existence of hydrostatic and/or colloid osmotic pressure differences between fetal and maternal vessels.[27] Placental water transfer between mother and fetus can serve as a reservoir to stabilize fetal ECF volume and blood pressure. The intravascular infusion of large volumes of crystalloid solutions in fetal sheep results in the transfer of large amounts of water and solute across the placenta to the mother, either against or in the absence of chemical concentration gradients.[28,29] These observations suggest that a normal fetus can protect itself against both volume and salt overloads by rapid transfer of excess to the mother. Reduced fetal blood pressure releases fetal angiotensin. This increases the resistance in the fetal placental precapillary vessels and reduces fetal placental blood flow, thereby promoting water transfer from mother to fetus to restore fetal blood pressure.[30] However, the placenta or any other single fetal structure does not control the amount of water that enters the fetus. The combined physiologic properties of the fetal heart, kidneys, somatic tissues, and placenta contribute to the control of the fetal volume status.[31]
2. Regulation of flow between the amniotic cavity and the fetus. Increasing or decreasing intramembranous absorption appears to be the main mechanism regulating flow between the amniotic cavity and fetus. Intramembranous water movement into the fetal circulation is driven by the large osmotic difference between fetal plasma and AF, because the fetal vessels on the placental surface are bathed in AF.[24] The primary mechanism that drives intramembranous volume flow is not passive osmosis. Instead, it has been suggested that AF with all its dissolved solutes is transported across the amniotic membrane via bulk flow transfer by a yet unspecified vesicular transport mechanism.[32] Aquaporins (AQPs) in the placental and fetal membranes may also play a role in AF absorption. AQP 1, 3, 8, and 9 are the major AQPs in the placental and fetal membranes. Fetal membrane AQP1, and placental AQP1 and AQP9 expression, were negatively correlated with AFV. Placental AQP3 expression was positively correlated with AFV in pregnant mice.[33]
3. Changes in maternal hydration: maternal oral hydration with water or intravenous hypotonic fluid significantly increases AFV in oligohydramnios[34] because of maternal osmotic changes, rather than maternal volume expansion.[35]

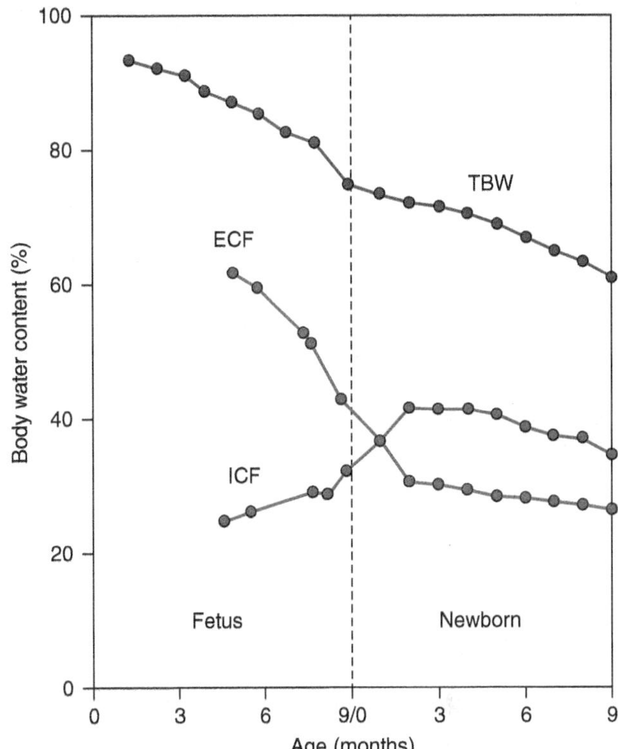

Fig. 105.5 Total body water *(TBW)* content and fluid distribution between intracellular fluid *(ICF)* and extracellular fluid *(ECF)* compartments in humans during fetal and neonatal development and during the first 9 months after birth. (Data from Friis-Hansen B. Body water compartments in children: changes during growth and related changes in body composition. *Pediatrics*. 1961;28:169.)

TOTAL BODY WATER

Friis-Hansen[36] in 1961 reported the developmental changes in the relative fluid volumes in humans from early in the fetal period through adulthood. As shown in Fig. 105.5, approximately 95% of the fetus is water in the early fetal period. The water proportion of total body weight gradually decreases throughout the fetal period to reach 86% at 27 weeks of gestation, of which the majority is in the ECF (60%), and 78% water with 44% in ECF, 34% in ICF at term.[36] This reduction in TBW is a result of the accumulation of body solids during growth. Body solids increase in the first two thirds of gestation because of the accretion of protein and minerals, but little fat deposition occurs. During the last trimester of gestation the proportion of body solids increases from 14% to 24% of body weight because of the deposition of body fat from 2% of body weight at 27 weeks of gestation to 10% to 15% of body weight at term.[37] The calculated body composition of the reference fetus for various gestational ages is indicated in Fig. 105.6.[37]

EXTRACELLULAR FLUID AND INTRACELLULAR FLUID COMPARTMENTS

Major changes occur in the body fluid distribution into ECF and ICF, which coincide with the reductions in TBW during fetal life. ECF volume is extremely large early in gestation, accounting for 62% of body weight, and is more than twice as large as the ICF volume. The large ECF space during fetal life is because growth occurs by cell division rather than by cell growth and results in tissues with small cells surrounded by a large ECF layer. Enlargement of cell size during normal intrauterine growth in the second half of gestation increases

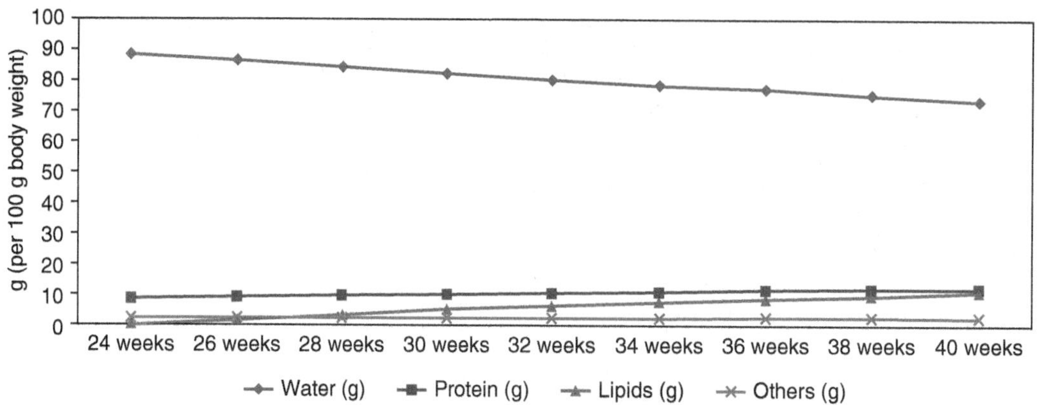

Fig. 105.6 During fetal growth, the reduction in total body water (TBW) is a result of the accumulation of body solids. Body solids increase in the first two-thirds of gestation because of the accretion of protein and minerals, but little fat deposition occurs. During the last trimester of gestation, the proportion of body solids increases from 14% to 24% of body weight because of the deposition of body fat from 2% of body weight at 27 weeks of gestation to 10% to 15% of body weight at term. (Data from Ziegler EE, O'Donnell AM, Nelson SE, Fomon SJ. Body composition of the reference fetus. *Growth*. 1976, Table 2. Body Composition of the Reference Fetus [per 100 g body weight]).

Table 105.2 Blood, Plasma, Red Blood Cell Volumes in Human Fetuses and Newborns (mL/kg).

	Age	Blood Volume (mL/kg)	Plasma Volume (mL/kg)	RBC volume (mL/kg)	Indicator	Reference
Fetus	16–22 wk GA	162[a] (FPV)			^{125}I (Volemetron)	44
	18–31 wk GA	101[b] (FPV; 18 wk, 117; 31 wk, 93)				45[e]
Newborn (at birth)	Preterm (<1500 g)	83[a]	46[a]		Sucrose (early clamp)	43
	Term	105 (CBV, 70.3[c]; PRBV, 34.7)		30.6	^{125}I	41
	Term 0 d	78.6[a]	40.5[a]	38.1[a]	^{125}I	176
	0–1 d	85[d]	41[a]	41[c]	Evans blue (PV), ^{32}P (RCV)	4

[a]Determined with plasma label.
[b]Determined with hematocrit changes during packed cell transfusion.
[c]Determined with RBC label.
[d]Determined with RBC plus plasma label.
[e]Data from fetuses with severe erythroblastosis.
BV, Blood volume; *CBV*, corrected blood volume; *FPV*, fetoplacental volume; *GA*, gestational age; *PRBV*, placental residual blood volume; *PV*, plasma volume, *RCV*, red blood cell volume.

the intracellular space from 25% to 32% of body weight from mid-gestation to term, whereas over the same interval ECF volume decreases from 62% to 43% of body weight.[36] Decreases in hyaluronan as gestation advances also contribute to reductions in ECF water content because it is major constituent of the extracellular matrix. Hyaluronan has a high water binding capacity and is the most abundant component of the fetal extracellular matrix during the early phase of rapid cell multiplication.[38] The reduction in ECF mainly results from loss of ISF because plasma volume per unit of body weight does not change at different gestational ages.[39] ICF increases approximately in proportion to body weight in the first few weeks of postnatal life. ICF continues to increase as a percent of body weight until it exceeds that of ECF, at three months of life. Hormonal, renal, and cardiovascular mechanisms are the main factors influencing ECF volume regulation in the fetus and neonate.[40]

BLOOD VOLUME

The circulating blood volume (CBV) in the fetus is considerably greater than in the newborn, because roughly one-third of the fetal blood volume is contained in the umbilical cord and fetal side of the placenta.[41] The total placental fetal blood volume in human neonates at term is 115 mL/kg, of which 70 mL/kg is in the fetus and 45 mL/kg in the placenta.[42] Reported values of blood, plasma, and RCV in the human fetus and neonate are summarized in Table 105.2.[4,41,43-45] These data should be interpreted cautiously because of the potential for methodologic errors, especially those related to plasma tracers, because capillary leak is greater in smaller fetuses.

Relationships among plasma volume, RBC, and blood volume have not been examined in the human fetus. Late-gestation chronically catheterized fetal sheep have plasma, RBC, and blood volumes under resting conditions that averaged 75, 36, and 111 mL/kg, respectively, and these were independent of fetal weight over the range of 1 to 4 kg.[46]

Human neonates with high blood volumes (weight normalized) have high RBC volumes but decreased plasma volumes.[4,47] The weight-normalized RBC volume also increases directly with venous hematocrit values, whereas plasma volume varies inversely with hematocrit.[47]

The relationship between hematocrit and true circulating red cell mass has received considerable attention because RBC volume measurements are not available in daily clinical practice and the hematocrit is used routinely to estimate RBC volume to guide transfusion practices. Correlations vary from weak ($r = 0.6$)[48] to strong ($r = 0.91$)[11] between venous hematocrits and RBC volumes in neonates. However, RBC volumes for individual neonates with a hematocrit of 30% ranged from 15 to 28 mL/kg, even when a strong correlation was present.[11] This range is of considerable clinical significance; this means that hematocrit is a relatively poor indicator of RBC volume.

FLUID DISTRIBUTION BETWEEN INTRAVASCULAR AND INTERSTITIAL COMPARTMENTS

Little is known about factors that reg ulate the distribution of fluid between the plasma and interstitial space in human fetuses. The best estimate of plasma volume is 76 mL/kg in late-gestation fetal sheep.[49] Interstitial volume has been estimated to average three times this volume, or 235 to 240 mL/kg of body weight.[50,51] The ratio of ISF volume to plasma volume (3:1) in the fetal sheep is similar to that of adults. However, when this ratio is corrected for the roughly 30% of the fetal plasma that circulates outside the fetal body (i.e., in the umbilical cord and placenta), the ratio of interstitial-to-plasma volume becomes 4.4:1 in the fetus. This clearly indicates that the interstitial space of the fetus is expanded relative to that of the adult. The elevated interstitial volume is consistent with the observation that interstitial compliance in the ovine fetus is roughly 10 times adult values.[51]

Considerable differences may exist in the ratio of interstitial to plasma volumes in the newborns of different species. Based upon interstitial volume calculated form ECF and plasma volume, the interstitial-plasma volume ratio was 6.8:1 in term baboon neonates (ECF 391 mL/kg and plasma volume 50 mL/kg),[52] 8.6:1 in human term neonates (ECF 377 mL/kg and plasma volume 44 mL/kg),[4,53] and 8.7:1 in human preterm neonates (<1500 g; ECF 444 mL/kg and plasma volume 46 mL/kg).[43] In contrast, the interstitial-plasma volume ratio (283 mL/kg vs. 54 mL/kg) is 5.2:1 in 1- to 3-week-old lambs,[12] which is significantly lower than that calculated for the human newborn infant.

The reason for the high ratio of interstitial to plasma volume in neonates appears to be related to differences in hematocrits at birth. For example, the high hematocrit of human neonates is associated with a low plasma volume, which, in turn, elevates the ratio of interstitial-to-plasma volume. In comparison, the much lower hematocrit in lambs produces a lower interstitial fluid-to-plasma volume ratio. Furthermore, methodologic differences could contribute to inter-study variability.

REGULATION OF PLASMA AND INTERSTITIAL VOLUMES

The detailed mechanisms that determine the distribution of fluid between the plasma and interstitial compartments in the fetus and neonate are not well understood. It is important to emphasize two facts: (1) Blood volume, not plasma volume, is regulated in the fetus, neonate, and adult. Hence, a major determinant of plasma loss across the body capillaries is the hydrostatic pressure of the circulating blood, which in turn depends upon the total blood volume rather than plasma volume. The interstitium is largely a volume reservoir for the vascular compartment. (2) Our understanding of the fluid volume regulatory mechanisms critically depends on the accuracy of methods used to measure the plasma and ISF volume, but it is somewhat inaccurate.

The distribution of fluid between the plasma and interstitial compartments depends on the balance between capillary permeability (filtration) and lymphatic function (lymph flow rate). There are several differences in fluid homeostasis across the capillary membrane between the human fetus or neonate and adult. The fetus and neonate operate at low intravascular hydrostatic and oncotic pressures, and high membrane permeability and lymphatic flows as summarized below: (1) The intravascular hydrostatic pressure, which favors fluid movement out of the intravascular space, is low in the fetus and neonate. The lower limit of mean blood pressure for extremely low-birth-weight infants is lower than that of more mature neonates and likewise increases over the first hours to days of life.[54] (2) The intravascular oncotic pressure is low because of low plasma albumin concentrations in the fetus and neonate, which increases from 2 g/dL at 24 weeks of gestation to approximately 3 g/dL at term.[55] Nonetheless, routinely increasing albumin concentrations in preterm infants has no therapeutic benefit.[56] (3) Capillary permeability: The capillary wall is much more permeable to albumin in the human neonate than in the adult. The transcapillary escape rate of albumin in term neonates is 18% to 20% per hour, which is approximately three to four times greater than in adults.[57] Capillaries in the ovine fetus have a filtration coefficient 5 to 10 times greater than adult values[51] and permeability for plasma proteins 15 times more than in the adult.[58] (4) Lymphatic: Subcutaneous tissue lymphatic flow in anesthetized puppies is approximately twice as high as in adult dogs when expressed in relation to body weight.[59] In addition, lung lymphatic flow is also higher in anesthetized newborn lambs than in adult sheep.[60] These observations support the concept that the local, as well as whole body, lymphatic flow rates corrected for body weight are significantly greater in the neonatal period than later in life.

ENDOTHELIAL GLYCOCALYX LAYER

The endothelial glycocalyx layer (EGL) is well-known intravascular structure in adults that is also found in the human placenta[61] and umbilical vein.[62] Movement of fluid, including proteins, between the intravascular and the ISF compartments is crucially dependent on the capillary endothelium and overlying capillary endothelial glycocalyx, which form the EGL.[63] The EGL is a major determinant of vascular permeability and plays a crucial role in movement of fluid between the intravascular and ISF compartments, which results in normal fluid homeostasis. The endothelial glycocalyx consists of glycoproteins and proteoglycans containing glycosaminoglycans attached to the endoluminal surface of the capillary endothelium. Albumin is contained within the glycocalyx layer, and the EGL requires a normal level of plasma albumin to function. The vascular endothelium/glycocalyx barrier is freely permeable to water, semipermeable to albumin, but impermeable to large protein molecules (>70 kDa) in plasma.

The hydrostatic and oncotic pressure gradients between the lumen of the blood vessel and the interstitial space depend largely on the endothelial glycocalyx. The oncotic pressure difference is not built up between the intravascular and the interstitial tissue spaces, but within a small protein-free zone beneath the glycocalyx surface layer (subglycocalyx space). The oncotic pressure difference is built up between the adsorbed albumin in the soluble EGL and a small protein-free zone (subglycocalyx space) leading to the revised Starling's equation.[64]

The traditional Starling equation follows: $J_v = K_f\,([P_c - P_i] - \sigma[\pi_c - \pi_i])$, where J_v is the net fluid movement between compartments and $([P_c - P_i] - \sigma[\pi_c - \pi_i])$ is the net driving force, P_c is the capillary hydrostatic pressure, P_i is the interstitial hydrostatic pressure, π_c is the capillary oncotic pressure, π_i is the interstitial oncotic pressure, K_f is the filtration coefficient—a proportionality constant—and σ is the reflection coefficient. Starling stated that these forces are balanced. Based on EGL, the revised Starling's equation incorporates π_g (glycocalyx oncotic

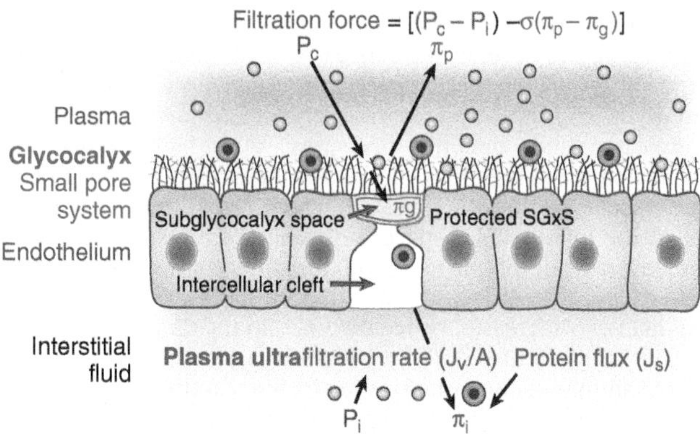

Fig. 105.7 The oncotic pressure difference is not built up between the intravascular and the interstitial tissue spaces, but within a small protein-free zone beneath the glycocalyx surface layer (subglycocalyx space). Therefore, the oncotic pressure difference is built up between the adsorbed albumin in the soluble endothelial glycocalyx layer (EGL) and subglycocalyx space (protein-free zone) in the intercellular cleft, leading to the revised Starling's equation. Based on EGL, the revised Starling's equation incorporates π_g instead of π_i and is stated as $J_v = K_f\,([P_c - P_i] - \sigma[\pi_p - \pi_g])$. J_v, Filtration from plasma to interstitial fluid; J_v/A, filtration rate per unit area; K_f, filtration coefficient; σ, reflection coefficient; P_c, capillary hydrostatic pressure; P_i, interstitial hydrostatic pressure; π_p, plasma oncotic pressure; π_i, interstitial oncotic pressure; π_g, glycocalyx oncotic pressure; *SGxS*, subglycocalyx space. (From Kundra P, Goswami S. Endothelial glycocalyx: role in body fluid homeostasis and fluid management. *Indian J. Anaesth.* 2019;63(1):6–14.)

pressure) instead of π_i, and is stated as $J_v = K_f([P_c - P_i] - \sigma[\pi_p - \pi_g])$ (Fig. 105.7).[64]

LYMPH AND LYMPH FLOW

There is a paucity of information regarding lymphatic function during fetal and neonatal life. Lymphatics must handle the increased ISF and, consequently, fetal lymphatic flow is five times higher than in adults. Lymphatic flow depends on outflow pressure. Fluid removal is dependent upon lung tidal volume and lung lymphatic flow in the lung.[39]

The ability of the thoracic duct to return lymph against an outflow pressure increases with maturation. However, lymphatic flow rate corrected for body weight is highest in immature animals. Thoracic duct lymph flow rates averaged 0.195, 0.123, and 0.038 mL/kg/min in fetal sheep, newborn lambs, and adult sheep, respectively.[65] This clearly demonstrates that basal lymphatic flow rates in the fetus and newborn are substantially higher than in adults. Thus, the lymphatic system in the fetus handles increased ISF and increased lymphatic flow. In addition, a slight increase in central venous pressure can result in a dramatic decrease in lymphatic flow rates. Therefore, the fetus is particularly susceptible to the development of edema.

On the other hand, the concentration of protein in the thoracic duct lymph exhibits an apparently uniform relationship to the plasma protein concentrations. At rest, the thoracic duct lymph protein concentration averages 50% to 75% of plasma protein concentrations in the fetus, newborn, and adult. This does not mean that the absolute protein concentrations are the same, because fetal plasma protein concentrations increase during gestation and average a little more than half the adult values at term.[66,67] Studies in the ovine fetus[68-70] have found that angiotensin II augments left thoracic duct lymph flow and atrial natriuretic factor suppresses lymph flow.

Table 105.3 summarizes the assumed range of estimated volumes of the body fluid compartments in the human full-term neonate.

Table 105.3 Assumed Range of Estimated Values of Plasma Volume, Blood Volume, Red Blood Cell Volume, and Total Extracellular Fluid in the Human Neonate At Term.

Compartment	Volume
Total body water (TBW = ICF + ECF)	700–850 mL/kg (70%–85% of BWt)
Intracellular fluid (ICF)	300–400 mL/kg (30%–40% of BWt)
Extracellular fluid (ECF = PV + ISV)	400–500 mL/kg (40%–50% of BWt)
Blood volume (BV = RCV + PV)	70–100 mL/kg
Red blood cell volume (RCV)	30–45 mL/kg
Plasma volume (PV)	40–65 mL/kg
Interstitial volume (ISV)	350–450 mL/kg
Ratio of PV : RCV	~3 : 2
Ratio of ISV : PV	~7.5–9.0 : 1
Placental transfusion	15–35 mL/kg

BWt, Total body weight.

PLACENTAL CIRCULATION

The placenta is a unique temporary organ that performs the functions of several adult organs for exchange of oxygen, nutrients, antibodies, hormones, and waste products between the mother and fetus. The placenta contains a low-resistance and high-flow vascular bed, which is composed of fetal (umbilicoplacental vascular bed) and maternal (uteroplacental vascular bed) components.[31] Although the placenta does not entirely control the amount of water that enters the fetus, almost all water that enters the fetus enters via the placenta. Fetal fluid volume control is dependent upon the combined physiologic properties of the fetal heart, kidneys, somatic tissues, and placenta.[31] The rate of fetal water acquisition depends upon the placental water permeability characteristics. Changes in the osmotic differences between the maternal and fetal sera can affect the volume of water flowing from the mother to the fetus.[71] Net water flux across the placenta is relatively small. In sheep, a bulk water flow to the fetus of 0.5 mL/min[72] is sufficient for fetal needs at term. By contrast, tracer studies suggest that the total water exchanged (i.e., diffusionary flow) between the ovine fetus and the mother is dramatically larger, up to 70 mL/min.[73] Most of this diffusionary flow is bidirectional, resulting in no net accumulation of water. Although the mechanisms regulating the maternal-fetal flux of water are speculative, the permeability of the placenta to water changes with gestation,[74] suggesting that placental water permeability may be a factor in regulating the water available to the fetus.

PERINATAL CHANGES IN BODY FLUID

PERIOD BEFORE LABOR

Several observations suggest that the fetus undergoes significant changes in its fluid status during the last few days, hours, and minutes before delivery. Studies have shown that lung fluid volume is reduced several days before the onset of labor,[26,75] mainly because the amount of fluid secreted by the lungs gradually decreases.[76] The reduction in fetal lung liquid secretion is mediated by increased expression of pulmonary epithelial sodium channels (ENaC) and sodium-potassium adenosine triphosphatase (Na^+,K^+-ATPase) near birth, which change epithelial cell ion transport from predominantly chloride secretion during fetal development to predominantly sodium absorption after birth. Epinephrine and other hormones (cyclic adenosine monophosphate, cortisol, and aldosterone), which are released just before and during labor, trigger the switch from liquid secretion to absorption.[77] Therefore, infants born after elective cesarean section without labor have an increased risk for postnatal respiratory disease such as transient tachypnea of the newborn.[78] Relatively large increases in fetal arterial pressure also occur in fetal sheep during the last few days before delivery and during delivery, especially associated with labor.[79] If this pressure were transmitted to the fetal lung capillaries, it would exert a major effect on the lung transcapillary transfer of fluid.

LABOR AND DELIVERY

Although it was once thought that the amount of water in the newborn infant varied by the mode of delivery, a study in full-term appropriate for gestational age (AGA) infants showed that there was no difference in TBW, ECF, and ICF in first 24 hours between infants delivered vaginally and by cesarean section before the onset of labor.[80] However, blood volume decreases in both human and animal fetuses during labor and delivery. Circulating fetal plasma and blood volumes decreased in fetal sheep during labor and delivery by 18% and 12%, respectively.[79] These results are consistent with studies in humans. The umbilical vein hematocrit averages 44% in infants delivered by elective cesarean section without labor[81] and 51% immediately after delivery if labor has occurred.[4,42,82] Assuming that RBCs are not released into the circulation during labor, this ratio of 44:51 demonstrates that the CBV is reduced by 14%. This corresponds to a reduction in plasma volume of 25%.

The mechanisms that mediate the loss of plasma during labor and delivery are multifactorial. Nonlabor uterine contractions in pregnant sheep produce a significant increases in fetal arterial and venous pressures during contractures, which are in excess of the rise in AF pressure.[83] This suggests that direct compression or conformational change of the fetus may cause fetal vascular changes during nonlabor uterine contractions.[84] Blood volume decreased by 0.6% to 3.6% during nonlabor uterine contractions in fetal sheep.[49] Furthermore, hypoxia, which can occur during labor, reduces CBV up to 14% in fetal sheep, resulting from a loss of plasma volume into the interstitial space.[85,86] In contrast, others have suggested that severe hypoxia may produce an in utero translocation of fetal blood out of the placenta into the fetal body, which increases capillary pressures and transcapillary filtration of fluid out of the fetal circulation.[87] In addition, major changes in the plasma concentrations of many vasoactive hormones occur during labor and delivery. Although the effects of a only a few hormones have been investigated, arginine vasopressin,[88] norepinephrine,[89] cortisol,[90] and atrial natriuretic factor[50,91] have the ability to reduce the circulating blood and plasma volume when acutely infused into the circulation of fetal sheep at low to moderate rates. The umbilical cord concentrations of each of these hormones are elevated after vaginal delivery in humans, suggesting that these hormones may indeed play a role in mediating the shift of fluid from the plasma into the interstitial compartment at the time of labor and delivery.

PLACENTAL TRANSFUSION: DELAYED CORD CLAMPING

A placentofetal transfusion, which displaces blood from the placenta into the fetus, is augmented by uterine contractions, delayed cord clamping (DCC), cord milking, and increases in maternal uterine blood flow. A fetoplacental transfusion that displaces blood from the fetus to the placenta, however, is augmented by maternal hypotension, cord compression, holding of the newborn infant above the level of the placenta, or cesarean section.[42]

The distribution of blood volume between neonate and placenta after delivery is influenced by a number of perinatal events. The single most important factor determining blood and plasma volumes in the newborn during the first few days of life is the quantity of the blood transfused from the placenta to the infant at delivery.[4,41,42,92] The amount of blood that is transferred to the infant between birth and cord clamping is termed the *placental transfusion*. The timing of cord clamping markedly influences the quantity of placental transfusion and, consequently, neonatal blood volume. Infants receive an increased placental transfusion when the clamping of the umbilical cord is delayed and, consequently, have higher blood and RBC volumes (Table 105.4).[92-95] The placental transfusion is usually complete by 2 minutes, but sometimes continues for up to 5 minutes. The placental transfusion contributes between one-third and one-fourth of the total potential blood volume after birth in full-term infants.[96]

Table 105.4 Comparisons of Blood, Plasma, and Red Blood Cell Volumes Between Early and Delayed Cord Clamping in Human Newborns.

Gestation	Age (Days)	Cord Clamping	Blood Volume (mL/kg)	Plasma Volume (mL/kg)	RBC Volume (mL/kg)	Reference
Preterm (24–32 wk)	0	Early Delayed	62.7[b] (Biotin) 74.4[b] (Biotin) $P < 0.001$			93
Preterm (<37 wk)		Early Delayed			36.8[c] (Biotin) 42.1[c] (Biotin) $P = 0.04$	95
Term (38–42 wk)	0	Early Delayed	78.0 98.6 $P < 0.001$ (¹³¹I Volemetron)	45.9 48.0 NS	32.1 50.6 $P < 0.001$	92
Term (38–42 wk)	0	Early Delayed	76.9[a] 102.5[a] $P < 0.001$ (¹³¹I Volemetron)	42.7 48.8 NS	34.6 49.4 $P < 0.001$	94

[a]Determined with plasma label.
[b]Determined with RBC label.
[c]Determined with RBC label. Difference was not reflected by concurrent blood hematocrit values of 54% for delayed cord clamping and 53.6% for immediate cord clamping.
( ), Indicator; *NS*, not significant; *RBC*, red blood cell.

Delaying cord clamping for 3 minutes results in an essentially complete placental transfusion, along with stepwise increments in CBV and RCV in full-term infants born to healthy mothers. Although the increases in the CBV and RCV from <5 seconds to 3 minutes after birth were 32% and 57.8%, respectively, the residual placental blood volume decreased by 60.2%. The close correlation between the increase in RCV after DCC at 3 minutes (57.8%) and the associated decrease in residual placental blood volume (60%) supports the contention that the RCV is a better guide than CBV to quantify the amount of placental transfusion.[41]

The hematocrit in the full-term infant averages 48% to 51% and remains unchanged over a period of days when the umbilical cord is clamped immediately after delivery.[82,92] However, if the umbilical cord is not clamped immediately and placental blood is gradually transfused into the infant, it reaches a maximum volume by 3 to 4 minutes after delivery.[82,92] The peripheral or umbilical venous hematocrit in full-term infants with DCC gradually increases over 30 minutes to 4 hours from an estimated 48% at birth to 59% by 30 minutes and 64% by 4 hours.[92] Then, the hematocrit values decrease to 61.5% and 60% by 24 and 72 hours, respectively.[92] This placental transfusion of 25 to 50 mL/kg represents 50% increases in RBC and blood volumes within the neonate.[41,92]

DCC in preterm infants between 24 and 37 weeks of gestation results in hematocrit values ranging from 44% to 56% compared with infants exposed to immediate cord clamping, whose values at 4 hours of life range from 40% to 52%.[97] Umbilical cord milking in infants less than 28 weeks of gestation resulted in hematocrit values at 12 hours of age that were 47% compared with 42% after immediate cord clamping.[98]

DCC was more effective in increasing neonatal blood volume after vaginal delivery than after cesarean section.[93] Milking of the umbilical cord five times in full-term infants after cesarean section resulted in mean hematocrit values at 36 to 48 hours of age of 57%, compared with 51% after immediate umbilical cord clamping.[99] The increase in hematocrit is due to both an increase in RBC volume as well as a loss of plasma from the circulation. The reduction in plasma volume is mainly due to a shift of fluid from the intravascular into the interstitial space. However, urine flow is also significantly higher in infants after DCC.[100]

Placental transfusion has significant circulatory effects and increases neonatal blood pressure, central venous pressure, renal blood flow, and urine flow.[42] Hemodynamic studies after DCC have demonstrated improved measures of systemic blood flow over the first few days of life compared with immediate cord clamping.[98,101] DCC or umbilical cord milking at delivery appears to have beneficial effects for both full-term and preterm infants. A meta-analysis in full-term infants showed that DCC reduced the incidence of anemia in early infancy because of early increases in hemoglobin and iron store in infants.[102,103] A meta-analysis in preterm infants also showed that DCC for 30 to 120 seconds was associated with less need for blood transfusions, improved circulatory stability, less intraventricular hemorrhage (all grades), and lower risk for necrotizing enterocolitis.[97] The American College of Obstetricians and Gynecologists recommended a delay in umbilical cord clamping in vigorous term and preterm infants for at least 30 to 60 seconds after birth,[104] which was endorsed by American Academy of Pediatrics.[105]

POSTNATAL CHANGES IN BODY WATER DURING TRANSITION TO THE EXTRAUTERINE ENVIRONMENT

The fetus remains in an aquatic environment during intrauterine life. The lungs are filled with liquid, the skin is porous and lacks a keratin layer, urine output is high, and renal concentrating ability is limited. The transition to extrauterine life is associated with a transition from an aquatic to a terrestrial environment; metabolic, circulatory, and endocrine adaptations; gas exchange from the placenta to lungs; clearance of fetal lung fluid; reductions in pulmonary vascular resistance; and cardiovascular adaptations from the fetal to neonatal circulation. These factors contribute to postnatal changes in body fluid distribution and homeostasis.

POSTNATAL CLEARANCE OF LUNG FLUID

Birth marks a remarkable transition of gas exchange from the mother-dependent placental circulation to independent air breathing. Clearing the fluid-filled lungs is an important component of this transition. Physiologic events beginning days before delivery are accompanied by changes in the hormonal milieu including surges in fetal catecholamines, corticosteroids, and thyroid hormone. These changes facilitate a smooth neonatal transition, which includes clearance of the large body of lung fluid. Lung liquid removal begins before birth, is accelerated immediately after birth, and is normally complete within the 2 to 4 hours of life.[106] Respiratory morbidities resulting from failure to clear the lung fluid are common and can be particularly problematic in infants delivered prematurely or when delivery occurs operatively before the onset of spontaneous labor.[107]

Both the rate of lung liquid production and the lung liquid volume within the lumen of the fetal lung decrease before birth, most notably during labor.[108] Lung water content is about 25% greater after premature delivery than after term delivery. Cesarean section delivery without labor results in higher lung liquid than either vaginal delivery or operative delivery after the onset of labor.[108]

The lung epithelium changes from Cl^- secretion before birth to Na^{2+} absorption after birth.[109] Alveolar expression of highly selective Na^+ channels in the lung epithelia is regulated by the lung microenvironment, the presence of glucocorticoids, air interface, and increases in oxygen concentration.[109,110] Na^+ reabsorption is a two-step process in the lung. First, there is passive movement of Na^+ from the lumen across the apical membrane into the cell through epithelial sodium channels (ENaC). The second step is active extrusion of Na^+ from the cell across the basolateral membrane (Na^+,K^+-ATPase) into the serosal space. The osmotic gradient created from net ion movement directs water transport either through AQP and or by diffusion.[111] Mechanism(s) responsible for fetal lung fluid clearance have shown that active Na^{++} transport across the pulmonary epithelium drives liquid from lung lumen to the interstitium, with subsequent absorption into the vasculature.

Removal of liquid from the lung interstitium by both the vascular and lymphatic channels. The estimated size of lymphatics is lower for animals in labor[112] than for animals not in labor.[113] There is likely a redundancy in the lymphatic and vascular mechanisms because the pulmonary lymphatic system can cope with fivefold increases in pulmonary filtration.[106]

The combined effects of low-protein oncotic pressure, high pulmonary hydrostatic pressure, and large transpulmonary pressure gradients favor movement of water out of the vascular space into the interstitium. These same factors also impair lymphatic drainage. Lung ventilation is extremely important in regulating lung lymph flow in the newborn.[114] Both increases and decreases in ventilation cause rapid changes in lung lymph flow, which are not related to changes in lung weight. A decrease in tidal volume results in decreased lung lymph flow, suggesting that decreased tidal volume might act by increasing the downstream lymphatic resistance.[115]

NEONATAL INITIAL PHYSIOLOGIC WEIGHT LOSS: ECF CONTRACTION

Weight loss is universal in infants soon after birth. The weight loss reflects a decrease in TBW primarily resulting from a contraction of the ECF volume.[116] Early postnatal weight loss results from water losses rather than catabolic loss of body solids.[117-121] The reductions in ECF are a consequence of isotonic fluid loss from the interstitial space without changes in blood or plasma volumes.[43,94]

The contraction of ECF related to body weight loss during the first week of life is universal. An abrupt contraction of ECF shortly after birth is superimposed upon steady gradual reductions ECF reduction throughout life.[94,118,122-125] Body weight is similar to birth weight by the second week of life when urinary water and salt losses decrease. However, the ECF volume does not return to the 35% to 45% of body weight that are observed at birth. In contrast, the intracellular space remains at, or is restored to, its volume at birth, and the ratio of extracellular to intracellular water is closer to that observed later in infancy and childhood.[43,117-119,121] Although the mechanism(s) of the contraction in ECF are not known, it is associated with an increase in insensible water loss via skin, lung fluid absorption, an increase in the GFR, diuresis,[126] and natriuresis,[127] all of which predispose to the weight loss.

ECF loss is initiated by postnatal cardiopulmonary adaptation, principally by decreases in pulmonary vascular pressure. These changes are most likely determined by loss of the placental vascular bed and changes in the synthesis and metabolism of vasoactive agents (prostaglandins, atrial natriuretic peptide, and vasopressin) predisposing to dramatic increases in the pulmonary circulation, systemic circulatory hemodynamics, closure of the ductus arteriosus, and increases in renal blood flow.[120,128-131] The physiologic changes associated with the adaptation of the cardiorespiratory and renal systems to the extrauterine environment and the acute redistribution of body water appear to obligate the water loss that should not be replaced.[40]

Sodium and water balance is negative during postnatal adaptation phase because ECF is principally Na and water. The magnitude of ECF contraction is inversely proportional to gestational age (GA). More immature infants exhibit greater weight loss (term infants: 5% to 7%, preterm infants: 10% to 15%). Fractional excretion of sodium (FENa) and urine sodium excretion are inversely related to gestational age at birth and postnatal age.[132]

Urinary output is very low in preterm infants during the first day of life (*prediuretic phase*). The diuresis and natriuresis occur with or without increases of fluid intake (*diuretic phase*) during the second and third days of life. The GFR and FENa were low during the prediuretic phase, increase markedly during the diuretic phase, and then decreased to intermediate levels during the postdiuretic phase.[133] By the fourth or fifth day of life, urine output begins to vary appropriately in response to changes in fluid intake (*postdiuretic phase*). The principal management of fluid balance in very immature infants during postnatal initial weight loss period is by high humidification, to minimize evaporative water losses from the skin, restricting fluid without replacing salt before the end of the diuretic phase, and monitoring daily changes in body weight, serum sodium, and urine volume.[134]

Early fluid management, during the period of postnatal adaptation, should permit an isotonic contraction of the ECF and a brief period of negative sodium and water balance. Limiting the normal ECF contraction by high fluid and excess sodium intake significantly increases the incidences of patent ductus arteriosus, bronchopulmonary dysplasia, and necrotizing enterocolitis in low-birth-weight infants.[135-139]

SPECIAL CONSIDERATIONS

EFFECT OF ANTENATAL STEROIDS IN PRETERM INFANTS

Maternal treatment with antenatal corticosteroids (ACSs) before anticipated preterm birth is the worldwide standard of care for fetal maturation.[140] Maternal treatment with ACS has significant effects on the fluid balance because premature infants that were exposed to ACS in utero have lower insensible water loss (IWL), decreased incidences of nonoliguric hyperkalemia[141] and hypernatremia, and an earlier diuresis and natriuresis in extremely low-birth-weight neonates.[142] Preterm infants exposed to ACS exhibited higher urine outputs and GFRs, lower fractional sodium excretion, lower IWL, and less hyponatremia.[143,144] Glucocorticoid exposure also increases three distinct subunits (α, β, γ) of pulmonary epithelial Na^+ channels (ENaC) playing a critical role in the regulation of fluid reabsorption from airspaces of late-gestation fetal lung[145] and also increases renal cortical Na^+,K^+-ATPase activity and α1-expression.[146] These results suggest that ACS accelerates maturation of not only fetal lung but also skin, renal tubules resulting in earlier postnatal reabsorption of fetal lung fluid, lower IWL, and early diuresis.

INFANTS OF DIABETIC MOTHERS

Infants of diabetic mothers (IDMs) are often large for gestational age, particularly after the beginning of the third trimester. TBW (the ECF and the ICF) in these infants is generally lower per unit of body weight when compared to those of AGA. Most of the added weight of an IDM is a result of increased body fat.[147]

INTRAUTERINE GROWTH RESTRICTION

Intrauterine growth restriction (IUGR) appears to have little influence on the distribution of TBW between the ECF and ICF compartments unless it is severe. However, TBW content can be up to 15% higher in infants with severe IUGR compared with AGA infants. The increase is caused by decreased deposition of body solids (fat, protein, and mineral) with substantially lower fat contents,[53] rather than by excess water accumulation.[148] Table 105.5 contains comparisons of TBW, ECV, CBV, PV, RCV, and BV between AGA and small for gestational age (SGA) infants.[47,53,116,149-151] The TBW content was higher in both preterm and full-term SGA compared with AGA infants.[53,116,152] TBW content measured by bioelectrical impedance was also higher in SGA than AGA neonates.[153]

Although the higher body water content in preterm SGA infants reflects the reduced lean mass (protein and minerals), the increase in body water content in full-term SGA neonates reflects mainly lower fat content.[154] Fat deposition primarily occurs during the third trimester in normally grown fetuses.[154] SGA neonates have been shown to have reduced total body fat by multiple different methods.[155-158] In contrast, IUGR is not necessarily associated with increased plasma volume or red cell mass.[47] Nonetheless, blood volume calculated from changes in hematocrit in neonates requiring exchange transfusions was higher in polycythemic SGA compared with AGA infants.[151] The increased RBC volume in SGA neonates could be a result of adaptations to chronic intrauterine hypoxemia or the consequence of an acute placentofetal transfusions.[159]

Postnatal weight loss in SGA neonates differs somewhat from that of AGA infants because weight loss in SGA preterm neonates was only 5% and resulted from proportional reductions in body water and solids suggesting a component of catabolism.[14] Preterm SGA neonates had a maximal postnatal weight loss of only 2% compared 8% in AGA at 35 weeks of gestation. SGA neonates regain birth weight on days 4 to 6 of life without changes in TBW or body solids.[160] In contrast, TBW and body weight in AGA neonates at the same postnatal age was significantly lower than at birth despite the similar daily fluid and energy intakes during the first week of life between the AGA and SGA infants.[160] However, the AGA infants exhibited a higher urine outputs during this time interval. Possible explanations for the attenuated postnatal increase in urine output in SGA preterm neonates is altered hemodynamic adaptations because SGA preterm neonates do

Table 105.5 Total Body Water and Extracellular Volume in Appropriate for Gestational Age and Small for Gestational Age Human Neonates.

Fluid Compartment	Gestation	AGA	SGA	*P*-value	Dilution Indicator	Reference
TBW (mL/kg)	Preterm (25–30 wk)	906	844	0.019	$H_2{}^{18}O$	152
	Term	754–790	824–859	<0.02	^2H_2O (Deuterium oxide)	116
		688	790	<0.001	Antipyrine	53
ECV (mL/kg)	Preterm (25–30 wk)	505	511	NS	Bromide	152
	Term	376	419	<0.025	Bromide	150
		361	395	NR	Bromide	116
CBV (mL/kg)	Preterm and term	86.5	106	<0.001	Calculated from Hct	151
PV (mL/kg)	Term	37.1	36.5	NS	Evans Blue	47
RCV (mL/kg)	Term	63	69	NS	Calculation (BV – PV)	47
BV (mL/kg)	Term	101	105	NS	Calculation [PV×100/(100 – Hct)]	47

AGA, Appropriate for gestational age; *BV*, blood volume; *CBV*, circulating blood volume; *ECV*, extracellular volume; *Hct*, hematocrit; *NR*, not reported; *NS*, not significant; *PV*, plasma volume; *RCV*, red blood cell volume; *SGA*, small for gestational age; *TBW*, total body water.
Term, ≥37 weeks of gestation.

not exhibit a postnatal increase in cardiac output observed in AGA neonates,[161] and/or that stress in utero could have already accelerated renal function before birth.

RESPONSES TO VOLUME LOADING

Rapid intravascular infusions of isotonic solutions, such as saline or Ringer's lactate, expand blood volume by only a fraction of the infused volume because the infused fluid is lost mainly into the interstitial spaces. Intravascular infusions of isotonic crystalloid in the adult of several species resulted in intravascular retention averaging from 20% to 50% of the infused volumes at 30 to 60 minutes after rapid infusions. This finding is similar to the 30% to 40% intravascular retention observed in anesthetized newborn sheep after intravascular saline infusions.[162] In contrast, similar infusions increased the blood volume by only 6% to 7% of the infused volume in the unanesthetized ovine fetus.[163] The reduced intravascular retention of crystalloid during fetal life is due largely to the high interstitial-to-vascular compliance ratio and high capillary filtration coefficient.[51] The increased capillary filtration coefficient permits very rapid fluid movements across the capillary membrane, and the high interstitial-to-vascular compliance ratio allows for extensive fluid movements.

Left thoracic duct lymph flow increases after isotonic saline vascular volume expansion both in fetal and newborn sheep.[162,164] Lymph flow rate increases to a maximum of 3.5 times normal after extensive vascular volume loading; external drainage of the thoracic duct causes a rapid reduction in the fetal blood volume by 10% within 2 to 3 hours.

The plasma and interstitial protein concentrations are affected differently in the fetus than in the adult by volume expansion with crystalloid. The lymph-to-plasma protein concentration ratio decreased in the fetus after volume expansion,[164] whereas this protein concentration ratio increased transiently in adult subjects[29,66] and newborn sheep.[162] The diminished intravascular retention of fluid in the fetus compared with the adult may account for the urinary flow rate responses to volume loading. Normal adults excrete the entire volume load through their kidneys within several hours after receiving a volume load. In contrast, the fetus and neonate of several species, including human, have a reduced capacity to excrete volume loads. This reduced excretory capacity can be in part attributed to the reduced intravascular fluid retention.[165,166] In the adult, plasma renin activity and plasma arginine vasopressin and atrial natriuretic factor concentrations all change in a direction appropriate for increasing urine flow (because of the higher intravascular retention in the adult). However, in the ovine fetus, plasma arginine vasopressin and renin activity are unchanged, and atrial natriuretic factor exhibits only a transient increase as a result of the low intravascular retention.[166] Therefore, fetal urine flow rapidly returns to baseline after rapid vascular volume expansion because the hormonal stimuli that promote urinary output are not sustained.[166] However, the mechanism responsible for the diminished response to volume loading in human newborn infants remains to be determined.

Similarly, a small percentage of the transfused volume remains intravascular space after blood transfusions. Thirty-one percent of the transfused volume was lost in human fetuses of 19 to 36 weeks of gestation with anemia that received intravascular transfusions mainly into the fetal interstitial space, with minor amounts through the placenta, because of a loss of plasma from the circulation.[167]

Crystalloid (isotonic saline) solution is the initial treatment of choice to treat hypotension in preterm infants because it has comparable effects to colloid, less fluid retention in the first 48 hours, is less expensive and readily available.[168]

RESPONSES TO HEMORRHAGE

Perinatal blood loss of the fetus or neonate can occur after umbilical cord rupture, placental abruption, fetomaternal transfusion, twin-to-twin transfusion, or internal organ bleeding such as intracranial or intraabdominal hemorrhage. Twenty-four to 48 hours is required for blood volume to return to normal after blood loss in adults of several species, including humans, dogs, rats, cats, and sheep. This restoration of volume occurs as plasma volume returns to or rises above normal, whereas RBC volume remains reduced. The time required for full volume restoration after hemorrhage in the fetus or neonate is shorter than in the adult. The ovine fetus begins to restore twice the average blood volume as that of the adult within 30 minutes after rapid hemorrhage,[169] and also restores its blood volume to normal within 3 to 4 hours after a 30% hemorrhage,[170] which is one-tenth the time required in the adult.[171] This rapid restoration is mediated by a translocation of fluid and protein from the interstitial space into the vascular space but does not appear to result from a net movement of fluid across the placenta.[169] Neonatal kittens[172] and rabbits[173] were also better able to tolerate blood loss than adults were, in that more blood had to be removed before arterial pressure decreased. This was attributed to a more rapid mobilization of ISF in the young animals in the first week of life. Neonatal lambs also rapidly restore their blood volume to normal after hemorrhage.[174]

RESPONSES TO HYPOXIA

Reductions in blood volume occur rapidly and are linearly related to the reductions in arterial oxygen tension, such that for each 1 mm Hg decrease in arterial Po_2 there is a 1% decrease in blood volume in the ovine fetus.[85,86] The loss of plasma is undoubtedly a result of increases in capillary pressure within the fetal body. This phenomenon occurs without changes in fetal arterial or venous pressures during mild hypoxia, presumably because of vasodilation in selected organs, and is accompanied by increases in arterial and venous pressures with moderate to severe hypoxia.[86]

Newborns with a history of fetal distress and birth asphyxia have elevated blood, RBC, and plasma volumes.[159,175] These observations suggest that prenatal hypoxia or asphyxia induces a placental transfusion before delivery. This is consistent with the observation that acute hypoxia promotes a translocation of fetal blood out of the placenta in sheep.[87] In addition, Yao and colleagues[159] have shown that 10 to 20 minutes of hypoxia immediately before delivery in ewes elevates plasma, RBC, and blood volumes in the newborn lamb, compared with normal lambs with early cord clamping. Linderkamp and colleagues[176] also observed that intrauterine hypoxia, defined as abnormal fetal heart rate pattern, is associated with an elevated RBC volume in the newborn but that acute, intrapartum asphyxia, defined as 1 minute Apgar score of less than or equal to 5, is not associated with a predelivery placental transfusion. Thus, evidence is ample to support the concept that prenatal hypoxia causes a partial placental transfusion in utero, but its time course, exact extent, and reversibility remain unclear. Hypoxia that occurs postnatally reduces blood volume in the human neonate because of a loss of plasma and proteins from the circulation,[177] but the causes of the reduced blood volume remain to be determined.

CONCLUSION

Knowledge of physiologic changes in the fluid distribution of fetus and neonate are critical to the care of fetus and neonate. The distribution of body-fluid spaces, such as TBW, ICF, and ECF, including intravascular and ISF, in the fetus and neonate changes with age and a variety of clinical conditions. The transition from the intrauterine aquatic fetal to the terrestrial neonatal environment is affected by fetal maturation and various maternal and fetal conditions. Fluid distribution in the neonate is affected by gestational age, birth weight, adaptation to extrauterine environment, and postnatal age. Appropriate management of fluids and electrolytes in the preterm neonate can attenuate the development of many untoward complications of prematurity.

A complete reference list is available at www.ExpertConsult.com.

SELECT REFERENCES

4. Mollison PL, Veall N, Cutbush M. Red cell and plasma volume in newborn infants. *Archiv Dis Childhood*. 1950;25(123):242-253.
7. Anthony MY, Goodall SR, Papouli M, Levene MI. Measurement of plasma volume in neonates. *Archive Dis Childhood*. 1992;67(1 Spec No):36-40.
12. Longo LD, Allen WW, Niswonger JWH, Longo L, RDD D. The interrelations of blood and extracellular fluid volumes and cardiac output in the newborn lamb. In: *Fetal and Newborn Cardiovascular Physiology: Fetal and Newborn Circulation*. New York: Garland STPM Press; 1978:345-367.
13. Coulter DM. Postnatal fluid and electrolyte changes and clinical implications. In: Robert A, Brace MGR, Robillard JE, eds. *Fetal and Neonatal Body Fluids: The Scientific Basis for Clinical Practice*. Vol. 11. Ithaca, NY: Perinatology Press; 1989.
14. vd Wagen A, Okken A, Zweens J, Zijlstra WG. Composition of postnatal weight loss and subsequent weight gain in small for dates newborn infants. *Acta Paediatrica Scandinavica*. 1985;74(1):57-61.
15. Bauer K, Versmold H, Prolss A, De Graaf SS, Meeuwsen-Van der Roest WP, Zijlstra WG. Estimation of extracellular volume in preterm infants less than 1500 g, children, and adults by sucrose dilution. *Pediatr Res*. 1990;27(3):256-259.
19. Brace RA, Wolf EJ. Normal amniotic fluid volume changes throughout pregnancy. *Am J Obstetr Gynecol*. 1989;161(2):382-388.
20. Brace RA. Physiology of amniotic fluid volume regulation. *Clin Obstetr Gynecol*. 1997;40(2):280-289.
29. Brace RA. Fetal blood volume, urine flow, swallowing, and amniotic fluid volume responses to long-term intravascular infusions of saline. *Am J Obstetr Gynecol*. 1989;161(4):1049-1054.
31. Faber JJ, Anderson DF. The placenta in the integrated physiology of fetal volume control. *Intl J Develop Biol*. 2010;54(2-3):391-396.
33. Beall MH, Wang S, Yang B, Chaudhri N, Amidi F, Ross MG. Placental and membrane aquaporin water channels: correlation with amniotic fluid volume and composition. *Placenta*. 2007;28(5-6):421-428.
36. Friis-Hansen B. Body water compartments in children: changes during growth and related changes in body composition. *Pediatrics*. 1961;28:169-181.
37. Ziegler EE, O'Donnell AM, Nelson SE, Fomon SJ. Body composition of the reference fetus. *Growth*. 1976;40(4):329-341.
39. Bellini C, Boccardo F, Bonioli E, Campisi C. Lymphodynamics in the fetus and newborn. *Lymphology*. 2006;39(3):110-117.
42. Linderkamp O. Placental transfusion: determinants and effects. *Clin Perinatol*. 1982;9(3):559-592.
47. Brans YW, Shannon DL, Ramamurthy RS. Neonatal polycythemia: II. Plasma, blood and red cell volume estimates in relation to hematocrit levels and quality of intrauterine growth. *Pediatrics*. 1981;68(2):175-182.
51. Brace RA, Gold PS. Fetal whole-body interstitial compliance, vascular compliance, and capillary filtration coefficient. *Am J Physiol*. 1984;247(5 Pt 2):R800-R805.
52. Brans YW, Kuehl TJ, Hayashi RH, Andrew DS. Body water estimates in intrauterine-growth-retarded versus normally grown baboon neonates. *Biol Neonate*. 1986;50(4):231-236.
57. Parving HH, Klebe JG, Ingomar CJ. Simultaneous determination of plasma volume and transcapillary escape rate with 131 I-labelled albumin and T-1824 in the newborn. *Acta Paediatrica Scandinavica*. 1973;62(3):248-252.
58. Gold PS, Brace RA. Fetal whole-body permeability-surface area product and reflection coefficient for plasma proteins. *Microvascul Res*. 1988;36(3):262-274.
60. Boston RW, Humphreys PW, Reynolds EO, Strang LB. Lymph-flow and clearance of liquid from the lungs of the foetal lamb. *Lancet*. 1965;2(7410):473-474.
62. Chappell D, Jacob M, Paul O, et al. The glycocalyx of the human umbilical vein endothelial cell: an impressive structure ex vivo but not in culture. *Circ Res*. 2009;104(11):1313-1317.
65. Johnson SA, Vander Straten MC, Parellada JA, Schnakenberg W, Gest AL. Thoracic duct function in fetal, newborn, and adult sheep. *Lymphology*. 1996;29(2):50-56.
79. Comline RS, Silver M. The composition of foetal and maternal blood during parturition in the Ewe. *J Physiol*. 1972;222(1):233-256.
82. Yao AC, Lind J. Placental transfusion. *Am J Dis Child*. 1974;127(1):128-141.
83. Brace RA, Brittingham DS. Fetal vascular pressure and heart rate responses to nonlabor uterine contractions. *Am J Physiol*. 1986;251(2 Pt 2):R409-R416.
84. Shields LE, Brace RA. Fetal vascular pressure responses to nonlabor uterine contractions: dependence on amniotic fluid volume in the ovine fetus. *Am J Obstetr Gynecol*. 1994;171(1):84-89.
85. Brace RA. Fetal blood volume responses to acute fetal hypoxia. *Am J Obstetr Gynecol*. 1986;155(4):889-893.
87. Oh W, Omori K, Emmanouilides GC, Phelps DL. Placenta to lamb fetus transfusion in utero during acute hypoxia. *Am J Obstetr Gynecol*. 1975;122(3):316-322.
93. Aladangady N, McHugh S, Aitchison TC, Wardrop CA, Holland BM. Infants' blood volume in a controlled trial of placental transfusion at preterm delivery. *Pediatrics*. 2006;117(1):93-98.
94. Oh W, Blankenship W, Lind J. Futher study of neonatal blood volume in relation to placental transfusion. *Ann Paediatr*. 1966;207:147.
95. Strauss RG, Mock DM, Johnson K, et al. Circulating RBC volume, measured with biotinylated RBCs, is superior to the Hct to document the hematologic effects of delayed versus immediate umbilical cord clamping in preterm neonates. *Transfusion*. 2003;43(8):1168-1172.
97. Rabe H, Diaz-Rossello JL, Duley L, Dowswell T. Effect of timing of umbilical cord clamping and other strategies to influence placental transfusion at preterm birth on maternal and infant outcomes. *Cochrane Database Systemat Rev*. 2012;8:CD003248.
98. Katheria A, Blank D, Rich W, Finer N. Umbilical cord milking improves transition in premature infants at birth. *PloS One*. 2014;9(4):e94085.
100. Oh W, Oh M, Lind J. Renal function and blood volume in newborn infant related to placental transfusion. *Acta Paediatrica Scandinavica*. 1966;56:197-210.

103. McDonald SJ, Middleton P, Dowswell T, Morris PS. Effect of timing of umbilical cord clamping of term infants on maternal and neonatal outcomes. *Cochrane Database Systemat Rev*. 2013;7:CD004074.
113. Humphreys PW, Normand IC, Reynolds EO, Strang LB. Pulmonary lymph flow and the uptake of liquid from the lungs of the lamb at the start of breathing. *J Physiol*. 1967;193(1):1-29.
116. Cheek DB, Wishart J, MacLennan AH, Haslam R. Cell hydration in the normally grown, the premature and the low weight for gestational age infant. *Early Human Develop*. 1984;10(1-2):75-84.
118. Shaffer SG, Bradt SK, Hall RT. Postnatal changes in total body water and extracellular volume in the preterm infant with respiratory distress syndrome. *J Pediatr*. 1986;109(3):509-514.
127. Ross B, Cowett RM, Oh W. Renal functions of low birth weight infants during the first two months of life. *Pediatr Res*. 1977;11(11):1162-1164.
133. Lorenz JM, Kleinman LI, Ahmed G, Markarian K. Phases of fluid and electrolyte homeostasis in the extremely low birth weight infant. *Pediatrics*. 1995;96(3 Pt 1):484-489.
135. Stonestreet BS, Bell EF, Warburton D, Oh W. Renal response in low-birth-weight neonates. Results of prolonged intake of two different amounts of fluid and sodium. *Am J Dis Child*. 1983;137(3):215-219.
152. Hartnoll G, Betremieux P, Modi N. Body water content of extremely preterm infants at birth. *Archiv Dis Childhood Fetal Neonatal Ed*. 2000;83(1):F56-F59.
157. Petersen S, Gotfredsen A, Knudsen FU. Lean body mass in small for gestational age and appropriate for gestational age infants. *J Pediatr*. 1988;113(5):886-889.
158. Lapillonne A, Braillon P, Claris O, Chatelain PG, Delmas PD, Salle BL. Body composition in appropriate and in small for gestational age infants. *Acta Paediatrica*. 1997;86(2):196-200.
159. Yao AC, Lu T, Castellanos R, Matanic BP. Effect of prenatally and postnatally induced hypoxia on blood volume of newborn lambs. *Life Sciences*. 1978;22(11):931-936.
160. Bauer K, Cowett RM, Howard GM, vanEpp J, Oh W. Effect of intrauterine growth retardation on postnatal weight change in preterm infants. *J Pediatr*. 1993;123(2):301-306.
162. Harake B, Power GG. Thoracic duct lymph flow: a comparative study in newborn and adult sheep. *J Develop Physiol*. 1986;8(2):87-95.
176. Linderkamp O, Versmold HT, Messow-Zahn K, Muller-Holve W, Riegel KP, Betke K. The effect of intra-partum and intra-uterine asphyxia on placental transfusion in premature and full-term infants. *Euro J Pediatr*. 1978;127(2):91-99.
177. Towell ME. Blood volume of the fetus and the newborn infant. In: Goodwin JW, Godden JO, WC G, eds. *Perinatal Medicine: The Basic Science Underlying Clinical Practice*. Baltimore: Williams & Wilkins; 1976:209-222.

106 Regulation of Acid-Base Balance in the Fetus and Neonate

Timur Azhibekov | Philippe S. Friedlich | Istvan Seri

INTRODUCTION

The majority of the existing information on the regulation of acid-base homeostasis in mammals and humans was obtained from studies in adult subjects. Revolution in micromethodology and advances in developmental physiology and molecular biology provided additional insights and improved our understanding of the key mechanisms of fetal and neonatal regulation of acid-base balance.

In general, acid-base homeostasis is tightly regulated by extracellular and intracellular buffer systems and respiratory and renal compensatory mechanisms of the organism. Under physiologic circumstances, volatile and fixed acids generated by normal metabolism are excreted and the pH remains stable.[1] The normal range of H^+ ion concentration in the extracellular fluid is 35 to 45 nEq/L (nanoequivalents per liter) corresponding to a pH of 7.45 and 7.35, respectively.[2] Volatile carbonic acid is produced in the largest amounts and is readily excreted by the lungs in the form of carbon dioxide. Fixed acids, which include lactic acid, ketoacids, phosphoric acid, and sulfuric acid, are buffered principally by extracellular bicarbonate. The bicarbonate used in this process is then regenerated by the kidneys in a series of transmembrane transport processes resulting in the excretion of H^+ ions in the form of titratable acids and ammonium.[2]

EXTRACELLULAR BUFFER SYSTEM

Using various acid-base pairs, the extracellular buffer system responds immediately to alterations in pH in a fashion represented by the Henderson-Hasselbalch equation. The carbonic acid-bicarbonate system is the most important component of this buffer system. Based on the isohydric principle, changes in the concentrations of a single acid-base pair can be used as an indicator of acid-base homeostasis for the entire system.[1] Therefore serial measurements of the carbonic acid–bicarbonate buffer system have been used to describe accurately the changes in both the experimental and the clinical settings.

INTRACELLULAR BUFFER SYSTEM

The most important components of the intracellular buffer system are the hemoglobin and intracellular proteins and phosphates acting as an intracellular H^+ sink and reservoir attached to the extracellular buffers. This system provides buffering at a slower rate compared with extracellular buffers and requires several hours to reach maximum capacity.[3]

RESPIRATORY COMPENSATORY MECHANISM

Because of the open nature of the carbonic acid–bicarbonate system, normal gas exchange in the lungs serves as an immediate regulator of acid-base homeostasis by maintaining a normal $Paco_2$, thus eliminating the excess carbon dioxide generated by an acid load. However, activation of the respiratory compensatory mechanism is necessary to return pH further toward normal.

Changes in pH and $Paco_2$ activate both central and peripheral chemoreceptors, with predominance of central activation. Because low steady-state bicarbonate values in the cerebrospinal fluid (CSF), but not the plasma, are thought to affect central respiratory drive,[4] in metabolic acidosis, full activation of the respiratory compensation is delayed by a few hours. In contrast, carbon dioxide moves freely across the blood-brain barrier.[4] As a consequence, in respiratory acidosis, hypercarbia alters H^+ ion concentrations in CSF and cerebral interstitial fluid rapidly, leading to immediate activation of the respiratory compensatory mechanism.

Earlier reports suggested active transport of bicarbonate across the blood-brain barrier.[5] However, a substantial body of evidence in animal models has demonstrated that generation of bicarbonate via hydroxylation of dissolved CO_2 during CSF formation comprises the primary mechanism of bicarbonate production in the CSF.[6-8] Almost two-thirds of bicarbonate synthesis is catalyzed by carbonic anhydrase, predominantly in the choroid plexus and glial cells. Plasma bicarbonate appears to affect CSF levels only when significant changes in serum bicarbonate levels take place.[9] A number of ion transporters (Na^+, HCO_3^- cotransporters, Cl^-/HCO_3^- exchanger) have been suggested as molecular mechanisms for such transport across the blood-brain barrier.[10]

RENAL COMPENSATORY MECHANISM

By altering renal H^+ excretion in response to changes in extracellular pH, renal compensation is the ultimate mechanism to adjust H^+ content in the body. Although full activation of this system usually requires 2 to 3 days, alterations in renal acidification may be seen as early as a few hours after the development of the acid-base disturbance.

Urine acidification and bicarbonate reabsorption take place in several segments of the nephron: proximal tubule, loop of Henle, distal tubule, and collecting ducts where most acidification occurs. Active secretion of H^+ ions into the tubular lumen is the primary mechanism responsible for urinary acidification. Filtered bicarbonate combines with secreted H^+, forming carbonic acid that then dissociates into CO_2 and H_2O. Catalyzed by the luminal carbonic anhydrase IV enzyme, this reaction allows bicarbonate to enter tubular epithelial cells in the form of CO_2. In the cytoplasm, CO_2 undergoes reverse transformation by the cytosolic carbonic anhydrase II enzyme forming bicarbonate and H^+. The regenerated bicarbonate then enters the bloodstream via transmembrane transporters in the basolateral membrane.[11]

Net H^+ ion secretion in the distal nephron continues even after the reabsorption of virtually all bicarbonate. Based on data from animal experiments, it appears that the type A intercalated cells in the distal and collecting tubules are responsible for the active H^+ secretion via apical H^+-ATPase.[11] The secreted H^+ ions are excreted in the urine in the form of titratable acids (phosphate and sulfate salts) and as ammonium salts.[12] In addition to the excretion of H^+ ions, renal ammoniagenesis also results in the generation of bicarbonate.

In alkalosis, type B and non-A, non-B intercalated cells increase HCO_3^- excretion via Na^+-independent, electroneutral Cl^-/HCO_3^- exchanger, also known as *pendrin*, in their apical membrane.[13]

REGULATION OF ACID-BASE BALANCE IN THE FETUS

FETAL EXTRACELLULAR AND INTRACELLULAR BUFFER SYSTEMS

The fetus has an intact extracellular buffer system with the carbonic acid-bicarbonate buffer system serving as the predominant buffer system. For the fetus, the placenta is the organ of respiration and quickly eliminates the excess carbon dioxide generated by the development of fetal metabolic acidosis, provided that placental function, uterine and umbilical blood flows, and maternal respiratory status are uncompromised.[14]

Intracellular buffering capacity is considerably larger than the extracellular one[14] despite the fact that the fetus has a significantly smaller intracellular compartment compared with a child or adult.

FETAL RESPIRATORY AND RENAL COMPENSATORY MECHANISMS

The respiratory and renal compensatory mechanisms of the fetus are limited by immaturity and the surrounding maternal environment. The placentomaternal unit performs most of the effective compensatory functions.[14] Interestingly, hormones such as prostaglandins produced by the placenta suppress fetal breathing movements.[15-17] Fetal breathing movements are first noted late in the first trimester as sporadic and irregular. With advancing gestational age, fetal breathing movements attain a more consistent pattern and become better regulated. However, their critical role is likely to promote differentiation and proliferation of the developing lung tissue[18] rather than participation in acid-base balance regulation. In contrast, the fetal kidney has the ability to contribute to the maintenance of fetal acid-base balance.[19,20] For instance, ammonium excretion and thus generation of bicarbonate and possibly sodium excretion have been noted to increase during the recovery period from hypocapnic hypoxia in the fetal sheep.[19]

FETAL METABOLIC ACIDOSIS

The most frequent cause of fetal metabolic acidosis is fetal hypoxemia due to abnormalities of uteroplacental function, blood flow, or both. Primary maternal hypoxemia or maternal metabolic acidosis secondary to maternal diabetes mellitus, sepsis, or renal tubular abnormalities are unusual causes of fetal metabolic acidosis. During the course of fetal hypoxemia, metabolism becomes anaerobic, and large quantities of lactic acid accumulate. H^+ ions are buffered by the extracellular and intracellular buffering systems, and pH drops as plasma bicarbonate decreases. Because of the unhindered diffusion of carbon dioxide through the placenta,[21] restoration of fetal pH toward normal initially occurs through elimination of the volatile element of the carbonic acid-bicarbonate system via the maternal lungs. However, lactate and other fixed acids cross the placenta more slowly,[14] resulting in a delay of effective maternal renal compensation of fetal metabolic acidosis. If fetal oxygenation improves, the products of anaerobic metabolism are also metabolized by the fetus.

As described earlier, the respiratory compensatory mechanism in utero does not contribute to effective compensation of fetal metabolic acidosis. However, in the absence of fetal hypercarbia or hypoxemia, isolated metabolic acidosis still stimulates fetal breathing movements, with significant delay in the onset of activation.[22]

Several lines of evidence indicate that the fetal kidney is able to excrete acid[20,23,24] and organic acids[25] and to reabsorb more bicarbonate.[26] Studies in fetal sheep have found age-dependent increases in glomerular filtration rate (GFR), urinary titratable acid, ammonium, and net acid excretion.[23] Furthermore, a positive relationship has been demonstrated between changes in GFR and bicarbonate, sodium, and chloride excretions.[23,24] However, the fetal kidney has a developmentally regulated limited ability to adapt to changes in fetal acid-base balance. In fetal sheep, in response to metabolic acidosis induced by the infusion of hydrochloric acid, systolic blood pressure increases but the GFR does not change. Urinary titratable acid, ammonium, and net acid excretion increase without significant changes in renal bicarbonate absorption.[20] Evidence also indicates that the fetal kidney has the ability to increase bicarbonate reabsorption, at least during periods of volume depletion.[26] With regard to the human fetus, only limited information is available concerning renal acidification.[27] However, the physiologic importance of these adaptive fetal renal responses is limited when compared with those in the postnatal period because the acid load excreted in the fetal urine remains within the immediate fetal environment and still has to be eliminated by the placenta or metabolized by the fetus.

FETAL RESPIRATORY ACIDOSIS

Fetal respiratory acidosis develops when prolonged maternal hypoventilation occurs with maternal asthma, airway obstruction, narcotic overdosing, maternal anesthesia, severe hypokalemia, and magnesium sulfate toxicity. Depending on the neurophysiologic state of the fetus, fetal breathing movements increase in response to increasing $Paco_2$,[28] and the fetal kidney exerts a maturation-dependent limited response by reclaiming more bicarbonate in an attempt to restore the 20:1 bicarbonate to carbonic acid ratio and thus increase the pH toward normal.[14] Obviously, only the renal compensation has some limited physiologic significance for the fetus in cases of respiratory acidosis.

FETAL METABOLIC ALKALOSIS

Metabolic alkalosis rarely affects the fetus, but it may occur in women with hyperemesis gravidarum. As a result of the significant maternal hydrogen chloride losses, bicarbonate is retained by the mother to maintain the anionic balance with extracellular sodium. Because bicarbonate is transported slowly across the placenta, the development of fetal metabolic alkalosis lags behind that of the mother. Compensatory maternal hypoventilation tends to restore normal pH in the fetus as a result of the rapid movement of carbon dioxide across the placenta.

FETAL RESPIRATORY ALKALOSIS

The physiologic hyperventilation of the pregnant woman causes a compensatory decrease in her serum bicarbonate concentration to approximately 22 mM.[14] In fetal sheep, maternal respiratory alkalosis due to hyperventilation results in hypocapnia with increased pH in the umbilical venous blood, while maternal metabolic alkalosis does not affect fetal pH or Pa_{CO_2}, at least in the short term.[29] However, a decrease in umbilical vein P_{O_2} occurs with the decrease in maternal Pa_{CO_2} levels. In addition, severe acute maternal hyperventilation results in decreased umbilical arterial flow and the development of fetal hypoxia and metabolic acidosis.[30] In humans, maternal hyperventilation also results in fetal acidosis, decreased oxygen saturation in the umbilical blood vessels, and perinatal depression at birth.[31] These findings are thought to be due to uterine vasoconstriction. In addition, a decrease and even cessation of fetal breathing movements have been observed with maternal hyperventilation.[32,33] Whether the inhibition of fetal breathing movements is due to fetal hypocapnia or resulted from the acute fetal hypoxia secondary to uterine vasoconstriction remains to be determined. Experimental models support the transient suppression of fetal breathing movements in response to fetal hypoxia.[34,35] Finally, restoration of maternal carbon dioxide levels to normal has been proposed to correct both the abnormal uterine blood flow and the acid-base abnormality in the fetus.

REGULATION OF ACID-BASE BALANCE IN THE NEONATE

The neonate continues to undergo maturation of the overall adaptive responses to changes in acid-base homeostasis. An abrupt increase in the sensitivity of the central respiratory control system to changes in pH and Pa_{CO_2} occurs at the time of delivery, augmented by the catecholamine surge and change in the environmental temperature during labor and immediately postnatally.[18] Regulation of acid-base balance becomes tighter after birth; however, the cellular mechanisms responsible for the increased sensitivity of the acid-base balance regulation system are not fully understood.

NEONATAL EXTRACELLULAR AND INTRACELLULAR BUFFER SYSTEMS

The neonate has well-functioning extracellular and intracellular buffering systems. Postnatally, the gradual increase in the size of the intracellular compartment further enhances the overall buffering capacity.

NEONATAL RESPIRATORY COMPENSATORY MECHANISM

With postpartum establishment of the functional residual capacity, the neonatal lungs become the end organ of the respiratory compensatory mechanism to changes in acid-base balance. The effectiveness of respiratory compensation depends on the maturity of the central respiratory control system[36] and pulmonary function. Ventilatory responses to changes in Pa_{CO_2} via peripheral and central chemoreceptors are developmentally regulated and thus related to gestational and postnatal age. Preterm infants exhibit a decrease in CO_2 sensitivity.[37] The physiologic mechanisms responsible for this phenomenon remain unclear. In addition, interaction between CO_2 responses and the level of oxygenation differs from that in adults.[38,39]

Pulmonary function itself determines the ultimate effectiveness of the postnatal respiratory response. Indeed, neonates with parenchymal lung disease, especially if they are born prematurely, have a limited ability to increase ventilation in response to acidosis.

NEONATAL RENAL COMPENSATORY MECHANISM

The renal compensatory mechanisms of the neonate are immature, resulting in a developmentally regulated decreased ability to maintain acid-base balance.[40,41] Both renal microhemodynamic and tubular epithelial factors play a role in the limited renal compensatory capacity of the newborn.

Following a decrease in renal blood flow immediately after delivery, renal blood flow significantly increases in the postnatal period and the renal vasodilatory mechanisms appear to be functionally mature as early as 24 weeks of gestation.[42] GFR is also low in the immediate postnatal period, and it increases as a function of both gestational and postnatal age.[43-45] The low GFR is one of the most important factors limiting the ability of the preterm and term infant to handle an acid load adequately.[40,41] Net renal acid excretion also depends on several gestational and postnatal age-dependent tubular epithelial functions.[46]

Under physiologic conditions, three main transport mechanisms regulate active acid extrusion and transepithelial bicarbonate reabsorption by the proximal tubular epithelia (Fig. 106.1): (1) the H^+-ATPase and (2) the Na^+-H^+ antiporter in the apical membrane and (3) the electrogenic Na^+-$3HCO_3^-$ cotransporter in the basolateral membrane.[11] The apical membrane H^+-ATPase is responsible for the primary active transport of hydrogen ions into the tubular lumen, while the secondary active transport of H^+ via the Na^+-H^+ antiporter is driven by the low intracellular Na concentration that is maintained by the Na, K^+-ATPase in the basolateral membrane. The apical membrane Na^+-H^+ antiporter mediates most of the $NaHCO_3$ absorption in the proximal tubule. In the basolateral membrane, the electrogenic Na^+-$3HCO_3^-$ cotransporter represents the key mechanism for base efflux into the interstitium.

Available evidence suggests that up to 80% of the filtered bicarbonate is reabsorbed in the proximal tubule.[47] Therefore the function of the proximal tubular transporters essentially determines the renal threshold for bicarbonate reabsorption. The bicarbonate threshold for reabsorption has been reported to be approximately 18 mEq/L in the premature infant[48,49] and approximately 21 mEq/L in the term infant.[48] The bicarbonate threshold reaches adult levels (24 to 26 mEq/L) only after 1 year of age.[50] However, in the extremely premature neonate in the early postnatal period, the renal bicarbonate threshold may be as low as 14 mEq/L.[49] Renal carbonic anhydrase is present and active during fetal life (at least by 26 weeks of gestation),[51] and its activity is similar to that of the adult kidney.[52] Therefore it is most likely that developmentally regulated immaturity of the expression, molecular structure, membrane assembly, or second-messenger[53] and, to less extent, third-messenger function of the proximal tubular transporters is responsible for the low bicarbonate threshold during early development. Indeed, reduced activity of the Na^+-$3HCO_3^-$ cotransporter was observed in an animal model during neonatal period.[54] Activity of the Na^+-H^+ antiporter has been reported to be approximately one third of the adult activity,[54] corresponding to the decrease of bicarbonate

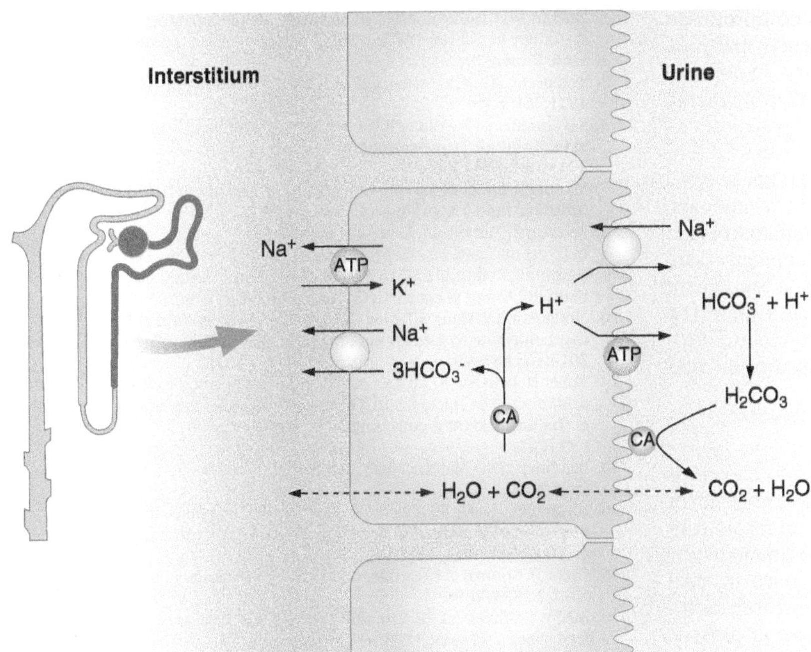

Fig. 106.1 Main transport mechanisms of hydrogen ion secretion and bicarbonate reabsorption in the proximal tubule. In the apical membrane, the H^+-ATPase uses metabolic energy (ATP) to actively secrete hydrogen ions into the luminal fluid (primary active transport). The apical membrane Na^+-H^+ antiporter extrudes H^+ in exchange for Na^+, and its function relies on the low intracellular Na concentration that is controlled by the basolateral membrane Na, K^+-ATPase (secondary active transport). Most of the regenerated bicarbonate exits the cell into the interstitium via the Na^+-$3HCO_3^-$ cotransporter in the basolateral membrane. *ATP*, Adenosine triphosphate; *CA*, carbonic anhydrase.

reabsorption of a similar magnitude in the proximal tubule.[55] In addition, both the activity and the hormonal responsiveness of the proximal tubular Na^+, K^+-ATPase are decreased in younger animals.[56]

Medications used in the treatment of critically ill neonates may also affect proximal tubular bicarbonate reabsorption. For example, dopamine administration may potentially decrease the low bicarbonate threshold of the neonate[57] because the drug inhibits the activity of the proximal tubular Na^+/H^+ antiporter.[58,59] Carbonic anhydrase inhibitors decrease proximal tubular bicarbonate reabsorption by limiting intracellular bicarbonate formation and H^+ ion availability for the Na^+-H^+ antiporter. These drugs also reduce carbonic acid dissociation into CO_2 and H_2O in the tubular lumen.[60] Finally, furosemide, acting on several transport proteins along the nephron, directly increases urinary excretion of titratable acids and ammonium.[61]

Under physiologic circumstances, the loop of Henle, particularly the thick ascending limb, reabsorbs approximately 15% of the filtered bicarbonate,[62] and the distal tubule reabsorbs the remainder. Both segments use transport mechanisms similar to those of the proximal tubule except for the presence of the HCO_3^--Cl^- antiporter that transports bicarbonate across the basolateral membrane only in the distal nephron.[11]

Urinary excretion of titratable acid and ammonium increases as a function of gestational and postnatal age.[41,45] However, distal tubular H^+ ion secretion appears to be inducible independent of the gestational age, because the ability to effectively acidify the urine is acquired by the age of 1 month even in very premature infants.[63,64]

It has been well established that $H_2PO_4^-$ is the major constituent of titratable acid in the urine. Therefore drugs that decrease proximal tubular phosphate reabsorption and thus increase the delivery of phosphate to the distal nephron may increase the renal acidification capacity of the neonate. Indeed, by inhibiting proximal tubular phosphate reabsorption, dopamine has been shown to increase the excretion of titratable acids in preterm infants.[65]

Among the endocrine factors influencing distal tubular acidification, aldosterone is one of the most important hormones. By affecting the function of several different transport mechanisms, aldosterone stimulates net H^+ ion excretion in the distal nephron.[11] However, the distal nephron of the premature neonate has a developmentally regulated relative insensitivity to aldosterone.[66,67]

NEONATAL METABOLIC ACIDOSIS

The most frequent causes of increased anion-gap (most often lactic) metabolic acidosis in the neonate are hypoxemia or ischemia secondary to perinatal asphyxia, severe lung disease, volume depletion, vasoregulatory disturbances, or myocardial dysfunction caused by immaturity, sepsis, or asphyxia. Severe metabolic acidosis caused by a neonatal metabolic disorder is rare but should always be considered. Interestingly, the type of anesthesia used during caesarean section has also been suggested to influence neonatal acid-base status. Indeed, according to a meta-analysis of the findings of 27 studies, cord pH was lower and base deficit was higher in newborns whose mothers received spinal anesthesia compared with those receiving general and epidural anesthesia.[68] Therefore, when assessing a neonate born via caesarean section who presents with metabolic acidosis in the immediate postnatal period, the type of anesthesia needs to be considered when searching for the etiology of the acid-base disturbance.

As discussed earlier, preterm neonates frequently present with a mild to moderate normal anion-gap acidosis that in extremely preterm infants typically peaks by day 4 of life, and subsequently resolves during the second week of life.[69] This metabolic acidosis has been attributed both to the low renal bicarbonate threshold of the premature kidney[41,48,50] and reduced ability to secrete titratable acid and ammonium.[63,70] In addition, the use of carbonic anhydrase inhibitors, as well as the maturation-related decreased sensitivity to aldosterone, may also contribute to the development of normal anion-gap acidosis in the neonate.[2,66,67] Parenteral nutrition, namely early use of amino acids in premature infants, does not appear to significantly affect acid-base balance[71]; however, increased risk of metabolic acidosis is associated with increased amino acid and lipid intake during the first week of life in extremely preterm infants.[72]

In metabolic acidosis caused by the accumulation of lactic acid, H^+ ions are buffered by the extracellular and intracellular buffering systems; pH drops as plasma bicarbonate concentration decreases. Initial restoration of pH toward normal through elimination of the CO_2 by the lungs may be severely compromised in the sick preterm and term neonate with parenchymal lung disease or conditions associated with pulmonary hypoplasia such as prolonged amniotic fluid leak, congenital diaphragmatic hernia, or cystic pulmonary adenomatoid malformation. As described earlier, the renal compensatory mechanisms are also less effective because of the immaturity of neonatal renal function. The main elements of the response of the neonatal kidney to metabolic acidosis in the immediate postnatal period are the attenuated increases in GFR, proximal tubular bicarbonate reabsorption, and distal tubular net acid secretion. A significant improvement in the overall renal response occurs after the first month of postnatal life even in the premature infant.[48,63,64] However, complete maturation does not occur until after the first year of age.

NEONATAL RESPIRATORY ACIDOSIS

In the clinical setting, neonatal respiratory acidosis develops most frequently in newborns with respiratory distress and/or failure. In premature infants, stimulation of the central respiratory center by the elevated interstitial carbon dioxide immediately increases respiratory rate with only minor increases in tidal volume. However, term newborns respond to hypercapnia with an increase in the tidal volume first.[73] Overall, carbon dioxide elimination by the lungs is usually limited because of immaturity and/or parenchymal lung disease.

In response to respiratory acidosis, the kidneys also reclaim more bicarbonate, especially during the first few weeks of postnatal life. However, renal compensation is limited by the developmentally regulated immaturity of proximal and distal tubular functions.

NEONATAL METABOLIC ALKALOSIS

Metabolic alkalosis most frequently develops in the preterm neonate who receives prolonged diuretic treatment for bronchopulmonary dysplasia. The respiratory response is a decrease in the rate and depth of breathing to increase carbon dioxide retention. This response may not be effective if the intubated neonate is being overventilated with a mechanical ventilator. In response to a metabolic alkalosis, urinary bicarbonate reabsorption and distal tubular net acid excretion decrease, resulting in a return of the extracellular pH toward normal.

NEONATAL RESPIRATORY ALKALOSIS

Neonatal respiratory alkalosis occurs most frequently secondary to fever and iatrogenic hyperventilation of the intubated preterm and term infant. Rarely, respiratory alkalosis may be the presenting sign of a urea cycle disorder during the first days after delivery because rising ammonia levels may initially stimulate the central respiratory center. Renal compensation plays an important, although limited role, in cases of neonatal respiratory alkalosis.

CONCLUSION

The fetus and the neonate exhibit a limited ability to maintain and regulate acid-base homeostasis. However, regardless of the state of maturity, an abrupt increase in the sensitivity of acid-base regulation occurs with delivery. The exact mechanisms for this accelerated maturation remain incompletely understood.

 A complete reference list is available at www.ExpertConsult.com.

SELECT REFERENCES

1. Masoro EJ. An overview of hydrogen ion regulation. *Arch Intern Med.* 1982;142:1019.
2. Brewer ED. Disorders of acid-base balance. *Pediatr Clin North Am.* 1990;37:429.
3. Kaehny WD. Pathogenesis and management of respiratory and mixed acid-base disorders. In: Schrier RW, ed. *Renal and Electrolyte Disorders.* 3rd ed. Boston: Little Brown; 1986:187.
4. Sorensen SC. The chemical control of ventilation. *Acta Physiol Scand.* 1971;361:1.
5. Severinghaus JW, Mitchell RA, Richardson BW, Singer MM. Respiratory control at high altitude suggesting active transport regulation of CSF pH. *J Appl Physiol.* 1963;18:1155-1166.
7. Maren TH. Effect of varying CO2 equilibria on rates of HCO3- formation in cerebrospinal fluid. *J Appl Physiol.* 1979;47:471-477.
8. Javaheri S, Nardell EA, Kazemi H. Role of PCO2 as determinant of CSF [HCO-3] in metabolic acidosis. *Respir Physiol.* 1979;36:155-166.
9. Nattie EE, Romer L. CSF HCO3- regulation in isosmotic conditions: the role of brain PCO2 and plasma HCO3-. *Respir Physiol.* 1978;33:177-198.
10. Mokgokong R, Wang S, Taylor CJ, et al. Ion transporters in brain endothelial cells that contribute to formation of brain interstitial fluid. *Pflüg Arch Eur J Physiol.* 2014;466:887-901.
13. Amlal H, Petrovic S, Xu J, et al. Deletion of the anion exchanger Slc26a4 (pendrin) decreases apical Cl(-)/HCO3(-) exchanger activity and impairs bicarbonate secretion in kidney collecting duct. *Am J Physiol Cell Physiol.* 2010;299(1): C33-C41.
14. Blechner JN. Maternal-fetal acid-base, physiology. *Clin Obstet Gynecol.* 1993;36:3.
16. Alvaro RE, Hasan SU, Chemtob S, et al. Prostaglandins are responsible for the inhibition of breathing observed with a placental extract in fetal sheep. *Respir Physiol Neurobiol.* 2004;144:35-44.
18. Greer JJ. Control of breathing activity in the fetus and newborn. *Compr Physiol.* 2012;2:1873-1888.
20. Kesby GJ, Lumbers ER. The effects of metabolic acidosis on renal function of fetal sheep. *J Physiol.* 1988;396:65-74.
22. Molteni RA, Melmed MH, Sheldon RE, et al. Induction of fetal breathing by metabolic acidemia and its effect on blood flow to the respiratory muscles. *Am J Obstet Gynecol.* 1980;136:609.
23. Kesby GJ, Lumbers ER. Factors affecting renal handling of sodium, hydrogen ions, and bicarbonate in the fetus. *Am J Physiol.* 1986;251:226.
27. Blechner JN, Stenger VG, Eitzman DV, Prystowsky H. Effects of maternal metabolic acidosis on the human fetus and newborn infant. *Am J Obstet Gynecol.* 1967;9:46.
30. Motoyama EK, Rivard G, Acheson F, Cook CD. Adverse effect of maternal hyperventilation on the foetus. *Lancet.* 1966;1:286-288.
31. Moya F, Morishima HO, Shnider SM, James LS. Influence of maternal hyperventilation on the newborn infant. *Am J Obstet Gynecol.* 1965;91:76.
32. Connors G, Hunse C, Carmichael L, et al. Control of fetal breathing in the human fetus between 24 and 34 weeks' gestation. *Am J Obstet Gynecol.* 1989;160: 932-938.
33. Connors G, Hunse C, Carmichael L, et al. The role of carbon dioxide in the generation of human fetal breathing movements. *Am J Obstet Gynecol.* 1988;158:322-327.
36. Darnall RA. The role of CO2 and central chemoreception in the control of breathing in the fetus and the neonate. *Respir Physiol Neurobiol.* 2010;173:201-212.
37. Abu-Shaweesh JM. Maturation of respiratory reflex responses in the fetus and neonate. *Semin Neonatol.* 2004;9:169-180.
38. Albersheim S, Boychuk R, Seshia MM, et al. Effects of CO2 on immediate ventilatory response to O2 in preterm infants. *J Appl Physiol.* 1976;41:609-611.
39. Wolsink JG, Berkenbosch A, DeGoede J, et al. The effects of hypoxia on the ventilatory response to sudden changes in CO2 in newborn piglets. *J Physiol.* 1992;456:39-48.
40. Guignard JP, John EG. Renal function in the tiny premature infant. *Clin Perinatol.* 1986;13:377.
41. Jones DP, Chesney RW. Development of tubular function. *Clin Perinatol.* 1992;19:33.
42. Seri I, Abbasi S, Wood DC, Gerdes JS. Regional hemodynamic effects of dopamine in the sick preterm infant. *J Pediatr.* 1998;133:728.
43. Fawer CL, Torrado A, Guignard JP. Maturation of renal function in full-term and premature neonates. *Helv Paediatr Acta.* 1979;34:11.
44. Guignard JP, Torrado A, Da Cunha O, Gautier E. Glomerular filtration rate in the first three weeks of life. *J Pediatr.* 1975;87:268.
45. Arant BS. Developmental patterns of renal functional maturation compared in the human neonate. *J Pediatr.* 1978;92:705-712.
47. Quigley R, Baum M. Neonatal acid base balance and disturbances. *Semin Perinatol.* 2004;28:97-102.
48. Svenningsen NW. Renal acid-base titration studies in infants with and without metabolic acidosis in the postneonatal period. *Pediatr Res.* 1974;8:659-672.
50. Edelmann CM, Soriano JR, Boichis H, et al. Renal bicarbonate reabsorption and hydrogen ion excretion in normal infants. *J Clin Invest.* 1967;46:1309-1317.
52. Lonnerholm C, Wistrand PJ. Carbonic anhydrase in the human fetal kidney. *Pediatr Res.* 1983;17:390.
53. Bobulescu IA, Moe OW. Luminal Na(+)/H (+) exchange in the proximal tubule. *Pflüg Arch Eur J Physiol.* 2009;458:5-21.

56. Fryckstedt J, Svensson LB, Lindén M, Aperia A. The effect of dopamine on adenylate cyclase and Na^+, K^+-ATPase activity in the developing rat renal cortical and medullary tubule cells. *Pediatr Res*. 1993;34:308.
59. Bobulescu IA, Quiñones H, Gisler SM, et al. Acute regulation of renal Na+/H+ exchanger NHE3 by dopamine: role of protein phosphatase 2A. *Am J Physiol Ren Physiol*. 2010;298:1205–1213.
61. Hropot M, Fowler N, Karlmark B, Giebisch G. Tubular action of diuretics: distal effects on electrolyte transport and acidification. *Kidney Int*. 1985;28:477.
62. Capasso G, Unwin R, Agulian S, Giebisch G. Bicarbonate transport along the loop of Henle. I. Microperfusion studies of load and inhibitor sensitivity. *J Clin Invest*. 1991;88:430–437.
63. Kerpel-Fronius E, Heim T, Sulyok E. The development of the renal acidifying processes and their relation to acidosis in low-birth-weight infants. *Biol Neonate*. 1970;15:156–168.
64. Sulyok E, Heim T. Assessment of maximal urinary acidification in premature infants. *Biol Neonate*. 1971;19:200–210.
65. Seri I, Rudas G, Bors Z, et al. Effects of low-dose dopamine on cardiovascular and renal functions, cerebral blood flow, and plasma catecholamine levels in sick preterm neonates. *Pediatr Res*. 1993;34:742.
66. Sulyok E, Németh M, Tényi I, et al. Relationship between maturity, electrolyte balance and the function of the renin-angiotensin-aldosterone system in newborn infants. *Biol Neonate*. 1979;35:60.
68. Reynolds F, Seed PT. Anesthesia for caesarian section and neonatal acid-base status: a meta-analysis. *Anesthesia*. 2005;60:636.
69. Bourchier D, Weston PJ. Metabolic acidosis in the first 14 days of life in infants of gestation less than 26 weeks. *Eur J Pediatr*. 2015;174(1):49–54.
70. Sato T, Takahashi N, Komatsu Y, et al. Urinary acidification in extremely low birth weight infants. *Early Hum Dev*. 2002;70(1-2):15–24.
71. Trivedi A, Sinn JK. Early versus late administration of amino acids in preterm infants receiving parenteral nutrition. *Cochrane Database Syst Rev*. 2013;7:CD008771.
72. Bonsante F, Gouyon J-B, Robillard P-Y, Gouyon B, Iacobelli S. Early optimal parenteral nutrition and metabolic acidosis in very preterm infants. *PloS One*. 2017;12(11):e0186936.
73. Bodegård G. Control of respiration in newborn babies. III. Developmental changes of respiratory depth and rate responses to CO2. *Acta Paediatr Scand*. 1975;64:684–692.

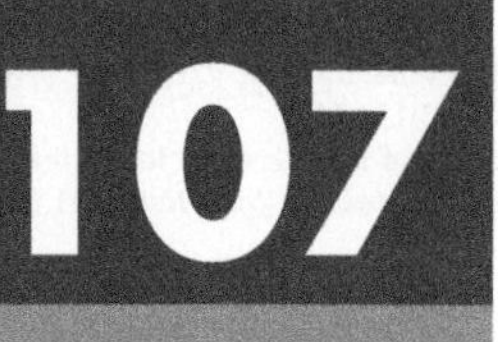

Developmental Biology of Hematopoietic Stem Cells

Amélie Collins

INTRODUCTION

The hematopoietic system is made up of all of the blood cells, including red blood cells, platelets, myeloid cells such as granulocytes, monocyte-macrophages, and dendritic cells (DC), and lymphoid cells such as T, B, and natural killer (NK) cells. Together, these cells function to provide oxygen-carrying capacity, hemostasis, innate and adaptive immune function, and tissue regeneration and repair. Hematopoiesis is the process by which these lineage-committed blood cells are produced from hematopoietic stem and progenitor cells (HSPCs). In adults, hematopoietic stem cells (HSCs) sit at the top of the hematopoietic hierarchy and are functionally defined as cells capable of both self-renewal and differentiation into all the lineages of the blood system, giving rise to approximately 10^{12} cells daily.[1] Adult hematopoiesis takes place in the bone marrow in specific microenvironmental areas called *niches*. During development, transient waves of hematopoiesis supply the embryo with blood cells tailored to the needs of the developing organism, with the production of these cells occurring in distinct anatomic locations. This chapter will focus on the emergence of the hematopoietic system during embryogenesis, the establishment of "definitive," or adult-like, hematopoiesis, and developmental regulation of HSC function during fetal and neonatal life. Basic concepts in stem cell biology will be introduced, including the recent development of induced pluripotent stem cells (iPSCs) and their use in further investigating developmental hematopoiesis.

METHODOLOGIES TO STUDY HEMATOPOIESIS

Our understanding of human developmental hematopoiesis has been shaped by the availability (or lack thereof) of human embryonic and fetal specimens that are accessible for investigation and, just as important, by the methodologies that have been available to study them. Phenotypic definition of HSCs that would allow for their prospective identification, by microscopy or flow cytometry, is imperfect. Our best definition of HSCs still only identifies a heterogeneous population of cells, only 1 in 10 of which possesses HSC activity (see below).[2] HSCs remain defined functionally, on the basis of both their multi-lineage potential (multipotency) and their long-term reconstitution (self-renewal). As such, our ability to identify HSCs has only been as good as the assays available at the time that allow determination of these features of HSC function. Early experiments used in vitro colony-forming assays as surrogates for HSC activity, with the formation of cobblestone areas under stromal support cells (cobblestone area forming cells, CAFCs) or colony formation in semisolid methylcellulose medium (colony-forming unit cell, CFU-C, posited to be generated by long-term culture-initiating cells, LTC-ICs) being representative of HSC function.[3] It is important that these measures of HSC activity are by definition retrospective, in that progenitor activity can only be inferred after differentiation has occurred, and heterogeneous populations of cells are identified.[4,5] In vitro colony formation can also be used to assay multipotency. In methylcellulose, HSCs and their derivatives are categorized on the basis of the characteristics of the colonies that they form. A single hematopoietic colony consists of more than 50 hematopoietic cells and may include hundreds or even thousands of cells. The more immature (early) progenitor cells are highly proliferative and form colonies consisting of more than two kinds of cell types; thus a colony containing cells for several lineages is considered to be derived from a multipotent progenitor (MPP) cell, such as a CFU-GEMM (granulocyte, erythrocyte, monocyte, megakaryocyte) or CFU-mix. A progenitor cell that forms a colony consisting of granulocyte and macrophages is called a *CFU-GM*. Later committed progenitor cells that form a single lineage are called *CFU-G* (for *granulocyte*), or *CFU-M* (for *macrophage*). In the erythroid lineage, early erythroid progenitors are proliferative and form burst colonies and are called *erythroid burst-forming units (BFU-E),* whereas late erythroid progenitors form relatively small colonies and are called *CFU-E.*

While methylcellulose has been the standard for years, it has some important limitations. It does not support the development of colonies from cells isolated from early embryonic tissues, thus precluding an analysis of the hematopoietic potential of these cells. To overcome this limitation, explant cultures were developed,[6] in which undissociated regions of early human embryos are cultured in toto on a mouse stromal cell line (MS-5) that supports the further differentiation of hematopoietic precursors. Subsequent to this short undissociated culture period, cells are dissociated to yield a single-cell suspension and then seeded in methylcellulose for standard colony formation assessment. Such an approach allowed for the identification of hematopoietic potential at the earliest embryonic timepoints (see below). Another limitation is that methylcellulose only supports the development of megakaryocytic, erythrocytic, and myeloid cells. Identification of mouse stromal cell lines (including MS-5) that also support the differentiation of human hematopoietic differentiation has allowed for the refinement of in vitro assays to reveal megakaryocytic, erythroid, myeloid, and lymphoid potential from a single sorted progenitor cell.[7,8]

Perhaps the most significant advance in assessing human HSC function arose with the advent of immune-deficient mice that allow for xenotransplantation of human cells. These efforts were facilitated by the discovery of severe combined immune-deficient *(Scid)* mice that lack B and T cells, allowing for partial engraftment of human cells. *Scid* mice were found to allow infused human peripheral blood cells to produce antibodies specific to tetanus toxin (*Scid*-PBL model),[9,10] and also could sustain long-term production of human B and T cells when surgically grafted with human fetal tissue and human fetal liver cells (*Scid-hu* model).[11,12] Myeloid reconstitution was achieved by transplanting human bone marrow cells into *Scid* mice that also received myeloid-promoting cytokines.[13,14]

The functional unit responsible for *Scid* mouse repopulation was thus referred to as the "*Scid*-repopulating cell" or SRC, and to this day reconstitution in immune-deficient mice remains a gold standard for proof of "stemness." Improvements to the *Scid* model came when *Scid* mice were crossed to nonobese diabetic mice (NOD-*Scid* mice) that supported higher levels of human cell engraftment due to a mutation in the *Sirpa* gene that promotes host macrophage tolerance of transplanted human cells.[15,16] NOD-*Scid* mice with a mutation in the IL2R common γ chain (NSG mice)[17,18] are completely devoid of B, T, and NK cells and support fivefold higher engraftment of human $CD34^+$ cells than NOD-*Scid* mice. Finally, NSG mice engineered to express human cytokines are allowing for an even more robust evaluation of human hematopoiesis.[19,20] The most stringent definition of self-renewal activity is reserved for cells that when transplanted into an immunodeficient recipient give rise not only to multiple hematopoietic lineages over the long term (generally longer than 12 to 20 weeks is considered long term) but can also reconstitute a secondary immunodeficient recipient upon harvest from the primary recipient bone marrow, so-called *serial transplantation*. Although transplantation into immunodeficient mice remains the gold standard for "stemness" in the field, it should be remembered that this represents the activity of a stem cell removed from its native microenvironment and may thus not be representative of unperturbed hematopoiesis.

DEVELOPMENTAL HEMATOPOIESIS IN THE HUMAN EMBRYO AND FETUS

Hematopoiesis starts in the extraembryonic yolk sac (YS) of the human embryo. The human embryonic period encompasses the time from the moment of fertilization to the end of the eighth week of embryonic age (tenth postmenstrual week). Human hematopoiesis during the embryonic period comprises a period of primitive hematopoiesis in the YS, HSC emergence in the aorta-gonad-mesonephros (AGM) region from the hemogenic endothelium, and the seeding of HSCs from the AGM into the liver. During the fetal period (8 weeks until birth), HSCs and their progenitors exist in the placenta and circulation, expand in the fetal liver, and subsequently move into the bone marrow during the second trimester, where hematopoiesis resides throughout adult life. This is summarized in Fig. 107.1.

YOLK SAC HEMATOPOIESIS

The YS forms outside of the embryo in a balloon-like structure 7 to 8 days after implantation. Within the YS, mesodermal cells aggregate in initially homogeneous solid clusters. The cells at the periphery of these clusters acquire the characteristics of endothelial cells while the internal cells regress to form vessel lumens. Groups of mesodermal cells remain associated to newly formed endothelial cells, forming "blood islands" by embryonic day 16.[21] Within this early YS vascular network, prior to the onset of circulation at embryonic day 21, are found primarily large primitive nucleated erythrocytes (megaloblasts),[22] with scarce interspersed macrophages and megakaryocytes.[23]

Early functional studies of human YS hematopoiesis from 4.5 week embryos has demonstrated the presence of clonogenic progenitors including early (BFU-E) and late (CFU-E) erythroid, granulo-macrocytic (CFU-GM), and mixed (CFU-GEMM) progenitors.[24] A subsequent study confirmed the presence of progenitors with both erythroid and myeloid clonogenic potential as early as 25 days.[25] The frequency of these progenitors drops sharply after about the sixth week of development, a time

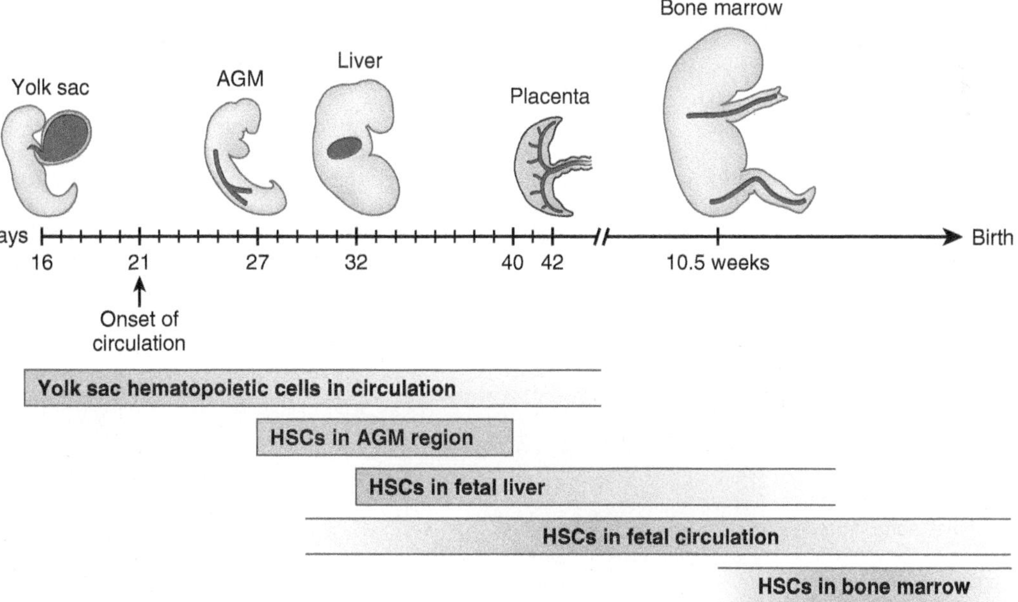

Fig. 107.1 Discrete temporal and anatomic waves of hematopoietic development in the human embryo and fetus. Hematopoietic cells are found in the yolk sac as early as day 16, and persist in both the yolk sac and the intraembryonic circulation and organs until the yolk sac disappears. Definitive hematopoiesis emerges from the floor of the dorsal aorta in the aorta-gonad-mesonephros *(AGM)* region, with $CD34^+CD45^+$ cells capable of giving rise to the hematopoietic system present from days 27 to 40. $CD34^+CD45^+$ cells with hematopoietic potential are first detected in the fetal liver on day 30. While the hematopoietic compartment is thought to transition to the bone marrow cavity during the second trimester, with hematopoietic cells present as early as gestational week 10.5 and cells with hematopoietic stem cell *(HSC)* activity detectable by gestational week 15 to 16, it is unclear when the fetal liver stops supporting hematopoiesis. Hematopoietic cells including HSCs are also found in the circulation and placenta starting at day 42 and persisting until delivery. The bone marrow cavity is thought to be the primary hematopoietic organ by the time of delivery and throughout childhood and adult life.

at which hematopoiesis is leaving the YS and transitioning to the embryo proper, primarily taking up residence in the liver rudiment (see below). This period is also marked by the switch, in the liver, from embryonic to fetal hemoglobin (ξ-globin → α-globin and ε- globin → γ-globin) and the transition from primitive (nucleated) megaloblasts to definitive (enucleated) macrocytes.[26] These studies were initially taken as supporting a monoclonal model of human hematopoiesis, in which cells arising in the YS give rise first to primitive cells of the erythroid and myeloid (primarily macrophage) lineage, then migrate to the liver where definitive hematopoiesis (including the appearance of definitive HSCs) is established. However, these studies were done in specimens obtained after the onset of circulation (day 21). It is now generally accepted that definitive hematopoiesis originates in the embryo proper (within specialized regions of the aorta, see below), and that any long-term reconstituting HSCs found in the YS have migrated from intra-embryonic tissues where they originate.[27] The only study to have examined the hematopoietic potential of the YS and intra-embryonic tissues prior to the onset of circulation (2 specimens at 19 days) demonstrated that YS explants generate few CD34+ cells that decrease rapidly in numbers as ex vivo culture progress, and only give rise to myeloid and NK cells in vitro. In contrast, intra-embryonic tissues from the same specimen give rise to larger numbers of CD34+ cells that survive longer in culture and have myeloid, NK, B and T cell potential,[6] suggestive of discrete waves of hematopoiesis with a restriction in the hematopoietic potential of YS progenitors to primitive cells. In agreement with the findings of this study, a spatiotemporal analysis of HSC activity from early human embryonic tissues found that cells capable of long-term hematopoietic reconstitution in NSG mice are present in the AGM region as early as 32 to 33 days, 5 days prior to detection of this activity in the YS,[27] supporting the hypothesis that any cell with long-term reconstituting activity in the YS has arrived there via the circulation but originated in the embryo proper.

DEFINITIVE HEMATOPOIESIS EMERGES FROM ENDOTHELIAL CELLS WITHIN THE AORTA-GONAD-MESONEPHROS

The cells that will ultimately give rise to self-renewing adult HSCs arise within the ventral wall of the dorsal aorta between embryonic days 27 to 40.[28,29] This area of the vessel wall is thus referred to as hemogenic endothelium. The paired dorsal aortae appear on day 21 and start fusing from day 25 onward. In the caudal region of the embryo, the aorta does not fuse completely, giving rise to the left and right umbilical arteries. On day 30, the vitelline artery appears and connects the embryonic blood vessels with those of the YS. Endothelial cells express CD34 (which will subsequently mark adult HSCs) as early as embryonic day 19.[6,28-30] Clusters of cells expressing both CD34 and CD45 (a pan-hematopoietic cell surface marker) are found in the periumbilical region of the aorta as early as day 27, as well as in the vitelline artery between days 30 and 36.

The intra-aortic hematopoietic clusters (IAHCs) increase in size to reach several hundred by day 36 and decrease in size gradually by day 40 (Fig. 107.2).[28,29] IAHCs express known early hematopoietic transcription factors such as T-cell acute lymphocytic leukemia 1/stem cell leukemia (Tal/SCL), myeloblastosis oncogene (c-Myb), and GATA-binding protein 2 (GATA2) (shown by in situ hybridization).[31] The mesenchymal cells underlying the ventral wall of the aorta express *GATA3* or bone morphogenetic protein 4 *(BMP4)*,[32] consistent with a hypothesis that HSCs emerge from the subaortic mesenchymal region and migrate into the blood vessel lumen.[29] Whether these GATA3+ or BMP4+ cells are precursors or inducers of human HSCs remains to be resolved.[33,34] IAHCs also express angiotensin-converting enzyme (ACE; CD143), which is expressed by HSCs from fetal liver, umbilical cord blood, and adult hematopoietic tissues.[35] Additionally, ACE marks rare CD34− CD45− cells in the hemogenic region of the embryo at embryonic days 23 to 26 that have 40 times the hematopoietic colony generating capacity of ACE-negative cells, suggesting that ACE may be a marker for the mesodermal precursors that give rise to IAHCs and definitive hematopoiesis.[36] In fact, sections of intra-embryonic splanchnopleura from embryonic day 19 specimens, before the aorta has even begun to form, also contains hematopoietic potential, demonstrating that mesodermal cells fated for hematopoietic differentiation are already present within the region of the embryo that will subsequently give rise to the aorta. Explant culture of defined portions of the aorta between embryonic days 24 and 58 confirmed that only the median region of the aorta, encompassing the periumbilical region and origin of the vitelline artery, gives rise to hematopoietic colonies,[29] and furthermore that cells contained within this region are multipotent, being able to give rise to myeloid as well as lymphoid cells in vitro[6] and all lineages (erythroid, myeloid, lymphoid) in vivo.[27] Cells in this region can also self-renew, as demonstrated by the ability of AGM-derived bone marrow cells in recipient NSG mice to reconstitute the hematopoietic system of secondary NSG recipient mice.[27] Based on the numbers of cells transplanted, this allowed for the calculation that one HSC from the isolated AGM region was capable of generating at least 300 daughter HSCs on transplantation. Further refinement in the location and marker expression has shown that cells with

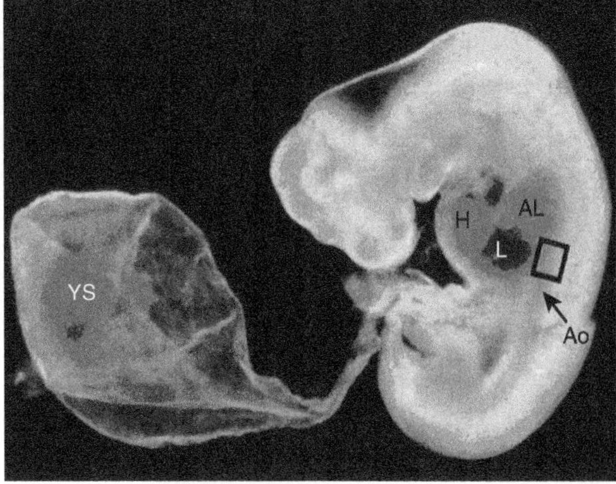

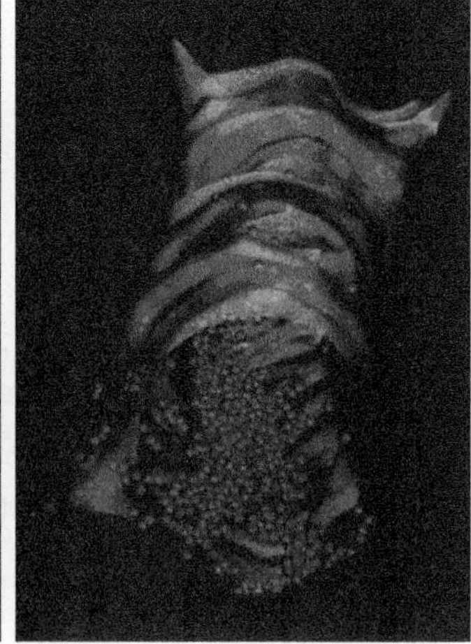

Fig. 107.2 Computer-assisted reconstruction of the dorsal aorta from a 5-week human embryo. Seventy-two 5-μm sections made in the preumbilical region (framed on the picture of the whole embryo on the left) were immunostained for CD34. The CD34+ intraaortic hematopoietic cells are in green color. *AL*, Anterior limn rudiment; *Ao*, dorsal aorta; *H*, heart; *L*, liver; *YS*, yolk sac. (From Tavian M, Coulombel L, Luton D, et al. Aorta-associated CD34+ hematopoietic cells in the early human embryo. *Blood.* 1996;87:67–72.)

the phenotype CD45$^+$cKit$^+$Thy1$^+$Endoglin$^+$Runx1$^+$CD38$^{-/lo}$ CD45RA$^-$ localized within the ventral wall of the dorsal aorta are enriched up to 1000-fold for hematopoietic activity compared to the total AGM region,[37] a surface marker phenotype that fits well with our current understanding of the human hematopoietic hierarchy (see below).

HEMATOPOIESIS EXPANDS IN THE EMBRYONIC AND FETAL LIVER

The liver rudiment develops from the floor of the foregut around embryonic day 22. From embryonic days 22 to 26, rare CD34$^-$CD45$^+$ cells are found scattered throughout the liver. These cells express the monocyte/macrophage marker CD68, do not possess the ability to form hematopoietic colonies in vitro, and cannot reconstitute an immunodeficient mouse.[6,27] As such, they have been hypothesized to represent a first hepatic colonization with yolk-sac-derived primitive cells that do not have HSC function. CD34$^+$CD45$^+$ cells are first detected in the liver on day 30, in close proximity to the endothelium of capillaries, and increase rapidly in number. By day 42, the liver is the major hematopoietic organ in the embryo, as cells with hematopoietic potential are no longer found within the dorsal aorta.[29] This is consistent with studies showing a rapid upswing in the BFU-E, CFU-E, and CFU-GM forming capacity of liver cells starting at the fifth week of gestation.[24] Based on careful temporal analysis of the hematopoietic colony forming capacity and long-term reconstitution in immunodeficient mice, it is currently accepted that the liver is colonized by hematopoietic cells that originate in the AGM. HSCs that can engraft in NOD/SCID mice are detected as early as week 7 in the human embryonic liver. In addition to CD34 and CD45, a subset of these HSCs express VE-cadherin, an endothelial cell marker. The VE-cadherin$^+$ HSCs possess a higher frequency of high-proliferative-potential colony-forming cells and long-term-culture-initiating cells compared with the VE-cadherin$^-$CD34$^+$CD45$^+$ hematopoietic progenitor cells. They are detectable between 6 and 10 weeks and completely absent by 23 weeks, suggesting that the surface marker of embryonic liver HSCs transits from VE-cadherin$^+$ to VE-cadherin$^-$.[38] The transient expression of an endothelial cell marker on hematopoietic precursors in the liver points to the endothelial origin of hematopoietic cells, although it is unknown whether VE-cadherin$^+$ HSCs persist in other hematopoietic compartments. Although the VE-cadherin$^+$ cells disappear from fetal liver by 23 weeks gestational age, hematopoietic potential has been detected in the fetal liver up until then,[30,39] and investigations at later gestational ages are limited by the availability of fetal tissues after that time. Although it appears that the bone marrow becomes a site of hematopoiesis starting at 15 to 16 weeks (see below), it is currently unknown when the fetal liver stops supporting hematopoiesis.

HEMATOPOIESIS MOVES TO THE BONE MARROW

The transition of the hematopoietic compartment to the bones follows the development of the bone marrow cavity. In the long bones, this has been divided into 5 stages.[40] During weeks 6.5 to 8 of gestation, the long bones are entirely cartilaginous, with no marrow cavity, but contain many CD68$^+$ monocyte-macrophage lineage cells concentrated along the diaphyseal shaft alongside a rich network of capillaries organized parallel to the bone rudiment. These phagocytic cells appear to then participate in active chondrolysis, which proceeds rapidly during 8.5 to 9 weeks. During this period, the forming marrow cavity is colonized with vascular, osteoblast, and osteoclast precursors. The development of the vascular bed occurs from 9 to 10.5 weeks with the appearance of primary logettes containing an arteriole lined with an intima of CD34$^+$ endothelial cells and a media of α SM actin$^+$ smooth muscle cells. At this time, there are no round CD34$^+$ hematopoietic cells present. Hematopoietic cells appear in the marrow cavity from 10.5 weeks, although from this time until around 15 weeks, CD15$^+$ granulocytes are the predominant hematopoietic cell present, with a smaller fraction of glycophorin A$^+$ erythroblasts. This is similar to what has been described in fetal vertebral bones from 13 to 17 weeks gestation, in which the first hematopoietic cells to be visualized are of the granulocytic lineage and are presumed to be required for chondrolysis and cavity formation.[41] The final organization of the marrow cavity in the long bones occurs after 16 weeks' gestation. Up until 16 weeks, histologic observation of rounded CD34$^+$ hematopoietic cells that could represent more primitive stem or progenitor cells is exceedingly rare. This is consistent with a report that did not detect any stem cell activity, defined as cells capable of giving rise to CFU-GEMM, in fetal bone marrow until 15 to 16 weeks of gestation.[39] Once established in the bone marrow, the hematopoietic compartment increases in size,[42] although due to the inaccessibility of bone marrow samples after 24 weeks gestation, it remains unclear what further shifts occur prior to birth and in the immediate postnatal period.

CIRCULATING HEMATOPOIETIC CELLS (SPLEEN, PLACENTA)

Inherent in the model that hematopoietic cells arise in distinct parts of the developing embryo and subsequently seed hematopoietic organs is the notion that hematopoietic cells must be capable of homing from one site to another, that these migrations take place in the blood vessels, and thus that hematopoietic cells are found in the circulation throughout fetal life. Analysis of highly vascularized organs during fetal development has revealed the presence of hematopoietic activity, although it is unknown if this activity is representative of the transient presence of circulating hematopoietic cells or their de novo emergence (see below). In the placenta, CD34^{++}CD45^{lo} cells can be identified as early as 5.4 weeks gestation and are present throughout gestation up to and including term (39.5 weeks) placentas.[43] Within this population is a fraction that contains multilineage erythroid, myeloid, and lymphoid potential as measured by in vitro assays.[43] Sorted placental cells from both CD34$^+$ and CD34$^-$ fractions of 6-week gestation specimens can repopulate immunodeficient mice,[44] although no secondary transplantations were performed. These data are thus inconclusive with regard to whether the placenta truly contains cells with self-renewal activity or instead acts as a reservoir for intermediate progenitors. The fetal spleen also contains hematopoietic activity, with CFU-GEMM potential cells arising later than in both the liver and bone marrow at 18 to 19 weeks gestation.[39]

Direct measurement of hematopoietic activity in fetal blood confirms that HSPCs circulate throughout gestation. As early as 12.5 weeks, cells with CFU-GM and BFU-E activity are detected, and this activity is significantly higher than what is measured in adult blood.[45] Multilineage potential as measured by CFU-GEMM can also be detected at these early timepoints, at levels that are as high if not higher than that found in bone marrow, liver, and spleen from the same fetal specimen.[39] Fetal blood at this time also has the capacity to repopulate NOD-*Scid* mice.[46] When compared to term umbilical cord blood, blood from fetuses aged 12 to 18 weeks is enriched for the more immature CD34$^+$CD38$^-$Lin$^-$ cells, the fraction known to contain reconstituting activity. When mononuclear cells from either fetal blood or cord blood are transplanted into immunodeficient mice, even when correcting for the higher frequency of immature cells in fetal blood by transplanting correspondingly more cord blood cells, fetal blood cells result in higher levels of reconstitution. This remains true even when purified CD34⁺CD38⁻Lin⁻ cells are transplanted, which suggests that either fetal blood HSCs have intrinsically higher reconstitution capacity, or that within the purified immature CD34⁺CD38⁻Lin⁻ fraction, the frequency of "true" HSCs is higher in fetal compared to cord blood. Regardless, the use of full-term umbilical cord blood as a source of CD34⁺ HSCs for transplantation confirms that human HSCs continue to circulate and seed the marrow even up to the time of birth. Primitive hematopoietic progenitor cells capable of forming hematopoietic colonies in vitro were first detected in full-term human umbilical cord blood in 1982.[47] This observation was extended by others,[48] and subsequently the first umbilical cord blood transplantation was successfully performed in a patient with Fanconi anemia in 1988.[49] Since then, umbilical cord blood has been extensively used to treat patients with hematologic disease and malignancies.[50]

HEMOGENIC ENDOTHELIAL CELLS IN THE HUMAN EMBRYO

It appears that long after the emergence of HSCs from the hemogenic endothelium of the AGM region, endothelial cells in hematopoietic organs maintain the potential to generate hematopoietic cells throughout embryonic and fetal life. Oberlin and colleagues sorted CD34⁺CD45⁻ endothelial cells from human YS, AGM region, embryonic liver, and fetal bone marrow and analyzed their hematopoietic potential.[30] CD34⁺CD45⁻ endothelial cells in each tissue do not have colony-forming ability in methylcellulose culture, grow in endothelial growth medium 2 (EGM2) endothelial medium, and express endothelial markers such as CD31, *Ulex europaeus*, and von Willebrand factor. However, when those CD34⁺CD45⁻ endothelial cells from the YS (26 to 40 days), AGM region (28 to 44 days), liver (36 to 54 days), and fetal bone marrow (16 to 24 weeks) were co-cultured on MS5 stromal cells, all produced cobblestone area-forming cells, followed by CD33⁺ myeloid, CD56⁺ natural killer, and CD19⁺ B lymphoid cells, indicating that these CD34⁺CD45⁻ cells are hemogenic endothelial cells. The persistence of hematopoietic potential in endothelial cells in fetal bone marrow as late as 24 weeks gestation may contribute to the massive expansion of the early hematopoietic compartment in prenatal life. However, an examination of the hemogenic potential of endothelial cells in adult bone marrow has not been performed, so it remains unresolved whether this is a unique feature of endothelial cells in prenatal hematopoietic organs or instead represents a source of hematopoietic potential throughout development and into adult life.

COMPARISON OF HEMATOPOIETIC POTENTIAL ACROSS ONTOGENY

A consistent theme in the field of developmental hematopoiesis is that ontologically younger cells have a higher proliferative capacity, higher repopulating capacity, and higher sensitivity to growth factors. Many of the studies that have compared hematopoietic potential across ontogeny have used bulk populations of cells, either without any enrichment or isolated based on surface markers that enrich for HSPCs but still represent heterogenous populations. Fetal blood has higher CFU activity per 10^5 input cells than does adult blood.[45] Direct comparison of the ability of human fetal liver, term umbilical cord blood, and adult bone marrow cells to repopulate NOD-*Scid* mice revealed the FL cells have the highest SRC activity, followed by UCB and then adult BM, decreasing by a factor of 100 over ontogeny. Furthermore, FL cells give rise to the highest number of immature CD34⁺CD38⁻ cells in vivo as well as the highest frequency of erythroid lineage cells. In contrast, UCB was found to generate larger numbers of cells, and more granulocytes were derived from UCB and ABM than FL.[51,52] CD34⁺ umbilical cord blood cells have also been shown to start dividing earlier and have a higher proliferative potential than CD34⁺ adult bone marrow cells,[53] and proliferative potential of CD34⁺CD45RA^{lo} cells declines significantly from fetal liver to umbilical cord blood to adult bone marrow.[54] These findings can be explained by the fact that the frequency of immature progenitors is higher in ontologically younger tissues, an observation that remains valid even when applying the most stringent definition of HSCs (see below).[55] Nevertheless, there is also compelling evidence than on a per cell basis, younger cells are more proliferative and have intrinsically higher regenerative capacities. Single sorted CD34⁺CD38⁻ cells from umbilical cord blood have higher cloning efficiency, form colonies of at least 100 cells within 7 days of culture, and give rise to 7 fold more cells as compared to single sorted CD34⁺CD38⁻ cells from adult cord blood, which take 21 days to form 100-cell colonies.[56] The cloning efficiency of single sorted cells from fetal liver or fetal bone marrow is also greater than that of umbilical cord blood, adult bone marrow, or adult mobilized peripheral blood cells, regardless of surface marker phenotype.[57] Such ontologically distinct functional behavior is consistent with the shifting needs of the developing human embryo and fetus, in which hematopoiesis is geared at expansion and establishment of the hematopoietic compartment along with the primary need for oxygen carrying capacity, to that of the adult, in which HSC quiescence and protection from potentially leukemogenic insults take priority. Analysis of telomere length suggests that this shift from rapid cycling of HSCs to a more quiescent phenotype occurs in the first year of life.[58]

ISOLATION OF HUMAN HEMATOPOIETIC STEM CELLS AND THE HUMAN HEMATOPOIETIC HIERARCHY

As has already been described, most phenotypic characterizations of human HSCs include expression of CD34. Anti-human CD34 antibody was first described to enrich human myeloid progenitor cells from bone marrow cells.[59] Since then, human CD34 has been used to isolate HSCs in both experimental and clinical settings. However, approximately 1% of adult bone marrow cells are CD34⁺ and true HSCs are known to be far rarer. Thus, investigations into the HSC potential of populations of cells defined solely on the basis of surface expression of CD34 are by definition looking at heterogeneous populations of cells where only the minority of cells actually contain HSC activity. Thus, as seen above, comparisons of HSC activity in populations of cells isolated from different hematopoietic organs and across different timepoints of ontogeny may reflect nothing more than altered frequencies of "true HSCs" in these organs at specific developmental timepoints.

Significant efforts have been spent refining the surface markers that identify true human HSCs, to allow for prospective isolation. Ninety-nine percent of adult bone marrow CD34⁺ cells express the surface antigen CD38, with expression of most mature lineage markers on CD38⁺ cells. Further subfractionation of adult BM into CD34⁺CD38⁺ and CD34⁺CD38⁻ subsets revealed that blast colony-forming cells were significantly enriched in the CD38⁻ fraction.[60] The enrichment of in vitro colony-forming potential and in vivo repopulation activity in the Lin⁻CD34⁺CD38⁻ fraction of fetal liver,[61] fetal bone marrow,[62] and umbilical cord blood[56] has been confirmed. While all human HSCs are exclusively found within the Lin⁻CD34⁺CD38⁻ population, limiting dilution analysis has revealed that only 1 in 617 such cells possess true

HSC activity.[63] Further refinement of $Lin^-CD34^+CD38^-$ cells based on expression of CD45RA and Thy1 has revealed that HSCs are contained within the $CD45RA^-$ fraction, and further hinted at the existence of MPPs that retain multilineage potentiality and even short-term repopulating activity in immunodeficient mice, but lack self-renewal on the basis of lack of long-term reconstitution and/or ability to reconstitute immunodeficient mice upon serial transplantation; thus they are not true HSCs.[64] One in 100 $Lin^-CD34^+CD38^-CD45RA^-Thy1^-$cells contain long-term repopulating activity, compared to 1in 20 $Lin^-CD34^+CD38^-CD45RA^-Thy1^+$ cells. Comparison of these two subsets suggested that differential expression of integrin α 6 (CD49f) accounted for the difference in repopulating activity; addition of this marker to the phenotypic characterization of HSCs revealed that 1 in 10.5 $Lin^-CD34^+CD38^-CD45RA^-Thy1^+CD49f^+$ cells are "true" HSCs.[2] Previous work has also shown that high efflux of the mitochondrial dye rhodamine-123 (Rho) can enrich for HSCs within the $Lin^-CD34^+CD38^-$ fraction.[65] Combining both enrichment strategies with an experimental design that allowed for the prospective isolation and transplantation of single cells into immunodeficient mice resulted in long-term reconstitution in 14% to 28% of recipient NSG mice, confirming that $Lin^-CD34^+CD38^-CD45RA^-Thy1^+CD49f^+Rho^-$ cells are indeed true human HSCs. In contrast, $Lin^-CD34^+CD38^-CD45RA^-Thy1^+CD49f^-$ cells give rise to all the major hematopoietic lineages in vivo, but engraftment peaks 2 to 4 weeks post-transplantation and none of the recipient mice exhibited long-term (>20 weeks) reconstitution, confirming that this population contains bona fide MPPs but not HSCs.

The hematopoietic hierarchy has classically been conceived of as a pyramid, with true HSCs located at the apex and giving rise sequentially to short-term HSCs and MPPs with limited self-renewal capacity, followed by increasingly lineage-restricted progenitors (Fig. 107.3A). In this model, erythroid/megakaryocytic, myeloid, and lymphoid potential is thought to be strictly segregated to respective progenitor populations, each of which is generated directly from HSCs. With the refinement in the phenotypic definition of true HSCs based on additional surface markers, it has become clear that within the heterogeneous population of cells previously considered to be HSCs are progenitors that retain multipotent lineage potential but have largely lost the capacity for self-renewal. Concurrently, it is also now appreciated that progenitors previously thought to be strictly lineage-restricted in fact may be lineage-biased but retain the capability to give rise to more than one lineage. In particular, myeloid and lymphoid cell fates have been revealed to be more intertwined than previously appreciated, with intermediate cells known as *multilymphoid progenitors (MLPs)* retaining the capacity for monocyte/macrophage/DC potential as well as lymphoid potential (see Fig. 107.3B).[66] By applying the most rigorous definition of HSCs, MPPs, and more downstream progenitors and using single-cell in vitro assays and in vivo reconstitution in NSG mice, John Dick and colleagues have revealed that there are significant differences in the hematopoietic hierarchy across ontogeny.[55] In adult bone marrow, the hematopoietic stem and progenitor compartment is composed of two tiers: a top tier containing HSCs and MPPs that retains multipotency for erythroid (Er), megakaryocyte (Mk), and myeloid (My) lineages, and a bottom tier of largely unipotent progenitors committed to either My or Er lineages, whereas in fetal liver a third tier of oligopotent progenitors retaining Er/Mk/My and Er/Mk potential is evident between the multipotent HSC/MPP top tier and the unipotent bottom tier. In addition, they found that in fetal liver, megakaryocyte potential was distributed throughout all the tiers of the hierarchy while in adult bone marrow it was largely restricted to the multipotent top tier.

As the field of hematopoiesis has moved toward an appreciation that previously defined populations of stem and progenitor cells based on a limited number of surface markers are heterogeneous, the natural extension of this logic has been the application of single-cell technologies to the study of hematopoiesis.[67,68] In particular, single-cell RNA sequencing technology has allowed for the large-scale sequencing of the transcriptomes of 1000s of individual cells without the need for a priori isolation based on cell surface markers. This has resulted in a shift in our understanding of hematopoiesis from one in which early stem and progenitor cells exist in discrete cellular states and differentiation is the process of switching from one state to another, to the notion that differentiation is a continuum with gradual transitions along a multitude of differentiation trajectories. Using such technology, Steinmetz and colleagues[69] showed that adult bone marrow cells in the $Lin^-CD34^+CD38^-$ fraction cannot be resolved into the classically defined clusters (HSC, MPP, MLP) that surface marker phenotyping would suggest, and that they instead exist in a continuum of undifferentiated HSPCs. In contrast, cells in the $Lin^-CD34^+CD38^+$ fraction clustered into populations with good correspondence to previously established unipotent progenitor types. These authors suggested that, rather than a tree composed of obligate intermediate progenitor states with discrete branching points where binary cell fate decisions are made, early hematopoiesis instead is a cellular continuum from which individual lineage trajectories emerge without passing through a series of discrete stable progenitors, represented graphically as a Waddington's landscape (see Fig. 107.3C).

Single-cell RNA sequencing has also been applied to the study of hematopoiesis in the fetal liver.[70] By sequencing all human fetal liver cells from 7 to 17 weeks' gestation, Popescu and colleagues found that there was an early bias toward erythroid lineages, with the appearance of myeloid and lymphoid lineages later in gestation. Furthermore, no granulocytes (neutrophils, basophils, or eosinophils) were present in fetal liver, consistent with reports of granulocytes emerging only in fetal bone marrow.[71] The authors inferred trajectories of hematopoietic development all stemming from the central node of clustered HSC/MPP cells. Three major trajectories emerged: a megakaryocyte-erythroid-mast cell trajectory, a myeloid trajectory including monocytes, macrophages, and dendritic cells, and a lymphoid trajectory comprised of B, T, NK, and innate lymphoid cells. Radiating from the central HSC cluster were trajectories of MPP cells with gradually shifting transcriptomic landscapes toward each major lineage, consistent with the notion of early hematopoiesis as a continuum of differentiation. This analysis was paired with single-cell in vitro culture assays, which demonstrated that $Lin^-CD34^+CD38^-CD45RA^-$ cells from early (7 to 8 weeks' gestation) timepoints had the highest trilineage potential (erythroid, myeloid, and lymphoid) and were enriched for erythroid-containing colonies, while cells from later gestational ages shifted to more unipotent colonies and had increasing numbers of lymphoid-containing colonies. The authors also found an increase in the frequency of $CD34^-CD38^+$ cells in G_0 (resting phase of the cell cycle) with advancing gestational age, suggesting that even within fetal liver, prior to migration to the bone marrow, the early hematopoietic compartment is moving toward the adult profile of quiescence.

While significant progress has been made in understanding the broad outlines of human developmental hematopoiesis, much is unknown. In particular, the period from 24 weeks gestation to term, whether experienced as a fetus in utero or as a premature infant in the NICU, remains largely unexplored, as does the immediate postnatal period. In addition, very little attention has been paid to how the challenges common to the perinatal period (inflammation, infection) affect the function of the early hematopoietic compartment. Single-cell approaches are only just now allowing us to hope that we will be able to prospectively identify cells that definitively represent true HSCs. This will undoubtedly pave the way for more precise investigations into differences in regenerative capacity, lineage potential, and response to external stress and stimuli throughout ontogeny and development.

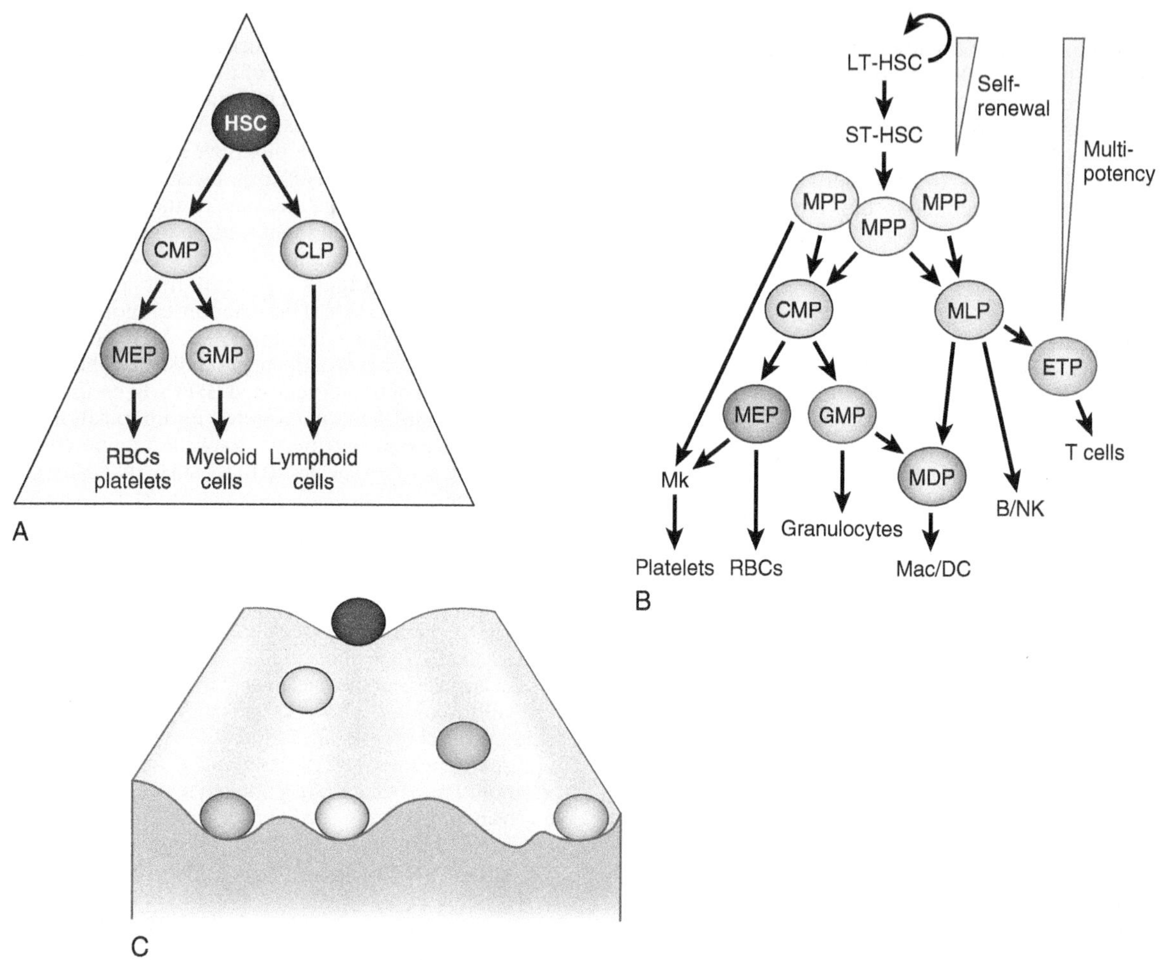

Fig. 107.3 Evolving views of the human hematopoietic hierarchy. (A) The hematopoietic hierarchy was initially conceived of as a pyramid with hematopoietic stem cells *(HSCs)* located at the apex, giving rise to increasingly lineage restricted progenitors. (B) Refinement in the identification of hematopoietic progenitors has caused that hierarchy to be substantially revised, with the appreciation that self-renewal is lost before multipotency, and that lineage fates are much more intertwined. (C) More recent single-cell profiling approaches suggest that early hematopoiesis is a cellular continuum from which individual lineage trajectories emerge without passing through a series of discrete stable progenitors. *CLP*, Common lymphoid progenitor; *CMP*, common myeloid progenitor; *ETP*, early thymic progenitor; GMP, granulocyte-monocyte progenitor; *LT-HSC*, long-term HSC; *MDP*, macrophage-DC progenitor; *MEP*, megakaryocyte-erythrocyte progenitor; *MLP*, multilymphoid progenitor; *MPP*, multipotent progenitor; *RBC*, red blood cell; *ST-HSC*, short-term HSC.

BASIC CONCEPTS IN STEM CELL BIOLOGY

INTRODUCTION

Stem cells play fundamental roles in development as the building blocks of the organism, of all organs (organogenesis), and throughout development and adult life as the mediators of organ homeostasis. Stem cells are generally divided into pluripotent stem cells, including embryonic stem cells (ESCs) and iPSCs, and somatic stem cells. The term *pluripotent* is used for ESCs and iPSCs, as they can give rise to all three embryonic germ (EG) layers: endoderm, ectoderm, and mesoderm. In contrast, somatic stem cells are referred to as *multipotent* and are understood to be able to give rise only to the multitude of cell types that comprise one tissue or organ system, derived from one germ layer (e.g., HSCs are mesoderm-derived cells that can give rise to all hematopoietic lineage cells but are not thought to be able to generate ectoderm-derived neural cells or endoderm-derived intestinal cells). Self-renewing stem cells can undergo symmetric cell division, splitting into two identical daughter cells that are themselves stem cells when the stem cell pool must be expanded rapidly, such as during the first stages of organogenesis or in the first response to extrinsic stimuli such as stress or injury. Stem cells can also undergo asymmetric cell division, giving rise to a more specialized daughter cell and only one new stem cell, when the stem cell pool simply needs to be maintained at a constant size. Very often, this cell division can be quite slow, such that the stem cell largely exists in a quiescent state. In some organ systems, it is hypothesized that, when tissue turnover is required to be at its zenith, the stem cell gives rise to an even more rapidly dividing *transient amplifying cell*. Normal development of the organism requires that there be a balanced switching between a stem cell's symmetric and asymmetric proliferation.[72]

EMBRYONIC STEM CELLS

A 3- to 5-day-old preimplantation human embryo known as the *blastocyst* contains the inner cell mass (ICM) and the trophectoderm.[73] The trophectoderm lacks stem cells but contains *trophoblastic precursor cells* that later become the fetal side of the placenta. The ICM consists of approximately 30 pluripotent cells that can give rise to all tissue types of the fetus. Implantation of the embryo (days 7 to 12 in humans) is associated with further cellular differentiation and the impending disappearance of the pluripotent state. This is followed by the establishment of the *primitive endoderm* that contains precursors to cells of the embryonic YS.

ESCs are derived from the in vitro expansion of ICM cells from the pre-implantation blastocyst stage (Fig. 107.4). Human

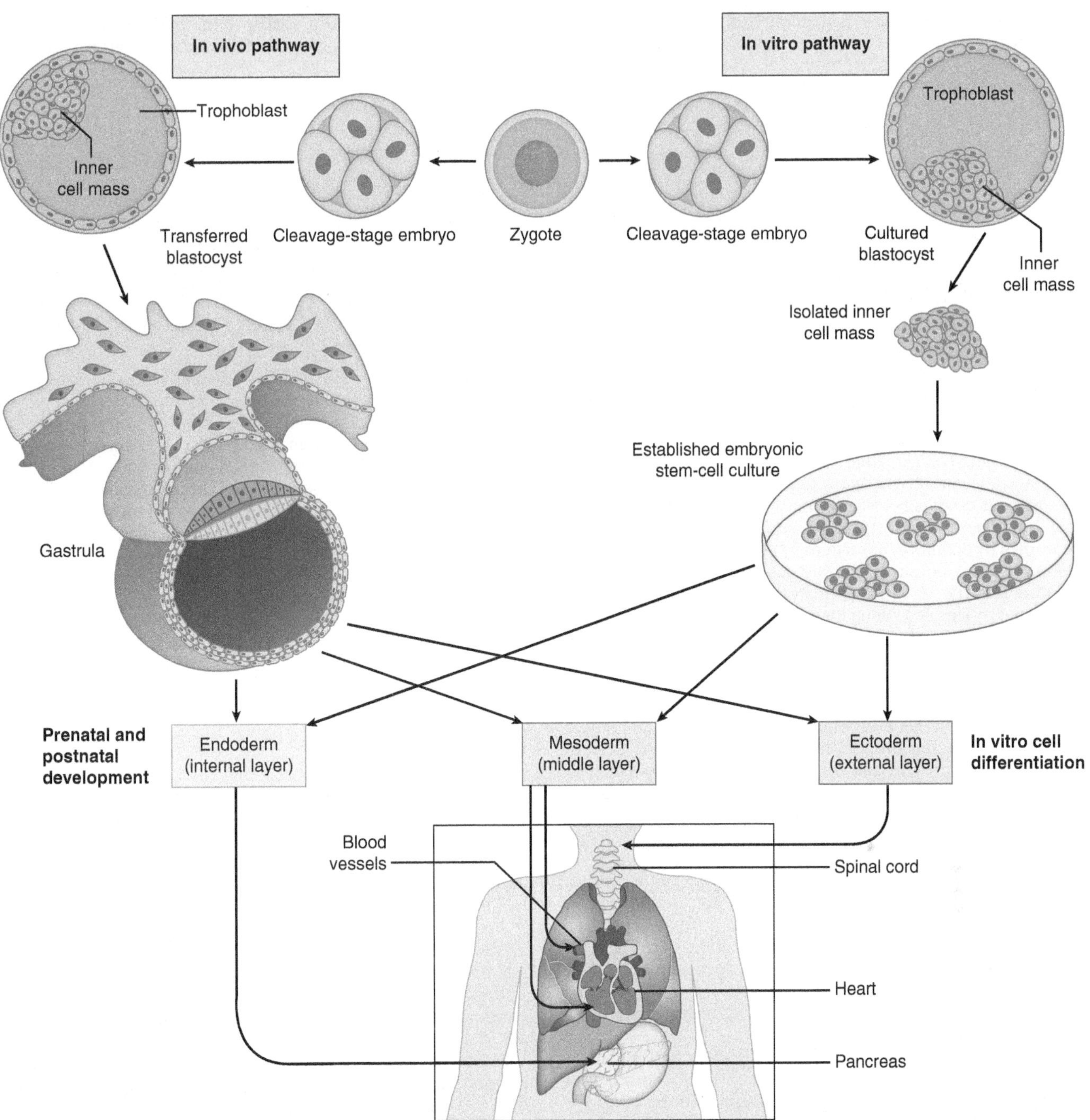

Fig. 107.4 Alternative fates for an in vitro-fertilized zygote: intrauterine versus in vitro development. There are two possible developmental pathways for an embryo generated by in vitro fertilization (IVF). When an embryo is transferred to the uterus at the cleavage or blastocyst stage, its development can result in the birth of a child. When an embryo is cultured exclusively in vitro, it can result in the derivation of stem cells. These two divergent pathways could converge ultimately in the use of stem cells and their derivatives for cell-based transplantation therapies. IVF is used primarily as a treatment for infertility, a procedure in which the resulting embryos are transplanted to the uterus at the early cleavage or blastocyst stage. This in vivo pathway can result (in approximately one third of cases) in the implantation of the embryo into the wall of the uterus, where it undergoes gastrulation and subsequent prenatal development. The ability to isolate human embryonic stem cells (hESCs) from the inner cell mass (ICM) has given biologic and potentially therapeutic utility to blastocysts that are either inappropriate for implantation (because they are imperfect or carry a lethal disease) or are left over following IVF and would simply be discarded. Isolation and culture of the ICM can result (in up to 50% of cases) in the prolonged growth of cells that have the capacity to differentiate into all three cell types of the body, endoderm, mesoderm, and ectoderm. hESCs have been shown to be capable of differentiating in vitro into insulin-producing cells, heart cells, blood-vessel cells, and nerve cells, as have their mouse counterparts. Therefore hESCs are a promising source of tissue for the study of or the treatment of (following transplantation) such diseases as diabetes, lung disease, cardiovascular disease, anemia, and other diseases of the blood, and diseases or injuries of the central nervous system. (From Bradley JA, Bolton EM, Pedersen RA. Stem cell medicine encounters the immune system. *Nat Rev Immunol.* 2002;2:859–871.)

ESCs (hESCs) are typically generated from excess, abnormal, or nonviable blastocysts that have been left over and are to be discarded following fertility treatment. The isolation, growth, and characterization of the first hESCs was reported in 1998.[74] Establishment of ESC lines is classically accomplished by plating the cells on specialized feeder cell layers, often mouse or human embryonic fibroblasts, or by culturing them under entirely defined conditions, including without need of a feeder layer, by supplying, along with other factors, members of the transforming growth factor-β superfamily. If the ICM cells begin to divide and maintain their undifferentiated state (marked by the presence of a panel of proteins consisting of Oct-4, Nanog, SSEA-4, Tra-1-81, Tra-1-60, alkaline phosphatase), for at least 12 passages, they are considered ESCs. If allowed to differentiate, true ESCs will begin to generate daughter cells that become partitioned to one of the three germ layers: *ectodermal, mesodermal,* or *endodermal.* This is most classically promoted experimentally by allowing the ESCs to aggregate in a floating clump of cells called an *embryoid body* (EB), so termed because it mimics—albeit in a very haphazard, random, and disorganized fashion—the emerging cell types of the embryo in vivo. The ability to form EBs containing all three germ layers is one of the ways that a true ESC line has been established is classically tested. The other is that the cells should yield teratomas when implanted into immunodeficient mice (teratomas, by definition, contain representatives of all three germ layers). However, because of its cost, labor intensity, invasiveness, and duration, the teratoma formation test is more commonly supplanted by simply looking for a threshold expression of genes marking the pluripotent state.[75,76]

Once established, ESCs should be capable of being maintained and expanded in an undifferentiated state in the laboratory indefinitely as stable cell lines. At this point, the goal becomes to differentiate the ESCs in a more controlled, lineage-specific manner. Typically, this process involves removing the ESCs from a feeder layer if present and often omitting mitogens (such as basic fibroblast growth factor) from the medium while adding such inducing molecules as retinoic acid or Sonic hedgehog. Novel protocols are constantly being devised for efficiently directing ESCs toward becoming different cell types. It is important to know that the ability to properly generate specific cell lineages from hESCs relies on a thorough knowledge of the presumed differentiation of that lineage in vivo. A corollary to this observation is that knowledge about the in vivo differentiation of specific lineages has also been acquired based on improvements in the in vitro generation of those cells. This has certainly been true for attempts to differentiate HSCs in vitro (see below).

Significant cross-pollination of knowledge and technical expertise occurs between the fields of hESC research and the rapidly evolving area of assisted reproductive research, especially in vitro fertilization (IVF). The rapid development of preimplantation genetic diagnosis (PGD) at the eight-cell blastomere stage is an example of the union between scientific and technical advances. PGD represents a significant advance in the prenatal diagnosis of genetic diseases.[77] Often, PGD indicates that a blastocyst generated by IVF in the context of assisted reproduction bears a lethal or devastating disease, rendering it morally unacceptable to implant the blastocyst. The defective blastocysts, however, can be used to generate hESC lines that then might faithfully model cellular aspects of that human disease. Such cellular models are particularly useful for conditions in which no good representative and predictive animal model exists. The resultant disease lines can then be used to test pharmaceuticals, to identify novel drug targets, to gain mechanistic insights at the cellular and molecular levels, and to identify better prognostic or diagnostic markers. This use of hESCs is potentially quite powerful and offers prospects for therapeutic applications apart from direct cell-mediated repair. In a similar vein, hESCs may serve as an in vitro model or surrogate for dissecting the earliest stages of human embryogenesis that, for obvious ethical reasons, cannot be directly observed in situ.

As described below, the entire disease-modeling role for hESCs is now starting to be assumed by a new type of pluripotent stem cell, the so-called *induced pluripotent stem cells (iPSCs),* which are ostensibly differentiated somatic cells that can be obtained from a diseased patient and "reprogrammed" to act like hESCs for the purposes described previously. These cells can be obtained from living adult patients (and even their family members) and can be differentiated to yield formerly inaccessible cell types.

INDUCED PLURIPOTENT STEM CELLS AND DIRECT CELL REPROGRAMMING

Although culturing the ICM of a blastocyst to create ESCs is the gold standard of a pluripotent cell, other modalities for creating pluripotent cells have come to dominate much of the last decade of stem cell research. Using a variety of techniques, they all are predicated on the reprogramming of an ostensibly end-differentiated, lineage-committed nucleated somatic cell (e.g., a skin or blood cell)[78-80] back to a more primitive pluripotent stem cell state from which multiple lineages can be derived, all genetically related to the original founder cell.

The most prominent of these techniques is the use of a combination of transcription factors that are necessary and sufficient to confer pluripotency onto a non-pluripotent cell. The identification in 2007 of at least 4 such factors, the so-called *Yamanaka cocktail,* has revolutionized this field.[81-87] From a list of 24 genes found to be highly differentially expressed between differentiated and undifferentiated hESCs, an empiric trial-and-error unbiased approach identified that a combination of four from that list (*Oct3/4, Sox2, c-Myc,* and *Klf4*) was sufficient to turn back the clock on murine and then human somatic cells (adult, neonatal, and fetal skin fibroblasts; gastric epithelium; hepatocytes; and peripheral blood mononuclear cells, including lymphocytes).[81-85,88-92] The introduction of these four factors, even transiently, was found to trigger resetting of the genome and epigenome, with the final reprogramming process actually being effectuated by the endogenous versions of these genes.[93-98] Because the reprogrammed somatic cells not only expressed genes associated with pluripotency but also could form both teratomas and EBs and self-renew, they were called *induced pluripotent stem cells.* Once the iPSC field challenged the long-entrenched notion that lineage commitment and differentiation are not end-stage or immutable, it was further shown that somatic cells do not need to be reprogrammed all the way back to pluripotency to derive another desired cell type, but that somatic cells of one lineage (generally fibroblasts) can be directly reprogrammed to an alternative fate without going through a pluripotent intermediate.[99-103]

By and large, the value of a PSC is not in its undifferentiated state, but rather in the differentiated cell types it can become. Obtaining a desired specialized cell type of a particular organ—a neuron, pancreatic β cell, pulmonary alveolar cell, cardiomyocyte, blood cell, osteocyte, or endothelial cell—has been predicated on understanding and recapitulating in vitro lineage development as it transpires in the actual embryo or fetus and is still an area of intense investigation. In other words, the field makes the assumption that the hESC (or cells that emulate the hESC) models the epiblast and therefore should be manipulated to emulate lineage commitment in the epiblast. Again, as for the efforts geared toward differentiating somatic cells (stem or more differentiated) from ESCs, efforts to direct iPSCs to a specific cell lineage are both predicated on, and have contributed to the advancement of, our understanding of the endogenous transcriptional regulation of these differentiation pathways in situ.

RECAPITULATION OF HUMAN HEMATOPOIETIC DEVELOPMENT USING EMBRYONIC STEM CELLS AND INDUCED PLURIPOTENT STEM CELLS

With this context in mind, we will examine how ESCs and iPSCs have advanced the study of human developmental hematopoiesis. Because the blood system is derived from mesoderm, early attempts to generate hematopoietic cells from hESCs focused on known mesoderm-inducing signals. In vivo, mesoderm is patterned by fibroblast growth factor (FGF), BMP4, activin, and canonical Wnt signals.[104] FGF2- and vascular endothelial growth factor (VEGF)-dependent colonies can be generated from hESC-derived mesoderm after 2 to 4 days of in vitro culture.[105,106] These blast colonies are capable of giving rise to multiple mesoderm lineage cells including hematopoietic cells, endothelial cells, and smooth muscle cells, but the hematopoietic cells appear to be limited to primitive erythrocytes, megakaryocytes, and macrophages only.[107] Further differentiation gives rise to $CD34^+$ cells after 4 to 6 days, which are now restricted to endothelial and hematopoietic lineages. Emergence of hematopoietic-restricted cells occurs by 6 to 8 days and is marked by the expression of CD43.[108] These $CD34^+CD43^+$ cells are only capable of giving rise to erythroid and myeloid lineage cells, and have no long-term repopulating activity as measured by xenotransplantation.[109–111] Thus, initial attempts to generate HSCs from hESCs gave rise to YS-like hematopoietic progeny, as occurs during embryogenesis. It was subsequently realized that mesoderm-specifying signals were required in specific temporal sequences for the suppression of primitive hematopoiesis as well as the induction of definitive hematopoiesis. BMP4-based mesoderm induction followed by either activin inhibition,[110] Wnt stimulation,[112] or both[111] was shown to result in the inhibition of an erythroid-biased primitive hematopoietic program and instead promote generation of definitive hematopoietic lineages, as measured primarily by the ability to generate T cells. Generation of definitive hematopoiesis was tied to upregulation of *HOXA* genes.[111] Concurrently, lack of upregulation of *HOXA* genes was found to distinguish poorly engrafting YS-like hESC-HSCs from FL-HSCs, and knockdown of *HOXA7* in FL-HSCs resulted in disruption of their function and reversion to an hESC-derived HSC-like transcriptomic profile.[113] This example nicely demonstrates the way in which in vitro generation of HSCs has informed our understanding of embryonic hematopoiesis, and vice versa.

Since the discovery of iPSCs, much effort has been directed at reprogramming cells from multiple different sources to HSCs. Many groups have focused on using established hiPSC lines as a starting point. By screening 27 candidate transcription factors known to play a role in hESC-derived mesodermal and vascular patterning, two pairs of transcription factors (*ETV2/GATA2* and *GATA2/SCL*) were found to activate myeloid/erythroid/megakaryocytic and restricted erythro-megakaryocytic gene programs, respectively, and result in generation of these differentiated cell types.[114] Generation of these lineages progressed through endothelial intermediates, consistent with what is known about hematopoietic emergence in the embryo, but no long-term repopulating cells were generated. Similar results were obtained when hiPSC-derived $CD45^+CD34^+$ myeloid progenitor cells were transduced with the combination of transcription factors *HOXA9/ERG/RORA/SOX4/MYB*,[115] which had been previously identified as distinguishing an HSC-enriched population from more mature progenitors in human UCB.[66,116] The resulting cells showed robust myeloid, erythroid, and megakaryocytic differentiation potential and modest lymphoid differentiation capacity in vitro, but only resulted in short-term engraftment of myeloid and erythroid cells at low levels in NSG mice. Intriguingly, the erythroid cells generated in vitro maintained embryonic (ε globin) and fetal (γ globin) hemoglobin expression patterns, whereas the erythroid cells generated in xenotransplanted mice had largely suppressed ε globin expression and significantly upregulated adult β hemoglobin, suggesting that critical microenvironmental factors lacking in vitro were contributing to hematopoietic maturation. Thus, similar to the studies investigating the generation of HSCs from hESCs, the first hematopoietic cells to be generated from ontologically younger sources, even reprogrammed, display ontologically younger patterns of hematopoietic differentiation. Long-term repopulating HSCs were successfully generated from hiPSCs by first achieving the generation of hemogenic endothelium-like cells and subsequently directing them to the hematopoietic lineage. A combination of 7 transcription factors (*ERG/HOXA5/HOXA9/HOXA10/LCOR/RUNX1/SPI1*) was found to be sufficient to direct hPSC-derived $CD34^+Flk1^+$ $CD43^-CD235A^-$ hemogenic endothelial cells to cells capable of long-term multilineage reconstitution in NSG mice.[117] Bona fide HSC generation was confirmed by secondary transplantation of hPSC-derived cells, which again gave rise to multilineage hematopoietic reconstitution, and evidence of definitive hematopoiesis was supported by the globin expression pattern of human erythroid cells generated in vivo. Reprogramming of cells to the hematopoietic lineage without a pluripotent intermediate stage has also been achieved.[103,118] As part of the reprogramming protocol to derive iPSCs from human fibroblasts, intermediate states lacking pluripotency were noted to have the ability to give rise to hematopoietic cells (primarily myeloid cells) when cultured in the presence of hematopoietic cytokines, and were able to transiently give rise to myeloid and erythroid cells in xenotransplantation models but limited repopulating activity upon secondary transplantation, suggesting that hematopoietic progenitors but not bona fide HSCs were generated.[103] Finally, multilineage and long-term repopulating activity upon primary and secondary transplantation in NSG mice was achieved by reprogramming human umbilical vein endothelial cells (HUVECs) or adult dermal microvascular endothelial cells with a combination of four transcription factors (*FOSB/GFI1/RUNX1/SPI1*) in addition to a defined culture on instructive vascular niche monolayers,[118] again reinforcing the intertwined fate of endothelium and hematopoietic cells.

These studies have leveraged our understanding of the cellular and molecular regulation of hematopoietic development to advance stem cell approaches that could one day be translated into clinical practice. In turn, hESC and hiPSC investigations have shed light on novel aspects of the molecular regulation of primitive and definitive hematopoiesis in ways that had not previously been appreciated. It is likely that significant progress in these areas will continue to be made in the years to come, and it is to be hoped that this will have greater impact on the care of neonates in the perinatal period.

CONCLUSION

Recent advances in understanding the biology of stem cells, as well as the molecular controls of cellular pluripotency, have significantly extended current understanding of the fundamental biology, with obvious practical implications. Stem cells, endowed with their special biologic characteristics, provide an invaluable tool for the study of developmental cell biology. Even in therapeutic transplantation paradigms, their beneficial actions typically derive from their simply performing their core functions. Indeed, any therapeutic use of stem cells should be viewed as translational developmental biology. And, of course, this melds nicely with the view that neonatologists and perinatologists are clinical developmental biologists.

A complete reference list is available at www.ExpertConsult.com. 

SELECT REFERENCES

2. Notta F, Doulatov S, Laurenti E, Poeppl A, Jurisica I, Dick JE. Isolation of single human hematopoietic stem cells capable of long-term multilineage engraftment. *Science*. 2011;333(6039):218–221. https://doi.org/10.1126/science.1201219.
6. Tavian M, Robin C, Coulombel L, Péault B. The human embryo, but not its yolk sac, generates lympho-myeloid stem cells: mapping multipotent hematopoietic cell fate in intraembryonic mesoderm. *Immunity*. 2001;15(3):487–495. https://doi.org/10.1016/S1074-7613(01)00193-5.
9. Mosier DE, Gulizia RJ, Baird SM, Wilson DB. Transfer of a functional human immune system to mice with severe combined immunodeficiency. *Nature*. 1988;335(6187):256–259. https://doi.org/10.1038/335256a0.
10. Mosier D, Gulizia R, Baird S, Wilson D, Spector D, Spector S. Human immunodeficiency virus infection of human-PBL-SCID mice. *Science (80-)*. 1991;251(4995):791–794. https://doi:10.1126/science.1990441.
11. McCune JM, Namikawa R, Kaneshima H, Shultz LD, Lieberman M, Weissman IL. The SCID-hu mouse: murine model for the analysis of human hematolymphoid differentiation and function. *Science*. 1988;241(4873):1632–1639. https://doi.org/10.1126/science.2971269.
12. Namikawa R, Kaneshima H, Lieberman M, Weissman I, McCune J. Infection of the SCID-hu mouse by HIV-1. *Science (80-)*. 1988;242(4886):1684–1686. https://doi:10.1126/science.3201256.
13. Kamel-Reid S, Dick JE. Engraftment of immune-deficient mice with human hematopoietic stem cells. *Science*. 1988;242(4886):1706–1709. https://doi.org/10.1126/science.2904703.
14. Lapidot T, Pflumio F, Doedens M, Murdoch B, Williams DE, Dick JE. Cytokine stimulation of multilineage hematopoiesis from immature human cells engrafted in SCID mice. *Science*. 1992;255(5048):1137–1141. https://doi.org/10.1126/science.1372131.
21. Luckett WP. Origin and differentiation of the yolk sac and extraembryonic mesoderm in presomite human and rhesus monkey embryos. *Am J Anat*. 1978;152(1):59–97. https://doi.org/10.1002/aja.1001520106.
22. Bloom W, Bartelmez GW. Hematopoiesis in young human embryos. *Am J Anat*. 1940;67(1):21–53. https://doi.org/10.1002/aja.1000670103.
23. Fukuda T. Fetal hemopoiesis. I. Electron microscopic studies on human yolk sac hemopoiesis. *Virchows Arch B, Cell Pathol.* 1973;14(3):197–213.
24. Migliaccio G, Migliaccio AR, Petti S, et al. Human embryonic hemopoiesis. Kinetics of progenitors and precursors underlying the yolk sac—liver transition. *J Clin Invest*. 1986;78(1):51–60. https://doi.org/10.1172/JCI112572.
27. Ivanovs A, Rybtsov S, Welch L, Anderson RA, Turner ML, Medvinsky A. Highly potent human hematopoietic stem cells first emerge in the intraembryonic aorta-gonad-mesonephros region. *J Exp Med*. 2011;208(12):2417–2427. https://doi.org/10.1084/jem.20111688.
28. Tavian M, Coulombel L, Luton D, Clemente H, Dieterlen-Lievre F, Peault B. Aorta-associated CD34+ hematopoietic cells in the early human embryo. *Blood*. 1996;87(1):67–72. https://doi.org/10.1182/blood.V87.1.67.67.
29. Tavian M, Hallais MF, Péault B, Péault B. Emergence of intraembryonic hematopoietic precursors in the pre-liver human embryo. *Development*. 1999;126(4):793–803.
30. Oberlin E, Tavian M, Blazsek I, Péault B. Blood-forming potential of vascular endothelium in the human embryo. *Development*. 2002;129(17):4147–4157.
37. Ivanovs A, Rybtsov S, Anderson RA, Turner ML, Medvinsky A. Identification of the niche and phenotype of the first human hematopoietic stem cells. *Stem Cell Reports*. 2014;2(4):449–456. https://doi.org/10.1016/j.stemcr.2014.02.004.
38. Oberlin E, Fleury M, Clay D, et al. VE-cadherin expression allows identification of a new class of hematopoietic stem cells within human embryonic liver. *Blood*. 2010;116(22):4444–4455. https://doi.org/10.1182/blood-2010-03-272625.
39. Hann I, Bodger M, Hoffbrand A. Development of pluripotent hematopoietic progenitor cells in the human fetus. *Blood*. 1983;62(1):118–123. https://doi.org/10.1182/blood.V62.1.118.118.
40. Charbord P, Tavian M, Humeau L, Peault B. Early ontogeny of the human marrow from long bones: an immunohistochemical study of hematopoiesis and its microenvironment [see comments]. *Blood*. 1996;87(10):4109–4119. https://doi.org/10.1182/blood.V87.10.4109.bloodjournal87104109.
44. Robin C, Bollerot K, Mendes S, et al. Human placenta is a potent hematopoietic niche containing hematopoietic stem and progenitor cells throughout development. *Cell Stem Cell*. 2009;5(4):385–395. https://doi.org/10.1016/j.stem.2009.08.020.
51. Holyoake TL, Nicolini FE, Eaves CJ. Functional differences between transplantable human hematopoietic stem cells from fetal liver, cord blood, and adult marrow. *Exp Hematol*. 1999;27(9):1418–1427. https://doi.org/10.1016/S0301-472X(99)00078-8.
52. Nicolini FE, Holyoake TL, Cashman JD, Chu PPY, Lambie K, Eaves CJ. Unique differentiation programs of human fetal liver stem cells shown both in vitro and in vivo in NOD/SCID mice. *Blood*. 1999;94(8):2686–2695. https://doi.org/10.1182/blood.V94.8.2686.420k15_2686_2695.
55. Notta F, Zandi S, Takayama N, et al. Distinct routes of lineage development reshape the human blood hierarchy across ontogeny. *Science*. 2016;351(6269):aab2116. https://doi.org/10.1126/science.aab2116.
66. Doulatov S, Notta F, Eppert K, Nguyen LT, Ohashi PS, Dick JE. Revised map of the human progenitor hierarchy shows the origin of macrophages and dendritic cells in early lymphoid development. *Nat Immunol*. 2010;11(7):585–593. https://doi.org/10.1038/ni.1889.
67. Laurenti E, Göttgens B. From haematopoietic stem cells to complex differentiation landscapes. *Nature*. 2018;553(7689):418–426. https://doi.org/10.1038/nature25022.
68. Watcham S, Kucinski I, Gottgens B. New insights into hematopoietic differentiation landscapes from single-cell RNA sequencing. *Blood*. 2019;133(13):1415–1426. https://doi.org/10.1182/blood-2018-08-835355.
69. Velten L, Haas SF, Raffel S, et al. Human haematopoietic stem cell lineage commitment is a continuous process. *Nat Cell Biol*. 2017;19(4):271–281. https://doi.org/10.1038/ncb3493.
70. Popescu D-M, Botting RA, Stephenson E, et al. Decoding human fetal liver haematopoiesis. *Nature*. 2019;574(7778):365–371. https://doi.org/10.1038/s41586-019-1652-y.
74. Thomson JA, Itskovitz-Eldor J, Shapiro SS, et al. Embryonic stem cell lines derived from human blastocysts. *Science (80-)*. 1998;282(5391):1145–1147. https://doi:10.1126/science.282.5391.1145.
81. Takahashi K, Yamanaka S. Induction of pluripotent stem cells from mouse embryonic and adult fibroblast cultures by defined factors. *Cell*. 2006;126(4):663–676. https://doi.org/10.1016/J.CELL.2006.07.024.
82. Wernig M, Meissner A, Foreman R, et al. In vitro reprogramming of fibroblasts into a pluripotent ES-cell-like state. *Nature*. 2007;448(7151):318–324. https://doi.org/10.1038/nature05944.
83. Takahashi K, Tanabe K, Ohnuki M, et al. Induction of pluripotent stem cells from adult human fibroblasts by defined factors. *Cell*. 2007;131(5):861–872. https://doi.org/10.1016/J.CELL.2007.11.019.
84. Yu J, Vodyanik MA, Smuga-Otto K, et al. Induced pluripotent stem cell lines derived from human somatic cells. *Science (80-)*. 2007;318(5858):1917–1920. https://doi:10.1126/science.1151526.
96. Yamanaka S, Blau HM. Nuclear reprogramming to a pluripotent state by three approaches. *Nature*. 2010;465(7299):704–712. https://doi.org/10.1038/nature09229.
103. Szabo E, Rampalli S, Risueño RM, et al. Direct conversion of human fibroblasts to multilineage blood progenitors. *Nature*. 2010;468(7323):521–526. https://doi.org/10.1038/nature09591.
105. Kennedy M, D'Souza SL, Lynch-Kattman M, Schwantz S, Keller G. Development of the hemangioblast defines the onset of hematopoiesis in human ES cell differentiation cultures. *Blood*. 2007;109(7):2679–2687. https://doi.org/10.1182/blood-2006-09-047704.
106. Vodyanik MA, Yu J, Zhang X, et al. A mesoderm-derived precursor for mesenchymal stem and endothelial cells. *Cell Stem Cell*. 2010;7(6):718–729. https://doi.org/10.1016/J.STEM.2010.11.011.
107. Yu QC, Hirst CE, Costa M, et al. APELIN promotes hematopoiesis from human embryonic stem cells. *Blood*. 2012;119(26):6243–6254. https://doi.org/10.1182/blood-2011-12-396093.
108. Vodyanik MA, Thomson JA. Slukvin II. Leukosialin (CD43) defines hematopoietic progenitors in human embryonic stem cell differentiation cultures. *Blood*. 2006;108(6):2095–2105. https://doi.org/10.1182/blood-2006-02-003327.
109. Choi K-D, Vodyanik MA, Togarrati PP, et al. Identification of the hemogenic endothelial progenitor and its direct precursor in human pluripotent stem cell differentiation cultures. *Cell Rep*. 2012;2(3):553–567. https://doi.org/10.1016/J.CELREP.2012.08.002.
110. Kennedy M, Awong G, Sturgeon CM, et al. T lymphocyte potential marks the emergence of definitive hematopoietic progenitors in human pluripotent stem cell differentiation cultures. *Cell Rep*. 2012;2(6):1722–1735. https://doi.org/10.1016/j.celrep.2012.11.003.
111. Ng ES, Azzola L, Bruveris FF, et al. Differentiation of human embryonic stem cells to HOXA+ hemogenic vasculature that resembles the aorta-gonad-mesonephros. *Nat Biotechnol*. 2016;34(11):1168–1179. https://doi.org/10.1038/nbt.3702.
112. Sturgeon CM, Ditadi A, Awong G, Kennedy M, Keller G. Wnt signaling controls the specification of definitive and primitive hematopoiesis from human pluripotent stem cells. *Nat Biotechnol*. 2014;32(6):554–561. https://doi.org/10.1038/nbt.2915.
113. Dou DR, Calvanese V, Sierra MI, et al. Medial HOXA genes demarcate haematopoietic stem cell fate during human development. *Nat Cell Biol*. 2016;18(6):595–606. https://doi.org/10.1038/ncb3354.
114. Elcheva I, Brok-Volchanskaya V, Kumar A, et al. Direct induction of haematoendothelial programs in human pluripotent stem cells by transcriptional regulators. *Nat Commun*. 2014;5(1):4372. https://doi.org/10.1038/ncomms5372.
115. Doulatov S, Vo LT, Chou SS, et al. Induction of multipotential hematopoietic progenitors from human pluripotent stem cells via respecification of lineage-restricted precursors. *Cell Stem Cell*. 2013;13(4):459–470. https://doi.org/10.1016/J.STEM.2013.09.002.
116. Laurenti E, Doulatov S, Zandi S, et al. The transcriptional architecture of early human hematopoiesis identifies multilevel control of lymphoid commitment. *Nat Immunol*. 2013;14(7):756–763. https://doi.org/10.1038/ni.2615.
117. Sugimura R, Jha DK, Han A, et al. Haematopoietic stem and progenitor cells from human pluripotent stem cells. *Nature*. 2017;545(7655):432–438. https://doi.org/10.1038/nature22370.
118. Sandler VM, Lis R, Liu Y, et al. Reprogramming human endothelial cells to haematopoietic cells requires vascular induction. *Nature*. 2014;511(7509):312–318. https://doi.org/10.1038/nature13547.

Neutrophil Granulopoiesis and Homeostasis

108

Shelley M. Lawrence | Victor Nizet

INTRODUCTION

From their initial emergence in the yolk sac at the beginning stages of embryogenesis to their vast proliferation in the bone marrow at the end of term gestation, the differentiation of the pluripotent hematopoietic stem cell into a mature, segmented neutrophil is a tightly controlled process where the transcriptional regulators C/EBP-α and C/EBP-ε have essential roles. Despite their relatively short life span, these intriguing cells are not only vital for pathogen elimination during early infection, but also link innate and adaptive immune responses to promote resolution of inflammation and wound healing. In this chapter, neutrophil granulopoiesis, commencing at the earliest stages of embryogenesis, will be examined. Mechanisms controlling granular sorting, trafficking, and degranulation, as well as neutrophil homeostasis and specific differences between neonatal and adult neutrophil biology will also be discussed.

DEVELOPMENT

HEMATOPOIESIS

During human development, the creation of all blood cells, or fetal hematopoiesis, is an evolutionarily conserved process that transpires over three distinct stages (Fig. 108.1).[1] Commencing in the extra-embryonic yolk sac around the third week of embryogenesis, the first, or primitive, stage is marked by the production of a transient population of primordial erythroid cells, macrophages, and megakaryocytes.[2] The second, or pro-definitive, stage is discernable close to the fifth week of fetal growth by the appearance of the hemogenic endothelium within the yolk sac. This early phase of hematopoiesis is marked by differentiation of visceral yolk sac mesoderm into endothelial cells of the vitelline vessels and hematopoietic cells.[3] The transcription factor stem cell leukemia (SCL) is essential for this stage of fetal hematopoiesis, as *Scl* null mice failed to develop yolk sac hematopoietic colonies and lacked expression of essential hematopoietic transcription factors GATA-1, GATA-2, and PU.1.[3] This dedicated hemogenic endothelium generates a greater variety of transitory myeloid lineage precursors in addition to primitive megakaryocytes and erythrocytes.[4,5] It is not until the third, or definitive, stage of fetal hematopoiesis around the seventh to eighth weeks of human gestation, however, that genuine pluripotent hematopoietic stem cells (HSCs) are detected. These multifaceted cells co-express hematopoietic and endothelial markers, including CD34, CD144 (VE-cadherin), CD45, and RUNX1,[6–11] and originate from specialized intra-embryonic endothelial cells located within the ventral wall of the descending aorta in a process that has been termed *endothelial-to-hematopoietic transition* (EHT).[12,13]

Within the distinctive hematopoietic niches of the dorsal aorta and yolk sac, the successful completion of EHT, as well as the survival and maturation (but not proliferation) of pre-HSCs, is dependent upon the production of Kit ligand (Kitl).[14] Mice deficient for Kitl demonstrated critical reductions of yolk sac erythro-myeloid progenitors (EMPs), leading to severe anemia and late embryonic or early perinatal lethality due to a loss of fetal liver erythroid cells prior to HSC-derived erythropoiesis.[14,15] Notch-1 signaling[16,17] and GATA-2 transcription factor induction[18] also function as essential regulators of EHT and subsequent HSC production, with inhibition of either signaling pathway resulting in serious disruptions of definitive hematopoiesis.[18]

A common stem/progenitor pool, rather than two independent lineages of germinal and HSC cells, has also been proposed. Primordial germ cell (PGC) populations, which are first observed in the epiblast, and then within the allantois at the base of the yolk sac around the fifth week of fetal development, may link the traditional second and third stages of fetal hematopoiesis.[19] PGCs will eventually settle in the aorta-gonad-mesonephros (AGM) region of the developing fetus. Here these cells maintain their differentiation plasticity and continue to undergo extensive proliferation and genome reprogramming as long as their expression of the transcription factor Oct3/4 remains low.[19] PGCs destined to differentiate into gametes within the emerging gonads will ultimately express high levels of Oct3/4, while a subset of these mesodermal progenitors with continued low Oct3/4 concentrations will enter various lineages, including the hematopoietic pathway.[19] PGCs destined to become pluripotent HSCs, therefore, show distinct expression of PGC markers (BLIMP-1, AP, TG-1, and STELLA), co-expressed proteins (CD34, CD41, and FLK-1), and genes (*Brachyury, Hox-B4, Scl/Tal-1,* and *GATA-2*), but remain weakly positive for Oct3/4.[19]

Irrespective of mechanisms by which HSCs come to occupy the AGM region of the ventral wall of the descending aorta, these self-renewing cells will subsequently come to seed the liver, thymus, and spleen, where hematopoiesis will continue until the third trimester of human pregnancy.[13,20] Within the fetal liver, specialized hematopoietic tissue-derived endothelial cells lining the walls of hepatic sinusoids, known as *fetal liver sinusoidal endothelial cells (FLSECs)*, secrete principal growth factors and Notch receptors to expedite HSC proliferation and expansion.[21] In neonates less than 32 weeks' gestational age (GA), fetal liver HSCs generate oligopotent progenitors with myeloid-erythroid-megakaryocyte and erythroid-megakaryocyte activities.[13] During this developmental stage in mice and humans, myeloid lineages generally originate from HSC/multipotent progenitors (MPPs) via three intermediates including (1) a neutrophil-myeloid progenitor expressing CD34, SPINK2 (serine protease inhibitor Kazal-type 2), AZU1 (azurocidin), PRTN3 (proteinase 3), ELANE (neutrophil elastase), MPO (myeloperoxidase), and LYZ (lysozyme), (2) monocyte precursors, and (3) dendritic cell precursors.[22] Although these early progenitors maintain a high proliferation potential, the fraction of fetal liver HSC/MPPs becoming quiescent steadily rises throughout fetal development.[20,22] This transformation occurs in conjunction with a surge in heat shock protein 1 (HSPA1A) expression, which may function to maintain cellular genome and proteome integrity.[22] Concurrent to the surge in HSPA1A, MHC-1 (HLA-B) levels decline and may potentially cause impaired antigen-presenting potential in fetal liver–derived (compared with cord blood or adult bone marrow) HSC/MPPs.[22] As fetal development progresses, hematopoietic composition of the fetal liver exhibits a coinciding shift away from predominately erythroid production, with a parallel escalation in the differentiation potential of HSCs/MPPs.[22] By the end of term gestation, hematopoiesis transitions to the bone marrow, which becomes the only site for platelet, red, and white blood cell development during one's lifetime.[13,20]

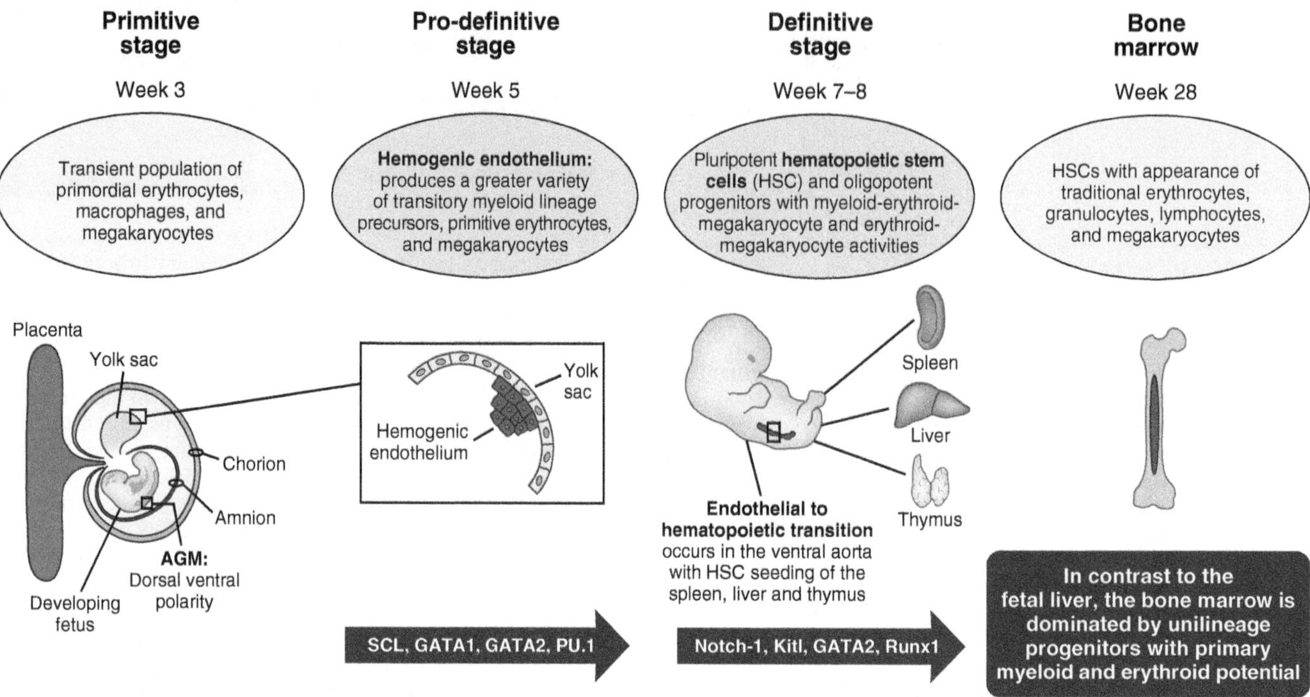

Fig. 108.1 Ontogeny of hematopoiesis. The origin of human blood cells begins in the mesoderm of the extra-embryonic yolk sac around the third week of embryogenesis and is known as the primitive stage. Differentiation of visceral yolk mesoderm into endothelial cells of the vitelline vessels and hematopoietic cells and the emergence of hemogenic endothelium within the yolk sac around the fifth week of gestation marks the pro-definitive (second) stage of fetal hematopoiesis. The second stage is regulated by the transcription factor stem cell leukemia *(SCL)*, dorsal-ventral polarity, and Notch signaling. Blood cell production then transitions to the ventral wall of the aorta, or aorta-gonad-mesonephros (AGM) region, around the seventh to eighth week during the definitive stage and is regulated by the transcription factor Runx1 in a process known as *endothelial-to-hematopoietic transition (EHT)*, where genuine hematopoietic stem cells (HSCs) are first identified. After the eighth week of gestation, early blood cells seed the liver, thymus, and spleen until the seventh month of gestation, when hematopoiesis transitions to the bone marrow. After this time, the bone marrow becomes the sole site for traditional platelet, red, and white blood cell formation.

The bone marrow, in contrast to the fetal liver, is dominated by unilineage progenitors with primary myeloid and erythroid potential.[13]

Even though in situ genetic labeling and barcoding of HSCs enable direct quantitative and qualitative measurements to illustrate the origins of blood cells from the common progenitor HSC, the initiating factors that determine whether a HSC will differentiate into a myeloid or lymphoid precursor remain controversial.[23] In the **"classical" or "hierarchical model,"** all HSCs have equal multi-lineage differentiation potential, but the fate of the HSC is predetermined prior to single lineage commitment and differentiation (Fig. 108.2). In this model, bone marrow HSCs can transform into either common lymphoid progenitor (CLP) or a common myeloid progenitor (CMP), but after this transformation the cell loses its ability to differentiate into any other blood cell type.[23,24] CLP precursors will become either T or B lymphocytes, NK cells, or dendritic cells, while CMPs will differentiate into either granulocyte monocyte progenitors (GMPs) or megakaryocyte erythroid progenitors (MEPs).[25] In contrast, the **"alternative model"** postulates that common myeloid and lymphoid progenitor cells have mixed lineage potential with transcriptional and functional heterogeneity, and cell fate is principally determined by the availability of differentiation and survival factors (Fig. 108.3).[24] This model of HSC differentiation is supported by observations that HSCs can directly differentiate into CMPs, MEPs, megakaryocytes, or lymphoid-primed multipotent progenitors (LMPPs). In addition, CMPs and LMPPs can subsequently transform into CLPs or GMPs but lack the potential of becoming megakaryocytes or erythrocytes.[13,25]

DIFFERENTIATION OF NEUTROPHILS FROM HEMATOPOIETIC STEM CELLS

Irrespective of which hematopoietic pathway is correct, the differentiation of myeloid cells from HSCs is a well-described, closely regulated process dependent upon several transcription factors, including CCAAT/enhancer binding proteins (C/EBP), GATA-1, and PU.1.[26,27] C/EBPs consist of a family of six transcription factors (-α, -β, -γ, -δ, -ε, -ζ) that function to modulate numerous biologic processes involving cell motility, proliferation, differentiation, growth arrest, and cell death, in various tissues, including central nervous system, lung, adipose, and bone marrow.[28] Once destined to become a myeloid cell, the HSC will develop into both megakaryocyte/erythroid and granulocyte/macrophage lineages from a pluripotent CMP cell.[26,27] Whereas C/EBP-α and PU.1 will induce CMPs to differentiate into monocytes and macrophages, C/EBP-ε and Gfi1 will generate neutrophils and eosinophils.[26,29] Differentiation of CMPs into neutrophils instead of eosinophils, however, ultimately depends upon the acetylation of C/EBP-ε at specific lysines (K121 and K198) and absence of GATA-1.[26,30] The importance of C/EBPs -α, -β, and -ε in neutrophil development is demonstrated by mutations of C/EBP-α and -β that lead to a variety of lymphocytic and myeloid leukemias,[30] and absence of C/EBP-ε, which is associated with inhibition of neutrophil differentiation and maturation out of the progenitor compartment.[31] In contrast, high levels of C/EBP-δ and PU.1 are observed only in mature and circulating neutrophils.[32]

Posttranscriptional regulators of hematopoiesis are also necessary. For example, microRNAs (miRNAs), or small, non-coding, single-stranded RNA molecules measuring approximately 19 to 25 nucleotides in length, are involved in most aspects of

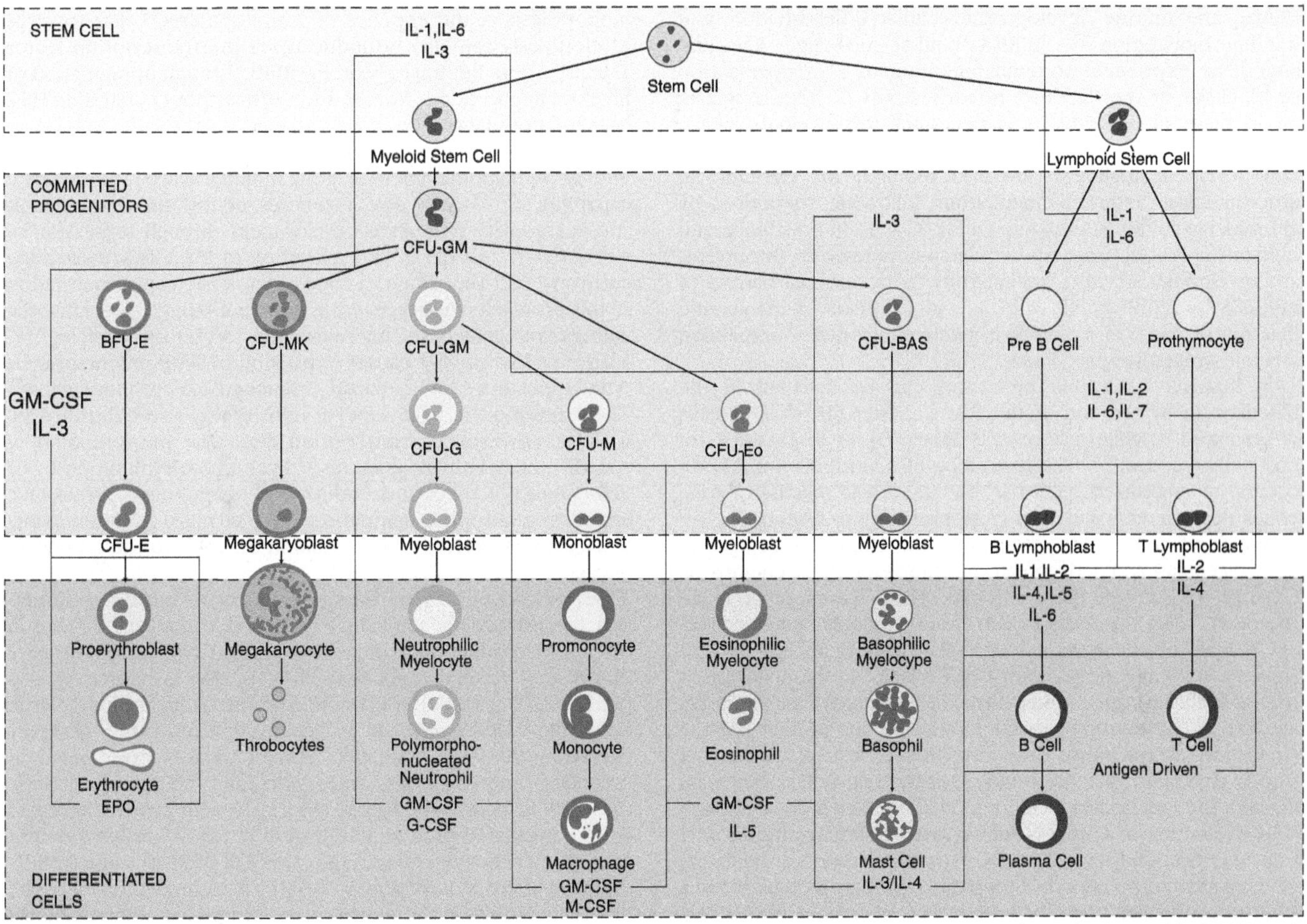

STEM CELL
IL-1,IL-6
IL-3
Stem Cell
Myeloid Stem Cell
Lymphoid Stem Cell
COMMITTED PROGENITORS
CFU-GM
IL-3
IL-1
IL-6
BFU-E
CFU-MK
CFU-GM
CFU-BAS
Pre B Cell
Prothymocyte
GM-CSF
IL-3
CFU-G
CFU-M
CFU-Eo
IL-1,IL-2
IL-6,IL-7
CFU-E
Megakaryoblast
Myeloblast
Monoblast
Myeloblast
Myeloblast
B Lymphoblast
T Lymphoblast
IL-1,IL-2
IL-4,IL-5
IL-6
IL-2
IL-4
Proerythroblast
Megakaryocyte
Neutrophilic Myelocyte
Promonocyte
Eosinophilic Myelocyte
Basophilic Myelocype
Throbocytes
Polymorpho-nucleated Neutrophil
Monocyte
Eosinophil
Basophil
B Cell
T Cell
Antigen Driven
Erythrocyte
EPO
GM-CSF
G-CSF
GM-CSF
IL-5
Macrophage
GM-CSF
M-CSF
Mast Cell
IL-3/IL-4
Plasma Cell
DIFFERENTIATED CELLS

Fig. 108.2 Classic hematopoietic development. *BFU-E,* Burst-forming unit—erythroid; *CFU-BAS,* colony-forming unit—basophil; *CFU-E,* colony-forming unit—erythroid; *CFU-Eo,* colony-forming unit—eosinophil; *CFU-G,* colony-forming unit—granulocyte; *CFU-GM,* colony-forming unit—granulocyte-macrophage; *CFU-M,* colony-forming unit—macrophage; *CFU-MK,* colony-forming unit—megakaryocyte; *EPO,* erythropoietin; *G-CSF,* granulocyte colony-stimulating factor; *GM-CSF,* granulocyte-macrophage colony-stimulating factor; *IL,* interleukin; *M-CSF,* macrophage colony-stimulating factor.

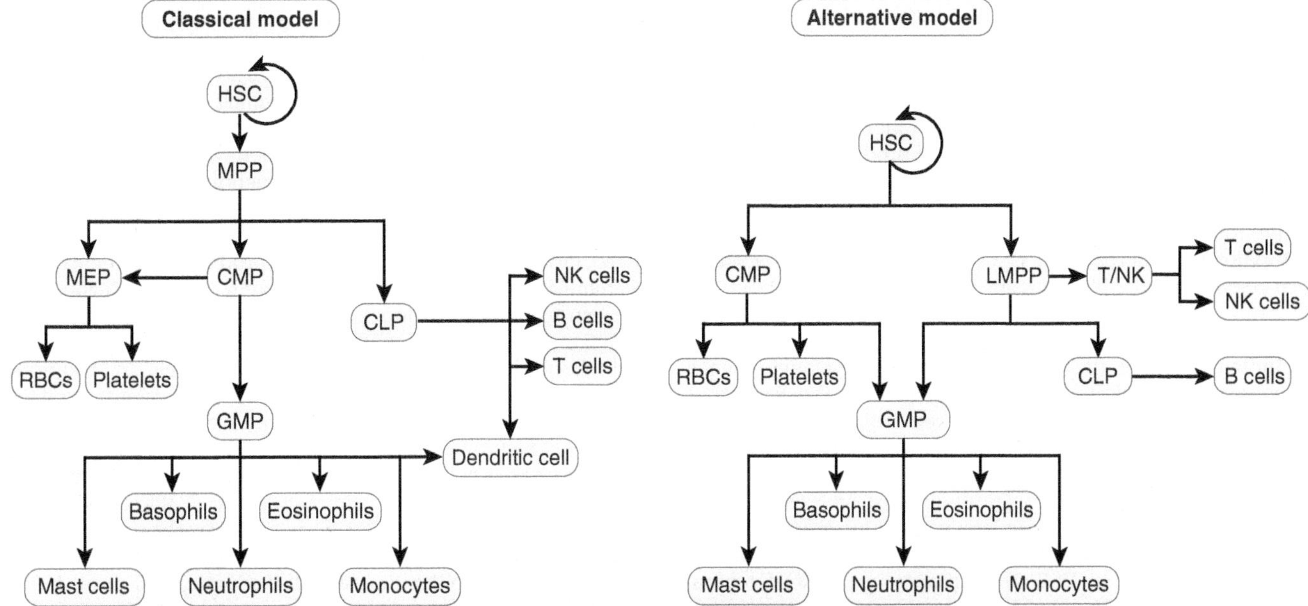

Fig. 108.3 Classical versus alternative hematopoiesis. *CLP,* Common lymphoid progenitor; *CMP,* common myeloid progenitor; *GMP,* granulocyte monocyte progenitor; *HSC,* hematopoietic stem cell; *LMPP,* lymphoid-primed multipotent progenitors; *MEP,* megakaryocyte erythroid progenitor; *MPP,* multipotent progenitor; *NK,* natural killer T cell; *RBC,* red blood cell (erythrocyte).

human and murine development, cellular differentiation, and immune modulation.[33,34] miRNAs bind to messenger RNA and alter gene expression through inhibition of RNA degradation or blockage of translation.[34] In early stages of hematopoiesis, an increase in miR-142-3p is necessary for myeloid lineage differentiation,[35] while miR-16 is essential for erythropoiesis.[36] Low levels of mi-R125b are also required for granulocytic differentiation and cell maturation following induction by granulocyte-colony stimulating factor (G-CSF) in both mice and humans.[33] Proper regulation of granulopoiesis erythropoiesis and myelopoiesis is also facilitated by transcriptional control of miR-223 by C/EBP-β, NFI-A, PU.1, and C/EBP-α,[37] with genetic deletion of miR-223 resulting in neutrophilia due to expanded myeloid progenitor precursors.[38]

In humans, neutrophil precursors can be detected in the bloodstream by the end of the first trimester (10 to 11 weeks of gestation),[39] while mature cells appear by 14 to 16 weeks of postmenstrual age.[40,41] The generation of neutrophils from HSCs occurs in specialized niches in the trabecular regions of long bones near the endosteum in close proximity to osteoblasts.[39,42] Retention of neutrophils within the bone marrow is dependent upon osteoblast and perivascular cell expression of the chemokine CXCL12, a ligand for the neutrophil cell membrane chemokine receptor CXCR4.[43] As the neutrophil matures, simultaneous declines of CXCR4 levels and increased expression of the chemokine CXCL2, and its cell membrane receptor CXCR2, facilitate the neutrophil's release from the bone marrow as the cell becomes less responsive to CXCL12.[44] Neutrophils become available for release into the circulation after a transit time through the post-mitotic pool of 4 to 6 days.[45] To exit the bone marrow, neutrophils must pass through the cell bodies of the endothelium, rather than through cell-cell junction, in a process known as *transcellular migration*.[46] Conventional dendritic cells (cDCs) are also important regulators of neutrophil homeostasis between the bone marrow, bloodstream, and organs through controlled production of chemokines CXCL1, CCL2, and CXCL10 and growth factor G-CSF.[47] Although the exact mechanism of their involvement remains unclear, depletion of cDCs in murine models causes a surge in neutrophil numbers, while cDC expansion leads to low circulating neutrophil numbers, or neutropenia, due to bone marrow neutrophil loss.[47,48]

To summarize, neutrophil differentiation from progenitor cells involves an intricate interaction between modulators and transcription factors, including C/EBPs, PU.1, and Gfi1.[49] Generation, regulation, and maintenance of HSCs is supported by osteoblasts and perivascular cells within dedicated niches within the trabecular regions of long bones and their secretion of growth factors, such as angiopoietin, thrombopoietin, and stem cell factor.[15] A delicate interplay between production of CXCL12 by perivascular cells and osteoblasts and its receptor, CXCR4, on the neutrophil cell membrane confines developing neutrophils to the bone marrow. Declining CXCR4 levels during neutrophil maturation and increases in CXCL2/CXCR2, however, facilitate their release into the bloodstream.[43,44]

NEUTROPHIL GRANULOPOIESIS

Beginning between the myeloblast and promyelocyte stages of neutrophil development, granulopoiesis, or the formation of granules within the developing neutrophil, occurs over approximately 4 to 6 days (Fig. 108.4).[50] High concentrations of C/EBP-α and low amounts of PU.1 in myeloblasts favor granulocytic rather than monocytic differentiation.[51] Other major transcription factors that regulate neutrophil granulopoiesis include Runx1, Gfi-1, and C/EBP-ε.[52] In murine models, Runx1 plays a crucial role in HSC development in the AGM region, with fetal *runx1* murine knockouts exhibiting impaired endothelial to EMP/HSC transition prior to liver colonization and subsequent blockage of myeloid hematopoiesis.[53,54] Deletion of the *runx1* gene in adult mice also leads to primary monopoiesis at the expense of granulopoiesis.[55] Bias towards myelopoiesis can also be induced via the transcription factor Trim 27, a zinc Ret finger protein (RFP), through upregulation of myeloid master genes *Runx1* and *Cbfb* without expanding HSC baseline populations.[56]

Gfi-1 is required to maintain the functional integrity of HSCs, with *gfi-1* ablation in mice resulting in impaired HSC self-renewal capabilities.[57-59] Gfi-1 also promotes neutrophil development and antagonizes monocyte development through repression of *c-FOS, Egr-1, and Egr-2,* and inhibition of the ERK1/2 signaling pathway.[57] Gfi-1knockout in mice hinders neutrophil maturation at the promyelocyte stage, with cells exhibiting developmental failures of gelatinase granules and secretory vesicles.[52,60] Moreover, loss of *gfi-1* causes expansion of GMP precursor cells with appearance of immature monocyte-like myeloid cells.[57] The promyelocyte to myelocyte transition is also controlled by C/EBP-ε, an essential transcription factor for the formation of specific and gelatinase granules.[32] Even though inhibition of C/EBP-ε does not affect initial neutrophil commitment, its absence impedes neutrophil maturation and terminal differentiation, leading to an aberrant differentiation of GMPs to the monocyte lineage.[31,32]

Severe congenital neutropenia (SCN), or Kostmann syndrome, is a life-threatening congenital condition caused by defects in neutrophil production. Mainly characterized by recurrent invasive fungal and bacterial infections, SCN is also associated with a predisposition for acute myeloid leukemia and myelodysplastic syndrome, with a rate of malignant transformation generally exceeding 20%.[61,62] More than half of all SCN cases occur as secondary mutations in genes encoding neutrophil elastase (*ELA2*).[63] SCN is, however, also associated with genetic defects in HCLS1 associated protein X-1 (*HAX1*),[64] *GIF1*,[60] or inhibition of secretory leukocyte protease inhibitor (SLPI).[61] Many causes of SCN originate at the earliest phases of GMP commitment to neutrophil differentiation, or at the myeloblast-to-promyelocyte maturational stage.[65] Defects of *ELA2*, for example, lead to neutrophil elastase mis-folding, prompting its intracellular accumulation and mis-localization. This anomaly subsequently causes endoplasmic reticulum stress and induction of apoptosis through activation of the unfolded-protein response (UPR).[63] For cases resulting from SLPI disruption, G-CSF phosphorylation of STAT5, ERK1/2, and lymphoid enhancer-binding factor-1 (LEF-1) is blocked in bone marrow myeloid progenitor cells, leading to downstream inhibition of LEF-1 target genes that are essential for neutrophil survival and proliferation, such as *c-myc, survivin,* and *cyclin D1*.[61,66] LEF-1 also induces C/EBP-α binding to the *SLPI* promotor to boost *SLPI* gene expression and neutrophil differentiation.[61] Inhibition or loss of LEF-1 blocks neutrophil maturation and proliferation, even though the production of red blood cells and monocytes remain unhindered due to a decline in C/EBP-α and heightened c-Myc levels.[61] The *HAX1* gene, on the other hand, directly controls mitochondrial proteases that regulate the accumulation of BL-2-associated X protein (BAX), a proapoptotic protein in the outer mitochondrial membrane.[64] Mitochondrial functions, indispensable for cell survival, are abrogated when cytoplasmic levels of BAX exceed that of their anti-apoptotic counterparts MCL-1.[64] This facilitates BAX oligomerization and the formation of pores in the outer mitochondrial membrane, which enables cytochrome c release into the cytoplasm and cell death through caspase activation via the *intrinsic cell death pathway*.[67]

To summarize, the transformation of CMPs to GMPs is dependent upon the suppression of c-Myc by the differentiation factor C/EBP-α.[68] Conversely, c-Myc is primarily involved in progenitor cell proliferation, which if silenced will result in the absence of all hematopoietic lineages except megakaryocytes.[69] Failure to appropriately repress the *c-myc* gene at the correct maturational state may, therefore, elicit the development of myeloid leukemias.[68]

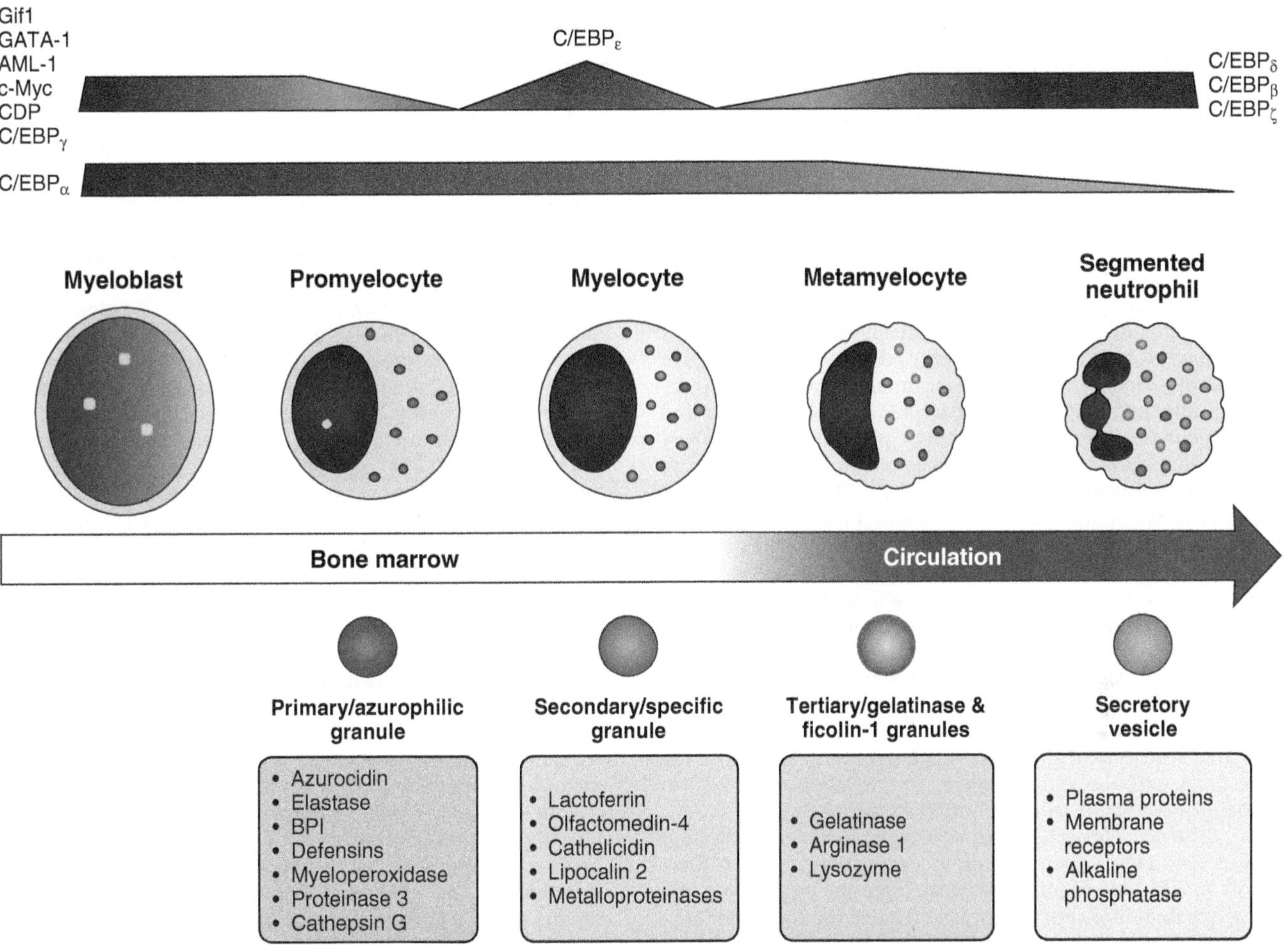

Fig. 108.4 Neutrophil granulopoiesis. Granulopoiesis begins with the development of azurophilic granules in myeloblasts and early promyelocytes and ends after creation of secretory vesicles in mature, segmented cells. Gene expression of GATA-1, C/EBP-ζ, AML-1, and c-Myc are imperative for azurophilic granule formation. Creation of specific granules occurs in conjunction with declining AML-1, c-Myc, and CDP concentrations. Reductions in CDP levels relieve its repression of C/EBP-ε genes, allowing for C/EBP-ε-induced transcription of both C/EBP-δ and specific granule proteins. Once the neutrophil matures into a metamyelocyte, it can no longer proliferate, marking the beginning of terminal neutrophil differentiation. This change results from the inhibition of proliferative genes, AML-1, C/EBP-γ, and CDP, and the emergence of anti-proliferative factors such as C/EBP-δ and C/EBP-ζ. The transcription factor C/EBP-ε becomes down-regulated as the gene expression for C/EBP-β, C/EBP-δ, and C/EBP-ζ are enhanced to form gelatinase granules. Myeloblasts, promyelocytes, and myelocytes comprise the proliferative pool and are primarily located within the bone marrow. In contrast, metamyelocytes, bands, and mature, segmented neutrophils are contained within the marginating and circulating neutrophil pools within the bloodstream. *AML-1*, Acute myeloid leukemia-1; *BPI*, Bactericidal/permeability-increasing protein; *C/EBP*, CCAAT/enhancer binding proteins; *CDP*, CCAAT displacement protein.

STEADY STATE AND EMERGENCY GRANULOPOIESIS

An estimated 10^{11} neutrophils, or 10^{9} cells/kg of body weight, are generated every day to maintain neutrophil homeostasis, or the delicate balance between granulopoiesis, bone marrow storage and release, intravascular margination, and migration into peripheral tissues.[48] Neutrophil production in the bone marrow involves five main stages of differentiation, beginning with (1) myeloblasts that maintain proliferative capabilities for nearly 1 week prior to maturation,[50] (2) promyelocytes/myelocytes, (3) metamyelocytes, (4) band forms, and (5) segmented neutrophils. The regulation of neutrophil production has been described in terms of steady-state versus emergency granulopoiesis and is directly dependent upon, and impacts, the individual's health.

In steady state, human neutrophils are short-lived cells with an estimated half-life of approximately 19 hours.[70] Aged and dying neutrophils are continually replenished by mature, segmented neutrophils, located within bone marrow reserve pools.[32,71] Turnover and replenishment of quiescent neutrophils follows the ingestion of apoptotic cells by tissue macrophages, which triggers the transcription of C/EBP-α and factors of the LXR family to suppress proinflammatory cytokine production and, in turn, diminish G-CSF levels.[72,73] Under baseline conditions in humans and mice, the transformation of a promyelocyte to mature, segmented neutrophil is accompanied by a drastic decline in transcripts and proteins related to general cellular processes, including DNA replication and repair, RNA transcription and processing, protein translation, and mitochondrial energy metabolism.[32,65,71] Concurrent with this decline in cellular proteins is a drop in cell-cycle, transcriptional, mitochondrial, and metabolic activity.[65] Despite an overall reduction in transcription and translation, components related to immune system functions and vesicle transport processes are preserved or become upregulated,[71] including those necessary for cellular response to microbial stimuli,[32] G-protein cell receptor (GPCR) signaling to facilitate chemotaxis, and cytoskeletal rearrangements to enable direct motility.[65,71] Finally, only modest contributions are made in histone modifications and epigenetic profiles during neutrophil development.[71]

In contrast, emergency granulopoiesis is activated following a microbial or inflammatory challenge and results a surge of both immature and mature neutrophil forms from bone marrow storage pools into the peripheral circulation. This process leads to a clinical neutrophilia with a "left-shift," or increased number of bloodstream neutrophils composed of a greater proportion of immature forms. This neutrophilia occurs in response to host-induced mechanisms (i.e., induction of C/EBP-β and early inflammatory mediators, such as interleukin [IL]-1β, tumor necrosis factor [TNF]-α, G-CSF, and GM-CSF) and pathogen-mediated factors, such as lipopolysaccharide (LPS) and other microbial products.[72,74]

The abrupt biologic switch from steady-state to emergency granulopoiesis requires high energy demands, which have only recently been elucidated using murine models of Gram-negative infection.[75] Although anaerobic glycolysis is favored by quiescent HSCs, exposure to host or pathogen inflammatory or infectious etiologies quickly shifts metabolic demands to mitochondrial oxidative phosphorylation.[75] This transformation is facilitated by the transfer of mitochondria from bone marrow stromal cells (BMSCs) directly to specific HSCs, targeted to undergo proliferation and differentiation. This energy switch is triggered by elevations in reactive oxygen species (ROS) levels in response to infection-associated stressors.[75] Mitochondrial transfer from BMSC to HSCs is controlled by phosphoinositide 3-kinase (PI3K) signaling and transpires through connexin 43 gap junctions.[75] This interplay between cells of the bone marrow microenvironment, therefore, enables pluripotent HSCs to rapidly cycle and differentiate into key innate immune cells, including neutrophils, without being subjected to critical delays related to intracellular activation of mitochondrial biogenesis.[75]

The detection of conserved pathogen-associated molecular patterns (PAMPs) by host pattern recognition receptors (PRRs), such as Toll-like receptors (TLRs), may unite the steady-state and emergency granulopoietic pathways.[47] Under routine conditions, the interplay between direct or indirect activation of PRRs on HSCs and/or progenitor cells may function to maintain steady-state granulopoiesis. Following acute infection or inflammation, however, increased activation of PRRs on HSCs and HSC exposure to proinflammatory chemokines, including keratinocyte chemoattractant (KC), macrophage inflammatory protein (MIP)-2, G-CSF, and TNF-α,[74,76,77] act as powerful stimulators for neutrophil proliferation and differentiation.[78] Moreover, induction of nicotinamide adenine dinucleotide phosphate (NADPH) oxidase by bone marrow myeloid cells boosts the production of ROS, which acts locally to trigger oxidation and deactivation of phosphate and tensin homolog (PTEN) in resident myeloid cells, leading to increased levels of G-CSF, upregulation of PtIns(3,4,5) P3 signaling, and induction of emergency granulopoiesis.[78]

NEUTROPHIL GRANULES AND SECRETORY VESICLES

AZUROPHILIC GRANULES

The transcription factors acute myeloid leukemia-1 (AML-1) and c-Myc are essential for azurophilic granule formation.[79] In particular, AML-1 and c-Myc regulate the expression of MPO and elastase,[79] as well as cell membrane receptors for IL-6 and G-CSF.[51,80] Azurophilic granule production is also dependent upon the upregulation of GATA-1 and C/EBP-ζ expression.[51]

Although azurophilic (primary) granules are packed with microbicidal proteins and acidic hydrolases, these granules are typically distinguished by their abundance of myeloperoxidase (MPO), which accounts for nearly 5% of the cell's dry weight.[81,82] Azurophilic granules are also critical for the production of ROS that enable neutrophil-mediated pathogen killing. Once engulfed by an activated neutrophil, pathogens are held in cellular structures known as *phagosomes*, which fuse with azurophilic granules to become phagolysosomes. An essential neutrophil organelle, phagolysosomes provide a small, confined space for oxidative reactions, such as the respiratory burst, to kill engulfed microorganisms while protecting host tissue against harmful metabolites.[83]

ROS are created when NADPH oxidase, localized on the phagolysosome membrane, triggers the conversion of oxygen (O_2) to superoxide (O_2^-).[83] Superoxide (O_2^-) is then converted by superoxide dismutase into hydroxydioxylic acid (HO_2) and hydrogen peroxide (H_2O_2), which are both weakly bactericidal and contribute considerably to phagolysosome acidification.[83] MPO then catalyzes the oxidation reaction between H_2O_2 and chloride (Cl^-) to form hypochlorous acid (HOCl),[84] hydroxyl radicals (–OH), and chloramines, which are all potent oxidants that further contribute to the neutrophil's microbicidal capabilities.[85] The voltage-gated proton channel Hv1/VOSP extrudes protons, accumulated during NADPH oxidase activity, to prevent excessive plasma membrane depolarization and cytosolic acidification that may occur during these reactions.[86,87]

While the NADPH oxidase complex can be detected at the metamyelocyte stage of neutrophil maturation following stimulation with cell-permeable phorbol ester (PMA), it is not until the band stage onward that this complex can be activated by cell-impermeable agents such as *N*-formylmethionyl-leucyl-phenylalanine (fMLP).[32,65,71] The timeline for fMLP neutrophil responsiveness coincides with the initiation of FPR1 expression and full maturation of the fMLP signaling cascade that enables fMLP-induced degranulation.[65,71] Therefore even though the neutrophil's cytotoxic capabilities are established early, signaling components necessary to activate these antimicrobial mechanisms are transcribed at later stages, outside the bone marrow. This functions to protect the bone marrow niche against toxic neutrophil cytosolic and granular contents.[71] A devastating clinical condition known as *chronic granulomatous disease (CGD)* can occur with inactivating mutations of NADPH oxidase. Characterized by recurrent bacterial and fungal infections, patients with CGD also develop detrimental granulomas from the neutrophils' inability to completely kill and eliminate pathogens.[88]

A cationic glycoprotein, MPO can also bind to the surface of neutrophils[89] and platelets[90] via electrostatic carbohydrate-dependent mechanisms, thereby triggering pro-inflammatory functional activities.[91] MPO can also be liberated by activated neutrophils by inflammatory mediators, including TLR ligands,[92] GM-CSF,[93] tumor necrosis factor (TNF)-α, and Ig/Fc receptor-mediated signaling,[94] with extracellular release through both degranulation or necrotic cell death pathways.[81] Once in the extracellular space, MPO can bind to the plasma membrane via CD11b/CD18 (Mac-1) receptors, provoking azurophilic and specific granule degranulation of substances such as elastase, lysozyme, and lactoferrin in a dose-dependent manner via induction of tyrosine kinase, PI3K, and calcium signaling pathways.[91,95]

Azurophilic granules also contain serprocidins (serine proteases) including elastase, cathepsin G, proteinase 3, and neutrophil serine protease 4 (NSP4),[96] which display proteolytic enzymatic activity against extracellular matrix components, such as type IV collagen, fibronectin, elastin, vitronectin, and laminin.[97] Even though azurophilic proteins are produced and stored during the promyelocyte to myelocyte stage of neutrophil development, the protease release machinery is not available until the neutrophil is almost fully matured, or after the band stage.[71] The serprocidins, excluding NSP4, are potent antimicrobial substances that can induce the activation of endothelial cells, macrophages, lymphocytes, and platelets.[97] Serine proteases are normally synthesized as zygomens, or inactive proteins, and require two separate processing steps to become activated: (1) cleavage of the signal peptide by cathepsin C, which is necessary to initiate enzymatic activity[98] and (2) carboxy-terminal processing that enables interaction with adaptor protein 3 to facilitate the correct trafficking to their granular compartment.[99]

Table 108.1 Differences in Neonatal Compared to Adult Neutrophils.

Variable	Preterm	Term	Matures	Comment
Immature granulocytes in circulation	↑↑	↑	Yes	Neutrophil composition approximates that of adults by 72 h of life[186]
Neutrophils in circulation	↑↑	↑	Yes	Increases noted for all GA infants in the first 24 h after birth. Quantities return to adult levels by 72 h of life. The highest levels are found in neonates <28 wk GA.[185]
Storage Pool	↓↓	↓	Yes	Reduced storage pools lead to increased risks for neutropenia if infection occurs postnatally[169,175]
Neutrophil cell mass (per gram BW)	↓↓	↓	Yes	Adult levels achieved by 4 wk of age[169,192]
Chemotaxis	↓	↓	No	Factors include reduced mobilization of intracellular calcium[193] and anomalies in cytoskeletal organization[194]
Rolling and firm adhesion	↓↓	↓	Yes	Functional differences result from gestational age-related reductions in neutrophil membrane L-selectin levels and shedding,[195] in addition to decreased levels of P- and E-selectins located on endothelial cells of the vasculature[196]
Transmigration	↓↓	↓	Yes	Decreased due to diminished release of chemokines and cytokines from tissue neutrophils and macrophages[180,196]
Granule Protein Levels				
BPI	↓↓	↓	Yes	Decreased in unstimulated neonatal compared with adult neutrophils.[114] Demonstrates age-dependent maturational effects.[118] During sepsis[116] or pneumonia,[117] term neonates can secrete similar BPI levels as adults, while preterm neonates produce less[114]
Lactoferrin	↓↓	↓	Yes	Term neonatal neutrophils are half of adult concentrations, while even lower quantities are found in neutrophils from preterm infants[131]
Myeloperoxidase[114]	N	N	No	
Defensin		N	Unknown	Only documented for term newborns[114]
Degranulation	↓	N	Yes	Only known for BPI, elastase, and lactoferrin[118,179]
Respiratory burst	N / ↑	N / ↑	No	Decreased in stressed neonates or those with perinatal distress[197]
Chemiluminescence	N / ↓	N / ↑	No	Reduced in critically ill neonates and those challenged with large bacterial loads[198,199]

↑, Increased; ↓, decreased; *BPI*, bactericidal permeability-increasing protein; *GA*, gestational age; *N*, normal (similar to adult).

Except NSP4, whose inhibition does not result in significant neutrophil function loss, serine proteases have specific pathogen-mediated killing capabilities.[96] Cathepsins G is known to target *Staphylococcus aureus*,[100] while elastase has particular antimicrobial activity gram-negative bacteria.[101] Both cathepsin G and elastase, however, have potent microbicidal activity against fungal organisms.[100] Alternatively, mutations of the gene encoding neutrophil elastase, *ELA2*, is implicated in the pathogenesis of SCN and cyclic neutropenia at the earliest phases of neutrophil differentiation, or the myeloblast to promyelocyte maturational stage.[63]

Several membrane proteins have been identified in azurophilic granules including CD63,[102] CD68,[102] presenilin1,[103] stomatin,[104] and vacuolar-type H^+-ATPase.[105] Azurophilic granules also contain a variety of important microbicidal peptides, including α-defensin, azurocidin, and bactericidal/permeability-increasing protein (BPI). Making up at least 5% of the protein content of neutrophils,[106] α-defensin has antimicrobial activity against bacteria, enveloped viruses, fungus, and protozoa through the creation of multimeric transmembrane pores in the microbial outer membrane.[107,108] Following extracellular exocytosis, α-defensins also activates the chemotaxis of $CD4^+$ T-helper cells, $CD8^+$ T-cytotoxic cells,[109] and monocytes.[110]

Azurocidin, an inactive serine protease homologue with broad microbicidal capabilities, can foster vascular permeability during neutrophil extravasation[111] and is an effective chemoattractant for monocytes, fibroblasts, and T cells.[112] BPI is a potent antimicrobial substance that specifically targets the obliteration of Gram-negative bacteria at nanomolar concentrations.[113] BPI neutralizes Gram-negative bacteria by binding with high affinity to the lipid A portion of LPS located in the bacteria's outer cell membrane.[114] BPI also enhances the neutrophil's phagocytic and intracellular killing of Gram-negative bacterium by acting as an opsonin.[114,115]

Healthy, term neonatal and adult neutrophils contain equal concentrations of MPO and α-defensin, but neonates exhibit a threefold decrease of BPI in unstimulated neutrophils compared to adult controls (Table 108.1).[114] In term infants with early onset sepsis (EOS), however, plasma levels of BPI can rise to concentrations similar to older children and adults with sepsis[116] and/or pneumonia.[117] BPI mobilization, though, exhibits an age-dependent maturational effect,[118] which may help explain why *Escherichia coli* is the leading cause of EOS in preterm infants, while group B *Streptococcus* remains the leading cause of EOS in term neonates.[119]

SPECIFIC GRANULES

The creation of specific granule proteins is activated by the termination of azurophilic granule protein gene expression, or via acute reductions in AML-1 and c-Myc concentrations. Production of specific granule proteins is also supported by declines in active CDP levels, which lifts its repression of C/EBP-ε genes (i.e., gp91^{phox}) to promote C/EBP-ε-mediated transcription of C/EBP-δ.[51,120] Gene expression of C/EBP-ε also rises throughout neutrophil maturation, with peak levels observed in myelocytes/metamyelocytes when the cell stops proliferating. Although concentrations of C/EBP-ε messenger RNA begin to decline as the cell continues to mature, C/EBP-ε protein is only detected in myelocytes/metamyelocytes.[121]

Mutations in *CEBPE* cause an autosomal recessive immunodeficiency disorder known as *neutrophil-specific granule deficiency (SGD),* which blocks terminal differentiation of neutrophils beyond the myelocyte stage of neutrophil maturation.[122] SGD is characterized by atypical bilobed nuclei, lack of expression of granule proteins, abnormal respiratory burst, impaired chemotaxis, diminished bactericidal activity, and frequent bacterial infections.[123] Additionally, microRNAs have also been shown to regulate C/EBP-ε protein expression in granulocytic precursors.[121] In particular, overexpression of miRNA-130a caused decreased translation of C/EBP-ε and downregulated the expression of lactoferrin, cathelicidin antimicrobial peptide, and lipocalin-2,[121] giving rise to neutrophils with a similar immature phenotype as that observed in *Cebpe*$^{-/-}$ murine models.[121] C/EBP-ε is, therefore, a critical transcription factor that regulates cell-cycle protein expression and ensures a robust and irreversible exit from cell proliferation by the metamyelocyte stage of neutrophil development.[52]

Specific (secondary) granules are loaded with antibiotic substances that contribute to the neutrophil's microbicidal activities, either upon mobilization with the phagosome or through release into the extracellular milieu. A primary specific granule protein, lactoferrin, directs bacteriostatic and bactericidal activities against viruses, gram-positive bacteria, gram-negative bacilli, and fungi.[124] Lactoferrin disrupts and destabilizes microbial cell membranes by sequestering vital iron in biologic fluids.[125] In addition, lactoferrin can modulate adaptive immune responses by boosting immature B cell differentiation into antigen-presenting cells[126] and accelerating the maturation of T-cell precursors into competent $CD4^+$ T-helper cells.[127] Moreover, lactoferrin can enhance cathepsin G activation and serine proteases in activated neutrophils to promote innate immune responses during acute inflammation.[128] Lactoferrin can, conversely, inhibit pro-inflammatory pathway activation and subsequent tissue injury by impairing ROS production[129] and sequestering LPS and CD14.[130] Notably, lactoferrin concentrations in term neonatal neutrophils are half of adult concentrations, while even lower quantities are found in neutrophils from preterm infants (see Table 108.1).[131]

Specific granules contain other vital antimicrobial proteins. Neutrophil gelatinase-associated lipocalin, NGAL, can sequester iron chelators produced by pathogens, in coordination with lactoferrin, when iron availability is low, to inhibit bacterial growth and proliferation.[132] NGAL may also be able to bind small lipophilic inflammatory mediators such as platelet activating factor, leukotriene B4, and LPS to facilitate neutrophil innate responses.[133] The cytokine, resistin, which localizes to the neutrophil's cell membrane, can counterbalance the neutrophil's proinflammatory responses by decreasing the cell's oxidative burst capacity. Moreover, resistin can impair the neutrophil's chemotactic capabilities to inhibit their accumulation at inflamed sites by a dose-dependent induction of nuclear factor (NF)-κB activity.[134] In addition, signal regulatory protein alpha (SIRPα) is a cell surface glycoprotein that is rapidly mobilized to the neutrophil cell surface and functions to limit neutrophil aggregation at inflamed sites together with resistin.[135] Finally, olfactomedin-4 (OLFM-4) can attenuate neutrophil killing of *S. aureus* and *E. coli* by hindering cathepsin C-mediated protease activities.[136] OLFM-4 is unique among neutrophil granule proteins as it is only recovered from 20% to 25% of mature adult neutrophils.[137]

GELATINASE GRANULES/FICOLIN-1 RICH GRANULES

Gelatinase and ficolin-1 granules form between the transition of metamyelocytes to band neutrophils, marking the beginning of terminal differentiation when the developing neutrophil can no longer proliferate. This transformation is caused by the inhibition of proliferative genes, AML-1, C/EBP-γ, and CDP, and the emergence of anti-proliferative factors such as C/EBP-δ and C/EBP-ζ.[51] Additionally, the transcription factor C/EBP-ε, which was vital for specific granule formation, becomes down-regulated as the gene expression for C/EBP-β, C/EBP-δ, and C/EBP-ζ are enhanced.[51]

Gelatinase (tertiary)[138] and ficolin-1 rich granules[139] are mobilized when the neutrophil establishes primary rolling contact with activated endothelium. Components of these granules are primarily involved in neutrophil locomotion, firm adhesion, and transendothelial migration.[139–141] These granules contain matrix-degrading enzymes, such as gelatinase, membrane receptors including CD11b/CD18, CD67, CD177, fMLF-R, SCAMP, and VAMP2, and several cytoskeleton-binding proteins, which are important in the earliest phases of the neutrophil inflammatory responses and extravasation into inflamed tissues.[52,141] Arginase 1, for example, is a critical gelatinase protein that metabolizes arginine and diminishes its availability as a substrate for nitric oxide synthase (NOS). The enhanced metabolism of arginine leads to endothelial dysfunction due to impaired nitric oxide (NO) synthesis. Arginase 1, however, can also foster tissue regeneration and dampen pro-inflammatory immune responses by promoting ornithine production.[142]

SECRETORY VESICLES

Secretory vesicles are significantly smaller than neutrophil granules and are an important reservoir of membrane-associated receptors, including CD10, CD11b/CD18, CD15, CD16, CD35, MMP-25, SCAMP, VAMP2, NRAMP2, LFA-1, MAC-1, as well as actin, actin-binding proteins, and alkaline phosphatase, which are required at the earliest phases of neutrophil-mediated inflammatory responses.[52,139] Secretory vesicles are not considered to be true neutrophil granules and are the easiest and most exocytosed cell organelle in the neutrophil. Cell membrane receptors contained within these organelles are important for neutrophil's ability to complete: (1) slow rolling, (2) establish firm contact to the activated vascular endothelium, (3) complete diapedesis into inflamed tissue, and (4) undergo chemotactic-directed migration within the inflamed tissues to locate and eradicate the offending microorganisms.[139,141]

NEUTROPHIL GRANULE PROTEIN TRAFFICKING AND SORTING

Neutrophil granules display heterogeneity with an overlap of protein content due to a process described by the *targeting by timing model,* whereby the timing of protein synthesis is dependent only upon cell maturity. In this model, granule protein production occurs in a continuum during all stages of neutrophil development and proteins are simply packed into granules as they are produced.[50,143] Thus azurophilic granule proteins are synthesized only at the promyelocyte developmental stage, specific granule proteins at the myelocyte stage, and gelatinase and ficolin-1-rich granule proteins at the metamyelocyte and band stages of neutrophil maturation, after which granule formation concludes and secretory vesicles form.[144]

Proper shuttling and packaging of potentially noxious granule proteins is vital for neutrophil maturation and development. Several cellular processes ensure this process is correctly performed, such as the anionic proteoglycan serglycin that packages and safely shuttles cationic azurophilic granule proteins, including MPO,[145] defensin, and elastase.[146–148] In addition, the synthesis of inactive granule enzymes, or zymogens, allows safe cytosolic passage to their final destination, where proteolytic cleavage of their pro-domains triggers their activation.[149] Although not well defined in neutrophils, complex co- and post-translational processing of granule proteins may also be expedited by multi-subunit adaptor protein complexes (APs), particularly AP1, AP3, and AP4, and the monomeric Golgi-localized γ-adaptin ear homology (GGA) ARF-binding protein. Together these complexes may enable the proper organization and trafficking of granule proteins from the *trans*-Golgi network to their respective neutrophil granule compartments in a manner similar to that exhibited by lysosomal sorting in other cell types.[149,150] Protein mis-sorting between the different neutrophil granules can occur and cause alterations of the cell's function. This typically leads to premature activation and degradation of granule substances by catalytically active azurophilic proteases, making them biologically active.[151]

DEGRANULATION AND EXOCYTOSIS OF NEUTROPHIL GRANULES

Neutrophils can rapidly mobilize to inflamed sites and deploy their potent chemical and enzymatic arsenal, which is critical for neutrophil-mediated innate immune responses. Extracellular release, or degranulation, of neutrophil granule substances, however, occurs in a hierarchical fashion that is inversely related to the order of granule production.[97,151] While only minimal cellular activation or stimulation is sufficient to incite secretory vesicle exocytosis, increasing stimulus strength is required to release of ficolin-1-rich, gelatinase, specific, and finally azurophilic granules.[97,139,151-153] Therefore, mediators required during early infection or inflammation are contained in secretory vesicles and gelatinase/ficolin-1 granules and function to enable chemotaxis, slow rolling, and transmigration. Conversely, toxic microbicidal proteins and enzymes that kill invading micro-organisms and contribute tissue injury are stored in specific and azurophilic granules. Notably, term neonatal and adult neutrophils have similar degranulation capabilities, while those from preterm infants have considerable impairments in the release of bactericidal/permeability-increasing protein (BPI), elastase, and lactoferrin when compared to either term neonatal or adult cells (see Table 108.1).[118,154]

Unique among the neutrophil granules, azurophilic granules can release a small amount of their content extracellularly, but the bulk of their granular contents are released into phagosomes[155,156]. This process not only facilitates ROS production and pathogen death, but also functions to initiate efferocytosis, which couples microbial killing to accelerated neutrophil clearance.[157,158] Neutrophil programmed death by efferocytosis dampens the inflammatory response by rendering the cell unresponsive to extracellular stimuli, enables the recognition and clearance of dying cells by professional phagocytes, and promotes wound healing.[159]

The order of neutrophil granule exocytosis is in part due to variations in insoluble *N*-ethylmaleimide-sensitive factor attachment protein receptor (SNARE) complexes: whereas all neutrophil granules contain syntaxin 4 and SNARE complexes, azurophilic granules have SNARE complexes with high levels of VAMP-1 and VAMP-7, while specific and gelatinase granules have increased levels of VAMP-1, VAMP-2, and 23-kDa synaptosome-associated protein (SNAP-23).[156,160] Gelatinase granules are also regulated by syntaxin 3, which controls the extracellular release of cytokines IL-1α, IL-1β, IL-12b, and CCL4 during early inflammatory responses.[161,162] SNARE-interacting Sec1/Munc18 (SM) family members, mainly MUNC18-2 and MUNC18-3, are also important for enabling selective vesicular shuttling in neutrophils. While MUNC18-2 and its respective SNARE-binding partner syntaxin 3 are preferentially associated with regulation of azurophilic granule exocytosis, MUNC18-3 and its SNARE-binding partner syntaxin 4 controls extracellular membrane fusion and degranulation of specific and gelatinase granules.[162]

Azurophilic granules are also controlled by MUNC13-4, a RAB27A effector and key coordinator of azurophilic granular exocytosis, that functions to direct phagosomal maturation and regulates intracellular and extracellular production of ROS through p22*phox* induction.[163,164] Even though RAB27A is a master organizer of vesicular shuttling, RAB27A-deficient neutrophils maintained normal phagosomal maturation, including normal delivery of azurophilic and specific granule proteins to the phagosomal membrane.[163] Impairment of MUNC13-4, however, inhibits phagosomal maturation and results in defective trafficking of azurophilic granule components.[163] Deficiencies of either RAB27A or MUNC13-4 can lead to a medical condition known as *hemophagocytic lymphohistiocytosis*, where patients produce an abundance of activated immune cells and may suffer from fever, enlargement of the spleen, and neurologic abnormalities.[163,165,166]

NEUTROPHIL DISTRIBUTION

Nearly sixty percent of all leukocytes in the bone marrow comprise neutrophil precursors, with the largest percentage of hematopoiesis committed to the production of these cells.[70] This results in the generation of a staggering 100 billion neutrophils every day by the average human adult.[70] Neutrophil homeostasis is maintained through a meticulous balance between neutrophil development, bone marrow storage and release, migration into vascular compartments and peripheral tissues, cell aging, and death. In general, neutrophils reside in three different groups, or pools, known as the *proliferative*, *circulating*, and *marginating pools*, with numbers in each influenced by the maturational development of the cell and the individual's state of health.

PROLIFERATIVE POOL

Located within the bone marrow, the proliferative, or storage, pool comprises early neutrophil precursors, including myeloblasts, promyelocytes, and myelocytes, which maintain the ability to multiply in order to replenish neutrophil numbers.[167] The proliferative pool in the average human adult is between 4 and 5 × 10^9 cells/kg body weight, as extrapolated from data using rodent models (Fig. 108.5).[168] Term, healthy newborns, in contrast, have significantly smaller proliferative neutrophil pools, estimated to be only 10% of adult values, with nearly 75% of these cells residing in an active cell cycle, leading to significant cell turnover (Fig. 108.6 and see Table 108.1).[169]

The coevolution of mammals and their microbiota have also led to the reliance on microbiota-derived signals to provide tonic stimulation to the systemic innate immune system, which functions to maintain vigilance against infection but to also control the size of the proliferative pool.[170] This concept is well demonstrated in adult mice, where the size of the bone marrow mitotic pool strongly correlates with the complexity of the intestinal microbiota. Studies have also shown delayed pathogen clearance in germ-free mice following a systemic challenge with apathogenic bacteria.[170] Thus, the establishment of a healthy neonatal microbiome after birth is essential for maintaining neutrophil homeostasis and proper cell functioning.

Neutrophil production within the bone marrow is also enhanced by microbial induction of TLR-4 and activation of myeloid differentiation factor 88 (Myd88), which stimulates the production of IL-17 by group 3 innate lymphoid cells in the intestine to enhance circulating G-CSF levels.[171] Therefore, continuous TLR signaling by microbial antigens and TLR ligands at extremely low levels (below the threshold required for induction of adaptive immune responses) may control the size of the proliferative pool in steady-state granulopoiesis.[76,170] Emergency granulopoiesis, in contrast, may be activated by TLR detection of PAMPs from invading microorganisms, leading to an acute rise in pro-inflammatory cytokines IL-1β, TNF-α, G-CSF, and GM-CSF.[72,77] This surge of inflammatory mediators stimulates neutrophil proliferation and differentiation, resulting in an acute and drastic rise in the number of circulating neutrophils available to combat the ensuing infection. Common medical interventions that decrease the natural development of the newborn's microbiota, such as cesarean sections or exposure to intrapartum or postpartum antimicrobials, may therefore not only prolong their length of stay in the NICU but place the infant

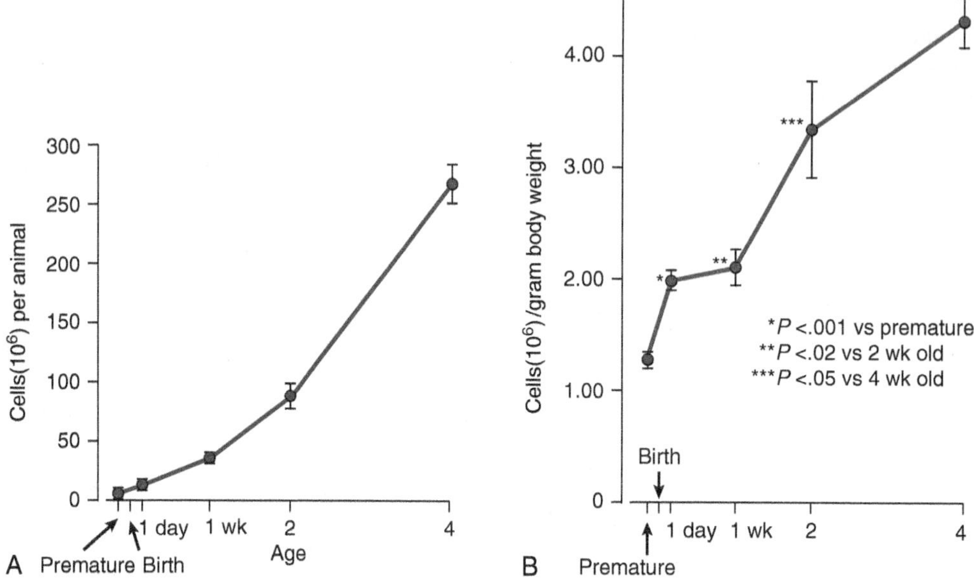

Fig. 108.5 (A) Neutrophil storage pool size at various ages in the developing rat. Each point represents the mean of eight to 12 animals ± the standard error. (B) Neutrophil storage pool size per gram of body weight at various ages in the developing rat. Each point represents the mean of eight to 12 animals ± the standard error. (From Erdmann SH, Christensen RD, Bradley PP, et al. Supply and release of storage neutrophils: a development study. *Biol Neonate*. 1982;41:132.)

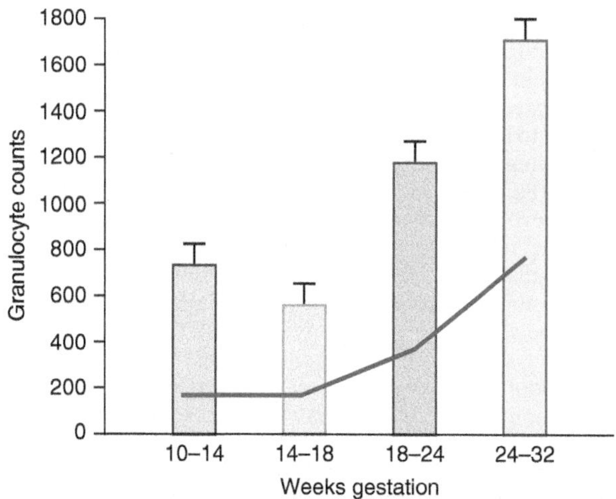

Fig. 108.6 Mean and range of neutrophil counts at 10 to 14, 14 to 18, 18 to 24, and 24 to 32 weeks' gestational age. (From Thomas DB, Yoffey JM. Human foetalhaemopoiesis. I. The cellular composition of foetal blood. *Br J Haematol*. 1962;8:290.)

at an increased risk for late onset sepsis, necrotizing enterocolitis, or even death.[172-174]

In healthy adults, the proliferative pool contains high numbers of quiescent progenitors that can be quickly recruited into the cell cycle during times of infection or inflammation.This process produces an influx of immature and mature neutrophil forms into the bloodstream to combat the infection, and is clinically referred to as a *left-shift*. Human adults maintain a large reserve pool that can be rapidly mobilized in acute infection, estimated at nearly 20 times more cells than that found in circulation.[168] In contrast, term newborns experience substantial reductions in their absolute neutrophil cell mass per gram of body weight; this is projected to be only 25% of adult values, while infants born prematurely display even lower numbers at approximately 20% of adult levels (see Table 108.1).[169] Reduced proliferative storage pools and the limited ability to rapidly recruit or produce increased neutrophil numbers during infection predispose newborn infants to the development of severe neutropenia, or very low circulating neutrophil numbers, and substantially raises their risk of sepsis-associated morbidity and mortality.[169,175]

Higher rates of neutropenia (absolute neutrophil count of <1000/mL) are observed in neonates who are born small for gestational age (SGA), or have a birth weight less than 10th percentile for their GA at birth.[176] SGA neutropenia is directly linked to the number of circulating red blood cells and is often associated with thrombocytopenia in more than 60% of infants.[176] Persisting for the first week of life, SGA neutropenia is caused by *in utero* growth restriction and relative hypoxia, which promotes production of hemoglobin-rich red blood cells at the expense of other blood cell types.[176] Reduced production, rather than increased utilization or turnover, is the primary cause of this transient neutropenia, as demonstrated by diminished bone marrow neutrophil proliferative and storage pools, decreased concentrations of granulocyte-macrophage progenitors, and lack of evidence for excessive margination.[176,177] Neutropenic SGA newborns have a higher risk of developing late onset sepsis, or infection after 72 hours of life, and have a fourfold increased risk of being diagnosed with necrotizing enterocolitis.[176] Surprisingly, the highest frequency of neutropenia is found in extremely low birth weight infants (ELBW or those <1000 g at birth).[178] Although the underlying etiology of this neutropenia remains unknown, neutropenic ELBW infants do not experience elevated sepsis risks, unlike their older GA counterparts who are admitted to the neonatal intensive care unit (NICU). Fortunately, neutropenia in neonates, irrespective of their GA or intrauterine growth, is transient, with levels rising significantly over the first week of life and reaching adult values around four weeks of age.[178]

CIRCULATING AND MARGINATING POOLS

Once neutrophils leave the bone marrow, they exist in equilibrium between the circulating and marginating pools.[179] While the circulating pool represents free-flowing neutrophils in the bloodstream, the marginating pool is composed of cells that

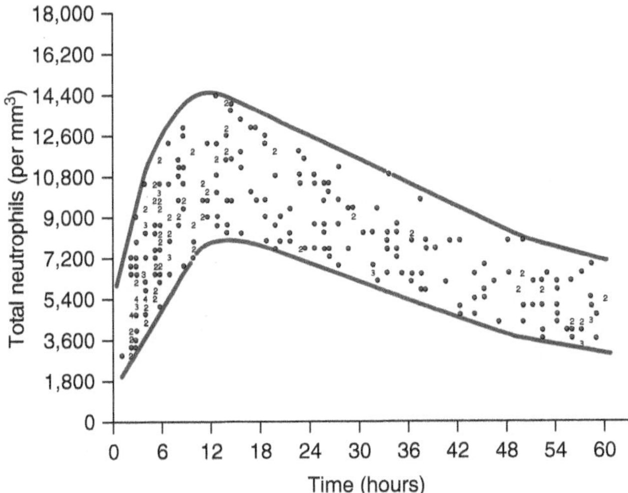

Fig. 108.7 The total neutrophil count reference range in the first 60 hours of life. (From Manroe BL, Weinberg AG, Rosenfeld CR, et al. The neonatal blood count in health and disease. *J Pediatr.* 1979;95:89.)

cannot be readily retrieved by routine blood sampling.[179] These post-mitotic pools consist of more mature neutrophils, including metamyelocytes, bands, and segmented forms.[179,180] First identified in the 1960s, marginating neutrophils were discovered following autologous transfusion of ex vivo radiolabeled neutrophils in healthy adult volunteers.[181] Following the transfusion, nearly half of the labeled neutrophils immediately disappeared from circulation, but could be recovered following a dose of adrenalin. In contrast, close to 87% of the originally transfused cells could be retrieved from subjects following several hours of exercise after the transfusion.[181] Although the lungs and pulmonary vasculature are the primary source of marginating neutrophils, the liver, spleen, and bone marrow also demonstrate rapid accumulation of neutrophils following labeled transfusion experiments.[182]

Marginating, mature neutrophils differ phenotypically between the pulmonary bed and the bone marrow. While bone marrow neutrophils demonstrate declines in CXCR4, the ligand for CXCL12 that enables their escape from the bone marrow, cells confined to the pulmonary vascular bed have enhanced expression of CXCLR12.[183] These pulmonary vascular bed neutrophils were readily recruited back to the bloodstream following CXCR4 inhibition via the drug plerixafor, without concomitant mobilization from the bone marrow.[184] In neonates, marginating neutrophils may be recruited into the bloodstream following birth due to the surge in stress-associated hormones such as epinephrine, norepinephrine, and cortisol, although the exact mechanisms are not well defined. This rapid accumulation of circulating neutrophils leads to high numbers that will never again be encountered in their lifetime while healthy. Peak neutrophil levels around 25 to 28,000 cells/μL are typically observed in newborns ≥28 weeks GA within the first 6 to 12 hours of life, while neutrophil counts as high as 40,000 cells/μL have been documented around 24 hours of life in neonates less than 28 weeks GA.[185] Following their peak, neutrophil levels in all gestational-aged infants will gradually decline to reach normal adult levels by 72 hours of life (Fig. 108.7).[185]

Neonates also have an abundance of immature circulating granulocytes, compared to adults, after birth (12% vs. 5%, respectively), including promyelocytes, myelocytes, and metamyelocytes (see Table 108.1).[186] These early neutrophil precursors generally lack gelatinase/ficolin-1 granules and secretory vesicles, which may impair early pro-inflammatory responses and increase the newborn's susceptibility to infection by preventing neutrophils from transmigrating into inflamed tissues.[186] Alternatively, this loss may also balance the necessity to protect the infant from an acute inflammatory response, as they become colonized with their microbiome postpartum.[186] Further investigation is necessary to determine significance of these findings.

Once neutrophils are released into the bloodstream from bone marrow stores, they begin the aging process and become progressively more pro-inflammatory.[187] Neutrophil aging is regulated by the circadian-related gene *Bmal1* through the expression of chemokine CXCL2, which induces chemokine receptor CXCR2-dependent diurnal changes in both transcriptional and migratory properties of circulating neutrophils.[187,188] Cell membrane expression of integrin $\alpha_M\beta_2$ (MAC-1) steadily increases, allowing them to be more proficient at combating pathogens during acute inflammatory conditions through enhanced chemotaxis, transmigration, and production of neutrophil extracellular traps (NETs).[189] Under steady-state conditions, observed changes in the cell's membrane receptor repertoire functions to prevent the aggregation of "primed," aged neutrophils into inflamed tissue at night, where their presence could exacerbate tissue damage. Their ability to migrate into naïve tissues, however, is not impeded, and they retain their capacity to quickly mount a robust pro-inflammatory response against infectious stimuli.[187] Mice engineered with constitutive neutrophil aging through deletion of *Cxcr4*, a negative regulator of CXCR2 signaling, exhibit unrestrained neutrophil aging. Even though these mice have improved survival against infection, they are predisposed to thrombo-inflammation and untimely death.[187]

CONCLUSION

From the earliest stages of embryogenesis when neutrophils first appear, to their continual production in large quantities from the bone marrow throughout postnatal life, the differentiation of a pluripotent HSC into a mature, segmented neutrophil is a highly orchestrated process in which the transcriptional regulators C/EBP-α and C/EBP-ε serve central functions.[141] Deficiencies of neutrophil differentiation or maturation can result in clinical conditions, including CGD, SCN, and neutrophil-specific granule deficiency (SGD), emphasizing the vital role neutrophils play in host defense against infectious disease. While neonatal neutrophils are often mischaracterized as "dysfunctional" when compared to adult cells, distinct differences between fetal and adult physiology must be considered.[190] Functional and phenotypic variances between fetal, neonatal, and adult neutrophils are important to allow natural immunologic processes to occur, such as postpartum colonization of the infant's microbiome without eliciting a pro-inflammatory immune response. As with other organ systems, postnatal neutrophil deficits are exacerbated in the most immature neonates, resulting in a 10-fold greater risk for infection compared to their term counterparts.[191] Further investigation must be dedicated to unraveling the mysteries of neutrophil biology during fetal development and postnatal life, taking into account environmental and compositional influences.

ABBREVIATIONS

AGM: Aorta-gonad-mesonephros region
AP: Adaptor protein complex
BMSC: Bone marrow stromal cells
BPI: Bactericidal/permeability-increasing protein
cDC: Conventional dendritic cell
CDP: CCAAT displacement protein
C/EBP: CCAAT/enhancer binding proteins
CGD: Chronic granulomatous disease
CLP: Common lymphoid progenitor
CMP: Common myeloid progenitor
ELBW: Extremely low birth weight
EOS: Early onset sepsis

FLSEC: Fetal liver sinusoidal endothelial cell
GA: Gestational age
GGA: Golgi-localized γ-adaptin ear homology ARF binding protein
GMP: Granulocyte monocyte progenitor
GPCR: G protein-coupled receptors
HSC: Hematopoietic stem cell
HSPA1A: Heat shock protein 1
KC: Keratinocyte chemoattractant
LAD: Leukocyte adhesive deficiency
LMPP: Lymphoid-primed multipotent progenitor
LPS: Lipopolysaccharide
LXA4: Lipoxin A4
MEP: Megakaryocyte erythroid progenitor
MIP: Macrophage inflammation protein
MPO: Myeloperoxidase
MPP: Multipotent progenitor
Myd88: Myeloid differentiation factor 88
NADPH: Nicotinamide adenine dinucleotide phosphate
NET: Neutrophil extracellular trap
NICU: Neonatal intensive care unit
NOD: Nod-like receptors
NSP4: Neutrophil serine protease 4
OLFM-4: Olfactomedin 4
PAMP: Pathogen-associated molecular pattern
PGC: Primordial germ cells
PIK3: Phosphoinositide 3-kinase
PRM: Pattern recognition molecules
PRR: Pattern recognition receptors
PTEN: Phosphate and tensin homolog
ROS: Reactive oxygen species
SCN: Severe congenital neutropenia
SGA: Small for gestational age
SGD: Neutrophil-Specific Granule Deficiency
SLPI: Secretory leukocyte protease inhibitor
SNAP-23: 23-kDA synaptosome-associated protein
SNARE: Soluble *N*-ethylmaleimide-sensitive factor attachment protein receptor
TLR: Toll-like receptor
TNF: Tumor necrosis factor
UPR: Unfolded-protein response

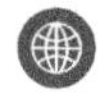 A complete reference list is available at www.ExpertConsult.com.

SELECT REFERENCES

6. Easterbrook J, Rybtsov S, Gordon-Keylock S, et al. Analysis of the spatiotemporal development of hematopoietic stem and progenitor cells in the early human embryo. *Stem Cell Reports*. 2019;12(5):1056-1068.
8. Ivanovs A, Rybtsov S, Anderson RA, Turner ML, Medvinsky A. Identification of the niche and phenotype of the first human hematopoietic stem cells. *Stem Cell Reports*. 2014;2(4):449-456.
13. Notta F, Zandi S, Takayama N, et al. Distinct routes of lineage development reshape the human blood hierarchy across ontogeny. *Science*. 2016;351(6269):aab2116.
22. Popescu DM, Botting RA, Stephenson E, et al. Decoding human fetal liver haematopoiesis. *Nature*. 2019;574(7778):365-371.
23. Höfer T, Rodewald HR. Differentiation-based model of hematopoietic stem cell functions and lineage pathways. *Blood*. 2018;132(11):1106-1113.
51. Bjerregaard MD, Jurlander J, Klausen P, Borregaard N, Cowland JB. The in vivo profile of transcription factors during neutrophil differentiation in human bone marrow. *Blood*. 2003;101(11):4322-4332.
52. Cowland JB, Borregaard N. Granulopoiesis and granules of human neutrophils. *Immunol Rev*. 2016;273(1):11-28.
65. Hoogendijk AJ, Pourfarzad F, Aarts CEM, et al. Dynamic transcriptome-proteome correlation networks reveal human myeloid differentiation and neutrophil-specific programming. *Cell Rep*. 2019;29(8):2505-2519.
71. Grassi L, Pourfarzad F, Ullrich S, et al. Dynamics of transcription regulation in human bone marrow myeloid differentiation to mature blood neutrophils. *Cell Rep*. 2018;24(10):2784-2794.
75. Mistry JJ, Marlein CR, Moore JA, et al. ROS-mediated PI3K activation drives mitochondrial transfer from stromal cells to hematopoietic stem cells in response to infection. *Proc Natl Acad Sci USA*. 2019:201913278.
139. Rørvig S, Østergaard O, Heegaard NH, Borregaard N. Proteome profiling of human neutrophil granule subsets, secretory vesicles, and cell membrane: correlation with transcriptome profiling of neutrophil precursors. *J Leuko Biol*. 2013;94(4):711-721.
141. Lawrence SM, Corriden R, Nizet V. The ontogeny of a neutrophil: mechanisms of granulopoiesis and homeostasis. *Microbiol Mol Biol Rev*. 2018;82(1): e00057-00017.
143. Le Cabec V, Cowland JB, Calafat J, Borregaard N. Targeting of proteins to granule subsets is determined by timing and not by sorting: the specific granule protein NGAL is localized to azurophil granules when expressed in HL-60 cells. *Proc Natl Acad Sci USA*. 1996;93(13):6454-6457.
157. Morioka S, Maueröder C, Ravichandran KS. Living on the edge: efferocytosis at the interface of homeostasis and pathology. *Immunity*. 2019;50(5):1149-1162.
171. Deshmukh HS, Liu Y, Menkiti OR, et al. The microbiota regulates neutrophil homeostasis and host resistance to Escherichia coli K1 sepsis in neonatal mice. *Nat Med*. 2014;20(5):524-530.
173. Cotten CM, Taylor S, Stoll B, et al. Prolonged duration of initial empirical antibiotic treatment is associated with increased rates of necrotizing enterocolitis and death for extremely low birth weight infants. *Pediatrics*. 2009;123(1):58-66.
174. Greenwood C, Morrow AL, Lagomarcino AJ, et al. Early empiric antibiotic use in preterm infants is associated with lower bacterial diversity and higher relative abundance of Enterobacter. *J Pediatr*. 2014;165(1):23-29.
176. Christensen RD, Yoder BA, Baer VL, Snow GL, Butler A. Early-onset neutropenia in small-for-gestational-age infants. *Pediatrics*. 2015;136(5):e1259-1267.
177. Koenig JM, Christensen RD. Incidence, neutrophil kinetics, and natural history of neonatal neutropenia associated with maternal hypertension. *N Engl J Med*. 1989;321(9):557-562.
178. Christensen RD, Henry E, Wiedmeier SE, Stoddard RA, Lambert DK. Low blood neutrophil concentrations among extremely low birth weight neonates: data from a multihospital health-care system. *J Perinatol*. 2006;26(11):682-687.
185. Schmutz N, Henry E, Jopling J, Christensen RD. Expected ranges for blood neutrophil concentrations of neonates: the Manroe and Mouzinho charts revisited. *J Perinatol*. 2008;28(4):275-281.
187. Adrover JM, Del Fresno C, Crainiciuc G, et al. A neutrophil timer coordinates immune defense and vascular protection. *Immunity*. 2019;50(2):390-402.
188. Winter C, Silvestre-Roig C, Ortega-Gomez A, et al. Chrono-pharmacological targeting of the CCL2-CCR2 axis ameliorates atherosclerosis. *Cell Metab*. 2018;28(1):175-182.
189. Zhang D, Chen G, Manwani D, et al. Neutrophil ageing is regulated by the microbiome. *Nature*. 2015;525(7570):528-532.
190. Lawrence SM, Corriden R, Nizet V. Age-appropriate functions and dysfunctions of the neonatal neutrophil. *Front Pediatr*. 2017;5(23):1-15.

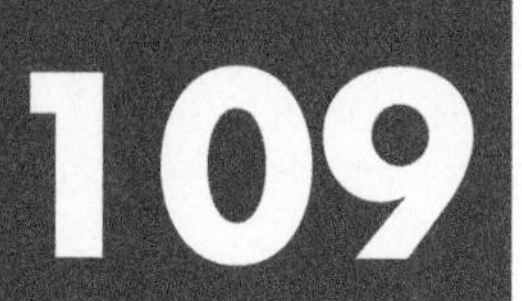

109 Developmental Erythropoiesis

Timothy M. Bahr | Robin K. Ohls

ERYTHROCYTE KINETICS

SITES AND STAGES OF FETAL RED BLOOD CELL PRODUCTION

EXTRAEMBRYONIC ERYTHROPOIESIS

Extraembryonic erythropoiesis begins in the fetal yolk sac by 14 days' gestation. Small nests of nucleated blood cells are present in the mesenchymal and endodermal layers of the yolk sac.[1] These red blood cells, or hematocytoblasts, are the product of primitive megaloblastic erythropoiesis,[2] and they differ from erythrocytes formed later in gestation when definitive normoblastic erythropoiesis occurs. Primitive erythroblasts are nucleated and macrocytic (20 to 25 μm in diameter). They have a mean corpuscular volume (MCV) of more than 180 fL and have a characteristic fine nuclear chromatin pattern and a polychromatophilic cytoplasm containing abundant hemoglobin.[2,3] Red blood cells enter the embryonic circulation at 3 to 4 weeks' gestation, coincident with joining of the vitelline and umbilical circulations.[4]

INTRAEMBRYONIC ERYTHROPOIESIS

Definitive normoblastic erythropoiesis of the fetus begins in the liver during the early first trimester.[5] By 6 to 8 weeks' gestation, the liver replaces the yolk sac as the primary site of red blood cell production, and by 10 to 12 weeks' gestation, extraembryonic erythropoiesis has essentially ceased. Red blood cell production occurs in the liver throughout the remainder of gestation, although production begins to diminish during the second trimester as bone marrow erythropoiesis increases (Fig. 109.1). Erythroblasts are first noted in the marrow at 8 to 9 weeks' gestation.[5] By the end of the third trimester, almost all erythropoiesis is occurring in the bone marrow, although residual erythropoiesis may continue in the liver and may be found in other sites. In rodents, the spleen is also a site of erythropoiesis before the onset of marrow red blood cell production. As with the liver, this site ceases production shortly after birth.[6] It is unclear whether the spleen contributes to erythropoiesis in the human fetus. Although erythroid precursors have been identified as early as 6 to 7 weeks' gestation in human splenic tissue,[7] it is not clear whether such cells are actually developing within splenic tissue or whether they are simply part of the circulation.[8]

ONTOGENY OF STEM CELLS

Red blood cell precursors in the yolk sac are extremely primitive cells, and they may either disappear or seed other areas where erythropoiesis later becomes prominent. The *unicentric theory* proposes that all hematopoietic stem cells originate from the yolk sac, then migrate from one hematopoietic site to another. Moore and Metcalf[9] demonstrated circulating pluripotent stem cells in the peripheral blood just before the development of liver erythropoiesis. They suggested that the development of intraembryonic hematopoiesis requires an intact yolk sac, and migration of stem cells from the yolk sac to hematopoietic tissue is necessary for the development of intraembryonic hematopoiesis. The development of other organ systems via migration of cells (such as neural crest tissue) gives credence to this theory.

The *multicentric theory* suggests that a new clonal formation of hematopoietic stem cells occurs at different sites of hematopoiesis

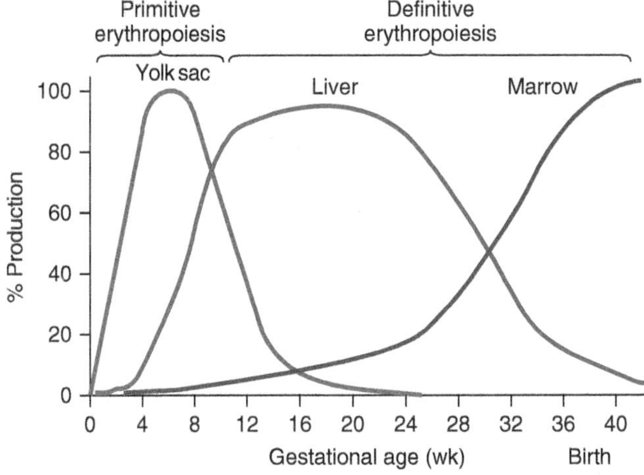

Fig. 109.1 Sites and stages of fetal erythropoiesis. Primitive erythropoiesis begins in the yolk sac at 2 to 3 weeks after conception. By the end of the first trimester the liver has become the primary erythroid organ. The liver is the primary source of red blood cells during the second trimester, whereas the bone marrow is the primary source of red blood cells during the last trimester.

during fetal development. Yolk sac cells are capable of producing granulocytic, megakaryocytic, and erythroid colonies when transplanted into adult irradiated recipients and in conditioned newborn recipients,[9,10] a finding that supports the view that fetal stem cells possess the capacity to be pluripotent and their differentiation is controlled by microenvironmental factors.

MARROW, LIVER, AND BLOOD DIFFERENTIALS

Table 109.1 describes the differential counts in fetal liver, marrow, and circulating blood according to gestational age.[11-14] The liver of the second-trimester human fetus is the primary organ for erythropoiesis, with a myeloid-to-erythroid ratio ranging from 0.07 at 14 to 17 weeks' gestation to 0.2 at 21 to 24 weeks' gestation.[11] By 24 weeks the composition of the fetal bone marrow begins to resemble that of adult bone marrow, differing by the presence of a large number of stromal elements, the absence of plasma cells and lymph follicles, and an overall increased cellularity in the fetal bone marrow. Unlike adult bone marrow, large fat cells are not present in fetal bone marrow. Between 18 and 22 weeks' gestation, the mitotic index of the fetal bone marrow becomes virtually identical to that of adult bone marrow. The fetal bone marrow myeloid-to-erythroid ratio starts to exceed the normal adult bone marrow ratio (1.5 ± 0.4) early in midgestation and remains elevated even at the time of birth.

PROGENITOR CELL CONCENTRATIONS

Studies of bone marrow cells in tissue culture have identified specific committed red blood cell precursors, termed *erythroid progenitors,*[15-18] on the basis of their characteristic growth in vitro. When bone marrow cells are placed in semisolid media culture systems for 5 to 7 days, an erythropoietin *(EPO)*-sensitive erythroid progenitor cell, termed *colony-forming unit-erythroid* (CFU-E), clonally matures into a single cluster containing 30 to 100 normoblasts (Fig. 109.2). An erythroid-specific progenitor that is less differentiated than a CFU-E (and therefore a more primitive cell) is termed a *burst-forming unit-erythroid* (BFU-E). Twelve to 14 days after cultures of bone marrow cells are initiated, a BFU-E develops into a large, multicentered colony of normoblasts, in which each center contains 200 to 10,000 normoblasts. Finally, the most primitive erythroid progenitor cell identifiable through in vitro culture is termed a *colony-forming unit-granulocyte, erythrocyte, macrophage, megakaryocyte* (CFU-GEMM, or CFU-MIX). Twelve to 14 days after marrow cells are placed in culture, this multipotent progenitor develops into a mixed colony of both normoblast clusters and granulocyte-macrophage clusters.

The ability of an organ to produce red blood cells is based on the number of progenitor cells it contains, as well as the growth factors stimulating those cells to proliferate. Determination of erythroid progenitor numbers obtained from cell suspensions of liver, marrow, spleen, and blood of second-trimester human fetuses (Table 109.2) showed twice the number of multipotent progenitors and erythroid progenitors in the fetal liver compared with marrow.[8,11,12] Erythroid progenitors from fetal liver also appeared to be more sensitive to *EPO* (the primary erythroid growth factor) than were progenitors from fetal marrow. Progenitor cell concentrations in the spleen were nearly identical to concentrations in the circulation.[8-12] Whether the progenitors isolated from liver and marrow represent different subpopulations of progenitors (e.g., populations that express different erythroid growth factor receptors, different receptor numbers, different receptor affinity, or different cycling rates) is not known.

REGULATION OF ERYTHROPOIESIS

Erythropoietic regulation in the human fetus differs markedly from that in the adult. In the adult, erythropoietic regulation primarily involves maintaining the red blood cell mass. In contrast,

Table 109.1 Differential Counts in Liver, Marrow, and Blood During Gestation.

Differential Counts (Percentage ± SD) of Liver Cell Suspensions From Fetuses at a Gestational Age of 14–24 wk

	Gestational Age (wk)		
Cells	**14–17 (*n* = 5)**	**18–20 (*n* = 7)**	**21–24 (*n* = 8)**
Normoblast			
Pronormoblast	3.1 ± 1.4	3.4 ± 1.0	2.9 ± 1.8
Basophilic	18.4 ± 7.6	13.7 ± 1.6	13.7 ± 4.7
Polychromatophilic	57.5 ± 12.6	55.3 ± 7.5	51.1 ± 5.5
Orthochromic	13.9 ± 5.2	15.9 ± 3.7	14.2 ± 5.0
Total erythroid cells	9.3 ± 6.3	87.8 ± 4.8	81.9 ± 5.0
Neutrophil			
Promyelocyte	0 ± 0	0.2 ± 0.2[a]	1.2 ± 0.4[a,b]
Myelocyte	0 ± 0	0 ± 0	0.2 ± 0.2[a,b]
Metamyelocyte	0 ± 0	0 ± 0	0 ± 0
Band	0 ± 0	0 ± 0	0 ± 0
Segmented	0 ± 0	0 ± 0	0 ± 0
Total neutrophils	0 ± 0	0.2 ± 0.2	1.4 ± 0.5[a,b]
Undifferentiated blast	0.5 ± 0.6	3.1 ± 1.8[a]	2.2 ± 0.7[a]
Macrophage	0.5 ± 0.6	1.2 ± 4.0[a]	1.3 ± 5.0
Lymphocyte	5.4 ± 2.6	3.9 ± 3.6	11.3 ± 4.2[a,b]
Eosinophil	0 ± 0	0 ± 0	0 ± 0
Other[c]	0.8 ± 0.8	3.4 ± 2.4	1.9 ± 2.4

Differential Counts (Percentage ± SD) of Marrow Cell Suspensions From Fetuses at a Gestational Age of 14–24 wk

	Gestational Age (wk)		
Cells	**14–17 (*n* = 6)**	**18–20 (*n* = 6)**	**21–24 (*n* = 8)**
Normoblast			
Pronormoblast	0.3 ± 0.2[d]	1.1 ± 0.4[d]	0.5 ± 0.2[d]
Basophilic	1.4 ± 0.6[d]	3.1 ± 0.8[d]	1.7 ± 1.0[d]
Polychromatophilic	9.2 ± 5.0[d]	12.9 ± 6.2[d]	12.3 ± 5.2[d]
Orthochromic	12.1 ± 11.1	20.7 ± 12.2	8.1 ± 4.4
Total erythroid cells	23.0 ± 13.3[d]	37.8 ± 16.8[d]	22.6 ± 9.0[d]
Neutrophil			
Promyelocyte	5.9 ± 2.9[d]	5.8 ± 2.6[d]	5.0 ± 1.7[d]
Myelocyte	2.7 ± 1.4[d]	3.4 ± 1.6[d]	2.1 ± 1.0[d]
Metamyelocyte	2.1 ± 1.0[d]	2.5 ± 1.8[d]	1.7 ± 1.0[d]
Band	3.1 ± 1.8[d]	3.2 ± 2.7[d]	1.6 ± 1.2[d]
Segmented	1.2 ± 1.3[d]	1.1 ± 1.3[d]	0.4 ± 0.2[d]
Total neutrophils	13.8 ± 6.1[d]	16.1 ± 8.0[d]	10.7 ± 5.0[d]
Undifferentiated blast	8.9 ± 12.4[d]	11.4 ± 5.4[d]	11.6 ± 3.6[d]
Macrophage	5.4 ± 3.8[d]	4.2 ± 2.4[d]	3.1 ± 1.6[d]
Lymphocyte	35.3 ± 15.8[d]	28.8 ± 8.0[d]	50.3 ± 6.8[d]
Eosinophil	0.5 ± 0.6	1.1 ± 1.2	1.2 ± 0.8[d]
Other[e]	0.8 ± 0.4	0.5 ± 0.4	0.4 ± 0.2

Differential Counts (Percentage ± SD) of Umbilical Cord Blood Samples From Fetuses at a Gestational Age of 18–29 wk

	Gestational Age (wk)		
Cells	**18–21 (*n* = 186)**	**22–25 (*n* = 230)**	**26–29 (*n* = 144)**
Normoblast (%WBCs)	45.0 ± 86.0	21.0 ± 23.0	21.0 ± 67.0
Basophilic	0.5 ± 1.0	0.5 ± 1.0	0.5 ± 1.0
Neutrophil	6.0 ± 4.0	6.5 ± 3.5	8.5 ± 4.0
Lymphocyte	88.0 ± 7.0	87.0 ± 6.0	85.0 ± 6.0
Eosinophil	2.0 ± 3.0	3.0 ± 3.0	4.0 ± 3.0
Monocyte	3.5 ± 2.0	3.0 ± 2.5	3.0 ± 2.5

[a]$P < .05$ versus 14 to 17 weeks.
[b]$P < .05$ versus 18 to 20 weeks.
[c]Hepatocyte, megakaryocyte, or cell of undetermined origin.
[d]$P < .05$ versus fetal liver.
[e]Megakaryocyte or cell of undetermined origin.
WBCs, White blood cells.

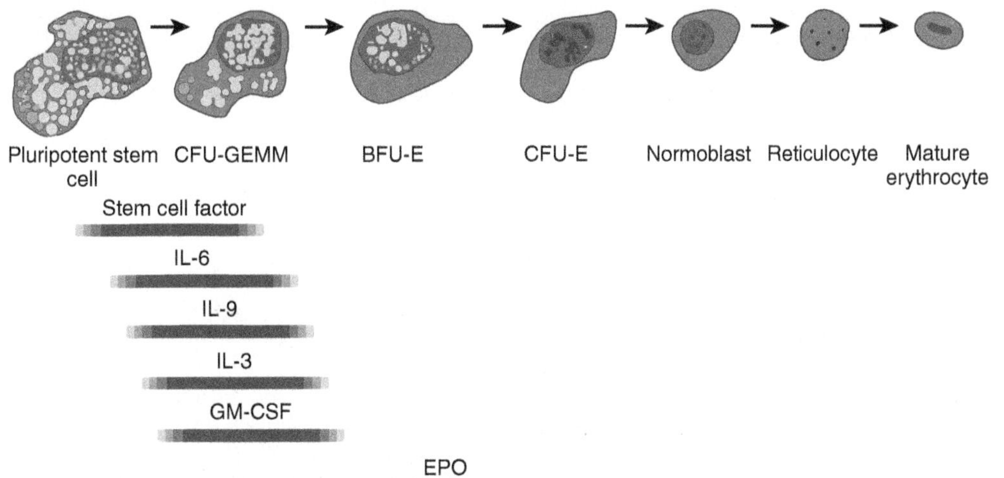

Fig. 109.2 Erythropoietic progenitors and the growth factors influencing erythropoiesis. *BFU-E,* Burst-forming unit–erythroid; *CFU-E,* colony-forming unit–erythroid; *CFU-GEMM,* colony-forming unit–granulocyte, erythrocyte, macrophage, and megakaryocyte; *EPO,* erythropoietin; *GM-CSF,* granulocyte-macrophage colony-stimulating factor; *IL-3,* interleukin-3; *IL-6,* interleukin-6; *IL-9,* interleukin-9.

Table 109.2 Progenitor Cell Concentrations in Fetal Liver, Marrow, Spleen, and Blood.

	CFU-MIX	BFU-E
Liver	12.7 ± 2.1	20.7 ± 3.1
Marrow	6.7 ± 1.4[a]	9.3 ± 2.7[a]
Spleen	4.2 ± 2.7[a]	5.9 ± 3.7[a]
Blood	–	8.0 ± 5.4[a]

[a] $P < .05$ versus liver.
Numbers represent cell concentrations per 5 × 10^3 cells plated.
BFU-E, Burst-forming unit–erythroid; *CFU-MIX,* colony-forming unit–granulocyte, erythrocyte, macrophage, and megakaryocyte.

constant and dramatic changes characterize erythropoiesis in the embryo and fetus. The incredible rate of somatic growth and the resultant need to constantly increase the fetal red blood cell mass necessitate an extraordinary erythropoietic effort. Moreover, the relatively low oxygen tensions but high metabolic rates of fetal tissues require a system of oxygen delivery that differs significantly from the adult system.

ERYTHROID GROWTH FACTORS

The production of erythrocytes, from pluripotent stem cell to mature red blood cell, is governed by various growth factors. These erythropoietic growth factors are produced by accessory cells such as liver macrophages and marrow stromal cells, and they stimulate maturation, growth, and differentiation at various stages of red blood cell production. The progenitors involved in red blood cell production and the factors that stimulate their cellular maturation are depicted in Fig. 109.2. Although these growth factors all facilitate production of red blood cells, none plays a more important regulatory role than *EPO*. *EPO* is a 30- to 39-kDa glycoprotein that binds to specific receptors on the surface of erythroid precursors and stimulates their differentiation and clonal maturation into mature erythrocytes.[19,20] The *EPO* gene *(EPO)* is located on chromosome band 7q21-22.[21] During fetal erythropoiesis, *EPO* is produced principally by cells of monocyte/macrophage origin residing in the liver. Postnatally, *EPO* is produced almost exclusively by peritubular cells of the kidney.

Other growth factors besides *EPO* play a role in the differentiation and clonal expansion of erythroid progenitors. These include granulocyte-macrophage colony-stimulating factor (GM-CSF),[15] stem cell factor (also known as *c-kit ligand*),[22] and interleukin (IL)-3, IL-6, IL-9, and IL-12.[23-26] Thrombopoietin, a growth factor involved in platelet production whose receptor is similar in structure to the *EPO* receptor, also stimulates erythroid colony formation.[27] IL-3 and GM-CSF were the first growth factors noted to have erythroid-stimulating properties, initially described as "burst-promoting activity." In combination with *EPO,* these factors synergistically stimulate differentiation and proliferation of BFUs-E and CFUs-GEMM.

Stem cell factor is a multipotent growth factor that, in combination with other factors, supports clonal maturation of hematopoietic progenitors. Murine studies indicate that stem cell factor may be expressed during embryogenesis, thereby affecting embryonic and fetal erythropoiesis. In vitro studies show that stem cell factor alone stimulates clonal maturation of fetal (but not adult) multipotent progenitors. Erythroid progenitors isolated from term umbilical cord blood are more responsive to stem cell factor, alone and in synergism with GM-CSF and IL-3, than are adult marrow progenitors.[22]

Term circulating erythroid progenitors are also more sensitive to IL-6 and IL-9 than are adult progenitors.[24] IL-6 is a multifunctional, 22- to 26-kDa glycoprotein cytokine involved in B-cell stimulation and immunoglobulin production, acute-phase reactions, and induction of hematopoietic progenitors from a noncycling (G_0) phase into an active cycling (S) phase. IL-6 alone supports clonogenic maturation of newborn umbilical cord blood BFUs-E and CFUs-GEMM and induces progenitor cell cycling.[24] IL-9 is also a multipotent cytokine and is similar to IL-6 in its ability to stimulate primitive erythroid progenitors and multipotent progenitors isolated from umbilical cord blood.[25] Insulin-like growth factor 1 has been shown to cause clonal expansion of erythroid progenitors isolated from adult marrow[28,29] and on erythroid and mesenchymal-like cells in the fetal spleen. A recently identified growth factor termed *regulator of human erythroid cell expansion* is an erythroid growth factor that promotes formation of hemoglobinizing erythroblasts.[30] It comprises a new *EPO/EPO* receptor target and regulator of human erythroid cell expansion that additionally acts to support late-stage erythroblast development.

UNIQUE FEATURES OF FETAL PROGENITORS

Fetal erythroid progenitors respond in a slightly different fashion than do adult erythroid progenitors. In addition to the features noted earlier, fetal progenitors appear more sensitive to *EPO* than adult erythroid progenitors.[31] Specifically, BFUs-E of fetal origin develop more rapidly into erythroid colonies, and the colonies generally contain significantly more normoblasts. In addition, BFUs-E from adult bone marrow require a combination of *EPO* plus another factor, such as IL-3 or GM-CSF, to mature clonally;

Table 109.3 Blood Cell Indices During Gestation.

Gestational Age (wk)	White Blood Cells[a] (×10⁹/L)	Total White Blood Cells (×10⁹/L)	Platelets (×10⁹/L)	Red Blood Cells (×10¹²/L)	Hemoglobin (g/dL)	Hematocrit (%)	Mean Corpuscular Volume (fL)
18–21 (*n* = 760)	4.68 ± 2.96	2.57 ± 0.42	234 ± 57	2.85 ± 0.36	11.69 ± 1.27	37.3 ± 4.3	131.1 ± 11.0
22–25 (*n* = 1200)	4.72 ± 2.82	3.73 ± 2.17	247 ± 59	3.09 ± 0.34	12.2 ± 1.6	38.6 ± 3.9	125.1 ± 7.8
26–29 (*n* = 460)	5.16 ± 2.53	4.08 ± 0.84	242 ± 69	3.46 ± 0.41	12.91 ± 1.38	40.9 ± 4.4	118.5 ± 8.0
>30 (*n* = 440)	7.71 ± 4.99	6.40 ± 2.99	232 ± 87	3.82 ± 0.64	13.64 ± 2.21	43.6 ± 7.2	114.4 ± 9.3

[a]Including normoblasts.
From Forestier F, Daffos F, Catherine N. Developmental hematopoiesis in normal human fetal blood. *Blood*. 1991;77:2360.

however, many fetal BFUs-E mature in the presence of *EPO* alone.[32] Studies have shown that fetal clones produce GM-CSF and IL-3, which may explain their unique capability for growth factor independence and auto-stimulation.[33]

CONTROL OF ERYTHROPOIETIN PRODUCTION

Erythropoiesis in utero is controlled by erythroid growth factors produced by the fetus, not the mother. *EPO* is the primary regulator of erythropoiesis in adults and appears to be the controlling factor for fetal erythropoiesis, especially during late gestation. *EPO* does not cross the placenta in humans,[34,35] monkeys, or sheep,[36] although it has been reported to do so in mice.[37] In the mouse, suppression of maternal erythropoiesis by hypertransfusion does not suppress fetal erythropoiesis.[38] In humans, stimulation of maternal *EPO* production does not result in stimulation of fetal red blood cell production.[39]

The expression of *EPO* is thought to be controlled by an oxygen-sensing mechanism in the liver and kidney.[40] Both hypoxia and anemia stimulate erythropoiesis by stimulating messenger RNA (mRNA) transcription and *EPO* production.[41] Two factors, hepatic nuclear factor 4 and hypoxia-inducible factor 1 (HIF-1), serve as transcription factors for *EPO* as well as other hypoxia-inducible genes. Hepatic nuclear factor 4 binds to the *EPO* promoter and enhancer regions of the gene. HIF-1 is a basic helix-loop-helix transcription factor composed of HIF-1α and HIF-1β subunits that bind to *cis*-acting hypoxia-response elements and induce *EPO* transcription. HIF-1 is expressed in many cells and is involved in up-regulating a variety of oxygen-regulated proteins, including vascular endothelial growth factor. HIF-1α appears to be constitutively expressed and rapidly degraded under normoxic conditions. RNA stability depends on the ubiquitin proteasome degradation system; inhibition of this system leads to increased levels of HIF-1 and *EPO*, even under normoxic conditions. Promoter and enhancer elements within the *EPO* gene are responsive to hypoxia, as well as to cobalt exposure in vitro.[42] In animal models, the liver-sensing mechanism has a decreased sensitivity to hypoxia, producing one tenth the amount of *EPO* in response to comparable stimuli in the kidney.[43,44] The liver also appears to require more prolonged hypoxia to achieve an *EPO* response.[45,46] Other substances, including testosterone,[47] estrogen,[48] thyroid hormone,[49] prostaglandins,[50] vitamin E,[51] and lipoproteins,[52] have been shown to enhance *EPO* production or its effects, both in vivo and in vitro.[53,54]

It is not known what factors regulate the switch of *EPO* production from the liver to the kidney. Renal production of *EPO* is not necessary for normal fetal erythropoiesis.[55] The lack of a renal contribution to *EPO* production is illustrated by the normal serum *EPO* concentrations and normal hematocrits of anephric fetuses.[56] In the sheep, *EPO* production in both the liver and the kidney is highest at 60 days' gestation (term being 140 days).[57] *EPO* production in the fetal liver decreases by 90 days' gestation; however, increased renal production of *EPO* continues until 130 days' gestation, when production falls to levels seen in adult sheep.[58]

Studies in human fetal and neonatal kidney obtained from postmortem specimens also report measurable quantities of *EPO* mRNA,[59] and quantitative mRNA studies in second-trimester human fetuses reveal that the fetal kidney produces approximately 5% of the amount of *EPO* mRNA that the fetal liver produces during the second trimester.[60] Thus it appears that regulation of *EPO* gene transcription differs between the liver and the kidney in utero.

One mechanism by which gene expression can be differentially regulated is through methylation of promoter and enhancer regions of a gene, and another is through deacetylation of histones.[61-65] Increased methylation generally results in decreased gene expression, whereas histone deacetylation causes relaxation of DNA structures and allows gene expression to occur. These two mechanisms may be involved in developmental *EPO* gene expression. For example, methylation of the enhancer region (leading to decreased expression) of the *EPO* gene in developing human kidney during the second trimester was much greater than in the liver.[66]

EPO levels have been measured in umbilical cord blood during the third trimester, and these levels gradually increase throughout later development.[67-69] From *EPO* measurements made in umbilical cord blood from infants of laboring and nonlaboring mothers[70] and from infants undergoing labor stress,[71-75] it seems likely that individual umbilical cord *EPO* levels primarily reflect hypoxic stress during labor and delivery. Serum *EPO* concentrations at birth normally range from 5 to 100 mU/mL. For comparison, serum *EPO* concentrations in anemic, nonuremic adults may be as high as 300 to 400 mU/mL.[76,77]

RED BLOOD CELL INDICES IN THE FETUS AND NEONATE

RED BLOOD CELL CONCENTRATIONS AND HEMATOCRIT

Red blood cell indices change during gestation and continue to change through the first year of life. Circulating red blood cell concentrations gradually increase during the second trimester, from (2.85 ± 0.36) × 10^6/μL at 18 to 21 weeks to (3.82 ± 0.64) × 10^6/μL at 30 weeks (Table 109.3).[12] At term gestation, circulating red blood cell concentrations range from 5.0 × 10^6 to 5.5 × 10^6/μL.[78] In parallel with increasing red blood cell concentrations, hematocrits increase from 30% to 40% during the second trimester and continue to increase to term values over the latter part of the third trimester.[78] Changes in hematocrit from 22 to 42 weeks' gestation can be seen in Fig. 109.3.[79] Term hematocrits range from 50% to 63%, with some variability noted because of delayed clamping of the umbilical cord.[80] Values are also dependent on the sampling site. Capillary hemoglobin concentrations are as much as 3.5 g/dL higher than venous hemoglobin concentrations.[81]

HEMOGLOBIN

The hemoglobin concentration gradually rises during gestation.[82] At 10 weeks gestation the average hemoglobin concentration is approximately 9 g/dL.[83] By 22 to 24 weeks' gestation, fetal

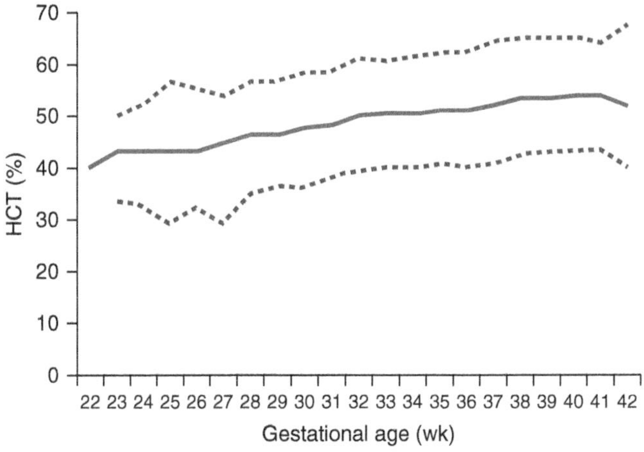

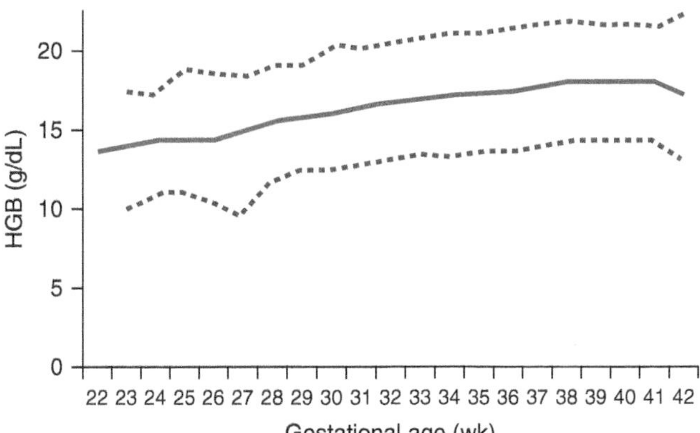

Fig. 109.3 Reference ranges for hematocrit and hemoglobin from 22 to 42 weeks' gestation. Reference ranges are shown for hematocrit *(HCT; upper panel)* and hemoglobin concentration *(HGB; lower panel)* at 22 to 42 weeks' gestation. Tests were done during a 6.5-year period on more than 20,000 neonates. Values were excluded when the diagnosis included abruption, placenta previa, or known cases of fetal anemia or when a blood transfusion was given before the first hematocrit was measured. The *solid line* represents the mean value, and the *dashed lines* represent the 5% and 95% reference range. (From Christensen RD, Jopling J, Henry E, et al. The erythrocyte indices of neonates, defined using data from over 12,000 patients in a multihospital system. *J Perinatal.* 2008;28:24–28.)

hemoglobin values reach 11 to 12 g/dL, and by 30 weeks the hemoglobin concentrations are 13 to 14 g/dL.[12] Premature male infants reach term umbilical cord hemoglobin values earlier than premature female infants,[84] possibly because of the erythropoietic effects of testosterone.[47] Hemoglobin concentrations are relatively constant during the last 6 to 8 weeks of gestation (see Fig. 109.3); at term the average hemoglobin concentration is approximately 16 to 17 g/dL.[85-87] An increase in hemoglobin concentration by 2 hours of postnatal life occurs in most infants, resulting from a decrease in plasma volume. By 8 to 12 hours after birth, the hemoglobin concentration achieves a relatively constant level. Red blood cell production decreases significantly at birth, so that hemoglobin concentrations gradually decline by the end of the first postnatal week.[80] The decrease in red blood cell production after birth is predominantly the result of increased availability of oxygen in the extrauterine environment, which greatly reduces *EPO* production and endogenous erythropoiesis. The continued fall in hemoglobin concentration over the next several weeks results from (1) decreased red blood cell production, (2) a shortened red blood cell life span of the fetal/neonatal erythrocyte, and (3) plasma dilution and an increase in blood volume related to growth. Multiple groups have also hypothesized that a process termed *neocytolysis* (the selective lysis of young erythrocytes) contributes to excessive hemolysis after birth, and thus a rapid decrease in hematocrit as the neonate adapts to its new, relatively hyperoxic environment.[88-90]

The nadir of hemoglobin concentration in term infants occurs at approximately 8 weeks, with an average hemoglobin concentration of 11.2 g/dL.[78,83] Hemoglobin values gradually rise such that, by 6 months, the average term infant has a hemoglobin concentration of 12.1 g/dL. Altitude may have a modest effect on the postnatal changes in hemoglobin concentration; infants living at 1600 m had higher hemoglobin concentrations (by 0.4 g/dL) by 6 months of age than infants living at sea level.[91,92]

The average decline in the hemoglobin concentration of preterm very low-birth-weight infants (<1500 g) is remarkably different from that of term infants, in part due to phlebotomy losses that invariably occur in preterm infants, as well as the effects of transfusions on endogenous erythropoiesis. Very low-birth-weight infants reach a nadir of hemoglobin concentration of 8 g/dL at 4 to 8 weeks of age.[93] Fig. 109.4 and Table 109.4 demonstrate relationships among birth weight, chronologic age, and red blood cell indices in term and preterm infants.[78,79,83,92-96]

Red blood cell indices may differ from normal ranges in infants born small for their gestational age, in whom placental insufficiency and secondary polycythemia are common.[91-98] Infants of diabetic mothers, infants of mothers who smoke, and infants born at higher altitudes also tend to have higher hemoglobin concentrations at birth.[91-96,98-100] In growth-restricted infants born to hypertensive mothers, the blood supply to the placenta and the capacity to deliver oxygen to the fetus are diminished. Accelerated erythropoiesis is likely part of a compensating mechanism that raises oxygen-carrying capacity, maintaining an adequate supply to the fetus. In infants of diabetic mothers, increased metabolic demands of the fetus (resulting from increased glucose availability) may account for higher fetal oxygen needs and compensatory increase in hemoglobin concentration by the fetus. The increased red blood cell mass in infants of diabetic mothers does not result from higher maternal levels of hemoglobin A_{1C} (a high-affinity hemoglobin capable of decreasing the oxygen transferred to the fetus). In mothers who smoke, the increase in fetal carbon monoxide and the subsequent decrease in available oxygen are the likely causes of the compensatory increase in hemoglobin levels in the fetus.

MEAN CORPUSCULAR VOLUME

The size of the red blood cell gradually decreases during development. The MCV is more than 180 fL in the embryo, falls to 130 fL by midgestation, and decreases to 115 fL by the end of pregnancy (Fig. 109.5). By 1 year of age, the MCV reaches an average of 82 fL.[95] Similar to cells of other organs in infants born prematurely, the red blood cell MCV declines quickly after birth, and the postpartum changes in MCV appear to be related to chronologic age rather than postmenstrual age.[94] The mean corpuscular hemoglobin concentrations remain relatively constant, and the mean corpuscular hemoglobin decreases slightly.[100]

BLOOD VOLUME

The placenta and umbilical cord contain 75 to 125 mL of blood at term, or approximately one fourth to one third of the fetal blood volume.[78] Umbilical arteries constrict shortly after birth, but the umbilical vein remains dilated, and blood flows in the direction of gravity. Infants held at or below the level of the placenta can receive half of the placental blood volume (30 to 50 mL) in 1 minute. Blood can also travel from the neonate into

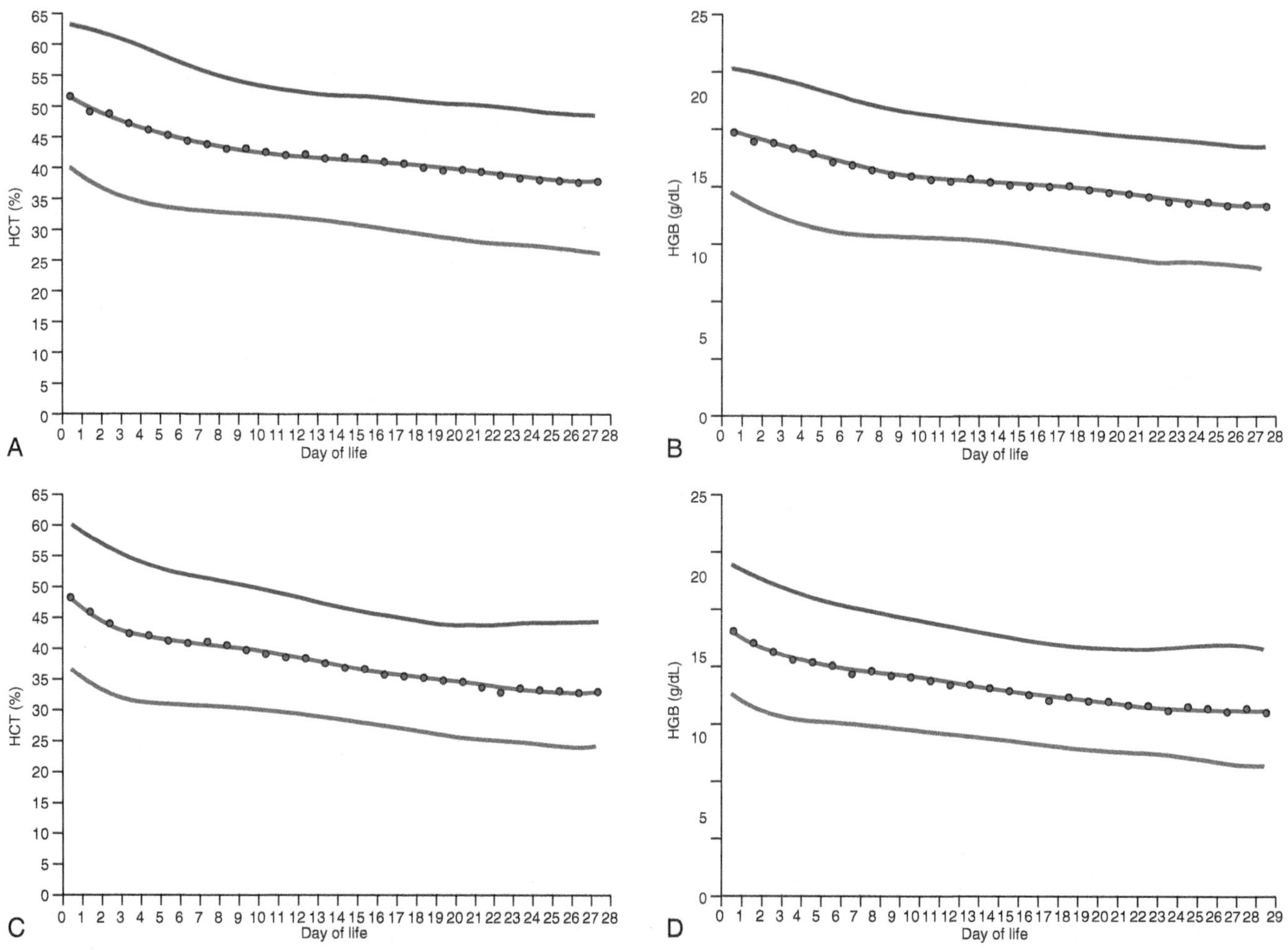

Fig. 109.4 Hematocrit and hemoglobin reference ranges for term and preterm infants in the first month of life. (A) Hematocrit *(HCT)* over the first 28 days of life for neonates born at 35 to 42 weeks' gestation. (B) Blood hemoglobin *(HGB)* concentration over the first 28 days of life for neonates born at 35 to 42 weeks' gestation. (C) HCT over the first 28 days of life for neonates born at 29 to 34 weeks' gestation. (D) Blood HGB concentration over the first 28 days of life for neonates born at 29 to 34 weeks' gestation. (Reprinted with permission from Henry E, Christensen RD. Reference intervals in neonatal hematology. *Clin Perinatol.* 2015;42:483–497.)

Table 109.4 Mean Hemoglobin Values (± 1 SD; g/dL) in Low-Birth-Weight Infants.

	Age (wk)				
Birth Weight (g)	**2**	**4**	**6**	**8**	**10**
800–1000	16.0 (14.8–17.2)	10.0 (6.8–13.2)	8.7 (7.0–10.2)	8.0 (7.1–9.8)	8.0 (6.9–10.2)
1001–1200	16.4 (14.1–18.7)	12.8 (7.8–15.3)	10.5 (7.2–12.3)	9.1 (7.8–10.4)	8.5 (7.0–10.0)
1201–1400	16.2 (13.6–18.8)	13.4 (8.8–16.2)	10.9 (8.5–13.3)	9.9 (8.0–11.8)	9.8 (8.4–11.3)
1401–1500	15.6 (13.4–17.8)	11.7 (9.7–13.7)	10.5 (9.1–11.9)	9.8 (8.4–12.0)	9.9 (8.4–11.4)
1501–2000	15.6 (13.5–17.7)	11.0 (9.6–14.0)	9.6 (8.8–11.5)	9.8 (8.4–12.1)	10.1 (8.6–11.8)

Data from Williams ML, Shoot RJ, O'Neal PL, et al. Role of dietary iron and fat in vitamin E deficiency anemia of infancy. *N Engl J Med.* 1975;292:887.

the placenta if there is a significant gradient, resulting in 20 to 30 mL of blood loss per minute.[101] Studies evaluating the benefits of delayed cord clamping or cord milking showed improvements in blood volume, hematocrit, decreased transfusions, decreased intraventricular hemorrhage (IVH), decreased late onset sepsis, and improved iron stores.[102]

The blood volume of infants with early umbilical cord clamping averages 72 mL/kg, while the blood volume of infants with delayed umbilical cord clamping averages 93 mL/kg. Preterm infants have slightly larger blood volumes (89 to 105 mL/kg), owing to an increased plasma volume. By 1 month of age, blood volumes in term infants average 73 to 77 mL/kg.

NUCLEATED RED BLOOD CELLS

Though nucleated red blood cells (NRBCs) are rarely observed in healthy adults and children, they are often observed in term and preterm neonates.[103-105] Multiple studies have hypothesized that high concentrations of NRBCs at birth (or within the first hours to days of life) are a marker of in utero hypoxia. Indeed, a high concentration of NRBCs at birth has been associated with an increased risk of developing IVH and/or retinopathy of

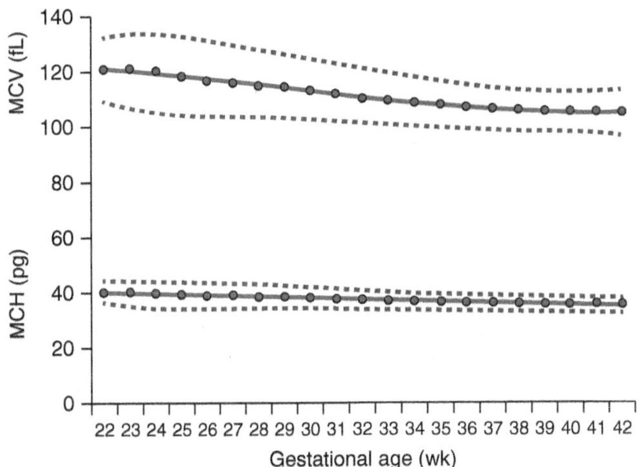

Fig. 109.5 Mean corpuscular volume *(MCV)* and mean corpuscular hemoglobin reference ranges from 22 to 42 weeks. Reference ranges are shown for the (MCV; *upper set of lines,* measured in femtoliters) and the mean corpuscular hemoglobin *(MCH)* concentration (*lower set of lines,* measured in picograms) at 22 to 42 weeks' gestation. Tests were done during a 6.5-year period on more than 20,000 neonates.

prematurity.[106-108] Placental abruption, intraamniotic infection, and intrauterine growth restriction have also been associated with significantly higher NRBCs at birth.[108] NRBCs are measured as either NRBC/μL or NRBC per 100 white blood cells (WBC; NRBC/100 WBC). The normative patterns of NRBCs are similar, regardless of units used. The number of NRBCs on the day of birth decreases from a median of ~25 NBRC/100 WBC for a neonate born at 23 to 28 weeks gestation to a median of 7 NRBC/100 WBC for a term neonate (Fig. 109.6).[108]

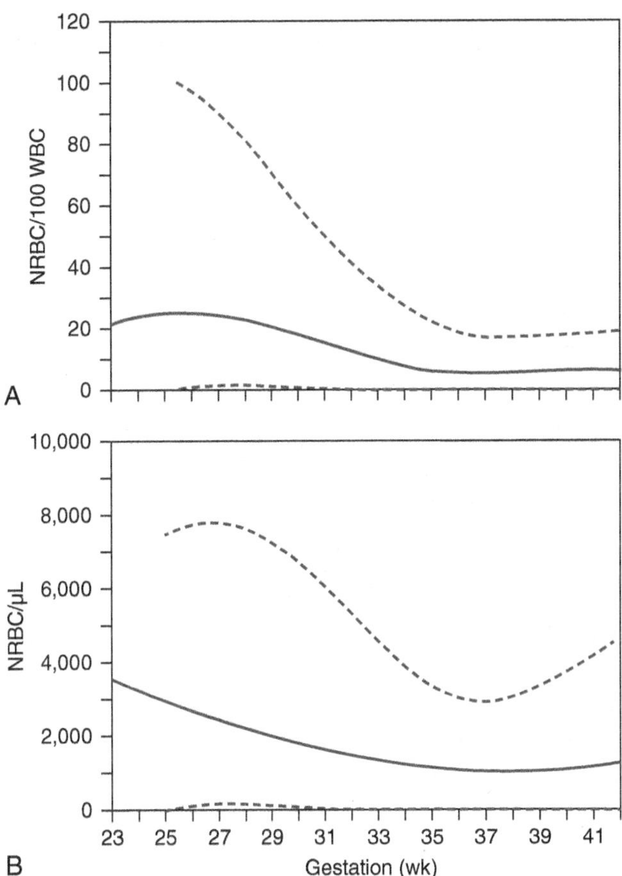

Fig. 109.6 Reference ranges for blood concentrations of nucleated red blood cell *(NRBC)* on the day of birth by gestational age. The *lower and upper lines* represent the 5th and 95th percentile limits. The *middle line* represents the mean value. (A) Data expressed as NRBC/100 white blood cell *(WBC)*. (B) Data expressed as NRBC/μL. (From Christensen RD, Henry E, Andres RL, et al. Reference ranges for blood concentrations of nucleated red blood cells in neonates. *Neonatology*. 2011;99[4]:289–294.)

RETICULOCYTE INDICES

Erythrocytes are released from the marrow into the blood as reticulocytes. The cytoplasmic organelles (e.g., ribosomes, mitochondria, Golgi apparatus) persist for 1 to 2 days after release before involution. Special staining detects elements of the residual organelles and allows for a manual reticulocyte count. Automated hematology counters that utilize flow cytometry have made more accurate reticulocyte enumeration possible because much larger samples of cells are evaluated than in a manual count. These analyzers also make it possible to identify subpopulations of reticulocytes that appear to be clinically helpful.

The reticulocyte count reflects the rate of effective erythropoiesis. Because *EPO* production and endogenous erythropoiesis falls dramatically after birth, the number of reticulocytes in circulation also falls. In an otherwise well neonate, the low number of reticulocytes in circulation persists through the first 90 days of life until the physiologic nadir of hemoglobin concentration is reached.[109]

The immature reticulocyte fraction (IRF) quantifies the proportion of reticulocytes that are particularly high in RNA as a ratio to total reticulocytes, and is an early and sensitive index of marrow erythropoietic activity. Because flow cytometric gating on automated hematology analyzers is not standardized, the IRF may vary among analyzer manufacturers for any given sample.

RED BLOOD CELL INDICES IN NEONATES WITH ANEUPLOIDY

Neonates with aneuploidy have consistent differences in their RBC indices. This phenomenon has been best described in neonates with trisomy 21.[110,111] Polycythemia at birth is common among this population. Henry and colleagues estimated that 33% of neonates with trisomy 21 have hematocrits over 65% during the first 3 days of life, and 14% have hematocrits over 70%.[112] Widness and colleagues reported elevated *EPO* concentrations in umbilical cord blood samples of neonates with trisomy 21, speculating that hypoxemia in utero resulted in elevated *EPO* and consequent polycythemia. In addition, neonates with trisomy 21 have an elevated MCV in the first 3 days of life.[112]

Less data is available on the hematologic abnormalities in neonates with trisomy 18 and trisomy 13. Like neonates with trisomy 21, platelet and leukocyte abnormalities are more pronounced. Wiedmeier and colleagues observed anemia in 40% and polycythemia in 17% of neonates with trisomy 18. Only 1 of 22 neonates in their cohort with trisomy 13 had abnormal erythrocyte findings.[113]

FETOMATERNAL RED BLOOD CELL TRANSFER

Maternal and fetal circulating cells may, at different times, cross the placental barrier. Fetal contamination of the maternal circulation can occur before delivery, as evidenced by studies of maternal blood group immunization. About 50% to 75% of pregnancies are associated with some degree of fetomaternal transfer of blood. This event is uncommon in the first trimester (3%). The volumes of fetal transplacental transfer are relatively small, usually on the order of 0.01 to 0.1 mL, but on occasion they may be much greater. About one pregnancy in 400 is associated with fetal transplacental bleeding of 30 mL or greater, and about one pregnancy in 2000 is associated with a potential fetal transplacental hemorrhage of 100 mL or more.[114] The overall risk of Rh immunization occurring in an Rh-incompatible pregnancy is 16% if the fetus is Rh positive and ABO compatible with its mother. This risk decreases to 1.5% if the fetus is Rh positive and ABO incompatible. Fetal transfer of cells to the mother occurs during abortions as well (about a 2% incidence of such a transfer with spontaneous abortion and a 4% to 5% rate if abortion is induced).[115] Because fetal hemoglobin is resistant to acid elution, cells containing fetal hemoglobin can be distinguished from cells containing hemoglobin A. The Kleihauer-Betke stain of peripheral maternal blood uses this characteristic of fetal hemoglobin to detect fetal cells in the maternal circulation,[116] although results from mothers with increased fetal hemoglobin synthesis (i.e., sickle cell disease, thalassemia, and hereditary persistence of fetal hemoglobin) are not reliable. Diagnosis of fetomaternal hemorrhage may also be missed when the mother and infant are ABO compatible. In these cases, the fetal cells are rapidly cleared from the maternal circulation by maternal anti-A or anti-B antibodies.

ERYTHROCYTE BIOCHEMISTRY

During fetal erythropoiesis, an orderly evolution of the production of different hemoglobins occurs. Eight globin genes direct the synthesis of six different polypeptide chains, designated α, β, γ, δ, ε, and ζ. These globin chains combine in the developing erythroblast to form seven different hemoglobin tetramers: hemoglobin Gower 1 (ζ_2-ε_2), hemoglobin Gower 2 (α_2-ε_2), hemoglobin Portland I (ζ_2-γ_2), hemoglobin Portland II (ζ_2-β_2), fetal hemoglobin (α_2-γ_2), hemoglobin A (α_2-β_2), and hemoglobin A_2 (α_2-δ_2).

GLOBIN GENES

The globin genes are organized into two clusters (Fig. 109.7). The α-like genes are located along a 20-kb distal segment of the short arm of chromosome 16. The cluster contains three functional genes (α_1, α_2, and ζ_2), three pseudogenes (evolutionary remnants of genes that are not expressed because of inactivating mutations that prevent production of a functional globin protein), and one gene of undetermined function (a globin-like gene without inactivating mutations). The β-like gene cluster is located along a 60-kb segment of the short arm of chromosome 11 and contains five functional genes (β, δ, $^G\gamma$, $^A\gamma$, and ε) and one pseudogene. Within each complex, the genes are all in the same 5′ to 3′ orientation and are arranged in the order in which they are expressed during development.[117]

The α genes are duplicated in humans. Each α gene is approximately 4 kb long, interrupted by two small nonhomologous regions. The exons and first introns of the two α-globin genes have identical sequences, but the second intron of α_1 is nine bases longer and differs by three bases from that of the α_2 gene. Despite the high degree of homology between these two genes, the sequences diverge in the 3′ untranslated regions, 13 bases beyond the TAA stop codon. Because of these sequence differences, the relative output of the two genes can be measured: α_2 mRNA is produced 2 to 3 times more abundantly than α_1 mRNA in fetal liver and marrow and in fetal and adult erythrocytes.[117]

The ζ gene appears critical to normal fetal development. In a murine model, both α-gene and ζ-gene expression can be measured from the onset of erythropoiesis in the yolk sac.[118] In addition, expression of both genes occurs concomitantly within the same cells. Expression of the ζ gene occurs predominantly through the first 6 to 8 weeks of gestation, although minute quantities of ζ-globin can be measured in fetal and neonatal red blood cells.[119]

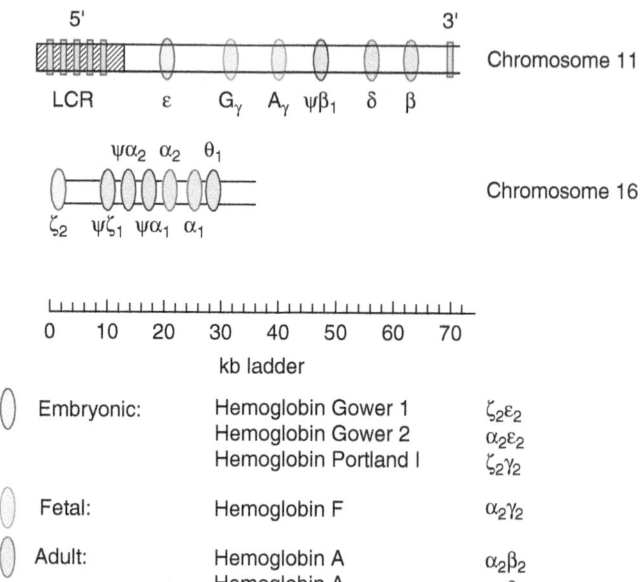

Fig. 109.7 Organization of the globin genes. Transcription of messenger RNA occurs from the 5′ to the 3′ end, and for both chromosomes the genes are arranged in order of their developmental activation. The *upper segment* represents the β-like globin genes on the short arm of chromosome 11, and the *lower segment* represents the α-like genes on the distal part of the short arm of chromosome 16. Regions of the gene that code for primary globin proteins are shown as *shaded ovals*, and regions that code for pseudogenes (ψ-nonexpressed remnants, which have a number of inactivating mutations that prevent transcription and translation into functional globin protein) are shown as *open ovals*. θ_1 is a globin-like gene without inactivating mutations. The locus control region *(LCR)* is shown as a *hatched segment* and contains five DNase I hypersensitivity sites, represented by *rectangles*. A downstream hypersensitivity site known as *3′ hypersensitivity site 1* is shown at the 3′ end. The composition of embryonic, fetal, and adult hemoglobins is listed.

Like the α_1 and α_2 genes, the $^G\gamma$ and $^A\gamma$ genes appear to be virtually identical over a span of 1.5 kb, suggesting a mechanism for gene matching during evolution. Amino acid sequencing of normal umbilical cord blood has shown that either glycine ($^G\gamma$) or alanine ($^A\gamma$) is present at the 136 position in the γ chain.[120] Short-chain organic acids, such as butyrate and acetate, increase γ-gene promoter activity. This activity can be enhanced even further by incorporation of sections of the β-gene locus control region.[121,122]

The β-globin gene cluster occupies a region of approximately 17 kb on the short arm of chromosome 11.[117] Each of its constituent genes, their flanking regions, and large stretches of the regions between them have been sequenced. Studies suggest that the transcription factor NF-E1 regulates increased β-globin gene expression during erythroid maturation. Deletion of the NF-E1 binding site in the upstream segment of the β-globin promoter blocks induction of transcription in murine leukemia cells.[123]

δ-Globin gene expression occurs early at the erythroid progenitor stage. By the reticulocyte stage, no δ-globin mRNA synthesis can be detected. The δ-globin gene promoter functions at a much lower level than the β-globin gene promoter, resulting in significantly lower levels of δ-globin mRNA production. In addition, decreased expression occurs because of a globin promoter–specific silencer element located upstream of the δ-globin gene.[124] Moreover, δ-globin mRNA is less stable than β-globin mRNA, which likely accounts for the early cessation of

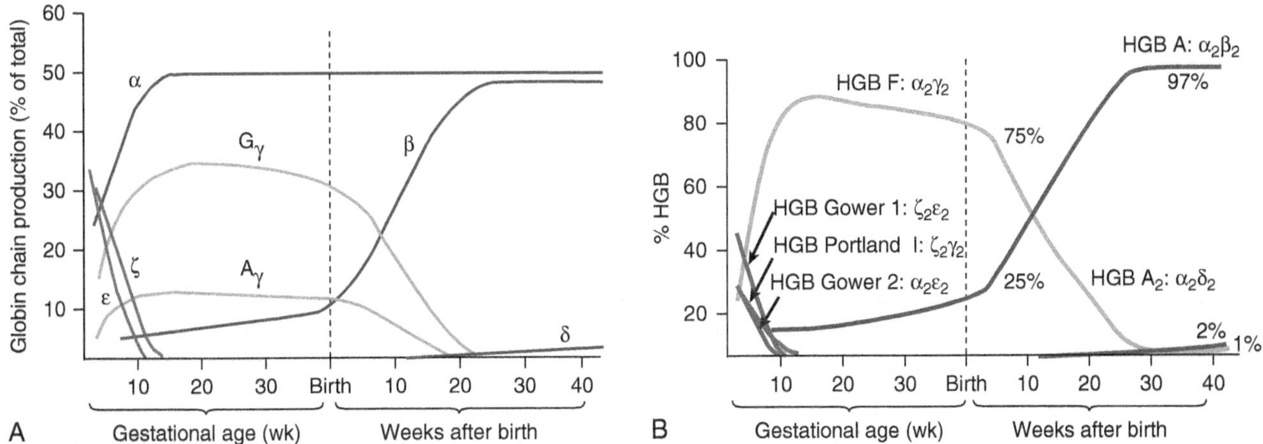

Fig. 109.8 Changes in globin subunits (A) and hemoglobin tetramers (B) during human development from the embryo to early infancy. *HGB*, Hemoglobin. (Data collated from Bunn HF, Forget BG. *Hemoglobin: Molecular, Genetic and Clinical Aspects.* Philadelphia: WB Saunders; 1986:68.)

δ-globin synthesis and significantly lower levels of hemoglobin A_2 compared with hemoglobin A.

The ε gene is located 5′ of the other β-like genes, and it is expressed during embryonic development. The ε gene is similar in sequence to the γ genes. A silencing element of the promoter region may be responsible for inactivating gene expression after the embryonic stage.[125] The only known mutation that results in persistent expression of this globin gene occurs in trisomy 13, in which there is a delay in the switch from ε-globin to γ-globin production.[126]

GLOBIN CHAIN SYNTHESIS

It has been possible to analyze the patterns of globin chain production at early ages of embryonic development during the transition from yolk sac (primitive) to hepatic (definitive) erythropoiesis. It is unknown why primitive erythroid progenitors programmed to produce one type of hemoglobin, such as hemoglobin Gower 1, give way to definitive progenitors programmed to produce a different type of hemoglobin, such as fetal hemoglobin. Quantification of globin gene synthesis reflects production by numerous red blood cells, and production of a specific hemoglobin is usually reported as a percentage of the total hemoglobin measured. Studies evaluating hemoglobin production by erythroid colonies in culture, however, show that individual cells in a colony produce predominantly one type of hemoglobin.[127]

During the fourth to fifth week, ζ, δ, and ε chains are the main globin chains synthesized (Fig. 109.8). During the sixth to seventh week, α, δ, ε, $^{G}\gamma$, and $^{A}\gamma$ chains are produced in the remaining primitive erythroblasts, and α, ε, $^{G}\gamma$, and $^{A}\gamma$ chains are produced in definitive erythrocytes. By the seventh to eighth week, ε- and ζ-chain synthesis is no longer detectable, and the main globin chains produced are α, $^{G}\gamma$, and $^{A}\gamma$. Production of the β chain is just barely detectable at this time and gradually increases, such that by 10 weeks, it makes up 10% of total non-α-chain production. As soon as β-chain production occurs, genetic disorders associated with β-chain synthetic or structural abnormalities may be detected in utero, a finding suggesting an asynchronous transition from ζ-chain to α-chain production as compared with ε-chain to γ-chain production, with the ζ-α switch occurring slightly earlier.[128]

From the 10th week to about the 33rd week of gestation, the main globin chains synthesized are α, $^{G}\gamma$, $^{A}\gamma$, and β. Assessment of the output of the two linked α-globin genes by mRNA analysis suggests that they are expressed in a ratio ranging from 1.5:1 to 3.0:1 (α_2/α_1) throughout fetal life. This does not appear to change during development and is the same as that observed in normal adults. The relative rates of $^{G}\gamma$-chain and $^{A}\gamma$-chain production are also constant throughout fetal life at a $^{G}\gamma/^{A}\gamma$ ratio of approximately 3:1.[120] It is not known whether these pairs of genes are initially activated at this ratio; however, this production ratio is reached early in development.

Somewhere between the 32nd week and the 36th week of gestation, the relative rate of β-chain synthesis increases and that of γ-chain production declines such that at birth β-chain synthesis makes up 30% to 50% of non-α-chain synthesis. It is generally held that the transition from fetal to adult erythropoiesis starts at 30 to 36 weeks after conception, but the rate of the transition has been controversial. A gradual transition from fetal to adult hemoglobin synthesis occurs, starting in the first trimester.[128,129] Considerable variation among infants occurs, however, because many infants show prolonged dependence on fetal hemoglobin. After birth the level of γ-chain production steadily declines and that of β-chain production increases, so by the end of the first year, γ-chain synthesis reaches the low level characteristic of adult life. The normal range of postnatal fetal hemoglobin production can be seen in Fig. 109.8. During the first few months of life, the $^{G}\gamma/^{A}\gamma$ ratio changes from 3:1 to 2:3, although this ratio is variable in adults.[130,131]

Production of the δ chain has been observed as early as 32 weeks. Activation of the δ gene lags β-gene activation, so the adult β/δ synthesis ratio is not reached until 4 to 6 months after birth.

HEMOGLOBIN PRODUCTION

Developmental changes in the production of the various hemoglobins are noted in Fig. 109.8. Before the onset of formation of other chains, unpaired globin chains may form tetramers, resulting in the presence of ε_4.[132] Almost immediately thereafter, α-chain and ζ-chain production begins, and hemoglobins Gower 1 (ζ_2-ε_2), Gower 2 (α_2-ε_2), and Portland I (ζ_2-γ_2) are formed.[133] By 5 to 6 weeks' gestation, hemoglobins Gower 1 and Gower 2 constitute 42% and 24% of the total hemoglobin, respectively, with fetal hemoglobin (α_2-γ_2) making up the remainder. By 14 to 16 weeks, hemoglobin F constitutes 50% of the total hemoglobin, and by 20 weeks, it forms more than 90% of the hemoglobin.[131,134] Small quantities of hemoglobin A (α_2-β_2) are found, beginning at 6 to 8 weeks' gestation. The increase in β-chain production occurring between 12 and 20 weeks' gestation accounts for the sudden rise in the amount of hemoglobin A found at the end of the first trimester of pregnancy. Tetramers of γ chains (γ_4, or hemoglobin Barts) and β-chains (β_4, or hemoglobin H) can be found in conditions in which α-chain synthesis is impaired or absent, such as the α-thalassemia syndromes.

Fetal hemoglobin is easily distinguished immunologically and biochemically from adult hemoglobin. The most significant physiologic characteristic of fetal hemoglobin is the decreased interaction with 2,3-diphosphoglycerate (2,3-DPG). 2,3-DPG binds to deoxyhemoglobin in a cavity between the β chains and stabilizes the deoxy form of hemoglobin, resulting in a reduced hemoglobin-oxygen affinity. 2,3-DPG binds less effectively to the γ-globin chains, because of the differing amino acid sequence in the non-α chain. Consequently, 2,3-DPG does not reduce the oxygen affinity of hemoglobin F as much as that of hemoglobin A.

Other differences in physical properties exist between fetal and adult hemoglobin. Hemoglobin F is more soluble in strong phosphate buffers than hemoglobin A.[116] Hemoglobin F is oxidized to methemoglobin more easily than is hemoglobin A, and it has a considerably greater affinity for oxygen than does adult hemoglobin as a result of differences in binding to 2,3-DPG. Fetal hemoglobin is resistant to acid elution, which allows differentiation of cells containing fetal hemoglobin from cells containing hemoglobin A.[116]

The total γ chains in the blood of the fetus and newborn comprise 70% to 80% of $^{G}\gamma$ chains. This fraction falls to about 40% by 5 months of age. This unique difference in $^{G}\gamma$ chain production found in the fetus helps to distinguish fetal hematopoiesis from that found in later life. Under stress, the older infant and adult revert to this intrauterine form of fetal hemoglobin structure. This often occurs in leukemic states in children and adults, and in other conditions as well.[135,136] The delay in the switch of hemoglobin F to hemoglobin A has been noted in conditions of maternal hypoxia,[137] in infants small for their gestational age,[138] and in infants of diabetic mothers.[139,140] Elevated levels of fetal hemoglobin may have protective effects in some disease states, and much research has gone into identifying fetal to adult hemoglobin transition, in order to "switch on" γ-globin gene expression and increase fetal hemoglobin production.[141] The regulators implicated in hemoglobin F production include B-cell lymphoma/leukemia 11A, myeloblastosis protooncogene protein, and Krüppel-like factor 1. In addition, microRNAs 15a and 16-1 play a role in gene regulation.[142]

The postpartum decline of fetal hemoglobin production and of the intercellular distribution of fetal and adult hemoglobins has been extensively examined during the first few months of life. Immediately after birth, there is a brief rise in hemoglobin F concentration, followed by a steady decline (Fig. 109.9). Studies of the intercellular distribution of hemoglobin F, using the relatively insensitive acid-elution technique, have shown that during the first few months of life the distribution of hemoglobin F is quite heterogeneous. At 3 months the distribution of hemoglobin F becomes bimodal, with populations of cells that contain acid-resistant hemoglobin F and populations of adult "ghost" cells. These observations have suggested that fetal hemoglobin-containing cells are replaced by a population of cells containing adult hemoglobin.

Profound changes occur in the rates of red blood cell production immediately before birth and during the first few months after birth. On a body-weight basis, red blood cell production during the latter months of gestation is significantly greater compared with that in adult life. Immediately after birth, erythropoiesis is considerably reduced, presumably as an adaptation to the extrauterine environment, and red blood cell production occurs at a low level for the first few weeks of life. It is clear from globin-chain synthetic studies that there is a steady and linear decline in γ-chain synthesis during the period of reduced neonatal erythropoiesis. Newly synthesized red blood cells appearing in the circulation when erythropoiesis resumes contain predominantly adult hemoglobin. These observations may explain the short plateau in the proportion of fetal hemoglobin (but not absolute levels) after birth and the appearance of predominantly adult hemoglobin-containing cells during the second and third months of life. These findings, together with the results of analyses of the intercellular distribution of fetal and adult hemoglobin by sensitive immunologic methods, suggest, although they do not prove, that the transition from fetal to adult hemoglobin production occurs in the same erythrocyte population. This conclusion is also consistent with the patterns of fetal and β-chain production in red blood cell colonies grown from neonatal blood.[143]

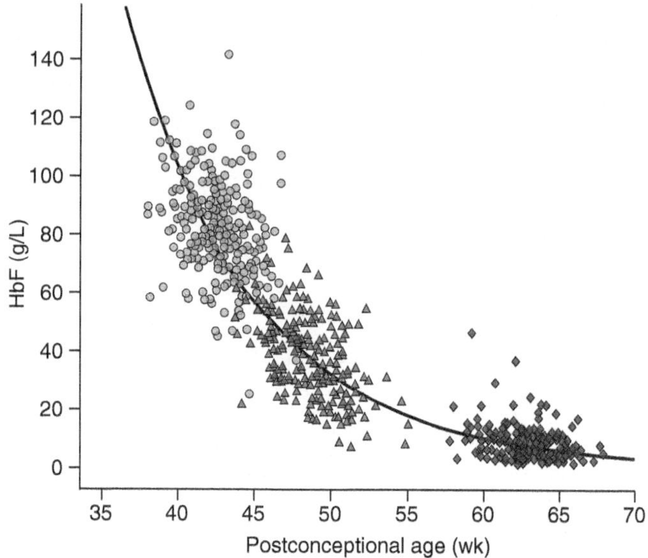

Fig. 109.9 Correlation between postconceptional age and absolute levels of fetal hemoglobin. Postnatal fetal hemoglobin concentrations *(HbF)* are shown for 280 infants, examined at postnatal ages of 6 weeks *(circles)*, 12 weeks *(triangles)*, and 6 months *(diamonds)*. (From Berglund SK, Lindberg J, Westrup B, et al. Effects of iron supplements and perinatal factors on fetal hemoglobin disappearance in LBW infants. *Pediatr Res.* 2014;76:477–482.)

Studies show that the type of globin chains produced at different stages of development are not closely related to the site of erythropoiesis. It appears that ζ and ε chains are synthesized in both primitive and definitive cell lines. Moreover, the switch from γ-chain to β-chain production occurs synchronously throughout the liver and bone marrow during the later stages of fetal development. The transition from γ-chain to β-chain synthesis is most closely related to postconceptional age and not chronologic age.[135] Thus premature infants continue to synthesize relatively large quantities of γ chains (and fetal hemoglobin) until 40 weeks' gestation.

ERYTHROCYTE METABOLISM

The mature red blood cell differs from other cells in the body in that it has no nucleus; it consequently lacks the ability to engage in de novo protein synthesis. It has no mitochondria or ribosomes, no nucleic acid or deoxyribonucleic acid synthesis, no Krebs cycle of intermediary metabolism, and no electron transport system for oxidative phosphorylation. Thus cellular metabolism is dependent on a limited supply of preexisting enzymes. These enzymes, coenzymes, and the substrates of glucose metabolism interact with hemoglobin and the red blood cell membrane to perform all the primary functions of the red blood cell, the most important being oxygen transport.

Other important functions of red blood cell metabolism include maintaining adequate amounts of energy in the form of adenosine triphosphate (ATP), producing reducing substances to act as antioxidants, and maintaining appropriate amounts of red

Box 109.1 Metabolic Characteristics of Neonatal Erythrocytes

Carbohydrate Metabolism

Glucose consumption increased
Galactose more completely utilized as a substrate both under normal circumstances and for methemoglobin reduction[a]
Decreased activity of sorbitol pathway[a]
Decreased triokinase activity[a]

Glycolytic Enzymes

Increased activity of hexokinase, phosphoglucose isomerase,[a] aldolase, glyceraldehyde 3-phosphate dehydrogenase,[a] phosphoglycerate kinase,[a] phosphoglycerate mutase, enolase,[a] pyruvate kinase, lactate dehydrogenase, glucose 6-phosphate dehydrogenase, 6-phosphogluconic dehydrogenase, galactokinase, and galactose 1-phosphate uridyltransferase
Decreased activity of phosphofructokinase[a]
Distribution of hexokinase isoenzymes differs from that of adults[a]

Nonglycolytic Enzymes

Increased activity of glutamic oxaloacetic transaminase and glutathione reductase
Decreased activity of NADP-dependent methemoglobin reductase,[a] catalase,[a] glutathione peroxidase, carbonic anhydrase,[a] adenylate kinase,[a] and glutathione synthetase[a]
Presence of α-glycerol-3-phosphate dehydrogenase[a]

Adenosine Triphosphate and Phosphate Metabolism

Decreased phosphate uptake,[a] slower incorporation into ATP and 2,3-diphosphoglycerate[a]
Accelerated decline of 2,3-diphosphoglycerate into red blood cell incubation[a]
Increased ATP levels
Accelerated decline of ATP levels during brief incubation

Storage Characteristics

Increased potassium efflux and greater degrees of hemolysis during short periods of storage
More rapid assumption of altered morphologic forms on storage or incubation[a]

Membrane

Decreased ouabain-sensitive ATPase[a]
Decreased potassium influx[a]
Decreased permeability to glycerol and thiourea[a]
Decreased membrane filterability[a]
Increased sphingomyelin content, decreased lecithin content of stromal phospholipids
Decreased content of linoleic acid[a]
Increase in content of lipid phosphorus and cholesterol per cell
Greater affinity for glucose[a]

Other

Increased methemoglobin content[a]
Increased affinity of hemoglobin for oxygen[a]
Glutathione instability[a]
Increased tendency for Heinz body formation in the presence of oxidant compounds[a]

[a] Appears to be a unique characteristic of the newborn's erythrocytes and not merely a function of the presence of young red blood cells.
From Oski FA, Naiman JL. *Hematologic Problems in the Newborn*. 3rd ed. Philadelphia: WB Saunders; 1982:107.
ATP, Adenosine triphosphate; *NADP*, nicotinamide adenine dinucleotide phosphate.

blood cell 2,3-DPG to assist in the modulation of hemoglobin's oxygen affinity. Energy metabolism is largely a function of the Embden-Meyerhof pathway. This pathway also regulates the quantity of red blood cell 2,3-DPG within the cell. The pentose phosphate pathway, among other functions, has a vital role in the production of reducing substances such as reduced nicotinamide adenine dinucleotide phosphate (NADPH). Box 109.1 lists the metabolic characteristics of neonatal erythrocytes. A few of the variations seen in comparison with adult red blood cells are clinically significant in that they affect the life span of neonatal red blood cells.

GLYCOLYSIS

Red blood cells need a constant supply of carbohydrate to maintain adequate levels of ATP. Although glucose is the preferred carbohydrate, the red blood cell metabolizes fructose or mannose almost as readily. Galactose is metabolized more slowly. Intracellular glucose concentrations equilibrate immediately with changes in plasma glucose concentrations. Glucose enters the human erythrocyte by facilitated transfer, and it is either converted to glucose 6-phosphate or reduced to its polyol derivative, sorbitol, which is then converted to fructose.[144] Once formed, glucose 6-phosphate is metabolized by one of three pathways. The Embden-Meyerhof pathway converts glucose 6-phosphate to lactate or pyruvate and in the process generates ATP. Metabolism by way of the pentose phosphate pathway produces reduced intermediates and a phosphorylated pentose sugar (ribulose 5-phosphate). This sugar ultimately returns to the Embden-Meyerhof pathway. Finally, glucose 6-phosphate may be converted to glucose 1-phosphate and then to glycogen, although less than 1% of glucose is metabolized to glycogen within the red blood cell.[145]

EMBDEN-MEYERHOF PATHWAY

At least 90% of glucose is metabolized via the Embden-Meyerhof pathway.[146,147] Two moles of ATP are produced for every mole of glucose catabolized, yielding two moles of lactic acid. This potential for the production of ATP is not fully achieved because approximately 20% of metabolized glucose traverses the 2,3-DPG cycle, thus bypassing one of the kinase steps, which is a site of ATP generation.[148]

The Embden-Meyerhof pathway has several unique characteristics with respect to fetal and newborn cells. These cells consume greater quantities of glucose than do the red blood cells of adults.[149] Galactose metabolism in the newborn red blood cell also differs.[150] Galactokinase activity is three times greater in the erythrocytes of newborns, and these cells consume galactose more rapidly than do those of the adult. The glycolytic enzymes phosphoglycerate kinase and enolase are much more active in the cells of the fetus and newborn infant than would be anticipated from their young cell age.[151,152] In contrast, the activity of phosphofructokinase (a rate-controlling enzyme in glycolysis) is lower than normal in the erythrocytes from newborn infants.[151,153,154] Developmental changes in the activities of these three enzymes towards normal adult values during the first year of life appear to be independent of red blood cell age and reflect a transition from fetal to adult erythropoiesis. The decreased phosphofructokinase activity of fetal cells may be a consequence of accelerated decay of an unstable enzyme. The relative deficiency of this enzyme appears to result in alterations in glucose metabolism, and it could be functionally significant. Several of the other enzymes of the Embden-Meyerhof pathway have shown differences in the staining intensity of certain isoenzyme zones as compared with adult controls, although the significance of this observation is not known.

The ATP generated via the Embden-Meyerhof pathway is necessary for the maintenance of the normal biconcave shape of the erythrocyte.[155] It is also necessary for pyrimidine nucleotide synthesis, completion of purine nucleotide synthesis and glutathione synthesis,[156] incorporation of fatty acids into membrane phospholipids,[157] active cation transport,[154] and the initial step in the phosphorylation of glucose by the enzyme hexokinase. Not all these synthesizing functions are important in the mature red blood cell, which lacks a nucleus. However, loss of red blood cell ATP produces a marked decrease in red blood cell deformability. As the cell ages, ATP levels fall, and older cells have lower glucose utilization, greater osmotic fragility on incubation, lower membrane lipid content, lower potassium concentration, and greater sodium concentration. They are less deformable and have a shorter life span. The red blood cells of term and preterm infants, when studied in the first several days of life, contain higher levels of ATP than do cells from adults.[158,159] The small premature infant has even higher ATP levels.[158]

Newborn red blood cells seem to demonstrate a transient immaturity in their metabolism. This results in a slower uptake of phosphorus, a delayed incorporation into 2,3-DPG, and a marked decline in 2,3-DPG levels, as well as ATP levels, during short periods of incubation in vitro. The precise reason for this relatively transient immaturity is not known, but it may explain why the newborn red blood cell loses potassium at an accelerated rate and undergoes marked morphologic alteration during short incubations in vitro.

Pyruvate kinase deficiency is a well-known enzymopathy that affects the normal function of the Embden-Meyerhof pathway and results in clinically significant erythrocyte pathology. Deleterious mutations in the *PKLR* (pyruvate kinase L/R) gene result in low levels of pyruvate kinase. This results in abnormal erythrocyte morphology (echinocytes, anisocytes, poikilocytes) and a lifelong hemolytic anemia. The exact mechanisms of hemolysis are not known. Though other Embden-Meyerhof pathway enzymopathies have been described in the literature, they are even more rare than pyruvate kinase deficiency.

PENTOSE PHOSPHATE PATHWAY

Glucose 6-phosphate undergoes oxidative decarboxylation through the pentose phosphate pathway, consuming oxygen and producing carbon dioxide. The pentose pathway requires NADPH as a cofactor. In the first step, oxidation of glucose 6-phosphate to 6-phosphogluconolactone is catabolized by glucose 6-phosphate dehydrogenase (G6PD), generating NADPH. This step is followed by enzymatic hydrolysis of 6-phosphogluconolactone to 6-phosphogluconate, which is then oxidized (in the presence of 6-phosphogluconic dehydrogenase) to ribulose 5-phosphate, with the production of carbon dioxide. Approximately 3% to 10% of all glucose metabolized by the cell is cycled through the pentose phosphate pathway. Hypoxia and acidosis increase the proportion of glucose metabolism shunted through this pathway.

The pentose phosphate shunt results in the production of two important products, ribose 5-phosphate and NADPH. Ribose 5-phosphate is a vital constituent of the pyridine nucleotides nicotinamide adenine dinucleotide phosphate and NADPH and the purine nucleotides adenosine diphosphate and ATP. There is no pathway for de novo purine formation inside the red blood cell; however, the mature red blood cell does retain the ability for pyridine nucleotide formation. NADPH is critical for preservation of cell integrity because it is necessary for methemoglobin reduction, the reduction of glutathione, and the stabilization of certain enzymes.[160] NADPH serves as a hydrogen donor in the presence of the enzyme glutathione reductase, resulting in reduction of glutathione. Reduced glutathione ultimately serves as a substrate for the enzyme glutathione peroxidase, which is responsible for the detoxification of hydrogen peroxide. Hydrogen peroxide is a byproduct of the conversion of oxyhemoglobin to methemoglobin, which is a naturally occurring reaction inside the red blood cell in the presence of oxidative stress. The absence of NADPH (or anything that interferes with the production of reduced glutathione), the synthesis of glutathione, or the inability to detoxify hydrogen peroxide severely impairs the viability of the red blood cell. This is the case in G6PD deficiency. Patients with this condition can experience hemolytic crises when they experience oxidative stress from illness, certain foods, and certain drugs.

The pentose phosphate pathway in the newborn red blood cell differs from that in the adult red blood cell. Two enzymes of the pentose pathway, G6PD and 6-phosphogluconic acid dehydrogenase, are active at levels higher than those seen in adult red blood cells.[161] Carbon dioxide production by erythrocytes of term and preterm infants is equal to or greater than that seen in red blood cells of adults.

Although there are suggestions that the pentose phosphate pathway activity in the newborn is normal, there is also evidence that newborn infants are more susceptible to oxidant-induced injury, leading to glutathione instability, Heinz body formation, and the development of methemoglobinemia.[162,163] This oxidant vulnerability may be caused by factors unrelated to the pentose phosphate pathway. For example, the red blood cell membrane in the fetus and newborn may have a decreased number of membrane sulfhydryl groups, making these cells more susceptible than mature red blood cells to Heinz body formation.[163] Additionally, NADPH-methemoglobin reductase activity is decreased in neonatal red blood cells, and the plasma of newborn infants appears to have a diminished antioxidant capacity.[164] The precise mechanisms surrounding the newborn red blood cell vulnerability to oxidant injury are not known. Fetal and newborn red blood cells have diminished levels of glutathione peroxidase, which may render the cells more vulnerable to hydrogen peroxide–induced oxidant injury. In addition, the newborn red blood cell may have a diminished capacity for handling other activated oxygen radicals, such as singlet oxygen and the superoxide radical.[165] The latter is converted to hydrogen peroxide in the presence of the enzyme superoxide dismutase. Superoxide dismutase levels differ widely among infants. Diminished activity of superoxide dismutase could result in accumulation of superoxide radicals. Free radicals are generally detoxified by antioxidants such as α-tocopherol (vitamin E). However, if superoxide dismutase levels are increased (as has been described in some infants), the hydrogen peroxide presented to reduced glutathione may not be adequately detoxified. Therefore a delicate balance appears to exist between enzymes involved in production and detoxification of free radicals and oxidative intermediates. The use of inhaled nitric oxide as treatment for pulmonary hypertension in sick neonates may affect this balance, and further studies are required to determine its impact on oxidant injury beyond an increase in methemoglobin formation.

2,3-DIPHOSPHOGLYCERATE METABOLISM

The affinity of a hemoglobin solution for oxygen can be decreased by interaction of hemoglobin with certain organic phosphates.[166] Among the organic phosphates tested, 2,3-DPG and ATP are the most effective in lowering oxygen affinity. The highly charged anion 2,3-DPG binds to deoxyhemoglobin but not to oxyhemoglobin. Various conditions increase the amount of 2,3-DPG present within the red blood cell, as regulated in the Embden-Meyerhof pathway. Once formed, each molecule of 2,3-DPG binds reversibly to one deoxyhemoglobin tetramer under physiologic conditions of solute concentration and pH. Fetal deoxyhemoglobin does not possess as great an affinity for 2,3-DPG as does adult deoxyhemoglobin, and therefore it cannot bind 2,3-DPG to the same degree as adult hemoglobin. Thus the fetal leftward-shifted hemoglobin-oxygen dissociation curve is not easily modulated by the presence of 2,3-DPG. The half-saturation pressure (P_{50}) of fetal blood is 19 to 21 mm Hg, some 6 to 8 mm Hg lower than that of adult blood. As the fetal hemoglobin concentration declines (see Fig. 109.9), the increasing percentage of adult hemoglobin and increasing red blood cell 2,3-DPG content produce a marked rightward shift in the hemoglobin-oxygen equilibrium curve. Infants with a greater proportion of adult hemoglobin but less 2,3-DPG may have the same P_{50} as those with increased quantities of fetal hemoglobin but a high red blood cell 2,3-DPG content.

ERYTHROCYTE PHYSIOLOGY

PHYSICAL PROPERTIES OF NEONATAL ERYTHROCYTES

The fetal and neonatal red blood cell differs from the mature red blood cell of the older infant, child, and adult in various ways. Specific characteristics of fetal red blood cells include a shortened life span, macrocytosis, high fetal hemoglobin content with a $^{G}\gamma/^{A}\gamma$ ratio of 3:1, the presence of i antigen,[167] and low carbonic anhydrase enzyme activity.[49]

LIFE SPAN

The differences in physical properties of red blood cells derived from term and preterm infants may in part account for the decreased life span of neonatal red blood cells within the circulation. The average life span for a neonatal red blood cell is 60 to 90 days,[168] approximately half to two thirds that of an adult red blood cell. When neonatal red blood cells are transfused into adults, they exhibit a shortened life span, owing to alterations intrinsic to the neonatal red blood cell.[169] In contrast, cells transfused from adult donors appear to survive normally in newborns.[169] With increasing degrees of prematurity, remarkably shorter red blood cell life spans (35 to 50 days) are found. Fetal studies using [^{14}C] cyanate-labeled red blood cells in sheep revealed an average red blood cell life span of 63.6 ± 5.8 days.[170] The mean red blood cell life span increased linearly from 35 to 107 days as the fetal age increased from 97 days (midgestation) to 136 days (term).

The shortened red blood cell life span of the preterm and term neonate may be explained by some of the characteristics specific to newborn cells—namely, a rapid decline in intracellular enzyme activity and ATP levels,[171] loss of membrane surface area by internalization of membrane lipids, decreased levels of intracellular carnitine,[172] increased susceptibility of membrane lipids and protein to peroxidation,[173] and increased mechanical fragility resulting from increased membrane deformability.[174]

SIZE

Red blood cell dimensions change markedly during fetal and neonatal development. Early in embryogenesis, cell diameters range from 20 to 25 μm, and the MCV averages 150 to 180 fL.[3] During fetal development red blood cells gradually decrease in size and volume (see Fig. 109.5); at term the average cell is 8 to 10 μm in diameter, with an MCV between 108 and 118 fL. During the first year of life red blood cells continue to diminish in size, and at 1 year of life they resemble adult red blood cells (Table 109.5).

SHAPE AND DEFORMABILITY

Just as there is variation in the size of newborn red blood cells, there is variation in shape. Irregularly shaped cells are present in much greater numbers in the peripheral blood of newborn infants than in that of adults.[175] Target cells, acanthocytes, puckered immature erythrocytes, and other irregular projections may normally be found. For example, a greater percentage of neonatal red blood cells have membrane surface pits, which are most likely the sites of formation of endocytic vacuoles. In normal adults, 2.6% of erythrocytes appear to have surface pits or craters ranging in size from 0.2 to 0.5 μm in diameter, demonstrated by interference-contrast microscopy.[176] In contrast, pits can be found in almost half of the erythrocytes of preterm infants and in one fourth of the erythrocytes of term infants.

Red blood cell deformability is principally governed by three factors: the surface area to volume relationship of the red blood cell, the viscosity of the cytoplasm of the cell, and intrinsic red blood cell membrane rigidity.[174] The deformability of erythrocytes is important for several reasons. First, red blood cell deformability appears to be an important determinant of red blood cell life span in vivo. The removal of a red blood cell from the circulation is thought to be a consequence of declining deformability, making the red blood cell susceptible to sequestration in the spleen and other organs, where it must negotiate extraordinarily narrow passages. Second, red blood cell deformability directly influences blood flow in the peripheral circulation. Third, red blood cell deformability affects whole blood viscosity, which, in turn, affects peripheral vascular resistance and cardiac workload.[177]

Neonatal red blood cells with the greatest density (representing the oldest cells in the circulation) lose more volume than adult red blood cells, have a higher mean corpuscular hemoglobin concentration than adult red blood cells, and are less deformable than the oldest red blood cells seen in adults. This suggests an accelerated decrease in deformability of aging red blood cells related to a more pronounced increase in the mean corpuscular hemoglobin concentration, the principal determinant of the internal viscosity of the red blood cell. Neonatal red blood cell membranes deform more readily to a given shear force than do adult red blood cell membranes, resulting in greater susceptibility of neonatal cell membranes to yield and fragment.[177] These mechanical properties may lead to accelerated membrane loss and a decreased life span. Recent studies evaluating the red blood cell deformability of preterm infants receiving recombinant *EPO* reported that erythrocyte deformability was significantly related to the reticulocyte count, indicating that the improvement of erythrocyte deformability with recombinant *EPO* therapy was due to the formation of well-deformable young erythrocytes.[178]

SURFACE CHARGE

The surface charge of newborn red blood cells is more negative than that of adult red blood cells. The negative charge at the red blood cell surface is largely responsible for the electrophoretic mobility of the cell, and it appears to reflect the sialic acid content of the red blood cell membrane.[179,180] Proteases expose more negative sites on neonatal red blood cells than on adult red blood cells and increase the electrophoretic mobility to a greater degree.[181] The sialic acid content of the newborn infant's erythrocyte membrane shows a gradual but significant decrease in the first several weeks of life.[182] Most studies, however, have shown that the electrophoretic mobility of the neonatal cell is similar to that of the adult cell.[180] The more negative surface charge of the neonatal red blood cell membrane is one of the many characteristics that results in a decreased sedimentation rate in newborns.[183]

OSMOTIC FRAGILITY

The osmotic fragility of red blood cells is a composite index of their shape, hydration, and, within certain limitations, proneness to in vivo destruction.[174,184] Preterm and term infants have an increased osmotic resistance.[185] The osmotic fragility of neonatal cells begins to revert towards adult values shortly after birth, and

Table 109.5 Postnatal Changes in Red Blood Cell Indices in Term Infants.

	Days			Weeks			Months					
RBC Indices	**Birth (Umbilical Cord Blood)**	**1**	**3**	**1**	**2**	**4**	**2**	**3**	**4**	**6**	**9**	**12**
Hemoglobin (g/dL)	16.5 (13.0)	18.5 (14.5)	18.6 (16.5)	17.5 (13.5)	16.6 (13.4)	13.9 (10.7)	11.2 (9.4)	11.5 (9.5)	12.2 (10.3)	12.6 (11.1)	12.7 (11.4)	12.7 (11.3)
Hematocrit (%)	51 (42)	56 (45)	55 (42)	54 (41)	53 (33)	44 (28)	35 (29)	35 (32)	38 (31)	36 (32)	36 (33)	37
Red blood cells ($\times 10^{12}$/L)	4.7 (3.9)	5.3 (4.0)	5.6 (3.9)	5.1 (3.9)	4.9 (3.3)	4.3 (3.1)	3.7 (3.1)	3.8 (3.5)	4.3 (3.9)	4.7 (4.0)	4.7 (4.1)	4.7
Mean corpuscular volume (fL)	108 (98)	108 (95)	110 (104)	107 (88)	105 (88)	101 (91)	95 (84)	91 (74)	87 (76)	76 (68)	78 (70)	78 (71)
MCH (pg)	34 (31)	34 (31)	36.7	34 (28)	33.6 (30.0)	32.5 (29)	30.4 (27)	30 (25)	28.6 (25)	26.8 (24)	27.3 (25)	26.8 (24)
MCHC (g/dL)	33 (30)	33 (29)	33.1	33 (28)	31.4 (28.1)	31.8 (28.1)	31.8 (28.3)	33 (30)	32.7 (28.8)	35 (32.7)	34.9 (32.4)	34.3 (32.1)

The values are the means (values in parentheses are −2 standard deviations).
MCH, Mean corpuscular hemoglobin; *MCHC,* mean corpuscular hemoglobin concentration; *RBC,* red blood cell.
Data from Saarinen UM, Siimes MA. Developmental changes in red blood cell counts and indices of infants after exclusion of iron deficiency by laboratory criteria and continuous iron supplementation. *J Pediatr.* 1978;92(3):412–416; and Dallman PR. In: Rudolph A, ed. *Pediatrics.* 16th ed. New York: Appleton-Century-Crofts; 1977:1111.

osmotic resistance reaches adult values by 4 to 6 weeks of age. There is no known advantage to the increased osmotic resistance seen in the neonatal red blood cell. However, studies of osmotic fragility in neonates have practical implications. It has been suggested that the diagnostic criteria for hereditary spherocytosis used in adults and older children are unreliable in newborn infants. For example, spherocytes are not regularly seen in all infants with hereditary spherocytosis. Indeed, spherocytes may be frequently found in ABO incompatibility. When one is performing an osmotic fragility test, a neonatal osmotic fragility curve must be used rather than an adult curve.[186] A relatively new diagnostic test for hereditary spherocytosis, eosin-5-maleimide (EMA)-flow cytometry, quantifies the erythrocyte membrane band 3 complex using an eosin-5-maleimide dye flow cytometric analysis.[187,188] A reduction in band 3 complex is consistent with hereditary spherocytosis. This test appears to perform very well in neonates even in the first days of life.[189,190]

SURFACE RECEPTORS AND ANTIGENS

The neonatal red blood cell differs from the adult red blood cell in its ability to bind various substances. For example, the neonatal red blood cell binds more insulin than the adult red blood cell because of the presence of greater numbers of insulin receptors per cell.[191,192] Newborn red blood cells have approximately 2.5 times the number of digoxin receptors in comparison with adult red blood cells,[193] and as a consequence they have erythrocyte-to-plasma digoxin ratios three times those of adults. This may explain the greater tolerance of newborns who are receiving maintenance digoxin therapy.

Another unique characteristic of the fetal red blood cell is the manifestation of the i antigen on the cell surface (adult red blood cells express i antigen). Membrane i antigen is a carbohydrate moiety located on protein membrane band 3, which, during development, is converted from a linear polylactosamine to a branched carbohydrate chain of *N* -acetyllactosamine units.[167] Red blood cells bearing the i antigen are usually not detectable by the first year of age. It has been suggested that the switch from fetal to adult hemoglobin and the transformation of i antigen expression that occur during the first year of life are governed by a common control mechanism; therefore the presence of i antigen can serve as a marker of fetal hematopoiesis.

Red blood cell antigens in the ABO, MN, Rh, Kell, Duffy, and Vel systems are well developed in early intrauterine life.[194] They are easily demonstrated in the fifth to seventh gestational weeks and remain constant through the remainder of intrauterine development. Other antigens, such as the Lutheran and Xg systems, develop more slowly but are present at birth. Lewis antigens are lacking in the newborn. By approximately 2 years of age, the child's red blood cell and plasma antigens have developed a pattern that is seen throughout the remainder of life.[78]

Although A and B antigens are present early in utero, A and B isoagglutinin production occurs much later.[195] By 30 to 34 weeks' gestation, however, about 50% of infants have some measurable anti-A or anti-B antibodies. The fetal production of such antibodies is not related to maternal ABO blood type. Intrauterine exposure to gram-negative organisms, whose antigens are chemically related to those of blood groups A and B, is a potent stimulus for the development of these antibodies. Isohemagglutinin antibodies ultimately are demonstrable in normal infants by 6 months of age and approach adult values at 2 years of age. Low to absent titers after this time are suggestive of immune deficiency.[196]

OXYGEN TRANSPORT

At no other time of life are the mechanisms controlling oxygen transport more complicated than in utero and during the immediate postpartum period. During prenatal life the fetal arterial oxygen tension (Po_2) is approximately 30 mm Hg, and the venous Po_2 is approximately 15 mm Hg (Fig. 109.10). This low Po_2 contributes to the development of relative polycythemia in the fetus. After birth, numerous factors affect oxygenation, including the inspired gas mixture, pulmonary function, the arterial oxygen dissociation curve, and the ability to extract oxygen at the tissue level.[197,198] It has been speculated that the actual amount of oxygen released to tissues may be greater in utero, given the characteristics of the hemoglobin-oxygen dissociation curve (Fig. 109.11).

If pulmonary function is normal, there will be a rise in the Po_2 of pulmonary blood in adults and neonates, from the 40 mm Hg of pulmonary arterial blood to the 100 mm Hg of pulmonary venous blood. Because of the shape of the hemoglobin-oxygen dissociation curve, these Po_2 values permit 95% saturation of hemoglobin by oxygen. Further increases in Po_2 produce little additional rise in saturation. In the normal adult (see Fig. 109.10), approximately 50% of hemoglobin will be saturated with oxygen when the Po_2 has fallen to 27 mm Hg (P_{50} = 27). In situations in which the hemoglobin-oxygen dissociation curve has shifted to the right, the affinity of hemoglobin for oxygen is reduced. Thus at any given Po_2, more oxygen is released to tissues. Conversely, if the curve is shifted to the left, the affinity of hemoglobin for oxygen is increased. Thus at any given Po_2, less oxygen is released to the tissues.

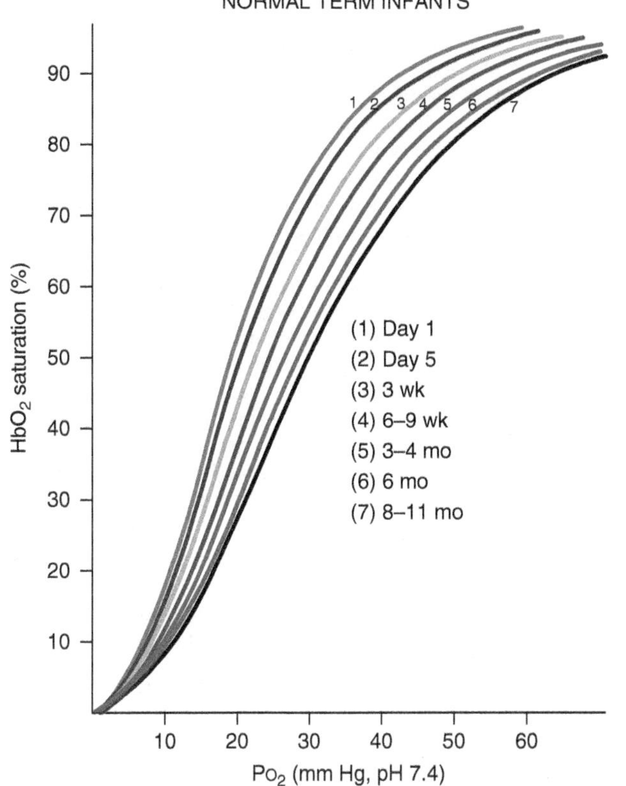

Fig. 109.10 Oxygen equilibrium curve of blood from term infants at different postnatal ages. The oxygen half-saturation pressure of hemoglobin (P_{50}) on day 1 is 19.4 ± 1.8 mm Hg and has shifted to 30.3 ± 0.7 at age 11 months (normal adult 27.0 ± 1.1 mm Hg). (From Oski FA, Naiman JL. *Hematologic Problems in the Newborn*. 3rd ed. Philadelphia: WB Saunders; 1982:250.)

Certain factors are known to alter hemoglobin's affinity for oxygen (Box 109.2). The most important of these are the fetal hemoglobin concentration and the red blood cell 2,3-DPG content. The level of red blood cell 2,3-DPG gradually increases with gestation. By the end of the first postnatal week, the 2,3-DPG levels are considerably higher than they are at birth (Table 109.6). After the first week, red blood cell 2,3-DPG levels remain relatively unchanged for the next 6 months. In term infants the hemoglobin-oxygen dissociation curve gradually shifts to the right, and by 4 to 6 months of age, the P_{50} values approximate those of the adult.

The situation is somewhat different in preterm infants. Fetal hemoglobin synthesis is still quite active; therefore, increases in P_{50} seen in term infants as a result of the switch from fetal to adult hemoglobin do not occur. The red blood cell 2,3-DPG concentrations are slightly lower in preterm infants as well.[96] These concentrations can be increased with the use of *EPO,* thereby shifting the hemoglobin-oxygen dissociation curve to the right.[199]

A precise relationship between the decrease in oxygen affinity of a neonate's blood and the progressive decline in the concentration of fetal hemoglobin does not exist.[198] Rather, changes in P_{50} reflect the interplay between the levels of red blood cell 2,3-DPG, the decline in fetal hemoglobin levels, and the subsequent increase in hemoglobin A levels. A unifying concept has emerged consisting of a "functioning 2,3-DPG fraction,"[96] which determines how well hemoglobin is able to release oxygen to tissues. The functioning 2,3-DPG fraction (expressed as nanomoles per milliliter of red blood cells) is calculated by multiplying the red blood cell 2,3-DPG content by the percentage of adult hemoglobin[93]:

$$[2,3\text{-DPG}]_{\text{functional}} = [2,3\text{-DPG}]_{\text{observed}} \times [100 - \%\ \text{hemoglobin}\ F] \quad [109.1]$$

If P_{50} cannot be measured directly, it may be calculated from the following equation[86] after determining the functioning 2,3-DPG fraction:

$$P_{50} = 18.4 + 0.0016[2,3\text{-DPG}]_{\text{functional}} \quad [109.2]$$

Table 109.6 illustrates the expected changes in hemoglobin concentration, 2,3-DPG concentration, functional 2,3-DPG fraction, and P_{50} during the first 3 months of life in low-birth-weight infants.[96] In low-birth-weight infants, the amount of oxygen released by hemoglobin can be determined (on the basis

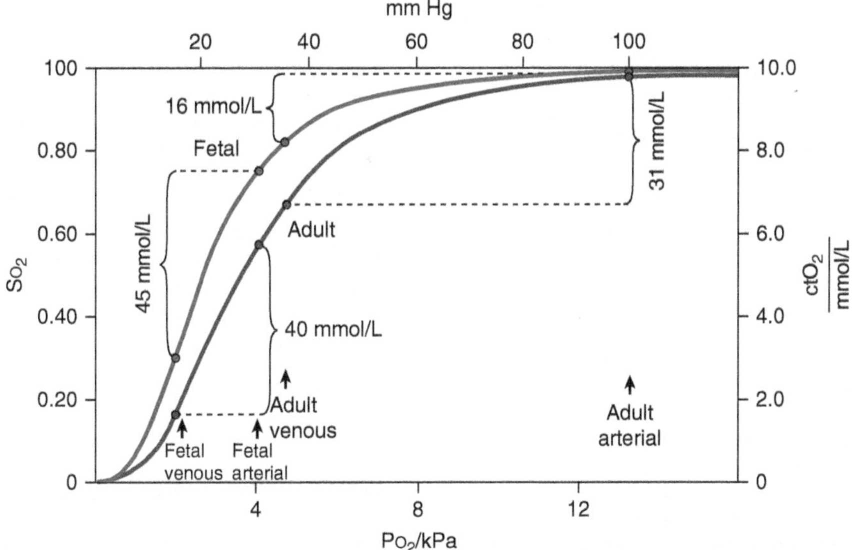

Fig. 109.11 Differences in the hemoglobin-oxygen dissociation curve between the newborn and the adult. This figure demonstrates the effects of these differences on oxygen tension (ctO_2) and oxygen saturation (SO_2). (From Stockman JA. Fetal Hematology. In: Eden RD, Boehm J, eds. *Assessment and Care of the Fetus*. Norwalk, CT: Appleton & Lange; 1989:124.)

Box 109.2 Factors Affecting Hemoglobin-Oxygen Affinity

Increased Amount of Red Blood Cell 2,3-Diphosphoglycerate, Increased P_{50}

Adaptation to high altitude
Hypoxemia associated with chronic pulmonary disease
Hypoxemia associated with cyanotic heart disease
Anemia
 Secondary to iron deficiency
 Secondary to chronic renal disease
 Caused by sickle cell anemia
Decreased red blood cell mass
Chronic liver disease
Hyperthyroidism
Red blood cell pyruvate kinase deficiency

Decreased Amount of Red Blood Cell 2,3-Diphosphoglycerate, Decreased P_{50}

Septic shock
Severe acidosis
Following massive transfusions of stored blood
Neonatal respiratory distress syndrome

Increased P_{50}, No Consistent Alteration in Amount of Red Blood Cell 2,3-Diphosphoglycerate

Abnormal hemoglobins (Kansas, Seattle, Hammersmith, Tacoma, E)
Vigorous exercise

Decreased P_{50}, No Consistent Alteration in Amount of Red Blood Cell 2,3-Diphosphoglycerate

Abnormal hemoglobins (Kempsey, Chesapeake, J Cape Town, Yakima, Rainier)

of unloading from a normal arterial Po_2 adjusted for age to an arbitrary central venous Po_2 of 40 mm Hg).[93] Although oxygen-carrying capacity (hemoglobin concentration × percentage of oxygen saturation × 1.36 mL oxygen per gram of hemoglobin) decreases during the first few months of life as a consequence of a decline in hemoglobin concentration, the amount of oxygen capable of being delivered to tissues actually increases. For example, a newborn weighing 1000 g with a hemoglobin concentration of 15 g/dL, a P_{50} of 19, and a central venous Po_2 of 40 mm Hg will unload 1 mL of oxygen to tissues for every 100 mL of blood that passes through the capillary bed. At 10 weeks of age, the P_{50} has shifted to the right and is now 24 mm Hg. This same infant will now deliver 2.1 mL of oxygen per 100 mL of blood, even though the hemoglobin concentration has declined to 8 g/dL (see Fig. 109.11).

These calculations emphasize the importance of understanding an infant's ability to deliver oxygen to tissues when one is determining whether to administer an erythrocyte transfusion. The decision to transfuse erythrocytes should not be based on hemoglobin concentration alone. Transfusions significantly affect an infant's endogenous erythropoiesis. For infants who undergo exchange transfusion or multiple transfusions, both *EPO* concentrations and reticulocyte counts are lower at any given hemoglobin concentration (Fig. 109.12).[93,200]

It is often assumed that oxygen delivery is decreased in newborns because of the presence of high-affinity hemoglobin. In fact, a leftward shift in the hemoglobin-oxygen dissociation curve resulting from high levels of fetal hemoglobin may better maintain oxygen delivery during episodes of severe hypoxemia. Fig. 109.13 illustrates the arterial Po_2 below which shifts to the right in the neonatal hemoglobin-oxygen dissociation curve are no longer advantageous. The gas tension at which this occurs is known as the *crossover Po_2*.[201] The crossover Po_2 is dependent on how low the venous Po_2 falls before oxygen delivery ceases. Wimberley[202] calculated that if the arterial Po_2 fell to less than 32 mm Hg, and if the venous Po_2 fell to 10 mm Hg (a value found in the cerebral venous blood of some sick newborns), the infant would achieve better oxygen delivery with a fetal hemoglobin-oxygen dissociation curve than with an adult curve. Conversely, if arterial Po_2 can be maintained at a higher value, better oxygen delivery would exist if the hemoglobin-oxygen dissociation curve were shifted to the right.

In neonates with hypoxemia (e.g., infants with cyanotic congenital heart disease), a shift to the right (a higher P_{50}) in the hemoglobin-oxygen dissociation curve tends to lower the arterial and venous oxygen saturation at any given Po_2. It has been documented that if arterial hypoxemia results from right-to-left shunting, shifts to the right in the hemoglobin-oxygen dissociation curve always tend to increase the arterial-venous oxygen difference and improve oxygen delivery.[201]

After intrauterine transfusion, infants have oxygen-unloading properties characteristic of those of adult blood. Despite the decrease in oxygen affinity that accompanies intrauterine transfusion, no deleterious effects of this procedure with respect to oxygen uptake by the fetus have been documented.[203] The physiologic significance of manipulating the hemoglobin-oxygen affinity of fetuses and extremely preterm infants remains to be fully studied.

PHYSIOLOGIC ANEMIA IN NEONATES AND THE ANEMIA OF PREMATURITY

A gradual decrease in hemoglobin concentration occurs during the first 2 to 3 months of life in term and preterm infants. The hemoglobin concentration remains stable during the next several weeks and then slowly rises. In term infants the fall in red blood cell production after birth is the result of improved oxygenation and occurs as a natural adaptation to extrauterine life. Because of this, the decrease in hemoglobin concentration has been termed a *physiologic nadir* rather than *true anemia*. However, in preterm infants, adaptive mechanisms may not be complete. Preterm infants generally decrease hemoglobin concentration to values lower than those seen in term infants, and the nadir varies with the degree of prematurity. Fig. 109.4 illustrates the decline in hemoglobin concentration in the first month of life on the basis of birth weight and gestational age. Hemoglobin values as low as 7 g/dL are common in preterm infants who have not undergone phlebotomies.[94,204]

Assessment of the factors that characterize oxygen supply and oxygen demand has provided insight into the adaptive changes occurring in preterm infants in response to low hemoglobin concentrations. In preterm infants, a low central venous Po_2 correlates with a mild increase in *EPO* production (Fig. 109.14).[205] The decline in central venous Po_2 may indicate the presence of anemia, representing the integration of variables that determine oxygen supply and demand: hemoglobin concentration, red blood cell and oxygen affinity, intravascular volume, oxygen consumption, heart rate, cardiac stroke volume, and arterial oxygenation. The hemoglobin concentration is only one of many important variables ensuring adequate oxygen delivery in both term and preterm infants.[186]

ANEMIA OF PREMATURITY

CHARACTERISTICS

Despite the slight increase in *EPO* production that occurs in response to declining central venous Po_2 values, *EPO*

Table 109.6 Changes in Hemoglobin Concentration, Hematocrit, and Other Markers of Oxygen Delivery During the First 3 Months of Life in Low-Birth-Weight Infants.

Age	Total Hemoglobin Blood (g/dL)	Hematocrit (%)	MCHC (%)	O_2 Capacity Blood (mL/dL)	P_{50} at pH 7.40 (mm Hg)	2,3-Diphosphoglycerate (nmol/mL)	Fetal Hemoglobin (% of Total)	FFDPG (nmol/mL)
Group I (<1000 g)[a]								
2 wk	17.2	47.0	36.6	23.9	18.0	6255	83.0	1002
4 wk	8.5	26.0	32.7	11.8	15.0	3923	81.0	761
9 wk	7.2	22.0	32.7	10.0	15.0	4636	87.1	974
11 wk	7.7	22.5	34.2	10.7	17.0	5867	78.0	1290
Group II (1001–1500 g)[b]								
1–2 days	15.1 ± 1.3	45.7 ± 3.7	33.0 ± 0.7	21.0 ± 1.8	18.0 ± 1.7	4124 ± 1562	86.6 ± 3.1	580 ± 287
5–8 days	13.4 ± 1.1	41.4 ± 3.2	33.5 ± 2.9	18.7 ± 1.5	18.9 ± 3.0	4501 ± 1919	84.4 ± 3.8	903 ± 689
2–3 wk	12.6 ± 3.1	33.6 ± 6.0	34.2 ± 1.1	15.9 ± 3.1	21.2 ± 1.9	5721 ± 1375	83.3 ± 5.1	1119 ± 557
4–5 wk	8.8 ± 0.9	25.3 ± 1.8	34.9 ± 1.7	12.3 ± 1.3	20.5 ± 1.7	6095 ± 2081	85.2 ± 2.3	931 ± 456
6–9 wk	9.1 ± 1.7	24.5 ± 5.8	35.1 ± 2.2	11.8 ± 2.4	23.4 ± 1.1	8734 ± 1834	77.2 ± 1.9	1995 ± 480
9–10 wk[c]	8.2	24.0	34.0	11.1	24.0	9000	77.0	2070
Group III (1501–2000 g)[b]								
1–2 days	16.1 ± 0.9	47.8 ± 1.9	33.7 ± 1.9	22.4 ± 1.2	19.3 ± 0.9	4475 ± 1174	87.2 ± 3.6	703 ± 331
5–8 days	16.8 ± 3.3	48.5 ± 10.0	34.7 ± 0.5	25.3 ± 4.7	19.8 ± 1.3	5489 ± 1428	79.4 ± 5.0	1056 ± 590
2–3 wk	13.6 ± 3.0	40.4 ± 9.8	34.4 ± 1.5	18.8 ± 4.0	21.3 ± 1.8	6002 ± 998	80.6 ± 5.8	1184 ± 329
4–5 wk	11.2 ± 2.8	31.9 ± 9.9	35.5 ± 2.2	15.5 ± 3.8	20.8 ± 1.6	5841 ± 839	75.8 ± 7.8	1569 ± 577
6–9 wk	8.0 ± 0.7	22.1 ± 1.7	35.9 ± 0.7	11.1 ± 1.0	24.0 ± 0.9	7290 ± 634	67.5 ± 6.2	2457 ± 575
Group IV (2001–2500 g)[b]								
1–2 days	15.9 ± 0.9	46.2 ± 5.8	35.8 ± 1.9	21.9 ± 1.5	20.2 ± 1.6	5306 ± 1075	76.8 ± 5.43	1258 ± 392
5–8 days	15.6 ± 1.7	47.0 ± 5.0	34.2 ± 1.1	21.5 ± 2.4	21.3 ± 3.3	6417 ± 1527	77.7 ± 6.3	1457 ± 603
2–3 wk	12.3 ± 1.1	35.1 ± 3.2	34.9 ± 0.5	17.1 ± 1.5	22.0 ± 1.3	7145 ± 1737	76.9 ± 4.7	1666 ± 472
6–9 wk[c]	14.0	44.0	34.0	19.5	25.5	7100	43.0	3212

[a]Only one patient.
[b]Values are given as the mean ± the standard deviation.
[c]Fewer than five infants.
FFDPG, Functioning fraction of 2,3-diphosphoglycerate; *MCHC,* mean corpuscular hemoglobin concentration; *RBC,* red blood cell.
From Delivoria-Papadopoulos M, Roncevic N, Oski FA. Postnatal changes in oxygen transport of term, preterm and sick infants: the role of red cell 2,3 diphosphoglycerate in adult hemoglobin. *Pediatr Res.* 1971;5:235.

concentrations in preterm infants are still significantly low, given the degree of anemia (Fig. 109.15).[76,111,205,206] This anemia, termed the *anemia of prematurity,* affects infants born at less than approximately 32 weeks gestation, and it is the most common anemia encountered in the neonatal period. It is a normocytic, normochromic anemia, generally associated with hemoglobin concentrations less than 10 g/dL and low reticulocyte counts. Some infants may be asymptomatic, whereas others demonstrate signs of anemia that are alleviated by transfusion. These signs traditionally include tachycardia, increased episodes of apnea and bradycardia, poor weight gain, an increased oxygen requirement, and elevated serum lactate concentrations that decrease after transfusion.[207–210]

Anemia of prematurity was first described by Schulman,[211] who divided the anemia into three phases. *Early anemia* was marked by an initial fall in hemoglobin concentration. The second, or *intermediate,* phase was characterized by maintenance of low hemoglobin concentrations. The third phase, *late anemia of prematurity,* resulted in hemoglobin concentrations that continued to fall, despite symptoms of anemia. The anemia of prematurity usually resolved spontaneously by 3 to 6 months of life.

Although much information has accumulated since the 1970s, detailed mechanisms responsible for the anemia of prematurity remain to be determined. Shortened erythrocyte survival,[212] hemodilution associated with a rapidly increasing body mass,[213] and the transition from fetal to adult hemoglobin[96] have all been implicated. Despite diminished levels of oxygen available to tissues[93] and the appearance of signs of anemia,[206] serum *EPO* concentrations remain low.[206] However, erythroid progenitors are highly sensitive to *EPO,*[214,215] and the concentrations of other erythropoietic growth factors, including IL-3 and GM-CSF, appear to be normal.[216]

Infants born prematurely lack a normal response to anemia and fail to increase *EPO* production despite an apparent need for improved tissue oxygenation.[217] This occurs regardless of the cause of anemia, whether it is the early anemia of phlebotomy loss or the later anemia of prematurity. Possible molecular and cellular mechanisms responsible for this lack of responsiveness include defects in transferring the hypoxic signal to the nucleus, diminished or defective binding of transcription factors to the promoter or enhancer regions of the gene, decreased production or stability of the transcriptional factors, decreased production or stability of *EPO* mRNA, diminished or unstable protein production, or increased production of counterregulatory proteins such as IL-1 and tumor necrosis factor. The inability of the kidney or liver in the premature infant to produce *EPO* mRNA with magnitude equal to that seen in the fetus may also involve a developmental delay in expression of transcriptional factors responsible for increasing *EPO* production, or in persistence of fetal *EPO* gene methylation patterns. Because *EPO* produced by the liver is indistinguishable from that produced by the kidney, it is unknown whether preterm infants rely on *EPO* produced by the liver, the kidney, or a combination of the two. However, macrophages from preterm infants generate *EPO* mRNA and protein as effectively as do those from term infants and adults.[218] The anemia of prematurity likely involves some sort of delay in activation of *EPO* gene expression, from prenatal (liver) to postnatal (kidney) sites of production.

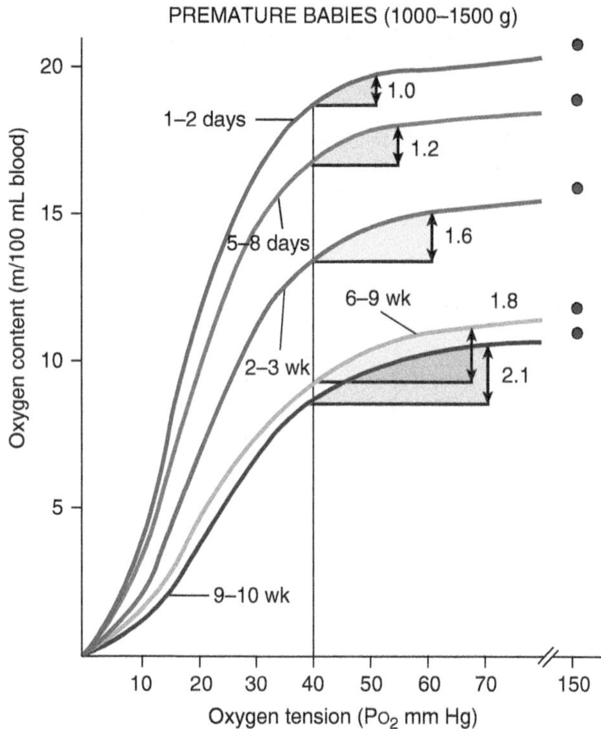

Fig. 109.12 Oxygen equilibrium curves of blood from premature infants (1000 to 1500 g) at different postnatal ages. *Double-headed arrows* represent the oxygen unloading capacity between a given arterial and venous Po_2. Points corresponding to 150 mm Hg on the abscissa are the oxygen capacities. Each curve represents the mean value of the infants studied in each group. (From Delivoria-Papadopoulos M, Roncevic N, Oski FA. Postnatal changes in oxygen transport of term, preterm and sick infants: the role of red cell 2,3 diphosphoglycerate in adult hemoglobin. *Pediatr Res.* 1971;5:235.)

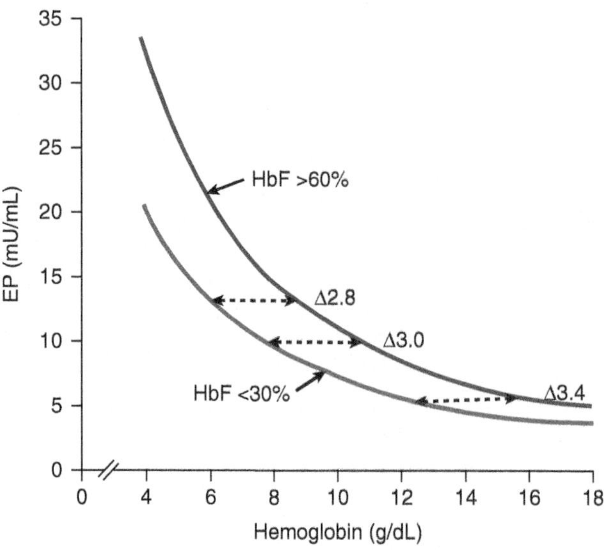

Fig. 109.13 Relationship between erythropoietin concentrations and postnatal hemoglobin. In infants born prematurely who have undergone exchange transfusion or multiple transfusion (fetal hemoglobin *[HbF]* <30%), the hemoglobin concentration may fall several grams per deciliter before resumption of erythropoietin production *(EP)*. (From Stockman JA, Garcia JF, Oski FA. The anemia of prematurity: factors governing the erythropoietin response. *New Engl J Med.* 1977;296:647.)

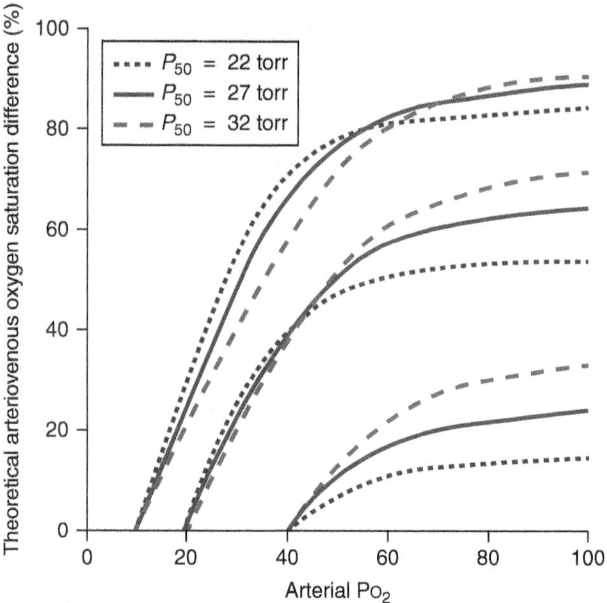

Fig. 109.14 The effect of arterial partial pressure of oxygen (Po_2) on theoretical arteriovenous oxygen content difference when venous partial pressure of oxygen is 40 mm Hg *(bottom set of curves)*, 20 mm Hg *(middle set of curves)*, or 10 mm Hg *(top set of curves)* at various oxygen half-saturation pressures of hemoglobin *(P_{50})*. (From Woodson RD. Physiological significance of oxygen dissociation curve shifts. *Crit Care Med.* 1979;7:368.)

CLINICAL TRIALS

Multiple clinical studies have been performed that have evaluate *EPO* administered to preterm infants.[219] Randomized controlled studies using *EPO* dosages greater than 500 U/kg/week for at least 2 weeks[220-233] have been reviewed elsewhere. A randomized placebo-controlled study of darbepoetin and *EPO* evaluated infants with a birth weight of 500 to 1250 g and 48 hours of age or younger who were randomized to receive darbepoetin (10 µg/kg, once per week subcutaneously), *EPO* (400 U/kg, three times per week subcutaneously), or placebo (sham dosing) through 35 weeks' gestation.[234] Infants in the darbepoetin and *EPO* groups received significantly fewer transfusions ($P = 0.015$) and, importantly, were exposed to fewer donors ($P = 0.044$) than the placebo group (darbepoetin, 1.2 ± 2.4 transfusions and 0.7 ± 1.2 donors per infant; *EPO*, 1.2 ± 1.6 transfusions and 0.8 ± 1.0 donors per infant; placebo, 2.4 ± 2.9 transfusions and 1.2 ± 1.3 donors per infant). Morbidities were similar among groups, including the incidence of retinopathy of prematurity. In this population of preterm infants, darbepoetin and *EPO* successfully serve as adjuncts to transfusions in maintaining red blood cell mass.

Recently published trials evaluating higher doses of *EPO* administered to extremely preterm infants evaluated potential neuroprotective effects, with varied outcomes.[235,236] It is clear from the most recent trials that *EPO* administration to preterm infants significantly decreases transfusions and improves hematocrit during the initial neonatal intensive care unit (NICU) hospitalization. Further evaluation regarding potential neuroprotection is ongoing.

PHARMACOKINETICS

Pharmacokinetic studies in newborn monkeys and sheep indicate that neonates have a larger volume of distribution and a faster elimination of *EPO*,[237,238] necessitating the use of doses higher than those required for adults.[239] These pharmacokinetic differences apply to preterm infants as well.[240,241] Although

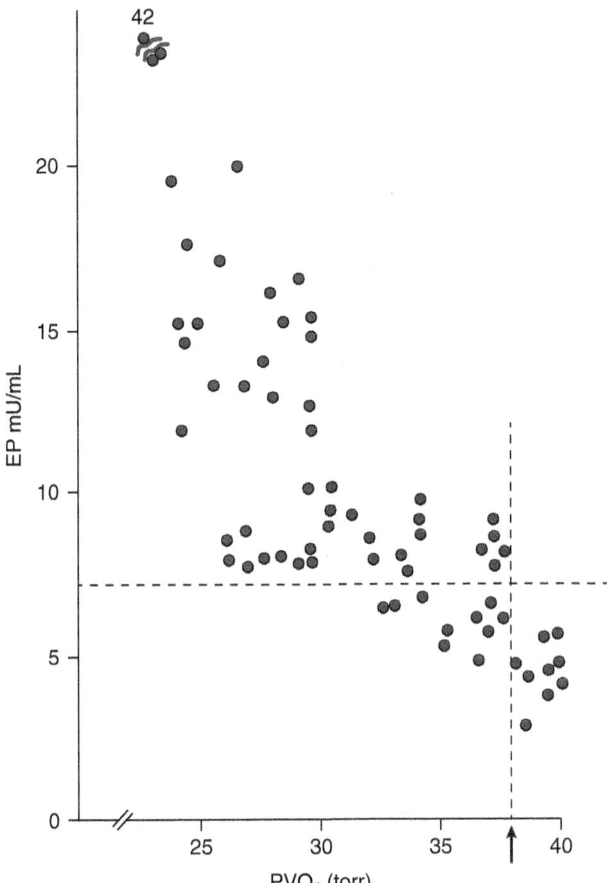

Fig. 109.15 Changes in plasma erythropoietin concentrations in response to declines in central venous oxygen tension (*PVO*$_2$) in preterm neonates. The *arrow* represents the position of 38 mm Hg, which for the purpose of this figure is the lower limit of normal for venous oxygen tension. The *horizontal dashed line* is the upper limit of normal for erythropoietin when venous oxygen tension of 38 Torr or greater is taken as normal. *EP,* Erythropoietin production. (From Stockman JA, Graeber JE, Clark DA, et al. Anemia of prematurity: determinants of the erythropoietin response. *Pediatr.* 1984;105:786.)

various *EPO* doses and dosing schedules have been evaluated in preterm infants, the erythrokinetics of *EPO* (the interaction between erythroid progenitors and their growth factors) in preterm infants are still being explored.

The route of administration also influences the effectiveness of *EPO*. Rapid intravenous administration of *EPO* generates peak serum concentrations that far exceed physiologic concentrations.[242] This may result in wasted drug via increased renal excretion. Dosing strategies that achieve lower peak serum concentrations over a more prolonged period may be more effective. Dosages in the range of 500 to 1400 U/kg/week, with administration subcutaneously every day or every other day, result in an adequate erythropoietic response. Newer, long-acting erythropoiesis-stimulating agents such as darbepoetin are currently being studied.[243,244] Data from preterm infants (considering half-life, volume of distribution, and clearance) suggest that higher doses will be required, but dosing intervals may be as great as once every 2 to 3 weeks.

SIDE EFFECTS OF ERYTHROPOIESIS-STIMULATING AGENTS

Side effects in neonates receiving erythropoiesis-stimulating agents have been rare. A side effect unique to neonates, transient neutropenia, was noted in early studies but has not been reported in the last decade.[245-247] The neutropenia was not associated with depletion of either neutrophil reserves or colony-forming unit-granulocyte-macrophage concentrations, but it appeared to involve reduced production of neutrophils from granulocytic progenitors[248,249]; it resolves after discontinuation of *EPO* administration. In newborn mice, neutropenia occurs after administration of very high doses of recombinant *EPO* as a result of decreased production of neutrophils from progenitors.[248]

Overall, the side effects of *EPO* administration in preterm infants have been minimal compared with those reported in adults (hypertension, bone pain, rash, and, rarely, seizures). None of these effects were reported in preterm infants involved in clinical trials. Moreover, no studies have reported differences between placebo and *EPO* recipients in the incidence of neonatal morbidities such as chronic lung disease, IVH, necrotizing enterocolitis, or late-onset sepsis. Meta-analyses first published in 2006 reported that, compared with late *EPO* administration, early (first week of life) *EPO* administration increased the incidence of retinopathy of prematurity (ROP) greater than stage 2.[250,251] Revised meta-analyses corrected a previous misclassification of a single-center *EPO* study into the late *EPO* administration group. The association between retinopathy of prematurity and *EPO* is no longer statistically significant.[252,253] No differences were seen in recently completed multicenter trials evaluating *EPO* administered to over 2000 extremely preterm infants.[235,236,254] In fact, when those infants are included in updated meta-analyses, the trend in greater than stage 2 ROP is greater in those infants randomized to placebo or control groups. Close ophthalmologic evaluation for retinopathy of prematurity continues to be a priority in clinical trials in preterm infants. Although there have been few long-term follow-up studies, it appears that the administration of *EPO* has no adverse effect on developmental outcome or growth, measured at 18 to 22 months.[255]

NUTRITIONAL SUPPLEMENTATION

Functional iron deficiency has frequently been reported in pediatric and adult patients receiving *EPO,* and it likely limited the success of some of the early *EPO* trials in preterm infants. Studies evaluating iron stores in *EPO* recipients[220,221] noted increased iron requirements in infants receiving *EPO,* as evidenced by diminished ferritin concentrations and elevated numbers of hypochromic red blood cells, despite iron doses of 6 mg/kg/day. Infants receiving *EPO* are likely at greater risk for iron deficiency than for iron overload and increased oxidant stress. However, further evaluation is still required to determine the optimal dose and most effective route of administration of iron in preterm infants receiving *EPO*.

Vitamin E is an antioxidant, inhibiting peroxidation of polyunsaturated fatty acids in the lipid bilayers of all cell membranes. Vitamin E requirements may be increased secondary to increased iron supplementation, because iron promotes oxidation of polyunsaturated fatty acids. Pathak and colleagues[228] evaluated high-dose vitamin E in preterm infants receiving *EPO* and found it showed no benefit compared with doses of 50 IU/kg/day. Further study is needed to determine the optimal dose of vitamin E in preterm infants receiving *EPO*.

Folate and vitamin B_{12} have recently been evaluated in combination with *EPO* and iron, and have shown significant promise.[232,256] In an evaluation of preterm infants weighing 800 g or less, Haiden and colleagues[232] achieved significantly greater success (38% of infants did not receive transfusion) when vitamin B_{12} at a dosage of 21 mg/kg/week subcutaneously was added to a regimen of *EPO,* iron, vitamin E, and folate.[239] When combined with limited phlebotomy losses, this therapy shows great promise in extremely low-birth-weight infants.

Regardless of the treatment strategy, a critical understanding of the developmental, physiologic, and pathologic influences affecting oxygen delivery in term and preterm infants is important in determining the optimal strategy in maintaining or altering the hematocrit through the administration of an erythrocyte transfusion or the administration of an erythropoiesis-stimulating agent.

CONCLUSION

The fetal and neonatal periods mark a time when erythrocyte indices and characteristics differ remarkably from indices of children and adults. The stages of erythropoiesis move from yolk sack to liver to marrow, whereas production of erythrocyte growth factors migrates from liver to marrow and kidney. Infants born prematurely have altered production of erythrocytes; the ability to deliver oxygen to tissues based on fetal and adult hemoglobin concentrations varies greatly during the early months of life in extremely low-birth-weight infants. A detailed understanding of erythrocyte physiology and the nutritional and growth factor needs of preterm and term infants will aid the clinician in caring for neonates in the first weeks of life.

ACKNOWLEDGMENTS

Parts of this chapter were adapted from sections of Chapter 134 by authors James A. Stockman III and Pedro A. DeAlarcon in the first edition of this book. We thank Erin Adair for assistance with illustrations.

 A complete reference list is available at www.ExpertConsult.com.

SELECT REFERENCES

9. Moore MAS, Metcalf D. Ontogeny of the haemopoietic system: yolk sac origin of *in vivo* and in vitro colony forming cells in the developing mouse embryo. *Br J Haematol*. 1970;18(3):279–296. https://doi.org/10.1111/j.1365-2141.1970.tb01443.x.
10. Yoder MC, Hiatt K. Engraftment of embryonic hematopoietic cells in conditioned newborn recipients. *Blood*. 1997;89(6):2176–2183. https://doi.org/10.1182/blood.V89.6.2176.
12. Forestier F, Daffos F, Catherine N, Renard M, Andreux JP. Developmental hematopoiesis in normal human fetal blood. *Blood*. 1991;77(11):2360–2363.
19. Spivak JL. The mechanism of action of erythropoietin. *Int J Cell Cloning*. 1986;4(3):139–166. https://doi.org/10.1002/stem.5530040302.
21. Jacobs K, Shoemaker C, Rudersdorf R, et al. Isolation and characterization of genomic and cDNA clones of human erythropoietin. *Nature*. 1985;313(6005):806–810. https://doi.org/10.1038/313806a0.
34. Zanjani ED, Pixley JS, Slotnick N, MacKintosh R, Ekhterae D, Clemons G. Erythropoietin does not cross the placenta into the fetus. *Pathobiology*. 1993;61(3-4):211–215. https://doi.org/10.1159/000163796.
40. Goldberg MA, Dunning SP, Bunn HF. Regulation of the erythropoietin gene: evidence that the oxygen sensor is a heme protein. *Science*. 1988;242(4884):1412–1415. https://doi.org/10.1126/science.2849206.
41. Peschle C, Marone G, Genovese A, Cillo C, Magli C, Condorelli M. Erythropoietin production by the liver in fetal-neonatal life. *Life Sci*. 1975;17(8):1325–1330. https://doi.org/10.1016/0024-3205(75)90146-0.
44. Erslev AJ, Caro J, Kansu E, Silver R. Renal and extrarenal erythropoietin production in anaemic rats. *Br J Haematol*. 1980;45(1):65–72. https://doi.org/10.1111/j.1365-2141.1980.tb03811.x.
55. Zanjani ED, Poster J, Burlington H, Mann LI, Wasserman LR. Liver as the primary site of erythropoietin formation in the fetus. *J Lab Clin Med*. 1977;89(3):640–644.
60. Ohls RK. Erythropoietin and hypoxia inducible factor-1 expression in the midtrimester human fetus. *Acta Paediatr*. 2002;91(9):27–30. https://doi.org/10.1080/080352502320764166.
76. Erslev AJ, Wilson J, Caro J. Erythropoietin titers in anemic, nonuremic patients. *J Lab Clin Med*. 1987;109(4):429–433.
79. Christensen RD, Jopling J, Henry E, Wiedmeier SE. The erythrocyte indices of neonates, defined using data from over 12 000 patients in a multihospital health care system. *J Perinatol*. 2008;28(1):24–28. https://doi.org/10.1038/sj.jp.7211852.
88. Song J, Sundar K, Gangaraju R, Prchal JT. Regulation of erythropoiesis after normoxic return from chronic sustained and intermittent hypoxia. *J Appl Physiol Bethesda Md*. 2017;123(6):1671–1675. https://doi.org/10.1152/japplphysiol.00119.2017. 1985.
93. Stockman JA, Garcia JF, Oski FA. The anemia of prematurity. Factors governing the erythropoietin response. *N Engl J Med*. 1977;296(12):647–650. https://doi.org/10.1056/NEJM197703242961202.
96. Delivoria-Papadopoulos M, Roncevic NP, Oski FA. Postnatal changes in oxygen transport of term, premature, and sick infants: the role of red cell 2,3-diphosphoglycerate and adult hemoglobin. *Pediatr Res*. 1971;5(6):235–245. https://doi.org/10.1203/00006450-197106000-00001.
101. Oh W, Lind J. Venous and capillary hematocrit in newborn infants and placental transfusion. *Acta Paediatr*. 1966;55(1):38–48. https://doi.org/10.1111/j.1651-2227.1966.tb15207.x.
108. Christensen RD, Henry E, Andres RL, Bennett ST. Reference ranges for blood concentrations of nucleated red blood cells in neonates. *Neonatology*. 2011;99(4):289–294. https://doi.org/10.1159/000320148.
111. Christensen RD, ed. *Hematologic Problems of the Neonate*. Philadelphia: Saunders; 2000.
120. Masala B, Manca L, Formato M, Pilo G. A study of the switch of fetal hemoglobin in newborn erythrocytes fractionated by density gradient. *Hemoglobin*. 1983;7(6):567–572. https://doi.org/10.3109/03630268309027937.
128. Peschle C, Mavilio F, Carè A, et al. Haemoglobin switching in human embryos: asynchrony of $\zeta \rightarrow \alpha$ and $\varepsilon \rightarrow \gamma$-globin switches in primitive and definitive erythropoietic lineage. *Nature*. 1985;313(5999):235–238. https://doi.org/10.1038/313235a0.
135. Bard H, Lachance C, Widness JA, Gagnon C. The reactivation of fetal hemoglobin synthesis during anemia of prematurity. *Pediatr Res*. 1994;36(2):253–256. https://doi.org/10.1203/00006450-199408000-00018.
143. Peschle C, Condorelli M. Regulation of fetal and adult erythropoiesis. In: Porter R, Fitzsimons DW, eds. *Ciba Foundation Symposium 37 – Congenital Disorders of Erythropoiesis*. Chichester, UK: John Wiley & Sons, Ltd.; 2008:25–47. https://doi.org/10.1002/9780470720196.ch3.
177. Linderkamp O, Stadler AA, Zilow EP. Blood viscosity and optimal hematocrit in preterm and full-term neonates in 50- to 500-μm tubes. *Pediatr Res*. 1992;32(1):97–102. https://doi.org/10.1203/00006450-199207000-00019.
203. Novy MJ, Frigoletto FD, Easterday CL, Umansky I, Nelson NM. Changes in umbilical-cord blood oxygen affinity after intrauterine transfusions for erythroblastosis. *N Engl J Med*. 1971;285(11):589–595. https://doi.org/10.1056/NEJM197109092851101.
204. Williams ML, Shoot RJ, O'Neal PL, Oski FA. Role of dietary iron and fat on vitamin E deficiency anemia of infancy. *N Engl J Med*. 1975;292(17):887–890. https://doi.org/10.1056/NEJM197504242921704.
205. Stockman JA, Graeber JE, Clark DA, McClellan K, Garcia JF, Kavey RE. Anemia of prematurity: determinants of the erythropoietin response. *J Pediatr*. 1984;105(5):786–792. https://doi.org/10.1016/s0022-3476(84)80308-x.
206. Brown MS, Garcia JF, Phibbs RH, Dallman PR. Decreased response of plasma immunoreactive erythropoietin to "available oxygen" in anemia of prematurity. *J Pediatr*. 1984;105(5):793–798. https://doi.org/10.1016/s0022-3476(84)80309-1.
208. Bifano EM, Smith F, Borer J. Relationship between determinants of oxygen delivery and respiratory abnormalities in preterm infants with anemia. *J Pediatr*. 1992;120(2 Pt 1):292–296. https://doi.org/10.1016/s0022-3476(05)80447-0.
209. Keyes WG, Donohue PK, Spivak JL, Jones MD, Oski FA. Assessing the need for transfusion of premature infants and role of hematocrit, clinical signs, and erythropoietin level. *Pediatrics*. 1989;84(3):412–417.
215. Rhondeau SM, Christensen RD, Ross MP, Rothstein G, Simmons MA. Responsiveness to recombinant human erythropoietin of marrow erythroid progenitors from infants with the "anemia of prematurity. *J Pediatr*. 1988;112(6):935–940. https://doi.org/10.1016/s0022-3476(88)80223-3.
216. Ohls RK, Liechty KW, Turner MC, Kimura R, Christensen RD. Erythroid "burst promoting" activity in serum of patients with the anemia of prematurity. *J Pediatr*. 1990;116(5):786–789. https://doi.org/10.1016/s0022-3476(05)82672-1.
220. Maier RF, Obladen M, Scigalla P, et al. The effect of epoetin beta (recombinant human erythropoietin) on the need for transfusion in very-low-birth-weight infants. European Multicentre Erythropoietin Study Group. *N Engl J Med*. 1994;330(17):1173–1178. https://doi.org/10.1056/NEJM199404283301701.
222. Shannon KM, Keith JF, Mentzer WC, et al. Recombinant human erythropoietin stimulates erythropoiesis and reduces erythrocyte transfusions in very low birth weight preterm infants. *Pediatrics*. 1995;95(1):1–8.
223. Ohls RK, Osborne KA, Christensen RD. Efficacy and cost analysis of treating very low birth weight infants with erythropoietin during their first two weeks of life: a randomized, placebo-controlled trial. *J Pediatr*. 1995;126(3):421–426. https://doi.org/10.1016/s0022-3476(95)70462-0.
225. Donato H, Vain N, Rendo P, et al. Effect of early versus late administration of human recombinant erythropoietin on transfusion requirements in premature infants: results of a randomized, placebo-controlled, multicenter trial. *Pediatrics*. 2000;105(5):1066–1072. https://doi.org/10.1542/peds.105.5.1066.
226. Ohls RK, Ehrenkranz RA, Wright LL, et al. Effects of early erythropoietin therapy on the transfusion requirements of preterm infants below 1250 grams birth weight: a multicenter, randomized, controlled trial. *Pediatrics*. 2001;108(4):934–942. https://doi.org/10.1542/peds.108.4.934.
227. Maier RF, Obladen M, Müller-Hansen I, et al. Early treatment with erythropoietin beta ameliorates anemia and reduces transfusion requirements in infants with birth weights below 1000 g. *J Pediatr*. 2002;141(1):8–15. https://doi.org/10.1067/mpd.2002.124309.
235. Juul SE, Comstock BA, Wadhawan R, et al. A randomized trial of erythropoietin for neuroprotection in preterm infants. *N Engl J Med*. 2020;382(3):233–243. https://doi.org/10.1056/NEJMoa1907423.
239. Eschbach JW, Egrie JC, Downing MR, Browne JK, Adamson JW. Correction of the anemia of end-stage renal disease with recombinant human erythropoietin. Results of a combined phase I and II clinical trial. *N Engl J Med*. 1987;316(2):73–78. https://doi.org/10.1056/NEJM198701083160203.

Developmental Megakaryopoiesis

110

Martha C. Sola-Visner | Patricia Davenport

INTRODUCTION

Megakaryocytes (MKs), among the rarest and most unusual hematopoietic cells in the human bone marrow, comprise 0.02% to 0.1% of the total nucleated marrow cells.[1,2] Over the past decades, the study of these cells lagged behind that of other hematopoietic lineages, partly because of the rarity and fragility of MKs in the bone marrow, and partly because of the lack of a potent thrombopoietic factor to stimulate the growth of these cells in culture. The cloning of thrombopoietin (Tpo) in 1994 broke many of these barriers and led to major advances in our understanding of megakaryopoiesis. The first part of this chapter is dedicated to reviewing the biology of MK progenitors, the differentiation and maturation of MKs, the effects of thrombopoietic cytokines (particularly Tpo), and how these processes differ between fetal, neonatal, and adult megakaryopoiesis. The second part of the chapter summarizes our current understanding of neonatal thrombocytopenia, with an emphasis on the factors underlying the predisposition of ill neonates to develop severe and prolonged thrombocytopenia. Although many questions in this field remain unanswered, it is now clear that fetal and neonatal MKs have cellular and molecular features clearly different from those of their adult counterparts. These developmental differences have implications for the pathogenesis of common and less common platelet disorders, and expand beyond neonatal hematology into the field of cord blood (CB) transplantation, a therapy frequently complicated by delayed platelet engraftment.

MEGAKARYOPOIESIS

In a very schematic fashion, the complex process of platelet production can be represented as consisting of four main steps (Fig. 110.1): (1) the production of thrombopoietic factors (mainly Tpo), (2) the proliferation of MK progenitors, (3) the differentiation and maturation of MKs through a unique process of endomitosis, and finally (4) the production and release of platelets into the circulation. The first part of this section is dedicated to reviewing the biology of adult megakaryopoiesis. The second half is focused on fetal and neonatal megakaryopoiesis, highlighting the key developmental differences.

ADULT MEGAKARYOCYTE PROGENITORS

The development of the megakaryocytic lineage from pluripotent hematopoietic stem cells (HSCs) is not clearly understood. The classical model states that HSCs give rise to a common lymphoid progenitor, which produces lymphocytes, and a common myeloid progenitor, which gives rise to the myeloid, macrophage, eosinophil, erythroid, and megakaryocytic lineages.[3] In this model, the erythroid and MK lineages arise from a common oligopotent MK-erythroid progenitor (MEP).[4,5] However, this classical pathway of hematopoiesis has been challenged by several recent discoveries. Studies examining the heterogeneity within the human hematopoietic progenitor/stem cell ($CD34^+$) compartment found that the blood hierarchy in adult BM was mainly composed of two tiers: a top tier containing multipotent cells such as HSCs and multipotent progenitors (MPPs), and a bottom tier composed of committed unipotent progenitors with primarily myeloid or erythroid potential.[6] Interestingly, this study found that the MK lineage in the adult BM emerged directly from the HSC compartment, supporting the hypothesis that MK branching in the adult human BM occurs directly from a multipotent cell and that there might be a subset of human HSCs primed for platelet production, similar to the von Willebrand factor (vWF)-positive platelet-primed stem cells described in the mouse.[7,8] The specific signals that regulate the separation into the different lineages are not well understood and are the subject of active research efforts.

The first cells fully committed to the MK lineage are the MK progenitors. By definition, these cells have proliferative potential and are characterized by their ability to form clusters of pure MKs (MK colonies) when cultured. Two different types of MK progenitors have been identified. The most primitive MK progenitor is the burst-forming unit–MK (BFU-MK). A later, more mature progenitor has been designated the colony-forming unit–MK (CFU-MK). These two progenitor types can be differentiated on the basis of their immunologic markers and the characteristics of the colonies that they form in vitro (Table 110.1). Overall, CFU-MK-derived colonies are smaller (usually <50 cells) and unifocal, compared with the large and multifocal appearance of BFU-MK colonies. CFU-MK progenitors are also the predominant MK progenitor type in the bone marrow, whereas BFU-MK progenitors predominate in the blood. Finally, although both progenitors express CD34, only CFU-MKs express the human leukocyte antigen (HLA)-DR.

Unlike MK progenitors, which possess a high proliferative potential, MKs are cells that have lost the ability to proliferate but instead undergo a unique process known as *endomitosis*, in which chromosomes duplicate without nuclear division, resulting in increased cell ploidy. The transition from MK progenitors to mature MKs is characterized by a significant level of overlap, which gives rise to a population of cells known as *transitional cells*, *MK precursors*, or *promegakaryoblasts*, which have increasing ploidy (4N to 8N) and decreasing proliferative potential. These cells are thought to represent the intermediate step between progenitors and MKs and are difficult to identify morphologically. Immunologic studies have suggested that transitional cells express both CD34 and CD61 (GPIIIa).[9] During maturation, the cells accumulate various α-granule proteins including platelet factor 4 (PF4), thrombospondin, β-thromboglobulin, and vWF, and accumulate surface markers such as platelet GPIb and the vWF receptor (Fig. 110.2).[10–15]

ADULT MEGAKARYOCYTES

MKs are cells that have lost their proliferative abilities and undergo a complex process of maturation. Through this process, they evolve from small, mononuclear cells that are indistinguishable from those of other lineages, to very large, polyploid cells that are easily recognized as MKs. The process of maturation involves both nuclear and cytoplasmic changes, as well as a corresponding increase in size. At the nuclear level, MKs undergo endoreduplication or endomitosis, which leads to increased ploidy. The ploidy level of MKs can be assessed on stained individual cells in a cytospin or by flow cytometry. Using the latter technique, the modal ploidy in adult marrow has

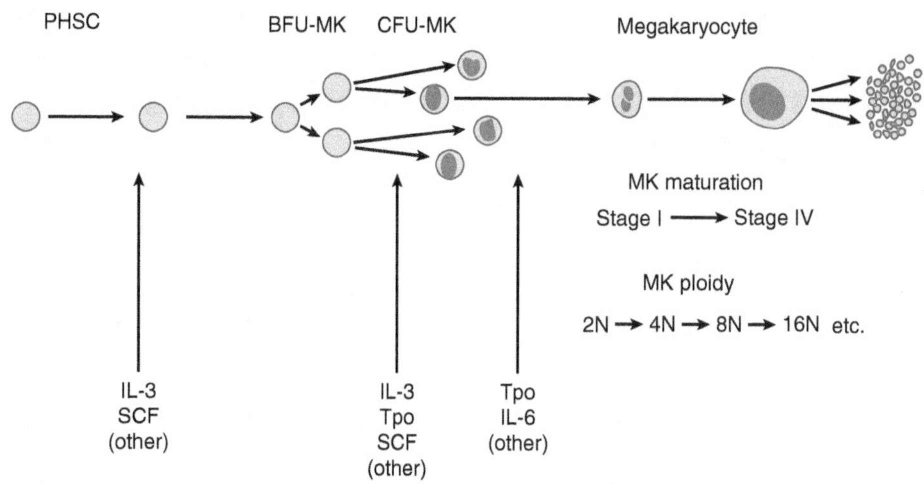

Fig. 110.1 Simplified scheme of megakaryocyte *(MK)* development. Many growth factors probably influence megakaryocytopoiesis at each stage. In some studies, the synergistic effect of interleukin-3 *(IL-3)* with stem cell factor (SCF) and thrombopoietin *(Tpo)* was demonstrated. IL-3 seems to be essential for early MK proliferation (especially fetal) from pluripotent hematopoietic stem cell *(PHSC)* through colony-forming unit, MK *(CFU-MK)*. *BFU,* Burst-forming unit; *IL-6*, interleukin 6.

Table 110.1 Comparison of Primitive Megakaryocyte Progenitors and Differentiated Megakaryocyte Progenitors.

Characteristic	BFU-MK	CFU-MK
Appearance in culture	Later	Earlier
Cells/colony	>50	3–50
Foci of development	≥2	1
Immunologic phenotype	CD34+, HLA-DR−	CD34+, HLA-DR+
Site of predominance	Peripheral blood and bone marrow	Bone marrow

BFU-MK, Burst-forming unit–megakaryocyte; *CFU-MK*, colony-forming unit–megakaryocyte; *HLA-DR*, human leukocyte antigen.
From Sola MC. Fetal megakaryocytopoiesis. In: Christensen R, ed. *Hematologic Problems of the Neonate*. Philadelphia: WB Saunders; 2000.

been shown to be 16N. Increasing ploidy levels correlate with increased platelet production by MKs, at least in vitro.[16]

The patterns of endomitosis are somewhat different between high and low ploidy MKs. In the transition from a 2N to a 4N MK, the cell elongates while creating two separated nuclear masses, forming a cleavage furrow; however, due to a halt in cytokinesis, the cells do not separate and instead move backwards to reassemble a 4N cell.[17] The clear cleavage furrow created through this process is seldom seen in higher ploidy MKs, as chromosomes segregate into 3 to 5 groups containing multiple territories, without exhibiting a clear furrow.[18]

Based on a combination of size and nuclear and cytoplasmic features, the maturational stages of the MKs have been classified as stages I to IV. This morphologic classification is often difficult, however, particularly because megakaryoblasts and stage I and II MKs can easily be missed on microscopic examination. For these reasons, other criteria have been established for MK differentiation, and for defining various maturational stages, including the development of surface glycoproteins and the appearance of specific granules.[11,13] For example, GPIIIa (CD61) and GPIIb/IIIa (CD41/61) are present in very early MKs, whereas GPIb (CD42b), GPIV (CD36), and the GP1b-V-IX (CD42) complexes appear later during MK maturation (see Fig. 110.2).[12,19–21] The development of the invaginated membrane system, formerly known as the *demarcation membrane system*, and of α-granules has been documented by electron microscopy. Contents of the α-granules, such as fibrinogen, thrombospondin, and vWF, also correlate with MK maturation.[12,13,15]

FETAL AND NEONATAL MEGAKARYOPOIESIS

In the course of human as well as murine development, hematopoiesis transitions from the yolk sac to the liver and then to the BM.[22] In humans, MKs have been observed in the yolk sac by 5 weeks' gestation,[23] and the first platelets appear in the circulation at 8 to 9 weeks.[24] The transition to hepatic hematopoiesis is thought to involve the migration of stem cells from the yolk sac to the liver.[25] MKs are first found in the human liver at 10 weeks' gestation.[26] Every stage of MK development is present in the fetal liver, although MKs at every stage are significantly smaller than their adult counterparts.[27,28] The transition from hepatic to BM hematopoiesis occurs progressively throughout gestation. BM hematopoiesis starts at 11 weeks' gestation,[29] and it becomes the dominant site of hematopoiesis by 20 weeks.[28,30–32] The contribution of the liver, in contrast, decreases throughout fetal development. At 16 weeks, 50% to 70% of all liver cells are hematopoietic cells, but this percentage decreases after 27 to 32 weeks' gestation to 25% to 30% at term.[33] Thus, in the human, the BM is the primary hematopoietic site in preterm and term neonates, but the liver is still active as a secondary hematopoietic site.

In the mouse, primitive MK/erythroid progenitors appear at embryonic day 7.25 (E7.25), along with pure MK and pure primitive erythroid progenitors, which indicates that primitive hematopoiesis is bilineal.[5] The first platelet-forming cells of the embryonic yolk sac are not polyploid MKs, but diploid platelet-forming cells (DPFCs),[34] similar to the 2N MKs that produce platelets in the human fetus (see "Fetal and Neonatal Megakaryocytes"). DPFCs appear in the yolk sac at E8.5 and produce the first platelets at E9.5. Highly polyploid MKs (achieving 8N) are first seen in the fetal liver at E11.5 and progressively achieve greater ploidy levels, a process associated with a significant expansion of the fetal platelet mass.[35] In contrast to humans, the liver is the main murine hematopoietic organ at birth, and the transition from liver to BM megakaryopoiesis occurs largely during the first 2 weeks of postnatal life, with the spleen providing hematopoietic support during this period.[36]

FETAL MEGAKARYOCYTE PROGENITORS

Recent studies challenging the traditional paradigms of hematopoiesis also unveiled important developmental differences between human fetal and adult hematopoiesis. Compared to the two-tier model in adult BM (see "Adult Megakaryocyte Progenitors), the fetal liver exhibits a three-tier hierarchy, composed of multipotent HSCs and MPPs at the top, oligopotent progenitors

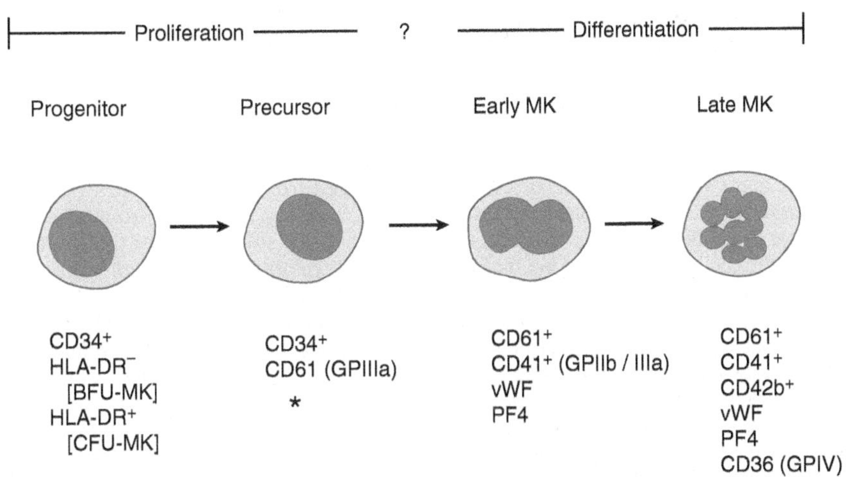

Fig. 110.2 Immunologic classification of megakaryocyte (MK) development. Burst-forming unit, MK *(BFU-MK)*, and colony-forming unit, MK *(CFU-MK)*, are considered progenitor cells. CFU-MK may transition into a precursor cell that still retains proliferative potential. Fragmentary data on various stages of MK differentiation suggest a chronologic appearance of specific platelet glycoproteins (GP) and other platelet antigens such as von Willebrand factor *(vWf)* and platelet factor 4 *(PF4)*. The *asterisk* indicates that MK antigens CD41 (GPIIb/IIIa) and CD41a (GPIIb) may be expressed on an earlier cell of the MK lineage that retains proliferative capacity. *HLA-DR*, Human leukocyte antigen-DR.

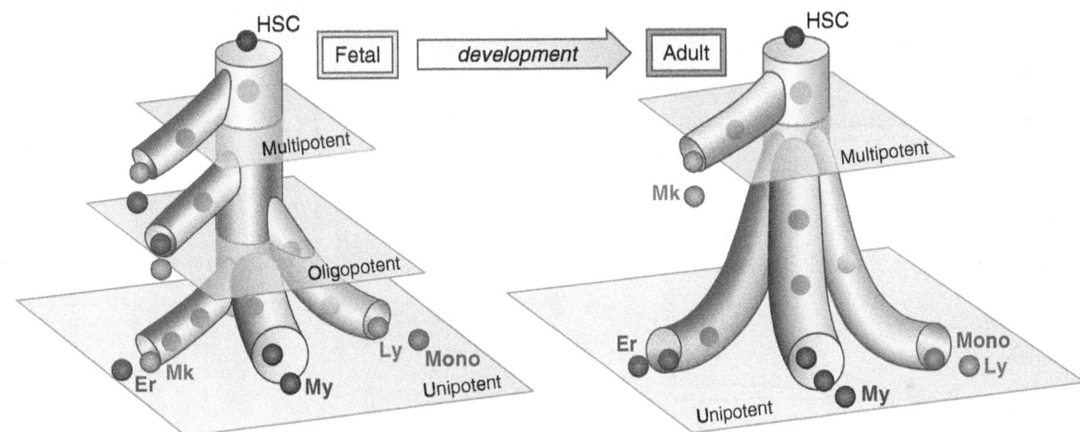

Fig. 110.3 Graphical representation of the redefined model showing the predominant lineage potential of the newly defined progenitor subsets. This redefined model envisions a developmental shift in the progenitor cell architecture, transitioning from a three-tier hierarchy in fetal life to a two-tier hierarchy by adulthood. *Er,* Erythrocytes; *HSCs*, hematopoietic stem cells; *Ly,* lymphocytes; *Mk,* megakaryocytes; *Mono,* monocytes. (Republished with permission from Notta F, Zandi S, Takayama N, et al. Distinct routes of lineage development reshape the human blood hierarchy across ontogeny. *Science.* 2016;351:aab2116.)

with myeloid-erythroid-MK and erythroid-MK activity in the middle, and unipotent progenitors in the bottom (Fig. 110.3).[6] An additional recent study investigating blood and immune cell development in the human liver between 7 and 17 weeks post-conception (when the liver is the main site of hematopoiesis), found that HSCs/MPPs in the fetal liver have different intrinsic potential according to gestational age, with samples from early stages exhibiting an erythroid lineage bias and lymphoid and myeloid lineages being more represented at later stages.[37] This study also supported the presence of a fetal liver-shared MK-erythroid-mast cell progenitor (MEMP) immediately downstream of the HSC/MPP cell, and identified *F11R, PBx1,* and *MEIS* as the genes dynamically modulated in the specification of the fetal MK lineage.

Most studies assessing the quantity and clonogenic potential of MK progenitors during fetal development have been performed using umbilical CB, from which large quantities of MK progenitors can be readily obtained. Olson and associates found a significantly higher concentration of CFU-MK progenitors in term and preterm CB than in adult peripheral blood (PB).[38] Furthermore, when stimulated with aplastic canine serum, CB CFU-MK-derived colonies contained significantly more MKs than adult colonies. Zauli and co-workers cultured hematopoietic progenitors ($CD34^+$ cells) obtained from the blood of fetuses between 18 and 22 weeks' gestation, or from adult bone marrow in a fibrin clot assay, and found that, as in adult blood, BFU-MKs predominate in fetal blood, with a CFU-MK/BFU-MK ratio of 0.4:1. Fetal and adult MK progenitors had similar immunologic profiles with regard to the expression of CD34 and HLA-DR.[39,40] However, there were significant differences in the morphology and size of the BFU-MK-derived colonies: the fetal BFU-MK-derived colonies were significantly larger than the adult colonies and were usually composed of only one or two foci of development, whereas the adult BFU-MK-derived colonies were always multifocal.

Other investigators have also reported the existence of a MK progenitor with an unusually high proliferative potential exclusively found in the human fetal bone marrow. Bruno and colleagues described a high proliferative potential cell–MK (HPPC-MK) in fetal bone marrow that gives rise to large, unifocal colonies with more than 300 cells.[41] This cell, not observed in adult bone marrow cultures, may represent a more primitive MK progenitor only present during fetal life. Nishihira and associates cultured CB hematopoietic progenitors (26 to 41 weeks' gestation) with optimal concentrations of recombinant Tpo (rTpo) and found that all colonies consisted of more than 50 cells and that 50% had more than 500 cells.[42] It is unclear whether these colonies should be classified as BFU-MK- or HPPC-MK-derived colonies.

Comparing circulating MK progenitors between preterm and term neonates, Murray and collaborators found that, in the first day of life, preterm neonates (24 to 36 weeks' gestation) had higher circulating concentrations of MK progenitors than those born at term.[43] This finding was in concordance with the previously described gestational age-related decrease in the concentration of other committed hematopoietic progenitors, deemed to reflect the migration of progenitors from the fetal liver to the bone marrow over gestation.[44] Saxonhouse and associates also observed an inverse relationship between the concentration of circulating MK progenitors and the postmenstrual age (gestational age + postnatal age in weeks) of growing preterm infants being cared for in the neonatal intensive care unit (NICU), suggesting that the decrease in circulating MK progenitors is a process that follows the same developmentally regulated pattern regardless of premature birth.[45]

In addition to these phenotypic differences, at the transcriptional level fetal and neonatal MK progenitors continue to express erythroid lineage markers, suggesting incomplete lineage separation in fetal/neonatal compared to adult progenitors. In a study comparing the gene expression profiles of purified MK progenitors from murine fetal livers and murine adult BM, 7 out of the 122 transcripts upregulated in fetal liver were erythroid transcripts.[46] Similarly, human CB-derived MKs (CD41$^+$ cells) express the erythroid antigen glycophorin A (GPA), while MKs derived from adult BM do not.[47,48]

FETAL AND NEONATAL MEGAKARYOCYTES

Using different cell sources and techniques, several investigators demonstrated that MKs in the fetal and neonatal BM, in CB, or cultured from CB progenitors were consistently smaller and of lower ploidy than MKs from adults,[30,49,50] and documented a progressive shift to higher ploidy classes and larger MKs during fetal development.[51,52] Despite this shift, however, 78% of MKs in the BM of fetuses at 7 to 8 months' gestation had a ploidy of 8N or less, compared with only 33% of the MKs in adult BM.[52]

Applying ultrastructural techniques, Hegyi and collaborators evaluated the maturational stage of small fetal liver MKs and found that, despite their low ploidy, they had all the cytoplasmic components of a mature cell, with multiple granules and a well-developed demarcation system.[51] Consistently, our group found that MK progenitors from CB cultured in liquid culture medium generated 10 times more MKs than progenitors from adult PB. The neonatal MKs, however, were significantly smaller and of lower ploidy than adult MKs, but were cytoplasmically mature based on surface markers, immunofluorescence, and electron microscopy (Fig. 110.4).[53] Taken together, these studies demonstrated a developmentally unique uncoupling of proliferation, polyploidization, and cytoplasmic maturation in neonatal MKs. In terms of platelet production,

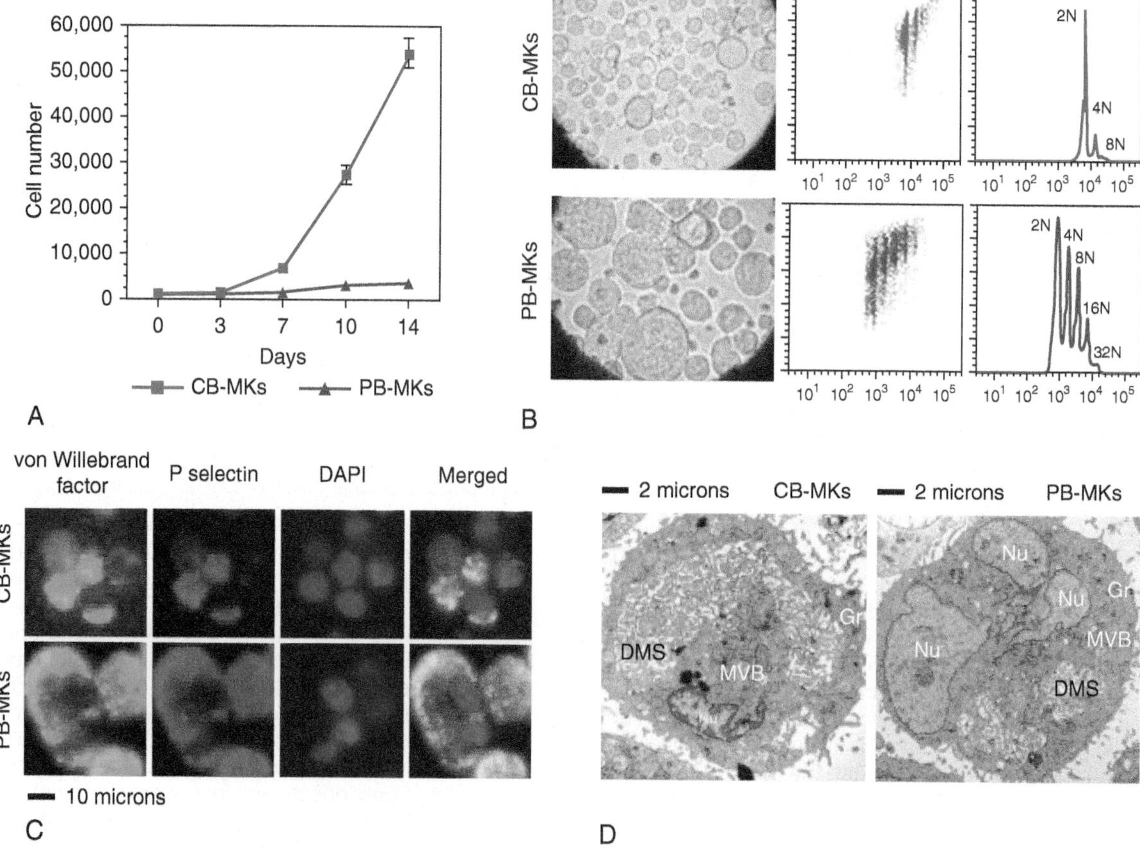

Fig. 110.4 Key features of neonatal megakaryopoiesis. Neonatal and adult MKs were generated in vitro by culturing CD34$^+$ cells obtained from cord blood *(CB)* or from adult mobilized peripheral blood *(PB)* in a serum-free liquid medium with 50 ng/mL of recombinant human Tpo as the only growth factor. (A) Number of cells derived from 1000 CD34+ cells over a 14-day culture period. CB-CD34+ cells generated approximately 10-fold more MKs than PB-CD34$^+$ cells. Each data point indicates the mean ± SEM of four independent samples. (B) Representative photomicrographs and ploidy levels by flow cytometry of CB- and PB-MKs at the end of the culture period, demonstrating the smaller size and lower ploidy levels of CB-MKs. Both pictures were taken at a magnification of 600×. (C) Despite their small size, CB-MKs exhibited abundant alpha granules, as demonstrated by immunofluorescent staining for von Willebrand factor and P-selectin. (D) Flow-sorted 2N/4N CB-MKs *(left)* were examined by transmission electron microscopy and found to contain abundant granules *(Gr)* and a well-developed demarcation membrane system *(DMS)*, consistent with mature MKs and similar to flow-sorted PB MKs with ploidy ≥8N *(right)*. *DAPI*, 4′,6-Diamidino-2-phenylindole; *MVB*, multivesicular bodies; *Nu*, nucleus; *Tpo*, Thrombopoietin. (Reproduced with permission from Davenport P, Liu ZJ, Sola-Visner M. Changes in megakaryopoiesis over ontogeny and their implications in health and disease. *Platelets*. 2020;1–8.)

however, the small size and low ploidy of CB MKs is associated with decreased levels of platelet production (per MK), compared to adult MKs.[16] Thus, the current evidence suggests that platelet production in fetuses and neonates is highly dependent on the increased proliferative rate of their MK progenitors.

The mechanisms underlying the small size of neonatal MKs are not clearly understood but likely involve a combination of cell-intrinsic factors and factors in the fetal and neonatal microenvironment. This was demonstrated by Slayton and associates, who transplanted neonatal liver cells or adult bone marrow cells from green fluorescent protein (GFP) transgenic mice into wild-type adult recipients and evaluated the size and ploidy of the donor-derived (GFP$^+$) MKs.[54] MKs derived from neonatal stem and progenitor cells, placed in an adult environment, were significantly larger and of higher ploidy than neonatal MKs in their original environment (neonatal liver). However, they were significantly smaller than post-transplantation MKs derived from adult bone marrow cells. In vitro studies culturing CB CD34$^+$ cells in adult bone marrow stromal cell–conditioned media also yielded MKs with higher ploidy levels than those cultured in fetal bone marrow stromal cell–conditioned or in unconditioned serum-free media.[55] Comparison of MK size in bone marrow biopsy specimens obtained from children transplanted with either CB - or adult bone marrow–stem cells revealed that MKs in the post-engraftment bone marrow samples were significantly smaller in the CB group than in the bone marrow group, demonstrating that the attainment of adult size in CB-derived MKs is delayed after human CB transplantation.[56] Taken together, these findings suggest that the environment influences the size and ploidy of MKs (with the adult environment being more conducive to MK maturation) but that cell-intrinsic factors limit the ultimate size and ploidy that neonatal MKs achieve.

To establish the timing of the transition from a neonatal to an adult phenotype, Fuchs and collaborators measured MK diameters (using a combination of immunohistochemistry and image analysis) in 72 BM samples from patients aged 3 days to 80 years.[57] This study found that neonates had MKs of uniform small sizes, which diverged into separate clusters of smaller and larger cells beginning at 2 years, and finally transitioned to larger (adult-like) MKs by 4 years.

TRANSCRIPTIONAL REGULATION OF MEGAKARYOPOIESIS

The process of megakaryopoiesis is carefully coordinated by a number of transcription factors and transcriptional regulators responsible for regulating the expression of MK-specific genes. Of current interest is how such factors may be responsible for stage-specific differences noted between neonatal and adult megakaryopoiesis. In the first comprehensive study comparing the transcriptome of MKs at different stages of development (human embryonic stem cells, fetal livers, full-term CB, and adult PB), 253 genes were found to be up-regulated in MKs through development, which revealed a progression toward increased polyploidization, proplatelet formation, and platelet function.[58] Genes enriched in fetal MKs, on the contrary, were mostly related to angiogenesis, the extracellular matrix, transforming growth factor receptor, and bone morphogenic protein (BMP) signaling. Some of the best studied transcription factors that play a role in megakaryopoiesis are summarized here.

THE GATA FAMILY

The GATA family of transcription factors plays key roles in normal hematopoiesis. GATA-1, a 47-kDa protein with the corresponding DNA sequence mapped to the X-chromosome, is required for terminal differentiation of both erythroid and megakaryocytic cell lines. GATA-1 contains three functional domains: two zinc fingers (N- and C-) and an N-terminal activating domain. The C-finger binds to GATA-1 binding sites. The N-finger provides stability during DNA binding and recruits the cofactor Friend of GATA-1 (FOG-1). Interaction with FOG-1 is necessary for normal hematopoiesis, as demonstrated by the presence of anemia and thrombocytopenia in individuals with *GATA1* mutations that interfere with the binding of FOG-1.[59] The N-terminal activating domain confers transcriptional activity.[60]

Specific GATA-1 knockout mice models have demonstrated the necessity of GATA-1 in normal hematopoiesis. GATA-1-null mice die during gestation from severe anemia. Mice with MK-specific deficiency of GATA-1 have thrombocytopenia without anemia, with platelet counts approximately 15% of normal. Morphologically, GATA1-deficient MKs are also abnormal, characterized by small size, large segmented nuclei, scant cytoplasm, and decreased ploidy compared with wild-type cells.[60,61] Several *GATA1* mutations have been described in patients with thrombocytopenia, usually characterized by the presence of large platelets (macrothrombocytopenia). Recently, Liu and colleagues showed a threefold increase in GATA-1 protein levels in CB—compared to PB-derived MKs.[53]

Calligaris and associates first described a short isoform of GATA-1, termed GATA-1 short (GATA-1s).[62] This isoform is 40 kDa in size, compared with the 47-kDa full-length protein, and is produced by the initiation of translation of the GATA-1 transcript at amino acid 84. The resultant protein lacks the N-terminal transactivation domain. Both full-length and short GATA-1 transcripts are normally found in murine fetal liver cells, in human MKs, and in K562 cells (a human erythroleukemia cell line with the ability to differentiate into erythroid and megakaryocytic cells). GATA-1s plays an important role in the pathogenesis of Down syndrome (trisomy 21)–associated transient myeloproliferative disorder (DS-TMD) and acute megakaryoblastic leukemia (DS-AMKL). DS-TMD is a disorder characterized by increased proliferation and maturational arrest of erythromegakaryocytic cells, which resolves spontaneously within the first few months of life, thus the name transient myeloproliferative disorder.[63] The abnormality in megakaryopoiesis is thought to originate in the fetal liver, as suggested by its spontaneous resolution within months of birth (as hematopoiesis in the fetal liver ceases) and by the progressive megakaryoblast infiltration of hepatocytes with relative sparing of the BM.[64] Two cytogenetic changes, or "hits," occur prenatally that are thought to give rise to this condition. The first is the presence of trisomy 21, which by itself is associated with increased frequency and clonogenicity of MEPs in the fetal liver,[65] and the second is a mutation in GATA-1 (within exon 2 of the *GATA-1* transcript) that results in the exclusive production of GATA-1s, which lacks the N-terminal transactivation domain.[62] Consistent with the transient nature of DS-TMD, a knock-in mouse engineered to exclusively express GATA-1s showed striking developmental stage-specific effects on megakaryopoiesis.[11] Specifically, murine MK progenitors from yolk sac and fetal liver were markedly hyperproliferative compared to wild-type progenitors, but this phenotype disappeared at later fetal stages and postnatally, even though the mice still exclusively produced GATA-1s. This observation indicated that the effects of GATA1s on MK hyperproliferation were sensitive to the molecular developmental differences between fetal and adult MK progenitors, potentially only affecting megakaryopoiesis from the fetal liver.

Two studies have shed light on the developmental stage-specific factors that mediate the unique sensitivity of fetal MK progenitors to GATA-1s. First, fetal (but not adult) MK progenitors are highly sensitive to insulin-like growth factor (IGF) signaling, which activates the E2F transcriptional network through mTOR. In normal fetal MK progenitors, full-length GATA-1 restricts the IGF-mediated activation of the E2F transcription network to coordinate proliferation and differentiation. In the absence of full-length GATA-1 (i.e., in mutated *GATA1s*) the overactive IGF signaling is "unchecked" and leads to unrestricted proliferation of fetal progenitors (Fig. 110.5).[66] In a separate study, type 1

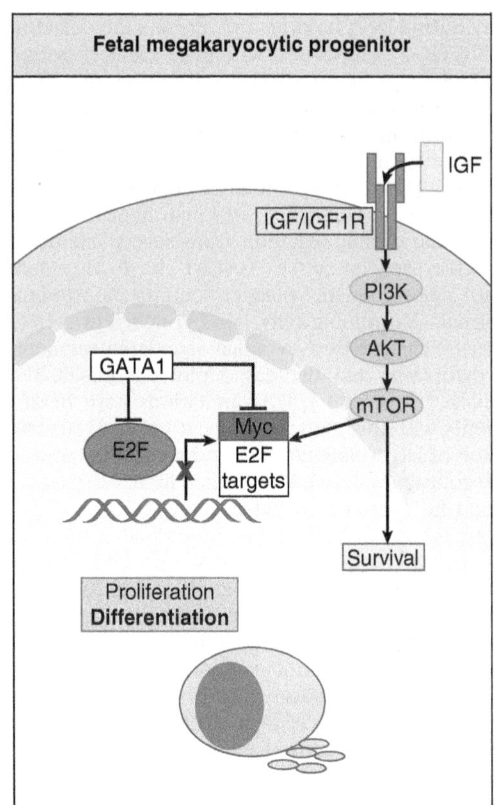

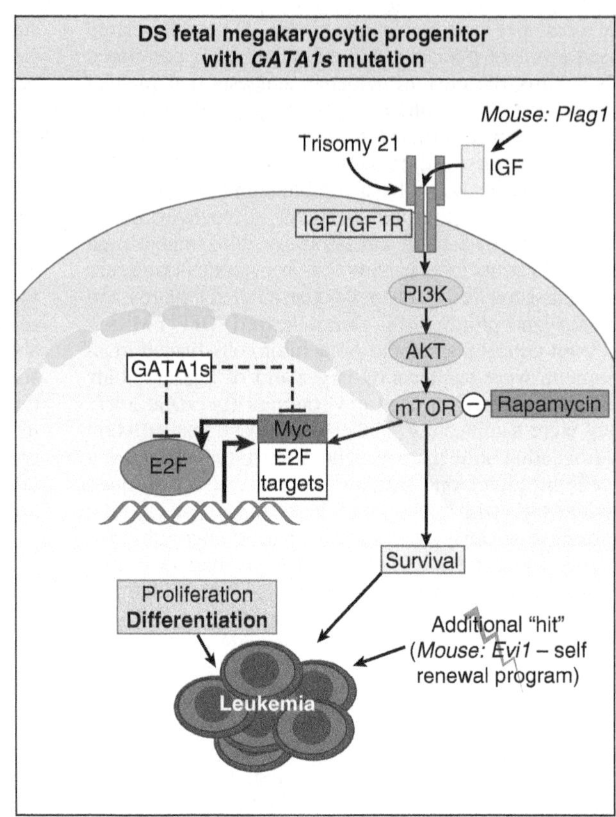

Fig. 110.5 GATA1 full-length protein restricts insulin-like growth factor *(IGF)* signaling-induced proliferation of fetal megakaryocytic progenitors. Full-length GATA1 represses E2F activity, coordinating terminal megakaryocytic differentiation and proliferation of IGF1/IGF1R signaling-dependent fetal progenitors. GATA1s fails to repress E2F activity, leading to their uncontrolled proliferation and increased survival. (Republished with permission from Klusmann J, Godinho F, Heitmann K, et al. Developmental stage-specific interplay of GATA1 and IGF signaling in fetal megakaryopoiesis and leukemogenesis. Genes Dev. 2010;24:1659–1672.)

interferon (IFN)-responsive genes were found to be upregulated in murine BM versus fetal liver-derived MK progenitors, as well as in human BM versus fetal liver MKs (thought to be secondary to production of IFN by osteoblasts and osteoclasts in the BM). Importantly, exogenous IFN-α markedly reduced the hyperproliferation of fetal liver MKs obtained from GATA-1s mice. Conversely, genetic or pharmacologic neutralization of IFN signaling increased the proliferation of MK progenitors in the BM of adult GATA-1s mice.[46] Taken together, these observations suggest that the insensitivity of adult MK progenitors to IGF signaling and the increased type 1 IFN signaling in the adult BM contributes to the spontaneous resolution of DS-TMD.

Despite 85% to 90% of newborns with DS-TMD demonstrating resolution of disease, approximately 20% to 30% subsequently develop acute megakaryoblastic leukemia (DS-AMKL), typically within 1 to 2 years after resolution of the TMD. Analysis of paired samples from patients with both TMD and DS-AMKL have found identical *GATA-1* gene mutations in both the TMD and DS-AMKL, suggesting that additional genetic and/or epigenetic transforming events or hits are involved in leukemic progression.[67] In one study, 44% of DS-AMKL samples showed additional genetic mutations aside from trisomy 21 and *GATA-1,* with major mutational targets involving multiple cohesin components and common signaling pathways, such as JAK family kinases, *MPL, SH2B3 (LNK),* and multiple RAS pathway genes.[68]

FOG-1

FOG-1 is an essential cofactor for proper megakaryopoiesis. Single-point mutations (V205M, D218G D218Y, G208S) have been described, which result in reduced GATA-1 and FOG-1 interaction and a phenotype of macrothrombocytopenia with anemia.[60] Mice engineered with complete absence of FOG-1 have a complete absence of MK progenitors. PF4 and GPIIb (early MK transcripts) are detectable in these models, implying an impaired differentiation and replication of early MK lineage cells. These data taken together suggest that FOG-1 plays multiple roles in megakaryopoiesis at both early and later stages.[60,69]

RUNX1

The core binding factor (CBF) is a group of heterodimeric transcription factors composed of a non-DNA-binding CBFβ chain and one of three DNA-binding CBFα chains: RUNX1, RUNX2, or RUNX3. RUNX1 is the predominant CBF expressed in hematopoietic cells. Knockout of RUNX1 in mice leads to a complete absence of all definitive hematopoiesis due to a failure of definitive HSCs to emerge from specialized hemogenic endothelium during mid-embryonic development. Hematopoietic selective deletion of RUNX1 in adult mice using a MX1-Cre model results in moderate thrombocytopenia, T cell defects, and a mild myeloproliferative disorder.[70] RUNX1-deficient MKs are small, contain scant cytoplasm, and have hypolobulated nuclei with low DNA ploidy compared to wild-type MKs. CBPβ deficiency likewise impairs MK development. In humans, germline haploinsufficiency of RUNX1 causes familial platelet disorder with propensity to develop AML (FPD/AML). This is a rare autosomal dominant disorder characterized by moderate thrombocytopenia, platelet dysfunction, and a high incidence of developing leukemia (approximately 35% lifetime risk). A number of RUNX1 MK direct target genes have been identified, including GPIIb, c-mpl, myosin light chain regulatory polypeptide (MYL9), PKC-theta, and platelet 12-lipoxygenase gene (ALOX12).

NF-E2

NF-E2 is a transcription factor found in erythroid, megakaryocytic, and mast cells. In MKs, NF-E2 regulates β-tubulin, a major component of microtubulin. Microtubulin formation is required for proplatelet formation and subsequent release of platelets from the MK. Loss of NF-E2 results in increased numbers of MKs with a disorganized internal membrane and impaired release of proplatelets, leading to thrombocytopenia and a lethal coagulopathy in the neonatal period, with only a mild decrease in erythropoiesis.[69,71]

THE ETS FAMILY

The Ets family of transcription factors is characterized by the presence of a highly conserved winged helix-turn-helix DNA binding domain (Ets domain) that allows recognition of purine-rich DNA sequences with a core GGA (A/T) consensus, designated EBS (Ets binding sequence). Ets-1 is up-regulated in megakaryopoiesis, and Ets binding sites have been identified in many MK-specific gene promoters. Overexpression of Ets-1 in cultured MK cells results in a state of increased proliferation with larger MKs that have an increased number of nuclear lobes. Gene expression studies in these same cells reveals increased GATA-2, GPIIb, and PF4, indicating that Ets-1 promotes MK differentiation.[72]

Friend leukemia integration-1 (Fli-1) is a member of the Ets family of transcription factors. It is expressed in hematopoietic cell lines as well as vascular endothelial cell lines and regulates expression of multiple MK proteins, including GATA-1, GPIb, IIb, VI, and XI, and c-mpl. In K-562 cells, expression of Fli-1 results in increased CD41 and CD61 expression. In murine knockout models, loss of Fli-1 results in embryonic death due to hemorrhage (related to a state of defective vasculature) as well as dysmegakaryopoiesis with immature-appearing MKs that express early genes (αIIb and c-mpl) but diminished expression of late genes (GPIX). Disruption of Fli-1 expression caused by a terminal deletion in chromosome 11 underlies Paris-Trousseau syndrome, which is characterized by thrombocytopenia with platelets that display large α-granules. This clinical phenotype can occur independently or as part of Jacobsen syndrome (platelet defects with cardiac anomalies, facial anomalies, and intellectual disability). In both instances, MKs are increased in number but have a diminished number of α-granules as well as a disorganized internal membrane.[69,73] In a recent study, induced pluripotent stem cell–derived MKs (iMKs) with a targeted heterozygous Fli-1 knockout *($FLI1^{+/-}$)* released fewer platelets per MK, and platelets released in vivo following infusion of these iMKs had shorter half-lives and poor functionality. Interestingly, Ets-1 was overexpressed in these Fli-1-deficient iMKs, suggesting that Fli-1 negatively regulates Ets-1 in megakaryopoiesis.[74] Furthermore, a study of 13 unrelated index cases of thrombocytopenia with dense granule secretion disorder revealed that six had novel alterations in Fli-1 or RUNX1, further strengthening the role of Fli-1 in thrombopoiesis.[75]

P-TEFB

A recent study identified a potential ontogenic master-regulator responsible for the phenotypic and molecular differences between neonatal and adult MKs. It is known that adult MK development is dependent on sustained, high-level activation of P-TEFb, which, along with CDK9 and cyclin T, form the complete kinase complex. This complex releases RNA polymerase II (RNAPII) from proximal stalling, thus accelerating transcriptional elongation to meet the high transcriptional demands of adult MKs.[76,77] In most non-MK cells, a feedback loop maintains P-TEFb sequestered in an inactive state within the 7SK snRNP complex. Adult MKs behave differently by employing a specialized activation pathway through down-regulation of 7SK stabilization factors (MePCE and LARP7), which allows the irreversible release and activation of P-TEFb.

Interestingly, neonatal MKs exhibit persistent inactivation of P-TEFb despite lineage-appropriate down-regulation of the 7SK stabilizing factors. In a recent study, Elagib and colleagues identified a fetal-specific 7SK stabilizing protein, IGF2BP3, responsible for the persistent inhibition of P-TEFb by 7SK despite down-regulation of MePCE and LARP7.[47] Genetic or pharmacologic knockdown of *IGF2BP3* in neonatal MKs caused down-regulation of 7SK, which led to enhanced P-TEFb activation and subsequent development of adult MK features, such as cellular enlargement, proliferation arrest, polyploidization, and erythroid suppression.[47] The mechanisms by which activated P-TEFb exerts these effects remain unknown.

miRNAS

miRNAs have been increasingly recognized as key regulators of multiple steps in the process of megakaryopoiesis. The previously mentioned study by Bluteau and colleagues comparing the transcriptome of MKs at different stages of development also found developmental differences in the expression of 32 micro-RNAs, including miR-9 and miR-224, both of which target *CXCR-4* (the SDF-1 receptor).[58] In a subsequent study, upregulation of miR-9 expression in the megakaryocytic cell line Meg-01 significantly downregulated CXCR-4 protein, supporting the hypothesis that miR-9 down-regulates CXCR-4 levels in MKs.[78] Fetal MKs express increased levels of miR-9 and show decreased CXCR-4 expression, which is associated with a failure to migrate in response to an SDF-1a gradient.[79] This is relevant because the SDF-1a/CXCR-4 axis promotes the interaction of MKs with the BM sinusoidal endothelial cells and is critical for progenitor homing to the BM and for Tpo-independent megakaryopoiesis.[80] It has been hypothesized that the low CXCR-4 levels in fetal/neonatal MKs could cause delays in the homing of MK progenitors to the BM following CB transplantation, which might contribute to the delayed platelet engraftment that frequently complicates CB transplants.

Another miRNA up-regulated in neonatal MKs is miR-99a, which is associated with decreased CTDSPL (a retinoblastoma [Rb] protein phosphatase), increased hyperphosphorylation of Rb, and E2F mediated induction of D-type cyclins. This suggests that the upregulation of miR-99a promotes cell cycle transition through the G1-S checkpoint in fetal MKs, possibly contributing to their hyperproliferative phenotype.[81] Other miRNAs have been found to be downregulated in the fetal/neonatal MK, including miR181a, predicted to target *LIN28B*, which in turn likely contributes to the decreased levels of Let-7 miRNAs found in fetal progenitors.[82] The exact pathways through which low miR181a and Let-7 contribute to the fetal/neonatal MK phenotype have not been elucidated. With the expansion of genetics-based technology, more miRNAs are expected to be found to play a role in the regulation of megakaryopoiesis.

CYTOKINE EFFECTS ON MEGAKARYOPOIESIS

THROMBOPOIETIN

Before the cloning of Tpo, CFU-MK proliferation was noted in the presence of serum from patients or animals with aplastic anemia, or when hematopoietic progenitor cells were cultured in media from human embryonic kidney cell cultures.[83,84] These therefore became widely used biologic sources of thrombopoietic factors. However, attempts to isolate and purify MK-CSF or Tpo from these sources failed, until the fortuitous discovery in the early 1990s of a viral myeloproliferative leukemia virus oncogene *(v-mpl)*, whose structure suggested that it was a member of the hematopoietic growth factor superfamily.[85] Surprisingly, the cellular homologue of this viral oncogene (termed cellular myeloproliferative leukemia virus, or *c-mpl*) was expressed almost exclusively in $CD34^+$ cells, MKs, and platelets.[86-89] These discoveries led to an active search for the c-mpl ligand, which culminated in 1994 with the almost simultaneous isolation of the new thrombopoietic growth factor by four different groups, each of which assigned the same protein a different name: MPL ligand,[90] Tpo,[91] MK growth and development factor (MGDF),[92] and megapoietin.[93]

The gene that encodes Tpo is localized in 3q26-27.[94-96] The *THPO* gene is composed of five coding exons, similar to the five erythropoietin exons.[97] The protein is composed of 332 amino acids, divided into two domains: an active amino-terminal half (153 amino acids) with marked homology to erythropoietin, and a carboxyl-terminal domain with 179 amino acids.[98] At all stages of development (i.e., during fetal, neonatal, and adult life), the main site of Tpo production is the liver,[91,99,100] although Tpo expression has also been identified in the kidneys, spleen, and bone marrow.[99,101] In response to severe thrombocytopenia, however, the usually low level of Tpo messenger RNA (mRNA) expression in bone marrow stromal cells increases greatly.[101] One study has shown that platelet-derived growth factor (PDGF) and fibroblast growth factor-2 (FGF-2) (both platelet α-granule proteins) might mediate this increase.[102]

The regulation of Tpo production has also been the object of extensive research. Early studies by several investigators demonstrated that, in steady-state and in noninflammatory conditions (i.e., idiopathic thrombocytopenia [ITP], aplastic anemia), hepatic Tpo production was constitutive; circulating Tpo levels were inversely related to the concentration of available c-mpl receptors and therefore to the platelet and MK mass, supporting a model of end receptor binding-mediated regulation.[103-106] Although this model seemed to apply to most conditions, it was challenged by the finding of elevated Tpo levels in patients with thrombocytosis associated with inflammatory conditions, such as infections or Kawasaki disease.[107] Later studies showed that hepatic Tpo expression was up-regulated in response to interleukin-6 (IL-6) both in vitro and in vivo.[108,109] Because an anti-Tpo antibody neutralizes the thrombopoietic effect of IL-6, it is now evident that this is the pathway responsible for inflammation-induced thrombocytosis.[107]

Recently, a mechanism through which platelets themselves regulate hepatic Tpo production was described. In this model, platelets become progressively desialylated as they age. Old, desialylated platelets are recognized by the Ashwell-Morell receptor located on hepatocytes and are phagocytosed, which triggers an increase in Tpo mRNA and protein expression via JAK2/STAT3 signaling, ultimately leading to increased platelet production (Fig. 110.6).[110] This model has implications in several disease processes, since platelets can also be desialylated in response to infections by neuraminidase-producing organisms, cooling, or in response to anti-GPIb alpha antibodies.[111-113]

Defects in the Tpo/c-mpl axis have also been recognized as the etiology of several human disorders. Specifically, *c-mpl* mutations causing frameshifts and early termination cause congenital amegakaryocytic thrombocytopenia (CAMT), a disorder typically characterized by severe thrombocytopenia and absence of MKs beginning in infancy.[114,115] In contrast, activating mutations in the Tpo gene promoter[116] or in the c-mpl receptor[117] have been found in subsets of patients with familial essential thrombocythemia.

In the years following the isolation of Tpo, multiple in vitro and in vivo studies were conducted to characterize the role of this cytokine. It quickly became evident that Tpo acted both as a potent proliferative factor (MK-CSF) and as a maturational factor on MKs.[118,119] The role of Tpo on the terminal stages of MK maturation and proplatelet formation has been less clearly established, and it is currently believed that this cytokine does not play a major role on those processes.[120,121] In vitro studies also have suggested that Tpo plays a role in platelet activation, mostly priming the platelets to the effects of other agonists.[122] However, these effects have not been confirmed in vivo.[123,124] *Tpo* and *c-mpl* knockout mice exhibit platelet counts equivalent to 10% to 15% of wild-type mice and greatly decreased marrow MKs,[125,126] but the mice are otherwise healthy and viable. This suggests that Tpo is the primary regulator of platelet production, but that alternative pathways exist for megakaryocytopoiesis. Further studies also have shown that the Tpo/c-mpl axis functions in early hematopoietic progenitors (including HSCs), disclosing an important role for Tpo in hematopoiesis in general, in addition to its megakaryopoietic functions.[127,128] These findings have significant

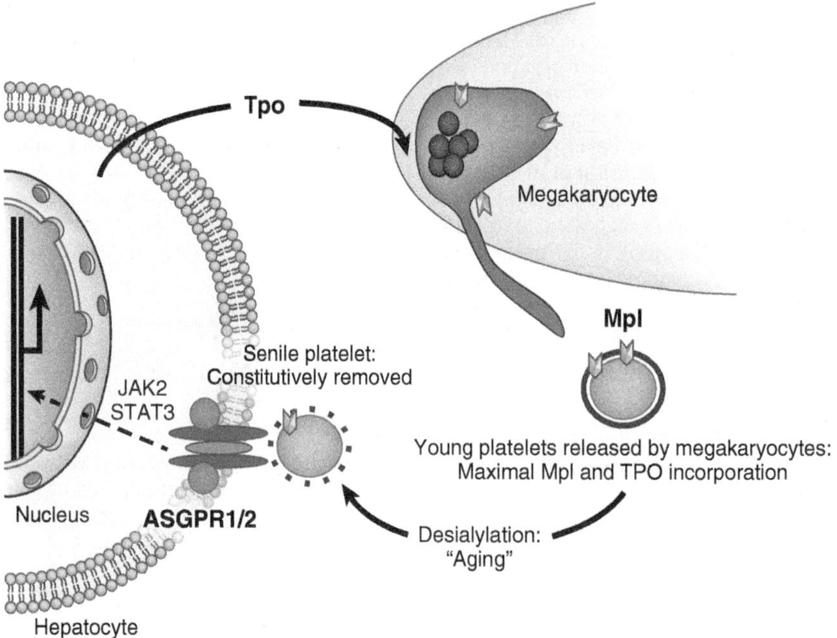

Fig. 110.6 Scheme of hepatic thrombopoietin *(Tpo)* production via JAK2-STAT3 signaling after desialylated platelet uptake by the Ashwell-Morrell (AMR) receptor. Bone marrow megakaryocytes produce and release young sialic acid (purple ring)-containing platelets into the blood stream. Young platelets maximally internalize Tpo via Mpl-mediated endocytosis. Circulating platelets become desialylated by active blood-borne sialidases as they age *(dashed purple ring)* and are recognized by the hepatic AMR. Desialylated platelet ingestion signaling positively stimulates hepatic Tpo mRNA expression via JAK2-STAT3 activation, releasing Tpo into plasma, thereby regulating bone marrow homeostasis and thrombopoiesis. (Republished with permission from Hoffmeister KM, Falet H. Platelet clearance by the hepatic Ashwell-Morrell receptor: mechanisms and biological significance. *Thromb Res.* 2016;141[suppl 2]:S68–S72.)

clinical implications for patients with disorders affecting this axis, such as in patients with CAMT, who frequently go on to develop aplastic anemia.

The cloning of Tpo in 1996 led to a flurry of studies that quickly progressed from bench research to animal studies and then to clinical trials, mostly using the full-length rTpo molecule or a recombinant human polypeptide that contains the receptor-binding N-terminal domain of Tpo (termed *MK growth and development factor*, or *rhMGDF*). When injected into normal animals, rTpo or rhMGDF induced significant thrombocytosis, with peak mean platelet counts up to 670% of baseline.[123,129-132] When administered to animals exposed to myelosuppressive chemotherapy, rhMGDF ameliorated or completely prevented the associated thrombocytopenia[129] and also accelerated red blood cell and neutrophil recovery.[133,134] Most human studies were conducted using a pegylated form of rhMGDF (PEG-rhMGDF, a molecule 5 to 10 times more potent in vivo than the unconjugated polypeptide).[123] In phase I and II clinical trials, rTpo and PEG-rhMGDF potently stimulated platelet production in non-thrombocytopenic adults[135,136] and in patients with chemotherapy-induced thrombocytopenia.[137,138] However, trials showed limited efficacy in the setting of thrombocytopenia associated with myeloablation and stem cell transplantation.[139] Unfortunately, a number of subjects treated with PEG-rhMGDF developed neutralizing antibodies against endogenous Tpo, which resulted in severe thrombocytopenia and aplastic anemia.[140] Ultimately, these complications led to the discontinuation of clinical trials involving any of these forms of rTpo.

As an alternative, much interest was directed to the development of Tpo-mimetic molecules. These are molecules that have no sequence homology to Tpo but bind to the Tpo receptor and have biologically comparable effects. The lack of homology represents a significant advantage over recombinant forms of Tpo because it should preclude the development of cross-reactive neutralizing antibodies against endogenous Tpo. At least five different Tpo receptor agonists have been described,[139-141] and three have been studied in human subjects.[142-145] Two Tpo mimetics are currently approved by the US Food and Drug Administration (FDA) for the treatment of adults and children greater than 1 year of age with chronic immune thrombocytopenic purpura (ITP) refractory to at least one other treatment: Romiplostim (AMG 531, Amgen) and eltrombopag (SB-497115, Glaxo-Smith-Kline). The six largest randomized controlled trials conducted in ITP have used one of these two agents, and all have demonstrated a platelet response rate between 50% and 90% and good safety and tolerability.[142,146,147]

Romiplostim is an engineered peptibody composed of a recombinant protein carrier FC domain linked to multiple c-mpl binding domains, and eltrombopag is an oral, nonpeptide Tpo receptor agonist. Eltrombopag is approved for two indications in addition to ITP: severe aplastic anemia refractory to first-line treatment and hepatitis C undergoing treatment with IFN-ribavirin.[147] However, no studies have used these agents in neonates. Of note, eltrombopag is also a potent iron chelator, and it has been shown in vitro that it can cross the blood-brain barrier and induce iron deficiency in developing murine hypocampal neurons.[148] Thus, it might be important to carefully monitor the iron status of neonates or young infants treated with eltrombopag.

THROMBOPOIETIN THROUGHOUT DEVELOPMENT

After the identification of Tpo as the primary regulator of megakaryopoiesis, several investigators evaluated Tpo concentrations in CB and in the blood of neonates.[99,149-154] Overall, median Tpo concentrations in neonates ranged between 76 and 191 pg/mL and were slightly higher in serum than in plasma. With the exception of the study by Albert and collaborators,[154] which reported higher Tpo concentration in preterm compared with term neonates, these studies found no obvious gestational age-related changes in plasma or serum Tpo concentrations and no correlation with platelet counts. However, all studies reported Tpo concentrations in neonates that were threefold to fourfold higher than in healthy adults. The reasons underlying this finding are unclear and might involve an increased rate of Tpo production, decreased Tpo clearance, alternative mechanisms of Tpo regulation, or a reduced number of c-mpl receptors.[155] In support of the last hypothesis, Kuwaki and associates described a significantly lower number of c-mpl receptors in MKs derived from CB cells than in those derived from adult bone marrow cells,[156] although other studies reported higher c-mpl concentrations in neonatal compared to adult MKs.[36] To determine when Tpo levels transitioned from normal neonatal to adult concentrations, Ishiguro and collaborators measured Tpo concentrations in healthy neonates, children, and adults.[153] In this study, Tpo concentrations increased shortly after birth, reached a peak on the second day of life, and returned to CB levels by the end of the first month. They then decreased gradually until adult levels were reached (Fig. 110.7).

Several investigators also evaluated Tpo concentrations in neonates with different varieties of thrombocytopenia,[154,157-161] and some correlated those with other measures of thrombopoiesis, such as marrow MKs[152,157,158] or circulating MK progenitors.[149,150,157,158] Overall, these investigators found great variability in Tpo concentrations among thrombocytopenic neonates and no strong correlation with platelet counts, possibly reflecting the different mechanisms underlying the different varieties of thrombocytopenia or possibly due to the different functions of c-mpl at different stages of development.

Three murine studies have provided evidence supporting the existence of different roles of c-mpl during development. First,

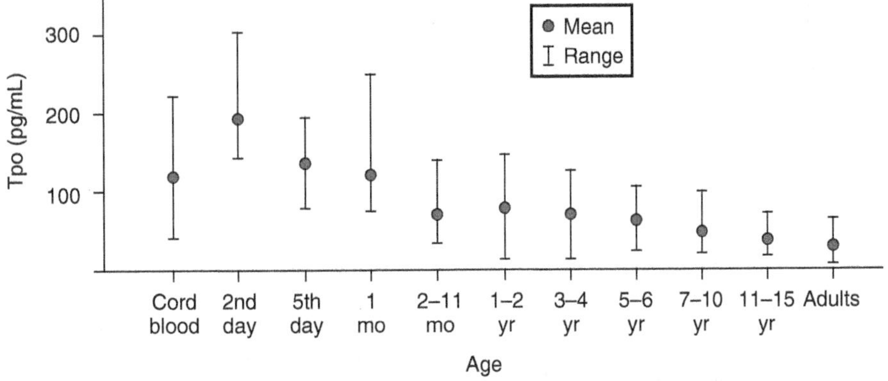

Fig. 110.7 Age-related changes in serum thrombopoietin *(Tpo)* levels in disease-free children. Tpo concentrations were measured in 254 serum samples, collected from 25 cord blood samples, 200 healthy children, and 29 healthy adults. *Filled circles* indicate the means; *bars* represent the ranges. (From Ishiguro A, Nakahata T, Matsubara K, et al. Age-related changes in thrombopoietin in children: reference interval for serum thrombopoietin levels. *Br J Haematol.* 1999;106:884–888; and Dame C. Thrombopoietin in thrombocytopenias of childhood. *Semin Thromb Hemost.* 2001;27:215–228.)

c-mpl(−/−) murine embryos were found to have completely normal diploid platelet-forming cells (DPFCs, see "Fetal and Neonatal Megakaryopoiesis") and circulating platelet numbers at E10.5, demonstrating that c-mpl is completely dispensable for DPFC formation and DPFC-derived thrombopoiesis during murine embryonic life.[35] At E14.5 to E16.5, *c-mpl(−/−)* fetuses developed thrombocytopenia, which was associated with normal MK numbers but a block in MK maturation at the 8N stage. This revealed that, opposite to adult life (when *c-mpl[−/−]* mice exhibit markedly decreased numbers of morphologically normal MKs), in fetal life c-mpl is required for normal MK polyploidization and maturation but not for proliferation. Interestingly, *c-mpl(−/−)* newborn mice have decreased MKs in the liver, which also exhibit ultrastructural defects consistent with abnormal maturation, likely representing an intermediate stage between the fetal and adult manifestations of absent c-mpl.[162]

The response to Tpo has also been shown to be substantially different in neonates than in adults. First, studies by several investigators demonstrated that neonatal MK progenitors generated significantly larger colonies with more MKs than adult BM cells in response to Tpo.[42,163] Furthermore, marrow cultures from either thrombocytopenic or non-thrombocytopenic neonates yielded three times more MK colonies that adult marrow cultures in response to Tpo.[164] These neonatal colonies also contained more MKs and were more sensitive to Tpo (i.e., the highest number of colonies was reached at a Tpo concentration of 10 ng/mL, compared with 50 ng/mL for adult cultures). Compared to adult PB-derived MKs, CB-derived MKs also had higher c-mpl protein levels and exhibited significantly upregulated JAK2 and mTOR signaling in response to Tpo, thus providing a mechanism for the increased sensitivity to this cytokine.[53] These findings were consistent with the pronounced increase in platelet counts observed in newborn rhesus monkeys treated with even low doses of PEG-rHuMGDF.[165]

Pastos and associates also evaluated the effects of Tpo on the ploidy of adult and neonatal MKs cultured in either serum-free media or adult bone marrow stromal cell-conditioned media with increasing concentrations of Tpo.[55] This study disclosed opposite effects of Tpo on the ploidy of neonatal compared with adult MKs. Although adult MKs reached highest ploidy levels when cultured in serum-free medium with maximal concentrations of rTpo, neonatal MKs reached their highest ploidy when cultured in marrow stromal cell-conditioned media in the absence of rTpo; the addition of supraphysiologic concentrations of rTpo (≥0.1 ng/mL) triggered rapid proliferation at the expense of polyploidization (Fig. 110.8). Consistent with these Tpo effects on polyploidization, a recent murine study found that administration of a single dose of the Tpo mimetic romiplostim induced a substantial increase in MK size in treated adult mice but not in newborn mice, which was associated with a blunted platelet count increase in newborn pups in response to romiplostim (approximately twofold increase vs. —fourfold to fivefold in adults).[166] These different responses were thought to represent a combination of possible pharmacokinetic differences between newborn and adult mice, and biologic differences in the ability of romiplostim to increase neonatal MK ploidy and size. Combined, these studies provided strong support for the hypothesis that neonatal and adult MKs have different biologic responses to Tpo.

INTERLEUKIN-11

Many other growth factors affect MK colony growth in vitro. IL-11 also increases MK proliferation in vitro, but not in the absence of other thrombopoietic stimulants.[167] Recombinant IL-11 (rIL-11) has been released for clinical use and is approved by the FDA as a thrombopoietic agent. Studies have shown that rIL-11 stimulates megakaryocytopoiesis in both adults and children.[168,169] However, it is also associated with significant flu-like symptoms and fluid retention. In addition, at least in one study involving patients with refractory ITP, rIL11 administration resulted in significant side effects combined with a lack of efficacy, leading to early termination of the trial.[170] Recently, rIL-11 has seen successful results in clinical trials for the treatment of dengue-associated thrombocytopenia, suggesting that short-term, low-dose regimens may serve a purpose in infectious disease scenarios.[171] In addition, the MK expanding properties of IL-11 may have a future in in vitro large-scale platelet production.[172]

GM-CSF, IL-3, AND IL 6

Granulocyte-macrophage CSF (GM-CSF) and IL-3 stimulate megakaryopoiesis, alone or in combination.[173,174] A synergistic effect of IL-3 and GM-CSF has also been documented.[174] IL-6 affects megakaryopoiesis in vitro, and MK maturation in particular.[175–177] IL-6 also promotes CFU-MK proliferation of in vitro human marrow cultures, although the effect is less than that seen with IL-3 or GM-CSF.[178] The IL-6 receptor has been identified on MKs, and the administration of IL-6 to suspension cultures increases ploidy.[179]

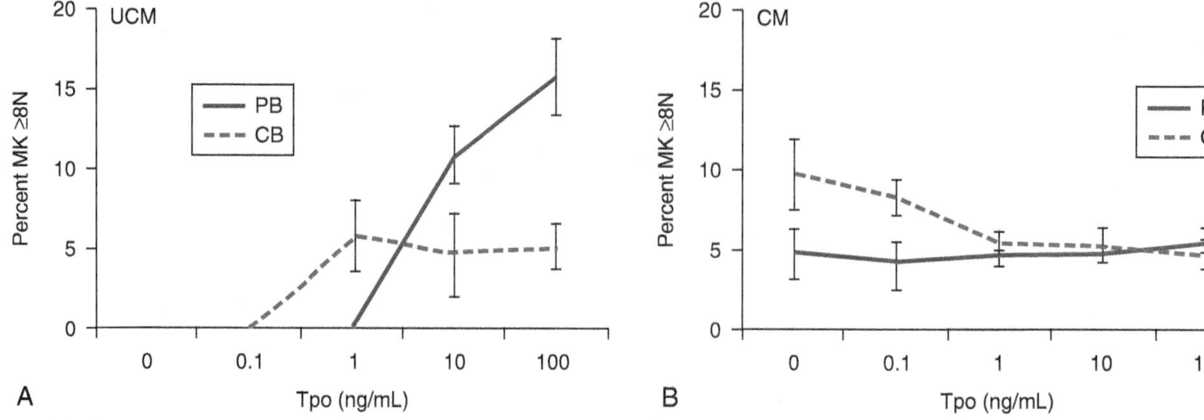

Fig. 110.8 The percentage of megakaryocytes (MKs) that were 8N or greater in peripheral blood *(PB)* and cord blood *(CB)* cultures differed depending on media source and recombinant thrombopoietin (rTpo) concentration. PB- and CB-CD34+ cells were cultured for 14 days in unconditioned media *(UCM)* (A) and conditioned media *(CM)* (B), with varying rTpo concentrations. PB-derived MKs *(solid lines)* cultured in UCM (A) exhibited a rTpo dose-dependent increase in ploidy levels, an effect inhibited by the presence of CM (B). CB-derived MKs *(dashed lines)* reached highest ploidy levels when cultured in CM with no rTpo, an effect that was reversed by rTpo concentrations of 1 ng/mL or greater (B). Data shown represent the means and standard error of the mean (SEM) of four separate experiments. *Tpo*, Thrombopoietin. (Republished with permission from Pastos KM, Slayton WB, Rimsza LM, et al. Differential effects of recombinant thrombopoietin and bone marrow stromal-conditioned media on neonatal versus adult megakaryocytes. *Blood.* 2006;108:3360–3362.)

In nonhuman primates, recombinant human IL-6 has been shown to affect megakaryopoiesis in vitro.[180-182] Recombinant IL-6 (5 to 80 μg/kg/day), injected twice daily for 14 days, caused dose-related increases in platelets and a shift to larger MKs in the bone marrow, indicating a maturational effect.[180] In a clinical phase 1 to 2 study, recombinant human IL-6 was administered to 20 patients with cancer.[183] Increases in platelet counts were observed but were associated with substantial side effects. Recombinant IL-6 is not clinically available.

STROMAL CELL–DERIVED FACTOR-1

Stromal cell–derived factor-1 (SDF-1) is a chemokine ligand for the receptor CXCR4 and has been shown to enhance HSC homing to the bone marrow.[184] Studies in Tpo-deficient mice demonstrated that increasing the levels of SDF-1 and/or FGF-4 resulted in a near normalization of the platelet counts, thus confirming the substantial Tpo-independent thrombopoietic effects of this pathway.[80] SDF-1 administration was also shown to increase the association of MKs with vascular niches, thereby increasing platelet production in radiation-induced thrombocytopenia.[185] These studies suggest that SDF-1 could be used as a therapy for thrombocytopenia, and its functional range is currently under study.

INTERFERON

Interferon-α (IFN-α) has long been known as a negative regulator of megakaryopoiesis, a property discovered through the development of thrombocytopenia in hepatitis patients receiving IFN therapy.[186] This led to the use of IFN-α in thrombocythemia, where MK proliferation must be reduced. The mechanism behind this may be the induction of SOCS-1 in IFN treated cells, which in turn inhibits Tpo signaling.[187] Similarly, the neutralization of IFN in GATA-1s mice increases MK progenitor proliferation (see "The GATA Family").[46]

It was also recently shown that the pro-inflammatory cytokine IFN-γ interferes with the binding of Tpo to its receptor c-mpl via steric occlusion of the low-affinity binding site, which perturbs Tpo-induced signaling pathways and causes decreased survival of human hematopoietic stem and progenitor cells. Importantly, eltrombopag binds to c-mpl at a position distinct from the extracellular binding site of Tpo, and is therefore able to bypass the inhibition of Tpo signaling caused by IFN-γ (Fig. 110.9).[188]

Numerous additional growth factors participate in the process of megakaryocytopoiesis, although their roles have been less extensively studied. These include erythropoietin,[189] stem cell factor,[190,191] vascular endothelial growth factor (VEGF),[192,193] IL-1,[194,195] basic FGF,[80,196] PDGF,[197] and nicotinamide.[198] Some factors have been shown to be potent inhibitors of thrombopoiesis, including transforming growth factor-beta (TGF-β)199 and PF4.[200,201]

NEONATAL PLATELETS

NEONATAL PLATELET COUNTS

Platelets are produced very early in the fetus, and platelet counts rise in a linear fashion throughout gestation.[202] Platelets in early fetal life are significantly larger than those in adults, with the size decreasing with advancing gestation. By the time fetuses approach 22 to 24 weeks' gestation, however, the mean platelet volume (MPV) is similar to that of full-term infants and adults, so that there is little difference between neonates of different gestational ages.[203] Premature infants, on average, have a slightly lower platelet count than term infants, but the mean platelet count remains within the same range observed in healthy older children and adults (i.e., 150,000 to 450 × 10^9/L).[204] Appleyard and Brinton evaluated platelet counts in low-birth-weight infants during the first 4 weeks of life.[205] In this study, platelet counts lower than 100 × 10^9/L were uncommon, and counts less than 50 × 10^9/L were usually associated with some clinical abnormality. In low-birth-weight infants platelet counts rose for several weeks after delivery, while in term infants platelet counts were equivalent to those in older children and adults.[205,206] Recently, Christensen and collaborators published epidemiologic reference ranges for platelet counts in the largest cohort to date, including over 47,000 infants of gestational ages ranging from 22 to 42 weeks (Fig. 110.10).[203]

The incidence of thrombocytopenia in neonates is extremely variable, depending on the population examined. Large studies evaluating platelet counts in thousands of unselected CB samples reported an incidence of neonatal thrombocytopenia of 0.7% to 0.9%, depending on the definition of the thrombocytopenia.[207,208] Severe thrombocytopenia (platelet count <50 × 10^9/L) was present at birth in approximately 0.1% of neonates, but the incidence increased to 0.28% if infants whose platelet counts dropped below that threshold during the first few days of life were included.[208,209]

The relatively low frequency of thrombocytopenia in the general population of neonates is in marked contrast with its high incidence among sick neonates. Mehta and co-workers reported an incidence of 35% among neonates admitted to the NICU.[210] Castle and colleagues evaluated platelet counts in 807 consecutive infants admitted to a regional NICU and found thrombocytopenia in 22%. Twenty percent of those infants had platelet counts below 50 × 10^9/L.[211] In a somewhat smaller study, Oren and associates observed an incidence of 18.2%

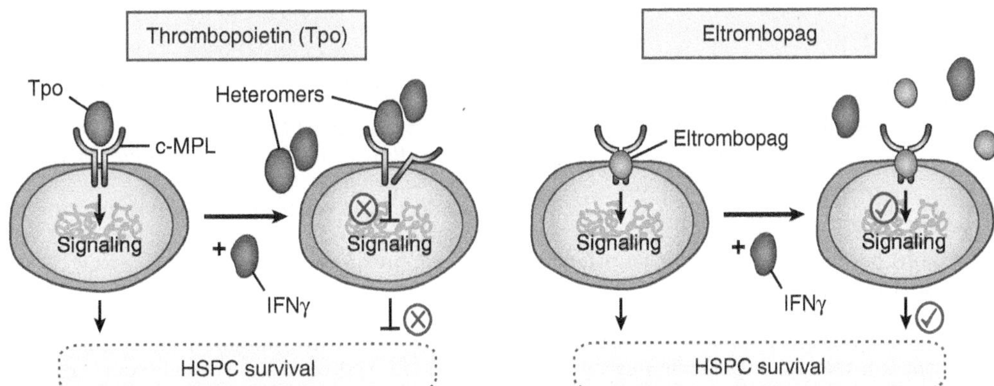

Fig. 110.9 Schematic representation of the effects of interferon-γ (IFN-γ) and eltrombopag on thrombopoietin signaling. *Left panel*: IFN-γ interferes with the binding of thrombopoietin *(Tpo)* to its receptor (c-mpl), which perturbs Tpo-induced signaling pathways and causes decreased survival of human hematopoietic stem (HS) and progenitor cells (PCs). *Right panel*: Eltrombopag binds to c-mpl at a position distinct from the extracellular binding site of Tpo and is therefore able to bypass the inhibition of Tpo signaling caused by IFN-γ. (Republished with permission from Alvarado LJ, Huntsman HD, Cheng H, et al. Eltrombopag maintains human hematopoietic stem and progenitor cells under inflammatory conditions mediated by IFN-gamma. *Blood.* 2019;133:2043–2055.)

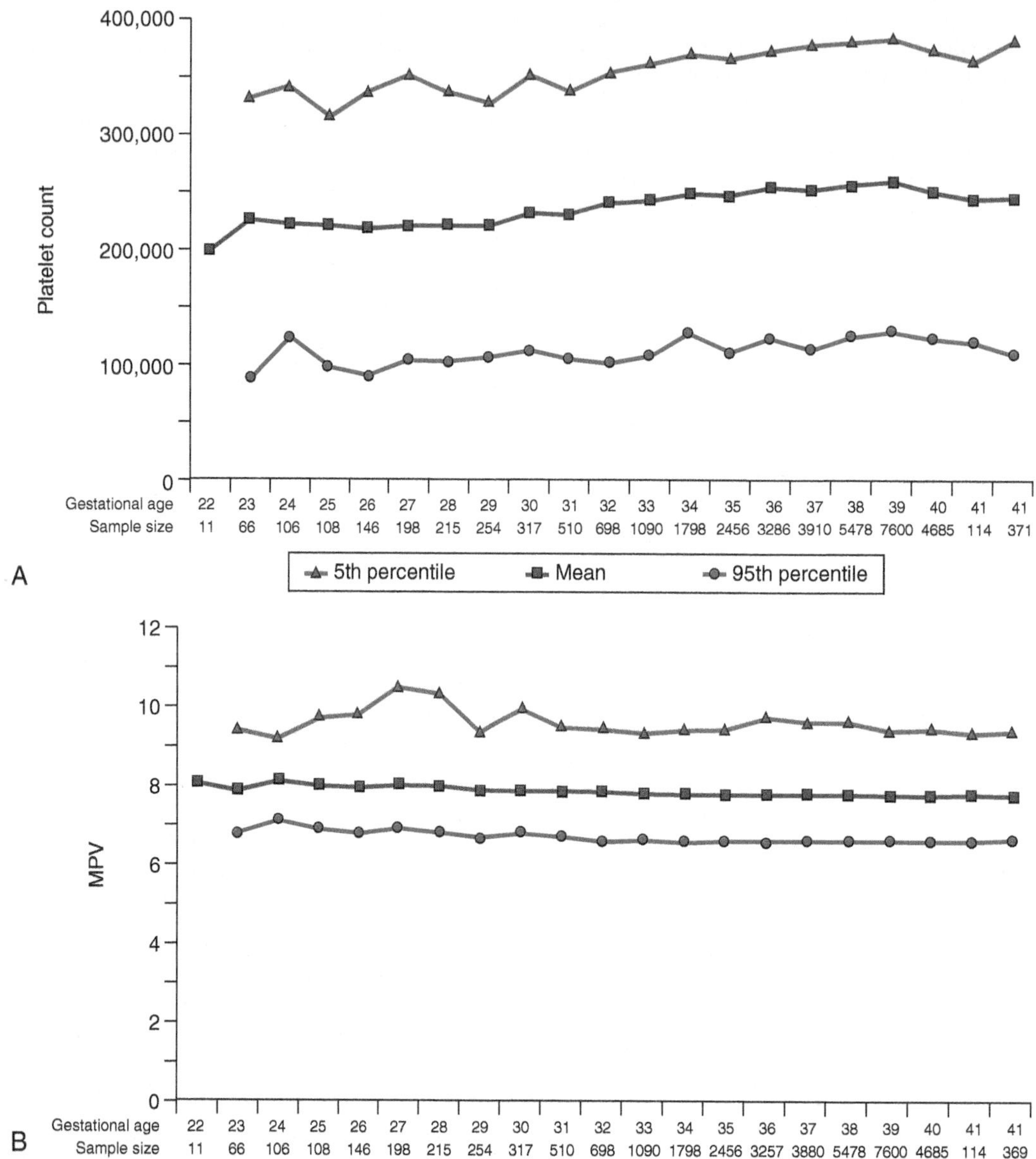

Fig. 110.10 Platelet counts and size in neonates according to gestational age. Reference ranges for both platelet count (A) and mean platelet volume *(MPV)* (B) during the first 90 days after birth. *Middle lines* represent the mean value while the lower and *upper lines* represent the 5th and 95th percentiles. (Republished with permission from Christensen RD, Henry E, Jopling J, et al. The CBC: reference ranges for neonates. *Semin Perinatol.* 2009;33:3–11.)

among preterm neonates and 0.8% among term neonates.[212] The incidence of thrombocytopenia is inversely proportional to gestational age and reaches 75% among those born with a weight less than 1000 g.[213]

NEONATAL PLATELET FUNCTION

Studies evaluating various aspects of platelet function (adhesion, aggregation, and activation) have shown that neonatal platelets are hyporesponsive in vitro to most agonists, compared with adult platelets,[214] and that this hyporeactivity is more pronounced in preterm infants.[215] Specifically, platelets from neonatal (full term) CB activate and aggregate less than adult platelets in response to traditional platelet agonists such as adenosine diphosphate (ADP), epinephrine, collagen, thrombin, and thromboxane analogues.[215,216] More recently, neonatal platelets were also found to exhibit a pronounced hyporesponsiveness to collagen-related peptide (CRP) and to the snake venom toxin rhodocytin, which activate the collagen receptor GPVI and C-type lectin-like receptor 2 (CLEC-2), respectively.[217] The same investigators also found developmental differences in platelet ***inhibitory*** pathways, specifically a hypersensitivity of neonatal platelets to inhibition by prostaglandin E1 (PGE_1) of ADP- and collagen-induced platelet aggregation, which might contribute to the hyporeactivity of neonatal platelets.[218]

Different mechanisms account for the developmentally unique responses of neonatal platelets to various agents: (1) the hyporesponsiveness to epinephrine is due to fewer α_2-adrenergic receptors (the binding sites for epinephrine); (2) the decreased responsiveness to thrombin is related to reduced expression of PAR-1 and PAR-4 in neonatal platelets[219]; (3) the decreased response to thromboxane results from reduced signaling downstream from the receptor[214]; (4) the reduced responses to collagen and rhodocytin result from mildly reduced expression of GPVI and CLEC-2 combined with a signaling defect evidenced by reduced Syk and PLCγ2 phosphorylation[217]; and (5) the hypersensitivity to PGE_1 inhibition of platelet aggregation is associated with a functionally increased PGE_1-cAMP-PKA axis.[218]

Surprisingly, while the hypofunctional in vitro platelet phenotype would predict a bleeding tendency, bleeding times (BTs) in healthy term neonates are paradoxically ***shorter*** than BTs in adults.[220] Similarly, studies using the Platelet Function Analyzer (PFA-100), an in vitro test of primary hemostasis that measures the time it takes to occlude a small aperture, or closure time (CT) found that CB samples from term neonates exhibited shorter CTs than samples from older children or adults.[221] The results of these studies suggest that full term neonates have enhanced platelet/vessel wall interaction, likely explained by their higher hematocrits, higher mean corpuscular volumes, and higher concentrations of vWF (particularly its ultralong polymers). Combined, these factors effectively counteract the intrinsic neonatal platelet hyporeactivity, suggesting that the in vitro platelet hyporeactivity of healthy full-term infants should be viewed as an integral part of a well-balanced unique neonatal hemostatic system, rather than a developmental deficiency.

These compensatory mechanisms might be less well developed in preterm infants, whose platelets are also more hyporeactive than those of full-term infants, probably leading to a more vulnerable hemostatic system. Specifically, BTs performed on the first day of life were longer in preterm compared with term infants, with neonates less than 33 weeks gestation exhibiting the longest BTs.[222] PFA-100 CTs from non-thrombocytopenic neonates were also inversely correlated to gestational age in both CB and neonatal PB samples obtained on the first day of life.[223] However, BTs and CTs in preterm neonates were still near or within the normal range for adults, suggesting that healthy preterm neonates also have adequate primary hemostasis. How disease processes perturb this delicate system, and whether these disturbances contribute to bleeding, are unanswered questions.

Neonatal platelet function improves significantly and nearly normalizes by 10 to 14 days, even in preterm infants.[224] Consistent with this, Del Vecchio and associates found that all infants had shorter BTs by day of life 10 than at birth, and that early gestational age–related differences disappeared by then.[222] Moreover, little or no further shortening occurred between days 10 and 30. While no causal association has been demonstrated, the first 10 days of life also constitute the period of highest bleeding risk in preterm neonates.

NEONATAL PREDISPOSITION TO THROMBOCYTOPENIA

Studies in thrombocytopenic adult patients and in animal models have shown that, under normal conditions, the adult BM responds to increased platelet demand by first increasing the MK size and ploidy and then the MK number.[225,226] These changes ultimately lead to a two- to eightfold increase in MK mass. To determine whether thrombocytopenic neonates can mount a similar response when facing increased platelet consumption due to illness, our group evaluated the MK concentration and size in BM samples from thrombocytopenic and non-thrombocytopenic neonates and adults. In this study, thrombocytopenic neonates (unlike thrombocytopenic adults) did not increase the size of their MKs.[50] Similar results were obtained in a study using a murine model of fetal immune thrombocytopenia.[227] Here, adult mice treated with an anti-platelet antibody (MWRReg30) increased the number and size of their MKs as expected, while newborn mice exposed in utero to the same antibody did not increase their MK size. Consistent with these observations, a recent study showed significant differences in the response of newborn and adult mice to a single dose of the Tpo mimetic romiplostim. While adult mice increased the number and size of MKs in the BM, newborn mice did not, resulting in an attenuated platelet increment.[166] Taken together, these observations support the notion that MKs in neonates have a limited ability to increase their size in response to increased platelet demand or Tpo stimulation, which decreases their ability to upregulate platelet production and likely contributes to the predisposition of sick neonates to develop thrombocytopenia. Furthermore, the evidence suggests that platelet production in neonates is dependent on the proliferative potential of their MK progenitors, thus making them highly susceptible to factors that affect MK proliferation.

COMMON CAUSES OF THROMBOCYTOPENIA IN NEONATES

Thrombocytopenia in the neonatal period can be caused by a large number of disease processes. Several different systems to classify neonatal thrombocytopenia have been proposed, some based on the suspected kinetic mechanism (increased platelet consumption versus decreased production),[228,229] and others based on the time of onset (early versus late thrombocytopenia).[230-232] One approach is to diagnose thrombocytopenic neonates based on recognizing typical patterns, which incorporate factors such as time of onset, severity, duration of thrombocytopenia, and suspected mechanism (Table 110.2).[233] These patterns are associated with specific pathophysiologic processes that can cause thrombocytopenia: immune, infectious, genetic, drug-induced, disseminated intravascular coagulation (DIC), placental insufficiency, and miscellaneous causes. Although not all-inclusive, this classification encompasses most common causes of neonatal thrombocytopenia.

IMMUNE-MEDIATED THROMBOCYTOPENIA

NEONATAL ALLOIMMUNE THROMBOCYTOPENIA

In 1953, Harrington and co-workers described a variety of thrombocytopenia that affects healthy neonates who have no other evidence of disease.[234] The pathogenesis of this type of thrombocytopenia, now known as *neonatal alloimmune thrombocytopenia (NAIT)*, resembles that of erythroblastosis fetalis; it is mediated by maternal antibodies directed against antigens on fetal platelets. When incompatibility between parental platelet antigens exists, the mother can become sensitized to an antigen (inherited from the father) expressed on the fetal platelets. These antibodies can then cross the placenta and coat the fetal platelets, which are then removed from the circulation by the fetal reticuloendothelial system. Unlike neonatal Rh disease, however, the first pregnancy can produce an affected fetus.

The study of NAIT has been complicated by the multiple antigens expressed on platelets and by the fact that the nomenclature for these antigens has undergone multiple changes during the past few decades. To standardize the nomenclature, platelet antigens have been now designated *human platelet antigens* (HPAs). Different allelic forms are distinguished by an "a" or "b" suffix, with "a" indicating the most common and "b" indicating the uncommon allele.[228,235] The most common cause of NAIT is alloantibodies against HPA-1a, formerly known as *PLA-1*, which accounts for 75% to 90% of all cases of NAIT. However, the frequency with which a particular antigen is responsible for cases of NAIT depends on the relative frequency of this antigen in that population. For example, although HPA-1a is the most common antigen responsible for NAIT in the Caucasian population (in which 68.9% of the population has the genotype HPA-1a/HPA-1a), HPA-4 is most frequently implicated among Asian subjects.[228] Cases mediated by antibodies against HPA-5,[236] HPA-3,[237] HPA-2,[238] and HPA-6[239] have also been described, although with much lower frequency. In addition, immunization against "low-frequency" or "private" platelet alloantigens might account for a higher percentage of NAIT than previously recognized, with HPA-9bw being by far the most commonly implicated of these rare antigens.[240]

Table 110.2 Classification of Etiologies of Thrombocytopenia, Including Severity, Onset, Time to Resolution, and Likely Mechanism.

Categories	Subtypes	Severity	Onset	Time to Resolution	Mechanism
Immune	Alloimmune	Severe	Early	Days to weeks	↑ Consumption
	Autoimmune	Moderate	Early	Weeks to months	↑ Consumption
Infections	Bacterial	Variable	Variable	1–7 days	Mixed
	Viral	Variable	Early	Variable	Mixed
	Fungal	Severe	Late	2–7 days	Mixed
Genetic Disorders	Chromosomal	Moderate	Early	Days to weeks	↓ Production
	Bone marrow failure	Severe	Early[a]	Variable[b]	↓ Production
	Familial thrombocytopenias	Mild to moderate	Early	Never	↓ Production
Drugs		Moderate to severe	Late	Median, 8 days[c]	Variable
DIC		Severe	Variable	Variable	↑ Consumption
PIH and IUGR		Mild to moderate	Early	7–10 days	↓ Production
NEC		Moderate to severe	Late	7–10 days	↑ Consumption

[a]Most congenital bone marrow failure syndromes are present at birth (i.e., congenital amegakaryocytic thrombocytopenia or thrombocytopenia-absent radii). However, the hematologic manifestations of Fanconi anemia usually do not appear until childhood.
[b]Thrombocytopenia associated with TAR syndrome usually resolves before school age. Other thrombocytopenias associated with bone marrow failure do not improve.
[c]After discontinuation of the offending agent.
DIC, Disseminated intravascular coagulation; *IUGR*, intrauterine growth restriction; *NEC*, necrotizing enterocolitis; *PIH*, pregnancy induced hypertension; *TAR*, thrombocytopenia and absent radii.
From Sola MC. Evaluation and treatment of severe and prolonged thrombocytopenia in neonates. *Clin Perinatol.* 2004;31:1–14.

Platelet antigens appear in the fetus early in gestation, and the maternal antibodies can cross the placenta early in the second trimester, thereby inducing severe fetal thrombocytopenia. Bussel and co-workers studied 107 fetuses who had siblings with NAIT, at a mean gestational age of 25 ± 4 weeks.[241] Fifty percent of them had initial platelet counts of 50 × 10^9/L or less, including 21 fetuses evaluated before 24 weeks' gestation. The only good predictive factor for severe thrombocytopenia was a history of antenatal intracranial hemorrhage in the sibling.

Overall, NAIT should be suspected in any neonate without obvious clinical illness or malformations, who presents with thrombocytopenia, which is typically severe. Intracranial hemorrhage is the most perilous complication and occurs in 10% to 30% of cases.[242-244] For that reason, neonates with NAIT and platelet counts lower than 50 × 10^9/L should be treated and should have a cranial ultrasonographic examination as soon as possible, to determine whether an intracranial hemorrhage occurred prior to delivery versus postnatally. For a long time, it was thought that infants with NAIT do not respond well to random donor platelet transfusions and needed to be transfused with antigen-negative platelets (obtained either from known HPA-1b platelet donors or from the mother). However, new evidence suggests that a significant percentage of neonates with NAIT respond to random donor platelet concentrates with a substantial increase in platelet counts, suggesting that transfusion of platelet concentrates from random donors is an appropriate strategy in the initial management of severe NAIT, pending the availability of antigen-compatible platelets.[245] High-dose intravenous immune globulin (IVIG, 1 g/kg/day for up to 2 days) has been reported to raise platelet counts to at least twice the baseline level in 48 hours.[246] Retreatment is occasionally required and subsequent pregnancies should be managed to limit the risk for fetal bleeding.[247,248] Typically, subsequent pregnancies are managed with administration of high-dose IVIG ± steroids to the mother, starting at different time points depending on whether the previous affected fetus had an intracranial hemorrhage or not. Intrauterine platelet transfusions are no longer recommended, due to the very high fetal mortality and morbidity associated with this procedure.

NEONATAL AUTOIMMUNE THROMBOCYTOPENIA

Neonatal autoimmune thrombocytopenia is similar to NAIT in that it is mediated by the transplacental passage of maternal antiplatelet antibodies. In contrast to NAIT, however, the antibody responsible for these cases binds both maternal and fetal platelets, causing thrombocytopenia in both the mother and neonate. In most cases, the underlying maternal disease is ITP, although other disorders (i.e., systemic lupus erythematosus) can also produce this syndrome. Thrombocytopenia (platelet count <150 × 10^9/L) is found in 13% to 64% of infants born to mothers with ITP.[249-255] Unlike in NAIT, however, the incidence of severe neonatal thrombocytopenia (platelet count <50 × 10^9/L) is relatively low, varying from 5% to 20% in different studies. These infants also have a very low rate of significant bleeding complications, particularly intracranial hemorrhages. In an analysis of 474 infants born to mothers with ITP, Cook and colleagues found an incidence of intracranial hemorrhage of 3% among infants with moderate or severe thrombocytopenia. Several subsequent studies have confirmed a very low fetal morbidity associated with maternal ITP.[256]

Several studies have tried to identify antenatal predictors of severe thrombocytopenia in the offspring of mothers with ITP. Unfortunately, the fetal or neonatal platelet count cannot be reliably predicted by maternal platelet count, platelet antibody levels, or history of maternal splenectomy. Neonates born to a mother with history of delivering an infant with thrombocytopenia are usually as affected as the first. Attempts to measure the fetal platelet count prior to delivery carry risk and are not recommended. There is also no evidence that cesarean section is safer for the fetus than uncomplicated vaginal delivery (although forceps or vacuum assist deliveries should be avoided), and thus the current recommendation is to treat the maternal ITP appropriately, but to use only obstetrical indications for cesarean delivery. Interestingly, a recent study reported the use of recombinant human Tpo to manage ITP during pregnancy. In this study of 31 patients, 74% responded. Furthermore, Tpo was well tolerated, and no problems were observed in the infants born to treated mothers.[257] This paved the way for the use of a new potential therapy to manage ITP during pregnancy.

While only a small percentage of neonates are born with severe thrombocytopenia in the setting of maternal ITP, mild to moderate thrombocytopenia is more common. Importantly, the platelet count typically decreases after birth, reaching a nadir between days 2 and 5.[251] For that reason, the recommendation is to obtain a platelet count immediately after delivery (from the cord or the baby) and to follow platelet counts in all infants with mild or moderate thrombocytopenia. A head ultrasound should be obtained on all infants with a platelet count less than 50 × 10^9/L at birth. Recommendations from the International Consensus Report on Management of ITP are to treat neonates with either clinical bleeding or a platelet count less than 20 × 10^9/L with a single dose of IVIG (1 g/kg), which can be repeated if necessary.[258] Major bleeding should be treated with platelet transfusions in addition to IVIG. Severe thrombocytopenia and major hemorrhage secondary to maternal ITP are rare, so evaluation for alloimmune thrombocytopenia or other causes of thrombocytopenia should be considered in those cases.[259]

Neonatal thrombocytopenia secondary to maternal ITP can last for months and requires long-term monitoring and occasionally a second dose of IVIG 4 to 6 weeks after birth. Interestingly, a recent study suggests that antiplatelet antibodies from ITP mothers are transferred to the fetus by breastmilk and are associated with neonatal thrombocytopenia persisting more than 4 months, which disappears following discontinuation of breastfeeding.[260]

INFECTION

The association of thrombocytopenia with neonatal bacterial sepsis has been described by several groups of investigators, although the reported incidence varies depending on the definition of thrombocytopenia. For example, Guida and collaborators defined thrombocytopenia as a platelet count less than 100 × 10^9/L and observed it in 54% of sepsis episodes,[261] while Manzoni and associates defined thrombocytopenia as a platelet count less than 80 × 10^9/L and detected it in 17.2% of septic infants.[262] Whether infections with certain organisms are more likely to induce thrombocytopenia than infections with other types (i.e., gram-positive vs. gram-negative organisms) is controversial,[261,262] but it appears that virtually any bacterial organism capable of causing sepsis in a neonate is also capable of inducing thrombocytopenia. In modern NICUs, late-onset sepsis is the most common clinical condition underlying severe thrombocytopenia in neonates.[263] If the infection is treated appropriately, the thrombocytopenia usually lasts an average of 6 days (range 1 to 10 days).[261,264] However, a number of neonates with sepsis develop severe thrombocytopenia that persists longer than 2 weeks,[263] and sepsis accounts for approximately one third of NICU patients who qualify as very-high platelet users (i.e., >20 transfusions).[265]

The etiology of thrombocytopenia in bacterial sepsis is an active area of research. Prior studies assessing platelet production in neonates with sepsis and/or necrotizing enterocolitis (NEC) showed a modest (twofold to threefold) elevation in Tpo levels, circulating MK progenitors and reticulated platelet percentages (a measure of newly released platelets), suggesting primarily a platelet consumptive etiology rather than decreased production.[266] Interestingly, however, neonates with gram-negative sepsis had only modest increases in thrombopoiesis, despite having more severe thrombocytopenia and more severe illness. This suggested that the thrombopoietic response in neonates can be dampened during severe illness, reaching a state of *relative hypoproliferation*, defined as a less than twofold increase in platelet production in response to consumptive thrombocytopenia.[266]

Traditionally, sepsis-induced platelet consumption has been attributed to DIC, increased platelet aggregation and adherence to the damaged endothelium with subsequent removal by the reticuloendothelial system, and/or immune mediated platelet destruction. With new research evidencing a central role of platelets in innate and adaptive immune responses, it is likely that the sepsis-induced consumption of platelets is more complex than previously thought. Platelets express and/or release multiple immune mediators, including cytokines, chemokines, and receptors known to be required for the initiation of the immune response to infection.[267,268] Andonegui and colleagues demonstrated the expression of TLR-4 (the LPS receptor) on platelets and showed that, in response to LPS, platelets accumulate in the lungs where they bind to adherent neutrophils.[269] Clark and colleagues studied this further and described that, once LPS-stimulated platelets adhere to neutrophils in the lungs, they induce robust neutrophil activation and the release of neutrophil extracellular traps (NETS) used to ensnare bacteria.[270] Furthermore, a recent study revealed that bacteria such as *Escherichia coli* and *Staphylococcus aureus* are able to induce apoptosis in platelets by producing α-hemolysin or α-toxin, respectively: both enzymes that induce rapid degradation of platelet Bcl-xL, an anti-apoptotic protein essential for platelet survival.[271] This in turn results in a rapid drop in platelet count.

Viral and parasitic infections also cause thrombocytopenia.The specific mechanisms of thrombocytopenia in these infections are unclear, but likely involve a mixture of platelet destruction and suppression of platelet production. Cytomegalovirus (CMV), the most common cause of congenital viral infection, affects megakaryopoiesis by directly infecting bone marrow stromal cells[272] and MKs.[273] In addition, CMV-infected infants frequently exhibit splenomegaly and require repeated transfusions due to platelet sequestration in the spleen. In regard to other viruses, herpes viruses can cause suppression of MK colony formation in vitro.[274] Parvovirus B19 usually causes severe anemia leading to hydrops fetalis, but it can also cause thrombocytopenia. In vitro parvovirus B19 suppresses MK colony formation,[275] and Forestier and coworkers found thrombocytopenia in 11 out of 13 fetuses with parvovirus B19 infection.[276] Neonatal enterovirus infection can also cause thrombocytopenia, especially in the presence of hepatitis and DIC.[277] HIV has also been recognized as a cause of thrombocytopenia in neonates. Like CMV and parvovirus, HIV can directly infect MKs and cause impaired platelet release, a phenomenon known as *ineffective platelet production*.[157] Among mothers infected with *Toxoplasma gondii* during pregnancy, 12 of 39 infected infants had low platelet counts.[278] Adenovirus, Epstein-Barr virus, and dengue virus have also been reported to cause neonatal thrombocytopenia, although these are rather uncommon infections in the neonatal period.

GENETIC CAUSES OF THROMBOCYTOPENIA

A variety of syndromes and congenital disorders are associated with neonatal thrombocytopenia. In some of these cases, there are associated features that are easily identified in the neonatal period, such as shortened or absent radii in the thrombocytopenia and absent radii (TAR) syndrome, or subtler physical findings, such as decreased ability to rotate the forearm due to radioulnar synostosis in the syndrome known as *amegakaryocytic thrombocytopenia and radioulnar synostosis (ATRUS)*.[158] Common chromosomal anomalies, such as trisomy 21, trisomy 18, trisomy 13, and Turner syndrome, are also associated with transient neonatal thrombocytopenia. In some congenital thrombocytopenias, there are no physical findings evident in the neonatal period, but the platelets are either abnormally small (microthrombocytopenias; MPV less than 7 fL) or abnormally large (macrothrombocytopenias, MPV greater than 11 fL). Geddis and associates classified congenital thrombocytopenias according to platelet size (Fig. 110.11), genetic mutations, and associated findings.[279] Hinckley and colleagues also outlined a widely encompassing group of thrombocytopenias associated with specific genetic disorders.[280] Certain inherited metabolic

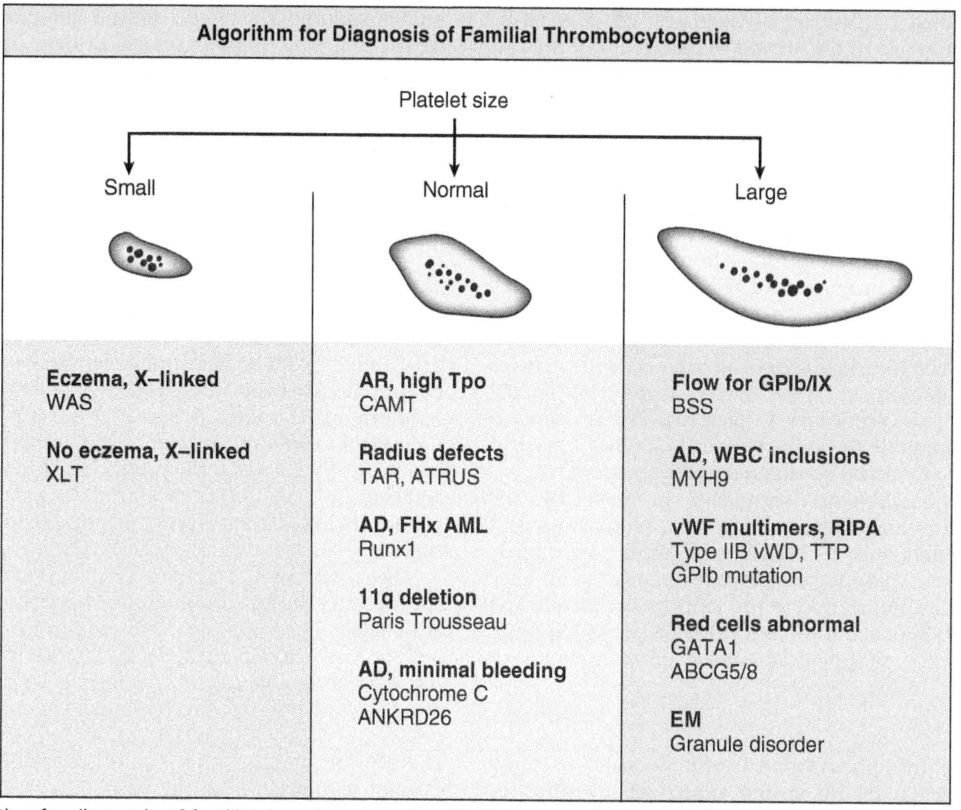

Fig. 110.11 Algorithm for diagnosis of familial thrombocytopenia. *AD,* Autosomal dominant; *AR,* autosomal recessive; *ATRUS,* amegakaryocytic thrombocytopenia with radio-ulnar synostosis; *BSS,* Bernard Soulier syndrome; *CAMT,* congenital amegakaryocytic thrombocytopenia; *EM,* electron microscopy; *FH$_X$ AML,* FOXJ2 acute myeloid leukemia; *RIPA,* ristocetin-induced platelet aggregation; *TAR,* thrombocytopenia with absent radii; *Tpo,* thrombopoietin; *TTP,* thrombotic thrombocytopenic purpura; *vWD,* von Willebrand's disease; *WAS,* Wiskott Aldrich syndrome; *XLT,* X-linked thrombocytopenia. (Republished with permission from Geddis AE. A potential new gene for thrombocytopenia. *Blood.* 2011;117:6406–6407.)

disorders can also present with thrombocytopenia, including methylmalonic acidemia, isovaleric acidemia, ketoglycinemia, and holocarboxylase synthetase deficiency.

THROMBOCYTOPENIA ABSENT RADIUS SYNDROME

TAR syndrome is a rare disorder involving thrombocytopenia and bilateral absence of the radius. Patients present in infancy with thrombocytopenia that often improves with age. Patients with TAR have decreased numbers of MK progenitors in the BM and exhibit defective Tpo signaling in their platelets. These defects in Tpo signaling result from decreased JAK2 phosphorylation. Interestingly, this defect corrected with age, with adult samples having normal JAK2 phosphorylation in response to Tpo signaling, suggesting a developmentally driven pathophysiology that has not yet been elucidated.[281] In regard to the genetic cause of TAR, early studies found a proximal microdeletion of 1.q21.1 that is present in all affected individuals, but the finding of multiple different patterns of inheritance suggested that the 1.q21.1 deletion is required but not sufficient to explain TAR.[282] Subsequent studies elucidated that TAR is caused by the compound inheritance of a rare null allele and one of two low-frequency SNPs in the regulatory regions of *RBM8A*, which encodes the Y14 subunit of the exon-junction complex. Of the 53 cases with this inheritance pattern, 51 carried a submicroscopic deletion of 1.q21.1 that had previously been associated with TAR. As expected, subjects with TAR had reduced Y14 expression in their platelets. However, the mechanism behind the developmental-stage specific manifestations of TAR syndrome is still not understood.[283]

CONGENITAL AMEGAKARYOCYTIC THROMBOCYTOPENIA

CAMT is a severe thrombocytopenic disorder with near-absence of MKs caused by mutations in the gene encoding *c-mpl*, the Tpo receptor. The severity of thrombocytopenia directly correlates to the degree of failure of the Tpo/c-mpl signaling axis. While the thrombocytopenic CAMT phenotype is consistent in adults, infants and children with type II CAMT (associated with reduced, but not absent c-mpl surface expression) can have near-normal platelet counts for a variable period of time, preceding the development of severe thrombocytopenia.[284,285] Alternatively, CAMT patients have been described who, as neonates, presented with severe thrombocytopenia despite appropriate numbers of immature-appearing MKs in their BM, suggesting that mechanisms other than reduced MKs might contribute to the thrombocytopenia in neonatal life.[286-288] The previously discussed studies supporting different functions of c-mpl throughout development (see "Thrombopoietin Throughout Development") suggest that defects in MK maturation can contribute to the thrombocytopenia in neonates with *c-mpl* mutations, thus providing a potential explanation for the finding of thrombocytopenia despite the presence of immature-appearing MKs in the BM of neonates later diagnosed with CAMT.

PLACENTAL INSUFFICIENCY AND CHRONIC INTRAUTERINE HYPOXIA

Chronic intrauterine hypoxia is the most frequent cause of early-onset thrombocytopenia (within the first 72 hours of life) in preterm neonates. Chronic intrauterine hypoxia is commonly seen in maternal conditions associated with placental insufficiency, such as pregnancy-induced hypertension and diabetes, and manifests in the fetus as intrauterine growth restriction resulting in small-for-gestational-age (SGA) neonates and hematologic abnormalities (i.e., thrombocytopenia, neutropenia, polycythemia). The thrombocytopenia associated with this condition is usually mild to moderate, with platelet counts between 50 and 100 × 10^9/L. In a large study of SGA neonates with thrombocytopenia presumably due to placental insufficiency and chronic intrauterine hypoxia (i.e., without other identifiable cause), which the authors termed *thrombocytopenia of SGA*, the mean nadir platelet count was 93 × 10^9/L.[289] In the same study, severely SGA neonates (birth weight <1st percentile for age) had lower platelet counts than less growth-restricted infants, and the nucleated red cell count elevation at birth correlated with the severity of the thrombocytopenia. Severe thrombocytopenia secondary to SGA is rare, however, and for that reason other causes of severe early onset thrombocytopenia (such as immune-mediated, infections, or genetic disorders) should be considered if the platelet count is less than 50 × 10^9/L. The thrombocytopenia associated with chronic intrauterine hypoxia and intrauterine growth restriction also follows a well-characterized natural course, reaching its nadir by day of life 4, and typically resolving by days of life 10 to 14. Thus, persistence of the thrombocytopenia beyond this period should also trigger an evaluation for other causes.

The pathophysiology of thrombocytopenia in fetuses and neonates exposed to chronic intrauterine hypoxia is not completely understood, but studies have implicated decreased platelet production. Murray and Roberts observed that preterm neonates with early-onset thrombocytopenia had decreased concentrations of circulating MK progenitors compared to their non-thrombocytopenic counterparts.[149,290] Similarly, Sola and collaborators reported decreased numbers of MKs in the BM of three thrombocytopenic preterm neonates born from pregnancies complicated by placental insufficiency.[152] Contrary to what would be expected, both groups of investigators reported that plasma Tpo concentrations in these neonates were normal to minimally elevated, suggesting that an inadequate up-regulation of Tpo production could contribute to the thrombocytopenia.

The effects of chronic hypoxia on thrombopoiesis in vivo have also been studied in animal models. These studies confirmed the association between chronic hypoxia and thrombocytopenia, and showed reduced MK differentiation of hematopoietic precursors resulting in decreased MK numbers in both adult and newborn animals exposed to hypoxia.[291,292] Subsequent in vitro studies demonstrated that MK progenitors are not directly damaged by hypoxia, but rather the effects seem to be mediated by non-progenitor cells.[293] Consistently, hypoxia was shown to alter the effects of cytokines on MK progenitors without damaging the MK cells directly.[294] Taken together, these findings suggest that chronic intrauterine hypoxia alters the MK response to cytokines leading to decreased MK production, which improves once the infant is exposed to the normoxic extrauterine environment. This explains the spontaneous resolution of this thrombocytopenia starting on day of life 4 to 5. Typically, no intervention is needed for the thrombocytopenia in affected infants, but it is important to document the normalization of the platelet count to rule out other possible causes.

NECROTIZING ENTEROCOLITIS

NEC is frequently associated with thrombocytopenia. In an early study published in 1976 assessing hematologic abnormalities in infants with NEC, as many as 90% of infants with NEC had platelet counts below 150 × 10^9/L, and 55% had platelet counts below 50 × 10^9/L.[295] Of the latter, 55% had bleeding complications, one-third of these serious enough to be considered contributory to the infant's death. Six of 14 infants studied had evidence of DIC and the mean duration of thrombocytopenia was 7 days (range 1 to 31 days). A more recent study found that neonates with NEC and severe thrombocytopenia (platelet count <60 × 10^9/L) had two-times more bleeding events than neonates with severe thrombocytopenia not related to NEC, but the bleeds were minor in severity.[296] In reviewing 58 cases of NEC treated in their institution, Ververidis and coworkers found that thrombocytopenia and/or a rapid fall in the platelet count was a poor prognostic factor, and that the degree of the thrombocytopenia correlated with the severity of the disease.[297]

The etiology of thrombocytopenia in NEC is an area of active research. The shortened survival of platelet transfusions in these infants suggests a platelet-consumptive process. This was corroborated in studies of both murine models and human neonates with NEC/sepsis, which found markers of increased megakaryopoiesis in association with thrombocytopenia.[266,298] Recently, platelet activation triggered by thrombin (induced by tissue factor produced in intestinal macrophages) was shown to be a contributory factor to the thrombocytopenia in an animal model of NEC. In the same model, platelet depletion or targeted inhibition of thrombin improved NEC survival, suggesting that platelets contribute to the pathogenesis of this disease.[299] However, a study by Cremer and co-workers found a reduced immature platelet fraction (IPF, a measure of platelet production) in *severely* thrombocytopenic neonates with NEC, suggesting decreased platelet production in these infants.[300] Interestingly, this subset of infants with NEC, severe thrombocytopenia and low IPF had the highest mortality, suggesting that decreased IPF in the setting of severe thrombocytopenia could be a marker of illness severity and poor prognosis in NEC.

Many pro-inflammatory cytokines are elevated in NEC, particularly platelet-activating factor (PAF), IL-1, and tumor necrosis factor (TNF).[301] PAF, in particular, has been strongly implicated in the pathogenesis of NEC, based on animal studies, demonstrating that the inhibition of PAF attenuates or prevents the development of NEC.[302] Interestingly, the levels of several pro-inflammatory cytokines (IL-1, IL-6, IL-8, TNF-α) increase in the supernatant of platelet units during storage in the blood bank, prior to platelets being transfused.[303-307] While most of these pro-inflammatory factors are released from leukocytes present in the platelet suspension, and thus levels are markedly reduced when the products are leukoreduced prior to storage, bioactive factors and cytokines are also released from the platelet granules during storage, which could potentially contribute to the pathophysiology of NEC and other neonatal pathology.[308,309] In that regard, at least two studies have suggested an association between higher number/volume of transfusions in patients with NEC and increased morbidity (short bowel syndrome and/or cholestasis)[310] or mortality (30.3 vs. 6.0 transfusions per 100 infant days in infants with NEC who died vs. survived in an unadjusted analysis).[308] Although the difference in number of platelet transfusions between infants who died and those who survived was no longer significant in the latter study after adjusting for birth weight and severity of illness, the results strongly suggested the potential for such association. Thus, platelet transfusions should be administered judiciously to infants with NEC.

ASPHYXIA

Several studies have established an association between perinatal asphyxia and thrombocytopenia.[211,311] The thrombocytopenia is typically self-limited and mild to moderate, with platelet counts between 50 and 100 × 10^9/L that improve spontaneously and normalize by days 19 to 21.[312] In a cohort of 171 neonates with perinatal asphyxia, Boutaybi and colleagues found early-onset thrombocytopenia (within the first 48 hours of life) in 51% of neonates. Multiple logistic regression analysis identified a significant independent association between early-onset thrombocytopenia and prolonged PT and higher lactate levels, suggesting a correlation between the severity of the asphyxia and the severity of thrombocytopenia.[313]

The mechanisms responsible for the decreased platelet count are not entirely clear. In a significant number of infants, severe perinatal asphyxia is associated with DIC, thus providing a reasonable explanation for the thrombocytopenia in these cases. However, some asphyxiated neonates develop thrombocytopenia in the absence of coagulopathy and the mechanisms underlying the thrombocytopenia in these cases are less clear. Findings in a rabbit model suggest that shortened platelet survival following exposure to transient hypoxia might lead to thrombocytopenia.[314] In contrast, a recent study by Christensen and associates described the thrombocytopenia of asphyxia as likely hyporegenerative and as a separate entity from, but also co-occurring with, DIC.[312]

Recently, total body cooling became a widely accepted intervention aimed at improving the neurodevelopmental outcome of neonates with moderate to severe perinatal asphyxia.[315] Multiple studies have described changes in coagulation and platelet function induced by hypothermia. Specifically, in response to hypothermia, there is an inhibition of platelet activation, adhesion, and aggregation as well as changes in the platelets' surface antigen composition, which can lead to their rapid removal from the circulation.[316-318] Boutaybi and co-workers compared thrombocytopenia due to asphyxia alone versus asphyxia treated with total body cooling and found there to be a three times higher incidence of thrombocytopenia in infants treated with hypothermia. Importantly, this increase was in infants with only mild to moderate thrombocytopenia.[313,319] Characterization of the time course of thrombocytopenia between the two cohorts showed that patients with asphyxia treated with hypothermia reached their nadir platelet count later than those with thrombocytopenia of asphyxia alone (day 5 vs. day 3). Christensen and associates also showed a significant lengthening of BTs and CTs measured with the PFA-100 (both measures of platelet function and primary hemostasis) during hypothermia, followed by rapid normalization after rewarming.[320] This study suggests that the platelet functional impairment in asphyxiated neonates undergoing therapeutic hypothermia is transient.

The dysregulation of coagulation, platelet function, and the development of thrombocytopenia induced by both asphyxia and therapeutic hypothermia manifests clinically with a higher incidence of bleeding and coagulopathy.[321-323] A few studies have aimed at determining the modifiable risk factors for bleeding during therapeutic hypothermia. One study using thromboelastography (TEG) as a comprehensive assessment of coagulation reported an increased risk of coagulopathy with hypothermia, which was associated with specific measures of TEG but not with platelet counts.[319] Two separate studies found that, while platelet counts below 130×10^9/L or below 100×10^9/L were associated with an increased risk of minor bleeding, coagulopathy, and hypofibrinogenemia were associated with severe bleeding.[319,324] Together, these studies suggest that thrombocytopenia in the setting of perinatal asphyxia and therapeutic hypothermia may put infants at increased risk of mild bleeding, but coagulopathy and hypofibrinogenemia may be more important risk factors for severe hemorrhage.

THROMBOSES

Neonatal thromboses can occur spontaneously (such as renal vein thrombosis or sagittal sinus thrombosis) or in association with an indwelling central catheter.[325] Thrombocytopenia is not a mandatory component of the clinical presentation of neonatal thromboses, but the presence of persistent thrombocytopenia with no clear etiology should raise suspicion for the potential of thrombus formation, particularly if predisposing factors are present (including perinatal asphyxia, congenital heart disease, maternal diabetes mellitus, polycythemia, dehydration, twin pregnancy, or presence of an indwelling catheter). In recent reviews, thrombocytopenia/anemia or both were present in 51% of cases of renal vein thrombosis,[326] but the classic triad of gross hematuria, palpable kidneys, and thrombocytopenia was found in only 13%.[327] Thus, a high index of suspicion is required to make an early diagnosis. While arterial thrombosis is less frequent than venous thrombosis in neonates,[328,329] a recent study in adults with consumptive platelet disorders, specifically heparin-induced thrombocytopenia (HIT) and thrombotic thrombocytopenic purpura, found that platelet transfusion increased the risk for arterial thromboses.[330] While this study did not include neonates, the findings suggest that further study is warranted in this population.

DISSEMINATED INTRAVASCULAR COAGULATION/ MALFORMATIONS

DIC is a thrombo-hemorrhagic disorder in which there is systemic activation of the coagulation system, simultaneously causing intravascular thrombi formation (compromising blood supply to organs) and depletion of platelets and coagulation factors, resulting in bleeding. DIC is not a primary pathologic process, it is always secondary to an underlying disorder such as sepsis, trauma, vascular abnormalities, or hypoxic ischemic encephalopathy.[331] Laboratory parameters associated with DIC include thrombocytopenia as well as deficits in coagulation factors that prompt frequent transfusions of blood products. The thrombocytopenia in DIC is secondary to thrombin-induced platelet aggregation.[332] Neonates have an increased incidence of DIC compared to pediatric or adult patients,[333-335] which has been attributed to their dynamically evolving hemostatic system after birth.[336-338]

Thrombocytopenia is one of the features of the Kasabach-Merritt syndrome (KMS), also known as *hemangioma thrombocytopenia syndrome*. It is now clear that the vascular tumors associated with the KMS are not true childhood hemangiomas, but rather hemangioendotheliomas.[339] Typically, the thrombocytopenia of KMS is preceded by enlargement and hardening of the vascular tumor. The primary mechanism is local consumption of platelets and clot formation, but platelets that have been damaged within the vascular abnormality are also removed in the spleen. KMS is refractory to transfused platelets and, if administered, they can result in painful tumor engorgement.[340] As a result, platelet transfusions are only indicated for active bleeding or immediately prior to surgery.[341]

DRUG INDUCED

A few drugs administered to pregnant women have been reported to cause thrombocytopenia in the mothers and their fetuses. However, only a small percentage of mothers who receive the particular drug have thrombocytopenia, thus making the firm establishment of this association difficult. Nevertheless, quinine, thiazide diuretics, hydralazine, and tolbutamide have been implicated as causes of fetal/neonatal thrombocytopenia when administered to pregnant women.

In addition, the development of moderate to severe late-onset thrombocytopenia in a well-appearing infant in whom infection, NEC, thromboses, and DIC have been ruled out should trigger suspicion for drug-induced thrombocytopenia. The literature regarding drug-induced thrombocytopenia in neonates mostly consists of isolated case reports. However, there is a significant number of medications known to cause drug-induced thrombocytopenia that are also commonly used in neonates, including antibiotics (penicillins, linezolid, ciprofloxacin, cephalosporins, metronidazole, vancomycin, and rifampin), ibuprofen, acetaminophen, famotidine, cimetidine, hydrochlorothiazide, phenobarbital, and phenytoin.[342] If a neonate develops thrombocytopenia shortly after one of these medications has been started, and if other (more common) etiologies of thrombocytopenia have been ruled out, removal of the suspected medication should be considered.

One of the medications most frequently associated with thrombocytopenia among hospitalized patients is heparin, particularly unfractionated heparin. HIT is an immune-mediated response to heparin administration. The incidence of HIT among neonates has been found to range from 0% to 1.5%.[343,344] The incidence is slightly higher in pediatric ICU patients, particularly among those receiving therapeutic doses of unfractionated heparin for the treatment of thromboses or following cardiac surgery.[345] Unfractionated heparin in prophylactic doses[342] and low-molecular weight heparin are rare causes of HIT in pediatric patients.[345]

HIT is a clinicopathologic syndrome, which means that both clinical and laboratory characteristics have to be fulfilled to make the diagnosis. These include the presence of heparin, a fall in the platelet count by 50% or more, the correct time of onset (approximately 5 to 10 days after the initial exposure to heparin), and the presence of heparin dependent antibodies. There are two types of antibody assays used to diagnose HIT: antigen assays, which simply determine the presence of antibodies directed against the HIT-specific epitopes on PF4, and functional assays, which determine the platelet-activating properties of the antibodies in a patient's serum. The latter represent the gold standard in HIT antibody testing, because they detect the clinically significant HIT antibodies. However, they are technically demanding and are only carried out by large laboratories. Furthermore, it is unclear whether these assays need to be modified for use in neonates.

If HIT is strongly suspected or confirmed, heparin therapy should be discontinued, and alternative anticoagulants such as lepirudin and argatroban should be considered to avoid the thrombotic manifestations of HIT. However, data regarding the use of these anticoagulants in the neonatal population is sparse,[346] and therefore their potential benefits need to be carefully balanced against the potential risks. For more information on HIT in neonates and children, the reader is referred to the excellent review by Risch and colleagues.[345]

LIVER FAILURE

At least two studies of neonatal thrombocytopenia have linked liver failure with prolonged thrombocytopenia,[347,348] and it has been suggested that neonates with this presentation would be good candidates for therapy with thrombopoietic factors. The main mechanism responsible for this thrombocytopenia is likely decreased platelet production secondary to insufficient Tpo production in the liver (the main site of Tpo production). In adults, this mechanism has been supported by the observation of increasing Tpo concentrations and reticulated platelet percentages following liver transplants.[349,350] A second proposed mechanism involves the loss of liver cell function causing a reduction in the hepatic vascular bed and increasing the splanchnic inflow, ultimately resulting in elevated portal venous pressure, splenomegaly, and platelet sequestration in the spleen.[351] Adult studies have questioned the importance of this mechanism since interventions that reverse the portal hypertension do not reliably correct the thrombocytopenia. The mechanism of thrombocytopenia in neonatal liver failure has never been specifically studied.

MISCELLANEOUS CAUSES OF THROMBOCYTOPENIA IN NEONATES

Other neonatal conditions in which thrombocytopenia occurs include polycythemia vera, extracorporeal membrane oxygenation, cyanotic congenital heart disease, congenital leukemia, osteopetrosis, and the histiocytoses, particularly hemophagocytic lymphohistiocytosis (HLH).

CONCLUSION

Over the last decade, numerous studies have begun to characterize the differences between adult and fetal/neonatal megakaryopoiesis. Multiple findings have opened the path for future research of developmental differences in cytokine production and transcription factor/receptor expression in megakaryopoiesis. Thrombocytopenia is a common problem among sick neonates, and the potential implementation of approaches that take into account developmental stage-specific aspects of thrombopoiesis may lead to better neonatal therapies in the future.

A complete reference list is available at www.ExpertConsult.com.

SELECT REFERENCES

6. Notta F, Zandi S, Takayama N, et al. Distinct routes of lineage development reshape the human blood hierarchy across ontogeny. *Science*. 2016;351:aab2116.
7. Yamamoto R, Morita Y, Ooehara J, et al. Clonal analysis unveils self-renewing lineage-restricted progenitors generated directly from hematopoietic stem cells. *Cell*. 2013;154:1112-1126.
8. Sanjuan-Pla A, Macaulay IC, Jensen CT, et al. Platelet-biased stem cells reside at the apex of the haematopoietic stem-cell hierarchy. *Nature*. 2013;502:232-236.
16. Mattia G, Vulcano F, Milazzo L, et al. Different ploidy levels of megakaryocytes generated from peripheral or cord blood CD34+ cells are correlated with different levels of platelet release. *Blood*. 2002;99:888-897.
17. Lordier L, Jalil A, Aurade F, et al. Megakaryocyte endomitosis is a failure of late cytokinesis related to defects in the contractile ring and Rho/Rock signaling. *Blood*. 2008;112:3164-3174.
34. Potts KS, Sargeant TJ, Markham JF, et al. A lineage of diploid platelet-forming cells precedes polyploid megakaryocyte formation in the mouse embryo. *Blood*. 2014;124:2725-2729.
35. Potts KS, Sargeant TJ, Dawson CA, et al. Mouse prenatal platelet-forming lineages share a core transcriptional program but divergent dependence on MPL. *Blood*. 2015;126:807-16.
37. Popescu DM, Botting RA, Stephenson E, et al. Decoding human fetal liver haematopoiesis. *Nature*. 2019;574:365-371.
46. Woo AJ, Wieland K, Huang H, et al. Developmental differences in IFN signaling affect GATA1s-induced megakaryocyte hyperproliferation. *J Clin Invest*. 2013;123:3292-3304.
47. Elagib KE, Lu CH, Mosoyan G, et al. Neonatal expression of RNA-binding protein IGF2BP3 regulates the human fetal-adult megakaryocyte transition. *J Clin Invest*. 2017;127:2365-2377.
50. Sola-Visner MC, Christensen RD, Hutson AD, et al. Megakaryocyte size and concentration in the bone marrow of thrombocytopenic and nonthrombocytopenic neonates. *Pediatr Res*. 2007;61:479-484.
53. Liu ZJ, Italiano Jr J, Ferrer-Marin F, et al. Developmental differences in megakaryocytopoiesis are associated with up-regulated TPO signaling through mTOR and elevated GATA-1 levels in neonatal megakaryocytes. *Blood*. 2011;117:4106-4117.
54. Slayton WB, Wainman DA, Li XM, et al. Developmental differences in megakaryocyte maturation are determined by the microenvironment. *Stem Cell*. 2005;23:1400-1408.
55. Pastos KM, Slayton WB, Rimsza LM, et al. Differential effects of recombinant thrombopoietin and bone marrow stromal-conditioned media on neonatal versus adult megakaryocytes. *Blood*. 2006;108:3360-3362.
58. Bluteau O, Langlois T, Rivera-Munoz P, et al. Developmental changes in human megakaryopoiesis. *J Thromb Haemost*. 2013;11:1730-1741.
66. Klusmann JH, Godinho FJ, Heitmann K, et al. Developmental stage-specific interplay of GATA1 and IGF signaling in fetal megakaryopoiesis and leukemogenesis. *Genes Dev*. 2010;24:1659-1672.
91. Lok S, Kaushansky K, Holly RD, et al. Cloning and expression of murine thrombopoietin cDNA and stimulation of platelet production in vivo. *Nature*. 1994;369:565-568.
110. Grozovsky R, Begonja AJ, Liu K, et al. The Ashwell-Morell receptor regulates hepatic thrombopoietin production via JAK2-STAT3 signaling. *Nat Med*. 2015;21:47-54.
114. Ballmaier M, Germeshausen M, Schulze H, et al. c-mpl mutations are the cause of congenital amegakaryocytic thrombocytopenia. *Blood*. 2001;97:139-146.
147. Ghanima W, Cooper N, Rodeghiero F, et al. Thrombopoietin receptor agonists: ten years later. *Haematologica*. 2019;104:1112-1123.
185. Niswander LM, Fegan KH, Kingsley PD, et al. SDF-1 dynamically mediates megakaryocyte niche occupancy and thrombopoiesis at steady state and following radiation injury. *Blood*. 2014;124:277-286.
187. Wang Q, Miyakawa Y, Fox N, et al. Interferon-alpha directly represses megakaryopoiesis by inhibiting thrombopoietin-induced signaling through induction of SOCS-1. *Blood*. 2000;96:2093-2099.
188. Alvarado LJ, Huntsman HD, Cheng H, et al. Eltrombopag maintains human hematopoietic stem and progenitor cells under inflammatory conditions mediated by IFN-gamma. *Blood*. 2019;133:2043-2055.
203. Christensen RD, Henry E, Jopling J, et al. The CBC: reference ranges for neonates. *Semin Perinatol*. 2009;33:3-11.
208. Dreyfus M, Kaplan C, Verdy E, et al. Frequency of immune thrombocytopenia in newborns: a prospective study. Immune Thrombocytopenia Working Group. *Blood*. 1997;89:4402-4406.
211. Castle V, Andrew M, Kelton J, et al. Frequency and mechanism of neonatal thrombocytopenia. *J Pediatr*. 1986;108:749-755.
213. Christensen RD, Henry E, Wiedmeier SE, et al. Thrombocytopenia among extremely low birth weight neonates: data from a multihospital healthcare system. *J Perinatol*. 2006;26:348-353.
217. Hardy AT, Palma-Barqueros V, Watson SK, et al. Significant hypo-responsiveness to GPVI and CLEC-2 agonists in pre-term and full-term neonatal platelets and following immune thrombocytopenia. *Thromb Haemost*. 2018;118:1009-1020.
221. Israels SJ, Cheang T, McMillan-Ward EM, et al. Evaluation of primary hemostasis in neonates with a new in vitro platelet function analyzer. *J Pediatr*. 2001;138:116-119.

224. Bednarek FJ, Bean S, Barnard MR, et al. The platelet hyporeactivity of extremely low birth weight neonates is age-dependent. *Thromb Res*. 2009;124:42-45.
241. Bussel JB, Zabusky MR, Berkowitz RL, et al. Fetal alloimmune thrombocytopenia. *N Engl J Med*. 1997;337:22-26.
243. Bussel JB, Zacharoulis S, Kramer K, et al. Clinical and diagnostic comparison of neonatal alloimmune thrombocytopenia to non-immune cases of thrombocytopenia. *Pediatr Blood Cancer*. 2005;45:176-183.
245. Kiefel V, Bassler D, Kroll H, et al. Antigen-positive platelet transfusion in neonatal alloimmune thrombocytopenia (NAIT). *Blood*. 2006;107:3761-3763.
248. Bussel JB, Berkowitz RL, McFarland JG, et al. Antenatal treatment of neonatal alloimmune thrombocytopenia. *N Engl J Med*. 1988;319:1374-1378.
257. Kong Z, Qin P, Xiao S, et al. A novel recombinant human thrombopoietin therapy for the management of immune thrombocytopenia in pregnancy. *Blood*. 2017;130:7.
258. Provan D, Stasi R, Newland AC, et al. International consensus report on the investigation and management of primary immune thrombocytopenia. *Blood*. 2010;115:168-186.
259. Samuels P, Bussel JB, Braitman LE, et al. Estimation of the risk of thrombocytopenia in the offspring of pregnant women with presumed immune thrombocytopenic purpura. *N Engl J Med*. 1990;323:229-235.
268. Semple JW, Italiano Jr JE, Freedman J. Platelets and the immune continuum. *Nat Rev Immunol*. 2011;11:264-274.
270. Clark SR, Ma AC, Tavener SA, et al. Platelet TLR4 activates neutrophil extracellular traps to ensnare bacteria in septic blood. *Nat Med*. 2007;13:463-469.
271. Kraemer BF, Campbell RA, Schwertz H, et al. Bacteria differentially induce degradation of Bcl-xL, a survival protein, by human platelets. *Blood*. 2012;120:5014-5020.
289. Christensen RD, Baer VL, Henry E, et al. Thrombocytopenia in small-for-gestational-age infants. *Pediatrics*. 2015;136:e361-e370.
299. Namachivayam K, MohanKumar K, Shores DR, et al. Targeted inhibition of thrombin attenuates murine neonatal necrotizing enterocolitis. *Proc Natl Acad Sci U S A*. 2020;117:10958-10969.
312. Christensen RD, Baer VL, Yaish HM. Thrombocytopenia in late preterm and term neonates after perinatal asphyxia. *Transfusion*. 2015;55:187-196.
320. Christensen RD, Sheffield MJ, Lambert DK, et al. Effect of therapeutic hypothermia in neonates with hypoxic-ischemic encephalopathy on platelet function. *Neonatology*. 2012;101:91-94.
342. Aster RH, Bougie DW. Drug-induced immune thrombocytopenia. *N Engl J Med*. 2007;357:580-587.
345. Risch L, Huber AR, Schmugge M. Diagnosis and treatment of heparin-induced thrombocytopenia in neonates and children. *Thromb Res*. 2006;118:123-135.

Developmental Hemostasis

111

Paul Monagle

INTRODUCTION

The presence of a complex hemostatic system is fundamental to all multicellular organisms with a blood circulatory system. Blood must remain in a fluid form to flow, and for survival, organisms must be able to stop that flow at sites of local injury, through the process of physiologic thrombus formation. However, under certain conditions, thrombus formation can become pathologic. In the mid-1800s Rudolf Virchow described a triad of factors that contributed to pathologic blood clotting: blood flow, blood vessel wall, and blood composition. The description is still relevant nowadays, and in fact is just as relevant to the development of bleeding as it is to abnormal clotting. Hemostasis involves complex interactions among the vascular endothelium, cellular elements within blood (particularly the platelets), and plasma proteins in the context of blood flow. Although developmental hemostasis is often discussed purely in terms of changes in plasma proteins, it is important to remember that all of the elements of the Virchow triad change with age. Furthermore, changes in plasma proteins are not restricted to the proteins that constitute the coagulation system but occur throughout the entire plasma proteome.[1-3] Although hemostasis is a dynamic, evolving process that is age dependent and begins in utero, there is arguably no greater time of change in the hemostatic system than around the time of birth.[4] Although evolving, the hemostatic system in healthy fetuses and infants must be considered physiologic. The evaluation of newborn infants for hemorrhagic or thrombotic complications presents unique problems that are not encountered in older children and adults.[5,6] For example, physiologic levels of many coagulation proteins in neonates are low, which makes the diagnoses of some inherited and acquired hemostatic problems difficult to establish. An understanding of developmental hemostasis in the broadest sense optimizes the prevention, diagnosis, and treatment of hemostatic problems during infancy and undoubtedly provides new insights into the pathophysiology of hemorrhagic and thrombotic complications for all ages.

THE COAGULATION SYSTEM

Our understanding of the hemostatic physiology in neonates and infants is poor compared with knowledge of this subject in adults. This deficiency is due to several factors: in neonates and infants, multiple reference ranges are required because these patients have rapidly evolving systems[4,7-9]; blood sampling in the young is technically difficult; only small blood samples can be obtained; microtechniques are required[10]; and greater variability in plasma concentrations of coagulation proteins necessitates the use of large patient numbers to establish normative data.

Coagulation proteins are independently synthesized by the fetus and do not cross the placenta.[11-23] By 10 weeks gestational age, plasma concentrations of most coagulation proteins are measurable, and they continue to increase gradually in parallel with gestational age. A number of studies have described normal values for hemostatic functional assays in fetuses or neonates (Table 111.1). Samples obtained during fetoscopy provide the best assessment of normal values for fetuses and, by extrapolation, very premature infants (Tables 111.2 and 111.3).[24] True reference ranges for extremely premature infants are not available because most of these infants have postnatal complications. Tables 111.4-111.7 provide reference ranges for coagulation proteins, inhibitors of coagulation, and components of the fibrinolytic system for premature (30 to 36 weeks gestational age) and term infants on day 1 after birth, as well as longitudinally during the first 6 months after birth.[4,7,8] Studies continue to demonstrate that samples obtained from umbilical cord blood may have considerable differences from samples obtained simultaneously from peripheral blood of the infant.[25]

In addition to the multitude reported studies of functional assays, Attard and colleagues described the antigenic levels of coagulation proteins in neonates compared with adults and confirmed that 10 proteins are quantitatively significantly different.[26] Further research is required to understand the role of posttranslational modifications and the correlations (or not) between quantitative levels and functional levels.

The factors controlling these changes remain unknown. Studies in mice have reported that, of the 41 microRNAs (miRNAs) that are overexpressed in newborn livers compared with adult livers, 21 have hemostatic messenger RNA (mRNA) as their targets.[27] miRNAs are an abundant class of small noncoding RNAs that are negative regulators in a number of physiologic and pathologic processes. Teruel and colleagues proposed that the miRNAs might have negative regulatory effects on the hemostatic proteins during the newborn period.[27] In a subsequent study, the same group showed a significant reduction of sialic acid content in neonatal antithrombin (AT) compared with adult AT in mice. The mRNA levels of St3gal3 and St3gal4, two sialyltransferases potentially involved in AT sialylation, were 85% lower in neonates in comparison with adults. In silico analysis of miRNAs overexpressed in neonates revealed that mir-200a might target these sialyltransferases.[28]

Previous studies have measured mRNA levels for factor (F) VII, FVIII, FIX, FX, fibrinogen, AT, and protein C in hepatocytes from 5- to 10-week-old human embryos and fetuses and in

Table 111.1 Studies Reporting Functional Hemostatic Parameters in Fetuses or Neonates.

Author, Year	Patients (n)	Assays/Proteins Reported	Age Groups
Perlman, 1975[141]	35 26 30	PT, TT, APTT, fibrinogen, FDP, platelet count, hematocrit, FV, FVIII, plasminogen, hemoglobin	Healthy infants Small-for-date infants Postmature infants
Beverley, 1984[99]	80	APTT, FII-VII-X, fibrinogen, α_2-antiplasmin, platelet count, MPV, megathrombocyte index, plasminogen	Cord blood Newborns (48 h)
Andrew, 1987[7]	28–75 samples per age group	PT, APTT, TCT, fibrinogen, FII, FV, FVII, FVIII, vWF, FIX, FX, FXI, FXII, PK, HMW-K, FXIIIa, FXIIIb, plasminogen, antithrombin, α_2-M, α_2-AP, C_1E-INH, α_1-AT, HCII, protein C, protein S	Day 1 newborn Day 5 newborn Day 30 newborn Day 90 newborn Day 180 newborn Adult
Andrew, 1988[8]	23–67 samples per age group	PT, APTT, TCT, fibrinogen, FII, FV, FVII, FVIII, vWF, FIX, FX, FXI, FXII, PK, HMW-K, FXIIIa, FXIIIb, plasminogen, antithrombin, α_2-M, α_2-AP, C_1E-INH, α_1-AT, HCII, protein C, protein S	Premature newborns (30–36 wk gestation) Day 1 Day 5 Day 30 Day 90 Day 180
Reverdiau-Moalic, 1996[24]	20 22 22 60 40	PT/INR, APTT, TCT, FI, FII, FVII, FVII, FIX, FX, FV, FVIII, FXI, FXII, PK, HMWK, AT, HCII, TFPI, protein C (Ag, Act), protein S (free and total), C4b-BP	Fetuses 19–23 wk gestation newborns 24–29 wk gestation newborns 30–38 wk gestation newborns Adults
Carcao, 1998[129]	17 57 31	PF-100 Hb Platelet count	Neonates Children Adults
Salonvaara, 2003[142]	21 25 34 45	FII, FV, FVII, FX, APTT, PT/INR, platelet count	24–27 wk gestation newborns 28–20 wk gestation newborns 31–33 wk gestation newborns 34–36 wk gestation newborns
Monagle, 2006[35]	Minimum of 20 samples per age group	APTT (4 reagents), PT/INR, fibrinogen, TCT, FII, FV, FVII, FVIII, FIX, FX, FXI, FXII, antithrombin, protein C, protein S, D dimers, TFPI (free and total), endogenous thrombin potential	Day 1 Day 3 <1 yr 1–5 yr 6–10 yr 11–16 yr Adults
Mitsiakos, 2009[143]	90 98	INR, PT, APTT, fibrinogen, FII, FV, FVII, FVIII, FIX, FX, FXI, FXII, antithrombin, protein C, protein S, APCr, TPA, PAI-1, vWF	Small-for-gestational-age newborns Appropriate for gestational age newborns
Boos, 1989[144]	57 (total)	PIVKA II, FVII, FII, FII:Ag	Day 1, 2, 3 neonates

α_1-AT, Alpha 1 antithrombin; *α_2-AP*, alpha 2 antiplasmin; *α_2-M*, alpha 2 macroglobulin; *APCr*, activated protein C resistance; *APTT*, activated partial thromboplastin time; *AT*, antithrombin; *C_1E-INH*, C1-esterase inhibitor; *C4b-BP*, C4b-binding protein; *F*, factor; *FDP*, fibrin degradation products; *FII:Ag*, factor II antigen; *HCII*, heparin cofactor II; *HMWK*, high-molecular-weight kininogen; *MPV*, mean platelet volume; *PAI-1*, plasminogen activator inhibitor-1; *PIVKA II*, protein induced by vitamin K absence; *PK*, prekallikrein; PT/INR, prothrombin time/international normalized ratio; *TCT*, thrombin-clotting time; *TFPI*, tissue factor pathway inhibitor; *TPA*, tissue plasminogen activator; *TT*, thrombin time; *vWF*, von Willebrand factor.

those from adults. Embryonic-fetal transcripts and adult mRNAs are similar in size; the nucleotide sequences of mRNA for FIX and FX are identical.[29,30] However, the expression of mRNA was variable, with adult values existing for some coagulation proteins but decreased for others. Similar concentrations of prothrombin mRNA were found in the livers of newborn and adult rabbits[31]; however, another study reported lower prothrombin mRNA concentrations in sheep.

In terms of understanding the controlling mechanisms of plasma protein concentrations, one of the most interesting studies demonstrated that, even with a transplanted adult liver in situ, children maintain plasma levels of certain coagulation proteins at their expected age-specific levels.[32] Thus the liver, despite being the site of production for most of the coagulation proteins and where control of levels may be exerted through miRNAs, is not the primary regulator of plasma levels. The authors hypothesized hormonal control, vascular endothelial control via an as-yet-unidentified mechanism, or control via variable clearance. However, whatever the mechanism, vascular endothelium seems a likely candidate as the primary regulator.[33]

The variable results for coagulation screening tests reflect the use of cord blood samples rather than samples from infants, differing ethnic populations, or use of different reagents.[34,35] Reference ranges for prothrombin time and activated partial thromboplastin times will differ with each different reagent and analyzer system, often significantly.[35,36] The thrombin-clotting time performed in the absence of calcium is prolonged because of the presence of the "fetal" form of fibrinogen at birth.[4,7,8] For Tables 111.3 and 111.4, the thrombin-clotting time was measured in the presence of calcium so that abnormal values secondary to the presence of heparin, as well as low levels of fibrinogen, could be detected.

COAGULANT PROTEINS

The vitamin K-dependent factors are the most extensively studied group of factors in infants, reflecting the clinical significance

Table 111.2 Coagulation Screening Tests and Coagulation Factor Levels in Fetuses, Term Infants, and Adults.

	Fetuses (Weeks Gestation)			Neonates	Adults
Parameter	19–23 (n = 20)	24–29 (n = 22)	30–38 (n = 22)	(n = 60)	(n = 40)
PT (s)	32.5 (19–45)	32.2 (19–44)[a]	22.6 (16–30)[a]	16.7 (12.0–23.5)[b]	13.5 (11.4–14.0)
PT (INR)	6.4 (1.7–11.1)	6.2 (2.1–10.6)[a]	3.0 (1.5–5.0)[b]	1.7 (0.9–2.7)[b]	1.1 (0.8–1.2)
APTT (s)	168.8 (83–250)	154.0 (87–210)[a]	104.8 (76–128)[a]	44.3 (35–52)[b]	33.0 (25–39)
TCT (s)	34.2 (24–44)[b]	26.2 (24–28)	21.4 (17.0–23.3)	20.4 (15.2–25.0)[a]	14.0 (12–16)
Factor I (g/L) von Clauss	0.85 (0.57–1.50)	1.12 (0.65–1.65)	1.35 (1.25–1.65)	1.68 (0.95–2.45)[a]	3.0 (1.78–4.50)
I Ag (g/L)	1.08 (0.75–1.50)	1.93 (1.56–2.40)	1.94 (1.30–2.40)	2.65 (1.68–3.60)[a]	3.5 (2.50–5.20)
IIc (%)	16.9 (10–24)	19.9 (11–30)[b]	27.9 (15–50)[a]	43.5 (27–64)[a]	98.7 (70–125)
VIIc (%)	27.4 (17–37)	33.8 (18–48)[b]	45.9 (31–62)	52.5 (28–78)[a]	101.3 (68–130)
IXc (%)	10.1 (6–14)	9.9 (5–15)	12.3 (5–24)[a]	31.8 (15–50)[a]	104.8 (70–142)
Xc (%)	20.5 (14–29)	24.9 (16–35)	28.0 (16–36)[a]	39.6 (21–65)[a]	99.2 (75–125)
Vc (%)	32.1 (21–44)	36.8 (25–50)	48.9 (23–70)[a]	89.9 (50–140)	99.8 (65–140)
VIIIc (%)	34.5 (18–50)	35.5 (20–52)	50.1 (27–78)[a]	94.3 (38–150)	101.8 (55–170)
XIc (%)	13.2 (8–19)	12.1 (6–22)	14.8 (6–26)[a]	37.2 (13–62)[a]	100.2 (70–135)
XIIc (%)	14.9 (6–25)	22.7 (6–40)	25.8 (11–50)[a]	69.8 (25–105)[a]	101.4 (65–144)
PK (%)	12.8 (8–19)	15.4 (8–26)	18.1 (8–28)[a]	35.4 (21–53)[a]	99.8 (65–135)
HMWK (%)	15.4 (10–22)	19.3 (10–26)	23.6 (12–34)[a]	38.9 (28–53)[a]	98.8 (68–135)

Data are mean (95% confidence intervals).
[a]$P < .01$.
[b]$P < .05$.
Ag, Antigen; *APTT*, activated partial thromboplastin time; *HMWK*, high-molecular-weight kininogen; *INR*, international normalized ratio; *PK*, prekallikrein; *PT*, prothrombin time; *TCT*, thrombin-clotting time.
From Reverdiau-Moalic P, Delahousse B, Body G, et al. Evolution of blood coagulation activators and inhibitors in the healthy human fetus. *Blood.* 1996;88:900.

Table 111.3 Blood Coagulation Inhibitor Levels in Fetuses, Term Infants, and Adults.

	Fetuses (Weeks Gestation)			Neonates	Adults
Parameter	19–23 (n = 20)[a]	24–29 (n = 22)	30–38 (n = 22)	(n = 60)	(n = 40)
AT (%)	20.2 (12–31)[b]	30.0 (20–39)	37.1 (24–55)[c]	59.4 (42–80)[c]	99.8 (65–130)
HCII (%)	10.3 (6–16)	12.9 (5.5–20)	21.1 (11–33)[c]	52.1 (19–99)[c]	101.4 (70–128)
TFPI (%)[a]	21.0 (16.0–29.2)	20.6 (13.4–33.2)	20.7 (10.4–31.5)[c]	38.1 (22.7–55.8)[c]	73.0 (50.9–90.1)
PC Ag (%)	9.5 (6–14)	12.1 (8–16)	15.9 (8–30)[c]	32.5 (21–47)[c]	100.8 (68–125)
PC Act (%)	9.6 (7–13)	10.4 (8–13)	14.1 (8–18)[b]	28.2 (14–42)[c]	98.8 (68–125)
Total PS (%)	15.1 (11–21)	17.4 (14–25)	21.0 (15–30)[c]	38.5 (22–55)[c]	99.6 (72–118)
Free PS (%)	21.7 (13–32)	27.9 (19–40)	27.0 (18–40)[c]	49.3 (33–67)[c]	98.7 (72–128)
Ratio of Free PS:Total PS	0.82 (0.75–0.92)	0.83 (0.76–0.95)	0.79 (0.70–0.89)[c]	0.64 (0.59–0.98)[c]	0.41 (0.38–0.43)
C4b-BP (%)	1.8 (0–6)	6.1 (0–12.5)	9.3 (5–14)	18.6 (3–40)[c]	100.3 (70–124)

Data are mean (95% confidence intervals).
[a]Twenty samples were assayed for each group but only 10 for 19- to 23-week-old fetuses.
[b]$P < .05$; [c]$P < .01$.
Act, Activity; *Ag*, antigen; *AT*, antithrombin; *HCII*, heparin cofactor II; *PC*, protein C; *PS*, protein S; *TFPI*, tissue factor pathway inhibitor.
From Reverdiau-Moalic P, Delahousse B, Body G, et al. Evolution of blood coagulation activators and inhibitors in the healthy human fetus. *Blood.* 1996;88:900–906.

of hemorrhagic disease of the newborn, currently known as ***vitamin K deficiency bleeding (VKDB)***.[35] Physiologically low levels of FII, FVII, FIX, and FX in Tables 111.4 and 111.5 are similar to those in other reports[4,7,8,37-47] and were measured in infants who received vitamin K prophylaxis at birth. The levels of the vitamin K–dependent factors and the contact factors (FXI, FXII, prekallikrein, and high-molecular-weight kininogen) gradually increase to values approaching adult levels by 6 months after birth.[4,7,8] Recently, low prothrombin levels were found to be associated with increased rates of intraventricular hemorrhage in very preterm infants. Both experimental and mathematical modeling studies have suggested that low prothrombin levels in neonates are the primary driver of reduced thrombin generation.[48,49]

Plasma levels of fibrinogen, FV, FVIII, FXIII, and von Willebrand factor (vWF) are not decreased at birth (see Tables 111.4 and 111.5). Fibrinogen levels continue to increase after birth.[50] Plasma levels of FVIII are skewed toward the high measurements, necessitating an adjustment of the lower limit of normal (see Tables 111.4 and 111.5). Levels of both vWF and high-molecular-weight multimers are increased at birth and for the first 3 months after birth.[4]

Differences in function and structure of fetal versus adult fibrinogen have been recognized for a number of years.[51,52] These differences have been primarily attributed to an increased sialic acid content of the fetal fibrinogen.[53] Posttranslational modification differences may be present in a number of coagulation proteins in neonates compared with adults. The functional and developmental significance of these changes remains to be determined.[54] Fibrinogen, whether of fetal or adult origin, is cleared more rapidly in newborn lambs than it is in sheep.[55] Similarly, clearance of fibrinogen is accelerated

Table 111.4 Reference Values for Coagulation Tests in Healthy Premature Infants (30–36 Weeks Gestation) During the First 6 Months After Birth.

Parameter	Day 1	Day 5	Day 30	Day 90	Day 180	Adults
PT (s)	13.0 (10.6–16.2)[a]	12.5 (10.0–15.3)[a]	11.8 (10.0–13.6)[a]	12.3 (10.0–14.6)	12.5 (10.0–15.0)[a]	12.4 (10.8–13.9)
INR	1.0 (0.61–1.70)	0.91 (0.53–1.48)	0.79 (0.53–1.11)	0.88 (0.53–1.32)	0.91 (0.53–1.48)	0.89 (0.64–1.17)
APTT (s)	53.6 (27.5–79.4)[b]	50.5 (26.9–74.1)	44.7 (26.9–62.5)	39.5 (28.3–50.7)	37.5 (27.2–53.3)	33.5 (26.6–40.3)
TCT (s)	24.8 (19.2–30.4)	24.1 (18.8–29.4)[a]	24.4 (18.8–29.9)	25.1 (19.4–30.8)	25.2 (18.9–31.5)	25.0 (19.7–30.3)
Fibrinogen (g/L)	2.43 (1.50–3.73)[a,b]	2.80 (1.60–4.18)[a,b]	2.54 (1.50–4.14)	2.46 (1.50–3.52)	2.28 (1.50–3.60)	2.78 (1.56–4.00)
II (U/mL)	0.45 (0.20–0.77)	0.57 (0.29–0.85)[b]	0.57 (0.36–0.95)	0.68 (0.30–1.06)	0.87 (0.51–1.23)	1.08 (0.70–1.46)
V (U/mL)	0.88 (0.41–1.44)[a,b]	1.00 (0.46–1.54)[a]	1.02 (0.48–1.56)[a]	0.99 (0.59–1.39)	1.02 (0.58–1.46)[a]	1.06 (0.62–1.50)
VII (U/mL)	0.67 (0.21–1.13)	0.84 (0.30–1.38)	0.83 (0.21–1.45)	0.87 (0.31–1.43)	0.99 (0.47–1.51)[a]	1.05 (0.67–1.43)
VIII (U/mL)	1.11 (0.50–2.13)	1.15 (0.53–2.05)[a,b]	1.11 (0.50–1.99)	1.06 (0.58–1.88)[a,b]	0.99 (0.50–1.87)[a,b]	0.99 (0.50–1.49)
vWF (U/mL)	1.36 (0.78–2.10)	1.33 (0.72–2.19)	1.36 (0.66–2.16)	1.12 (0.75–1.84)[a,b]	0.98 (0.54–1.58)[a]	0.92 (0.50–1.58)[a]
IX (U/mL)	0.35 (0.19–0.65)[b]	0.42 (0.14–0.74)[b]	0.44 (0.13–0.80)	0.59 (0.25–0.93)	0.81 (0.50–1.20)	1.09 (0.55–1.63)
X (U/mL)	0.41 (0.11–0.71)	0.51 (0.19–0.83)	0.56 (0.20–0.92)	0.67 (0.35–0.99)	0.77 (0.35–1.19)	1.06 (0.70–1.52)
XI (U/mL)	0.30 (0.08–0.52)[b]	0.41 (0.13–0.69)[b]	0.43 (0.15–0.71)[b]	0.59 (0.25–0.93)[a]	0.78 (0.46–1.10)	0.97 (0.67–1.27)
XII (U/mL)	0.38 (0.10–0.66)[b]	0.39 (0.09–0.69)[b]	0.43 (0.11–0.75)	0.61 (0.15–1.07)	0.82 (0.22–1.42)	1.08 (0.52–1.64)
PK (U/mL)	0.33 (0.09–0.57)	0.45 (0.25–0.75)	0.59 (0.31–0.87)	0.79 (0.37–1.21)	0.78 (0.40–1.16)	1.12 (0.62–1.62)
HMWK (U/mL)	0.49 (0.09–0.89)	0.62 (0.24–1.00)[b]	0.64 (0.16–1.12)[b]	0.78 (0.32–1.24)	0.83 (0.41–1.25)[a]	0.92 (0.50–1.36)
XIIIa (U/mL)	0.70 (0.32–1.08)	1.01 (0.57–1.45)[a]	0.99 (0.51–1.47)[a]	1.13 (0.71–1.55)[a]	1.13 (0.65–1.61)[a]	1.05 (0.55–1.55)
XIIIb (U/mL)	0.81 (0.35–1.27)	1.10 (0.68–1.58)[a]	1.07 (0.57–1.57)[a]	1.21 (0.75–1.67)	1.15 (0.67–1.63)	0.97 (0.57–1.37)

Data are mean (95% confidence intervals).
[a]$P < .05$; [b]$P < .01$.
APTT, Activated partial thromboplastin time; *HMWK,* high-molecular-weight kininogen; *INR,* international normalized ratio; *PK,* prekallikrein; *PT,* prothrombin time; *TCT,* thrombin-clotting time; *vWF,* von Willebrand factor.
From Andrew M, Paes B, Milner R, et al. Development of the human coagulation system in the healthy premature infant. *Blood*. 1988;72:1651.

Table 111.5 Reference Values for Coagulation Tests in Healthy Term Infants During the First 6 Months After Birth.

Parameter	Day 1	Day 5	Day 30	Day 90	Day 180	Adults
PT (sec)	13.0 (10.1–15.9)[a]	12.4 (10.0–15.3)[a]	11.8 (10.0–14.3)[a]	11.9 (10.0–14.2)[a]	12.3 (10.7–13.9)[a]	12.4 (10.8–13.9)
INR	1.00 (0.53–1.62)	0.89 (0.53–1.48)	0.79 (0.53–1.26)	0.81 (0.53–1.26)	0.88 (0.61–1.17)	0.89 (0.64–1.17)
APTT (sec)	42.9 (31.3–54.5)	42.6 (25.4–59.8)	40.4 (32.0–55.2)	37.1 (29.0–50.1)[a]	35.5 (28.1–42.9)[a]	33.5 (26.6–40.3)
TCT (sec)	23.5 (19.0–28.3)[a]	23.1 (18.0–29.2)	24.3 (19.4–29.2)[a]	25.1 (20.5–29.7)[a]	25.5 (19.8–31.2)[a]	25.0 (19.7–30.3)
Fibrinogen (g/L)	2.83 (1.67–3.99)[a]	3.12 (1.62–4.62)[a]	2.70 (1.62–3.78)[a]	2.43 (1.50–3.79)[a]	2.51 (1.50–3.87)[a]	2.78 (1.56–4.00)
II (U/mL)	0.48 (0.26–0.70)	0.63 (0.33–0.93)	0.68 (0.34–1.02)	0.75 (0.45–1.05)	0.88 (0.60–1.16)	1.08 (0.70–1.46)
V (U/mL)	0.72 (0.34–1.08)	0.95 (0.45–1.45)	0.98 (0.62–1.34)	0.90 (0.48–1.32)	0.91 (0.55–1.27)	1.06 (0.62–1.50)
VII (U/mL)	0.66 (0.28–1.04)	0.89 (0.35–1.43)	0.90 (0.42–1.38)	0.91 (0.39–1.43)	0.87 (0.47–1.27)	1.05 (0.67–1.43)
VIII (U/mL)	1.00 (0.50–1.78)[a]	0.88 (0.50–1.54)[a]	0.91 (0.50–1.57)[a]	0.79 (0.50–1.25)[a]	0.73 (0.50–1.09)	0.99 (0.50–1.49)
vWF (U/mL)	1.53 (0.50–2.87)	1.40 (0.50–2.54)	1.28 (0.50–2.46)	1.18 (0.50–2.06)	1.07 (0.50–1.97)	0.92 (0.50–1.58)
IX (U/mL)	0.53 (0.15–0.91)	0.53 (0.15–0.91)	0.51 (0.21–0.81)	0.67 (0.21–1.13)	0.86 (0.36–1.36)	1.09 (0.55–1.63)
X (U/mL)	0.40 (0.12–0.68)	0.49 (0.19–0.79)	0.59 (0.31–0.87)	0.71 (0.35–1.07)	0.78 (0.38–1.18)	1.06 (0.70–1.52)
XI (U/mL)	0.38 (0.10–0.66)	0.55 (0.23–0.87)	0.53 (0.27–0.79)	0.69 (0.41–0.97)	0.86 (0.49–1.34)	0.97 (0.67–1.27)
XII (U/mL)	0.53 (0.13–0.93)	0.47 (0.11–0.83)	0.49 (0.17–0.81)	0.67 (0.25–1.09)	0.77 (0.39–1.15)	1.08 (0.52–1.64)
PK (U/mL)	0.37 (0.18–0.69)	0.48 (0.20–0.76)	0.57 (0.23–0.91)	0.73 (0.41–1.05)	0.86 (0.56–1.16)	1.12 (0.62–1.62)
HMWK (U/mL)	0.54 (0.06–1.02)	0.74 (0.16–1.32)	0.77 (0.33–1.21)	0.82 (0.30–1.46)[a]	0.82 (0.36–1.28)[a]	0.92 (0.50–1.36)
XIIIa (U/mL)	0.79 (0.27–1.31)	0.94 (0.44–1.44)[a]	0.93 (0.39–1.47)[a]	1.04 (0.36–1.72)[a]	1.04 (0.46–1.62)[a]	1.05 (0.55–1.55)
XIIIb (U/mL)	0.76 (0.30–1.22)	1.06 (0.32–1.80)	1.11 (0.39–1.73)[a]	1.16 (0.48–1.84)[a]	1.10 (0.50–1.70)[a]	0.97 (0.57–1.37)

Data are mean (95% confidence intervals).
[a]Values that are indistinguishable from those of the adult.
APTT, Activated partial thromboplastin time; *HMWK,* high-molecular-weight kininogen; *INR,* international normalized ratio; *PK,* prekallikrein; *PT,* prothrombin time; *TCT,* thrombin-clotting time; *vWF,* von Willebrand factor.
From Andrew M, Paes B, Milner R, et al. Development of the human coagulation system in the full-term infant. *Blood*. 1987;70:165.

in premature infants with or without respiratory distress syndrome.[56] An increased basal metabolic rate in the young probably contributes to the accelerated clearance of proteins.[57]

REGULATION OF THROMBIN

Thrombin regulation is both delayed and decreased in newborn plasma compared with adult plasma and is similar to plasma from adults receiving therapeutic doses of warfarin or heparin.[58] Thrombin generation in newborn plasma is further decreased in the presence of endothelial cell surfaces but not to the same extent as adult plasma. The amount of thrombin generated is directly proportional to the prothrombin concentration,[48,49,59] whereas the rate of thrombin generation reflects the concentration of other procoagulants.

Thrombin is directly inhibited by AT, heparin cofactor II, and α_2-macroglobulin. In addition, a circulating physiologic anticoagulant in cord blood has properties similar to those of dermatan sulfate.[60] The fetal proteoglycan is present in plasma in concentrations of 0.29 μg/mL, has a molecular weight of 150,000 kDa, and catalyzes thrombin inhibition by means of the

Table 111.6 Reference Values for the Inhibitors of Coagulation in Healthy Infants During the First 6 Months After Birth.

Parameter	Day 1	Day 5	Day 30	Day 90	Day 180	Adults
Healthy Term Infants						
AT (U/mL)	0.63 (0.39–0.87)	0.67 (0.41–0.93)	0.78 (0.48–1.08)	0.97 (0.73–1.21)[a]	1.04 (0.84–1.24)[a]	1.05 (0.79–1.31)
2M (U/mL)	1.39 (0.95–1.83)	1.48 (0.98–1.98)	1.50 (1.06–1.94)	1.76 (1.26–2.26)	1.91 (1.49–2.33)	0.86 (0.52–1.20)
C1E-INH (U/mL)	0.72 (0.36–1.08)	0.90 (0.60–1.20)[a]	0.89 (0.47–1.31)	1.15 (0.71–1.59)	1.41 (0.89–1.93)	1.01 (0.71–1.31)
1AT (U/mL)	0.93 (0.49–1.37)[a]	0.89 (0.49–1.29)[a]	0.62 (0.36–0.88)	0.72 (0.42–1.02)	0.77 (0.47–1.07)	0.93 (0.55–1.31)
HCII (U/mL)	0.43 (0.10–0.93)	0.48 (0.00–0.96)	0.47 (0.10–0.87)	0.72 (0.10–1.46)	1.20 (0.50–1.90)	0.96 (0.66–1.26)
Protein C (U/mL)	0.35 (0.17–0.53)	0.42 (0.20–0.64)	0.43 (0.21–0.65)	0.54 (0.28–0.80)	0.59 (0.37–0.81)	0.96 (0.64–1.28)
Protein S (U/mL)	0.36 (0.12–0.60)	0.50 (0.22–0.78)	0.63 (0.33–0.93)	0.86 (0.54–1.18)[a]	0.87 (0.55–1.19)[a]	0.92 (0.60–1.24)
Healthy Premature Infants (30–36 Weeks Gestation)						
AT (U/mL)	0.38 (0.14–0.62)[b]	0.56 (0.30–0.82)	0.59 (0.37–0.81)[b]	0.83 (0.45–1.21)[b]	0.90 (0.52–1.28)[b]	1.05 (0.79–1.31)
2M (U/mL)	1.10 (0.56–1.82)[b]	1.25 (0.71–1.77)	1.38 (0.72–2.04)	1.80 (1.20–2.66)	2.09 (1.10–3.21)	0.86 (0.52–1.20)
C1E-INH (U/mL)	0.65 (0.31–0.99)	0.83 (0.45–1.21)	0.74 (0.40–1.24)[b]	1.14 (0.60–1.68)[a]	1.40 (0.96–2.04)	1.01 (0.71–1.31)
1AT (U/mL)	0.90 (0.36–1.44)[a]	0.94 (0.42–1.46)[a]	0.76 (0.38–1.12)[b]	0.81 (0.49–1.13)[a,b]	0.82 (0.48–1.16)[a]	0.93 (0.55–1.31)
HCII (U/mL)	0.32 (0.10–0.60)[b]	0.34 (0.10–0.69)	0.43 (0.15–0.71)	0.61 (0.20–1.11)	0.89 (0.45–1.40)[a,b]	0.96 (0.66–1.26)
Protein C (U/mL)	0.28 (0.12–0.44)[b]	0.31 (0.11–0.51)	0.37 (0.15–0.59)[b]	0.45 (0.23–0.67)[b]	0.57 (0.31–0.83)	0.96 (0.64–1.28)
Protein S (U/mL)	0.26 (0.14–0.38)[b]	0.37 (0.13–0.61)	0.56 (0.22–0.90)	0.76 (0.40–1.12)[b]	0.82 (0.44–1.20)	0.92 (0.60–1.24)

Data are mean (95% confidence intervals).
[a]Values that are indistinguishable from those of the adult.
[b]Values different from those of term infants.
1AT, Antitrypsin; *2M,* 2-macroglobulin; *AT,* antithrombin; *C1E-INH,* C1-esterase inhibitor; *HCII,* heparin cofactor II.
From Andrew M, Paes B, Johnston M. Development of the hemostatic system in the neonate and young infant. *Am J Pediatr Hematol Oncol.* 1990;12:95.

Table 111.7 Reference Values for the Components of the Fibrinolytic System in Healthy Infants During the First 6 Months After Birth.

Parameter	Day 1	Day 5	Day 30	Day 90	Day 180	Adults
Healthy Term Infants						
Plasminogen (U/mL)	1.95 (1.25–2.65)	2.17 (1.41–2.93)	1.98 (1.26–2.70)	2.48 (1.74–3.22)	3.01 (2.21–3.81)	3.36 (2.48–4.24)
TPA (ng/mL)	9.6 (5.0–18.9)	5.6 (4.0–10.0)[a]	4.1 (1.0–6.0)[a]	2.1 (1.0–5.0)[a]	2.8 (1.0–6.0)[a]	4.9 (1.4–8.4)
2AP (U/mL)	0.85 (0.55–1.15)	1.00 (0.70–1.30)[a]	1.00 (0.76–1.24)[a]	1.08 (0.76–1.40)[a]	1.11 (0.83–1.39)[a]	1.02 (0.68–1.36)
PAI-1 (U/mL)	6.4 (2.0–15.1)	2.3 (0.0–8.1)[a]	3.4 (0.0–8.8)[a]	7.2 (1.0–15.3)	8.1 (6.0–13.0)	3.6 (0.0–11.0)
Healthy Premature Infants (30–36 Weeks Gestation)						
Plasminogen (U/mL)	1.70 (1.12–2.48)[b]	1.91 (1.21–2.61)+	1.81 (1.09–2.53)	2.38 (1.58–3.18)	2.75 (1.91–3.59)+	3.36 (2.48–4.24)
TPA (ng/mL)	8.48 (3.00–16.70)	3.97 (2.00–6.93)[a]	4.13 (2.00–7.79)[a]	3.31 (2.00–5.07)[a]	3.48 (2.00–5.85)[a]	4.96 (1.46–8.46)
2AP (U/mL)	0.78 (0.40–1.16)	0.81 (0.49–1.13)[b]	0.89 (0.55–1.23)[b]	1.06 (0.64–1.48)[a]	1.15 (0.77–1.53)	1.02 (0.68–1.36)
PAI-1 (U/mL)	5.4 (0.0–12.2)[a b]	2.5 (0.0–7.1)[a]	4.3 (0.0–10.9)[a]	4.8 (1.0–11.8)[a,b]	4.9 (1.0–10.2)[a,b]	3.6 (0.0–11.0)

Data are mean (95% confidence intervals).
[a]Values that are indistinguishable from those of the adult.
[b]Values that are different from those of the term infant.
2AP, 2-Antiplasmin; *PAI-1,* plasminogen activator inhibitor-1; *TPA,* tissue plasminogen activator.
From Andrew M, Paes B, Johnston M. Development of the hemostatic system in the neonate and young infant. *Am J Pediatr Hematol Oncol.* 1990;12:95.

natural inhibitor heparin cofactor II. The fetal anticoagulant also is present in plasma from pregnant women and is produced by the placenta.[61] The length of time that the fetal anticoagulant circulates in neonates is not known. α_2-Macroglobulin is a more important inhibitor of thrombin in plasmas from neonates than it is in plasmas from adults.[62-64] α_2-Macroglobulin compensates, in part, for the low levels of AT in neonates, even in the presence of endothelial cell surfaces. The elimination half-life of AT is shorter in healthy infants than in adults.[57] Despite these differences, the rate of inhibition of thrombin is still slower in newborn infants than it is in adults.

At birth, plasma concentrations of protein C are very low, and they remain decreased during the first 6 months after birth.[4,7] Protein C in neonatal plasma has a twofold increase in the single-chain form compared with the double-chain form that is prominent in adults.[65-67] Neonatal protein C has increased *N*-linked glycosylation compared with that of adults. Overall, the generation of activated protein C appears to be reduced in neonatal plasma compared with adults.[68] Although total amounts of protein S are decreased at birth, functional activity is similar to that in the adult because protein S is completely present in the free, active form due to the absence of C4 binding protein.[69,70] Furthermore, the interaction of protein S with activated protein C in newborn plasma may be regulated by the increased levels of α_2-macroglobulin. Plasma concentrations of thrombomodulin are increased in early childhood and decrease to adult values by the late teenage years; however, the influence of age on endothelial cell expression of thrombomodulin has not been determined.[71-75]

Total tissue factor pathway inhibitor levels in newborn infants are reported as being similar to levels in older children or adults. However, free tissue factor pathway inhibitor is reported as being significantly lower in children.[35]

The capacity of newborn fibrin clots to bind thrombin has been assessed through the measurement of fibrinopeptide A production. Cord plasma clots generate significantly less fibrinopeptide A than do adult plasma clots because of the decreased plasma concentrations of prothrombin in cord plasma.[76] This observation suggests that thrombi in newborn infants may not have the same propensity to propagate as do thrombi in adult patients.

Recent studies have demonstrated that the fibrin clot nanostructure is different in adult compared with neonatal clots.[77] Fibrin properties have also been shown to differ.[78]

THE FIBRINOLYTIC SYSTEM

Though plasmin is generated and inhibited similarly in infants and adults, important differences do exist.[7] In neonates, plasminogen levels are only 50% of adult values, α_2-antiplasmin levels are 80% of adult values, and plasma concentrations of plasminogen activator inhibitor (PAI)-1 and tissue plasminogen activator (TPA) are significantly greater than adult levels.[4,7,8,37-45,47,79-81] Increased levels of TPA and PAI-1 on day 1 after birth are in marked contrast to values from cord blood, in which concentrations of these two proteins are significantly lower than they are in adults.[47,76,79] The discrepancy between newborn and cord plasma concentrations of TPA and PAI-1 can be explained by the enhanced release of TPA and PAI-1 from the endothelium shortly after birth. PAI-2 levels are detectable in cord blood but are significantly lower than they are in pregnant women.[82] Plasminogen, like fibrinogen, has a fetal form. Fetal plasminogen exists in two glycoforms that have increased amounts of mannose and sialic acid.[83] The enzymatic activity of "fetal plasmin" and its binding to cellular receptors for fetal plasminogen are decreased relative to the adult form.

Short whole-blood clotting times, short euglobulin lysis times, and increased plasma concentrations of the Bβ15-42 fibrin-related peptides suggest that the fibrinolytic system is activated at birth.[4,81] At the same time, the capacity of the fetal fibrinolytic system to generate plasmin in response to stimulation by a thrombolytic agent is decreased compared with that of adults; this reflects low levels of plasminogen.[84]

Over recent years, the majority of studies of fibrinolysis in neonates have used thromboelastography (TEG).[85-87] Premature infants are reported to have more active fibrinolysis than term infants using this methodology.[88]

PLATELETS

Classic platelet studies in newborn infants are inhibited by sample volume requirements. Flow cytometry is useful because of the small sample volume required for extensive platelet function studies. Differences in sample timing, method of collection, and concentrations and compositions of platelet agonists likely contribute to apparently conflicting reports on platelet function in the newborn.

Megakaryocytopoiesis has been difficult to study in the fetus and neonate because of the intrinsic low level of megakaryocyte production in the marrow and the lack of availability of marrow samples to study. Using microassay techniques, Murray and Roberts[89] have shown that megakaryocytopoiesis is likely increased at 24 to 36 weeks of gestation versus term gestation. Platelets appear at 5 weeks after conception, and megakaryocytes appear in the liver at 8 weeks. Fetal and neonatal megakaryocytes are smaller than adult megakaryocytes.[90]

MEGAKARYOCYTES

The cord blood of preterm babies has increased numbers of all megakaryocyte precursors compared with term infants. Furthermore, term infants have increased circulating megakaryocyte progenitor numbers at birth compared with adults.[91] The magnitude of cord blood megakaryocyte progenitors' proliferative and maturational responses to cytokines is related to developmental age.[89] Reticulated platelet counts are reported to be similar to adult levels in healthy neonates greater than 30 weeks gestational age but increased in neonates younger than 30 weeks gestational age.[92] However, a study by Joseph and colleagues[93] reported reduced reticulated platelet counts in neonates of all gestational ages compared with adults.

PLATELETS IN CORD BLOOD

Platelet counts and mean platelet volumes in neonates are similar to those in adults, with values of 150 to 450 × 10^9/L and 7 to 9 femtoliter (platelet volume), respectively.[47,94-101] Platelet counts in fetuses between 18 and 30 weeks gestational age also fall within the adult range, with the average value being 250 × 10^9/L.[11] Platelet survival has not been measured in healthy infants. Electron microscopy studies on cord platelets have demonstrated normal numbers of granules; however, serotonin and adenosine diphosphate, which are stored in dense granules, are present at concentrations that are less than 50% of adult values. Flow cytometry studies in whole blood without added agonists show that differences between neonates and adults in platelet binding of monoclonal antibodies for glycoprotein Ib or P-selectin are not significant; however, glycoprotein IIb/IIIa is significantly reduced.[102] Platelet adhesion at birth has not been assessed with sensitive and reproducible assays; this may explain the conflicting in vitro results.[103,104] Glycoprotein Ib is present on fetal platelet membranes in adult quantities.[105]

Both the plasma concentrations of vWF and the proportion of high-molecular-weight multimers (and therefore more active forms) of vWF are increased in neonates.[106,107] The cord multimeric pattern of vWF appears similar to the forms released by endothelial cells. This may be explained by the finding that newborn plasma has little if any detectable vWF cleaving protease.[106] The quantitative and qualitative differences in vWF at birth are likely responsible for the enhanced cord platelet agglutination to low concentrations of ristocetin.[107,108] Glycoprotein IIb/IIIa complexes are expressed on platelet membranes early in gestation[105]; however, the capacity of cord platelets to aggregate following exposure to a variety of agonists has been variable, with some observations being more consistent than others. Differences between the cord blood of premature and term infants have been described, with reduced aggregation in preterm infants.[109]

Epinephrine-induced aggregation of cord platelets is consistently decreased compared with that of adult platelets because of the decreased availability of α-adrenergic receptors.[110-117] Ristocetin-induced agglutination of cord platelets is consistently increased compared with that of adult platelets, likely because of quantitative and qualitative increases in the level of vWF. Aggregation of cord platelets induced by adenosine diphosphate, collagen, thrombin, and arachidonic acid is variable and may be moderately decreased or similar to that of adult platelets.[118-120] Thromboxane A2 production is reduced in neonates despite normal receptor binding, suggesting a postreceptor signal transduction problem.[121]

Inositol phosphate production and protein phosphorylation are normal, as are production of arachidonic acid and its metabolites.[120] In fact, cord platelets release more arachidonic acid than adult platelets in response to stimulation by thrombin.[110] This increased release may be due to the greater reactivity of platelet membranes induced by low levels of vitamin E.[122,123] Agonist receptors, with the exception of the α-adrenergic receptor discussed previously, do not appear to be decreased in number. Despite a poor response to collagen stimulation, cord platelets have normal numbers of the collagen receptor glycoprotein Ia/IIa present in platelet membranes.[105] Coupling of agonist receptors to phospholipases may be the site of this transient activation defect in response to collagen.[124]

PLATELET FUNCTION IN NEONATES

A few studies have assessed aggregation of newborn platelets obtained during the first few days after birth; other studies have evaluated platelets of older neonates.[117] There is strong evidence that platelets are activated during the birth process. Cord plasma levels of thromboxane B2, β-thromboglobulin, and platelet factor-4 are increased, the granular content of cord platelets is decreased, and epinephrine receptor availability is reduced, perhaps secondary to occupation.[125-127] Improved platelet aggregation was seen in platelets from newborns that were drawn 2 hours after birth, with normalization of platelet aggregation at 48 hours. Studies using whole-blood flow cytometry show that compared with adult platelets, neonatal platelets are hyporeactive to thrombin, a combination of adenosine diphosphate and epinephrine, and a thromboxane A2 analogue.[111,116,122,128]

Newborn infants have shorter closure times than adults, using the platelet function analyzer (PFA)-100 system (Siemens Healthcare Diagnostics, Washington, DC) that are not influenced by red or white blood cells.[129]

Neonatal platelet function has been recently summarized by Margraf and colleagues.[130] Table 111.8 summarizes the differences between platelet expression and response to stimulation in neonates and adults. Fig. 111.1 summarizes the differences in platelet associated receptors and ligands between preterm and term infants, respectively. In addition, the interactions of platelets with other cells in the blood have been shown to be different to those described in adults,[131] with potential novel mechanisms of interaction in neonates yet to be fully elucidated. The clinical significance of these observations remains unknown. This is in the context of a renewed focus on the implications of transfusing adult platelets into neonates during clinical care.[132]

BLOOD VESSEL WALL

The vessel wall profoundly influences hemostasis due to the procoagulant and anticoagulant properties of endothelial cells and extracellular matrix components. Each of these properties is significantly influenced by age. In a rabbit venous model, glycosaminoglycans by mass are significantly increased in inferior vena cavas from pups compared with adult rabbits. The AT-mediated anticoagulant activity of inferior vena cava glycosaminoglycans, especially heparin sulfate, is increased in pups compared with adult rabbits.[133] In a rabbit arterial model, total proteoglycan, chondroitin sulfate, and heparin sulfate content are increased in the intima and media of aortas from pups compared with adult rabbits. AT activity in aortas of pups due to heparin sulfate glycosaminoglycans is also increased.[134] The increased glycosaminoglycan-mediated vessel wall AT activity in pups compared with adult rabbits suggests that young blood vessels may have greater antithrombotic potential.

When measured directly, thrombin generation in cord plasma is decreased in the presence of human umbilical endothelial cells compared with plastic, owing to cell surface promotion of AT inhibition of thrombin.[135] Soluble levels of endothelial cell adhesion molecules and selectins are also age dependent, suggesting developmental differences in endothelial cell expression and secretion of these molecules.[136]

Nitric oxide is a labile humoral agent that modulates vascular tone in fetal and postnatal lungs and contributes to the normal decline in pulmonary vascular resistance at birth. Nitric oxide is a potent inhibitor of platelet adhesion and aggregation and stimulates disaggregation of platelet aggregates. Nitric oxide likely interacts with prostaglandin I_2 and other metabolites of the lipoxygenase pathway to modulate platelet function in a synergistic manner.[137]

It has been observed in sheep that vessel wall thickness increases in the perinatal period.[138] This is likely in response to increases in stress per vessel internal diameter. Contractility also increases with fetal development.[139] The endothelial cells of fetal vessels are larger and less uniform and protrude into the lumen.[140]

Table 111.8 Differences in Receptors/Ligands Important to Platelet Function Between Preterm and Term Infants.

Receptor	Ligand	Ligand Expression in Preterm Infants	Ligand Expression in Term Infants
GPIb	vWF (h)	Increased in preterm; unusually large vWF multimers	Increased
	Thrombin (h)	See PAR Thrombin below	
	P-selectin (m, h, r)	Reduced in fetal platelets and endothelial cells	Normal P-selectin content in unstimulated human samples but reduced surface expression in stimulated platelets
	Mac-1 (m, h)	Reduced on fetal neutrophils, related to gestational age	
GPIIb	Fibrinogen (h)	Slightly reduced in small-for- gestational-age and extremely premature infants	No difference (slight increase around day 5 postnatal)
	vWF (h)	See GPIb vWF above	
	Vitronectin (h)		Reduced
	Fibronectin (h)	Reduced	Reduced
GPVI; GPIa/IIa	Collagen (r, h)	Changing collagen types during fetal development	
PAR	Thrombin (h)	Thrombin generation similar between preterm and term infants; prothrombin activity below term neonates	Prothrombin ~50% of adult values (contradicting results for peak thrombin activity)
P2Y	ADP (h)		Reduced dense granules and ADP content
Thromboxane receptor	Thromboxane A2 (h)	Reduced platelet release upon collagen stimulation	Elevated thromboxane levels in plasma; reduced production by washed platelets

ADP, Adenosine diphosphate; *GP,* glycoprotein; *h*, human data; *m*, mouse data; *PAR,* protease activated receptor; *r*, rat data; *vWF,* von Willebrand factor.
Adapted from Margraf A, Nussbaum C, Sperandio M. Ontogeny of platelet function. *Blood Adv*. 2019;3(4):692–703.

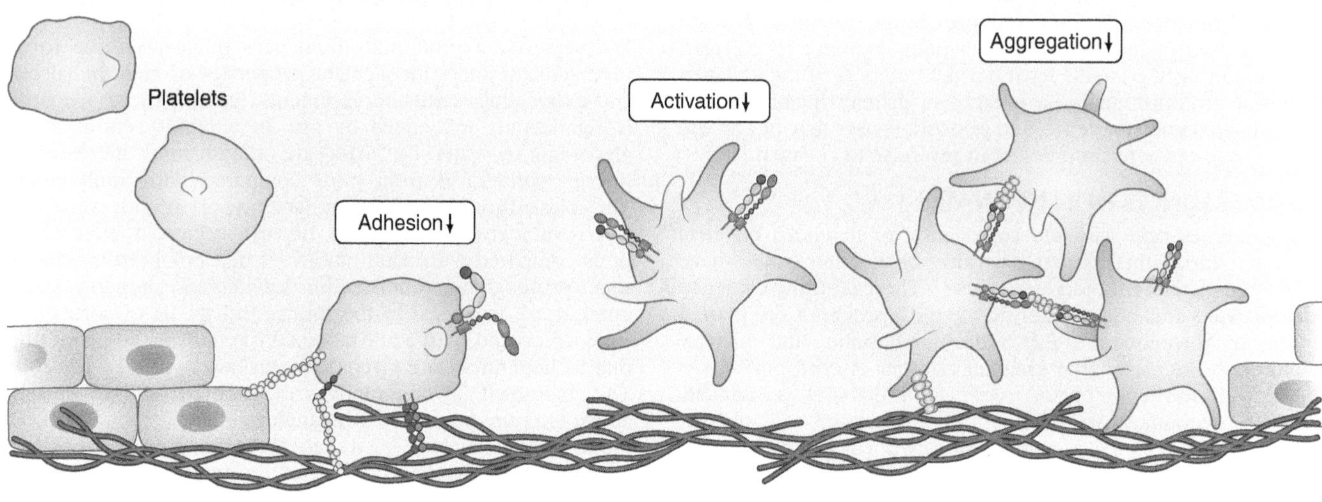

	Expression								Stimulation response					Activation response				
	Glycoprotein				PAR													
	Ib/V/IX	VI	Ia/IIa	IIb/IIIa	1	3	4	P-Sel	ADP	Thrombin	TxA2	Collagen	Epinephrine	Ca^{2+} influx	PS exposure	Granule release	High affinity GPIIb/IIIa	Spreading
Fetus Neonate murine	+	+		+++		++	++/+++	−	++	++	++	+					+	+
Neonate human	++	++	+/++	+	+		+	++	++	++	++	+	+	+	++	−	+	+
Adult	++	+++	++	++	+++	++	++	++	+++	+++	+++	+++	+++	+++	++	++	+++	+++

Fig. 111.1 Important platelet expression and activation responses in the neonate compared with adults. *ADP,* Adenosine diphosphate; *GP,* glycoprotein; *PAR,* protease activated receptor; *PS,* phosphatidylserine; *TxA2,* thromboxane A2; *vWF,* von Willebrand factor. (From Margraf A, Nussbaum C, Sperandio M. Ontogeny of platelet function. *Blood Adv.* 2019;3:692–703.)

CONCLUSION

The vascular and hemostatic systems of the fetus and neonate are continually evolving. One must take this into consideration when evaluating these systems for dysfunction. Adult normative data do not apply to the fetus or neonate. Although different in content and structure, these systems should be considered physiologically in the fetus and neonate. This is an important consideration when determining and monitoring therapeutic intervention.

 A complete reference list is available at www.ExpertConsult.com.

SELECT REFERENCES

1. Ignjatovic V, Lai C, Summerhayes R, et al. Age-related differences in plasma proteins: how plasma proteins change from neonates to adults. *PloS One.* 2011;6:e17213.
2. Bjelosevic S, Pascovici D, Ping H, et al. Quantitative age-specific variability of plasma proteins in healthy neonates, children and adults. *Mol Cell Proteomics.* 2017;16:924-935.
3. McCafferty C, Busuttil-Crellin X, Cai T, et al. Plasma proteomic analysis reveals age-specific changes in platelet- and endothelial cell-derived proteins and regulators of plasma coagulation and fibrinolysis. *J Pediatr.* 2020;221S:S29-S36.
4. Andrew M, Paes B, Johnston M. Development of the hemostatic system in the neonate and young infant. *Am J Pediatr Hematol Oncol.* 1990;12:95-104.
6. Chalmers EA. Neonatal coagulation problems. *Arch Dis Child Fetal Neonatal Ed.* 2004;89:F475-478.
7. Andrew M, Paes B, Milner R, et al. Development of the human coagulation system in the full-term infant. *Blood.* 1987;70:165-172.
8. Andrew M, Paes B, Milner R, et al. Development of the human coagulation system in the healthy premature infant. *Blood.* 1988;72:1651-1657.
11. Forestier F, Daffos F, Galactèros F, et al. Hematological values of 163 normal fetuses between 18 and 30 weeks of gestation. *Pediatr Res.* 1986;20:342-346.
24. Reverdiau-Moalic P, Delahousse B, Body G, et al. Evolution of blood coagulation activators and inhibitors in the healthy human fetus. *Blood.* 1996;88:900-906.
25. Raffaeli G, Tripodi A, Manzoni F, et al. Is placental blood a reliable source for the evaluation of neonatal hemostasis at birth? *Transfusion.* 2020;60:1069-1077.
26. Attard C, van der Straaten T, Karlaftis V, et al. Developmental hemostasis: age-specific differences in the levels of hemostatic proteins. *J Thromb Haemost.* 2013;11:1850-1854.
32. Lisman T, Platto M, Meijers JC, et al. The hemostatic status of pediatric recipients of adult liver grafts suggests that plasma levels of hemostatic proteins are not regulated by the liver. *Blood.* 2011;117:2070-2072.
35. Monagle P, Barnes C, Ignjatovic V, et al. Developmental haemostasis. Impact for clinical haemostasis laboratories. *Thromb Haemost.* 2006;95:362-372.
36. Ignjatovic V, Kenet G, Monagle P, et al. Developmental hemostasis: recommendations for laboratories reporting pediatric samples. *J Thromb Haemost.* 2012;10:298-300.
49. Kremers R, Wagenvoord RJ, de Laat HB, et al. Low paediatric thrombin generation is caused by an attenuation of prothrombin conversion. *Thromb Haemost.* 2016;115:1090-1100.
51. Witt I, Muller H, Kunzer W. Evidence for the existence of foetal fibrinogen. *Thromb Diath Haemorrh.* 1969;22:101-109.

59. Andrew M, Schmidt B, Mitchell L, et al. Thrombin generation in newborn plasma is critically dependent on the concentration of prothrombin. *Thromb Haemost*. 1990;64:027-030.
60. Andrew M, Mitchell L, Berry L, et al. An anticoagulant dermatan sulfate proteoglycan circulates in the pregnant woman and her fetus. *J Clin Invest*. 1992;89:321-326.
64. Ignjatovic V, Greenway A, Summerhayes R, et al. Thrombin generation: the functional role of alpha-2-macroglobulin and influence of developmental haemostasis. *Br J Haematol*. 2007;138:366-368.
67. Berry LR, Van Walderveen MC, Atkinson HM, et al. Comparison of N-linked glycosylation of protein C in newborns and adults. *Carbohydr Res*. 2013;365:32-37.
68. Chan AK, Patel S, Male C, et al. Activated protein C generation is greatly decreased in plasma from newborns compared to adults in the presence or absence of endothelium. *Thromb Haemost*. 2004;91:238-247.
76. Patel P, Weitz J, Brooker LA, et al. Decreased thrombin activity of fibrin clots prepared in cord plasma compared with adult plasma. *Pediatr Res*. 1996;39:826-830.
77. Ignjatovic V, Pelkmans L, Kelchtermans H, et al. Differences in the mechanism of blood clot formation and nanostructure in infants and children compared with adults. *Thromb Res*. 2015;136:1303-1309.
78. Nellenbach KA, Nandi S, Kyu A, et al. Comparison of neonatal and adult fibrin clot properties between porcine and human plasma. *Anesthesiology*. 2020;132:1091-1101.
79. Corrigan Jr JJ. Neonatal thrombosis and the thrombolytic system: pathophysiology and therapy. *Am J Pediatr Hematol Oncol*. 1988;10:83-91.
80. Corrigan Jr JJ, Sleeth JJ, Jeter M, et al. Newborn's fibrinolytic mechanism: components and plasmin generation. *Am J Hematol*. 1989;32:273-278.
83. Edelberg JM, Enghild JJ, Pizzo SV, et al. Neonatal plasminogen displays altered cell surface binding and activation kinetics. Correlation with increased glycosylation of the protein. *J Clin Invest*. 1990;86:107-112.
85. Schott NJ, Emery SP, Garbee C, et al. Thromboelastography in term neonates. *J Matern Fetal Neonatal Med*. 2018;31:2599-2604.
86. Sewell EK, Forman KR, Wong EC, et al. Thromboelastography in term neonates: an alternative approach to evaluating coagulopathy. *Arch Dis Child Fetal Neonatal Ed*. 2017;102:F79-F84.
89. Murray NA, Roberts IA. Circulating megakaryocytes and their progenitors (BFU-MK and CFU-MK) in term and pre-term neonates. *Br J Haematol*. 1995;89:41-46.
90. Allen Graeve JL, de Alarcon PA. Megakaryocytopoiesis in the human fetus. *Arch Dis Child*. 1989;64:481-484.
93. Joseph MA, Adams D, Maragos J, et al. Flow cytometry of neonatal platelet RNA. *J Pediatr Hematol Oncol*. 1996;18:277-281.
99. Beverley DW, Inwood MJ, Chance GW, et al. Normal' haemostasis parameters: a study in a well-defined inborn population of preterm infants. *Early Hum Dev*. 1984;9:249-257.
102. Rajasekhar D, Kestin AS, Bednarek FJ, et al. Neonatal platelets are less reactive than adult platelets to physiological agonists in whole blood. *Thromb Haemost*. 1994;72:957-963.
103. Mull MM, Hathaway WE. Altered platelet function in newborns. *Pediatr Res*. 1970;4:229-237.
109. Strauss T, Sidlik-Muskatel R, Kenet G. Developmental hemostasis: primary hemostasis and evaluation of platelet function in neonates. *Semin Fetal Neonatal Med*. 2011;16:301-304.
120. Israels SJ, Daniels M, McMillan EM. Deficient collagen-induced activation in the newborn platelet. *Pediatr Res*. 1990;27:337-343.
129. Carcao MD, Blanchette VS, Dean JA, et al. The Platelet Function Analyzer (PFA-100): a novel *in-vitro* system for evaluation of primary haemostasis in children. *Br J Haematol*. 1998;101:70-73.
130. Margraf A, Nussbaum C, Sperandio M. Ontogeny of platelet function. *Blood Adv*. 2019;3:692-703.
131. Yip C, Ignjatovic V, Attard C, et al. First report of elevated monocyte-platelet aggregates in healthy children. *PLoS One*. 2013;8:e67416.
132. Ferrer-Marin F, Chavda C, Lampa M, et al. Effects of *in vitro* adult platelet transfusions on neonatal hemostasis. *J Thromb Haemost*. 2011;9:1020-1028.
133. Nitschmann E, Berry L, Bridge S, et al. Morphologic and biochemical features affecting the antithrombotic properties of the inferior vena cava of rabbit pups and adult rabbits. *Pediatr Res*. 1998;43:62-67.
134. Nitschmann E, Berry L, Bridge S, et al. Morphological and biochemical features affecting the antithrombotic properties of the aorta in adult rabbits and rabbit pups. *Thromb Haemost*. 1998;79:1034-1040.
135. Ling X, Delorme M, Berry L, et al. Alpha 2-macroglobulin remains as important as antithrombin III for thrombin regulation in cord plasma in the presence of endothelial cell surfaces. *Pediatr Res*. 1995;37:373-378.
138. Pearce WJ, Longo LD. Developmental aspects of endothelial function. *Semin Perinatol*. 1991;15:40-48.

112 Platelet–Vessel Wall Interactions

Thomas G. Diacovo

INTRODUCTION

Platelets are the sentinels of the circulatory system; they recognize and rapidly respond to a disruption in vascular integrity, thereby preventing significant blood loss. This is achieved through the formation of a primary hemostatic plug, which requires platelets to undergo a highly regulated series of events including the adhesion, activation, generation, and release of thrombogenic agents and ultimately aggregation. The importance of these processes is underscored by the bleeding sequelae that result from a reduction in platelet numbers or function associated with various disease states and complications attributable to invasive monitoring and treatments for critically ill neonates. In fact, a significant proportion of newborns admitted to the neonatal intensive care unit (NICU) will present with or develop thrombocytopenia during their hospitalization. Consequently, an estimated 80,000 platelet transfusions are administered annually to NICU patients in the United States.[1] To complicate matters, neonatal platelets appear to be hyporesponsive to common activating stimuli as compared with those from healthy adults, which may further compromise their ability to adequately support hemostasis. To understand both the mechanisms that may predispose critically ill neonates to bleeding and the clinical relevance of the reported reduction in function of their platelets, it is necessary to have a broad overview of mechanisms that limit as well as promote platelet-vessel wall interactions.

VASCULAR ENDOTHELIUM

MECHANISMS PREVENTING PLATELET–VESSEL WALL INTERACTIONS

Vascular endothelium is strategically located at the interface between blood and tissues; as such it is ideally positioned to modulate platelet function. In fact, the role of endothelial cells far exceeds simply providing a boundary layer, as they actively generate substances that directly affect platelet reactivity (Fig. 112.1).[2] One such molecule is prostacyclin (PGI_2), which is a major metabolite of arachidonic acid and is constitutively produced by the cyclooxygenase system in vascular endothelium.[3] Cyclooxygenase expression can also be augmented by shear stress, cytokines, and mitogenic factors. Once released into the circulation, PGI_2 can bind to the thromboxane receptor, a G protein–coupled receptor (GPCR) on the surface of platelets, which in turn activates intracellular adenylyl cyclase. Consequently, this increases intracellular levels of cyclic adenosine monophosphate (cAMP), which ultimately leads to activation of protein kinase A and direct inhibition of Ca^{2+} mobilization and granule release.[4] These events limit the ability of platelets to respond to procoagulant stimuli, thereby preventing interactions with the intact vessel wall. Serum levels of prostacyclin tend to be higher in newborns than in adults, which is thought to aid in the postnatal reduction of pulmonary vascular resistance and may contribute to the reported hyporesponsive state of their platelets.[5]

Antithrombotic

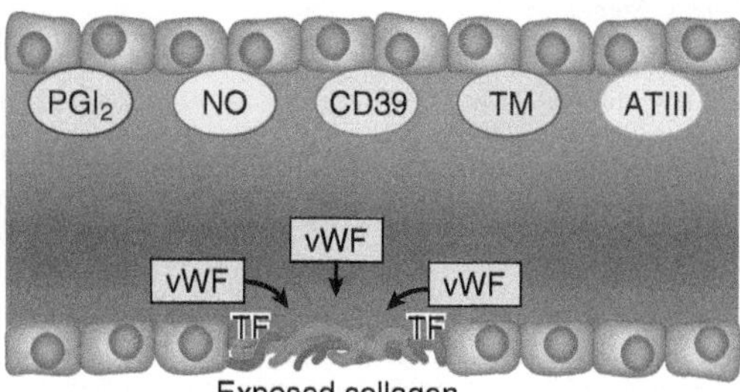

Prothrombotic

Fig. 112.1 Antithrombotic and prothrombotic properties of vascular endothelium. *Top,* Molecules that limit the activation of platelets and the coagulation cascade. *Bottom,* Consequences of disrupting the endothelial cell barrier, which include exposure of tissue factor *(TF)* and collagen, the latter serving as a binding surface for von Willebrand factor *(vWF)*. *ATIII,* Antithrombin III; *NO,* nitric oxide; *PGI*$_2$, prostacyclin; *TM,* thrombomodulin.

Nitric oxide (NO) is another essential molecule produced by endothelial cells that can prevent inappropriate platelet activation and aggregation. NO is short lived (with a half-life of a few seconds), highly reactive, and produced by nitric oxide synthase (NOS). Vascular endothelium NOS (eNOS) is constitutively expressed and active. In addition, production of NO can be enhanced by endothelial cell stimulation or in response to fluid shear stress.[6] Once produced, NO is able to diffuse rapidly into nearby platelets, where it binds to and activates guanylyl cyclase, which in turn catalyzes the conversion of GTP to cGMP. Consequently, levels of cGMP are increased, preventing the release of stored intracellular calcium, which is necessary for full platelet activation and aggregation. Of note, NO blunts the response of neonatal platelets to agonist-induced activation, suggesting that it can play a role in limiting their reactivity in newborns.[7]

Adenosine diphosphate (ADP) is a platelet activator that is released from platelet-dense granules during the formation of a hemostatic plug. To regulate the activity of this agonist, vascular endothelial cells express CD39/ecto-adenosine diphosphatase, a membrane-bound glycoprotein that converts ADP to AMP. Its importance in this process is supported by the ability of recombinant soluble CD39 to both inhibit ADP-induced platelet activation and significantly reduce the degree of ischemia-induced cerebral infarction in CD39-null mice.[8] Although the role of CD39 in contributing to thromboregulation in neonates is not known, human umbilical vein cells do express a functional form of this ecto-ADPase.

One of the most potent stimulators of platelets is thrombin, a serine protease generated at sites of vascular injury in response to activation of the coagulation cascade. It is also essential for promoting clot stability by supporting fibrin formation and the conversion of coagulation factors—notably V, VIII, and XIII—into their active forms.[9] However, the procoagulant activities of thrombin are mitigated by thrombomodulin (TM), a membrane-bound endothelial cell protein.[10] Upon binding to TM, thrombin undergoes a conformational change resulting in enhanced affinity for protein C, which plays a major role in inhibiting blood coagulation. Activated protein C forms a complex with protein S, which leads to inactivation of clotting factors VIIIa and Va. In addition, thrombin bound to TM has a reduced ability to convert fibrinogen to fibrin and to promote platelet aggregation. Although a deficiency in TM is known to result in embryonic lethality, it is not known whether differences in function exist between neonates and adults.[11]

In addition to TM, the plasma protein antithrombin III (ATIII) also regulates the activity of thrombin as well as other serine proteases such as factors Xa, IXa, and XIIa. It does so by preventing the active site of these proteases from binding to known substrates. Its activity is markedly potentiated by heparin, and this is the principal mechanism by which heparin administration promotes anticoagulation in patients.[12] In addition, a small fraction of antithrombin III is bound to heparan sulfate on the endothelial cell surface and thus is strategically located to inactivate thrombin generated at sites of vascular injury. The importance of this plasma protein in preventing clot formation is exemplified in patients with a congenital deficiency in ATIII. This rare autosomal disorder is classified into two major types and results in an increased risk of venous and arterial thrombosis. Type I deficiency is characterized by reduced antithrombin level and function, both at approximately 50% of normal. Type II deficiency results from the presence of a functionally inactive protein with almost normal antigen levels. More than half of all patients with type I disease will likely have a clotting event within their lifetimes.[13] In neonates, ATIII activity has been reported to be 50% to 60% of that found in adults but does not appear to increase their risk of thrombosis.[14] This may be due to the ability of other protease inhibitors, such as a2-macroglobulin, to partially compensate for the low levels of ATIII in neonates until they reach adult values by about 6 months of age.[15]

MECHANISMS PROMOTING PLATELET–VESSEL WALL INTERACTIONS

Vascular injury due to physical disruption or exposure to stimuli such as cytokines, microbial toxins, lipid mediators, and immunologic agents can result in the loss and/or dysfunction of endothelial cells and ultimately platelet deposition. This results not only in the loss of the aforementioned protective mechanisms but also in the exposure of a highly reactive surface that triggers the hemostatic process. In the latter case, disruption of the endothelium lining arterial blood vessels exposes collagen fibers that are the most thrombogenic macromolecular components of the extracellular matrix. Platelet interaction with collagen occurs via a two-step process: (1) indirect contact mediated by von Willebrand factor (vWF), followed by (2) direct contact, resulting in platelet activation and firm adhesion to the site of injury (see Fig. 112.1). However, it is the adhesive interaction between platelets and surface-immobilized vWF that is essential for initiating the formation of a primary hemostatic plug.

vWF is a large multimeric and multidomain glycoprotein produced by vascular endothelium and megakaryocytes. It not only functions as a carrier for factor VIII, protecting it from proteolysis, but also serves as homing beacon for platelets by directing their recruitment to the injured vessel wall. To accomplish this task, vWF adheres to components of the subendothelial matrix (e.g., collagen) and to receptors on the surface of platelets (e.g., GPIba), forming a bridge between them.[16] One remarkable feature of this plasma glycoprotein is its ability to support significant interactions with platelets only upon surface immobilization and under specific hemodynamic conditions, as encountered on the arterial side of the circulation.[17] This avoids the disastrous consequences of platelet–vWF aggregate formation in flowing blood.

vWF production by endothelium occurs through constitutive and inducible mechanisms, with the latter relying on storage and subsequent release from an intracellular, membrane-bound organelle known as a *Weibel-Palade body*, in response to vascular injury. The inducible pathway is most efficacious in terms of platelet recruitment, because it results in the release of predominantly high-molecular-weight multimers of vWF, which possess the greatest hemostatic properties.[18] vWF storage, however, is not limited to endothelial cells, because megakaryocytes and platelets also possess this capability (stored in organelles known as *α-granules*). Although platelet-derived vWF contributes minimally to plasma levels, it does play a role in promoting platelet-platelet interactions and thus accrual at sites of vascular damage. Interestingly, it has been reported that neonates have higher amounts of large vWF multimers and that these may support increased platelet deposition on exposed subendothelial matrix.[19]

PLATELETS

Platelets are small, disk-shaped objects that circulate in the blood for a period of 7 to 10 days. They are produced by the fragmentation of megakaryocytes, and although platelets do not possess nuclei, they can synthesize protein products from posttranscriptionally processed messenger RNAs through a process termed *signal-dependent translation*.[20] In addition, platelets store growth factors, coagulation proteins, adhesion molecules, cytokines, cell-activating agents, and angiogenic factors in secretory organelles known as α and *dense granules*[21]; these play a major role in hemostatic and thrombotic processes as well as in the modulation of immune and inflammatory events.[22] In the developing fetus, platelet production by the middle of the second trimester is sufficient to achieve and maintain counts between 150 and 450 × 10^9/L, which is within the normal range for adults.[23] Despite this similarity, it is believed that functional differences exist between newborn and adult platelets and that these may reduce the capacity of the former to maintain adequate hemostasis, especially in the context of increased blood vessel fragility, as is the case in premature infants or as a consequence of asphyxia or infection. To better understand the relevance of these observations, it is first necessary to have a basic knowledge of the adhesive and signaling pathways that promote platelet deposition at sites of vascular injury.

KEY ADHESION MOLECULES EXPRESSED ON PLATELETS

Platelets are uniquely poised to adhere to sites where the integrity of the vasculature has been compromised, as they not only travel in close proximity to the vessel wall but also express cell surface adhesion molecules that have distinct roles in the initiation and stabilization of a primary hemostatic plug (Fig. 112.2). For instance, the ability of platelets to rapidly attach to sites of vascular injury requires the participation of a glycoprotein complex (GP) known as *GPIb-IX-V*.[24] Each component of the complex is a member of the leucine-rich repeat family and includes GPIbα, GPIbβ, GPIX, and GPV. GPIbα plays the predominant role in this process due to its ability to bind to surface-immobilized vWF. As mentioned earlier, vWF serves as a bridge between platelets and components of the damaged vessel wall due to specialized regions within the molecule that can interact with collagen (e.g., the A3 domain) and GPIbα (e.g., the A1 domain). However, binding between GPIbα and the A1 domain of vWF is extremely labile in nature due to the unique kinetic and mechanical properties of the interaction and its response to disruptive shear forces generated by flowing blood.[25] The importance of this adhesion event is demonstrated by the perturbation in hemostasis that occurs in type 2M von Willebrand disease.[26] vWF from afflicted individuals has a reduced capacity to interact with GPIbα on platelets due to a loss-of-function point mutation contained within its A1 domain. This is borne out in genetically modified mice that developed a significant bleeding phenotype upon insertion of a loss-of-function mutation into the A1 of mouse vWF.[27] For platelets to be retained at sites of vascular injury, a second family of adhesion receptors must engage counterligands that are exposed or deposited in such areas. One such receptor is the integrin α2β1, which permits platelets to firmly adhere to exposed collagen.[28] As with other members of the integrin family, it exists in an

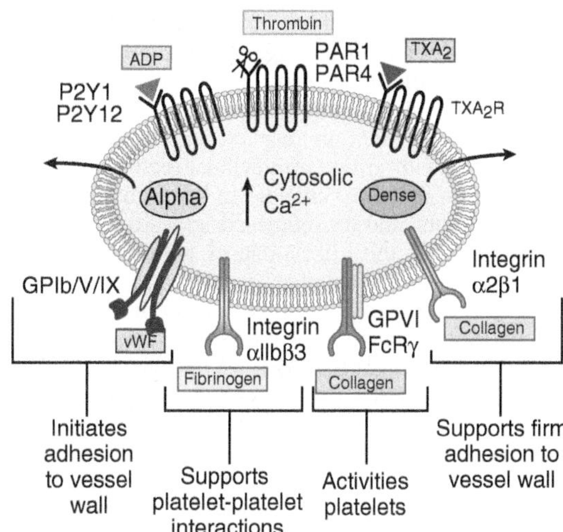

Fig. 112.2 Receptors critical for platelet adhesion and activation. The ability of platelets to initiate contact and subsequently adhere with the injured vessel wall relies on the adhesion receptors GPIb-IX-V and α2β1; whereas platelet-platelet interactions are dependent on αIIbβ3. Receptors that support signal transduction include P2Y1/P2Y12, PAR1/PAR4, TxA_2R, and GPVI, which contribute to the mobilization of intracellular calcium stores. Ligands or agonists that bind to platelet receptors are boxed. *ADP,* Adenosine diphosphate; *GP,* glycoprotein; *PAR,* protease-activated receptors; *TXA_2,* thromboxane A_2; *vWF,* von Willebrand factor.

inactive form on resting platelets and can bind to collagen only in response to various activating stimuli. Once engaged, α2β1-collagen interactions are thought to stabilize the formation of the initial layer of platelets covering the injured area. Of note, no differences in expression levels or ability of this integrin receptor to support adhesion to surface-immobilized collagen have been reported for platelets from neonates compared with those from adults.[29]

After the formation of an initial platelet layer, it is the role of the integrin αIIbβ3, the most abundant glycoprotein expressed on the surface of platelets, to further promote the growth and stability of the hemostatic plug.[30] It mediates this response by rapidly transitioning from a resting to an activated state where it can then serve as a receptor for several ligands (e.g., fibrinogen and vWF) that enable platelets to firmly adhere to each other. Its importance in this process is exemplified in the autosomal recessive disorder known as *Glanzmann thrombasthenia*, where absence or dysfunction of this integrin receptor results in a severe bleeding phenotype in humans. Alterations in αIIbβ3 function and possibly expression have been implicated as a potential mechanism for neonatal platelet hyporesponsiveness, but results are conflicting. That said, the reported defects in aggregation may have more to do with intracellular signaling events that convert this integrin to an activated state than to the actual numbers of receptors present on neonatal platelets.[31,32] However, the mechanisms proposed to contribute to clot strength appear to be intact in neonatal platelets.[33]

KEY SIGNALING PATHWAYS IN PLATELETS

The ability of platelets to form a stable hemostatic plug relies on series of progressive and overlapping signaling events that are essential not only for the activation of surface adhesion molecules but also for the release of stored granule contents. Multiple agonists are generated or exposed at the site of injury, and these can induce platelet activation through a series of intracellular reactions. This process involves both G protein–independent (initial phase of platelet-vessel wall interactions) and G protein–dependent (thrombus growth and stability) signaling events.[34]

G proteins (short for guanine nucleotide-binding proteins) are involved in second-messenger cascades that contribute to platelet activation by causing a rise in cytosolic calcium concentration.[35,36] In fact, previously documented abnormalities in neonatal platelet function may be largely due to impaired mobilization of this important intracellular mediator.[37] Ultimately, platelet activation results in changes in the cytoskeleton, release of granule contents, and an increased adhesiveness of integrin receptors (e.g. $\alpha2\beta1$ and $\alpha IIb\beta3$), all of which are essential for stabilizing platelet-extracellular matrix and platelet-platelet interactions. Platelets express several receptors that convert external environmental cues into biochemical signals in response to interactions with agonists such as collagen, thrombin, ADP, or thromboxane A_2 (TXA_2) (see Fig. 112.2). A brief description follows.

For platelets to adhere at sites where disruption of the endothelial lining of blood vessels occurs requires signal transduction through surface expressed proteins such the collagen receptor glycoprotein VI (GPVI). It is a member of the immunoglobulin superfamily and is noncovalently associated with a small immunoreceptor tyrosine-based activation motif (ITAM)-containing subunit, the FcRγ chain.[28] Although GPVI expression relies entirely on its association with the FcRγ chain, signaling can occur by Fc receptor–dependent or -independent pathways. In either case, engagement of GPVI results in increased adhesiveness of the integrins $\alpha2\beta1$ and $\alpha IIb\beta3$, enabling platelets to firmly attach to collagen and to one another.[38] It also results in release of storage granule contents that are critical for augmenting and maintaining platelet activation. GPVI deficiency has been reported in humans, causing a mild bleeding diathesis. However, its role in the observed hyporesponsiveness of neonatal platelets remains controversial because of conflicting results related to the ability of collagen to induce GPVI-mediated platelet aggregation in solution-based assays.

ADP also plays an essential role in hemostasis by supporting platelet accrual because of its ability to function in an autocrine and paracrine fashion. It is stored in organelles known as *dense granules* and is released from platelets in response to agonists such as collagen and thrombin. ADP binding to the G protein–coupled receptors P2Y1 and in particular P2Y12 on the surface of platelets is required for a full response to this agonist.[39,40] The reduced response of platelets to thrombin in the absence of these receptors, as well as observations that patients with deficiencies in either dense granules or the P2Y12 receptor have an increased propensity to bleed, provide evidence to support a role for ADP as a positive-feedback mediator required for sustained platelet activation.[41] It was initially thought that platelets from neonates were less responsive to ADP than those from their adult counterparts. However, an in-depth evaluation of platelets from full-term neonates using state-of-the-art in vitro technologies demonstrated that they have nearly identical surface expression of the P2Y12 receptor and response to ADP as do platelets isolated from adult volunteers.[42] Moreover, it was shown—using a unique avatar mouse model—that P2Y12 inhibition limited the ability of platelets isolated from neonates to support thrombus growth and vessel occlusion in vivo but did not abolish their initial attachment at sites of arterial injury. This is of considerable clinical significance, as administration of this class of antiplatelet agents to neonatal patients may prevent thrombosis while preserving hemostasis.[42]

As in the case of ADP, TXA_2 is a powerful activator of platelets that also functions in an autocrine and a paracrine manner.[43] TXA_2 is a biologically active lipid mediator that is produced by the metabolism of arachidonic acid through the cyclooxygenase pathway. Its effects on platelets and on other target cells are mediated via interaction with G protein–coupled thromboxane-prostanoid receptors. Consistent with the important role of TXA_2 signaling hemostasis is the ability of aspirin, a potent cyclooxygenase inhibitor, to reduce pathologic thrombus formation in cardiac patients and the prolonged bleeding times in mice lacking the thromboxane-prostanoid receptor.[44] In the case of neonatal platelets, they not only have an impaired response to this agonist but also produce less of this cyclooxygenase product compared with their adult counterparts because of a decreased conversion of arachidonic acid to TXA_2.[45] Because no differences in thromboxane-prostanoid receptor binding characteristics have been reported between neonatal and adult platelets, it appears that the reduced responsiveness of the former may be mediated by impairment in postreceptor signaling.[46]

As mentioned earlier, thrombin is the major protease of the hemostatic system and an effective activator of platelets. Although not stored in or secreted by platelets, thrombin is generated on the surface of activated platelets as part of the coagulation process. Thrombin activates platelets through GPCRs known as *protease-activated receptors (PARs)*. Of the four known receptors, only PAR1 and PAR4 are expressed on human platelets; the former has been shown to mediate platelet activation at low concentrations of thrombin and the latter in the presence of high concentrations of the agonist.[47] As with most platelet agonists, thrombin can trigger shape change, release of granule contents, and increased adhesiveness of integrin receptors. No reported bleeding disorders have been attributed to loss or dysfunction of PAR1 or PAR4 in humans, although inherited disorders in clotting factors demonstrate the requirement for thrombin in promoting effective hemostasis. Reports on neonatal platelet responsiveness to thrombin are conflicting, as is also the ability of plasma from newborns to generate this procoagulant substance.[48,49]

CONCLUSION

The ability of platelets to interact with the injured vessel wall on the arterial side of the circulation requires the exposure and generation of agonists that promote adhesion, as well as the activation of the clotting cascade. Based on previous in vitro studies suggesting that neonatal platelets are hyporesponsive to physiologic activators that promote hemostasis, it appears that critically ill neonates would be at increased risk of bleeding. Despite these findings, the hemostatic system of healthy newborns appears to be effective because they are not prone to spontaneous hemorrhage. Thus standardized testing and better methodologies are needed to assess platelet function in neonates before the clinical relevance of these observations can be fully ascertained. What may be of greater importance is the number of platelets in the circulation, because these anucleate cells can release proangiogenic cytokines and growth factors that are essential for enabling vascular endothelium to maintain an antithrombotic barrier in the absence of injury.[50] This is evidenced by the spontaneous extravasation of erythrocytes into surrounding tissues when platelet counts fall below a critical value due to loss of the integrity of the endothelial cell barrier. A better understanding of the role that platelets play in stabilizing the vessel wall is needed to aid clinicians in their decision as to when to transfuse the neonate with thrombocytopenia in the absence of overt bleeding.

SELECT REFERENCES

1. Sparger K, Deschmann E, Sola-Visner M. Platelet transfusions in the neonatal intensive care unit. *Clin Perinatol*. 2015;42:613–623.
2. Jin RC, Voetsch B, Loscalzo J. Endogenous mechanisms of inhibition of platelet function. *Microcirculation*. 2005;12:247–258.
3. Smyth EM, Grosser T, Wang M, et al. Prostanoids in health and disease. *J Lipid Res*. 2009;50(suppl):S423–S428.
4. Abrams CS. Intracellular signaling in platelets. *Curr Opin Hematol*. 2005;12:401–405.

5. Kaapa P, Viinikka L, Ylikorkala O. Plasma prostacyclin from birth to adolescence. *Arch Dis Child*. 1982;57:459-461.
6. Govers R, Rabelink TJ. Cellular regulation of endothelial nitric oxide synthase. *Am J Physiol Renal Physiol*. 2001;280:F193-F206.
7. Cheung PY, Salas E, Schulz R, et al. Nitric oxide and platelet function: implications for neonatology. *Semin Perinatol*. 1997;21:409-417.
8. Marcus AJ, Broekman MJ, Drosopoulos JH, et al. Role of CD39 (NTPdase-1) in thromboregulation, cerebroprotection, and cardioprotection. *Semin Thromb Hemost*. 2005;31:234-246.
9. Crawley JT, Zanardelli S, Chion CK, Lane DA. The central role of thrombin in hemostasis. *J Thromb Haemost*. 2007;5(suppl 1):95-101.
10. Weiler H, Isermann BH. Thrombomodulin. *J Thromb Haemost*. 2003;1:1515-1524.
11. Isermann B, Sood R, Pawlinski R, et al. The thrombomodulin-protein C system is essential for the maintenance of pregnancy. *Nat Med*. 2003;9:331-337.
12. Perry DJ. Antithrombin and its inherited deficiencies. *Blood Rev*. 1994;8:37-55.
13. Patnaik MM, Moll S. Inherited antithrombin deficiency: a review. *Haemophilia*. 2008;14:1229-1239.
14. Andrew M, Paes B, Milner R, et al. Development of the human coagulation system in the full-term infant. *Blood*. 1987;70:165-172.
15. Mongale P, Massicotte P. Developmental haemostasis: secondary haemostasis. *Semin Fetal Neonatal Med*. 2011;16:294-300.
16. Sakariassen KS, Bolhuis PA, Sixma JJ. Human blood platelet adhesion to artery subendothelium is mediated by factor VIII-von Willebrand factor bound to the subendothelium. *Nature*. 1979;279:636-6381979.
17. Savage B, Saldivar E, Ruggeri ZM. Initiation of platelet adhesion by arrest onto fibrinogen or translocation on von Willebrand factor. *Cell*. 1996;84:289-297.
18. Federici AB, Bader R, Pagani S, et al. Binding of von Willebrand factor to glycoproteins Ib and IIb/IIIa complex: affinity is related to multimeric size. *Br J Haematol*. 1989;73:93-99.
19. Shenkman B, Linder N, Savion N, et al. Increased neonatal platelet deposition on subendothelium under flow conditions: the role of plasma von Willebrand factor. *Pediatr Res*. 1999;45:270-275.
20. Zimmerman GA, Weyrich AS. Signal-dependent protein synthesis by activated platelets: new pathways to altered phenotype and function. *Arterioscler Thromb Vasc Biol*. 2008;28:s17-s24.
21. King SM, Reed RL. Development of platelet secretory granules. *Semin Cell Dev Biol*. 2002;13:292-302.
22. Herter JM, Rossaint J, Zarbock A. Platelets in inflammation and immunity. *J Thromb Haemost*. 2014;12:1764-1775.
23. Forestier F, Daffos F, Galacteros F, et al. Hematological values of 163 normal fetuses between 18 and 30 weeks of gestation. *Pediatr Res*. 1986;20:342-346.
24. Andrews RK, Lopez JA, Berndt MC. Molecular mechanisms of platelet adhesion and activation. *Int J Biochem Cell Biol*. 1997;29:91-105.
25. Doggett TA, Girdhar G, Lawshe A, et al. Selectin-like kinetics and biomechanics promote rapid platelet adhesion in flow: the GPIbα-VWF tether bond. *Biophys J*. 2002;83:194-205.
26. Sadler JE, Budde U, Eikenboom JC, et al. Update on the pathophysiology and classification of von Willebrand disease: a report of the subcommittee on von Willebrand factor. *J Thromb Haemost*. 2006;4:2103-2114.
27. Chen J, Zhou H, Diacovo A, et al. Exploiting the kinetic interplay between GPIbα-VWF binding interfaces to regulate hemostasis and thrombosis. *Blood*. 2014;124(25):3799-3807.
28. Farndale RW, Sixma JJ, Barnes MJ, de Groot PG. The role of collagen in thrombosis and hemostasis. *J Thromb Haemost*. 2004;2:561-573.
29. Israels SJ, Daniels M, McMillan EM. Deficient collagen-induced activation in the newborn platelet. *Pediatr Res*. 1990;27:337-343.
30. Bennett JS. Structure and function of the platelet integrin alpha IIb beta3. *J Clin Invest*. 2005;115:3363-3369.
31. Simak J, Holada K, Janota J, et al. Surface expression of major membrane glycoproteins on resting and trap-activated neonatal platelets. *Pediatr Res*. 1999;46:445-449.
32. Hezard N, Potron G, Schlegel N, et al. Unexpected persistence of platelet hyporeactivity beyond the neonatal period: a flow cytometric study in neonates, infants and older children. *Thromb Haemost*. 2003;90:116-123.
33. Israels SJ, Gowen B, Gerrard JM. Contractile activity of neonatal platelets. *Pediatr Res*. 1987;21:293-295.
34. Offermanns S. Activation of platelet function through G protein-coupled receptors. *Circ Res*. 2006;99:1293-1304.
35. Nesbitt WS, Giuliano S, Kulkarni S, et al. Intercellular calcium communication regulates platelet aggregation and thrombus growth. *J Cell Biol*. 2003;160:1151-1161.
36. Jardin I, Lopez JJ, Pariente JA, et al. Intracellular calcium release from human platelets: different messengers for multiple stores. *Trends Cardiovasc Med*. 2008;18:57-61.
37. Gelman B, Setty BN, Chen D, et al. Impaired mobilization of intracellular calcium in neonatal platelets. *Pediatr Res*. 1996;39:692-696.
38. Watson SP, Auger JM, McCarty OJ, et al. GPVI and integrin alphaIIb beta3 signaling in platelets. *J Thromb Haemost*. 2005;3:1752-1762.
39. Dorsam RT, Kunapuli SP. Central role of the P2Y12 receptor in platelet activation. *J Clin Invest*. 2004;113:340-345.
40. Ucar T, Gurman C, Arsan S, et al. Platelet aggregation in term and preterm newborns. *Pediatr Hematol Oncol*. 2005;22:139-145.
41. Mankin P, Maragos J, Akhand M, Saving KL. Impaired platelet-dense granule release in neonates. *J Pediatr Hematol Oncol*. 2000;22:143-147.
42. Kaza E, Egalka M, Zhou H, et al. P2Y12 Receptor function and response to cangrelor in neonates with cyanotic congenital heart disease. *JACC, BTS*. 2017;2:465-476.
43. Arita H, Nakano T, Hanasaki K. Thromboxane A2: its generation and role in platelet activation. *Prog Lipid Res*. 1989;28:273-301.
44. Thomas DW, Mannon RB, Mannon PJ, et al. Coagulation defects and altered hemodynamic responses in mice lacking receptors for thromboxane A2. *J Clin Invest*. 1998;102:1994-2001.
45. Stuart MJ, Dusse J, Clark DA, et al. Differences in thromboxane production between neonatal and adult platelets in response to arachidonic acid and epinephrine. *Pediatr Res*. 1984;18:823-826.
46. Israels SJ, Cheang T, Roberston C, et al. Impaired signal transduction in neonatal platelets. *Pediatr Res*. 1999;45:687-691.
47. Coughlin SR. Protease-activated receptors in hemostasis, thrombosis and vascular biology. *J Thromb Haemost*. 2005;3:1800-1814.
48. Andrew M, Schmidt B, Mitchell L, et al. Thrombin generation in newborn plasma is critically dependent on the concentration of prothrombin. *Thromb Haemost*. 1990;63:27-30.
49. Muntean W, Leschnik B, Baier K, et al. *In vivo* thrombin generation in neonates. *J Thromb Haemost*. 2004;2:2071-2072.
50. Nachman RL, Rafii S. Platelets, petechiae, and preservation of the vascular wall. *N Engl J Med*. 2008;359:1261-1270.

Host Defense Mechanisms Against Bacteria

Tobias R. Kollmann | Nicolas Dauby | Danny Harbeson | Mario Fidanza | Arnaud Marchant

INTRODUCTION

Globally, infections cause an estimated 1 million neonatal deaths annually, representing over 40% of all neonatal deaths.[1,2] Overwhelming host response to a microbial infection, or neonatal sepsis, is defined as infection in the first 28 days of life; for preterm infants, this period includes up to 4 weeks after the expected due date. This is further subdivided into early-onset neonatal sepsis (EOS), with an onset during the first 72 hours of age, and late-onset neonatal sepsis (LOS), where incidence peaks in the second to third week of postnatal life but includes events up to 1 month of age.[3]

It is difficult to clinically differentiate between serious bacterial infections (SBI) versus viral, fungal, or other causes without concomitant microbial identification.[4,5] Unfortunately, the incidence of culture-positivity in cases of clinically suspected bacterial sepsis is on average only 10% in the United States; this rate is substantially higher in prematurely born and/or very-low- birth-weight (VLBW) infants.[6] Available data suggest that in several populations around the world the rate of SBI in newborns may be orders of magnitude higher than in the United States.[7-10] However, few high-quality studies exist that examined culture-proven SBI in resource-restricted regions of the world, although this is where most neonatal deaths occur. In two studies, one from South Africa and another one from south Asia, pathogen detection succeeded in no more than approximately one-fourth of all cases of clinically suspected SBI (also known as possible SBI or pSBI), despite cutting-edge study design and methodology (including culture and molecular testing).[4,5] The fact that approximately three-fourths of all cases had no pathogen identified likely indicates that some pathogens were missed, but also that not all pSBI are related to a pathogen; it may be that some are driven by the host for yet unknown reasons.Among infectious pathogens identified, bacteria were the leading cause of neonatal infectious deaths. For example, a meta-analysis of studies between 2008 and 2018 highlighted *Staphylococcus aureus* (SA), *Klebsiella*, and *Escherichia coli* spp. as the dominant causes of culture-proven SBI in neonates (<28 days) in sub-Saharan Africa.[11] *Ureaplasma* spp. and Group B *Streptococcus* (GBS) were most frequently identified among pSBI cases in South Africa.[5] *Ureaplasma* spp. were also the most commonly identified pathogens in cases of pSBI in 60-day-old or younger infants in south Asia.[4]

Despite the development of potent antimicrobial agents, the mortality rate associated with neonatal bacterial sepsis remains very high, especially in preterm infants. In the pre-antibiotic era the case fatality rate of neonatal sepsis exceeded 80%; with the introduction of antibiotics and advances in perinatal care, the case fatality rate has dropped to under 20%.[3] However, this rate is still far higher than in the pediatric or young adult age groups.[12] Beyond mortality, neonatal sepsis also causes significant immediate and long-term morbidity in those that survive.[1] In particular, the risks for central nervous system injury leading to cerebral palsy, abnormal neurodevelopment, visual impairment, and poor growth are significantly elevated with each episode of sepsis. Lastly, neonatal sepsis also causes significant strain on the health care system. In North America alone, it is estimated that each episode of bacterial sepsis prolongs the duration of a neonate's hospital stay by about 2 weeks, resulting in an incremental cost of USD $25,000 per episode.[3]

The high prevalence of specific species associated with infection in early life, such as *Ureaplasma* spp. and several gram-negative bacteria, suggests that there are particular virulence factors peculiar to these pathogens, or to age-specific host responses to those microorganisms, which are centrally involved in the high morbidity and mortality of newborn bacterial sepsis. In this chapter, we will review virulence factors known to be involved for the most important bacterial pathogens in early life and what is known about the age-specific host response to bacterial infections, with a strong focus on those aspects presumed to be of relevance for protection from bacterial infection in early life.

BACTERIAL FACTORS CONTRIBUTING TO INFECTION IN EARLY LIFE

As causative agents of chorioamnionitis, preterm delivery, and neonatal sepsis, *Ureaplasma* species (*Ureaplasma* spp.) are a major contributor to maternal-fetal morbidity worldwide. *Ureaplasma* spp. are frequent commensals of the female lower genital tract; colonization rates are influenced by multiple factors, including ethnicity and age.[13] Clinical outcome of infection with *Ureaplasma* spp. is highly variable across human populations and also bacterial species (genotype- and even serovar)-dependent.[13,14] In vitro studies showed that some *Ureaplasma* spp. bind host cells and can actively suppress innate immune pathways, while in vivo (animal) infection demonstrated that *Ureaplasma* spp. can induce inflammatory responses in fetal immune cells.[13,15] Several virulence factors for *Ureaplasma* spp. have been identified, including the multiple band antigen (MBA). The N-terminal domain of the MBA is conserved among the 14 serovars of *Ureaplasma*; antigenic size variation has, however, been reported for the C-terminal region of MBA protein and is hypothesized to be involved in immune evasion, allowing chronic infection during pregnancy.[16] Variation of the size of the MBA protein also appears associated with distinct cord blood innate immune responses.[16]While MBA may be an important contributor to *Ureaplasma* spp. pathogenicity, much remains to be learned about how and why *Ureaplasma* spp. are so frequently linked to pSBI of the newborn, especially in low-resource settings.

Klebsiella pneumoniae has emerged has an important cause of morbidity and mortality in neonates.[17] Drug-resistant strains of *Klebsiella* that have been associated with outbreaks in neonatal intensive care units around the globe are especially problematic.[18] *K. pneumoniae* has developed multiple immune evasion strategies, including inhibition of complement activation, dampening of inflammatory response, and apoptosis of macrophages, which often appears to involve the capsular polysaccharide.[17] While *K. pneumoniae* is now considered as an "urgent threat to human health," surprisingly little is known about this important bacterial pathogen, not only in regards to its role in early life infections but overall.

E. coli has long been recognized as one of the leading bacterial agents for EOS and LOS, as well as neonatal meningitis.[19,20] *E. coli* contains several virulence factors, promoting translocation through the amniotic membrane and subsequent invasion of the fetal and newborn blood-brain barrier, which are likely to be responsible for its high prevalence in cases of newborn sepsis and meningitis.[19-21] The majority of *E. coli* strains causing meningitis belong to a specific capsular serotype (K1) that possesses type 1 pili and the outer membrane protein OmpA, promoting adhesion and penetration across endothelial layers.[21] In vitro, OmpA can also suppress dendritic cell (DC) maturation and function, dampen pro-inflammatory cytokine production, and increased production of anti-inflammatory cytokines such as interleukin (IL)-10 and transforming growth factor (TGF)-β.[22] Further emphasizing OmpA's importance in neonatal virulence is the finding that different portions of the extracellular loops of OmpA allow invasion and subsequent survival inside of the very host cells that should eliminate this pathogen, such as neutrophils.[23] Despite its long history as a neonatal pathogen, the precise molecular host-bacterial interactions that give *E. coli* this infamously prominent role in early life infections are barely understood.

Among the gram-positive bacteria, *Streptococcus agalactiae*, or GBS remains one of the important invasive pathogens for newborns, despite antibiotic prophylaxis regimens implemented in many parts of the world.[24] In North America and Europe, where GBS is a commensal of the human intestinal and vaginal tract in 15% to 30% of healthy adults, every 10th neonate acquires GBS vertically during passage through the birth canal or shortly thereafter. Yet, 99% of colonized infants will never develop invasive GBS disease. Some of the underlying mechanisms that lead to disease are beginning to emerge. For example, the ability of type III GBS in particular to adhere to the neonatal epithelium facilitates colonization and predominance in early-onset neonatal sepsis. Crossing the mucosal barrier and the blood-brain barrier seems to be mechanistically linked, as GBS serotype III is a particularly frequent isolate in neonatal meningitis. The high-level neurotropism is at least partially due to expression of the adhesion molecule hypervirulent GBS adhesin (HvgA). HvgA efficiently supports bacterial adhesion and transfer through to the intestinal wall and later across the blood-brain barrier, specifically the vascular endothelium of the choroid plexus. Expression levels of HvgA and other GBS virulence factors, such as pili and toxins, are regulated by the upstream two-component control system CovR/S. This in turn is modulated by acidic pH and high glucose levels, which the microbe encounters during the passage through the intestine. After invasion, GBS has the ability to subvert innate immunity by different mechanisms. The GBS enzyme glyceraldehyde-3-phosphate-dehydrogenase induces the production of IL-10 and thereby decreases the recruitment of neutrophils and limits their bactericidal activity.[24] GBS capsular polysaccharides, allowing the identification of 10 unique serotypes (Ia, Ib, II to IX), have a terminal sialic acid residue. This SIA residue binds to host inhibitory sialic acid binding immunoglobulin (Ig)-like lectins (SIGLECs 5, 9 and 14) and thereby dampens phagocytosis, oxidative burst, and platelet-mediated antimicrobial killing.[25,26] On the host side, sensing of GBS nucleic acids and lipopeptides by both Toll-like receptors (TLRs) and the inflammasome appears to be critical for host resistance against GBS; these host functions display age-dependent changes in function (see below).

Staphylococcus spp. and particularly *S. epidermidis* are other leading causes of sepsis in neonates (reviewed by Marchant and colleagues and Power Coombs and colleagues[3,27]). Newborns are often colonized via horizontal rather than vertical transfer. *S. epidermidis* produces a biofilm that favors its persistence on medical devices. Epidemic clones that display significant antibiotic resistance preferentially produce extracellular polymers, such as polysaccharide intercellular adhesion (PIA), that are part of the biofilm. PIA modulates host innate immune responses by different mechanisms, including inhibition of phagocytosis.[28] *Staphylococcus* spp. also evade clearance by the immune system by using exoenzymes such as protease and endopeptidase, and in part by generating adenosine.[28] Adenosine is an endogenous purine metabolite that acts via cognate seven-transmembrane receptors to induce immunomodulatory intracellular cyclic adenosine monophosphate (cAMP). cAMP enhances production of IL-6, which impairs neutrophil function while inhibiting production of tumor necrosis factor (TNF)α, which is important for neutrophil activation. Neonatal mononuclear cells are particularly sensitive to the effects of adenosine.

Protein toxins are another group of important virulence factors contributing to neonatal sepsis (reviewed in Sonnen and Henneke[29]). Most of the major pathogens responsible for neonatal sepsis, namely GBS, *E. coli*, and *S. aureus*, secrete toxins of different molecular natures, but each is key for defining the disease. These pore-forming exotoxins are expressed as soluble monomers prior to engagement of the target cell membrane with subsequent formation of an aqueous membrane pore. Membrane pore formation allows penetration of epithelial barriers as well as evasion of the immune system. In the process, pore formation contributes to inflammation and hence to the manifold manifestations of sepsis. *S. epidermidis* produces phenol-soluble modulin toxins that participate in biofilm formation and induction of pro-inflammatory responses that may be associated with necrotizing enterocolitis.[28]

AGE-DEPENDENT ASPECTS OF HOST DEFENSE CONTRIBUTING TO BACTERIAL INFECTION EARLY IN LIFE

Immune-mediated protection, in evolution as well as ontogeny, starts with a focus on primitive host defenses of single-cells, designated cell-autonomous immunity. This is followed by increasingly complex interactions, such as biochemical coordination in collections of cells via nutritional immunity, to increasingly specialized cells that provide barrier function and innate immunity. Only at the last stages of evolution and ontogeny is adaptive immunity, with its highly specialized tissues, readily identifiable. During fetal and early neonatal life, the host protective immune system undergoes profoundly rapid developmental changes; these changes occur in adaptation to specific functional demands as well as changes encoded in the host genome. The early life immune system is thus not simply stuck in a fixed state of "immaturity" but has in fact been shaped over millennia of human phylogeny to assure our survival as a species; yet it remains highly responsive to the rapidly changing demands of each individual's ontogeny. The increased risk for bacterial infection then must arise from this interphase between phylogenetically selected survival programs and extraordinary demands during ontogeny.

CELL AUTONOMOUS IMMUNITY

Cell autonomous immunity (CAI) is the most ancient and prevalent form of host protection, where individual cells try to protect against intracellular infection (reviewed by Randow and colleagues[30]). Given this focus on intracellular infection, CAI is primarily based upon intracellular compartmentalization. This involves sensory machinery such as pattern recognition receptors (PRRs) that detect pathogen-associated molecular patterns (PAMPs) and danger receptors that monitor danger-associated molecular patterns (DAMPs) at each intracellular border. For example, PAMP activation of interferon (IFN) pathways will trigger production of guanylate binding proteins (GBPs), which will rapidly coat intracellular bacteria, simultaneously damaging the bacterial membrane and recruiting a wide array of other host antimicrobial effectors.[31] Galectins, a family of cytosolic lectins with specificity for β-galactosides, detect membrane damage and upon activation induce autophagy of the damaged subcellular compartment. Galectins can also bind nonself glycans on the surface of pathogenic microbes and in doing so function as PRRs that can inhibit microbial adhesion or cell entry.[32] However, recent reports have also demonstrated the capacity for certain viruses and bacteria such as *Porphyromonas gingivalis*,[33] *Streptococcus pneumoniae*,[34] and *Chlamydia trachomatis*[35], to subvert and exploit this recognition pathway to facilitate cell adhesion and increase virulence.

Cytosolic PRRs targeting foreign nucleic acids (DNA, RNA) induce a potent antimicrobial state when activated. Infected cells increase expression of proton-dependent efflux pumps, such as natural resistance-associated macrophage protein-1 (NRAMP-1), that export iron from vacuoles to prevent access of captured microbes to this essential metal. This latter aspect functionally links CAI to the next and more complex stage of development, nutritional immunity. While CAI is likely operative throughout life, it may play an especially important role in the earliest stages of embryonic development. However, changes of CAI as a function of age have not yet been investigated, precluding an assessment of CAI as a contributor to the risk of SBI early in life.

NUTRITIONAL IMMUNITY

Nutritional immunity refers to another ancient evolutionary method of host protection from bacterial infection based on deliberate changes in essential nutrients.[36] One of the best-studied examples relates to essential metals, especially iron (Fe) (reviewed in Hood and Skaar[37]). All living organisms require Fe to survive. Human tissues represent a rich resource of Fe, but to reduce the risk for bacterial invasion, humans restrict access to Fe. The master-switch controlling free Fe is hepcidin. Hepcidin is produced in the liver, and its expression is increased in response to inflammation, danger, or pathogen recognition. Hepcidin restricts the availability of extracellular iron and therefore, serves as an important form of nutritional immunity.[38] In mammals, the physiologic drop in serum Fe around birth has been proposed as an evolutionary survival advantage, presumed to reduce the risk for neonatal sepsis.[38,39] Specifically, while cord blood is characterized by *hyper*ferremia (high Fe levels), within 6 to 12 hours of birth this changes to a profound *hypo*ferremic (low Fe) state.[40-42] It is currently not clear what drives this rapid postnatal drop in serum Fe, but serum Fe levels in human newborns have in fact been shown to be a sensitive, direct correlate of susceptibility to sepsis; that is, the higher the Fe level the higher the risk for sepsis.[39,43-46] Furthermore, supplemental Fe given to Fe-replete infants can increase the risk for sepsis and death.[46-49]

Sequestration of zinc (Zn) and manganese (Mn) represent other important facets of nutritional immunity.[50] Mn may be of particular relevance to the newborn; the heterodimeric S100A8/A9 alarmin complex (commonly known as calprotectin) inhibits the growth of both *S. aureus* and GBS in breast milk through Mn chelation. Calprotectin production is massively elevated in breast milk immediately after birth, corresponding with high levels in neonatal plasma, which slowly lower to adult levels around one month after birth.[50,51]

Microbes have developed several complex defense strategies in the "battle" for metal ions. These include employing metal ion scavenging siderophores that compete with host defenses to pirate metal ions.[52] Illustrating the critical nature of the metal ion battle, the siderophore gene clusters aerobactin *(iuc)* and salmochelin *(iro)* have been identified as key virulence factors for *K. pneumoniae*,[53] which is one of the most common causes of neonatal sepsis. Thus nutritional immunity likely is a key component of protection from bacterial infection in early life.

PHYSICAL AND FUNCTIONAL BARRIERS

Protective barrier functions such as physical and chemical components of placenta, skin, and mucous membranes are already in place during fetal life (reviewed in King and colleagues[54]). The placental layers also produce a range of antimicrobial proteins and peptides (APP) that can be detected in the amniotic fluid surrounding the embryo/fetus (reviewed in King and colleagues[55]). APPs include defensins, bactericidal/permeability-increasing protein, whey acidic protein (WAP) motif containing proteins, secretory leukocyte protease inhibitor (SLPI) and elafin (antiproteinase 3; skin derived antileuko-proteinase), lactoferrin, and lysozyme.[55] Human β-defensins (HBD) 1-3 and elafin can be found in abundance in many layers of the placenta. In cases of preterm premature rupture of membranes (PPROM) both SLPI and elafin are found at reduced levels in amniotic fluid and fetal membrane, but in cases of chorioamnionitis, elafin, HBD3, various α-defensins, and human neutrophil peptides (HNP) 1-3, all increase in maternal plasma and amniotic fluid.

The outermost layer of the skin (stratum corneum) acts as a physical barrier and first line of defense against bacterial invasion; however, the stratum corneum only fully matures over the first 2 weeks after birth, leaving the newborn infant vulnerable (reviewed in Marchant and colleagues[3]). The skin of the preterm newborn further lacks effective chemical barriers (acidic pH) until approximately 1 month after birth. This lower level of barrier function around birth appears balanced by the constitutively high production of APPs such as β-defensins and cathelicidins, especially in the vernix caseosa present at birth. However, the vernix caseosa is mainly formed during the last trimester of gestation, again leaving premature neonates more vulnerable. Underlying the dermis and epidermis is the dermal white adipose tissue (DWAT) layer that is further equipped with diverse immune functions coordinated by resident immune cells and parenchyma-derived cytokines. The DWAT is a particularly important source of cathelicidins.[56] It is thickest in neonates before gradually thinning over time as dermal fibroblasts transition from adipogenic to pro-fibrotic. This transition is coordinated by increased TGFβ signaling and dramatically reduces the cathelicidin production capacity and antimicrobial function of the DWAT.[56]

Growth factors and cytokines within the amniotic fluid contribute to development of fetal intestinal barrier function (reviewed by Hornef and Fulde[57]). Newborns from pregnancies complicated by oligohydramnios are at higher risk for intestinal infections. Specifically, in preterm neonates, the protective glycocalyx layer coating the intestinal epithelium is somewhat smaller.[3,57] The intestinal mucosa appears to pass through specific postnatal developmental stages. For example, the neonatal small intestinal epithelium already expresses the cathelicidin cathelin-related antimicrobial peptide (CRAMP), which exerts antibacterial activity against commensal and pathogenic bacteria. However, production of Paneth cell-derived APPs like cryptdins and cryptdin related sequences (CRS) peptides only starts after birth, reflecting the delayed appearance of small intestinal Paneth cells during the postnatal period. Intestinal epithelial CRAMP expression wanes after the postnatal period, which results in a switch in the peptide repertoire and production site from epithelial CRAMP expression in the neonate to Paneth cell–secreted cryptdins and CRS peptides after weaning. The lack of Paneth cell–derived defensins in the neonatal host might contribute the high susceptibility of infection with *Shigella* and *Salmonella.* Production of these APP is even lower in preterm infants.[3] Lastly, the gastrointestinal tract is also less acidic at birth than in later life, further compromising barrier function.

Physical protection of the respiratory tract includes the cilia found in the nasal mucosa and the passageways of the upper airways, bronchi, and bronchioles, as they impede respiratory invasion of microbial pathogens and remove or expel them; cilial function in early life appears similar to that of adults (reviewed in Zhang and colleagues[58]). Mucin glycoproteins contribute to protection of the airways by providing viscosity that physically impede microbial invasion.[59,60] The airway surface fluid also contains a variety of other APPs, such as lysozyme, lactoferrin, and defensins.[61,62] Lastly, the salt or fluid content at the airway surface helps protect against microbial invasion. The high salt content or the decreased airway fluid observed in patients with cystic fibrosis inhibits normal airway antibacterial activities and contributes to the persistent bacterial colonization and chronic infections seen in these patients.[62,63] Unfortunately, little is known about the changes during early development of these barrier functions in the respiratory tract.[64]

THE MICROBIAL BARRIER

The unique characteristics of neonatal skin and a general lack of exposure to the microbe-rich outside world contribute to a neonatal cutaneous microbiome distinct from that of adults (reviewed in Schoch and colleagues[65]). The cutaneous microbiome on the surface of the stratum corneum provides an additional layer of physical defense against invasive pathogens.[66] The urgent need to establish this cutaneous microbiome is reflected by a wave of regulatory T cells (T regs) that migrate to the skin immediately after birth; these T regs appear to establish a localized state of immune tolerance allowing colonization by commensal bacteria.[67] As with the intestinal microbiome, this layer of cutaneous microbes is likely critical to the development of healthy cutaneous immunity.

Within hours after birth, the neonate's intestinal tract is colonized by multiple species of bacteria (reviewed in Arrieta and colleagues[68]). While the microbial composition, or microbiota, changes during the first years of life, it is unique to the host and can be viewed as a personal fingerprint that emerges in early infancy. Development of the intestinal microbiome is influenced by a wide swath of factors including genetics, fetal swallowing, maternal lifestyle, maternal diet, antibiotic exposure, birth mode, feeding mode, and postnatal environment.[24,68,69] While disruptions to the intestinal microbiome in early life have been "associated with development of many pathologic states like infantile colic, inflammatory bowel disease, necrotizing enterocolitis, asthma, atopic diseases, celiac disease, diabetes, mood disorders, and autism spectrum disorders," proof of mechanistic cause-effect chains are still largely lacking.[70]

Bacterial colonizers of the human intestine are classified as *symbionts* that stabilize the intestinal homeostasis, or as pathobionts that under particular circumstances can cause severe local or systemic disease (reviewed by Landwehr-Kenzel and Henneke[24] and Arieta and colleagues[68]). Some of these microorganisms can suppress the overgrowth of true pathogens, via production of bacteriocins and other antimicrobial agents, but the protective role of microbial colonization extends far beyond inhibition of colonization with pathogens by commensal bacteria.[68] In some instances microbial colonization results in direct host-microbial interactions that increase host resistance to infection at mucosal surfaces and beyond.[68,71] For example, colonization of both the intestinal as well as respiratory mucosa with commensal bacteria is essential to initiate normal development of the mucosa-associated lymphoid tissue (MALT) as well as systemic immunity.[57,71] As a result, alteration of the microbiome by feeding or birth mode, or antibiotic exposure during time-restricted periods very early in life, can be associated with alteration of local as well as systemic immunity.[72,73] For example, the decreased diversity of the *Bacteroidetes* phylum in infants born by cesarean section is associated with lower serum levels of chemokine C-X-C motif ligands CXCL10 and CXCL11, two IFN-dependent chemokines that are important for white blood cell migration to sites of infection (reviewed in De Kleer and colleagues[74]).

Early nutrient availability is thought to be a critical variable dictating the compositional structure of the infant intestinal microbiome.[75] Since bacterial species grow at different rates under different nutrient conditions, nutrient availability directly shapes microbiome composition by shaping competitive niches where certain microbes with similar biochemical needs can flourish. This has been confirmed by the demonstration that early microbiome composition was fundamentally shaped by nitrogen bioavailability, further reinforcing the concept that what feeds the early microbiome determines its composition.[76] Factors that unfavorably influence nutrient status, and therefore likely microbiome composition, have been directly linked to early immunologic programming and function.[76-78] Not surprisingly, then, enteral probiotic supplementation significantly reduces the risk for infection (sepsis, pneumonia, diarrhea) and death early in life of rural Indian newborns weighing at least 2000 g and born after 35 gestational weeks: that is, a population considered full term and normal birth weight.[79,80] While the cellular and molecular mechanisms underlying these beneficial host-probiotic interactions have not yet been delineated in human newborns, it is known that monocytes and DCs isolated from the blood of mice treated with antibiotics have reduced expression of IFN-responsive genes, suggesting that signals derived from commensal bacteria can influence systemic innate responses.[74] Furthermore, this was shown to involve chromatin level changes, as DCs from germ-free or antibiotic-treated mice show reduced histone modification (specifically H3K4me3) deposits at specific inflammatory genes. As a result, despite normal activation of two key transcription factors in the immune system upon TLR stimulation—namely, nuclear factor (NF)-κB or interferon regulatory transcription factor (IRF) 3—direct recruitment of these to promoter regions was reduced in DCs from antibiotic treated mice. Tonic stimulation by commensals or probiotics might therefore enable rapid induction of specific defense genes upon infection.

INNATE IMMUNITY

Immunity becomes increasingly important for host protection of multicellular organisms, where the evolutionarily earliest forms are referred to as *innate immunity* (reviewed by Buchmann[81]). An innate immune system is present in all multicellular organisms, including plants, insects, and animals. Innate immune cells such as phagocytes are equipped with a wide range of PRRs recognizing PAMPs that upon ligation activate a complex cascade of cellular reactions, which in turn lead to production of a wide array of effector molecules. Innate immunity directly interfaces with the evolutionarily more ancient nutritional immunity, in that a shift to aerobic glycolysis through activation of the mammalian target of rapamycin (mTOR) pathway increases the activity of phagocytes and other innate effector cells.[82] This pathway also coordinates the memory-like function of innate immunity—that is, epigenetic changes that lead to long-lasting alteration of innate immune memory (also known as *trained immunity*).[82,83] Lastly, innate immune cells directly link to adaptive immunity, most importantly through antigen presentation, expression of co-stimulatory molecules, and cytokines. The activities of innate immunity are both rapid (preventing microbial spread) and nonspecific (protecting against multiple pathogens of diverse nature). The innate immune system exerts its function through soluble as well as cell-mediated aspects. We here highlight only some of the key aspects of soluble and cell-mediated innate immune ontogeny in relation to protection from bacterial infection; for more details, the reader is asked to consult the cited reviews.

SOLUBLE COMPONENTS OF INNATE IMMUNITY

The complement system consists of a cascade of enzymatic proteins found in the blood plasma and tissues (reviewed by Pettengill and colleagues[84]). Upon activation of this cascade, complement deposits various components on the surface of microbes, initiating opsonization and phagocytosis or direct lysis of target cells. The complement cascade can be activated via three pathways: the classical pathway, initiated by antibody binding; the mannose-binding lectin (MBL) pathway (reviewed by Auriti and colleagues[85]); and the alternative pathway. All three pathways finally lead to attachment of parts of C3 on the surface of their target, resulting in either opsonization or the assembly of a membrane-attack complex that damages the target membrane. Activity of the classical pathway (measured as CH50) is approximately 50% to 75% of adult controls for preterm subjects and 69% of adult controls for term subjects; activity of the alternate pathway (measured as AP50) is 49%, 53%, and 60% of adult controls for extreme preterm (28 to 33 weeks gestational age), preterm (34 to 36 weeks gestational age), and term subjects, respectively.[84] Studies of age-specific differences in MBL in plasma have produced somewhat contradictory findings; however, functional assessment via in vitro incubation of cord blood with recombinant mannose-binding lectin (rMBL) showed that high concentrations of exogenous rMBL provided little to no improvement in antibacterial or antifungal activity in either group.[86] While levels of many complement proteins are found to be lower in preterm and term cord blood plasma compared to adult peripheral blood plasma, the terminal membrane-attack complex proteins C8 and C9 have shown substantial age-dependency, with the lowest levels in the most prematurely born newborns. Of interest, complement proteins with an apparently strong age-dependent change in plasma concentration (i.e., most of them) are produced in the liver; only complement component C7 is produced in neutrophils and is found only modestly reduced in preterm infants and already at adult-like levels in term newborns. This suggests age-dependent differences in hepatic function may underpin the age-dependent differences in complement components.

APPs play an important role in fetal and neonatal innate immunity, helping to regulate colonization while enhancing resistance to infection (reviewed in Pettengill and colleagues[84]). Lactoferrin, which can bind iron as well as endotoxin, is found at very high concentrations in breast milk but is lower in newborn neutrophils. Similarly, bactericidal/permeability-increasing protein (BPI, which is potently active against gram-negative bacteria) and human cathelicidin antimicrobial peptide 18 (hCAP-18, also called *LL-37*) also display clear age-dependent concentration differences (reviewed in Pettengill and colleagues[84]); this may be important functionally, as exogenous addition of LL-37 significantly inhibited growth of *Staphylococcus epidermidis* (SE) and *Candida albicans* (CA) in both term and preterm cord blood, yet it only inhibited SA growth in term cord blood.[86] Clinically, lower serum levels of cathelicidin have been found associated with increased severity of acute bacterial respiratory infection in children aged 0 to 24 months. Lastly, among the α-defensins and β-defensins, which are functionally important APPs targeting bacteria, viruses, as well as fungi,[84] the α-defensins (predominately produced by neutrophils [HNP1-4]) appear at adult-like concentrations around birth, while β-defensins (predominately produced by epithelial cells, macrophages, and neutrophils) are lower in newborns compared with adult serum levels. Lower β-defensin-2 levels in particular appear to be associated with increased risk for sepsis in preterm neonates.[84]

Not all soluble innate molecules are found at lower concentration or function in the newborn. For example, soluble CD14 (sCD14 or presepsin) and sTLR2 are common components of human breast milk[87] and have higher serum concentrations in infants than adults.[88] These two soluble receptors have a variety of immunomodulatory functions and have been implicated in host recognition of and resistance against a variety of microbes.[89] There is substantial evidence that the response of TLRs to their respective ligands is regulated by sTLRs and sCD14, preventing potentially damaging responses and facilitating commensal tolerance.[89] For example, in some small pilot studies CD14 has been identified as a possible valuable diagnostic biomarker for late onset neonatal sepsis.[90] Neonatal cord blood plasma also has significantly higher levels than adults of soluble innate immune regulators, such as adenosine, an endogenous purine metabolite that inhibits TLR-mediated T cell responses.[27] Specifically, the neonatal adenosine system inhibits TLR-induced TNF production but not IL-6, leading to a higher basal IL-6/TNF ratio as compared to adults. Lastly, newborn neutrophils demonstrate impairment in production of nucleic acid–based neutrophil extracellular traps (NETs) that serve as scaffolds for APPs and are important for host defense.[27] Overall, reduced plasma levels of complement and APPs as well as impaired deployment of APPs on NETs may, in part, explain why neonates are more susceptible to infection.

CELLULAR COMPONENTS OF INNATE IMMUNITY

The cells of the innate immune systems, which have diverse effector and immunoregulatory functions, include the myeloid lineages (namely granulocytes, monocytes, macrophages, and (DCs) as well as innate lymphocytes, including natural killer (NK) cells and other innate lymphoid cells (ILCs), NK-T cells (NKT), and γδ-T cells. There appear to be developmentally restricted windows of immune cell development in which fetal cells, functionally distinct from their adult counterparts, arise from discrete hematopoietic stem and progenitor cells and seed specific anatomic locations. Immune ontogeny in humans then proceeds in a layered fashion, with a fetal system that predominates in utero and early life, and an adult system that predominates later in life (i.e., "layered innate immune hematopoiesis," reviewed by Krow-Lucal and McCune[91]).

Immune layering is perhaps best illustrated by tissue-resident macrophages. Mouse studies have demonstrated that tissue-resident macrophages arise from at least three different sources: the yolk sac, fetal liver, and bone marrow (reviewed in De Kleer and colleagues[74] and Hoeffel and Ginhoux[92]). During the primitive wave of hematopoiesis, macrophages arising from the yolk sac colonize various organs such as the brain, liver, skin, and lungs. Subsequently, definitive hematopoiesis is established and hematopoietic stem cells, which are initially stored in the fetal liver and later in the bone marrow, produce monocytes that differentiate into macrophages to supplement or replace yolk sac–derived tissue-resident macrophage populations. Depending on the tissue, yolk sac– and fetal monocyte–derived tissue-resident macrophages may persist and be maintained by self-renewal for extended periods, even throughout life, or may be replaced prior to or after birth by bone marrow-derived monocytes. In addition to these resident macrophage populations, which arise under steady-state conditions and at specific developmental time points, monocytes can also be recruited to sites of infection or injury and differentiate in situ into macrophages.

Granulocytes

Granulocytes (neutrophils, eosinophils, and basophils) represent the largest myeloid cell fraction in the blood throughout life. Of these, neutrophils are the most important for host protection from bacterial infection. Neutrophils are present in the liver parenchyma of human fetuses as early as 5 weeks' gestation and as of mid-gestation are generated in high numbers in the bone marrow.[74] Fetal blood contains relatively few mature neutrophils but abundant neutrophil progenitors. Levels of granulocyte-monocyte colony-stimulating factor (GM-CSF) and G-CSF, which drive neutrophil differentiation and promote neutrophil survival, are also low in fetal blood, but G-CSF and neutrophil numbers increase rapidly just before birth. Consistent with this, neonatal neutrophils have expression of surface G-CSF receptors similar to adult neutrophils.

Neutrophils extravasate from blood into tissues following inflammatory signals, and there combat microorganisms via phagocytosis, the release of microbicidal proteins, and by NET formation.[74] Compared to adult neutrophils, neutrophils from healthy infants exhibit differences in the expression of granule proteins important for bacterial defense.[93] For instance, neonatal neutrophils contain concentrations of the azurophilic granule proteins myeloperoxidase and α-defensin, which are similar to adult neutrophils, but have lower levels of BPI and lactoferrin. Degranulation is similar in neutrophils of healthy term infants and adults, but neutrophils from preterm infants exhibit impaired release of BPI, elastase, and lactoferrin.

While neutrophils of the newborn are as capable of phagocytosis as those of adults, they are somewhat less chemotactic, and exhibit a lower respiratory burst and an impaired ability to form extracellular traps important for capturing and killing extracellular bacteria (reviewed by Power Coombs and colleagues[27]). For extremely low-gestational-age newborns (ELGAN <28 weeks' gestation), this may in part relate to lower expression of key components of the pathogen-sensing machinery such as TLR2, TLR4, cluster of differentiation (CD)14, myeloid differentiation primary response 88 factor (MyD88), and myeloid differentiation factor (MD) 2. Moreover, while neutrophils of term infants express similar levels of TLRs and downstream signaling molecules, they also express higher levels of the inhibitory receptor leukocyte-associated immunoglobulin- (Ig-) like receptor-1 (LAIR-1) and siglec-9 than adults. Granulocytes that suppress T and NK cell responses, often referred to as granulocytic myeloid-derived suppressor cells (G-MDSCs), are also abundant in cord blood and neonatal blood, but decline over the first year of life.[94] They are thought to promote maternal-fetal tolerance during gestation, but likely also contribute to susceptibility to infection. Lastly, newborn neutrophils are more rapidly depleted following infection, which partly explains the high frequency of neutropenia during infectious episodes, especially in premature infants.[95-97]

Monocytes and Macrophages

Monocyte production and release into the fetal blood begins when self-renewing hematopoietic stem cells seed the fetal liver (reviewed by De Kleer and colleagues[74]). Although there likely are many more subsets of monocytes,[98] three major subsets of human monocytes have been described based on not only their phenotype but also their function. These include classical monocytes ($CD14^{++}CD16^{-}$, intermediate monocytes ($CD14^{++}CD16^{+}$) and nonclassical monocytes ($CD14^{dim}CD16^{+}$). Classical monocytes are mostly regarded as pro-inflammatory, while nonclassical monocytes are found to be anti-inflammatory/healing. Recent evidence supports a model of sequential development of intermediate and nonclassical monocytes from classical monocytes, with induction of CD16 followed by downregulation of CD14. However, only 1% of classical monocytes are thought to undergo this conversion.[99] Classical monocytes are rapidly recruited to sites of infection or injury, although this recruitment appears less efficient for newborn as compared to adult monocytes.[64] Depending on the local context, classical monocytes can differentiate in situ into inflammatory macrophages or monocyte-derived dendritic cells (Mo-DCs). Classical monocytes also produce a range of pro-inflammatory mediators, which are known to be essential for protection from several intracellular pathogens. Intermediate monocytes exhibit a pro-inflammatory response, especially to TLR4 stimulation, while nonclassical monocytes are often found around blood vessels and offer protection against harmful inflammation and promote healing through angiogenesis.

Reduced expression of TLR4 and a lower frequency of intermediate monocytes in cord blood compared to adult blood may further contribute to the decreased responsiveness of whole blood TLR4 stimulation. Age-dependent differences in the classical monocyte response may also relate to numeric differences (relative proportion of specific monocyte subsets) or cell-intrinsic quantitative as well as qualitative differences.[100] For example, upon TLR stimulation, classical monocytes in human cord blood are known to produce lower levels than adult monocytes of a range of pro-inflammatory mediators; this may be due to lower MyD88 expression and reduced NF-κB activity. Yet, in response to the same stimulation they produce similar or even higher amounts of IL-6 and IL-10 than adult classical monocytes, suggesting not so much a quantitatively lower but a qualitatively different response.[74,100]

Qualitative differences in the function of monocytes in early versus later life is further supported by the finding that fetal monocytes more strongly phosphorylate canonical and noncanonical signal transducers and activators of transcription (STATs) than adult monocytes in response to cytokines such as IFNγ, and upregulate genes associated with antimicrobial defense, but not genes involved in antigen presentation, co-stimulation, or inflammation. Tissue resident human macrophages are also less responsive to IFNγ in early life, with distinctly altered STAT1 phosphorylation. Furthermore, neonatal macrophages phagocytose *E. coli* less efficiently than adult macrophages, and this difference is more pronounced in prematurely born infants. The decreased capacity of circulating monocytes to produce inflammatory cytokines such as TNF-α or IL-1β, and the decreased capacity of tissue-resident macrophages to phagocytose, may thus contribute to the increased risk of bacterial infection in newborns.

Dendritic Cells

DCs are professional antigen-processing and antigen-presenting cells with key roles in initiating and regulating adaptive immune responses, and in the development of immunologic memory and tolerance (reviewed in De Kleer and colleagues[74,101]). DCs arise from BM progenitors, and distinct DC subsets differing in surface marker expression and developmental programming have been identified, namely conventional and plasmacytoid DCs (cDCs and pDCs, respectively). Under inflammatory conditions, DCs can also arise from monocytes (MoDCs), which share some functional properties with cDCs and pDCs despite having distinct origins.

Similar to monocytes, there likely are many subsets of DC.[98] However, most information currently is based on subdividing at least cDC into $CD141/BDCA3^{+}$cDCs (cDC1) and CD1c/$BDCA1^{+}$cDCs (cDC2). Both subsets are capable of activating $CD4^{+}$ T cells, but $CD141^{+}$cDCs appear to be more efficient than $CD1c^{+}$cDCs at cross-presenting cell-associated antigens to $CD8^{+}$ T cells. $CD1c^{+}$cDCs are more abundant and have recently been shown to be transcriptionally heterogeneous,[98,102] although the functions of the $CD1c^{+}$cDC subsets have not yet been thoroughly delineated and appear to vary between tissues. cDCs generally display a short half-life of approximately 3 to 6 days and are constantly replenished from BM precursors.[74] Plasmacytoid DCs are longer lived than cDCs and are present in the bone marrow and all peripheral organs.[74] They are particularly specialized to respond to viral and intracellular bacterial infection by producing type I IFNs.

Developmental and neonatal variation in human cDC subsets has not yet been characterized, but cDC2s dominate in adult mice, while cDC1s are the more abundant mouse cDC subset in early life.[103] The antigen presentation capacity of human DCs also remains to be characterized, although evidence from mouse studies demonstrates age-dependent differences, including lower basal expression of MHC II and co-stimulatory molecules by cDCs in early life.

Possibly related to the layered ontogeny of innate immune cells and/or changes in the microbiome,[74,91] responses of human cDCs to in vitro TLR stimulation vary with age.[100] Newborn cDCs produce less than their adult counterparts of the key Th1-promoting cytokine IL-12p70 (consisting of the IL-12p35 and IL-12p40), yet more of the Th17-promoting cytokine IL-23 (consisting of IL-12p40 and IL-23p19). This difference persists into early adolescence due to epigenetic changes at the IL-12p35 promoter, leading to weaker binding of the transcription factor IRF3, and in turn decreased transcription of IL-12p35. Together, this may relate to the clinically observed increased risk for newborns to suffer from infection with intracellular microbes.

The response of human cord blood pDCs to TLR stimulation is also different as compared to that of older children (reviewed by Macri and colleagues[101]). Specifically, cord blood pDCs display reduced capacity to produce type 1 IFNα and IFNβ in response to in vitro TLR7 and TLR9 stimulation or in vitro HCMV, HSV-1, and RSV exposure. The mechanisms behind this appears related to reduced nuclear translocation of IRF7, a transcription factor necessary for some of the type 1 IFNs. While similar differences have been described in murine pDC and were proposed to relate to downregulation of E2.2, a master transcriptional regulator of murine pDC, this was not confirmed in vivo, suggesting contextual (e.g., environmental) differences rather than age-dependent cell-intrinsic differences. The clinical relevance of the age-related differences identified for pDC thus remains to be determined.

Innate Lymphocytes

Innate lymphocytes are lymphoid cells with innate characteristics that distinguish them from conventional adaptive T and B lymphocytes. These characteristics include the recognition of molecular patterns, the rapid expression of effector functions, and the fact that they do not require clonal expansion to respond to pathogens.[104] Innate lymphocytes participate in the response to bacterial, viral, and parasitic infections and form an expanding family of cells. Some innate lymphocytes express somatically rearranged antigen receptors, but others lack T or B cell receptors and are called *ILCs*.[105] ILCs include cytotoxic NK cells and noncytotoxic ILC1, 2, and 3 subsets.

NK cells exhibit cytotoxic functions and produce inflammatory cytokines (such as TNFα and IFNγ) upon activation by cytokines produced by myeloid cells (such as IL-12 and IL-15).[106] Although NK cells are mostly known for their role in immunity against viruses and cancer, they also participate in the defense against intracellular bacteria such as *Listeria monocytogenes*.[107] NK cells are detectable in the fetal liver at 6 weeks of gestation. In term newborns, the number of circulating NK cells is similar or higher than in adults.[108] Newborn NK cells produce high levels of effector cytokines but have reduced cytotoxic responses to some viruses as compared to adult NK cells.[64]

Noncytotoxic ILCs are enriched at mucosal surfaces where they respond to signals provided by epithelial cells and myeloid cells following tissue damage or infection. ILC1s respond to similar signals and produce similar effector cytokines as NK cells and Th1 lymphocytes (see later) and could thereby contribute to the defense against intracellular bacteria.[109] ILC2s secrete IL-4, IL-5, and IL-13 in response to helminths and promote asthma and allergic inflammation.[110] ILC3s play an important role in the early defense against extracellular bacteria by producing IL-17 and IL-23, stimulating the production of antimicrobial peptides and promoting the integrity of mucosal barriers.[111] In addition to their role in antibacterial defense, ILCs also maintain immune homeostasis at mucosal surfaces by regulating inappropriate immune responses to commensal bacteria.[112,113] All three major subtypes of ILCs have been reported in the fetal liver, which is thought to be the primary site of ILC progenitors.[114] In mice, ILC development is influenced by the level of maternal retinoids, suggesting a link between maternal diet and bacterial defense in early life.[115,116]

In contrast to ILCs, several subsets of innate lymphocytes express rearranged T cell receptors. These include invariant NKT (iNKT) cells, mucosal-associated invariant T (MAIT) cells expressing invariant αβ T cell receptors, and T cells expressing semi-invariant γδ T cell receptors. iNKT cells recognize lipids derived from microbes, including bacteria, in the context of the MHC-class I-like CD1d molecule.[117] In humans, iNKT cells are abundant in the fetal thymus.[118] At birth, iNKT cells are able to produce inflammatory cytokines, including TNFα and IFNγ, and could thereby contribute to antimicrobial defense in the neonatal period.[119] MAIT cells are enriched at mucosal sites and recognize microbial riboflavin metabolites presented by the MHC-class I-like molecule MR1.[120] Functional MAIT cells can be detected in the mucosa of human fetuses, suggesting a role in antibacterial defense.[121]

γδ T cells develop early during human fetal life. At mid-gestation, the fetal γδ T cell repertoire is dominated by cells expressing a canonical Vγ9Vδ2 receptor recognizing intermediates of isoprenoid metabolism called *phosphoantigens*.[104,122] Phosphoantigens derived from microbes, including bacteria, are more potent activators of fetal and adult Vγ9Vδ2 T cells than host phosphoantigens, probably reflecting a mechanism of self, versus nonself, recognition.[104,123] On the other hand, a potent response of effector non-Vγ9Vδ2 T cells producing inflammatory cytokines, including TNFα and IFNγ, is detected in newborns infected in utero with cytomegalovirus, supporting the notion that, as observed in the mouse, γδ T cells play an important role in antimicrobial defense in early human life.[124]

Innate lymphocytes expressing rearranged B cell receptors include B1 cells and marginal zone (MZ) B cells. In the mouse, B1 cells are primarily located in the peritoneal cavity, whereas MZ B cells are found in the MZ of the spleen.[125,126] Innate B lymphocytes are programmed to produce the so-called natural antibodies, or Igs, independently of antigen stimulation, and to rapidly differentiate into antibody-secreting cells upon exposure to antigens without requiring the help of CD4 T lymphocytes. Antibodies produced by innate B lymphocytes are primarily of the IgM isotype and recognize polysaccharide and lipid antigens. Mouse studies indicate that natural antibodies play a critical role in antimicrobial defense.[127,128] Human B1 cells remain poorly characterized because of a lack of consensus on their markers. MZ B cells develop in the human fetus and undergo somatic hypermutations (see "αβ T Lymphocytes") of the IgM genes indicating a diversification of their repertoire in utero.[129] Children have a very low capacity to produce antibodies against polysaccharide antigens during the first 2 years of life, and this correlates with their susceptibility to encapsulated bacteria such as *Haemophilus influenzae* type b, pneumococcus, or meningococcus.[130] The fact that MZ B cells develop early during fetal life indicates that this reduced capacity is related to qualitative defects of this subset or of other cell types with which innate B cells interact.[64]

The early development of innate lymphocytes during fetal life indicates that the immune system of the human newborn is equipped with a number of effector cells that could contribute to the control of the pathogenic and commensal bacteria to which it will be exposed soon after birth. Recent studies demonstrated that innate lymphocytes maintain an effector cell program after their activation.[131] This process, called *trained immunity*, is analogous to the immunologic memory phenotype acquired by conventional T and B lymphocytes. The possibility that the innate effector lymphocytes activated by pathogens in early life could acquire a trained immunity phenotype and participate in the immune response to unrelated pathogens remains to be explored.[132]

ADAPTIVE IMMUNITY

The hallmarks of acquired, or adaptive, immunity are its specificity for structurally distinct antigens, the requirement of cell differentiation for the expression of mature effector functions, and the induction of memory following prior antigen exposure. Adaptive immune responses also involve the expansion of cells expressing T-cell receptors (TCRs) or B-cell receptors (BCRs) recognizing specific antigens that are present at low frequencies in the naïve T- and B-cell repertoires. Adaptive immune responses are the last to develop phylogenetically and the last to mature ontogenetically; they require close cooperation between cellular elements of the innate immune system and the αβ T and B lymphocytes. Adaptive immunity also interfaces with the evolutionarily more ancient nutritional immunity, in that the acquisition of effector functions by T lymphocytes involves a shift to aerobic glycolysis.[133]

αβ T LYMPHOCYTES

Conventional T lymphocytes express a TCR formed by an α and a β chain. αβ T lymphocytes are involved in the defense against all microbes, including bacteria. They develop in the thymus from bone marrow-derived progenitors and migrate as naïve cells in secondary lymphoid organs where they are stimulated by protein antigens presented by antigen-presenting cells. In the thymus, αβ T lymphocytes differentiate into either CD4 or CD8 T lymphocytes recognizing protein fragments, or peptides, presented in combination with MHC class II or MHC class I molecules, respectively. These two different pathways allow the presentation of peptides derived from proteins present in infected cells (MHC class I) or internalized by phagocytosis or endocytosis (MHC class II). Although naïve CD8 T cells have some functional plasticity, they primarily differentiate into cytotoxic cells when they are stimulated by antigen-presenting cells.[134] Therefore, they play a central role in the defense against intracellular pathogens. Naïve CD4, or helper, T cells have an important functional plasticity that allows them to express a variety of effector functions. As described for ILCs (see "Innate Lymphocytes"), several subsets of antigen-experienced CD4 T cells can be distinguished on the basis of the cytokines they produce.[135] The most relevant subsets to antibacterial defenses are T helper 1 (Th1) and Th17 cell lymphocytes, follicular helper T (TFH) cells, and Treg cells. Th1 cells produce a similar profile of cytokines to NK cells or ILC1s and promote immunity to intracellular pathogens. Th17 cells produce a similar profile of cytokines as ILC3s and promote immunity to extracellular pathogens.[136] TFH cells stimulate B lymphocytes and promote the production of diverse and high avidity antibodies against protein antigens that are therefore named T-dependent.[137] Treg cells control effector T-cell responses at multiple levels and prevent immunopathology. Natural Treg cells develop in the thymus, whereas induced Treg cells differentiate in the periphery following exposure to antigens.[138]

Mature αβ T lymphocytes can be detected in the fetus at around 14 weeks of gestation, several months later than a number of innate lymphocyte subsets.[64] During the second and third trimesters, αβ T cells diversify their TCR repertoire.[139] Natural Tregs develop in parallel with naïve T cells during fetal life.[64] Studies suggest that fetal Treg are preferentially induced by noninherited MHC molecules expressed by maternal cells crossing the placenta.[140] This process was proposed to be related to a specific program of fetal hematopoietic stem cells favoring the development of regulatory rather than effector immune responses.[141] In early human life, the majority of αβ T lymphocytes are recent thymic emigrants and have an increased turnover rate as compared to adult cells.[142] Newborns have a reduced capacity to develop Th1 type responses. This correlates with a limited capacity of newborn CD4 T cells to produce IFNγ and with a limited capacity of newborn antigen-presenting cells to produce cytokines promoting the differentiation of Th1 cells (see "Dendritic Cells").[135,143] However, this reduced capacity is not absolute, as newborns and young infants develop adult-type Th1 responses to BCG and whole cell pertussis vaccines and fetuses develop Th1 responses to CMV infection.[144] This indicates that the quality and magnitude of inflammatory signals present at the time of naïve CD4 T cell activation determine the development of immune responses against intracellular pathogens in early life. The profile of cytokines produced by newborn antigen-presenting cells, including IL-6 and IL-23 (see "Dendritic Cells"), suggest that newborns may be able to mount Th17 and TFH cells at similar or higher levels than adults, but this possibility remains to be investigated.[135] Recent studies suggest that some fetal αβ T lymphocytes can acquire a phenotype of memory cells programmed to produce Th1, Th2, or Th17 cytokines in utero.[145] Whether microbial antigens crossing the placenta contribute to the induction of these cells and whether they participate in the immune responses to microbes after birth remains to be explored.

B LYMPHOCYTES

Although B lymphocytes can exhibit a number of functions including cytokine production and immune regulation, their primary function is to produce antibodies. B lymphocytes develop in the bone marrow and migrate as immature B cells in secondary lymphoid organs where they are exposed to antigens. B cells recognizing polysaccharide or lipid antigens do not require T-cell help to produce antibodies (see "Innate Lymphocytes"). Adaptive B cells recognizing protein antigens function as antigen-presenting cells for CD4 T lymphocytes, and this interaction induces the formation of an organized structure, called the *germinal center*, where B cells acquire the capacity to produce high-quality antibodies. Soon after their activation, B cells produce IgM. The signals provided by CD4 T cells then promote a switch to the production of other isotypes, including IgG1 to 4, IgA or IgE, and the induction of somatic hypermutations, which favors the production of high-affinity antibodies. The early B-cell response induces the differentiation of short-lived antibody-secreting cells, or plasma cells. B-cell memory is formed by long-lived plasma cells spontaneously secreting antibodies in the bone marrow and by memory B cells differentiating into plasma cells upon re-encounter with their cognate antigen.

The heterogeneity of antibody isotypes allows the expression of different effector functions.[146] IgM complexed with antigens activates complement and thereby stimulates immune cells, including B lymphocytes during the early phase of their response. Complement activation by IgG is highest with IgG3 and lowest with IgG4. IgG subtypes also have different capacity to bind Fc receptors and thereby induce quantitatively different cellular responses. The binding to Fc receptors and thereby functional activity of IgG is also influenced by their level of glycosylation.[147] Recent studies indicate that the glycosylation profile of IgG dynamically evolves during childhood and suggest that aberrant glycosylation profiles may predispose to recurrent respiratory infections.[148] IgA antibodies are produced at the mucosal level and are transported across mucosal membranes by a secretory component to prevent invasion by pathogenic bacteria.[149] IgE antibodies bind to Fc receptors on mast cells and basophils and are primarily responsible for allergic reactions and for protection against parasites. IgD antibodies are expressed by naïve B cells. Their role in antimicrobial defense is not fully elucidated.[150]

Mature B lymphocytes can be detected in the fetal liver from 8 weeks' gestation.[64] Somatic hypermutation and isotype switch already occur in utero and favor the diversification of the B cell receptor repertoire before birth.[139] The capacity of the newborn to develop antibody responses appears to depend on the nature of the immune stimulus. Immunization schedules in low- and middle-income countries currently include the administration of hepatitis B and oral polio vaccines in newborns. Hepatitis B immunization induces at least equivalent antibody responses in newborns as compared to adults.[151] In contrast, antibody response to oral polio, measles and rubella vaccines increase with age at vaccination during infancy.[152] The mechanisms underlying this maturation of effector B lymphocyte responses remain unclear, but could involve a reduced expression of complement receptors and of T-cell co-stimulatory molecules by neonatal B lymphocytes or defective interactions between neonatal B and TFH cells.[152] Importantly, immunization at birth can induce potent memory B-cell responses. These memory B cells promote the response to booster immunizations and the induction of high titers of IgG against specific pathogens during the first months of life.[153]

MATERNAL ANTIBODIES

The time required to induce the production of high levels of high-quality antibodies by newborn B cells limits their impact on the control of pathogens during the first weeks after birth. This limitation is circumvented by the transfer of maternal antibodies during fetal life. As it is induced in the mother, the antigenic repertoire of maternal antibodies is adapted to the microbial antigens to which the newborn will be exposed. This principle is the basis for immunizing pregnant women against pathogens that their young infants will encounter.[154] Maternal immunization against tetanus and *Bordetella pertussis* has demonstrated high efficacy in protecting neonates and young infants. IgG, and not the other isotypes, are actively transported through the placenta by a receptor to the IgG Fc fragment, called the *neonatal Fc receptor (FcRn)*.[155] Serum concentrations of maternal IgG increase from mid-gestation until birth, when they can be higher than those of the mother. Higher levels of maternal antibodies are detected following immunization during the second as compared to the third trimester of pregnancy, a phenomenon likely related to the longer duration of transplacental transfer.[156] The efficiency of the transfer is highest for IgG1 and lowest for IgG2. As IgG2 is particularly involved in the recognition of polysaccharide antigens, the relatively low transfer of this isotype further limits immunity to encapsulated bacteria in early infancy.[157]

Recent studies demonstrated that maternal IgG transferred across the placenta is enriched in galactosylated isoforms with potent NK cell activation properties. This selective transfer probably involves the coordinated binding of maternal IgG to multiple Fc receptors expressed by placental cells.[158]

After birth, maternal antibodies are cleared and the levels of IgG progressively decrease, reaching a nadir around 3 to 4 months of age in term infants.[64] In premature infants, the reduced transfer of maternal antibodies probably plays an important role in the susceptibility to bacterial infections.[64] The transfer of maternal antibodies is also reduced by maternal HIV infection and by placental malaria.[159] Infants born to HIV-infected mothers, but who are themselves uninfected by the virus, are more susceptible to bacterial infections, including GBS.[160] Mechanisms are probably multifactorial and include decreased transfer of maternal antibodies, avoidance of breast-milk feeding, abnormal inflammatory responses, and colonization by virulent strains.[161] In parallel with their protective effect against infections during the first months of life, maternal antibodies also reduce antibody responses to vaccines in the young infants and thereby limit their capacity to rapidly develop their own antimicrobial immune responses.[162] Importantly, the induction of memory B- and T-cell responses to vaccines is much less affected by maternal antibodies, allowing the priming to booster immunization. Recent studies in mice demonstrated that maternal antibodies do not prevent activation of infant B cells but rather interfere with optimal germinal center reactions.[163]

Breastfeeding

Breastfeeding represents a second important process increasing immune defenses in the neonate. Breast milk contains maternal antibodies, including IgG and IgA, as well as maternal immune cells, including memory B cells and plasmablasts and a large number of other molecules with immunologic properties.[164,165] Maternal immunization against *S. pneumonia*, *Neisseria meningitis*, and *B. pertussis* is associated with high concentration of sIgA and IgG in breast milk of immunized mothers.[166] While studies suggest a protective role of anti-GBS sIgA and IgG against GBS colonization and disease,[167] and breast-feeding overall has a clear impact on the control of microbial pathogens and on the development of the infant immune system, the role of the individual components of breast milk and in particular of antibodies is not clearly established.[157]

A complete reference list is available at www.ExpertConsult.com. 

SELECT REFERENCES

1. Shane AL, Stoll BJ. Neonatal sepsis: progress towards improved outcomes. *J Infect*. 2014;68(suppl 1):S24-32.
2. Santos RP, Tristram D. A practical guide to the diagnosis, treatment, and prevention of neonatal infections. *Pediatr Clin North Am*. 2015;62:491-508.
3. Marchant EA, Boyce GK, Sadarangani M, et al. Neonatal sepsis due to coagulase-negative staphylococci. *Clin Dev Immunol*. 2013:586076.
4. Saha SK, Schrag SJ, El Arifeen S, et al. Causes and incidence of community-acquired serious infections among young children in south Asia (ANISA): an observational cohort study. *Lancet*. 2018;392:145-159.
5. Velaphi SC, Westercamp M, Moleleki M, et al. Surveillance for incidence and etiology of early-onset neonatal sepsis in Soweto, South Africa. *PLoS One*. 2019;14:e0214077.
6. Simonsen KA, Anderson-Berry AL, Delair SF, et al. Early-onset neonatal sepsis. *Clin Microbiol Rev*. 2014;27:21-47.
7. Hamer DH, Darmstadt GL, Carlin JB, et al. Etiology of bacteremia in young infants in six countries. *Pediatr Infect Dis J*. 2015;34:e1-8.
8. Zaidi AK, Thaver D, Ali SA, et al. Pathogens associated with sepsis in newborns and young infants in developing countries. *Pediatr Infect Dis J*. 2009;28:S10-18.
9. Murray CJ, Vos T, Lozano R, et al. Disability-adjusted life years (DALYs) for 291 diseases and injuries in 21 regions, 1990-2010: a systematic analysis for the Global Burden of Disease Study 2010. *Lancet*. 2012;380:2197-2223.
10. Muley VA, Ghadage DP, Bhore AV. Bacteriological profile of neonatal septicemia in a tertiary care hospital from western India. *J Glob Infect Dis*. 2015;7:75-77.
11. Okomo U, Akpalu ENK, Le Doare K, et al. Aetiology of invasive bacterial infection and antimicrobial resistance in neonates in sub-Saharan Africa: a systematic review and meta-analysis in line with the STROBE-NI reporting guidelines. *Lancet Infect Dis*. 2019;19:1219-1234.
12. Melamed A, Sorvillo FJ. The burden of sepsis-associated mortality in the United States from 1999 to 2005: an analysis of multiple-cause-of-death data. *Crit Care*. 2009;13:R28.
13. Sweeney EL, Dando SJ, Kallapur SG, et al. The human ureaplasma species as causative agents of chorioamnionitis. *Clin Microbiol Rev*. 2017;30:349-379.
14. Payne MS, Ireland DJ, Watts R, et al. *Ureaplasma parvum* genotype, combined vaginal colonisation with *Candida albicans*, and spontaneous preterm birth in an Australian cohort of pregnant women. *BMC Pregnancy Childbirth*. 2016;16:312.
15. Senthamaraikannan P, Presicce P, Rueda CM, et al. Intra-amniotic *Ureaplasma parvum*-induced maternal and fetal inflammation and immune responses in *Rhesus* macaques. *J Infect Dis*. 2016;214:1597-1604.
16. Sweeney EL, Kallapur SG, Meawad S, et al. Ureaplasma species multiple banded antigen (mba) variation is associated with the severity of inflammation in vivo and in vitro in human placentae. *Front Cell Infect Microbiol*. 2017;7:123.
17. Bengoechea JA, Sa Pessoa J. *Klebsiella pneumoniae* infection biology: living to counteract host defences. *FEMS Microbiol Rev*. 2019;43:123-144.

18. Johnson J, Quach C. Outbreaks in the neonatal ICU: a review of the literature. *CurrOpin Infect Dis*. 2017;30:395-403.
19. Soto SM, Bosch J, Jimenez de Anta MT, et al. Comparative study of virulence traits of *Escherichia coli* clinical isolates causing early and late neonatal sepsis. *J Clin Microbiol*. 2008;46:1123-1125.
20. Vila J, Saez-Lopez E, Johnson JR, et al. Escherichia coli: an old friend with new tidings. *FEMS Microbiol Rev*. 2016;40:437-463.
21. Kim KS. Current concepts on the pathogenesis of Escherichia coli meningitis: implications for therapy and prevention. *CurrOpin Infect Dis*. 2012;25:273-278.
22. Mittal R, Prasadarao NV. Outer membrane protein A expression in *Escherichia coli* K1 is required to prevent the maturation of myeloid dendritic cells and the induction of IL-10 and TGF-beta. *J Immunol*. 2008;181:2672-2682.
23. Mittal R, Krishnan S, Gonzalez-Gomez I, et al. Deciphering the roles of outer membrane protein A extracellular loops in the pathogenesis of Escherichia coli K1 meningitis. *J Biol Chem*. 2011;286:2183-2193.
24. Landwehr-Kenzel S, Henneke P. Interaction of Streptococcus agalactiae and cellular innate immunity in colonization and disease. *Front Immunol*. 2014;5:519.
25. Uchiyama S, Sun J, Fukahori K, et al. Dual actions of group B *Streptococcus* capsular sialic acid provide resistance to platelet-mediated antimicrobial killing. *Proc Natl Acad Sci U S A*. 2019;116:7465-7470.
26. Chang YC, Olson J, Beasley FC, et al. Group B *Streptococcus* engages an inhibitory Siglec through sialic acid mimicry to blunt innate immune and inflammatory responses *in vivo*. *PLoSPathog*. 2014;10:e1003846.
27. Power Coombs MR, Kronforst K, Levy O. Neonatal host defense against Staphylococcal infections. *Clin Dev Immunol*. 2013:826303.
28. Dong Y, Speer CP, Glaser K. Beyond sepsis: Staphylococcus epidermidis is an underestimated but significant contributor to neonatal morbidity. *Virulence*. 2018;9:621-633.
29. Sonnen AF, Henneke P. Role of pore-forming toxins in neonatal sepsis. *Clin Dev Immunol*. 2013:608456.
30. Randow F, MacMicking JD, James LC. Cellular self-defense: how cell-autonomous immunity protects against pathogens. *Science*. 2013;340:701-706.
31. Huang S, Meng Q, Maminska A, et al. Cell-autonomous immunity by IFN-induced GBPs in animals and plants. *CurrOpin Immunol*. 2019;60:71-80.
32. Johannes L, Jacob R, Leffler H. Galectins at a glance. *J Cell Sci*. 2018;131:jcs208884.
33. Tamai R, Kobayashi-Sakamoto M, Kiyoura Y. Extracellular galectin-1 enhances adhesion to and invasion of oral epithelial cells by Porphyromonas gingivalis. *Can J Microbiol*. 2018;64:465-471.
34. Nita-Lazar M, Banerjee A, Feng C, et al. Galectins regulate the inflammatory response in airway epithelial cells exposed to microbial neuraminidase by modulating the expression of SOCS1 and RIG1. *Mol Immunol*. 2015;68:194-202.
35. Lujan AL, Croci DO, GambarteTudela JA, et al. Glycosylation-dependent galectin-receptor interactions promote Chlamydia trachomatis infection. *Proc Natl Acad Sci U S A*. 2018;115:E6000-E6009.
36. Beisel WR. History of nutritional immunology: introduction and overview. *J Nutr*. 1992;122:591-596.
37. Hood MI, Skaar EP. Nutritional immunity: transition metals at the pathogen-host interface. *Nat Rev Microbiol*. 2012;10:525-537.
38. Recalcati S, Locati M, Cairo G. Systemic and cellular consequences of macrophage control of iron metabolism. *Semin Immunol*. 2012;24:393-398.
39. Bullen J, Griffiths E, Rogers H, et al. Sepsis: the critical role of iron. *Microbes Infect*. 2000;2:409-415.
40. Sturgeon P. Studies of iron requirements in infante and children. I. Normal values for serum iron, copper and free erythrocyte protoporphyrin. *Pediatrics*. 1954;13:107-125.
41. Szabo M, Vasarhelyi B, Balla G, et al. Acute postnatal increase of extracellular antioxidant defence of neonates: the role of iron metabolism. *Acta Paediatr*. 2001;90:1167-1170.
42. Hay G, Refsum H, Whitelaw A, et al. Predictors of serum ferritin and serum soluble transferrin receptor in newborns and their associations with iron status during the first 2 y of life. *Am J Clin Nutr*. 2007;86:64-73.
43. Wander K, Shell-Duncan B, McDade TW. Evaluation of iron deficiency as a nutritional adaptation to infectious disease: an evolutionary medicine perspective. *Am J Hum Biol*. 2009;21:172-179.
44. Nairz M, Haschka D, Demetz E, et al. Iron at the interface of immunity and infection. *Front Pharmacol*. 2014;5:152.
45. Johnson EE, Wessling-Resnick M. Iron metabolism and the innate immune response to infection. *Microbes Infect*. 2012;14:207-216.
46. Oppenheimer S. Iron and infection: narrative review of a major iron supplementation study in Papua New Guinea undertaken by the Department of Tropical Paediatrics, Liverpool School of Tropical Medicine, 1979-1983, its aftermath and the continuing relevance of its results. *Paediatr Int Child Health*. 2012;32(suppl 2):S21-29.
47. Roth AE, Benn CS, Ravn H, et al. Effect of revaccination with BCG in early childhood on mortality: randomised trial in Guinea-Bissau. *BMJ*. 2010;340:c671.
48. Sazawal S, Black RE, Ramsan M, et al. Effects of routine prophylactic supplementation with iron and folic acid on admission to hospital and mortality in preschool children in a high malaria transmission setting: community-based, randomised, placebo-controlled trial. *Lancet*. 2006;367:133-143.
49. Oppenheimer SJ. Iron and its relation to immunity and infectious disease. *J Nutr*. 2001;131:616S-633S; discussion 633S-635S.
50. Hennigar SR, McClung JP. Nutritional immunity: starving pathogens of trace minerals. *Am J Lifestyle Med*. 2016;10:170-173.

Host Defense Mechanisms Against Fungi 114

Melinda Erdős | László Maródi

INTRODUCTION

Fungal infections are commonly classified as either endemic or opportunistic.[1] An endemic fungal infection may occur in any individual living in a geographic area that is the natural habitat of that fungus. Histoplasmosis, coccidioidomycosis, and blastomycosis, which are usually acquired by inhalation, are examples.Although exposure to *endemic* fungi might be possible in the newborn period, it is unlikely under normal circumstances. Therefore we do not discuss mechanisms of resisting these organisms but rather focus on resistance to *opportunistic* fungi.

Opportunistic fungal infections occur primarily in immunocompromised individuals. Extensive investigation of host defense mechanisms in the immunocompromised newborn has indicated that multiple systems are partially blunted, and it is probably this combination of partial deficiencies that places the newborn at risk.[2] Among the opportunistic fungi, *Candida* species stand out as particularly threatening to the neonate, especially the extremely low-birth-weight infant.[3,4] Although our understanding of how the host resists fungal infection is incomplete, host-*Candida* interactions have been relatively well studied. For these reasons, this chapter focuses primarily on *Candida* and the mechanisms of host defense against candidal infections.

Perineal and oral thrush caused by *Candida* species is common in otherwise normal neonates. In neonatal intensive care units, all newborns are at risk for more serious invasive candidal disease, even those with birth weights above 2500 g.[5] *Candida albicans* remains the most common fungal species isolated in neonatal surveillance cultures and the most common cause of neonatal candidiasis, but non-*albicans* species such as *C. parapsilosis* and *C. glabrata* are also frequent causes of invasive neonatal infection, especially in low-birth-weight infants.[6] The frequency of serious candidal disease in newborns at present may be attributed to technical improvements in medical practices and intensive care measures on a backdrop of the newborn's blunted capacity to fight infection.[2,7] The prominence of neonatal candidal infections and the difficulties posed by the diagnosis and treatment of invasive candidiasis emphasize the importance of acquiring a better understanding of the mechanisms by which this species causes neonatal infection.

This chapter begins with a discussion of antifungal defense mechanisms thought to be active at body surfaces and how these may be related to mucocutaneous candidiasis; this is followed by a review of those mechanisms that are expected to defend the newborn against invasive candidal infection. In discussing both mucocutaneous and invasive forms of candidiasis, we use the experience of individuals with primary or acquired immunodeficiency diseases with fungal

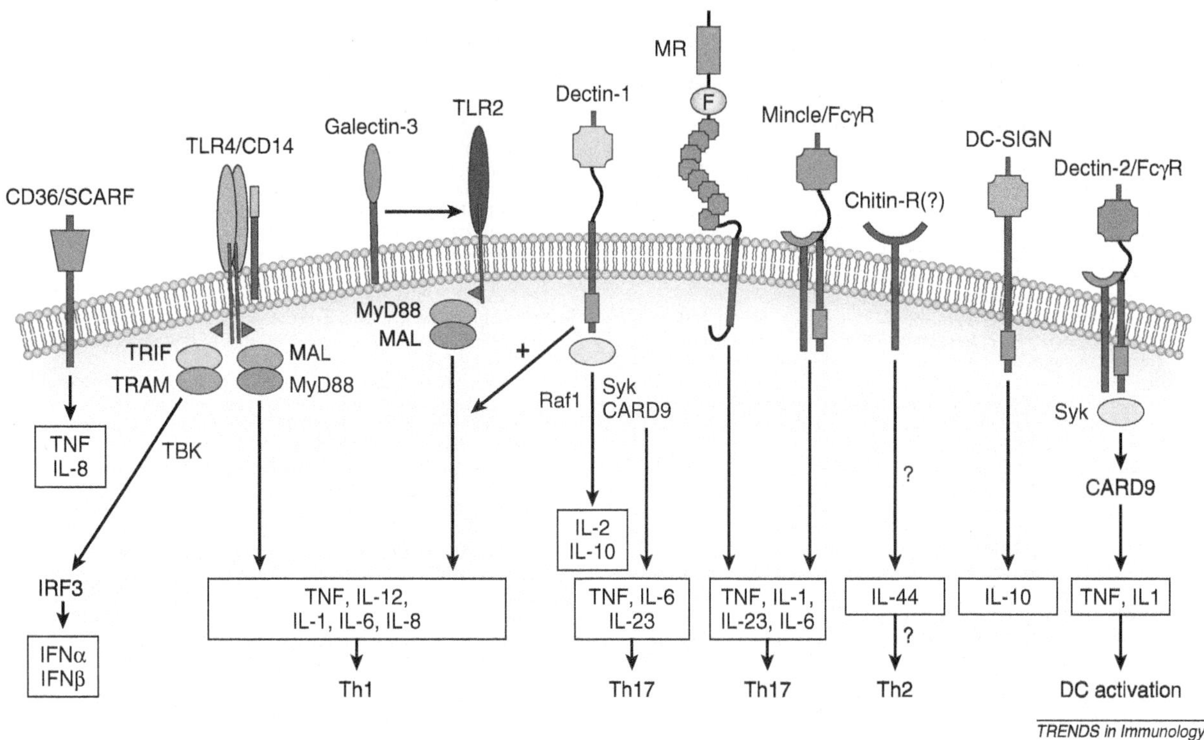

Fig. 114.1 Pattern recognition receptors sensing *Candida albicans* at the membrane level. Recognition of *C. albicans* is mediated by TLRs and lectin receptors. Both TLR4 and TLR2 can induce proinflammatory signals in monocytic cell types (monocytes, macrophages, and DCs) through the MyD88 and Mal-mediated pathways, as well as the TRIF pathway to initiate Th1 responses. The assembly of signaling complexes requires the activation of protein kinases (IRAK4, TRAF6, and TAK1). A second downstream effect of TLR4 signaling involves TRIF and TRAM adapter proteins that activate TBK1 and the IRF3 transcription factor required for the expression of type I interferon genes. TLR2 binding stimulates strong IL-10 and TGFβ and induces proliferation of regulatory T cells and immunosuppression but is also able to induce proinflammatory cytokines such as tumor necrosis factor (TNF) or IL-6. However, through an Erk and c-Fos-dependent pathway, TLR2 is also able to inhibit IL-12 synthesis and Th1 responses. The proinflammatory effects of TLR2 can be amplified by dectin-1 and Galectin-3. In addition to the amplification of TLR2 effects, the lectin-like receptor dectin-1 induces IL-2, IL-10, and Th17 responses through a Syk/CARD9 cascade, independent of its interaction with TLR2. The classical lectin-like receptor MR induces proinflammatory effects in monocytes and macrophages, whereas chitin-dependent stimulation induces mainly Th2 responses, although this effect still has to be demonstrated for *C. albicans* and the identity of its receptor is unknown. Other less well characterized pathways include stimulation of inflammatory cytokine release by dectin-2, Mincle, and CD36/SCARF lectin receptors, and of the immunosuppressive cytokine IL-10 by DC-SIGN in dendritic cells. *DC-SIGN*, DC-specific intracellular adhesion molecule-grabbing non-integrin; *IFN*, interferon; *IL*, interleukin; *IRAK*, interleukin-1 receptor-associated kinase; *IRF*, interferon response factor; *MAL*, MyD88 adapter-like; *MR*, mannose receptor; *Syk*, T-cell lineage-specific tyrosine kinase; *TAK*, tumor growth factor (TGF) β-activated kinase; *TBK*, TRAF family member-associated NF-κB activator-binding kinase; *Th*, T-helper cell; *TLR*, toll-like receptor; *TRAF*, TNF receptor-associated factor; *TRAM*, TRIF-related adapter molecule; *TRIF*, Toll–interleukin-1 receptor domain-containing adapter inducing interferon β. (From Netea MG, Maródi L: Innate immune mechanisms for recognition and uptake of *Candida* species. *Trends Immunol* 31:346–353, 2010)

infections as a guide to understanding basic host-fungal interactions and how these might be expressed in the newborn.

The first step in mounting a protective immune response is recognition of the fungal pathogen by cell surface receptors, which are located on professional phagocytes (granulocytes, monocytes/macrophages) and dendritic cells as well as non-immune cells (Fig. 114.1; reviewed by Szolnoky et al.[36]). In tissue macrophages and blood-derived monocytes cultured in vitro under specific experimental conditions, the macrophage mannose receptors appear to play a key role in sensing mannose-containing surface molecules on Candida (Fig. 114.2; see Maródi et al.[32]).

DEFENSE AGAINST MUCOCUTANEOUS CANDIDIASIS

CANDIDA VIRULENCE FACTORS AND SURFACE HOST DEFENSE

Candida species cause a broad range of infections involving the skin and mucous membranes.[8,9] *C. albicans* is part of the common commensal microbial flora of the oral cavity and the gastrointestinal and genitourinary tracts of healthy humans. Candidal vulvovaginitis occurs commonly in most women during pregnancy, and the body surfaces of newborns are colonized at birth. Overgrowth of these colonizing *Candida* species may lead to mucosal or cutaneous candidiasis, characterized by local signs of infection and, in the mouth, visible white patches.

Transformation from the yeast phase to the filamentous form (with pseudohyphae, hyphae, and germ tubes) appears to be essential for candidal pathogenicity.[10] Adhesins on blastospores and hyphae of *C. albicans*, like integrins on human leukocytes, can recognize arginine-glycine-aspartic acid (RGD) sequences on epithelial cells and several extracellular matrix proteins.[11] The *Candida* gene *INT1* encodes an adhesin, INT1p, that recognizes the RGD-containing proteins and promotes the growth of filaments. This candidal adhesin is homologous to mammalian integrins and itself contains an RGD site that may be recognized by integrins on human cells, further facilitating the adhesion of *Candida* to the cell surface.[11] These findings provide at least a

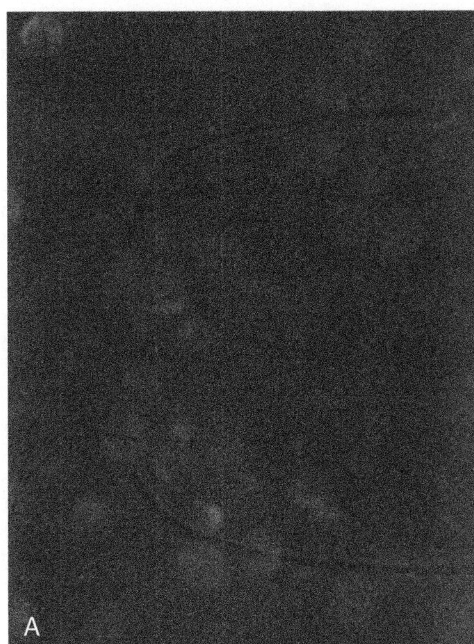

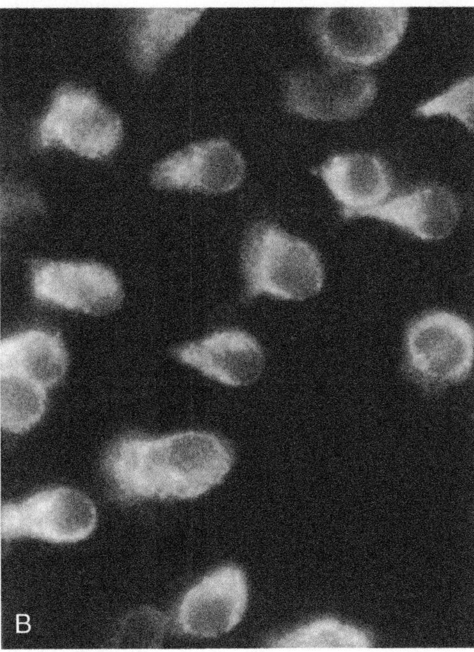

Fig. 114.2 Mannose receptor (MR) expression on blood monocytes (MO; A) and monocyte-derived macrophages (MDM; B). In an indirect immunofluorescence assay MDMs, in contrast with MOs, were shown to express clearly detectable MR expression after treatment with rabbit anti-human MR.

partial explanation for the symbiosis of *Candida* with humans and the tropism of these fungi to intestinal and mucosal epithelium.

On the host side, secretory antibodies—especially of the immunoglobulin (Ig) A class, mucous layer, and cilia—act to prevent adhesion to mucosal surfaces; in addition, a variety of antimicrobial peptides protect the skin and mucosae. These have the potential to prevent the penetration of commensal fungi such as *Candida*. Isolation of peptides with broad and potent antimicrobial properties from frog skin—the magainins—proved the principle.[12] These cationic peptides bind to anionic components of the microbial membrane and form pores that permeabilize the cell. Two major classes of cationic antimicrobial polypeptides have been described in human skin and epithelia, the β-defensins, and the cathelicidins.[12] Both can kill fungi. An additional peptide, dermcidin, which is secreted in sweat, can also kill fungi.[13] Nasal and lung secretions contain the antimicrobial polypeptide constituents lysozyme, lactoferrin, and secretory leukoprotease inhibitor as well as neutrophil and epithelial defensins.[14] The precise role of these proteins in defense against fungal (or any) infection is not yet fully defined. However, in the familial disorder Kostmann congenital neutropenia, patients' neutrophils are markedly deficient in antimicrobial peptides.[15] Normalizing neutrophil counts by treatment with colony-stimulating factor prevents systemic infections, but destructive periodontitis continues until the patient's neutrophils are replaced with normal myeloid cells through bone marrow transplantation.[15]

LESSONS FROM PRIMARY AND ACQUIRED IMMUNODEFICIENCY DISORDERS

The blunting of T cell-mediated immunity in newborns, even those born at full term, may play a part in the frequent mucocutaneous candidal infections seen in this age group. Persistent mucosal candidiasis and oropharyngeal thrush are common complications of primary T-cell deficiencies such as DiGeorge syndrome and severe combined immunodeficiency disease. Patients with autoimmune polyendocrinopathy-candidiasis-ectodermal dystrophy (APECED) syndrome and hyper-IgE syndrome, both of which are characterized by subtle defects in T lymphocytes, may have protracted candidal infections of the mucous membranes, nails, and skin.[16] These patients, however, are no more susceptible to life-threatening, generalized candidiasis than immunocompetent individuals. The specific susceptibility to the chronic mucocutaneous candidiasis (CMC) of APECED patients may be related to the production of neutralizing antibodies against interleukin (IL)-17-type cytokines, in particular, anti-IL-17A.[8]

Over the past decade, several primary immunodeficiency diseases characterized by CMC have been identified, including IL-12Rβ1 and IL-12p40 deficiencies, mutations in the gene encoding signal transducer and activator of transcription (STAT)-1, tyrosine kinase (TYK)-2 deficiency, and caspase recruitment domain (CARD)-9 deficiency.[8] CMC in these disorders and in APECED occurs in combination with other clinical defects. However, CMC may occur in isolation in patients with the gain-of-function *STAT-1* mutation, IL-17F cytokine and IL-17RA receptor deficiencies, and ACT1 deficiency.[9] Each of these genetic disorders may be associated with the impaired development or functioning of IL-17-producing T lymphocytes, suggesting a role for these cells and cytokines in defense against CMC.

Esophageal candidiasis is one of the diagnostic criteria of acquired immunodeficiency syndrome (AIDS). Oral and gastrointestinal candidiasis is a common manifestation of AIDS, presumably as a consequence of defective T cell-mediated host defense.[17] An adequate number of normally functioning T cells is required for the development of a secretory immune response to *Candida*, and T cells play an essential role in stimulating differentiation of IgA$^+$ B lymphocytes into plasma cells that produce secretory IgA.

Taken together, these observations support the concept that partial or selective T-cell deficiency is responsible for the development of mucosal candidiasis in a variety of conditions, including CMC, secretory IgA deficiency, AIDS, and the newborn. This concept is further supported by the observation in mice that recovery from oropharyngeal infection with *C. albicans* depends largely on CD4$^+$ T-cell augmentation of monocyte and neutrophil functions through the release of Th1-type cytokines (e.g., IL-12, and interferon [IFN]-γ). Fig. 114.3 indicates the primary role of T cell-mediated immunity in host defense against mucosal candidiasis in patients with primary deficiencies of T-cell immunity.

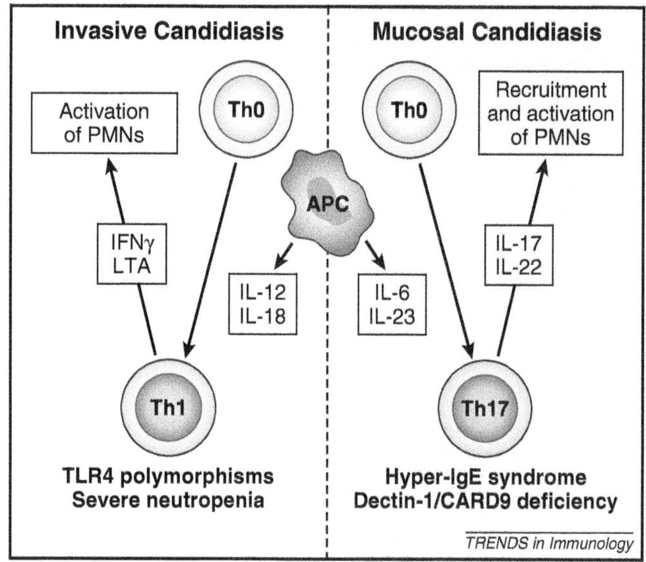

Fig. 114.3 Genetic susceptibility to fungal infections. Host defense against invasive and mucosal infections relies on the proper accumulation and function of neutrophils. However, an important difference appears to be present in terms of T-helper *(Th)* cell population responsible for activation of neutrophils in invasive candidiasis or mucosal candidiasis. In the case of systemic infection, the release of interferon-γ *(IFNγ)* and lymphotoxin-α *(LTA)* from Th1 cells is responsible for activation of the antifungal properties of neutrophils and macrophages in the deep tissues. During infection of the mucosa, the release of interleukin *(IL)*-17 and IL-22 from specific Th17 lymphocytes recruits and activates neutrophils for the elimination of infection. Importantly, IL-22 participates in host defense also through stimulation of the production of defensins by epithelial cells. Variability of the activation of the immune pathways can lead to an increased susceptibility to infection. TLR4 is an important PPR driving Th1 responses, and an increased susceptibility to invasive candidiasis is seen in patients with functional TLR4 polymorphisms. Defects of IL-17 production such as that in patients with hyper-immunoglobulin E (IgE) syndrome or dectin-1/CARD9-deficiency are associated with an increased susceptibility to mucosal forms of Candida infections. *APC*, Antigen-presenting cell; *PMN*, polymorphonuclear neutrophil; *TLR*, toll-like receptor. (From Netea MG, Maródi L: Innate immune mechanisms for recognition and uptake of Candida species. *Trends Immunol* 31:346–353, 2010.)

DEFICIENT T CELL–MEDIATED IMMUNITY IN NEWBORNS

Neonatal T-cell responses are compromised at several steps, including deficient production of cytokines by CD4+ T cells. Deficient IFN-γ production by neonatal T cells has been well documented[18] and may be attributed to lymphocyte immaturity with decreased production of IL-12 by cord blood-mixed mononuclear cells and dendritic cells.[19] This apparent downregulation of Th1 responses in human neonates,[20] including impaired IL-17+ T helper-cell differentiation and function, may play a part in the developmental immaturity of the immune system on mucosal surfaces and the susceptibility of newborns to candidiasis.

DEFENSE AGAINST INVASIVE CANDIDIASIS

Invasive candidal disease may arise from translocation of the gut flora and may be propagated by the ability of *Candida* to adhere to nonbiologic materials such as intravenous catheters.[21] Electron microscopy has shown that *Candida* can burrow into the catheter and form a surrounding biofilm. The use of heparin to prevent blood clot formation in newborns with intravascular catheters may accidentally promote invasive candidal disease. It has been proposed that heparin might facilitate the cleavage of the *C. albicans* surface adhesion protein INT1p, with release of the fungi from the catheter and generation of a cleavage product that stimulates release of inflammatory cytokines.[22]

Once in the bloodstream, *Candida* are able to adhere to the vascular endothelium. Adherence of *C. albicans* exceeds that of less virulent species, and germinated *C. albicans* adheres better than do yeast-phase organisms. INT1p appears to play an essential role in both adhesion and development of filamentous forms.[11] In mice, administration of broad-spectrum antibiotics and glucocorticoids, known risk factors for disseminated candidiasis in newborns,[7] accentuated the pathogenesis of *C. albicans* infection through an INT1p-influenced mechanism.[23]

Pulmonary surfactant protein-D (SP-D) has been implicated in host defense against *C. albicans* in pulmonary alveoli.[24] SP-D may facilitate mucociliary clearance by agglutinating *C. albicans* into large complexes and by decreasing hyphal outgrowth. Decreased concentration of SP-D in surfactant-deficient neonates or alteration in its levels because of lung disease and mechanical ventilation could disrupt local host defense and contribute to the development of pulmonary candidal infection.

Pseudomonas aeruginosa can form a dense biofilm on *C. albicans* filaments and kill the fungi.[25] This example of a bacterial antifungal-suppressive mechanism emphasizes the risk for dectin-1infection posed by giving broad-spectrum antibiotic therapy to a neonate.[7]

ROLE OF PHAGOCYTES IN PROTECTION AGAINST INVASIVE CANDIDIASIS

In contrast to the importance of T cell–mediated adaptive immunity in protecting against mucocutaneous candidiasis, the innate immune system, particularly phagocytic cells, plays the key role in eliminating *Candida* that have entered the bloodstream and reached tissues.[26,27] Neutropenia from any cause and genetic defects of phagocytic activity, as experiments of nature, have illustrated this essential function. Patients with chronic granulomatous disease, whose phagocytes cannot convert oxygen to toxic oxidants as well as patients with primary or secondary neutropenia have an increased susceptibility to invasive infections by *C. albicans* and other fungi. This predisposition exists in the absence of antibiotic or corticosteroid therapy, depressed cell-mediated immunity, or intravenous lines.[28]

A few individuals with diabetes mellitus and complete deficiency of neutrophil myeloperoxidase (MPO), which combines with hydrogen peroxide to generate microbicidal oxidants, have developed systemic candidiasis,[29] and neutrophils from patients with MPO deficiency have an impaired ability to kill ingested *C. albicans*. An important role for MPO-derived oxidants in the killing of *Candida* is supported by the in vitro findings that MPO-rich human monocytes killed *C. albicans* significantly better than monocyte-derived macrophages, which have little MPO,[30] and that recombinant human MPO significantly enhanced the killing of *C. albicans* by macrophages in a concentration-dependent manner.[31] Relative resistance to MPO-derived oxidants appears to explain at least partially the greater pathogenicity of *C. albicans* compared with other *Candida* species.[30,32]

In vitro studies have suggested that antibody-mediated immunity can protect against invasive candidal disease.[33,34] Optimal phagocytosis of *Candida* species by human mononuclear phagocytes requires opsonization by human serum, which supports this hypothesis.[32] However, no clinical observation suggests that patients with immunodeficiency disorders other than quantitative or functional phagocytic cell defects have increased susceptibility to invasive candidiasis. It is notable that patients with X-linked agammaglobulinemia or other severe hypogammaglobulinemias do not exhibit an increased susceptibility to either mucocutaneous or invasive candidal infections.

In patients with hypogammaglobulinemia, T cells, natural killer cells, and antimicrobial peptides may suppress *Candida* at the surface. In addition, macrophages and keratinocytes, which phagocytize and kill candidal yeasts through the mannose receptor,[32,35,36] might protect without the need for antibody opsonization. Mouse macrophages can mediate nonopsonic recognition of *C. albicans* and consequent release of cytokines through a complex of Toll-like receptor (TLR)-2 and dectin-1. The latter is a phagocytic receptor that functions as a transmembrane pattern-recognition receptor. It binds to the fungal-derived β-glucan, which comprises an inner skeletal layer of the candidal cell wall.[37] *C. albicans* cell-wall mannan can mediate binding to macrophages and release of cytokines through TLR-4 and its MyD88-dependent signaling pathway as well as through the mannose receptor.[38] Neonatal monocytes and mononuclear leukocytes have been reported to have blunted TLR-4 responses to endotoxin and decreased MyD88 levels.[39,40] Furthermore, cord blood mononuclear cells produced significantly less IFN-γ, IL-12, and IL-18 than adult cells following exposure to group B streptococci.[41] These abnormalities would be expected to predispose newborns to disseminated candidiasis.

DEFICIENT ANTICANDIDAL ACTIVITIES OF NEONATAL MONOCYTES AND MACROPHAGES

The extent of phagocytosis and killing of serum-opsonized *Candida* by resident monocytes and monocyte-derived macrophages has been reported to be comparable in newborns and adults.[41] In the absence of serum, ingestion and killing by cord and adult cells were reduced by half but were still equivalent. Mannan inhibited ingestion of unopsonized *Candida* by macrophages in a concentration-dependent manner, indicating a role for the mannose receptor. However, exposure of cord and adult macrophages to IFN-γ gave quantitatively different results in *Candida* killing as well as in release of superoxide anion. Maximal increase in these functions with adult macrophages was achieved with 100 U/mL IFN-γ. No enhancement with cord macrophages could be detected after treatment with 100 U/mL, and 500 U/mL of IFN-γ; killing and superoxide release by cord macrophages were still significantly lower compared with adult cells.[41] A similar blunted response of cord macrophages to IFN-γ-induced activation and increased killing was found by using group B streptococci as the target organism.[42] It is noteworthy that the number and binding capacity of IFN-γ receptors were greater on newborn than adult mononuclear phagocytes.[41] These data suggest that neonatal macrophages have a normal baseline capacity to ingest and kill both opsonized and unopsonized *Candida* but cannot be fully activated by IFN-γ, a finding that could not be attributed to lower expression of IFN-γ receptors on neonatal cells.[41]

What is the mechanism for the decreased activation of cord macrophages by IFN-γ? In response to IFN-γ, phosphorylation of STAT-1 was significantly decreased in neonatal monocytes and macrophages.[43] The STAT family are a group of key signaling molecules linking cytokine binding to the macrophage proinflammatory responses. These proteins are phosphorylated by Janus kinases that are activated by the binding of IFN-γ to its receptors. Expression of STAT-1 protein was equivalent in cord and adult monocytes and macrophages, but STAT-1 phosphorylation was deficient in cord cells.[43] Thus defective signal transduction might explain the decreased capacity of cord macrophages to activation by IFN-γ, but further experimentation is needed.

Candida have evolved a variety of mechanisms to evade innate immune phagocytic killing by macrophages. These include a thick glycoprotein cell wall composed of mannoprotein and covalently linked chitin-glucan components that resist degradation by lysosomal enzymes.[44] Phagocytosis of *C. albicans* by mouse macrophages reportedly induces rapid fusion of the phagolysosome membrane with late endosomes and lysosomes.[45] The ensuing phagolysosome acidification promotes germ tube formation, distention of the phagocyte's membranes, and eventual escape of the organism.

Ingestion of *Candida* by macrophages can induce genes of the organism's glyoxylate cycle, an important upregulation of the organism's metabolism shown to promote candidal virulence.[46] In *C. albicans* isolated from macrophage phagolysosomes, the principal enzymes of the glyoxylate cycle, isocitrate lyase and malate synthase, were upregulated. *C. albicans* mutants lacking isocitrate lyase were markedly less virulent in mice than wild-type *Candida*.[46] These findings illustrate the complexity of the host-parasite interactions that have the potential to influence the outcome of invasive candidal disease in the newborn infant.

CONCLUSION

Newborns, especially those born very prematurely, are at serious risk for fungal infections, most often those due to *C. albicans*. In an immunocompromised individual, candidal infections of the skin and mucous membranes can become chronic, and *Candida* can invade the bloodstream and tissues. Newborns are immunocompromised even at term. The younger the gestational age at birth, the greater of immunocompromise and the more likely that advanced life-saving practices will be needed. The necessary use of intravenous lines and antibiotics will then greatly increase the risk of invasive candidiasis. We have reviewed candidal virulence factors and the antifungal defense mechanisms active at body surfaces (T-cell–dependent adaptive immunity and antimicrobial peptides) and those most active against candidal invasion (innate defenses mediated by neutrophils, mononuclear phagocytes, and dendritic cells). Much of our understanding of the host defense mechanisms relevant to candidal infections derives from study of the experiments of nature represented by certain genetic immunodeficiency diseases. The basic premise underlying this review has been the hope that we might stimulate the research needed to better protect newborn infants from serious surface or life-threatening invasive candidal disease.

ACKNOWLEDGMENTS

The authors wish to thank Richard B. Johnston, Jr., MD, PhD, who remarkably contributed to this chapter in previous editions of *Fetal and Neonatal Physiology*.

SELECT REFERENCES

1. Pfaller MA. Epidemiology and control of fungal infections. *Clin Infect Dis*. 1994;19(suppl 1):S8–13.
2. Maródi L. Innate cellular immune responses in newborns. *Clin Immunol*. 2006;118:137–144.
3. Baley JE, Kleigman R, Fanaroff A. Disseminated fungal infections in very low-birth-weight infants: clinical manifestations and epidemiology. *Pediatrics*. 1984;73:144–152.
4. Aliaga S, Clark RH, Laughon M, et al. Changes in the incidence of candidiasis in neonatal intensive care units. *Pediatrics*. 2014;133:236–242.
5. Kaufman DA, Gurka MJ, Hazen KC, et al. Patterns of fungal colonization in preterm infants weighing less than 1000 grams at birth. *Pediatr Infect Dis J*. 2006;25:733–737.
6. Fairchild KD, Tomkoria S, Sharp EC, et al. Neonatal *Candida glabrata* sepsis: clinical and laboratory features compared with other *Candida* species. *Pediatr Infect Dis J*. 2002;21:39–43.
7. Maródi L. Local and systemic host defense mechanisms against *Candida*: immunopathology of candidal infections. *Pediatr Infect Dis J*. 1997;16:795–01.
8. Maródi L, Cypowyj S, Tóth B, et al. Molecular mechanisms of mucocutaneous immunity against *Candida* and *Staphylococcus* species. *J Allergy Clin Immunol*. 2012;130(5):1019–1027.

9. Puel A, Cypowyj S, Bustamante J, et al. Chronic mucocutaneous candidiasis in humans with inborn errors of interleukin-17 immunity. *Science*. 2011;332:65-68.
10. Lo HJ, Kohler JR, DiDominico B, et al. Nonfilamentous *C. albicans* mutants are avirulent. *Cell*. 1997;90:939-949.
11. Hostetter MK. RGD-mediated adhesion in fungal pathogens of humans, plants and insects. *Curr Opin Micro*. 2000;3:344-348.
12. Zasloff M. Defending the epithelium. *Nat Med*. 2006;12:607-608.
13. Schittek B, Hipfel R, Sauer B, et al. Dermcidin: a novel human antibiotic peptide secreted by sweat glands. *Nat Immunol*. 2001;2:1133-1137.
14. Ganz T. Antimicrobial polypeptides in host defense of the respiratory tract. *J Clin Invest*. 2002;109:693-697.
15. Putsep K, Carlsson G, Boman HG, et al. Deficiency of antimicrobial peptides in patients with morbus Kostmann: an observation study. *Lancet*. 2002;360:1144-1149.
16. Jiao H, Tóth B, Erdős M, et al. Novel and recurrent *STAT3* mutations in hyper-IgE syndrome patients from different ethnic groups. *Mol Immunol*. 2008;46:202-206.
17. Whelan WL, Kirsch DR, Kwon-Chung KJ, et al. *Candida albicans* in patients with the acquired immunodeficiency syndrome: absence of a novel hypervirulent strain. *J Infect Dis*. 1990;162:513-518.
18. Wilson CB, Westall J, Johnston L, et al. Decreased production of interferon gamma by human neonatal cells. *J Clin Invest*. 1986;77:860-867.
19. Lee SM, Suen Y, Chang L, et al. Decreased interleukin-12 (IL-12) from activated cord versus adult peripheral blood mononuclear cells and upregulation of interferon- γ, natural killer, and lymphokine-activated killer activity by IL-12 in cord blood mononuclear cells. *Blood*. 1996;88:945-954.
20. Maródi L. Down-regulation of Th1 responses in human neonates. *Clin Exp Immunol*. 2002;128:1-2.
21. Klotz SA, Drutz DJ, Zajic JE. Factors governing adherence of *Candida* species to plastic surfaces. *Infect Immun*. 1985;50:97-101.
22. Stephenson J. Can a common medical practice transform *Candida* infections from benign to deadly? *JAMA*. 2001;286:2531-2532.
23. Bendel CM, Wiesner SM, Garni RM, et al. Cecal colonization and systemic spread of *Candida albicans* in mice treated with antibiotics and dexamethasone. *Pediatr Res*. 2002;51:290-295.
24. van Rozendaal BA, van Spriel AB, van De Winkel JG, et al. Role of pulmonary surfactant protein D in innate defense against *Candida albicans*. *J Infect Dis*. 2000;182:917-922.
25. Hogan DA, Kolter R. *Pseudomonas-Candida* interactions: an ecological role for virulence factors. *Science*. 2002;296:2229-2232.
26. Netea MG, Brown GD, Kulberg BJ, et al. An integrated model of the recognition of *Candida albicans* by the innate immune system. *Nat Rev Microbiol*. 2008;6:67-68.
27. Gazendam RP, van Hamme JL, Tool ATJ, et al. Two independent killing mechanisms of *Candida albicans* by human neutrophils: evidence from innate immunity defects. *Blood*. 2014;124:590-597.
28. Johnston Jr RB. Clinical aspects of chronic granulomatous disease. *Curr Opin Hematol*. 2001;8:17-22.
29. Nauseef WM. Myeloperoxidase deficiency. *Hematol Oncol Clin North Am*. 1988;2:135-147.
30. Maródi L, Forehand JR, Johnston Jr RB. Mechanisms of host defense against candida species. II. Biochemical basis for the killing of *Candida* by mononuclear phagocytes. *J Immunol*. 1991;146:2790-2794.
31. Maródi L, Tournay C, Káposzta R, et al. Augmentation of human macrophage candidacidal capacity by recombinant human myeloperoxidase and granulocyte-macrophage colony-stimulating factor. *Infect Immun*. 1998;66:2750-2754.
32. Maródi L, Korchak HM, Johnston Jr RB. Mechanisms of host defense against *Candida* species: I. Phagocytosis by monocytes and monocyte-derived macrophages. *J Immunol*. 1991;146:2783-2789.
33. Han Y, Cutler JE. Antibody response that protects against disseminated candidiasis. *Infect Immun*. 1995;63:2714-2719.
34. Han Y, Kanbe T, Cherniak R, et al. Biochemical characterization of *Candida albicans* epitopes that can elicit protective and nonprotective antibodies. *Infect Immun*. 1997;65:4100-4107.
35. Maródi L, Schreiber S, Anderson DC, et al. Enhancement of macrophage candidacidal activity by interferon-gamma. Increased phagocytosis, killing, and calcium signal mediated by a decreased number of mannose receptors. *J Clin Invest*. 1993;91. 2596-01.
36. Szolnoky G, Bata-Csorgo Z, Kenderessy AS, et al. A mannose-binding receptor is expressed on human keratinocytes and mediates killing of *Candida albicans*. *J Invest Dermatol*. 2001;117:205-213.
37. Brown GD, Herre J, Williams DL, et al. Dectin-1 mediates the biological effects of β-glucans. *J Exp Med*. 2003;197:1119-1124.
38. Netea MG, Maródi L. Innate immune mechanisms for recognition and uptake of *Candida* species. *Trends Immunol*. 2010;31:346-353.
39. Levy O, Zarember KA, Roy RM, et al. Selective impairment of TLR-mediated innate immunity in human newborns: neonatal blood plasma reduces monocyte TNF-alpha induction by bacterial lipopeptides, lipopolysaccharide, and imiquimod, but preserves the response to R-848. *J Immunol*. 2004;173:4627-4634.
40. Yan SR, Qing G, Byers DM, et al. Role of MyD88 in diminished tumor necrosis factor alpha production by newborn mononuclear cells in response to lipopolysaccharide. *Infect Immun*. 2004;72:1223-1229.
41. Maródi L, Kaposzta R, Campbell DE, et al. Candidacidal mechanisms in the human neonate: impaired IFN-γ activation of macrophages in newborn infants. *J Immunol*. 1994;153:5643-5649.
42. Maródi L, Kaposzta R, Nemes E. Survival of group B *Streptococcus* type III in mononuclear phagocytes: differential regulation of bacterial killing in cord macrophages by human recombinant gamma interferon and granulocyte-macrophage colony-stimulating factor. *Infect Immun*. 2000;68:2167-2170.
43. Maródi L, Goda K, Palicz A, et al. Cytokine receptor signaling in neonatal macrophages: defective STAT-1 phosphorylation in response to stimulation with IFN-γ. *Clin Exp Immunol*. 2001;126:456-460.
44. Marquis G, Garzon S, Montplaisir S, et al. Histochemical and immunochemical study of the fate of Candida albicans inside human neutrophil phagolysosomes. *J Leukoc Biol*. 1991;50:587-589.
45. Káposzta R, Maródi L, Hollinshead M, et al. Rapid recruitment of late endosomes and lysosomes in mouse macrophages ingesting Candida albicans. *J Cell Sci*. 1999;112:3237-3248.
46. Lorenz MC, Fink GR. The glyoxylate cycle is required for fungal virulence. *Nature*. 2001;412:83-86.

115 Host Defense Mechanisms Against Viruses

James E. Crowe, Jr. | Fabienne Willems | Arnaud Marchant

OVERVIEW OF INNATE AND ADAPTIVE ANTIVIRAL IMMUNITY

Viral host defense mechanisms of humans depend on a combination of tightly integrated innate and adaptive immune mechanisms. Key innate immune mechanisms include antiviral and proinflammatory cytokines, such as type I interferon (IFN), IFN-γ, and tumor necrosis factor (TNF)-α, which have pleiotropic immunoregulatory effects and multiple potential cellular sources, including mononuclear phagocytes, dendritic cells (DCs), and natural killer (NK) cells. DCs are key for initiating the adaptive immune response and efficiently take up viral material in various forms, such as necrotic or apoptotic cellular debris. Some viral pathogens, such as human immunodeficiency virus (HIV), also may directly infect DCs. DCs process viral proteins and present these in the form of peptides bound to class I (human leukocyte antigen [HLA]-A, -B, and -C in humans) and class II (HLA-DR, -DP, and -DQ in humans) major histocompatibility complex (MHC) molecules for activation of CD8+ and CD4+ T cells, respectively.

As a result of clonal expansion and differentiation, virus-specific CD8+ and CD4+ effector T cells that carry out direct and indirect antiviral immune functions are generated. CD4+ T cells provide key help to B cells for the production of antiviral antibodies, and to CD8+ T cells. They are a major source of cytokines with antiviral activity, and they can also play a role in cell-mediated cytotoxicity. Effector CD8+ T cells are the key cells involved with

Table 115.1 Viruses Commonly Causing Disease in the Fetus or Neonate.

Virus Classification			Common Disease Pattern		
Family	**Subfamily; Genus**	**Virus**	**Congenital**	**Perinatal**	**Early Postnatal**
Herpesviridae	Alphaherpesvirinae; *Simplexvirus*	Herpes simplex virus 1 and 2	+	+	+
	Herpesviridae; Alphaherpesvirinae; *Varicellovirus*	Varicella-zoster virus	+	+	+
	Herpesviridae; Betaherpesvirinae; *Cytomegalovirus*	Cytomegalovirus	+	+	+
Retroviridae	Orthoretroviridae; *Lentivirus*	Human immunodeficiency virus	+	+	+
Hepadnaviridae	*Orthohepadnavirus*	Hepatitis B virus	+	+	
Flaviviridae	*Hepacivirus*	Hepatitis C virus	+	+	
Parvoviridae	*Erythroparvovirus*	Parvovirus B19 (also referred to as erythrovirus B19 or primate erythroparvovirus 1)	+		
Togaviridae	*Rubivirus*	Rubella virus	+		
Picornaviridae	*Enterovirus*	Echoviruses	+		
		Coxsackie virus	+		
		Enteroviruses	+		+
Paramyxoviridae	Paramyxovirinae; *Pneumovirus*	Respiratory syncytial virus			+
	Paramyxovirinae; *Metapneumovirus*	Metapneumovirus			+
Coronaviridae	*Betacoronavirus*	SARS-CoV-2			+

CoV, Coronavirus; *SARS*, severe acute respiratory syndrome.

the clearance of virally infected cells from infected tissues by cell-mediated cytotoxicity, which is triggered when their T cell receptors (TCRs) recognize viral peptide–class I MHC complexes on the surfaces of target cells. B cells provide antiviral antibody that can neutralize viral attachment and entry into cells. Viruses, particularly herpes viruses, can block antigen presentation and may down-regulate the overall level of class I MHC expression on the cell, potentially thwarting $CD8^+$ T cell recognition. As a countermeasure, NK cells recognize and immediately kill cells with reduced class I MHC expression, providing innate and early protection against viral infection before the appearance of differentiated T cells and B cells. NK cell–mediated killing also is augmented by virus-specific antibody produced by B cells, a further example of the linkage of innate and adaptive immunity. Although innate immune mechanisms can exhibit some capacity for memory,[1] T cell- and B cell-specific viral immunity persists for years or for a lifetime. The durability of immunity varies by pathogen, for reasons that are poorly understood.[2]

The neonate is at risk of severe or rapidly progressive infection with many, but not all, viruses (Table 115.1), most notably herpes simplex virus (HSV) type 1 and type 2 (HSV-1 and -2, which are often fatal or severe),[3,4] HIV, and enteroviruses.[5] Another herpes virus, human cytomegalovirus (HCMV), is the most common congenital infection. Most congenital CMV infections are asymptomatic at birth, with only about 13% being detected on routine neonatal examination,[6] but long-term consequences may follow both asymptomatic and symptomatic infection. Congenital CMV infection is the leading cause of sensorineural hearing loss of nongenetic origin and occurs in 10% to 15% of infected neonates.[6–8] CMV can also cause severe disease in the premature neonate. Neonatal infection with varicella zoster virus (VZV) often causes serious systemic illness, with mortality rates up to 30%. Newborns of mothers who were exposed to VZV or who have clinical disease manifestations within 2 weeks of delivery are at the highest risk of perinatal infection. The risk of neonatal infection and neonatal case fatality rates are highest when infected mothers exhibit symptoms less than 5 days before delivery.[9] In contrast, neonatal VZV infection between 10 and 28 days after birth is usually mild, but neonates still exhibit a higher risk of severe disease than older infants.[10] Viral infections that primarily involve mucosal surfaces also have the potential to cause disease that is more severe in neonates than in older individuals. For example, respiratory syncytial virus (RSV) is the most common viral cause of severe lower respiratory tract illness in infants, with a peak incidence of hospitalization in the first 2 months of life. Early, severe RSV infection may result in early immunologic and physiologic imprinting that is associated with long-term reactive airway disease or asthma.[11]

The immune effectors that regulate barrier function and detection of danger and infection (innate immune components) differ from those that resolve established infection or prevent reinfection. Cellular immune responses, typically including T cells and NK cells, are central to control of viral replication and elimination of infected cells, through mechanisms that control or block intracellular viral replication, spread of virus from cell to cell, or both. Antibody and complement may also modify viral infection, especially by preventing spread of virus systemically and into tissues such as those in the central nervous system (CNS). Prevention of viral reinfection following a primary infection or series of vaccinations depends principally on antibodies at the mucosa and in the systemic compartment. However, none of these major components of the immune system is siloed; rather, these systems are intricately intertwined and interdependent.

This chapter presents a systematic review of the key components of human innate and adaptive antiviral immunity against viruses such as HSV, HCMV, HIV, RSV, and enterovirus, including considerations specific to the role of these components in the neonate. In addition to being "unprimed" as a consequence of lack of previous exposure to antigen, the neonatal immune system exhibits a high level of regulation, with resulting differences in both speed and magnitude of innate and adaptive immune responses to viruses as compared to older children or adults.

OVERVIEW OF IMMUNOLOGIC DEVELOPMENT IN FETUSES AND NEONATES

Development of the immune system begins very early in life. There are limited studies of the specificity and complexity of the fetal immune system in humans. However, recent studies have begun to elucidate significant milestones along the path to development of immunologic maturity.[12] The placenta mediates hormonal, nutritional, and oxygen support of the fetus while also playing an important immunomodulatory role. Fetal syncytiotrophoblasts, which form the surface of the chorionic villi and are bathed by maternal blood, release various-sized vesicles of numerous functions. For example, placenta-derived exosomes impair T cell signaling, down-regulate the NK cell receptor NKG2D, stimulate apoptosis by means of the Fas ligand (FasL)- and TNF-related apoptosis-inducing ligand (TRAIL)-mediated pathways, and promote an immunosuppressive environment via the cytokine transforming growth factor (TGF)-β and costimulatory molecule PD-L1, which primes regulatory T cells.[13] Modulation of the maternal immune system during fetal gestation and postnatal microbial colonization may play fundamental roles in the induction, training, and function of the host immune system. Increasingly it is appreciated that the maternal microbiome affects early immunologic patterning in fetuses and neonates.[12,14-16]

Although fetuses ideally do not encounter viruses during development, foreign antigens clearly do cross the placenta.[17,18] Maternal viral infections that have a viremic component, such as CMV, herpes virus type 1 and 2, and rubella, may cross the placenta into fetal tissues. These infections can significantly disrupt both immunologic and overall physiologic development of fetuses.[14-16,19]

Both the T cell and B cell lymphocyte compartments exhibit age-dependent maturation, with low numbers of memory-effector T and B cells detectable after birth into early infancy.[20] Regulatory T cells with suppressive function are present in the fetus, and they establish functional tolerance to foreign antigens (including noninherited maternal antigens [NIMA]) present during development in utero. Regulatory T cells have been observed in fetal lymph nodes at 18 to 22 weeks of gestation, and these cells facilitated the presence of maternal cells in the fetus (maternal microchimerism) in 15 of 18 lymph node samples studied.[21] Intriguingly, tolerance to NIMA and maternal microchimerism may facilitate reproductive fitness across generations.[22]

At birth, neonates begin to encounter an extraordinarily diverse set of antigens, a subset of which is found in viruses that have the potential for causing severe disease. A switch from tolerization to recognition of and response to viral pathogens must occur very rapidly, but it is not instantaneous. Neonates of all gestations remain in an immunologic transition for a significant period. Studies of human neonates show that they continue to exhibit features of tolerance, associated with significant levels of B cell tolerance[23] and persistence of long-lived regulatory T cells.[21] Some viral infections are either more severe or more prolonged when they happen in the fetus and neonate. This observation suggests that there are persisting quantitative or qualitative differences in immune responses to foreign pathogens compared to later in life. Overall, however, the evidence suggests that, although the developmental program controlling the fetal immune system promotes a relatively high level of tolerance, the fetal and neonatal immune system has significant capacity for functional activity in response to infection.

Studies of responses to viral infections have revealed that functional immune responses can already develop in utero.[24] As compared to the adult immune system, qualitative differences may underlie differences in the control of viral replication. Most studies have focused on the major adaptive immune system components of B cell and T cell responses, which have been characterized qualitatively and quantitatively in addition to their underlying molecular characteristics.

GUT MICROBIOME

Before birth, the intestine is generally sterile. The intestinal tract becomes colonized soon after birth with a variety of ingested environmental and maternal microorganisms. This process is influenced by many factors, including mode of delivery, diet, environment, and use of antibiotics.[25,26] For example, a breast-fed, term infant normally has an intestinal microbiota in which bifidobacteria predominate over potentially harmful bacteria, whereas in formula-fed infants, enterococci, bacteroides, and clostridia predominate.[27] Experiments in mice demonstrate that the beneficial effects of commensal bacteria are mediated via Toll-like receptors (TLRs).[28] The recognition of commensal bacterial-derived molecules by TLRs represents a critical component of the symbiosis between the host and indigenous microflora and is important for protection against gut injury and associated mortality.[19,29,30]

GUT IMMUNE SYSTEM DEVELOPMENT

The development of the gut immune system is initiated before birth by a genetic program that drives the formation of Peyer patches and mesenteric lymph nodes, but its postnatal maturation depends on the establishment of a balanced indigenous microbiota.[31] Intestinal commensal microorganisms provide signals that foster normal immune system development and influence the ensuing immune responses.[32] Signals delivered by these commensal microorganisms drive the development of isolated lymphoid follicles, stimulate maturation of Peyer patches, and initiate migration of IgA-producing plasma cells, innate lymphoid cells, and mature T lymphocytes into the mucosa.[32-34]

MODELS OF STUDY OF FETAL AND NEONATAL IMMUNITY

Due to obvious safety and ethical issues, studies involving tissue and blood sampling of fetuses and neonates are limited. Most immunology studies in adult humans have been developed and performed with large-volume samples, but the volume of blood that can be acquired from neonates is typically on the order of a few milliliters at most. Amniotic fluid collection, used clinically for prenatal genetic diagnosis, can also give information about fetal inflammation and stress. Placentas may be obtained from elective terminations of pregnancy in the first trimester or after delivery in preterm or term infants. Tissue acquisition from fetuses and neonates is limited to fetal tissues obtained after medical termination of pregnancy, neonatal tissues from cases of sudden and unexpected infant death (SUID),[35] or occasionally from small surgical biopsies.[36] Maternal-embryo interactions in the first 8 weeks of gestation following embryo implantation probably are foundational in establishing immune system parameters, and this period of development likely differs significantly from later stages, but there is very little detailed or reliable information on tissues from this period in humans.[37] Preliminary studies performed in the 1980s showed that cells involved in innate immune responses develop as early as the fourth week of gestation in humans, and mature fetal T and B lymphocytes can be detected by the end of the first trimester of gestation.

For these reasons, animal models are frequently used to investigate early immune development, but these models may not reliably recapitulate human immune development. Modeling of in utero development is challenging because of anatomic and physiologic differences between humans and animals. For example, no other species has a placental structure and function identical to that of humans. Postnatal animal models of neonatal immune development and response are also complicated by differences from humans. Neonatal mice are used often because of the ease of breeding and the availability of reagents that facilitate elegant mechanistic studies. The gestational period of mice (about 3 weeks) is quite short, and postnatal development is very rapid compared with humans. In contrast to humans, mouse T lymphocytes only develop after birth. It is difficult to identify days of life in neonatal mice that temporally correspond appropriately to weeks or months of human postnatal life. A variety of molecular characteristics of the immune response are significantly different between young mice and humans. For example, variation in TLR structure between species drives different responses to TLR agonists, which result in species-specific pathogen recognition.[38] Therefore, mouse models often poorly mimic human inflammatory diseases and immune responses.[39] Nonhuman primate models of immune development during pregnancy and the neonatal period are being investigated and have some promise, but they are expensive and require very special facilities and expertise.

MECHANISMS OF ADAPTIVE IMMUNITY: B CELLS/ANTIBODIES AND T CELLS

B CELLS/ANTIBODIES

The antigen-specific receptor of B cells is formed by recombination of variable (V), diversity (D), and joining (J) genes. Recombining V, D, and J genes achieves a diverse repertoire of antigen receptors that can recognize the myriad foreign antigens in a highly regulated process consistent with ability to respond to pathogens without causing autoimmune phenomena. Although neonatal mice use different dominant antibody variable genes compared with adult mice, it appears that the general makeup of human neonatal repertoires is similar to that of adults. In the human fetus, early B cell development is associated with progressive diversification of the antibody gene repertoire.[40] At term, the antibody gene repertoire possesses mature levels of junctional diversity, including nontemplated (N) and palindromic (P) type of additions at the V/D and D/J gene junctions. Furthermore, the average amino acid length of the complementarity-determining regions (antibody-variable loops) appears to be similar to that of adults.[41] In contrast to adult antibody gene sequences, however, neonatal sequences have lower levels of somatic mutations.[40,41] This finding is presumably due to lack of extensive prior exposure to foreign antigens that drives terminal center formation, which is associated with B cell proliferation and differentiation in concert with the molecular program of somatic hypermutation. Using unmutated recombined antibody gene sequences to encode antiviral antibodies leads to the secretion of antibodies with low affinity for virus antigens, and consequently low antiviral function.[42] Somatic hypermutation is a complex process that requires antigen presentation, CD4 T lymphocyte help via soluble factors and cell surface receptor expression, and interaction with B cells. In a robust germinal center reaction, stimulation of B cells leads to expression of activation-induced cytidine deamidase (AID) and error-prone DNA polymerases. It is possible that there is a lower level of intrinsic response in neonatal B cells in the germinal center milieu. However, human cord blood B cells do up-regulate the transcription of genes involved in somatic hypermutation, including AID and polymerases, following stimulation with CD154 and cytokines (mimicking T helper cell interaction).[43] Human newborns can develop potent antibody responses to T cell–dependent vaccine antigens.[44] Infants exhibit a profound deficiency in antibody response to polysaccharides, which is most pertinent in response to the capsular polysaccharides of some pathogenic bacteria including *Streptococcus pneumonia*, *Neisseria meningitides*, and *Haemophilus influenzae*; it is not clear whether this deficiency also pertains to the response to glycans present on the surface glycoproteins of many pathogenic viruses.

ANTIBODIES

Respiratory viruses are the most common cause of hospitalization of infants in the developed world, and thus they are interesting models for probing development of antibody-mediated immunity. The most common viral causes of serious lower respiratory tract disease in humans are RSV; parainfluenza virus (PIV) types 1, 2, and 3; and influenza viruses. The mechanisms by which antibodies contribute to resolution of or protection against infection or disease caused by respiratory viruses have been increasingly elucidated over the last decade through in vitro studies of neutralization and in vivo studies of protection. Antibodies neutralize respiratory viruses in vitro using a wide variety of molecular mechanisms. The cell substrate used for neutralization assays matters greatly, because the level of expression of membrane receptors and intracellular restriction factors varies among continuous cell lines. Important antibody characteristics that regulate neutralization potency include the Fab affinity for viral antigen, avidity of multivalent interactions, immunoglobulin (Ig) isotype (IgM, IgG, or IgA) and subclass (IgG1, IgG2, IgG3, or IgG4), concentration, molar ratio of antibody combining sites to epitopes on the surface of viral particles, state of polymerization (monomeric/polymeric IgA or IgM regulated by joining J chain), ability to bind the polyimmunoglobulin receptor (pIgR), ability of certain antibodies to fix complement, and virus protein and epitope specificity. Immunity is also affected by many viral factors, such as replication cycle features including use of diverse host molecules as attachment factors, mode of entry into the cell, pH dependence of fusion (neutral or low pH), and the natural site of replication. Individual characteristics of a specific virus strain can alter the antigenic recognition capacity of antibodies (corresponding to diverse serotypes, clades, antigenic subgroups, and amino acid sequences of viral surface proteins). Some of the major mechanisms of antibody-mediated virus neutralization (Table 115.2) are reviewed next.

AGGREGATION

Antibodies possess the potential for bivalent or higher valency interactions, depending on isotype, allowing one antibody molecule to bind more than one copy of an epitope. Recognition of quaternary structures through binding of multiple epitope copies on a single oligomer[45] or multiple oligomers[46] can be associated with high potency of virus neutralization. If a multivalent antibody directed against viral surface proteins crosslinks multiple free virions in solution, however, these particles can be aggregated. It is thought that aggregation of multiple infectious virions into a single particle reduces the number of those virions to a single infectious particle, because size constraints suggest that a single particle usually attaches only to one cell. Aggregates caused by IgM, IgG, or IgA to influenza virus have been visualized directly in electron microscopy studies.[47-49]

BLOCKING OF ATTACHMENT

Antibodies can inhibit virus attachment to cell surface receptors or attachment factors; virion particles that cannot attach to cells do not initiate infection. The principal target of neutralizing antibodies for influenza virus is the hemagglutinin (HA) protein, which mediates both virus attachment to its cellular receptor (a glycoconjugate terminating in sialic acid) and fusion with an intracellular membrane at low pH. Some of the most potent anti-HA antibodies bind directly to the recessed receptor-binding site (RBS) for sialic acid on the head domain of HA, by inserting an antibody hypervariable loop (complementarity-determining region) into the site.[50] Interestingly, there are canonical molecular modes of interaction of these antibody loops with the HA RBS that use either a charge-based interaction with an antibody loop aspartate or pi-pi stacking of aromatic residues to mimic the molecular interactions with sialic acid.[50] The stacking of aromatic residues between attachment-blocking antibodies and virus RBS regions has also been observed in other families of viruses, such as neutralizing antibodies to filoviruses,[51] and thus may be a very common and important mechanism of virus receptor blocking. Anti-HA IgA and IgG antibodies inhibit influenza virus attachment to both mammalian cell culture monolayers and tracheal cell

Table 115.2 Mechanisms of Viral Inhibition by Antibodies.

Effectors	Mechanism	Comments
Immunoglobulin (Ig) alone	Aggregation	Before attachment. Aggregating multiple infectious particles into one complex reduces infectious units
	Blocking of attachment	Binding to the receptor-binding domain on virus attachment factors abrogates binding of the virions to cell receptors or co-receptors
	Blocking entry	Typically accomplished by binding to a virus surface protein that mediates fusion and inhibiting complex conformational changes required for fusion of virion and host cell membranes ("fusion inhibition")
	Postattachment inhibition	Inhibition of viral uncoating even after entry of particles into the cell
	Inhibition of egress	Antibodies bind to newly expressed viral proteins on the cell surface, blocking assembly or budding of infectious particles from infected cells
Viral clearance is aided by additional molecules or cells	Complement-enhanced inhibition	Aggregation by complement fixation on multiple Ig molecules bound to virion particles
		Complement receptor uptake by phagocytic cells bearing complement receptors
	Fc receptor (FcR)–mediated action	FcRγ-mediated uptake of antigen-antibody immune complexes by phagocytic cells
	Polymeric immunoglobulin receptor	IgA- or IgM-mediated recycling of complexes of polymeric antibodies and virions
	FcR neonatal (FcRn)	Recycling of antigen-antibody immune complexes in FcRn-bearing cells
	Antibody-dependent cell-mediated cytotoxicity (ADCC)	Lysis of a host cell displaying antibodies bound to viral integral membrane antigens by natural killer cells, macrophages, neutrophils or eosinophils
	Antibody-dependent cell-mediated virus inhibition	A measure of FcRγ-mediated antiviral activity due in part to ADCC and in part to noncytolytic mechanisms such as β-chemokine release from the effector cells

epithelia.[49,52,53] The basis for the conventional hemagglutination inhibition test, often used for serologic assays of functional antiinfluenza antibodies, is blockade of virus attachment to sialic acid on the surface of red blood cells. Influenza is not unique in this regard. The HN (HA-neuraminidase [NA]) glycoprotein of PIV mediates attachment to sialic acid-containing host-cell receptors.[54] Antibodies to several of the major antigenic sites on PIV3 HN are neutralizing.[55] RSV does not use sialic acid as receptor; the cellular receptors for RSV are poorly defined, but the RSV G (glycosylated) glycoprotein is considered to be the virus surface glycoprotein that mediates attachment.[56] Interestingly, antibodies to the RSV G protein typically possess a low level of neutralizing activity in vitro, and most monoclonal antibodies (mAbs) directed to the RSV G protein mediate only partial neutralization, even at maximal concentrations. This incomplete neutralization effect likely is due to heterogeneity in glycosylation of the virus protein.

FUSION INHIBITION

Even if viruses attach to cells, some antibodies can neutralize the tethered virion particles at the cell surface before cell entry, especially if they inhibit fusion of virus particles with cell membranes. RSV can be inhibited in vitro by the presence of immune serum during the first 60 minutes after inoculation.[57] This finding suggests that some neutralizing antibodies inhibit events that follow virion attachment to host cells. The role of fusion proteins varies depending on the type of virus (especially enveloped versus nonenveloped virion particles). Fusion proteins of enveloped viruses merge the virus lipid membrane with that of the host cell, either at the cell surface or for some viruses in the endosome. The fusion (F) protein of paramyxoviruses, for example, mediates direct fusion of the viral envelope with the cell membrane after attachment at neutral pH. Many antibodies directed to RSV or PIV3 F glycoproteins are effective at virus neutralization. The three-dimensional structure of paramyxovirus F proteins and the function of diverse regions of the F proteins during fusion of viral and cellular membranes have been defined recently.[58-60] F proteins require cleavage from an F_0 precursor to F_1 and F_2 subunits for infectivity, and a highly conserved hydrophobic region near the cleavage site functions as a fusogenic peptide. Some paramyxovirus-neutralizing anti-F antibodies inhibit fusion at the cell surface membrane. Fusion inhibition (FI) activity often is measured by inhibition of multinucleate giant cell (syncytium) formation caused by cell-to-cell fusion after productive infection of cell monolayer cultures. Because viral surface proteins traffic to the cell surface during the processes of assembly and budding (which are necessary for egress from the cell), antibodies can inhibit virus egress. Some anti-F antibodies appear to inhibit the release of progeny paramyxoviruses from infected cells. The epitope of binding to the F protein is important to the extent and mechanism of function observed, because some RSV or PIV F antibodies bind to F but do not neutralize virus, some of these antibodies bind to F protein and neutralize virus in vitro, and still others exhibit both in vitro neutralization *and* FI properties.[61,62] Major neutralizing sites have been defined for these fusion proteins by competition-binding assays, determination of the nucleotide sequence of the F proteins of mAb escape mutants, crystallography of mAb-virus protein complexes, and other techniques. Such studies have facilitated the first successful "reverse vaccinolog" studies to design structure-based epitope vaccines,[63] using as a starting point the atomic resolution structure of a neutralizing antibody (motavizumab) in complex with the epitope derived from RSV F protein.[64]

Other viruses, including influenza virus as a prototype, do not fuse with host cell membranes at neutral pH at the cell surface; instead, the attached virus particles enter the cell by endocytosis, then fuse with endosomal membranes when the pH of the vesicle drops (typically to a pH of about 5.2). Postattachment inhibition of endocytosis of influenza has been reported.[49] Polymeric IgM appears to be especially effective in this setting, likely due to the large amount of steric hindrance associated with the 5 or 6 copies of IgM in such complexes.

INHIBITION OF UNCOATING

Even after endocytosis, antibodies that remain bound to viral protein targets may mediate neutralization. Some influenza HA-specific neutralizing antibodies prevent uncoating of virus due to low-pH membrane fusion.[52,65] Some anti-HA IgGs appear to mediate neutralization of influenza virus replication at steps even later than primary uncoating, although the mechanism of such effects is unclear.[52,65]

COMPLEMENT-ENHANCED ANTIBODY-MEDIATED NEUTRALIZATION

The complement system comprises about 30 proteins and protein fragments that are part of the innate immune system. Most complement components are synthesized as inactive precursors in the liver and distributed by systemic circulation. Complement protein levels are low in neonates, especially the terminal elements of the complement cascade. As a result, neonates cannot form the membrane attack complex that is necessary for some antimicrobial responses. Certain isotypes of antibodies fix complement by interaction in the CH2 domain of antibodies, in the Fc region of the Ig molecule. The complement system mediates diverse immune functions, including aggregation of pathogens (as discussed previously for antibodies), chemotaxis-enhancing properties for neutrophils and macrophages, opsonization to enhance phagocytosis of virions by Fc receptor (FcR)–bearing phagocytic cells, and lysis of cells and virions by assembly of a membrane attack complex. Complement fixation (the combining of complement with antigen-antibody complexes) is mediated by certain isotypes of antibodies, and this activity often enhances viral neutralization. Without complement, antibody function is reduced. Complement is also necessary for optimal recruitment of immune factors during local responses, and it plays a role in antigen presentation by enhancing uptake of foreign antigens into antigen-presenting cells (APCs) through various complement receptors.

ANTIBODY-DEPENDENT CELL-MEDIATED CYTOTOXICITY

Many of the FcRs bind antigen-antibody complexes and thereby induce a phagocytic cell-mediated mechanism of immunity termed *antibody-dependent cell-mediated cytotoxicity (ADCC)*. Antibodies in human serum and some monoclonal antibodies have been shown to trigger ADCC activity. Antibodies mediating ADCC against influenza virus–infected cells were detected in serum samples obtained from young children after natural infection or after vaccination with inactivated and live attenuated viruses,[66] recognizing HA and NA proteins. Cord blood lymphocytes, monocytes, and neutrophils from neonates can mediate ADCC against influenza virus–infected cells, and antibodies capable of mediating ADCC activity were detected in cord plasma.[67] Human RSV–specific antibodies mediating ADCC have been detected in adults, including in colostrum, and also have been detected in serum of infants.[68,69] Mucosal antibodies that mediate ADCC also have been seen in nasopharyngeal secretions collected after primary RSV infection.[70,71] These data suggest that the functional components required to mediate ADCC against virus-infected cells are present in neonates.

CD4+ T CELLS

Optimal antiviral antibody responses require CD4+ T cell help. Most experts feel that T cells exhibit a higher level of functional maturity than B cells early in life, but significant skewing of neonatal T cell responses has been described repeatedly. Mouse studies of cytokine secretion patterns demonstrated a T_H2-dominant phenotype in most neonatal responses, due to generally reduced magnitude of T_H1-type cytokines in the neonatal response.[72] Human vaccine studies confirmed the limited ability of young infants to develop adult-type Th1 responses, except when challenged with BCG or whole cell pertussis.[24] Upon challenge with immune stimuli, infants under the age of 2 months express an innate T_H2 and T_H17 cell polarization, weak T_H1 polarization, and low innate antiviral type I IFN responses.[73] Several in vitro and ex vivo studies have demonstrated impaired ability of neonatal leukocytes to produce T_H1-polarizing cytokines, such as IL-12p70 and TNFα, compared with adult leukocytes.[74-77] Whether reduced T_H1 responses in human neonates are associated with a corresponding increase in T_H2 or T_H17 responses has not been clearly demonstrated. Neonatal T cells exhibit an unusual phenotype in that a substantial number of CD4+ T cells from human newborns respond to activation by expressing high levels of CXC-chemokine ligand 8 (CXCL8; also known as IL-8).[78] CXCL8 enhances IFN-γ expression in γδ T cells, which are considered to be important producers of effector cytokines in newborns and can activate human neutrophils. CXCL8 secretion may be a proinflammatory immunoprotective function of neonatal T cells despite the overall antiinflammatory state of the neonatal immune system.

The original bimodal phenotype of T_H1 versus T_H2 CD4+ T cell responses has been revised in recent years to reflect much greater complexity (Table 115.3). Additional T_H cell subsets, such as T_H17, T_H9, T_H22, T_{FH}, Tr1, and Treg cells, have been described in detail. Careful studies in model systems suggest that there is a high degree of functional heterogeneity of the human CD4+ T cell response, suggesting that polarized responses result from preferential expansion of cells with a particular phenotype rather than a deterministic mode of priming.[79] Naïve T_H cells express retinoic acid–related orphan receptor (ROR)γt in the presence of IL-1 and IL-23 in humans and differentiate into T_H17 cells that produce a host of cytokines, including IL-17. Human inborn errors of immunity mediated by the cytokines IL-17A and IL-17F (IL-17A/F) are responsible for mucocutaneous candidiasis; inborn errors of IFN-γ immunity underlie mycobacterial disease, and biallelic RAR-related orphan receptor C (RORC) loss-of-function mutations are associated with both candidiasis and mycobacteriosis.[80] When stimulated with IL-4 and TGF-β, T_H2 cells further differentiate into T_H9 cells, which produce IL-9 and IL-10. Naïve T_H cells also can differentiate into T_H22 cells that express the aryl hydrocarbon receptor and secrete IL-22 when stimulated with TNF-α and IL-6.

The molecular and cellular basis for skewing of the phenotype of neonatal T_H cells is under study. T_H1 cells appear to undergo apoptosis during early responses in a process driven by the prototypic T_H2 cytokine IL-4.[81] Interestingly, neonates appear to possess cells capable of rapidly expressing IL-4 in a nonclassic program.[82] Epigenetic factors in the T_H2 genomic locus appear to promote T_H2 cytokine gene expression and thus the prominent development of T_H2 cells.[83] In contrast, neonatal human monocyte-derived DCs (moDCs) possess a repressive chromatin state that reduces *IL-12p35* gene transcription, resulting in a defect in IL-12p70 secretion.[84] In mice, neonatal regulatory T cells reduce CD4+ and CD8+ T cell antiviral function during neonatal herpes virus infection.[85] Human neonatal T CD4+ T cells possess altered microRNA patterns that result in different patterns of immune regulation.[86] Fetal T cells may arise from different populations of hematopoietic cells than do adult T cells, and fetal T cell lineages appear to be biased toward immune tolerance.[87]

ROLE OF CD4+ T CELL RESPONSES IN INCREASED SUSCEPTIBILITY TO VIRAL INFECTIONS

The distinct neonatal pattern of regulation of T cells with increased regulatory T cell function and reduced T_H1 cell responses is likely to play an important role in the more severe or more prolonged viral infections in the fetus and young infant.[88,89] In pediatric HIV infection, this T cell functional pattern is associated with higher viral loads and more rapid disease progression.[90] Studies of congenital CMV infection indicate that high frequencies of antiviral CD4+ and CD8+ T cells can be induced early during fetal life.[91] However, CMV-specific fetal effector cells express an exhausted phenotype, with increased expression of inhibitory receptors and reduced production of antiviral cytokines as compared to adult cells.

Table 115.3 CD4+ T Cells and Their Subsets.

Subset of Cells	Factors That Drive Their Differentiation	Lineage-Defining Factors	Common Cytokines They Produce
T_H1	Interleukin (IL)-12	Signal transducers and activators of transcription (STAT)-4 T-bet	Interferon (INF)- γ Tumor necrosis factor (TNF)-α IL-2 IL-10
T_H2	IL-4 IL-25 IL-33	STAT-6 GATA-3	IL-4 IL-5 IL-13
T_H22	IL-23 IL-12 IL-6 TNF-α Agonists of aryl hydrocarbon receptor (AhR)	c-Maf repressor function	IL-22
Tfh	IL-6 IL-21	Bcl-6 transcription repressor	IL-21 IL-10 Il-4
T_H19	IL-4 TGF-β IL-2 IL-9	STAT6	IL-9
T_H17	Pathogenic subtype IL-1 IL-6 IL-23 Transforming growth factor (TGF)-β3	STAT-3 Retinoic acid-related orphan receptor (ROR)γt Runx1/2 T-bet	IL-17A IFN-γ IL-22
	Nonpathogenic subtype TGF-β1 IL-6	STAT-3 RORγt	IL-17A IL-10
Induced regulatory T cell (iTreg)	IL-2 TGF-β		
Natural regulatory T cell (nTreg)	Direct thymic export	STAT-3 Foxp3	IL-10 IL-35 TGF-β

These regulated responses may be important to prevent immunopathology, at the expense of viral replication and prolonged viral shedding. Similarly, the frequent development of chronic carriage following hepatitis B virus infection in young infants may be related to increased regulation of inflammatory responses.[92] On the other hand, T_H2 and T_H17 biased responses may limit control of RSV replication and cause enhanced inflammatory disease during infection early in life.[93]

ANTIGEN-PRESENTING CELLS

Neonatal antigen-presenting cells include DCs, monocytes, and macrophages. Reduced frequency of CD14+CD16+ intermediate monocytes in cord blood compared to adult blood was found to contribute to lipopolysaccharide (LPS) hyporesponsiveness in newborns.[94] Upon stimulation with IFN-γ, fetal (8 to 12 gestational weeks) monocytes fail to up-regulate costimulatory and antigen presentation genes but instead up-regulate many genes that mediate innate pathogen responses.[95] Down-regulation of TLR-mediated NLRP3 inflammasome activity is associated with impaired IL-1-β production in human fetal monocytes, which is restored to adult levels during the neonatal period.[96] Cord blood and adult monocytes have similar ability to process antigen, but neonatal monocytes are less able to present antigen to T cells, due to the lower expression of CD40 and CD86 costimulatory molecules on newborn as compared to adult monocytes.[97] Neonatal macrophages exhibit similar phagocytic capacity to *C. albicans* or *Escherichia coli*.[98] Human neonatal macrophages are less capable of responding to IFN-γ stimulation, leading to defective STAT1 signaling and impaired clearance of intracellular pathogens such as group B *Streptococcus*.[99] Recently, unbiased transcriptomic, metabolic, and polysome profiling studies showed that fetal monocytes are metabolically skewed and lack translation of key immune response genes in a gestational age-dependent manner.[100]

DCs are antigen-presenting cells crucial for the innate and adaptive immune response to infections and for maintaining immune tolerance to self tissues.[101] In response to pathogens recognized by PRR or danger signals, DCs migrate to lymph nodes and undergo maturation. DC maturation is necessary for effective antigen loading and priming of naïve T cells and is characterized by up-regulation of MHC and CD40, CD80, CD86, CD83 co-stimulatory molecules and by their production of inflammatory cytokines for T-cell polarization.

The DC subtypes found in a steady state in the mouse and in humans include plasmacytoid DCs (pDCs) and conventional DCs (cDCs) in nonlymphoid tissues, in circulation, and in lymphoid tissues.[102] In addition, DCs can develop after infection or inflammation and include the moDCs[103] that can be differentiated from human monocytes upon in vitro culture in presence of granulocyte-macrophage colony-stimulating factor (GM-CSF) and IL-4.[104] Within human peripheral blood, two populations of DCs can be classified: myeloid CD11c+ cDCs whose main function is to prime and functionally polarize naïve T cells, and pDCs that lack CD11c but express CD123 and are one of the major sources of type I IFNs during viral infections.[105]

Most of our current understanding of the biology of DCs in early life comes from studies on cord blood DCs and on moDCs. Following PRR stimulation, human newborn monocytes and DCs including cDCs and moDCs produce a cytokine profile that differs substantially from those of their adult counterparts. Specifically, upon in vitro stimulation of most TLR ligands, cord blood cells produce less T_H1 cell-polarizing cytokines (such as IL-12p70, TNF-α type I IFN), but more IL10 and T_H17 cell-polarizing cytokines (such as IL-6, IL-23, and IL-1β) than adult blood cells.[106,107] The response of neonatal monocytes to TLR-8 ligand is an exception to this profile as TLR-8 stimulation of DCs induces increased TNF and IL-12 relative to the adults.[108] As described in the paragraph below, various immunosuppressive mechanisms have been implicated in the distinct functional properties of monocytes/DCs in early life. Besides the role of external factors, evidence indicates that cord blood moDCs exhibit an intrinsic defect in their capacity to produce IL-12p70.[109,110] The transcription of the p35 subunit of IL-12p70 in neonatal moDCs stimulated with LPS is limited by epigenetic regulation owing to a nucleosome remodeling impairment[84] and diminished DNA-binding activity and interaction between IRF3 and its co-activator CREB-binding protein, which is a transcription factor required for IL-12p35 synthesis.[111]

Taken together, these data derived from in vitro experiments suggest that neonatal monocytes and DCs in humans are not simply less responsive but functionally different from those of an adult. Their reduced ability to produce T_H1-supporting cytokines correlate with limited T_H1-type responses to some vaccines and pathogens in newborns. This may contribute to the increased risk of infection with intracellular pathogens such as *Listeria monocytogenes* and HSV in early life. Conversely, at birth human APCs have an enhanced capacity to promote T_H17-type immune responses involved in the defense against extracellular pathogens. It appears that the first year of life represents an important period for the acquisition of "adult-like" responsiveness to TLR ligands by circulating monocytes/DCs[112] and that functional programming of immune cells is likely regulated by commensal microbes that begin to colonize the gastrointestinal tract at birth.[113,114]

IMMUNE REGULATION

The general immunologic milieu in the fetal environment appears to be shaped by regulatory factors that reduce robust responses. Both soluble and cellular factors appear to promote fetal immune homeostasis. Soluble factors regulating T cell responses in fetal and neonatal life include a wide variety of molecules, such as cytokines, adipokines, complement, antibodies, lipid-type molecules, vitamins, and purine adenosine.[115] As an example, components of complement contribute to proinflammatory responses to pathogens but are produced in reduced levels in fetuses and neonates.

The basis for the profile of the neonatal response likely stems not only from different functional programming compared with adults but also from active suppression or regulation of immune responses. Adenosine promotes regulatory T cell responses and is present in elevated levels early in development. Suppressive cytokines likely play a prominent role in neonatal responses. Regulatory B cells have been described, and they may be especially active in neonates.[116] Neonatal B cells secreting the inhibitory cytokine IL-10 have been shown to regulate DC responses following stimulation of TLRs.[117,118] Transcriptional profiling and biologic network analysis identified TGF-β and associated signaling molecules as differentially regulated in cord blood cells versus adult cells; TGF-β1 was decreased in RSV-infected adult blood DCs but increased in RSV-infected cord blood DCs.[119] Cellular factors also contribute to immune regulation—for instance, myeloid-derived suppressor cells are present in high frequency during fetal life. An immune environment programmed toward regulation may have an important impact on the susceptibility of the fetus and the young infant to infectious pathogens and on their responses to vaccines. Neonates exhibit high numbers of circulating $CD71^+$ erythroid precursor cells (nucleated red blood cells), which express the enzyme arginase-2 and exert immunosuppressive properties.[120] These cells mediate the beneficial effect of protection against undesirable inflammatory cell activation and immunopathology during transition to postnatal life, but they also inhibit active responses to pathogens resulting in increased susceptibility to infection. The immunosuppressive effects of $CD71^+$ erythroid cells were demonstrated using adoptive transfer of those cells into adult mice, leading to an immunosuppressive effect mediated by the enzyme arginase-2.[120] Conversely, depletion of $CD71^+$ cells in neonatal mice increases resistance to neonatal pathogens.[120] Human cord blood cells also may contain a high number of $CD71^+$ cells,[120] and premature infants exhibit a higher frequency of nucleated red blood cells in cord blood.[121]

MATERNAL ANTIBODIES AND ANTIBODY FEEDBACK REGULATION

Animals and humans respond differently when antigens are administered together with virus-specific antibodies than when the virus or virus antigen is delivered alone. This biologic phenomenon has been termed *antibody feedback regulation,* and it is associated with either marked enhancement or suppression of the virus-specific antibody responses.[122-125] In some cases both occur, such as suppressed primary antibody secretion responses to RSV following passive transfer of RSV immune globulin, but markedly enhanced RSV-neutralizing responses after secondary infection.[126]

Transplacental transfer of maternal antibodies is a special case of antibody feedback regulation. Maternal antibodies protect against viruses for which the mother has been infected or immunized, but these antibodies in the infant also can reduce the active immune response of infants to viral vaccines or infections.[127] The principal route of transfer of antibodies from human mothers to infants is transplacental. In contrast, in some animal models there is little transfer across the placenta but rather large-scale acquisition of maternal antibodies in milk transferred in the intestine. This makes animal modeling of this phenomenon challenging. The IgG1 subclass of antibody is transferred preferentially in humans, with little or no IgM, IgA, or IgE transferred. The placenta is a complex tissue with multiple cell layers and cell types that use regulated molecular transport mechanisms to provide oxygen, nutrients, and regulatory signals to the fetus. Although the term *passive transfer* is often used for transfer of antibodies from one individual to another (as opposed to active immunization), the actual molecular transfer of antibodies across the placenta does not simply occur by passive diffusion. Transfer of Igs to the fetus is mediated by active transport using specialized types of FcRs. Although the placenta contains a number of proteins that bind antibodies, the principal molecule that mediates Ig transfer is the human homolog of the neonatal rat FcR (FcRn). This nonclassic major MHC class I molecule is a heterodimer that binds and releases Igs in a pH-dependent manner.[128] Maternal IgG is carried to fetal tissues by a pH gradient from acidic endosomes to the pH-neutral basolateral surface of the syncytiotrophoblast and across the fetal blood vessel endothelium. The FcRn also has emerged as an important molecule in postnatal life because it regulates IgG concentrations and half-life in serum and tissues by controlling IgG circulation, transport, and catabolism.[128] Other IgG-binding FcRs, such as FcγRI, FcγRII, and FcγRIII on cells in the stroma and FcγRII on endothelial cells, also appear to clear maternal antibodies complexed with fetal antigens and could contribute to the transplacental transfer (Fig. 115.1).[129]

Transfer of antibody in significant amounts begins at about 28 weeks of gestation in humans, and the amount of maternal IgG antibodies found in fetal blood increases from that point until birth. In premature infants, levels of both total Igs and virus-specific antibodies are lower than those in term infants.[130] In general, titers of virus-specific antibodies are similar in human term infants and their mothers, suggesting that active transport does not usually target particular specificities. Antibodies of the IgG1 isotype are the principal Igs that are transferred across the placenta, although all subclasses of IgG cross to some degree.[131,132] For most viruses, IgG1 antibodies are capable

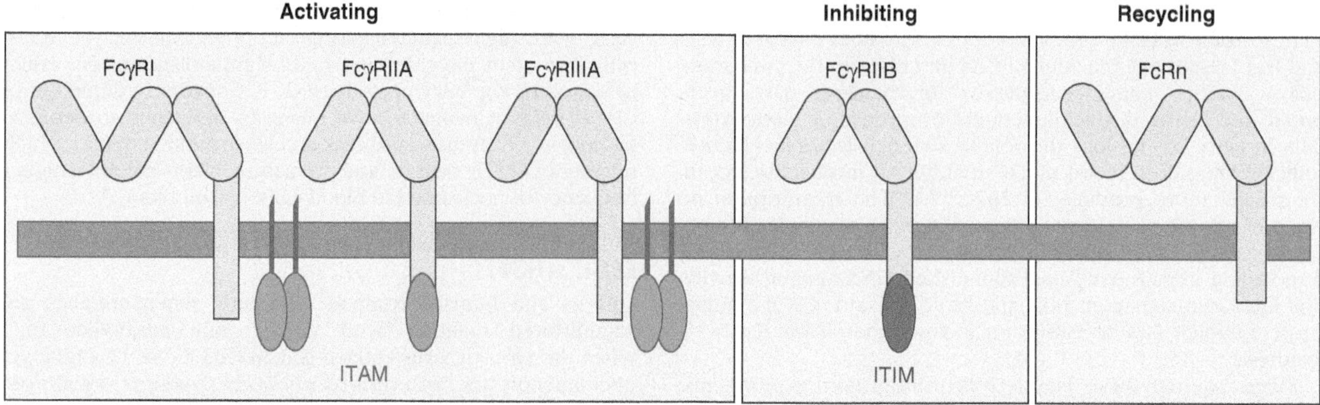

Fig. 115.1 Fc receptors (FcRs). Members of the FcγR family of receptors for the Fc portion of immunoglobulin (Ig)G molecules are present on the surface myeloid cells, with three principal members FcγRI, FcγRII, and FcγRIII. The Ig-binding α-subunit in the high-affinity IgG receptor (FcγRI) possesses three extracellular Ig-like domains, while the low-affinity receptors FcγRII and FcγRIII possess two. FcγRI can bind to monomeric IgG but FcγRII and FcγRIII only bind strongly to antigen-antibody complexes. Receptors that activate cells following Ig binding contain an immunoreceptor tyrosine-based activation motif *(ITAM)* sequence. FcγRI and FcγRIII require the common γ chain for ITAM-mediated signaling. FcγRIIB is an inhibitory receptor with an immunoreceptor tyrosine-based inhibitory motif *(ITIM)* sequence. Binding FcγRIIB counteracts ITAM-mediated signaling. The neonatal Fc receptor *(FcRn)* recycles, extending the half-life of IgG, binding strongly to IgG at lower pH, and releasing it on return to the cell surface.

of effective neutralization, so preferential transport of IgG1 transfers a maternal level of functional serum antibody-mediated immunity. For example, the highest titers of RSV-specific antibodies depend on IgG1 subclass antibodies.[133] In contrast, for microbial pathogens in which there is a strong association of immunity with other isotypes (such as IgG2 with polysaccharide bacterial antigens), the IgG1 transfer preference may be more limiting.[132]

BREAST MILK ANTIBODIES

Breast milk contains a high concentration of antibodies, especially secretory IgA molecules that are dimeric or higher-order forms. Polymeric Igs are actively transported into breast milk by transcytosis facilitated by the polymeric Ig receptor.[134] There is strong evidence from large-scale observational studies that breast-feeding is associated with reduced incidence of viral infection or reduced severity of disease following infection, but this literature is confusing. This type of study is confounded by many environmental, genetic, and behavioral variables. For instance, early population studies suggested that breast-feeding protects against RSV- or PIV-associated severe lower respiratory tract infection,[135,136] but this effect was not replicated in all studies. One factor affecting the discrepancies could be that studies performed in low- and middle-income countries generally show protection, whereas studies conducted in high income countries often do not. More recent studies using multivariate analysis found that breast-feeding was associated with a very strong protective effect against RSV disease in female infants but not in males.[137] These findings suggest that there are breast milk protective factors other than Igs. Breast milk may contribute to protection against respiratory viruses by activating innate antiviral mechanisms in the host. For example, higher rates and levels of type I IFN production were detected in breast-fed infants infected with influenza virus.[138] Breast-milk antibodies may regulate the presence of commensals and control allergic responses.[139,140]

MATERNAL ANTIBODIES CAN BE INHIBITORY

Many classic human studies demonstrated the inhibitory effect of passively acquired antibodies on active immune responses to measles virus vaccines.[141] Indeed, measles virus immunization still is not recommended in the first year of life because of the inhibitory effect of maternal antibodies on measles virus immunogenicity. Live attenuated measles virus vaccine is delivered by intramuscular inoculation, which exposes the vaccine virus to neutralizing antibodies in serum and tissue fluid. This results in a stronger inhibition of the immune response than occurs with the response to viruses that predominately infect the airway and lack a viremic phase. In monkeys, as little as 0.1 IU of monkey measles virus-neutralizing antibody per milliliter of serum blocked the induction of measles virus-serum IgM or IgG or neutralizing antibodies after inoculation with live attenuated measles virus.[142] The live attenuated measles virus vaccine is highly protective because it induces neutralizing antibodies in seronegative individuals, but a low level of maternal antibodies in infant serum can interfere with the induction of protective responses in humans.[143,144] This effect depends on the level of serum antibodies, which varies between mothers; therefore the precise age at which maternal antibody-mediated inhibition of active immunization can be surmounted varies. In addition, the epidemiology of this suppression is changing, because the mean levels of these antibodies are lower in infants whose mothers received vaccine than they were in infants whose mothers were exposed to natural measles virus in decades past.[145]

Many typical neonatal and infant respiratory viral pathogens enter the body by infecting the respiratory tract mucosal epithelia, and they cause disease at the portal of entry without causing viremia. Even in these situations, there is evidence from human studies of antibody-mediated immune suppression of the response to naturally acquired infection, for instance with wild-type RSV, PIV, or influenza viruses. The same observation is true for experimental infection with live attenuated RSV, PIV, or candidate influenza vaccine viruses.[146,147]

EVIDENCE OF IMMUNE SUPPRESSION FROM EXPERIMENTAL VACCINE STUDIES

Experimental methods for measuring effects of passive antibodies on active immune responses in infants include carefully conducted vaccine trials and animal model studies of the same vaccine candidates. In these settings, passive antibodies are especially suppressive of active immune responses of infants to virus subunit vaccine candidates administered by the parenteral route.[148] Passively acquired antibodies also inhibit responses to the recombinant viral vaccine antigens expressed by live virus vectors, such as poxviruses expressing the RSV or PIV surface glycoproteins.[149,150] Because systemically acquired antibodies are highest in concentration in the serum and tissue fluids, one strategy to overcome the inhibitory effect of such antibodies is by inoculation with live virus–vectored vaccines on mucosal surfaces.[151]

The immunosuppressive effect of maternal antibodies also has been modeled in passive antibody studies in nonhuman primates such as chimpanzees, in which inhibition of the replication of live wild-type or attenuated respiratory viruses has been observed.[152,153] In these studies, there was a beneficial effect of antibodies (reduced wild-type virus infection), but an inhibitory effect on the active immune response induced in the subject by infection or vaccination. The suppressive effects of maternal antibodies observed in studies of the systemic compartment also may also affect mucosal immune responses. Passive antibodies have been observed to inhibit the number of mucosal antibody-secreting cells and level of mucosal antibodies in both animals and humans.[152,154]

The mechanisms of antibody-mediated immune suppression are not completely understood.[155] It is thought that a major component of the antigen-specific suppression stems from blocking recognition of the B cell epitopes by passive antibodies (epitope masking). Some antigen may be simply eliminated by clearance via immune complexes that are degraded following receptor-mediated phagocytosis by FcγR$^+$ cells. There are also likely immune regulatory effects of a more global nature, mediated by differential effects upon binding of different types of human FcγRs for IgG.[156] Differences in the cytoplasmic domain of these receptors, with some molecules containing immunoreceptor tyrosine-based activation motifs (ITAMs) and others inhibition motifs (ITIMs), affect the functions of different FcγRs in antigen-presenting cells, including B cells. FcγRIIB, the only inhibitory FcγR, binds IgG in immune complexes and possesses an ITIM in its cytoplasmic domain. Crosslinking of FcγRIIB by immune complexes causes ITIM phosphorylation, with resulting inhibition of activating signaling. FcγRIIB appears to play a central role in limiting immunogenic responses, and it likely plays a critical role in the suppressive effect of passive maternal antibodies in neonates. Some Fc-FcR interactions are not suppressive; instead they play critical roles in active antiviral immunity.[157] There are five FcγRs with ITAMs and activating functions. FcγRI is the high-affinity activating receptor that binds monomeric IgG, and there are four low-affinity IgG receptors (designated FcγRIIA, FcγRIIC, FcγRIIIA, and FcγRIIIB), which only bind IgG in immune complexes. The members of this family of FcγRs differ in affinity of binding of the Fc fragment of antibody and their patterns of expression in diverse cell types.

Most studies of passive antibodies suggest there is a much less prominent suppressive effect on T cell responses. Studies with measles virus, influenza virus, or RSV in animals do not demonstrate significant inhibition of cytolytic T lymphocyte (CTL) responses by passive antibodies.[152,158] Presentation of T cell epitopes for hepatitis B antigens is enhanced by the presence of antibodies to hepatitis B surface antigen, consistent with a model in which antibody enhances antigen uptake in presenting cells using Fc-FcR interactions.[159,160] Antibodies may enhance some diseases in settings where the antimicrobial functional activity of the antibodies is low and FcR-bearing cells are susceptible to productive infection. In that circumstance, binding of noninhibitory antibodies may facilitate enhanced entry of pathogens via Fc-mediated uptake. Dengue virus reinfection is the classical example in which severe disease on reinfection with a dengue virus of a heterologous type may result in severe dengue disease. Passive transfer of some maternal antibodies to a fetus also might simulate prior infection for the infant. Reduced fucosylation (afucosylation) of passively transferred antidengue IgGs has been associated with symptomatic dengue infections in infants, possibly by both increased uptake and promotion of FcγRIIIa signaling in monocytes.[155]

MUCOSAL SITES

The mucosal barrier in the intestine must accomplish complex tasks of nutritional uptake while detecting and excluding pathogens. The inflammatory set point of the gut must be highly regulated during developmental and adaptive changes associated with the enormous exposure to diverse microbial species and foreign antigens in food. Indeed, failure to regulate gut homeostasis in the face of massive exposure to foreign antigens leads to necrotizing enterocolitis, a severe condition most common in premature infants and one of the most common causes of mortality in them. Unbalanced features of the gut microbiome early in life may be associated with the development of longer-term health effects characterized by chronic inflammation, such as inflammatory bowel diseases and asthma. Successful regulatory changes associated with host-microbial homeostasis likely facilitate the establishment of a stable and non-inflammatory milieu, but they also probably contribute to increased susceptibility to enteric pathogens, including viruses.[161] In addition to the microbiome, many other environmental factors including nutrients, chemicals, and infectious pathogens probably affect immune development in the gut during fetal and early postnatal life.[162] Observations of a wide diversity of responses in populations with similar exposures suggest that gene-environment interactions add to the complexity of these phenomena.[163]

Gut homeostasis is critically dependent on the presence of antibodies, especially polymeric forms of secretory (s)IgA and sIgM, which are transcytosed in a basolateral to apical direction across polarized epithelial cells onto the gut lumen. The actively transported dimeric IgA or pentameric IgM that contain joining (J) chain forms the first line of defense against such viruses as enteroviruses and rotaviruses in the intestine. Neonates have only a few IgA-secreting cells in the blood, reflective of the overall low level of IgA-secreting cells in the body at birth. After a few weeks, however, the newly established microbiome stimulates gut-associated lymphoid tissues to induce IgA-secreting cells.[164] In low socioeconomic areas with exposure to heavy microbial loads, such as in many developing countries, IgA-secreting cells accumulate more rapidly. The incidence of atopy is lower in these populations,[165] leading to the hygiene hypothesis, which proposes that recent increases in the incidence of atopic disorders stem from a lower incidence of infection in early childhood.[166] Consistent with this hypothesis, mice kept in germ-free conditions develop increased susceptibility to allergy.[167–170] This susceptibility appears to occur during a developmental period early in childhood.[171,172] The mechanisms underlying this altered programming are still under investigation, but are likely to be complex, such as regulation of T_H2 immunity by microbiota though RORγt$^+$ T cells.[173]

INNATE ANTIVIRAL IMMUNITY

The antiviral immune response generally can be divided into an early, nonspecific phase (typically the first 5 to 7 days of infection) involving innate immune mechanisms, followed by a later, antigen-specific phase involving adaptive immunity by T and B cells.[174] The early phase is critical, because infection may be either successfully contained or disseminated throughout the host. A closer look at the neonatal antiviral response is provided in the following discussion, which describes host recognition of viral infection, identifies the inflammatory mediators produced in response, and summarizes the cells participating in these processes.

After recognition of pathogens (principally by DCs), mediators such as IFNs, cytokines, chemokines, and surfactant proteins are necessary in signaling the antiviral state within the cell and activating and attracting other immune cells such as neutrophils, macrophages, and NK cells to orchestrate an effective antiviral response at the site of infection. The induction of the innate immune mechanisms is not pathogen-specific but depends on interactions between pathogenic factors and host cell determinants. The aim of this early innate response is to either eliminate the pathogen or to avoid spread of the

Table 115.4 Pattern Recognition Receptors.

Location	Type	Receptors	Characteristics
Membrane bound	Toll-like receptors (TLRs)	TLR1–TLR11	Interaction of TLRs with their specific pathogen-associated molecular patterns (PAMPs) induces NF-κB signaling and the MAP kinase pathway, resulting in expression of costimulatory molecules and proinflammatory cytokines.
	C-type lectin receptors (CLRs)	Group I and II CLRs	Group I CLRs: The mannose receptors. Mannose receptors recognize and bind to repeated mannose units on the surfaces of viruses. Their activation triggers endocytosis and phagocytosis of the virus via the complement system, involving the C5 convertase and the membrane attack complex (MAC). Group II CLRs: Asialoglycoprotein receptor family.
Cytoplasmic	NOD-like receptors (NLRs)		NLRs are cytoplasmic proteins that regulate inflammatory and apoptotic responses; there is a large family of cytosolic PRRs (34 members in mice, 23 in human), which are able to recognize various PAMPs and danger-associated molecular patterns and thereby initiate innate immune response toward invading pathogens and cellular damage.
		Nucleotide-binding oligomerization domain-containing protein 1 and 2 (NOD 1 and 2)	NOD2 binds to the mitochondrial antiviral signaling protein in response to viral RNA treatment and activates the interferon response.
		NACHT, LRR, and PYD domain-containing proteins (NALPs)	NALPs are involved in the activation of caspase-1 by TLRs during response to microbial infection.
		RIG-I-like receptors (RLRs)	RNA helicases that recruit factors via twin N-terminal caspase activation and recruitment domains to activate antiviral gene programs. RIG-I recognizes 5′ triphosphate-RNA while MDA5 recognizes double-stranded RNA.
Secreted	Diverse	Many types of molecules including pentraxins (e.g., C-reactive protein), complement receptors, collectins (e.g., mannan-binding lectin [MBL]), ficolins, and peptidoglycan recognition proteins.	MBL recognizes sugars, phospholipids, nucleic acids, and proteins on pathogens and initiates the lectin pathway of complement activation.

infection until elimination is achieved through the adaptive immune response. Additionally, the innate immune system serves to shape and regulate the developing immune response by promoting or inhibiting development of specific downstream effector mechanisms. This function is exemplified by the ability of innate cytokines to improve the efficiency of antigen-presenting cells and to direct the development of naïve T cells into different subtypes expressing distinct immune responses. Overall, regulation is important to a successful immune response, because many immune mechanisms can cause disease if they are unregulated or remain inappropriately activated.

PATTERN RECOGNITION RECEPTORS

Before mounting an antiviral response, the host must first recognize the infection. Unlike the adaptive immune system, which uses remarkably specific receptors and circulating factors to recognize highly variable antigens such as proteins, the receptors and factors of the innate immune system react more broadly to less variable structures. The task of innate immune recognition is to identify key molecular signatures borne by pathogens, termed *pathogen-associated molecular patterns (PAMPs)*[175] by pathogen-recognition receptors (PRRs), leading to a cascade of intracellular signaling and ultimately the mobilization of soluble defense molecules, killing of infected cells, acquisition of specialized functions by sentinel cells, and priming of the adaptive immune response (Table 115.4). These cells also express PRRs that can detect what have been termed *damage-associated molecular patterns (DAMPs)*, typically byproducts of cellular damage such as reactive oxygen species (ROSs) or released ATP.[176] The process of PRR-mediated recognition starts with the identification of virions or viral products by extracellular and intracellular receptors. At least six main classes of PRRs have been identified, including TLRs, C-type lectin receptors (CLRs), macrophage scavenger receptor (MSRs), retinoic acid inducible gene protein-1 (RIG-1)-like receptors, nucleotide oligomerization and binding domain (NOD)-like receptors (NLRs), and the Pyrin-HIN (PYHIN) domain-containing family. TLRs and CLRs are expressed on the cell surface and in endosomes, while NLRs, RLRs, and PYHINs sense PAMPs and DAMPs in intracellular compartments.[177-179]

TLR3, TLR7, TLR8, TLR9, and to a lesser extent TLR2 and TLR4[180-182] have been associated with viral recognition by the innate immune system and subsequently acquired antiviral properties such as IFN production (Fig. 115.2). pDCs recognize HSV (e.g., by TLR9) expressed on endosomes to sense viral material. TLR9 identifies the HSV DNA because it contains abundant, unmethylated deoxycytidylate-phosphate-deoxyguanylate (CpG) motifs. These CpG motifs are underrepresented in mammalian DNA, where they generally are methylated. In response, pDCs secrete high levels of IFN-α and represent the so-called natural IFN-producing cells of the body.[183] Consistent with this recognition mechanism for HSV, human pDCs express very high levels of TLR9 compared with other DC populations, such as most myeloid DCs.[183] The secretion of high levels of IFN-α by pDCs probably results in a systemic antiviral state, because receptors for type I IFNs are essentially ubiquitous. Exposure of secondary lymphoid tissue to IFN-α also may enhance local adaptive immune

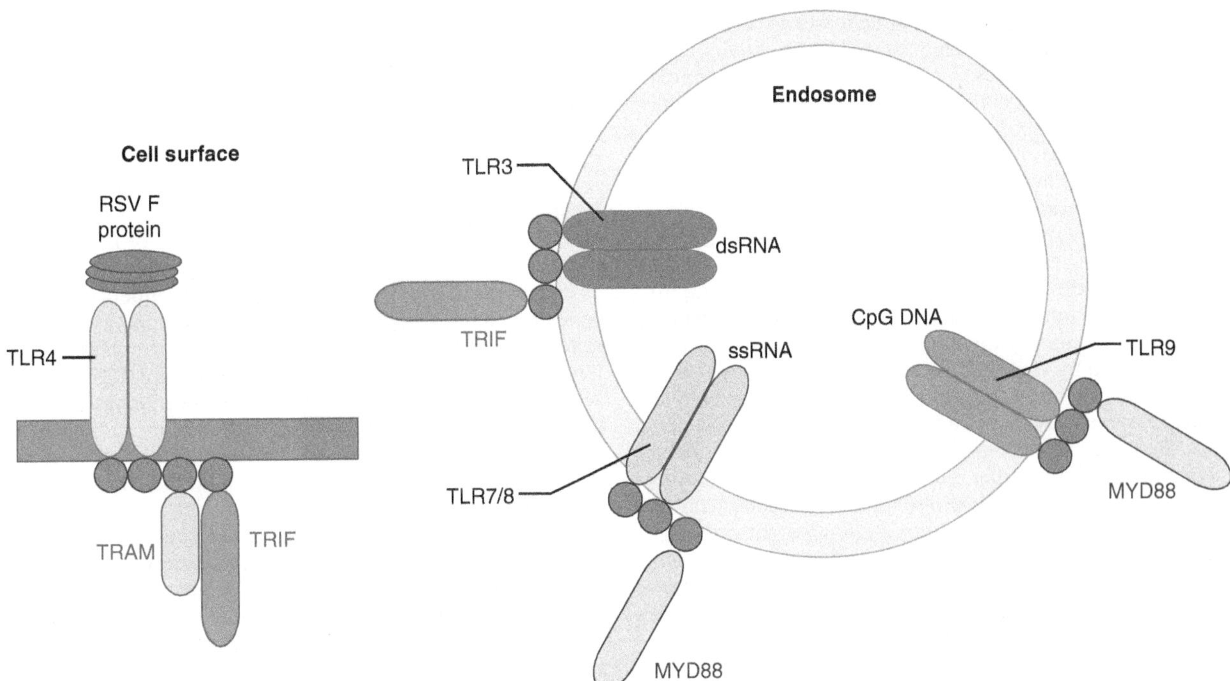

Fig. 115.2 Toll-like receptors *(TLRs)* recognizing viruses. TLRs are a family of integral membrane protein receptors in cells of the innate immune system receptors such as macrophages and dendritic cells that recognize structurally conserved molecules. A subset of TLRs recognize viral components. TLR4 recognizes the fusion *(F)* protein of respiratory syncytial virus *(RSV)*, the most common respiratory pathogen of neonates and infants. TLRs in the endosome recognize viral nucleic acids, such as single-stranded RNA *(ssRNA)*, double-stranded RNA *(dsRNA)*, and unmethylated CpG dinucleotide sites in DNA *(CpG DNA)*. *TRAM*, TRIF-related adaptor molecule; *TRIF*, TIR-domain-containing adapter-inducing interferon-β.

responses.[184] Although in vitro studies of pDCs in knockout mice deficient in TLR9 and MyD88 demonstrate a poor IFN response, no significant differences in morbidity or mortality were noted after HSV infection in these mice in vivo. This observation demonstrates that the presence of TLR9- and MyD88-independent pathways in cells other than pDCs can effectively compensate for defective IFN production by pDCs in response to HSV.[185] Mouse TLR7 and human TLR7/8 recognize single-stranded (ss) RNAs oligonucleotides rich in guanosine or uridine derived from ssRNA viruses such as HIV, influenza virus, and vesicular stomatitis virus.

Upon engagement with nucleic acid ligands, TLR9 and TLR7 deliver intracellular signals through the cytosolic adapter MyD88, which acts as a docking site for IRAK1/4, TRAF3, IKKα, and IRF7. IRF7 is then phosphorylated and translocated into the nucleus to induce the transcriptional activation of the type I IFN genes. IRF7 is constitutively expressed by pDCs and serve as a master regulator of IFN-α/β gene expression.[186] MyD88 also recruits IRF5, a transcription factor that cooperates with nuclear factor-κB (NF-κB) in activating the transcription of genes encoding proinflammatory cytokines and chemokines.[187] TLR7 and TLR9 signaling pathways also induce the maturation of pDCs, which consists of increased expression of MHC class II and costimulatory molecules (CD80, CD86 and CD40), resulting in the capacity to present antigens.

TLR3 also functions to recognize viral infection. TLR3, a known ligand for double-stranded (DS) RNA, also has been shown to initiate IFN production after viral infection in a MyD88-independent manner. This is done through an adapter protein named Toll/IL-1 receptor domain-containing adapter, inducing IFN by activation of IFN transcription regulatory factor-3 (IRF-3). IRF-3 is produced constitutively in most cell types and, in the absence of activation, is present in the cytoplasm in an inactive form. Activation occurs by means of two kinases: IκB kinase-ε (IKK-ε) and TANK-binding kinase-1 (TBK-1). Upon phosphorylation, IRF-3 dimerizes and translocates to the nucleus, where it interacts with coactivators CAAT-binding protein and p300. This complex serves as an enhanceosome complex that transactivates *IFN-β* gene expression in cooperation with activator protein-1 (AP-1) and NFκB. Infected cells secrete mainly IFN-β as an initial response to infection then switch to IFN-α during subsequent amplification of the IFN response.[188,189] Mice deficient in TLR9 or TLR3 displayed significant abrogation in IFN production when challenged with murine cytomegalovirus (MCMV) and were susceptible to MCMV infection.[190]

Besides TLRs, other extracellular receptors exist to identify pathogens within the innate immune system. Mannan-binding lectin, which activates the complement system, C-reactive protein, serum amyloid protein, and the macrophage mannin receptor are pattern recognition molecules that mediate phagocytosis of microorganisms, primarily bacteria and fungi. Another phagocytic pattern recognition receptor expressed on macrophages, MSR, has a broader role in host defense including recognition of viruses. Belonging to the scavenger receptor family (type A), it has specificity for a variety of polyanionic ligands, including dsRNA, LPS, lipoteichoic acid, and acetylated low-density lipoproteins. MSR-deficient mice have an increased susceptibility to HSV infection (as well as to other infections such as listeriosis and malaria).[175]

Extracellular receptors and TLRs are not the sole receptors controlling the innate immune response. Recognition of other families of molecules that play a key role in the sensing of infectious microorganisms is emerging. The existence of specific innate immunity receptors in the cytosol illustrates the topologic problem posed by the cellular location of TLRs: These transmembrane receptors have access only to ligands that are either extracellular or are in the lumen of endosomes and are blind to microorganisms or their products that have penetrated the cytosol. Two such cytoplasmic receptors of dsRNA have been identified as members of a family of DExD/H box RNA helicases:

RIG-1 and MDA5. The DExD/H box RNA helicases are defined by their ability to unwind dsRNA with intrinsic ATPase activity. Both RIG-I and MDA5 contain a caspase recruitment domain, which serves to activate NFκB and IRF-3, critical regulators of innate immune responses, in response to cytoplasmic dsRNA.

Other well-described cytosolic sensors of viruses include protein kinase RNA-activated (PKR), the 2-5A system, and the Mx proteins. PKR normally is inactive, but on binding dsRNA it undergoes autophosphorylation and subsequent dsRNA-dependent phosphorylation of substrates, including the α subunit of eukaryotic initiation factor 2 (eIF2-α), leading to rapid inhibition of translation. The oligoadenylate synthetase (OAS) system is a multienzyme pathway in which IFN-inducible OASs are stimulated by viral dsRNAs to produce a series of short 2′,5°-oligoadenylates ("2-5A") that activate the 2-5A–dependent RNase ligand, which cleaves ssRNA halting viral and cellular processes. Similarly, the Mx proteins are IFN-inducible GTPases in the dynamin superfamily that interfere with viral transcription on encountering a wide range of ssRNA virus targets, such as influenza virus genomic RNA. Another large family of cytosolic receptors is the group of nucleotide-binding domain, leucine-rich repeat-containing proteins (NLRs).[191] A large number of viruses have been shown to have NLRP3-activating properties, including pathogens affecting fetuses and neonates such as enterovirus 71, HSV-1, and RSV.[192]

INTERFERONS

The IFN system is indispensable for vertebrates to control viral infections. Knockout mice with deletions in IFN receptors quickly succumb to viral infections despite having a normal adaptive immune system.[193] Likewise, children with genetic defects in the IFN-α/β system die in infancy from viral infection, such as HSV.[194] Animal studies modeling specific knockout genes of effector molecules within this pathway also have revealed extreme susceptibility to various viral infections, demonstrating the significant power of this antiviral system.[193,195-200]

During viral infections, IFNs are some of the most prominent cytokines produced. Named for their ability to interfere with viral replication,[201] IFNs are a large family of multifunctional secreted proteins involved in antiviral defense, cell growth regulation, and immune activation. They are classified into three dominant types. Type I IFNs (IFN-α and IFN-β) are produced in direct response to viral infection and consist of the products of the IFN-α multigene family, which are synthesized predominantly by leukocytes, and the product of the *IFN-β* gene, which is synthesized by most cell types but especially fibroblasts. Type II IFN consists of the products of the *IFN-γ* gene and, rather than being induced directly by viral infection, is synthesized in response to the recognition of infected cells by activated T lymphocytes ($CD4^+$ T helper 1 cells and $CD8^+$ cytotoxic T cells) and NK cells.[202] More recently, molecules called *IL-29, IL-28A,* and *IL-28B* have been classified as the type III IFN group, designated IFN-λ molecules 1, 2, and 3, respectively. RIG-I–like receptors induce type III IFN expression in a variety of human cell types, and peroxisomes appear to be a primary site of initiation of type III IFN expression. As intestinal epithelial cells differentiate, peroxisome biogenesis up-regulates and promotes strong type III IFN responses in human cells.[203]

IFNs stimulate an antiviral state in target cells, whereby the replication of virus is blocked or impaired owing to IFN receptor signaling and the subsequent synthesis of a number of enzymes that interfere with cellular and viral processes. Additionally, IFNs make cells more susceptible to apoptosis, further limiting spread of virus. Finally, IFN molecules have profound immunomodulatory effects and stimulate the adaptive response. However, although both IFN-α/β and IFN-γ influence immune effector cells, they have significant functional differences that probably account for the different spectrums of antiviral activities of the two types of IFN.

The signaling pathways for the IFN response circuit are well characterized and have been reviewed.[189,195,202,204,205] The biologic activities of IFNs are initiated by binding of IFN-α/β and IFN-γ to their cognate receptors on the surface of cells, which results in activation of distinct but related signaling pathways, known as the *Janus kinase/signal transducer and transcriptional activator (Jak/STAT)* pathways. The ultimate outcome of this signaling is the transcription of target genes that previously were quiescent or expressed at low levels. The regulatory sequences of IFN-α/β genes contain a variation of the upstream consensus sequence called the IFN-stimulated response element (ISRE), whereas IFN-γ–inducible genes contain the upstream IFN-γ activation sequence (GAS). STATs are latent transcription factors that become tyrosine phosphorylated by Jaks. After binding to their receptor (IFNAR), type I IFNs activate intracellular signaling, including Jak1, Tyk2, STAT1, STAT2, and STAT3. Jaks activate (phosphorylate) STATs, which dimerize, translocate to the nucleus, and induce IFN-simulated genes (ISGs). STAT1-STAT2 heterodimers complex with cofactor nuclear protein p48, forming a heterotrimeric complex known as ISGF3 that binds the ISRE sequence in the promoters of ISGs, influencing the transcription of a distinct group of genes.[206] These include the gene for IRF-7, which amplifies type I IFN production if viruses infect cells that previously have been exposed to type I IFN.[207] STAT1 homodimers and STAT1-STAT3 heterodimers activate GAS sequences.[208] Because STAT-1, but not other STATs, is tyrosine-phosphorylated by IFN-γ binding to its specific receptor,[208] the potential exists for type I IFN to induce genes that are characteristic of IFN-γ responses, but not vice versa.

Patients who have genetic defects in STAT-1 that compromise the GAS pathway, but not the ISRE pathway of gene regulation, are not prone to severe viral infections.[209] This point argues that the regulation of the GAS pathway by type I IFNs, and the induction of certain gene products such as IRF-1,[210] are dispensable for antiviral immunity in humans. By contrast, complete lack of STAT-1 function and, as a result, loss of the ISRE-mediated pathway of signal transduction in humans resulted in recurrent HSV-1 encephalitis and death.[193] The critical importance of the ISRE pathway also is supported by the observation that mice genetically deficient in the type I IFN receptor are highly susceptible to HSV.[211]

IFNs can induce more than 300 cellular proteins.[212] However, the exact pattern of induction varies by cell type and type of IFN. The IFN-induced proteins include enzymes, signaling proteins, chemokines, antigen presentation proteins, transcription factors, heat shock proteins, and apoptotic proteins. Several of the cellular systems already discussed in the detection of viruses (PKR, Mx proteins, and the 2-5A system) also are IFN-driven, allowing for a positive reinforcement of these antiviral systems. Moreover, loss of any of these three systems leads to increased susceptibility to viral infection in mice.[213,214] Interestingly, despite their potency, knockout mice lacking PKR, Mx, and OAS still exhibit a limited IFN-induced antiviral state, indicating that additional pathways exist.[215]

Of note, ISG56 encodes *P56,* which is one of the most strongly induced genes among all of the IFN-stimulated genes. *P56* binds to the large multimeric complex of eIF-3 through p48 and blocks its function in initiating protein synthesis. Of interest, ISG56 also is strongly induced by non-IFN pathways after viral infection (dsRNA).[216]

IFNs also have a profound effect on cells of the immune system that mediate innate and adaptive immunity. Members of the P200 family of structurally related proteins are strongly induced by type I IFNs and encoded by a gene cluster. The P202 protein impairs cell proliferation by inhibiting the functions of many cellular factors, including NFκB, E2F, TP53, c-Fos, c-Jun, MyoD, myogenin, c-Myc, and Rb.[217]

IFN-γ is the major immunomodulator and activator of macrophages. Consequently, mice defective in *IFN-γ*, *IFN-γ receptor*, or *STAT1* genes are highly susceptible to infection with a number of microorganisms, mostly bacterial.[218] IFN-γ has an important role in the development of CD4+ helper T cells by directing CD4+ T cells toward the T_H1 direction and, by blocking IL-4 production, away from T_H2. This shift is facilitated by enhancing the synthesis of IL-12 in APCs, an effect that also promotes development of T_H1 cells. IFN-γ also up-regulates CD4+ T cell expression of IL-12 receptors.

Both types I and II IFNs promote expression of MHC class I molecules and development of CD8+ T cell responses.[219] MHC class II induction occurs in mononuclear phagocytes, endothelial cells, epithelial cells, and T cells, where it enhances CD4+ responses. The positive role of IFNs in enhancing antigen presentation (besides up-regulating MHC molecules) is augmented by regulating the expression of many proteins responsible for generating antigenic peptides. This is accomplished through IFN-γ induction of three proteasome subunits—LMP2, LMP7, and MECL1. IFN-γ also induces the expression of PA28, the nonenzymatic subunit of the proteasome, and TAP1 and TAP2 (transporter associated with antigen-processing proteins), which transfer the proteasome-mediated peptides to the endoplasmic reticulum, where they bind nascent MHC class I proteins.[219]

INTERFERING WITH INTERFERONS

Shortly after the recognition that heat-inactivated influenza viruses induce IFN, it was discovered that infection of cells with live virus inhibited the subsequent induction of IFN by an inactivated virus—"inverse interference."[201] The key role of both type I (α and β) and II (γ) IFNs as one of the first antiviral defense mechanisms is highlighted by the fact that anti-IFN strategies are present in most viruses.[202,220] Viruses have been reported to block nearly all aspects of the IFN regulatory pathway.[221-223] Some of the medically relevant viral interactions with the neonatal host are summarized here. Viruses counteract the host IFN response in a number of ways, including by inhibiting IFN production or signaling and by circumventing IFN-induced antiviral effector molecules.

Substantial amounts of type I IFN are found in the tissues of HSV-infected animals and humans.[224,225] Although HSV efficiently induces the secretion of type I IFN, the virus is relatively resistant to their antiviral effects. HSV attempts to block synthesis and function of type I IFN in infected cells by several mechanisms. In cells infected with HSV, viral DNA replication leads to the activation of another cytoplasmic receptor, PKR, that phosphorylates the α subunit of translation initiation factor 2 (eIF-2α) and thereby inhibits translation initiation.[190] As a countermeasure, the ICP34.5 protein is expressed by HSV to prevent the shutoff of protein synthesis. ICP34.5 interacts with cellular protein phosphatase 1 and redirects its activity to dephosphorylate eIF-2α.[226] Recent data demonstrate that in HSV-infected cells, eIF-2α dephosphorylation mediated by the ICP34.5 protein is tightly coupled with viral resistance to IFN.[226] As expected, ICP34.5-minus recombinant HSVs are attenuated in the host. Interestingly, the phenotype can be reestablished by extragenic mutations in the herpes genome, resulting in earlier expression of US11 protein. If the US11 protein binds PKR before its phosphorylation, US11 is able to fully compensate, demonstrating that HSV has utilized at least two ways to overcome PKR.[227]

ICP34.5 and US11 protein effectively negate a major effect of the type I IFNs. Second, HSV blocks the phosphorylation of STAT1, STAT2, and Janus kinases induced by IFNs.[228] This observation may account for the limited ability of type I IFNs to treat recurrences of established HSV infections, such as of the eye. A combination of IFN types I and II is effective in the control of HSV infection, at least in mice,[229] suggesting that cellular sources of IFN-γ in vivo (T_H1 CD4+ T cells, CD8+ T cells, γδ T cells, NK cells, or NK T cells) play an important role in host defense against HSV by acting in concert with type I IFN.

The OAS (2-5A RNase L) pathway also is inhibited by HSV-infected cells by generation of substituting 2′,5′-oligoadenylate derivatives that inhibit RNase L.[230] HCMV has complex interactions with the IFN system. HCMV binding of the cell by its gB glycoprotein activates type I IFN; at the same time, however, the virus disarms downstream effectors involved in the induction of the antiviral state. It does this by reducing the expression of Jak1 and IRF-9, thereby disrupting IFN signaling.[231]

Adenoviruses also encode several mechanisms to antagonize IFNs. Adenovirus-infected cells express VAI viral RNA, which, like dsRNA, binds to PKR; however, unlike dsRNA, it does not activate PKR but in fact inhibits it. Additionally, adenovirus produces E1A protein, which inhibits ISGF3 complex by down-regulating the expression of STAT1 and IRF-9 and by directly binding to STAT1.[232] Influenza viruses counteract IFNs through production of a nonstructural protein, NS1. NS1 binds to dsRNA, prevents dsRNA-mediated activation of PKR and OAS, and prevents synthesis of IFN. NS1 achieves this inhibitory effect through disruption of dsRNA-stimulated *IFN* gene transcription of IRF-3, IRF-7, and NFκB and activation of cellular protein (p58IPK), which inhibits PKR. NS1 also binds another IFN-induced protein, ISG15, and blocks its action.[233] PIVs encode proteins that inhibit IFN signaling by degradation of the Jak/STAT pathway.[234]

Hepatitis B capsid protein specifically inhibits *MxA* gene expression through an unknown mechanism.[202] Its open-reading frame C product and the viral terminal protein inhibit IFN production at the transcription level by sequestering dsRNA.[235] The sequestration of dsRNA by viral proteins probably has a wider role in protecting the virus from antiviral mechanisms, because dsRNA-activated PKR can activate NFκB and induce synthesis of immunomodulatory genes, in addition to IFN.

HIV type I (HIV-1) RNA transcripts contain stem bulge loop structures, called *transactivating response* (TAR) elements, in the 5′-untranslated region, which are readily detected by PKR. Its transcriptional transactivation protein (Tat) is able to compete with PKR for binding to eIF2-α, allowing protein synthesis and viral replication to proceed.[236] Of interest, the use of PKR-phosphorylated Tat by HIV-1 has been shown to increase the interaction with its TAR-containing RNAs, thereby enhancing transcription.[237] HIV down-regulates RNase L (OAS) by inducing the expression of the RNase L inhibitor, which antagonizes 2-5A binding to RNase L, preventing its activation.[238]

INNATE CELLULAR MECHANISMS

Herpes viruses induce and combat many of the cardinal immune programs of the innate and T cell response in humans. Here, we will focus on examples of innate and then T cell responses to herpes viruses, as a paradigm of responses to all fetal and neonatal virus infections.

MONONUCLEAR PHAGOCYTES AND INDUCIBLE NITRIC OXIDE SYNTHASE

Mononuclear phagocytes are widely distributed in tissues as macrophages and are likely to play an important role in the local containment of viral infections such as HSV before activation of the adaptive immune response. In experimental models of HSV and MCMV infection (intraperitoneal and corneal), macrophages have been identified as the predominant cell type involved and demonstrate HSV-instigated production of TNF-α. TNF-α has direct anti-HSV effects, particularly in combination with IFN-γ,[239] and these two cytokines may act synergistically to increase expression of leukocyte adhesion molecules and inducible nitric oxide synthase (iNOS) expression by mononuclear phagocytes. HSV infection of mononuclear phagocytes also acts synergistically with IFN-γ to promote expression of iNOS,[240] which has anti-HSV effects in vitro,[241] and for production of TNF-α.[242] Systemic depletion of mononuclear phagocytes (by administration of liposomes containing dichloromethylene diphosphonate) or of γδ T cells (which produce IFN-γ), or inhibition of TNF-α, IFN-γ, or iNOS activity in the HSV corneal infection model, results in increased HSV-1 replication within the ganglion.[243,244] Specific inhibition of iNOS in mice challenged with intranasal aminoguanidine causes a dose-dependent increase in pneumonitis compared with that in control animals.[245] These complex interactions illustrate the importance of cellular and cytokine components in local antiviral host defense. An antiviral role for iNOS also is suggested by the increased susceptibility of mice with complete genetic deficiency of iNOS to HSV infection following a footpad injection. These mice also demonstrate exaggerated T_H1 responses, indicating that iNOS may have key antiviral effects, as well as inhibitory effects on T_H1 differentiation.[246]

However, innate antiviral immune mechanisms mediated by mononuclear phagocytes, such as iNOS induction, may not necessarily be beneficial in all contexts of HSV infection. In a murine model of HSV pneumonia, inhibition of iNOS activity markedly reduced pulmonary inflammation and improved survival, despite increases in the lung tissue HSV viral titer.[247] Inhibition of iNOS activity also was of clinical benefit in experimental HSV-1 encephalitis in rats and was not associated with increased viral load.[248]

DENDRITIC CELLS

DCs play a pivotal role in the development of $CD4^+$ and $CD8^+$ T cell responses to a variety of viruses. When the virus is able to overcome the immune response, it permits persistence of viral infection within the host. Direct infection of DCs is one such strategy and has been used by a number of viruses, including influenza virus, HIV, and HSV-1 and -2, to block the amplification of the immune response by DCs. Indeed, myeloid DCs generated from peripheral blood monocytes express HSV entry receptors Hve-A and Hve-B. Although attack of mature DCs by HSV-1 generally results in a nonproductive or aborted infection, the mature cells generally are not found at the sites of HSV infection. Immature DCs are, however, readily infected by HSV and subsequently down-regulate their costimulatory and adhesion molecules; expression of MHC molecules is largely unaffected.[226] The inability of HSV ICP47 to interfere with MHC class I expression probably is the consequence of innately high levels of the "transporter associated with antigen processing" (TAP) protein in DCs. Down-regulation of other molecules does have an impact on its stimulatory ability; for example, down-regulation of CD40 expression on HSV-infected DCs may lead to decreased production of IL-12 on contact with T cells. Observed down-regulation of CD54 on the surface of immature DCs may also effect generation of anti-HSV immunity. CD54/ICAM-1 is a surface glycoprotein that binds leukocyte function antigen-1 (LFA-1), facilitating a number of cellular events, including antigen-specific T cell activation and leukocyte transendothelial migration. Binding of CD54 to LFA-1 appears to be of critical importance for the activation of naïve T lymphocytes, especially at low antigen concentrations.[249] Infected DCs subsequently are compromised in their ability to carry out their function in stimulating effector cells and may undergo rapid apoptosis. Although this destructive process removes a pool of cells that present antigen, thereby potentially giving a "head start" to viral infection, neighboring uninfected DCs readily take up apoptotic cell debris for antigen presentation through MHC class I (an example of cross-presentation of antigen) and stimulate effector cells such as HSV-specific $CD8^+$ T cells. Transfer of viral peptide antigens from infected cells to neighboring bystanders through gap junctions also has been proposed.[250] pDCs are key players in the early antiviral responses, notably by their ability to produce a large amount of type I IFN and type III IFN. Their response is rapid and triggered mainly by the endosomal sensors TLR7 and TLR9, which recognize viral nucleic acids (RNA and DNA, respectively).[251] Despite comparable levels of TLR9 and TLR7 expression in adult and neonatal human pDCs, cord blood pDCs have a strong limitation in their capacity to produce IFN-α in response to TLR9 and TLR7 ligation, HCMV, or HSV exposure.[252] This decreased production is associated with a reduced nuclear translocation of IRF7.[253] In contrast another report indicates that purified cord blood pDCs are responsive to CpG and a variety of virus.[254] Despite such discrepancy, impaired type I IFN production was also demonstrated both ex vivo in cord blood mononuclear cells infected with RSV and in vivo upon primary RSV infection in neonatal mice.[255,256] Similarly, in mouse, neonatal pDCs exhibit dampened IFN-α and IRF7 translocation during lymphocytic choriomeningitis virus (LCMV) infection.[257]

The limitations of DC function in early-life antiviral immunity include the decreased capacity of cord blood cDCs to produce IL12p70 and their lower expression of MHC and costimulatory molecules as previously described. A thorough understanding of neonatal DC responses during viral infection must consider local lung-migratory DC populations, namely in mice, $CD103^+$ and $CD11b^+$ DCs subsets, known to induce adaptive T cell responses. Both $CD103^+$ and $CD11b^+$ DCs of neonatal mice are less efficient at antigen uptake and processing, and have lower costimulatory molecule expression than their adult counterparts.[258] Type 2 innate lymphoid immune cells (ILC2s) are also involved, as shortly after birth, ILC2s accumulate in an IL-33-dependent manner in the developing lung. Interleukin-33 furthermore boosts the function of neonatal DCs to promote long-lasting T_H2-cell-mediated immunity.[259] Although cDCs and pDCs exhibit relative defects in their capacity to synthesize IL-12p70 and type I IFN, it appears that antiviral immune responses can be induced under specific conditions. Indeed, treatment of neonatal mice with Flt-3 ligand and growth factors, which enhances the number and maturation of peripheral cDCs and pDCs, increases resistance of neonatal mice to HSV infection.[260,261] Collectively, these observations suggest that early life cDCs and pDCs responses to virus are tightly regulated in vivo, which may be beneficial to avoid potentially harmful inflammatory reactions and result in increased vulnerability to viral pathogens such as influenza, RSV, HSV-1 or CMV.

NATURAL KILLER CELLS

NK cells are important in conferring protection from viral infections and in immunosurveillance of transformed cells. NK cells are bone marrow–derived lymphocytes that lack the antigen-specific TCRs and Igs that are characteristic of T and B cells, respectively. They make up approximately 5% to 20% of lymphocytes in the spleen, liver, and peripheral blood and are present in lower frequencies in the thymus, lymph nodes, and bone marrow.[261] In humans, a minority population of $CD56^{hi}$ NK cells is primarily involved in producing large amounts of cytokines such as TNF-α, IFN-γ and chemokines. Their production of IFN-γ early in an immune response promotes the development of T_H1 cell immunity. $CD56^{low}$ NK cells that predominate in peripheral blood and inflamed tissues display lower cytokine production, but potent cytotoxicity either by direct lysis of virus-infected cells and tumors or through ADCC due to their high expression of low-affinity FcR for IgG (FcγRIII) (also known as *CD16*). Unlike CTLs, NK cells do not require antigen-specific recognition to kill their targets. NK cell reactivity is regulated by a complex array of surface receptors delivering either inhibitory or activating signals in combination with cytokines.[262]

The two major groups of inhibitory NK receptors are the killer inhibitory receptors (KIRs) and CD94/NKG2A. The KIRs bind to portions of HLA-B and HLA-C molecules located outside the peptide-binding groove recognized by the TCR, whereas CD94/NKG2A binds to HLA-E, a nonclassic and nonvariable MHC molecule that requires hydrophobic leader peptides from HLA-A, -B, and -C for its surface expression. These NK cell receptors help counteract the ability of viruses to decrease surface expression of class I MHC molecules, thereby limiting $CD8^+$ T cell–mediated viral clearance. For example, both HSV and HCMV have been shown to induce NK cell cytotoxicity by down-regulating HLA-C molecules engaged in triggering of KIRs.[263]

NK cells also express activating receptors,[264] such as 2B4 (CD244), NKG2D, NKp30, NKp44, NKp46, and NKR-P1A (CD161), that are important for killing. NKG2D may be activated by binding to MHC class I chain A (MICA) or chain B (MICB) or UL-16–binding proteins (ULBPs) on target cells. These molecules are induced by cell stress. Direct activation by viral products is also possible. For example, the Ly49H-activating receptor of murine NK cells specifically recognizes a MCMV-encoded protein, m157.[265] Viruses, including herpes viruses, use a wide variety of strategies to inhibit NK cell–mediated cytotoxicity, indicating the importance of this antiviral mechanism in vivo.[266,267] HCMVs interfere at multiple steps of cellular MHC-I production. For example, they cause sequestration of MHC-I before they reach the surface by interfering with peptide chaperones. Then they produce their own MHC-I viral homologues (HCMV UL18).

NK cells are a particularly important restraint on viral replication and dissemination before the appearance of adaptive immune responses mediated by T and B cells. They play a key role in settings in which class I MHC expression is down-regulated and $CD8^+$ T cell recognition of virus-infected target cells is hampered. NK cell depletion in HSV-infected mice was shown to result in decreased early viral control. Humans genetically deficient in NK cells are particularly susceptible to herpes viruses including HSV, HCMV, and VZV.[268] Although the initial disease is severe, these patients are able eventually to clear virus, presumably by means of T cell–mediated immunity.[268,269] Studies with MCMV also suggest that NK cells are important in the early control of herpes virus infection[270] and that IFN-γ produced by NK cells is more important for this protection than is NK cell–mediated cytolytic activity.[271]

NK cells have been observed to interact with DCs in a number of experimental and in vivo settings including studies with herpes viruses. The bidirectional crosstalk between DCs and NK cells can occur in the periphery or in secondary lymphoid tissues where they interact with each other through cell-cell contact and soluble factors. Interaction of NK cells with DCs results in maturation, activation, and cytokine production by both cells and is implicated in fine-tuning the adaptive immune response to viral infections.[272]

The proportions of circulating $CD56^{hi}$ NK and $CD56^{low}$ NK are rather stable over time between birth and adult life, though $CD56^{hi}$ NK cell numbers were reported to be slightly higher in newborns.[273] The cytotoxic function of NK cells increases progressively during fetal life to reach values at term gestation approximately 50% (range, 15% to 60%) of those for adult cells.[274-284] An important point is that decreased cytotoxic activity by neonatal NK cells compared with adult cells is consistently observed with HSV-infected[285-287] and HCMV-infected target cells,[288] but not with HIV-1–infected cells.[289,290] It is clear that reduced neonatal NK cell activity is not determined at the level of the hematopoietic stem cell or later precursor cells of the NK cell lineage, because donor-derived NK cells appear early after cord blood transplantation and mediate robust cytotoxicity by way of the perforin/granzyme and Fas/Fas ligand cytotoxic pathways.[291]

Similar to their effects on adult NK cells, cytokines such as IL-2, IL-12, IL-15, type I IFN, and IFN-γ can augment the cytotoxic activity of neonatal NK cells within a few hours.[292-294] However, neonatal NK cells are less responsive to activation by the combination of IL-12 and IL-15 than are adult NK cells, as reflected in the induction of CD69 surface expression.[295]

Reduced NK cell cytotoxic activity and cytokine production may be an important contributor to the pathogenesis of neonatal HSV infection. In the murine neonatal model in which human cells are adoptively transferred, the age-related maturation of NK cell function parallels the development of resistance to HSV.[296,297] Neonatal mice, which like human neonates are more susceptible to HSV infection, can be protected by adoptive transfer of human blood mononuclear cells from adults but not those from neonates. As in adults, expansion of $NKG2C^+$ NK cells have also been observed in young children infected in utero with CMV.[298] The role of NK cells in the control of CMV infection in early life is supported by the report of a 3-month-old $T^-B^+NK^+$SCID infant who presented a CMV gastroenteritis that resolved spontaneously without antiviral treatment.[299] These data show that CMV infection in early life can activate NK cells with antiviral properties.

ANTIVIRAL T CELL IMMUNITY: AN OVERVIEW

The lymphoid stem cell derives from the pluripotent hematopoietic stem cell and differentiates into three types of cells—the T lymphocyte, the B lymphocyte, and the non-T, non-B NK cell progenitor, discussed previously. The lymphoid stem cells destined to be T lymphocytes undergo positive and negative selection principally within the thymus and undergo development into descendant cells with rearranged α and β (or γ and δ) genes of its TCR. T cell surface expression of the TCR depends on coexpression with the CD3 molecule, which is a cluster of γ-, δ-, ε-, and ζζ-chains. Together, the TCR and CD3 molecules form the TCR complex. These early T cells are capable of distinguishing between self- and nonself-antigens in the context of self-MHC molecules and circulate within the bloodstream, the lymphatic system, and tissues. For the most part, three populations of T cells leave the thymus: TCR-αβ/$CD4^+$ T cells, TCR-αβ/$CD8^+$ T cells, and (as a minority) TCR-γδ T cells, which are predominantly $CD4^-$/$CD8^-$. All bear the TCR complex; thus CD3 represents a universal T cell marker.

Although $CD4^+$ T cells are referred to as helper T cells and $CD8^+$ T cells as CTLs, they can have diverse functions and should be understood on the basis of their respective phenotypes and their response to MHC molecules. $CD8^+$ T cells recognize peptides in the context of class I MHC (displayed on virtually all nucleated cells), and $CD4^+$ T cells recognize antigens as presented in the context of class II MHC molecules, found on APCs such as monocytes, macrophages, B cells, and DCs.

T cells play the critical role in resolution of active HSV infection and maintenance of viral latency.[300,301] Studies in mice suggest $CD4^+$ and $CD8^+$ T cells contribute to clearance of HSV after acute infection, but B cells alone are not able to provide full protection. The importance of T cells in the control of human HSV and other herpes virus infections is indicated by the increased susceptibility of those with quantitative (purine nucleoside phosphorylase deficiency,[302] late HIV infection) or qualitative T cell and antigen presentation defects (Wiskott-Aldrich syndrome). Murine studies also suggest that $CD4^+$ T cells are more important than $CD8^+$ T cells in the control of HSV infections of the skin and peripheral nervous system,[303] suggesting that the relative importance of $CD4^+$ versus $CD8^+$ T cells in antiviral control is tissue-specific.

Comparison of newborn and adult T lymphocyte function explains some of the increased susceptibility to viral infections such as HSV infection in neonates. Although the mean T lymphocyte count is higher in neonates, neonatal T cells do not proliferate well in response to antigen, do not function efficiently as B cell helpers, and produce cytokines IFN-γ and IL-4 in significantly lesser amounts.[304] Additionally, neonatal T cell cytotoxicity may be limited in comparison with that of adult T cells. The specific role of T cell immaturity in severe clinical HSV infection in neonates is further suggested by the observation that neonates infected with HSV showed delayed antigen-specific cellular responses (including decreased proliferation and IFN-γ production) compared with adults who had primary HSV infection.[305]

CD4+ T CELL–MEDIATED ANTIVIRAL IMMUNITY

CD4+ T cells appear to play a key role in protection from HSV and have been identified in the circulation[306] and in multiple sites of recurrent human HSV infection, such as the skin,[307,308] cervix,[309] cornea,[310] and retina.[311] Natural infection results in CD4+ T cell recognition of peptide epitopes from a variety of HSV proteins, including those of the envelope, tegument, and capsid.[274,312] A number of mechanisms are likely to be important, reflecting the central and diverse roles of CD4+ T cells in mediating and regulating antigen-specific immunity in HSV infection.

T CELL ACTIVATION AND T_H1/T_H2 DIFFERENTIATION

In response to microbial pathogens, CD4+ T cells differentiate into a T_H1 or T_H2 phenotype. On the one hand, T_H1 cells principally produce IFN-γ and induce B cells to release IgG2 isotype mouse antibodies, which are responsible for phagocyte activation of ADDC, and defend against intracellular pathogens. On the other hand, T_H2 cells produce IL-4, IL-5, and IL-10 and induce IgE antibodies, which are responsible for immunity against parasitic infections.

As discussed previously, TLRs are important for innate immunity and activation of many cell types in response to recognition of pathogens through pattern recognition receptors. For example, the uptake of microorganisms by DCs through TLRs induces the up-regulation of costimulatory and MHC molecules, expression of chemokines, and migration of the DC to draining lymph nodes. There they prime and activate the adaptive immune response through interaction with T cells. The activation of T cells by APCs results from (1) T cell recognition of MHC class II-bound pathogen peptide, (2) activation of costimulatory molecules (such as CD28/CD80/86 or CD154/CD40), and (3) an initiation signal from specific cytokines, such IL-12 driving a T_H1-type response or IL-4/IL-10 driving a T_H2-type response.

After activation of T cells, a crucial step in tailoring adaptive immunity is determining the T_H1 versus T_H2 phenotype.[313,314] Factors such as the density of peptides presented, the types of costimulatory molecules expressed, and the state of APC activation influence whether the CD4+ T cells differentiate into either a T_H1 or T_H2 phenotype. However, the most important signal is the cytokine milieu present at the time of T cell stimulation, with either a T_H1-inducing profile represented by IL-12 family members and IFN-α or T_H2-inducing profile represented by IL-4 and IL-10.

Because presentation of antigen in the absence of costimulatory signals leads to anergy instead of activation, the stimulation of CD80 or CD86 by TLR-mediated signals is an important step in the activation of adaptive immunity.[315] In this way, TLRs participate in the translation of nonspecific information contained in conserved PAMPs into antigen-specific information and clonal expansion of T cells.

In vitro models of activation have shown that neonatal CD4+ T cells differ from adult CD4+ T cells in tending to become anergic (permanently nonresponsive to antigenic stimuli) unless antigen is presented by primed or mature DCs expressing costimulatory molecules and cytokines.[316–319] This anergic tendency may apply to CD4+ T cells that are expanded when neonates are infected with bacteria that express superantigen toxins, such as toxic shock syndrome toxin-1.[317]

T_H1 CYTOKINE PRODUCTION

The HSV-specific CD4+ T cell response of humans is characterized by a predominant T_H1 response.[284] The differentiation of naïve CD4+ T cells into T_H1 effector cells is favored by production of cytokines, such as IL-12, IL-23, and IL-27,[320] which are induced as part of HSV infection in vivo. These cytokines also can directly induce differentiated T_H1 cells to produce IFN-γ. HSV infection also may promote T_H1 immunity by inducing the production of osteopontin by T cells at an early stage of activation and differentiation. This cytokine may act on APCs by interacting with $β_3$ integrins to maintain IL-12 production and with CD44 to inhibit IL-10 production, thereby favoring a T_H1 adaptive immune response.[321] Osteopontin is required for the development of delayed-type hypersensitivity responses (characteristic of T_H1 immunity) to HSV, and of HSV-induced corneal inflammation, which is T_H1-dependent.[321]

IFN-γ is a key immunoregulatory cytokine that is produced in substantial amounts by CD4+ T cells of the T_H1 subset, CD8+ T cells, γδ T cells, and NK cells. It is a key component in appropriately regulating adaptive and innate cellular mechanisms of antiviral control. The potential cellular sources of this cytokine and their temporal appearance (e.g., NK and γδ T cell–derived IFN-γ production preceding CD4+ and CD8+ T cell–mediated production), as well as their location, need to be considered when evaluating the importance of IFN-γ in vivo. IFN-γ acts to increase the antiviral state of many cell types, such as mononuclear phagocytes. In addition, this cytokine enhances the expression of the class I heavy chain, $β_2$-microglobulin, and TAP transporter. These effects help counteract the negative effects of HSV on class I MHC antigen presentation and increase the ability of infected cells to be lysed.[282] CD40 ligand expression by CD4+ T cells also is key for antibody production by B cells and isotype switching.

Administration of neutralizing antibodies to IFN-γ increases the severity of HSV-1 infection in mice.[322] Likewise, knockout mice lacking IFN-γ or its receptor are impaired in their ability to control HSV infection, as measured by higher mortality, prolonged infection, and more frequent reactivations. IFN-γ is a poor inhibitor of HSV replication in vitro. This is not a biologically relevant situation, however, because T_H1 cells do not secrete IFN-γ in environments devoid of other cytokines. In vivo, the secretion of other proinflammatory cytokines and chemokines occurs before and during the recruitment of T cells into sites of viral infection. In addition, IFN-γ has been found to act in concert with other cytokines such as type I IFNs to effect potent inhibition of HSV in vitro.[229]

Virus-specific T_H1 cells also are major sources of TNF-α. TNF-α has direct antiviral effects, particularly in conjunction with IFN-γ, and also proinflammatory effects (e.g., by increasing adhesion molecule expression by nonhematopoietic cells, such as endothelium, and production of chemokines). In human corneal infection with HSV, the combination of TNF-α and IFN-γ exerts a synergistic antiherpes effect within the corneal fibroblasts, chiefly attributed to the induction of IFN-β.[323] In the case of MCMV infection, some of these antiviral effects mediated by IFN-γ may be cell type-specific—for example, they may be operative for mononuclear phagocytes but not fibroblasts—and involve novel mechanisms that are shared with type I IFN.[324] Some of these T_H1 cells also are a rich source of IL-17, which is found at sites of HSV infection, such as the cornea. IL-17 may contribute to local inflammation by increasing the production of proinflammatory cytokines and neutrophil chemotactic proteins, such as chemokines.[325]

Some of the best-documented limitations in neonatal adaptive immunity come from two studies comparing T cell responses in neonates and adults with primary HSV or HCMV infection.[305,326] HSV-specific proliferation of peripheral blood mononuclear cells and production of both IFN-γ and TNF-α were diminished and delayed in neonates compared with adults. The neonates did not achieve adult levels of these responses for 3 to 6 weeks after clinical presentation, whereas the adults all exhibited robust responses by 2 weeks. These studies used ultraviolet light-irradiated viral preparations to stimulate peripheral blood mononuclear cells, in which viral proteins are processed mainly by the class II rather than the class I MHC antigen presentation pathway. Therefore they assayed mainly $CD4^+$ and not $CD8^+$ T cell function.

These results suggest a profound lag in the development of adaptive immunity to HSV in normal neonates, during which viral replication and cell lysis could continue. Because $CD4^+$ T cells provide multiple critical effector mechanisms that may be important for the resolution of HSV infection (including direct antiviral cytokine production and help for $CD8^+$ T cell and B cell responses), these findings suggest that a lag in T cell immunity may be a key contributor to the tendency of HSV infection to disseminate and cause prolonged disease in neonates.

Studies of the responses of neonates and infants to viral vaccines support the idea that the development of $CD4^+$ T cell immunity to viruses may be limited early in life. Peripheral blood mononuclear cells from neonates given oral poliovirus vaccine (OPV) at birth and at 1, 2, and 3 months of age exhibited decreased OPV-specific proliferation, IFN-γ production, and IFN-γ-positive cells in comparison with cells from immunized (but not reimmunized) adults.[327] By contrast, antibody titers of neonates and infants were higher than those of adults. As noted above, effector $CD4^+$ T cell responses are induced by congenital HCMV infection. HCMV-specific fetal T cells express high levels of transcription factors typical of T_H1 cells, including Tbet and Eomes, indicating no fundamental defect in T_H1 cell differentiation.[328] However, fetal T_H1 cells produced markedly lower levels of antiviral cytokines as compared to adult cells; this defect was associated with the expression of high levels of inhibitory receptors, suggesting functional exhaustion. Whether similar cell intrinsic regulatory processes limit T_H1 responses to other viruses or viral vaccines in early life remains to be established.

Antigenically naïve $CD4^+$ T cells initially show a very limited capacity to express cytokines other than IL-2; in contrast, distinct subsets of memory $CD4^+$ T cells express particular cytokines. T_H1 and T_H2 cells produce IFN-γ and IL-4, respectively.[329] Thus the essential absence of memory $CD4^+$ T cells in the circulation of neonates accounts for the limited ability of neonatal $CD4^+$ T cells to produce IFN-γ compared with adult $CD4^+$ T cells.[304] If naïve $CD4^+$ T cells are activated in vitro, they differentiate into effector-like cells that acquire the capacity to produce IFN-γ (T_H1 effectors) or IL-4 (T_H2 effectors), depending on the cytokine milieu and APC populations.[330-332] As mentioned earlier, however, studies suggest that neonatal naïve $CD4^+$ T cells have a decreased capacity to become IFN-γ-producing cells compared with adult naïve $CD4^+$ T cells in response to short-term (i.e., 24 to 48 hours) stimulation by allogeneic DCs.

This decreased expression of IFN-γ by neonatal $CD4^+$ T cells is likely to be due to several factors. First, neonatal $CD4^+$ T cells are less effective than adult naïve cells at inducing the cocultured adult DCs to produce IL-12, a key cytokine for promoting IFN-γ production. Second, as discussed earlier, neonatal APCs, such as DCs, may have a decreased capacity to produce IL-12 and related cytokines that are key for T_H1 differentiation.[109] It is interesting that this decreased capacity for IL-12 production by mononuclear cells may continue into early childhood, at least for certain stimuli, such as LPS.[333] Third, neonatal naïve $CD4^+$ T cells exhibit a decreased expression of certain transcription factors that may play a role in the induction of *IFN-γ* gene expression, such as the NFATc2 protein.[334,335] Fourth, the greater methylation of DNA of the IFN-γ genetic locus in neonatal T cells also may contribute to a reduced and delayed acquisition of IFN-γ production after activation in vitro.[336] Some or all of these mechanisms are likely to contribute to the delay in the appearance of IFN-γ production by antigen-specific $CD4^+$ T cells after viral infections in the neonatal period.

CD154/CD40 INTERACTIONS

CD154 (CD40 ligand) is a member of the TNF ligand superfamily and is expressed abundantly on the surface of activated but not resting $CD4^+$ T cells. CD154 engages CD40, a molecule expressed by "professional" APCs,[337] including DCs, mononuclear phagocytes, B cells, and possibly $CD8^+$ T cells. Engagement of CD40 on DCs is a potent maturation signal and an inducer of IL-12. This engagement also counteracts the inhibitory effect of other cytokines, such as IL-10.[338] The CD154/CD40 interaction is essential for many events in adaptive immunity, including the generation of memory $CD4^+$ T cells of the T_H1 phenotype and memory B cells, as well as most Ig isotope switching.[339]

The role of CD154 in viral host defense appears to vary with different pathogens but in general correlates with the particular requirement for $CD4^+$ T cells, indicating that $CD4^+$ T cells and CD154 are linked in mediating such help. CD154 deficiency in mice results in decreased $CD4^+$ and $CD8^+$ T cell responses to viral antigens and increased mortality after HSV-1 footpad infection. In studies of HSV corneal infection, the numbers of $CD4^+$ and $CD8^+$ T cells and B cells within draining lymph nodes dramatically expand within the first 7 days. However, no IFN-γ-secreting $CD4^+$ cells can be seen immediately. IFN-γ and a full T_H1 response do not appear until after 7 days after expression of CD154. These findings suggest that CD154 is not required for the initial expansion of HSV-1-specific $CD4^+$ T cells in the draining lymph node, but it is important for their differentiation into mature T_H1 effector cells. Exogenous IL-12 can at least partially relieve the requirement for CD154 in the T_H1 differentiation of HSV-1-specific T cells, consistent with the known capacity of CD40 signaling to induce IL-12 production in DCs.[340]

Mice lacking CD154 as a result of selective gene disruption or that had CD154/CD40 interactions neutralized by monoclonal antibody demonstrated an increased frequency of CNS infection and paralysis compared with wild-type mice after footpad inoculation with HSV.[325] These abnormalities correlated with reductions in $CD4^+$ but not $CD8^+$ T cell responses. The absence of CD154/CD40 interactions eliminates most antiviral antibodies and results in severe disease in viral infections in which antibody plays a critical role, such as in the dissemination of vesicular stomatitis virus to the CNS. In humans, CD154 also appears to play an important role in the expansion of $CD8^+$ T cells in recognizing viral peptide antigens, such as from influenza A virus and HIV-1.[341]

Freshly isolated monocytes from neonates or adults express low levels of CD40,[342] but whether they have a similar capacity to produce cytokines in response to CD154 (CD40 ligand) engagement remains unclear. Using more physiologically relevant stimulation, neonatal $CD4^+$ T cells co-cultured with DCs increase their expression of CD154[343] and induce IL-12 production by DCs.[344] CD154 expression by purified neonatal naïve $CD4^+$ T cells co-cultured with adult allogeneic DCs was substantially less than by adult naïve CD4+ T cells after 24 to 48 hours of stimulation. This reduced CD154 production was accompanied by reduced IL-12 production (by moDCs) and IFN-γ production (by naïve CD4+ T cells).[109] These observations suggest that CD154 surface expression is at least initially more limited for neonatal T cells, but that with continued priming in vitro, this limitation can be overcome. A likely consequence is that the differentiation of naïve CD4+ T cells into T_H1 effector cells by an IL-12-dependent and DC-dependent process may be delayed.

The generation of CD4+ T effector cells is a complex process, involving antigen presentation by DCs to naïve CD4+ T cells and multiple steps of T cell clonal expansion and differentiation; compromise of any of these steps could result in limited T_H1 immunity. Myeloid DCs are essential to the differentiation of naïve CD4+ T cells to T_H1 effector and memory T cells. Key events promoting T_H1 differentiation include the elaboration by DCs of cytokines, such as IL-12, IL-23, and IL-27, and their binding to specific receptors on CD4+ T cells.[320] CD154 is expressed by naïve CD4+ T cells after the T cell recognizes peptide antigen/MHC complexes through the αβ-TCR and receives costimulation through CD28 binding to CD80 and CD86. The engagement of CD40 on the DC by CD154 on the T cell enhances the DC production of these T_H1-promoting cytokines and also increases the expression of CD80 and CD86, which helps sustain T cell activation. In persons who are genetically deficient in CD40 ligand[345] or in the ability to respond to IL-12 and IL-23,[346] antigen-specific T_H1 responses are absent or severely depressed, supporting the validity of this model.

The basis for the delayed development of HSV antigen-specific CD4+ T cells in neonates is not known; it could reflect limitations at one or more of the steps just described. Historical studies suggested that neonates have a lower frequency of precursor T cells capable of responding to HSV and HCMV.[347] This finding is unlikely to be due to a limitation in the diversity of the αβ-TCR repertoire[348–350] and is more likely to reflect intrinsic regulation or limitations in T cell function. Indeed, studies of fetal T cell responses to congenital HCMV infection demonstrated large expansions of virus-specific cells and revealed that functional regulation rather than defective effector cell differentiation underlies defective antiviral cytokine responses.[328,351]

CYTOLYTIC CD4+ T CELL–MEDIATED MECHANISMS

CTLs use two main pathways in executing cytotoxicity: (1) exocytosis of perforin and granzyme granules and (2) death receptor signaling through Fas/Fas ligand (CD95/CD95L) or TNF/TNF-R signaling. Both pathways trigger the apoptotic cascade and programmed cell death involving activation of caspase-3 and cleavage of apoptotic substrates. Gene knockout studies in mice defective in key elements of these pathways revealed that MHC-restricted cytolysis by murine CD4+ T cells is mediated predominantly by the death receptor system, whereas MHC-I-restricted cytolysis by CD8+ CTLs relies on perforins and granzymes. Human CD4+ CTLs use both pathways.[352]

CD4+ CTLs make up a sizable minority of CD4+ T cells in murine HSV infection (around 30%) and recognize HSV-specific antigens presented on MHC class II molecules.[283] In fact, early efforts to clone CTLs specific for HSV resulted in CD4+ instead of CD8+ CTL clones.[353] Studies evaluating the CD4+ CTL response suggest that activated CD4+ T cells express perforin and granzyme A and B, in a fashion similar to that for CD8+ cells; however, CD4+ T cells express substantially lower amounts of perforin and granzymes in both cell numbers and amounts per cell, compared with CD8+ T cells.[354] Human CD4+ cytotoxic cells can recognize peptides derived from viral glycoproteins found in the HSV lipid envelope,[300,355,356] such as gB, gC, and gD,[357] and it is likely that these viral glycoproteins enter into the class II antigen-processing endocytic pathway by first fusing with the host cell membrane.

Although class II MHC normally is expressed by APCs, such as B cells, mononuclear phagocytes, and DCs, a wide variety of cell types can express class II MHC and, in most cases, present antigen after exposure to IFN-γ, GM-CSF, or TNF-α. These cell types, which include endothelial cells, enterocytes, renal epithelial cells, thyroid epithelial cells, microglial cells, epidermal keratinocytes, myoblasts, eosinophils, NK cells, and T cells themselves, might then become potential targets for cytotoxic CD4+ T cells. However, the importance of CD4+ T cell–mediated cytotoxicity in the control of infection has been questioned, given that substantial CD8+ T cell responses to HSV are generated in humans and that HSV-specific CD8+ T cells constitute a prominent part of the viral response in tissues such as skin and cervix. Additionally, HSV-1 renders infected cells resistant to CTL-induced apoptosis[358] by mechanisms such as the down-regulation of MHC class II through the virion host shutoff (vhs) protein and the viral protein encoded by the $\gamma_1 34.5$ gene.[359]

An expanded target cell range is possible, however, because class II MHC expression is up-regulated on many non-APC types in response to cytokines, such as IFN-γ. Thus it is plausible that CD4+ cytolytic T cells play an important role in the resolution of HSV infection in humans. A major trigger of cytolytic CD4+ T cells in humans is CMV infection. CMV-specific cytolytic CD4+ T cells express high levels of perforins and granzymes and express an advanced stage of differentiation characterized by the down-regulation of the CD27 and CD28 receptors.[360] Following congenital HCMV infection, fetal CD4+ T cells acquire the expression of perforin and granzymes, alongside their differentiation in Th1 cells.[328]

CD8+ T CELL–MEDIATED ANTIVIRAL IMMUNITY

CD8+ CTLs are important in effective clearance of viral infections, including CMV and HSV,[308,361–363] and are found at sites of local recurrence of such infection such as the skin adjacent to the genital tract,[308,364] cervix,[309] and cornea.[365] CD8+ T cells, when first activated by antigen, are not effective killers, but subsequently, under the influence of cytokines such as IL-2 and IL-15, proliferate and differentiate into an effector cell lymphoblast population that efficiently kills. They kill target cells by exocytosing cytotoxic molecules such as perforin, granzymes, or granulysin. Fas/Fas ligand and TRAIL/DR interactions also may play a part in this killing. This differentiation includes increased expression of molecules involved in cytotoxicity, such as perforin, granzymes, Fas ligand, and granulysin, as well as an increased capacity to produce cytokines, such as IFN-γ and TNF-α. The mature virus-specific CD8+ CTL looks conspicuously different from the unprimed, naïve CD8+ T cell.

CD8+ T cell differentiation also results in cell surface changes that reflect the stage of maturation and nomenclature of this population (Table 115.5). For example, in contrast with naïve CD8+ T cells, which uniformly express CD45RA, HCMV-specific CD8+ T cells exhibit CD45RO surface expression early in infection. CD45 is a transmembrane phosphatase that regulates signaling through TCR CD3, and distinct isoforms of the molecule are generated through alternative splicing of amino-terminal (N-terminal) exons A, B, and C. The high-molecular-weight form (CD45RA) contains A, B, or C (or all three), whereas CD45RO does not. Similarly, patterns of CCR7 expression change, indicating activated CTL homing signals. Chemokine receptor CCR7 binds CCL19 and CCL21 and directs the migration of lymphocytes to the lymph node. CD127 (IL-7R-α) is expressed by naïve T cells and

Table 115.5 CD8⁺ T Cells and Their Subsets.

Exposure Status	Subset	Markers[a]	Features
Naïve	Naïve	KLRG1 low CD62L hi LY6C low IL7R lo	Naïve cells before exposure or activation
Antigen experienced	Terminally differentiated short-lived effector T cells (activated)	KLRG1 low CD62L hi LY6C hi	Generally short-lived; secrete interferon (IFN)-γ, granzyme B and perforin.
	Long-lived effector (memory) T cells	CCR7 lo CD62L lo KLRG1 hi CD62L low LY6C hi IL7R hi	Produce cytokines and cytolytic molecules, but also persist in the host once antigen has been cleared.
	Long-term (central) memory	CCR7 hi CD62L hi KLRG1 low CD62L hi LY6C hi IL7R hi	Do not exhibit immediate effector functions; must undergo proliferation and further differentiation in order to reach full cytotoxic capacity.

[a]**KLRG1** is a C-type lectin-like receptor that contains an immune receptor tyrosine-based inhibitory motif. **CD62L (L-selectin)** is a homing receptor for lymphocytes to enter secondary lymphoid tissues via high endothelial venules. **Ly6C** is a GPI-anchored cell surface glycoprotein involved in target cell killing by cytotoxic cells and regulates CD8 T cell homing in vivo. The **IL7 receptor (IL7R)** consists of two subunits, interleukin-7 receptor-α (CD127) and the common-γ chain receptor (CD132). **CCR7** is a G protein-coupled receptor that controls the migration of memory T cells to secondary lymphoid organs, such as lymph nodes.

disappears for the most part during active infection but reappears in a subset of virus-specific CD8⁺ cells within the memory pool with the ability to respond to cytokine IL-7, enabling reactivation.

Thus the functionality of human CD8⁺ T cells can be analyzed along at least two dimensions—one defined by the expression of cell surface marker (such as CD45RA, CCR7, CD28, and CD27) and the other marked by distinct expression levels of transcription factors such as T-bet and others that determine the functional profile of antigen-experienced cells.[366]

Studies using class I MHC/viral peptide tetramers, which allow direct detection of CD8⁺ T cells based on their TCR specificity, have documented that virus-specific CD8⁺ T cells undergo a dramatic expansion in vivo during viral infection. In some instances, such as with primary EBV infection, more than 40% of circulating CD8⁺ T cells may be reactive with a single viral peptide epitope.[367] Most CD8⁺ effector T cells have a relatively short life span and are probably eliminated by apoptosis after antigen clearance. CD4⁺ T cells may aid directly in the generation of CD8⁺ cytolytic T cells by the production of several cytokines, including IL-2 and IFN-γ. In addition, CD4⁺ T cells may indirectly influence this process by enhancing DC function through a CD154/CD40 interaction; DCs, in turn, may then help promote CD8⁺ cytolytic T cell generation by secreting cytokines and engaging costimulatory molecules. In animal models, CD8⁺ T cells also appear to be key in resolving HSV lytic infection of ganglia during primary infection,[346,368] and in preventing reactivation of virus from latency in sensory neurons.[369] This latter function may involve an IFN-γ-dependent mechanism.[370] Direct recognition of infected ganglion cells by CD8⁺ T cells is likely, because HSV infection induces detectable class I MHC expression by sensory neurons.[371] Noncytolytic mechanisms,[372] such as the production of cytokines with antiviral activity (e.g., IFN-γ)[373] or the secretion of granzyme A,[374] may be key for CD8⁺ T cells to maintain latency and to prevent viral spread. By contrast, cytolytic mechanisms, such as those mediated by perforin, may not be necessary for control of HSV infection at particular tissue sites, such as the cornea or brain, and may even contribute to inflammatory disease.[375,376]

VIRAL INHIBITION OF ANTIGEN PRESENTATION AND EFFECT ON THE T CELL IMMUNE RESPONSE

In view of the importance of class I MHC-restricted cytotoxicity in the control of viral infection, it is perhaps not surprising that a number of viruses, including HSV and HCMV,[375] have developed mechanisms to inhibit class I MHC antigen presentation. First, the virus can establish latency in sensory ganglia, an immunoprivileged site in which viral proteins are not expressed. During lytic replication, however, the HSV ICP47 protein (gene *US12*) blocks the MHC class I antigen presentation pathway by inhibiting the transporter associated with antigen presentation (i.e., TAP); this transporter translocates peptides across the endoplasmic reticulum membrane.[323,377-380] The vhs protein degrades host cell mRNA, preventing synthesis of new HLA class I.[358] The combination of these two proteins is responsible for poor recognition of infected cells by CD8⁺ CTLs; however, CTL toxicity is restored somewhat by exposure of those cells to IFN-γ, which up-regulates class I antigen processing and presentation. Certainly, the high levels of IFN-γ isolated from clinical lesions suggest that this effect occurs in vivo in addition to in vitro.[381]

CTL cytotoxicity also is inhibited by HSV products US3 kinase, ICP22, ICP27, ICP4, gJ, and gD, which confer apoptosis resistance to infected cells.[358] When IFN-γ is present and the effects of ICP47 are not as evident, the second-line defense effects of US3 (US3 kinase) and US5 (gJ) become more apparent. They both partially block CTL-induced chromium release. US3 kinase blocks the cleavage of Bid by granzyme B. In addition, gJ prevents the activation of caspase-3 by granzyme B.

Despite these inhibitory mechanisms, class I MHC-restricted human CD8⁺ T cells that can lyse HSV-infected targets have been be isolated from HSV-2 lesions of patients with genital disease[239,301] or from the blood of HSV-immune individuals.[382,383] The CD8⁺ T cell response in humans appears to be dominated by recognition of HSV proteins that are internal structural components of the virion, such as those of the tegument and nucleocapsid, or those that are rapidly induced upon viral entry, such as certain immediate-early genes.[384,385] These proteins apparently can be processed into peptides and presented on class I MHC molecules before the inhibitory effect of either the vhs or TAP inhibitor proteins. Similarly, immediate-early gene products and tegument and nucleocapsid proteins also may be important targets of the human CD8+ T cell response against HCMV by interacting with CD8+ T cells before the onset of mechanisms that interfere with class I MHC antigen presentation. By contrast, viral glycoproteins that are found in the HSV lipid envelope do not appear to be important antigens for class I MHC-restricted responses, probably because they fuse with the host cell membrane and do not enter the cytoplasm in substantial amounts.[323]

Inhibition of viral replication also can occur without killing of the infected cell. Studies using fibroblasts inoculated with HSV for 2 hours before exposure to CTLs, under conditions in which less than 10% lysis was observed, resulted in a 50% decrease in production of infectious virus.[372] Similarly, control of viral replication and reactivation from latency in infected neurons is controlled by nonlytic mechanisms.[369] Studies using US12-deleted HSV (ICP47−) led to a decrease in virus yield, especially when CTL attack occurred at early stages of viral replication. In vivo, the effect of ICP47 probably serves to open a short window of time in which infected cells are spared from recognition and attack by CTLs. ICP47 is not present in the virions but is one of the first proteins to be made in infected cells. Therefore, early on, before sufficient ICP47 is present, antigen is presented on the surface of the cells, permitting recognition by CTLs. At intermediate time points, the effect of ICP47 prevents recognition of infected cells, but once IFN-γ is up-regulated within lesions, recognition of infected cells is restored. At that time, the second lines of defense, such as inhibition of apoptosis, come to the fore.

HCMV also encodes proteins that inhibit class II MHC antigen presentation,[386] and the same has been found to be true of HSV, with vhs and γ134.5.[359] Infection of mice with virulent HSV strains results in CNS lesions in which class II MHC expression remains intracellular, thereby avoiding any chance of detection by CD4+ T cells.[387]

CD8+ T cells can be sensitized in vitro for cytotoxicity using allogeneic (MHC other than self) stimulator cells, followed by testing for cytotoxic activity against allogeneic target cells. With this approach, most studies have found that neonatal T cells are moderately less effective than adult T cells as cytotoxic effector cells.[388-391] More substantial defects in T cell–mediated cytotoxicity by neonatal T cells after allogeneic priming are observed when no exogenous cytokines, such as IL-2, are added.[392,393] This finding suggests that such decreased cytolytic activity could be of physiologic significance in vivo if CD4+ T cell help also was limited.

The mechanism for reduced neonatal T cell–mediated cytotoxicity remains poorly understood. In vitro studies demonstrated that antigen-specific neonatal CD8+ T cells can be differentiated in cytolytic cells when stimulated in vitro with DCs, suggesting that there is intrinsic defect in their capacity to become effector cells.[394]

Many in vivo studies of cytolytic CD8+ T cells to date have focused on congenital and perinatal HIV-1 infection. In congenital HIV-1 infection, an expansion of HIV-specific cytotoxic T cells was detected at birth, indicating that fetal T cells were activated by viral antigens.[395] In another case of in utero HIV infection, HIV-specific T cell–mediated cytotoxicity was detected at 4 months of age and persisted for several years despite a high HIV viral load.[396] Cytotoxic responses to HIV in perinatally infected infants suggest that, although CD8+ T cells capable of mediating cytotoxicity have undergone clonal expansion in vivo (as early as 4 months of age),[397] their cytotoxicity may be reduced and delayed in appearance compared with that of adults.[398] In many cases, HIV-1–specific cytotoxic lymphocyte responses were not detectable during the first few months of life.[395,398] When evaluated beyond infancy, cytolytic activity directed to HIV envelope proteins was commonly detected, but that directed against *gag* or *pol* proteins was rarely detected.[399] Also noted was decreased HIV-specific CD8+ T cell production of IFN-γ by young infants with perinatal HIV infection,[400] along with an inability to generate HIV-specific cytotoxic T cells after antiretroviral therapy.[401] Together, these results point to the possibility of a delay in the development of CD8+ T cell–mediated responses in comparison with that in adults and suggest that the nature of the target antigens recognized by neonatal CD8+ T cells may be more limited. These developmental limitations in CD8+ T cell function may not necessarily be limited to HIV-1, at least in early infancy. For example, one study of RSV-specific cytotoxicity found that it was more pronounced and frequent in infants 6 to 24 months of age than in younger infants.[402]

HIV-1 infection is characterized by a number of severely immunosuppressive features that may not apply to most other viral infections. These include impairment of antigen presentation,[403] decreasing thymic T cell output,[404] and promotion of T cell apoptosis.[405] Of note, these suppressive effects of HIV-1 on cytotoxic responses may be relatively specific for HIV-1, because HIV-infected infants who lack HIV-specific cytotoxic T cells may maintain CD8+ T cell responses against EBV and CMV.[400,401] Also, large expansions of cytolytic CD8+ T cells are detected following congenital HCMV infection.[351] These cells express perforin-dependent cytolytic activity ex vivo. As observed in CD4+ T cells, fetal CD8+ T cells express high levels of inhibitory receptors and produce lower levels of antiviral cytokines as compared to adult cells.[328]

CD28/CD80–86 CO-STIMULATION

In addition to engagement of the αβ-TCR by peptide/class II MHC antigen, full naïve T cell activation is thought to require costimulation, such as occurs with engagement of CD28 on the T cell by CD80 or CD86 on the APC. Murine studies indicate that such costimulation is critical for the development of an effective adaptive immune response to HSV. CD28/CD80–86 interactions appear critical for paralysis-free survival, as well as for the generation of both HSV-specific CD4+ and CD8+ T cell responses in the footpad injection model.[325] This was demonstrated using mice with selective genetic disruption of CD28 and in normal mice in which CD28/CD80–CD86 interactions were neutralized in vivo by administration of CTLA-4-Ig (cytotoxic T lymphocyte antigen-4-Ig),[325] a soluble fusion molecule that effectively competes with T cell–associated CD28 for CD80–86 binding. In an intravaginal HSV murine model, mice lacking both CD80 and CD86 were prone to severe local and disseminated disease and death[406] and, as in the other study, were unable to mount effective CD4+ or CD8+ T cell responses and exhibited more severe disease and increased mortality.[407]

Neonatal T cells express levels of CD28 similar to those in adult T cells and produce IL-2 and proliferate as well as adult T cells do in response to mouse APCs expressing human CD80 or CD86 and to anti-CD3 monoclonal antibody, indicating that CD28-mediated signaling is intact.[408] This finding also is supported by a study showing that anti-CD28 monoclonal antibody treatment of neonatal T cells markedly augments their ability to produce IL-2 and proliferate in response to anti-CD2 monoclonal antibody.[409] However, these results do not exclude the possibility that neonatal T cell costimulation by CD28 could be limited because of decreased expression of CD80 or CD86 by key APCs, such as neonatal myeloid DCs.

CHEMOTACTIC AND HOMING RECEPTOR EXPRESSION BY VIRAL ANTIGEN-SPECIFIC T CELLS

The differential expression of chemokine and homing receptors by T cells is important in their selective trafficking, either to sites at which naïve T cells may potentially encounter antigen for the first time, such as the spleen and lymph nodes, or to inflamed tissues for effector functions.[410] The homeostatic chemokines CCL19 and CCL21 have been shown to be essential in the transmigration of lymphocytes across high endothelial venules (HEVs) (highly specialized postcapillary venules within the lymph nodes and Peyer patches), allowing the passage of lymphocytes bearing their shared receptor CCR7 from the blood compartment into secondary lymphatic organs. CCR7 is uniformly expressed on naïve T cells, as well as a subset of resting memory T cells known as *central memory T cells*. CCL21 is constitutively expressed within the lumen of HEVs, whereas CCL19 is produced by other cells within the lymph node but becomes displayed on the HEV lumen after transcytosis across the endothelial barrier.

Naïve T cells also express CCR9 and CXCR4. CCR9 ligand is CCL25 and may help traffic T cells into the gastrointestinal lymphatics. The ligand of CXCR4 is CXCL12 and is involved in transendothelial migration across HEVs. These are the principal chemokine receptors expressed on naïve lymphocytes; this is in contrast with the numerous chemokine receptors expressed on effector T cells.

Primed $CD4^+$ T cells briefly express CXCR5, which is a chemokine receptor otherwise expressed principally on B cells. Its ligand CXCL13 is produced within the B cell–rich follicular compartment of secondary lymphoid tissues but is absent from the adjacent T zone. The acquisition of CXCR5 by recently primed $CD4^+$ T cells temporarily relocates these cells to the outer follicle, where they can interact with B cells during antibody production. CXCR5 is rapidly lost during T cell proliferation, indicating that the homing program is an early and transient step in the T cell activation and differentiation process.[411] There has been a recent explosion of interest and research in the study of these cells. They are the principal mediators of B cell help and are now designated *T follicular helper cells* (T_{FH}).

Affinity maturation and isotype switching of B cells in the germinal center depends on T_{FH} cells, and therefore this T cell subset appears critical in protective antiviral immunity. T_{FH} cells have been essential for control in model systems of LCMV[412,413] SIV[414] and other viruses. A lot of focus in this field has centered on HIV responses because of the high interest in understanding broad and potent HIV neutralizing antibodies. Investigators have found that impaired T_{FH} cell help for B cells is found in HIV-infected individuals[415], but elevated frequencies of highly functional memory T_{FH} cells ($PD1^{lo}CXCR3^-CXCR5^+$) in certain HIV-infected individuals are associated with induction of higher levels of broadly neutralizing antibodies against HIV.[416] There is limited research on neonatal T_{FH} cells. Studies in neonatal mice suggest these cells can be induced in neonatal mice after antigenic stimulation, but their magnitude and function is reduced compared to mature animals.[417,418]

Effector T cells are equipped with receptors for inflammatory cytokines and adhesion molecules that are greatly up-regulated during inflammation, so these cells efficiently home to sites of pathogen entry and disease. By contrast, memory T cells are believed to confer rapid and superior protection against pathogens that they have encountered during previous immune responses. They are divided into two subsets based on their different migratory and functional properties. The subset $CCR7^+CD62L^+$ memory T cells, termed *central memory T (T_{CM}) cells,* far outnumber the memory subset lacking these lymph node-homing receptors, termed *effector memory T (T_{EM}) cells*. The utility of these T_{CM} cells in responding to recurrent herpes virus infection is unclear, because a recent study did not indicate accelerated proliferation kinetics or tissue infiltration of T_{CM} cells when compared with naïve T cells. A more brisk effector (T_{EM}) response was demonstrated.[419]

In established HSV infection, most recurrences of viral replication occur in keratinocytes found at epithelial sites, such as the skin and genitourinary mucosa. Trafficking of T cells into this location is controlled by the expression of cutaneous lymphocyte-associated antigen (CLA), which is a fucose-containing carbohydrate that can decorate P-selectin glycoprotein ligand-1 on T cells. CLA is expressed from most T cells recovered from the skin and is on approximately 5% to 10% of circulating $CD8^+$ T cells. During symptomatic recurrences of virus at these cutaneous sites, virus-specific $CD4^+$ T cells and NK cells may infiltrate within 48 hours after the appearance of lesions. This is followed several days later by infiltration by virus-specific $CD8^+$T cells, which are associated with viral clearance.[308] Consistent with the importance of $CD8^+$T cell immunity at these local sites of replication, a majority of $CD8^+$ T cells that recognize a particular HSV peptide express CLA.[307]

It is likely that HSV-specific T cells that enter sites of viral replication, such as the CNS during HSV encephalitis, utilize a distinct combination of homing and chemotactic receptors to achieve selective trafficking. As indicated by studies in mice using other neurotropic viruses, expression of CXCR3, CCR2, and CCR5 chemokine receptors may regulate $CD8^+$T cells trafficking into the CNS.[420] Other chemokine and homing receptor combinations are likely to be important for trafficking of HSV-specific T cells to the liver and gastrointestinal tract in cases of disseminated disease.

As discussed earlier, down-regulation of CCR7 and up-regulation of other chemokine receptors by effector T cells probably are important for redirecting these cells from secondary lymphoid tissue to other sites of tissue inflammation, where they can carry out their effector functions. A restriction of CMV-specific T_H1 effector function to $CCR7^{low}$ cells has been observed after primary CMV infection in both adults and young children as well in congenital infection.[328]

Human neonatal naïve T cells differ from those of adults in that they do not increase CXCR3 expression, which favors trafficking to inflamed tissues that have been exposed to IFN-γ, and they decrease CCR7 expression after activation by way of anti-CD3 and CD28 monoclonal antibodies.[421,422] The CCR7 expressed on neonatal T cells is functional and mediates chemotaxis of these cells in response to CCL19 and CCL21.[423] Neonatal T cells can increase the surface expression of CCR5 by treatment with either mitogen or IL-2[424] or after differentiation in vitro in a cytokine milieu that favors T_H1 development.[410,425,426] Whether CCR5 expression by T cells, which probably is important for their homing to the CNS, is up-regulated in cases of neonatal or postnatal HSV encephalitis is not known. Up-regulation of CCR5 by fetal $CD4^+$ and $CD8^+$T cells is observed following congenital HCMV infection, indicating that this pathway can contribute to T cell homing to tissues in early life.[328]

γδ T CELLS

The γδ T lymphocytes are one of the first T cells to emigrate from the thymus and express a TCR heterodimer consisting of a γ-chain and a δ-chain, in association with CD3. A majority of these γδ T cells take up residence in epithelial tissues including the skin, intestines, lung, and reproductive tracts. Their nomenclature is based on their TCR gene rearrangements; for example, the three γ genes are *Vγ1* to *Vγ3*. Vδ1 T cells are found principally in the skin and are known as *dendritic epidermal T cells* (DETCs) and are maintained by expression of zeta (ζ)-chain–associated protein 70 (ZAP-70) signaling molecule within the epidermis.[427] $V\gamma5^+$ γδ T cells, known as *intestinal intraepithelial lymphocytes* (IELs), are found predominantly in the intestines and are dependent on thymus IL-15 for development. The γδ T cells have multiple functions including tissue homeostasis and wound repair, facilitated by γδ expression of insulin-like growth factor-1 (IGF-1) and keratinocyte growth factor-1 (KGF-1), respectively. γδ T cells also regulate local inflammation. KGF-1 produced by DETCs, for example, induces expression of hyaluronan by keratinocytes, which recruits inflammatory cells such as macrophages. γδ IELs also influence neighboring epithelial cells to produce proinflammatory factors such as chemokine IL-8 and IFN-γ-inducible protein-10.[428] γδ T cells also are able to recognize and lyse (perforin-mediated) cancerous epithelial cells and lymphoma cells, and they are able to recognize and fight infection.[429]

In contrast to conventional αβ T cells, γδ T cells are not dependent on classical MHC molecules presenting peptides. Based on the ligands that have been identified, it appears that some γδ TCRs can recognize antigens in an antibody-like fashion, while the TCR of other γδ T cell subsets can bind to the MHC-like protein CD1d loaded with lipids.[430]

T cells expressing the TCR variable region pair Vγ9Vδ2 are the predominant γδ T cell subset in human peripheral blood. The Vγ9Vδ2 subset has been shown to react specifically toward nonpeptide low-molecular-weight phosphorylated metabolites (so-called *phosphoantigens*).[431]

In contrast to adult peripheral blood γδ T cells, human neonatal cord blood γδ T cells express diverse Vγ and Vδ chains. There is increasing evidence that γδ T cells make a critical contribution to immunologic protection in early life.

A central role of γδ T cells in immunity in early life has been demonstrated in a mouse model of intestinal parasite infection.[432] Placental malaria, which can produce phosphoantigens, increases the percentage of central memory Vγ9Vδ2 T cells.[433] Congenital CMV infection elicits a marked response of fetal public/invariant Vγ8Vδ1 TCR-expressing subset.[434] Fetal blood (before 30 weeks) contains high levels of Vγ9Vδ2 T cells known to react to a set of pathogen-derived small molecules (phosphoantigens). These fetal T cells are functionally preprogrammed as they exhibit features of adult blood γδ T cells such as the ability to produce IFN-γ and granzymes.[435]

NATURAL KILLER T CELLS

A small population of circulating human T cells express αβ TCRs, lack expression of both CD4 and CD8, and express NKR-P1A, the human ortholog of the mouse NK1.1 protein. These features, as well as others (such as CD56 and CD57 surface expression, along with a dependence on the cytokine IL-15 for their development[436]), are characteristic of NK cells. For this reason, these cells frequently are referred to as *NK T cells,* or *natural T cells*. Like murine T cells expressing NK1.1, human NK T cells have a restricted TCR repertoire and mainly recognize antigens presented by the nonclassic MHC molecule CD1d, rather than by class I or class II MHC molecules. These CD1d-restricted antigens that can be recognized by NK T cells include certain lipid molecules, as well as hydrophobic peptides. NK T cells also have the ability to secrete high levels of IL-4 and IFN-γ and to express death-inducing ligands (Fas ligand and TNF-related apoptosis-inducing ligand [TRAIL]) on their cell surface on primary stimulation—a capacity not observed with most antigenically naïve αβ T cells.[437,438] This suggests that they could play a role in the early stages of the immune response. Additionally, NK T cells help B cells to produce antibody. Murine NK T cells have been implicated in the control of zosteriform HSV infection[439] but the antiviral mechanisms involved remain to be defined.[440]

In contrast to previous reports showing that cord blood NKTs are functionally immature,[441,442] a more recent report showed that they were capable of significant cytokine production after stimulation with PMA/Ionomycin including IFN-γ and TNF.[443] Also fetal NKT can mature in the second trimester fetus, especially in the fetal intestine, thus before microbial exposure.[444] The role of NKT cells in early-life viral infections requires further investigation.

A complete reference list is available at www.ExpertConsult.com. 

SELECT REFERENCES

2. Amanna IJ, Carlson NE, Slifka MK. Duration of humoral immunity to common viral and vaccine antigens. *N Engl J Med*. 2007;357(19):1903-1915.
12. Park JE, Jardine L, Gottgens B, Teichmann SA, Haniffa M. Prenatal development of human immunity. *Science*. 2020;368(6491):600-603.
15. Tourneur E, Chassin C. Neonatal immune adaptation of the gut and its role during infections. *Clin Dev Immunol*. 2013;2013:270301.
16. Belkaid Y, Hand TW. Role of the microbiota in immunity and inflammation. *Cell*. 2014;157(1):121-141.
19. Yockey LJ, Lucas C, Iwasaki A. Contributions of maternal and fetal antiviral immunity in congenital disease. *Science*. 2020;368(6491):608-612.
20. Zhivaki D, Lo-Man R. *In utero* development of memory T cells. *Semin Immunopathol*. 2017;39(6):585-592.
21. Mold JE, Michaelsson J, Burt TD, et al. Maternal alloantigens promote the development of tolerogenic fetal regulatory T cells *in utero*. *Science*. 2008;322(5907):1562-1565.
24. Kollmann TR, Kampmann B, Mazmanian SK, Marchant A, Levy O. Protecting the newborn and young infant from infectious diseases: lessons from immune ontogeny. *Immunity*. 2017;46(3):350-363.
30. Fulde M, Sommer F, Chassaing B, et al. Neonatal selection by Toll-like receptor 5 influences long-term gut microbiota composition. *Nature*. 2018;560(7719):489-493.
32. Hooper LV, Littman DR, Macpherson AJ. Interactions between the microbiota and the immune system. *Science*. 2012;336(6086):1268-1273.
34. Li N, van Unen V, Hollt T, et al. Mass cytometry reveals innate lymphoid cell differentiation pathways in the human fetal intestine. *J Exp Med*. 2018;215(5):1383-1396.
40. Rechavi E, Lev A, Lee YN, et al. Timely and spatially regulated maturation of B and T cell repertoire during human fetal development. *Sci Transl Med*. 2015;7(276):276ra225.
44. Kollmann TR, Marchant A, Way SS. Vaccination strategies to enhance immunity in neonates. *Science*. 2020;368(6491):612-615.
72. Zaghouani H, Hoeman CM, Adkins B. Neonatal immunity: faulty T-helpers and the shortcomings of dendritic cells. *Trends Immunol*. 2009;30(12):585-591.
73. Kollmann TR, Levy O, Montgomery RR, Goriely S. Innate immune function by Toll-like receptors: distinct responses in newborns and the elderly. *Immunity*. 2012;37(5):771-783.
78. Gibbons D, Fleming P, Virasami A, et al. Interleukin-8 (CXCL8) production is a signatory T cell effector function of human newborn infants. *Nat Med*. 2014;20(10):1206-1210.
81. Li L, Lee HH, Bell JJ, et al. IL-4 utilizes an alternative receptor to drive apoptosis of Th1 cells and skews neonatal immunity toward Th2. *Immunity*. 2004;20(4):429-440.
84. Goriely S, Van Lint C, Dadkhah R, et al. A defect in nucleosome remodeling prevents IL-12(p35) gene transcription in neonatal dendritic cells. *J Exp Med*. 2004;199(7):1011-1016.
87. Mold JE, Venkatasubrahmanyam S, Burt TD, et al. Fetal and adult hematopoietic stem cells give rise to distinct T cell lineages in humans. *Science*. 2010;330(6011):1695-1699.
93. Lambert L, Sagfors AM, Openshaw PJ, Culley FJ. Immunity to RSV in early-life. *Front Immunol*. 2014;5:466.
95. Krow-Lucal ER, Kim CC, Burt TD, McCune JM. Distinct functional programming of human fetal and adult monocytes. *Blood*. 2014;123(12):1897-1904.
101. Steinman RM. Decisions about dendritic cells: past, present, and future. *Ann Rev Immunol*. 2012;30:1-22.
106. Kollmann TR, Crabtree J, Rein-Weston A, et al. Neonatal innate TLR-mediated responses are distinct from those of adults. *J Immunol*. 2009;183(11):7150-7160.
110. Tonon S, Goriely S, Aksoy E, et al. Bordetella pertussis toxin induces the release of inflammatory cytokines and dendritic cell activation in whole blood: impaired responses in human newborns. *Eur J Immunol*. 2002;32(11):3118-3125.
111. Aksoy E, Albarani V, Nguyen M, et al. Interferon regulatory factor 3-dependent responses to lipopolysaccharide are selectively blunted in cord blood cells. *Blood*. 2007;109(7):2887-2893.
114. Gensollen T, Iyer SS, Kasper DL, Blumberg RS. How colonization by microbiota in early life shapes the immune system. *Science*. 2016;352(6285):539-544.
130. Pou C, Nkulikiyimfura D, Henckel E, et al. The repertoire of maternal anti-viral antibodies in human newborns. *Nat Med*. 2019;25(4):591-596.
134. Telemo E, Hanson LA. Antibodies in milk. *J Mammary Gland Biol Neoplasia*. 1996;1(3):243-249.
140. Ohsaki A, Venturelli N, Buccigrosso TM, et al. Maternal IgG immune complexes induce food allergen-specific tolerance in offspring. *J Exp Med*. 2018;215(1):91-113.
141. Gans HA, Arvin AM, Galinus J, Logan L, DeHovitz R, Maldonado Y. Deficiency of the humoral immune response to measles vaccine in infants immunized at age 6 months. *JAMA*. 1998;280(6):527-532.
147. Crowe Jr JE. Immune responses of infants to infection with respiratory viruses and live attenuated respiratory virus candidate vaccines. *Vaccine*. 1998;16(14-15):1423-1432.
152. Crowe Jr JE, Firestone CY, Murphy BR. Passively acquired antibodies suppress humoral but not cell-mediated immunity in mice immunized with live attenuated respiratory syncytial virus vaccines. *J Immunol*. 2001;167(7):3910-3918.

155. Thulin NK, Brewer RC, Sherwood R, et al. Maternal anti-dengue IgG fucosylation predicts susceptibility to dengue disease in infants. *Cell Rep*. 2020;31(6):107642.
167. Lathrop SK, Bloom SM, Rao SM, et al. Peripheral education of the immune system by colonic commensal microbiota. *Nature*. 2011;478(7368):250–254.
251. Colonna M, Trinchieri G, Liu YJ. Plasmacytoid dendritic cells in immunity. *Nat Immunol*. 2004;5(12):1219–1226.
252. De Wit D, Olislagers V, Goriely S, et al. Blood plasmacytoid dendritic cell responses to CpG oligodeoxynucleotides are impaired in human newborns. *Blood*. 2004;103(3):1030–1032.
268. Biron CA, Byron KS, Sullivan JL. Severe herpesvirus infections in an adolescent without natural killer cells. *N Engl J Med*. 1989;320(26):1731–1735.
273. Guilmot A, Hermann E, Braud VM, Carlier Y, Truyens C. Natural killer cell responses to infections in early life. *J Innate Immun*. 2011;3(3):280–288.
293. Nguyen QH, Roberts RL, Ank BJ, Lin SJ, Thomas EK, Stiehm ER. Interleukin (IL)-15 enhances antibody-dependent cellular cytotoxicity and natural killer activity in neonatal cells. *Cell Immunol*. 1998;185(2):83–92.
299. Kuijpers TW, Baars PA, Dantin C, van den Burg M, van Lier RA, Roosnek E. Human NK cells can control CMV infection in the absence of T cells. *Blood*. 2008;112(3):914–915.
329. Lewis DB, Prickett KS, Larsen A, Grabstein K, Weaver M, Wilson CB. Restricted production of interleukin 4 by activated human T cells. *Proc Natl Acad Sci U S A*. 1988;85(24):9743–9747.
333. Upham JW, Lee PT, Holt BJ, et al. Development of interleukin-12-producing capacity throughout childhood. *Infect Immun*. 2002;70(12):6583–6588.
343. Matthews NC, Wadhwa M, Bird C, Borras FE, Navarrete CV. Sustained expression of CD154 (CD40L) and proinflammatory cytokine production by alloantigen-stimulated umbilical cord blood T cells. *J Immunol*. 2000;164(12):6206–6212.
351. Marchant A, Appay V, Van Der Sande M, et al. Mature CD8(+) T lymphocyte response to viral infection during fetal life. *J Clin Invest*. 2003;111(11):1747–1755.
363. Klenerman P, Oxenius A. T cell responses to cytomegalovirus. *Nat Rev Immunol*. 2016;16(6):367–377.
398. Pikora CA, Sullivan JL, Panicali D, Luzuriaga K. Early HIV-1 envelope-specific cytotoxic T lymphocyte responses in vertically infected infants. *J Exp Med*. 1997;185(7):1153–1161.
413. Harker JA, Lewis GM, Mack L, Zuniga EI. Late interleukin-6 escalates T follicular helper cell responses and controls a chronic viral infection. *Science*. 2011;334(6057):825–829.
432. Ramsburg E, Tigelaar R, Craft J, Hayday A. Age-depende nt requirement for gammadelta T cells in the primary but not secondary protective immune response against an intestinal parasite. *J Exp Med*. 2003;198(9):1403–1414.
435. Dimova T, Brouwer M, Gosselin F, et al. Effector Vgamma9Vdelta2 T cells dominate the human fetal gammadelta T-cell repertoire. *Proc Natl Acad Sci U S A*. 2015;112(6):E556–E565.
444. Loh L, Ivarsson MA, Michaelsson J, Sandberg JK, Nixon DF. Invariant natural killer T cells developing in the human fetus accumulate and mature in the small intestine. *Mucosal Immunol*. 2014;7(5):1233–1243.

T-Cell Development 116

Melinda Erdős | László Maródi

INTRODUCTION

Hematopoietic stem cells give rise to committed progenitors of multiple lineages. Whereas maturation along myeloid, erythroid, and megakaryocytic cell lineages occurs within the bone marrow, and differentiation into B lymphocytes initiates in the bone marrow and is completed in the periphery, T-lymphocyte development occurs within the thymus, where bone marrow–derived common lymphoid progenitors migrate. In particular, interaction of lymphoid progenitors with thymic stromal cells permits differentiation of $CD4^-$ and $CD8^-$, double-negative cells into $CD4^+$ and $CD8^+$, double-positive (DP) thymocytes within the thymus cortex. Subsequently, DP cells lose expression of either CD4 or CD8, becoming functionally active single-positive cells that populate the thymic medulla (Fig. 116.1).

Although the thymus is particularly active early in life, it ensures lifelong generation of a pool of newly generated T cells. Of importance, the thymus also plays a critical role in purging self-reactive T lymphocytes. Therefore T cells produced in the thymus carry a seemingly unrestricted antigen receptor repertoire, whose reactivity is largely restricted to foreign antigens and is tolerant to self-antigens.[1]

T-CELL PHENOTYPES AND ANTIGEN RECEPTORS

T-cell development in the human thymus starts at approximately 7 weeks of gestation[2] with the entry of precursors with the leukocyte antigens CD7 and CD45 on their surface. These cells mature to express first the CD2 co-stimulatory molecule and then, at around 8.5 weeks gestation, CD3. By 9.5 weeks, 32% of the $CD3^+$ cells have the β-chain of the T-cell receptor (TCR) in the cytoplasm, and at 10 weeks, many of the cells also have the α-chain the cytoplasm. The proportion of cells expressing the δ-chain of the γδ TCR is highest at 9.5 weeks gestation (11%) and rapidly diminishes to 4% at 10 weeks and 1% at 12 weeks. CD1a, CD4, and CD8 appear on lymphocytes in the thymus by 10 weeks gestation, and the high-density CD3 phenotype (associated with mature antigen receptor expression) appears on these cells at approximately 12 weeks. A population of immature $CD7^+$ cells with potential for multiple differentiation pathways is present in cord blood.[3] The T-cell antigen receptor αβ heterodimer has a molecular mass of approximately 90 kDa. The complete αβ or γδ heterodimer is expressed on the T-cell surface in association with five invariant chains, which constitute the CD3 complex.

Some estimate of the time and rate of T-cell export from the human fetal thymus comes from the measurement of T cells in the blood and spleen. $CD3^+$ cells are present in blood from the end of week 12 of gestation, their proportion rising from 20% to 30% at 14 weeks to 50% or more by 22 weeks. Studies suggest that the range of *VDJ* recombination that occur before 14 weeks gestation is limited.[4] The mechanism for limited diversity during fetal life may relate to a limited use of N region diversification, secondary to low levels of the terminal deoxynucleotidyl transferase enzyme in the thymus. It is interesting that the diversity of the fetal B cell repertoire is also limited, although a selective preference for certain *VH* genes appears to be the explanation in this case.[5] Because the T-cell diversity is limited, the fetus may have much less ability to respond to antigens (or to reject foreign grafts) than might be predicted from the presence of CD3 cells in the blood. Much remains to be learned about the range of *TCR* gene recombinations that can be made at different gestational ages.[6]

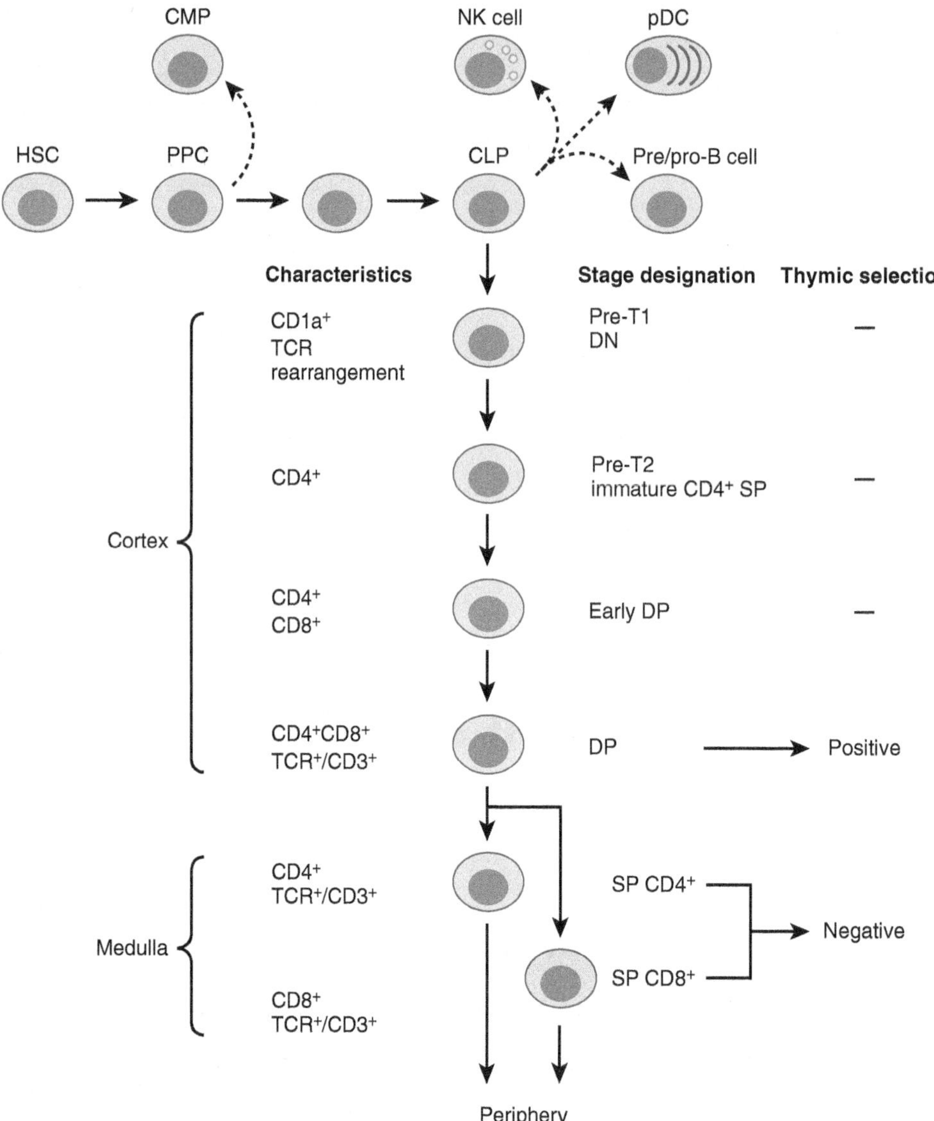

Fig. 116.1 T-cell development and selection in the thymus. Hematopoietic stem cells *(HSCs)* with self-renewing capacity give rise to pluripotent progenitor cells *(PPCs)* that may differentiate to common myeloid progenitors *(CMPs)* or common lymphoid progenitors *(CLPs)*. CLPs, in turn, differentiate into T-cell-restricted precursors (indicated in *green*), in addition to giving rise to natural killer *(NK)* cells, plasmacytoid dendritic cells *(pDCs)*, and B cells. T-cell lineage-restricted cells then pass through pre-T1, pre-T2, early double-positive *(DP)*, DP, and single-positive *(SP)* stages in the thymic cortex and medulla. T cells at the pre-T1 differentiation stage express CD1a and initiate T-cell receptor *(TCR)* rearrangement. Next, they express CD4 but not CD8 and are referred to as CD4+ immature cells. Further maturation gives rise to cells expressing both CD4 and CD8 markers, in addition to *TCR/CD3*. These cells are subjected to positive selection in the thymic cortex. DP thymocytes then differentiate into CD4+ or CD8+ *SP* cells. After post-selection maturation in the medulla, T cells are exported to the periphery.

Of fetal $CD3^+$ cells in blood and spleen, 90% to 96% use αβ heterodimers, and the proportion of γδ receptor-positive cells is between 2% and 8% at 20 to 40 weeks of gestation; this subunit distribution is similar to that found in adults.[7] Fetal T cells resemble adult lymphocytes in expressing either CD4 or CD8 but not both. T cells also appear in the intestinal epithelium and lamina propria by 14 weeks gestation.[8] Cells carrying γδ TCRs populate the epithelium more slowly than do αβ TCR^+ cells and may arise in part through local differentiation, rather than exclusively from thymic sources. Gut-associated γδ lymphocytes increase rapidly in the fed neonate,[9] suggesting that local antigenic stimulation may be responsible for the expansion of this population.

By analogy with studies in animals, it seems likely that T cells accumulate in the blood and lymph nodes of fetuses during the second half of gestation, principally as a result of thymic emigration. This view is supported by studies of CD45 isoforms, which distinguish between naïve and memory T cells. More than 99% of the lymphocytes in the cord blood of neonates express high-molecular-weight isoforms of CD45 ($CD45RA^+$ and $CD45RB^+$)[10] in association with low levels of LFA-1 (CD11a/CD18) and other integrins; this expression pattern is characteristic of the naïve T-cell phenotype. When stimulated, naïve cells of newborn infants switch to express the $CD45R0^-$ isoform of CD45. This isoform is present on the surface of adult circulating T cells that respond to recall antigens. The low number of $CD45R0^-$ cells in the blood of healthy term neonates suggests that little antigen-driven expansion of T cells occurs before birth.

FUNCTIONAL RESPONSES OF FETAL T CELLS

In vitro tests indicate that several components of a T-cell response (proliferation to mitogens or to alloantigens and interleukin [IL]-2 production) exist beginning at approximately 12 weeks gestation. In addition to these ligand-driven proliferative responses, T cells of neonates also can be maintained in culture using a combination of IL-4 and IL-2 or of IL-4 and IL-12.[11] Evidence that fetal T cells can make antigen-specific responses comes from their proliferation in mixed lymphocyte culture, together with the generation of antigen-specific cytotoxic cells.[12] Other stimuli, such as *Staphylococcus* enterotoxins and anti-TCR antibodies, tend to elicit lesser responses by neonatal than by adult cells.[13] This difference is accounted for, at least in part, by the lower proportion of CD45R0+ cells in neonates than in adults.[14]

The maturation of naïve cells to the memory cell phenotype most likely follows an encounter with an antigen presented on a specialized antigen-presenting cell, such as B lymphocytes or dendritic cells (DCs) in the lymph nodes. Several studies suggest that naïve T cells that encounter antigen in the absence of co-stimulation enter a pathway that leads to unresponsiveness, also known as *anergy,* which may be temporary or permanent.[15] A polyclonal population of CD4+ and CD8+ T cells with a memory (CD45R0+) phenotype makes up 25% of human fetal spleen cells; these T cells express high-affinity IL-2 receptors and proliferate in response to exogenous IL-2 but not to anti-CD2 or anti-CD3 antibodies.[16] Some of these cells may be autoreactive T cells destined to become unresponsive. Finally, umbilical cord blood contains a population of T cells with reduced in vivo responsiveness following ligation of cell surface CD47.[17]

Production of soluble mediators, or cytokines, by T cells that respond to antigen stimulation is essential for host defense.[18] Naïve and memory T cells make similar amounts of IL-2, which is required for T-cell proliferation, whereas other cytokines, including IL-4, IL-10, IL-12, and interferon-γ (IFN-γ), are made largely by memory T cells. Consequently, T cells of newborns make little IFN-γ or IL-4 unless they first undergo several cycles of proliferation and maturation.[19] These differences are likely to be important because T cells show functional specialization regarding their predominant cytokine production.[20] The cells making IL-4 and IL-10 are described as type 2 helper T (T_H2) cells. These cells have an essential role in promoting B-cell replication and increasing the production of immunoglobulin (Ig) E isotype antibodies. T_H1 cells make mainly IFN-γ, and they promote local inflammatory responses and stimulate B cells to make IgG. The specialization of cells into a T_H1 or T_H2 phenotype from T_H0 cells is determined in part by the cytokine environment in which stimulation occurs. The presence of IFN-γ, for example, biases responses toward a T_H1 phenotype, whereas IL-4 tends to suppress IFN-γ production and to promote differentiation toward a T_H2 phenotype. Naïve cells from human newborns can mature into those making IL-4 apparently in the absence of preexisting IL-4.[21] IL-13, an important cytokine in the T_H2 pathway, is produced by newborns' CD8+ T cells even when production of IL-4, IL-10, and IFN-γ remains low.[22] Different specificities of cytokine receptors on the surface of T_H1 and T_H2 cells cause them to have different homing patterns. Responses to immunization can be markedly altered by deliberate manipulation of the cytokine milieu in which immunizing antigens are presented to the immune system. This strategy may be useful in the design of future vaccines.[23]

The extent of signaling through the TCR-CD3 complex also can be modified by simultaneous interactions of receptor–ligand pairs of costimulatory molecules on the surface of T cells and antigen-presenting cells. Interaction of CD28 molecules on the T-cell surface with its ligands B7-1 and B7-2 on B cells, macrophages, and DCs markedly enhances the proliferation and cytokine production of "naïve" T cells in response to specific antigen-MHC complexes. Other surface molecules with costimulatory function include LFA-1, the inducible co-stimulator ICOS (another CD28/B7 family member), and tumor necrosis factor family members such as OX40. These membrane-bound receptors carry amino acid residues in their cytoplasmic tails that allow recruitment of activating kinases that can amplify intracellular signaling. On the other hand, other members of the CD28 family of molecules, such as CTLA-4, contain intracytoplasmic inhibitory sequences that can activate a series of intracellular phosphatases with opposite function. CTLA-4 also can bind B7-1 and B7-2 molecules on the surface of antigen-presenting cells, and its affinity for these molecules is higher than that of CD28; accordingly, interaction of CTLA with B7-1 (or with B7-2) actively suppresses intracellular TCR signaling. The balance of positive and negative co-stimulation shapes the final T-cell repertoire by regulating both clonal expansion and differential cytokine production of the responding T cells. Interruption of these costimulatory and regulatory interactions can markedly alter the development of antigen-specific T-cell responses. The effectiveness of blocking CD28 interactions with B7-1 and B7-2 in limiting or reversing rejection of allogeneic tissue grafts is a potential treatment option in patients with graft-versus-host disease.[24]

POSTNATAL DEVELOPMENT OF MEMORY T CELLS

Approximately 70% of naïve T cells—the predominant population in human newborn infants—contain T-cell receptor excision circles (TRECs) that identify recent thymic emigrants.[25] The TREC does not replicate in parallel with nuclear DNA, so counting TRECs in blood T cells gives an indirect estimate of T-cell production from the thymus that also is affected by cell division. Indeed, the measurement of TRECs on dried blood spots at birth has been introduced in newborn screening for severe combined immunodeficiency. Recirculation of naïve T cells through the specialized venules of lymph nodes and other lymphoid tissues allows them to migrate to the T-cell-dependent areas of lymph nodes. T cells that do not encounter antigen leave the node in the efferent lymph and return to the bloodstream through the thoracic duct. By contrast, naïve T cells, whose surface antigen receptors are cross-linked by antigen in the context of self-MHC molecules, enter a response cycle that is accompanied by expression of a surface receptor for IL-2. In the presence of a co-stimulator signal (e.g., binding of B7-1 or B7-2 to CD28), the T cells themselves release IL-2. This autocrine loop permits cell division of IL-2-dependent T cells for as long as the antigen stimulus persists. The development of a useful repertoire of T cells in the circulation is therefore best thought of as a consequence of antigenic experience stimulating T-cell proliferation. Specialized DCs play a key role in capturing antigens in tissues and at body surfaces and in transporting them through lymphatics to the draining lymph nodes. The migration of DCs is regulated by chemokine gradients (particularly that for CCR7), and their handling of antigens is affected by receptors for bacterial products such as lipopolysaccharides and certain unmethylated dinucleotides.[26] DCs are likely to contribute to the specialization of T cells along T_H1 or T_H2 pathways (described earlier). B lymphocytes also can present antigens, albeit at low concentrations, and hence may participate in T-cell activation.

The response of naïve T cells to antigen stimulation depends largely on the costimulatory environment.[27] Stimulation results in an increase in the proportion of CD45R0+ cells from less than 5% at birth to 35% to 45% by age 16 years. This increase occurs mainly during the first years of life[14]; and one attribute of memory cells—the production of IFN-γ—is mature around the age of 2 years. The expansion of populations with defined specificities has been documented for only a few antigens. For example, the frequency of lymphocytes in blood responding to the varicella-zoster virus (VZV) antigen is less than 1 in 10^6 before immunization or infection.[28] After a varicella infection, VZV-responsive cells do not appear in the blood for approximately 10 days. At 1 month into convalescence, the responder cell frequency is approximately 1:20,000

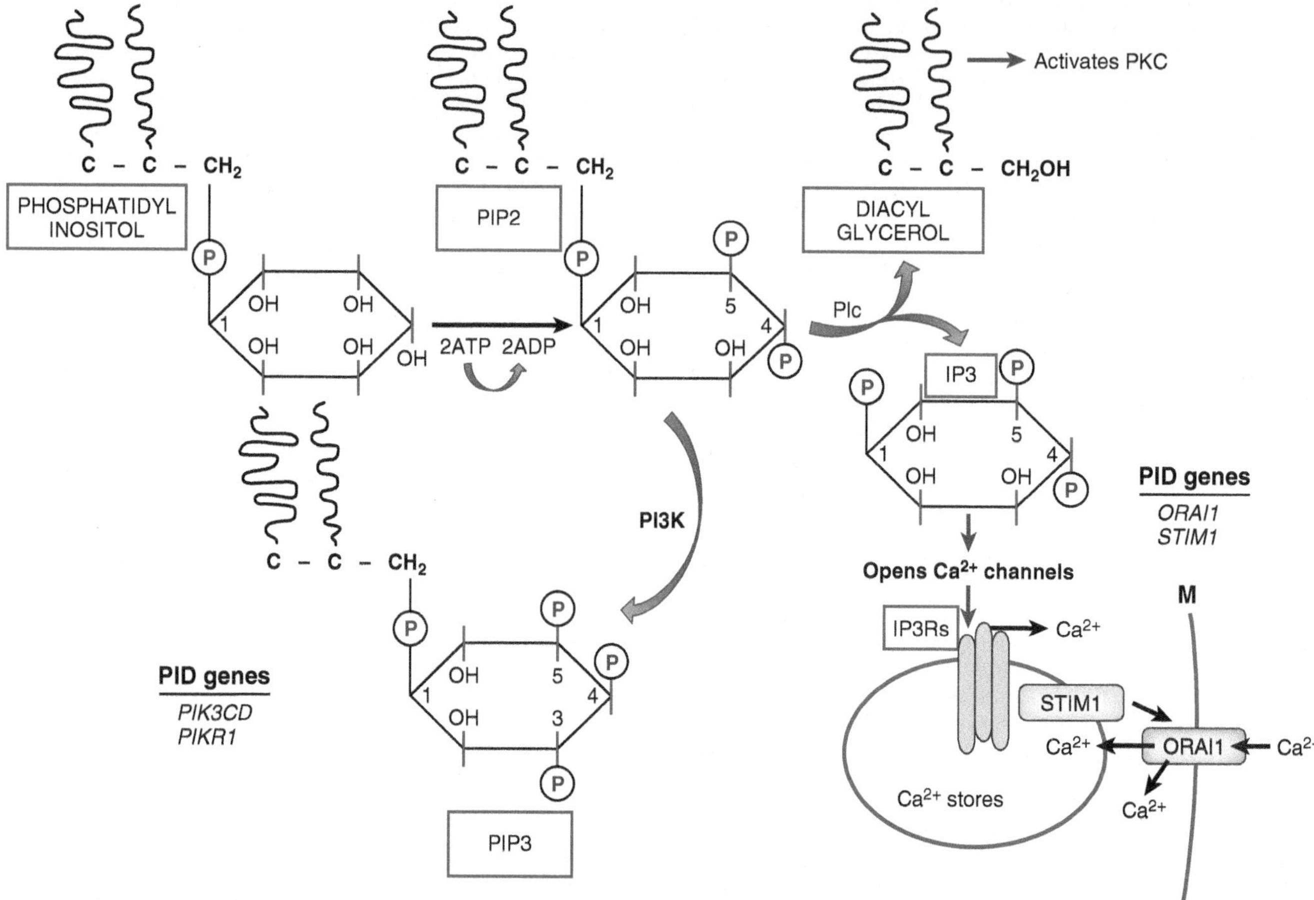

Fig. 116.2 During T-cell activation the phosphoinositide cascade mediated by G proteins evokes many cellular responses by converting extracellular signals into intracellular ones. The intracellular messengers, inositol 1,4,5 triphosphate *(IP3)* and diacyl glycerol (DAG), formed during the activation of this cascade arise from the plasma membrane lipid phosphatidyl inositol 4,5 diphosphate *(PIP2)* cleaved by phospholipase C (Plc). IP3, a short-lived molecule, binds to its receptor expressed in the endoplasmic reticulum (ER) membrane, which initiates the release of Ca^{2+} to the cytoplasm. Next, ER-membrane-located *STIM1* and cell-membrane-located *ORAI1* interact to replace intracellular Ca^{2+} from the extracellular space. The other major second messenger, DAG, activates many target proteins by the promotion of protein kinase C *(PKC)* and phosphorylation of serine and threonine residues. The importance of this activation pathway is underlined by the description of combined primary immunodeficiencies in patients with *STIM1* and *ORAI1* mutations. The phosphoinositide 3-kinase δ gene (*PIK3CD*) mutation characterized by decreased circulating T cell and B cell number and severe, recurrent respiratory tract infections and airway damage has also been reported. *CRAC*, Ca^{2+} release-activated Ca^{2+} channel.

cells, rising to 1:10,000 after 3 months.[29] VZV is latent and responder cell frequencies in the range of 1:10,000 to 1:20,000 are maintained through the age of 50 years, when they start to decline. The frequency of T cells with specificity for a nonreplicating antigen—tetanus toxoid—fluctuates directly in relation to immunization. Before infants receive tetanus toxoid, they have fewer than 1:10^5 cells that respond to this antigen. Six weeks after the first immunization, the responder cell frequency is still less than 1:40,000. With completion of the course of three injections by the age of 6 months, the frequency of responder cells increases to 1:10,000 cells, and this falls to less than 1:40,000 1 year later.

NOVEL SUBSETS OF CD4⁺ T CELLS

An effector population of CD4⁺ cells is defined as T_H17 T cells, because they secrete several IL-17 cytokines. The generation of these T-cell subsets requires IL-6 and IL-1 in humans, and differentiation is amplified by IL-21 and IL-23.[30] Severe depletion of T_H17 cells was found in patients with *STAT-3* deficiency and sporadic hyper-IgE syndrome.[31,32]

Negative selection in the thymic medulla delete many self-reactive T lymphocytes as potential sources of autoimmunity. However, self-reactive T cells slipping past negative selection require a different strategy to restore their naïve status. This strategy involves CD4⁺CD25⁺ regulatory T cells (Treg cells), which express the transcription factor Foxp3. Scurfy mice lack detectable Treg function as a consequence of mutations of the *Foxp3* gene.[33] In humans, immune dysregulation-polyendocrinopathy-enteropathy X-linked (IPEX) syndrome is a primary immunodeficiency disease characterized by defective Treg function secondary to mutation in the *FOXP3* gene.[34]

IL-22-producing helper T cells (T_H22 cells) also have been proposed as a CD4⁺ T lymphocyte subset.[35] T_H22 cells are characterized not only by producing IL-22 but also by their propensity to express skin-homing chemokine receptors.

HELP FOR B LYMPHOCYTES

B cells, which bind antigen through their surface Ig receptors, enter a pathway that leads either to self-destruction by apoptosis[36] or, if a T-cell signal is received, to proliferation and differentiation. The T-cell signal for B-cell proliferation is supplied by cytokines and is delivered mostly at the T cell–B cell interface in lymph nodes. T cells control the switch from IgM to IgG (isotype switching) as well as proliferation. The switch signal is supplied by binding a 39,000-kDa glycoprotein, termed *CD40 ligand (CD40L)*, to the CD40 receptor, which is constitutively expressed on the B-cell surface. Resting memory T cells express CD40L within a few hours of a response to antigens, whereas naïve T cells take longer to become CD40L-positive. In vitro experiments suggest that delay in CD40L expression on naïve T cells is an important factor limiting the ability of human newborns to make antibodies.[37] T_H1 cells help with certain IgG responses, and IL-4 from T_H2-type cells promotes IgA and IgE responses. As noted previously, T_H2 cells are most efficiently generated in an environment already containing IL-4 and IL-13. IL-21 is a very important T-cell-derived cytokine, which is secreted by helper T cells in the lymph node follicles, the so-called follicular helper T cells (T_{FH}), and promotes B-cell maturation and Ig secretion. The transcriptional factor, Bcl6, is critically important to induce T_{FH} differentiation in addition to other molecules such as CXCR5 and PD-1.[38] Studies in mice showed that $CD4^+CXCR5^+PD\text{-}1^+$ T_{FH} cells are present and functional in newborn animals.[39] However, the expression of Bcl6 and IL-21 was lower in neonatal mice compared with that of cells from adult animals. In addition, these cells were poorly localized to germinal centers but were present mostly in interfollicular areas.

CONCLUSION

T-cell development occurs in multiple discrete steps, beginning with lineage commitment by hematopoietic stem cells in the specialized environment of the thymus. Progression through the developmental pathway in the thymus is controlled by soluble cytokine growth factors and cellular interactions between the maturing thymocytes and the local stromal cell compartment (Figs. 116.1 and 116.2). The repertoire of antigen-specific TCRs expressed on mature thymocytes before export to the periphery results from both positive and negative selection of receptor specificities generated by a random association of variable regions for TCR heterodimers and the addition of N region diversity through random nucleotide deletions or additions during recombination events. After export from the thymus, the mature T-cell pool is further shaped by antigen exposure and the local production of cytokines during initial activation and clonal expansion in the lymph nodes, spleen, and epithelial structures such as skin and intestine. Although mature T cells are present in significant numbers by mid-gestation in humans, a fully mature T-cell population develops slowly after birth in response to antigen exposure.

ACKNOWLEDGMENT

The authors wish to thank Marcia McDuffie, MD, Anthony R. Hayward, MD, PhD, and Luigi Notarangelo, MD, PhD, who contributed exceptionally to previous editions of this chapter in the third edition of *Fetal and Neonatal Physiology*.

SELECT REFERENCES

1. Holländer GA, Peterson P. Learning to be tolerant: how T cells keep out of trouble. *J Intern Med*. 2009;265:541.
2. Royo C, Touraine JL, de Bouteiller O. Ontogeny of T lymphocyte differentiation in the human fetus: acquisition of phenotype and functions. *Thymus*. 1987;10:57.
3. Hao QL, Zhu J, Price MA, et al. Identification of a novel, human multilymphoid progenitor in cord blood. *Blood*. 2001;97:3683.
4. Raaphorst FM, Kaijzel EL, van Tol MJ, et al. Non-random employment of Vβ6 and Jβ gene elements and conserved amino acid usage profiles in CDR3 regions of human fetal and adult TCR β chain rearrangements. *Int Immunol*. 1994;6:1.
5. Pascual V, Verkruyse L, Casey ML, Capra JD. Analysis of Ig H chain gene segment utilization in human fetal liver. Revisiting the "proximal utilization hypothesis." *J Immunol*. 1993;151:4164.
6. Schultz C, Reiss I, Bucsky P, et al. Maturational changes of lymphocyte surface antigens in human blood: comparison between fetuses, neonates and adults. *Biol Neonate*. 2000;78:77.
7. Lobach DF, Hensley LL, Ho W, Haynes BF. Human T cell antigen expression during the early stages of fetal thymic maturation. *J Immunol*. 1985;135:1752.
8. Machado CS, Rodrigues MA, Maffei HV. Assessment of gut intraepithelial lymphocytes during late gestation and the neonatal period. *Biol Neonate*. 1994;66:324.
9. Spencer J, Isaacson PG, Walker-Smith JA, MacDonald TT. Heterogeneity in intraepithelial lymphocyte subpopulations in fetal and postnatal human small intestine. *J Pediatr Gastroenterol Nutr*. 1989;9:173.
10. Bofill M, Akbar AN, Salmon M, et al. Immature $CD45RA^{low}RO^{low}$ T cells in the human cord blood. I. Antecedents of $CD45RA^+$ unprimed T cells. *J Immunol*. 1994;152:5613.
11. Wu CY, Demeure CE, Gately M, et al. In vitro maturation of human neonatal CD4 T lymphocytes. I. Induction of IL-4-producing cells after long-term culture in the presence of IL-4 plus either IL-2 or IL-12. *J Immunol*. 1994;152:1141.
12. Rayfield LS, Brent L, Rodeck CH. Development of cell-mediated lympholysis in human foetal blood lymphocytes. *Clin Exp Immunol*. 1980;42:561.
13. Horgan KJ, Van Seventer GA, Shimizu Y, Shaw S. Hyporesponsiveness of "naive" ($CD45RA^+$) human T cells to multiple receptor-mediated stimuli but augmentation of responses by co-stimuli. *Eur J Immunol*. 1990;20:1111.
14. Hayward AR, Lee J, Beverley PC. Ontogeny of expression of UCHL1 on $TcR\text{-}1^+$ (CD4/8) and $TcR\text{-}delta^+$ T cells. *Eur J Immunol*. 1989;19:771.
15. Durie FH, Foy TM, Masters SR, et al. The role of CD40 in the regulation of humoral and cell-mediated immunity. *Immunol Today*. 1994;15:406.
16. Byrne JA, Stankovic AK, Cooper MD. A novel subpopulation of primed T cells in the human fetus. *J Immunol*. 1994;152:3098.
17. Avice MN, Rubio M, Sergerie M, et al. Role of CD47 in the induction of human naive T cell anergy. *J Immunol*. 2001;167:2459.
18. Leonard WJ. Cytokines and immunodeficiency diseases. *Nat Rev Immunol*. 2001;1:200.
19. Maródi L. Down-regulation of Th1 responses in human neonates. *Clin Exp Immunol*. 2002;128:1.
20. Mosmann TR, Coffman RL. Th1 and Th2 cells: different patterns of lymphokine secretion lead to different functional properties. *Annu Rev Immunol*. 1989;7:145.
21. Kaliński P, Hilkens CM, Wierenga EA, et al. Functional maturation of human naive T helper cells in the absence of accessory cells. Generation of IL-4-producing T helper cells does not require exogenous IL-4. *J Immunol*. 1995;154:3753.
22. Ribeiro-do-Couto LM, Boeije LC, Kroon JS, et al. High IL-13 production by human neonatal T cells: neonate immune system regulator? *Eur J Immunol*. 2001;31:3394.
23. Silva RA, Pais TF, Appelberg R. Evaluation of IL-12 in immunotherapy and vaccine design in experimental *Mycobacterium avium* infections. *J Immunol*. 1998;161:5578.
24. Jacobsohn DA, Vogelsang GB. Novel pharmacotherapeutic approaches to prevention and treatment of GVHD. *Drugs*. 2002;62:879.
25. Hassan J, Reen DJ. Human recent thymic emigrants—identification, expansion, and survival characteristics. *J Immunol*. 2001;167:1970.
26. Krieg AM. CpG motifs in bacterial DNA and their immune effects. *Annu Rev Immunol*. 2002;20:709.
27. Fadel S, Sarzotti M. Cellular immune responses in neonates. *Int Rev Immunol*. 2000;19:173.
28. Chilmonczyk B, Levin MJ, McDuffy R, Hayward AR. Characterization of the newborn response to herpes virus antigens. *J Immunol*. 1985;134:4184.
29. Rotbart HA, Levin MJ, Hayward AR. Immune responses to varicella zoster virus infections in healthy children. *J Infect Dis*. 1993;167:195.
30. Wilson NJ, Boniface K, Chan JR, et al. Development, cytokine profile and function of human interleukin-17 producing helper T cells. *Nat Immunol*. 2007;8:950.
31. Jiao H, Tóth B, Erdős M, et al. Novel and recurrent STAT3 mutations in hyper-IgE syndrome patients from different ethnic groups. *Mol Immunol*. 2008;46:202.
32. Milner JD, Brenchley JM, Laurence A, et al. Impaired T(H)17 cell differentiation in subjects with autosomal dominant hyper-IgE syndrome. *Nature*. 2008;452:773.
33. Brunkow ME, Jeffery EW, Hjerrild KA, et al. Disruption of new forkhead/winged-helix protein, scurfin, results in the fetal lymphoproliferative disorder of the scurfy mouse. *Nat Genet*. 2001;27:68.
34. Bennett CL, Christie J, Ramsdell F, et al. The immune dysregulation, polyendocrinopathy, enteropathy, X-linked syndrome (IPEX) is caused by mutations in FOXP3. *Nat Genet*. 2001;27:20.
35. Duhen T, Geiger R, Jarrossay D, et al. Production of interleukin 22 but not interleukin 17 by a subset of human skin-homing memory T cells. *Nat Immunol*. 2009;10:857.
36. Punnonen J, Aversa GG, Vandekerckhove B, et al. Induction of isotype switching and Ig production by $CD5^+$ and $CD10^+$ human fetal B cells. *J Immunol*. 1992;148:3398.
37. Brugnoni D, Airò P, Graf D, et al. Ontogeny of CD40L [corrected] expression by activated peripheral blood lymphocytes in humans. *Immunol Lett*. 1996;49:27.
38. Choi YS, Kageyama R, Eto D, et al. ICOS receptor instructs T follicular helper cell versus effector cell differentiation via induction of the transcriptional repressor Bcl6. *Immunity*. 2011;34:932.
39. Debock I, Jaworski K, Chadlaoui H, et al. Neonatal follicular Th cell responses are impaired and modulated by IL-4. *J Immunol*. 2013;191:1231.

117 B-Cell Development

Sandra C.A. Nielsen | Scott D. Boyd

INTRODUCTION

Mammalian B-cell development occurs via a series of sequential developmental transitions that culminate in the establishment of a protective antibody repertoire that is essential for the host's immunity to microbial pathogens. Primary antibody deficiencies can result from mutations in genes that are expressed in B-lineage cells and are critical for normal development and function. This chapter focuses on the developmental biology of human B-lineage cells, the mechanisms by which B cells generate their diverse B-cell receptor (BCR) and antibody repertoires, and gene mutations that block the development of antibody-mediated immunity.

SITES OF HUMAN B-CELL DEVELOPMENT

Similar to all blood cells that reside in the periphery, B lymphocytes are derived from hematopoietic stem cells (HSCs). The liver and omentum are the initial sites of B lymphopoiesis in the human fetus, beginning at approximately 8 weeks' gestation.[1] Between 12 and 15 weeks' gestation, HSCs begin to home to the bone marrow, at which time multiple stages of B-lineage cells are present. Human B-cell development continues in the marrow from the midtrimester of fetal development through at least the eighth decade of life,[2] in contrast to T cells, which appear to develop primarily until the fourth decade of life.[3]

STAGES OF MARROW B-CELL DEVELOPMENT

Development of mammalian blood cells from HSCs is mediated by cytokines that regulate survival, proliferation, and differentiation; transcription factors that regulate gene expression; and the microenvironment of primary lymphoid organs such as fetal liver and marrow.[4] The stages of mammalian B-cell development have historically been defined by two methods: (1) detection of the rearrangement and expression of immunoglobulin (Ig) gene segments and (2) measurement of cell-surface molecules, termed *cluster of differentiation* (CD) markers, using monoclonal antibodies.

B-lineage cells in primary lymphoid tissue are derived from lymphohematopoietic progenitors. Multilymphoid progenitors have the capacity to develop into all T, B, and/or natural killer (NK) cells, with limited fitness to develop into myeloid cells.[4] As shown in Fig. 117.1, one model suggests that multilymphoid progenitors can differentiate into early thymic progenitors, which develop into all T-lineage cells, or a common B/NK progenitor, which develops into B-lineage or NK cells.

Rearrangement of genomic deoxyribonucleic acid (DNA) at the Ig heavy (IgH) and light (IgL) chain loci[5,6] distinguishes B-lineage cells from all other cells in the body and is thus a signature event in commitment to the B-lineage. The Ig loci are located on three human chromosomes: heavy chain (IGH) is at 14q32, the kappa (κ) light chain (IGK) at 2p11, and the lambda (λ) light chain (IGL) at 22q11; each of these loci contains arrays of variable (V), diversity (D; only for IGH), and joining (J) gene segments, followed by constant (C) region genes. Fig. 117.2 illustrates the rearrangement of V(D)J genes from germline DNA, which together with heavy and light chain constant region genes encode the BCR and antibody proteins. IgH genes are the first to be assembled: first, an IGHD gene segment is joined to an IGHJ gene segment in the $CD34^+/CD10^+/CD22^+/CD19^-$ progenitor (pro-B) cell.[7] Pro-B cells with IGHD to IGHJ rearrangements on both copies of chromosome 14 then progress to pro-B-1 cells by selecting an IGHV gene segment to join to the DJ rearrangement and expressing the B-lineage-specific cell surface molecule CD19 with continued expression of CD34 and CD10. The next differentiation step to pre-B-cell phenotype includes stopping expression of CD34. Pre-B-1 cells that fail to produce in-frame VDJ rearrangements (i.e., rearrangements that encode a μ heavy chain protein) undergo apoptosis and are eliminated from further development.

If the VDJ rearrangement on either chromosome is in frame, pre-B-1 cells then differentiate into $CD34^-/CD10^+/CD19^+$ large pre-B-2 cells, defined by transient cell surface and constitutive cytoplasmic expression of the rearranged μ heavy chain protein. The cell surface μ heavy chain pairs with the surrogate light chain (a heterodimer of two proteins originally designated VpreB and λ5 in the mouse) as well as associating with anchoring molecules CD79α (Igα) and CD79B (IgB); the complex is referred to as the pre-B-cell receptor (pre-BCR).[8,9] Pre-BCR expression is required for normal human B-cell development (see further on). A point of considerable debate since the initial discovery of the pre-BCR is whether it has a natural ligand in the marrow microenvironment. Although the structure of the pre-BCR is compatible with a ligand-independent signaling function, compelling evidence in human and mouse studies has revealed that the soluble lectin produced by marrow stromal cells, Galectin-1, can function as a pre-BCR ligand.[9] Cell-surface pre-BCR signals the large pre-B-2 cells to undergo substantial proliferation (estimated to be four to six cell divisions), thereby expanding the number of cells with in-frame VDJ rearrangements.[10] Large pre-B-2 cells eventually cease expression of the surrogate light chain (and hence the pre-BCR) and exit the cell cycle. At this stage they are designated small pre-B-2 cells and undergo V-to-J rearrangement at the IGK locus. If the small pre-B-2 cell makes an in-frame VJ κ rearrangement, it expresses cell-surface μ/κ Ig. If rearrangement of both κ alleles is out of frame, the small pre-B-2 cell can undergo rearrangement at the λ LC locus. Immature B cells harboring in-frame IgL rearrangements express the κ or λ chain in complex with a μ or δ heavy chain on the cell surface as the BCR. Both IgM and IgD with the same VDJ-encoded sequences are expressed on the surface of these cells via alternative splicing of primary ribonucleic acid (RNA) transcripts to join the VDJ gene rearrangement to either IgM or IgD constant region genes. Several B-lineage-restricted cell-surface markers—including CD20, CD21, CD22, and CD40—are expressed at high levels in immature B cells.[11]

Orderly expression of the genes that mediate recombination and diversification of the Ig loci is essential for normal B-cell development. The protein products of recombination activating genes (RAG)1 and RAG2 are required for initiation of Ig germline rearrangement and generation of DNA strand breaks at recognition signal sequences 5′ or 3′ of Ig gene segments.[10,12] RAG proteins are also essential for rearrangement

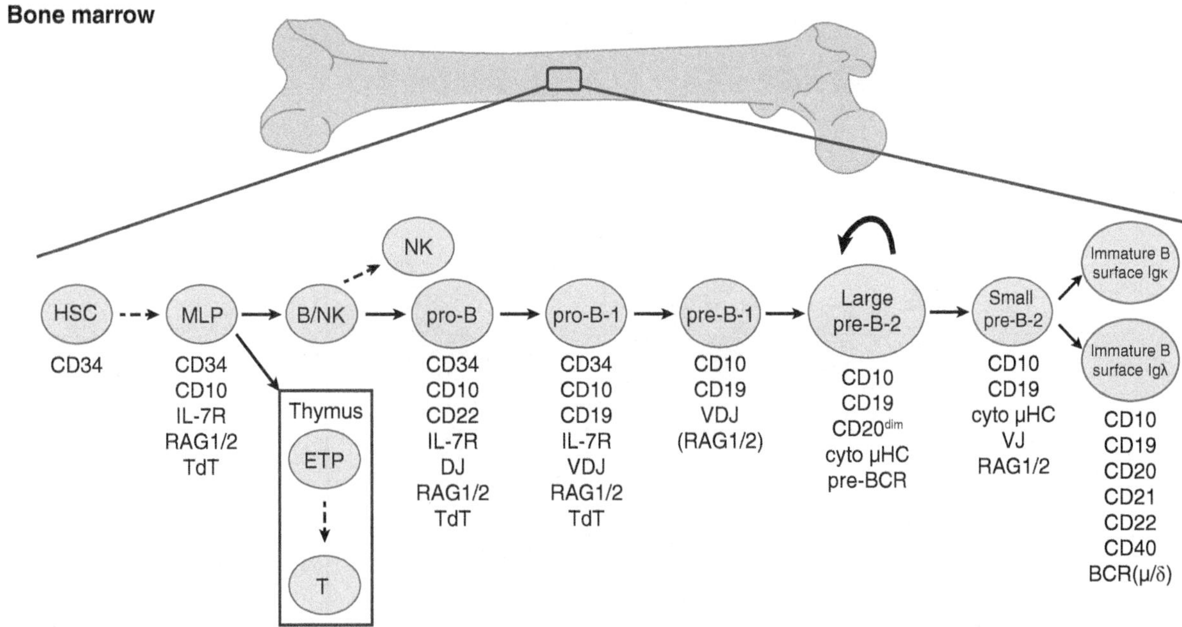

Fig. 117.1 B-cell development in the bone marrow. Hematopoietic stem cells *(HSCs)* differentiate into multipotent lymphoid progenitors *(MLPs)* that represent cells committed to the lymphoid lineages, at the exclusion of myeloid/erythroid lineages. Some MLPs likely migrate to the thymus, where they undergo development into early thymic progenitors *(ETPs)*, followed by development into T lymphocytes. Alternatively, MLPs differentiate into a B/natural killer *(NK)* cell progenitor in the marrow. Commitment to the B-lineage is initiated when the immunoglobulin (Ig) heavy chain locus undergoes D-to-J (pro-B) and then V-to-DJ (pro-B-1) rearrangement. Large pre-B-2 cells that have successfully rearranged the IgH locus express the μ heavy chain protein paired with the surrogate light chain as the pre-B-cell receptor (pre-BCR). Large pre-B-2 cells undergo several rounds of cell division *(curved arrow)*. Rearrangement of the Ig light chain at either the κ or λ loci occurs in small pre-B-2 cells, which then express functionally rearranged IgH and IgL genes as the BCR to become immature B cells. Most immature B cells express IgM and IgD. B-lineage cells that fail to make successful (i.e., in-frame) IgH and IgL rearrangements undergo apoptosis in the marrow (not shown). *Dashed lines* indicate that more than one developmental stage exists between two cell types. *IL,* Interleukin; *RAG,* recombination activating gene; *TdT,* terminal deoxynucleotidyl transferase. Other gene products with a critical role in and/or useful for characterizing developmental stages by flow cytometry are shown.

of T-cell-receptor genes during T-cell development in the thymus. RAG expression is initiated in $CD10^+/CD19^-$ pro-B cells, undergoes downregulation in pre-B-1 cells following in-frame heavy chain rearrangements, and is reinduced at the small pre-B-2 cell stage during IGK/L rearrangement.[13] Terminal deoxynucleotidyl transferase (TdT) is another enzyme expressed in early B- and T-cell development. TdT contributes to repertoire diversification by adding random nucleotides in a template-independent manner to the 3′ overhangs during the formation of the VD and DJ junctions of IgH, and at the VJ junction of the IgL chain.[14] Therefore, the combined actions of RAG and TdT are required to form the most diverse parts of the Ig heavy and light chain repertoires, the VDJ and VJ junctional regions that encode the complementarity-determining region-3 (CDR3) loops that are often involved in antigen-binding contacts.

A complex interplay of transcription factors is essential in mediating the continuing restriction that locks B-lineage cells into their developmental fate; these include PU.1 and Ikaros, which function at the myeloid/lymphoid cell junction and the transcription factor E2A (E2A), early B-cell factor (EBF), and paired box protein 5 (PAX5; also known as *BSAP*), which regulate irreversible specification and commitment to the B-lineage. Whereas E2A and EBF are essential for the formation of pro-B cells with EBF appearing only after E2A expression, PAX5 is necessary for final commitment to B-cell differentiation and is expressed throughout B-cell development.[15] Other transcription factors (discussed later) that play key roles in terminal B-cell development and differentiation into plasma cells include B-cell lymphoma 6 (BCL-6), B-lymphocyte-induced maturation protein 1 (BLIMP1), X-box-binding protein 1 (XBP1), and interferon regulatory factor 4 (IRF4). A summary of the patterns of gene expression characterizing the individual stages of B-cell development in the marrow is shown in Fig. 117.1.

It is clear that there are selective pressures on B cells during their development prior to leaving the bone marrow for the peripheral blood. Comparison of BCR sequence features between bone marrow B-cell precursors and mature naïve B cells in human blood show fewer long CDR3 sequences in the heavy chain of naïve B cells, and lower rates of autoreactivity or polyreactivity of the antibodies expressed, consistent with a selection against autoreactive B cells.[16] Other checkpoints may also act at earlier stages in B-cell development.

POSTMARROW B-CELL DEVELOPMENT

Following egress from the marrow, human peripheral B-cell development proceeds through multiple stages (Fig. 117.3).[17] Immature/transitional B cells express cell surface IgM and IgD, are $CD24^{hi}/CD38^{hi}$, and most express CD5.[18] These cells are transiting via the blood between the marrow and secondary lymphoid organs, such as spleen and lymph node. They constitute approximately 5% of adult peripheral blood B cells but up to 50% of B cells present in cord blood. Naïve/mature B cells circulate in peripheral blood or reside in primary follicles in lymph nodes to form the naïve follicular B-cell compartment. They generally express a $CD24^+/CD38^+$ phenotype that distinguishes them from immature/transitional B cells. These cells have not been stimulated by foreign antigen in either a thymic-dependent or thymic-independent manner.

Antigen-induced activation of B-cell differentiation in the lymph node and other secondary lymphoid tissue encompasses a series of transitions collectively referred to as the *germinal center (GC) reaction.*[19] These transitions include clonal expansion, class switch recombination (CSR) at the IgH locus, somatic hypermutation (SHM) of IgH V genes, and affinity maturation

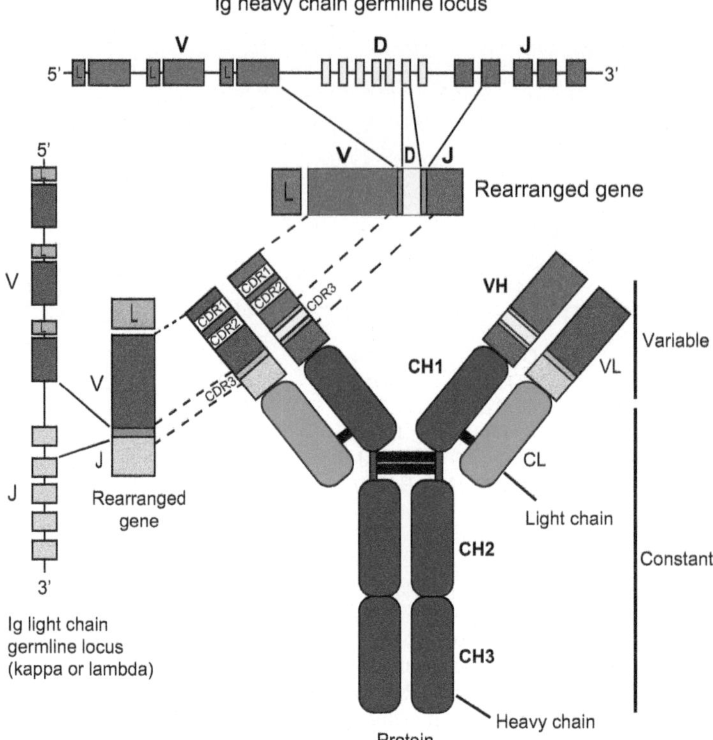

Fig. 117.2 Schematic representation of antibody structure showing contributions of germline gene segments in immunoglobulin *(Ig)* heavy *(top)* and light *(left side)* chain loci. IgH D and J gene segments are first selected and joined together, followed by rearrangement of a V segment to the DJ product. During rearrangement, the ends of the gene segments are subject to exonuclease digestion and insertion of random nucleotides creating sequence diversity at the *V-D-J* junctional regions. A similar process of rearrangement takes place for light chain V and J segments. These junctional regions encode the complementarity-determining region 3 (CDR3) loops, which are often involved in antigen binding. Ig constant region exons (IgH domains: CH1, CH2, and CH3; IgL domain: CL) are located downstream of V(D)J gene segments and are joined to the rearranged V(D)J region by mRNA splicing. *L*, Leader (signal sequence) sequence that encodes a peptide required for entry into the endoplasmic reticulum during protein synthesis but is removed from the final protein.

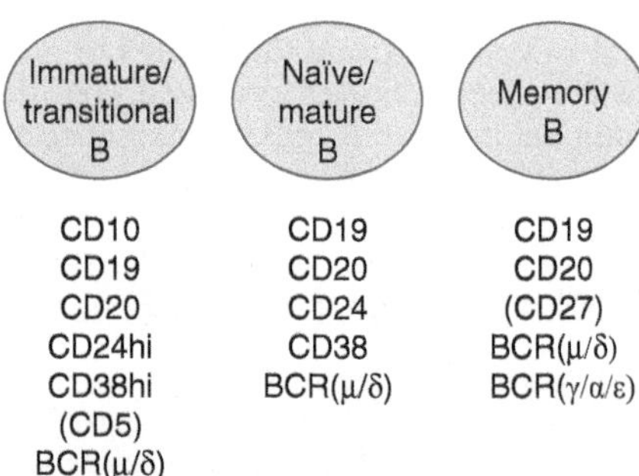

Fig. 117.3 B cells in peripheral blood. After exiting the marrow, immature/transitional B cells circulate in the blood and/or migrate to secondary lymphoid organs such as spleen and lymph node. These immature/transitional B cells represent approximately 5% of total peripheral blood B cells and can be distinguished from the naïve/mature B cells by expression of CD10 and high levels of CD24 and CD38. Most also express CD5. Most memory B cells are identified by CD27 expression and are divided into non-class-switched cells expressing immunoglobulin (Ig)M, IgD, or both, and class-switched cells expressing IgG, IgA, or more rarely, IgE. These can circulate in the peripheral blood following development in the germinal center reaction, or may reside in local tissues. A number of activated B-cell phenotypes have been described in the blood following antigen stimulation; these are not shown. Gene products with a critical role in and/or useful for characterizing developmental stages by flow cytometry are shown. *BCR*, B-cell receptor;

of the IgH V sequences that recognize antigen. As shown in Fig. 117.4, the GC reaction is initiated when naïve B cells are triggered by antigen-driven BCR crosslinking in the presence of costimulatory signals from helper T cells. Naïve B cells undergo robust proliferative expansion; the proliferating larger B cells in the GC are referred to as *centroblasts*. Populations of centroblasts can be morphologically identified in the so-called *dark zone* of the GC, and these cells are undergoing SHM of their IgH V genes. The master transcriptional regulator at this developmental stage is BCL-6.[20,21] After exiting the cell cycle, centroblasts differentiate into centrocytes, and the latter form the so-called *light zone* of the GC. Multiparameter fluorescence activated cell sorting of tonsillar B-cell subpopulations and subsequent DNA sequencing of VDJ rearrangements demonstrated that SHM is initiated in centroblasts.[22] Centrocytes are highly enriched for mutated IgH V genes and undergo selection by virtue of binding to cognate antigen presented by follicular dendritic cells and T cells. The affinity of the interaction dictates whether centrocytes will undergo apoptosis (low-affinity interaction) or be selected for further differentiation (high-affinity interaction) into memory B cells or plasma cells. Some centrocytes also undergo CSR and shift from expression of cell surface IgM and IgD to expression of cell surface IgG, IgA, and possibly IgE. Following selection in the light zone, some centrocytes reenter the dark zone for additional rounds of cell division and SHM diversification of their BCR sequences before returning to be selected again in the light zone.[23] Memory B cells may reenter the GC upon reactivation and go through additional rounds of mutation and selection thus driving and optimizing B-cell memory.[24,25]

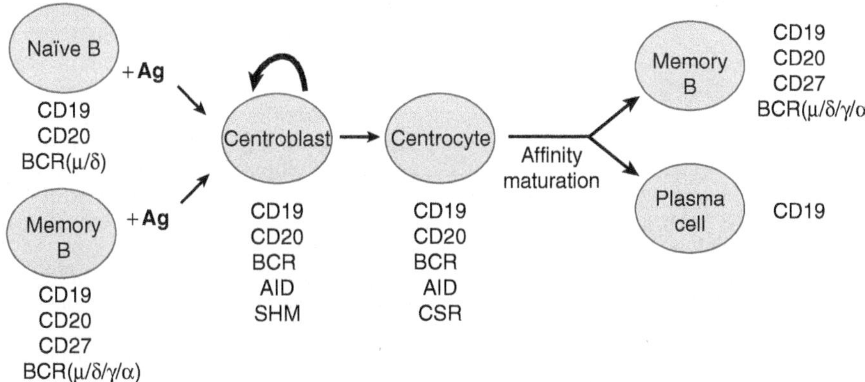

Fig. 117.4 B-cell maturation in the germinal center. Naïve B cells encounter antigen in secondary lymphoid organs and, in cooperation with signals from CD4+ helper T cells (not shown), up-regulate markers of proliferation (e.g., Ki67) and the cellular machinery (e.g., activation-induced cytidine deaminase *[AID]*) necessary for induction of somatic hypermutation. These highly proliferative *(curved arrow)* B-cell populations undergoing somatic mutation of their antibody genes are designated centroblasts and occupy the "dark zone" of the germinal center. Centroblasts differentiate into centrocytes, which enter the "light zone" of the germinal center where B cells expressing higher-affinity B-cell receptors *(BCRs)* have a selective advantage. Antigen-stimulated B cells differentiate into either CD27+ memory B cells or antibody-secreting plasma cells. The latter down-regulate all major surface markers with the exception of CD19 and home to the bone marrow. Gene products with a critical role in and/or useful for characterizing developmental stages by flow cytometry are shown.

Expression of the tumor necrosis factor receptor family member CD27 correlates with the presence of somatically hypermutated *IgH V* genes in B-lineage cells.[26] Four separate CD27+ memory B-cell populations have been described: IgM+/IgD+, IgM+/IgD−, IgM−/IgD+, and class switched (IgG+, IgA+, and IgE+). Newborn infants have very few memory B cells, but memory and naïve B-cell populations represent approximately 40% and 60% of peripheral blood B cells in adults, respectively. However, not all circulating memory B cells (i.e., cells with SHM) express CD27.[26]

A distinct population of B cells with attributes of both naïve and memory cells are the splenic marginal zone (MZ) B cells.[27] MZ B cells are a first line of defense against encapsulated bacteria in rodents and primates, but the stage of development and function of MZ B cells in humans is not completely resolved. This partially reflects the fact that the microscopic anatomy of the human splenic MZ differs substantially from that of rodents.[27]

The mechanism underlying CSR and SHM was a protracted mystery in immunology for many years, but the mystery was solved by the discovery of an enzyme designated activation-induced cytidine deaminase (AID).[28] Originally proposed to be an RNA-editing enzyme, AID functions by deaminating cytidines to uridines, which in combination with DNA-modification processes including base excision and mismatch repair, makes AID a natural mutator.[29] As might be expected of an enzyme with this function, AID expression is induced in GC centroblasts, where CSR and SHM occur. In addition, AID is also expressed in immature B cells, and it has been proposed that constitutive expression of this enzyme is necessary for autoreactive B-cell removal and hence central B-cell tolerance.[30] Interestingly, aberrant AID activity is now known to contribute to the development of B-cell lymphomas by inducing point mutations or translocations in known oncogenes.[31]

As discussed elsewhere in this book, neonates are vulnerable to infection with selected pathogens (e.g., encapsulated bacteria) and respond poorly to immunization compared with children. Compared to adults, infant Ig repertoires differ in gene segment usage frequencies and CDR3 features, as well as isotype proportions in class-switched B cells. However, maturation of other elements in the immune system, such as GCs, could also contribute to the susceptibility to infection.[32]

REGULATORY B CELLS

A large number of studies during the last several years have described a subpopulation of mouse and human B cells that secrete interleukin (IL)-10 and have substantial immunosuppressive properties.[33,34] These cells have been designated *B10 cells* or *regulatory B cells* (Bregs). Bregs can modulate T-cell function and appear to protect against a number of autoimmune pathologies, including multiple sclerosis, rheumatoid arthritis, inflammatory bowel disease, and systemic lupus erythematosus. Considerable effort has gone into determining the origin, development, and function of these cells. There is no evidence that Bregs are a distinct lineage of B cells based on cell surface marker analysis. Bregs are present at a frequency of approximately 1% of the lymphocytes in human peripheral blood. Bregs themselves are regulated by the cytokines IL-21 and IL-35[35] and are yet another example of a layered regulatory network within the immune system.

PLASMA CELL DEVELOPMENT

Plasma cells are terminally differentiated B-lineage cells that secrete copious quantities of Ig central to the protective antibody response. Cells differentiating toward a plasma cell phenotype following vaccination or during the response to an infection are sometimes referred to as *plasmablasts* or *antibody-secreting cells (ASCs)* in the literature. Plasma cell differentiation can be stimulated by either T-cell-dependent or T-cell-independent antigen stimulation.[36] Several transcription factors work in concert to regulate the potential of an activated B cell to differentiate into a memory B cell or a plasma cell.[37] The transcription factors BCL-6 and PAX5 suppress plasma cell development, thereby favoring development of memory B cells. A prominent target gene of BCL-6 is BLIMP1, a transcription factor whose function is central to driving activated B cells into plasma cells. Signaling events received at the surface of B-lineage cells may trigger a reduction in BCL-6 levels, which in turn may relieve suppression of BLIMP1. A negative feedback loop then ensues, involving BLIMP1 suppression of BCL-6 that, when coupled with the action of two other transcription factors designated XBP1 and IRF4, promotes differentiation to the plasma cell stage.[37]

Many plasma cells generated in the spleen or lymph nodes during post-GC reactions migrate to the bone marrow, where they serve as a major source of antibody production.

CYTOKINES AND CHEMOKINES IN B-CELL DEVELOPMENT

B-cell development occurs in a complex microenvironment consisting of other lymphohematopoietic cells, stromal cells, and extracellular matrix components such as fibronectin and type IV collagen.[38] B-lineage cells develop in the extravascular compartment of the marrow and, upon differentiation to the immature B cell stage, migrate to medullary vascular sinuses as a prelude to entering the bloodstream. The term *stromal cell* is a generic term encompassing multiple cell types, including adipocytes, endothelial cells, osteoblasts, and fibroblastic reticular cells. Marrow stromal cells secrete cytokines and chemokines such as IL-7 and CXCL12 that mediate development of B-lineage cells and regulate adhesion of early B-lineage cells to stromal cells, respectively.[39] However, these cytokines and chemokines optimally function at short distances, requiring that B-lineage cells and stromal cells be in physical apposition to one another. In vitro studies using human marrow-derived fibroblastic reticular cells indicated that vascular cell adhesion molecule-1 (VCAM-1) plays an important role in the adherence of normal human B-lineage cells via interaction with CD49d on the surface of B-lineage cells.[40] A study of the physical disposition of human B-lineage cells and marrow stromal cells in situ indicated that B-lineage cells were prominently juxtaposed to CD10$^+$ stromal cells and that B-cell differentiation was spatially oriented with the most mature cells progressing toward marrow sinusoids.[41]

INTERLEUKIN-7

The roles of IL-7 and its receptor subunits the IL-7 receptor (IL-7R) α chain and the γ_c chain have been extensively studied in mouse lymphopoiesis.[42,43] The physiologic importance of IL-7 was elucidated by the demonstration that targeted disruption of the IL-7 or IL-7Rα chain genes leads to profound disruption of B-cell (and T-cell) development in adult mice. In contrast, IL-7-deficient mice have a severe disruption of adult B-cell development but undergo normal fetal and perinatal B-cell development. Targeted disruption of the genes encoding the γ_c subunit of the receptors for IL-2, -4, -7, -9, -15, and -21 and the JAK3 tyrosine kinase also leads to severe disruptions in B-cell development. This is consistent with the known structure of IL-7R and the activation of JAK3 following IL-7 stimulation.[44] In contrast, mice doubly deficient for the cytokine receptor FLT3 and the IL-7Rα chain fail to develop fetal and neonatal B-lineage cells. Thus, IL-7 and FLT3-ligand (FLT3-L) are cytokines that collectively orchestrate fetal and adult mouse B-cell development.

Insight into the role of IL-7 in human B-cell development has been gleaned from analysis of patients with rare types of immune deficiency as well as clinical studies wherein IL-7 is administered in the setting of immune reconstitution clinical protocols.[45] Studies of children with severe combined immune deficiency (SCID) have been particularly informative. Patients with X-linked SCID harboring mutations in the γ_c subunit and patients with autosomal recessive mutations in the JAK3 tyrosine kinase have severe defects in T and NK cell development, but have normal or even elevated numbers of peripheral blood B cells. Mutations in the IL-7Rα chain are now the third most common cause of SCID.[46] An increase in percentage or absolute number of peripheral blood B cells occurred in essentially all of these patients. Thus, the presence of circulating B cells in these SCID patients indicates that an absolute requirement of IL-7 signaling for their development does not exist. However, a normal peripheral blood B-cell count does not necessarily equate to normal B-cell development in these patients with SCID.[47] The requirement of IL-7 signaling could vary in humans as a function of ontogeny, with fetal/neonatal B-cell development being relatively IL-7 independent, as it is in the mouse. Interestingly, no cases have been reported of a patient with a mutation in the IL-7 gene coding sequence or within the IL-7 gene locus, and so the potentially most informative clinical experiment of nature, wherein a patient makes no IL-7 protein, is not available to shed light on the role of the cytokine itself in human B-cell development.

Studies of patients with non-SCID immune deficiency provide a separate perspective on the possible role of IL-7 in human B-cell development.[45] In a study evaluating whether IL-7 administration could restore T cell numbers in patients with lymphopenic cancer, marrow biopsies performed before and after IL-7 administration revealed a three- to eightfold increase in the percentage of CD19$^+$/CD10$^+$ B-lineage cells in four of six patients after IL-7 administration. Administration of IL-7 may therefore have induced the expansion of B-cell precursors in the marrow of some patients. Studies in patients with human immunodeficiency virus (HIV) and patients with idiopathic CD4$^+$ T lymphocytopenia (an HIV-independent syndrome) revealed a positive correlation between serum levels of IL-7 and the existence of circulating CD10$^+$/CD27$^-$ immature/transitional B cells. In vitro studies have shown that IL-7 transduces a replicative signal to normal human B-lineage cells that is complemented by additional stromal cell-derived signals that cooperate with IL-7 to promote normal human B-cell development.[48] These collective studies suggest a role for IL-7 in human B-cell development but potentially on a cellular scale that is more limited or functionally distinct from that of the mouse.

PRIMARY ANTIBODY IMMUNODEFICIENCIES

Given the unique and critical functional role of gene products essential for full competency of early B-cell development, it is no surprise that mutations in some of these genes can have dire consequences on the development and function of human B cells, culminating in primary antibody deficiencies.[49] If a genetic disease affecting B cells deserves the title of a "classic," it would be X-linked agammaglobulinemia. The pediatrician O. C. Bruton[50] originally described an 8-year-old boy with recurrent respiratory bacterial infection and no detectable serum gamma globulins. Subsequent studies showed that the disease was inherited in an X-linked pattern[51] and was characterized by an absence of circulating B cells,[52] hence the designation X-linked agammaglobulinemia. Two landmark reports[53,54] identified the gene mutated in X-linked agammaglobulinemia, and it was christened Bruton tyrosine kinase (BTK). BTK plays a critical role in a variety of biochemical signaling pathways in B-lineage cells.[49] Notably, pre-BCR and BCR crosslinking result in activation of the tyrosine kinases SYK and LYN, which in turn phosphorylate BTK and the adaptor protein B-cell linker (BLNK).[55] BTK and BLNK then cooperate to activate phospholipase Cγ2 and the phosphoinositide 3-kinase pathway, culminating in a sustained calcium flux central to proliferation. Hundreds of distinct mutations in BTK have been identified in patients with X-linked agammaglobulinemia, and most result in a lack of BTK protein. A strict relationship between a specific mutation and severity of the disease has not been identified, but mutations that do not adversely affect BTK protein levels may yield a somewhat milder phenotype. Approximately 85% of agammaglobulinemias are X-linked, but rare cases of autosomal recessive agammaglobulinemia have also been described. This heterogeneous cohort includes patients with mutations in the μ heavy chain, the λ5 subunit of the surrogate light chain, the pre-BCR/BCR-associated signaling molecules Igα and IgB, the p85α chain of PI3-kinase, and the adapter signaling molecule BLNK. These patients have similar clinical characteristics to patients with X-linked agammaglobulinemia, and gamma globulin replacement therapy must be administered throughout life.

A COMMENT ABOUT METHODS

Many of the discoveries of B-cell development pathways have been highly dependent on the development of new technologies for analyzing single cells. Analytic multiparameter flow cytometry has been a valuable tool for cellular phenotyping for more than 30 years. In this method, cells in suspension are stained with fluorescently labeled monoclonal antibodies or other specific reagents targeting particular cell antigens and then forced to flow one at a time through a series of laser light paths and fluorescence emission detectors, thus revealing the markers expressed by each cell. Improvements in laser technology and the development of novel fluorescent probes have resulted in the ability to routinely stain cell populations with 5 to 10 and, in specialized cases, over 20 different monoclonal antibodies. Flow cytometry is often coupled with sorting or recovering the heterogenous mixture of cells into cell populations of interest for further analysis or manipulation (e.g., RNA-sequencing or cell culture). Mass cytometry is a relatively new technology that greatly expands on the classical method of flow cytometry for phenotyping single cells by using metal isotopes, instead of fluorophores, conjugated to ligands or monoclonal antibodies. A major constraint of fluorescent dyes is their overlapping light absorption or emission spectra. Mass cytometry circumvents this limitation due to the nonoverlapping nature of mass-to-charge ratios for the metal isotopes used, enabling more markers to be measured in each experiment. As in traditional fluorescent flow cytometry, intracellular molecules can also be detected in permeabilized cells, including signal transduction molecules that are phosphorylated on critical functional sites. One important drawback of mass cytometry is that the cells analyzed are destroyed during the process; therefore no subsequent sorting or analyses are possible. In a remarkable study, 44 markers were simultaneously used to characterize human B-cell development occurring in normal bone marrow.[56] Several important conclusions were drawn from this study: (1) the overall ordering of marrow B-lineage populations identified with fluorescence flow cytometry were confirmed; (2) the makeup of the B-cell developmental compartments varied little among marrow donors; and (3) several very rare subpopulations were identified, including one at a frequency of 0.007% of normal bone marrow mononuclear cells that responded to IL-7 stimulation by undergoing signal transducer and activator of transcription 5 (STAT5) phosphorylation.

Within the last decade, advancements in DNA sequencing technology have greatly improved researchers' ability to examine the complex BCR gene rearrangements and track clonal populations of B cells in human specimens. BCRs from B-cell cancers, several B-lineage cell stages, and B cells responding to changes or stimuli—such as infections and vaccines or autoimmune conditions—have been sequenced.[32,57-62]

CONCLUSION

Human B-cell development consists of a series of cellular transitions that begins in fetal liver or marrow with the development of lymphoid cells from HSCs and culminates in the seeding of secondary lymphoid tissue with naïve B cells. The establishment of a diverse Ig repertoire encoded by rearrangement of Ig gene segments provides the basis for subsequent recognition of any potential pathogens encountered during the individual's lifetime. The repertoire is shaped by mutational mechanisms and selection processes that occur in the GC reaction. Mutations in B-lineage-specific genes that encode proteins essential for normal B-cell development can prevent the formation of antibody-producing cells, thereby resulting in profound immune deficiency and a requirement for gamma globulin replacement therapy.

ACKNOWLEDGMENTS

The authors would like to acknowledge Tucker LeBien for portions of this chapter derived from the previous edition.

A complete reference list is available at www.ExpertConsult.com. 

SELECT REFERENCES

1. Cooper MD. Current concepts. B lymphocytes. Normal development and function. *N Engl J Med*. 1987;317:1452.
2. Rossi MI, Yokota T, Medina KL, et al. B lymphopoiesis is active throughout human life, but there are developmental age-related changes. *Blood*. 2003;101:576.
3. Kumar BV, Conners TJ, Farber DL. Human T cell development, localization, and function throughout life. *Immunity*. 2018;48:202.
4. Doulatov S, Notta F, Laurenti E, Dick JE. Hematopoiesis: a human perspective. *Cell Stem Cell*. 2012;10:120.
7. van Zelm MC, van der Burg M, de Ridder D, et al. Ig gene rearrangement steps are initiated in early human precursor B-cell subsets and correlate with specific transcription factor expression. *J Immunol*. 2005;175:5912.
8. Nagata K, Nakamura T, Kitamura F, et al. The Igα/IgB heterodimer on μ-negative ProB cells is competent for transducing signals to induce early B cell differentiation. *Immunity*. 1997;7:559.
10. Spicuglia S, Franchini DM, Ferrier P. Regulation of V(D)J recombination. *Curr Opin Immunol*. 2006;18:158.
11. LeBien TW, Tedder TF. B lymphocytes: how they develop and function. *Blood*. 2008;112:1570.
12. Schatz DG, Oettinger MA. Baltimore D: the V(D)J recombination activating gene, RAG-1. *Cell*. 1989;59:1035.
13. Ghia P, ten Boekel E, Sanz E, et al. Ordering of human bone marrow B lymphocyte precursors by single-cell polymerase chain reaction analyses of the rearrangement status of the immunoglobulin H and L chain gene loci. *J Exp Med*. 1996;184:2217.
14. Thai TH, Kearney JF. Isoforms of terminal deoxynucleotidyl transferase: developmental aspects and function. *Adv Immunol*. 2005;86:113.
15. Matthias P, Rolink AG. Transcriptional networks in developing and mature B cells. *Nat Rev Immunol*. 2005;5:497.
16. Wardemann H, Yurasov S, Schaefer A, Young JW, Meffre E, Nussenzweig MC. Predominant autoantibody production by early human B cell precursors. *Science*. 2003;5:1374.
18. Sims GP, Ettinger R, Shirota Y, Yarboro CH, Illei GG, Lipsky PE. Identification and characterization of circulating human transitional B cells. *Blood*. 2005;105:4390.
19. Victora GD, Nussenzweig MC. Germinal centers. *Annu Rev Immunol*. 2012;30:1429.
20. Klein U, Tu Y, Stolovitzky GA. Transcriptional analysis of the B cell germinal center reaction. *Proc Natl Acad Sci Unit States Am*. 2003;100:2639.
22. Pascual V, Liu YJ, Magalski A, et al. Analysis of somatic mutation in five B-cell subsets of human tonsil. *J Exp Med*. 1994;180:329.
23. Rajewsky K. Clonal selection and learning in the antibody system. *Nature*. 1996;381:751.
24. Bende RJ, van Maldegem F, Triesscheijn M, Wormhoudt TAM, Guijt R, van Noesel CJM. Germinal centers in human lymph nodes contain reactivated memory B cells. *J Exp Med*. 2007;204:2655.
25. Seifert M, Przekopowitz M, Taudien S, et al. Functional capacities of human IgM memory B cells in early inflammatory responses and secondary germinal center reactions. *Proc Natl Acad Sci Unit States Am*. 2015;112:E546.
26. Klein U, Rajewsky K, Kuppers R. Human immunoglobulin (Ig)M+IgD+ peripheral blood B-cells expressing the CD27 cell surface antigen carry somatically mutated variable region genes: CD27 as a general marker for somatically mutated (memory) B-cells. *J Exp Med*. 1998;188:1679.
27. Steiniger B, Timphus EM, Barth PJ. The splenic marginal zone in humans and rodents: an enigmatic compartment and its inhabitants. *Histochem Cell Biol*. 2006;126:641.
28. Muramatsu M, Kinoshita K, Fagarasan S, Yamada S, Shinkai Y, Honjo T. Class switch recombination and hypermutation require activation-induced cytidine deaminase (AID), a potential RNA editing enzyme. *Cell*. 2000;102:553.
30. Cantaert T, Schickel J-N, Bannock JM, et al. Activation-induced cytidine deaminase expression in human B cell precursors is essential for central B cell tolerance. *Immunity*. 2015;43:884.
31. Shaffer AL, Young RM, Staudt LM. Pathogenesis of human B-cell lymphomas. *Annu Rev Immunol*. 2012;30:565.

32. Nielsen SCA, Roskin KM, Jackson KJL, et al. Shaping of infant B cell receptor repertoires by environmental factors and infectious disease. *Sci Trans Med.* 2019;11:eaat2004.
34. van de Veen W, Stanic B, Wirz OF, Jansen K, Globinska A, Akdis M. Role of regulatory B cells in immune tolerance to allergens and beyond. *JACI.* 2016; 138:654.
35. Tedder TF, Leonard WJ. Autoimmunity: regulatory B-cells—IL-35 and IL-21 regulate the regulators. *Nat Rev Rheumatol.* 2014;10:452.
36. Shapiro-Shelef M, Calame K. Regulation of plasma cell development. *Nat Rev Immunol.* 2005;5:230.
37. Nutt SL, Taubenheim N, Hasbold J, et al. The genetic network controlling plasma cell differentiation. *Semin Immunol.* 2011;23:341.
38. Nagasawa T. Microenvironmental niches in the bone marrow required for B-cell development. *Nat Rev Immunol.* 2006;6:107.
39. Glodek AM, Honczarenko M, Le Y, et al. Sustained activation of cell adhesion is a differentially regulated process in B lymphopoiesis. *J Exp Med.* 2003; 197:461.
40. Dittel BN, McCarthy JB, Wayner EA, LeBien TW. Regulation of human B-cell precursor adhesion to bone marrow stromal cells by cytokines that exert opposing effects on the expression of vascular cell adhesion molecule-1 (VCAM-1). *Blood.* 1993;81:2272.
41. Torlakovic E, Tenstad E, Funderud S, Rian E. $CD10^+$ cells form B-lymphocyte maturation niches in the human bone marrow. *J Pathol.* 2005;205:311.
43. Corfe FA, Paige CJ. The many roles of IL-7 in B-cell development; mediator of survival, proliferation and differentiation. *Semin Immunol.* 2012;24:198.
44. Mazzucchelli RI, Riva A, Durum SK. The human IL-7 receptor gene: deletions, polymorphisms, and mutations. *Semin Immunol.* 2012;24:225.
45. Lundstrom W, Fewkes NM, Mackall CL. IL-7 in human health and disease. *Semin Immunol.* 2012;24:218.
46. Giliani S, Mori L, de Saint Basile G, et al. Interleukin-7 receptor a (IL-7Ra) deficiency; cellular and molecular bases: analysis of clinical, immunological, and molecular features in 16 novel patients. *Immunol Rev.* 2005;203:110.
47. Liao C-Y, Yu H-W, Cheng C-N, et al. A novel pathogenic mutation on Interleukin-7 receptor leading to severe combined immunodeficiency identified with newborn screening and whole exome sequencing. *J Microbiol Immunol Infect.* 2018;53:99-105.
48. Johnson SE, Shah N, Panoskaltsis-Mortari A, LeBien TW. Murine and human IL-7 activate STAT5 and induce proliferation of normal human pro-B-cells. *J Immunol.* 2005;175:7325.
49. Durandy A, Kracker S, Fischer A. Primary antibody deficiencies. *Nat Rev Immunol.* 2013;13:519.
51. Good RA. Clinical investigations in patients with agammaglobulinemia. *J Lab Clin Med.* 1954;44:803.
52. Siegal FP, Pernis B, Kunkel HG. Lymphocytes in human immunodeficiency states: a study of membrane associated immunoglobulins. *Eur J Immunol.* 1971;1:482.
53. Vetrie D, Vorechovsky I, Sideras P, et al. The gene involved in X-linked agammaglobulinemia is a member of the src family of protein tyrosine kinases. *Nature.* 1993;361:226.
54. Tsukada S, Saffran DC, Rawlings DJ, et al. Deficient expression of a B-cell cytoplasmic tyrosine kinase in human X-linked agammaglobulinemia. *Cell.* 1993;72:279.
55. Tsukada S, Baba Y, Wantanabe D. Btk and BLNK in B-cell development. *Adv Immunol.* 2001;77:123.
56. Bendall SC, Davis KL, Amir el- AD, et al. Single-cell trajectory detection uncovers progression and regulatory coordination in human B-cell development. *Cell.* 2014;157:714.
57. Logan AC, Zhang B, Narasimhan B, et al. Minimal residual disease quantification using consensus primers and high-throughput IGH sequencing predicts post-transplant relapse in chronic lymphocytic leukemia. *Leukemia.* 2013;27:1659.
59. Stern JN, Yaari G, Vander Heiden JA, et al. B cells populating the multiple sclerosis brain mature in the draining cervical lymph nodes. *Sci Trans Med.* 2014;6:248ra107.
61. Davis CW, Jackson KJL, McElroy AK, et al. Longitudinal analysis of the human B cell response to Ebola virus infection. *Cell.* 2019;177:1370.
62. Nielsen SCA, Boyd SD, et al. New technologies and applications in infant B cell immunology. *Curr Opin Immunol.* 2019;57:53.

118 Mononuclear Phagocyte System

Pascal M. Lavoie | Ofer Levy

OVERVIEW OF THE MONONUCLEAR PHAGOCYTE SYSTEM

The mononuclear phagocyte system (MPS) refers to a network of cells that share the ability to engulf (i.e., internalize) and digest large particles such as whole microbes (e.g., bacteria, fungi, and viruses) or dying cells, but also tumor cells and toxic metabolic products. Mononuclear cells have a single, round nucleus. Neutrophils and other granulocytes also share phagocytic functions, but they are morphologically distinct, polynuclear, and have historically been excluded from the MPS. Neutrophils are covered in Chapter 119.

Mononuclear phagocytes are located throughout different organs and tissues, in large numbers in the spleen, but also in organs such as the lungs, brain, liver, peritoneal cavity, and placenta, as well as the connective tissues. They are highly evolutionarily conserved in multicellular animals and plants and are a fundamental component of cellular immune defenses.[1] In addition to their phagocytic capability, these cells can sense and migrate toward gradients of microbial products, secrete chemokine and cytokine mediators resulting in the migration and activation of other leukocytes, and present antigens to the adaptive immune system. They also accomplish other important homeostatic functions related to tissue repair, remodeling, angiogenesis, and neural networking during embryonic, fetal, and postnatal development.[2]

The innate immune system is the first line of defense against microbes, whereas the adaptive immune system is most typically known for its capacity to develop immunologic memory upon pathogen encounters. Invertebrates and plants do not possess a traditional adaptive immune system.[3] In vertebrates, mononuclear phagocytes are also endowed with functions related to the presence of an adaptive immune system, including phagocytosis of pathogens that have been marked via antibody opsonization and the production of specific T and B lymphocyte differentiation cytokines.

ONTOGENY OF MONONUCLEAR PHAGOCYTES

The MPS is composed of monocytes, macrophages, and dendritic cells (DCs). Monocytes predominate in blood, whereas macrophages and DCs reside in tissues. DCs are generally much less abundant compared with monocytes. They are the most efficient of the antigen-presenting cells. Thus they usually migrate into lymph nodes after sensing pathogens to present a fragment of this pathogen to T and B lymphocytes.[4]

Mononuclear phagocytes are generated through a process called *myelopoiesis*. They arise in early embryogenesis, from at least two distinct hematopoietic waves: (1) a *primitive* wave that begins during the third week of gestation *in the yolk sac* (also called *umbilical vesicle*), until gestational week 10 to 12 in humans[5]; this wave gives rise to red blood cells and *embryonic macrophages*, and (2) a *definitive* wave that begins during the fourth week of gestation and gives rise to all hematopoietic cell types, continuing into postnatal life.[6] During primitive hematopoiesis, erythromyeloid progenitors (EMPs) emerge, to produce blood islands and establish a primitive circulation (Fig. 118.1), and to produce embryonic macrophages that migrate into peripheral tissues such as the central nervous system (CNS).[7] Embryonic macrophages retain a long-term capacity for self-renewal and cell survival, likely for years.[8] Following the establishment of the blood circulation, primitive yolk sac–derived EMPs start seeding the fetal liver and spleen around the fifth week of gestation.[1] In the second, definitive wave of hematopoiesis, lymphomyeloid progenitors (LMPs) migrate from the yolk sac to the liver (also called *transient definitive* wave).

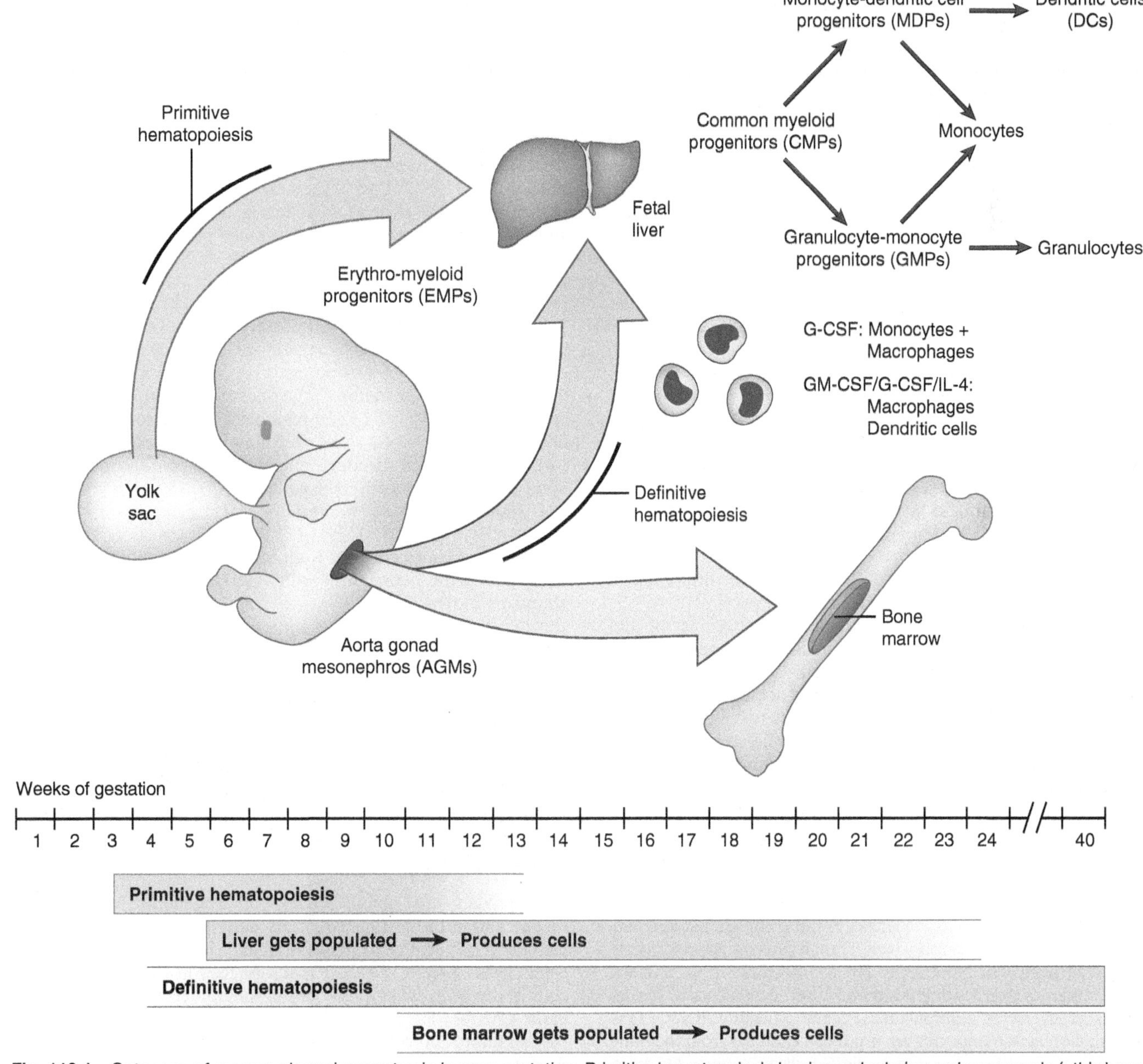

Fig. 118.1 Ontogeny of mononuclear phagocytes in human gestation. Primitive hematopoiesis begins early during embryogenesis (~third gestational week in humans), in the yolk sac, with the production of erythrocytes and embryonic macrophages. Later (~5 gestational week), CD34-expressing hematopoietic stem cells appear in the aorta-gonad-mesonephros *(AGM)* region, giving rise to hematopoietic progenitors that then will go on to populate other, more definitive hematopoietic organs such as the liver and bone marrow. *G-CSF,* Granulocyte colony-stimulating factor; *GM-CSF,* granulocyte-macrophage colony-stimulating factor; *IL,* interleukin; *M-CSF,* macrophage colony-stimulating factor. (Courtesy Kristin Johnson, Boston Children's Hospital.)

Pluripotent CD34-expressing hematopoietic stem cells (HSCs) that can give rise to all blood cells autonomously[9] also begin to emerge around the fourth week of gestation in humans, in a region called the *aortogonad mesonephros (AGM)* situated in the endothelium of the dorsal aorta.[10] Until approximately 22 weeks of gestation, the fetal liver and spleen remain the dominant sources of hematopoiesis. At approximately 8 to 10 weeks of gestation, HSCs start populating the bone marrow. During the third trimester of gestation the bone marrow becomes the main source of hematopoietic cells, continuing into postnatal life, and as hematopoiesis in the fetal liver gradually wanes.[11]

Differentiation of progenitor cells into monocytes, macrophages, and DCs is guided by a highly coordinated epigenetic program involving chemical modifications of deoxyribonucleic acid (DNA), and reconfiguration of the chromatin and the structure of histones.[12] Monocytes, macrophages, and DCs originate from common myeloid progenitors (CMPs). CMPs give rise to two main progenitor lineages: granulocyte-monocyte progenitors (GMPs), which give rise to granulocytes and monocytes, and monocyte-DC progenitors (MDPs), which give rise to another common DC progenitor (CDP, for DCs), but also to monocytes (see Fig. 118.1).[13-15]

Monocytes are most abundant in blood, whereas macrophages are found in tissues. Once blood monocytes reach the tissues, they rapidly differentiate into macrophages, and monocyte-derived DCs (MoDCs) under certain inflammatory conditions.[16,17] In humans, development and differentiation of monocytes and macrophages from progenitors depend on the macrophage colony-stimulating factor (M-CSF, also known as *CSF-1*). Its receptor counterpart, the M-CSF receptor (MCSFR), is expressed on all three cell types of the MPS, as well as their precursors. M-CSF is part of a family that also includes granulocyte-macrophage colony-stimulating factor (GM-CSF) and interleukin (IL)-3. GM-CSF, granulocyte colony-stimulating factor (G-CSF), IL-4, and FMS-related tyrosine kinase 3 ligand (Flt3L) are particularly important for the development and homeostasis of macrophages and DCs.[16,18] In humans, in vitro protocols to differentiate blood cells from pluripotent stem cells have been extremely invaluable to understand hematopoiesis and validate data from mice. Based on this type of studies, requirements for the differentiation of monocyte-derived macrophages and DCs differ between adult and neonatal monocytes.[19,20] In addition, the reduced production of macrophages and DCs in response to GM-CSF in preterm neonates may underlie the reduced myelopoietic responses that occur upon infection in these babies.[21]

Stress (including corticosteroids and catecholamines) and inflammation increase the production and differentiation of myeloid progenitors during embryonic and postnatal life and can provoke a demarginalization of monocytes, thereby increasing counts in circulating blood.[22] Therefore leukocytosis, an augmentation of white blood cell counts (particularly neutrophils but also monocytes), is frequently observed in sepsis and in inflammatory situations such as chorioamnionitis. Moderate leukocytosis is also a favorable prognostic factor. In contrast, an inappropriately low leukocyte count is associated with a worse outcome in newborn sepsis.

MONOCYTES

Monocytes are the most abundant mononuclear phagocyte and third most abundant leukocyte subset in the complete blood count, after neutrophils and lymphocytes. They represent approximately 10% of all nucleated blood cells. Their concentration in neonatal blood ranges from 300 to 3300 (mean 1400) cells/μL at 40 weeks, approximately twice as abundant as counts in healthy adults.[23] One to 10 million new monocytes are produced each day from the bone marrow in a healthy adult in a cyclic (~5 days) manner. Of these, approximately 20% are free flowing in the circulation, and the rest are "marginalized" (i.e., adherent and rolling on the endothelium surface of the blood vessels).[24] Monocytes generally reside only for a short period in blood (<48 hours) after being produced in the bone marrow, following which they rapidly transmigrate to peripheral tissues (e.g., lung, kidney, peritoneum, and gastrointestinal or reproductive tracts), where a majority of them differentiate into macrophages or DCs.[25,26] In tissues, a minority of monocytes conserve their original phenotype (so-called *tissue monocytes*) and may play an important and specific role in vascular remodeling.[27,28]

Monocytes have been studied for more than a century and were originally identified based on morphologic criteria. However, with the use of flow cytometry, three main, functionally distinct subsets have been defined in human blood, based on their expression of cell surface CD14, a co-receptor for the gram-negative cell wall component lipopolysaccharide (LPS), and CD16, the immunoglobulin (Ig)G Fc receptor FcγR-III (Fig. 118.2).[29,30] The subset composition and function of human monocytes have been comprehensively reviewed[31] and vary considerably across development, suggesting distinct physiologic roles during fetal ontogeny.[32,33]

Classical monocytes express high levels of the CD14 surface receptor but lack expression of the receptor CD16; thus they are commonly referred to as $CD14^{high}/CD16^{-}$ monocytes. They are efficient at phagocytosis and produce high amounts of IL-10 upon stimulation with LPS.[34] They represent the main monocyte subset and make up the majority (>80%) of monocytes in adult blood. However, they are less predominant in neonatal blood (<40% to 60%).[35,36]

Nonclassical monocytes express CD16 but only low levels of CD14 ($CD14^{low}/CD16^{+}$). They are capable of efficient antigen presentation and express high levels of the human leukocyte antigen (HLA)-DR molecule.[30] They are particularly responsive to intracellular nucleic acids such as those from single-stranded viruses, due to high expression of certain pattern recognition receptors (PRRs), Toll-like receptor (TLR) 7 and TLR8 (see later).[36] They are smaller in size and represent 5% to 10% of the monocytes in adult blood. In neonatal blood, they are relatively more abundant earlier in gestation, representing up to 40% of monocytes less than 32 weeks of gestation.[35,33] Nonclassical monocytes are also potent producers of IL-1β and tumor necrosis factor (TNF)-α.[34,37] Because of their specific role patrolling the vascular endothelial surface, nonclassical monocytes may also play an important role as immediate responders in neonatal sepsis.[38]

A third subset of *intermediate* monocytes express high levels of CD14 and CD16 ($CD14^{high}/CD16^{+}$).[39] This subset represents a minority of monocytes in adult blood (<5% of all monocytes) compared with neonatal (cord) blood where they are more abundant (~10% to 20%,[33] up to 30% of monocytes based on another study[35]). Intermediate monocytes play an important role in the resolution of inflammation.[40,41] Although little is known regarding their specific in vivo role during fetal life, they appear to differentiate directly from fetal liver embryonic stem cells rather than from classical monocytes as reported in mature, adult individuals.[42] Their high production of proangiogenic factors such as endoglin and vascular endothelial growth factor (VEGF) receptor 2 and their unique ability to induce the generation of capillary networks suggest that these cells may play a distinct, important role in angiogenesis and vascular remodeling.[39,43]

MACROPHAGES

Macrophages are phenotypically heterogeneous, existing in several different specialized forms depending on the tissue of residence. Specialized tissue-specific macrophages include osteoclasts in bone, alveolar macrophages in the lung, Kupffer cells in the liver, Langerhans cells in the epidermis, and microglia in the CNS (see Fig. 118.2). In the placenta, decidual macrophages play an important role ensuring immunologic tolerance between the fetus and its mother.[44]

As discussed earlier, macrophages originate from EMPs during the primitive hematopoiesis wave from the yolk sac or during the definitive hematopoietic wave from liver- or bone marrow-derived monocytes.[45] Therefore the embryonic wave of tissue-resident macrophage is independent from the pool of monocyte-derived

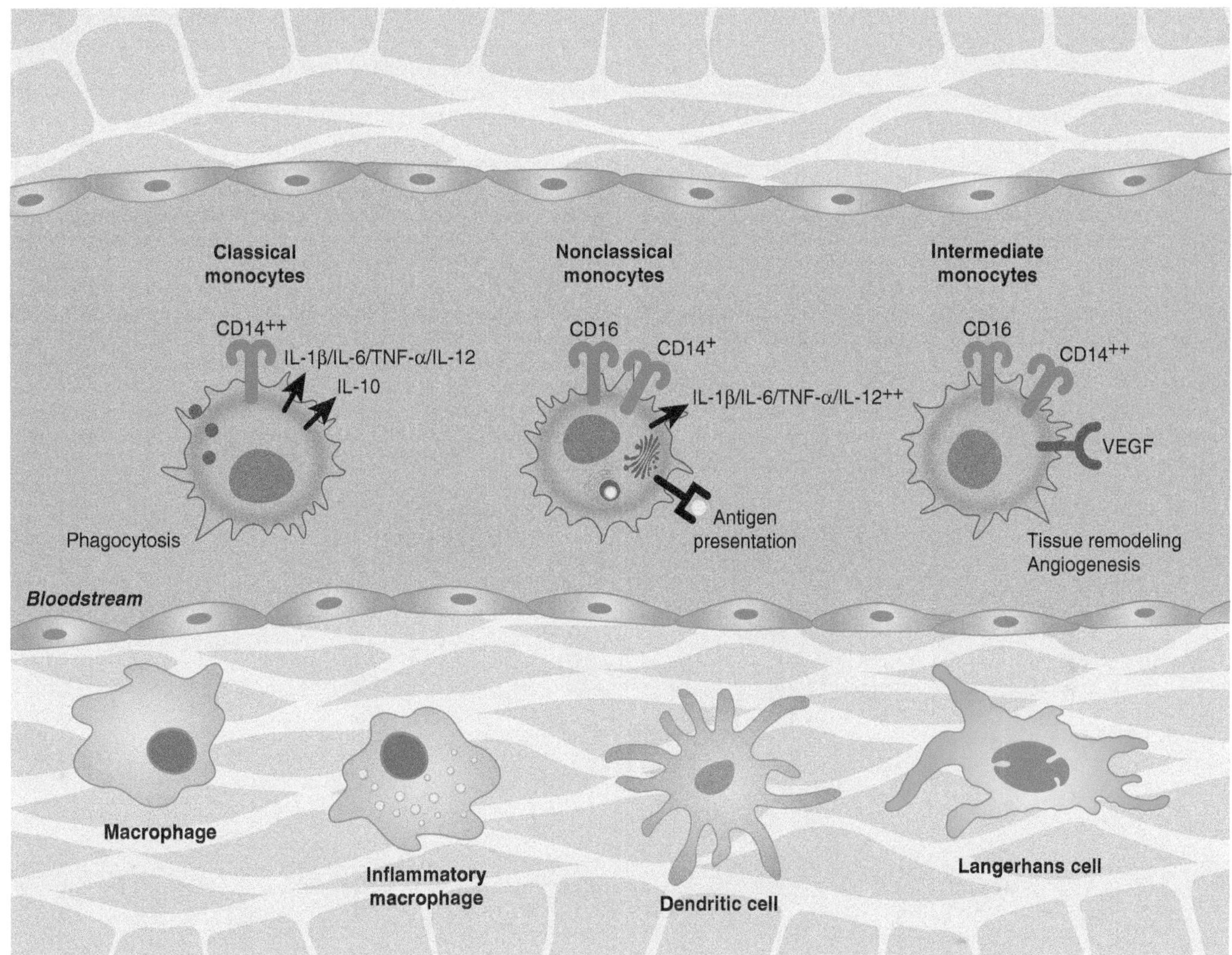

Fig. 118.2 Subsets of monocytes, macrophages, and dendritic cells. Illustration of circulating monocyte subsets in a blood vessel, whereas macrophages, dendritic cells, and Langerhans cells are generally located in tissues. The function of each subset of monocytes is also indicated (see text). *IL,* Interleukin; *TNF,* tumor necrosis factor; *VEGF*, vascular endothelial growth factor. (Courtesy Kristin Johnson, Boston Children's Hospital.)

macrophage originating from the bone marrow.[46-48] In addition, tissue-resident macrophages can also be produced from the differentiation of a distinct type of EMPs that express the transcription factor c-MYB[a] and that seed the liver from the yolk sac during embryogenesis to give rise to fetal monocytes that then will become macrophages in tissues.[49] Based on fate-mapping studies where the traveling of labeled cells can be followed over periods in mice, the proportion of macrophages directly originating from embryonic versus embryonic liver-derived versus definitive liver- or bone marrow derived–monocytes vary considerably among tissues. Monocyte-derived macrophages are most abundant in tissues such as the spleen, skin, gut, lungs, and heart,[50] whereas in the CNS, the vast majority of macrophages and DCs may originate from the self-renewal of tissue-resident embryonic macrophages that were produced during embryonic life.[7,51,52]

The proinflammatory or antiinflammatory function of macrophages can be polarized by cytokine milieu, referred to also as M1 and M2 macrophages, respectively. GM-CSF–derived macrophages are able to carry out highly efficient antimicrobial functions and promote adaptive cellular T-cell responses through the production of proinflammatory cytokines, high expression of costimulatory molecules (for antigen presentation), and production of enzymes such as the inducible nitric oxide synthase (iNOS) (at least in mice) and nicotinamide adenine dinucleotide phosphate (NADPH) oxidase. M-CSF–differentiated macrophages are relatively anergic to inflammatory stimuli and are well adapted for the clearance of debris through phagocytosis in the promotion of wound healing and resolution of inflammation. This function is mediated by the production of antiinflammatory cytokines, immunosuppressive arginase (in mice), and scavenger receptors.[53]

DENDRITIC CELLS

DCs specialize in presentation of antigens to T lymphocytes and therefore express high levels of major histocompatibility complex (MHC) class II molecules such as HLA-DR. At least three main subsets of DCs are recognized, according to the expression of surface markers, functional characteristics, ontogeny, and tissue localization.[54,55] Two subsets of conventional (or myeloid) DCs (cDCs) can be distinguished based on the high expression of the surface markers CD141 and CD1c,[29] whereas a third subset of plasmacytoid dendritic cells (pDCs) more distinctively expresses the cell surface marker CD123. These two main DC subsets are present in high proportions from early in the third trimester of gestation throughout adult life.[56,57] Immature DCs are also found in blood and can give rise to tissue DCs.[29] The ontogeny of DCs in human fetuses and neonates has been much less studied than monocytes, in part because of their low abundance in blood makes them difficult to obtain in large enough numbers. pDCs are the main producer of interferon (IFN)-α, a key cytokine in antiviral defense, and neonatal pDCs generally produce relatively low amounts of this cytokine in response to most stimuli.[58-61] During gestation,

[a] MYC was discovered as viral gene that transforms cells into a myeloblast phenotype. The *c* in c-MYC stands for "conserved" and denotes the host homolog of the gene as opposed to the viral homology v-MYC.

DCs that highly express arginase 2 promote tolerance to maternal and fetal antigens.[62,63]

NEONATAL MATURATION OF PHAGOCYTES

Mononuclear phagocytes show major functional changes during gestation and early postnatal life. Knowledge of these maturation stages is important to fully appreciate the immunocompromised state of very low-birth-weight neonates and their vulnerability to bacterial and fungal infections.[64,65] Detection and elimination of pathogens by the MPS depend on a number of functions, whose developmental changes throughout fetal and postnatal life are detailed later.

PATTERN RECOGNITION RECEPTORS

A main function of phagocytes is surveillance, which consists in patrolling organs to provide a rapid, early detection and clearance of microbial pathogens by the innate immune system. This is particularly relevant in neonates, whose adaptive immune system is largely naïve and thus unable to respond quickly.[66,67] This surveillance is achieved through a series of microorganism-recognizing receptors, termed *PRRs*. PRRs are highly conserved among species. Each PRR targets a different structurally conserved motif uniquely present on bacteria, fungi, or viruses, termed *pathogen-associated molecular patterns (PAMPs)*. PRRs can be intracellular or extracellular, and include TLRs, nucleotide-binding oligomerization domain-containing protein (NOD), and NOD-like receptors (NLRs), C-type lectin receptors (CLRs) such as the dectin-1 receptor (see later), and the retinoic acid-inducible gene I (RIG-I) and RIG-I-like receptors (RLRs). Stimulation of PRRs results in a cascade of cellular events leading to the activation of phagocytes and production of cytokines and chemokines (Fig. 118.3).

Before the third trimester of gestation, the function of most PRRs is profoundly diminished. At birth, most PRRs are already

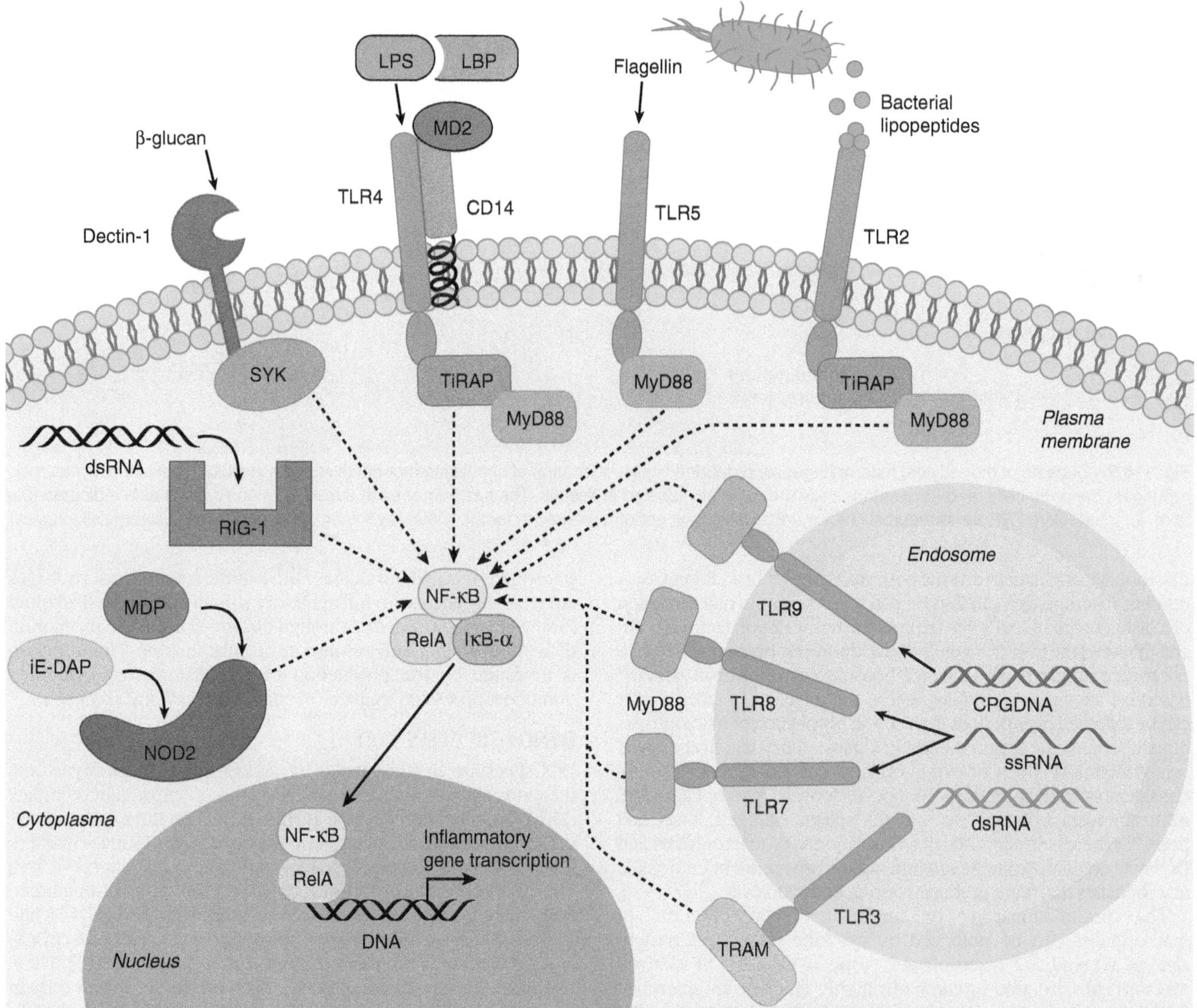

Fig. 118.3 Cellular localization of main pattern-recognition receptors and their ligands (pathogen-associated molecular patterns). *ASC,* Apoptosis-associated speck-like protein containing CARD; *ATP,* adenosine triphosphate; *CARD,* caspase recruitment domain; *dsRNA,* double-stranded ribonucleic acid; *iE-DAP,* D-glutamyl-meso-diaminopimelic acid; *LPS,* lipopolysaccharide; *LBP,* lipopolysaccharide binding protein; *MDP,* muramyl dipeptide; *NOD,* nucleotide-binding oligomerization domain-containing protein; *NLRP,* NOD-like receptor family pyrin domain; *RIG,* retinoic acid-inducible gene; *ssRNA,* single-stranded ribonucleic acid; *TiRAP,* Toll-interleukin 1 receptor domain containing adaptor protein; *TLR,* Toll-like receptor; *TRAM,* Toll-interleukin 1 receptor (TIR)-domain-containing adapter-inducing interferon-β factor (TRIF)-related adaptor molecule. (Courtesy Kristin Johnson, Boston Children's Hospital.)

functional, although some adopt an adult phenotype only later in postnatal life. In between, PRRs do not become responsive all at once, but rather, mature sequentially during the early third trimester of gestation, following an hierarchy, with intracellular PRRs maturing earlier than extracellular PRRs.[68-70] Authors have hypothesized that this hierarchical maturation of PRRs follows corresponding selective advantages and requirements during the establishment of self-tolerance to maternal and fetal self-antigens as the adaptive immune system is deployed.[47] For example, in the skin, the strength of inflammatory response determines whether the body considers microorganisms to be commensal versus pathogenic during the neonatal period.[71] Suppression of PRR activity in early fetal life may also serve to limit potentially harmful inflammatory responses prior to the fetus reaching a viable stage.[65] Intriguingly, PRR functions are naturally dampened in adult bats, making them more tolerant to disease rather than able to fight infection.[72]

TOLL-LIKE RECEPTORS

Humans have 10 known TLRs, whose biologic responses are dictated by their structural characteristics, cell-specific expression, and cellular localization profiles.[73] TLR-1, -2, -4, -5, and -6 are extracellular (surface) receptors specialized in the recognition of bacterial products, whereas TLR-3, -7, -8, and -9 are intracellular (endosomal) receptors specialized in the detection of viral or bacterial nucleic acids.[74] No natural ligand has been identified for TLR-10 as of yet, although activation of this receptor with synthetic ligands suppresses inflammation.[75]

The function of most TLRs is profoundly attenuated in neonatal monocytes and DCs before 29 to 32 weeks of gestation. This is reflected in markedly reduced cytokine responses to in vitro stimulation of mononuclear cells using single TLR agonists or whole microorganisms.[33,56,68,76-82] After birth, TLR-mediated cytokine responses mature within a few weeks even in extremely low-birth-weight infants.[83,84] This delayed postnatal maturation may be in part responsible for the reduced response to conventional vaccine adjuvants observed in these infants.[85,86] In some studies, greater attenuation in TLR-stimulated proinflammatory compared with antiinflammatory cytokine responses have been reported at lower gestational ages, consistent with a relative antiinflammatory state of mononuclear cells during early fetal life.[56,76,77,80,84,87]

NUCLEOTIDE-BINDING OLIGOMERIZATION DOMAIN–CONTAINING PROTEIN AND NOD-LIKE RECEPTORS

NLRs include three main subtypes (NODs, NLR family pyrin domain-containing proteins [NLRPs], and NLR family caspase recruitment domain-containing proteins [NRLCs]) with several subfamily members.[88] NLRs mainly sense intracellular microorganisms. Like other intracellular PRRs, activity of NOD1 and NOD2 develops early in gestation compared with extracellular TLRs.[89] However, this does not appear to be the case for all NLRs. For example, activity of NLRP3 remains suppressed until the middle of the third trimester of gestation.[33] NLRP3 plays a major role in the cellular production of IL-1β, a main pyrogenic cytokine that is also distinct in that activation of cells in presence of this cytokine amplifies responses to other PRR stimulation. Systemic production of IL-1β leads to fever and at high levels can induce profound metabolic disturbances; hence it requires tight regulation. The importance of NLRP3 in the recognition of group B *Streptococcus* by mononuclear phagocytes may underlie the increased risk of infection with this pathogen in premature infants of lower gestational age.[90]

C-TYPE LECTIN RECEPTORS (DECTIN-1, MANNOSE RECEPTOR)

The PRRs dectin-1, mannose, CD206, and DC-SIGN are classic members of the family of CLRs. The dectin-1 receptor is the most studied CLR, and this receptor is particularly relevant to the immune recognition of *Candida* species through recognizing the fungal cell wall component β-1,3-glucan. Intracellular signaling through stimulation of dectin-1 leads to the activation of the intracellular receptor adaptor molecule SYK. This is followed by the activation of the paracaspase intracytoplasmic multiprotein complex constituted of mucosa-associated lymphoid tissue lymphoma translocation protein 1 (MALT1), caspase recruitment domain-containing protein 9 (CARD9), and B-cell lymphoma/leukemia 10 (BCL-10). Humans with genetic mutations impairing CARD9 or MALT1 functions are highly vulnerable to invasive fungal infections.[91] Accordingly, the greatly diminished activity of the dectin-1-paracaspase complex in mononuclear phagocytes before 32 weeks likely contributes to the gestational-dependent increase in the vulnerability of extremely low-birth-weight preterm neonates to invasive fungal infections.[65]

RETINOIC ACID-INDUCIBLE GENE I-LIKE RECEPTORS

Less is known about the maturation of RLRs in neonatal mononuclear phagocytes. RLRs are helicase enzymes that sense double-stranded ribonucleic acid (RNA) viruses (e.g., influenza A and respiratory syncytial virus [RSV]).[92-94] As with other PRRs, RIG-I activation in virus-infected cells leads to the production and release of cytokines, particularly type I IFNs.[95-97] Neonates display impaired RIG-I-dependent activity even at term, which may contribute to their high vulnerability to RSV infections.[61]

MECHANISMS UNDERLYING FUNCTIONAL MATURATION OF PATTERN RECOGNITION RECEPTORS IN NEONATES

The mechanisms underlying the graded maturation of PRR functions across development in human neonates are not completely understood. Some investigators have attributed the attenuation in neonatal TLR function to a gestational age–dependent reduction in surface expression of TLRs or their co-receptors (e.g., CD14[98-100]) or to reduced expression of signaling adaptor molecules, which are key components of the TLR signaling cascade, such as MyD88, IRF5, and ERK.[100-102] Lack of these molecules has been linked to a functional impairment in the activity of MAP kinases p38 and JNK, and nuclear translocation of nuclear factor (NF)-κB, a major and central inflammatory transcription factor.[100,102] However, because attenuation in PRR pathways in early fetuses is broad, involving receptors with distinct signaling pathways, it is unlikely that the functional differences between neonatal and adult MPS cells can simply be ascribed to reductions in the expression of these receptors and/or their signaling pathways. For example, term monocytes express levels of TLRs similar to those of their adult counterparts, yet they have a highly divergent cytokine response characterized by low production of proinflammatory and T helper (Th)1-polarizing cytokines (e.g., TNF-α, IL-12p70) and high production of Th2/Th17 and antiinflammatory cytokine responses.[103] Rather, more upstream mechanisms are likely involved; two recent articles demonstrated suppression of mammalian target of rapamycin (mTOR), a central regulator of cellular energy metabolism and protein synthesis, linked to a global impairment in activation in fetal mononuclear phagocytes.[65,104] Soluble mediators also modulate PRR responsiveness in the perinatal period.[105] Immediately after birth, high plasma concentrations of S-100–alarmin prevent hyperactivation of PRR responses, which become more similar to adult responses over the first year of life.[106,107]

INHIBITORY RECEPTORS AND SUPPRESSOR CELLS

In addition to activating receptors, phagocytes express inhibitory receptors. More than 40 inhibitory immune receptors have been reported in humans,[108] but very few have been investigated in human neonates. Significantly lower expression of the immune receptor expressed on myeloid cells 1 (IREM-1), an inhibitory receptor of the Ig superfamily of receptors expressed on myeloid cells, has been shown on CD14^{high}/CD16^{-} monocytes from cord blood compared with monocytes from adults.[109] Human neonatal blood plasma features relatively high concentrations of adenosine, an endogenous purine metabolite, that together with a heightened sensitivity of neonatal mononuclear cells to adenosine receptor-mediated accumulation of cyclic adenosine monophosphate (cAMP), inhibits TNF-α production by neonatal monocytes.[110-113] In addition, specific cells can actively suppress neonatal phagocytes, including myeloid-derived suppressor cells and nucleated red blood cells.[114,115]

PHAGOCYTOSIS

Phagocytosis is the process by which cells engulf cells or particulate matter. From an immunologic perspective, phagocytosis is critical for the clearance of infections, killing of pathogens, and activation of host defenses.[116] Phagocytosis is mediated by contraction of actin-myosin structures, leading to the migration of phagosomes with lysosomes. Macrophages are capable of engulfing particles up to 3 times greater than their own volume. Phagocytosis involves opsonic and nonopsonic mechanisms. Opsonic phagocytosis relies on the binding of antibodies (IgG) or complement proteins to mark a particle or pathogen for internalization via the Fc or complement receptors; in contrast, nonopsonic pathways use PRRs such as dectin-1 or TLRs.

Complement-mediated and opsonic activities are well developed in term infants.[117] In addition, compared with PRRs, phagocytosis mechanisms appear to be functional earlier during fetal life.[67,118-125] This may be due to the overlapping functions of multiple phagocytic receptors, which can complement each other.[65] On the other hand, preterm neonates lack maternal antibodies normally transferred during the third trimester of gestation and serum complement proteins; as such, they may be more reliant on nonopsonic mechanisms of phagocytosis.[126] Moreover, early in vitro studies have indicated that phagocytosis may proceed more slowly in neonatal monocytes with decreasing gestational age. Whether these differences impact the risk of infection in a clinically relevant way is undertermined.[127]

Phagocytosis plays an important role in the induction of labor. Phagocytes are activated following the onset of labor, characterized by a heightened production of IL-6 that accelerates parturition and resulting in up-regulation of PRR responsiveness in term infants within 72 hours after birth.[128-131] Other effects of labor on phagocyte function have generated conflicting results, likely because the small size of studies predisposes to type I errors. Impaired recruitment and migration of neutrophils may be in part due to the polarization of newborn mononuclear cells to high production of IL-6, which inhibits tissue neutrophilia, and low production of proinflammatory/Th1-polarizing cytokines such as TNF.[132,133]

CHEMOTAXIS AND OXIDATIVE KILLING

Another important characteristic of professional phagocytes is their propensity to migrate towards chemokine gradients and recruit other cells through chemotaxis. Phagocytes also share a high efficiency at oxidative-mediated killing of microbial pathogens, which is achieved through an oxidative burst within the controlled microenvironment of the phagosome. Chemotaxis is more limited in neonatal phagocytes, possibly due to a difference in signals present in adult cells.[125] As an illustration of this, data suggest that human neonates express distinct developmental-specific isoforms of chemokines.[134] Naïve CD4 T lymphocytes that most recently egressed from the thymus are abundant in neonates and express high levels of the CXCL8 (IL-8) chemokine, which may favor the preferential recruitment of neutrophils in the period of life preceding establishment of classic immunologic memory.[135-137]

Two broad types of redox molecules mediate oxidative bursts: nitric oxide and its derivatives, and reactive oxygen species (ROS; e.g., superoxide anion: O_2^-, peroxide: H_2O_2). In addition to their role in microbial killing, redox molecules are important regulators of immune pathways. In the phagosome, nitric oxide is mainly produced from arginine by iNOS, whereas ROS is produced by oxidases, including NADPH oxidase.[138] Oxidative-mediated killing is reduced in neonates, particularly in preterm neonates and under conditions of stress.[139,140] The susceptibility of neonatal pathogens to ROS and nitric oxide greatly depends on the specific sequence of the redox molecules produced within the phagosome. For example, little bactericidal activity is observed against *Escherichia coli* unless both nitric oxide and peroxides are produced. In the case of *Staphylococcus aureus*, superoxide/ROS followed by nitric oxide is most effective in eradicating these bacteria, whereas *Listeria monocytogenes* is relatively resistant to oxidative-mediated killing.

ANTIGEN PROCESSING AND PRESENTATION

Another important function of phagocytes is their ability to cleave exogenous molecules such as proteins into smaller peptides in specialized vesicles called *endosomes* and present these small molecules to T lymphocytes through MHC class II surface molecules. DCs are specialized in this matter. Antigen presentation to Th lymphocytes is critical to the development of immunologic memory by the adaptive immune system. Neonatal phagocytes generally display a gestational age-dependent reduction in the surface expression of HLA.[141]

The IL-12 and IL-23 cytokines are particularly important during antigen presentation and promotion of the differentiation of Th1 and Th17 lymphocytes, respectively. In general, neonatal DCs produce little of the IL-12p70 heterodimeric cytokine due to a lack of production of its IL-12p35 subunit.[142] In full-term newborns this may be compensated for by production of IL-27, which can regulate humoral (antibody) responses,[143,144] as well as IL-23, which regulates mucosal immune responses by promoting the differentiation of IL-17-producing Th cells.[145] Production of IL-23 by neonatal DCs may help to compensate for the intrinsic lack of Th17 differentiation in neonates and young infants.[146] Monocytes and DCs from neonates born before 29 weeks of gestation also lack production of both IL-12 and IL-23 cytokines.[56] Due to an important role of the IL-12/IL-23 family of cytokines in the control of fungal mucocutaneous infections, the deficit in both cytokines in extremely low-birth-weight infants may contribute to their susceptibility to these infections. In mice, a developmental change in production of IL-12 p70 occurs in CD8α-expressing DCs, restoring Th1 responses approximately 1 week after birth.[147] In humans, ontogeny is prolonged and this change occurs over several months after birth.

CLINICAL DEFECTS IN THE MONONUCLEAR PHAGOCYTE SYSTEM

INHERITED DEFECTS

A detailed review of inherited defects affecting the function of mononuclear phagocytes is outside the scope of this chapter. However, it is worth mentioning a few of these defects that are the most relevant to the MPS.

Chédiak-Higashi syndrome (CHS) is a rare (<1 in 100,000 individuals) autosomal recessive condition resulting in decreased phagocytosis due to altered lysosomal trafficking. Infants with CHS present with recurrent pyogenic infections (particularly in the respiratory tract and dermis), a mild coagulation defect due to defective platelets, and hypopigmentation of the skin (partial albinism). Mutations in the CHS1/LYST lysosomal trafficking regulator gene also result in varying neurologic problems, including weakness, ataxia, and progressive neurodegenerative/neurosensory losses.[148]

Chronic granulomatous disease (CGD) occurs in approximately 1 in 200,000 individuals and is a genetically heterogeneous condition, resulting in reduced oxidative killing due to a defect in the NADPH oxidase complex that impairs formation of ROS.[149] The most frequent form of CGD is X-linked, whereas other, more rare forms are transmitted in an autosomal recessive manner. CGD usually presents in infancy (<2 years of age) with lymphadenitis, pneumonia, gastroenteritis and colitis, skin abscesses, and hepatomegaly. The hallmark of CGD is the formation of granulomas. Infections mostly involve catalase-producing bacteria (e.g., *S. aureus*, *Pseudomonas aeruginosa*).

Several mutations have been described in PRRs. Mutations in the TLR signaling pathways increase susceptibility to pyogenic infections in humans, especially in neonates and young infants.[150] Of note, patients with defects in the TLR signaling axis (i.e., IRAK4 or MyD88; see Fig. 118.3) are at greatest risk in early life and tend to have fewer infections as they age, suggesting that the TLR system is particularly important in early life before other compensatory responses become more fully mature.[151] Mutations in NLRP3 also cause neonatal-onset multisystem inflammatory disease (NOMID, also known as *chronic infantile neurologic cutaneous and articular [CINCA] syndrome*), a rare genetic disorder presenting in the newborn period with uncontrolled inflammation characterized by skin rashes, severe arthritis, and chronic meningitis that can lead to neurologic damage.[152] Genetic defects in NLRs also result in other rare inflammatory disorders, including hereditary periodic fever syndromes.[88] Mutations in NLRC4 cause neonatal-onset enterocolitis, periodic fever, and fatal or near-fatal episodes of autoinflammation.[153] Inherited genetic defects in components of the paracaspase and C-type lectin (e.g., dectin-1) profoundly increase vulnerability to invasive candidiasis.[154-156] So far, no homozygous genetic defects have been reported with RIG-I in humans. In mice, complete loss of function of RIG-I is lethal. However, heterozygous human carriers of common variants appear to be more susceptible to viral infections.[157,158]

Leukocyte adhesion deficiency (LAD) occurs as an autosomal recessive disorder, with an estimated prevalence of 1 per 100,000 live births. Three subtypes exist. The most common (LAD1) involves a mutation in the β_2 integrin receptor that leads to impaired extravasation of neutrophils to sites of infections. Children with LAD present early during the neonatal period with recurrent life-threatening infections such as omphalitis, pneumonia, and spontaneous peritonitis. Cure can be achieved only with a bone marrow transplant.[159]

IMPACT OF NEONATAL CONDITIONS

Epidemiologic studies have frequently shown a strong association of preterm labor with chorioamnionitis. Chronic inflammation modulates the gene expression program of phagocytes[160] and attenuates phagocyte responses, although the extent of this effect in very low-birth-weight infants is debated.[68] In lamb models, an intraamniotic injection of proinflammatory stimuli (e.g., LPS) induced the differentiation of monocytes into macrophages. It also resulted in a hyporesponsive state to subsequent PRR stimulation in monocytes from preterm animals.[161] Although the concept of endotoxin tolerance following sepsis is more established in the adult sepsis literature, the effect of chorioamnionitis on neonates' phagocyte immune functions may be more difficult to establish, in part due to a lack of precise, consistent histologic definitions. Hyperoxia induces inflammatory cytokine responses in tissues and circulating monocytes.[162-164] Consequently, high circulating levels of inflammatory cytokines have been observed in preterm neonates in the absence of overt sepsis, suggesting ongoing immune stimulation.[165]

During sepsis, phagocytes are an important source of pyrogenic cytokines. Endogenous pyrogens (e.g., IL-1, IL-6, and TNF) act on the vasculosum lamina terminalis in the anterior hypothalamus to stimulate production of prostaglandins (e.g., PGE_2) that in turn act on thermoregulatory neurons to reset the body's thermoregulatory setpoint and produce fever.[166] Premature neonates are unable to mount a strong febrile response to infection or tissue injury, likely due to diminished production of pyrogenic cytokines by phagocytes.[167]

Nutrients, particularly vitamin D, vitamin A, minerals such as zinc, and long-chain polyunsaturated fatty acids, play important roles in the regulation of phagocytic responses, stressing the importance of an adequate caloric and dietary intake in newborns, particularly those affected by a serious illness.[168-173] Recent compelling data have also highlighted the importance of breast milk and the early life microbiome in modulating immune responses and phagocytic functions, and these are two important emerging areas in neonatal immunology.[174,175] Effects of nutritional deficits on phagocytic defenses are worthy of further investigation.

IMPACT OF PERINATAL DRUG EXPOSURES

Several drugs used in neonatal medicine have the potential to affect the function of immune cells, including phagocytes, based on neonatal studies in vitro and adult studies in vivo. However, for most of these drugs, scant data regarding effects in human neonates are available.

The use of antenatal corticosteroids (ANSs) in mothers of preterm infants delivered before 34 weeks of gestation is standard practice in perinatal medicine.[176] In sheep models, a short-term intrauterine exposure to ANSs blunted endotoxin-stimulated cytokine responses, and hydrogen peroxidation in monocytes, when measured within 2 days after birth.[177] Phagocytes exposed in vitro to corticosteroid equivalents comparable with levels measured in serum of pregnant women after a single-course ANS treatment demonstrate significant functional alterations. Furthermore, functional immune differences have also been observed in infants exposed to ANSs.[178-187] In contrast, when comparing responses in cord blood from infants who were exposed or were not exposed to ANSs using rigorous, standard immune function tests, no major functional differences were observed.[68,83] These data raise questions about the significance of the effect of ANS observed in animal models, when applied to populations of preterm human neonates. In addition, large randomized clinical trials of a single-course exposure to ANSs have not demonstrated any measurable impact on the ability of the preterm infant to defend against common neonatal pathogens, because these studies have demonstrated a reduction (rather than an increase) in the incidence of neonatal sepsis in neonates born to mothers who received ANSs.[176]

Magnesium sulfate also reversibly inhibits phagocyte cytokine responses at doses currently used in vivo for intrapartum neuroprotection in the context of preterm labor. The mechanism appears to be mediated through reduction in NFκB activation.[188] Its effects on the neonatal immune system have been incompletely studied. Based on small studies and on the mechanisms of inhibition, it appears that these effects may be only transient.[83,188,189]

The macrolide antibiotic azithromycin blocks NF-κB activation in adult monocytes and may suppress proinflammatory responses to microbial stimuli at doses given to human infants.[190,191] Exogenous (but potentially also endogenous) catecholamines, including epinephrine, can inhibit endotoxin-induced proinflammatory cytokine production in adult humans,[192] but we are not aware of similar studies in preterm or term newborns.

Caffeine is routinely given to preterm neonates for prevention of apnea of prematurity and bronchopulmonary dysplasia.[193] Protective effects of caffeine in the neonatal lung may be mediated, at least in part, by reduction of pulmonary inflammation.[194]

Lactoferrin has been shown to mitigate high inflammatory responses produced by human neonatal phagocytes in vitro.[195] Supplementation of preterm infants with exogenous lactoferrin has yielded conflicting results.

CONCLUDING REMARKS

Cells of the MPS share major immune and nonimmune roles during embryogenesis, fetal development, and early postnatal life. Important functional changes occur also during this period, underlying the rapid growth and development of the neonate. The ontogeny of mononuclear phagocytes is currently an intense, exciting research area of research that offers the potential for guiding the discovery of novel cell-based therapies. As our understanding of the heterogeneity and plasticity of the cells of the MPS improves, it becomes clear that this knowledge offers great possibilities for its targeted therapeutic manipulation.

Early life ontogeny of PRR function has important implications in our understanding of neonatal pathogen susceptibilities and vaccine responses at different ages. Historically, phagocytes have been viewed as unable to "learn" from previous encounters with pathogens, contrary to lymphocytes. However, multiple recent studies have changed this conception, and it is increasingly accepted that these cells are also capable of an immunologic memory, termed *trained immunity.* Immune training provides long-term enhancement of innate immune responses to subsequent pathogen encounters[196,197] and may explain why certain vaccines, such as bacille Calmette-Guérin (BCG), comprised of live attenuated *Mycobacterium bovis*, seem to have major heterologous protective effects, apparently decreasing all infectious-cause mortality in low-birth-weight neonates.[198]

Myelopoiesis shares common features across species and mouse models have advanced understanding of the ontogeny of the MPS. However, it is also important to recognize major differences between mice and humans that limit interpretation of data from animal models and mandate more direct studies in human neonates. Cord blood is a relatively noninvasive source of blood cells and has enabled studies of the neonatal immune system. Although it is difficult to completely exclude the possibility that functional differences observed on cord blood may be due to the conditions that resulted in the premature birth of these infants, in general data suggest that these functional differences arise from developmental factors rather than from exogenous factors (e.g., chorioamnionitis or use of corticosteroids). Moreover, recent data suggest that cord blood has distinct features from immune cells during postnatal life[199] and studies examining events that occur beyond cord blood will be important. Similarly, although study of blood cells can provide important insights, it does not capture important events occurring in specialized immune organs such as the gut, spleen, or lymphoid organs.[200] High-throughput molecular assays and bioinformatics analytic approaches that can capture changes at the systems and single-cell levels, including all genes, proteins, and metabolites, using small volumes of biologic material has dramatically improved our capacity to study and understand the developing neonatal immune system.[107]

Future studies will assess how the microbiome, breast milk, and nutritional factors regulate the developing human neonatal immune system, particularly at the mucosal lung and intestinal interfaces. Translational studies will characterize how mechanisms regulating phagocyte maturation can be exploited to improve vaccine responses and reduce the risk of infections. A promising area is discovery and development of vaccine adjuvants that more effectively activate neonatal phagocytes.[201-203] For conditions that involve overexuberant inflammation, a range of agents that limit inflammation or enhance its resolution are under investigation for potential clinical benefit, including antimicrobial proteins and peptides such as bactericidal/permeability-increasing protein and lactoferrin, arachidonic acid derivatives such as proresolving lipid mediators, as well as metabolic agents that reprogram monocyte cytokine production such as pentoxifylline.[204-206] Multiple clinical trials are ongoing to test such agents.[204,207] These translational efforts may be derisked and accelerated via use of age-specific animal studies in vivo and human assay platforms to assess monocyte, macrophage, and DC function in vitro.[208]

A complete reference list is available at www.ExpertConsult.com. 

SELECT REFERENCES

1. Ginhoux F, Schultze JL, Murray PJ, et al. New insights into the multidimensional concept of macrophage ontogeny, activation and function. *Nat Immunol.* 2016;17:34-40.
2. Hume DA. The mononuclear phagocyte system. *Curr Opin Immunol.* 2006;18:49-53.
4. Guilliams M, Ginhoux F, Jakubzick C, et al. Dendritic cells, monocytes and macrophages: a unified nomenclature based on ontogeny. *Nat Rev Immunol.* 2014;14:571-578.
5. Frame JM, McGrath KE, Palis J. Erythro-myeloid progenitors: "definitive" hematopoiesis in the conceptus prior to the emergence of hematopoietic stem cells. *Blood Cells Mol Dis.* 2013;51:220-225.
7. Ginhoux F, Greter M, Leboeuf M, et al. Fate mapping analysis reveals that adult microglia derive from primitive macrophages. *Science.* 2010;330:841-845.
8. Meuret G. The kinetics of mononuclear phagocytes in man. *Haematol Blood Transfus.* 1981;27:11-22.
9. Tavian M, Biasch K, Sinka L, et al. Embryonic origin of human hematopoiesis. *Int J Dev Biol.* 2010;54:1061-1065.
10. Tavian M, Coulombel L, Luton D, et al. Aorta-associated CD34+ hematopoietic cells in the early human embryo. *Blood.* 1996;87:67-72.
11. Golub R, Cumano A. Embryonic hematopoiesis. *Blood Cells Mol Dis.* 2013;51:226-231.
12. Alvarez-Errico D, Vento-Tormo R, Sieweke M, Ballestar E. Epigenetic control of myeloid cell differentiation, identity and function. *Nat Rev Immunol.* 2015;15:7-17.
13. Varol C, Landsman L, Fogg DK, et al. Monocytes give rise to mucosal, but not splenic, conventional dendritic cells. *J Exp Med.* 2007;204:171-180.
14. Lee J, Breton G, Oliveira TY, et al. Restricted dendritic cell and monocyte progenitors in human cord blood and bone marrow. *J Exp Med.* 2015;212:385-399.
16. Auffray C, Sieweke MH, Geissmann F. Blood monocytes: development, heterogeneity, and relationship with dendritic cells. *Annu Rev Immunol.* 2009;27:669-692.
17. Krutzik SR, Tan B, Li H, et al. TLR activation triggers the rapid differentiation of monocytes into macrophages and dendritic cells. *Nat Med.* 2005;11:653-660.
18. Santiago-Schwarz F, Divaris N, Kay C, Carsons SE. Mechanisms of tumor necrosis factor-granulocyte-macrophage colony-stimulating factor-induced dendritic cell development. *Blood.* 1993;82:3019-3028.
19. Liu E, Tu W, Law HK, Lau YL. Decreased yield, phenotypic expression and function of immature monocyte-derived dendritic cells in cord blood. *Br J Haematol.* 2001;113:240-246.
20. Romani N, Gruner S, Brang D, et al. Proliferating dendritic cell progenitors in human blood. *J Exp Med.* 1994;180:83-93.
21. Schibler KR, Liechty KW, White WL, Christensen RD. Production of granulocyte colony-stimulating factor *in vitro* by monocytes from preterm and term neonates. *Blood.* 1993;82:2478-2484.
22. Li Y, Esain V, Teng L, et al. Inflammatory signaling regulates embryonic hematopoietic stem and progenitor cell production. *Genes Dev.* 2014;28:2597-2612.
23. Christensen RD, Jensen J, Maheshwari A, Henry E. Reference ranges for blood concentrations of eosinophils and monocytes during the neonatal period defined from over 63000 records in a multihospital health-care system. *J Perinatol.* 2010;30:540-545.
24. Meuret G. Origin, ontogeny, and kinetics of mononuclear phagocytes. *Adv Exp Med Biol.* 1976;73:71-81. PT-A.
25. Lord BI. Myeloid cell kinetics in response to haemopoietic growth factors. *Baillieres Clin Haematol.* 1992;5:533-550.
26. Meuret G, Bammert J, Hoffmann G. Kinetics of human monocytopoiesis. *Blood.* 1974;44:801-816.
27. Avraham-Davidi I, Yona S, Grunewald M, et al. On-site education of VEGF-recruited monocytes improves their performance as angiogenic and arteriogenic accessory cells. *J Exp Med.* 2013;210:2611-2625.

28. Jakubzick C, Gautier EL, Gibbings SL, et al. Minimal differentiation of classical monocytes as they survey steady-state tissues and transport antigen to lymph nodes. *Immunity*. 2013;39:599-610.
29. Ziegler-Heitbrock L, Ancuta P, Crowe S, et al. Nomenclature of monocytes and dendritic cells in blood. *Blood*. 2011;116:e74-e80.
30. Passlick B, Flieger D, Ziegler-Heitbrock HW. Identification and characterization of a novel monocyte subpopulation in human peripheral blood. *Blood*. 1989;74:2527-2534.
32. Krow-Lucal ER, Kim CC, Burt TD, McCune JM. Distinct functional programming of human fetal and adult monocytes. *Blood*. 2014;123:1897-1904.
33. Sharma AA, Jen R, Kan B, et al. Impaired NLRP3 inflammasome activity during fetal development regulates IL-1β production in human monocytes. *Eur J Immunol*. 2015;45:238-249.
34. Frankenberger M, Sternsdorf T, Pechumer H, et al. Differential cytokine expression in human blood monocyte subpopulations: a polymerase chain reaction analysis. *Blood*. 1996;87:373-377.
36. Cros J, Cagnard N, Woollard K, et al. Human CD14^{dim} monocytes patrol and sense nucleic acids and viruses via TLR7 and TLR8 receptors. *Immunity*. 2010;33:375-386.
37. Ziegler-Heitbrock HW, Ströbel M, Kieper D, et al. Differential expression of cytokines in human blood monocyte subpopulations. *Blood*. 1992;79:503-511.
38. Fingerle G, Pforte A, Passlick B, et al. The novel subset of CD14+/CD16+ blood monocytes is expanded in sepsis patients. *Blood*. 1993;82:3170-3176.
39. Zawada AM, Rogacev KS, Rotter B, et al. SuperSAGE evidence for CD14++CD16+ monocytes as a third monocyte subset. *Blood*. 2011;118:e50-e61.
40. Ziegler-Heitbrock L. Blood monocytes and their subsets: established features and open questions. *Front Immunol*. 2015;6:423.
41. Ziegler-Heitbrock L. The CD14+ CD16+ blood monocytes: their role in infection and inflammation. *J Leukoc Biol*. 2007;81:584-592.
42. Klimchenko O, Di Stefano A, Geoerger B, et al. Monocytic cells derived from human embryonic stem cells and fetal liver share common differentiation pathways and homeostatic functions. *Blood*. 2011;117:3065-3075.
43. De Palma M, Venneri MA, Galli R, et al. Tie2 identifies a hematopoietic lineage of proangiogenic monocytes required for tumor vessel formation and a mesenchymal population of pericyte progenitors. *Cancer Cell*. 2005;8:211-226.
44. van Furth R. The mononuclear phagocyte system. *Verh Dtsch Ges Pathol*. 1980;64:1-11.
46. Katsumoto A, Lu H, Miranda AS, Ransohoff RM. Ontogeny and functions of central nervous system macrophages. *J Immunol*. 2014;193:2615-2621.
47. Kan B, Razzaghian HR, Lavoie PM. An immunological perspective on neonatal sepsis. *Trends Mol Med*. 2016;22(4):290-302.
48. Chorro L, Geissmann F. Development and homeostasis of 'resident' myeloid cells: the case of the Langerhans cell. *Trends Immunol*. 2010;31:438-445.
50. Guilliams M, De Kleer I, Henri S, et al. Alveolar macrophages develop from fetal monocytes that differentiate into long-lived cells in the first week of life via GM-CSF. *J Exp Med*. 2013;210:1977-1992.
52. Kierdorf K, Erny D, Goldmann T, et al. Microglia emerge from erythromyeloid precursors via Pu.1- and Irf8-dependent pathways. *Nat Neurosci*. 2013;16:273-280.
53. Hamilton TA, Zhao C, Pavicic Jr PG, Datta S. Myeloid colony-stimulating factors as regulators of macrophage polarization. *Front Immunol*. 2014;5:554.
55. Dudziak D, Kamphorst AO, Heidkamp GF, et al. Differential antigen processing by dendritic cell subsets *in vivo*. *Science*. 2007;315:107-111.
56. Lavoie PM, Huang Q, Jolette E, et al. Profound lack of interleukin (IL)-12/IL-23p40 in neonates born early in gestation is associated with an increased risk of sepsis. *J Infect Dis*. 2010;202:1754-1763.
57. Schibler KR, Georgelas A, Rigaa A. Developmental biology of the dendritic cell system. *Acta Paediatr Suppl*. 2002;91:9-16.
66. Serbina NV, Jia T, Hohl TM, Pamer EG. Monocyte-mediated defense against microbial pathogens. *Annu Rev Immunol*. 2008;26:421-452.
209. Houser BL. Decidual macrophages and their roles at the maternal-fetal interface. *Yale J Biol Med*. 2012;85:105-118.

Normal and Abnormal Neutrophil Physiology in the Newborn

119

Joyce M. Koenig | Joseph M. Bliss | Markus Sperandio

INTRODUCTION

The response of the immune-competent host to invasive pathogens includes a variety of local and systemic mechanisms. Among these are humoral elements, such as complement or immunoglobulins (Igs), as well as cellular defenses that involve both innate (nonspecific but immediate) and adaptive (antigen-specific, programmed) immune responses. Neutrophils, or polymorphonuclear cells, comprise a critical arm of the innate immune system (reviewed by Nauseef and colleagues[1] and Nemeth and colleagues[2]) and are the most abundant cell type in the circulating pool of immune cells. Inadequate numbers of circulating neutrophils can compromise host defense, which increases the risk of infection-associated morbidity and mortality. However, in addition to adequate circulating numbers, proper functioning of neutrophils is required to mount an effective antimicrobial defense. Individuals with dysfunctional neutrophils are at risk for severe local and systemic bacterial and fungal infections despite having normal numbers of circulating neutrophils or even neutrophilia in some patients.[3,4]

During ontogeny, the fetus develops in a protected environment. Accordingly, aggressive innate immune defense mechanisms are unnecessary and would be maladaptive for proper fetal growth and development. Conversely, neonates and particularly preterm neonates are at considerable risk for bacterial and fungal infections after birth, necessitating a transitional period that promotes the adaptation of immune function to life outside the protective uterus.[5,6] This chapter discusses the role of neutrophils in host defense and inflammation during fetal life and in the neonate, with a specific emphasis on the functions modulated by host immaturity.

NEUTROPHIL HOMEOSTASIS

Neutrophils, the major class of leukocytes in the blood, are the host's "first responders" against invading pathogens. Neonates with abnormally low neutrophil numbers *(neutropenia)* are at increased risk for infection, and a failure to rapidly replenish neutrophils during sepsis contributes to mortality.[7] Neutrophil homeostasis is a finely tuned process that orchestrates the balance between neutrophils lost by attrition (apoptosis, programmed cell death) and the production of adequate numbers of new cells to protect the health of the host.[8]

After birth, the bone marrow is the primary site of neutrophil production and storage. (See Chapter 108 for a detailed discussion of this process.) Under stable, noninfected conditions, neutrophil progenitors and their developing progeny are retained in bone marrow niches, in part through interactions between the chemokine receptor CXCR4 and its ligand CXCL12 (Fig. 119.1).[9] Under homeostatic conditions, neutrophils undergo a

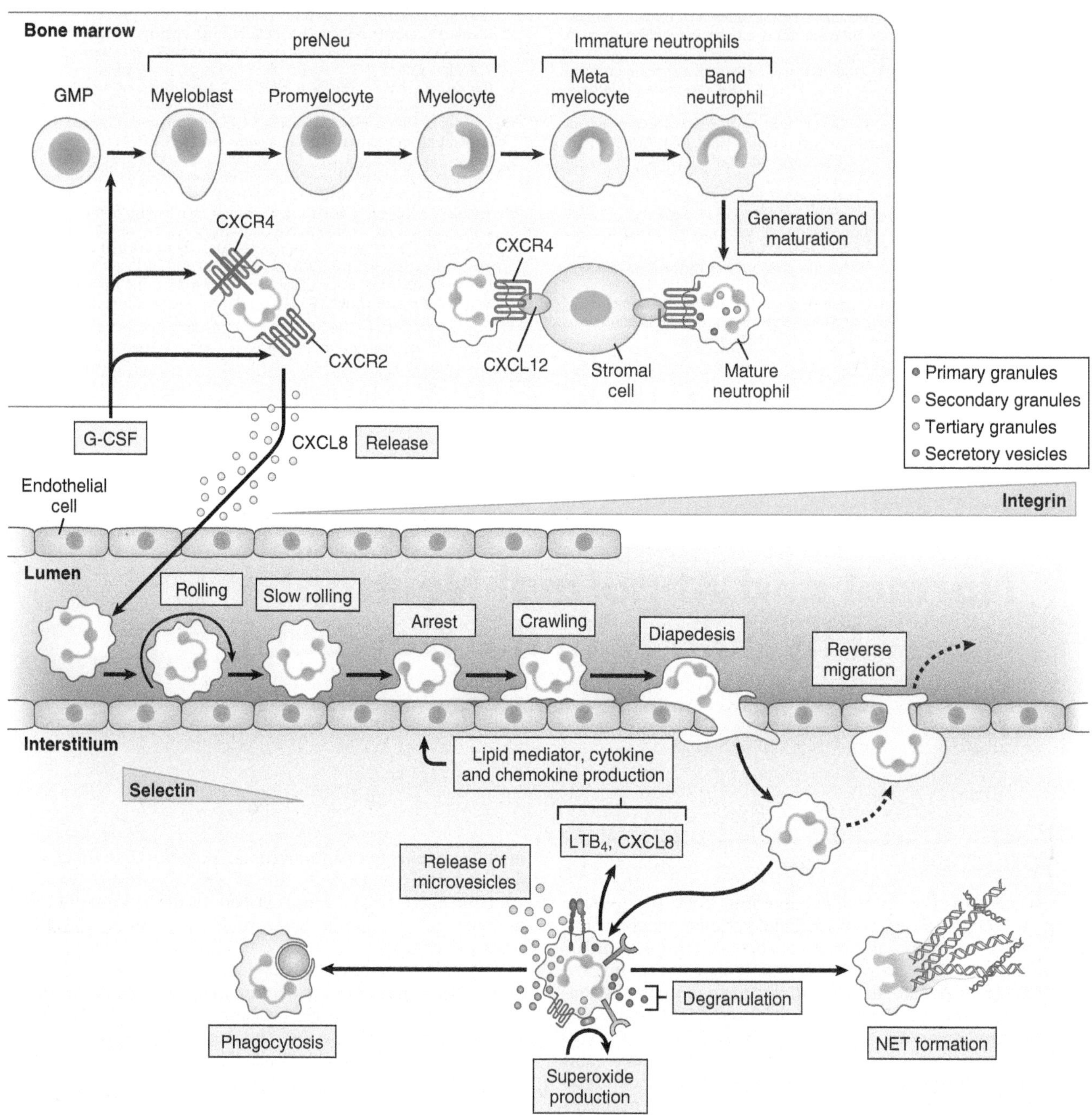

Fig. 119.1 Neutrophil development and function. Neutrophils are generated in the bone marrow, where they mature before their release into the blood circulation. This process is critically dependent on granulocyte colony-stimulating factor *(G-CSF)*. Under homeostatic conditions neutrophils circulate in the bloodstream in a quiescent state. During an inflammatory response, neutrophils are activated on the inflamed endothelium and extravasate to the site of tissue injury. Extravasation follows a multistep recruitment process, which includes tethering, rolling, firm adhesion, crawling, and transendothelial migration into tissue. At the site of inflammation, neutrophils exert various effector functions through degranulation, resulting in the release of pro-inflammatory mediators, antimicrobial molecules, vesicles, and reactive oxygen species. In addition, neutrophils are able to phagocytose invaded pathogens and form neutrophil extracellular traps *(NETs)*. *CXCL*, CXC-chemokine ligand; *CXCR*, CXC-chemokine receptor; *GMP*, granulo-monocytic progenitor; *LTB4*, leukotriene B4. (Adapted with permission from Nemeth T, Sperandio M, Mocsai A. Neutrophils as emerging therapeutic targets. *Nat Rev Drug Discov.* 2020;19[4]:253–275.)

differentiation pathway in the bone marrow. Along this pathway, several neutrophil subsets with distinct molecular signatures and proliferation rates have been defined, which eventually lead to the formation of mature neutrophils that gradually egress from the bone marrow into the circulation to maintain enough circulating neutrophils for immune surveillance.[10] The migration of aging neutrophils back to the bone marrow appears to be a critical factor in neutrophil homeostasis.[9,11] Recent evidence also suggests an important regulatory role of the intestinal microbiome and homeostatic neutrophil trafficking into peripheral tissues in this process.[12]

In contrast, under conditions of stress, pro-inflammatory signaling releases cytokines and chemokines into the bloodstream. This process is driven in part by T-cell-mediated release of interleukin (IL)-17, which increases circulating levels of granulocyte-colony stimulating factor (G-CSF).[13] G-CSF is a cytokine important to neutrophil production as well as their mobilization from the bone marrow into the vasculature, in part through inhibitory actions on CXCL12 (C-X-C motif chemokine 12, or stromal cell-derived factor-1, SDF-1).[14] Under normal circumstances, resolution of inflammatory processes involves macrophage-mediated phagocytosis *(efferocytosis)* and clearance of apoptotic tissue neutrophils.[15] Efferocytosis of senescent neutrophils promotes antiinflammatory mechanisms in macrophages, including a decrease in IL-23 release, which leads to a reduction in IL-17 secretion and hence G-CSF release.[16]

NEUTROPHIL ACTIVATION MECHANISMS

OVERVIEW

Under homeostatic conditions, mature neutrophils released by the bone marrow traverse the circulatory system in an inactivated, quiescent form. Alterations in the environment, such as those induced by microbial invasion of tissues, exposure to circulating microbial products, or tissue damage *(sterile inflammation)*, can initiate the activation of neutrophils and their recruitment to the site of injury.[17,18] As a result, neutrophils migrate through the vascular wall into inflamed tissues and enter a state of readiness to initiate their immune functions. However, neutrophil-mediated inflammation is a double-edged sword: dysregulation of the activating mechanisms so critical to host protection can incidentally lead to exaggerated or persistent inflammatory responses that contribute to tissue injury and chronic diseases.[2]

A variety of inflammatory mediators, alone or in combination, can engage surface receptors on neutrophils and induce their activation, either directly or through priming (Fig. 119.2). These include bacterial products such as lipopolysaccharide (LPS, an endotoxin) and the bacterial peptide *formyl*-methionyl-leucyl-phenylalanine (*f*MLP), complement factors (C5a), inflammatory cytokines, leukotriene B_4, and platelet-activating factor (PAF).[2] Here, we will provide a short overview on how these factors interact with receptor systems on the neutrophil surface. In addition, we will also describe signal transduction processes

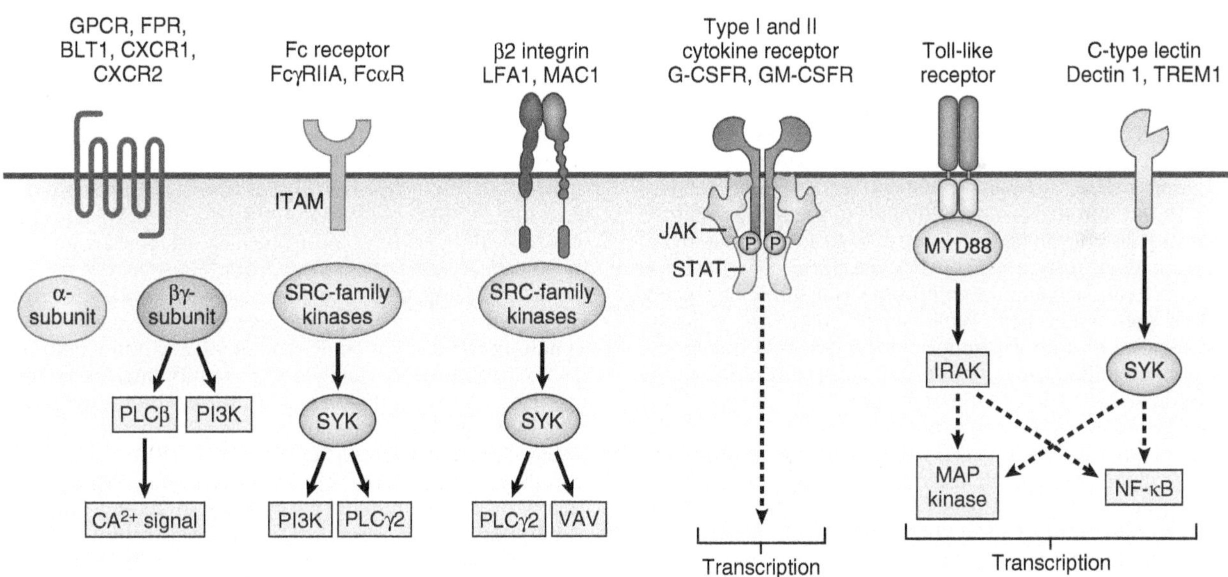

Fig. 119.2 Neutrophil cell surface receptors. Neutrophils express a variety of cell surface receptors that activate various intracellular signaling pathways. These pathways trigger the execution of specific effector functions. G protein-coupled receptors *(GPCRs)* signal through phospholipase Cβ *(PLCβ)* and an increase in intracellular calcium levels. The immunoreceptor tyrosine-based activation motif *(ITAM)* tyrosines of Fcγ and Fcα receptors (FcγRIIA and FcαR) are phosphorylated by Src family kinases. This leads to the recruitment of the nonreceptor tyrosine kinase SYK and downstream PLCγ2/caspase recruitment domain-protein 9 *(CARD9)* activation triggering activation of NF-κB-dependent gene expression. Fcγ receptors and β_2 integrins use similar signal transduction pathways. Type I and type II cytokine receptors activate Janus kinases *(JAKs)* leading to the nuclear translocation of signal transducer and activator of transcription *(STAT)* molecules and respective transcription. Toll-like receptors and C-type lectins use MyD88 and IL-1 receptor-associated kinases *(IRAKs)* or SYK in their pathways, leading to mitogen-activated protein *(MAP)* kinase/NF-κB activation. *BLT1*, leukotriene B4 receptor 1; *CXCR*, CXC-chemokine receptor; *FPR,* formyl peptide receptor; *G-CSFR*, granulocyte colony-stimulating factor receptor; *GM- CSFR*, granulocyte–macrophage colony-stimulating factor receptor; *LFA1*, lymphocyte function-associated antigen 1; *PI3K*, phosphoinositide 3-kinase; *PKC*, protein kinase C. (Adapted with permission from Nemeth T, Sperandio M, Mocsai A. Neutrophils as emerging therapeutic targets. *Nat Rev Drug Discov.* 2020;19[4]:253–275.)

through activation of these receptor systems, which are instrumental for mounting an effective immune response. Finally, we will discuss how these receptor systems work in the fetus and neonate, although much remains unknown in this regard.

G PROTEIN-COUPLED RECEPTORS

Contact of neutrophils with bacterial peptides and various inflammatory molecules such as leukotriene LTB4, *f*MLP, complement fragment C5a, and chemokines including CXCL8 (IL-8) or CCL2 induce the engagement of inhibitory G ($G_{\alpha i}$)-protein-coupled receptors (GPCRs).[19] According to the stimulus, the following $G_{\alpha i}$-protein-coupled receptors are involved (respective ligands are in parenthesis): leukotriene receptor BLT1 (LTB4), *formyl* peptide receptors FPR1 and 2 (*f*MLP), complement receptor C5aR (C5a), and chemokine receptors CXCR1 and 2 (CXCL8). Upon ligand binding, $G_{\alpha i}$-protein-coupled receptors trigger intracellular signaling processes leading to respective effector responses by the activated neutrophil. Signaling through $G_{\alpha i}$-coupled receptors follows characteristic cell signaling pathways including activation of neutrophil-specific *Src* tyrosine kinase family members Hck, Fgr, and Lyn, nonreceptor tyrosine kinase Syk, phospholipase Cβ (triggering an increase in intracellular Ca^{2+}), and phosphatidylinositol 3-kinases (PI3K) (see Fig. 119.2). Depending on the stimulus, engagement of respective $G_{\alpha i}$-coupled receptors can induce all aspects of neutrophil effector functions including integrin activation and adhesion, chemotaxis, phagocytosis, granule release, and the production of reactive oxygen species (ROS).

TYPE I AND TYPE II CYTOKINE RECEPTORS

Several type I and type II cytokine receptors expressed on the neutrophil surface (see Fig. 119.2) bind to a diverse group of cytokines. Type I cytokine receptors on neutrophils include granulocyte colony-stimulating factor receptor (G-CSFR), which binds to G-CSF, and granulocyte-macrophage colony-stimulating factor receptor (GM-CSFR), which binds to GM-CSF. These receptors (particularly G-CSFR) are primary mediators of neutrophil production, differentiation, and function.[20] Type II cytokine receptors on neutrophils include those for type I interferons, IFN-α and IFN-β, which bind to (IFN)-α/β receptor; the type II interferon, IFN-γ, which binds to the IFN-γ receptor; and the type III interferon, IFN- λ, which binds to the IFN- λ receptor. Type I and II interferon signaling are critical for acute antiviral and inflammatory responses. The balance between type I and type II interferon signaling in neutrophils is a subject of recent interest in the cancer field. While type I interferon signaling shifts the balance to an antitumor *(neutrophil N1)* phenotype with increased killing capacity of tumor cells, activation of type II interferon signaling favors tumor supporting *(neutrophil N2)* functions including production of proangiogenic factors (vascular endothelial growth factor [VEGF], matrix metalloproteinase-9 [MMP9]).[21] Recently, type III interferon signaling through the IFN- λ receptor in neutrophils has been reported to be crucial during infection with *Aspergillus fumigatus*.[22] Interestingly, engagement of both type I and type II cytokine receptors primarily activate signaling through members of the JAK and STAT family, although other signaling pathways involving MAPK or PI3K can also be involved (see Fig. 119.2).

PATTERN RECOGNITION RECEPTORS IN NEUTROPHILS

Functioning as an integral part of the innate immune system, *pattern-recognition receptors* (PRRs) on neutrophils interact with ligands expressed by microbial pathogens or generated as endogenous danger signals. All these ligands carry common structural motifs termed *pathogen-associated molecular patterns* (PAMPs) for microbial-derived factors (e.g., LPS, bacterial DNA, or double-stranded viral RNA) and *damage-associated molecular patterns* (DAMPs) for endogenous danger signals (e.g., HMGB1, S100A8/A9).[23,24] Among PRRs, *Toll-like receptors* (TLRs) play a predominant role in neutrophils (see Fig. 119.2). Nearly all TLRs (with the exception of TLR3 and possibly TLR7) are expressed at basal levels in neutrophils and interact with microbial DNA and RNA, as well as lipids, carbohydrates, and proteins. Engagement of TLRs primes neutrophils for enhanced activation in response to secondary stimuli.[25] In addition, recent work demonstrated that TLR2 and TLR4 stimulation can also induce rapid induction of neutrophil effector functions through MyD88-dependent processes, which do not require transcriptional activity.[26,27] Specific TLRs are responsible for recognizing different sources of PAMPs or DAMPs. In general, engagement of TLRs activates downstream signaling pathways, particularly those involving NFκB (nuclear factor *kappa* B), p38 MAPK, and JNK, all of which respond to cellular stress. Besides TLRs, several other groups of pattern recognition receptors on neutrophils have been described. These include retinoic acid inducible gene I-like receptors (RLRs), nucleotide-binding oligomerization domain-like receptors (NLRs), AIM2-like receptors, and DNA sensors such as the recently described transcription factor Sox2.[28] In addition, some members of the *C-type lectin receptor family* including Dectin-1 and TREM-1 (Triggering Receptor Expressed on Myeloid cells 1) also belong to the PRR family. Through its binding to β-glucans, commonly found in various fungi, Dectin-1 is involved in antifungal defense mechanisms and signals via an immunoreceptor tyrosine-based activation motif (ITAM) in its cytoplasmic tail.[29] The other C-type lectin, TREM-1, synergizes with additional activating receptors on neutrophils during inflammatory responses and has recently been reported to influence neutrophil chemotaxis, ROS production, and transepithelial migration.[30]

NEUTROPHIL FC RECEPTORS

Neutrophils express several receptors that recognize the constant region (Fc) of IgG or IgA (see Fig. 119.2). This enables neutrophils to bind IgG- and IgA-opsonized particles and pathogens reacting against it, resulting in various proinflammatory responses including phagocytosis and degranulation. The following Fc receptors are expressed in neutrophils (see Fig. 119.2): FcαRI (CD89), which binds to IgA; and FcγRIA (CD64A), FcγRIIA (CD32A), and FcγRIIIB (CD16B), all of which bind to IgG. FcαRI, FcγRIA, and FcγRIIA are *classical activation* receptors. These carry an ITAM at the cytoplasmic tail, as in the case of FcγRIIA, or they are associated with the ITAM-bearing signaling unit Fc receptor γ chain in the case of FcαRI and FcγRIA. Upon ligand binding, ITAMs are phosphorylated by Src family kinases, triggering a signaling cascade involving the nonreceptor tyrosine kinase Syk, PI3K, and phospholipase Cγ (PLCγ) (see Fig. 119.2). Similar to stimulation of FcγRIA and FcγRIIA by IgG,[31] FcαRI stimulation of neutrophils by multimeric IgA triggers a variety of proinflammatory functions including phagocytosis, degranulation, ROS production, and neutrophil extracellular trap (NET) formation.[32] Multimeric IgA also induces the release of leukotriene LTB4, which attracts additional neutrophils.[33] In contrast, the binding of FcαRI to monomeric serum IgA exerts antiinflammatory responses.[34]

NEUTROPHIL ACTIVATION MECHANISMS IN NEONATES

In contrast to the extensive body of work defining activation mechanisms in adult neutrophils, the influence of developmental stage on neutrophil activation processes and associated pathology in neonates is less understood. Neonatal neutrophils, even in preterm infants, have the capacity for activation under conditions of stress, such as respiratory distress or sepsis.[35,36] However, neonatal inflammatory responses may be excessive relative to those of adults. Neonatal animals exhibit exaggerated inflammatory reactions in response to injury, such as intestinal ischemia-reperfusion,[37,38] which are findings that recapitulate the exaggerated inflammatory responses observed in human neonates.[39]

In vitro studies also suggest that neonatal neutrophils may be intrinsically "primed for action" even under basal conditions. Neonatal neutrophils exhibit constitutive activation of the transcription factor NF-κB, which is associated with increased generation of proinflammatory mediators such as IL-8 or expression of anti-apoptotic proteins such as FLICE.[40,41] Pertinently, NF-κB activation is a critical component of inflammatory injury in neonates.[42,43] Neutrophil activation of NF-κB in neonates is also linked to basal activity of signaling mechanisms that promote cell survival, such as Akt, a gatekeeper for DNA damage response/repair.[41]

While the aforementioned studies indicate that neonatal neutrophils are hyperreactive and constitutively activated, others suggest a relative resistance of neonatal neutrophils to certain activation pathways, such as those involving TLR4 or the Src kinase, Lyn.[44,45] These findings are supported by in vivo studies investigating neutrophil recruitment in the mouse fetus, which showed a strong fetal age-dependent inability of neutrophils to extravasate into inflamed tissue.[46] Similar results were found in an in vitro flow chamber study where an ontogenetically regulated reduction in rolling and adhesion of cord blood neutrophils was observed.[47] How can we explain these presumably conflicting reports on hyper- and hypoactive neutrophils? Potential reasons for the observed differences in studies of ex vivo neutrophils might be related to mode of delivery (cesarean section vs. vaginal delivery), blood source (placental cord blood vs. postnatal peripheral blood sampling), and processing techniques (isolation and treatments). In a recent exciting study by the Viemann group, it became evident that the innate immune system, including its pattern recognition receptors, are well prepared for the transition from intrauterine life to the challenges of postnatal life.[48] This transition brings about rapid changes in innate immune cell function and programming. Future work in this area is urgently warranted to more completely define neonatal neutrophil inflammatory responses and to distinguish these from inflammatory responses by fetal neutrophils. Clarifying these issues will certainly also help in identifying new potential age-adjusted therapeutic strategies for premature and mature infants suffering from severe infections or from other inflammatory conditions.

NEUTROPHIL RECRUITMENT

OVERVIEW: THE NEUTROPHIL RECRUITMENT CASCADE

Neutrophil recruitment is an important immunologic process that enables neutrophils to leave the circulating pool of blood-resident cells and extravasate into inflamed tissue in order to fulfill their task of host defense. Neutrophil recruitment follows a well-defined cascade of adhesion and activation events (see Fig. 119.1), consisting of initial neutrophil capture *(tethering)* and rolling along the inflamed endothelium, followed by firm arrest. Subsequently, neutrophils strengthen their adhesive bonds and spread over the underlying endothelial surface (to better withstand shear forces exerted by the flowing blood) before they start "crawling" along the endothelial lining to find an appropriate spot for *transmigration* into inflamed tissues.[49,50] Neutrophil transmigration, that is passage through the endothelial lining, occurs mostly in a paracellular fashion and is followed by penetration of the underlying vascular basement membrane before the neutrophil reaches the inflamed tissue.[51,52]

Neutrophil recruitment is primarily mediated by groups of adhesion molecules that include the selectins and selectin ligands, integrins, and the Ig gene superfamily. Each serves a specific purpose related to the recruitment process.

SELECTINS AND SELECTIN LIGANDS

The selectin (CD62) family constitutes a group of *C-type lectins* that bind to specific carbohydrate moieties on selectin ligands in a calcium-dependent manner.[53,54] Members of this family include leukocyte-expressed *L-selectin* (CD62L); *E-selectin* (CD62E), expressed on inflamed endothelial cells; and *P-selectin* (CD62P), found on activated endothelial cells and activated platelets. Selectin ligand activity depends on critical posttranslational glycosylation steps during selectin ligand synthesis including α2,3 sialylation and α1,3 fucosylation leading to the generation of the tetrasaccharide sialyl Lewis^X (sLe^X) found at the terminus of core2-decorated O-glycans.[54,55]

The most prominent selectin ligand, the sialomucin *P-selectin glycoprotein ligand-1* (PSGL-1), is expressed on the neutrophil surface and binds to all three selectins.[56] Besides PSGL-1, L-selectin can function as a selectin ligand by interacting with E-selectin. Notably, this interaction has been observed in the human system but not in the mouse.[57,58] Initially considered as part of a braking system to slow down circulating neutrophils when interacting with the inflamed endothelium, more recent work has identified important signaling functions of selectin/selectin ligand interactions. Signaling through PSGL-1 relies on the adapter molecules DAP12 and FcRγ and induces the activation of β_2 integrins.[59] Interestingly, the engagement of PSGL-1 (or L-selectin) by E-selectin mediates the release of the DAMP molecule S100A8/A9 from neutrophils. Released S100A8/A9 in turn binds to TLR 4 in an autocrine fashion and stimulates β_2 integrin activation, suggesting that an additional extracellular activation loop is necessary for β_2 integrin activation during the recruitment process.[27,58]

INTEGRINS

Neutrophil-expressed *integrins* including the β2 integrins LFA-1 (αLβ2) and Mac-1 (αMβ2) are crucial players in neutrophil recruitment and involved in all steps of the recruitment cascade (see Figs. 119.1 and 119.2). Integrins not only provide an adhesive platform critical for firm neutrophil arrest on the endothelium in a microenvironment, where pulling forces are exerted constantly on the attached neutrophil,[60] but neutrophil integrins also exhibit critical signaling functions during the recruitment process.

In general, β2 integrins on circulating neutrophils are kept in a bent, inactive conformation, which strongly impairs interactions of integrins with their ligands in *trans*, although ligand binding, as recently reported, is possible in *cis,* leading to inhibition of leukocyte adhesion.[61] During the recruitment process neutrophils make intimate contact with endothelial cells, providing neutrophils the opportunity to interact with adhesion and activation molecules bound to the endothelial surface (see Fig. 119.1). There are a number of surface receptors on neutrophils, which upon ligation with their specific ligands (mostly found on the luminal surface of endothelial cells) mediate activation of β2 integrins, a process called *inside out signaling*.[62] Surface receptors inducing β2 integrin activation with relevance during the recruitment phase include GPCR such as chemokine receptors, *formyl* peptide receptors, receptors for LTB4, PAF, and C5a.[2] In addition, and as mentioned above, selectin ligands such as PSGL-1 have been shown to activate β2 integrins in neutrophils[27,63] Recently, several inhibitors of integrin activation have been reported, including developmental endothelial locus-1 (Del-1), fibroblast growth factor 23 (FGF23), and growth-differentiation factor-15 (GDF-15), which add to the complexity of how neutrophil recruitment is regulated.[64-66]

In contrast to inside-out signaling, *outside-in signaling* refers to signaling events following the engagement of integrins with their ligands and associated integrin clustering. As outside-in signaling during the recruitment process often occurs at the same time as inside-out signaling events, and because it uses at least in part the same kinases and adaptor molecules (including

Src kinases, Syk, Talin, and Kindlin3), these two processes are often difficult to differentiate.[50] In the context of neutrophil recruitment, adhesion strengthening, spreading, and crawling are typical events related to outside-in signaling. These processes require extensive rearrangement of the actin cytoskeleton and are regulated by a complex network of signaling events aiming to prepare the attached neutrophil for its migratory journey into tissue.[62,67] Besides β2 integrins, recent work has elucidated that the β1 integrins VLA3 and VLA6, which are laminin-binding integrins, are involved in the penetration of neutrophils through the vascular basement membrane. For this step, neutrophil VLA3 and VLA6 are mobilized from intracellular storage granules to the cell surface, where they become available for binding to laminins, key components of the vascular basement membrane.[68,69]

IMMUNOGLOBULIN GENE SUPERFAMILY

Similar to integrins, members of the *Ig gene superfamily* are involved in all steps along the recruitment cascade.[55] Endothelial members include ICAM-1 (CD54), ICAM-2 (CD102), VCAM-1 (CD106), PECAM-1 (CD31), MAdCAM-1, and junctional adhesion molecule (JAM) family members. Endothelial ICAM-1 binds to LFA-1 and Mac-1 on neutrophils and firmly anchors neutrophils to the inflamed endothelium. ICAM-1 is upregulated on the endothelium following stimulation by inflammatory cytokines, including tumor necrosis factor-α (TNF-α), IL-1, and IFN-γ. Interestingly, engagement of endothelial ICAM-1 by β2 integrins also leads to signaling events inducing the phosphorylation of VE-cadherin, an important molecule at endothelial junctions. PECAM-1, present on neutrophils and other hematopoietic cells as well as on platelets and the endothelium, is critical for neutrophil extravasation.[56] Structurally, PECAM-1 is a member of the *Ig immunoreceptor tyrosine-based inhibitory motif* (Ig-ITIM) family. Phosphorylation of its ITIM domain can promote cell proliferation and activation as well as inhibit signaling events related to adhesion and migration. JAM-A, -B, and -C contribute to cell-cell contact integrity; their expression at tight junctions of endothelial and epithelial cells influences barrier permeability during inflammation.[57] JAM molecules are involved in neutrophil transendothelial migration. In addition, cleavage of JAM-C by neutrophil elastase has been demonstrated to be critical in triggering *reverse neutrophil transmigration*, a process describing the return of extravasated neutrophils into the blood circulation.[70] Although the function of reverse neutrophil transmigration is not completely clear, it may potentially expand inflammatory activity to other tissues.

ONTOGENETIC REGULATION OF NEUTROPHIL RECRUITMENT

GENERAL CONSIDERATIONS

Comparative studies between neutrophils of adults and those of fetuses and neonates have shown developmental impairments of neutrophil recruitment that can adversely affect their capacity to protect the host against invasive pathogens. These impairments affect all steps along the inflammatory cascade.[71] Studies in fetal and neonatal animal models as well as in human neonates have shown that diminished neutrophil capacity for rolling and firm adherence under flow conditions is directly related to gestational age.[46,47]

Specific Impairments of Neutrophil Adhesion Molecules in Neonates

Studies in fetal and neonatal animal models have shown that neutrophil capacity for rolling and firm adherence under flow conditions is influenced by ontogenetic alterations.[46,72] Ex vivo studies of human preterm and term neonates have confirmed these findings.[47] Neutrophil adherence defects are related to low intrinsic levels or functional capacities of neutrophil and/or endothelial adhesion molecules, as described below. These impairments appear to be developmentally programmed because the "recruitability" of neutrophils isolated from the placental cord blood of preterm infants matched those of their postconception age-matched already born counterparts.[47,73]

Selectin Impairments in Neonates. Selectin-dependent rolling of neutrophils has been studied in flow chamber assays using neutrophils isolated from human preterm and term neonates. To test L-selectin dependent rolling, flow chambers were coated with human umbilical vein endothelial cells stimulated with IL-1. Treatment with neutralizing antibody to L-selectin inhibited the tethering and rolling of adult neutrophils to the activated endothelium while this treatment had a minimal effect on neonatal neutrophils, consistent with diminished L-selectin function.[73] Additional in vitro studies revealed that neutrophils from mature neonates showed reduced levels of L-selectin while fetal neutrophils express surface levels of L-selectin similar to those of adults.[74,75] P- and E-selectin-dependent neutrophil rolling has been investigated in flow chambers coated with P- or E-selectin. For both selectins, neutrophil rolling was diminished in preterm infants but increased with advancing gestational age.[47] This can be explained, at least in part, by developmentally regulated PSGL-1 expression on neutrophils and E-selectin expression on the endothelium.[47,76] As mentioned above, selectin/selectin-ligand interactions together with chemokine-dependent activation mediate the transition of neutrophils from rolling to β_2 integrin-mediated arrest/firm adhesion on endothelial cells. Using flow chambers and cord blood neutrophils from premature and mature infants, a strong reduction in the induction of firm neutrophil arrest and adhesion under flow was observed in flow chambers coated with E-selectin, ICAM-1, and CXCL1, suggesting that the induction of adhesion is impaired in neutrophils from term and preterm infants.[47]

β2 Integrin Impairments in Neonates. Stimulated cord blood neutrophils exhibit variable defects in integrin-dependent adhesion, chemotaxis, and transmigration compared to adult neutrophils.[27,47,77-81] This can be explained in part by diminished surface and total Mac-1 expression in neutrophils of term and preterm infants. In contrast, expression of LFA-1, the other prominent β_2 integrin on neutrophils, does not change significantly during fetal ontogeny.[47]

Neonatal neutrophils are also impaired in their capacity to localize to inflammatory sites.[46,82] In immature animals, neutrophil accumulation is delayed in response to experimentally inflamed peritoneum or following lung injury. Decreased functional expression of Mac-1 appears to contribute to deficits in neonatal recruitment and accumulation, while other functions such as phagocytosis remain intact.

Specific Impairments of Endothelial Adhesion in Neonates

The influence of ontogeny on endothelial adhesion molecule expression and function remains incompletely understood. Much of our current understanding has been based on extensive studies utilizing in vitro models of cultured human endothelial cells from umbilical veins (HUVECs) or foreskin, or in vivo animal models. LPS-stimulated HUVEC showed reduced upregulation of E-selectin and ICAM-1 surface expression, indicating that the endothelial compartment also contributes to impaired neutrophil recruitment during ontogeny.[47] Neonatal neutrophils exhibit impaired transendothelial migration as a result of abnormal CD11b-ICAM-1 interactions,[82,83] findings confirmed by intravital microscopy of fMLP-stimulated yolk sac vessels in the mouse.[46] Deficient P- and E-selectin expression in fetal and neonatal animals has also been linked to impaired leukocyte accumulation and localization.[46] Similarly, human preterm neonates exhibit decreased endothelial P-selectin surface expression.[84]

Specific Impairments in Transendothelial Migration and Chemotaxis in Neonates

Previous studies in neonatal humans and in animal models indicate an age-dependent response of neutrophil localization to inflammatory stimuli.[85,86] Compared to adults, neonates exhibit decreased neutrophil accumulation in various organs, such as the lungs, in response to inflammatory stimuli.

Neonatal leukocyte functional impairments are related to both structural differences as well as to alterations in adhesive capacity. Preterm and term neutrophils exhibit inadequate migration responses to chemoattractants in a gestational age-dependent manner.[6,77] Neonatal neutrophils exhibit decreased random *(chemokinesis)* and directed *(chemotaxis)* migration.[87] In the first weeks of life, neutrophil chemotactic function is only 50% of that observed in adult neutrophils. This impairment is related to adhesive or activation defects, as suggested by lower intracellular free calcium levels and decreased generation of filamentous (F)-actin.[88,89] Extrinsic factors such as sepsis, antenatal steroids, maternal magnesium therapy, and delivery by cesarean section may further reduce chemotaxis.[89-92] While these functional impediments increase the neonatal risk for infection, particularly in preterm infants, they may also represent a teleologic mechanism to limit excessive inflammatory responses in utero. In fact, intravital observations of leukocyte extravasation following local stimulation with fMLP has been performed in murine yolk sac vessels of the living fetus still connected to the mother. These experiments showed an ontogenetically regulated increase in myeloid cell extravasation,[46] supporting the concept that age-limited inflammatory responses might be beneficial for proper fetal growth and development.

ANTIMICROBIAL FUNCTIONS OF NEUTROPHILS

Inflammatory neutrophils recruited to tissue sites of microbial invasion engage a variety of attack mechanisms. These processes include phagocytosis, oxidative metabolism, degranulation, and the formation of NETs.

PHAGOCYTOSIS

OVERVIEW

The process of *phagocytosis*, or leukocyte ingestion of foreign particles, has been recognized since the 19th century. The earliest descriptions of phagocytosis were published by Joseph Richardson and William Osler in 1869 and 1875, respectively[93]; although credit for the term and its discovery are commonly attributed to Élie Metchnikoff, who shared the 1908 Nobel Prize in Physiology or Medicine with Paul Ehrlich. Phagocytosis is so crucial to host defense that two categories of leukocytes are classified as "professional phagocytes" and neutrophils lead the charge in that regard.

A preparatory step for phagocytosis is *opsonization,* the process of "tagging" the targeted pathogens by coating them with opsonins. An opsonin may be an Ig (especially IgG), fibronectin, and complement-derived cleavage products (C3b and C3bi). This coating prepares pathogens for ingestion by phagocytes, including neutrophils.[94] Opsonized pathogens bind to neutrophils through specific surface receptors such as CD11b. Adhesive contact between opsonized particles and inflammatory neutrophils initiates both phagocytosis and the neutrophil *respiratory burst*, a process that generates reactive oxygen intermediates (ROIs) that mediate intracellular killing and degradation of ingested pathogens.[95]

Neutrophil receptors for Ig opsonins include *Fc receptors* that recognize and bind the Fc portion of the IgG molecule. Neutrophils possess three distinct Fc receptors: FcγRI (CD64), FcγRII (CD32), and FcγRIII (CD16).[96] FcγRI is the high-affinity receptor for IgG. It is not expressed at high levels on the cell surface until the neutrophil undergoes activation, and it lacks a direct role in promoting phagocytosis. However, it may potentiate phagocytosis mediated by other receptors.[97] FcγRII and FcγRIII are constitutively expressed lower-affinity Fc receptors that are important to the efficiency of neutrophil phagocytosis.

Perhaps the most important receptor for phagocytosis is *complement receptor 3* (CR3, also known as *Mac-1*). CR3 is a β_2-integrin, a heterodimer of CD18 (common to all members of this integrin family) and CD11b, which contains the C3bi binding site and has a recognition domain for other matrix proteins including fibrinogen. CR3 also contains a lectin-like binding site that can bind bacteria independent of opsonization.[98] When C3bi binds to CR3, it initiates two pathogen-killing mechanisms: phagocytosis and the respiratory burst (described below).[99]

Binding of an opsonized target to the neutrophil cell surface through any of the aforementioned mechanisms activates intracellular microfilaments that enable pseudopods to extend and surround the target, capturing it inside the cell. This membrane-bound vacuole contains the target, or "phagosome," and fuses with intracellular granules. Granule release of toxic contents into the vacuole facilitates pathogen killing and removal.

NEONATAL IMPAIRMENTS IN PHAGOCYTOSIS

Phagocytosis is a complex process that is impacted by multiple factors including the involved surface receptors, the opsonization status of the target, and the properties of the target itself. As such, phagocytosis of neonatal neutrophils is impacted by the developmental stage and setting of the infant. Neonatal neutrophils have reduced CR3 receptor pools relative to adults, and neutrophils from preterm infants have reduced FcγRII and FcγRIII.[100] Phagocytic activity of neonatal neutrophils can also be impaired by reduced availability of opsonins. Maternal Ig is actively transported across the placenta, but the majority of such transfer occurs in the third trimester, leaving preterm infants with considerably less than term infants. A number of studies have investigated neonatal neutrophil phagocytosis covering a range of targets including bacteria and fungi. Some suggest defects, particularly in preterm infants, where others did not, likely reflecting variability in assay technique and conditions, as well as the numerous variables that impact the process.[101,102]

OXIDATIVE MICROBIAL KILLING

OVERVIEW

Neutrophil activation is accompanied by a marked increase in oxygen consumption and glucose utilization known as the *respiratory burst*, a reaction that is crucial in enabling phagocytes to degrade internalized pathogens. This process, catalyzed by the membrane-bound phagocyte oxidase complex, generates an array of ROIs that are toxic to surrounding microbial targets. Among these ROIs are hydrogen peroxide (H_2O_2) and superoxide anion (O_2^-). The phagocyte oxidase complex comprises a 91-kDa flavoprotein and a 22-kDa heme protein, collectively referred to as flavocytochrome b_{558}.[103] In resting states, flavocytochrome b_{558} is mostly sequestered in the membranes of secretory vesicles and specific granules, where it can be rapidly activated through degranulation.

NADPH is required for generating O_2^-, and the binding sites of flavocytochrome b_{558} provide the cognate ligand. In a carefully orchestrated, highly regulated process, soluble cytoplasmic components including p47^{phox}, p67^{phox}, p40^{phox}, and the GTPase, Rac1 help "build" the cluster of proteins called the NADPH oxidase complex and catalyze electron donation from NADPH to O_2 to produce superoxide.[104] Chronic granulomatous disease (CGD), manifested by an increased susceptibility to infection secondary to an inability to mount the respiratory burst, results from deficiencies in flavocytochrome b_{558}, p47^{phox}, or p67^{phox}.[105]

After the phagocytic oxidase generates O_2^-, superoxide dismutase rapidly converts it to H_2O_2. Further reactions involving O_2^- and H_2O_2 in the presence of iron produce a hydroxide ion and a hydroxyl radical. Because oxidative killing carries a high threat for damage to healthy tissue, processes are in place to control and limit the reaction. Other neutrophil products including catalase and glutathione peroxidase help to neutralize these reactive molecules and prevent potential injury to healthy tissue.

Neutrophil azurophilic granules utilize two additional mechanisms of oxidative killing. Myeloperoxidase (MPO) from the granules can catalyze the formation of chloramines and hypochlorous acid (the active component in bleach) from H_2O_2 and chloride. Inducible nitric oxide synthase (iNOS) is also present in azurophilic granules. When induced, the synthase produces the highly reactive molecule nitric oxide (NO).[106] NO production generates reactive nitrogen intermediates that complement the antimicrobial activity of ROS.

NEONATAL RESPIRATORY BURST

The respiratory burst in neonatal neutrophils has been studied extensively since the 1970s.[100] Most evidence suggests that, at birth, neutrophils of full-term infants elicit a respiratory burst equivalent to that in adult neutrophils. In contrast, preterm infants are deficient in this response. This holds true for both spontaneous and fMLP-stimulated neutrophil respiratory burst in neonates with or without signs of infection.[107] Additionally, "stressed" preterm infants with sepsis or respiratory distress can exhibit severe impairments in neutrophil-mediated antibacterial function[108] and delayed maturation of the respiratory burst. Other perinatal variables also affect the respiratory burst. Cord blood neutrophils collected after labor and vaginal delivery generate more ROS in response to stimulation with *Escherichia coli* and have higher CD11b expression than those collected after cesarean section.[107]

In addition to quantifiable differences between neonatal and adult respiratory burst responses, qualitative characteristics differ as well. Compared to adult cells, neonatal neutrophils generate more O_2^- from the initial stage of the respiratory burst both at baseline and in response to stimulation. This may be related to the altered content of membrane-associated flavocytochrome b_{558} relative to cytoplasmic phox components.[109] However, bactericidal oxidants generated later in the pathway, such as hydroxyl radicals, are reduced in neonates. The reduced neonatal content of MPO, which generates chloramines and hypochlorous acid from H_2O_2, and lactoferrin, which enhances hydroxide ion production when saturated with iron, are thought to contribute to the deficiencies in generating these bactericidal constituents.[100]

Finally, there is evidence that the oxidative burst is sensitive to therapy with dexamethasone used in the treatment of bronchopulmonary dysplasia (BPD) in premature infants.[110] Although respiratory burst activity increases with postnatal age in very low-birth-weight infants, exposure to dexamethasone diminishes responses relative to age-matched controls. Lower levels of antioxidant enzymes, such as glutathione, in neonates compared with adults,[111] may also contribute to neutrophil-mediated toxicity in the local tissue environment.

DEGRANULATION

Neutrophils are categorized as *granulocytes* based on the diverse array of densely packed granules and secretory vesicles highly visible within these cells. All of these components are key players in the antimicrobial defenses mediated by neutrophils. Additionally, these granules contain receptors, adhesion molecules, and inflammatory mediators that play vital roles in nearly every aspect of neutrophil function.[112]

Following neutrophil activation, intracellular granules and secretory vesicles translocate to the neutrophil surface.[112,113] Precise control of granule release is essential not only in transforming these cells from innocuous patrollers to deadly effector cells, but also in limiting their potential for causing collateral damage to healthy tissues.

OVERVIEW: NEUTROPHIL GRANULES

Neutrophil granules and vesicles are variably formed at specific steps during the process of myeloid differentiation; thus, their individual expression is a function of neutrophil maturity (see Fig. 119.1). During neutrophil differentiation, ***primary granules*** are formed first, at the myeloblast and promyelocyte stages. These granules contain large amounts of MPO, which has an affinity for the basic dye, azure A; hence, their designation as "azurophilic granules." Because MPO synthesis stops as development continues beyond the promyelocyte stage, the remaining granules are peroxidase negative.

Later-developing granules can be divided into *specific* ("secondary") and *gelatinase* ("tertiary") granules. Specific granules are rich in lactoferrin and low in gelatinase, while gelatinase granules have the opposite composition. Again, their contents reflect the timing of their development: lactoferrin is highly expressed in myelocytes and metamyelocytes; gelatinase is chiefly expressed in "bands" and "segs" (immature and mature segmented neutrophils, respectively). The application of subcellular fractionation techniques suggests that this classical categorization can be further subdivided based on levels of individual components.[114]

Finally, secretory vesicles form in mature cells and contain plasma proteins and membrane-associated receptors. Upon receiving an inflammatory stimulus, these vesicles are rapidly mobilized and become incorporated into the neutrophil surface membrane, where they display receptors that orchestrate neutrophil antimicrobial responses.[114]

AZUROPHILIC GRANULES

Azurophilic granules contain peptides that confer potent antimicrobial activity through both oxidative and nonoxidative pathways. Important peptides include MPO, α-defensins, bactericidal/permeability-increasing protein (BPI), elastase, proteinase-3, and cathepsin G. These granules primarily target and release their contents into the phagosome rather than extracellular pathways.[115] MPO is critical for oxidative killing; it reacts with H_2O_2 to form toxic reactive oxygen and nitrogen intermediates.[116]

The cationic antimicrobial peptides, *α-defensins* and *cathelicidins* (e.g., LL-37), form another major component of azurophilic granules, comprising approximately 5% of the total protein content in neutrophils. These two groups of small peptides mediate killing by forming transmembrane pores in a broad range of bacteria, fungi, protists, and enveloped viruses.[114] BPI is a cationic protein that kills gram-negative bacteria by binding to the negatively charged LPS contained in the outer membrane of those bacteria. BPI-LPS binding also neutralizes the potent pro-inflammatory properties of LPS. The C-terminal domain of this protein facilitates phagocytosis by mediating attachment of bacteria to neutrophils and monocytes.[117]

Elastase, *proteinase-3*, and *cathepsin G* are serine proteases with microbicidal activity and are collectively referred to as *serprocidins*.[115] These proteins help neutrophils detach after initial cell adhesion and facilitate transmigration.[118]

SPECIFIC AND GELATINASE GRANULES

The peroxidase-negative specific and gelatinase granules differ in content and function. While specific granules contain abundant antimicrobial proteins that can be directed to the phagosome or to the neutrophil exterior, gelatinase granules have a strong tendency for exocytosis and contain membrane receptors and enzymes that degrade the extracellular matrix.[119,120]

Lactoferrin is found primarily in specific granules. Its N-terminal region binds bacterial membranes and causes cell lysis to both gram-positive and gram-negative bacteria.[121] It also inhibits bacterial growth by binding iron, making this essential nutrient less available to microbes.

Human cationic antimicrobial protein (hCAP-18), a member of the cathelicidin family of antimicrobial peptides,[122] like lactoferrin contains a domain with broad-spectrum antibacterial properties. *Neutrophil gelatinase-associated lipocalin* (NGAL), a third antimicrobial component of specific granules, works primarily to inhibit bacterial growth by interfering with iron acquisition through bacterial iron-binding siderophores.[123]

Several proteins, including *lysozyme* and the MMPs, are more widely distributed among the granule subtypes. Lysozyme has the capacity to degrade the peptidoglycan that provides structural stability to bacterial cell walls, thereby promoting cell lysis.[124] Lysozyme also has affinity for the lipid A moiety of LPS and can alter its pro-inflammatory properties.[125] The MMPs expressed in neutrophils include MMP-8 (neutrophil collagenase, primarily in specific granules), MMP-9 (gelatinase, primarily in gelatinase granules), and MT6-MMP/MMP-25 (leukolysin, widely distributed). These proteins are activated following exocytosis and degrade a number of extracellular matrix proteins to facilitate neutrophil migration.[115] A regulatory feedback loop by *tissue inhibitors of the MMPs* (TIMPs) limits the damaging effects of MMPs on surrounding tissues.[126]

NEONATAL NEUTROPHIL GRANULES

Reduced levels of granule components are among the functional deficiencies that have been described in newborns and infants. While neutrophils of term neonates and adults contain similar amounts of MPO and defensins, MPO is reduced in neutrophils of preterm infants.[127,128] In contrast, lactoferrin and BPI are reduced in neutrophils from term infants to 50% and 30% of adult levels, respectively.[128]

GALECTIN-3

OVERVIEW

Galectin-3 (gal3) is a member of the family of β-galactoside-binding animal lectins. Widely distributed among tissues and cell types, gal3 has been studied for its role in diverse diseases including malignancy, heart failure, and asthma (reviewed by Sciacchitano and colleagues[129]). Gal3 plays a prominent role in the inflammatory response, and its numerous effects on neutrophils are well described.[130] Gal3 promotes neutrophil adhesion to endothelial cells, triggers the respiratory burst in primed or transmigrated neutrophils, and increases phagocytic activity.[131] Potential neutrophil receptors for gal3 that may mediate these events (CD66a, CD66b) have been identified.[132] There is also evidence for a role of gal3 in phagocytosis of diverse microorganisms including *Haemophilus influenza* and *Candida* spp.[133,134]

NEONATAL ALTERATIONS IN GAL3

Evidence suggests that gal3 expression and activity may be altered in neonates, although some data are conflicting. Several studies have shown decreased serum or whole blood gal3 expression in preterm and term neonates relative to levels in adults.[135,136] In contrast, higher serum gal3 expression in neonates was associated with robust gal3-induced oxidative burst that was independent of a priming stimulus.[137] These observations led the authors to conclude that neutrophils in newborn infants are pre-primed at delivery and therefore have enhanced reactivity to gal3 at baseline. Despite inconsistencies in reported gal3 expression in neonates, evidence collectively points to an influence of this lectin on neutrophil function and its likely important contribution to neonatal innate immunity.

NEUTROPHIL EXTRACELLULAR TRAPS

Whereas phagocytosis, degranulation, and oxidative killing mechanisms have been studied for decades and are now considered classical features of neutrophil biology, the production of NETs is a more recent discovery. First described by Zychlinsky and colleagues in 2004, this process involves the extrusion of chromatin fibers outside the cell to form a "mesh" adorned with antimicrobial peptides and enzymes including elastase and MPO.[138]

OVERVIEW

The production of NETs was first described as "NETosis," a pathogen-induced cell death in which the nuclear and granule membranes break down, releasing decondensed chromatin and associated granule contents into the extracellular space. Compared to degranulation or the oxidative burst as an antimicrobial strategy, in its original description NETosis was noted to be considerably slower, occurring over 2 to 4 hours. This process was stimulated by a variety of inflammatory mediators and a wide range of microbes, and required activation of the NADPH oxidase and production of ROS. Since its initial description, studies of NET formation have uncovered considerable complexity in this process.[139] NET release can occur much more rapidly, is not always associated with cell lysis, and can occur independently of NADPH oxidase and ROS production. It can be initiated by a number of different stimuli and by more than a single pathway.[140] Varied subtypes of NETs have been described that are associated with different triggers for their release.[141] "Cloudy" NETs have been associated with stimulation with LPS or crystals, in contrast to "spiky" NETs triggered by stimulation with C5a. "Aggregated" NETs (aggNETS) occur in the setting of high neutrophil densities. Their large size has been associated with vascular occlusion is some studies. In addition to a potential role in pathogen clearance, aggNETs may also degrade pro-inflammatory mediators to promote resolution of inflammation and wound healing. Evidence has also emerged that mitochondrial DNA can contribute to NET formation in addition to nuclear DNA.[140]

The role of NETs in neutrophil antimicrobial function is an area of ongoing investigation. Numerous reports suggest that this meshwork of DNA, histones, and antimicrobial enzymes derived from granule components trap microorganisms to limit their dissemination and provide a locally concentrated source of antimicrobial activity to promote killing. They have been proposed as an alternate defense mechanism when the capacity for phagocytosis is limited by number or size of the target.[142] Many bacteria and fungi bind to NETs; however, some *Streptococcus* and *Staphylococcus* strains elaborate endonucleases that may free them from NETs.[139] NETs also have a role in inflammation and host tissue damage including autoimmune and other inflammatory conditions that are not infectious in nature. They have been suggested to have both detrimental and beneficial roles in maintenance of inflammation.[142] Considerable controversy remains in part due to the heterogeneity of research methods, models of disease, and the intricate biology of this process that differs based on disease setting, triggers, and mechanisms of release. Interest in further elucidating the role of these structures is driven by the potential to modify their activity in disease settings ranging from sepsis to thrombosis and autoimmune diseases in which they likely play a role.

NEONATAL NEUTROPHIL EXTRACELLULAR TRAPS

In the first study of NETs in neonatal neutrophils, Yost and colleagues[143] found that in vitro stimulation of neutrophils from term and preterm infants with NET-inducing agents including LPS, platelet activating factor, phorbol myristate acetate, or bacteria (*Staphylococcus aureus* and *E. coli*) resulted in NETs only rarely or not at all, while adult neutrophils exhibited NET formation within 60 minutes. This study also correlated a deficiency in NET production with impaired killing of extracellular bacteria in vitro. A subsequent study suggested that NET formation does occur in neonatal neutrophils, with a response that is delayed beyond 60 minutes.[144] This delay was less apparent when neutrophils were stimulated with agonists of TLR5, TLR8, and TLR9, suggesting that pathways of NET generation other than those mediated by TLR2 and TLR4 are intact. Another study demonstrated NET generation equivalent to adult cells by term infant neutrophils stimulated by fibronectin together with *Candida albicans* hyphae or β-glucan in a ROS-independent manner.[145] These observations underscore the complexity of NET generation and the distinctive features associated with different triggers and pathways.

The finding of delayed NET formation in neonatal neutrophils prompted investigations into regulators of NET generation that may be at play in the neonatal period. Indeed, comparisons of LPS-induced NET formation in cord blood neutrophils to neutrophils from venous samples collected from infants after birth demonstrated that the capacity to generate NETs appeared within days after birth in both term and preterm infants.[146] Further, adult or 60-day-old preterm infant neutrophils lost their capacity to generate NETs when tested in the presence of cord blood plasma suggesting that cord blood had NET inhibiting factors. The authors utilized proteomic analyses of cord blood to identify neonatal NET inhibitory factor (nNIF) and nNIF-related peptides that are potent inhibitors of NET formation. They are effective against a wide variety of microbial, host-derived, and pharmacologic triggers of NET formation while leaving other antimicrobial neutrophil functions intact. Importantly, they inhibited NET formation in vivo and had beneficial effects in models of infection and sterile inflammation. These findings support the presence of a fetal regulatory mechanism to limit NET formation and raise the possibility that nNIF peptides could be clinically useful antiinflammatory agents.

A role for NETs in the setting of necrotizing enterocolitis (NEC) has been suggested. Reductions in mortality, tissue damage, and other markers of inflammation were reported in a mouse model of NEC with inhibition of the enzyme PAD4.[147] PAD4 is highly expressed in neutrophils, and by mediating the conversion of arginine to citrulline in histones contributes to the decondensation of chromatin.[148] However, the dependence of NET formation on PAD4 is controversial.[140] Additionally, fecal calprotectin is a marker of intestinal inflammation that has been investigated as a biomarker for NEC.[149] This antibacterial protein makes up a large proportion of neutrophil cytoplasmic proteins and colocalizes with NETs in necrotic bowel specimens resected in the setting of NEC. Thus, NET formation may be one source for fecal calprotectin.[150]

NEUTROPHILS AND INFLAMMATION RESOLUTION

Following the process of microbial killing, spent neutrophils undergo structural cell changes associated with *apoptosis* (programmed cell death) and are subsequently ingested by resident macrophages *(efferocytosis)*.[151] These last steps are critical to the resolution of inflammation and the resumption of cellular homeostasis.[152]

RESOLUTION OF INFLAMMATION

Neutrophils resolve acute inflammation using approaches that both prevent "collateral damage" to neighboring cells and that limit the development of chronic inflammation (the reader is referred to recent elegant reviews[153,154]). Resolution of inflammation involves the initial suppression of inflammation *(antiinflammatory phase)* followed by a *proresolving phase*. The initial phase involves the down-regulation of inflammatory responses, such as through anti-inflammatory cytokine release, the production of cytokine inhibitors (IL1-RA), and inhibited signaling mediated by NFκB.[155] The second phase is mediated by the release of mediators such as lipoxin A4, protectins and resolvins, all of which inhibit neutrophil accumulation in tissues.[156] In addition, neutrophils release MPO, a bactericidal enzyme that can also suppress inflammatory responses.[157]

APOPTOSIS

Under stable conditions, neutrophils released into circulation undergo apoptosis or programmed cell death within 48 hours after egressing from the bone marrow.[158] Structural changes on senescent neutrophils, including the surface exposure of membrane phosphatidyl serine, initiate their ingestion by tissue phagocytes. The mechanisms regulating neutrophil apoptosis are complex, primarily involving pathways mediated by Fas-Fas ligand interactions as well as others (reviewed in Cabrini and colleagues[159] and Caielli and colleagues[160]). The removal of these spent, senescent neutrophils is critical for proper neutrophil homeostasis and resolution of inflammatory processes.[16] Conversely, neutrophils that have reentered the vasculature (reverse transmigration) are ultimately cleared in the bone marrow.[154]

In contrast to neutrophils under homeostatic conditions, neutrophils activated by inflammatory conditions can also exhibit prolonged life spans.[161] Such neutrophils retain their inflammatory functions, which initially facilitate the clearance of invasive pathogens. However, surviving neutrophils that evade the structural changes associated with apoptosis fail to be ingested by macrophages and thus cannot be removed by the reticuloendothelial system. Thus, their persistence in tissues in the absence of an infectious nidus potentially perpetuates inflammatory processes that contribute to chronic disorders.

APOPTOSIS IN NEONATAL NEUTROPHILS

Neonatal neutrophils constitutively exhibit delayed apoptosis compared to adult neutrophils.[162-164] Neonatal neutrophils that survive apoptotic conditions in culture retain inflammatory and cytotoxic functions to a greater degree than adult neutrophils.[164,165] In one study, impaired efferocytosis of apoptotic neonatal neutrophils was observed to result in continued monocyte IL-8 release while this process was inhibited in adult co-cultures, suggesting a mechanism to perpetuate inflammation in neonates.[166]

The mechanisms contributing to the prolonged survival of neonatal neutrophils are associated with decreased expression of pro-apoptotic proteins, including caspase-3, and the persistence of anti-apoptotic proteins such as FLICE-inhibitory protein (FLIP) relative to their levels in adult neutrophils.[167,168] Both of these proteins are key common components of the major caspase-mediated cell death pathways. Other studies have shown a contribution of survival pathways such as NF-κB and Akt/PI3K to both longevity and inflammatory functions of neonatal neutrophils.[40,167]

Neonates are developmentally hampered by inadequate neutrophil stores and impaired neutrophil function. Thus, the intrinsic survival bias of neonatal neutrophils could plausibly provide a protective advantage in guarding against infection. Conversely, however, the persistence of activated neutrophils in post-infectious tissue, such as in the lungs, could potentiate injury and promote chronic inflammation, particularly in preterm infants. This possibility is supported by evidence of decreased neutrophil apoptosis or apoptotic activity in tracheal aspirates of preterm neonates who later developed BPD.[169,170] The antiinflammatory effects of pentoxifylline treatment in preterm neonates could be partially attributed to the induction of neutrophil apoptosis.[171,172] In contrast, glucocorticoids promote the survival of neutrophils and impede their clearance, effects that could potentially subvert the intended goal of suppressing inflammatory responses.[173]

In contrast to the potential pro-inflammatory properties of surviving mature neutrophils, some evidence suggests that granulocytic myeloid derived suppressor cells (G-MDSCs), an immature neutrophil subset with antiinflammatory capacity,[174] are resistant to *E. coli*-induced apoptosis.[175] This observation suggests a potential role for surviving G-MDSCs in modulating neonatal inflammatory responses following bacterial infection, although more investigations in this area are needed.

NEONATAL NEUTROPHILS AND INFLAMMATORY DISORDERS

Clinically significant inflammation occurs commonly in neonates, particularly when infection and the inflammatory response are associated with preterm labor and delivery. The neonatal inflammatory cascade is commonly initiated by maternal infection, maternal or fetal chorioamnionitis, or postnatal infections that occur during the neonatal period.The effects and outcomes of systemic inflammation manifest in neonates in ways that are distinct from older children or adults, and is a subject of intensive study. Regardless of the trigger, potentially maladaptive inflammatory activities mediated by neutrophils are crucial contributors to neonatal outcomes.

LUNG INFLAMMATION

The best-studied inflammatory neutrophil conditions that arise from complications of prematurity are respiratory distress syndrome (RDS) and BPD. Both small and large animal models have been developed to study this process; additionally, human studies using autopsy specimens or endotracheal aspirates/lavage have contributed a great deal to our understanding of these mechanisms. Culprits that initiate the inflammatory cascade resulting in these conditions include sepsis, lung infections, and mechanical ventilation. In the latter, positive pressures and exposure to high oxygen concentrations can trigger inflammatory cascades mimicking that of infection, alluding to the possibility of a common pathway to lung injury.[176] Notably, even exposure to ambient oxygen concentrations could be considered "hyperoxic" in a premature infant, as exposure to oxygen is much lower in utero and antioxidant mechanisms are not yet fully developed.

In RDS, damage to epithelial and endothelial cells leads to interstitial and alveolar edema, increased lung permeability, and localized accumulation of large numbers of leukocytes that are predominantly neutrophils. The severity of lung injury is associated with the extent of neutrophil accumulation in the lung, and persistence of lung neutrophils is notable in infants with RDS who later develop BPD.[177] Not surprisingly, elevated lung levels of cytokines and chemokines that attract and sustain neutrophils are present in infants with RDS. High concentrations of these mediators, along with increased expression of adhesion molecules such as L-selectin, CD11b, and ICAM-1, are associated with the development of BPD.[178] Neutrophil release of the protease, elastase, breaks down elastin fibers, which may contribute to simplification of alveolar structure that is characteristic of BPD. Inflammatory neutrophils can release MMPs, including collagenase and gelatinase, that damage the extracellular matrix and break down basement membranes. An imbalance between these proteases and protease inhibitors has been demonstrated in infants developing BPD.[178]

Byproducts of the respiratory burst can also induce oxidative damage to neonatal lung tissue and likely contribute to the pathogenesis of BPD.[179] This injury is due in part to immaturity of antioxidant mechanisms such as superoxide dismutase. Additionally, as discussed in Section VI, neonatal neutrophils resist apoptosis, and their prolonged survival can perpetuate chronic inflammation and lung injury.[165]

BRAIN INJURY

Neutrophils are a critical component of the host defense against neonatal meningitis.[180] However, a small but growing body of indirect evidence in animal studies supports a contributory role of neutrophils to neonatal brain injury.[181–183] In one study, administration of chemerin, an adipokine that reduces neutrophil infiltration, to neonatal rats with intraventricular hemorrhage suppressed neuroinflammation and promoted neurologic recovery.[184] Studies in human infants have also correlated neutrophil-associated neuroinflammation with the pathogenesis of injury due to hypoxia-ischemia,[182] meningitis,[185] and encephalopathy.[186]

Abundant evidence shows that systemic inflammation early in life is strongly associated with brain injury and adverse neurodevelopmental outcomes.[187,188] The most common lesion associated with white-matter injury is periventricular leukomalacia (PVL). Adverse outcomes related to PVL are linked to systemic inflammation associated with culture-negative clinical infections, culture-proven sepsis, meningitis, and NEC with or without positive blood cultures. This association persists, even when considering "less virulent" organisms such as coagulase-negative *Staphylococcus*. Although neutrophils are a prominent cell type in the central nervous system (CNS) when meningitis is present, other inflammation-associated brain injuries can lead to marked abnormalities in neurodevelopment without apparent direct involvement of neutrophils within the CNS. Thus, the extent to which neutrophils directly contribute to white-matter injury in the brain remains to be fully defined.

NECROTIZING ENTEROCOLITIS

The intestinal microbiome plays a critical role in modulating neutrophil homeostasis. In a murine model of antibiotic exposure, simplification of the neonatal microbiome was associated with neutropenia and decreased resistance to gram-negative infection.[12] Conversely, neutrophils may be important to the pathogenesis of NEC. In a rat model of experimental inflammatory NEC, neutrophil depletion was protective against bowel necrosis.[189] Elevated vascular endothelial expression of P-selectin in infants with NEC correlated with the degree of intestinal injury, and neutrophil infiltration paralleled P-selectin expression.[190] In a more recent study, neutropenic newborn mice were infected with *Cronobacter sakazakii* to induce NEC.[191] Experimental pups had increased the recruitment of dendritic cells (DCs) accompanied by enhanced bacterial load and cytokine production, all of which exacerbated NEC injury. These studies suggest that while neutrophils are important for surveillance and protection against bacterial exposure in the gut, they may also potentiate the pathology of NEC after it is established.

ADHESION MOLECULES AS INFLAMMATORY MARKERS

NEUTROPHIL CELL ADHESION MOLECULES

Neutrophil activation leading to upregulated neutrophil expression of CD11b has been observed in preterm and term infants with sepsis or in association with mechanical ventilation.[192,193] Under basal conditions, L-selectin expression is highest in neutrophils newly released from the bone marrow; levels decrease during the neutrophil ageing process.[194] However, surface levels of L-selectin may be acutely downregulated on activated neutrophils, and expression is decreased in neutrophils of septic neonates.[195] Given that selectins provide the initial "tether" to initiate neutrophil-endothelial adhesion, as reviewed earlier, a quantitative or functional loss of selectin receptors on neutrophils can inhibit downstream antimicrobial activities of this leukocyte.

The normal shedding of L-selectin during marrow release depresses surface L-selectin levels on circulating neutrophils.[196] Surface L-selectin levels also can be modulated by a number of endogenous inflammatory mediators; in addition, glucocorticoids, IL-6, and G-CSF have also been shown to induce shedding of L-selectin.[197]

SOLUBLE CELL ADHESION MOLECULES

Shedding of membrane-associated selectins can result in increased levels of the soluble forms. Plasma levels of soluble (s)L-selectin were lower in the cord blood of term infants compared to adults, consistent with lower overall expression levels.[198] Soluble L-selectin levels were higher in bronchoalveolar lung fluid but not in plasma of preterm infants who ultimately developed BPD. In contrast, plasma soluble E-selectin levels correlated with later BPD.[199,200] Serum levels of several soluble cell adhesion molecules (CAMs), including ICAM-1, VCAM-1, L-selectin, and P-selectin, were also found to be elevated in neonates with possible or proven infection, and correlated with infection severity,[201] although none of these soluble adhesion molecules have apparent utility in predicting infection. Dexamethasone may dampen inflammatory responses by inhibiting levels of soluble CAMS.[202]

MYELOID-DERIVED SUPPRESSOR CELLS AND NEONATAL INFLAMMATION

Myeloid-derived suppressor cells (MDSCs), of granulocytic or monocytic origin, characteristically feature the capacity to suppress adaptive immune responses (reviewed by Gabrilovich and Nagaraj[203]). While these cell subsets are typically of low frequency, their numbers are enhanced during pathologic conditions such as inflammation and cancer.[204] Recent studies have also shown a prominence of granulocytic (G)-MDSCs during pregnancy and in umbilical cord blood,[205-207] suggesting their contribution to fetal tolerance mechanisms. However, the persistence of MDSC in neonates[208] could be a factor underlying the increased infectious risk and inadequate vaccine responses often observed in this population.[173,209,210] Supportive of this premise, cord blood granulocytic MDSC have been shown to inhibit protective Th1 but promote antiinflammatory Th2 and Treg responses.[205] Conversely, neonatal granulocytic MDSCs infected with *E. coli* had prolonged survival and retained innate immune host defense mechanisms.[174] Recent data in a neonatal mouse model showed a correlation between low MDSC frequencies and increased risk for NEC.[211] In addition, lactoferrin induced the conversion of mature neutrophils or monocytes to MDSC that were strongly antiinflammatory and protective against death from NEC-associated inflammation.[212] While these observations point to MDSC as a cell type that may be influential in modulating immune and inflammatory homeostasis in newborns, much remains to be learned about these unique immune cells.

NEONATAL NEUTROPENIA

Neutropenia is defined as an absolute decrease in the expected number of circulating neutrophils based on established reference ranges. In neonates, the normal circulating neutrophil concentration is a function of both gestational and postnatal age.[213-215] A diagnosis of neutropenia can be made if the absolute neutrophil count is less than 1.1×10^9/L in the first 48 hours after birth or less than 1.5×10^9/L thereafter. Neutropenia that presents in the newborn period may be immune-mediated, -acquired, -inherited, or -idiopathic. As in adults, the severity of the neutropenia, particularly in its inherited forms, correlates with an infant's susceptibility to life-threatening infections. Neutropenic disorders are generally grouped according to the primary mechanistic defect: decreased production/abnormal maturation *or* increased destruction/decreased survival of circulating cells.

NEUTROPENIA DUE TO DECREASED PRODUCTION OR ABNORMAL DIFFERENTIATION

ACQUIRED IN UTERO

Pregnancy-Induced Hypertension/Preeclampsia

Maternal hypertension and preeclampsia can lead to neutropenia that lasts for several days to weeks in affected infants; such neutropenia is associated with low circulating numbers of colony forming unit-granulocyte monocyte (CFU-GM) and diminished neutrophil storage pools.[216] While most infants have a transient neutropenia lasting less than 60 hours, prolonged neutropenia in a few affected infants can persist for days to weeks. This type of neutropenia resolves naturally, although in some cases it may be severe enough to consider treatment with G-CSF or GM-CSF.[217] Studies have variably shown an association between this form of neutropenia and an enhanced risk for later infection, even after the neutropenia resolves.[216,218,219] In addition, a higher incidence of death in low-birth-weight neonates born after preeclampsia has been reported.[220] The mechanism underlying this variety of neonatal neutropenia is related to an inhibition of myelopoiesis by an as-yet-undefined transplacental factor.[221]

Rh Hemolytic Disease

A self-limiting, benign postnatal neutropenia has been described in neonates born with Rh hemolytic disease.[222] A possible mechanism may involve down-modulation of neutrophil production in concert with high levels of erythropoietin and increased erythropoiesis.[223,224] Similarly, neutropenia is a reported complication in infants receiving recombinant human erythropoietin to treat the anemia of prematurity.[225]

Intrauterine Growth Restriction

Neutropenia is commonly associated in neonates who are small for gestational age. A recent retrospective analysis of over 8000 mother-infant pairs showed that neutropenia in small for gestational age neonates is a self-resolving disorder that may be due to transiently decreased granulopoiesis and that responds to treatment with G-CSF.[226]

Birth Depression

Neutropenia can occur in infants who are born with severely depressed vital signs subsequent to a variety of antenatal or peripartum events, particularly in association with therapeutic hypothermia.[227] Intraventricular hemorrhage at or soon after birth has also been associated with neonatal neutropenia; however, whether this is causal or only an association is unclear.[228]

CONGENITAL NEUTROPENIA

This varied group of heterogeneous, rare disorders is characterized by severe neutropenia due to specific genetic defects (reviewed in Spoor and colleagues[229]). While heritable neutropenias can present in the neonatal period, infants with severe congenital neutropenia (SCN) typically exhibit recurring or unusual infections early in the first year of life. In both cyclical neutropenia (CyN) and SCN, germline mutations involve defects in the neutrophil elastase gene (*ELANE* or *ELA2*).[230,231] These and other genetic defects associated with congenital neutropenia disorders have been reviewed recently.[232] The best studied of the SCNs include *cyclical neutropenia* and SCN type I *(Kostmann syndrome)*.[233] The primary underlying genetic defect in both disorders involves ELANE, the gene encoding the neutrophil granule elastase. A mutation in this gene is more common with CyN, although the majority of individuals with SCN also have this mutation. Neutropenic episodes are associated with marrow myeloid hypoplasia related to apoptosis of myeloid progenitors or an arrest of neutrophil maturation.[231] Some evidence suggests that CyN and SCN, rather than being separate disorders, are part of the same spectrum.[234]

Cyclic Neutropenia

In this autosomal dominant disorder, neutropenia occurs periodically in an approximately 21-day cycle, often in association with fever. The accompanying neutropenia is severe, in some cases including absence of circulating neutrophils but a monocytosis, typically lasting for several days.[233] Although the risk for infection with CyN is generally low, recurrent, self-limited mucosal and soft tissue infections in association with neutropenic episodes have been observed. Systemic infections during the nadir of this cycle can be fatal. Treatment with G-CSF may improve the neutrophil counts and reduce the number of infectious episodes. Unlike patients with SCN, CyN has not been associated with an increased risk for leukemia.[235]

Severe Congenital Neutropenia (Kostmann Syndrome)

Kostmann first described a neonatal neutropenia that was severe (absolute neutrophil counts $<0.2 \times 10^9/L$) and persistent, occurring in less than 10 cases per million individuals.[236] This genetically heterogenous, primarily autosomal dominant, disorder is due to a variety of genetic defects, with involvement of the neutrophil elastase gene, *ELANE,* in over half of affected individuals.[231] In addition to severe neutropenia, neutrophils from affected individuals may have defective microbicidal function.[237] Affected individuals develop frequent episodes of fever, and systemic infections may be lethal. Exogenous treatment with rhG-CSF is generally successful, although "nonresponders" may require stem cell transplantation and are at higher risk for malignant transformation. In contrast to CyN, up to 30% of individuals with SCN are reportedly at increased risk for conversion to acute myeloid leukemia or myelodysplastic syndrome.[236] While some evidence suggests a link between leukemic transformation and cumulative G-CSF dose, this association remains controversial.

NEUTROPENIA DUE TO OTHER CAUSES

Benign Chronic Neutropenia

This mild to moderate neutropenia is an autosomal recessive disorder of unclear genetic etiology. It has been observed in approximately 5% in populations of African ancestry.[238] This type of neutropenia is not associated with either bone marrow abnormalities or increased risk for infection. One form of this disorder has been associated with altered function of the Duffy blood group chemokine receptor gene *(DARC)*, a mechanism that may be protective against malaria.[238]

Neutropenia Associated With Other Inherited Disorders

Mild to severe persistent neutropenia may accompany a variety of other inherited disorders. Heterogeneous in their origins, the mechanistic etiologies of the associated neutropenias are varied. Some may result from imbalances in the positive and negative regulators of hematopoiesis, leading to decreased production, while others involve accelerated apoptosis or destruction.[239] Equally variable is how these disorders can affect organs in addition to the hematopoietic system. Disorders in this grouping include glycogen storage disease Ib, Wiskott-Aldrich syndrome, Barth syndrome, Hermansky-Pudlak syndrome, Chédiak-Higashi syndrome (CHS), and Shwachman-Diamond syndrome, among others (reviewed in Skokowa and colleagues[230] and Walkovich and Connelly[240]).

NEUTROPENIA RESULTING FROM INCREASED UTILIZATION OR DESTRUCTION

Sepsis

Infection is the most common cause of neutropenia in newborns.[7] Human studies and animal models suggest several factors that promote septic neutropenia in infected infants (reviewed in Chapter 108. During the last trimester of pregnancy, granulopoiesis becomes the main hematopoietic focus in the bone marrow.[5,71] This emphasis leads to increased numbers of circulating neutrophils, a high proportion of proliferating myeloid cells, and the generation of a postmitotic, nearly mature bone marrow neutrophil storage pool. The fetal bone marrow may be restricted in its capacity to generate new neutrophils despite increased demand, such as during infection; in addition, it has a diminished storage pool compared to that of adults. Neutrophil egress from the bone marrow in response to stimulation proceeds in a dysregulated fashion in neonates, which can rapidly deplete postmitotic neutrophil stores, causing severe neutropenia.[101] Additional factors that increase the demand for circulating neutrophils include massive recruitment into the infected areas, increased neutrophil destruction/decreased survival at inflammatory sites, and increased neutrophil margination along inflamed vessels.[241] All of these factors diminish the supply of functional neutrophils available to infected infants, which may be reflected in decreased circulating neutrophil numbers.[213,241] Severe neutropenia combined with depletion of the postmitotic neutrophil bone marrow storage pool are associated with a poor prognosis in the septic newborn.[7]

IMMUNE-MEDIATED NEUTROPENIAS

In contrast to a variety of neonatal neutropenias, those that are immune-mediated are relatively rare. These primarily include neonatal alloimmune and rarely autoimmune neutropenias. The pathogenesis of *neonatal alloimmune neutropenia (NAIN)* involves transplacental transfer of maternal antibodies against a specific fetal or neonatal neutrophil antigen, a result of sensitization of the maternal immune system to an inherited paternal antigen (reviewed in Black and Maheshwari[242] and Porcelijm and de Haas[243]). Maternal anti-neutrophil antibodies that have crossed into the fetal circulation induce neutropenia by destroying neutrophils and possibly by inhibiting neutrophil production. NAIN has been detected in less than 1% of births, although the true incidence is unclear since asymptomatic babies may not have been tested; in addition, the detection of circulating anti-neutrophil antibodies in mothers does not necessarily correlate with neonatal neutropenia.[243] While this type of neutropenia is typically diagnosed in healthy babies, it has been associated with a spectrum of disorders that range from mild skin infections to omphalitis, sepsis, and meningitis.[244] Affected infants typically present with neutropenia in the first week of life, and this may persist for up to 6 months. NAIN responds well to G-CSF therapy except in cases associated with anti-HNA-2a antibodies.[245] Although neutropenia is common in the neonatal intensive care unit, the diagnosis of immune-mediated neutropenia should be a consideration in a neonate whose neutrophil counts fail to normalize within several days in the absence of common etiologies. Genotyping of the human neutrophil antigen (HNA) by polymerase chain reaction has replaced serologic HNA typing as an effective diagnostic tool for NAIN.[243]

Autoimmune neutropenia of infancy (AIN), due to self-directed antibodies against neutrophil antigens, is rare in the neonatal period but typically presents between 5 and 15 months of age in healthy infants.[246] This neutropenia is not usually associated with severe infection and resolves in 90% of cases before the age of 2 years. Like NAIN, AIN responds well to G-CSF. The pathogenesis, diagnosis, and treatment of this group of neutropenias has been reviewed.[246,247]

NEONATAL NEUTROPHILIA

Neutrophilia is defined as an elevation in the absolute number of circulating neutrophils relative to established values. Absolute neutrophil counts as high as 14.4×10^9/L have been measured in full-term infants at 12 hours of age, in association with the rapid postnatal increase of circulating blood cells at birth.[214,241] After 72 hours of age, absolute neutrophil counts ranging from 5.4 to 7.0×10^9/L for both full-term and premature infants constitute the upper limits of normal during the first week of life, values equivalent to adult subjects.[214,215] Neutrophil counts vary with the site of collection; neutrophil counts are higher (approximately 20%) in capillary blood samples compared to those obtained by venous or arterial sampling.[248]

PERINATAL AND ACQUIRED NEUTROPHILIA

Peripartum complications associated with neutrophilia in newborn infants include sepsis, chorioamnionitis, hypoglycemia, stressful labor, seizures, pneumothorax, and meconium aspiration syndrome.[249] In the majority of these instances, increased neutrophil counts are related to enhanced release from the marginated pool, increased mobilization from the bone marrow storage pool, or decreased egress from the circulating pool (reviewed by Koenig and Yoder[250]). The administration of steroids, commonly used as a treatment for chronic lung disease, can also increase peripheral neutrophils, in part through augmented release of marginated neutrophils or possibly through a potentiating effect on myelopoiesis.[251] Enhanced neutrophil production may account for the neutrophilia commonly observed in neonates born after exposure to chorioamnionitis, an inflammatory gestational disorder.[252,253] A persistent neutrophilia, especially if associated with recurrent bacterial infections or a delayed separation of the umbilical cord, should prompt the investigation of leukocyte adhesion deficiency (LAD) as a possible diagnosis.[254]

NEUTROPHILIA AND GENETIC DISORDERS

On occasion, infants with trisomy 21 have neutrophil counts that are so high as to be indistinguishable from the leukocyte counts of infants with acute leukemia.[255,256] Organomegaly, a high percentage of myeloid blast forms in peripheral blood, and persistent elevation of the leukocyte count for weeks may also be seen in these infants. Bone marrow examination may assist in distinguishing between leukemia and a transient myeloproliferative disorder. Infants with leukocyte adhesion deficiencies classically present with marked neutrophilia, as discussed below.

DISORDERS OF NEONATAL NEUTROPHIL FUNCTION

A simple way to understand qualitative disorders of neutrophil function is to categorize them according to the step(s) that go awry in recruiting neutrophils to an infection and/or of neutrophil ingestion or killing of invasive microorganisms. Most of the inherited disorders are rare. Although acquired neutrophil function disorders are more common than inherited disorders, the mechanisms accounting for the former are not as well characterized. The following section describes current knowledge of acquired and inherited neutrophil disorders.

ACQUIRED DISORDERS

A variety of environmental factors can influence neutrophil function and may have an especially profound impact on the developmentally immature host. Both magnesium sulfate, a common tocolytic used to manage preterm labor, as well as antenatal steroids can dampen expression of endothelial adhesion molecules and negatively influence certain neutrophil functions.[202,257] While sepsis risk is enhanced as a result of neutrophil dysfunction, sepsis itself can mediate deleterious effects on neutrophil functions (reviewed by Melvan and colleagues[258]). Mode of delivery or exposure to labor can also influence in vitro neutrophil inflammatory function; vaginal delivery has been shown to increase neutrophil Mac-1 levels and IL-8 release in neonates, while relative dampening of neutrophil inflammatory function has been observed after cesarean section.[92,259] Conversely, alterations of the microbiome related to caesarean section and other perinatal factors have been linked to an increased risk for chronic inflammatory disorders in later life.[260]

LEUKOCYTE ADHESION DEFICIENCIES

LAD is a heterogenous group of rare inherited disorders characterized by adhesion defects associated with neutrophilia and recurrent infections.[50] In general, LAD I and III involve low expression or functional deficiencies in leukocyte β_2 integrins (CD18), while LAD II represents a defect in fucose availability that affects selectin-mediated leukocyte rolling. These disorders typically present in the first year of life but may on occasion be diagnosed in the newborn period.[261]

LEUKOCYTE ADHESION DEFICIENCY I

LAD I is a rare autosomal recessive disorder, with an incidence of 2 cases per 1,000,000 individuals.[50] The affected gene, *ITGB2*, encodes the common β2-chain of the β_2 integrin family of adhesion molecules. Individuals with this disorder are characterized by neutrophilia and variably deficient expression of leukocyte β_2 integrins. Affected neutrophils exhibit impaired adhesion to endothelial cells and extracellular matrix proteins, ineffective chemotaxis, and defective phagocytosis of complement-coated microorganisms. As a result, individuals with classical LAD I can have profoundly impaired neutrophil mobilization to tissue inflammatory sites, which are typically devoid of neutrophils even during marked neutrophilia, and exhibit delayed wound healing. Severe gingivitis is pathognomonic of this disorder and may be the presenting symptom.

Infants with the severe LAD I phenotype may present with delayed umbilical cord separation, often associated with omphalitis and neutrophilia. However, delayed cord separation is not a universal finding in LAD I. Normal separation of the cord is typically observed in the first 2 weeks of life; however, a range from 3 to 67 days has been reported.[262] Overwhelming bacterial infections are associated with high mortality rates in infants with the severe phenotype, while viral infections are typically normal in severity.[263]

Persistent, marked neutrophilia associated with recurrent infections in the newborn period or in early infancy should prompt suspicion of the LAD I disorder. Classic, severe LAD I is associated with marked deficiency or absence of β_2 integrins on circulating leukocytes, as determined by flow cytometric analysis; functional assays show normal neutrophil rolling, but defective adhesion and migration.[262] Current therapeutic approaches include antibiotics for recurring bacterial infections; in severe cases granulocyte transfusions may be required. Bone marrow transplant may be therapeutic, and the success of gene therapy (introduction of a normal β_2 subunit gene [ITGB2] into hematopoietic stem cells) in animal studies suggests a potential curative approach.[263]

LEUKOCYTE ADHESION DEFICIENCY II

The primary functional abnormality in this very rare disorder is related to impaired selectin-mediated leukocyte (neutrophil) rolling.[50] Defective rolling in LAD II is due to a loss of function mutation of the gene SLC35C1. SLC35C1 encodes for the GDP-fucose transporter 1, which is critical for transferring GDP-fucose into the Golgi network where fucose is used for posttranslational fucosylation of glycoproteins. Loss of posttranslational fucosylation as observed in LAD II leads to the absence of sialyl Lewis X, a specific fucose-containing carbohydrate determinant on selectin ligands, which binds to all three selectins with low affinity and is critical for leukocyte rolling.[54] Accordingly, neutrophils of affected patients exhibit strongly impaired selectin-dependent leukocyte rolling leading to a severe defect in neutrophil recruitment into inflamed tissue.[264] In contrast, neutrophil CD18 expression and integrin-mediated endothelial adhesion are normal.

Affected neonates may present with extreme neutrophilia, with neutrophil counts reportedly as high as 150.0×10^9/L during infection. Recurrent infections, gingivitis, growth restriction, mental retardation, characteristic facies, and the rare Bombay blood group are typical of this disorder. In contrast to LAD I and LAD III, delayed separation of the umbilical cord is not a characteristic feature. Flow cytometric analysis of circulating leukocytes and specific functional assays are essential diagnostic tools. Acute infections, which are not typically severe, can be managed with antibiotic therapy. Fucose supplementation has yielded variable results.[265]

LEUKOCYTE ADHESION DEFICIENCY III

Patients with LAD III constitute a third, very rare group of autosomal recessive immune disorders that exhibit dysfunctional leukocyte characteristics similar to those of LAD I.[266] Studies have identified mutations in the kindlin-3 gene in this syndrome.[267] While the expression of β_2 integrins, including Mac-1 and LFA-1, are within normal values, integrin function in response to stimulation is abnormal. Specifically, neutrophils of affected patients have normal selectin-mediated rolling, but exhibit defective arrest and extravasation. Affected infants typically have delayed umbilical cord separation and altered wound healing and can develop abnormal bone density; however, severity of these complications and infections vary among individuals.[50] Stem cell transplantation is the only curative approach.

DEFECTS IN PHAGOCYTOSIS AND BACTERIAL KILLING

CHRONIC GRANULOMATOUS DISEASE

CGD is the most common inherited disorder of neutrophil dysfunction, with an incidence of 1:200,000 (reviewed by Dinauer[105] and Holland[268]). Phagocytes of individuals with CGD exhibit defects in the NADPH oxidase complex. Defects in oxidase function are associated with ineffective killing of microbes, particularly catalase positive organisms that produce low levels of hydrogen peroxide. The degree of functional oxidase activity in neutrophils depends on which of the four main subunits ($gp91^{phox}$, $gp22^{phox}$, $p47^{phox}$, $p67^{phox}$) are affected. The most common CGD variant, involving deficiency of $gp91^{phox}$ (NOX2), has an X-linked inheritance, while other subunit mutations are autosomal recessive. As with other disorders of neutrophil function, individuals with CGD are plagued by recurrent infections with bacteria and fungi. However, a hallmark of CGD is granuloma formation, which is associated with exaggerated neutrophil-mediated inflammatory responses.

The most severe CGD-related complications involve defects of $p22^{phox}$ or $p67^{phox}$, while those with the $p47^{phox}$ mutation tend to have milder symptoms. Recurrent deep-tissue and bone infections, abscesses, lymphadenopathy, and draining lymph nodes may be the presenting symptoms in infants or in young children. Infections classically involve *S. aureus* but may also include unusual bacteria and fungi. Enlargements of lymphoid tissues or organs including lymph nodes and the spleen (as well as the liver) have been reported. Chronic granulomas may lead to obstructive or inflammatory symptoms in the gastrointestinal or urinary tracts.

Diagnosis of CGD is relatively straightforward.[105] The nitroblue tetrazolium test (NBT), based on the formation of a purple formazan precipitate following neutrophil-mediated reduction of the NBT dye, historically has been the commonly used method to test for neutrophil respiratory burst activity. Quantitative measures of neutrophil respiratory burst are increasingly determined by flow cytometry, using dihydrorhodamine (DHR) expression to confirm the diagnosis. The absence of ROS production when no other abnormalities in neutrophil function are present is indicative of CGD; however, the milder $p47^{phox}$ deficiency variant may still produce a weak positive signal with testing. Prenatal diagnosis of CGD utilizes these tests combined with advances in molecular techniques to diagnose CGD mutations in fetal neutrophils or by chorionic villus sampling.[269]

Stem cell transplantation is the treatment of choice for CGD, and supportive therapy includes antibiotic and antifungal therapy.[270] Gene therapy approaches have met with mixed results, but new knowledge in this area suggests its curative potential.[271]

CHÉDIAK-HIGASHI SYNDROME

CHS is a rare autosomal recessive disorder of lysozymal storage: neutrophils exhibit giant cytoplasmic granules, a result of fusion of azurophilic granules.[272] CHS involves various abnormalities of the *CHS1/LYST* gene. Affected individuals exhibit oculocutaneous albinism (hypopigmentation of the skin, eyes and hair), a feature shared with the equally rare Hermansky-Pudlak syndrome.[273] CHS is associated with frequent soft tissue infections most commonly involving *S. aureus*, although reported pathogens include other organisms as well. Functional neutrophil defects involve abnormalities in chemotaxis and microbicidal function, although phagocytosis may be normal. CHS can involve dysfunction of lymphocytes and platelets as well as neurologic abnormalities, particularly peripheral neuropathies.[273] Management of associated infections includes aggressive antibiotic therapy and surgical drainage. Neurologic symptoms are progressive; however, stem cell transplantation resolves the hematologic and immune abnormalities.

OTHER INHERITED DISORDERS

MYELOPEROXIDASE DEFICIENCY

Deficiency of the neutrophil granule MPO is an inherited autosomal recessive disorder caused by missense mutations.[116] It is a relatively common phagocyte disorder, with an incidence of 1:2000 to 1:4000. Although this disorder is generally considered to be benign, neutrophil killing of certain *Candida* species may be impaired in certain individuals.[274]

RAC2 MUTATION

The Rho family of GTPases include guanosine triphosphate proteins that are important in multiple signal transduction pathways.[275] Deficiency of Rac2, associated with defects of neutrophil adhesion and migration, has been reported.[275,276] Both children presented with neonatal omphalitis associated with neutrophilia and absence of pus. Neutrophils exhibited functional defects in chemotaxis, migration, F-actin formation, and the respiratory burst (NADPH oxidase activity). Both children were afflicted with repetitive, serious bacterial infections; neutrophil functions and clinical status improved following stem cell transplantation.

MST1 DEFICIENCY

Several patients with a loss of function mutation of the gene mammalian sterile 20-like kinase 1 (*MST1*, also named STK4) have been described.[277,278] These patients have a complex immunologic deficiency disorder affecting adaptive and innate immune functions. Patients presented in the first year of life with recurrent bacterial, viral, and/or fungal infections mostly affecting the lung and the skin. Some patients also showed human papillomavirus infections (cutaneous warts). Using *MST1* deficient mice, Kurz and colleagues subsequently demonstrated that neutrophils of *MST1* knockout mice showed a severe impairment in neutrophil recruitment into inflamed tissue at the level of vascular basement membrane penetration.[68] This process is dependent on *MST1*, which controls the necessary mobilization of intracellular vesicles containing neutrophil elastase and the integrins VLA3 and VLA6 to the neutrophil surface.

NEUTROPHILS AND ADAPTIVE IMMUNITY

The primary and critical role of neutrophils as a first line of defense in protecting the host from extracellular microbes is firmly established. However, mounting evidence also points to the diversification of neutrophil functions and phenotypes, a heterogeneity that contributes to immune pathophysiology.[279] A discussion of neutrophils would be incomplete without addressing their increasingly appreciated contributions to immune responses against viruses and intracellular pathogens in collaboration with the adaptive immune system. Neutrophils can interact with a variety of both innate and adaptive immune cells to amplify protective and inflammatory responses. Several elegant reviews of this subject have been published.[280-282]

NEUTROPHIL INTERACTIONS WITH ADAPTIVE IMMUNE CELLS

Mounting evidence indicates a supportive role for neutrophils in the education and function of the adaptive immune system in addition to their critical role in innate immunity.[282,283] Neutrophils invade the marginal zones in the spleen during fetal life, a process augmented shortly after birth following exposure to commensal bacteria.[284] These splenic neutrophils interact with marginal zone B cells to function as B helper cells, including the promotion of antibody production in a T-cell-independent manner; these cells have been aptly named *B-cell helper neutrophils*.[285] Pertinently, individuals with congenital neutropenia have lower serum levels of Ig, underscoring the importance of neutrophils to humoral immunity.

Neutrophil interactions with T cells are incompletely defined, although studies suggest a relationship that may be either activating or inhibitory.[286] Neutrophils can directly present antigens to T cells[287] as well as activate antigen-specific T cells.[288] Neutrophil actions on DC can indirectly modulate T-cell immune function (reviewed by Yang and colleagues[289] and van Gisbergen and colleagues[290]). Neutrophils release factors such as IL-12 to promote the DC maturation and activation necessary to induce T-cell responses. Conversely, a subset of myeloid cells with neutrophil properties, MDSCs, can limit T-cell function during systemic inflammation or infection.[291] Cord blood contains higher number of MDSCs relative to adult blood, which could contribute to maternal-fetal tolerance by dampening T-cell responses[206] or promote neonatal antibacterial host defense mechanisms by suppressing T-cell proliferation.[175]

Neutrophils have been shown to potentiate inflammatory responses through their interactions with T cells. Co-localization of neutrophils and the pro-inflammatory T-cell subset, Th17, has been observed at various inflammatory tissue sites.[292,293] Neutrophils release chemokines that specifically attract Th17 cells.[294] Reciprocally, Th17 cells indirectly recruit neutrophils by releasing IL-17, a cytokine that induces the release of neutrophil-activating IL-8 and G-CSF from environmental cells.[295] In addition to activating neutrophils and potentiating their function, the IL-17 induced release of G-CSF promotes bone marrow production of neutrophils, augmenting neonatal neutrophil pools.[12] Conversely, neonatal neutrophils activated by Group B *Streptococcus* were shown to promote the in vitro propagation of Th17 cells.[296] Studies in infant mice born after antenatal inflammation and in human neonates exposed to chorioamnionitis have shown enrichment of Th17 populations that parallel neutrophil prominence.[297-299] Furthermore, a unique T-cell subset in human neonates, rare in adults, may directly attract and act on neutrophils through the release of IL-8.[300]

NEUTROPHILS, T CELLS, AND INFECTION

Neutrophil-lymphocyte interactions are important in the host response to infections. Neutrophil infiltration of infected tissues is accompanied by the recruitment and activation of DC, a process that is critical to the formation of protective Th1 responses.[301] Infected neutrophils, through their expression of MHC-I and the co-stimulatory molecules CD80 and CD86, can also directly present antigens to $CD8^+$ T cells to promote antiviral activity.[302] Lung infections with respiratory syncytial virus or influenza are associated with robust neutrophil responses that can activate virus specific $CD8^+$ T-cells.[303,304] The neutrophil mediated inflammatory microenvironment of infected tissue may also induce a "bystander response" through the cytokine-mediated activation of nonspecific T cells.[305] Neutrophils have also been shown to migrate to lymph nodes and the spleen during infection-induced inflammation.[306,307] Lymphoid recruitment of neutrophils may occur via migration from the blood through high endothelial venules or by way of the lymphatic system.

Neutrophils can counteract the effects of viruses, such as HIV-1, on T-cell infectivity through NET formation and extrusion of extracellular DNA.[308] Neutrophils can also assist specific antiviral actions of T cells.[302,309] Neutrophil-depleted mice exhibit pathologic immune responses to viral infections, findings that highlight the key modulatory role for neutrophils in this context.[304,310] Conversely, granulocytic MDSCs may limit immune-mediated injury associated with viral infection through the arginase-dependent suppression of T cells.[311]

Neutrophils play a critical role in protecting the host against bacteria (elegantly reviewed by Nauseef and Borregaard[1]). However, in cases of ineffective microbicidal killing, ingested bacteria can utilize neutrophils as "Trojan horses" as a means of systemic dissemination and transport to lymphatic tissue.[312,313] The inflammatory tissue infiltration of neutrophils is primarily associated with the recruitment of γδT cells, a subset that can amplify inflammatory responses through crosstalk with neutrophils; however, conversely, neutrophils may suppress γδT cell function.[314,315] Neutrophils also appear to be critical for the development of protective Th1 responses to infection.[316]

Severe infection and sepsis have been associated with suppression of immune responses.[317] Under these conditions, certain neutrophils, particularly granulocytic MDSCs, have been shown to express arginase, which may suppress T-cell function through the depletion of L-arginine.[318] The release of IFNγ during sepsis may induce the expression of PD-L1 on neutrophils and subsequent T-cell apoptosis.[319]

CONCLUSION

In summary, neonates exhibit a variety of physiologic alterations in neutrophil function that are influenced by both gestational age and postnatal maturity. Functional neutrophil abnormalities that suppress host protective mechanisms in neonates may be instrumental in modulating neonatal susceptibility to infection, especially when the host is delivered prematurely. In addition, mounting evidence indicates an important role for suppressive neutrophil subsets in modulating immune responses that can increase risk for infection. In contrast, neutrophils of neonates (relative to those of adults) can exhibit exaggerated inflammatory responses to infectious stimuli, or they can amplify interactions with adaptive immune cells that may be pathogenic for disorders associated with chronic inflammation, such as BPD and NEC. Intrauterine or postnatal exposure to an inflammatory environment may additionally augment abnormalities in neonatal neutrophils that not only affect innate immune function, but also could influence the "education" of the adaptive immune system, with potentially lifelong effects.

 A complete reference list is available at www.ExpertConsult.com.

SELECT REFERENCES

2. Nemeth T, Sperandio M, Mocsai A. Neutrophils as emerging therapeutic targets. *Nat Rev Drug Discov*. 2020;19(4):253–275.
3. Dinauer MC. Inflammatory consequences of inherited disorders affecting neutrophil function. *Blood*. 2019;(20):2130–2139.
5. Christensen RD. Neutrophil kinetics in the fetus and neonate. *Am J Pediatr Hematol Oncol*. 1989;11(2):215–223.
10. Evrard M, Kwok IWH, Chong SZ, et al. Developmental analysis of bone marrow neutrophils reveals populations specialized in expansion, trafficking, and effector functions. *Immunity*. 2018;48(2):364–379.
12. Deshmukh HS, Liu Y, Menkiti OR, et al. The microbiota regulates neutrophil homeostasis and host resistance to Escherichia coli K1 sepsis in neonatal mice. *Nat Med*. 2014;20(5):524–530.
39. Wennekamp J, Henneke P. Induction and termination of inflammatory signaling in group B streptococcal sepsis. *Immunol Rev*. 2008;225:114–127.
46. Sperandio M, Quackenbush EJ, Sushkova N, et al. Ontogenetic regulation of leukocyte recruitment in mouse yolk sac vessels. *Blood*. 2013;121(21):e118–e128.
47. Nussbaum C, Gloning A, Pruenster M, et al. Neutrophil and endothelial adhesive function during human fetal ontogeny. *J Leukoc Biol*. 2013;93(2):175–184.
48. Ulas T, Pirr S, Fehlhaber B, et al. S100-alarmin-induced innate immune programming protects newborn infants from sepsis. *Nat Immunol*. 2017;18(6):622–632.
49. Margraf A, Ley K, Zarbock A. Neutrophil recruitment: from model systems to tissue-specific patterns. *Trends Immunol*. 2019;2019(7):613–634.
52. Filippi MD. Neutrophil transendothelial migration: updates and new perspectives. *Blood*. 2019;2019(20):2149–2158.
56. McEver RP. Selectins: initiators of leucocyte adhesion and signalling at the vascular wall. *Cardiovasc Res*. 2015;107(3):331–339.
79. McEvoy LT, Zakem-Cloud H, Tosi MF. Total cell content of CR3 (CD11b/CD18) and LFA-1 (CD11a/CD18) in neonatal neutrophils: relationship to gestational age. *Blood*. 1996;87(9):3929–3933.
82. Mariscalco MM, Vergara W, Mei J, Smith EO, Smith CW. Mechanisms of decreased leukocyte localization in the developing host. *Am J Physiol Heart Circ Physiol*. 2002;282(2):H636–H644.
94. Baehner RL. Microbe ingestion and killing by neutrophils: normal mechanisms and abnormalities. *Clin Haematol*. 1975;4(3):609–633.
100. Carr R. Neutrophil production and function in newborn infants. *Br J Haematol*. 2000;110(1):18–28.
101. Lawrence SM, Corriden R, Nizet V. Age-appropriate functions and dysfunctions of the neonatal neutrophil. *Front Pediatr*. 2017;5:23.
105. Dinauer MC. Disorders of neutrophil function: an overview. *Methods Mol Biol*. 2014;1124:501–515.
112. Masgrau-Alsina S, Sperandio M, Rohwedder I. Neutrophil recruitment and intracellular vesicle transport: a short overview. *Eur J Clin Invest*. 2020;50:e13237.
114. Hager M, Cowland JB, Borregaard N. Neutrophil granules in health and disease. *J Intern Med*. 2010;268(1):25–34.
128. Levy O. Innate immunity of the newborn: basic mechanisms and clinical correlates. *Nat Rev Immunol*. 2007;7(5):379–390.
134. Linden JR, Kunkel D, Laforce-Nesbitt SS, Bliss JM. The role of galectin-3 in phagocytosis of Candida albicans and Candida parapsilosis by human neutrophils. *Cell Microbiol*. 2013;15(7):1127–1142.
138. Brinkmann V, Reichard U, Goosmann C, et al. Neutrophil extracellular traps kill bacteria. *Science*. 2004;303(5663):1532–1535.
139. Yipp BG, Kubes P. NETosis: how vital is it? *Blood*. 2013;122(16):2784–2794.
143. Yost CC, Cody MJ, Harris ES, et al. Impaired neutrophil extracellular trap (NET) formation: a novel innate immune deficiency of human neonates. *Blood*. 2009;113(25):6419–6427.
146. Yost CC, Schwertz H, Cody MJ, et al. Neonatal NET-inhibitory factor and related peptides inhibit neutrophil extracellular trap formation. *J Clin Invest*. 2016;126(10):3783–3798.
147. Vincent D, Klinke M, Eschenburg G, et al. NEC is likely a NETs dependent process and markers of NETosis are predictive of NEC in mice and humans. *Sci Rep*. 2018;8(1):12612.
152. Matute-Bello G, Martin TR. Science review: apoptosis in acute lung injury. *Crit Care*. 2003;7(5):355–358.
154. Liew PX, Kubes P. The neutrophil's role during health and disease. *Physiol Rev*. 2019;99(2):1223–1248.
159. Cabrini M, Nahmod K, Geffner J. New insights into the mechanisms controlling neutrophil survival. *Curr Opin Hematol*. 2010;17(1):31–35.
170. Kotecha S, Mildner RJ, Prince LR, et al. The role of neutrophil apoptosis in the resolution of acute lung injury in newborn infants. *Thorax*. 2003;58(11):961–967.
179. Jobe AH, Ikegami M. Mechanisms initiating lung injury in the preterm. *Early Hum Dev*. 1998;53(1):81–94.
187. Malaeb S, Dammann O. Fetal inflammatory response and brain injury in the preterm newborn. *J Child Neurol*. 2009;24(9):1119–1126.
206. Rieber N, Gille C, Kostlin N, et al. Neutrophilic myeloid-derived suppressor cells in cord blood modulate innate and adaptive immune responses. *Clin Exp Immunol*. 2013;174(1):45–52.
209. Dowling DJ, Levy O. Ontogeny of early life immunity. *Trends Immunol*. 2014;35(7):299–310.
211. He YM, Li X, Perego M, et al. Transitory presence of myeloid-derived suppressor cells in neonates is critical for control of inflammation. *Nat Med*. 2018;24(2):224–231.
213. Engle WD, Rosenfeld CR, Mouzinho A, Risser RC, Zeray F, Sanchez PJ. Circulating neutrophils in septic preterm neonates: comparison of two reference ranges. *Pediatrics*. 1997;99(3):E10.
214. Manroe BL, Weinberg AG, Rosenfeld CR, Browne R. The neonatal blood count in health and disease. I. Reference values for neutrophilic cells. *J Pediatr*. 1979;95(1):89–98.
215. Mouzinho A, Rosenfeld CR, Sanchez PJ, Risser R. Revised reference ranges for circulating neutrophils in very-low-birth-weight neonates. *Pediatrics*. 1994;94(1):76–82.
216. Koenig JM, Christensen RD. Incidence, neutrophil kinetics, and natural history of neonatal neutropenia associated with maternal hypertension. *N Engl J Med*. 1989;321(9):557–562.
230. Skokowa J, Dale DC, Touw IP, Zeidler C, Welte K. Severe congenital neutropenias. *Nat Rev Dis Primers*. 2017;3:17032.
236. Kostmann R. Infantile genetic agranulocytosis; agranulocytosis infantilis hereditaria. *Acta Paediatr Suppl*. 1956;45(suppl 105):1–78.
242. Black LV, Maheshwari A. Immune-mediated neutropenia in the neonate. *NeoReviews*. 2009;10:446–453.
248. Christensen RD, Rothstein G. Pitfalls in the interpretation of leukocyte counts of newborn infants. *Am J Clin Pathol*. 1979;72(4):608–611.
258. Melvan JN, Bagby GJ, Welsh DA, Nelson S, Zhang P. Neonatal sepsis and neutrophil insufficiencies. *Int Rev Immunol*. 2010;29(3):315–348.
260. Munyaka PM, Khafipour E, Ghia JE. External influence of early childhood establishment of gut microbiota and subsequent health implications. *Front Pediatr*. 2014;2:109.
281. Mocsai A. Diverse novel functions of neutrophils in immunity, inflammation, and beyond. *J Exp Med*. 2013;210(7):1283–1299.
298. Rito DC, Viehl LT, Buchanan PM, Haridas S, Koenig JM. Augmented Th17-type immune responses in preterm neonates exposed to histologic chorioamnionitis. *Pediatr Res*. 2017;81(4):639–645.
299. Jackson CM, Wells CB, Tabangin ME, Meinzen-Derr J, Jobe AH, Chougnet CA. Pro-inflammatory immune responses in leukocytes of premature infants exposed to maternal chorioamnionitis or funisitis. *Pediatr Res*. 2017;81(2):384–390.
300. Gibbons D, Fleming P, Virasami A, et al. Interleukin-8 (CXCL8) production is a signatory T cell effector function of human newborn infants. *Nat Med*. 2014;2014(10):1206–1210.
317. Hotchkiss RS, Monneret G, Payen D. Sepsis-induced immunosuppression: from cellular dysfunctions to immunotherapy. *Nat Rev Immunol*. 2013;13(12):862–874.

120 The Complement System of the Fetus and Newborn

Melvin Berger

INTRODUCTION

The complement system is composed of more than 30 soluble proteins, cell surface regulatory factors, and receptors that work together to accomplish a wide variety of functions.[1-3] These are important not only in host defense and inflammatory responses but also in normal physiologic homeostasis. By facilitating proper disposal of apoptotic cells and antigens from infectious agents, complement plays an important role in preventing autoimmune and immune complex deposition diseases. During infection, complement fragments rapidly activate and attract leukocytes and macrophages and provide opsonins that facilitate clearance and killing of invading organisms. Complement also bridges the innate and adaptive immune systems in both directions. Besides its traditionally understood roles in amplifying the effector functions of antibodies, it also has important influences on antigen presentation and B-cell activation, giving it a key role in the afferent limb of antibody responses. As expected of a system with so many different physiologic activities, disorders of complement can have wide-ranging effects.[2]

Complement activation involves a series of elegant biochemical processes by which individual circulating proteins are transformed into complex multisubunit enzymes, come together to form multichain membrane channels that insert into cells from the outside, provide address tags that direct trafficking of a wide variety of targets, and stimulate vigorous inflammatory responses. These transformations are mainly achieved by limited proteolytic cleavage and/or conformational changes.[3,4] At each stage of activation, newly revealed conformations are accompanied by new enzyme activities and/or markedly increased affinity for other components or cell surface receptors. Newly formed enzymes can cleave many molecules of the next component in the sequence, providing potent forward amplification. For this reason, the activation pathways are considered "cascades," in analogy with the cascades of the clotting or contact activation systems. Understanding how the complement proteins are activated is the first step towards understanding this system.

ACTIVATION PATHWAYS

Complement activation can be initiated by three major pathways. Because the complement system was originally discovered as a set of heat-labile serum proteins that could lyse erythrocytes sensitized with antibody, the antibody-dependent or "classical" pathway has been best studied. Although it is phylogenetically the newest pathway, its activation is easiest to describe and is presented first (Fig. 120.1).

THE CLASSICAL PATHWAY

C1, its first component, is composed of 22 peptide chains arranged into three subcomponents termed *C1q, r,* and *s.* C1q itself contains six sets of trimers, each of which has a collagen-like stalk and a globular head[5,6] that can bind the Fc domain of immunoglobulin (Ig) G or IgM. Electron micrographs show the six stalks together in parallel and the globular heads all at the same end, giving the appearance of a bunch of tulips. Around the bunch of stalks are wrapped two molecules each of C1r and C1s, which are latent proteases.[7] Classical pathway activation can be initiated when two or more of the six globular Ig-binding heads become attached to Fc domains of antigen-bound IgM or IgG molecules, but will be most efficient when all six are engaged by Fc domains in close proximity.[8] Engagement of the heads of C1q induces internal rearrangements, leading to activation of latent proteolytic activity of C1r, which then cleaves and activates the C1s subunits.[5,6] Because of the requirement for two or more of the globular heads of C1q to be engaged for activation to begin, IgM, which has five Fc domains attached together, is a very efficient activator of the classical pathway. In contrast, many molecules of IgG must be bound to the surface of a target cell or bacterium for two or more IgG molecules to be close enough together to bridge a single C1q. The other classes of Igs—IgD, IgA, and IgE—do not bind to C1q and hence do not activate the classical pathway. C1s, when activated, has proteolytic activity and can also cleave synthetic esters in vitro; hence it is often referred to as *C1 esterase*. Its physiologic role is to carry out limited proteolytic cleavage of the next two components in the reaction sequence: C4 and C2.[1,4-7] (The components were numbered in the order in which they were discovered rather than the order in which they act; hence C4 comes before C2.[1,4]) C1s cleaves the largest of the three chains of C4 at a single site, liberating a 9-kDa peptide (C4a) and leaving the larger fragment (C4b) with a transient ability to form a covalent bond with the target.[7] The C4b takes on a new conformation in which it can bind C2 and promote its cleavage by C1s as well. Again, a small fragment is released and diffuses away, and the conformation and activity of the larger fragment are changed. With C2, the larger fragment is called *C2a*, which also has a newly exposed proteolytic active site. Together with C4b, which can also hold onto a C3 molecule, C2a forms an enzyme that can cleave and activate C3. This C4bC2a complex is therefore called *C3 convertase*.[1-4,7] This classical pathway C3 convertase, composed of one molecule of C4b covalently attached to the target and loosely bound to one molecule of C2a,[7] is capable of cleaving many molecules of C3. C3 is homologous with C4, and on cleavage, its larger fragment (C3b) also transiently acquires the ability to bind covalently to the Ig molecule, surface, or target on which activation is occurring.[3,4,9,10] Many molecules of C3 can be cleaved by a single convertase, but the convertase eventually loses activity when the C2a subunit diffuses or is pushed away, and/or if C4b is degraded. Some of the newly cleaved C3b molecules diffuse away before they can bind to the surface. Many others bind to the surface at short distances around the convertase; these may serve to opsonize (facilitate phagocytosis of) the target. Some of the C3b molecules may deposit close enough to C4b2a to join with it and provide a binding site for C5 molecules, which will be cleaved by the proteolytic active site on C2a.[7,11] Thus the complex C4b2a3b serves as the *classical pathway C5 convertase*.[11] Like C4 and C3, the cleavage of C5 liberates a small fragment (C5a), but unlike C4 and C3, C5 cannot form a covalent bond with the surface. The larger fragment, C5b, however, undergoes a conformational change that allows it to bind to C6. This starts formation of the lipophilic membrane attack complex (MAC), discussed later.

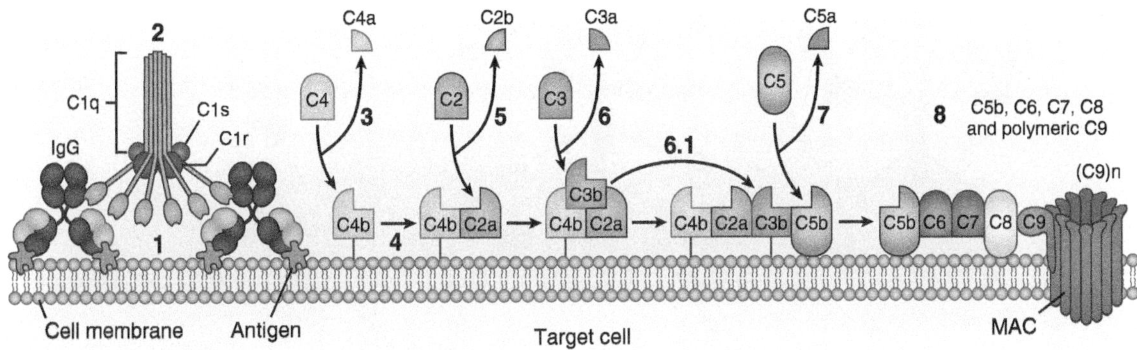

Fig. 120.1 Detailed schematic representation of the classical complement pathway, showing initiation by binding of the *C1q* component of *C1* to the Fc domains of two or more immunoglobulin G *(IgG)* antibody molecules bound to antigen on the surface of a target cell. The numbers in bold indicate sequential steps that are involved in the activation of each of the components leading to the final lytic event carried out by the membrane attack complex *(MAC)*. (Some sources now use a revised nomenclature for the fragment of *C2*, in which *C2a* is the small fragment which diffuses away and *C2b* is the larger fragment that binds with *C4b* and acts in the *C3* convertase, *C4b2b*.)

1. Binding of multiple IgGs or multiple Fabs of IgM to antigen.
2. Binding of C1q to multiple Fcs of IgG or IgM activates C1r, which activates C1s.
3. Cleavage of C4 by C1s. C4b becomes covalently attached to target.
4. C2 binds to C4b.
5. C2 bound to C4b is cleaved by C1s. C2a remains with C4b, while C2b diffuses away.
6. C3 binds to C4b2a, the classical pathway C3 convertase. C2a cleaves C3, and C3b becomes covalently attached to target.

6.1. Some C3b molecules may remain associated with C4b2a, forming the C5 convertase: C4b2a3b.

7. C5 is cleaved by the convertase. C5a, a potent chemoattractant and anaphylotoxin, diffuses away. C5b is lipophilic and associates with lipids in the cell membrane.
8. C6, C7, C8, and multiple molecules of C9 associate sequentially and form the membrane attack complex, a pore in the membrane lined by unfolded C9 molecules. Note that these steps do not involve enzymatic cleavage. (Modified From Bellanti JA. *Immunology IV: Clinical Applications in Health and Disease*. Bethesda, MD: I Care Press; 2012. Fig. 4.2)

THE LECTIN PATHWAY

Activation by this route begins with the protein *mannan-binding lectin* (MBL) (Fig. 120.2, *center*). Like C1q, MBL is a multimer of collagen-like stalks, each composed of three protein chains that also form a globular binding domain at one end.[12,13] In the case of MBL, however, the binding sites recognize polysaccharides containing mannose, hence its name. Because MBL, C1q, and other similar molecules have collagen-like domains and lectin-like binding sites for polysaccharides, they are often considered to be members of the same family of collagen-like lectins, or *collectins*.[14] Lung surfactant proteins A and D are also members of this collectin family.

Different isoforms of MBL may contain between two and eight of the basic trimer subunits. Because many bacteria and fungi are coated with mannose-containing polysaccharides, the MBL pathway is considered part of the innate immune system, as is the alternative pathway, which is discussed later. Phylogenetically, the alternative and lectin pathways likely originated earlier than the classical pathway. In that sense, C1q may be seen as an adaptor protein that allowed this important part of the innate immune system to be recruited to enhance the activity of antibodies produced by the adaptive (or cognate) immune system. The ability of the lectin and alternative pathways to activate complement in the absence of antibody may be particularly important in the neonate, in whom the adaptive immune system is immature. Similarly, early in the course of infections, before antibodies and other specific effector mechanisms of the adaptive immune system are brought to bear, the lectin and alternative pathways provide an important innate system for distinguishing non-self from self. Like the binding of C1q to the Fc regions of IgG or IgM, the binding of MBL to mannose-containing polysaccharides leads to activation of latent protease subunits. In this pathway, the proteases that are analogous to C1r and C1s are termed *MBL-associated serine proteases (MASPs)*.[7,13,15] Two major MASPs have been identified and may circulate in the plasma as a large complex together with MBL and other minor protein components. When MBL is engaged with polysaccharides, MASP1 becomes activated and cleaves MASP2.[7,13,15] Both MASP1 and MASP2 have been shown to be capable of cleaving C3, but some studies suggest that they actually act more like C1r and C1s in cleaving C4 and C2.[7,13,15] Just as in the classical pathway, C2a and C4b generated by MASPs go on to form a C3 convertase, and the addition of a molecule of C3b confers C5 convertase activity on the complex.[11] The physiologic importance of the lectin pathway is illustrated by an increased susceptibility to infections and also to autoimmune diseases like systemic lupus erythematosus (SLE) in patients with MBL deficiency.[16]

THE ALTERNATIVE PATHWAY

The alternative pathway, also known as the *properdin pathway*, shares with the lectin pathway the ability to activate complement without antibody (see Fig. 120.2, *right*). Alternative pathway activation is initiated by C3b, which may be formed by one of the other pathways, by nonspecific proteolytic cleavage of C3, or after the spontaneous activation of C3 by water molecules[1,3,17–19] (see later). Most investigators visualize native C3 in the circulation as a kind of coiled spring, which holds a unique structure called a *thioester* in an internal hydrophobic pocket.[3,10,18,19] This highly unusual chemical structure is formed by the binding of a thiol on the side chain of a cysteine residue with the carboxyl on the side chain of glutamate three residues away in the largest (α) polypeptide chain.[9,10]

```
                                            H              OH
                                            |              |
S--------------C=O                          S              C=O
|              |                            |              |
-Gly-Cys-Gly-Glu-Glu-Asn-Met    -Gly-Cys-Gly-Glu-Glu-Asn-Met
```

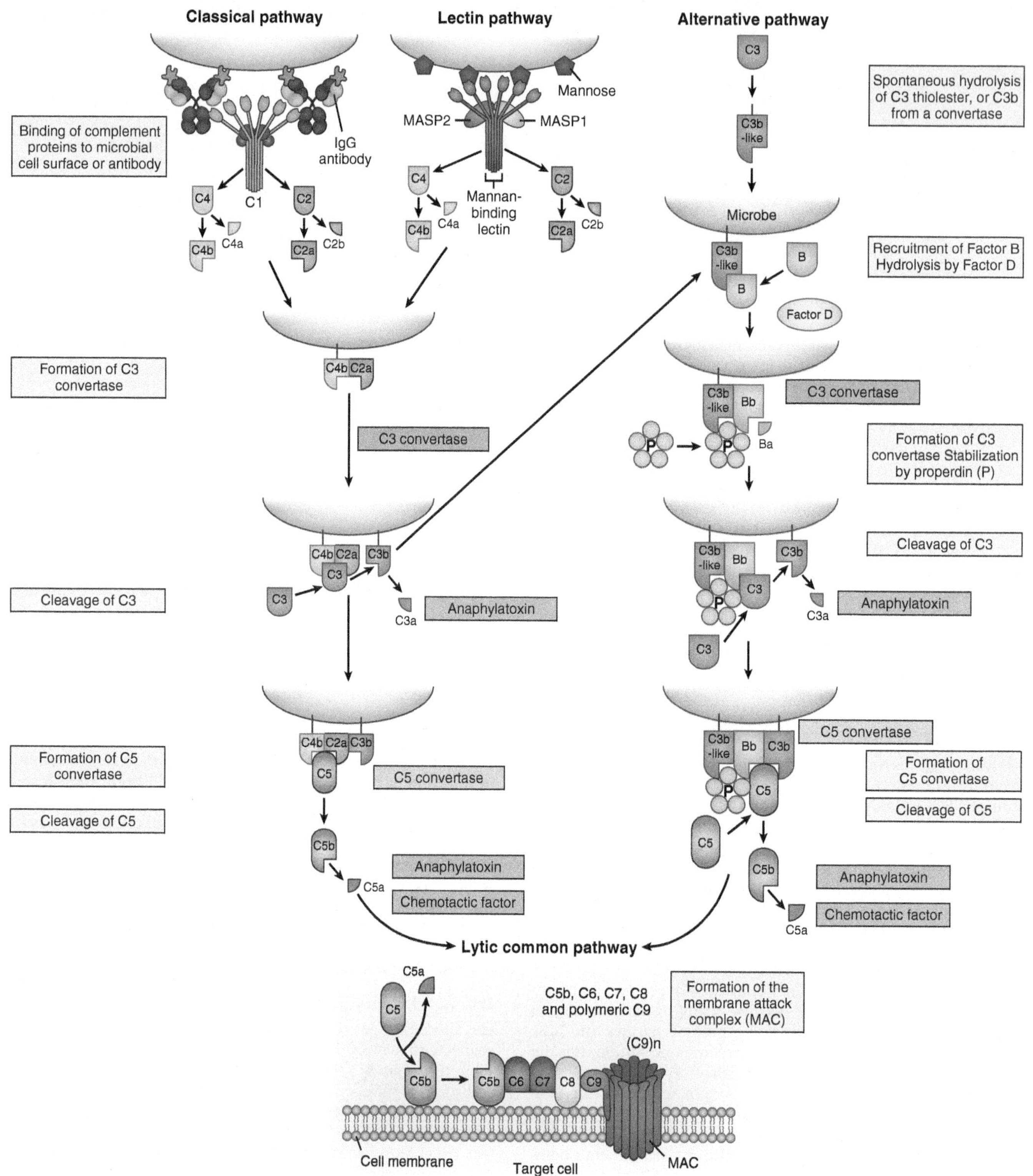

Fig. 120.2 Diagram of complement activation drawn to emphasize homology between different pathways. The classical pathway *(left)* is activated when C1q in the C1 complex binds to antigen-bound immunoglobulin *(Ig)* G or M. C1r then activates C1s. The lectin pathway *(middle)* is activated when the mannan-binding lectin *(MBL)*-MBL associated serine protease *(MASP)* complex binds to mannose residues of a polysaccharide. MASP1 activates MASP2. C1s or MASP2 cleave C4 and C2, which form a C3 convertase, C4b2a. The inactive C4a and C2b fragments diffuse away. The convertase cleaves C3 into C3a, an anaphylotoxin that diffuses, and the major fragment C3b, which attaches covalently to the target. The alternative pathway *(right)* is activated when Factor B binds to "C3b-like"-C3 or to C3b deposited by one of the other pathways. Factor B is analogous to C2- when bound to C3b or "C3b-like" C3, Factor D cleaves B just as C1s or MASPs cleave C2. The alternative pathway C3 convertase is thus C3bBb, which is homologous with C4b2a. Because it can be initiated by C3b generated by the other pathways, the alternative pathway is often described as an "amplification loop." Activation of C5 and formation of the membrane attack complex *(MAC)*: Addition of another molecule of C3b to either convertase provides a binding site for C5 and changes the C3 convertase into a C5 convertase. C5 can be cleaved by the classical/lectin pathway convertase C4b2a3b or the alternative pathway convertase C3bBb3b (shown here in the form stabilized by properdin, *P*). The smaller fragment, C5a, is an anaphylotoxin and chemoattractant that diffuses. The larger fragment binds to C6, forming a lipophilic complex that may insert into cell membranes. C5b6 binds C7 and then C8 without proteolytic cleavage, and this complex activates and binds multiple molecules of C9, forming the complete MAC. (Modified From Bellanti JA. *Immunology IV: Clinical Applications in Health and Disease*. Bethesda, MD; I Care Press; 2012:fig. 4-1)

C4 and α_2-macroglobulin also contain this internal thioester. Cleavage of a short peptide (C3a) from the amino-terminal end of the α chain, distant from the thioester, causes conformational changes in which the coiled spring is released, the thioester is transiently exposed, and the carbon on the glutamate can transfer one of its bonds from the sulfur of the cysteine to another acceptor.[1,3,4,9,10] It is the ability of C3b and C4b to transfer a carbon bond to a hydroxyl or amino group on another protein or to a sugar chain that allows covalent attachment. If the transfer to another protein or sugar does not occur within milliseconds, the bond will transfer to the hydroxyl group of a water molecule, whose other hydrogen atom will bind to the sulfur of the cysteine to create a free thiol (–SH).

Transfer of the internal thioester is greatly accelerated by the conformational changes that follow cleavage of the protein chain.[3,18,20] However, water molecules may occasionally penetrate into the hydrophobic pocket and hydrolyze this bond even in intact molecules of C3. Once that occurs, the same sequence of conformational changes in the protein chains will follow,[18-20] even though no cleavage fragment has been removed. Thus, the thioester can be visualized as an internal latch, which keeps the spring coiled. Hydrolysis of the thioester by water and the subsequent conformational changes occur spontaneously at a slow continuous rate; hence there is always some basal rate of generation of C3 molecules with hydrolyzed thioester bonds. These molecules have a conformation similar to that of C3b and are thus called *C3b-like C3 molecules*.[1,3,4,17] This constant low-grade "tick-over" of C3 into C3b-like molecules[19] may be thought of as the idling of a car engine—the system is always running at a slow rate and is ready to accelerate at any time. This allows the alternative pathway to play an important role in recognition of foreign invaders as part of the innate immune system and also allows it to play a role in eliminating dead or damaged body cells. However, it also means that the system must be carefully regulated, as discussed in Control of Complement Activation.

C3 and C4 are highly homologous. Similarly, the alternative and lectin pathway C3 convertases are also highly homologous with the classical pathway convertase and are formed in an analogous way.[1,7,17] Activation of the alternative pathway can be initiated when a molecule of "C3b-like C3," or C3b itself, which acts like C4b in the classical pathway, binds with a molecule called *factor B*, which is homologous with C2.[1,17] The factor B is then cleaved by factor D, a proteolytic enzyme that seems to be constitutively activated by a third MASP.[21] Factor D can act on factor B only when it is held in the proper configuration by C3b. Cleavage of factor B by D is analogous to cleavage of C2 by C1s, but the large fragment is named Bb.[1,7,17] Like C2, factor B has latent protease activity.[7] The Bb resulting from cleavage by factor D has its proteolytic active site exposed and can cleave C3 and C5. The C3b or C3b-like C3 molecule that initiated the pathway also serves the same role as C4b in the classical pathway C3 convertase, that is, holding additional molecules of C3 substrate in place, so they can be cleaved by Bb. Just as in the classical pathway, some of the newly cleaved C3b molecules will deposit sufficiently close to the C3bBb enzyme to join with it as a subunit that provides a binding site for C5, which can then be cleaved by Bb. Thus, the addition of this new C3b molecule changes the alternative and lectin pathway C3 convertase C3bBb into the *alternative pathway C5 convertase* C3bBb3b.[7,11,17]

The alternative pathway depends on an additional molecule called *properdin*, or *factor P*, which is not found in the classical or lectin pathways.[1,22,23] The discovery of this molecule led to the elucidation of the alternative pathway, so it is sometimes called the *properdin pathway*.[22] P stabilizes the alternative pathway convertases, which would otherwise lose activity when Bb, with its proteolytic active site, diffuses away.[1,17,23] Thus, surfaces or targets that favor binding of P favor activation of the alternative pathway.[23] Stabilization of the convertase may also occur pathologically in the presence of C3 nephritic factor, an autoantibody with properdin-like properties found in some patients with glomerulonepritis[24] and in patients with gain-of-function mutations, which confer increased stability on the convertase (see below).

ACTIVATION OF C5 AND FORMATION OF THE MEMBRANE ATTACK COMPLEX (MAC)

One of the most dramatic features of complement activation is the conversion of individual, water-soluble, circulating proteins into a large multichain lipophilic assembly that can insert itself into plasma membranes,[1,4] forming a pore that spans both leaflets, compromising its barrier function. Insertion of just one of these channels into an erythrocyte allows enough water to rush into the cell to cause explosive lysis. This ability of a heat-labile fraction of plasma proteins to lyse erythrocytes sensitized by heat-stabile antibodies was recognized more than 100 years ago and led to the elucidation of the complement reaction sequence, because the liberated hemoglobin provided a convenient end point for assays. Arguably, however, complement-mediated lysis is not the most important function of the complement system in vivo, because nucleated cells can internalize or shed bits of membrane bearing C5 through C9 complexes. The transmembrane pore formed by the assembly of C5 through C9 is called the *MAC* and its formation begins with activation of C5 by proteolytic cleavage.

Regardless of the pathway by which C5 is cleaved, the remaining steps of activation of C6 through C9 follow the same sequence (see Fig. 120.2). Unlike the early activation pathways, however, activation beyond C5 and formation of the MAC do not involve proteolytic cleavages. C5 does not contain the same internal thioester as its homologues C3 and C4, and C5b cannot bind covalently to the target. However, just after cleavage, C5b gains the ability to interact with C6. Binding with C6 stabilizes and increases the lipophilicity of C5b, and the C5b6 complex can insert into lipid membranes at some distance from the C5 convertase or even on nearby cells.[25] This phenomenon can lead to *bystander lysis* of normal cells in the vicinity of soluble immune complexes or bacteria on which complement is being activated. C5b6 can also bind a molecule of C7. The complex of C5b67 is highly lipophilic and, if formed in the fluid phase, will rapidly insert into plasma membranes, where it serves as a binding site for C8. Binding of C8 to C5b67 creates a complex that can disrupt the phospholipids of target cell membranes and can cause slow lysis of erythrocytes, even without the addition of C9. The C5b8 complex also induces conformational changes in soluble C9 molecules.[26,27] These include elongation and unfolding of the C9 molecules, exposing previously protected hydrophobic regions and potential sites for disulfide bonds between chains.[26,27] In turn, additional C9 molecules change conformation, polymerize and join the complex. Isolated C9 can also be induced to undergo these conformational changes and polymerize in vitro under carefully defined chemical conditions. C9 polymers may contain up to 12 molecules linked in dimers by disulfide bonds. Electron micrographs of these C9 polymers look very similar to MACs isolated from cells or artificial membranes that have been attacked by complement. They appear like grommets or donuts, with a top rim 15 to 20 nm in diameter sitting above a slightly narrower cylinder 15 to 16 nm in length, which span the plasma membrane.[27,28] The conformational changes that accompany C9 polymerization are recognized by monoclonal antibodies that do not bind to native, circulating C9 molecules.[29] These antibodies to the C9 "neoantigen" formed upon activation may be used to identify sites of MAC deposition in tissue sections.[29] Antibody sandwich assays against the soluble C5b-9 complex (sC5b-9) are now widely used in enzyme-linked immunosorbent assays of complement activity.

CONTROL OF COMPLEMENT ACTIVATION

Besides the ability to lyse cells, complement activation liberates C3a and C5a, which are potent mediators of inflammation. The deposition of large amounts of C3b can opsonize, or target, our own cells for attack by neutrophils and/or destruction by macrophages in the reticuloendothelial system, just as it can opsonize invading microorganisms. The apparent dichotomy between complement's role as a part of the innate immune system that is always turned on to detect foreign invaders and its potential for damage and destruction of host cells and tissues requires that a delicate balance be maintained at all times. This balance depends on a set of control mechanisms no less intricate than the activation pathways.[30]

CONTROL OF THE ALTERNATIVE PATHWAY

The need to control alternative pathway activation becomes apparent when one considers the fact that the alternative pathway can be initiated whenever and wherever C3b is formed, whether by any of the activation pathways, by nonspecific action of a serine protease, or even when C3b-like molecules are formed spontaneously as the thioester is lysed by water.[1,17,20] The alternative pathway is often visualized as an amplification loop that can feed forward whenever C3b is formed (see Fig. 120.2). The danger of uncontrolled alternative pathway activation is illustrated by observations in a patient with congenital homozygous deficiency of the complement regulatory protein *factor H* (see later).[31] This patient lacked detectable C3 activity in his serum because most of the C3 was consumed as fast as it was produced, by continuous nonspecific activation of the alternative pathway. The lack of C3 caused increased susceptibility to infection. Incongruously, some of the C3b deposited on his red blood cells caused a mild but chronic hemolytic anemia.[31]

First of all, the activity of complement is limited by the low circulating concentrations of most of its components. However, C3, C4, and other components are acute-phase reactants, whose synthesis by hepatocytes and other types of cells increases rapidly in response to cytokines, hormones, and other signals.[32] Thus, local synthesis and changes in vascular permeability determine the amounts of the components available at any site or time. The activation cascades are inherently limited by the instability of the multisubunit convertases. In these bimolecular and trimolecular complexes, the proteolytic active sites are on the C2a and Bb fragments, which are not covalently bound to the target or to the other subunits of the convertases. These proteolytically active subunits have relatively weak, noncovalent interactions with C4b and/or C3b and can easily dissociate and diffuse away. The mechanism by which P facilitates activation of the alternative pathway is by holding together the two subunits of the noncovalent C3bBb enzyme so that it will maintain activity.[17,23] In contrast, dissociation of the proteolytically active subunit (C2a or Bb, respectively, in the classical/lectin vs. alternative pathways) causes loss, or *decay*, of the convertase activity. Decay may occur spontaneously, or it may be accelerated by proteins that bind to the covalently attached member of the convertase and push away the loosely held enzymatically active subunit.[33] Several proteins have this function; some are soluble and some are membrane bound (Table 120.1). Many of these proteins share homology with each other, as expected because they all bind to C3, C4, or both, which are themselves homologous. These proteins belong to the *regulators of complement activation* (RCA) family and are encoded by genes in a cluster on chromosome 1q32.[34,35] Members of this family are all composed of variable numbers of short homologous repeats, each of which has 60 to 65 amino acids and two internal disulfide bonds, which give it a double-looped structure. These are further grouped into long homologous repeats, which form the binding sites for C4b and C3b.[35,36] A prototypic member of this family is called *decay accelerating factor (DAF)* (CD55).[30,33,35-37] DAF is bound to the plasma membrane by a glycolipid anchor, which is believed to increase its mobility in the membrane, to better prevent attack of complement on our own cells.[37] The major function of DAF is to bind to C3b and C4b molecules and push off Bb or C2a. Besides the ability to bind to and push off (or block binding of) the active subunits of convertases, some of these regulatory proteins can also facilitate or serve as *cofactors* for degradation of the C4b or C3b to which they bind. A circulating protease, called *C3b/C4b inactivator (factor I)*, can cleave C3b and C4b into forms that no longer bind other components of the convertases.[38] Factor I can cleave C3b and C4b only in the presence of an additional cofactor that renders C3b and C4b susceptible to cleavage.[30,38] Soluble *cofactors* include C4-binding protein (C4bp) and complement factor H (CFH, formerly termed *β-1-H globulin*). Although it can bind to C3b, DAF does not have cofactor activity. However, several other membrane proteins have this kind of cofactor activity, including *complement receptor type 1* (C3b receptor, CR1, CD35)[36] and a separate *membrane cofactor protein* (MCP) (CD46).[39] DAF and MCP bind only to C3b and C4b that have been deposited on the same cell on which they reside, so they are considered important in protecting our own cells from becoming activators or targets of complement.[30] C4bp, CFH, and CR1 can also bind to C3b on other cells or circulating complexes, so they have an important role in processing these complexes.[30] The enzymatically inactive fragments are termed *iC4b* and *iC3b*, respectively. The latter still serves as an important opsonin, however, by binding to its own receptor, termed *CR3*.

From the viewpoint of a C3b molecule, regulation of the alternative pathway might be seen as a competition between binding of factor B, which would lead to additional activation, and factor H, which would lead to inactivation.[1,40,41] The enzymes that execute those actions, factor D and factor I, respectively, both circulate in their active forms. An important determinant of the fate of any given C3b molecule is the chemical nature of the surface on which it is bound, which plays a critical role in influencing the binding of B versus H. Surfaces that are rich in sialic acid, like our own cells, favor the binding of H and thus promote the action of I.[40,41] These surfaces are thus poor activators of the alternative pathway. In contrast, many bacteria and cells from some other species of mammals lack sialic acid. On these surfaces, binding of B is favored. Those cells are good activators of the alternative pathway. Thus, the binding of P and H versus B serves to distinguish non-self from self, even in the absence of a specific antibody or T-cell receptors. Interestingly, bacteria such as K12 *Escherichia coli*[42] and type III group B *Streptococcus*[43] have adapted by adding terminal sialic acid residues to their surfaces or capsular polysaccharides, making them dangerous pathogens, particularly for newborns who lack specific antibody. Related bacteria without the sialic acid are much less virulent. Antibody molecules provide good acceptor sites for C3b deposition, because B is favored over H, and bound C3b is protected against inactivation.[44] This allows the alternative pathway to strongly and rapidly amplify initial signals generated by antibodies and the classical pathway. Besides their coating with sialic acid, most of our own cells are protected from amplification of the alternative pathway by DAF and MCP. Some cell types, including erythrocytes, are also similarly protected by CR1.

The importance of these protein-protein interactions that regulate the alternative pathway, particularly on our own cells, is illustrated by the occurrence of the atypical hemolytic-uremic syndrome (aHUS) in patients in whom the alternative complement pathway escapes from control because of loss-of-function mutations in factor H, factor I, or MCP, or gain-of-function mutations in C3 or factor B. More than 300 disease-causing

Table 120.1 Regulators of Complement Activation Proteins.

Protein[a]	Abbreviation	Molecular Weight	No. of Short Consensus Repeats (SCRs)	Dissociation of C3 and C5 Convertases		Factor I Cofactor Activity on	
				Alternative	Classical	C3b	C4b
Factor H, β_{1H}	H	150,000	20	+	–	+	–
C4-binding protein	C4bp	570,000 (Octamer)	8	–	+	–	+
Decay accelerating factor (CD55)	DAF	70,000–80,000	4	+	+	–	–
Membrane cofactor protein (CD46)	MCP	45,000–70,000	4	–	–	+	+
Complement receptor type 1 C3b/C4b receptor (CD35)	CR1	205,000–250,000	22–30	+	+	+	+
Complement receptor type 2 C3d receptor (CD21)	CR2	145,000	15/16	–	–	–	–

[a]Factor H and C4bp are soluble. All others are membrane proteins indicated by CD number in parentheses.
DAF, Decay accelerating factor; *MCP*, membrane cofactor protein.
Modified from Ahearn JM, Fearon DT. Structure and function of the complement receptors, CR1 (CD35) and CR2 (CD21). *Adv Immunol*. 1989;46:183–219; and Weisman HF, Bartow T, Leppo MK, et al. Soluble human complement receptor type 1: *in vivo* inhibitor of complement suppressing post-ischemic myocardial inflammation and necrosis. *Science*. 1990;249:146–151.

mutations in these proteins have been described.[45-47] Clinically, aHUS includes the triad of microangiopathic hemolytic anemia, thrombocytopenia, and renal failure.[45-47] Rarely, aHUS may present in the first weeks or months of life, even without infectious diarrhea or another trigger.[48] Exogenous triggers are more typical in hemolytic-uremic syndrome caused by toxin-producing *E. coli.*[49] There have even been reports of perinatal asphyxia due to anemia caused by aHUS.[50] The damage to the red cells and consumption of platelets are believed to be consequences of excessive complement activation and MAC formation on the endothelial cells. Endothelial cell damage in the mother may occur when complement control protein mutations are present in women who develop antiphospholipid or other autoantibodies. This type of endothelial damage likely contributes to many cases of preeclampsia; the HELLP syndrome (hypertension; hemolysis, elevated liver enzymes, and low platelets; intrauterine growth restriction (IUGR); and even some cases of recurrent fetal loss (see below).[51]

CONTROL OF EARLY STEPS OF THE CLASSICAL AND LECTIN PATHWAYS

Besides these critical mechanisms of regulation of the activation of the alternative pathway, there is a specific plasma protein, called *C1 inhibitor (C1 INH)* or *C1 esterase inhibitor*, that can complex with C1r and C1s (and also the homologous MASPs) and terminate their activity.[52,53] All of these enzymes contain serine in their active sites,[7] and C1 INH is a member of the serine protease inhibitor or *Serpin* family of proteins. C1 INH can also inhibit serine proteases in the contact, clotting, and kallikrein-kinin systems. Heterozygous deficiency of this protein results in the autosomal dominant condition hereditary angioedema, which may be a cause of colic in affected babies but is most often manifest clinically in repeated episodes of swelling, including potentially fatal attacks of laryngeal edema.[47,52]

CONTROL OF MEMBRANE ATTACK COMPLEX FORMATION

Activation of complement beyond C5 involves conformational changes in individual soluble proteins that expose hydrophobic domains and lead to assembly of a multimeric lipophilic complex. Several circulating proteins can interact with the newly developing lipophilic sites on the C5b67 complex and prevent their attachment to plasma membranes. Some of these proteins may also interfere with binding of C8 or C9 and may bind to nascent MACs forming on cells, preventing their completion. Soluble proteins with these properties include some of the lipoproteins, *clusterin* (apolipoprotein J)[54] and *S-protein* or *vitronectin*,[55,56] which also inhibit the blood-clotting system. Besides these circulating proteins that inhibit the formation of MACs before they insert into cells, there are membrane proteins that protect the cells on which they reside.[57-59] These include *homologous restriction factor*, also known as *protectin* (CD59), which inhibits polymerization and incorporation of C9.[58,59] Like DAF (CD55), CD59 is not a true integral transmembrane protein but is linked to the cell by a phosphatidyl inositol glycolipid anchor that allows high lateral mobility in the plasma membrane.[57-59] Mutations in the enzymes that produce this type of anchor lead to the disease paroxysmal nocturnal hemoglobinuria, in which there can be spontaneous complement lysis of the unprotected erythrocytes.[57]

PHYSIOLOGIC EFFECTS OF COMPLEMENT ACTIVATION AND DEPOSITION

ANAPHYLOTOXINS: C3A AND C5A

C3a is a 9.6-kDa fragment released from the N terminus of the α chain of C3 when it is cleaved by convertases or nonspecifically by other serine proteases. C5a is similarly released on cleavage of C5, but C5a is heavily glycosylated and has a molecular weight of approximately 11 kDa. Both of these peptides can bind to specific receptors on several types of cells, including mast cells, causing non-IgE-mediated degranulation with release of histamine and other mediators. Thus, the actions of C3a and C5a mimic anaphylaxis, and they are known as *anaphylotoxins*.[60] C4a is a homologue but has only weak anaphylotoxin activity. Expression of g-protein coupled receptors[61] for C3a and C5a on glands and smooth muscle in the lung likely contributes to non-histamine-mediated mucus secretion and bronchoconstriction. The anaphylotoxins can also induce interleukin-6 production,[62] providing a mechanism by which local complement activation contributes to the systemic response to infection. All three of these peptides end with a carboxyl-terminal arginine. Removal of this residue by the enzyme carboxypeptidase N (an *anaphylotoxin inactivator*) markedly decreases the ability of the des-Arg forms of the anaphylotoxins to activate their receptors.[63]

The carbohydrate moiety is important in the binding of C5a to its receptor (CD88) on myeloid cells, making this peptide one of the most potent known chemoattractants and activators of neutrophils, monocytes, and macrophages.[64] The des-Arg form of C5a has reduced, but still very potent, chemoattractant and proinflammatory activity. Exposure of neutrophils to C5a or C5a des-Arg causes rapid up-regulation and activation of surface CD11/CD18 (CR3, Mac1), which allows the cells to adhere to surfaces and/or aggregate with each other.[65] Neutrophil aggregates formed in response to C5a or C5a des-Arg generated by intravascular complement activation may plug pulmonary capillaries, which can cause transient pulmonary dysfunction or acute respiratory distress syndrome.[65] This may occur in sepsis, burns, and ischemia-reperfusion injury, in which damaged tissues activate multiple complement pathways. This also occurs when blood comes into contact with artificial membranes in extracorporeal oxygenators and during hemodialysis.[65] It has been hypothesized that part of the pulmonary dysfunction that accompanies amniotic fluid embolism may actually be caused by neutrophil aggregation induced by C5a produced intravascularly when complement is activated by fetal antigens and intracellular debris from the placenta that have entered the maternal circulation.[66]

BOUND C3 FRAGMENTS AND THEIR RECEPTORS

C3 has a higher serum concentration than any other complement protein (approximately 100 mg/dL in normal adults) (Table 120.2). On activation, C3b can become covalently bound to its target, whether that is a bacterium, human cell, or soluble antigen. Subsequent processing of bound C3b involves an orderly sequence of limited proteolytic cleavages, resulting in conformationally distinct fragments that bind to different receptors on different types of cells.[20,30,67,68] The stage of degradation of C3 fragments on any target of complement activation thus plays a major role in determining the fate of that target and the host's response to it.[30,67,68]

When the α chain of C3 is cleaved or when the internal thioester is opened, the resulting C3b or "C3b-like" molecule undergoes conformational changes that markedly increase its affinity for CR1 (CD35), the C3b receptor.[36,69] Uncleaved, native C3 does not bind to this receptor,[69] but C4b can also bind, so it is often termed the *C3b/C4b receptor*.[36] This receptor is a member of the RCA family, but its cytoplasmic domain is short and usually does not activate cells.[70] Hence its main function is to hold onto C3b-bearing immune complexes and C3b-opsonized bacteria and cells, although it also has cofactor and decay-accelerating activity. The internalization phase of phagocytosis[70,71] usually requires a second signal, such as that generated by binding of IgG to certain Fc_γ receptors.[70,71]

Conversion of bound C3b to iC3b (i.e., by H and I) is accompanied by conformational changes similar in magnitude to those that accompany conversion of C3 to C3b.[18,20,67] Cleavage to iC3b greatly reduces the affinity for CR1 (CD35) but increases the affinity for CR3 (CD11b/CD18), a multifunctional molecule that is also a leukocyte β 2 integrin and important adhesion protein. Mutations in CD18 interfere with expression of this class of molecules, resulting in the condition known as *leukocyte adherence deficiency type 1*.[72] Reduced intracellular pools of this molecule likely contribute to decreased chemotactic and phagocytic responses of neonates' neutrophils.[73] Because there are fewer CR3 molecules on neutrophils from newborn infants, more iC3b must be on the opsonized target to promote adherence and phagocytosis.[74]

Further cleavage of iC3b results in the release of a large soluble fragment termed *C3c,* which contains fragments of the cleaved α chain and the entire β chain.[67] A small piece of the α chain around the original thioester site remains covalently bound to the target. This fragment is termed *C3dg* or *C3d,*[75] depending on whether additional cleavages occur, and it binds to another distinct receptor, CR2 (CD21), also a member of the RCA family.[67,68] CD21 is most notably expressed on B lymphocytes and follicular dendritic cells. Simultaneous engagement of CR2 by C3d on an antigen and the specific receptor for that antigen (surface Ig) markedly enhances the B-cell response to the antigen.[76] Persistence of C3d-bearing antigen complexes on the surface of dendritic cells and costimulation of B cells by additional bound C3d fragments is a major mechanism by which complement stimulates immunologic memory and contributes to the afferent arm of adaptive immune responses (see below).

C3 AND DISPOSAL OF IMMUNE COMPLEXES AND APOPTOTIC AND NECROTIC CELLS

Although the activities of complement in host defense against infection usually receive the greatest emphasis, observations in patients and animals with complement mutations suggest that the role of complement in eliminating our own cells when they become damaged or senescent is critical for preventing self-sensitization and autoimmune disease. Complement prevents tissue pathology by promoting solubilization and clearance of antigen-antibody complexes, apoptotic cells, and intracellular constituents of necrotic cells.[77] Activation of complement results in deposition of many C4b and C3b molecules onto antigen-antibody precipitates. The covalent binding of these water-soluble polypeptides disrupts the lattice-like structure of the antigen-antibody precipitate, forming smaller, soluble C3b-bearing complexes, which circulate and are readily phagocytosed in the reticuloendothelial system. Thus, large antigen-antibody aggregates that might otherwise be trapped in tissues and/or bound by ionic interactions with basement membranes (e.g., in the kidney) can be solubilized and cleared by complement. C3b-bearing complexes adhere to CR1 on the surface of erythrocytes (in primates only), and the erythrocytes carry the complexes on their surfaces through the narrow sinusoids of the liver and spleen.[78] This *immune adherence* of the C3b-bearing complexes to CR1 on the nonphagocytic erythrocytes slows transit of the complexes through the reticuloendothelial organs and allows macrophages to strip them off the erythrocyte's surface. Studies in patients with deficiencies of C3 or other early complement components demonstrate the importance of these mechanisms in normal immunologic homeostasis: patients with congenital C3 deficiency have persistent circulating immune complexes after infections and an increased incidence of glomerulonephritis, due to a lack of reticuloendothelial clearance of antigen-antibody complexes that routinely result from common infections.[79] The inability to solubilize and opsonize antigen-antibody complexes allows their accumulation in the kidneys, where they induce pathology by other pathways.[79]

Patients with deficiencies of the early components of the classical pathway or MBL have a markedly increased incidence of autoimmune diseases like SLE.[2,16,80-83] C1q can bind to proteins that are usually intracellular but become exposed when cells undergo apoptosis or necrosis.[80-83] Such cells can also bind "natural antibodies" and MBL, and can activate complement by the classical and/or lectin pathways.[82,83] C3b deposited on apoptotic cells and debris enhances their phagocytosis in situ by tissue macrophages, thus facilitating disposal of this cellular waste.[1,80,81] It is hypothesized that the failure to efficiently clear cellular debris, nucleic acids, and proteins that would normally be hidden from the immune system allows potentially antigenic material to accumulate, and epitopes that are not normally exposed may then stimulate autoimmune responses. Viewed in this way, a properly functioning complement system actually plays an important role in preventing inappropriate inflammatory and immune responses.[1,83]

Table 120.2 Properties of Complement Components and Inhibitors.

Component	Molecular Weight	Serum Concentration (μg/mL)	Chain Structure
Classical Pathway			
C1q	390,000	190	6 each α, β, γ
C1r	95,000	100	s[a]
C1s	85,000	80	s
C4	209,000	430	α, β, γ
C2	117,000	30	s
C3	190,000	1400	α, β
C5	206,000	75	α, β
C6	95,000	60	s
C7	120,000	55	s
C8	163,000	80	α, β, γ
C9	79,000	160	s
Alternate Pathway			
P (properdin)	223,000	25	4 identical chains
D	25,000	1–5	s
B	100,000	200	s
Mannan-Binding Lectin Pathway			
Mannan-binding lectin	32,000	0.5 ng–5 μg/mL	3 identical chains per unit circulates as assembly of 2–8 units
MASP1	90,000	1.6–7.5 μg/mL	s
MASP2	74,000	0.4 μg/mL	s
Control Proteins			
Soluble Control Proteins			
C1 esterase inhibitor (C1EI, C1 INH)	105,000	180	s
C4-binding protein	570,000	150	6–7 α chains, 1 β chain
I (C3b/C4b inactivator, C3 INA)	100,000	50	α, β
H (β_{1H} globulin)	150,000	520	s
Clusterin (apolipoprotein J)	80,000	50–100	2
S protein (vitronectin)	80,000	600	s
Membrane-Bound Control Proteins[a]		**CD Designation**	
Decay accelerating factor (DAF)	70,000–80,000	CD55	s
Membrane cofactor protein (MCP)	48,000–68,000	CD46	s
Complement receptor type 1 (CR1)	190–220,000	CD35	s
Protectin, homologous restriction factor	20,000	CD59	s

[a]Single chain.
MASP, Mannan-binding lectin–associated serine protease.

COMPLEMENT IN HOST DEFENSE AGAINST INFECTIOUS AGENTS

VIRUSES

Because viruses require specific protein-protein interactions to adhere to and enter host cells, binding of antibody or complement directly to or nearby these proteins on the virus surface can block these interactions, neutralizing the viruses' infectivity.[84] With enveloped viruses, insertion of the MAC can disrupt or lyse the envelope.[85] With some viruses, however, specific antibody may be required to direct the complement to critical sites. Retroviruses may activate the classical pathway directly by interacting with C1 without antibody, but this does not usually lead to neutralization or lysis of the envelope.[86] C3b or C3d may actually facilitate entry of the virus into host macrophages that express CR1 or CR2.[86] Many other pathogens may also employ similar strategies of subverting complement-receptor or regulatory protein interactions to increase their virulence (see below).[87]

BACTERIA

The most important functions of complement in host defense are its contributions to control of bacteria, as seen in the increase in bacterial infections in patients with complement deficiencies.[88] Gram-positive bacteria have thick cell walls and must be phagocytosed and killed intracellularly to be eradicated.[87,89] The MAC cannot penetrate the cell wall to reach the cell membrane, which is why phagocytosis is so important. Although the cell walls themselves often activate the alternative pathway, many organisms express polysaccharide capsules surrounding the cell wall. The capsule is permeable to proteins but holds other cells at a distance. Thus, with encapsulated gram-positive organisms, C3 fragments may become bound to the cell wall, but phagocytes cannot reach them. Capsules that lack sialic acid are generally good activators of the alternative pathway, and complement will easily limit the pathogenicity of those organisms. On the other hand, organisms with sialic acid on their capsules do not activate the alternative pathway. With these types of organisms, which include group B *Streptococcus*, K12 *E. coli*, and others, anticapsular antibody plays a critical role by binding to the capsule, activating the classical pathway, and providing good acceptor sites for C3b.[87,89] Phagocytes, attracted and activated by the C5a generated during complement activation, will then rapidly phagocytose the C3b-opsonized organisms, especially if the anticapsular antibody is IgG. The synergistic roles of IgG antibody and complement in clearance of circulating bacteria from the bloodstream, preventing sepsis, are similar to those in phagocytosis of the bacteria at peripheral sites of tissue invasion.[71]

Efficient killing of gram-negative bacteria requires insertion of the C5 through C9 MAC into their cell membranes, which lack thick cell walls and are therefore more accessible than the membranes of gram-positive organisms.[87,89] Patients deficient in C5 to C9 thus have an increased susceptibility to serious infection with *Neisseria* species[87-89] but may not present until their teenage years.

PROTOZOANS

The cell membranes of protozoans are generally susceptible to MAC lysis,[90,91] but several protozoans have adapted elements of the complement system to their own advantage. For example, *Plasmodium falciparum* has a surface protein that binds CR1 and other cell surface proteins, allowing it to adhere to and enter erythrocytes and endothelial cells and avoid destruction in the liver or spleen.[92] There is some evidence suggesting that different allotypes of CR1 correspond with differences in susceptibility to malaria.[92] Some types of leishmanial promastigotes may also be killed by complement, but deposition of C3 fragments on their surfaces promotes phagocytosis via complement receptors on macrophages, in which they may survive by altering trafficking of lysosomes and inhibiting microbicidal mechanisms.[90] Other protozoans, including *Trypanosoma cruzi,* protect themselves by producing complement regulatory proteins that function like DAF.[93] Many protozoans produce extracellular proteases that may degrade complement proteins, protecting the organisms.[94] In addition, some protozoans and bacteria produce enzymes that can transfer sialic acid onto their surfaces in mammalian hosts, preventing alternative pathway attack.

MOLECULAR MIMICRY AND COMPLEMENT-EVASION STRATEGIES OF PATHOGENS

Many clinically important pathogens have either adapted elements of the complement system to facilitate invasion of the host or have developed adaptations to evade complement attack.[87,89,95] For example, adenoviruses, human herpesvirus type 6, measles virus, and other pathogens use CD46 (MCP) and other cell surface proteins as attachment sites to facilitate their entry into a variety of host cell types.[96] The surface protein GP350/220 of Epstein-Barr virus (EBV) contains a nine-residue sequence that is similar to the sequence on C3d that interacts with CR2.[97] This allows EBV to bind to B lymphocytes, leading to infection of those cells and induction of polyclonal activation. Deposition of C3d onto the surface of human immunodeficiency virus serves to hold the virus (via CR2) on the surface of follicular dendritic cells in lymph nodes, accounting for a major reservoir of the virus.[98] Mycobacteria may become coated with complement without being damaged. The mycobacteria are then phagocytosed via complement receptors on macrophages. However, they can survive and replicate intracellularly.[99]

Besides putting sialic acid on their capsules to inhibit alternative pathway activation, many other adaptations help pathogenic bacteria evade complement.[87,89] The side chains of some gram-negative bacterial lipopolysaccharides are able to hold active complement components at a distance from the cell membrane or cause shedding of the nascent MAC as it is being formed. Many gram-positive bacteria have surface proteins that mimic or bind complement control factors. For example, streptococcal M proteins and similar proteins on pneumococci and some meningococci can bind C4 binding protein or factor H from serum in configurations that inhibit complement activation on the bacteria.[95] A similar strategy has been developed by *Borrelia burgdorferi,*[100] the Lyme disease spirochete, and by the blood forms of treponemes, protozoans, and parasitic worms. In addition, some bacteria secrete enzymes that can degrade the complement components in their milieu.[101] Orthopoxviruses, including both variola and vaccinia, code for proteins that are homologous with RCA family members and protect virus-infected cells from attack.[102] In yet another variation, cytomegalovirus infection increases host cell expression of CD46 (MCP), protecting infected cells from complement attack and increasing pathogenicity of the virus.[103]

ROLE OF COMPLEMENT IN ANTIBODY RESPONSES

Complement plays a major role in localization and persistence of antigen on follicular dendritic cells in germinal centers, most importantly by the interaction of C3d with CR2.[104] Complement-bearing antigens are much more efficient in activating B cells than are non-complement-bearing antigens because simultaneous co-engagement of CR2 and antigen receptor (surface Ig) increases processing and expression of major histocompatibility complex (MHC) class II-antigen peptide complexes on the B cells, which enhances T-cell activation.[76] Some T cells themselves have complement receptors, so locally synthesized and activated complement may provide costimulation.[105] These effects, particularly promotion of antigen persistence and localization, likely explain observations that depletion of complement in mice decreases secondary antibody responses, particularly to T cell-dependent antigens.[106] Similar results are found in humans and guinea pigs congenitally deficient in C4.[107] Primary IgM responses are only minimally affected, but on reimmunization, the secondary IgG response is markedly diminished.[107] Thus, by directing antigen localization and by increasing B-cell activation and co-stimulation, bound C3d fragments play a major role in formation of immunologic memory and Ig class switching.

COMPLEMENT GENES AND THEIR ORGANIZATION

The genes for each of the complement proteins, receptors, and control proteins have been identified and sequenced.[108] As expected, because many of the proteins are homologous with each other (i.e., C1r with C1s and the MASPs; C2 with factor B; C3, C4, and C5 with each other), the structures and locations of their genes suggest that the homologies arose by gene duplication then divergence. The three different polypeptides in each subunit of C1q are encoded by different genes that are clustered together on the short arm of chromosome 1. The homologous genes for MBL, surfactant proteins A and D, and other members of the collectin family are on chromosome 10.[108] C1r and C1s, which share approximately 40% homology, are encoded by separate but adjacent genes on chromosome 12. The homologous genes for MASP1 and MASP2 are on chromosomes 3 and 1, respectively. The genes for C2, its homologue, factor B, and C4 are on chromosome 6 and are considered MHC class III gene products.[109] Although less diverse than MHC class I and II proteins, these and many other complement proteins also have different allotypes, which correlate with susceptibility to different autoimmune diseases, although the reasons for this have not been clearly elucidated. There are two separate loci for C4, with multiple allotypes at each.[110] The proteins encoded by the different genes differ slightly in their tendencies to form amide versus ester bonds, and they may have different activities in hemolytic versus other types of assays.[110] It is possible to have homozygous null mutations at one locus but still produce the other type of C4. The two slightly different gene products are distinguished as the Chido and Rodgers blood group antigens when their fragments are displayed on red cells. Like its homologues C3 and C5, C4 is synthesized as a single-chain precursor, pro-C4, which is cleaved to the mature form that predominates in plasma. However, as much as 5% may circulate as the large single-chain pro-C4 form.[111] Unlike the other multichain components, the three chains of C8 are the products of two separate genes. Most of the genes for the homologous proteins that regulate complement activity by binding to C3 and/or C4 are found in the RCA gene cluster on chromosome 1q32.[34] CR1, the C4b/C3b receptor, has structural allotypes and genetically determined quantitative differences in expression.[112] Allotypic differences in specific components' functions, as well as in receptor expression and function, may lead to differences in the efficiency of clearance of immune complexes and therefore to the susceptibility to autoimmune and inflammatory diseases.

Factor H itself contains 20 short consensus repeats and serves as the prototype of a whole family of proteins with common structural elements: *factor H-like protein 1* arises from the same gene as CFH by alternative splicing, and there are at least five distinct genes within the RCA locus on chromosome 1 that code for different factor H–related proteins (FHR 1 to 5). Each has four to nine different short consensus repeats and different glycosylation sites. Different short consensus repeats may differentially bind C3b, heparin, other glycosaminoglycans, and other proteins. Thus, these related proteins may differ in the relative specificity for the surface on which they regulate the fate of C3b.[113]

COMPLEMENT SYNTHESIS

Complement synthesis by fetal tissues has been observed as early as the 6th week of gestation, and most of the components are detectable in fetal serum by the 10th to 12th weeks.[114-116] Studies of maternal-fetal pairs that express different allotypes of C3 and other components, and studies in babies of complement-deficient mothers indicate minimal placental transfer, suggesting that fetal synthesis accounts for the complement components easily measurable in cord blood.[116-118] Complement synthesis has been documented in kidney and other fetal tissues,[115,117] but the liver is the major site of production of most of the complement proteins in adults.[118] The colon may be the major site of production of C1 in fetal life[119] and continues to be an important site of synthesis in the adult. Various components can also be synthesized by myeloid and other types of cells, and local synthesis may play important roles in inflamed joints, lung, and sites of infection.[119,120] The levels of most components increase with gestational age and by term reach 50% to 75% of the levels in maternal serum.[121-124] However, the levels of most of the complement proteins in maternal serum also increase during pregnancy, so the levels in the term newborn are actually approximately 80% of normal adult levels. The levels of C8 and C9 in term babies are lower, at only approximately 10% of the level in maternal serum.[125] The addition of C9 in vitro increases the hemolytic activity and the ability of neonatal sera to kill gram-negative bacteria.[125] In contrast to the active components, C1 INH reaches the same concentration as in adult serum by the 28th week of gestation.[114]

As expected, because the concentrations of most components increase progressively during gestation, preterm babies have lower levels of complement activity than term babies.[123,124] The concentrations usually climb to within the normal adult range by 3 months of postnatal life. The difference between the actual functional amount of complement at a site of infection in a baby compared with an adult, however, may be greater than the difference in the serum levels because synthesis in the baby may not increase in the same way as in the adult.[32,120] However, it is not clear whether this is due to differences in the regulation of the complement genes themselves or deficiencies in signaling proteins, such as interferon-γ, whose production in response to infection and other stimuli is reduced in newborns.[32] The relatively lower levels of C3 and factor B in neonates' sera, together with the decreased CR3 in neonate's neutrophils, combine to compromise phagocytic defenses,[126] even in term newborns.

COMPLEMENT IN MATERNAL-FETAL MEDICINE

Fetal as well as maternal proteins are present in the placenta, and expression of the regulatory proteins DAF (CD55), MCP (CD46), and protectin (CD59) on trophoblasts has been documented.[127,128] Multiple lines of evidence suggest that these membrane-bound regulators, as well as soluble control proteins, play important roles in protecting both the fetus and mother from deleterious effects of excessive complement activation. Several studies suggest ongoing low-level complement activation during normal pregnancy, but higher-level activation in pregnancies complicated by severe preeclampsia[129,130] and/or recurrent fetal loss. Indeed, increased concentrations of C3a, C5a, Bb, and/or C5b9 complexes have been reported in the circulation[131-134,] and/or urine[133,135] of mothers with severe preeclampsia as compared with matched control mothers. Denny and colleagues and Hoffman et al. also reported significantly higher C5a and Bb concentrations in cord blood from babies of preeclamptic mothers.[132,134] A study from the Netherlands reported deposition of C4d on syncytiotrophoblasts in 50% of placentas from preeclamptic women versus only 3% of placentas from controls ($P < .001$).[128] Diffuse placental C4d staining correlated with significantly lower gestational age at delivery in these preeclamptic women.[136] Previous reports suggested increased risk for preeclampsia in women with a low expressing allele of CR1 compared with those with medium- or high-level CR1 expression,[137] and a recent multicenter study of 10 women with personal or family histories of multiple preterm births, including two mother-daughter pairs, showed that half had at least one novel missense variant in CR1 or another complement regulatory gene.[138] Animal studies support the hypothesis that excessive complement activation/dysregulated control are major factors contributing to maternal and fetal pathology.[139-142] Multiple case reports and a recent review suggest that inhibiting C5 with the monoclonal antibody eculizumab may be beneficial in preeclampsia.[143,144]

Clearly, maternal auto- and allo-antibodies can cause excessive complement activation in the placenta. Elegant studies in mice show that passive transfer of antiphospholipid antibodies from women with recurrent pregnancy losses or other signs of antiphospholipid antibody syndrome causes fetal loss.[140-142] Furthermore, there may be complement-fixing antitrophoblast or antiendothelial cell antibodies in the serum of women with recurrent fetal losses who do not have antiphospholipid antibodies per se.[145,146] Analysis of the PROMISSE cohort of 250 women with SLE and/or antiphospholipid antibodies revealed 40 who had preeclampsia. Sequencing of the genes for the complement control proteins MCP, factor I, and factor H in these 40 women showed that 7 (18%) had mutations,[147] 5 of which had previously been identified in patients with aHUS, which is also associated with endothelial injury. A confirmatory analysis in a separate cohort of women with preeclampsia but not autoimmunity revealed that 5 of 59 had heterozygous mutations in MCP or factor I.[147] Excessive complement activation could contribute to the pathophysiology of preeclampsia and/or placental pathology by increasing endothelial damage and/or by increasing C5a, resulting in excessive neutrophil activation.[141]Activation of neutrophils by intravascular C5a induces formation of aggregates that can occlude capillaries. In addition, local complement activation, deposition of the MAC on endothelial cells, and release of mediators like tumor necrosis factor from complement-activated leukocytes is likely to lead to prothrombotic changes in endothelial cells and microthromboses.[148] The resulting restriction of blood flow could contribute to hypertension in the mother and IUGR in the fetus.[149,150] An alternative but not exclusive hypothesis is that activation of C5a contributes to an imbalance of angiogenic and antiangiogenic factors affecting both the mother and fetus.[141] Recognition of the role of complement in preeclampsia and HELLP syndrome has led to use of the C5 inhibitor eculizumab to ameliorate symptoms in the mother-to-be and to prolong the pregnancy.[143,144,149-153] Eculizumab does not appear to inhibit the complement system of the fetus, perhaps because of poor placental transfer.[153,154]

COMPLEMENT AND PATHOLOGY IN THE NEWBORN

Meconium is a potent activator of the alternative pathway, and the severity of lung damage after instillation of meconium into the lungs of piglets correlates with complement activation.[155] Addition of meconium to whole blood initiates leukocyte activation, which can be inhibited by blocking the alternative pathway with antibody to factor D or against C5.[155] C5a likely plays an important role in leukocyte activation and lung damage in this situation. However, phospholipase A_2 in meconium may produce potent arachidonic acid metabolites, and meconium can activate Toll-like receptor pathways and NF-kB, resulting in production of many proinflammatory cytokines and chemokines. These may further contribute to a vigorous local and systemic inflammatory response.[156] Because multiple proinflammatory signaling pathways are activated simultaneously, it seems unlikely that complement inhibition alone would have a major impact on the severity of meconium aspiration syndrome.

Complement does not play a major role in Rh(D) hemolytic disease of the newborn because D antigens on erythrocytes are too few and far apart for the IgG antibodies to attach to and activate C1 molecules.[157] In this situation, the fetal red cells are likely destroyed by FcγR-mediated macrophage phagocytosis. In other conditions caused by maternal antibodies crossing the placenta and affecting the fetus, the possible involvement of complement must always be considered because the IgG subclasses that are transported across the placenta by FcRn are the most potent activators of the classical complement pathway.

THERAPEUTIC MANIPULATION OF COMPLEMENT ACTIVITY

In many diseases that involve auto- or alloantibodies formed by the mother against antigens expressed by the fetus, complement may be physiologically activated. However, because the antigen in these situations is a normal body constituent, the complement activation causes pathology. In addition, complement is activated by multiple pathways during ischemia-reperfusion injury.[158] C5a-induced neutrophil aggregates can plug capillaries, deposition of C3 fragments may lead to attack on cells and basement membranes, and deposition of MACs may cause endothelial or parenchymal cell damage. Thus, there are many conditions in which it may be desirable to inhibit complement activation therapeutically. Augmentation of normal C1 esterase inhibitor activity may be beneficial because it selectively inhibits the classical and lectin pathways, leaving the alternative pathway intact for host defenses.[159] Small molecule inhibitors of the complement convertases and analogues of CR1 are in development, but they have not yet come into use clinically. One of the most promising complement inhibitors in use clinically is eculizumab, a humanized monoclonal antibody against C5 that prevents cleavage of C5 and generation of C5a and MAC by all of the activation pathways.[160] Eculizumab has been approved by the United States Food and Drug Administration (FDA) to reduce erythrocyte lysis in paroxysmal nocturnal hemoglobinuria and to inhibit complement-mediated thrombotic microangiopathy in aHUS.[160,161] Although its use in pregnancy is classified as category C, several publications describe its off-label use in a variety of conditions that may affect the mother and/or fetus.[144,149,151-154,162] Because eculizumab inhibits MAC formation by all of the complement pathways, it is associated with an increased risk for meningococcal and other *Neisseria* infections. Therefore, patients should be immunized with meningococcal vaccine before eculizumab is administered.[161]

As mentioned earlier, IgG antibody molecules provide very good acceptors for the nascent covalent binding site that is exposed during C3 activation. Excess soluble IgG can therefore divert C3b and decrease its deposition onto targets. In vitro, excess nonspecific IgG can prevent complement-mediated cell lysis.[163] Therapeutically, administration of high doses of intravenous immune globulin (IVIG) (1 to 2 g/kg) has this effect in vivo,[164] and inhibition of complement deposition and reticuloendothelial clearance may be major mechanisms by which IVIG treatment acts in autoantibody- or alloantibody-mediated diseases, such as thrombocytopenia due to maternal alloantibodies. By saturating the FcRn, which transports IgG across the placenta, it is likely that administering high-dose IVIG to the mother may decrease transfer of maternal auto- or alloantibodies, which could potentially harm the fetus,[165] but this has not been extensively studied, and IVIG is classified as category C by the FDA.

CONCLUSION

Complement is an important part of the innate immune system, which may be particularly important in neonates, who have low IgM concentrations and do not produce much of their own IgG. When antibody is present, complement can serve as a major amplification and effector pathway for the adaptive immune system. As with other complement activities, its ability to attract and activate leukocytes is a double-edged sword that is necessary for normal host defense but can cause serious pathology when activated inappropriately or insufficiently regulated. Complement plays important roles in limiting inflammatory responses by removing infectious agents and noxious stimuli and supports normal homeostasis by directing trafficking and disposal of apoptotic cells and immune complexes. However, complement can contribute to local pathology when these mechanisms are overwhelmed or function imperfectly. Fortunately, an elaborate set of soluble and cell surface regulatory molecules usually keeps this system in delicate balance.

A complete reference list is available at www.ExpertConsult.com. 

SELECT REFERENCES

1. Walport MJ. Complement. First of two parts. *N Engl J Med*. 2001;344:1058-1066.
3. Ricklin D, Hajishengallis G, Yang K, Lambris JD. Complement: a key system for immune surveillance and homeostasis. *Nat Immunol*. 2010;11:785-797.
4. Gros P, Milder FJ, Janssen BJ. Complement driven by conformational changes. *Nat Rev Immunol*. 2008;8:48-58.
7. Forneris F, Wu J, Gros P. The modular serine proteases of the complement cascade. *Curr Opin Struct Biol*. 2012;22:333-341.
13. Kjaer TR, Thiel S, Andersen GR. Toward a structure-based comprehension of the lectin pathway of complement. *Mol Immunol*. 2013;56:413-422.
16. Holers VM. Complement deficiency states, disease susceptibility and infection risk in systemic lupus erythematosus. *Arthritis Rheum*. 1999;42:2023-2025.
18. Janssen BJ, Christodoulidou A, McCarthy A, et al. Structure of C3b reveals conformational changes that underlie complement activity. *Nature*. 2006;444:213-216.
19. Nilsson B, Nilsson Ekdahl K. The tick-over theory revisited: is C3 a contact-activated protein? *Immunobiology*. 2012;217:1106-1110.
23. Kemper C, Hourcade DE. Properdin: new roles in pattern recognition and target clearance. *Mol Immunol*. 2008;45:4048-4056.
27. Sonnen AF, Henneke P. Structural biology of the membrane attack complex. *Subcell Biochem*. 2014;80:83-116.

28. Bhakdi S, Tranum-Jensen J. Membrane damage by channel forming proteins. *Trends Biochem Sci*. 1983;8:134.-146.
30. Zipfel PF, Skerka C. Complement regulators and inhibitory proteins. *Nat Rev Immunol*. 2009;9:729-740.
35. Herbert A, O'Leary J, Krych-Goldberg M, et al. Three-dimensional structure and flexibility of proteins of the RCA family: a progress report. *Biochem Soc Trans*. 2002;30:990-996.
33. Krych-Goldberg M, Atkinson JP. Structure-function relationships of complement receptor type 1. *Immunol Rev*. 2001;180:112-122.
36. Nilsson SC, Sim RB, Lea SM, et al. Complement factor I in health and disease. *Mol Immunol*. 2011;48:1611-1620.
40. Fearon DT, Austen KF. The alternative pathway of complement: a system for host resistance to microbial infection. *N Engl J Med*. 1980;303:259-263.
41. Fearon DT. Regulation by membrane sialic acid of β1H-dependent decay dissociation of amplification C3 convertase of the alternative complement pathway. *Proc Natl Acad Sci U S A*. 1978;75:1971-1975.
46. Joseph C, Gattineni J. Complement disorders and hemolytic uremic syndrome. *Curr Opin Pediatr*. 2013;25:209-215.
48. Çakar N, Ozcakar ZB, Ozaltin F, et al. Atypical hemolytic uremic syndrome in children aged <2 years. *Nephron*. 2018;139:211-218.
51. Fang CJ, Fremeaux-Bacchi V, Liszewski MK, et al. Membrane cofactor protein mutations in atypical hemolytic uremic syndrome (aHUS), fatal Stx-HUS, C3 glomerulonephritis, and the HELLP syndrome. *Blood*. 2008;111:624-632.
52. Davis 3rd AE. Biological effects of C1 inhibitor. *Drug News Perspect*. 2004;17:439-446.
53. Petersen SV, Thiel S, Jensen L, et al. Control of the classical and the MBL pathway of complement activation. *Mol Immunol*. 2000;37:803-811.
58. Morgan BP, Meri S. Membrane proteins that protect against complement lysis. *Springer Semin Immunopathol*. 1994;15:369-396.
65. Jacob HS, Craddock PR, Hammerschmidt DE, Moldow CF. Complement induced granulocyte aggregation. *N Engl J Med*. 1980;302:789-794.
66. Benson MD. A hypothesis regarding complement activation and amniotic fluid embolism. *Med Hypotheses*. 2007;68:1019-1025.
75. Fishelson Z. Complement C3: a molecular mosaic of binding sites. *Mol Immunol*. 1991;28:545-552.
80. Mevorach D. Clearance of dying cells and systemic lupus erythematosus: the role of C1q and the complement system. *Apoptosis*. 2010;15:1114-1123.
86. Huber G, Bánki Z, Lengauer S, Stoiber H. Emerging role for complement in HIV infection. *Curr Opin HIV AIDS*. 2011;6:419-426.
87. Moffitt MC, Frank MM. Complement resistance in microbes. *Springer Semin Immunopathol*. 1994;15:327-344.
88. Skattum L, van Deuren M, van der Poll T, Truedsson L. Complement deficiency states and associated infections. *Mol Immunol*. 2011;48:1643-1655.
106. Pepys MB. Role of complement in the induction of immunological responses. *Transplant Rev*. 1976;32:93-120.
108. Degn SE, Jensenius JC, Thiel S. Disease-causing mutations in genes of the complement system. *Am J Hum Genet*. 2011;88:689-705.
113. Zipfel PF, Skerka C, Hellwage J, et al. Factor H family proteins: on complement, microbes and human diseases. *Biochem Soc Trans*. 2002;30:971-978.
114. Gitlin D, Biasucci A. Development of gamma G, gamma A, gamma M, beta IC-beta IA, C 1 esterase inhibitor, ceruloplasmin, transferrin, hemopexin, haptoglobin, fibrinogen, plasminogen, alpha 1-antitrypsin, orosomucoid, beta-lipoprotein, alpha 2-macroglobulin, and prealbumin in the human conceptus. *J Clin Invest*. 1969;48:1433-1446.
126. Berger M. Complement deficiency and neutrophil dysfunction as risk factors for bacterial infection in newborns and the role of granulocyte transfusion in therapy. *Rev Infect Dis*. 1990;12:S401-S409.
128. Tedesco F, Narchi G, Radillo O, et al. Susceptibility of human trophoblast to killing by human complement and the role of the complement regulatory proteins. *J Immunol*. 1993;151:1562-1570.
131. Tincani A, Cavazzana I, Ziglioli T, et al. Complement activation and pregnancy failure. *Clin Rev Allergy Immunol*. 2010;39:153-159.
133. Burwick RM, Fichorova RN, Dawood HY, et al. Urinary excretion of C5b-9 in severe preeclampsia: tipping the balance of complement activation in pregnancy. *Hypertension*. 2013;62:1040-1045.
136. Buurma A, Cohen D, Veraar K, et al. Preeclampsia is characterized by placental complement dysregulation. *Hypertension*. 2012;60:1332-1337.
140. Holers VM, Girardi G, Mo L, et al. Complement C3 activation is required for antiphospholipid antibody-induced fetal loss. *J Exp Med*. 2002;195:211-220.
141. Girardi G, Berman J, Redecha P, et al. Complement C5a receptors and neutrophils mediate fetal injury in the antiphospholipid syndrome. *J Clin Invest*. 2003;112:1644-1654.
145. Girardi G, Bulla R, Salmon JE, Tedesco F. The complement system in the pathophysiology of pregnancy. *Mol Immunol*. 2006;43:68-77.
149. Girardi G. Complement inhibition keeps mothers calm and avoids fetal rejection. *Immunol Invest*. 2008;37:645-659.
150. Ahmed A, Ramma W. Unravelling the theories of preeclampsia: are the protective pathways the new paradigm? *Br J Pharmacol*. 2015;172:1574-1586.
153. Sarno L, Tufano A, Maruotti GM, et al. Eculizumab in pregnancy: a narrative overview. *J Nephrol*. 2019;32:17-25.
155. Mollnes TE, Castellheim A, Lindenskov PHH, et al. The role of complement in meconium aspiration syndrome. *J Perinatol*. 2008;28:S116-S119.
156. Salvesen B, Stenvik J, Rossetti C, et al. Meconium-induced release of cytokines is mediated by the TRL4/MD-2 complex in a CD14-dependent manner. *Mol Immunol*. 2010;47:1226-1234.
157. Zawodnik SA, Bonnard GD, Gautier AE, Macdonald HR. Antibody-dependent cell-mediated destruction of human erythrocytes sensitized in ABO and rhesus fetal-maternal incompatibilities. *Pediatr Res*. 1976;10:791-796.
158. Gorsuch WB, Chrysanthou E, Schwaeble WJ, Stahl GL. The complement system in ischemia-reperfusion injuries. *Immunobiology*. 2012;217:1026-1033.

Cytokines and Inflammatory Response in the Fetus and Neonate

121

Scott M. Gordon | Lakshmi Srinivasan | Mary Catherine Harris | Laurie E. Kilpatrick

CLINICAL RELEVANCE OF INFLAMMATION IN THE FETUS AND NEONATE

Thanks to skilled clinicians and cutting-edge technologies, care of the critically ill neonate has advanced significantly since the inception of neonatology. However, interventions presently employed by neonatologists to sustain patients' lives, including ventilators, antibiotics, and vasoactive medications, to name a few, represent only types of supportive care. Mounting evidence suggests that disturbed homeostasis of the immune system is at the core of many common and devastating disorders affecting the fetus and neonate. With rare exception, our field has yet to develop the knowledge or tools required to treat the dysregulated inflammation underlying necrotizing enterocolitis (NEC), bronchopulmonary dysplasia (BPD), or sepsis, among others.

Cytokines are endogenous mediators of inflammation. Tightly regulated inflammation is essential under conditions of homeostasis and in response to infections and tissue injury. Uncontrolled inflammation can exacerbate tissue injury and lead to severe organ dysfunction. To promote understanding of how the fetal and neonatal immune response is regulated, we provide an overview of the biology of inflammation and cytokines, with particular attention paid to review of clinically relevant primary data (Table 121.1).

INTRODUCTION TO INFLAMMATION

Inflammation is a host organism's response to such immune stimuli as infection or tissue injury. The inflammatory response is characterized by the delivery of leukocytes and plasma proteins systemically or locally to affected tissues.[1,2] Often, this response is initiated when tissue parenchyma, stroma, or immune cells are exposed to "danger" signals—pathogen-associated molecular patterns (PAMPs) or tissue damage-associated molecular patterns (DAMPs).

PAMPs are microbe-specific molecular signatures, such as cell wall or flagellar components (e.g., lipopolysaccharide [LPS],

Table 121.1 Summary of Cytokines—Immune and Clinical Effects, Pathology Related to Imbalance.

	Mediator	Immune Effects	Clinical Effects	Endogenous Counter-Regulatory Molecules	Pathology Linked to Unbalanced Response
Proinflammatory Classical	**TNF**	Initiation/amplification of inflammatory cascades Indirectly promotes recruitment of neutrophils Control of cell life and death – Cell survival and proliferation – Cell death via apoptosis or necroptosis Procoagulation and antifibrinolysis	All contribute directly or indirectly to: — Fever (IL-6 most potent endogenous pyrogen) — Anorexia — Lethargy Enhance production of acute phase reactants	Soluble TNFRs (can act as decoy receptors)	Elevated levels associated with IUGR, preeclampsia, and preterm birth Damage to fetal oligodendrocytes in the context of fetal inflammation Enhanced activity associated with increased mortality in sepsis
	IL-1	Initiation/amplification of inflammatory cascades – Activation of IL-6 and acute-phase response – Promotes recruitment of neutrophils Procoagulation and antifibrinolysis		IL-1Ra (competitive inhibitor of IL-1) IL-1R2 (can act as a decoy receptor) IL-1R8 (tempers response to IL-1)	Associated with preterm labor and prolonged rupture of membranes Prenatal exposure mediates end organ damage and neonatal mortality IL-1α effects associated with increased mortality in neonatal sepsis
	IL-6	Initiation/amplification of inflammatory cascades – Main driver of acute phase response			Associated with fetal inflammatory response syndrome — Levels in amniotic fluid correlate with brain injury in preterm infants Mixed data on IL-6 production by preterm neonates — Reduced IL-6 in sepsis may predispose to impaired bacterial clearance — Enhanced IL-6 in sepsis may drive organ damage
Type 1	**IL-12** **IL-18**	Stimulation and fate determination of lymphocytes Mediate immunity to viruses and intracellular bacteria Procoagulation		IL-18-binding protein (soluble antagonist) IL-1R8 (tempers response to IL-18)	Fetus and neonate with impaired production of type 1 cytokines – May contribute to fetal/neonatal susceptibility to viruses and intracellular bacteria Enhanced IL-18 activity contributes to mortality in neonatal sepsis
	IFNγ	Stimulation of lymphocytes and phagocytes – Amplification of inflammatory cascades – Promotes chemotaxis of multiple leukocytes – Promotes antimicrobial function of phagocytes	May indirectly cause fever Contributes to acute-phase response		Elevated levels associated with development of severe, chronic inflammation – Promotes tissue damage and cell death
Type 2	**IL-4** **IL-5** **IL-13**	Determination of fate and function in innate and adaptive immune cells – Promote tissue repair – Oppose type 1 proinflammatory cytokines Antihelminth immunity	IL-4 can oppose acute phase reactants	IL-13Ra2 (can act as a decoy receptor)	Bias of fetal and neonatal immune response toward type 2 cytokines Enhanced levels of type 2 cytokines associated with severe RSV bronchiolitis and asthma IL-4 promotes brain inflammation and damage to oligodendrocytes in setting of IUGR
	IL-33	Modulates mucosal immune responses Determination of fate and function in innate and adaptive immune cells		Soluble ST2 (can act as a decoy receptor) IL-1R8 (tempers response to IL-33)	Elevated levels of IL-33 promote severe lung inflammation – Associated with development of BPD, severe RSV bronchiolitis, and asthma Impaired activity of IL-33 may lead to mortality in sepsis
Antiinflammatory	**IL-10**	Downmodulates innate and adaptive immune responses – Reduction in chemotaxis – Reduction in antimicrobial function of phagocytes – Impairs synthesis of proinflammatory cytokines Opposes coagulation and promotes fibrinolysis	Antipyretic		Elevated levels impair bacterial clearance in neonatal sepsis Genetic mutation in IL-10 receptors lead to very early-onset IBD in the neonatal period Impaired production of IL-10 linked with development of NEC and BPD
Chemokines	**IL-8/CXCL8**	Main driver of neutrophil chemotaxis to site of infection or tissue injury Promotes degranulation of neutrophils and production of ROS			Elevated levels in amniotic fluid associated with intrauterine inflammation and preterm birth – Levels correlate with chorioamnionitis, also with RDS and CLD

CLD, Chronic lung disease; *IL-1*, interkeulin-1; *IL-1R2*, type II IL-1 receptor; *IL-1ra*, interleukin-1 receptor antagonist; *IL-6*, interleukin-6; *ROS*, reactive oxygen species; *RSV*, respiratory syncytial virus; *TNF*, tumor necrosis factor; *TNFR*, tumor necrosis factor receptor.

β-glycan, flagellin).[3] In contrast, DAMPs are components of host cells. To maintain immune quiescence in the steady state, DAMPs are sequestered intracellularly and hidden from immune cells. Upon tissue stress or injury, DAMPs are released.[2-7] Examples of DAMPs include a variety of cytosolic, nuclear, mitochondrial, endoplasmic reticular, and granule-associated proteins, heat shock proteins, nuclear and mitochondrial DNA, and fragments of extracellular matrix.

PAMPs and DAMPs bind to pattern recognition receptors (PRRs), including toll-like receptors, C-type lectin receptors, nucleotide-binding oligomerization domain (NOD)-like receptors, retinoic acid-inducible gene I-like (RIG I-like) receptors, scavenger receptors, and purinergic receptors. PRRs are expressed mainly, but not exclusively, by innate immune cells, such as macrophages, dendritic cells, and neutrophils. Subsequent to engagement of a PRR by its cognate ligand, numerous inflammatory pathways are activated.[1-3,6-8]

INTRODUCTION TO CYTOKINES

Cytokines are produced by various immune and nonimmune cell types in response to multiple stimuli.[9-12] Cytokines are potent mediators of the immune system that act in minute quantities (nano- to pico-molar range). Thus, synthesis and secretion of cytokines are carefully controlled. Once these proteins are released, their half-life is relatively short, further limiting their biologic activity. Cytokines bind to specific receptors that drive alterations in cellular physiology and gene expression.

In other words, signaling by cytokines on target cells represents a mode of cell-to-cell communication, which may occur in an autocrine, paracrine, or endocrine fashion.[3,9,10,12] Some cytokines act locally by simple diffusion or by direct cell-to-cell contact. Others may leave the local environment, enter the circulation, interact with more distant immune cells and organ systems, and alter host physiology.

Proinflammatory cytokines are produced to signal the presence of infection or tissue injury.[1,3,12] They serve to initiate and amplify immune responses. Once proinflammatory cytokines disseminate systemically, they can have profound effects on systemic physiology in the host. For instance, interleukin (IL)-1, tumor necrosis factor (TNF), and IL-6 mediate common clinical signs of infection, such as fever, anorexia, somnolence, and the acute phase reaction.[1,13] Proinflammatory cytokines can be further subdivided by the type of response they promote and the type of immune cells they stimulate. We discuss several different types of proinflammatory cytokines in this chapter, with each cytokine exerting unique effects on the host.

Unchecked, a proinflammatory response can cause substantial damage to host tissues, even though it may effectively clear a pathogen from the body. Thus, inflammatory stimuli also trigger the synthesis and release of *antiinflammatory* cytokines and endogenous inhibitors of proinflammatory cytokines that serve to balance the host immune response.[13-15] Antiinflammatory cytokines limit inflammation by a number of mechanisms, including by inhibiting synthesis of proinflammatory cytokines. Similarly, naturally occurring inhibitors of proinflammatory cytokines block cytokine–cytokine receptor interactions by consuming a cytokine itself or by binding its specific receptor. This chapter will examine several endogenous inhibitors, including soluble "decoy" receptors, antagonists of cytokine receptors, and cytokine-binding proteins. As with proinflammatory molecules, the antiinflammatory response must not be out of balance. An inappropriate abundance of antiinflammatory signals may spare bystander tissues but allow a microbe to overwhelm the host. In summary, a complex inflammatory milieu determines the nature, strength, and duration of the immune response.

PROINFLAMMATORY CYTOKINES

TUMOR NECROSIS FACTOR

MOLECULAR MECHANISMS

TNF is a pleiotropic cytokine that is a key regulator of the inflammatory response and has a critical role in orchestrating the local inflammatory response through cell activation and initiation of a cytokine cascade. TNF also activates diverse homeostatic or pathogenic signaling pathways that mediate a wide range of downstream effects that include cell-cell communication, proliferation, differentiation, and cell death.[16,17] TNF synthesis is triggered by multiple stimuli, including PAMPs, DAMPs, viruses, ischemia/hypoxia, trauma, cytokines, and TNF itself.[13,18,19] Monocytes and tissue macrophages are the primary producer cells for TNF. TNF is also produced by lymphocytes, natural killer (NK) cells, neutrophils, mast cells, endothelial cells, keratinocytes, smooth muscle cells, and astrocytes. TNF is synthesized as a 26-kDa transmembrane protein, which is processed to the mature soluble 17-kDa form following cleavage by a membrane-bound disintegrin metalloproteinase, TNF-converting enzyme (TACE/ADAM 17).[20,21] Both the soluble (sTNF) and membrane associated form of TNF (mTNF) are active, with mTNF regulating local inflammatory responses.[21]

TUMOR NECROSIS FACTOR RECEPTORS

TNF binds to two structurally related receptors. TNFR1, a 55- to 60-kDa receptor, is expressed on most cell types, while TNFR2, a 75- to 80-kDa receptor, is expressed principally on immune and endothelial cells (Fig. 121.1).[22-24] TNFR1 binds both sTNF and mTNF, while TNFR2 is preferentially activated by mTNF.[25] TNF signaling is tightly regulated through ubiquitination and phosphorylation, which produce distinct signaling complexes that control different functional outcomes, such as inflammation, cell survival, apoptosis, and necroptosis.[17,24] TNFR1 activation leads to the assembly of complex I or II (see Fig. 121.1). Complex I is largely responsible for proinflammatory and anti-apoptotic cellular responses through activation of mitogen-activated protein kinases and transcription factors such as nuclear factor κB (NFκB) and activator protein.[9,18,26,27] Complex I regulates inflammation, host defense, and cell survival.[9,17,18,26-30] Other complexes can also be formed, termed *complex IIa, IIb*, and *IIc*, which lead to cell death. Formation of complex IIa or IIb leads to apoptosis, while formation of complex IIc results in necroptosis and inflammation.[17] Factors such as cell type and presence of other cytokines and inflammatory mediators may shift TNF-mediated signaling either towards or against cell death. In contrast, TNFR2, which is activated primarily by mTNF, does not contain a death domain and cannot elicit cell apoptosis or necroptosis. TNFR2 is important for cell–cell communication and assembles complex I that induces cell survival, proliferation, and tissue regeneration.[16,17,31]

TUMOR NECROSIS FACTOR IN THE FETUS AND NEONATE

TNF is produced by human fetal Kupffer cells, as well as placental mononuclear cells, in response to stimulation by the PAMP LPS.[32,33] Although pregnancy is generally biased away from T helper 1 (T_H1) responses and rejection of the fetus, TNF can be found in amniotic fluid during the second and third trimesters, with levels rising throughout pregnancy.[34] Further, elevated TNF levels have been related to pregnancy complications including growth restriction, preeclampsia, and preterm birth.[34-36] Although animal studies show conflicting effects on neonatal immune development, there remains a paucity of human clinical data on the safety of anti-TNF biologic agents for the growing fetus.[37,38]

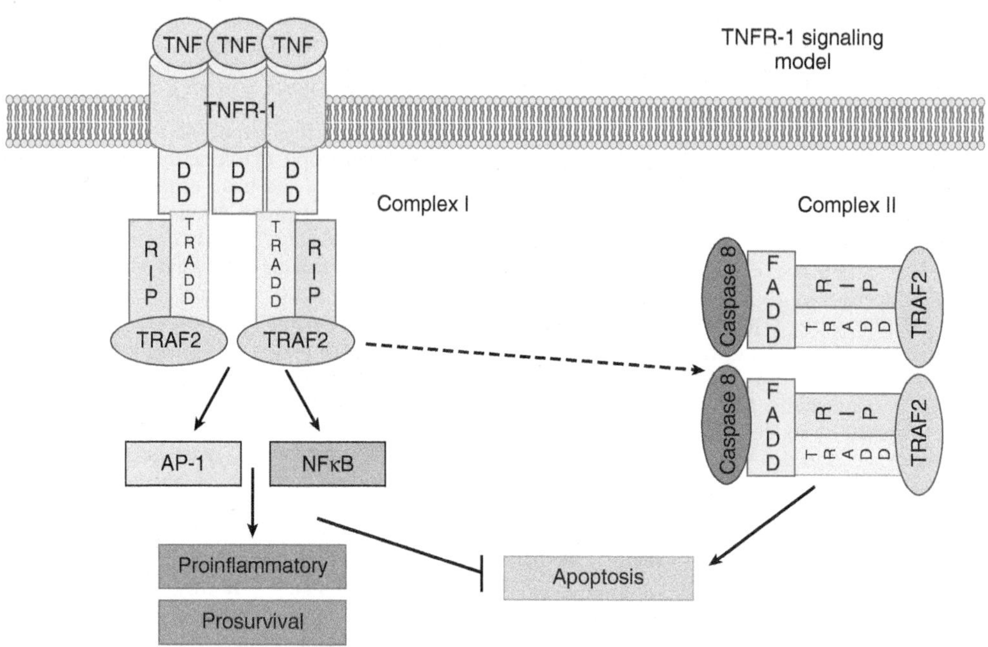

Fig. 121.1 The tumor necrosis factor receptor 1 *(TNFR-1)* signaling complex. Binding of tumor necrosis factor *(TNF)* to TNFR1 results in the recruitment and formation of a TNFR-1 signaling complex. TNFR-1-associated death domain *(TRADD)* associates with TNFR-1 through death domain *(DD)* interactions and serves as a platform for the recruitment of other adaptor proteins, including TNF receptor–associated factor 2 *(TRAF2)* and receptor-interacting protein *(RIP)* to form complex I. These adapter proteins recruit additional components necessary for the activation of proinflammatory and antiapoptotic pathways through the activation of transcription factors, such as nuclear factor κB *(NFκB)* and activator protein 1 *(AP-1)*. Complex II is formed when TRADD-RIP-TRAF2 disassociates from TNFR-1. Subsequent recruitment of Fas-associated death domain *(FADD)* and caspase 8 to this complex initiates TNF-mediated apoptosis.

Several (but not all) investigators have demonstrated significantly decreased TNF production by umbilical cord blood monocytes.[39-44] In addition, preterm infants born before 30 weeks' gestation demonstrated significantly diminished LPS-stimulated TNF secretion when compared with neonates of later gestational ages or adults.[41-43] When analyzed in culture, monocytes and macrophages derived from newborn infants also secreted diminished amounts of TNF when compared with adult cells.[43,45] Kwak and colleagues examined TNF production by umbilical cord blood mononuclear cells in response to several stimuli.[46] In contrast with the immediate response to LPS (in which TNF, IL-1β, IL-6, and IL-8 appeared almost simultaneously), stimulation by group B streptococci resulted in increased TNF production but a delayed appearance of the other cytokines. Additional investigations by Levy and colleagues demonstrated that impaired perinatal TNF production was mediated by the purine metabolite, adenosine.[47] TNFR expression may also be diminished. Using flow cytometry and a human recombinant TNF that binds to the 75- and 55-kDa receptors, Chheda and colleagues demonstrated reduced expression of TNFRs on umbilical cord blood monocytes when compared with that of adult cells.[45] Thus abnormalities of TNF production, release, and dissociation from the production of other cytokines may protect the fetus from excessive inflammatory responses. On the other hand, excessive TNF production, such as in the setting of a fetal inflammatory response to chorioamnionitis, may mediate oligodendrocyte injury at a vulnerable period in development.[38]

INTERLEUKIN-1

MOLECULAR MECHANISMS

The IL-1 ligand superfamily includes IL-1α (or IL-1F1), IL-1β (or IL-1F2), IL-18, IL-33, IL-36α, IL-36β, IL-36γ (agonists), IL-1 receptor antagonist (IL-1ra; or IL-1F3), IL-36 receptor antagonist, IL-38 (see "Inhibitors of Proinflammatory Cytokines"), and IL-37 (antiinflammatory cytokine).[48-51] IL-1α and IL-1β are important mediators of local and systemic inflammation. The two molecules share little sequence homology (22% to 26%) but have similar tertiary structures, bind to the same receptors, and share biologic activities.[50]

IL-1α and IL-1β are synthesized as 31-kDa precursor proteins (proIL-1α and proIL-1β).[48,52] IL-1α is constitutively expressed in healthy individuals in multiple cell types including epithelial and mesenchymal cell types.[53] Most of IL-1α remains in the cell cytosol in the pro-form, where it can function in an autocrine fashion or be transported to the cell surface and participate in cell-to-cell communication.[48] IL-1α is also biologically active when it is cleaved to the 17.5-kDa mature protein by membrane-associated cysteine protease calpains and then released from the cell. IL-1α is rarely observed in the circulation and appears systemically only during severe disease, where it is released following cell necrosis and functions as a DAMP.[54,55]

By contrast, IL-1β is produced principally by cells of the innate immune system such as monocytes, macrophages, and dendritic cells. IL-1β is active only in its cleaved mature form, and after secretion, it is the principal mediator of the systemic effects of IL-1 and is an important regulator of host defense.[54] Activation and release of the mature biologically active 17-kDa form is tightly regulated and requires cleavage by caspase 1 following inflammasome activation.[56,57] Non–inflammasome-mediated activation of IL-1β can also occur, mediated by proteases derived from neutrophils or pathogens themselves.[58] IL-1 synthesis is triggered by many of the same stimuli that activate TNF production (i.e., PAMPs and DAMPs).

INTERLEUKIN-1 RECEPTORS

Two different receptors bind IL-1: the type I IL-1 receptor (IL-1R1) and the type II IL-1 receptor (IL-1R2) (Fig. 121.2). Both receptors are members of the IL-1 receptor/toll-like receptor superfamily.[50,59,60] IL-1R1 is found on most cell types and requires the recruitment of IL-1 receptor accessory protein to the receptor to form a high-affinity receptor complex, a requirement for optimal signal transduction and the activation of NFκB and proinflammatory

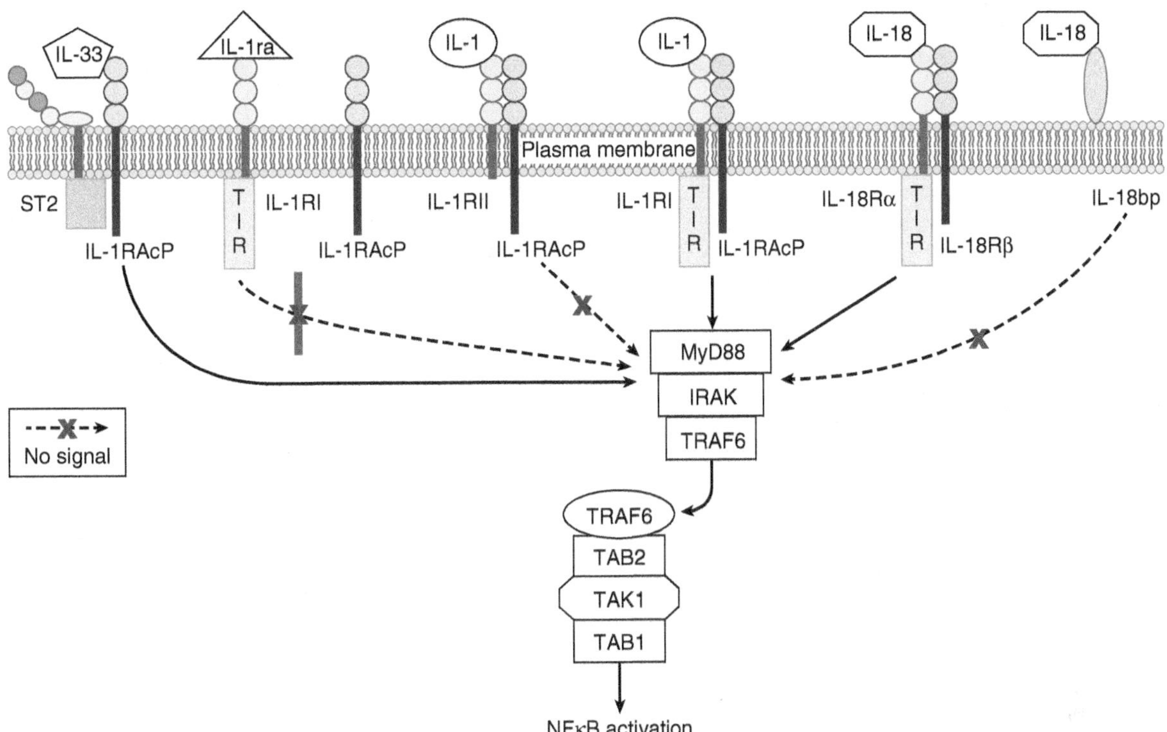

Fig. 121.2 Interkeulin-1 *(IL-1)* and interkeulin-18 *(IL-18)* receptor family. The IL-1 and IL-18 receptors are members of the IL-1/toll-like receptor family. IL-1 can bind to either the type I IL-1 receptor *(IL-1RI)* or the type II IL-1R *(IL-1RII)*. IL-1 binding to IL-1RI results in the association of IL-1R accessory protein *(IL-1RAcP)* to form a complex that recruits the myeloid differentiation protein 88 *(MyD88)* to the toll/IL-1 receptor *(TIR)* domain, activation of the MyD88 signaling cascade, and subsequent activation of nuclear factor κB *(NFκB)* and proinflammatory gene transcription. Members of the IL-1RI signaling complex include MyD88, IL-1R-associated kinase *(IRAK)*, tumor necrosis factor receptor–associated factor 6 *(TRAF6)*, transforming growth factor β-kinase *(TAK-1)*, TAK-1-binding protein 1 *(TAB-1)*, and TAK-1-binding protein 2 *(TAB-2)*. IL-1 receptor antagonist (IL-1ra) also binds to IL-1RI but does not trigger the association of IL-1RAcP and activation of the MyD88 signaling cascade. IL-1RII can bind IL-1, but binding does not result in the formation of a signaling complex. IL-1RII lacks the TIR domain and may act as a decoy receptor. IL-18 is also a member of the IL-1/toll-like receptor family. IL-18 binding to IL-18Rα triggers the association of IL-18Rβ and activation of the MyD88 signaling cascade. IL-18 can also bind to IL-18 binding protein *(IL-18bp)*, a soluble inhibitor that prevents IL-18 interaction with the IL-18 receptor. Interleukin-33 *(IL-33)* binds to the ST2 receptor, which associates with IL-1RAcP and activates the MyD88 signaling pathway.

gene transcription.[60-62] However, IL-1α and IL-1β binding to IL-1R2 does not trigger signal transduction. This receptor may serve as a decoy receptor to decrease the availability of IL-1 to bind to the functionally active IL-1R1 (see "Inhibitors of Proinflammatory Cytokines").[60] Although IL-1 and TNF share many of the same post-receptor signaling pathways, they are not entirely redundant cytokines. IL-1, unlike TNF, cannot activate programmed cell death pathways. IL-1β, known as *endogenous pyrogen*, has hypothalamic effects, including the induction of fever. It plays an important role in activating IL-6, as well as inducing C-reactive protein, an important acute-phase reactant.

INTERLEUKIN-1 IN THE FETUS AND NEONATE

Similar to TNF, IL-1 is produced by fetal Kupffer cells in response to LPS.[33] IL-1 is present in amniotic fluid and increases with premature rupture of membranes.[35] In the context of preterm labor or prolonged rupture of membranes, fetal IL-1 initiates a robust systemic inflammatory response that may progress to multiorgan system damage and death.[63]

Production of IL-1 by umbilical cord blood monocytes is comparable with that of adult controls, even in monocytes obtained from preterm infants.[39,40,64-68] However, in preterm infants with bacterial sepsis, monocyte IL-1 secretion is lower during acute infection but improves significantly during convalescence.[69] When studying the role of IL-1 signaling, Benjamin found that IL-1α rather than IL-1β determined murine sepsis related mortality.[70] After stimulation with LPS or TNF, Contrino and colleagues demonstrated significantly increased expression of IL-1 by umbilical cord blood neutrophils compared with cells from adults suggesting that neutrophil IL-1 secretion may be important in the amplification of the early inflammatory response.[71] IL-1 signaling in mice also stimulates production of neutrophil chemoattractants and recruitment to sites of group B streptococcal infection.[72] Presicce and colleagues further reported that IL-1 blockade decreases concentrations of proinflammatory mediators, secretion of neutrophil chemoattractants, and accumulation of neutrophils at sites of inflammation.[73] Recent evidence from a murine model suggests that antenatal exposure to IL-1 is associated with preterm birth and increased neonatal mortality.[74] Surviving neonates demonstrated elevated levels of multiple proinflammatory cytokines in placental and fetal tissues and morphologic alterations in brain, lung, and intestine.

INTERLEUKIN-6

MOLECULAR MECHANISMS

IL-6 is a pleiotropic cytokine with a wide range of biologic functions and is an important regulator of inflammation, immune responses, oncogenesis, and hematopoiesis.[75-77] IL-6 is a potent inducer of the acute-phase response, as well as specific cellular and humoral immune responses, including B-cell differentiation and T-cell activation, including T helper 17 (T_H17) cells.[75-77] IL-6 is also an important regulator of the transition from acute to chronic inflammation and of the shift from neutrophil to mononuclear cell infiltration.[78] IL-6 is not expressed constitutively,

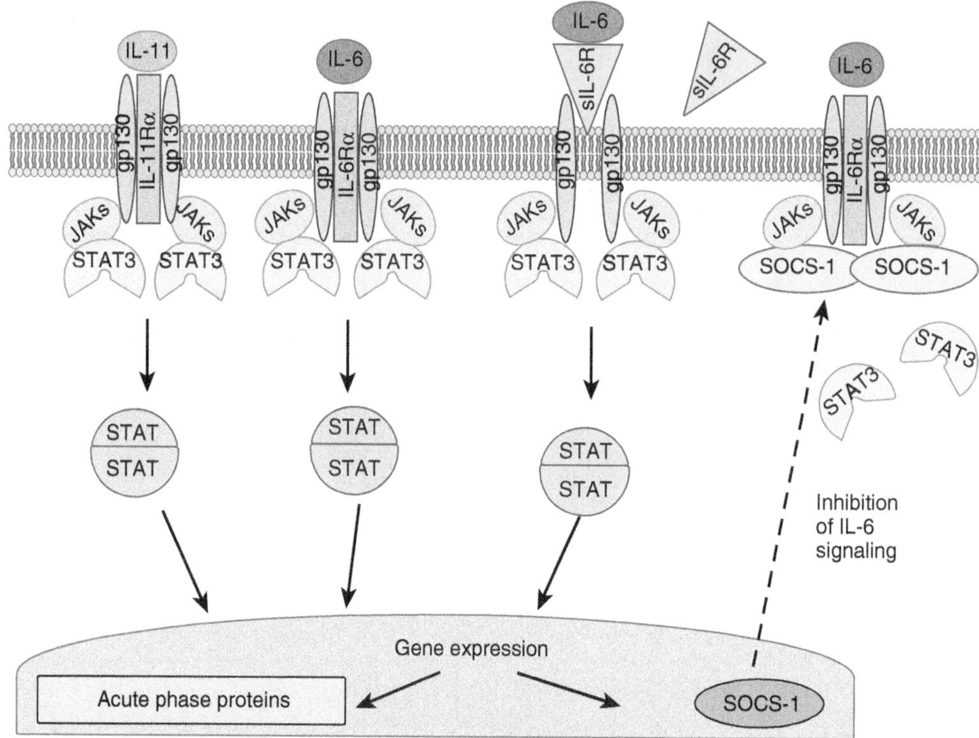

Fig. 121.3 Interleukin-6 *(IL-6)* and interleukin-11 *(IL-11)* receptors are members of the IL-6 receptor family and utilize a common signal transducing subunit glycoprotein 130 *(gp130)*. IL-6 and IL-11 bind to unique receptor-α chains, IL-6Rα and IL-11Rα, respectively. A soluble form of IL-6 receptor *(sIL-6R)* can also bind IL-6, and this complex can then associate with gp130 and initiate IL-6 signaling through a process termed *trans signaling.* Receptor binding triggers association of gp130, activation of Janus kinases *(JAKs)* and signal transducer and activator of transcription 3 *(STAT3)*, and the subsequent activation of gene transcription. STAT3 induces transcription of multiple genes, including toe encoding acute-phase proteins and suppressor of cytokine signaling 1 *(SOCS-1)*. SOCS-1 acts as a negative feedback regulator of IL-6 signaling by preventing JAK/signal transducer and activator of transcription *(STAT)* signaling.

and its production is triggered in response to infection and tissue injury, as well as other cytokines, such as TNF, IL-1β, and interferon (IFN)-γ. IL-6 is produced by a variety of cells, including monocytes, macrophages, endothelial cells, fibroblasts, B and T cells, and some tumor cells.[75,79]

INTERLEUKIN-6 RECEPTORS

The IL-6 receptor system consists of two components: a ligand-binding molecule IL-6R and a nonligand binding signal transducer glycoprotein 130 (gp130) (Fig. 121.3).[75,80] GP130 is also the common signal-transducing subunit for other members of the cytokine receptor family, including IL-11, oncostatin M, ciliary neurotrophic factor, cardiotrophin 1, leukemia inhibitory factor, IL-27, and IL-31, leading to redundancy in cytokine activity.[11,75,81] Although the membrane IL-6R is expressed on hepatocytes, monocytes, macrophages, neutrophils, and some types of lymphocytes, a naturally occurring soluble form of IL-6R (sIL-6R) is also present in most body fluids.[81–83] IL-6 binding to sIL-6R triggers the association with the signal-transducing gp130 component in cells that do not express the membrane-bound form of IL-6R.[81] Thus, unlike most other soluble cytokine receptors, sIL-6R can act as an agonist and through *trans* signaling can activate cell types that do not express IL-6R. A third type of IL-6 signaling, termed IL-6 transpresentation, occurs in the context of antigen specific interactions of dendritic cells with T cells.[82,83] IL-6 bound to IL-6R on dendritic cells is presented to membrane bound gp130 on T cells leading to the development of pathogenic Th17 cells.

INTERLEUKIN-6 IN THE FETUS AND NEONATE

After stimulation with LPS, IL-6 is produced by human fetal Kupffer cells as early as 13 weeks after conception.[33] This cytokine is now recognized as an important marker of the fetal inflammatory response syndrome and subsequent neonatal morbidity and mortality.[84] In a cohort of pregnancies between 34 and 37 weeks gestation, Musilova found that intraamniotic infection and microbial invasion was associated with the highest cord blood IL-6 levels compared to controls.[85] Furthermore, elevated levels of IL-6 in amniotic fluid were predictive of brain injury in preterm infants.[86] Hadley and colleagues reported an increase in IL-6, IL-8, TNF, and IL-1β in term labor, providing evidence of their role in promoting labor with antiinflammatory cytokines notably absent.[87] In addition, Mir recently demonstrated that elevations of IL-6 and Il-8 during parturition were most likely of fetal origin and modulated by placental clearance.[88] Recent studies also noted the effectiveness of a point of care IL-6 determination in the identification of intra-amniotic inflammation.[89,90]

Several studies have evaluated IL-6 production by monocytes from newborn infants.[41,42,64,91–93] Liechty and others demonstrated equivalent IL-6 production by fetal and maternal mononuclear cells after stimulation with IL-1.[91] Angelone and colleagues demonstrated robust LPS-stimulated umbilical cord blood IL-6 production and higher IL-6 to TNF ratios than in adult peripheral blood.[42] However, IL-6 production was reduced in preterm neonates, perhaps contributing to their enhanced susceptibility to overwhelming bacterial infection.[91,94,95] Using flow cytometry and LPS stimulation, Schultz and colleagues demonstrated that both term and preterm monocytes demonstrated enhanced synthesis of IL-6 compared to monocytes from adults, suggesting an enhanced inflammatory response.[96] A recent study by Reuschel and colleagues investigated cytokine profiles of cord blood monocytes stimulated with LPS from several gram negative species.[97] IL-6 and IL-8 responses were greatest following stimulation with *Escherichia coli* and *Enterobacter aerogenes,* while stimulation with *Pseudomonas aeruginosa* showed the weakest response.

INTERLEUKIN-8 AND CHEMOKINES

MOLECULAR MECHANISMS

IL-8 (also termed *CXCL8*) is a member of the chemokine supergene family, which is composed of approximately 50 members.[98-101] Chemokines are critical regulators of immune cell activation and trafficking.[102,103] Chemokines also play an important role in homeostasis, proliferation, differentiation, and survival.[102,103] CXCL8 is the prototype chemokine that orchestrates the recruitment of leukocytes to sites of inflammation. CXCL8 is produced by monocytes, macrophages, fibroblasts, endothelial cells, epithelial cells, hepatocytes, keratinocytes, synovial cells, chondrocytes, and some tumor cells.[104] LPS, TNF, and IL-1, but not IL-6, trigger production of CXCL8. IL-3, granulocyte-macrophage colony-stimulating factor, lectins, immune complexes, and phagocytosis also stimulate CXCL8 production.

The chemokine family is divided into four structural groups characterized by the number and spacing of conserved cysteine residues: CXC, CC, C, and CX_3C. The CXC chemokine group contains one amino acid between the first two cysteine residues. The CXC chemokine subgroup is further divided into two groups based on the presence or absence of a Glu-Leu-Arg (ELR) motif located before the first cysteine residue and termed *ELR^+CXC* and *ELR^-CXC chemokines*.[105] ELR^+CXC chemokines act primarily on neutrophils, whereas ELR^-CXC chemokines interact with mononuclear leukocytes. The ELR^+CXC family includes several chemokines with biologic activity similar to that of CXCL8 such as CXCL1 (GRO-α), CXCL2 (GRO-β), CXCL3 (GRO-γ), CXCL7 (neutrophil-activating peptide 2), CXCL5 (epithelial cell–derived neutrophil-activating protein 78), and CXCL6 (granulocyte chemotactic protein 2).[98]

CC chemokines—the second structural group—contain adjacent cysteine residues. CC chemokines act principally on monocytes, basophils, eosinophils, and some lymphocyte subpopulations.[98,100] The best-characterized CC chemokine is CCL2 (monocyte chemotactic protein 1). Other members of the CC chemokine family include CCL8 (monocyte chemotactic protein 2), CCL7 (monocyte chemotactic protein 3), CCL5 (RANTES), CCL3 (macrophage inflammatory protein 1α), and CCL4 (macrophage inflammatory protein 1β).

The C chemokine structural group has a single amino-terminal cysteine and contains two highly related chemokines, XCL1 (lymphotactin) and XCL2 (single cysteine motif 1β).[99] The last subgroup, CX_3C, contains a single member, CX3CL1 (fractalkine), which is characterized by separation of the first two cysteine residues by three amino acids. CX3CL1, as well as CXCL16, is present in two forms: a membrane-bound form, which acts as a leukocyte adhesion receptor, and a cleaved form, which is secreted and acts as a soluble chemoattractant.[98,101]

CHEMOKINE RECEPTORS

Chemokine receptors are a family of G protein–coupled receptors composed of at least 10 CC chemokine receptors, six CXC chemokine receptors, one CX_3C chemokine receptor, and one C chemokine receptor.[98,106] An unusual feature of this receptor family is the ability to bind more than one chemokine within a particular subclass. An exception is Duffy antigen receptor for chemokines, located on erythrocytes and endothelial cells, which will bind both CC and CXC chemokines. Engagement of this receptor does not appear to activate signal transduction, and Duffy antigen receptor for chemokines may limit leukocyte activation by serving as a chemokine sink.

Two distinct CXCL8 receptors, CXCR1 and CXCR2, have been characterized.[107,108] CXCR1 binds CXCL8 with high affinity and CXCL1 and CXCL7 with low affinity, whereas CXCR2 binds most ELR^+CXC chemokines.[106] Binding of CXCL8 to neutrophil CXCR1 and CXCR2 triggers degranulation and cell migration, but only activation of CXCR1 induces reactive oxygen species (ROS).[102] CXCL8 binding also triggers receptor phosphorylation and desensitization, a process thought to be important for continued cellular ability to detect chemotactic gradients.[109]

INTERLEUKIN-8 IN THE FETUS AND NEONATE

IL-8 in amniotic fluid is associated with intrauterine inflammation and preterm birth as well as the development of neonatal complications including respiratory distress syndrome and chronic lung disease (CLD).[110] Similarly, Taniguchi and colleagues found that fetal mononuclear cell IL-8 production was significantly greater in women with chorioamnionitis than in fetuses of healthy women.[111] In addition to a robust proinflammatory response following microbial invasion of the amniotic cavity, IL-8 induces the infiltration of neutrophils to the site of inflammation.[112] Furthermore IL-1 blockade of IL-8 responses during chorioamnionitis significantly reduces neutrophil activation and intrauterine inflammation.[73] Hadley further noted increased levels of IL-8 in gestational tissues at term labor.[87] Most recently Oh and colleagues reported the utility of a point of care IL-8 assay in prediction of intra-amniotic inflammation.[113]

Although early studies suggested deficiencies in IL-8 production by neonatal mononuclear cells, more recent literature indicates an intact proinflammatory cytokine pathway.[114-116] After LPS stimulation of whole-blood cultures, IL-8 production by neonates exceeded adult levels.[96,117,118] Moreover, IL-8 production was independent of gestational age although gender significant differences have been observed.[94,119]

INTERLEUKIN-12 FAMILY

MOLECULAR MECHANISMS

IL-12 is a potent proinflammatory cytokine that plays a major role in linking innate and adaptive immune responses.[120-122] IL-12 is a member of the IL-12 cytokine family, which comprises structurally related but functionally disparate cytokines, including IL-12, IL-23, IL-27, and IL-35.[120,123,124] IL-12 is a heterodimer composed of two subunits, an α-chain (p35 subunit) and a β-chain (p40 subunit).[121,125] The p40 subunit of IL-12 contains the receptor binding site, whereas the p35 subunit is required for signal transduction. The p40 chain of IL-12 can also associate with another molecule termed *p19* to form a distinctive heterodimeric cytokine, IL-23.[126] A homologue of IL-12p40, Epstein-Barr virus–induced gene 3 *(EBI3)*, forms a noncovalent association with another homologue of IL-12p35 (p28) to produce IL-27, whereas *EBI3* in association with IL-12p35 produces a related cytokine, IL-35.[124,127]

IL-12 is produced in response to inflammatory stimuli by phagocytic cells, such as monocytes, macrophages, and neutrophils, and by microglial and dendritic cells. IL-23 and IL-27 are produced primarily by macrophages and dendritic cells.[120,123] IL-12 induces production of IFN-γ and regulates T_H1-type inflammatory responses. IL-27 also promotes T_H1 cell differentiation and IFN-γ production but preferentially acts on naïve $CD4^+$ T cells.[120] By contrast, IL-23 acts on several T-cell types, plays a key role in T_H17 subset maturation, and promotes synthesis of IL-17, a proinflammatory cytokine involved in neutrophil-mediated inflammation.[123,124] Both IL-12 and IL-27 act to suppress the development of IL-17-secreting T cells and limit IL-17-mediated proinflammatory acti ons.[120,123,124] The most recent addition to this group, IL-35, induces regulatory T cells, and thus is antiinflammatory in its actions.

INTERLEUKIN-12 RECEPTORS

IL-12 receptors are expressed primarily on NK and T cells. The receptor is composed of two subunits, IL-12Rβ1 and IL-12Rβ2, and is a member of the gp130 cytokine receptor superfamily.[124,128] IL-12 signaling is through the Janus kinase (JAK)/signal transducer and activator of transcription (STAT) family signal transduction pathway leading to the synthesis of IFNγ.[121,123,129] IL-23 binds to a receptor composed of the IL-12Rβ1 subunit and an IL-23 receptor subunit and activates a similar pattern of JAKs and STATs.[121] The IL-27 receptor is also located on NK and T cells but is composed of an orphan receptor subunit WSX1/TCCR linked to a gp130 subunit.[124] IL-35 is able to bind to IL-12Rβ2-gp130, IL-12Rβ2-IL-12Rβ2, and gp130-gp130, and activates STAT1 and STAT3.[130] IL-12 and IL-27 signaling is mediated principally through STAT4, whereas IL-23 signaling is mediated through STAT3.[121,123]

INTERLEUKIN-12 IN THE FETUS AND NEONATE

Decreased expression of IL-12, a key cytokine involved in T_H1 up-regulation, has been observed in pregnancy.[131] IL-12 levels are therefore very low in the fetus and neonate.[132] IL-12p70 synthesis is impaired in cord blood mononuclear cells, which is reflective of adenosine-induced cAMP accumulation.[47,133] Further, both murine and human studies have demonstrated reduced expression of IL-12p70 following infectious challenge.[134] Additional studies have shown impaired nucleosome remodeling and deficient IL-12p35 expression.[133,135]

INTERFERON-γ

MOLECULAR MECHANISMS

IFN-γ is a pleiotropic cytokine that modulates antiviral and antimicrobial immunity. IFN-γ is predominantly produced by T_H1 cells, $CD8^+$ T cells, γδ T cells, NK T cells, NK cells, and macrophages in response to IL-12, IL-27, and IL-18; production is inhibited by IL-4, IL-10, and transforming growth factor β (TGFβ).[11,136,137] IFN-γ is a central effector of cell-mediated immunity and a critical mediator of T-cell recruitment and phagocyte-mediated clearance of pathogens.[138] In macrophages, IFN-γ triggers cytokine (including TNF) and chemokine synthesis, enhanced oxygen radical generation, nitric oxide (NO) production, and induction of major histocompatibility complex class II expression.[137] IFN-γ synthesis is tightly regulated as dysregulated production can result in chronic inflammation, tissue damage, and cell death.[138]

INTERFERON-γ RECEPTORS

Similarly to other cytokine receptor systems, the receptor is composed of two subunits, IFN-γR1, which is necessary for ligand binding, and IFN-γR2, which is involved in signal transduction.[12,136,137] The cellular targets of IFN-γ are numerous as IFN-γ receptors are expressed on virtually every cell type, and most of the biologic effects mediated by IFN-γ are through transcriptional regulation of approximately 500 genes.[136,137,139]

INTERFERON-γ IN THE FETUS AND NEONATE

The T_H1 to T_H2 imbalance of the fetus and neonate is associated with low to undetectable IFN-γ levels in neonatal cells from infected and healthy neonates.[140] This is mediated by a reduction in IL-12 P70 production by neonatal mononuclear cells and other T_H1 inducers of NK cell production of IFN-γ.[44,135] In a study of the developmental trajectory of multiple cytokines during the first week of life, Lee and colleagues demonstrated increasing levels of IFN -γ and IL-17 with simultaneous decreasing levels of IL-6 and IL-10.[141] Furthermore, Corbett and colleagues found that IFN-γ levels rose slowly after birth to adult levels by 1 year of age.[142]

INTERLEUKIN-18

MOLECULAR MECHANISMS

IL-18 is an important regulator of both innate and acquired immune responses. IL-18 is a member of the IL-1 family and shares structural homology with IL-1β.[143,144] Similarly to IL-1β, IL-18 is synthesized in a pro form with an unusual signal peptide that lacks the amino acid sequence necessary for secretion.[145,146] Unlike IL-1β, the precursor form of IL-18 is constitutively expressed and has no biologic activity.[146] ProIL-18 is also cleaved by caspase 1 to an 18-kDa protein. IL-18 is produced by a wide range of cell types, including macrophages, monocytes, T and B cells, dendritic cells, epithelial cells, and keratinocytes.[50,147,148]

INTERLEUKIN-18 RECEPTORS

The IL-18 receptor system is similar to that of the multicomponent IL-1β receptor system and is expressed in a variety of cells, including macrophages, neutrophils, NK cells, smooth muscle cells, and dendritic cells.[50,147,148] The IL-18 receptor is composed of two subunits, an IL-18-binding component (IL-18Rα) and a signal-transducing component (IL-18Rβ), which is a homologue of IL-1 receptor accessory protein (see Fig. 121.2).[50,147,148] IL-18 binding to the IL-18 receptor complex activates signaling pathways that stimulate the synthesis of several proinflammatory proteins, including other cytokines and cytokine receptors, chemokine and chemokine receptors, NO synthase, adhesion molecules, and the Fas ligand.[50,147] Although several similarities between the biologic properties of IL-1 and IL-18 have been identified, significant differences are recognized. Unlike IL-1, IL-18 is not able to induce fever but can stimulate IFN-γ synthesis in T cells and NK cells.[147–149]

INTERLEUKIN-18 IN THE FETUS AND NEONATE

Although an early study found diminished umbilical cord blood mononuclear IL-18 production in response to stimulation with group B streptococci, more recent studies have reported increased levels of IL-18 in preterm infants compared to those born at term with levels inversely related to gestational age.[150,151] Wynn and colleagues reported that IL-18 increased mortality in neonatal sepsis through induction of IL-17A, which, in turn, is dependent on IL-1 receptor 1(IL-1R1) signaling.[152]

INTERLEUKIN-33

MOLECULAR MECHANISMS

IL-33 is among the more recently described members of the IL-1 superfamily, its discovery generating considerable interest over the past decade due to its pleiotropic effects on inflammation in several important human diseases. IL-33 is known as an *alarmin*, constitutively expressed by a host of cells, processed and released when the cells are damaged or exposed to inflammatory stimuli.[153–156] In the steady state, IL-33 is concentrated in nuclei of endothelial cells and epithelial cells of mucosal barriers.[157,158] Not surprisingly, IL-33 plays important roles in modulating both mucosal and systemic immune responses.[159]

MEMBRANE-BOUND AND SOLUBLE INTERLEUKIN-33 RECEPTOR

The heterodimeric IL-33 receptor is composed of a unique subunit, ST2, and the IL-1-receptor accessory protein (IL-1RAcP), which is shared with other IL-1 superfamily members (see Fig. 121.2).[160–162] A variety of immune and nonimmune cell types can express ST2. Classically, ST2 is found on eosinophils, basophils, mast cells, type 2 innate lymphoid cells, and T_H2 cells, all type 2 inflammatory cells that mediate immunity to helminths, tissue repair, and pathologic allergic immune responses.[163,164]

Like other IL-1 receptor superfamily members, ST2 also exists as a soluble isoform (sST2) that lacks the transmembrane and intracellular domains of membrane-bound ST2 (see Fig. 121.2).[165] Induced by IL-33 itself, sST2 acts as a "decoy" receptor to consume free IL-33, preventing it from continually acting on target cells.[166,167] This regulatory mechanism balances proinflammatory effects of IL-33, which, left unchecked, lead to rapid pathologic changes at mucosal surfaces, including the lung and gastrointestinal tract.[160] The lungs of mice treated with excess IL-33 show vascular inflammation and epithelial hypertrophy in larger airways with mucus plugging. The animals also exhibit splenomegaly with extramedullary hematopoiesis, significant esophagitis, and intestinal goblet cell hypertrophy and hyperplasia with increased production of mucus.

INTERLEUKIN-33 AXIS IN THE FETUS AND NEONATE

Given its predominance at mucosal surfaces, IL-33 may provide a link between environmental exposures during the fetal and neonatal period and priming of later allergic disorders. In a

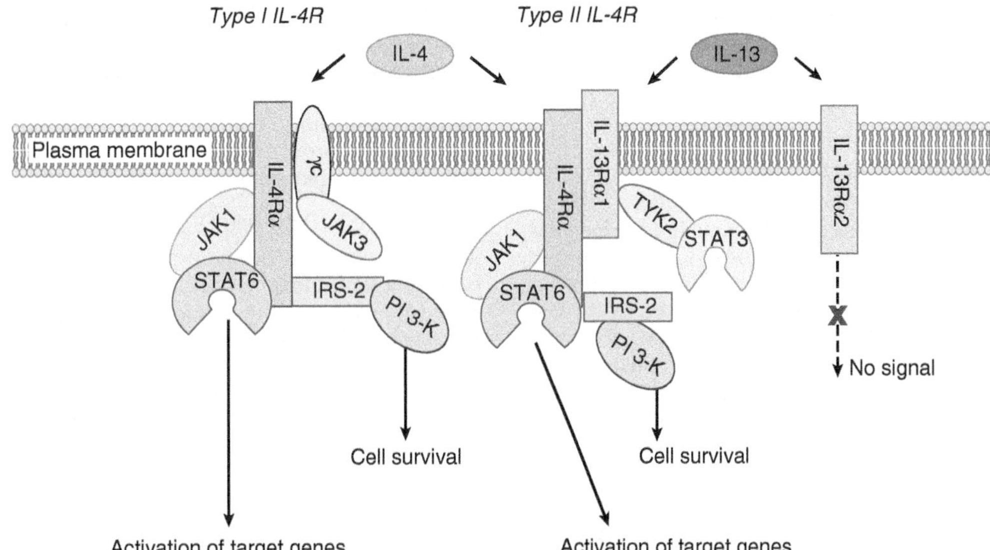

Fig. 121.4 Interleukin (IL)-4 and IL-13 receptor complexes. IL-4 can bind to two different receptors: type I IL-4 receptor *(IL-4R)* and type II IL-4R. Type I IL-4R is composed of IL-4Rα and the common γ subunit (γc), whereas type II IL-4R contains both IL-4Rα and IL-13Rα subunits. IL-4 binds to both type I IL-4R and type II IL-4R by way of the common IL-4Rα chain. By contrast, IL-13 binds only to type II IL-4R by way of the IL-13Rα1 subunit. Both receptors activate signal transducer and activator of transcription 6 *(STAT6)* and insulin receptor substrate 2 *(IRS-2)* signaling pathways, resulting in the induction of gene expression and cell survival pathways. IL-13 also binds to IL-13Rα2 with high affinity. However, this receptor does not initiate signaling and may serve as a decoy receptor to suppress IL-13 signaling. *JAK*, Janus kinase; *PI 3-K*, phosphoinositide 3-kinase; *STAT3*, signal transducer and activator of transcription 3; *TYK2*, tyrosine kinase 2.

prospective cohort study of pregnant women in Canada, IL-33 levels in cord blood (with thymic stromal lymphopoietin, another cytokine associated with epithelial type 2 inflammation) directly correlated with maternal allergy status and heavy exposure to street traffic.[168] Basic investigations in mice revealed that IL-33 naturally accumulates in the lung during the early alveolar phase of development, a time during which neonates are susceptible to significant type 2 inflammation caused by allergens.[169] In this animal model, blockade of IL-33 at the time of initial sensitization to house dust mite antigen prevents airway inflammation and mucus production upon reencountering this allergen later in life. Like some human infants with BPD, wild-type neonatal mice exposed to hyperoxia during the late saccular phase of lung development develop airway hyperresponsiveness and express many genes associated with type 2 inflammation and asthma.[170] However, mice deficient in IL-33 or ST2 do not upregulate such genes upon exposure to hyperoxia and do not develop BPD-like histopathology.[170,171] A recent nested case-control study from Turkey found that while cord blood levels of IL-33 were similar in control premature infants and those eventually diagnosed with moderate to severe BPD, serum IL-33 at 36 weeks post-menstrual age was significantly higher in the BPD group.[172]

The IL-33/ST2 axis may also play roles in the neonatal response to infection. As opposed to those of adult mice, lungs of wild-type infant mice secrete large amounts of IL-33 and develop severe inflammation after infection with respiratory syncytial virus (RSV).[173] In contrast, infant mice lacking ST2 were protected from RSV-induced disease of the airways. Consistent with these data in mice, IL-33 is rapidly elevated in nasal aspirates of human infants infected with RSV. Similarly, sST2 is significantly elevated in nasopharyngeal aspirates of infants requiring mechanical ventilation due to RSV bronchiolitis, relative to infants with less severe bronchiolitis, in a multi-center cohort study in the Netherlands.[174] As sST2 is induced by IL-33 in a negative feedback loop, these data suggest that unrestrained activity of IL-33 may contribute to severe RSV bronchiolitis in infants. In the same study, a polymorphism in *Il1rl1*, encoding ST2, was determined to be significantly associated with severe bronchiolitis, though the underlying mechanism remains unclear.

IL-33 can amplify mucosal inflammation to the detriment of the host. Conversely, IL-33 can also limit severe systemic inflammation. While these studies remain to be performed in neonates, adult mice treated with recombinant IL-33 more readily recruit neutrophils to the site of infection and are protected from death in a model of severe polymicrobial sepsis.[175] Additional research into IL-33/ST2 in neonates may lead to novel therapies to treat a variety of disorders of inflammation seen commonly in the neonatal intensive care unit (NICU).

INTERLEUKIN-4 AND INTERLEUKIN-13

MOLECULAR MECHANISMS

The products of numerous innate and adaptive immune cells, IL-4 and IL-13 are type 2 inflammatory cytokines with some overlapping biologic properties.[14,176–178] Expression of these functionally-related cytokines is linked, as the genes encoding IL-4 and IL-13, and another type 2 inflammatory cytokine, IL-5, are neighbors at the same genomic locus with similar regulatory elements.[179,180] Classically, both IL-4 and IL-13 are necessary for proper antihelminth immunity.[179] They also induce macrophages to adopt an "M2" phenotype associated with tissue repair and type 2 immune responses.[181] IL-4 and IL-13 are also key drivers of allergic airway inflammation and hyperreactivity. While related, the two cytokines do not share all biologic properties, though. For instance, IL-4 uniquely drives TH2 differentiation of $CD4^+$ T cells.[178,182] Additionally, IL-4 promotes antibody class-switching in B cells to IgE.

INTERLEUKIN-4 AND INTERLEUKIN-13 RECEPTORS

The overlapping biologic properties of these two cytokines are the result of a common component in their respective receptors. IL-4 can bind to two receptor complexes.[178,183,184] The type I IL-4 receptor, consisting of a ligand-binding chain (IL-4Rα) and the common γ-signaling chain (γc), binds only IL-4 (Fig. 121.4). It is expressed predominantly by lymphoid and myeloid immune cells. The type II IL-4 receptor, composed of IL-4Rα and an IL-13Rα1 subunit, binds both IL-4 and IL-13 (see Fig. 121.4). It is expressed by some myeloid cells, but in contrast to the type I receptor, the type II receptor is expressed mainly by nonhematopoietic cells, like epithelial cells. A second IL-13 binding component has been identified, IL-13Rα2, which can signal a pro-fibrotic program in macrophages or act as a decoy receptor to down-modulate IL-13 activity in some contexts.[185]

INTERLEUKIN-4 AND INTERLEUKIN-13 IN THE FETUS AND NEONATE

Several lines of evidence suggest that neonatal immunity is biased toward type 2 inflammation. Minimally differentiated CD4+ T cells in the neonate readily produce IL-4 and IL-13, especially compared to adult CD4+ T cells.[186,187] Indeed, naïve neonatal CD4+T cells express and sequester IL-4 intracellularly even prior to encountering antigen.[187] These data are supported by the fact that the gene encoding IL-4 is epigenetically poised for rapid expression.[188] Further, the gene encoding IL-13 remains in an open, or accessible, chromatin state in neonatal CD4+T cells, even when cultured under the same conditions that render the locus inaccessible in adult CD4+ T cells.[189] While T_H1 and T_H2 cells are generated in response to immune challenge in the neonate, IL-4 and IL-13 produced during a recall response to the same antigen will selectively kill T_H1 cells.[190,191]

Such an unbalanced immune response with a T_H2 bias can lead to inappropriate responses to pathogens and predisposition to develop exaggerated allergic or atopic inflammation. Herberth and colleagues noted a link between low IFN-γ levels, high IL-4 levels, and subsequent risk for atopy.[192] IL-13 is produced as early as 27 weeks gestation by fetal mononuclear cells, and elevated umbilical cord blood IL-13 levels are associated with later atopic disease of childhood.[181,193] A large genomic study revealed polymorphisms predicted to result in over-activity of the genes encoding IL-4 and IL-13 are associated with development of severe RSV bronchiolitis in newborns and infants.[194] In nasal aspirates of infants suffering from RSV bronchiolitis, it was found that a predominance of type 2 cytokines, including IL-4 and IL-13, combined with a relative paucity of type 1 cytokines, including IFNγ, predicted more severe disease.[195] Finally, a recent report detailed a surprising role for IL-4 in promoting deleterious inflammation in the brain of fetal and neonatal rats born under conditions of intrauterine growth restriction.[196] In this model, neutralization of IL-4 prevents the accumulation of macrophages and protects oligodendrocytes. Altogether, these data support a model in which unchecked type 2 inflammation can put the fetus and neonate in danger of adverse outcomes, both short term and long term.

ANTIINFLAMMATORY CYTOKINES AND ENDOGENOUS INHIBITORS OF PROINFLAMMATORY CYTOKINES

INTERLEUKIN-10

MOLECULAR MECHANISMS

IL-10 was first described as a product of T_H2 cells that inhibited production of IFN-γ by T_H1 cells.[197] It is now recognized that IL-10 possesses diverse and potent immunomodulatory properties in many contexts. Expressed by numerous immune and nonimmune cells, IL-10 inhibits synthesis of a wide range of proinflammatory cytokines, including TNF, IL-1, IL-6, IFN-γ, IL-12, IL-18, and CXC and CC chemokines.[14,198-201] IL-10 also stimulates production of natural proinflammatory cytokine inhibitors such as IL-1RA and soluble TNFRs, discussed elsewhere in this chapter.[14,198-200] IL-10 further modulates innate and adaptive immune responses by down-regulating expression of class II major histocompatibility complex and intercellular adhesion molecule (ICAM)-1, production of oxygen radicals, and synthesis of NO. Thus, IL-10 maintains immune homeostasis in the steady state and regulates the magnitude of inflammatory responses in the setting of infection.[198-200]

INTERLEUKIN-10 RECEPTOR

IL-10 receptors are members of the class II cytokine receptor family and are expressed predominantly on immune cells.[198,202] The IL-10 receptor is composed of IL-10R1, a ligand-binding subunit, and IL-10R2, an accessory subunit required for signaling. Signal transduction downstream of IL-10R inhibits synthesis of proinflammatory cytokines and also enhances mRNA degradation of proinflammatory cytokines.[198,203] Further, IL-10 promotes expression of proteins that suppress proinflammatory signaling cascades at the biochemical level.[201,204]

INTERLEUKIN-10 IN THE FETUS AND NEONATE

During pregnancy, mechanisms preventing maternal "rejection" of a semi-allogeneic fetus remain incompletely described. Cytotrophoblasts of the developing fetal placenta produce IL-10 capable of inhibiting T-cell activation in vitro.[205] Further, placental extracts produce soluble factors capable of enhancing the expression of IL-10 by cultured macrophages, as well as generating immunosuppressive CD4+Foxp3+ regulatory T cells.[206] However, in mouse models in vivo, pregnancy and delivery proceed normally in mattings in which IL-10 is completely absent from the maternal-fetal interface.[207] In fact, larger litter sizes and larger fetuses and neonates are seen in such mattings, though the mechanisms underlying these observations remain to be elucidated.

An imbalance of pro- and antiinflammatory signals in the neonate may contribute to the observation that neonates are highly susceptible to infections. Soluble factors in cord blood plasma enhance production of IL-10 by adult blood mononuclear cells.[208] Conflicting data exist regarding the intrinsic ability of neonatal immune cells to produce IL-10 when stimulated in culture, but the most comprehensive report to date showed that neonatal cells make enhanced IL-10 to a variety of stimuli, compared to their counterparts in the adult.[44] Interestingly, though, neonatal immune cells respond less robustly to IL-10 than do adult immune cells. While high-dose IL-10 completely inhibits the expression of proinflammatory cytokines by adult blood immune cells stimulated in vitro, IL-10 only partially prevents neonatal cells from elaborating the same cytokines.[209] In mouse models, the challenge of neonates with *Listeria monocytogenes* or Group B *Streptococcus* results in robust increases in levels of plasma IL-10 early in the immune response.[210-214] The blockade of IL-10/IL-10R just prior to infection with either organism enhances neutrophil migration to infected organs, bacterial clearance, and survival.

As the IL-10 axis maintains antiinflammatory "tone," disturbed homeostasis of IL-10 can result in unchecked inflammation, compromising barrier integrity. Mutations in the genes encoding IL-10, IL-10R1 *(Il10RA)*, and IL-10R2 *(Il10RB)* in humans have all been associated with very early-onset inflammatory bowel disease, which can be especially severe when it presents in the neonatal period.[215] Consistent with these observations, mice lacking IL-10 or the IL-10R spontaneously develop colitis.[216,217] Similarly, several studies in rodent models of NEC revealed that IL-10 was essential to protect neonates from severe intestinal pathology.[218] Further, intestinal IL-10 was enhanced by feeding with mother's milk, compared with formula feeding. Indeed, IL-10 itself can be detected in human milk, with some data linking lower IL-10 levels in breastmilk with the development of NEC. Finally, in preterm neonates who went on to develop BPD, circulating levels of IL-10 were significantly lower at 24 hours of life than preterm neonates not diagnosed with BPD.[219] Taken together, these data highlight the need to better understand how to manipulate IL-10 to benefit neonates clinically.

INHIBITORS OF PROINFLAMMATORY CYTOKINES

SOLUBLE TUMOR NECROSIS FACTOR RECEPTORS

In response to various proinflammatory stimuli, including TNF itself, TNFR-1 and TNFR-2 can be proteolytically cleaved and the extracellular cytokine binding domains released.[220-223] Both forms of the soluble TNF receptors (sTNFRs) retain their ability to bind TNF and compete with membrane-bound TNFRs, leading to decreased availability of circulating TNF.[223] Conversion of membrane-bound TNFRs to sTNFRs, or "shedding" of receptors from the cell surface, also serves to decrease responsiveness to TNF by decreasing the number of cell-surface receptors. Classically, sTNFRs represent a negative feedback loop to regulate TNF bioactivity and promote balanced inflammation. However, in some contexts, sTNFRs are believed to enhance the half-life and bioactivity of circulating TNF.[220] Studies of adult sepsis support that both TNF and sTNFRs increase rapidly in sepsis, with some investigators associating increased TNF and/or sTNFRs ratios with increased mortality, while others suggest that ratios of TNF to sTNFRs drive outcomes.[224-227] Fewer data in neonates exist, but one study showed significantly but modestly elevated serum levels of sTNFRs in preterm and term neonates with confirmed or suspected sepsis or pneumonia, compared to uninfected infants.[228] Concentrations of cord blood sTNFR1 were elevated in a small cohort of infants of 28 or fewer weeks gestation who went on to develop CLD, relative to gestational age-matched infants who did not develop CLD.[229] Finally, urinary levels of sTNFRs were elevated in infants diagnosed with posterior urethral valves and appeared to directly correlate with clinical laboratory markers of renal dysfunction.[230] These data support that sTNFRs are released under conditions of inflammation, but the complex biology merits further study in the fetus and neonate.

INTERLEUKIN-1 RECEPTOR ANTAGONIST

As IL-1 is so powerfully proinflammatory, numerous endogenous mechanisms exist to balance its effects. Interleukin-1 receptor antagonist (IL-1ra) and type II interleukin-1 receptor (IL-1R2) are two natural regulators of IL-1 biologic activity.[14,51,231-233] Creating a negative feedback loop, synthesis of IL-1ra is triggered by the same stimuli that trigger IL-1 production. IL-1ra is a competitive inhibitor and binds to IL-1R1 with similar affinity as IL-1α and IL-1β, but it has no agonist activity. During the inflammatory response, IL-1ra levels tend to increase later than IL-1 levels, suggesting that IL-1ra functions to block further IL-1 activity and has a role in the termination of the inflammatory response.[234] IL-1ra has been studied in a variety of contexts in the neonate. Neonatal-onset multisystem inflammatory disease (NOMID), a rare but deadly disorder of infancy characterized by severe immune dysregulation and overproduction of active IL-1, has been successfully treated with recombinant IL-1ra (anakinra).[235,236] In rodent models of BPD, administration of recombinant IL-1ra protected animals from hyperoxia- and inflammation-induced histologic and functional BPD and pulmonary hypertension.[237-239] Finally, as mounting evidence suggested IL-1 is a major player in mediating perinatal brain injury, IL-1ra has shown substantial promise in protecting the neonatal brain from injury in numerous animal models.[240]

TYPE II INTERLEUKIN-1 RECEPTOR

Expressed by a variety of myeloid and lymphoid cells, IL-1R2 is a decoy receptor for IL-1 with both a membrane-bound and as a truncated, soluble form.[51,232,233,241,242] IL-1R2 is able to bind IL-1 but does not signal. Not only does IL-1R2 bind active IL-1 forms, it also binds pro-IL-1a and b, preventing them from being cleaved into active IL-1. While production of IL-1R2 is inhibited by proinflammatory mediators, including TNF and IFNγ, IL-1R2 can be induced by a variety of antiinflammatory cytokines and type 2 inflammatory cytokines, such as IL-4, IL-13, and IL-10.[242] Circulating levels of soluble IL-1R2 are increased during systemic inflammation, presumably serving to modulate systemic IL-1 activity.[242-244] Indeed, IL-1R2 is sharply upregulated in the setting of neonatal sepsis, though the specific roles for IL-1R2 in the fetus and neonate have yet to be determined.[245]

INTERLEUKIN-1 RECEPTOR 8

IL1R8, also known as *Toll/IL-1R (TIR) 8* or *SIGIRR* (single-immunoglobulin interleukin-1 receptor-related molecule), tempers signaling by a variety of proinflammatory Toll-like receptors and IL-1R family members, such as the IL-1, IL-18, and IL-33 receptors.[242] It is widely expressed by numerous immune and nonimmune cells, including epithelial cells at mucosal barriers. Given its immunomodulatory role and expression pattern, it is perhaps not surprising that mutations in the gene encoding IL1R8 have been associated with development of severe NEC in premature infants.[246] Indeed, relative to wild-type mice, mice lacking IL-1R8 exhibit exaggerated production of proinflammatory cytokines in the intestine, along with more severe histopathology after induction of NEC.[246,247] On the other hand, transfer of IL1R8-deficient natural killer cells to newborn mice provided enhanced protection against infection with murine cytomegalovirus, compared to transfer of wild-type NK cells. Thus, manipulation of IL1R8 may alter the course of dysregulated inflammation associated with NEC, while also modulating immunity of newborns to pathogens.

INTERLEUKIN-18-BINDING PROTEIN

IL-18, similarly to IL-1 and TNF, has a naturally occurring circulating inhibitor.[148] However, unlike sTNFR or IL-1R2, IL-18-binding protein (IL-18bp) is not a truncated form of the extracellular domain of the IL-18 receptor. Rather, IL-18bp is a naturally occurring, secreted antagonist of IL-18 that binds to IL-18 with high affinity and prevents binding to the IL-18 receptor.[147,148] IL-18bp is constitutively produced and is present at high levels in the serum in the steady state.[148] It is further induced by interferons, including IFNγ, as part of a negative feedback loop that limits IFN-mediated inflammation.[148,248] Current data support a model in which a disturbed ratio of IL-18 to IL-18bp promotes excessive inflammation and tissue damage. Recently, a cohort of infants have been described with genetic mutations causing hyperactivation of "inflammasomes," protein complexes that promote rapid release of proinflammatory cytokines, including active IL-18.[249-251] One such infant developed an overwhelming immune response to a parainfluenza infection, characterized by a great excess of IL-18 and inadequate levels of IL-18bp.[250] Her disease was refractory to a host of immunosuppressives, but she rapidly improved after addition of recombinant IL-18bp to the immunomodulatory regimen. These data underscore the importance of balanced immune activation, as well as the need to investigate roles for IL-18 in the fetus and neonate.

THE COMPLEX, MULTI-SYSTEM INFLAMMATORY RESPONSE

CROSSTALK BETWEEN LEUKOCYTES AND ENDOTHELIUM

The accumulation of specific subpopulations of leukocytes at the site of inflammation is the result of a series of events: (1) endothelial cell activation and the expression of adhesion molecules; (2) leukocyte expression of adhesion molecules and leukocyte-endothelial cell adhesion; (3) leukocyte transendothelial migration; (4) leukocyte migration along a chemotactic gradient; and (5) the release of reactive oxidants, proteinases, and antimicrobial polypeptides at the site of inflammation.[252,253] As inflammation progresses, a transition occurs to antiinflammatory mediators, which is crucial to contain the inflammatory response, limit host tissue damage, and promote tissue remodeling. Cytokines are involved at each step of this process and act both locally and systemically to initiate, maintain, and finally resolve the inflammatory response, or alternatively, mediate the transition to a chronic inflammatory state.

Leukocytes and endothelial cells have key roles in the initiation of local inflammation. At the site of inflammation, the local release of TNF and IL-1 and other cytokines, including IL-8, IL-4, IL-13, IL-18, IL-6, and IFN-γ, leads to activation of endothelial cells and expression or up-regulation of adhesion molecules such as selectins, ICAMs, platelet–endothelial cell adhesion molecule 1, and vascular cell adhesion molecule 1.[252,253] Cytokines, ROS, and reactive nitrogen species also induce degradation of the endothelial glycocalyx. This event exposes adhesion molecules to circulating leukocytes and initiates leukocyte-endothelial cell interaction. Increased endothelial cell surface expression of the adhesion molecules E-selectin and P-selectin, in conjunction with the constitutively expressed L-selectin on leukocytes, mediates the initial adhesive interaction resulting in the trapping and rolling of leukocytes along the endothelium.[254]

The endothelium is also a source of cytokines such as TNF, IL-1, IL-4, IL-11, IL-8, and IL-18.[255] These cytokines, as well as IFN-γ, promote glycocalyx degradation, leukocyte activation, surface expression of the adhesion molecules β integrins, and the shedding of L-selectins.[106,253,254] The interactions between leukocyte β_2 integrins and endothelial counterligands such as ICAM-1, ICAM-2, and ICAM-3 mediate the firm attachment of the leukocytes to the endothelium and subsequent migration. Activated endothelium also produces CC and CXC chemokines, which are released or localized on the luminal surface of the endothelium to further enhance leukocyte adhesion.[253-255] Transmigration occurs by migration through endothelial junctions (paracellular transmigration) or through the endothelial cell itself (transcellular migration).[182,254,256,257] Paracellular migration involves the release of endothelium-expressed VE-cadherin and involves platelet–endothelial cell adhesion molecule 1, ICAM-1, ICAM-2, CD99, endothelial cell–selective adhesion molecule, and junctional adhesion molecules. The specific adhesion molecules involved in transmigration are both stimulus dependent and cell dependent. Endothelial cell dysfunction in inflammation varies widely between different blood vessel types and different organs.

Movement of leukocytes to the inflammatory site is directed along a chemotactic gradient, where the strongest concentration of chemoattractants is at the site of inflammation. Local production of chemokines by both immune and nonimmune cells serves as a source for long-lasting chemoattractants. The movement of specific populations of leukocytes into the inflammatory site depends on the specific stimuli and the resultant type of chemokines synthesized (i.e., CXC chemokines vs. CC chemokines).[182,253,254] Thus, the movement of leukocytes is a cytokine-mediated process and the result of coordination of endothelial expression of adhesion molecules, leukocyte adherence, and specific chemotactic gradients.

Cytokines are also directly involved in the activation of cells at the inflammatory site. After recruitment of inflammatory cells to the site of inflammation, cytokines can further amplify the inflammatory response through the activation of transcription factors, such as NFκB, which regulate proinflammatory gene expression. Both TNF and IL-1 increase the expression of the genes for proinflammatory cytokines, chemokines, adhesion molecules, inducible NO synthase, matrix metalloproteinases, and cyclooxygenase 2.[2] Cytokines and chemokines can also affect the activation of resident and recruited phagocytic cells. Both CXC and CC chemokines are capable of triggering the generation of oxygen radicals in their specific target cells, as well as exocytosis of secretory vesicles and release of specific granules, resulting in an outpouring of enzymes and other soluble proteins.[106,258] In adherent neutrophils, TNF triggers the release of oxygen radicals and degradative granule enzymes such as elastase; TNF also promotes cytoskeleton reorganization.[259,260] IFN-γ acts directly on phagocytic cells and enhances bactericidal activity, phagocytosis, NO synthesis, and oxygen radical production.[137] Proinflammatory cytokines such as TNF, IL-1, and IFN-γ stimulate the release of potent lipid mediators such as platelet-activating factor, leukotrienes, thromboxane, and prostaglandins.[261] IL-18 has a direct role in neutrophil activation and can induce cytokine and chemokine release, increased β_2 integrin expression, and degranulation.[262] Antiinflammatory cytokines modulate local activation of phagocytic cells. IL-10, IL-4, and IL-13 can inhibit proinflammatory cytokine synthesis, suppress oxygen radical production, and down-regulate NO synthesis, thereby further limiting the local inflammatory response.[178,198,199,263,264]

Mature neutrophils are end-stage cells and have a relatively short life span. Once released into the circulation, neutrophils undergo constitutive apoptosis, or programmed cell death. Enhanced neutrophil survival at the site of inflammation not only promotes increased bactericidal activity but also may play a role in acute inflammatory damage through excessive release of oxygen radicals, proteases, lipid mediators, and cytokines. TNF and other proinflammatory cytokines are important regulators of neutrophil function during the inflammatory response through activation of proinflammatory signaling and suppression of neutrophil apoptosis.[259,265,266] Thus cytokines are involved both in trafficking specific populations of leukocytes to the site of inflammation and in the activation process once the leukocytes arrive at their destination.

INTERPLAY BETWEEN INFLAMMATION AND COAGULATION

The coagulation system is activated during the inflammatory response and is an essential component of the host response. Coagulation is initiated by the expression of tissue factor on the surface of endothelium and monocytes.[267] The proinflammatory cytokines TNF, IL-1, and IL-6 promote the expression of tissue factor and activation of the extrinsic pathway of coagulation resulting in thrombin production and ultimately fibrin deposition.[268,269] Studies have also implicated IL-12, IL-8, and the chemokine CCL2 as procoagulation mediators.[268,270] TNF and IL-1 further enhance the procoagulation state by also inhibiting key anticoagulation pathways. TNF and IL-1 inhibit the synthesis and release of thrombomodulin, resulting in the impairment of thrombin-mediated protein C activation and the subsequent inhibition of that anticoagulation pathway.[268]

Fibrinolysis is suppressed by TNF through the inhibition of tissue-type plasminogen activator release.[271] Tissue-type plasminogen activator is essential for the conversion of plasminogen to the active protease plasmin. Plasmin can dissolve the fibrin network in thrombi. Fibrinolysis is also limited by TNF and IL-1-mediated release of plasminogen activator inhibitors (e.g., plasminogen activator inhibitor 1), which further inhibit the conversion of plasminogen to plasmin.[271,272] The stimulation of the extrinsic coagulation pathway, coupled with the inhibition of fibrinolysis, is thought to promote containment and localization of the inflammatory site. However, the activation of the coagulation pathway can further up-regulate the inflammatory response through crosstalk between the two pathways. For example, thrombin binding to its receptor triggers the activation of NFκB, the synthesis of proinflammatory cytokines, and the release of NO.[268,271]

Antiinflammatory cytokines also regulate coagulation. In vivo administration of IL-10 reduced LPS activation of the coagulation pathway and modulated the fibrinolytic system.[271,273] Although the coagulation system is critical for the maintenance of homeostasis and the containment of inflammatory stimuli, if not adequately regulated, it can lead to the development of disseminated intravascular coagulation and multiple organ failure.[269]

CLINICAL MONITORING OF INFLAMMATION

FEVER

IL-1β (previously known as *endogenous pyrogen*), TNF, and IL-6 are able to raise the temperature setpoint of an organism and cause fever.[274,275] These cytokines stimulate production of inducible cyclooxygenase (i.e., cyclooxygenase 2), which induces the hypothalamic production of prostaglandins, particularly prostaglandin E_2. Prostaglandin E_2 stimulates the release of neurotransmitters such as cyclic adenosine monophosphate and increases body temperature.[51,275] Other proinflammatory cytokines, such as IFN-γ, may indirectly cause fever through induction of IL-1 and TNF synthesis. Cytokines that are members of the same receptor families as those of pyrogenic proinflammatory cytokines do not necessarily trigger fever. IL-18 receptor is a member of the IL-1/toll-like receptor superfamily, but unlike IL-1, IL-18 does not trigger prostaglandin E_2 synthesis in vitro or cause fever when it is administered in vivo.[149,275] IL-10 is an endogenous antipyretic cytokine and probably modulates fever through inhibition of proinflammatory cytokine synthesis.[276] IL-1ra production is elevated slightly later than IL-1 production, and by competing with IL-1 for receptor sites, IL-1ra likely modulates the extent and duration of the febrile response.[277,278]

ACUTE-PHASE REACTION

The synthesis and release of hepatic acute-phase proteins constitute an important mechanism in modulating the inflammatory response and the restoration of homeostasis. Acute-phase proteins have diverse biologic activities and include antiproteases, antioxidants, activators of the complement system, blood-clotting agents, and immune response modulators.[76,277,279] In some cases, acute-phase proteins can be conveniently measured to aid in clinical decision making.

The hepatic acute-phase response is regulated principally by IL-6.[76,279] TNF, IL-1, IFN-γ, and possibly IL-8 also induce synthesis of various hepatic acute-phase proteins.[76,277,279] The acute-phase reaction is terminated indirectly through the inhibition of proinflammatory cytokine synthesis by IL-4, IL-13, and IL-10.[280] Natural inhibitors of TNF, IL-1, and IL-6, including soluble receptors and receptor antagonists, can also remove excess IL-6, IL-1, and TNF. IL-4; in contrast with other antiinflammatory cytokines, these inhibitors can inhibit synthesis of select hepatic acute-phase proteins.[281] Acute-phase proteins themselves are also capable of modulating the proinflammatory response through the induction of cytokine antagonists such as IL-1ra.[282] Thus crosstalk between cytokines and the hepatic acute-phase response contributes to the resolution of the inflammatory response.

IMBALANCE OF INFLAMMATION AND THERAPEUTIC STRATEGIES IN THE FETUS AND NEONATE

In most cases the inflammatory response is successfully resolved. However, overzealous production of cytokines or the inability to shut down proinflammatory cytokine production can lead to increasing concentrations of cytokines in the systemic circulation ("cytokine storm").[12] This continued cytokine production can have a deleterious effect on the host, with the development of hypotension, intravascular thrombosis, pulmonary edema, and hemorrhage; if this process is left unchecked, it can lead to multiple organ failure and death. This condition often is referred to as the *systemic inflammatory response syndrome* (SIRS).[283] This term describes the clinical manifestations of widespread endothelial inflammation that leads to increased vascular permeability.[271,284,285] This condition is the initiating pathologic process in a group of diverse disorders, such as bacterial sepsis, ischemia, burn injury, trauma and tissue injury, and hemorrhagic shock.

Studies suggest a genetic predisposition that determines the balance of proinflammatory and antiinflammatory cytokines and, hence, susceptibility to disease.[9,14,286-288] Various polymorphisms have been identified within cytokine and cytokine receptor genes that alter their expression. These cytokine and cytokine receptor gene polymorphisms may determine the balance of proinflammatory and antiinflammatory cytokines in the inflammatory response.

To date, therapeutic strategies targeting proinflammatory cytokines such as TNF and IL-1β have proved ineffective in the treatment of SIRS—multiple clinical trials of antagonists of proinflammatory mediators demonstrated no improvement, and in some cases, worsened survival.[10,289-291] Proinflammatory cytokines are critical to the initiation of the inflammatory response; however, their levels may have peaked before the clinical signs and symptoms of SIRS become apparent. Furthermore, although a hyperinflammatory response may be responsible for some cases of sepsis-related death, a predominant antiinflammatory response or global cytokine suppression may be the cause in many other instances, especially in populations with weakened immune systems such as neonates or the elderly.[292] As a result, recent therapeutic approaches have focused more on immunomodulatory or immune-stimulatory mediators, such as granulocyte-monocyte colony-stimulating factor or IL-7, which has an important role in lymphocyte replenishment.[290,291,293-295]

Furthermore, mediators that appear later in disease progression may also hold promise for therapeutic intervention in uncontrolled inflammation in the context of severe sepsis and autoimmune disorders. DAMPs such as HMGB1, mitochondrial DNA and heat shock proteins, and mitochondrial formyl peptide are important late proinflammatory mediators.[296]

HMGB1, originally identified as a DNA-binding protein, is now recognized as a late mediator of sepsis and SIRS.[297] HMGB1 is actively released by macrophages and endothelial cells during the inflammatory response, as well as passively from necrotic cells. HMGB1 mediates numerous proinflammatory actions both locally and systemically.[298] Antibodies or antagonists directed against HMGB1 are protective in animal models of sepsis and SIRS.[299,300]

Another late proinflammatory mediator, macrophage inhibitory factor, was originally identified as a modulator of macrophage migration; it is now recognized to be a critical regulator of the inflammatory response.[301] In animal models of infection and sepsis, anti-macrophage inhibitory factor therapy significantly improved survival.[301] Thus these "late" proinflammatory mediators may provide novel therapeutic targets for the treatment of SIRS.[302-304] Strategies that selectively target DAMP-related inflammatory responses, while allowing appropriate immune response to PAMPs, are of especial interest in the context of SIRS and sepsis.[297]

The fetus and newborn infant are unique from the standpoint of immunity and infection. The fetus lives in an environment with limited microbial interaction. However, it is during this time that the development of the immune system is initiated—a highly complex process mediated, at least in part, by the expression of cytokines.[305,306] Fetal cytokines are known to play a role in the regulation of hematopoiesis and to protect the fetus against rejection. Cytokine crosstalk across maternal and fetal surfaces is essential for maternal-fetal immunotolerance.[307] Placental and fetal cytokines also protect against infection.[305,306]

The newborn period represents a time of increased risk for the development of bacterial infection and increased mortality from sepsis.[308,309] Among other factors known to increase this risk is a functional immaturity of newborn immune mechanisms. Both immunoglobulin and complement levels are low, and leukocyte functions, including the secretion of inflammatory mediators, may be deficient.[310,311]

CONCLUSION

Evidence suggests that alterations in cytokine profiles in the fetus and neonate play a role in the pathophysiology of preterm labor, as well as severe neonatal diseases, including sepsis, bronchopulmonary dysplasia, and necrotizing enterocolitis.[96,312-316] Several critical aspects of the innate and adaptive immune response appear to be down-regulated in the neonate as compared with older age groups.[317] In the past, therapeutic strategies were aimed exclusively at killing the bacteria that caused neonatal infection. However, it has become evident that many infants die despite the sterilization of blood cultures with antimicrobial agents.[114,318] It is now appreciated that the physiologic derangements that occur during sepsis are secondary to the host response induced by pathogenic microorganisms. During overwhelming sepsis, the host produces proinflammatory cytokines that initiate a cascade of events resulting in tissue injury at distant sites and generalized multiorgan system failure.[114,319] The balance of proinflammatory and antiinflammatory cytokines may ultimately determine the outcome of sepsis and other inflammatory conditions in newborn infants. This inflammatory response may have its origins during the fetal period.[305,306] Thus the heightened morbidity and mortality in neonatal sepsis result from physiologic differences in immune function, as well as the pathophysiologic alterations produced by PAMPs.[114,318] Therapeutic strategies for neonatal sepsis involving immunomodulation have been unsuccessful to date, possibly because they do not take into account how the neonatal immune response differs from older populations in which similar therapies may have met with some success.[320,321] Further research into the unique nature of the fetal and neonatal immune response is desperately needed to limit morbidity and mortality in this vulnerable population.

 A complete reference list is available at www.ExpertConsult.com.

SELECT REFERENCES

1. Medzhitov R. Origin and physiological roles of inflammation. *Nature*. 2008;454(7203):428–435. https://doi.org/10.1038/nature07201.
2. Medzhitov R. Inflammation 2010: new adventures of an old flame. *Cell*. 2010;140(6):771–776. https://doi.org/10.1016/j.cell.2010.03.006.
3. Medzhitov R. Recognition of microorganisms and activation of the immune response. *Nature*. 2007;449(7164):819–826. https://doi.org/10.1038/nature06246.
4. WG. L. Oxidative injury-induced, damage associated molecular pattern molecules and their pattern recognition receptors. In: WG. L, ed. *Innate Alloimmunity: Part II—Innate Immunity and Rejection*. Baskent University-Pabst Science Publishers; 2011:229–337.
5. Mondrinos MJ, Kennedy PA, Lyons M, Deutschman CS, Kilpatrick LE. Protein kinase C and acute respiratory distress syndrome. *Shock*. 2013;39(6):467–479. https://doi.org/10.1097/SHK.0b013e318294f85a.
6. Tolle LB, Standiford TJ. Danger-associated molecular patterns (DAMPs) in acute lung injury. *J Pathol*. 2013;229(2):145–156. https://doi.org/10.1002/path.4124.
7. Piccinini AM, Midwood KS. DAMPening inflammation by modulating TLR signalling. *Mediators Inflamm*. 2010;2010:672395. https://doi.org/10.1155/2010/672395.
8. Mogensen TH. Pathogen recognition and inflammatory signaling in innate immune defenses. *Clin Microbiol Rev*. 2009;22(2):240–273, Table of Contents. https://doi.org/10.1128/CMR.00046-08.
9. Dinarello CA. Proinflammatory cytokines. *Chest*. 2000;118(2):503–508. https://doi.org/10.1378/chest.118.2.503.
10. Dinarello CA. Historical insights into cytokines. *Eur J Immunol*. 2007;37(suppl 1):S34–S45. https://doi.org/10.1002/eji.200737772.
11. Kopf M, Bachmann MF, Marsland BJ. Averting inflammation by targeting the cytokine environment. *Nat Rev Drug Discov*. 2010;9(9):703–718. https://doi.org/10.1038/nrd2805.
12. Tisoncik JR, Korth MJ, Simmons CP, Farrar J, Martin TR, Katze MG. Into the eye of the cytokine storm. *Microbiol Mol Biol Rev*. 2012;76(1):16–32. https://doi.org/10.1128/MMBR.05015-11.
13. Boontham P, Chandran P, Rowlands B, Eremin O. Surgical sepsis: dysregulation of immune function and therapeutic implications. *Surgeon*. 2003;1(4):187–206. https://doi.org/10.1016/s1479-666x(03)80018-5.
14. Opal SM, DePalo VA. Anti-inflammatory cytokines. *Chest*. 2000;117(4):1162–1172. https://doi.org/10.1378/chest.117.4.1162.
15. van der Poll T, van Deventer SJ. Cytokines and anticytokines in the pathogenesis of sepsis. *Infect Dis Clin North Am*. 1999;13(2):413–426, ix. https://doi.org/10.1016/s0891-5520(05)70083-0.
16. Holbrook J, Lara-Reyna S, Jarosz-Griffiths H, McDermott M. Tumour necrosis factor signalling in health and disease. *F1000Res*. 2019;8:F1000 Faculty Rev-111. https://doi.org/10.12688/f1000research.17023.1.
17. Kalliolias GD, Ivashkiv LB. TNF biology, pathogenic mechanisms and emerging therapeutic strategies. *Nat Rev Rheumatol*. 2016;12(1):49–62. https://doi.org/10.1038/nrrheum.2015.169.
18. Aggarwal BB. Signalling pathways of the TNF superfamily: a double-edged sword. *Nat Rev Immunol*. 2003;3(9):745–756. https://doi.org/10.1038/nri1184.
19. MacEwan DJ. TNF receptor subtype signalling: differences and cellular consequences. *Cell Signal*. 2002;14(6):477–492. https://doi.org/10.1016/s0898-6568(01)00262-5.
20. Pennica D, Nedwin GE, Hayflick JS, et al. Human tumour necrosis factor: precursor structure, expression and homology to lymphotoxin. *Nature*. 1984;312(5996):724–729. https://doi.org/10.1038/312724a0.
21. Black RA, Rauch CT, Kozlosky CJ, et al. A metalloproteinase disintegrin that releases tumour-necrosis factor-alpha from cells. *Nature*. 1997;385(6618):729–733. https://doi.org/10.1038/385729a0.
22. Loetscher H, Pan YC, Lahm HW, et al. Molecular cloning and expression of the human 55 kd tumor necrosis factor receptor. *Cell*. 1990;61(2):351–359. https://doi.org/10.1016/0092-8674(90)90815-v.
23. Schall TJ, Lewis M, Koller KJ, et al. Molecular cloning and expression of a receptor for human tumor necrosis factor. *Cell*. 1990;61(2):361–370. https://doi.org/10.1016/0092-8674(90)90816-w.
24. Varfolomeev E, Vucic D. Intracellular regulation of TNF activity in health and disease. *Cytokine*. 2018;101:26–32. https://doi.org/10.1016/j.cyto.2016.08.035.
25. Delgado ME, Brunner T. The many faces of tumor necrosis factor signaling in the intestinal epithelium. *Genes Immun*. 2019;20(8):609–626. https://doi.org/10.1038/s41435-019-0057-0.
26. Chen G, Goeddel DV. TNF-R1 signaling: a beautiful pathway. *Science*. 2002;296(5573):1634–1635. https://doi.org/10.1126/science.1071924.
27. Grivennikov SI, Kuprash DV, Liu ZG, Nedospasov SA. Intracellular signals and events activated by cytokines of the tumor necrosis factor superfamily: from simple paradigms to complex mechanisms. *Int Rev Cytol*. 2006;252:129–161. https://doi.org/10.1016/S0074-7696(06)52002-9.
28. Ting AT, Pimentel-Muiños FX, Seed B. RIP mediates tumor necrosis factor receptor 1 activation of NF-kappaB but not Fas/APO-1-initiated apoptosis. *EMBO J*. 1996;15(22):6189–6196.
29. Kelliher MA, Grimm S, Ishida Y, Kuo F, Stanger BZ, Leder P. The death domain kinase RIP mediates the TNF-induced NF-kappaB signal. *Immunity*. 1998;8(3):297–303. https://doi.org/10.1016/s1074-7613(00)80535-x.
30. Devin A, Cook A, Lin Y, Rodriguez Y, Kelliher M, Liu Z. The distinct roles of TRAF2 and RIP in IKK activation by TNF-R1: TRAF2 recruits IKK to TNF-R1 while RIP mediates IKK activation. *Immunity*. 2000;12(4):419–429. https://doi.org/10.1016/s1074-7613(00)80194-6.
31. Szondy Z, Pallai A. Transmembrane TNF-alpha reverse signaling leading to TGF-beta production is selectively activated by TNF targeting molecules: therapeutic implications. *Pharmacol Res*. 2017;115:124–132. https://doi.org/10.1016/j.phrs.2016.11.025.
32. Kutteh WH, Rainey WE, Carr BR. Regulation of interleukin-6 production in human fetal Kupffer cells. *Scand J Immunol*. 1991;33(5):607–613. https://doi.org/10.1111/j.1365-3083.1991.tb02532.x.
33. Kutteh WH, Rainey WE, Beutler B, Carr BR. Tumor necrosis factor-alpha and interleukin-1 beta production by human fetal Kupffer cells. *Am J Obstet Gynecol*. 1991;165(1):112–120. https://doi.org/10.1016/0002-9378(91)90237-l.
34. Alijotas-Reig J, Esteve-Valverde E, Ferrer-Oliveras R, Llurba E, Gris JM. Tumor necrosis factor-alpha and pregnancy: focus on biologics. An updated and comprehensive review. *Clin Rev Allergy Immunol*. 2017;53(1):40–53. https://doi.org/10.1007/s12016-016-8596-x.
35. Romero R, Mazor M, Sepulveda W, Avila C, Copeland D, Williams J. Tumor necrosis factor in preterm and term labor. *Am J Obstet Gynecol*. 1992;166(5):1576–1587. https://doi.org/10.1016/0002-9378(92)91636-o.
36. Challis JR, Lockwood CJ, Myatt L, Norman JE, Strauss JF, Petraglia F. Inflammation and pregnancy. *Reprod Sci*. 2009;16(2):206–215. https://doi.org/10.1177/1933719108329095.
37. Arsenescu R, Arsenescu V, de Villiers WJ. TNF-α and the development of the neonatal immune system: implications for inhibitor use in pregnancy. *Am J Gastroenterol*. 2011;106(4):559–562. https://doi.org/10.1038/ajg.2011.5.
38. Feldhaus B, Dietzel ID, Heumann R, Berger R. Effects of interferon-gamma and tumor necrosis factor-alpha on survival and differentiation of oligodendrocyte progenitors. *J Soc Gynecol Investig*. 2004;11(2):89–96. https://doi.org/10.1016/j.jsgi.2003.08.004.
39. Seghaye MC, Heyl W, Grabitz RG, et al. The production of pro- and anti-inflammatory cytokines in neonates assessed by stimulated whole cord blood culture and by plasma levels at birth. *Biol Neonate*. 1998;73(4):220–227. https://doi.org/10.1159/000013980.
40. Peters AM, Bertram P, Gahr M, Speer CP. Reduced secretion of interleukin-1 and tumor necrosis factor-alpha by neonatal monocytes. *Biol Neonate*. 1993;63(3):157–162. https://doi.org/10.1159/000243926.
41. Förster-Waldl E, Sadeghi K, Tamandl D, et al. Monocyte toll-like receptor 4 expression and LPS-induced cytokine production increase during gestational aging. *Pediatr Res*. 2005;58(1):121–124. https://doi.org/10.1203/01.PDR.0000163397.53466.0F.
42. Angelone DF, Wessels MR, Coughlin M, et al. Innate immunity of the human newborn is polarized toward a high ratio of IL-6/TNF-alpha production in vitro and in vivo. *Pediatr Res*. 2006;60(2):205–209. https://doi.org/10.1203/01.pdr.0000228319.10481.ea.
43. Burchett SK, Weaver WM, Westall JA, Larsen A, Kronheim S, Wilson CB. Regulation of tumor necrosis factor/cachectin and IL-1 secretion in human mononuclear phagocytes. *J Immunol*. 1988;140(10):3473–3481.
44. Kollmann TR, Crabtree J, Rein-Weston A, et al. Neonatal innate TLR-mediated responses are distinct from those of adults. *J Immunol*. 2009;183(11):7150–7160. https://doi.org/10.4049/jimmunol.0901481.

45. Chheda S, Palkowetz KH, Garofalo R, Rassin DK, Goldman AS. Decreased interleukin-10 production by neonatal monocytes and T cells: relationship to decreased production and expression of tumor necrosis factor-alpha and its receptors. *Pediatr Res*. 1996;40(3):475–483. https://doi.org/10.1203/00006450-199609000-00018.
46. Kwak DJ, Augustine NH, Borges WG, Joyner JL, Green WF, Hill HR. Intracellular and extracellular cytokine production by human mixed mononuclear cells in response to group B streptococci. *Infect Immun*. 2000;68(1):320–327. https://doi.org/10.1128/iai.68.1.320-327.2000.
47. Levy O, Coughlin M, Cronstein BN, Roy RM, Desai A, Wessels MR. The adenosine system selectively inhibits TLR-mediated TNF-alpha production in the human newborn. *J Immunol*. 2006;177(3):1956–1966. https://doi.org/10.4049/jimmunol.177.3.1956.
48. Dinarello CA. The IL-1 family and inflammatory diseases. *Clin Exp Rheumatol*. 2002;20(5 suppl 27):S1–S13.
49. Dinarello C, Arend W, Sims J, et al. IL-1 family nomenclature. *Nat Immunol*. 2010;11(11):973. https://doi.org/10.1038/ni1110-973.
50. Sims JE, Smith DE. The IL-1 family: regulators of immunity. *Nat Rev Immunol*. 2010;10(2):89–102. https://doi.org/10.1038/nri2691.

Immunology of Human Milk

122

Armond S. Goldman | Sadhana Chheda | Susan E. Keeney

INTRODUCTION

In 1891, it was discovered in experimental animals that immunity was transmitted through breast-feeding.[1,2] In the second decade of the 20th century, the incidence of diarrheal diseases was found to be much lower in breast-fed infants than cow's milk-fed infants.[3] Those observations were confirmed in developing and industrialized countries.[4-14] Subsequently it was discovered that breast-feeding protected against many bacterial and viral enteric pathogens.[8-15] Three explanations for the protection were advanced: (1) because human milk was less contaminated with pathogenic microorganisms than formula feedings, breast-fed infants were exposed to fewer infectious agents; (2) increased birth-spacing due to contraceptive effects of lactation decreased the number of children who transmit common contagious agents to susceptible siblings[16]; and (3) breast-fed infants were less likely to be in group care and thus were less exposed to children harboring communicable diseases. However, these propositions did not completely explain the protection provided by breast-feeding when breast-fed infants were found to be asymptomatic even when *Shigella* contaminated the mother's nipples.[6] Evidence then emerged that breast-fed infants were more resistant to certain respiratory infections.[17-20]

Many antimicrobial agents in human milk and their features were discovered in the latter half of the 20th century.[21,22] They were found to be a heterogeneous array of biochemical agents and live leukocytes, which are more prominent in human milk than in other milk products used in human infants. They are common in mucosal sites and are adapted to persist in the gastrointestinal tract. They often inhibit or kill certain microbial pathogens synergistically and are frequently multifunctional. They protect without triggering inflammation, and their production is often inversely related to production in the infant. This last feature suggests a close evolutionary relationship between the immune system in human milk and development of the infant's immune system.[23-25] The concept of an immune system in human milk was subsequently expanded by the discovery of many antimicrobial, antiinflammatory,[26,27] and immunomodulating agents[27] in human milk. The key features of the immune functions of human milk are summarized in Box 122.1.

ANTIMICROBIAL FACTORS

Antimicrobial agents in human milk include a number of proteins or polypeptides, oligosaccharides, glycoconjugates, and lipids. The agents and their functions are listed in Table 122.1.

ANTIBODIES

Human milk contains immunoglobulin (Ig)M, IgG, IgD, and IgA. The concentration of IgM is much lower in human milk than in serum.[28] IgM molecules in blood and milk are pentamers. However, unlike serum IgM, most human milk IgM is bound to a secretory component, and the antibody specificities are often similar to those of human milk secretory IgA (SIgA). Concentrations of IgG in human milk are lower than those for IgM and are much lower than serum IgG levels.[28] All IgG subclasses are found in human milk,[29] but the proportion of IgG4 is higher in milk.[29] Very little IgD is present in human milk.[30] IgE is undetectable.[31]

In contrast, SIgA comprises more than 95% of human milk immunoglobulins.[28] Most SIgA consists of two identical IgA monomers united by a 15-kDa polypeptide called the *joining chain* and complexed to secretory component, a 75-kDa glycopeptide fragment of the polymeric Ig receptor on the mammary gland epithelium.[32,33] SIgA is assembled when dimeric IgA produced by plasma cells in the stroma of the mammary gland binds to the first domain of polymeric Ig receptors on the basolateral surface of the mammary gland epithelium.[34] The complex is internalized, the cytoplasmic part of the receptor is cleaved off, and the remaining protein (SIgA) is transported into milk.

SIgA antibodies in human milk are principally directed against foreign enteric and respiratory microbial antigens (Table 122.2). Antibody-producing cells in the mammary gland originate from those mucosal sites, where their precursors are released by antigen stimulation.[35] During lactation, antigen-stimulated B cells from Peyer patches (aggregated lymphoid nodules) in the lower small intestines switch from producing IgM to dimeric IgA and then migrate to the mammary gland.[36,37] A similar B-cell pathway links bronchial lymphoid tissues to the mammary gland.[38]

The switch from IgM$^+$ to dimeric IgA$^+$ in B cells in Peyer patches requires cytokines produced by local mononuclear leukocytes.[39-41] These isotype-switched B cells migrate sequentially into local lymphatics, mesenteric lymph nodes, the cisterna chyli, the thoracic duct, and blood. CCL28 and its receptor CCR10 are crucial to this process. CCL28 is up-regulated in the murine mammary gland epithelium during lactation.[42] Most dimeric IgA$^+$ B cells in the enteromammary gland pathway display CCR10, the receptor for that chemokine.[42] CCL28 expressed by mammary gland epithelium is a chemoattractant for dimeric IgA$^+$ CCR10$^+$ B cells.[43]

After entering the mammary gland, dimeric IgA$^+$ B cells differentiate into dimeric IgA-producing plasma cells in the

Box 122.1 Key Concepts in Immune Functions of Human Milk

1. Certain postnatal developmental delays in the immune system are compensated by those same agents in human milk.
2. Other postnatal delays in the immune system are offset by other agents in human milk.
3. Some agents in human milk alter the physiologic state of the alimentary tract from one suited for fetal life to one appropriate for extrauterine life.
4. Defense agents in human milk protect against microbial pathogens without provoking inflammation.
5. Many agents in human milk inhibit inflammation.
6. Cells that produce antibodies in human milk originate in the maternal small intestines and bronchi.
7. Defense agents in human milk are resistant to enzymatic digestion and thus function in the recipient's gastrointestinal tract.
8. Certain defense agents are created by partial digestion of substrates in milk in the infant's gastrointestinal tract.
9. When defense agents in human milk interact with some pathogens, symptomatic infections are prevented and immune responses to those pathogens develop in the infant.
10. Agents in human milk augment the growth of commensal enteric bacteria that protect against bacterial pathogens, interfere with the attachment of certain pathogens to epithelium, and convey other immunologic benefits.

lamina propria. IgA dimers produced by those plasma cells principally contain λ-light chains, whereas κ-light chains predominate in serum immunoglobulins.[44] IgA dimers bind to polymeric Ig receptors on the basolateral external membranes of mammary gland epithelial cells.[32,33,45,46] The resultant complex is transported to the apical side of an epithelial cell where the original intracytoplasmic portion of the receptor is cleaved away. The resultant molecule, SIgA, is secreted into milk. Thus enteromammary and bronchomammary pathways protect the infant against pathogens in the environment of the dyad (see Table 122.2). This is important because SIgA antibodies and the antigen-binding repertoire of immunoglobulins are not optimally produced during early infancy.[47] Further, antiidiotypic SIgA antibodies in human milk elicit an immune response as though they were the original foreign antigens.[48]

Some of the natural SIgA antibodies in human milk, which arise without antigenic stimuli, are directed against CCR5, the co-receptor for R5-tropic strains of human immunodeficiency virus (HIV)-1. Via CCR5, macrophages and immature dendritic cells become infected with HIV-1.[49] Antibodies from HIV-1-infected women bind to the second extracellular loop of CCR5 and thus reduce HIV-1 infection of macrophages and dendritic cells. In addition, SIgA antibodies to DNA enzymatically cleave DNA.[50,51] Therefore, the DNA is recognized not only as an autoantigen but also as a substrate by the antibody-enzyme that hydrolyzes free nucleic acids in the recipient's intestinal and respiratory tracts.

The quantity of SIgA in human milk gradually declines as lactation proceeds, but considerable SIgA is transmitted to the infant throughout breast-feeding.[52-55] Concentrations of SIgA in human milk are highest in colostrum[48] and gradually plateau later in lactation.[54] The approximate mean daily intake of SIgA in healthy, term, breast-fed infants is 600 mg/day at 1 month and 500 mg/day by 4 months.[55]

The pattern of immunoglobulins in human milk differs from that in other mammals except for closely related primates.[25]

Table 122.1 Principal Antimicrobial Agents in Human Milk.

Agents	Main Functions
Proteins and peptides	Microbiostatic and microbiocidal
Lactoferrin	Lyses siderophilic pathogens by chelating Fe^{+3}
Lysozyme	Lyses certain bacteria by degrading exposed cell wall peptidoglycans
Human milk secretory immunoglobulin A	Binds adherence sites, toxins, virulence factors on intestinal and respiratory pathogens
α-Lactalbumin	Kills *Streptococcus pneumoniae*
CCL28	Kills *Candida albicans* and many gram-positive and gram-negative bacteria
MUC1	Blocks binding of S-fimbriated *Escherichia coli* to epithelium
Lactadherin	Blocks attachment of rotavirus to mucosa
C3 and fibronectin	Augment phagocytosis of pathogens
Pentraxin	Facilitates phagocytosis of *Pseudomonas*
β-Defensin-1 and α-defensin1,2,3	Lyses bacteria and inhibits human immunodeficiency virus (HIV)-1, respectively
Oligosaccharides glycoconjugates	Receptor analogues inhibit binding to epithelium and facilitate growth of protective enteric bacteria
GM1 gangliosides	*Vibrio cholerae* and *E. coli*
Globotriaosylceramide Gb3	Shiga toxin B subunits
Fucosyloligosaccharides	*E. coli* stable toxin, *Campylobacter jejuni*
G1cNAc(β1-3) Gal-disaccharide	*Streptococcus pneumoniae*
Sulfated glycolipids	HIV-1
Glycosaminoglycans	HIV-1
Lewis X component	HIV-1
Monoglycerides and fatty acids from digested milk lipids	Disrupt enveloped viruses, certain bacteria, *Giardia lamblia,* and *Entamoeba histolytica*

Table 122.2 Antigen-Binding Repertoire of Human Milk Secretory Immunoglobulin A Antibodies in Human Milk.

Bacteria	Viruses
Escherichia coli	Adenoviruses
Helicobacter pylori	Cytomegalovirus
Clostridium botulinum	Polioviruses and other enteroviruses
Klebsiella pneumoniae	Rotaviruses
Campylobacter sp.	Respiratory syncytial virus
Shigella sp.	**Parasites**
Salmonella sp.	*Giardia lamblia*
Vibrio cholerae	**Autoantigens**
Streptococcus pneumoniae	DNA
Group B *Streptococcus*	RNA
Haemophilus influenzae	CCR5
Fungi	
Candida sp.	

For example, IgG is the dominant immunoglobulin in bovine colostrum, and much of it is absorbed by the calf, whose IgG production is developmentally delayed. Without colostrum, calves are IgG-deficient and susceptible to intestinal infections.

Human SIgA is resistant to intestinal proteases including pancreatic trypsin.[56] Bacterial proteases attack the hinge region of IgA1,[57] but IgA2 is resistant to those proteases and is disproportionally increased in human milk.[28] Furthermore, SIgA antibodies against bacterial IgA proteases are in human milk.[57] Consequently, the amount of SIgA excreted in stools of low-birth-weight infants fed human milk is approximately 30 times that in infants fed a cow's milk formula.[58] In addition, urinary excretion of SIgA rises as a result of human milk feedings.[59,60] It is unlikely that the antibodies are from human milk, because there is no mechanism for their transport from the gastrointestinal tract to the blood. The mechanism responsible for SIgA antibodies in the infant's urinary tract remains unclear.

LACTOFERRIN

Lactoferrin is a glycoprotein with two globular lobes, each of which displays a binding site for ferric iron.[61] In 90% of lactoferrin in human milk,[62] iron-binding sites are free to compete with siderophilic bacteria and fungal enterochelin for ferric iron.[63-65] Iron chelation disrupts proliferation of those pathogens. Lactoferrin also kills by damaging outer membranes of many gram-positive and gram-negative bacteria and filamentous fungi[66-68] by a peptide comprised of 18 amino acid residues from the N-terminal region formed by pepsin digestion (lactoferricin).[67,68] Furthermore, lactoferrin inhibits certain viruses in a chelation-independent manner.[69-72] With free secretory component, lactoferrin interferes with the adhesion of *Escherichia coli* to epithelial cells.[73]

The mean concentration of lactoferrin in human colostrum is between 5 and 6 mg/mL.[52] The concentration falls to approximately 1 mg/mL at 2 to 3 months of lactation.[53] The mean intake of milk lactoferrin in healthy breast-fed term infants is approximately 1200 mg/day at 1 month and 700 mg/day by 4 months.[55] Because human lactoferrin resists proteolysis[74] and the concentration of lactoferrin is much greater in human than bovine milk,[25] the excretion of lactoferrin in the stools is higher in infants fed human milk than in those fed cow's milk.[58,75] The quantity of lactoferrin excreted in stools of low-birth-weight infants fed human milk is approximately 185 times that excreted by infants fed cow's milk.[58] However, that estimate may be too high because fragments of lactoferrin, which may be biologically active, are present in stools of human milk-fed infants.[76] There is also a significant increment in urinary excretion of intact and fragmented lactoferrin as a result of human milk feedings.[60,76] The increase is due to absorbed human milk lactoferrin and its fragments.[77]

LYSOZYME

Lysozyme, a 15-kDa single chain protein, lyses susceptible bacteria by hydrolyzing β-1,4 linkages between *N*-acetylmuramic acid and 2-acetylamino-2-deoxy-D-glucose residues in cell walls.[78] High concentrations of lysozyme are in human milk throughout lactation.[52-54] Longitudinal changes in lysozyme during lactation are unlike most other agents in human milk. The mean concentration of lysozyme is approximately 70 µg/mL in colostrum,[52] 20 µg/mL at 1 month, and 250 µg/mL by 6 months of lactation.[53] The reason why the concentration rises by 6 months is not understood. The high content of lysozyme in human milk and its resistance to proteolysis lead to an eight-fold increase in lysozyme excreted in the stools of low-birth-weight infants fed human milk as compared to infants fed cow's milk.[58] However, urinary excretion of lysozyme is not increased in infants fed human milk.[60]

α-LACTALBUMIN

α-Lactalbumin is expressed only in the lactating mammary gland. A folding variant of the protein kills *Streptococcus pneumoniae*.[79] Furthermore, multimeric α-lactalbumin kills certain tumor cells in vitro by inducing apoptosis.[80,81]

CCL28

CCL28 kills *Candida albicans* and many gram-positive and gram-negative bacteria. The killing is mediated by its 28 amino acid carboxyl terminus.[82]

MACROPHAGE MIGRATION INHIBITORY FACTOR

Macrophage migration inhibitory factor, a constituent of human milk,[83] is a proinflammatory cytokine (see later) that also up-regulates TLR-4[84] and aids in killing *Mycobacterium tuberculosis* in macrophages.[85]

FIBRONECTIN

Fibronectin, which is found in human milk, facilitates uptake of bacteria and certain other particulates by mononuclear phagocytes.[86] Its in vivo effects in human milk are unknown.

COMPLEMENT

All components of the classic and alternative pathways of complement are in human milk, but their concentrations are much lower than those in serum.[87-89] In vitro experiments[90] suggest that C3 in human milk augments phagocytosis of microbial pathogens in the gastrointestinal and respiratory tracts.

HUMAN MILK MUCINS

Milk mucins are high-molecular-weight, highly glycosylated proteins.[91] Approximately two-thirds of them are bound to milk fat globules. The concentration of human milk mucin is between 50 and 90 mg/mL. Human milk fat globules and mucin from their membranes inhibit binding of S-fimbriated *E. coli* to human epithelium[92] and inhibit rotavirus replication.[93] The most prominent human milk mucin, MUC1, resists intragastric digestion in preterm infants.[94] Major fragments of MUC1 are detected in feces of breast-fed infants.[95] Mucins from such feces inhibit adhesion of S-fimbriated *E. coli* to epithelium more than feces from formula-fed infants.[96]

LACTADHERIN

A human milk mucin complex defends against rotavirus in mice.[97] Rotavirus binds not only to the complex, but also to its 49-kDa component. That component, the glycoprotein lactadherin,[98] resists intragastric digestion.[94] Murine milk fat globules contain MFG-E8, a protein analogous to human lactadherin.[99] MFG-E8 on murine macrophages links to phosphatidyl serine on outer leaflets of external membranes of apoptotic cells.[100,101] In turn, MFG-E8 binds to α1β3 and α1β5 integrins on macrophages in the spleen and lymph nodes and elicits peritoneal macrophages via a tripeptide (RDG) motif within the second of its two EGF repeats. When those apoptotic cells are phagocytized by macrophages, less inflammation is produced. Human lactadherin may have a similar effect.

PROTOTYPIC LONG PENTRAXIN

Prototypic long pentraxin, which facilitates phagocytosis of *Pseudomonas aeruginosa* and *Aspergillus fumigatus*, is present in human milk during early lactation.[102] Concentrations in human milk are approximately 30- to 40-fold those in adult blood. It is produced by cultured human mammary gland epithelium and CD11b-positive cells in human colostrum. The concentration of prototypic long pentraxin in human umbilical cord blood is approximately half that of adult blood. Therefore, this agent in human milk compensates for a developmental delay in its production in newborns.

LOW-MOLECULAR-WEIGHT ANTIMICROBIAL PEPTIDES

Cysteine-rich, cationic, low-molecular-weight peptides in human milk include β-defensin-1[103] and the α-defensins-1, -2, and -3 (HNP-1, -2, and -3).[102] β-defensin-1[104] disrupts *E. coli*. The α-defensins inhibit HIV-1 replication and may interfere with postpartum transmission of HIV-1.[104]

OLIGOSACCHARIDES AND GLYCOCONJUGATES

Oligosaccharides in human milk are produced by mammary gland glycosyltransferases. Their concentrations in colostrum and mature milk are approximately 20 mg/dL and 12 mg/dL, respectively.[105] Over 200 structural types of oligosaccharides are in human milk,[106,107] and they differ from those in cow's milk. For example, human milk contains much more monosialoganglioside 3 and GM1 gangliosides.[106,108] The types of oligosaccharides in human milk vary according to the woman's Lewis blood group antigens and the secretor gene FUT2.

Oligosaccharides in human milk are receptor analogues that inhibit the binding of certain enteric or respiratory bacterial pathogens and their toxins to epithelial cells.[106,108,109] For example, GM1 gangliosides are receptor analogues for *Vibrio cholerae* and *E. coli* toxins[110] while globotriaosylceramide Gb3 binds to B subunits of Shigatoxin.[111] A fucosyloligosaccharide inhibits the stable toxin of *E. coli*[112]; a different one inhibits *Campylobacter jejuni*.[113] Human milk oligosaccharides interfere with attachments of *Haemophilus influenzae* and *Streptococcus pneumoniae* to respiratory epithelium.[114] GlcNAc(β1-3) Gal-disaccharide subunits block attachment of *Streptococcus pneumoniae* to respiratory epithelium.[115]

Human milk α1,2-linked fucosylated glycans are receptors for caliciviruses, *Campylobacter*, and the stable toxin of enteropathogenic *E. coli*. In that respect, the severity of *Campylobacter* or calicivirus enteritis in breast-fed infants is inversely proportional to concentrations of certain 2-linked fucosyloligosaccharides in milk.[115]

Sulfated glycolipids, glycosaminoglycans,[116] and Lewis X component[117] in human milk inhibit in vitro infection by HIV-1. Polymers of Lewis X component interact with a dendritic cell-specific ICAM-3-grabbing nonintegrin (DC-SIGN) that facilitates the transfer of HIV-1 from dendritic cells to CD4⁺ T cells. Consequently, gp120 on the envelope of HIV-1 is unable to bind to those T cells. There also appears to be a relationship between the concentrations of non-3′sialyllactose and protection against HIV transmission via breast-feeding.[107]

Certain human milk oligosaccharides survive passage throughout the alimentary tract,[118] and some of the carbohydrates are absorbed and excreted into the urinary tract.[119] This may account for part of the protection by human milk against urinary tract infections.[120] Sugars in the glycoconjugates, mucins, lactadherin, and SIgA also interfere with binding of bacterial pathogens to epithelium.[91,92,121]

At the same time, nitrogen-containing oligosaccharides, glycoproteins, and glycopeptides in human milk are growth promoters for *Lactobacilli* and *Bifidobacilli*.[122,123] For example, the growth-promoter activity associated with caseins may reside in the oligosaccharide moiety of those complex molecules.[123] Consequently, *Lactobacilli* and *Bifidobacilli* predominate in the bacterial flora of the large intestine of breast-fed infants. The commensal bacteria produce acetic acid, which aids in suppressing multiplication of enteropathogens. The *Lactobacillus* strain GG may also aid in the recovery from rotavirus infections[124] and may enhance the formation of specific circulating antibodies during those enteric infections.[124] In addition, enteric commensal bacteria may stimulate the production of low-molecular-weight, antibacterial peptides such as defensins.[125] These defense mechanisms may contribute to the comparative paucity of bacterial pathogens such as P-fimbriated *E. coli* in stools of breast-fed infants.[126]

Human milk oligosaccharides inhibit rotavirus infections in newborn piglets.[127] Human milk oligosaccharides increase the pH of colonic contents, enhance the abundance of unclassified *Lachnospiraceae*, which contains numerous butyrate-producing bacteria, and augment the production of interferon-gamma and IL-10 in the ileum. As a result, the duration of rotavirus infections in those piglets is reduced.

Finally, in ex vivo human fetal intestinal tissue, oligosaccharides from human colostrum inhibited the production of certain proinflammatory cytokines, including IL-8, and promoted the production of antiinflammatory agents.[128] It is unknown whether those events occur in vivo.

LIPIDS

Certain medium-chain saturated and long-chain unsaturated fatty acids and monoglycerides generated by enzymatic digestion of lipids in human milk disrupt enveloped viruses.[129,130] These antiviral lipids may also defend against intestinal parasites such as *Giardia lamblia* and *Entamoeba histolytica*.[131,132] Monoglycerides from milk-lipid hydrolysis also inactivate certain gram-positive and gram-negative bacteria.[133] These lipids may act synergistically with one another or with antibacterial peptides.[133] Hydrolysis of milk lipids occurs in infants because of lingual lipase and activation of human milk–bile salt-stimulated lipase in the duodenum. Thus, products of lipid digestion defend breast-fed infants against enteric infections in the proximal gastrointestinal (GI) tract.

CELLS IN HUMAN MILK

During early lactation, human milk contains living leukocytes,[134,135] virtually all of which are activated.[136-138] The highest concentrations of leukocytes in human milk occur in the first few days of lactation (1 to 3 × 10^6/mL). The types (Fig. 122.1) and major features of those leukocytes are as follows.

LYMPHOCYTES

The relative frequencies of T cells and B cells among lymphocytes in early human milk are 83% and 6%, respectively.[134] The low cytotoxic activity of human milk[139] reflects the small number of natural killer cells in human milk.[134] The small number of B cells in human milk results from transformation of most B cells that enter the mammary gland into sessile plasma cells.

Human milk contains both CD4⁺ (helper) and CD8⁺ (cytotoxic/suppressor) T cells[137]; the proportion of CD8⁺ T cells in human milk is greater than that in blood.[137] It is striking that a higher percentage of T cells in human milk bear γ/δ T cell antigen receptors than their counterparts in blood. Moreover, CD4⁺ and CD8⁺ T cells in human milk display markers of cellular activation including CD45RO[136,137] and HLA-DR.[137] In addition, a greater percentage of human milk CD8⁺ T cells (compared to blood T cells) express the intestinal homing receptor (integrin αE also known as *CD103*), which binds to E-cadherin on epithelial cells and the mucosal homing receptor, C-C chemokine receptor type 9 (CCR9), which binds to CCL25.[140] T cells in human milk also are more motile than those in blood. The increased motility is due to an agent in human milk.[141] T cells in human milk produce certain cytokines such as interferon γ.[142] Additional cytokines are produced by human milk leukocytes.[143] The extent of the cytokine production by those cells is undetermined.

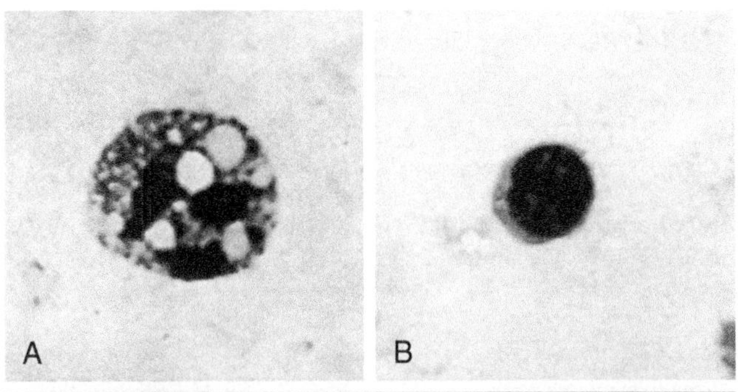

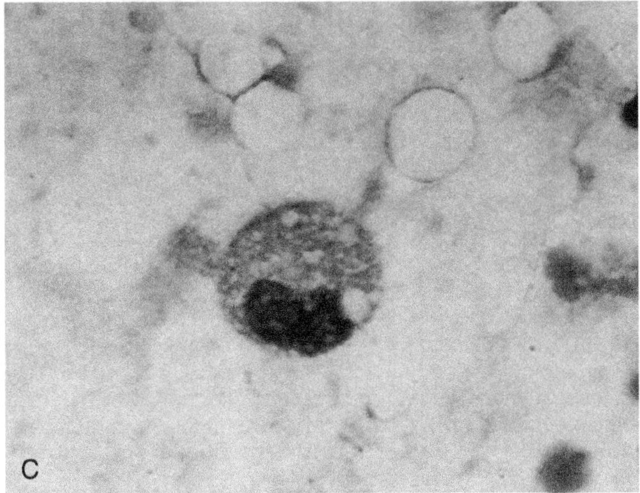

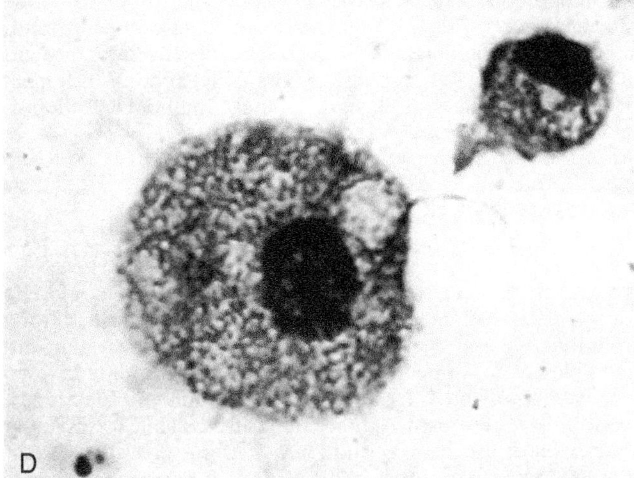

Fig. 122.1 Photomicrographs of living activated leukocytes in human milk. (A) Neutrophil. (B) Lymphocyte. (C) Macrophage. (D) Macrophage (the larger cell) and a lymphocyte (the smaller cell).

NEUTROPHILS AND MACROPHAGES

Neutrophils and macrophages in human milk are laden with milk fat globules and other phagocytized membranes. Because of these intracytoplasmic bodies, the cells are difficult to recognize by common staining methods. They can be identified by myeloperoxidase in neutrophils[143] or by nonspecific esterase and CD14 or MHC class II molecules in macrophages.[143] Those cells in human milk are phagocytic. A respiratory burst occurs in milk macrophages after stimulation.[144,145] Superoxide anion generation by those cells is more marked after exposure to mannose-receptor ligands.[145] The macrophages also process and present antigens to T cells.[146]

After exposure to chemoattractants, human milk neutrophils (compared with blood neutrophils) do not increase adherence, polarity, directed migration,[147] or deformability.[148] That may be due to agents in human milk. For example, the decreased calcium influx found in human milk neutrophils can be replicated by incubating blood neutrophils in human milk.[149]

Unlike human milk neutrophils, the motility of macrophages in human milk is increased compared with blood monocytes.[150,151] That is likely due to cellular activation, because they display phenotypic features of activation.[138]

Macrophages in human milk produce prototypic long pentraxin[102] and granulocyte macrophage-stimulating factor.[147] Furthermore, IL-4 stimulates human milk macrophages to transform into dendritic cells, which have the most marked abilities to process and present protein antigens to T cells.

The fate and role of human milk leukocytes in the infant are poorly understood. Do human milk leukocytes enter the alimentary and respiratory tracts? Because only small numbers of memory T cells are detected in infancy,[152] memory T cells in human milk may compensate for that developmental delay in the infant. In experimental animals, milk lymphocytes enter neonatal tissues,[143] but that has not been demonstrated in humans. However, that possibility is suggested by the finding that cellular immunity may be transferred by breast-feeding.[153]

EPITHELIAL CELLS

Many epithelial cells are in human milk.[154] Although their in vivo functions are undetermined, some are likely stem cells.[155]

ANTIINFLAMMATORY PROPERTIES

Inflammatory agents and their precursors, such as coagulation factors, kallikrein-kininogen, complement, IgE, basophils, mast cells, eosinophils, and cytotoxic lymphocytes, are poorly represented in human milk.[26] Human milk contains a few proinflammatory cytokines, but there is no evidence that they generate inflammation in the recipient.[26] In contrast antiinflammatory agents are abundant in human milk (Table 122.3).[26] They include epithelial growth promoters that strengthen mucosal barriers, antioxidants, lactoferrin that interferes with some complement components,[26,156] enzymes that degrade inflammatory mediators, protease inhibitors,[157] agents that bind to proinflammatory substrates such as lysozyme to elastin[158] and lactoferrin to lipopolysaccharide, lipid A,[159] cytoprotective agents (prostaglandins E_1, E_2, and $F_2\alpha$[160,161]), and agents that inhibit inflammatory leukocytes[26] such as binding of LPS to CD14 by lactoferrin.[159] Furthermore, many are adapted to survive and function in the alimentary tract.

The main antioxidants in human milk include an ascorbate-like compound,[162] uric acid,[162] α-tocopherol[163,164] and β-carotene.[164] Blood levels of α-tocopherol and β-carotene are higher in breast-fed than unsupplemented formula-fed infants.[164] Mucosal growth factors in human milk include epithelial growth factor,[165] lactoferrin,[9,166] cortisol,[167] and polyamines.[168] Other hormones and growth factors in human milk[169] may accelerate growth and differentiation of epithelium,[170,171] limiting penetration of antigens and pathogens into the intestines through earlier achievement of more mature, adult-like epithelial barriers.[172,173]

Enzymes in human milk degrade inflammatory mediators. Platelet-activating factor (PAF) that plays a role in intestinal injury in rats induced by endotoxin and hypoxia[174] is degraded by a human milk acetylhydrolase.[175] That correlates with the developmental delay in the production of human PAF-acetylhydrolase[176] and the lessened intestinal permeability in human infants fed human milk.[177-178]

Table 122.3 Antiinflammatory Agents in Human Milk.

Categories	Examples
Cytoprotectives	Prostaglandins E_1, E_2, $F_{2\alpha}$
Epithelial growth factors (EGFs)	EGF, lactoferrin, polyamines
Maturational factors	Cortisol
Enzymes that degrade inflammatory mediators	PAF-acetylhydrolase
Binders of enzymes	α_1-Antichymotrypsin
Binders of substrates of enzymes	Lysozyme to elastin
Binders of toxins	Lactoferrin to lipid A of LPS
Modulators of inflammatory leukocytes	IL-10, TGF-β1
Antioxidants	Uric acid, α-tocopherol, β-carotene, ascorbate

Table 122.4 Cytokines in Human Milk.

Biologic Effects	Cytokine Mediators
T-cell production augmentation	IL-7, CCL27
Cellular immunity enhancement	Interferon-γ, TNF-α, IL-12, IL-18
Humoral immunity enhancement	IL-4, IL-10
Macrophage stimulation	IL-1β, IL-6, MIF, M-CSF
Chemokine activities	IL-8, RANTES, eotaxin, MIP-1, CCL28, osteopontin
Interferon-inducible proteins	IP-10, MIG
Antiinflammatory actions	TGF-β1, TGF-β2, IL-4, IL-10
Growth stimulation	EGF, G-CSF, M-CSF, hepatic growth factor, IL-4, erythropoietin
CCR5 receptor ligands (block HIV binding)	MIP-1, MIP-1s, RANTES

TNF-α, Tumor necrosis factor-alpha.

IMMUNOMODULATING AGENTS

Many clinical observations suggested the presence of immunomodulating agents in human milk. Epidemiologic studies showed that children breast-fed during infancy were at less risk for certain diseases mediated by immunologic, inflammatory, or oncogenic mechanisms, including type 1 and 2 diabetes mellitus,[179-181] childhood leukemia and lymphoma,[182-184] and ulcerative colitis and Crohn disease.[185-187] Increased levels of certain immune factors in breast-fed infants could not be accounted for by passive transfer of them from human milk. For example, breast-feeding primes the recipient to produce higher blood levels of interferon-α in response to respiratory syncytial virus infections.[188] That likely aids in preventing wheezing episodes in older children following a respiratory syncytial infection earlier in life.[189] Also, increments in blood levels of fibronectin achieved by breast-feeding cannot be accounted for by the quantities of that protein in human milk. Moreover, breast-feeding leads to a more rapid development of systemic[190]and secretory[191] antibody responses and of SIgA in external secretions[58-60] including urine,[59,60] which are far removed from the site of ingestion, so those increments are not due to absorption of those same factors from human milk.

When Jacques Miller discovered an immunologic role of the thymus in thymectomized neonatal mice in 1962,[192] the mice seemed normal until they were weaned. Afterwards they became lymphopenic, could not reject allografts, and often died. In contrast, mice thymectomized later in life were not immunodeficient. The possibility that the delay was due to agents in murine milk. It is now known that thymic growth[193] and function,[194] T-cell emigration from the thymus,[195] and T-cell maturation and function[192] are increased in breast-fed compared to non-breast-fed human infants.

CYTOKINES

After it was ascertained that human milk leukocytes were activated, activating agents in human milk were sought. It was found that human milk enhanced the movement of blood monocytes in vitro and that increased motility was abrogated by antibodies to tumor necrosis factor-alpha (TNF-α).[196] Subsequently, TNF-α in human milk was detected immunochemically.[197] Since then, many different cytokines and growth factors that likely have important effects have been found in human milk (Table 122.4).[198-219]

OTHER MODULATORS

Other immunomodulating agents in human milk include β-casomorphins,[220] prolactin,[221] antiidiotypic antibodies,[48] α -tocopherol,[161,162] nucleotides that enhance natural killer (NK)-cells, macrophage and Th1 activities,[222-224]cell adhesion molecules ICAM-1, VCAM-1, and E and L-selectin,[225] mannan-binding lectin, which activates complement by the lectin pathway after recognizing surface saccharide motifs on micro-organisms,[226] and CD14, a B-cell mitogen.[227] In addition, some oligosaccharides are immunomodulatory. Lacto-N-fucopentaose III and lacto-N-neotetraose increase the production of murine IL-10.[228] Human milk acidic oligosaccharides increase the number of interferon-producing $CD4^+$ and $CD8^+$ T cells, IL-13 production by $CD8^+$ T cells, and CD25 expression on $CD4^+$ T cells.[229]

Osteopontin, which plays an important role in bone mineralization and remodeling, is also a chemotaxin for neutrophils and macrophages, increases the expression of some integrins, and enhances certain Th1 responses.[230] Its concentration in human milk is approximately 138 mg/L, whereas the concentration in bovine milk is approximately one-tenth of that.[231]

IMMUNE SYSTEM IN HUMAN MILK AND THE RECIPIENT INFANT

The complementary relationship between the infant's immune status and defense agents in human milk appears to have a strong evolutionary basis. Many aspects of the immune system are incompletely developed at birth and even more so in very low-birth-weight infants. These include mobilization and function of neutrophils,[232-234] maturation of dendritic cells,[235,236] mucosal production of lysozyme[237] and SIgA,[238,239] memory T cells that bear CD45RO,[152] full expression of the antibody repertoire,[139] and production of numerous cytokines (including TNF-α,[240-242] IL-4,[243,244] interferon-γ,[244-246] IL-6,[241,247] IL-10,[240,248] IL-12,[249,250] IL-18,[250] G-CSF,[251] GM-CSF,[252] IL-3,[251] and RANTES[253]). Human milk contains significant quantities of many of these immune defense products (Table 122.5). For instance, SIgA antibodies in milk compensate for low production of SIgA during early infancy.[254] Human milk antibodies are directed against protein and polysaccharide antigens. This is important because infants display a more restricted antibody clonality[255] and do not produce sufficient quantities of IgG antibodies to polysaccharides.[256] Moreover, antibody responses to conjugate vaccines are higher in breast-fed than cow's milk-fed infants.[257]

An additional example is the interrelationship between the production of lysozyme by the infant and the mammary gland. High lysozyme levels in human milk[53] are coupled with low production of the protein by tracheobronchial mucosal cells during infancy.[237] Indeed, achievement of normal intraluminal concentrations of lysozyme in infancy may depend on breast-feeding.

Table 122.5 Immune Factors in Human Milk Whose Production Is Delayed in the Recipient.

Immune Functions	Representative Agents
Antimicrobial	Human milk SIgA
	Lactoferrin
	Lysozyme
Antiinflammatory	IL-10
	PAF-acetylhydrolase
	Lactoferrin
	Lysozyme
Immunomodulatory	Memory T cells
	IL-4
	IL-10
	IL-12
	G-CSF
	TNF-α
	Interferon-γ
	RANTES

TNF-α, Tumor necrosis factor-alpha.

Function of human milk immune factors in the infant depends on maintenance of their structural integrity, or survival, after ingestion by the infant. Ingested proteins may affect the epithelium, leukocytes, or other cells of the proximal GI or respiratory tracts where proteolytic enzymes are not produced. Proteins also may escape digestion because of developmental delays in production of gastric acid and pancreatic proteases,[258] shielding of acid-labile components by the buffering capacity of milk, antiproteases in human milk,[258] inherent resistance of many defense agents in human milk to digestive processes, or compartmentalization of some defense agents in human milk.[83,91,259] For example, human milk TNF-α is protected by binding to its soluble receptors in human milk.[259] This binding may influence the action of that agent. It has also been found that complexes of human milk lactoferrin and osteopontin are more resistant to in vitro proteolysis.[260] That may promote an in vivo proliferation and differentiation of certain intestinal epithelial cells.

PROTECTION OF PREMATURE INFANTS BY HUMAN MILK

Maturational delays of the immune system are more profound in premature infants. In contrast to mature epithelium, neonatal intestinal epithelium overexpresses certain innate inflammatory genes.[261] The problem is compounded by the shortened placental transfer of IgG in premature infants[262] and medical problems unrelated to the infant's immune system.

Preterm milk contains many antimicrobial factors found in term milk.[263] Concentrations of some defense agents are higher in preterm than term milk, which may be due to a lower production of milk by those women. However, that may not be the total explanation. The patterns of concentrations of some antimicrobial agents in preterm and term milk are not the same.[263] Moreover, it is unclear whether most antiinflammatory and immunomodulating factors in mature milk are in preterm milk and whether the inverse relationships between the production of immune agents by the infant and the maternal mammary gland also occur in premature infants and preterm milk. Furthermore, donor milk is not the same as a mother's own milk and may not confer the same advantages to preterm infants.[264]

BACTERIAL SEPSIS

In addition to the protection against enteric and respiratory infections, several studies indicate that human milk feedings protect premature infants against systemic infections to which such infants may be prone, including late-onset sepsis.[264-267]

NECROTIZING ENTEROCOLITIS

Human milk protects against necrotizing enterocolitis (NEC),[268,269] but the factors responsible for this protection are unclear. Because NEC in human preterm infants is likely generated by a complex train of inflammatory processes, protection against NEC may involve many human milk agents working additively or synergistically. Human and experimental animal studies suggest that SIgA,[270] erythropoietin,[271,272] lactoferrin,[273] PAF-acetylhydrolase,[175,176] and IL-10[203,274,275] are likely possibilities. In each case, endogenous production is developmentally delayed, but the agent is well represented in human milk.

One animal model suggests that IL-10 in human milk may prevent intestinal inflammation. Mice homozygous for IL-10 null genes develop a fatal enterocolitis that begins soon after weaning and is dependent on an enteric bacterial flora.[274,275] The enterocolitis is prevented by intraperitoneal injections of IL-10 given when weaning begins.[275] Other gene-knockout models might provide further clues to the function of other agents in protection against NEC.

One clinical study suggests that low concentrations of IL-10 in human milk may increase the risk of NEC in premature infants.[204] Women were found to fall into two distinct populations with respect to the concentrations of IL-10 in their milk, with 72% being high producers and 28% being very low producers. In more than 90% of the infants who developed NEC while receiving their own mother's milk, IL-10 was barely detected or undetected in their mother's milk.[204]

An additional possibility is that human milk growth factors help establish a safe intestinal bacterial flora and alter mucosal immunity. Animal studies indicate that commensal enteric bacteria initiate a complex chain of events that profoundly affect mucosal immunity.[276] Agents from intestinal commensal bacteria have been shown to stimulate resident macrophages in the lamina propria to release IL-1β. That in turn promotes the release of granulocyte-macrophage colony-stimulating factor from intestinal lymphoid cells that controls the number and function of mucosal dendritic cells and macrophages. Consequently, retinoic acid from dendritic cells enhances the production of regulatory T cells and IL-10 from macrophages, inhibiting production of proinflammatory cytokines. Similar events in breast-fed infants seem likely.

LUNG DISEASE

Although it is unknown whether human milk protects against pulmonary and vascular effects of hyperoxia, α_1-antitrypsin prevents many of those features in a hyperoxic neonatal rat model, including elevated pulmonary elastolytic activity.[277] This is germane because α_1-antitrypsin is prominent in human milk.[278] Other agents in human milk may protect against pulmonary inflammation. For example, a murine model suggests that TGF-β1 in human milk protects against pulmonary inflammation.[275-277] Mice homozygous for the TGF-β1 null gene display infiltrations of macrophages and T cells in the lungs and other sites.[279,280] Further, the effects of TGF-β1 deficiency are mitigated by ingestion of that cytokine in murine milk.

ATOPIC DISEASE AND HUMAN MILK

Some studies suggest that human milk protects against atopic dermatitis[281,282] and asthma[213,282] and that the protection against asthma is mediated by TGF-β1[213] and soluble CD14 in human milk.[282] However, there is no consensus that breast-feeding protects against atopic diseases.[8,283,284] The disagreements may be due to variations in genetic predisposition to atopic disorders[281] and the sufficiency of breast-feeding. Further, the degree of exposures to infectious agents might be a determinant because increased exposures facilitate Th1 responses that lead to cellular immunity. In contrast, lower exposures engender

Th2 responses that lead to antibody formation and hence to a possible IgE-mediated hypersensitivity.[285] Thus, the effects of breast-feeding on atopic diseases may depend on factors that are not equally represented in all investigated populations.

A further confusing factor is that atopic diseases are probably multiple discrete diseases. As more genetic errors responsible for allergic diseases are discovered, it will be possible to ascertain which of them are prevented, minimized, or not affected by breast-feeding.

Foreign food antigens in human milk[286] trigger allergic reactions in some infants.[287] To test whether a breast-fed infant reacts to a foreign food antigen in human milk, the suspected food should be eliminated from the mother's diet to determine if the infant improves and then added back to determine if the infant becomes symptomatic.[288,289] The early introduction of peanuts to infants prevents the onset of that allergy.[290] It is unclear whether that pertains to other food allergens including cow's milk.[291]

Finally, the entire matter of atopic diseases and breast-feeding should be considered in the context of biologic evolution. There have been myriads of changes in our diets and exposures to environmental agents. Thus, there has been little time for humans to adapt to environmental alterations not encountered during our evolution.[23,25,288]

IMMUNOLOGIC TOLERANCE

Evidence for induction of immunologic tolerance by breast-feeding comes from studies of alloreactivity. Maternal renal allografts are better tolerated in children from women who breast-fed transplant recipients during infancy than in those who did not.[291,292] The difference in alloreactivity is also shown with blood lymphocytes from mothers and their children. Less alloreactivity occurs when lymphocytes from the mother (stimulators) and her breast-fed child (reactors) are co-cultured.[293] The tolerance may be induced by HLA-DR antigens on fat globules[294,295] and cells in human milk.

CONCLUSION

The immune system in human milk is adapted to function at mucosal sites and in some cases systemically. Consequently, the recipient is protected against certain infections, inflammatory processes, and some diseases such as otitis media that occur long after weaning. Much is to be learned about the immune system in human milk, including (1) undiscovered agents, (2) new functions for known ones, (3) regulation of immune factor production, (4) factor interactions, (5) the role of compartmentalized and soluble-receptor bound agents, (6) the in vivo fate of human milk cells, (7) relationships among milk, the enteric microbial flora, and mucosal immunity, (8) benefits of mother's own milk and donor human milk in the premature infant, and (9) the spectrum of and basis for disease prevention by breast-feeding.

Although much remains to be discovered,[296] it is known that the immune system in human milk is more complex than other human secretion, and that the human milk immune system and its relationship to the immunologic status of the developing infant is an outcome of many millions of years of experiments in nature.[25] Thus, in some ways, non-breast-fed infants are immunodeficient. As a result, human milk is superior to other types of feeding for human infants.

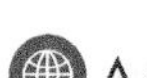
A complete reference list is available at www.ExpertConsult.com.

SELECT REFERENCES

1. Ehrlich P. Experimentelle untersuchangen über immunität. I. Ueber ricin. *Dtsch Med Wochenschr*. 1891;17:976-979.
2. Ehrlich P. Experimentelle untersuchangen über immunität. II. Üeber abrin. *Dtsch Med Wochenschr*. 1891;17:1218-1219.
3. Woodbury RM. The relation between breast and artificial feeding and infant mortality. *Am J Hygiene*. 1922;2:668-687.
4. Grulee CG, Sanford HN, Herron PH. Breast and artificially feeding of infants. Influence on morbidity and mortality of twenty thousand infants. *JAMA*. 1934;103:735-739.
5. Grulee CG, Sanford HN, Schwartz H. Breast and artificially fed infants. A study of the age incidence in the morbidity and mortality in twenty thousand cases. *JAMA*. 1935;104:1986-1988.
6. Wyatt RG, Mata LJ. Bacteria in colostrum and milk of Guatemalan Indian women. *J Trop Pediatr*. 1969;15:159-162.
7. Mata LJ, Urrutia JJ, Gordon JE. Diarrhoeal disease in a cohort of Guatemalan village children observed from birth to age two years. *Trop Geogr Med*. 1967;19:247-257.
8. Mata LJ, Urrutia JJ, García B. Shigella infection in breast-fed Guatemalan Indian neonates. *Am J Dis Child*. 1969;117:142-146.
9. Glass RI, Stoll BJ. The protective effect of human milk against diarrhea: a review of studies from Bangladesh. *Acta Paediatr Scand Suppl*. 1989;351: 131-136.
10. Clemens JB, Stanton B, Stoll B, et al. Breast-feeding as a determinant of severity in shigellosis: evidence for protection throughout the first three years of life in Bangladeshi children. *Am J Epidemiol*. 1986;123:710-720.
11. Glass RI, Svennerholm AM, Stoll BJ, et al. Protection against cholera in breast-fed children by antibodies in breast milk. *N Engl J Med*. 1983;308:1389-1392.
12. Totterdell BM, Chrystie IL, Banatvala JE. Rotavirus infection in a maternity unit. *Arch Dis Child*. 1976;51:924-928.
13. McLean BS, Holmes IH. Effects of antibodies, trypsin and trypsin inhibitors on susceptibility of neonates to rotavirus infections. *J Clin Microbiol*. 1981;13:22-29.
14. Duffy LC, Riepenhoff-Talty M, Byers TE, et al. Modulation of rotavirus enteritis during breastfeeding. Implications on alterations in the intestinal bacterial flora. *Am J Dis Child*. 1986;140:1164-1168.
15. Sabin AB, Fieldsteel AH. Antipoliomyelitic activity of human and bovine colostrum and milk. *Pediatrics*. 1962;29:105-115.
16. Thapa S, Short RV, Potts M. Breast feeding, birth spacing and their effects on child survival. *Nature*. 1988;335:679-692.
17. Downham MA, Scott R, Sims DG, et al. Breast-feeding protects against respiratory syncytial virus infections. *Br Med J*. 1976;2:274-276.
18. Pullan CR, Toms GL, Martin AJ, et al. Breast-feeding and respiratory syncytial virus infection. *Br Med J*. 1980;281:1034-1036.
19. Howie PW, Forsyth JS, Ogston SA, et al. Protective effect of breastfeeding against infection. *Br Med J*. 1990;300:11-16.
20. Hamosh M, Dewey KG, Garza C, et al. *Infant Outcomes. In Institute of Medicine. Subcommittee on Nutrition during Lactation. Nutrition During Lactation*. Washington, DC: National Academy Press; 1991:152-196.
21. Goldman AS. The immunological system in human milk: the past—a pathway to the future. *Adv Nutr Res*. 2001;10:15-37.
22. Goldman AS, Smith CW. Host resistance factors in human milk. *J Pediatr*. 1973;82:1082-1090.
23. Goldman AS, Chheda S, Garofalo R. Evolution of immunologic functions of the mammary gland and the postnatal development of immunity. *Pediatr Res*. 1998;43:155-162.
24. Goldman AS. Modulation of the gastrointestinal tract of infants by human milk. Interfaces and interactions. An evolutionary perspective. *J Nutr*. 2000;130(25 Suppl):426S-431S.
25. Goldman AS. Evolution of the mammary gland defense system and ontogeny of the immune system. *J Mammary Gland Biol Neoplasia*. 2002;7:277-289.
26. Goldman AS, Thorpe LW, Goldblum RM, et al. Anti-inflammatory properties of human milk. *Acta Paediatr Scand*. 1986;75:689-695.
27. Garofalo RP, Goldman AS. Expression of functional immunomodulatory and antiinflammatory factors in human milk. *Clin Perinatol*. 1999;26: 361-377.
28. Goldman AS, Goldblum RM. Immunoglobulins in human milk. In: Atkinson SA, Lonnerdal B, eds. *Protein and Non-Protein Nitrogen in Human Milk*. Boca Raton: CRC Press; 1989:43-51.
29. Keller MA, Heiner DC, Kidd RM, et al. Local production of IgG4 in human colostrum. *J Immunol*. 1983;130:1654-1657.
30. Keller MA, Heiner DC, Myers AS, et al. IgD—a mucosal immunoglobulin? *Pediatr Res*. 1984;18:258A.
31. Underdown BJ, Knight A, Papsin FR. The relative paucity of IgE in human milk. *J Immunol*. 1976;116:1435-1438.
32. Brandtzaeg P. Polymeric IgA is complexed with secretory component (SC) on the surface of human intestinal epithelial cells. *Scand J Immunol*. 1978;8:39-52.
33. Mostov KE, Blobel G. A transmembrane precursor of secretory component. The receptor for transcellular transport of polymeric immunoglobulins. *J Biol Chem*. 1982;257:11816-90011821.
34. Bakos M-A, Kurosky A, Goldblum RM. Characterization of a critical binding site for human polymeric Ig on secretory component. *J Immunol*. 1991;147:3419-3426.
35. Goldblum RM, Ahlstedt S, Carlsson B, et al. Antibody forming cells in human colostrum after oral immunisation. *Nature*. 1975;257:797-798.
36. Roux ME, McWilliams M, Phillips-Quagliata JM, et al. Origin of IgA secreting plasma cells in the mammary gland. *J Exp Med*. 1977;146:1311-1332.
37. Weisz-Carrington P, Roux ME, McWilliams M, et al. Hormonal induction of the secretory immune system in the mammary gland. *Proc Natl Acad Sci U S A*. 1978;75:2928-2932.
38. Fishaut M, Murphy D, Neifert M, et al. Broncho-mammary axis in the immune response to respiratory syncytial virus. *J Pediatr*. 1981;99:186-191.

39. Beagley KW, Fujihash K, Aicher W, et al. Mucosal homeostasis: role of interleukins, isotype-specific factors and contrasuppression in the IgA response. *Immunol Invest*. 1989;18:77-89.
40. Schultz CL, Coffman RL. Control of isotype switching by T cells and cytokines. *Immunol Invest*. 1991;3:350-354.
41. Kono Y, Beagley KW, Fujhash K, et al. Cytokine regulation of localized inflammation. Induction of activated B cells and IL-6-mediated polyclonal IgG and IgA synthesis in inflamed human gingiva. *J Immunol*. 1991;146:1812-1821.
42. Wilson E, Butcher EC. CCL28 controls immunoglobulin (Ig)A plasma cell accumulation in the lactating mammary gland and IgA antibody transfer to the neonate. *J Exp Med*. 2004;200:805-809.
43. Hieshima K, Ohtani H, Shibano M, et al. CCL28 has dual roles in mucosal immunity as a chemokine with broad-spectrum antimicrobial activity. *J Immunol*. 2003;170:1452-1461.
44. Molé CM, Montagne PM, Béné MC, et al. Sequential assay of human milk immunoglobulins shows a predominance of lambda chains. *Lab Invest*. 1992;67:147-151.
45. Crago SS, Kulhavy R, Prince SJ, et al. Secretory component of epithelial cells is a surface receptor for polymeric immunoglobulins. *J Exp Med*. 1978;147:1832-1837.
46. Brown WR, Isobe Y, Nakane PK. Studies on translocation of immunoglobulins across intestinal epithelium. II. Immunoelectronmicroscopic localization of immunoglobulins and secretory component in human intestinal mucosa. *Gastroenterology*. 1976;71:985-995.
47. Adderson EE, Johnston JM, Shackerford PG, et al. Development of the human antibody repertoire. *Pediatr Res*. 1992;32:257-263.
48. Hahn-Zoric M, Carlsson B, Jeansson S, et al. Anti-idiotypic antibodies to polio virus in commercial immunoglobulin preparations, human serum, and milk. *Pediatr Res*. 1993;33:475-480.
299. Kaila M, Isolauri E, Soppi E, et al. Enhancement of the circulating antibody secreting cell response in human diarrhea by a human Lactobacillus strain. *Pediatr Res*. 1992;32:141-144.
300. Duggan C, Gannon J, Walker WA. Protective nutrients and functional foods for the gastrointestinal tract. *Am J Clin Nutr*. 2002;75:789-808.

Neonatal Pulmonary Host Defense

123

Misty Good | Jay K. Kolls | Kerry M. Empey

INTRODUCTION

Like the skin and gastrointestinal (GI) tract, the lung is a mucosal organ with a large surface area exposed to the external environment. Unlike the skin and GI tract, the lung is considered to be largely sterile below the glottis, whereas the skin and GI tract are colonized with bacteria termed *commensal flora*. Despite the lower airway being sterile, the upper airway becomes rapidly colonized with bacteria that can be aspirated into the lower airway; thus the lung has evolved an array of host defense mechanisms to prevent development of infection in the air space. This robust development of pulmonary host defense mechanisms was an essential step in the evolution of air-breathing animals. The major physiologic aspect of the lung is to perform gas exchange—namely the exchange of oxygen and carbon dioxide across the alveolar capillary membrane. To maintain this function, the lungs must have buffering capacity in the airway and alveolar space to neutralize potentially injurious agents including pathogens. In a 3.5-kg neonate with a minute ventilation ranging from 100 to 150 mL/(kg/min), the lungs are required to filter approximately 30 L of inhaled air hourly. This is a problematic task in that the alveolar surface area requiring protection is 20 times the average neonatal body surface area.[1] In addition to normal tidal breathing or gas exchange, the lung must be able to handle larger insults because of what may occur upon aspiration of oropharyngeal or gastric contents.

Available pulmonary host defenses can be broadly categorized as either structural or immunologic. Examples of structural defenses include the larynx and epiglottis (which are anatomically situated to minimize aspiration of oropharyngeal material), airway angulation, mucus secretion, and mucociliary clearance mechanisms, including the cough reflex. These mechanisms result in progressive filtering of approximately 99% of inhaled particles as they pass through the conducting airways so that overall level of antigen exposure at a given site is inversely related to its depth within the respiratory tree.

Immunologic mechanisms can be divided into innate immune response and adaptive immune response. Innate immunity is highly conserved from lower-order species such as worms *(Caenorhabditis elegans)* and fruit flies *(Drosophila melanogaster)*. Innate immunity is rapid (within minutes to hours) and generally lacks specificity toward the pathogen. Adaptive immunity takes longer to develop (days as opposed to minutes to hours), is more pathogen specific, and is characterized by recombination of cell surface receptors to achieve pathogen specificity in both B-lymphocytes and T-lymphocytes. Adaptive immunity is present in higher-order eukaryotes such as fish and mammals. Although innate immune responses are thought to be nonspecific, they often rely on host recognition of pathogen-associated molecular patterns (PAMPs) or specific molecules such as peptidoglycans, lipopeptides, lipopolysaccharides (LPSs), flagellin, fungal glucans, or specific nucleic acid structures such as single-stranded RNA or unmethylated CpG DNA (Fig. 123.1).[2] These receptors are expressed on both blood-derived cells such as lung dendritic cells (DCs) and alveolar macrophages and on nonmyeloid cells such as the lung epithelial cell.[3,4] Ligation of Toll-like receptors (TLRs) can initiate early alarm cytokines such as tumor necrosis factor (TNF)-α and interleukin (IL)-1β in the lung, and these can, in turn, stimulate lung endothelial expression of adhesion molecules, which augments binding of inflammatory cells to endothelium.[5] Additionally, TLR signaling and the alarm cytokines can amplify the production of specific chemokines such as C3a, CXCL1, CXCL2, and CXCL8, which can augment neutrophil recruitment into the air space. Mice deficient in CXCR2, which is the receptor for CXCL1, CXCL2, and CXCL5 in the mouse, have significantly attenuated neutrophil recruitment in response to bacteria and hence have markedly reduced survival as a result of an inability to control bacterial growth in the lung.[6]

The lung is unique among mucosal organs in that it expresses surfactant proteins (SPs). Although surfactant was originally described as the critical phospholipid component of the alveolar lining fluid that reduces surface tension and allows successful transition from liquid breathing in the fetus to air breathing in the neonate, surfactant also plays critical roles in innate immunity.[7] Specifically, the SPs A and D have collagen stalks with lectin-binding domains termed *collections*. SP-A and SP-D can act as opsonins and have been shown to be critical for host defense against bacterial, fungal, and viral pathogens.[8,9] These proteins can interact with carbohydrates on pathogens to directly neutralize the pathogen or augment macrophage-mediated uptake of these pathogens. Macrophages express a variety of phagocytic receptors to ingest and kill pathogens including Dectin-1, macrophage

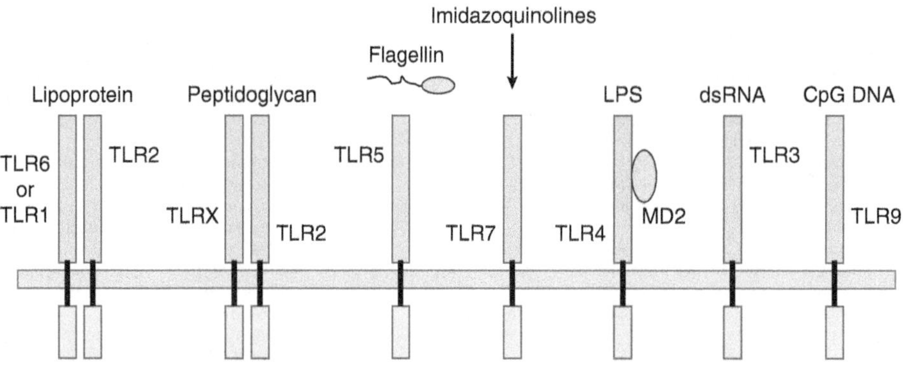

Fig. 123.1 Toll-like receptors *(TLRs)* and their ligands. TLRs function as molecular recognition receptors with specific ligand recognition motifs encoded by their leucine-rich repeat domains *(horizontal lines)*. The TLR2/6 heterodimer recognizes bacterial lipoproteins, and *TLR2* also recognizes peptidoglycans. *TLR5* recognizes flagellin, whereas *TLR7* recognizes molecules such as imiquimod. *TLR4* in conjunction with *MD2* recognizes lipopolysaccharide *(LPS)*, but *TLR4* is critical for signaling induced by LPS stimulation. TLR3 recognizes double-stranded *(ds) RNA*, and *TLR9* recognizes hypomethylated *CpG DNA*.

mannose receptors, and scavenger receptors.[10] Immature dendritic cells (iDCs) are also capable of ingesting pathogens-antigens, and when activated, iDCs can become mature DCs that express high levels of class II major histocompatibility complex (MHC) for antigen presentation and costimulatory molecules such as CD80 and CD86. In addition, maturation leads to up-regulation of CCR7, a G-coupled chemokine receptor that is critical for migration of DCs to lymphoid tissue for antigen presentation to CD4$^+$ T cells. Furthermore, it has been shown that cytokines, specifically IL-12p40, are required for DC migration to lymph nodes, possibly through regulation of CCR7.[11] It is partly through these mechanisms that innate immunity can markedly drive adaptive immunity. For example, antigen presentation to CD4$^+$ T cells in the absence of costimulation (via CD80 or CD86) can lead to anergic T cell responses that may be a key mechanism of achieving antigen tolerance in the lung. This is important because the delicate lining of the lung cannot afford to have strong immune reactions to all inhaled particles (such as ubiquitous mold spores) because the inflammation could adversely affect gas exchange. Thus, the lung comprises macrophages and DCs, which likely respond to specific thresholds of stimulus that are important in regulating decision points of antigen-specific tolerance versus antigen-specific immunity.

In addition to macrophages, DCs, and epithelial cells, the lung also contains cells that are capable of bridging immunity. These cells include γδ T cells and natural killer (NK) T cells that often respond to canonical antigens (and cytokines). Thus, these cells can secrete cytokines that control mucosal immunity, but undergo limited T cell receptor (TCR) rearrangement compared with classic αβ T cells, which orchestrate more specific adaptive immunity. In addition a new class of cells have been characterized—innate lymphoid cells (ILCs) that derive from lymphoid progenitors but do not express TCRs.[12] These cells can differentiate into lineages that secrete effector cytokines including interferon (IFN)-γ, IL-5, IL-13, IL-17, and IL-22 analogous to T helper 1 (Th1), Th2, and Th17 cells among the αβ T cell lineage. The recruitment of αβ T cells and B cells heralds the onset of the adaptive immune response. These cells express T cell and B cell receptors that undergo genetic reengagement so that the receptor has high affinity for peptides that are antigen specific. These cells consist of an effector population and a memory population. The latter population is capable of responding much more rapidly than naïve cells if the antigen is reencountered by the host. Adaptive immunity thus initiates a targeted response aimed at containment and clearance of a specific antigen, allowing titration of nonspecific—and potentially host-injurious—alveolar inflammation. Although it is convenient to think of innate and adaptive immunity as innate immunity occurring proximal to adaptive immunity, complex pulmonary immune responses, as seen in pneumonia, require interplay between innate and adaptive elements.

STRUCTURAL MECHANISMS OF HOST DEFENSE

Structural defense exists throughout the respiratory tract. During air entry, the nose performs humidification of entrained air and also serves as an important filter. Particle filtration occurs through nasal hairs and through nasal turbinates. The turbulent airflow that exists in the upper airway facilitates particle deposition in the upper airway. These structures can filter particles as small as 10 μm. The next barrier to protect the lower airway is the larynx, which consists of the epiglottis, aryepiglottic folds, and glottis. Innervation of these structures provides a gag and cough reflux, which minimizes oropharyngeal aspiration. Particles smaller than 10 μm can be inhaled into the lower respiratory tract, and particle deposition is greatest at areas of airway bifurcation. An important clearance mechanism in the lower airways is cough and mucociliary clearance, which is coordinated by specialized epithelial cells.

EPITHELIAL CELLS

Airway epithelial cells consist of both ciliated and non-ciliated cells. The cells in the large airways exist as a pseudostratified epithelium with each cell having contact with the basement membrane. These cells express apical-tight junctions that restrict passive diffusion or pathogen movement across the lateral intracellular space, augmenting local mechanical barriers.[13] The cilia extend apically from the epithelium into the airway surface liquid (ASL), which has been estimated to be 7 to 8 μm in height.[14] On top of this liquid layer there is a mucous layer, which is the site of particle deposition. The height of the ASL can markedly affect mucociliary clearance and is regulated by both sodium and chloride transport across the epithelium. Excluding regions of the larynx and pharynx where squamous epithelium predominates, ciliated epithelium is present from the upper respiratory tract to the level of the respiratory bronchioles. In addition to the ciliated epithelium, there are a variety of different non-ciliated cell types including mucus-producing goblet cells, serous cells, club cells, neuroendocrine cells, and basal cells.[15,16] Ciliated cells are in physical contact at tight junction desmosomes and in physiologic communication via gap junctions.[17] Columnar ciliated cells may carry up to 200 cilia, ranging from 4 μm in the distal airways to 6 μm centrally. Ciliogenesis commences in the upper trachea early in gestation (week 7) and proceeds distally; by week 24 of gestation, the fetal airway epithelium resembles that of the mature trachea.[18] Although fetal cilia are motile, the function of ciliary activity in utero is unknown.

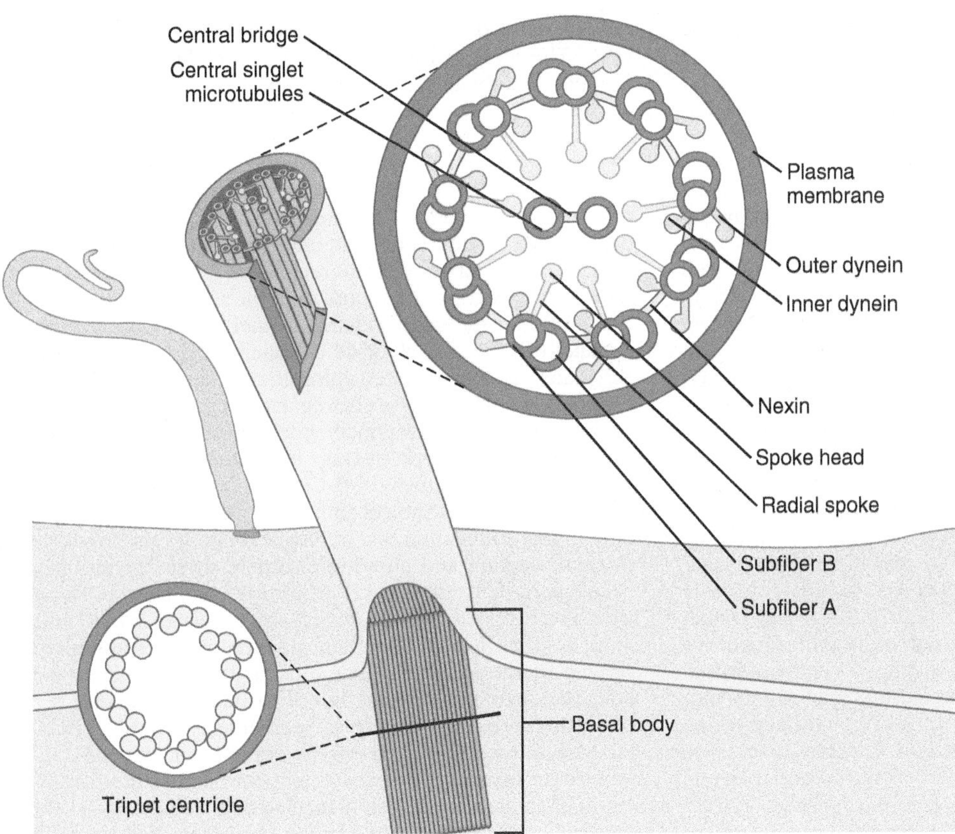

Fig. 123.2 Schematic diagram of a cilium. Note the relationship of dynein projections from one subfiber with the adjacent subfiber *(inset)*. Adenosine triphosphate hydrolysis results in conformational changes of the dynein arm, inducing subfiber movement and ultimately ciliary movement.

Epithelial cell types responsible for mucus production include the goblet cells, serous cells, and club cells. Goblet cells are found predominantly in large airways and are the principal source of mucus. Club cells are found only in small airways and produce watery secretions; serous cells have similar location and function but have been identified only in fetal tissues. Club cells also serve as a likely stem cell for regeneration of ciliated epithelium.[19,20] A novel population of lineage-negative epithelial stem/progenitor cells has been found to repopulate the epithelium after influenza or bleomycin lung injury.[21] These cells require NOTCH signaling that acts through a splice variant of p63 that regulates cell proliferation. Submucosal glands located in the cartilaginous portion of the airways also contribute to overall mucus secretion and express high levels of the chloride transporter cystic fibrosis (CF) transmembrane conductance regulator (CFTR). Recently, studies using single cell RNAseq have shown that CFTR expression is concentrated in specialized secretory cells termed *ionocytes*.[22,23]

There is hierarchy of cell populations when traveling from the large airways to the alveolar ducts. In the trachea and large airways, ciliated columnar epithelium forms an essentially continuous epithelium, with a ratio of ciliated cells to goblet cells of 5:1.[24] In the lower airways, ciliated and goblet cell numbers are reduced, a ciliated cuboidal epithelium predominates, and club cells become the only secretory cells present.[25] Single cell technology has identified novel cells in the airway and will likely greatly inform lung repair in response to injury.

As alluded to previously, particle deposition occurs in the mucus layer and the apical situated glycocalyx layer, which consists of mucins tethered to the epithelial cell surface.[26] The epithelium expresses both tethered and nontethered mucins.[26] *MUC1*, *MUC4,* and *MUC16* are genes that encode tethered mucins, which are highly glycosylated and extend up to 1500 nm into the airway lumen.[27] These mucins and other glycoproteins in the glycocalyx can bind particles and bacteria, facilitate clearance, and form an anatomic barrier between the particle and the epithelial cell. The glycocalyx has also been shown to be a critical barrier to prevent infection of the epithelium by various respiratory viruses.[28]

CILIARY FUNCTION

Human cilia are composed of nine doublet microtubules (subfibers) surrounding two microtubules. The major microtubular axonemal proteins are dynein, adenosine triphosphatase (ATPase), and tubulin.[29] At the tip of the cilium, the nine subfibers simplify into nine single fibers that insert into a common cytoplasmic extension (Fig. 123.2) through which they mechanically engage the overlying mucus sheet during the effective ciliary stroke.[30-32] At the base of the cilium, the nine subfibers end in the basal body, which is anchored to the cytoskeleton.[32] Because all basal bodies of a cell are oriented in approximately the same direction, the effective strokes of all cilia of a given cell have a similar orientation; however, neither the orientation of these structures nor the orientation of the ciliary beats is necessarily identical in adjacent cells.[33,34] During ciliary motion, dynein projections from one subfiber transiently interact with the non-dynein-containing subfiber of an adjacent microtubule doublet and, using energy from dynein-mediated adenosine triphosphate (ATP) hydrolysis, induce a conformational change resulting in subfiber movement. Repetition of this process in adjacent doublets, in a unidirectional front circumferentially, causes the sequential movement of fibers that affect cilia motion.[35] From a resting state, a cilium in its recovery stroke swings close to the cell 180 degrees backward, then fully extends and moves through its effective stroke, an arc of approximately 110 degrees in a plane perpendicular to the cell surface.[36] During the effective stroke, the ciliary tip engages the overlying mucus, advancing it in the same direction. Following this, the cilium rests and then repeats this sequence.As a cilium swings backward into its recovery stroke, it engages other resting cilia, stimulating them to begin a recovery stroke; this mechanical recruitment is pivotal for the coordinated beating of airway cilia.[37]

Cilia of human nasal, tracheal, and bronchial mucosa beat at 11 to 15 Hz at body temperature, with progressively slower frequencies noted in proximal bronchi and bronchioles.[32] Because the combined surface areas of the distal airways are exponentially greater than those of the central airways, this differential ciliary beat frequency allows efficient handling of the relatively large mucus loads eventually delivered to the trachea. Endogenous mechanisms that allow such local ciliary beat modulation have been described. Local physiologic loads to airway epithelium, such as increased quantities of mucus, can mechanically stimulate increased ciliary beating in vivo; this effect appears to be mediated by increased cytosolic calcium and can be reproduced pharmacologically by agents that modulate intracellular calcium levels.[38,39] Ciliary beat frequency is also exquisitely sensitive to alterations in temperature; cilia of the small airways beat optimally near body temperature, decreasing and increasing their beat frequencies in response to decreased and increased body temperatures, respectively.[39] Increased ciliary beat frequency in response to increased ambient air concentrations of nitric oxide (NO) has been described, suggesting that local cellular production of this bioactive substance may modulate ciliary function.[39] These observations are consistent with in vitro data demonstrating that ciliated epithelium produce NO, which regulates ciliary beat frequency in an autocrine manner via a cyclic guanosine monophosphate signaling pathway.[40] In addition to the dynein ATPase, a cyclic adenosine monophosphate (cAMP)-dependent kinase also facilitates control of ciliary beating.[39] Whether intrinsic neural control of ciliary beat frequency exists is unclear. Although acetylcholine increases ciliary beat frequency in vitro, suggesting a potential role for cholinergic regulation of ciliary tone, there is no cholinergic efferent innervation of the superficial airway epithelium, making it unlikely that neural mechanisms regulate lung mucus transport.[41] Finally, recent interest has focused on autocrine and paracrine airway epithelial signals generated by local purinergic pathways.[39,42] In this model, luminal ATP and uridine triphosphate (UTP) induce increased ciliary beat frequency by binding to G protein-coupled purinoreceptors on the epithelial apical membrane. Nucleotide-hydrolyzing enzymes of the airway surface liberate adenosine, which acts through a separate receptor to sustain the ciliostimulatory effects of ATP, while cilia-derived phosphatases hydrolyze ATP and UTP, down-regulating ciliary beat frequency. Nucleotide release by airway epithelia is induced by shear stress and possibly other stimuli so that local mechanical or metabolic perturbations may modulate ciliary activity.[39]

Ciliary function may also be affected by a variety of exogenous substances introduced into the airway. Inhaled β-adrenergic agonists may increase ciliary beat frequency by increasing cellular cAMP.[43] Inhaled NO, via metabolism to S-nitrosothiols, may increase ciliary motility.[44] Conversely, ciliary activity may be diminished by a number of anesthetic gases or by exposure to high concentrations of inspired oxygen or ethanol exposure.[39,45] Finally, ciliary function may be impaired by infection. Specific pathogens, including *Pseudomonas aeruginosa, Streptococcus pneumoniae, Haemophilus influenzae, Mycoplasma pneumoniae,* and *Chlamydia pneumoniae,* produce soluble products inhibiting ciliary function.[39] These products may induce ciliary beat slowing, ciliary beat disorientation, ciliostasis, or frank ciliary lysis. Some of these substances are directly ciliotoxic, whereas others act by inducing local macrophages to generate hydrogen peroxide, which has a local cilioinhibitory effect. Lipid-derived inflammatory mediators, such as platelet-activating factor (PAF), induce dose-dependent slowing of ciliary beat, whereas proteins released into the airway lumen during inflammation, such as leukocyte elastase and neutral protease, are also ciliotoxic.[39] Although other inflammatory mediators stimulate ciliary beating in vitro, overall mucociliary function is typically diminished during inflammation in vivo.[39]

AIRWAY SURFACE LIQUID

ASL is a thin, nonviscous secretion lying just between the epithelial cell and overlying mucus, bathing the basal portion of the cilia and providing an environment of low resistance for the cilia to move during the backstroke portion of the movement cycle. The level of the ASL is critical for effective mucociliary function.[14] If the fluid level is too high, the ciliary tips will not be able to engage the overlying mucus and effect its movement. If the fluid level is too low, as occurs in CF, the cilia will not be able to disengage from the mucus layer during the recovery stroke and ciliary beating will be impeded.[14,46]

As mentioned, ASL is regulated by active ion transport across the epithelial cells with concomitant fluid movement that is either passive or aquaporin regulated.[14,46] The bulk of fluid transport is regulated by both sodium and chloride transport. The predominant apical sodium channel is the epithelial sodium channel (ENaC), and chloride conductance is regulated by the CFTR and calcium-activated chloride channels (Fig. 123.3). These channels are subject to precise regulation by environmental stress such as particle deposition or infection. ENaC is regulated by proteases, as proteolytic cleavage of ENaC subunits can markedly augment channel activity.[47,48] CFTR is regulated by cAMP, and thus this channel is subject to influences such as osmotic stress or cytokine stimulation that influence cAMP levels.[49] In addition to these sodium and chloride channels, there are bicarbonate exchangers that regulate ASL pH.[50] Large-animal models of CF have also revealed that CFTR itself also regulates ASL pH and the more acidic pH in CFTR mutant tracheas reduces antimicrobial activity of the ASL.[51] Passive efflux of water across the apical epithelial membrane results in cell shrinkage, triggering release of epithelial-derived mediators, including NO; these mediators increase blood flow and water content of the submucosa. Movement of water from the submucosa across the basolateral epithelial membrane, possibly regulated by aquaporin 4, restores epithelial cell volume.[52] In contrast, fetal lung fluid results from active secretion of Cl^- by all respiratory tract epithelia, with passive cation and fluid transit into the airway lumen.[53] In the distal airways these mechanisms persist, providing a source of periciliary fluid and mucus hydration for the rest of the lung. Conversely, tracheobronchial epithelium gradually transitions postnatally from Cl^- secretion to Na^+ absorption, and Na^+ absorption eventually predominates in the larger airways under basal conditions.[14] At the same time, production of mucus components transiently increases. Mucociliary clearance is reduced in neonates, presumably the result of increased ASL secretion and impaired ciliary tip engagement of mucus. It has also been shown that the reduced ASL in CF results in enhanced mucous adherence and reduced detachment,[54] which would impair mucous transport.

MUCINS AND MUCUS

Mucins are high-molecular-weight, heavily glycosylated proteins that contribute to the gel-like qualities of mucus and are critical for mucosal host defense. Multiple mucin genes are expressed in the airways, but the primary gene products in mucus are MUC5AC and MUC5B.[55] Mucins are formed in the Golgi apparatus, concentrated in vesicles, and released by exocytosis from goblet cells and mucus cells of submucosal glands. Once secreted, condensed mucin polymers are hydrated, increasing their volume exponentially.[56,57] Mucin proteins typically exhibit several hundred sugar side chains that contribute to their structural and barrier functions. As a result of their extensive glycosylation and their long carbohydrate side chains, mucins are capable of binding virtually any inhaled particle they encounter, facilitating particle entrapment within the mucus layer. Both MUC5AC and MUC5B show extensive regulation by both Th2 cytokines, including IL-9[58] and IL-13,[59] and Th17 cytokines, namely by IL-17.[60] Additionally, proinflammatory molecules such as histamine, prostaglandins, leukotrienes (LTs), platelet-activating factor (PAF), and TNF-α can regulate mucin expression.

Mucus also contains proteoglycans, other proteins, lipids, water, and DNA. DNA is found in significant concentrations only

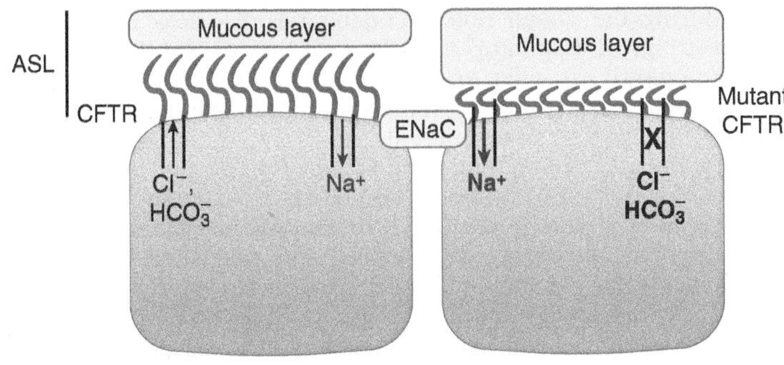

Fig. 123.3 Regulation of the airway surface liquid *(ASL)* by cystic fibrosis transmembrane conductance regulator *(CFTR)*. The ASL is regulated by active ion transport across the epithelial cells with concomitant fluid movement that is either passive or aquaporin regulated. CFTR regulates both *Cl⁻* and *HCO_3^-* transport, and along with the epithelial sodium channel *(ENaC)* regulates the height of the ASL. Disease-causing mutations of the CFTR result in defective Cl^- and HCO_3^- conductance and reduction of the ASL. This leads to ciliary dysfunction and mucous impaction.

during infection or inflammation of the airways originating from dead leukocytes or denuded epithelium; large amounts of DNA markedly increase mucus viscosity.[61,62] DNA is an important component of neutrophil extracellular traps (NETs), which consist of products of degranulated neutrophils such as granular proteases and antimicrobial peptides.[63] NETs have been shown to serve as traps for bacteria and possibly as a way to concentrate antimicrobial peptides at the host pathogen interface.[63] Other antimicrobial proteins, including lysozyme, lactoferrin, human β defensin-2 (HB-2), and immunoglobulin A (IgA), are secreted into the ASL-mucus layer.[64] Mucus rheology is determined by mucus hydration and by polyionic interactions between mucin molecules. These factors, in turn, depend on the pH and salt content of the ASL, and this may explain the thick, relatively immobile mucus seen with the impaired transepithelial Cl^- secretion and accelerated Na^+ absorption characteristic of CF.[51,65]

MUCOCILIARY FUNCTION

Optimal mucociliary function depends on complex interactions among cilia, the mucus layer, and the intervening ASL. Both the mucus layer and the ASL are moved unidirectionally along airway surfaces by ciliary action; cilia effect movement of the mucus layer through direct contact, while frictional interaction with the mucus layer drags periciliary fluid. Beyond their propulsive function, cilia also impart vertical movements within the mucus layer; inhaled particles deposited within the airways are effectively churned into the mucus layer, facilitating binding by mucins and retention within the mucus layer until forced removal by mucociliary transport occurs.[66] Using aerosols of technetium-labeled albumin, one can measure mucociliary clearance in humans.[67] Mucociliary transport has been estimated to be 4 to 5 mm/min in the trachea, decreasing in the smaller airways to less than 0.4 mm/min in the bronchioles. Overall mucociliary clearance of the lung is achieved in two phases: (1) an initial rapid phase (half-life of approximately 4 hours) representing mucociliary clearance of the tracheobronchial tree and (2) a simultaneous slow phase lasting weeks to months, which represents alveolar clearance by non-mucociliary transport mechanisms.[68] Humans exhibit a wide range of mucociliary clearance rates, implying some endogenous control of this process. As noted earlier, purinergic regulatory mechanisms have been postulated, given the demonstrated effect of secreted nucleotides on ciliary beat frequency, goblet cell degranulation, and periciliary fluid secretion.[69] Mucociliary function continues to develop postnatally, gradually becoming adult-like over several weeks.

Mucociliary function can be perturbed by alterations in ciliary activity, changes in ASL composition, pH, mucus secretion, or mucociliary interactions. Relevant environmental influences include temperature and humidity. Ciliary beat frequency and mucus transport rates are diminished at conditions below body temperature. Environmental tobacco smoke also reduces mucociliary clearance.[70] High inspired concentrations of oxygen can also damage the respiratory epithelium and impair mucociliary clearance.

Bacterial exotoxins can also perturb mucociliary clearance. Cholinergic agonists increase mucus clearance by increasing rates of mucus secretion and ciliary beat frequency, whereas atropine decreases mucociliary clearance and transport rates.[71] β-Adrenergic agonists increase intracellular cAMP levels, which increase ciliary beating ion and fluid secretion and mucus elaboration, resulting in the expected increase in mucociliary transport rates.[39,71] Methylated xanthines also enhance mucociliary clearance, presumably through similar actions on epithelial cell cAMP levels. Hypertonic saline has also been shown to enhance mucociliary clearance in patients with CF.[72]

The critical role of cilia in mucosal host defense in humans has been clearly demonstrated by disorders that disrupt ciliogenesis or result in impaired ciliary function. These patients often lose sterility of the lower respiratory tract and suffer from sinusitis, bronchitis, and ultimately bronchiectasis. Primary ciliary dyskinesia (PCD) is a group of genetic disorders that result in a congenital ciliary dysmotility state. At least 30 disease-causing mutations in different genes have been reported to date.[73,74] Some mutations result in an absence of an intermediate-chain dynein, which is important in assembly and coordination of heavy-chain dyneins of the ciliary shaft.[75] A subgroup of PCD is manifested by the triad of sinusitis, bronchiectasis, and situs inversus and is termed *Kartagener syndrome*.[76] Other structural defects such as abnormal cilia length and orientation have been described in association with bronchiectasis and recurrent pulmonary infection. There is an ongoing effort to establish a clearer phenotype of these patients to allow better gene association studies to advance the gene-based diagnosis of these disorders. In addition to congenital disorders, many respiratory infections including both viral and bacterial infections can impair ciliary function. It is important to note that PCD can present as respiratory distress in the newborn period.[77] Adenovirus infection, particularly serotype 7, has been shown to cause marked damage to lung epithelium resulting in impaired ciliary function and the development of bronchiectasis.[78] As a result of marked decrease in blood flow to the damaged lung, the patient may develop a hyperlucent lung, as described by Swyer and James.[79]

Another important cause of acquired ciliary dysfunction is the use of positive pressure ventilation in the neonate. Ventilator-associated lung injury and bronchopulmonary dysplasia (BPD) can impair mucociliary clearance. The airway epithelium is exquisitely sensitive to mechanical injury, and manipulations such as endotracheal intubation and/or the use of suction catheters have been shown to cause flattening or denuding of the epithelium in concert with a local inflammatory response. Prolonged mechanical ventilation has been shown to result in squamous metaplasia of the respiratory epithelium. Additionally, BPD is associated with bronchomalacia, which may further impair regional mucociliary clearance.[80]

AIRWAY REFLEXES

INTEGRATION OF BREATHING AND SWALLOWING

Shared upper pathways for breathing and swallowing require that these functions be closely coordinated to prevent pulmonary contamination with oropharyngeal contents. In the neonate, multiple protective processes functionally separate the respiratory and alimentary tracts during swallowing.[81] The more cranial position of the larynx provides closer approximation of the epiglottis and soft palate, better isolating the oral cavity from the rest of the upper airway. Because newborns have lower resistance across the nasal passage than across the oral passage, owing to deficient control of oropharyngeal musculature, nasal breathing is favored, especially by preterm newborns; this may also facilitate functional separation between the upper tracts. Finally, it is well documented that neonatal breathing is interrupted by airway closure during nutritive sucking.[82]

Swallowing occurs early in fetal life, and three distinct stages have been identified: oral, pharyngeal, and esophageal. In neonates, the oral stage is coincident with nutritive sucking. During the pharyngeal stage, the bolus moves through the pharynx into the esophagus; the larynx is elevated and pulled forward; the epiglottis covers the laryngeal opening, which is further sealed by contraction of the laryngeal adductors; and inhibition of breathing occurs. At the end of the swallow, the airway reopens, and the esophageal phase follows.[83] This transient apneic response is also seen in nonfeeding swallows, which allow the infant to clear the airway of oral secretions or regurgitated materials before resuming breathing.[84,85] Premature infants typically exhibit incomplete integration of swallowing and breathing functions, such that oral feeding may result in pronounced apneic pauses.

When studied, intact cough reflexes were found in only 50% of term infants and only 25% of preterm infants; therefore, when challenged by a swallowing misadventure, neonates are more likely to defend the airway by sustained laryngeal closure than by coughing. Reflex laryngeal closure is mediated by stimulation of receptors in the laryngeal mucosa innervated by branches of the superior laryngeal nerves.[86] Although potentially pathologic, this response is also adaptive because attempts to breathe against an obstructed airway are reduced. Conversely, failure of laryngeal closure and premature termination of the apnea before airway clearance has occurred may result in aspiration. As maturation occurs, coughing replaces apnea as the primary response to stimulation of these receptors.[87]

COUGH AND FORCED EXHALATION

In addition to mucociliary transport, cough is an important mechanism to accelerate the transport of inhaled or aspirated particulates out of the lung. The accessory muscles of expiration are used for coughing and sneezing. Contraction of the internal intercostal muscles decreases the anteroposterior diameter of the thorax, aiding in expiration. The abdominal muscles aid in forceful expiration (such as coughing) by increasing intraabdominal pressure; the increased pressure is transmitted through the diaphragm to the pleural space. To move the mucus in the direction of the large airways, the shear force generated by the airflow must overcome mucus viscosity and gravitational forces. At high airflow velocities (2500 cm/s), mucus is rendered off the surface as droplets, producing the mist flow characteristic of sputum expectoration from the trachea; such airflow velocities can be reached in the small airways during cough or forced exhalation.[87]

For a cough maneuver, rapid inhalation of a supranormal is followed by tidal volume glottal closure, an intrathoracic pressure increase (50 to 100 mm Hg), and glottal opening with rapid exhalation. Although the cough reflex is quite effective in older children and adults, the cough is not as effective in neonates. This is the result of the markedly enhanced compliance of the chest wall and cartilaginous airways that impairs the ability to transfer pleural pressure to transpulmonary pressure. In addition, as the airways are more compliant, the neonate is subject to more airway collapse during the cough reflex. Coughing is also less effective in settings of respiratory muscle weakness or inability to close the glottis (as when endotracheally intubated). A coordinated cough maneuver relies on local chemoreceptors and mechanoreceptors, vagal afferents, signal integration in the dorsal medulla, and efferent innervation to relevant muscles of inspiration and expiration. The receptors inducing cough are poorly characterized but may be activated by local mediators, including histamine, tachykinins, and substance P.[88] Cough can also be induced by stimulation of other vagally innervated sites such as the external auditory canal or esophagus. The afferent limb involves the vagus nerve and vagally innervated structures such as the larynx and conducting airways. Of these, the larynx and upper airways seem more sensitive to mechanical stimulation, whereas the lower airways are more chemosensitive.[88] Vagal afferents from these sites synapse in the nucleus tractus solitarius of the dorsal medulla, the putative cough center. Efferent pathways include the recurrent laryngeal nerve, which stimulates glottal closure, and spinal nerves from C3 to S2, which innervate intercostal, abdominal, and pelvic muscles required to achieve sufficient tidal volume and expiratory pressure. As noted earlier, the cough reflex of premature neonates tends to be immature or absent, which is attributed to incomplete myelination of vagal afferents.[57]

In the absence of effective cough, additional airway protective reflexes exist. Mechanical irritation of the epipharynx via the glossopharyngeal nerve elicits the snifflike aspiration reflex by which foreign particles can be removed from the back of the nose and then swallowed or expelled by mucociliary clearance. Mechanical stimulation of the vocal folds by means of the superior laryngeal nerve elicits a brief expiratory effort without preceding inspiration (the expiration reflex).

INNATE IMMUNE MECHANISMS OF HOST DEFENSE

Despite barriers to microbial colonization and invasion discussed earlier, particles of 2 to 10 μm in diameter may still infiltrate the lower airways and alveoli. Furthermore, anatomic barriers may be inadequate in situations of overwhelming pathogen inoculum via the airstream or ineffective in the situation of lung microbial invasion through hematogenous routes. Immune-protective mechanisms are therefore frequently employed to contain penetrant microorganisms. Such mechanisms may be broadly characterized as either innate or adaptive. Adaptive immunity relies on specialized antigen-presenting cells to activate T cells and B cells, resulting in clonal expansion of lymphocyte pools unique for a specific antigen. Although advantageous for their specificity and capacity for long-term memory, such responses are also delayed, owing to the multiple cellular interactions required. This is especially true in the setting of an immunologically naïve host such as the newborn. Because delay in this setting may be deleterious to survival, the capacity for a more immediate immune response must also exist. The soluble and cellular components of this immediate host response constitute innate immunity.

Innate immunity is phylogenetically primitive, nonspecific, immediate, and the primary antimicrobial defense of the naïve host. Innate immune responses recognize and target structurally conserved molecular sequences shared among groups of pathogens; these include LPS of gram-negative bacteria, lipoteichoic acid of gram-positive bacteria, bacterial lipoproteins or peptidoglycans, mycobacterial glycolipids, fungal mannans or β-glucans, unmethylated bacterial DNA sequences, and double- or single-stranded viral RNAs. The structures may vary subtly from one organism to another, but the essential elements are conserved, forming the template for what is referred to collectively as *pathogen-associated molecular patterns*. In addition to patterns generated as the result of invading organisms, the innate immune system also recognizes molecular patterns released by cells undergoing necrotic death. These molecules are referred to as *damage-associated molecular patterns* (DAMPs) and include different families of proteins and nonproteinaceous substances such as uric acid microcrystals.[89] Both PAMPs and DAMPs are recognized and ligated by pattern recognition receptors (PRRs) of the innate immune system. PRRs are nonclonal and do not depend on immunologic memory because they are germline encoded. These receptors are expressed on barrier and effector cells—such as epithelial cells, endothelium, and phagocytes—of innate immunity where binding and activation induce either direct phagocytosis or cellular signals, culminating in leukocyte recruitment and nonspecific inflammation.[90] Alternatively, PRRs are also components of soluble or secreted humoral proteins. When present in the airway lining fluid, they constitute an additional chemical barrier and complement mucociliary clearance.[26,91]

SOLUBLE ELEMENTS OF INNATE IMMUNITY

As noted earlier, bacterial clearance from peripheral airways by mucus transport may require up to 6 hours; because bacteria can exhibit doubling times of less than 20 minutes, forced mucociliary clearance alone is potentially inadequate to maintain alveolar and airway sterility. Therefore, concurrent mechanisms to contain bacterial growth must be present. Products of the neonatal lung that confer innate, or nonspecific, antimicrobial protection include complement, other opsonins such as fibronectin, antimicrobial peptides (defensins, cathelicidins), lysozyme, collectins, and NO, though evidence shows these mechanisms do not all function at adult levels in early life, leaving the infant airway susceptible to more severe infections.[92] As cells are continuously regenerating, the identification and removal of dying cells, either self or nonself, is a function duplicated throughout immunity. Included in this group are soluble innate immune pattern-recognition proteins, which identify nonself and altered-self molecular patterns and include such proteins as collectins, ficolins, and pentraxins.[19]

COMPLEMENT

The complement system is essential for innate and acquired immune responses. Deficiencies in complement proteins may result in greater susceptibility to infections and/or to the development of autoimmune diseases. As a sentinel limb of innate immunity, it can be directly activated by component recognition of PAMPs. As such, it is a potentially important neonatal host defense mechanism providing direct bacterial lysis in the absence of optimal cellular immune responses. Specific complement components also function as microbial opsonins to facilitate phagocytosis, and as chemotaxins to facilitate granulocyte recruitment.[93-96] The complement system consists of more than 20 proteins synthesized by cells of the liver or the reticuloendothelial system. Once activated, most components exhibit a proteolytic function responsible for activation of subsequent components in orderly series. Although normally quiescent, circulating and local complement components may be activated by any one of three major pathways.

The classic complement pathway is initiated by the binding of C1q to the Fc portion of either IgG or IgM complexed to antigen. This results in an amplified cascade leading sequentially to activation of C4b2a (C3 convertase), generation of C3a and C3b, and formation of the C4b2a3b complex that cleaves C5 into its split components C5a and C5b. The mannose-binding lectin (MBL) pathway is mediated by MBL, an acute phase protein of the collectin family structurally similar to C1q.[97-100] MBL possesses domains that recognize and bind membrane glycoproteins of bacteria, yeast, mycobacteria, and certain viruses.[101,102] Pathogen binding induces an MBL conformational change, exposing two MBL serine proteases that activate C4, ultimately generating classic C3 convertase.[103-106] The alternative pathway is initiated by a number of substances, including endotoxin, complex polysaccharides, immune complexes, and surface components of intact cells such as certain bacteria and fungi.[107-111] Binding of nascent C3b fragments to these substances protects C3b from inactivation by serum factors H and I. Subsequent cleavage and binding of factor B and the stabilizing protein properdin yield C3bBb, alternative pathway C3/C5 convertase, which enzymatically cleaves C5 into the active components C5a and C5b. Each pathway ultimately activates terminal components of the complement system to form C5b-9, which inserts into lipid bilayers to form a transmembrane pore, permitting bidirectional solute flow and ultimately cell wall lysis.

Complement is an essential part of the immune system, but its lack of full functionality in newborns may contribute to the increased risk for severe infections among neonates and unfortunately is not compensated for by a mature adaptive immune system.[112,113] Advances in technology have allowed for premature infants surviving birth at earlier gestational ages than ever before. However, we are only beginning to understand the functional capacity of these infants' immune systems. A study examining the complement system at different gestational ages revealed functional impairment in the classic pathway as measured by CH50 in premature infants, with levels increasing in term infants.[114] Specific components of the classic pathway, including C8 and C9, have shown marked deficiencies, and they are linked with poor killing of gram-negative bacteria in vitro.[115,116] Poor crosslinking of C3 may also contribute to decreased lytic and opsonic activity.[117,118] Grumach and colleagues showed that the alternative pathway, as measured by properdin, was lower at birth, reaching only 25% of adult levels in preterm and term infants compared with adults.[114] Finally, whereas MBL serum levels of term neonates approach those of adults, values in preterm neonates are approximately 60% of levels in term infants; the absence of increased morbidity or infection suggests only an adjunctive role for the MBL pathway in this population.[119] Taken together, preterm neonates have more consistent impairment of classic and alternative pathways, which improves steadily postnatally and reaches adult levels by 12 to 18 months of age; in contrast, MBL appears ontologically conserved.[114,117,118,120,121]

Aside from MBL, ficolins and collectins are also involved in lectin pathway activation.[103,122] Among these, L-ficolin is a serum lectin, which stands out as a ficolin with the greatest capacity for antimicrobial activity. It recognizes and binds various microorganisms, including gram-negative and gram-positive bacteria, DNA, and 1, 3-β-glucans, as well as apoptotic cells.[103,123-125] It is postulated that L-ficolin may confer protection from microorganisms that exacerbate allergic inflammation in the lung, whereas deficiency of L-ficolin may contribute to enhanced susceptibility to respiratory infections.[126] Recent findings revealed that acute-phase pentraxins, including C-reactive protein, serum-amyloid P, and long pentraxin 3, which are capable of selectively opsonizing bacteria, fungi, and viruses,[127] are involved in complement activation and regulation.[122,128] Among these, the antibody-like features of long pentraxin 3 (PTX3) enable interaction with MBL, resulting in communication with C1q to boost complement activation.[122] In addition to enhancing activation, PTX3 is able to bind the main fluid-phase regulator of the classical and lectin pathways, C4BP, to avoid overwhelming activation.[129]

Complement components are found throughout the lower respiratory tract and are produced locally by alveolar macrophages, pulmonary fibroblasts, and type II epithelial cells (Fig. 123.4).[130-132] In this milieu, complement activation can be initiated by PAMPs or in the immune host by microbial binding to IgM or IgG. Each pathway results in binding of component C3b, which is recognized by specific receptors on neutrophils and macrophages, facilitating phagocytosis. C3a and C5a are potent

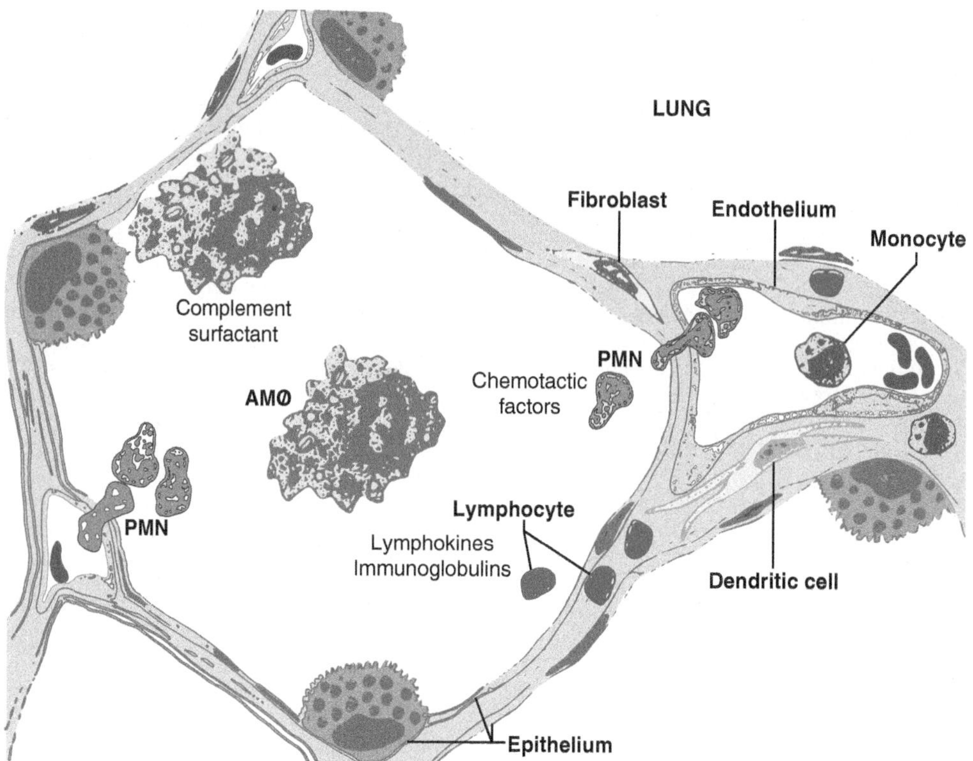

Fig. 123.4 Normal alveolar architecture. Note specifically the relative location of structural cells (fibroblasts, epithelial cells, endothelial cells), which may be stimulated to participate in modulating local immune-inflammatory events. As noted in the text, vascular endothelial cells are strategically located to directly facilitate immune cell recruitment to the alveolar space. *AMØ,* Alveolar macrophage; *PMN,* polymorphonuclear neutrophil. (From Toews GB. NIH conference. Respiratory disease in the immunosuppressed patient. In Shelhamer JH (moderator). *Ann Intern Med.* 1992;117:415.)

neutrophil chemoattractants, whereas C5b initiates the membrane attack complex effecting direct, non-leukocyte-mediated bacterial killing. Data from experimental animal models of acquired and inherited hypocomplementemia indicate that complement is critical in clearance of *S. pneumoniae* and *P. aeruginosa*.[133-135]

While deficiencies among individual components of the complement system may fail to effectively defend the infant airway against foreign pathogens, overproduction of activated complement fragments have been implicated in the pathogenesis of asthma.[136,137] Asthma is a chronic inflammatory disease of the bronchi caused by inappropriate immunologic responses to common antigens in genetically predisposed individuals.[138] Asthma is typically characterized by T_H2-skewed inflammation with elevated pulmonary levels of IL-4, IL-5, and IL-13 levels.[139] The discovery of IL-17 in the lungs of asthmatic persons has led to important new research linking IL-17 with airway constriction and neutrophil recruitment associated with asthma pathology.[140] Both T_H2 CD4 T cells and IL-17-producing Th17 cells engage C3 or C5 complement components, resulting in the induction of airway hyperresponsiveness.[139]

FIBRONECTIN

Fibronectins are extracellular matrix glycoproteins capable of interacting with a number of macromolecules and cells bearing specific fibronectin receptors.[141] The ability of specific mesenchymal cells such as fibroblasts to elaborate fibronectin during embryogenesis is critical to thoracic development. After birth, basal expression of fibronectin is limited primarily to hepatocytes, which produce circulatory fibronectin, and to the respiratory tract, where fibronectin is present in saliva produced by bronchoepithelial cells and constitutively secreted by alveolar macrophages.[142] Serum concentrations of fibronectin are diminished in neonates (particularly in preterm infants), whereas bronchoalveolar lavage (BAL) levels appear inducible in settings of lung injury.[143-145] Enhanced fibronectin production by pulmonary fibroblasts, alveolar macrophages, and epithelial cells is induced by local production of macrophage-derived cytokines associated with acute inflammation, TNF-α, IL-1β, transforming growth factor-β (TGF-β), and platelet-derived growth factor.[146] In acute lung injury, fibronectin stimulates fibroblast and epithelial cell recruitment and endothelial cell proliferation to facilitate tissue reparative processes. However, the ability of fibronectin to bind certain bacteria and to augment leukocyte adherence and migration suggests an additional role for this molecule in lung antimicrobial defense.

Fibronectin is bound by a number of pathogenic bacteria (*Staphylococcus aureus, Streptococcus pyogenes, Escherichia coli,* and *P. aeruginosa*) as well as *Mycobacterium* species, *Pneumocystis,* and fungi.[147-152] Because fibronectin binds multiple microorganisms, it was originally thought to promote phagocytosis and destruction of the invasive organism before the onset of a specific immune response; studies demonstrating increased neutrophil and macrophage binding of *S. aureus* supported this theory.[153-155] Opposing studies suggested that fibronectin by itself may possess only weak opsonic activity.[156,157] More recent data indicate that fibronectin-binding proteins (FnBPs) present on the surface of *S. aureus* and streptococcal organisms promote adhesion of the bacteria to host tissue, leading to increased colonization and infection.[158-160] This would be particularly problematic in cases of impaired mucociliary clearance or epithelial cell damage, yielding a partial explanation of pulmonary microbial tropism in these settings. In vitro studies have demonstrated that *S. aureus* can be internalized by a variety of nonphagocytic cells including epithelial and endothelial cells, fibroblasts, osteoblasts, keratinocytes, and kidney cells.[161-165] Furthermore, recent studies have shed light on a newly discovered mode of internalization through FnBPs, which may avoid fusion with the degrading lysosomes of phagocytic cells.[166-169] In the normal lung, the most important host defense role of fibronectin may be to facilitate binding of, and local colonization by, nonpathogenic organisms. New information is needed to better understand the role of fibronectin in pulmonary tropism and infection, particularly as it pertains to the newborns who possess one-third to one-half the level of fibronectin found in adults.[170]

IRON-BINDING PROTEINS

The availability of iron in the host environment and its effect on bacterial growth is one of the best studied aspects in pathogenicity.[171,172] Iron is an essential element for bacterial growth and survival; thus, pathogens have evolved various ways to compete for the host's iron. In response, host defenses have developed several mechanisms to restrict bacterial colonization or invasion by sequestering elemental iron either in cells or complexed to transport proteins.[173]

There are currently five known iron-binding proteins that have been described in human innate immunity: lipocalin, hepcidin, natural resistance-associated macrophage protein (Nramp), the transferrin family of proteins (lactoferrin and transferrin), and ferritin (cytosolic and plasma).[174-188] Siderophilins are glycoproteins, made up of lactoferrin and transferrin, that are increasingly identified as playing important roles in the regulation of infectious diseases. Transferrin transports iron between cells and is the predominant human siderophilin found in plasma and lymphatic fluids. Transferrin is also found in BAL fluid in concentrations between 1 and 2 times greater than those in matched serum. Transferrin iron saturation is similar in healthy adults and children at approximately 33%, although in times of iron depletion or anemia, transferrin saturation may drop below 10%.[189]

In contrast to transferrin, lactoferrin is the predominant iron-binding protein of airway secretions and is rarely present in deep alveolar lavage unless inflammation is actively occurring; it is also stored in neutrophil granules in addition to its secretion on mucosal surfaces.[171] It binds with high affinity to lipid A and may play an antimicrobial role by depriving invading microorganisms of iron.[179,180] Similar to transferrin, lactoferrin transports extracellular iron between cells with high affinity, but unlike transferrin, lactoferrin is usually less than 10% iron saturated.[190]

Iron-binding proteins effectively complex free iron available in mucosal secretions and alveolar lining fluid, thereby limiting the growth of most iron-dependent pathogens; notable exceptions include *Moraxella* and *Neisseria* species, which are able to obtain iron from these proteins.[191] In addition to iron binding, human lactoferrin has other antimicrobial activity against specific bacteria, including *E. coli*, *S. pneumoniae*, and *Legionella pneumophilia*.[104,192] Lactoferrin binds to LPS, disrupting gram-negative bacterial membranes, and this effect may be synergistic with the effects of other soluble components of the mucociliary layer such as lysozyme.[193] Lactoferrin also demonstrates antiviral activity, binding to human immunodeficiency virus and cytomegalovirus (CMV), preventing their uptake by host cells.[194] Cleavage of lactoferrin by either proteases or pepsin yields a small cationic peptide, lactoferricin, with structure and antimicrobial activity similar to those of the defensins.[195] Finally, recent work suggests a unique role for lactoferrin in prevention of bacterial biofilms. Biofilm formation is a growth mode specialized for long-term bacterial colonization of surfaces, as is seen in chronic *Pseudomonas* infection; once established, organisms within biofilms are notoriously resistant to host eradication.[196] By chelating iron, lactoferrin stimulates twitching, a pili-mediated bacterial motility that deters biofilm formation. Once a biofilm has been established, however, sensitivity to this lactoferrin effect is lost.[180] However, recent evidence shows that US Food and Drug Administration–approved iron chelators given in combination with aminoglycosides such as tobramycin dramatically reduce *P. aeruginosa* biofilm formation on CF airway epithelial cells.[197] For reasons that are largely unknown, the iron concentration in the ASL of CF patients is 400-fold greater than in non-CF patients, making iron chelation a viable and important therapeutic target.[198,199]

Beyond these antimicrobial effects, lactoferrin also plays a role in the modulation of local immune responses. As a component of neutrophil secondary granules, lactoferrin is delivered to sites of inflammation. Here, lactoferrin binds LPS, effectively competing with LPS-binding protein (LBP) and minimizing endotoxin presentation to immune cells.[200] Similarly, lactoferrin also recognizes and binds recurrent motifs of bacterial DNA, potentially dampening the broad proinflammatory immune responses that would ordinarily be triggered.[201] Teleologically, this may allow lactoferrin to limit excess immunostimulatory activity at mucosal surfaces with microbial exposure. Most recently, human recombinant lactoferrin was shown to induce human DC maturation via TLRs 2 and 4, suggesting that endogenous lactoferrin may also regulate similar aspects of innate immunity.

In addition to the siderophilins, lactoferrin and transferrin, recent studies have provided insight into the antimicrobial roles of lipocalin, hepcidin, and Nramp. Using a mouse model, host lipocalin has been shown to bind bacterial siderophores, thereby preventing iron acquisition by invading pathogens.[174,202] The human analogue of lipocalins, siderocalin demonstrates a dramatic up-regulation following bacterial colonization with *S. pneumoniae* to potentially bacteriostatic levels, strongly indicating its role as a host defense mechanism in the upper respiratory tract.[175]

Hepcidin, first discovered by Park and colleagues,[177] is a key regulator of iron homeostasis as well as an acute-phase reactant with a critical role in inflammation. It contributes to host defense by blocking the microorganism's access to iron.[203] Originally, only hepatocytes were thought to produce this iron regulatory protein; however, recent evidence has shown that alveolar macrophages produce hepcidin in addition to expressing the iron importer divalent metal transport and iron exporter ferroportin1 (FPN1) proteins.[204] Further studies suggest that upon exposure to LPS, iron mobilization by alveolar macrophages is reduced and is mediated by hepcidin-induced degradation of the FPN1; as such, less iron becomes less available to the pathogen.[204] This mature iron regulatory system, however, maneuvers its iron stores primarily based on localization of the invading pathogen. In the case of extracellular bacteria, hepcidin targets FPN1 on the cell surface, resulting in its degradation and subsequently reducing macrophage iron release. IFNγ produced during an inflammatory state also inhibits FPN1 through its support of hepcidin production. Iron availability is then reduced for extracellular bacteria, while intracellular iron is incorporated into ferritin. In the event of intracellular bacterial infections, iron stores are shifted out of the cytoplasm and phagolysosome through hepcidin-mediated increases in FPN1 as well as Nramp.[205]

More than 30 years ago, Nramp was discovered to possess antimicrobial properties. It is now widely accepted that the expression of Nramp1 (also called *Slc11a1*) confers innate immune defense against certain bacterial infections. It is thought to work by sequestering iron from bacteria within the phagosome or through a reaction in which iron catalyzes the production of toxic hydroxyl radicals.[206] Nramp1 has further been shown to play a role in early macrophage activation, and its expression is up-regulated by IFN-γ, LPS, and granulocyte-colony-stimulating factor (G-CSF).[107,207-210]

ANTIMICROBIAL PEPTIDES (DEFENSINS, CATHELICIDINS, LYSOZYME)

One form of host defense, found in both plants and animals and therefore predating the separation of the plant and animal lineages, is the production of antimicrobial peptides. These endogenous peptides complement the activity of the larger opsonizing or nutrient-binding proteins in maintaining airway sterility (Table 123.1). They act by disrupting cell membranes of a wide range of pathogens including bacteria, viruses, and fungi; each peptide manifests a broad but fixed spectrum of activity, underscoring the need for multiple peptide classes within the airway lining fluid.[211-213] Within the respiratory tree they are either produced by epithelial cells (where their expression is both constitutive and inducible) or delivered to vulnerable loci by circulating

Table 123.1 Antimicrobial Products in the Mucosa (Partial Listing).

Product	Relative Concentration	Source
SLPI	μg/mL	Epithelia, Paneth cells, macrophages
Lactoferrin	μg/mL	Epithelia, Paneth cells, neutrophils
SP-A, SP-D	ng-μg/mL	Epithelia, type II pneumocyte
α-Defensins	ng-mg/mL	Paneth cells, neutrophils
β-Defensins	ng-mg/mL	Epithelia, neutrophils, glands
Reg3γ/Reg3 β	ng-mg/mL	Paneth cells
Lipocalin-2	ng/mL	Epithelia, neutrophils
CCL20	ng/mL	Epithelia, neutrophils, macrophages
PGLYRP-1	μg-mg/mL	Neutrophils, M cells
PGLYRP-3, PGLYRP-4	μg/mL	Epithelia, glands
Cathelicidins (LL37)	μg/mL	Epithelia, neutrophils

leukocytes. Apart from their direct antimicrobial activity, which is nearly immediate in onset, these peptides can also activate cellular immunity, amplifying host response as necessary. The major human antimicrobial peptides are lysozyme, cathelicidins, and the defensins.

Defensins are small (3 to 6 kDa, 29 to 40 amino acids) cationic peptides containing six conserved cysteine residues. They are divided into α and β subclasses on the basis of their secondary structure, but their gene locations imply a common evolutionary origin.[214] Structurally, they share a β-sheet conformation that spatially segregates their cationic and hydrophobic amino acid clusters into an amphipathic motif.[215] When secreted, defensins are driven into anionic phospholipid bilayer membranes by electromotive forces where they multimerize into channels, disrupt normal membrane function, and induce cell lysis.[215,216] Although host cells are potential bystander targets, their lower anionic lipid content and the presence of cholesterol as a membrane stabilizer imbue significant protection.[217,218] Apart from their structural differences, the α and β defensins differ in their sites of expression and roles in airway defense.

The human α-defensins constitute a subclass of six members: four human neutrophil peptides (HNP-1 through HNP-4) and two human defensins (HD-5 and HD-6). HD-5 and HD-6 are secreted by Paneth cells of the small intestine and epithelia of the female urogenital tract and are presumed to attenuate local commensal burden; respiratory epithelium is not a source of α-defensins.[219,220] HNPs 1 through 4 are abundant (up to 50% of total protein) in primary granules of neutrophils, where they assist in nonoxidative killing, and are also found in NK cells, monocytes, and lymphocytes.[221,222] Individual α-defensins have unique spectra of antibacterial activity against gram-positive and gram-negative species, as well as activity against enveloped viruses (including Herpes species) and against *Candida*.[212,214,223] The α-defensins also exhibit both pro- and antiinflammatory activities. As discussed later, they are chemotactic and induce chemotaxins for a variety of immune cells. They also bind to serine protease inhibitors, amplifying polymorphonuclear neutrophil (PMN)–derived elastase activity.[224] Conversely, they can inhibit complement activation by binding to C1q and participate in local wound repair by stimulating epithelial cell proliferation.[225,226] Extracellular α-defensins are scavenged by α2-macroglobulin, which minimizes cytotoxicity to host cells and down-regulates defensin concentration at inflammatory sites.[227] Immunohistochemical analysis has demonstrated HNPs on bronchial epithelial surfaces and in mucinous exudate in the air spaces, presumably derived from PMN granule release within the airway.[228] In adults, α-defensins have been found in BAL fluid of patients with pneumonitis, correlating with chemotaxin concentration and PMN counts.[229]

Unlike the α-defensins, the β-defensins are produced by airway epithelium. This subclass contains four identified human β-defensins (HBD-1 through HBD-4), although more than 20 genes are postulated to exist.[230] As a group, these peptides demonstrate antimicrobial activity against several gram-positive and gram-negative organisms, as well as *Candida* and *Aspergillus* species; however, differences in antimicrobial spectra exist between individual peptides.[220,231] Histologically, β-defensins are expressed in the epithelia of airways and lung and in the serous cells of submucosal glands.[231,232] HBD-1 is found in the BAL specimens of healthy adults; its expression in the airways appears to be constitutive and noninducible.[233] In contrast, the remaining β-defensins are all inducible, with HBD-2 the best characterized. Endotoxin, *Pseudomonas,* and the cytokines TNF-α and IL-1β each induce HBD-2 expression, and this induction may be amplified further by concurrent alveolar macrophage stimulation. Apart from this interaction with alveolar macrophages, HBDs further interface with cellular immunity by functioning as chemoattractants. HBD-1 and HBD-2 are each chemotactic for iDCs, as well as memory T cells by binding to the chemokine receptor CCR6. Sustained β-defensin induction by noncontained microbial stimuli may thus invoke cellular and adaptive immune responses. Tracheal aspirates of term and preterm newborns demonstrate similar levels of HBD-2, with increased levels seen in local and systemic infections. These data imply that β-defensin responses are intact even in preterm infants and that neonates may up-regulate some facets of pulmonary innate immunity in the context of a systemic inflammatory response.[234] More recent information confirms that HBD-2 is the predominant β-defensin in human neonatal lung; however, its abundance in neonatal tracheal aspirates increases as a function of gestational age. Compared with HBD-2, HBD-1 had a lower level of expression, and HBD-3 expression was absent in neonatal airway epithelial cultures.[235] Although no direct correlations have been made, it is likely that the lower levels of HBD-2 in infants may contribute to the increased susceptibility of premature infants to pulmonary infections. More recently, plasma levels of HBD2 have been studied for their potential as a prognostic biomarker for patients with community-acquired pneumonia, whereby lower HBD2 plasma levels on admission predicts worse outcomes in adults. Based on studies showing that HBD increases as a function of age, combined with more recent data demonstrating increased HBDs in neonatal tracheal aspirates during infection, it is postulated that low levels of HBD during infection may contribute to severity of disease and worse outcomes.[234,236,237]

Cathelicidins are a diverse family of vertebrate antimicrobial proteins found in leukocytes and on epithelial surfaces where they function like defensins. They are produced as preproproteins, stored as inactive proforms, and require enzymatic cleavage for bioactivity. The sole known human cathelicidin is hCAP-18, which requires proteolytic activation by proteinase 3 to liberate the antibacterial peptide LL-37. LL-37 is a 37-amino acid molecule whose amphiphilic α-helical structure facilitates affinity to and disruption of bacterial membranes. Human LL-37 displays a range of antimicrobial activities. It is a broad-spectrum antimicrobial with effects against *Actinobacillus, E. coli, P. aeruginosa, Enterococcus faecalis,* and *S. aureus,* and it demonstrates synergy with the defensins. Though typically considered to have antibacterial activity, LL-37 was recently shown to have activity against respiratory syncytial virus (RSV) in vitro,[238] a virus that typically infects all children by the age of 2 years. LL-37 prevented RSV-induced cell death of epithelial cultures and inhibited the production of new infectious particles.[238] LL-37 also directly binds endotoxin and is chemotactic for eosinophils, neutrophils, monocytes, and T lymphocytes.[239] LL-37 is found in primary granules of neutrophils and has also been shown in NK cells, lymphocytes, and monocytes. Expression of LL-37 in the lung is seen in cells of the submucosal glands and surface epithelia of the proximal airway, where its elaboration can be induced by up to 50-fold in states of inflammation. IFN-γ has been shown to induce LL-37 release, but it concurrently down-regulates gene transcription, perhaps balancing antimicrobial effects against host cytotoxicity.[231] At high concentrations, LL-37 can manifest cytotoxicity toward eukaryotic cells, and hosts have scavenging mechanisms, as exist for the defensins. Comparable levels of LL-37 are found in the tracheal aspirates of term and preterm newborns, with increased levels seen in local and systemic infections. A recent study demonstrated that LL-37 is present in the airway secretions of newborns, but there was no association between concentration and gestational age. A more in-depth look at the structure and function of LL-37 can be found in the detailed review by Wang and colleagues.[240]

Lysozyme is a 14-kDa cationic enzyme that hydrolyzes glycosidic bonds of bacterial cell wall peptidoglycan. This peptide is found in the granules of neutrophils and mononuclear phagocytes and is also secreted by airway epithelial cells of the pulmonary tract where it confers nonspecific antimicrobial protection. Lysozyme is highly active against many streptococci, but resistance to its enzymatic activity is common among other gram-positive organisms and nearly universal among gram-negative organisms. This is likely caused by variable accessibility of vulnerable glycosidic bonds within the cell wall matrix with the outer membrane of gram-negative bacteria providing an additional barrier to the penetration of lysozyme. However, in the presence of other membrane-targeting substances such as complement or hydrogen peroxide, lysozyme enhances the destruction of *E. coli* and other gram-negative bacteria. Lysozyme is also capable of direct antimicrobial activity toward *Streptococcus sanguinis* and *Streptococcus faecalis* species by virtue of its cationic properties and possesses fungicidal activity against *Candida albicans* by targeting the glycosidic bonds of fungal chitin. Although lysozyme may appear redundant in the presence of other antimicrobial peptides, emerging data suggest otherwise. In a transgenic murine model of lysozyme overexpression, increased resistance to pulmonary infection from either *P. aeruginosa* or group B *Streptococcus* (GBS) was observed. Furthermore, lysozyme exhibits important antimicrobial synergy with HBD-2, LL-37, and lactoferrin. More recently, immunodepletion studies have suggested that lysozyme is a major antibacterial component secreted by submucosal glands within the tracheobronchial airways.[236] Moreover, several studies have examined lysozyme's potential as an exogenously delivered biotherapeutic. Bhavsar and colleagues administered aerosolized recombinant hamster lysozyme to hamsters infected with pulmonary *P. aeruginosa.*[241] Following aerosolized delivery for 2 hours on 3 consecutive days, the bacterial burden in lung homogenate and bronchoalveolar lavage fluid (BALF) was reduced.[241]

Similar to other antimicrobial peptides, short palate, lung, nasal epithelium clone 1 (SPLUNC1) has demonstrated antimicrobial activity against *P. aeruginosa, S aureus, M. pneumonia,* and *K. pneumonia.*[242,243] SPLUNC1 is also considered to have antibiofilm activity that functions to reduce of the surface tension by regulating the ASL volume.[244] SPLUNC1 is expressed in serous cells within the airway and has bactericidal/permeability increasing protein (BPI)-like activity to mediate gram-negative bacteria endotoxin LPS-induced bacterial killing.[245,246] Similar to BPI, SPLUNC1 can also bind LPS and is thought to scavenge LPS to minimize its inflammatory properties.[245-247]

LIPOPOLYSACCHARIDE-BINDING PROTEIN

LBP is a soluble 60-kDa glycoprotein that recognizes and binds the lipid A moiety of LPS, enhancing host immune response to endotoxin. LBP is homologous to other phospholipid transport proteins and functions as a transport protein that disaggregates soluble LPS and presents it to targets on cellular membranes. Membrane-bound CD14 is a PRR for LPS; however, it does not contain a cytoplasmic domain and cannot transduce activating signals across the cell membrane.[248] Instead CD14 complexes with TLR4 to form the cellular PRR for LPS, with TLR4 acting as the transmembrane signal-transducing portion of the receptor. LPS-induced signaling through the CD14/TLR4 complex, expressed on inflammatory cells, is distinctly enhanced by the presence of LBP, resulting in the production of early response cytokines TNF-α and IL-1β.[249,250] LBP is produced primarily in the liver as an acute-phase protein, and its plasma concentration increases exponentially during acute inflammatory responses. LBP is also a normal constituent of lung fluid, with alveolar concentrations estimated at 1 μg/mL; these concentrations also increase exponentially with pulmonary inflammation, likely owing to capillary leak of plasma LBP and enhanced local generation. The relevance of LBP to pulmonary host defense is suggested by murine transgenic models of LBP deficiency, which exhibit blunted alveolar bacterial clearance with increased bacteremia and lethality in response to pneumonia. Human alveolar type II epithelial cells demonstrate capability ex vivo to up-regulate LPB production in response to mediators (TNF-α, IL-1β, IL-6) that similarly induce hepatic acute-phase production of LBP. Additionally, animal models suggest that, in the neonate, alveolar macrophages may be a concurrent source of LBP in the lung. Although elevated serum levels of LBP have been reported in neonatal sepsis, pulmonary LBP expression in response to respiratory infection remains uncertain in this population. The most recent studies of infant LBP suggest its use as a viable diagnostic tool for neonatal bacterial infections.[251]

PULMONARY COLLECTINS

Pulmonary surfactant is a bioactive material that bathes the alveolar surfaces and keeps alveoli from collapsing during expiration by reducing surface tension at the air-liquid interface.[252] It is a mixture of lipids and proteins, whereby dipalmitoylphosphatidylcholine (DPCC) functions as the primary lipid for lowering surface tension. The four known SPs are SP-A, SP-B, SP-C, and SP-D. Together, they have several important functions including regulation of surfactant lipid metabolism, lipid membrane organization, and pulmonary host defense.[233] As with the lipid components of pulmonary surfactant, SP-B and SP-C are extremely hydrophobic and function primarily to reduce surface tension and maintain pulmonary homeostasis after birth.[253] The role of pulmonary host defense rests with SP-A and SP-D, which along with mannan-binding lectin, make up a family of carbohydrate-binding proteins known as *collagenous C-type lectins* or *collectins*. These proteins are characterized by a discrete, four-domain primary structure consisting of a cysteine-containing amino terminus, a subsequent collagen-like region, a coiled neck region, and a carboxyl terminus carbohydrate recognition domain (CRD).[254] Collectins function as soluble scavenger receptors, interacting through their lectin CRDs with microbial carbohydrate and glycolipid PAMPs to enhance phagocytosis and pathogen clearance; through this mechanism, collectins exhibit activity against a broad range of bacterial, viral, and fungal pathogens. Beyond these opsonizing qualities, SP-A and SP-D each exerts specific immunomodulatory effects that titrate the magnitude of inflammation and influence pulmonary immune responses.[116,255]

SP-A and SP-D share many characteristics related to their synthesis and bioactivity. Both collectins are produced by type II alveolar epithelium and club cells and are secreted into the alveoli and distal airways. Production and secretion of both proteins increase dramatically during the third trimester of fetal lung development and appear to be further inducible in utero in response to dexamethasone; both proteins are also up-regulated in response to acute lung injury or epithelial activation by microbial products such as LPS. The pulmonary collectins directly interact with a variety of microorganisms.[256-258] Both SP-A and SP-D bind with broad specificity to bacteria including *Klebsiella pneumoniae, P. aeruginosa, H. influenza, S. pneumoniae, S. aureus, E. coli, M. tuberculosis,* and *M. avium.* Pathogen encounter with lung collectins results in agglutination and/or opsonization. Agglutination impedes microbial invasion and colonization and facilitates clearance by the mucociliary escalator, whereas agglutination of viruses enhances their internalization by neutrophils. Alternatively, SP-A or SP-D may act as opsonins by bridging between PAMPs on the microbial surface and collectin receptors on phagocytes. The pulmonary collectins also enhance specific leukocyte functions. Both SP-A and SP-D are chemotactic for neutrophils and macrophages, although SP-D is more potent in this regard. SP-A and SP-D both enhance alveolar macrophage phagocytic function and oxyradical production. Induction of this latter effect requires the collectin CRD(s) to concurrently engage ligand; this presumably minimizes spurious up-regulation of potentially injurious mediators. Finally, although earlier studies suggested a direct inhibition of T cell proliferation by SP-A and SP-D, recent evidence demonstrates that this inhibition may be a result of the presence of TGF-β in SP preparations.[259] Although the relationship between SP-A and TGF-β has not been fully described, it is postulated that SP-A acts as a storage site for latent TGF-β in the lung, thereby indirectly participating in the control of inflammation.[259] Recent evidence indicates that SP-A functions in a more purposeful manner to maintain homeostasis in the airway through TGF-β-mediated induction of regulatory T cells (Tregs).[260] Work by d'Alessio and colleagues recently reported that Tregs are important in the recovery of acute lung injury via TGF-β, a cytokine known to induce Treg function.[261-263] Mukherjee and colleagues showed that SP-A-/- mice have impaired expression of Foxp3 Treg cells ex vivo compared with wild-type mice, which could be fully restored with the addition of exogenous SP-A.[260] Despite their many shared functions, SP-A and SP-D exhibit several biochemical differences that result in distinctive, unshared activities in vivo. Relevant differences include solubility, CRD specificity, length of collagen domain, and affinity for available collectin receptors.

Approximately 30% of the pulmonary collectin pool is made up of SP-D, the product of a single gene. SP-D exists primarily in a cruciform structure: four homotrimeric subunits radiating from a disulfide-linked hub. Unlike SP-A, it is relatively impervious to proteolytic or elastase degradation. Its up-regulation secondary to LPS-induced cytokines confirms its role in innate host defense. SP-D binds specifically to carbohydrates containing glucopyranosides, resulting in affinity for the core oligosaccharides of LPS, the mannose-rich oligosaccharides of influenza A hemagglutinin, and fungal cell wall glycoconjugates of *Candida* and *Pneumocystis carinii.* SP-D binds to the putative collectin opsonin receptor, gp-340, a macrophage scavenger receptor, and CD14 via interactions between the CRD and the N-linked oligosaccharides on CD14; SP-D inhibits the interactions between CD14 and LPS.[9,264] Attempts to further clarify the role of SP-D in host defense have led to the development of transgenic murine models of SP-D deficiency. Such mice exhibit a phenotype of pulmonary alveolar proteinosis, with foamy activated macrophages, hypertrophy of alveolar type II cells, and increased inducible inflammatory responses.[265] SP-D-deficient mice show impaired functions of host defense against *H. influenzae,* GBS, influenza type A virus, and RSV, but lack of SP-D does not affect newborn survival from infection.[266-268] A recent study by Kotecha and colleagues, conducted in premature and newborn infants, demonstrated sizeable and functionally relevant variation in the expression of SP-D between preterm and term newborn lung secretions. Moreover, the percent of neonatal SP-D capable of binding zymosan rarely surpassed 50% in BALF samples and was 3.5 times lower in preterm infants than in term infants on the first day of life.

In contrast, approximately 70% of the pulmonary collectin pool is made up of SP-A, the product of two genes, SP-A1 and SP-A2, each producing different chain types. The SP-A subunit can therefore exist as a homotrimer or heterotrimer, introducing heterogeneity to this protein. Differential tissue expression has been reported, with SP-A1 expressed in the lower respiratory tract and SP-A2 expressed in the tracheal and bronchial epithelium and submucosal glands. Its production is up-regulated by IFN-γ and other LPS-induced cytokines. Its short collagen domain and preferred hexameric structure result in a "flower bouquet" pattern, and this clustering of CRDs influences ligand selectivity. SP-A binds specifically to carbohydrates including fungal wall glycoconjugates and some capsular polysaccharides. It also binds a variety of lipids including the lipid A moiety of LPS. Leukocyte receptors for SP-A include the C1q receptor, SPR210 (the 210-kDa receptor specific for SP-A), the gp-340 receptor, and CD14. Multiple studies suggest that SP-A influences LPS-CD14 binding; however, reports disagree on whether SP-A promotes or inhibits this interaction.[264,269,270] SP-A-deficient mice exhibit increased susceptibility to many pathogens including GBS, *H. influenza,* RSV, *P. aeruginosa,* and *Pneumocystis jirovecti.*[267,271-273]

SP-A exhibits a variety of immunoregulatory activities within the alveolus. It suppresses IFN-γ, an activator of leukocyte and macrophage inflammatory activity and an essential mediator for transition to a lymphocyte-mediated adaptive immune response. SP-A may also dampen LPS-dependent cellular activation by competing with LBP. Taken together with the reported SP-A/TGF-β inhibition of T cell proliferation, these functions suggest that SP-A acts, at least in part, by tempering inflammation that might induce alveolar injury. Such a host-protective role would be consistent with transgenic models of SP-A deficiency, where microbial challenge results in delayed pathogen clearance, increased pathogen dissemination, and enhanced inflammation with increased production of TNF-α, IL-1β, and IL-6. This paradigm, however, is complicated by contradictory data regarding SP-A induction of proinflammatory cytokines and up-regulation of inducible NO synthase (iNOS). These disparate findings are reconciled by recent observations that the response to SP-A is determined by the state of cell activation and concurrent stimuli. Thus SP-A up-regulates iNOS in alveolar macrophages primed by IFN-α and stimulated by LPS, but conversely inhibits LPS-induced iNOS if IFN-γ priming has not occurred. SP-A, therefore, augments an inflammatory response already under way but dampens similar responses evolving de novo. In this context, SP-A induction of iNOS also exerts host protective effects. In a murine model of tuberculosis, exogenous SP-A enhanced pathogen entry into alveolar macrophages by almost five-fold. This enhanced entry resulted from SP-A ligation of the SPR210 receptor with increased endocytosis of the SP-A:BCG complex. Furthermore, SP-A-mediated up-regulation of NO and TNF-α production enhanced mycobacterial killing.

SP-A and SP-D exhibit only partial redundancy of their bacterial specificities, owing to their distinct structures and their differing affinities for specific carbohydrates and lipids. These differences may result in complementary functions that enhance the antimicrobial activity of surfactant in total. One example of such synergy is illustrated by collectin interactions with *Klebsiella,* a pulmonary pathogen that can reversibly switch between encapsulated and unencapsulated phenotypes. Unencapsulated forms of this organism allow optimal adhesion to the epithelial surface, facilitating colonization; these forms predominate early in infection. As noted earlier, SP-A binds to lipid A of LPS, whereas SP-D preferentially binds to the LPS core sugars. Because lipid A is embedded within the bacterial cell wall and inaccessible to SP-A, SP-D is the primary collectin ligand for LPS expressed on the surface of unencapsulated forms. Encapsulation limits interaction of SP-D with the underlying LPS, but invokes significant binding by SP-A, which recognizes the capsular polysaccharides expressed by this pathogen. In this scenario, SP-A and SP-D thus fulfill distinct but complementary opsonizing roles in the innate host response

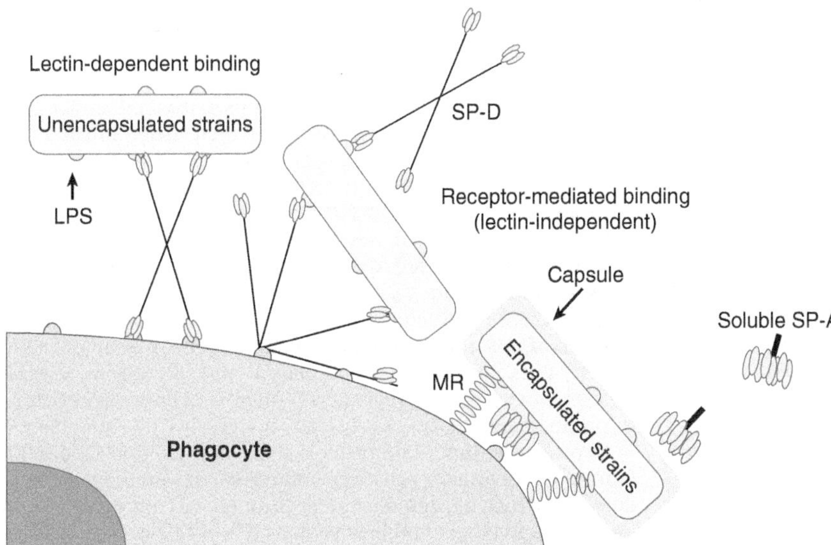

Fig. 123.5 Surfactant protein *(SP)-A* and *SP-D* are complementary opsonins for gram-negative bacteria. SP-D binds to lipopolysaccharide *(LPS)* core sugars exposed by nonencapsulated variants, the phenotype required for colonization and invasion. Encapsulation increases pathogenicity and limits SP-D binding, but allows SP-A recognition and binding of capsular polysaccharides. Subsequent phagocytosis may occur through SP binding to phagocyte surface carbohydrates (lectin-dependent) or may be receptor mediated (lectin-independent), as depicted by SP-A engagement of mannose receptors. (Reprinted with permission of the American Thoracic Society. Copyright © 2015 American Thoracic Society. From Crouch EC. Collectins and pulmonary host defense. *Am J Respir Cell Mol Biol.* 1997;19:177–201. The American Journal of Respiratory Cell and Molecular Biology is an official journal of the American Thoracic Society.)

(Fig. 123.5). Similar complementary function is illustrated by collectin interaction with influenza A virus (IAV). SP-D binds viral envelope glycoproteins (hemagglutinin and neuraminidase) through its CRD and induces massive agglutination of IAV particles; this agglutination is facilitated by higher-order oligomerization, most achievable by SP-D by virtue of its longer collagen domain. Such agglutination generates particle size sufficient for mucociliary clearance and also directly enhances neutrophil uptake and respiratory burst. Alternatively, SP-A activity results from IAV recognition and binding of sialic acid residues on this collectin. SP-A has much less agglutinating capacity but interacts with a broader range of IAV strains including those that are highly resistant to inhibition by SP-D or serum collectins. SP-A forms much smaller aggregates, resulting in less augmented neutrophil uptake but enhanced uptake by alveolar macrophages. As before, the differing collectin structures and binding affinities result in a broader range of antimicrobial activity and immune cell activation, which ultimately prove to be beneficial to the host.

IMMUNOMODULATING ROLE OF SURFACTANT

Apart from the specific actions of its collectins, surfactant also exerts a host of immunomodulatory effects within the alveolus. Surfactant enhances phagocytosis by means of a mechanism separate from the actions of SP-A. Interestingly, this prophagocytic effect is more pronounced for resident alveolar macrophages than for recruited peripheral blood monocytes. Whole surfactant reportedly suppresses mononuclear cell oxyradical production by inhibiting the intracellular assembly of nicotinamide adenine dinucleotide phosphate (NADPH) oxidase, impairing hydrogen peroxide generation. However, specific lipid components of surfactant may exert different modulatory effects. Therefore, macrophage oxidative burst is blunted by phosphatidylglycerol moieties; however, it is enhanced by phosphatidylcholine components. Enhanced microbicidal function of phagocytes and down-regulation of Fc receptors have each been reported and attributed to the lysophospholipid and free fatty acid components of surfactant. Whole surfactant also modulates phagocyte chemotaxis. Macrophage movement into the alveolus postnatally coincides with increased surfactant synthesis, suggesting a chemotactic effect, which is possibly SP-A mediated. Conversely, DPCC treatment of alveolar macrophages in vitro decreases their migration in response to serum chemotaxins; this is consistent with a teleologically preferred default attenuation of inflammatory response designed to preserve alveolar function. Lastly, surfactant reportedly modulates lymphocyte function as well. Lymphocytes exposed in vitro to surfactant are less responsive to mitogens and exhibit depressed function; under similar conditions, cytotoxic T cells, B cells, and NK cells are all inhibited to various degrees. As discussed earlier, however, some lipid components (DPCC, phosphatidylglycerol) are more suppressive, whereas less abundant components (cholesterol, sphingomyelin) stimulate lymphocyte proliferation. This suggests that conditions that alter these phospholipids ratios may alter adaptive immune responses. Additionally, the differing effects of SP-A and surfactant lipids on lymphocyte proliferation are consistent with the hypothesis that, in some scenarios, surfactant lipids and proteins may be counterregulatory.

In contrast to whole surfactant, conventional surfactant analogues (e.g., beractant, calfactant, poractant) contain neither SP-A nor SP-D. Thus, collectin-mediated immune effects are not provided by exogenous replacement therapies. Moreover, the surfactant replacements are generally immunosuppressive, presumably owing to their nonphysiologic lipid/protein ratios. These products inhibit production of the early-response cytokines TNF-α, IL-1β, and IL-6 by stimulated alveolar macrophages, putatively by depressing activation of nuclear factor kappa B (NF-κB). Similar suppression of fibroblast-derived IL-6 and prostaglandin E2 (PGE2) has also been described, suggesting impairment of those inflammatory responses up-regulated by alveolar cytokine networks. During shorter (10 minutes to 2 hours) exposures, regulation of human macrophage responses by SP-A occurs through reduced kinase activity required for proinflammatory cytokine production. Nguyen and colleagues recently showed that long-term surfactant-mediated suppression of proinflammatory cytokine production in response to TLR 4 activation was regulated by IL-1 receptor-associated kinase M (IRAK-M), a negative regulator of TLR-mediated NF-κB activation. Exposure to beractant, the natural bovine lung extract lacking SP-A, also enhanced IRAK-M expression, but at a lower magnitude and for a shorter duration than SP-A. In response to surfactant, IRAK-M is up-regulated in macrophages thereby suppressing TLR4-mediated TNF-α and IL-6 production in response to LPS.[274] Additionally, beractant has been shown to blunt lymphocyte proliferation, killer cell cytotoxicity, and adhesion molecule expression, possibly through down-regulation of lymphocyte receptors for IL-2. Much of this is in vitro data and must therefore be interpreted cautiously. However, it suggests that available surfactant replacement therapies, although efficacious in normalizing pulmonary compliance, may concomitantly attenuate normal alveolar immune cell responses. For a detailed review of surfactant replacement therapy, including modes of administration and clinical practice standards, refer to the recently published review by Hentschel and colleagues.[275]

NITRIC OXIDE

NO is a short-lived, oxyradical-related bioactive mediator with potent vasodilatory actions. It mediates and modulates pulmonary transition from fetal to postnatal life and plays a role in both immune regulation and innate host defense. NO is synthesized by three isoforms of NO synthase (NOS-1, -2, and -3), all of which are expressed in the airway epithelium from the bronchus to the distal air space.[276] Thus NO is produced along the entire length of the human airway,[276] and its metabolic product, nitrite, is present in airway-lining fluid at concentrations of approximately 15 μM.[277] NO isoforms exist in either constitutive (NOS-1, NOS-3) or inducible (NOS-2) forms; cells with constitutive NOS include neurons, vascular endothelium, neutrophils, and platelets. Cells with inducible NOS (iNOS, NOS-2) include mononuclear phagocytes, alveolar macrophages, vascular smooth muscle cells, epithelial cells, type II pneumocytes, and hepatocytes.[278-283] All NOS isoforms are detected early in lung development, and ontogeny shows no significant changes in abundance or distribution with advancing gestational age.[276]

NO exerts potent cytotoxic and inflammatory effects, which support its role as an antimicrobial molecule during host response to infection. NO production from cells containing iNOS is induced by microbial products such as lipoteichoic acid, endotoxin, and bacterial DNA. Locally produced NO inhibits sodium uptake from the apical surface of airway epithelial cells, increasing airway hydration and enhancing mucociliary clearance. Specific NO products such as nitrosylated thiols exert antimicrobial activity by killing the pathogen directly or by inhibiting the pathogens' replication. NO inhibits the growth of a wide variety of organisms including viruses, bacteria, parasites, and fungi, presumably by targeting microbial DNA and cysteine proteases, which are critical for virulence or replication of these pathogens.[284-286] NO appears to be particularly important in the innate immune response to intracellular organisms such as *Listeria monocytogenes*, *Salmonella*, and *M. tuberculosis*.[287] NO products also inhibit viral RNA synthesis, inactivate a broad range of microbial proteins by S-nitrosylation, and induce membrane damage through lipid peroxidation. By up-regulating inflammatory cell function; NO augments macrophage motility, up-regulates surface expression of complement and immunoglobulin Fc receptors, and stimulates leukocyte respiratory burst. Concurrent synthesis of NO increases microbicidal activity of the leukocyte respiratory burst by generating additional cytotoxic radicals such as peroxynitrite, which generates potent activity against bacteria and *Candida*. In vitro, phagocytes demonstrate diminished microbicidal activity after NOS inhibition, and this correlates with in vivo models in which diminished NOS activity impairs microbial clearance.

The role of NO in pulmonary microbial clearance is consistent with recent data from neonates. BAL specimens from preterm (≤32 weeks estimated gestational age) infants exposed to intrauterine infection demonstrated a strong association between inability to express iNOS or up-regulate NO and subsequent development of fulminant pneumonia. Conversely, newborns of similar age and risk who did not develop pneumonia exhibited iNOS up-regulation and increased NO products on BAL analysis, relative to either their pneumonic cohorts or noninfected control subjects. A separate retrospective analysis of lung tissue from neonatal autopsies yielded similar findings; alveolar macrophage-derived iNOS could not be detected in specimens from fulminant pneumonia patients but was demonstrable in control subjects. Taken together, these data suggest that delayed or diminished macrophage-derived NO in the setting of neonatal pulmonary infection correlates with increased morbidity. Etiology of this impaired response is speculative but may result from a paucity of mediators (TNF, IFN-γ) known to up-regulate iNOS expression. Based on the important antimicrobial function of NO, recent studies have evaluated the role of inhaled NO on pulmonary infections in humans. These studies have generated mixed results; however, it is likely that infections caused by intracellular organisms will be more likely to benefit from inhaled NO therapy.[288-291]

In general, NO exerts antimicrobial effects; however, not all pathogens are inhibited by NO, and in some instances, NO may contribute to injury to the host. In an influenza pneumonia mouse model, targeted deletion of iNOS or treatment with NOS inhibitors led to less severe disease compared with control mice.[292] Similar observations were made in mouse models of *M. avium* pneumonia and herpes simplex virus encephalitis.[293,294] It is postulated that in these disease processes, cytotoxic effects of NO on host cells may contribute to pathogenesis.

Beyond the functions just detailed, NO exhibits additional immunomodulatory activities relevant to pulmonary host defense, which is demonstrated through its up-regulation by immune activating cytokines such as IFN-γ, TNF-α, IL-1, and IL-2. NO has been shown to reduce T helper 1 (Th1) proliferation and IL-2 synthesis while increasing IL-4 synthesis by T helper 2 (Th2) cells.[295-297] Th1 cells produce IFN-γ, which is an essential cytokine in viral cell-mediated immune responses. Alternatively, Th2 cells selectively produce IL-4 and IL-5 that participate in the development of humoral immunity. NO-induced imbalance in the Th2/Th1 ratio may promote inflammation in allergic diseases like asthma while inhibiting the inflammatory response to viral and bacterial pathogens.[298] RSV is a common pulmonary infection in infants, which has been linked to a large Th2/Th1 cytokine immune response; it has been associated with the pathogenesis of RSV bronchiolitis and the severity of infection in infants.[299-301] Several studies have associated poor IFN-γ production to greater disease severity and subsequent development of allergic asthma. Although IFN-γ induces NO production, no studies have directly linked NO with RSV disease outcomes. However, a recent study by Gadish and colleagues showed reduced levels of exhaled NO among infants with acute RSV bronchiolitis, possibly secondary to reduced IFN-γ production.[302]

NK cells are specialized cytotoxic lymphocytes and a primary source of IFN-γ within the alveolus; they are normally activated by IL-12. Transgenic iNOS deficiency induces a phenotype of IL-12 deficiency despite normal IL-12 levels. This phenotype is characterized by diminished IFN-γ and increased TGF-β, a cytokine milieu suppressing local macrophage function. Analysis of these data subsequently identified iNOS-derived NO as an essential co-signal for IL-12 signal transduction and activation of NK cells. In this model, the signaling role of NO was therefore critical in maintaining a cytokine microenvironment that allowed normal immune cell function. NO exerts a biphasic effect on NF-κB activity, which is dependent on local NO concentrations. Therefore, NO is able to both up- and down-regulate the expression of a number of inflammatory mediators. In this paradigm, immune activation up-regulates iNOS, generating increased NO. Initial NO activation of NF-κB promotes expression of adhesion molecules and proinflammatory cytokines, facilitating immune cell recruitment. NF-κB up-regulation of iNOS amplifies NO production, eventually generating local NO concentrations sufficient to inhibit NF-κB activity. At this point, both inflammatory cytokine and adhesion molecule expression are down-regulated, effectively dampening the component of inflammation sensitive to modulation by NO. In summary, the putative actions of NO in immune cell signal transduction suggest a sentinel role for this molecule in both the initiation and suppression of cellular immunity. It is reasonable to consider that disruption of NO homeostasis, elicited by a pulmonary-tropic organism such as RSV at a very early age, would break down the barriers against infection and decrease mitigators of inflammation, leading to prolonged infection and increased inflammation.

CARBON MONOXIDE

As with NO, evolving data suggest a potential role for carbon monoxide (CO) in pulmonary host defense. Endogenous CO derives from degradation of heme from molecules such as hemoglobin, myoglobin, and cytochromes by the enzyme heme oxygenase (HO). HO immunoreactivity is found throughout the airway in respiratory epithelium, alveolar macrophages, seromucous glands, and nose and paranasal sinuses. Like NOS, HO exists in constitutive (HO-2) and inducible (HO-1) isoforms. Whereas HO-2 is basally expressed in most tissues, HO-1 is identified as a heat shock protein inducible by a variety of stimuli including microbial toxins, proinflammatory cytokines, and reactive oxygen or nitrogen species; both isoforms are substantially expressed in human lungs. HO-1 is a cryoprotective and antiinflammatory enzyme that plays a critical role in defending the body against oxidant-induced injury during inflammatory processes.[303] It catalyzes the first and rate-limiting step in the oxidative degradation of heme to CO and two other molecules (biliverdin and ferrous iron) with cytoprotective properties.[304-306] The antiinflammatory properties of HO-1 are related to inhibition of adhesion molecule expression and reduction of oxidative stress, while exogenous CO gas treatment decreases the production of inflammatory mediators such as cytokines and NO.[307] Like iNOS, HO is induced by many infectious agents, and levels of carboxyhemoglobin and/or exhaled CO are reportedly elevated in patients with viral or bacterial respiratory tract infections. Unlike NO, however, the direct effects of CO appear less microbicidal and more antiinflammatory, or host cytoprotective. In vitro and in vivo, CO has been shown to inhibit endotoxin-induced proinflammatory cytokines, including TNF, IL-1β, and macrophage inflammatory protein-1β (MIP-1β) while concurrently up-regulating antiinflammatory IL-10. Furthermore, in a murine model of influenza A pneumonitis, overexpression of HO-1 resulted in diminished respiratory epithelial cell apoptosis and decreased lung inflammation. Interestingly, HO appears to counteract the cytotoxicity caused by excessive production of NO.[308-311] The up-regulation of iNOS in inducible pulmonary cells upon exposure to LPS results in a burst of NO generation that is essential for bactericidal effects. However, increased amounts of NO are also associated with deleterious effects such as tissue damage.[312] Thus induction of HO-1 significantly reduces NO production and potentially restores cellular homeostasis.[303,313] It is well accepted that HO-1 and CO play an important role in minimizing injurious inflammatory processes during infection and other inflammatory states. Recent evidence, however, has identified an antimicrobial role for CO during infection. In vitro and in vivo studies have demonstrated that CO increases macrophage and neutrophil phagocytosis of the pathogenic organisms *E. coli* and *E. faecalis,* respectively.[314,315] Based on its anti-inflammatory properties, particularly in patients with chronic obstructive pulmonary disease, inhaled CO is currently being investigated in a phase I study to assess its pharmacologic potential to reduce acute airway inflammation (NCT00094406). Due to concerns regarding poor precision in the delivery of CO in the form of a gas, chemical carriers known as *CO-releasing molecules (CO-RMs)* have been developed.[316,317] Recent studies by Murray and coworkers demonstrated that CO-RM-2, a ruthenium-containing CO-RM soluble in dimethyl sulfoxide, attenuated biofilm formation and planktonic growth of the majority of both mucoid and nonmucoid strains of *P. aeruginosa* isolates.[318]

IMMUNOLOGICALLY RECRUITABLE PULMONARY STRUCTURAL CELLS

ENDOTHELIUM

Because of its anatomic location at the interface between the vascular and alveolar compartments, the endothelium is uniquely situated to regulate pulmonary immune responses requiring recruitment and facilitated passage of intravascular inflammatory cells. Vascular endothelial cells express MHC class II molecules and may present antigens to T cells.[319] Endothelial cells also participate in immune processes by elaborating or responding to cytokines in the local microenvironment. For example, TNF-α is an endogenous mediator of inflammatory immune responses secreted by alveolar macrophages in response to bacterial endotoxin. Endothelial cells manifest a pleiotropic response to TNF-α, including increased expression of adhesion molecules, increased prostaglandin production, increased MHC antigen expression, and increased cytokine release including IL-1, IL-6, IL-8, granulocyte-macrophage colony-stimulating factory (GM-CSF), and monocyte chemotactic protein-1 (MCP-1).[111,320,321] The net effect of these signals is an increased chemotactic recruitment and activation of inflammatory cells at the interface of the vascular space and the interstitium; the TNF-induced increase in endothelial cell-leukocyte adhesion further enhances this response. Endothelial cells also express the TLRs TLR4 (constitutive) and TLR2 (inducible by IFN-γ or TNF-α); this allows a direct response to endotoxin, manifested by up-regulation of adhesion molecule expression and induction of IL-1, IL-8, MCP-1, and GM-CSF expression.[322-327] By responding either to endotoxin directly or to endotoxin-induced macrophage-derived TNF-α, the endothelial cell may either generate an initial immune response or participate in amplifying a local inflammatory cascade. The up-regulation of adhesion molecules on the endothelium allows for neutrophil attachment, rolling, firm attachment, and ultimately diapedesis.[328]

FIBROBLASTS

Whereas most studies of fibroblasts have focused on their production of structural and matrix proteins, it is now evident that fibroblasts may also function as important immune-effector cells at sites of inflammation. When appropriately stimulated, fibroblasts may generate bioactive amounts of multiple cytokines, including IL-6, IL-8, IL-1α, IL-11, colony-stimulating factors (CSFs), and growth factors such as TGF-β.[329] TNF-α or IL-1 can each induce fibroblast-derived IL-6, IL-1, IL-8, and IL-11, and their combined action synergistically further up-regulates fibroblast elaboration of these cytokines.[330,331] Although fibroblasts and alveolar macrophages are often capable of elaborating the same inflammatory cytokine(s), maximal production of these cytokines typically occurs in response to different signals. This is illustrated by the distinct response of these cells to endotoxin. Endotoxin is a potent stimulator of macrophage-derived TNF-α and IL-1 but exerts little direct stimulation of fibroblasts. Conversely, pulmonary fibroblasts elaborate inflammatory cytokines in response to IL-1 and TNF-α, whereas macrophage response to these cytokines is more diverse.[332-334] This suggests that, although classic immune cells such as alveolar macrophages produce inflammatory cytokines in a stimulus-specific fashion, fibroblasts produce inflammatory cytokines in response to macrophage-derived TNF-α or IL-1, independent of the precipitating stimulus. This response serves to amplify local pulmonary inflammation and illustrates the potential immunologic role of the fibroblast, transcending its putative structural function. IL-17 can induce chemokine generation by lung fibroblasts, which also may be important in establishing chemokine gradients with lung tissue.[335]

EPITHELIUM

Pulmonary epithelial cells serve multiple functions including maintenance of solute fluxes, production of surfactant, and providing a surface for gas transfer. Beyond these metabolic and barrier functions, pulmonary epithelial cells are capable of augmenting and regulating local innate immunity in response to environmental signals. The airway epithelium senses bacterial exposure and responds by increasing the release of antimicrobial peptides, chemokines, and cytokines.[336] This inflammatory reaction results in recruitment of phagocytes, DCs, and lymphocytes, which aid in the innate immune response and prepare an adaptive immune response if necessary. Epithelial cell recognition of invading pathogens is a key initiating factor in mounting an adequate immune response to microbial pathogens. The mechanism by which this occurs is through the expression of a variety of PRRs including TLR1-10, CD14, and the CFTR.[94,337-342] Additionally, alveolar type II epithelial cells have collectin receptors, allowing them to internalize microbes opsonized by SP-A or SP-D.[255] Endotoxin or the early response cytokines TNF-α or IL-1β each may up-regulate epithelial-derived defensins such as human-β defensin 2 (HBD-2) by binding to cells expressing CD14 and TLR2.[342,343] IL-17, a cytokine produced by T cells and ILCs, can induce the expression of chemokines[344] and HBD-2.[60] These effects can be augmented by IL-22,[345] which increases epithelial repair and augments barrier function of the epithelium.[345] Airway epithelial cells also exhibit tonic, high-level expression of iNOS leading to cytotoxic NO production.[346] The cyclooxygenase and lipoxygenase pathways are expressed at high levels in epithelial cells, resulting in production of lipid mediators including PGE2 and the neutrophil chemoactivator LTB_4.[347,348] Infection with RSV can directly induce epithelial-derived IFN-β, IL-1α, and the chemokines IL-8 and RANTES.[94,349] Alternatively, pulmonary epithelial cells can also secrete several cytokines in response to various stimuli including TGF-β, GM-CSF, IL-5, IL-6, IL-8, and MCP-1; release of these cytokines facilitates chemotaxis and activation of multiple immune cells including PMNs, mononuclear phagocytes, and T lymphocytes.[350-355] Indeed, epithelial CXCL5 had been shown to be important in neutrophil emigration in response to pneumococcal pneumonia.[356] Airway epithelial cells can titrate local cytokine signals by shedding soluble TNF-α receptor; this adsorbs available TNF-α and diminishes its bioactivity.[357] Airway and alveolar epithelial cells in vivo also express intercellular adhesion molecule-1 (ICAM-1), a natural ligand for complementary adhesins of PMNs and monocytes induced in response to IFN-γ, TNF-α, or IL-1. Increased epithelial expression of ICAM facilitates inflammatory cell migration along epithelial barriers. Moreover, antimicrobial activity of phagocytes in vitro is enhanced by ICAM-mediated interactions with the alveolar epithelium.[358] Finally, airway epithelial cells, in response to specific cytokine stimulation, can express MHC antigens, allowing them to interact directly with T lymphocytes, possibly as antigen-presenting cells.[359] Together, these data suggest that in response to appropriate local stimuli, pulmonary epithelial cells may effect complex immune modulation within the milieu of the alveolus and airway.

CELLULAR MECHANISMS OF HOST IMMUNE DEFENSE

Adaptive immunity requires sensitization to individually encountered antigens; once sensitization occurs, these immune responses are characterized by their high antigen specificity and long-lasting memory. Although many soluble and cellular components of host defense may link aspects of innate and adaptive immunity, adaptive immune responses are executed by lymphocytes.

Lymphocytes (T cells, B cells, and NK cells) are normally present at multiple sites in the lungs and may participate in complex immune responses to encountered antigens or act directly as effector cells against local microorganisms. Lung interstitial lymphocytes are plentiful, with numbers comparable to those of the circulating blood pool, and they possess a characteristic size, distribution, subset composition, and cytokine production profile.[360] Large numbers of NK cells are also found in the interstitial space.[360] Moreover γδ T cells are elicited in response to bacterial infection[361] and can proliferate rapidly in lung tissue.[362]

T CELLS

The pulmonary lymphocyte population is made up primarily of T cells.[360,363] Fetal and neonatal T cells express markers found on thymocytes,[364] suggesting that these T cells represent an immature transitional population; alternatively, this may reflect stress-induced release of cortical thymocytes into the circulation.[364] The neonatal T cell phenotype corresponds closely to that of antigenically naïve T cells in the adult.[365] These findings likely reflect a combination of the limited exposure of the neonate to foreign antigens and the limitations of neonatal DC function, rather than intrinsic neonatal T cell dysfunction. T cells recognize foreign peptides that have been modified by antigen-presenting cells and expressed in the context of MHC proteins. $CD4^+$ T cells differentiate upon antigen stimulation in the context of class II MHC and can differentiate along several lineages including Th1, Th2, Th17, or T_{Reg} subsets. Important immunoregulatory functions provided by pulmonary T cell subsets include cytokine production, enhancement of immunoglobulin production, and direct T cell cytotoxicity.

Cytotoxic T cells mainly express the CD8 co-receptor and act to lyse host cells infected with intracellular pathogens.[366] In distinction to the $CD4^+$ T cell that recognizes peptide antigen in the context of class II MHC, these T cells recognize small peptide antigens that are presented by MHC class I molecules (signal I). Like other T cells, these cells require a second signal to develop effective cytotoxicity, which is performed by costimulatory interaction between the T cell CD28 molecule and B7 ligands (CD80 and CD86) expressed by the antigen-presenting cell. In the absence of costimulation, the $CD8^+$ T cell is rendered either anergic or apoptotic.[366] Activated cytotoxic T cells can lyse and kill infected target cells through Fas-mediated apoptosis or through the release of cytolytic mediators. The latter process involves the exocytosis of granules containing perforin, granzyme, and granulysin.[367] Perforin is a glycoprotein that induces pore formation in the target cell membrane, facilitating both osmotic lysis and entry of granzymes and granulysin.[367] Granzymes are serine esterases that activate the caspase cascade, inducing target cell apoptosis. Granulysin is an antimicrobial peptide with broad-spectrum activity against bacteria, mycobacteria, and fungi.[368] Cytotoxic lymphocytes are particularly important in host defense against nonlytic viruses such as CMV and also appear to be critical in host response to mycobacteria.[369,370] $CD8^+$ T cells have also been shown to have activity against *P. carinii* by up-regulating macrophage-mediated killing of the organism.[371] T lymphocytes from newborns are capable of developing into cytotoxic T cells during natural infections postnatally. Furthermore, in utero infection may induce a profound CD8 cytotoxic response.[372] In general, however, the development of neonatal cytotoxic lymphocytes and the overall magnitude of the response tend to be diminished relative to that in older children.

$CD4^+$ helper T cells, or Th cells, function to orchestrate B cell and T cell responses. These CD4 cells recognize antigen presented by the MHC class II-dependent pathway and, on activation, may be induced to differentiate into specific Th phenotypes depending on the concurrent costimulatory signal (signal II) and cytokine stimulation (signal III) they receive. Undifferentiated naïve T cells are called *Th0 cells* and can differentiate along specific T cell subsets as outlined later.

TH1 CELLS

Th1 cells differentiate from Th0 cells in the presence of macrophage-derived IL-12p70, a heterodimeric cytokine consisting of IL-12p35 and IL-12p40, which are encoded by separate genes. IL-12 was the first heterodimeric cytokine discovered[373] and is the founding member of the IL-12 family of cytokines that consists of IL-12, IL-23, IL-27, and IL-35 (Fig. 123.6).[374] IL-12 directs Th1 differentiation by the phosphorylation of *Stat4*.[373,375] Th1 lymphocytes are controlled by the

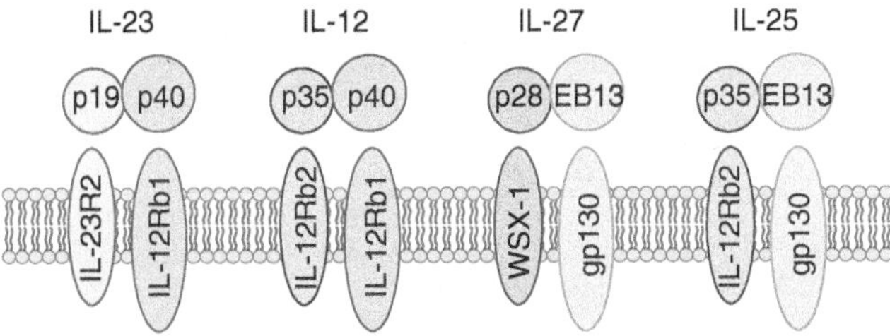

Fig. 123.6 Interleukin *(IL)*-12, IL-23, IL-27, and IL-35 cytokines and receptor complexes. IL-23 consists of a heterodimer of IL-12p40 and IL-23 p19, which is similar in structure to the IL-12 p35 subunit. IL-12 is comprised of the IL-12p40 subunit and a p35 subunit. IL-27 consists of EBI3 and p28. IL-35 consists of p35 and EBI3. IL-12p40 and EBI3 are group 3 soluble cytokine receptors. IL-23p19, p35, and p28 are members of the IL-6 subfamily of type I cytokines. The IL-23 receptor consists of the IL-12Rβ1 and IL-23R subunits. The IL-12 receptor consists of the IL-12Rβ1 and IL-12Rβ2 subunits. The IL-12Rβ2 and IL-23R are structurally similar. The IL-27 receptor consists of a gp130 and WSX-1 subunit and the IL-35 receptor consists of gp130 and 12Rβ2.

transcription factor T-bet and characterized by their expression of IL-2, IL-12, TNF-α, and IFN-γ.[376] Th1 cells function to activate macrophages and neutrophils and are critical for host defense against intracellular pathogens such as *M. tuberculosis.*[377,378] In support of this, patients with defects in IL-12p40 production, IFN-γ production, or IFN-γ receptor signaling have an increased risk of TB.[379,380] Th1 cells can also influence the development of cytotoxic $CD8^+$ T cells as well as facilitating class switching of B cells to produce IgG2a. In this context, the Th1 response has been shown to be critical for host resistance against a variety of pulmonary pathogens, including *M. tuberculosis, Legionella pneumophila, Chlamydophila pneumoniae,* and *P. carinii.*[381-383]

IFN-γ activates mononuclear phagocytes, augmenting phagocytosis and inducing production of reactive oxygen species, NO, and cytokines such as TNF-α, IL-1, and IL-6. IFN-γ up-regulates pulmonary epithelial cell and endothelial cell expression of adhesion molecules, with resultant enhanced PMN adherence.[384-387] This cytokine also increases expression of MHC molecules on epithelial cells and monocytes, enhancing their ability to function as antigen-presenting cells.[388] Finally, IFN-γ promotes proliferation of antigen-stimulated T cells, generation of cytotoxic T cells, and enhanced cytotoxic activity.[389] The net result of these effects is enhanced leukocyte recruitment and macrophage antimicrobial activity and amplified inflammatory tone. The enhanced antigen presentation induced by IFN-γ may facilitate later transition from macrophage-driven inflammation to a lymphocyte-executed adaptive immune response. As a sentinel mediator of the Th1 response, IFN-γ is antagonized by the Th2 cytokines IL-4 and IL-13. IL-4 and IL-13 also inhibit the expression of many IFN-γ inducible genes, as well as the ability of IFN-γ to augment microbicidal activities such as superoxide production. IL-10 is similar to IL-4 in its inhibition of IFN-γ synthesis by Th1 cells, NK cells, and macrophages. At the receptor level, Th1 and Th2 cells exhibit different responses to IFN-γ through differential expression of a specific IFN-γ receptor subunit that transduces suppressive signals.[390]

IFN-γ-activated macrophages are capable of restricting the growth of a number of microbes, such as *Legionella,* mycobacteria, *P. carinii,* pathogenic fungi, and *Chlamydia,* that parasitize macrophages.[378,391,392] In vivo, IFN-γ replacement or overexpression has been shown to enhance bacterial clearance in murine model of *L. pneumophila, P. aeruginosa,* and *K. pneumoniae.*[393-395] IFN-γ has been demonstrated in the BAL specimens of neonates with RSV, and gene polymorphisms in IFN-γ are linked to longer hospital lengths of stay and increased illness severity in infants with RSV infection.[396,397] Most likely, the diminished ability of neonatal lymphocytes to generate this cytokine (capacity less than 10% of adults) limits optimal alveolar macrophage activation, compromising the neonatal pulmonary immune response.[398]

TH2 CELLS

Alternatively, in the absence of IL-12, activated Th0 cells are induced by IL-4 to adopt the Th2 phenotype, characterized by secretion of IL-4, IL-5, IL-6, IL-9, and IL-13. Th2 cells develop under control of *Stat6* and the transcription factor Gata-3.[399,400] Th2 lymphocytes are required for expulsion of helminth parasites and also function to generate humoral immune responses and antibody production, particularly IgG1, IgA, and IgE.[401] The Th1 cytokine IFN-γ acts on Th0 cells to induce Th1 differentiation and inhibit Th2 differentiation. Conversely, the Th2 cytokine IL-4 inhibits Th1 differentiation (Fig. 123.7).

Mature T cells are capable of enhancing antibody secretion by regulating the proliferation and immunoglobulin isotype expression of B cells; this regulation is provided both through contact-dependent mechanisms and through secretion of specific cytokines. Contact-dependent interactions include cognate recognition through MHC antigens or receptor-ligand interactions primarily between the B cell CD40 molecule and the T cell CD40 ligand.[402] Activated Th cells markedly up-regulate their surface expression of CD40 ligand, a membrane-bound cytokine with homology to TNF.[403] Subsequent engagement with the B cell-surface CD40 molecule triggers the expression of B cell of cytokine receptors. At this point, activated Th cells can begin to secrete cytokines in a directional fashion within the immunologic synapse. Signals delivered to the B cell (via CD40 binding) markedly enhance immunoglobulin production and promote immunoglobulin class switching in the presence of co-activation signals provided by specific cytokines; relevant examples include IL-2, which promotes IgM secretion; IL-4 or IL-13, which facilitates IgE synthesis; IL-10, which induces IgG1 and IgG3 production; and IFN-γ, which promotes IgG2 production.[404-406] Patients with mutations in CD40L cannot undergo antibody class switching and thus have an abundance of B cells that stain positively for surface IgM. Measurement of antibodies in serum reveals mainly IgM, and thus this syndrome is named *hyper IgM syndrome*. These patients are at risk for infection from encapsulated bacteria as well as opportunistic fungi such as *P. carinii.*[407]

IL-5 is a major product of Th2 cells.[408] In humans, IL-5 is thought to be specific for promoting eosinophil and basophilic maturation and eosinophil survival and chemotaxis.[409] IL-5 appears to be critical for producing tissue eosinophilia and is thus of primary interest for its role in asthma. Indeed, anti-IL-5 appears to be beneficial in patients with asthma with elevated blood eosinophils.[410] Eosinophilia is reportedly common among premature neonates and considered a marker of occult infection. Roux and colleagues evaluated the role of IL-5 in the neonatal host response by comparing the ability of neonatal and adult lung explants to produce IL-5.[411] Indeed, neonatal explants subjected to treatment with anti-CD3 mAb secreted more IL-5 than adult explants.[411]

IL-4 is an 18-kDa cytokine produced by activated T cells of the Th2 subset, γδ T cells, mast cells, and basophils. IL-4 has two receptors: a high-affinity receptor that shares signaling components with IL-2 and IL-7 and an alternate receptor that shares components of the IL-13 receptor; cells expressing either receptor can transduce the IL-4 signal. IL-4 stimulation of naïve T cells induces their differentiation into Th2 cells, initiating the Th2 response. Concurrently, IL-4 exhibits a number of important functions related to humoral immunity, including B cell activation and induction of B cell isotype switching necessary for production of IgE and some IgG subclasses.[412] Consistent with the Th2 cellular response, IL-4 facilitates the migration

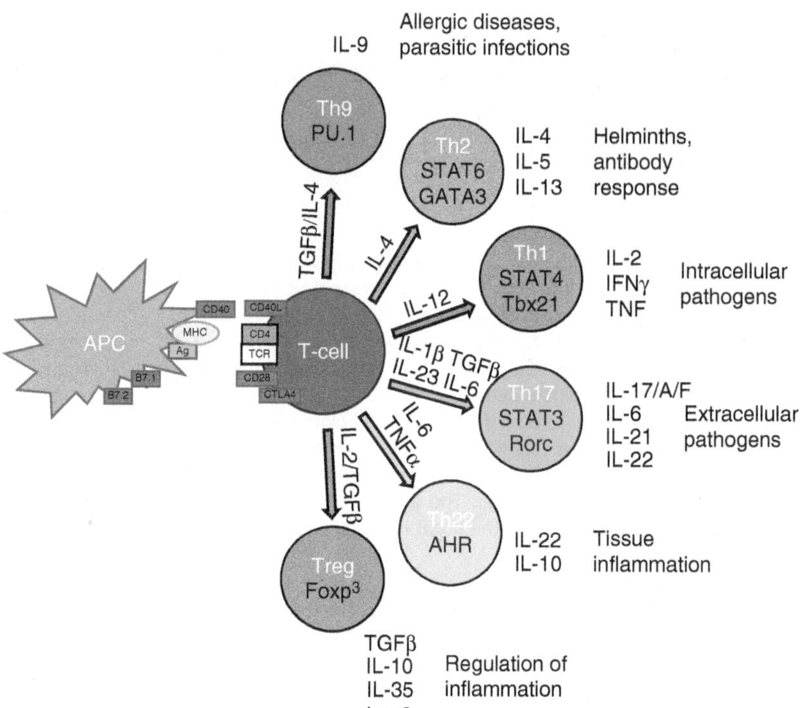

Fig. 123.7 Differentiation of CD4+ into effector T cell subsets. T helper 1 *(Th1)* cells develop after antigen presentation via class II major histocompatibility complex *(MHC)* (signal I), costimulation (signal II), and under cytokine control of interleukin *(IL)-12* (signal III). Th1 cells produce interferon *(IFN)*-γ and are critical for intracellular pathogens as well as immunoglobulin (Ig) G2A production. In the absence of IL-12 and under control of *IL-4*, Th2 cells can differentiate and produce IL-4, *IL-5*, and *IL-13*. These cells are critical for host dense against helminths as well as IgG1 production. Both IFN-γ and IL-4 show reciprocal inhibition of Th2 and Th1 responses, respectively. Th17 cells can differentiate under transforming growth factor *(TGF)β* and IL-6 as well as IL-1b. IL-23 regulates the terminal differentiation of Th17 cells. These cells mediated host defense against extracellular bacteria and fungi. Naïve T cells in the presence of TGFβ alone can differentiate into regulatory T cells *(Tregs)*.

of eosinophils, basophils, and monocytes by up-regulating endothelial expression of vascular cell adhesion molecule (VCAM).[413] Neonatal leukocyte production of IL-4 is estimated to be less than 10% of adult capacity, and this correlates with in vivo data, in which IL-4 is undetectable in tracheobronchial aspirates of preterm and term newborns.[414,415]

IL-13 shares sequence homology (≈30%) and biologic activities with IL-4.[416,417] Part of the activities shared by IL-4 and IL-13 results from a shared receptor subunit IL-4Rα. However, IL-13-mediated effects are more restricted, and IL-13 is generally less potent than IL-4, owing to competitive inhibition resulting from the higher affinity of IL-4 for its receptor.[418] Although IL-13 does not stimulate T cells as IL-4 does, IL-13 can stimulate B cell proliferation and immunoglobulin isotype switching synergistically with IL-4.[418] IL-13 is also a potent inducer of mucins in lung epithelium.[418,419] Recent studies have shown efficacy of an antil-IL-13 antibody in adults with asthma that were classified as likely responders based on high periostin levels, a gene that is regulated by IL-13.[420] Normal pregnancy is associated with the production of appreciable quantities of IL-13, initially by the placenta and subsequently by the fetus; IL-13 is inducible from cord blood cells by 27 weeks' gestation.[421] Postnatally, higher levels of inducible IL-13 from cord lymphocytes may identify neonates at risk for later development of atopic or Th2 response-associated disease processes.[422]

TH9 CELLS

Th9 cells secrete IL-9 and are the most recently described subset of Th cells. Th9 cells have been implicated in allergic diseases, including food allergy, and can promote inflammation in parasitic infections and inflammatory bowel disease.[423] Th9 cells were first described in 1994, but their phenotype and functions have only been recently further characterized.[424] Differentiation of Th9 cells requires transcription factors STAT5, STAT6/IL-4, and TGF-β signaling. Other signaling pathways such as NF-κB or STAT1-mediated induction of interferon-regulatory factor (IRF1) all can increase IL-9 production.[425] Other important transcription factors responsible for Th9 differentiation include PU.1, IRF4, BATF, GATA3, and ETV5.[423,425,426]

The IL-9 secreted from Th9 cells can contribute to the pathology of diseases or mediate protection depending on the context. For example, several Th9-related genes have been implicated in development of asthma, atopic dermatitis, and food allergies.[427-431] Myeloid DCs obtained from patients with allergic asthma and primed with thymic stromal lymphopoietin (TSLP) were found to promote polarization of CD4+ T cells into Th9 cells and was dependent on TGF-β.[431] Notably, retinoic acid has been shown to inhibit Th9 differentiation by modifying the epigenome via retinoic acid receptor α (RARα). Treatment with retinoic acid attenuated Th9-mediated pulmonary inflammation in mice, and this effect was independent of Foxp3.[432] These data suggest that inhibition of Th9-induced inflammation may play a role in other pulmonary diseases.

TH17 CELLS

Th17 cells are a lineage that develops from naïve T cells under the control of TGF-β and IL-6. Th17 cell development requires phosphorylation of *Stat3* and the transcription factors RORγ and RORα.[433,434] Once established, the IL-12 family member IL-23 regulates their proliferation and survival, as well as the expression of specific effector cytokines.[435] The effector cytokines produced by Th17 cells include, IL-17A, IL-17F, IL-22, and TNF-α. In fact IL-23 is required for IL-22 production, whereas TGF-β and IL-6–directed differentiation is sufficient for IL-17A and IL-17F expression.[436] Experiments in animal models demonstrate that the Th17 lineage is critical for host defense against extracellular bacteria such as *K. pneumoniae*, as well as organisms such as *Mycoplasma pulmonis* and *Citrobacter rodentium*, an enteric pathogen.[345,436,437] This lineage controls several aspects of mucosal immunity. IL-17R signaling has also been shown to be important for control of disseminated *C. albicans* infection,[438] as well as mucocutaneous candidiasis.[439] IL-17 and IL-17R signaling has been shown to critical for regulating granulopoiesis in response to infection, as well as the regulation of local chemokines such as CXCL1 and CXCL2, which are important for the recruitment of neutrophils to the infected tissue site. Humans with mutations in IL-17RA or mutations that affect IL-17R signaling develop chronic mucocutaneous candidiasis.[440,441] IL-22 synergizes with IL-17 to regulate the expression of antimicrobial peptides at epithelial surfaces.[345,442,443] IL-22 regulation of antimicrobial proteins has been shown to exist at several mucosal surfaces including the skin, gut, and lung.[444] Interestingly, although there is some overlap with types of genes induced in skin keratinocytes and lung epithelium, such as HBD-2, IL-22 appears to regulate organ-specific genes in the gut. IL-22 regulates the expression of Reg proteins in GI epithelium, which are soluble lectin-binding proteins that have direct antimicrobial activity.[445,446] It has recently been shown that patients with Job syndrome or autosomal dominant hyper IgE syndrome have mutations in *Stat3* and thus lack antigen-specific Th17 cells in their peripheral blood.[447] These patients develop cutaneous infections with *S. aureus* and *C. albicans.* The individual contributions of IL-17, IL-22, and non-myeloid STAT3 in this phenotype remain to be determined. This T cell lineage has also been implicated in diseases of autoimmunity such as rheumatoid arthritis, Crohn disease, multiple sclerosis, and psoriasis.[448]

T FOLLICULAR HELPER CELLS

T follicular helper (Tfh) cells respond to the chemokine CXCL13 via the chemokine receptor CXCR5.[449] This allows homing of Tfh cells to germinal centers in secondary lymphoid tissues. Here these cells activate B cell proliferation and class switching. One of the key cytokines that mediate this effect is IL-21. Patients with IL-21R deficiency have been reported, and these children present in infancy with disseminated cryptosporidiosis causing biliary disease, as well as *Pneumocystis* pneumonia. Functional IL-21R deficiency was identified in two separate cohorts.[450] The reported patients had reduced class-switched B cells, reduced T cell proliferative responses, and reduced IL-17F and IL-22 production from T cells.[450] Both cohorts of patients showed an elevated IgE but reduced antigen-specific IgGs.

T CELL IMMUNITY IN NEONATES

As mentioned previously, most neonatal T cells are naïve cells with reduced expression of the TCR, decreased adhesion molecule expression, and diminished expression of the CD40 ligand.[451] Neonatal T cells also exhibit diminished cytokine production (notably IL-4, IFN-γ, IL-12, IL-15, GM-CSF), putatively owing to labile posttranscriptional regulation and markedly shortened mRNA half-life.[452,453] Although normal levels of cytokine elaboration are inducible by sustained TCR triggering, the decreased adhesion molecule expression by neonatal T cells impairs interaction with antigen-presenting cells, resulting in costimulatory signals, which are insufficient to achieve levels of adult functioning. Similarly, diminished expression of the T cell CD40 ligand precludes optimal contact-dependent activation of B cells. Finally, neonatal T cell differentiation appears biased toward a Th2 or Th0 profile under neutral conditions. Whether neonatal T cells are capable of Th17 differentiation is unclear. Studies suggest that in the presence of IL-21, neonatal T cells exhibit a defect in Th17 differentiation.[454] However, neonatal γδ T cells can produce IL-17 and IL-22.[455] Additionally, in transcriptional analyses of skin lesions in early onset pediatric atopic dermatitis, skewing of Th17/Th22 was demonstrated, without the up-regulation of Th1 that is characteristic of adult onset atopic dermatitis.[456]

Factors favoring such a Th2 bias include the low MHC-peptide density of neonates (favors priming of Th2 cells), relative dearth of the Th1-inducing cytokines IFN-γ and IL-12, and the greater costimulation required to elicit Th1 differentiation.[457,458] Factors favoring a Th0 state include paucity of the Th2-inducing cytokines IL-4 and IL-10. Interestingly, pregnancy is also associated with a state of T cell tolerance with several factors (IL-4, IL-10, TGF-β) present at the maternal-fetal interface that can induce a shift from a Th1 to a Th2 profile.[459] Additionally, TGF-β can also result in differentiation of regulatory T cells, which have been shown to be critical for antigen-specific tolerance.[460,461] The importance of this T cell lineage in humans has been demonstrated in patients with immune dysregulation, polyendocrinopathy, enteropathy, X-linked syndrome, which is result of mutations in *FOXP3*—the transcription factor that controls the development of regulatory T cells.[462,463] This is an X-linked disorder that can present with neonatal diabetes mellitus, immune dysregulation with extremely high concentrations of IgE, and intractable diarrhea.[463,464] These patients also show exaggerated immune responses to viral infections.

γδ T CELLS

T cells expressing the γδ receptor are present at mucosal surfaces including the skin, gut, and lung.[465] These cells likely do not recirculate; they appear to be resident pulmonary lymphocytes. γδ T cells can develop by thymic-independent pathways and can recognize small molecules and intact proteins without the requirement for antigen processing that other T cells exhibit.[465] Small-molecule recognition by γδ cells requires cell-cell contact, suggesting that non-MHC molecules may present small antigens to these cells, or that costimulation from neighboring cells is required.[465,466] A germline-encoded phosphoantigen binding site enables these cells to respond to mycobacterial pyrophosphate, but they are also activated by antigen from disparate pathogens such as *L. monocytogenes.*[467] In vitro, γδ T cells can be induced to generate IFN-γ, TNF, IL-17, and IL-4 in a stimulus-specific fashion similar to Th0 cells.[468] In models of pulmonary fibrosis, γδ T cells appear to be protective.[469] The precise function of these cells in host defense remains unclear, but their anatomic locale and potential for cytotoxicity suggest a role in rapid initiation of immune reactions at mucosal surfaces of the airway. They are a rapid source of IL-17 in response to *K. pneumoniae*[362] and *M. tuberculosis*[361] infection. In the gut, γδ T cells may regulate granulopoiesis through IL-17 elaboration, which subsequently controls the expression of G-CSF.[470] Neonatal γδ T cells have also been shown to be an important source of the chemokine CXCL8, suggesting that these cells can directly mediate neutrophil recruitment.[471] This capacity of these cells to make CXCL8 declines with age.

B CELLS

B cells make up only a small percentage (≤2%) of the lung lymphocyte population, and this proportion of B cells or their precursors is attained in the fetal lung by 18 to 22 weeks of gestation.[472] In more mature subjects, B cells of the lung interstitium participate in local humoral responses through elaboration of immunoglobulins in response to specific antigenic stimuli. In the neonate, however, this capacity is limited, attributed in part to the inability of neonatal T cells to provide either the contact-dependent help or cytokine factors required to induce B cell differentiation into memory B cells.[415] A higher percentage of neonatal B cells are so-called B-1 cells, characterized by production mainly of polyreactive, low-affinity IgM, rather than the specific, high-affinity antibodies generated by B-2 cells.[473] Natural antibodies (nAbs) are immunoglobulins existing in individuals before specific antigenic stimulation and include specificities present in cord blood or germ-free mice. The predominant nAb isotype is IgM, and in germ-free mice quantities of IgM in the serum are unchanged; in contrast, IgG and mucosal IgA are significantly diminished, suggesting that production of IgM and IgG-IgA isotypes differs in their requirements for exogenous antigens.[474-476] The nAb display low-level broad cross-reactivity with self-antigens such as erythrocyte phospholipids and double-stranded DNA; however, selective pressures on the repertoire may relate to the role of nAb in host defense, as nAbs recognize various pathogen molecules, such as bacterial phosphorylcholine, α-1,3-dextran, and influenza hemagglutinin. Further, they have been shown to directly neutralize viruses such as varicella-zoster virus. As these antibodies are present at the earliest stages of infections and significantly earlier than the adaptive immune response, it is hypothesized that they play a critical role in the limitation of infection. Additionally, as IgM contains unique effector functions, it is thought that the early role of IgM nAb in host defense likely contributes to the quality and quantity of the emerging adaptive host immune response to infection. In addition to direct antimicrobial activity, the functions of IgM nAb appear to regulate disease processes at mucosal surfaces and adaptive immune responses. It has been shown that mice unable to secrete IgM have decreased survival and clearance of infection in response to influenza challenge. Interestingly, these mice had delayed production of influenza-specific IgG1 and IgG2a, suggesting that IgM immune complexes with the virus may influence aspects of antigen presentation to B cells.[477]

Receptor ligation of neonatal B cells induces minimal up-regulation of MHC class II molecules and fails to induce CD86, impairing antigen presentation by these cells.[478] B cells from preterm neonates also exhibit diminished expression of the complement receptor CD21, limiting their capacity to be stimulated by complement.[479] Although capable of local immunoglobulin production (primarily IgM and IgA), neonatal B cells remain unable to generate antibodies to bacterial capsular polysaccharides; this results in particular vulnerability to organisms such as *H. influenzae* and GBS.[480] Neonatal B cell function and lung humoral defense mechanisms are discussed in further detail later.

NATURAL KILLER CELLS

NK cells are large granular lymphocytes with cytotoxic function, comprising up to 15% of circulating lymphocytes, but less than 2% of the lung lymphocyte pool. They share a common progenitor with T cells but lack the TCR required for specific antigen recognition.[481] Within the lung, they are found on epithelial surfaces and in the interstitium, and they are also recruitable from the circulation in response to locally generated chemokines.[482] Activated NK cells contribute to early innate defense by lysing infected cells and generating cytokines that stimulate T cells and alveolar macrophages.[483] IL-12p70 is a key cytokine that up-regulates NK-cell perforin and granzyme, enhancing activated NK-cell lysis of infected cells.[481] As opposed to T cells, which recognize their target cells through MHC-restricted peptide expression, NK cells recognize the absence or very low levels of MHC class I antigen expressed on infected cells.[481] This has been termed the *missing self-hypothesis* and is described as the ability of NK cells to attack other cells within the host that express decreased MHC class I antigen.[484] Activating receptors on NK cells include NKG2D and DAP10. DAP12 can activate or inhibit NK-cell activation, and these negative regulatory adaptor proteins may avoid indiscriminate lysis of noninfected cells.

Early in infection, activated NK cells may be a primary source of IFN-γ within the lung.[485] NK cell-derived IFN-γ and TNF-α from multiple sources synergistically enhance alveolar macrophage killing of intracellular pathogens. In addition, NK cell-derived IFN-γ may initiate alveolar T cell-mediated immunity by inducing differentiation of Th0 cells into a Th1 phenotype.[486] The capacity to produce IFN-γ, augment immunity against intracellular pathogens, and effect cytotoxic responses without prior sensitization all imply a sentinel role for NK cells in neonatal host defense. Indeed, NK-cell precursors appear early in gestation by thymic-independent mechanisms and reach adult levels by term.[487] NK cytolytic function, however, remains diminished (≤50% of adult NK cells) for much of the first year of age, with more pronounced depression in premature neonates.[488] This diminished function corresponds to an immature NK-cell subset with impaired perforin-granzyme delivery;[489] this may predispose the neonatal lung to infections with agents such as herpes simplex virus and CMV.[489]

INNATE LYMPHOID CELLS

ILCs are a lineage of cells that likely arise from a subset of common lymphoid progenitor cells that do not express linage markers (such as CD19, Ly6G, CD3, CD11B, CD11C) or T cell or B cell receptors, but express CD127 or the IL-7 receptor. ILC progenitors express the transcription factor Id2 and the integrin α4β7.[12] These cells can develop into conventional cytolytic NK cells or noncytolytic INF-γ-producing ILC1 cells. ILC2 cells populate some mucosal tissues like the fetal intestine during development.[490] They also populate the lung during fetal development.[491] In murine studies, ILC2 cells can be found in fetal lung as early as ED17.5 and contribute to the ILC2 in adults. It is still unclear when this occurs in humans and whether preterm neonates may have reduced numbers of ILCs. Recently, it was discovered in the developing mouse lung that pulmonary ILC3s were derived from fibroblast ILC precursors.[492] Furthermore, premature infants with BPD had reduced lung ILC3s in their BAL fluid compared to infants without BPD.[492] These ILC3s can also populate the placenta and may also play key roles in the maternal-fetal interface.[493] Group 2 ILCs express receptors for IL-33 and IL-7 and can produce IL-5 and IL-13. As IL-13 is a major driver of mucin expression, these cells could be key sources of IL-13-driven mucin expression in neonates.[494] ILC3 cells express IL-23 receptor and IL-1RA and produce IL-17A and IL-22, two molecules important in host defense against extracellular pathogens. These cells are also found in the intestine, and there are emerging reports of their presence in the lung. They can respond to both environmental and cytokine cues and can be an early source of cytokines that we classically associate with mature T cells. However, these cells can respond in an antigen-independent fashion and thus can provide a source of T cell cytokines such as IFNγ, IL-5, IL-13, IL-17, or IL-22 early, in response to infection or injury, before the development of an adaptive T cell response.

HUMORAL IMMUNE RESPONSES

B lymphocytes bearing surface Ig of the IgA, IgG, and IgD isotypes appear early in gestation. Although the B cell Ig repertoire expands during gestation, at birth it remains limited relative to older hosts.[495,496] Immunoglobulin-secreting plasma cells appear later in gestation than B cells, between weeks 15 and 30.[497] Typically, neonatal B cells can differentiate into IgM-secreting plasma cells as efficiently as in the adult, but do not differentiate into IgG- or IgA-secreting cells until these functions fully mature.[498] As previously discussed, the relative inability to achieve isotype switching in the neonate results at least in part from inadequacy of mutual signaling between neonatal T cells and B cells. The antibody response of neonatal B cells to specific antigens develops sequentially, with responsiveness to antigens requiring contact-dependent T cell help (e.g., protein antigens) preceding the development of responses not requiring such cognate help (for example, capsular polysaccharides). Although infection of neonates elicits a protective response to most protein antigens, the response to polysaccharide antigens is absent or severely blunted. This has been postulated to result from decreased surface expression of CD21 and to decreased complement levels, resulting in suboptimal signal transduction via CD21 and inability to achieve the CD21/B cell receptor synergy required for B cell activation.[479,499] Alternatively, humoral responses to bacterial capsular polysaccharides are enhanced by specific T cell-derived cytokines such as IFNγ, IL-12, and GM-CSF, all of which are relatively deficient in the neonate.[500,501] The limited capacity of naïve neonatal T cells to provide these cytokines may contribute to the poor antibody responses of neonates to encapsulated bacteria such as group B streptococci. This T cell immaturity combined with differences in antibody repertoire and functional immaturity of B cells limits the capacity of the fetus or neonate to produce antibodies to certain antigens.

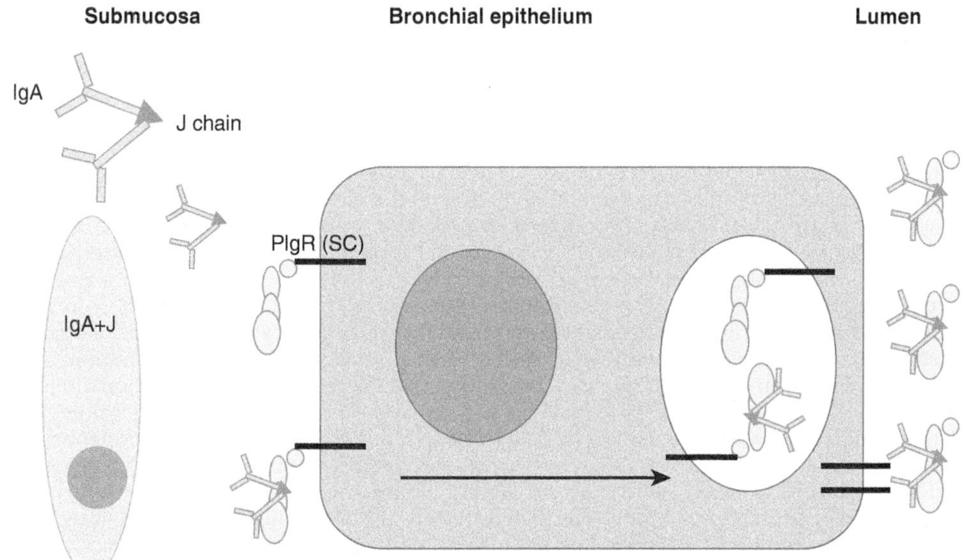

Fig. 123.8 Transport of immunoglobulin *(Ig)A* across secretory epithelium. Dimeric IgA binds to the polymeric Ig receptor *(PlgR)*, also known as membrane secretory component *(SC)*. After transport and export via PlgR, secretory IgA *(SIgA)* consists of dimeric IgA with J chain (IgA+J), which can function as blocking antibodies at mucosal surfaces.

SECRETORY IMMUNOGLOBULINS

Secretory component is an epithelial-derived glycoprotein that facilitates transfer of immunoglobulins from subepithelial sites into epithelial-lined lumina by transepithelial transport and secretion.[502] IgA and IgM constitute the primary secreted immunoglobulin subclasses of the lung. IgM is more abundant in secretions of neonates than in adults.[503-505] IgM is the first immunoglobulin class to be produced in a primary response to an antigen and is the only immunoglobulin other than IgG that fixes and activates complement. It is secreted as a pentamer, and the resultant 10 antigen-binding sites render it a superb agglutinin. Whereas serum concentrations are low at birth, postnatal IgM concentrations rise rapidly in the first month, reflecting increased antigen exposure; IgM concentrations in premature infants remain lower for the first 6 months of life. Secretory IgA is undetectable at birth but found by 1 to 2 weeks in saliva and nasopharyngeal secretions. The earlier expression of secretory IgA relative to serum IgA presumably reflects increased local production in response to encountered antigen[506] Serum IgA largely consists of monomeric IgA, whereas transported IgA is largely homodimeric. Transport occurs from the basolateral epithelial surface to the apical surface through the basolateral polymeric immunoglobulin receptor (PIGR) (Fig. 123.8). Both IL-17 and IL-22 can up-regulate the expression of PIGR and may facilitate IgA transport during inflammation.[507]

OTHER IMMUNOGLOBULINS

IgG is the predominant immunoglobulin isotype at all ages, and passively derived cross-placental transfer of maternal IgG is the primary source of all IgG subclasses detected in the normal fetus and neonate. These levels fall postnatally, reaching a nadir between 2 and 4 months of age (depending on gestational age) when nascent IgG production by the infant is unable to keep pace with utilization of maternally derived IgG. Preterm infants have proportionally lower IgG concentrations at birth compared with term infants, demonstrate lower serum IgG nadirs, and manifest lower serum IgG levels throughout the first year of life. Although IgG is not actively transported into secretions like IgA, significant quantities of IgG may be found in fluids obtained from bronchoalveolar and airway lavage, presumably by passive transfer.[508] A critical role of IgG in the lung has been shown in patients with various IgG deficiencies, such as common variable hypogammaglobulinemia and Bruton *X*-linked agammaglobulinemia, who suffer from pulmonary infections with encapsulated bacteria. This phenotype illustrates the critical role of IgGs in mediating opsonization and complement fixation.

MOLECULES INVOLVED IN THE RECRUITMENT OF LUNG IMMUNE CELLS

LIPID MEDIATORS

Lipid mediators of inflammation constitute a diverse group of biologically active products liberated from cellular membranes in response to local immune and nonimmune stimuli.[509] As opposed to cytokine synthesis, which often requires transcription, translation, and posttranslational processing steps, lipid mediators can be generated within minutes. Eicosanoids are a class of lipid mediators that are important in the recruitment of immune cells.[510] Endotoxin directly stimulates leukocyte membrane-associated phospholipase A_2 (PLA_2), which metabolizes adjacent membrane phospholipids to release free fatty acid products such as lysophosphatidylcholine and arachidonic acid.[511] Arachidonic acid can be metabolized by cyclooxygenase or lipoxygenase pathways to generate a number of bioactive lipid products, including thromboxane A_2 (TXA_2), prostacyclin (PGI_2), prostaglandins, and LTs, while lysophosphatidylcholine may be acylated to produce the potent mediator, PAF.[512]

PAF is synthesized by a number of cells, including mononuclear phagocytes, neutrophils, endothelial cells, platelets, eosinophils, and mast cells, and it has demonstrable biologic effects at nanomolar concentrations.[513] Known for its induction of platelet aggregation and degranulation, PAF also stimulates activation of PMNs, macrophages, and chemotaxis and augments PMN adhesion to endothelial cells.[514] Animal models of gram-negative infection implicate PAF in mediating endotoxin-induced inflammation, as well as having a role in the impaired hypoxic pulmonary vasoconstriction and alveolar capillary leak associated with severe pneumonitis.[515] Other studies have linked PAF to transfusion-associated lung injury and reperfusion lung injury.[516] In neonates, PAF is implicated in the pathogenesis of septic complications such as disseminated intravascular coagulation and necrotizing enterocolitis.[517,518] Premature infants with necrotizing enterocolitis have elevated plasma and stool PAF levels compared with control subjects.[519,520] Additionally, elevated PAF levels are documented in the tracheal aspirates of infants in association with meconium aspiration, pneumonia, and intrauterine infection, suggesting a role in neonatal pulmonary inflammation.[521]

Arachidonic acids are released from cell-membrane phospholipids in response to a variety of inflammatory stimuli.[513] Once liberated, they are primarily metabolized by either the lipoxygenase or the cyclooxygenase pathway. The lipoxygenase pathway produces LTs, including the potent PMN chemotactic activator LTB_4, and LTC_4 and its cysteinyl degradation products LTD_4 and LTE_4.[513] LTB_4 is a potent neutrophil chemoattractant, whereas the cysteinyl LTs are potent bronchoconstrictors. In addition, the cysteinyl LTs up-regulate macrophage Fc receptor expression and phagocytic activity. LTC4 and LTD4 are increased in the lung lavage fluids from hypoxemic neonates with persistent pulmonary hypertension (PPHN) versus ventilated infants without PPHN.[522] Although LT activity in the human neonatal lung has not been well characterized, animal models suggest that neonatal alveolar macrophages may have diminished capacity to synthesize LTB_4 compared with adults. This presumably results in part from lower inducible levels of IFN-γ and less capacity to up-regulate lipoxygenase pathway enzymes.[523] The important role of LTs in host response has been further suggested by a transgenic animal model of LT deficiency; in this model, alveolar macrophage phagocytic function was impaired, intratracheal inoculation of bacteria resulted in increased bacteremia and lethality, and alveolar macrophage function was restorable in vitro by exogenous LTB_4.[524]

Products of the cyclooxygenase pathway include PGI_2, TXA_2, and prostaglandins. Although TXA_2 increases microvascular tone and activates inflammatory cells, prostaglandin species, particularly the PGE series, are known to block transcription of TNF, suppress leukocyte adhesion, and blunt the generation of other proinflammatory arachidonic acid metabolites.[525] In meconium aspiration syndrome (MAS) of the newborn, airway epithelial cell exposure to meconium can induce complement activation and the release of TXA_2[526] and TNF-α.[527] Cellular constituents of the lung appear specialized in their generation of arachidonic acid products, with LTB_4, PGE_2, and TXA_2 being the primary ones generated by alveolar macrophages. Because inflammatory actions of these mediators may be conflicting, and because alveolar macrophages may produce varying amounts of these mediators at different stages of the inflammatory process, this suggests another mechanism by which the alveolar macrophage may regulate local inflammatory events.

PROTEINS

Complement

Activation of the complement cascade, by either classic or innate means, results in the eventual generation of multiple components with potent inflammatory activity. C3a, C4a, and C5a all have functions as anaphylatoxins, capable of inducing histamine release and increased vascular permeability; there is evidence that C3a and C5a mediate some of these effects by inducing local production of arachidonic acid metabolites.[528,529] C3a and C5a stimulate PMN lysosomal enzyme release, while C5a is also a potent neutrophil chemoattractant.[528]

C3a and C5a may regulate a broad range of inflammatory functions by binding their cognate receptors C3aR and C5aR. Previously recognized only on myeloid cells, both receptors have been demonstrated on human alveolar epithelium and alveolar macrophages.[530] C5a has also been shown to be involved in the development of acute respiratory distress syndrome[531] and in neonates with BPD.[532] In a murine model of sepsis, putative activation of toll pathways by endotoxin increased C3aR and C5aR expression on alveolar epithelium.[533] In this model, C5a activation of C5aR was implicated in increased expression of TNF-α and IL-6. Conversely, C3a has been shown to depress TNF-α and IL-6 secretion and hence blunt evolution of polyclonal immunity.[528] In a newborn piglet model of MAS, complement activation correlated with lung dysfunction, raising the possibility that an anticomplement therapy may be beneficial in the treatment of MAS.[534]

Neurokinins

The autonomic nervous system may participate in some aspects of airway inflammation, because stimulated or injured sensory nerves can initiate or amplify leukocyte responses. Local axonal reflexes play a role through stimulation of afferent nerve fibers, leading to the release of neurokinins. Neurokinins, such as substance P, are stored in unmyelinated nerve fibers (C fibers) as well as intrinsic airway neurons and are released as part of a nociceptive response.[535] Airway surface epithelium and submucosal glands are in proximity to sites of neurokinin release. Once secreted, neurokinins activate the neurokinin-1 receptor (NK-1R), mediating local increases in vascular permeability and leukocyte adherence to airway epithelial surfaces; the ensuing plasma extravasation and leukocyte infiltration constitute neurogenic inflammation.[536] The duration and intensity of this response are determined by the rate of neurokinin breakdown by neutral endopeptidase (NEP), an enzyme produced by epithelial cells.[537] Epithelial damage, as caused by inflammation, mechanical injury, or viral infection, reduces NEP availability, leading to sustained inflammatory effects of the neurokinins.

Beyond the classic model of neurogenic inflammation, studies have identified other neurokinin sources within the lung. Resident lung macrophages, as well as circulating leukocytes, have been found to express neurokinin receptors, as well as the *preprotachykinin A (PPT-A)* gene encoding neurokinins such as substance P.[538] This suggests that lung immune cells may use neurokinins for paracrine or autocrine signaling, propagating inflammation beyond the distribution of C fibers and intrinsic neurons. Animal models of either *NK-1R* or *PPT-A* deletion support such a role. The injury normally induced by antigen-antibody complexes within the airway is attenuated in a transgenic murine model of *NK-1R* deletion, suggesting an essential, rather than complementary, function of neurokinins in this type of inflammation.[539] Similarly, *PPT-A* deficiency blunts immune complex-mediated inflammation, yielding additional important insights. First, neurokinins intervene very proximally in the inflammatory cascade, because airway TNF-α levels are essentially undetectable in *PPT-A*-deficient mice. Second, reconstitution of leukocyte *PPT-A* expression does not alter the blunted inflammatory response in *PPT-A*-deficient mice; however, transplantation of *PPT-A*-deficient bone marrow into wild-type mice is protective, underscoring the essential role of leukocyte-derived *PPT-A* in neurogenic inflammation.[540] These data, taken together, suggest a paradigm in which subepithelial sensory neurons interact synergistically with resident immune cells of the lung to initiate neurogenic inflammation. Secreted neuropeptides are potent chemotaxins and can recruit leukocytes directly or by the induction of cytokines by local interstitial and immune cells.

Apart from their inflammatory actions, other relevant effects of airway neuropeptides relate to alterations in mucus secretion. Substance P stimulates mucin elaboration and increases mucus secretion by stimulating serous cells and goblet cells.[541] Both substance P and vasoactive intestinal peptide stimulate epithelial cell chloride secretion, increasing the periciliary fluid level.[542] The net effect is increased local production of mucus, with increased periciliary fluid secretion to maintain mucus hydration and normal viscosity. It has also been shown that neurokinins play a critical role in lung inflammation mediated by RSV infection.[543] It is not important, however, in the airway hyperreactivity associated with BPD.[544] Activation of the NK1 receptor and excitation of the serotonin neurons may be critical during the neonatal period. For example, mice deficient in serotonin neurons or with NK1 receptor inhibition demonstrate severe apneas and increased mortality in the neonatal period.[545] This may be one of the underlying causes seen in infants with sudden infant death syndrome.[546]

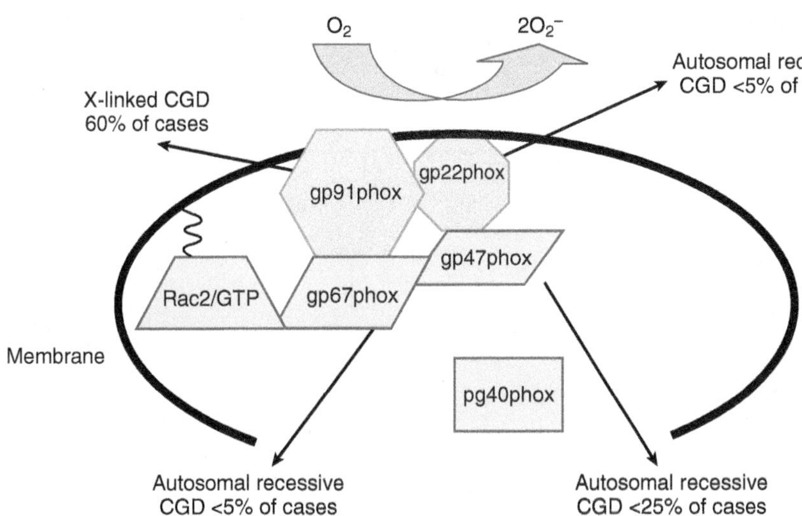

Fig. 123.9 Structure of functional nicotinamide adenine dinucleotide phosphate (NADPH) oxidase. NADPH oxidase consists of six subunits that are separated in different locations in the cell. *p22phox* and *gp91phox* are integral membrane proteins and form a heterodimeric structure that constitutes the catalytic core of the enzyme. *Rac GTPase* and *p47phox, p67phox*, and *p40phox* are cytosolic members of the complex. *CGD*, Chronic granulomatous disease.

Defensins

Apart from their primary antimicrobial activity, defensins also exhibit properties facilitating pulmonary inflammation. In vitro, α-defensins have been shown to induce the neutrophil chemoattractant IL-8 from airway epithelial cells and stimulate alveolar macrophage production of LTB_4 and IL-8.[547] α-Defensins can protect the host against many bacteria, fungi, and some viruses[548] and are produced by neutrophils, type I cells of the lung,[549] and enterocytes (specifically the Paneth cells within the intestine).[550] Additionally, HNP-1 and HNP-2 are each directly chemotactic for monocytes and can induce monocyte-derived TNF and IL-1.[551,552] Finally, α-defensins have been shown to induce T cell–derived IFN-γ, IL-6, and IL-10, whereas β-defensins have chemoattractant effects on immature DCs and naïve T cells. This suggests that beyond their antimicrobial and proinflammatory effects, defensins may also facilitate the local transition from innate to adaptive immune response.[553,554] Furthermore, in term and preterm infants, antimicrobial peptides are present in airway secretions and are increased in the presence of systemic or pulmonary infection, suggesting a role in the defense against the inflammatory response.[234]

Proteases. Phagocytic cells (PMNs, mononuclear leukocytes) contain a number of proteolytic enzymes capable of both microbial killing and proteolytic degradation of lung structural elements.[555] PMN primary (azurophilic) granules contain serine protease homologues with cytocidal activity (serprocidins); these include neutrophil elastase, cathepsin G, proteinase-3, and azurocidin. The serprocidins are structurally related to the granzymes of cytotoxic lymphocytes and exhibit broad-spectrum microbicidal activity against bacteria, fungi, and protozoa. Proteases contained in primary granules have the capacity to degrade a number of extracellular proteins, including collagen (types I to IV), elastin, fibronectin, laminin, proteoglycans, and complement, contributing to microbicidal action[556,557]; alternatively, many proteases possess antimicrobial activity unrelated to their proteolytic effects.[556] PMN secondary (specific) granules contain matrix metalloproteinase 9 (MMP9) and possibly gelatinase, which facilitate PMN migration.[555,556,558] MMP9 has been demonstrated to be elevated in the tracheal aspirates of infants with BPD,[559,560] as well as in a model of hypoxia-induced IFN-γ–mediated murine lung injury.[561] Furthermore, stored proteases are released extracellularly in response to various stimuli. Migration of PMN through tissues results in release of specific granule contents; this may be due to the interaction of complement receptors on the specific granule membrane with local complement components directing PMN chemotaxis. The local proteolytic actions of secreted proteases are regulated by extracellular antiproteases such as α1-antitrypsin, α1-antichymotrypsin, and α1-protease inhibitor.[562,563] Under conditions of homeostasis, a balance between proteolytic activity and antiprotease activity exists. However, when antiproteases are deficient or overwhelmed by the degree of the inflammatory response, diminished regulation of protease activity may ensue. Subsequent proteolytic generation of chemotactic extracellular matrix fragments and complement components can lead to further recruitment of phagocytic cells and intensified local inflammation.

REACTIVE OXYGEN SPECIES

A key component of pulmonary host defense is the generation of reactive oxygen species including superoxide and hydrogen peroxide, which can combine to form peroxynitrite. These molecules are often confined to the phagolysosome of PMNs and macrophages to minimize damage to host tissues.[564,565] This process is characterized by a rapid uptake of molecular oxygen by the phagocyte (the oxidative burst) that is triggered by cell membrane signaling before particle ingestion. Activation of cell membrane-associated NADPH oxidase results in shuttling of electrons from cytosolic NADPH to molecular oxygen—thereby initiating a series of reactions responsible for producing multiple oxyradical species. NADPH oxidase consists of six subunits that are separated in different locations in the cell (Fig. 123.9). p22phox and gp91phox are integral membrane proteins and form a heterodimeric structure that constitutes the catalytic core of the enzyme.[566] Rac GTPase and p47phox, p67phox, and p40phox are cytosolic members of the complex.[566,567] In the presence of activated-membrane NADPH oxidase, molecular oxygen accepts a single donated electron, becoming superoxide ion (O_2^-). Because this radical can either accept or donate an electron, it may be subsequently oxidized or reduced; when two such radicals interact, in the presence of superoxide dismutase, one is oxidized and one is reduced, such that $O_2^- + O_2^- + 2H^+ \rightarrow O_2 + H_2O_2$, generate hydrogen peroxide.[568] Transfer of a second electron to the superoxide ion, via NADPH oxidase, also generates H_2O_2. Neutrophil granules contain myeloperoxidase, an enzyme capable of generating further antimicrobial oxyradicals. Hydrogen peroxide reacts with myeloperoxidase and available halide species (primarily chloride in vivo) to generate hypochlorous acid (HOCl).[569] HOCl is an extremely powerful oxidant, analogous to bleach. Because it is highly reactive, it does not accumulate and is rapidly consumed in further reactions producing new oxidants. An important interaction may occur with primary or secondary amines to produce chloramines; although chloramines are weaker oxidants than HOCl, they tend to be longer lived and remain able to oxidize multiple potential targets.[570] Mutations in gp91-phox or other NADPH oxidase components result in chronic granulomatous disease, and patients with this disorder suffer from both bacterial infections and infections with *Aspergillus fumigatus*.[571] In addition, it has been suggested that NADPH oxidase isoforms play a key role in the pathogenesis of influenza A infection due to ROS production[568]; specifically, inhibition of NOX2 oxidase resulted in decreased lung viral titers.[572,573]

CYTOKINES

Cytokines play a sentinel role in the recruitment, proliferation, and survival of inflammatory cells within the lung. Cytokines are soluble proteins transiently synthesized by an appropriately stimulated immune or nonimmune effector cell and whose effects are mediated by binding to specific receptors on target cells. A cytokine may have autocrine effect when it modulates the properties of the cell producing it, paracrine effects when modulating the properties of cells proximally, and endocrine effects when it mediates its effects distally. Some cytokines may remain cell-associated or membrane-bound and exert their effects through cell-to-cell contact; this may facilitate more specific regulation of local inflammatory events. A single cytokine may be produced by many cell types, and a single cell type may produce many cytokines.[574] In general, cytokines are multifunctional molecules, participating in a wide spectrum of immune and nonimmune processes, including inflammation, metabolism, morphogenesis, fibrosis, and hemostasis. The action of a given cytokine may vary depending on its dose, receptor availability, the state of activation of the target cell, and the presence of other cytokines in the local milieu. Additionally, cytokines frequently stimulate target tissues to produce other bioactive cytokines. Accordingly, the biologic effects of cytokines result from their direct effects on target tissues and their ability to interact with one another in regulating target cell function; the eventual response of a cell to these mediators will depend on the sum of the signals received and the cell's state of responsiveness to each of these signals.

TUMOR NECROSIS FACTOR

TNF is a phylogenetically primitive mediator, based on its high degree of homology across species. It is produced primarily by monocytes and macrophages in response to LPS, as well as in response to enterotoxin, mycobacterial cell wall products, and components of complement.[575] TNF is also produced by T cells and NK cells.[575] Its local half-life is approximately 6 minutes, with peak levels at 1 to 2 hours after LPS exposure, defining its role as an early response mediator in endotoxin-induced inflammatory cascades.[576] It is now clear that TNF is a key mediator of host defense against a wide range of pulmonary pathogens, including *Pseudomonas, Legionella, Klebsiella, S. aureus, S. pneumoniae,* and *Mycobacterium* species.[577-580] Alveolar macrophage-derived TNF remains compartmentalized within the alveolus, where it exerts protean inflammatory effects.[112] TNF acts on PMNs to increase phagocytosis, adhesion molecule expression, and respiratory burst capacity.[581,582] TNF acts on epithelial and vascular endothelial cells to similarly up-regulate adhesion molecule expression, thereby facilitating inflammatory cell migration.[581] TNF induces IL-1 generation by endothelial cells and local mononuclear phagocytes, which augments the initial inflammatory signal[583] and can directly induce production of the potent neutrophil-activating factor IL-8 from multiple cell types, further amplifying inflammation. TNF also induces IL-6 production by fibroblasts, epithelial cells, and endothelial cells, initiating an acute-phase response.[584] Neonatal monocytes and T cells have diminished (50% to 60%) capacities to generate TNF relative to adult cells, and these limitations are further pronounced in preterm neonates (25% adult capacity).[585,586]

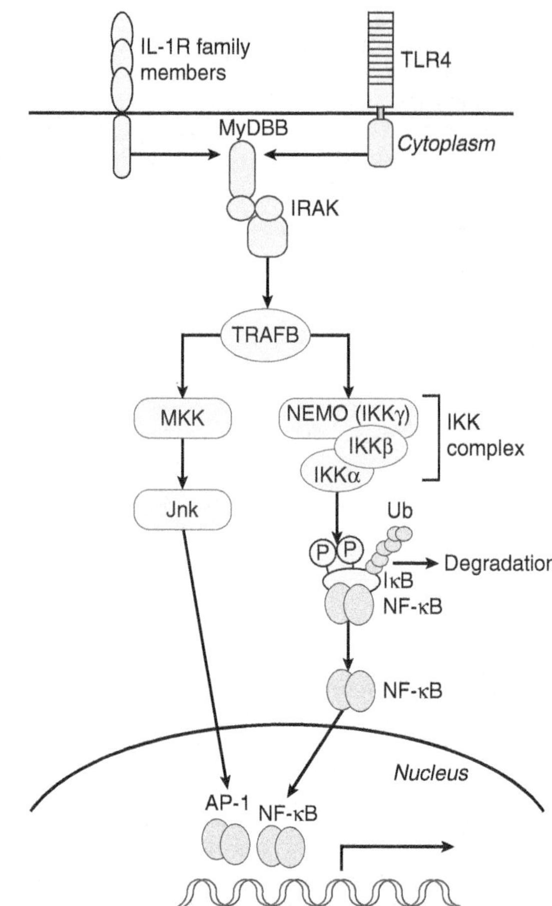

Fig. 123.10 Interleukin *(IL)-1R1*/toll-like receptor *(TLR)* signaling. To illustrate the shares signaling pathway, the molecular components involved in IL-1R and *TLR4* signaling are shown. Both IL-1R1 and TLR4 (as well as TLR1, 2, 6, 7, 8, and 9) can associate with a cytoplasmic adaptor molecule, *MyD88*. This interaction occurs between the TIR domains. *MyD88* encodes a death domain that mediates association with a serine-threonine kinase, *IRAK*. TRAF6 serves as scaffold protein can activate MAP kinases *(MKKs)* as well as the *IKK* complex. MKK can also lead to AP-1 activation via Jnk. The IKK complex induces phosphorylation of *IκB*, which allows ubiquitination of IκB followed by proteasomal degradation. This allows nuclear translocation of *NF-κB* and gene expression. (From Akira S, Takeda K, Kaisho T. Toll-like receptors: critical proteins linking innate and acquired immunity. *Nat Immunol.* 2001;2:675–680.)

INTERLEUKINS

Interleukin-1

The IL-1 family consists of several proinflammatory agonists. This chapter will focus on two, IL-1α and IL-1β, and the antiinflammatory IL-1 receptor antagonist protein (IL-1ra). IL-1α is primarily membrane bound, while IL-1β is secreted. IL-1α and IL-1β are encoded by separate genes but share the same receptor by virtue of a 23% homology, and thus they can elicit similar effects. These receptors are ubiquitously expressed, so the effects of this cytokine are pleiotropic.[587,588] Ligation of the receptor IL-1R1 activates IRAK, which culminates in liberation, and nuclear translocation, of NF-κB.[588] Of note is that the IL-1R1 signaling cascade shares MyD88 and IRAK with the pathways for TLRs 1, 2, 4, 5, 6, 7, 8, and 9 (Fig. 123.10).[589] IL-1 shares many properties with TNF, including enhancement of adhesion molecule expression by PMNs and endothelial cells, up-regulation of NOS, and neutrophil priming. IL-1 acts on fibroblasts, epithelial cells, and endothelial cells to induce IL-6 and IL-8 production, thereby modulating both enhanced PMN chemoactivation and initiation of the acute phase response.[588] IL-1 is an endogenous pyrogen and within the central nervous system can elicit fever.[588,590] Other actions of IL-1 include stimulation of T cell proliferation, increased IL-2 receptor expression on T and B cells, and increased release of T cell–derived IL-2.[588] IL-1β has been implicated in the differentiation of both murine and human Th17 cells.[591,592] Regulation of IL-1 occurs by either direct IL-1ra antagonism or sequestration of IL-1 by its decoy receptor, the IL-1R2.[588] Engagement of this receptor by IL-1 does not induce signal transduction. Furthermore, cleavage of this receptor from cell surfaces by metalloprotease releases a soluble receptor that blocks IL-1–mediated effects.

Mononuclear phagocytes do not produce IL-1 constitutively, but its production is induced by multiple stimuli, including viruses, microbial products (endotoxin, peptidoglycans, teichoic acid, yeast cell walls), C5a, TNF, and IL-1 itself.[588] However, secretion of IL-1β requires cleavage by caspase-1.[588] This enzyme is activated by proinflammatory stimuli through a series of cytosolic molecules that detect lipopeptides. Similar to TLRs these proteins encode leucine-rich repeats, which are critical for ligand recognition. These NOD and NALP proteins sense microbial products and activate the inflammasome, which is critical for cleavage of IL-1β.[593,594] Both term and preterm neonates possess adult capacity to produce monocyte-derived IL-1 and exceed adult capacity to produce PMN-derived IL-1.[585,595]

IL-1ra is an endogenous IL-1 inhibitor that competitively binds to the IL-1R1 without inducing signal.[596] It exists in two intracellular isoforms found in epithelial cells and as a third isoform secreted by monocytes.[597] IL-1ra is synthesized by alveolar macrophages (and other mononuclear cells) in response to LPS or adherent IgG.[598] Animal models of endotoxin-induced pneumonitis demonstrate profound antiinflammatory response to intratracheally instilled IL-1ra, whereas murine models of IL-1ra deficiency show exaggerated and persisting inflammatory response.[599,600] These data, along with known in vitro actions, suggest that IL-1ra may function as an endogenous down-regulator of inflammatory cytokine cascading within the alveolar space. IL-1ra is found in tracheal aspirates of preterm infants at risk for BPD,[601,602] but this may represent release from injured epithelium rather than de novo immune cell production.[603] Serum IL-1ra levels are elevated in healthy newborns, decline within days of birth, and increase in response to infection, indicating capacity for stimulus-specific IL-1ra production.[604] Strikingly, in a murine model of BPD, IL-1 receptor antagonist prevented BPD, which was induced with perinatal inflammation and hyperoxia.[605] The effects in humans need to be further investigated.

Interleukin-6

IL-6 is primarily produced by mononuclear phagocytes. It is also produced by T and B cells and may be produced by endothelial cells, epithelial cells, and fibroblasts in response to TNF and IL-1.[606,607] IL-6 production by stimulated neonatal mononuclear cells matches or exceeds that of adults, although diminished production is noted with marked prematurity.[608,609] IL-6 is able to exert effects on a wide range of cells, owing to the unique properties of its receptor. When activated by IL-6, the IL-6 receptor complexes with the gp130 membrane protein, which is required for intracellular signal transduction through the phosphorylation of *Stat3*. IL-6R also circulates in a soluble (sIL-6R) form, which binds secreted IL-6.[606] The IL-6:IL-6R complex can then activate any cell bearing the gp130 membrane protein, allowing IL-6 to activate a wide range of cell types. Functions of IL-6 include providing costimulatory signals to enhance T cell responses and differentiation of Th17 cells[436,461] and stimulation of B cell differentiation and antibody production.[610] IL-6 also induces the acute phase response, characterized by hepatocyte production of such proteins as fibrinogen, α_2-macroglobulin, and α_1-antitrypsin and also up-regulates local acute-phase protein production by mononuclear phagocytes.[611] IL-6 is found in BAL specimens of adults with pulmonary inflammation, as well as in BAL specimens of mechanically ventilated, premature neonates. However, it remains unclear whether IL-6 is a marker, or mediator, of inflammation in either of these scenarios.[612,613] Furthermore, elevated umbilical cord levels of IL-6 are associated with an increased risk of respiratory distress syndrome and BPD in the presence of intrauterine infection.[614]

Interleukin-10

IL-10 is a critical cytokine produced by T cells, B cells, and mononuclear phagocytes in response to stimuli, including LPS and TNF-α.[615] IL-10 augments proliferation and differentiation of activated B cells while up-regulating their MHC class II expression.[615] IL-10 inhibits the generation of oxyradicals and NO by macrophages and PMNs, impairing their microbicidal functions.[616,617] IL-10 also suppresses macrophage expression of MHC class II and costimulatory molecules CD80 and CD86, diminishing their capacity to present antigen.[615] Finally, IL-10 inhibits macrophage-dependent T cell proliferation and Th1 cytokine production by macrophages, PMNs, Th1 cells, and NK cells.[615] Mice deficient in IL-10 develop spontaneous colitis.[405,618] These data along with the observation that IL-10 is expressed by regulatory T cells suggest that IL-10 is critical as a negative regulator of the immune response.

There is evidence that IL-10 production in the lungs may be protective in some types of inflammatory injuries, and animal models of pneumonia have helped to clarify this role of IL-10 in vivo.[619] Exogenous IL-10, preceding intratracheal bacterial challenge, reduced lung TNF and IFN-γ responses, but increased lung bacterial counts, systemic bacteremia, and morbidity in a murine model of *S. pneumoniae* infection.[620] IL-10 neutralization in this same model resulted in increased lung TNF, diminished lung bacterial counts, and increased survival rates. Similar outcomes have been shown in a murine model of *Klebsiella* pneumonia, treated with systemic anti-IL-10 antibody.[621] Given these data, it is thus presumed that in the context of pneumonia, IL-10 acts to modulate the local inflammatory response initiated by the offending pathogen; this preserves alveolar structure, pulmonary gas-exchange function, and host survival. The data regarding the ability of neonates to produce IL-10 are somewhat contradictory but do allow some broad generalizations. First, stimulated neonatal monocytes exhibit only 20% to 40% of the IL-10 production inducible from stimulated adult monocytes.[622,623] Second, available BAL data from mechanically ventilated infants indicate that IL-10 expression in the lung is diminished in preterm infants but increases with advancing gestational age.[624,625] Third, IL-10 expression in the cord blood of infants with congenital diaphragmatic hernia (CDH) is higher than in healthy term neonates; infants with CDH who required extracorporeal membrane oxygenation had even higher levels of IL-10 than those infants with a milder form of CDH.[626] These age-related findings parallel data suggesting differential IL-10 production by lung macrophages ex vivo from term and preterm infants.[627] Such differences, if true in vivo, suggest that premature infants may be less able to attenuate alveolar inflammation in the setting of a pneumonitis or other inflammatory insult.

Interleukin-15

IL-15 is a 15-kDa peptide that shares β-and γ-receptor components with IL-2, resulting in overlapping immune functions including induction of T cell proliferation and increased T cell cytotoxic activity.[628,629] Like IL-2, IL-15 binding requires a distinct α-chain receptor component (IL-15Ra); this component is expressed in a variety of tissues, conferring pleiotropic immune activities distinct from those of IL-2. IL-15 induces NK-cell–derived TNF-α, GM-CSF, and IFN-γ and augments IL-12 up-regulation of T cell-derived IFN-γ.[630,631] IL-15 also induces NK-cell differentiation, activation, and supports prolonged NK-cell survival. Beyond these effects, IL-15 induces IL-8 expression by T cells and monocytes, as well as up-regulating monocyte-derived MCP-1 and MIP-1β, facilitating phagocyte recruitment and a proinflammatory milieu.[632] Finally, IL-15 also directly activates PMNs, inducing membrane stiffening, enhancing phagocytosis, and delaying apoptosis.[629] Although macrophages are the primary cellular source of IL-15, gene expression of this cytokine has also been identified in lung fibroblast and epithelial cells, DCs, and endothelial cells in response to a variety of bacterial and viral stimuli, indicating a role for IL-15 in pulmonary immune regulation.[629] IL-15 is critical for homeostatic proliferation of T cells and regulates the generation of memory T cells.[633] IL-15 production has not been characterized in the neonatal air space, but stimulated neonatal monocytes in vitro exhibit diminished IL-15 mRNA stability and protein expression of only approximately 30% relative to adult controls.[634] Given this finding, it is reasonable to speculate that attenuated IL-15 production by the neonate may contribute to impaired pulmonary cellular immunity.

Interleukin-17

IL-17 is a proinflammatory cytokine, produced by activated memory CD4 T cells of the Th17 subset, that facilitates granulopoiesis and pulmonary PMN recruitment in response to local bacterial infection.[443] It is the prototypical member of a cytokine cohort collectively designated IL-17A-F, which also includes IL-25 (IL-17E).[635] IL-17A signals through the adaptor proteins Act1 to induced NF-κB and AP-1.[636,637] IL-17 stabilizes transcripts for CXCL1 and G-CSF and therefore synergizes with other inducers of NF-κB such as TNF-α.[443,638] The target cells of IL-17's actions are mainly epithelial cells, fibroblasts, and endothelial cells.[443,635] In neonatal mice deficient in IL-17 receptor A, the number of circulating neutrophils was significantly lower than in age-matched controls.[639] The concentration of IL-17 in cord blood of premature infants was found to have no association with premature birth.[640] Pulmonary IL-17 has not as yet been quantified in neonatal cohorts, but it may be negligible given the relative paucity of memory T cells in this population. IL-17E is the most divergent IL-17 family member showing only 25% homology with IL-17A. Interestingly IL-17E or IL-25 potently induces IL-4 and IL-13 and is involved in Th2 T cell differentiation.[641,642]

Interleukin-18

Initially identified as IFN-γ-inducing factor, IL-18 is an approximately 18-kDa protein that enhances IFN-γ production and exhibits other proinflammatory functions.[643] IL-18 is similar to IL-1β both in secondary structure and in its secretion as an inactive precursor requiring cleavage by IL-1β-converting enzyme (caspase-1) to become bioactive.[643] IL-18 also shares receptor components and signal transduction mechanisms with IL-1.[643] Binding of IL-18 to its receptor, the IL-1 receptor–related protein (IL-1Rrp), triggers a signaling pathway that requires IRAK and eventually culminates in the nuclear translocation of NF-κB and gene transcription. IL-18 may also bind to its alternative ligand, IL-18 binding protein (IL-18bp), an endogenous soluble decoy receptor that inhibits IL-18 activity; IL-18 bioactivity may thus be titrated either by regulation of cleavage activation or by modulation of IL-18bp levels.[644] IL-18 is present constitutively within the lung, primarily derived from alveolar macrophages, although also inducible in vitro from pulmonary fibroblasts.[645] Like other macrophage-derived cytokines, IL-18 is up-regulated in response to microbial products (LPS, gram-positive bacterial exotoxins) and is also induced by exposure to TNF-α, chemokines (IL-8, MCP-1, MIP-1α), and mycobacteria.[643] As suggested earlier, IL-18 has important IFN-γ-inducing activity. By direct activation of the IFN-γ promoter, IL-18 achieves potent synergy with IL-12 for IFN-γ production by T cells, B cells, and NK cells, but only modest induction of IFN-γ in the absence of IL-12; this augmented IFN-γ production may favor a Th1 response within the alveolus.[643] IL-18 is protective against fungal, bacterial, and viral pathogens.[646-648] Such a role has been demonstrated in vivo in a transgenic model of IL-18 deficiency, where impaired lung bacterial clearance and fulminant progression to systemic infection resulted from intratracheal inoculation with *S. pneumoniae*.[649] In neonates, however, the pulmonary expression of IL-18 remains incompletely characterized. A study evaluating the presence of IL-18 polymorphisms in the genetics of premature birth and BPD found that IL-18 did not play a critical role in either of these events in the neonatal population.[650]

Interleukin-22

IL-22 is one of the IL-10 family cytokines, which also include IL-10, IL-19, IL-20, IL-24, IL-26, as well as more distantly related IL-28 and IL-29. The IL-26 gene is conserved across vertebrate species but is not expressed in mice.[651] IL-22 was first identified as an IL-10–related T cell-derived inducible factor from a lymphoma cell line treated with IL-9.[652] IL-22R and IL-10R2 were soon identified as the heterodimeric receptor complex for the function of IL-22.[443] As mentioned, one biologic function of IL-22 is that it synergizes with IL-17 to regulate the expression of antimicrobial peptides at epithelial surfaces.[345,442] IL-22 regulation of antimicrobial proteins has been shown to exist at several mucosal surfaces including the skin, gut, and lung (Fig. 123.11).[345,443,653] Mice exposed to hyperoxia as neonates were reported to have less IL-22$^+$ lung NK cells after an influenza infection as an adult, demonstrating the potential of oxygen exposure in the neonatal period to have a long-lasting impact on the host response to infections later in life.[654]

Interleukin-25

IL-25, also known as IL-17E, is a member of the IL-17 family. IL-25 injection is involved in mediating a type 2 immune response, eosinophilia.[641] Rhinovirus infection in the neonatal period leads to airway hyperresponsiveness and mucous metaplasia via IL-25 and type 2 ILCs (ILC2s).[655] Mice with rhinovirus in the early neonatal period were noted to have asthma related to this IL-25-mediated response.[655]

Interleukin-33

IL-33 is an innate cytokine expressed in airway smooth muscle and the epithelium, which can also induce airway hyperresponsiveness.[656] IL-33 has the ability to activate ILC2s, but also requires thymic stromal lymphoprotein, IL-2, or IL-7 for the activation and is synergistic with IL-4.[657] ILC2 activation by IL-33 leads to allergic airway inflammation due to the innate type 2 response.[657] IL-33 has also been known to promote ILC2 activation in other disease processes including fungal infections,[658] viral infections due to H1N1 and other influenza strains,[659] and animal models of pulmonary fibrosis.[660]

CHEMOKINES

IL-8 and several other structurally homologous proteins comprise the family of cytokines known as chemokines. The chemokine family consists of more than 40 small (70 to 130 amino acid) cytokines divided into four subfamilies based on the position of one or two conserved cysteine residues located near the N terminus defining four structural motifs: CXC, CC, C, and CX3C.[661,662] Different leukocyte subsets express a unique chemokine receptor profile that defines the response potential of each type of cell. In turn, chemokines can be modified by proteases in the extracellular milieu to become more active or inert.[663] Although most chemokine receptors bind more than one chemokine, CC receptors bind only CC chemokines and

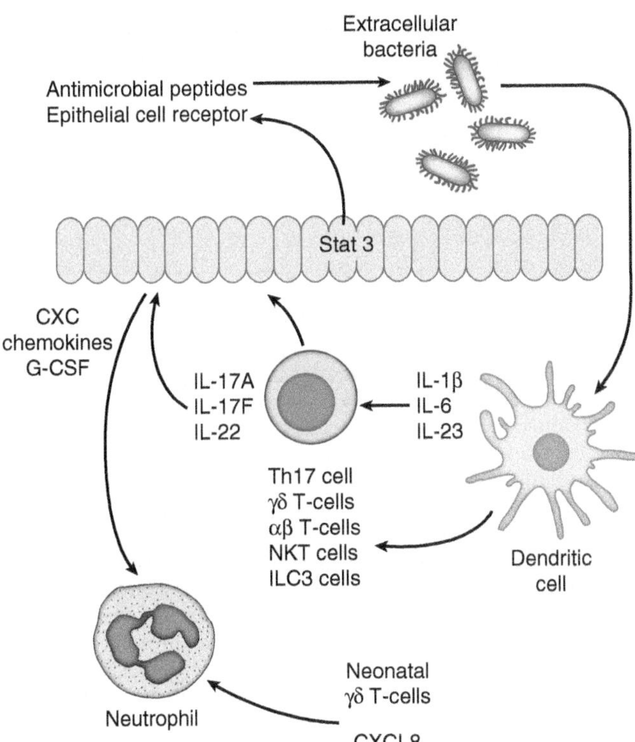

Fig. 123.11 Schematic of type 17 immune responses in the lung. Interleukin *(IL)-17* and *IL-22* are induced rapidly in experimental bacterial pneumonia and produced by several T cell populations in the lung includingγδ-T cells, NK T cells, group 3 innate lymphoid cells, as well as effector memory αβ CD4+ T cells. IL-17 signaling regulates granulopoiesis through the regulation of and granulocyte–colony-stimulating factor *(G-CSF)* as well as neutrophil recruitment via the regulation of *CXC* chemokines by epithelial cells. IL-22 and IL-17 induce the expression of antimicrobial peptides from target cells and can augment epithelial repair. This cooperative induction of neutrophil recruitment and antimicrobial peptide production augments epithelial barrier function and is critical for mucosal host defense against bacteria and fungi. Neonatal γδ T cells can produce CXC chemokines like IL-8 themselves to regulate neutrophil responses, but this capacity appears to be lost as the immune system develops from infancy to adulthood.

CXC receptors bind only CXC chemokines. Chemokines play a critical role in recruitment and activation of inflammatory cells at sites of infection. Both CC and CXC chemokines have positively charged C-terminus residues that bind to negatively charged glycosaminoglycans on matrix proteins in the interstitium and on cell surfaces; this provides a mechanism to stabilize chemokines near sites of generation, achieving relatively fixed local chemotactic gradients. Proteolytic cleavage of glycosaminoglycans such as syndecan can also modify the amount of free chemokine available to serve as a chemoattractant.[664] The spectrum of action of a given chemokine is thus a function of its local concentration, its posttranslational processing, and the temporal expression of chemokine receptor(s) on putative target cells. Important representative chemokines implicated in the regulation of pulmonary immune responses include members of the CXC and CC subfamilies.

CXC Chemokine Subfamily

CXC chemokines can be further subdivided into two groups based on the presence or absence of three amino acids (Glu-Leu-Arg: the ELR motif) preceding the first cysteine residue.[665] The ELR+ CXC chemokines are potent neutrophil chemoattractants and angiogenic agents, which may be mediated by the chemokine receptors CXCR1 and CXCR2.[665] However, the ELR− CXC chemokines, such as CXCL4, CXCL9, CXCL10, and CXCL11, are chemoattractant for mononuclear leukocytes and are angiostatic.[665] CXCL8 (IL-8), the prototypical ELR+ CXC chemokine, is produced by a number of pulmonary cells, including mononuclear phagocytes, endothelial cells, fibroblasts, epithelial cells, mesothelial cells, and T cells.[666,667] Chemokine production by these cells can be induced by multiple stimuli, including viruses, bacterial products, TNF, IL-1, C5a, LTB_4, IL-17, and IFN.[666,667] Actions of IL-8 on PMNs include potent chemoattraction, up-regulation of adhesion molecule expression, and enhancement of PMN respiratory burst and degranulation.[666-668] IL-8 is a major activating factor of neutrophils in humans[471,665,669] and also stimulates PMN production of the inflammatory lipid mediators LTB_4 and PAF.[666,667] It is important to keep in mind that IL-8 is only one ligand for CXCR2 and that CXCL1, CXCL2, CXCL5, and CXCL6 can each serve as ligands for CXCR2.

IL-8 is locally expressed in patients with pneumonia, and its critical role in host response is further supported by animal models of bacterial pneumonitis; in these models, depletion of CXC chemokines or blockade of CXC receptors attenuates PMN recruitment and blunts pulmonary bacterial clearance.[395,670-672] A similar role likely exists for IL-8 in neonates, but data regarding IL-8 production in this population are somewhat contradictory. In vitro stimulation of neonatal immune cells has typically demonstrated IL-8 production well below adult levels.[673,674] However, neonatal IL-8 production exceeding adult response has been shown using flow cytometric analysis in an ex vivo model of neonatal sepsis or neonatal stress.[608,675] Although against conventional wisdom, these findings are consistent with other emerging data showing the presence of significant, inducible IL-8 in the BAL specimens of term and preterm newborns with lung insults such as MAS or hyaline membrane disease.[676] In addition, IL-8–producing T cells were found to be present in very premature infants as early as 23 weeks' gestation.[471] IL-8 should therefore be considered as a likely relevant mediator both in neonatal pulmonary host defense as well as in inflammatory lung pathology. CXCL9, CXCL10, and CXCL11 are all ligands for CXCR3, which is preferentially expressed on Th1 cells. Therefore, these chemokines have been shown to be critical for recruitment of Th1 cells to the lung and granuloma formation.[677,678]

CC Chemokine Subfamily

CCL3 (MIP-1α), CCL2 (MCP-1), and other members of the CC chemokine subfamily are derived from multiple pulmonary cells, including PMNs, mononuclear phagocytes, lymphocytes, NK cells, endothelium, fibroblasts, epithelial cells, and mesothelium.[679-681] Stimuli that induce production of the CC chemokines include viruses, bacterial products, TNF, IL-1, C5a, LTB4, and IFN, whereas IL-10 is a potent CC chemokine suppressor. The CC chemokines have specific chemotactic activity for monocytes, lymphocytes, eosinophils, and basophils and tend to have proinflammatory properties.[665,682,683] Binding of CC chemokines to their corresponding receptors on monocytes produces an increased respiratory burst and induces rapid release of arachidonic acid metabolites.[681,683] CCL3 and CCL2 regulate monocyte expression of adhesion molecules, preferentially increasing monocyte expression of the β2 integrin CD11/CD18 normally associated with PMNs, rather than the usual monocyte adhesion VLA-4.[684] This enhanced expression of β2 integrins results in augmented monocyte adhesion to endothelium, putatively enhancing monocyte migration to inflammatory loci. The CC chemokines have also been identified in the recruitment of T cells, B cells, and NK cells; however, they appear to lack significant effects on PMNs.[681,685,686]

There have been a handful of atypical chemokine receptors identified, including CXCR7, CCBP2, CCRL1, CCRL2, and Duff antigen receptor for chemokines (DARC),[665] whose functions may include being a chemokine scavenger or decoy receptor.[687,688] DARC has also been called a silent receptor or interceptor (internalizing receptors) and can bind inflammatory chemokines from the CC or CXC subfamilies.[689] Chemokine binding to DARC can prevent their diffusion from blood into the lungs and possibly other tissues[689] and may be important in maintaining plasma chemokine levels.[690] While early in vitro work demonstrated neonatal monocytes to have decreased inducible CCL3 relative to adults, recent data have challenged these findings.[691] Basal serum levels of CCL3 are found to be similar in neonatal and adult cohorts, and monocyte-derived CCL3 is comparably inducible in these two age groups.[692] Levels of CCL3 are increased in airway fluids of infants with inflammatory pulmonic processes including severe RSV infection, *Ureaplasma* infection, and respiratory distress syndrome, suggesting local inducibility of this chemokine in response to infection or insult.[693-697] Neonatal levels of MCP-1, in both serum and airway fluid, are found to be similarly inducible in response to appropriate stress. Taken together, these data suggest that the CC chemokines, like IL-8, should be considered relevant mediators of both pulmonary host defense and inflammatory lung injury in the neonate.

TRANSFORMING GROWTH FACTOR-β

TGF-β is a cytokine primarily associated with tissue repair and fibrosis, but one that also exerts important immunomodulatory effects. This cytokine is secreted as an inactive disulfide bond-linked dimer, and liberation of the 25-kDa active form occurs in response either to proteolytic activation or acidic conditions.[698-700] TGF-β is produced by multiple cell lines, including platelets, T cells, PMNs, mononuclear cells, fibroblasts, epithelial cells, and endothelial cells, and exerts pleiotropic effects relevant to host immune response.[700] TGF-β can induce production of acute-phase proteins via IL-6 and also controls the development of Th17 cells.[461,701] In the absence of IL-6, TGF-β can induce the development of regulatory T cells.[461] TGF-β can also act as a potent chemoattractant for monocytes and macrophages and can induce these cells to produce TGF-β, thereby amplifying its local effects.[702] Although TGF-β can induce monocyte-derived IL-1 and TNF-α, it inhibits LPS induction of macrophage-derived IL-1, TNF-α, and IFN-γ, thus exhibiting antiinflammatory activity in settings of immune activation.[699] TGF-β can also down-regulate macrophage NO production and MHC II expression and suppress the macrophage respiratory burst.[703] Beyond macrophage deactivation, TGF-β also down-regulates IL-2 receptors, inhibiting IL-2–dependent T cell proliferation and IL-1–dependent lymphocyte proliferation. The net result of TGF-β activity is impairment of IL-2 effects and inhibition of Th1 response. Within the alveolus, this manifests as impaired antigen presentation and a general suppression of inflammation. Data defining the role of TGF-β in neonatal pulmonary defense remain incomplete. In vitro, TGF-β production from stimulated neonatal monocytes is only 35% to 40% of that from adult monocytes; this may suggest compromised ability of the neonate to titrate inflammation through TGF-β production.[691] This is supported by in vivo data showing lower TGF-β levels in the BAL specimens of infants progressing to states of chronic lung disease.[704] Finally, additional studies have shown elevated neonatal BAL levels of TGF-β, suggesting that expression of this cytokine may be more inducible than indicated by in vitro data.[613]

CLUB CELL SECRETORY PROTEIN (CC10, CC16)

Club cell secretory protein (CCSP) is one of the most abundant proteins of the airway lining fluid. It is secreted by club cells, as well as by serous and goblet cells of the proximal airways.[705] Structurally, CCSP is a small homodimeric protein consisting of two 8-kDa subunits aligned by disulfide links to form a hydrophobic pocket.[706] This pocket can bind phosphatidylcholine and phosphatidylinositol, and CCSP was originally postulated to participate in surfactant metabolism. CCSP has been noted to modulate inflammatory responses, suggesting a potential immunoregulatory role within the airways and alveoli. In vitro, CCSP has been shown to inhibit PMN chemotaxis, as well as macrophage phagocytosis.[706] Its hydrophobic pocket allows CCSP to scavenge PLA_2 within the milieu, further limiting PMN activation.[706] CCSP has also been shown to inhibit the production and bioactivity of IFN-γ.[706] Murine models of CCSP deficiency have attempted to further clarify the in vivo role of this protein. In a hyperoxic model of lung injury, CCSP-deficient animals exhibited higher lung levels of IL-1β, IL-6, and IL-3, increased lung inflammation, and decreased survival rates.[707] In a model of adenoviral lung infection, CCSP deficiency resulted in an earlier and increased inflammatory response; this was accompanied by increased expression of TNF, IL-1β, IL-6, and chemokines (CCL3 and CCL2).[708] CCSP-deficient animals receiving an antigenic challenge showed increased levels of Th2 cytokines with exacerbated eosinophilic inflammation.[709] Finally, CCSP-deficient mice demonstrate increased expression of IgA.[710] The exaggerated cellular response seen in each of these models is consistent with the putative role of CCSP as an antiinflammatory molecule. LPS depresses *CCSP* gene expression in a dose-dependent fashion, suggesting that potent signals of infection may dampen CCSP secretion as required to allow an appropriate inflammatory response.[711] In newborns, CCSP levels are detected in tracheal/alveolar aspirates obtained at birth and correlate with gestational age. Neonates with clinical signs of infection have increased CCSP levels, correlating inversely with tracheoalveolar fluid leukocyte counts.[712] Similarly, infants who subsequently develop BPD demonstrate diminished inducibility of CCSP and generally lower CCSP levels in their airway fluid, possibly contributing to the increased lung inflammation seen in this process.[713,714] In a study with newborn piglets who received surfactant and a recombinant human club cell protein, pulmonary compliance was improved.[715,716] In summary, CCSP appears to serve a homeostatic role in titrating inflammatory activity within the air spaces of the lung. Although not classically viewed as a cytokine, CCSP meets these criteria because it exhibits receptor-mediated signaling, regulates other cytokines and immune cell function, and is regulated in dose-dependent fashion by relevant biologic stimuli such as IFN and LPS.

COLONY-STIMULATING FACTORS

CSFs such as GM-CSF are also identified as participants in pulmonary host defense. These factors, including G-CSF and macrophage colony-stimulating factor, are generated by a number of relevant pulmonary cells, including endothelial cells, epithelial cells, fibroblasts, mononuclear phagocytes, and T lymphocytes; production of these factors may be induced by an array of microbial products and pathogens.[717,718] Once elaborated at a site of potential infection, these factors exert pleiotropic effects on local immune cells, including increased membrane expression of receptors and adhesion molecules, enhanced motility, increased microbiocidal function of phagocytic cells, enhanced phagocyte survival, and stimulation of cytokine secretion by mononuclear phagocytes.[717,718] GM-CSF also acts on macrophages to stimulate their antigen presentation capabilities and directs DC differentiation and distribution in the lung.[719,720] Within the lung, GM-CSF is produced by alveolar macrophages, bronchial epithelial cells, and vascular endothelium. It is a potent stimulus for PMN degranulation, and its production by endothelial cells has been implicated in PMN-mediated alveolar injury.[721] GM-CSF deficiency results in a phenotype of pulmonary alveolar proteinosis.[722] Although the precise mechanism of this phenotype remains unclear, GM-CSF–deficient macrophages show reduced expression of the transcription factor PU.1 and reduced phagocytic capacity.[723,724] Furthermore, the alveolar macrophages of GM-CSF knockout mice possess a unique mix of M1 and M2 macrophages.[725] Although the capacity of neonatal T cells to generate GM-CSF is only 50% of adult T cells, mononuclear cells from neonates possess adult capacity for production of this cytokine and may thus be able to induce local responses dependent on GM-CSF elaboration. This premise is supported by data from newborns demonstrating alveolar macrophage generation of GM-CSF.[726] Of note, GM-CSF is increased in the bronchiolar lavage fluid of premature infants who have gone on to develop BPD.[727]

Of the CSFs, G-CSF appears to be most critical in pulmonary host defense against bacteria. Alveolar macrophages are potent secretors of G-CSF in response to LPS, or when stimulated by TNF or IL-1. Alveolar macrophage–derived G-CSF acts locally to recruit, activate, and delay apoptosis of PMNs while acting systemically to induce granulopoiesis and increase the circulating neutrophil count. The importance of G-CSF in this context is underscored by animal studies, where antibody neutralization of G-CSF results in profoundly suppressed PMN recruitment and diminished bactericidal activity against aerosolized *P. aeruginosa*.[728,729] Of note, G-CSF also induces antiinflammatory mediators such as IL-1ra and soluble TNF receptors, locally titrating the inflammatory response.[730] Neonatal monocytes can be stimulated to generate near-adult amounts of G-CSF. Preterm infants, however, appear much more compromised in their ability to up-regulate G-CSF production (10% to 30% of adult response), and this may constitute yet another deficiency of pulmonary host defense in this cohort.[731] However, a meta-analysis reviewing the efficacy and safety of either G-CSF or GM-CSF in neonates as prophylaxis to reduce the incidence of systemic infection or as means to prevent mortality concluded that there was insufficient evidence to support introduction of G-CSF or GM-CSF into clinical practice.[732]

ADHESION MOLECULES

Leukocyte migration from the intravascular space to an eventual inflammatory locus within the lung is a multistep process, dependent on mechanisms directing cell movement to the appropriate site; leukocytes must marginate and adhere to the vascular endothelium, followed by diapedesis between endothelial cells and movement from the vascular space.[733,734] Directed movement along concentration gradients of chemotaxins is one mechanism, while another is haptotaxis, or directed migration along gradients of endothelial adhesiveness. This latter process requires the presence of both leukocyte- and endothelial-derived adhesion molecules and is mediated by three families of molecules: the integrins, the immunoglobulin gene superfamily, and the selectins.

The integrins are a family of proteins involved in cell adhesion and motility. Present on leukocyte membranes, these molecules adhere to specific endothelial ligands and various components of connective tissue matrix. The integrins are expressed as heterodimers, each containing one α and one β chain; subclassification of these adhesins is based on specific α/β chain content.[735,736] The α4 integrins are expressed at high levels on monocytes, lymphocytes, and eosinophils. Although typically absent from neutrophils, α4 integrin is present on immature PMNs, or on mature forms under conditions of transendothelial migration or chemokine stimulation.[737,738] The β1 integrins include VLA-4, found on lymphocytes and monocytes.[739] The β2 integrins include CD11a/CD18, constitutively expressed on all leukocyte subsets, and CD11b/CD18 and CD11c/CD18, which are prominent adhesins of PMNs.[740] Because the PMN must deform to navigate the narrow alveolar capillary space, the PMN surface membranes are brought into close contact with those of the vascular endothelium, inviting adherence interactions.[741] CD11/CD18 is therefore maintained in an inactive state, until chemotactic activation occurs.[742] PMN activation results in a CD11/CD18 conformational change to an activated form that recognizes its corresponding endothelial ligand.[743] PMN activation also results in mobilization of a significant intracellular stored pool of CD11/CD18, facilitating additional rapid surface expression of this molecule,[740] although the constitutively smaller pool in neonatal PMNs may tend to blunt this response.

The immunoglobulin gene superfamily includes ICAM-1 and ICAM-2, VCAM-1, and platelet-endothelial cell adhesion molecule (PECAM). ICAM-1, the endothelial ligand for CD11/CD18, is expressed on endothelial cells constitutively and up-regulated in response to endotoxin, TNF-α, or IL-1β; ICAM-1 is also expressed on the surface of fibroblasts and epithelial cells.[744] VCAM is similarly up-regulated by TNF-α and IL-1β, recognizes VLA-4 (and other β1 integrins), and binds monocytes and lymphocytes.[745] PECAM is present constitutively and in the pulmonary vasculature it may up-regulate in response to hyperoxia.[746] Its primary counterreceptor is the P-selectin glycoprotein ligand-1 (PSGL-1), found on a variety of leukocytes, including PMNs. PECAM-mediated adhesion may be important in transendothelial cell diapedesis of PMNs from the intravascular space.[747]

The selectin family includes L-selectin, P-selectin, and E-selectin. L-selectin is expressed on the surface of PMNs and is shed shortly after activation in vitro.[748] P-selectin is stored in endothelial cells and rapidly mobilized to the surface after initial endothelial activation.[749] E-selectin (endothelial-leukocyte adhesion molecule) is expressed on the surface of endothelial cells only after activation by bacterial products or mediators including C1q, TNF-α, IL-1β, and IL-10.[750,751] PMN receptors for the endothelial selectins include PSGL-1 and sialyl Lewis X antigen (sLe^x), an oligosaccharide present on many proteins including the PMN adhesins L-selectin and CD11/CD18.[752] The initial step in leukocyte migration to extravascular sites is a slowing of leukocyte movement through the area of inflammation by a series of loose, transient, leukocyte-endothelial cell adhesions, characterized as "rolling." This step is mediated through interaction of endothelial selectins with PSGL-1 and L-selectin on the PMN surface.[753] Low L-selectin and sLe^x concentrations on neonatal PMN surfaces have been implicated in impaired chemotaxis but are likely not relevant in the pulmonary circulation, where the constrained vascular space obviates the need for this receptor-ligand interaction.[754] The next step entails binding of local chemotactic activators (C3a, C5a, IL-8, PAF) to the rolling PMN, inducing expression and activation of CD11/CD18 and shedding of L-selectin.[753] Subsequently, the leukocytes firmly attach to the endothelium via a CD11/CD18 to ICAM-1 interaction (PMNs) or by means of a VLA-4 to VCAM-1 interaction (mononuclear cells, lymphocytes).[755,756] The final step is diapedesis of the adherent leukocyte through the vessel wall and migration along a chemotactic gradient to the site of inflammation. Although this process remains incompletely characterized, transendothelial migration appears mediated by the adhesion molecules PECAM and the integrin-associated protein CD47.[757] Once extravasated, neutrophils appear to follow a fixed chemotactic gradient laid down in the extracellular matrix, migrating along interstitial fibroblasts and eventually squeezing between type I and type II epithelial cells to reach the air spaces of the lung.[758]

GENERATION OF A LOCAL IMMUNE RESPONSE

In animal models of bacterial pneumonia, the influx of inflammatory cells follows a well-orchestrated sequence. First, neutrophils enter the lung within minutes to hours of airway inoculation. This early neutrophil recruitment is partly dependent on TNF-α, IL-1β (which can up-regulate ICAM-1), and induction CXCL1, XCL2, and CXCL5. PMN accumulation is maximal within 2 days, with cell clearance primarily through apoptosis. Later PMN recruitment is in part regulated by IL-17, which stabilizes CXC chemokine expression as well as induced G-CSF.[443,635] By day 2 to 3, monocytes are recruited, with maximal accrual by day 5 to 7 in resolving inflammation. Lymphocyte influx begins by 5 days, often occurring despite clearance of the organism. Although the timing of events is not consistently this rigid, the sequential appearance of each cell type is characteristic, consistent with a transition from acute inflammation to a more specific immune response. Factors unique to the lung that regulate this coordinated host response are now considered.

INTRAPULMONARY NEUTROPHIL TRAFFICKING

Most marginated neutrophils (up to 50% of intravascular PMN) reside in lung capillaries; thus, compared with other organs, the lungs enjoy a large, readily mobilized granulocyte pool.[735] The narrow caliber of these vessels (diameter 5 to 9 μm) does not allow leukocyte rolling but rather requires neutrophils (diameter 6.5 to 8 μm) to deform and slowly squeeze through this vascular space; this imposes sustained PMN-endothelial contact, independent of adhesion molecules.[759] The small distance between pulmonary capillaries and their alveoli facilitates brisk PMN response to alveolar-derived inflammatory signals. In this setting, mediator activation of neutrophils induces cytoskeletal changes that reduce PMN deformability, thereby increasing duration of capillary transit and neutrophil-endothelial contact.[760] Of note, the impaired deformability of neonatal neutrophils may engender a larger marginated pool of these cells within the newborn lung. Once activated, "stiffened" neutrophils are retained briefly (4 to 7 minutes in vivo) near inflammatory sites, until appropriate adhesins can be expressed to facilitate firm attachment and eventual transendothelial diapedesis.[761]

Beyond the rheologic conditions promoting neutrophil margination, neutrophil trafficking in the pulmonary capillary differs from other vascular sites in the repertoire of adhesive interactions invoked. P-selectin is not expressed on pulmonary capillary endothelium, consistent with spatial constraints that obviate selectin-initiated rolling as an initial step in PMN recruitment.[762] However, once activated, neutrophils are sequestered only transiently and return to the circulation unless firm adhesion to the endothelium occurs. Available data suggest that this adhesion is mediated first by L-selectin, then by CD11/CD18.[763] Firm adhesion mediated by CD11/CD18 is temporally associated with resolution of neutrophil "stiffening," allowing sufficient PMN surface area to flatten and engage the endothelium.[760] Once firmly adhered, neutrophil emigration from the vascular space then proceeds in a manner that is either CD11/CD18-dependent or CD11/CD18-independent, depending on the specific stimulus. *P. aeruginosa*, *E. coli* (or its endotoxin), IgG immune complexes, and IL-1 each induce PMN emigration mediated by CD11/CD18; because these stimuli also up-regulate endothelial ICAM expression, CD11/CD18-dependent migration may result from critical availability of this counter ligand.[764] Alternatively, stimuli including hyperoxia, C5a, IL-8, LTB_4, and the organisms *S. pneumoniae*, *S. aureus*, and GBS induce PMN emigration, which is CD11/CD18-independent.[764,765]

ALVEOLAR MACROPHAGE REGULATION OF INFLAMMATION

The ability of the alveolar macrophage to recruit and regulate other inflammatory cells is the major attribute allowing alveolar macrophages to locally regulate pulmonary host defenses. In addition to their phagocytic function, the alveolar macrophage can recruit PMNs, eosinophils, interstitial and airway macrophages, and peripheral blood monocytes to the alveolar space; once present in the alveolus, these cells are either activated or suppressed by alveolar macrophage–derived mediators.

Mediators that up-regulate inflammation within the alveolus are not constitutively expressed by alveolar macrophages; their release therefore requires alveolar macrophage activation. Activation typically occurs through engagement of macrophage PRRs and can be titrated by competitive interactions with soluble PRRs within the alveolar milieu. One example of this is the interaction between SP-A and the CD14 ligand LBP. In the basal (uninflamed) state, SP-A is present at much higher concentrations than the acute-phase protein LBP and therefore is the primary ligand for any LPS inadvertently deposited from the air stream into the ASL. This prevents initiation of the LBP/CD14 pathway and dampens inflammatory tone within the alveolus. However, under conditions of inflammation, SP-A concentrations may fall dramatically, owing to degradation by PMN-derived proteases and elastases, whereas LBP is concurrently up-regulated as an acute-phase protein. Under these conditions, LBP becomes the dominant LBP in the alveolus; this facilitates alveolar macrophage activation via the CD14 receptor, amplifying the bioactivity of LPS and subsequent inflammation several-fold.[766] Alternatively, alveolar macrophage activation can occur in response to GM-CSF elaborated by activated alveolar epithelium or in response to IFN-γ elaborated by local NK or T cells.

The activated alveolar macrophage effects PMN emigration to the alveolus through its production of multiple neutrophil chemotaxins, including the lipid mediators PAF and LTB_4, complement components C3a and C5a, and IL-8. Activated alveolar macrophages also produce TNF-α and IL-1β, which, although not directly chemotactic, can activate PMN and up-regulate local endothelial cell surface adhesins; they may thereby facilitate PMN recruitment from the intravascular space. Additionally, alveolar macrophages have the capacity to recruit and activate other inflammatory cells. Alveolar macrophages can induce chemotaxis and activation of monocytes by secretion of the chemokines MCP-1 and MIP-1α. In pneumonia this resulting monocyte infiltration typically peaks between days 5 and 7. Mononuclear cell response to either MCP-1 or MIP-1α includes increased respiratory burst, increased chemotaxis, increased monocyte expression of β2 integrins, and increased generation of arachidonic acid products; MCP-1 has also been shown to prime macrophages to respond to LPS, resulting in a proinflammatory amplifying loop. NK cells are also recruited and activated by these chemokines, and alveolar macrophage–derived IL-12 increases NK cell cytotoxicity and induces NK-derived IFN-γ, generating another proinflammatory amplifying loop.

Consistent with its role in regulating intraalveolar immune responses, the alveolar macrophage also induces or expresses several mediators capable of honing or down-regulating local inflammatory processes. IL-6 derived directly from alveolar macrophage or from alveolar cells (fibroblasts, endothelium, epithelium) in response to alveolar macrophage–derived IL-1 induces T and B cell proliferation but down-regulates subsequent alveolar macrophage production of TNF or IL-1. More directly, alveolar macrophage–derived IL-1ra, produced in response to endotoxin or adherent IgG, inhibits local IL-1β effects by competitive binding of the IL-1 receptor. Alveolar macrophage release of PGE_2 suppresses chemotaxis and release of inflammatory LTs by PMNs and alveolar macrophages, further down-regulating TNF and IL-1 production. Alveolar macrophage–secreted TGF-β blunts further alveolar macrophage response to LPS and serves to dampen the proinflammatory amplifying loops noted earlier. Additionally, alveolar macrophages can be induced to generate IL-10, although the most prominent alveolar source of this cytokine may actually be the recruited peripheral monocytes. This cytokine exhibits protean antiinflammatory activity. It suppresses a variety of proinflammatory cytokines and facilitates transition to a T cell–mediated adaptive immune response. Finally, alveolar macrophages down-regulate inflammation in the air space through clearance of apoptotic neutrophils; this activity is enhanced by the effects of IL-10, which diminishes phagocyte killing capability but up-regulates phagocytic function. This constitutes an antiinflammatory function because failure to clear necrotic PMNs results in protease release, local cell injury, sustained inflammation, and parenchymal destruction, as demonstrated in animal models of pneumonia.[767] Alveolar macrophages are poor at antigen presentation because they express low levels of costimulatory molecules. Thus it is thought that DCs play a key role in initiating of adaptive immunity in the lung.

DENDRITIC CELLS AND ADAPTIVE IMMUNE RESPONSES

DCs are distributed throughout the airways of the respiratory tract. Moreover, their numbers can be greatly augmented within a short time by TLR agonists such as LPS.[768,769] Airways contain intraepithelial DCs that can extend dendritic processes into the ASL to sample antigens from the airway surface.[768,769] DCs of the myeloid subset express TLR2, 4, 5, and 9 and are critical for recognizing many extracellular pathogens. Plasmacytoid DCs enriched for TLRs such as TLR7, which can recognize viral RNAs, are critical for induction of type I interferons in response to RSV infection.[770] As mentioned, IDCs are endocytic and upon TLR activation mature and migrate to regional lymph nodes via the up-regulation of CCR7. For *M. tuberculosis,* the induction of IL-12p40 is also critical for this migration.[11] Once there, antigen presentation to T cells can occur. Naïve T cells develop under control of both costimulation and cytokine signals to Th1, Th2, Th17, or Treg cells. It has been shown that inhaled antigen that lacks PRR or TLR activation does not lead to anergy in the lung. In contrast, pure antigen that lacks TLR or other PRR activators can induce a population of Foxp3 regulatory T cells that express surface TGF-β, and this T cell population is critical for the development of tolerance in the lung.[771] This mechanism is very important, as the lung encounters a lot of inhaled particulate and cannot afford to generate robust immune responses to each particle or risk the development of chronic lung inflammation. Once an effector T cell is generated, however, it recirculates back to the site of infection along chemokine gradients. This is also the basis of mucosal vaccination to generate a pool of effector memory T cells that can rapidly respond to a pathogen challenge.

The mucosal IgA response is regulated by T cells, which provide an initial contact-dependent signal to the B cell and subsequently secrete TGF-β, resulting in B cell switching of IgM expression to IgA expression.[772] The T cell cytokines IL-5 and IL-6 are necessary for final differentiation of surface IgA-expressing B cells to IgA-secreting plasma cells. Similarly, elaboration of other cytokines during T cell–mediated activation induces B cell switching to other immunoglobulin classes.

In the neonate, however, effective pulmonary adaptive immune response is impaired at multiple levels. As noted previously, the phenotype of neonatal T cells is essentially that of antigenically naïve adult T cells, presumably caused by limited antigen exposure. These T cells exhibit decreased surface density of TCRs and decreased adhesion molecules. They require sustained receptor stimulation for activation, as well as greater costimulation to achieve a Th1 phenotype. Additionally, whereas memory T cells tend to home to specific organs based on prior antigenic exposure, neonatal T cells preferentially reside in distal lymphoid tissues, resulting in delayed recruitment. The net effect is a neonatal lymphocyte response that is more delayed, less facile in terms of accessory cell activation, less able to rapidly evolve a Th1 cellular immune response, less focused in regard to specific antibody production, and possibly less efficient in terms of dampening inflammatory responses once initiated.

RESOLUTION OF INFLAMMATION

Because inflammation due to cellular responses may induce local tissue injury, the capacity to appropriately down-regulate inflammation is essential to preserve lung function. One mechanism of counterbalancing T cell immunity is provided by networks involving Treg and Th2 cytokines. As mentioned previously, both IL-10 and TGF-β can regulate Th1 immune response. It has been shown, that depletion of Tregs markedly enhances lung inflammation and lung injury in response to *P. carinii* lung infection.[773] IL-4 can suppress the development of both Th1 and Th17 cells.[436] It has also been shown that another IL-12 family member, IL-27, signaling via *Stat1,* can suppress Th17 development and thus may also be another critical negative regulator of IL-17–induced inflammation in the lung.[774,775] Many cytokines can also induce suppressor of cytokine signaling proteins such as SOCS3 that can antagonize cytokine receptor signaling to dampen inflammation.

SYSTEMIC CYTOKINE NETWORKING

Pulmonary cytokines generated in response to a local infection ideally, but rarely, remain confined to the alveolar space. Inflammatory disruption of alveolar epithelial integrity allows movement of locally generated cytokines into the intravascular space; this results in systemic cytokine networking, which may be either beneficial or deleterious to the host, depending on the specific cytokine and the context of the infection. For instance, it is likely that lung IL-6 generated during alveolar inflammation reaches the systemic circulation, where it stimulates the hepatic acute-phase response. Another example of systemic cytokine networking is provided by alveolar-derived CSFs, which are generated as part of the amplification response in pulmonary inflammation. GM-CSF and G-CSF are produced by alveolar macrophages in response to LPS, TNF-α, or IL-1β, whereas GM-CSF is also produced by stimulated epithelial cells and endothelial cells. Alveolar macrophages recovered from patients with pneumonia spontaneously release G-CSF, which acts locally to activate recruited PMNs and delay their apoptosis.[776] In animal models of pneumonia, levels of G-CSF rise rapidly in the lungs and are measurable in the serum within 24 hours; this response is virtually ablated by antibody neutralization of TNF, underscoring the role of cytokine networking in generating alveolar G-CSF.[777] Quinton and colleagues have shown that in the first few hours of pneumonia the lung is the principal source of G-CSF.[777] Parallel studies have demonstrated that intratracheal deposition of G-CSF induces systemic neutrophilia. Taken together, these data suggest a model in which the lung, when challenged by bacteria, produces G-CSF in response to locally generated early response cytokines. Alveolar G-CSF easily reaches the circulation, stimulates granulopoiesis, and amplifies the PMN recruitment response. This response is associated with higher PMN counts in BAL specimens, more rapid bacterial clearance, and increased host survival.[728]

A complete reference list is available at www.ExpertConsult.com. 

SELECT REFERENCES

1. Longo LD. Fetal gas exchange. In: Crystal RG, West JB, eds. *The Lung: Scientific Foundations*. New York: Raven Press; 1991:1699-1710.
2. Beutler B. Not "molecular patterns" but molecules. *Immunity*. 2003;19:155-156.
3. Vermaelen KY, Carro-Muino I, Lambrecht BN, et al. Specific migratory dendritic cells rapidly transport antigen from the airways to the thoracic lymph nodes. *J Exp Med*. 2001;193:51-60.
4. Muir A, Soong G, Sokol S, et al. Toll-like receptors in normal and cystic fibrosis airway epithelial cells. *Am J Respir Cell Mol Biol*. 2004;30:777-783.
5. Guo RF, Ward PA. Mediators and regulation of neutrophil accumulation in inflammatory responses in lung: insights from the IgG immune complex model. *Free Radic Biol Med*. 2002;33:303-310.
6. Tsai WC, Strieter RM, Mehrad B, et al. CXC chemokine receptor CXCR2 is essential for protective innate host response in murine *Pseudomonas aeruginosa* pneumonia. *Infect Immun*. 2000;68:4289-4296.
7. Avery ME. Surfactant deficiency in hyaline membrane disease: the story of discovery. *Am J Respir Crit Care Med*. 2000;161:1074-1075.
8. Kuroki Y, Takahashi M, Nishitani C. Pulmonary collectins in innate immunity of the lung. *Cell Microbiol*. 2007;9:1871-1879.
9. Kingma PS, Whitsett JA. In defense of the lung: surfactant protein A and surfactant protein D. *Curr Opin Pharmacol*. 2006;6:277-283.
10. Palecanda A, Kobzik L. Receptors for unopsonized particles: the role of alveolar macrophage scavenger receptors. *Curr Mol Med*. 2001;1:589-595.

11. Khader SA, Partida-Sanchez S, Bell G, et al. Interleukin 12p40 is required for dendritic cell migration and T cell priming after *Mycobacterium tuberculosis* infection. *J Exp Med*. 2006;203:1805-1815.
12. Artis D, Spits H. The biology of innate lymphoid cells. *Nature*. 2015;517:293-301.
13. Gumbiner B. Structure, biochemistry, and assembly of epithelial tight junctions. *Am J Physiol*. 1987;253:C749-C758.
14. Donaldson SH, Boucher RC. Update on pathogenesis of cystic fibrosis lung disease. *Curr Opin Pulm Med*. 2003;9:486-491.
15. Plopper CG, Mariassy AT, Lollini LO. Structure as revealed by airway dissection. A comparison of mammalian lungs. *Am Rev Respir Dis*. 1983;128:S4-S7.
16. Breeze RG, Wheeldon EB. The cells of the pulmonary airways. *Am Rev Respir Dis*. 1977;116:705-777.
17. Sanderson MJ, Chow I, Dirksen ER. Intercellular communication between ciliated cells in culture. *Am J Physiol*. 1988;254:C63. -C74.
18. Gaillard DA, Lallement AV, Petit AF, et al. *In vivo* ciliogenesis in human fetal tracheal epithelium. *Am J Anat*. 1989;185:415-428.
19. Giangreco A, Reynolds SD, Stripp BR. Terminal bronchioles harbor a unique airway stem cell population that localizes to the bronchoalveolar duct junction. *Am J Pathol*. 2002;161:173-182.
20. Johnson NF, Hubbs AF. Epithelial progenitor cells in the rat trachea. *Am J Respir Cell Mol Biol*. 1990;3:579-585.
21. Vaughan AE, Brumwell AN, Xi Y, et al. Lineage-negative progenitors mobilize to regenerate lung epithelium after major injury. *Nature*. 2015;517:621-625.
22. Rhodin JA: The ciliated cell. Ultrastructure and function of the human tracheal mucosa. *Am Rev Respir Dis*. 93(suppl 15):1966.
23. Widdicombe JG, Pack RJ. The Clara cell. *Eur J Respir Dis*. 1982;63:202-220.
24. Knowles MR, Boucher RC. Mucus clearance as a primary innate defense mechanism for mammalian airways. *J Clin Invest*. 2002;109:571-577.
25. Kim KC. Role of epithelial mucins during airway infection. *Pulm Pharmacol Ther*. 2012;25:415-419.
26. Pickles RJ, Fahrner JA, Petrella JM, et al. Retargeting the coxsackievirus and adenovirus receptor to the apical surface of polarized epithelial cells reveals the glycocalyx as a barrier to adenovirus-mediated gene transfer. *J Virol*. 2000;74:6050-6057.
27. Hastie AT, Marchese-Ragona SP, Johnson KA, et al. Structure and mass of mammalian respiratory ciliary outer arm 19S dynein. *Cell Motil Cytoskeleton*. 1988;11:157-166.
28. Benali R, Tournier JM, Chevillard M, et al. Tubule formation by human surface respiratory epithelial cells cultured in a three-dimensional collagen lattice. *Am J Physiol*. 1993;264:L183-L192.
29. Foliguet B, Puchelle E. Apical structure of human respiratory cilia. *Bull Eur Physiopathol Respir*. 1986;22:43-47.
30. Zariwala MA, Knowles MR, Omran H. Genetic defects in ciliary structure and function. *Annu Rev Physiol*. 2007;69:423-450.
31. Sanderson MJ, Sleigh MA. Ciliary activity of cultured rabbit tracheal epithelium: beat pattern and metachrony. *J Cell Sci*. 1981;47:331-347.
32. Holley MC, Afzelius BA. Alignment of cilia in immotile-cilia syndrome. *Tissue Cell*. 1986;18:521-529.
33. Gibbons IR. Cilia and flagella of eukaryotes. *J Cell Biol*. 1981;91:107s-124s.
34. Marino MR, Aiello E. Cinemicrographic analysis of beat dynamics of human respiratory cilia. *Prog Clin Biol Res*. 1982;80:35-39.
35. Sleigh MA, Blake JR, Liron N. The propulsion of mucus by cilia. *Am Rev Respir Dis*. 1988;137:726-741.
36. Sanderson MJ, Charles AC, Dirksen ER. Mechanical stimulation and intercellular communication increases intracellular Ca2+ in epithelial cells. *Cell Regul*. 1990;1:585-596.
37. Salathe M. Regulation of mammalian ciliary beating. *Annu Rev Physiol*. 2007;69:401-422.
38. Li D, Shirakami G, Zhan X, et al. Regulation of ciliary beat frequency by the nitric oxide-cyclic guanosine monophosphate signaling pathway in rat airway epithelial cells. *Am J Respir Cell Mol Biol*. 2000;23:175-181.
39. Ingels KJ, Meeuwsen F, Graamans K, et al. Influence of sympathetic and parasympathetic substances in clinical concentrations on human nasal ciliary beat. *Rhinology*. 1992;30:149-159.
40. Kim CH, Kim SS, Choi JY, et al. Membrane-specific expression of functional purinergic receptors in normal human nasal epithelial cells. *Am J Physiol Lung Cell Mol Physiol*. 2004;287:L835-L842.
41. Devalia JL, Sapsford RJ, Rusznak C, et al. The effects of salmeterol and salbutamol on ciliary beat frequency of cultured human bronchial epithelial cells, *in vitro*. *Pulm Pharmacol*. 1992;5:257-263.
42. Gaston B. Nitric oxide and thiol groups. *Biochim Biophys Acta*. 1999;1411:323-333.
43. Elliott MK, Sisson JH, Wyatt TA. Effects of cigarette smoke and alcohol on ciliated tracheal epithelium and inflammatory cell recruitment. *Am J Respir Cell Mol Biol*. 2007;36:452-459.
44. Tarran R, Button B, Boucher RC. Regulation of normal and cystic fibrosis airway surface liquid volume by phasic shear stress. *Annu Rev Physiol*. 2006;68:543-561.
45. Bruns JB, Carattino MD, Sheng S, et al. Epithelial Na+ channels are fully activated by furin- and prostasin-dependent release of an inhibitory peptide from the gamma-subunit. *J Biol Chem*. 2007;282:6153-6160.
46. Myerburg MM, Harvey PR, Heidrich EM, et al. Acute regulation of the epithelial sodium channel in airway epithelia by proteases and trafficking. *Am J Respir Cell Mol Biol*. 2010;43:712-719.
47. Kunzelmann K. The cystic fibrosis transmembrane conductance regulator and its function in epithelial transport. *Rev Physiol Biochem Pharmacol*. 1999;137:1-70.
48. Ng AW, Bidani A, Heming TA. Innate host defense of the lung: effects of lung-lining fluid pH. *Lung*. 2004;182:297-317.
49. Pezzulo AA, Tang XX, Hoegger MJ, et al. Reduced airway surface pH impairs bacterial killing in the porcine cystic fibrosis lung. *Nature*. 2012;487:109-113.
50. Matsui H, Davis CW, Tarran R, et al. Osmotic water permeabilities of cultured, well-differentiated normal and cystic fibrosis airway epithelia. *J Clin Invest*. 2000;105:1419-1427.

Development of the Nervous System

124

Christopher J. Yuskaitis | Scott L. Pomeroy

INTRODUCTION

The human brain arises from a restricted population of embryonic cells to become the most complex organ system known during the brief 280 days of human gestation. The newborn brain is comprised of billions of neurons and glia arranged and interconnected in an exquisitely precise three-dimensional network. Unfortunately, minor changes have profound implications for postnatal development and function. Overlapping genetic and epigenetic events during neurodevelopment are tightly regulated in both time and space, transforming a thin disk of undifferentiated neuroepithelium into a complex multilayered system. The brain, with its massive prefrontal cortex and ability to investigate and reflect on its own nature and function, primarily differentiates human fetal development from that of other species. In this chapter we review the major temporal events in prenatal nervous system development together with several common disorders and anomalies that result from perturbations of these pathways. An overview of significant stages of central nervous system (CNS) development and the disorders associated with their interruption in fetal life is provided in Table 124.1.

EMBRYOGENESIS AND EARLY FORMATION OF THE NERVOUS SYSTEM

The fertilized human ovum divides symmetrically into identical totipotent blastomeres, and within a few cell divisions a blastocyst forms, uterine implantation occurs, and the inner cell mass contains cells committed to formation of the embryo. The progressive specialization of cells is highly dependent on extrinsic factors in the surrounding environment and intrinsic genomic expression. The temporal and spatial sequence of events during early development is tightly regulated. The nervous system is sensitive to genetic mutation (inherited or de novo) and local, epigenetic disruptions that may lead to similar or overlapping anomalies.[1,2]

One of the first steps in successful brain development occurs in the third week of gestation when the bilaminar inner cell mass, composed of the epiblast and the hypoblast, undergoes gastrulation to form the three embryonic germ layers (endoderm, mesoderm, and ectoderm).[1] The process begins with the appearance of the primitive streak (Fig. 124.1) on the epiblast surface and a defined cephalic pole, the primitive node. Formation of the streak is controlled primarily by the activation of the Wnt pathway. The epiblast gains the ability to migrate towards the primitive streak through the process of epithelial-to-mesenchymal transformation. Epithelial-to-mesenchymal transformation and migration towards the streak occurs under control of the Wnt pathway, the transforming growth factor β family member Nodal, and fibroblast growth factor 8, a growth factor synthesized by streak cells. Zinc finger transcription factors, SNAI1 and SNAI2, are mediated by fibroblast growth factors to down-regulate E-cadherin, the molecule responsible for epiblast binding. Decreased cell adhesion allows migrating epiblast cells to invaginate in the region of the node and streak, and delaminate and displace hypoblast cells to form the endoderm and mesoderm. Remaining epiblast cells differentiate into ectoderm.[3] The dorsal mesoderm gives rise to the notochord. The notochord then induces the overlying ectoderm to thicken and form the neural plate and subsequently gives rise to neuroectoderm, marking the end of gastrulation and the beginning of neurulation.

Gastrulation also marks the visible establishment of primary axes of the embryo and nervous system: lateral, anteroposterior, and dorsoventral. The future complex shape and three-dimensional structure of the fetal brain is determined by patterning events that begin with the establishment of the neural placode and plate. Two sets of polarity are required. The first is anteroposterior regional differentiation into future forebrain, midbrain ("neuromeres"), hindbrain (subsegmented into "rhombomeres"), and spinal cord, due to initial clonal restriction and refinement under the influence of local neural plate "organizers" and anteroposterior regionally restricted regulatory transcription factors.[4] The second is establishment of the dorsoventral polarity that sequestrates motor neurons from sensory neurons in the developing spinal cord, and eventually cerebral cortical regionalization into recognizable functional areas such as motor or visual cortex. Further, positional cues are conferred by mesodermal structures such as notochord and prechordal mesoderm. Intricate timing and precise localization of intracellular and extracellular factors are key in the establishment of the fetal brain.

Three major steps are required in the formation of the prospective forebrain. Ectodermal cells must acquire neural identity, rostral neural tissue must adopt anterior character, and regional patterning must occur within the rostral neural plate. In addition to the multiple feedback and feed-forward loops that exist, many factors are expressed several times throughout development, adding to the complexity of the system.

Neural induction is the process by which embryonic cells in the ectoderm acquire a neural fate (to form the neural plate) rather than giving rise to other structures such as epidermis or mesoderm.[5]

Ectodermal cells will acquire an anterior neural fate without extracellular cues. However, multiple extracellular signaling molecules are involved in the establishment of the rostral-caudal axis. Fibroblast growth factors, Wnts, retinoic acid, Nodals, and bone morphogenetic proteins (BMPs) are among the signaling molecules that have been proposed as caudalizing factors, which inhibit neuronal fate. Localized expression of the caudalizing factors, localized expression of caudalizing factor antagonists in rostral tissue, and morphogenetic movements keeping the anterior neural plate out of the range of the factors are the mechanisms by which the axis is formed.

BMPs and the transforming growth factor β signaling pathway promotes an epithelial fate and are potent inhibitors

Table 124.1 Neurology of the Newborn.

Development Event	Peak Time	Anomaly
Primary and secondary neurulation	3–4 wk	Craniorachischisis/anencephaly Encephalocele Myeloschisis Myelomeningocele Dysraphic states
Prosencephalic cleavage (ventral induction) and midline development	5–6 wk	Holoprosencephaly Agenesis of the corpus callosum Septo-optic dysplasia
Neuronal Proliferation		
Cerebral	2–4 mo	Micrencephaly and macrencephaly Hemimegalencephaly Tuberous sclerosis Polymicrogyria
Cerebellar	2–10 mo postnatally	Dandy-Walker malformation Vermian and cerebellar hypoplasias
Neuronal Migration		
Cerebral	3–5 mo	Schizencephaly Lissencephaly-pachygyria Heterotopias
Cerebellar	4–10 mo postnatally	Joubert syndrome Rhombencephalosynapsis
Neuronal Differentiation		
Axon outgrowth	3 mo to birth	Agenesis of the corpus callosum
Dendritic growth and synapse formation	6 mo–1 yr postnatally	Developmental disability Autism Angelman syndrome
Synaptic rearrangement	Birth to years postnatally	Down syndrome Rett syndrome Fragile X syndrome
Myelination	Birth to years postnatally	Cerebral white matter hypoplasia 18q syndrome Cerebral white matter disease of prematurity Nutritional and metabolic disturbances Leukodystrophies

Data from Volpe JJ, ed. *Neurology of the Newborn*. 5th ed. Philadelphia: WB Saunders; 2008.

of neural differentiation. If the BMP signal is blocked by one of many extracellular antagonists derived from adjacent cells, the Smad pathway is inhibited, allowing expression of the Sox proteins that activate transcription of proneural basic helix-loop-helix class genes. These genes code for a class of more than 20 transcription factors necessary and sufficient for nervous system formation, some expressed throughout the developing nervous system, others specific to regions such as the forebrain and spinal cord. Overall, if BMP signaling is too high, nonneural fates are promoted, whereas if it is too low, then more medial neural plate fates are promoted.[3,6]

Similarly, ectodermal cells acquire a neural identity through expression of antagonists of the canonical Wnt. Antagonism of the Wnt pathway occurs by extracellular proteins, such as the secreted frizzled-related protein, and intracellular factors—for example, the scaffolding protein axin 1 and the transcriptional repressor transcription factor 3. In addition, the transcription factors SIX3 and IRX are expressed in anterior and posterior regions of the neural plate, respectively, and act in a mutually repressive fashion in response to Wnt activity.[6]

The Notch/Delta signaling pathway allows delamination of ectodermal cells to become neuroblasts (i.e., committed neural progenitors) while laterally inhibiting other ectodermal cells from following this fate.[6] As a result of these signals, cells destined to form the neural plate elongate in an apical-basal direction to form the neural placode, broader at its cranial end and narrowing caudally.

Homeobox gene clusters encode transcription factors that establish an anteroposterior axis and control body segmentation through formation of somites. Within the homeobox clusters, forebrain and midbrain are specified by the OTX (orthodenticle homologue) gene family. OTX genes are expressed before the EMX (empty spiracles homologue) genes, which are expressed only in the forebrain. The hindbrain is specified by expression of the earliest HOX genes, *HOXA1*, *HOXA2*, and *HOXB2*. Expression and repression of these patterning genes is controlled primarily by gradients of the multiple extracellular signaling molecules.[7]

Our understanding of early neuronal patterning has been refined due to novel genetic techniques and the development of mammalian embryonic stem cell systems. The number of factors impinging upon the BMP, Wnt, and Notch/Delta signaling pathways has grown. Recent studies have added to the complexity of early patterning that demonstrates epigenetic chromatin-remodeling events that preconfigure epiblast cells to respond to these extracellular cues.[8] The precise interaction across these pathways and the contribution of epigenetic control mechanisms remain to be fully elucidated.

NEURULATION AND FORMATION OF THE SPINAL CORD

Neurulation is the process of formation of the hollow neural tube by folding of the epithelial neural plate (Fig. 124.2). Neurulation in humans occurs in two distinct phases: primary neurulation during weeks 3 and 4 of gestation leading to development of the brain and spinal cord (Fig. 124.3), and secondary neurulation during weeks 5 and 6, with formation of the lower sacral and coccygeal cord. Defects of neurulation are the earliest abnormalities of brain development that are clinically detectable in fetal life and extend into postnatal life.

The neural plate elongates into a drop-shaped structure, broader at its cranial end and narrower in the future spinal regions. This morphogenetic event, known as *convergent extension*, is under the control of the noncanonical Wnt pathway and downstream proteins such as VANGL1, CELSR1, SCRB1, and Dishevelled.[9-11]

The neural plate is further shaped by bending at the median hinge point overlying the notochord at the future upper spinal cord and at the paired dorsolateral hinge points at the levels of the brain and lower spinal cord. This differential bending appears to be under the control of signals diffusing from the notochord, including the signal transduction molecule sonic hedgehog (SHH), which is also the major determinant of ventral neural progenitor identity in embryonic spinal cord and forebrain.[12,13] Differential gradients of expression between the ventral SHH expression and BMPs in the dorsal ectoderm not only establish a dorsoventral plane but also lead to the later establishment of distinct classes of neurons with the spinal cord.[14,15] The neural plate rotates by elevation and convergence around the median and dorsal hinge points. This bending appears to be dependent on apical constriction of columnar neural tube cells to become wedge-shaped under the control of actin-related genes, such as *ARHGAP35* (a negative regulator of Rho GTPase), *MARCKS* (a protein kinase C

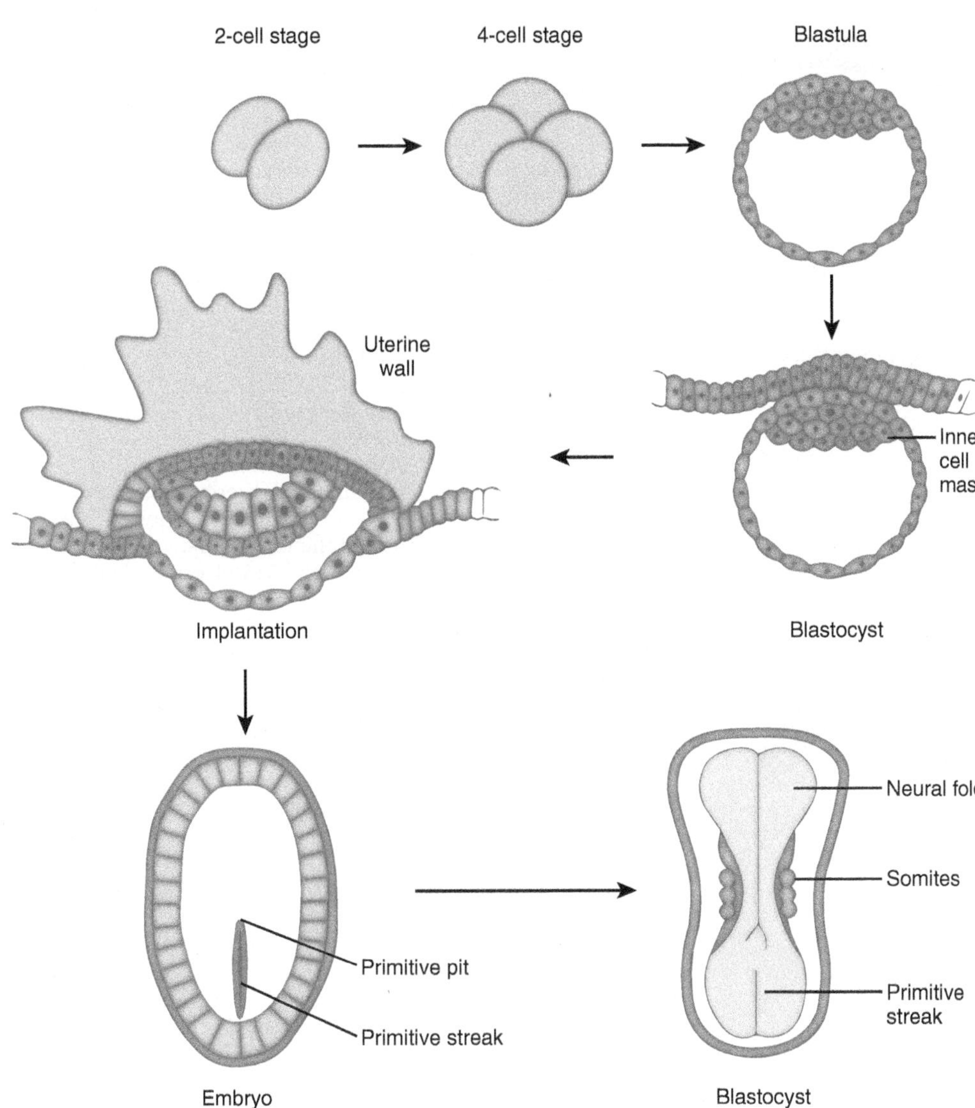

Fig. 124.1 Early development of the human embryo. Initial symmetric cell divisions are followed by multiple cleavage events to produce a distinct inner cell mass. This is followed by elongation of the embryo and development of the primitive streak. Cells migrate through the primitive streak to form the mesoderm. The overlying ectoderm forms the neural tube that will roll to form the brain and spinal cord. (Adapted from Sanes DH, Reh TA, Harris WA, eds. Neural induction. In: *Development of the Nervous System*. San Diego, CA: Academic Press; 2006.)

target), shroom genes (which encode an actin-associated protein family), and *VCL* (which encodes the actin-binding protein vinculin). Cytoskeletal proteins appear to regulate only cranial neurulation, whereas the spinal neural tube closes normally despite defects in several cytoskeleton-related genes.[9]

Neural tube closure appears to continue by the development of bilateral folds at its junction with nonneural ectoderm.[16] These folds elevate and become opposed in the midline, with fusion occurring by interdigitation of cellular protrusions from apical cells and the formation of permanent cell contacts. Membrane-bound ephrin ligands and their Eph tyrosine kinase receptors have been implicated in this process. Maintenance of proliferation by Notch signaling and apoptotic programmed cell death play important but poorly understood roles in the process as well.

Neural tube closure is a discontinuous process occurring at two invariant sites in humans, with a third variable site representing a potential factor for neural tube defects (NTDs). The open neural folds between initiation closure sites are known as *neuropores.* As closure progresses, the neuropores gradually shorten and close, leading to an intact closed neural tube. This is subsequently covered by ectoderm-derived epidermis.

Secondary neurulation is initiated after primary neurulation is complete and the posterior neuropore closes. The tail bud, a pluripotent mass of cells, a remnant of the caudal primitive streak, proliferates and condenses, followed by cavitation and fusion with the central canal of the neural tube. As this process of canalization progresses during ensuing weeks, neurons and ependymal cells differentiate to form the caudal end of the spinal cord. Resorption of the tail bud and other cells of the caudal cell mass leaves the filum terminale, which often contains ependymal cell nests along its length. These nests of ependymal cells can begin to proliferate later in life as a monoclonal population of glial cells. These ependymomas, uncommon glial cell tumors, are among the most common tumors of the cauda equina and filum terminale.

The closed neural tube consists of a thick pseudostratified epithelium of neuroepithelial cells that begin to divide rapidly immediately after closure and give rise to a second cell type, the neuroblast. These cells form the mantle layer, the future gray matter of the spinal cord. This further gives rise to an outermost layer, the marginal layer that will become myelinated and form the future white matter of the spinal cord. As neuroblast proliferation continues, the neural tube develops dorsal and ventral thickenings that become the alar and basal plates that will give rise to the sensory and motor areas of the spinal cord, respectively. A longitudinal groove, the sulcus limitans, demarcates the boundary between the two.

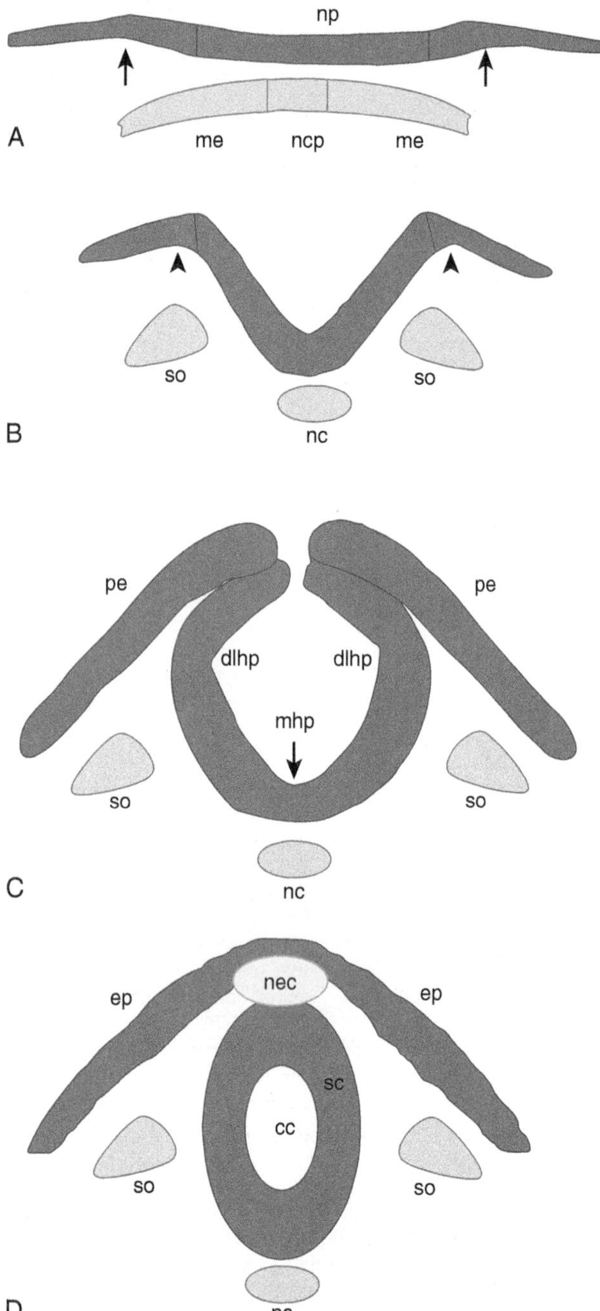

Fig. 124.2 A simplified diagram of neural tube closure. Neural folds form at the lateral extremes of the neural plate (A, *arrows*), elevate (B, *arrows*) and converge toward the dorsal midline (C), and fuse at their dorsal tips to form the closed neural tube (D). Bending or hinge points form at two sites: the median hinge point *(mhp)* overlying the notochord and the paired dorsolateral hinge points *(dlhp)* at the lateral sides of the folds. *cc,* Central canal; *ep,* epidermis; *me,* mesoderm; *nc,* notochord; *ncp,* notochordal plate; *nec,* neural crest; *np,* neural plate; *pe,* presumptive epidermis; *sc,* spinal cord; *so,* somites. (From Bassuk AG, Kibar Z. Genetic basis of neural tube defects. *Semin Pediatr Neurol.* 2009;16:102.)

As the neural tube closes, cells at the edge of the neural plate separate from the neural epithelium and migrate into the extracellular matrix to become neural crest cells. Neural crest migration is required for complete closure of the cranial neural tube but not for spinal neural tube closure. Although cell adhesion molecules were previously thought to play a role in neurulation, more recent studies have shown mice with null mutations in neural cell adhesion molecule (NCAM) or N-cadherin undergo normal neurulation. Down-regulation of cell adhesion molecules, transition from tight junction to gap junction molecules, and an increased expression of matrix metalloproteinases play an important role in neural crest migration.[9]

Neural crest cells migrate widely to become neurons and glia in dorsal root and autonomic ganglia. The fate of neural crest-derived cells is also to provide innervation for the gastrointestinal tract and to become neurons in the sensory ganglia of the cranial nerves (also formed in part by ectodermal placodes) and to become melanocytes, cartilage of the bone and face, and a variety of endocrine and structural tissues.[17]

The ultimate phenotypic and developmental fate of neural crest cells is tied to the timing, mode, and pattern of migration and is in large part controlled by the environment in which they reside. In addition to various permissive versus inhibitory signaling molecules including Eph/ephrin, semaphorin/neuropilin, and Robo/Slit, a complex relationship exists between neural crest cells and the developing vasculature. The dorsal aorta, the first major blood vessel established during embryogenesis, expresses BMP signals to direct migration and lineage segregation of neural crest cells into adrenal medulla or sympathetic ganglia. Schwann cells, neural crest-derived glia that ensheath peripheral nervous system neurons, direct patterning of arterial vasculature parallel to sensory nerves through the expression of *CXCL12* (also known as *SDF1*).[18] Neural crest cells retain a relatively broad developmental potential as they begin migration and their ultimate fate is strongly influenced by local factors.

NEURAL TUBE DEFECTS

NTDs are collectively the most common malformation of the nervous system, with an incidence of 1 to 2 per 1000 births, although there is significant geographic and historic variation in prevalence.[19] This variation hints at the complex cause of these disorders, in which both genetic and environmental factors appear to be significant, including maternal age and diet, maternal diabetes and obesity, teratogen exposure, and socioeconomic class. Pathologically, NTDs are characterized by a failure of closure of the neural tube at any level. Failures of primary neurulation frequently lead to "open" NTDs, in which the neural defect is exposed to the environment, whereas failures of secondary neurulation frequently lead to "closed" defects, in which the defect is covered by skin and integuments.[9,11] Open NTDs are usually associated with other CNS anomalies, in contrast to closed NTDs, where associated CNS anomalies are rare.

CRANIORACHISCHISIS AND ANENCEPHALY

These disorders represent the most severe failures of primary neurulation. Craniorachischisis is a rare and lethal condition manifested by essentially total failure of neurulation with a neural plate-like structure present but no skeletal or dermal elements overlying it. The incidence is unknown. Mutants of the Wnt/Frizzled pathway have been shown to result in craniorachischisis.[9] The equally rare disorder of failure of posterior neuropore closure known as *myeloschisis* is the inverse of craniorachischisis, where a neural plate-like structure without overlying vertebrae or dermis replaces large portions of the spinal cord.[20]

Anencephaly is primarily thought to be a defect of anterior neural tube closure and includes failure of formation of elements from the rostral portion of the neural tube anywhere to the foramen magnum caudally. There is also an absence of the frontal, parietal, and squamous occipital bones and scalp. The forebrain and upper brain stem are usually involved, resulting in a formless mass of degenerated, hemorrhagic neuronal and glial tissue. The risk of the

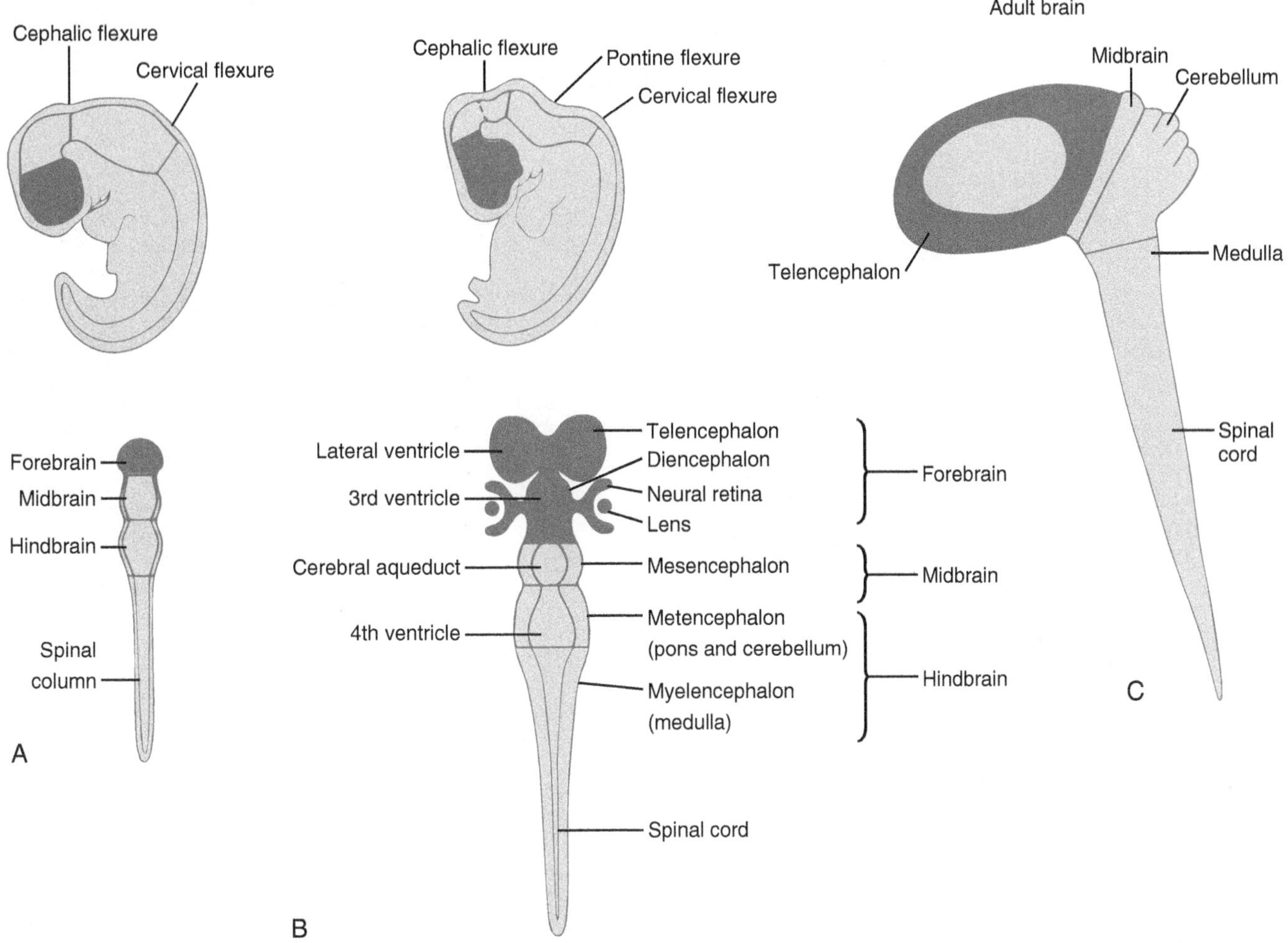

Fig. 124.3 Development of the brain and spinal cord from the neural tube. (A–C) The primary divisions of the brain. (A) The initial divisions of the three brain vesicles and spinal cord. (B) The next stage in development result in further subdivision of the brain which are related to the corresponding structures of (C) the adult brain. (Adapted from Sanes DH, Reh TA, Harris WA, eds. Polarity and segmentation. In: *Development of the Nervous System*. San Diego, CA: Academic Press; 2006.)

disorder varies considerably among geographic location, race, sex, ethnic group, maternal age, and socioeconomic status. The risk is higher in Irish and Mexican ethnicities, in very young and very old mothers, in those of lower socioeconomic status, in females, and in those with a history of previously affected siblings. The incidence showed a secular decline in the United States from 0.5 per 1000 live births in 1970 to 0.12 per 1000 births in 2011, likely due to mandatory food fortification with folic acid in 1998.[21] The onset of anencephaly is estimated to be no later than 24 days of gestation. Polyhydramnios is a frequent prenatal finding, and the malformation is now commonly diagnosed in the first trimester during routine obstetric screening, allowing elective termination of pregnancy.

MYELOMENINGOCELE

Failure of posterior neural tube closure results in a malformation of the spinal cord, myelomeningocele. This is the most commonly encountered NTD in pediatric practice because most infants born with this anomaly survive. Valproic acid exposure increases the risk 10-fold, and diabetic mothers are at increased risk as well.[9] The lesion consists of neural plate or rudimentary neural tube tissue herniating through a defect in the vertebra (spina bifida) in the form of a sac containing meninges, cerebrospinal fluid (CSF), nerve roots, and spinal cord. The dorsal part of the cord is most affected, and there may be some dermal coverings. The vast majority of myelomeningoceles occur in the lumbar region (Fig. 124.4B), and 10% may contain no neural tissue and are known as *meningoceles*. Spinal cord lesions above the myelomeningocele, such as syringomyelia, hydromyelia, and split cord, are common. Hydrocephalus, Arnold-Chiari malformations, and cortical dysplasias are frequent associations.[22] Fetal closure of a lumbosacral NTD is associated with better long-term outcomes,[23] suggesting that secondary effects of a prolonged open NTD can be assuaged.

ENCEPHALOCELE

This group of disorders represents herniation of the brain or meninges through the skull. The underlying pathogenesis is unknown but may relate to a disturbance in the separation of neural and surface ectoderm at the anterior neuropore. It is relatively uncommon, with an estimated incidence of 1 to 3 per 10,000 live births and is increasingly detected antenatally.[24] More than 70% of encephaloceles herniate through the occipital part of the skull (see Fig. 124.4A), although nasofrontal encephaloceles are relatively more common in Southeast Asia. Basilar, temporal, and parietal encephaloceles are unusual. The herniated mass may comprise one or more of meninges, CSF, or neural tissue—in some cases surprisingly well organized. Hydrocephalus occurs in 50% of occipital encephaloceles, and other malformations are common, including agenesis of the corpus callosum, Chiari III malformation, and subependymal nodular heterotopia.[22] Encephaloceles are found in a number of multiple congenital anomaly syndromes and are associated with first-trimester maternal hyperthermia, folate deficiency, and environmental factors.[24]

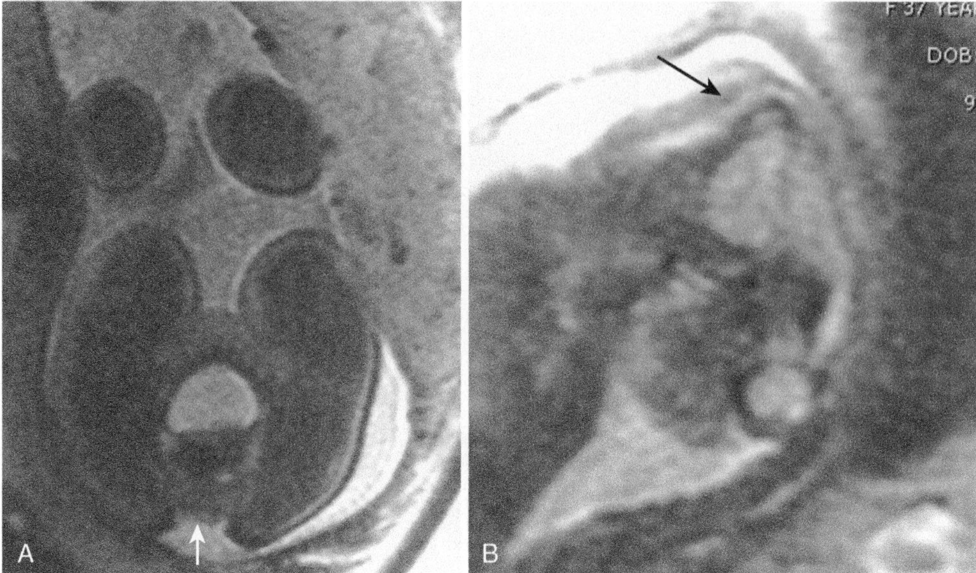

Fig. 124.4 Fetal magnetic resonance imaging at 18 gestational weeks. (A) Occipital encephalocele *(arrow)*. (B) Lumbosacral myelomeningocele *(arrow)*.

OCCULT DYSRAPHISMS

Disorders of secondary neurulation involve the caudal spinal cord and its coverings. The occult dysraphic states are commonly associated with vertebral anomalies and are usually covered with skin. Elongation of the conus medullaris and shortening and thickening of the filum terminale with "tethering" of these structures may result in traction injuries to the spinal cord. The occult dysraphic states are commonly associated with vertebral anomalies and are usually covered with skin. A *myelocystocele* is a localized dilation of the central canal in the caudal spinal cord often associated with severe malformations, including cloacal exstrophy and vertebral anomalies. The caudal cord in *diastematomyelia* is divided by a septum arising from a vertebral body. *Diplomyelia* is a divided, and at times duplicated, spinal cord with no septum. *Meningocele* is an extrusion of the subarachnoid space with no gross abnormality of either the brain or the spinal cord; when associated with a lipoma, the abnormality is referred to as a *lipomeningocele* and other tumors such as *teratomata, neuroblastomata,* and *ganglioneuromata* may occur and extend into the dural space. A cutaneous dimple in the lumbosacral region may be contiguous with a *dermal sinus* and a *dermal (dermoid)* or *epidermal (epidermoid) cyst* or may extend into the vertebral canal. Lipoma and dermal sinus are the most common of the occult dysraphic states.[25]

CAUSE OF NEURAL TUBE DEFECTS

NTDs have a heterogeneous cause; syndromic associations are recognized, as are a wide range of aneuploidies.[19] Specific teratogens are associated with NTDs, in particular thalidomide, carbamazepine, and valproic acid. Other maternal susceptibility factors include hyperthermia, low vitamin B_{12} levels, diabetes mellitus, and obesity. First-trimester ultrasound scans and increased α fetoprotein levels result in early pregnancy detection of NTDs. Periconceptual folate supplementation has been shown to significantly reduce the incidence of NTDs (up to 83% reductions with 4 mg of supplemental folate).[26] Additionally, susceptibility factors related to folate metabolism have been identified; polymorphisms in the gene methylenetetrahydrofolate reductase *(MTHFR)* have a significant increased risk of NTDs. Nonetheless, primary genetic variants in folate-related genes do not seem to account for the overall genetic contribution to NTD incidences.[9]

Studies in animal models, in particular the mouse, have identified a large list of candidate genes for human NTDs, in particular genes involved in convergent extension and the tissue polarity pathway. These include *ALDH1A2, CYP26A, MSX2, NCAM1, PAX* genes, *PDGFRA, PRKCA, SNAI2,* and *ZIC2*. Of particular interest is the gene *VANGL1*, the human homologue of the mouse gene *Vangl2,* which is mutated in the severe murine craniorachischisis loop tail mutant. Sequencing of *VANGL1* has identified a number of missense mutations in both sporadic and familial human NTDs.[9,21]

DISORDERS OF NEURAL CREST-DERIVED CELLS

Defects in neural crest development are known as *neurocristopathies.* Many of the neurocutaneous disorders are a result of defects in neural crest tissue.[27] Tuberous sclerosis and neurofibromatosis will be discussed later in this chapter but are a result of overgrowth of cells originating from the neural crest. In Waardenburg syndrome, children have hypoganglionosis, congenital megacolon, abnormalities of the great vessels, sensorineural deafness, and abnormalities of skin, hair, and iris pigmentation. Congenital aganglionosis (Hirschsprung disease) is characterized by a lack of neurons in the enteric plexus of the colon as a result of either failure of migration or failure of differentiation of neural crest cells. A mutation in *L1CAM*, a gene that encodes a neural cell adhesion molecule, has been described in newborn males with congenital hydrocephalus, aqueductal stenosis, and/or agenesis of the corpus callosum and Hirschsprung disease, suggesting a role for cell adhesion mediated by L1 cell adhesion molecule.[28]

Disorders of the spinal and autonomic ganglia are rare. Congenital insensitivity to pain with anhidrosis is an autosomal recessive disorder resulting from defective neural crest differentiation. The presence of multiple coincident neurocristopathies has been reported, specifically with the association between congenital central hypoventilation, Hirschsprung disease, and autonomic dysfunction, with *PHOX2B* the main disease-causing gene identified.[29]

EMBRYONIC DEVELOPMENT OF THE BRAIN AND VENTRICULAR SYSTEM

The brain forms from three vesicles that develop in the cranial neural tube: the forebrain (prosencephalon), midbrain (mesencephalon), and hindbrain (rhombencephalon). This process occurs at weeks 4 and 6 of gestation in humans shortly after closure of the anterior neuropore. Inductive interactions between the rostral notochord-prechordal mesoderm and the most cranial portion of the neural tube initiate formation of the fetal forebrain. As this process occurs in the ventral surface of the rostral neural tube, it is often known as *ventral induction*. This induction influences the formation of much of the face and forebrain, thus disruption of this process leads to severe brain disorders and accompanied facial anomalies. Ventral induction is followed by the cleavage of the forebrain in three planes: horizontally, to give rise to the paired optic vesicles, olfactory bulbs, and tracts; transversely, to separate the diencephalon from the telencephalon; and finally, sagittally, to form the paired cerebral hemispheres, lateral ventricles, and basal ganglia.

During the fifth week of gestation the cerebral hemispheres develop as symmetric invaginations of the lateral wall of the prosencephalon. The median portion of the prosencephalon forms the diencephalon, giving rise ultimately to the third ventricle, thalamus, hypothalamus, and mammillary bodies. The cavities of the hemispheres form the lateral ventricles and communicate with the lumen of the diencephalon through the foramina of Monro. The basal parts of the hemispheres begin to grow and bulge into the floor of the foramina to form the ganglionic eminence and ultimately the caudate and lentiform nuclei. Clusters of neurons along the midline begin to form nuclei of the brain stem, thalamus, and hypothalamus. The remarkable expansion of the cerebral hemispheres follows during the remainder of gestation.[30]

Transcription factors, such as FOXG1, GLI3, and PAX6, among others, play significant roles in dividing the telencephalon into dorsal and ventral sections.[31,32] FOXG1 is expressed in the anterior plate cells and induces the expression of fibroblast growth factor 8 to positively regulate ventral telencephalic development. PAX6 is essential for setting up the sharp border between the dorsal and ventral telencephalon. GLI3 expression is important for dorsal telencephalic development and induction of the Wnt and BMP signaling pathways. BMP signaling appears to be required for formation of the dorsal midline structures through the nodal pathway and induction of transcriptional regulators TGIF, TDGFI, and FASTI. Interaction between BMP and Wnt signaling appears to be important for hippocampal formation.[31] The transcription factors discussed and others, such as COUPTF1, EMX2, and LHX2, are responsible for cortical and subcortical development and regionalization.[32]

The SHH signaling pathway, activated by secretion of SHH proteins from the prechordal mesoderm, is critical to the development of the ventral prosencephalon.[12] SHH is a secreted signaling molecule that undergoes cleavage into amino-terminal and carboxyl-terminal domains. The amino-terminal domain binds to the patched 1 receptor to suppress its repression of the G protein–coupled receptor Smoothened, which activates downstream signaling. A key role for SHH is to antagonize GLI3-mediated repression of ventral telencephalic and spinal cord gene expression and thus promote ventral identities. For example, SHH is critical for thalamic patterning[33] and hypothalamus formation, because all hypothalamic tissue is absent in mice lacking SHH activity.[31] This requirement is observed for most ventral neuronal populations throughout the neuraxis, such as motor neurons of the hindbrain and spinal cord.[34]

These events are followed by midline prosencephalic development with formation of the commissural, chiasmatic, and hypothalamic plates, giving rise to the corpus callosum and septum pellucidum, optic nerve chiasm, and the hypothalamus, respectively. The earliest component of the corpus callosum appears at approximately 9 weeks, and by 12 weeks an independent corpus callosum is definable at the commissural plate. Axonal guidance following preexisting axon tracts from pioneering axons is critical in the formation of the corpus callosum. Mutations in *VAX1*, *GAP43*, heparan sulfate genes, and other genes are involved in a common phenotype where cortical neurons fail to reach the midline but continue to grow in swirled bundles of axons called *Probst bundles*.[35]

Glial structures such as the glial wedge, midline zipper glia, indusium griseum glia, and subcallosal glial sling are present at the midline and are necessary for corpus callosum formation. Guidance by the glial wedge occurs through Slit/Robo signaling. Callosal axons are attracted through Netrin family chemoattractants and then repelled from recrossing by Slit-activated Robo molecules. Dorsal to the developing corpus callosum, the glia of the indusium griseum express Slit2. Nuclear factor I family transcription factors appear to regulate the development of midline glia and commissural development. Multiple additional signaling molecules, including ephrins, semaphorins, and neuropilins, are also involved in axonal guidance and are critical for proper brain development.[35] As for neuronal precursors, emerging evidence indicates that radial glia undergo patterning by SHH and other organizational cues to generate restricted domains of precursors for astrocytes and myelinating oligodendrocytes.[36]

DISORDERS OF FOREBRAIN DEVELOPMENT

HOLOPROSENCEPHALY

Disorders of this group are the result of different degrees of failure of prosencephalic cleavage and are distinguished by the severity of failed cleavage of the cerebral hemispheres and deep nuclear structures. The most severe form is *alobar holoprosencephaly*, in which there is a single spherical cerebral structure and monoventricle with fusion of the thalami and deep nuclei, together with absence of the corpus callosum and olfactory bulbs. Neuronal migration and cortical organization are severely disordered. In *semilobar holoprosencephaly* there is failure of separation of the anterior cerebral cortex and absence of the anterior corpus callosum (Fig. 124.5). The least severe form

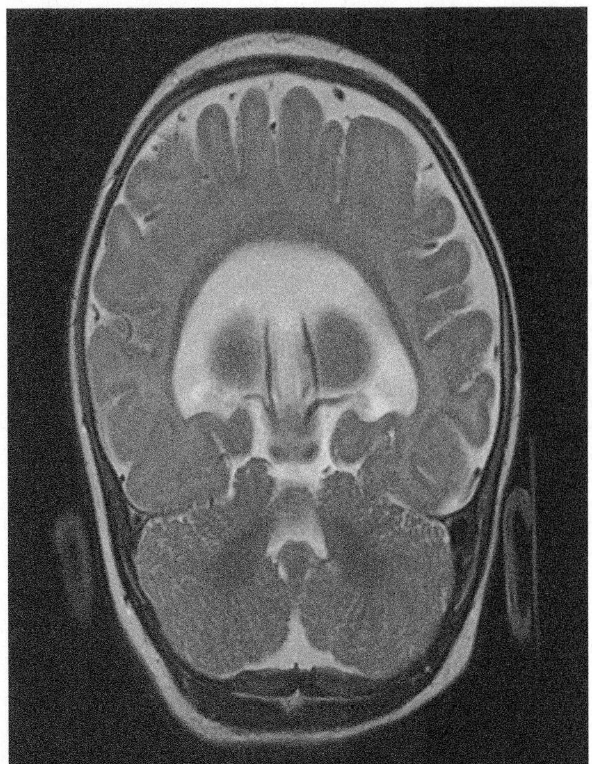

Fig. 124.5 Coronal magnetic resonance imaging of a 5-day-old infant demonstrating semilobar holoprosencephaly. Note the single ventricle.

is *lobar holoprosencephaly*, in which the cerebral hemispheres are nearly fully separated and the deep nuclei are partially or completely separated. In the *middle interhemispheric variant* only the posterior frontal and parietal regions fail to separate. Hydrocephalus is present in most infants with alobar holoprosencephaly due to fusion of the thalami and impaired drainage of CSF through the aqueduct. Infants with semilobar and lobar forms are usually microcephalic. Endocrine abnormalities are common due to disruption of hypothalamic development. Facial anomalies are usual and range from severe cyclopia with proboscis through ocular hypotelorism with a flat single-nostril nose (cebocephaly) to mild hypotelorism with or without cleft palate.[37]

The disorder occurs in 1 per 10,000 live births, but the incidence is 50-fold greater in conceptuses examined after miscarriage or abortion. Both genetic and cytogenetic causes are involved, as are teratogens. More than two-thirds of cases are related to full or partial chromosomal aneuploidies, in particular trisomy 13. Maternal diabetes and exposure to teratogens are significant risk factors, as are several identified genes and genetic loci listed in Table 124.2.[38,39]

AGENESIS OF THE CORPUS CALLOSUM AND SEPTUM PELLUCIDUM

Disorders of this group are characterized by various degrees of failure of midline prosencephalic development. Agenesis of the corpus callosum may be complete or partial and is associated with deformation of the lateral ventricles to give a parallel ventricular arrangement known as *colpocephaly* (Fig. 124.6). This is usually accompanied by abnormally formed Probst bundles coursing along the medial aspect of the hemispheres. Agenesis of the corpus callosum may be isolated or in up to 40% to 50% of cases associated with other cerebral abnormalities, in particular cerebellar malformation and cortical migration anomalies. It is one of the most common anomalies, occurring in up to 7 per 1000 live births and 3% of children with developmental delay. It may be completely asymptomatic; however, there is a strong risk of cognitive and neuromotor impairment when agenesis of the corpus callosum is associated with other anomalies. Agenesis of the corpus callosum is associated with more than 65 known genetic syndromes (Box 124.1).[40]

Absence of the septum pellucidum is another common anomaly and is frequently associated with more diffuse cerebral malformations such as schizencephaly, septo-optic dysplasia (or de Morsier syndrome), agenesis of the corpus callosum, holoprosencephaly, and hydrocephalus. Failure of fusion of the septal leaflets is known as *cavum septum pellucidum* and includes septo-optic dysplasia, in which absent septal leaflets are associated with optic nerve hypoplasia and disturbances of the hypothalamic-pituitary axis. Although most cases of septo-optic dysplasia are sporadic, mutations in several SHH signaling molecules (e.g., SOX2, SOX3) and a reduction in SHH expression in the hypothalamus can cause septo-optic dysplasia.[41] Remnants of Rathke pouch may give rise to craniopharyngiomas, suprasellar tumors that may cause hydrocephalus, visual field loss, and hypothalamic and pituitary dysfunction.

Table 124.2 Syndromic and Genetic Loci Associated With Holoprosencephaly.

Syndrome	Chromosomal Locus	Gene
CHARGE	8q12	*CHD*
Pallister-Hall	7p13	*GLI3*
Rubenstein-Taybi	16p11.3	*CREBBP*
Smith-Lemli-Opitz	11q12-13	*DHCR7*
Meckel		
Pseudotrisomy 13		
Ring chromosome disorders	ch13, ch18	
Velocardiofacial	22q11	*TBX1*
HPE and fetal akinesia	X	
HPE with ectrodactyly	X	
HPE1	21q22.3	
HPE2	2p21	*SIX3*
HPE3	7q36	*SHH*
HPE4	18q11.3	*TGIF1*
HPE5	13q32	*ZIC2*
HPE6	2q37.1-q37.3	
HPE7	9q22.1-q31	*PTCH1*
HPE8	14q13	
HPE9	2q14.2	*GLI2*
HPE10	1q41-q42 deletion	
HPE11	11q24.2	*CDON*
HPE12	16q21	*CNOT1*
	3p23-p21	*TDGF1*
	5p deletion	
	6q26	
	8q24.3	*FOXH1*
	20p13	

HPE, Holoprosencephaly.

FETAL BRAIN DEVELOPMENT

The embryonic events of the first 6 weeks of development establish the three-dimensional pattern of the brain and spinal cord and determine the fate of the first neural cells. Further developmental stages are characterized by massive proliferation and differentiation of neurons and glia, migration and organization of the cerebral and cerebellar cortex, dendritic growth and synaptogenesis, and finally, ensheathment of neurons with myelin. A common plan of cell layers, types, and connections is modified by regional variations in cellular architecture.[13] The result is an intricately laminated structure with a vast diversity of neurons with trillions of connections that underpin the unique cognitive and behavioral capacity of humans.[42] Although there is a limited capacity for regeneration and repair, neurons must remain dynamic and responsive to the external environment for decades.

Somatic mutations are being identified as important causes of neurodevelopmental disorders. Somatic mutations arise after fertilization during mitotic cell divisions in the developing zygote (Fig. 124.7). Post-zygotic somatic mutations lead to an individual who is mosaic, with only a subset of cells harboring the mutation. Somatic mutations often occur in genes that would otherwise be lethal if it occurred in the germline. For example, X-linked *FLNA* and *DCX* mutations are typically lethal in males, but males with somatic mutations in these genes survive and exhibit the typical disease seen in those affected. Late mutations in a subset of neurons may lead to an isolated defect of cortical development. Somatic mutations have been identified in genes associated with all aspects of brain development from neuronal proliferation and migration to cortical organization.

NEURONAL AND GLIAL PROLIFERATION

All neurons and glia are derived from the specialized proliferative centers close to the pial surface, the ventricular, subventricular, and the more recently described outer subventricular zones (Fig. 124.8).[43] Brain growth is characterized by neuronal proliferation between 8 and 15 weeks (Fig. 124.9) and generation of radial glia switching to primarily glial multiplication in the

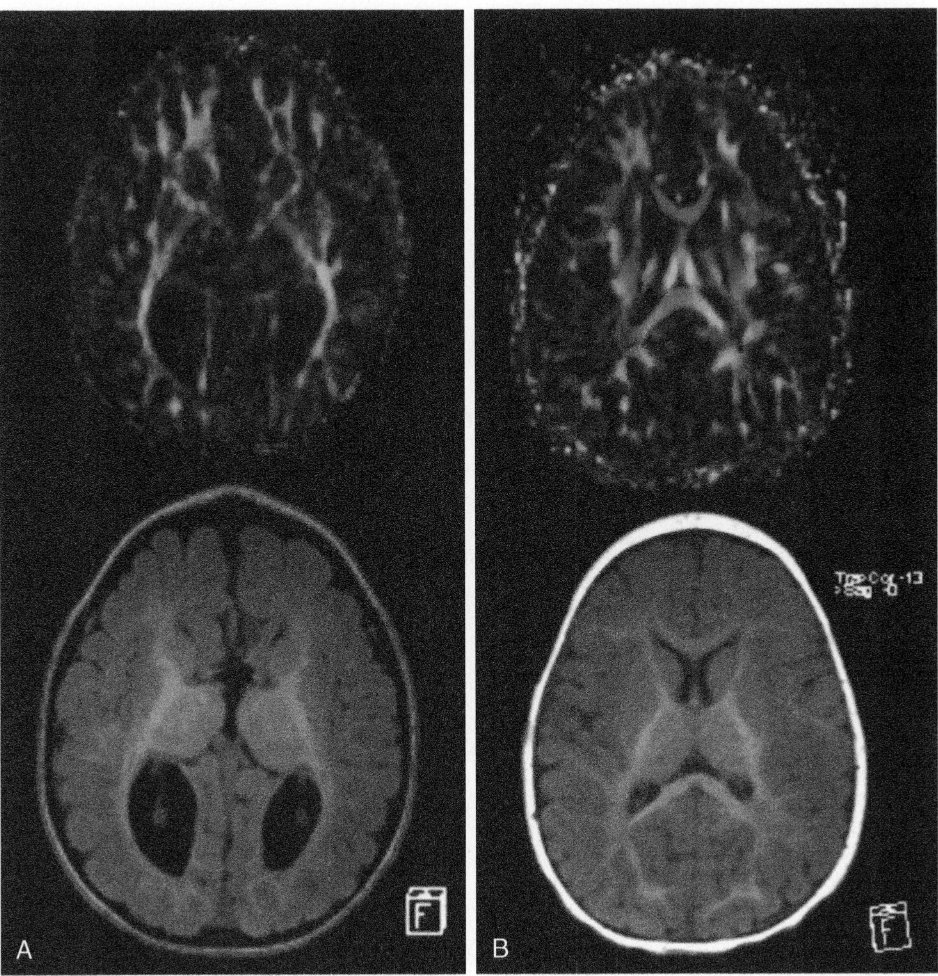

Fig. 124.6 Diffusion tensor imaging *(top)* showing white matter tracts and T1 magnetic resonance imaging sequences *(bottom)* in a brain with agenesis of the corpus callosum and microcephaly (A) and a normal brain for the age with an intact corpus callosum (B). Note the lack of crossing fibers in A that are seen in B colored *red/yellow*.

middle of the second trimester and extending into postnatal life. Some neuronal proliferation does occur later in gestation, primarily in the external granule cell layer of the cerebellum and the subventricular zone.

The cortical primordium is composed of dividing pluripotent neural stem cells and more restrictive neural progenitor cells that collectively form the ventricular zone. These neural cells divide through the unique process of interkinetic nuclear movement. As the nucleus moves in concert with the cell cycle, the environment along the apical-basal axis exposes the nuclei to different, proliferative versus neurogenic signals.[44] These early proliferative events dramatically increase the thickness and surface area of the ventricular zone, particularly in the forebrain. Derived from the ventricular zone, radial glia remain more pluripotent and are capable of producing both neurons and glial cells—astrocytes and oligodendrocytes. Radial glial cells are elongated nonneuronal cells that serve two functions: as a guidance scaffold for later migration of neurons and as neurogenic and glial progenitors.[45]

After the onset of neurogenesis, intermediate progenitors appear above the ventricular zone in a region known as the *subventricular zone*. (Conventionally, the ventricular surface is considered the top of the proliferative zone and layers described downward. *Apical* thus refers to the ventricular surface and *basal* refers to areas away from the ventricular surface, towards the pial surface.) The subventricular zone and its outer region are distinctively large and active in humans compared with other species and are the principal source of cortical neurons.[46] Increasing literature suggests that a select population of progenitor cells retain the ability to proliferate into adulthood.[47]

Given the link to multiple neurologic conditions and the interest in using neural stem cells therapeutically, there is growing interest in understanding the molecular mechanisms of neurogenesis and differentiation of neural progenitor cells. Proneural factors such as the transcription factor *ASCL1* and neurogenins 1 and 2 induce neural differentiation and activate the Notch signaling pathway. Notch signaling maintains the population of neural stem cells and distinguishes them from the progenitor cell population.[48] Regulation during development and adult neurogenesis is controlled by both intracellular and extracellular signals, ultimately choreographed by epigenetic changes. The mechanisms by which this process occurs include RNA-mediated feedback pathways, DNA methylation, and histone H3K27 methylation.[47]

The proliferative events involving the radial glial cell as a neuronal progenitor are modulated by several key signaling pathways involving the Notch receptor, the ErbB receptor via the ligand neuregulin, fibroblast growth factor receptor, and β-catenin.[45] Calcium waves propagating through connexin channels of the radial glial cell also appear to be important in the regulation of radial glial production of neurons.

Box 124.1 Partial List of Syndromes Associated With Agenesis of the Corpus Callosum (Known Genes in Parentheses)

ACC with spastic paraparesis *(SPG11)*
ACC with fatal lactic acidosis *(MRPS16)*
Acrocallosal *(KIF7)*
Anophthalmia-esophageal-genital syndrome *(SOX2)*
Aicardi
Andermann *(KCC3)*
Baraitser-Winter *(ACTB)*
Chudley-McCullough *(GPSM2)*
Cerebrooculofacialskeletal *(ERCC6)*
Craniofrontonasal dysplasia *(CFND)*
De Morsier *(HESX1)*
Donnai-Barrow *(LRP2)*
FG/Opitz-Kaveggia *(MED12)*
Fryn
Marden-Walker *(PIEZO2)*
Meckel-Gruber *(MKS1)*
Mental retardation–spasticity–adducted thumbs *(L1CAM)*
Mowat-Wilson *(ZFHX1B)*
Pyruvate decarboxylase deficiency (PDHA1)
Rubenstein-Taybi *(CREBBP)*
Sotos *(NSD1)*
Taybi-Linder *(RNU4ATAC)*
Toriello-Carey
Warburg micro *(RAB3GAP2)*
Wolf-Hirschhorn (deletion of 4p)
XLAG *(ARX)*

ACC, Agenesis of the corpus callosum; *XLAG*, X-linked lissencephaly with abnormal genitalia.

DISORDERS OF NEURONAL PROLIFERATION

MICROCEPHALY

Disorders related to impaired neuronal proliferation are categorized by the term *primary microcephaly*, or *micrencephaly*. This distinguishes the disorder from the more common microcephalies secondary to hypoxic-ischemic, infectious metabolic, or other destructive events. *Micrencephaly vera* refers to a group of autosomal recessive disorders characterized by small brain size because of a derangement of proliferation (Fig. 124.10). Radial microbrain is a rare disorder of particular interest because it appears to provide a clear example of a disturbance in a number of proliferative units without marked gyral abnormalities. At least 16 gene loci have been identified for autosomal recessive primary micrencephaly, or micrencephaly vera. *MCPH1* is crucial for cell cycle control, chromosome condensation, and DNA repair with mutations resulting in microcephaly in females. *CDK5RAP2* encodes for a centrosomal protein involved in microtubular function necessary for formation of the mitotic spindle. *ASPM* is also necessary for microtubular function at the poles of the mitotic spindle, and *CENPJ* similarly is involved in formation of the mitotic spindle.[49] Recent advances in genetic sequencing have identified several additional genes related to microcephaly that encode proteins required for proper functioning of the mitotic spindle and biogenesis of the centriole.[50]

Microcephaly can be caused by familial, teratogenic, and syndromic disorders (Box 124.2). In addition to the autosomal recessive group, inherited varieties include autosomal dominant and X-linked recessive types. The best-documented teratogenic agent producing microcephaly is irradiation (e.g., from an atomic bomb or by radiation therapy), particularly before 18 weeks' gestation. Maternal alcoholism and cocaine abuse are associated with micrencephaly. Micrencephaly, usually with developmental disability, occurs in as many as 75% to 90% of nonphenylketonuric children of women with phenylketonuria. Other teratogens responsible for microcephaly include anticonvulsant drugs and vitamin A toxicity. Fetal infections that may cause micrencephaly include rubella, cytomegalovirus, HIV, and the recently identified Zika virus.[51] A vast array of syndromes feature microcephaly as one of a number of fetal anomalies, in particular those associated with aneuploidies and chromosomal rearrangements.[52] Studies suggest that microcephaly genes are favored targets of natural selection during human evolution to drive evolutionary enlargement of the human brain.[53]

MEGALENCEPHALY

Megalencephaly (also known as *macrencephaly*) is characterized by a large brain greater than two standard deviations from the age-related mean and may relate to either excessive proliferation or abnormally prolonged windows for otherwise normal proliferation during development. Megalencephaly may be isolated or associated with severe neurologic findings, in particular epilepsy and developmental disability, or with other anomalies of somatic growth and some neurocutaneous disorders.[54] Megalencephaly is restricted to enlargement of the brain parenchyma and should be distinguished from macrocephaly, enlargement of the head size overall. In addition to megalencephaly, macrocephaly can also be caused hydrocephalus, ventriculomegaly, enlarged extraaxial spaces, and thickened skull bones.[55]

The cause of megalencephalies is classified as either anatomic or metabolic in nature. The metabolic megalencephalies encompass multiple disorders featuring accumulation of abnormal metabolites, whereas anatomic megalencephaly was described as increased size and/or number of cells without an identifiable metabolic abnormality. Both forms of megalencephaly have underlying genetic etiologies, and identification of causative single gene defects in these disorders has largely supported the original classification system.

Although metabolic diseases can be associated with both microcephaly and macrocephaly, there are several that are clearly associated with macrocephaly. Leukodystrophies, disorders of the white matter, with macrocephaly as a prominent feature, include Canavan disease, Alexander disease, and megalencephalic leukoencephalopathy with subcortical cysts. Most inborn errors of metabolism are not associated with macrocephaly, with the exception of glutaric aciduria type 1, where macrocephaly is present in the neonatal period.[56]

The most benign anatomic causes of macrocephaly are isolated sporatic or familial macrocephaly. Benign, familial macrocephaly is an autosomal dominant condition in which the head is unusually large at birth (greater than the 90th percentile in approximately 50% of cases) and continues to grow rapidly in early postnatal life. Neurologic findings are usually minor, and parental head size is also usually above the 90th percentile.

Macrencephaly may be associated with generalized disorders of growth, such as Beckwith-Wiedemann syndrome, Cowden syndrome, Fragile X syndrome, Marshall-Smith syndrome, Simpson-Golabi-Behmel syndrome, Sotos syndrome, and Weaver syndrome.[56] The function of genes associated with these disorders are implicated in either cellular growth or proliferation pathways. As an example, the gene mutated or deleted in Sotos syndrome, *NSD1*, encodes a nuclear receptor binding protein that may be involved in proliferative events.

Several neurocutaneous disorders are associated with evidence of excessive cellular proliferation within the CNS, sometimes with overt macrencephaly and evidence of excessive

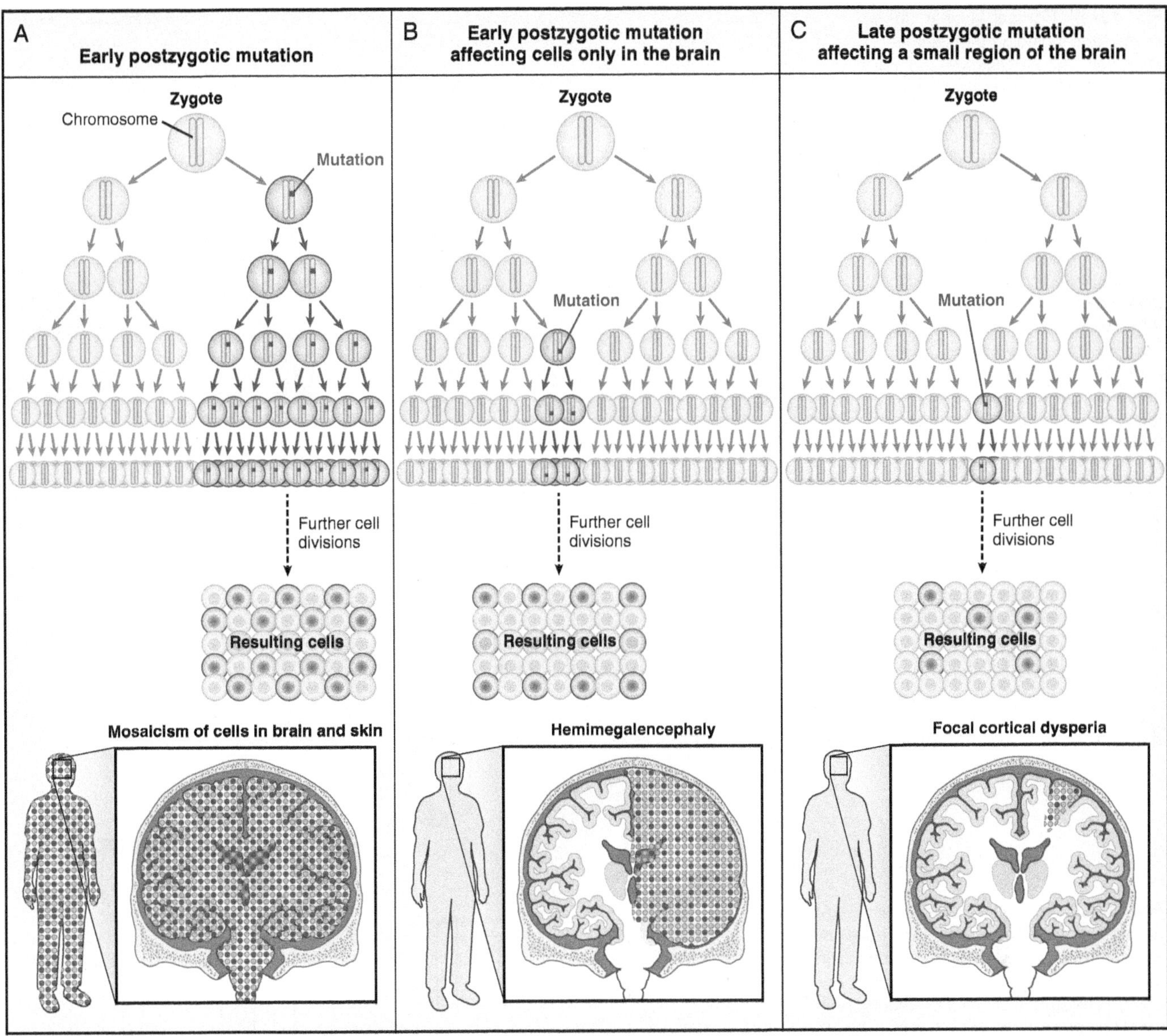

Fig. 124.7 The effect of timing of somatic/postzygotic mutations on the extent of the effect on the brain. *Panel A* shows a mutation (in *pink*) early in postzygotic development affecting half of the cells in the body. *Panel B* shows a mutation in a more differentiated cell type restricting the mutated gene expression to one hemisphere of the brain. *Panel C* shows a mutation in an isolated neural progenitor cell resulting in localized cortical disruption, such as seen in focal cortical dysplasia (discussed later). (From Poduri A, Pomeroy SL. Tracking the fate of cells in health and disease. *N Engl J Med.* 2016;375[25]:2494–2496.)

proliferation of mesodermal structures. Macrencephaly occurs most consistently in this context in the *PTEN*-related hamartoma syndromes and rarely in conditions such as megalencephaly-cutis marmorata syndrome and megalencephaly-polymicrogyria-polydactyly-hydrocephalus syndrome. Cowden syndrome, Bannayan-Riley-Ruvalcaba syndrome, Proteus syndrome, and Proteus-like syndrome are all associated with germline mutations in the tumor suppressor gene *PTEN*.[57] *PTEN* mutations are also one of the most common single gene mutations found in patients with autism and macrocephaly.[58]

Type 1 neurofibromatosis is an autosomal dominant neurocutaneous disorder characterized by abnormal glial cell proliferation. The megalencephaly relates primarily to increases in cerebral white matter. The gene responsible for this disorder, *NF1*, has been shown to encode a protein involved in the negative regulation of a key signal transduction pathway, the Ras pathway, which transmits mitogenic signals to the nucleus. Loss of the neurofibromatosis protein neurofibromin leads to increased mitogenic signaling, causing the proliferative abnormalities characteristic of the disorder.

Sturge-Weber disease is a neurocutaneous disorder primarily affecting the leptomeningeal blood vessels that also results in macrocephaly. Postzygotic mutations in the *GNAQ* gene are responsible for the formation of abnormal vascular channels and lack of proper cerebral vessel development. The characteristic features of Sturge-Weber disease are a facial port-wine stain on the affected side, cerebral calcifications, leptomeningeal angiomatosis, and congested deep cerebral veins.

Tuberous sclerosis complex (TSC) is neurocutaneous syndrome with abnormal proliferation of both neurons and glia resulting from dysfunction of the genes *TSC1* or *TSC2*, which encode the proteins hamartin and tuberin, respectively

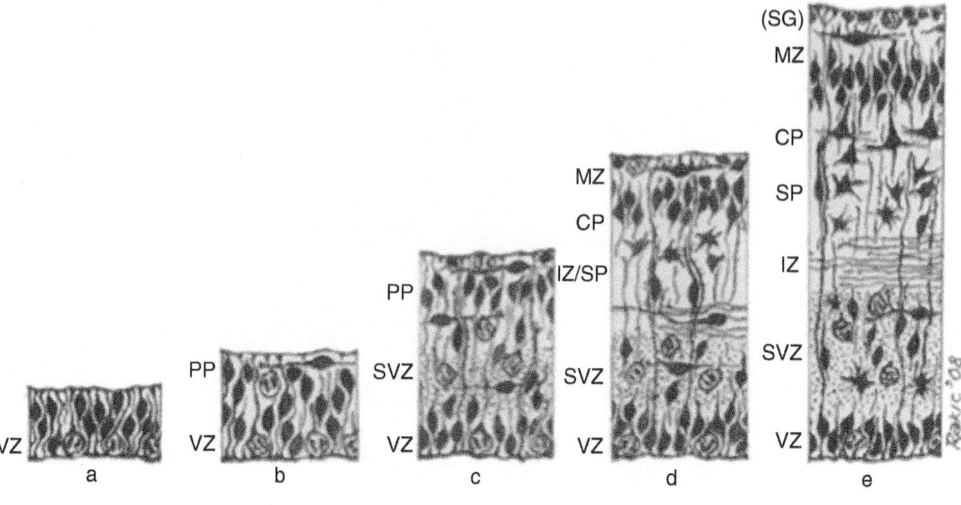

Fig. 124.8 Cortical laminar development, including transient fetal zones. The panels correspond to the following approximate ages (for the lateral part of the dorsal telencephalon): *a:* embryonic day (E) 30; *b:* E31–E32; *c:* E45; *d:* E55; *e:* gestational week 14. *CP,* Cortical plate; *IZ,* intermediate zone; *MZ,* marginal zone; *PP*, preplate; *SG,* subpial granular layer (part of the marginal zone); *SP*, subplate; *SVZ,* subventricular zone; *VZ,* ventricular zone. (Adapted from Bystron I, Blakemore C, Rakic P. Development of the human cerebral cortex: Boulder Committee revisited. *Nat Rev Neurosci.* 2008;9:110–112.)

Fig. 124.9 Neuronal development. (A) General anatomic overview of the developing cerebral cortex. Higher magnification diagram *(right)* of inset *(left)* illustrates ongoing proliferation of neural precursors in the VZ *(circles),* initial departure from the VZ *(light gray),* active migration into the cortical plate *(dark gray),* and subsequent arrest and differentiation into neurons *(black).* (B) Temporal progression of human cerebral cortical development. During the first 8 to 16 weeks of development, neural progenitors undergo proliferation, with the period of neuronal migration extending over 8–20 weeks. By 16–40 weeks, regional specification with clear formation of sulci and gyri is apparent. Earlier-born neurons *(black)* become situated in deeper cortical layers (V/VI), with later-born neurons *(light gray)* positioned more superficially in layers II/III. *CP,* Cortical plate; *CR,* Cajal-Retzius cells; *IZ,* intermediate zone; *MZ,* marginal zone; *SP,* subplate; *SVZ,* subventricular zone; *VZ,* ventricular zone; *WM,* white matter. (From Lian G, Sheen V. Cerebral developmental disorders. *Curr Opin Pediatr.* 2006;18[6]:614–620.)

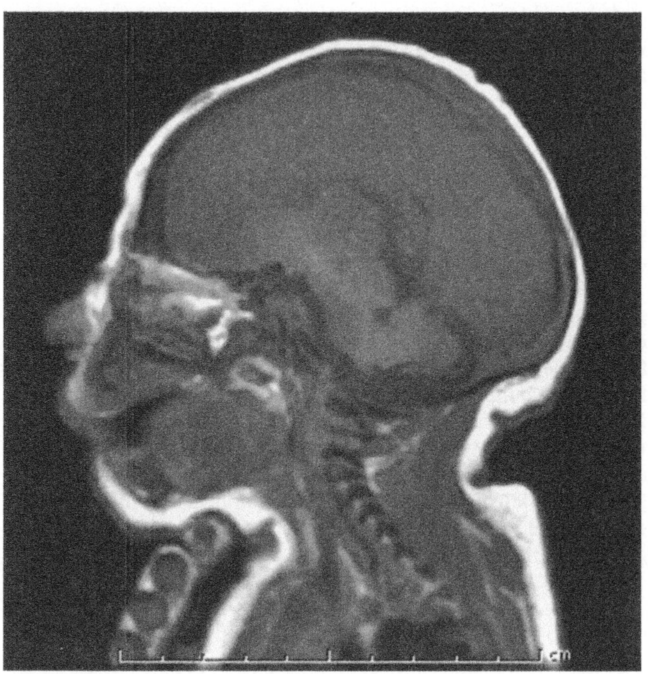

Fig. 124.10 Magnetic resonance imaging of a newborn infant with micrencephaly vera. Note the disproportion between the cranium and the face.

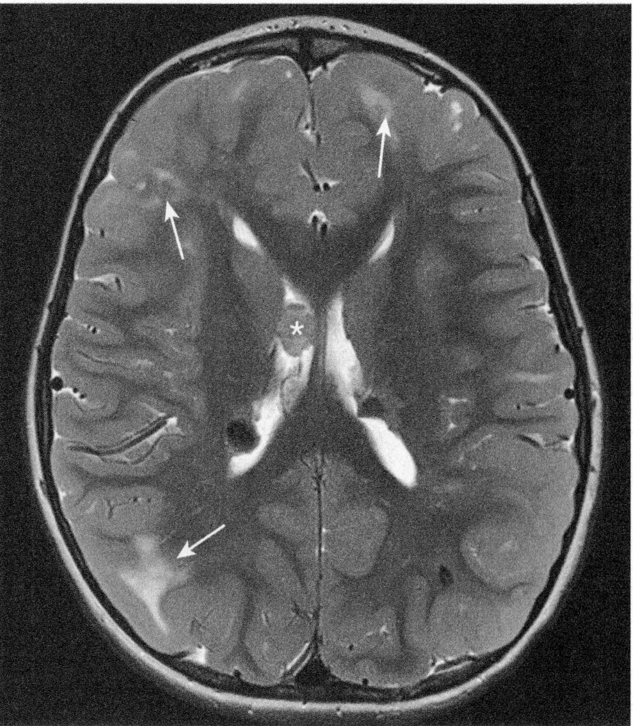

Fig. 124.11 Magnetic resonance imaging of a patient with tuberous sclerosis and a *TSC2* mutation. Note the cortical tubers *(arrows)* and subependymal giant cell astrocytoma *(asterisk)*.

Box 124.2 Partial List of Genetic Causes of Micrencephaly

Isolated[a]

AR micrencephaly
AD micrencephaly
XL micrencephaly

Chromosomal

Trisomy 21
Trisomy 13
Trisomy 18
4p deletion (Wolf-Hirschhorn)
5p deletion (Cri du chat)
7q11.23 deletion (Williams)
17p13.3 deletion (Miller-Dieker)

Syndromic

Angelman *(UBE3A)*
Cockayne (*ERCC6*, *ERCC8*)
Cornelia de Lange *(NIPBL, SMC1A, SMC3, RAD21)*
Fanconi
Mowat-Wilson
Pseudo-TORCH
Seckel
Rett
Rubenstein-Taybi
Smith-Lemli-Opitz

[a] For additional details refer to Jayaraman D, Bae BI, Walsh CA. The genetics of primary microcephaly. *Ann Rev Genomics Hum Genet.* 2018;19:177–200.

AD, Autosomal dominant; *AR*, autosomal recessive; *XL*, X-linked.

(Fig. 124.11). Hamartin and tuberin form a molecular signaling system critical for cell proliferation, cell growth, and cell adhesion/migration and lie as part of the phosphoinositide 3-kinase (PI3K), AKT, a mechanistic target of the rapamycin (mTOR) pathway.[55] Hemimegalencephaly is characterized by enlargement of part or all of one hemisphere, large and sometimes bizarre neurons, heterotopic neurons in subcortical white matter, and increased number and size of astrocytes. Although primarily due to an excessive proliferation of both neurons and astrocytes, defects in subsequent migration and cortical organization also occur. Patients often have early-onset intractable epilepsy. This abnormality may be sporadic or syndromic. Recent evidence has recognized the role of somatic mutations, a postzygotic event, in brain malformations and may explain the overlap seen between syndromic causes of hemimegalencephaly and megalencephaly.[55,59]

mTOR pathway genes are identified in a number of malformations of cortical development. Activating mutations of *MTOR*, PIK3CA, *PIK3R2*, or *AKT3*, or loss of function mutations of *TSC1, TSC2, PTEN, DEPDC5, NPRL2*, or *NPRL3* lead to activation of the mTOR pathway and disorders of proliferation or downstream events such as focal cortical dysplasia, as discussed below. The importance of the mTOR pathway is underscored by the fact that disruption of this pathway leads to conditions spanning the spectrum from neurodevelopmental to neurodegenerative disorders.

NEURONAL MIGRATION

Between 12 and 20 weeks' gestation, millions of postmitotic neurons move from their sites of origin in the ventricular zone and subventricular zone to the developing cortex and deep nuclei, where they will reside for life, taking up specific positions to form the six-layered cortex clearly observable by 28 weeks' gestation. The timing and direction of these many simultaneous migrations are tightly regulated, and disorders of this remarkable process are surprisingly uncommon; yet when they do occur, they have significant consequences for fetal and neonatal well-being.

Before the neural tube even closes, specialized neurons known as *predecessor cells,* unique to humans, arrive at the pial surface of the forebrain, invading it tangentially to form the preplate.[60] These bipolar cells have a variety of molecular signatures, principally neuron specific beta III tubulin, and lack axons. They have long horizontal processes and may act as a scaffold for axonal navigation. These cells are largely transient and destined to die. The preplate then begins to subcompartmentalize with the appearance of reelin-expressing Cajal-Retzius cells. These transient bipolar cells arise from radial migration from the local ventricular zone, as well as by tangential migration from more distant extracortical sites. These cells take up a superficial subpial position as the marginal zone. Reelin terminates further migration, and these cells therefore mark the pial limit of neuronal migration, the upper boundary of the protocortex, the cortical plate.[61]

The cortical plate is a critical developmental phase in the formation of the human brain, progressively thickening with a clear temporal gradient. Radially migrating neurons accumulate in the cortical plate in an inside-out sequence, the earliest-born neurons becoming the deeper layer (V/VI) and later-born neurons becoming the more superficial layer (II/III). GABAergic interneurons migrate tangentially from the basal telencephalon, as well as locally from the subventricular zone. Between the ventricular proliferative zones and the postmigratory neurons towards the pial surface is a heterogeneous compartment, the intermediate zone. This contains radially and tangentially migrating cells, as well as extrinsic axons. Eventually, the invasion of corticocortical fibers and myelination transforms the intermediate zone into the white matter.

Between the cortical plate and the intermediate zone is a distinct neuronal compartment, the subplate, which contains heterogeneous cell populations. These include radially migrating glutamatergic neurons that extend subcortical pioneer axons and express the transcription factors TBR1 and EMX1 and the p75 neurotrophin receptor. Interneurons within the subplate express transcription factors associated with GABAergic neurons such as DLX1/2 and LHX6. The subplate expands dramatically during gestation to become four times thicker than the cortical plate by 6 months' gestation, then gradually decreases in size, leaving only cell-sparse white matter by 6 months of postnatal life.[61] The function of the subplate remains unclear, but silver staining and dye tracing studies suggest that it acts as a waiting compartment for thalamic axons arrested until the cortical plate becomes growth permissive and allows thalamocortical fibers to reach their target. The prolonged existence of this transient fetal zone into the third trimester and early postnatal life has profound implications for perturbations of sensory input related to premature birth or an aberrant neonatal experience such as asphyxia or exposure to drugs.

As they migrate along radial glia, many neurons within the cerebral wall extend processes that are soon recognizable as axons. The formation and maintenance of axonal and dendritic arbors are largely under the control of environmental cues. The tip of each process is composed of a specialized motile structure, a growth cone, which resembles the head of a club, with microspikes (filopodia) extending in all directions. Living growth cones, when viewed in a microscope, are constantly moving by local extension and retraction. When in contact with an appropriate substrate, they crawl forward and leave behind the elongating axon.[62]

In the developing nervous system, a variety of molecules within the extracellular matrix have been shown to provide this substrate for axon outgrowth. Two of the most active promoters of growth cone migration, laminin and fibronectin, have been shown to be expressed transiently as components of the extracellular matrix in cortical regions that have particularly active axon growth. Responsiveness to laminin may be developmentally regulated and enhanced by activation of integrins. Administration of exogenous laminin favors neuronal migration and neurite growth, whereas inhibition or neutralization of laminin results in inhibition of neurite outgrowth. Proteoglycans such as chondroitin sulfate, which are macromolecules composed of core polypeptide and glycosaminoglycan chains, can modulate neurite outgrowth along with laminin. Matrix metalloproteinases, proteases that degrade extracellular matrix molecules, are thought to be involved in stabilization of laminin and cell-matrix interactions. Extracellular matrix proteins, such as collagen, have also been shown in cell culture to suppress apoptosis, or programmed cell death, and thus to provide a more nurturing substrate for neuronal survival and differentiation.

Although extracellular matrix substrates promote axon outgrowth, they alone do not provide all the directional signals required during axon outgrowth. As growth cones advance, their filopodia extend and appear to explore the local environment to find the path most favorable for continued axon growth. Growth-associated protein 43 (GAP43) is a major growth cone protein whose phosphorylation in response to extracellular guidance cues can secondarily regulate microtubule behavior. Mice lacking GAP43 fail to form the anterior commissure, hippocampal commissure, and corpus callosum.[63] Growth of axons along voltage gradients or diffusible chemical gradients also occurs in the developing brain.

A growing body of evidence indicates that axon guidance is directed by the integrated and summed influence of both attractant and repulsive cues. These cues may be expressed in gradients, and they ultimately lead to the establishment of axon projection maps as found in the projection from the retina to the midbrain tectum. In fact, a family of axon-repulsive molecules, ligands of the Eph family of receptor tyrosine kinases, has been identified as the probable positional labels for the retinotectal projection. Additional signaling pathways regulating migration include Notch signaling through the downstream brain lipid-binding protein.[35]

DISORDERS OF NEURONAL MIGRATION

Neuronal proliferation, migration, and organization are not temporally separate but rather continually overlap during development. Classification of disorders is best at the earliest abnormal step, given that cells with proliferative defects often do not migrate or organize properly.

Migrational disorders are a large and complex group of conditions characterized by relative impairments in the radial migration of neurons into the cerebral cortex and tangential migration of interneurons into the cortex. Magnetic resonance imaging is the most useful initial investigation when a migrational disorder is suspected, with the hallmark finding of gyral abnormalities and occasionally abnormalities of the corpus callosum.[64] Cortical malformations are now classified by causative gene rather than phenotype, with the largest number of causative genes associated with migration defects.[65]

Lissencephaly-pachygyria represents a spectrum of disorders marked by underdevelopment or absence of normal gyrification. In lissencephaly there are absent gyri and an immature cerebral mantle with disorganized and heterotopic neuronal layering (Fig. 124.12). Cobblestone complex disorders, of which Walker-Warburg syndrome is one, are characterized by clustered, whorled arrays of neurons separated by glia and large heterotopic formations of neurons, often migrating into the pia, giving a characteristic "cobblestone" appearance. Pachygyria is demonstrated by thickened simple gyri that are underdeveloped and is a continuum of lissencephaly. The known causes of these types of lissencephalies are listed in Table 124.3 together with salient clinical features and diagnostic indicators.[64,65] Disruption in growing number of tubulin genes, *TUBA1A*, *TUBA8*, *TUBB2B*, *TUBB3*, *TUBB5* and *TUBG1*, lead to a "tubulinopathy" phenotype associated with cortical dysgenesis and often abnormalities of the basal ganglia, corpus callosum, and posterior fossa.[66]

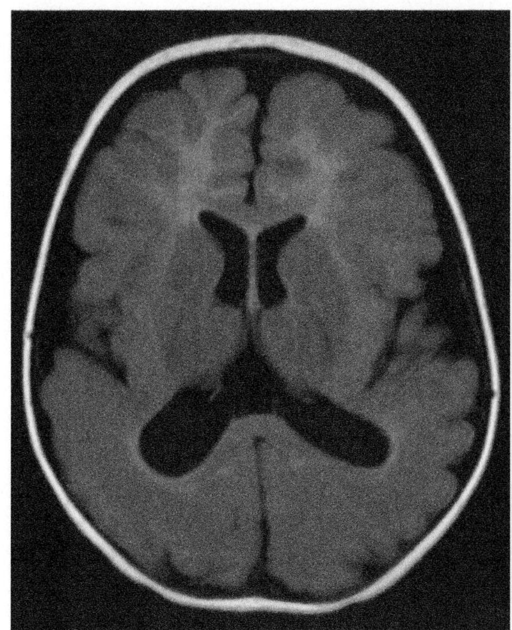
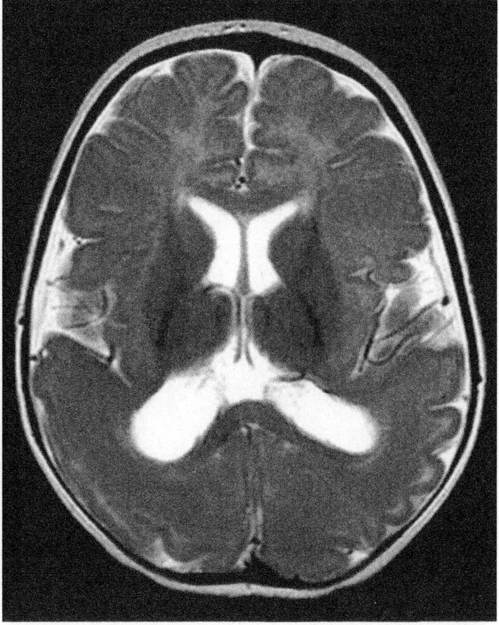

Fig. 124.12 Magnetic resonance imaging of posterior dominant lissencephaly. Note the decreased gyrification and smooth cerebral surface in the posterior lobes with a normal gyral pattern in the frontal lobes.

Table 124.3 Causes of Type 1 and Type 2 Lissencephaly With Characteristic Magnetic Resonance Imaging or Clinical Findings.

Gene	Cytogenetic Location	Phenotype
Lissencephaly Three-Layered With Agenesis of Corpus Callosum		
ARX	Xp22.1	XLAG
Lissencephaly Reelin Type With Anterior-to-Posterior Gradient		
RELN	7q22.1	LCH, reelin type
VLDLR	9p24.2	LCH, reelin type
Lissencephaly Two-Layered and Four-Layered With Anterior-to-Posterior Gradient		
ACTB	7p22.1	BWS lissencephaly
ACTG1	17q25.3	BWS lissencephaly
DCX (female)	Xq23	Subcortical band heterotopia
DCX (male)	Xq23	ILS, lissencephaly
Lissencephaly Two-Layered and Four-Layered With Posterior-to-Anterior Gradient		
DYNC1H1	14q32.31	ILS, lissencephaly
KIF2A	5q12.1	ILS, lissencephaly
LIS1	17p13.3	ILS, lissencephaly
Deletion *LIS1* and *YWHAE*	17p13.3	MDS, lissencephaly
TUBA1A	12q13.12	ILS, lissencephaly; LCH, lissencephaly; polymicrogyria-like
TUBB2B	6p25.2	ILS, lissencephaly; LCH, lissencephaly; polymicrogyria-like
TUBG1	17q21.2	ILS, lissencephaly

BWS, Baraitser-Winter syndrome; *ILS*, isolated lissencephaly sequence; *LCH*, lissencephaly with cerebellar hypoplasia; *MDS*, Miller-Dieker syndrome; *XLAG*, X-linked lissencephaly with abnormal genitalia.
Adapted from Guerrini R, Dobyns WB. Malformations of cortical development: clinical features and genetic causes. *Lancet Neurol*. 2014;13(7):710–726.

Neuronal heterotopias represent arrest of migration of neurons. These may be located close to the ventricular surface in the subependyma after arrest in early radial migration (Fig. 124.13). These are usually nodular and multiple. The most common mutation is that of the X-linked *FLNA* gene, which encodes an actin crosslinking protein. *FLNA* mutations primarily affect females and result in bilateral periventricular nodular heterotopia. Other genetic causes of heterotopias are seen in varying areas of the subcortical white matter or can also be seen in subcortical bands of neurons.[64]

DISORDERS OF ORGANIZATION

Polymicrogyria is characterized by numerous small folds of gyri that may have a basic four-layered anatomy or may be unlayered with a poorly laminated heterotopic collection of neurons below the cerebral mantle (Fig. 124.14). The causes of polymicrogyria include extrinsic factors, such as in utero cytomegalovirus infection or vascular insults, and intrinsic factors, such as single-gene mutations, copy-number variants, and metabolic conditions.

Schizencephaly is a severe restricted disorder of cortical formation resulting in a cleft, often extending from the ependymal surface to the pial surface (see Fig. 124.14). The cleft is lined by polymicrogyria and may be unilateral or bilateral, usually in the frontal or perirolandic region. The edges of the pial surface may be opposed ("closed lip") or more commonly widely separated ("open lip"). As stated above, the diverse processes resulting in polymicrogyria and schizencephaly suggest many different mechanisms yet to be elucidated.[64,65]

Focal cortical dysplasias represent abnormalities of both proliferation and organization. Focal cortical dysplasias with balloon cells, large dysplastic multipotent cells, are a disorder of proliferation rather than migration. Focal cortical dysplasias without balloon cells are disorders of cortical organization.[65] Regardless of the cause, focal cortical dysplasias often result in intractable epilepsy but are often amenable to epilepsy surgery. Focal cortical dysplasias are suspected to be caused by somatic mutations, given the funnel-shaped appearance suggesting that they arise from a single mutated neural progenitor cell (see Fig. 124.7).[59]

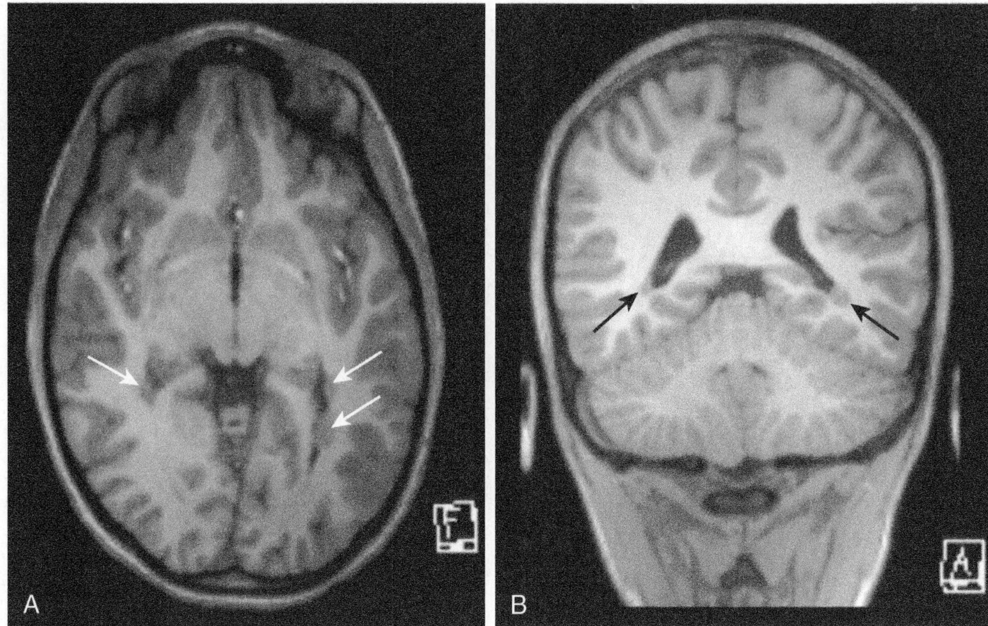

Fig. 124.13 Axial (A) and coronal (B) magnetic resonance imaging showing bilateral periventricular heterotopia *(arrows)* in a 14-year-old child with epilepsy.

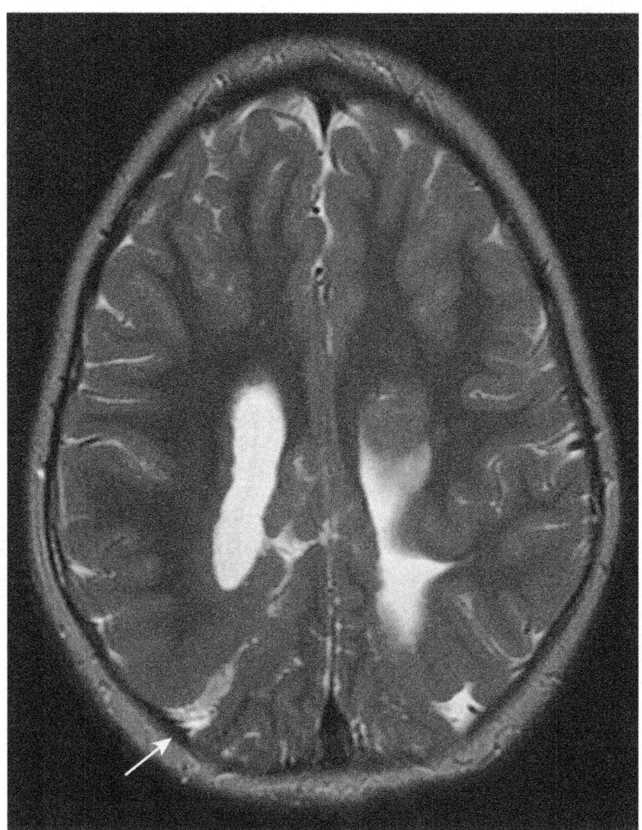

Fig. 124.14 Axial magnetic resonance imaging demonstrating schizencephaly *(arrow)* lined with polymicrogy ria in a 4-year-old patient with a duplication of chromosome band 11p15. Also note the lateral ventricle lined with periventricular heterotopia. (Courtesy Kristina Julich.)

NORMAL DEVELOPMENT OF THE CEREBELLAR CORTEX

The cerebellum is one of the first structures of the brain to differentiate but does not achieve the mature configuration until many months after birth. The primordia of the cerebellar territory, the cerebellar anlage, is located at the border between the mesencephalon and rhombencephalon, the future midbrain-hindbrain junction. The cerebellar hemispheres appear in the fifth gestational week as bilateral thickenings in the lateral aspects of the dorsal surface of the rhombencephalon, the rhombic lips. An updated view of cerebellar development finds that the cerebellar vermis and hemispheres originate from a single cerebellar anlage.[67] Regulation of early patterning is critically important for the formation of the vermis, a midline expanded region of the cerebellum unique to mammals. The primitive vermis and cerebellar anlage become apparent by 12 to 13 weeks.[68]

During the initial stage of development, around week 8, neurons migrate from the ventricular germinal matrix radially to form deep cerebellar nuclei followed by GABAergic Purkinje cells and other interneurons of the cerebellum. Cerebellar granule neurons arise from the rhombic lip directly and migrate tangentially to form glutamatergic neurons of the external granular layer.[69] During the next 3 months the external granular layer increases to a maximum thickness of about nine rows of cells and continues to generate neurons well into the first postnatal year. During this time, approximately 45 billion granule neurons are produced, which constitutes approximately half the neurons in the entire human brain.[70] The major driver of granule neuron precursor proliferation is SHH signaling.[71] As postmitotic neurons of the external granular layer are generated, they assume a deeper position within the layer. The migrating neurons pass through Purkinje cell dendrites in the molecular layer and then past the Purkinje cell bodies. After crossing the lamina dissecans, a layer just below the Purkinje cells that is rich in axon terminals of cerebellar afferents, such as the mossy fibers, the migrating neurons form the internal granular layer. Horizontal processes establish synapses with Purkinje cells and become parallel fibers, which are ordered within the molecular layer so that more recently generated fibers lie more superficially.[69]

Many of the same genetic and environmental cues that control other aspects of neural development are important in the establishment of cerebellar cortical organization. SHH is expressed in the cerebellum throughout life, although it promotes proliferation of developing cerebellar granule cells only in the early postnatal period, suggesting that downstream regulators may be important gatekeepers for the proliferative environment of the external granular layer. The Notch signaling pathway is also important for neuronal differentiation and expansion of granule cell progenitors in the cerebellum, which appears to be regulated by SHH.[72] BMP and Wnt secreted from the fourth ventricle roof plate also influence cerebellar development. Zinc finger proteins appear to have a role in granule cell proliferation. Brain-derived neurotrophic factor and other trophic factors appear to play an important role in survival and modulation of apoptosis for both Purkinje cells and granule cells. In addition, interaction between Purkinje and granule cells is important for proliferation of external granular layer precursors. Netrin receptors are differentially expressed on neurons as they reach successive phases of migration and axonal projection. The reelin pathway is important for timely arrest of migration of Purkinje cells. Finally, neurotransmitters, such as *N*-methyl-D-aspartate, may be important in the regulation of proliferation and migration of precursor cells via developmentally regulated, ligand-gated ion channel receptors.[69] These pathways and cerebellar growth might be negatively impacted in preterm infants who have a high incidence of cerebellar hypoplasia.[73]

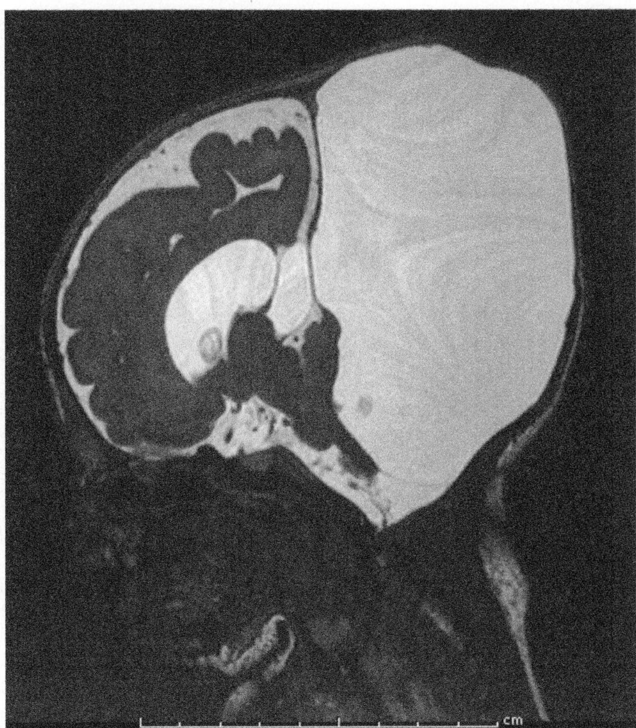

Fig. 124.15 Magnetic resonance imaging of a newborn with Dandy-Walker elevation. Note the rudimentary cerebellum and massive retrocerebellar cyst.

DISORDERS OF CEREBELLAR FORMATION

Medulloblastoma, the most common malignant childhood brain tumor, arises from cerebellar granule neuron precursors, rhombic lip cells, or neural stem cells. Recent work on genomic features of medulloblastomas has identified distinct molecular subgroups, each requiring different therapeutic approaches. The Wnt subgroup of tumors arise from the rhombic lip progenitors and currently have the best overall prognosis, with more than 95% survival. Most of these tumors harbor somatic mutations of *CTNNB1*, which promotes stabilization of nuclear β-catenin and drives Wnt signaling. The SHH tumor subgroup represents an intermediate prognosis. SHH tumors are usually a result of germline or somatic mutations of SHH signaling genes in external granular layer precursors. *PTCH1* is the gene most commonly mutated and encodes an inhibitor receptor protein for SHH. Patched 1 constitutive inhibition of downstream signaling is relieved by binding SHH, which stimulates mitosis of the granule cell precursors. Inactivating mutations of *PTCH1* may therefore lead to the persistent proliferation of granule cell precursors. The other two subgroups result in mutations in protooncogenes driving tumorigenesis.[74]

Cerebellar malformations include malformations of the vermis and hemispheres, typically absence or fusion, as well as abnormalities of CSF flow through the aqueduct of Sylvius, draining the third ventricle into the fourth ventricle or through the medial and lateral CSF foramina in the posterior fossa. Hydrocephalus is frequently associated with cerebellar malformations.

Dandy-Walker malformation is the most common congenital malformation of the human cerebellum and consists of four major abnormalities: (1) complete or partial agenesis of the cerebellar vermis, (2) cystic dilation of the fourth ventricle, (3) enlargement of the posterior fossa with a resulting high position of the tentorium and torcula, and (4) hydrocephalus.[75] Associated abnormalities of the CNS occur in as many as 70% of cases, with the clinically most important examples being agenesis of the corpus callosum and a variety of neuronal migration defects. Dandy-Walker malformation appears to be primarily failure of cavitation of the posterior membranous area of the developing roof of the fourth ventricle, allowing a buildup of CSF and cystic dilation of the fourth ventricle (Fig. 124.15).[24] In contrast, *Blake pouch cyst* is benign variant increasingly recognized by prenatal ultrasound and MRI. The cyst formation is due to failure of perforation of the lining of the fourth ventricle around 9 to 10 weeks gestation. The majority of these resolve spontaneously during term gestation without long-term sequelae.

Joubert syndrome and related disorders (JSRD) are a group of autosomal recessively inherited conditions with cerebellar vermis hypoplasia, hypotonia, ataxia, cognitive impairment, abnormal eye movements, and/or respiratory arrhythmia. The neuroradiologic hallmark of this cerebellar midbrain-hindbrain malformation on axial magnetic resonance images is a triangular ("bat-wing"-shaped) fourth ventricle, the small cerebellar vermis, and large uncrossed cerebellar peduncles giving rise to the "molar tooth" sign (Fig. 124.16). Over 25 gene mutations have been implicated in the JSRD spectrum. Several identified genes, *NPHP1*, *CEP290*, *RPGRIP1-like,* and *AHI1*, encode proteins mediating cilia function. Many of these genetic causes lead to additional defects outside of the cerebellum, such as malformations of cortex, brainstem, or corpus callosum. Furthermore, multiple overlapping features exist between JSRD and other primary ciliopathy disorders outside of the CNS.[76]

Rhombencephalosynapsis is a rare disorder characterized by hypoplasia of the vermis, fusion of the cerebellar hemispheres, and fusion of the dentate nuclei and cerebellar peduncles. *Pontocerebellar hypoplasias* (PCH) are a spectrum of autosomal

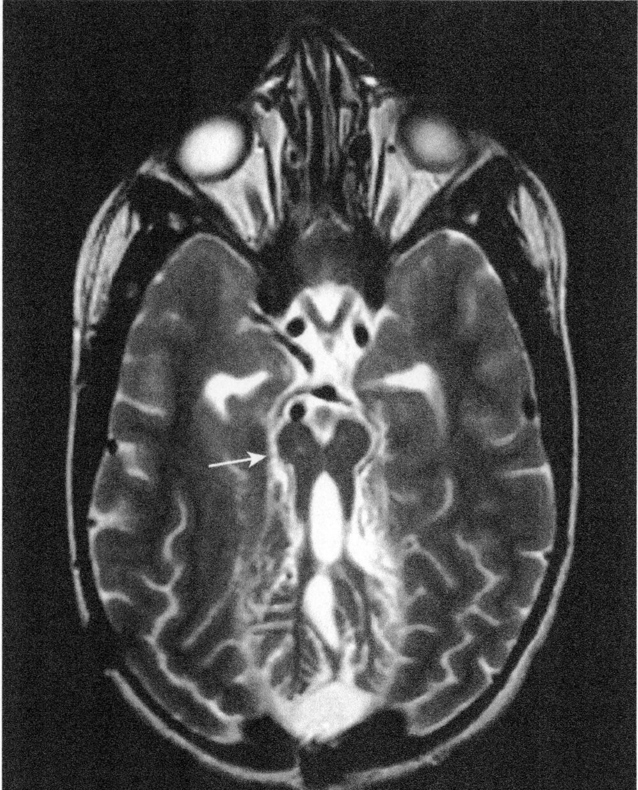

Fig. 124.16 Magnetic resonance imaging of an 11-year-old with Joubert syndrome. Note the "molar tooth sign" *(arrow)* with deep midbrain fossa anteriorly, thin and elongated superior cerebellar peduncles, and cerebellar vermis hypoplasia.

recessive anomalies characterized by a small pons and various degrees of cerebellar hypoplasia, thought to be related to a rhombic lip defect.[50,75] To date, 10 types of PCH have been described caused by a number of genes (e.g., *AMPD2, CLP1, CHMP1A, COASY, EXOSC3, EXOSC8, EXOSC9, PCLO, RARS2, SEPSECS, SLC25A46, TBC1D23, TSEN2, TSEN15, TSEN34, TSEN54, VPS51, VSP53, VRK1*) but invariably they often result in severe and progressive global delays, with or without seizures. The cerebellum is extremely vulnerable to developmental disruption during the second half of gestation, as this is a time of major cerebellar growth and proliferation. There is increasing awareness of the potential impact on cerebellar development from exposure to opioids, neurosteroids, other drugs (e.g., phenytoin), or irradiation. In addition, vascular insults and infections can selectively impact the cerebellum. Premature infants may spend part of this critical period in an extrauterine environment exposed to a number of intrinsic and extrinsic factors that may negatively impact normal cerebellar development.[77]

SYNAPTOGENESIS

The timing of synapse formation varies throughout the developing brain. The basic principles of synaptogenesis are the formation of the earliest synapses in the marginal and subplate zones, an increase in the number of synapses in the cortical plate to a peak that exceeds the adult number, and a subsequent period of synapse elimination. In the cerebrum, synapses are observed initially on neurons of the subplate and the marginal zone. Initially, dendrites appear as thick processes with only a few fine branches. As development progresses, a great number and variety of dendritic spines appear. Synapse elimination then begins, and a large proportion of synapses are lost.[70]

The factors that stimulate synapse formation and development in developing brain include both activity-independent events and activity-dependent events occurring after the development of receptors on target neurons and the generation of electrical activity.[32] Many signaling pathways are involved in synapse formation and dendritic spine development and remodeling.[78] The two principal themes are modulation of ion channels by neurotransmitters, especially *N*-methyl-D-aspartate and glutamate, and alteration of cell-surface receptors by a variety of ligands. These intracellular events lead to effects on actin-binding proteins and the actin cytoskeleton, with resulting changes in spine shape, size, and motility.[79]

APOPTOSIS AND SYNAPTIC PRUNING

Cell death and selective elimination of neuronal processes and synapses, or pruning in brain development, are critical to normal postnatal behavior. Typically about half of the neurons in the cortical region die before final maturation. This process of programmed cell death, apoptosis, is initiated and sustained by the expression of specific genes. Critical in the final phases of the sequence to cell death is the activation of caspases. Apoptosis appears to be fundamentally triggered by neuronal competition for limited amounts of trophic factors, generated by the target, afferent input, or associated glia, allowing numeric matching of interconnecting populations of neurons and elimination of projections that are aberrant or otherwise incorrect.[80]

Neural organization is refined further by selective pruning of neuronal processes and synapses. This causes the removal of terminal axonal branches and their synapses. The ratio of excitatory and inhibitory inputs varies throughout development and by location.[81] Activation of the *N*-methyl-D-aspartate receptor appears to be an important step in synapse elimination during development. In addition, microglia and astrocytes are emerging as key contributors to synaptogenesis and neuronal plasticity.[82]

DISORDERS OF SYNAPTOGENESIS

Abnormalities in synaptogenesis and synaptic pruning are implicated in myriad conditions from mild learning disabilities, attention-deficit/hyperactivity disorder, and autism spectrum disorders (ASDs) to profound intellectual disability.[83] Several studies have identified single-gene mutations in children with intellectual and developmental disability.[84] Some gene mutations include *ARHGEF6*, *OPHN1*, *PAK3*, and *FGD1* encoding proteins that directly interact with Rho GTPases to regulate neuronal outgrowth and spine formation through cytoskeletal dynamics. Other gene mutations, such as mutations in *L1CAM*, *DLG3*, neuroligin genes, and *TSPAN7*, are involved in other signaling pathways to regulate the actin cytoskeleton. Deletions in the postsynaptic neuroligin gene *NLGN4X* are associated with autism, Tourette syndrome, attention-deficit/hyperactivity disorder, learning disorders, anxiety, and depression. SHANK3 is a synaptic scaffolding protein that interacts with neuroligins. Mutations in *SHANK3* are associated with ASD and intellectual disability in humans, and abnormal synaptic transmission and plasticity in animal models. Disturbances of cytoskeletal structures cause dendritic abnormalities, altered neuronal function, and ultimately a variety of neurologic conditions.[84-86]

Rett syndrome is one of the most common causes of intellectual disability and autism in females. It is characterized clinically by onset of deceleration of the rate of head growth in the first months of life, loss of purposeful hand movement near the end of the first year, and development of stereotypic hand movements, ataxia, microcephaly, seizures, developmental

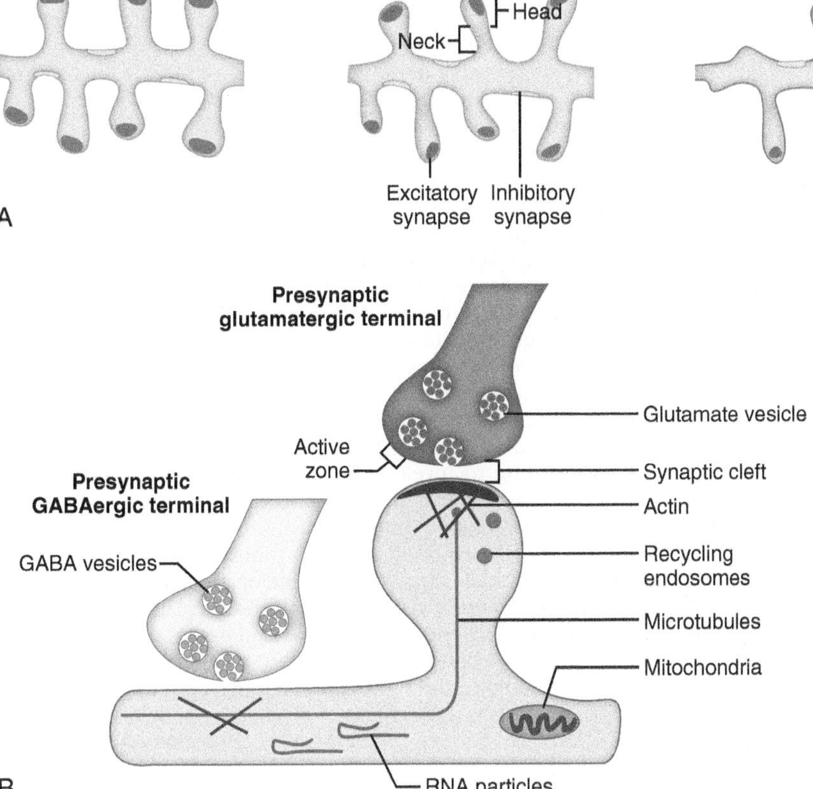

Fig. 124.17 (A) Dendritic morphology with examples of increased and decreased spine density in fragile X syndrome and Rett syndrome, respectively. (B) Localization of excitatory (glutamatergic) and inhibitory (GABAergic) synapses in neuronal dendrites. (Adapted from Spooren W, Lindemann L, Ghosh A, et al. Synapse dysfunction in autism: a molecular medicine approach to drug discovery in neurodevelopment disorders. *Trends Pharmacol Sci.* 2012;33[12]:669–684.)

disability, and often autism, all occurring before the age of 5 years. The underlying molecular defect is principally loss of function of the *MECP2* gene, encoding for a transcriptional repressor expressed throughout the brain.[87] Neuropathologic features of Rett syndrome include a small brain with an apparent disturbance of neuronal development, characterized by dendritic spine abnormalities (Fig. 124.17) and small, densely packed neurons. Animal studies suggest a fundamental perturbation in the ability to form stable synapses despite repeated experience-dependent stimulation.

Abnormalities of dendritic and axonal development have been described in infants with Down syndrome, including alterations in cortical lamination, reduced dendritic branching, diminished numbers of dendritic spines and synapses, giant spines, and abnormal spine shape. Abnormalities are not apparent before 22 weeks' gestation, at which point the rapid progression of organizational events occur. In the first months of postnatal life an excess in dendritic branching precedes a decrease in dendritic branching observed after approximately 6 months of age. Animal models of impaired dendritic branching also demonstrate this sequence of excessive initial branching followed by deficits in dendritic branching.

Fragile X syndrome is the most common inherited cause of autism and developmental disability mainly affecting males. The cause of fragile X syndrome is an amplification of a trinucleotide CGG repeat sequence in the *FMR1* gene. Neuropathologic features of fragile X syndrome include abnormal dendritic spine morphology, including long dendritic spines, fewer short spines, more immature-appearing spines, and fewer mature-appearing spines.[83] The brain otherwise has no overt abnormalities. Similarly abnormal dendritic spines are seen in *Fmr1*-knockout mice. Increasing evidence from a number of other disorders, both congenital and acquired, suggests the profound influence of abnormalities of dendritic formation and pruning in the genesis of severe neurologic deficits, including developmental disability and epilepsy.[86]

ASD is the leading cause of neurodevelopmental impairment, with an incidence of more than 1 in 100 children in the United States. ASD is a heritable disorder, but in only 25% of cases is there an identified underlying genetic disorder. Many distinct autism loci with de novo copy-number variants and single-gene mutations have been identified mainly in synaptic, transcriptional, and chromatin remodeling pathways. Mounting evidence continues to accumulate that ASD reflects fundamental failures of synaptic function or organization.[86] The overlap of related conditions such as Rett syndrome, fragile X syndrome, and ASD suggests multiple convergent pathways resulting in perturbations of dendritic spine morphology, pruning of synapses, or stability of synapses (see Fig. 124.17). It is likely that this stage of fetal and neonatal brain development will become the most critical for understanding the major postnatal neurologic disorders of childhood.

NORMAL DEVELOPMENT OF MYELINATION

Myelination occurs after neuronal maturation in a coordinated fashion. Myelination peaks in postnatal life (Fig. 124.18). Oligodendrocytes originate from progenitors in the subventricular zone and radial glial progenitors. The early-phase cells are generated from mid-gestation to early postnatal life. As these

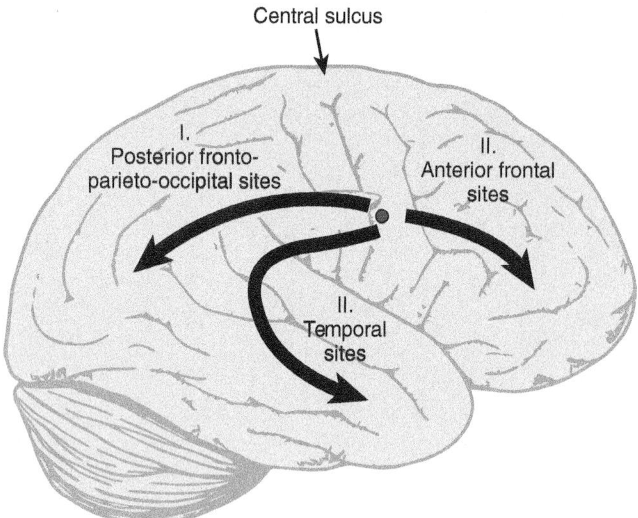

Fig. 124.18 Progress of myelination. The progression of myelination in telencephalic sites starts from the central sulcus outward to the poles, with the posterior sites preceding the anterior frontal and temporal sites. (From Volpe JJ, editor. Neuronal proliferation, migration, organization, and myelination. In: *Neurology of the Newborn*. 5th ed. Philadelphia: WB Saunders; 2008.)

oligodendrocyte precursors migrate, they respond to internal cues, as well as to the local influences of the other neurons and glia.[88] The progression of maturation continues as preoligodendrocytes, then immature oligodendrocytes, and finally mature oligodendrocytes.

Much of oligodendrocyte precursor development occurs through transcriptional, posttranscriptional, and epigenetic mechanisms. The initial specification of the oligodendrocyte lineage is reliant on the transcription factor OLIG2. Transcription factors ID2/4, HES5, and SOX6 are active in maintaining oligodendrocyte precursors in their undifferentiated state and repress myelin gene expression. Chromatin remodeling and microRNAs appear to promote oligodendrocyte differentiation by targeting and inhibiting these inhibitory transcription factors. Relief from inhibitory signals allows the induction of transcription factors such as SOX10, OLIG1, and myelin gene regulatory factor to promote differentiation and myelin formation.[89]

The extracellular factors involved in myelination include a number of growth factors, hormones, cytokines, and other secreted factors. Neurotrophin-3, nerve growth factor, ephrins, and semiphorins are examples of secreted factors while axonal expression of nonsecreted ligands also play an important role: Jagged, neural cell adhesion molecule, Nogo receptors, Eph receptors, and LINGO-1. Paradoxically, many of these factors are inhibitory, preventing oligodendrocyte differentiation and myelination. In the peripheral nervous system, expression of nectin-like adhesion molecules and axonal expression of neuregulins are the main signals for the inducing of correct Schwann cell myelination.[90] Myelination is also driven by neuronal activity, although the mechanisms remain to be fully elucidated. Oligodendrocyte precursors receive synaptic input directly from neurons, which has been observed in the context of remyelination in the adult CNS and is lost after cells differentiate into mature oligodendrocytes.[88]

These cues determine when progenitor cells exit the cell cycle, begin to proliferate, and differentiate into mature oligodendrocytes. The waves of migration of these cells may be the anatomic correlate of the periventricular bands visualized on magnetic resonance images of the premature infant. Cell death is an important feature of oligodendroglial development, with approximately 50% of oligodendroglia undergoing apoptosis during development.

In the third trimester of gestation, the immature oligodendrocytes develop linear extensions as they ensheath axons in preparation for myelination. In the CNS, oligodendrocytes form as many as 40 separate myelin segments on multiple axons, in contrast to the peripheral nervous system, where Schwann cells myelinate single axons.

This process is followed by differentiation to the mature oligodendrocyte, which might be triggered in part by axonal activity-dependent cues.[91] Mature oligodendrocytes become the predominant oligodendroglial stage in the months after term birth and give rise to myelination. After initiation of myelination, intracellular processes begin to ramp up to create the lipid-rich composition of myelin. Cholesterol, phospholipids, and glycosphingolipids account for 70% of the dry weight of the myelin membrane. These cells have developed a highly effective system to maintain the optimal ratio of lipid classes in the tightly wrapped membrane to perform its insulating function during nerve conduction. The increase in cell surface area from premyelinating to myelinating oligodendrocyte is estimated to be 6500-fold, which implies there must be adequate access to substrate from blood vessels.[92]

Similarly to cortical organization, myelination exhibits pronounced regional variation. The regional features have been defined well in the human cerebrum and anticipate the functional developmental milestones of the human infant. Caudal and posterior areas of the brain myelinate before rostral and anterior brain regions. In addition, the earliest myelin is detected within the roots of motor and then sensory nerves. Myelination soon occurs within the neuraxis, where central sensory systems generally myelinate before central motor systems and primary projection systems begin to myelinate before associative systems. The cerebral commissures and other corticocortical projections begin to myelinate and continue to do so into late adolescence.[93] In addition, there is evidence of ongoing differentiation of oligodendrocyte precursors into myelinating oligodendrocytes in the adult CNS,[88] which is required for the learning of complex motor tasks.[94]

DISORDERS OF MYELINATION

Leukoencephalopathies are a heterogeneous group of conditions characterized by developmental abnormalities or degeneration of white matter. White matter disorders are subdivided into hypomyelinating disorders, dysmyelinating disorders, leukodystrophies, disorders related to myelin splitting, and secondary disorders of white matter.

Hypomyelinating disorders are due to primary disturbance in myelin formation.[95] Pelizaeus-Merzbacher disease is caused by altered expression of the proteolipid protein, resulting in hypomyelination and clinical features such as nystagmus, ataxia, hypotonia, and developmental delay. Inborn metabolic errors that cause abnormal neuronal storage, such as GM1 gangliosidosis, have been associated with hypomyelination. *Dysmyelinating disorders* are described in a variety of organic and aminoacidopathies, hypothyroidism, phenylketonuria, and some chromosomal anomalies (in particular 18q deletion and Down syndrome).[96]

Leukodystrophies are progressive demyelinating diseases due to altered myelin composition or metabolism, such as *ABCD1* gene mutations in X-linked adrenoleukodystrophy resulting in incorrect incorporation of very-long-chain fatty acids into the myelin membrane instead of the normal shorter-chain fatty acids. Mitochondrial disorders and a few other rare disorders, such as Canavan disease, are related to myelin splitting and cystic degeneration. Despite the recent increase in identifying genetic mutations, the cause of approximately 50% of leukoencephalopathies remains unknown.[96]

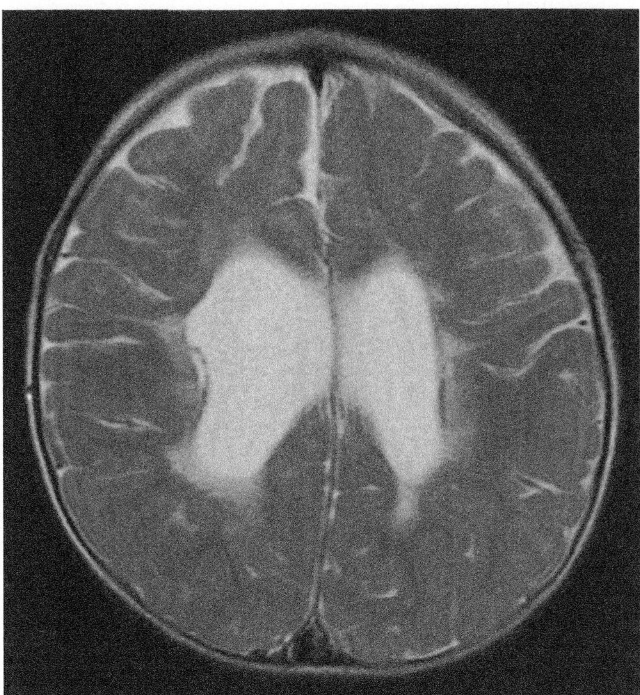

Fig. 124.19 Magnetic resonance imaging of a former 28-week premature baby at term-corrected age demonstrating periventricular leukomalacia.

Evidence continues to accumulate regarding the involvement of white matter in learning and development, cognition, and psychiatric disorders.[97] Novel noninvasive brain imaging, including diffusion tensor imaging, is providing new insights into structural differences in white matter tracts throughout normal and abnormal development.[98] Without doubt, the most significant anomaly of myelination in current neonatal practice remains periventricular leukomalacia (Fig. 124.19) and cerebral white matter injury of prematurity.[99] This clinical and neuropathologic syndrome reflects the exquisite vulnerability of the myelinating nervous system to external perturbations. Oligodendrocyte injury increasingly appears to have deleterious consequences for neuronal growth and development.[100] The profound effects of the damage to the immaturely myelinated nervous system are reflected in the high incidence of motor, visual, and cognitive-behavioral abnormalities in survivors of preterm birth.

CONCLUSION

The development of the human nervous system is arguably the most remarkable sequence of events observable in nature. In 40 weeks a few embryonic cells give rise to one of the most complex structures imaginable. Tightly regulated gene expression interacts with local and distant epigenetic factors to produce trillions of functional connections that continue to grow and develop decades after birth. It is not clear when brain development truly ends because there is evidence of positive morphologic and functional changes well into adulthood.

Inevitably, such a complex network of events is sensitive to damage and intrinsic perturbation, the consequences of which are at least in part determined by the phase of development in which they occur. These may represent massive failure, as in anencephaly, or subtler aberrations, such as cognitive disability and disorders of attention and executive control. Understanding the anatomic scaffold on which the nervous system is built allows us to predict, prevent, and potentially intervene in some of the most challenging disorders in medicine.

A complete reference list is available at www.ExpertConsult.com. 

SELECT REFERENCES

2. Moore KL, Persaud TVN, Torchia MG. *The Developing Human: Clinically Oriented Embryology*. 10th ed. Philadelphia, PA: Elsevier; 2016.
3. Arnold SJRobertson EJ. Making a commitment: cell lineage allocation and axis patterning in the early mouse embryo. *Nat Rev Mol Cell Biol*. 2009;10(2): 91-103.
5. Stern CD. Neural induction: 10 years on since the 'default model'. *Curr Opin Cell Biol*. 2006;18(6):692-697. https://doi.org/10.1016/j.ceb.2006.09.002.
6. Wilson SW, Houart C. Early steps in the development of the forebrain. *Dev Cell*. 2004;6(2):167-181.
7. Tan W, Gilmore EC, Baris HN. Chapter 15- human developmental genetics. In: Rimoin DL, et al., ed. *Emery and Rimoin's Principles and Practice of Medical Genetics*. 6th ed. Philadelphia, PA: Churchill Livingstone Elsevier; 2013.
8. Metzis V, Steinhauser S, Pakanavicius E, et al. Nervous system regionalization Entails axial allocation before neural differentiation. *Cell*. 2018;175(4): 1105-1118. e1117. https://doi.org/10.1016/j.cell.2018.09.040.
9. Copp AJ, Stanier P, Greene ND. Neural tube defects: recent advances, unsolved questions, and controversies. *Lancet Neurol*. 2013;12(8):799-810.
11. Wallingford JB, Harland RM. Xenopus Dishevelled signaling regulates both neural and mesodermal convergent extension: parallel forces elongating the body axis. *Development*. 2001;128(13):2581-2592.
15. Tanabe Y, Jessell TM. Diversity and pattern in the developing spinal cord. *Science*. 1996;274(5290):1115-1123.
16. Massarwa R, Ray HJ, Niswander L. Morphogenetic movements in the neural plate and neural tube: mouse. *Wiley Interdiscip Rev Dev Biol*. 2014;3(1): 59-68.
19. Wallingford JB, Niswander LA, Shaw GM, Finnell RH. The continuing challenge of understanding, preventing, and treating neural tube defects. *Science*. 2013;339(6123):1222002.
22. Gilbert JN, Jones KL, Rorke LB, et al. Central nervous system anomalies associated with meningomyelocele, hydrocephalus, and the Arnold-Chiari malformation: reappraisal of theories regarding the pathogenesis of posterior neural tube closure defects. *Neurosurgery*. 1986;18(5):559-564.
26. MRC Vitamin Study Research Group. Prevention of neural tube defects: results of the medical research council vitamin study. *Lancet*. 1991;338(8760): 131-137.
30. Sidman R, Rakic P. Development of the human central nervous system. In: Haymaker W, Adams RD, eds. *Histology and Histopathology of the Nervous System*. Springfield, IL: Charles C Thomas; 1982:3-145.
31. Hébert JM, Fishell G. The genetics of early telencephalon patterning: some assembly required. *Nat Rev Neurosci*. 2008;9(9):678-685.
32. Sur M, Rubenstein JL. Patterning and plasticity of the cerebral cortex. *Science*. 2005;310(5749):805-810.
35. Plachez C, Richards LJ. Mechanisms of axon guidance in the developing nervous system. *Curr Top Dev Biol*. 2005;69:267-346.
36. Rowitch DH, Kriegstein AR. Developmental genetics of vertebrate glial-cell specification. *Nature*. 2010;468(7321):214-222.
40. Paul LK, Brown WS, Adolphs R, et al. Agenesis of the corpus callosum: genetic, developmental and functional aspects of connectivity. *Nat Rev Neurosci*. 2007;8(4):287-299.
42. Rakic P. Specification of cerebral cortical areas. *Science*. 1988;241(4862): 170-176.
51. Mlakar J, Korva M, Tul N, et al. Zika virus associated with microcephaly. *N Engl J Med*. 2016;374(10):951-958. https://doi.org/10.1056/NEJMoa1600651.
52. Volpe JJ. *Neurology of the Newborn*. 6th ed. Philadelphia: Elsevier; 2018.
54. Winden KD, Yuskaitis CJ, Poduri A. Megalencephaly and macrocephaly. *Semin Neurol*. 2015;35(3):277-287. https://doi.org/10.1055/s-0035-1552622.
59. Poduri A, Evrony GD, Cai X, Walsh CA. Somatic mutation, genomic variation, and neurological disease. *Science*. 2013;341(6141):1237758.
60. Bystron I, Rakic P, Molnar Z, Blakemore C. The first neurons of the human cerebral cortex. *Nat Neurosci*. 2006;9(7):880-886. https://doi.org/10.1038/nn1726.
61. Bystron I, Blakemore C, Rakic P. Development of the human cerebral cortex: Boulder Committee revisited. *Nat Rev Neurosci*. 2008;9(2):110-122.
64. Guerrini R, Dobyns WB. Malformations of cortical development: clinical features and genetic causes. *Lancet Neurol*. 2014;13(7):710-726.
65. Barkovich AJ, Kuzniecky RI, Jackson GD, et al. A developmental and genetic classification for malformations of cortical development. *Neurology*. 2005;65(12):1873-1887.
67. Butts T, Green MJ, Wingate RJ. Development of the cerebellum: simple steps to make a 'little brain'. *Development*. 2014;141(21):4031-4041. https://doi.org/10.1242/dev.106559.
74. Northcott PA, Jones DT, Kool M, et al. Medulloblastomics: the end of the beginning. *Nat Rev Cancer*. 2012;12(12):818-834.
77. Volpe JJ. Cerebellum of the premature infant: rapidly developing, vulnerable, clinically important. *J Child Neurol*. 2009;24(9):1085-1104. https://doi.org/10.1177/0883073809338067.

78. Garner CC, Zhai RG, Gundelfinger ED, Ziv NE. Molecular mechanisms of CNS synaptogenesis. *Trends Neurosci*. 2002;25(5):243-251.
82. Haydon PG. GLIA: listening and talking to the synapse. *Nat Rev Neurosci*. 2001;2(3):185-193.
84. Krumm N, O'Roak BJ, Shendure J, Eichler EE. A de novo convergence of autism genetics and molecular neuroscience. *Trends Neurosci*. 2014;37(2):95-105.
87. Chahrour M, Zoghbi HY. The story of Rett syndrome: from clinic to neurobiology. *Neuron*. 2007;56(3):422-437.
91. Fields RD. Myelin formation and remodeling. *Cell*. 2014;156(1-2):15-17.
93. Lebel C, Beaulieu C. Longitudinal development of human brain wiring continues from childhood into adulthood. *J Neurosci*. 2011;31(30):10937-10947.
95. Pouwels PJ, Vanderver A, Bernard G, et al. Hypomyelinating leukodystrophies: translational research progress and prospects. *Ann Neurol*. 2014;76(1):5-19.
99. Volpe JJ. Brain injury in premature infants: a complex amalgam of destructive and developmental disturbances. *Lancet Neurol*. 2009;8(1):110-124.

125 Mechanisms of Cell Death in the Developing Brain

Claire Thornton

INTRODUCTION

When the brain is exposed to stress, a number of adaptive responses can act to reestablish homeostasis.[1] However, when the stress is severe and/or the endogenous protective processes are not sufficiently effective, the cell will die.[2,3] Cell death can be initiated by numerous organelles (e.g., nucleus, mitochondrion, endoplasmic reticulum/lysosome, cytoskeleton, plasma membrane) and mitochondria, in particular, play a key role in the initiation and execution of cell death mechanisms in the immature brain.[4,5] Once triggered, cell death can proceed via a variety of routes, including the well-characterized apoptosis pathway, as well as by lesser-known necroptosis, ferroptosis, parthanatos, and autophagy-dependent cell death mechanisms (Fig. 125.1).[6] Which cell death mechanism predominates will depend on the metabolic state, severity and type of insult, cell type, developmental age, and other factors.[3,6] The traditional classification of cell death by morphology is no longer used, as mixed morphologic phenotypes are often detected in many pathologic situations.[7,8] Classification now favors the use of molecular markers indicative of particular cell death pathways.[6] Indeed, for effective neuroprotective intervention, understanding the biochemical route(s) to cell death is critical, considering that when one route is inhibited, cell death may occur via an alternative mechanism.[9,10] Long-term functional cell recovery following genetic alteration and/or pharmacologic intervention often yields significant information concerning the essential components in a specific route of cell death and any alternative routes triggered. More recently, unbiased proteomics approaches have provided a more comprehensive identification of the major players in a variety of cell death paradigms.[7,11,12]

Cell death can be classified into *accidental* and *regulated* (see Fig. 125.1).[10] Accidental cell death is evoked by severe insults (such as severe trauma, core of an ischemic infarct, high temperature), which cause immediate cellular demise that does not involve a specific molecular mechanism and cannot be prevented or modulated.[13] However, cellular contents released following accidental cell death act as damage-associated molecular patterns (DAMPs) often having direct toxic effects on surrounding cells that survived the initial insult. Exposure to DAMPs may extend the primary injury, as they have immunogenic properties, contributing to an inflammatory response that may cause injury and aggravate the situation further.[14,15] Various interventions that attenuate DAMP-induced cellular actions can provide protective effects.[16] So even if accidental cell death cannot be targeted directly, its consequences can be intercepted and bystander injury prevented to some extent. For example, therapeutic hypothermia is used in mitigation of the effects of hypoxic-ischemic injury. In contrast, regulated cell death involves the coordinated molecular machinery of the cell (see Fig. 125.1), and its course can be modulated by pharmacologic and genetic means.[6,17] Regulated cell death usually occurs with a delay, in situations when endogenous protective mechanisms fail to restore cellular homeostasis.

In the developing brain, cell damage can be induced by a variety of insults, such as hypoxia,[18] hypoxia-ischemia (HI),[19] trauma,[20] and infections.[21] While definitive studies using human neonatal brain tissues are lacking, substantial knowledge of the mechanisms of cell death in the immature central nervous system has emerged from in vitro studies in cell cultures (exposed to toxins or oxygen/glucose deprivation) and in vivo, in models of HI in rodents and to some extent larger animals (e.g., piglets, rabbits, or fetal sheep).[22] Exposure to HI results in an initial depletion of high-energy phosphates, in particular ATP and phosphocreatine. The levels of these phosphates return transiently to the baseline, but this is followed by a second, more prolonged depletion of cellular energy reserves accompanied by progression of brain injury (see Chapter 167).[4,23] These disturbances in energy metabolism trigger a number of pathophysiologic responses that ultimately lead to cell death, with mechanisms including initial necrosis, and subsequently apoptosis,[24-26], necroptosis[27-29] or autophagy-dependent cell death.[30-33]

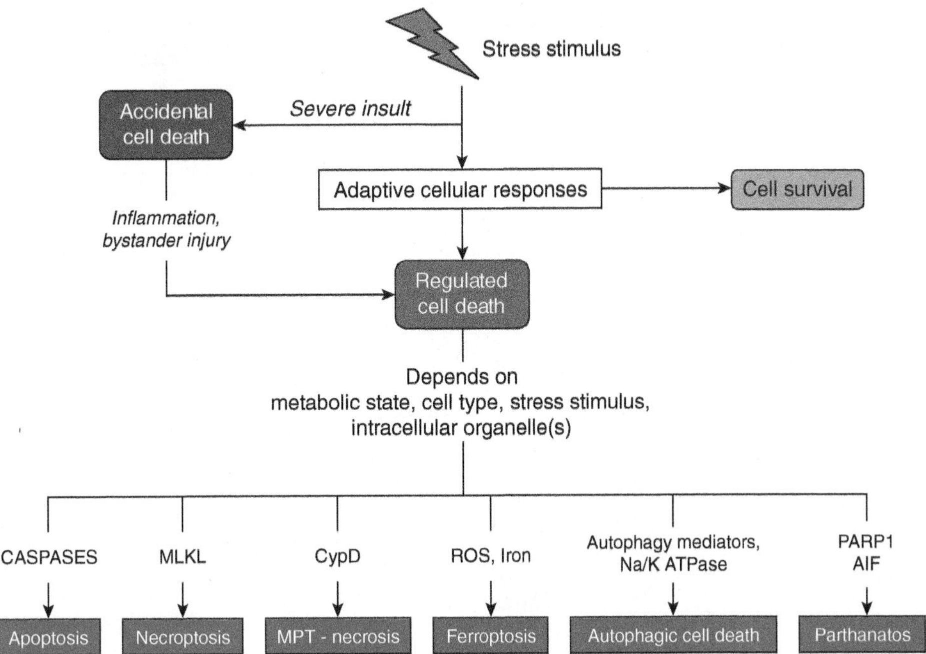

Fig. 125.1 Overview of cell death pathways. In response to mild stress stimuli, a number of compensatory mechanisms will be activated, most often leading to cell survival. Moderate-to-severe insults may trigger regulated cell death. Depending on several factors such as the metabolic situation, cell type, nature of the stress stimulus, and which intracellular organelle(s) are affected, the cell undergoes apoptosis (caspase activation), necroptosis (mixed lineage kinase domain–like *[MLKL]* activation), opening of the mitochondrial permeability transition *(MPT)* pore (regulated by cyclophilin D *[CypD]*), ferroptosis (iron- and ROS-dependent lipid peroxidation), autophagic cell death (autophagy/Na^+,K^+-ATPase), or parthanatos (poly(ADP-ribose) polymerase 1 *[PARP1]*, apoptosis-inducing factor *[AIF]*). Severe insults cause accidental cell death that cannot be modulated genetically or by pharmacologic means. However, accidental cell death leads to the release of factors (damage-associated molecular patterns) that initiate systemic effects, as well as inflammation and (regulated) secondary brain injury in neighboring tissue. *ROS*, Reactive oxygen species.

This chapter will describe the mechanisms underlying the most common forms of regulated cell death and then summarize the evidence for their involvement in cell death in the immature brain exposed to hypoxic-ischemic insult.

THE APOPTOTIC CELL DEATH MACHINERY

The apoptosis pathway triggered depends on whether the stimulus is intracellular (intrinsic, mitochondrial) or extracellular (extrinsic), although both converge at the activation of caspases-3 and -7 (Fig. 125.2). The **intrinsic** pathway relies on mitochondrial outer membrane permeabilization (MOMP) resulting in the release of a number of proapoptotic proteins into the cytosol.[34] This permeabilization is tightly controlled by the pro- and antiapoptotic members of the B cell lymphoma 2 (BCL2) family. MOMP is directly executed by BCL2-associated X protein (BAX) and BCL2-antagonist/killer 1 (BAK1) that oligomerize to form outer membrane pores (see Fig. 125.2). The opening of the BAX/BAK1 pore is regulated by the balanced action of antiapoptotic BCL2 family proteins such as BCL2 itself, BCL2-like 1 (BCL-XL), and myeloid cell leukemia 1, and proapoptotic "sensitizers" such as BCL2 binding component 3 (PUMA), BCL2-like 11 (BIM), and BH3-interacting domain death agonist (BID), which can initiate the pathway.[35] Initiation of MOMP can also be controlled by p53, c-Jun N-terminal kinase (JNK), and caspase-2.[36] Once MOMP is initiated, leakage of proapoptotic proteins from the mitochondrial intermembrane space occurs, most notably cytochrome *c* (Cyt *c*). Cyt *c* forms an apoptosome complex with deoxy-ATP, and apoptotic peptidase-activating factor 1 (APAF-1), which recruits and activates caspase-9, leading to the downstream activation of the executioner caspase-3.[37,38] Additional proapoptotic proteins released from the mitochondrion include Smac/DIABLO and Omi/HtrA2, proteases that cleave X-linked inhibitor of apoptosis (XIAP), preventing XIAP-mediated inhibition of caspase activation.[36] Finally, apoptosis-inducing factor (AIF) is also released from the mitochondrion, translocating to the nucleus where it facilitates chromatinolysis and cell death in a caspase-independent manner.[39] MOMP is not only very rapid[40] but also extensive; once initiated in a limited number of mitochondria, MOMP swiftly proceeds through all mitochondria within the cell.[41]

In the **extrinsic** pathway, binding of extracellular ligands to a death receptor leads to activation of caspase-8 and cleavage of either BID (to crossover with the intrinsic pathway) or directly to caspase-3.[42] Over 20 ligand-receptor pairings are now included in the death receptor ligand tumor necrosis factor (TNF) superfamily.[43] These TNF-receptor (TNFR) and TNFR-like molecules are similar in structure to TNF and function as trimers (both ligands and receptors).[43] Because of the similarity of their structure, multiple ligands are able to bind and induce signaling through one receptor, or a single ligand is able to bind multiple receptors. Receptors containing the so-called death domain in their intracellular domain (e.g., TNFR1, DR4, DR5, Fas) are able to trigger apoptosis when activated by the binding of the corresponding ligand (e.g., TNF-α, TNF-related apoptosis inducing ligand [TRAIL], FasL). This extrinsic pathway of apoptosis continues with the activation of a death-inducing signaling complex (DISC) adjacent to the death domain of the receptor. DISC comprises Fas-associated death domain protein (FADD) and procaspase-8; binding results in caspase-8 homodimerization and activation by proteolytic cleavage (see Fig. 125.2).[44] Activated caspase-8 either directly activates caspase-3 or mediates cleavage of BID to

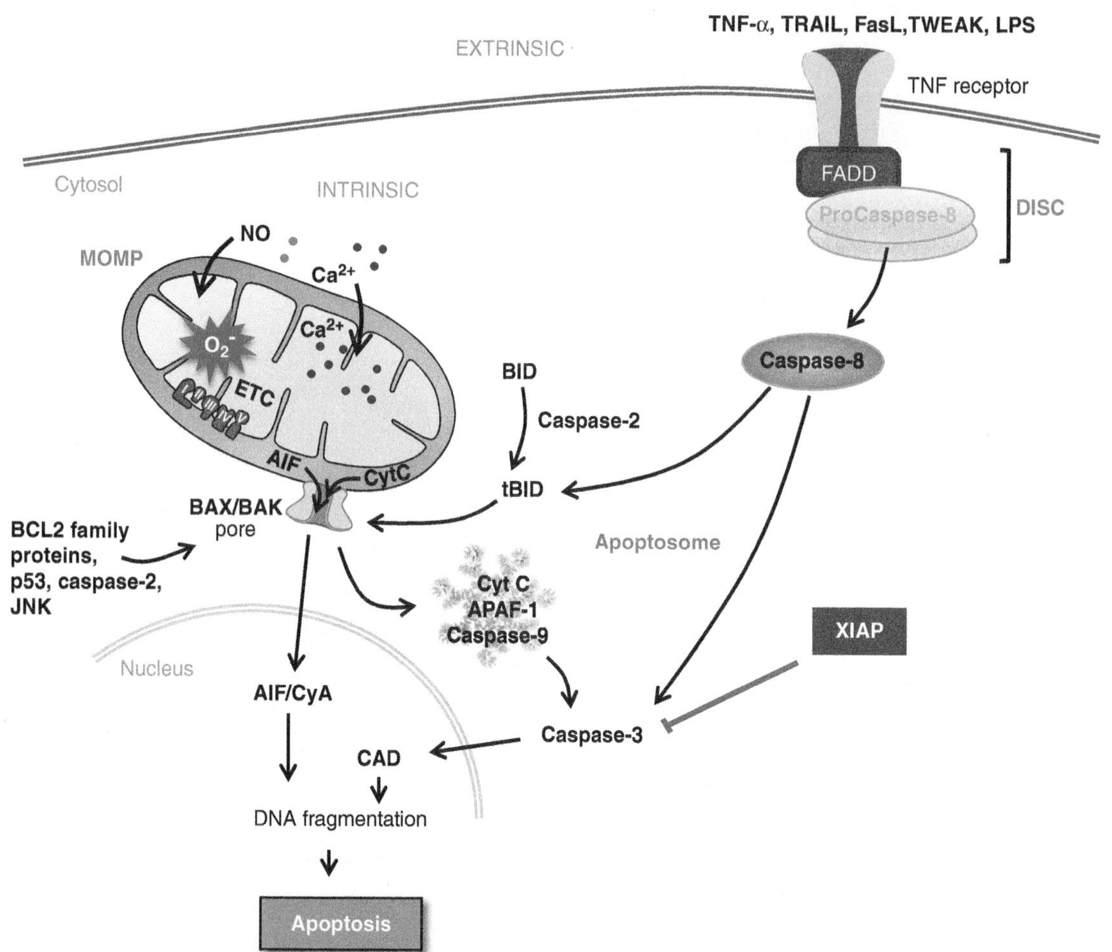

Fig. 125.2 Apoptotic mechanisms. Apoptosis can be induced via the intrinsic or the extrinsic pathway. The intrinsic pathway can be triggered by mitochondrial impairment related to excessive intracellular Ca^{2+} accumulation or accumulation of NO and reactive oxygen species. Such intramitochondrial alterations can trigger a shift in localization of proapoptotic proteins such as Cyt c from the inner mitochondrial membrane to the intermembrane space. In addition, perturbation in the nucleus, endoplasmic reticulum, or other organelles can increase the proapoptotic versus antiapoptotic B cell lymphoma 2 *(BCL2)* protein family balance, caspase-2 activity, or p53 expression at the level of the mitochondrial outer membrane. Such changes trigger mitochondrial outer membrane permeabilization *(MOMP)* and release of proapoptotic proteins into the cytosol. Cyt c initiates the assembly of the apoptosome, leading to the activation of caspase-9 and subsequently the executioner caspase-3 and DNA cleavage through activation of caspase-activated DNase *(CAD)*. Apoptosis-inducing factor *(AIF)* binds to cyclophilin A *(CyA)*, and the complex translocates to the nucleus and triggers chromatinolysis. The extrinsic pathway is activated by death receptor ligation and formation of the death-inducing signaling complex *(DISC)*, which activates caspase-8 leading to downstream activation of executioner caspases. Caspase-8 can also cleave and activate BH3-interacting domain death agonist *(BID)*, forming truncated BID *(tBID)*, which can trigger MOMP. Inhibitors of apoptosis (e.g., X-linked inhibitor of apoptosis *[XIAP]*) block caspases 3 and 9. *APAF-1,* Apoptotic peptidase-activating factor 1, *BAX,* BCL2-associated X protein; *BAK,* BCL2-antagonist/killer; *ETC,* electron transport chain; *FADD,* Fas-associated Death Domain protein; *FasL,* Fas ligand; *JNK,* c-Jun N-terminal kinase; *LPS,* lipopolysaccharide; *TNF,* tumor necrosis factor; *TRAIL,* TNF-related apoptosis inducing ligand; *TWEAK,* TNF-like weak inducer of apoptosis.

truncated BID (tBID), which integrates different death pathways at the mitochondria.[45] Truncated BID translocates to mitochondria, where it interacts with other proapoptotic proteins and triggers the release of apoptogenic factors, leading to caspase-dependent and caspase-independent cell death.[42] Death receptors can also trigger necroptosis, particularly under conditions when caspase-8 is inactive[2] (see the section "Necrosis and Necroptosis").

APOPTOSIS IN THE IMMATURE BRAIN

Apoptosis is critical for normal brain development and determines the size and shape of the central nervous system.[46] In some regions more than half of all neurons initially formed undergo apoptotic cell death,[47] with data from mouse brain suggesting that cell death peaks just after birth.[48] Similarly, oligodendrocytes are produced in excess and then pruned to needed numbers by apoptosis.[49] Many of the proteins involved in apoptosis, such as caspase-3,[26] APAF-1,[50] and BCL2-family proteins,[51,52] are upregulated during brain development. Mice devoid of caspase-3 or caspase-9 exhibit hyperplastic disorganized brains,[53,54] whereas other organs such as the thymus (with ongoing apoptosis) develop normally, supporting the concept that caspases are of particular importance in shaping the developing brain. Thus, several components of the intrinsic pathway are already markedly up-regulated in the postnatal brain because of physiologic apoptosis as part of central nervous system development.

ROLE OF THE INTRINSIC PATHWAY IN PERINATAL BRAIN INJURY

Mitochondria in the developing brain are prone to permeabilization in response to HI.[55,56] The timing of mitochondrial permeabilization is debated, but most study findings suggest that it happens 3 to 24 hours after HI—that is, starting during the latent phase and proceeding into the secondary phase of injury depending on the severity of insult, the animal model, and the brain region.[4,57-60] These proposed timings are also supported by evidence from interventions that block mitochondrial permeabilization, which are effective if given up to 6 hours after HI.[61-64]

Proapoptotic proteins (e.g., Cyt *c* and AIF) are released from mitochondria, the apoptosome forms, and downstream executioner caspases (particularly caspase-3) are activated after hypoxic-ischemic insult.[24,58] Pathways dependent on AIF[65,66] and caspases seem to be more strongly activated in the immature brain than in the adult brain,[59,67] and mitochondrial permeabilization has been proposed to mark the point of no return in hypoxic-ischemic injury of the immature brain.[68,69] Furthermore, studies that ablate the effects of BAX-mediated MOMP (e.g., knockout models of *BIM* and *BCL2-associated death promoter* (*BAD*),[70] Tat-BCL-XL–mediated neuroprotection,[71] *Bcl-XL* transgenic mice[72]) consistently reduce brain injury after neonatal HI. Indeed, BAX-inhibitory peptides[61,73] and BAX deficiency[74] substantially protect the immature brain in mice. Following HI insult in neonatal rats, a peak of caspase-3 activity is observed 24 hours after the insult,[58] and caspase-3 activity remains elevated in excess of 6 days.[24] Caspase inhibitors have therefore been shown to be neuroprotective in models of immature brain injury following HI.[58,75]

MITOCHONDRIAL PERMEABILITY TRANSITION

The molecular mechanisms of mitochondrial permeabilization under pathologic conditions are still not completely understood. Mitochondria can permeabilize through either BAX-BAK–dependent MOMP (see earlier) or opening of the mitochondrial permeability transition (MPT) pore at the junction of the inner and outer mitochondrial membranes.[68,76] The pore opens in response to increased matrix calcium concentration (as might be experienced during excitotoxicity) dissipating mitochondrial membrane potential, resulting in depolarization and mitochondrial swelling.[77] Although the nature of the MPT pore components is still debated (candidates include Fo F1 ATP synthase[78]), cyclophilin D appears to be critical for the regulation of MPT.[77,79] Cell death mediated by the MPT pore opening occurs in adult brain ischemic injury, because deficiency of the cyclophilin D gene *Ppid* and cyclophilin D inhibitors are neuroprotective.[80] However, in the immature brain, *Ppid* deficiency aggravates rather than lessens HI injury, and cyclophilin D inhibitors do not reduce injury.[61,81] These data suggest that BAX-dependent permeabilization (see above), rather than cyclophilin D–mediated opening of the MPT pore, is the more common pathway in the developing brain.

PARTHANATOS

AIF is normally tethered to the inner mitochondrial membrane; on pathologic stimuli AIF is cleaved and migrates through the permeabilized outer mitochondrial membrane where it accumulates in the cytosol.[39] This release from the mitochondrion is dependent on activation and binding of poly(ADP-ribose) polymerase 1 (PARP1) to AIF and as such, this specific route of cell death is often referred to as parthanatos (see Fig. 125.1) rather than apoptosis, as it morphologically resembles aspects of necrosis.[2,82] AIF can interact with a number of cytosolic proteins including cyclophilin A, and translocates to the nucleus where it facilitates DNA fragmentation and chromatin condensation, resulting in caspase-independent cell death.[39] In the immature brain, AIF also translocates to the nucleus after neonatal HI,[83] and mice with lower expression of AIF are less vulnerable to HI, especially in combination with administration of a caspase inhibitor.[66] Conversely, in models in which AIF expression is increased (e.g., by compensation following ablation of brain-specific AIF isoform,[84] or by AIF knock-in[85]), there is an increased cell death and infarct size, suggesting that mitochondrial AIF release contributes to neonatal brain injury.

UPSTREAM REGULATORS OF MITOCHONDRIAL OUTER MEMBRANE PERMEABILIZATION

Protein **p53** is a tumor suppressor that triggers apoptosis via multiple pathways, including cell cycle arrest and the regulation of autophagy through transactivating proapoptotic genes and repressing antiapoptotic genes.[86] It is highly conserved and regulates cell death resulting from a wide variety of both physiologic and pathologic stimuli. Protein p53 also has cytoplasmic actions at the mitochondrial level and can promote BAX/BAK-dependent mitochondrial permeabilization.[87,88] In unstressed neurons, p53 expression is generally low, limited by its association with its negative regulator MDM2, which functions as a ubiquitin ligase, targeting polyubiquitinated p53 for degradation.[89] Cellular stress displaces p53 from MDM2, and subsequently p53 expression is stabilized through substantial posttranslational modification.[90] The classic role of p53 is as an activator of transcription, and on stabilization, it accumulates in the nucleus, where it up-regulates the transcription of proapoptotic genes such as *PUMA* and *NOXA*.[91] Indeed, p53 expression is up-regulated and accumulates in the nucleus and mitochondria in an in vivo rat model of neonatal HI.[92,93] In consequence, there is an up-regulation of apoptotic pathways, leading to activation of caspase-3. Targeting pathways upstream of p53 with an nuclear factor (NF)κB inhibitor peptide resulted in a decreased accumulation of p53, increasing neuronal survival in response to neonatal HI.[92-94] However, the therapeutic benefit of reducing p53 in neonatal brain injury is still unclear,[62,95] highlighting the complex regulation of signaling required by a p53-BAX–dependent pathway.

JNKs are members of the mitogen-activated protein kinase family and, as such, are activated in response to stress. There are three mammalian JNK genes and 10 expressed isoforms as the result of alternative splicing; however, it is JNK3 that is predominantly active in the brain.[96] In a mouse model in which JNK3 expression is ablated, both adult and neonatal animals were partially protected against hypoxic-ischemic insult, and in newborn animals compared with wild-type animals, levels of c-jun were reduced.[97,98] In rat pups exposed to HI, activation of JNK3 is accompanied by translocation of the transcription factor FOXO3a to the nucleus and upregulation of proapoptotic Bim and caspase-3.[99] Pharmacologic inhibition of FOXO3a decreased cell death and infarct in this model.[99] Inhibition of JNK (either by TAT-JBD[100] or by D-JNKi[63]) in neonatal mice after HI resulted in reduced infarct size, preservation of mitochondrial integrity, and a more favorable behavioral outcome. JNK3 is hypothesized to act upstream of the proapoptotic BCL2 family as JNK3-mediated increases in BIM and PUMA expression were absent in *JNK3* gene-knockout mice.[98] In addition, activation of caspase-3 was also decreased, suggesting that activation of JNK3 in response to hypoxic-ischemic insult results in caspase-dependent apoptosis.

Caspase-2 is a member of the initiator subgroup of caspases, and is developmentally regulated.[101] Canonical activation of caspase-2 is dependent on its dimerization and subsequent cleavage, facilitated through interaction with p53-induced death domain–containing protein (PIDD) and RIP-associated ICH-1/CED3 homologous protein with a death domain (RAIDD) in some cellular systems.[102] In addition, caspase-2 activation can be triggered by nuclear DNA damage or endoplasmic reticulum (ER) or Golgi apparatus stress via a mechanism not dependent on PIDD/RAIDD.[103] Once activated, caspase-2 promotes BID cleavage, resulting in BAX translocation and release of Cyt *c*.[104] Notably, neonatal *caspase-2*-null mice are partially protected from excitotoxic and HI injury,[105,106] in contrast with adult *caspase-2*-knockout mice.[107] High expression of caspase-2 was found in neonatal mice and rats and in postmortem human tissue from neonates[105]; TRP601, a group II caspase inhibitor targeting caspase-2 and caspase-3, provided significant protection against white and gray matter loss in neonatal animals subjected to excitotoxicity, arterial stroke, or HI.[64]

EXTRINSIC PATHWAY AND DEATH RECEPTORS IN PERINATAL BRAIN INJURY

During inflammation initiated by perinatal brain injury, activation of immune cells will produce reactive oxygen species (ROS) and release excitatory amino acid agonists, proinflammatory cytokines (e.g., interleukin [IL]-1β, IL-18, TNF-α), chemokines, and TNFs (e.g., TNF-α, TNF-β, FasL, TRAIL, TNF-like weak inducer of apoptosis [TWEAK]) that may contribute to cell death.[108-110] TNF-α activity is mediated through activation of two receptors: low-affinity TNFR1 (p55) and high-affinity TNFR2 (p75),[111] found in both neuronal[112,113] and glial cell populations.[114] Although the extracellular domains of both receptors have a high degree of homology, their intracellular domains differ significantly; TNFR2 lacks the death domain present in TNFR1.[115] This leads to complex signal transduction pathways that can be triggered and may result in activation of the antagonistic functions of these two receptors.[111,116] When activated, TNFR1 (containing the death domain) triggers apoptosis,[117] by recruiting FADD and Caspase-8, forming the DISC, whereas TNFR2 initiates neuroprotection through activation of NF-κB.[118] There are several pieces of evidence that suggest the involvement of the TNF pathway in the development of white matter damage. Placental and postnatal inflammation in infants born extremely preterm result in increased TNFα and other markers of inflammation, correlating with an increased risk of white matter damage and cerebral palsy.[119] Children who develop cerebral palsy also show increased blood levels of TNF-α,[120,121] and TNFR1 is critical for lipopolysaccharide-mediated sensitization to oxygen/glucose deprivation in vitro.[122] Moreover, deletion of the TNF gene cluster abolishes lipopolysaccharide-mediated sensitization of the neonatal brain to HI insult.[123] TNF-α treatment appears to be toxic for oligodendroglial precursor cells[124] and potentiates the interferon γ toxicity on those cells in vitro.[125] TNF is also implicated in brain neuroprotection. Neuronal damage after ischemic and excitotoxic insults are enhanced in *TNFR*-knockout mice.[126] The neuroprotective role for TNF in cerebral ischemia is at least partly attributed to TNFR2 activity.[127,128]

FasL is able to bind with Fas death receptor (triggering apoptosis) and with decoy receptor (DcR) 3.[129] HI activates Fas death receptor signaling in the neonatal brain,[130] and hypoxic-ischemic brain injury is reduced in mice lacking Fas death receptors.[131] Fas expression in primary oligodendroglial precursor cells is higher than in mature oligodendrocytes,[125] implying higher susceptibility to FasL at earlier developmental stages. Two TRAIL receptors in humans contain cytoplasmic death domains (DR4 and DR5) and have the capacity to induce apoptotic cell death,[132,133] whereas DcR1 (TRAIL receptor 3) and DcR2 (TRAIL receptor 4) lack functional death domains and thus are considered to act as decoy receptors.[134,135] In mice, two membrane decoy receptors mDcTRAILR1 and mDcTRAILR2 have been reported[121,136]; there is one death-mediating TRAIL receptor, mDR5, which has the highest homology with the human TRAIL receptor DR5.[137] Expression of TRAIL, mDR5, and mDcTRAILR2 is significantly increased after HI.[138] TRAIL protein was expressed primarily in microglia and astroglia, whereas DR5 colocalized with neurons and oligodendroglial precursors in vivo. Recombinant TRAIL exerted toxicity alone or in combination with oxygen/glucose deprivation and TNF-α/interferon γ exposure in primary neurons, suggesting that the elevated TRAIL levels after HI may aggravate brain injury during the recovery phase.[138] Injection of soluble DR5 significantly reduces infarct volume after ischemia, at least in adult rodent models.[139]

The only receptor for TWEAK identified to date in both humans and rodents is fibroblast growth factor inducible 14 (Fn14).[140] The Fn14 cytoplasmic tail does not contain a canonical death domain, and TWEAK binding to Fn14 can induce multiple cell death pathways in different cellular contexts.[141,142] Expression of both TWEAK and Fn14 increases significantly in male mice following exposure to neonatal HI and male *Fn14* knockout mice have a reduced infarct size following HI.[143]

NECROSIS AND NECROPTOSIS

Another major form of cell death is necrosis, which is traditionally defined as accidental or uncontrolled cell death characterized by cell swelling and membrane rupture.[144] After insult, an initial depletion of ATP disrupts the action of plasma membrane transporters such as Na^+,K^+-ATPase, causing an influx of Na^+ and Cl^-, accompanied by increases in intracellular Ca^{2+} and water.[145] The subsequent increase in intracellular volume results in the release of cell contents into the extracellular space (in contrast with apoptosis) triggering the host's inflammatory response caused by exposure to DAMPs such as mitochondrial DNA (see Fig. 125.1).[146,147]

However, within the last 30 years, it has become obvious that in response to ligands such as TNF-family cytokines, a tightly regulated series of events is triggered with a morphology resembling that of necrosis. Necroptosis, or programmed necrosis,[6,148,149] is a form of highly regulated cell death that occurs in an environment that is dramatically depleted of ATP[150,151] or in which caspases are inhibited.[152-154]

THE CELLULAR MECHANISM OF NECROPTOSIS

Necroptosis is a proinflammatory cell death mechanism commonly induced by death receptor ligands such as TNF-α, Fas/CD95, and TRAIL, or by Toll-like receptor (TLR) 3 and 4 signaling.[155] Binding of the ligand to the death receptor initiates the assembly of a plasma membrane–associated complex (Complex I) comprising the receptor, its adaptor protein (e.g., TRADD, TRIF, and DAI, for TNFR, TLR, and T cell receptors, respectively), and receptor-interacting protein kinase (RIP) 1 (also known as *RIPK1*) (Fig. 125.3).[156-158] Interaction occurs through common death domains on the activated receptor and RIP1, and the resulting complex I is stabilized by the recruitment of cellular inhibitor of apoptosis proteins (cIAPs[159]). RIP1 initiates numerous signaling pathways, including NF-κB activation[160] and therefore is implicated in the development of the inflammatory response and prosurvival mechanisms. How then is its signaling diverted to the induction of cell death? The answer lies in the rapid polyubiquitination of RIP1 by cIAP1 and cIAP2, which occurs as complex I forms at the membrane and pushes RIP1 function toward NF-κB activation and mitogen-activated protein kinase signaling.[159,161] However, degradation of cIAPs by autoubiquitination assisted by the action of SMAC[162] results in release of RIP1 from the complex and removal of the Lys63-linked ubiquitin chain by deubiquitinating enzymes cylindromatosis (CYLD) and A20.[163,164] This marks the point at which the cell commits to a cell death outcome, but even here RIP1 signaling can still be diverted from necroptosis to the induction of apoptosis if caspase-8 is present in the cell.[165] RIP1 can form a complex with Fas-associated death domain and caspase-8 (complex IIa), initiating the latter's conversion to its active form and subsequently triggering apoptosis (see Fig. 125.2).[165,166] In the absence of caspase-8, as might occur by viral inhibition[153,154] or if the related kinase RIP3 is expressed above a threshold level within the cell,[167] necroptosis will occur.[168] RIP1 and RIP3 interact through their RIP homotypic interaction motif (RHIM) domains, resulting in the formation of the necrosome (complex IIb), a fibrillar, amyloid-like structure,[169] and further recruitment of RIP3 to the necrosome occurs.[170] RIP3 autophosphorylates, and binds its substrate pseudokinase, mixed

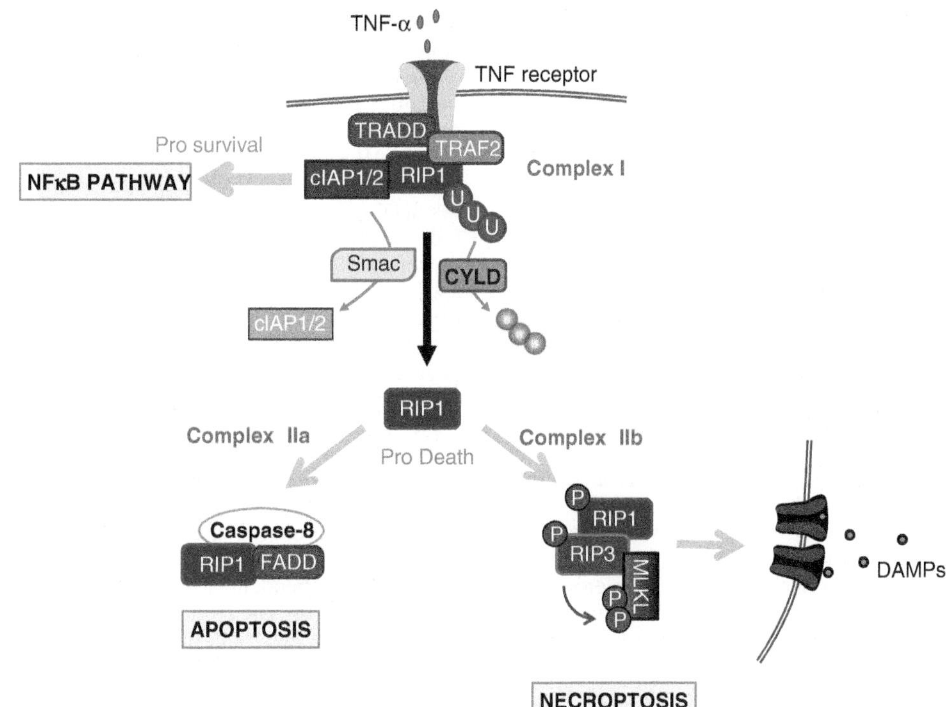

Fig. 125.3 Induction of necroptosis. Brain injury, including hypoxic-ischemic injury, results in an increase in the levels of circulating death receptor ligands such as tumor necrosis factor *(TNF)*α, Fas, and TNF-related apoptosis-inducing ligand (TRAIL). In response to ligand-receptor binding, complex I is formed at the membrane and comprises the receptor, adaptor protein, and receptor-interacting protein kinase 1 *(RIP1)*, which is rapidly polyubiquitinated by cellular inhibitor of apoptosis protein *(cIAP)*. This complex can trigger the nuclear factor κB *(NFκB)* pathway and a prosurvival response. However, deubiquitinating enzymes such as CYLD and second mitochondria-derived activator of caspases (Smac; which degrades cIAPs) release RIP1 from complex I and commit the cell to a cell death pathway. In the presence of caspases, RIP1 forms complex IIa with active caspase-8 and Fas-associated death domain *(FADD)*, triggering apoptosis. Caspase-8 can also prevent the induction of necroptosis by cleaving key proteins. In the absence of caspases, RIP1 interacts with receptor-interacting protein kinase 3 *(RIP3)*, which autophosphorylates (at Ser227) and subsequently recruits mixed lineage kinase domain–like *(MLKL)* to the necrosome complex. Phosphorylated MLKL (Thr357, Ser358) will target the necrosome to membrane lipid–rich regions such as mitochondrial or plasma membranes, forming pores allowing influx of ions, efflux of DAMPs, and cell swelling. *CYLD,* Cylindromatosis; *DAMPs*, damage-associated molecular patterns; *TRADD,* TNF receptor 1–associated death domain protein; *TRAF2,* TNF receptor-associated factor 2.

lineage kinase domain–like (MLKL), into the necrosome, where it is phosphorylated by RIP3 (see Fig. 125.3). Phosphorylation and activation of MLKL results in its oligomerization, and in this form it can bind membrane lipids such as phosphatidylinositol phosphate or the mitochondrially located cardiolipin to form pores.[171] These activated necrosomes orchestrate the permeabilization of both organelle and cell membranes, resulting in the release of DAMPs.[172,173]

Necroptosis can also be induced by alternative routes that bypass the need for RIP1. Activation of necroptosis by TLR3 and TLR4 results in the RHIM-domain-containing protein TRIF interacting with RIP3 to recruit MLKL to the necrosome.[174,175] Infection by murine cytomegalovirus can also trigger interaction between the RHIM domain protein DNA-dependent activator of interferon regulatory factors (DAI) and RIP3, resulting in virus-induced necroptosis.[176]

The presence of RIP3 and MLKL is pivotal for the execution of necroptosis, and it is worth noting that only RIP3 and MLKL are true markers of necroptosis, as RIP1 can participate in both prosurvival and apoptotic mechanisms.[6]

NEGATIVE REGULATION OF NECROPTOSIS

As can be inferred from the preceding discussion, there are a number of stages at which necroptosis can be inhibited,[177] both by endogenous events and by addition of pharmacologic reagents. The formation of the necrosome relies on the removal of ubiquitin from RIP1, and therefore up-regulation of cIAPs or down-regulation of SMADs will prevent complex formation.[178] Necroptosis and apoptosis are fundamentally linked, as certain ligands (e.g., TNFs) can trigger both pathways. In this situation, caspase-8 activation state sits at the divergence point. Contributing to the prolonged ubiquitination of RIP1, CYLD is a substrate for cleavage by active caspase-8, which can also cleave RIP1 and RIP3; therefore necroptosis is inhibited.[179] In addition, caspase-8 homodimers promote apoptosis, whereas caspase-8-FLIP (FLICE [FADD-like interleukin-1beta converting enzyme]-like inhibitory protein) heterodimers actively inhibit necroptosis.[180] Depletion of RIP3 or its substrate MLKL can also prevent necroptosis from occurring, favoring the apoptosis route.[166,181]

Pharmacologic inhibitors of necroptosis continue to be identified. During the search for substrates of RIP3, necrosulfonamide, a small molecule inhibitor, was identified; it targets MLKL, preventing formation of the necrosome.[182,183] A chemical inhibitor of RIP1, necrostatin, and its derivatives have also been instrumental in dissecting the necroptosis pathway, but as with many pharmacologic compounds, care should be taken in the interpretation of the results.[184,185] More recently, DNA-encoded library screening methods have identified GSK2982772 (derived from GSK418), a first-in-class RIP1 inhibitor that completed phase I clinical trial as a prelude for treatment of chronic inflammatory disease.[186,187]

NECROPTOSIS AND THE MITOCHONDRION

Data implicating mitochondrial dysfunction in the execution of necroptosis are still somewhat contradictory. Activation of RIP3 in cells depleted of mitochondria (through upregulation of mitophagy) resulted in MLKL-mediated necroptosis; no significant protection was observed.[188] However, mitochondrial ROS production is known to facilitate necroptosis.[167] Increasing ROS concentrations are sensed by RIP1, which can then autophosphorylate and recruit RIP3 to the necrosome.[189] In addition, activated RIP3 reportedly increases aerobic respiration and the production of ROS via phosphorylation of pyruvate dehydrogenase complex.[190] Interestingly, RIP3 activation of pyruvate dehydrogenase complex is dependent on the presence of MLKL.[190]

Mitophagy is a process of autophagic recycling of mitochondria, mediated most notably by the actions of PINK1 and Parkin. Lines of evidence suggest that mitophagy and necroptosis are linked, although whether positively or negatively remains an open question. Inhibiting mitochondrial division or genetic ablation of PINK1, resulted in a decrease in necroptosis in an in vivo model of chronic obstructive pulmonary disease.[191] In microglia, loss of Parkin also reduced necroptosis, but propagated neuroinflammation through survival of activated microglia.[192] Clearly, further work is required to determine whether injury, stimulus, or cell type alters the involvement of mitochondria in the development of necroptosis.

NECROPTOSIS AND HYPOXIC-ISCHEMIC INJURY

Knockout mouse models of *RIP3* and *MLKL*, the key genes involved in necroptosis, are both viable and fertile and have permitted the analysis of pathologic necroptosis in a wide variety of injury models.[181] A role for necroptosis-mediated cell death has been suggested in infection,[154] inflammation,[193] pancreatitis,[181] atherosclerosis,[194] and ischemia-reperfusion injury.[195,196] Furthermore, necroptosis can occur after ischemic injury to both the adult and the immature brain. The original work describing the discovery of necrostatin-1 found that after middle carotid artery occlusion generating a transient focal ischemia in rats, necrostatin-1 treatment reduced infarct size, whether it was administered before or after injury.[197] This was recapitulated in a subsequent study where necrostatin-1 was combined with antiapoptotic drugs and showed protection in both in vitro oxygen/glucose deprivation experiments and in middle carotid artery occlusion.[198] After intracerebral hemorrhage, both hematoma volume and neurovascular damage were also reduced by necrostatin-1.[199]

The role of necroptosis in immature brain injury has only recently been explored and was based on observations by Northington and colleagues[8] suggesting that the morphologic and molecular landscape of neonatal brain death is more of a "continuum," ranging from apoptosis through necroptosis to necrosis. In a neonatal mouse model of hypoxic-ischemic injury, injection of necrostatin-1 after insult blocked progression of the injury, prevented RIP1-RIP3 interaction, and inhibited NF-κB and caspase 1 signaling.[28] However, apoptotic signaling is also widespread after injury in neonatal mouse models,[200] and necrostatin treatment not only inhibits necroptosis, but also alters cell death to a more apoptotic phenotype,[28] supporting the idea that a continuum of cell death occurs depending on the injury environment. Necrostatin-1 also decreased the accumulation of oxidants, prevented the decline in mitochondrial complex I activity and improved ATP levels 24 and 96 hours after HI,[201] supporting the hypothesis that execution of necroptosis in the immature brain depends on mitochondria. The involvement of necroptosis in the development of infarct may also be dependent on severity of insult. There was a significant increase in necroptosis in the peri-infarct region in immature rats exposed to severe, rather than mild-moderate hypoxic-ischemic injury.[202] In line with this, reduction of MLKL expression by in vivo siRNA in neonatal rats reduced infarct size and restored behavioral deficits following HI.[27] A follow-up of this study showed that oligodendrocyte precursor cells were also protected from necroptosis after MLKL knockdown in vivo and hypoxia-ischemia-disrupted myelin formation was partially restored by inhibition of RIP3-MLKL interaction.[203] In the immature brain, necroptotic signaling is prevalent when hypoxia-ischemic injury occurs in neonatal mouse pups on a background of hyperglycemia[204]; indeed, there is a shift from apoptosis to necroptosis in the presence of high glucose, even in the presence of an active apoptotic pathway. Infarct size is increased, which is sensitive to treatment with the necroptosis inhibitor nec-1.[205]

FERROPTOSIS

Ferroptosis is an iron-dependent, pro-inflammatory cell death mechanism, which is triggered following system Xc- or glutathione-dependent peroxidase 4 inhibition and increases in lipid peroxidation and accumulation of ROS.[6] While conclusive evidence for a key role of ferroptosis in neonatal brain injury is still required, a number of independent observations can be linked by an explanation of ferroptosis. The requirement of iron for myelination necessitates iron concentrations in the neonatal brain and cerebrospinal fluid to be significantly higher than in the adult, making the immature brain more susceptible to iron-induced cell death.[206] Indeed, premyelinating oligodendrocytes can exhibit ferroptosis in certain neurogenetic disorders.[207] Following HI brain injury in rat pups, there was increased and persistent iron staining in the grey matter[208,209] and periventricular white matter.[209] Non-protein-bound iron was also increased in the serum and cerebrospinal fluid of infants with HIE, and increased iron correlated with poor outcome.[210] Lipid peroxidation is a hallmark of periventricular white matter injury in babies born preterm[211] and injury was aggravated by iron supplementation in an excitotoxic mouse model of preterm brain injury.[212] Another scenario of likely ferroptosis is intraventricular hemorrhage (see Chapter 131). Thus, ferroptosis may be a mechanism for targeting of new therapies in neonatal brain injury and certain neurodevelopmental disorders.[213]

AUTOPHAGY AND AUTOPHAGIC CELL DEATH

Autophagy is normally considered a prosurvival mechanism, as it is the method by which intracellular macromolecules are recycled; inhibitors of autophagy usually enhance cell death.[214,215] The criteria surrounding autophagic cell death are has been strongly debated,[216] as traditionally, it has been difficult to distinguish causal events from secondary events,[6] but under certain pathophysiologic conditions, autophagic signaling culminates in cellular demise.

AUTOPHAGY

Macroautophagy (subsequently referred to as *autophagy*) is observed in a variety of physiologic and pathologic events, such as normal development, nutrient deprivation, neurodegeneration, immunity, and aging.[217] Autophagy is a highly conserved process (indeed, more than 35 autophagy-related (ATG) proteins have been identified in yeast[218-220]) and is classically triggered following nutrient deprivation. In response to such stimuli, a series of highly choreographed steps is initiated, governed by a regulated interplay of phosphorylation and dephosphorylation (Fig. 125.4).

First, the process is initiated by the formation of the initiation complex comprising the UNC-51-like kinase (ULK) 1, autophagy-related protein (ATG) 13, and ATG101. Complex formation is promoted by activation of AMP-activated protein kinase (AMPK) in response to a reduction in cellular ATP and inhibited by mammalian target of rapamycin (mTOR).

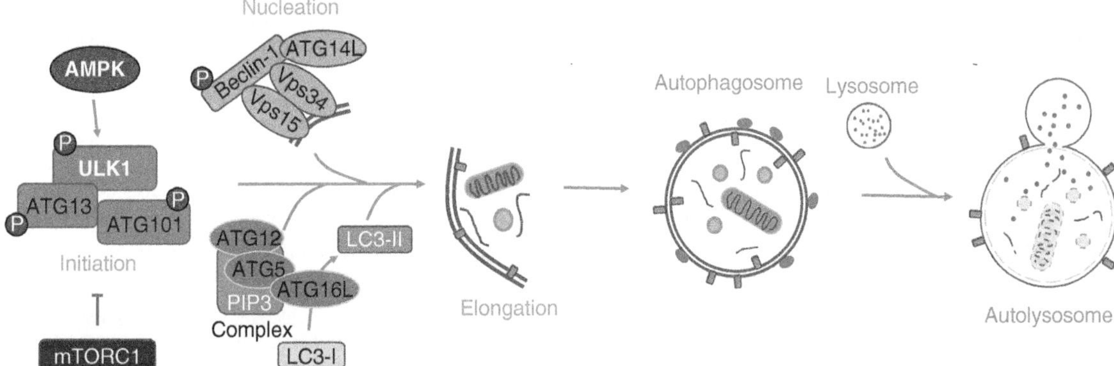

Fig. 125.4 Autophagy. In response to nutrient deprivation, inhibition of the UNC-51-like kinase 1 *(ULK1)* initiation complex by mammalian target of rapamycin complex 1 *(mTORC1)* is removed. ULK1 autophosphorylates and activates ATG13 and ATG101. AMP-activated protein kinase *(AMPK),* activated in response to starvation, contributes by phosphorylating and inhibiting components of mTORC1 and phosphorylating and further activating ULK1. ULK1 subsequently phosphorylates beclin 1 and Vps34, resulting in nucleation of the isolation membrane. Lipids are recruited to the growing phagophore, and two ubiquitin-like conjugation pathways are triggered, resulting in an autophagy-related 12 *(ATG12)*-autophagy-related 5 *(ATG5)*-autophagy-related 16 *(ATG16)* complex at the autophagosome and light-chain 3 *(LC3)* II insertion into the membrane, where it recruits cargo. Lysosomes dock to the outer membrane of the autophagosome, forming an autolysosome, and allowing hydrolases to degrade its contents *PIP3,* Phosphatidylinositol-3-phosphate.

The second step is the initiation and formation of a U-shaped double-membrane phagophore from an isolation membrane, in which the autophagic cargo is eventually sequestered. A phosphatidylinositol 3-(PI3) kinase complex comprising the lipid kinase VPS34, VPS15, beclin 1, and ATG14,[221] drives the nucleation of the isolation membrane and beclin 1-interacting transmembrane proteins such as VMP1 and ATG9 likely play a role in recruiting lipids into the forming membrane.[222,223] Further recruitment of ATG proteins is achieved through a PI3-phosphate (PI3P) binding complex.The PI3P complex interacts with ATG16L, ATG5, and ATG12, which facilitate the cleavage and conjugation of LC3 from LC3-I to LC3-II and its subsequent incorporation into the growing membrane.This represents the third step, resulting in phagophore extension, until an autophagosome is formed and the autophagic cargo is completely engulfed. Conversion from LC3-I to LC3-II, along with its subsequent relocalization into the membrane, is often used as an experimental marker for autophagy, as LC3-II remains membrane-associated until the end of the process. Lysosomes dock to the outer membrane of the autophagosome in the fourth step, mediated by SNARE (soluble NSF attachment protein [SNAP] receptor) proteins resulting in formation of the autolysosome. Finally, influx of acid hydrolases from the lysosome degrade the engulfed contents.[224]

AUTOPHAGIC CELL DEATH

Although the prosurvival function and benefits of autophagy are clear, extreme levels of autophagy have been proposed to trigger cell death. However, in some experimental systems it has been hard to distinguish between autophagy causing cell death by triggering other cell death pathways (e.g., apoptosis, necrosis) and autophagy causing cell death itself.[225] The definition of autophagic cell death has been refined to move away from a classification simply based on morphology, as accumulation of autophagosomes and autophagic vacuoles are also observed in response to apoptosis and necrosis. Therefore autophagic cell death is now described as cell death reliant on the components of the autophagic machinery itself.[6] Furthermore, two components of the pathway need to be targeted, as individually, a number of autophagy proteins act in other, nonautophagic pathways.[6] Even with these stricter criteria, a number of examples of autophagic cell death can be observed. For example, embryonic fibroblasts from mice lacking the apoptosis regulators BAX and BAK underwent cell death after treatment with apoptosis-inducing agents (etoposide and staurosporine). However, this cell death was autophagic in nature, was prevented by autophagy inhibitors, and was characterized by autophagosome formation.[226,227] Knockdown of *ATG5* expression in HeLa cells results in resistance to cell death induced by interferon γ treatment, and conversely, overexpression results in autophagic cell death, even in the presence of a functioning apoptotic pathway.[228] A subcategory of autophagic cell death, autosis, has also been identified, with a distinct morphology consisting of early nuclear convolutions, increased autolysosomes, and later, perinuclear swelling.[33,229] This form of autophagic cell death is regulated by Na^+,K^+-ATPase because autosis can be inhibited by treatment with cardiac glycosides.

AUTOPHAGIC CELL DEATH AND HYPOXIC-ISCHEMIC INJURY

Not only is autophagy activated by neonatal nutrient deprivation,[230] but acute cellular events that occur during hypoxic-ischemic injury, such as calcium influx[231] and ROS production,[232] are also triggers for autophagy. It is thus not surprising that increases in autophagic flux and markers of autophagy are observed in rodent models of adult and neonatal HI.[29,59,233-235] However it remains unclear as to the extent of the contribution of autophagic cell death to neonatal brain injury paradigms. Histologic assessment of the brains of asphyxiated term newborns provided evidence of enhanced autophagic flux in thalamic neurons, coupled with increased levels of apoptotic markers.[236,237] In a rat neonatal model, pretreatment with an mTOR inhibitor, rapamycin, promoted autophagy rather than the apoptosis usually observed after insult.[238] In addition, overactivation of autophagy has been implicated as a neuroprotective mechanism after neonatal HI, by reducing ER stress.[239] The neuroprotective effects of erythropoietin in the neonatal brain may act through increasing autophagic flux, as reported in a neonatal seizure model.[240] Autophagy was also rapidly increased in a piglet model of neonatal HI, but this increased autophagic flux decreased following subsequent impaired autophagosomal clearance.[30]. Rapid increases in LC3-II have also been observed following neonatal HI injury in rodents, which was region- and sex-specific.[32,233] Ablation of *ATG7* mice resulted in significant neuroprotection and reduction in infarct size following HI injury.[31,237] In an excitotoxicity rat model of preterm periventricular leukomalacia, autophagic flux was increased 24 hours following injury and neuroprotection was observed on pharmacologic inhibition of autophagy.[241] Evidence also suggests that the lack of efficacy of NMDA receptor inhibitors for preventing excitotoxicity in the immature mouse brain may be due to induction of autophagic cell death mechanisms in GABAergic neurons.[242] Furthermore, autosis, dependent on Na^+,K^+-ATPase, was detected regionally in the hippocampus after neonatal HI, potentially exerting its effects through interaction with beclin 1.[33,243] This is in line with other studies suggesting brain region–specific and sex-specific differences in induction of autophagic cell death after neonatal brain injury.[32,59,233,244]

STRESS RESPONSE PATHWAYS CAN PREVENT CELL DEATH MECHANISMS

As described above, cell death pathways can be induced by a variety of stresses, including nutrient deprivation, environment, and infection/inflammation. However, before the cell commits to cell death, there are stress response pathways that can mitigate a catastrophic outcome. These pathways may therefore represent avenues for therapeutic intervention.[245]

UNFOLDED PROTEIN RESPONSE

The ER regulates protein folding of specialized proteins as well as storage of intracellular calcium. ER stress has been identified in rodent models of neonatal HIE leading to the toxic buildup of misfolded proteins in the ER.[246,247] The unfolded protein response (UPR) mechanism acts through glucose-regulated protein (GRP)78 (also known as *binding immunoglobulin protein*). The accumulation of unfolded proteins in the ER lumen removes GRP78 from its inhibitory interactions with UPR sensors, initiating ER-mediated degradation (ERAD), autophagy, and/or protein synthesis of chaperones and antioxidants. However, if the unfolded protein load generates a severe or prolonged stress, intrinsic and extrinsic cell death pathways are triggered.[248,249]

INTEGRATED STRESS RESPONSE

The integrated stress response (ISR) is an integrated series of responses to both extracellular (hypoxia, nutrient deprivation) and intracellular (ER stress, ROS) stresses.[245] Although the stimuli can be varied, pathways converge at the phosphorylation and activation of eukaryotic translation initiation factor 2 (eIF2α), which reduces protein synthesis and up-regulates prosurvival mechanisms, including induction of autophagy and inhibition of apoptosis by cIAP1/2 expression.[250] Once cellular homeostasis is reinstated, eIF2α is dephosphorylated and normal protein synthesis is restored.[251] As with the UPR, if the cellular environment does not recover, cell death pathways can be triggered, usually through apoptosis.

CONCLUSION

Previously it was believed that cells died either through accidental necrosis or regulated (programmed) apoptotic cell death. Today it is becoming generally accepted that there are numerous forms of regulated cell death and these are required to be defined by biochemical hallmarks rather than morphologic features. Indeed, experimental studies suggest that accidental cell death pathways and the types of regulated cell death pathways discussed in this chapter are important in the context of immature brain injury, depending on the intensity and type of insult, cell type, brain region, sex, and developmental age. Further insights into these cell death cascades will result in novel and more efficient strategies for neuroprotection.

A complete reference list is available at www.ExpertConsult.com.

SELECT REFERENCES

4. Hagberg H, Mallard C, Rousset CI, Thornton C. Mitochondria: hub of injury responses in the developing brain. *Lancet Neurol*. 2014;13(2):217-232.
6. Galluzzi L, Vitale I, Aaronson SA, et al. Molecular mechanisms of cell death: recommendations of the nomenclature committee on cell death 2018. *Cell Death Differ*. 2018;25(3):486-541.
8. Northington FJ, Zelaya ME, O'Riordan DP, et al. Failure to complete apoptosis following neonatal hypoxia-ischemia manifests as "continuum" phenotype of cell death and occurs with multiple manifestations of mitochondrial dysfunction in rodent forebrain. *Neuroscience*. 2007;149(4):822-833.
17. Tang D, Kang R, Berghe TV, Vandenabeele P, Kroemer G. The molecular machinery of regulated cell death. *Cell Res*. 2019;29(5):347-364.
19. Rice 3rd JE, Vannucci RC, Brierley JB. The influence of immaturity on hypoxic-ischemic brain damage in the rat. *Ann Neurol*. 1981;9(2):131-141.
20. Bittigau P, Sifringer M, Felderhoff-Mueser U, Ikonomidou C. Apoptotic neurodegeneration in the context of traumatic injury to the developing brain. *Exp Toxicol Pathol*. 2004;56(1-2):83-89.
21. Strunk T, Inder T, Wang X, Burgner D, Mallard C, Levy O. Infection-induced inflammation and cerebral injury in preterm infants. *Lancet Infect Dis*. 2014;14(8):751-762.
22. Millar LJ, Shi L, Hoerder-Suabedissen A, Molnar Z. Neonatal hypoxia ischaemia: mechanisms, models, and therapeutic challenges. *Front Cell Neurosci*. 2017;11:78.
23. Blumberg RM, Cady EB, Wigglesworth JS, McKenzie JE, Edwards AD. Relation between delayed impairment of cerebral energy metabolism and infarction following transient focal hypoxia-ischaemia in the developing brain. *Exp Brain Res*. 1997;113(1):130-137.
25. Edwards AD, Yue X, Cox P, et al. Apoptosis in the brains of infants suffering intrauterine cerebral injury. *Pediatr Res*. 1997;42(5):684-689.
31. Koike M, Shibata M, Tadakoshi M, et al. Inhibition of autophagy prevents hippocampal pyramidal neuron death after hypoxic-ischemic injury. *Am J Pathol*. 2008;172(2):454-469.
32. Ginet V, Puyal J, Clarke PG, Truttmann AC. Enhancement of autophagic flux after neonatal cerebral hypoxia-ischemia and its region-specific relationship to apoptotic mechanisms. *Am J Pathol*. 2009;175(5):1962-1974.
34. Bock FJ, Tait SWG. Mitochondria as multifaceted regulators of cell death. *Nat Rev Mol Cell Biol*. 2020;21(2):85-100.
35. Cosentino K, Garcia-Saez AJ. Bax and bak pores: are we closing the circle? *Trends Cell Biol*. 2017;27(4):266-275.
39. Bano D, Prehn JHM. Apoptosis-inducing factor (AIF) in physiology and disease: the tale of a repented natural born killer. *EBioMedicine*. 2018;30:29-37.
45. Tummers B, Green DR. Caspase-8: regulating life and death. *Immunol Rev*. 2017;277(1):76-89.
46. Yamaguchi Y, Miura M. Programmed cell death in neurodevelopment. *Dev Cell*. 2015;32(4):478-490.
57. Northington FJ, Ferriero DM, Flock DL, Martin LJ. Delayed neurodegeneration in neonatal rat thalamus after hypoxia-ischemia is apoptosis. *J Neurosci*. 2001;21(6):1931-1938.
61. Wang X, Han W, Du X, et al. Neuroprotective effect of Bax-inhibiting peptide on neonatal brain injury. *Stroke*. 2010;41(9):2050-2055.
73. Wang X, Carlsson Y, Basso E, et al. Developmental shift of cyclophilin D contribution to hypoxic-ischemic brain injury. *J Neurosci*. 2009;29(8):2588-2596.
74. Gibson ME, Han BH, Choi J, et al. BAX contributes to apoptotic-like death following neonatal hypoxia-ischemia: evidence for distinct apoptosis pathways. *Mol Med*. 2001;7(9):644-655.
79. Baines CP, Kaiser RA, Purcell NH, et al. Loss of cyclophilin D reveals a critical role for mitochondrial permeability transition in cell death. *Nature*. 2005;434(7033):658-662.
85. Li T, Li K, Zhang S, et al. Overexpression of apoptosis inducing factor aggravates hypoxic-ischemic brain injury in neonatal mice. *Cell Death Dis*. 2020;11(1):77.
87. Chipuk JE, Kuwana T, Bouchier-Hayes L, et al. Direct activation of Bax by p53 mediates mitochondrial membrane permeabilization and apoptosis. *Science*. 2004;303(5660):1010-1014.
93. Nijboer CH, Heijnen CJ, Groenendaal F, May MJ, van Bel F, Kavelaars A. A dual role of the NF-kappaB pathway in neonatal hypoxic-ischemic brain damage. *Stroke*. 2008;39(9):2578-2586.
105. Carlsson Y, Schwendimann L, Vontell R, et al. Genetic inhibition of caspase-2 reduces hypoxic-ischemic and excitotoxic neonatal brain injury. *Ann Neurol*. 2011;70(5):781-789.
116. Fontaine V, Mohand-Said S, Hanoteau N, Fuchs C, Pfizenmaier K, Eisel U. Neurodegenerative and neuroprotective effects of tumor necrosis factor (TNF) in retinal ischemia: opposite roles of TNF receptor 1 and TNF receptor 2. *J Neurosci*. 2002;22(7):RC216.
117. Hsu H, Xiong J, Goeddel DV. The TNF receptor 1-associated protein TRADD signals cell death and NF-kappa B activation. *Cell*. 1995;81(4):495-504.
121. Nelson KB, Grether JK, Dambrosia JM, et al. Neonatal cytokines and cerebral palsy in very preterm infants. *Pediatr Res*. 2003;53(4):600-607.
126. Bruce AJ, Boling W, Kindy MS, et al. Altered neuronal and microglial responses to excitotoxic and ischemic brain injury in mice lacking TNF receptors. *Nat Med*. 1996;2(7):788-794.
146. Scaffidi P, Misteli T, Bianchi ME. Release of chromatin protein HMGB1 by necrotic cells triggers inflammation. *Nature*. 2002;418(6894):191-195.

147. Zhang Q, Raoof M, Chen Y, et al. Circulating mitochondrial DAMPs cause inflammatory responses to injury. *Nature*. 2010;464(7285):104-107.
153. Kaiser WJ, Upton JW, Long AB, et al. RIP3 mediates the embryonic lethality of caspase-8-deficient mice. *Nature*. 2011;471(7338):368-372.
154. Cho YS, Challa S, Moquin D, et al. Phosphorylation-driven assembly of the RIP1-RIP3 complex regulates programmed necrosis and virus-induced inflammation. *Cell*. 2009;137(6):1112-1123.
161. Lalaoui N, Vaux DL. Recent advances in understanding inhibitor of apoptosis proteins. *F1000Res*. 2018;7:F1000.
165. Wang L, Du F, Wang X. TNF-alpha induces two distinct caspase-8 activation pathways. *Cell*. 2008;133(4):693-703.
167. Zhang DW, Shao J, Lin J, et al. RIP3, an energy metabolism regulator that switches TNF-induced cell death from apoptosis to necrosis. *Science*. 2009;325(5938):332-336.
168. Khoury MK, Gupta K, Franco SR, Liu B. Necroptosis in the pathophysiology of disease. *Am J Pathol*. 2020;190(2):272-285.
177. Weinlich R, Oberst A, Beere HM, Green DR. Necroptosis in development, inflammation and disease. *Nat Rev Mol Cell Biol*. 2017;18(2):127-136.
197. Degterev A, Huang Z, Boyce M, et al. Chemical inhibitor of nonapoptotic cell death with therapeutic potential for ischemic brain injury. *Nat Chem Biol*. 2005;1(2):112-119.
201. Chavez-Valdez R, Martin LJ, Flock DL, Northington FJ. Necrostatin-1 attenuates mitochondrial dysfunction in neurons and astrocytes following neonatal hypoxia-ischemia. *Neuroscience*. 2012;219:192-203.
211. Back SA, Luo NL, Mallinson RA, et al. Selective vulnerability of preterm white matter to oxidative damage defined by F2-isoprostanes. *Ann Neurol*. 2005;58(1):108-120.
213. Wu Y, Song J, Wang Y, Wang X, Culmsee C, Zhu C. The potential role of ferroptosis in neonatal brain injury. *Front Neurosci*. 2019;13:115.
215. Galluzzi L, Bravo-San Pedro JM, Levine B, Green DR, Kroemer G. Pharmacological modulation of autophagy: therapeutic potential and persisting obstacles. *Nat Rev Drug Discov*. 2017;16(7):487-511.
224. Longatti A, Tooze SA. Vesicular trafficking and autophagosome formation. *Cell Death Differ*. 2009;16(7):956-965.
230. Kuma A, Hatano M, Matsui M, et al. The role of autophagy during the early neonatal starvation period. *Nature*. 2004;432(7020):1032-1036.
236. Ginet V, Pittet MP, Rummel C, et al. Dying neurons in thalamus of asphyxiated term newborns and rats are autophagic. *Ann Neurol*. 2014;76(5):695-711.
237. Xie C, Ginet V, Sun Y, et al. Neuroprotection by selective neuronal deletion of Atg7 in neonatal brain injury. *Autophagy*. 2016;12(2):410-423.
241. Descloux C, Ginet V, Rummel C, Truttmann AC, Puyal J. Enhanced autophagy contributes to excitotoxic lesions in a rat model of preterm brain injury. *Cell Death Dis*. 2018;9(9):853.
243. Fernandez AF, Liu Y, Ginet V, et al. Interaction between the autophagy protein Beclin 1 and Na+,K+-ATPase during starvation, exercise, and ischemia. *JCI Insight*. 2020;5(1):e133282.
248. Karagoz GE, Acosta-Alvear D, Walter P. The unfolded protein response: detecting and responding to fluctuations in the protein-folding capacity of the endoplasmic reticulum. *Cold Spring Harb Perspect Biol*. 2019;11(9).

Development of the Blood-Brain Barrier 126

Clémence Disdier | Susan S. Cohen | Mariella Errede | Daniela Virgintino | Barbara S. Stonestreet

INTRODUCTION

The blood-brain barrier (BBB) is a selective diffusion barrier that maintains central nervous system (CNS) homeostasis and limits the entry of substances that could potentially alter neuronal function. The main anatomic substrate of the BBB is the specialized cerebral microvascular endothelium. It and associated astrocytes, pericytes, microglia, neurons, and the extracellular matrix components constitute the classical components of the neurovascular unit (NVU) (Figs. 126.1 and 126.2).[1] In addition, oligodendrocyte lineage cells that can express NG2 chondroitin sulfate proteoglycan have been demonstrated to also contribute to the NVU.[2,3] In contrast with other endothelium in the body, properties specific to the cerebral vascular endothelium include the presence of tight cell-cell junctions between the endothelial cells, a lack of fenestrations across the endothelial surface, specific transporters, and low exchange by transcytosis. The NVU is essential in coupling neuronal activity with other vascular/barrier functions in the CNS throughout development and in the adult.[1] Although systematic measurements of BBB function in the fetus and newborn have been limited to date, understanding of the development of the barrier continues to increase.

This chapter reviews the basic concepts of the BBB, summarizes the molecular biology of the BBB, introduces the concept of the NVU, and places these concepts in the context of the developing fetus and neonate. Finally, the BBB is discussed with special emphasis on the relevance of the barrier to select aspects of perinatal medicine.

HISTORICAL PERSPECTIVES

In 1878, Paul Ehrlich, a German microbiologist, demonstrated in a seminal publication that there was a barrier between the vascular system supplying the peripheral circulatory system and the brain.[4] Later experiments by Edwin Goldmann, an associate of Ehrlich, further established that this barrier was truly selective and not a result of the binding properties of the dye.[5] Lewandowsky in 1900 introduced the descriptive term *blood-brain barrier* in this context.[6] Although the concept of the BBB has been refined over the past few decades, the current understanding of its basic structure is built on the work of Reese, Karnovsky, and Brightman in the late 1960s.[7,8] Their work confirmed the presence of epithelial-like "tight junctions" that physically seal the interendothelial cleft, forming a continuous, impermeable membrane that constitutes the primary anatomic substrate of the BBB.[7,8] Reese and Karnovsky in 1967 proposed that the capillary lumen bridged by tight junctions formed a continuous, impermeable membrane that constituted the primary anatomic substrate of the BBB.[7,8] Studies by Brightman and Reese showed that horseradish peroxidase injected into the brain could diffuse through the approximately 20-nm gaps between the astrocyte end feet to the abluminal surface of the endothelium, indicating that astrocytes do not form the physical barrier.[7,8] Recent developments suggest that the BBB represents a dynamic interface devoted to the bidirectional control of the exchange of molecules and ions between the bloodstream and CNS, which also provides surveillance of immune-cell trafficking into the brain.[9,10] The BBB is now considered a component of a

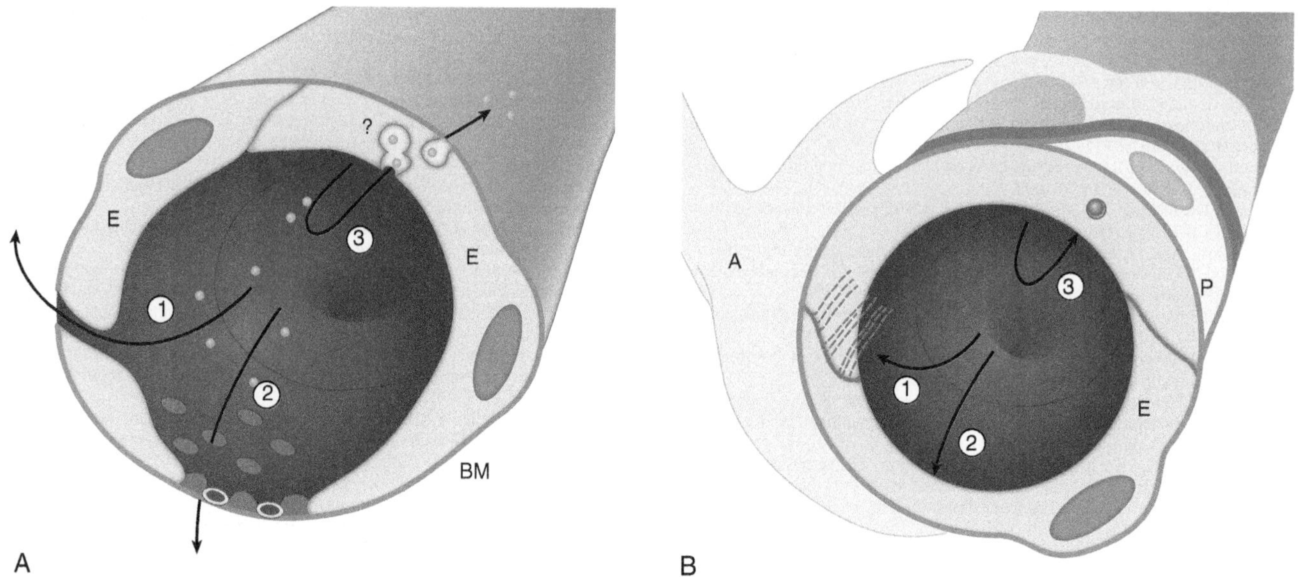

Fig. 126.1 Comparative anatomic features of nonbarrier and blood-brain barrier capillaries. (A) Peripheral capillaries and nonbarrier capillaries of the central nervous system lack an effective barrier to blood-borne polar molecules because of diffusion between endothelial cells *(1)*, diffusion through endothelial fenestrations *(2)*, and vesicular-tubulovesicular transport *(3)*. (B) Barrier capillaries are ensheathed by astrocytic foot processes, develop complex interendothelial tight junctions that block paracellular diffusion of polar substances, lack fenestrations, and contain a sparse vesicular transport system. A relatively thick basement membrane *(BM)* is interposed between the endothelial cells *(E)*, astrocytic foot processes *(A)*, and pericytes *(P)*.

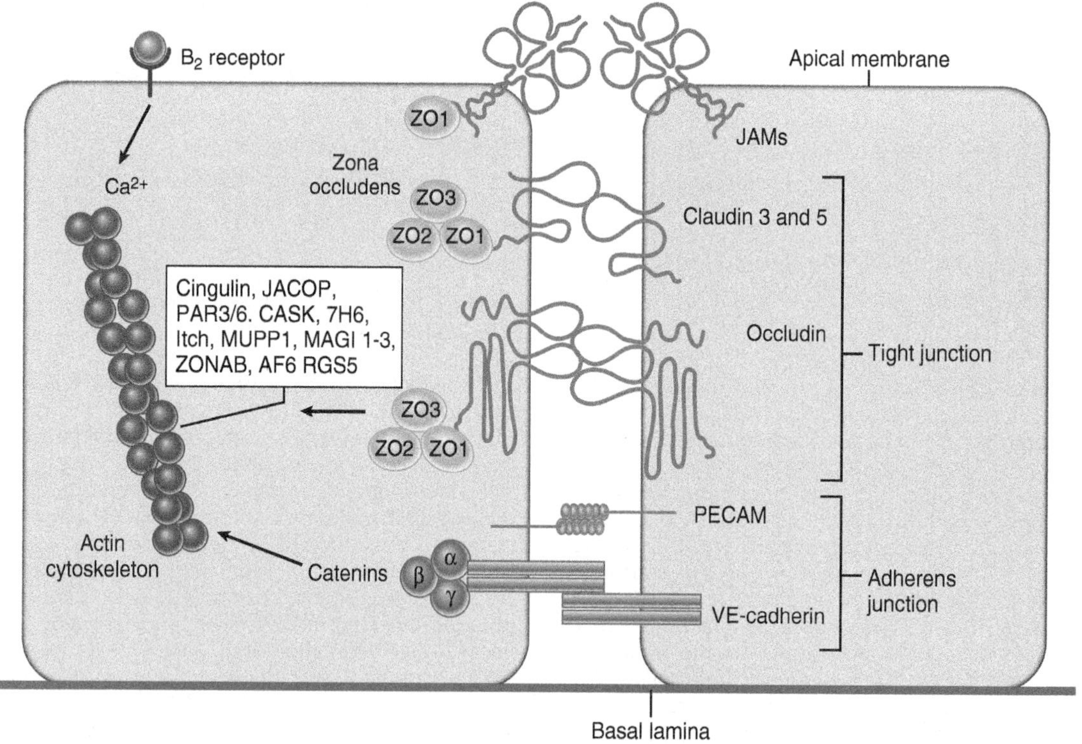

Fig. 126.2 Neurovascular unit: The cell associations at the blood-brain barrier (BBB). The cerebral endothelial cells form tight junctions at their margins, which seal the aqueous paracellular diffusional pathway between the cells. Pericytes are distributed discontinuously along the length of the cerebral capillaries and partially surround the endothelium. Both the cerebral endothelial cells and the pericytes are enclosed by and contribute to the local basement membrane, which forms a distinct perivascular extracellular matrix (basal lamina 1 [BL1]), different in composition from the extracellular matrix of the glial end feet bounding the brain parenchyma (BL2). Foot processes from astrocytes form a complex network surrounding capillaries, and this close cell association is important for the induction and maintenance of the barrier's properties. Axonal projections from neurons onto arteriolar smooth muscle contain vasoactive neurotransmitters and peptides and regulate local cerebral blood. BBB permeability may be regulated by the release of vasoactive peptides and other agents from cells associated with the endothelium. Microglia are the resident immunocompetent cells of the brain. The movement of solutes across the BBB is either passive, driven by a concentration gradient from plasma to brain, with more lipid-soluble substances entering most easily, or it may be facilitated by passive or active transporters in the endothelial cell membranes. Efflux transporters in the endothelium limit the central nervous system penetration of a wide variety of solutes. *JAMS*, junctional adhesion molecules; *PECAM*, platelet–endothelial cell adhesion molecule. (Modified from Abbot NJ, Patabendige AAK, Dolman DEM, et al. Structure and function of the BBB. *Neurobiol Dis.* 2010;37:13–25)

larger physiologic unit termed the *neurovascular unit*, which contributes to the dynamic function of this vital interface between the systemic circulation and the brain.[1,11,12]

DEFINITION OF THE BLOOD-BRAIN BARRIER AS A CONSTITUENT OF THE NEUROVASCULAR UNIT

In peripheral microvessels and in limited nonbarrier capillaries of the CNS, blood-borne polar molecules diffuse across the vessel wall into tissues through spaces between adjacent endothelial cells and through transcellular routes—specifically "endothelial fenestrations" and/or vesicular or tubulovesicular structures (see Fig. 126.1A). In contrast, the BBB capillary is primarily formed by a "continuous" endothelium that is present in several other anatomically distinct structures. However, there are specialized junctional complexes found only in the brain that selectively prevent blood-borne molecules from freely passing through the interendothelial clefts. This endothelium, along with other perivascular cells, maintains an optimal microenvironment that couples neuronal activity with vascular-barrier function within the NVU (see Fig. 126.1B). The BBB at the level of the endothelial cells is composed of three main features[1]:

1. The "physical barrier," formed by tight junctions between endothelial cells, prevents paracellular diffusion.
2. The "transport barrier" controls the movement of nutrients, ions, and toxins across the endothelium via specific metabolic transporters and efflux pumps located on the luminal and abluminal membranes of endothelial cells.[1,12] For example, the ATP-binding cassette (ABC) superfamily multidrug *efflux pumps* located on the luminal (apical) membrane serve as "gatekeepers" to extrude mainly xenobiotic lipophilic substances from the endothelial cytoplasm.[13,14]
3. The "metabolic barrier" represents a combination of intracellular and extracellular enzymes, such as cytochromes P450 and monoamine oxidase that metabolize molecules capable of penetrating cerebral endothelial cells. This barrier-specific endothelial phenotype is determined by complex interactions of endothelial cells with other members of the NVU, including astrocytes, pericytes, smooth muscle cells, microglial cells, neurons, and the extracellular matrix molecules (see Fig. 126.2).[1,15,16] Moreover, the components of the NVU contribute to the dynamic regulation of microvascular permeability and therefore regulate the function of the endothelial *physical and transport barrier* during normal and pathologic BBB activity.[1,15,16]

MAIN MOLECULAR CONSTITUENTS OF THE BLOOD-BRAIN BARRIER

THE PHYSICAL BARRIER: TIGHT JUNCTIONS

The endothelia of the brain's blood vessels are interconnected by a continuous network of complex tight junctions that functionally fuse plasma membranes of adjacent endothelial cells and are responsible for the physical barrier of the BBB (Fig. 126.3).[7,8] Tight junctions restrict the movement to small ions, such that the transendothelial electrical resistance can be as high as 1000 ohm/cm^2 in brain endothelium compared with 2 to 20 ohm/cm^2 in peripheral capillaries.[1,17]

Tight junctions form a continuous circumferential belt separating apical and basolateral plasma membrane domains, thus

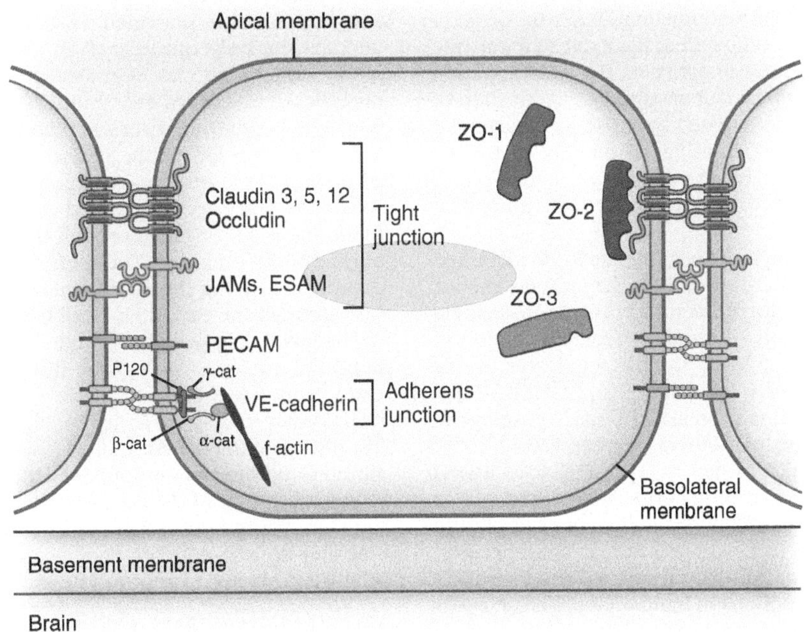

Fig. 126.3 Structure of the blood-brain barrier's tight junctions. The tight junctional complex comprises occludin, claudin 3 and 5, and possibly other claudins. Cadherins of the adherens junctions provide structural integrity and attachment between the cells and are necessary for the formation of tight junctions. The barrier to diffusion and the high electrical resistance of the blood-brain barrier appear to be largely due to the properties of claudin 3 and 5. The claudins associate and bind to each other across the intercellular cleft. A different ratio of the claudin mix may subtly alter tight junctional properties and the strength of the junction. Occludin has similar associations across the cleft but does not form the restrictive pore to small ions. The claudins and occludin are linked to the scaffolding proteins ZO-1, ZO-2, and ZO-3 and, in turn, via cingulin dimers to the actin/myosin cytoskeletal system within the cell. The role of the junction-associated molecules (junctional adhesion molecules [JAMs], members of the immunoglobulin superfamily) is unclear. JAM-A is localized on the lateral membrane of brain endothelial cells. *ESAM*, Endothelial cell-selective adhesion molecule; *PECAM*, platelet–endothelial cell adhesion molecule.

working as a barrier within the intercellular space and as a fence within the plasma membrane to define cell polarity.[1,18,19] The structural characteristics of these junctions were confirmed by transmission electron microscopy and freeze-fracture studies. They appear by transmission electron microscopy as focal contacts between membranes of adjacent cells.[7] Freeze-fracture electron microscopy showed that these contacts correspond to branching fibrils of transmembrane particles.[20] The main protein components of the tight junctions are transmembrane proteins that can be classified into three distinct groups: (1) the claudin family (encompassing 27 members in humans); (2) the tight junction–associated MARVEL proteins (TAMPs), including occludin; and (3) the junctional adhesion molecules (JAMs) (see Fig. 126.3).[1,12,16,18]

Claudins and occludin have four membrane-spanning domains and two extracellular loops. Occludin was identified in 1993 as the first integral protein localized in the tight junction.[21] It is a 60- to 65-kDa protein with a carboxyl-terminal domain.[21] The main function of occludin appears to be in the regulation of tight junctions.[1,12,16,22] Likewise, the family of claudin proteins are 22-kDa phosphoproteins that have four transmembrane domains and contribute to the high electrical resistance of the tight junctions.[1,16,18,23] Twenty-seven members of the claudin family have been identified.[1,18,23] Claudin-3, claudin-5, and claudin-12 are the main claudins that contribute to the high resistance of the BBB.[1,18,23] Together, claudins and occludins form the extracellular components of tight junctions, and both are required for the formation and proper functioning of the BBB.[24]

Transmembrane proteins are connected to the actin cytoskeleton by the submembranous junctional plaques. These are composed of adapter proteins that form multiple protein-protein interaction motifs.[20,25–27] These proteins are located at the cytoplasmic surface of endothelial cells and connect the transmembrane tight junction proteins to actin, which is the primary cytoskeleton protein for the maintenance of structural and functional integrity of the endothelium.[16] A ring of actin microfilaments underlies the complex and has a role in regulating the permeability and structural integrity of the tight junction complexes situated on the apical cell membrane.[20] Activation of the actin cytoskeleton may be initiated by a rise in intracellular calcium, for example, resulting from ligand binding to the B2 bradykinin receptor, which may change the configuration of claudins and occludin, thereby modifying the tight junctional properties.[12]

The first components of the junctional plaque to be identified were the zonula occludens (ZO-1, -2, and -3). ZO proteins anchor the tight junction complex to the actin cytoskeleton, making them essential for the assembly of claudins, occludins, and JAM-A.[28,29] Other examples of scaffolding proteins implicated in this protein network are symplekin, cingulin, 7H6, ZONAB (ZO-1-associated *n*ucleic *a*cid-*b*inding protein), AF-6 (*ALL1-f*used gene from chromosome *6* protein), and others (see Fig. 126.3).[12,20,25] Additionally, regulatory molecules such as G proteins (Gαi, RGS5) have been localized to the tight junction structure and play a major role in the regulation of BBB permeability. For example, the heterotrimeric G proteins (Gαi) were identified in association with ZO-1. This regulatory protein contributes to the formation and maintenance of tight junctions in brain endothelial cells[30,31] and is involved in lymphocyte extravasation.[32,33]

Adherens junctions are formed by junction-associated adhesion proteins (JAMs), members of the immunoglobulin (Ig) superfamily. JAMs are transmembrane proteins composed of two extracellular Ig domains and a short cytoplasmic domain. JAMs appear to regulate cell polarity and endothelial permeability, also acting as cell adhesion molecules for leukocytes.[12,34] In the resting state, JAM-A is typically localized on the lateral membrane of brain endothelial cells; under inflammatory conditions, tight junction complex remodeling results in JAM-A relocalization away from the lateral membrane.[35] Platelet-endothelial cell adhesion molecules (PECAMs) and vascular endothelial cadherins are the two important proteins involved in the adherens junctions and are critical for the promotion of close physical contact between endothelial cells so as to facilitate the formation of tight junctions.[18,36] They also contribute to the high electrical resistance of tight junctions and play a role in inflammatory cell transmigration through junctional complexes.[36] The disruption of adherens junctions leads to impaired BBB function, extravasation of blood components, and the influx of water, thereby predisposing to the formation of vasogenic edema.[37]

TRANSPORTERS IN THE ENDOTHELIUM

Paracellular diffusion is prevented by tight junctions between endothelial cells; only small lipophilic molecules with molecular weights less than 400 Da can access the brain parenchyma *by* diffusion across the endothelial wall. Specific transporters for larger molecules are present in the endothelial cells that constitute the "transport barrier" of the BBB (Fig. 126.4C). They are located on the luminal and abluminal membranes of endothelia and control nutrients, ions, and toxins crossing between the bloodstream and brain. The solute carrier (SLC) family of transporters mainly regulates substrate uptake, whereas the ABC transporter family regulates efflux out of the brain parenchyma. However, some SLC transporters function both as uptake and efflux transporters.

A total of 395 members of the SLC superfamily have been identified and classified into 52 families.[38,39] The glucose transporter 1 (GLUT 1), monocarboxylate transporters 1 and 2 (MCT1 and MCT2), and the L-system neutral amino acid transporter 1 (LAT 1) belong to the SLC family and supply the brain parenchyma with glucose, ketone bodies, and neutral amino acids, respectively. Forty-eight known ABC transporters have been identified in humans. They are classified into seven subfamilies (A through G). They bind and hydrolyze ATP to translocate lipid-soluble molecules across the endothelial plasma cell membrane of the brain and therefore are classified as active transporters. This family includes the P-glycoprotein (P-gp, also termed the *ABCB1 transporter*), the breast cancer resistance protein (BCRP, also termed the *ABCG2 transporter*),[12] multidrug resistance-associated proteins (MRPs), and transporters belonging to the C family. P-gp is commonly considered the primary transporter in the ABC family because it is responsible for transporting a large variety of substrates. P-gp is concentrated on the luminal membrane and functions as a barrier, preventing the entry of drugs and xenobiotics into the brain.[40,41] These efflux transporters maintain tight control, restricting the substances that are allowed to enter the CNS through the endothelial cell barrier.[37]

High-molecular-weight solutes (e.g., large proteins and peptides) are able to cross the BBB to enter the intact CNS via endocytotic mechanisms called *receptor-mediated transcytosis (RMT)*; they transport larger molecules such as insulin or act by adsorptive-mediated transcytosis (AMT), which transports albumin and similar compounds. Macromolecules bind to specific receptors during RMT. These receptors cluster with their ligands into vesicular caveolae that are internalized into the endothelial cell; they are subsequently transported across the cytoplasm and finally exocytosed at appropriate locations within the cell.

ENZYMATIC SYSTEMS AND METABOLISM

Brain endothelial cells express different systems responsible for the metabolism of drugs typically found in the liver, including the cytochromes P450 and phase II enzymes of metabolism.[42] These drug and toxin-metabolizing enzymes contribute, along with the efflux transporters, to the detoxification activity of the BBB and participate in drug pharmacodynamics. In addition, enzymes regulate the concentration of signaling molecules and metabolize endogenous substrates such as fatty acids, hormones, steroids, and vitamins. Brain endothelial cells also express several enzymes

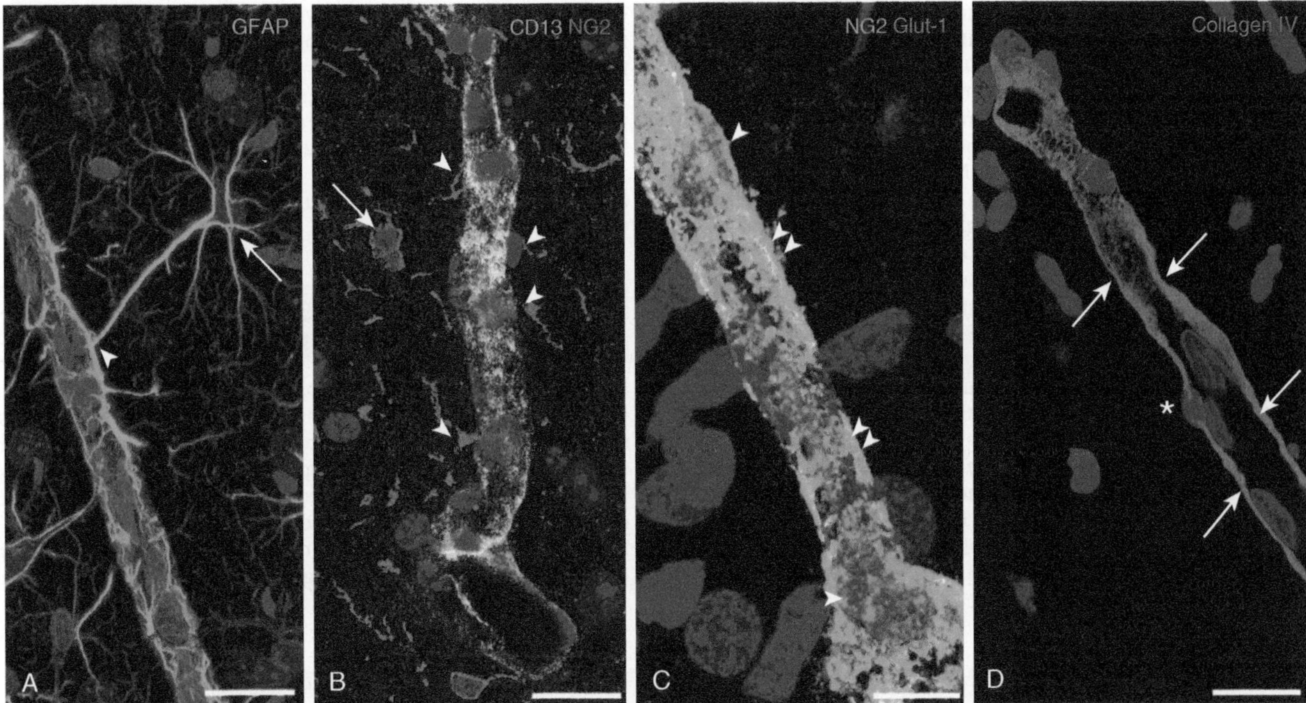

Fig. 126.4 Cellular (A–C) and noncellular (D) components of the neurovascular unit as detected in human fetal telencephalon at 20 weeks of development. (A) A perivascular astrocyte *(arrow)* is revealed by the astroglia-specific marker GFAP, which sends a process to the microvessel wall *(arrowhead)*. (B) Perivascular NG2-expressing oligodendroglial cells *(arrows)*, marked by the expression of proteoglycan NG2, send processes and terminal ends *(arrowhead)* to the wall of a microvessel enveloped by NG2+CD13+ pericytes *(yellowish)*. (C) The marker Glut-1. Specific to the blood-brain barrier, reveals endothelial cells *(red)* that appears to be extensively covered by bodies *(arrowhead)* and processes *(double arrowheads)* of NG2+ pericytes. (D) The microvessel basal lamina, revealed by its content of collagen IV molecules *(arrows)*, completely embeds pericytes, revealing their typically prominent nuclei *(asterisk)*. Scale bars = 20 μm in A, B, D and 10 μm in C.

that metabolize neurotransmitters such as monoamine esterases, cholinesterases, γ-aminobutyric acid (GABA), transaminases, aminopeptidases, and endopeptidases.

GLIAL CELL REGULATION OF THE BLOOD–BRAIN BARRIER

Astrocytes, pericytes, and, more recently, oligodendroglial cells[2] have been shown to regulate barrier properties at the level of the capillary, although the list of the regulative pathways remains far from complete.

Astrocytes

Astrocytic end feet surround the entire brain capillary and are an important constituent of the NVU (see Figs. 126.2 to 126.4). Astrocytes modulate regional cerebral blood flow in response to brain activity and metabolic demand. They also regulate several critical aspects of BBB function, including the tightness of the interendothelial junctions[1,43,44] and the expression and polarization of specialized enzyme and nutrient transporter systems.[1,45-47] The significance of astrocytes in the maturation and maintenance of various BBB properties has mostly been investigated using in vitro methods.[3,48,49]

There are multidirectional communications between endothelium, astrocytes, and pericytes as follows: (1) Astrocytes secrete a wide range of molecules including transforming growth factor β (TGFβ), basic fibroblast growth factor (bFGF), glial-derived neurotrophic factor (GDNF), and angiopoietin 1, which induce the BBB phenotype in the endothelium in vitro.[50] (2) Endothelium-derived leukemia inhibitory factor (LIF) induces astrocyte differentiation because astrocyte end feet exhibit specialized orthogonal array particles (OAPs) containing AQP4 after astrocyte exposure to LIF. (3) Likewise, factors released by astrocytes and endothelia affect pericyte properties such as TGFβ, which induces pericyte proliferation and migration.[51,52]

Oligodendroglia and Pericytes

Although cells of oligodendrocyte lineage are classically known for roles in myelination, roles for immature NG2-expressing oligodendrocyte precursors in angiogenesis and BBB regulation are reported in developing and normal adult brain as well as in pathologic conditions by several recent studies (see Fig. 126.4B).[2,3,52a] Vessel-associated NG2-glia, which also include pericytes, may exert part of their biologic functions within the NVU via the trans activity of proteoglycan NG2 and/or by interactions of NG2 with the vascular basal lamina molecules.[53]

Pericytes are completely embedded in the vascular basal lamina.[54] Each pericyte extends two primary major processes that parallel the capillary axis. These processes, in turn, extend flattened secondary processes, which possess orthogonal radiations that intimately embrace the entire endothelial tube (see Figs. 126.2 and 126.4). It is important to emphasize that the amount of pericyte coverage in brain microvessels is greater than for the microvasculature of any other organ.[54]

The importance of pericytes in fetal and adult brain BBB formation, vessel stabilization, barrier maintenance, and the regulation of capillary blood flow has become increasingly apparent.[16,50,55-58] Vessels with reduced numbers of pericytes or lacking pericytes exhibit vascular abnormalities including microaneurysms, compromised barrier function, and abnormal astrocytic end foot polarity during the development of the NVU.[51,52,59,60] The crosstalk between pericytes and the other components of the NVU result from cell-cell contacts and the production of soluble factors. Various signaling pathways are involved in pericyte-endothelial interactions; these include (1) platelet-derived growth factor receptor-β (PDGFR-β)/PDGF-B in pericyte proliferation and migration along the vascular tree; (2) TGF-βR/TGFβ and Notch/N-cadherin signaling in pericyte attachment to endothelium; (3) Notch3 in combination with PDGFR-β in pericyte survival[52]; (4) pericyte-derived angiopoietin in enhancement of endothelial tight junction formation as well as the downregulation of transcytosis and of leukocyte adhesion molecules[16,50,61]; and (5) NG2 proteoglycan/α3β1 integrin signaling in the stabilization of tight junctions (TJs) and BBB integrity.[62]

Basal Lamina

The basal lamina is the noncellular support of the BBB and plays a significant role in BBB permeability maintenance (Fig. 126.5; see Figs. 126.4D). The structural proteins of the basal lamina are secreted by astrocytes, pericytes, and endothelial cells. Hyaluronic acid, one of the major components of the basal lamina, has been shown to influence neuroimmune processes, in part by activating toll-like receptors.[63] Laminins alpha α1, α2, α4, and α5 have also been involved in the control of leukocyte blood-brain extravasation during neuroinflammation (see Fig. 126.5A).[64] Disruption of these NVUs' molecular components is associated with increased BBB permeability in pathologic states.[16,65,66] Recognition of the complex interactions among the components of the NVU continues to provide a basis for understanding the multiple mechanisms by which cerebral microvascular permeability may potentially be influenced by development, medications, and disease sta tes.[1,12,16,18,50]

DEVELOPMENTAL ASPECTS OF THE BLOOD-BRAIN BARRIER

Knowledge regarding the development of the BBB in vertebrates is derived from experiments in a wide spectrum of organisms ranging from jawless hagfish to sheep. Although information more recently derived from autopsy material from human fetuses and premature infants has become available,[67-70] information on barrier function in human fetuses and premature infants is lacking. Most functional studies of BBB have been carried out in rodents, and comparisons among vertebrate classes indicate that

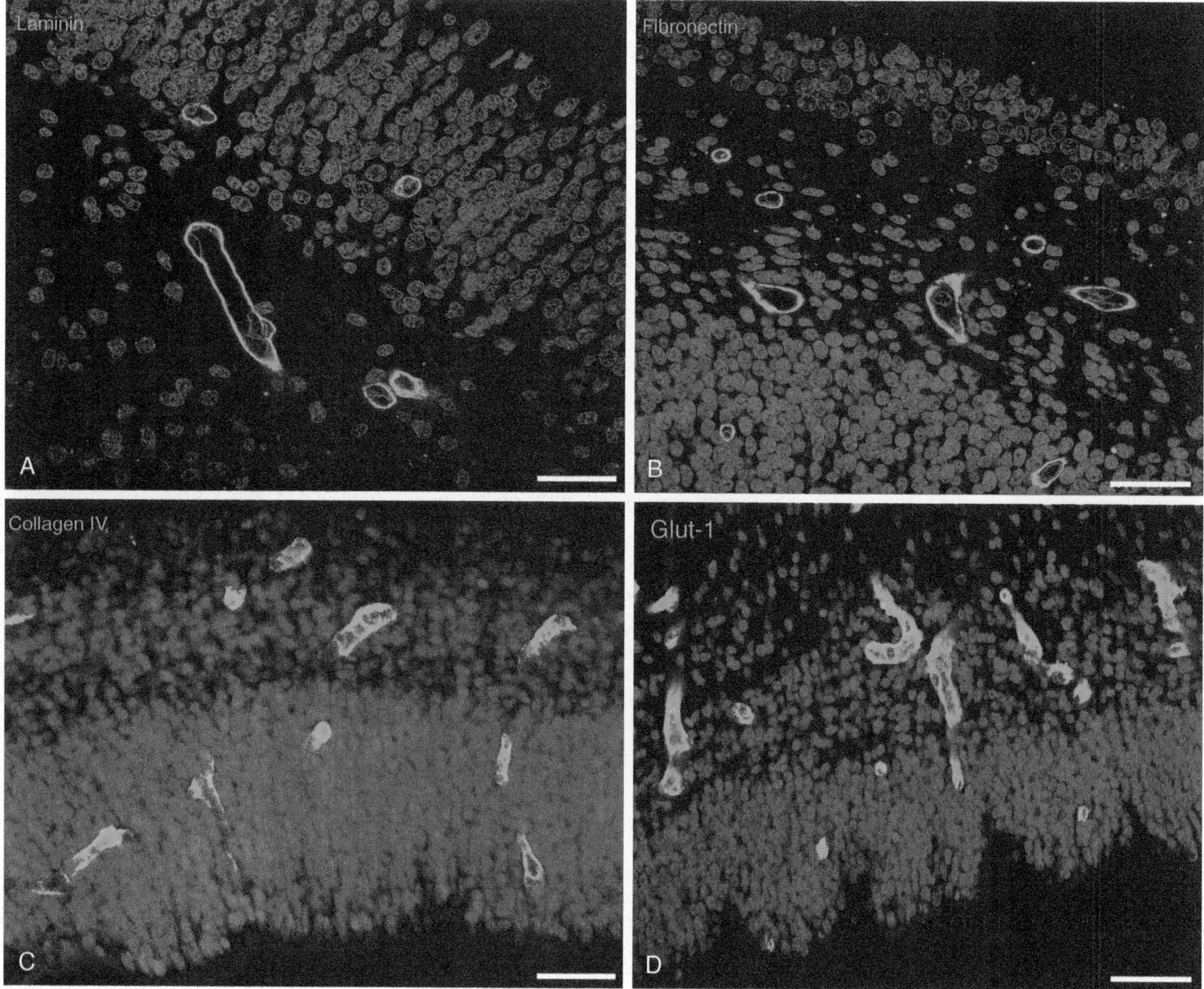

Fig. 126.5 Human fetal telencephalon at 10 (A, C) and 12 (B, D) weeks of development. (A to C) Molecules of the vascular basal lamina, laminin, fibronectin, and collagen IV are already expressed by the penetrated, growing microvessels. (D) Endothelial cells already express the blood-brain barrier's endothelial marker Glut-1. Scale bars =20 μm.

the structural and functional aspects of the BBB are remarkably conserved.[71,72] Nonetheless, caution must be exercised in analyzing experimental data on the temporal aspects of prenatal or postnatal barrier development because the timing of brain growth and differentiation relative to the timing of birth differs considerably among species.[73,74]

ANGIOGENESIS: CAPILLARY FORMATION AND PROPERTIES OF THE BLOOD-BRAIN BARRIER

The development of the CNS vasculature begins during embryogenesis, when angioblasts arise in the mesoderm of the head region and form a perineural vascular plexus by a process called *vasculogenesis,* a mechanism of in situ differentiation of endothelial cells.[75] The perineural vascular plexus covers the entire surface of the neural tube by day 9 in rodent embryos[76-78] and by week 8 in embryonic human development.[79] Vascular sprouts arise from the perineural plexus with a mechanism termed *angiogenesis,* the origin of new vessels from preexisting ones; these sprouts invade the proliferating neuroepithelium by day 11 of the third month in rodent and human embryonic development, respectively.[80] During angiogenesis, newly forming vessels radially invade the neuroectodermal tissue, elongate, give rise to manifold branches, and finally anastomose with adjacent sprouts to form a plexus of undifferentiated capillaries in the ventricular zone of the developing brain.

Endothelial cells begin to develop the BBB phenotype with presence of the tight junction proteins (occludin, claudin-5, and ZO1) and some influx transporters such as GLUT1 as early as embryonic day 12 in rodents. Interestingly, pericyte recruitment to the CNS correlates temporally with the maturation of BBB function.[59] Studies have shown that PDGF-B activation of PDGFRβ is critical to pericyte generation and survival.[51,52,59] In addition, TGF-β released by pericytes contributes to endothelial cell differentiation and BBB maturation.[50-52] Endothelial cells later become invested with astrocytic end feet. The perivascular basal lamina between astrocytes and endothelial cells becomes more prominent gradually from birth through the third to fourth postnatal week in the mouse and rat. During this period in the mouse, vessel wall thickness decreases by 60%, and the basal lamina thickens from undetectable levels to 71 nm by electron microscopic criteria.[81] Moreover, there is strong evidence from in vitro experiments showing that astrocytes contribute to the final maturation of BBB properties, resulting in increases in tight junction proteins and specific transporters such as P-glycoprotein 1 (P-gP) and GLUT 1. Paracellular diffusion diminishes during these latter stages in the formation of the capillary-astrocytic complex, basal lamina and perivascular consolidation. Nonbarrier vessels in the circumventricular organs (i.e., area postrema) do not develop these differentiated features.

DEVELOPMENT OF TIGHT JUNCTIONS

Development of the BBB begins during the embryonic period with the formation of tight junction complexes between endothelial cells.[82-86] The exact timing of the maturation of these barrier components remains controversial. However, evidence suggests the importance of contributions from pericytes and radial glial cells in this process.[50,53,87] Pericytes are now thought to play a critical role in early embryonic endothelial differentiation before the astrocytes are present.[51,52,59] This concept is supported by in vivo studies in rodents; these have demonstrated pericyte recruitment by PDGF signaling in E12 mice and shown that signaling molecules such as TGFβ and angiopoietin promote barrier maturation and the acquisition of tight junctions. These findings are also supported by similar work in models of the human BBB in vitro, suggesting that the WNT pathway is stimulated by pericytes, which contribute to increases in tight junction proteins at the endothelial barrier.[51,52,59] Moreover, a cooperative effect has been suggested during human brain development between Wnt/β-catenin signalling and the CXCL12/CXCR4 chemokine axis in neurovascular patterning and barrier differentiation that is mediated by radial glial cells.[53]

An important concept is that the BBB does not "switch" to a tight barrier at a specific time during angiogenesis but rather that the tightness of the barrier gradually increases in a region-dependent manner at the same time as angiogenesis is ongoing.[88] Wnt 7a and Wnt 7b appear to mediate the regulation of vascular development in the embryonic and postnatal mouse brain.[89,90] These and possibly other Wnt family members appear to promote the formation and differentiation of the CNS vasculature through a canonical Wnt signaling pathway.[89]

Vascular fenestrae disappear, pinocytosis decreases, and vessels decrease in diameter between embryonic days 11 to 17 in rodents.[86,91] The onset of tight junction formation is detectable by day 15, but tight junctions continue to increase in complexity through postnatal day 1.[17,92-95] However, some features of the tight junctions appear to continue to mature with brain development.[83] The expressions of the complex array of the tight junction transmembrane and cytoplasmic proteins[1,16,83] are developmentally regulated in rodents.[94,96,97] Occludin expression is low in rat brain endothelial cells at postnatal day 8 but clearly increases by day 70,[96] and ZO-1 protein expression increases between fetal days 15 and 19 and after birth in mouse brain microvessels.[94] BBB tight junction development has been reported in other animal models including nonhuman primate,[98] opossum,[99,100] and sheep.[101] In contrast to the rodent, in which development of the BBB occurs primarily after birth, the human barrier and its tight junction protein complex develop mainly in utero.[17,97,102] Evidence confirms that the proteins of the tight junction complex are present very early during human fetal brain development.[67-70]

The first stage of human fetal intracortical vascularization is characterized by the development of radially penetrating stem vessels in fetuses from 10 to 12 weeks of gestation, which is associated with the appearance of vascular basal lamina components including endothelium-specific markers and barrier-specific transporters (see Fig. 126.5).[69,70,103] The second stage of intracortical vascularization spans the period of midgestation and is characterized by vascular branching, increasing microvessel density, and barrier differentiation demonstrated by the detection of tight junction molecules, barrier-specific metabolic transporters, and efflux carriers (Fig. 126.6).[69,70,103]

Pericytes play an early strategic role in the process of angiogenesis.[104] They appear to be the principal cells during vascular sprouting, facilitating the interactions with endothelial cells during angiogenesis.[64] In fact, it has been demonstrated that endothelial cells of growing microvessels already display the BBB phenotype as revealed by the expression of tight junction molecules and specific transporters.[105,106] These observations suggest the possibility that pericytes could be relevant to the timing of tight junctional protein expression during development in human fetuses and premature infants. Two studies have reported maturational changes in the expression of these proteins,[67,69] whereas a third study did not find similar changes.[68] The primary endothelial tight junction molecules that have thus far been identified in the developing human brain include occludin, claudin-5, JAM-1, and ZO-1.[67,69,70,82] Occludin and claudin-5 are already expressed in the primary vessels of the telencephalon by week 12 of gestation, and by midgestation (18 weeks) they show dramatic changes (Fig. 126.7).[69] The most critical change occurs between 12 and 14 weeks of gestation, when occludin and claudin-5 immunoreactivity shifts from the endothelial cytoplasm to the endothelial borders and concentrates in linear, discontinuous tracts that may correspond to simple incomplete networks of tight junctional strands (see Fig. 126.7).[69] Soon thereafter, a nearly continuous staining

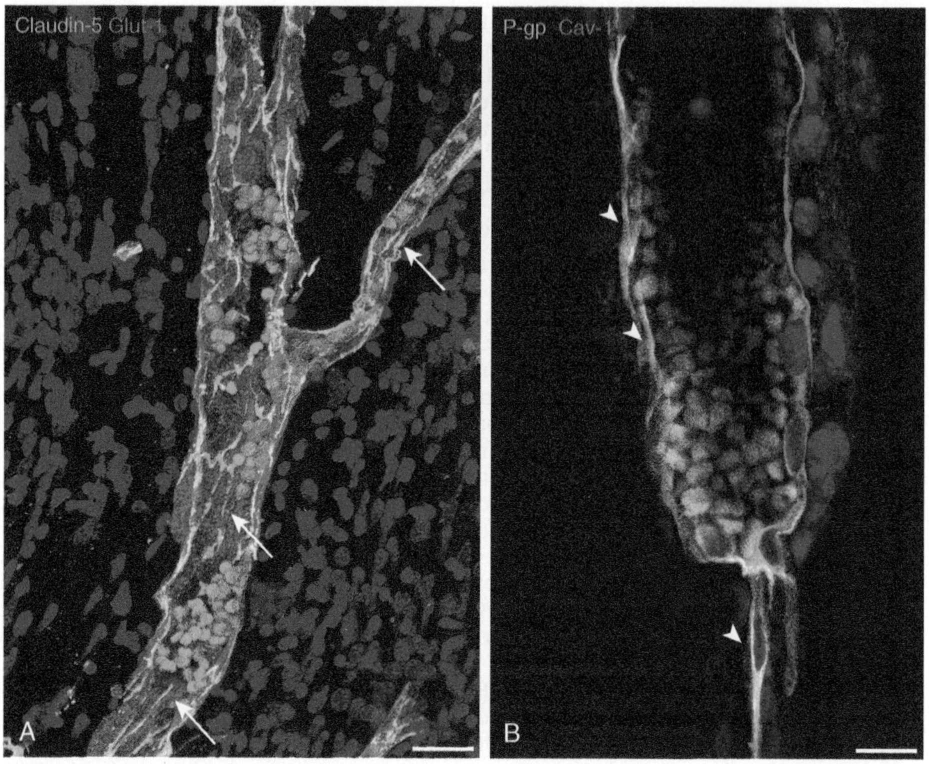

Fig. 126.6 Human fetal telencephalon at 18 weeks of development. (A) At the time of microvessel collateralization, endothelial cells express the blood-brain barrier's metabolic transporter Glut-1 and are sealed by tight junctions, here revealed by claudin-5 *(arrows)*. (B) At the same fetal age, endothelial cells revealed by caveolin-1 (Cav-1) also express the efflux transporter P-glycoprotein (P-gp) *(arrowheads)*. Scale bars = 30 μm in A and 10 μm in B.

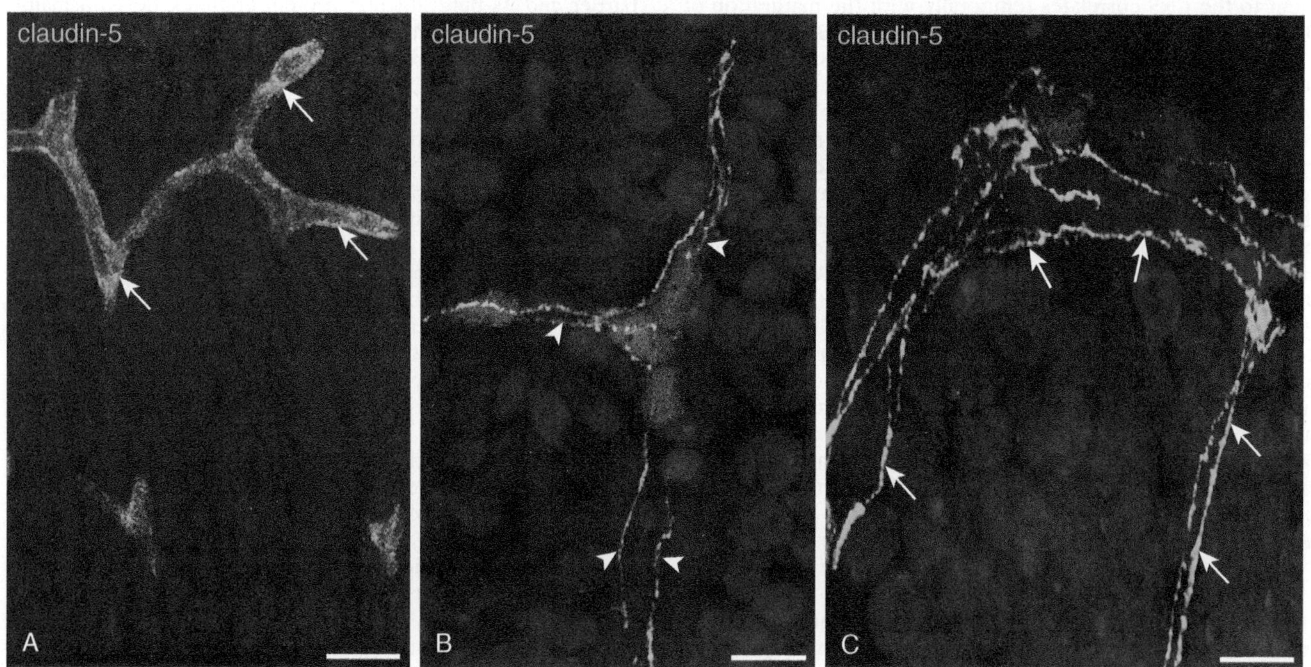

Fig. 126.7 Human fetal telencephalon at 12 (A), 14 (B), and 18 (C) weeks of development. At 12 weeks, a claudin-5 punctate staining pattern is detected in the endothelial cytoplasm *(arrows)*. At 14 weeks, the punctate pattern starts to form interrupted linear tracks *(arrowheads)* that, at 18 weeks (C), appear as nearly continuous thick bands *(arrows)*. Scale bars = 15 μm in A and B and 10 μm in C.

pattern is detectable and more extended and complex strands form, resembling those observed in mature tight junctions (see Fig. 126.7).[69] Therefore human endothelial tight junction development appears to begin earlier and proceed faster than that in other vertebrate species.[93,107-109]

Consistent with the maturational changes in the tight junctional proteins during very early in fetal development,[69] occludin, claudin-5, and ZO-1 immunoreactivity was detected in the germinal matrix and cortical vessels of premature infants with postconceptual ages ranging from 24 to 42 weeks.[67] Although the immunoreactivity of occludin, claudin-5, and ZO-1 in the cortical vessels appears to increase with increasing postconceptual age, increases in the immunoreactivity of these proteins appear to be greater with maturation of the germinal matrix.[67] Therefore the structural elements of the germinal matrix vascular endothelial tight junctional complexes appear to accumulate from 24 weeks until term, suggesting that the tight junctions in the germinal matrix mature during the third trimester.[67] Nonetheless, in another detailed study, the primary tight junction molecules—occludin, claudin-5, and JAM-1—were shown to be expressed in the BBB as early as 16 weeks of gestation but did not show significant differences in expression in the vasculature of the germinal matrix, white matter, or cortex between 16 and 40 weeks of gestation.[68]

DEVELOPMENT OF THE TRANSPORT BARRIER

The expression of some ABC transport carriers at the BBB exhibit maturational differences between the neonatal and adult brain during a similar period when the tight junctional proteins exhibit an effective physical barrier in the developing brain. This may reflect the specific nutrient transport requirements of the developing brain. However, the efflux transporters exhibit both increases and decreases during development.[98,110-117] Although P-gp immunoreactivity has been detected as early as 8 to 12 weeks of gestation in the fetal brain, the expression remains relatively low until birth and progressively increases to reach adult levels by approximately 3 to 6 months of age (see Fig. 126.6B).[111,118-120] The relatively low expression of the P-gp efflux transporter in the fetal and neonatal brain could be of considerable consequence with regard to potential exposures as well as the bioavailability and distribution of drugs and toxins in the developing brain. Consequently the immature brain could be more vulnerable to drugs and toxins. Thus the lower expressions of transporter systems must be considered when pregnant women, neonates, or infants are being treated with pharmaceutical agents.

MATURATION OF THE BLOOD-BRAIN BARRIER'S PERMEABILITY

As summarized earlier for the development of the tight junctions, the functional development of the fetal and neonatal BBB has been the subject of some controversy.[77,121,122] Some investigators have claimed that a barrier to proteins is present as early as when blood vessels form in the fetal brain,[121] although this is contended.[122] This controversy[77,121,122] appeared to have been based on a paucity of quantitative BBB permeability measurements in the same species from early fetal through later neonatal development up to maturity in adults. As described earlier, comparisons between species are difficult because of differences in rates of brain development.[74] BBB function was first investigated in developing fetal sheep by examining steady-state brain-to-plasma sucrose ratios in anesthetized exteriorized acutely studied fetal sheep.[123] The brain-to-blood sucrose ratios exhibited rapid decreases in early gestation, followed by smaller decreases later in gestation through the first week of postnatal life.[123] The ontogeny of BBB permeability was later quantified with the rate constant for influx (K_i) across the BBB using α-aminoisobutyric acid (AIB), a low-molecular-weight (103 Da) synthetic inert hydrophilic amino acid. These studies were performed in a non-anesthetized chronically instrumented sheep model at three different points in development during the last 2 months of fetal life, in the first months of postnatal life, and at full maturation (i.e., in adult sheep) (Fig. 126.8).[124] The K_i measured with AIB was significantly lower in all brain regions of the adult sheep and in most brain regions of newborn and older lambs than in the brains of fetuses at 60% and 90% of gestation. However, the BBB was relatively impermeable to AIB in all age groups and brain regions because the magnitude of the changes from 60% of gestation to maturity was not large. Although the permeability of the barrier to AIB was relatively low during fetal and neonatal development, the ovine fetus and neonate exhibited ontogenic decreases in barrier permeability (see Fig. 126.8).[124]

The low permeability to AIB suggests that a functionally tight barrier may be present from very early in gestation, which

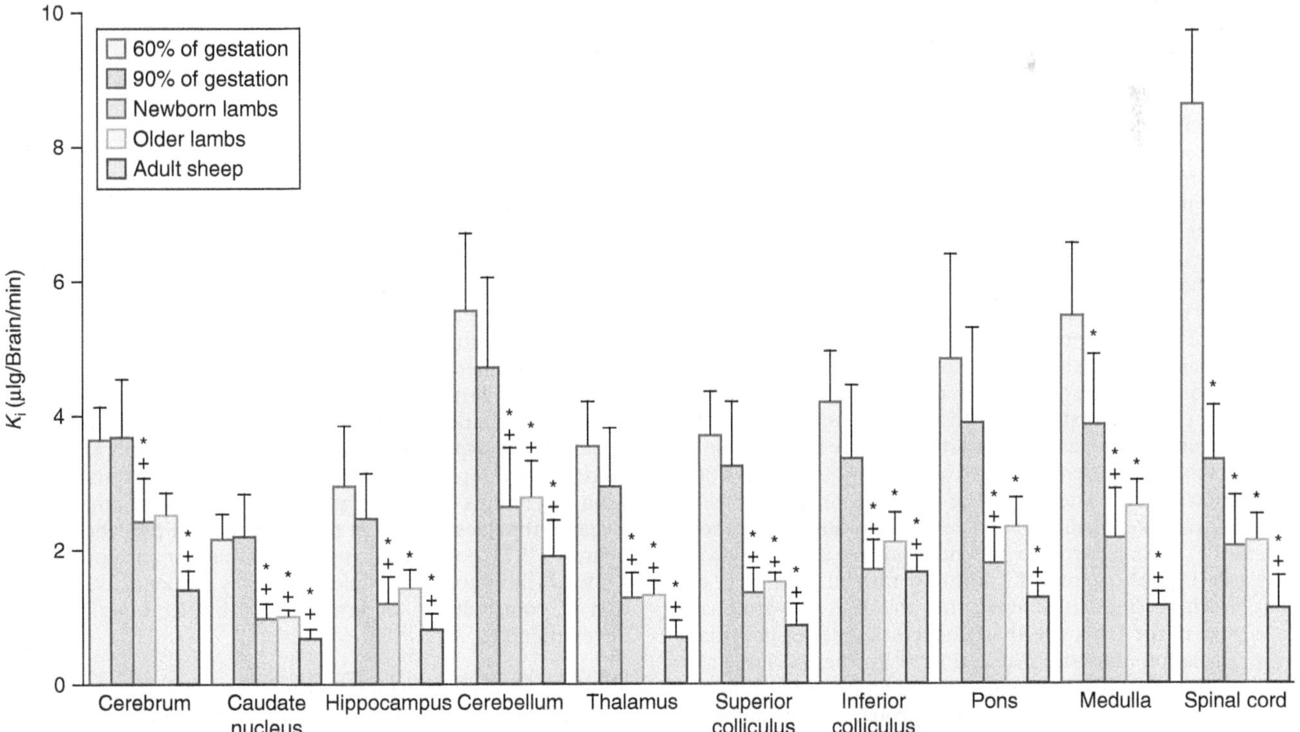

Fig. 126.8 Regional blood-to-brain transfer constants for influx (K_i) to α-aminoisobutyric acid (AIB), an amino acid used extensively to measure total and regional barrier permeability, which is decreased with development in sheep. The magnitude of the changes from 60% of gestation to maturity was not large. The low permeability to AIB suggests the presence of a functionally tight blood-brain barrier from very early in gestation, which probably serves to isolate the developing brain from systemic blood constituents. *$P<0.05$ versus fetus at 60% of gestation and + $p<0.05$ versus fetus at 90% of gestation. (Modified from Stonestreet BS, Patlak CS, Pettigrew KD, et al. Ontogeny of BBB function in ovine fetuses, lambs, and adults. *Am J Physiol.* 1996;271:R1594–R1601.)

probably serves to isolate the developing brain from systemic blood constituents. Inspection of the regional K_i values for AIB (see Fig. 126.8) reveals that the cerebrum exhibits the smallest differences in the K_i between the fetuses at 60% of gestation and the adult sheep. By contrast, the more caudal brain regions, including the cerebellum, medulla, and spinal cord, exhibit relatively larger developmental decreases in permeability between fetuses at 60% of gestation and adult sheep. These findings suggest that the cerebral cortex represents a relatively privileged site because of its unique neuronal composition and function. These measures of barrier function early in sheep gestation are consistent with results suggesting very precocious barrier differentiation in the human fetal cerebral cortex, as described earlier.[69,70]

The decreases in permeability to AIB in sheep[124] were similar to developmental changes in barrier permeability measured quantitatively in rats, using potassium.[125] Permeability to potassium was higher in 21-day fetal than in newborn or adult rats.[125] Taken together, the findings in sheep[124] and in developing rats[125] suggest that barrier permeability to both a cation and low-molecular-weight hydrophilic molecules decreases from fetal to adult life.[124]

The ontogenic decreases in permeability in sheep[124] were also similar to postnatal reductions in permeability to AIB in rabbits[126] and to inulin, sucrose, mannitol, and urea in rats.[127-130] However, in contrast to the findings in rabbits, which exhibited 80% to 90% postnatal reductions in permeability from day 1 of postnatal life to adulthood, the sheep exhibited 39% to 45% reductions in permeability from day 3 to adulthood.[124] The timing and schedule of brain growth are probably critical to maturation of the BBB.[125] Comparison of barrier development among species requires consideration of brain growth differences. The sheep brain develops mostly before birth, the rabbit brain develops perinatally, and the rat brain develops after birth.[76] The prenatal brain development in sheep may account for the more modest differences in permeability between newborn lamb and adult sheep.

ROLE OF GLUCOCORTICOIDS IN MATURATION OF THE BLOOD-BRAIN BARRIER

Antenatal glucocorticoid therapy is the standard of care for pregnancies at risk of preterm delivery and represents one of the most striking successes in perinatal medicine to enhance fetal maturation.[131] Evidence in adult subjects suggests that the BBB is under hormonal control.[132-135] Adrenalectomy increases BBB permeability, and corticosterone replacement reverses this effect on the barrier in adult rats.[133] These findings suggest that the pituitary-adrenal-cortical axis may function as a physiologic regulator of barrier function.[133] It is well known that the pituitary-adrenal-cortical axis matures during fetal development and that endogenous cortisol concentrations increase particularly in the latter part of gestation.[136] In sheep, maternally administered exogenous antenatal glucocorticoids have been shown to reduce blood-brain permeability early (at 60%, 70%, and 80% of gestation) but not late (at 90% of gestation) in fetal development or in the neonatal period.[137-139] In addition, endogenous increases in plasma cortisol concentrations are associated with decreases in BBB permeability during normal fetal development.[140] These findings suggest that the BBB is hormonally responsive in the fetus and that glucocorticoids are important in the regulation of barrier maturation.[140] Furthermore, the age-related differential responsiveness of the fetal barrier to maternally administered glucocorticoids is probably attributable to the fact that the barrier is still responsive to exogenous glucocorticoids early in gestation as it has not yet been exposed to the increases in endogenous glucocorticoids.[139,140] Later in gestation[140] and in the newborn,[139] endogenous increases in cortisol will have already accelerated the maturation of the BBB, so it is no longer responsive to the exogenously administered glucocorticoids.[139,140] These findings are important because during the perinatal period, when the brain potentially may be exposed to systemic elevations in neurotoxic substances, increases in endogenous cortisol serve to protect the fetal and neonatal brain by reducing its own permeability.[139,140]

The site of action of glucocorticoids on the BBB in the fetus[137,138,141] is most likely mainly the capillary endothelial cells, because physiologic hydrocortisone concentrations have been shown to increase transendothelial resistance and to decrease permeability in cerebral capillary endothelial cells in vitro.[142] Consistent with these findings, glucocorticoids also have been shown to increase transendothelial electrical resistance in conjunction with increases in occludin and claudin-5 expression in a microvascular endothelia cell line[143] and to regulate the human occludin gene via a glucocorticoid response element.[144] In addition, maternal glucocorticoid treatment increases the expressions of claudin-5, occludin, claudin-1, and zonula occludens (ZO)-1 in vivo in multiple brain regions of the preterm fetal sheep, and these increases in claudin-1, claudin-5, and ZO-2 expression are associated with decreases in BBB permeability.[145]

Glucocorticoids also affect other elements of the NVU that could impact BBB function. Recent work demonstrates beneficial effects of glucocorticoids on the balance between matrix metalloproteinases (MMPs) and their endogenous inhibitors, tissue inhibitors of metalloproteinases (TIMPs). Hydrocortisone application selectively upregulates TIMP-3; downregulates TIMP-1, TIMP-2, and TIMP-4; and enriches the extracellular matrix with TIMP-3. Consequently hydrocortisone targets TIMP-3 at the BBB and appears to have a protective role against matrix disruption, thereby improving barrier integrity.[146] Glucocorticoids also contribute to stabilization of the barrier by increasing angiopoietin-1 and decreasing vascular endothelial growth factor (VEGF) in astrocytes and pericytes.[147] Therefore glucocorticoids appear to stabilize barrier function via effects on multiple constituents in the NVU.

ALTERATIONS IN BLOOD-BRAIN BARRIER DEVELOPMENT AND FUNCTION: CLINICAL IMPLICATIONS

Abnormalities in the BBB are associated with several brain disorders and neurodegenerative diseases in adults including stroke, multiple sclerosis, and both Parkinson and Alzheimer disease.[16] However, factors predisposing to alterations in BBB function in the fetus and premature infant have not been extensively investigated. The relatively impermeable BBB in the fetus and neonate protect the developing brain from insults that could impair neuronal function during fetal life as well as during delivery and neonatal development.[124] However, emerging evidence suggests that a number of pathologic states (e.g., inflammation), prenatal-perinatal abnormalities, circulating factors, and treatment strategies could be predisposing factors for BBB dysfunction at different stages of development.[148] Elucidation of the mechanisms underlying alterations in BBB function during development could suggest strategies to protect the brain in both pre- and full-term infants.[149] The conditions summarized further on represent just a few of the factors that could potentially influence barrier function or contribute to abnormalities of barrier function during development.

INFLAMMATION AND INFECTION

Systemic and local inflammatory mediators can impair the barrier function of the NVU.[11] Various circulating inflammatory ligands, such as lipopolysaccharide (LPS), can activate locally produced proinflammatory cytokines such as IL-1, IL-6, and TNF-α, which bind to corresponding receptors on various elements of the NVU and alter the integrity of the BBB.[148-151] One of the mechanisms by which inflammation can alter BBB integrity is by directly disruption of the expression and localization of tight junction proteins and other components of the NVU.[152-154] Proinflammatory cytokines such as interleukin-6 (IL-6) can downregulate the expression of tight junction proteins in microvessels isolated from young and adult sheep.[151] Exposure to inflammation (LPS) in fetal sheep results in decreased cerebral cortical and white matter vascular density and astrogliosis, reduced pericyte and astrocytic microvascular coverage, and induce perivascular microglial activation.[154a] Furthermore, these alterations in the NVU could predispose to neuronal injury as well as impaired brain growth and maturation. Recent work has demonstrated that there is "crosstalk" between the cellular constituents of the BBB, secreted cytokines, and cellular interactions could also result in cytoarchitectural changes in tight junction proteins.[155] Nonetheless, despite increasing information regarding the effects of inflammation on the BBB, the precise effects of inflammation on signaling between the constituents of the NVU require further investigation in the developing brain.[153]

Several lines of evidence suggest that proinflammatory cytokines may gain access to the fetal brain after being produced during maternal inflammation or chorioamnionitis.[156-158] The uterus, fetal circulation, and brain represent three compartments separated by boundaries made up of the placenta and amniotic membranes and the BBB.[156] It has been postulated that cytokines originating in the uterus, amniotic fluid, or placenta could enter the fetal circulation or be produced because of inflammatory conditions within the fetal circulation.[156] As a result, proinflammatory cytokines originating from each of these sources could potentially damage the fetal BBB or gain access to the fetal brain by crossing the barrier. In this regard, interleukin-1β has been shown to cross the intact fetal BBB, and its transfer is accentuated by ischemia-reperfusion related injury to the fetal BBB.[101] Once cytokines cross the BBB, they can directly damage the brain.[154,156,157]

Systemic inflammation induced by a single dose of LPS administered intravenously to fetal sheep has been shown to be associated with increases in albumin concentrations in the brain parenchyma, suggesting that BBB permeability may also increase after exposure of the fetus to endotoxin.[159] Infusion of LPS into the maternal uterine artery results in plasma albumin extravasation in the cerebellum of fetal sheep, suggesting compromise to the BBB in the cerebellum.[160] One of the mechanisms by which LPS induces damage to the BBB is by stimulation of several proinflammatory cytokine receptors in astrocytes such as TNF-α.[161] This process varies as a function of the stages of development, specific brain regions, and localization of key receptors such as intercellular adhesion molecule 1 (ICAM-1).[153] Moreover, systemic inflammation increases the permeability of the BBB with predilection for specific vessels within the periventricular white matter tracts.[162] However, there is a paucity of information regarding the potential effects of inflammation on BBB and NVU dysfunction in the fetus and neonate. This remains an important area of investigation because systemic inflammation is known to impair neurodevelopmental outcomes in premature infants, and BBB dysfunction can potentially contribute to these adverse outcomes.[163,164]

Microorganisms can cause systemic inflammation and gain direct access into the brain parenchyma by breaching the BBB.[165-167] K1 type *Escherichia coli, Listeria monocytogenes,* and type III group B streptococci are some of the specific bacterial pathogens representing the leading causes of severe disease in perinatal medicine. These organisms penetrate the cerebrovascular endothelium and increase BBB permeability as compared with other organisms.[165-168] The K1 type *E. coli* has been shown to have specific genetic virulence determinants that contribute to brain microvascular endothelial cell adhesion and invasion.[168-173] Moreover, increases in TNF-α in cerebrospinal fluid appear to correlate with increases in barrier permeability in experimental meningitis.[165] Inflammation, systemic infections, and meningitis during the fetal and perinatal period have been shown to seriously interfere with normal CNS function and development.[174] Thus, abnormalities in the BBB most likely contribute to the brain injury associated with systemic inflammation and infection in premature and full-term infants.

HYPOXIA, ISCHEMIA, AND REPERFUSION INJURY

Hypoxic-ischemic brain injury is the most common neurologic problem in the perinatal period.[175-177] Evidence suggests that impaired BBB function represents an important component of hypoxic-ischemic brain injury, particularly early after ischemic insults to the fetal brain.[178] Therefore barrier dysfunction could potentially exacerbate brain damage by facilitating the entry of blood-borne substances into the brain. The expression and localization of various tight junction proteins as well as nutrient and electrolyte transporters are altered in the brain after exposure to hypoxic or ischemic insults.[178-180] The mechanisms underlying these changes include the direct effects of energy failure resulting from oxygen and metabolite deprivation, damaging effects of oxygen free radicals, cessation of shear blood flow with invasion of the NVU by static leukocytes adhering to the blood vessel walls, induction of local inflammatory cascades associated with hypoxic-ischemic injury to the tissues, and alterations in the molecular composition of tight junction proteins.[178,181,182] Hypoxic-ischemic related alterations in BBB function could represent a potential therapeutic target to attenuate the related parenchymal brain injury. The proinflammatory cytokines interleukin-1β and interleukin-6 (IL-1β and IL-6) have been shown to contribute to impaired BBB function after ischemia in fetal sheep.[149,183] Furthermore, systemic infusions of specific anti-IL-1β and anti-IL-6 monoclonal antibodies after ischemia result in antibody uptake into the fetal brain and diminish the ischemia-related increases in BBB permeability across brain regions in the fetal sheep.[149,183,184] Moreover, specific anti-IL-1β antibodies also reduce IL-1β transport across the BBB after ischemia in the ovine fetus.[184]

The need for cardiopulmonary resuscitation is one of the most common scenarios potentially associated with barrier dysfunction and hypoxic-ischemic brain injury. BBB permeability was investigated in young anesthetized pigs during and after cardiopulmonary resuscitation. After 8 minutes of cardiac arrest followed by either 10 or 40 minutes of continuous sternal compressions, the BBB transfer coefficient did not increase. However, after 8 minutes of arrest, 6 minutes of cardiopulmonary resuscitation, and 4 hours of spontaneous circulation, the BBB transfer coefficient increased by 59% to 107% in 10 of 11 regions rostral to the pons. Thus, after an 8-minute period of complete ischemia, the BBB remained intact during and immediately after resuscitation but not after several hours of recirculation. These findings contrast with previous work in adult animals in which no delayed increase in permeability was demonstrated.[185]

In a model of cerebral ischemia-reperfusion injury in newborn piglets, the blood-to-brain transfer of urea, sodium, and sucrose was measured at 30 minutes and again after 2 hours of reperfusion.[186] The blood-to-brain transfer constants for the two lower-molecular-weight tracers, sodium and urea, increased by 30 minutes after ischemia, followed by a subsequent increase for the largest tracer, sucrose, at 2 hours. These findings in neonatal piglets are consistent with the effects of hypoxia-ischemia in adults, specifically formation of a paracellular leak across the BBB with a pore diameter, which increases with time and the severity of the insult.[186-188] In contrast to these findings, the barrier was found to be relatively impermeable to sodium and mannitol in newborn piglets exposed to 60 minutes of systemic hypoxia and hypercapnia and 20 minutes of hypotension either immediately after the insult or 24 hours later.[188] Taken together, these studies suggest that the amount of damage to the barrier in the newborn is probably a function of the duration and severity of the insult.[186-188]

Studies in rodents have shown that albumin extravasation increased in injured adult rat brain 5- to 25-fold but only 2-fold in neonatal rats.[189] Interestingly, gene and protein expression of several tight junction components and basement membrane proteins showed greater preservation after ischemic stroke in neonates than in adults.[189] There are also developmental differences with regard to immune cell infiltration into the brain. Neutrophils infiltrate into the brain and contribute to BBB abnormalities after brain ischemia in adults.[189] In contrast, neutrophil infiltration is more limited after stroke in neonates.[189] Although the molecular mechanisms that restrict neutrophil infiltration in newborns have not yet been elucidated, differences in the patterns of expression of adhesion molecules, metalloproteinases, and chemokines between neonatal and adult rodents could potentially contribute to some of these developmental differences.[189] Taken together, these findings suggest that BBB dysfunction after hypoxia-ischemia differs with respect to the stage of brain development, severity of the insult, and timing of the barrier permeability measurements after the insults.

Pericytes are among the first cells to respond to hypoxia. They migrate away from blood vessels, resulting in decreased vascular support within hours after hypoxia in adults.[190,191] Pericytes express VEGF, which can exacerbate BBB dysfunction after hypoxia.[191,192] Therefore migration of pericytes away from regions of injured BBB and/or increases in pericyte VEGF expression could potentially contribute to vascular fragility in fetal or neonatal subjects. Pericytes have also been shown to contract after hypoxic insults, leading to capillary occlusion and BBB abnormalities that limit reperfusion and potentially exacerbate injury.[193] Moderate inflammation and hypoxia result in pericyte loss mediated by caspase-3 in an in vitro immature cerebral cortical model.[194] The role of pericytes in barrier dysfunction requires further investigation in the fetus and neonate because pericytes are important contributors to BBB integrity.

Edema formation is often associated with BBB disruption. The water channel aquaporin 4 (AQP4) is present in the astrocytic end feet and is associated with the development of brain edema in adults.[195] Increases in AQP4 observed on astrocytic end feet at the margin of ischemic lesions have been shown to limit the development of ischemic injury in rats.[196] Vessel coverage by astrocytic end feet begins before birth and continues during the first weeks after birth; the amount of AQP4 expression increases concomitantly with BBB maturation.[197] Therefore increased amounts of AQP4 could also contribute increases in BBB resistance to metabolic abnormalities and diminish the amount of edema formation in immature subjects.[195,196]

During hypoxia or ischemia and nutrient deprivation, alternate energy fuels such as ketone bodies and lactate substitute for glucose, thereby protecting the immature brain from hypoglycemia.[175] The expression of GLUT proteins at the BBB and on neuronal and nonneuronal elements in the brain parenchyma shows similar maturational patterns.[175] These findings suggest that the immature brain may be better able to withstand episodes of decreased nutrient supply during hypoxic-ischemic episodes because the immature BBB may be more efficient than that of the adult in the transport of certain alternative substrates.[198,199]

HYPERBILIRUBINEMIA

Hyperbilirubinemia has been associated with acute bilirubin encephalopathy and kernicterus in both pre- and full-term infants.[200] Evidence indicates that the unconjugated fraction of bilirubin in the serum is more directly related to bilirubin neurotoxicity than total bilirubin concentrations.[201] These findings suggest that the higher the level of unconjugated bilirubin in the serum, the more likely it is for bilirubin to cross the BBB and result in bilirubin-related neurotoxicity. At any given concentration of unconjugated serum bilirubin, conditions that decrease BBB permeability to bilirubin are less likely to be associated with bilirubin-related neurotoxicity.

Experimental evidence has shown that hyperbilirubinemia induced by comparable bilirubin infusions resulted in higher brain bilirubin contents and brain-to-blood distribution ratios for bilirubin in 2-day-old piglets than in those who were 2 weeks old. These ratios were higher in subcortical regions—namely, the cerebellum and brain stem—than in the cerebral cortex.[202] The results of this study suggest that postnatal maturation of the barrier for unconjugated bilirubin is probable and that the permeability for bilirubin is relatively greater in subcortical than in cortical regions of the developing brain.[201-203] These maturational changes in the permeability to bilirubin during development serve to protect the more mature brain from bilirubin toxicity. These findings also provide a basis for the clinical observation that newborn infants are at a higher risk for kernicterus at lower bilirubin concentrations in the first few hours after birth than later in postnatal life.[204]

Conversely, conditions that adversely affect blood-brain permeability to unconjugated bilirubin could be associated with higher risks for bilirubin-related neurotoxicity. Disruption of the BBB by inflammation, hypoxia–ischemia, or hyperosmolality could also facilitate transport of bilirubin into brain.[205,206] Premature infants are frequently exposed to systemic fetal and neonatal inflammation and to recurrent episodes of hypoxia and ischemia-reperfusion. These insults, combined with immaturity of the BBB for bilirubin, places very early preterm and late-preterm infants at a higher risk for bilirubin-related neurotoxicity compared with full-term newborns.[207]

Studies have elucidated the multifaceted effects of unconjugated bilirubin directly upon the BBB and important components of the NVU.[208,209] Elevated levels of unconjugated bilirubin impair the integrity of confluent monolayers of human brain microvascular endothelial, as demonstrated in vitro in a BBB model, by increasing oxidative stress and proinflammatory cytokine release.[210] Sustained exposure of human brain microvascular endothelial cells to unconjugated bilirubin reduces transendothelial electrical resistance and increases paracellular permeability. This was associated with a reduction in zonula occludens (ZO)-1 and β-catenin levels and thus of TJs strands and cell-to-cell contacts.[210,211] Consequently unconjugated bilirubin damages the endothelium of the BBB and facilitates its own entry into and accumulation in the brain parenchyma, where it can result in neurologic dysfunction.[208,210-212] In addition, unconjugated bilirubin also stimulates other components of the NVU, including astrocytes and microglia, to release proinflammatory cytokines and glutamate, which can further augment neurotoxicity.[213,214] Therefore hyperbilirubinemia exerts multiple effects on the NVU to create a proinflammatory-excitotoxic state that damages the BBB and facilitates its own entry into the brain parenchyma.

HYPEROSMOLAR STRESS

The phenomenon of hyperosmotic opening of the BBB has been extensively investigated in adults.[215] The degree of barrier opening varies with the concentration of the solute and the type of hyperosmotic solution used. Cserr et al.[216] has shown barrier opening with degrees of hyperosmolality comparable to those encountered clinically in sick premature infants.[216-219] The effects of a hyperosmolar stress on BBB function was determined quantitatively during the last 2 months of fetal development and in the first month of postnatal life in sheep. The results demonstrated that BBB permeability increases with increases in plasma osmolality in fetal sheep and lambs.[220] The experiments also demonstrated that the barrier became more resistant to the effects of hyperosmotic stress during development; consequently the immature fetuses were more vulnerable to osmotic stress than were older subjects.[220]

Numerous pathologic conditions can predispose premature and full-term neonates to dysregulation of glucose homeostasis, potentially resulting in the untoward effects of hyperosmolality.[221] Hyperglycemic-hyperosmotic and mannitol-induced hyperosmotic stress has similar effects on the BBB in fetal and neonatal subjects.[220,221] The BBB becomes more resistant to glucose-induced hyperosmolality during brain development in two select brain regions, the superior colliculus and the pons.[221] The thresholds for osmolar opening of the BBB were higher during glucose- than mannitol-induced hyperosmolality in the thalamus, superior colliculus, inferior colliculus, and medulla of premature lambs and the cerebrum and cerebellum of newborn lambs.[221] However, it is important to point out that in contrast to mannitol, glucose is actively transported at the BBB into the brain parenchyma by facilitative GLUTs.[222] Although the molecular mechanisms for the higher thresholds during glucose- versus mannitol-induced hyperosmolality have not yet been determined, the quantity of GLUTs increases with maturation.[223] Therefore it is possible that increases in the GLUTs with maturation could have contributed to the greater resistance of the BBB to glucose- than mannitol-induced hyperosmolality because of the greater active transport of glucose into the brain during increasing development.[221]

The precise mechanism underlying impairment of the BBB in response to hyperosmolality remains to be determined. However, previous work suggests that pores created between adjacent endothelial cells resulting from the opening of tight junctions contribute to the development of water-filled channels at the blood-brain interface.[216] AQP4s are water channels expressed on astrocyte end feet that increase when the BBB becomes more resistant to hyperosmotic stress.[195–197] Increased AQP4 in astrocyte end feet during development might contribute to improved water homeostasis within the NVU as well as accounting for the improved ability of the brain to exhibit volume regulation during development in sheep.[224,225]

INTRAVENTRICULAR HEMORRHAGE

Infants born preterm are at increased risk for intraventricular and intraparenchymal hemorrhage, which adversely affects their neurodevelopmental outcomes.[67,226] Extravasation of blood normally contained within the cerebral intravascular space into the parenchymal–ventricular space represents complete disruption of the BBB. Hence, understanding the pathophysiology of impaired BBB function is of vital importance in perinatal medicine because premature infants are at high risk for brain hemorrhage.

Germinal matrix hemorrhage progressing to intraventricular or intraparenchymal hemorrhage is the prototype of intracranial hemorrhage encountered in preterm infants.[227] Germinal matrix capillaries have large diameters and thin basement membranes; they lack direct contact with perivascular structures along a large proportion of their circumference, in contrast with capillaries within the cerebral cortex at the same gestational age.[228] The blood vessel density and the percentage of blood vessel area are larger in the germinal matrix vessels than in those of adjacent gray and white matter in autopsy material from fetuses and preterm infants born between 16 and 40 weeks of gestation, potentially predisposing to hemorrhage in the germinal matrix.[229]

The periventricular germinal matrix exhibits rapid angiogenesis, which results in high metabolic demand, rapid endothelial turnover, and high vascularity.[230] Deficiencies in any of the components of the BBB can weaken this vasculature and increase the propensity for hemorrhage. Current understanding suggests that paucity of pericytes, low fibronectin levels in the basal lamina, and reduced key intermediate filaments of the astrocytic end feet contribute to the fragility of the germinal matrix BBB, rendering this area of the brain vulnerable to hemorrhage.[230]

Pericytes are particularly important in the development of intraventricular hemorrhage because they play a key role in angiogenesis, providing structural support to the vasculature, maintaining the BBB, and controlling the remaining cells of the NVU.[60,231,232] Pericyte recruitment is regulated by ligand-receptor systems that include platelet-derived growth factor, sphingosine-1 phosphate, angiopoietin, and TGF-β.[233] TGF-β expression is reduced in the germinal matrix microvasculature, resulting in pericyte paucity and increased fragility of the germinal matrix microvasculature.

The basal lamina is comprised of several constituents including fibronectin that contribute to the structural integrity of vasculature by virtue of its anchoring function.[234–236] Fibronectin levels are significantly reduced in the germinal matrix vasculature compared with the cerebral cortex and white matter in premature infants.[237] TGF-β upregulates fibronectin. Consequently, low levels of TGF-β in the germinal matrix result in decreased fibronectin germinal matrix levels. Thus reduced fibronectin in the basal lamina of the germinal matrix may also contribute to vascular fragility in this brain region.[238,239]

Astrocytes also contribute to BBB development, regulate its function, provide structural integrity, and contribute to barrier permeability.[234] Glial fibrillary acidic protein (GFAP) is a key intermediate filament of the astrocytic end foot cytoskeleton.[240–242] GFAP provides structural integrity and mechanical strength to astrocytic end feet. Consequently, reduced GFAP expression in germinal matrix astrocytic end feet in conjunction with a paucity of pericytes and reduced basal lamina fibronectin contribute to the fragility of the of the germinal matrix vasculature and its vulnerability to hemorrhage in premature infants.[243]

Glucocorticoids are among the most widely used prenatal pharmacologic treatments to accelerate fetal maturation.[244] Several studies have confirmed that prenatal glucocorticoids reduce both severity and incidence of intraventricular hemorrhage.[244–246] The beneficial effects of prenatal glucocorticoids include stabilization of the microvasculature of the germinal matrix. Prenatal glucocorticoids suppress angiogenesis in the germinal matrix microvasculature and trim the nascent and fragile vasculature stabilizing the BBB, thereby reducing the vulnerability to hemorrhage. Infants treated with prenatal glucocorticoids exhibit improved pericyte coverage of the germinal matrix vasculature, higher fibronectin levels, and larger amounts of GFAP in the astrocytic end feet of germinal matrix blood vessels compared with those of untreated infants.[237,247,248]

Prenatal corticosteroid administration also results in decreased permeability of the BBB early in the ovine gestation.[137,138,140] The decrease in permeability was associated with increased expression in key tight junction proteins such as claudin-1, claudin-5, and zona occludin-2.[145] Taken together, the decreased incidence of intraventricular hemorrhage in premature infants after prenatal glucocorticoid treatment[249] and the decreased permeability of the BBB in the ovine fetus after glucocorticoid treatment of the ewes[137,138,141] suggest that glucocorticoids may accelerate microvascular maturation with a beneficial effects on BBB function in the human fetus and premature infant. In addition, endogenous increases in glucocorticoids also may contribute to accelerated maturation of the endothelial vasculature of the fetus and premature infant.[140]

MECHANICAL VENTILATION

The rates of neurodevelopmental impairment are very high among premature infants exposed to prolonged ventilation.[250] Abnormalities in the BBB may potentially contribute to the associated brain injury by allowing circulating toxic substances greater access to the brain parenchyma. Elevation in mean airway pressure during positive-pressure ventilation in newborn piglets selectively alters blood-to-brain transport of small water-soluble molecules.[251] Hence, increased cerebral venous pressures during ventilation cause the increases in the blood-to-brain transport of these low-molecular-weight tracers.[251] Increases in the duration of positive-pressure ventilation also predispose premature lambs to increases in regional BBB permeability measured using a low-molecular-weight tracer (i.e., AIB). These alterations in barrier function were shown to occur over relatively short time intervals (minutes to hours) and were not a result of changes in mean airway pressure.[141] Therefore both increases in mean airway pressure and increases in the duration of ventilation each contribute to altered blood-to-brain transport, which could adversely affect neuronal function during ventilation.[141,251] It is important to point out that the duration ventilation in the experimental studies[141,251] was relatively short compared with the potential durations of ventilation in premature neonates.

A recent study in ventilated growth-restricted fetal sheep showed that they were more likely to develop increased apoptosis (caspase-3), BBB dysfunction (albumin extravasation), activated microglia (Iba-1), and increased expression of cellular oxidative stress compared with ventilated fetal sheep that were appropriate for gestational age.[252] Evidence also suggests that ventilation of premature infants for more than 2 weeks is accompanied by elevated blood concentrations of proinflammatory proteins indicative of systemic inflammation including proinflammatory cytokines (IL-1β, and TNF-α), chemokines (IL-8, MCP-1), an adhesion molecule (ICAM-1), and a matrix metalloprotease (MMP-9).[253] Therefore the potential exists that increases in systemic circulating proinflammatory proteins in conjunction with ventilation-related impaired BBB function could permit inflammatory-related molecules to enter the brain of premature infants. This could represent one of the factors contributing to the ventilation-related neurodevelopmental impairment in premature infants.[140,250,251,253]

Information suggests that the glymphatic system could provide a pathway to remove small molecules from cerebral perivascular spaces via potentially passive networks that are regulated directly by intracerebral venous pressure.[254] Inspiration increases and exhalation reduces venous outflow from the brain in the low-pressure venous drainage system.[255] These finding potentially suggest that the respiratory pulsations act as a low-pressure counterpulsating system that could drive accumulated waste products into the perivenous areas and subsequently out of the brain.[254,255] Therefore prolonged ventilation in premature infants may interfere with the removal of potentially toxic waste products and contribute to neurodevelopmental impairment.[250]

CONCLUSION

The BBB, a complex, dynamic barrier at the level of the microvascular endothelium, has a critical role in maintaining the health and function of the brain. The tight junctional complex plays a critical role in regulating paracellular permeability. The NVU provides a framework for understanding how the endothelium, astrocytes, neurons, oligodendroglia, pericytes, and extracellular matrix function together to form a protective barrier for the brain. The development of the BBB is an important area of inquiry with a significant impact on the neurodevelopmental outcomes of pre- and full-term infants. A variety of perinatal disorders and related therapies can directly affect the properties of the BBB complex and the NVU. Abnormalities in the BBB and NVU associated with perinatal disorders and their therapies can, in turn, affect the neurodevelopmental outcomes of premature infants. Further understanding of this important barrier may lead to identification of clinically useful neuroprotective strategies during development.

ACKNOWLEDGMENTS

Some of the work on which this chapter is based was supported by National Institutes of Health (NIH) grants R01-HD34618 and 1R01-HD-057100.

A complete reference list is available at www.ExpertConsult.com.

SELECT REFERENCES

1. Abbott NJ, Ronnback L, Hansson E. Astrocyte-endothelial interactions at the blood-brain barrier. *Nat Rev Neurosci*. 2006;7:41-53.
9. Engelhardt B, Coisne C. Fluids and barriers of the CNS establish immune privilege by confining immune surveillance to a two-walled castle moat surrounding the CNS castle. *Fluids Barriers CNS*. 2011;8:4.
10. Abbott NJ. Blood-brain barrier structure and function and the challenges for CNS drug delivery. *J Inherit Metab Dis*. 2013;36:437-449.
11. Abbott NJ, Friedman A. Overview and introduction: the blood-brain barrier in health and disease. *Epilepsia*. 2012;53(suppl 6):1-6.
12. Abbott NJ, Patabendige AA, Dolman DE, Yusof SR, Begley DJ. Structure and function of the blood-brain barrier. *Neurobiol Dis*. 2010;37:13-25.
13. Loscher W, Potschka H. Blood-brain barrier active efflux transporters: ATP-binding cassette gene family. *NeuroRx*. 2005;2:86-98.
16. Hawkins BT, Davis TP. The blood-brain barrier/neurovascular unit in health and disease. *Pharmacol Rev*. 2005;57:173-185.
18. Forster C. Tight junctions and the modulation of barrier function in disease. *Histochem Cell Biol*. 2008;130:55-70.
42. Shawahna R, Uchida Y, Decleves X, et al. Transcriptomic and quantitative proteomic analysis of transporters and drug metabolizing enzymes in freshly isolated human brain microvessels. *Mol Pharm*. 2011;8:1332-1341.
48. Cecchelli R, Berezowski V, Lundquist S, et al. Modelling of the blood-brain barrier in drug discovery and development. *Nat Rev Drug Discov*. 2007;6:650-661.
50. Obermeier B, Daneman R, Ransohoff RM. Development, maintenance and disruption of the blood-brain barrier. *Nat Med*. 2013;19:1584-1596.
53. Errede M, Girolamo F, Rizzi M, Bertossi M, Roncali L, Virgintino D. The contribution of cxcl12-expressing radial glia cells to neuro-vascular patterning during human cerebral cortex development. *Front Neurosci*. 2014;8:324.
59. Daneman R, Zhou L, Kebede AA, Barres BA. Pericytes are required for blood-brain barrier integrity during embryogenesis. *Nature*. 2010;468:562-566.
60. Armulik A, Genove G, Mae M, et al. Pericytes regulate the blood-brain barrier. *Nature*. 2010;468:557-561.
63. Banks WA, Gray AM, Erickson MA, et al. Lipopolysaccharide-induced blood-brain barrier disruption: roles of cyclooxygenase, oxidative stress, neuroinflammation, and elements of the neurovascular unit. *J Neuroinflammation*. 2015;12:223.
67. Anstrom JA, Thore CR, Moody DM, Brown WR. Immunolocalization of tight junction proteins in blood vessels in human germinal matrix and cortex. *Histochem Cell Biol*. 2007;127:205-213.
69. Virgintino D, Errede M, Robertson D, et al. Immunolocalization of tight junction proteins in the adult and developing human brain. *Histochem Cell Biol*. 2004;122:51-59.
70. Virgintino D, Girolamo F, Errede M, et al. An intimate interplay between precocious, migrating pericytes and endothelial cells governs human fetal brain angiogenesis. *Angiogenesis*. 2007;10:35-45.
71. Cserr HF, Bundgaard M. Blood-brain interfaces in vertebrates: a comparative approach. *Am J Physiol*. 1984;246:R277-288.
72. Bundgaard M, Abbott NJ. All vertebrates started out with a glial blood-brain barrier 4-500 million years ago. *Glia*. 2008;56:699-708.
73. Dobbing J. The development of the blood-brain barrier. *Prog Brain Res*. 1968;29:417-427.
74. Dobbing J, Sands J. Comparative aspects of the brain growth spurt. *Early Hum Dev*. 1979;3:79-83.
83. Saunders NR, Knott GW, Dziegielewska KM. Barriers in the immature brain. *Cell Mol Neurobiol*. 2000;20:29-40.
84. Mollgard K, Saunders NR. The development of the human blood-brain and blood-CSF barriers. *Neuropathol Appl Neurobiol*. 1986;12:337-358.
85. Saunders NR, Habgood MD, Dziegielewska KM. Barrier mechanisms in the brain, I. Adult brain. *Clin Exp Pharmacol Physiol*. 1999;26:11-19.
87. Engelhardt B. Development of the blood-brain barrier. *Cell Tissue Res*. 2003;314:119-129.
98. Ek CJ, D'Angelo B, Lehner C, Nathanielsz P, Li C, Mallard C. Expression of tight junction proteins and transporters for xenobiotic metabolism at the blood-CSF barrier during development in the nonhuman primate (p. Hamadryas). *Reprod Toxicol*. 2015;56:32-44.
112. Ek CJ, Wong A, Liddelow SA, Johansson PA, Dziegielewska KM, Saunders NR. Efflux mechanisms at the developing brain barriers: ABC-transporters in the fetal and postnatal rat. *Toxicol Lett*. 2010;197:51-59.
115. Strazielle N, Ghersi-Egea JF. Efflux transporters in blood-brain interfaces of the developing brain. *Front Neurosci*. 2015;9:21.
116. Mollgard K, Dziegielewska KM, Holst CB, Habgood MD, Saunders NR. Brain barriers and functional interfaces with sequential appearance of ABC efflux transporters during human development. *Sci Rep*. 2017;7.
120. Virgintino D, Robertson D, Errede M, et al. Expression of p-glycoprotein in human cerebral cortex microvessels. *J Histochem Cytochem*. 2002;50:1671-1676.
124. Stonestreet BS, Patlak CS, Pettigrew KD, Reilly CB, Cserr HF. Ontogeny of blood-brain barrier function in ovine fetuses, lambs, and adults. *Am J Physiol Regul Integr Comp Physiol*. 1996;271:R1594-R1601.
137. Sadowska GB, Patlak CS, Petersson KH, Stonestreet BS. Effects of multiple courses of antenatal corticosteroids on blood-brain barrier permeability in the ovine fetus. *J Soc Gynecol Invest*. 2006;13:248-255.
140. Stonestreet BS, Sadowska GB, McKnight AJ, Patlak C, Petersson KH. Exogenous and endogenous corticosteroids modulate blood-brain barrier development in the ovine fetus. *Am J Physiol Regul Integr Comp Physiol*. 2000;279:R468-R477.

145. Sadowska GB, Malaeb SN, Stonestreet BS. Maternal glucocorticoid exposure alters tight junction protein expression in the brain of fetal sheep. *Am J Physiol Heart Circ Physiol*. 2010;298:H179-H188.
153. Stolp HB, Liddelow SA, Sa-Pereira I, Dziegielewska KM, Saunders NR. Immune responses at brain barriers and implications for brain development and neurological function in later life. *Front Integr Neurosci*. 2013;7:61.
155. Banks WA, Kovac A, Morofuji Y. Neurovascular unit crosstalk: pericytes and astrocytes modify cytokine secretion patterns of brain endothelial cells. *J Cereb Blood Flow Metab*. 2018;38:1104-1118.
157. Malaeb S, Dammann O. Fetal inflammatory response and brain injury in the preterm newborn. *J Child Neurol*. 2009;24:1119-1126.
162. Stolp HB, Dziegielewska KM, Ek CJ, et al. Breakdown of the blood-brain barrier to proteins in white matter of the developing brain following systemic inflammation. *Cell Tissue Res*. 2005;320:369-378.
174. Hagberg H, Mallard C. Effect of inflammation on central nervous system development and vulnerability. *Curr Opin Neurol*. 2005;18:117-123.
177. Vannucci SJ, Hagberg H. Hypoxia-ischemia in the immature brain. *J Exp Biol*. 2004;207:3149-3154.
178. Chen X, Threlkeld SW, Cummings EE, et al. Ischemia-reperfusion impairs blood-brain barrier function and alters tight junction protein expression in the ovine fetus. *Neuroscience*. 2012;226:89-100.
200. Dennery PA, Seidman DS, Stevenson DK. Neonatal hyperbilirubinemia. *N Engl J Med*. 2001;344:581-590.
205. Wennberg RP. The blood-brain barrier and bilirubin encephalopathy. *Cell Mol Neurobiol*. 2000;20:97-109.
216. Cserr HF, DePasquale M, Patlak CS. Volume regulatory influx of electrolytes from plasma to brain during acute hyperosmolality. *Am J Physiol*. 1987;253:F530-F537.
220. Stonestreet BS, Sadowska GB, Leeman J, Hanumara RC, Petersson KH, Patlak CS. Effects of acute hyperosmolality on blood-brain barrier function in ovine fetuses and lambs. *Am J Physiol Regul Integr Comp Physiol*. 2006;291:R1031-R1039.
225. Stonestreet BS, Oen-Hsiao JM, Petersson KH, Sadowska GB, Patlak CS. Regulation of brain water during acute hyperosmolality in ovine fetuses, lambs, and adults. *J Appl Physiol*. 2003;94:1491-1500.
226. Vohr B, Allan WC, Scott DT, et al. Early-onset intraventricular hemorrhage in preterm neonates: incidence of neurodevelopmental handicap. *Semin Perinatol*. 1999;23:212-217.
243. El-Khoury N, Braun A, Hu FR, et al. Astrocyte end-feet in germinal matrix, cerebral cortex, and white matter in developing infants. *Pediatr Res*. 2006;59:673-679.

Trophic Factor, Nutritional, and Hormonal Regulation of Brain Development

127

David Pleasure

INTRODUCTION

This chapter reviews advances in our understanding of the roles of neurotrophic proteins, retinoids, folate, lipids, and thyroid and steroid hormones in neural development. These molecules play central roles in the regulation of neuronal and glial lineages; when they are not maintained at optimal levels in the developing nervous system, neural structural abnormalities and permanent neurologic dysfunction may result. For example, maternal folate deficiency increases the frequency of neural tube defects (NTDs), particularly in genetically susceptible fetuses, and maternal folate prophylaxis sharply reduces the frequency of these defects.[1,2]

The development of the nervous system entails the most complex array of cellular migrations and interactions of any organ system. The actions of neural morphogens, neurotrophic proteins, retinoids, folate, and thyroid and steroid hormones must be appreciated within this dynamic context. Actions of these molecules on the nervous system not only depend on their concentrations but are also specific to stage and location.[3,4] Altered actions of these molecules by mutations or environmental perturbations may delay brain development or cause irreversible brain injuries.[5]

NEURAL DEVELOPMENT

Induction of neuroectoderm, which occurs in the region of ectodermal contact with dorsal mesoderm, is the third major event of embryogenesis, after the establishment of embryonic dorsoventral and anteroposterior axes and the formation of mesoderm during gastrulation. The subsequent formation of the forebrain is induced by mesoderm anterior to the notochord, whereas Sonic hedgehog (Shh) secreted by notochord induces ventral structures of the hindbrain and spinal cord.[6]

The neural plate, composed of multipotential neuroectodermal cells destined to form both the central nervous system (CNS) and peripheral nervous system, appears in the human embryo 18 days after fertilization, and genes begin to be transcribed in this structure that encode adhesion molecules, including neural cell adhesion molecule (NCAM), L1CAM, and N-cadherin. Mutations affecting one of these genes, *L1*, cause X-linked aqueductal stenosis and agenesis of the corpus callosum, which occurs approximately once in 20,000 births.[7]

The dorsal aspect of the embryo develops lateral furls, and then invagination of the neural plate forms a fold (Fig. 127.1). A tube appears along the length of the fetus by fusion of this fold, proceeding both forward and backward. The anterior neuropore closes at day 24, and the posterior neuropore closes at days 26 to 28. The neural tube initially consists of a single layer of neuroectodermal cells, which proliferate and generate neuroepithelial progenitors for neurons and neuroglial cells. Radial glial cells appear early during neural tube formation and stretch across the wall of the neural tube. Neurons originate at the inner luminal border of the neural tube from these radial glial cells and then migrate outward along the radial glial cells.[8] In the cerebral cortex, which is highly laminated, early-born neurons

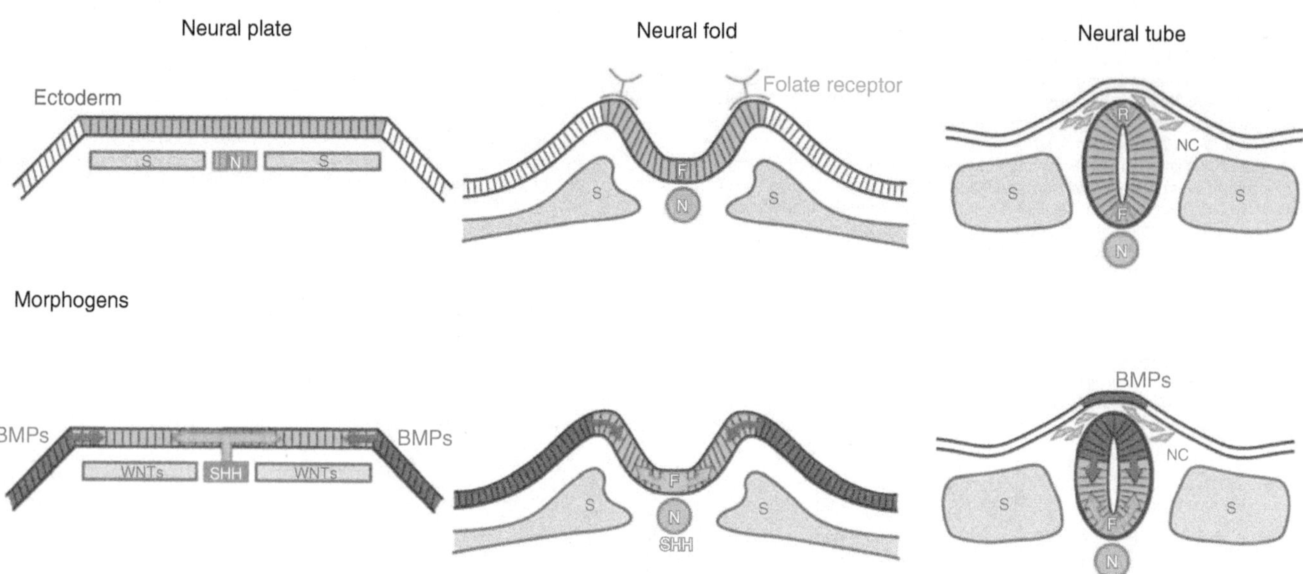

Fig. 127.1 Bone morphogenetic protein *(BMP)*, sonic hedgehog *(SHH)*, and *Wnt* gradients induce neural plate folding and neural tube formation they also specify neural tube and neural crest cells *(NC)*. Notochord *(N)* and floorplate *(F)* are sources for SHH. *S,* Somite. Folate signals via folate receptor 1 to drive redistribution of neural plate adhesion molecules, neural plate cell elongation, neural plate folding, and neural tube closure.[2]

occupy the deeper cortical layers and later-born neurons migrate past the deep layers to establish new superficial layers. Thus the deepest cortical region contains the ontogenically oldest neurons.[9]

Neural crest cells are derived from neuroectoderm of the dorsolateral neural tube and form the peripheral and enteric nervous systems. The neural crest cells migrate from the neural tube into the surrounding mesenchyme at about the time of neural tube closure. The cephalic neural crest contributes to the formation of the facial skeleton, branchial arches, and, in conjunction with placode-derived cells, the lower cranial nerves. Neural crest cells migrating from the dorsolateral aspects of the spinal neural tube serve as progenitors for the peripheral and enteric nervous systems, the adrenal medulla, and melanocytes.[4,10]

Our understanding of human brain development has recently been enhanced by methods for the single-neural-cell transcriptomic analyses of human postmortem fetal brain cells and for guiding human-induced pluripotent stem cells (hiPSCs) to form brain organoids.[11-13] However, most experimental studies of neural development have used rodent and other experimental animal models. The mouse CNS at birth is at a developmental stage similar to that of the human CNS at 5 to 6 months' gestation. By 10 days postpartum, the mouse CNS has matured to a stage equivalent to that of the human brain at term. Cerebral cortical neurogenesis is largely completed by birth in both human and mouse, although some new neurons continue to be generated throughout life from neural stem cells that persist in both the mouse and human CNS, particularly in the hippocampus and the subventricular zone bordering the cerebral ventricles.[14,15] CNS myelination in humans commences during the third trimester of gestation; in rats and mice, differentiated oligodendroglial cells first appear around the time of birth, and myelination is an entirely postnatal process.[16,17]

NEUROTROPHIC PROTEINS

Various terms—including *hormone, trophic protein, morphogen, growth factor, cytokine,* and *chemokine*—are applied to proteins present in extracellular fluids that modulate the behavior of cells. Hormones are secreted proteins and other molecules that circulate in the bloodstream and act on distant tissues, whereas trophic proteins act on neighboring cells (paracrine factors) or on the synthetic cells themselves (autocrine factors). Concentration gradients of morphogenic proteins provide epigenetic control of cellular specification and commitment during early development and contribute to axonal guidance at a later stage in development.[18] Examples of neural morphogens are Shh, the Wnts, and the bone morphogenetic proteins (BMPs). The categorization of these factors is somewhat operational, because factors that act as hormones in one context may act as neurotrophic factors in other contexts. Likewise, the main development morphogens have also been found to have distinct signaling roles.

The phrase *neurotrophic protein* is usually used to refer to proteins that influence cell survival and differentiation (e.g., nerve growth factor [NGF]). Proteins that enhance the proliferation of target cells are referred to as *growth factors,* but many exert morphogenetic and trophic as well as mitogenic effects. The term *cytokine* was initially applied to bioactive proteins released by lymph node- and bone marrow-derived cells, but it is now clear that other cell types, including those derived from neuroectoderm (neurons, astrocytes, and oligodendrocytes) and embryonic yolk sac (microglia) also synthesize cytokines. Chemokines, cytokines that exert chemotactic (migration enhancing) effects on cells, are involved both in the recruitment of cells of the immune system from the bloodstream to the CNS during CNS infectious and autoimmune disorders and in the migration of neural progenitors and microglia within the CNS.[14,19,20]

Rather than attempting a global description of the many neurotrophic protein classes, this chapter briefly considers three morphogens that govern dorsoventral patterning during CNS development: Shh, the BMPs, and the Wnts. Then three neurotrophic protein families that regulate neural cell proliferation, differentiation, and survival are discussed: the fibroblast growth factors (FGFs), the platelet-derived growth factors (PDGFs), and the neurotrophins. A concentration gradient of Shh, a morphogen secreted by the notochord and floor plate, signals by activation of Patched (Ptc) receptors and

Gli transcription factors and stimulates production from the ventral spinal cord's neural stem cells of motor neurons and oligodendroglial cells. In opposition to this ventralizing action of Shh, members of the BMP and Wnt families, produced by the roof plate and the ectoderm above it, inhibit the generation of motor neurons and oligodendrocytes while stimulating the production of sensory neurons and astroglia.[21] Inactivating and activating mutations in Shh signaling pathways give rise to holoprosencephaly and medulloblastoma, respectively.[22,23] Mutations in Wnt signaling pathways are responsible for some NTDs,[24] and BMP signaling mutations can cause cerebral malformations.[25]

FGF signaling pathways interact with signaling by the Wnts during the early development of the CNS and later are important in regulating formation of the corpus callosum.[26] FGF receptor mutations cause craniosynostosis and achondroplasia.[27] The PDGFs, like the FGFs, signal by activating plasma membrane protein tyrosine kinase receptors. Platelet-derived growth factor subunit A (PDGFA) exerts trophic and proliferative effects on oligodendroglial progenitors.[28]

Much of what is known about the regulation of the early stages of neural development by neurotrophic proteins pertains to the neural crest, which originates as a population of pluripotent stem cells that arises between nonneural and neural ectoderm. At the stage of development where the neural tube closes, these stem cells generate migratory progenitors that give rise to lineage-restricted progenitors for neuronal, glial, melanogenic, endocrine, cartilage, and bone cells.[4,10] The neurotrophins (i.e., NGF, brain-derived neurotrophic factor [BDNF], NT-3, and NT-4/5), which play leading roles in governing the fates and survival of neural crest neuronal progenitors, are synthesized as precursor proteins (proneurotrophins) that signal by activating the p75 neurotrophin receptor (p75NTR). However, after proteolytic processing to mature neurotrophins, their primary receptors are members of the Trk family of protein tyrosine kinases. Activation of p75NTR often leads to target-cell apoptosis, whereas activation of the Trks enhances neuronal survival and regulates the neuronal transmitter phenotype.[29] Pioneering in vivo experiments by Hamburger and Levi-Montalcini have demonstrated that excess NGF during development causes sympathetic neuronal hyperplasia, whereas NGF depletion results in partial sympathectomy.[30] Inactivating mutations of the TrkA NGF receptor cause congenital insensitivity to pain with anhidrosis (hereditary sensory and autonomic neuropathy type IV).[31]

VITAMIN A AND OTHER RETINOIDS

Three forms of vitamin A are biologically active. Retinol (vitamin A_1 alcohol) maintains mucous membrane structure and function and is the circulating form of the vitamin. Retinal (vitamin A_1 aldehyde) plays a role in retinal development through conversion to a derivative that is incorporated into rhodopsin. Retinoic acid (RA) contributes to the regulation of pattern formation in the early embryo. Most abundant in the body are retinol and retinyl esters, the latter basically inactive except as precursors for the visual chromophore. At least five natural biologically active forms of RA are known: all-trans-RA (by definition vitamin A); 9-cis-RA; 3,4-didehydro-RA; 14-hydroxy-4,14-retroretinol; and 4-oxo-RA.[32]

Retinoid-binding proteins are primarily intracellular: chief among them are CRABPI and CRABPII, which bind RA, and CRBPI and CRBPII, which bind retinol and retinal. These transporters stabilize the retinoids for delivery and metabolism.[33] Observations that correlated retinoid exposure with CNS malformations have led to recognition of the retinoid receptors and homeodomain-encoded transcription factors as effectors for retinoid actions.[34] Megadoses of retinol and therapeutic oral doses of isotretinoin (13-cis-RA), its analogue, elicit teratogenic effects in the human fetus, causing both microcephaly and hydrocephalus. After maternal dietary manipulation to expose rats to RA at embryonic day 10, myelomeningocele developed in 60% of the fetuses.[35] The teratogenic potential of retinoids is powerful and persistent: malformations resembling RA embryopathy have occurred up to a year after discontinuance of the oral use of the RA analogue etretinate, which is stored in fat and slowly released into the circulation.[36]

The retinoids play important roles during normal neural development at the earliest stages of neurogenesis, at the time of neural plate formation, and also later, when the form of the mature nervous system has already been established. The neural plate binds retinol, is the site for its most efficient conversion to RA, and—by generating an RA gradient—regulates right-left patterning during somitogenesis.[37]

Much of the impetus to pursue RA as an important signaling molecule in the CNS came from observations of the startling and diverse patterns of defects in both deficiency and excess of retinoid signaling. RA exposure, for instance, inhibits migration of cranial neural crest cells in the cultured mouse embryo, and mutant mice deficient in RA synthesis fail to develop neural crest derivatives, including enteric ganglia and pharyngeal pouch derivatives.[38]

RA regulates CNS segmentation by inducing the orderly patterns of expression of members of a superfamily of *Hox* and *Hox*-related genes that contain a conserved homeodomain. The *Hox* genes occur in four separate clusters (*Hox* a,b,c,d), encoding transcription factors that control embryonic segmentation and organogenesis in part by regulating the expression of NCAM, which modulates cell movement.[39] Later in brain development, RA and members of the Wnt and BMP families of morphogens presenting or originating in the meninges and skin regulate cortical neurogenesis and axonal guidance.[19,40]

FOLATE

Human NTDs were first closely linked to folate deficiency in 1965 by Hibbard and Smithells, who reported that folate deficiency occurred in 69% of mothers of children with CNS abnormalities compared with 17% of control women. Subsequent studies suggesting the important role of diet in the prevention of NTDs, including the increased occurrence of anencephaly and myelomeningocele in the offspring of women who had inadequate nutrition or who used folic acid inhibitors during pregnancy.

Folate plays an essential role in methyl group transfer reactions. Methylation is cyclic, involving the interchange of methyl groups between homocysteine and methionine mediated by the enzyme methionine synthase (5-methyltetrahydrofolate-homocysteine S-methyltransferase). Methionine is activated by adenosine triphosphate to S-adenosylmethionine (SAM), a central source for methyl group transfer to proteins, lipids, and nucleic acids. One product of methyl transfer is S-adenosylhomocysteine, which is then hydrolyzed to homocysteine. In most cells, homocysteine is remethylated to methionine by vitamin B_{12}-dependent methionine synthase. This remethylation reaction is the only enzymatic step in humans that requires both folic acid and vitamin B_{12} as cofactors.[41] Two folate transporters, reduced folate carrier (RFC) and proton-coupled folate transporter (PCFT), participate in the absorption of dietary folate and the entry of folate into cells. PCFT mutations are responsible for hereditary folate malabsorption, a recessive disorder that may present with seizures or immunodeficiency.[42]

In mice, mutations in 240 genes are thus far known to cause NTDs. Interacting effects of RA and folate on NTDs in these mutant mice are often complex. For example, although RA increases the incidence of exencephaly in four of these mutant mouse strains, it also decreases the incidence of caudal spina bifida in several of the same strains. In many of these mutant mouse strains, folate deficiency increases the frequency of NTDs by impairing de novo nucleotide biosynthesis, whereas in nonmutant (wild-type) mice, simple maternal folate deficiency is not sufficient to induce NTDs. These observations lend support to the hypothesis that the majority of human NTDs result from a combination of heightened genetic susceptibility owing to genetic polymorphisms and the teratogenic effects of folate deficiency.[43]

Epileptic mothers with fetal malformations have low folate levels. Administration of folate reduces the incidence of valproic acid (VPA)-induced NTDs in mice. VPA is a potent teratogen, exposure to which yields an estimated 20-fold increase in the frequency of NTDs in offspring.[44] Mechanisms that have been proposed to explain the teratogenic effect of VPA include inhibition of high-affinity folate receptors and histone deacetylase as well as perturbations of Wnt and planar cell polarity signaling.[45]

It has been estimated that 300,000 to 400,000 children with spina bifida or anencephaly are born yearly worldwide. Holmes estimated that the prevalence of NTDs in New England in 1994 was 1.2 per 1000. Among the 146 cases in his 15-year survey, 54 infants had spina bifida, 74 had anencephaly, and 19 had encephalocele. Approximately 75% of affected fetuses died in utero, 7.5% were infants of insulin-dependent diabetic mothers, and only 1 child (0.7%) had been exposed to anticonvulsants in utero.[46]

The effect of early folic acid supplementation in women to prevent recurrent NTDs was reported in 1991. Administration of 4 mg of folic acid daily before conception and during early gestation resulted in a sixfold decrease in risk (0.6% vs. 3.6%) for recurrent NTDs and an overall diminution in NTD occurrence of 50% to 70%. Based on those observations, folic acid has been recommended to reproductive-age women since the 1990s at 0.4 mg/d starting well before conception and extending until 3 months of gestation for the general population and 4 mg/d for women who have already had children with NTDs.

Yet another means of folate prophylaxis was begun in 1996 with the folic acid enrichment of flour, breads, cereals, and rice. This means of supplementation became mandatory in the United States in January 1998, with the minimum addition designed to be 0.14 mg of folic acid/100 g of cereal grain, which was calculated to increase intake by an average of 0.1 mg/day. This approach was shown to be effective in a southern California study, which demonstrated that levels of serum and red cell folate greatly exceeded minimal acceptable levels in both socioeconomically disadvantaged and advantaged women. In a survey of multiple states in the United States, NTD prevalence after grain fortification with folate decreased by approximately 19% to 30.5 per 100,000 live births; however, no decrease occurred among patients with either no or only late prenatal care, confirming the strong desirability of early folate prophylaxis. In addition, several large studies have noted that Hispanic women have a higher incidence of children with NTDs. Children of those who have not acculturated, in particular regarding language, have a higher risk of NTDs due to lack of awareness of folic acid recommendations.

A genetic variant in 5,10-methylenetetrahydrofolate reductase (MTHFR), estimated to be present in 5% to 15% of the general population, is associated with defective transfer of a methyl group to homocysteine to form methionine. Two mutations in the *MTHFR* gene, C677T and A1298C, which lead to increased homocysteine levels, significantly increase risks of NTD in offspring. Homocysteine levels in women with these *MTHFR* variants can be normalized with large doses of folate.

FATTY ACIDS AND CHOLESTEROL

The brain is rich in lipids, and studies in animal models show that brain lipids are changed by alterations in the intake of essential fatty acids. The transfer of long-chain polyunsaturated fatty acids (LC-PUFAs) to the fetus occurs through the placenta before birth and to the newborn through breast milk after birth. Premature birth interrupts placental transfer of LC-PUFAs. The essential fatty acids of the diet are linoleic (C18:2*n*-6) and linolenic (C18:3*n*-3) acids. Premature and growth-restricted infants are born with essential fatty acid deficiency, and studies in experimental animals indicate that such deficiency is associated with cognitive and visual impairments. Supplementing human maternal intake of docosahexaenoic acid, the most abundant long-chain omega-3 polyunsaturated fatty acid found in retina and brain, yields improved childhood visual and psychomotor development.[47]

Some inborn errors of cholesterol metabolism perturb embryonic development. The first-described and prototypic example is Smith-Lemli-Opitz syndrome (SLOS), induced by any of more than 100 recessive mutations of the 7-dehydrocholesterol reductase gene *(DHCR7)* located on chromosome 11q13.4. The incidence of SLOS is approximately 1 per 10,000 to 1 per 60,000 live births and is most common in populations of northern European heritage. Affected infants have plasma cholesterol concentrations as low as 1 mg/dL (2% of the newborn norm) in tandem with high 7- and 8-dehydrocholesterol levels. This low cholesterol availability interferes with adrenal steroid production, yielding treatable adrenal insufficiency. Other clinical manifestations are variable, including dysmorphic facies, cognitive delay, hypotonia, and various anomalies of the heart, lungs, intestine, kidneys, genitalia, and limbs. Cardinal signs of the disease are hypospadias, a small or proximally placed thumb, syndactyly of the second to third toes, and microcephaly with agenesis of the corpus callosum and holoprosencephaly (the latter occurring in 5% to 6% of these infants).

The brain is particularly affected in SLOS owing to limitations in the rate of cholesterol transport from the maternal circulation via placental adenosine triphosphate (ATP)–binding cassette transporter A1 (ABCA1) and apolipoprotein E (Apo E). Postnatally, the brain is also unable to utilize cholesterol derived from the diet or from systemic metabolism owing to limitations of transport across the blood-brain barrier. Genetic polymorphisms that influence the transport capabilities of ABCA1 and Apo E influence the severity of SLOS.[48] Present attempts at SLOS therapy center on cholesterol supplementation and statin treatment.[49]

Other disorders of postsqualene cholesterol synthesis that affect development include lathosterolosis, desmosterolosis, sterol-C-4 methyl oxidase-like (SC4MOL) deficiency, dominant chondrodysplasia punctata (CDPX2) and congenital hemidysplasia with ichthyosiform erythroderma and limb defects (CHILD) syndrome, Antley-Bixler syndrome, and hydrops-ectopic calcification-moth-eaten (HEM) skeletal dysplasia. Some degree of cholesterol deficiency occurs in all of these syndromes, but specific precursor sterols that accumulate likely contribute to the specific clinical features of each.[50]

HORMONES

Although the effects of hormonal deficiency or excess on neural function in the adult may be profound, they are in general reversible. By contrast, perturbations in the availability of hormones during critical periods of neuronal and glial cell development often result in permanent and profound abnormalities in synaptogenesis and myelination.[5] This section focuses on thyroid and steroid hormones with emphasis on the special vulnerability of the immature nervous system to deficiencies of these hormones.

Thyroid disorders are the most prevalent endocrine derangements in the world, even more common than diabetes mellitus. According to World Health Organization (WHO) estimates from 1990, endemic hypothyroidism primarily resulting from low dietary iodine intake affected approximately 750 million people in the world, largely in Asia and Africa, and approximately

43 million were affected by brain damage secondary to low iodine intake either prenatally, in infancy, or in early childhood. Maternal iodine deficiency can be exacerbated by environmental pollutants including nitrate, thiocyanate, and perchlorate.[51]

The sodium-iodide symporter (NIS) mediates iodide absorption by the stomach and duodenum as well as active uptake by the thyroid gland. NIS is also expressed in lactating breast tissue, concentrating iodine in colostrum and breast milk. The thyroid usually contains 10 to 20 g of iodine, depending on the adequacy of the diet. Maternal iodine requirements increase in early pregnancy. An approximately 50% increase in thyroid hormone (TH) output occurs in early pregnancy in relation to several mechanisms: stimulation by thyroid-stimulating hormone (TSH), stimulation by human chorionic gonadotropin (hCG) (peaking at 9 to 11 weeks' gestation, binding to and stimulating the TSH receptor in the thyroid), and high estrogen levels that increase serum thyroxine-binding globulin concentration 1.5-fold. Approximately 90% of thyroid iodine is organically bound to thyroglobulin, the large glycoprotein secreted by and residing in thyroid follicular cells. Once in the thyroid gland, iodide is oxidized by thyroid peroxidase (TPO) to iodine. TPO also iodinates tyrosine residues of thyroglobulin to form monoiodotyrosine (MIT) and diiodotyrosine (DIT) and allows the coupling of MIT and DIT to form T_3 and T_4. The matrix for both the synthesis and storage of T_3 and T_4 is thyroglobulin. The molar ratio of secreted T_4 to T_3 is 11:1 owing to intrathyroidal deiodination of T_4 to T_3 by type 1 and 2 deiodinases (D1 and D2). T_3 and T_4 are released into the bloodstream, following pinocytosis and lysosomal digestion of thyroglobulin by peptidases. Another deiodinase, type 3 deiodinase (D3), inactivates THs by removing the inner-ring iodine from T_3 and T_4. D3 is high in concentration in the placenta, thus promoting the ready crossing of iodine to the fetus. D2, the only 5′ deiodinase in the adult human CNS, is highly expressed in ependymal cells of the third ventricle, in the mediobasal hypothalamus, and in astrocytes. D2 in these cells likely provides T_3 for neighboring neurons that have thyroid receptors but cannot generate T_3. D3 is the main inactivator of THs, converting T_3 and T_4 into inactive compounds. In humans, D3 messenger RNA or protein has been detected in the fetal cerebral cortex where, unlike D2, it is found predominantly in neuronal cells.[52,53]

Delivery TH to the brain requires that the hormone cross the blood-brain barrier and brain target-cell plasma membranes. An example of a TH cell membrane transporter that is associated with a significant human illness is the monocarboxylate transporter 8 (MCT8, encoded by *SLC16A2*). Mutations in this molecule block T_3 transport, causing the Allan-Herndon-Dudley syndrome. This X-linked disease, first described clinically in 1944, is characterized by hypotonia, myopathic facies, early feeding problems, and motor and speech delays. Hearing and vision are unaffected, but the children eventually develop spasticity, contractures, dystonia, and sometimes seizures and delayed CNS myelination. Affected children have a high T_3, low rT_3, low or low-normal T_4, and normal or slightly high TSH. More than 100 affected families have been described, with more than 70 mutations in the gene. Some female carriers are symptomatic owing to random X inactivation but have normal thyroid function and neurodevelopment. Diiodothyropropionic acid (DITPA) and 3,3′,5-tri-iodothyroacetic acid (tiratricol) have some therapeutic efficacy in the Allan-Herndon-Dudley syndrome.[54]

Iodine deficiency is of greatest consequence for pregnant women and their fetuses, with deleterious outcomes including goiter, cretinism, intellectual impairments, growth retardation, neonatal hypothyroidism, increased pregnancy loss, and infant mortality. If adequate iodine is not available to produce TH during pregnancy, TSH rises and maternal and fetal goiter develop. Because the human thyroid is not fully developed until 10 to 12 weeks' gestation, most of the fetal THs in the first half of human gestation are provided transplacentally by the mother. The fetus requires iodine for endogenous TH production beginning at approximately 20 weeks' gestation. Dietary iodine deficiency is the most common cause of congenital hypothyroidism worldwide. With exclusive breastfeeding, women lose approximately 75 to 200 μg of iodine daily in breast milk. Therefore increased dietary iodine intake is needed; recommendations for dietary iodine intake during lactation range from 250 to 290 μg/day, higher than the 150 μg/day recommended for nonpregnant and nonlactating individuals. Mothers living in iodine-deficient areas may be unable to meet the increased demands for iodine intake for normal neurodevelopment of nursing infants.

The neurologic consequences of early hypothyroidism vary with the degree of maternal, fetal, and neonatal hypothyroidism. Sporadic hypothyroidism occurs in approximately 1 in 4000 live births in the United States. Screening programs for this abnormality are widespread among developed countries. Knowledge gained from these programs has shown that the fetus is usually unaffected by intrinsic in utero hypothyroidism, even when athyrotic. Prompt treatment of these children often prevents retardation. Causes of congenital hypothyroidism include genetic defects in factors involved in TH synthesis.[55]

Fetal neurogenesis is dependent on maternal TH. Maternal TH deficiency alters expression of multiple transcription factors, most notably downregulating the radial glia transcription factor Pax6, thus suppressing forebrain neurogenesis and neuronal migration and leading to reduced cortical thickness and cognitive deficits.

Nuclear thyroid hormone receptors (TRs) bind with 10- to 15-fold greater affinity to T_3 than T_4. The THs bind to specific deoxyribonucleic acid sequences (response elements) within promoters of target genes and act as transcriptional regulators. The T_3 receptor genes TR-α and TR-β encode four receptors: TR-α_1, TR-β_1, TR-β_2, and TR-β_3. These receptors occupy target response elements usually as heterodimers with the retinoid X receptor. TR-α1 is constitutively expressed in embryonic development, and TR-β is expressed later on. TR-α1 and TR-α2 predominate in the brain, bone, heart, and intestine, and TR-β1 is the major form in the liver, kidney, and thyroid. TR-β_2 is expressed in the hypothalamus, pituitary, cochlea, and retina and is involved in regulating the hypothalamic-pituitary-thyroid axis as well as in neurosensory development. Classical hypothyroidism with only borderline abnormal hormone values and a spotty response of some physical abnormalities to thyroxine therapy can be caused by TR mutations.[56]

Environmental toxins may exert thyromimetic or thyroid-suppressive effects. The polychlorinated biphenyls (PCBs) and related substances are known as developmental endocrine disruptors. The toxic potential of these molecules was highlighted in 1968, when 1000 western Japanese became symptomatic from ingesting PCB-contaminated rice oil. A similar epidemic occurred in Taiwan in 1979. Symptoms and signs included skin and neurologic changes. Infants born to these PCB-exposed women were often of low birth weight and showed varying degrees of hyperpigmentation of the skin and mucous membranes, gingival hyperplasia, and abnormal skull calcification. Other polyhalogenated aromatic hydrocarbon environmental toxins include dichlorodiphenyl-trichloroethane (DDT), dichlorodiphenyl dichloroethene (DDE), polychlorinated dibenzodioxins (PCDDs or simply dioxins), polybrominated diphenylethers (PBDEs), and hexachlorobenzene. These have persisted in the environment despite the banning of DDT and PCBs in the United States and most Western nations since the 1970s. In vivo elimination is slow, with a mean half-life varying from 1.2 to 10 years, depending on the specific congener and initial concentration. Once ingested—for example, from contaminated fish, dairy products, meat, or water—these compounds are stored in the liver and fat tissues, including the breast and breast milk. Some of these molecules are similar to THs in structure, some have higher affinity for transthyretin than T_4, and some bind to thyroxine-binding globulin. Decreased neonatal T_4 has been observed in humans exposed to these environmental toxins in utero. Studies of neurodevelopmental sequelae in children after in utero exposure to these contaminants have thus far been limited by inadequate cohort size and nonuniformity of exposures but have pointed to some intellectual impairments.[57]

Glucocorticoids, estrogens, progesterone, and androgens also influence CNS development. Their actions are transduced by cytosolic receptors that, on binding of their ligand steroid, are released from complexes with other cytosolic proteins and move to the nucleus, where they modulate the transcription of target genes. The expression of these receptors is regulated by transcriptional, translational, and posttranslational mechanisms, and the activity of each of these receptors is modulated via interactions with other receptors. Glucocorticoid receptors (GRs) are expressed by both neurons and glia. The enzymes 11β-hydroxysteroid dehydrogenases type 1 and type 2 (HSD1 and HSD2) determine access of the glucocorticoids to their receptors. There are time- and locus-dependent windows for the various adrenal steroid hormone actions on fetal brain. For example, fetuses and newborns are exposed to maternal estradiol and to their own gonadal and brain-synthesized estradiol. Estradiol affects neurotrophin secretion and the morphology and survival of neurons and astrocytes. Type I adrenal corticosteroid receptors, concentrated in the hippocampus, bind both mineralocorticoids and glucocorticoids with high affinity, whereas type II corticosteroid receptors are distributed throughout the brain and bind glucocorticoids with high affinity. In the developing nervous system, glucocorticoids regulate the frequency with which nascent neurons undergo apoptosis. Excess glucocorticoid, by stimulating cholinergic neurotransmission and eliciting neuronal loss, has complex effects on the immature brain.[58,59] Several studies have reported deleterious effects of postnatal glucocorticoid therapy on cerebellar development. Animal experiments have shown that glucocorticoids speed the loss of neuroblasts from the cerebellar external granule layer, the region responsible for the production of the vast majority of cerebellar neurons. This finding is likely due to inhibition of Shh signaling by glucocorticoids.[60]

CONCLUSIONS AND FUTURE PROSPECTS

The end of the last century was marked by substantial advances in our knowledge of environmental influences on neural development. Those advances, generated largely by epidemiologic studies, included recognition of the ill effects of various toxins, such as methylmercury and lead, and the validation of iodized salt- and folate-supplemented flour as prophylaxis against gestational hypothyroidism and NTDs. The decreases in the incidence of neonatal hypothyroidism and spina bifida that followed the introduction of those dietary manipulations helped investigators to focus on kindreds in which mutations, rather than environmental influences, were responsible for abnormalities in neural development. Now, in the 21st century, progress in molecular medicine will enhance our capacity to prevent and treat early-onset neurologic diseases.

 A complete reference list is available at www.ExpertConsult.com.

SELECT REFERENCES

1. Molloy AM, Pangilinan F, Brody LC. Genetic risk factors for folate-responsive neural tube defects. *Annu Rev Nutr*. 2017;37:269-291.
2. Balashova OA, Visina O, Borodinsky LN. Folate action in nervous system development and disease. *Dev Neurobiol*. 2018;78:391-402.
3. Haushalter C, Asselin L, Fraulob V, et al. Retinoic acid controls early neurogenesis in the developing mouse cerebral cortex. *Dev Biol*. 2017;430:129-141.
4. Soldatov R, Kaucka M, Kastriti ME, et al. Spatiotemporal structure of cell fate decisions in murine neural crest. *Science*. 2019;364:eaas9536.
5. Penn AA, Gressens P, Fleiss B, et al. Controversies in preterm brain injury. *Neurobiol Dis*. 2016;92:90-101.
6. Fucillo M, Joyner AL, Fishell G. Morphogen to mitogen: the multiple roles of hedgehog signaling in vertebrate neural development. *Nature Rev Neurosci*. 2006;7:772-783.
7. Adle-Biassette H, Saugier-Veber P, Fallet-Biano C, et al. Neuropathological review of 138 cases genetically tested for X-linked hydrocephalus: evidence for closely related clinical entities of unknown molecular bases. *Acta Neuropath*. 2013;126:427-442.
8. Pollen AA, Nowakowski TJ, Chen J, et al. Molecular identity of human outer radial glia during cortical development. *Cell*. 2015;163:55-67.
9. Noctor SC, Flint AC, Weissman TA, et al. Neurons derived from radial glial cells establish radial units in neocortex. *Nature*. 2001;409:714-720.
10. Crane JF, Trainor PA. Neural crest stem and progenitor cells. *Annu Rev Cell Dev Biol*. 2006;22:267-286.
11. Boldog E, Bakken TE, Hodge RD, et al. Transcriptomic and morphophysiological evidence for a specialized human cortical GABAergic cell type. *Nature Neurosci*. 2018;21:1185-1195.
12. Di Lullo E, Kriegstein AR. The use of brain organoids to investigate neural development and disease. *Nat Rev Neurosci*. 2017;18:573-584.
13. Tao Y, Zhang S-C. Neural subtype specification from human pluripotent stem cells. *Cell Stem Cell*. 2016;19:573-586.
14. Choe Y, Pleasure SJ, Mira H. Control of adult neurogenesis by short-range morphogenic-signaling molecules. *Cold Spring Harb Perspect Biol*. 2016;8:a018887.
15. Obernier K, Cebrian-Silla A, Thomson M, et al. Adult neurogenesis is sustained by symmetric self-renewal and differentiation. *Cell Stem Cell*. 2018;22:221-234.
16. Dean JM, Moravec MD, Grafe M, et al. Strain-specific differences in perinatal rodent oligodendrocyte lineage progression and its correlation with human. *Dev Neurosci*. 2011;33:251-260.
17. Forbes TA, Gallo V. All wrapped up: environmental effects on myelination. *Trends Neurosci*. 2017;40:572-587.
18. Charron F, Tessier-Lavigne M. Novel brain wiring functions for classical morphogens: a role as graded positional cues in axon guidance. *Development*. 2005;132:2251-2262.
19. Choe Y, Pleasure SJ. Meningeal Bmps regulate cortical layer formation. *Brain Plast*. 2018;4:169-183.
20. Moreno M, Bannerman P, Ma J, et al. Conditional ablation of astroglial CCL2 suppresses CNS accumulation of M1 macrophages and preserves axons in mice with MOG peptide EAE. *J Neurosci*. 2014;34:8175-8185.
21. Cayuso J, Ulloa F, Cox B, et al. The Sonic hedgehog pathway independently controls the patterning, proliferation and survival of neuroepithelial cells by regulating Gli activity. *Development*. 2006;133:517-528.
22. Hong M, Kraus RS. Modeling the complex etiology of holoprosencephaly in mice. *Am J Med Genet*. 2018;178C:140-150.
23. Suzuki H, Kumar SA, Shuai S, et al. Recurrent noncoding U1 snRNA mutations drive cryptic splicing in SHH medulloblastoma. *Nature*. 2019;574:707-711.
24. Lopez-Escobar B, Caro-Veja JM, Vijayraghavan DS, et al. The non-canonical Wnt-PCP pathway shapes the mouse caudal neural plate. *Development*. 2018;145:1-15.
25. Klingensmith J, Matsui M, Yang Y-P, Anderson RM. Roles of bone morphogenetic protein signaling and its antagonism in holoprosencephaly. *Am J Med Genet*. 2010;154C:43-51.
26. Lindwall C, Fothergill T, Richards LJ. Commissure formation in the mammalian forebrain. *Curr Topic Neurobiol*. 2007;17:3-14.
27. Di Rocco F, Duplan MB, Heuze Y, et al. FGFR3 mutation causes abnormal membranous ossification in achondroplasia. *Human Mol Genet*. 2014;23:2914-2925.
28. Grinspan JB, Stern JL, Pustilnik SM, Pleasure D. Cerebral white matter contains PDGF-responsive precursors to O2A cells. *J Neurosci*. 1990;10:1866-1873.
29. Barker PA. High affinity not in the vicinity? *Neuron*. 2007;53:1-4.
30. Cowan WM, Hamburger V, Levi-Montalcini R. The path to the discovery of nerve growth factor. *Annu Rev Neurosci*. 2001;24:551-600.
31. Franco ML, Melero C, Sarasola E, et al. Mutations in TrkA causing congenital insensitivity to pain with anhidrosis (CIPA) induce misfolding, aggregation, and mutation-dependent neurodegeneration by dysfunction of the autophagic flux. *J Biol Chem*. 2016;291:21363-21374.
32. O'Byrne SM, Blaner WS. Retinol and retinyl esters: biochemistry and physiology. *J Lipid Res*. 2013;54:1731-1743.
33. Lefebvre P, Benomar Y, Staels B. Retinoid X receptors: common heterodimerization partners with distinct functions. *Trends Endocrin Metab*. 2010;21:676-683.
34. Adams J. The neurobehavioral teratology of retinoids: a 50-year history. *Birth Defects Res (Part A)*. 2010;88:895-905.
35. Danzer E, Schwarz U, Wehrli S, et al. Retinoic acid induced myelomeningocele in fetal rats: characterization by histopathological analysis and magnetic resonance imaging. *Exp Neurol*. 2005;194:467-475.
36. Geiger J-M, Baudin M, Saurat J-H. Teratogenic risk with etretinate and acitretin treatment. *Dermatology*. 1994;189:109-116.
37. Sirbu IO, Duester G. Retinoic-acid signalling in node ectoderm and posterior neural plate directs left-right patterning of somatic mesoderm. *Nat Cell Biol*. 2006;8:271-277.
38. Williams AL, Bohnsack BL. What's retinoic acid got to do with it? Retinoic acid regulation of the neural crest in craniofacial and ocular development. *Genesis*. 2019;57:e23308.
39. Nolte C, De Kumar B, Krumlauf R. *Hox* genes: downstream "effectors" of retinoic acid signaling in vertebrate embryogenesis. *Genesis*. 2019;57:e23306.

40. Siegenthaler JA, Ashique AM, Zarbalis K, et al. Retinoic acid from the meninges regulates cortical neuron development. *Cell*. 2009;139:597-609.
41. Blom HJ, Smulders Y. Overview of homocysteine and folate metabolism. With special references to cardiovascular disease and neural tube defects. *J Inherit Metab Dis*. 2011;34:75-81.
42. Zhao R, Diop-Bove N, Visentin M, Goldman ID. Mechanisms of membrane transport of folates into cells and across epithelia. *Annu Rev Nutr*. 31:177-201.
43. Burren KA, Scott JM, Copp AJ, Greene NDE. The genetic background of the *Curly Tail* strain confers susceptibility to folate-deficiency-induced exencephaly. *Birth Defects Res (Part A)*. 2010;88:76-83.
44. Weston J, Bromley R, Jackson CF, et al. Monotherapy treatment of epilepsy in pregnancy: congenital malformation outcomes in the child. *Cochrane Database Syst Rev*. 2016;11:CD010224.
45. Copp AJ, Stanier P, Greene NDE. Neural tube defects: recent advances, unsolved questions, and controversies. *Lancet Neurol*. 2013;12:799-810.
46. Holmes LB, Driscoll SG, Atkins L. Etiologic heterogeneity of neural-tube defects. *New Engl J Med*. 1976;294:365-369.
47. Shulkin M, Pimpin L, Bellinger D, et al. n-3 Fatty acid supplementation in mothers, preterm infants, and term infants and childhood psychomotor and visual development: a systematic review and meta-analysis. *J Nutr*. 2018;148:409-418.
48. Nowaczyk MJM, Irons MB. Smith-Lemli-Opitz syndrome: phenotype, natural history, and epidemiology. *Am J Med Genet*. 2012;160C:250-262.
49. Svoboda MD, Christie JM, Eroglu Y, et al. Treatment of Smith-Lemli-Opitz syndrome and other sterol disorders. *Am J Med Genet*. 2012;160C:285-294.
50. Porter FD, Herman GE. Malformation syndromes caused by disorders of cholesterol synthesis. *J Lipid Res*. 2011;52:6-34.

Developmental Aspects of Pain

128

Manon Ranger | Simon Beggs | Ruth E. Grunau

INTRODUCTION

Pain is an intrinsic experience which is processed early in life by the maturing nervous system. However, for an individual to experience fully mature pain, sophisticated assimilation at higher cortical levels of sensory discriminatory and emotional or motivational dimensions is necessary, as is the involvement of neuronal activation of integrated central subcortical and cortical brain regions. However, in the very immature infant, pain can be considered as a more primitive experience involving the processing of nociceptive activity at the lower level of the central nervous system (CNS) (i.e., spinal cord and brain stem). Although thalamocortical connections begin around 24 weeks gestation, these are functionally immature.[1,2] Thus as the nervous system develops, the nociceptive signal reaches higher-order processing and can be discriminated from other types of sensory inputs. Moreover, understanding the development of ascending nociceptive and descending modulatory pain pathways, as well as these systems' plasticity, is essential to appreciate the lasting impact early exposure to pain and stress may have on the immature neurologic system of the neonate.

Evidence in rodents suggests that early sensory experience can influence the development of nociceptive pathways,[3] and tissue injury during this critical time of development may prime adult pain perception.[4] Exposure to painful and stressful stimuli is inherent to high-technology neonatal intensive care for infants born very sick and/or prematurely. Infants born very preterm (<33 weeks gestational age) are exposed to an average of 7 to 17 invasive procedures per day[5] during a period of rapid brain development and programming of the hypothalamic-pituitary-adrenal (HPA) axis. Notably, throughout this critical phase of immaturity, the nervous system shows heightened neuronal activation to sensation[6] and less descending inhibitory input.[7] The negative effects of pain on brain development and behavioral outcomes have been reported in both rodents[8,9] and humans (for a review see Ranger and Grunau[10])—for example, in two Canadian cohorts, short- and long-term adverse effects on brain development, the functional trajectory of activity of the HPA axis, and neurodevelopment.[11-24]

This chapter reviews the development of pain sensation and processing, as well as long-term effects of early pain exposure on the developing infant. Because of the physiologic immaturity of the nervous system and extensive brain development and programming of the HPA axis in the preterm infant hospitalized in the neonatal intensive care unit (NICU), these infants are particularly vulnerable to pain exposure early in life. Research in rodents is especially relevant because rats and mice are born neurologically immature; the first week of life provides a good model for human prematurity and is physiologically "similar" to late second trimester preterm human neonates.[25] Thus, both animal and clinical studies will be considered, with a particular focus on pain in the developing very preterm neonate.

DEVELOPMENT OF PERIPHERAL AND CENTRAL NOCICEPTIVE PATHWAYS

Noxious stimuli are detected by sensory neurons throughout the body, and these nociceptive signals transmit via the spinal cord to the brain where the perception of pain is generated. Modulation of these signals can occur at any point on this journey involving interactions between neurons, glia, and the immune system.[26] Physical interaction with the external world is detected by free nerve endings and specific peripheral end organs of primary sensory afferent fibers that respond to particular stimulus modalities. They transform mechanical, thermal, or chemical stimuli into electrical signals to be transmitted to the CNS. These primary afferent fibers arise from neurons within the sensory (dorsal root and trigeminal) ganglia during embryonic development. This gives rise to four main classes of sensory afferent based on their threshold and conduction velocity: thickly myelinated Aα and Aβ fibers that are low-threshold and transmit proprioception and touch, thinly myelinated Aδ and unmyelinated C fibers that are primarily high-threshold and are associated with transmitting noxious stimuli.[27] These different classes of sensory neurons not only transmit distinct sensory modalities, but also undergo unique developmental trajectories.[1]

Cutaneous receptive fields are large in the newborn rat and preterm neonate, and peripheral sensory fibers have a heightened sensitivity to tissue injury.[28-30] Moreover, discrimination between noxious and non-noxious stimuli is imperfect for the neonate due to a combination of the transient overlapping between axon terminals in the superficial laminae of the spinal cord and low-threshold tactile inputs[3] and an underdeveloped local and descending inhibitory influence.[31,32]

Although reflex behaviors and autonomic and hormonal responses to pain exist early in development due to nociceptive transmission through the spinal cord, brain stem, and subcortical midbrain regions, this is not enough to generate a comprehensive perception and awareness of pain. The development of thalamocortical afferents in the human is characterized by colossal connection growth and discrimination: in the infant younger than 24 weeks gestational age, thalamocortical afferents are temporarily in "standby" in the subplate (SP) zone; between 24 and 26 weeks gestational age, axons start to enter the cortical plate and begin to form functional synapses with cortical neurons in layer IV; from 33 to 35 weeks gestational age, the SP region commences to wane, followed by a significant development of massive associative connections with the cortex after 36 weeks gestation.[2] Fig. 128.1 illustrates this critical stage of maturation. During fetal life, general development and myelination of pain pathways occur in parallel with cortical maturation, dendritic arborization, and thalamocortical fiber synaptogenesis.[32]

Noxious information is not processed in the brain in the same way as other sensory modalities. There is no dedicated primary "pain" cortex analogous to the primary somatosensory or visual cortices; rather, noxious stimulation evokes a diffuse pattern of activity in many brain areas. The current view of pain is that it arises from a distributed network of brain activity, and that the conscious experience of pain arises from a dynamic change in a distributed network of brain activity,[33,34] but how does this network develop? Sensory networks in the visual and auditory systems require modality-specific input for their functional maturation, but nociceptive circuits do not require noxious sensory experience in order to develop normally. Instead their development occurs through a cross-modality mechanism requiring spontaneous tactile input during a critical period of early life.[35,36]

How and when this complex brain network develops to encode noxious stimuli distinct from tactile stimuli and create the experience of pain is an important and ongoing area of research. This information has clear clinical implications for the developing infants and also how noxious input at an early stage of development might affect the maturation of the nociceptive system. Sensory system connectivity and functioning are established during specific developmental time windows called *critical periods*, during which deprivation of that normal modality-specific input or disruption of neuronal activity causes long-lasting disruption of sensory cortical maps and consequent sensory impairment. While this phenomenon has been well characterized in animal models for the visual, auditory, and somatosensory systems,[37] it is difficult to define for nociception because nociceptive stimuli are normally absent during development. However, both pre-clinical animal models and clinical studies have shown that early exposure to noxious procedures causes long-term alterations of pain perception, and brain structure and function.[10,38-41]

NEUROIMMUNE INTERACTIONS AND PAIN

The nervous and immune systems are inextricably linked and the degree of complexity of their interactions continues to be discovered. Mechanisms involving elements of the immune system are crucial throughout normal nervous system development.[42] Dysfunction of these interactions has been implicated in many neurodevelopmental and psychiatric disorders.[43] Any exploration of neuronal function and development in health or disease requires consideration of the impact of the immune system.

For nociception, the spinal cord dorsal horn is the first site of processing within the CNS. Transmission of the nociceptive information from the periphery to the spinal cord is via sensory primary afferent neurons as previously discussed; subsequent transmission to the brain is also a neuronally mediated process. However, the processing of the nociceptive signal within the spinal cord is more complex. It is here that the immune system of the CNS becomes important, specifically the actions of microglia.[44]

It is now well documented that microglia are intrinsically active in the normal development of the CNS.[42] Not simply reactive to injury or disease, microglia have an instructive role in synaptic maturation and the refinement of neuronal circuitry perinatally.[45] Microglia sculpt immature neuronal circuits, engulfing and eliminating excessive synaptic structures, all under the control of the classical complement cascade.[46] This function of microglia is important in the development of spinal nociceptive circuitry where considerable postnatal refinement of connectivity occurs, as well as the strengthening and maturation of developmentally appropriate synaptic connectivity (Beggs, unpublished observations).[1] An intriguing prospect is that microglia may be driving these developmental processes in preference to the defined immune role they play in the adult, preventing the risk of an autoinflammatory response to the clearance of axonal debris.[47] The complex molecular machinery underlying this process remains unclear, and it is likely that other molecules are working in tandem with complement to control spatial and temporal aspects of pruning. However, evidence is accumulating that suggests aberrant pruning during critical periods of postnatal development contributes to neurodevelopmental disorders.[42]

Immune activation in early life has the potential to impact both neuronal maturation and the normal developmental influence of microglia on circuit formation, disrupting both basal nociceptive function and, as is discussed in the next section, responses to painful stimuli in later life. Neuroimmune responses occur not only to direct immune activation but also to tissue-damaging injury (e.g., surgical incision). If an injury occurs within the critical period of plasticity that spans the first postnatal week in the rodent (which likely maps onto preterm infancy in humans), the immune response appears muted in terms of microglial reactivity, in comparison to the adult, but there is a priming of microglia such that they mount a greater response to reinjury in later life, resulting in an amplified behavioral pain response.[4,48] A surprising discovery is that this microglial-mediated priming is specific to males, and while the same behavioral priming occurs in females, it is a microglia-independent phenomenon.[48]

Sexual dimorphism is highly prevalent in pain epidemiology, and it is perhaps not surprising that the neuroimmune interactions that underlie the long-term consequences of early-life painful events is sexually dimorphic. The development of microglia is influenced by extrinsic factors including sex.[49] Microglial responses to inflammation and microbiota-derived signals differ between males and females, as do pain responses, both to injury in adulthood and, as described, the long-term consequences of injury in early life.[49,50] Although the reason why this occurs is not clear, there are a few clues to where differences lie. Male and female microglia have a different transcriptomic profile in early life[51] that persists into adulthood[52] and is independent of sex hormonal control, suggesting the differences are established in early life. Following preterm birth, male sex is a risk factor for adverse neurodevelopmental outcome,[53] while repeated exposure to potentially painful procedures has a greater impact

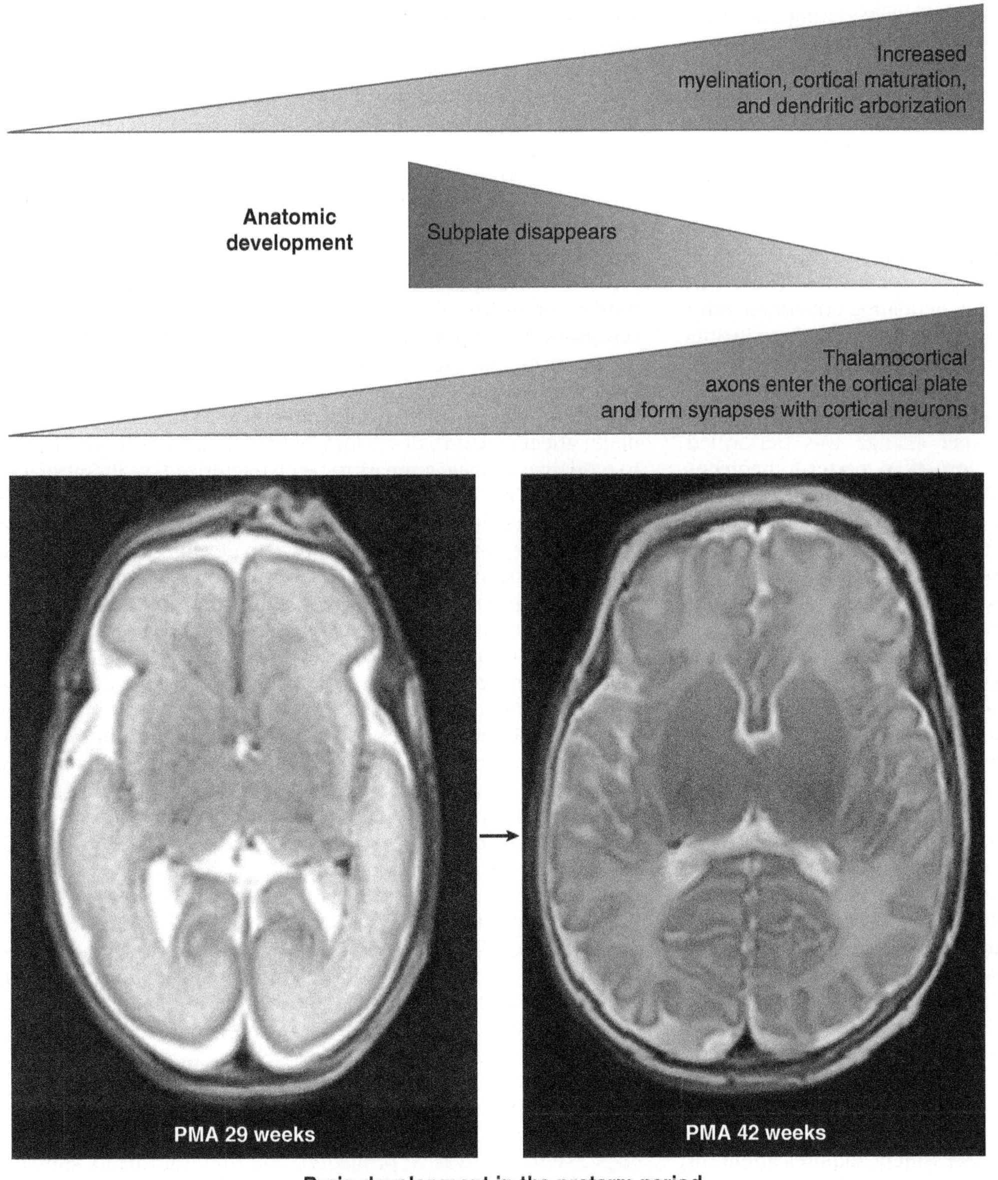

Fig. 128.1 Brain development in the preterm period. Changes in the anatomic development *(red)* and evoked cortical activity *(blue)* in the preterm period. Magnetic resonance imaging (MRI) shows the development of the brain from the preterm period (29 weeks; *left*) to term (42 weeks; *right*). See text for full details. *PMA,* Postmenstrual age. (MRI images courtesy Dr. Steven P. Miller, Hospital for Sick Children, Toronto.)

on brain development in females.[54] Both males and females born extremely preterm demonstrate altered but different somatosensory function and pain experience.[55]

Neuroimmune interactions are central to CNS circuit formation and immune cell function, with long-term implications for CNS homeostasis. How microglia function impacts health across the lifespan and how their dysfunction contributes to disease is only just beginning to be understood. For the study of pain, what is becoming apparent is that the long-lasting effects of pain in early life are partly a consequence of a disruption in the interactions of developing nervous and immune systems. This is a fascinating development and opens new vistas of research opportunities to investigate the translational potential leading to a better understanding and treatment of pain.

PAIN IN THE HUMAN IMMATURE NERVOUS SYSTEM

In the immature infant, facial and motor responses to pain appear to be predominantly mediated at the spinal and subcortical levels, combined with physiologic hormonal and autonomic reactions.[56]

However, specific responses vary substantially among individual infants and differ depending on numerous factors including gestational age, postnatal age, length of NICU hospitalization, and extent and timing of preceding procedures.[57,58]

Preterm neonates are more sensitive to pain compared with term infants, as demonstrated by lower tactile thresholds and sensitization to repeated touch and invasive stimulation, with confirmatory studies in rat pups.[2] Reduction in cutaneous withdrawal response, rise in pain threshold, and reduction in receptive field size with increased postnatal age are clear indicators of the maturation of pain pathways. Thus, this lower tactile threshold in preterm neonates, combined with sensitization to repeated tactile stimulation, renders these infants to be particularly vulnerable to repetitive handling and invasive procedures.[59]

Physiologic and behavioral reactivity can be altered by prior events. For example, when a diaper change was performed 30 minutes before blood collection, very preterm neonates displayed a greater pain response to blood collection by heel lance compared with infants left undisturbed for 1 hour before the invasive procedure.[58] Conversely, in a crossover design, when the same group of infants underwent blood collection first, they responded adversely—and to a similar degree—to a diaper change 30 minutes after the invasive procedure itself.[57] Also, among extremely preterm neonates, reactivity may manifest only after the procedure ends.

Multimodal assessment of pain reactivity is recognized as essential.[60,61] However, although use of a single score summed from multiple indicators (combining behavioral and physiologic indices) is widely used,[62] currently the value of examining behavioral, autonomic, and hemodynamic parameters independently to evaluate the effect of pain on specific systems is advocated, especially for research purposes.[10,61,63] Behavioral, autonomic, and hormonal responses are evident following invasive procedures,[64] yet none of these indicators are specific to pain; in addition, these responses can be evoked by distress or agitation or, in the case of physiologic biomarkers, may signal clinical changes in the infant's health status rather than pain. Facial responses can be subdued or lacking at low gestational ages and become more pronounced with increasing postnatal age.[65] Moreover, cortical somatosensory evoked responses can be observed in the absence of a facial response in some infants.[66,67] The inherent variability in pain responses has led to a general recognition that pain assessment requires attention to multiple modalities, but the assessment and consideration of different response systems separately, rather than use of a single multidimensional pain score, are important. This approach allows the effect of stimulation or management to be fully evaluated because some interventions may reduce pain behaviors but not physiologic responses, leaving the infant at risk of hemodynamic and other adverse events.[63] Because the pain response is complex in very preterm infants, it remains challenging to distinguish pain behaviorally or physiologically from stress. Although a comprehensive consideration of assessment is beyond the scope of this chapter, it is discussed elsewhere.[61]

LONG-TERM EFFECTS OF PAIN

VULNERABILITY OF THE DEVELOPING PRETERM BRAIN

The cytoarchitecture of the brain undergoes rapid development during the late second and third trimesters of fetal life. Infants born very preterm undergo NICU care during a critical developmental window. Rapid neuronal proliferation, development of oligodendrocytes, differentiation of SP neurons, formation and pruning of synapses, cerebellar neuronal proliferation and migration, and cerebral axonal development are all processes that could be vulnerable to external stimulation and circumstances related to the NICU environment and neonatal disease (for a review see Volpe[68]). In rodents, early pain exposure affects neuronal survival due to enhanced vulnerability of immature neurons to excitotoxic damage, and effects of early pain were demonstrated in the rodent brain.[8-69,70] SP neurons establish a temporary connection between axons projecting from the thalamus and their progression to the final target in the cerebral cortex,[71] which render them to be particularly sensitive to excitotoxic damage.[72] Another process vulnerable to unanticipated environmental stressors is the phase of development of the myelin sheath surrounding axons, which proceeds from preoligodendrocytes to the mature oligodendrocyte (for a review see Back and Miller[73]). Finally, late migration of young interneurons to focal areas of cortex continues in the human brain at term and at later stages.[74] Procedural stress and pain induces inflammatory responses, and oxidative stress might affect neuronal development in several ways. Injury related to oxidative damage appears to be characterized by alterations in the complexity of the dendritic branches rather than cell death.[75] These processes may contribute to the distinctive pattern of white matter injury of the very preterm developing brain.[76,77]

Another source of vulnerability is immaturity of autoregulation of cerebral blood flow. Stress and pain from procedures in the NICU induce alterations in cerebral blood flow.[78] Suctioning and endotracheal tube repositioning, which are relatively minor and quite frequent procedures, lead to changes in systemic and cerebral hemodynamic disturbances.[78,79] Similarly, tracheal intubation (which is known to cause significant discomfort in adults) causes decreased transcutaneous oxygen tension measurements, as well as increased arterial blood pressure and intracranial pressure, in both term and preterm infants.[80] Infants born very preterm are particularly susceptible to major fluctuations in mean arterial blood pressure and thereby to disturbances in cerebral blood flow due to immature autoregulation.[81] Impaired cerebrovascular autoregulation would increase the likelihood for changes in cerebral blood flow, as evidenced by near-infrared spectroscopy (NIRS).[82] Studies using NIRS, electroencephalography (EEG), and magnetic resonance imaging (MRI) have demonstrated that infants display cortical responses to stress and procedural pain as early as 25 weeks gestation.[66,67,78,83-88]

Importantly, key differences in evoked cortical responses across development have been reported.[86] In that study, whereas term infants displayed a specific somatosensory-evoked response to an invasive procedure, the preterm infants showed widespread diffuse "delta brush" responses. The delta brush pattern is the typical response of preterm neonates to all sensory stimulation. The widespread responses suggest vulnerability to developmentally unexpected sensory stimulation, far beyond nociceptive or somatosensory processes. Conversely, supportive human touch-based interventions, such as skin-to-skin, maternal care/touch, and care bundles, can have a powerful effect not only at blunting the detrimental effects of pain but also in helping to prevent brain injury in the case of care bundles[59] and support brain maturation in infancy.[89-92]

In summary, adverse effects of early exposure to nociceptive stimulation of the developing brain do not depend on pain perception or memory. Rather, hemodynamic and excitotoxic processes instigated during stressful or painful procedures and handling of the very preterm neonate can directly alter the immature brain structures and developing networks.

PAIN AND THE DEVELOPING BRAIN

In human preterm neonates, repetitive pain (quantified as the number of invasive procedures) during NICU care is associated with altered grey and white matter maturation of cerebral microstructure as measured by diffusion tensor imaging and magnetic resonance spectroscopic imaging.[12] In a series of studies, NICU pain was associated with altered brain development in the neonatal period and at school age, after adjusting for multiple clinical risk factors of prematurity. In the neonatal brain, altered white matter maturation and volumes and metabolism in subcortical brain regions, as well as delayed corticospinal tract development were associated with greater exposure to pain/stress.[12,93] Long-term associations between repetitive exposure to neonatal procedural pain/stress and brain development persist on MRI at age 8 years, in altered cortical thickness,[19] white matter maturation,[21] cerebellar regional volumes,[18] and regional volumes in the thalamus and limbic system.[14] Moreover, the pain-related effects on brain (after accounting for clinical factors related to prematurity) were associated with poorer cognitive functions.

The thalamocortical pathway has a key role in nociceptive signaling; therefore the thalamus is a primary target of interest in understanding mechanisms of long-term effects of pain on brain dysmaturation. Greater exposure to neonatal pain (beyond clinical risk factors) in children born very preterm is associated with thalamic growth, metabolism, and microstructure in the neonatal period[13,54] and, in turn, is related to later poorer cognitive and motor outcomes. Importantly, when windows of pain exposure were examined, more procedural pain during 24 to approximately 31 weeks post-menstrual age, not later pain, accounted for poorer thalamic maturation.[13]

Cortical oscillations generated in the thalamocortical system are related to attention, memory, and cognition. These oscillations are mediated by intrinsic cellular mechanisms. Greater cumulative neonatal pain was related to spontaneous oscillatory brain activity using magnetoencephalography at school age, which was associated with cognitive function.[23,94,95] The link between neonatal pain and brain oscillatory activity was primarily in children born extremely preterm (24 to 28 weeks gestation). Moreover, sex differences were evident in extent of alterations in the resting neurophysiologic network.[96] It is well established that there are progressive changes in the maturation of oscillatory brain activity throughout the preterm period. The finding that neonatal pain was associated with brain oscillatory activity in infants born at 24 to 28 weeks, but not later, may reflect the distinct phases of development of the thalamocortical pathway occurring within this "fetal" period.[23,95]

Repeated pain exposure is only one of many neonatal factors that influence development of brain microstructure, connectivity, and processing.[42,97] Infection, hypotension, and exposure to medications such as midazolam and postnatal dexamethasone have all been implicated in adverse brain development.[98-100] While neonatal morphine is not related to major impairments,[101] associations with poorer brain function[94-96] and more symptoms of internalizing behaviors (anxiety/depressive symptoms)[15] have been reported in preterm children. Therefore, pharmacologic pain management needs to be evaluated in the context of protecting the developing brain to avoid possible unintended adverse consequences.

ALTERATION IN PROGRAMING OF THE STRESS AXIS

Stress responses reflect a range of hormonal and metabolic changes associated with physical and psychologic trauma.[102-104] This includes the release of pituitary, pancreatic, and adrenal hormones that affect metabolic balance.[102] Furthermore, fetuses of 24 to 34 weeks gestation displayed increases in cortisol and β-endorphin levels in response to intrauterine abdominal needling.[105] One key aspect of the HPA axis response is the end-product release of cortisol, which is the primary stress hormone in humans. In the NICU, cortisol variations are related to numerous clinical factors,[106,107] including procedural pain and stress.[108] In very preterm infants, greater cumulative exposure to neonatal pain-related stress has been associated with altered cortisol levels long after NICU discharge, in infancy and at school age.[20,22,24,109-111] Notably, in very preterm school-age children, greater neonatal pain exposure predicted *lower* salivary cortisol during the study visit day, which was found mainly in boys, and *lower* overall diurnal salivary cortisol (at home),[20] as well as *lower* hair cortisol (cumulative stress).[22] Altered cortisol levels may be a result of early stress-induced programming of the HPA axis.[112,113] But moreover, dampened HPA axis activity at school age may reflect adrenal fatigue in a population exposed to ongoing chronic stress.

CONSEQUENCES ON PAIN REACTIVITY

Clinical observations of differences in reactivity to later pain exposure, such as during immunization, in infants exposed to noxious and stressful experiences as neonates compared with healthy newborns has led researchers to investigate this phenomenon in clinical studies. Research findings support that neonatal exposure to noxious insults and surgical procedures during NICU stay is in fact associated with altered basal nociceptive processing in infancy.[108,114-116] Specifically, recurring pain-related stress in preterm infants has been shown to have short- and long-term effects on these children's somatosensory processing,[117-119] sensitivity to pain,[115,119,120] and response to pain.[16,121,108,114,122]

There is evidence that prematurity and NICU experience influences cortical pain processing at term age and before hospital discharge. The level of evoked potential measured, in contrast to non-noxious touch stimulation, was significantly greater in the preterm infants compared with term age-matched controls.[123] Lower thresholds to mechanical touch on "primed" heels from repeated heel lances for blood sampling during NICU stay have been described in preterm infants during the first year of life compared with term controls.[114] During the first year of life, more days in the NICU, possibly indicating greater pain and stress exposure, was associated with amplified pain expression in response to immunization in former very preterm infants.

GENETIC AND EPIGENETIC FACTORS: FUTURE DIRECTION

Basic experimental and clinical research shows that genetics influence pain sensitivity; however, this has received little attention in pediatric pain. It is now evident that innate factors, such as sex and genetic makeup, influence how nociceptive stimuli are processed and how the brain interprets these different types of pain messages (e.g., peripheral injury, inflammatory, visceral or neuropathic pain).[124] Notably, adverse life events, such as pain, stress, or disease, can alter the system at many levels (for a review see Denk et al.[125]).[41] In a series of studies, genetic factors that moderate long-term effects of early pain in children born very preterm have begun to be identified. Environmental stress, the HPA-axis, and the immune system interact and are involved in brain development and function.[126] Therefore, altered stress regulation and inflammatory factors provide yet another route whereby neonatal pain/stress may be related to long-term altered neurodevelopment in children born very preterm. Inflammatory cytokines were higher in very preterm compared to full-term children at age 7 years, but the relationship between neonatal pain/stress and cytokine levels depended on genetic vulnerability to inflammatory response and was sex-specific.[22] In very preterm boys but not girls, presence of the minor allele of nuclear factorκB inhibitor α (*NFκBIA*), an inflammatory regulator, was associated with higher secretion of inflammatory cytokines, supporting the hypothesis that neonatal pain-related stress may act as a proinflammatory stimulus that induces long-term immune cell activation.

Brain-derived neurotrophic factor (BDNF), a widely expressed neurotrophin in the brain, is essential for neuronal survival, development, and synaptic plasticity.[127] The *BDNF* genotype moderated the association between neonatal pain and cortisol (levels and reactivity) in very preterm boys, but not girls, at 7 years of age.[24] Moreover, in very premature children with the catechol-O-transferase *COMT val158 met/met* genotype, greater neonatal invasive procedures was associated with lower brain volumes in the amygdala, thalamus, and subregions in the hippocampus.[14] These smaller volumes were in turn differentially related to poorer cognitive, visual-motor, and behavioral outcomes.

It is now evident that analgesic effects of exogenous opioids are influenced by genetic factors.[128] New genes are being identified in rodents that show promise for future treatments to provide better targeted pain relief for patients.[123] In human preterm infants, genetic markers related to morphine metabolism may identify infants highly sensitive to adverse effects of morphine on behavior problems.[129] Decreased opioid-induced pain relief has been observed in preterm intubated infants with the *COMT* Val/Val alleles compared with the Val/Met or Met/Met alleles.[130]

Epigenetic phenomena (i.e., deoxyribonucleic acid [DNA] methylation and histone modifications) can change how genes are expressed and function without affecting the sequence itself. Modification of DNA by methylation is a critical epigenetic mechanism regulating gene expression, whereby increased methylation can inhibit gene expression and decreased methylation can increase it. With the rising interest in the field of pain epigenetics, linking early pain-related stress exposure and changes in gene expression provides a novel avenue to better understand mechanisms underlying interindividual differences in later developmental outcomes, as well as the susceptibility of individuals to develop certain pain conditions.[131]

Alterations in DNA methylation and in gene expression have been associated with early-life adversity and stress exposure,[132-134] changes that may be already arising long before birth.[135] DNA methylation has been suggested as a possible molecular mechanism contributing to the diversity in behavioral outcomes that follow exposure to early-life stressful events.[133,136,137] This critical epigenetic mechanism regulating gene expression offers a promising direction in understanding how exposure to adverse or stressful early-life events, such as pain, may lead to enduring changes in neuronal function.[138] In very preterm infants, an increase of methylation percentage in the *SLC6A4* promoter was observed from birth to discharge but only in very preterm infants exposed to high levels of pain-related stress during their NICU admission, compared to those with low levels.[139] Moreover, in the same cohort of very preterm infants, pain-related increase in *SLC6A4* transporter gene methylation at NICU discharge was found to be associated with higher anger response to emotional stress at 4.5 years of age.[140] In a different study, children born very preterm were found to have higher *SLC6A4* promoter methylation compared with term children, and exposure to procedural pain-related stress, after controlling for clinical confounding factors, appeared to be one of the contributing factors to the higher *SLC6A4* methylation.[17] Interestingly, early repeated procedural pain-related stress exposure was associated with altered methylation of the *SLC6A4* promoter only in children born very preterm with the *COMT* 158 Met/Met genotype.

It is through complex multisystem approaches that a better understanding may arise of how pain may differentially impact the organism depending on genetic variation, and also how the environment (e.g., early pain-stress exposure) may modulate relationships through epigenetic modifications. Importantly, it is essential that future studies incorporate sex into the design. Basic research has established the importance of sex differences in effects of early pain, and a handful of clinical cohort studies have identified differential sex effects in the impact of early pain exposure. However, the role of sex on specific systems, potentially varying in developmental windows of pain exposure, remains largely unknown.

CONCLUSION

Although efforts to minimize exposure to pain in the NICU have been advocated over the last 20 years, infants in this setting are still exposed to high levels of pain-related stress during a particularly vulnerable period of brain development. This is especially important when it comes to those born very preterm. Current evidence indicates that neonatal pain and possibly some pain treatment strategies have short- and long-term effects, including on brain development and neurodevelopmental outcomes in children born very preterm, after accounting for clinical confounders associated with prematurity. Specific effects of procedural pain on brain structure and function, behavioral outcomes, as well as stress hormone regulation of fragile preterm infants have been demonstrated in longitudinal cohort studies. Additionally, noxious-specific brain activity has previously been identified in EEG recordings of newborn infants older than 35 weeks gestation in response to a medically required invasive procedure. Although fMRI has been widely used in adults to understand pain-evoked brain activity, it remains challenging to use and interpret in infants but is an emerging research area. Finally, recent investigations focusing on the gene by environment interactions highlight the complexity that interplays when examining how exposure to early-life pain may impact the developing infant. New insight is emerging on possible avenues of research to discover brain-protective treatments to improve the care of the most fragile infants, leading to improved cognitive, behavioral, and mental health outcomes.

ACKNOWLEDGMENTS

Ruth Grunau's research is supported by the Canadian Institute of Health Research (CIHR) and a Senior Scientist salary award from the BC Children's Hospital Research Institute. Simon Beggs' research is supported by the Medical Research Council (MRC, UK) and National Institute of Academic Anaesthesia (NIAA).

A complete reference list is available at www.ExpertConsult.com. 

SELECT REFERENCES

1. Fitzgerald M. The development of nociceptive circuits. *Nat Rev Neurosci*. 2005;6:507-520.
2. Brewer CL, Baccei ML. The development of pain circuits and unique effects of neonatal injury. *J Neural Transm*. 2020;127:467-479.
3. Beggs S, Torsney C, Drew LJ, Fitzgerald M. The postnatal reorganization of primary afferent input and dorsal horn cell receptive fields in the rat spinal cord is an activity-dependent process. *Eur J Neurosci*. 2002;16:1249-1258.
4. Beggs S, Currie G, Salter MW, et al. Priming of adult pain responses by neonatal pain experience: maintenance by central neuroimmune activity. *Brain*. 2012;135:404-417.
8. Duhrsen L, Simons SHP, Dzietko M, et al. Effects of repetitive exposure to pain and morphine treatment on the neonatal rat brain. *Neonatology*. 2013;103.
10. Ranger M, Grunau RE. Early repetitive pain in preterm infants in relation to the developing brain. *Pain Manag*. 2014;4(1):57-67.
12. Brummelte S, Grunau RE, Chau V, et al. Procedural pain and brain development in premature newborns. *Ann Neurol*. 2012;71(3):385-396.
13. Duerden EG, Grunau RE, Guo T, et al. Early procedural pain is associated with regionally-specific alterations in thalamic development in preterm neonates. *J Neurosci*. 2018;38(4):878-886.
14. Chau CM, Ranger M, Bichin M, et al. Hippocampus, amygdala, and thalamus volumes in very preterm children at 8 years: neonatal pain and genetic variation. *Front Behav Neurosci*. 2019;13:51.
17. Chau CM, Ranger M, Sulistyoningrum D, et al. Neonatal pain and COMT Val158Met genotype in relation to serotonin transporter (SLC6A4) promoter methylation in very preterm children at school age. *Front Behav Neurosci*. 2014;8:409.
18. Ranger M, Zwicker JG, Chau CMY, et al. Neonatal pain and infection relate to smaller cerebellum in very preterm children at school age. *J Pediatrics*. 2015;167(2). 292-298.e1.

19. Ranger M, Chau CMY, Garg A, et al. Neonatal pain-related stress predicts cortical thickness at age 7 years in children born very preterm. *Plos One*. 2013;8(10):e76702.
20. Brummelte S, Chau CM, Cepeda IL, et al. Cortisol levels in former preterm children at school age are predicted by neonatal procedural pain-related stress. *Psychoneuroendocrinology*. 2015;51:151-163.
21. Vinall J, Miller SP, Bjornson BH, et al. Invasive procedures in preterm children: brain and cognitive development at school age. *Pediatrics*. 2014;133(3):412-421.
22. Grunau RE, Cepeda IL, Chau CM, et al. Neonatal pain-related stress and NFKBIA genotype are associated with altered cortisol levels in preterm boys at school age. *PloS One*. 2013;8(9):e73926.
23. Doesburg SM, Chau CM, Cheung TP, et al. Neonatal pain-related stress, functional cortical activity and visual-perceptual abilities in school-age children born at extremely low gestational age. *Pain*. 2013;154(10):1946-1952.
24. Chau CMY, Cepeda IL, Devlin AM, et al. The Val66Met brain-derived neurotrophic factor gene variant interacts with early pain exposure to predict cortisol dysregulation in 7-year-old children born very preterm: implications for cognition. *Neuroscience*. 2015;342(7):188-199.
30. Fitzgerald M, Walker SM. Infant pain management: a developmental neurobiological approach. *Nat Clin Pract Neurol*. 2009;5:35-50.
40. Schwaller F, Fitzgerald M. The consequences of pain in early life: injury-induced plasticity in developing pain pathways. *Eur J Neurosci*. 2014;39:344-352.
42. Walker SM. Long-term effects of neonatal pain. *Semin Fetal Neonatal Med*. 2019;24:1-6.
43. Salter MW, Stevens B. Microglia emerge as central players in brain disease. *Nat Med*. 2017;23:1018-1027.
44. Hammond TR, Robinton D, Stevens B. Microglia and the brain: complementary partners in development and disease. *Ann Rev Cell Dev Biol*. 2018;6(34):523-544.
45. Beggs S, Trang T, Salter MW. P2X4R+ microglia drive neuropathic pain. *Nat Neurosci*. 2012;15:1068-1073.
51. Mapplebeck JCS, Beggs S, Salter MW. Sex differences in pain: a tale of two immune cells. *Pain*. 2016;157(suppl 1):S2-S6.
55. Schneider J, Duerden EG, Guo T, et al. Procedural pain and oral glucose in neonates: brain development and sex-specific effects. *Pain*. 2018;159(3):515-525.
56. Walker SM, et al. Somatosensory function and pain in extremely preterm young adults from the UK EPICure cohort: sex-dependent differences and impact of neonatal surgery. *Br J Anaesth*. 2018;121:623-635.
69. Volpe JJ. Brain injury in premature infants: a complex amalgam of destructive and developmental disturbances. *Lancet Neurol*. 2009;8:110-124.
70. Anand KJ, Coskun V, Thrivikraman KV, et al. Long-term behavioral effects of repetitive pain in neonatal rat pups. *Physiol Behav*. 1999;66:627-637.
78. Limperopoulos C, Gauvreau KK, O'Leary H, et al. Cerebral hemodynamic changes during intensive care of preterm infants. *Pediatrics*. 2008;122:e1006-e1013.
83. Slater R, Cantarella A, Gallella S, et al. Cortical pain responses in human infants. *J Neurosci*. 2006;26:3662-3666.
84. Verriotis M, Chang P, Fitzgerald M, Fabrizi L. Review - The development of the nociceptive brain. *Neuroscience*. 2016;338:207-219.
86. Fabrizi L, Slater R, Worley A, et al. A shift in sensory processing that enables the developing human brain to discriminate touch from pain. *Curr Biol*. 2011;21:1552-1558.
87. Verriotis M, Jones L, Whitehead K, et al. The distribution of pain across the human neonatal brain is sex dependent. *NeuroImage*. 2018;178:60-77.
88. Goksan S, Hartley C, Emery F, et al. fMRI reveals neural activity overlap between adult and infant pain. *eLife*. 2015;4:e06356.
93. Zwicker JG, Grunau RE, Adams E, et al. Score for neonatal acute physiology-II and neonatal pain predict corticospinal tract development in premature newborns. *Pediatr Neurol*. 2013;48. 123-129.e1.
96. Kozhemiako N, Nunes AS, Vakorin VA, et al. Sex differences in brain connectivity and male vulnerability in very preterm children. *Hum Brain Mapp*. 2019;41:388-400.
101. McPherson C, Grunau RE. Neonatal pain control and neurologic effects of anesthetics and sedatives in preterm infants. *Clin Perinatol*. 2014;41:209-227.
108. Grunau RE, Holsti L, Haley DW, et al. Neonatal procedural pain exposure predicts lower cortisol and behavioral reactivity in preterm infants in the NICU. *Pain*. 2005;113:293-300.
110. Grunau RE, Haley DW, Whitfield MF, et al. Altered basal cortisol levels at 3, 6, 8 and 18 months in infants born at extremely low gestational age. *J Pediatr*. 2007;150:151-156.
111. Brummelte S, Grunau RE, Zaidman-Zait A, et al. Cortisol levels in relation to maternal interaction and child internalizing behavior in preterm and full-term children at 18 months corrected age. *Dev Psychobiol*. 2011;53:184-195.
114. Allegaert K, Devlieger H, Bulckaert D, et al. Variability in pain expression characteristics in former preterm infants. *J Perinat Med*. 2005;33:442-448.
118. Walker SM, Franck LS, Fitzgerald M, et al. Long-term impact of neonatal intensive care and surgery on somatosensory perception in children born extremely preterm. *Pain*. 2009;141:79-87.
119. Hermann C, Hohmeister J, Demirakca S, et al. Long-term alteration of pain sensitivity in school-aged children with early pain experiences. *Pain*. 2006;125:278-285.
121. Walker SM, O'Reilly H, Beckmann J, et al. Conditioned pain modulation identifies altered sensitivity in extremely preterm young adult males and females. *Br J Anaesth*. 2018;121(3):636-646.
123. Slater R, Fabrizi L, Worley A, et al. Premature infants display increased noxious-evoked neuronal activity in the brain compared to healthy age-matched term-born infants. *Neuroimage*. 2010;52:583-589.
126. Zouikr I, Bartholomeusz M, Hodgson D. Early life programming of pain: focus on neuroimmune to endocrine communication. *J Transl Med*. 2016;14(1):123.
129. Chau MYC, Ross CJD, Chau V, et al. Morphine biotransformation genes and neonatal clinical factors predicted behaviour problems in very preterm children at 18 months. *EBioMedicine*. 2019;40:655-662.
139. Provenzi L, Fumagalli M, Sirgiovanni I, et al. Pain-related stress during the neonatal intensive care unit stay and *SLC6A4* methylation in very preterm infants. *Front Behav Neurosci*. 2015;9:99.
140. Provenzi L, Fumagalli M, Scotto di Minico G, et al. Pain–related increase in serotonin transporter gene methylation associates with emotional regulation in 4.5–year–old preterm–born children. *Acta Paediatrica*. 2020;109:1166-1174.

Cerebellar Development—The Impact of Preterm Birth and Comorbidities 129

Emily W.Y. Tam | Manon J.N.L. Benders | Vivi M. Heine

INTRODUCTION

It is well known that preterm birth is associated with increased risks of brain injury and impaired brain development resulting in impairments in motor, cognitive, and behavioral function. However, the focus has traditionally been on brain injury patterns in the cerebrum, such as intraventricular hemorrhage (IVH) and periventricular leukomalacia (PVL). In recent years, it has become evident that the cerebellum is another major target for injury and developmental impairment associated with prematurity. Such primary injuries can include cerebellar hemorrhage or ischemia, with long-term outcomes dependent on the size and location of the lesions. Secondary impairments in cerebellar development are more prevalent and may be associated with a number of clinical risk factors in the early postnatal period (Table 129.1). Thus, to comprehensively understand brain injury after preterm birth and optimize long-term outcomes, it is important to not only consider supratentorial brain injury, such as IVH and PVL, but also injury to the infratentorial cerebellar structure.

NORMAL FETAL AND NEONATAL CEREBELLAR DEVELOPMENT

CEREBELLAR ORGANIZATION

The human cerebellum is formed by the anterior, posterior, and the flocculonodular lobes and shows a surface with fine parallel folia/gyri along the sagittal axis. Functional structures of the cerebellum structures include (1) the medial section, the spinocerebellum with the vermis; (2) the lateral sections, the cerebrocerebellum; and (3) the most posterior section, the vestibulocerebellum (flocculonodular lobe). The spinocerebellum is involved in direction and rate of intended movements, the cerebrocerebellum plans and modifies motor output to muscles, and the vestibulocerebellum regulates balance, posture, and eye movements. Although the cerebellum is traditionally thought to coordinate movements, it is now generally accepted to also play a role in higher-order functions like cognition[1]; however, the specific cerebellar structures involved are unclear.[2,3]

Anatomically, the cerebellum consists of the cortex, white matter, deep cerebellar nuclei, and the fourth ventricle. The cortex represents most of the volume and can be divided in the most medial granule layer, the intermediate Purkinje layer, and the outer molecular layer (Fig. 129.1). The granule layer is packed with granule (the most abundant neuronal cell type in the brain), Golgi, Lugaro, and unipolar brush cells. The Purkinje layer is a thin layer of Purkinje cells and Bergmann glia cells. The molecular layer contains the dendritic trees of the Purkinje cells, as well as the stellate and basket interneurons. The Purkinje and granule cells are the two major neuronal cell types in the cerebellar circuit. Underneath the cortex lies the cerebellar white matter, which also contains gray matter deep nuclei structures. The cerebrospinal fluid–filled fourth ventricle is located between the brain stem and cerebellum.

The cerebellum receives information from the motor cortex, the proprioceptors, vestibular organs, and other brain stem nuclei. Information enters the cerebellum via the mossy fibers, which project onto the granule cells and the deep cerebellar nuclei, or via the climbing fibers, which project onto the Purkinje cells (see Fig. 129.1). All climbing fibers originate from the inferior olivary nucleus, and the mossy fibers originate from multiple sources. Before entering the cerebellar cortex, climbing fibers also give off collaterals to the deep nuclei. Next to the input from one climbing fiber, the Purkinje cells receive input from numerous granule cells via the parallel fibers onto their distal dendrites. The Purkinje cells in turn innervate other parts of the cerebellar cortex, including other Purkinje, Golgi, Lugaro, and basket cells, and project onto the deep cerebellar nuclei. Four deep nuclei reside in the cerebellar white matter and are from lateral to medial: dentate, emboliform, globose, and fastigii. The dentate nucleus belongs to and communicates only with the lateral cerebrocerebellum. The other three deep nuclei belong to the spinocerebellum and communicate with different regions of the cerebellum and cerebrum. The deep nuclei integrate the inhibitory (gamma-aminobutyric acid [GABA]-ergic) input from the Purkinje cells and the excitatory input (glutamatergic) from the mossy and climbing fibers. Next to the vestibular nuclei, the deep cerebellar nuclei give the sole output of the cerebellum.

Table 129.1 Classification of Preterm Cerebellar Pathologies.

Classification	Mechanism
Preterm cerebellar injury	Large cerebellar hemorrhage (>4 mm diameter) Small cerebellar hemorrhage (<4 mm diameter) Cerebellar infarct
Cerebellar hypoplasia of prematurity (CHOP)	Cerebral injury (e.g., periventricular hemorrhagic infarction, periventricular leukomalacia) Intraventricular hemorrhage Postnatal glucocorticoid exposure Postnatal opioid exposure and pain Cardiorespiratory instability Nutrition and growth Socioeconomic factors

EARLY CEREBELLAR DEVELOPMENT

Development of the human cerebellum starts during early embryonic development and continues into postnatal life.[4,5] Using magnetic resonance imaging (MRI), the gross anatomic changes of the cerebellum during development have been monitored. The cerebellar primordium is formed at the border of the mid- and hindbrain and can be identified as thickenings on the lateral sites of the alar plate facing the fourth ventricle, as early as gestational week 6. Around gestational weeks 8 and 9, the vermis starts to fuse, and after gestational week 12, the vermis and cerebellar hemispheres begin to grow rapidly. The formation of the white matter of the cerebellum becomes apparent between gestational weeks 32 and 37.[6] Growth of the cerebellum, however, peaks

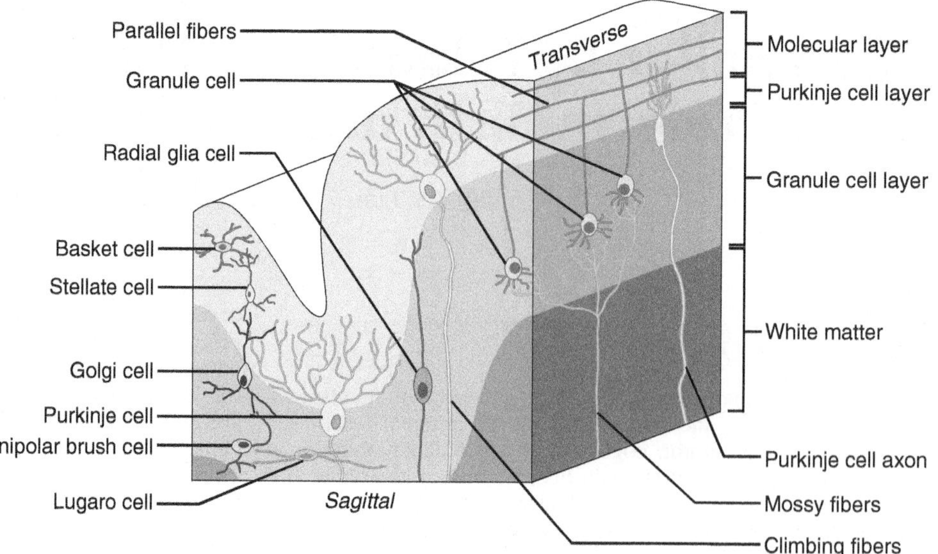

Fig. 129.1 Transverse and sagittal planes of the mammalian cerebellar cortex organization. (From Schulman JA, Bloom FE. Golgi cells of the cerebellum are inhibited by inferior olive activity. *Brain Res.* 1981;210:350–355.)

after birth,[7] which most likely can be explained by the growth of the cerebellar cortex. Growth of the cerebellum continues until at least 2 years postnatally in humans.[8]

Anatomic and histologic studies in humans and fate-map studies in mouse models have yielded insight into the development of the cerebellar primordium. Two germinative neuroepithelia—the ventricular zone and the rhombic lip, which become anatomically apparent around gestational day 57[9]—generate the different cerebellar cell types.[10-14]

The ventricular zone lies adjacent to the fourth ventricle and gives rise to cells of the deep cerebellar nuclei around gestational week 8[15] and to Purkinje cells during the fourth fetal month.[16] At later stages, the ventricular zone produces Golgi cells that will reside in the granule layer and basket and stellate interneurons that will locate to the molecular layer.[10]

Of these cell types, the development of the Purkinje cells is best understood. The Purkinje cells migrate along the fibers of the radial glial cells, past the deep nuclei. They create a scaffold for the granule cells to form the final layer of granule cells, the internal granule cell layer (IGL). Between gestational weeks 12 and 20, the Purkinje precursor cell population drastically reduces in number.[17] This coincides with the radial migration of granule cell precursors and with the formation of a single layer of Purkinje cells. During late gestational stages and early neonatal life, the Purkinje cells create their final characteristic morphology, a flattened dendritic tree in a perpendicular plane to the folia. Shortly after reaching their maturity, the Purkinje cells receive a layer of myelin around their axons.

The rhombic lip gives rise to the granule cells, the pontine nuclei, the inferior olive, and the unipolar brush cells.[5,10,18] The cerebellar granule cell precursors (CGNPs) are generated in the upper rhombic lip. The proliferating CGNPs migrate in the outer region of the cerebellum, creating the external granule cell layer (EGL),[5,19] which can be identified around gestational day 51.[9] Once the EGL is formed, CGNPs migrate radially along Bergmann glia past the Purkinje layer into the cerebellar primordium to form the IGL.[13] The CGNPs in the superficial EGL are small and round, whereas CGNPs in the deeper layers show radially oriented bipolar cells ready to migrate. The IGL starts to shape around gestational week 15 and shows a clear layer by gestational week 30, but it continues to form in early postnatal life.[20]

GENETIC REGULATION

Genetic studies in the fruit fly, *Drosophila,* as well as chick, mouse, and human embryos, have informed our knowledge base of the regulatory genes involved in the development of the cerebellum. Although human development shows differences, many mechanisms are highly conserved between species. The specification of the mesencephalic and metencephalic structures, giving rise to the cerebellum, is regulated by their boundary, the isthmus organizer (IO).[21,22] The formation of the IO, as well as early cerebellar structures, is under the influence of fibroblast growth factors (FGFs), Wnt and bone morphogenic proteins (BMPs),[11,23] and transcription factors, including Engrailed1/2 (En), PAX2/5/8, OTX2, and GBX2 (Fig. 129.2). Loss-of-function mutations in the genes encoding these signaling pathways and transcription factors result in abnormal cerebellar development.[24,25] Wnt1 and FGF8 are critical early regulators of IO formation. Wnt1, expressed anterior of the IO, is a secreted glycoprotein and plays an important role in patterning of the mesencephalon and the most posterior rhombomere, r1.[26] FGF8, expressed posterior of the IO, patterns the hindbrain by limiting *Hox* gene expression.[27] R1, the only hindbrain segment structure that does not express Hox, gives rise to the cerebellum, and inactivation of FGF8 leads to the disappearance of the cerebellum.[28] Hence FGF8 is a key regulator in the inductive activity of the IO. Next to Wnt1 and FGF8, many other factors are involved in the development of the cerebellum.[29] GBX2 and OTX2 are expressed very early in the central nervous system (CNS) and play a role in the positioning of the IO (see Fig. 129.2).[30] PAX2 is necessary for regulating FGF8 expression.[31] Additionally, the *En* genes are involved in maintenance of Wnt1 and FGF8 expression and have important functions in patterning of mid- and hindbrain regions.[32,33] Transcriptional regulation of these and other genes involved in the human IO needs to be confirmed, in which recent human stem cell technologies show great prospects.[34]

The ventricular zone gives rise to its GABAergic derivatives in different waves. However, knowledge about genetic control of the generation of the different cerebellar cell types from the ventricular zone is limited. In mice, basic helix-loop-helix (bHLH) transcription factor, Ptf1a, is expressed during early embryonic stages and contributes to all GABAergic neurons in the cerebellum.[35] However, when downstream target of Ptf1a, Neph3, is expressed in combination with E-cadherin, it specifically locates the Purkinje cells progenitors in the ventricular zone.[36] Regional expression of proneural genes *Ngn1, Ngn2,* and *Mash1* in the ventricular zone and the early stage cerebellar nuclei indicates selective involvement in the generation of the different GABAergic derivatives.[37] PAX2 expression is specifically involved in the generation of GABAergic interneurons. PAX2-positive progenitors first give rise to the interneurons in the deep nuclei, then to the Golgi and Lugaro cells in the granule cell layer, and finally, to the basket and stellate interneurons in the molecular layer.[38] More research is necessary to understand how the generation of the different cerebellar cell types in the ventricular zone is genetically regulated.

Under the influence of signals of the IO, the rhombic lip arises and expands.[5,39] *Math1* (i.e., *ATOH1*), expressed in the germinal epithelium, is involved in the proper formation of the rhombic lip and in the generation of the CGNPs from this germinal layer.[40,41] *Math1* mutations lead to disappearance of several cell types generated by the rhombic lip.[15] When the proliferating CGNPs

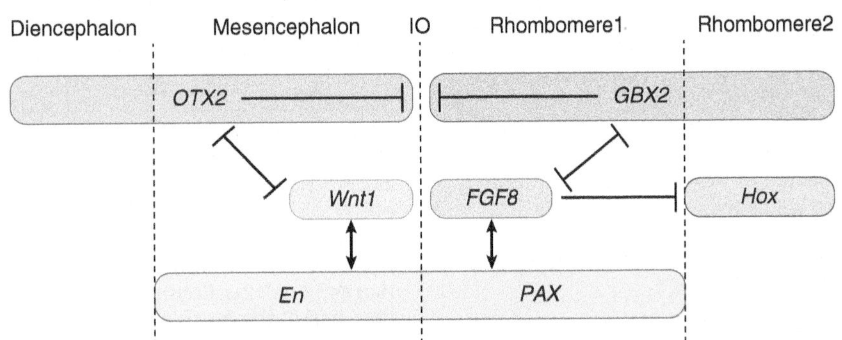

Fig. 129.2 Gene expression pattern domain during early specification of the mesencephalic and metencephalic structures giving rise to the cerebellum. (From Wurst W, Bally-Cuif L. Neural plate patterning: upstream and downstream of the isthmic organizer. *Nat Rev Neurosci.* 2001;2:99–108.)

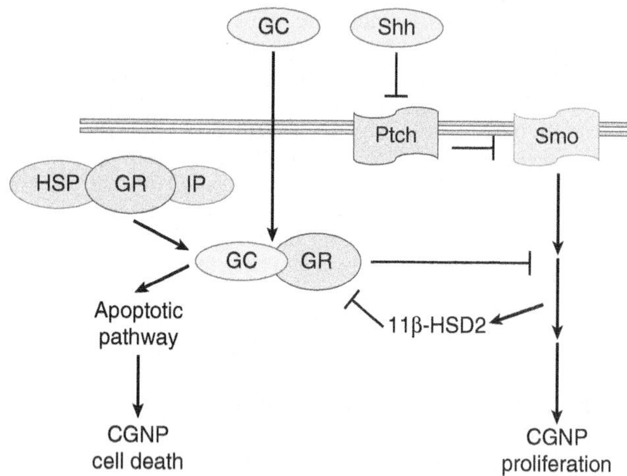

Fig. 129.3 Model for cross-antagonistic interactions of Sonic hedgehog signaling and acute/chronic glucocorticoid signaling in developing cerebellar granule cell precursors. Sonic hedgehog *(Shh)*-Smoothened *(Smo)* activation in proliferating cerebellar granule cell precursors *(CGNPs)* promotes cell cycle progression and induces 11β-hydroxysteroid dehydrogenases type 2 *(11β-HSD2)* expression through regulation of its downstream activators. *GC*, Glucocorticoid; *GR*, glucocorticoid receptor; *HSP*, heat shock protein; *IP*, immunophilin; *Ptch*, Patched. (From Heine VM, Rowitch DH. Hedgehog signaling has a protective effect in glucocorticoid-induced mouse neonatal brain injury through an 11betaHSD2-dependent mechanism. *J Clin Invest.* 2009;119:267–277.)

populate the EGL, they begin to express zinc finger proliferation 1 and 3 (Zic1 and Zic3).[19,40,42] Defects in *Zic1* and *Zic3* lead to neural tube defects and aberrant generation of CGNPs.[42,43] When CGNPs are ready to migrate to form the EGL, they start to express mature markers, like tubulin-associated glycoprotein 1 (Tag1), and become dependent on Sonic hedgehog (Shh). Shh is the most important mitogenic factor for CGNPs. Shh binds the transmembrane receptor Patched (Ptch), which relieves the inhibition on transmembrane protein G-coupled receptor Smoothened (Smo; Fig. 129.3).[44] Then Smo is free to accumulate in the cilia[45] and to activate the expression of the downstream transcription factors, including N-Myc and G1 cyclins Gli1, Gli2, and Gli3, which results in a proliferative response of the CGNPs.[46-50] Before Shh is active, it needs to be modified by cholesterol. Patients with Smith-Lemli-Opitz syndrome, who have a reduced cholesterol metabolism, show a hypoplasmic cerebellum.[51] In contrast, gain-of-function mutations in the Shh pathway (SAG) (e.g., loss of Ptch) are associated with sporadic medulloblastoma[52] and familial basal cell nevus (also known as *Gorlin*) syndrome.[53] Mouse studies have shown that Shh is secreted by the Purkinje cells. In humans, however, there is an early stage of Shh signaling, before the Purkinje cells start to secrete Shh.[54] Bergmann glia also show expression of Ptch and Gli1 and are affected by Shh signaling.[46,55] Although it is unclear how Shh signaling regulates Bergmann glia differentiation, their fibers are malformed when Gli2 is mutated.[56] Overall, Shh has an important function in cerebellar development and growth. As such, it has become a focus of studies that seek to understand the molecular mechanisms affected by developmental injuries to the cerebellum in human preterm neonates.

PRETERM CEREBELLAR INJURY

CEREBELLAR HEMORRHAGE

Cerebellar injury, such as cerebellar hemorrhage, ischemia/infarction, and secondary cerebellar hypoplasia, are now commonly diagnosed in preterm infants[57,58] because of improved posterior fossa neuroimaging, including both cranial ultrasound (CUS) and MRI. Preterm infants have a high risk of developing cerebellar hemorrhage, resulting from damage to the vulnerable germinal matrix present in the fourth ventricle and the external granular layer covering the surface of the cerebellum. This is a highly vascularized region of the brain, with immature vascular walls prone to hemorrhage.[59]

The ventral surface of the posterior lobe of the cerebellum is often involved, together with the deep cerebellar cortex or related cerebellar white matter. Postmortem analysis shows that cerebellar hemorrhage is often multifocal, bilateral, and variable in size in various ages of preterm infants,[60] although this observation is based on a biased population of the most severely ill babies. Pathology in the deep cerebellar nuclei, such as dentate nuclei, as well as the inferior olivary, often occurs in association with cerebellar hemorrhage. Cerebellar hemorrhage in surviving preterm infants is usually unilateral and is often associated with supratentorial lesions, primarily IVH,[59] suggesting they might share common pathogenetic mechanisms. Such hemorrhages are sometimes followed by cerebellar atrophy. In large cerebellar hemorrhages, a reduction in contralateral cerebral volume has been found, which might be because of impaired remote trans-synaptic trophic effects.[61]

Cerebellar hemorrhage can be divided into different patterns, varying from a focal form, which is a milder form with small multiple punctate lesions or a larger hemorrhagic lesion in one cerebellar hemisphere, to a most severe form, which comprises large bilateral cerebellar hemorrhages (Fig. 129.4). One study described six types of cerebellar hemorrhages using CUS and speculated on underlying pathogenetic mechanisms: (1) subarachnoid, due to extension of subarachnoid hemorrhage into the cerebellum; (2) small folial hemorrhages; (3) large lobar hemorrhages due to bleeding of the germinal matrix; (4) bilateral lobar involvement; (5) giant lobar hemorrhage involving the vermis, originating from bleeding of the subependymal germinal matrix or dissection of blood from the fourth ventricle into the vermis; and (6) contusional hemorrhage mainly related to birth trauma and occipital osteodiastasis.[62] The vermis is involved in almost one third of patients.[63] Large cerebellar hemorrhages or subarachnoid blood in the cisterna magna or underneath the tentorium may compress the fourth ventricle. This may cause ventricular dilatation by cerebral spinal fluid circulation disturbances (Fig. 129.5).[62]

IMAGING OF CEREBELLAR HEMORRHAGE

The increased use of MRI has improved the detection of lesions in the cerebellum. Focal cerebellar injury can be detected by CUS only when lesions are large enough (>4 mm), with better results obtained in the mastoid fontanel. Smaller lesions can be diagnosed only by MRI.[64]

Using CUS via the anterior fontanel, it is rather difficult to visualize the posterior fossa because of the highly echogenic tentorium and the cerebellar vermis.[65] High-frequency transducers with superficial focal zones of penetration make it even more difficult.[66] This may have played a role in missing cerebellar pathology. Advances in CUS and serial scanning via the posterior and mastoid fontanel as an acoustic window identify these lesions better (Fig. 129.6A). When the mastoid fontanel is used as additional acoustic window, the transducer is closer to the posterior fossa structures, providing better detection of cerebellar injury (see Fig. 129.6B).[66,67] Steggerda and colleagues[68] found almost 10% posterior fossa hemorrhage in their preterm population (<32 weeks). Routine anterior fontanel view detected fewer than half of these cases.[68]

An advantage of ultrasound is that it is particularly sensitive to hemorrhage. Furthermore, MRI tends to be undertaken later due to the logistics of transporting unstable infants to the scanner, despite this being the highest-risk group. It is important

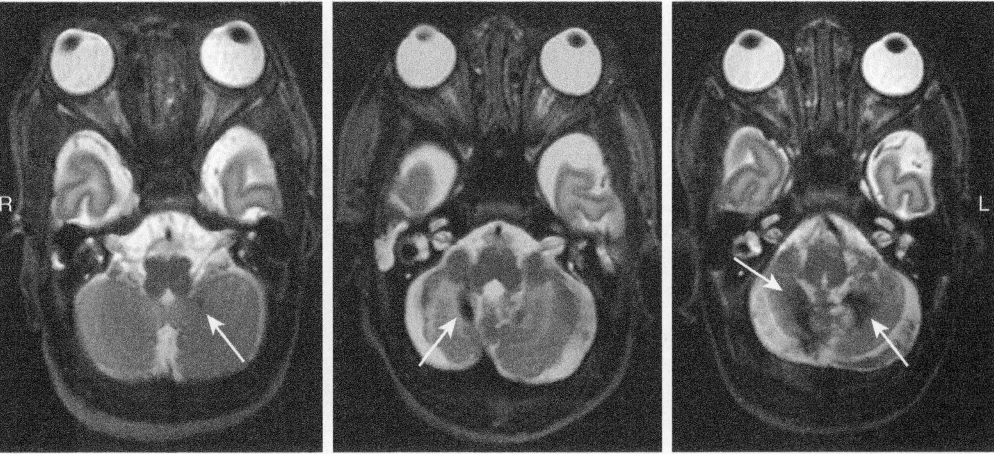

Fig. 129.4 Cerebellar hemorrhages. Cerebellar hemorrhage can be divided into different patterns: focal, small multiple punctate lesions, larger hemorrhagic lesion in one cerebellar hemisphere, or large bilateral cerebellar hemorrhages. *White arrows* indicate the cerebellar lesions. (From Van Kooij BJ, Benders MJ, Anbeek P, et al. Cerebellar volume and proton magnetic resonance spectroscopy at term, and neurodevelopment at 2 years of age in preterm infants. *Dev Med Child Neurol.* 2012;54:260–266.)

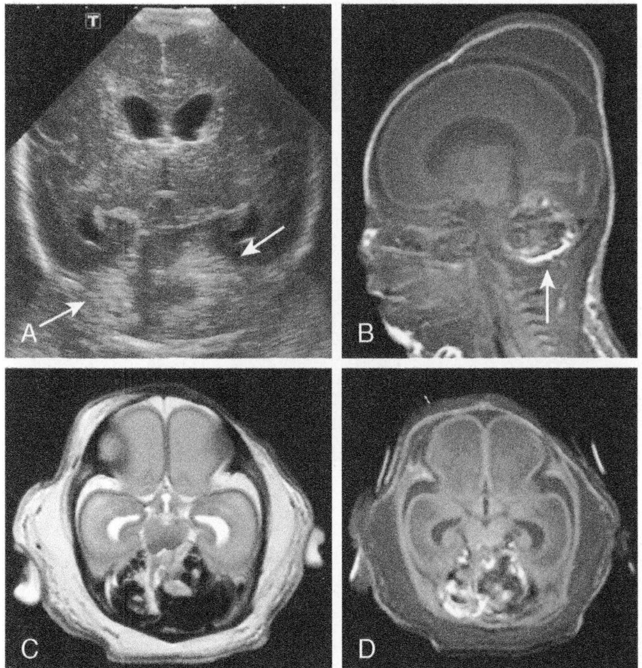

Fig. 129.5 Ventricular dilatation in combination with cerebellar hemorrhage. Baby girl, 24 weeks. Cranial ultrasound: a large bilateral cerebellar hemorrhage *(arrows)*: (A) Magnetic resonance imaging a few days later confirmed cerebellar hemorrhage *(arrow)*; illustrated on a sagittal T1 (B), axial T2 (C), and axial T1 (D) images. The cerebellar structure has been completely destroyed by the hemorrhages. Ventricular dilatation was probably caused by obstruction of the cerebral spinal fluid circulation around the level of the fourth ventricle and aqueduct because minimal amount of intraventricular blood was visible.

to perform the CUS, including via the mastoid fontanel, in particular to evaluate the cerebellum, because this might aid in guiding parental counseling. Several studies showed the higher rate of cerebellar hemorrhage when using the acoustic mastoid window.[63,67-69] Thus, considering its relatively high prevalence, systematic serial ultrasound screening via anterior and mastoid fontanel should be part of every CUS in extremely preterm babies, especially those with other supratentorial pathology. Serial scanning is especially important to evaluate changes (see Fig. 129.6B).

MRI demonstrates the size and extent of hemorrhages more precisely,[70] especially in the posterior fossa. MRI confirms CUS findings in all cases. However, in studies MRI showed punctate hemorrhage of 1 to 3 mm in diameter in the cerebellum in 20% of the cases, which were not detected on CUS.[64,68] Because these punctate lesions are small (1 to 3 mm), the slice thickness of the MRI needs to be taken into account to evaluate the accuracy of the MRI. Susceptibility-weighted imaging (SWI) seems to increase the sensitivity in identifying hemorrhagic foci in the brain, especially in the cerebellum (Fig. 129.7).[71]

Considering that preterm infants with cerebellar hemorrhage have fivefold increased odds for neurologic deficits, MRI is essential to screen for cerebellar hemorrhages in this patient population.[72] Additionally, with serial CUS it is still possible to miss the diagnosis of even severe cerebellar hemorrhages, especially because the approach via the mastoid might be complicated with the use of continuous positive airway pressure (CPAP) caps. A vanishing cerebellum may be seen at term-equivalent age, which is better to know beforehand to guide in deciding which infants need close follow-up and may in the future help in selecting those infants for neuroprotective interventions.

INCIDENCE OF CEREBELLAR HEMORRHAGE

Cerebellar hemorrhage is now commonly reported, perhaps from increased survival of preterm infants with younger gestational age[57,58] and improved resolution in neuroimaging with coverage of the posterior fossa. The incidence is different depending on the gestational age of the preterm baby of the investigated cohort, mode of assessment, and type of study (retrospective or prospective). Thus, estimating the incidence is difficult, and cerebellar hemorrhage might be underdiagnosed without the use of MRI.

The reported incidence with CUS ranges from 2% to 9% depending on gestational age or birth weight (Table 129.2). Nearly 60% of hemorrhages occurred in infants weighing less than 750 g at birth, with a significant positive trend over time: 2% to 19% in a 5-year period,[63] perhaps because of improved neuroimaging techniques. The highest incidence was 19% in infants examined with both CUS and MRI.[68] Another difficulty in incidence estimation is selection bias. In the Wilhelmina Children's Hospital's population, the incidence was almost 18% on term-equivalent MRI in a population of 210 preterm infants with a gestational age younger than 28 weeks, without selection of patients, between 2008 and 2012. These numbers have general implications because in this study routine MRI was performed in

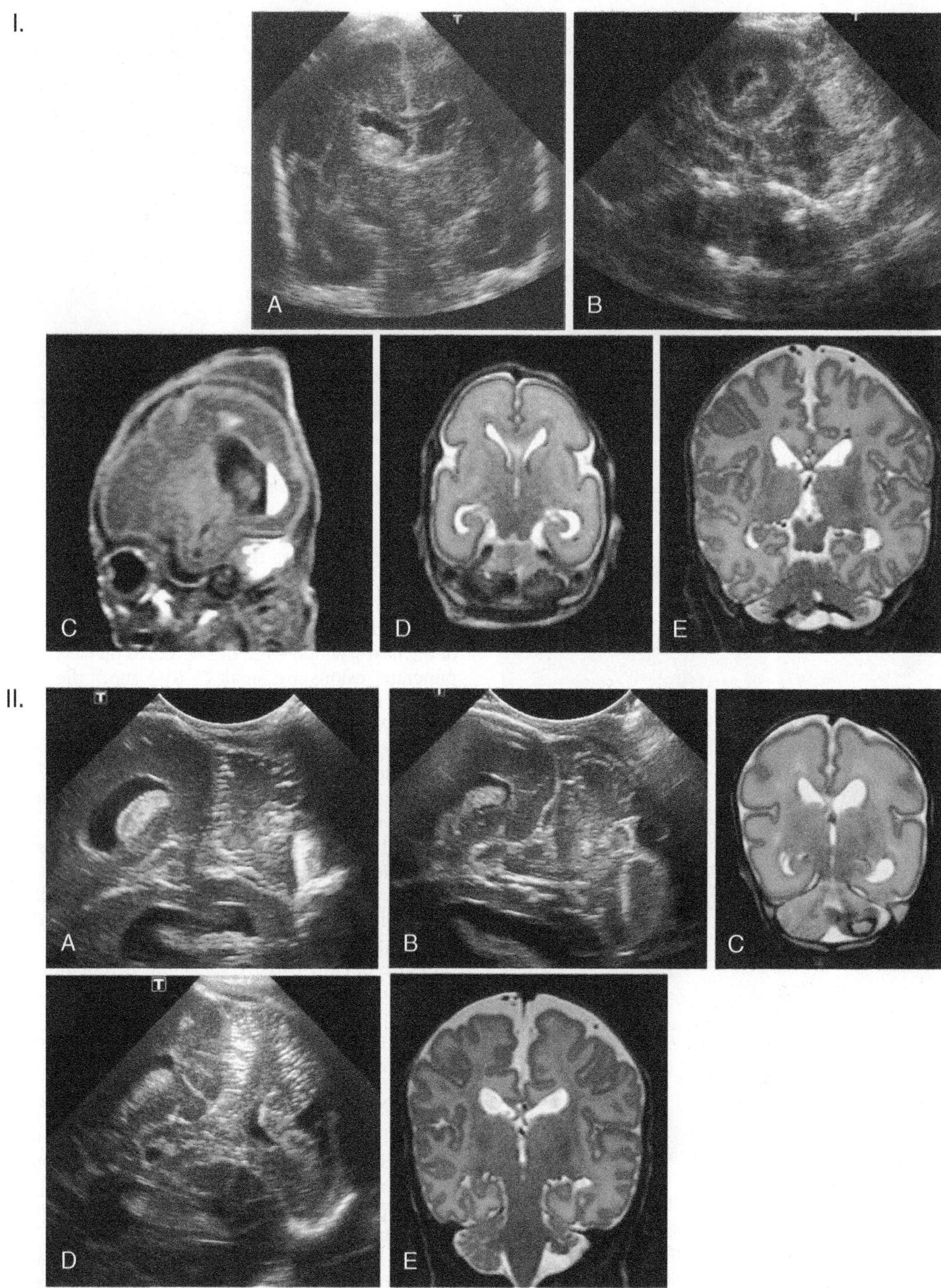

Fig. 129.6 (I) Large cerebellar hemorrhage on ultrasound. The large cerebellar hemorrhage is difficult to recognize on coronal view (A); however, there is a high suspicion for a large cerebellar hemorrhage on mastoid view (B). This was confirmed on sagittal magnetic resonance imaging (MRI) (C) and axial T2-weighted imaging (D) at 30 weeks corrected age. The MRI at term-equivalent age shows resorption hemorrhage and bilateral volume loss (E). (II) Serial scanning via the mastoid view detecting cerebellar hemorrhage. Via the mastoid fontanel, cerebellar hemorrhage is clearly visible (A). After 10 days, change in signal intensity due to resorption of blood (B). Hemorrhage is confirmed on early preterm MRI (C). At term-equivalent age, mastoid view shows atrophy of the affected cerebellar hemisphere (D), confirmed on MRI (E).

all surviving preterm infants younger than 28 weeks as standard clinical care (unpublished data). However, the incidence in non-surviving preterm infants was not taken into account, for whom autopsy studies found an incidence of 10% to 25%.[60,73] In a retrospective study, Johnsen and colleagues[74] reviewed brain MRI of children with cerebral palsy born before 28 weeks gestation, showing an incidence of 30%. Grunnet and Shields[75] found 8% cerebellar injury in an autopsy series of premature babies born between 20 and 32 weeks gestation.

RISK FACTORS FOR CEREBELLAR HEMORRHAGE

Large cerebellar hemorrhage affects the sickest and most immature infants.[63] The pathogenesis of large and small cerebellar hemorrhages may be different. For large cerebellar hemorrhage, circulatory factors are important, including patent ductus arteriosus and need for inotropic support, especially because of impaired cerebrovascular autoregulation. This might cause fluctuations in arterial pressure and increased risk of rupture of immature vessels in the capillary beds of the germinal matrix.[63] Circulatory risk factors have not been found for small cerebellar hemorrhages.

The pathogenesis of lesions of the cerebellum is multifactorial, as with IVH. Identified risk factors are emergency cesarean section, patent ductus arteriosus, and low pH during the first days of life. Vaginal delivery has also been described in preterm infants as a risk factor.[64,76] Furthermore, coagulopathy or an increase in venous pressure have been implicated.[62] Autopsy data have suggested that cerebellar hemorrhagic injury might be caused by alterations in venous drainage.[60]

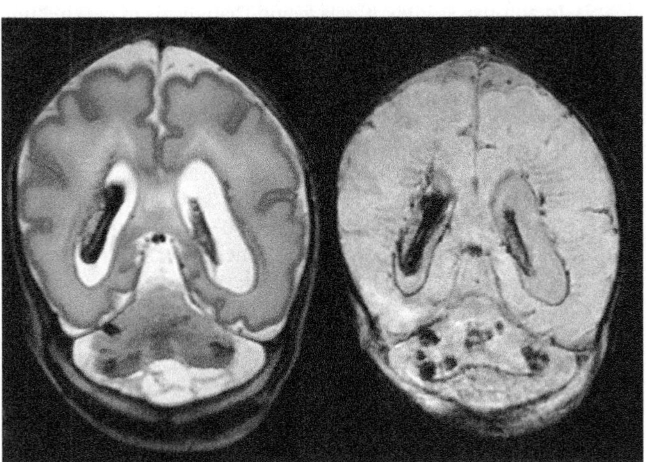

Fig. 129.7 Susceptibility-weighted imaging. Susceptibility-weighted imaging increases the sensitivity for hemorrhagic foci in the brain, especially in the cerebellum, compared with T2-weighted imaging alone. (Republished with permission from Brouwer AJ, Groenendaal F, Benders MJNL, de Vries LS. Early and late complications of germinal matrix-intraventricular haemorrhage in the preterm infant: what is new? *Neonatology.* 2014;106:296–303.)

The mechanisms underlying cerebellar hemorrhage are poorly understood. By injection of collagenase into the adult rat,[77-78] intracerebellar hemorrhage can be modeled. If this procedure could be modified for newborn rats, it could provide a valuable model to study therapeutic interventions and underlying mechanisms after cerebellar hemorrhages in human neonates.

CEREBELLAR ISCHEMIA

There is relatively little evidence for arterial ischemia in the preterm cerebellum. One cohort study reviewing neuroimaging findings of infants born before 28 weeks gestation with a diagnosis of cerebral palsy showed cerebellar abnormalities in 32 of 94 children with MRI studies. These included major destruction of the inferior vermis or cerebellar hemisphere in 23 children and focal or unilateral loss of cerebellar tissue in 4. The pattern of injury and lack of hemosiderin deposition were noted to be suggestive of vascular insult.[79] Cohort studies of preterm newborns with early postnatal MRI studies have not commonly reported cerebellar ischemia.

CEREBELLAR HYPOPLASIA OF PREMATURITY

Although direct injury to the cerebellum results in volume loss, longitudinal studies have also shown that preterm birth is associated with smaller cerebellar volumes even in the absence of direct hemorrhagic or ischemic insult. First reported in 2001 in a study of 14- to 15-year-old children, including 67 children born before 33 weeks gestation and 50 age-matched children born at term, those born preterm were found to have on average 8 cm^3 smaller cerebellar volumes.[80] These differences remained significant even after adjustment for whole brain volume, gender, and socioeconomic status.

More recently, a cohort of 38 preterm infants studied using brain MRI were compared to 38 postmenstrual age-matched healthy fetuses in the third trimester using fetal MRI. Preterm infants were found to have smaller cerebellar hemispheric volumes, but increased anterior, neo-, and posterior vermian regional volumes compared to the healthy fetuses. At term-equivalent age, smaller neovermian volume was associated with birth weight, sex, and supratentorial brain injury.[81] Comparing

Table 129.2 Incidence of Cerebellar Hemorrhages Diagnosed by Cranial Ultrasound and Magnetic Resonance Imaging.

	Window	Gestational Age or Birth Weight	*N*	Percentage
CUS				
Merill et al., 1998[65]	Mastoid	Low birth weight	250	2.8
Sehgal et al., 2009[185]	Mastoid	<30 wk	497	2.6
Limperopoulos et al., 2005[63]	Mastoid	<750 g	230	8.7
Muller et al., 2007[186]	Anterior	<33 wk	260	2.3
O'Shea et al., 2008[187]	Anterior	<28 wk	1017	1.4
Correa et al., 2004[188]	Posterior	<2000 g	164	1.2
Claris et al., 1996[189]	Posterior	<28 wk	199	2
MRI				
Steggerda et al., 2009[68]	MRI/CUS	<32 wk	77	18.6
Dyet et al., 2006[73]	MRI	<30 wk	199	6.7
Tam et al., 2011[72]	MRI	<34 wk	133	10
Van Kooij et al., 2012[174]	MRI	<31 wk	112	15.2
Kersbergen et al., in preparation	MRI	<28 wk	210	17.6

CUS, Cranial ultrasound; *MRI,* magnetic resonance imaging.
From Hou D, Shetty U, Phillips M, Gray PH. Cerebellar haemorrhage in the extremely preterm infant. *J Paediatr Child Health*. 2011;48:350–355.

preterm newborns at term-equivalent age to term-born controls, microstructural abnormalities in the cerebellum have also been noted, with higher fractional anisotropy in the dentate nuclei and middle cerebellar peduncle, and lower diffusivity in the vermis.[82] Following a cohort of 36 preterm newborns to school age (6 to 12 years) demonstrated that lasting changes are seen in the cerebellum, with reduced cerebellar white matter volume, surface area, and fractional anisotropy.[83]

Cerebellar hypoplasia of prematurity is believed to be due to impaired development of the cerebellum, as opposed to primary injury.[84] Characterization of the patterns of cerebellar growth impairment led to an observation of several patterns of cerebellar hypoplasia, including (1) symmetric hemispheric volume loss with preservation of the shape of the vermis; (2) symmetric hemispheric volume loss with a small, deformed vermis; and (3) normal cerebellar shape with overall size reduction. Associated with cerebellar hypoplasia is also flattening of the anterior pons and loss of supratentorial white matter.[85] In addition to volume loss, microstructural differences are noted, with changes in mean diffusivity in the cerebellar hemispheres and vermis associated with preterm birth.[86] Neuropathologic study comparing 19 preterm and stillborn brains showed preterm birth and ex utero development to be associated with decreased thickness and increased packing density of the external and internal granular layers of the cerebellum, reduced density of the Bergmann glial fibers, and reduced expression of Shh in the Purkinje cell layer.[87]

Recent prospective cohort studies of preterm newborns with neuroimaging have provided important insight into the risk factors and mechanisms for this hypoplasia. The strongest independently associated risk factors include cerebral brain injury and postnatal glucocorticoid exposure, with increasing evidence for other risk factors, including opioid and pain exposure, cardiorespiratory instability, nutrition, and somatic growth. Understanding of cerebellar development and control by Shh have provided insights into the possible molecular basis of such postnatal insults in preterm infants. For example, postnatal glucocorticoids are potent antagonists of Shh mitogenic effects on CGNPs and cerebellar growth.[88] Glucocorticoids such as hydrocortisone and prednisone are metabolized and inactivated by 11β-hydroxysteroid dehydrogenases type 2 (11β-HSD2), which is expressed in CGNPs (see Fig. 129.3). Moreover, mutations that activate Smo or treatment with a small molecule agonist of the SAG up-regulates 11β-HSD2 in CGNPs and thus protects against neurotoxic effects of these glucocorticoids in neonatal cerebellum.[88-90] In contrast, glucocorticoids like dexamethasone (and betamethasone) are not inactivated by 11β-HSD2 and need to be used with caution in the postnatal period in human neonates. This issue is discussed further below (see "Glucocorticoids").

SUPRATENTORIAL BRAIN INJURY

Nearly all infants with cerebellar hemorrhages (30% to 80%) also had a supratentorial hemorrhage.[76] Cerebellar hemorrhage and IVH do often coexist; this is confirmed by autopsy studies.[60] These hemorrhagic lesions probably share a common pathophysiologic mechanism.[91,92] Impaired autoregulation makes the preterm brain susceptible during episodes of hypoperfusion and/or hypoxia, which can weaken blood vessels, especially in the germinal matrix. The germinal layer is highly perfused and is well represented in the cerebellum in the roof of the fourth ventricle and over the cerebellar surface, forming the transient external granular layer. The blood vessels are prone to rupture during episodes of perfusion disturbances leading to hemorrhages in preterm infants.[60] Additionally, hemosiderin deposition on the developing cerebellar surface in preterm infants may be a crucial factor for cell death and developmental arrest of the granule cells because these cells normally grow inside the cerebellum molecular layer, the Purkinje layer, and into the internal granular layer to form the white matter. This might cause a subsequent decrease in production of the neurons with a decrease of cerebellar volume.[93] Other mechanisms are that hemosiderin deposition is related to the generation of free radicals, especially reactive oxygen species. Cerebellar subarachnoid hemorrhage in the preterm infant shows a decrease in the glutamate transporters in Purkinje cell dendrites, leading to an increase in extracellular glutamate and excitotoxic Purkinje cell death.[94]

A strong correlation between hypoxia-ischemia and inflammation with cerebellar injury has also been described, mainly in relation with PVL. The frequency of PVL related with cerebellar hemorrhage is high, approximately 26% to 34%.[92] This seems to be mainly related to perinatal events, such as hemodynamically significant patent ductus arteriosus and severe hypotension and mechanical ventilation. In relation to the degree of periventricular white matter damage, the size of the cerebellum and pons was found to be smaller in preterm infants. In autopsy studies, it was found that gliosis in cerebellum and cerebellar nuclei was more common in the presence of PVL. The incidence of gliosis was 43% in dentate, 29% in cerebellar cortex, 100% in the pons, and 92% in inferior olive compared with a group of preterm infants without PVL (who showed an incidence of only 5% to 15%).[92]

The cerebral cortex and cerebellum are connected by polysynaptic circuits, with feed-forward and feed-back limbs, forming functionally coupled networks. The feed-forward limb projects in the cerebellum, via the pontine nuclei, from a specific region of the cerebral cortex. These cerebral cortical regions in turn become the feed-back projection from the dentate nucleus, the cerebellar output center.[95] It is unclear how the cerebellum affects neurologic function within loops. Within the circuits, the cerebellum's role seems to be coordinating, integrating, and modulating neural activity.[1,57,96] If so, injury to the cerebellum might cause a functional disconnection with cerebral cortex and potentially affect subsequent development of remote regions of the cerebral cortex. This phenomenon, known as *diaschisis,* represents the loss of a function and/or tissue in a brain area connected to, but remote from, the brain lesion.[76]

Bilateral cerebellar hemorrhages result in decreased cerebellar volume; however, a decrease in supratentorial cerebral volume has also been described.[61] Unilateral cerebellar hemorrhages show (in addition to an expected decrease in the ipsilateral cerebellar volume) a significant decrease in the contralateral cerebral volume.[61] Conversely, in supratentorial unilateral periventricular hemorrhagic infarction, loss in volume of the contralateral cerebellar hemisphere has been described, so called *crossed cerebellar atrophy* (Fig. 129.8). The interconnections between

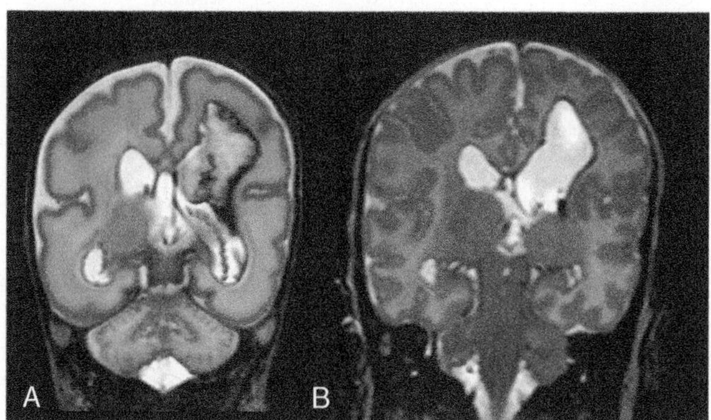

Fig. 129.8 Diaschisis. Supratentorial, unilateral periventricular hemorrhagic infarction on early preterm magnetic resonance imaging at 30 weeks corrected age (A), and expected porencephalic cyst at term-equivalent age (B), now also showing marked crossed cerebellar "atrophy."

cerebellum and cerebral cortex are built over a short period of the time, mainly during the third trimester of gestation. Thus, either cerebellar or cerebral pathology might delay or impede the establishment of critical neuroanatomic connections[97] and contribute to long-term neurodevelopmental deficits.[60] Indeed, the patterns of growth impairment in the preterm cerebellum vary based on whether hemorrhage occurs in the supratentorial intraventricular space versus directly in the cerebellum.[98] The crossed cerebellar diaschisis is suggested to be caused by the loss of excitatory input from cerebrum via corticopontine tracts, which synapse on pontine nuclei; the fibers cross the pons and ascend in the contralateral cerebellar peduncle to the contralateral cerebellar hemisphere (*green lines,* Fig. 129.9).[59] This schematic overview also explains the loss of feedback from the cerebellar hemisphere via the crossed dentato-rubro-thalamic-cortical pathway to the contralateral cerebral cortex in case of cerebellar injury (*red lines,* see Fig. 129.9).

The structural volumetric cerebellar growth deficits after supratentorial injury in extremely preterm infants appear to be considerably greater and more frequent than the mild cerebellar atrophy observed only in a minority of adults. A possible reason for this maturation-distinctive diaschisis in the small preterm infant may relate to the phase of rapid cerebellar development. Moreover, the fact that apoptosis is a more active process in developing than in adult neurons suggests that the apoptotic stimulus could have more profound effects on the rapidly developing cerebellum of the small premature infant than on the adult cerebellum.

Although cerebellar growth impairment in very preterm infants was found in association with supratentorial lesions, some studies showed that cerebellar volume of very preterm infants without supratentorial lesions did not differ from term control infants.[99,100] However, Limperopoulos and colleagues[101] showed a decrease in cerebellar volume in preterm infants without supratentorial cerebral injury, albeit the differences in cerebellar volume between preterm children without cerebral injury and term control infants were smaller than between preterm children with cerebral injury and the term control group. Adverse effects of perinatal events on cerebellar development may be smaller than the effects of cerebro-cerebellar diaschisis.

A diffusion MRI study confirmed the interaction between supratentorial and cerebellar injury by showing that infants with IVH have significant diffusivity changes in the cerebellar cortex compared with control infants.[102] More advanced imaging studies may provide more information about abnormal cerebellar development in preterm neonates in relation to supratentorial injury. However, because there are no monosynaptic connections between the cerebral cortex and the cerebellum, conventional tract-tracing techniques have been unable to map the relationship between the cortex and its projection zones in the cerebellum. However, more advanced diffusion tensor imaging (DTI) studies, such as high angular resolution diffusion imaging and constrained spherical deconvolution analysis, might be able to illustrate cerebro-cerebellar connectivity. In conjunction with a large porencephalic cyst after large periventricular hemorrhagic infarction, asymmetry in the peduncles and a decreased contralateral cerebellar hemisphere can be seen (Fig. 129.10). Additionally, there is an expected interruption of the ipsilateral corticospinal tracts, next to an impressive, reduced fiber density in the contralateral hemisphere of the cerebellum (Fig. 129.11). This interruption may lead to loss of neuronal activation from supratentorial corticopontine tracts, with subsequent impaired development of the cerebellum, suggesting that neuronal activation is crucial for brain development.[103] Future work is necessary to improve the possibility to reconstruct the developing cerebellar connectivity in relation to the cerebral cortex.

GLUCOCORTICOIDS

Glucocorticoids have played an important role in the management of preterm newborns, with antenatal treatment to accelerate lung maturation and postnatal treatment to address hypotension and to aid extubation in the case of subglottic stenosis. Despite the success of these medications on infant survival and cardiorespiratory stabilization, their impact on the developing brain, and particularly the preterm cerebellum, remains a significant concern for their use.

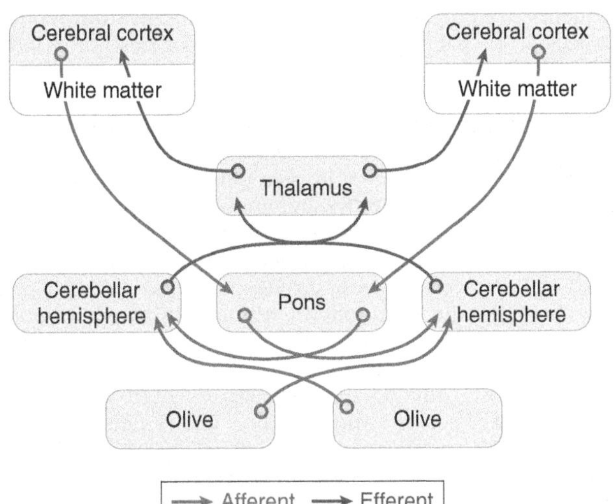

Fig. 129.9 Schematic overview of the main connections between cerebrum and cerebellum. (From Volpe JJ. Cerebellum of the premature infant: rapidly developing, vulnerable, clinically important. *J Child Neurol.* 2009;24:1085–1104.)

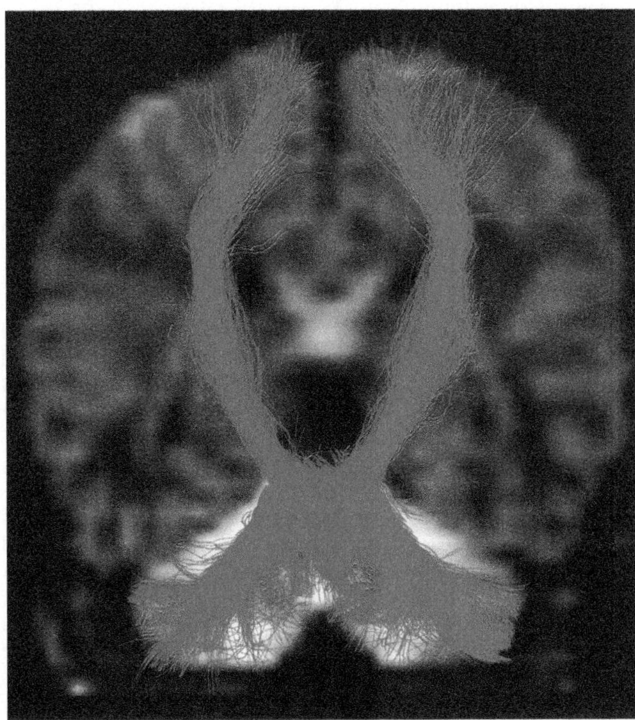

Fig. 129.10 Cerebro-cerebellar connectivity. Tractography illustrates how cortical spinal tracts are related to local tract organization in the cerebellum by in vivo diffusion imaging and tractography methods. (Courtesy Prof. S. Counsell and Dr. K. Pieterman.)

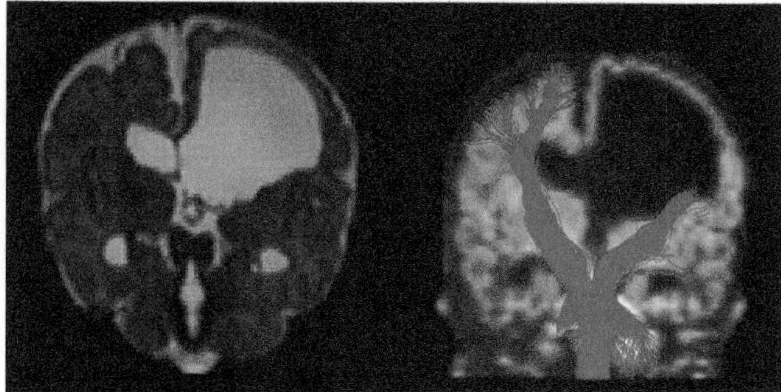

Fig. 129.11 Cerebro-cerebellar connectivity and porencephalic cyst caused by periventricular hemorrhagic infarction *(left)*. Interruption of ipsilateral cortical spinal tracts in the left hemisphere with subsequent reduced fiber density of the contralateral cerebellum *(right)*. (Courtesy Prof. S. Counsell and Dr. K. Pieterman.)

Studies in multiple animal models have suggested negative effects of glucocorticoids on the developing cerebellum. The neonatal cerebellum has the highest levels of glucocorticoid receptors in the brain,[104] localized to the external granular layer.[105] First reported in the 1970s, hydrocortisone treatment of neonatal rats slowed the normal increase in body and brain weight, with most pronounced effects in the cerebellum.[106,107] Histologic analysis of the cerebellum showed delay in secondary foliation and reduction in mitosis and final number of cells in the external granular layer.[108] Further study in neonatal mice treated with dexamethasone showed that doses higher than 0.1 mg/kg resulted in increased apoptosis in the external granular layer, with a window of vulnerability between postnatal days 4 and 10, corresponding to the human period of 20 weeks gestation to 6.5 weeks after term age.[105] Comparing the toxicity of dexamethasone and hydrocortisone in chicken embryos, apoptosis in the cerebellum was seen in a dose-dependent fashion, with doubling of the apoptosis rate at a dose of 5 mg/kg of dexamethasone and 1 mg/kg of hydrocortisone.[109]

Although both dexamethasone and hydrocortisone show toxicity in newborn rodents and chickens, differences in metabolism of these two drugs suggest there may be potential differences in level of toxicity. The fetal brain has high expression of 11β-HSD2, an endogenous enzyme capable of metabolizing hydrocortisone but not dexamethasone.[110] In addition, hydrocortisone has a greater mineralocorticoid effect than dexamethasone. Despite animal models suggesting toxicity with both drugs, these differences have resulted in the suggestion that hydrocortisone may be a safer alternative drug in newborns.

Multiple studies have suggested negative effects of postnatal dexamethasone on the preterm cerebellum. One observational study comparing 11 newborns exposed to postnatal dexamethasone with 30 untreated newborns found smaller overall brain volumes at term-equivalent age, including 20% smaller cerebellar volumes.[111] In an observational cohort study including 235 infants exposed to postnatal dexamethasone, increasing the duration of exposure to dexamethasone was associated with increasing deficits in both the mental and psychomotor developmental indices of the Bayley Scales of Infant Development second edition at 6 to 8 months of age.[112]

The association between postnatal hydrocortisone and preterm cerebellar development is less clear. One prospective cohort study of 172 preterm newborns showed 1.88 cm^3 (95% confidence interval [CI], −2.91 to −0.86; $P < .001$) smaller cerebellar volumes associated with postnatal hydrocortisone exposure and 2.31 cm^3 (95% CI, −3.52 to −1.10; $P < .001$) smaller volumes associated with postnatal dexamethasone exposure, after adjusting for confounding factors. This translated to an 8% smaller volume associated with hydrocortisone and a 10% smaller volume associated with dexamethasone.[113] Another study comparing 73 preterm newborns exposed to hydrocortisone with matched controls reported no significant difference in cerebellar volume, with a coefficient of −0.53 cm^3 (95% CI, −1.8 to 0.7; $P = .39$).[114] Thus although both studies reported overlapping confidence intervals, only one found a statistically significant association between postnatal hydrocortisone exposure and cerebellar development. Differences in the two studies may be related to differences in glucocorticoid dosing or other management differences. In a cohort study including 80 infants exposed to hydrocortisone, developmental outcomes were found to be negatively affected only if the duration of exposure to hydrocortisone was longer than 7 days.[115]

Aside from the importance of glucocorticoid type and exposure, timing also seems to be an important factor. Although postnatal glucocorticoids have been associated with adverse cerebellar development, antenatal glucocorticoids have not been shown to have such effects. In a cohort study of 172 preterm newborns, of which 85% were exposed to antenatal betamethasone, antenatal exposure to glucocorticoids was not found to be associated with cerebellar development, even after adjusting for confounders.[113]

With the usefulness of glucocorticoids in preterm newborns and evidence for cerebellar toxicity, multiple attempts have been made to identify drugs to circumvent the associated neurologic side effects. *N*-Methyl-D-aspartate (NMDA) receptor antagonists have been found to block dexamethasone-induced cell death in rat cerebellar granule cell culture.[116] Lithium pretreatment has been shown to be protective against neurotoxic effects of dexamethasone treatment both in vivo and in vitro in neonatal mice.[117] Interestingly, SAG has also been found to result in protection of the expansion of the external granular layer with exposure to dexamethasone or prednisolone,[89] especially due to its effects on the Shh signaling pathway, which is known to be involved in external granular layer expansion in the preterm cerebellum (see Fig. 129.3).[88] SAG is also protective in a dual injury model involving hypoxia and glucocorticoids.[90] However, no studies have yet been conducted in humans to test the efficacy of these treatments.

OPIOIDS AND PAIN

Preterm newborns in the neonatal intensive care unit (NICU) undergo significant amounts of stress and pain during hospitalization. Multiple studies have reported on the high frequency of painful procedures in the NICU. One study reported a mean of 14 painful procedures a day for newborns in the NICU.[118] Another study showed that preterm newborns younger than 32 weeks of gestational age at birth experienced a median of 74 skin-breaking procedures during their hospitalization.[119] Painful stress has been found to be associated with impairments in brain development,[119,120] in pain perception detectable into childhood,[121] and in cognitive and motor outcomes.[122]

Following a cohort of 56 preterm-born children to 7 years of age with neuroimaging, higher neonatal procedural pain was found to be associated with smaller cerebellar volumes in the posterior VIIIA and VIIIB lobules, resulting in poorer cognition and visuo-motor integration.[123] Thus pain is associated with poor cerebellar growth.

As the most common opioid analgesic used in the NICU, morphine has been the most studied for its effects on brain development and outcome. In the large NEOPAIN trial, 898 preterm newborns were randomized to either masked placebo or morphine infusions for preemptive analgesia for up to 14 days. Preemptive morphine infusions did not change the frequency of severe IVH, PVL, or death. However, additional intermittent boluses of open-label morphine were associated with increased risk of severe IVH, PVL, or neonatal death.[124] Conversely, other studies have suggested lower incidences of IVH after morphine infusions.[125,126] However, these studies did not investigate specific effects in the cerebellum. When looking at long-term outcome, although one study found adverse motor outcomes associated with morphine exposure,[122] other studies did not find developmental sequelae after morphine treatment.[127-130]

Looking specifically at the cerebellum in a cohort of 136 preterm newborns with serial neuroimaging, a 10-fold increase in morphine exposure was associated with a 5.5% decrease in cerebellar volume by term-equivalent age, with no corresponding changes to cerebral brain volume. In this study, greater morphine exposure was also associated with worse motor and cognitive outcomes by 18 months corrected age.[131]

Studies in animals have shown that opioids, including morphine, can affect cerebellar development.[132-135] Morphine administration before and during pregnancy, as well as during the lactation period, affects the number of Purkinje cells in young-adult mice.[133] However, the number of studies investigating opioid analgesia in the cerebellum and the underlying mechanisms is limited. Although voltage-dependent calcium channels are involved in the mechanisms underlying morphine administration,[136] their role in morphine-induced changes in the developing cerebellum is unclear. Mice studies have suggested that G-protein-activated inwardly rectifying K+ (GIRK) channels are involved in opioid-induced analgesia in the cerebellum.[137-139] Opioid receptor activation results in activation of inhibitory regulative (Gi) proteins, which in turn inhibit activity of enzymes or other downstream pathways. Various Gi proteins regulate neuronal excitability and are associated with GIRK channels, which are highly expressed in the brain.[140-142] A mutation in the GIRK 2 subunit in the weaver mouse results in reduced Gi protein activation and reduced analgesia after opioid administration.[139] The weaver mouse shows, among other defects, predominantly cerebellar abnormalities caused by failure of the granule cells to differentiate and migrate into the IGL and reduced numbers of Purkinje cells and neurons in the deep cerebellar nuclei.[143,144] The weaver mouse could therefore be a useful research tool to investigate GIRK channel involvement in opioid-induced analgesia in the developing cerebellum in more detail. Thus, although animal evidence suggests potential effects of opioids on preterm cerebellar development, further research is needed to assess its effects in humans.

CARDIORESPIRATORY FACTORS

Preterm newborns are at risk of multiple cardiorespiratory issues, including the need for prolonged ventilator support, chronic lung disease, hypotension, and patent ductus arteriosus. Although it is well known that such factors affect supratentorial brain injury and development, including IVH and PVL, the effects of these factors on the cerebellum are not well studied or understood.

Multiple observational studies in preterm newborns have identified these as important factors associated with cerebellar hypoplasia. In a study comparing 33 preterm newborns born between 26 and 36 weeks gestational age without overt brain injury and 27 term controls, MRI from 0.4 to 5.5 years showed reduced volumes in the vermis, cerebellum, and pons associated with duration of mechanical ventilation, severe hypotension (<30 mm Hg), and large patent ductus arteriosus with bounding pulses.[92] Another cohort study of 47 infants born before 27 weeks gestational age without overt brain injury showed specific volume losses in the cerebellum associated with the need for patent ductus arteriosus ligation.[145] A cohort study of 172 infants born before 32 weeks gestational age with serial MRI studies in the neonatal period looked at a range of potential associated factors. Aside from postnatal glucocorticoids and IVH, other factors found to be associated with cerebellar hypoplasia included duration of intubation, hypotension, and patent ductus arteriosus (Fig. 129.12).[113]

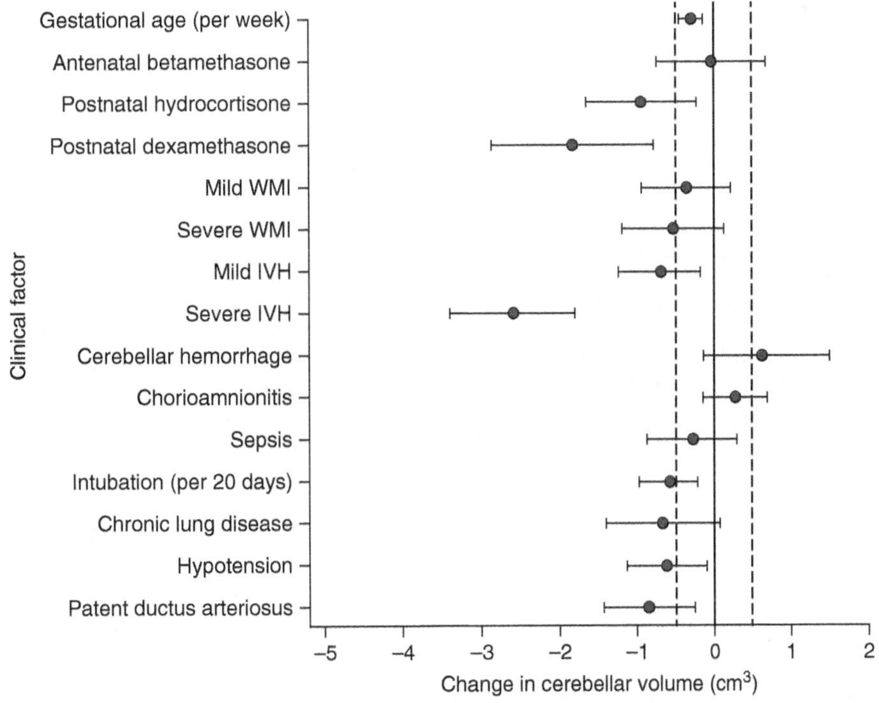

Fig. 129.12 Change in cerebellar volume associated with various clinical factors. Significant factors include postnatal glucocorticoid exposure, mild and severe intraventricular hemorrhage *(IVH)*, duration of intubation, hypotension, and patent ductus arteriosus. *WMI,* White matter injury. (From Tam EW, Chau V, Ferriero DM, et al. Preterm cerebellar growth impairment after postnatal exposure to glucocorticoids. *Sci Transl Med.* 2011;3:105ra105.)

More recently, assessing cerebellar metabolites using magnetic resonance spectroscopy in 53 preterm newborns, cerebellar injury was found to be associated with lower cerebellar N-acetyl aspartate, choline, and creatine concentrations. Meanwhile, these alterations in cerebellar metabolites were found to be associated with necrotizing enterocolitis, infection, and bronchopulmonary dysplasia, implicating these infectious and respiratory factors with metabolic abnormalities in the cerebellum.[146]

Although studies in neonatal rats show that hypoxia causes damage to all developing cerebellar structures,[147,148] cerebellar involvement after cardiorespiratory casualties and their underlying mechanisms is poorly studied in animals.

Thus, although it may be difficult to tease out the contribution of each of these factors on cerebellar growth and although the exact mechanisms for these effects are not well understood, it is clear that cardiorespiratory factors contribute to cerebellar hypoplasia of prematurity.

NUTRITION AND GROWTH

With the dramatic growth of the cerebellum in the third trimester and the impact of preterm birth, it seems likely that nutrition and somatic growth would be important factors regulating development of the cerebellum. However, there is surprisingly little research so far regarding this issue.

Evidence for the importance of nutrition and somatic growth on the cerebellum can be inferred from research on intrauterine growth restriction. In fetal sheep, intrauterine growth restriction has been found to be associated with changes in synaptogenesis, mitochondrial formation, and development of the Purkinje cell dendritic tree in the cerebellar cortex.[149,150] In human studies, intrauterine growth restriction has been associated with impairments in overall brain development,[151] including cerebellar development.[152,153]

Increasingly, recent literature has demonstrated the importance of perinatal and postnatal nutritional factors and cerebellar outcome. Studying a cohort of 42 preterm newborns from birth until term, overall weight gain, weight, length, fat mass, and fat-free mass were all positively correlated with cerebellar volumes by term.[154] In a cohort study of 49 preterm newborns assessed with serial neuroimaging from preterm until term-equivalent age, greater energy and lipid intake was shown to be associated with increased total brain volume, and more specifically increased cerebellar volume.[155] Thus, overall growth and nutrition has beneficial impacts on cerebellar development.

Looking more specifically at the types of lipids, one recent study of 60 preterm newborns with serial blood samples studying polyunsaturated fatty acids and neuroimaging demonstrated that higher red blood cell membrane docosahexaenoic acid levels near term-equivalent age were associated with larger cerebellar volumes and improved motor outcomes by 36 months corrected age.[156] From the same cohort of 60 preterm newborns with serial blood samples, higher early postnatal plasma cholesterol levels were also reported to be associated with improved cerebellar volumes. The authors note that cholesterol is a necessary factor in the Sonic hedgehog signaling pathway, highlighting its potential impact on preterm cerebellar development.[157] Thus, more specific nutritional factors, particularly docosahexaenoic acid and cholesterol, seem to play important roles in preterm cerebellar development.

POSTNATAL FACTORS

Although perinatal factors may be critical, the cerebellum continues to develop past term-equivalent age, with the external granular layer continuing to play a role until the age of 2 years.[8] As a result, an understanding of the risk factors for impaired cerebellar development would require not only a study of the early postnatal period, but continued analysis of the factors affecting development in the first few years of life. Unfortunately, although prospective studies maintain excellent records of factors occurring in the NICU, most put very little emphasis on the factors affecting the infant after discharge. Socioeconomic status, including family stress, infant exposures, and parental education, are becoming increasingly recognized factors affecting long-term outcome after brain injury or preterm birth. There is a breadth of literature showing that socioeconomic status is associated with a range of cognitive outcomes, including memory, cognition, executive function, and language.[158-160] Increasing evidence exists regarding how early social environments and experiences can affect the course of human development.[161] Specifically in the cerebellum, a study of 42 healthy adult males (not preterm) showed that both early life socioeconomic status and current socioeconomic status were correlated with cerebellar grey matter volumes.[162]

One study has investigated the impact of postnatal environmental exposure on cerebellar development after prematurity. In a cohort study of 26 preterm newborns with serial neuroimaging at birth, near term, and again at 2 years of age, parental education was assessed. Maternal postsecondary education was not associated with near-term cerebellar volumes. Cerebellar volumes at 2 years were found to be associated with near-term volumes, with this relationship confounded by maternal postsecondary education, with higher education associated with improved cerebellar volumes by 2 years.[163] Thus, while cerebellar hypoplasia seems to persist later in life, postnatal factors can positively influence these outcomes. While maternal education seems to modify the outcomes after preterm cerebellar hypoplasia, more research is needed to confirm and clarify how socioeconomic status impacts these long-term outcomes.

LONG-TERM OUTCOME AFTER CEREBELLAR INJURY AND IMPAIRED DEVELOPMENT

LARGE AND SMALL CEREBELLAR HEMORRHAGE

Traditionally diagnosed via head ultrasound, large cerebellar hemorrhages are associated with a high risk of morbidity and mortality. In a retrospective study of 1242 preterm infants, 35 (3%) were identified to have cerebellar hemorrhage on head ultrasound, with a mortality rate of 14%.[63] Median age at death was 6 days (ranging from 4 to 15 days). In a cohort study of 119 preterm infants born before 30 weeks gestational age, 8 were found to have large cerebellar hemorrhages, of which 3 (38%) died in the neonatal period. Of the survivors, those with cerebellar hemorrhage were found to be microcephalic compared with normal peers, and another 3 (60% of survivors) had severe developmental delay.[73] In a case series of six preterm infants born between 24 and 28 weeks gestational age diagnosed with large cerebellar hemorrhages, three died during the neonatal period, and the remaining three had severe neurologic sequelae. These sequelae included microcephaly, hypotonia, and developmental delay.[164] However, because infants with cerebellar hemorrhage often have concurrent injury in other brain regions, it is important to study the outcome of isolated cerebellar hemorrhage. In a larger group of 35 preterm infants with isolated cerebellar hemorrhagic injury, 66% were found to have neurologic abnormalities by 2.5 years of age. Compared with 35 age-matched controls, these infants had significantly lower mean scores on all tested measures, including motor, expressive language, receptive language, and cognitive testing, with findings more severe when injury was present in the cerebellar vermis. Also prevalent were abnormalities on autism screening and internalizing behavioral problems.[165] Thus, large cerebellar hemorrhages are associated with a high risk of early mortality and broad deficits in motor and cognitive skills in survivors, especially in those with involvement of the cerebellar vermis.

Smaller cerebellar hemorrhages not detectable on head ultrasound have a generally more favorable prognosis, with no risk of mortality in the neonatal period. In one cohort study of 131 preterm newborns younger than 34 weeks gestational age, 10 infants were found to have small cerebellar hemorrhage. These children, when assessed at 5 years of age, were found to have fivefold increased odds of abnormalities on neurologic examination, including lower-limb hypertonia and hyperreflexia. Conversely, all of these children were ambulatory and had no differences in cognitive testing compared with their peers. In addition, no differences were noted in outcome when comparing the location of the hemorrhages.[72] In another cohort study of 108 preterm newborns younger than 32 weeks gestational age, 16 infants were found to have small cerebellar hemorrhage, with no differences in neurodevelopmental testing identified at 2 years of age compared with peers.[166] Yet another cohort of 24 preterm infants with punctate cerebellar hemorrhage were not found to have differences in neurodevelopmental outcome at 2 years corrected age compared to term control infants.[167] In a large multicenter study of 2018 preterm infants with cerebellar hemorrhage, increasing size of hemorrhage was found to be associated with worse outcomes on neurodevelopmental testing, particularly those with at least one-third of the cerebellar hemisphere affected.[168] As a result, although not associated with mortality or cognitive deficits, smaller cerebellar hemorrhages appear to be associated with motor impairments detectable on neurologic examination by school age.

CEREBELLAR HYPOPLASIA OF PREMATURITY

Unlike cerebellar hemorrhage, where there is significant emphasis on mortality and severe motor deficits, sequelae from cerebellar hypoplasia are less severe, albeit significant. Studies have shed light on the complex deficits that can occur. Some studies have used an easily reproducible measure of transcerebellar diameter to assess cerebellar hypoplasia. In a study of 83 preterm newborns assessed at 3 months of age, smaller cerebellar diameter was found to be associated with abnormal generalized movements.[169] Another study of 166 preterm infants demonstrated smaller transcerebellar diameter by term age associated with 17% lower Bayley mental developmental index scores.[170]

Focusing on the neurologic examination, a longitudinal study of 98 preterm infants found that reduced volume of the cerebellum by term equivalent age was associated with complex minor neurologic dysfunction on the Touwen neurologic examination or a diagnosis of cerebral palsy.[171] Looking at specific deficits on neurologic examination, one study of 119 preterm newborns demonstrated that a cerebellar volume of less than $19cm^3$ by term-equivalent age is associated with specific abnormalities by 19 months corrected age including 8-fold odds of truncal hypotonia, 9-fold odds of postural instability on standing, and 10-fold odds of patellar hyperreflexia. Using deformation-based morphometry, this study demonstrated postural instability specifically associated with decreased volumes in the paramedian regions of the cerebellum.[172] Another study of cerebellar microstructure using DTI by term-equivalent age in a cohort of 64 preterm newborns demonstrated that lower fractional anisotropy in the superior and middle cerebellar peduncles was associated with a diagnosis of cerebral palsy by the age of 2 years corrected.[173] Thus, macrostructural and microstructural abnormalities in the cerebellum by term-equivalent age is associated with motor impairments in follow-up.

By 24 months of age, smaller cerebellar volumes on structural MRI and lower N-acetylaspartate/choline ratios on MR spectroscopy were also found to be associated with impaired scores on cognitive testing in 112 infants born before 31 weeks gestational age.[174] When 31 preterm newborns with impaired cerebellar development were compared with 31 age-matched controls, worse outcomes were noted by 24 months of age in both motor and cognitive domains, with 48% of the affected children diagnosed with mixed cerebral palsy, including spastic-ataxic, spastic-dyskinetic, and dyskinetic-ataxic subtypes.[175] In another cohort study of 164 very low-birth-weight infants with MRI scans at term-equivalent age and follow-up assessments at 24 months, volumes of various brain tissues were assessed. Smaller volumes in total brain tissue, cerebrum, frontal lobes, basal ganglia and thalami, and cerebellum were associated with neurodevelopmental impairment, including cerebral palsy, hearing loss, blindness, or significantly delayed cognitive performance. Even without neurodevelopmental impairment, smaller cerebellar volumes were associated with poorer developmental scores.[176]

By 6.5 years, in a cohort of 107 preterm children, decreased cerebellar volume was found to be associated with poorer fine motor skills.[177] Another study following preterm children to 9 years showed correlations between smaller cerebellar volumes and deficits in attention and executive function scores.[178] In longer follow-up to 13 years, smaller cerebellar volumes in a cohort of children born under 30 weeks were found to be associated with poorer goal setting performance.[179] At 14 to 15 years of age, children born before 33 weeks gestational age with smaller cerebellar volumes were not found to have motor deficits but did have significant cognitive deficits compared with term-born controls.[80] Additionally, these children were found to have reduced self-reported measures of well-being.[180] Specific outcome deficits seem to be associated with the region of injury in the cerebellum. In the same study at 14 to 15 years of age, hypoplasia of the lateral lobes was found to be associated with reduced executive, visuospatial, and language functions.[181] In a cohort of preterm-born children assessed from 9 to 17 years of age, impaired microstructure of the cerebral peduncles was associated with impaired reading comprehension.[182] Studying specifically eyeblink conditioning as a marker of cerebellar dysfunction in children and young adults without cerebellar hemorrhage, those born preterm were found to have significantly less conditioned responses and slower learning rates.[183] Thus, in the absence of early childhood deficits on developmental testing, long-lasting impairments in cerebellar function, including motor and cognitive functions, continue throughout life.

In addition to motor and cognitive deficits, others have studied the impact of cerebellar hypoplasia on mental health. In a cohort of 30 preterm newborns and 37 controls assessed through adolescence, smaller cerebellar volumes of preterm-born subjects at 15 and 19 years was associated with poorer psychosocial function and inattention. Poorer development of the cerebellum from age 15 to 19 years in the preterm-born subjects was also associated with a higher frequency of psychiatric diagnosis on testing.[184]

In summary, cerebellar hypoplasia of prematurity has been demonstrated to be associated with early and lasting deficits in not only motor and cognitive domains, but also deficits in overall well-being and psychiatric diagnoses.

CONCLUSION AND FUTURE DIRECTIONS

The cerebellum has relatively recently been identified as a major target for injury and impaired development after preterm birth. With increasing evidence that injury to this part of the brain has an important role in long-term motor and cognitive outcomes, identification of key risk factors, causal injury pathways, and new treatment approaches are obviously important. Aside from supratentorial brain injury, hemorrhage, and postnatal glucocorticoid exposure, we need to improve our understanding of how other factors, such as opioid exposure, cardiorespiratory factors, nutrition, and postnatal factors, affect the development of this critical brain structure. Identifying targets for improving neonatal care, such as pharmacologic targets to minimize the effects of postnatal glucocorticoids on the cerebellum, may result in improvements in motor and cognitive outcomes after preterm birth.

 A complete reference list is available at www.ExpertConsult.com.

SELECT REFERENCES

1. Schmahmann JD. The cerebellum and cognition. *Neurosci Lett*. 2019;688:62-75.
2. Voogd J, Ruigrok TJH. Cerebellum and precerebellar nuclei. In: Mai JK, Paxinos G, eds. *The Human Nervous System*. 3rd ed. San Diego, CA: Academic Press; 2012:471-545.
3. White JJ, Sillitoe RV. Development of the cerebellum: from gene expression patterns to circuit maps. *Wiley Interdiscip Rev Dev Biol*. 2013;2:149-164.
4. Ashwell KWS, Mai JK. Fetal development of the central nervous system. In: Mai JK, Paxinos G, eds. *The Human Nervous System*. 3rd ed. San Diego, CA: Academic Press; 2012:31-79.
5. Wingate RJ. The rhombic lip and early cerebellar development. *Curr Opin Neurobiol*. 2001;11:82-88.
11. Millen KJ, Gleeson JG. Cerebellar development and disease. *Curr Opin Neurobiol*. 2008;18:12-19.
15. Wang VY, Zoghbi HY. Genetic regulation of cerebellar development. *Nat Rev Neurosci*. 2001;2:484-491.
22. Hatten ME, Heintz N. Mechanisms of neural patterning and specification in the developing cerebellum. *Annu Rev Neurosci*. 1995;18:385-408.
29. Wurst W, Bally-Cuif L. Neural plate patterning: upstream and downstream of the isthmic organizer. *Nat Rev Neurosci*. 2001;2:99-108.
30. Liu A, Joyner AL. Early anterior/posterior patterning of the midbrain and cerebellum. *Annu Rev Neurosci*. 2001;24:869-896.
44. Ho KS, Scott MP. Sonic hedgehog in the nervous system: functions, modifications and mechanisms. *Curr Opin Neurobiol*. 2002;12:57-63.
46. Dahmane N, Altaba A. Sonic hedgehog regulates the growth and patterning of the cerebellum. *Development*. 1999;126:3089-3100.
59. Volpe JJ. Cerebellum of the premature infant: rapidly developing, vulnerable, clinically important. *J Child Neurol*. 2009;24:1085-1104.
60. Haines KM, Wang W, Pierson CR. Cerebellar hemorrhagic injury in premature infants occurs during a vulnerable developmental period and is associated with wider neuropathology. *Acta Neuropathol Commun*. 2013;1:69.
61. Limperopoulos C, Soul JS, Haidar H, et al. Impaired trophic interactions between the cerebellum and the cerebrum among preterm infants. *Pediatrics*. 2005;116:844-850.
62. Ecury-Goossen GM, Dudink J, Lequin M, et al. The clinical presentation of preterm cerebellar haemorrhage. *Eur J Pediatr*. 2010;169:1249-1253.
63. Limperopoulos C, Benson CB, Bassan H, et al. Cerebellar hemorrhage in the preterm infant: ultrasonographic findings and risk factors. *Pediatrics*. 2005;116:717-724.
64. Steggerda SJ, De Bruïne FT, van den Berg-Huysmans AA, et al. Small cerebellar hemorrhage in preterm infants: perinatal and postnatal factors and outcome. *Cerebellum*. 2013;12:794-801.
65. Merrill JD, Piecuch RE, Fell SC, et al. A new pattern of cerebellar hemorrhages in preterm infants. *Pediatrics*. 1998;102:E62.
66. Steggerda SJ, Leijser LM, Walther FJ, van Wezel-Meijler G. Neonatal cranial ultrasonography: how to optimize its performance. *Early Hum Dev*. 2009;85:93-99.
67. Enriquez G, Correa F, Aso C, et al. Mastoid fontanelle approach for sonographic imaging of the neonatal brain. *Pediatr Radiol*. 2006;36:532-540.
68. Steggerda SJ, Leijser LM, Wiggers-de Bruïne FT, et al. Cerebellar injury in preterm infants: incidence and findings on US and MR images. *Radiology*. 2009;252:190-199.
69. Di Salvo DN. A new view of the neonatal brain: clinical utility of supplemental neurologic US imaging windows. *Radiographics*. 2001;21:943-955.
71. Intrapiromkul J, Northington F, Huisman TA, et al. Accuracy of head ultrasound for the detection of intracranial hemorrhage in preterm neonates: comparison with brain MRI and susceptibility-weighted imaging. *J Neuroradiol*. 2013;40:81-88.
72. Tam EW, Rosenbluth G, Rogers EE, et al. Cerebellar hemorrhage on magnetic resonance imaging in preterm newborns associated with abnormal neurologic outcome. *J Pediatr*. 2011;158:245-250.
73. Dyet LE, Kennea N, Counsell SJ, et al. Natural history of brain lesions in extremely preterm infants studied with serial magnetic resonance imaging from birth and neurodevelopmental assessment. *Pediatrics*. 2006;118:536-548.
74. Johnsen SD, Bodensteiner JB, Lotze TE. Frequency and nature of cerebellar injury in the extremely premature survivor with cerebral palsy. *J Child Neurol*. 2005;20:60-64.
75. Grunnet ML, Shields WD. Cerebellar hemorrhage in the premature infant. *J Pediatr*. 1976;88:605-608.
76. Fumagalli M, Bassi L, Sirgiovanni I, et al. From germinal matrix to cerebellar haemorrhage. *J Matern Fetal Neonatal Med*. 2015;28(suppl 1):2280-2285.
80. Allin M, Matsumoto H, Santhouse AM, et al. Cognitive and motor function and the size of the cerebellum in adolescents born very pre-term. *Brain*. 2001;124:60-66.
85. Messerschmidt A, Brugger PC, Boltshauser E, et al. Disruption of cerebellar development: potential complication of extreme prematurity. *AJNR Am J Neuroradiol*. 2005;26:1659-1667.
86. Hart AR, Whitby EH, Clark SJ, et al. Diffusion-weighted imaging of cerebral white matter and the cerebellum following preterm birth. *Dev Med Child Neurol*. 2010;52:652-659.
87. Haldipur P, Bharti U, Alberti C, et al. Preterm delivery disrupts the developmental program of the cerebellum. *PloS One*. 2011;6:e23449.
88. Heine VM, Rowitch DH. Hedgehog signaling has a protective effect in glucocorticoid-induced mouse neonatal brain injury through an 11betaHSD2-dependent mechanism. *J Clin Invest*. 2009;119:267-277.
89. Heine VM, Griveau A, Chapin C, et al. A small-molecule smoothened agonist prevents glucocorticoid-induced neonatal cerebellar injury. *Sci Transl Med*. 2011;3:105ra104.
91. Tam EW, Miller SP, Studholme C, et al. Differential effects of intraventricular hemorrhage and white matter injury on preterm cerebellar growth. *J Pediatr*. 2011;158:366-371.
92. Argyropoulou MI, Xydis V, Drougia A, et al. MRI measurements of the pons and cerebellum in children born preterm; associations with the severity of periventricular leukomalacia and perinatal risk factors. *Neuroradiology*. 2003;45:730-734.
95. Limperopoulos C, Chilingaryan G, Sullivan N, et al. Injury to the premature cerebellum: outcome is related to remote cortical development. *Cereb Cortex*. 2014;24:728-736.
107. Bohn MC, Lauder JM. Cerebellar granule cell genesis in the hydrocortisone-treated rats. *Dev Neurosci*. 1980;3:81-89.
111. Parikh NA, Lasky RE, Kennedy KA, et al. Postnatal dexamethasone therapy and cerebral tissue volumes in extremely low birth weight infants. *Pediatrics*. 2007;119:265-272.
112. Needelman H, Evans M, Roberts H, et al. Effects of postnatal dexamethasone exposure on the developmental outcome of premature infants. *J Child Neurol*. 2008;23:421-424.
113. Tam EW, Chau V, Ferriero DM, et al. Preterm cerebellar growth impairment after postnatal exposure to glucocorticoids. *Sci Transl Med*. 2011;3:105ra105.
114. Kersbergen KJ, de Vries LS, van Kooij BJ, et al. Hydrocortisone treatment for bronchopulmonary dysplasia and brain volumes in preterm infants. *J Pediatr*. 2013;163:666-671.e1.
115. Needelman H, Hoskappal A, Roberts H, et al. The effect of hydrocortisone on neurodevelopmental outcome in premature infants less than 29 weeks' gestation. *J Child Neurol*. 2010;25:448-452.
122. Grunau RE, Whitfield MF, Petrie-Thomas J, et al. Neonatal pain, parenting stress and interaction, in relation to cognitive and motor development at 8 and 18 months in preterm infants. *Pain*. 2009;143:138-146.
124. Anand KJ, Hall RW, Desai N, et al. Effects of morphine analgesia in ventilated preterm neonates: primary outcomes from the NEOPAIN randomised trial. *Lancet*. 2004;363:1673-1682.
135. Zagon IS, McLaughlin PJ. Increased brain size and cellular content in infant rats treated with an opiate antagonist. *Science*. 1983;221:1179-1180.
148. Biran V, Heine VM, Verney C, et al. Cerebellar abnormalities following hypoxia alone compared to hypoxic-ischemic forebrain injury in the developing rat brain. *Neurobiol Dis*. 2011;41:138-146.
153. Sanz-Cortes M, Egana-Ugrinovic G, Zupan R, et al. Brainstem and cerebellar differences and their association with neurobehavior in term small-for-gestational-age fetuses assessed by fetal MRI. *Am J Obstet Gynecol*. 2014;210:452.e1-452.e8.
162. Cavanagh J, Krishnadas R, Batty GD, et al. Socioeconomic status and the cerebellar grey matter volume. Data from a well-characterised population sample. *Cerebellum*. 2013;12:882-891.
165. Limperopoulos C, Bassan H, Gauvreau K, et al. Does cerebellar injury in premature infants contribute to the high prevalence of long-term cognitive, learning, and behavioral disability in survivors? *Pediatrics*. 2007;120:584-593.
174. Van Kooij BJ, Benders MJ, Anbeek P, et al. Cerebellar volume and proton magnetic resonance spectroscopy at term, and neurodevelopment at 2 years of age in preterm infants. *Dev Med Child Neurol*. 2012;54:260-266.
175. Messerschmidt A, Fuiko R, Prayer D, et al. Disrupted cerebellar development in preterm infants is associated with impaired neurodevelopmental outcome. *Eur J Pediatr*. 2008;167:1141-1147.

Electroencephalography in the Preterm and Term Infant

130

Maria Roberta Cilio | Francesco Pisani

INTRODUCTION

Despite the evolution of new technologies for assessing neonatal brain function, electroencephalography (EEG) remains one of the most valuable diagnostic and prognostic tools. It is considered the gold standard for distinguishing epileptic seizures from nonepileptic paroxysmal events and for detecting subclinical seizure activity in high-risk babies. In babies who are severely ill, EEG is a more efficient predictive test than the neurologic examination. Background patterns, more than the presence or absence of seizures, correlate significantly with the long-term outcome. The prognostic value of neonatal EEG has long been recognized in term and preterm infants, and its value can be increased by obtaining early recording (e.g., within the first 48 hours of life and prior to administration of antiepileptic drugs [AEDs]), prolonged recording to include samples of different activity states, and serial EEGs at short intervals to assess rapid changes that are likely to occur in high-risk infants. Different drugs currently used in the neonatal intensive care unit (NICU), especially if in the toxic range, can alter the EEG background. Those effects need to be considered in the interpretation of neonatal EEG. It is important to distinguish neonatal seizures from neonatal-onset epilepsies and epilepsy syndromes. Both benign and severe neonatal epilepsy syndromes exist. Benign familial neonatal seizures represent a neonatal syndrome with benign outcome, whereas early myoclonic encephalopathy (EME) and Ohtahara syndrome (OS) are severe epilepsy syndromes.

In the past decade, neonatal EEG has faced a phase of renewal due to increased possibilities of data elaboration and display because of digital acquisition allowing for continuous video-EEG (vEEG) monitoring. The use of vEEG has now entered everyday clinical practice in many NICUs, leading to improved diagnosis and prognostication ability, brain function assessment, and neonatal seizure diagnostic rate.

Conventional EEG with simultaneous video recording is now considered the standard of care in many institutions.[1] It is used for routine examination, usually lasting 30 to 90 minutes, and well as for continuous monitoring. It is considered the gold standard for seizure diagnosis, seizure characterization, and quantification of seizure burden in newborns. It allows clinicians to determine the exact localization of seizure onset and of their propagation[2] and can provide detailed information on brain maturation, acute or remote brain injury, prognosis, and response to AEDs. However, not every institution has ready access to it, or at least not on a 24-hour basis,[3] and there is limited availability of expertise in performing and interpreting EEG in the neonatal period. On the other hand, with the development of new therapeutic strategies for hypoxic-ischemic encephalopathy (HIE), such as hypothermia, there has been great interest in generating alternative strategies for the continuous assessment of brain function in the neonate, including trend analysis of EEG recordings such as amplitude-integrated EEG (aEEG). aEEG is a simplified method of continuous cerebral function monitoring that has become common clinical practice in the NICU, as it can be easily interpreted by neonatologists and bedside nurses.

aEEG is an EEG-based bedside brain-monitoring tool.[4] It displays one or two channels of EEG data after filtering, rectification, and smoothing, on a semilogarithmic scale.[5] Studies have demonstrated reliability in assessing background activity and degree of HIE, with good correlation with outcome[6]; however, its use for seizure detection is debated, and it is generally agreed that it has to be considered as a screening, complementary tool[2,7] and that reference to conventional or "raw" EEG should be made in order to increase sensitivity and specificity.[8,9] In fact, aEEG has a number of limitations (e.g., seizures of short duration and focal seizures remote from the recording electrodes might be missed), and these must be taken into account.[1,9]

The combined use of both of these techniques provides complementary benefits of (1) displaying aEEG on the bedside monitor to assist neonatologists in prompt decision making and (2) allowing full revision and interpretation by neonatal neurologists or neurophysiologists for subsequent diagnostic confirmation or useful refinements.[2]

In this chapter we will focus on conventional EEG, its technical aspects and major indications, behavioral states, characteristics of physiologic and pathologic EEG patterns according to postmenstrual age (PMA), and principal electrographic features of common clinical disorders, including seizures. Finally, we will give an overview of the EEG patterns seen in neonatal-onset epilepsies and epileptic encephalopathy and provide information for early diagnosis.

TECHNICAL ASPECTS

Neonatal EEG recordings should cause the least possible distress to the newborn in order to reduce interference with behavior.

To properly assess the neonatal EEG, it is necessary to interpret it in light of the PMA at the time of the recording, the behavioral state, the clinical data including medication history,[10] and the presence and depth of therapeutic hypothermia. Furthermore, the recording should include a complete cycle of wakefulness, active sleep, and quiet sleep in infants aged at least 30 weeks of conceptional age (CA), or include the most continuous and most discontinuous pattern and last at least 40 minutes in infants aged less than 30 weeks CA, in whom indeterminate sleep is the most consistent behavioral state.[11,12] The American Clinical Neurophysiology Society (ACNS) recommends[2] the application of 11 scalp electrodes according to the International 10 to 20 System modified for neonates (Fp1, C3, T3, O1; Fp2, C4, T4, O2; Fz, Cz, Pz; Fig. 130.1).

The standard recommended bipolar montages are the longitudinal and the transverse.[13]

Because the current gold standard for correct state classification and differential diagnosis of paroxysmal events is represented by polygraphic vEEG, the following noncerebral signals should also be simultaneously recorded: (1) electrooculogram, (2) electromyography, (3) electrocardiogram, and (4) pneumogram;[2,10] in addition, a video camera should be synchronized with the EEG.[2] Along with the information derived from polygraphic vEEG recording, careful annotations from the attending technologist are very useful in describing the patient's activity (e.g., eye opening/closing, subtle movements, hiccup, sucking), handling by ward personnel, beginning and end of drug administration, and artifacts when difficult to remove. With

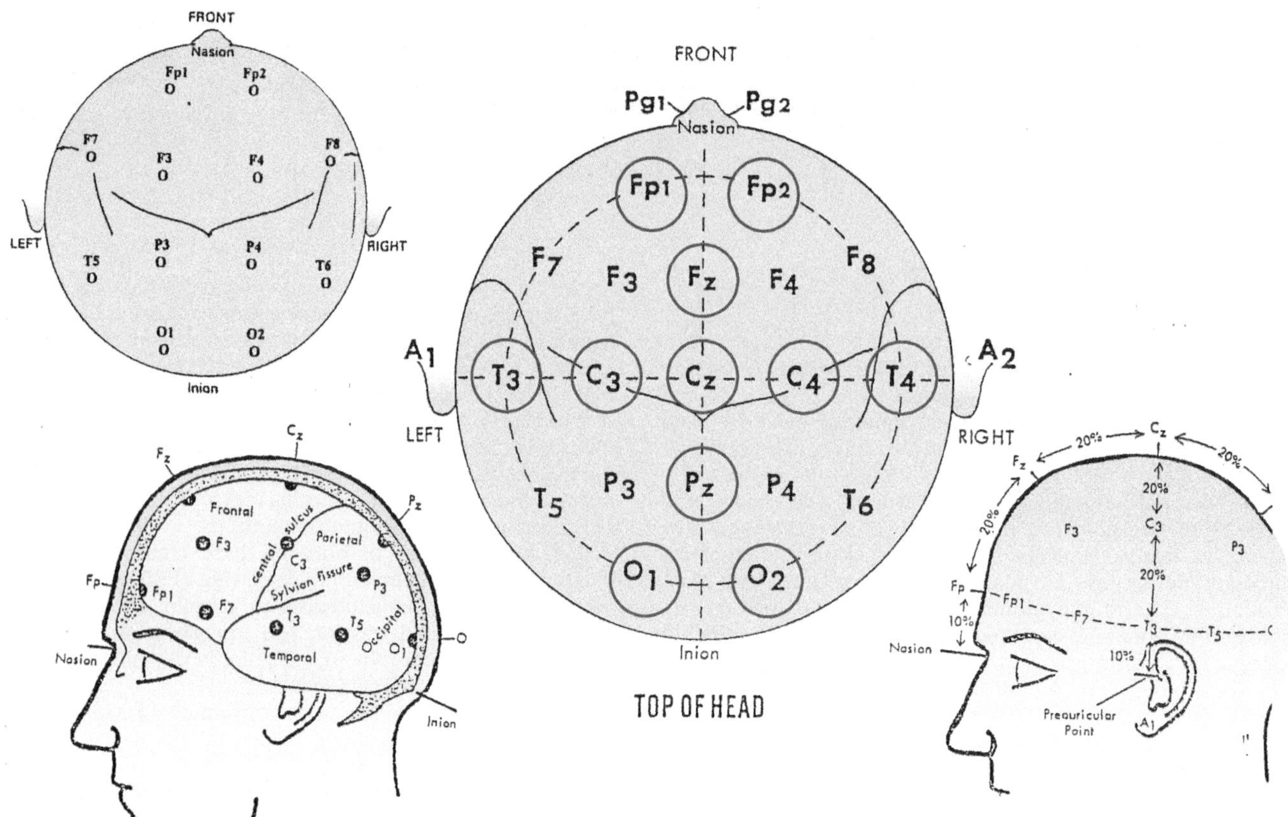

Fig. 130.1 The International 10 to 20 System for electrode placement, modified for neonates. Electrode positions circled in *red* are included in the typical neonatal montage.

digital tracings it is also important to remember the importance of sampling frequency, which is recommended to be at least of 256 Hz.

INDICATIONS AND AIMS

EEG recording should be considered as an important part of the neurologic evaluation of the critically ill newborns admitted to the NICU, as these patients constitute a group at high risk of neurologic sequelae in whom assessment of brain function exclusively by means of neurologic examination might prove challenging, for example because of iatrogenic paralysis.[2] EEG should be considered for concerns about the neonate's neurologic status or the possibility of seizures, and when specific risk factors exist (e.g., fetal distress, central nervous system infection, HIE, preterm birth, intracranial hemorrhage, cardiac surgery).[1] The literature has widely demonstrated that only a small percentage of neonatal seizures have a clinical correlate,[14,15] and therefore vEEG monitoring is recommended to diagnose subclinical siezures.[1] According to the ACNS, monitoring should be performed for a period of 24 hours,[2] although some research has proven an increased risk in the first 36-hour period, and some centers monitor for longer durations.[16–18]

In the presence of suspicious clinical events, EEG is necessary in the differential diagnosis of abnormal movements,[2] such as myoclonic jerks, lip-smacking, pedaling, or boxing, and other paroxysmal events or fluctuating autonomic signs[9] to exclude or confirm a diagnosis of neonatal seizures and possibly avoid unnecessary prescription of anticonvulsant therapy. When this constitutes the indication for conventional EEG, its duration should primarily depend on the ability to record multiple typical clinical events.[2]

Once the diagnosis of neonatal seizures is confirmed, prolonged or continuous monitoring is used to assess seizure burden and diagnose neonatal status epilepticus,[19,20] which has therapeutic and prognostic significance. EEG is mandatory to monitor effectiveness of antiseizure drugs (ASDs) as well as in the differential diagnosis between true response and uncoupling, which has been reported in 58% of newborns with persistent seizures after either phenobarbital or phenytoin.[21] Once the true response, which is absence of EEG seizures, has been achieved, it is recommended to continue EEG monitoring until the patient has been seizure-free for 24 hours; it is also advisable to monitor for seizure recurrence during and after discontinuation of ASDs.[2]

EEG helps assess the functional extent of brain injury by evaluating the degree of abnormality of background EEG patterns and, especially with serial recordings, predict neurologic outcome according to its dynamic evolution over time.[2] Proper evaluation of background activity includes recording of wakefulness, active sleep, and quiet sleep and usually requires at least 1 hour for recording,[2] or longer in case of disruption of sleep rhythms after the acute phase of encephalopathy.[22] This has been extensively studied in the context of acute HIE but holds true for different etiologies. For example, in newborns with meningitis, the degree of background abnormality and the presence of seizures have been demonstrated to be outcome predictors.[23] In the context of HIE, even a brief EEG assessment can be useful in predicting neurologic outcome[24] and short-term risk of neonatal seizures in the following 18 to 24 hours, depending on the background activity.[16] However, several studies conducted during hypothermia treatment for HIE demonstrated that continuous EEG monitoring provides the most accurate information.[25,26] Monitoring of a burst-suppression (BS) pattern with conventional EEG is also advisable when the aim is to quantify interburst intervals (IBIs), for example in the course of metabolic encephalopathies, in which progressive shortening of IBI has been correlated with medical correction of hyperammonemia,[27] or when the BS is drug-induced in the context of treatment of refractory status epilepticus. In this second scenario, conventional EEG would also allow for the detection of ongoing seizure activity.[2] In preterm newborns, EEG can help in determining the most likely timing of a brain insult by distinguishing between acute- and chronic-stage abnormalities, whereas with serial EEGs beginning immediately after birth the degree of severity can also be estimated.[28]

vEEG can allow for the early detection of electroclinical features that can suggest a focal cerebral injury,[29] for example in the context of perinatal ischemic stroke or in case of subarachnoid or subdural hemorrhage.[30] EEG might point to a focal structural etiology by identifying focal electrographic seizures, focal sharp waves, or focal attenuation of background activities,[1] which would prompt neuroimaging (Fig. 130.2). A study on perinatal arterial ischemic stroke confirmed suppression over the infarcted side, together with the presence of unilateral theta bursts intermixed with sharp or spike waves. Seizure patterns characteristically consisted of focal sharp/spikes/polispikes at 1 to 2 Hz and a predominance of electrographic-only seizures.[31] Even if other methods for detection of seizures in the newborn such as aEEG are becoming readily available, vEEG remains the gold standard for the diagnosis of neonatal-onset epilepsies and epileptic encephalopathies. Finally, EEG monitoring can contribute to NICU decisions to continue medical care, offer supportive care,[29] or, in countries where this decision is applicable, withdraw care.

BEHAVIORAL STATES

The term *behavioral states* describes a series of physiologic and behavioral variables[32] that when interpreted together provide the basis for identification of wakefulness and/or sleep states required for the correct interpretation of EEG. The ACNS Critical Care Monitoring Committee established that a behavioral state should be considered as present when its features are recognizable for at least 1 minute.[33]

Wakefulness is defined by the presence of eyes open, a condition that is not possible before 24 weeks PMA, when eyelids are still fused together.[34] In the preterm newborn, at around 32 to 34 weeks PMA, other polysomnographic signs (e.g., irregular respiratory pattern, phasic or tonic chin electromyographic (EMG) activity, the presence of body movements) can reliably contribute to the wakefulness definition.[33] In the healthy term infant, wakefulness is defined by the association of the above-stated behavioral condition with the presence of the *activité moyenne* as the background activity (Fig. 130.3).[33] This is a typical EEG pattern of the full-term newborn corresponding to wakefulness or to active sleep state characterized by continuous electric activity with prevalent delta-theta frequencies, with an amplitude between 25 and 50 μV, with superimposed beta activity.

Two different types of eyes-open wakefulness can be recognized: active (distinguished by the presence of agitation) and quiet wakefulness.

To recognize sleep states, it is necessary to combine data from observation of the clinical state of the newborn together with EEG and polygraphic information, especially linked to the presence of rapid eye movements (REMs), which represent a hallmark of REM sleep (also known as *active sleep* in the newborn). Periods in which the various characteristic physiologic parameters cannot be unequivocally identified correspond to *indeterminate or undifferentiated sleep*, which is also called *transitional* when separating two periods of well-identifiable sleep states. The first appearance of the sleep-wake cycle has been reported in neonates between 25 and 30 weeks PMA.[35] By 30 weeks gestation the concordance between electrographic and clinical indicators of behavioral states begins to arise, although this is not consistent. Between 24 and 27 weeks PMA, neonates typically remain in an indeterminate sleep, characterized by few ocular movements and poorly variable heart rate.[36] More recently, it has been argued that criteria developed in term or near-term neonates are not applicable to extremely preterm newborns and that a differentiation between states based on REM and EEG activity alone should be used instead, as body movements are not reliable in defining sleep states in this population.[37] Following this approach, rudimentary REM (high-voltage, more continuous EEG activity) and non-REM (more discontinuous EEG) sleep states can be recognized as early as 25 weeks CA.[38]

Sleep onset in the neonatal period is marked by the appearance of active sleep, which is characterized by the presence of REM, small and large body movements, irregular respiration, and, in the term infant, continuous activity on the EEG. Beyond 35 weeks CA, two different types of active sleep can be recognized: active sleep 1 (AS 1), which precedes quiet sleep and is characterized by high-amplitude mixed pattern, and active sleep 2 (AS 2), which follows quiet sleep and is characterized by a low-voltage irregular pattern. Active sleep in the preterm infant is initially characterized by a *tracé discontinu* (discontinuous tracing) on the EEG (predominating before 28 weeks CA), and movements tend to include segmental myoclonus or generalized myoclonic and tonic posturing. Continuous EEG activity is observed by 34 weeks CA. By 28 to 31 weeks CA, periods of concordance can be recorded (eyes closed, REM, irregular respirations, body movements, and continuous EEG).[33]

In the preterm, quiet sleep is initially characterized by a *tracé discontinu* (emerging at around 28 weeks CA and recorded only during quiet sleep by 34 to 36 weeks CA).[39] The pattern of quiet sleep is fully developed at 36 to 37 weeks CA and is defined by absent REM, increased EMG tone, regular respiration, absent body movements and possibly chin movements, occasional sucking activity, and generalized myoclonic startles.[33,40] At term, two different types of quiet sleep activity can be distinguished: tracé alternant (TA) and high-voltage slow (HVS) pattern, the latter of which is first recorded at 36 weeks CA and replaces TA at 44 to 45 weeks CA.[41] Finally, by 4 to 8 weeks post-term, sleep spindles appear.[33,40]

At term, a complete sleep and waking cycle typically lasts 3 to 4 hours[11] with a sleep cycle of 50 to 60 minutes,[42] in contrast to 30 to 50 minutes in preterm infants less than 35 weeks CA.[33] In extremely preterm infants born at 24 to 26 weeks CA, the duration of those periods varies widely from approximately 9 to 55 minutes.[38] The percentage of time the newborn spends in quiet sleep increases with age: at 27 to 34 weeks CA, 40% to 45% of sleeping time is spent in active sleep, 25% to 30% in quiet sleep, and 30% in indeterminate sleep, whereas at term, approximately 50% to 60% of a sleep cycle is spent in active sleep, 30% to 40% in quiet sleep, and 10% to 15% in transitional sleep.[43,44] Quiet sleep is an important state to record because of the higher frequency of EEG abnormalities[10] and because an increase in indeterminate sleep at the expense of quiet sleep may be a sign of encephalopathy, even in the presence of a normal waking or active sleep tracing.[45]

To acknowledge the presence of a liability of the background activity in infants with disrupted EEG features that make recognition of definite specific sleep states impossible, the ACNS has defined the condition of unspecified state changes in which a cycling between different EEG patterns can be recognized due to modifications in the amount of discontinuity, voltage, or frequencies of a minimum duration of 1 minute each.[33]

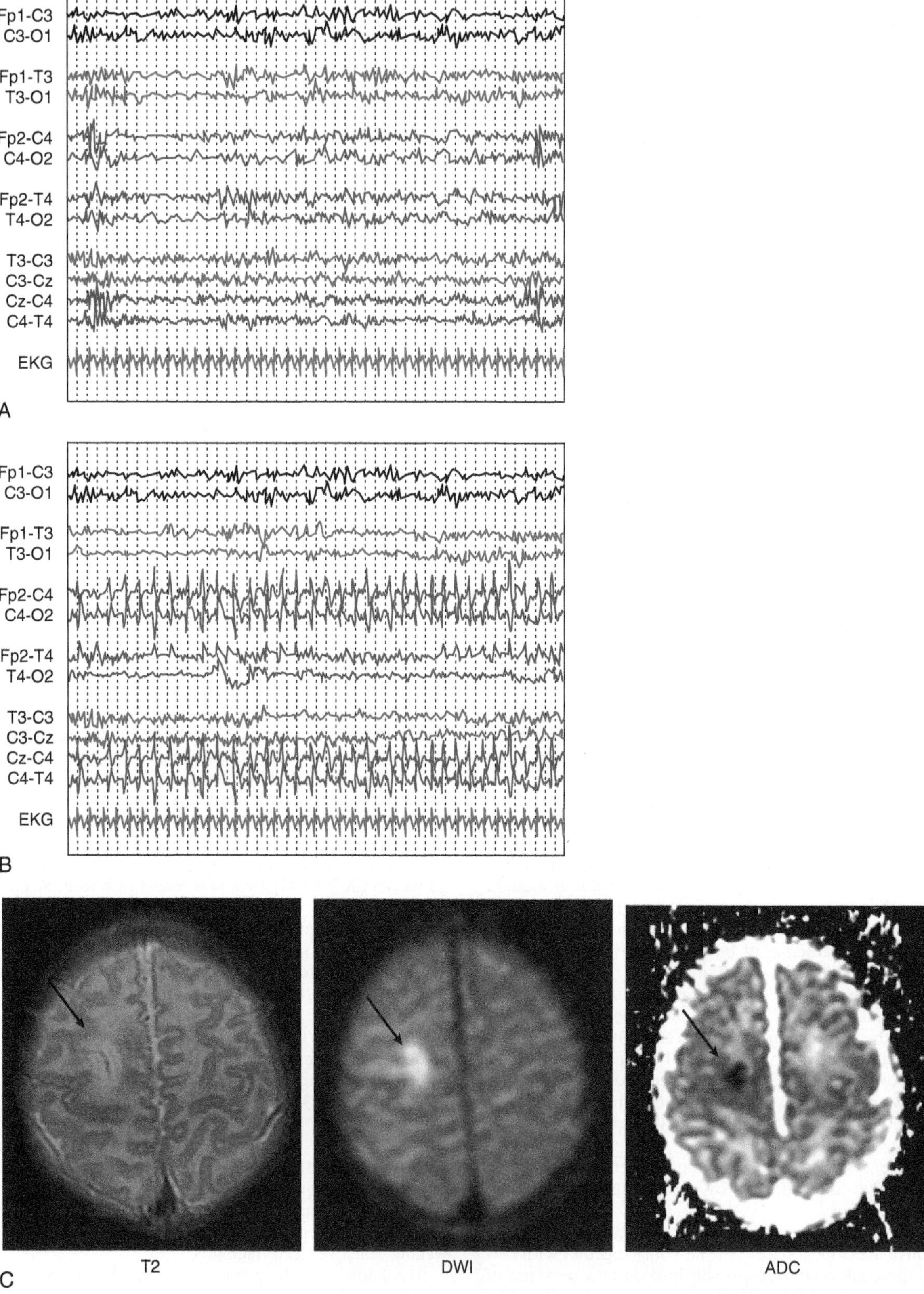

Fig. 130.2 One-day-old term neonate presenting with prolonged focal clonic jerking of the left arm. (A) Interictal spikes are seen over the right central region over a normal background. (B) Ictal discharge characterized by rhythmic spikes followed by slow waves with the spikes being time-locked with the clonic jerks. Gain, 10 μV/mm; high frequency filter, 70 Hz; paper speed, 15 mm/s. (C) MRI showing a focal ischemic stroke on the right central region concordant with the location of the interictal and ictal discharges on electroencephalography. *ADC*, Apparent diffusion coefficient; *DWI*, diffusion-weighted imaging.

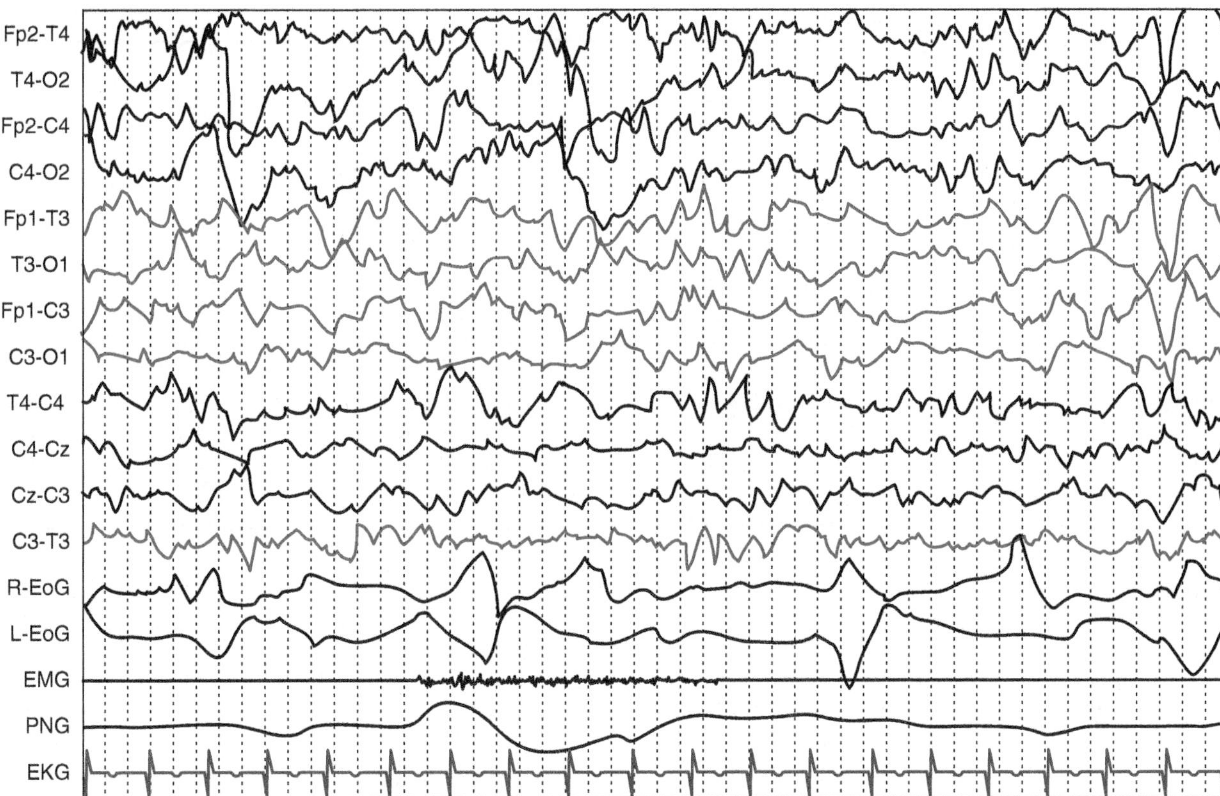

Fig. 130.3 Healthy term newborn. Quiet wakefulness. Delta-theta medium-to-high voltage continuous background activity with intermixed low voltage fast rhythms *(activité moyenne)*. Note the presence of ocular movements, muscular activity, and irregularity of the respiratory pattern. Polygraphic video-electroencephalography (EEG, EOG: electro-oculogram, EMG: right deltoid, PNG: pneumogram, EKG). Gain, 7 µV/mm; high-frequency filter, 70 Hz; paper speed, 10 mm/s.

PHYSIOLOGIC ELECTROENCEPHALOGRAPHY TRACINGS

The major characteristics of neonatal EEG comprise its reactivity, the temporal organization (defined by continuity, symmetry, and synchrony), and spatial organization (mainly defined by the presence of physiologic features constituting maturational hallmarks, which characteristically appear at a certain CA, peak to a period of maximum expression, and then progressively decline).

REACTIVITY

Reactivity represents the ability of the functional activity of the brain to modify in response to internal and external stimuli. This includes changes in continuity, amplitude, and/or frequencies accompanying changes in behavioral state[40] and changes in background activity after a provocative stimulus. Reactivity is PMA- and state-dependent and should be distinguished from clinical reaction to stimulation. It is best evaluated during quiet sleep[46] and is detectable, although still variable, from 28 to 29 weeks PMA,[47] becoming more consistent at 30 to 31 weeks PMA, when stimulation during quiet sleep provokes the transient appearance of a continuous activity, whereas if performed during active sleep, it elicits a decrease in amplitude. At 35 to 36 weeks CA, reactivity can be more clearly visualized as a general transient decrease in background activity during active sleep and in the appearance of a high-amplitude continuous slow wave activity if performed during quiet sleep. At term, auditory, tactile, or painful stimuli can induce either attenuation or reinforcement of the background EEG activity.[10]

TEMPORAL ORGANIZATION

The first hallmark of an EEG is its degree of continuity. Continuity is defined as the uninterrupted presence of electrical activity, with minimal amplitude of 25 µV and less than 2 seconds of voltage attenuation below this value, lasting at least 1 minute.[10,33] Extremely preterm newborns (24 to 28 weeks PMA) have almost exclusively discontinuous tracings (Fig. 130.4).[48-50] Continuity is present in active sleep beginning at approximately 28 weeks PMA. By 32 weeks of gestational age, continuous EEG dominates over discontinuous activity,[34] and it is constant in both sleep states in healthy term newborns (at least 39 weeks PMA).[10] One experimental study found normal EEG continuity to correlate with measures of cortical sulcation and surface and longer periods of inactivity in the first day of life to relate to less cortical surface and lower total brain volume.[51]

In the normal neonatal EEG in term infants, amplitude, frequencies, and distribution of transients should be equally represented on both hemispheres. In other words, the EEG should be symmetrical. However, in premature newborns, asymmetry is not considered pathologic unless it exceeds 50% over one hemisphere and is persistent.[33]

Synchrony, defined as the onset of bursts of activity that occur nearly simultaneously between hemispheres,[33] changes with PMA in a nonlinear fashion, being almost complete for high-amplitude bursts up to 28-weeks PMA, when it transiently decreases until approximately 30 weeks PMA and finally gradually increases to become almost complete at term.[10,33] From 35 to 43 weeks PMA, asymmetry, asynchrony, and transient flattening, frequently unilateral, can be seen at the onset of quiet sleep with no pathologic implications.[52] One proposed operational definition implies a delay longer than 1.5 seconds between bursts of identical waveforms.[53]

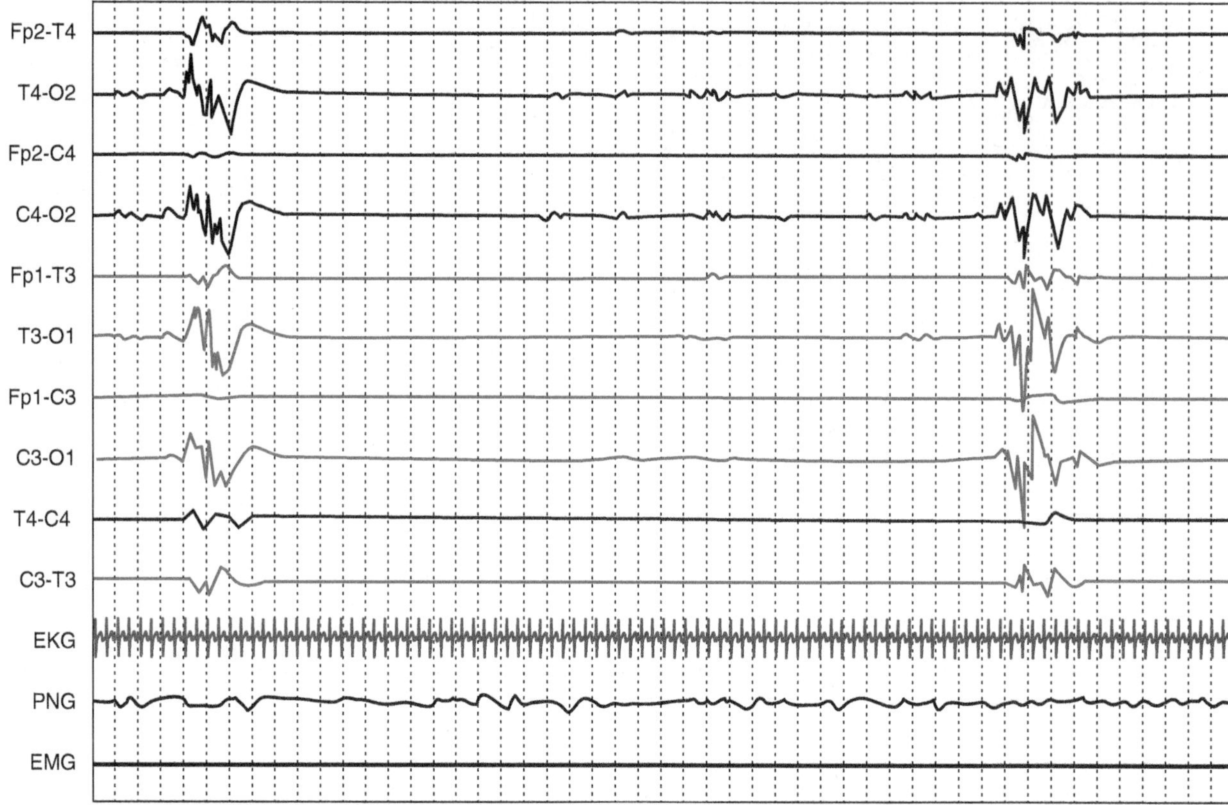

Fig. 130.4 Polygraphic electroencephalography tracing recorded at 1 week of age (25 weeks postmenstrual age) in a preterm neonate born at 24 weeks. Discontinuous tracing. Delta bursts of 3 seconds duration, intermixed with interburst interval of 25 seconds (EEG, EKG, PNG: pneumogram, EMG: right deltoid). Gain, 15 μV/mm; high frequency filter, 70 Hz; paper speed, 120 mm/s.

Physiologic features, which are the main element determining spatial organization, will be described separately.

BACKGROUND PATTERNS

The evolution of EEG patterns in the immature brain is the expression of ongoing cornerstone maturational processes. In fact, during early phases of development, the increase in the complexity of EEG waveforms parallels that of gyration, whereas spatial synchrony is related to the growth in thalamocortical and corticocortical connections.[54] Early electrical activity in neuronal networks has a fundamental role in trophism and guidance for activity-dependent neuronal wiring.[55,56] Through experimental models, it has been possible to demonstrate that spontaneous and intermittent ("discontinuous") activity is highly conserved during maturation in different species[57] and is already present before sensory mechanisms become active.[55,58] Furthermore, the development of a more continuous tracing is temporally linked to the maturation of γ-aminobutyric acid (GABA) receptors toward an inhibitory function.[59,60]

TERM NEWBORN

The background EEG activity of the term newborn is characterized by a continuous tracing, corresponding to *activité moyenne* in wakefulness, to the "mixed frequency tracing" during AS 1, and to the "low-voltage irregular pattern" in AS 2.[40] *Activité moyenne* consists of irregular delta-theta activity, generally with amplitudes of 25 to 50 μV (but up to 100 μV), being higher over the posterior regions. Rhythmic, mainly theta, activity is usually superimposed, especially over the central regions, whereas irregular alpha and beta rhythms up to 30 μV are superimposed over all areas.[10,61] During "low-voltage irregular pattern," EEG is dominated by low-voltage fast theta over all scalp regions, together with slower components.[40]

During quiet sleep, the EEG of the term infant can either show a *tracé alternant* (alternating tracing) or to "high-voltage slow" patterns. The former usually predominates between 37 weeks PMA, when it first appears, and 44 weeks PMA, and is characterized by bilateral synchronous and symmetrical bursts of delta waves of 50 to 150 μV over a continuous theta activity of 25 to 50 μV, in which the two approximately show the same duration, from 3 to 8 seconds (Fig. 130.5).[10] This pattern is reactive to stimuli and alternates with the continuous pattern of active sleep. It can be distinguished from the pathologic BS pattern by the presence of HVS wave activity alternating with periods of low voltage, which is higher compared with the very low, suppressed, interburst activity of the BS pattern. The HVS pattern (or *tracé lent continu*) first appears at 38 weeks PMA and is characterized by a continuous delta activity predominating over occipital areas with an amplitude between 50 and 150 μV (Fig. 130.6).[10]

PRETERM NEWBORN

The EEG undergoes relevant changes in preterm babies, with gradual transition from a discontinuous to a more continuous tracing, a decrease in amplitude of ongoing activities, and a reduction in the total amount of delta waves with the appearance of a polyrhythmic pattern. With advancing PMA, the percentage of time showing discontinuous background patterns significantly diminishes. Hayakawa and colleagues found a mean percentage of discontinuous activity of 69% at 21 to 22 weeks PMA and of 48.4% at 25 to 26 weeks PMA.[62] At 32 weeks PMA, discontinuous activity corresponds to 50% and by approximately 35 weeks PMA the EEG is continuous during the awake state. This increase in the length of periods of activity and reduction in the length of periods of inactivity can be seen in relation to a maturation in

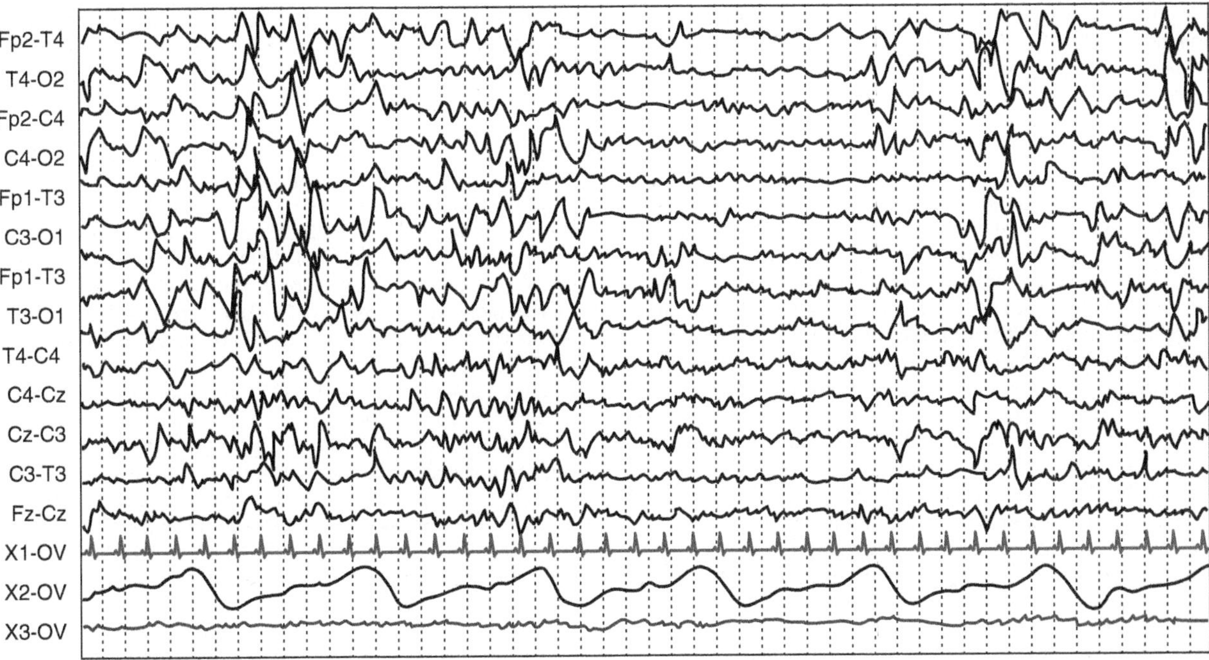

Fig. 130.5 Ten-day-old term newborn. Pattern of *tracé alternant* during quiet sleep characterized by bilateral synchronous and symmetrical bursts of delta waves of high amplitude alternating with theta activity of lower amplitude. Gain, 10 μV/mm; high frequency filter, 70 Hz; paper speed, 15 mm/s.

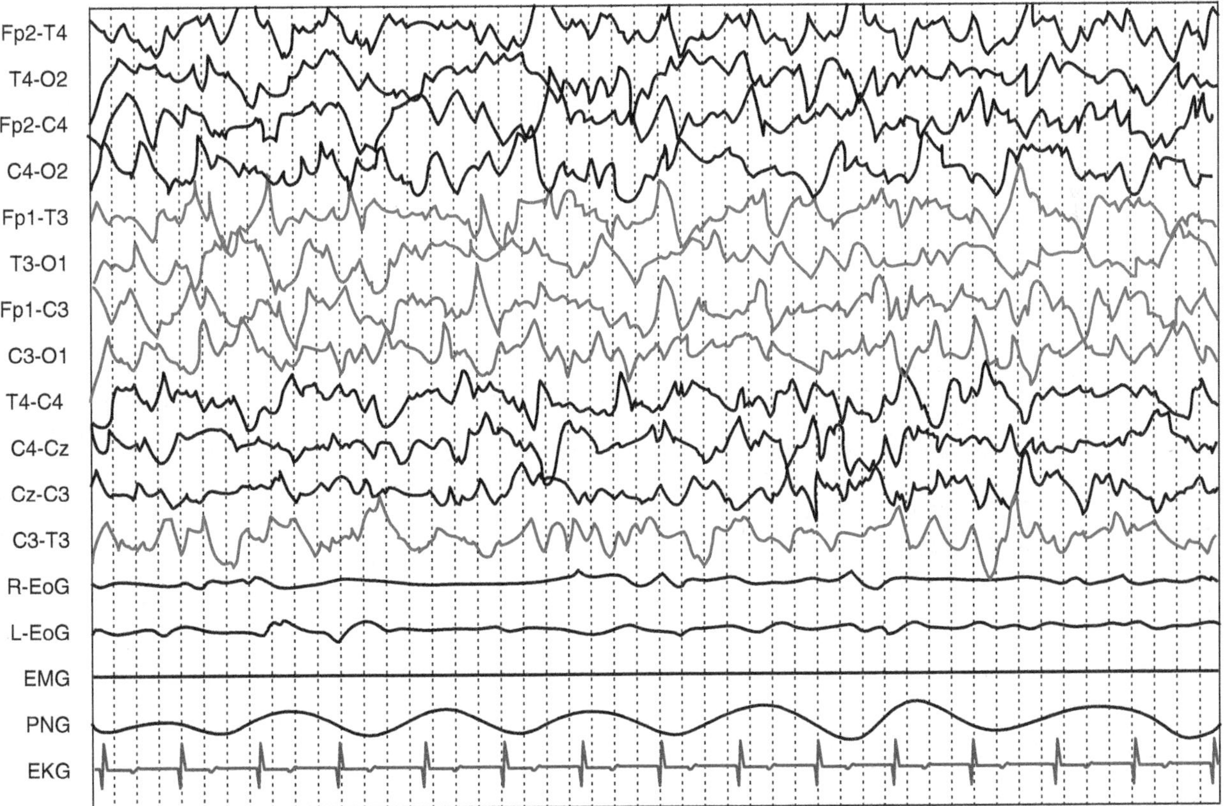

Fig. 130.6 Term newborn. Quiet sleep, high-voltage slow pattern, characterized by continuous delta activity of high-medium voltage. Behavioral state is confirmed by the regularity of the respiratory pattern and the absence of rapid ocular movements. Polygraphic video-electroencephalography (R-EoG: right electro-oculogram, L-EoG: left electro-oculogram, EMG, PNG: pneumogram, EKG). Gain, 7 μV/mm; high frequency filter, 70 Hz; paper speed, 30 mm/s.

the excitatory synapses; a reduced drive from subcortical areas responsible for the abrupt bihemispheric inhibition of cortical activity is also related. This is also considered to play a prominent role in the high synchrony of the bursts before 30 weeks PMA, when it constitutes an important maturational criterion.[38,63–65] It has been shown that neuronal networks seem to express a different development in posterior and frontal areas, as frontally prominent networks emerge only in term newborns.[56]

Discontinuous tracing, which is the hallmark of preterm EEG,[66] is defined as an EEG pattern of bursts of physiologic activity appropriate for the gestational age separated by intervals of variably defined amplitudes (<25 µV[10] or 10 µV[66]), with a duration of more than 3 seconds. The duration of both the bursts and the intervals of lower amplitude vary according to gestational age; they not appear to be consistent in the different studies.[10] There is a growing interest in understanding early neuronal activity functioning, which is profoundly different from what is found in the mature brain.[56,57,67] In a study of preterm infants of less than 30 weeks PMA, the maximum duration of IBI significantly correlated with the degree of cortical folding.[68]

Although EEG features in near-term neonates are better known, it is difficult to describe normal features in extremely preterm neonates due to the poor concordance between studies regarding the amplitude of bursts and duration of IBI, the number of electrodes on which activity must be present, and the limited number of healthy subjects without brain injury or neurotropic medications.[66]

Among the most precocious recordings reported was that of Hayakawa and coworkers, who described the characteristics of EEGs undertaken at 21 to 22 weeks PMA and found a mean and a maximum IBI duration of 25.8 and 18.4 seconds, respectively (with wide ranges), and a mean burst duration of 4.3 seconds.[62] However, the whole sample size was small and the differences between the group of preterm infants of 21 to 22 weeks and preterms of 23 to 24 weeks PMA were not statistically significant, although there were statistical differences when those were compared with preterm infants aged 25 to 26 weeks PMA.[62]

Between 24 and 27 weeks PMA, bursts constitute close to 35% of the recording.[38] At 28 to 29 weeks, longer reported bursts can last up to 10 minutes.[66] IBIs represent approximately 45% of the recording at 24 to 27 weeks, and the cutoff for the longest discontinuity considered physiologic is 60 seconds or less at 24 weeks,[38] and it decreases to 20 seconds or less at 30 weeks.[69]

In younger newborns, amplitudes are higher (100 to 300 µV) and frequencies are lower (0.5 to 1 Hz), with some superimposed faster rhythms of 5 to 9 Hz.[66] Maturation mainly consists of a progressive displacement of delta waves to the central-occipital areas. Those are initially mainly synchronous and smooth, then increasingly superimposed by fast activities.[47] Occipital delta waves are recorded as soon as 25 weeks PMA,[38] whereas frontal delta waves are the least frequent in this extremely low PMA.[38] Rudimentary REM and non-REM sleep states have been identified as early as 25 weeks PMA, provided that concordance among EEG, eye movements, and body movements is not consistent: rudimentary REM sleep is associated with a high-voltage more continuous EEG activity, whereas non-REM sleep is characterized by more discontinuous epochs of recordings.[38,70]

Theta bursts are initially diffuse, then predominate over the occipital and then temporal areas. Two different types of theta bursts have been recognized between 26 and 28 weeks CA: high or very high rhythmic and sharp waves over the temporal areas and lower amplitude bursts predominantly located over the occipital regions,[49] also known as *sharp theta rhythm on the occipital areas of prematures (STOP)*.[49,66] The maturation of theta rhythms from 26 to 28 weeks PMA[49] seems to reflect the posterior-anterior gradient in cerebral maturation that has been documented with magnetic resonance imaging (MRI).[65] Temporal theta rhythms are mainly recorded during sleep.[49,71]

From 24 to 27 weeks PMA, temporal slow waves occur either isolated or in short sequences, more often unilaterally, whereas occipital and central slow waves appear monophasic, smooth, or with superimposed fast rhythms (Fig. 130.7). Frontal slow waves are also present at this stage, although less abundant, either with

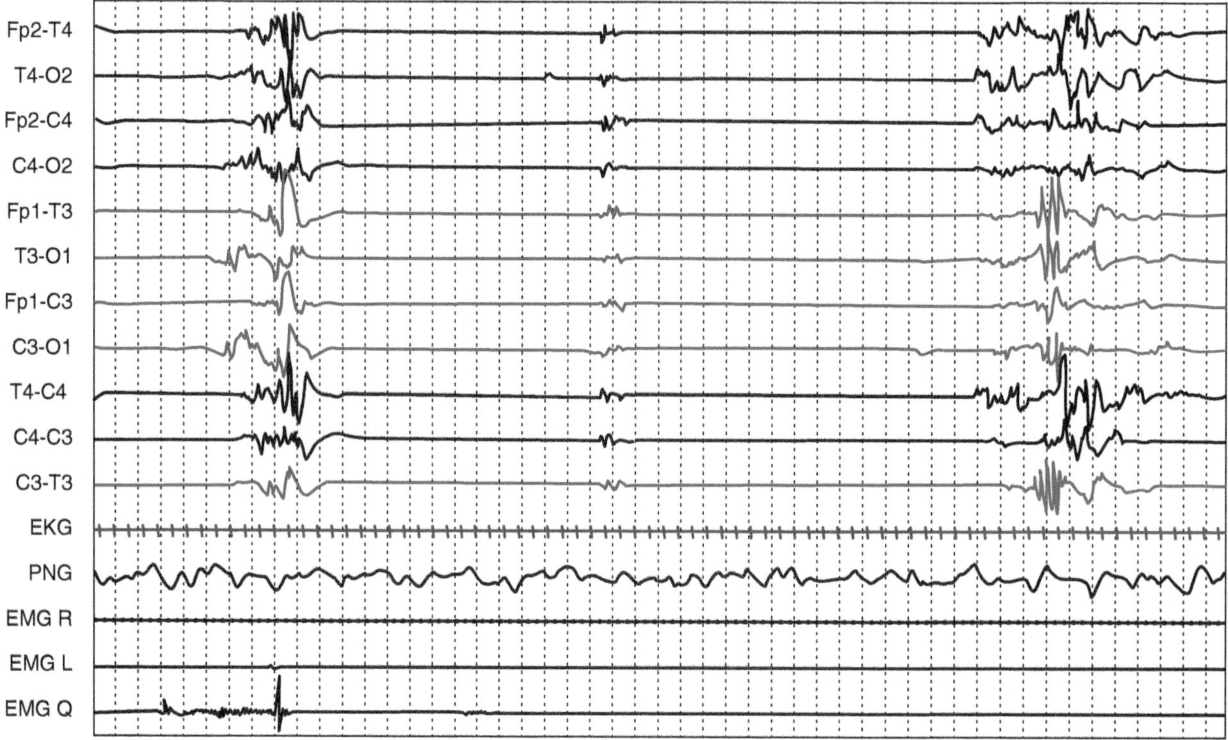

Fig. 130.7 Preterm newborn born at 24 weeks postmenstrual age (PMA), recorded at 4 weeks of age (28 weeks PMA). Interburst intervals of 9 and 12 seconds, respectively. Polygraphic electroencephalography recording (EKG, PNG: pneumogram; EMG R: right deltoid; EMG L: left deltoid; EMG Q: quadriceps). Gain, 30 µV/mm; high frequency filter, 70 Hz; paper speed, 120 mm/s.

a sharp and rapid morphology or slower and smoother.[38] At 24 to 25 weeks, short bursts of synchronous HVS waves are also observed,[38] disappearing before 28 weeks.[66] At 28 to 29 weeks, the temporal slow waves are of intermediate amplitude, whereas the occipital ones show the highest voltages and the lowest frequency, and there are abundant central slow waves of low amplitude and duration of greater than 1 second. Waves of higher frequency are also superimposed.[66]

At 30 weeks PMA, bursts of delta waves have slightly lower amplitude and are more frequent over the occipital area. They can show a superimposed fast activity with the morphology of delta brushes, which, at younger PMAs, are called *spindle-like fast rhythms* and can be recorded at as soon as 27 weeks.[49] Bursts of theta rhythm, either diffuse or predominant over the temporal areas, can be recorded from 24 weeks, become more abundant at 26 to 27 weeks, and appear more localized over the temporal and occipital areas. At 30 weeks, these theta bursts are observed mainly during quiet sleep and over the temporal areas.[66] Delta waves, mainly synchronous, with superimposed theta, are predominant in the occipital-temporal areas, especially during active sleep, whereas theta activity predominates over the temporal areas, mainly in quiet sleep. Between 32 and 34 weeks, delta brushes are most abundant, and temporal theta activity completely declines (Fig. 130.8). Physiologic duration of IBI corresponds to 15 seconds or less at 32 weeks and 10 seconds or less at 34 weeks CA. At 36 weeks, it is possible to differentiate between AS 1 and AS 2, whereas quiet sleep appears discontinuous or, according to some authors, semi-discontinuous, with periods of low amplitude activity lasting less than 10 seconds.[10]

NORMAL GRAPHOELEMENTS

Important developmental features of neonatal EEG are summarized in Tables 130.1 and 130.2 and are described in the section below.

Monorhythmic Occipital Delta Activity

In healthy preterm newborns, the posterior regions are dominated by runs of HVS bioccipital monorhythmic positive polarity delta activity, lasting 2 to 60 seconds and often being synchronous on the two hemispheres. While they are present at earlier stages, they show a pick between 30 and 33 weeks, decreasing by 34 weeks of age.[38,49,72] It is a highly conservative rhythm, usually still recordable even in the context of severe encephalopathies.[34]

Central-Temporal Delta Activity

This is constituted by sustained trains of semirhythmic delta activity, recorded in the extremely preterm infant, and fading by 34 weeks CA.[34]

Frontal Sharp Transients (Encoches Frontales)

Diphasic (small negative deflection followed by a positive deflection), usually synchronous, they first appear at 35 weeks CA, although immature broad, incomplete, and asymmetrical sharp transients may be seen from 33 weeks CA[10] and disappear after 44 weeks CA.[33] They are often present in transitional phases, especially from active to quiet sleep.[40,73]

Anterior Slow Dysrhythmia

It is represented by monomorphic/polymorphic delta waves over the frontal areas in short runs of a few seconds, appearing at 36 to 37 weeks CA, typically synchronous and symmetric. They tend to markedly decline during wakefulness in the first week in term newborns but persist in sleep throughout the first month.[40]

Delta Brushes

Delta waves (50 to 200 μV, 0.3 to 1 Hz) with superimposed fast activity (8 to 30 Hz, 20 to 200 μV) are first observed at 28 weeks CA, have a maximum expression at 32 to 34 weeks CA

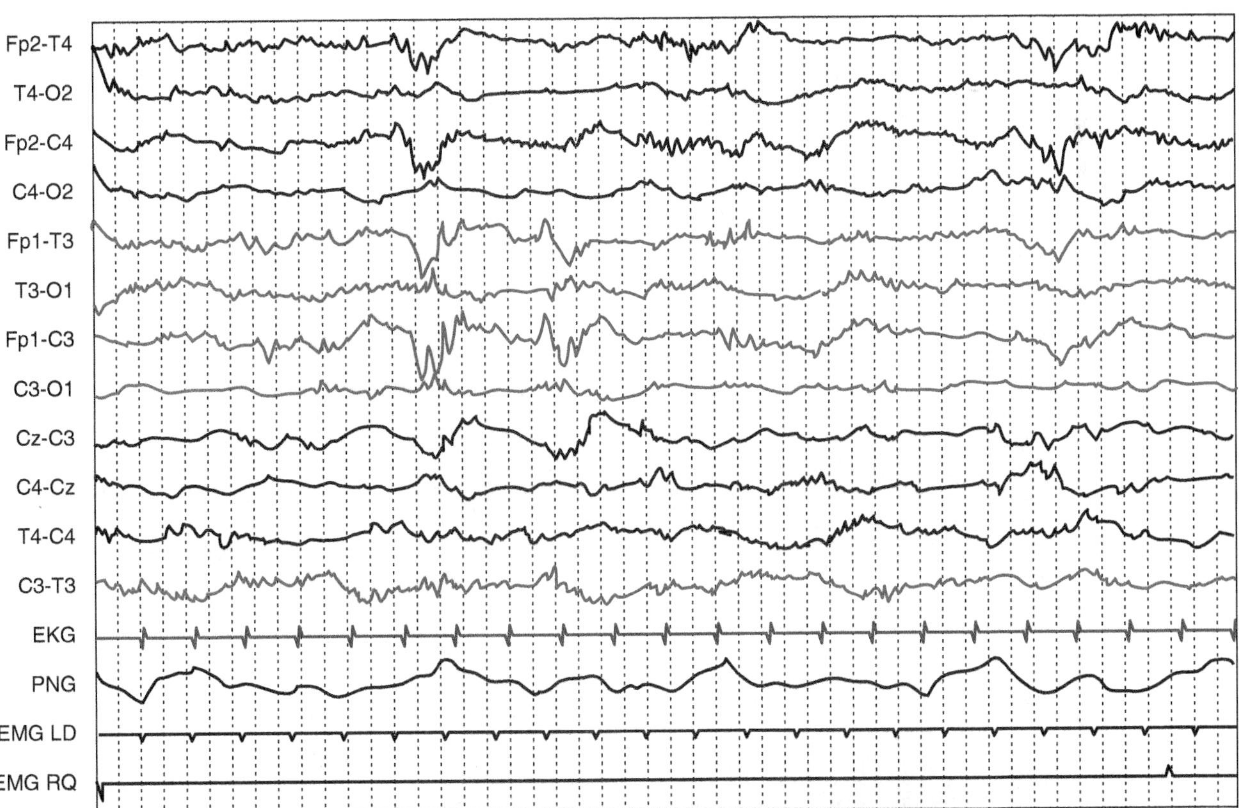

Fig. 130.8 Preterm newborn, 32 weeks gestational age. Active sleep. Continuous tracing with abundant bilateral delta brushes. Polygraphic electroencephalography recording (EKG, PNG: pneumogram, EMG LD: left deltoid; EMG RQ: right quadriceps). Gain, 15 μV/mm; high frequency filter, 70 Hz; paper speed, 30 mm/s.

Table 130.1 Behavioral States, Background Activity, Lability, and Reactivity According to Postmenstrual Age, Based on Developmental Features.

	Postmenstrual Age							
Parameter	**24–25 wk**	**26–27 wk**	**28–29 wk**	**30–31 wk**	**32–34 wk**	**35–36 wk**	**37–38 wk**	**39–41 wk**
Organization and Behavioral States	Activity and rest Association EEG-behavior: inconsistent	AW AS QS Inconsistent	AW AS QS Inconsistent	AW AS QS Rare QW Concordance between EEG and behavioral criteria	AW AS QS Rare QW	AW QW QS AS (from 36 wk CA: AS 1 AS 2)	AW QW QS AS 1, AS 2	AW QW QS AS 1, AS 2
Background Activity	Very discontinuous	Very discontinuous Brief semicontinuous periods	Discontinuous Very variable IBI (≤30 s), longer periods of continuity	AS: continuous/ semidiscontinuous QS: discontinuous (bursts ≥3 s; IBI ≤20 s)	AW: continuous (frequent artefacts) QW: continuous AS: continuous QW: discontinuous (IBI ≤15 s at 32 and ≤10 s at 34 wk CA)	AW, QW: *activité moyenne* (36 wk CA) AS 1: high amplitude continuous AS 2: continuous, lower amplitude, > rapid activity QS: discontinuous/ semidiscontinuous IBI <10 s	AW, QW, AS 2: *activité moyenne* AS 1: high amplitude mixed frequency QS: semidiscontinuous; TA	AW, QW, AS 2: *activité moyenne* AS 1: mixed frequency tracing QS: TA and/ or slow continuous tracing
Lability	Present	Present	Present	Present	Present	Present	Present	Present
Reactivity	Not visible on the EEG Painful stimuli → limb withdrawal	Barely visible with tactile stimulations	Inconstant, variable	AS: decrease in amplitude QS: transiently continuous activity	AS: diffuse decrease in EEG activity QS: transient appearance of continuous slow activity	AS: diffuse transient decrease in background activity QS: continuous high amplitude slow waves	AS: general transient decrease QS: lengthening of slow wave bursts or IBI	Auditory, tactile, and painful stimuli → attenuation of background activity

AS, Active sleep; *AS 1*, active sleep type 1; *AS 2*, active sleep type 2; *AW*, active wakefulness; *CA*, conceptional age; *EEG*, electroencephalography; *IBI*, interburst interval; *QS*, quiet sleep; *QW*, quiet wakefulness; *s*, seconds; *TA*, tracé alternant; *wk*, weeks.

Table 130.2 Spatial and Temporal Organization, and Postmenstrual Age–Dependent Graphoelements, Based on Developmental Features.

Parameter	Postmenstrual Age							
	24–25 wk CA	**26–27 wk CA**	**28–29 wk CA**	**30–31 wk CA**	**32–34 wk CA**	**35–36 wk CA**	**37–38 wk CA**	**39–41 wk CA**
PMA-Dependent Graphoelements	Mono/diphasic delta, >smooth Sharp theta bursts	Diphasic delta (smooth/ theta-alpha superimposed) Sharp theta waves > in bursts (+)	High amplitude mono/diphasic delta Theta waves in isolated bursts (++) Delta brushes (+)	Delta waves with superimposed theta ↑ Theta activity Diffuse delta brushes 31 > 30 wk CA (++)	Temporal theta disappears in AS at 32 and in QS at 33–34 wk CA Delta brushes (+++) Immature frontal transients at 34 wk (>smooth, incomplete, asymmetric)	Diffuse theta waves (AS 2 > AS 1) Delta brushes (AS 1 > AS 2, QS) Immature frontal transients; more mature at the onset of QS ASD in AS 1	Delta waves (> in AS 2) Delta brushes in all behavioral states Clear frontal transients (AS 1; QS onset) ASD in AS 1	Delta brushes only in QS Frontal transients and ASD at 37–38 wk CA Short runs of alpha and delta over rolandic areas
Spatial and Temporal Organization	T slow waves: isolated/in sequences O and C slow waves: bilaterally synchronous/ unilateral Bursts of sharp theta: diffuse/>T	Delta waves (> in central areas) High amplitude delta bursts (>synchronous) over occipital areas Theta waves (temporal > diffuse)	↓ Diffuse delta waves, posterior predominance in AS and QS ↓ Synchrony (persisting over occipital areas) ↓↓ Temporal delta bursts Abundant central delta waves Synchronized diffuse bursts of theta rhythms (> T and O)	Delta waves with theta >O/O-T Delta mainly synchronous, > in AS Theta (>T) > in QS	Delta brushes: O-T at 32, O at 33–34 wk CA	Delta waves > O in AS, diffuse in QS Constantly synchrony in AS Possible asynchrony at the onset of QS	Delta brushes > O in AS and QS Interhemispheric synchrony ↑ Theta waves over C areas in AS 1 and AS 2	Constant symmetry and synchrony (possible asynchrony at the onset of QS) Slow continuous tracing precedes TA in a single QS period

AS, Active sleep; *AS 1*, active sleep type 1; *AS 2*, active sleep type 2; *ASD*, anterior slow dysrhythmia; *C*, central; *CA*, conceptional age; *O*, occipital; *QS*, quiet sleep; *T*, temporal; *TA*, tracé alternant; *wk*, weeks; ↑, increasing; ↓, diminishing; ↓↓, disappearing; (+), present; (++), abundant; (+++), maximal.

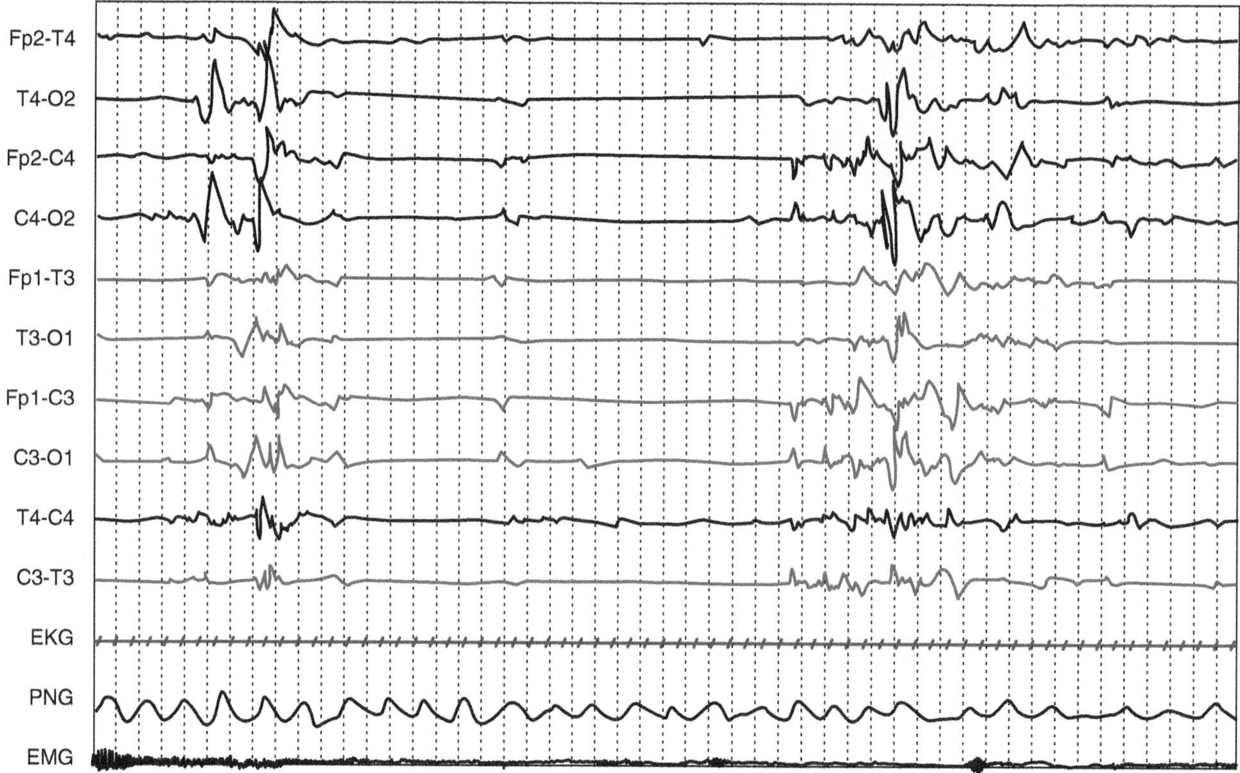

Fig. 130.9 Indeterminate state, recorded at 2 weeks of age (27 weeks postmenstrual age) in a preterm neonate born at 25 weeks. Polygraphic electroencephalography recording (EMG of the right upper limb, EKG, and PNG). Discontinuous tracing. Bursts of high-voltage delta waves with superimposed fast rhythms are separated by interburst interval of 19 seconds. Gain, 15 μV/mm; high frequency filter, 70 Hz; paper speed, 120 mm/s.

(after which it decreases), and show progressively reduced amplitude and higher frequencies with maturation as well as an evolution in location from diffuse[40] or localized over the rolandic regions in the very premature, to the temporal and then occipital areas, until they become exclusively occipital at 36 weeks CA.[48] Immature delta brushes (spindle-like fast rhythms) superimposed on slow waves are recorded as soon as 27 weeks CA and are predominantly localized on the occipital and central areas (Fig. 130.9).[49] They disappear first in wakefulness and active sleep, and then in quiet sleep.[40] Their persistence in the term newborn, a persistently focal or hemispheric location, or a unilateral attenuation in the preterm infant are abnormal and might reflect structural lesions.[40,69] From a physiologic point of view, delta brushes are thought to play an important role in the development of thalamocortical connections.[74,75] In the immature rat, spindle bursts, considered homologous to delta brushes, are abolished after removal of subplate neurons, resulting in reduced thalamocortical connections.[75] Spindle bursts and delta brushes can be spontaneous or triggered by sensory stimuli.[74,76–78]

Premature Temporal Theta (Temporal Sawtooth)

It consist of rhythmic bursts of 4.5 to 6 Hz theta activity over temporal areas,[52] usually bilateral and asynchronous, more frequent during active sleep, recorded from 24 weeks of gestational age, maximally expressed between 29 and 31 weeks, with a rapid disappearance after 32 weeks (Fig. 130.10).[69] Both their delayed appearance[71] and their persistence after 33 weeks should be considered as abnormal.[79] A delay in their appearance has been linked to the presence of intraventricular hemorrhage.[71] Temporal sawtooth is an immature pattern: they have been found to correlate with low-to-intermediate scores of cortical folding,[68] and they are maximally encountered at a time when cortical folding has started in the occipital lobes but not yet in the temporal one.[80]

Occipital Theta Rhythms/Occipital Sawtooth

Monorhythmic theta activities in the occipital regions can be seen in newborns of less than 28 weeks gestational age.[69] They are also known as *STOP rhythm*,[81] and they are reported to predominate in neonates from 25 to 26 weeks of gestational age according to Kuremoto and colleagues.[82] This finding has been debated, however.

Midline Theta or Alpha Activity

This activity is present in both preterm and term newborns, especially during transitional and quiet sleep. It is characterized by a low to moderate amplitude and a spindle-like, sometimes sharply contoured, morphology.[69]

Alpha and Theta Rolandic Activity

Runs of alpha and theta waves of short duration can be seen rarely over rolandic areas in active sleep and quiet sleep in term and late preterm newborns.[83]

Negative Sharp Wave Transients

Physiologic negative sharp waves are a frequent finding in the EEG of healthy term and preterm newborns, especially in the midtemporal, central, and central-temporal regions, symmetrically distributed and most frequently isolated.[33] They are considered abnormal if persistently concentrated over one area or if abundant, especially if in atypical locations, such as the occipital or frontal areas. Occipital sharp waves have been considered pathologic when they have a negative polarity and an amplitude of greater than 150 μV. Frontal sharps have been considered pathologic when they have a positive polarity and an amplitude of greater

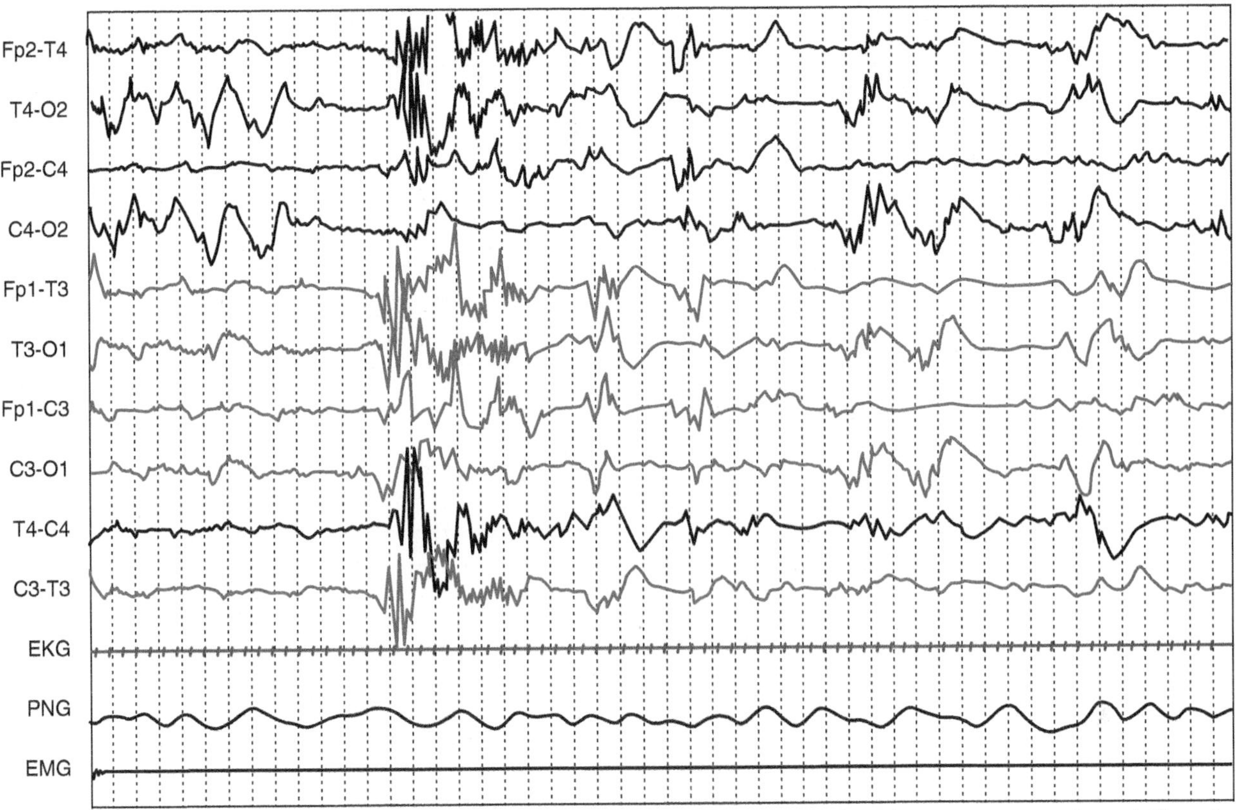

Fig. 130.10 Indeterminate state, electroencephalography recorded at 27 weeks postmenstrual age in preterm neonate born at 25 weeks. Periods of higher continuity are seen, characterized by runs of repetitive delta waves with some superimposed fast activity and temporal sawtooth waves. Polygraphic recording (EMG of the right upper limb, EKG, PNG: pneumogram). Gain, 15 μV/mm; high frequency filter, 70 Hz; paper speed, 60 mm/s.

than 100 μV.[84] They tend to be present in the context of an abnormal background activity and are more likely to recur in runs or trains.[85] Occipital sharp transients are considered as precursors of lambda waves, and they can be seen rarely from the second postnatal week onward in infants in response to visual stimuli.[86]

Spikes

Sporadic spikes can be considered normal if bilateral, confined to the bursts in the *tracé alternant,* or seen during quiet sleep over rolandic areas. On the contrary, they are definitely abnormal if persistently focal, excessively frequent, or present in wakefulness or active sleep after the second week of life in newborns born at 36 to 41 weeks of gestation.[40]

PATHOLOGIC ELECTROENCEPHALOGRAPHY PATTERNS

PATHOLOGIC BACKGROUND ACTIVITY

Background abnormalities in newborns can be classified according to different criteria. Some authors proposed classifications based on the presence of abnormalities in amplitude, continuity, frequency, symmetry, interhemispheric synchrony, sleep states, maturation, and presence of "non-ictal paroxysmal patterns."[87] These are the most relevant variables to evaluate, although it must be noted that single newborns often have multiple abnormalities and that the conclusive interpretation of findings depends on a critical synthesis of all EEG features, in light of the clinical context and of the dynamic evolution of neonatal EEG according to CA. Therefore, abnormal background activity EEG findings will be presented separately for the term and preterm neonate.

TERM NEWBORN

In the term infant, a wide series of different pathologic EEG patterns have been described and associated to subsequent outcome. Among continuous background activities, the hyperactive rapid tracing and the abnormal slow tracing need to be mentioned.[10] The first is defined as continuous background activity consisting of normal features associated to abundant high-amplitude waves in the theta-alpha range: diffuse, asynchronous, and frequently sharp.[88,89] The second one is characterized by continuous diffuse low-voltage delta waves, with little reactivity and no lability, present during both wakefulness and quiet sleep.[90] An abnormal pattern of alternating tracing is known as *sharp alternating theta tracing*, consisting predominantly of theta activity, alternating or discontinuous, which is diffuse, nonreactive, and scarcely labile, and lacks the physiologic features of EEG in term newborns.[91] Finally, different patterns of discontinuous EEG tracings have been described: discontinuous (divided into types A and B), BS, periodic, paroxysmal, and low-voltage plus theta.[10] The discontinuous type A tracing consists of bursts lasting 10 to 30 seconds and separated by intervals of less than 10 seconds of activity of less than 10 μV, in which lability can be present even though definite sleep cycles cannot be identified, and spatial organization is present. On the other hand, the discontinuous type B tracing lacks both temporal and spatial organization and shows little lability.[88,92]

The BS pattern has been variably defined in the literature.[33] Cornerstone elements for its definition are the presence of bursts of activity separated by periods of inactivity and the lack of lability and reactivity; identification of these elements enables correct interpretation of this pattern and its prognostic implications.[33] It is an invariant and unreactive pattern characterized by

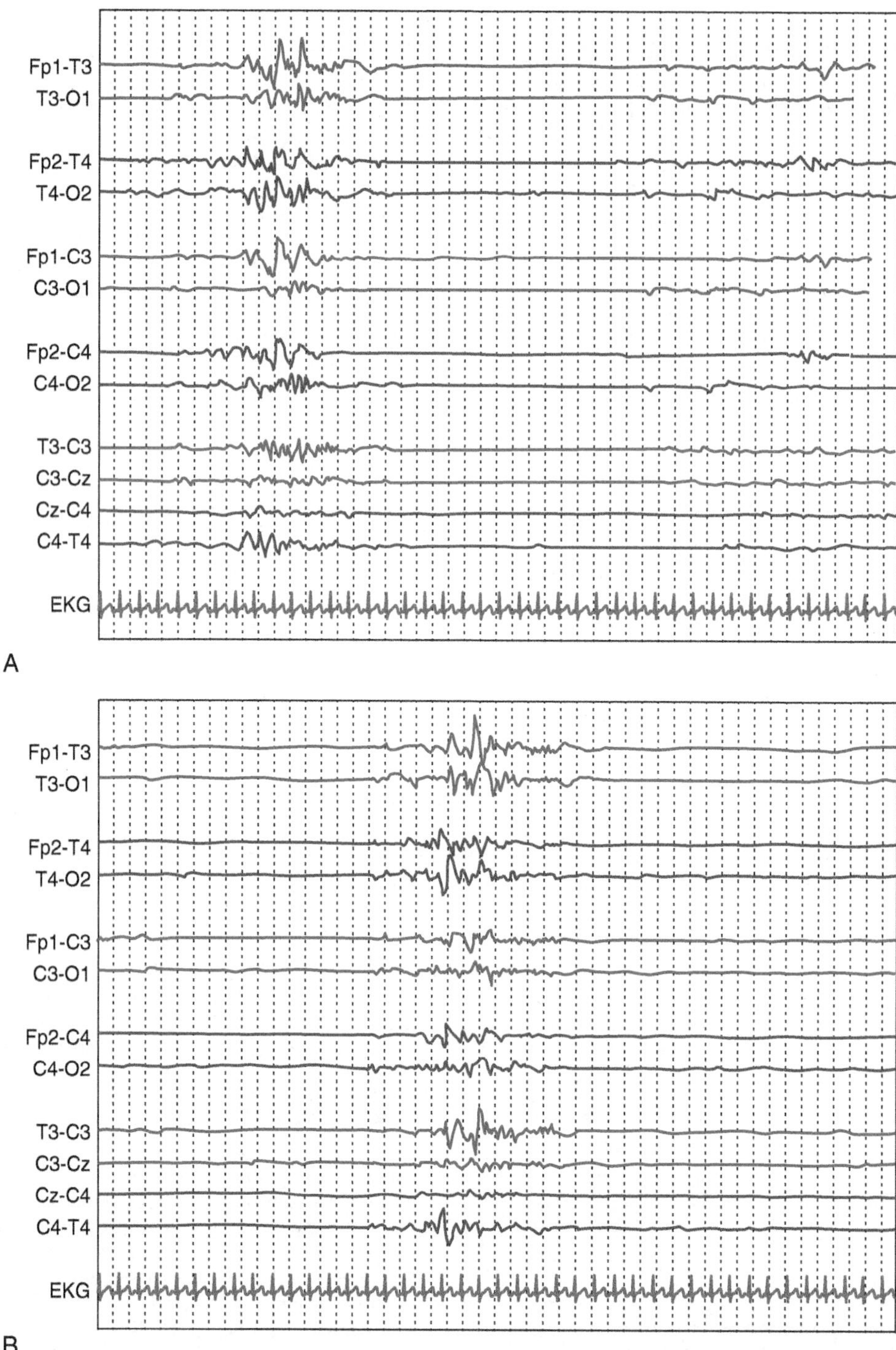

Fig. 130.11 Burst-suppression pattern recorded at 24 hours of life in a term infant with severe hypoxic-ischemic encephalopathy during therapeutic hypothermia. Sequential pages of the EEG (A and B) showing bursts of synchronous activity consisting of spikes, sharp and slow waves but no age-appropriate activity alternating with prolonged periods of marked background attenuation. Gain 7 μV/mm; high frequency filter, 70 Hz; paper speed, 15 mm/s.

synchronous bursts of activity, lasting 0.5 to 10 seconds, interrupted by periods of generalized isoelectric background lasting between 2 and 10 seconds (Fig. 130.11).[93] This pattern can be observed in severe central nervous system disorders, such as HIE, inborn errors of metabolism, malformations, or as a result of pharmacologic interventions.[87,94] It also represents the hallmark of specific epileptic neonatal syndromes such as OS and EME.[95] Death or severe developmental disability have been reported in 80% to 100% of cases[96-98] and have been associated with significant neuropathologic findings.[99] Aside from BS, other discontinuous abnormal tracings have been described, especially by the French school: periodic, paroxysmal, and low-voltage plus theta tracing.

Periodic tracing consists of repetitive medium-amplitude stereotyped activity, lacking both temporal and spatial organization, separated by low-amplitude intervals of approximately fixed duration,[100-102] while paroxysmal tracing shows a pattern of short bursts (1 to 10 seconds), with variable morphology separated by periods of activity of less than 5 μV lasting 10 to 60 seconds. Periodicity, lability, and reactivity are absent.[103]

A low-voltage plus theta consists of theta activities between 5 and 30 μV, either continuous or discontinuous over an inactive or very-low-amplitude tracing (<15 μV), usually nonreactive.[83] In a retrospective review of excessively discontinuous EEGs in term newborns, it was found that patients with a predominant IBI duration longer than 30 seconds had a 100% probability of severe neurologic disability and 86% probability of developing subsequent epilepsy.[104] A final category of abnormal EEG patterns comprises low-voltage and inactive tracings. A low-voltage tracing in the term newborn is characterized by amplitude between 5 and 15 μV during wakefulness and active sleep and between 10 and 25 μV during quiet sleep.[83]

Finally, inactive EEG or electrocerebral inactivity[33] consists of an isoelectric tracing such as the absence of any discernible cerebral electrical activity over 2 μV when reviewed at a sensitivity of 2 μV/mm[87] or, according to Lamblin and André, tracings of amplitude of less than 5 μV.[46]

PRETERM NEWBORN

In preterm babies between 24 and 30 weeks CA, the most important parameter to assess is continuity, evaluated by taking into account the proportion of burst and IBI and the changes in this proportion during the recording time. The presence of sleep-states cycling is also an important parameter.[79] Nevertheless, issues arise when comparing literature data because of differences in bursts and IBI definitions regarding their duration and the threshold values for amplitude. After reviewing the available literature data, Nguyen The Tich and colleagues proposed, in standard recordings without sedative drugs, the following values to be considered as pathologic: at 26 to 27 weeks PMA, IBI greater than 60 seconds and burst less than 60 seconds; at 28 to 29 weeks PMA, IBI greater than 30 seconds and the burst less than 2 minutes; at 30 to 32 weeks PMA, IBI greater than 20 seconds and bursts less than 10 minutes.[79] Values recommended by the ACNS are as follows: in the age group less than 30 weeks PMA, a maximum IBI of 35 seconds with an interburst voltage of less than 25 μV; between 30 and 33 weeks PMA, a maximum IBI of 20 seconds and the same voltage as above; between 34 and 36 weeks PMA, a maximum IBI duration of 10 seconds (and a voltage of approximately 25 μV); and more than 36 weeks, an IBI maximal duration of 6 seconds with an amplitude of more than 25 μV.[33]

Abnormally long IBIs tend to correlate with poor neurologic prognosis and, together with other parameters, identify subjects at high neurologic risk.[105,106] Decreased maximum and mean burst duration are both associated with brain lesions.[107] As far as sleep-states cycling is concerned, even though indeterminate sleep predominates before 30 weeks gestation, fluctuations in discontinuity can be recorded as early as 25 weeks PMA.[35,37] The percentage of indeterminate sleep is higher in newborns with cerebral lesions even at less than 29 weeks PMA.[108]

According to Nguyen The Tich and colleagues,[79] the severity of recorded abnormalities in preterm infants of less than 30 weeks PMA can be divided into moderate severity, including immature pattern for PMA, low voltage with normal background activity, excessive asynchrony for PMA, or poorly developed occipital delta; and major severity, including isoelectric tracing, positive rolandic sharp waves, ictal discharges, paroxysmal tracing, interhemispheric asynchrony, persistent asymmetry, and excessively slow background without age-appropriate transients. Watanabe and coworkers have proposed an alternative classification of EEG findings in preterm newborns according to the time lag between the brain insult and the recording.[12] Acute-stage abnormalities reflect the acute phase of brain injury, in which the EEG is dominated by changes in continuity, amplitude, and frequencies, according to the increasing degrees of severity. In order to assess continuity, these authors did suggest evaluating the percentage of continuous and discontinuous tracing as well as the maximal and mean IBI. Changes in frequency mainly consist of the attenuation of faster frequency, comprising delta brushes and temporal theta bursts when appropriate for PMA. Cutoff values for amplitude are modified according to PMA (a mildly low voltage corresponds to an amplitude of delta waves of less than 200 μV before 30 weeks, and less than 150 μV at 30 to 33 weeks; a moderately low voltage is defined as a amplitude of 20 to 50 μV with intermixed 50 to 100 μV delta waves; a markedly low voltage corresponds to an amplitude of <20 μV).[12] Chronic-stage abnormalities are seen when an abnormal EEG does not show markers of acute "depression." Two different patterns can be distinguished: the dysmature and the disorganized pattern. A dysmature pattern is defined as the presence of EEG features that would be physiologic in an infant at least 2 weeks younger compared with the PMA of the infant.[79,109] A persistently dysmature pattern is associated with an increased risk of abnormal neurologic outcome.[87,110] A disorganized pattern in premature newborns describes a background activity characterized by distorted delta waves associated with abnormal sharp waves and cogwheel-shaped brushes (mechanical brushes).[109]

PATHOLOGIC ASYMMETRY

Persistent asymmetry may indicate focal lesions (arterial ischemic stroke, sinovenous thrombosis, abscess, or focal hemorrhage).[33]

PATHOLOGIC TRANSIENTS

Positive Rolandic Sharp Waves Type A

These are surface-positive broad-based sharp waves of less than 500 ms duration, with an amplitude between 20 and 200 μV, localized over C3, C4, and Cz, unilateral or bilateral, usually more abundant and sometimes isolated over Cz.[79] They can either occur in isolation or in runs.[79] When occurring more frequently than 1 to 2 per minute, they have been associated with white matter lesions and subsequent development of motor impairments.[10] They are mainly observed in premature newborns born before 34 weeks PMA.[10]

Periodic Lateralized Epileptiform Discharges

Rarely encountered in term infants, they can have a variable morphology (slow waves, sharp waves or spikes, either di-, tri-, or polyphasic) and last between 200 and 400 ms, with amplitude between 100 to 200 μV. They tend to recur at regular intervals of 1 to 10 seconds, in the same location and with constant morphology, without evolution.[111,112]

Cogwheel-Shaped Brushes or Mechanical Brushes

Defined as spindle-like, fast, spiky wave bursts with maximum amplitude higher than 40 μV and frequencies between 13 and 20 Hz, they lack smoothness and have a wider basis and increased peak-to-peak amplitude than observed in physiologic delta waves and delta brushes.[113] They can be difficult to identify before 28 weeks PMA,[79] although this task is made easier by using a 30 mm/s speed and a low cutoff filter set at 10 Hz to eliminate slow waves.[114] They represent, together with abnormal sharp waves, chronic-stage abnormalities, usually recorded within disorganized patterns (Fig. 130.12).[113]

TRANSIENTS OF UNCERTAIN SIGNIFICANCE

Positive Temporal Sharp Waves

They are surface-positive monophasic, diphasic, or triphasic transient sharp waves, located over temporal regions, with a duration of 400 ms or less, and an amplitude over 50 μV.[115] They peak at 31 to 33 weeks PMA, and some authors consider them a maturational pattern frequently seen in preterm infants born between 31 and 34 weeks PMA. They tend to persist until term-equivalent age even if with decreasing incidence, possibly representing a sign of maturational delay.[115] They are also reported in term newborns and indicate lesions, if repeated in serial recordings.[79]

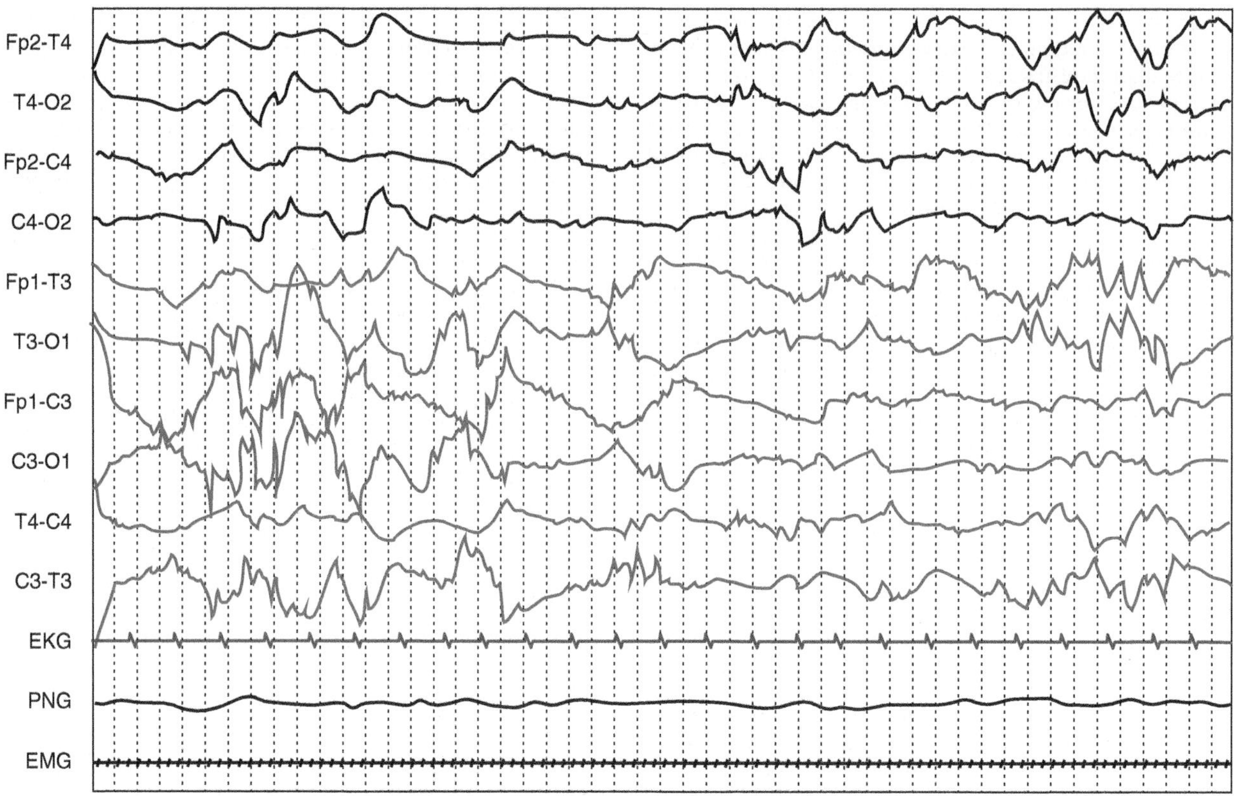

Fig. 130.12 Preterm baby born at 23 weeks postmenstrual age (PMA) and recorded at 28 weeks PMA. Disorganized tracing, showing on the left high-voltage distorted delta waves with superimposed sharp fast rhythms (mechanical brushes), while on the right positive temporal sharps can be seen. Polygraphic EEG (EMG: right deltoid; PNG: pneumogram EKG). Gain, 10 µV/mm; high frequency filter, 70 Hz; paper speed, 30 mm/s.

Positive Rolandic Sharp Waves Type B

They have a lower amplitude than type A and tend to occur in short runs of 3 to 7 seconds' duration, at a repetition rate of 1 to 4 Hz. They are particularly present after 34 weeks PMA, and their prognostic value is uncertain at present.[79]

Long Alpha/Theta Bursts

These are long—3 to 12 seconds—bursts of theta or alpha activity over rolandic regions, of constant frequency in single individuals.[116,117]

ELECTROENCEPHALOGRAPHY FEATURES IN SELECTED CLINICAL CONDITIONS

HYPOXIC-ISCHEMIC ENCEPHALOPATHY

The usefulness of EEG in newborns with HIE relies on the correlation between EEG, severity of encephalopathy, and subsequent outcome.[46,118] EEG has been reported to have a higher predictive value than neurologic examination.[119] Time-appropriate evaluation of background EEG activities can assist in the correct planning of subsequent recordings, with an increase in prognostic accuracy,[33] whereas recordings undertaken at the wrong time could be misleading due to lower sensitivity, as background EEG activity tends to improve in all newborns as a function of time.[83] Outcome prediction accuracy is particularly high for normal and severely abnormal background patterns.

When evaluating clinical studies regarding the role of EEG in HIE, a significant heterogeneity in background pattern definitions must be acknowledged.[120] Very abnormal tracings implying a very severe prognosis[87] which usually cannot be modified by hypothermia[121] include inactive tracing, paroxysmal tracing, "low-voltage plus theta" tracing, BS, and "constantly discontinuous" pattern, which are almost always recorded only during the first week of life.[46,87] It must be emphasized that, although inactive tracings imply a severe prognosis, particularly when recorded after the first 48 hours of life,[46] a favorable evolution has been exceptionally reported when the first EEG was recorded very early after birth (within the first 6,[122] 8,[26] or 10[88] hours) and was followed by prompt improvement of background activities by 12 to 24 hours or by 2 to 3 days.[88]

Other EEG patterns can provide prognostic information only if confirmed over serial recordings and if one takes into consideration their temporal evolution. Slow continuous tracing has a prognostic value only if recorded beyond the first week of life and low-voltage EEG after the second.[46] In case of a hyperactive tracing or of a discontinuous tracing, abnormalities observed within the first 48 hours of life have an uncertain significance.[46] One study established that discontinuous tracings diagnosed within 48 hours of life are significant in terms of prognosis only if they are confirmed with a second recording undertaken within the first week.[123]

Based on literature data, Lamblin and André[46] have proposed an algorithm for the EEG surveillance of term newborns with HIE, guided by the characteristics of background activity. The time point at which a normal background EEG is best predictive of normal outcome varies between studies: a time interval between hypoxia-ischemia and EEG of at least 24 hours is recommended by Tharp,[124] circumscribed by[26] a range of 24 to 36 hours, whereas Lamblin and André suggest recording in the first 12 hours of life.[46] In any case, one single normal EEG obtained more than 1 week after the hypoxic-ischemic event has no prognostic value.[83] On the contrary, if the EEG is severely abnormal, an unfavorable outcome can be foreseen from 12 hours of life, even if a follow-up EEG after 24 hours is recommended in order to rule out potential confounders.[46] Finally, if the initial EEG reports intermediate findings, a control EEG during the first week of life documenting normalization would be reassuring, whereas persistently uncertain EEG findings are likely to be followed by neurologic deficits, even if difficult to specify.[46] Apart from the background activity, additional EEG features can have a complementary role in assessing the severity of hypoxic-ischemic injury: the presence or absence of sleep-wake cycle, of neonatal seizures, and of pathologic transients.[46] The presence of a normal sleep-wake cycle in the first 6 to 24 hours is associated with favorable outcomes,[26,88] whereas if this is absent at 48 hours of life a negative outcome can be predicted, because it reflects higher grades of encephalopathy.[26] Following HIE, a reduction in active sleep and an increase in quiet sleep were demonstrated.[26] The severity of sleep-wake cycle disruption shows good correlation with that of background activity.[125,126]

Among pathologic transients, alpha-like rhythms, the persistence of anterior slow dysrhythmia, and *encoches frontales* after the first week of life,[46] as well as the presence of positive temporal spikes (PTS), appearing 2 to 3 days after clinical signs and regressing with the clinical signs, have been reported.[127] With the advent of therapeutic hypothermia as standard of care for HIE, there has been a great development of the aEEG, and its usefulness in prognostication has been evaluated in clinical trials, leading to the discovery that hypothermia determines a slower recovery of background activity compared with normothermia,[128] even if the exact pathophysiologic mechanisms leading to this phenomenon have not been elucidated.[129] For example, the time to recovery of a normal background activity on aEEG within 24 hours reliably predicts favorable outcome in the normothermic group, whereas this same cutoff point for newborns with hypothermia is 48 hours. Similarly, although the reappearance of a sleep-wake cycle is a marker of good prognosis if taking place within 36 hours, in the hypothermic group this was found to be true up to 60 hours after birth, even if with a wide range.[128] Nevertheless, continuous vEEG monitoring remains the gold standard for brain function evaluation and detection of electrographic seizures in newborns with HIE.[25,26] Nash and colleagues have shown that conventional continuous vEEG monitoring during hypothermia for neonatal HIE is associated with short-term outcome as assessed by brain MRI.[110] In this study, a normal EEG was associated with the absence of brain injury or mild brain injury on MRI, especially in the beginning of cooling, whereas a severely abnormal background activity was most predictive for moderate to severe brain injury at midcooling.[110] Additionally, this study better highlighted a prognostic significance of an excessively discontinuous EEG background activity during hypothermia (Fig. 130.13) compared with normothermic series. However, it must be acknowledged that the definition of this type of pattern

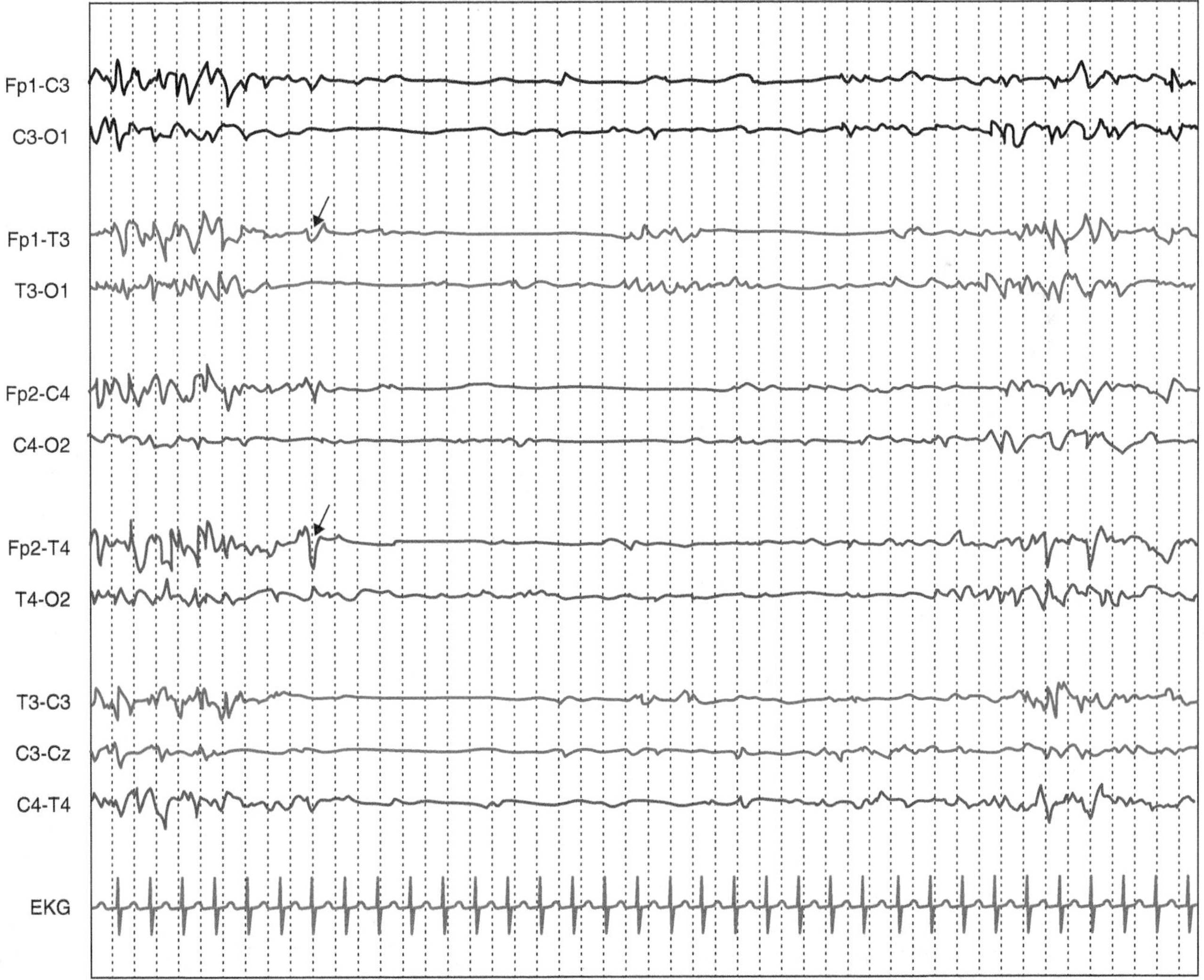

Fig. 130.13 Excessively discontinuous pattern recorded in a 2-day-old term neonate with hypoxic-ischemic encephalopathy during therapeutic hypothermia. Although the bursts contain some normal patterns and graphoelements (see *arrows* indicating encoche frontales), the interburst interval is too prolonged and low voltage. Gain, 7 μV/mm; high frequency filter, 70 Hz; paper speed, 15 mm/s.

in the literature encompasses a wide range of IBI durations, resulting in a generally poor predictive value.[130] Another study evaluating the prognostic value of EEG background patterns in term newborns with severe HIE found an inactive pattern at 48 hours is associated with a high mortality risk.[121]

PRETERM INFANTS AND WHITE MATTER DAMAGE

By using the above-mentioned distinction into acute- and chronic-stage abnormalities,[12] EEG interpretation in preterm infants offers useful clues for diagnostic and prognostic purposes and allows assessment of both severity and timing of brain injury. However, it might be difficult to differentiate between acute- and chronic-stage abnormalities before 30 weeks PMA.[66] Serial recordings can significantly increase the information that can be derived from a one-time recording for both diagnostic and prognostic purposes. Starting with a first recording in the immediate postnatal period, it is possible to establish the timing of injury (prenatal, perinatal, or postnatal),[131] depending on the presence and timing of the appearance of acute- versus chronic-stage abnormalities, even if repetitive insults can also occur. Both the severity of acute-stage abnormalities and the type and severity of chronic-stage abnormalities[131] can assist prognostication.

Similarly to what has been shown in term newborns concerning the prognostic value of EEG, tracings with increased discontinuity and decreased amplitude are associated with unfavorable prognosis,[63,107] and their best diagnostic and prognostic value is observed when the EEG is performed soon after birth, especially in the first 2 days of life, whereas afterwards they show a low sensitivity.[105] Decreased maximum and mean duration of the bursts has been associated with cerebral lesions,[12,107,115,132] and, even in preterm infants of less than 29 weeks PMA, the percentage of indeterminate sleep is higher in subjects with brain damage.[107,130]

A so-called dysmature pattern usually persists for some time during the neonatal period, being present around term-equivalent age, but its usefulness as a prognostic tool has also been reported in the preterm neonate of 28 to 34 weeks PMA.[110] It has been recorded in newborns suffering from bronchopulmonary dysplasia[133] and tends to follow prolonged mild acute-stage abnormalities without ultrasonographic changes,[134] or intraventricular hemorrhage without parenchymal involvement.[109] It has been associated with the later occurrence of mental retardation[134] rather than motor deficits. Based on the frequent finding of a maturational delay upon reaching term-equivalent age, especially in preterm infants born before 29 weeks[107] and very low-birth-weight newborns,[135] some authors suggested that the general assumption that the maturation of sleep-wake cycle and EEG patterns is independent of gestational age and birth weight[136] might not apply to these extremely preterm infants. In this respect, the finding of a suppressive effect of preterm birth on neurogenesis might represent an interesting field for further research.[137] On the other hand, a disorganized pattern is mostly found in infants between 32 and 36 weeks CA and might be difficult to recognize in younger preterm infants or in term infants.[12] It is often preceded by severe acute-stage abnormalities and associated with white matter injury and the subsequent development of cerebral palsy.[12,113] Transients commonly encountered in the context of an abnormal background pattern consist of positive rolandic sharp waves, mechanical brushes, and positive temporal sharp waves.

Positive rolandic sharp waves are generally considered as an example of chronic-stage abnormality, although some authors have also interpreted them as acute/subacute signs.[115] They represent a marker of white matter injury, namely, periventricular leukomalacia,[138,139] and can be recorded on EEG even before ultrasound scans yield positive findings.[138,140] They have been shown to predict motor disability with high sensitivity and specificity.[138] Of note, they were recorded more frequently on Cz than C3 or C4, highlighting the usefulness of midline recordings.[140] Finally, studies assessing the presence and prognostic value of positive rolandic sharp waves used a density/minute cutoff (2/min[138] or 1/min[139]), and suggested that under 0.1/min the risk of unfavorable neurologic outcomes is significantly lower.[141]

Mechanical (or cogwheel) brushes are more frequently expressed over the occipital, temporal, and central regions. They correlate with periventricular leukomalacia when appearing with a high density (especially >1/min over the temporal and occipital region), and their topography correlates with the extent of underlying white matter damage and the severity of subsequent motor impairment.[114] In contrast, positive temporal sharp waves have a less definite relationship with outcome.[115] They are considered abnormal when they are frequent (density cutoff values have been proposed),[115] high amplitude, and/or persistent on serial recordings.[79] Their increased expression is mostly associated with EEG patterns suggestive of chronic central nervous system dysfunction,[115] in which case, they correlate with severe ultrasound abnormalities, and their maximum expression has been found even to precede ultrasound evidence of periventricular leucomalacia.[115] However, they cannot be considered specific for a single type of brain injury, as they have also been described in the context of HI damage and metabolic disease.[142] They could possibly represent an expression of the peculiar sensitivity of temporal lobes to various injuries.[143,144] The persistence of sawtooth beyond 34 weeks CA is considered a sign of maturational lag.[65] A higher incidence of sawtooth at 34 to 36 weeks CA was reported in preterm neonates born between 24 and 36 weeks CA and associated with intraventricular hemorrhage, cystic periventricular leukomalacia, and persistent ventricular dilatation.[107]

SEIZURES AND STATUS EPILEPTICUS

A seizure is defined as a sudden, repetitive, stereotyped episode of abnormal electrographic activity with a peak-to-peak amplitude of at least 2 μV, a minimum duration of 10 seconds, and evolution with clear beginning, middle, and end.[145] Seizures in newborns occur mainly during active sleep, if sleep cycle is maintained.[146-148] The onset of electrographically confirmed seizures tends to occurs earlier in term than preterm newborns: it has been reported within the first 48 hours from birth in 49% of term infants versus 27.5% of preterm ones.[19] Furthermore, it was found to occur within 48 hours from birth in only approximately 10% of preterm newborns younger than 29 weeks PMA and in 50% of those 30 weeks or older. Mean onset time in the first age group was 8.3 days versus 3.2 days in the second.[19] One study addressing the temporal evolution of seizures in term infants with HIE found that the maximum seizure burden was reached at a mean of 22.7 hours of life, and the last seizure was recorded at a mean of 55.5 hours.[149]

The average duration of seizures in neonates, as studied in different populations and etiologies, tends to range from 1 to 5 minutes, with the majority lasting less than 3 minutes.[145,150-152] Scher and colleagues found that the duration of seizures is longer in term newborns given the higher incidence of status epilepticus compared with preterms.[153] It must be emphasized that these studies were conducted on populations of term and preterm newborns of different gestational ages, in some cases prior to and in others after anticonvulsant administration, which might limit comparison. Additionally, they were based on routine short-term EEGs.[3] Subsequent studies with continuous EEG monitoring have confirmed those findings but have also highlighted a high occurrence of seizures lasting up to 40 minutes.[15,149,154,155]

By definition, each seizure has to be separated from another by at least 10 seconds to be considered as a distinct event,[7] even though this cutoff has not been chosen on the basis of physiologic implications.[7] Scher and colleagues found longer interictal durations in preterm newborns older than 32 weeks estimated gestational age compared with the age group between 23 and 31 weeks estimated gestational age.[153] The mean frequency per hour likely depends on the monitored time frame and was found to correspond to 7 per hour[151]; the mean percent time seizing equaled 25%, with remarkable variability (0.7% to 87%).[151] A study conducted exclusively on preterm infants found a 23.5% rate of status epilepticus among all cases of seizures.[18] According to topography and considering the focus onset and the region involved at the time of the maximal spread, seizures have been divided into localized, lateralized, and diffuse, or into unifocal, multifocal, and bilaterally independent.[7] Typical phenomena of the immature brain are migration (defined as a change of seizure focus within one hemisphere) and shifting of ictal discharges (defined as a change of focus from one hemisphere to the other),[152] which is indicated as flip-flop when discharges finally shift back to the original hemisphere.[148]

A focal onset is present in the majority of cases in term newborns, whereas for preterm newborns either a regional[156] or focal[152] onset have been reported as most frequent. In any case, generalized onset is exceptional.[157] Description of seizure onset has important clinical implications, as the consistent presence of a single-onset focus is suggestive of focal injury (e.g., stroke), whereas multifocal or varying foci suggest a diffuse dysfunction (e.g., infection or global brain injury)[158]; however, focal seizures in the neonatal period do not necessarily indicate corresponding anatomic lesions, and diffuse insults can manifest as focal discharges.[156]

The most frequent onset focus is the central-temporal[13,148,151] or vertex region,[151] without any significant difference between term and preterm infants.[156] A different study on preterm newborns found a higher prevalence of onset over the posterior regions.[159] In contrast, seizure foci over the frontal or occipital regions should prompt investigations for a focal lesion, as these regions are rarely involved in seizure onset.[158] In another study, multiple independent areas of discharges at seizure onset were observed in 55% of newborns.[159] Propagation of the discharges can be present in both preterm and term newborns, and some authors found it to be mainly ipsilateral for seizures with a focal onset and contralateral or bilateral for regional-onset seizures.[156] Although several reports failed to correlate seizure manifestation and ictal foci or propagation in preterm newborns,[152] more recently it has been suggested that the description of the seizure spread might enable correlation with evolving clinical signs.[158] Furthermore, it can provide prognostic information, as a spread from a lateralized onset to the contralateral hemisphere has been associated with adverse outcome.[159]

Several qualitative seizure morphology classification systems have been proposed. In some cases only EEG discharges topography and morphology were considered: focal spike/sharp wave discharges, focal low-frequency discharges, focal rhythmic discharges, and multifocal discharges.[160] Other authors also considered background activity: focal ictal patterns with normal background, focal patterns with abnormal background, focal monorhythmic patterns with normal background, focal patterns with abnormal background, focal monorhythmic periodic patterns, and multifocal ictal patterns.[161] Repetitive spikes, sharp waves, stereotyped wave complexes, and alpha, theta, or delta discharges are frequent.[162] Alpha seizure activity is characterized by a sudden transient appearance of rhythmic activity, more typically in the temporal or central region.[163,164] In a study conducted on both term and preterm newborns, spikes and sharp waves were recorded in 34% of cases and pseudorhythmic activity in 32%; these patterns were seen associated in 34% of patients.[159]

Different types of paroxysmal discharges might be present during a given seizure, and frequently independent seizures are recorded, occurring simultaneously over different areas of both hemispheres.[146] Term newborns tend to have sharp waves and delta or sharp and slow waves at the onset of seizures, whereas preterm newborns are more likely to show rhythmic alpha or delta. In the study by Nagarajan, in which all recorded newborns were older than 34 weeks CA, sharp or slow sharp waves were the most frequent EEG pattern seen at the onset of the seizure.[148] Spike potentials often present with a slower rate and a longer duration compared with older ages, and this phenomenon has been referred to as *burnt-out spikes*.[94] The ability to generate well-formed spikes at high discharge rates tends to improve with increasing PMA and is reduced in the context of severe brain injury.[116]

Evolution of discharges during the seizure usually consists of a decrease in frequency and an increase in amplitude.[152] During the ictal discharge, delta and sharp waves were the most frequent finding in both term and preterm infants.[156]

Seizures in severely affected newborns may lack a clear field and pattern of evolution, the amplitude may be low, the frequency is often slow,[1] and the ictal discharges tend to be prolonged.[165] In those cases, discharges are more likely to remain confined to a single EEG channel or alternate between hemispheres, making the diagnosis particularly challenging (Fig. 130.14).[1]

The hypothesis that different ictal characteristics may have a different impact on brain physiology or on outcome is still unproved,[7] although it has been suggested that alpha discharges imply a worse prognosis.[163] Similarly, no correlation between seizure characteristics and specific etiologies has been reported.[152,156]

There is no clear association between clinical semiology and characteristics of EEG discharges, and the same type of discharges can be associated with different types of clinical seizures in different patients.[162] However, Okumura and colleagues in a cohort of preterm newborns found that the duration of seizures was relatively shorter when motor phenomena were present, in comparison to apneic or electrographic seizures.[152] There is a tendency for neonates with severely abnormal background to

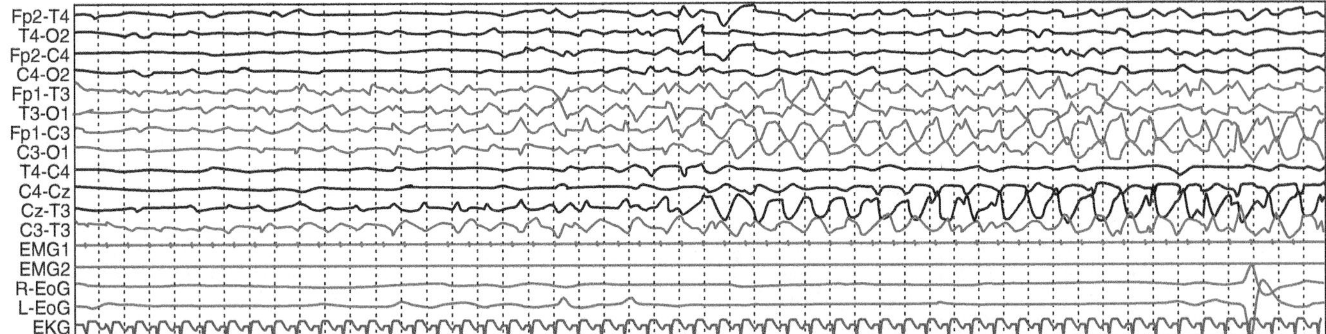

Fig. 130.14 Left central neonatal seizure in a 1-day-old term neonate with hypoxic-ischemic encephalopathy consisting of repetitive rhythmic positive rolandic sharp waves evolving in amplitude and frequency. Gain, 7 μV/mm; high frequency filter, 70 Hz; paper speed, 30 mm/s.

present with electrographic-only seizures.[148,156] In her work, Nagarajan found electroclinical seizures to be more likely associated with bilateral discharges, higher frequency, and minimum and maximum amplitude of discharges.[148]

Prognostic implications of ictal discharges are limited, but low-amplitude maximal amplitude of ictal discharges is associated with higher mortality, and average maximal ictal EEG frequency of less than 2 Hz (notably associated with moderate to severe background EEG abnormalities) has been associated with the later development of cerebral palsy.[148,160] Of note, the presence of multiple independent foci also correlated with a worse outcome.[166,167] Although it has been shown that seizure frequency[168] and overall seizure duration correlate with subsequent outcome, it is also known that the simple count of total seizure number is a poor index of prognosis,[158] as it is prone to biases related to recording time and monitoring modality. To overcome such limitations, the use of the "ictal fraction" parameter has also been proposed, corresponding to the total seizure duration/total EEG duration per hour, and a correlation with the subsequent neurodevelopmental outcome has been demonstrated in cases in which the ictal fraction it exceeds 10 minutes.[159] Interestingly, the presence of spreading toward the contralateral hemisphere has been demonstrated to imply a detrimental effect on outcome; it was present in all of the newborns who later developed epilepsy, suggesting that the recruitment of neurons over a wider area might be associated with more severe brain injury.[159]

The occurrence of neonatal status epilepticus is rather frequent in neonates with variable figures between 14% and 43%, even if heterogeneity in study designs makes comparison difficult.[19,151,155] The definition of neonatal status epilepticus is subject to even more controversies than in the adult population. It has been usually defined as either continuous seizures lasting for more than 30 minutes or seizure present for at least 50% of the recording time, with no return to the baseline neurologic condition.[169] It was demonstrated that this clinical scenario is associated with the severest brain damage and is more detrimental than the occurrence of recurrent seizures in terms of death and neurologic sequelae[19]; furthermore, it is independently predictive of the later development of remote symptomatic epilepsy.[170] Alternative, operational definitions with a shorter cut-off time have also been proposed,[7] even if a specific threshold has yet to be found. For this reason, a more generic term has also been used in the literature, referring to *seizure burden* to indicate the percentage of the EEG recording with ictal activity at any location.[151]

EPILEPSIES AND EPILEPTIC ENCEPHALOPATHIES

The last decade has witnessed a major transformation in our understanding of epilepsies presenting in the neonatal period, resulting from two advances. First, the advent of long-term vEEG monitoring in the nursery provided an opportunity for neurologists to be more involved in the clinical evaluation of seizing newborns. A result of this experience was the rejection of the notion that seizure phenomenology in neonates is essentially different from those of older children and adults.[1] Second, advances in neuroimaging and metabolic testing, together with readily available sophisticated genetic analysis, has allowed for the identification of an increasing proportion of epilepsies presenting in the nursery, among the large number of newborns with seizures resulting from acute brain insults.[2] Although most seizures in the neonatal period reflect acute, acquired brain dysfunction such as HIE, stroke, or infection, in about 15% of patients they represent the presenting symptom of a neonatal epilepsy.[171] This early distinction is important in terms of both treatment and prognosis.[172] An epilepsy syndrome is defined by the combination of age at onset, seizure types, interictal and ictal pattern, and etiology. The recognition of epileptic syndromes allows an accurate diagnosis, management, and prognosis and provides useful information for research for discovery of new treatments and etiologies, including the genetic ones. The identification of epilepsy syndromes is based mainly on clinical and EEG criteria, and advances in neuroimaging and genetics have by no means contradicted this concept.[173] Currently, three epilepsy syndromes with onset in the neonatal period have been recognized by the International League Against Epilepsy (ILAE):[174] Benign familial neonatal epilepsy (BNFE), EME, and OS. However, the last decade has witnessed a major transformation in our understanding of epilepsies presenting in the neonatal period, resulting from two advances. First, the implementation of long-term vEEG monitoring in the nursery provided an opportunity for neurologists to be more involved in the clinical evaluation of seizing newborns. Second, advances in neuroimaging and metabolic testing together with readily available sophisticated genetic analysis has allowed for the identification of an increasing proportion of epilepsies presenting in the nursery from among the large number of newborns with seizures resulting from the acute brain injury.[2] The consequence of these developments has been an appreciation of the nuanced differences among patients previously lumped together under broad umbrella syndromes—OS and EME—allowing for the recognition of new distinct electroclinical phenotypes, reflecting discrete etiologic entities (e.g., STXBP1 encephalopathy, KCNQ2 encephalopathy, CDKL5 deficiency disorder [CDD], encephalopathy, SCN2A encephalopathy). Indeed, OS and EME were first described in 1976 and 1978[3] respectively, when neuroimaging was in its infancy and gene sequencing was in the process of being developed.

EME and OS share the important feature of BS on EEG associated with clinical signs of encephalopathy, although there has been much discussion concerning specific differences of the BS pattern in each of these syndromes.[175] BS consists of short periods of high-voltage activity with mixed features but no age-appropriate activity alternating with periods of marked background attenuation (Fig. 130.15).

This pattern is typically unreactive and unaltered by exogenous or endogenous stimuli. Although neonates presenting with BS may have different underlying etiologies, the pathophysiology of BS is a fascinating question that has been addressed in research studies. Steriade and colleagues showed that suppression epochs are due to absence of synaptic activity among cortical neurons.[176] Interestingly, at variance with cortical neurons, only 60% to 70% of thalamic cells ceased firing and were completely silent during the suppressed periods of EEG activity. The remaining 30% to 40% of thalamic cells discharged rhythmic (1 to 4 Hz) spike bursts during periods of cortical silence.

EME is characterized by a BS pattern associated with erratic, fragmentary myoclonus and the eventual development of focal seizures and infantile spasms. Onset of symptoms occurs almost always in the first days of life. The neurologic status is always abnormal at onset:[175] neonates are hypotonic and poorly responsive. The outcome of infants with EME is poor.[177] There is a high incidence of death in the first few years of life. In the survivors, there is virtual absence of psychomotor development.[175] Erratic myoclonias shift typically from one part of the body to another in a random and asynchronous fashion. They are often restricted in a finger, a toe, the eyebrows, eyelids, or lips, occurring in the same muscle group and often migrating elsewhere. The EEG recording demonstrates that myoclonias are brief, single or repetitive, can be very frequent, and nearly continuous. Massive, usually bisynchronous, axial myoclonic jerks may start from the onset of the disease or occur later, often interspersed with erratic myoclonias. Simple focal seizures are usually subtle, with eye deviation or autonomic symptoms such as flushing of the face or apnea, but they can be focal clonic, involving any part of the body. Epileptic spasms are rare and

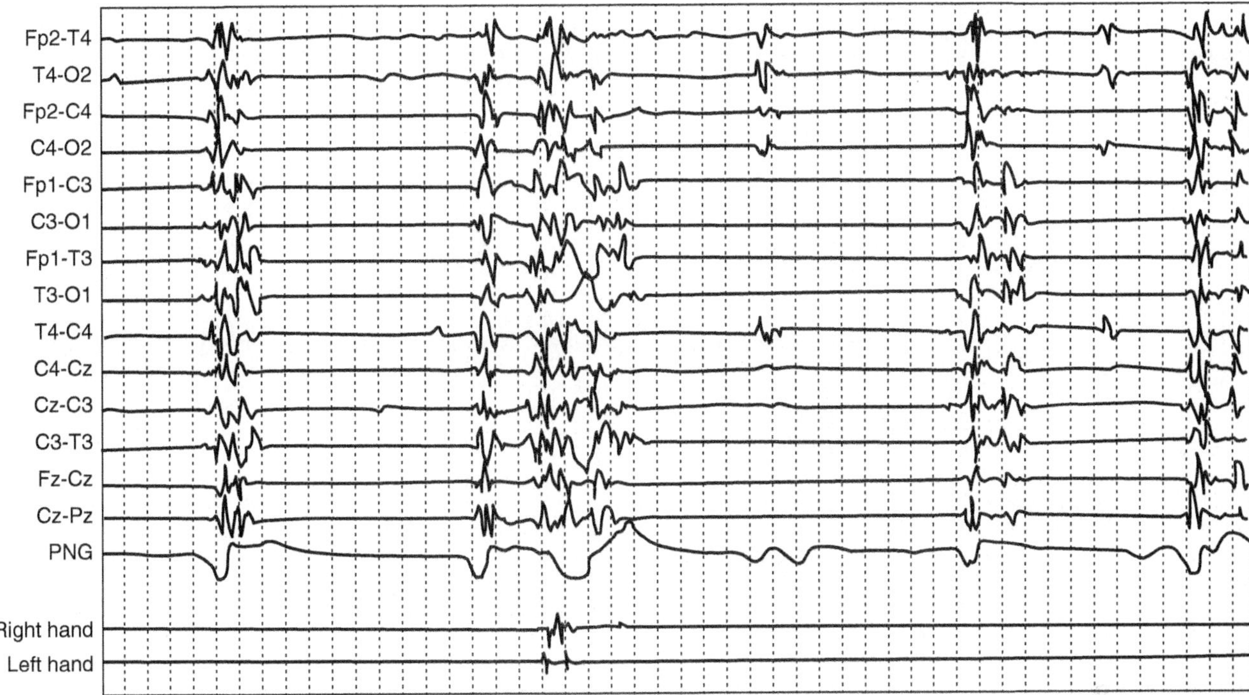

Fig. 130.15 Burst-suppression pattern in a 7-day-old term newborn with early myoclonic encephalopathy. The bursts last 2 to 3 seconds and appear synchronously and asynchronously on the two hemispheres. Polygraphic recording shows an altered respiratory pattern with chest movements occurring almost exclusively during the bursts phase. The polygraphic recording demonstrates fragmentary low-amplitude myoclonic jerks involving both extremities and shifting randomly from one side to another. Gain, 15 μV/mm; high frequency filter, 70 Hz; paper speed, 15 mm/s.

generally appear late in the course of the disease, usually at around 3 to 4 months of age. A metabolic etiology is highest on the differential, including glycine encephalopathy, propionic academia, D-glyceric acidemia, and methylmalonic aciduria.[178] Numerous cases of pyridoxine dependency presenting as EME have been reported, supporting an early therapeutic trial with pyridoxine in this condition.[179]

OS, first reported by Ohtahara in 1976,[180,181] is also characterized by onset within the first 3 months of life (most often in the neonatal period), persistent SB pattern on EEG, and encephalopathy. The distinctive seizure type in this condition consists of tonic spasms, isolated or in cluster, symmetric or asymmetric. Partial seizures may also be present, whereas myoclonic seizures are very rare.[182] The SB pattern, as described by Ohtahara and colleagues,[180,181,183] is consistently observed in both wake and sleep states, and it is characterized by high-voltage bursts alternating with nearly isoelectric periods at an approximately regular rate. Bursts of 1 to 3 seconds comprise 150- to 350-microvolt HVS waves intermixed with multifocal spikes. The duration of the suppression phase ranges from 2 to 5 seconds. Similar to EME, the prognosis of infants with OS is poor: developmental delay and evolution into West syndrome is common. Structural brain abnormalities, such as hemimegalencephaly (see Fig. 130.15) and large focal cortical dysplasias, represent the most frequent etiology of OS, whereas metabolic disorders have been reported in only a few cases. More recently, a main focus of investigation regarding pathophysiology of OS has been on genetic mutations, including aristaless-related homeobox *(ARX)* gene,[184] and syntaxin-binding protein 1 *(STXBP1)* gene.[185]

BENIGN FAMILIAL NEONATAL EPILEPSY

BFNE is an autosomal dominant epilepsy syndrome of the newborn. Typically, seizures occur on day 2 or 3 of life, with the majority in the first week of life. Seizures are brief (1 to 2 minutes in duration) but can occur up to 30 times/day, sometimes evolving into status epilepticus.[186] Family history often reveals other members with seizures in the neonatal period.[187]

The seizure semiology is characterized by initial asymmetric tonic posturing, often accompanied by autonomic features (apnea), sometimes with progression to unilateral or bilateral clonic jerks. Myoclonic seizures and epileptic spasms have not been reported. The ictal EEG is characterized by an electrodecremental pattern with superimposed muscle artifact during the tonic phase, and then rhythmic focal spike and wave discharges during the clonic phase (Fig. 130.16). Interestingly, a distinct ictal aEEG pattern has been described in neonates with KCNQ2-related epilepsies,[188] characterized by a sudden rise in in the upper and lower margin followed by a marked reduction of the electrical activity (Fig. 130.17). The interictal EEG may show some bilateral independent epileptiform abnormalities mainly over the central regions but is otherwise normal. Poor prognostic patterns, such as BS, have never been reported. Seizures show a rapid response to oral sodium-channel blockers such as carbamazepine in a high percentage of cases.[186] The genes associated with BFNE are *KCNQ2* on chromosome 20q13.3 and *KCNQ3* on chromosome 8q24 and encode the voltage-gated potassium channel subunits KV 7.2 (Q2) and KV 7.3 (Q3), which play a key role in repolarizing action potentials by allowing flow of potassium out of the cell; the reduction of the activity of these channels will cause increased neuronal excitability.

KCNQ2 ENCEPHALOPATHY

More recently, the genetic screening for *KCNQ2/KCNQ3* mutations of patients with unexplained neonatal-onset epileptic encephalopathy led to the recognition of de novo *KCNQ2* mutations in patients with severe neonatal epileptic encephalopathy. This new entity has been named *KCNQ2* encephalopathy and is characterized by intractable seizures of neonatal onset and severe psychomotor impairment. Within the last 2 years, a number of studies with several dozen patients

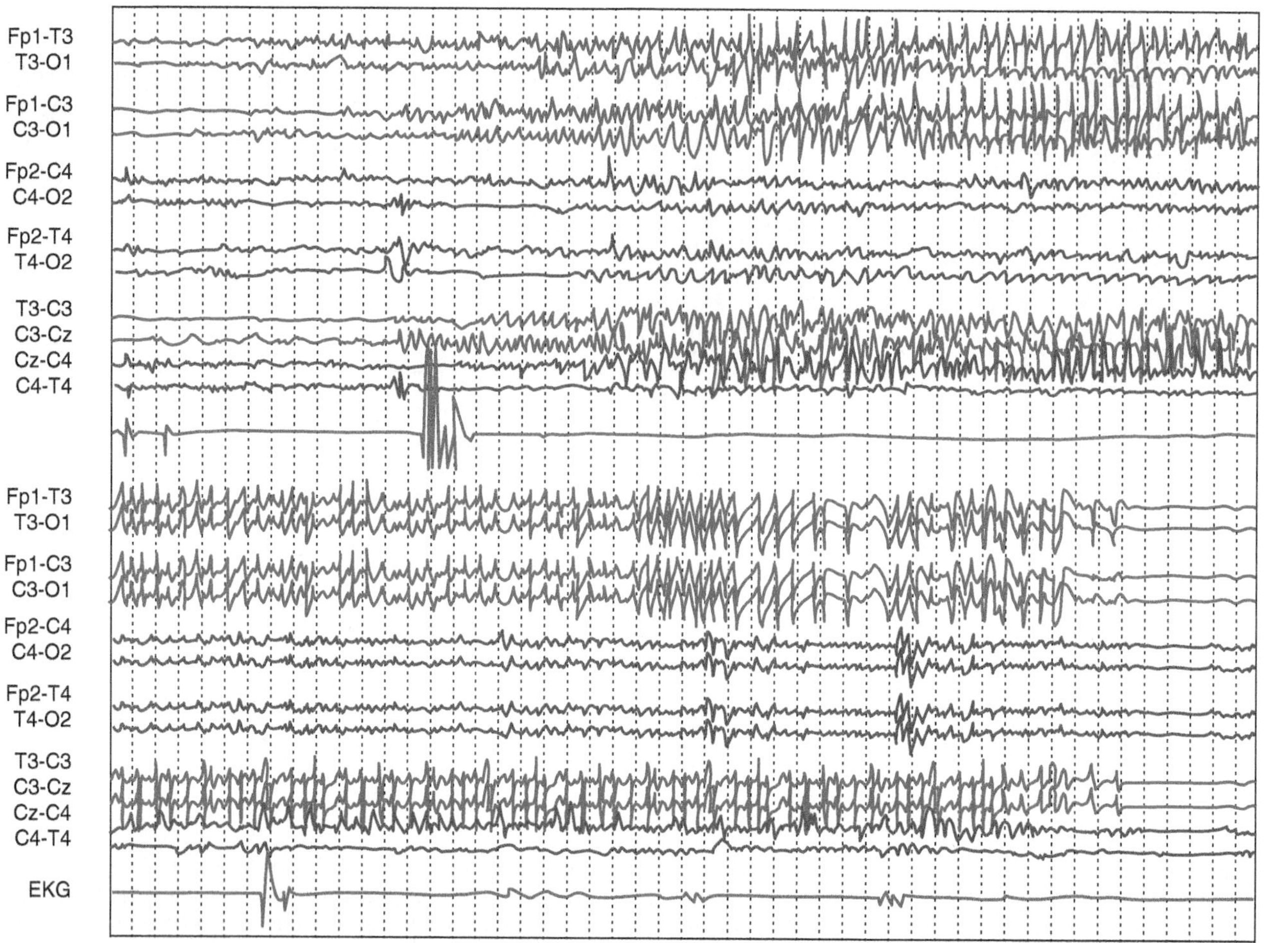

Fig. 130.16 One hundred-twenty-second epoch of ictal recording in a 4-day-old term neonate with benign familial neonatal seizures showing a left focal seizure, which starts with a tonic phase of asymmetric tonic posturing correlating with the initial low-amplitude fast activity, followed by a focal clonic phase correlating with rhythmic, high-amplitude spikes over the left hemisphere. At the end of the ictal discharge, asymmetric postictal attenuation is seen over the right hemisphere. Gain, 7 μV/mm; high frequency filter, 70 Hz; paper speed, 15 mm/s.

have been reported.[189-193] Several common features are seen in patients with *KCNQ2* encephalopathy when compared with BFNS. The onset of seizures occurs in the first week of life, most often the very first days. The seizure semiology also is very similar to that of BFNE—a prominent tonic component, with or without associated clonic jerking of the face or limbs—and is often associated with autonomic features such as apnea and desaturation. However, the seizure frequency in *KCNQ2* encephalopathy is quite high, with multiple seizures per day or even per hour. Similar to BFNS, seizures are particularly sensitive to sodium channel blockers, including carbamazepine and phenytoin.[194] In the long term, there is a tendency for seizure remission after the first years of life. All babies will have a severely abnormal interictal EEG pattern, either of BS or multifocal epileptiform activity.

More recently, the analysis of vEEG findings in patients with *KCNQ2* encephalopathy diagnosed in the neonatal period allowed the description of a distinct electroclinical phenotype, as well as a dramatic response to oral carbamazepine[192] and/or phenytoin.[194] The ictal EEG is characterized by initial low-voltage fast activity over a single hemisphere followed by focal spike and wave complexes. Although the seizures are quite short, the postictal phase is characterized by marked and prolonged diffuse voltage attenuation (Fig. 130.18). Although both age at onset and seizure semiology are similar to those of BFNS, the interictal EEG and clinical examination in babies with *KCNQ2* encephalopathy are very different and show lack of physiologic patterns and multifocal epileptiform abnormalities, intermixed with random, asynchronous attenuations (Fig. 130.19).

EPILEPSY OF INFANCY WITH MIGRATING FOCAL SEIZURES

EIMFS, first described by Coppola and Dulac in 1995,[195] is characterized by polymorphous, migrating, almost continuous, highly intractable, focal seizures associated with arrest of development, resulting in profound disability. Mutation of *KCNT1*, which encodes for a voltage-dependent and intracellular sodium-activated potassium channel, is tightly associated.[196]

EEG ictal discharges arise randomly from various areas of both hemispheres and migrate from one region to another, conferring the main feature and name to this syndrome. Most affected infants start to have seizures in the first few weeks of life, and all start having seizures by 6 months of age.[197] At onset, interictal EEG background varies from normal to diffuse slowing, and epileptiform discharges may be rare, with unifocal or multifocal interictal patterns. The multifocal character of the seizures may become evident only with prolonged vEEG monitoring, which plays an important role in the diagnosis of this disease. EEGs reflect the escalation of seizure activity, as no infant continues to have a normal EEG. The location of the ictal onset varies not only from side to side but also within a hemisphere. Electrographically, the single ictal event shift from one region to another and from one hemisphere to the other and additional seizures beginning in other areas in either

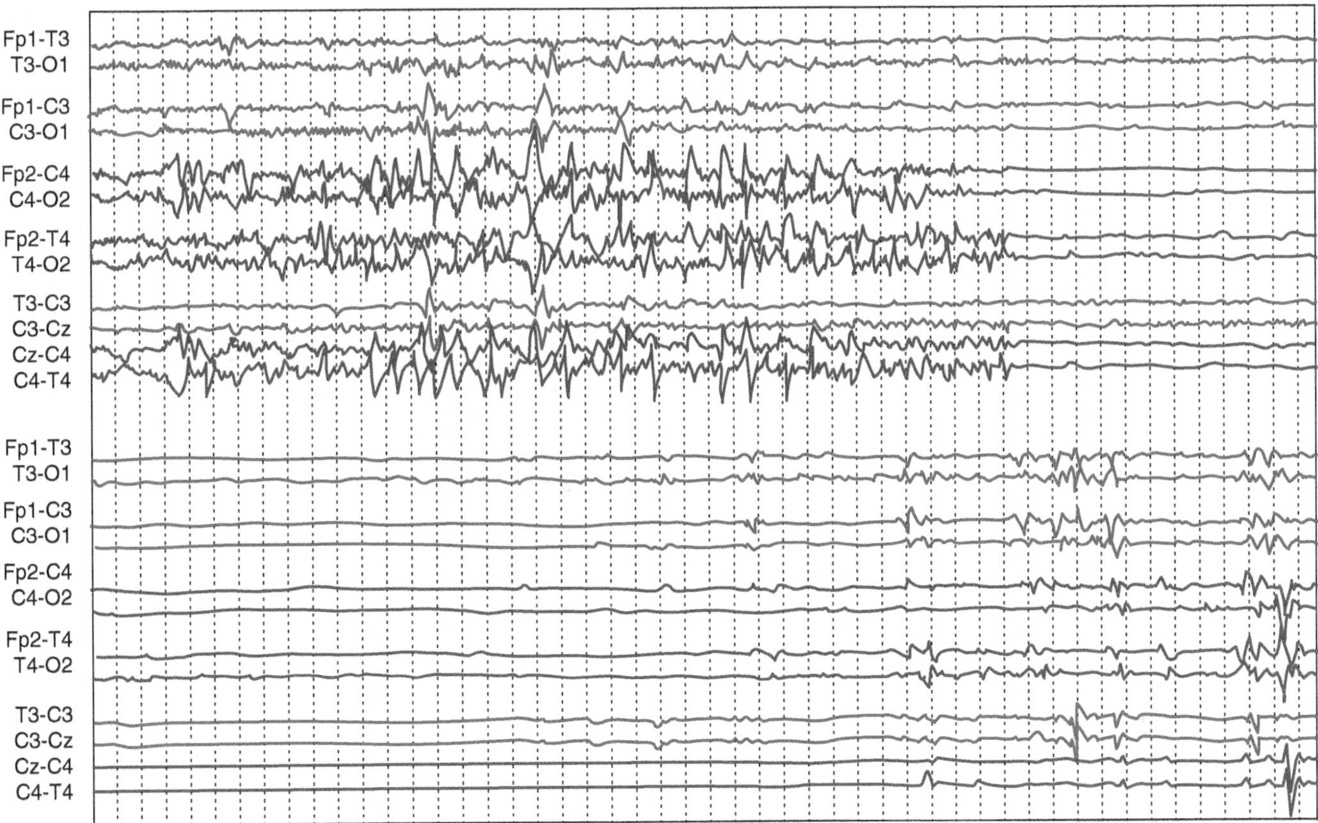

Fig. 130.17 One hundred-twenty-second epoch of ictal recording in a 6-week-old infant (ex-preterm born at 34 weeks, 40 weeks postmenstrual age at the time of this recording) with *KCNQ2* encephalopathy showing a short focal seizure starting with focal low-voltage fast activity over the right hemisphere with superimposed muscle artifacts corresponding to the asymmetric tonic posturing phase, followed by focal rhythmic high-amplitude spikes corresponding to the brief clonic phase. Although the duration of the seizure is only approximately 40 seconds, there is a severe, diffuse, postictal attenuation lasting approximately 75 seconds with slow recovery of the background activity. Gain, 7 μV/mm; high frequency filter, 70 Hz; paper speed, 15 mm/s.

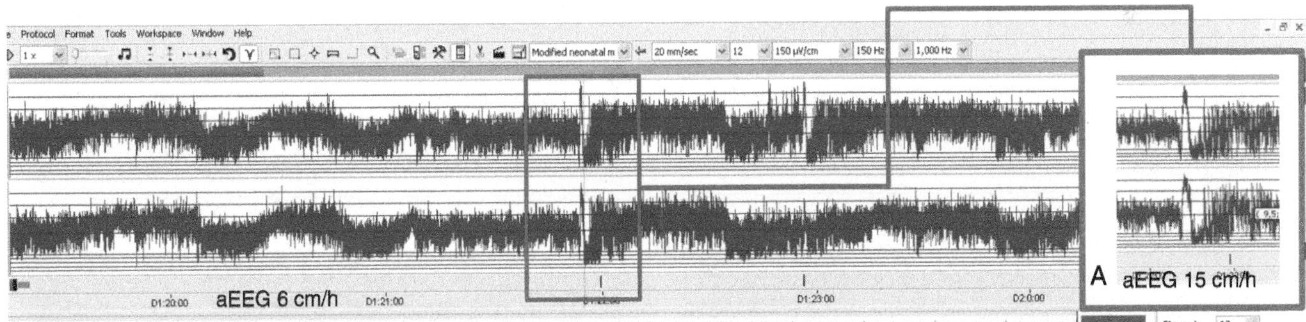

Fig. 130.18 Amplitude-integrated electroencephalography (aEEG) seizure pattern in term neonate with benign familial neonatal epilepsy. aEEG at 6 cm/h and shows an ictal discharge over a continuous background pattern, identified by a brief and rise in amplitude followed by a marked reduction of electrocortical activity. This is more easily seen in less time compressed recording at 15 cm/h (A). *aEEG,* Amplitude-integrated EEG.

hemisphere could start before the end of the first event or may immediately follow it (Fig. 130.20). The clinical semiology of seizures begins with focal motor movements that can alternate from one side of the body to another with lateral deviation of the head and eyes, eye jerks, twitching of the eyelids, limb myoclonic jerks, and increased tone of one or both limbs. The focal motor component is often accompanied by autonomic signs, including flushing of the face, salivation, and apnea. Truly generalized tonic-clonic seizures are very rare, even later in life. Prolonged observation soon shows that both sides are alternatively affected, which demonstrates the involvement of the whole brain cortex. Given the unique clinical and EEG features exhibited by children with EMFSI, it is extremely unlikely that this condition could be mistaken for one of the severe epileptic syndromes of neonatal period, such EME and OS, as the above entities display the typical BS interictal EEG pattern. In addition, differently from OS, spasms are lacking in EIMFS. A EEG quantitative analysis of patients with EIMFS showed that the migrating EEG pattern is not a random process. Seizures began localized predominantly in temporal and occipital areas and evolved with a stable frequency of 4 to 7 Hz. Inter- and intrahemispheric migration were present in 60% of EIMFS seizures. Interhemispheric migrating seizures spread in 71% from temporal and occipital channels to the homologous contralateral ones, while intrahemispheric seizures involved mainly frontotemporal, temporal, and occipital channels.[198]

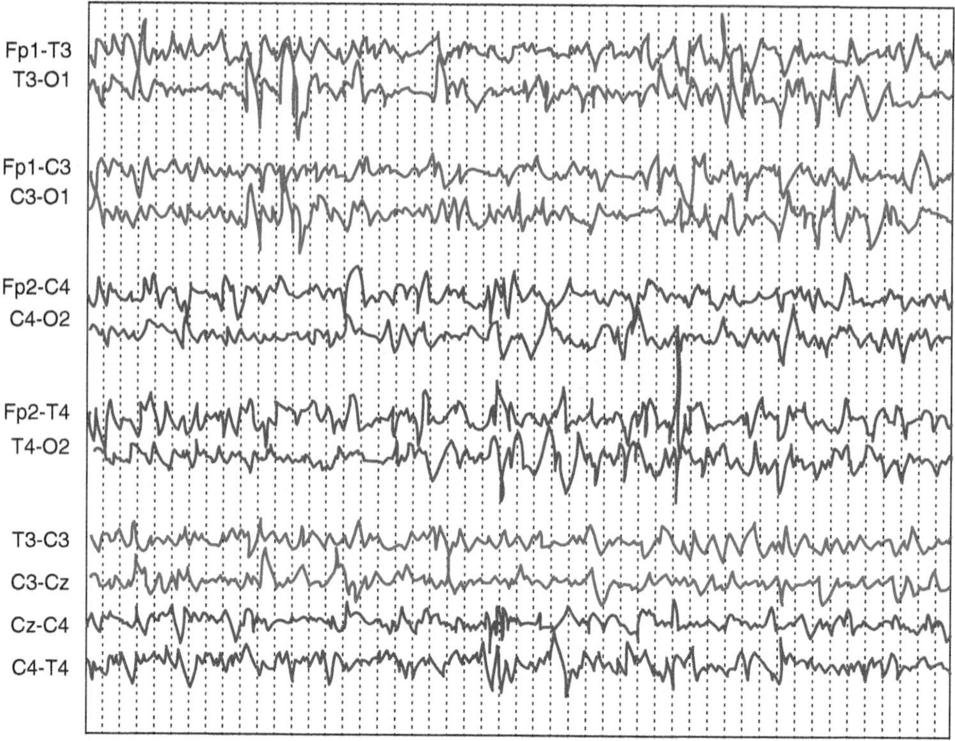

Fig. 130.19 Interictal electroencephalography in the same patient as Fig. 130.18, characterized by multifocal spikes, sharp waves, and slow waves with short 1-second periods of asynchronous random attenuation. Gain, 7 μV/mm; high frequency filter, 70 Hz; paper speed, 15 mm/s.

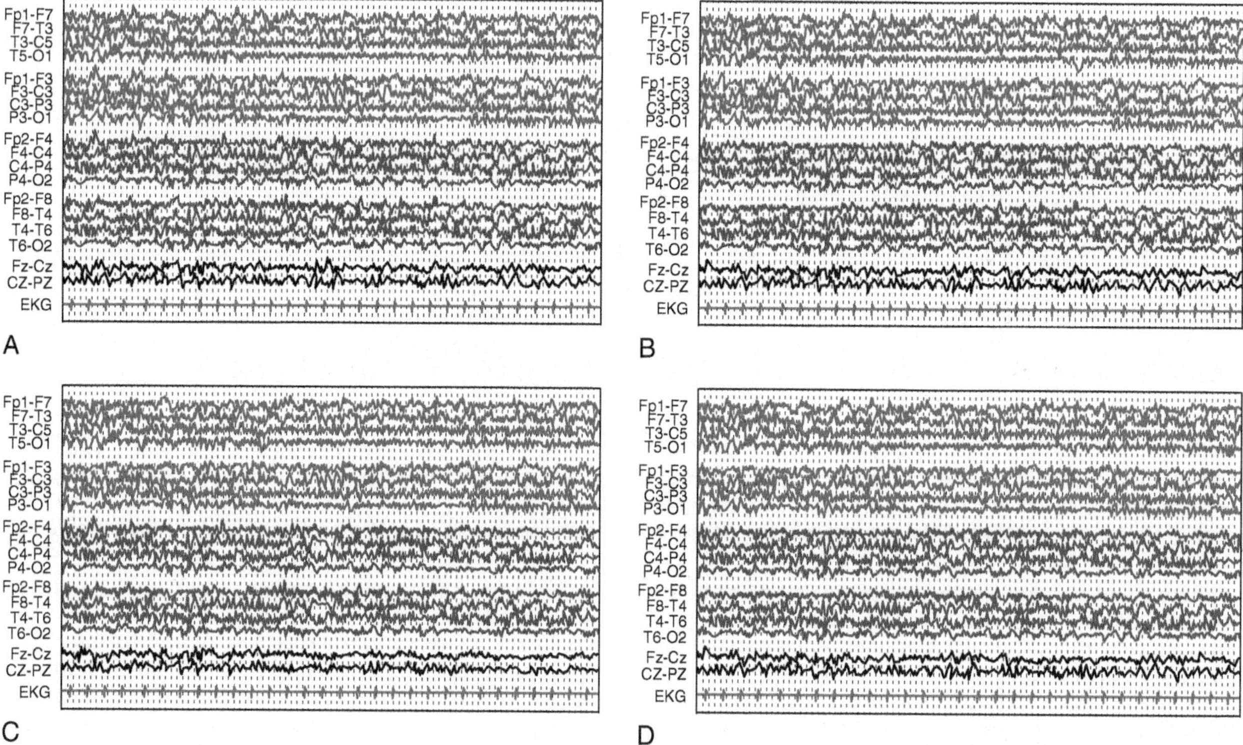

Fig. 130.20 Ictal recording in a 2-month-old term infant with neonatal-onset epilepsy with migrating focal seizures and *KCNT1* mutation. Note the random onset of prolonged ictal discharges migrating from one hemisphere to the other. (A) A low-amplitude fast activity seizure starts over the posterior regions of the left hemisphere. (B) Simultaneous independent ictal discharges involving two different cortical regions: while the ictal discharge over the left posterior region is ending, another ictal discharge starts over the central-temporal regions of the right hemisphere. (C and D) The seizure over the left hemisphere is over, while the ictal discharge over the right hemisphere now involves the frontal-central-temporal regions. Gain, 15 μV/mm; high frequency filter, 60 Hz; paper speed, 15 mm/s.

EPILEPTIC AND DEVELOPMENTAL ENCEPHALOPATHY ASSOCIATED WITH CDKL5 DEFICIENCY DISORDER

In this X-linked condition most frequently observed in females (12:1 female-to-male ratio) the epileptic encephalopathy associated with *CDKL5* mutations can arise in the neonatal period, with the majority of patients having onset of seizures within the first 3 months of life. At onset, the interictal EEG can be normal. A three-stage electroclinical course was described by Bahi-Buisson and colleagues.[199] Initially, affected individuals show frequent, albeit brief, seizures. Some of these children may reach seizure control after several weeks to months, with some even achieving a "honeymoon period" of seizure freedom. Regardless of ultimate epilepsy course, all patients at this stage already exhibit hypotonia and poor eye contact. The second stage is characterized by a failure of developmental progression and the appearance of epileptic spasms with or without hypsarrhythmia on EEG. Finally, in the third stage, at approximately 2 to 3 years of age, children with CDD suffer from severe refractory epilepsy with multiple seizure types, including tonic, myoclonic, and spasms. By then, EEG is abnormal, with high-amplitude slow waves and bursts of spikes and polyspikes (Fig. 130.21). A distinctive seizure type seen during the course of this epileptic encephalopathy is the hypermotor-tonic-spasms sequence.[200] However, recognizing CDD at onset, in the very first weeks of life, can be challenging, and most patients are diagnosed only later in life. Nevertheless, the onset of brief tonic-spasm seizures in an infant, particularly a girl, with no interictal EEG abnormalities should suggest a CDD (Fig. 130.22).[200]

TOWARD STRATIFIED DIAGNOSIS OF NEONATAL EPILEPSIES

Historically, studies on neonatal seizures have lumped all etiologies together. The past few years have seen the recognition of neonatal epilepsies as a separate from acute symptomatic neonatal seizures. Many neonatal epilepsies have a genetic origin and some of them are amenable to specific treatment. Therefore, early distinction is essential for appropriate clinical management and counseling. However, many unresolved questions remain. The electroclinical presentation in the neonatal period of neonatal-onset epilepsies is not yet well defined because many patients are diagnosed later in life, and clinical and EEG findings related to the neonatal period may be scarce. Additionally, mutations in the same gene can be associated with both benign and severe epilepsies. Early diagnosis of neonatal epilepsies enables effective treatment to be established before the damaging effect of seizures on the developing brain have taken place and improve the long-term outcome. Precise characterization of the neonatal presentation raises the index of diagnostic suspicion, prioritizing patients with rare conditions for targeted investigations, reducing the exposure to unnecessary procedures. The introduction of whole-genome diagnostics in NICU should resolve these issues.[201] Collaboration among multiple subspecialists and care providers should allow

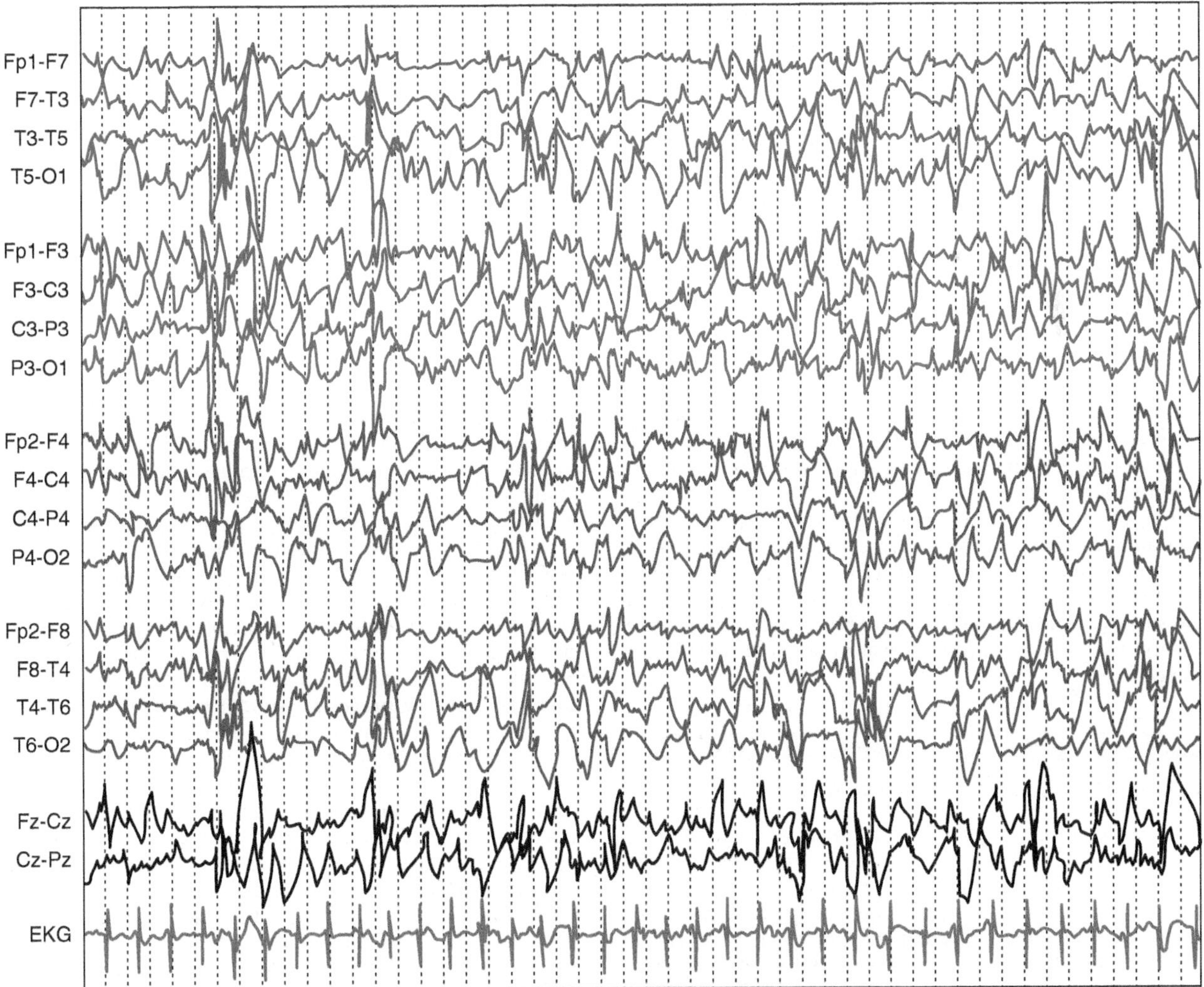

Fig. 130.21 Electroencephalography (EEG) recorded in a 2-year-old girl with CDKL5 deficiency disorder. Interictal EEG recorded during sleep and showing diffuse slowing with intermixed frequent high-amplitude generalized bursts of polyspikes, spikes, and waves. Gain, 20 μV/mm; high frequency filter, 70 Hz; paper speed, 15 mm/s.

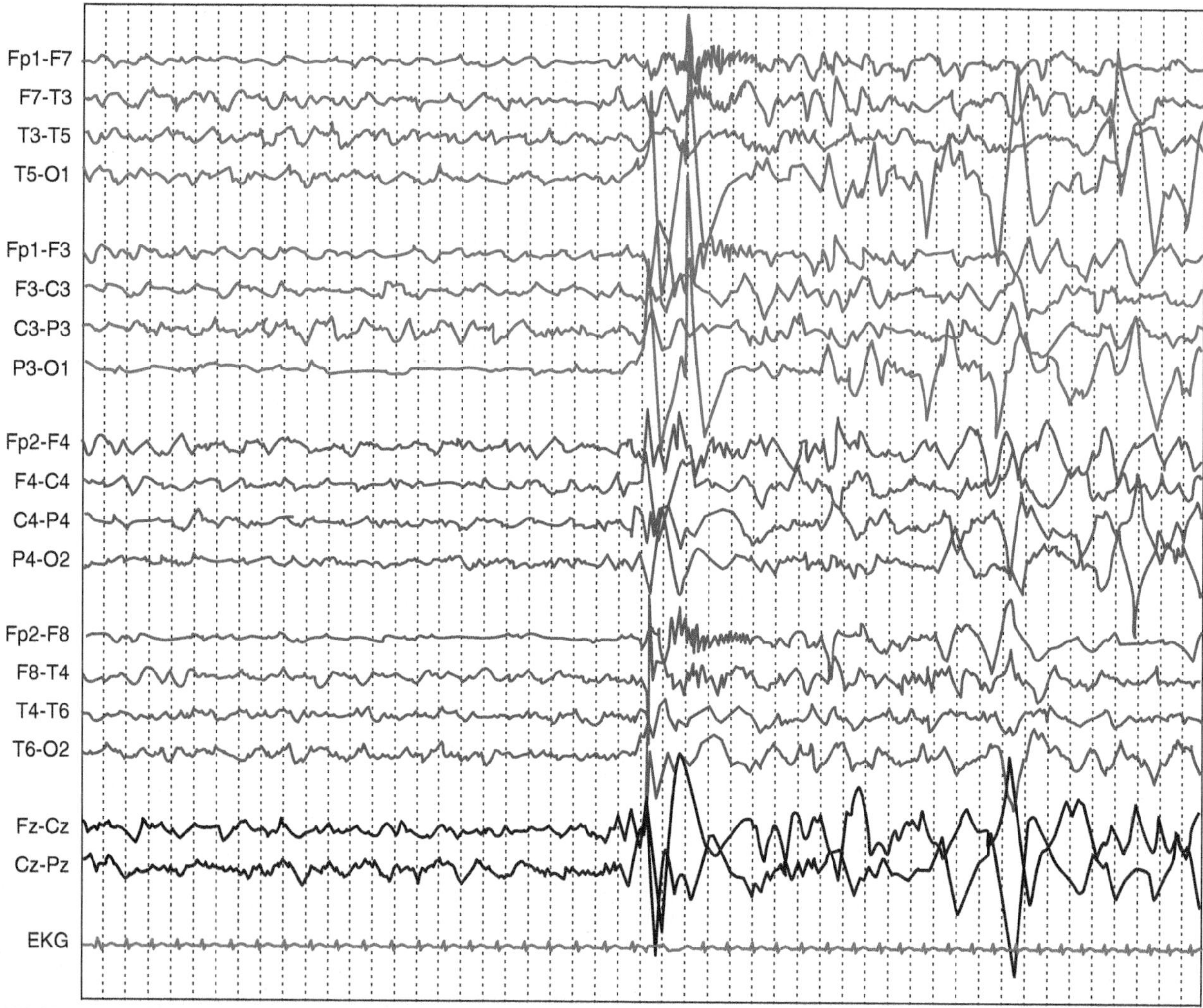

Fig. 130.22 Electroencephalography recorded at 3 weeks of age in the same patient as Fig. 130.21 showing the ictal pattern of a brief tonic seizure characterized by diffuse low-amplitude fast activity preceded by a normal background. Gain, 7 μV/mm; high frequency filter, 70 Hz; paper speed, 15 mm/s.

for the integration of clinical and vEEG findings into the process of interpretation of whole-exome and whole-genome data, as it is likely that whole-genome sequencing will standard of care in the NICU in the near future.[202]

In conclusion, the definition of the electroclinical phenotype remains an important piece for a correct diagnosis, management, and prognosis. In the context of precision medicine, an accurate characterization of the neonatal epilepsy phenotype is essential for the success of new treatment strategies, especially when the goal is not only seizure control but also a normal developmental outcome.

EFFECT OF DRUGS AND HYPOTHERMIA ON NEONATAL ELECTROENCEPHALOGRAPHY

Although there are few studies documenting the effect of drugs on the neonatal EEG, it is evident that, as with older children, drugs (especially if in the toxic range) can alter background activity. Prolonged periods of inactivity on the EEG recording usually occur following a loading dose of phenobarbital and may last longer than 1 hour following administration. Staudt and colleagues[203] argued that infants with phenobarbital plasma levels above 6 mg/dL show significant background suppression. Other authors also reported the appearance of isoelectric[204] or invariant discontinuous recording[88] after treatment with phenobarbital. Levels greater than 25 μg/mL in neonates were reported to suppress EEG activity.[204] In their study, Ashwal and Schneider found a discordance between EEG activity and radionuclide uptake in infants with phenobarbital levels between 25 and 35 μg/mL. The lack of EEG activity with presence of cerebral blood flood suggested that phenobarbital suppressed EEG activity. In the same study, one infant who met the clinical criteria for brain death had absent cerebral activity with a level of 30 μg/mL. However, he developed some cerebral activity when the phenobarbital level fell to zero.[204] These are important observations that should be taken into account by electroencephalographers, as phenobarbital therapy is frequently administered to the neonate on a clinical basis, prior to the first EEG recording. However, this correlation was not confirmed in preterm infants. Benda and colleagues by studying 46 preterm infants found that a mean serum level of phenobarbital of 34.5 μg/mL with a range of 14 to 64 μg/mL did not prolong IBI during *tracé discontinu* in preterm infants.[205] Among medications other than AEDs that may also affect the EEG tracing, morphine has been found to produce profound, largely reversible alteration of neonatal EEG as recorded in preterm and term infants.[206] Conversely, when Bye and colleagues investigated the effect of morphine and midazolam on background EEG of a group of neonates undergoing extracorporeal membrane oxygenation, they noted that despite midazolam and morphine serum levels that were sufficient to produce adequate sedation, no patients had burst-suppressed or inactive EEG backgrounds.[207] In addition, these authors pointed out that prolonged immobility due to sedation may lead to artifacts due to scalp edema and subsequent false attenuation of EEG background.

Hypothermia has become the standard of care for neonates with HIE and in many NICUs patients are monitored with continuous vEEG. The effect on the neonatal EEG varies depending on the level of hypothermia. Deep hypothermia such as 30°C and lower, significantly alters the EEG background. Studies in infants on cardiopulmonary bypass have shown slowing and decreased amplitude followed by discontinuous activity.[208,209] However, hypothermia to 33.5°C to 34.5°C does not seem to cause significant changes in EEG background activity. Newborns undergoing extracorporeal membrane oxygenation and cooling to 34°C showed no change in aEEG voltage.[210] However, therapeutic hypothermia does change the time at which background patterns are predictive of MRI injury.[130] Interestingly, in one study predicted seizure burden from neonatal stroke was decreased in infants undergoing hypothermia.[211] While a normal EEG at the beginning of cooling predicts a favorable MRI, the prognostic value of BS or extremely low voltage patterns is higher at mid-cooling or thereafter.[130,212]

FUTURE PERSPECTIVES

Additional monitoring strategies that need to be more extensively studied in the neonatal period include digital trend analysis (DTA), envelope trend, and spectrogram.[213] In brief, the raw EEG signal is mathematically treated to present information that can be more readily interpreted by bedside clinicians. Density spectral array gives an expression of how much of the power in the EEG signal falls into the different frequency ranges. It can be used as an adjunct to conventional EEG, but further studies in the newborn period are requested to better understand its diagnostic contribution.[2] Experience with envelope trend is even more limited,[213] but one study found that for prolonged seizures its sensitivity approached that of aEEG.[214] It displays the median amplitude of successive EEG epochs, with a significant ability to detect brief and slowly evolving seizures.[2] Alongside these methods, integrated research groups are working on development and validation-automated detection systems for seizure recognition and background grading algorithms.[7,215,216] For the time being, however, the gold standard of real-time detection of seizures with continuous full EEG monitoring remains unfeasible in usual clinical practice. The chief obstacles remain starting a recording, and resourcing the real-time specialist review of suspect seizures.[217] Remote EEG reporting in large international networks has also been used for research purposes as a strategy to overcome the paucity of experts in the field of neonatal neurophysiology.[3]

Some research is also being directed to establish to what extent high-density EEG could improve information acquisition on the immature brain and how much this could affect future research projects or even clinical practice.[218] All the cited technologic improvements may also represent a step forward in the understanding of neonatal brain physiology, in order to move from electroclinical correlations and pattern recognition toward a deeper knowledge of the basis of maturational processes.

Finally, the new classification of the epilepsies of the ILAE,[219] which applies to older children and adults, incorporates etiology at each stage of the diagnostic process, such as the diagnosis of the seizure type, the epilepsy type, and the epilepsy syndrome. From the moment that the patient presents with the first epileptic seizure, the clinician should be aiming to determine the etiology, with emphasis on those that have implications for treatment. However, the early diagnosis and personalized treatment in the neonate is lagging behind. In the era of precision medicine, implementation of multimodal diagnostic approaches, including continuous vEEG, MRI, metabolic screen, and whole genome-wide sequencing with rapid turnaround time, will enable early detection, stratified diagnosis (i.e., brain injury, stroke, metabolic disease, brain malformation, or rare neonatal epilepsies), and appropriate treatment, including drug repurposing, for neonatal seizures, epilepsies, and epileptic encephalopathies.

CONCLUSION

Neonatal EEG is the gold standard to assess brain maturation, encephalopathy, and seizure recognition and classification, to make epilepsy syndrome diagnoses in neonates. Interpreting neonatal EEG is very helpful in ensuring that neonatologists and child neurologists gain as much information as possible from this helpful, noninvasive bedside investigation. Continuous EEG monitoring lies at the forefront of neonatal neurocritical care. While neonatal EEG had previously been limited at many centers to brief routine studies, there is an increasing demand for long-term continuous vEEG in the nursery for a wide spectrum of patients. Expanding the use of vEEG in neonates has greatly improved the management of neonates, from extreme preterm to the term baby, at risk of neurologic dysfunction, and has allowed the delineation of neonatal epilepsy electroclinical phenotypes. Finally, as neonatal EEG is increasingly used in the NICU, the demand will strengthen for reliable methods of automated seizure detection to facilitate timely seizure identification and treatment.

A complete reference list is available at www.ExpertConsult.com. 

SELECT REFERENCES

1. McCoy B, Hahn CD. Continuous EEG monitoring in the neonatal intensive care unit. *J Clin Neurophysiol*. 2013;30:106.
2. Shellhaas RA, Chang T, Tsuchida T, et al. The American Clinical Neurophysiology Society's Guideline on continuous electroencephalography monitoring in neonates. *J Clin Neurophysiol*. 2011;28:611.
3. Boylan GB, Stevenson NJ, Vanhatalo S. Monitoring neonatal seizures. *Semin Fetal Neonatal Med*. 2013;18:202.
10. André M, Lamblin MD, d'Allest AM, et al. Electroencephalography in premature and full-term infants. Developmental features and glossary. *Neurophysiol Clin*. 2010;40:59.
11. Scher MS. Electroencephalography of the newborn: normal and abnormal features. In: Niedermeyer E, Lopes da Silva FH, eds. *Electroencephalography: Basic Principles, Clinical Applications, and Related Fields*. 5th ed. Philadelphia: Lippincott Williams and Wilkins; 2005:937-989.
12. Watanabe K, Hayakawa F, Okumura A. Neonatal EEG: a powerful tool in the assessment of brain damage in preterm infants. *Brain Dev*. 1999;21:361.
18. Pisani F, Barilli AL, Sisti L, et al. Preterm infants with video-EEG confirmed seizures: outcome at 30 months of age. *Brain Dev*. 2008;30:20.
19. Pisani F, Cerminara C, Fusco C, Sisti L. Neonatal status epilepticus vs recurrent neonatal seizures: clinical findings and outcome. *Neurology*. 2007;69:2177.
21. Scher MS, Alvin J, Gaus L, et al. Uncoupling of EEG-clinical neonatal seizures after antiepileptic drug use. *Pediatr Neurol*. 2003;28:277.
33. Tsuchida TN, Wusthoff CJ, Shellhaas RA, et al. American Clinical Neurophysiology Society standardized EEG terminology and categorization for the description of continuous EEG monitoring in neonates: report of the American Clinical Neurophysiology Society critical care monitoring committee. *J Clin Neurophysiol*. 2013;30:161.
38. Vecchierini MF, d'Allest AM, Verpillat P. EEG patterns in 10 extreme premature neonates with normal neurological outcome: qualitative and quantitative data. *Brain Dev*. 2003;25:330.
46. Lamblin MD, André M. Electroencephalogram of the full-term newborn. Normal features and hypoxic-ischemic encephalopathy. *Neurophysiol Clin*. 2011;41:1.
51. Benders MJ, Palmu K, Menache C, et al. Early brain activity relates to subsequent brain growth in premature infants. *Cereb Cortex*. 2015;25:3014.
55. Khazipov R, Luhmann HJ. Early patterns of electrical activity in the developing cerebral cortex of humans and rodents. *Trends Neurosci*. 2006;29:414.
56. Omidvarnia A, Fransson P, Metsäranta M, Vanhatalo S. Functional bimodality in the brain networks of preterm and term human newborns. *Cereb Cortex*. 2014;24:2657.

62. Hayakawa M, Okumura A, Hayakawa F, et al. Background electroencephalographic (EEG) activities of very preterm infants born at less than 27 weeks gestation: a study on the degree of continuity. *Arch Dis Child Fetal Neonatal Ed*. 2001;84:F163.
66. Vecchierini MF, André M, d'Allest AM. Normal EEG of premature infants born between 24 and 30 weeks gestational age: terminology, definitions and maturation aspects. *Neurophysiol Clin*. 2007;37:311.
69. Scher MS. Ontogeny of EEG sleep from neonatal through infancy periods. *Handb Clin Neurol*. 2011;98:111.
74. Colonnese M, Khazipov R. Spontaneous activity in developing sensory circuits: implications for resting state fMRI. *Neuroimage*. 2012;62:2212.
76. Khazipov R, Sirota A, Leinekugel X, et al. Early motor activity drives spindle bursts in the developing somatosensory cortex. *Nature*. 2004;432:758.
77. Milh M, Kaminska A, Huon C, et al. Rapid cortical oscillations and early motor activity in premature human neonate. *Cereb Cortex*. 2007;17:1582.
81. Hughes JR, Miller JK, Fino JJ, Hughes CA. The sharp theta rhythm on the occipital areas of prematures (STOP): a newly described waveform. *Clin Electroencephalogr*. 1990;21:77.
83. Monod N, Pajot N, Guidasci S. The neonatal EEG: statistical studies and prognostic value in full-term and pre-term babies. *Electroencephalogr Clin Neurophysiol*. 1972;32:529.
104. Menache CC, Bourgeois BF, Volpe JJ. Prognostic value of neonatal discontinuous EEG. *Pediatr Neurol*. 2002;27:93.
118. Biagioni E, Bartalena L, Boldrini A, et al. Constantly discontinuous EEG patterns in full-term neonates with hypoxic-ischaemic encephalopathy. *Clin Neurophysiol*. 1999;110:1510.
122. Pressler RM, Boylan GB, Morton M, et al. Early serial EEG in hypoxic ischaemic encephalopathy. *Clin Neurophysiol*. 2001;112:31.
130. Nash KB, Bonifacio SL, Glass HC, et al. Video-EEG monitoring in newborns with hypoxic-ischemic encephalopathy treated with hypothermia. *Neurology*. 2011;76:556.
143. Marret S, Parain D, Ménard JF, et al. Prognostic value of neonatal electroencephalography in premature newborns less than 33 weeks of gestational age. *Electroencephalogr Clin Neurophysiol*. 1997;102:178.
148. Nagarajan L, Ghosh S, Palumbo L. Ictal electroencephalograms in neonatal seizures: characteristics and associations. *Pediatr Neurol*. 2011;45:11.
149. Lynch NE, Stevenson NJ, Livingstone V, et al. The temporal evolution of electrographic seizure burden in neonatal hypoxic ischemic encephalopathy. *Epilepsia*. 2012;53:549.
151. Shelhaas RA, Clancy RR. Characterization of neonatal seizures by conventional EEG and single-channel EEG. *Clin Neurophysiol*. 2007;118:2156-2900.
159. Pisani F, Copioli C, Di Gioia C, et al. Neonatal seizures: relation of ictal video-electroencephalography (EEG) findings with neurodevelopmental outcome. *J Child Neurol*. 2008;23:394.
170. Pisani F, Piccolo B, Cantalupo G, et al. Neonatal seizures and postneonatal epilepsy: a 7-y follow-up study. *Pediatr Res*. 2012;72:186.
171. Shellhaas RA, Wusthoff CJ, Tsuchida TN, et al. Profile of neonatal epilepsies: characteristics of a prospective US cohort. *Neurology*. 2017;89(9):893-899.
172. Cornet MC, Sands TT, Cilio MR. Neonatal epilepsies: clinical management. *Semin Fetal Neonatal Med*. 2018;23(3):204-212.
174. Berg AT, Berkovic SF, Brodie MJ, et al. Revised terminology and concepts for organization of seizure and epilepsies: report of the ILAE Commission on Classification and Terminology, 2005-2009. *Epilepsia*. 2010;51:676.
175. Aicardi J, Ohtahara S. Severe neonatal epilepsies with suppression-burst. In: Roger JB, Dravet M, Genton C, et al., eds. *Epileptic Syndromes in Infancy, Childhood and Adolescence*. Paris: John Libbey Eurotext; 2005:39-50.
178. Dulac O. Epileptic encephalopathy with suppression-bursts and nonketotic hyperglycinemia. *Handb Clin Neurol*. 2013;113:1785.
181. Ohtahara S, Yamatogi Y. Epileptic encephalopathies in early infancy with suppression-burst. *J Clin Neurophysiol*. 2003;20:398.
185. Saitzu H, Kato M, Mizuguchi T, et al. De novo mutations in the gene encoding STXBP1 (MUNCH-18) cause early infantile epileptic encephalopathy. *Nat Genet*. 2008;40:782.
186. Sands TT, Balestri M, Bellini G, et al. Rapid and safe response to low-dose carbamazepine in neonatal epilepsy. *Epilepsia*. 2016;57(12):2019-2030.
188. Vilan A, Mendes Ribeiro J, Striano P, et al. A distinctive ictal amplitude-integrated electroencephalography pattern in newborns with neonatal epilepsy associated with KCNQ2 mutations. *Neonatology*. 2017;112(4):387-393.
189. Weckhuysen S, Mandelstam S, Suls A, et al. KCNQ2 encephalopathy: emerging phenotype of a neonatal epileptic encephalopathy. *Ann Neurol*. 2012;71:15.
192. Numis AL, Angriman M, Sullivan JE, et al. KCNQ2 encephalopathy: delineation of the electroclinical phenotype and treatment response. *Neurology*. 2014;82:368.
194. Pisano T, Numis AL, Heavin SB, et al. Early and effective treatment of KCNQ2 encephalopathy. *Epilepsia*. 2015;56:685.
196. Barcia G, Fleming MR, Deligniere A, et al. De novo gain-of-function KCNT1 channel mutations cause malignant migrating partial seizures of infancy. *Nat Genet*. 2012;44:1255.
197. Cilio MR, Dulac O, Guerrini R, Vigevano F. Migrating partial seizures in infancy. In: Engel JJ, Pedley T, Aicardi J, eds. *Epilepsy: A Comprehensive Textbook (International Textbook of Medicine, vol 3)*. 2nd ed. Philadelphia: Lippincott William & Wilkins; 2008:2323-2328.
198. Kuchenbuch M, Benquet P, Kaminska A, et al. Quantitative analysis and EEG markers of KCNT1 epilepsy of infancy with migrating focal seizures. *Epilepsia*. 2019;60(1):20-32.
201. French CE, Delon I, Dolling H, et al. Whole genome sequencing reveals that genetic conditions are frequent in critically ill children. *Intensive Care Med*. 2019;45:627-636.
219. Scheffer IE, Berkovic S, Capovilla G, et al. ILAE classification of the epilepsies: position paper of the ILAE commission for classification and terminology. *Epilepsia*. 2017;58:512-521.

131 Intraventricular Hemorrhage in the Neonate

Brian H. Walsh | Terrie E. Inder

INTRODUCTION

Germinal matrix hemorrhage-intraventricular hemorrhage (IVH) is the commonest form of intracranial hemorrhage in the newborn and is characteristic of the premature infant.[1] The incidence of IVH in premature infants was documented to decline from very high rates of 34% to 49%[2-4] in the 1970s to approximately 20% in the late 1980s.[5,6] There has also been a modest reduction in the rates of severe IVH (grades III and IV), with a decline from 19% in 1993 to 15% by 2012. This decline, however, has not been consistent for all preterm infants, with minor reductions in severe IVHs only occurring among those of 26 weeks' gestation or greater (Fig. 131.1).[7]

Unfortunately in the past decade the incidence of IVH has remained static, with an overall incidence of 25% (Fig. 131.2). In one of the largest series, 535,682 very low-birth-weight infants were observed between 2009 and 2018 from 1022 neonatal intensive care units (NICUs) as part of the Vermont Oxford Network Very Low Birth Weight database (data provided from 2009 to 2018 from the Vermont Oxford Network database; see Figs. 131.2 and 131.3). The incidence of all grades of IVH remained static during this 9-year period at 24% to 26%, with the incidence of the severest forms of IVH (grades III and IV) being approximately 7%. It has been hypothesized that the rates of IVH may not be improving because of the greater number of extremely immature infants, with a higher risk of IVH, who are surviving. However, the data from the Vermont Oxford Network database from 2009 to 2018 demonstrate that the percentage of preterm infants weighing less than 750 g across this 9-year period remained at 16%.

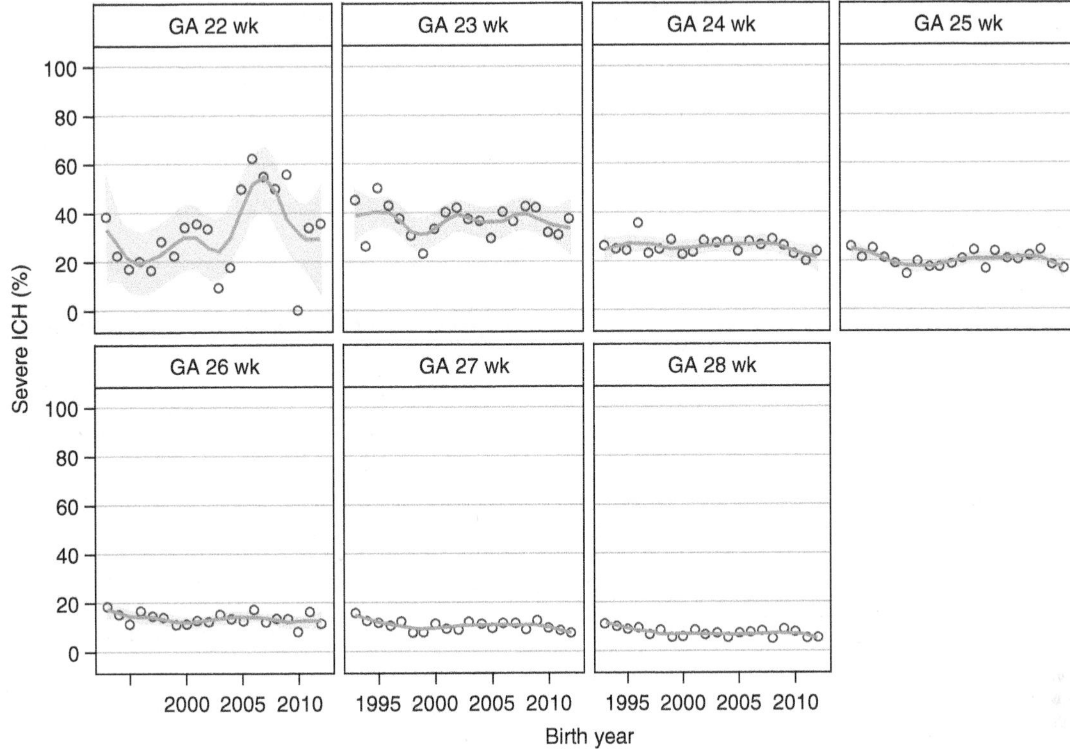

Fig. 131.1 Annual incidence of severe intracranial hemorrhage *(ICH)* for infants born from 22 to 28 weeks gestational age between 1993 and 2012. (Published with permission from Stoll BJ, Hansen NI, Bell EF, et al. Trends in care practices, morbidity, and mortality of extremely preterm neonates, 1993–2012. *JAMA*. 2015;314[10]:1039–1051.)

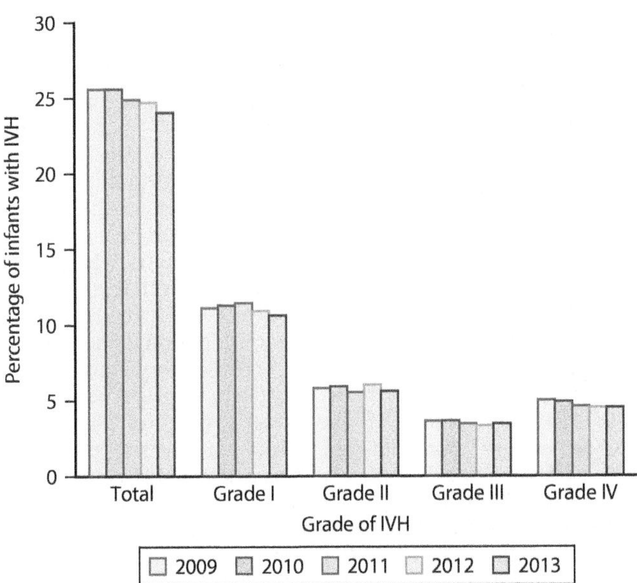

Fig. 131.2 The incidence of (percentage of all infants with) all grades of intraventricular hemorrhage *(IVH)*, grade I IVH, grade II IVH, grade III IVH, and grade IV IVH in the Vermont Oxford Network Very Low Birth Weight database from 2009 to 2013 (*n* = 247,392). The incidence of IVH is static across all grades and across the 5-year period. (From Horbar JD. *Vermont-Oxford Network Database Summary*. Burlington, VT: Vermont-Oxford Network; 2014.)

The Vermont Oxford Network database data also highlights the strong association between birth weight and risk for IVH (see Fig. 131.3).[8] For infants weighing less than 750 g, the risk of any IVH is approximately threefold higher than for a preterm infant weighing more than 1250 g (44% vs. 16%), with a 10-fold higher risk of grade III–IV IVH (20% vs. 2%; see Fig. 131.3). For an infant weighing less than 750 g, an equal risk (approximately 10%) exists for developing grade I through grade IV IVH, while an infant weighing more than 1250 g has a 10% risk of grade I IVH but only a 1% risk of grade III or grade IV IVH (see Fig. 131.3). Thus, IVH remains a significant problem in the preterm infant, particularly for the most immature infants. Currently, in the United States approximately 57,000 very low-birth-weight infants are born each year,[9] of whom approximately 14,000 will have IVH, and more than 2000 infants will have periventricular hemorrhagic infarction.

In this chapter, we briefly discuss the background of diagnosis and clinical presentation for IVH before a more detailed discussion of the neuropathology and pathogenesis of the lesion, highlighting both experimental and human study findings.

CLINICAL FEATURES

The most common clinical presentation for IVH is a *clinically silent* syndrome occurring in up to 50% of infants in whom even careful and serial clinical assessments may fail to reveal any abnormal signs indicative of the lesion.[10–12] The timing of onset of IVH by clinical recognition is limited. From cranial ultrasound studies, it appears that the *onset of IVH* is by the first day of life in at least 50% of affected infants, with up to 90% of lesions present by 72 hours[5,13] and all lesions visible by 7 days.[14] However, further *progression of an initial IVH* occurs in 20% to 40% of the affected infants, with the maximal extent of the lesion generally seen by 3 to 5 days after the initial diagnosis.[15,16]

DIAGNOSIS

The diagnosis of IVH is most commonly established at the bedside of the sick preterm infant with use of portable cranial

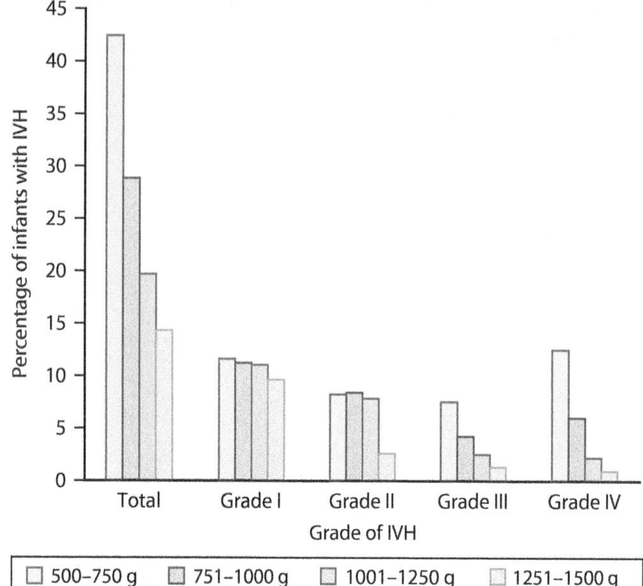

Fig. 131.3 The incidence of (percentage of all infants with) all grades of intraventricular hemorrhage *(IVH)*, grade I IVH, grade II IVH, grade III IVH, and grade IV IVH in the Vermont Oxford Network Very Low Birth Weight database in 2013 (n = 51,019) for each grouping of birth weight from 500 to 750 g, from 751 to 1000 g, from 1001 to 1250 g, and from 1251 to 1500 g. (From Horbar JD. *Vermont-Oxford Network Database Summary*. Burlington, VT: Vermont-Oxford Network; 2013.)

ultrasonography, and vast experience demonstrates the reliability and versatility of cranial ultrasonography for the diagnosis of IVH.[2,17-22] The determination of blood in the germinal matrix is best made on the coronal ultrasound scan at the level of the caudothalamic notch, whereas the determination of the amount of blood in the lateral ventricles is most accurate on the parasagittal ultrasound scan (Fig. 131.4).

In comparison with the bedside technique of cranial ultrasonography, computed tomography (CT) and magnetic resonance imaging (MRI) have the major disadvantage of requiring the sick premature infant to be transported to another site. Historically, CT played a role in the early diagnosis of IVH and clearly defined the site and extent of IVH in the premature infant.[3,4,23,24] However, concerns about the potential effects of ionizing radiation on the developing nervous system suggest that one should restrict the use of CT to neurosurgical emergencies in the newborn.[25] MRI provides excellent images of IVH, but the major advantage of MRI lies in its superior ability to demonstrate the nature and severity of any parenchymal injury[26-29] (Fig. 131.5) alongside a more extensive evaluation of the cerebral white matter, deep nuclear gray matter, cerebellum, and gyral development as indicators of additional neuropathology, which aids in prognosis.[30-32]

In addition to imaging for the diagnosis of IVH, *lumbar puncture* can provide a characteristic cerebrospinal fluid (CSF) profile consisting initially of increased red blood cell count and elevated protein content, followed shortly by xanthochromia and depressed glucose content. The degree of elevation of CSF protein content correlates approximately with the severity of the hemorrhage.[33] Exploratory work has analyzed the ability of various maternal and neonatal biomarkers for the early prediction and identification of IVH. These studies have analyzed a range of candidate markers, including S-100 β, activin A, and erythropoietin, but the most commonly studied analytes have been proinflammatory cytokines (interleukin [IL]-6, IL-8, tumor necrosis factor [TNF]α).[34-37] Results from different groups have been conflicting, however, and none of the findings from these studies have been validated as being specific for IVH, which limits their potential usefulness.[38-40]

During the last decade, amplitude-integrated electroencephalography has been used to study the vulnerable period of the first week of life, revealing the association of abnormal patterns with high-grade IVH.[41-44] Amplitude-integrated electroencephalography may serve as a useful tool to assist in understanding the presence of IVH.

CLASSIFICATION OF INTRAVENTRICULAR HEMORRHAGE

The grading system most commonly used for IVH in the infant was first reported by Papile and colleagues[4] and is based on the presence and amount of blood in the germinal matrix and the lateral ventricles seen on any form of neuroimaging (Table 131.1 and Fig. 131.4). Grade I represents hemorrhage confined to the subependymal germinal matrix, grade II represents hemorrhage within the lateral ventricles without ventricular dilatation, grade III represents hemorrhage with ventricular dilatation and/or hemorrhage occupying more than 50% of the ventricle, and grade IV represents parenchymal hemorrhage. Although grade IV IVH is now recognized principally as a periventricular hemorrhagic infarction rather than a simple extension of IVH, most reports continue to classify the cranial ultrasonography findings according to this earlier established classification system, and because of its common pathway of pathogenesis (as discussed further below).

CLINICAL RISK FACTORS

The clinical risk factors for IVH have been studied using two scientific approaches: first, by experimental and case-control studies outlining factors related to the pathogenesis in a preterm infant; and second, by epidemiologic or registry-type studies that may also identify factors related to therapeutic or NICU factors. Clinical variables commonly identified as contributing to the risk of IVH include lower gestational age, lack of corticosteroids antenatally, clinical chorioamnionitis, male sex, significant delivery room resuscitation, mechanical ventilation, and hypotension requiring multiple inotropes,[45-50] among other variables. A study across the Canadian Neonatal Network of 19,507 preterm infants admitted to 17 NICUs during an 18-month period demonstrated that on Bayesian hierarchic logistic regression modeling, 30% of the risk of high-grade IVH was related to baseline population risks (male sex, gestational age, initial severity of illness, and outborn status).[51] An additional 14% of the risk was associated with admission-day therapies, such as acidosis and hypotension that require intervention, and another 31%, the largest fraction of variation, was related to NICU characteristics. NICUs with greater patient volumes and neonatology staffing had lower rates of severe IVH. These findings that NICU structure and care practices may influence the risk of IVH are supported by other findings[52] and suggest that high patient load and neonatal physician experience may be associated with improved care practices and reduction in the risk of severe IVH. The variation between NICUs in registry data in the incidence of IVH does not appear to relate to differences in the interpretation of cranial ultrasound scans.[53]

More recently, routine nursing care interventions have been proposed to avoid (rapid) fluctuations in cerebral blood flow (CBF) during routine care, resulting in reductions in IVH. These interventions are especially important during the first 72 postnatal hours and include positioning the head in a midline position to enable optimal cerebral venous drainage and elevating the head of the incubator 15 to 30 degrees upwards to facilitate cerebral venous outflow by promoting hydrostatic cerebral

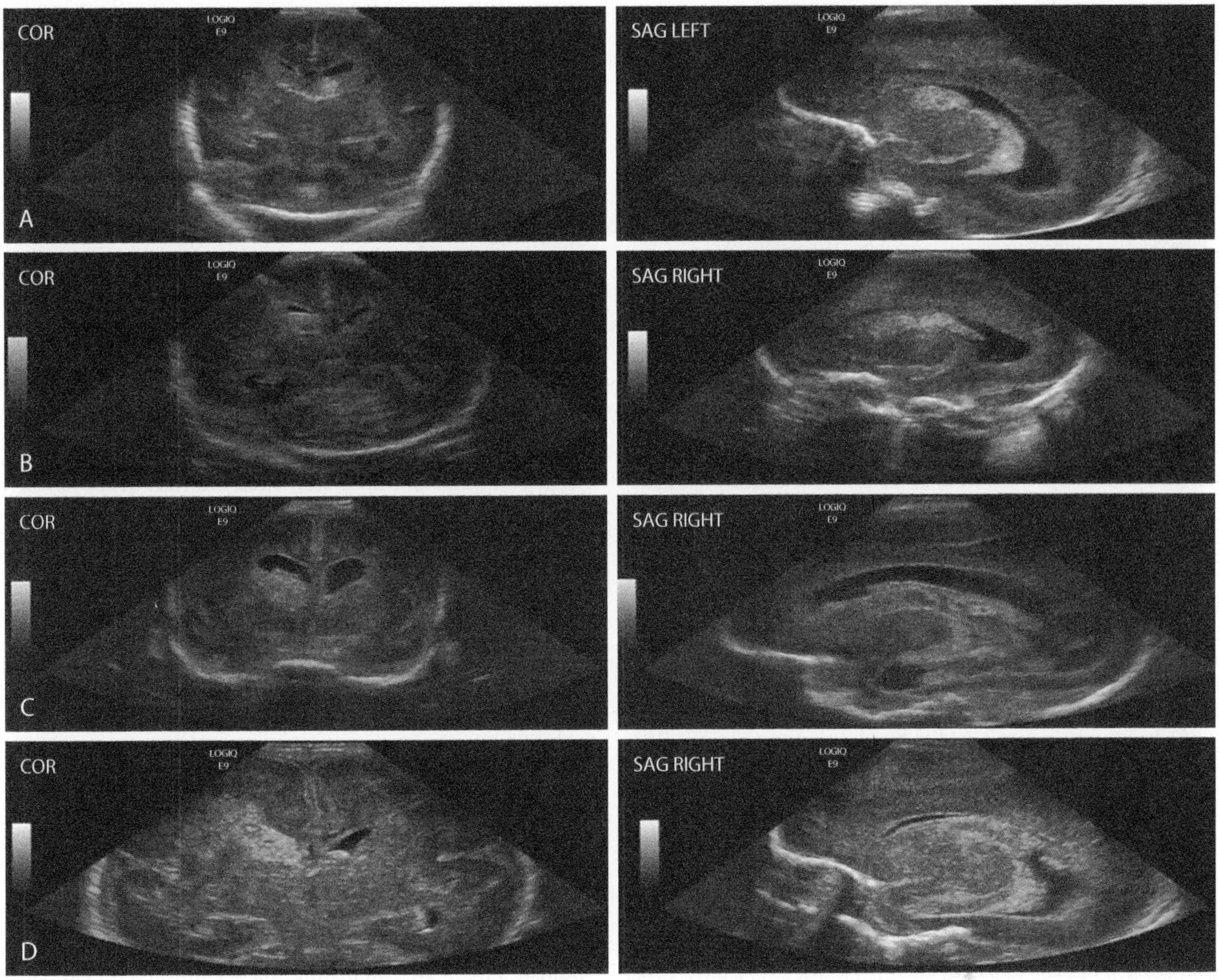

Fig. 131.4 Grading of the severity of germinal matrix hemorrhage–intraventricular hemorrhage (IVH). Coronal *(COR)* and parasagittal *(SAG)* ultrasound scans: (A) germinal matrix hemorrhage, grade I; (B) IVH (filling <50% of the ventricular area), grade II; (C) IVH with ventricular dilatation, grade III; (D) large IVH with associated parenchymal echogenicity (hemorrhagic infarct), grade IV.

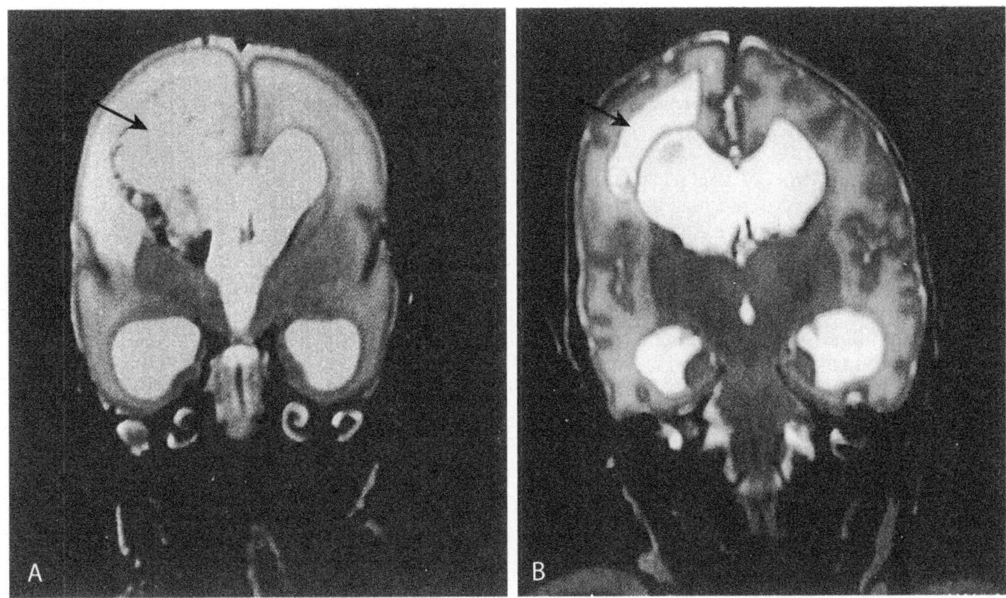

Fig. 131.5 Coronal T2-weighted magnetic resonance imaging scans of acute periventricular hemorrhagic infarction. (A) Note the fan-shaped distribution of increased signal in the parenchyma *(arrow)* and the generalized increased signal in the white matter in the area surrounding the infarct. (B) Later image of the same infant with cystic transformation of the infarct *(arrow)*. Note the ventriculomegaly present in both images.

Table 131.1 Grading of Severity of Germinal Matrix Hemorrhage–Intraventricular Hemorrhage by Ultrasound Scanning.

Severity	Description
Grade I	Germinal matrix hemorrhage with no or minimal intraventricular hemorrhage (10% of ventricular area on parasagittal view)
Grade II	Intraventricular hemorrhage (10%–50% of ventricular area on parasagittal view)
Grade III	Intraventricular hemorrhage (>50% of ventricular area on parasagittal view; usually distends lateral ventricle)

venous drainage. The results of a recently published randomized controlled trial (RCT) indicate that maintaining an elevated head position during the first four postnatal days was associated with a lower risk of developing a germinal matrix and intraventricular hemorrhage (GMH-IVH).[54] Other nursing interventions include avoidance of elevation of the legs during diaper change and slow arterial/intravenous flushing and slow arterial blood withdrawal. In a recent published RCT using all four of these interventions as a bundle, there was a lower risk of developing a GMH-IVH (any degree), cystic periventricular leukomalacia, and/or mortality (adjusted odds ratio [OR] 0.42, 95% confidence interval [CI] 0.27 to 0.65). In the group receiving the bundle, also severe GMH-IVH, cystic periventricular leukomalacia, and/or death were less often observed (adjusted OR 0.54, 95% CI 0.33 to 0.91 HYPERLIN[55]).

Controversy remains over the role of indomethacin in reducing the risk of IVH. In a number of clinical trials, indomethacin treatment has been shown to reduce the incidence of IVH.[56,57] Secondary analyses of a multicenter study based on sex have shown that indomethacin treatment reduces the rate of IVH in male infants but not in female infants.[58] Despite these early encouraging findings, across all of the 19 RCTs that have used indomethacin treatment, it was not demonstrated to improve neurodevelopmental outcomes in preterm infants.[59-61] Thus, indomethacin prophylaxis has immediate benefits of reduction in symptomatic patent ductus arteriosus and severe IVH; however, this does not appear to impact long-term neurodevelopmental outcomes. Given these findings, variable practices remain across NICUs in relation to the use of prophylactic indomethacin.

NEUROPATHOLOGY

The neuropathology of IVH is considered best in terms of the site of origin, that is, primarily the germinal matrix, the spread of the hemorrhage throughout the ventricular system, the neuropathologic consequences of the hemorrhage, and the neuropathologic accompaniments not necessarily related directly to the IVH.

The basic lesion in germinal matrix hemorrhage-IVH is bleeding into the subependymal germinal matrix. During the final 12 to 16 weeks' gestation, this matrix becomes less and less prominent and is essentially absent by term. This region is highly cellular, gelatinous in texture, and richly vascularized, as would be expected for a structure with active cellular proliferation. Moreover, studies show that massive numbers of neurons transit through the germinal matrix, raising the possibility that this process is impeded by even low-grade IVH.[62]

SITE OF ORIGIN

The site of origin of IVH characteristically is the *subependymal germinal matrix*. This region is comparable to that often referred to as the *median ganglion eminence*. This cellular region immediately ventrolateral to the lateral ventricle serves initially as a source of cerebral neuronal precursors between approximately 10 and 20 weeks' gestation. The region also gives rise to later-migrating neurons, primarily GABAergic interneurons, destined for the thalamus in the third trimester.[63] The subventricular zone dorsal and lateral to the angle of the lateral ventricle gives rise to the late migratory neurons destined for the cerebral cortex. Later in the third trimester, the matrix generates glial precursors that will become cerebral oligodendroglia and astrocytes.[64] The germinal matrix undergoes a progressive decrease in size, from a width of 2.5 mm at 23 to 24 weeks, to 1.4 mm at 32 weeks, to nearly complete involution by approximately 36 weeks.[65,66] The many thin-walled vessels in the matrix are vulnerable to bleeding. Hemorrhage from the choroid plexus occurs in nearly 50% of infants with germinal matrix hemorrhage and IVH,[67] and in more mature infants especially, it may be the exclusive site of origin of IVH. It is important to additionally note that these interneurons transit through GM until well after the third trimester in what becomes the subventricular zone.[68]

The vascular *site of origin* of germinal matrix hemorrhage within the microcirculation of this region appears to be the prominent endothelial-lined vessels of the matrix and not the arterioles or arteries.[69-72] The vessels in free communication with the venous circulation appear to be of particular importance, such as the capillary-venule junction or small venules. This has been shown by histochemical studies of germinal matrix vessels at the site of hemorrhage[70] and by the emergence of solution into the germinal matrix hemorrhage from postmortem injection into the jugular veins but no emergence of solution into the germinal matrix hemorrhage from injection into the carotid artery.[69]

Finally, there are key structural differences in the germinal matrix that may increase the vulnerability of the immature vasculature. These include the extracellular matrix of the cerebral vasculature that contains laminin, fibronectin, collagen IV, and perlecan for structural stability of blood vessels. In both human fetuses and premature infants, fibronectin expression is lower in the germinal matrix than in the cortical mantle or white matter anlagen. Low-dose prenatal betamethasone treatment, which is known to reduce the risk of IVH by 50%, enhances fibronectin level by 1.5-fold to twofold. Because fibronectin provides structural stability to the blood vessels, its reduced expression in the germinal matrix may contribute to the fragility of germinal matrix vasculature and its propensity to hemorrhage in premature neonates. In addition, the expression of collagen type IV α_1 and α_2 chains increases with advancing gestational age.[73] Some studies have suggested that accumulated collagen in the blood vessels themselves does not differ in the immature germinal matrix.[74] Cytoskeletal vascular stabilizing influences from both pericytes[75] and astrocyte end feet[76] seem to be lacking in the immature germinal matrix, which may also contribute to the fragility of the germinal matrix vasculature and its propensity to hemorrhage. Finally, the molecular features that may underlie the fragility of germinal matrix microvasculature have been described.[77]

SPREAD OF INTRAVENTRICULAR HEMORRHAGE

In approximately 80% of patients with germinal matrix hemorrhage, blood enters the lateral ventricles and spreads throughout the ventricular system.[72-78] Blood proceeds through the foramina of Magendie and Luschka and tends to collect in the basilar cisterns in the posterior fossa. With substantial collections, the blood may incite an obliterative arachnoiditis over days to weeks, with impairment of CSF flow. Other sites at which particulate blood clot may lead to impaired CSF dynamics are the aqueduct of Sylvius and the arachnoid villi.

NEUROPATHOLOGIC CONSEQUENCES OF INTRAVENTRICULAR HEMORRHAGE

Several major neuropathologic states occur as apparent consequences of IVH, including, in temporal order of occurrence, germinal matrix destruction, periventricular hemorrhagic infarction, and post-hemorrhagic hydrocephalus.

GERMINAL MATRIX DESTRUCTION

The destruction of germinal matrix and, perhaps most important, of its glial precursor cells is an associated consequence of germinal matrix hemorrhage.[71,72] The hematoma is replaced frequently by a cyst, the walls of which include hemosiderin-laden macrophages and reactive astrocytes. Destruction of glial precursor cells in the germinal matrix[66] may have a deleterious influence on subsequent brain development and neurodevelopmental outcomes (see later).

PERIVENTRICULAR HEMORRHAGIC INFARCTION

Approximately 15% of infants with IVH also exhibit a characteristic parenchymal lesion, *periventricular hemorrhagic infarction.* The incidence of this lesion increases with decreasing gestational age, such that in infants weighing 500 to 750 g, periventricular hemorrhagic infarction accounts for approximately one-quarter of all cases of IVH (see Fig. 131.3), with an absolute incidence among these infants of approximately 10%.[79-81] The neuropathology of periventricular hemorrhagic infarction consists of a relatively large region of hemorrhagic necrosis in the periventricular white matter, just dorsal and lateral to the external angle of the lateral ventricle. The necrosis is strikingly *asymmetric*—in the largest series reported, 67% of such lesions were exclusively *unilateral,* and, in virtually all of the remaining cases, they were grossly asymmetric, even though bilateral.[82] Approximately half of the lesions are extensive and involve periventricular white matter from the frontal to the parietooccipital regions. Approximately 80% of cases are associated with large IVH, and commonly (and mistakenly), the parenchymal hemorrhagic lesion is described as an "extension" of the hemorrhage. That simple extension of blood into cerebral white matter from germinal matrix or lateral ventricle does *not* account for the periventricular hemorrhagic necrosis that has been shown clearly by several neuropathology studies.[67,79,80,82-84] Microscopic study of this periventricular hemorrhagic necrosis indicates that the lesion is a *hemorrhagic infarction.*[82-85] The studies of Gould and colleagues[83] and Takashima and colleagues[85] emphasize that the hemorrhagic component of the infarction tends to be most concentrated near the ventricular angle, where the medullary veins draining the cerebral white matter become confluent and ultimately join the terminal vein in the subependymal region. Thus it appears that periventricular hemorrhagic necrosis occurring in association with large IVH is, in fact, a *venous infarction.*

The pathogenesis of periventricular hemorrhagic infarction appears to be related directly to the associated germinal matrix hemorrhage-IVH, as the association of large asymmetric germinal matrix hemorrhage-IVH and progression to *ipsilateral* periventricular hemorrhagic infarction has been clearly documented.[82,86,87] These data raise the possibility that the IVH or its associated germinal matrix hemorrhage may lead to obstruction of the terminal or collecting veins with secondary hemorrhagic venous infarction.[82,83,88] This pathogenetic formulation has received further support from imaging studies. Doppler determinations of blood flow velocity demonstrated obstruction of flow in the terminal vein by the ipsilateral germinal matrix hemorrhage during the evolution of the infarction in a living premature infant.[89] In addition, an MRI study of acute periventricular hemorrhagic infarction showed an appearance consistent with a combination of intravascular thrombi and perivascular hemorrhage along the course of the medullary veins within the area of infarction.[90] A pathogenetic scheme illustrating most examples of periventricular hemorrhagic infarction is shown in Fig. 131.6.

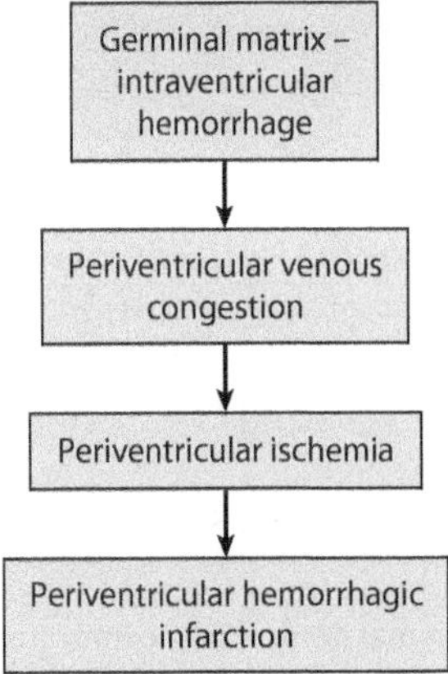

Fig. 131.6 Pathogenesis of periventricular hemorrhagic infarction. The formulation indicates a central role for germinal matrix hemorrhage–intraventricular hemorrhage in causation of the periventricular venous infarction.

Finally, atypical cases of periventricular hemorrhagic infarction have been described, with atypical timing with fetal or very late presentation without a related deteriorating clinical condition. In these cases, a high proportion (>50%) carried either the factor V Leiden (G1691A) mutation, or variants in the *MTHFR* or *COL4A1* genes.[91]

POST-HEMORRHAGIC VENTRICULAR DILATATION

A third neuropathologic consequence of IVH is progressive post-hemorrhagic ventricular dilatation (PHVD) (i.e., *hydrocephalus*). The likelihood of and the speed of evolution of hydrocephalus after IVH is related directly to the quantity of intraventricular blood. Thus, with large IVH, hydrocephalus may evolve over days (*acute* hydrocephalus), and with smaller IVH, the process usually evolves over weeks (*subacute-chronic* hydrocephalus).

Acute hydrocephalus is accompanied by particulate blood clots, which may impair CSF absorption by obstruction of the arachnoid villi. This mechanism may be likely in the newborn because of the presence of only microscopic arachnoid villi and not the larger, later-appearing arachnoid granulations.[92] Other contributing factors to the development of acute hydrocephalus may include an impaired ability to mediate clot lysis due to extremely low plasminogen levels and elevations in plasminogen activator inhibitor levels in the CSF of infants with recent IVH.[93]

Subacute-chronic hydrocephalus relates most commonly either to obliterative arachnoiditis in the posterior fossa resulting in obstruction of fourth ventricular outflow or flow through the tentorial notch or to aqueductal obstruction by blood clot, disrupted ependyma, and reactive gliosis.[71,94,95]

NEUROPATHOLOGIC ACCOMPANIMENTS OF INTRAVENTRICULAR HEMORRHAGE

Several neuropathologic states are commonly associated with but not directly caused by IVH. The most common findings include periventricular leukomalacia, pontine neuronal necrosis, and loss of cerebellar volume.

PERIVENTRICULAR LEUKOMALACIA

Periventricular leukomalacia was observed in 75% of one series of infants who died with IVH.[67] Although all of the infants in this series had an IVH, only 42% died secondary to cerebral hemorrhage. The remaining causes of mortality included infection, respiratory failure, and circulatory insufficiency. In

Table 131.2 Periventricular White Matter Lesions of the Premature Infant.

Term Disturbance	Symmetry	Gross Hemorrhage	Probable Site of Circulatory Insult
Periventricular leukomalacia	Predominantly symmetric	Uncommon	Arterial
Periventricular hemorrhagic infarction	Predominantly asymmetric	Invariable	Venous

contrast to parenchymal hemorrhagic infarction, periventricular leukomalacia is a generally symmetric, nonhemorrhagic, and associated with apparent ischemic white matter injury in the arterial end zones (Table 131.2). The frequent association of periventricular leukomalacia with IVH has also been emphasized in three other neuropathology reports.[85,96] Takashima and colleagues[85] suggested periventricular hemorrhagic infarction and hemorrhagic periventricular leukomalacia may be distinguishable in part on the basis of topography. Hemorrhagic periventricular leukomalacia has a predilection for periventricular arterial border zones, particularly in the region near the trigone of the lateral ventricles. Venous infarction is particularly prominent anteriorly, as the lesion radiates from the periventricular region at the site of confluence of the medullary and terminal veins and assumes a roughly triangular, fan-shaped appearance in periventricular white matter. The mechanism of injury is not fully defined but is associated with the complex interaction of ischemia and inflammation, with some studies highlighting the importance of injury to preoligodendrocytes secondary to these processes.[97,98] Injury to the white matter axons and subplate neurons is a frequent accompaniment of periventricular leukomalacia.[99] A potential role for activated microglia in the process is suggested by the demonstration in brains with IVH of CD68 microglia and damaged axons in cerebral white matter.[100] Another study showed that oligodendrocyte precursors have critical roles in regulation of angiogenesis in developing white matter tracts, and that inactivation of hypoxia-inducible factor signaling within such precursors resulted in cystic lesions reminiscent of periventricular leukomalacia.[101]

CEREBELLAR DYSMATURATION

IVH, in addition to other supratentorial brain injuries, has been shown to be associated with reductions in cerebellar volume.[31,102-104] Two key mechanisms have been proposed for the association of IVH with reduced cerebellar lesions.[105] The first is the direct toxicity of hemosiderin over the surface of the cerebellum, impairing the proliferation of the external granular layer. This hypothesis was initially raised by Messerschmidt and colleagues,[106] who described acquired cerebellar growth failure in a series of 35 premature infants who had prominent hemosiderin over the cerebellar surface. In that study, all of the infants had IVH and two thirds developed post-hemorrhagic hydrocephalus. Consistent with this hypothesis of IVH-associated hemosiderin influencing cerebellar growth, a more recent study of 172 preterm infants found an association between IVH and smaller cerebellar volumes on both sides, suggesting a global impact from surface-based hemosiderin associated with the IVH.[102] A second mechanism potentially involved in the cerebellar underdevelopment in association with IVH involves the loss of remote transsynaptic effects from cerebral neural connections. This mechanism represents a maturation-distinctive form of diaschisis, characterizing a loss of function in a brain area neutrally connected to but remote from a separate lesioned brain area. A relationship between IVH and contralateral connected cerebellum has been demonstrated, supporting this hypothesis. In a study of 74 infants born at less than 32 weeks with an MRI scan at term, it was found that a unilateral IVH was significantly associated with a smaller cerebellar hemisphere on the contralateral side. In the crossed cerebellocerebral deficits, the loss of cortical input could disturb both primarily the cerebellum and the dentatorubrothalamic cortical pathway.[105] For further information on cerebellar hypoplasia, see Chapter 129.

Box 131.1 Pathogenesis of Germinal Matrix Hemorrhage

Intravascular Factors

- Fluctuating blood pressure in pressure-passive circulation
- Increase in cerebral blood flow—systemic hypertension in the setting of a pressure-passive circulation, rapid volume expansion, hypercarbia, decreased hematocrit, decreased blood glucose level
- Increase in cerebral venous pressure—venous anatomic arrangement, labor and vaginal delivery, respiratory disturbance, head positioning
- Decrease in cerebral blood flow (followed by reperfusion)—systemic hypotension
- Platelet and coagulation disturbance

Vascular Factors

- Tenuous capillary integrity—the germinal matrix is an involuting remodeling capillary bed with deficient vascular lining and a large vascular and luminal area
- Vulnerability of matrix capillaries to hypoxic-ischemic injury—the area has a high requirement for oxidative metabolism and lies at a vascular border zone

Extravascular Factors

- Deficient vascular and extracellular matrix support
- Excessive fibrinolytic activity

PATHOGENESIS

The pathogenesis of IVH is considered best in terms of intravascular, vascular, and extravascular factors.[1] Clearly, the pathogenesis of IVH is multifactorial, and thus different combinations of these factors are operative in different patients.

INTRAVASCULAR FACTORS

Intravascular factors are those that relate primarily to the regulation of blood flow, pressure, and volume in the microvascular bed of the germinal matrix (Box 131.1, Fig. 131.7).

FLUCTUATING CEREBRAL BLOOD FLOW

Significant fluctuations in *CBF* appear important in the pathogenesis of IVH. A *fluctuating pattern* of arterial blood pressure, characterized by marked and continuous alterations in both systolic and diastolic flow velocities in the systemic circulation, was shown to be associated with similar trends in CBF velocity and high risk of subsequent IVH. Smaller fluctuations in arterial pressure of less than 10% (coefficient of variation) did not appear to produce this adverse outcome.[107-109] The cause of the fluctuations in both the systemic circulation and the cerebral circulation was related

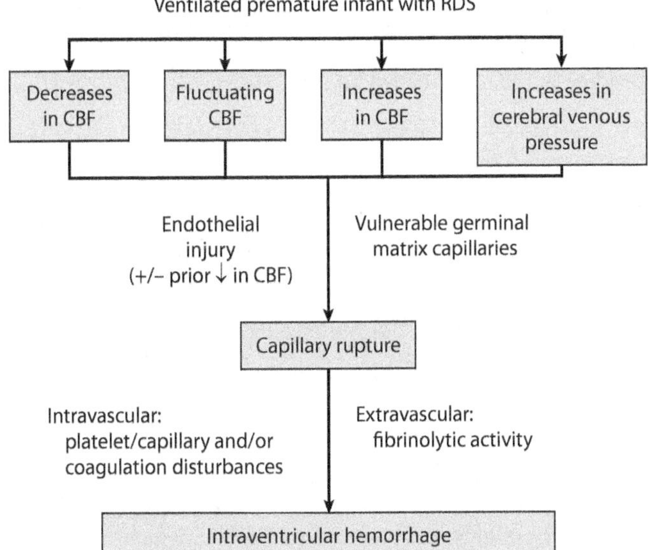

Fig. 131.7 Interaction of the major pathogenetic factors for the occurrence of germinal matrix hemorrhage–intraventricular hemorrhage in the premature infant. *CBF,* Cerebral blood flow; *RDS,* respiratory distress syndrome.

to the mechanics of ventilation[110,111] and the severity of illness, with contributing factors including hypercarbia, hypovolemia, hypotension, "restlessness," patent ductus arteriosus, and relatively high inspired oxygen concentrations.[108,111-113]

INCREASES IN CEREBRAL BLOOD FLOW

The close temporal correlation between the occurrence of IVH and abrupt increases in arterial blood pressure, increases in CBF, and increases in CBF velocity[114-117] supports the earlier hypothesis[117] that increases in CBF play an important pathogenetic role in IVH. Using near-infrared spectroscopy to continuously monitor infants born at less than 32 weeks for the first 72 hours Alderliesten and colleagues[118] found a decrease in cerebral fraction tissue oxygen extraction, which is consistent with increased CBF, before severe IVH. Additionally, they found reduced cerebral autoregulation in infants who developed IVH. A pressure-passive cerebral circulatory state in an unstable preterm infant is considered a major contributing factor for dangerous elevations of CBF.[119-125]

Pressure-Passive Cerebral Circulation and Elevations of Arterial Blood Pressure

Whereas an intact cerebrovascular autoregulation is present in clinically stable preterm infants, a pressure-passive cerebral circulation is present in sick preterm infants in whom IVH develops.[121,126-130] In a study in 57 preterm infants with ultrasonographic signs of IVH, severe IVH developed only in infants with earlier evidence of a pressure-passive cerebral circulation.[120] In those infants with intact cerebrovascular autoregulation, no, or only mild, hemorrhage developed.[120,123] Similarly, an analysis of CBF with continuous transcranial Doppler ultrasonography in 15 critically ill extremely low-birth-weight infants with adverse short-term outcomes (early death or severe IVH) found that there was a corresponding increase in CBF associated with increased blood pressure.[131] Among all preterm infants, it is thought that the range of blood pressures over which the cerebral autoregulation remains intact is limited relative to that in older patients.[132,133] Both the narrow range of blood pressure over which cerebral autoregulation remains intact and the propensity for pressure passivity in unstable infants may explain the relationship between maximum systolic blood pressure above a threshold and the subsequent occurrence of IVH.[134] The limit for the highest tolerable peak systolic blood pressure is markedly lower for smaller infants.[134]

Causes of Increased Arterial Blood Pressure in the Human Newborn

It is clearly important to detect and, whenever possible, prevent abrupt elevations in arterial blood pressure, which may be accompanied by increased CBF velocity. These causes of elevated arterial blood pressure include the following: such "caretaking" concomitants as inadvertent noxious stimulation, abdominal examination, handling, instillation of mydriatics, and tracheal suctioning; systemic complications including pneumothorax, exchange transfusion, and rapid infusion of colloid; and neurologic complications such as seizures.[114,115,117,135-141] Pneumothorax has been frequently associated with an elevated risk of IVH.[142,143] In a study of nine infants, pneumothorax was uniformly accompanied by abrupt elevations of systemic blood pressure and CBF velocity, and these circulatory changes were followed within hours by IVH.[144] Studies in newborn dogs documented abrupt increases in arterial blood pressure on rapid evacuation of pneumothorax.[142]

Relevant Experimental Studies: Role of Hypertension

The importance of abrupt increases in systemic blood pressure and CBF in the pathogenesis of IVH was demonstrated in *experimental* studies in the newborn beagle puppy[144-148] and in the preterm sheep fetus.[149] A highly predictable pattern of germinal matrix hemorrhage-IVH clinically similar to that of the human premature infant is produced in the beagle puppy by a sequence of hypotension and hypertension produced by blood removal and volume reinfusion.[150]

Hypercarbia

Careful studies in preterm infants receiving mechanical ventilation show a pronounced reactivity of CBF to changes in arterial carbon dioxide tension ($Paco_2$), with an approximately 30% increase in CBF per kilopascal increase in $Paco_2$ after the first 24 hours of life.[121,151,152] However, in the first 24 hours of life, the period of greatest risk of IVH, this reactivity is more attenuated, with an approximately 10% increase in CBF per kilopascal increase in $Paco_2$ in very premature infants, and, most strikingly, this reactivity is *absent* in infants with subsequent severe IVH.[120] Using multivariate analysis, Szymonowicz and colleagues[153] were the first to report an association between hypercarbia and the risk of IVH in extremely low-birth-weight infants. Van de Bor and colleagues[154] demonstrated that elevated $Paco_2$ preceded the development of IVH in premature infants. Kaiser and colleagues[155] documented an association between the maximum $Paco_2$ and the risk of grade III–IV IVH in a study in 574 very low-birth-weight (VLBW) infants between 1999 and 2004. On multivariate logistic modeling controlling for gestational age, sex, 1-minute Apgar score, multiplicity, and inotrope use, maximum $Paco_2$ during the first 72 hours of life was related to the risk of severe IVH in a dose-dependent manner, with the risk increasing with a $Paco_2$ greater than 56 mm Hg. The adjusted odds ratio for severe IVH was nearly fivefold greater when the maximum $Paco_2$ was greater than 75 mm Hg.

More recently, Fabres and colleagues[156] demonstrated that it is not just an increased $Paco_2$ that is associated with severe IVH, but also a low $Paco_2$. On their multivariate modeling, Fabres and colleagues found a twofold increase in the risk of severe IVH if the $Paco_2$ was greater than 60 mmHg, and a 2.5-fold increase in risk if it was less than 39 mm Hg. In light of the trend in newborn medicine towards more permissive hypercapnia, clinicians should be aware of this increased risk of IVH associated with a higher $Paco_2$. Encouragingly, however, Hagen and colleagues[157] found no increased risk of IVH with permissive hypercapnia when $Paco_2$

was maintained within the range 45 to 55 mm Hg, compared with normocapnia. Taken in conjunction with the findings of Kaiser and colleagues and Fabres and colleagues, this suggests that permissive hypercapnia does not significantly increase the risk of IVH if the $Paco_2$ is maintained within appropriate parameters.

Decreased Hemoglobin Concentration

An inverse correlation exists in the human infant between hemoglobin concentration and CBF.[121,158,159] In one study in premature infants in the first days of life, CBF increased by 12% per 1 mmol/L decrease in hemoglobin concentration.[121] CBF presumably increases to maintain constant cerebral delivery, but with increasing CBF, the risk of IVH will be higher in those premature infants born with anemia. Recently an increased risk of severe IVH among VLBW infants after a red cell transfusion within the first 72 hours of birth has been reported. This remained significant after confounding variables had been controlled for (relative risk 2.02, 95% CI 1.54 to 3.33).[160] Baer and colleagues[160] were unable to determine the underlying mechanism given the retrospective nature of the review, but one possibility for the increased risk is concomitant anemia requiring transfusion, rather than the transfusion itself. These associations and that of total blood volume being related to the risk of IVH are further supported by studies of the timing of umbilical cord clamping. Delayed umbilical cord clamping (30 seconds) compared with immediate umbilical cord clamping (6 to 7 seconds) is associated with a slightly higher baseline hematocrit (49% vs. 46%), higher mean blood pressure (33.8 mm Hg vs. 31.9 mm Hg), increased superior vena cava flow, and a significantly reduced risk of IVH (14% vs. 36%).[161,162] This reduction in the risk for IVH with delayed umbilical cord clamping is supported by a meta-analysis of the randomized trials in preterm infants.[163,164] While delayed cord clamping would appear to be protective, it is worth noting that a recent trial comparing delayed cord clamping to umbilical cord milking was terminated early, due to an increased rate of severe IVH among those in the milking group. It is postulated that the milking was associated with a rapid fluctuation in the CBF, which as discussed earlier is a risk for IVH, particularly in the presence of a pressure passive circulation.[165]

Blood Glucose Levels

Decreased blood glucose concentration should be considered in the evaluation of pathogenetic factors for IVH in view of the observation that CBF increases twofold to threefold when blood glucose concentration declines to levels lower than 1.7 mmol/L in the premature infant.[121,151] Blood glucose levels lower than 1.7 mmol/L in premature infants are not rare in the first days of life in many NICUs. More data are needed on a potential contributory role for low blood glucose concentrations in the pathogenesis of IVH.

Increased blood glucose concentration has been evaluated as a potential risk factor for IVH. A case-control study compared 70 infants with high-grade IVH with 108 infants without IVH.[166] The IVH group had significantly more hyperglycemic events (2.9 ± 1.7 events vs 2.4 ± 1.8 events, $P < .05$) with longer duration (22.2 ± 14.2 hours vs. 14.1 ± 12.5 hours, $P < .001$) and a higher hyperglycemic index (1.0 ± 0.9 vs. 1.4 ± 1.0, $P = .003$) compared with the non-IVH controls. Respiratory distress syndrome, hypotension, and thrombocytopenia increased the adjusted odds ratio for IVH. Hypoglycemia was not independently associated with IVH. Conversely, the increase in hyperglycemic duration most prominently increased the adjusted odds ratio for severe IVH (OR 10.33, 95% CI 10.0 to 10.6, $P = .033$). To avoid hyperglycemia, insulin therapy is often initiated. However, an important RCT of "tight" glycemic control with insulin versus standard care has been undertaken and documented a nonsignificant trend toward an increased risk of grade III to IV IVH in the insulin-treated group (14% vs. 7% for standard care).[167] The insulin-treated group had more episodes of hypoglycemia. Thus avoidance of both protracted hyperglycemia or hypoglycemia would appear most prudent in reducing the risk of IVH.

INCREASES IN CEREBRAL VENOUS PRESSURE

Elevations of cerebral venous pressure may contribute to the occurrence of IVH.[168] The potential importance of venous factors is suggested by the demonstration that with postmortem injection of different-colored barium solutions into the carotid artery or jugular vein in infants with germinal matrix hemorrhage, the injected material entered the hemorrhage only by venous injections.[69] The *most important causes* of such increases are labor and delivery, asphyxia, and respiratory complications. Additionally, it has been suggested that alterations in the osmotic gradient, leading to an increase in the intravascular pressure relative to pressure in the surrounding tissue, may predispose to IVH.[169] Several cohort studies have shown that the development of states associated with an alteration in the osmotic balance such as hyperglycemia, hypernatremia, and even high sodium intake in the absence of hypernatremia is associated with increased risk of IVH.[166,170-172] However, the retrospective nature of these studies cannot delineate the underlying mechanism for this increased risk.

Importance of Venous Anatomy

The importance of increased venous pressure in the pathogenesis of IVH relates in part to the *venous anatomy* in the region of the germinal matrix. The direction of deep venous flow takes a peculiar U-turn in the subependymal region at the level of the foramen of Monro, which is the most common site of germinal matrix hemorrhage.

Labor and Delivery

During labor and delivery, marked increases in cerebral venous pressure may occur. Measurement of "fetal head compression pressure" by a compression transducer positioned between the fetal head and the wall of the uterus during labor revealed an overall mean pressure of 158 mm Hg.[173] Consistent with this hypothesis of increased venous pressure during labor, initial studies found an increased risk of the occurrence of IVH in the premature infant with vaginal delivery.[87,174-177] More recent studies have produced conflicting results, with several finding no association with the method of delivery.[178-181] A study of 158 infants born weighing less than 1500 g found that there was an increased risk of mild IVH among infants with vaginal delivery compared with cesarean delivery before the second stage of labor, but not with cesarean delivery during the second stage.[182] That study was limited by small numbers, but its findings are compatible with those of the previous studies described above, which found the risks of IVH to be greatest with prolonged labor.[176] The studies that did not report an association between the mode of delivery and IVH did not comment on the duration of labor or the stage during which the cesarean delivery was performed, possibly explaining the discrepancies in the literature. Another explanation for the discrepancies is that there may be genetic variants that predispose to injury during vaginal delivery. A mouse model of mutation of *COL4A1*, coding for collagen type IV in the basement membrane, found that mutant pups delivered vaginally all had cerebral hemorrhages, whereas those delivered surgically did not.[183] Human studies have found *COL4A1* mutations associated with IVH in preterm infants. However, even among those with IVH, it is a rare genetic variant.[184] It is possible, though, that other genetic variants could also increase the risk of IVH.

Head position, both before delivery and in the neonatal nursery, may also alter cerebral venous drainage. One study using near-infrared spectroscopy documented that cerebral venous drainage may be impaired in prone or side positions.[185]

Asphyxia

The importance of increased venous pressure in association with asphyxia in the causation of IVH has been shown in experimental studies of preterm fetal sheep.[149]

Respiratory Disturbances

Data suggest that such factors as positive pressure ventilation with relatively high peak inflation pressure, tracheal suctioning, abnormalities of the mechanics of respiration, and pneumothorax may be major causes of increased cerebral venous pressure in the premature infant.[168,186–188] Doppler measurements of blood flow velocity in the superior sagittal sinus demonstrated a striking sensitivity of the venous circulation to the level of peak inflation pressure, with the smallest infants exhibiting the most marked effects.[168,189]

Tracheal suctioning and pneumothorax have also been shown to produce pronounced changes in venous pressure.[107,168,190,191] Studies of the method of ventilation in premature infants have raised concerns because of associations between the method of ventilation and increased rates of IVH, particularly high-grade IVH. The proposed mechanism of increased IVH in premature infants receiving positive pressure ventilation is an increased intrathoracic pressure with decreased cerebral venous return.[192] Current practice frequently involves the early use of noninvasive ventilatory support, typically with continuous positive airway pressure, which is capable of generating high intrathoracic pressures. A meta-analysis found no difference in IVH when comparing these noninvasive strategies with conventional methods.[193] For conventional ventilation, two meta-analyses comparing volume-targeted versus pressure-limited ventilation found a reduction in the incidence of severe IVH, and the composite outcome of severe IVH or periventricular leukomalacia when volume-targeted rather than pressure-limited ventilation was used. This finding may reflect reduced intrathoracic pressures associated with volume-targeted techniques.[194,195]

There have been similar concerns regarding high frequency oscillatory ventilation (HFOV),[196] with one RCT of HFOV documenting an increased rate of IVH among infants who were switched from conventional ventilation to HFOV.[197] These findings have led some authors to recommend that conventional ventilation should remain the ventilatory method of choice in premature infants with respiratory distress syndrome.[197,198] However, a premature baboon model comparing HFOV and low-volume positive pressure ventilation strategies found no increased risk of neuropathology with HFOV.[199] Additionally a meta-analysis of the 17 randomized controlled studies comparing elective HFOV and conventional ventilation demonstrated no significant increase in the risk of grade III or grade IV IVH or adverse neurodevelopmental outcome.[198]

DECREASES IN CEREBRAL BLOOD FLOW

Importance of Pressure-Passive Cerebral Circulation

Decreases in CBF may play an important role in the pathogenesis of IVH. The principal consequence of the decreased CBF is injury of germinal matrix vessels, which rupture subsequently on reperfusion. As indicated earlier, hemorrhagic hypotension preceding volume re-expansion is the optimal means to produce IVH experimentally in the newborn beagle puppy. Noori and colleagues[200] performed an interesting observational study in a cohort of 22 extremely premature infants. They performed sequential echocardiogram, head ultrasound scans, and continuous near-infrared spectroscopy monitoring for the first 72 hours of life and found that infants who developed an IVH initially had cerebral hypoperfusion, with a low left ventricular output, with a low cerebral regional oxygen saturation ($rsCO_2$) and high cerebral fraction tissue oxygen extraction. Then immediately before the IVH, perfusion increased, with a higher left ventricular output, higher $rsCO_2$, and reduced cerebral fraction tissue oxygen extraction, supporting the hypoperfusion/reperfusion model of IVH development. Fig. 131.8 outlines the potential mechanism of cerebral ischemia and reperfusion resulting in IVH.

In the premature infant, decreases in CBF are most likely with systemic hypotension and perinatal events. Because of the pressure-passive cerebral circulation in sick premature infants, hypotension can lead to a parallel decrease in CBF.

Perinatal Hypoxic-Ischemic Events

Perinatal hypoxic-ischemic events presumably explain, at least in part, the relationship among low Apgar scores, early acidosis, the early use of bicarbonate, and the subsequent occurrence of IVH, particularly cases that develop in the first 12 hours.[201,202] Several studies of delivery-room management have demonstrated a significant increase in IVH among preterm infants who required significant resuscitation.[47] In one study of approximately 25,000 very low-birth-weight infants, severe IVH was three times more common in those infants requiring cardiopulmonary resuscitation at delivery (15.3%) than in those not requiring resuscitation (4.9%).[203] The mechanism for provocation of IVH with perinatal asphyxia is complex and includes increases in cerebral venous pressure, and changes in CBF associated with impaired vascular autoregulation, such as decreases in CBF associated with hypotension, with resulting injury to matrix capillaries. Studies of the concentrations of brain-specific creatine kinase isoenzymes in umbilical cord blood, or in blood samples obtained early in the postnatal period, or concentrations of the hypoxanthine metabolite uric acid in blood samples obtained on the first postnatal day in preterm infants in whom IVH later developed, support the notion that late intrauterine events (perhaps asphyxia) may be involved in at least some cases of IVH.[204–206] Moreover, the possibility of a perinatal hypoxic-ischemic insult to the brain as a predecessor to IVH is also suggested by the finding of electroencephalographic abnormalities before the occurrence of IVH.[207–210]

Postnatal Ischemic Events

A relationship between postnatal arterial hypotension and increased risk of IVH has been frequently documented.[211,212] However, currently, there is debate over the significance of isolated hypotension in preterm infants. Dempsey and colleagues[213] found no difference in short-term outcome (death, or composite short-term outcome of severe IVH and cystic periventricular leukomalacia or surgical necrotizing enterocolitis) among extremely low-birth-weight infants who were normotensive or hypotensive with good perfusion. Similarly, Lightburn and colleagues[126] found no difference in either CBF velocities using near-infrared spectroscopy or IVH rates between stable hypotensive and normotensive extremely low-birth-weight infants. The differences in findings associated with hypotension can likely be explained by the presence or absence of cerebral autoregulation. As a pressure-passive cerebral circulation develops, hypotension would be associated with reduced CBF and increased risk of IVH. Near-infrared spectroscopy in the first 24 hours of life in preterm infants has shown that CBF is significantly lower in infants in whom IVH subsequently developed (median 7.0 mL/100 g per minute) than in those without IVH (median 12.2 mL/100 g per minute).[214] In addition, supportive of a relation between postnatal ischemic events and the occurrence of IVH is the demonstration of decreased cardiac output in the first 36 hours of life in infants in whom the lesion developed, especially severe IVH.[215] Finally, the potential importance of ischemic injury in pathogenesis is supported further by the demonstration of a beneficial effect of

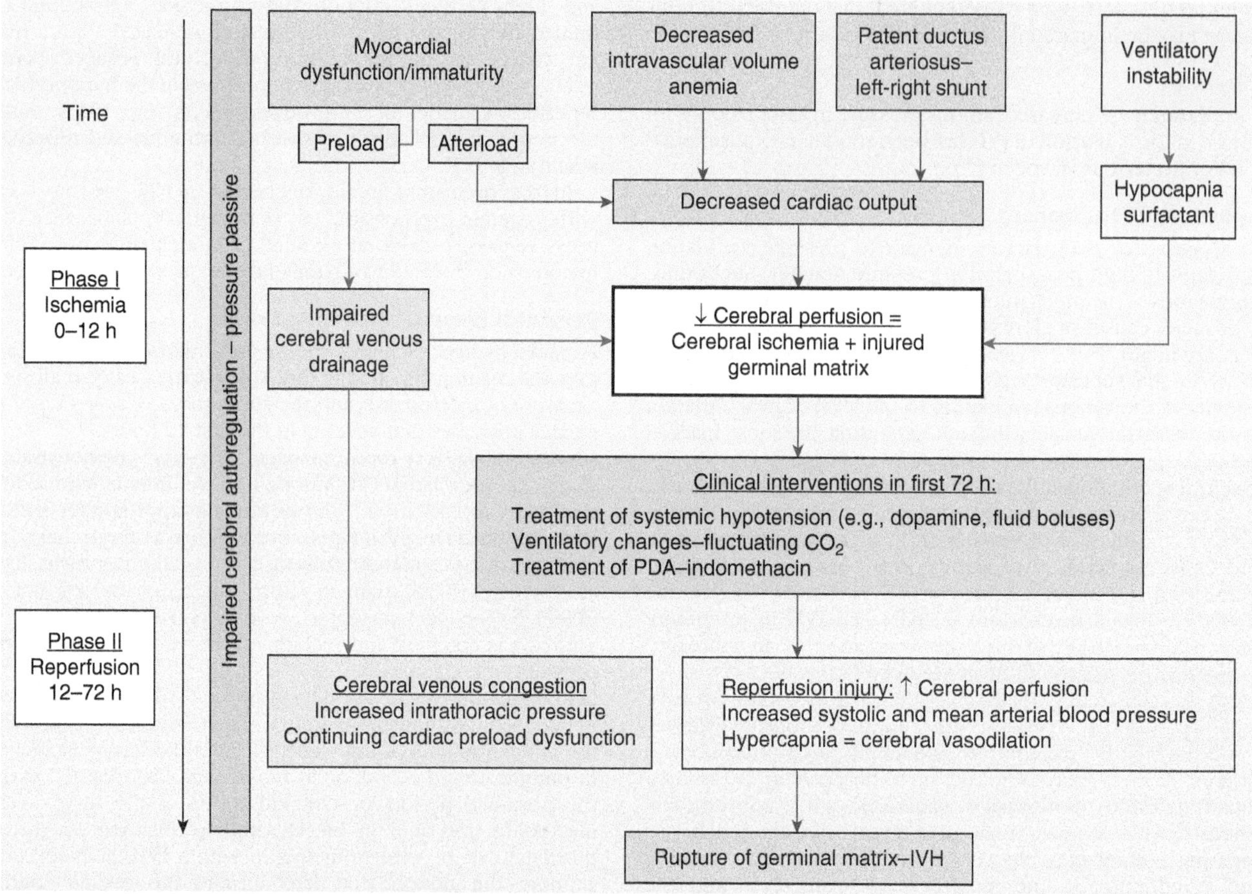

Fig. 131.8 Mechanisms of cerebral ischemia and reperfusion in the pathogenesis of germinal-matrix-intraventricular hemorrhage. *IVH*, Intraventricular hemorrhage; *PDA*, patent ductus arteriosus.

administration of superoxide dismutase in prevention of IVH in the beagle puppy model.[216] This enzyme is critical in the defense against free radicals, the formation of which is provoked by hypoxic-ischemic insult.

PLATELET AND COAGULATION DISTURBANCES

Disturbances of platelet-capillary function and coagulation may contribute to the pathogenesis of IVH, although uniformity is lacking in results of studies designed to investigate the pathogenetic role of such disturbances.

PLATELET-CAPILLARY FUNCTION

Forty percent of infants with a birth weight less than 1500 g in one study[204] exhibited platelet counts of less than 100,000/mm^3, and most of these infants with thrombocytopenia had abnormal bleeding times. The incidences of IVH in infants with thrombocytopenia versus those without thrombocytopenia were 78%, versus 48% for those weighing less than 1000 g. Thus it was concluded that the presence of thrombocytopenia appeared to be an independent pathogenetic factor for causation of IVH. Subsequent work has both confirmed and refuted a role for thrombocytopenia in the pathogenesis of IVH.[217-219] The most recent studies have tended to support an association.[220,221] The largest of these studied 655 infants born at 32 weeks' gestational age, 44% of whom had thrombocytopenia. Within this cohort there was a 30% (85/286) incidence of IVH in those with thrombocytopenia versus 14% (53/369) in those with a normal platelet count.[221] No correlation existed between the severity of thrombocytopenia and incidence of IVH; rather, it was the presence or absence of any thrombocytopenia that affected the rate of IVH occurrence.[220,221] Similarly, no protective effect was demonstrated with increased platelet transfusion.[221] In an a cohort of 251 neonates, Rastogi and colleagues[222] found no significant difference in the odds of a severe IVH between a reference group of preterm infants with a normal static platelet count and those with stable thrombocytopenia in isolation, but the odds of a severe IVH were increased fourfold if there was a sudden drop in the platelet count, and the odds increased to 14 times the baseline level if this drop occurred on a baseline of thrombocytopenia. The exact mechanism linking IVH and thrombocytopenia has not been elucidated. The timing of the thrombocytopenia in the relationship with the IVH is also unclear and could also be a result of a large IVH. Some evidence suggests that premature infants demonstrate elevated levels of prostacyclin before the occurrence of IVH.[223] Because prostaglandins have an impact not only on platelet function but also on factors such as CBF and free radical production that may also be important in pathogenesis of IVH, it is not clear to what extent the effects on platelet-capillary function are independently related to causation of IVH.

COAGULATION

Disagreement exists concerning the role of coagulopathy in the causation of IVH.[217,224-227] Because disturbances of coagulation are not uncommon in preterm infants with other provocative factors for IVH (e.g., serious respiratory distress syndrome, asphyxia) or they may occur *secondary* to major hemorrhage, it has been difficult to establish an independent pathogenetic role for such disturbances. Although administration of fresh frozen plasma was shown in one study to decrease the incidence of IVH,[228] no effect on coagulation measures accompanied the apparent beneficial effect. Moreover, later investigations have failed to show a beneficial effect of prophylactic early fresh frozen plasma in premature infants.[229-231]

Recent reports have examined the potential role of mutations in coagulation proteins as possible risk modifiers for IVH. Several common mutations in coagulation proteins are associated with increased tendency for thrombotic events. Factor XIII stabilizes the fibrin clot, and thus it is hypothesized that low levels of factor XIII may predispose to IVH. Low factor XIII levels in preterm infants may contribute to the relatively higher fibrinolytic activity that occurs in preterm infants.[232] Two studies, however, failed to find any association between factor XIII V34L mutation and IVH.[233,234] Factor V Leiden is a common mutation in the white population associated with thrombotic events, with decreased inactivation of factor V leading to greatly increased thrombin generation. The role of factor V Leiden in the risk of IVH is unclear. Results have been conflicting, with some studies suggesting a significant role for factor V Leiden in the risk of IVH,[235-237] and others suggesting no role,[233,238] or a mixed pattern, whereby the mutation is associated with low-grade IVH (grade I or II) but a reduced risk of severe IVH.[234,239] There have been similarly conflicting findings for prothrombin G20210A mutations and the development of IVH.[233,235]

Two mutations (C677T and A1298C) in the *MTHFR* gene are known to cause hyperhomocysteinemia under conditions of decreased folate or vitamin B_{12} concentrations. This leads to an increased risk of thrombosis. Although no consistent association has been found with either mutation and IVH,[232,239] Ment and colleagues[240] did find a significantly increased association of this polymorphism among preterm infants, specifically with grade II to IV IVH.

VASCULAR FACTORS

Vascular factors that may predispose the blood vessels of the germinal matrix to hemorrhage include the tenuous integrity of matrix capillaries and the vulnerability of these vessels to hypoxic-ischemic injury.

TENUOUS CAPILLARY INTEGRITY

Anatomic and histologic evidence suggests that the capillary integrity is tenuous in the germinal matrix. First, these vessels, like the germinal matrix itself, are in a process of involution. Pape and Wigglesworth[241] characterized the elaborate capillary bed of the germinal matrix as "a persisting immature vascular rete," an immature microvascular network that is remodeled into a mature capillary bed when the matrix disappears. This involuting remodeling capillary bed may be expected to be more susceptible to rupture than more mature vessels. Second, many studies have emphasized that the matrix microcirculation is composed of simple endothelial-lined vessels that are often larger than capillaries but cannot be categorized as arterioles or venules because of absence of muscle and collagen.[70,71,78,241] Studies have documented the absence of muscle[242] and type VI collagen.[243] It has been postulated that such vessels are likely to be more susceptible to rupture. Third, an electron-microscopic study of cortical and germinal matrix vessels shows a twofold to fourfold greater diameter of both the vessels and vessel lumens of the germinal matrix in comparison with those of the cortical plate in infants of 25 to 33 weeks' gestation.[244] Thus in the age range of greatest propensity for the occurrence of IVH, the diameters are unusually large, a finding of potential pathogenetic importance because of Laplace's law, which states that the larger the vessel diameter, the greater the total force on the wall at any given pressure. Finally, immunomicroscopy of neuropathology specimens has shown that staining for tight junction proteins (zona occludens 1, claudin, and occludin) in the germinal matrix vessels at 24 weeks revealed reduced and immature staining patterns. Immature tight junctions between endothelial cells would impact the functionality of the blood-brain barrier, and could predispose the vessels to hemorrhagic rupture.[245]

Box 131.2 Mechanisms of Brain Injury With Germinal Matrix Hemorrhage—Intraventricular Hemorrhage

- Preceding hypoxic-ischemic injury, especially periventricular leukomalacia
- Destruction of glial and neuronal/interneuronal precursors in germinal matrix
- Destruction of periventricular white matter (i.e., periventricular hemorrhagic infarction) and subsequent impairment of cortical organization
- Periventricular white matter injury resulting from intraventricular, parenchymal, or subarachnoid blood products with vasoconstriction and generation of free radical products
- Alteration in cerebellar development
- Intracranial hypertension and impaired cerebral perfusion
- Post-hemorrhagic hydrocephalus

The possibility should be considered that effects of these maturational deficiencies of germinal matrix vessels underlie the interesting observation that women with preeclampsia exhibit a much lower risk for an infant with IVH (2.5%) than do women without preeclampsia (17%).[246] This lower risk of IVH has been confirmed.[247,248] Infants born to women with preeclampsia exhibit a variety of features suggestive of accelerated maturation of the brain and other organs.[227,249] A maturational acceleration in the germinal matrix may be mediated in a manner similar to that found with the administration of antenatal steroids.[73]

MECHANISMS OF BRAIN INJURY

MAJOR FACTORS

The principal mechanisms of brain injury in the premature infant with IVH relate to one or more of at least the following six major factors (Box 131.2): (1) hypoxic-ischemic injury that may precede the IVH; (2) destruction of germinal matrix with its neuronal and glial precursors; (3) destruction of periventricular white matter (i.e., periventricular hemorrhagic infarction); (4) periventricular white matter injury resulting from activation of microglia or intraventricular blood products or both; (5) a marked increase in intracranial pressure and concomitant defects in cerebral perfusion at the time of severe IVH; and (6) post-hemorrhagic hydrocephalus.

PRECEDING HYPOXIC-ISCHEMIC INJURY

Post-mortem neuropathology studies indicate that infants with IVH exhibit two principal lesions related to hypoxic-ischemic insults: periventricular leukomalacia and a subtype of selective neuronal necrosis, pontine and subicular neuronal necrosis.[96] Periventricular leukomalacia has been reported in neuropathology series in as many as 75% of cases of IVH, and pontine neuronal necrosis is noted in nearly 50%. Moreover, the finding that ventricular dilatation correlates strongly with subsequent neurologic and cognitive deficits after IVH,[250] in the absence of progressive hydrocephalus or periventricular hemorrhagic infarction,[251-254] further suggests that concomitant periventricular leukomalacia and cerebral white (and concomitant gray) matter atrophy are common and important in the outcome of infants with IVH.

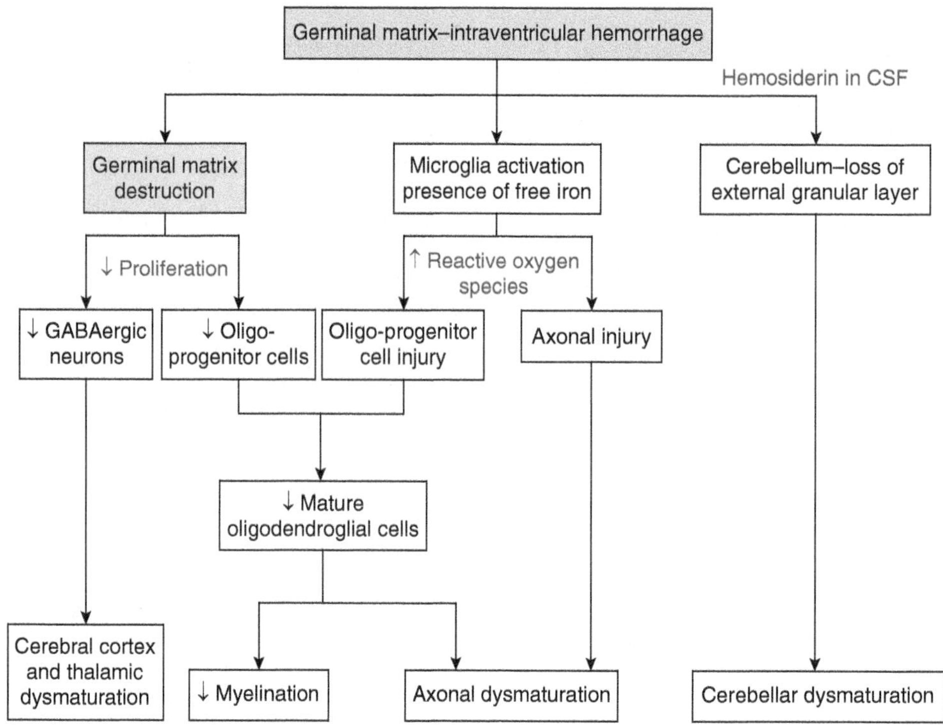

Fig. 131.9 Neuropathologic consequences of intraventricular hemorrhage on cerebral white and gray mater, and cerebellum. *CSF*, Cerebrospinal fluid.

DESTRUCTION OF GERMINAL MATRIX AND THE NEURONAL AND GLIAL PRECURSORS

One[255] of the consistent neuropathologic consequences of IVH is destruction of germinal matrix with its neuronal and glial precursor cells (Fig. 131.9). The glial precursor cells are destined to give rise to both oligodendroglia and astrocytes. The neuronal precursors are principally GABAergic interneurons destined for the thalamus.[256] These cells preferentially populate the association thalamic nuclei that are anatomically related to the association cerebral cortices involved in higher cognitive function and language.[257] Thus loss of these neurons could have important deleterious functional effects. The loss of the glial precursor cells may affect subsequent cerebral development through the loss of oligodendroglia or astrocytes. Loss of mature oligodendroglia through either apoptosis or arrest of maturation of preoligodendrocytes may lead to a subsequent impairment of myelination after germinal matrix destruction.[256,258] A rabbit model of preterm IVH found both apoptosis and reduced proliferation of oligodendrocyte progenitor cells after IVH, consistent with the human studies.[259,260] However, a study in mouse brain shows that oligodendrocyte progenitor populations proliferate robustly in response to widespread cellular death,[261] suggesting that IVH might inhibit reparative mechanisms. The loss of glial precursor cells may also impair subsequent development of astrocytes. Gressens and coworkers[262,263] showed that astrocytes destined for supragranular (upper) cortical layers originate and migrate after the occurrence of neuronal migration and are crucial for normal organizational development of the supragranular cerebral cortex. These astrocytic precursors are likely to be destroyed by germinal matrix hemorrhage, a finding raising the possibility of a subsequent disturbance in cortical development.[263]

The ependymal/subependymal destruction caused by germinal matrix hemorrhage-IVH could lead to impaired glial and neuronal development by adversely affecting primary cilia in this region, which have been shown to be critical for neural progenitor cell survival and proliferation.[260]

DESTRUCTION OF PERIVENTRICULAR WHITE MATTER: PERIVENTRICULAR HEMORRHAGIC INFARCTION

Numerous follow-up studies have correlated cranial ultrasonographic findings in the neonatal period in patients with IVH with the occurrence of subsequent neurologic deficits. Del Bigio[66] has demonstrated in premature infants with germinal matrix hemorrhage-IVH, studied post mortem, a marked decrease in cell proliferation, and a subsequent decrease in the number of oligodendrocytes. These studies confirm the presence of periventricular hemorrhagic infarction as the single most important determinant of neurologic outcome. Of all survivors of IVH, this lesion accounts for the largest proportion of subsequent severe neurologic deficits. The deleterious neurologic effects of periventricular hemorrhagic infarction may relate not only to destruction of cerebral white matter per se but also to the effects of the white matter injury on cerebral cortical development. A post-mortem neuropathology study of cerebral cortical organization in infants with a history of major hemorrhagic white matter lesions has shown marked alterations in neuronal axonal and dendritic ramifications in areas overlying the white matter destruction.[264] These abnormalities are postulated to be caused by disturbances of afferent input to and efferent input from the areas of cortex through disruption of the respective white matter axon. These critical connections may also have disturbed thalamocortical connectivity, which is increasingly recognized as a factor determining cognitive outcomes in preterm children.[265] Another potential cause of the cortical abnormalities is destruction of subplate neurons by the white matter infarction.[266] These neurons are critical for cerebral cortical organization and are abundant in subcortical white matter in the human premature infant. Whatever the mechanism, these *cerebral cortical* abnormalities with periventricular hemorrhagic infarction could be important in determination of subsequent cognitive deficits and seizure disorders.

Table 131.3 Short-Term Outcome of Germinal Matrix Hemorrhage–Intraventricular Hemorrhage as a Function of the Severity of the Hemorrhage.

	Deaths in First 14 Days		PVD in Survivors 14 Days Old		Surgery and Late Death			
Grade	**<750 g (*n* = 173)**	**751–1500 g (*n* = 75)**	**<750 g (*n* = 165)**	**751–1500 g (*n* = 56)**	**<750 g (*n* = 165)**	**751–1500 g (*n* = 56)**	**Mortality**	**Surgery in Survivors**
I (*n* = 104)	3/24 (12%)	0/80 (0%)	1/21 (5%)	3/80 (4%)	(0 + 4)/21 (19%)	(0 + 3)/80 (4%)	10/104 (10%)	0/94 (0%)
II (*n* = 65)	5/21 (24%)	1/44 (2%)	1/16 (6%)	6/43 (14%)	(0 + 5)/16 (31%)	(1 + 2)/43 (7%)	13/65 (20%)	1/52 (2%)
III (*n* = 45)	6/19 (32%)	2/26 (8%)	10/13 (77%)	18/24 (75%)	(3 + 2)/13 (38%)	(7 + 4)/24 (42%)	14/45 (31%)	10/31 (32%)
IV (*n* = 34)	5/11 (45%)	5/23 (22%)	5/6 (83%)	12/18 (66%)	(1 + 3)/6 (66%)	(7 + 4)/18 (61%)	17/34 (50%)	8/17 (47%)

PVD, Progressive ventricular dilatation.

PERIVENTRICULAR WHITE MATTER INJURY CAUSED BY BLOOD PRODUCTS

The presence of blood products may have a direct pathogenetic role in the evolution of periventricular white matter injury, as demonstrated by the observation that the presence of IVH is associated with a fivefold to ninefold increased risk of ultrasonographic correlates (e.g., echolucencies) of white matter injury.[17] Experimental studies suggest that two interacting mechanisms could be operative to produce white matter injury in the presence of IVH: impairment of CBF and increased generation of free radicals. Parenchymal or subarachnoid blood has been demonstrated to result in disturbances of cerebral blood flow. Proposed mechanisms for this include the local release of vasoconstricting potassium from hemolyzed red blood cells,[267] prostanoids,[268] or 5-hydroxytrptamine.[268,269] However, as the walls of cerebral parenchymal vessels do not contain the smooth muscle cell layer necessary for vasospasm in the human premature infant,[242] it seems unlikely that local CBF could be affected by this mechanism. However, subarachnoid blood potentially could cause vasoconstriction of major leptomeningeal cerebral vessels, which do contain a smooth muscle cell layer in the human premature infant.

Perhaps a more likely mechanism of white matter injury with intraventricular or parenchymal blood involves *increased free radical formation,* provoked by local release of iron from the blood.[270] The presence of blood products is particularly dangerous in the premature infant because the expression of heme oxygenase is especially high in the immature cerebral white matter,[271] thus enhancing formation of Fe^{2+} when hemorrhage is present. The Fe^{2+} could then catalyze the generation of the highly reactive and dangerous hydroxyl radical through the Fenton reaction. The early differentiating oligodendroglia have been shown to be exquisitely vulnerable to free radical attack,[272] and thus the enhanced hydroxyl radical generation could accelerate cerebral white matter injury. Indeed, neuropathology studies of preterm infants have described increased numbers of microglia, expression of the proinflammatory mediator TNF-α, and evidence of free radical damage in premyelinating oligodendrocytes (lipid peroxidation and positive immunoreactivity for nitrotyrosine) associated with IVH and periventricular leukomalacia.[98,100] Additionally, studies in the early postnatal period have documented elevated levels of free radical products in the CSF of premature infants who are later found to have cerebral white matter injury on MRI at term.[269,273] Finally, it has been proposed that blood products may also have direct toxic effects to oligodendroglial progenitor cells (OPCs). Cell culture of rat subventricular cells and OPCs demonstrated that blood products, and in particular thrombin, is directly toxic to both. Furthermore, thrombin may lead to reduced differentiation and migration of OPCs.[274]

COMPLICATIONS OF INTRAVENTRICULAR HEMORRHAGE

POST-HEMORRHAGIC VENTRICULAR DILATATION

INCIDENCE AND DEFINITION

PHVD is the progressive ventricular dilatation resulting from a disturbance in CSF dynamics, and encompasses other terms such as post-hemorrhagic hydrocephalus. PHVD is a frequent sequela of IVH (Table 131.3).[2,3,275-279] As could be expected, the incidence of PHVD is related closely to the severity of the initial hemorrhage. A clear clinical distinction between ventriculomegaly resulting from periventricular cerebral atrophy and ventriculomegaly resulting from hydrocephalus with attendant impairment of CSF dynamics can be difficult, but it is critical for the formulation of appropriate management decisions. In general, the development of ventriculomegaly resulting from atrophy occurs slowly, over several weeks, is not associated with the development of increased intracranial pressure or rapid head growth, and evolves to a state of stable ventricular size—that is, ventricular size neither decreases, as in transient hydrocephalus, nor continues to increase, as in persistently progressive hydrocephalus. The evaluation of PHVD after IVH can be best undertaken with cranial ultrasonography, particularly for the systematic evaluation of ventricular size. Cranial ultrasound images have been typically evaluated qualitatively for ventricular size. Although this strategy has proved useful, it would appear more informative to evaluate ventricular size in a quantitative fashion, on the basis of established norms.[280] Multiple different quantitative measurements have been developed, including measurement of ventricular index, ventricular height, anterior horn width (AHW), and thalamooccipital distance. No single measurement has been proven to be superior to the others (Fig. 131.10).[281] The Levene index has traditionally been the most commonly performed measurement, and one that clinicians are most familiar with, while the occipital horn is the first parameter to enlarge after IVH, and the anterior horn the first to change with increased intracranial pressure.[281,282] Thus utilizing a combination of measurements, including the Levene index, the thalamo-occipital distance,[280] and the AHW, potentially provides the clinician with a more robust assessment. Frequent monitoring of the ventricular dimensions by cranial ultrasonography, particularly in the acute period, may assist in assessing the infant's course and determining the need for intervention with ventricular drainage. It may also guide the frequency and volume of CSF drainage necessary to decrease ventricular size. Finally, recent data have suggested a strong relationship between the maximal measures on cranial ultrasonography and later neurodevelopmental outcomes.[250]

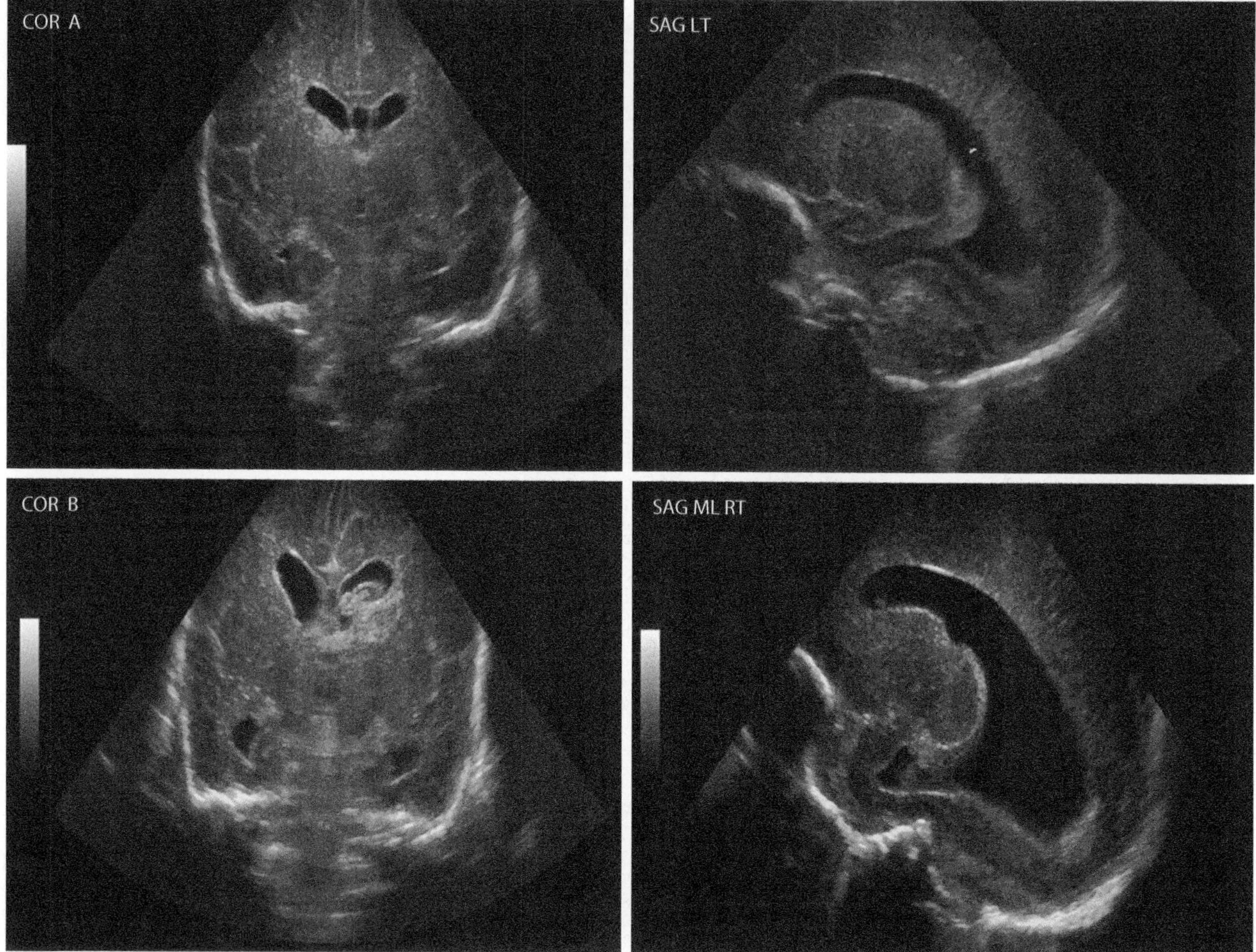

Fig. 131.10 Ventricular dilatation. Coronal *(COR)* and parasagittal *(SAG)* ultrasound scans: (A) mild dilatation; (B) moderate dilatation (note residual intraventricular hemorrhage is still present).

PATHOGENESIS

The pathogenesis of PHVD can be considered in terms of either the acute process, apparent within days, or the subacute-chronic process, apparent within weeks. Acute hydrocephalus appears to be a result of an impairment of CSF absorption caused by particulate blood clot and demonstrable by ultrasound scan (Fig. 131.11).[283] Subacute-chronic hydrocephalus is presumably related to obliterative arachnoiditis in the posterior fossa, where the blood tends to collect.[71] The ventricular dilatation may begin essentially with the hemorrhage, especially with marked IVH. More often, definite ventricular dilatation and, particularly, the progression thereof begin within 1 to 3 weeks of the hemorrhage.

RELATION OF VENTRICULAR DILATATION TO BRAIN INJURY

The precise relation of progressive PHVD to brain injury is not fully defined and likely represents a complex multifactorial process. The injury likely relates to a combination of (1) the release of blood products into the CSF (in particular free iron) that lead to both a proinflammatory response and ventricular dilatation, and (2) the ventricular dilatation then exacerbating the injury by impairing cerebral hemodynamics with associated tissue hypoxia-ischemia and further neuroinflammation. This issue is discussed in the following sections.

Experimental Studies

Animal models have demonstrated that the injection of blood and hemoglobin into the ventricles generates a proinflammatory cascade with free radical formation, leading to white mater injury and neuronal loss.[284] This has been well documented, and is discussed in detail in the previous section.

In addition to this direct injury, *experimental studies* have shown the development of ventriculomegaly following the injection of blood, hemoglobin, or iron into CSF.[285-289] In neonatal rats, intraventricular injection of hemoglobin led to acute ventricular enlargement, development of gliosis, increased inflammatory cytokines in cerebral white matter, impaired myelination, reduced hippocampal volumes, and periventricular "cell death."[285,286] The importance of iron has been particularly highlighted in these studies. When iron-deficient protoporphyrin, rather than iron-rich hemoglobin, was injected into the CSF, the ventricles did not enlarge. Furthermore, the addition of deferoxamine, an iron chelator, after injection of hemoglobin ameliorated both the ventricular enlargement and the inflammation.[286]

The deleterious effects of ventriculomegaly itself on the brain may include disturbances of cerebral white matter, cerebral blood vessels, and cerebral cortex. Experimental models of hydrocephalus, utilizing kaolin injection in neonatal rat pups, has provided insight into the impact of the ventriculomegaly independent of the associated injury due to the intraventricular blood. These studies have demonstrated that ventriculomegaly is associated with white matter edema, periventricular hypoxia, reactive astrogliosis, and axonal disruption.[290,291] The degree of ventriculomegaly is also directly associated with severity of cognitive impairment demonstrated in the animal models.[290]

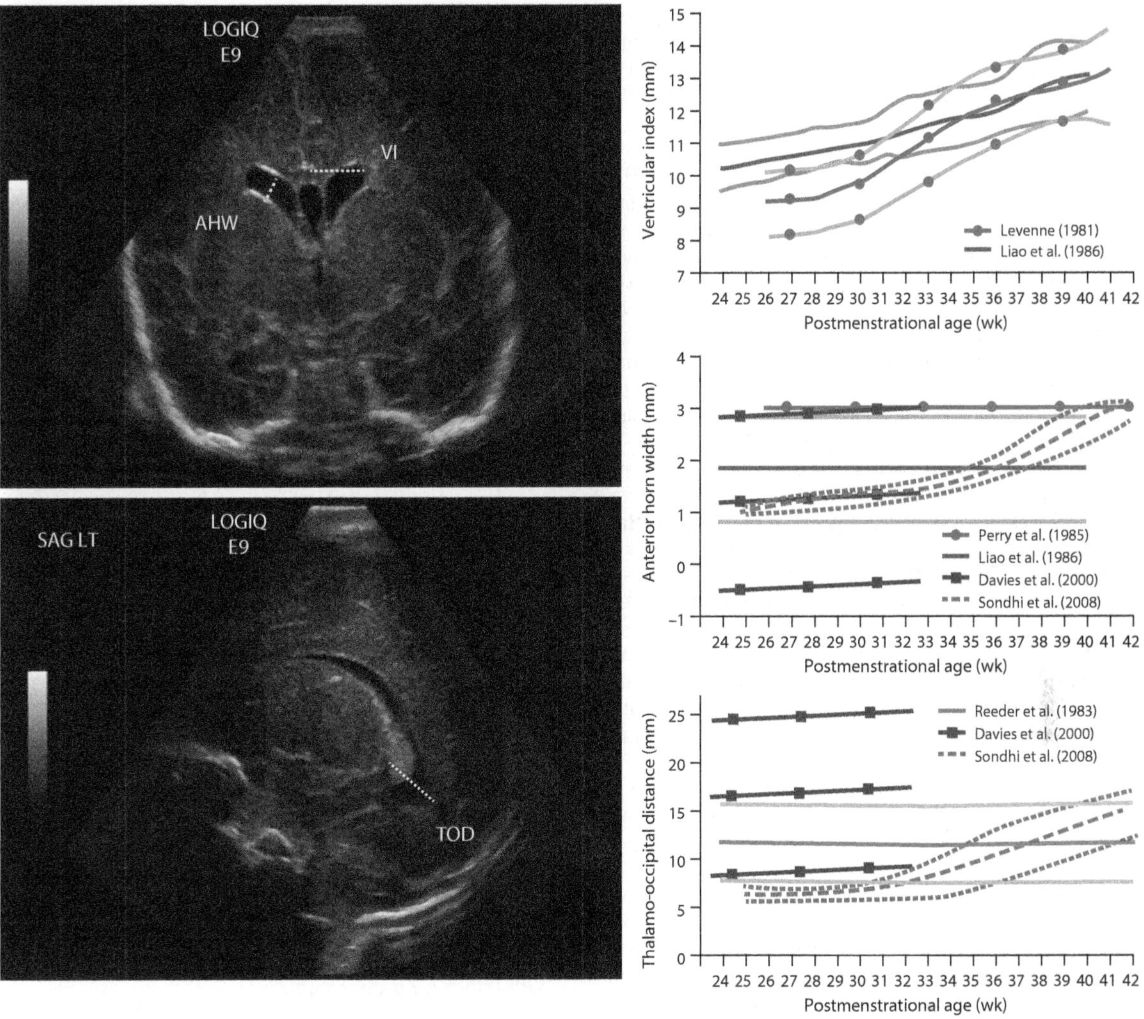

Fig. 131.11 Methods of ventricular measurement on coronal (at the level of the third ventricle) and parasagittal *(SAG)* ultrasound views. *AHW,* Anterior horn width; *TOD,* thalamooccipital distance; *VI,* ventricular index. (Adapted from Brouwer MJ, de Vries LS, Pistorius L, et al. Ultrasound measurements of the lateral ventricles in neonates: why, how and when? A systematic review. *Acta Paediatr.* 2010;99[9]:1298–1306.)

The earliest changes in the *cerebral white matter* are seen within 1 week after induction of experimental hydrocephalus, with a decrease in the levels of myelin-associated enzymes (e.g., ceramide galactosyltransferase) and structural proteins (e.g., myelin basic protein). Later, after several weeks, axonal loss and impaired myelination are apparent. Shunting at 1 week but not at 4 weeks, when axonal loss had occurred, has been shown to allow recovery of myelination and improved behavioral testing.[292,293] The late occurrence of axonal loss with hydrocephalus was noted in earlier studies.[294-296] Thus intervention should occur before this stage in an attempt to ameliorate these permanent structural deficits.

A potential role for *cerebral vascular changes and ischemia* in the genesis of the white matter injury in experimental hydrocephalus is demonstrated by morphologic studies that show an alteration in the caliber of major cerebral vessels with a decrease in the caliber of secondary and tertiary vessels in the cerebral white matter.[297,298] These changes may explain, at least in part, the decrease in CBF and energy metabolism in hydrocephalic animal models.[299-301] Further supportive of cerebral ischemia are the findings in cerebral white matter of increased rates of glucose metabolism (presumably anaerobic glycolysis), elevated lactate levels, decreased levels of high-energy phosphates, and elevated levels of free radicals.[302-304] Enhanced free radical production is particularly relevant, in view of the particular vulnerability of differentiating oligodendroglia to free radical attack.[227] These biochemical changes and neurochemical signs of axonal loss have been shown to be prevented by early shunting in the various experimental models.[301,302]

Of additional interest are the documented alterations in *cerebral cortical neurons* in hydrocephalic animal models. Disturbances in catecholaminergic and serotonergic neurotransmitter development and in synaptogenesis with evidence of neuronal degeneration have been delineated.[305-314] These effects may reflect disturbance to ascending and descending axons in cerebral white matter, with secondary anterograde and retrograde effects on organizational development of cerebral cortex. Again, these deleterious effects have been shown to be reversible when the hydrocephalic state is corrected early.

Human Studies

Data from studies in infants concerning the deleterious effect of progressive PHVD relate to cerebral hemodynamics, neurophysiologic function, morphologic disturbances, biochemical indicators of hypoxia, and clinical outcome. The data are difficult to interpret conclusively because details such as the rate of progression, degree and duration of ventriculomegaly, intracranial pressure, preceding parenchymal injury, and neurologic outcome are often not provided.

Concerning *cerebral hemodynamics*, post-hemorrhagic hydrocephalus was initially demonstrated to be associated with *impaired blood flow velocity*,[115,315-317] which can be reversed with therapy to correct the hydrocephalic state.[115] This disturbance of CBF velocity appears to correlate more closely with ventriculomegaly than with increased intracranial pressure. In two small observational studies of preterm infants with PHVD, infants with PHVD had lower $rsCO_2$ values than preterm infants without PHVD;[318] however, following decompression with placement of an external ventricular drain, the $rsCO^2$ among infants with PHVD increased from a mean of 42.6 ± 12.9% to 55 ± 12.2%.[319] These results indicate that PHVD impacts cerebral hemodynamics, which may improve following treatment.

Concerning *neurophysiologic function,* visual evoked potentials, brain stem auditory evoked potentials, somatosensory evoked responses, and amplitude-integrated electroencephalography recordings have all been shown to be altered by PHVD. The studies have demonstrated prolonged latencies of these evoked potentials with PHVD in the premature infant.[320-323] Improvement in latencies was demonstrated after CSF removal by placement of a ventriculoperitoneal (VP) shunt or direct removal of ventricular fluid.[320-323] These data suggest that an axonal disturbance is caused by ventricular distention, and this disturbance can be reversed by effective therapy.

Concerning *morphologic evidence of brain injury* with PHVD, a paucity of data exists from studies of autopsies of human infants who did not have markedly advanced disease. Studies of biopsy specimens taken at the time of VP shunt placement have shown four major findings: (1) disruption of ependyma, (2) direct evidence of axonal injury ("axonal ballooning"), (3) lipid-laden microglia, and (4) diminished numbers of myelinated axons.[295,324-327] These findings are consistent with the experimental models of hydrocephalus.

Biochemical evidence of hypoxia has been observed and suggests injury to the brain that is reversible by therapy.[328] *Elevated CSF levels of hypoxanthine,* a marker for hypoxic tissue, have been found in infants with post-hemorrhagic hydrocephalus, but these have declined significantly after successful treatment.[328] Although the morphologic effects of hydrocephalus on cerebral vessels, and the resulting deleterious cerebral hemodynamic effects, are a probable explanation for tissue hypoxia, elevated levels of vasoconstricting eicosanoids (e.g., thromboxanes) or edema-producing eicosanoids (e.g., leukotrienes) appear important. The levels of these eicosanoids have been shown to be elevated in CSF of infants with PHVD.[329] The source of these compounds remains unclear, and their specific relation to the PHVD remains to be established. Biochemical evidence of oxygen deficiency at the mitochondrial level is found with the demonstration by near-infrared spectroscopy of an increase in *brain levels* of *oxidized cytochrome* aa_3 after lumbar puncture in infants with PHVD accompanied by increased intracranial pressure.[330,331] This observation is consistent with the demonstration by positron emission tomography of increases in cerebral metabolic rate for oxygen in several infants (one newborn) after treatment of hydrocephalus.[332] More data are needed on these issues.

NATURAL HISTORY

Management of PHVD must begin with recognition of the natural history of the disorder. We undertook a large study in premature infants to investigate the natural history of PHVD.[333] In this cohort of 248 very low-birth-weight infants with IVH (mean gestational age 27 weeks), 25% of the infants exhibited PHVD (see Fig. 131.11). Arrest of PHVD occurred without treatment in one-third of infants. Of the remaining two-thirds of infants who did not have arrested PHVD and thus had persistent PHVD, most received nonsurgical therapy consisting of pharmacologic therapy or drainage of CSF by serial lumbar punctures only. Half of the patients with persistent PHVD received surgical therapy with insertion of a VP reservoir or shunt, and one-third of the infants with persistent PHVD died (Fig. 131.12). The development of PHVD after IVH and the occurrence of an adverse short-term outcome, such as the requirement for surgical therapy, were predicted most strongly by the severity of IVH (see Table 131.3 and Fig. 131.12).

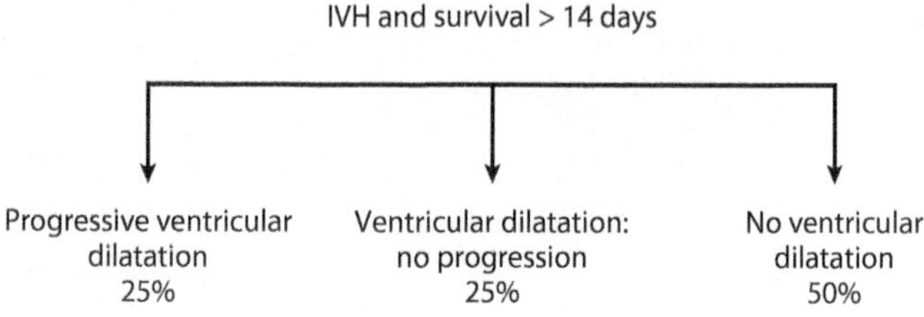

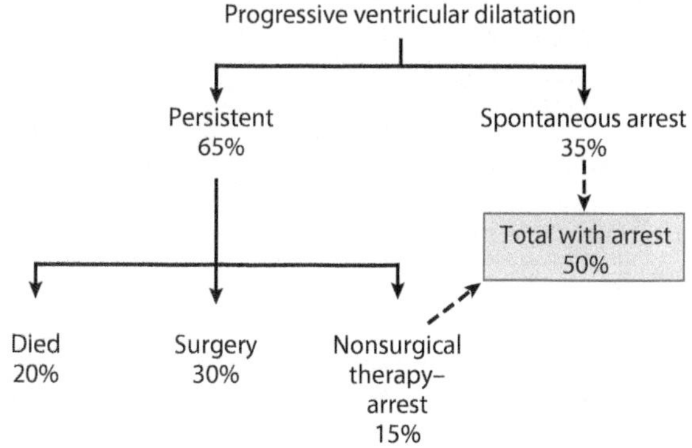

Fig. 131.12 Natural history of very low-birth-weight infants with post-hemorrhagic ventricular dilatation. *IVH,* Intraventricular hemorrhage.

MANAGEMENT OF POST-HEMORRHAGIC VENTRICULAR DILATATION

Management approaches for PHVD have focused on reducing CSF, either through the use of medications to reduce production, or by draining the CSF. Acetazolamide, in combination with furosemide, has been trialed to reduce CSF production in neonates with PHVD. However rather than indicating benefit, infants in the acetazolamide and furosemide group actually had worse outcomes than those receiving standard care, and therefore this management cannot be recommended at this time.[334,335]

An alternate and novel approach to management that has been proposed was DRIFT—ventricular *dr*ainage, *i*rrigation, and *f*ibrinolytic *t*herapy. This involved the placement of two ventricular reservoirs, instillation of tissue-type plasminogen activator into the ventricle, and then, after 8 hours, irrigation with artificial CSF. The hypothesis was that this would enhance removal of blood and blood products from the ventricles, thereby reducing the noxious impact of the blood products and attenuating the proinflammatory cascade. Unfortunately the randomized trial demonstrated an increase in secondary IVH among those in the intervention arm compared to standard care, necessitating stopping the trial early, called for by the data safety monitoring group. However, it should be noted that infants in the intervention arm had improved outcomes at both 2 and 10 years of age compared to those in standard care.[336,337] Therefore, while DRIFT itself is not recommended, it supports the hypothesis that removal of the blood products could improve the ultimate outcome for these infants.

Serial lumbar punctures are often the first management step in attempting to remove CSF fluid to arrest PHVD progression. If the PHVD continues to progress, this approach may be followed by neurosurgical intervention, including temporizing procedures such as ventricular reservoirs or ventriculosubgaleal shunts, or ultimately insertion of a VP shunt. While the use of endoscopic third ventriculostomy with or without choroid plexus cauterization is an appealing alternative to a VP shunt, due to the lack of indwelling hardware, the data to date does not support its use over the placement of a VP shunt or PHVD.[338]

There has been considerable debate over whether the presence of ventricular dilatation independent of the original IVH results in brain injury and worsening of neurodevelopmental outcomes. To address this one must consider the literature relating the association of ventricular size with neurodevelopmental outcome. The association between the maximal size of ventricular measurements and neurodevelopmental outcomes has been supported by more than one report.[250,339,340] Similarly, retrospective and observational studies have demonstrated that earlier intervention with serial LPs, or temporizing surgical procedures to reduce ventriculomegaly, was associated with improved neurodevelopmental outcome at 18 to 24 months.[339,341] Following this, a multicenter prospective randomized trial of early versus late ventricular intervention (ELVIS) was conducted. Infants with PHVD were randomized to early intervention (Levene index >97th percentile, and AHW >6 mm, and/or TOD >25 mm) or late intervention (Levene index >97th percentile + 4 mm, and AHW >10 mm). Intervention consisted initially of serial LPs (maximum of 3) followed by placement of a ventricular reservoir if further drainage was required, and ultimately a shunt if still progressing. For the primary composite outcome of death or need for VP shunt, there was no difference between study arms.[342] There was, however, reduced brain injury demonstrated on MRI among those with early intervention.[343] The 2-year outcome data, which is currently submitted for publication, did not demonstrate a significant difference between study arms; however, this may reflect the relatively small differences in AHW measurements between study arms and the relatively aggressive management even among those in the late intervention arm.[340] This is demonstrated in Fig. 131.13 where the relationship of maximal AHW during the NICU period following PHVD is plotted against neurodevelopmental outcomes at 18 to 24 months on Bayley II assessment. The bars overlaid represent the data reported from the two arms of the ELVIS trial, early intervention (red) and late intervention (blue), and a single center North American observational study (yellow bar), which intervened based primarily on clinical signs of raised ICP.[339] The figure demonstrates that the observational study typically intervened later than both arms of ELVIS, at a much increased AHW. The mean cognitive scores between the three groups were 93 (early intervention ELVIS: red bar), 90 (late intervention ELVIS: blue bar), and 68 (observational study: yellow bar).[340] This data taken together further supports the association between increased ventricular dilatation and worse developmental outcome. A randomized trial found that only brain volume, but not ventricular volume, correlated with early developmental outcome. But that study was conducted in full-term infants treated for postnatal postinflammatory hydrocephalus prior to 6 months of age, whereas the situation may well be different in the preterm brain.[71,72,344]

Clinical studies and practices based on interventions for PHVD performed after a substantial increase in ventricular size or following detection of clinical signs and symptoms of increased ICP do not show significant improvement in short- or long-term outcomes. This lack of benefit could be related to the late nature of such interventions, as well as the use of more invasive procedures such as ventricular taps and VP-shunt placement. By contrast, the ELVIS trial, as well as similar practice approaches that relied on sequential ultrasound measurements of ventricular size and early interventions based on the ventricular measurements, were associated with less injury on brain MRI and better outcomes, with the degree of ventricular dilatation inversely correlating

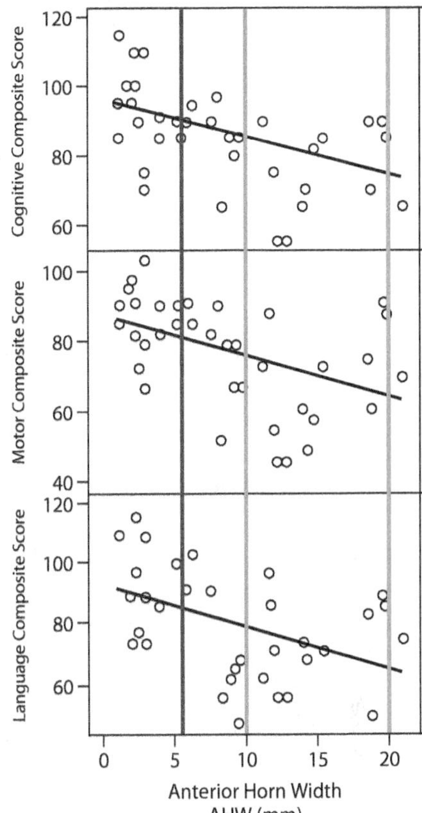

Fig. 131.13 Association between Anterior Horn Width *(AHW)* and neurodevelopmental outcome at 18 to 24 months. *Red bar*, Early arm of ELVIS trial; *blue bar*, late arm of ELVIS trial; *yellow bar*, observational cohort that intervened based on signs of raised ICP.

with neurodevelopmental outcome. Taken together, these results suggest that early interventions can prevent or ameliorate brain injury in PHVD, especially when temporizing measures such as LP, VR, and ventriculosubgaleal shunt are used.

Recently, an expert international group representing neonatologists, neurologists, and neurosurgeons have proposed a management pathway that utilizes a combination of both imaging and clinical findings to stratify risk and recommend method and timing of intervention (Fig. 131.14).[345]

PROGNOSIS

The prognosis of patients with IVH is considered best in terms of the short-term outcome (mortality rate and development of PVD) and the long-term outcome (neurologic sequelae). The *short-term outcome* relates clearly to the severity of the hemorrhage. The mortality rates and incidences of progressive PVD (see Table 131.3) are strongly related to the severity of the hemorrhage, documented primarily by ultrasound scan.[3,17,346-349] With small lesions confined to the germinal matrix or accompanied by small amounts of intraventricular blood, mortality rates are low, and the likelihood of PVD in survivors is rare. In contrast, infants with severe lesions (i.e., blood filling the ventricles) have high mortality rates (approximately 20%), and more than half of the survivors exhibit PVD.[350] The *long-term neurodevelopmental outcome* of the infant with IVH depends particularly on the degree of parenchymal injury. A large body of literature describes associations between cranial ultrasonography findings and neurologic outcome (Table 131.4). The EPIPAGE study enrolled 1954 infants born at less than 32

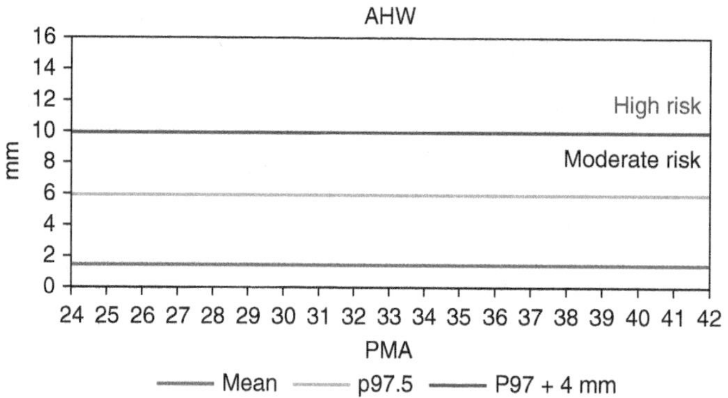

Green zone

Key criteria:
Ventricular size with the following
- VI ≤ 97th percentile
 and
- AHW ≤ 6 mm

And
All the following clinical criteria:
- HC growth < 2 cm/wk
- No separated suture
- No bulging fontanelles

Additional considerations:
No evidence of alteration of:
- NIRS
- Doppler

Management:
- Observation in NICU
- cUS twice a week until stable for 2 wk then every 1–2 wk till 34 wk PMA
- MRI at term equivalent

Yellow zone

Key criteria:
Ventricular size with the following
- VI > 97th percentile
 and
- AHW > 6 mm and/or TOD > 25 mm

And
All the following clinical criteria:
- HC growth < 2 cm/wk
- No separated suture
- No bulging fontanelles

Additional considerations:
No evidence of alteration of:
- NIRS
- Doppler

Management:
- Referral to a regional center for neurosurgical review
- Consider LP 2–3 times
- cUS 2–3 times a week until stable for 2 wk then every 1–2 wk till 34 wk PMA
- Neurosurgical intervention when no stabilization occurs
- MRI at term equivalent

Red zone

Key criteria:
Ventricular size with the following
- VI > 97th percentile + 4 mm
 and
- AHW > 10 mm and/or TOD > 25 mm

Or
Any of the following clinical criteria
- HC growth > 2 cm/wk
- Separated sutures
- Bulging fontanelles

Additional considerations:
Any evidence of alteration of:
- NIRS
- Doppler

Management:
- Consider LP 2–3 times
- Neurosurgical intervention including either temporizing measures or VP shunt
- MRI at term equivalent

Fig. 131.14 Proposed risk stratification and management pathway for infants with post-hemorrhagic ventricular dilatation. *AHW,* Anterior horn width; *HC,* head circumference; *LP,* lumbar puncture; *MRI,* magnetic resonance imaging; *NICU,* neonatal intensive care unit; *NIRS,* near infrared spectroscopy; *PMA,* postmenstrual age; *TOD,* thalamooccipital distance; *VI,* ventricular index; *VP,* ventriculoperitoneal.

Table 131.4 Long-Term Outcome: Neurologic Sequelae With Germinal Matrix Hemorrhage–Intraventricular Hemorrhage as a Function of the Severity of the Hemorrhage.

Severity of Hemorrhage	Incidence of Neurologic Sequelae (%)
Mild	5–10
Moderate	15
Severe	35
Severe and apparent periventricular hemorrhagic infarction	50–100

weeks' gestation[351] and described a clear relationship between worsening IVH and an increased risk of adverse outcome. Even in isolated grade I-II IVH, the rates of cerebral palsy increased substantially from 5.5% to 8.1% for grade I IVH (n = 229) and to 12.2% for grade II IVH (n = 168). Notably, cerebral palsy rates with isolated grade I-III IVH also rose with immaturity from 5% at 31 to 32 weeks to 10% to 15% at 27 to 30 weeks and 33% at 24 to 26 weeks. Patra and colleagues[352] also reported that grade I-II IVH was associated with a twofold increase in the risk of lower cognitive performance (Mental Developmental Index) and a 2.6-fold increase in the risk of neuromotor abnormalities (cerebral palsy and tone) after social and neonatal factors (sex, bronchopulmonary dysplasia, sepsis, necrotizing enterocolitis, maternal marital status, race, and education) had been controlled for. There were similar findings in two recent independent cohorts, with grade I-II IVH being associated with worse Mental Developmental Index and Psychomotor Developmental Index scores.[352-354] These findings persisted after gestational age had been corrected for only at less than 28 to 29 weeks' gestation. For school-age outcomes, Sherlock and colleagues[355] examined 298 preterm infants weighing less than 1000 g at age 8 years to determine the impact of IVH in relation to neuromotor and cognitive outcomes. They documented that no IVH was associated with cerebral palsy rates of 6.7%, with no rise in association with grade I IVH (6.4%) but a marked elevation with grade II IVH to 24%. Finally, an ultrasonography-based study evaluated 338 preterm adolescents (birth weight 600 to 1250 g) for intelligence, executive function, and memory tasks, comparing them to an age-matched cohort of term controls. The preterm population was grouped into 251 preterm infants with no hemorrhage, 31 with grade I hemorrhage, and 44 with grade II hemorrhage. All subgroups of the preterm cohort demonstrated lower full-scale IQ scores, lower verbal IQ scores, and lower performance IQ scores compared with term controls. An inverse relationship between severity of hemorrhage and the IQ score existed, with the higher the grade of hemorrhage the lower the score. Tests of memory and executive function in infants with grade II hemorrhage demonstrated consistently higher deficit rates of verbal intelligence, receptive vocabulary, phonemic fluency, cognitive flexibility, and phonologic fluency than term controls, while preterm infants with either no hemorrhage or grade I hemorrhage had more variable outcomes in these domains. Vohr and colleagues[356] concluded that preterm adolescents born in the early 1990s with isolated grade II hemorrhage are at increased risk of learning challenges, including cognitive and executive function deficits.

There continues to be disagreement concerning the significance of low-grade IVH, with two of the largest and most recent studies having directly conflicting results. Payne and colleagues[357] enrolled 1472 infants, all born at less than 27 weeks' gestation. Comparing infants with no IVH and infants with low-grade IVH, they found no difference in the rates of cerebral palsy (8% vs. 9%) and neurodevelopmental impairment (10% vs. 10%), with similarly no increased risk on multivariate analysis. Bolisetty and colleagues[358] enrolled a different cohort of 1472 infants, all born at less than 29 weeks' gestation. They found a consistent association between low grades of IVH and both cerebral palsy (no IVH versus grade I-II IVH, 6.5% vs. 10.4%) and moderate-severe neurosensory impairment (no IVH vs. grade I-II IVH, 12% vs. 22%). On multivariate analysis there remained a 1.5 times increased risk of moderate-severe neurosensory impairment with low-grade IVH, when gestation, sex, small for gestational age, chronic lung disease, retinopathy of prematurity, and periventricular leukomalacia were controlled for. The notable differences between these studies were that Payne and colleagues had a 1 to 2-week lower mean gestational age for all subgroups, with slightly worse outcomes among infants without IVH, and had fewer infants with a low-grade IVH (270 vs. 336). All of these studies have been limited by the necessity to combine grade I and grade II IVH into a composite for statistical purposes, and the inability to truly distinguish by adequate neuroimaging the key neuropathologies that may be leading to the subsequent impairment of neurodevelopmental outcome. Cranial ultrasonography has been demonstrated to have poor diagnostic utility for diffuse white matter injury, which has been shown to occur in most preterm infants. The cerebral white matter is also the commonest site of neuropathologic impact for IVH, as described earlier. Thus low-grade IVH may be merely a visible marker on cranial ultrasonography for the more critical neuropathology of cerebral white matter injury, which on MRI has been shown to be highly predictive of both motor and cognitive deficits.[359] Of note, the elevation of the risk of poor outcomes with low-grade IVH with increasing immaturity also suggests an independent role for the loss of the neuronal and glial precursors from the immature germinal matrix.

A complete reference list is available at www.ExpertConsult.com.

SELECT REFERENCES

1. Volpe JJ, Inder TE, du Plessis AJ, et al., eds. *Volpe's Neurology of the Newborn*. 6th ed. Philadelphia: Elsevier; 2018.
3. Ahmann PA, Lazzara A, Dykes FD, et al. Intraventricular hemorrhage in the high-risk preterm infant: incidence and outcome. *Ann Neurol*. 1980;7:118-124.
4. Papile LA, Burstein J, Burstein R, et al. Incidence and evolution of subependymal and intraventricular hemorrhage: a study of infants with birth weights less than 1,500 gm. *J Pediatr*. 1978;92:529-534.
5. Paneth N, Pinto-Martin J, Gardiner J, et al. Incidence and timing o germinal matrix/intraventricular hemorrhage in low birth weight infants. *Am J Epidemiol*. 1993;137:1167-1176.
7. Stoll BJ, Hansen NI, Bell EF, et al. Trends in care practices, morbidity, and mortality of extremely preterm neonates, 1993-2012. *J Am Med Assoc*. 2015;314(10):1039-1051.
12. Kadri H, Mawla AA, Kazah J. The incidence, timing, and predisposing factors of germinal matrix and intraventricular hemorrhage (GMH/IVH) in preterm neonates. *Childs Nerv Syst*. 2006;22(9):1086-1090.
13. Perlman JM, Volpe JJ. Intraventricular hemorrhage in extremely small premature infants. *Am J Dis Child*. 1986;140(11):1122-1124.
14. de Vries LS, Van Haastert IL, Rademaker KJ, et al. Ultrasound abnormalities preceding cerebral palsy in high-risk preterm infants. *J Pediatr*. 2004;144:815-820.
17. Kuban K, Sanocka U, Leviton A, et al. White matter disorders of prematurity: association with intraventricular hemorrhage and ventriculomegaly. *J Pediatr*. 1999;134:539-546.
20. Kuban K, Adler I, Allred EN, et al. Observer variability assessing US scans of the preterm brain: the ELGAN study. *Pediatr Radiol*. 2007;37(12):1201-1208.
30. Dyet LE, Kennea N, Counsell SJ, et al. Natural history of brain lesions in extremely preterm infants studied with serial magnetic resonance imaging from birth and neurodevelopmental assessment. *Pediatrics*. 2006;118(2):536-548.
31. Kidokoro H, Neil JJ, Inder TE. New MR imaging assessment tool to define brain abnormalities in very preterm infants at term. *AJNR Am J Neuroradiol*. 2013;34(11):2208-2214.
39. Leviton A, Allred EN, Dammann O, et al. Systemic inflammation, intraventricular hemorrhage, and white matter injury. *J Child Neurol*. 2013;28(12):1637-1645.
45. Carlo WA, McDonald SA, Fanaroff AA, et al. Association of antenatal corticosteroids with mortality and neurodevelopmental outcomes among infants born at 22 to 25 weeks' gestation. *J Am Med Assoc*. 2011;306(21):2348-2358.
50. Shankaran S, Lin A, Maller-Kesselman J, et al. Maternal race, demography, and health care disparities impact risk for intraventricular hemorrhage in preterm neonates. *J Pediatr*. 2014;164(5):1005-1011.e1003.
55. de Bijl-Marcus K, Brouwer AJ, De Vries LS, Groenendaal F, Wezel-Meijler GV. Neonatal care bundles are associated with a reduction in the incidence of intraventricular haemorrhage in preterm infants: a multicentre cohort study. *Arch Dis Child Fetal Neonatal Ed*. 2020;105(4):419-424.
62. Paredes MF, James D, Gil-Perotin S, et al. Extensive migration of young neurons into the infant human frontal lobe. *Science*. 2016;354(6308):aaf7073.
63. Xu G, Broadbelt KG, Haynes RL, et al. Late development of the GABAergic system in the human cerebral cortex and white matter. *J Neuropathol Exp Neurol*. 2011;70(10):841-858.
66. Del Bigio MR. Cell proliferation in human ganglionic eminence and suppression after prematurity-associated haemorrhage. *Brain*. 2011;134(Pt 5):1344-1361.
68. Sanai N, Nguyen T, Ihrie RA, et al. Corridors of migrating neurons in the human brain and their decline during infancy. *Nature*. 2011;478(7369):382-386.
85. Takashima S, Mito T, Ando Y. Pathogenesis of periventricular white matter hemorrhages in preterm infants. *Brain Dev*. 1986;8:25-30.
88. Dudink J, Lequin M, Weisglas-Kuperus N, et al. Venous subtypes of preterm periventricular haemorrhagic infarction. *Arch Dis Child Fetal Neonatal Ed*. 2008;93(3):F201-F206.
99. Kinney HC, Haynes RL, Xu G, et al. Neuron deficit in the white matter and subplate in periventricular leukomalacia. *Ann Neurol*. 2012;71(3):397-406.
102. Tam EW, Miller SP, Studholme C, et al. Differential effects of intraventricular hemorrhage and white matter injury on preterm cerebellar growth. *J Pediatr*. 2011;158(3):366-371.
105. Volpe JJ. Cerebellum of the premature infant -- rapidly developing, vulnerable, clinically important. *J Child Neurol*. 2009;24:1085-1104.
106. Messerschmidt A, Prayer D, Brugger PC, et al. Preterm birth and disruptive cerebellar development: assessment of perinatal risk factors. *Eur J Paediatr Neurol*. 2008;12:455-460.
118. Alderliesten T, Lemmers PM, Smarius JJ, et al. Cerebral oxygenation, extraction, and autoregulation in very preterm infants who develop peri-intraventricular hemorrhage. *J Pediatr*. 2013;162(4):698-704.e692.
123. Tsuji M, Saul JP, du Plessis A, et al. Cerebral intravascular oxygenation correlates with mean arterial pressure in critically ill premature infants. *Pediatrics*. 2000;106(4):625-632.
155. Kaiser JR, Gauss CH, Pont MM, et al. Hypercapnia during the first 3 days of life is associated with severe intraventricular hemorrhage in very low birth weight infants. *J Perinatol*. 2006;26(5):279-285.
165. Katheria A, Reister F, Essers J, et al. Association of umbilical cord milking vs delayed umbilical cord clamping with death or severe intraventricular hemorrhage among preterm infants. *J Am Med Assoc*. 2019;322(19):1877-1886.
166. Auerbach A, Eventov-Friedman S, Arad I, et al. Long duration of hyperglycemia in the first 96 hours of life is associated with severe intraventricular hemorrhage in preterm infants. *J Pediatr*. 2013;163(2):388-393.
171. Lim WH, Lien R, Chiang MC, et al. Hypernatremia and grade III/IV intraventricular hemorrhage among extremely low birth weight infants. *J Perinatol*. 2011;31(3):193-198.
179. Riskin A, Riskin-Mashiah S, Bader D, et al. Delivery mode and severe intraventricular hemorrhage in single, very low birth weight, vertex infants. *Obstet Gynecol*. 2008;112(1):21-28.

200. Noori S, McCoy M, Anderson MP, et al. Changes in cardiac function and cerebral blood flow in relation to peri/intraventricular hemorrhage in extremely preterm infants. *J Pediatr*. 2014;164(2):264-270.e261-e263.
213. Dempsey EM, Al Hazzani F, Barrington KJ. Permissive hypotension in the extremely low birthweight infant with signs of good perfusion. *Arch Dis Child Fetal Neonatal Ed*. 2009;94(4):F241-F244.
221. von Lindern JS, Hulzebos CV, Bos AF, et al. Thrombocytopaenia and intraventricular haemorrhage in very premature infants: a tale of two cities. *Arch Dis Child Fetal Neonatal Ed*. 2012;97(5):F348-F352.
240. Ment LR, Aden U, Lin A, et al. Gene-environment interactions in severe intraventricular hemorrhage of preterm neonates. *Pediatr Res*. 2014;75(1-2):241-250.
250. Srinivasakumar P, Limbrick D, Munro R, et al. Posthemorrhagic ventricular dilatation-impact on early neurodevelopmental outcome. *Am J Perinatol*. 2013;30(3):207-214.
256. Volpe JJ. Brain injury in premature infants: a complex amalgam of destructive and developmental disturbances. *Lancet Neurol*. 2009;8(4):110-124.
281. Brouwer MJ, de Vries LS, Pistorius L, et al. Ultrasound measurements of the lateral ventricles in neonates: why, how and when? A systematic review. *Acta Paediatr*. 2010;99(9):1298-1306.
293. Del Bigio MR, Kanfer JN, Zhang YW. Myelination delay in the cerebral white matter of immature rats with kaolin-induced hydrocephalus is reversible. *J Neuropathol Exp Neurol*. 1997;56(9):1053-1066.
333. Murphy BP, Inder TE, Rooks V, et al. Posthemorrhagic ventricular dilatation in the premature infant - natural history and predictors of outcome. *Arch Dis Child*. 2002;87:F37-F41.
337. Luyt K, Jary S, Lea C, et al. Ten-year follow-up of a randomised trial of drainage, irrigation and fibrinolytic therapy (DRIFT) in infants with post-haemorrhagic ventricular dilatation. *Health Technol Assess*. 2019;23(4):1-116.
338. Warf BC, Campbell JW, Riddle E. Initial experience with combined endoscopic third ventriculostomy and choroid plexus cauterization for post-hemorrhagic hydrocephalus of prematurity: the importance of prepontine cistern status and the predictive value of FIESTA MRI imaging. *Childs Nerv Syst*. 2011;7:1063-1071.
340. Cizmeci MN, Groenendaal F, Liem KD, et al. Randomized controlled early versus late ventricular intervention study (ELVIS) in post-hemorrhagic ventricular dilatation: outcome at 2 years. *J Pediatr*. 2020;S0022-3476(20):30996-31003. Epub ahead of print.
342. de Vries LS, Groenendaal F, Liem KD, et al. Treatment thresholds for intervention in posthaemorrhagic ventricular dilation: a randomised controlled trial. *Arch Dis Child Fetal Neonatal Ed*. 2019;104(1):F70-F75.
345. El-Dib M, Limbrick Jr DD, Inder T, et al. Management of post-hemorrhagic ventricular dilatation in the infant born preterm. *J Pediatr*. 2020;S0022-3476(20):30978-30981. Epub ahead of print.
350. Brouwer A, Groenendaal F, van Haastert IL, et al. Neurodevelopmental outcome of preterm infants with severe intraventricular hemorrhage and therapy for post-hemorrhagic ventricular dilatation. *J Pediatr*. 2008;152(5):648-654.
353. Vavasseur C, Slevin M, Donoghue V, et al. Effect of low grade intraventricular hemorrhage on developmental outcome of preterm infants. *J Pediatr*. 2007;151(2):e6;author reply e6-7.

132 Pathophysiology of Neonatal White Matter Injury

Steven P. Miller | Stephen A. Back

WHITE MATTER INJURY IN THE PRETERM NEONATE

Preterm birth is a major public health issue affecting an estimated 13 million babies worldwide; one in eight deliveries in the United States are now preterm.[1] Over the past two decades, improved neonatal intensive care unit (NICU) therapies have reduced the mortality and increased the survival of preterm newborns.[2] Despite these advances in neonatal intensive care, preterm birth remains a leading cause of childhood and lifelong disability.[3] These disabilities place enormous burdens on the children and their families.[4-7] Even with modern intensive care, more than half of very preterm infants will have serious neurodevelopmental challenges that often follow severe intraventricular hemorrhage (IVH) and white matter injury (WMI).[8-10] Here we focus on the pathophysiology and consequence of WMI, the most significant brain injury in contemporary cohorts of children born preterm.

Injury to the preterm developing brain leads to functional consequences in several domains: motor, cognition, language, behavior, mental health, vision, and hearing. Impairments in these domains often co-occur.[11] For example, the consequence of severe WMI, cystic periventricular leukomalacia (PVL), includes spastic diplegic cerebral palsy often with associated impairments in vision, cognition, and learning. Importantly, the cognitive and behavior issues that are prevalent in children born preterm most often occur in the absence of PVL and remain evident through young adulthood.[12-17] These prevalent neurocognitive impairments point to widely distributed brain abnormalities or problems with brain connectivity.[18] Increasing evidence suggests that the normal trajectory of brain maturation is disrupted by common systemic illnesses such as recurrent infections and exacerbated further by pain and stress.[19-21] The diverse spectrum of neurocognitive and motor outcomes following preterm birth points to widespread cellular maturational disturbances that target cerebral gray and white matter.

Historically, the prevalent pattern of WMI in the preterm neonate was destructive white matter lesions that resulted in cystic PVL. PVL was accompanied by secondary cortical and subcortical gray matter degeneration. Fortunately, contemporary cohorts of preterm neonates with WMI typically have less severe injuries that do not appear to involve gross glial or neuronal loss. However, even this milder form of WMI can be accompanied by diffuse gliosis and reduced cerebral and cerebellar growth. In this chapter, we will review human and experimental studies that indicate how impaired brain growth is related to distinct responses in gray and white matter. More specifically, we cover cerebral white matter myelination abnormalities related to aberrant regeneration and repair responses of the oligodendrocyte (OL) lineage.

We will review studies of the response to premyelinating oligodendrocyte (preOL) death, whereby early OL progenitors rapidly proliferate and differentiate, as well as evidence for OL precursor maturation arrest in the setting of hypoxia and human WMI. Despite these responses to injury, potentially regenerative preOLs fail to mature along normal pathways to become the myelinating cells critical to normal white matter maturation (Fig. 132.1). We will also address the response of immature neurons in the preterm brain to hypoxia and hypoxia-ischemia, which includes widespread disturbances in maturation of their dendritic arbors. Together, the maladaptive responses

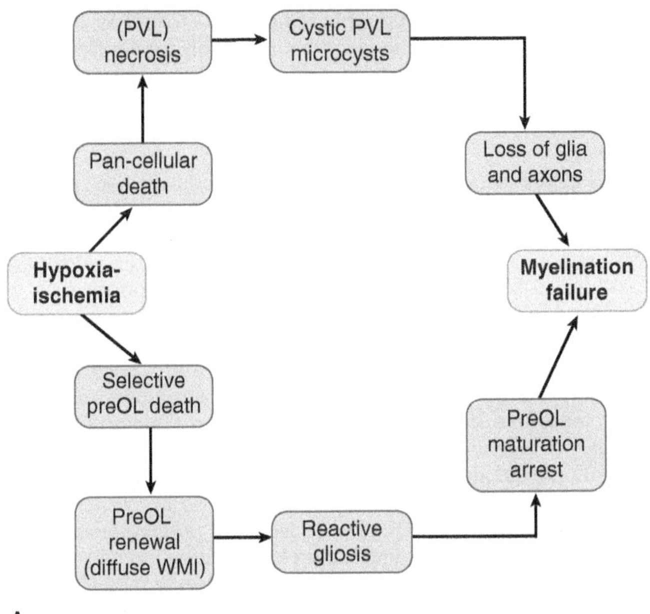

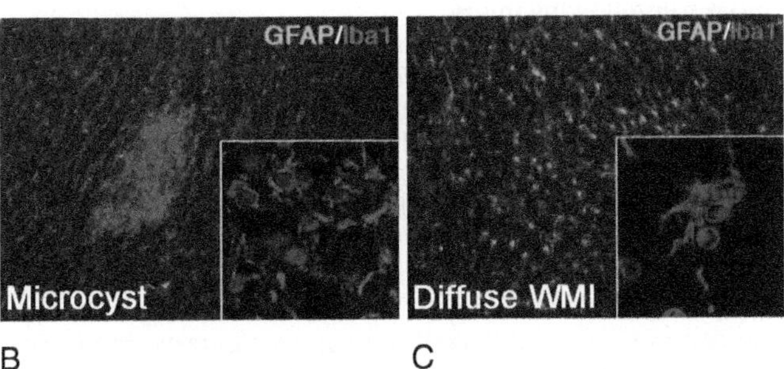

Fig. 132.1 (A) Distinctly different pathogenetic mechanisms mediate abnormal myelination in necrotic lesions (periventricular leukomalacia *[PVL]; upper pathway)* compared with lesions with diffuse white matter injury *(WMI; lower pathway)*. Hypoxia-ischemia (H-I) is illustrated as one potential trigger for WMI. More severe H-I triggers white matter necrosis *(upper pathway)* that depletes the white matter of all cells. Severe necrosis results in cystic PVL, whereas milder necrosis results in microcysts. Milder H-I *(lower pathway)* selectively triggers death of premyelinating oligodendrocyte *(preOLs)* that are rapidly regenerated but blocked from maturation by astrocytes-derived factors. Note that the lower pathway is the dominant one in most contemporary preterm neonates, whereas the minor upper pathway reflects the declining burden of white matter necrosis that has accompanied advances in neonatal intensive care. (B) A typical microscopic necrotic lesion containing reactive microglia and macrophages *(red cells and inset)* and rare astrocytes *(green cells)*. Nuclei are *blue*. (C) Diffuse WMI is notable for reactive astrocytes *(green cells)* and a lesser population of microglia/macrophages *(red cells)*.

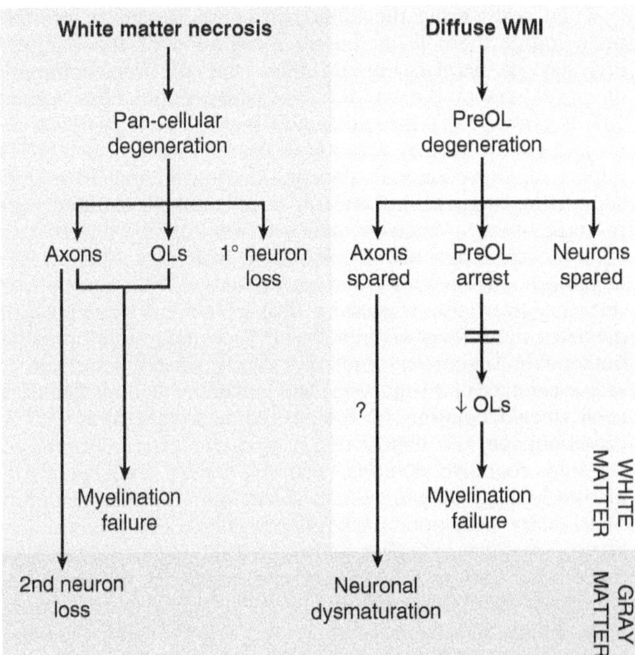

Fig. 132.2 In the preterm premyelinated white matter, the cellular mechanisms of cerebral white matter injury *(WMI)* and gray matter injury are distinct for necrotic and diffuse WMI. White matter necrosis (cystic periventricular leukomalacia *[PVL]*/microcysts; *left panel*) is characterized by death of all cells. Degeneration of axons and/or oligodendrocytes *(OLs)* both can lead to myelination failure. Degeneration of axons can lead to secondary neuronal loss in cerebral gray matter. Diffuse WMI *(right panel)* involves selective death of premyelinating oligodendrocytes *(preOLs)* with sparing of axons and neurons. Myelination failure is related to preOLs that fail to differentiate to OLs that make myelin. (Adapted from Back SA, Miller SP. Brain injury in premature neonates: a primary cerebral dysmaturation disorder? *Ann Neurol.* 2014;75:469–486.)

of immature oligodendroglia and neurons to injury involves a widespread failure of normal maturation during a critical window in the development of brain circuitry (Fig. 132.2). This contemporary spectrum of WMI, with abnormal maturation of cerebral gray and white matter, raises new diagnostic challenges for clinicians and opens new potential avenues for therapies to promote optimal brain health and improve neurodevelopmental outcomes.

NEONATAL BRAIN HEALTH PREDICTS FUNCTIONAL OUTCOMES

The functional consequences of preterm brain injury affect several domains that are essential to quality of life: motor, cognition, behavior, mental health, vision, and hearing.[22] Cognitive and behavior problems in preterm-born children persist to young adulthood and impact function in family, school, employment, and society.[12-16] Impairments in cognition and motor skills (e.g., cerebral palsy) have been described extensively. More recently, it is recognized that preterm children with broadly normal IQ nonetheless have processing deficits including problems in attention and executive functions (e.g., cognitive flexibility, working memory),[23-25] visually based information processing and language.[15,26,27]

Considerable progress has been made to define the structural and functional consequences of preterm birth with magnetic resonance imaging (MRI). MRI is currently the "gold-standard" diagnostic test for the safe and reliable clinical identification of injury in the developing brain.[28] Brain injuries (e.g., WMI) are indicated by discrete (focal) areas of MRI signal abnormalities. WMI occurs in a characteristic topology, with most lesions occurring in the periventricular central region, followed by posterior and frontal regions. WMI is most readily evident on MRI early in life rather than at term-equivalent age.[29] Quantitative mapping of MRI-defined punctate WMI demonstrates that lesion volume and location are important contributors to the prognostic significance of WMI, with frontal lesions being of particular concern.[10] The predictive value of frontal WMI volume highlights the importance of lesion location when considering the neurodevelopmental significance of WMI. This imaging classification tool that considers location is useful to predict preschool age outcomes in children born preterm.[29]

When considering the functional consequences of preterm brain injury, there is increasing recognition of the complex interplay of neonatal brain injury and the socioeconomic circumstances of the child. In normative populations, among children from lower-income families, small differences in income predict relatively large differences in brain surface area.[30] The impact of socioeconomic status is most prominent in regions supporting language and executive functions. In children born preterm, speech, language, and communication concerns are common and independently associated with increasing levels of neighborhood deprivation and gestational age.[31] This is especially relevant given the suggestion that epigenetic dysregulation mediates the effects of preterm birth on neurodevelopmental outcome.[32] Among extremely preterm neonates, moderate to severe neonatal brain injury predicts impaired cognitive functions even when accounting for the level of maternal education.[33] At preschool age, in a cohort of 170 very and extremely preterm children, cognitive outcome was comparably associated with maternal education and neonatal brain injury. The association of brain injury with poorer cognition was attenuated in children born to mothers of higher education level, indicating the need to consider the implications of neonatal brain health in the context of the child's environment.[34] The neurobiology of these relationships, and the long-term impact of both higher and lower socioeconomic status, need to be determined.

As early as the newborn period, sophisticated imaging methods can also detect and quantify developmental abnormalities of brain structure or function as they evolve from the acute to longer-term recovery phases. Observations with advanced MRI techniques indicate that WMI and some common clinical conditions impede brain maturation in areas that appear normal on conventional (T1 and T2) MRI.[5,35-37]

Several brain MRI measures can now be applied in the research and clinical setting to measure white matter dysmaturation in the preterm neonate: volumetrics, diffusion tensor imaging (DTI), magnetic resonance spectroscopic imaging (MRSI), functional connectivity MRI (fcMRI), and magnetoencephalography (MEG). *Structure*: High-resolution MRI analyzed with deformation-based morphometry can quantify volumetric growth of cortical and subcortical brain structures. *Microstructure*: DTI measures regional brain microstructure reflected in parameters such as fractional anisotropy (FA), a measure of the directionality of water diffusion in each pixel of the DTI image. Using these MRI tools, brain dysmaturation is increasingly recognized as the component of WMI critical to brain health for preterm neonates.

Despite the widespread use of diagnostic MRI in clinical practice, it is nonetheless important to recognize the limitations of MRI at regularly used clinical field strengths (e.g., 1.5 or 3 T). This is particularly relevant for detection of the full spectrum of WMI because MRI currently has limited sensitivity for imaging microscopic foci of necrosis, and conventional imaging may not fully define early diffuse WMI.[38] The definition of diffuse WMI by MRI is of particular interest, given that these lesions correspond to foci of dysmaturation with preOL maturation arrest and abnormal myelination.

WHITE MATTER INJURY AND BRAIN DYSMATURATION: AN OVERVIEW

Patterns of injury in the neonatal brain result from "selective vulnerability" of certain cell populations during distinct times in development.[39] In the preterm neonate's brain, some types of OL progenitors (i.e., late progenitors; preOLs) are vulnerable to insults that do not affect mature myelin-forming OLs.[40] This selective preOL vulnerability in the developing white matter is a central feature of the propensity for WMI in preterm neonates. WMI in preterm neonates is linked to ischemia (e.g., hypotension), infections, and inflammation.[5,19,41-44] After preOL death has occurred, the primary mechanism of myelination failure in the human preterm neonate involves a dysmaturation process where preOLs fail to differentiate in diffuse chronic lesions enriched in reactive astrocytes (i.e., preOL maturation arrest).[45]

As noted earlier, multifocal WMI predominates in preterm neonates and predicts later visual, motor, and cognitive dysfunction.[5,43,46] Yet, WMI is the tip of the iceberg in regards to brain abnormalities.[43,47,48] Punctate white matter lesions are associated with widespread neuroanatomic abnormalities as revealed by multimodal MRI.[46] The changes in white matter FA, a metric derived from DTI, are associated with brain maturation and correspond with maturation of the OL lineage.[49] WMI is followed by diffusely abnormal microstructural (e.g., FA) and metabolic brain maturation, as preterm neonates grow to term.[5,35,37,50] Abnormalities in brain maturation persist through childhood and are associated with adverse neuro-developmental outcomes.[17,48,51-53] The adverse outcomes do not appear to be due to a loss of the preOL pool. In fact, glial progenitors respond to WMI by partially, but incompletely, mounting a repair process that regenerates and expands the preOL pool, which is then blocked from maturation and myelination.[38,45,54] Ultimately, this brain dysmaturation disrupts the brain's capacity for regeneration and repair following injury.

Abnormalities in gray matter structures such as the thalamus, cortex, hippocampus, and cerebellum are also increasingly recognized in association with WMI by MRI.[50,55-58] For example, delayed maturation of the cerebral cortex is detected with DTI in preterm neonates with impaired postnatal growth.[56] Importantly, in a preterm sheep model, cortical growth impairments measured with DTI following moderate hypoxia-ischemia were associated with diffuse disturbances in the dendritic arbor and synapse formation of cortical neurons.[59] This simplification of the dendritic arbor of immature neurons contrasts sharply with mature neurons in the full-term neonate that degenerate from activation of excitotoxic and apoptotic pathways.[60]

Subplate neurons (SPNs) are a transient cell population important for developing thalamocortical connections.[61] Similar to other neuronal populations, SPNs degenerate in more severe lesions arising from perinatal hypoxia-ischemia in rodents[62,63] and human PVL.[64] Notably, in association with less severe multifocal WMI, fetal ovine SPNs did not degenerate, but rather displayed functional maturation disturbances. Given the central role of SPNs in establishing thalamocortical connectivity, this dysmaturation response may contribute to aberrant thalamocortical connections in the visual cortex of preterm neonates with WMI, for whom visual dysfunction is common.[65]

Preterm neonates at term age also exhibit reduced functional thalamocortical connectivity on fcMRI, particularly with WMI.[66-68] MRI studies of preterm neonates from 25 to 45 postmenstrual weeks suggest more effective use of impaired white matter reserve, as short-range corticocortical connections and connectivity involving thalamus, cerebellum, superior frontal lobe, and cingulate gyrus and were related to the severity of prematurity.[69] Furthermore, cognitive scores at 2 years are correlated with structural connectivity between the thalamus and extensive cortical regions at term.[70] Altered functional connectivity in children and adolescents born preterm is a critical risk factor for adverse cognitive outcomes.[53,71] There is altered cortical activation and functional connectivity during language and visual processing in preterm-born children and adults who have *normal* cognitive function, highlighting the important role of brain imaging, neurophysiology, and neuroscience to fully understand the spectrum of injury in this population.[18,71-74] Studies have shown late postnatal migration of cortical interneurons in human brain,[75,76] suggesting another vulnerable population, critical to neural circuit formation, in preterm brain injury. Indeed, because the majority of such interneurons traffic through the subventricular zone, a prediction is that even focal IVH would prevent them from reaching their intended targets.

Taken together, recent data support that brain dysmaturation (1) involves white matter and gray matter and (2) disrupts an essential developmental window characterized by rapid brain growth and the enhancement of neuronal connectivity through myelination, elaboration of the dendritic arbor, and synaptogenesis. Furthermore, disturbances in brain maturation appear to be multifactorial and related to clinical factors such as malnutrition, infections, and lung disease.

SPECTRUM OF INJURY AND DYSMATURATION IN PRETERM WHITE MATTER INJURY

The spectrum of WMI seen in human preterm neonates is very similar to that generated by cerebral ischemia in a preterm fetal sheep model. This model has provided access to ex vivo ultra-high field (12 T) MRI images that were aligned at high resolution with WMI visualized in the same brains by histopathology.[38] At this ultra-high field strength, MRI defined three types of subacute lesions that correspond to distinct forms of human necrotic or diffuse WMI:

1. **Cystic necrotic WMI**: Cystic PVL describes foci of necrosis that are typically larger than one millimeter in diameter with degeneration of all cell types including glia and axons on pathologic examination.[77-85] Pronounced necrotic WMI is visualized on MRI as hyperintense signal abnormalities on T2-weighted (T_2W) images or as volume loss of major white mater tracts such as the corpus callosum or optic radiations. These large necrotic lesions are highly enriched in macrophages.
2. **Microscopic necrotic WMI**: Despite the pronounced reduction in incidence of cystic PVL on MRI,[86] these small foci of necrosis (less than a millimeter in diameter) are evident on neuropathologic examination (i.e., microcysts).[87] Similar to cystic PVL, microcysts are also enriched in cellular debris, degenerating axons, and phagocytic macrophages.[45] The extent to which microcysts contribute to functional impairments or are clinically silent is unclear, because they are poorly visualized by MRI at clinical field strengths. In preterm fetal sheep[38] and human autopsy cases,[45] microcysts were observed in at least one third of cases imaged at 12 T. Yet, because of their size and extent, microcysts comprise only a small proportion, less than 5%, of lesion burden, highlighting the importance of diffuse WMI.
3. ***Diffuse WMI:*** The imaging characteristics of diffuse WMI differ substantially at clinical field strengths compared with those at higher field strengths. Diffuse WMI is visualized by ultra-high field MRI as diffuse hypointense signal abnormalities on T_2W images. Early subacute signal changes correspond to reactive astrogliosis and myelination disturbances arising from maturation arrest of preOLs. In diffuse WMI, there is selective degeneration of preOLs, while axonal degeneration is initiated at foci of microscopic necrosis.[84,85] Diffuse WMI is not as directly evident on diagnostic MRI. At clinical MRI field strengths, WMI is indicated by discrete focal or multifocal areas of MR signal abnormalities. Structural or metabolic abnormalities related to diffuse WMI may also be detected by advanced MRI techniques such as DTI and spectroscopic imaging. Disturbances in DTI parameters such as FA correspond in part to maturation of the OL lineage[49] consistent with the role of preOL arrest in the myelination disturbances in diffuse WMI. The importance of diffuse WMI must be stressed because this is the most common form of WMI in autopsy studies of contemporary human cohorts. In fetal sheep, diffuse WMI comprised nearly 90% of the total volume of WMI.

Although the extent of diffuse WMI is difficult to define, these lesions display a robust inflammatory reaction that extends considerably beyond the apparent lesion boundaries defined by conventional neuropathology.[45] Although the chronic inflammatory reaction is incompletely understood, it occurs in response to early WMI, which targets the human OL lineage and axons via oxidative damage[88] of a severity consistent with hypoxia-ischemia.[89,90]

Advances in imaging science are providing a new window on diffuse WMI and white matter maturation. For example, pixel-based analysis is a novel imaging framework that reveals alterations in microstructural and macrostructural changes in axonal fiber populations within regions of crossing fibers. It is sensitive to the effect of preterm birth and aspects of neonatal intensive care such as days on ventilation and total parenteral nutrition.[91] It will be interesting and important to further evaluate such MRI biomarkers against pathologic analysis in suitable cases using the latest tools, such as immunohistochemical and mRNA markers of neural precursors, mature cell types, and signaling pathways in situ.

CLINICAL RISK FACTORS FOR THE SPECTRUM OF WHITE MATTER INJURY IN THE PRETERM NEONATE

The conditions that contribute to both focal and diffuse WMI are multifactorial. There is greater recognition of the importance of clinical factors as predictors of brain dysmaturation, the critical lesion in diffuse WMI. Postnatal illness severity is a better predictor of brain health than gestational age at birth.[39,92] Postnatal illness severity is also a stronger predictor of focal and diffuse WMI than are several prenatal factors.[5,19,37,56,93] Such conditions include infection, bronchopulmonary dysplasia (BPD), and chronic hypoxemia, as well as repetitive exposure to painful procedures.

1. **Infection.** In preterm neonates, complex systemic illness contributes to the risks of brain injury and adverse outcomes. For example, recurrent postnatal infections in preterm neonates predict a significantly increased risk of WMI.[5,20,42] These neonates are also at risk for "progressive WMI," where the punctate lesions of WMI are more readily evident on MRI scans at term equivalent age rather than on earlier scans.[41] In addition, preterm neonates with postnatal infections show evidence of altered white matter pathway development[37] and even more widespread impairments in brain development.[19] Postnatal infections, even without positive cultures, predict impaired neurodevelopmental outcome consistent with the neonatal brain imaging findings of widespread delayed brain maturation.[42,94]
2. **BPD,** requiring prolonged treatment with mechanical ventilation and supplemental oxygen, is strongly associated with adverse cognitive outcome, even after accounting for other morbidities.[95] In cohorts of preterm neonates studied with MRI, BPD, and days of ventilation are associated with impaired white matter and cortical development.[96-98] BPD in preterm neonates is associated with hypoxic episodes.[99] This is especially concerning given observations that brief hypoxic episodes induce robust structural and functional disturbances in the dendritic maturation of CA1 neurons in an ovine experimental model.[100] BPD treatment with corticosteroids is also associated with impaired growth of the cerebellum.[101] Notably, extremely preterm neonates born at U.S. academic centers over the past 20 years display increased rates of BPD despite modest improvements in other neonatal morbidities.[2]
3. **Exposure to Pain and Analgesics.** During a period of rapid brain development, preterm neonates are exposed to

multiple painful and stressful procedures as part of their life-saving NICU care (see Chapter 128). Pain is a central factor that predicts dysmaturation[21]; neonates with infections are exposed to more painful procedures, and these painful procedures predict poor somatic growth and altered brain maturation from preterm early life to term age.[21,102-104] The amount of procedural pain and stress to which a preterm neonate is exposed is particularly linked to altered maturation of sensory regions of the thalamus.[21] Early pain exposure, especially in the youngest preterm neonates, has the most robust relationship with dysmaturation of the thalamus.[21] Analgesic and sedative practices vary considerably among hospitals, even for infants with similar characteristics and illness severity. Medications commonly used to provide analgesia or sedation include opiates, benzodiazepines, and sucrose, but their use varies considerably across sites.[105,106] At least 70% of preterm neonates receive narcotics or benzodiazepines.[102,107] Reports suggest that some medications regularly used for analgesia and sedation in the NICU have unanticipated harmful effects with regional specificity.[105,108] Midazolam is associated with slower growth of the hippocampus, a finding congruent with experimental rodent models in which Midazolam results in widespread neurodegeneration, impairments in synapse formation, and long-term memory deficits.[109,110] In addition, morphine is associated with slower growth of the cerebellum, and glucose for analgesia with slower growth of the basal ganglia.[104,111] Future work is needed in relevant experimental models and clinical trials to determine the analgesia strategies that best promote brain maturation and neurodevelopmental outcome in this population.

Consistent with neonatal brain imaging observations, the increasing amount of pain to which a preterm neonate is exposed during NICU care predicts poorer neurodevelopment, a relationship moderated by parent-child interaction.[112,113] The influence of parent-child interaction on outcomes indicates how factors that follow the NICU period, including parental stress, may also contribute to cognitive and behavioral outcomes of preterm survivors.[114] Preterm-born infants exposed to a parental intervention for sensitivity training demonstrated enhanced maturation and connectivity on MRI at term equivalent age.[115] A longer time-horizon for potential interventions to improve brain development and outcomes is suggested by experimental and clinical evidence that parent-infant interactions may modify early brain maturation.[113,116-119] Future work is needed in relevant experimental models and clinical cohorts to define the evolution of cerebral white matter lesions *over years* to define the period over which WMI may be repaired and optimal brain development promoted.

MECHANISMS OF INJURY IN PRETERM WHITE MATTER INJURY

WHITE MATTER DEGENERATION AND DYSMATURATION OF GLIAL PROGENITORS

In diffuse WMI, several lines of evidence indicate that abnormal myelination is associated with maturation arrest of OL precursors or degeneration of preOLs that are normally prevalent in the white matter during the early third trimester of gestation corresponding to the high-risk period for WMI.[120] The magnitude and distribution of acute ischemic injury in several experimental models of WMI correspond to the spatial distribution of these susceptible OL lineage cells. Unlike other stages of OL lineage cells, preOLs are highly vulnerable to hypoxia-ischemia and inflammation.[40,121,122]

Genetic contributors to the interindividual vulnerability to WMI are currently being identified. DLG4 (PSD95), a hub protein in the microglial inflammatory response, is synthesized in the preterm mouse and human brain. Genetic variations in DLG4 predict structural differences in the preterm neonate brain.[123] Furthermore, microglial regulators through Wnt/β-catenin signaling are also recognized as a pathway to drive a microglial phenotype of maturation arrest causing hypomyelination.[124] Interestingly, genomic variation in the Wnt pathway is also associated with levels of connectivity found in preterm neonatal brains.[124]

Despite the pronounced selective degeneration of preOLs in acute diffuse WMI, abnormal myelination is defined by a more complex process of cellular dysmaturation. Findings support that myelination disturbances involve a potentially reversible process linked to arrested pre-OL maturation rather than an irreversible loss of pre-OLs. This process involves initial preOL degeneration followed by proliferation of progenitors, which replenishes depleted preOLs at sites of WMI[125] or cortical injury.[126] A robust expansion of human preOLs is also observed in chronic lesions[48] despite the significant loss of these cells during the acute phase of WMI.[88] However, these newly generated preOLs fail to myelinate intact axons and display persistent arrested differentiation, whether in human lesions or experimental models. Thus diffuse WMI is characterized by an aberrant response to acute injury, whereby preOLs are regenerated but fail to mature.

Maturation arrest of PreOLs contributes to white matter dysmaturation in a number of ways. Viable OLs and myelination are critical for axon survival.[127] Functional integrity of axons in chronic lesions may be disrupted by preOL arrest. Oligodendrocyte progenitor cells (OPCs), which give rise to preOLs, express hypoxia-inducible factor (HIF), which plays a role in oxygen tension-mediated regulation of postnatal myelination. Thus, through HIF signaling, OPCs link postnatal white matter angiogenesis, axon integrity, and the onset of myelination.[128] In rodents, preOL maturation-arrest expanded the developmental window of vulnerability for WMI, because this expanded population of preOLs was highly vulnerable to recurrent hypoxia-ischemia.[125] This may be relevant to human preterm infants who are at risk for recurrent insults, such as hypoxia-ischemia that may occur in the setting of infections.[5,39,41,129,130]

MOLECULAR MECHANISMS OF PREOL MATURATION ARREST

As shown in Fig. 132.1, preOL arrest is a complex process that involves aberrant proliferation of OPCs and arrested OL lineage progression that disrupts myelination through mechanisms that may involve intrinsic, extrinsic, and epigenetic factors.[131-135] Proliferation and differentiation of OL progenitors are blocked by inhibitors of voltage-activated potassium channels and membrane depolarization block.[136,137] The OL progenitor cell cycle exit is partly regulated by Sox17, and enhanced Sox17 expression is evident in active remyelinating lesions.[138] Oxidative stress activates several genes that regulate OL maturation and promotes global histone acetylation, which in turn blocks OL differentiation.[139-143] PreOL maturation and normal myelination is also blocked by multiple molecules that are linked to reactive astrogliosis, a distinct pathologic feature of diffuse WMI.[45,144,145] In diffuse WMI, myelination is disrupted by a diffuse chronic inflammatory response that involves the extracellular matrix (ECM), which is a rich source of high-molecular-weight forms of hyaluronic acid (HA).[45] In human WMI,[45] reactive astrocytes synthesize high-molecular-weight HA that accumulates in the ECM.[146] These high molecular weight forms of HA contribute to arrest of preOL maturation via a mechanism that involves digestion of HA to a variety of HA fragment sizes. A bioactive HA fragment was identified that selectively blocks preOL maturation via an immune tolerance pathway involving Toll-like receptor 4, which potently blocks preOL differentiation.[147] This pathway potently suppressed white matter repair by chronically blocking promyelination signaling mediated by brain-derived neurotrophic factor (BDNF).[147] Other promyelination signals that may be similarly blocked include astrocyte-derived bone morphogenetic proteins, which inhibit OL progenitor differentiation while promoting astrocyte differentiation and regulating myelin protein expression.[148-151] In addition, epidermal growth factor receptor (EGFR) is constitutively expressed by astrocytes and promotes proliferation of OL progenitors.[152] Intranasally administered EGF following chronic neonatal hypoxia promoted OL maturation and myelination and functional improvement.[153] Dysregulation of WNT/β-catenin signaling in OPCs also leads to preOL arrest, resulting in delayed myelination and disrupted remyelination.[154-159]

ROLE OF AXONAL INJURY IN WHITE MATTER INJURY

Necrotic lesions are a minor component of WMI in both human and experimental models (detailed earlier).[38,45] Yet, in these necrotic lesions, axonal injury is prominent with dystrophic axons and axonal spheroids, which degenerate during the early phase of coagulative necrosis.[45,77,87,160-163] Thus complete myelination failure occurs in areas of necrosis because of a degeneration of all cellular elements including axons. Glutamate-mediated maturation-dependent mechanisms underlie the susceptibility of developing axons to oxidative stress and hypoxia-ischemia.[164-166] The axons that are most susceptible to injury appear to be larger caliber axons that are preparing to myelinate, rather than more resistant smaller caliber unmyelinated axons.[167]

Axonal degeneration does not appear to be a major contributor to human diffuse WMI. While axonal injury is observed in regions of diffuse WMI adjacent to necrosis,[84] these dystrophic axons are likely to be structurally continuous with the degenerating axons in necrotic foci. Similarly, in preterm fetal sheep, acute axonal injury was rare during the acute phase of diffuse WMI,[90] and in the chronic phase, significant axonal degeneration or loss was not observed by quantitative electron microscopy.[38,85]

MECHANISMS OF INJURY IN PRETERM WHITE MATTER INJURY: GRAY MATTER

GRAY MATTER DYSMATURATION IN PRETERM WHITE MATTER INJURY

The concept of an *encephalopathy of prematurity* was first proposed by Volpe and highlights how brain injury in the preterm neonate involves both destructive and developmental disturbances of the cerebral gray matter and white matter.[44] It is now apparent that gray matter abnormalities are prevalent among preterm neonates and must be considered as an important component of diffuse brain injury in this population. Reduced volumes of cortical and subcortical gray matter structures, which include the basal ganglia, thalamus, hippocampus, and cerebellum, are now recognized in preterm-born children, even in the absence of significant overt focal WMI.[50,51,55,56,168] With advances in neonatal care, impaired cerebral growth appears to less commonly arise from widespread primary degeneration of neurons in cortical and subcortical gray matter structures. The burden of secondary neuronal degeneration related to axonal injury in foci of white matter necrosis remains unclear due to the limitations of MRI to detect microscopic foci of necrosis. An alternative mechanism of impaired cerebral growth may involve disrupted neuronal maturation of large populations of neurons in cortical and subcortical structures. One emerging tool to define neuronal dysmaturation may be neurite orientation dispersion and density imaging (NODDI). When this advanced diffusion MRI method is applied to the cerebral cortex in preterm neonates, findings suggest that cortical development between 25 and 38 weeks postmenstrual age involves a predominant increase in dendritic arborization and neurite growth, whereas increasing cellular and organelle density predominates from 38 to 47 weeks.[169]

In addition, altered cortical activation and functional connectivity during language and visual processing is evident in children and adults born preterm, even among those with normal neurocognitive function.[18,71-73,170] Alterations in connectivity are now also recognized as a critical risk factor for adverse neurocognitive outcomes in children born preterm.[53,71,170,171] Recent brain imaging studies indicate that the experience of extrauterine life in preterm neonates modulates network development, altering the maturation of networks thought to support salience, executive, and cognitive functions.[171] These alterations in functional connectivity between the cortex and thalamus on fcMRI indicate that gray matter abnormalities extend beyond destructive brain lesions visualized with clinical MRI.[66]

NEURONAL DEGENERATION IN PRETERM WHITE MATTER INJURY

Neurons in the neonatal brain at term are highly vulnerable to hypoxic-ischemic death that is mediated by excitotoxic neuronal necrosis and apoptosis.[172-177] In contrast, neuronal loss at more preterm ages appear to involve more severe insults associated with concurrent WMI. Significant white matter necrosis is often accompanied by degeneration of neurons in cerebral gray and white matter. In experimental models, the severity and extent of neuronal degeneration in the preterm brain increases with the duration of hypoxia-ischemia; prolonged hypoxia-ischemia triggers widespread neuronal death concurrent with cystic necrotic WMI.[90] In the human preterm brain, necrotic WMI may be accompanied by primary neuronal loss in the cortex, basal ganglia, thalamus, and cerebellum,[64,87,178,179] as well as secondary neuronal loss from retrograde axonal degeneration.[84,85]

In contrast, nonnecrotic diffuse WMI spares axons. In preterm fetal sheep, diffuse WMI was also accompanied by preservation of gray matter and SPNs, despite similar degrees of ischemia in the superficial cortex and periventricular white matter.[90,180] In human preterm autopsy cases with early diffuse WMI, no significant degeneration of neurons or axons was observed, despite evidence of oxidative stress comparable with that observed in term neonates with severe hypoxic-ischemic encephalopathy.[88] Thus, in the preterm neonate, neuronal loss is primarily associated with destructive WMI, whereas neuronal loss does not appear to be a prominent feature when diffuse WMI predominates. However, a note of caution seems appropriate because of studies showing axon protective roles of myelin,[181] implying that axons in lesions of chronic neonatal WMI could be at risk of injury or loss.

NEURONAL DYSMATURATION IN PRETERM WHITE MATTER INJURY

Neuronal maturation can be disrupted in the absence of significant neuronal loss. In preterm fetal sheep, diffuse WMI was accompanied by cortical volume loss that was unrelated to neuronal loss. Rather it arose from an increased packing density of neurons,[59] as explained by a significant reduction in the complexity of the dendritic arbor of cortical projection neurons. During preterm development, cortical projection neurons are normally immature with a simplified arbor. However, in near term animals, the dendritic arbor becomes highly arborized, which results in a marked increase in cortical volume. Similar reductions in dendritic arbor complexity have been observed in the subplate, basal ganglia, and hippocampus.[100,182] For example, following ischemia in preterm sheep, the caudate nucleus displayed reduced growth without any apparent loss of γ-aminobutyric acid γ (GABA)ergic projection neurons or interneurons.[180]

DTI has been applied in preterm neonates to noninvasively characterize normal cortical maturation. A progressive decline in cortical FA accompanies normal cortical maturation in human[183] and nonhuman primates.[184-186] This normal loss of FA is proposed to reflect the loss of radial glial cells and the maturation of the dendritic arbor of cortical neurons with normal cortical development.[183] The decline in FA has been shown to coincide with the progressive maturational complexity of the process arbor of cortical neurons.[187] The normal progressive loss of

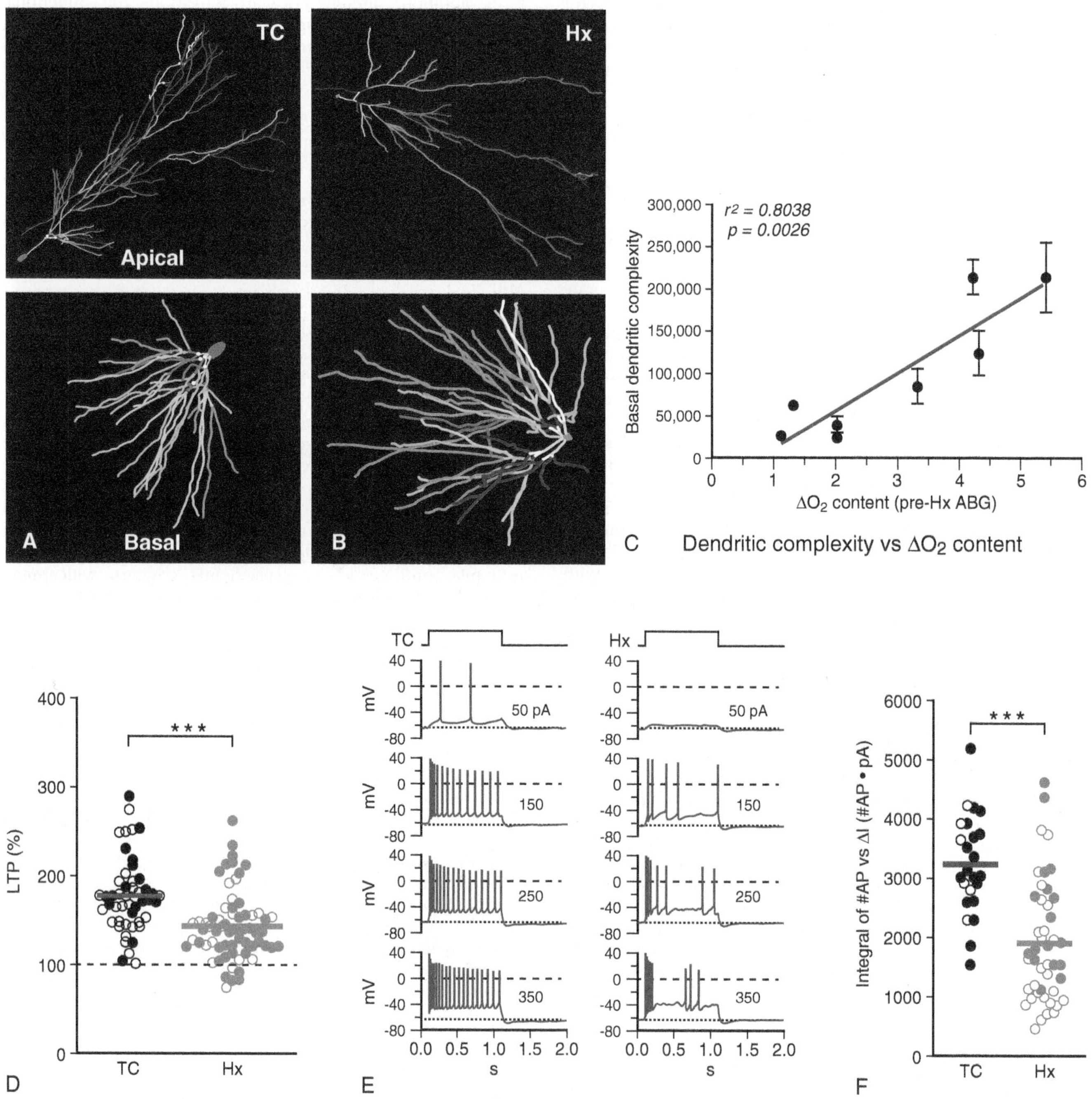

Fig. 132.3 A brief 30-minute episode of systemic hypoxia *(Hx)* causes persistent disturbances in the structural and functional maturation of hippocampal CA1 pyramidal neurons, which play an integral role in learning and memory mechanisms.[100,182] Typical three-dimensional (3D) reconstructions of apical and basal dendrites of CA1 hippocampal neurons from control (A; *TC*) versus Hx-exposed (B) preterm fetal sheep. Hx caused a significant decrease in apical arbors and an apparent compensatory increase in basal arbors, consistent with homeostatic plasticity. (C) The increase in basal dendritic complexity was significantly associated with the magnitude of the fall in fetal systemic oxygenation during Hx (delta O_2 content). Hx reduced both long-term potentiation *(LTP)* (D) and synaptic firing rates in CA1 neurons (E) from which intrinsic excitability (IE) was determined. (F) Summary scatter plots of IE measured as the integral of the number of action potentials fired as a function of current injection (δI). ***p <0.001.

cortical FA is delayed in human preterm neonates with impaired postnatal growth[56] or reduced cortical growth.[188] These FA disturbances were postulated to reflect disrupted maturation of cortical pyramidal neurons. Notably, in preterm fetal sheep, global cerebral ischemia led to impaired cortical growth and higher cortical FA values (i.e., less mature) relative to controls.[59] To explain this observation, a mathematical model was developed to calculate FA based on the morphology of control and ischemic cortical neurons defined by Golgi stain. An increase in FA in the ischemic fetuses was related to the decreased complexity of the dendritic arbor of projection neurons. Interestingly, in human neonates, abnormal microstructural cortical growth was related to impaired somatic growth (weight, length, and head circumference), even after accounting for WMI and other aspects of systemic illness such as infection.[56] Impaired cortical growth and function is also observed after repeated stressful procedures during neonatal intensive care.[73,102,189] Hence, even in the absence of significant neuronal loss, multiple factors may contribute to the pathogenesis of cortical neuronal dysmaturation in preterm neonates.

NEURONAL DYSMATURATION AND DISTURBANCES IN SYNAPTIC ACTIVITY

Very preterm neonates are at increased risk for serious developmental problems including cognitive, language, behavioral, sensory, or motor deficits, as well as more subtle abnormalities including motor dyspraxias and disturbances in attention and executive function. Neuronal dysmaturation in the preterm neonate occurs during a sensitive window in the establishment of neuronal connections and may thus have long-lasting consequences. In preterm fetal sheep, cerebral ischemia caused persistent abnormalities in excitatory synaptic activity mediated by NMDA and AMPA receptors on projection neurons in the caudate, consistent with reductions in spine density.[180] Chronic disturbances in spine density and excitatory synaptic activity suggested several potential mechanisms for cerebral dysmaturation and disrupted connectivity. Reduced excitatory inputs to caudate projection neurons was associated with a shorter time window for integration of multiple synaptic inputs. Furthermore, disturbances in NMDA receptor–mediated synaptic activity may alter neuronal migration, synapse formation, and dendritic pruning.[190-193] Thus neuronal dysmaturation may precipitate a vicious cycle with further alteration of neuronal circuitry maturation. The resultant widespread disturbances in neuronal maturation may contribute to the global disturbances in cerebral connectivity and the diverse spectrum of neurodevelopment impairment seen in preterm-born children.

Experimental studies in preterm fetal sheep support that neuronal dysmaturation can by triggered by transient hypoxic exposures alone, without ischemia.[100,182] Hypoxemia did not cause pronounced degeneration of subplate or hippocampal neurons. Rather, clinically relevant episodes of brief fetal hypoxia of only 30 minutes produced persistent neuronal dysmaturation (Fig. 132.3). Notably, the severity of dysmaturation was significantly associated with the severity of fetal systemic hypoxemia. In the hippocampus, transient hypoxia caused persistent functional disturbances, which included decreased synaptic firing rates and significant disruptions in synaptic plasticity (long-term potentiation) intrinsic to learning and memory mechanisms. Hence preterm neurons are remarkably sensitive to transient disturbances in cerebral oxygenation. Such insults have the potential to disrupt thalamocortical connectivity by targeting SPNs and to disrupt hippocampal circuitry integral to learning and memory. Future studies are needed to determine the impact of brief repetitive episodes of hypoxemia, as commonly occur with apnea of prematurity or more chronic exposure to hypoxemia as occurs in congenital heart disease or BPD.

CONCLUSION

Advances in neonatal intensive care have resulted in a marked reduction in the severity and extent of destructive brain injury. Our understanding of the pathogenesis of brain injury in contemporary cohorts of preterm neonates has been significantly redefined through the application of enhanced brain imaging and longitudinal MRI studies, which provide better resolution of brain injury and development. Preterm survivors currently appear to sustain a reduced burden of irreversible destructive lesions and a broader spectrum of injury that is accompanied by diffuse cerebral dysmaturation involving glia and neurons. Experimental studies suggest that disturbances in cerebral plasticity may be triggered by relatively mild brief insults similar to those commonly encountered during neonatal care. Further study is urgently needed to determine if the burden of neurodevelopmental disabilities might be reduced in preterm survivors by reducing exposure to factors that trigger dysmaturation. Chronic disabilities in preterm survivors may ultimately be amenable to therapies directed at promoting normal brain maturation. Therapies required to promote or normalize cellular dysmaturation will likely differ for gray and white matter—either in regard to timing or mechanism. Pharmacologic interventions aimed at inhibiting the pathways that sustain preOL maturation arrest may ultimately prevent myelination failure, thereby promoting optimal brain connectivity. The data reviewed regarding risk factors for vulnerability suggest that improving infant nutrition, reducing neonatal stress, preventing infections, and optimizing the external environment may all have a future in this therapeutic armamentarium to promote healthy brain maturation.

To develop therapies that will improve long-term neurologic and developmental outcomes, clinical MRI sequences at routine field strengths must achieve greater sensitivity to detect early diffuse WMI and microcysts. The ability to define these lesions on routine clinical exams will support the earlier diagnostic detection of WMI and provide an early surrogate measure for counseling families regarding outcome and monitoring therapeutic trials. The opportunity to optimize brain maturation and growth is currently especially relevant because destructive processes and encephalomalacia are the minority of cerebral injury in the preterm neonate.

A complete reference list is available at www.ExpertConsult.com. 

SELECT REFERENCES

4. Miller SP, Ferriero DM, Leonard C, et al. Early brain injury in premature newborns detected with magnetic resonance imaging is associated with adverse early neurodevelopmental outcome. *J Pediatr*. 2005;147:609-616.
5. Chau V, Poskitt KJ, McFadden DE, et al. Effect of chorioamnionitis on brain development and injury in premature newborns. *Ann Neurol*. 2009;66:155-164.
7. Back SA, Miller SP. Brain injury in premature neonates: a primary cerebral dysmaturation disorder? *Ann Neurol*. 2014;75:469-486.
10. Guo T, Duerden EG, Adams E, et al. Quantitative assessment of white matter injury in preterm neonates: association with outcomes. *Neurology*. 2017;88:614-622.
19. Chau V, Brant R, Poskitt KJ, Tam EW, Synnes A, Miller SP. Postnatal infection is associated with widespread abnormalities of brain development in premature newborns. *Pediatr Res*. 2012;71:274-279.
20. Glass TJA, Chau V, Grunau RE, et al. Multiple postnatal infections in newborns born preterm predict delayed maturation of motor pathways at term-equivalent age with poorer motor outcomes at 3 years. *J Pediatr*. 2018;196:91-7.e1.
21. Duerden EG, Grunau RE, Guo T, et al. Early procedural pain is associated with regionally-specific alterations in thalamic development in preterm neonates. *J Neurosci*. 2018;38:878-886.
22. Johnson S, Marlow N. Growing up after extremely preterm birth: lifespan mental health outcomes. *Semin Fetal Neonatal Med*. 2014;19:97-104.

24. Marlow N, Wolke D, Bracewell MA, Samara M. Neurologic and developmental disability at six years of age after extremely preterm birth. *N Engl J Med.* 2005;352:9-19.
29. Cayam-Rand D, Guo T, Grunau RE, et al. Predicting developmental outcomes in preterm infants: a simple white matter injury imaging rule. *Neurology.* 2019;93:e1231-e1240.
30. Noble KG, Houston SM, Brito NH, et al. Family income, parental education and brain structure in children and adolescents. *Nat Neurosci.* 2015;18:773-778.
34. Benavente-Fernandez I, Synnes A, Grunau RE, et al. Association of socioeconomic status and brain injury with neurodevelopmental outcomes of very preterm children. *JAMA Netw Open.* 2019;2:e192914.
36. Miller SP, McQuillen PS, Hamrick S, et al. Abnormal brain development in newborns with congenital heart disease. *N Engl J Med.* 2007;357:1928-1938.
38. Riddle A, Dean J, Buser JR, et al. Histopathological correlates of magnetic resonance imaging-defined chronic perinatal white matter injury. *Ann Neurol.* 2011;70:493-507.
40. Back SA, Rosenberg PA. Pathophysiology of glia in perinatal white matter injury. *Glia.* 2014;62:1790-1815.
41. Glass HC, Bonifacio SL, Chau V, et al. Recurrent postnatal infections are associated with progressive white matter injury in premature infants. *Pediatrics.* 2008;122:299-305.
44. Volpe JJ. Brain injury in premature infants: a complex amalgam of destructive and developmental disturbances. *Lancet Neurol.* 2009;8:110-124.
45. Buser JR, Maire J, Riddle A, et al. Arrested preoligodendrocyte maturation contributes to myelination failure in premature infants. *Ann Neurol.* 2012;71:93-109.
46. Tusor N, Benders MJ, Counsell SJ, et al. Punctate white matter lesions associated with altered brain development and adverse motor outcome in preterm infants. *Sci Rep.* 2017;7:13250.
47. Woodward LJ, Anderson PJ, Austin NC, Howard K, Inder TE. Neonatal MRI to predict neurodevelopmental outcomes in preterm infants. *N Engl J Med.* 2006;355:685-694.
48. Counsell SJ, Edwards AD, Chew AT, et al. Specific relations between neurodevelopmental abilities and white matter microstructure in children born preterm. *Brain.* 2008;131:3201-3208.
49. Drobyshevsky A, Song SK, Gamkrelidze G, et al. Developmental changes in diffusion anisotropy coincide with immature oligodendrocyte progression and maturation of compound action potential. *J Neurosci.* 2005;25:5988-5997.
52. Ment LR, Kesler S, Vohr B, et al. Longitudinal brain volume changes in preterm and term control subjects during late childhood and adolescence. *Pediatrics.* 2009;123:503-511.
54. Segovia KN, McClure M, Moravec M, et al. Arrested oligodendrocyte lineage maturation in chronic perinatal white matter injury. *Ann Neurol.* 2008;63:520-530.
56. Vinall J, Grunau RE, Brant R, et al. Slower postnatal growth is associated with delayed cerebral cortical maturation in preterm newborns. *Sci Transl Med.* 2013;5:168ra8.
57. Beauchamp MH, Thompson DK, Howard K, et al. Preterm infant hippocampal volumes correlate with later working memory deficits. *Brain.* 2008;131:2986-2994.
58. Thompson DK, Wood SJ, Doyle LW, et al. Neonate hippocampal volumes: prematurity, perinatal predictors, and 2-year outcome. *Ann Neurol.* 2008;63:642-651.
59. Dean J, McClendon E, Hansen K, et al. Prenatal cerebral ischemia disrupts MRI-defined cortical microstructure through disturbances in neuronal arborization. *Sci Transl Med.* 2013;5:101-111.
61. Kanold PO, Luhmann HJ. The subplate and early cortical circuits. *Annu Rev Neurosci.* 2010;33:23-48.
65. Counsell SJ, Dyet LE, Larkman DJ, et al. Thalamo-cortical connectivity in children born preterm mapped using probabilistic magnetic resonance tractography. *Neuroimage.* 2007;34:896-904.
66. Smyser CD, Inder TE, Shimony JS, et al. Longitudinal analysis of neural network development in preterm infants. *Cereb Cortex.* 2010;20:2852-2862.
73. Doesburg SM, Chau CM, Cheung TP, et al. Neonatal pain-related stress, functional cortical activity and visual-perceptual abilities in school-age children born at extremely low gestational age. *Pain.* 2013;154:1946-1952.
77. Banker B, Larroche J. Periventricular leukomalacia of infancy. A form of neonatal anoxic encephalopathy. *Arch Neurol.* 1962;7:386-410.
89. Back SA, Han BH, Luo NL, et al. Selective vulnerability of late oligodendrocyte progenitors to hypoxia-ischemia. *J Neurosci.* 2002;22:455-463.
90. Riddle A, Luo N, Manese M, et al. Spatial heterogeneity in oligodendrocyte lineage maturation and not cerebral blood flow predicts fetal ovine periventricular white matter injury. *J Neurosci.* 2006;26:3045-3055.
91. Pecheva D, Tournier JD, Pietsch M, et al. Fixel-based analysis of the preterm brain: disentangling bundle-specific white matter microstructural and macrostructural changes in relation to clinical risk factors. *Neuroimage Clin.* 2019;23:101820.
100. McClendon E, Wang K, Degener-O'Brien K, et al. Transient hypoxemia disrupts anatomical and functional maturation of preterm fetal ovine CA1 pyramidal neurons. *J Neurosci.* 2019;39:7853-7871.
101. Tam EW, Chau V, Ferriero DM, et al. Preterm cerebellar growth impairment after postnatal exposure to glucocorticoids. *Sci Transl Med.* 2011;3:105ra.
102. Brummelte S, Grunau RE, Chau V, et al. Procedural pain and brain development in premature newborns. *Ann Neurol.* 2012;71:385-396.
107. Chau V, Synnes A, Grunau RE, Poskitt KJ, Brant R, Miller SP. Abnormal brain maturation in preterm neonates associated with adverse developmental outcomes. *Neurology.* 2013;81:2082-2089.
108. McPherson C, Miller SP, El-Dib M, Massaro AN, Inder TE. The influence of pain, agitation, and their management on the immature brain. *Pediatr Res.* 2020;88:168-175.
110. Duerden EG, Guo T, Dodbiba L, et al. Midazolam dose correlates with abnormal hippocampal growth and neurodevelopmental outcome in preterm infants. *Ann Neurol.* 2016;79:548-559.
120. Back SA, Luo NL, Borenstein NS, Levine JM, Volpe JJ, Kinney HC. Late oligodendrocyte progenitors coincide with the developmental window of vulnerability for human perinatal white matter injury. *J Neurosci.* 2001;21:1302-1312.
123. Krishnan ML, Van Steenwinckel J, Schang AL, et al. Integrative genomics of microglia implicates DLG4 (PSD95) in the white matter development of preterm infants. *Nat Commun.* 2017;8:428.
124. Van Steenwinckel J, Schang AL, Krishnan ML, et al. Decreased microglial Wnt/beta-catenin signalling drives microglial pro-inflammatory activation in the developing brain. *Brain.* 2019;142:3806-3833.
125. Segovia K, McClure M, Moravec M, et al. Arrested oligodendrocyte lineage maturation in chronic perinatal white matter injury. *Ann Neurol.* 2008;63:517-526.
147. Srivastava T, Diba P, Dean JM, et al. A TLR/AKT/FoxO3 immune tolerance-like pathway disrupts the repair capacity of oligodendrocyte progenitors. *J Clin Invest.* 2018;128:2025-2041.
180. McClendon E, Chen K, Gong X, et al. Prenatal cerebral ischemia triggers dysmaturation of caudate projection neurons. *Ann Neurol.* 2014;75:508-24.
182. McClendon E, Shaver DC, Degener-O'Brien K, et al. Transient hypoxemia chronically disrupts maturation of preterm fetal ovine subplate neuron arborization and activity. *J Neurosci.* 2017;37:11912-11929.
185. Kroenke C, Van Essen D, Inder T, Rees S, Bretthorst G, Neil J. Microstructural changes of the baboon cerebral cortex during gestational development reflected in magnetic resonance imaging diffusion anisotropy. *J Neurosci.* 2007;14:12506-12515.
187. Jespersen SN, Leigland LA, Cornea A, Kroenke CD. Determination of axonal and dendritic orientation distributions within the developing cerebral cortex by diffusion tensor imaging. *IEEE Trans Med Imaging.* 2012;31:16-32.
188. Ball G, Srinivasan L, Aljabar P, et al. Development of cortical microstructure in the preterm human brain. *Proc Natl Acad Sci U S A.* 2013;110:9541-9546.

133 Cellular and Molecular Mechanisms of Neonatal Brain Injury and Neuroprotection

Panagiotis Kratimenos | Joseph Scafidi | Vittorio Gallo

INTRODUCTION

Brain injury in neonates remains a leading cause of neurodevelopmental delays, long-term morbidity, and death.[1-6] The effects of injury in the newborn brain are evident in domains related to motor function, social, behavioral, cognitive, and mental health.[1,5] While the long-term results of neonatal brain injury are clear, a new mechanistic understanding of the specific neural cell populations and regions vulnerable to injury is necessary in order to define rational therapies. Due to the in utero and ex utero dynamic state of the developing brain, the patterns of damage in different central nervous system (CNS) regions may vary significantly.[7-10] The premature nervous system is vulnerable to injurious events that potentially alter its framework and functions. Early loss of placental support, hypoxia, emboli, substance exposure, inflammation, and hormonal dysregulation are some of the known predisposing factors to neonatal brain injury.[11,12] The susceptibility of the developing brain to injurious insults is multifactorial and depends on the anatomic location and the developmental event that is affected by the insult.[13] Neurons and glial cells are also differentially susceptible to injury.[13-15] Due to maturational changes (neurogenesis and neural circuit formation, glial cell differentiation and myelination) occurring in different developmental epochs, one could anticipate patterns of injury that correspond to specific neural cell types and the developmental trajectories to be affected.[14]

Acute causes of neonatal brain injury in the neonatal intensive care unit (NICU) include hypoxia, ischemia, inflammation, hemorrhage, infection, metabolic disorders, and any combination of these events. Importantly, insults may occur during the prenatal period and have a role in initiating or regulating perinatal brain injury. Finally, different causes of brain injury, either in the term or preterm neonate, eventually converge into common cellular and molecular pathways that we will describe and discuss in this chapter.

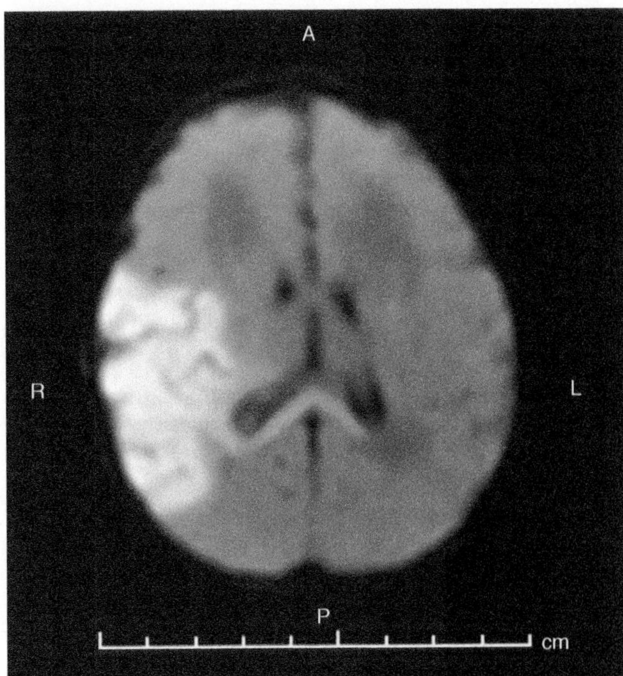

Fig. 133.1 Diffusion-weighted magnetic resonance imaging (DW-MRI) shows neonatal stroke in a term infant. The infant displayed seizures at 16 hours of life. Patient exam revealed an encephalopathic infant with left sided hypotonia and hyporeflexia—arm greater than leg. Electroencephalogram (EEG) demonstrated attenuated signal on the right and multifocal seizures emanating from the right central-temporal region. MRI demonstrates large right middle cerebral artery ischemic stroke and magnetic resonance angiography (MRA) revealed focal narrowing in the M2 artery. An interesting finding is the restricted diffusion in the splenium of the corpus callosum, often observed in neonates with seizures. This may be accounted by the abundance of glutamate receptors in the corpus callosum of the developing brain, as well as homotopic axon projection from the right cerebral hemisphere to the left cerebral hemisphere.

IMPACT OF NEONATAL BRAIN INJURY

Both term and preterm born neonates are susceptible to severe brain injury, although the classic causes vary. For term infants, neonatal hypoxic-ischemic encephalopathy (HIE), has an incidence of 1 to 8/1000 live births worldwide with a high risk of death (85% in severe HIE), cerebral palsy (CP), and developmental disabilities (Fig. 133.1).[1,2,5] Preterm birth, occurring in 1 in 10 infants in the United States (approximately 15 million of all births worldwide per year), and its associated complications are important causes of mortality in children under 5 years of age.[2] Neurodevelopmental impairments include CP, learning disabilities, neuropsychiatric disorders, and potentially, autism spectrum disorder (ASD).[6,16-19] Several studies have documented a strong correlation between prematurity and deficits in auditory, visual, and tactile sensory domains.[2,20] The prevalence of neuropsychiatric diseases, including diagnosis of ASD, attention-deficit/hyperactivity disorder (ADHD), schizophrenia, anxiety, and behavioral disorders, is four to five times higher in children and adults who were born prematurely.[16,17,21] Indeed, because very few long-term studies of preterm infants have been carried out, the behavioral and psychiatric impact may be underestimated.[20,22] In addition, the financial burden associated with premature birth in the United States, including the inability to work due to lack of independence or ability, is estimated at $26.2 billion each year.[23]

BRAIN DEVELOPMENT AND INJURY

To delineate the mechanisms of neonatal brain injury, it is important to consider the basic principles of brain development (also see Chapters 125, 126, and 132). The degree to which neuropsychiatric disease and neurodevelopmental disorders have a placental origin has been underestimated in the past.[11,24] Emerging evidence supports the concept of placental programming of conditions—including neuropsychiatric disease—that will be apparent in the postnatal and even adult life.[25] Therefore, identifying the physiologic cellular trajectories of different types of neural cells in the developing brain will allow us to understand how the effect of multiple injurious insults might converge on a specific developmental time point vulnerable to conferring long-term disease impact.

The developmental processes of neuronal and glial cell lineage generation and maturation during gestation and neonatal life are complex and evolve during each gestational phase, peaking with rapid brain growth in the third trimester.[26-29] During this critical period, the rapid cellular dynamics that contribute to the development of the brain also expose the vulnerability of maturational processes to injury. The brain weight, volume, and cortical surface increase rapidly during gestation, mainly between 23 and 35 weeks of gestation, with the formation of gyri and sulci.[14,30] The cerebellum lobules and folia are formed mostly during the last trimester of pregnancy.[8,15,31] Indeed, third-trimester cerebellar growth is driven by sonic hedgehog (SHH) signaling, which can be directly inhibited by neonatal insults such as hypoxia and glucocorticoid exposure leading to cerebellar hypoplasia.[32-34] Numerous fetal neuroimaging studies have highlighted the developmental changes and the complexity of the cerebral connectome during the last trimester of gestation. During this time and continuing into the first few years after birth, the brain undergoes several key events that lead to telencephalic organization.[8,31] These events include alignment, orientation, and lamination of cortical neurons; gyral development; dendritic arborization; synapse development; cell death; and elimination of specific neuronal processes and synapses that precede the formation of mature neural circuits.[14,29,35]

Myelination is a critical process, initiated during fetal development and continuing postnatally into young adulthood.[14] Myelin—the lipid-rich, tightly wrapped membranous extensions that ensheath axons—is essential for rapid communication within neural circuits and between different brain regions. The myelination process begins in the second trimester in caudal structures, such as the brain stem, and progresses rostrally towards the telencephalon in the third trimester.[9,36-38] Myelination requires the proliferation, migration, and subsequent differentiation of oligodendroglial cells, whose maturation culminates with myelin formation and wrapping around axons.[13,39-41] Oligodendrocyte progenitor cells (OPCs) and pre-oligodendrocytes (pre-OLs) proliferate (19 to 20 weeks), differentiate to mature OLs, which myelinate axonal processes (24 to 32 weeks) during different developmental waves.[27,29] Importantly, along with early-stage OLs, OPCs represent half of the total OL lineage cells at birth (40 weeks).[29] Diseases that target myelin include multiple sclerosis (autoimmune) and Pelizaeus-Merzbacher disease (genetic), and both are associated with profound neurologic disability due to the lack of myelin function.[42] Interestingly, work shows that myelin also includes channel proteins that help maintain axon integrity,[39] suggesting that hypomyelination in preterm brain injury could be a secondary cause of axon and white matter volume decrease.[43]

ETIOLOGY OF BRAIN INJURY IN THE NEWBORN

Brain injury in the fetal and neonatal period may be caused by numerous prenatal, perinatal, or postnatal factors (Table 133.1) that manifest differently in neonates born at term or preterm. As most clinical signs are nonspecific, particularly during immediate postnatal presentation, differential diagnosis is often challenging. The following sections discuss:

1. **Mechanisms of brain injury**, outlining the basic cellular and molecular mechanisms involved in neuronal injury following hypoxia-ischemia and inflammation. We will describe in detail the events following brain injury to include energy failure, excitotoxicity, free radical generation, growth factors, and other intracellular signaling leading to cell death.
2. **Clinical considerations** in the neonate. We will review mechanistic perspectives related to specific clinical scenarios in the fetus and neonate starting in utero and extending into the neonatal period and infancy. We review the placental programming and the effect of prematurity on the developing brain. We will conclude this chapter by reviewing the mechanisms of injury in the neonatal brain caused by infection and inflammation, necrotizing enterocolitis (NEC), hyperbilirubinemia, and metabolic disorders, including hypoglycemia. We will also provide insights into future directions for neonatal brain research.

MECHANISMS OF BRAIN INJURY

Despite the multifactorial etiology of perinatal brain injury, with the exemption of the congenital and/or syndromic developmental brain malformations, many pathways converge to a common signaling cascade culminating in neuronal cell death. Therefore, in this chapter, we will be focusing on the cellular and molecular mechanisms of injury that follow specific pathologic events (Fig. 133.2).

ENERGY FAILURE

The developing brain requires a constant supply of energy to initiate and complete developmental programs that include cell division, migration, differentiation, and biosynthesis of lipids, nucleotides, and proteins. While the mature brain primarily relies on glucose for its source of energy, the high metabolic demands of the rapidly developing brain utilize many substrates such as glucose, ketone bodies, lactate, fatty acids, and amino acids.[44-46]

Table 133.1 Etiology of Neonatal Brain Injury.

Etiology of Neonatal Brain Injury	Clinical Pearls
1. Hypoxic-ischemic encephalopathy (HIE) and asphyxia	Total body hypothermia may improve neurodevelopment outcomes if initiated <6 h. Clinical trials on adjunctive therapies are underway
2. Infection (mainly meningitis and encephalitis)	Chorioamnionitis is a significant factor and is associated with poor neurodevelopment, often due to vertical transmission of neurotrophic viruses
3. Intraventricular hemorrhage (IVH)	Decreased incidence of IVH following various preventative measures in the NICU
4. Developmental brain malformations (neurulation, proliferation, migration defects)	Prenatal diagnostics, including fetal MRI, allow parents to engage in early decision making
5. Genetic syndromes	Advancements in preimplantation genetic testing (including free DNA testing) have increased the detection of genetic syndromes
6. Neonatal hypoglycemia	Insufficient evidence to support specific serum glucose levels associated with risk for brain injury, especially in the first 2 days of life
7. Birth trauma	Skull fracture, subdural, and subarachnoid or epidural hemorrhages associated with high morbidity
8. Placental insufficiency	Poor placental perfusion may be associated with IUGR and compromised neurodevelopment
9. Seizures	An acute sign of brain injury such as HIE, intracranial hemorrhage, or infection. Increasing evidence that seizures can worsen brain injury
10. Maternal stress	Preclinical and clinical evidence suggests an association with premature birth, epigenetic alterations in the placenta, IUGR, and poor neurodevelopment
11. Perinatal ischemic stroke (arterial or venous)	Unexplained etiology (>90%) with placental/cord infection a common suspect. Most commonly presents in the neonatal period (60%) or during early childhood (40%). If no underlying condition (e.g., cardiac disease, neural tube defect, or other), the recurrence risk <1%. Anticoagulation therapy remains controversial
12. Inborn errors of metabolism	Most present with pathognomonic patterns of brain injury using advanced imaging techniques, which may assist with early diagnosis and prompt initiation of treatments. In the majority of the acidemias the injury occurs after birth when maternal compensation is no longer possible. Neurodegenerative disorders can have onset in utero resulting in prenatal and progressive postnatal brain injury
13. Environmental toxicity (prenatal or postnatal)	Effects of lead toxicity well described—unclear impact of noise or benefit of private room configuration in the NICU on neurodevelopmental outcomes
14. Noxious substances	For example, alcohol (fetal alcohol syndrome), opiates, marijuana, cocaine (neonatal abstinence syndrome), SSRI (neonatal adaptive syndrome)

IUGR, Intrauterine growth restriction; *MRI*, magnetic resonance imaging; *NICU*, neonatal intensive care unit; *SSRI*, selective serotonin reuptake inhibitor.

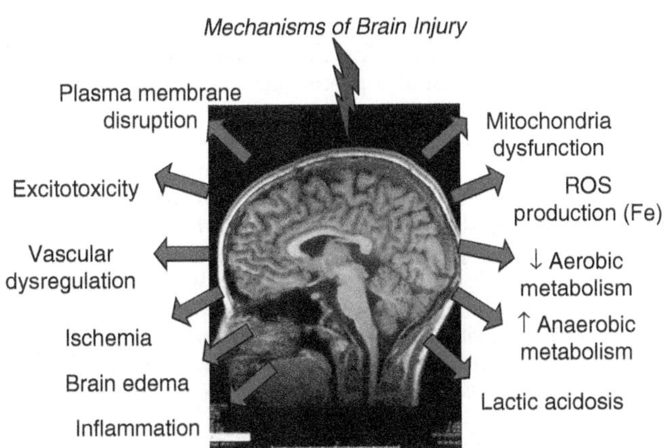

Fig. 133.2 Multifactorial causes and pleotropic effects characterize neonatal injury in the developing brain. The figure illustrates upstream causes, cascade events, and the impact in brain regions and at different developmental stages. The end result is either cell death of different neural cell populations, altered developmental trajectories, and/or brain circuits and function. *ROS,* Reactive oxygen species.

During early development, there are high circulating levels of lactate, ketone bodies, and glucose. The uptake and utilization of these substrates require transporters that are developmentally and regionally regulated.[47,48] Rodent studies have demonstrated that enzyme levels responsible for the oxidative metabolism of glucose exponentially increase during the first month after birth, while the proteins responsible for ketone metabolism are highly expressed in the first week and gradually decrease with age.[49,50]

Brain injury during the neonatal period is superimposed on the high metabolic demands of the developing brain. Acute injury, whether due to hypoxia, hypoxia-ischemia, or inflammation, can halt or interfere with normal developmental processes due to alterations in bioenergetic substrate availability, modifications in the expression of proteins/enzymes responsible for metabolism, and/or depletion of antioxidant capacity. The resulting energy failure can halt or delay normal maturation processes, contributing to neurodevelopmental delays.

Lactate and ketones enter the brain via specific monocarboxylate transporters (MCTs) and provide acetyl-CoA moieties that can directly enter the tricarboxylic acid (TCA) cycle. This process can provide more than half of the energy required during the first few weeks of life in rodents.[44] Besides being a substrate for energy in the developing brain, ketones such as β-hydroxybutyrate may also decrease inflammatory cytokine release.[45] Glucose enters the brain via specific glucose transporters that are also developmentally regulated.[48,51] As glycolysis provides a limited number of ATP molecules, the expression of enzymes necessary for oxidative metabolism—a significant contributor to ATP synthesis—exponentially increases during development. While glucose may not necessarily contribute to all of the cellular energy demands during the early stages of development, it does provide the carbon-backbone critical for nucleotide and NADPH synthesis via the pentose phosphate pathway (PPP). Studies have shown that the neonatal brain has a higher glucose flux into the PPP than the adult, which is consistent with the higher biosynthetic demands of early brain development.[52,53]

During the initial phase of a perinatal event, such as hypoxia, decreased oxygen, and glucose delivery, there is a switch in cellular anaerobic respiration. An initial decrease in phosphocreatine—the principal storage of high energy phosphate in the brain—first occurs, followed by decreased levels of ATP.[54-56]

The accumulation of lactate and a decrease in pH initially lead to an increase in cerebral blood flow. However, a reduction in pH inhibits phosphofructokinase activity, resulting in decreased generation of ATP from glycolysis. Injured cells also experience an accumulation of excitotoxic amino acids—such as glutamate—and an increase in cytosolic Ca^{2+}, combined with mitochondrial dysfunction and mitochondrial membrane permeabilization. The impact of the insult on mitochondria is clearly evident in changes in their dynamics—involving a balance between fission, mitophagy, fusion, and biogenesis—which normally ensure an adequate amount of ATP in the active cells.[57,58]

During periods of high energy ATP demands, including early development, fusion is necessary to create larger mitochondria and the mixing of mitochondrial contents. Following insult, such as oxygen-glucose deprivation, the balance of mitochondrial dynamics favors fission.[59,60] Damaged mitochondria undergo mitophagy (selective autophagy) through an autophagosomal-lysosomal pathway.[61] The increased fission and mitophagy of mitochondria result in marked upregulation of mitochondrial DNA and proteins in the border zone regions of cortical infarcts at 24 hours after infarct.[62]

After the initial phase of energy failure, there is a recovery of phosphocreatine levels with reduced lactate levels in the region. Using magnetic resonance (MR) spectroscopy, a few studies demonstrated that another decline in phosphocreatine occurs several hours later.[63,64]

Immunohistochemical studies also showed that this decline is preceded by a significant decrease in different neuronal cell populations.[65] Therefore, evidence suggests that the observed decrease in phosphocreatine levels may be a consequence of events occurring during the primary energy failure phase, resulting in cell death.

The role of mitochondria in oxidative metabolism is not only to provide energy through ATP production, as the intermediate metabolites of the TCA cycle can produce either pro- or anti-inflammatory signals, and thus change the production of reactive oxygen species.[61] The function of microglia, the nascent immune cells in the brain, may also be dictated by mitochondria and their dynamic state. In models of infection using lipopolysaccharide (LPS), an increase in mitochondrial-dependent oxidative phosphorylation in microglia was observed.[66] However, prolonged LPS exposure decreased oxidative metabolism and increased glycolysis.[66,67]

Damaged mitochondria can also be pro-inflammatory because the released mitochondrial DNA acts as damage-associated molecular pattern (DAMP) molecules or binds to NLRP3.[61,68-70] These pathways promote autophagy, apoptosis, and disruption of glycolysis.[61]

In conclusion, the maintenance of adequate energy levels is crucial for cell development and homeostasis. Without appropriate levels of energy substrates, the metabolic demands of a cell cannot be met, and a cascade of events occurs, which ultimately triggers the eventual demise of the cell. The developing brain is unique in that substrates other than glucose can be utilized, unlike the adult brain, where glucose is the primary source. Therefore, targeting metabolic pathways and mitochondria may lead to potential treatment regimens that restore energy balance during times of excessive metabolic demand imposed by neonatal brain injury.

EXCITOTOXICITY

Whether excitotoxicity follows hypoxia-ischemia or inflammation, there is an increase in glutamate release from presynaptic terminals and failure in the reuptake of glutamate.[71,72] Glutamate is the major excitatory amino acid neurotransmitter in the brain and acts on the excitatory receptors for AMPA, kainate, and N-methyl-D-aspartate (NMDA). Glutamate synthesis is dependent on glucose metabolism, as the carbon backbone of glutamate is derived from α-ketoglutarate, an intermediate of the TCA cycle in the mitochondria. During injury, such as hypoxia, there is an increase in glutamate released from the presynaptic neurons into the synaptic clefts, as well as decreased reuptake both at these presynaptic terminals and by astrocytes.[73] This excess glutamate results in hyperactivation of NMDA receptors, leading to a sustained intracellular calcium increase in neurons.[74-76] In addition, energy failure (described above) due to mitochondrial dysfunction and decreased substrate availability causes a collapse in energy-dependent pumps that are responsible for removing excess intracellular calcium and sodium.[77,78] As a consequence of this dysfunction, cytosolic phosphatases are deactivated by increased calcium concentration, while phospholipases, proteases, and endonucleases are overactivated. This cascade of biochemical events results in neuronal disruption and extensive cell death.[73,79]

FREE RADICAL GENERATION

Several preclinical studies in rodents and large animal models provided unambiguous evidence of increased free radical generation during hypoxic insults in the newborn brain. These studies demonstrate increased free radical production during hypoxia in the cerebral cortex of the fetus and the newborn.[76,77] Alkoxyl radical appears to be the predominant free radical species identified during hypoxia, indicating that free-radical-mediated lipid peroxidation is an ongoing event during cerebral hypoxia and a significant cause of hypoxic neuronal injury.[78] During hypoxia, the increased accumulation of intracellular Ca^{2+} from excessive activation of NMDA and non-NMDA receptors plays a crucial role in cellular excitotoxicity.[77,80] Increased intracellular Ca^{2+} will trigger a sequence of events that result in the genesis of free radicals and cell death, including the activation of:

- Phospholipase A2, cyclooxygenase, and lipoxygenase pathways.
- Nitric oxide synthase (NOS).
- Proteases, leading to the conversion of xanthine dehydrogenase to xanthine oxidase.
- Phospholipase C1 leading to IP3 formation, which increases the release of intracellular Ca^{2+}.

The generation of free radicals triggers the release of additional excitatory amino acids neurotransmitters and modulates NMDA receptor ion-channel activity through the redox site.[76-78,80,81]

In addition to Ca^{2+}-induced mechanisms of free radical generation during hypoxia, other events also occur, including compromise of the electron transport chain elements, increased release of ferritin, and increased breakdown of ATP, resulting in increased free radical production.[75,76,78,80-82]

While the focus of this section has been on hypoxia and hypoxia-ischemia as a cause of free radical generation, it should be noted that inflammation is also a significant contributor. The perinatal infection triggers an innate immune systemic response, resulting in increased cytokines secretion and activation of the biochemical pathways described above.

GROWTH FACTORS

Growth and trophic factors regulate the development of all neural cell types, including neurons and oligodendrocytes. OPC development, proliferation, migration, and differentiation are regulated by several growth factors that act in concert to modulate all these phases of oligodendrocyte generation and maturation. The levels and biologic effects of these factors are also regulated by perinatal injury. Fibroblast growth factor 2 (FGF2), epidermal growth factor (EGF), and leukemia inhibitory factor (LIF)—which promote OPC development under normal physiologic conditions—are upregulated in the major postnatal neurogenic niche, the subventricular zone (SVZ), after hypoxic insult.[26,83,84] Insulin-like growth factor-1 (IGF-1) plays a crucial role in promoting oligodendrogenesis and myelination in early brain development.[36,38] IGF-1 treatment after neonatal brain injury recapitulates some of its developmental effects and promotes OL regeneration. Consistent with its role also in regeneration after injury, IGF-1 administration after hypoxia-ischemia (HI) had multiple effects, including preventing immature OL death, enhancing myelination, and protecting OPCs in the SVZ and in white matter regions.[85,86]

Other growth factors, such as EGF, may also play a very important role after perinatal brain injury. It is known that EGF receptor (EGF-R) is expressed in the developing neonatal brain in many regions, including the white matter.[36,84,87,88] In rodent models of neonatal brain injury, such as hypoxia and hypoxia-ischemia, there was an increase in endogenous EGF in the white matter and in the SVZ.[84,87,88] It has been shown that noninvasive intranasal EGF delivery during a critical developmental time window immediately after a hypoxic injury caused a significant expansion of the OPC pool in the white matter and promoted oligodendrocyte proliferation and maturation. The end result was functional and behavioral recovery.[84] In this study, it was demonstrated that one of the molecular mechanisms that contributed to the beneficial effects of EGF treatment on oligodendrocyte regeneration was inhibition of hypoxia-induced Notch activation, as this pathway is known to prevent differentiation of OPCs.[84]

Another important growth factor, platelet-derived growth factor (PDGF), has also been associated with embryonic development, cell proliferation, and differentiation, involving multiple organs, as well as the brain and spinal cord.[89-94] The PDGF-receptor (PDGFR) and its subunits (A, B, C, and D) play a critical physiologic role in the developing nervous system as well as in pathologic conditions, where they regulate oligodendrogenesis and the permeability of the blood-brain barrier.[92-94] PDGFR appears to be a promising neuroprotective target for hypoxic brain injury and pathologic conditions leading to hypomyelination.[27,90,93-95]

Preclinical evidence supports the notion that hypoxia also results in the activation of regulatory enzymes in the nucleus and the cytosol, including Src kinase, calcium calmodulin kinase 4 (CaMK4), and members of the receptor tyrosine kinase (RTK) group, as well as leakage of the Second mitochondria-derived activator of caspase/direct inhibitor of apoptosis-binding protein with low pI (Smac/DIABLO) from the mitochondrial membrane.[96,97] Activation of these enzymes by hypoxia resulted in increased apoptotic cell death in the cerebral cortex of newborn piglets.[74,79,98,99] Concurrent treatment with hypothermia and selective inhibition with small molecules resulted in improved neuropathology in a piglet model of HIE.[97]

Hypoxia induces hypoxia-inducible factor 1-alpha (HIF-1α), a basic helix-loop-helix transcription factor, and a master regulator of cellular homeostatic responses to hypoxia.[100] HIF-1α activates transcription of genes involved in energy metabolism, angiogenesis, apoptosis, and cell differentiation.[101] HIF-1α is a DNA binding protein that binds to a hypoxia-inducible enhancer in the 3′ flanking sequence of the erythropoietin *EPO* gene, and displays a broad expression pattern in different tissues, but is rapidly degraded under normoxic conditions.[101] Under normoxic conditions, HIF-1α is regulated post-transcriptionally by prolyl hydroxylases and rapidly degraded by proteasomes.[101] However, accumulating data indicate that HIF-1α may be regulated not only by hypoxia but also in response to inflammatory stimuli in an NF-κB–dependent manner. NF-κB activation is controlled by I kappa-B kinases (IKK), mainly IKK-β, which was found to be activated in hypoxic cell cultures and is also deficient in some forms of severe combined immunodeficiencies (SCID).[102,103] NF-κB is a critical transcriptional activator of HIF-1α. Minimal NF-κB activity is required for HIF-1α protein accumulation under hypoxic conditions.[103] The interplay between hypoxia and inflammation, along with its pathologic role in acute and chronic inflammatory disease states, such as atherosclerosis, has emerged as a subject of significant scientific interest for neonatal brain injury.

The human body responds to hypoxic conditions by producing more oxygen-carrying red blood cells. One mechanism is through the increased expression of HIFs, which result in the upregulation of *EPO* in the kidney and erythropoiesis.[104] EPO is an important trophic factor of the brain that plays a significant role in neonatal brain injury. EPO has been shown to exert a neuroprotective effect in preclinical models of neonatal brain injury[105-108] as well as in preclinical models and patients with psychiatric diseases and multiple sclerosis.[104,108-112] Phase I trials have also suggested some efficacy in neonates born at term who sustained some degree of HIE, in particular for high doses of erythropoietin used as an adjuvant to hypothermia.[106,113] In a randomized control trial, the Preterm Erythropoietin Neuroprotection Trial (PENUT), 941 extremely premature neonates received a high dose of erythropoietin or placebo; it was demonstrated that a high-dose erythropoietin treatment that was initiated 24 hours from birth until 32 weeks of postmenstrual age was not associated with improved neurodevelopment or decreased mortality by 2 years of age.[105] One explanation might be the feedback loop inhibition of HIF-1α from the accumulated prolyl hydroxylase domain protein 2 (PHD2) that causes degradation of HIF-1α.[114]

OTHER INTRACELLULAR PATHWAYS

A variety of other intracellular pathways have been identified as important mediators of neonatal brain injury. AMP-activated protein kinase (AMPK) is activated by increased levels of intracellular calcium and increased free radicals and reactive oxygen species via liver kinase 1 (LKB1) and Ca^{2+}/calmodulin-dependent protein kinase kinase-β (CAMKKBeta).[115] AMPK has been shown to inhibit energy consumption and increase energy production, thus contributing to metabolic imbalance during development.[116] Other intracellular signals that play a significant role in propagating injury at the cellular level include time- and cell-dependent increase in extracellular-signal-regulated kinase (ERK) phosphorylation resulting in neuronal cell death.[117]

Molecular pathways that contribute to axonal development are also affected by hypoxia. MCT1 is a protein that is encoded by the *SLC16A1* gene and, with others, plays a significant role in axonal metabolism.[118] In a recent preclinical study, environmental enrichment (EE) following hypoxia resulted in improved behavioral outcomes and attenuated cellular and molecular alterations induced by injury.[119]Transcriptomic analysis revealed the upregulation of *SLC16A1* in OLs after EE exposure. OL-specific inhibition of MCT1 causes axonal degeneration and motor neuron death, highlighting its potential importance in EE-induced recovery from hypoxia. MCT1 may, therefore, represent a novel therapeutic target for premature brain injury.[119] Additionally, other experience-dependent changes in OL mRNAs may be candidates for future therapy, although further studies investigating differential gene expression over time are required before we fully appreciate the role of OLs in neurodevelopment and plasticity, especially after a perinatal injury.[119]

A major regulator of organogenesis and brain development, including the proliferation of glia, is the SHH protein. This protein is encoded by the *SHH* gene.[120-122] Experimental evidence supports a major role of steroids in modulating the *SHH* pathway in the developing human brain.[123] Premature neonates often receive multiple doses of corticosteroids for the treatment of pressor-resistant hypotension (mainly hydrocortisone), or as a prevention and treatment of chronic lung disease (dexamethasone).[124-126] However, the off-target effects of corticosteroids in neurodevelopment are not fully understood.[127-129] The mechanism by which corticosteroids cause brain injury is thought to be through their interaction with SHH. Heine and Rowitch reported that steroids could modulate the SHH pathway in postnatal mice and suppress SHH-induced proliferation of cerebellar progenitor cells.[123] Conversely, SHH signaling is protective against glucocorticoid-induced neonatal cerebellar injury by inducing the enzyme 11βHSD2. Of note, 11βHSD2 inhibits hydrocortisone and prednisolone, but not dexamethasone, indicating that the former agents would be expected to have less neurotoxicity.[123]

Neonatal brain injury also causes abnormalities in the timing of neural cell proliferation and differentiation in the brain. Using a mouse model, Jablonska and colleagues demonstrated that neonatal brain injury caused by chronic perinatal hypoxia elevates OPC proliferation and delays OL maturation in the white matter through activation of the Cdk2/Rb/E2F1 and p27Kip1/FoxO1 pathways, respectively.[130] The histone deacetylase Sirt1 was identified as a crucial regulator of OPC development in response to hypoxia.[131] Downregulation of Sirt1 expression suppressed both basal and hypoxia-induced OPC proliferation. Importantly, inhibition of Sirt1 with sirtinol, a potent inhibitor of Sirt1 activity, prevented the effects of hypoxia on OPC proliferation and promoted OPC differentiation. Altogether, these molecular studies demonstrate that hypoxia-induced delays in OPC development occur through the Cdk2/Rb/E2F1 pathway and that HIF1α-dependent post-translational modifications of Cdk2 and Rb play a crucial modulatory role.[130,131]

In conclusion, the intracellular molecular pathways described in this section are important regulators of neural cell development in the normal brain; however, injury causes either sustained activation or inhibition of these pathways, thereby contributing to the altered developmental trajectory of specific cell populations and overall developmental delay of the brain.

CELL DEATH

Necrosis and apoptosis are the two main types of cell death occurring in all tissues, including the developing brain. Necrosis (early cell death) is usually the consequence of a brief and severe insult, and is due to failure of the ATP-dependent Na^+/K^+ pump, followed by sodium and water influx into the cell, ultimately resulting in cell swelling, membrane fragmentation, and death (Fig. 133.3).[73,132] Apoptosis (delayed cell death) is usually the result of a relatively longer and milder insult that leads to membrane depolarization, glutamate release, calcium influx, cell shrinkage, and DNA fragmentation.[74,132] It has been proposed that neuronal cell death occurs in hybrid forms, generating a cell death continuum, ranging from apoptosis to necrosis—and that this may occur with significant regional variability in different cell types of the developing brain.[73,132]

Following the abovementioned energy failure and free radical formation in the cytosol, several enzyme complexes of focal adhesions (FAs) localized in the cytosol, such as Src and EGFR kinase, become activated and enter the nucleus through phosphorylation of calmodulin and calcium/calmodulin kinase IV (CaM kinase IV).[74,97,133,134] At the same time, mitochondrial apoptotic proteins are released into the cytosol and re-activate the initiator and effector caspases by releasing inhibitor of apoptosis proteins (IAP)-mediated inhibition. Under physiologic conditions, IAP is bound to caspases 3, 7, and 9 and prevents their activation.[135] The inhibition of IAPs allows for increased caspase activity, resulting in apoptotic cell death.[135] Apoptosis-inducing factor (AIF) is released upon loss of mitochondrial membrane potential and is translocated to the nucleus where it activates the caspases leading to apoptosis. It has been previously demonstrated that hypoxia results in increased expression of AIF in the cerebral cortex, which results in increased caspase activation, DNA fragmentation, and cell death.[10,96,136]

Proteins of the Bcl-2 family are important regulators of apoptotic cell death and are expressed in neurons of the central and peripheral nervous system.[137] The anti-apoptotic Bcl-2 protein enhances cell survival following a broad range of deleterious stimuli.[138] Bcl-2 proteins reside in the nuclear envelope, endoplasmic reticulum, cytoplasm, and mitochondria. Pro-apoptotic proteins, such as Bax, have been demonstrated to induce cell death by activating caspases.[74] Both Bax and Bcl-2 are important key players in cell signaling following brain hypoxia.

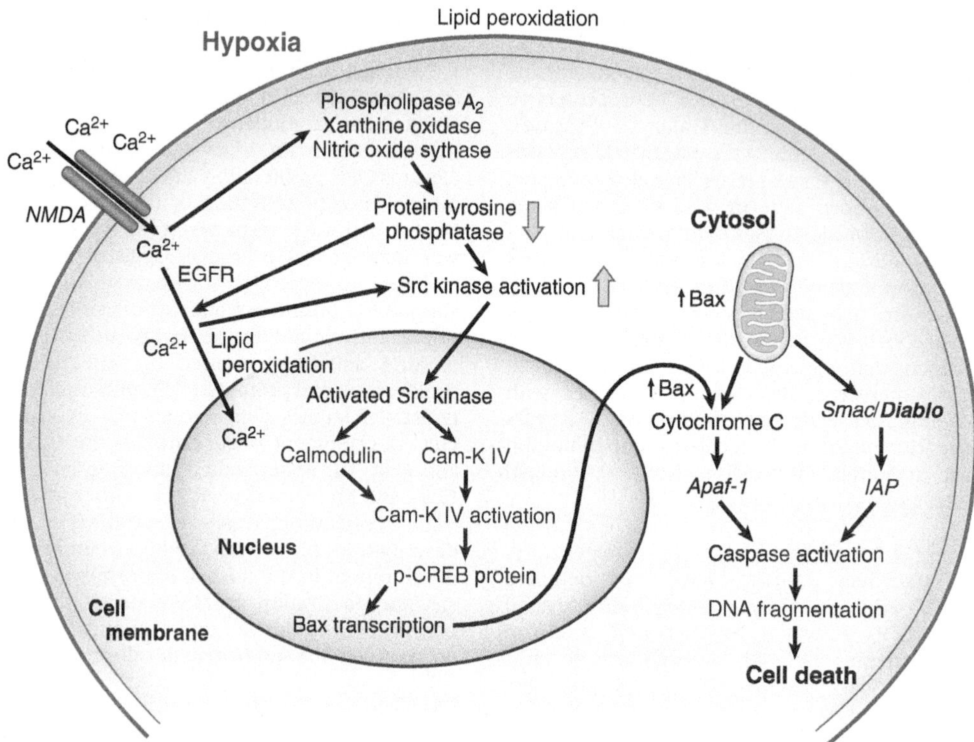

Fig. 133.3 Intracellular pathways that contribute to cell death in the developing brain as a consequence of neonatal brain injury. Such pathways function differently in a variety of cell types and subcellular domains, including the cell membrane, cytosol, mitochondria, and cell nucleus, providing a challenge to finding systemic drug therapies. *EGFR*, Epidermal growth factor receptor; *IAP*, Inhibitor of apoptosis proteins; *NMDA*, *N*-methyl-D-aspartate.

Bcl-2 prevents apoptosis by regulating nuclear Ca^{2+} concentrations and a cascade of Ca^{2+}-dependent events that culminate in cell injury and death.[139,140] Nuclear calcium signaling also controls several other neural cell functions, including gene transcription, DNA replication, and nuclear envelope breakdown.[135,139]

CLINICAL CONSIDERATIONS

PLACENTAL PROGRAMMING

There are important and specific time-points in which the embryo and fetus are more vulnerable to stressful events, and the impact of such events will vary depending on when they occur during gestation. Maldevelopment of the brain may also be influenced by genetic factors. Several genes associated with neuropsychiatric disease and neurodevelopmental deficits are highly expressed in both the placenta and the brain.[12,25,141-143] In utero, the placenta is responsible for providing a protective barrier between the fetus and the mother, and for preventing the exposure of the fetus to maternal insults. Fetal stress due to hypoxia, inflammation, or malnutrition may directly impact the fetal brain by altering gene expression, inducing placental malperfusion,[144,145] and elicit a sterile inflammatory response.[146,147] Maternal conditions, such as obesity or malignancy, may potentiate the inflammatory response in the fetus and glucocorticoid release.[24] High levels of maternal cortisol due to stress or impaired activity of placental 11βHSD2 isoform due to stressors (e.g., hypoxia or other insults) may lead to fetal tissues being exposed to higher than normal glucocorticoid levels, suppressing cell proliferation, and inducing epigenetic changes.[148-150] As maternal cortisol is released, placental corticotropin-releasing hormone (CRH) increases steroid hormone production, exposing the fetal brain to high glucocorticoid levels that may be deleterious to early development.[151] When infection and inflammation occur during gestation, they place the offspring at higher risk for brain disorders, including severe learning disabilities.[152]

Recent work by Ursini and colleagues[25] has linked a multitude of insults, defined broadly as early life complications (ELC), with placental genomic signatures that may increase the risk of schizophrenia. Genetic risk for schizophrenia was defined as polygenic risk scores (PRS) derived from genome-wide association studies (GWAS) done in independent populations from the United States, Europe, and Japan. The report of ELCs significantly increased the association of PRS with schizophrenia.[25] The gene loci linked to schizophrenia risk were highly expressed in the placenta, were increased in male placenta compared to females, and were differentially expressed in placentas from complicated pregnancies compared to normal. In addition to a fetal genetic contribution to schizophrenia risk via placental gene expression, a maternal contribution also likely exists. Abnormal brain levels of kynurenic acid (KYNA), an endogenous antagonist of NMDA, and of α7 nicotinic acetylcholine receptors have been associated with schizophrenia-like phenotypes in animal models.[153] It was recently reported that genetic alteration of maternal kynurenine 3-monooxygenase, and thus fetal KYNA exposure, may lead to the increased placenta and brain KYNA, suggesting that maternal placental genotype may also contribute to schizophrenic pathology.[154]

PREMATURITY

Very premature birth is considered a risk factor for brain injury and neurodevelopmental disabilities, even without considering the associated prenatal and postnatal complications, such as infection, inflammation, and hypoxia (Fig. 133.4; see Table 133.1), which are described above. Prematurely born children are at higher risk for developmental delays and neuropsychiatric disorders, as well as motor learning deficits.[16,17] Prematurity is associated with increased risk for both white matter injury (WMI) and cortical gray matter injury.[37,155] In a very recent study including 63 10-year-old children who were born prematurely

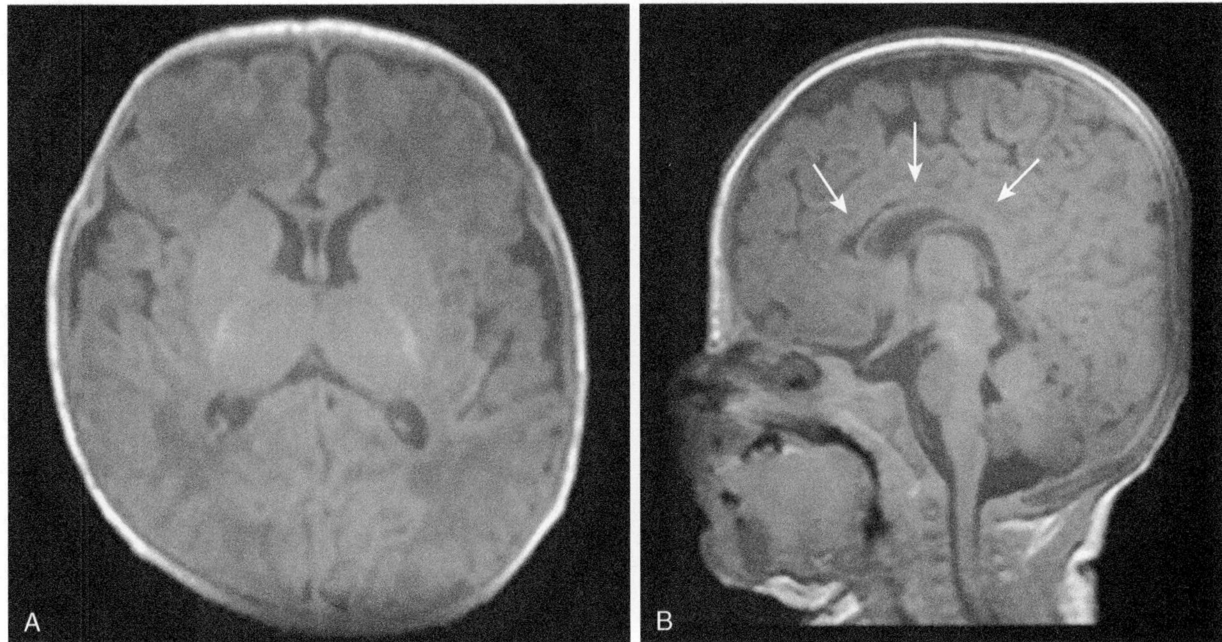

Fig. 133.4 Term-equivalent brain magnetic resonance imaging (MRI) of a 24-week preterm infant who was born due to uterine incompetence and chorioamnionitis with subsequent chronic lung disease. Neurologic exam at term was unremarkable. The infant's term-equivalent brain MRI demonstrates decreased white matter volume (A) and thinned corpus callosum *(arrows)* (B). During the third trimester of gestation, oligodendrocytes in the telencephalon undergo extensive proliferation, migration, and maturation towards myelin-producing cells. The stressors associated with premature birth—such as inflammation, hypoxia, and hypoxia-ischemia—are known to inhibit oligodendrocyte progenitor cell maturation. Because myelin has axon trophic effects, it is possible that hypomyelination leads to long-term axonal and white matter volume loss. The long-term consequence of these cellular abnormalities is white matter dysmaturity and increased risk of neurodevelopmental delays.

(<32 weeks of gestation and without major comorbidities), language functions were significantly worse than vocabulary scores and verbal intelligent quotients.[19] Also, their verbal intelligent quotient was strongly associated with language scores, suggesting that children with low verbal intelligent quotient scores may be at risk for speech delays and long-term compromised academic performance.[19]

Impaired cerebral autoregulation has been associated with brain injury in premature and term-born neonates in preclinical and clinical studies.[156-161] Interventricular hemorrhage (IVH) and post-hemorrhagic hydrocephalus (PHH) often complicate the course of premature neonates resulting in further injury.[161] Malnutrition, NEC, exposure to surgeries and general anesthesia and chronic hypoxia due to chronic lung disease or pulmonary hypertension are only a fraction of the numerous factors that can affect brain development and result in brain injury.[162] Infants born very premature characteristically have WMI and altered cortical, hippocampal, and cerebellar microstructure. The cerebellar alterations due to prematurity appear to be associated with the gestational age, prenatal and postnatal steroid administration, and the presence of cerebellar hemorrhage.[14,31,163]

INFECTION AND INFLAMMATION

Multiple studies have highlighted immune involvement in developmental disabilities, suggesting a model of brain immune dysregulation, which begins in utero. One possibility is that maternal inflammation, a known risk factor for ASD, sets this immune activation in motion.[164] This hypothesis is being investigated using several animal models.[165] There is also histopathologic evidence that among subjects with developmental delays, those associated with maternal inflammation are characterized by specific pathology, which suggests that diverse causes for those disorders may explain some of their heterogeneity. Approximately 10% of term and 35% of premature pregnancies are complicated by chorioamnionitis.[166]

During infection, there is robust activation of pro-inflammatory cytokines and microglial cells, which in turn express more inflammatory mediators. Cytokine-activated cells secrete reactive oxygen species and other toxic cellular products. Pro-inflammatory cytokines can result in the activation of cytotoxic T cells, natural killer cells, and lymphokine-activated killer cells, leading to tissue damage. This results in changes in cell proliferation and differentiation, possibly leading to cell death. Since all these events occur at a critical time of oligodendrocyte development, white matter damage is often the result, contributing to long-term neurologic injury among both the preterm and term neonates.

Clinical or histologic chorioamnionitis is strongly associated with poor fetal outcomes. The placenta can identify and respond to pathogens. Studies have shown that maternal immune activation during gestation alone is sufficient to cause behavioral, motor, and sensory abnormalities in offspring.[164,167,168] Neuropathologic analysis of postnatal or adult brains of offspring revealed alterations following the prenatal insult.[167-170] The placenta has been shown to have a role in mediating the extent of injury following infectious processes of viral etiology such as influenza.[167,171,172]

NECROTIZING ENTEROCOLITIS

Deaths attributed to NEC have increased significantly—almost doubled—over the last 2 decades, as shown in two large multicenter trials in the United States and the United Kingdom.[3,4] This increase in mortality attributed to NEC is postulated to be due to an improvement in the early survival of extremely premature infants.[3,4]

Although the intestine is initially inflamed, the brain is affected as well.[35,173-177] The connection between the brain and microbiome of the gastrointestinal tract—the brain-gut axis (BGA)—consists of several direct or indirect routes of bidirectional communication between the intestine and the nervous system.[178-182] Evidence supports the notion of a connection between the brain and the intestine through the immune, endocrine, and nervous systems.[176,178,183-190] Microbiome alterations create an abnormal equilibrium of neurotransmitters and active metabolites, and alter brain plasticity.[191] The role of the vagus nerve is also vital in sensing the inflamed bowel locally or centrally through inflammatory cytokine secretion.[192-194]

Experimental animal models of NEC, as well as analysis of human postmortem tissue, have been used by several research groups to elucidate the mechanisms underlying brain injury induced by the inflamed and ischemic gut, supporting the idea that the severity of intestinal injury in the ileum correlates with the severity of brain injury involving multiple brain regions, such as the hippocampus, cerebral cortex, and the subcortical white matter.[174,175,195-198] Recent work highlights the role of the Toll-like receptor 4 (TLR4) in NEC. TLR4, a bacterial receptor associated with gram-negative organisms (typically involved in NEC), appears to be a key factor in the mechanism of NEC-induced brain injury.[198-200] The overabundance of TLR4 in preemies as compared to term neonates may explain why term-born neonates are less prone to developing NEC.[197,199,201,202]

HYPERBILIRUBINEMIA-INDUCED BRAIN INJURY

The term *kernicterus* was initially used to describe a characteristic pattern of central yellow staining seen in postmortem brains of infants with hyperbilirubinemia. Bilirubin is an end product of heme breakdown and is transported in plasma bound to albumin before it is conjugated in the liver and secreted in stool and urine. Physiologically, there is a constant exchange of small amounts of bilirubin through an intact blood-brain barrier. However, large influxes of bilirubin in the brain can cause neuronal injury.[203,204] Both in vitro and in vivo studies have shown that neurons are more susceptible than glia to bilirubin-induced injury, which is mediated through many different pathways. An important initial step in bilirubin neurotoxicity is its injurious effect on neuronal cell membranes.[204] Damage in the cell membrane promotes the entry of bilirubin into the cells, which in turn causes injury to other intracellular structures such as mitochondria, endoplasmic reticulum, and nuclei. The resultant energy failure leads to neuronal swelling and cell death.[205] Other potential mechanisms for bilirubin neurotoxicity include impairment of myelination, DNA synthesis, protein synthesis, neurotransmitter synthesis, and alterations in excitatory amino acid homeostasis. Although bilirubin is toxic to both myelinated and unmyelinated neurons, unmyelinated neurons are likely to be more susceptible.[205] The typical clinical findings in an infant with kernicterus suggest susceptibility of some regions of the brain to bilirubin-induced injury.[206]

The findings from neuropathologic and neuroradiologic examination suggest that the areas of the brain most frequently affected are basal ganglia, particularly the globus pallidus and subthalamic nucleus, and auditory pathways, including vestibular and cochlear nuclei.[207] Other areas affected are the hippocampus, substantia nigra, cerebellum, parts of midbrain and pons, as well as other brain stem nuclei. Magnetic resonance imaging (MRI) can help in the diagnosis of an affected infant. The most characteristic finding on MRI is a bilateral, symmetric, high-intensity signal (a sign of demyelination) in the region of the globus pallidus.[207]

METABOLIC DISORDERS

Metabolic disorders typically affect the brain. Hypoglycemia is the most common abnormality of metabolism in the newborn period and may result, when severe, in brain injury. Glycolytic flux is decreased in hypoglycemia, contributing to a decreased cerebral metabolic rate for glucose. Oxaloacetate increases due to the decrease of acetate, resulting in decreased citrate within the Krebs cycle.[208] Hypoglycemia is characterized by the activation of cell death pathways, including necrosis.[208] Neuropathologic findings from newborns with severe hypoglycemia described diffuse brain injury involving the cerebral cortex, deep nuclear gray matter, and cerebral white matter. Neuroimaging studies have shown that hypoglycemia-induced brain injury in neonates has a predilection for the occipital tracts and lobes.[209] It is unclear what degree of hypoglycemia may result in brain injury in neonates. A very recent multicenter, randomized, noninferiority trial involving 689 otherwise healthy newborns born at 35 weeks of gestation—or later—compared two threshold values for treatment of asymptomatic moderate hypoglycemia.[210] The authors reported that in otherwise healthy neonates with asymptomatic moderate hypoglycemia, a lower glucose treatment threshold (36 mg/dL) was not less effective to a traditional threshold (47 mg/dL) regarding psychomotor development at 18 months.[210]

Inborn errors of metabolism (IEM), although rare, can result in brain injury through various mechanisms. About one-quarter of these conditions become symptomatic in the newborn period, and chemical analysis of cerebrospinal fluid, blood, and urine is the mainstay of the diagnostic evaluation.[7,209] There is a spatial pattern of vulnerability in the majority of IEM that cannot be easily understood, given that the whole brain is exposed to the metabolic condition. Neuroimaging (in particular MRI) is crucial in narrowing the differential diagnosis, especially considering that clinical symptoms can be nonspecific (encephalopathy) and similar to other conditions.[7,209]

In maple syrup urine disease (MSUD), rapid accumulation of branched-chain amino acids (valine, leucine, and isoleucine) displaces other essential amino acids, resulting in neurotransmitter depletion and disruption of normal brain growth and development.[7,211,212] Damage is especially noted along the corticospinal tracts and in the brain stem, but not in the frontal lobes, which lack myelin in newborns.[212] In the urea cycle defects (UCD), acute hyperammonemia selectively affects the white matter of the brain. Uptake of ammonia in the astrocyte and its conversion to glutamine results in swelling of these cells. Glutamine is osmotically active and can lead to astrocytic swelling, ultimately leading to cytotoxic edema.[7]

FUTURE DIRECTIONS

As our shared goal is to better understand human neonatal brain injury, the need for more studies in humans is crucial. The development of the NIH NeuroBioBank has contributed to validating preclinical data and identifying patterns of injuries in human tissues. Efforts are made by multiple hospitals to develop institutional neurobiobanks and eventually develop consortia for the exchange of samples and collaborative studies. Research involving human postmortem tissues is difficult and complex, due to the heterogeneous clinical scenarios and the challenge in capturing specific cases to serve as appropriate controls. However, careful interpretation of the data obtained from such studies can contribute largely to our understanding of human neurobiology and to the development of more complete and precise animal models. A combination of large-scale high-throughput gene expression profiling studies and the use of brain tissue organoids are gradually emerging as cutting-edge experimental approaches and as tools to define cell-type-specific injury-induced abnormalities and are aiding in the development of new therapeutic approaches that target specific mechanisms of developmental brain injury.

CONCLUSION

As the phenotypic profile of premature and critically ill neonates continuously changes, the pathobiology of neonatal brain injury is a rapidly evolving field of discovery-based and clinical research. A clearer picture is emerging that links the dynamic and delicate balance of perinatal brain development to long-term neurodevelopmental outcome. During the perinatal period, there are crucial time-points and milestones in which the newborn is more vulnerable to stressful events. During these critical developmental periods, clinicians aim to optimize oxygenation and nutrition, decrease inflammation, implement necessary pharmacotherapies, and provide an enriched environment. All these factors will contribute to the fine-tuning of clinical management based on good-quality evidence and will optimize neurodevelopmental outcome later in life.

ACKNOWLEDGMENTS

We thank Drs. Billie Short, Nickie Andescavage, and Nneka Nzegwu (Division of Neonatology, Children's National Hospital); Dr. Taeun Chang (Neonatal Neurology Program, Division of Epilepsy, Neurophysiology & Critical Care, Children's National Hospital); and Dr. Hideo Jinno (Center for Neuroscience Research, Children's National Hospital and Department of Pediatrics and Neonatology, Nagoya City University Graduate School of Medical Sciences) for critically reading this chapter. The research program of the authors of this chapter is supported by award numbers R37NS109478 (Javits Award) and R01NS105138 from NINDS (V.G.), R01NS099461 (J.S.) and by an award from the Board of Visitors of Children's National Hospital (P.K.). The authors' work is also supported by the District of Columbia Intellectual and Developmental Disabilities Research Center U54HD090257 (V.G.) from Eunice Kennedy Shriver National Institute of Child Health and Human Development (NICHD). This content is solely the responsibility of the authors and does not necessarily represent the official views of the National Institutes of Health.

 A complete reference list is available at www.ExpertConsult.com.

SELECT REFERENCES

8. Haldipur P, Aldinger KA, Bernardo S, et al. Spatiotemporal expansion of primary progenitor zones in the developing human cerebellum. *Science*. 2019;366:454–460.
11. Bierstone D, Wagenaar N, Gano DL, et al. Association of histologic chorioamnionitis with perinatal brain injury and early childhood neurodevelopmental outcomes among preterm neonates. *JAMA Pediatr*. 2018;172:534–541.
14. Volpe JJ. Dysmaturation of premature brain: importance, cellular mechanisms, and potential interventions. *Pediatr Neurol*. 2019;95:42–66.
20. O'Reilly H, Johnson S, Ni Y, et al. Neuropsychological outcomes at 19 years of age following extremely preterm birth. *Pediatrics*. 2020;145:e20192087.
24. Mina TH, Raikkonen K, Riley SC, et al. Maternal distress associates with placental genes regulating fetal glucocorticoid exposure and IGF2: role of obesity and sex. *Psychoneuroendocrinology*. 2015;59:112–122.
25. Ursini G, Punzi G, Chen Q, et al. Convergence of placenta biology and genetic risk for schizophrenia. *Nat Med*. 2018;24:792–801.
27. Kessaris N, Fogarty M, Iannarelli P, et al. Competing waves of oligodendrocytes in the forebrain and postnatal elimination of an embryonic lineage. *Nat Neurosci*. 2006;9:173–179.
32. Nguyen V, Sabeur K, Maltepe E, et al. Sonic hedgehog agonist protects against complex neonatal cerebellar injury. *Cerebellum*. 2018;17:213–227.
33. Tam EW, Chau V, Ferriero DM, et al. Preterm cerebellar growth impairment after postnatal exposure to glucocorticoids. *Sci Transl Med*. 2011;3:105ra105.
34. Heine VM, Griveau A, Chapin C, et al. A small-molecule smoothened agonist prevents glucocorticoid-induced neonatal cerebellar injury. *Sci Transl Med*. 2011;3:105ra104.
36. Carson MJ, Behringer RR, Brinster RL, et al. Insulin-like growth factor I increases brain growth and central nervous system myelination in transgenic mice. *Neuron*. 1993;10:729–740.
40. Hughes AN, Appel B. Oligodendrocytes express synaptic proteins that modulate myelin sheath formation. *Nat Commun*. 2019;10:4125.
44. McKenna MC. Substrate competition studies demonstrate oxidative metabolism of glucose, glutamate, glutamine, lactate and 3-hydroxybutyrate in cortical astrocytes from rat brain. *Neurochem Res*. 2012;37:2613–2626.
46. Sperringer JE, Addington A, Hutson SM. Branched-chain amino acids and brain metabolism. *Neurochem Res*. 2017;42:1697–1709.
59. Baburamani AA, Hurling C, Stolp H, et al. Mitochondrial optic atrophy (OPA) 1 processing is altered in response to neonatal hypoxic-ischemic brain injury. *Int J Mol Sci*. 2015;16:22509–22526.
62. Yin W, Signore AP, Iwai M, et al. Rapidly increased neuronal mitochondrial biogenesis after hypoxic-ischemic brain injury. *Stroke*. 2008;39:3057–3063.
70. Shimada K, Crother TR, Karlin J, et al. Oxidized mitochondrial DNA activates the NLRP3 inflammasome during apoptosis. *Immunity*. 2012;36:401–414.
73. Chavez-Valdez R, Martin LJ, Northington FJ. Programmed necrosis: a prominent mechanism of cell death following neonatal brain injury. *Neurol Res Int*. 2012;2012:257563.
75. Mishra OP, Delivoria-Papadopoulos M. Nitric oxide-mediated Ca^{++}-influx in neuronal nuclei and cortical synaptosomes of normoxic and hypoxic newborn piglets. *Neurosci Lett*. 2002;318:93–97.
78. Numagami Y, Zubrow AB, Mishra OP, et al. Lipid free radical generation and brain cell membrane alteration following nitric oxide synthase inhibition during cerebral hypoxia in the newborn piglet. *J Neurochem*. 1997;69:1542–1547.
80. Torres L, Anderson C, Marro P, et al. Cyclooxygenase-mediated generation of free radicals during hypoxia in the cerebral cortex of newborn piglets. *Neurochem Res*. 2004;29:1825–1830.
85. Lin S, Fan LW, Rhodes PG, et al. Intranasal administration of IGF-1 attenuates hypoxic-ischemic brain injury in neonatal rats. *Exp Neurol*. 2009;217:361–370.
93. Pringle NP, Mudhar HS, Collarini EJ, et al. PDGF receptors in the rat CNS: during late neurogenesis, PDGF alpha-receptor expression appears to be restricted to glial cells of the oligodendrocyte lineage. *Development*. 1992;115:535–551.
95. Barres BA, Raff MC. Axonal control of oligodendrocyte development. *J Cell Biol*. 1999;147:1123–1128.
97. Kratimenos P, Koutroulis I, Jain A, et al. Effect of concurrent Src kinase inhibition with short-duration hypothermia on Ca^{2+}/calmodulin kinase IV activity and neuropathology after hypoxia-ischemia in the newborn swine brain. *Neonatology*. 2018;113:37–43.
98. Chiang MC, Ashraf QM, Ara J, et al. Mechanism of caspase-3 activation during hypoxia in the cerebral cortex of newborn piglets. *Neurosci Lett*. 2007;421:67–71.
104. Haase VH. Regulation of erythropoiesis by hypoxia-inducible factors. *Blood Rev*. 2013;27:41–53.
106. Fischer HS, Reibel NJ, Buhrer C, et al. Prophylactic early erythropoietin for neuroprotection in preterm infants: a meta-analysis. *Pediatrics*. 2017;139:e20164317.
109. Adamcio B, Sargin D, Stradomska A, et al. Erythropoietin enhances hippocampal long-term potentiation and memory. *BMC Biol*. 2008;6:37.
113. Wu YW, Mathur AM, Chang T, et al. High-dose erythropoietin and hypothermia for hypoxic-ischemic encephalopathy: a phase II trial. *Pediatrics*. 2016;137:e20160191.
115. Woods A, Dickerson K, Heath R, et al. Ca^{2+}/calmodulin-dependent protein kinase kinase-beta acts upstream of AMP-activated protein kinase in mammalian cells. *Cell Metab*. 2005;2:21–33.
116. Hill JL, Kobori N, Zhao J, et al. Traumatic brain injury decreases AMP-activated protein kinase activity and pharmacological enhancement of its activity improves cognitive outcome. *J Neurochem*. 2016;139:106–119.
120. Yu K, McGlynn S, Matise MP. Floor plate-derived sonic hedgehog regulates glial and ependymal cell fates in the developing spinal cord. *Development*. 2013;140:1594–1604.
122. Nusslein-Volhard C, Wieschaus E. Mutations affecting segment number and polarity in *Drosophila*. *Nature*. 1980;287:795–801.
124. Halliday HL, Ehrenkranz RA, Doyle LW. Early (< 8 days) postnatal corticosteroids for preventing chronic lung disease in preterm infants. *Cochrane Database Syst Rev*. 2009:CD001146.
131. Jablonska B, Gierdalski M, Chew LJ, et al. Sirt1 regulates glial progenitor proliferation and regeneration in white matter after neonatal brain injury. *Nat Commun*. 2016;7:13866.
132. Northington FJ, Chavez-Valdez R, Martin LJ. Neuronal cell death in neonatal hypoxia-ischemia. *Ann Neurol*. 2011;69:743–758.
133. You LH, Li Z, Duan XL, et al. Mitochondrial ferritin suppresses MPTP-induced cell damage by regulating iron metabolism and attenuating oxidative stress. *Brain Res*. 2016;1642:33–42.
135. Deveraux QL, Takahashi R, Salvesen GS, et al. X-linked IAP is a direct inhibitor of cell-death proteases. *Nature*. 1997;388:300–304.
140. Southwell DG, Paredes MF, Galvao RP, et al. Intrinsically determined cell death of developing cortical interneurons. *Nature*. 2012;491:109–113.
143. Winn VD, Haimov-Kochman R, Paquet AC, et al. Gene expression profiling of the human maternal-fetal interface reveals dramatic changes between midgestation and term. *Endocrinology*. 2007;148:1059–1079.
163. Haines KM, Wang W, Pierson CR. Cerebellar hemorrhagic injury in premature infants occurs during a vulnerable developmental period and is associated with wider neuropathology. *Acta Neuropathol Commun*. 2013;1:69.
166. Wu YW, Escobar GJ, Grether JK, et al. Chorioamnionitis and cerebral palsy in term and near-term infants. *J Am Med Assoc*. 2003;290:2677–2684.
175. Brunse A, Abbaspour A, Sangild PT. Brain barrier disruption and region-specific neuronal degeneration during necrotizing enterocolitis in preterm pigs. *Dev Neurosci*. 2018;40:198–208.
177. Jiang ZD, Wang C, Chen C. Neonatal necrotizing enterocolitis adversely affects neural conduction of the rostral brainstem in preterm babies. *Clin Neurophysiol*. 2014;125:2277–2285.
179. Lu J, Claud EC. Connection between gut microbiome and brain development in preterm infants. *Dev Psychobiol*. 2019;61:739–751.
193. Gaykema RP, Dijkstra I, Tilders FJ. Subdiaphragmatic vagotomy suppresses endotoxin-induced activation of hypothalamic corticotropin-releasing hormone neurons and ACTH secretion. *Endocrinology*. 1995;136:4717–4720.
199. Egan CE, Sodhi CP, Good M, et al. Toll-like receptor 4-mediated lymphocyte influx induces neonatal necrotizing enterocolitis. *J Clin Invest*. 2016;126:495–508.
200. Carlisle EM, Poroyko V, Caplan MS, et al. Gram negative bacteria are associated with the early stages of necrotizing enterocolitis. *PloS One*. 2011;6:e18084.
206. Morioka I, Iwatani S, Koda T, et al. Disorders of bilirubin binding to albumin and bilirubin-induced neurologic dysfunction. *Semin Fetal Neonatal Med*. 2015;20:31–36.
211. Zinnanti WJ, Lazovic J, Griffin K, et al. Dual mechanism of brain injury and novel treatment strategy in maple syrup urine disease. *Brain*. 2009;132:903–918.

134 Neuroprotective Therapeutic Hypothermia

Alistair J. Gunn | Joanne O. Davidson | Laura Bennet

INTRODUCTION

Moderate to severe hypoxic-ischemic encephalopathy (HIE) continues to be a significant cause of acute neurologic injury at birth, occurring in approximately 1 to 2 cases per 1000 term live births in the developed world.[1] The risks are approximately 10-fold higher in the developing world.[1] The possibility that hypothermia may alleviate asphyxial brain injury is a "dream revisited."[2] Early experimental studies, mainly in precocial animals such as kittens, demonstrated that hypothermia during postnatal hypoxia greatly extended the "time to last gasp" and improved neurologic recovery.[3] This finding led to a series of small uncontrolled studies in the 1950s and 1960s in which infants who were not breathing spontaneously at 5 minutes after birth were immersed in cold water until respiration began and then allowed to rewarm spontaneously over many hours.[4] Although outcomes were said to be better than for historical controls, this experimental approach was overtaken by two major developments: the introduction of active ventilation and resuscitation of infants exposed to asphyxia and the recognition that even mild hypothermia is associated with greater mortality in preterm newborns.[5] Thus resuscitation guidelines for the newborn exposed to asphyxia have, until recently, simply emphasized keeping the newly born infant warm—that is to say, avoiding hypothermia.[6]

The early experimental studies already noted focused entirely on the effects of cooling *during* severe hypoxia, which is now well established to be associated with potent dose-related long-lasting neuroprotection.[7] The central clinical question is, of course, whether cooling *after* asphyxial or hypoxic-ischemic injury is beneficial. This chapter reviews the recent development and clinical translation of mild postresuscitation cooling, or therapeutic hypothermia, to improve outcomes.

PATHOPHYSIOLOGIC PHASES OF CEREBRAL INJURY

The key advance was the clinical and experimental observation in term fetuses, newborns, and adults that injury to the brain is not a single "event" occurring at or just after an insult but rather an evolving process that leads to a significant proportion of cell death well after the end of acute hypoxia-ischemia.[8] Using magnetic resonance spectroscopy, Wyatt and coworkers showed that infants with evidence of moderate to severe asphyxia often had normal cerebral oxidative metabolism shortly after birth, but many then went on to develop energy failure 6 to 15 hours later.[9] Those infants who did not show transient recovery had a very high mortality, whereas in survivors the degree of secondary energy failure after 24 to 48 hours was closely associated with impaired neurodevelopmental outcome at 4 years of age.[10] An identical pattern of initial recovery of cerebral oxidative metabolism followed by secondary energy failure was seen after hypoxia-ischemia in the piglet.[8] Greater recovery of cerebral phosphocreatine levels after hypoxia-ischemia was associated with more favorable outcomes.[11] In turn, the severity of subsequent secondary loss of oxidative metabolism was closely correlated with the severity of neuronal loss.[12] This delay between insult and injury raised the tantalizing possibility that asphyxial cell death may be prevented even well after the insult.

Distinct pathophysiologic phases of evolving injury may be distinguished, as illustrated in Fig. 134.1. The actual period of hypoxia-ischemia is the *primary* phase of cell injury. During this phase, progressive hypoxic depolarization of cells leads to severe cytotoxic edema, with failure of reuptake, leading to the extracellular accumulation of excitatory amino acids (*excitotoxins*).[8] Excessive levels of excitatory amino acids cause activation of their ion channels and promote further excessive entry of salt, water, and calcium into the cells. After the return of cerebral circulation during resuscitation, the initial hypoxia-induced cytotoxic edema may transiently resolve over approximately 30 to 60 minutes, with partial or even complete recovery of cerebral oxidative metabolism in a *latent phase*.[11] This latent phase is characterized by continuing suppression of electroencephalographic (EEG) activity, with a delayed onset of cerebral hypoperfusion associated with suppressed cerebral metabolism.[13] This is followed by a *secondary phase* of deterioration (~6 to 15 hours later) that may extend over many days. At term gestation, this secondary phase is characterized by delayed onset seizures, secondary cytotoxic edema (see Fig. 134.1), extracellular accumulation of excitotoxins, progressive failure of cerebral oxidative energy metabolism, and ultimately neuronal and oligodendrocyte death.[8]

The studies discussed in this chapter strongly suggest that it is the early recovery, or latent phase, that represents the key window of opportunity for intervention with therapeutic hypothermia.

FACTORS DETERMINING EFFECTIVE NEUROPROTECTION WITH HYPOTHERMIA

Experimentally, the efficacy of neuroprotection with hypothermia is critically dependent on the timing of initiation of cooling, its depth, and its duration.

COOLING DURING RESUSCITATION AND REPERFUSION

Brief hypothermia, for 1 to 2 hours, appears to be modestly neuroprotective provided that it is initiated immediately after the insult. For example, after 15 minutes of reversible ischemia in the piglet, mild hypothermia (a reduction of brain temperature of 2°C to 3°C from the normal basal temperature of 38°C in the piglet) for 1 to 3 hours significantly improved recovery and reduced neuronal loss 3 days later.[14,15] Critically, protection was lost if the brief interval of hypothermia was delayed by as little as 15 to 45 minutes after the primary insult.[16-19] This extreme sensitivity to delay is consistent with the hypothesis that brief, resuscitative hypothermia can suppress damage secondary to oxygen free radical production during reperfusion.[20,21] Alternatively, this strategy may in effect represent intervention at the end of the primary phase, when cerebrovascular perfusion is being reestablished, cell function is just starting to recover, and levels of excitatory amino acids are still high.[22]

Even if immediate cooling at birth was consistently effective, it is simply not possible at present to identify reliably the few infants requiring resuscitation who will go on to develop significant encephalopathy until some hours after birth.

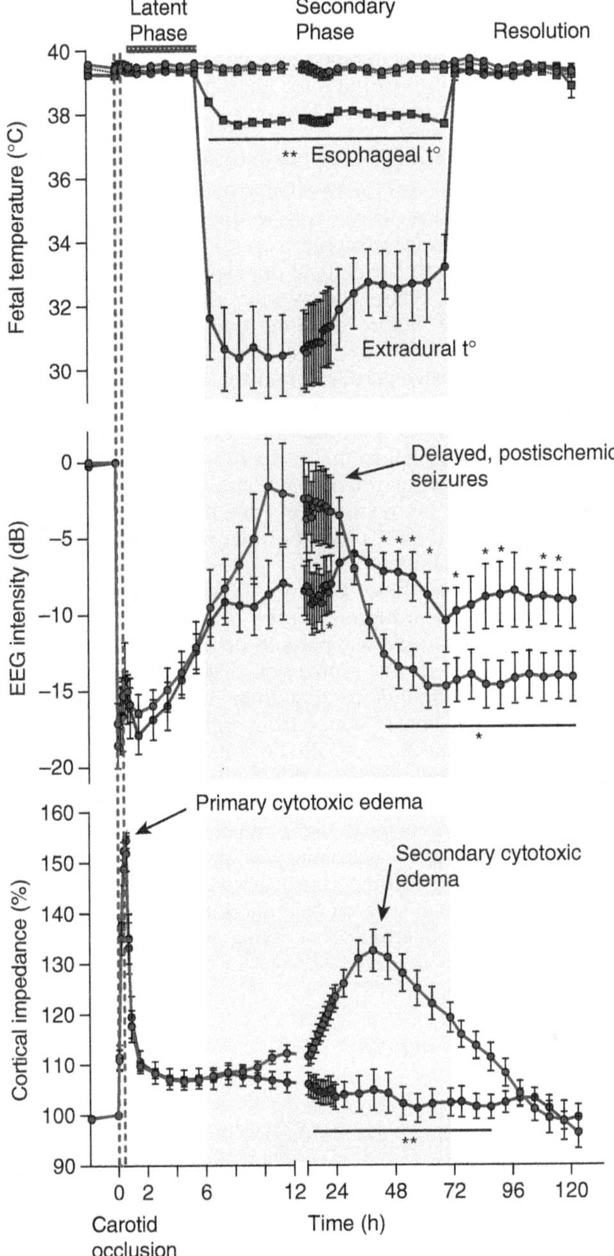

Fig. 134.1 The effect of hypothermia started 5.5 hours after reperfusion following 30 minutes of cerebral ischemia in near-term fetal sheep. The period of ischemia is shown by *dotted lines*, whereas cooling is shown by the *bar*. The *top panel* shows changes in extradural *(solid circles)* and esophageal *(solid squares)* temperature in the hypothermia group and extradural *(open circles)* and esophageal *(open squares)* temperature in the sham-cooled group. The *lower two panels* show changes in electroencephalographic (EEG) intensity and cortical impedance (expressed as percentage of baseline) in the hypothermia *(solid circles)* and sham-cooled *(open circles)* groups. Impedance is a measure of cytotoxic edema (cell swelling). The hypothermia group shows greater recovery of EEG intensity after resolution of delayed seizures and complete suppression of the secondary rise in impedance. Mean ± SEM, * $P < .05$, ** $P < .001$ hypothermia versus sham-cooled fetuses. (Data from Gunn et al.[43]

PROLONGED COOLING

Subsequent studies examined the strategy of suppressing secondary encephalopathic processes by maintaining hypothermia throughout the course of the secondary phase. Such extended periods of cooling of between 5 and 72 hours appear to be more consistently effective.[23–25] For example, in a study of reversible middle cerebral artery occlusion in the adult rat, 21 hours but not 1 hour of mild hypothermia reduced the area of infarction after 48 hours of recovery.[26] After severe global ischemia in the adult gerbil, 12 hours of mild hypothermia was ineffective, whereas extending the interval to 24 hours did afford protection.[24]

Studies in newborn animals support these data. In unanesthetized infant rats subjected to moderate hypoxia-ischemia, mild hypothermia (2°C to 3°C reduction in brain temperature from 37°C in normothermic controls) for 72 hours from the end of hypoxia prevented cortical infarction, whereas 6 hours of cooling had only intermediate, nonsignificant results.[27] In the same model, a greater reduction in body temperature (by 5°C) for 6 hours, starting immediately after the insult, gave significant neuroprotection as well as neurobehavioral improvement after both 1 and 6 weeks' survival.[28] Finally, in the anesthetized piglet exposed either to hypoxia with bilateral carotid ligation or to hypoxia with hypotension, 12 to 48 hours of moderate whole-body hypothermia or head cooling with mild systemic hypothermia (started immediately after hypoxia) prevented delayed energy failure,[25,29] reduced neuronal loss,[30–32] and suppressed posthypoxic seizures.[31]

IF SOME IS GOOD, IS MORE BETTER? A CRITICAL DEPTH OF COOLING

A critical depth of cerebral hypothermia of between 32°C and 34°C appears to be required for effective neuronal rescue. In the fetal sheep cooled from 90 minutes after ischemia, substantial neuroprotection was seen only in fetuses that had a sustained fall of the extradural temperature to less than 34°C (normal temperature in the fetal sheep is 39.5°C).[33] In the adult gerbil, cooling to a rectal temperature of 32°C (vs. 37°C in controls) was associated with greater behavioral and histologic neuroprotection than a temperature of 34°C.[34] More recently, in 7-day-old rat pups that were cooled immediately after hypoxia-ischemia, cooling to 33.5°C for 5 hours was neuroprotective compared with 37°C, with no additional protection with cooling to deeper temperatures of 32°C, 30°C, 26°C, or 18°C.[35] Similarly, in neonatal piglets, whole-body hypothermia with a reduction in body temperature of either 3.5°C or 5°C was associated with significant (and highly similar) overall neuroprotection after global cerebral ischemia, whereas a reduction of 8°C was associated with less neuroprotection.[36]

In part this loss of neuroprotection is likely related to the adverse systemic effects of cooling, which increase below a core temperature of approximately 33°C to 34°C.[37] In particular, after hypoxia-ischemia in newborn piglets, cooling to 30°C was associated with greater metabolic acidosis, increased blood glucose levels, and a greater risk of cardiac arrest and deaths compared with cooling to 33.5°C or 35°C.[38] Similarly, in adult dogs, deep hypothermia (to a rectal temperature of 15°C) after cardiac arrest was detrimental, whereas mild hypothermia (34°C to 36°C), from 10 minutes until 12 hours after cardiac arrest was beneficial.[39]

A WINDOW OF OPPORTUNITY FOR TREATMENT WITH HYPOTHERMIA?

At present, the window of opportunity for any particular therapy can only be determined empirically. However, some general principles can be discerned. For example, initiation of neuronal degeneration is accelerated by more severe insults. DNA fragmentation in the hippocampus can be detected as early as 10 hours after a 60-minutes of hypoxia-ischemia in the rat, but in the same paradigm, after 15-minutes of hypoxia-ischemia, DNA fragmentation in the hippocampus is detectable only at 3 to 5 days.[40] The appearance of DNA fragmentation and classic ischemic cell change represents only the terminal events of this cascade and is thus not a good guide to determining when cell death may still be reversible. In vitro studies have distinguished latent and active or execution phases during the process of programmed or apoptotic cell death.[41] Whereas the active phase involves downstream factors that could induce DNA fragmentation and chromatin condensation within previously normal nuclei, the preceding latent phase is characterized by caspase activation (a large family of enzymes that mediate and amplify apoptosis) confined to the cytoplasm, without activation of downstream factors.[42] These data suggest that it is the activation of intranuclear pathways of cell death that is the critical step corresponding to the transition from the latent to the execution phases of programmed neuronal death. Thus, in principle, it seems far more likely that intervention would be protective if it were applied during the initial, latent phase of programmed cell death rather than during the execution phase, even though the latter still precedes DNA fragmentation and cell death.[41]

Systematic in vivo studies support that the latent phase defines the window of opportunity for treatment with therapeutic hypothermia. In near-term fetal sheep, moderate hypothermia induced 90 minutes after reperfusion (i.e., in the early latent phase) and continued until 72 hours after ischemia prevented secondary cytotoxic edema and improved EEG recovery.[33] There was a concomitant substantial reduction in parasagittal cortical infarction and improvement in neuronal loss scores in all regions. When the start of hypothermia was delayed until just before the onset of secondary seizures in this paradigm, 5.5 hours after reperfusion, only partial protection was seen (Fig. 134.2).[43] With further delay (until after seizures were established, 8.5 hours after reperfusion), there was no electrophysiologic or overall histologic protection with cooling.[44] Similarly, in 7-day-old rat pups, mild (33.5°C) hypothermia for 5 hours was protective after a "moderate" (90-minute) duration of hypoxia-ischemia,[45] such that immediate induction of hypothermia after moderate hypoxia-ischemia significantly reduced the area of cortical infarction, with partial protection after 3 hours and loss of protection after 6 hours of delay. It is important to note that in that study, immediate hypothermia did not improve outcomes after very prolonged hypoxia-ischemia (150 minutes), illustrating that the window of opportunity for therapeutic hypothermia is dependent on the severity of hypoxia-ischemia.

HOW LONG IS SUFFICIENT FOR NEUROPROTECTION?

There is now detailed animal evidence that delayed hypothermia initiated during the latent phase must be continued for approximately 72 hours to achieve optimal neuroprotection.[46,47] Broadly, and critically for clinical practice, the greater the delay within the latent phase (i.e., within the first 6 hours after hypoxia-ischemia) before starting cooling, the greater the duration of cooling required to achieve some neuroprotection. For example, in adult gerbils, when the delay before initiating a 24-hour period of cooling was increased from 1 to 4 hours, neuroprotection in the CA1 region of the hippocampus after 6 months of recovery fell from 70% to 12%.[48] Critically, when the start of cooling was delayed until 6 hours after cerebral ischemia, protection could be restored by extending the duration of moderate (32°C to 34°C) hypothermia to 48 hours plus slow rewarming over 6 hours.[49]

Consistent with these findings, in near-term fetal sheep, delayed cerebral hypothermia, started 3 hours after ischemia and continued until 48 hours, was partially protective but significantly less effective both for the recovery of EEG power and neuronal survival than continuing cooling from 3 hours to 72 hours.[47] Given this compelling evidence from animals—that for optimal protection, hypothermia should be continued for at least 72 hours—there has been interest in whether further prolongation of the hypothermia might be associated with greater benefit. However, in near-term fetal sheep, when delayed hypothermia starting 3 hours after ischemia was prolonged from 3 to 5 days, there was no further improvement in electrophysiologic recovery or neuronal survival or reduction in cortical microglial induction.[46] Indeed, extended cooling was associated with a small reduction in neuronal survival in the parasagittal cortex and dentate gyrus.

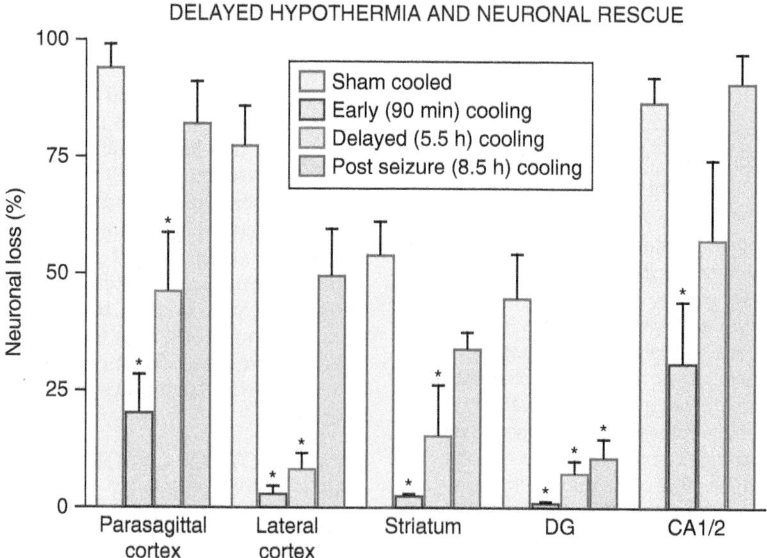

Fig. 134.2 Comparison of the effect of cerebral cooling in the fetal sheep started at different times after reperfusion and continued until 72 hours on microscopically assessed neuronal loss in the neuronal regions of cortex after 5 days of recovery from 30 minutes of cerebral ischemia. Compared with the sham-cooled group (n = 13), cooling that was started 90 minutes after reperfusion (n = 7) or just before the end of the latent phase (5.5 hours after reperfusion, n = 11) was protective, whereas cooling started shortly after the start of the secondary phase (8.5 hours after reperfusion, n = 5) was not. Only cooled fetuses in which the extradural temperature was successfully maintained at less than 34°C have been included. DG = dentate gyrus. *P < .005 compared with sham-cooled (control) fetuses, Mann-Whitney U test. Mean ± SEM. (Data from References 37, 38, and 39).

IS NEUROPROTECTION MAINTAINED OVER THE LONG TERM?

Studies in 7-day-old rats and in adults of other species have confirmed that a sufficiently prolonged phase of moderate cooling is associated with persistent behavioral and histologic protection for many weeks and months.[8,28] A few reports have suggested that hypothermia may only delay, rather than prevent, neuronal degeneration after global ischemia in the adult rat[50,51] and after hypoxia-ischemia in the 7-day-old rat.[52] The most likely explanation is that the duration or depth of hypothermia was insufficient to provide optimal neuroprotection, as suggested by the finding that 5°C of cooling for 6 hours,[28] or 2°C to 3°C for 72 hours in infant rats,[27] after carotid occlusion plus hypoxia, were both associated with long-term improvement.

An additional issue may have been rebound hyperthermia after early cooling. Even short periods of hyperthermia, 24 hours after either global or brief focal ischemia in the adult rat, exacerbated injury.[53,54] Similarly, in 10-day-old rat pups, a 1.5°C increase in brain temperature for several hours during induced seizures after hypoxia-ischemia was associated with exacerbation of neural injury up to 20 days later.[55] Further, when moderate hypothermia 2 to 9 hours after global ischemia in the adult rat was combined with the prevention of spontaneous delayed pyrexia with antipyretics, histologic protection was seen after 2 months of recovery.[51] Each intervention alone had essentially short-term benefit only. Whether mild hypothermia could have had additional benefit compared with normothermia in this late interval is, regrettably, unknown.

IS IT POSSIBLE TO COOL THE HEAD "SELECTIVELY"?

To provide adequate neuroprotection with minimal risk of systemic adverse effects in sick, unstable neonates, ideally only the brain would be cooled. Although this has been demonstrated experimentally using cardiac bypass procedures,[56] it is clearly impractical in routine practice. Pragmatically, partially selective cerebral cooling can be achieved using a cooling cap applied to the scalp while the body is warmed by some method such as an overhead heater to limit the degree of systemic hypothermia.[57] Mild systemic hypothermia is desirable during head cooling, first to limit the steepness of the intracerebral gradient that would otherwise be needed (avoiding excessively cold cap temperatures) and second to provide greater cooling of the brain stem. This approach was demonstrated in studies in the piglet to achieve a substantial (median 5.3°C), sustained decrease in deep intracerebral temperature at the level of the basal ganglia compared with the rectal temperature.[58] Similar results from studies of brief head cooling have been reported in the newborn rat.[59] Although direct temperature measurements are not feasible in the newborn infant, head cooling increased the gradient between nasopharyngeal and rectal temperature by nearly 1°C.[60]

In many ways, this approach is an extension of normal physiology. Even in the healthy neonate, there is no single cerebral temperature but a gradient from the warmer deep regions to the cooler surface.[61] The brain is a major source of heat production and is cooled by a combination of surface radiation and blood flow convection. Thus the deep brain temperature is approximately 1°C to 2°C higher than the surface of the head, 0.7°C higher than core body temperature, and increased during reduced perfusion, as occurs after severe asphyxia.[61]

MECHANISMS OF ACTION OF HYPOTHERMIA

The mechanisms of hypothermic neuroprotection are only partially understood. This does not affect its pragmatic clinical use, but it is critical to efforts to develop more effective strategies such as combining hypothermia with other treatments.[62] Broadly, it is now well established that cooling suppresses many of the pathways leading to delayed cell death. As well as reducing cellular metabolic demands, hypothermia reduces the excessive accumulation of cytotoxins such as glutamate and oxygen free radicals, suppresses the postischemic inflammatory reaction, and inhibits the intracellular pathways leading to programmed (i.e., apoptosis-like) cell death.[8] This suppression of delayed cell death pathways needs to be continued until the cell environment has recovered, in order to actively support cell survival.[63]

CEREBRAL METABOLISM, EXCITOTOXINS, AND FREE RADICALS DURING THE PRIMARY AND REPERFUSION PHASES

The combination of hypoxic depolarization and extracellular excitotoxin accumulation is a key factor in the initiation of neuronal injury in the primary phase. Hypothermia produces a graded reduction in cerebral metabolism of about 5% for every degree of temperature reduction, which delays the onset of anoxic cell depolarization.[64] However, the protective effects of hypothermia are strikingly disproportionate to the reduction in metabolism, and cooling improves cell survival even when the absolute duration of depolarization is controlled.[65] Cooling potently reduces the postdepolarization release of numerous toxins, including excitatory amino acids, nitric oxide, and other free radicals.[8]

Similarly, cooling begun during reperfusion reduces levels of extracellular excitatory amino acids and nitric oxide production in the piglet.[21] It is critical to appreciate that extracellular levels of excitatory amino acids rapidly return to baseline values after reperfusion.[21,22] Nevertheless, despite this rapid normalization of extracellular glutamate, a study of 10-day-old rats showed evidence of the pathologic hyperexcitability of glutamate receptors for many hours after HI, indicating that receptor blockade improved neuronal survival.[66] Similarly, in preterm fetal sheep, despite the suppression of background EEG activity for many hours after asphyxia, transient epileptiform activity was seen in the latent phase and correlated with the severity of neuronal loss in the striatum and hippocampus.[67,68] Suppression of these EEG transients with a glutamate receptor antagonist partially reduced neuronal cell loss.[69] Further, in the same paradigm, neuroprotection with postasphyxial moderate cerebral hypothermia was associated with marked suppression of epileptiform transient activity in the first 6 hours after asphyxia.[70] However, the combination of glutamate receptor antagonist infusion and hypothermia after severe asphyxia did not further improve hypothermic neuroprotection, consistent with the hypothesis that therapeutic hypothermia is partly protective by attenuating glutamate receptor hyperactivity.[71]

INTRACELLULAR PATHWAYS IN THE LATENT PHASE

The effects of hypothermia on pathways distal to cell membrane ion channels are likely to be more important. For example, intrainsult hypothermia did not prevent intracellular accumulation of calcium during cardiac arrest in vivo or during glutamate exposure in vitro.[8] Indeed, in adult rats, the apparent neuroprotective effect of NBQX, a glutamate antagonist administered from 1 hour after mild ischemia, was actually mediated by mild, drug-induced hypothermia rather than glutamate blockade per se.[50] Conversely, in vitro studies show that neuronal degeneration can be prevented by cooling initiated after the excitotoxins have been washed out.[8] Thus the ability of hypothermia to reduce the release of excitotoxins does not appear to be central to its postinsult neuroprotective effects. Rather, these data suggest that the critical effect of hypothermia is to block the intracellular consequences of HI.

Study or Subgroup	Hypothermia Events	Hypothermia Total	Normothermia Events	Normothermia Total	Weight	Risk Ratio M-H, Fixed, 95% CI	Year
NICHD 2005	32	102	22	106	16.0%	1.51 [0.94, 2.42]	2005
CoolCap 2005	29	108	20	110	14.7%	1.48 [0.89, 2.44]	2005
TOBY 2009	71	163	45	162	33.4%	1.57 [1.16, 2.12]	2009
Neo.nEURO 2010	21	33	8	25	6.7%	1.99 [1.06, 3.72]	2010
China Study Group 2010	32	59	15	49	12.1%	1.77 [1.09, 2.87]	2010
ICE 2011	42	106	22	97	17.0%	1.75 [1.13, 2.70]	2011
Total (95% CI)		**571**		**549**	**100.0%**	**1.63 [1.36, 1.95]**	
Total events	227		132				

Heterogeneity: $Chi^2 = 0.91$, df = 5 (P = 0.97); $I^2 = 0\%$
Test for overall effect: Z = 5.35 (P < 0.00001)

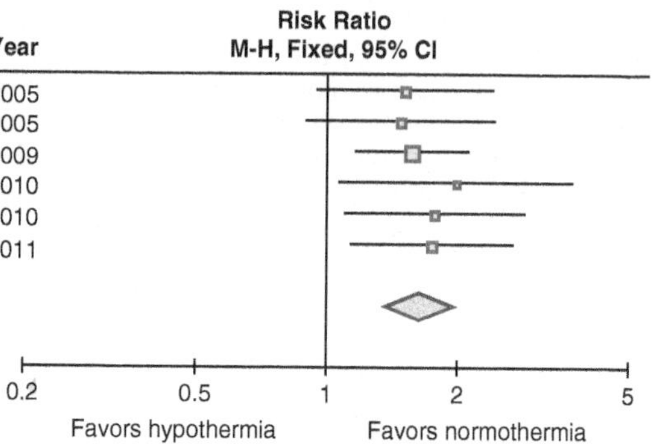

Fig. 134.3 Forest plot of survival with normal neurologic outcome at 18 months of age.[81–86] The diamond shows the overall summary estimate (the width of the diamond = 95% CI). *CI,* Confidence interval; *M-H,* Mantel-Haenzel test.

SUPPRESSION OF INFLAMMATORY SECOND MESSENGERS

Brain injury leads to induction of the inflammatory cascade with increased release of cytokines and interleukins.[72] These compounds are believed to exacerbate delayed injury, either by direct neurotoxicity and induction of apoptosis or by promoting stimulation of capillary endothelial cell proinflammatory responses and leukocyte adhesion and infiltration into the ischemic brain. There is good evidence that cooling can suppress this inflammatory reaction. As reviewed,[8] in vitro hypothermia potently inhibits proliferation, superoxide production, and nitric oxide production by microglia. In the adult rat, hypothermia suppresses the posttraumatic release of interleukin-1β and accumulation of polymorphonuclear leukocytes. Similarly, hypothermia reduces microglial activation after transient ischemia in the term-equivalent fetal sheep.[8] Thus these data suggest that the hypothermic protection against postischemic neuronal damage may be partly the result of suppression of microglial activation.

DOES HYPOTHERMIA SPECIFICALLY PREVENT OR SUPPRESS PROGRAMMED CELL DEATH?

There is now considerable evidence that hypothermia has a particular role in suppressing multiple programmed cell death pathways. In the developing brain, apoptosis is particularly prominent,[8] but pathways leading to delayed necrotic cell death are also involved, and studies in adult animals show that hypothermia can also prevent delayed necrosis.[73] As previously reviewed,[8] moderate hypothermia was associated with inhibition of apoptotic cell death and the expression of apoptotic factors after freezing-induced and ischemic brain injury in adult rats. Similarly, in the piglet, hypothermia begun after severe hypoxia-ischemia reduced apoptotic cell death, and hypothermic neuroprotection in the near-term fetal sheep was closely linked with suppression of activated caspase-3.[74]

SUMMARY

The experimental studies discussed in this chapter suggest that mild to moderate (32°C to 34°C) cerebral hypothermia continued for 72 hours and started as soon as possible (within approximately 6 hours) after hypoxic-ischemic injury could improve long-term neural outcomes. Based on these findings, a number of clinical trials were undertaken.

CLINICAL TRIALS OF HYPOTHERMIA

PILOT STUDIES

A number of small controlled trials of head cooling with mild hypothermia[57,60,75,76] or whole-body cooling[77] have reported that the cooling asphyxiated newborns was both feasible and apparently safe. Although none of these studies were powered to evaluate long-term outcome, there were apparent trends toward improved outcomes.[75,78,79]

LARGE RANDOMIZED CONTROLLED TRIALS

These encouraging safety data supported a series of large randomized controlled trials (RCTs). A Cochrane meta-analysis identified 11 RCTs involving 1505 infants that compared mild induced hypothermia with normothermia.[80] Overall, hypothermia was associated with a substantial reduction in death or neurodevelopmental disability to 18 months of age (RR 0.75; 95% confidence interval [CI] 0.68 to 0.83), number needed to treat 7 (5 to 10); from a total of 1344 infants in eight studies. The components of this combined outcome were also improved. Cooling was associated with both reduced mortality (relative risk [RR] 0.75; 95% CI 0.64–0.88) among 1468 infants in 11 studies, and with reduced risk of neurodevelopmental disability in survivors (RR 0.77; 95% CI 0.63 to 0.94) from 917 infants in eight studies. The effects of whole-body cooling and head cooling were extremely similar. In six trials involving 1120 infants that reported survival with normal neurologic function,[81–86] hypothermia was associated with a significant increase in normal survival (RR 1.63; CI 1.12 to 2.7; Fig. 134.3). The outcomes were strikingly similar among trials.

These RCTs were very similar in design. All involved the initiation of cooling within 6 hours of birth by either head cooling with mild systemic hypothermia or mild whole-body cooling for up to 72 hours. For example, in the CoolCap trial, infants with moderate to severe HIE were randomized to head cooling with mild systemic hypothermia, defined as a rectal temperature of 34°C to 35°C ($n = 116$) or conventional care ($n = 118$).[81] Death or disability at 18 months was reduced in infants with less severe EEG changes at trial entry ($n = 172$, odds ratio 0.42; 95% CI 0.22 to 0.80, $P = .009$). By contrast, however, there was no benefit in those with the combination of seizures and profound suppression of the amplitude-integrated electroencephalogram (aEEG) recording before cooling was started. The improvement was primarily due to a reduction in motor disability with a more than 50% reduction in severe neuromotor disability in survivors and improved continuous Bayley Scales of Infant Development (BSID)-II scores and no change in early neonatal mortality. The only consistent minor adverse effects were scalp edema under the cap, which resolved rapidly before or after removal of the cap, transient hyperglycemia from 4 to 24 hours compared with controls (mean ± SD, 7.6 ± 4.4 vs. 5.4 ± 3.1 mmol/L, at 4 hours, $P < .001$), and sinus bradycardia (a well-known physiologic response to hypothermia[87]) that did not require treatment. Conversely, there was an apparent reduction in the incidence of elevated serum transaminase levels in the cooled group (38% of cooled infants vs. 53% of controls, $P = .02$).

Similarly, in a further large multicenter trial of whole-body cooling from the National Institutes of Child Health and Human Development (NICDH), 208 infants were enrolled based on clinical and laboratory criteria consistent with exposure to severe perinatal hypoxia plus moderate or severe HIE.[82] Infants in the experimental group (n = 102) were cooled to a rectal temperature of 33.5°C ± 0.5°C for 72 hours using a cooling blanket. The incidence of death and/or moderate to severe disability at 18 months of age was significantly reduced in the cooled infants (45%) compared with the normothermic group (62%, RR 0.72; 95 % CI, 0.55 to 0.93). There was no difference for death or disability alone.

Subsequent trials had similar results. The Total Body Cooling trial (TOBY) in England compared cooling of the body to 33.5°C ± 0.5°C for 72 hours (n = 163) to standard care (n = 162).[83] There was no significant effect on death or disability (RR 0.86; 95% CI 0.68 to 1.07; P = .17) at 18 months of age but improved survival without neurologic abnormality (RR 1.57; 95% CI 1.16 to 2.12; P = .003), with reduced risk of cerebral palsy in survivors (RR 0.67; 95% CI 0.47 to 0.96; P = .03) as well as improvement in the Mental Developmental Index and Psychomotor Developmental Index of the BSID II. Similarly, the European neo.nEURO. network trial compared term neonates with HIE randomized to cooling to 33.5°C ± 0.05°C with a cooling blanket for 72 hours (n = 53) followed by slow rewarming or to standard care with normothermia (core temperature 37°C ± 0.5°C, n = 58). All infants were given prophylactic analgesia with morphine or fentanyl. There was a significant reduction in death or severe disability (51% in the hypothermia group vs. 83% in those with normothermia, P = .001; OR 0.21 [95% CI 0.09 to 0.54]) and fewer clinical seizures in the hypothermia group. It is unknown whether the routine use of sedation contributed to the apparent improvement seen in this trial.

The China Study Group reported a study of selective head cooling with mild systemic hypothermia initiated within 6 hours after birth to a nasopharyngeal temperature of 34°C ± 0.2°C and rectal temperature of 34.5°C to 35.0°C for 72 hours (n = 100) compared with standard care, with rectal temperature maintained at 36.0°C to 37.5°C (n = 94).[84] Head cooling was associated with a risk of death or disability of 31% compared with 49% after standard care (OR 0.47; 95% CI 0.26 to 0.84; P = .01).

Finally, the Infant Cooling Evaluation (ICE) RCT recruited from neonatal intensive care units in Australia, New Zealand, Canada, and the United States.[86] This study involved whole-body cooling induced by turning off the radiant warmer and then applying refrigerated gel packs to achieve 33.5°C ± 0.5°C for 72 hours (n = 110) or standard care (37°C, n = 111). Cooling was associated with a reduced risk of death or major sensorineural disability at 2 years of age (RR 0.77; 95% CI 0.62 to 0.98; P = .03). This study is particularly interesting because it showed that a very simple method could be used within strict protocols to induce hypothermia in nontertiary neonatal settings before transport.

An important observation from these studies is that in infants with HIE, mild hypothermia delayed recovery both of sleep state cycling on amplitude-integrated EEG monitoring[88] and neurologic recovery.[89] In the CoolCap study, for example, infants with moderate encephalopathy on day 4, after rewarming, had a higher rate of favorable outcome than those who received standard care; there was no effect of treatment on those with continuing severe encephalopathy.[89] By contrast, several clinical studies have confirmed that improved functional outcomes with treatment were associated with reduced structural damage on magnetic resonance imaging (MRI) and that the predictive value of the MRI was not affected by hypothermia.[90,91]

LONG-TERM FOLLOW-UP

There is increasing evidence that improved outcomes at 18 to 24 months of age are sustained at school age. The TOBY trial found a greater frequency of survival with an IQ score of 85 or higher at 6 to 7 years of age after treatment with mild hypothermia (75/145 children, 52%), than with standard care (52 of 132, 39%, RR 1.31; P = .04).[92] Further, more children treated with mild hypothermia survived without neurologic abnormalities (45% vs. 28%; RR 1.60; 95% CI 1.15 to 2.22), including a reduced risk of cerebral palsy (21% vs. 36%, P = .03) and moderate or severe disability (22% vs. 37%, P = .03).

Other studies have reported supportive outcomes. Follow-up of the NICHD trial showed a strong trend to reduced risk of death or an IQ score below 70 at 6 to 7 years of age, in 46 (47%) of infants in the hypothermia group and 58 (62%) after standard care (P = .06).[93] Similarly, follow-up of 62 of 135 surviving patients from the CoolCap trial suggested that functional outcome at 7 to 8 years was strongly associated with the previous 18-month neurodevelopmental assessment.[94] Thus these studies support the long-term predictive value of a favorable outcome at 18 months of age.

LONGER, DEEPER COOLING IS NOT BETTER

Consistent with the experimental data discussed earlier, a subsequent clinical trial of prolonged duration and increased depth of therapeutic hypothermia was abandoned due to lack of effect as well as safety concerns.[95,96] The adjusted risk ratio for death in the neonatal intensive care unit after cooling for 120 hours compared with 72 hours was 1.37 (95% CI 0.92–2.04) and for the 32°C compared with 33.5°C was 1.24 (CI 0.69–2.25). Further, there was no significant overall effect of longer or deeper cooling on death or disability at a mean age of 18 months.[96] Thus the current protocols for therapeutic hypothermia are essentially optimal. To further improve outcomes and awaiting the results of further research, it is important not to forget that the most effective way to optimize treatment with hypothermia is to avoid pyrexia and start treatment as soon as possible after resuscitation.[97] EEG recordings and other early biomarkers can help to identify patients who would benefit from treatment in this short time frame.[98]

SYSTEMIC EFFECTS OF HYPOTHERMIA

The RCTs discussed earlier show that mild hypothermia is generally safe. Meta-analysis suggests that hypothermia is associated with a significant increase in thrombocytopenia but no increase in hemorrhagic complications.[80] One small study did report an increase in systemic hemorrhage, although it was possible to manage this clinically.[99] It is unclear at this time whether this difference was due to deeper cooling, to a rectal temperature of 33°C as in the study from Eicher et al.,[99] or just a chance finding in a small study. It is reassuring that in piglets, where the cortex was cooled to less than 30°C after hypoxia-ischemia, no hemorrhagic changes were seen in the brain.[100]

The trials also highlighted the clinical importance of understanding the physiologic changes associated with hypothermia. In particular, a significant increase in blood pressure has been reported at the initiation of cooling both experimentally[43] and clinically.[101] This response is mediated by rapid peripheral vasoconstriction (i.e., centralization of blood flow).[102] Further, hypothermia slows the atrial pacemaker and intracardiac conduction. Consequently hypothermia to less than approximately 35.5°C is associated with mild but sustained sinus bradycardia not requiring treatment.[80] This relationship between heart rate and core temperature likely mainly reflects decreased metabolic demand with decreasing temperature. Some infants show marked prolongation of the QT interval above the 98th percentile (corrected for age and heart rate) without arrhythmia and during cooling that resolves with rewarming.[103] Although such isolated prolongation of the QT interval does not seem to be associated with an increased risk of ventricular arrhythmias, other therapies that lengthen the QT interval (such as macrolide antibiotics) should be avoided. A consistent metabolic effect associated with hypothermia was transient, mild hyperglycemia, both in adults[104] and infants,[81] but no change in the rate of hypoglycemia. A similar transient rise in glucose concentrations has been observed in the piglet and near-term fetal sheep[33,38] and likely reflects hypothermia-induced catecholamine release.

It is important to appreciate that although there was no increase in the rate of complications such as infection in the newborn studies, this must in part reflect the routine screening and treatment for possible infection included in the trials.[81,82] Hypothermia has profound antiinflammatory effects and in older adults seems to increase the risk of infective complications such as pneumonia and bacteremia[37,105]; thus this potential risk should continue to be carefully monitored in clinical use.

Finally, it is important to note that all these clinical trials involved term infants. It is unknown whether, in the setting of modern intensive care, selected late preterm infants with evidence of acute metabolic acidosis on cord blood and clinical encephalopathy would also benefit from hypothermia.[106] Studies in preterm fetal sheep at an equivalent stage of neural maturation now suggest that head cooling, started 90 minutes after profound asphyxia, can reduce the loss of white and gray matter.[68] Thus cautious clinical studies are in progress for late preterm infants with evidence of HIE (NCT01793129).

SHOULD WE COOL INFANTS WITH "MILD" HYPOXIC-ISCHEMIC ENCEPHALOPATHY?

The large RCTs of therapeutic hypothermia excluded infants who had "mild" HIE in the first 6 hours of life in order to increase the rates of unfavorable outcome; thus the potential benefit of treating these infants with therapeutic hypothermia is unknown. Meta-analysis of published studies suggests that approximately 25% of infants with mild HIE as defined using the trial criteria in the first 6 hours of life have abnormal neurodevelopmental outcomes.[107] Adverse outcome was defined as death, cerebral palsy, or neurodevelopmental test scores that were more than one standard deviation below the mean. Although most of these studies recruited on clinical criteria, a prospective cohort study of infants who were not treated with therapeutic hypothermia suggested that infants with mild HIE, determined by both early EEG and clinical examination, had adverse cognitive and neuromotor outcomes at 5 years of age compared with heathy controls.[108] Although intact survival was much greater after mild than moderate or severe HIE, survivors showed no significant difference in cognitive outcomes between those who had had mild compared to moderate HIE. It is critical to appreciate that some of these infants would very likely have been classified as having evolved to stage II (moderate) encephalopathy by Sarnat and Sarnat by 24 hours[109] based on longitudinal assessment of neurologic progress until hospital discharge or death plus multimodal assessment, typically including a formal EEG and imaging. Thus, it is not really possible to accurately define mild HIE in the first 6 hours of life.

Given that this population of infants with mild HIE in the first 6 hours is heterogeneous, the balance of clinical risk and benefit is unclear. Treating all cases of mild HIE would lead to a considerable increase in numbers of infants being separated from their parents for at least 3 days, receiving invasive treatments such as central lines, invasive respiratory support, sedation, and delayed oral feeding. Nevertheless, it is reasonable to reflect that there is evidence from young rodents that therapeutic hypothermia seems to be more protective after milder hypoxia-ischemia.[8] Taken as a whole, these data suggest that therapeutic hypothermia is likely to effectively reduce cell loss in infants with milder clinical HIE in the first 6 hours of life than in those who were included in the trials. Given that there are roughly as many infants with mild HIE as there are with moderate to severe HIE, it is critical that the benefits of treatment for this groups should now be formally tested.

CONCLUSION

There is now overwhelming clinical and experimental evidence that mild to moderate postasphyxial cerebral cooling can be associated with long-term neuroprotection. The key preclinical requirements for neuroprotection are that hypothermia be initiated as soon as possible in the latent phase, within the first 6 hours, before secondary deterioration, and that it be continued for a sufficient period in relation to the evolution of delayed encephalopathic processes, typically 72 hours.[8] These findings are now supported by large randomized trials of both head cooling combined with mild systemic hypothermia and whole-body cooling. It was also found that cooling is safe in the intensive care environment and associated with a significant improvement in survival without disability. These studies show that hypothermia is an important advance; as currently applied, approximately 15% of infants will have better outcomes after cooling compared with standard care.[80]

To further improve neonatal outcomes, it is vital to find ways of optimizing cooling protocols—for example, by combining hypothermia with adjunctive therapies. Several combination protocols are now in clinical trials.[110] Further, the CoolCap study suggested that EEG monitoring could identify a subgroup of infants with profound suppression of amplitude and onset of seizures at the time of randomization who did not respond.[81] It will be vital to refine these initial findings in focused experimental and clinical studies.

Thus although many questions remain regarding the optimal protocol for hypothermia, there is now strong evidence that mild, early hypothermia does improve outcomes, and we can now hope that a greater understanding of the determinants of protection with ongoing studies will yield further improvements in outcome.

ACKNOWLEDGMENTS

Our work reported in this chapter is supported by the Health Research Council of New Zealand, the National Institutes of Health, the Lottery Health Board of New Zealand, the Auckland Medical Research Foundation, and the Neurological Foundation of New Zealand.

A complete reference list is available at www.ExpertConsult.com. 

SELECT REFERENCES

8. Wassink G, Gunn ER, Drury PP, et al. The mechanisms and treatment of asphyxial encephalopathy. *Front Neurosci*. 2014;8:40.
10. Roth SC, Baudin J, Cady E, et al. Relation of deranged neonatal cerebral oxidative metabolism with neurodevelopmental outcome and head circumference at 4 years. *Dev Med Child Neurol*. 1997;39:718-725.
11. Iwata O, Iwata S, Bainbridge A, et al. Supra- and sub-baseline phosphocreatine recovery in developing brain after transient hypoxia-ischaemia: relation to baseline energetics, insult severity and outcome. *Brain*. 2008;131:2220-2226.
13. Jensen EC, Bennet L, Hunter CJ, et al. Post-hypoxic hypoperfusion is associated with suppression of cerebral metabolism and increased tissue oxygenation in near-term fetal sheep. *J Physiol*. 2006;572:131-139.
24. Colbourne F, Corbett D. Delayed and prolonged post-ischemic hypothermia is neuroprotective in the gerbil. *Brain Res*. 1994;654:265-272.
25. Thoresen M, Penrice J, Lorek A, et al. Mild hypothermia after severe transient hypoxia-ischemia ameliorates delayed cerebral energy failure in the newborn piglet. *Pediatr Res*. 1995;37:667-670.
28. Bona E, Hagberg H, Loberg EM, et al. Protective effects of moderate hypothermia after neonatal hypoxia- ischemia: short- and long-term outcome. *Pediatr Res*. 1998;43:738-745.
46. Davidson JO, Wassink G, Yuill CA, et al. How long is too long for cerebral cooling after ischemia in fetal sheep? *J Cereb Blood Flow Metab*. 2015;35:751-758.
47. Davidson JO, Draghi V, Whitham S, et al. How long is sufficient for optimal neuroprotection with cerebral cooling after ischemia in fetal sheep? *J Cereb Blood Flow Metab*. 2018;38:1047-1059.

48. Colbourne F, Corbett D. Delayed postischemic hypothermia: a six month survival study using behavioral and histological assessments of neuroprotection. *J Neurosci*. 1995;15:7250-7260.
74. Roelfsema V, Bennet L, George S, et al. The window of opportunity for cerebral hypothermia and white matter injury after cerebral ischemia in near-term fetal sheep. *J Cereb Blood Flow Metab*. 2004;24:877-886.
75. Battin MR, Dezoete JA, Gunn TR, et al. Neurodevelopmental outcome of infants treated with head cooling and mild hypothermia after perinatal asphyxia. *Pediatrics*. 2001;107:480-484.
80. Jacobs SE, Berg M, Hunt R, et al. Cooling for newborns with hypoxic ischaemic encephalopathy. *Cochrane Database Syst Rev*. 2013;1:CD003311.
81. Gluckman PD, Wyatt JS, Azzopardi D, et al. Selective head cooling with mild systemic hypothermia after neonatal encephalopathy: multicentre randomised trial. *Lancet*. 2005;365:663-670.
82. Shankaran S, Laptook AR, Ehrenkranz RA, et al. Whole-body hypothermia for neonates with hypoxic-ischemic encephalopathy. *N Engl J Med*. 2005;353:1574-1584.
83. Azzopardi DV, Strohm B, Edwards AD, et al. Moderate hypothermia to treat perinatal asphyxial encephalopathy. *N Engl J Med*. 2009;361:1349-1358.
84. Zhou WH, Cheng GQ, Shao XM, et al. Selective head cooling with mild systemic hypothermia after neonatal hypoxic-ischemic encephalopathy: a multicenter randomized controlled trial in China. *J Pediatr*. 2010;157:367-372.
85. Simbruner G, Mittal RA, Rohlmann F, et al. Systemic hypothermia after neonatal encephalopathy: outcomes of neo.nEURO.network RCT. *Pediatrics*. 2010;126:e771-e778.
86. Jacobs SE, Morley CJ, Inder TE, et al. Whole-body hypothermia for term and near-term newborns with hypoxic-ischemic encephalopathy: a randomized controlled trial. *Arch Pediatr Adolesc Med*. 2011;165:692-700.
88. Thoresen M, Hellstrom-Westas L, Liu X, et al. Effect of hypothermia on amplitude-integrated electroencephalogram in infants with asphyxia. *Pediatrics*. 2010;126:e131-e139.
89. Gunn AJ, Wyatt JS, Whitelaw A, et al. Therapeutic hypothermia changes the prognostic value of clinical evaluation of neonatal encephalopathy. *J Pediatr*. 2008;152:55-58.
91. Rutherford M, Ramenghi LA, Edwards AD, et al. Assessment of brain tissue injury after moderate hypothermia in neonates with hypoxic-ischaemic encephalopathy: a nested substudy of a randomised controlled trial. *Lancet Neurol*. 2010;9:39-45.
92. Azzopardi D, Strohm B, Marlow N, et al. Effects of hypothermia for perinatal asphyxia on childhood outcomes. *N Engl J Med*. 2014;371:140-149.
93. Shankaran S, Pappas A, McDonald SA, et al. Childhood outcomes after hypothermia for neonatal encephalopathy. *N Engl J Med*. 2012;366:2085-2092.
94. Guillet R, Edwards AD, Thoresen M, et al. Seven- to eight-year follow-up of the CoolCap trial of head cooling for neonatal encephalopathy. *Pediatr Res*. 2012;71:205-209.
96. Shankaran S, Laptook AR, Pappas A, et al. Effect of depth and duration of cooling on death or disability at age 18 months among neonates with hypoxic-ischemic encephalopathy: a randomized clinical trial. *JAMA*. 2017;318:57-67.
106. Salhab WA, Perlman JM. Severe fetal acidemia and subsequent neonatal encephalopathy in the larger premature infant. *Pediatr Neurol*. 2005;32:25-29.
107. Conway JM, Walsh BH, Boylan GB, et al. Mild hypoxic ischaemic encephalopathy and long term neurodevelopmental outcome - A systematic review. *Early Hum Dev*. 2018;120:80-87.
108. Murray DM, O'Connor CM, Ryan CA, et al. Early EEG grade and outcome at 5 years after mild neonatal hypoxic ischemic encephalopathy. *Pediatrics*. 2016;138. e20160659.

135 Early Development of the Human Auditory System

Kelsey L. Anbuhl | Kristin M. Uhler | Lynne A. Werner | Daniel J. Tollin

EARLY MORPHOLOGY AND PHYSIOLOGY

This section reviews the course of morphologic development of the auditory system and the physiologic correlates of these events in both humans and nonhumans. In studies of nonhumans, the function of the auditory system is primarily measured as electrical potentials recorded at the site of generation, such as single-neuron physiologic responses. Gross, scalp-recorded evoked potentials that result from auditory stimulation have also been used as an objective measure of auditory function.[1] Many of the same auditory capacities—sensitivity, frequency resolution, and temporal resolution—have also been measured in human fetuses and neonates. In the case of humans, these measurements are largely based on noninvasive, scalp-recorded evoked potentials. Although the same capacities can be measured in this way, it is more difficult to fully characterize auditory maturation when evoked potentials are used; in addition, a satisfactory approach to assessing auditory function in fetuses in utero has yet to be developed. Fortunately, despite these difficulties, many of the developmental trends that have been observed in nonhumans have also been observed in human fetuses and neonates.

PERIPHERAL AUDITORY SYSTEM: THE EAR

The ear is generally divided into three regional sections: the external ear, including the pinna and ear canal; the middle ear, including the tympanic membrane (eardrum) and ossicles (malleus, incus, stapes) suspended in the tympanic cavity; and the inner ear, including the semicircular canals, vestibule, and cochlea (Figs. 135.2 and 135.3). Sound waves enter the external ear and travel through the ear canal, where they reach the middle ear. The tympanic membrane and middle ear ossicles vibrate and amplify the sound, transmitting the sound energy to the cochlea—a snail-shaped structure that contains the sensory organ of hearing. Within this organ are sensory cells known as *auditory hair cells* that are responsible for transforming the sounds into neural signals. This occurs when deflection of the hairlike bundles of the hair cells (known as *stereocilia*) due to the incoming mechanical sound waves results in a pattern of electrical excitation that can be encoded by sensory neurons in the spiral ganglion for transmission to the brain (Fig. 135.4). A detailed account of current understanding of sound conduction and transduction in the auditory system can be found in Musiek and Baran.[2] Several classic texts describe the embryology and later morphologic development of the peripheral auditory system.[3,4] Texts on this topic are also widely accessible.[5] See Fig. 135.3 for an overview of the developmental time course of the peripheral system.

CONDUCTIVE APPARATUS

The external ear canal begins to form early in gestation, becoming easily identifiable by 6 weeks of gestation. The canal originates from the ectoderm that makes up the dorsal end of the first branchial groove. Initially, the ectoderm thickens and grows medially towards the tympanic cavity, resulting in the formation of a meatal plug or plate. The inner cells of the meatal plug subsequently degenerate, forming the ear canal. The distal end of the ear canal remains closed as it elongates and does not reopen until approximately 24 to 35 weeks of gestation. In addition, at around 6 weeks of gestation, six mesenchymal protuberances—the auricular hillocks—appear at the edges of the first branchial groove. The auricular hillocks fuse to form the pinnae, achieving adult form by approximately 18 weeks of gestation. Although the ear canal and the pinnae are well developed and fully functional at birth, both structures continue to grow in childhood with changes continuing into adult life. The tympanic membrane is also derived from the first branchial groove, where the most medial cells of the meatal plug eventually become the outer layer of the tympanic membrane. The mesenchyme, developing between the endoderm lining the presumptive tympanic cavity and the surface ectoderm, eventually differentiates into the collagenic fibers that give the tympanic membrane its elasticity. The developing tympanic membrane becomes thinner while expanding in surface area. The area of the membrane is largely adultlike by approximately 28 weeks of gestation.[6] The ratio of the large tympanic membrane surface area to the small area of the stapes footplate (the portion of the stapes attached to the oval window of the cochlea) allows the middle ear to overcome the impedance mismatch between the air-filled ear canal to the fluid-filled cochlea, resulting in efficient transmission of sound. Although this ratio has not been followed during development in humans, it is known that in cats there is little change in the ratio following the onset of hearing function.[7]

The mesenchyme that will form the middle ear ossicles is first identifiable at approximately 5 weeks of gestation. As the ossicles grow and begin ossification, the surrounding tympanic cavity expands and eventually suspends the small bones. The tympanic cavity continues to increase in size well into childhood. Between 21 and 40 weeks of gestation, the linear dimensions and mass of the ossicles are still increasing and continue to grow somewhat into the postnatal period.[8]

The conductive mechanism has several characteristics that appear to be common to all mammals through the development of the neonate, particularly at the point in development when responses to sound can first be recorded.[9] In general, the ear canal and pinna are relatively small; at birth, the human ear canal is only 14 to 15 mm long, whereas the adult canal length is approximately 23 mm long.[10] In some mammals, the ear canal may not be completely open at birth, and the walls of the canal of young animals are generally more compliant than those of adults. The middle ear cavity is also small, with partial ossification of the ossicles resulting in middle ear bones that are somewhat smaller and lighter than in the adult. In addition, the tympanic membrane of young animals tends to be less rigid than their adult counterparts.

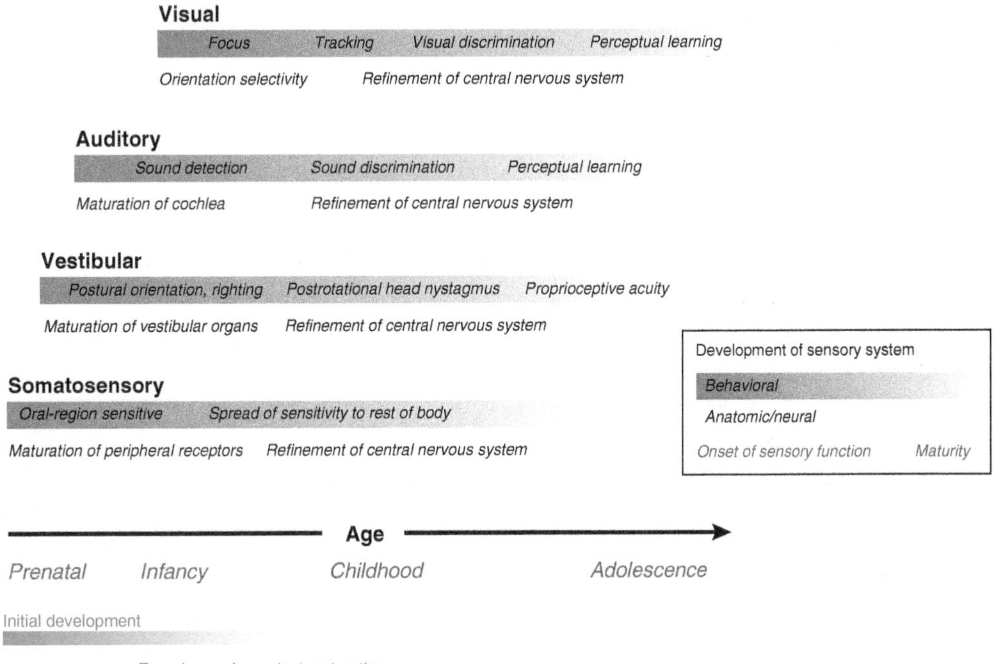

Fig. 135.1 The ontogenetic sequence of development of four sensory systems. (Adapted from Gottlieb G. Ontogenesis of sensory function in birds and mammals. In: Tobach E, Aronson LR, Shaw ES, eds. *The Biopsychology of Development.* New York: Academic Press; 1971:69.)

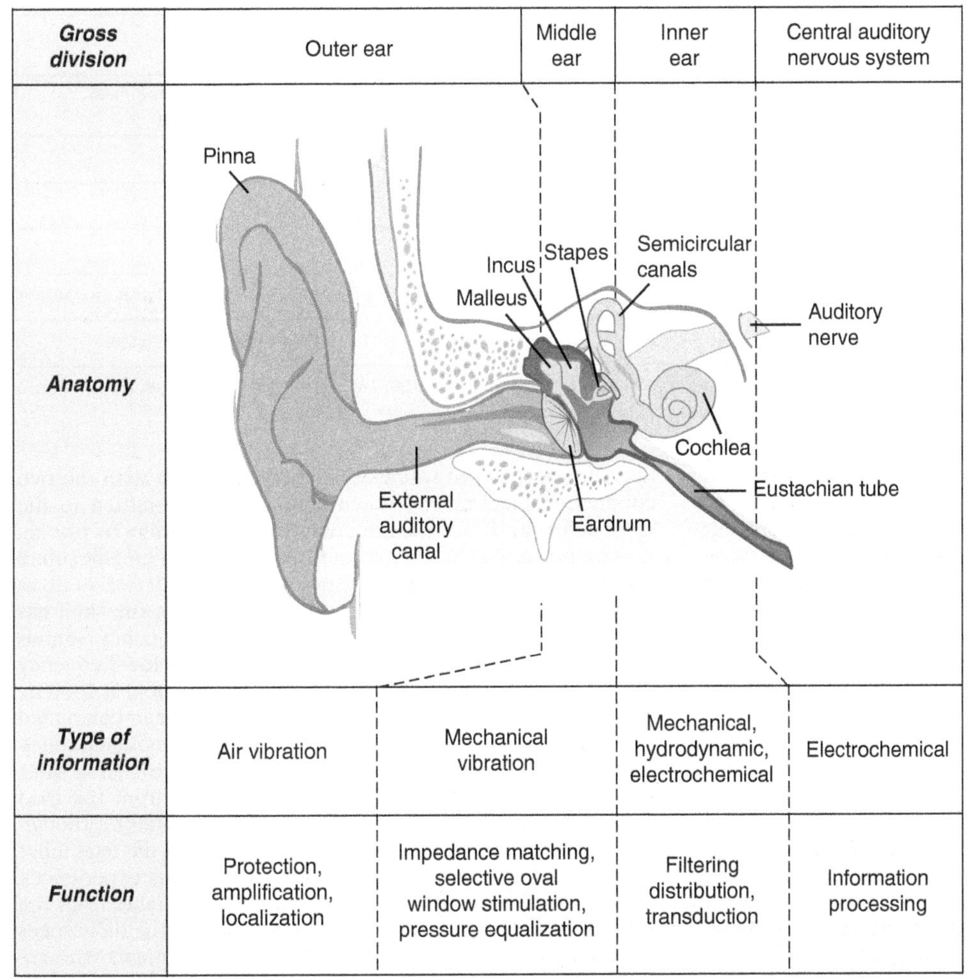

Fig. 135.2 Cross-section of the human ear, showing the external, middle, and inner ear and the major functions of each subdivision. (Adapted from Yost W. *Fundamentals of Hearing.* New York: Academic Press; 1994:62.)

Week of Development	Outer ear	Middle ear	Inner ear
3			Auditory (otic) placode; auditory pit (ectoderm)
4	First and second pharyngeal arches and grooves emerge (all germ layers)	Tubotympanic recess begins to develop (pharyngeal pouch; ectoderm)	Auditory vesicle (otocyst); utricular and saccular divisions emerge
5	Four well-defined arches and grooves are visible; first pharyngeal groove begins inward migration to form the external auditory meatus (ectoderm)	First pharyngeal groove and pouch approximate, initiating first and third layer of TM (ectoderm and endoderm); mesoderm grows between groove and pouch, initiating second layer of TM	
6	Auditory hillocks develop on the pharyngeal arches and surround first pharyngeal groove; external ear canal is identifiable	Development of ossicles initiated from pharyngeal arches; first Meckel's cartilage	Semicircular canal development begins
7	As mandible develops, auricles begin to migrate to side of head		One cochlear coil present; sensory cells in utricle and saccule
8	Cartilage of external auditory meatus formed (first pharyngeal groove; mesoderm)	Incus and malleus apparent (first pharyngeal arch; Meckel's cartilage)	Sensory cells develop in ampullae of semicircular canals
9		TM shows all three layers (all germ layers)	Afferent processes of spiral ganglion cells grow into the presumptive cochlea; stria vascularis appears; tectorial membrane rests on stereocilia of hair cells; inner and outer hair cells have differential developmental gradients
11			2½ cochlear turns present; nerve VIII attaches to cochlear duct
12			Sensory cells in cochlea; membranous labyrinth complete; otic capsule begins ossification (mesoderm)
15–16		Cartilaginous stapes present (second pharyngeal arch; Reichert's cartilage); malleus and incus begin to ossify	
18	Auricle shows adult shape; continues to grow in childhood	Stapes begins to ossify	
20			Inner ear is completely formed and adultsized
21	Meatal plug disintegrates	TM is exposed	
28		Surface area of TM is adultlike	
30		Middle ear pneumatization begins	
32		Malleus and incus ossified	
34			Stria vascularis is adultlike

Fig. 135.3 Overview of milestones in human development of the outer, middle, and inner ear structures. *TM*, Tympanic membrane. (From Moore KL. *The Developing Human Clinically Oriented Embryology.* Philadelphia: WB Saunders; 1998.)

Unlike humans, there are several species of mammals that have altricial hearing, where auditory function develops only after birth. The functional implications of conductive development are quite different for animals with altricial hearing than for those that begin to hear in utero. Perhaps the greatest difference in the development of the conductive ear is the environment in which the peripheral auditory system matures. In the case for neonatal animals that begin to hear after birth, the external and middle ears transform the spectrum of sounds reaching the inner ear in *air,* whereas for animals that begin to hear in utero, the external and middle ears are surrounded in a *fluid-filled* environment. Not surprisingly, this fluid-filled environment alters the normal conductive route to the inner ear. It is likely that sounds reach the inner ear via bone conduction through the skull instead of traditional conductive mechanisms (although how much sound reaches the fetus is a separate issue considered in a later section). Nonetheless, the cochlea responds similarly whether a sound arrives via air conduction through the middle ear or bone conduction through the skull. However, it is important to note that the spectrum of sounds is shaped differently with the two conduction mechanisms. When sounds are transmitted to the adult inner ear by bone conduction (this can be done by placing a vibration device on the mastoid process), much greater sound energy is required to elicit a response, on the order of 40 dB at 1000 Hz. Furthermore, bone conduction through the skull has a "high-frequency emphasis," where higher-frequency sounds travel much more efficiently through bone than low-frequency sounds. For example, in adults, the detection threshold at 1000 Hz is approximately 15 dB lower than that at 250 Hz for air-conducted tones but approximately 22 dB lower for bone-conducted tones. Of course, the fetal skull is not as well ossified as the adult skull, and in utero sound is transmitted to the skull from the fluid surrounding the fetus, not from a mechanical vibrator. Although it is clear that the route of sound transmission to the fetal inner ear will have substantial effects on what the fetus experiences, the nature of these effects is not entirely predictable from the adult bone conduction. One clear implication of the differences between air- and bone-conducted sound is that infants who are

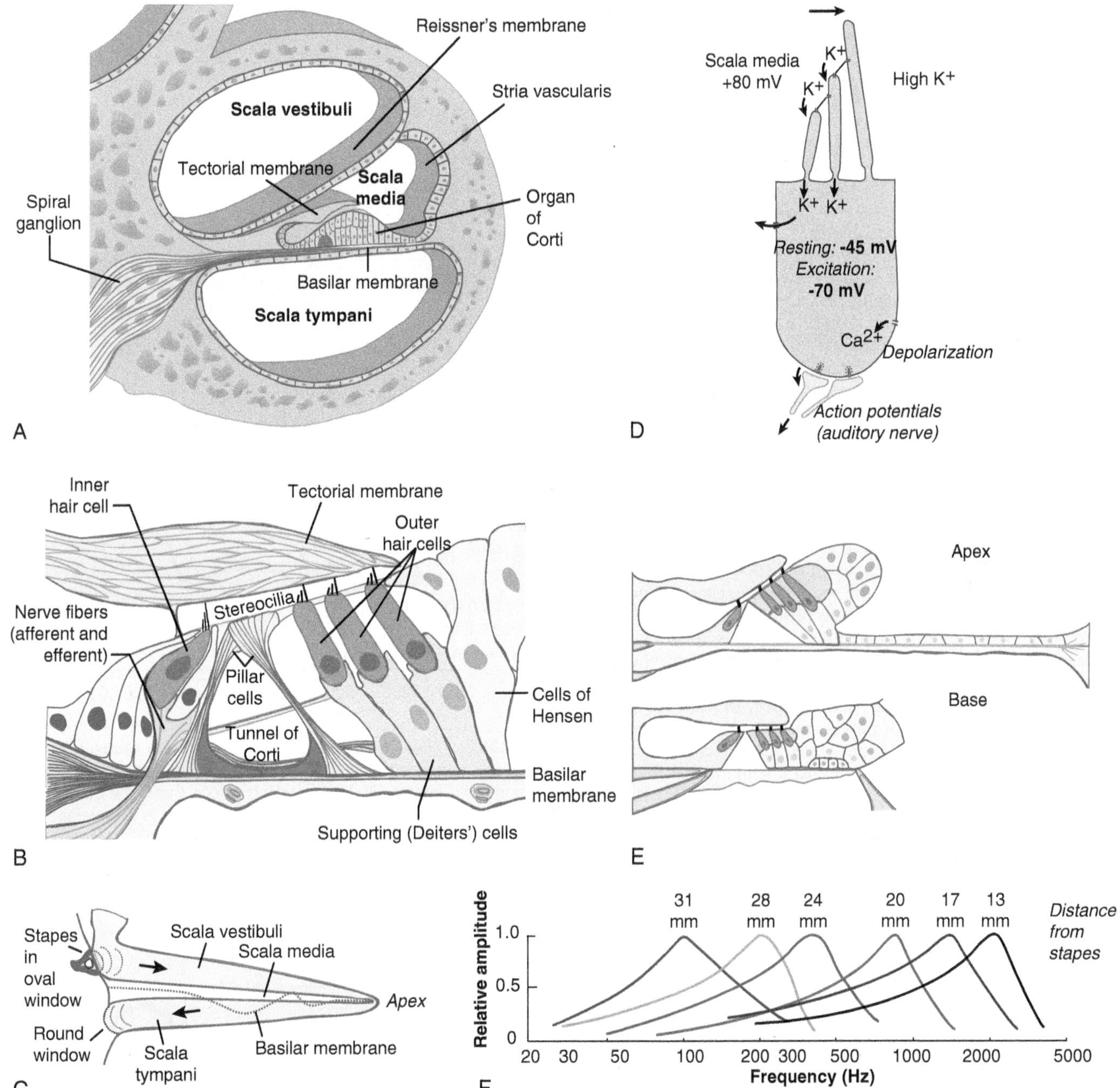

Fig. 135.4 Series of drawings illustrating the process by which sound energy is transduced into a neural response by the inner ear. (A) Schematic cross-section of the cochlear duct. (B) Cross-section through the organ of Corti. The hair cells are the auditory receptors responsible for transforming the sounds into neural signals. (C) Longitudinal cross-section through the uncoiled cochlea. Sound coming through the external and middle ear causes movement of the stapes in the oval window, which results in a traveling wave along the basilar membrane. (D) Movement of the basilar membrane causes deflection of the hair cell stereocilia, which opens ion channels in the stereocilia tips, depolarizing the hair cell and leading to a response in the auditory nerve fiber. (E) Schematic cross-sections through the organ of Corti near the apex and the base of the cochlea. The basilar membrane is wider and floppier near the apex and narrower and stiffer near the base. (F) The amplitude of basilar membrane displacement as a function of frequency at various locations along the basilar membrane, specified in distance from the stapes (cochlear base). The structural differences along the length of the basilar membrane result in maximum displacement for higher frequencies near the base of the cochlea and maximum displacement for lower frequencies near the apex of the cochlea. Thus the position of maximum activity along the length of the cochlea provides information about a sound's frequency. (Adapted from Pickles JO. *An Introduction to the Physiology of Hearing*. New York: Academic Press; 1988:28–30, 39, 60.)

born prematurely will be exposed to a qualitatively different set of sounds than they would have in utero.

The implications of having an immature conductive apparatus after birth lead to some predictions as to how sounds can be transformed by the developing structures. The resonance characteristics of a small ear canal and pinna suggest that for sounds of equal amplitude approaching the listener, high frequencies will reach the middle ear at relatively higher amplitude than low frequencies. If the ear canal is not fully open, of course, significantly less sound energy will reach the middle ear. The amount of attenuation due to a closed ear canal may be comparable to the attenuation due to another type of physical obstruction, such as earplugs; this has been described in detail by Lupo and colleagues.[11] In addition, the immature tympanic membrane and ossicles may decrease the efficiency of the middle ear in transmitting sound to the inner ear, resulting in a biasing of the sound toward lower frequencies. Studies of the acoustic response of the conductive apparatus in nonhuman species confirm these predictions.[12-14]

The acoustics of the external and middle ear have not been described in premature human infants, although data exist for 1-month postterm infants. The external ear data are in the form of sound-field-to-ear-canal transfer functions. These transfer functions show the level of sound in the ear canal as a function of frequency, when the intensity level of sound in the surrounding field is equal at all frequencies. In adults, this function shows a broad peak of approximately 10 dB between approximately 2000 and 5000 Hz as a result of the resonance of the ear canal and pinna (Fig. 135.5A). The peak resonance frequency of the adult external ear is typically given as 2700 Hz. Keefe and colleagues[15] characterized the acoustic response of the infant external ear, with the youngest infants being 1 month of age. The average resonance frequency in this age group was 4000 to 5000 Hz (see Fig. 135.5B), consistent with physical measurements of ear canal length. Thus, relative to adults, the level of sound reaching the neonatal middle ear at frequencies in the 1000 to 3000 Hz range is lower. They also found that the sound-field to ear-canal transfer function is not mature by 24 months postnatal age, and the age at which the transfer function becomes adultlike is not yet known.

Keefe and colleagues[16,17] have also published comprehensive studies of the acoustic properties of the infant middle ear. They have estimated the acoustic conductance, or flow of sound energy, in the middle ear of newborns and 1- to 24-month-olds. The results for newborns, 1-month-olds, and adults are shown in Fig. 135.6. The conductance of the infant's middle ear is smaller than that of adults for frequencies greater than 500 Hz, with the greatest difference at higher frequencies. For frequencies greater than 1000 Hz, some improvement in conductance occurs in the first postnatal month, but at approximately 4000 Hz, infants would be expected to lose 10 to 15 dB relative to adults. The combined effects of external and middle ear immaturity could account for the loss of sound intensity at higher frequencies. Conversely, at frequencies lower than 500 Hz, both neonates and 1-month-olds appear to generate higher levels of sound intensity in the middle ear than in adults. In fact, conductance for low frequencies appears to decline between birth and 1 month and again between 1 month and adulthood. This result is consistent with the presence of a low-frequency resonance in the neonatal ear canal, perhaps resulting from the greater compliance of the ear canal walls. Although this could further explain why tympanometry is not the optimal diagnostic tool in young infants,[18,19] it can still be used as a screening method.

It is often not appreciated that the growth of the pinna, ear canal, and head also has important implications for sound localization. The primary cues used to locate a sound source in the horizontal plane are differences in the timing and intensity of the sound arriving at the two ears.[20] Measurements in both human and nonhuman species indicate that smaller head dimensions produce smaller interaural differences.[21,22] Clifton and colleagues[22] measured head diameter longitudinally in a group of infants from birth to 22 weeks of age. From these measurements, they estimated that the largest interaural time difference (ITD) that an infant's head could produce increased from 420 microseconds at birth to 520 microseconds at 22 weeks of age. The average adult head, however, produces an ITD of approximately 700 microseconds.

Thus, for any sound source location, the infant experiences a smaller cue (Fig. 135.7). Similar effects would be expected for

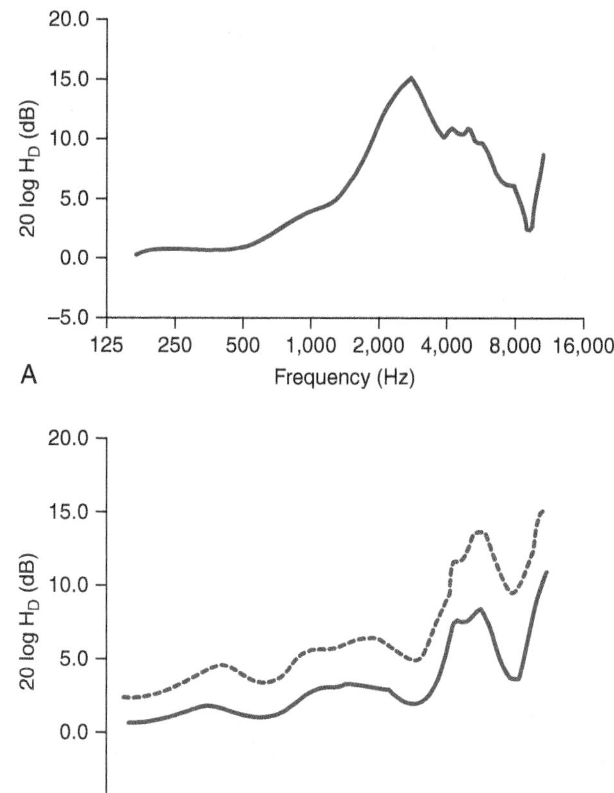

Fig. 135.5 Diffuse field sound-source to eardrum acoustic transfer functions measured in a KEMAR human adult manikin (A) and for 1-month-old infants (B). In panel (B) the *solid line* is the across-subject average transfer function and the *dashed line* is the average plus 1 SD. H_D, Diffuse field transfer function magnitude. (Adapted from Keefe D, Bulen JC, Campbell SL, Burns EM. Pressure transfer function from the diffuse field to the human infant ear canal. *J Acoust Soc Am.* 1994;95:355–371.)

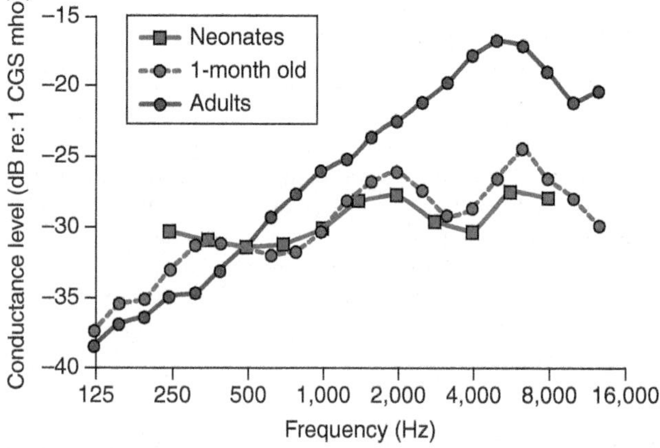

Fig. 135.6 Ear canal conductance level, indicating energy flow into the middle ear, as a function of frequency for adults, neonates, and 1-month-old infants. *CGS*, Centimeter-gram-second. (Adapted from Keefe D, Bulen JC, Arehart KH, Burns EM. Ear-canal impedance and reflection coefficient in human infants and adults. *J Acoust Soc Am.* 1993;94:2617–2638; and Keefe D, Folsom RC, Gorga MP, et al. Identification of neonatal hearing impairment: ear-canal measurements of acoustic admittance and reflectance in neonates. *Ear Hear.* 2000;21:443–461.)

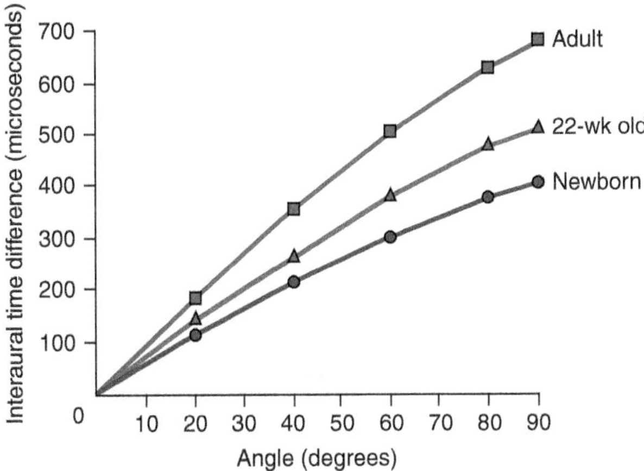

Fig. 135.7 Interaural time differences produced by sounds as a function of their position in azimuth, for adults, 22-week-old infants, and newborns. (Adapted from Clifton RK, Gwiazda J, Bauer J, et al. Growth in head size during infancy: implications for sound localization. *Dev Psychol.* 1988;24:477–483.)

interaural intensity differences. Interaural differences would also vary with sound frequency differently when the head is small: interaural intensity differences would be available at higher frequencies than in the adult, but interaural intensity differences in the midfrequency range would be relatively small.[21] Finally, the transformation of the sound spectrum, due to the pinna and the ear canal, changes with the position of the sound source relative to the ear. These "spectral cues" are used to localize sounds in elevation and to distinguish sound source locations behind the head from those in front of the head.[12] One would expect that smaller pinnae and ear canals would produce poor spectral cues for the localization of sound sources in the midfrequency range. However, the relative contributions of conductive, cochlear, and neural maturation to the development of sound localization remain to be established (although for a review, see Tollin[20]).

COCHLEA

The earliest structures that can be identified as external, middle, and inner ear arise in close temporal proximity. The otic placode, a thickening of the surface ectoderm at the level of the caudal hindbrain, can be seen early in the fourth week of gestation. The placode invaginates, closes off, and detaches from the epidermal surface to form the otocyst, or otic vesicle, a few days later. Shortly thereafter, the precursors of the spiral ganglion migrate out of the otocyst and orient at a location ventromedial to the developing inner ear. As the precursors of the specialized support cells and hair cells are born, the otocyst elongates, and the older cells are "pushed" towards the distal end of the presumptive cochlea.[23] The undifferentiated cells form a mass along the dorsal wall of the tube. The otocyst coils as it elongates, eventually forming two and a half turns of the cochlea by the 25th week of gestation. These events are illustrated schematically in Fig. 135.8.

The bony labyrinth that contains the cochlea begins to ossify at approximately 16 weeks of gestation, a process that is closely coordinated with cochlear growth and innervation. The growth, ossification, and differentiation of the inner ear structures require a complex series of regulatory interactions between epithelial and mesenchymal tissues. See Fig. 135.3 for an overview of the developmental milestones of the outer, middle, and inner ears (for a more comprehensive review also see Rubel[24]).

Studies describing the early development of the cochlea report similar developmental milestones in both human and nonhuman species.[24,25] As described in many vertebrates, the afferent processes of the spiral ganglion grow into the presumptive cochlea and make contact with undifferentiated

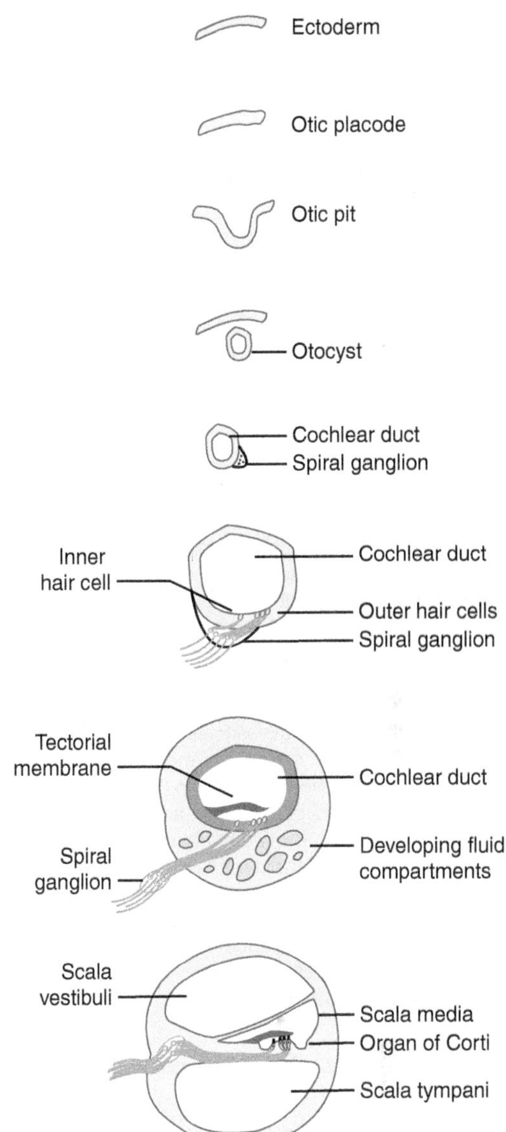

Fig. 135.8 Major events in the development of the inner ear. The otic placode, originating from the ectoderm, gives rise to the otocyst, which eventually gives rise to the membranous labyrinth of the inner ear that houses the auditory sensory organ.

cells by 9 weeks of gestation. Cells that will become auditory hair cells then separate from their basement membrane and migrate toward the luminal surface of the epithelium. Once the cells have reached the luminal surface, stereocilia form, and other features of hair cells become evident. Efferent processes are not identified in the cochlea until some time later, approximately 12 weeks of gestation in humans.[26] The stria vascularis, a highly vascularized tissue in the lateral wall of the cochlea, is responsible for maintaining the unique ionic composition within the cochlea necessary for hair cell mechanotransduction. The stria vascularis appears at 9 weeks of gestation and matures slowly between 14 and 20 weeks, becoming adultlike at 34 weeks.[27] The tectorial membrane, which rests on the stereocilia of hair cells, also appears at approximately 9 weeks of gestation. The inner and outer hair cells have differential developmental gradients: inner hair cells tend to differentiate and mature before outer hair cells, and innervation and differentiation of hair cells and their supporting cells tend to occur earlier near the base of the developing cochlea.[24] These developmental gradients have later functional implications because inner and outer hair cells play

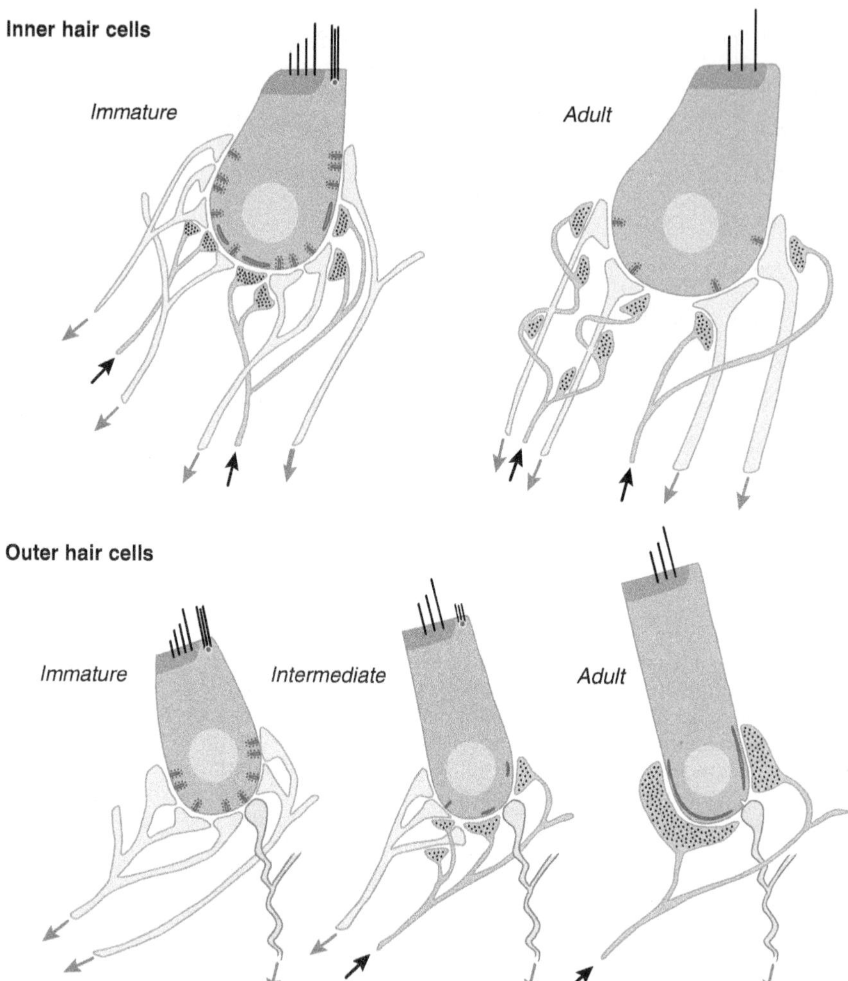

Fig. 135.9 Changes in the innervation patterns of inner and outer hair cells around the time that the cochlea begins to function. Efferents are dark gray fibers with vesiculated profiles and *inward arrows*. Afferents are light gray fibers with *outward arrows*. Inner hair cells *(top panel)* at the immature stage are characterized by a branching of radial afferents that make multiple contacts with the cell. In adulthood, the afferents are represented with their respective efferent synapses. Outer hair cells *(bottom panel)* at the immature stage only have afferent innervation (two types—radial: *light gray*; spiral: *white*). In adulthood, only spiral afferent and efferents forming large synapses are seen. (Adapted from Pujol R, Lavigne-Rebillard M, Lenoir M. Development of sensory and neural structures in the mammalian cochlea. In: Rubel EW, Fay RR, Popper AN, et al, eds. *Development of the Auditory System*. New York: Springer; 1998:146–192.)

different roles in the transduction process and because of the tonotopic organization of the cochlea, in which high-frequency information is coded at the basal end of the cochlea and low-frequency information is coded at the apex.

When responses to sound can first be measured in utero, the inner ear is largely immature in several respects. The fluid spaces within the cochlea are not well developed, the basilar membrane is thick, and the physical arrangement of the support cells and hair cells is immature (Fig. 135.9). In addition, the innervation of the hair cells is also immature.[26] In mature mammals, afferent endings predominate on inner hair cells, and efferent fibers synapse on afferent fibers, whereas in the developing mammal both afferent and efferent synapses can be found on the inner hair cell membrane. Mature outer hair cells are encapsulated by massive efferent endings at their basal membrane with a few small afferent endings. At the onset of hearing, the number of afferent and efferent endings contacting outer hair cells is roughly equal, and both types of endings are rather small and bouton-shaped (see Fig. 135.9). As with the other inner ear structures, the stria vascularis in utero differs from the adult in several respects, suggesting that the endocochlear potential, the "battery" that drives the transduction process, is immature. All of these factors contributing to immaturity are likely to limit the mechanical response of the cochlea. Although the cochlea has an adultlike appearance at the end of the second trimester, full cochlear maturity is not attained until just a few weeks before birth.

One implication of structural immaturity of the cochlea at this stage of development is that sensitivity to sound will be quite poor. More acoustic energy will be required to set the basilar membrane in motion, and energy will be transferred to the stereocilia less efficiently. Although inner hair cells are able to transmit their message to the central nervous system (CNS), the outer hair cells may be less efficient. The outer hair cells are known to act as effectors, mechanically amplifying the basilar membrane response and increasing the frequency specificity of the response. Without functional outer hair cells, hearing thresholds can be elevated by as much as 50 dB in mammals.[28]

It is well documented in nonhumans that the combination of conductive and cochlear immaturity is reflected in cochlear responses[29]; in single-unit responses in the auditory nerve, brain stem, and cortex[30,31]; and in gross evoked potentials.[32] When responses to sound are first observable, thresholds are quite high, on the order of 100 dB sound pressure level (SPL). Although the precise time course varies across species, sensitivity improves quite dramatically in the subsequent days or weeks. In humans, this rapid maturation of auditory sensitivity likely occurs between 24 and 35 weeks of gestation. Unfortunately, no data document the course of auditory physiologic development before approximately 28 weeks of gestation in humans.

Otoacoustic emissions (OAEs) are tiny sounds generated from the motility of cochlear outer hair cells that can be measured in the ear canal. The presence of spontaneous OAEs indicates normal function of cochlear amplification, and OAEs have been recorded in infants as young as 30 weeks postmenstrual age.[33] Two types of click-evoked OAEs are clinically available: transient-evoked OAEs (TEOAEs)[34] and distortion product OAEs (DPOAEs).[35] Click-evoked OAEs have been recorded in nearly all infants by 33 weeks postmenstrual age at a threshold 10 to 15 dB higher than that of adults.[36] The amplitude of OAEs to a fixed-level click also increases between 30 and 40 weeks postmenstrual age.[37] DPOAEs are frequency specific and can be recorded when two tones close in frequency, f_1 and f_2 (lower and higher in frequency, respectively), are presented to the ear; in this case, the emission is a pure tone with a frequency equal to $2f_1-f_2$. Lasky[38,39] recorded DPOAEs in preterm infants, term infants, and adults, finding that the minimum stimulus level required to elicit a DPOAE was similar across age groups, at least for stimulating tones at approximately 4000 Hz. Lasky concluded that nearly all of the observed age-related differences in DPOAEs could be accounted for by developmental differences in the resonance characteristics of the outer and middle ears.

The auditory brain stem response (ABR) is a scalp-recorded potential reflecting the summative response of neurons in the auditory nerve and brain stem. The ABR is typically characterized by five to seven "waves" approximately corresponding to different contributions of the ascending auditory pathway. For example, wave I of the ABR is known to arise from the auditory nerve, and wave V is largely thought to arise from the inferior colliculus. Adult ABR thresholds for a click are approximately 10 dB normal adult hearing level (nHL).[32] The ABR can first be reliably elicited from preterm infants at approximately 28 weeks postmenstrual age, although a few reports exist of responses at 26 or 27 weeks.[40,41] Lary and colleagues[41] reported that the average click intensity required to elicit an ABR decreased from approximately 55 dB nHL at 27 weeks postmenstrual age to 21 dB nHL at 38 weeks postmenstrual age. Subsequent studies have confirmed this result.[42,43] This pattern is consistent with an improvement in auditory sensitivity on the order of 25 to 30 dB between the onset of the response and term birth, but the relative contributions of conductive, cochlear, and neural sensitivity to the ABR threshold are not known. In addition, the latency of wave I has been shown to decrease between 33 and 44 weeks postmenstrual age.[40]

One result that is consistent across studies is that by the time of term birth, thresholds for cochlear responses elicited by broadband sounds are within 10 or 15 dB of adult values. This is the case for wave I of the ABR,[32] OAEs,[36] and electrocochleograms (scalp-recorded cochlear potentials).[44] Because a threshold shift of that magnitude can easily be accounted for by conductive factors,[19] these reports suggest that the cochlea is most likely mature by 40 weeks postmenstrual age.

Coincident with the improvement in sensitivity, a dramatic improvement occurs in the frequency selectivity of the cochlear response just after hearing begins in nonhumans. In the mature mammal, each inner hair cell and the afferent fibers connected to it respond over a range of approximately one third of an octave. When the cochlea begins to respond to sound, many auditory nerve fibers are essentially "untuned," and the best fibers respond over a range as broad as three octaves (Fig. 135.10).[45] Frequency specificity is closely correlated with sensitivity during development, and its maturation is likely the result of both mechanical maturation of the basilar membrane and the outer hair cells. Reduced frequency selectivity would likely result in many behavioral consequences, such as poor sensitivity in noise[46] and difficulty distinguishing similar frequencies. This is perhaps due to a "fuzzy" internal representation of the spectrum of complex sounds for naïve listeners.

Frequency selectivity at the cochlear level has been studied with DPOAE. It has been shown that the amplitude of DPOAE can be reduced by presenting external sounds that are close to the emission in frequency. In fact, the narrower the range of frequencies that will "suppress" the emission, the better the cochlear frequency selectivity. This can be visualized by generating a suppression tuning curve, which depicts the level of an external tone required to reduce the emission by a criterion amount as a function of the tone frequency. Abdala[47] has found that preterm and term infants demonstrate sharper suppression tuning curves, or better frequency selectivity, than adults (Fig. 135.11). Abdala argued that early in development, the human cochlea "overshoots" the amplification required; this has also been observed in young gerbils.[48] However, it is also true that suppression tuning curves measured at lower intensity are generally sharper than those measured at higher intensity. Thus, attenuation of the sound reaching the infant cochlea via an immature middle ear could be responsible for the age difference in tuning. This has since been supported by several findings.[49-51] Of course, neural limitations may also effectively limit the frequency selectivity of the system, as discussed later.

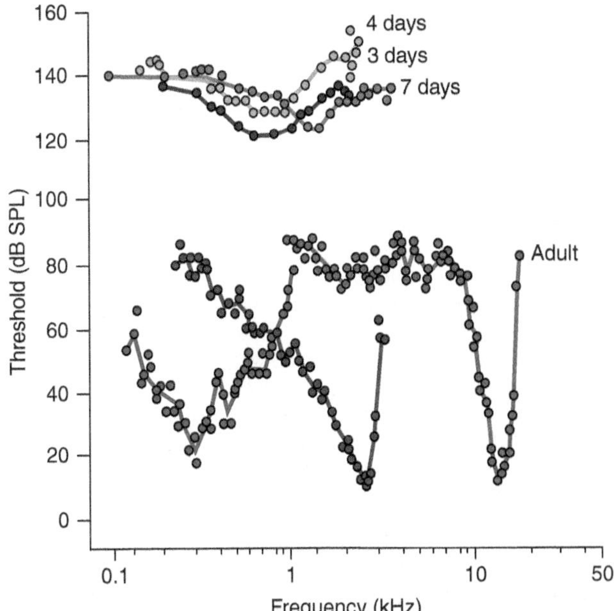

Fig. 135.10 Sound level required to produce a threshold response in fibers of the cat auditory nerve as a function of frequency. Each curve represents the response of a single nerve fiber. Adult responses are generally more "tuned" and tend to respond to very low sound levels within a restricted frequency range. Responses of 3- to 7-day-old kittens require very high sound levels and are not well tuned. *SPL*, Sound pressure level. (Adapted from Walsh EJ, McGee J. Postnatal development of auditory nerve and cochlear nucleus neuronal responses in kittens. *Hear Res.* 1987;28:97–116.)

As noted earlier, many events in cochlear development tend to occur in structures located at or near the base of the cochlea before they occur in structures located at the apex. Because the mass and stiffness vary along the length of the basilar membrane, different regions can produce greater responses based on the frequency of the incoming sound. For example, in mature vertebrates, high-frequency sounds produce greater responses at the base of the cochlea, whereas low-frequency sounds produce greater responses at the apex. Thus, one might predict that responses to high-frequency sounds might appear and mature earlier than those to low-frequency sounds. However, just the opposite is typically observed: the initial responses to sound are limited to the low or low-to-middle section of the mature animal's range of hearing. Then the range of frequencies that elicit responses gradually increases as sensitivity improves during development. The most likely explanation for this apparent paradox is that the basal cochlea is most responsive to relatively low frequencies at the time that it begins to respond.[52] Studies suggest that the immature frequency response of the basal cochlea is the result of mechanical properties of the basilar membrane.[48] Although such effects have yet to be demonstrated

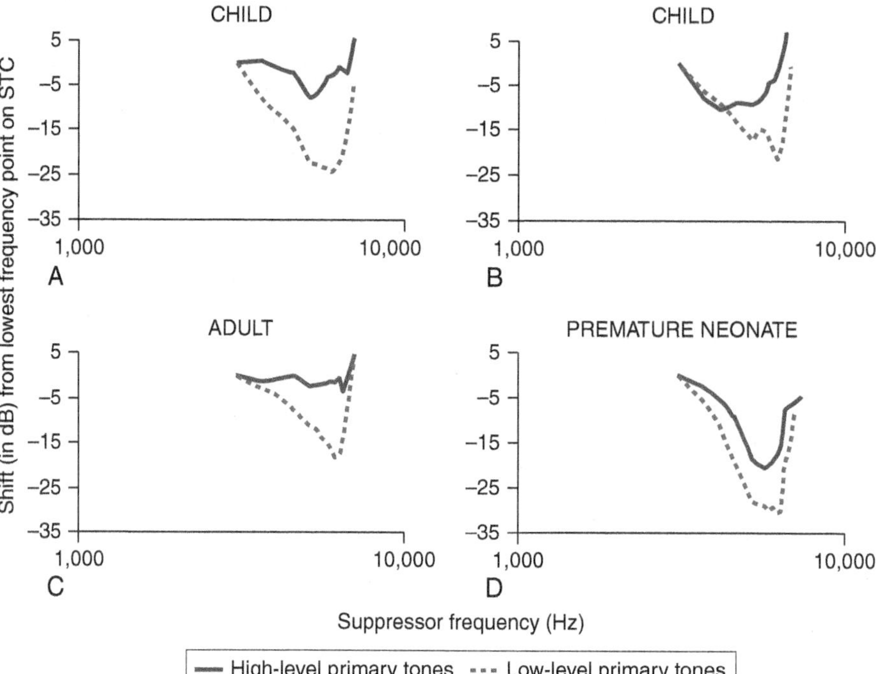

Fig. 135.11 Relative level of a suppressor tone required to suppress a distortion product otoacoustic emission, as a function of the frequency of the tone, so-called *suppression tuning curves (STC),* for high- and low-level stimulating ("primary") tones. Each emission tends to be suppressed with low-level tones close to its own frequency. (A and B) Responses from children 8 to 12 years of age. (C) Response from an adult. (D) Response from a premature infant. The premature infant's response is sharper than those of other subjects, and the sharpness is maintained at high levels of stimulation. (Adapted from Abdala C. DPOAE suppression tuning: cochlear immaturity in premature neonates or auditory aging in normal-hearing adults? *J Acoust Soc Am.* 2001;110:3155–3162.)

in humans, the refinement of frequency selectivity would be predicted to occur between 24 and 37 weeks of gestation.

Because cochlear responses can be readily assessed in neonates, OAE and ABR measurements are often used in newborn hearing screens. Congenital hearing loss occurs in 2 or 3 per 1000 neonates[53]; thus it is essential to use these measures to ensure early detection of hearing loss and institute proper course of rehabilitation.

EARLY HEARING DETECTION AND INTERVENTION PROGRAMS

TEOAE, DPOAE, and ABR have been shown to be equally sensitive screening measures with similar referral rates.[53] Concurrent measurement of middle-ear function may allow distinction between transitory or permanent conductive impairment and cochlear impairment.[17] Ideally, infants who fail the initial hearing screen undergo a comprehensive diagnostic hearing assessment before 3 months of age, and early intervention services (e.g., hearing aids, early language intervention) are implemented before 6 months. Early intervention is associated with near-normal language development by the preschool period. Early cochlear implantation is now a good option for infants with severe-to-profound hearing loss. It should be noted, however, that children with mild-to-moderate or unilateral hearing loss may be missed by early hearing detection and intervention (EHDI) programs. Furthermore, if OAE is considered in isolation, hearing disorders that result from auditory neuropathy/dyssynchrony will also not be identified.[54]

More than half of infants born with congenital hearing loss have genetic causes, with the remainder resulting from infection, exposure to ototoxic drugs, prematurity, or other environmental causes.[55] Hearing loss is associated with several hereditary syndromes, including Waardenburg, branchio-oto-renal, Stickler, Pendred, and Usher, among others. The majority of genetic deafness, however, is nonsyndromic. Tremendous progress has been made in the last decade in identifying the genes responsible for many types of nonsyndromic hearing loss. More than 70% of nonsyndromic congenital hearing losses are autosomal recessive; approximately half of these result from mutations of *GJB2* and/or *GJB6*. Approximately 1 in 33 people of northern European descent in the United States is a carrier of a recessive deafness-causing mutation of *GJB2*.[55] *GJB2* and *GJB6* encode Connexin 26 and Connexin 30, respectively. These proteins form the gap junctions that provide intercellular bridges for the recirculation of potassium ions into the cochlear endolymph necessary for the establishment and maintenance of the endocochlear potential. The other cases of nonsyndromic congenital hearing loss result from mutations of numerous other genes, and some of these occur in only one or two families.[55] Some types of genetic hearing loss, particularly syndromic and autosomal dominant types, have their onset later in childhood or in adulthood.[56]

CENTRAL AUDITORY NERVOUS SYSTEM

The limited data concerning the development of the human auditory nervous system are often found in articles dealing with the development of the whole brain.[57] Although this situation has begun to be remedied,[58–60] the available information with respect to human auditory neural development remains sparse. The available data do suggest, however, that substantial differences do not exist between the human and nonhuman development of the primary auditory pathways. The neurons of the auditory pathways in all vertebrates undergo final mitosis, migrate to their mature locations, and form appropriate connections in parallel with developmental events at the periphery; by the time that the cochlea begins to respond to sound, gross evoked responses can be recorded in primary auditory cortex.[61]

Between the 9th and 13th fetal weeks, all of the brain stem structures have formed their basic configuration, even though they will continue to increase in size.[62] However, brain stem structures are still immature at birth and may limit early sensitivity to sound. Sininger and Abdala[63] estimated newborns' frequency-specific ABR threshold, calibrating their stimuli in the ear canal to control for age differences in ear canal size. Their data show that newborns are close to adultlike in sensitivity at 500 Hz but are 20 to 25 dB less sensitive than adults at levels greater than 4000 Hz. The high-frequency age difference is greater than can be accounted for by middle-ear immaturity alone, suggesting an immature central auditory system.

Neural immaturities appear to limit the frequency selectivity of the auditory system early in human development. Two studies show that the ABR to a high-frequency sound is affected by a broader range of interfering frequencies, or "maskers," in 3-month-old infants than in adults.[64] This suggests that the frequency selectivity of the infant brain stem response is poorer at high frequencies. Because the cochlear response is largely mature by this age,[65] the source of the immaturity in frequency selectivity is likely to be neural. In premature infants, these immaturities may be more pronounced and extend to lower frequencies. Of course, at younger ages, cochlear immaturities may also be present, and it is not known how cochlear and neural immaturities may interact.

The work of Sanes and his colleagues has been important to understanding how neural maturation and experience with sound contribute to the development of frequency resolution. Sanes and Constantine-Paton[66] reported that young mice exposed to repetitive clicks displayed significantly broader frequency tuning curves than did normally reared mice, indicating that click-reared mice had a reduction in neural frequency selectivity. Sanes also ruled out the possibility that the periphery was compromised. Thus, acoustic environment that guides the selectivity of neural connections can affect frequency selectivity. This study and others indicate that immature animals must be exposed to a normal acoustic environment for the central auditory system to accurately represent different frequencies at the mature state. Moreover, Sanes and Rubel[67] noted that fine frequency selectivity was not characteristic of all neurons in the auditory brain stem. Within a single frequency region, both neurons with mature selectivity and neurons with very immature selectivity could be found in the developing animal. It was consistently found that frequency selectivity was significantly poorer in younger animals than in adult animals. Because all of these neurons receive their afferent input from the same brain stem location, it is still unclear why variability exists in the maturity of some neural responses. In other studies, Sanes and colleagues[68,69] directly measured the increasing specificity of developing neural connections in one auditory brain stem nucleus and showed that maturation of neuronal morphology correlated with maturation of neural response specificity. Finally, it should be noted that although some neural response patterns appear mature when described on a relative scale (i.e., when data are normalized by age-specific maximum responsiveness), they appear quite immature on an absolute scale (i.e., adult neural responses are more robust and reliable than those in immature animals). Thus, it is becoming increasingly evident that neural immaturities impose a fundamental limitation on early auditory function (for a review of mechanisms underlying development of ascending auditory pathways see Tollin[20]). In humans, structural maturation of auditory cortex continues until 11 or 12 years of age.[60,62]

Commonly reported characteristics of immature auditory neurons include being unable to sustain a continuous response[70] and a low maximum response rate.[71] Such response characteristics would have profound influences on all aspects of acoustic neural coding. These include a reduction in the range of sound intensities that could be processed, a diminished ability to distinguish changes in sound intensity, and a general reduction in acoustic sensitivity. The weak and "fatigued" responses of young neurons are almost certainly not a result of cochlear limitations, although they may play a role in the reduction of intensity sensitivity. Although no data are available in this regard for preterm infants, Durieux-Smith and colleagues[72] have reported a similar limitation in the neonatal ABR. In adults, the amplitude of the ABR increases with increasing sound intensity of the click presentation, whereas in term neonates, the response amplitude does not increase to the same degree as in adults (Fig. 135.12). Cornacchia and colleagues[73] reported that sensitivity to sound intensity in ABR measurements is adultlike by 6 months after term.

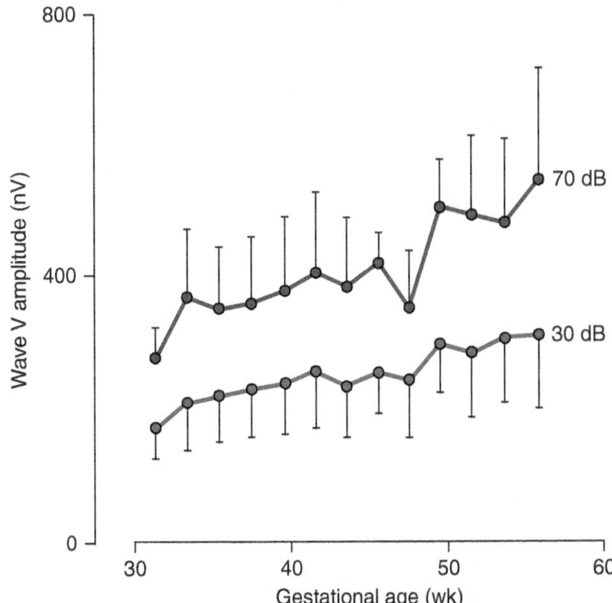

Fig. 135.12 Amplitude of wave V of the auditory brain stem response as a function of gestational age for two sound intensities. The effects of increasing intensity are greater at later gestational ages. (Adapted from Durieux-Smith A, Edwards CG, Picton TW, McMurray B. Auditory brain stem responses to clicks in neonates. *J Otolaryngol.* 1985;14:12–18.)

A means of rapidly conducting neural impulses over long distances is crucial for normal nervous system activity. In vertebrates, this is achieved by surrounding neuronal axons with myelin, which is largely produced by oligodendrocytes in the developing CNS. Myelination sheaths can be seen up to the glial junction, where the nerve exits the temporal bone.[62] The nuclei of the auditory pathway are well formed early in the second trimester with recognizable, yet immature, dendrites.[74] Between the 22nd and 26th weeks, anatomic staining can be done to identify the descending axons from the superior olivary complex of the brain to the organ of Corti in the cochlea. This staining illustrates the first of higher-level control of cochlear efferents.[75] Also during this time in development, the number of axons entering the cortex, presumably from the reticular formation, is increasing. During the 27th fetal week (the beginning of the third trimester), myelination occurs from the cochlea through the brain stem and up to the auditory thalamus.[62]

Increasing myelination increases the speed with which information is transmitted through the auditory system. Not surprisingly, the acquisition of myelin is a major step in CNS maturation and is reflected in the development of temporal aspects of the neural response. This is demonstrated by the decreasing latency of both single-unit responses and of gross evoked potentials during development, with greater changes in response latencies in more central nuclei.[31,70] Increased myelination might also be expected to produce improvements in auditory functions that depend on a precise temporal representation of the stimulus, such as with sound localization. Variability in the latencies of action potentials, both within and between neurons, would be reduced in nerve fibers that become well myelinated.

Response latency is the most frequently studied characteristic of evoked potentials in humans, and it is one of the few measures that has been made extensively for both preterm and term neonates. Gorga and colleagues,[40] for example, reported that between 33 and 44 weeks postmenstrual age, wave I latency of the ABR (corresponding to the auditory nerve) in response

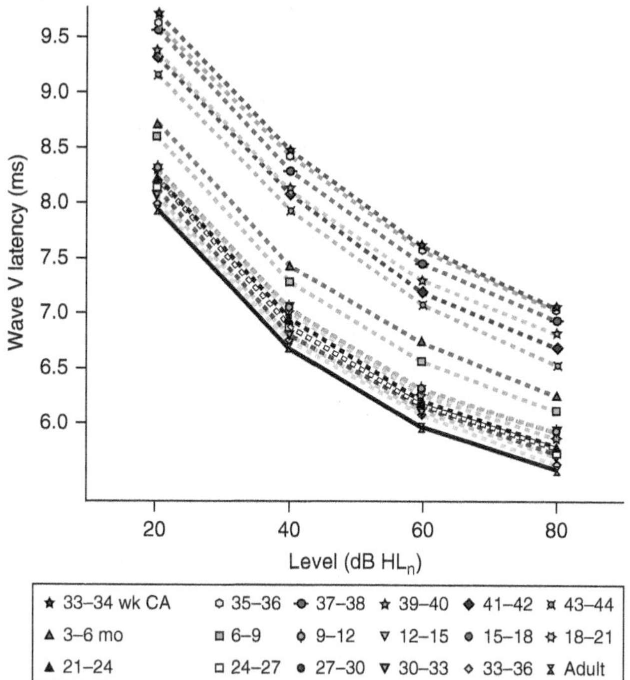

Fig. 135.13 Latency of wave V of the auditory brain stem response as a function of sound intensities at various ages. The curves are more or less parallel. *CA*, Conceptional age; *HL*$_n$, Hearing level re: normal. (Adapted from Gorga MP, Kaminski JR, Beauchaine KL, et al. Auditory brain stem responses from children three months to three years of age: normal patterns of response II. *J Speech Hear Res.* 1989;32:281–288.)

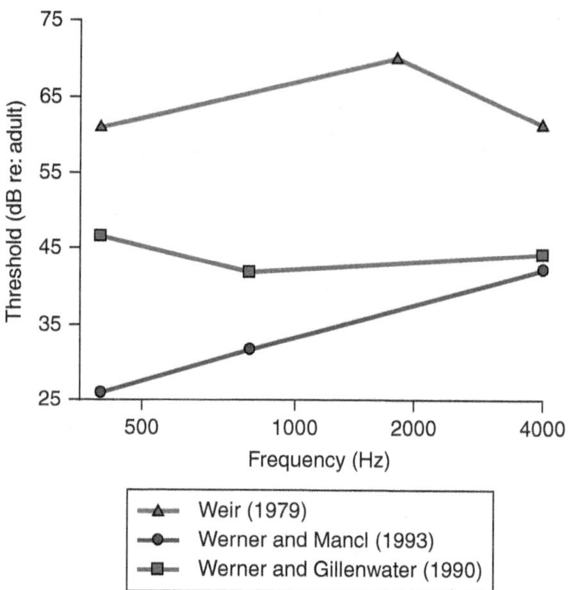

Fig. 135.14 Comparison of detection thresholds, expressed relative to adult threshold, at three frequencies from 0- to 1-month-old infants in three studies. (Adapted from Werner LA, Marean GC. *Human Auditory Development*. Boulder, CO: Westview Press; 1995.)

to 80 dB nHL clicks decreased from approximately 1.8 ms to approximately 1.6 ms. Wave V latency (largely corresponding to the inferior colliculus) decreased from 7.0 to 6.5 ms over the same period. It is thought that the greater decrease in latency for wave V is mainly due to greater neural maturation at this site. One interesting aspect of these results is that the effects of increasing sound intensity were no different for the youngest (33 to 34 weeks postmenstrual age) and oldest (43 to 44 weeks postmenstrual age) infants (see also Zimmerman and colleagues[76]). In fact, the effects of sound level on wave V latency were adultlike in the youngest preterms examined (Fig. 135.13). By 40 weeks postmenstrual age, wave I latency is close to adult values, but wave V latency continues to decrease into the second postnatal year (see also Hall[32]).

Two issues concerning the infant ABR have both developmental and clinical implications. First, some reports exist of rapid improvements in ABR detectability, amplitude, and latency in the first 48 hours after birth.[77-79] Explanations for these rapid postnatal changes vary. The typical explanation is that early postnatal changes result from clearing of fluid or other material from the middle ear,[80,81] although some argue that cochlear adaptation to extrauterine life is responsible.[82,83] Yamasaki and colleagues[77] found that the interwave interval between waves I and V, the so-called *central conduction time,* also decreased in the immediate postnatal period. It is not clear how differences in central conduction time could result from either conductive or cochlear factors. Although the reason for rapid changes in the ABR after birth is not conclusive, the general consensus is that stable ABRs are most readily obtained after 48 postnatal hours.

The second issue concerns the use of the ABR in the preterm population. It is not entirely clear whether extrauterine experience affects ABR parameters independently of postmenstrual age. In other words, it is unclear whether the ABR of a 40-week postmenstrual age infant whose gestational age is 32 weeks differs from the ABR of a 40-week postmenstrual age infant who was born yesterday. Although some studies report no differences between preterm and term infants of equal postmenstrual age,[84] Eggermont and Salamy[85] found that preterm infants tended to have longer wave latencies but equivalent interwave latencies. They propose that this difference arises from the higher incidence of otitis media in the preterm population. Collet and colleagues,[86] in contrast, report shorter interwave intervals among preterm infants and conclude that the smaller head size of preterm infants is responsible. In any case, the differences between term and preterm infants of the same postmenstrual age are small, and little evidence exists of a direct effect of extrauterine experience on the development of the ABR.

At least three factors influence the latency of evoked potentials and are possible explanations for developmental changes. First, sensitivity at sites peripheral to the generator of a given wave contributes to its latency. For example, latencies of all ABR waves are longer for lower intensities of sound and in cases of conductive or sensorineural hearing loss.[32] The changes in wave I latency with postmenstrual age are consistent with approximately a 20-dB conductive immaturity at 33 to 34 weeks postmenstrual age and a 10- to 15-dB conductive immaturity at term birth, as suggested by the middle-ear data.[16] To achieve a wave V latency of 7.5 ms, however, the data of Gorga and colleagues[87] indicate that a term infant requires a level approximately 25 dB higher than an adult (Fig. 135.14). It is clear that neither conductive nor cochlear factors can account for such a large difference. Second, myelination of the auditory pathway would increase conduction velocity; it is well established that myelination of the auditory pathways progresses through the postnatal period and into childhood.[57,88] This is the most clearly established contribution to ABR latency development, and by some accounts, conduction time improvements can completely account for changes in the latency of the ABR during development.[89] Third, synaptic efficiency may play a role. The number of synapses in the auditory brain stem continues to increase throughout childhood and into adulthood,[90] although synapse number does not necessarily equate to synapse efficiency. One finding does suggest that synaptic efficiency may be important as the ABR thresholds were positively correlated with behavioral thresholds at certain frequencies in early infancy.[91] No evidence exists that neural latency directly affects sensitivity; in fact, latencies can be very abnormal while sensitivity remains normal.[44] A loss of information resulting from inefficient synaptic transmission could very well affect both sensitivity and evoked response latency.

Other evoked responses, such as the middle and long latency responses that originate from the midbrain and cortex, have not been studied extensively in neonates (for a review see Hall[32]). It appears that the difference between infants and adults in threshold for the middle latency response (MLR), for example, is greater than the difference in ABR threshold,[92,93] and MLR latencies take longer to reach adult values.[94] Cortical responses have been recorded even in preterm infants,[61] but again the developmental course of such responses is prolonged. Although the factors that contribute to the delayed maturation of MLRs and late responses have not been delineated, their later development is consistent with the later myelination of the midbrain and cortical pathway.

Of course, latency is not the only temporal characteristic of neural responses. Because of the characteristics of the auditory transduction process, some auditory neurons tend to fire at the same phase of the stimulus on each cycle of a periodic sound; this neural response is said to be *phase-locked*. Mature neurons that exhibit phase locking are robust and precise, which allows for accurate estimation of the frequency of a sound on the basis of the interval between the phase-locked action potentials. The precision of neural phase locking is in part due to both the efficiency of synaptic transmission and the extent of myelination of nerve fibers. Phase locking is believed to contribute to pitch perception, among other things, and is the basis of ITD processing in sound localization. Of the basic auditory neural response properties, phase locking is the one that takes longest to develop. Brugge and colleagues[95] reported that phase locking in the auditory nerve of the cat developed over a 2-week period, with maturation first beginning with fibers responding to low frequencies. The development of phase locking at the level of the cochlear nucleus (the next "step" in the ascending auditory pathway following the auditory nerve) followed the same frequency gradient but took as long as 2 months to develop.[96] The course of phase-locking development in nuclei beyond the cochlear nucleus has not been described. The relative contributions of synaptic maturation and increased myelination (see later) to the development of phase locking have also not been assessed. One evoked measure of phase locking is the frequency-following response (FFR), a scalp-recorded response generated by continuous presentation of low-frequency tone stimuli. The FFR reflects the sustained phase locked activity in neural populations within the auditory nerve and brain stem.[32] Studies have examined the FFR in term neonates, and in general the response appears to be adultlike at birth.[97,98] Similar measures of phase locking at more central locations in the nervous system have not yet been developed. Again, no data on the development of temporal processing are available for preterm infants.

Another property of neurons that has implications for temporal coding is adaptation. Auditory nerve fibers show a characteristic high response rate at stimulus onset, followed by a rapid decrease in response rate to a lower, steady rate; this decrease in response over time is known as *adaptation*. After the offset of the stimulus, a recovery period occurs during which it is difficult to elicit responses from the neuron; even spontaneous activity is absent during recovery. Evidence exists that the immature auditory system is more susceptible to adaptation and takes longer to recover from its effects than the mature system. In human infants, increasing the rate of presentation of clicks used to elicit the ABR response has a greater effect on response latency for newborns.[80,99,100] The size of the latency shift with increasing stimulus rate decreases progressively between 28 and 50 weeks postmenstrual age.[101] This effect is more pronounced for wave V than it is for wave I, suggesting a neural contribution to the effect on wave V (largely thought to arise from the inferior colliculus). By 3 months of age, the ABR shows "rate effects" similar to those seen for adults. Responses originating at more central locations, such as from MLR and cortical responses, continue to be more susceptible to increased stimulation rate well into childhood.[102,103]

In a series of studies summarized by Altman and Bayer,[104] the first neurons to undergo their final mitosis, in nearly all auditory nuclei, were the neurons that in adulthood would respond to high-frequency sounds. The same gradient has been reported for at least some aspects of neural differentiation.[105] Although the first cochlear hair cells to undergo final mitosis are likely the ones that respond to low-frequency sounds,[23] the gradient in neural development mirrors the near basal to apical gradient of cochlear differentiation and innervation. Thus, the most mature cochlear hair cells would appear to be connected to the most mature neurons in each auditory nucleus. Interestingly, two studies of the frequency-specific ABR of human infants revealed a similar frequency gradient. ABR wave I-V interwave interval appears to mature first at mid to high frequencies of 2 to 4 kHz and later at both lower and higher frequencies.[106,107] ABR responses first start to mature for lower-frequency sounds between 1 and 2 years of age and mature for higher-frequency sounds between 2 and 3 years.

BEHAVIORAL DEVELOPMENT

An important, yet difficult, question to resolve is how the morphologic and physiologic properties of the fetal and neonatal auditory system are reflected in auditory behavior. Our current understanding of auditory sensitivity, sound localization, and speech perception are described in the following sections.

SENSITIVITY

In the last several decades, many studies of fetal motor or cardiac responses to external "sounds" have been published[108-113]; however, there are numerous methodologic difficulties with these studies. Many of these studies use an artificial larynx stimulator that is applied to the maternal abdomen. Because these devices deliver sound energy that is in the frequency range to which tactile receptors are sensitive,[114] it is possible that the fetus is responding to the tactile stimulation. In addition, the mother is often aware of when the stimulus presentations are occurring, so fetal responses to sound may actually represent the response to a change in the maternal physiologic state. In any case, the actual sound intensity delivered to the fetus can be estimated only in a very broad fashion, and it is difficult to estimate the level of intrauterine noise.[109]

Despite the technical difficulties, the general consensus is that the first fetal motor responses to sound occur at approximately 26 weeks of gestation. This is the case even in studies that use tighter controls on the stimulus and stimulus-delivery system.[110] The proportion of fetuses demonstrating responses increases progressively with gestational age,[108,110] and some indication is seen that older fetuses (34 to 39 weeks of gestation) respond to lower sound intensities than younger fetuses (26 to 28 weeks of gestation).[108,109] In general, the external SPL required to elicit a fetal response is on the order of 90 to 110 dB SPL. Lecanuet and colleagues,[111] however, reported late-gestation heart rate responses to a syllable played at an external level of only 80 to 90 dB SPL. They also showed that late-gestation fetuses responded most often to high-intensity, high-frequency (5000 Hz) sounds.[113] Although responses were recorded to 500- and 2000-Hz stimuli, these were less frequent and tended to occur only at the highest intensities presented. This finding is puzzling in that mammals that begin to hear after birth respond first to low- to middle-frequency sounds.[24] Differences in the transfer of sound through the maternal abdomen cannot account for the discrepancy as the maternal abdomen appears to attenuate frequencies greater than 1000 Hz rather dramatically.[109] The spectrum of intrauterine noise, however, is weighted towards low frequencies[109] and so may mask other low-frequency sounds. Perhaps the most important factor is that the spectrum of sound delivered to the fetal inner ear is shaped by the skull, rather than by the external and middle ears (see discussion earlier), so that the effective level of the high-frequency sound entering the system is higher than that of low frequencies. The apparent sensitivity differences across frequency could easily be accounted for by the acoustic properties of the skull.[115]

If the frequency dependence of the fetal response to sound is determined by how sound is transmitted to the inner ear, then one might predict that preterm infants' responses would be different. However, Gerber and colleagues[116,117] reported that both term and 29- to 37-week postmenstrual age neonates have a motor response to approximately only 25% of the presentations of a wide-band noise of 90 dB SPL centered at approximately 3000 Hz. Although Schulman[118] showed that preterm infants' heart rates changed in response to a doorbell with a level estimated at approximately 80 dB SPL, no information about the frequency dependence of the response is available.

Our knowledge of the fetal behavioral response to sound, then, is summarized as follows: fetuses begin to respond to intense external sounds at approximately 26 weeks of gestation. Late-gestation fetuses appear to respond to somewhat lower intensities, particularly for an appropriate stimulus, and to be more sensitive to high-frequency external sounds. High sound intensities are also required to elicit a motor response from preterm infants at the same postmenstrual age, but the frequency dependence of the preterm response is unknown.

Some studies have estimated thresholds for frequency-specific sounds among term neonates. These data are summarized in Fig. 135.14. Weir[119] used a combination of respiratory and motor responses to assess 1- to 8-day postterm infants' sensitivity to pure tones. She found that few infants would respond consistently to the stimuli, but those who did respond consistently had thresholds on the order of 30 to 70 dB higher than those of adults. Thresholds were more adultlike at lower frequencies. Subsequent studies in 2- to 4-week-olds using more sensitive measures of behavior have reported more realistic thresholds of 25 to 35 dB higher than those of adults between 0.5 and 4 kHz.[120]

Early threshold immaturity is at least partly accounted for by conductive immaturity. Immature brain stem pathways are also involved, as suggested by the similarity of the behavioral thresholds to those reported for the ABR by Sininger and Abdala.[63] Furthermore, Werner and colleagues[91] demonstrated a moderately high correlation (approximately 0.7) between behavioral threshold and ABR wave I-V interwave latency among 3-month-olds, suggesting that some factor such as synaptic efficiency is at least partially responsible for threshold immaturity in early infancy.

Regardless of the mode of sound transmission in utero, it is clear that fetuses hear and are affected by the sounds they hear. For example, newborn infants recognize their mother's voice very soon after birth and even recognize sounds and speech patterns to which they were exposed only in utero (for a review see Saffran[120]).[121] Additionally, during the beginning of the third trimester, ultrasound imaging can demonstrate infant responses to vibroacoustic stimulation.[108,122] These responses become consistent between the 28th and 29th weeks of gestation.

SOUND LOCALIZATION

Among the most widely studied of infant auditory capacities is the ability to localize a sound source. Interest in this topic stems from the observation that the cues to sound location, which are dependent on the physical size and shape of the head and the external ears, change after birth as the head and ears grow. It is thought that the central auditory system undergoes a developmentally sensitive period during which it adapts to this changing acoustical environment and accommodates the physical changes that are crucial for mature spatial hearing. In fact, the precision with which changes in sound source location can be detected improves progressively between term birth and approximately 5 years of age.[120,121]

Despite some early controversy on this topic,[123] it is now well established that term neonates are able to orient their head and eyes towards the direction of a sound source within hours after birth and even as early as 32 weeks postmenstrual age.[124] Neonates orient towards a sound source slowly, and their heads must be supported to allow the response to occur.[124] The frequency, duration, and repetition rate of the stimulus are important in determining whether a response will occur.[125]

Sound location is typically specified in terms of angle in azimuth—the horizontal plane intersecting the ears—and angle in elevation above or below that plane. Although nearly all studies of newborns' orientation to sound sources have asked infants to make only left-right discrimination choices, Muir[126] reported that the extent of the neonate's head turn towards a sound source was largely related to the position of the sound source in azimuth. Although infants can display excellent left-right discrimination of sounds, the precision with which they do so is not well established; however, by 1 month of age, infants respond to a change in azimuth on the order of 27 degrees.[120] The angle of separation needed to perceive a left-right change in sound source decreases progressively through infancy and early childhood to a value of 1 to 2 degrees.[120] Similarly, Muir[126] reported that neonates would turn their heads up or down appropriately towards sound sources above or below azimuth. Morrongiello and colleagues[127] have reported that infants can detect a change in elevation on the order of 15 degrees at 6 months of age; this value progressively decreases to 4 degrees among adults, similar to the developmental time course of left-right discrimination measures. Finally, although neonates are able to discriminate left and right sound source locations, they have difficulty in identifying sound source locations in reverberant environments.[124] Five-year-olds also have difficulty in localizing in reverberant environments,[121] whereas adults perform better at these auditory tasks.

The sources of early immaturity of sound localization are only beginning to be understood. Although physical limitations on head and ear size modify and limit the cues available for localization, it is clear that other factors are involved. According to head size measurements by Clifton and colleagues,[22] a newborn would need a change in sound source azimuth of 20 degrees to produce an ITD similar to that produced by a 10-degree change for adults. Recall that adults can detect changes in azimuth of 1 to 2 degrees, whereas newborns can only detect changes in azimuth of at least 20 degrees. Ashmead and colleagues[128] compared infant localization ability in free field with their ability to detect ITDs over headphones (a lateralization task). They found that infants could detect ITDs substantially better over headphones than in the free-field task. If sensitivity to ITDs were a constraining factor on the free-field localization studies, then the discrimination ability over headphones would be the same (lateralization tasks utilize a single cue only). Because they are not, this suggests that free-field sound localization uses other cues (interaural level differences, spectral cues) and that the ability to perform this task is a cue-integrative process. Thus far, infant sensitivity to interaural level differences is not well described.

To summarize, neonates as young as 1 month are capable of distinguishing the location of a sound source on the basis of auditory cues alone to an accuracy of approximately 25 degrees in both azimuth and elevation. Although the physical size of the head and ears limits the acoustic information available to neonates,[20] perhaps the greater limitation is the accuracy with which acoustic cues are encoded in the infant central auditory system and the precision with which the central system is able to extract, process, and combine acoustic cue information to generate an internal representation of source location.

SPEECH PERCEPTION

Some of the most interesting studies of infant auditory perception are those describing the infant's ability to discriminate between speech sounds. Eimas and colleagues[129] demonstrated that 1-month-old infants discriminated between /b/ and /p/, speech sounds differing in only one phonetic feature. Since that demonstration, the development of speech perception has been one of the most active areas of infant research. The results of these studies are easily summarized, although their interpretation may be more complicated than initially thought.A major finding is that even newborn infants appear to be capable of discriminating between all of the pairs of speech sounds that have been examined to date.[130] Furthermore, this ability appears to extend to the sounds of all spoken languages.[131] Second, although it is clear that the newborn can represent speech sounds sufficiently well to discriminate between sounds under many conditions, the newborn's representation of speech sounds may be less detailed than that of adults or older infants. The ability to make fine distinctions among speech sounds continues to develop into childhood.[120] Abnormal experience with sound may impair this process of refinement.[132] Third, infants appear to be sensitive to many aspects of speech besides phonemic distinctions. For example, they are sensitive to changes in intonation that signal clause boundaries.[120] Newborns are capable of distinguishing between different languages, although this ability depends on the native language to which the infant was exposed before birth, as well as the specific languages under consideration.[133]

The major events in the development of speech perception during the first year of life involve a progressive specification of native language sounds, sometimes at the cost of losing the ability to discriminate nonnative speech sounds (for review, see Werker and Hensch[134]). By 2 months of age, infants appear to recognize the predominant stress pattern that occurs in their native speech.[135] By 6 months of age, they tend to categorize the vowels of their native language in a broader way than they categorize the vowels of other languages.[136] The extent to which these tendencies depend on prenatal experience with speech sounds is not clear, and the age when infants first demonstrate these aspects of language-specific perception has not been determined.

By 12 months of age, infants have lost the ability to discriminate among many nonnative consonants.[120] Some nonnative consonants appear to be discriminable by infants and remain discriminable into adulthood, such as Zulu "clicks" by American speakers of English.[137] This appears to occur when the nonnative sound is so different acoustically from native sounds that the specification of native speech sounds has no effect on the nonnative speech category. Other speech sounds are discriminable by 6-month-olds, not discriminable by 12-month-olds, and remain very difficult for adults to discriminate, such as Nthlakampx (a native American language) or glottal stops by Canadian speakers of English.[120] In this case it appears that, as native speech sounds are specified, native speech categories "absorb" acoustically similar nonnative speech categories. Finally, some nonnative vowel sounds are discriminable by 6-month-olds and not discriminable by 12-month-olds but can be discriminated by adults, such as German back rounded vowels by Canadian speakers of English.[138] These observations suggest that the refinement of speech perception that occurs during childhood can redefine a native speech category in such a way that it no longer includes nonnative speech sounds that it may have "absorbed" early in development.

An important issue for future research in this area is the significance of specific language experience on both the initial specification of native language sounds and the subsequent refinement of speech sound categories. In particular, it is not clear what, how much, and when experience is necessary to properly learn language. Although these issues are difficult to address, they are very important ones for certain populations—preterm infants, infants with congenital hearing loss, infants with chronic otitis media—whose early experience with sound is abnormal to varying degrees. Preliminary findings by Uhler and colleagues[139] found no difference in the performance of new cochlear implant (CI) users and their normal hearing (NH) age-matched peers evaluated at the same time intervals. Uhler and colleagues conducted three longitudinal case studies in young children with hearing loss who received CIs and a cohort of NH children. These case studies found that a modified version of conditioned head turn paradigm could successfully evaluate the abilities of these newly implanted toddlers. These three toddlers could discriminate three out of five phoneme contrasts (i.e., /a-i/, /a-u/, /ta-da/, /pa-ta/, and /sa-ma/) presented at 60 dB by 3 months after initial activation of their CI. Further examination is needed to allow further insight on the impact of congenital hearing loss and speech-perception abilities.

A final note with respect to the development of speech perception is that despite the extraordinary ability of infants in processing speech, immature primary auditory processing remains an important constraint on speech processing. Six-month-olds require just as much of a boost in SPL to detect and discriminate speech sounds as they do to detect and discriminate pure tones.[120,140] In general, newborn infants are less sensitive to sound and may be particularly vulnerable to interference from noise, and their representations of the spectral shape of speech sounds may be "fuzzier" than those of older infants and adults. Newborn infants may be less capable of following rapid changes in a sound (but see Jusczyk and colleagues[141]). It is not surprising that their representations of speech are not detailed[130] or that adults exaggerate many acoustic properties of speech when they speak to infants.[142] In future studies, it will be essential to determine precisely how immature sensory processing limits early speech perception. In particular, it will be important to pinpoint the effects of early auditory deprivation on subsequent auditory perception and language-learning abilities and perhaps explore ways to amend these deficits.

CONCLUSION

Between the time that the cochlea begins to function during gestation and the neonatal period, the auditory system undergoes dramatic development. Although few data from humans exist, all indications from the available data are that the auditory system of a 28-week fetus is immature indeed: sensitivity is known to be poor, and both spectral and temporal representations of suprathreshold sounds are less precise. By term birth, hearing has improved dramatically; neonates are capable of discriminating among many complex sounds. Nonetheless, the term neonate is still less sensitive and less able to process the details of a stimulus than an adult. During very early development, the major contributor to improvements in hearing is likely the maturation of the cochlea. The central auditory system, however, continues to mature through adolescence, imposing limitations on hearing in the neonatal period. Beyond the neonatal period, as the central auditory system matures, higher cognitive-level processes such as attention and memory are also slow to mature, contributing to auditory perceptual immaturity until well after infancy.

ACKNOWLEDGMENTS

Preparation of this chapter was supported by grants from the National Institute on Deafness and Other Communication Disorders (R01DC011555 and R01DC017924 [DJT], F32DC018195 [KLA], and K23DC013583 [KMU]).

 A complete reference list is available at www.ExpertConsult.com.

SELECT REFERENCES

1. Moller A. *Hearing: Anatomy, Physiology, and Disorders of the Auditory System*. 2nd ed. Boston: Academic Press; 2006.
2. Musiek FE, Baran JA. *Auditory System: Anatomy, Physiology, and Clinical Correlates*. Boston: Allyn & Bacon; 2007.
5. Gulya JA. Anatomy and embryology of the ear. In: Hughes GB, Pensak ML, eds. *Clinical Otology*. New York: Thieme Publishers; 2007:3–35.
9. Pujol R, Hilding D. Anatomy and physiology of the onset of auditory function. *Acta Otolaryngol*. 1973;76:1-10.
11. Lupo JE, Koka K, Thornton JL, Tollin DJ. The effects of experimentally induced conductive hearing loss on spectral and temporal aspects of sound transmission through the ear. *Hear Res*. 2011;272:30-41.
12. Tollin DJ, Koka K. Postnatal development of sound pressure transformations by the head and pinnae of the cat: monaural characteristics. *J Acoust Soc Am*. 2009;125:980-994.
15. Keefe DH, Bulen JC, Campbell SL, Burns EM. Pressure transfer function from the diffuse field to the human infant ear canal. *J Acoust Soc Am*. 1994;95:355-371.
16. Keefe DH, Bulen JC, Arehart KH, Burns EM. Ear-canal impedance and reflection coefficient in human infants and adults. *J Acoust Soc Am*. 1993;94:2617-2638.
17. Keefe DH, Folsom RC, Gorga MP, et al. Identification of neonatal hearing impairment: ear-canal measurements of acoustic admittance and reflectance in neonates. *Ear Hear*. 2000;21:443-461.
19. Thornton JL, Chevallier KM, Koka K, et al. Conductive hearing loss induced by experimental middle-ear effusion in a chinchilla model reveals impaired tympanic membrane-coupled ossicular chain movement. *J Assoc Res Otolaryngol*. 2013;14:451-464.
20. Tollin DJ. The development of sound localization mechanisms. In: Blumberg MS, Freeman JH, Robinson SR, eds. *Oxford Handbook of Developmental Behavioral Neuroscience*. Oxford, England: Oxford University Press; 2010:262-282.
21. Tollin DJ, Koka K. Postnatal development of sound pressure transformations by the head and pinnae of the cat: binaural characteristics. *J Acoust Soc Am*. 2009;126:3125-3136.
22. Clifton RK, Gwiazda J, Bauer J, et al. Growth in head size during infancy: implications for sound localization. *Dev Psychol*. 1988;24:477-483.
24. Rubel EW, Fritzsch B. Auditory system development: primary auditory neurons and their targets. *Annu Rev Neurosci*. 2002;25:51-101.
25. Pujol R, Lavigne-Rebillard M, Lenoir M. Development of sensory and neural structures in the mammalian cochlea. In: Rubel EW, Fay RR, Popper AN, eds. *Development of the Auditory System*. New York: Springer; 1998:146-192.
29. Jones HG, Koka K, Tollin DJ. Postnatal development of cochlear microphonic and compound action potentials in a precocious species, Chinchilla lanigera. *J Acoust Soc Am*. 2011;130:38-43.
32. Hall JW. *New Handbook of Auditory Evoked Responses*. New York: Pearson; 2007.
33. Probst R, Harris FP. Otoacoustic emissions. In: Alford BR, Jerger J, Jenkins HA, eds. *Electrophysiologic Evaluation in Otolaryngology*. Basel, Switzerland: Karger; 1997:182-204.
34. Norton SJ, Gorga MP, Widen JE, et al. Identification of neonatal hearing impairment: evaluation of transient evoked otoacoustic emission, distortion product otoacoustic emission, and auditory brain stem response test performance. *Ear Hear*. 2000;21:508-528.
40. Gorga MP, Reiland JK, Beauchaine KA, et al. Auditory brainstem responses from graduates of an intensive care nursery: normal patterns of response. *J Speech Hear Res*. 1987;30:311-318.
41. Lary S, Briassoulis G, de Vries L, et al. Hearing threshold in preterm and term infants by auditory brainstem response. *J Pediatr*. 1985;107:593-599.
43. Guerit JM. Applications of surface-recorded auditory evoked potentials for the early diagnosis of hearing loss in neonates and premature infants. *Acta Otolaryngol*. 1985;421:68-76.
45. Walsh EJ, McGee J. Postnatal development of auditory nerve and cochlear nucleus neuronal responses in kittens. *Hear Res*. 1987;28:97-116.
47. Abdala C. DPOAE suppression tuning: cochlear immaturity in premature neonates or auditory aging in normal-hearing adults? *J Acoust Soc Am*. 2001;110:3155-3162.
51. Abdala C, Keefe DH. Effects of middle-ear immaturity on distortion product otoacoustic emission suppression tuning in infant ears. *J Acoust Soc Am*. 2006;120:3832-3842.
55. Toriello HV, Smith SD. *Hereditary Hearing Loss and its Syndromes*. Oxford, England: Oxford University Press; 2013.
60. Moore JK, Guan YL. Cytoarchitectural and axonal maturation in human auditory cortex. *J Assoc Res Otolaryngol*. 2001;2:297-311.
62. Moore JK, Linthicum FH. The human auditory system: a timeline of development. *Int J Audiol*. 2007;46:460-478.
63. Sininger Y, Abdala C. Auditory brainstem response thresholds of newborns based on ear canal levels. *Ear Hear*. 1996;17:395-401.
71. Sanes DH, Rubel EW. The development of stimulus coding in the auditory system. In: Jahn AF, Santos-Sacchi JR, eds. *Physiology of the Ear*. New York: Raven Press; 1988:431-455.
72. Durieux-Smith A, Edwards CG, Picton TW, et al. Auditory brainstem responses to clicks in neonates. *J Otolaryngol*. 1985;14:12-18.
73. Cornacchia L, Martini A, Morra B. Air and bone conduction brain stem responses in adults and infants. *Audiology*. 1983;22:430-437.
85. Eggermont JJ, Salamy A. Maturational time course for the ABR in preterm and full term infants. *Hear Res*. 1988;33:35-48.
87. Gorga MP, Kaminski JR, Beauchaine KL, et al. Auditory brainstem responses from children three months to three years of age: normal patterns of response II. *J Speech Hear Res*. 1989;32:281-288.
88. Moore JK, Perazzo LM, Braun A. Time course of axonal myelination in human brainstem auditory pathway. *Hear Res*. 1995;87:21-31.
91. Werner LA, Folsom RC, Mancl LR. The relationship between auditory brainstem response latencies and behavioral thresholds in normal hearing infants and adults. *Hear Res*. 1994;77:88-98.
108. Birnholz JC, Benacerraf BR. The development of human fetal hearing. *Science*. 1983;222:516-518.
109. Querleu D, Renard X, Versyp F, et al. Fetal hearing. *Eur J Obstet Gynecol Reprod Biol*. 1988;29:191-212.
119. Weir C. Auditory frequency sensitivity of human newborns: some data with improved acoustic and behavioral controls. *Percept Psychophys*. 1979;26:287-294.
120. Saffran J, Werker J, Werner LA. The infant's auditory world: hearing, speech and the beginnings of language. In: Kuhn D, Siegler RS, eds. *Handbook of Child Psychology*. Vol 2. 6th ed. New York: John Wiley & Sons; 2006:58-108.
121. Litovsky RY. Developmental changes in the precedence effect: estimates of minimum audible angle. *J Acoust Soc Am*. 1997;102:1739-1745.
122. Abrams RM, Gerhardt KJ. The acoustic environment and physiological responses of the fetus. *J Perinatol*. 2000;20:S31-S36.
126. Muir D. The development of infants' auditory spatial sensitivity. In: Trehub SE, Schneider BA, eds. *Auditory Development in Infancy*. New York: Plenum Press; 1985:51-84.
129. Eimas PD, Siqueland ER, Jusczyk P, Vigorito J. Speech perception in infants. *Science*. 1971;171:303-306.
132. Clarkson RL, Eimas PD, Marean GC. Speech perception in children with histories of recurrent otitis media. *J Acoust Soc Am*. 1989;85:926-933.
133. Mehler J, Jusczyk PW, Lambertz G, et al. A precursor of language acquisition in young infants. *Cognition*. 1988;29:143-178.
137. Best CT, McRoberts GW, Sithole NM. Examination of perceptual reorganization for nonnative speech contrasts: Zulu click discrimination by English-speaking adults and infants. *J Exp Psychol Hum Percept Perform*. 1988;14:345-360.
138. Werker JK, Polka L. Developmental changes in speech perception: new challenges and new directions. *J Phon*. 1993;21:83-101.
139. Uhler K, Yoshinaga-Itano C, Gabbard SA, et al. Longitudinal infant speech perception in young cochlear implant users. *J Am Acad Audiol*. 2011;22:129-142.
141. Jusczyk PW, Pisoni DB, Reed MA, et al. Infants' discrimination of the duration of a rapid spectrum change in nonspeech signals. *Science*. 1983;222:175-177.

Development of Olfaction and Taste in the Human Fetus and Neonate

136

Harvey B. Sarnat

OLFACTION

Perception of odorous molecules is the oldest special sense in both phylogeny and ontogeny. Olfaction is the earliest special sense in evolution; even polyps and jellyfishes, possessing only a loose neural net without a brain or even a ganglion, can perceive noxious odors and chemicals in their surrounding water and retract in response, or respond positively to attractants (i.e., food), noted as early as 1849 by Thomas Huxley.[1] However, it is difficult to know whether perception of soluble molecules in seawater should be designated olfactory or gustatory. The human fetus can perceive odors in the amniotic fluid that circulates through the nasal passages as soon as the nasal epithelial plug resolves in the early second trimester. Though olfaction and taste are mediated by different cranial nerves in remote parts of the brain, their functional distinction is blurred. Even the adult enjoyment of food and wine combines smell and taste.[2,3]

A primordial olfactory bulb appears at 41 days gestation as a ventrorostral outgrowth of the newly formed telencephalic hemispheres after prosencephalic cleavage.[4,5] It is a prominent structure of the ventral telencephalon with the volume ratio becoming relatively less as gestation progresses (Fig. 136.1). The mature olfactory bulb exhibits laminar architecture unlike that of the cerebral, cerebellar, or other cortices. Its unique organization is, in part, because none of its neurons arise from the intrinsic neural tissue of the olfactory bulb itself during ontogenesis; neuroblasts stream into the olfactory bulb from the rostral telencephalon and then secondarily migrate radially. This *rostral migratory stream* is present in all vertebrate embryos.[6-10] The olfactory tract also is unlike any other white matter fasciculus and is much more than a simple bundle of axons. It includes as much grey as white matter because granular neurons extend into it from the olfactory bulb at one end as do pyramidal neurons of the anterior olfactory nucleus from the other. In addition, resident progenitor "stem" cells capable of neuronal differentiation are present in the olfactory bulb and tract of both the fetus and the adult; the only other reservoir of such progenitor cells in the mature brain is in the polymorphic layer beneath the hippocampal dentate gyrus. Primary olfactory neurons residing in the nasal epithelium exhibit continuous turnover and extraordinary regenerative capacity in both the fetus and adult, unmatched in any other structure of the nervous system. If primary olfactory neurons could not regenerate, irreversible anosmia might ensue after a severe upper respiratory tract infection.

Olfaction is the only special sensory system in vertebrates without synaptic relay via the thalamus, because the olfactory bulb incorporates its own thalamic equivalents: (1) the core of intrinsic granular neurons that lack axons and form dendrodendritic synapses, (2) the periglomerular inhibitory interneurons, and (3) the anterior olfactory nucleus, which serves as a relay to the amygdala (to govern behavior in response to odors) and to the entorhinal cortex (part of the parahippocampal gyrus).[3,11-13] Granular and periglomerular neurons are gamma-aminobutyric acid (GABA)-ergic, and the latter coexpress dopamine. Neurons of the anterior olfactory nucleus are mostly glutamatergic, but a minority are GABAergic.

DEVELOPMENTAL NEUROBIOLOGY OF THE OLFACTORY SYSTEM

An understanding of olfactory function during development can only be fully understood in correlation with morphogenesis of the anatomic olfactory structures.[3] Immunocytochemical reactivities and histochemical stains have greatly enhanced the microscopic observations of anatomic maturation, particularly in documenting synaptogenesis in the olfactory bulb, the maturation of individual neuronal types, and the distribution of progenitor "stem" cells within the olfactory bulb. Despite early conclusions based on histology that the human olfactory bulb is mature by 11 weeks gestation,[14] and the functional evidence that neonates and fetuses respond to olfactory stimuli (see later), more recent immunocytochemical studies in our laboratory demonstrate that the olfactory bulb is far from mature at birth. Neuronal maturation, synapse formation, and myelination are incompletely developed at term. The transitory fetal olfactory recess of the lateral ventricle persists and does not involute until after birth.[15] Even the nasal olfactory epithelium is not yet fully mature at birth.[16] Secondary telencephalic sites of olfactory projections, such as the amygdala and entorhinal neocortex, also are not yet mature at birth, particularly in synaptic circuitry.

OLFACTORY EPITHELIUM

Olfactory epithelium lines the roof of the nasal cavities, part of the nasal septum, and the superior (and sometimes extending to the middle) turbinate bones.[17,18] Epithelial plugs obstruct the external nares in the first trimester but regress between 16 and 24 weeks gestation, a finding that was demonstrated as early as 1910.[19] Volatile molecules must penetrate an aqueous mucus layer covering the olfactory epithelium to reach receptor sites on the cilia of primary olfactory dendrites.[17] The number of bipolar primary olfactory neurons increases greatly with the formation of the turbinates, beginning at approximately 8 weeks gestation, which enables a greatly enlarged surface area of olfactory epithelium in the nasal cavity (Fig. 136.2).

An active process of apoptosis occurs simultaneously with the generation of new neurons in the olfactory epithelium.[20] The β-secretase enzyme BACE-1 is essential for axonal guidance of olfactory sensory neurons and for formation of synaptic glomeruli of the olfactory bulb.[21] Neural precursors in the developing olfactory epithelium give rise to three major neuronal classes: olfactory receptors, vomeronasal receptors, and gonadotropin-releasing hormone secretory neurons, each associated with a variety of genes.[22] These neuronal types are mixed rather than anatomically segregated, but different gene-expressing neurons reside in the medial and lateral portions.[23] Specific olfactory marker proteins are identified in the human olfactory epithelium from 28 weeks gestation[24,25] and also in that of the fetal rat.[26] Novel DNA microarrays recognize human olfactory receptor gene families and classes of neural precursors in the olfactory epithelium.[27,28] The olfactory epithelium with its primary olfactory receptor neurons is well characterized by transmission and scanning electron microscopy in humans[16,29] and is immature until near term.

Primary olfactory neurons have a high turnover rate throughout life. This regenerative capacity replaces cells lost

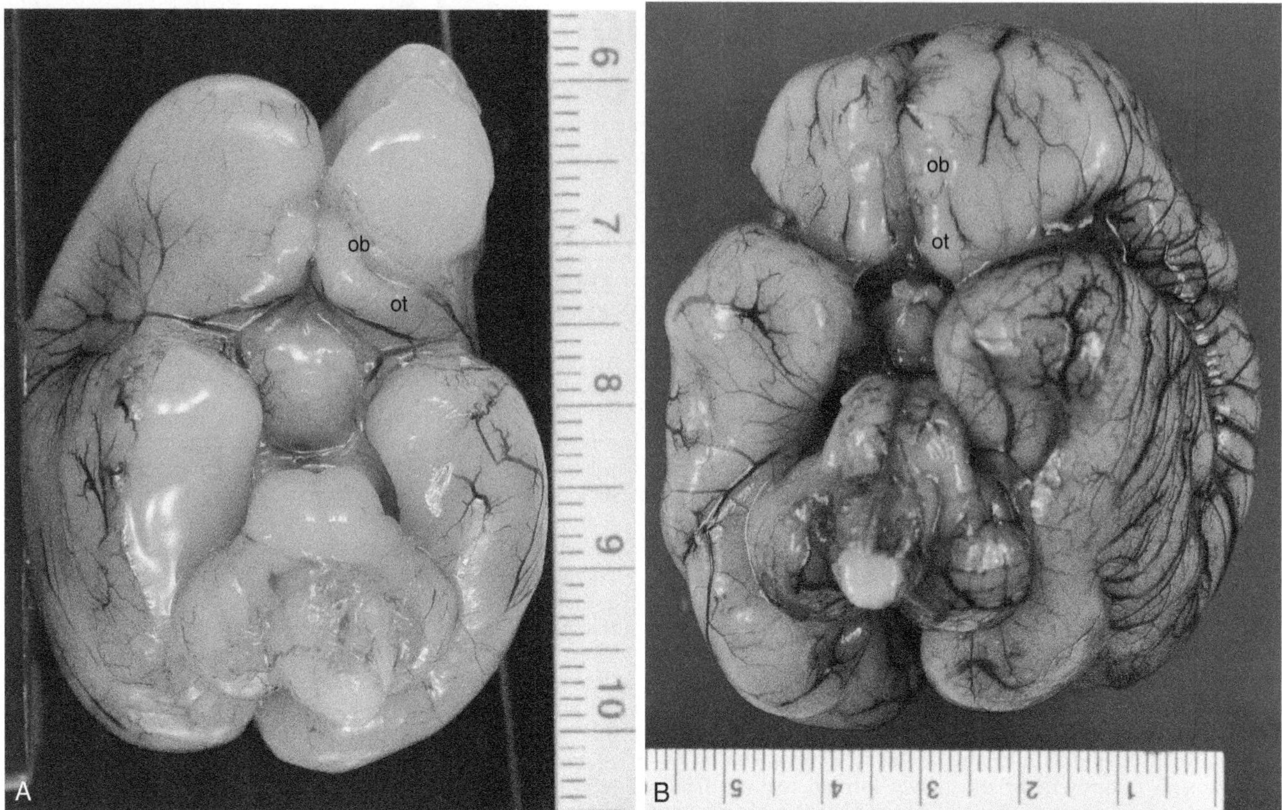

Fig. 136.1 Ventral surface of the brain of (A) a 17-week fetus and (B) a 25-week fetus to show the olfactory bulb *(ob)* and olfactory tract *(ot)*. These structures are relatively large compared with their ratio to the telencephalic hemisphere in adult brains. The ventral surface of the olfactory bulbs seen here is the site of the synaptic glomeruli because it faces the cribriform plate, through which olfactory nerve axons pass from the olfactory epithelium lining the superior part of the nasal cavities.

during severe upper respiratory tract infections, for example, so the subject is not left anosmic afterward.The life span of olfactory neurons is modulated by activity-dependent histones.[30] Olfactory ensheathing cells are specialized glial cells that secrete a large number of neurotrophic factors and cover the entire length of the olfactory nerve and bulb and are essential to preserve the structural integrity of the olfactory nerve, serving as do Schwann cells in other peripheral nerves, and also olfactory resident stem cells for neuroblast proliferation in physiologic turnover and regeneration.[31,32]

OLFACTORY VENTRICULAR RECESS

The outgrowth of the incipient olfactory bulb includes a rostral extension of the primordial frontal horn of the lateral ventricle, the *olfactory ventricular recess*.[4,12,13] This transitory structure begins to involute in the third trimester but is still present at term (Fig. 136.3). It is not always located in the exact middle of the core of the olfactory bulb but sometimes is eccentric, though it remains within the granular layer and never lies superficial to the mitral cell layer. The olfactory recess initially is lined by primitive neuroepithelium but acquires an ependyma at midgestation, arresting neuroepithelial mitotic activity at the luminal surface as in other parts of the lateral ventricles. Its ependyma is a pseudostratified columnar epithelium that does not become a simple cuboidal even at term; it continues to exhibit reactivity to vimentin and glial fibrillary acidic protein even in the term neonate, unlike the mature permanent ventricular ependyma of the lateral, third, and fourth ventricles, in which these reactivities disappear with maturation in the third trimester.[33,34] Humphrey reported that the olfactory recess begins to involute by growth of its ependymal cells into the lumen starting at 14 weeks and completes this process by 18 weeks,[14] but we found a well-formed recess with an ependymal-lined lumen even in the term neonate,[15] though it no longer is evident within a few weeks postnatally. Magnetic resonance imaging (MRI) demonstrated remnants of this recess in 72 of 122 (59%) normal adult subjects.[35] These adult remnants are confirmed histologically either as glial-lined microcysts[35] or as small clusters of residual ependymal cells.

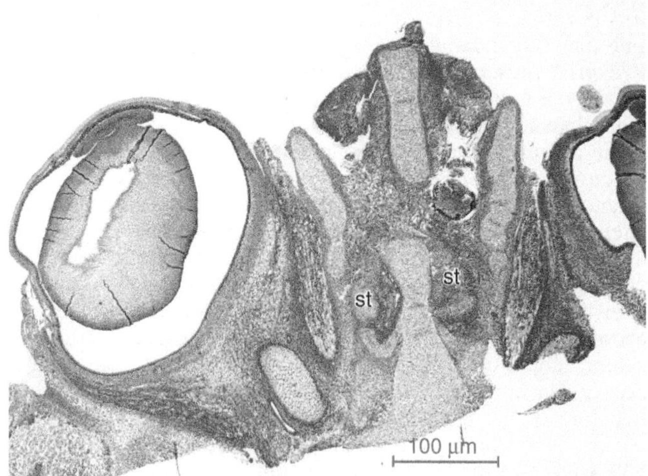

Fig. 136.2 Horizontal section through the face of a 10-week human fetus to show the cartilages forming the superior turbinate *(st)* bones in relation to the developing nasal cavity and orbits. These cartilages will later ossify. The olfactory epithelium extends to cover the superior and part of the middle turbinates, thus greatly increasing the area in which primary olfactory neurons can proliferate. Vimentin immunoreactivity.

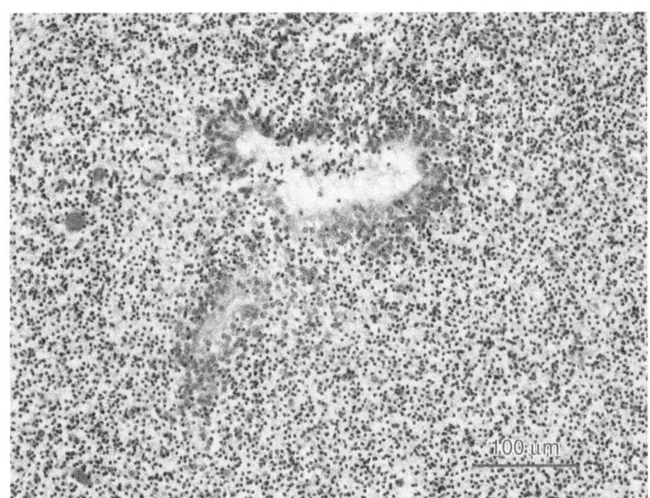

Fig. 136.3 Olfactory ventricular recess in the core of the olfactory bulb of a 38-week human fetus. The lumen is patent and contains a few desquamated cells. The ependymal lining is a pseudostratified columnar epithelium. The olfactory recess regresses in the postnatal period, and only residual clusters of ependymal cells or glial-lined microcysts are occasionally found in the child or adult. Hematoxylin-eosin staining.

ARCHITECTURE AND MORPHOGENESIS OF THE OLFACTORY BULB

The olfactory bulb lacks the molecular zone, Cajal-Retzius neurons, a subplate zone, and a subpial granular glial layer of Brun that characterize the developing neocortex.[36] Synaptic glomeruli lie superficial to the layer of large mitral cells, unlike the synaptic glomeruli of the internal granular layer of cerebellar cortex. The concentric laminar architecture of the mature olfactory bulb is well characterized, and the histology of the fetal olfactory bulb during development also is documented.[37-42] The cortex of the olfactory bulb consists of six layers parallel to the surface of the bulb, none of which corresponds to those of the hexalaminar cerebral neocortex, the layers of the cerebellar cortex, the hippocampus, or even the loose lamination of the midbrain superior colliculus. Fig. 136.4 is the first Golgi depiction of the olfactory bulb by Golgi in 1875, and Fig. 136.5 illustrates a histologic comparison of olfactory, neocortical, and cerebellar cortices. The constituents of each layer are described as follows:

1. The most superficial layer of the olfactory bulb is acellular and composed of unmyelinated olfactory receptor cell axons that have passed through the bony cribriform plate. In rodents, a zonal organization of the olfactory epithelium is preserved in its somatotopic distribution in the olfactory bulb, as determined by zone-specific markers.[43] Axonal transport of synaptophysin molecules within unmyelinated axons in this layer is well demonstrated by antisynaptophysin antibodies throughout the late first and second trimesters.[15] These glycoproteins are thus immunocytochemically evident from their site of biosynthesis in the cytoplasm of the neuronal soma to their final site in the axonal terminal, where they contribute to the structure of the synaptic vesicular membrane. Late in gestation and the neonatal period they become reduced in the intensity of their reactivity, and only presynaptic terminals are strongly reactive.
2. The glomerular layer contains the prominent synaptic glomeruli, generally arranged in a single layer but possibly two or three cells thick in some places. Periglomerular interneurons also occur in this layer. Small periglomerular neurons often form sheet-like processes that envelop other small periglomerular neurons.[44] Spine-laden dendrites of periglomerular cells ramify within two, or occasionally more, glomeruli. Their axons extend across as many as six glomeruli as they contact local interneurons. These periglomerular neurons are heterogeneous in morphology, neurochemistry, and physiology; approximately 10% lack synapses with olfactory

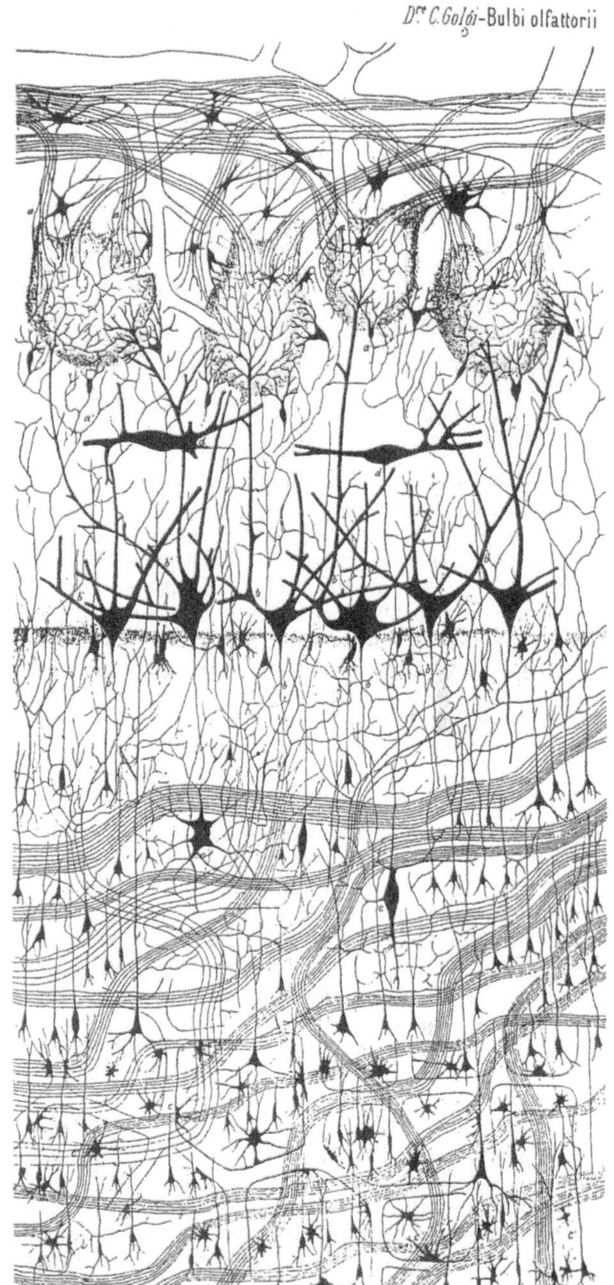

Fig. 136.4 Original camera lucida drawing of the olfactory bulb by Camillo Golgi in 1875.[76] Note the meticulous detail of the synaptic glomeruli but that they are illustrated as a syncytium rather than as synaptic contacts, corresponding to the belief of Golgi about the architecture of the central nervous system. Periglomerular neurons, which we now know are gamma-aminobutyric acid (GABA)-ergic inhibitory interneurons, also are illustrated. The olfactory glomerular surface faces ventrally, but the figure was purposely demonstrated upside-down so that it could be compared with the cerebral and cerebellar cortices that conventionally are illustrated in this way. This was the first depiction of any part of the human brain as seen microscopically by Golgi silver impregnation.

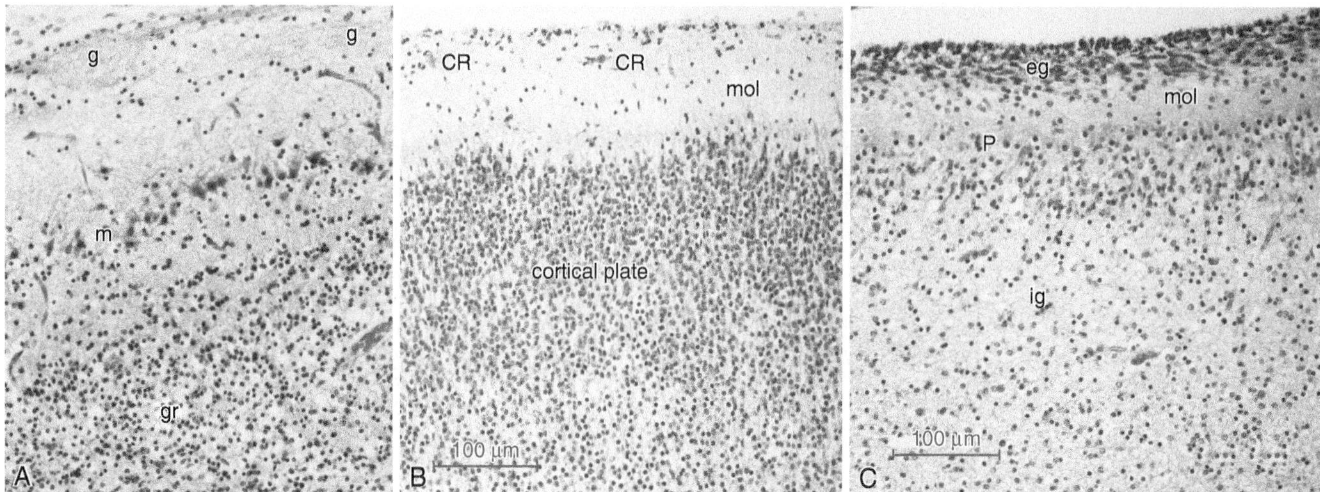

Fig. 136.5 Comparison of the histologic architecture of three laminar cortices of a 21-week human fetus. (A) Olfactory bulb; (B) cerebral neocortex; (C) cerebellar cortex. (A) The surface layers of the olfactory bulb lacks the molecular zone *(mol)* of the cerebral and cerebellar cortices, the external granular (neuronal) layer *(eg)*, Purkinje cell layer *(P)* and internal granular layer *(ig)* of the cerebellar cortex, and the subpial granular glial layer of Brun of the cerebral cortex. In the olfactory bulb, the layer of fine unmyelinated axons of primary olfactory neurons in the olfactory epithelium coalesce as the superficial layer, corresponding to a compact cranial nerve I. A series of large synaptic glomeruli *(g)* on the ventral surface of the olfactory bulb is where these primary axons form synapses with dendrites of the single row of mitral neurons *(m)*, whose somata are deep to the synaptic glomeruli. The synaptic glomeruli correspond to ganglia along the course of other sensory cranial nerves. The deepest layer of the olfactory bulb consists of granular neurons *(gr)* that lack axons and form dendrodendritic synapses and functionally serve as the principal component of an intrinsic olfactory thalamus, extending into the olfactory tract. None of the axons of the olfactory bulb or tract are myelinated until the postnatal period (not shown).

neurons.[40] Periglomerular cells synthesize GABA and dopamine as transmitters, and these molecules are colocalized[45,46]; these neurons also contain one of two calcium-binding proteins, calbindin or parvalbumin.[45-48] Axons of primary olfactory neurons in the mucosa and dendrites of mitral cells form synapses within the glomeruli. Each glomerulus receives as many as 25,000 axons of olfactory nerve neurons (rabbit).[49] A convergence of approximately 1000 receptor cell axons upon every second-order neuron (rabbit) results in major summation or amplification of olfactory stimuli. The olfactory bulb thus exhibits mathematical precision in its intrinsic synaptic relations. More than 20 known neurotransmitters or modulators have been identified in the olfactory bulb.[50] It is not surprising, therefore, that a large array of genes is expressed during fetal life. The glomerular layer is one of the last layers of the olfactory bulb to develop, beginning at approximately 14 weeks. Other layers appear earlier, except for the concentric lamination of the granular zone of the core. Specific odor receptors project their axons to specific glomeruli, thus creating a topographic odor map within the olfactory bulb (zebrafish), programmed by the genes *Robo2/Slit*; without these gene expressions from as early as the olfactory placode, growing olfactory axons are misrouted.[51] Each primary olfactory neuron in the epithelium expresses only one specific receptor because all others are suppressed by a G-protein that couples to membrane receptors.[52] These morphologic relations and constant ratios of cells and synapses suggest functional modules in the olfactory bulb,[53] analogous to the functional columns (barrels; radial units) of visual (striate), somatosensory, motor, and insular neocortices.[54-61] Indeed, a columnar arrangement with only limited lateral connectivity also is demonstrated in the olfactory bulb.[62-64]

3. An external plexiform layer is cell-sparse and formed largely by primary dendrites of granule cells and secondary dendrites of mitral and tufted neurons. Tufted neurons reside in this layer. These cells are similar to mitral neurons in morphology (though smaller), synaptic connections, and transmitter synthesis (glutamate). Approximately 80% of synaptic contacts between neurons are organized as reciprocal pairs: mitral-to-granule cell synapses are excitatory and granule cell-to-mitral neuronal synapses are inhibitory.[40]
4. This is a single layer of large mitral neurons. There is heterogeneity in the neurochemistry and electrophysiologic functions amongst several classes of mitral neurons.[65,66] During development, mitral neurons can be identified as early as 8 weeks gestation, at which time neuronal differentiation and cytoplasmic growth of these large neurons occurs. Tufted neurons are similar to mitral neurons, though smaller and found only in the most rostral regions of the olfactory bulb and more superficially than the mitral cells. They also project their axons caudally into the olfactory tract. The mitral cell layer is initiated at 9.5 weeks, is well developed by 11 weeks, and is more prominent at 18.5 weeks than in the adult.[14]
5. An internal plexiform layer of neurites but with few synapses.
6. The innermost cellular layer of the olfactory bulb consists of granule cells in a ratio of approximately 50 to 100 granule cells for each mitral cell. These small interneurons are GABAergic and possess no extrinsic connections; they are unique in lacking a definite axon, but rather form dendrodendritic synapses with mitral and tufted neurons. Lamination in the granular layer, and also in the mitral cell layer, is at least partly regulated in fetal mice by the zinc-finger gene *Fex* in olfactory neurons.[67] The neuroepithelium surrounding the olfactory ventricular recess shows proliferative activity. Massive apoptotic cellular death occurs in the murine olfactory bulb, especially amongst granular neurons, if thiamine is deficient.[68]

The intrinsic thalamic equivalent of the olfactory bulb is in its granule cells and periglomerular interneurons, which "modulate" intrinsic olfactory bulb synaptic circuits but have no extrinsic afferent or efferent connections. They are GABAergic interneurons intensely immunoreactive in tissue sections with calcium-binding soluble proteins such as calretinin and parvalbumin. The anterior olfactory nucleus also contributes to thalamic-like function in serving as a

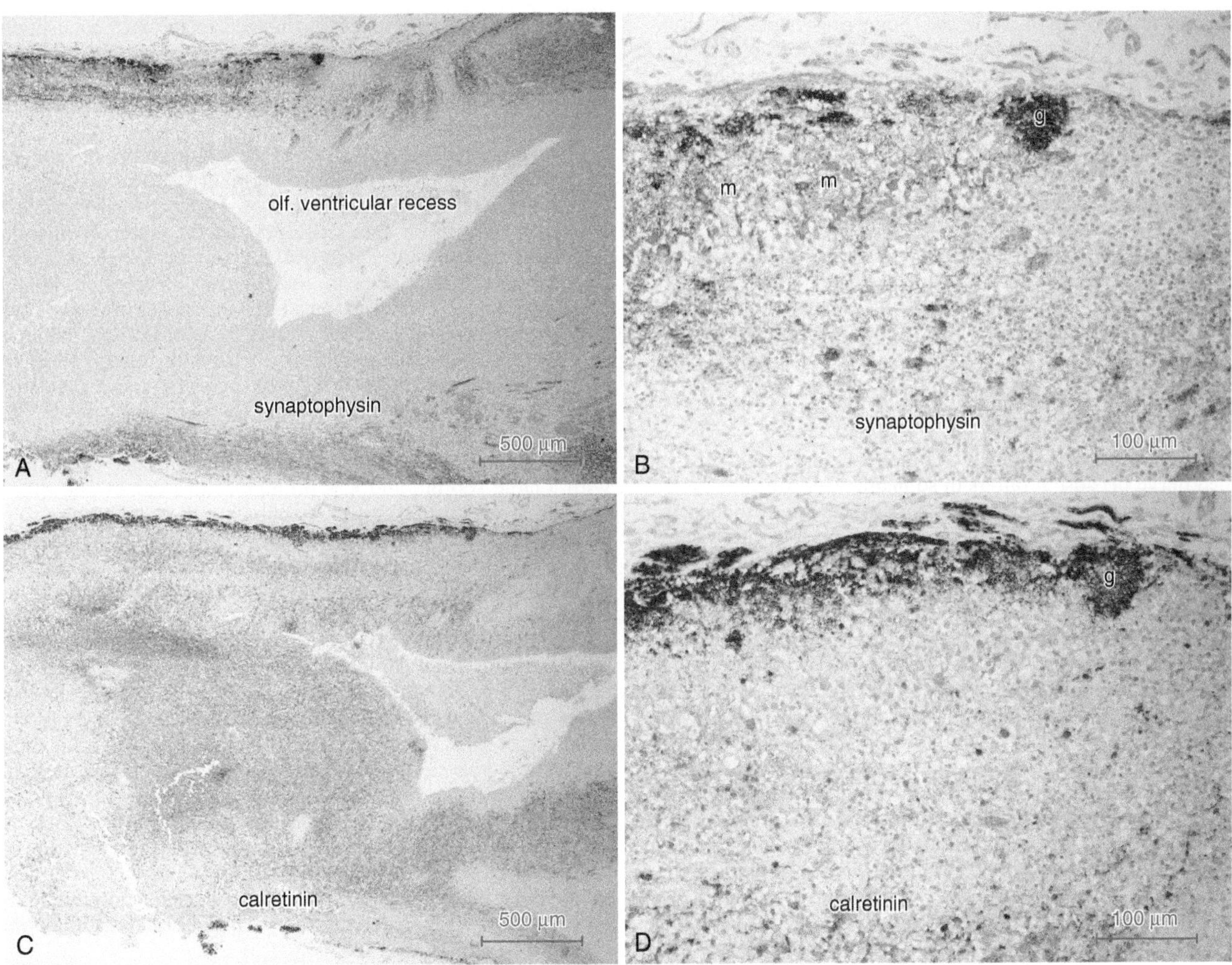

Fig. 136.6 Immunoreactivity demonstrates cytologic maturation of neurons of the olfactory bulb. (A and B) At 16 weeks gestation, there is strong synaptophysin reactivity in the superficial layer of primary olfactory axons; this axoplasmic reactivity is consistent with immaturity. A few synaptic glomeruli *(g)* are formed. Initiation of synapse formation also is seen in the mitral cell layer *(m)* and in some synaptic glomeruli. Reactivity is seen within the somatic cytoplasm of immature mitral cells. There is no synaptophysin reactivity in the immature granular layer surrounding the olfactory ventricular recess and in the deep core of the bulb. (C and D) Calretinin immunoreactivity (which selectively demonstrates gamma-aminobutyric acid (GABA)-ergic interneurons) of sections from the same blocks as (A and B) shows a striking contrast to synaptophysin by its strong reactivity in immature granular neurons of the core. Calretinin also is seen in primary olfactory axons in the superficial zone, including some olfactory axons in the meninges that are just entering the olfactory bulb and in some but not all synaptic glomeruli, similar to synaptophysin.

relay between the olfactory bulb and telencephalic targets, particularly the amygdala and entorhinal cortex.[11,39,69,70] Portions of the anterior olfactory nucleus extend into the olfactory tract (see later).

Olfaction also is rare amongst sensory systems because the primary receptors are naked dendritic endings within an epithelium, though pain receptors in the skin share this characteristic. The ganglion cells of these primary olfactory neurons lie outside the central nervous system (CNS), as with sensory ganglia of other cranial nerves and spinal dorsal roots. Axonal terminals of these primary olfactory neurons enter the olfactory bulb and form *synaptic glomeruli* (*glomerulus* = Greek; *ball of threads*) with dendrites of the layered mitral and tufted cells that give origin to long axons that extend into the olfactory tract and project to diencephalic structures in the hypothalamus and telencephalic structures.

The deepest core of the mature olfactory bulb corresponds to subcortical white matter and contains the axons of mitral and tufted neurons that pass caudally to form the olfactory tract and project to other structures of the brain. However, it also contains many granular cells and progenitor cells that extend into the olfactory tract (see below). The immunocytochemical profile of synaptophysin and calretinin in the maturing olfactory bulb in the human fetus is illustrated in Fig. 136.6.

OLFACTORY TRACT

The olfactory tract is much more complex than a simple fasciculus of longitudinal ascending and descending axons. The axonal bundles are surrounded by granule cells that extend caudally from the olfactory bulb. At the other end of the olfactory tract, there is an extension rostrally of pyramidal neurons of the anterior olfactory nucleus and one to several clusters of such neurons within the olfactory tract, which are separated parts of the anterior olfactory nucleus.[71,72] In addition, long, slender processes of bipolar progenitor cells residing mainly in the granular layer of the olfactory bulb extend caudally within the olfactory tract in parallel with the descending axonal pathway.[15]

Axons of the tufted and mitral neurons form the olfactory tract and pass caudally to terminate mainly in the anterior olfactory nucleus but also directly to other telencephalic and diencephalic regions. One of the principal telencephalic centers for processing of odors is the amygdala.[11] Postsynaptic axons of anterior olfactory neurons enter the anterior commissure, as shown by

DiI axonal transport in the rat fetus.[71] Some presynaptic olfactory tract axons also cross the midline in the anterior commissure. Olfactory contributions form the peripheral rim of fibers of the anterior commissure, with axons of the anterior temporal neocortex forming most of the deep core; these olfactory fibers of the anterior commissure myelinate postnatally, the sharpest contrast with unmyelinated anterior commissural axons seen at approximately 4 months of age using Luxol fast blue myelin stain.[73]

Cortical areas of olfactory perception are poorly defined and are not assigned a Brodmann area number (unlike the gustatory system) but mainly are localized to the insula and nearby ventral part of the postcentral gyrus, where they may be integrated with gustatory input.

IS THE OLFACTORY (CRANIAL NERVE I) A "TRUE" CRANIAL NERVE?

Some authors have questioned whether the olfactory is really a cranial nerve because it differs in so many ways from the lower special sensory cranial nerves: its axons are separated individually rather than as a compact bundle; there is no peripheral ganglion in the course of the nerve; it remains unmyelinated throughout life. However, the individual axons that pass through the cribriform plate then coalesce into a bundle that forms layer 1 of the olfactory bulb; the synaptic glomeruli on the ventral surface of the olfactory bulb as layer 2 serve as the peripheral ganglion; many autonomic axons of lower cranial nerves also remain unmyelinated throughout life. Hence the olfactory nerve is a true cranial nerve but has a more primitive structure both ontogenetically and phylogenetically, perhaps related to the lack of neural crest migration into the area of the olfactory bulb, except for extension of the leptomeninges.[74] Nevertheless, an important difference between the olfactory and every other special sensory system is the turnover of primary sensory neurons in the olfactory mucosa and a population of resident progenitor cells in the olfactory bulb and tract that throughout life can generate new neurons; the only other site of perpetual resident stem cells is beneath the dentate gyrus of the hippocampus.

HISTORICAL PERSPECTIVE

Contact of peripheral olfactory nerve fibers with processes of mitral cells extending into the glomeruli of the olfactory bulb was described by Owsjannikow in 1860[75] and Walter in 1861[72] and was further defined in the 1890s and early 1900s by several distinguished developmental neuroanatomists of the late 19th and early 20th centuries. The olfactory bulb was the first structure of the human brain in which the intrinsic architecture was first elucidated by Golgi impregnations, indeed by Camillo Golgi himself in 1875[76] (see Fig. 136.4). The olfactory bulb thus served as an important template for demonstrating architecture of the CNS in general. Studies of olfactory bulb architecture confirm the microscopic findings of the early investigators and expand upon them, including Golgi impregnations; they enable correlations with clinical disorders of olfaction and developmental anomalies of the olfactory bulbs.[15,36,37,77-79]

PHYLOGENETIC PERSPECTIVE

An olfactory system is present in all animals. In vertebrates, the large size and prominence of the olfactory bulb relative to the rest of the forebrain in simple vertebrates such as the lamprey and the shark contrasts with its relatively smaller size ratio to the forebrain in birds and primates, although it is relatively large in rodents and dogs, who have a keener sense of smell than humans. The interspecific differences do not correlate with total brain size or complexity. Animals with a relatively poorer sense of smell include birds, cetaceans (whales, dolphins), and primates. Nevertheless, it is estimated that humans can discriminate more than one trillion olfactory stimuli.[80]

Phylogenetic development or evolution often provides clues to understanding embryonic development.[81,82] The 1887 adage of Haeckel, "Ontogeny recapitulates phylogeny,"[83] has had many detractors over more than a century, but the general principle is recognized as having much truth despite some exceptions.[81] Despite wide differences in size of the olfactory bulb and functional acuity of smell amongst various classes of vertebrates and species within each class, the basic histologic laminar architecture of the olfactory bulb—with a peripheral sheet of synaptic glomeruli, a sheet of mitral neurons, and an internal layer of granule cells—is constant in all vertebrates.[49,81,84] Afferent and efferent connections also are similar, except that the projection to the septum is more prominent in animals with a large septum and less prominent in humans and other animals in which the septum atrophies or is reduced to a thin membrane in the adult, the *septum pellucidum*. The olfactory recess of the rostral lateral ventricle is a transitory fetal and neonatal structure in mammals but persists into adult life in sharks and amphibians.[81]

Comparative electron microscopy further confirms at the ultrastructural level an almost identical organization of the olfactory bulb in all vertebrates, comparing even primitive fishes such as cyclostomes (lamprey, hagfish) and mammals; the structure of synapses in the olfactory bulb are specific for each connection type in all.[84,85] However, a few minor differences do occur; for example, mitral cells usually contact several olfactory glomeruli in nonmammalian vertebrates but project to only one glomerulus in mammals. This comparative neuroanatomic study indicates that the olfactory bulb was one of the earliest structures of the brain to develop phylogenetically and has retained a constant structural and synaptic stability throughout vertebrate evolution.

FETAL AND POSTNATAL MATURATION OF THE OLFACTORY BULB

Though it was stated by early developmental neuroanatomists that the human olfactory bulb is mature by 14 weeks gestation, based upon histologic architecture,[14] modern immunocytochemical methods demonstrate that the olfactory bulb is still immature in the term neonate by criteria of (1) expression of individual neuronal proteins, (2) synaptogenesis, (3) complete lack of myelination until the postnatal period, and (4) persistence of the transitory fetal olfactory ventricular recess.[12] Conclusions regarding olfactory bulb maturation thus cannot be based solely upon microscopic sections stained with hematoxylin-eosin, Nissl stain, or other general histologic stains, but should encompass immunocytochemical markers of neuronal maturity.[15]

Immunocytochemical antibodies against specific neuronal proteins not only denote a neuronal lineage of cells and in some cases are even specific for types of neurons but also identify maturation of neuroblasts to neurons by their timing of expression (see Fig. 136.6).[86-88] Some, such as calretinin, are expressed very early, even in early differentiating neuroepithelial cells, whereas others, such as NeuN, are expressed only late, at the time of terminal maturation of the neurons. Synaptophysin is a structural glycoprotein of the synaptic vesicular membrane in axonal terminals and is similar regardless of the site of the synapse (axosomatic, axodendritic, dendrodendritic), function of the synapse (excitatory, inhibitory), or the nature of the chemical neurotransmitter contained within.

CLINICAL CORRELATIONS OF OLFACTORY SYSTEM ONTOGENESIS

Preterm neonates do not reliably respond to olfactory stimuli before 28 weeks gestation.[23] Olfactory reflexes are described as a reliable test in the neurologic examination of the term neonate.[2,89] Olfaction can even be semiquantitated in gradients, and sensitivity increases in the first few postnatal days.[90] Olfactory development exemplifies a general neuro-ontogenetic principle that full anatomic maturation is not required for function to begin.[2]

The test substance for olfaction must be aromatic and not primarily an irritant that also stimulates pain receptors of the ethmoid and nasopalatine branches of the trigeminal nerve, which also are present in the olfactory epithelium and responsive from 10 weeks gestation. There are no truly "pure" aromatic molecules; even ammonia, primarily an irritant, also has a distinctive pungent odor. Peppermint extract is an excellent test substance for neonates[89,90]; anise (licorice), cloves, and garlic are other acceptable test substances.[91,92] Preterm neonates also respond to pure olfactory stimuli after 28 to 30 weeks gestation.[93] Vanilla odor did not influence resting energy expenditure compared with controls, however.[94] Even brief exposure to specific odors immediately after birth is sufficient for the development of olfactory "learning" (i.e., conditioning).[95] The intensity (including concentration) of an odor that provokes a response is more difficult to quantify in the olfactory than in most other special sensory systems and to localize at the various neuroanatomic sites of olfactory processing, in part because of the extreme plasticity of the olfactory system in terms of axonal targeting.[89-98] In the fetal mouse, there is a critical period during development of axonal targeting.[99] Olfactory memory requires an intact CA2 sector of the hippocampal Ammon's horn.[100] Enriched neonatal exposure to odors increases the number of neurons in the adult olfactory bulb and enhances olfactory memory.[101-105] Rodents deprived early of olfactory stimuli exhibit deficient synaptogenesis in the olfactory bulb.[106] In aging, by contrast, there is a gradual loss of mitral neurons and synaptic glomeruli, contributing to hyposmia in the elderly.[107,108]

A continuous turnover of amniotic fluid takes place through the fetal nasal passages, and the fetus can detect odors in amniotic fluid of foods ingested by the mother, particularly foods with strong aromas such as garlic and onion.[91-93,109,110] Neonates also detect the odor of their mother's breast milk, axilla, and other body odors and thus can recognize their mother within hours after birth.[111]

In normal school-age children, a novel, noninvasive approach to examining olfactory perception and distinction is by functional MRI (fMRI), which shows activation in secondary and tertiary sites of olfactory circuits.[112]

In focal epilepsy in children and adults, the primary source of olfactory auras is generally attributed to entorhinal cortex, amygdala, or the insula, but in some cases might arise in the olfactory bulb itself and then be propagated by the amygdala or temporal lobe neocortical structures to be brought to conscious awareness.[113]

OLFACTORY BULB DYSGENESIS

Neuropathologic reports of dysgenesis of the olfactory bulb are sparse, even in autopsies of patients with major cerebral malformations. Postmortem descriptions of the olfactory bulb are usually limited to its gross presence or absence, as in holoprosencephaly and Kallmann syndrome. The dysgeneses that have been described include dilatation of the olfactory ventricular recess in fetal hydrocephalus,[15] pathologic fusion of the two olfactory bulbs,[15] enlargement, dysplasia, and an abnormal longitudinal sulcus in hemimegalencephaly.[12,15,114,115] Hypoplasia of the olfactory bulbs, as occurs in half of patients with septo-optic-pituitary dysplasia, and enlargement of the hemimegalencephalic olfactory bulb also may be demonstrated in life by MRI[2,114] and pathologically, the latter also showing dysplasia.[12,15,115] In tuberous sclerosis complex, the human olfactory bulb may exhibit hamartomata.[116] Specific genetic mutations are known to be associated with agenesis of the olfactory bulbs and anosmia.[117-121]

RESIDENT PROGENITOR STEM CELLS OF THE OLFACTORY BULB AND REGENERATION

The olfactory bulb has an importance beyond its function in detecting odors. It is one of only two permanent repositories in the mature brain in which resident multipotential progenitor "stem" cells are generated; the other repository is the dentate gyrus of the hippocampus. Migratory cells from the periventricular zone of the lateral ventricles of the mouse continue to stream into the olfactory bulb even in adult life to form more neuronal precursor cells, mediated by the chemoattractant activity of the *Sonic hedgehog (SHH)* gene.[122] The olfactory bulb and the olfactory mucosal epithelium are sites of resident stem cells in both the mature rodent and human.[123,124]

Olfactory afferents regenerate following olfactory bulbectomy in neonatal mice; these regenerating axons are capable of innervating neocortex directly, bypassing the intermediate synapses in their missing normal target in the olfactory bulb.[125,126] Homotopically transplanted olfactory bulbs in neonatal rats after bulb removal are able to mature and reestablish relations with both the brain and the periphery.[126] Early olfactory deprivation greatly modifies the synaptic organization within the olfactory bulb.[127]

ACCESSORY OLFACTORY BULB AND VOMERONASAL SYSTEM

A small secondary olfactory system also exists in most vertebrates. In cartilaginous fishes, such as sharks, it may be the principal olfactory sense.[128] The paired accessory olfactory bulbs receive input from the same olfactory epithelium as the principal bulbs[129,130] and project axons to the amygdala for relay to accessory olfactory cortex, rather than directly to entorhinal cortex.[131,132] The histologic structure of the accessory bulb is similar to that of the primary olfactory bulb but usually not as well developed (Fig. 136.7).[14,132] Some immunocytochemical

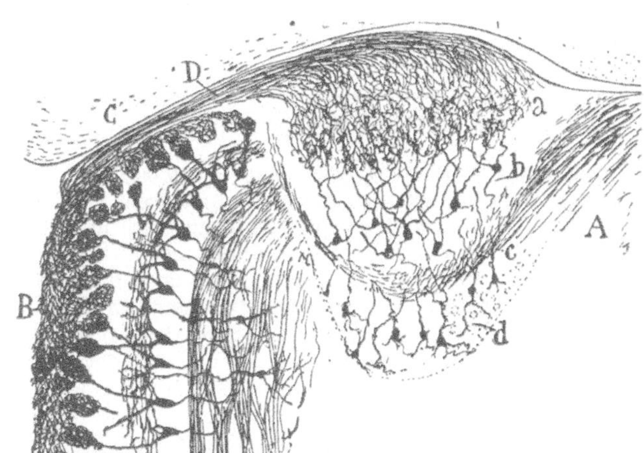

Fig. 136.7 Camera lucida drawing of Golgi silver impregnation of the accessory olfactory bulb, adjacent to the principal olfactory bulb, in an 11-week human fetus, published by Ramón y Cajal, 1901. The accessory bulb is a miniature olfactory bulb with similar architecture, though less well organized and more compressed. (Ramón y Cajal SR de. La corteza olfativa del cerebro. *Trab d Laborat d Investig Biol* 1, 1901).

and genetic markers may distinguish the human vomeronasal system, including the epithelium and the accessory bulb.[133] The accessory bulb is on the medial side of the principal olfactory bulb in early fetuses, is at the dorsal surface of the primary bulb at 15.5 weeks gestation, and is dorsolateral at 18.5 weeks gestation, a shift in position probably due to rotation of the primary olfactory bulb during its growth and development.[14] Neuronogenesis and apoptosis continue in the vomeronasal epithelium in the adult mouse as in the fetus.[134]

Accessory olfactory nerves are called the *nervus terminalis,* sometimes termed *cranial nerve 0* or *cranial nerve 13.*[135] DiI fiber tracing in the rat embryo shows that axons of the nervus terminalis project to the telencephalic septal nuclei.[71] On the dorsoposterior surface of the human fetal olfactory bulb is the diminutive accessory olfactory bulb with similar architecture that represents a parallel olfactory system arising from a distinct chemoreceptor olfactory epithelium called the *vomeronasal (Jacobson) organ.*[136,137] It projects to the amygdala rather than to entorhinal cortex or the septum.[138-141] The nasal olfactory epithelium of the nervus terminalis is shared with the epithelium for the principal olfactory bulb and is not anatomically distinct.[142]

The accessory olfactory bulbs in humans are asymmetric; the left is larger and better formed than the right and is retained longer in older fetuses.[14] A similar asymmetry was noted between the left and right vomeronasal organ in 1905.[143] The function of this small secondary olfactory system in humans is poorly understood; however, in rodents and nonmammalian vertebrates, it is related to the olfactory perception of pheromones and perhaps some steroid molecules used to identify other members of the same species or of the opposite sex, and it participates in higher neural circuits identifying the initiation of instinctive behaviors such as aggression, sexuality, mating, and protectiveness of their young.[136,137,144] More than 250 putative pheromone receptors, which can be divided into two major classes, have been identified in the murine vomeronasal organ.[145,146]

The vomeronasal organ is rudimentary or vestigial in adult humans and contains no recognizable neuroepithelium, but a transitory vomeronasal organ forms in early fetal life and atrophies by 28 weeks gestation. This tubular structure is located superiorly, adjacent to the paraseptal cartilages, and in higher primates including humans consists of a homogeneous pseudostratified columnar epithelium with ciliated regions and mucus-producing structures.[129] The accessory olfactory bulb may be absent in adult humans, or a vestigial bulb is sometimes identified.

GUSTATORY SENSATION (TASTE)

As mentioned, distinction between olfaction and taste is difficult in simple species of animals and even in humans at times. The functional development of taste probably begins early in fetal life because of the early differentiation of taste receptors and the early onset of swallowing of amniotic fluid. As with olfaction, humans are capable of appreciating thousands of different flavors despite a fundamental few basic tastes. Taste perception may be influenced by hormonal changes or other physiologic or epigenetic phenomena. An example is pregnancy. In early gestation in particular, some tastes that were previously enjoyed become repugnant, and cravings may develop for other foods or tastes to which the individual previously was indifferent or did not much enjoy. Prior experience with different tastes also influences the preferences of young infants, such as a change from breast milk to formula or nondairy products such as soy. Some medications may alter taste perception as a secondary effect.

TASTE RECEPTORS OR "TASTE BUDS"

Taste receptors are modified elongated epithelial cells found throughout the oral cavity on hard and soft palates, tonsils, pharynx, and epiglottis, but they are most numerous on the tongue. Taste pores are openings in the epithelium for chemical substances to enter, and regional gene expression surrounding taste buds regulates their formation and is partially controlled by innervating nerves.[147] Peripheral sensory innervation is through branches of three cranial nerves: facial (VII), glossopharyngeal (IX), and vagal (X). Of the four morphologically distinct types of lingual papillae, only three bear taste receptors: the fungiform, foliate, and circumvallate papillae.[17,148]

Specialized taste cells first appear in the human fetus at 7 to 8 weeks gestation and are morphologically mature at 13 to 15 weeks.[149] Chemicals in the amniotic fluid may stimulate fetal taste receptors. The fetus begins to swallow amniotic fluid episodically at the 12th week of gestation,[150] and by term even anencephalic fetuses can swallow 200 to 760 mL/day.[151] Amniotic fluid contains glucose, fructose, lactic acid, pyruvic acid, citric acid, fatty acids, phospholipids, creatinine, urea, uric acid, various amino acids, polypeptides, proteins, and salts.[152] The composition may change during gestation and is altered by fetal urination into this fluid.[153]

Traditionally, four fundamental tastes are identified: salty, bitter, sweet, and sour. More recently it was discovered that the artificial flavor enhancer monosodium glutamate (MSG; umami) also has specific glutamate receptors and hence must be regarded as a fifth fundamental taste that can be detected even in the newborn.[154,155] None of these specific tastes are segregated within the gustatory nuclei of the brain stem or in the cortical gustatory regions. Nevertheless, each taste is detected by dedicated taste receptor cells in the taste buds, and there is fine selectivity in taste preference in ganglion cells and specific transfer of taste information between taste cells and the brain.[156]

GUSTATORY CENTERS OF THE BRAIN

Multiple gustatory nuclei are located within the brain stem, corresponding to the three cranial nerves. The most prominent gustatory nucleus is the enlarged rostral cap of the nucleus solitarius at the ponto-medullary junction; the portion of this nucleus caudal to the gustatory nucleus is the pneumotaxic center. The gustatory portion of the nucleus solitarius receives special visceral afferent taste fibers from the facial and glossopharyngeal nerves. Unlike the olfactory system, the gustatory system projects to the thalamus for relay to the insular cortex.[157] Brodmann area 43, the most ventral (opercular) part of the postcentral gyrus, is another nearby cortical primary gustatory region. Gustatory nuclear projections to the superior colliculus are documented, though how and why they integrate with visual signals in the optic tectum of the midbrain are poorly understood. Brain stem gustatory nuclei also project to the hypothalamus and to the amygdala, where they integrate with olfactory projections.[39,69,158] Orexin receptors in the amygdala reinforce various tastes and may be important in taste learning and aversion.[158] These G-protein-coupled receptors bind the neuropeptides orexin-A and -B,[159] found in cholinergic neurons of the basal forebrain from the hypothalamus and alter both olfactory and gustatory discrimination.[160]

Apparent absence of the olfactory bulbs by MRI but with clinical odor perception occurs in 0.6% of women but not in men.[161] This phenomenon might be due to hypoplastic but still partially functional olfactory bulbs below the resolution of neuroimaging, or perhaps by enhanced gustatory receptors of the tongue that perceive odorous molecules in the air of the mouth. Neuropathologic confirmation of olfactory bulb status is not available.

GENETIC ASPECTS AND NEUROTROPHIC FACTORS

Brain-derived neurotrophic factor and neurotrophin-4 are two neurotrophic molecules that have distinct and interchangeable roles in the survival of taste sensory neurons, target innervations, and taste bud formation. These two neurotrophins both bind to the tropomyosin-related kinase B (TrkB) receptor and the pan-neurotrophin receptor p75, which can play interchangeable roles.[162,163] The p75 receptor regulates gustatory axonal branching and innervation of taste buds of the tongue.[164] Pathways downstream of TrkB regulate specific taste receptors by distinct signaling pathways.[165] The gene *Mash1* is required in mice for the expression of GAD67 (related to GABA) and the gene product of *Dlx5* in taste buds.[166] Another essential gene for embryonic taste bud progenitor cells is *Pax9*.[167] Bitter taste receptors can participate in the regulation of thyroid function by negatively influencing thyroid-stimulating hormone.[168] Expansion of the bitter taste receptor gene spectrum has occurred during the evolution of mammals.[169] Wilms tumor-1 protein is a transcription factor important for taste bud development.[170]

During ontogenesis, *SHH* negatively regulates taste bud patterning, such that inhibition of *SHH* causes the formation of more and larger taste bud primordia, including ectopic buds in lingual sites where they normally are absent.[171] The ectopic buds can detect all types of gustatory types: salty, sweet, bitter, sour, and umami. A principal process in the homeostatic control of sodium ion levels is salt intake; in sheep and rats, the peripheral nerve responses to sodium chloride are of low magnitude during early development, but with maturation an increasing proportion of fibers respond maximally.[172] Sodium aspartate is a specific enhancer of salty taste perception.[173]

CLINICAL CORRELATES OF GUSTATORY ONTOGENESIS

Odorous molecules from strong foods ingested by the mother (e.g., onion, garlic, curry, and other spices) cross the placenta and become dissolved in the amniotic fluid and perceived by the fetus after 28 to 30 weeks of gestation[174-177] as well as by postnatal preterm infants of the same conceptional age. Differential fetal swallowing patterns after injections of sweet or bitter substances into the amniotic fluid of pregnant women suggests that fetuses in the third trimester may show a preference for sweet and rejection of bitter.[152,178] A similar preference for sweet, including changes in facial expression and cessation of crying, was demonstrated postnatally in preterm and term infants.[179-183] In both the infant and adult, bitter receptors on the tongue and indeed distributed in many tissues serve as a defense against microbial invaders.[184]

CONCLUSION

The olfactory and gustatory systems are closely interrelated despite their mediation through different cranial nerves and processing in different parts of the brain. Detection of dissolved chemical substances is the oldest special sense, both phylogenetically and ontogenetically. The olfactory system is unique in the CNS of vertebrates because (1) it is the only system to not project to the thalamus because it has its own intrinsic thalamic equivalent; (2) the architecture of the olfactory bulb is unlike any other cortex; (3) neurons of the olfactory bulb stream into it from outside the bulb; (4) the bulb includes an olfactory recess from the lateral ventricle, a transitory structure that involutes postnatally; (5) synaptic glomeruli on the ventral surface of the olfactory bulb are the equivalent of peripheral ganglia on lower sensory cranial nerves; (6) an accessory olfactory bulb and vomeronasal nerves are other transitory fetal structures that begin to involute in the second trimester; and (7) the olfactory bulb and dentate gyrus of the hippocampus are reservoirs of progenitor stem cells even in the adult brain. The olfactory bulb is still immature at birth, though functional. Fetuses can perceive odors and tastes in amniotic fluid in the late second and third trimesters and develop fondness and aversion to specific odors and tastes, especially related to their mothers and altered by their mothers' dietary content.

A complete reference list is available at www.ExpertConsult.com. 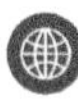

SELECT REFERENCES

4. Pearson A. The development of the olfactory nerve in man. *J Comp Neurol*. 1941;75:199-217.
5. Müller F, O'Rahilly F. Olfactory structures in staged human embryos. *Cells Tissues Organs*. 2004;178:93-116.
6. O'Rourke NA. Neuronal chain gangs: homotypic contacts support migration into the olfactory bulb. *Neuron*. 1996;16:1061-1064.
7. Rousselot P, Lois C, Álvarez-Bullya A. Embryonic (PSA) N-CAM reveals chains of migrating neuroblasts between the lateral ventricle and the olfactory bulb of adult mice. *J Comp Neurol*. 1994;351:51-61.
8. Lois C, García-Verdugo JM, Varez-Bullya A. Chain migration of neuronal precursors. *Science*. 1996;271:978-981.
9. Lledo P-M, Merkle FT, Álvarez-Buylla A. Origin and function of olfactory bulb interneuron diversity. *Trends Neurosci*. 2008;31:392-400.
10. Kishi K, Peng JY, Kakuta S, et al. Migration of bipolar subependymal cells precursors of granule cells of the rat olfactory bulb with reference to the arrangement of the radial glial fibers. *Arch Histol Cytol*. 1990;53:219-226.
11. Root CM, Denny CA, Hen R, Axel R. The participation of cortical amygdala in innate, odour-driven behaviour. *Nature*. 2014;515:269-273.
14. Humphrey T. The development of the olfactory and the accessory olfactory formations in human embryos and fetuses. *J Comp Neurol*. 1940;73:431-468.
15. Sarnat HB, Yu W. Maturation and dysgenesis of the olfactory bulb. *Brain Pathol*. 2015;26:301-318.
16. Pyatkina GA. Development of the olfactory epithelium in man. *Z Mikrosk-Anat Forsch (Leipz)*. 1982;96:361-372.
17. Cowart BJ, Beauchamp GK, Mennella JA. Development of taste and smell in the neonate. In: Polin RA, Fox WW, Abman SH, eds. *Fetal and Neonatal Physiology*. Ed 4. Philadelphia: Elsevier Saunders; 2011:1899-1907.
19. Schaffer JP. The lateral wall of the cavum nasi in man with special reference to the various developmental stages. *J Morphol*. 1910;21:613-707.
20. Magrassi L, Graziadei PPC. Cell death in the olfactory epithelium. *Anat Embryol*. 1995;192:77-87.
22. Tucker ES, Lehtinen MK, Maynard T, et al. Proliferative and transcriptional identity of distinct classes of neural precursors in the mammalian olfactory epithelium. *Dev*. 2010;137:2471-2481.
27. Zhang X, de la Cruz O, Pinto JM, et al. Characterizing the expression of the human olfactory receptor gene family using a novel DNA microarray. *Genome Biol*. 2007;8:R86.
29. Kimura M, Umehara T, Udagawa J, et al. Development of olfactory epithelium in the human fetus: scanning electron microscopic observations. *Congenit Anom (Kyoto)*. 2009;49:102-107.
33. Sarnat HB. Regional differentiation of the human fetal ependyma: immunocytochemical markers. *J Neuropathol Exp Neurol*. 1992;51:58-75.
37. Patel RM, Pinto JM. Olfaction: anatomy, physiology and disease. *Clin Anat*. 2014;27:54-60.
40. Kratskin IL, Belluzi O. Anatomy and neurochemistry of the olfactory bulb. In: Doty RL, ed. *Handbook of Olfaction and Gustation*. New York: Marcel Dekker; 2003:139-164.
41. Nakashima T, Kimmelman CP, Snow Jr JB. Structure of human fetal and adult olfactory epithelium. *Arch Otolaryngol*. 1984;110:641-646.
42. Treloar HB, Miller AM, Ray A, Greer CA. Development of the olfactory system. In: Menini A, ed. *The Neurobiology of Olfaction*. Boca Raton, Florida: CRC Press; 2010:131-155.
43. Mori K, Nagao H, Yoshihara Y. The olfactory bulb. Coding and processing of odor molecule information. *Science*. 1999;286:711-715.
46. Gall CM, Hendry SH, Seroogy KB, et al. Evidence for coexistence of GABA and dopamine in neurons of the rat olfactory bulb. *J Comp Neurol*. 1987;266:307-318.
53. Kauer JS, Cinelli AR. Are there structural and functional modules in the vertebrate olfactory bulb? *Microsc Res Tech*. 1993;24:157-167.
63. Kim DH, Phillips ME, Chang AY, et al. Lateral connectivity in the olfactory bulb is sparse and segregated. *Front Neural Circuits*. 2011;5:5.
69. Crosby EC, Humphrey T, Lauer EW. *Correlative Anatomy of the Nervous System*. New York: MacMillan; 1962.
70. Crosby EC, Humphrey T. Studies of the vertebrate telencephalon. II. The nuclear pattern of the anterior olfactory nucleus, tuberculum olfactorium and amygdaloid complex in adult man. *J Comp Neurol*. 1941;74:309-352.
71. Marchand R, Bélanger MC. Ontogenesis of the axonal circuitry associated with the olfactory system of the rat embryo. *Neurosci Lett*. 1991;129:285-290.
76. Golgi C. Sulli fina struttura dei bulbi olfattorii. *Riv Sper Freniat Reggio-Emilia*. 1875;1:66-78.

80. Bushdid C, Magnasco MO, Vosshall LB, Keller A. Humans can discriminate more than 1 trillion olfactory stimuli. *Science*. 2014;343:1370-1372.
81. Sarnat HB, Netsky MG. *Evolution of the Nervous System*. Ed 2. New York: Oxford University Press; 1981:329-338.
87. Sarnat HB. Clinical neuropathology practice guide 5-2013: markers of neuronal maturation. *Clin Neuropathol*. 2013;32:340-369.
89. Sarnat HB. Olfactory reflexes in the newborn infant. *J Pediatr*. 1978;92: 624-626.
90. Lipsitt LP, Engen T, Kaye H. Developmental changes in the olfactory threshold of the neonate. *Child Dev*. 1963;34:371-376.
93. Marlier L, Gaugler C, Astruc D, Messer J. La sensibilité olfactive du nouveau-né prématuré. *Arch Pediatr*. 2007;14:45-53.
105. Rochefort C, Gheusi G, Vincent ID, Lledo PM. Enriched odor exposure increases the number of newborn neurons in the adult olfactory bulb and improves odor memory. *J Neurosci*. 2002;22:2679-2689.
109. Schaal B, Marlier L, Soussignan R. Olfactory function in the human fetus: evidence from selective neonatal responsiveness to the odor of amniotic fluid. *Behav Neurosci*. 1998;112:1438-1449.
136. Grus WE, Zhang J. Origin of the genetic components of the vomeronasal system in the common ancestor of all extant vertebrates. *Mol Biol Evol*. 2009;26:407-419.
141. Halpern M, Martínez-Marcos A. Structure and function of the vomeronasal system. An update. *Prog Neurobiol*. 2003;70:245-318.
149. Bradley RM, Stern IB. The development of the human taste bud during the foetal period. *J Anat*. 1967;101:743-752.
156. Barretto RP, Gillis-Smith S, Chandrashekar J, et al. The neural representation of taste quality at the periphery. *Nature*. 2014;517:373-376.
158. Risco S, Mediavilla C. Orexin-1 receptor antagonist in central nucleus of the amygdala attenuates the acquisition of flavour-taste preference in rats. *Pharmacol Biochem Behav*. 2014;126C:7-12.
163. Huang T, Krimm RF. BDNF and NT4 play interchangeable roles in gustatory development. *Dev Biol*. 2014;386:308-320.
165. Koudelka J, Horn JM, Vatanashevanopakorn C, Minichiello L. Genetic dissection of TrkB activated signalling pathways required for specific aspects of taste. *Neural Dev*. 2014;9:21.
167. Kist R, Watson M, Crosier M, et al. The formation of endoderm-derived taste sensory organs requires a Pax9-dependent expansion of embryonic taste bud progenitor cells. *PLoS Genet*. 2014;10:e1004709.
168. Clark AA, Dotson CD, Elson AE, et al. TAS2R bitter taste receptors regulate thyroid function. *FASEB J*. 2014;29:164-172.
171. Castillo D, Seidel K, Salcedo E, et al. Induction of ectopic taste buds by *SHH* reveals the competency and plasticity of adult lingual epithelium. *Dev*. 2014;141:2993-3002.
172. Hill DL, Mistrella CM. Developmental neurobiology of salt taste sensation. *Trends Neurosci*. 1990;13:188-195.
181. Rosenstein D, Oster H. Differential facial responses to four basic tastes in newborns. *Child Dev*. 1988;59:1555-1568.

The Growth Plate: Embryologic Origin, Structure, and Function

137

Emmanouil Grigoriou | John P. Dormans

INTRODUCTION

Skeletal formation and growth occur as a process of sequential morphologic and biochemical events that take place during fetal development. During development, bone tissue is formed and grows through one of two processes. Bone can form directly from mesenchymal tissue, which is called *intramembranous ossification*. This occurs at the periosteal surfaces of all bones and in parts of the pelvis, scapula, clavicles, and skull. Alternatively, bone tissue can form by replacement of a cartilaginous model, which is referred to as *endochondral ossification*. Endochondral ossification occurs at the base of the skull, the vertebrae, and at the growth plates of the appendicular skeleton.

Proliferating cartilage constitutes the basis for much of the size increase of bones as organs, because bone tissue itself does not grow interstitially. In the long bones of the limbs the proliferating cartilage is located at the ends, in the form of what is known as a *growth plate, physeal plate,* or *physis*. The cartilage in the growth plate has a unique zonal structure, biochemistry, process of matrix mineralization, and blood supply that differs markedly from hyaline or articular cartilage. Other areas of the body that have proliferating cartilage of various configurations include the skull (sutures and the base), the spine (end plates and synchondroses), the pelvis (triradiate cartilages), and the carpus and tarsus.

DEVELOPMENT OF THE GROWTH PLATE

Limb development has been studied in various organisms. Chick studies provided a wealth of information in the past because of the accessibility of the limb bud in ovo. However, molecular studies have focused largely on the mouse embryo. Cross-species transplants have indicated that many of the same signals control limb formation in both organisms. Additional information about limb patterning has been derived from the study of regenerating amphibian limbs.

The formation of the developing limb bud in vertebrates is initiated by the mesenchyme. Somites give rise to all limb muscle cells, whereas the lateral plate mesoderm gives rise to connective tissue and cartilage and thus determines the primary limb pattern.[1,2] In the absence of somites, the lateral plate mesoderm forms a limb with normal skeletal structure and tendons, which is devoid of any musculature.

The embryonic limb bud formation is initiated during the fourth week of gestation by the lateral plate mesoderm as a small projection on the ventrolateral body wall.[3] This mesenchymal projection is covered by ectoderm, the tip of which thickens and becomes what is known as the *apical ectodermal ridge* (AER) (Fig. 137.1), which drives limb outgrowth and proximodistal patterning. Underlying the AER are rapidly proliferating, undifferentiated mesenchymal cells that form what is known as the *progress zone* (PZ). Proliferation of these cells causes limb outgrowth. The events in upper and lower limb buds are similar in character and sequence. However, a slight craniocaudal time gradient exists, with the upper limb bud appearing and progressing 1 to 2 days before the lower limb bud. The molecular interaction between the AER and the underlying undifferentiated mesenchymal cells (PZ) drives limb development. Once the process of differentiation of all limb elements is complete, the AER disappears. Clinically, limb bud development is first identifiable by transvaginal ultrasound at 8 weeks.

As the limb bud grows, three major limb axes appear at different times and by different mechanisms (Fig. 137.2). The limb bud develops asymmetries along the proximodistal (flank to digit tip), anteroposterior (thumb to small finger), and dorsoventral (back of hand to palm) axes. Some of the important signals for initiating and maintaining these axes have been described in literature and will be discussed later in this chapter. The genes that initiate and potentiate signals in different axes often interact and are regulated via feedback mechanisms, resulting in effects in multiple planes of growth.

LIMB BUD OUTGROWTH (PROXIMODISTAL PATTERNING)

Limb bud outgrowth (proximodistal patterning) is dependent on signals emanating from the AER. The first signaling center to appear is AER and fibroblast growth factors (FGFs) produced in the AER stimulate cell proliferation in the underlying mesenchyme of the PZ. The expression of FGF-10 and FGF-8 is necessary to initiate limb bud outgrowth. The expression of each supports and promotes the expression of the other.[4] This FGF-8/FGF-10 loop is mediated by Wnt-2b, a mammalian homologue of *Drosophila* segment polarity gene-wingless and Wnt-8c proteins, through a β-catenin (Wnt/β-catenin) pathway.[5] FGF-2, FGF-4, FGF-8, FGF-9, and FGF-17 are expressed in the AER, and each is able to sustain limb bud outgrowth. A graft of an AER to an ectopic site on the bud leads to extra limb growth in the ectopic location. Removal of the AER or an abnormality in the AER stops limb bud growth and leads to proximal limb truncation. Similarly, disrupted FGF signaling leads to arrested limb development. Clinical examples of this are cleft hand and radial clubhand. However, limb bud outgrowth can be sustained after excision of the AER if FGF-impregnated beads are inserted in place of the AER.[6,7]

Cell growth and proliferation of the mesenchyme are maintained through a regulatory loop, with FGFs and a protein called *sonic hedgehog (Shh)*, which maintains the integrity of the AER. The formin gene, which encodes several proteins that function as cytokines, is required to establish this Shh/FGF-4 feedback loop. Bone morphogenetic proteins (BMPs), members of the transforming growth factor-β (TGF-β) superfamily, play a complex role in the regulation of the AER (also in dorsoventral patterning).[8,9] BMPs are necessary to the induction of the AER.[8] However, BMP signaling must be moderated by Gremlin (a BMP antagonist) to maintain the Shh/FGF-4 feedback loop necessary for limb outgrowth and patterning.[10] The activation of Gremlin is dependent on the expression of the formin gene.[11]

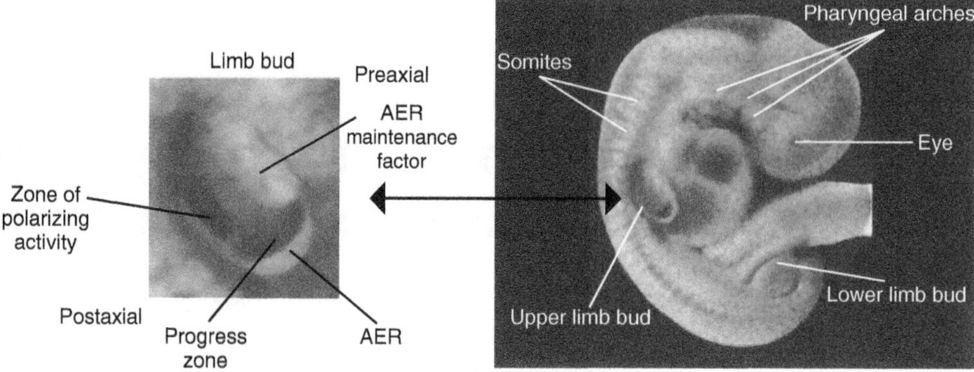

Fig. 137.1 A 5-week-old human embryo and enlargement of the upper and lower limb buds. The limb bud at this time is a jacket of ectoderm (apical ectodermal ridge *[AER]*) covering undifferentiated mesenchymal cells (progress zone). The zone of polarizing activity, which is involved in anteroposterior patterning of the limb, is localized in a small area of mesoderm along the posterior border of the limb bud.

ANTEROPOSTERIOR AXIS DETERMINATION

Anteroposterior axis determination is under the control of the zone of polarizing activity (ZPA), which is an area of tissue in the posterior aspect of the limb bud (see Fig. 137.1).Anteroposterior limb growth is also called *radioulnar* with ulnar signifying posterior and radius anterior location. Early chick studies showed that a mirror image digit duplication pattern developed when tissue from the posterior area was transplanted to the anterior portion of another wing bud.[12] The number of these additional digits developed depended on the strength (number of cells) and duration of transplant (16 hours for 2 digits, 20 hours for 3 digits). This observation led to the development of the morphogen gradient model whereby anteroposterior patterning was determined by diffusion of a signal. The *Shh* gene is an important regulator of anteroposterior patterning.[13] Normally there is a high concentration of Shh on the posterior (ulnar) side for small finger development and low concentration of Shh on anterior (radial) side for thumb development. Although early studies showed that exogenous application of retinoic acid to the anterior border of a normal limb could mimic results from ZPA transplant studies, this effect is now thought to occur via activation of the *Shh* gene.[14] *Shh* represses Gli3R activity in the posterior limb bud, thus affecting the precise balance of Gli3A and Gli3R, which may be the basis for the graded response to Shh signaling.[13]

Other genes important in anteroposterior patterning under investigation include the 5′Hoxd genes, Tbox, and Sall family genes (specifically Tbx2, Tbx3, Sall1, and Sall4), and defects in these genes cause digital alterations in humans.[15-17] Clinically, abnormal upregulation of Shh in the ZPA results in polydactyly on the ulnar (posterior) side, while upregulation of Shh in the anterior aspect of the limb bud (where Shh concentration should be low) leads to an absent thumb.

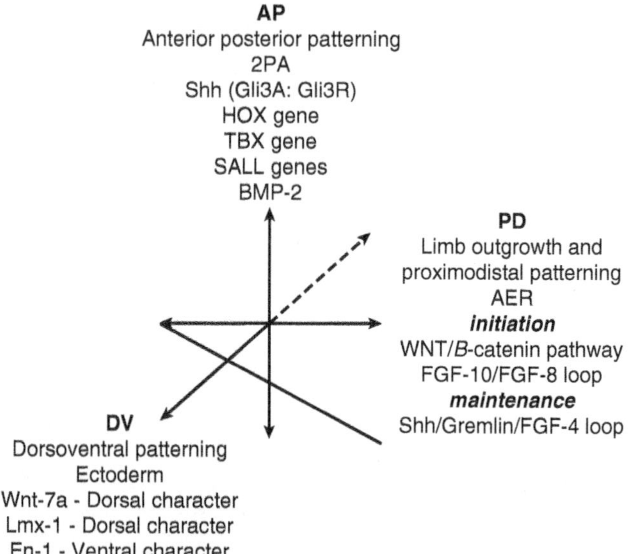

Fig. 137.2 Three major limb axes. As the limb bud grows, it develops asymmetries along the proximodistal *(PD)*, anteroposterior *(AP)*, and dorsoventral *(DV)* axes. The genes encoding the important signals that initiate and maintain these axes often interact and feedback, resulting in effects that are not confined to one direction of growth. *AER,* Apical ectodermal ridge; *BMP,* bone morphogenetic protein; *En,* engrailed; *FGF,* fibroblast growth factor; *GLI3A,* GLI3 activate; *GLI3R,* GLI3 repress; *Hox,* homeobox-containing gene; *SALL,* Sal-like gene; *Shh,* sonic hedgehog; *TBX,* T-box genes; *Wnt,* wingless; *ZPA,* zone of polarizing activity.

DORSOVENTRAL AXIS DETERMINATION

The dorsoventral axis is under the control of both the mesoderm and ectoderm of the limb bud at different stages of development. The mesoderm specifies the axis initially, but very early after limb bud formation, the ectodermal orientation becomes prominent. Wnt-7a, a secreted signaling protein, confers the dorsal character to the ectoderm and stimulates Lmx-1.[18] Lmx-1 is a HOX gene that encodes a transcription factor (LMX-1) that dorsalizes the mesoderm. In this way, Wnt-7a is responsible for all dorsal features including nails. The ventral ectoderm limb expresses a transcription factor called *engrailed-1 (EN-1) protein*, which suppresses Wnt-7a expression, thereby limiting such expression, and consequently LMX-1 activity to the area of the dorsal mesenchyme.[19] Studies on BMP function have shown that BMP signaling is both necessary and sufficient to regulate EN1 expression, and consequently plays a role in dorsoventral patterning.[8]

Both the AER and the ZPA activate *HOXA* and *HOXD* genes. *HOX* genes have specifically been shown to affect the growth of cartilage and precartilaginous condensations. They are likely to be important in determining the length, segmentation, and branching of limb elements. *HOX* genes are not expressed strictly along anteroposterior or dorsoventral axes, and their position of expression differs in various areas of the limb.

BONE AND GROWTH PLATE DEVELOPMENT

The first sign of potential bone formation occurs in the early embryonic period as a localized condensation of the mesenchyme. Cellular condensations arise as a result of either increased mitotic activity or an aggregation of cells drawn toward a specific site.[20] As the mesenchyme begins to condense, the cells become more rounded, a process that occurs concomitantly with a reduction in the amount of intercellular substance. This stage is referred to as the *precartilage blastema.* As the tissue continues to mature, the mesenchymal condensations differentiate into

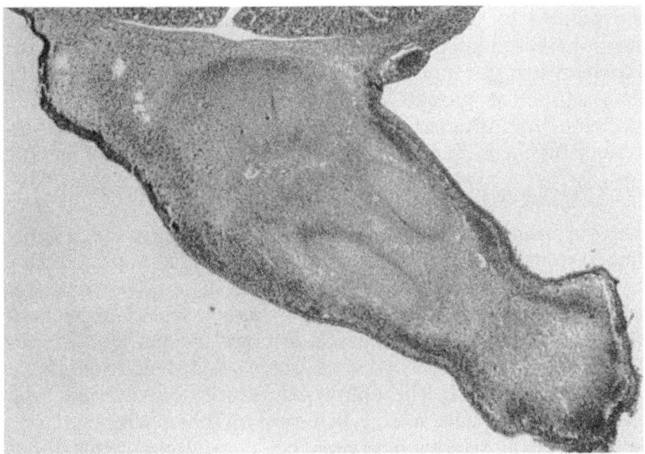

Fig. 137.3 Longitudinal section of the developing hindlimb from a 13-day mouse embryo (hematoxylin and eosin,×40). Mesenchymal condensations of the skeletal anlagen have begun to form.

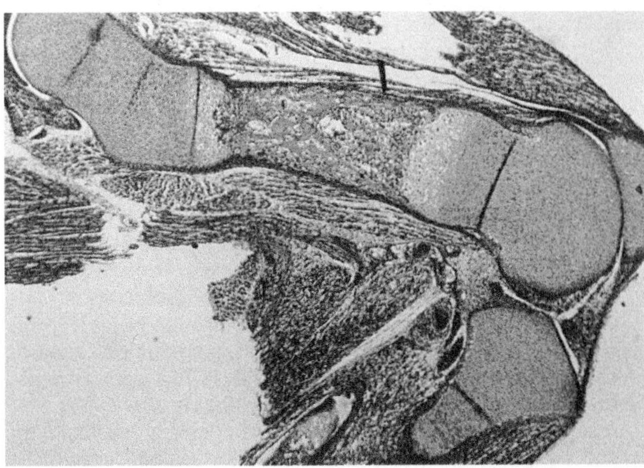

Fig. 137.4 Longitudinal section of the femur and proximal tibia from an 18-day mouse fetus (hematoxylin and eosin,×40). The primary center of ossification has formed at the midshaft of the femur. The proximal (*left*, hip) and distal (*right*, knee) chondroepiphyses are visible, as are part of the cartilaginous patella and the proximal tibial chondroepiphysis.

chondrocytes, which are characterized by specific molecular markers, such as aggrecan and type II collagen. These extracellular matrix (ECM) proteins distinguish differentiating chondrocytes from the undifferentiated mesenchymal cells remaining at the periphery of the skeletal element that form a structure called the *perichondrium*.[21] Chondrocytes proliferate in parallel columns to form a template, or anlagen (skeletal anlagen), of the future bone (Fig. 137.3). This transformation occurs during the sixth week of gestation. During the seventh week of gestation, the innermost chondrocytes of the anlagen further differentiate into hypertrophic chondrocytes. At the same time as the chondrocytes hypertrophy, perichondrial cells start to differentiate into osteoblasts to form a mineralized structure around the cartilaginous core, termed the *bone collar*.[22,23] Once fully differentiated, hypertrophic chondrocytes become surrounded by a calcified ECM that favors vascular invasions from the bone collar through a vascular endothelial growth factor-dependent pathway. This process brings in chondroblasts that will degrade the ECM surrounding the hypertrophic chondrocytes and provides progenitors of osteoblasts derived from the bone collar.[24] The osteoblasts produce an osteoid matrix on the surfaces of the calcified cartilaginous bars and form the primary trabeculae; this process is called *endochondral ossification*. This initial site of ossification is known as the *primary ossification center*, and most of these appear in the late fetal period (Fig. 137.4).

This sequential process of chondrocyte proliferation, hypertrophy, and replacement by osteoblasts becomes organized into the growth plate at each end of the expanding bone. The growth plates are apposed to the metaphyses at either end of the long bone. The histologic elements of the growth plate are well defined. Chondrocyte division is well organized into zones that can be demonstrated using autoradiography and tritiated thymidine.[25-27] Once the growth plate has been formed, longitudinal growth of the bone occurs by appositional growth of cells from within the growth plate, and new bone is formed at the metaphyseal side of each growth plate through a process that recapitulates the stages that occurred in the central portion of the original cartilaginous anlage. The rate at which this growth occurs varies at different anatomic positions; proliferating cartilage is arranged differently at different anatomic locations. This process continues until closure of the growth plates at skeletal maturity.

At specific times in the postnatal development of each long bone, a secondary center of ossification (epiphysis) forms at the end of each bone. The secondary center of ossification is another zone of proliferating cartilage underneath the articular cartilage and is responsible for growth of the chondro-epiphyseal cartilage surrounding the epiphysis (Fig. 137.5).[28] The processes of chondrocyte proliferation and hypertrophy, matrix calcification, vascular invasion, and osteoblastic new bone formation occur in the same sequence as in the growth plate associated with the primary ossification center. However, the epiphyseal end of the long bone enlarges as a result of radial apposition of cells around the secondary ossification center. Although not essential, the proinflammatory cytokine interleukin-1 (IL-1) is necessary for normal growth plate and bone development. IL-1 receptor deficiency is associated with a narrower growth plate and abnormal proteoglycan content.[29]

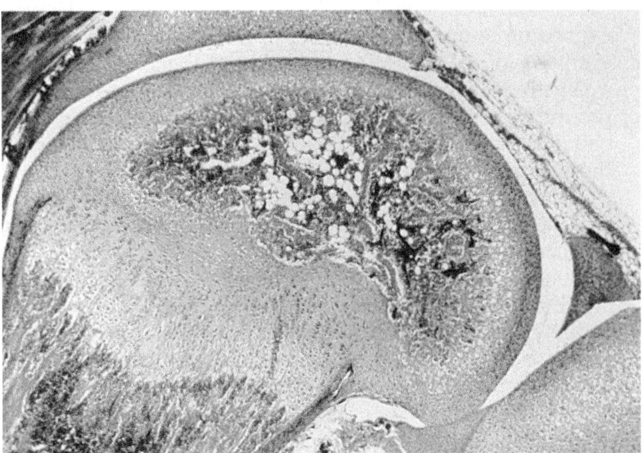

Fig. 137.5 Longitudinal section of the distal femur from a 10-day postnatal mouse (hematoxylin and eosin,×40). The secondary center of ossification has formed within the distal femoral chondroepiphysis. The growth plate or physis is clearly defined between the secondary center of ossification and the metaphysis.

MOLECULAR BIOLOGY OF CHONDROCYTE DIFFERENTIATION

The growth plate is made up of highly organized chondrocytes at different stages of differentiation. Several growth factors, transcription factors, ECM proteins, and cell-matrix interactions control nonhypertrophic chondrocyte differentiation and proliferation. Transcriptional factors, including Sox9 and Sox5, control chondrogenesis.[30,31] Runx2, also called *core-binding factor-α subunit 1 (CBFA1)*, is a member of the runt family of transcription factors and is necessary for osteoblast-specific gene expression.[32] Runx2 is expressed in prehypertrophic chondrocytes and its constitutive expression in nonhypertrophic chondrocytes induces differentiation to hypertrophic chondrocytes, Indian hedgehog (Ihh) expression, and eventually, endochondral bone formation.[33] These functions, along with its role during osteoblast differentiation and vascular invasion, identify CBFA1 as the most pleiotropic regulator of skeletogenesis. Genetic deletion of various transcriptional factors can lead to severe skeletal malformation and will be discussed at the last section of this chapter.

There are a number of mediators involved in chondrogenesis:

- FGF signaling regulates chondrocyte proliferation and differentiation. FGFs activate signaling through FGF receptors (FGFRs). FGF receptor 3 (FGFR3) is expressed in proliferating chondrocytes, while FGF receptor 1 (FGFR1) is expressed in prehypertrophic and hypertrophic chondrocytes. FGF receptor 2 (FRFR2) is expressed in condensing mesenchyme and by perichondrial cells. The FGFR3 inhibits growth by restraining chondrocyte division.[34] A genetic mutation leading to constitutive activation of FGFR3 is the cause of achondroplasia, a dwarfing condition in which short stature is the result of continuous inhibition of chondrocyte proliferation in the growth plate.[35,36]
- Ihh promotes nonhypertrophic chondrocyte proliferation. Parathyroid-hormone (PTH) related protein (PTHrP) expression is under the control of Ihh; Ihh up-regulates the synthesis of PTHrP by prehypertrophic chondrocytes via a negative feedback loop, thereby indirectly slowing down the process of chondrocyte hypertrophy and promoting chondrocyte proliferation.[22,32,37] An interesting link between the Ihh pathway and the FGF pathway is indicated by data showing that FGFR3 signaling can inhibit Ihh expression.[38] It is believed that the effects of FGF signaling are in part mediated by suppression of the Ihh/PTHrP signaling.[38,39]
- Insulin-like growth factor (IGF)-1 receptor signaling also plays a role in chondrocyte differentiation by interacting with the PTHrP/Ihh pathway. An absence of the anabolic growth factor IGR-1 results in reduced proliferation, increased apoptosis, and abnormal differentiation of chondrocytes.[40,41]
- C-type natriuretic peptide (CNP) signaling stimulates longitudinal growth of cartilage and promotes endochondral bone growth.[31]
- BMP signaling is complex. The BMP family of growth factors play a role in osteogenesis and chondrogenesis from commitment and condensation to terminal differentiation.[42] BMP receptors BMPR1B and BMPR1A are expressed in cartilage condensations and the embryonic mesenchyme, respectively, though their functions overlap in the early stages of chondrogenesis. BMP signaling acts to control specific aspects of chondrocyte proliferation and differentiation. BMPs also have a role in the regulation of the Ihh/PTHrP and FGF pathways.
- Wnt signaling also plays an important role in the regulation of hypertrophic chondrocyte biology. Studies have shown that misexpression of Wnt-4 accelerates the transition from nonhypertrophic chondrocyte to hypertrophic chondrocyte, and in doing so results in slightly advanced ossification, whereas misexpression of Wnt-5a causes a delay in the transition from prehypertrophic to hypertrophic chondrocyte and results in a mild delay in ossification.[34]
- Other growth factors include TGF-β, thyroid hormone, and connective tissue growth factor.

GROWTH PLATE

The growth plate of a long bone provides an exceptional example of seamless correlation among histology, ordered cytodifferentiation, molecular biology, and physical function. The growth plate is composed of a cartilaginous component surrounded by a fibrous component and bounded by a bony metaphyseal component. Each component has a unique structure, biochemistry, and function; together, these result in longitudinal and latitudinal growth and remodeling of the developing skeleton. The vascular supply of the growth plate results in unique biochemical properties and is integral to normal function.

VASCULAR SUPPLY

The normal growth and development of a bone are inextricably linked to its vascular, and in particular its arterial, supply. In fact, the onset and maintenance of ossification depend on a constant supply of nutrients. There are three major vascular suppliers to the growth plate: the epiphyseal arteries, the nutrient arteries (from the metaphyseal vascular system), and the perichondrial arteries (Fig. 137.6). The epiphyseal arteries are derived from periarticular vascular arcades that form on the nonarticular bone surfaces. These arteries send branches through the cartilaginous epiphysis within cartilage canals to supply the reserve and proliferative zones of the growth plate.[43] Thus the overall viability of the growth plate to maintain normal bone growth and development depends on the integrity of these vessels. Any damage to these arteries has the potential to result in growth arrest.

The metaphyseal supply is primarily derived from the nutrient arteries, also known as *diaphyseal arteries*. The nutrient arteries are generally derived from an adjacent major systemic artery. A nutrient artery enters a bone through its nutrient foramen, which leads into a nutrient canal, and once the vessel reaches the medullary cavity, it divides into ascending and descending medullary branches.[43,44] The ascending and descending medullary branches anastomose with the metaphyseal collaterals at the metaphyseal zone. The metaphyseal supply induces blood-borne precursors that promote ossification and remodeling at the hypertrophic zone (HZ) of the growth plate.[43,45] The physeal cartilage itself maintains a separation between these two circulations throughout normal human growth. The perichondrial arteries supply the ring of LaCroix and the groove of Ranvier (see later). Capillaries from this system communicate with the epiphyseal and metaphyseal capillaries in addition to the vessels of the joint capsule.

CARTILAGINOUS COMPONENT

Within the growth plate the various subpopulations of chondrocytes (zones)—reserve (resting), proliferative (proliferating), hypertrophic—are arranged in columns (see Fig. 137.6). These chondrocytes regulate longitudinal growth of the skeleton until their disappearance at the end of puberty in humans. Each zone has characteristic histologic and biochemical features that define its formation.[45-47]

The zone farthest away from the diaphysis and closest to the epiphysis is the *reserve zone* (RZ). In this zone the chondrocytes are small, round, and randomly distributed. The chondrocytes in the RZ rarely replicate; the ratio of matrix volume to cell volume is the highest of any layer of the growth plate.[47] The matrix contains randomly oriented fibrils of type II collagen, which inhibit calcification and act as a barrier to the advancing front of the secondary center of ossification.[21] The chondrocytes in this zone receive a vascular supply from the epiphyseal vessels; however, the epiphyseal vessels do not actually arborize in the RZ, and hence the oxygen tension in this zone is relatively low. The precise function of the RZ remains ill defined. Two likely functions are (1) physical separation between the osseous tissue of the secondary center and the remainder of the growth plate, and (2) synthesis and storage of nutrients and raw materials (i.e., glycogen, lipid, and proteoglycan aggregates) that will be used for matrix production and to replenish the pool of proliferative chondrocytes at the lower zones of the growth plate.[48] Gaucher's disease and multiple skeletal dysplasias (diastrophic dysplasia,

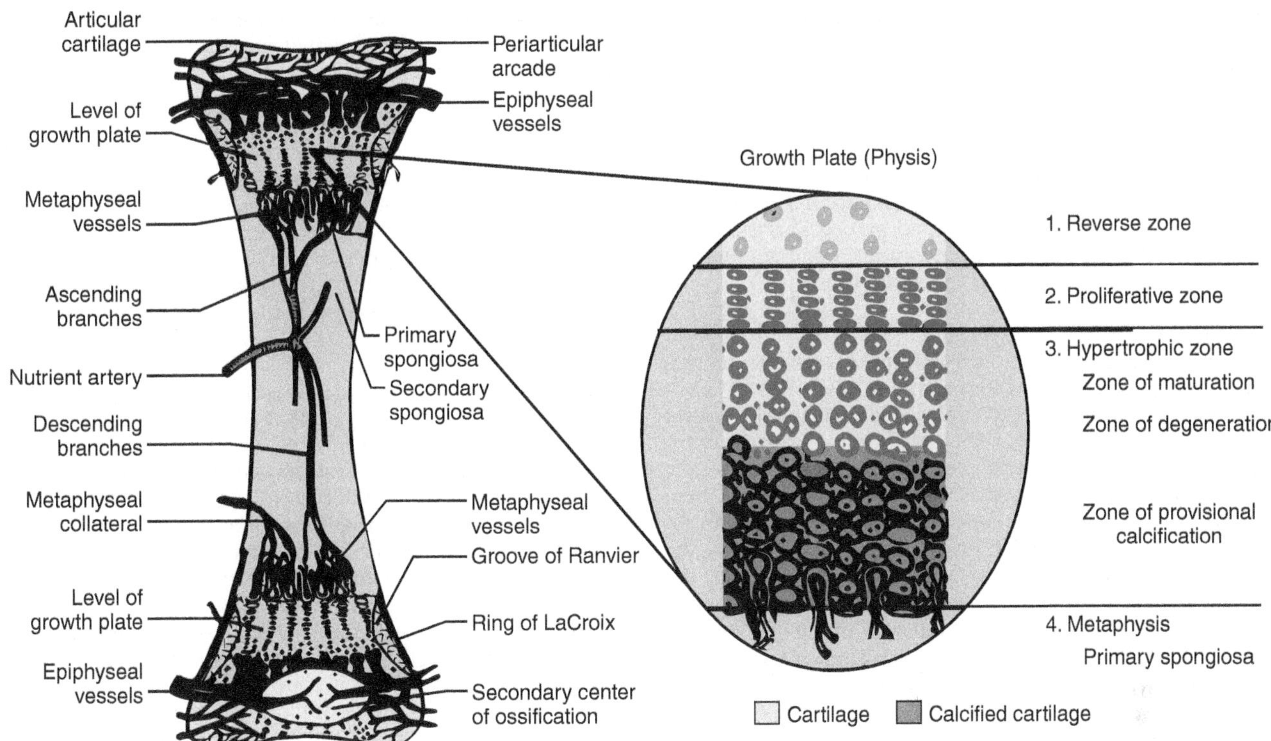

Fig. 137.6 Diagrammatic illustration of the blood supply and zones of the growth plate. (Modified from Scheuer L, Black S. Bone development. In: Scheuer L, Black S, editors. *Developmental Juvenile Osteology*. London: Academic Press; 2000:18–31.)

Kniest dysplasia, pseudoachondroplasia) have their anatomic basis of pathology at this zone.

In the adjacent *proliferative zone,* the chondrocytes are tightly bound in columns parallel to the axis of the length of the bone. The cytoplasm contains glycogen stores and is rich in endoplasmic reticulum, features suggesting a rich source of nutrients for aerobic glycolysis and a high capacity for protein synthesis. Of the three zones, this zone has the highest rate of proteoglycan synthesis and turnover. The proteoglycans (aggrecans) in this zone are large aggregates consisting of glycosaminoglycans attached to core proteins.[49] Such aggregates inhibit calcification. The chondrocytes replicate rapidly in the proliferative zone, and they become flattened and slightly irregular in shape. The rate of duplication of cells is closely regulated and usually constant.[50] The binding matrix is contiguous with the matrix of the RZ and has the same biochemical composition. The type II collagen fibrils are oriented longitudinally, surrounding the columns of chondrocytes. The epiphyseal vessels that crossed the RZ terminate in the proliferative zone, thereby resulting in the highest oxygen concentration in the growth plate. The presence of rich glycogen stores and a high oxygen tension supports aerobic metabolism in the proliferative zone chondrocyte. The functions of the proliferative zone—matrix production and cellular division—together contribute to longitudinal growth.[46,47] Achondroplasia, gigantism, and hereditary multiple osteochondromas affect this zone of the growth plate.

The HZ has traditionally been divided into two parts: the upper, or zone of maturation; and the lower, or zone of degeneration. The very lowest portion of the HZ, right at the metaphyseal border, is also called the *zone of provisional calcification.* In the zone of maturation, the chondrocytes start to hypertrophy. A change occurs in the proteoglycans of the matrix in this zone, which involves a decrease in the size of the aggrecan. This decrease results from an active degradation mediated by physeal enzymes, including metalloproteases (i.e., collagenase, stromelysin, and neutral growth plate proteases).[51,52] A marked decrease also occurs in type II collagen synthesis. In moving down the cellular column and away from the epiphyseal vessels, the chondrocytes are exposed to an environment of increasingly lower oxygen tension.

The major energy source for production of adenosine triphosphate (ATP) in the HZ chondrocytes is anaerobic glycolysis of glucose from endogenous glycogen stores. Glycogen is stored in the RZ and proliferative zone and is then consumed in the HZ. Metabolic activity in the HZ cells differs from that in most animal cells. In most cell types, glucose is oxidized to pyruvate in the cytoplasm, and the pyruvate then enters the mitochondria (by glycerol phosphate shuttle) to be further oxidized by the Krebs cycle. The Krebs cycle is an important additional energy source for most cells. In the growth plate, pyruvate continues to enter the mitochondria but at a much-reduced rate, and glycerol phosphate does not enter the mitochondria because the growth plate zones lack the glycerol phosphate shuttle. Thus, even in the presence of oxygen, the growth plate cartilage metabolizes glucose relatively anaerobically. The mitochondria of the chondrocytes in the proliferative zone are capable of conducting the Krebs cycle and generating ATP. However, in the HZ, owing to lower oxygen tension, a switch occurs in the function of the mitochondria from ATP production to calcium accumulation. These mitochondrial stores allow buffering of the ionized intracellular calcium in the already high concentrations of the HZ.[53,54]

In the zone of degeneration, a further diminution in proteoglycan size is observed. The proteoglycan, which in aggrecan form is an inhibitor of calcification, no longer serves such a role because it is increasingly degraded.[51,52] Biochemical analysis shows that the chondrocytes in this zone are very active metabolically. They synthesize alkaline phosphatase, neutral proteases, and type X collagen, thereby participating in matrix mineralization. The mitochondria of the chondrocytes here begin to disgorge the calcium previously accumulated. This calcium is apparently packaged in vesicles of cellular membrane and is deposited into the surrounding matrix.[53] The hypertrophic chondrocytes do not synthesize type II collagen in the lower HZ, but instead synthesize type X collagen, a unique protein associated with endochondral ossification.[55,56] Active changes in chondrocytic activity occur at this site and lead to degeneration and cell death at the last intact transverse septum forming the interface with the metaphysis.[57] The longitudinal septa begin to calcify in this region of the growth plate; hence this zone is also termed the *zone of provisional calcification*. This is where the last transverse septa are ultimately degraded. This is also the zone where physeal fractures, slipped capital femoral epiphysis (SCFE), rickets, and many skeletal dysplasias occur.

METAPHYSIS

The metaphysis begins distal to the last intact transverse septum of each cartilaginous cell column of the HZ (see Fig. 137.6). It functions in the removal of the mineralized cartilaginous matrix of the HZ and eventually in the formation of the *primary spongiosa*. Bone formation begins with the invasion of the hypertrophic lacunae by vascular loops, bringing with them osteoblasts that initiate the synthesis of bone.[58,59] The osteoblasts progressively lay down bone on the cartilage template, the cartilage bars produced by physeal expansion. Subsequently, the initial woven bone and cartilage bars of the primary spongiosa are resorbed by osteoblasts and are replaced by lamellar bone to produce the *secondary spongiosa*.[58]

PERICHONDRIAL RING OF LACROIX AND GROOVE OF RANVIER

Surrounding the periphery of the physis is a wedge-shaped structure known as the *groove of Ranvier* and a ring of fibrous tissue known as the *ring of LaCroix* (see Fig. 137.6). During the first year of life, this ring spreads over the adjacent metaphysis to form a fibrous circumferential ring bridging the epiphysis to the diaphysis. The cells in the groove of Ranvier are active in cell division and contribute to an increase in the diameter, or latitudinal growth, of the growth plate. Besides appositional bone growth, this ring also increases the mechanical strength of the physis. The basic structure of the perichondrial ring of LaCroix is a fibrous collagenous network that is continuous with the fibrous portion of the groove of Ranvier and the periosteum of the metaphysis. The perichondrial ring functions as a strong mechanical support at the bone-cartilage junction of the growth plate, and anchors and supports the physis through peripheral stability.

GROWTH AND ITS CONTROL

The endocrine control of the growth plate is a complex and important aspect of growth (Fig. 137.7). Numerous factors have been identified as important regulators of bone and cartilage (Table 137.1). Some of these factors (systemic hormones, vitamins, and growth factors) are produced at a site distant from the growth plate and therefore act on the chondrocytes through a classic endocrine mechanism. Other factors are produced and act within the growth plate and therefore function as paracrine or autocrine factors.[30] Each zone of the growth plate may be specifically targeted by one or more agents to affect a particular stage in the cell maturation phenomenon.

Growth hormone (GH) is a peptide hormone secreted by the pituitary gland; its deficiency or insensitivity leads to pituitary dwarfism while its excess (most commonly due to pituitary

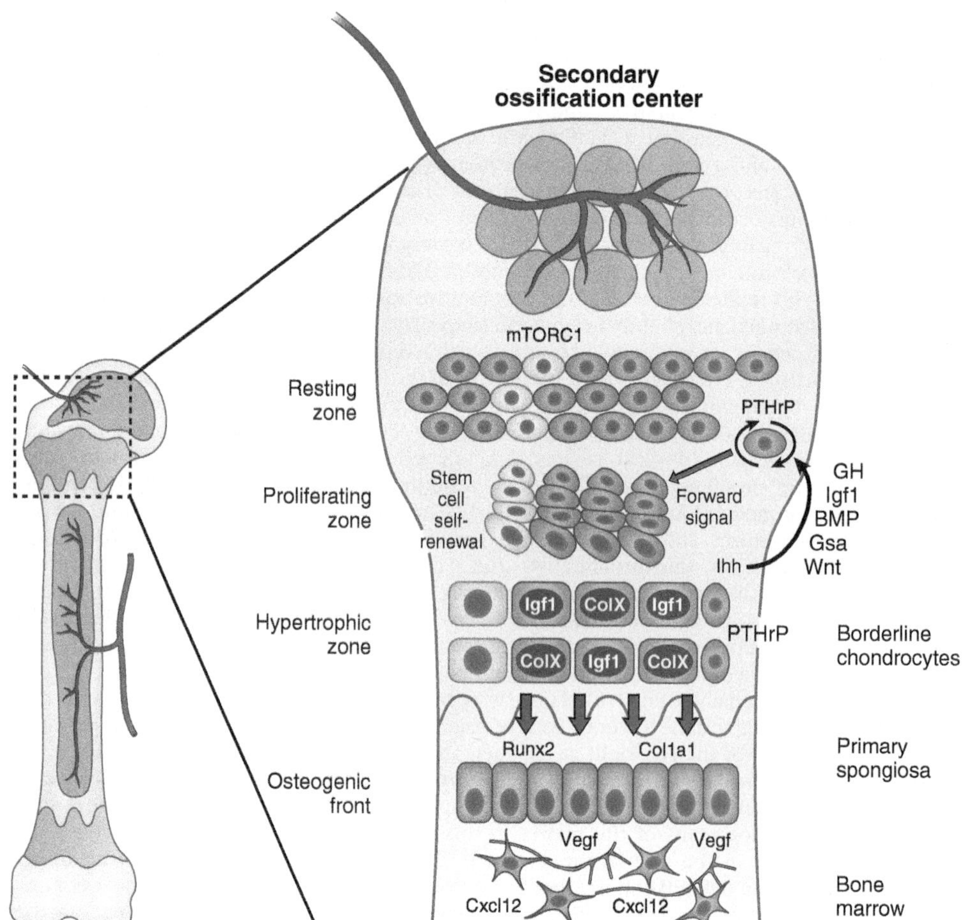

Fig. 137.7 Molecular characteristics of growth plate chondrocytes and their differentiation trajectories. *BMP*, Bone morphogenetic protein; *GH*, growth hormone; *IGF*, insulin-like growth factor; *Wnt*, wingless. (Modified from Hallett SA, Ono W, Ono N. Growth plate chondrocytes: skeletal development, growth and beyond. *Int J Mol Sci*. 2019;20:6009.)

adenomas in childhood) leads to gigantism. GH acts throughout the growth plate and primarily stimulates cellular proliferation. GH does not directly stimulate the growth plate; rather, it stimulates production of a group of peptide growth factors termed *somatomedin* or IGF. The effects of GH mainly result from the production of serum-derived IGF by the liver, but a direct GH effect also occurs that causes chondrocytes to produce IGF locally (paracrine or autocrine effect). IGF-I (somatomedin C) is the potent stimulator of postnatal growth mediating chondrocyte proliferation and matrix synthesis, whereas IGF-II is mainly the fetal somatomedin.[60] Immunohistochemical studies have localized the highest concentration of IGF-I receptors to the PZ of the growth plate.[61] IGF-I increases cellular proliferation, probably by two mechanisms: by direct IGF-I effects and, perhaps more importantly, through the modulation of other growth factor effects. The synergistic interactions of IGF-I with FGF and TGF-β are specific for DNA synthesis, a finding that confirms the central role of IGF-I on mitogenesis in the growth plate.[60]

The thyroid hormones thyroxine (T4) and triiodothyronine (T3) are peptide hormones produced by the thyroid gland. The thyroid hormones act on the PZ and upper HZ chondrocytes through a systemic endocrine mechanism that promotes chondrocyte maturation.[32,62,63] Thyroxine enhances cartilage growth by two functions: (1) it increases DNA synthesis in cells from the proliferative zone, and (2) it increases glycosaminoglycan and collagen synthesis and alkaline phosphatase activity. Its effect on cartilage growth is mediated by synergy between thyroxine and IGF-I. These two agents together modulate both growth and maturation. Triiodothyronine also increases cartilage growth by interacting with IGF-I. It promotes the cytodifferentiation from a proliferative to a hypertrophic chondrocyte; however, independently from IGF-I.

PTH is produced by the parathyroid glands. It acts primarily on the proliferative zone and upper HZ chondrocytes, and it has a direct agonist role in the cellular metabolism of the growth plate.[62,63] A complex relationship exists among PTH, the intracellular calcium concentration, and regulation of the growth plate.[37,64] In the growth plate chondrocyte, PTH stimulates the production of inositol triphosphate from phosphoinositol 4,5-biphosphate. Inositol triphosphate induces the release of calcium from an intracellular store, which causes a transient increase in the cytosolic ionized calcium concentration. PTH also mediates an increase in proteoglycan synthesis through the breakdown of membrane phosphoinositides and subsequent activation of protein kinase C. The regeneration of membrane phosphoinositides can result in the stimulation of prostaglandin synthesis, which also appears to have a small stimulatory effect on proteoglycan synthesis. PTHrP, secreted during fetal life by perichondrial cells at the ends of cartilage, acts on the same G-protein-coupled receptor used by PTH. PTHrP binds to the PTH/PTHrP receptor present in prehypertrophic chondrocytes and by delaying chondrocyte maturation keeps proliferating chondrocytes in the proliferative pool, ensuring the supply of proliferating chondrocytes necessary for skeletal growth is maintained.[32,37,64]

The effects of sex steroids (androgens and estrogens) on proliferating cartilage are complex.[63] Although androgens and estrogens may increase chondrocyte division, they may also interact with adrenal steroids and many other factors. Androgens function primarily in the lower portion of the growth plate to stimulate mineralization. Their anabolic effect is manifested as an increased deposition of glycogen and lipids in cells and an increase in proteoglycans in cartilage matrix. Androgens can also stimulate DNA synthesis in chondrocytes. Estrogen signaling is necessary for normal skeletal maturation and growth plate closure in late puberty, in both males and females. Premature exposure to high levels of estrogen (precocious puberty) causes premature growth plate closure and short stature, while males with genetic loss of estrogen receptors, or of the aromatase enzyme that converts androgen to estrogen, have delayed bone age and epiphyseal closure.[30,65]

Besides FGFs (see the earlier section, "Bone and Growth Plate Development"), several other growth factors have been demonstrated to contribute to the regulation of the growth

Table 137.1 Growth Plate Control.

Agent	Effect
Specific Endocrine Hormones	
1. Thyroid hormones	↑ Chondrocyte proliferation, ↑ chondrocyte maturation
2. Growth hormones	Secreted by pituitary; converted to somatomedin (IGF-I); IGF-I interacts with local factors
3. IGF-I	↑ Chondrocyte proliferation in resting and proliferative zones, regulate enchondral bone formation
4. Insulin	Interacts with IGF-I receptor, ↑ chondrocyte proliferation
5. PTH-related peptide	Binds to PTH receptor → ↑ cAMP → ↑ chondrocyte proliferation and matrix synthesis, also works through inositol triphosphate and protein kinase C. Negative feedback loop with Ihh.
6. Androgens	↑ Proliferation but pharmacologic doses may promote growth plate closure
7. Estrogens	↓ Proliferation in the proliferative zone and ↑ growth plate closure
8. Glucocorticoids	↓ Chondrocyte proliferation and ↓ growth plate closure
Local Agents	
1. Various growth factors	
2. Various cytokines	
3. Other small molecules	
Autocrine, paracrine	
- Fibroblast growth factor	↑ Chondrocyte proliferation, regulate enchondral bone formation, interact with IGF-I
- Transforming growth factor-β	Relatively variable effects depending on other agents present, ↑ chondrocyte proliferation and maturation, important in expression and maintenance of SOX9
- Interleukin-1	↑ Matrix degradation through metalloproteinases
- Prostaglandin	↑ Proteoglycan, ↓ collagen, alkaline phosphatase
Vitamins	
1. Vitamin A	Required for chondrocyte maturation, variable pathways
2. Vitamin C	Necessary cofactor for collagen synthesis
3. Vitamin D and metabolites	Required for calcification of matrix, deficiency, leads to failure of calcification and marked elongation of the hypertrophic zone (rickets)

cAMP, Cyclic adenosine monophosphate; *IGF*, insulin-like growth factor; *Ihh*, Indian hedgehog; *PTH*, parathyroid hormone.

plate. Platelet-derived growth factor stimulates DNA synthesis and cell replication of chondrocytes and protein synthesis. TGF-β is a multifunctional peptide that controls cell replication and differentiation. It is involved in cartilage formation during the first step of endochondral bone formation. Release of TGF-β is stimulated by PTH, but the overall effect of TGF-β appears to depend on constituent growth factors in the cell. Therefore its effects may be stimulatory or inhibitory, depending on the hormonal environment when TGF-β is introduced to the chondrocytes.[44] For example, TGF-β can inhibit progression of growth plate chondrocytes to the full hypertrophic phenotype, although this can be overcome by the thyroid hormones that drive maturation.[28] However, TGF-β is a potent inhibitor of a lymphocyte-activating factor called IL-1, which induces degradation in growth plate chondrocytes.[53]

The mammalian target of rapamycin (mTOR) pathway is a ubiquitous, central regulator of cell metabolism, which is critical for organismal growth and homeostasis, and recently has been implicated and further studied in the homeostasis of the growth plate. There are several studies that show its role in embryonic skeletal growth, and it was demonstrated recently that it promotes early stage chondrocyte proliferation and prevents later stage terminal differentiation.[66] It seems that mTOR signaling is an important coordinator of chondrocyte proliferation and hypertrophy and its disruption might affect growth plate homeostasis through disrupting other signaling pathways.[62]

Several vitamins are required for normal growth plate function.[67] The active metabolites of vitamin D (1,25- and 24,25-dihydroxyvitamin D3) are produced in the liver and kidney. The vitamin D metabolites are bound to cells in all growth plate zones except the HZ. The highest levels are found in the PZ. Vitamin D deficiency results in an elongation of the cell columns of the HZ and defective mineralization. Histologically, rickets—the clinically observed form of vitamin D deficiency—presents as failure of calcification of the matrix and marked elongation of the HZ. Histologically, the RZ and PZ are normal, but the HZ is greatly expanded, and this results in widening of the growth plate.[30,68] Vitamin C is a necessary cofactor for the synthesis of collagen. Deficiency of vitamin C leads to scurvy. The greatest deficiency in collagen synthesis is seen in the metaphysis. The microscopic appearance of the cartilaginous portion of the growth plate is normal, but that of the metaphysis is quite abnormal. The physeal-metaphyseal junction is particularly disrupted, with persistence of calcified cartilage and sparse bony trabeculae. Vitamin A is essential for epiphyseal cartilage cell metabolism. A deficiency state results in impairment of the chondrocyte maturation.

CORRELATED CLINICAL CONDITIONS

Review of the pathophysiology of some common skeletal dysplasias (osteochondrodysplasias) will allow better understanding of the physiology of the normal bone and growth plate development. Skeletal dysplasias are a group of genetic disorders characterized by abnormalities of growth and development of bone and cartilage. The generalized disturbance in the development of the skeleton affects the skull, the spine, and the extremities in varying degrees, resulting in disproportionate short stature (short-trunk or short-limb dwarfism). Because of the numerous endocrine and paracrine signaling pathways required for the physiologic function of the growth plate, it is not surprising that mutations in more than 400 genes have been described, causing more than 460 discrete skeletal dysplasias.[69,70] The pathogenesis of many of these conditions is slowly being discovered, teaching us little by little about the growth of the skeleton (Table 137.2). Future research in this area may lead to the development of therapeutic agents that target the genetic abnormalities that cause the following mentioned pathologies.

Achondroplasia, the most frequent form of short-limb dwarfism and the most common skeletal dysplasia, is an autosomal dominant condition. Two thirds of cases arise by spontaneous new mutations that have been mapped to chromosome 4, in a region encoding *Fgfr-3*.[35,36] The activating mutations in the *Fgfr-3* gene lead to a retardation in chondrocyte proliferation in the proliferative zone resulting in abnormal endochondral ossification. It is characterized by rhizomelic dwarfism with normal trunk and short arms and legs, and midface hypoplasia with macrocephaly and frontal bossing. *Hypochondroplasia* is an autosomal dominant allelic variant of achondroplasia with similar phenotypic and genotypic features while sometimes it is associated with intellectual disability and/or epilepsy. The mutation in the *Fgfr-3* gene occurs in a different region (in the tyrosine kinase domain in contrast to the transmembrane domain in achondroplasia).[35] A mutation in *Fgfr-2* results in *Crouzon syndrome,* in which the cranial sutures are disrupted.[71] *Pfeiffer syndrome* and *Jackson-Weiss syndrome* (both of which are characterized by craniosynostoses and limb defects) are mutations in both the *Fgfr-1* and *Fgfr-2 genes*.[72] The coordination of the various *Fgfrs* and receptors appears to be responsible for proportional growth.

Table 137.2 Molecular and Pathogenetic Basis of Selected Chondrodysplasias.

Condition	Molecular Basis	Defective
Achondroplasia Hypochondroplasia	FGFR3	Receptor/signal transduction
Various craniosynostosis syndromes (Apert, Crouzon, Pfeiffer)	FGFR2	Receptor/signal transduction
Diastrophic dysplasia Achondrogenesis 1B Autosomal recessive multiple epiphyseal dysplasia (MED)	Diastrophic dysplasia sulfate transporter (DTDST gene), SLC26A2	Sulphation/metabolic pathways
Spondyloepiphyseal dysplasia (SED) Stickler syndrome Kniest dysplasia	COL2A1	Type 2 collagen
MED Pseudoachondroplasia	COMP, COL9A1, COL9A2, COL9A3, COMP, MATN3	Extracellular structural proteins
Jansen's metaphyseal chondrodysplasia	PTH/PTHrP receptor	Receptor/signal transduction

COMP, Cartilage oligomeric matrix protein; *FGFR,* fibroblast growth factor receptor; *PTH/PTHrP,* parathyroid hormone/parathyroid-hormone related peptide.

Diastrophic dysplasia is a rare autosomal recessive condition characterized by short-limb dwarfism with spinal deformities and specific hand, foot, and ear abnormalities. The responsible gene has been mapped to chromosome 5 (DTDST gene) and encodes a sulfate transporter protein (diastrophic dysplasia sulfate transporter).[73] Impaired function of this protein is thought to lead to undersulfation of proteoglycans in the cartilage matrix, thus affecting hydration of the cartilage. Because it causes failure of formation of the secondary ossification center, it is associated with a progressive deformity.

Mutations in the gene encoding type II collagen, the predominant protein of cartilage, underlie several skeletal dysplasias: Stickler syndrome, spondyloepiphyseal dysplasia (SED), Kniest dysplasia, and Langer-Saldino achondrogenesis.[74,75] These conditions are characterized by short-trunk dwarfism (preferential shortening of the trunk as compared with the limbs) and severe involvement of the vertebrae and epiphysis of bones (Fig. 137.8). The gene defects have been linked to the *COL2A1* gene on chromosome 12.[75] In addition to the congenital autosomal dominant form of SED, an X-linked form presenting in boys in late childhood has also been described.[76,77]

Pseudoachondroplasia and *multiple epiphyseal dysplasia* are frequent autosomal dominant disorders characterized by short-limb dwarfism, and epiphyseal and additional metaphyseal changes. The gene responsible for these disorders has been localized to chromosome 19 and appears to encode the cartilage oligomeric matrix protein (COMP), a glycoprotein found in the matrix surrounding chondrocytes.[78,79]

Jansen metaphyseal chondrodysplasia is a rare autosomal dominant disorder characterized by abnormal growth plate maturation with metaphyseal changes but normal epiphyses and laboratory findings that are indistinguishable from hyperparathyroidism. This disorder is caused by activating mutations in PTH/PTHrP receptors.[80,81] These receptors are important both in calcium metabolism (leading to hypercalcemia, hypophosphatemia, and elevated urinary calcium) and in regulation of chondrocyte maturation.

CONCLUSION

Limb development is initiated during the fourth week of gestation and results in the formation of the limb bud. Three axes—the proximodistal, the anteroposterior, and the dorsoventral—are responsible for limb bud patterning. Endochondral bone formation begins early in the embryonic period when mesenchymal cells form condensations. These cell clusters differentiate into chondrocytes, which proliferate to form the growth plate or physis. This is a complex process that is regulated by a number of transcriptional factors and soluble mediators. The growth plate is responsible for longitudinal bone growth by the mechanism of endochondral ossification. Within the growth plate, chondrocyte proliferation, hypertrophy, and cartilage matrix secretion result in the formation of cartilage that is subsequently invaded by blood vessels and bone cells that remodel the cartilage into bone tissue. A complex network

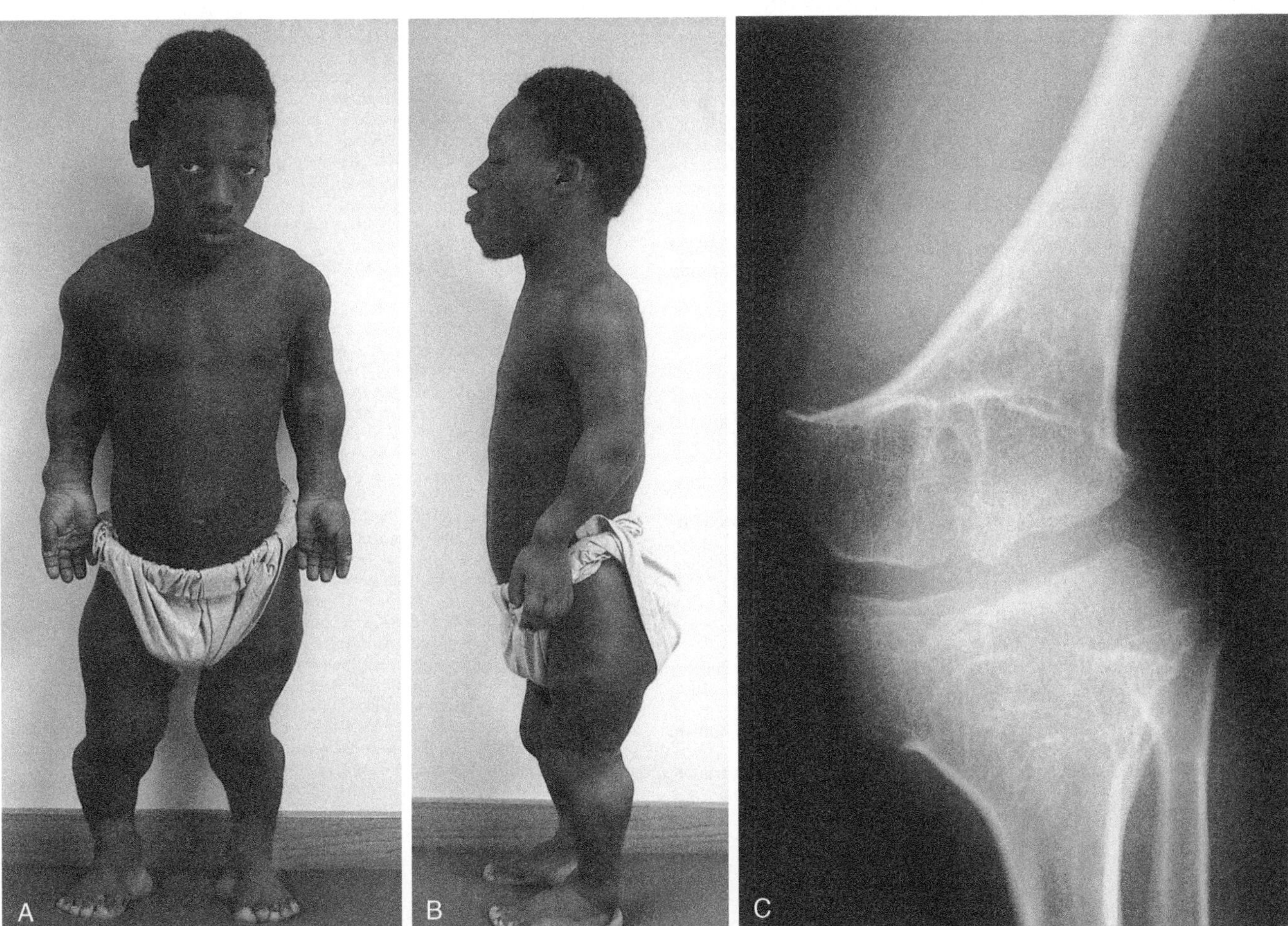

Fig. 137.8 A 19-year-old patient with spondyloepiphyseal dysplasia congenita (A and B). Note the markedly short stature with short trunk and limbs. There are angular deformities of the lower limbs. (C) An anteroposterior radiograph of the knee shows abnormally flattened and broad femoral and tibial epiphyses, causing angular deformities.

of endocrine signals—including GH, IGF-I thyroid hormones, estrogen, androgen, and vitamin D—work seamlessly to regulate longitudinal bone growth. Their action might occur locally on the growth plate chondrocytes, or by modulation of other endocrine signals in the network. Many human skeletal growth disorders are caused by abnormalities in the endocrine regulation of the growth plate, including achondroplasia, diastrophic dysplasia, and Jansen metaphyseal chondrodysplasia. The determinants of chondrocyte shape and the coordination of growth plate function with the development of joints, tendons, and ligaments are currently being studied and our understanding of this continually evolves.

ACKNOWLEDGMENTS

Disclosures: The authors report no conflict of interest, financial or otherwise, concerning the material or methods used in this study or the findings specified in this paper.

Funding: There were no sources of financial or material support for this report.

 A complete reference list is available at www.ExpertConsult.com.

SELECT REFERENCES

3. Sledge C, Zaleske D. Developmental anatomy of the joint 3rd ed. In: Resnick D, ed. *Diagnosis of Bone and Joint Disorders*. Philadelphia: Saunders; 1995.
5. Capdevila J, Izpisúa Belmonte JC. Patterning mechanism controlling vertebrate limb development. *Ann Rev Cell Biol*. 2001;17:87-132.
6. Cohn MJ, Izpisua-Belmonte JC, Abud H, et al. Fibroblast growth factors induce additional limb development from the flank of chick embryos. *Cell*. 1995;80:739-746.
8. Pizette S, Abate-Shen C, Niswander L. BMP controls proximodistal outgrowth, via induction of the apical ectodermal ridge, and dorsoventral patterning in the vertebrate limb. *Development*. 2001;128:4463-4474.
9. Robert B. Bone morphogenetic protein signaling in limb outgrowth and patterning. *Dev Growth Differ*. 2007;49:455-468.
10. Khokha MK, Hsu D, Brunet LJ, et al. Gremlin is the BMP antagonist required for maintenance of Shh and Fgf signals during limb patterning. *Nat Genet*. 2003;34:303-307.
11. Zuniga A, Haramis AP, McMahon AP, et al. Signal relay by BMP antagonism controls the SHH/FGF4 feedback loop in vertebrate limb buds. *Nature*. 1999;401:598-602.
13. Towers M, Tickle C. Growing models of vertebrate limb development. *Development*. 2009;136:179-190.
23. Kobayashi T, Soegiarto DW, Yang Y, et al. Indian hedgehog stimulates periarticular chondrocyte differentiation to regulate growth plate length independently of PTHrP. *J Clin Invest*. 2005;115:1734-1742.
24. Vu TH, Shipley JM, Bergers G, et al. MMP-9/gelatinase B is a key regulator of growth plate angiogenesis and apoptosis of hypertrophic chondrocytes. *Cell*. 1998;93:411-422.
28. Scheuer L, Black S. Bone development. In: Scheuer L, Black S, eds. *Developmental Juvenile Osteology*. San Diego: Academic Press; 2000:18-274.
29. Simsa-Maziel S, Zaretsky J, Reich A, et al. IL-1RI participates in normal growth plate development and bone modeling. *Am J Physiol Endocrinol Metab*. 2013;305:E15-E21.
30. Nilsson O, Marino R, De Luca F, et al. Endocrine regulation of the growth plate. *Horm Res*. 2005;64:157-165.
31. Michigami T. Regulatory mechanisms for the development of growth plate cartilage. *Cell Mol Life Sci*. 2013;70:4213-4221.
32. Adams SL, Cohen AJ, Lassova L. Integration of signaling pathways regulating chondrocyte differentiation during endochondral bone formation. *J Cell Physiol*. 2007;213:635-641.
35. Le Merrer M, Rousseau F, Legeai-Mallet L, et al. A gene for achondroplasia-hypochondroplasia maps to chromosome 4p. *Nat Genet*. 1994;6:318-321.
36. Shiang R, Thompson LM, Zhu YZ, et al. Mutations in the transmembrane domain of FGFR3 cause the most common genetic form of dwarfism, achondroplasia. *Cell*. 1994;78:335-342.
37. Kronenberg HM. Developmental regulation of the growth plate. *Nature*. 2003;423:332-336.
38. Ornitz DM, Marie PJ. FGF signaling pathways in endochondral and intramembranous bone development and human genetic disease. *Genes Dev*. 2002;16:1446-1465.
39. Minina E, Kreschel C, Naski MC, et al. Interaction of FGF, Ihh/Pthlh, and BMP signaling integrates chondrocyte proliferation and hypertrophic differentiation. *Dev Cell*. 2002;3:439-449.
40. Wang Y, Cheng Z, Elalieh HZ, et al. IGF-1R signaling in chondrocytes modulates growth plate development by interacting with the PTHrP/Ihh pathway. *J Bone Miner Res*. 2011;26:1437-1446.
41. Wang Y, Nishida S, Sakata T, et al. Insulin-like growth factor-I is essential for embryonic bone development. *Endocrinology*. 2006;147:4753-4761.
42. Yoon BS, Lyons KM. Multiple functions of BMPs in chondrogenesis. *J Cell Biochem*. 2004;93:93-103.
47. Robertson Jr WW. Newest knowledge of the growth plate. *Clin Orthop Relat Res*. 1990:270-278.
48. Abad V, Meyers JL, Weise M, et al. The role of the resting zone in growth plate chondrogenesis. *Endocrinology*. 2002;143:1851-1857.
49. Buckwalter JA. Proteoglycan structure in calcifying cartilage. *Clin Orthop Relat Res*. 1983:207-232.
51. Ehrlich MG, Armstrong AL, Mankin HJ. Partial purification and characterization of a proteoglycan-degrading neutral protease from bovine epiphyseal cartilage. *J Orthop Res*. 1984;2:126-133.
52. Ehrlich MG, Armstrong AL, Neuman RG, et al. Patterns of proteoglycan degradation by a neutral protease from human growth-plate epiphyseal cartilage. *J Bone Joint Surg Am*. 1982;64:1350-1354.
53. Iannotti JP, Naidu S, Noguchi Y, et al. Growth plate matrix vesicle biogenesis. The role of intracellular calcium. *Clin Orthop Relat Res*. 1994:222-229.
54. Simon SR. *Orthopaedic Basic Science*. Rosemont, IL: American Academy of Orthopaedic Surgeons; 1994:192.
55. Burgeson RE, Nimni ME. Collagen types. Molecular structure and tissue distribution. *Clin Orthop Relat Res*. 1992:250-272.
56. Sandell LJ, Sugai JV, Trippel SB. Expression of collagens I, II, X, and XI and aggrecan mRNAs by bovine growth plate chondrocytes *in situ*. *J Orthop Res*. 1994;12:1-14.
57. Breur GJ, VanEnkevort BA, Farnum CE, et al. Linear relationship between the volume of hypertrophic chondrocytes and the rate of longitudinal bone growth in growth plates. *J Orthop Res*. 1991;9:348-359.
58. Ballock RT, O'Keefe RJ. The biology of the growth plate. *J Bone Joint Surg Am*. 2003;85-A:715-726.
59. Roach HI, Baker JE, Clarke NM. Initiation of the bony epiphysis in long bones: chronology of interactions between the vascular system and the chondrocytes. *J Bone Miner Res*. 1998;13:950-961.
60. O'Keefe RJ, Crabb ID, Puzas JE, et al. Effects of transforming growth factor-beta 1 and fibroblast growth factor on DNA synthesis in growth plate chondrocytes are enhanced by insulin-like growth factor-I. *J Orthop Res*. 1994;12:299-310.
62. Hallett SA, Ono W, Ono N. Growth plate chondrocytes: skeletal development, growth and beyond. *Int J Mol Sci*. 2019;20:6009.
63. Samsa WE, Zhou X, Zhou G. Signaling pathways regulating cartilage growth plate formation and activity. *Semin Cell Dev Biol*. 2017;62:3-15.
64. Iannotti JP, Brighton CT, Iannotti V, et al. Mechanism of action of parathyroid hormone-induced proteoglycan synthesis in the growth plate chondrocyte. *J Orthop Res*. 1990;8:136-145.
66. Yan B, Zhang Z, Jin D, et al. mTORC1 regulates PTHrP to coordinate chondrocyte growth, proliferation and differentiation. *Nat Commun*. 2016;7:11151.
67. Mankin HJ, Mankin CJ. Metabolic bone disease: a review and update. *Instr Course Lect*. 2008;57:575-593.
68. Dean DD, Boyan BD, Schwart Z, et al. Effect of 1alpha,25-dihydroxyvitamin D3 and 24R,25-dihydroxyvitamin D3 on metalloproteinase activity and cell maturation in growth plate cartilage *in vivo*. *Endocrine*. 2001;14:311-323.
69. Rimoin DL, Cohn D, Krakow D, et al. The skeletal dysplasias: clinical-molecular correlations. *Ann N Y Acad Sci*. 2007;1117:302-309.
70. Mortier GR, Cohn DH, Cormier-Daire V, et al. Nosology and classification of genetic skeletal disorders: 2019 revision. *Am J Med Genet*. 2019;179:2393-2419.
71. Reardon W, Winter RM, Rutland P, et al. Mutations in the fibroblast growth factor receptor 2 gene cause Crouzon syndrome. *Nat Genet*. 1994;8:98-103.
72. Jabs EW, Li X, Scott AF, et al. Jackson-Weiss and Crouzon syndromes are allelic with mutations in fibroblast growth factor receptor 2. *Nat Genet*. 1994;8:275-279.
73. Hastbacka J, de la Chapelle A, Mahtani MM, et al. The diastrophic dysplasia gene encodes a novel sulfate transporter: positional cloning by fine-structure linkage disequilibrium mapping. *Cell*. 1994;78:1073-1087.
76. Gedeon AK, Tiller GE, Le Merrer M, et al. The molecular basis of X-linked spondyloepiphyseal dysplasia tarda. *Am J Hum Genet*. 2001;68:1386-1397.
79. Mabuchi A, Manabe N, Haga N, et al. Novel types of COMP mutations and genotype-phenotype association in pseudoachondroplasia and multiple epiphyseal dysplasia. *Hum Genet*. 2003;112:84-90.
80. Erlebacher A, Filvaroff EH, Gitelman SE, et al. Toward a molecular understanding of skeletal development. *Cell*. 1995;80:371-378.

Ontogenesis of Striated Muscle

138

Harvey B. Sarnat

INTRODUCTION

Embryology is the basis for understanding the intimate relation between structures in different organ systems, such as the nervous system and muscle, and is primordial for understanding pathogenesis in disorders of development that in the human may present as one of the congenital myopathies. Demonstration of a defective gene provides an etiology but does not define morphogenesis. The timing and sequence of striated muscle maturation are as precise and predictable as in the nervous system. Interest in neuromuscular ontogeny began with the studies of MacCallum[1] in the late nineteenth century. The account of histologic changes in developing human muscle published in 1917 by Tello[2] in Spain remains as accurate and valid today as any subsequent studies by light microscopy. Ultrastructural studies of developing muscle by transmission electron microscopy began in the 1950s and were supplemented by studies using the scanning electron microscope two decades later. Histochemical techniques to demonstrate biochemical constituents and enzymatic activities in developing muscle were introduced in the 1960s and 1970s; the 1980s was a decade for the introduction of immunocytochemistry to identify other molecules of subcellular components. The late 1980s and early 1990s saw a major breakthrough in the understanding of muscle differentiation by the discovery of myogenic regulatory genes and their transcription products. Studies of the complex interactions of these genes, their translated proteins, and the role of various trophic factors continue to be the focus of current investigations in muscle ontogenesis. Modern embryology, an integration of classic descriptive morphogenesis and the molecular genetic regulation of myogenesis, is the foundation for understanding the pathogenesis of congenital myopathies.[3]

EMBRYONIC ORIGIN OF MUSCLE

Muscle originates even before the three definitive germ layers have differentiated from the gastrula. The epiblast, the uppermost layer of the bilayered blastula, contains primordial mesodermal cells. Epiblastic cells migrate towards a line formed between parallel ridges that converge at one end; this line is known as the *primitive streak,* and the convergence of the parallel ridges is designated *anterior* and termed the *primitive node.* The axis thus formed establishes bilateral symmetry and a cephalocaudal gradient as the fundamental body plan.

From the primitive node and streak, epiblastic cells stream into the space between the two layers to form paired columns of prospective mesoderm. The primitive node is the future notochord. It is positioned beneath the future neural plate, which is of ectodermal origin. The mesodermal columns are composed of undifferentiated mesenchymal cells extending the entire length of the primitive streak. These cells migrate laterally and rostrally to fill the space between the overlying surface ectoderm, which includes the neural plate, and the deeper endodermal layer, except for an area on either side of the notochord beneath the neural plate.

Further development subdivides the layer of primitive mesenchyme. A thickened band of mesoderm condenses on either side of the primitive streak, from which primordial somites will differentiate. The myotomal plates within these still-unsegmented somite columns are anatomically distinct from the broad lateral expanse and a smaller intermediate strip of mesoderm. Elongation of the embryo is accompanied by regression of the primitive node (notochordal process) and streak caudally. As the node moves posteriorly, paired blocks of somites become segmentally condensed from the originally continuous somitic plate on either side of the developing neural tube. In addition, the lateral mesoderm splits into two layers: the upper layer, or *somatopleure,* forms the body wall, and the lower layer, or *splanchnopleure,* forms the mesenteries of the internal organs. A lateral palisading of paraxial mesenchyme against the lateral aspects of the notochord precedes overt segmentation, but once formed, the boundaries between somites are stable and provide no opportunity for cellular mixing.[4]

Segmentation of the myotomal plate occurs along a rostrocaudal gradient. As the more caudal segments are still in the process of separating, segregated anterior somites are already changing in size and arrangement. In transverse section, the somites are composed of high columnar cells arranged radially around a small central cavity. The dorsal part of the somite, the *dermatome,* retains this columnar structure and forms a flat plate beneath the surface ectoderm. Cells of the ventral portion of each somite disperse to form a loose network known as the *sclerotome.* The small myocele cavity of the somite is transitory and becomes obliterated by cellular proliferation.

The myotome that differentiates at the medial end of the dermatome as a ventral extension near the neural tube differentiates into the axial (i.e., paraspinal) muscles and also into the muscles of the extremities as the limb buds form. The contractile elements of the developing muscle are of somitic origin, whereas the tendons, interstitial connective tissue, blood vessels, and epimysial sheaths are somatopleural derivatives.

The notochord and floor plate ependyma of the neural plate synthesize retinoic acid[5] and express a gene known in vertebrates as *Sonic hedgehog.*[6] These factors are important in the dorsoventral patterning not only of the developing neural tube but also of the somites. Overexpression of these factors has a powerful ventralizing influence such that an ectopic length of notochord or a section of neural tube floor plate transplanted ventral to the newly formed segmental somite causes the excessive differentiation of sclerotome (the ventral part of the somite) and deficient formation of the myotome and dermatome, the dorsal part of the somite.[6-9] As the fetus matures, the loss of balanced antagonism between ventralizing genes, such as Sonic hedgehog, and dorsalizing genes, such as those of the bone morphogenetic protein and paired homeobox families, may result in segmental amyoplasia at the level of the notochordal or floor plate implant, a disturbance of *somitic induction.* Notochordal signals also regulate the transcriptional cascade of myogenic basic helix-loop-helix (bHLH) genes in the somite for myoblastic differentiation.[10] In a genetic mutant mouse in which somites form after notochordal degeneration, apoptosis of epaxial myotomes is accelerated.[11]

All nonmyofiber components of muscle, except for axons of intramuscular nerves, are derived from neural crest. These components include Schwann cells of nerves, capsules of muscle spindles, perimysial and endomysial collagenous connective and adipose tissues, and intramuscular blood vessels. Thermal stress induces progenitor adipocyte plasticity to produce a distinct form of thermogenic beige fat cell for energy homeostasis.[12]

MYOGENIC REGULATORY GENES

A family of four proto-oncogenes directs the differentiation of striated muscle from any undifferentiated or incompletely differentiated mesodermal cell by blocking the methylation of DNA.[13] The molecular mechanism of myoblast differentiation requires the activation and suppression of specific genes in a temporal and spatial sequence controlled by a complex array of regulatory transcription factors. Each of these genes can activate the expression of another and, under certain circumstances, can autoactivate as well.[14-17] The four myogenic regulatory genes are a "family" not only because of their closely related functions in myogenesis but also because they all share encoding transcription factors of the bHLH protein, a molecular structure so fundamental in evolution that it is even found in some bacteria. These four genes, or *myogenic regulatory factors (MRFs),* that control the specification and differentiation of striated muscle lineage are myogenic factor 5 *(Myf5),* myogenin, *Myf4* (also known as *herculin* and *Myf6*), and myoblast-differentiating factor, also known as *MyoD* or *MyoD1*.[14,18-28] Several other genes influence these MRFs or interact with them in ways that augment or impair their expression. Myogenin mainly mediates myoblast fusion, and without this factor an abundance of myoblasts may form, but they do not fuse to form myotubes. The expression of *Myf5* and *Myf4* is transient in early ontogenesis and returns much later in fetal life to persist into adult life.[24] Liver kinase B1 (a serine/threonine kinase) also provides a role in regulating division, self-renewal, proliferation, and differentiation of skeletal muscle progenitor cells.[29]

One of the most remarkable and complex features of all myogenic genes is their intimate interaction with one another. After the discovery of this family of genes, initially it was thought that they all were redundant and any could substitute for another if one were deleted. Some indeed do have overlapping functions, such as *Myf5* and *MyoD1*, which allow normal muscle development if one, but not both, of these two are defective.[30,31] A similar overlap or redundancy exists between *Myf4* and *MyoD1*.[32] In general, despite these partial redundancies, each gene regulates a different aspect of myogenesis, however, and they do not easily compensate for each other either in the embryo and fetus or in myoblast precursor cells in adults for the regeneration of muscle.[33] MyoD1 cannot compensate for an absence of myogenin expression.[34] MRF4, the human homolog to mouse myogenin (Myf4), but not MyoD1, can substitute for myogenin early in development.[36] Myf5 similarly may be redundant with myogenin but less efficiently.[37,38] In *Mrf4-* or myogenin-deficient mice, particularly severe impairments exist in the development of the thoracic myotomes for intercostal muscle development; rib fusions and sternal defects result, but these are probably secondary because neither of these genes is expressed in rib cartilage or sternum.[39] Immunoreactivity of MyoD1 is now available for application to human fetal and neonatal muscle and is useful for some diagnoses of congenital disorders, such as segmental amyoplasia.

Myf5 is the earliest muscle-specific bHLH gene activated in the developing embryo.[15,20] Its expression is restricted to the medial aspect of the myotome, adjacent to the least mature myocytes.[9] *Myf5* alone cannot support myogenesis without the other three bHLH genes, however.[40] *Myf5* also seems to be mitogenic in inducing the proliferation of myoblast precursors. *Myf5* requires some activation by *MRF4,* and murine *Myf4*-null mutants show extremely reduced expression of *Myf5,* similarly to *Myf5*-knockout mice.[31] Myogenin can substitute for *Myf5* but is less efficient in this function.[37]

Myogenin does not serve a proliferative function in the genesis of myoblasts but is essential to myoblast fusion in the formation of myotubes, and it is expressed before fusion begins.[41] Myogenin inactivation in mice results in a normal number of myoblasts, but they become arrested in terminal differentiation.[31] Wild-type myoblasts can rescue myogenin-null myoblasts and cause them to fuse in vivo.[42] Myogenin is a specific transcriptional target of mitochondrial activity, unlike *Myf5* and *MyoD1*.[43] Myogenin can be demonstrated by immunoreactivity in sections of human fetal and neonatal muscle (Fig. 138.1).

MyoD1 is the last of the genes to become activated.[24,25] *Myf5* expression is normally suppressed by *MyoD1*.[30] Despite its late expression, fetal mouse myoblasts express both myogenin and MyoD1 on day 1 in culture, but adult myoblasts (satellite cells) have a delay in expression of these genes and of myoblast fusion.[44] However, satellite cells coexpress proliferating cell nuclear antigen and MyoD1 on entering the mitotic cycle, and MyoD1 is critical for the programming of satellite cells into myogenin-differentiating cells.[45] The transition from proliferation to differentiation is delayed in mice lacking MyoD1. Though coexpressed, MyoD1 and Myf5 act at different times in the cell cycle: Myf5 is maximally expressed in G_2 phase and is minimally expressed in G_1 phase; MyoD1 is maximally expressed in G_1 phase and minimally expressed in S phase; it is reexpressed in G_2 phase but not as strongly as in G_1 phase.[46] Another bHLH muscle-restricted transcription factor, myogenic repressor (MyoR), which antagonizes MyoD1, has been identified.[47] MyoD1 and myogenin are expressed not only during fetal ontogenesis but also in adult life and are essential to the function of myogenic stem cells (i.e., satellite cells) in normal adults and also in the regenerating muscle in muscular dystrophies.[48,49] The myogenic regulatory genes, particularly MyoD1, are so dominant that they are able to convert fibroblasts, chondroblasts, and other partially differentiated mesodermal lineages into myoblasts.[50]

The human locus of the *MyoD1* gene is on chromosome 11, very near the domain associated with embryonal rhabdomyosarcoma.[26] The genes encoding *Myf5* and *Myf4* are on chromosome 12 and that for myogenin is on chromosome 1. MyoD1 and myogenin are strongly expressed in human rhabdomyosarcoma cell lines.[51-53] Furthermore, the *MyoD1* gene is closely related to the *NeuroD* gene, which may explain why some medulloblastomas of the cerebellum in children exhibit striated muscle fibers amongst the tumor cells.

In addition to the family of four bHLH genes, *Pax3* has important interactions. It is redundant with *Myf5*; an absence of both *Pax3* and *Myf5* in embryonic mice results in generalized total amyoplasia and death; an isolated *Myf5* mutation causes milder, partial amyoplasia. Up-regulation of *Pax3* in chick embryos, by contrast, leads to precocious muscle development and arrested migration of myoblast precursor cells. *Pax3* and *Lbx1* both induce myoblast proliferation.[54] Other genes that *Pax3* induces include *Dach2, Eya2,* and *Six1*.[55,56] Myogenin is another key regulator of *Six1*.[57] *Pax3* is essential for the migration but not differentiation of limb muscle precursors.[58] Additional important functions of *Pax3* are the development of the eyes and the differentiation and maintenance of Bergmann glial cells of the cerebellum. *Pax7* is critical for the normal function of satellite cells in mature muscle regeneration and is involved in fetal myogenesis as well.[59]

Other important genes or gene families that influence the bHLH myogenic genes are bone morphogenetic protein 2, which inhibits terminal differentiation of myogenic cells by suppressing MyoD1 and myogenin,[60] and LIM protein, which promotes myogenesis by enhancing the activity of MyoD1.[61] Wnt signaling is also essential to myogenesis, playing a role in regulating the functions of MyoD1 and myogenin.[62,63] *WNT3a* also up-regulates frizzled class receptor 7 (Fzd7) and induces

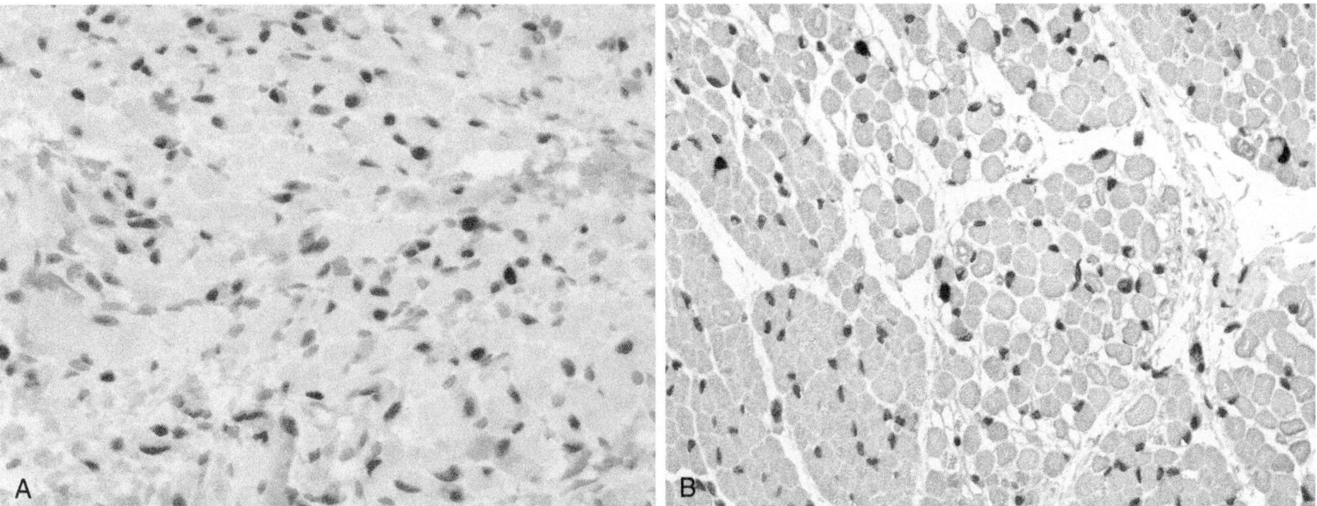

Fig. 138.1 Intranuclear myogenin immunoreactivity in (A) a term human neonate and (B) a 5-month-old boy with severe Duchenne muscular dystrophy. Normal neonatal muscle exhibits only occasional scattered nuclei that are marked; these are myoblasts or resident stem cells enclosed within the same basal lamina as their associated myofiber, also known as *satellite cells* in adult muscle. In muscular dystrophy, these myoblasts increase in number in an attempt to regenerate muscle; such extensive distribution as in this child resembles that of an 8- to 10-week fetus. (Original magnification ×250.)

symmetric expansion of satellite stem cells in developing and regenerating adult muscle.[63,64]

Myostatin is a negative regulator gene of muscle maturation.[65,66] It is a member of the transforming growth factor-β family, similar to bone morphogenetic protein. It has the latest expression in somites, after all other myogenic genes and desmin have been expressed. It is also coexpressed with MyoD1 but has a wider extent, also involving nonmuscular tissues such as the dermis. Myostatin inhibits transition from proliferation to differentiation but does not destroy myoblasts or alter mitotic cycling. Myostatin has received attention in the lay press because of its potential use to enhance athletic performance.[67,68] There is also a commercial interest in it to augment the muscular bulk of cattle and swine.

In later stages of muscle ontogenesis, the selective accumulation of MyoD1 and myogenin messenger RNA (mRNA) transcripts is not purely under genetic control but is modulated and modified by innervation of the muscle and by hormonal influences.[69-71] These effects begin earlier than the stage of histochemical differentiation of muscle fiber types at midgestation. Insulin-like growth factor (IGF) regulates normal myogenin expression[72] and influences muscle differentiation both upstream and downstream of myogenin.[73] IGF also augments proliferation that precedes differentiation.[74] Basic fibroblast growth factor similarly has a regulating influence on myoblast proliferation and differentiation.[75] Tumor necrosis factor-α, a cytokine, and basic fibroblast growth factor differentially inhibit expression of myogenin induced by IGF-I in myoblasts.[76,77] IGF-I has early inhibitory and late stimulatory effects on myogenin transcription.[78] Other families of genes the transcription factors that influence myodifferentiation include the POU homeodomain,[79] Rho proteins,[80] and Sox proteins.[81] A small number of neuroepithelial cells of the mouse neural tube coexpress neuronal markers and also *Myf5* and myosin in vitro, suggesting a potential for myogenesis from the neural tube itself.[82]

MicroRNA expression to detect the posttranscriptional modulation of cellular phenotypes in muscle and particularly in some of the congenital and degenerative diseases of muscle (muscular dystrophies) in humans is now feasible and promises to resolve many questions about the genetic regulation of muscle development, as well as the pathogenetic mechanisms of several developmental myopathies.[83] RNA interference libraries are being established in simple animals, such as the fruit fly *Drosophila,* which have genes that are phylogenetically conserved and include those of sarcomere formation in mammals.[84]

Other genes essential to muscle development and maintenance are the several genes that program sarcolemmal ion channels, particularly calcium channels. These channels form before innervation of the myofiber at 9 weeks' gestation. Several additional genes that undergo deletion or mutation are known to be the cause of congenital myopathies.[85] Conformational analysis of mutant proteins may be applied as a tool for the classification of myopathies.[86]

CYTODIFFERENTIATION OF MUSCLE CELLS

STRUCTURAL AND CONTRACTILE PROTEINS

The presumptive myoblast is a morphologically undifferentiated mesenchymal cell that divides mitotically, lacks the distinctive myofilaments of muscle cells, and does not fuse with neighboring cells of the same type.[87] The myoblast differs from its precursor, the presumptive myoblast, by synthesizing myosin and actin and assembling these proteins into thick and thin myofilaments, indicating a commitment to further differentiation as a muscle cell.[88] Although sarcomeres do not form in myoblasts, irregularly scattered clusters of myofilaments are loosely organized into interdigitating arrays. The cytoplasm of myoblasts is sparse. Adjacent myoblasts fuse by extending their contractile myofilaments across the plasma membranes of both cells and aligning the myofilaments produced by a row of several fused myoblasts (Fig. 138.2). Myoblast fusion is enhanced by isoforms of the neural cell adhesion molecule that mediates interactions of apposed plasma membranes.[89] The protein *myomaker* is a membrane activator of myoblast fusion.[90]

The multinucleated syncytium of the row of fused myoblasts forms the myotube. Early myotubes continue to fuse with myoblasts and also with other early myotubules (Fig. 138.3).[91] Circumferentially distributed myofilaments align themselves parallel to the longitudinal axis of the row of fused myoblasts as the filaments grow in length to extend through several fused myoblasts. Myotubular nuclei are enclosed within the center of the newly formed myotube as a single row within a central

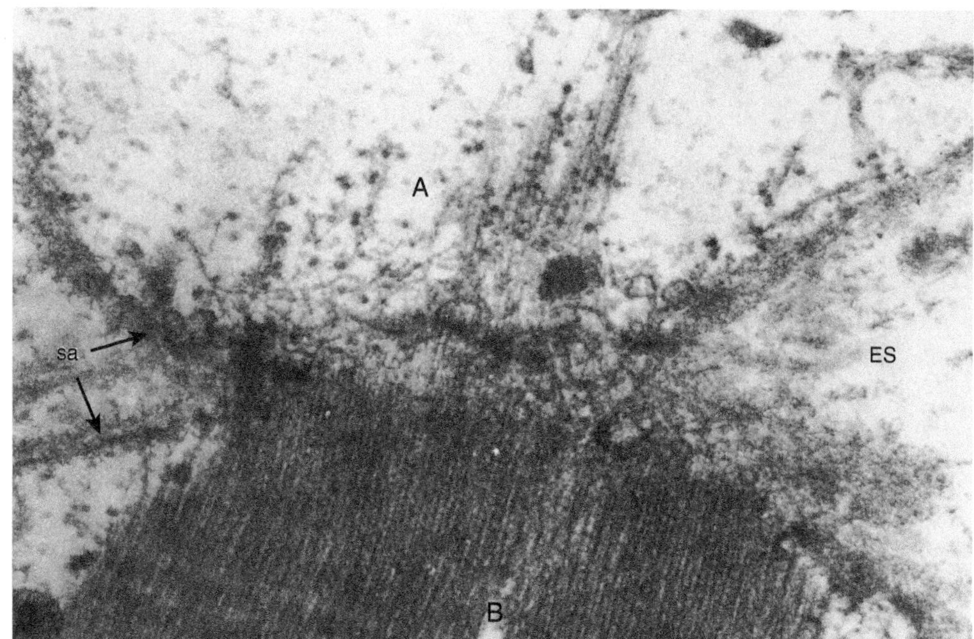

Fig. 138.2 Myoblast *(A)* fusing with early myotube *(B)* in the vastus lateralis muscle of a 12-week fetus. Filaments from the myotube are seen extending into the neighboring cell. *ES,* Extracellular space; *sa,* sarcolemma. (Original magnification ×50,000.) (From Tomanek RJ, Colling-Saltin AS. Cytologic differentiation of human fetal skeletal muscle. *Am J Anat.* 1977;149:227.)

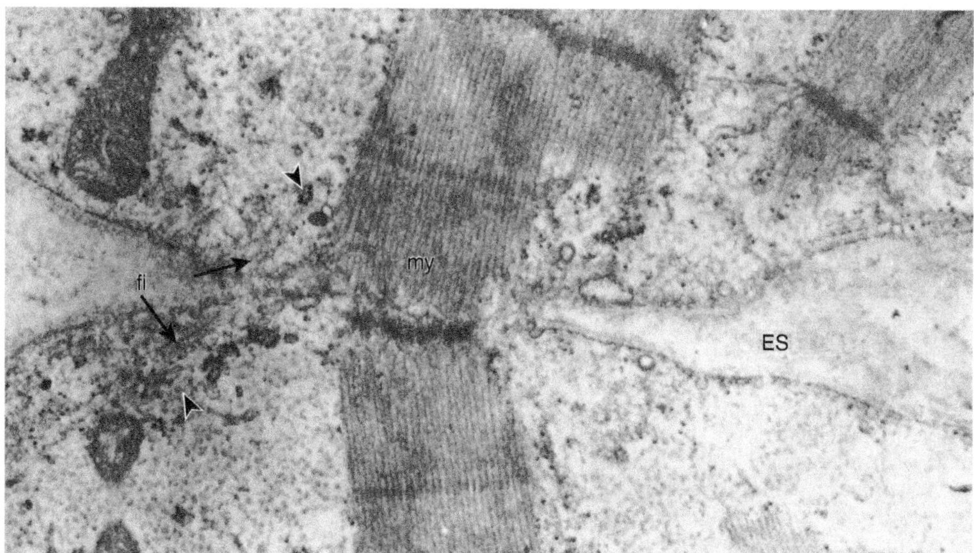

Fig. 138.3 Fusion of two myotubes, more advanced in development than the myocytes shown in Fig. 138.1, from the soleus muscle of a 16- to 17-week fetus. A well-formed myofibril *(my)* extends between two cells, which are joined by a narrow channel of sarcoplasm. Polyribosomes *(arrowheads)* and unassembled filaments *(fi)* are present in both cells. *ES,* Extracellular space. (Original magnification ×19,500.) (From Tomanek RJ, Colling-Saltin AS. Cytologic differentiation of human fetal skeletal muscle. *Am J Anat.* 1977;149:227.)

core of cytoplasm containing the membranous organelles and cytoplasmic particles. Cytoplasm is abundant, and contractile myofilaments are sparse in myotubes in comparison with more mature myocytes, but myofilaments and myofibrils are much more numerous in late myotubes than in early myotubes. Early myotubes predominate until the time of innervation at approximately 11 weeks' gestation, and late myotubes are dominant during the second half of the myotubular stage from 11 to 16 weeks' gestation.

Intermediate filaments, thinner but longer than the contractile myofilaments, appear in fusing myoblasts and myotubes.[92] These intermediate filaments, such as vimentin and desmin, are cytoskeletal proteins that help organize the cytologic structure of the muscle cell and spatial relationships of organelles, including the orientation and alignment of myofilaments (see later).

A basal lamina (i.e., basement membrane) appears as an indistinct, electron-dense thickening around the developing myotube. It usually encloses several myotubes and a number of less-differentiated myoblasts and presumptive myoblasts in the vicinity.[87,92,93] Mast cells, fibroblast-like cells, and other "unclassified" cells may also be included within the basal lamina.[94] Isolated myoblasts lack a basal lamina.[93] In this regard, they are similar to isolated fibroblasts and mast cells within the perimysium. Further maturation of the myotube to become a

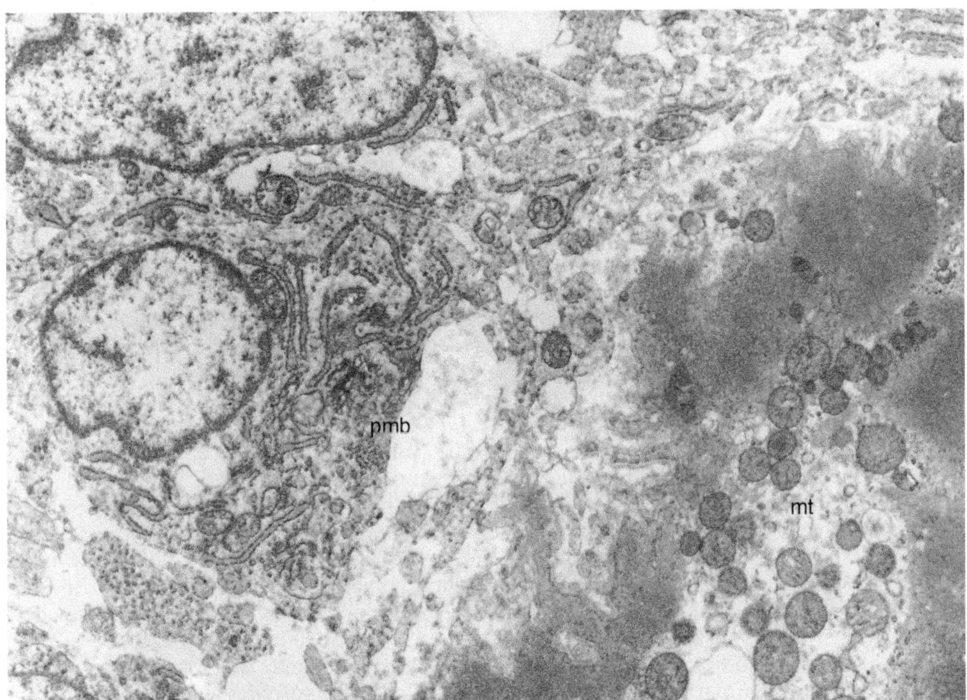

Fig. 138.4 Presumptive myoblast *(pmb)* associated with a myotube *(mt)* in the quadriceps femoris muscle of a 14-week human fetus. An extensive rough endoplasmic reticulum and many free ribosomes are present, but no contractile filaments or T tubules are developed. Mitochondria are also seen, both in the presumptive myoblast and in the central core of sarcoplasm of the adjacent myotube. (Electron micrograph, original magnification ×12,000.)

myocyte involves the synthesis of more contractile myofilaments and more numerous myofibrils, displacing the central nuclei to the peripheral subsarcolemmal region and dispersing the sarcoplasm (i.e., cytoplasm) and its organelles between myofibrils. The Z bands of several myofibrils within each maturing myotube are not "in register" with each other and do not become aligned consistently until approximately 30 weeks' gestation.[87] The sarcotubular system begins forming in the late myotube but is not mature until after 30 weeks' gestation.

After the myofiber has achieved morphologic maturity in the relative positions and orientations of the various subcellular components, the next phase consists of the myofiber achieving greater length, an increase in the number of myofibrils in a cross-sectional field of the myofiber, and the development of histochemical fiber types. Although the number of myofibers and their morphologic maturation are mainly genetically determined, metabolic differentiation into fiber types is principally under neural control. Metabolic fiber types also exhibit subtle morphologic differences in the relative number of mitochondria and glycogen granules and in variation in the width of the Z band. Single fiber proteomics by mass spectrometry now enables comparison, within the same myofiber, of proteins associated with different subcellular structures: plasma membrane, mitochondria, sarcoplasmic reticulum (SR), myofibrils, and nucleus.[95]

Spindle-shaped mononucleated cells with abundant polyribosomes and endoplasmic reticulum persist in close apposition to the myotube and myocyte (i.e., multinucleated myofiber) enclosed within the same basal lamina. Such cells are presumptive myoblasts (Fig. 138.4). In mature muscle, they are redesignated *satellite cells* (Fig. 138.5). Although they are dormant and inactive, they are capable of mitotic proliferation, migration, fusion, and myogenesis even in the adult and are the basis of regeneration of injured muscle.[96-101] In normal mature muscle, about 7% of the nuclei at the periphery of the myofiber are really satellite cells; this percentage is higher in immature muscle.[102]

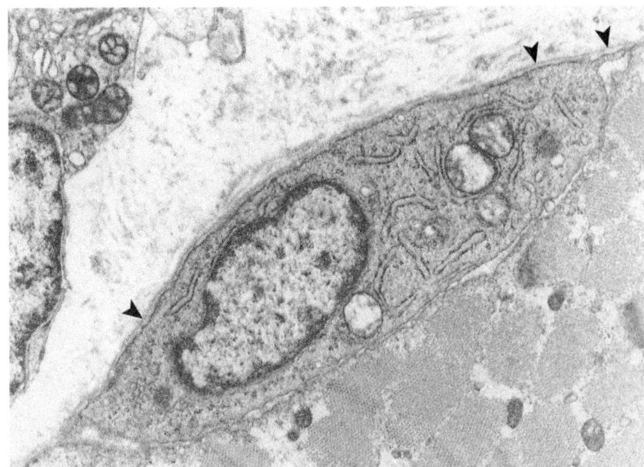

Fig. 138.5 Satellite cell of fully mature myofiber from quadriceps femoris muscle in a 7-year-old girl. As with the presumptive myoblast of fetal muscle (see Fig. 138.3), the satellite cell contains mitochondria, rough endoplasmic reticulum, and free ribosomes but no contractile proteins or T tubules and is enclosed within the same basal lamina *(arrowheads)* as the adjacent myofiber. The satellite cell is capable of mitosis and differentiation to become a true myoblast and then mature further and is the cell responsible for regeneration of injured muscle at any age. (Electron micrograph, uranyl acetate and lead citrate, original magnification ×20,000.)

No stage of fetal muscle development is "pure" in the sense of muscle cells exhibiting the same degree of maturation uniformly. Transitions among periods of development are gradual. At 5 to 8 weeks' gestation, presumptive and true myoblasts predominate, but scattered myotubes are already evident at 6 weeks' gestation. The period from 8 to 16 weeks' gestation is regarded as the myotubular stage of development, and myotubes are indeed the most numerous types of muscle cells. However, many myoblasts are still identified, presumptive myoblasts frequently undergoing mitosis are encountered, and a few maturing myocytes beyond the myotubular stage are scattered during the latter weeks of this period. From 16 to 20 weeks' gestation, a progressive maturation of myotubes to the cytologic structure of the mature myocyte occurs, but a few myotubes persist. Histochemical differentiation of muscle occurs mainly between 20 and 30 weeks gestation. From 30 weeks' gestation to term, myofibers undergo several more subtle morphologic adjustments to maturity, such as alignment of Z bands of adjacent myofibrils to attain "register" (i.e., parallel alignment) and further development of the sarcotubular system.

A 427-kDa cytoskeletal protein known as *dystrophin* is encoded by a large gene at the Xp21.2 locus. This subsarcolemmal protein attaches to the sarcolemmal membrane overlying the A band and M band of the myofibrils and consists of distinct regions or domains: the amino terminus contains 250 amino acids and is related to the binding site of α-actinin; the second domain is the largest, with 2800 amino acids, and contains many repeats, giving it a characteristic rod shape; a third domain is rich in cysteine and is related to the carboxyl-terminus domain of 400 amino acids, unique to dystrophin and to a dystrophin-related protein encoded by chromosome 6.[103] Dystrophin is part of a large tightly associated glycoprotein complex containing other proteins called *dystrophin-related proteins.*[104] Dystrophin may be demonstrated in striated muscle by its immunoreactivity, either by immunoperoxidase reaction (Fig. 138.6) or by fluorescence microscopy, and is detected in developing human fetal muscle at 11 weeks gestation.[105,106] Dystrophin mRNA is normally detected in cardiac and smooth muscle in striated muscle and in the brain. The dystrophin gene encodes a 14-kilobase mRNA of approximately 80 exons. Defective dystrophin is the biologic basis of Duchenne and Becker muscular dystrophies.

Several dystrophin-related glycoproteins also form in this same general period. α-Sarcoglycan (formerly *adhalin*) becomes expressed before 14 weeks gestation. The other sarcoglycans (β, γ, and δ) are expressed shortly thereafter. Dysferlin and caveolin 3 are other sarcolemmal membrane proteins at sites different from those of dystrophin and the sarcoglycans. Dysferlin deficiency is the basis of a well-documented progressive myopathy in children and adults, but dysferlin overexpression in striated muscle can also produce a progressive myopathy; hence the genetic regulation of expression, including its binding proteins, must be precise.[107] Caveolin 3 is first detected on day 10 in developing human somites.[108]

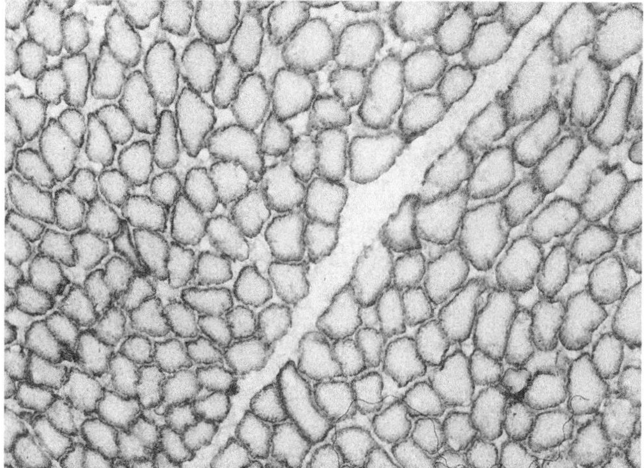

Fig. 138.6 Immunocytochemical stain demonstrating dystrophin outlining the sarcolemma of normal quadriceps femoris muscle fibers in a biopsy specimen of a term male neonate. The monoclonal antibodies shown are specific for the rod domain of the dystrophin molecule; other antibodies demonstrate only the carboxyl terminus or amino terminus. Dystrophin immunoreactivity is first detected in developing human muscle at 11 weeks gestation. (Original magnification ×250.)

α-Dystroglycan is another sarcolemmal regional protein. *O*-Glycosylation of this protein may be altered by mutations of several genes during development, and hypoglycosylation is the molecular basis for some of the congenital muscular dystrophies.[109]

The precise timing of the earliest expression of most sarcolemmal region proteins is uncertain, but collagen VI, which is deficient in a congenital muscular dystrophy known as *Ullrich disease*, is probably first detected at approximately 10 to 12 weeks,[110] which is similar to other proteins that attach to the sarcolemma. The principal source of collagen VI synthesis in striated muscle is the interstitial resident fibroblasts in the muscle.[111] It is noteworthy that this timing of the appearance of sarcolemmal regional proteins coincides with the time of innervation of muscle at 9 to 11 weeks' gestation. Knowledge of this timing is important in medicine because fetal muscle biopsies may now be performed during the course of pregnancy. Therefore if a fetus is at risk for one of these diseases because of involvement of a sibling, and the family wishes to know whether the present fetus is similarly involved, an accurate diagnosis can be confirmed as early as possible by immunoreactivity of sections of the fetal muscle or by haplotype analysis.[110] The various sarcolemmal regional proteins of striated muscle and their genetic defects in various myopathies were reviewed by Sewry.[112]

Cadherins are another group of transmembrane proteins that mediate calcium-dependent cell-cell adhesion by means of homophilic binding; M-cadherin is a cell type–specific member of this family. In regenerating muscle and in developing fetal muscle, reactivity for M-cadherin is restricted to the plasma membrane of myoblasts and satellite cells and is most intense at the membrane areas facing adjacent myotubes or myofibers.[113-115] M-cadherin is genetically expressed but appears to be neurally regulated[116]; it is not expressed in denervated muscle.[114] The mechanism by which increased cadherin expression promotes early steps in muscle differentiation is by up-regulation of myogenin.[117,118]

Merosin is an extracellular matrix protein forming the heavy chain of the skeletal muscle basement membrane protein laminin and is important for maintaining the integrity of the sarcolemma. Defective merosin is implicated in the pathogenesis of one form of congenital muscular dystrophy,[119-121] and the chromosomal site of the disease gene is at the 6q2 locus.[121] The merosin (laminin subunit α_2) gene maps to locus 6q22-23.[122,123] Merosin may be detected before birth in the human placenta.[124] Type XIX collagen is a transient extracellular matrix protein that contributes to the formation of fetal basal lamina and closely follows the expression of *Myf5*.[125] Extracellular matrix is required for muscle differentiation and for the fusion of myoblasts to form myotubes independently of myogenin.[126] Inhibition of fibrillar collagen production in avian and mammalian embryos results in abnormal somite formation and perturbed myogenesis.[127-129]

The nuclear envelop proteins Lamin-A and Lamin-C, encoded by the lamination's A/C *(LMAC)* gene, are normally expressed in both striated and cardiac muscle during development and modulate actin dynamics.[130] Their mutation results in Emery-Dreifuss muscular dystrophy with cardiomyopathy and a few other rarer myopathies.

The innervation of muscle fibers occurs at approximately 11 weeks' gestation, in the middle of the myotubular stage. Muscle spindles and Golgi tendon organs form after the myotubular stage as the general fascicular organization of the muscle evolves.

The development of joints in the extremities begins at approximately 5 weeks' gestation within the early mesenchymal condensations of precartilaginous bone. Joint spaces are already apparent by 7 weeks. Motion is probably essential for the development of joints, and some articular motion is evident as early as 8 weeks, before myotubes are innervated. These small-amplitude movements probably result from spontaneous contractions of newly formed sarcomeres. Active fetal movements are well established after 11 weeks, with the innervation of skeletal muscle, and increase progressively in both force and range of motion around articulations until birth.

CHAPERONE PROTEINS IN MUSCLE DEVELOPMENT

In addition to the various structural proteins of the myofiber and especially of the sarcolemma, certain "chaperone proteins" are essential for intracellular folding and assembly of polypeptides to achieve the final molecular structure of cellular structural proteins. However, they remain chaperones because they do not themselves become incorporated into the molecular structure of the protein they regulate in development. One of the most recognized of these chaperone proteins is the small heat shock protein α-B-crystallin, closely related to heat shock protein 27, which is found in all tissues and is phylogenetically very old, expressed even in bacteria and simple worms. It is demonstrated in both cytoplasm and nucleoplasm. It inhibits aggregation and precipitation of denatured proteins[131] and is up-regulated in a variety of tissues during various adverse or stressful conditions, such as fever, chronic ischemia, acidosis, X-irradiation, exposure to toxins, and in epileptic activity in the brain.[132,133] A close association of α-B-crystallin with the Z band of striated muscle implies that it is particularly important in protecting the Z band from the disintegration that results in myofibrillar breakdown and also protects myosin from thermal denaturation.[134]

In muscle, the natural form of α-B-crystallin is overexpressed in myofiber atrophy, associated with a decrease in the amount of the cytoskeletal microtubule protein tubulin.[135] It is also overexpressed, but as a mutant form, in certain diseases of muscle known as *myofibrillar myopathies*[136] and may cause severe weakness and muscle stiffness leading to early infantile death.[137] The α-B-crystallin may have an additional role in muscle in regulating connective tissue proliferation, as it does in the dermis of the skin during wound healing.[138] In normal human fetal muscle, this protein is not demonstrated by immunoreactivity at any gestational age, perhaps because the concentrations are too low to detect by this method.

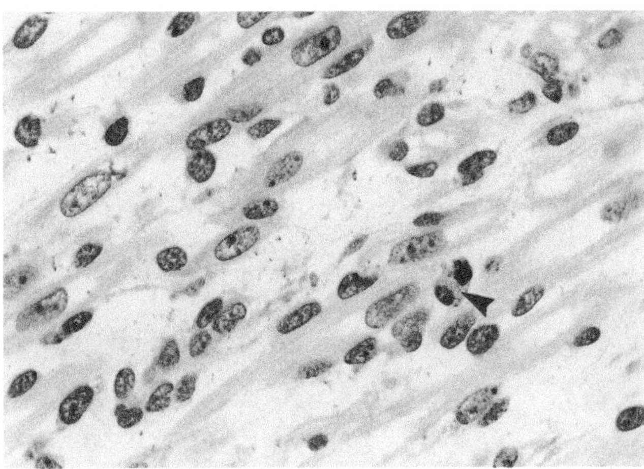

Fig. 138.7 Myotubes in the quadriceps femoris muscle of a 14-week human fetus. Nuclei are large and vesicular with finely dispersed chromatin and one or two prominent nucleoli. Mitotic figures of presumptive myoblasts *(arrowhead)* are common. (Hematoxylin and eosin, original magnification ×1000.)

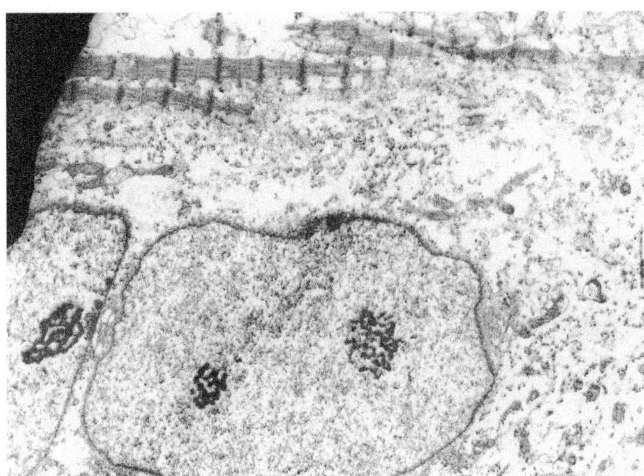

Fig. 138.8 Myotube in the quadriceps femoris muscle of a 14-week human fetus. Nuclei exhibit finely dispersed chromatin and strands of ribonucleoprotein-forming nucleoli. Newly formed sarcomeres of contractile proteins are seen at the *top*. The sarcoplasmic core contains many mitochondria. (Electron micrograph, uranyl acetate and lead citrate, original magnification ×10,000.)

MORPHOLOGIC STRUCTURE OF MYOTUBES AND MYOCYTES

SARCOLEMMAL NUCLEI

Myoblasts and myotubes have large, vesicular, ovoid nuclei. The chromatin is finely dispersed throughout the nucleoplasm, with a thin condensation against the nuclear membrane. One or often two prominent nucleoli are present (Fig. 138.7). Ultrastructurally, the ribonucleoprotein of these nucleoli forms coarse, electron-dense strands (nucleolonemata) rather than the more massive nucleolar sphere of the mature sarcolemmal nucleus (Fig. 138.8). These features of the nucleoli and of the finely dispersed DNA are characteristic of active transcription of RNA needed for the synthesis of contractile proteins. The nuclei of regenerating myofibers of children and adults have a similar appearance. The nuclear membrane of fetal myotubes contains pores, similarly to the mature state. In the term neonate, some sarcolemmal nuclei are still vesicular and ovoid as are seen in less mature stages, but most nuclei have acquired the elongated shape with dense chromatin that characterizes the mature state (Fig. 138.9). The nuclei of myotubes are arranged in a single-file row within the central core of sarcoplasm. Nuclei may be tightly packed and in contact with neighboring nuclei, or they may be separated by intermediate segments of sarcoplasm of variable lengths (Fig. 138.10). Both arrangements occur simultaneously within the same muscle, and contiguous as well as widely spaced nuclei occur within different segments along the same myofiber. Closely spaced nuclei are generally more characteristic of early myotubes than of late myotubes. Intranuclear lamin A/C is expressed in differentiating myoblasts.[139] Lamin A/C, lamin B1, and emerin are defective in certain hereditary myopathies, highlighting the importance of myonuclear membrane proteins, as well as sarcolemmal plasma membranes, in the integrity of normal muscle development and maintenance.

SARCOPLASMIC ORGANELLES

The abundant sarcoplasm (i.e., cytoplasm) within the core of the myotube between and around nuclei contains membranous organelles. These are mitochondria with well-formed cristae, Golgi apparatuses generally located at the end of a nucleus, and

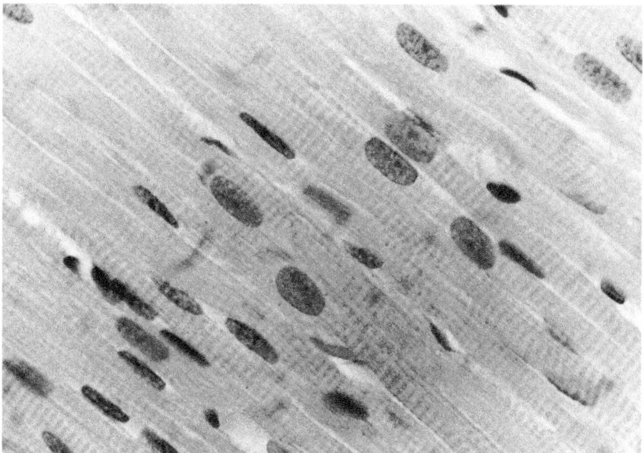

Fig. 138.9 Longitudinal section of the quadriceps femoris muscle from a term neonate. Many sarcolemmal nuclei retain the ovoid, vesicular appearance of the immature myofiber, but others are elongated and hyperchromatic, characteristic of mature myocytes. (Hematoxylin and eosin, original magnification ×1000.)

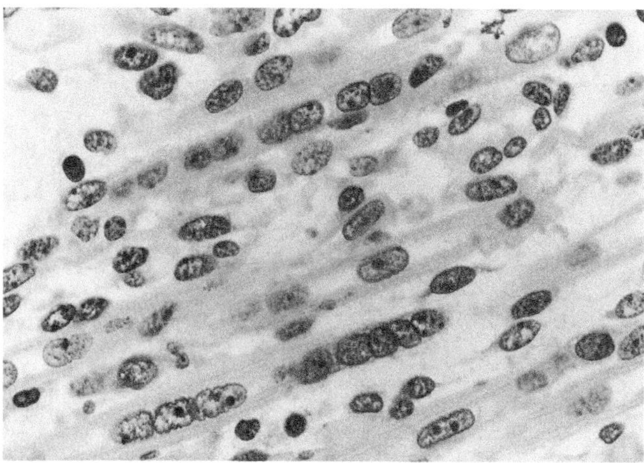

Fig. 138.10 Myotubes in the quadriceps femoris muscle of a 12-week human fetus. The spacing of central nuclei is variable. Rows of closely spaced, contiguous nuclei without intervening sarcoplasm are seen, or segments of internuclear sarcoplasm, often several nuclear diameters in length, are found. (Hematoxylin and eosin, original magnification ×1000.)

single-membrane vesicles. Most vesicles have dense cores and are probably lysosomes. Notably lacking from the core of sarcoplasm in myotubes are transverse tubules and SR (i.e., endoplasmic reticulum), including their dyads and triads that are so common in the intermyofibrillar sarcoplasm of more mature myocytes.

Mitochondria are almost the only organelles found in the subsarcolemmal sarcoplasm of myotubes. The septa of sarcoplasm that separate the myofibrils of myotubes contain few organelles, unlike the intermyofibrillar sarcoplasm of mature myofibers, although mitochondria may already begin to redistribute themselves between myofibrils of late myotubes.[93]

GLYCOGEN

Free glycogen particles are numerous in the central core of sarcoplasm and in the subsarcolemmal region of myotubes but are less concentrated between myofibrils. In older fetuses (after 30 weeks' gestation) and in the first postnatal month, double-membrane vesicles or membranous fragments containing glycogen are commonly seen in the intermyofibrillar sarcoplasm. These vesicles are probably derived from lysosomes. Free glycogen particles are notably lacking from the regions of vesicle-enclosed glycogen.[87] Several myopathies are glycogen-storage diseases, usually involving lysosomes.[140]

CONTRACTILE MYOFILAMENTS

In the myoblast, randomly oriented thin and thick myofilaments occur sparsely in the cytoplasm without parallel alignment or evidence of even rudimentary sarcomere formation. Z-band material is not condensed. The early myotube shows poorly aligned thin myofilaments in the periphery of the cytoplasm, near the inner cell membrane; clusters of thick myofilaments with their associated ribosomes are in close proximity.[87] Lattice formation involving alternating thick and thin filaments in a hexagonal array and Z bands become evident with the synthesis of even a small number of myofilaments. Haphazardly oriented thin filaments are peripheral to the lattice structure, suggesting their assembly even as new myosin filaments are synthesized. However, filament assembly and lattice formation may not depend on the presence of Z-band material because clusters of thin and thick filaments without associated Z-band material are commonly encountered. The Z bands that are seen always show fine filaments extending in either direction, and the earliest appearance of Z bands is consistently observed in foci of thin filament formation.[87] Z-band material may form when thick myofilaments are either present or lacking, and this formation appears to be unrelated to myosin.

Thick filaments are synthesized in sites of the early myotube cytoplasm different from those in which thin filaments are synthesized. Although thin filaments first appear in the periphery of the cytoplasm, thick filaments appear nearer the central core of sarcoplasm. Thin filaments also appear earlier than thick filaments.[141] Ribosomes are attached along the thick filaments but decrease in number as these myosin filaments are incorporated into the lattice structure of the sarcomere.

As more thin and thick myofilaments are assembled into a lattice structure, and repeating sarcomeres form as the myotube lengthens, the contractile filaments form a denser tubular structure enclosing the core of sarcoplasm and central nuclei (Fig. 138.11). The wall of this tube of contractile filaments thickens, and the diameter of the myotube increases. Progressive conversion of the myotube to a mature myofiber involves continued synthesis and arrangement of myofilaments, encroachment on the central sarcoplasmic core, and squeezing of the sarcoplasm between groups of myofilaments as the septa that isolate groups of myofilament lattices from adjacent groups. In addition, the central nuclei "migrate" between the forming myofibrils and the subsarcolemmal position that they occupy in the mature myofiber.

Growth of the myofiber near term and after birth involves mostly a continued synthesis of contractile proteins and an increased number of myofibrils, associated with a corresponding increase in the amount of sarcoplasm and organelles, as well as the addition of more sarcomeres as the muscle grows in length.

INTERMEDIATE FILAMENTS

Intermediate filaments are fibrous cytoskeletal polymers intermediate in size between 6-nm actin filaments and 23-nm microtubules that form the structural framework of nearly all eukaryotic cells. These scaffold proteins anchor cells against mechanical stress and function as bridges between linkage proteins and other cytoskeletal components.[141,142] Perinuclear regions of myotubes characteristically include nonoriented filaments, intermediate in diameter to thick 15-nm and thin 8-nm contractile filaments and measuring 10 to 12 nm.[87,92] Muscle intermediate filaments are also found distal to regions of sarcomere formation. These intermediate filaments are cytoskeletal proteins that help maintain the positions of nuclei and organelles in all cells and help organize the alignment of contractile elements

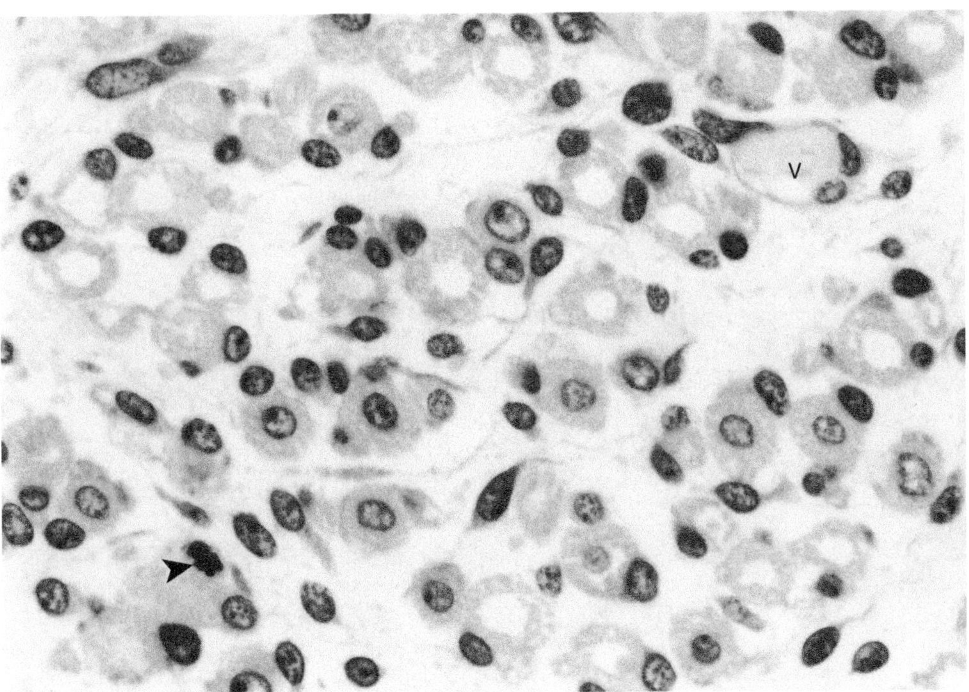

Fig. 138.11 Transverse section of the quadriceps femoris muscle in a 12-week human fetus. Late myotubes are a thick cylinder of myofibrils, surrounding central nuclei and the central core of sarcoplasm, seen as a clear space at levels between nuclei. Early myotubes have much thinner cylinders of myofibrils. The peripheral nuclei associated with some myotubes are myoblasts or presumptive myoblasts; one of the latter is undergoing mitosis *(arrowhead)*. Blood vessels *(V)* are a thin endothelium without smooth muscular walls. (Hematoxylin and eosin, original magnification ×1000.)

but are not contractile themselves. They may be important in determining the polarity of the early myotube.

Intermediate filament proteins have specific immunoreactivity in differentiating cells and mature cells of various types. The development of intermediate filaments has been less studied in muscle than in the nervous system, and most studies have focused on maturing muscle in tissue culture rather than on animal or human fetuses in vivo. Vimentin is largely a transitory fetal intermediate protein that disappears from most cells with maturation. In the fetal central nervous system (CNS), vimentin is demonstrated in primitive neuroectodermal cells but is replaced by either neurofilament protein or glial fibrillary acidic protein in cells differentiating along neuronal or glial lines, respectively. Vimentin is prominent in myoblasts,[143-146] and some investigators find that it disappears after myoblast fusion.[145] It continues to be expressed in fetal myotubes and has stronger immunoreactivity in late myotubes than in early myotubes (Fig. 138.12), but it is not demonstrated in mature striated muscle (see Fig. 138.12). However, even in adult life it persists in smooth muscle cells, including the muscular walls of blood vessels.

Another important muscular intermediate filament, desmin, is responsible for maintaining the register of Z bands between adjacent myofibrils by forming links between Z bands.[147] Desmin is thus the third protein, in addition to actinin and actin, to be localized at the Z band with use of immunocytochemical techniques. Desmin synthesis is initiated at the time of myoblast fusion and is prominent in fetal myotubes, especially late myotubes (Fig. 138.13A), having the same distribution as vimentin.[143,144] Early myotubes contain three times as much desmin as vimentin,[146] but this is difficult to demonstrate in mature muscle by immunocytologic reaction (see Fig. 138.13B). Desmin filaments begin to redistribute themselves transversely at the time of sarcomere formation.[145] Nevertheless, desmin is still demonstrated in adult muscle by electrophoretic and special immunologic methods.[144-150] The sparse strands of desmin in adult muscle connect myofibrils at the level of the Z bands to adjacent sarcolemma, mitochondria, and nuclei to maintain the relative positions of these structures, but they do not attach to the T-tubule systems.[150] Desmin is also associated with the neuromuscular junction site.[151] Immunocytochemical analysis demonstrates both vimentin and desmin in human striated muscle fibers until approximately 36 weeks' gestation, although neither is as strongly expressed as in myotubes.[152] In the term neonate, vimentin is not normally demonstrable in myofibers but is prominent in the endothelial cells of blood vessels. As with vimentin, desmin continues to be strongly expressed as evidenced by immunocytochemical methods in mature smooth muscle cells, in which these intermediate filaments appear to be associated with plasma membrane but are not connected to either actin or myosin filaments.[153] Desmin is closely associated with α-B-crystallin, and its abundance is augmented in certain human myopathies in a general category as "myofibrillar myopathies."[154]

MICROTUBULES

Microtubules that are approximately 25 nm in diameter are characteristic in regions of myofilament synthesis and early assembly, but they are lacking in regions of more advanced myofibril formation.[87] Their orientation is usually oblique, and they are situated near the ends of developing sarcomeres. A microtubular network is present in both mononucleated myoblasts (in which they radiate from a juxtanuclear center towards the cell periphery) and multinucleated myotubes, in which microtubules are numerous and are arranged in a parallel longitudinal orientation.[147,148]

RIBOSOMES

Ribosomes are abundant in regions of myofilament assembly and sarcomere formation.[92] They may be single and free in the cytoplasm, may occur in clusters as polyribosomes, or may be membrane associated. Ribosomes are structurally related

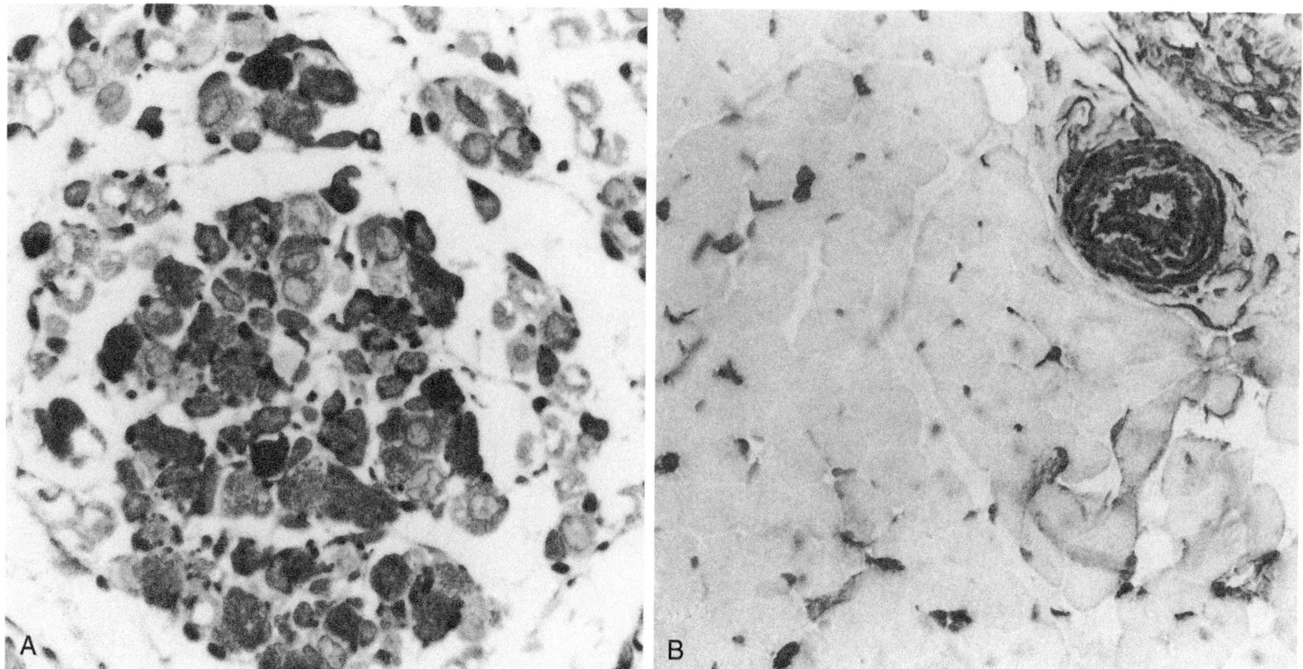

Fig. 138.12 Vimentin, a transient intermediate filament protein, is abundant in fetal myotubes (dark-staining immunoreactive product), particularly late myotubes, but is no longer seen in striated myofibers of the term neonate, although it is still strongly reactive in smooth muscle of vascular walls and also in endothelial cells. (A) Fourteen-week fetus. (B) Term neonate. (1:200 dilution; original magnification ×1000.)

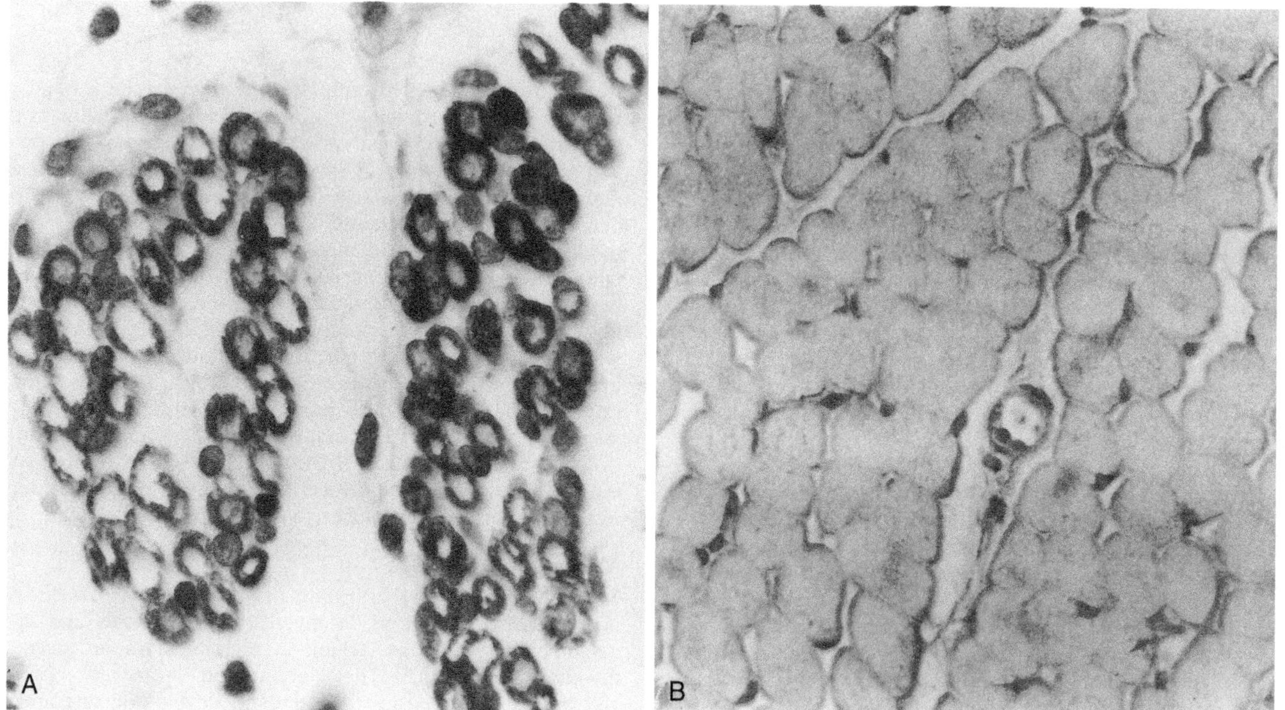

Fig. 138.13 Desmin (dark-staining product) is abundant in myotubes and has the same distribution as vimentin. It is no longer demonstrated by immunoreactivity in term neonatal muscle, although it persists in small amounts to maintain the registry of adjacent Z bands. (A) Fourteen-week fetus. (B) Term neonate. (1:800 dilution; original magnification ×1000.)

to the formation of thick myosin filaments but not to the formation of thin filaments. Polyribosomes of approximately 15 individual ribosomes are consistently clustered near both ends of the thick filaments, nearest to the I band, and single ribosomes also occur along the length of the myosin filament.[71] Ribosomes decrease in number and virtually disappear as the sarcomeres form, and they are rare in mature muscle. They reappear in regenerating myofibers at any age. The high RNA content in fetal myotubes and regenerating myofibers of injured mature muscle and the lack of demonstrable RNA in mature normal myocytes has been demonstrated by acridine orange fluorochrome studies.[155]

SARCOTUBULAR SYSTEM

In myotubes and mature myofibers, the endoplasmic reticulum of less differentiated myoblasts and presumptive myoblasts

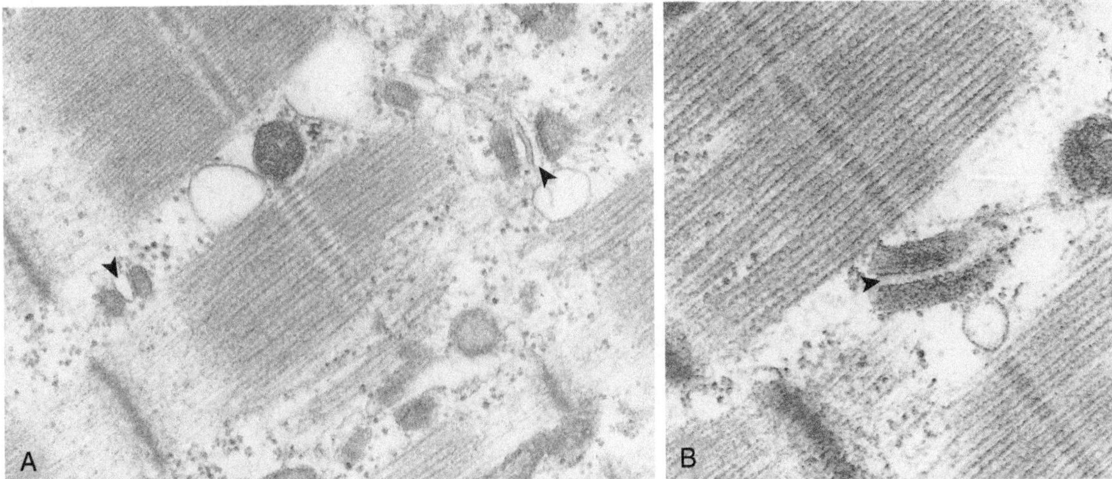

Fig. 138.14 Triad formation in term neonatal muscle. The triads *(arrowheads)* are formed by a T tubule with a pair of dilated terminal cisternae of sarcoplasmic reticulum. They generally occur at or near the Z band and are perpendicular to the long axis of the myofiber in the mature state (A), although they initially have a more parallel orientation in relation to the myofiber axis (B) until approximately 28 weeks gestation. (Electron micrographs, uranyl acetate and lead citrate. A, Original magnification ×25,000; B, original magnification ×35,000.)

is called the *SR*. Early myotubes exhibit multiple vesicular structures that probably are a primordial stage in the formation of SR. Irregular tubules show branching as the myotube matures, and these tubules are found in regions of cytoplasm containing myofilaments and forming sarcomeres. Numerous Z bands are in continuity with the SR, but this is not a constant feature. Some studies suggest that the SR tubules completely encircle the Z band,[93] but my laboratory's observations agree with those of Tomanek and Colling-Saltin[87] that this is an inconsistent feature. The SR does not appear essential in the assembly of myofilaments; however, the alignment of Z bands in register with those of adjacent myofibrils, a late development after 30 weeks' gestation, may be a function of SR tubules associated with Z bands.[87] The SR of both developing and mature myocytes is mostly smooth, without attached ribosomes. Short segments of rough endoplasmic reticulum are also encountered in myotubes but not in mature myofibers.

The T system develops by invaginations of the sarcolemma (i.e., cell membrane) of the myotube in cultured chick embryonic muscle.[156] Observations of human fetal muscle suggest a similar process of T-tubule formation.[87] Dyads, a close association of an SR tubule and a T tubule, and triads, a T tubule between a pair of dilated terminal cisternae of SR, are seen only in the periphery of myotubes, often associated with the sarcolemmal membrane (Fig. 138.14).[87,156-158] Dyads and triads occur in deeper regions of the myofiber only after sarcoplasmic septa separate the myofibrils as the central core of cytoplasm becomes dispersed with advanced maturation of the myotube. Membranes of SR and T tubules first become apposed with no visible structure between them; tenuous connections next traverse the space between apposed membranes, and well-developed bridges finally form.[158] Cisternae of the SR expand to form their characteristic structure after contacting T tubules.[156] SR cisternae contain electron-dense material that consists of mucopolysaccharides or glycoproteins to provide sites for calcium binding.

The observation that during early fetal development SR cisternae seldom show connections to other SR components suggests either that they develop independently or that they form on short fragments of SR that eventually unite with other SR tubules.[87] Triads have a predominantly longitudinal orientation relative to the long axis of the myofiber until approximately 28 weeks' gestation, after which time they rotate to the mature transverse orientation (see Fig. 138.14).[156-159]

Spherical vesicles with bristles on their outer surface in the periphery of the myotube are probably components of SR terminal cisternae rather than T tubules because they are also found in satellite cells. Presumptive myoblasts of fetal muscle and satellite cells of mature muscle possess an extensive endoplasmic reticulum, but T tubules are not evident and do not appear until the myotubular stage of development.[87]

MITOCHONDRIA

The mitochondria of striated muscle are similar to those in other types of cells but generally larger than in most cells and are very numerous because of the need to continuously generate energy. In the myotube, mitochondria are located in the central core of the myofiber between the row of central nuclei. With reorganization of the fiber after 15 weeks' gestation and relocation of the nuclei to the subsarcolemmal region, mitochondria become redistributed into the intermyofibrillar sarcoplasm throughout the fiber and in the subsarcolemmal region. They become particularly numerous and tightly clustered in the regions of motor end plates. Little difference is seen ultrastructurally between the cristae of mitochondria in immature and mature muscle. Because muscle is such a rich source of mitochondria, muscle obtained by biopsy is often the tissue of choice for the study of mitochondrial histochemical and ultrastructural features, for biochemical assay of respiratory chain enzymes, and for the study of mitochondrial DNA in suspected systemic mitochondrial diseases. In infantile mitochondrial cytopathies, the endothelial cells of capillaries within the muscle fascicles and in the subsarcolemmal region are often involved more severely and earlier than the mitochondria of adjacent myofibers.[160]

Normal mitochondria within myofibers and also in intramuscular endothelial cells are surrounded by granular endoplasmic reticulum, but a thin rim of cytoplasm separates them (Fig. 138.15A and B); in mitochondrial cytopathies, this layer of cytoplasm is obliterated and the endoplasmic reticulum becomes tightly adherent to the outer mitochondrial membrane.[160] These features can be demonstrated only by transmission electron microscopy, an obligatory part of a thorough pathology examination of muscle biopsy specimens for suspected mitochondrial disease.[102] Endothelial cells, including those of intramuscular capillaries, also have geometric parallel arrays of tubules that are normal structures known as *Weibel-Palade granules* (see Fig. 138.15C) that can be confused with the pathologic *paracrystalline structures* of compressed cristae in mitochondrial disease. Weibel-Palade bodies contain von Willebrand factor,[161] whereas mitochondrial paracrystalline structures are composed of creatine kinase.[102] Mitochondria

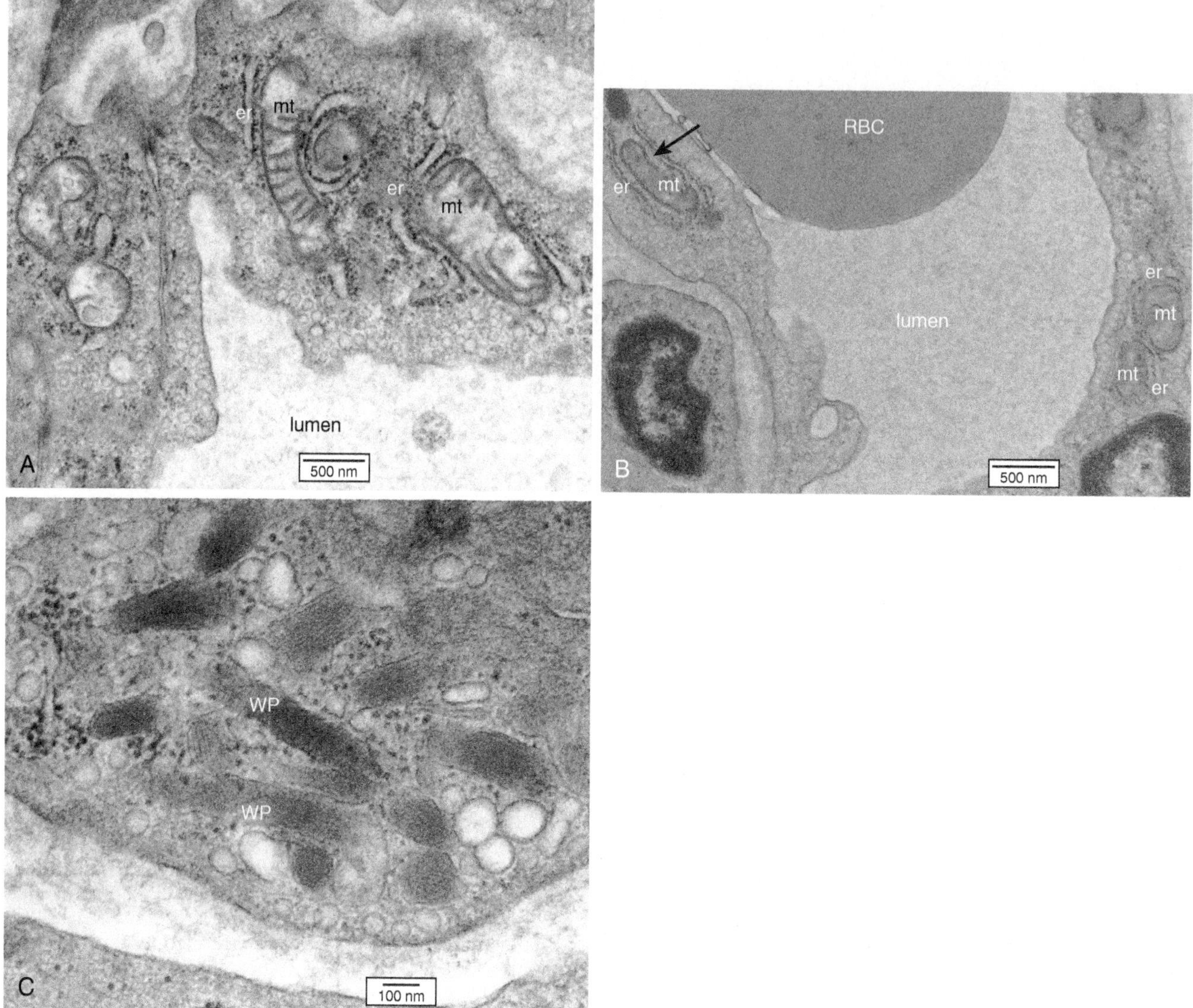

Fig. 138.15 (A and B) Transmission electron micrographs of endothelial cells of intramuscular capillaries in term neonates, showing normal relation of mitochondria *(mt)* with surrounding granular endoplasmic reticulum *(er)*. Normally there is always a thin layer of cytoplasm that separates the two (*arrow* in B), but in mitochondrial cytopathies this layer is obliterated and the endoplasmic reticulum is tightly adherent to the outer mitochondrial membrane (not shown). A red blood cell *(RBC)* is seen in the lumen of the capillary. (C) Weibel-Palade granules *(WP),* normal structures in endothelial cells that resemble abnormal mitochondrial paracrystalline structures. (Electron micrographs, uranyl acetate and lead citrate. See also Fig. 138.19 of a 14-week fetus for comparison of the same relation of mitochondrion to endoplasmic reticulum.) (From Sarnat HB, Flores-Sarnat L, Casey R, et al. Endothelial ultrastructural alterations of intramuscular capillaries in infantile mitochondrial cytopathies. *Neuropathology.* 2012;32:617–627.)

multiply by fusion and fission. Mitochondrial fusion proteins are regulated by proteases and ubiquitination; dynamins are inner mitochondrial membrane fusion factors and include the zinc protease Oma-1, which can cause changes in the structure of cristae.[162] Though it has been known for several decades that types I and II myofibers and their subtypes can be distinguished by histochemistry, including mitochondrial respiratory chain activities, mass spectrometry single fiber proteomics now also demonstrate mitochondrial specialization of fiber types.[95]

Mitochondria are essential to generate energy with calcium-mediated adenosine triphosphatase (ATPase). Patients with mitochondrial myopathies have altered mitochondria that often exhibit bizarre shapes and sizes and "paracrystalline" inclusion-like structures of lattice crystallin form that represent condensed creatine kinase.[163] In infants and toddlers, the more evident and severe changes are seen not in myofibers but rather in the endothelial cells of intramuscular capillaries[164]; they also occur in the subependymal region of the brain in severe infantile mitochondrial cytopathies such as Leigh encephalopathy, resulting in periventricular necrosis.[165] Pathologic paracrystalline structures must be distinguished from normal "Weibel-Palade granules" within endothelial cells that contain von Willebrand factor; they consist of parallel microtubules that, on oblique or longitudinal sections, have a repetitive pattern reminiscent of a crystal.[166] Additional inclusion-like structures are the small, electron-dense "spheroids," which occur in the cytoplasm in normally aging muscle of adults and in excess in children as well as adults with mitochondrial diseases. These spheroids are lipofuscin deposits in degenerating mitochondria and also can be demonstrated by fluorescence light microscopy because of their autofluorescent property.[155]

PHYSIOLOGIC CELL DEATH OF MYOTUBES

Degenerating myotubes occur singly or in small groups among normal myotubes in fetuses of 10 to 14 weeks' gestation.[167-169] Mononuclear phagocytic cells may be numerous around degenerating myocytes. Electron microscopy reveals nonartifactual extensive necrotic and degenerative changes both in nuclei and in sarcoplasm, loss of cell membranes, amorphous condensation of myofibrils, and extrusion of cellular contents into the endomysial extracellular space. This process of physiologic cell death is similar to that observed in the CNS and other body systems. An even earlier phase of apoptosis occurs among myoblasts still in the somitic myotome before they migrate into the sites of axial and appendicular muscles.[11]

Necrosis of a myofiber, by contrast, indicates pathologic degeneration, a loss of the ability to maintain homeostasis, and the generation of particulate debris that is carried away by phagocytic cells; this process generally begins focally in one segment of the fiber.[90]

GROWTH OF MYOFIBERS

The size of an individual muscle is determined by the number and size of its constituent myofibers and also by the amount of connective tissue that forms septa separating fascicles (i.e., perimysium). The diameter of individual muscle fibers is affected by many factors, including age, nutrition, exercise, and the effects of hormones, drugs, and disease. However, the number of muscle fibers in a particular muscle is relatively constant after birth and is genetically programmed.[170,171] A few studies have suggested a postnatal increase in the abundance of total myofibers of particular muscles such as those of mastication.[170] Protein-calorie malnutrition during fetal development may alter the final number of muscle fibers in animals,[172] but this phenomenon has not been adequately studied in human infants who have had intrauterine growth restriction or who are born to undernourished mothers. In contrast, the ratios of histochemical fiber types within the muscle are under neural control and are altered in either fetal or adult life by abnormal innervation patterns (see later). The average cross-sectional diameter of muscle fibers in the term neonate is 15 μm; the adult mean diameter of 65 μm is achieved at approximately 13 years of age. A standard curve plotted in 1969 for quantitative measurement in muscle biopsies of children remains valid and widely used by pathologists.[173]

Between 9 and 16 weeks' gestation in the human embryo, myotubes contain approximately 35 myofibrils in a transverse section of the tube of contractile filaments. Mature muscle fibers each contain approximately 80 to 110 myofibrils in a transverse section. Initially, myotubes are larger in cross-sectional diameter than other myofibers, but the situation is later reversed; as myotubes lengthen, their diameter actually decreases. Although the ratio of myotubes to maturing myofibers reverses, hypertrophy of individual myofibers replaces hyperplasia (i.e., increased number of myofibers) as the principal factor contributing to the total increase in the transverse area of the whole muscle.

Myofibril number is not related to myotube size, although it does increase at a declining rate. The total proliferation in the number of sarcolemmal nuclei with longitudinal growth of the myofiber is accomplished by mitosis of presumptive myoblasts and their conversion to true myoblasts, rather than by proliferation of existing sarcolemmal nuclei, because the latter are incapable of mitosis. This process slows in late gestation.[169]

Between 20 and 24 weeks gestation, approximately 10% of total myofibers in a cross-sectional field are noted to be approximately twice as large as the remaining 90%. These hypertrophic fibers are scattered uniformly throughout the fascicles and are never grouped. They were first identified by Wohlfart[174] in 1937 and were designated by him as *b-fibers*; the major population of smaller fibers were termed *a-fibers,* a terminology still used. The Wohlfart b-fibers were also later shown to be distinguishable from the a-fibers (see later) by histochemical reactivity. Between 24 and 30 weeks' gestation, as histochemical differentiation proceeds, the Wohlfart a-fibers increase in diameter to achieve the same size as the b-fibers, which do not grow as fast, until the two populations of myofibers can no longer be distinguished by size after 30 weeks.

Growth of myofibers during late gestation is mainly in length rather than diameter, but growth of the latter accelerates in the postnatal period. Some increase in the number of myofibers in late gestation and after birth may occur because of longitudinal splitting; an explanation of this splitting down the middle of the growing myofiber is that when a fiber achieves a critical size, the oblique pull of peripheral actin filaments is strong enough to cause the Z band to rupture.[175] After birth, linear growth of skeletal myofibers is greatest in the first 2 years and is accomplished mainly by addition of sarcomeres rather than by extension of the distance between Z bands.

METABOLIC DIFFERENTIATION OF MYOFIBERS

After nearly all fetal myotubes have become myocytes with peripheral sarcolemmal nuclei and an intermyofibrillar distribution of sarcoplasm and organelles, the next major maturational development is the differentiation of the uniform population of myofibers into a heterogeneous population of two distinct metabolic types and at least one subtype. Neural influence is first expressed in muscle maturation in the further growth and morphologic reorganization of myotubes and plays no role in the fusion of myoblasts to become myotubes. However, the expression of metabolic differences between muscle fibers is strongly controlled by innervation, and myofibers retain the capacity to change metabolic type with changes in innervation, as with denervation-reinnervation of muscle. This mutability is retained in human striated muscle, not only during fetal life and infancy but also in the adult. Since the 1970s it is known that innervation is the principal factor in determining whether individual myofibers are fast or slow in contractile rate.[176]

Metabolic differences between myofibers are expressed as relative differences in various enzymatic activities of the oxidative and glycolytic pathways, differences in calcium-mediated myofibrillar ATPase isozymes that are expressed maximally in various pH ranges, in heavy-chain myosin, and in the relative numbers or concentrations of mitochondria, lipid droplets, and glycogen particles within the sarcoplasm. These features are well demonstrated in frozen tissue section by histochemical methods and by immunocytochemical reactivity for heavy-chain myosin that distinguishes fiber types in formalin-fixed, paraffin-embedded sections.[177]

The period of histochemical differentiation is between 20 and 30 weeks' gestation in humans, but some differences among myofibers in their metabolic profiles may be seen as early as 18 weeks. Before that time, all myofibers appear histochemically uniform with all enzymatic stains; with use of myofibrillar ATPase stains, they correspond to type IIc fibers, which are considered the least differentiated subtype in mature muscle.

The early phase of histochemical differentiation, generally from 20 to 24 weeks, coincides with the appearance of Wohlfart b-fibers, the 10% of total myofibers that are larger than the rest and that are scattered evenly throughout the fascicles without being grouped.[174,178] These Wohlfart b-fibers are uniformly type I fibers (i.e., strong ATPase activity at acid pH of preincubation, strong oxidative enzymatic activity and weaker glycolytic activity, less glycogen than type II fibers); the 90% remaining Wohlfart a-fibers react histochemically as type II fibers (i.e., strongest ATPase activity at alkaline pH of preincubation, weaker oxidative and stronger glycolytic enzymatic activity, and more glycogen than type I fibers) and correspond almost exclusively to subtype IIc fibers of mature muscle (Fig. 138.16).

As maturation proceeds, and especially during the later phase of histochemical differentiation from 24 to 30 weeks' gestation,

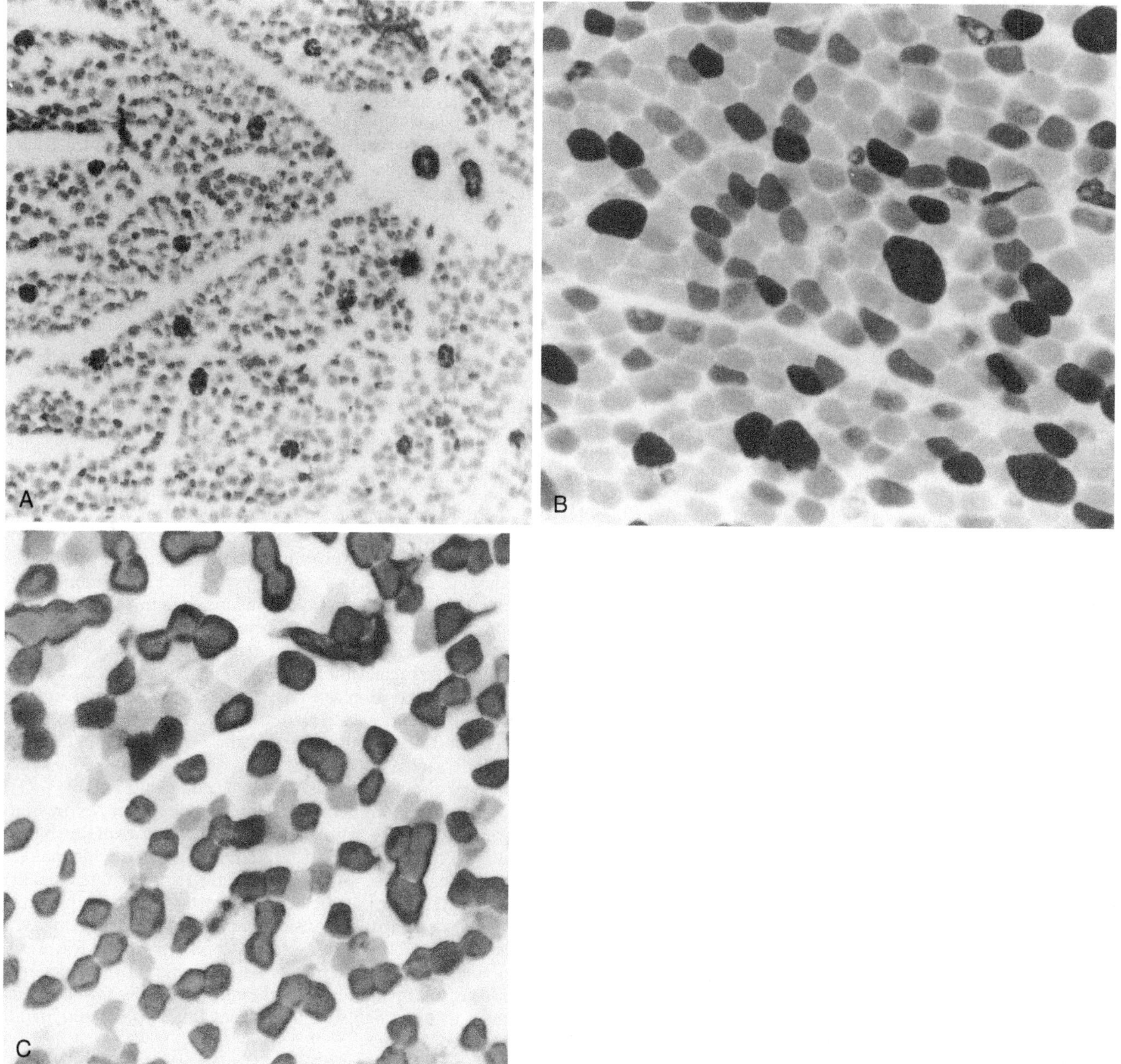

Fig. 138.16 Myofibrillar adenosine triphosphatase stain, preincubated at pH 4.3, in human fetuses at 24 weeks of gestation (A), 27 weeks gestation (B), and 40 weeks gestation *(term)* (C). In the early histochemical stage of development (A), approximately 10% of myofibers become larger than the others, are scattered in distribution and never grouped, and react as type I fibers, the "Wohlfart b-fibers." As maturation proceeds, more type II fibers become converted to type I fibers (B), until a relatively equal number of the two types exists at term (C). Still a greater proportion of subtype IIc fibers (intermediate intensity of staining) exists at birth than in the adult. (Original magnification ×250.)

progressive conversion of many type II fibers (Wohlfart a-fibers) to type I fibers occurs; however, growth of the population of smaller fibers at a greater rate than growth of the Wohlfart b-fibers obliterates the distinction of these populations by either size or their reactivity as type I fibers. By 30 weeks' gestation, most muscles of the human body have relatively equal numbers of type I and type II myofibers, and they are distributed in a mosaic or checkerboard pattern without large groups of either type, although small groups of three to five fibers of the same type may occur. Type II fibers may predominate in the single line of myofibers along the edges of fascicles.

During the later period of histochemical differentiation (after 30 weeks' gestation), type II fibers become distinguished by myofibrillar ATPase stains as subtypes defined by their degree of inhibition of reaction at differing pH of preincubation.[178] Thus at high pH, such as 9.8 or 10.4, all type II fibers are uniformly stained darker than type I fibers. At pH 4.6 or 4.7, type I fibers are dark, whereas some type II fibers are intermediate in intensity and others are totally inhibited and unstained. The inhibited fibers are designated *IIa,* and the intermediate fibers are designated *IIb* and *IIc.* At a still lower pH of preincubation (4.3), subtype IIa fibers remain completely inhibited, subtype IIb fibers are either totally inhibited or very light, and subtype IIc fibers are intermediate—darker than subtype IIb fibers but not as dark as type I fibers. At maturity, approximately 65% of total type II fibers are designated *IIa fibers,* 30% are designated *IIb fibers,* and only 5% are designated *IIc fibers.* In the term neonate, however, 15% to 20% of type II fibers are subtype IIc or "undifferentiated" fibers (see Fig. 138.16).[178-180] Differentiation of the soleus muscle, with a higher percentage of type I fibers, is not complete until 9 to 12

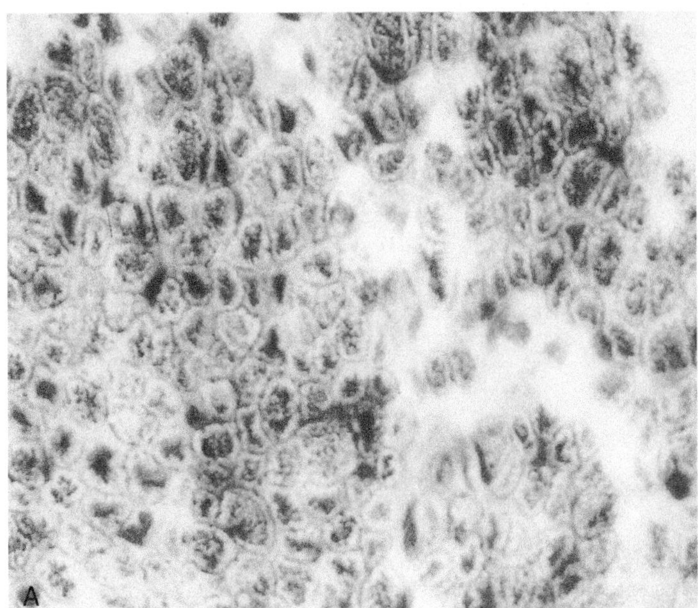
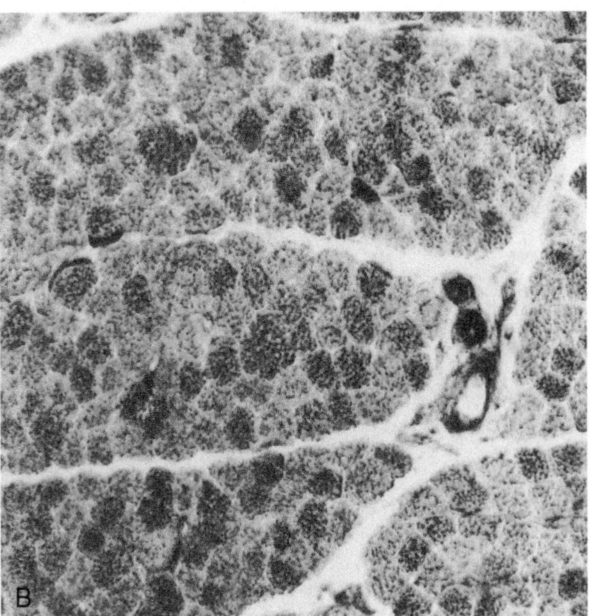

Fig. 138.17 (A) Oxidative enzymatic (mitochondrial) activity has a characteristic histochemical distribution in myotubes: intense staining confined to the central core of sarcoplasm and a thin rim in the subsarcolemmal region, the cylinder of myofibrils remaining unstained. Fiber types cannot be distinguished. (B) In term neonatal muscle, the oxidative enzymatic activity is now redistributed uniformly in the intermyofibrillar sarcoplasm. *Dark points* of activity are mitochondria. The *darker-stained fibers* are type I fibers, and the *lighter-stained fibers* are type II fibers, as in the adult. (Nicotinamide adenine dinucleotide tetrazolium reductase; A, original magnification ×1000; B, original magnification ×250.)

months of age in the human infant and is accompanied by slowing of contractile properties that correspond to the functional use of this muscle as the infant stands more and prepares to walk.[180]

The oxidative enzymatic activity of the mitochondria and SR has a characteristic histochemical distribution with use of stains of the electron transport chain (e.g., nicotine adenine dinucleotide [reduced form] tetrazolium reductase) and of the tricarboxylic acid (Krebs) cycle (e.g., succinate dehydrogenase, malate dehydrogenase, isocitrate dehydrogenase). In myotubes, the activity follows the distribution of mitochondria and is seen only in the central core of sarcoplasm and in the subsarcolemmal region (Fig. 138.17A). As the myofiber matures, the mitochondria become redistributed in the intermyofibrillar sarcoplasm. Therefore type I fibers, which have more mitochondria than type II fibers, appear darker (see Fig. 138.17B). Oxidative enzymatic stains used to be regarded only in a relative ratio of activity to glycolytic enzyme stains, but it is now recognized that each is a marker for the specific mitochondrial respiratory chain complexes, and they have assumed an even greater value in the interpretation of some muscle biopsy results, as well as in developmental studies of muscle. In mitochondrial myopathies, deficiencies in each and in combinations of respiratory chain complexes denote morphologic and phenotypical changes in the appearance of myofibers in the muscle biopsy, such as why some mitochondrial myopathies have ragged-red fibers and others do not.[181]

Myophosphorylase activity may also be histochemically demonstrated in unfixed frozen sections of striated muscle. A fetal form of myophosphorylase is replaced by the mature form of the enzyme after birth. In addition to myophosphorylase, phosphofructokinase and other enzymes of the glycolytic Embden-Meyerhof pathway may also be demonstrated in fetal muscle as early as the late myotubular stage. Distinction between histochemical fiber types is not evident until after 24 weeks' gestation, however. The myogenic genes may also play a role in muscle fiber-type differentiation, even though this phase of ontogenesis is considerably later than the primary period of expression of these genes. In transgenic mice, myogenin induces, or at least accompanies, a shift from glycolytic (type II fibers) to oxidative (type I fibers) metabolism.[182,183] With aging in adult life, changes in the levels of protein expression of myogenin and MyoD1 in muscle also occur.[184]

FASCICULAR ORGANIZATION OF DEVELOPING MUSCLE

As the paired longitudinal somitic plates on either side of the neural plate begin to segment into somites, the space between somites contains looser, less densely cellular mesenchyme than the more compact somites. The mesenchymal cells in this looser tissue differentiate into fibroblasts and soon secrete collagen into the intercellular space as the more compact mesenchymal cells of the somites predominantly become myoblasts and primordial dermal cells. During growth of the limb buds, the individual muscles of the extremities are derived from the somites, whereas the collagenous muscle capsules (i.e., epimysium), blood vessels, and tendons are somatopleural derivatives.

Individual muscles consist of loose arrays of presumptive and true myoblasts and differentiating myotubes without the connective tissue septa that subdivide more mature muscle into fascicles. During the myotubular stage of myogenesis, myotubes and myoblasts cluster in small groups of three to as many as eight cells, but mostly three to five myotubes, surrounded by a single common basal lamina.[179,185] Single myotubes enclosed within their own individual basal lamina and isolated myoblasts without a basal lamina also appear.[87] Independent myotubes become more numerous in later stages of development, and by the end of the myotubular stage, clusters of myotubes within a common basal lamina are no longer seen, although single myotubes continue to be closely associated with myoblasts and presumptive myoblasts.[185] Myoblasts and early myotubes tend to predominate at the periphery of the developing muscle, and maturation of the myotubes in the center of the muscle is more advanced (Fig. 138.18A).

Fibroblasts also are included within developing muscle and produce delicate reticular and collagen fibers. Thin collagenous

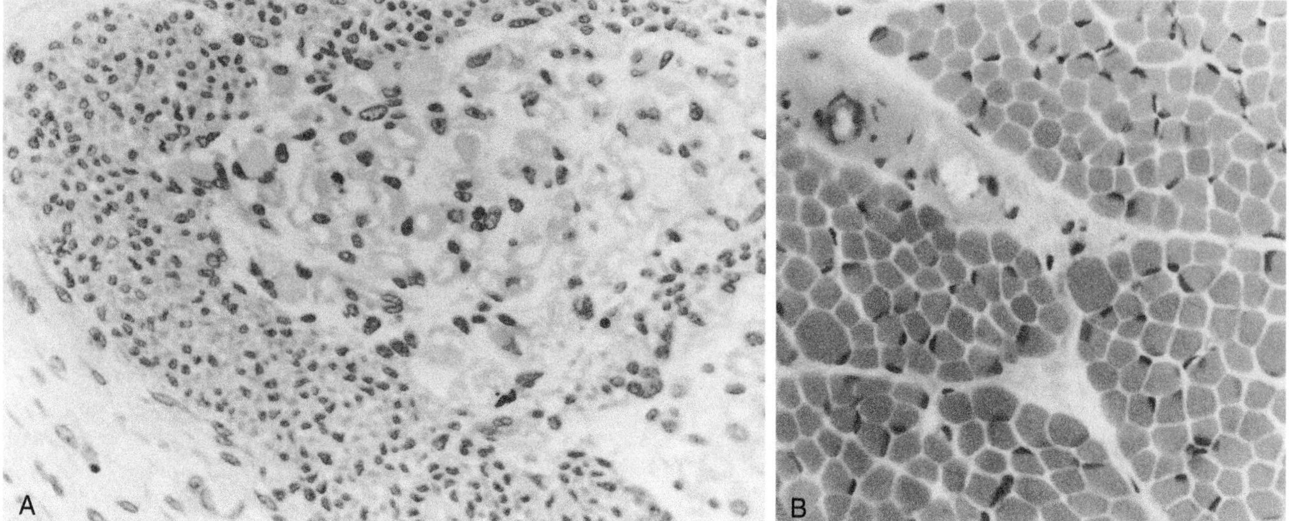

Fig. 138.18 (A) Soleus muscle of 12-week human fetus. Early myotubes and myoblasts tend to predominate at the periphery, and late myotubes are more frequent in the interior of the muscle. Perimysial connective tissue septa have not yet developed. (B) Term neonate, quadriceps femoris muscle. The fascicular organization of the muscle is well developed, with a well-defined perimysium that includes arterioles, venules, and intramuscular nerves. (Hematoxylin and eosin; A, original magnification ×400; B, original magnification ×250.)

septa (i.e., perimysium) divide the muscle into fascicles, particularly in association with the growth of blood vessels. This process begins in the late myotubular stage, occurring mainly as myotubes are converted to myocytes with peripheral nuclei and continuing during the early phase of histochemical differentiation. By 30 weeks' gestation, the fascicular organization of muscle is well established. Perimysial connective tissue then thickens and includes all arterioles, venules, and nerves that penetrate the muscle (see Fig. 138.18B). Endomysial collagen fibers between individual myofibers within a fascicle are thinner, sparser, and much more delicate in the term neonate than in the older child; the endomysium mainly develops after birth.

Blood vessels within developing muscle are seen as early as 6 weeks' gestation in humans. During the myotubular stage of development, vessels consist of delicate channels or sinuses with thin endothelial cells and wide lumina (Figs. 138.19 and 138.20). With growth of the perimysium, the feeding vessels develop smooth muscular walls and a thicker endothelium. The capillary network becomes denser as myofibers mature and contraction becomes more forceful. By term, both capillaries and larger arterioles and venules are well developed (see Fig. 138.18B).

Several resident inflammatory cells are seen scattered in the perimysium of muscle. At least two distinct populations of macrophages (M1 and M2) have differing roles in necrosis and regeneration in development and in myopathies.[186] Mast cells and scattered T and B lymphocytes are also present, even in fetal muscle, and can increase in number when signaled to do so. In addition, hematogenous arrival of additional inflammatory cells in response to injury occurs.

MUSCLE SPINDLES AND TENDON ORGANS

Intrafusal fibers are already forming during the myotubular stage of development, but they are difficult to recognize histologically because they closely resemble extrafusal fibers at this time. The distinctive connective tissue capsule of the spindle does not form until later.[187-189] Spindles may be readily identified after 20 weeks' gestation in humans, and they appear fully mature at 30 weeks, including well-developed nuclear bag and nuclear chain forms of intrafusal fibers (Fig. 138.21) with their mature histochemical characteristics.

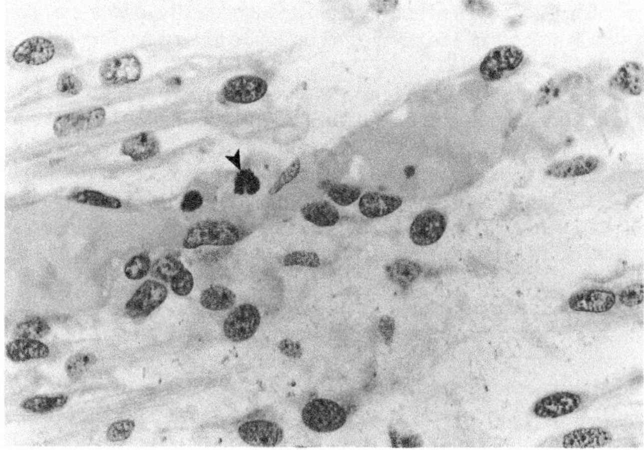

Fig. 138.19 Intramuscular blood vessel in quadriceps femoris muscle of a 14-week fetus. The vessel is thin walled, and the lumen is wide and dilated. The mitotic figure *(arrowhead)* may be an endothelial cell or a presumptive myoblast. (Hematoxylin and eosin, original magnification ×1000.)

Because intrafusal fibers enclosed by a delicate collagenous capsule may be recognized as early as 14 weeks' gestation in human fetuses, spindles actually begin forming late in the myotubular stages.

In the rat, the earliest detectable spindles in hindlimb muscles are seen less than 2 days before birth and consist of a single myotube bearing simple nerve terminals of the large primary afferent axon from nearby unmyelinated intramuscular nerve trunks. The capsule forms by an extension of the perineurium of the supplying nerve fasciculus and is confined initially to the innervated zone.[187-190] Myoblasts are present within the capsule of the spindle throughout its development and fuse to form a smaller and less differentiated myotube. This myotube matures in close association with the initial fiber, and by birth it has formed the smaller, intermediate nuclear bag fiber identified in the adult. Nuclear chain fibers develop in the same way, but myoblast fusion forms satellite myotubes in apposition to myoblasts of fibers that are more mature within the same basal lamina. By 4 days after

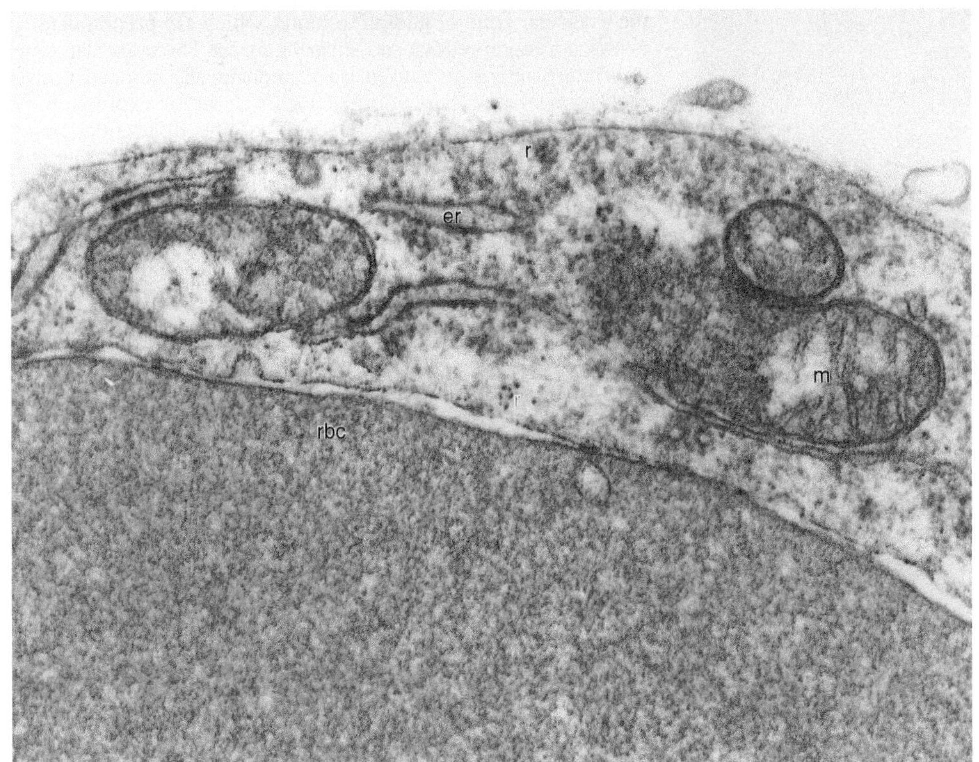

Fig. 138.20 Endothelial cell of intramuscular blood vessel of a 14-week fetus. Mitochondria *(m)*, rough granular endoplasmic reticulum *(er)*, and free ribosomes *(r)* are seen in the cytoplasm. Note the thin layer of cytoplasm separating the mitochondrion from nearby granular endoplasmic reticulum (compare with Fig. 138.15). A red blood cell *(rbc)* is seen in the lumen of the vessel. (Electron micrograph, uranyl acetate and lead citrate, original magnification ×25,000.)

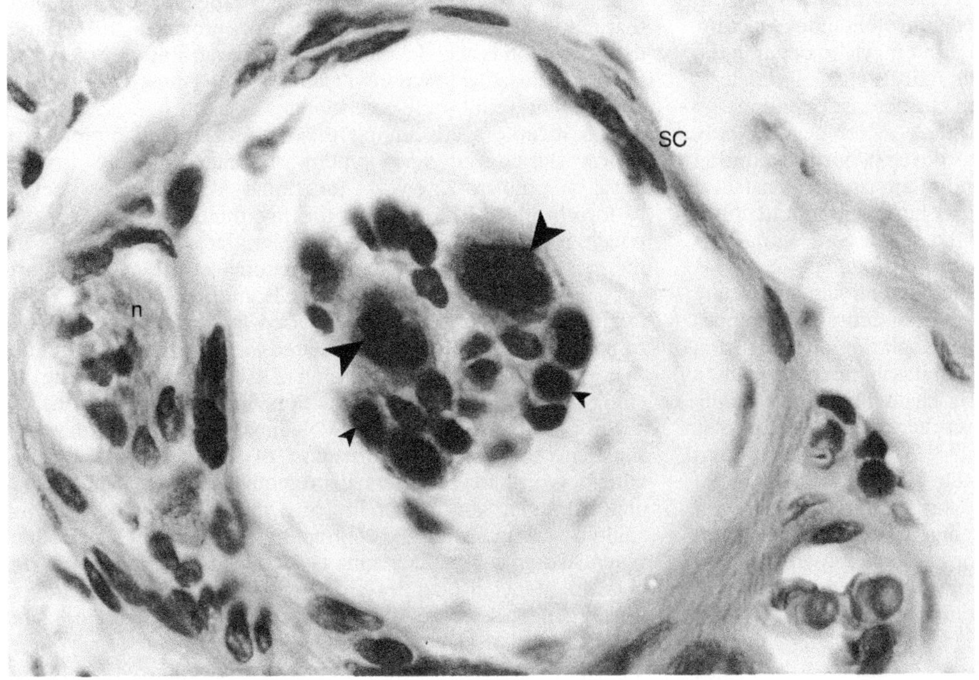

Fig. 138.21 Muscle spindle within the quadriceps femoris muscle of a term neonate. Both nuclear bag fibers *(large arrowheads)* and nuclear chain fibers *(small arrowheads)*, as well as the spindle capsule *(SC)* and associated nerve *(n)*, are well developed at birth. (Hematoxylin and eosin, original magnification ×1000.)

birth, the adult complement of four intramuscular muscle fibers is present. Fusiform innervation begins at birth and is not complete until the twelfth postnatal day (in the rat), when the myofibrillar ultrastructure is fully mature.[189] The periaxial space appears at the same time. Thus, afferent innervation precedes the efferent nerve supply to the intrafusal spindle fibers. Morphogenesis of the rat muscle spindle is complete at 25 days after birth.[190]

As with the differing morphologic features between extrafusal and intrafusal muscle fibers, mature intrafusal fibers exhibit histochemical characteristics that are unique and do not correspond to the histochemical types of extrafusal fibers.[190-194] These histochemical subpopulations appear somewhat later than the differentiation of fiber types of extrafusal myofibers, with some overlap.

Golgi tendon organs are stretch receptors found between muscle and tendon and less frequently within the tendon itself. They are also distributed in the intermuscular connective tissue and in the capsules of joints. Tendon organs are almost as numerous as muscle spindles, although they are infrequently seen in muscle biopsy specimens.[195] Because tendon organs

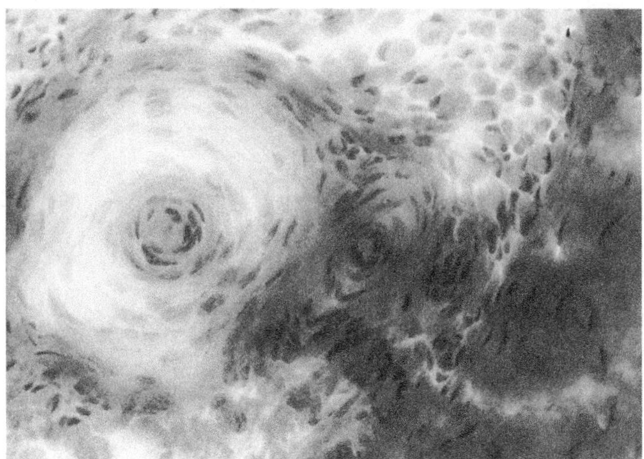

Fig. 138.22 Pacinian corpuscle near myotendinous insertion of the quadriceps femoris muscle in a 36-week premature infant. The fibrous epimysial muscle capsule is seen on the *right.* (Gomori trichrome, original magnification ×1000.)

lie in series with the main mass of muscle, they are sensitive to any sudden change in muscle length, active or passive, or to a summation of active and passive stretch. Their afferent nerve fibers all belong to group Ib, with widespread central connections that allow for patterned and sequential engagement of synergistic and antagonistic muscles as integrated movements. Golgi tendon organs develop after the myotubular stage and are well formed by 28 weeks' gestation. Numerous Pacinian corpuscles similar to those of the dermis also occur near the myotendinous junction, mainly within the tendon (Fig. 138.22), but they also occur in the perimysium between muscle fascicles at distal ends of muscles.

Unlike extrafusal myofibers, which characteristically undergo atrophy and disappear after loss of their motor nerve supply, intrafusal spindle fibers continue to develop normally during the first 3 weeks after deefferentation of immature neonatal rat muscle, but only if their afferent sensory nerve supply and dorsal root ganglia are preserved (even if the spinal cord segment is extirpated). Intrafusal fibers then actually proliferate at 3 to 5 weeks after denervation, with the supernumerary fibers forming from the fusion of myoblasts derived from activated intrafusal satellite cells and also from longitudinal splitting of preexisting intrafusal myofibers.[195-199] New intrafusal fibers originate from both nuclear bag and nuclear chain fibers but mainly from the latter.[196] The ratio of myosin heavy chain isoforms is altered under these circumstances.[192,199] The total efferent and afferent denervation of muscle spindles, by contrast, results in atrophy and numeric reduction of intrafusal myofibers.[199,200] In sum, intrafusal muscle fibers are much more dependent on sensory nerve supply than on motor nerve supply to preserve their integrity, and they proliferate as a delayed response to deefferentation rather than undergo atrophy.[191]

TENDON DEVELOPMENT

Tendons are dense fibrous bands that attach striated muscles to bones, as either the proximal origin or the distal insertion of the muscle. In *traction tendons,* in which the line of action corresponds to that of the muscle, few blood vessels are uniformly distributed within the tendon tissue. In *gliding tendons,* which change their direction of pull, an avascular zone normally forms in the region where the tendon wraps around the pulley.[201] The angiogenic peptide vascular endothelial growth factor is present in both endothelial cells and tenocytes (a fibroblast derivative) of human fetal tendons exposed to traction but not in the avascular zone of gliding tendons, which are predominantly exposed to compressive and shearing forces. The avascular zone of tendons might be caused by a mechanically induced down-regulation of vascular endothelial growth factor expression.[202] Tendons begin forming at the time of the differentiation of the fascicular organization of muscle. The transitional zone is a mixture of perimysial fibrous bands and myofibers that may show cytoarchitectural differences from the same fibers in the main belly of the muscle and hence can easily be misinterpreted as myopathic findings in muscle biopsy samples taken too near the insertion, as during "heel cord" (Achilles tendon)-lengthening procedures.

MEMBRANE EXCITABILITY AND INNERVATION OF FETAL MUSCLE

The resting membrane potential of mature muscle, approximately 90 mV, is actively maintained by continuous energy production derived from Na^+, K^+-ATPase (calcium-mediated ATPase and creatine kinase are the energy sources for the contractile mechanism of myofibrils). This energy-generating system for maintaining membrane excitability develops early in myogenesis; even early myotubes have a continuously polarized membrane. Spontaneous subthreshold potentials may be recorded anywhere along the sarcolemmal membrane, but their site of origin is in the middle of the fiber at the point at which end plates are eventually formed.[202] They resemble the miniature end-plate potentials of adult fibers but occur at a lower frequency and with a slower time course. The plasma membrane of myoblasts is also excitable, although it may easily fatigue. The compound that most strongly and consistently provokes membrane depolarization is acetylcholine (ACh), the transmitter secreted at the neuromuscular junction of mature striated muscle in humans, all vertebrates, and some invertebrates.

ACh receptors are among the first membrane proteins to appear during the development of striated muscle. In the larval amphibian *Xenopus,* functional ACh receptors begin to form within 2 hours after the myotomes begin to appear, which is much earlier than nerve contacts muscle.[203,204] In the rat, peripheral nerves and functional ACh receptors both appear when developing muscle cells are first identified[205] but functional innervation is not required for the development of ACh receptors, and myoblasts isolated in tissue culture continue to develop them.[206] The expression of ACh receptors in living rat embryos is unaltered after destruction of their motor neurons.[207]

Ion channels in the sarcolemmal membrane develop simultaneously with the formation of ACh receptors and, as with neurons, are an essential prerequisite for excitability and depolarization. The excitability of a muscle fiber, and thus its ability to generate force and contraction, depends on a high resting potential across its sarcolemma (−80 mV inside with respect to outside). Many myopathies are secondary to *channelopathies,* usually genetic defects of subunits of sodium, potassium, or calcium channels that produce either myotonia or periodic paralysis.[208] They may result from either gain or loss of function.[209]

Although innervation is not essential for the initial formation of functional ACh receptors, innervation of muscle leads to a major redistribution of receptors, eventually resulting in their aggregation at the points of nerve contact.[204,207,210] After concentration of receptors at the synapse point, a decrease occurs in the density of receptors in portions of the sarcolemmal membrane not directly contacted by nerve endings.[202,211,212] The decreased density of ACh receptors is accompanied by a low sensitivity of nonsynaptic membrane to ACh, a characteristic of adult muscle fibers. Aggregates of synaptic junction receptors remain after denervation; removal of the nerve results in a return of high levels of extrajunctional receptors.[213,214]

Innervation of human striated muscle occurs in the middle of the myotubular stage of development, maximally at approximately 11 weeks' gestation, but motor end plates begin to form as early as 9 weeks' gestation and continue to develop and mature until 20 weeks' gestation.[215] The primitive motor end plate contains a few axons always covered by one Schwann cell. It does not change either in number or in structure between 10 and 20 weeks' gestation, although continuous modification of the postsynaptic membrane is observed throughout this period.[216] The axon contains a few synaptic vesicles and is in close contact with the unfolded plasma membrane of the primary myotube. The first morphologic change indicative of end-plate formation is seen at the junction of the sarcolemma with the axolemma, the former having a distinct thickening in the small junctional zone. This thickening of the postsynaptic membrane may already be evident when the axon is 20 to 30 nm from the muscle cell.[216] At the mature myotubular stage, at approximately the fourteenth week of gestation, synaptic gutters and primary synaptic clefts form. Secondary synaptic clefts are first seen in the sixteenth week of gestation. The characteristic convolutions of the mature postsynaptic membrane are thus well established by midgestation and are fully mature at birth.

Myotubes are initially innervated from several nerves. The mature single-nerve supply to each myofiber results from retraction of all but one nerve as development proceeds. Fidziańska[216] found several synaptic axonal terminals grouped together and filled with synaptic vesicles at the motor end plate of human fetuses of 10 to 20 weeks' gestation; these axonal terminals did not seem to change in either ultrastructural appearance or number during this period and were always covered by a single Schwann cell. Silver impregnations of nerve fibers also show a single motor end plate on each fetal myofiber supplied by more than one axon.[217] It may be concluded from these data that each developing myofiber has just one end plate, but this end plate is supplied by two or more axons. This conclusion is consistent with other electrophysiologic and morphologic data indicating polyneural innervation of fetal muscle fibers. Scanning electron microscopy of nerve-muscle cultures also confirms that a single embryonic muscle fiber may be contacted by as many as five different nerves arising from different motor neurons.[218] Physiologic cell death of a spinal neuroblast is unrelated to the change from polyneuronal to mononeuronal innervation of muscle,[219] but functional neuromuscular innervation is probably one factor that regulates the natural process of cell death among embryonic motor neurons of the spinal cord, because the number of motor neurons undergoing natural cell death is closely related to muscular activity.[220] Development of the neuromuscular junction and its various disorders that cause congenital myasthenic syndromes were reviewed by Engel and colleagues.[221]

"Myotube satellite cells" with long cytoplasmic processes extending beyond the basal lamina into the endomysial space are seen in developing extraocular muscles. They contact free cells of similar appearance, as well as axon-surrounding Schwann cells, often forming an extensive network. These myotube satellite cells resemble Schwann cells in all respects except for the lack of an associated axon, and they may be Schwann cells disposed to promote axonal growth towards differentiating myofibers not yet innervated.[222]

Spinal motor nerve roots begin their myelination cycle at approximately 16 weeks of gestation, and roots and peripheral nerves are well myelinated by late gestation.[223] In the phrenic nerve, one and a half turns of myelin are seen around nerve fibers at 15 weeks' gestation[224]; the vagal nerve begins its myelination cycle at approximately 24 weeks' gestation in humans[225] and at a corresponding age in fetal lambs.[226] Myelination of axons innervating extraocular muscles is reported by some investigators as early as 18 weeks' gestation.[227]

SUPRASEGMENTAL NEURAL INFLUENCES ON MUSCLE MATURATION

The importance of innervation to muscle fiber maturation beyond the myotubular stage is well demonstrated both in vivo and in vitro. Neonatal neurectomy in rats prevents further development of the myocyte.[228] In humans the effects of perinatal denervation on the morphologic features of muscle are well demonstrated in progressive spinal muscular atrophy, a degenerative motor neuron disease beginning in fetal life and continuing after birth.[229]

Suprasegmental centers in the cerebrum, cerebellum, and brain stem may alter the discharge pattern of motor neurons and change the course of muscle maturation. Classic studies document that excessive nerve stimulation experimentally causes a conversion of type II fibers to type I fibers in the rat,[230,231] and abnormal suprasegmental stimulation of lower motor neurons in the human fetus may have a similar influence on histochemical differentiation.

Histochemical abnormalities in the muscle biopsy specimens from infants with cerebral malformations have been noted by several researchers.[232-235] Similar aberrations in the sizes and ratios of histochemical fiber types occur in the muscles of neonates with congenital contractures after fetal immobilization (i.e., arthrogryposis multiplex congenita).[235] Prospective study of the muscles of infants with various types of cerebral dysgenesis documented by imaging procedures or by postmortem examination demonstrates that three categories of disorders in muscle maturation may be identified: (1) delayed maturation in term infants, the muscle being morphologically normal but incompletely differentiated histochemically; (2) fiber-type predominance of more than 80% of either type I or type II fibers; and (3) the classic "congenital muscle fiber-type disproportion," defined as a predominance and uniform hypoplasia of type I fibers, often with secondary hypertrophy of type II fibers.[236,237]

An equally dramatic finding is the presence of normal and histochemically mature neonatal muscle in infants with normal spinal cords but severely hypoplastic brains, or with such severe dysplasias that few if any descending pathways exist to relay suprasegmental impulses.[236] This finding in the human is supported by observations in the stage 13 or 14 (day 2) chick embryo that extirpation of several cervical segments of spinal cord does not alter the development of motor end-plate distribution or histochemical differentiation by ATPase of muscles innervated by more caudal segments.[238] The relatively isolated human spinal cord with normal muscle maturation demonstrates that the motor unit is capable of maturing normally without cerebral influence, and the aberrant patterns found in infants with cerebral dysgenesis suggest that abnormal descending upper motor neuron influences may alter the course of muscle ontogenesis, probably by interfering with the discharge pattern of the lower motor neuron.

The most common malformation of the brain associated with abnormal muscle development is cerebellar hypoplasia as an isolated anomaly or in conjunction with cerebral dysplasias.[236,237] Abnormal development of brain stem structures is also associated with aberrant muscle maturation, but congenital lesions confined to suprasegmental structures, even when severe, do not seem to affect muscle development. Descending brain stem pathways become myelinated during the period of histochemical differentiation of muscle, between 20 and 30 weeks of gestation,[223] and are functional during this period. The corticospinal tract, by contrast, is unmyelinated until much later, after muscle maturation is complete, and probably subserves several functions in the term neonate.[239,240] It is therefore likely that suprasegmental influences on muscle maturation are mediated more by the numerous small bulbospinal (i.e., "subcorticospinal") pathways, such as the tectospinal, rubrospinal, olivospinal, vestibulospinal, and reticulospinal tracts, than by the much larger but late-myelinating corticospinal tract.

CONCLUSION

The embryonic origin of striated muscle is dual: myoblasts originate in the myotome portion of the somites, whereas the muscle matrix, including fibrous and adipose connective tissues, blood vessels, nerve sheaths, and spindle capsules, arise from neural crest cells. Several myogenic genes and other associated genes regulate development, including myoblast fusion to form multinucleated myofibers. Sarcolemmal membrane development includes the formation of ion channels for a resting membrane potential. Initially diffuse receptors for ACh later localize for neuromuscular junction formation. Innervation occurs at 9 to 11 weeks' gestation. Various intermediate filament proteins and other proteins exhibit changes with maturation. The development of an intramuscular capillary network and specialized organelles within endothelial cells are essential to mediate growth and conserve integrity of muscle. Satellite progenitor cells beneath the sarcolemma, but separate from the myofiber, can proliferate and differentiate for muscle growth and later for regenerative repair of injured muscle.

 A complete reference list is available at www.ExpertConsult.com.

SELECT REFERENCES

9. Venters SJ, Thorsteinsdóttir S, Duxson MJ. Early development of the myotome in the mouse. *Dev Dyn*. 1999;216:219.
27. Zammit PS. Function of the myogenic regulatory factors Myf5, MyoD, myogenin and MRF4 in skeletal muscle, satellite cells and regenerative myogenesis. *Semin Cell Dev Biol*. 2017;72:19-32.
28. Taylor MV. Skeletal muscle development on the 30th anniversary of MyoD. *Semin Cell Dev Biol*. 2017;72:1-2. https://doi.org/10.1016/j.semcdb.2017.11.019.
40. Valdez MR, Richardson JA, Klein WH, Olson EN. Failure of *Myf5* to support myogenic differentiation without myogenin, *MyoD* and *MRF4*. *Dev Biol*. 2000;219:287.
63. von Maltzahn J, Chang NC, Bentzinger CF, Rudnicki MA. *Wnt* signaling in myogenesis. *Trends Cell Biol*. 2012;22:602-609.
73. Tureckova J, Wilson EM, Cappalonga JL, Rotwein P. Insulin-like growth factor-mediated muscle differentiation: collaboration between phosphatidylinositol 3-kinase-Akt signaling pathways and myogenin. *J Biol Chem*. 2001;276:39264.
85. Gonorazky HD, Bonnemann CG, Dowling JJ. The genetics of congenital myopathies. *Handb Clin Neurol*. 2018;148:549-564.
90. Millay DP, O'Rourke JR, Sutherland LB, et al. Myomaker is a membrane activator of myoblast fusion and muscle formation. *Nature*. 2013;499:301-305.
91. Fidzianska A. Human ontogenesis. I. Ultrastructural characteristics of developing human muscle. *J Neuropathol Exp Neurol*. 1980;39:476.
100. Ali MA. Myotube formation in skeletal muscle regeneration. *J Anat*. 1979;128:553.
101. Yin H, Price F, Rudnicki MA. Satellite cells and the muscle stem cell niche. *Physiol Rev*. 2013;93:23-67.
102. Sarnat HB, Carpenter S. Muscle biopsy for diagnosis of neuromuscular and metabolic diseases. In: Darras BT, Jones Jr R, Ryan MM, De Vivo DC, eds. *Neuromuscular Disorders of Infancy, Childhood, and Adolescence. A Clinician's Approach*. Ed 2. Boston: Academic Press; 2015:46-65.
104. Darras BT, Menache-Starobinski CC, Hinton V, Kunkel LM. Dystrophinopathies. In: Darras BT, Jones Jr R, Ryan MM, De Vivo DC, eds. *Neuromuscular Disorders of Infancy, Childhood, and Adolescence. A Clinician's Approach*. Ed 2. Boston: Academic Press; 2015:551-592.
107. Glover LE, Newton K, Krishnan G, et al. Dysferlin overexpression in skeletal muscle produces a progressive myopathy. *Ann Neurol*. 2010;67:384-393.
109. Muntoni F, Brockington M, Godfrey C, et al. Muscular dystrophies due to defective glycosylation of dystroglycan. *Acta Myol*. 2007;26:129-135.
111. Zou Y, Zhang RZ, Sabatelli P, et al. Muscle interstitial fibroblasts are the main source of collagen VI synthesis in skeletal muscle: implications for congenital muscular dystrophy types Ullrich and Bethlem. *J Neuropathol Exp Neurol*. 2008;67:144-154.
112. Sewry CA. Muscular dystrophies: an update on pathology and diagnosis. *Acta Neuropathol*. 2010;120:343-358.
120. Tomé FM, Evangelista T, Leclerc A, et al. Congenital muscular dystrophy with merosin deficiency. *C R Acad Sci III*. 1994;317:351.
123. Mercuri E, Muntoni F. Congenital muscular dystrophies. In: Darras BT, Jones Jr R, Ryan MM, De Vivo DC, eds. *Neuromuscular Disorders of Infancy, Childhood, and Adolescence. A Clinician's Approach*. Ed 2. Boston: Academic Press; 2015:538-550.
124. Vuolteenaho R, Nissinen M, Sainio K, et al. Human laminin M chain (merosin): complete primary structure, chromosomal assignment and expression of the M and A chain in human fetal tissues. *J Cell Biol*. 1994;124:381.
128. Melo F, Carey DJ, Brandan E. Extracellular matrix is required for skeletal muscle differentiation but not myogenin expression. *J Cell Biochem*. 1996;62:227.
131. Markossian KA, Yudin IK, Kurganov BI. Mechanism of suppression of protein aggregation by alpha-crystallin. *Int J Mol Sci*. 2009;10:1314-1345.
134. Melkani GC, Cammarato A, Bernstein SI. α-B-crystallin maintains skeletal muscle myosin enzymatic activity and prevents its aggregation under heat-shock stress. *J Mol Biol*. 2006;358:635-645.
137. Del Bigio MR, Chudley AE, Sarnat HB, et al. α-B-crystallopathy of Canadian natives causes fatal infantile muscular dystrophy. *Ann Neurol*. 2011;69:866-871.
139. Muralikrishna B, Dhawan J, Rangaraj N, Parnaik VK. Distinct changes in intranuclear lamin A/C organization during myoblast differentiation. *J Cell Sci*. 2001;114:4001.
140. Oldfors A, DiMauro S. New insights in the field of muscle glycogenoses. *Curr Opin Neurol*. 2013;26:544-553.
146. Sarnat HB. Myotubular myopathy: arrest of morphogenesis of myofibres associated with persistence of fetal vimentin and desmin. Four cases compared with fetal and neonatal muscle. *Can J Neurol Sci*. 1990;17:109.
147. Lazarides E. Intermediate filaments as mechanical integrators of cellular space. *Nature*. 1980;283:249.
148. Tassin AM, Maro B, Bornens M. Fate of microtubule organizing centers during myogenesis *in vitro*. *J Cell Biol*. 1985;100:35.
149. Tokuyasu KT, Maher PA, Singer SJ. Distributions of vimentin and desmin in developing chick myotubes *in vivo*. II. Immunoelectron microscopic study. *J Cell Biol*. 1985;100:1157.
151. Askanas V, Bornemann A, Engel WK. Immunocytochemical localization of desmin at human neuromuscular junctions. *Neurology*. 1990;40:949.
152. Sarnat HB. Vimentin and desmin in maturing skeletal muscle and developmental myopathies. *Neurology*. 1992;42:1616.
154. Goebel HH, Warlo HT. Progress in desmin-related myopathies. *J Child Neurol*. 2000;15:565.
158. Edge MB. Development of apposed sarcoplasmic reticulum at the T-system and sarcolemma and the change in orientation of triads in rat skeletal muscle. *Dev Biol*. 1970;23:634.
160. Sarnat HB, Flores-Sarnat L, Casey R, et al. Endothelial ultrastructural alterations of intramuscular capillaries in infantile mitochondrial cytopathies. *Neuropathology*. 2012;32:617-627.
161. Valentijn KM, Sadler JE, Valentijn JA, et al. Functional architecture of Weibel-Palade bodies. *Blood*. 2011;117:5033-5043.
162. Van der Bliek AM, Shen Q, Kawajiri S. Mechanisms of mitochondrial fission and fusion. *Cold Spring Harb Perspect Biol*. 2013;5(6):a011072.
166. Sarnat HB, Carpenter S. Muscle biopsy for diagnosis of neuromuscular and metabolic diseases. In: Darras BT, Royden Jones Jr H, Ryan MM, De Vivo DC, eds. *Neuromuscular Disorders of Infancy, Childhood and Adolescence*. Ed 2. Amsterdam, NY: Elsevier; 2015:46-65.
169. Lindon C, Albagli O, Pinset C, Montarras D. Cell density-dependent induction of endogenous myogenin (*MRF4*) gene expression by *Myf5*. *Dev Biol*. 2001;240:574.
173. Brooke MH, Engel WK. The histographic analysis of human muscle biopsies with regard to fiber types. 4. Children's biopsies. *Neurology*. 1969;19:591.
178. Fenichel GM. The B fiber of human fetal skeletal muscle. *Neurology*. 1963;13:219.
182. Elder GCB, Kakulas BA. Histochemical and contractile property changes during human muscle development. *Muscle Nerve*. 1993;16:1246.
183. Hughes SM, Chi MM, Lowry OH, Gundersen K. Myogenin induces a shift of enzyme activity from glycolytic to oxidative metabolism in muscles of transgenic mice. *J Cell Biol*. 1999;145:633.
186. Tidball JG, Villalta SA. Regulatory interactions between muscle and the immune system during muscle regeneration. *Am J Physiol Regul Integr Comp Physiol*. 2010;298:R1173-R1187.
190. Kucera J, Walro JM, Reichler J. Motor and sensory innervation of muscle spindles in the neonatal rat. *Anat Embryol*. 1988;177:427.
204. Kullberg RW, Lentz TL, Cohen MW. Development of the myotomal neuromuscular junction in *Xenopus laevis*: an electrophysiological and fine-structural study. *Dev Biol*. 1977;60:101.
221. Engel AG, Shen X-M, Selcen D, Sine SM. Congenital myasthenic syndromes: pathogenesis, diagnosis and treatment. *Lancet Neurol*. 2015;14(4):420-434.
225. Sachis PN, Armstrong DL, Becker LE, Bryan AC. Myelination of the human vagus nerve from 24 weeks postconceptional age to adolescence. *J Neuropathol Exp Neurol*. 1982;41:466.
226. Hasan SU, Sarnat HB, Auer RN. Vagal nerve maturation in the fetal lamb: an ultrastructural and morphometric study. *Anat Rec*. 1993;237:527.
236. Sarnat HB. Cerebral dysgeneses and their influence on fetal muscle development. *Brain Dev*. 1986;8:495.

Hypothalamus: Neuroendometabolic Center

139

Adda Grimberg | Jessica Katz Kutikov

INTRODUCTION

Enabled by its strategic anatomy, the hypothalamus uniquely serves the interface between the neural and endocrine systems. It is at the same time a part of the brain, an intrinsic component of neural pathways, and an endocrine gland, specially connected to the pituitary gland to form the "master gland" unit of the body. The multiple functions of the hypothalamus ultimately involve regulation of the body's energy status and the maintenance of *homeostasis,* or bodily equilibrium. It has been long understood that, to refine this regulation, the hypothalamus responds both to information from the brain and to the levels of the peripheral hormones and body fluids it regulates. Appreciation has grown that the hypothalamus also receives input from the gut and fat stores, in essence closing the loop of metabolic regulation. All these incoming factors are compared with intrinsic setpoints, and outgoing messages are then released to enact modifications that will match the body to the appropriate setpoint. We have reviewed pediatric disorders of the neuroendocrine system, both congenital and acquired, elsewhere[1]; this chapter focuses on normal anatomy, embryology, and physiology of the hypothalamus.

ANATOMY

Despite the importance of the hypothalamus for multiple homeostatic functions, the structure is less than 1% of human brain volume; its various parts total approximately 4 g of the 1200 to 1400 g of an adult human brain[2] and measure less than 4 cm.[3] Many of the borders of the hypothalamus are difficult to distinguish and are semiarbitrary, although magnetic resonance imaging techniques for study of the hypothalamus are improving.[3] The hypothalamus lies at the base of the third ventricle, immediately posterior to the optic chiasm.[2-5]

Because of its many eminences, the hypothalamus is an irregular structure that roughly forms a diamond. It is composed of four main structures: the tuber cinereum, the median eminence, the infundibulum, and the mammillary bodies.[2] The tuber cinereum lies centrally on the inferior aspect of the hypothalamus. The median eminence, a central swelling located on the tuber cinereum, forms the floor of the third ventricle. The infundibulum is a stalk that connects the median eminence to the posterior lobe of the pituitary, and the mammillary bodies are two round protuberances at the posterior end of the inferior surface of the hypothalamus.[5]

The hypothalamus can be difficult to describe because of its lack of landmarks. Of the many systems devised to divide the hypothalamus into discrete areas, two are particularly helpful. One describes nine zones, determined by their mediolateral and anteroposterior locations[2,4]; it is shown in Fig. 139.1. The second system defines discrete clusters of cell bodies (nuclei) that have characteristic anatomic positions and functions (Table 139.1). Hypothalamic nuclei are not well circumscribed in adult brains. Examination of developing brains, in which cell groups are more discrete, has led to a greater understanding of hypothalamic architecture. Nonetheless, this schema is also semiarbitrary and is divided in many ways, depending on the source.

An area of particular controversy involves reports of sexual structural differences in several hypothalamic nuclei.[6] In both rats and human adults, the sexually dimorphic nucleus of the preoptic area is larger in males than in females.[7,8] Another preoptic cell group was found to be larger in men.[9-11] The bed nucleus of the stria terminalis is male predominant,[6,12] whereas the massa intermedia (interthalamic adhesion) is female predominant.[13] Age-related changes in neuronal health and sex hormone activity can affect these differences. For example, because the cell loss of human senescence in the sexually dimorphic nucleus of the preoptic area follows different time courses in men and women, the magnitude of the structural difference is age dependent.[6,14] Sexual functional differences have also been shown in the hypothalamus by immunocytochemical staining for various neuronal products (e.g., somatostatin and vasopressin, also known as *antidiuretic hormone* [*ADH*]) and hormone receptors (e.g., androgen and estrogen receptors) and may also be age dependent.[6] For example, the female dominance of neurokinin B immunoreactivity in the infundibular nucleus does not appear until puberty and progresses into adulthood.[15] Speculation and controversy surround the implications for sexually dimorphic behaviors and psychological phenomena. Most relevant to neonatologists is the debate about imprinting of the brain by androgens in utero and its consequences for therapeutic outcomes in patients with various disorders of sex development, including ambiguous genitalia.[16]

A final anatomic feature that is integral to hypothalamic functioning is blood supply. The hypothalamus communicates with the anterior pituitary gland through a special portal circulation that not only is fenestrated (the exception to the blood-brain barrier) but also transmits information bidirectionally. This feature enhances the ability of the hypothalamus to receive both signals from the general circulation and feedback from the pituitary. Furthermore, the hypothalamohypophysial portal system ensures that high concentrations of hypothalamic factors reach the pituitary, often at concentrations that far surpass those in the general circulation.[17]

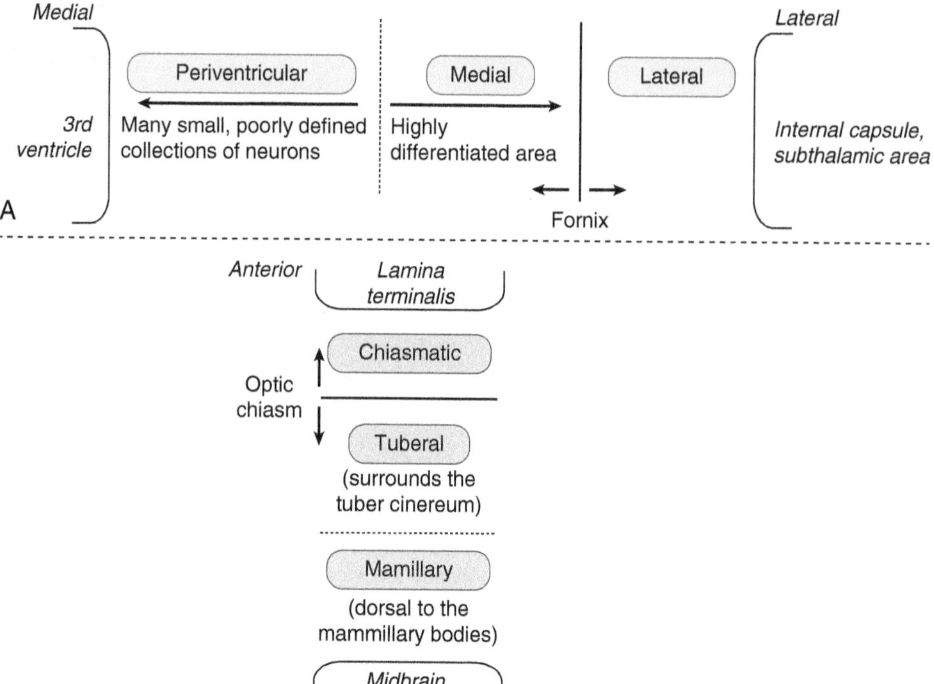

Fig. 139.1 Nine anatomic areas of the hypothalamus. Three mediolateral zones (A) and three anteroposterior zones (B) form a grid that divides the hypothalamus into nine anatomic areas. Defining features and boundaries of each zone are shown. The chiasmatic region can be further subdivided into preoptic (anterior to optic chiasm) and supraoptic (superior to optic chiasm) areas.

Table 139.1 Hypothalamic Nuclei.

Anteroposterior Region	Nuclei	Anatomy	Function
Chiasmatic	Preoptic area	Small nuclear groups, anterior to optic chiasm	Controls blood pressure, body temperature, hormonal release, reproductive activity
	Suprachiasmatic nucleus	Midline nucleus above optic chiasm	Sets circadian rhythm and sleep-wake cycles, regulates body temperature, hormonal control
	Paraventricular nucleus	Medial half = parvocellular neurons; lateral half = magnocellular neurons	Produces oxytocin and antidiuretic hormone (magnocellular neurons); regulates anterior pituitary function (parvocellular neurons); regulates autonomic responses
	Supraoptic nucleus	Superior to optic chiasm; also contains magnocellular neurons	Produces oxytocin and antidiuretic hormone
	Anterior nucleus	Between the paraventricular and supraoptic nuclei	Less differentiated; role ill-defined
Tuberal	Dorsomedial nucleus	Dorsal part of medial zone; projects locally and to periaqueductal gray matter	Feeding, growth, maturation, reproduction; parvocellular neurons regulate anterior pituitary function
	Ventromedial nucleus	Ventral part of medial zone; projects locally and to periaqueductal gray matter	Feeding, growth, maturation, reproduction; parvocellular neurons regulate anterior pituitary function
	Arcuate nucleus	Basal portion of tuber cinereum	Parvocellular neurons regulate anterior pituitary function; dopaminergic neurons
	Lateral hypothalamic nucleus	Large neurons lateral to ventromedial nucleus	Signals hunger
Mammillary	Posterior nucleus	Prominent nucleus, medial	Controls autonomic function
	Mammillary nuclei	Complex of three or four nuclei	Hippocampus → mammillary nuclei → thalamus; Papez circuit possibly involved in emotion and memory

EMBRYOLOGY

Early in nervous system development, three primary brain vesicles form from the neural tube: the prosencephalon or forebrain, the mesencephalon or midbrain, and the rhombencephalon or hindbrain.[18] Secondary vesicles then form from the prosencephalon during the fourth to fifth weeks of gestation. The secondary vesicles are termed the *telencephalon*, or *endbrain*, and the *diencephalon*. The telencephalon grows to cover all other brain structures and eventually becomes the cerebral hemispheres. The diencephalon also grows, forming a roof plate and two alar plates. During the sixth embryonic week, neuroblasts in the inferior portion of the alar plates of the diencephalon proliferate, forming the human hypothalamus.[18,19] Hypothalamic development occurs in two main stages: forebrain induction by early signals before or during gastrulation and then cell type differentiation by ventralizing and rostralizing signals from the axial mesendoderm. Axial mesendoderm induction of hypothalamic development is necessary for eye separation, and its failure causes holoprosencephaly.[20]

Distinct cell groups are easier to distinguish in the fetal hypothalamus than in the adult hypothalamus. The fetal hypothalamic nuclei become recognizable between 6 and 12 weeks of gestation. At this same time, the hypothalamic fiber tracts develop, and many hypothalamic factors become detectable.[21] For example, somatostatin, dopamine, and thyrotropin-releasing hormone are detectable as early as the 10th week of gestation.[19] At 9 to 10 weeks of gestation, little differentiation of the hypothalamic nuclei has occurred. By 24 to 33 weeks, the hypothalamus contains an increased number of better-defined structures and more closely resembles an adult hypothalamus. In the immediate postnatal period, the neonatal hypothalamic cell groups are remarkably similar to those structures in a mature adult.[22]

Information regarding the embryology of the hypothalamohypophysial portal system is limited. Evidence exists that the primary plexus begins to develop as early as 11.5 weeks of gestation.[19] Capillary penetrance of the median eminence is not evident until more than 16 weeks of gestation.[23] Further development throughout gestation is indicated by the greater number of capillary loops and the maturer vasculature present at birth.[19]

Our understanding of hypothalamic embryology has advanced from the morphologic to the genetic level. Development of the hypothalamus and pituitary gland is coordinated through parallel actions of genes expressed in both organs; extrinsic signals activate repertoires of transcription factors in a well-defined spatiotemporal pattern that leads to cellular differentiation into the various cell types that assume the distinct functions of the mature organs.[20,24,25] Some of these genes are summarized in Table 139.2.[20,24-30]

NEUROLOGIC FUNCTIONS

Like other brain centers, the hypothalamus participates in neural pathways by synthesizing and secreting neurotransmitters that are chemical messengers used for synaptic transmission, signaling, and neuromodulation. Different pathways control various functions of the hypothalamus, although for some functions, discrete areas or nuclei are not identifiable as the control centers. Some of the neurotransmitters are summarized in Table 139.3. For example, several hypothalamic nuclei project to the medulla oblongata to maintain homeostatic functions via the serotonergic system.[31] Other neurotransmitters are also involved in hypothalamic functioning, such as the excitatory amino acids in a pathway connecting to the hippocampus and limbic system, but their actions are less well understood.

Table 139.2 Genes in Hypothalamic Development.

Gene	Normal Function	Consequences of Mutation or Deletion
HESX1 (also known as *Rpx*)	Expressed during gastrulation in the midline endoderm-mesoderm (prechordal plate precursor), to induce anterior head structures Afterward, expression is restricted to Rathke pouch. Ventral → dorsal down-regulation of expression coincides with pituitary cell differentiation	Deletions: absence of infundibulum and Rathke pouch (severest); hypothalamic floor expansion and abnormal bifurcation of Rathke pouch Homozygous missense mutations (R53C) cause septooptic dysplasia, which is frequently associated with hypothalamic or pituitary dysfunction. Homozygous missense mutations (R160H) cause pan-hypopituitarism (anterior pituitary aplasia), thin pituitary stalk, but no midline defects (i.e., normal optic nerves)
Shh	Expressed by oral ectoderm Induces its own expression and that of other genes (e.g., *Nkx-2.1*) in ventral midline neural cells Suppresses *Pax6* expression in the midline Required for resolution of the single retinal field into 2 separate primordia	Holoprosencephaly Hypothalamic or pituitary absence or dysfunction
Six3	Transcription factor Expressed in Rathke pouch and hypothalamus Involved in early induction of the pituitary gland	Holoprosencephaly Hypothalamic or pituitary absence or dysfunction
Gli3	Represses *Shh* signaling	Pallister-Hall syndrome (hypothalamic hamartomas)
Nkx-2.1 (also known as *Tebp* and *TTF1*)	Dorsoventral gradient of expression (higher in ventral region and posterior pituitary; none in Rathke pouch). Required for development of Rathke pouch	Absence of entire pituitary gland. Absence of selective hypothalamic nuclei (premammillary nucleus, arcuate nucleus, mammillary body, supramammillary nucleus)
Brn2	Coexpressed with *Brn4* in presumptive paraventricular and supraoptic nuclei Required for terminal differentiation and survival of magnocellular and parvocellular neurons in these nuclei	Magnocellular and parvocellular neurons fail to project axons into the posterior pituitary Complete loss of posterior pituitary
Sim1	Expressed in paraventricular and supraoptic nuclei	Paraventricular and supraoptic nuclei fail to express *Brn2*, oxytocin, antidiuretic hormone, thyrotropin-releasing hormone, corticotropin-releasing hormone, and somatostatin Homozygous deletion: perinatal lethal from complete development defect of paraventricular nucleus Haploinsufficiency: isolated hyperphagia, severe early onset obesity, increased linear growth, no decrease in energy expenditure
Nhlh2	Expressed in developing hypothalamus Expressed in both embryonic and adult pituitary	Hypogonadism and progressive adult obesity Reduction of abundance of proopiomelanocortin-producing cells in the arcuate nucleus (increased leptin resistance)

Table 139.2 Genes in Hypothalamic Development.—cont'd

Gene	Normal Function	Consequences of Mutation or Deletion
SF1 (also known as *Ftzf1*)	Expressed in developing adrenal glands, gonads, and diencephalon Regulates both androgens and müllerian inhibiting factor (i.e., male differentiation)	Absence of adrenal glands. Absence of gonads Absence of pituitary gonadotropes (no luteinizing hormone, follicle-stimulating hormone, and gonadotropin-releasing hormone)
GSH1	Binds to growth hormone–releasing hormone promoter	Hypoplastic pituitary gland Dwarfism; growth hormone deficiency (from absence of growth hormone–releasing hormone in arcuate nucleus). Sexual infantilism and infertility
NDN	Paternal monoallelic expression in developing hypothalamus	Decreased number of oxytocin-producing cells in paraventricular nucleus Decreased number of gonadotropin-releasing hormone–producing cells in preoptic region Mutant mice show neonatal lethality with reduced penetrance Maps to the critical region of Prader-Willi syndrome
Peg3	Paternal monoallelic expression in developing hypothalamus	Decreased number of oxytocin-producing cells in paraventricular nucleus Abnormal maternal behavior leading to perinatal lethality of offspring mice
Sox2	Expressed in the developing central nervous system and placodes	Heterozygous mutations in humans: bilateral eye defects, anterior pituitary hypoplasia and hypogonadotropic hypogonadism, variable defects affecting the corpus callosum and mesial temporal structures, hypothalamic hamartoma, sensorineural hearing loss, esophageal atresia
SOX3	Expressed in infundibulum	X-linked hypopituitarism, infundibular hypoplasia, variable learning difficulties
KAL1	Encodes anosmin, a cell-surface protein that is proteolyzed to release a diffusible component that is incorporated into the extracellular matrix; promotes migration of olfactory axons and gonadotropin-releasing hormone neurons	X-linked Kallmann syndrome (hypoplasia of olfactory bulbs and absence of GnRH neurons from hypothalamus, leading to anosmia and hypogonadotropic hypogonadism)
PROKR2	Expressed in brain, testis, small intestine (ileocecum), ovary, thyroid, pituitary, and salivary gland	Heterozygous or homozygous mutations cause Kallmann syndrome; mutations also found in patients with congenital hypopituitarism and septooptic dysplasia *Prokr2*$^{-/-}$ mice: partially penetrant postnatal lethality; surviving mice were underweight, failed to breed, and were hypokinetic, with nocturnal locomotor activity unsynchronized from circadian night

Data from references Michaud JL. The developmental program of the hypothalamus and its disorders. *Clin Genet*. 2001;60:255; Kioussi C, Carrière C, Rosenfeld MG. A model for the development of the hypothalamic-pituitary axis: transcribing the hypophysis. *Mech Dev*. 1999;81:23; Kelberman D, Rizzoti K, Avilion A, et al. Mutations within Sox2/SOX2 are associated with abnormalities in the hypothalamo-pituitary-gonadal axis in mice and humans. *J Clin Invest*. 2006;116:2442; Woods KS, Cundall M, Turton J, et al. Over- and underdosage of SOX3 is associated with infundibular hypoplasia and hypopituitarism. *Am J Hum Genet*. 2005;76:833; Ramachandrappa S, Raimondo A, Cali AM, et al. Rare variants in single-minded 1 (SIM1) are associated with severe obesity. *J Clin Invest*. 2013;123:3042–3050; Costa-Barbosa FA, Balasubramanian R, Keefe KW, et al. Prioritizing genetic testing in patients with Kallmann syndrome using clinical phenotypes. *J Clin Endocrinol Metab*. 2013;98:E943–E953; McCabe MJ, Gaston-Massuet C, Gregory LC, et al. Variations in PROKR2, but not PROK2, are associated with hypopituitarism and septo-optic dysplasia. *J Clin Endocrinol Metab*. 2013;98:E547–E557.

CIRCADIAN RHYTHMS

The suprachiasmatic nucleus sets the clock for the body's circadian rhythms, adaptations to the reproducible 24-hour day-night cycle of life on Earth.[32] Neurons of the suprachiasmatic nucleus oscillate in a synchronized fashion in vitro with a period close to 24 hours.[33] In vivo, these oscillations become entrained to the solar day-night cycle by light; signals from the retina are transmitted by the retinohypothalamic tract to the suprachiasmatic nucleus. In the suprachiasmatic nucleus, these signals affect gene expression for at least four transcription factors that act in a transcription-transduction feedback loop to determine the oscillations.[32,33] Suprachiasmatic neurons contain somatostatin, vasoactive intestinal polypeptide, ADH, and neurotensin. Efferent pathways, including one that controls pineal function, then regulate various endocrine, cardiovascular, temperature, and behavioral circadian rhythms.[2,32,34]

In humans the suprachiasmatic nucleus is recognized by mid-gestation and the retinohypothalamic tract is recognized by the 80% point of gestation.[32,35] Fetuses show 24-hour rhythms in hormones, cardiovascular function, and behavior. Rather than being synchronized with the time of day, their rhythms are set by maternal signals, including the maternal cortisol rhythm.[32] Although the circadian system is responsive to light at premature stages in human and other primate infants, the system progressively matures after birth to achieve full entrainment after 2 months of age.[36] Different clock genes mature at different rates, so the postnatal light entrainment is a gradual process, and the ambient postnatal light environment can affect not only current but also future suprachiasmatic nucleus and circadian functions.[37]

The daily sleep-wakefulness cycle is the most obvious behavioral manifestation of the suprachiasmatic nucleus's activity and circadian rhythms. Human evolution as hunter-gatherers has led to the coordination of sleep with metabolic homeostatic mechanisms; hunger, vigilance, and food-seeking behaviors occur primarily during daylight hours, whereas satiety

Table 139.3 Hypothalamic Neurotransmitters.

Category	Neurotransmitter	Pathway	Function
Monoamines			
Catecholamines	Dopamine	Incertohypothalamic tract Mesencephalic tract Tuberoinfundibular tract Median eminence	Influences secretion of pituitary hormones Primary inhibitor of prolactin L-Dopa stimulates GH release
	Norepinephrine	Lateral tegmental system Dorsal tegmental system Can be localized to all hypothalamic nuclei; highest concentrations in the arcuate nucleus and median eminence	Regulates emotional and motivated behavior Stimulates GH and gonadotropin release Inhibits secretion of oxytocin, ADH, and corticotropin
	Epinephrine	Cell bodies near the locus ceruleus	Inhibits secretion of ADH and oxytocin
Indolamines	Serotonin	Most of the hypothalamic nuclei Highest concentrations in the arcuate and suprachiasmatic nucleus	Involved in cyclic release of some hypothalamic hormones Stimulates GH and prolactin release
	Histamine	Tuberomammillary nucleus in the posterior lateral hypothalamus	May help maintain arousal. Stimulates oxytocin, ADH, and GH release
Cholinergic	Acetylcholine	Large amount present in median eminence	Stimulates secretion of ADH, oxytocin, corticotropin, and gonadotropin. Inhibits somatostatin; stimulates GH release. Inhibits TSH release
Amino acids (inhibitory)	γ-Aminobutyric acid	Synthesized from glutamate. Basal ganglial system	In anterior hypothalamus, helps induce sleep. Inhibits oxytocin, ADH, corticotropin, prolactin, and TSH release. Stimulates GH and gonadotropin release
Peptides	Angiotensin II	Renin (from kidneys) cleaves angiotensinogen (made by liver) to angiotensin I; angiotensin I is cleaved by angiotensin-converting enzyme in lungs to angiotensin II	Stimulates secretion of ADH. Stimulates corticotropin and luteinizing hormone and inhibits prolactin and GH release. Induces thirst, drinking behavior. Involved in regulation of water balance
	Atrial natriuretic peptide	Left atrium Anterior tip of third ventricle Many neuronal endings in the median eminence	Opposes ADH secretion Involved in regulation of water balance
	β-Endorphins	Arcuate nucleus and basal tuberal area in the rat; project through the anterior hypothalamic area and innervate the median eminence	Released during stress. Stimulate corticotropin, prolactin, and GH release

ADH, Antidiuretic hormone; *GH*, growth hormone; *TSH*, thyroid-stimulating hormone.

and somnolence occur together for periodic rest.[38,39] Hypocretin (also called *orexin*) neurons in the lateral hypothalamus respond to metabolic signals of the body's nutritional status and to dark-light cues from the suprachiasmatic nucleus pacemaker to stimulate both alertness and appetite and feeding behaviors. Hypocretin deficiency, in both humans and animal models, causes narcolepsy.[40] Disturbances of the circadian cycle and long-term sleep deprivation have been implicated in hyperphagia and obesity, mainly via the hypocretin system,[38] and, with further contributions from unbalanced autonomic nervous system activity,[41] in metabolic syndrome (visceral obesity, type 2 diabetes mellitus, dyslipidemia, and hypertension).

AUTONOMIC NERVOUS SYSTEM FUNCTION

A topographic arrangement of autonomic function exists in the hypothalamus; parasympathetic control stems mainly from anterior and medial regions, whereas the lateral and posterior areas control sympathetic responses. Parasympathetic activity results in slowing of the heart rate, peripheral vasodilation, and increased gastrointestinal motility. Alternatively, sympathetic stimulation results in pupillary dilation, increased heart rate and blood pressure, and other responses associated with increased emotional stress.[2]

Heart rate, heart rate variability, and other cardiac measures are often used as markers when one is assessing fetal and neonatal autonomic function.[42,43] Fetuses at a gestational age of 20 weeks demonstrate heart rate stability and show differences among individuals. The fetal heart rate, beginning at 24 weeks of gestation, may be predictive of postnatal heart rate, but fetal heart rate variability does not become predictive of postnatal heart rate variability until 6 weeks later. This finding likely reflects a later maturation of the neuroregulatory system that controls heart rate variability.[42] The reduction in heart rate variability in fetuses with increasing gestational age also suggests that the autonomic nervous system continues to develop throughout gestation.[43]

Autonomic activity in fetuses varies over the course of a day. For instance, in normal fetuses, the fetal autonomic activity that controls heart rate follows a 12-hour cycle, as opposed to the maternal 24-hour rhythm. This 12-hour rhythm disappears immediately after birth, although the 24-hour circadian rhythm does not become established until 2 to 4 weeks later.[44]

TEMPERATURE REGULATION

Like autonomic control, temperature regulation occurs regionally, rather than in discrete nuclei. The preoptic anterior hypothalamus contains thermosensitive neurons that detect increases in blood temperature and cool the body by heat dissipation, whereas the posterior hypothalamus conserves heat when decreased body temperature is detected.[2,45] The temperature control centers of the hypothalamus coordinate behavioral, autonomic, and endocrine responses of the body to regulate body temperature, including panting and peripheral vasodilation in response to increased body temperature, shivering and peripheral vasoconstriction in response to decreased body temperature,[46] and modulation of thyroid hormone-stimulated thermogenesis.[47,48] Hypothalamic injury can produce prolonged hypothermia resulting from alterations in the temperature setpoint or defects in heat production mechanisms. Fever results from an elevation of the temperature setpoint by inflammatory cytokines, such as interleukin-1, that raise prostaglandin E levels in the hypothalamus; normal physiologic mechanisms then maintain body temperature at this elevated setpoint.[45]

The fetal environment is stable at approximately 37°C. The temperature gradient, wherein fetal temperature is approximately 0.5°C to 1.0°C higher than maternal temperature, results in fetal heat dissipation. Heat loss occurs through the placenta, fetal skin, amniotic fluid, and uterine wall. The hypothalamus most likely controls this higher fetal temperature in utero. After birth, the neonate has tremendous heat losses through the skin that require functioning thermoregulatory mechanisms to prevent hypothermia. Premature and low-birth-weight infants are often unable to maintain appropriate body temperature and behave like poikilotherms rather than homeotherms. How the hypothalamus matures to the environmental conditions after birth is still unknown.[49] A higher risk of complications is associated with hypothermia, and hyperthermia increases energy needs, so newborns should be placed in environments of thermal neutral temperature.[50]

EMOTIONAL EXPRESSION AND BEHAVIOR

Selective stimulation or lesions of various areas in the hypothalamus elicit different behavioral and emotional responses, such as aggression, anger, fear, pleasure, and sexual gratification. Although the hypothalamus is important for integrating and expressing emotion, other areas of the brain, including the cortex, limbic system, and thalamus, interact with the hypothalamus to bring about the varied types of responses.[2,51,52]

The hypothalamus participates in the two physiologic stress response systems: the sympathetic-adrenal-medullary system and the hypothalamic-pituitary-adrenal system. The sympathetic-adrenal-medullary system causes the well-known stress-induced release of epinephrine. Sympathetic-adrenal-medullary activation, which is dependent on characteristics of both the situation and the individual, occurs in response to challenges, with a faster onset than activation of the hypothalamic-pituitary-adrenal axis.[53] Hypothalamic-pituitary-adrenal axis function culminates in cortisol release, which is described in detail in Chapters 146 and 147. Stress induction of the hypothalamic-pituitary-adrenal axis is active in newborns, although it may be transiently blunted in extremely preterm infants.[54] When neonates are exposed to noxious stimuli (e.g., circumcision, heel stick blood sampling), cortisol levels rise and can be associated with how much the infant cries. Once the noxious stimulus has been removed, in healthy neonates cortisol levels quickly return to basal levels. Soothing procedures, such as the use of a pacifier, can reduce crying in response to noxious stimuli, but they do not affect the hypothalamic-pituitary-adrenal response to the stimuli.[55]

ENDOCRINE FUNCTIONS

The hypothalamus also serves as an endocrine organ, synthesizing and releasing hormones into the circulation to effect changes in target tissues. Hypothalamic endocrine activity can be divided into two distinct categories as established by the anatomy of the hypothalamopituitary unit. Because the posterior pituitary gland, or neurohypophysis, is composed of axonal projections from the hypothalamus, the hormones released into the circulation by the posterior pituitary are actually made in cell bodies of the hypothalamus. In contrast, the anterior pituitary gland, or adenohypophysis, is a distinct gland. The hypothalamus secretes various releasing and inhibiting factors that regulate anterior pituitary hormone synthesis and release. These factors are made in hypothalamic neurons and are carried down axons to the median eminence. They then reach the anterior pituitary by the special hypothalamohypophysial portal circulation, whereas the anterior pituitary hormones reach their target organs by the peripheral circulation.[34]

Hypothalamic hormone production and release are primarily regulated by humoral feedback. Three levels of feedback regulation to the hypothalamus exist. *First-order feedback* involves one hormone, as exemplified by oxytocin and ADH. These hormones act on target cells (breast, uterus, kidney) but do not stimulate the release of secondary hormones. Oxytocin and ADH levels, together with nonhormonal signals (e.g., plasma osmolality and hypovolemia or hypotension for ADH), directly regulate their own production and release. Close proximity of oxytocin and ADH neurons and colocalization of receptors for the hormones on the neurons that produce those hormones allow local concentrations of oxytocin and ADH within the supraoptic and paraventricular nuclei to refine further activity of the neurons that produce them.[56-58] *Second-order feedback* involves a second hormone produced by the pituitary, such as prolactin. Hypothalamic hormones stimulate or inhibit anterior pituitary release of a hormone, and the circulating levels of the pituitary hormone feed back to regulate hypothalamic hormone release. For example, increases in circulating prolactin concentrations stimulate hypothalamic secretion of dopamine (prolactin-inhibiting factor) into the hypothalamohypophysial portal circulation to prevent excessive prolactin release by the pituitary; high prolactin levels also inhibit hypothalamic release of vasoactive intestinal polypeptide, a hormone that stimulates prolactin release.[59] In a *third-order feedback* loop, a third endocrine gland (e.g., adrenals, gonads, thyroid) is involved in addition to the hypothalamus and pituitary. Within a third-order feedback pathway, multiple types of feedback loops exist: long, short, and ultrashort feedback. Long-loop feedback occurs when hormones from peripheral endocrine target cells or substances from tissue metabolism influence the production of hypothalamic hormones. This type of feedback is most often negative, although it can be positive. Short-loop feedback is second-order feedback within a third-order feedback system. For instance, certain pituitary hormones (e.g., corticotropin, luteinizing hormone, thyroid-stimulating hormone) not only stimulate target gland hormone production but also feed back to limit or terminate hypothalamic releasing hormone production (corticotropin-releasing hormone, gonadotropin-releasing hormone, and thyrotropin-releasing hormone, respectively). When hypothalamic hormone release affects its own synthesis, ultrashort feedback has occurred. This is similar to first-order feedback within a third-order system. The mechanism of this ultrashort feedback is either through neurotransmission between two cells in the hypothalamus or through pituitary tanycyte release of the hormone into cerebrospinal fluid, which can regulate hypothalamic activity because the hypothalamus is located at the base of the third ventricle.[34] The growth hormone pathway (reviewed in detail elsewhere[60,61]) is an excellent example of a third-order system and is shown in Fig. 139.2.

Two neurosecretory systems produce hypothalamic hormones (summarized in Table 139.4): magnocellular and parvocellular. The *magnocellular system* consists of specialized, large-celled (magnocellular) neurons, the hypothalamoneurohypophysial tract, and the neurohypophysis (posterior pituitary). Its principal products are ADH and oxytocin. Most of the magnocellular neurons are located in the supraoptic and paraventricular nuclei, but additional small nuclei also contain these neurons.[4] Apart from projections to the neurohypophysis, some magnocellular

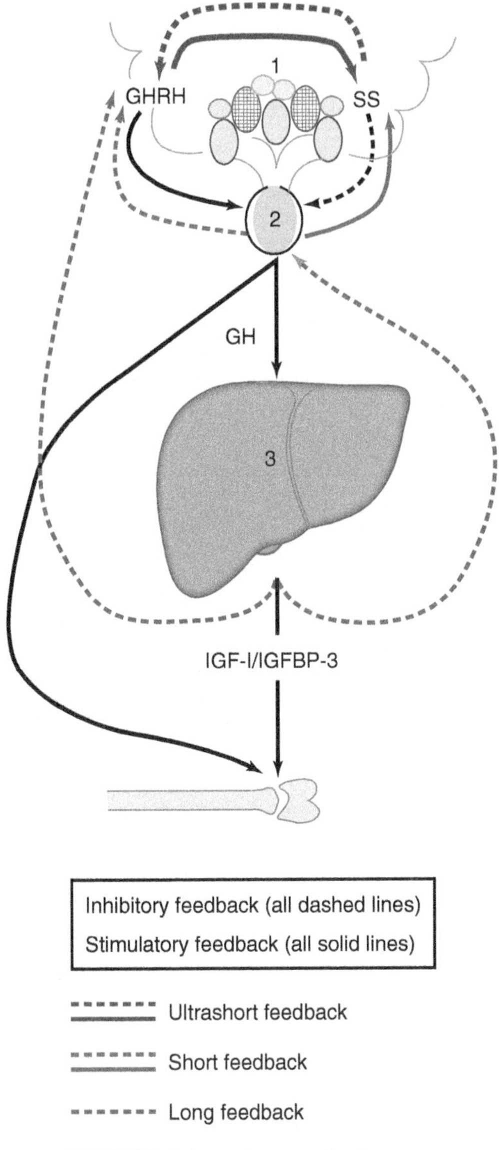

Fig. 139.2 The growth hormone *(GH)* axis exemplifies a third-order feedback loop. A third-order feedback loop involves hormonal production by three endocrine glands: *(1)* the hypothalamus produces growth hormone–releasing hormone *(GHRH)* and somatostatin *(SS)*; *(2)* the pituitary gland produces GH; and *(3)* the liver acts as an endocrine gland, producing insulin-like growth factor 1 *(IGF-1)* and its binding protein insulin-like growth factor binding protein 3 *(IGFBP-3)*. Stimulatory feedback is depicted as a *solid arrow,* and inhibitory feedback is depicted as a *dashed arrow.* Ultrashort feedback is colored in *red,* short feedback in *blue,* and long feedback in *black.* Primary hormonal action is shown in *green.* Among the final end organs of this system is the growth plate of growing bones.

neurons project to the median eminence and some ADH-containing fibers project to the choroid plexus in the lateral ventricles and brain stem regions.[17]

In contrast, the *parvocellular secretory cells* are small neurons, mostly in the region of the tuber cinereum below the third ventricle, that produce the hypophysiotropic hormones.[4] The parvocellular neurons are found in various hypothalamic nuclei, including the arcuate and paraventricular nuclei, and project to the median eminence.[34] Their hormonal products (all peptide hormones except dopamine) are carried by the hypothalamohypophysial portal system to the anterior pituitary, where they regulate adenohypophysial function. Because the hormonal systems of the anterior pituitary are reviewed in detail in Chapters 144 to 146 and 148, we focus on the magnocellular system.

Adult numbers of oxytocin- and ADH-producing cells in the supraoptic and paraventricular nuclei exist as early as the second half of gestation, which is earlier than development of some other nuclei.[62] Oxytocin and ADH can be detected as early as the tenth gestational week. Vasopressinergic neurons appear 1 week earlier in the supraoptic nucleus than in the paraventricular nucleus. Although an adult organization of vasopressinergic neurons can be identified early in the second trimester, the number of those neurons seems to increase until the twenty-sixth week of gestation. The vasopressinergic system of neurons is also highly active in the perinatal period.[63]

The synthetic pathways of oxytocin and ADH are very similar.[64] Both are synthesized from protein precursors (prohormones) that are encoded by single-copy genes located near each other on chromosome 20. Both genes are composed of three exons; the entire mature hormone is encoded within the first exon. The remainder of the oxytocin gene encodes neurophysin I, whereas the longer ADH gene also encodes neurophysin II and the glycoprotein copeptin.[65] The prohormones are transported down the axons and are stored in colloid-filled vesicles. Proteolytic enzymes in these neurosecretory granules cleave oxytocin and ADH from the neurophysins, which are presumed to primarily serve as their carriers during axonal transport. When the magnocellular cell bodies are properly stimulated, oxytocin, ADH, and the neurophysins are released from the axonal terminals by calcium-dependent exocytosis.[4] In addition to oxytocin and ADH, magnocellular secretory granules contain many other peptides but in much smaller amounts. These include dynorphin, enkephalins, galanin, and cholecystokinin, and, although they are secreted along with oxytocin and ADH, the role of many of these peptides is unknown.[66]

OXYTOCIN

Oxytocin secretion is prompted by mechanical vaginal distention and, in lactating women, by suckling and nipple stimulation; no recognized stimulus exists for its secretion in men. Cholinergic and α-adrenergic fibers carry the stimulatory inputs, whereas β-adrenergic fibers provide inhibition of oxytocin release. Oxytocin serves two physiologic functions: it aids in parturition by stimulating uterine contractions, and it facilitates nursing by stimulating contraction of myoepithelial cells in the lactating mammary gland (milk "let-down" reflex). In fact, nursing cannot occur without oxytocin, and maternal and fetal stress during labor and delivery can reduce oxytocin release, thereby impairing lactation.[67] Oxytocin action at parturition is primed by two major changes. Oxytocin release, which occurs in brief secretory bursts, increases in both the fetus and the mother during labor.[68,69] Meanwhile, the increase in the level of uterine oxytocin receptors at term makes the uterus particularly sensitive to the hormone.[68] Oxytocin secretion is suppressed by relaxin, an ovarian peptide that suppresses uterine contractions and relaxes pelvic connective tissue during parturition.[70] Therapeutically, oxytocin and its analogues are used to induce labor (or to augment labor in uterine dysfunction), to prevent postpartum uterine atony or hemorrhage, and to promote milk let-down in lactation.

ANTIDIURETIC HORMONE

The two names of this hormone, *vasopressin* and *ADH*, reflect its two main actions, which are mediated by two classes of receptors. V_1 receptors stimulate vasoconstriction, glycogenolysis, platelet aggregation, and vascular smooth muscle hypertrophy. A subclass of V_1 receptors (V_{1b}) is located in the anterior pituitary

Table 139.4 Hypothalamic Hormone Axes.

Neurosecretory System	Hormone	Hormone Gene Locus	Hypothalamic Nucleus of Origin	Secondary Pituitary Hormone	Pituitary Action	Final Axis Gland	Axis Function
Magnocellular	ADH	20p13	Supraoptic and paraventricular	NA	V_{1b} receptors: stimulate corticotropin release	NA	Enhances renal free water retention; vasoconstriction
	Oxytocin	20p13	Supraoptic and paraventricular	NA	NA	NA	Stimulates uterine contractions at parturition; milk let-down reflex for lactation
Parvocellular	GHRH	20q11.2	Arcuate	GH	Stimulatory	Liver	Somatic growth
	Somatostatin	3q28	Paraventricular; also in neocortex, basal ganglia, limbic system; endocrine pancreas and gut (D cells)	GH, prolactin, TSH, corticotropin	Inhibitory	Liver	Regulation of pituitary function, especially somatic growth; neurotransmitter; gut function and pancreatic endocrine regulation (locally produced somatostatin)
	CRH	8q13	Paraventricular	Corticotropin	Stimulatory	Adrenals	Maintenance of normal blood pressure and glucose; stress response
	TRH	3q13.3-q21	Paraventricular	TSH	Stimulatory	Thyroid	Regulates overall metabolic rate; effects on heart, bone, gut, and other organ functions
	GnRH	8p21-p11.2 (GnRH1); 20p13 (GnRH2)	Arcuate	LH, FSH	Stimulatory	Gonads	Reproduction
	Dopamine	—	Arcuate	Prolactin	Inhibitory	NA	Lactation

ADH, Antidiuretic hormone; *CRH*, corticotropin-releasing hormone; *FSH*, follicle-stimulating hormone; *GH*, growth hormone; *GHRH*, growth hormone–releasing hormone; *GnRH*, gonadotropin-releasing hormone; *LH*, luteinizing hormone; *NA*, not applicable; *TRH*, thyrotropin-releasing hormone; *TSH*, thyroid-stimulating hormone.

and stimulates corticotropin release. V_2 receptors increase water permeability of the renal collecting ducts by inducing aquaporins; this results in greater water retention and decreased urine volume. Neural input for ADH secretion can elicit newly synthesized hormone within 30 minutes, but it also exhibits fatigue with high frequencies or prolonged duration.[71] The main stimulus for the antidiuretic effects of ADH is an elevation in plasma osmolality, primarily the extracellular fluid concentration of sodium chloride, as detected by osmoreceptor cells within the hypothalamus. Baroreceptor (carotid sinuses, aortic arch, cardiac atria, and great veins) sensing of hypovolemia or hypotension leads to ADH levels superseding those required for maximal urine concentration and causes vasoconstriction.[17] In most cases, the two mechanisms act in concert; dehydration leads to both hypernatremia and hypovolemia. However, the two ADH responses may become dissociated in disease states involving intravascular volume depletion despite total body fluid overload and hyponatremia (e.g., congestive heart failure, cirrhosis, and nephrotic syndrome).[72] Deficiency of ADH production and resistance to ADH action cause central and nephrogenic diabetes insipidus, respectively;[73] both disorders are characterized by polyuria, polydipsia, and a tendency to dehydration. In contrast, the syndrome of inappropriate ADH secretion is characterized by diminished urine output and free water intoxication.

During development, ADH aids in regulating the proliferation and morphogenesis of target cells in the brain, pituitary, kidney, and liver. Because the fetus contributes significantly to modulation of fluid fluxes among the maternal, fetal, and amniotic fluid compartments, fetal ADH action is an important component of adaptive responses to changes in the environment in utero.[74] The ADH system also plays an essential role in fetal adaptation to the stresses of labor.[63,74] In the perinatal period, ADH is integral in establishing body fluid homeostasis, by providing the brain, pituitary, heart, and adrenals with increased blood flow and aiding in regulation of the cardiovascular system, water reabsorption, gluconeogenesis, and glycogenolysis after delivery.[63]

METABOLIC REGULATION

The hypothalamus plays a crucial role in regulating the body's metabolic state by controlling both feeding behavior and energy expenditure rates. The regulation is so precise that, under reasonably steady-state conditions, deflections in the body weight and fat mass of mammals remain within 0.5% to 1%.[75] The importance of the hypothalamus to this system has long been appreciated because of the hyperphagia and obesity syndromes that result from hypothalamic lesions. The ventromedial nucleus of the hypothalamus has been identified as a satiety center, whereas the lateral hypothalamic area stimulates feeding.[2,21] More recent investigations have focused on the peripheral hormones that feed metabolic information back to the hypothalamus.

LEPTIN

The *LEP* gene, located on chromosome band 7q32.1 and encoding the hormone leptin, was cloned and sequenced in 1994.[76] Leptin is produced by white adipose tissue and is secreted into the circulation in proportion to the body's fat mass.[77,78] Circulating both freely and protein bound, leptin crosses the blood-brain barrier and binds to leptin receptors in the central nervous system (CNS). Many of these receptors are located in the hypothalamus and control pathways involved in the regulation of appetite and thermogenesis.[77] Thus leptin serves as the hypothalamic index of body fat mass.[78,79] Leptin has other neuroendocrine functions, including regulation of fertility and the secretion of growth hormone, corticotropin-releasing hormone, thyrotropin-releasing hormone, and prolactin.[77,78]

The exact mechanism of leptin uptake into the CNS has yet to be elucidated, although it is inhibited by hypertriglyceridemia.[80] One possibility involves the neurons of the median eminence, which not only project outside the blood-brain barrier but also express leptin receptors. Once inside the CNS, leptin can bind to receptors present in many hypothalamic nuclei, especially the arcuate, dorsomedial, ventromedial, and ventral premammillary nuclei.[81] Leptin binding to its receptor signals the body's energy status to two opposing classes of neurons. Proopiomelanocortin (POMC) neurons (catabolic pathways) are stimulated by leptin, whereas neuropeptide Y (NPY) neurons (anabolic pathways) are inhibited.[79]

Leptin directly stimulates POMC neurons, which are located in the arcuate nucleus, as well as outside the hypothalamus in the nucleus of the tractus solitarius. POMC is a precursor to many polypeptides termed *melanocortins,* including α-melanocyte-stimulating hormone. When the hypothalamic melanocortin 3 receptors and melanocortin 4 receptors are stimulated by α-melanocyte-stimulating hormone, food intake is decreased and energy expenditure is increased.[75,79] Agouti gene–related peptide (AGRP) is an endogenous melanocortin system antagonist that is also expressed in the arcuate nucleus.[82]

AGRP messenger RNA (mRNA) is highly colocalized with mRNA of NPY,[83] the system opposing POMC. A member of the pancreatic polypeptide family, the anabolic, orexigenic hormone NPY is widely distributed in the human brain. NPY potently stimulates feeding, is capable of overriding the body's satiety and weight control mechanisms,[75] and reduces energy expenditure by decreasing nonshivering thermogenesis in brown adipose tissue.[75,77] Leptin inhibits NPY activity. NPY can inhibit POMC neurons directly at the cell body or postsynaptically through the release of AGRP.[75] Thus leptin stimulates POMC neurons both directly and indirectly, by eliminating the POMC inhibition by NPY,[79] and the two opposing systems are coordinated toward an overall negative effect on energy balance. Many other substances have been implicated in energy homeostasis but not all are understood as well as the POMC-NPY systems. Those also under leptin regulation include orexins,[75] cocaine- and amphetamine-regulated transcript, glucagon-like peptide 1, melanin-concentrating hormone, and cholecystokinin.[77,81]

Leptin is secreted in a rhythmic pattern that correlates with meals (leptin levels are reduced by fasting). Leptin's actions on the hypothalamus probably serve a long-term regulatory system that sets a point of satiety; it is likelier that short-term regulatory systems that control single meal intake are determined by leptin actions on the brain stem. Obesity more frequently results from leptin resistance than from leptin deficiency.[84] Leptin levels in females are almost double those in males with the same body mass index or fat reserve. This finding not only has implications for leptin physiology but also supports the role of leptin in reproductive and gonadal function.[77] A sex difference in leptin levels is found at birth, which suggests that the process begins in utero.[77,85] Circulating leptin levels are also higher during gestation than in nongravid individuals, and disturbances in leptin production have been found in several pathologic pregnancy states that alter fetal growth.[86]

The role of leptin in the fetus is unknown. Leptin has been identified in fetal umbilical cord blood in the eighteenth week of gestation. Adipose tissue development occurs during the second trimester; consistent with this finding, leptin levels dramatically increase at 34 weeks of gestation.[82] Leptin is also produced by the placenta but in very small amounts that are unlikely to contribute significantly to umbilical cord blood levels.[85] The level of leptin for body weight is disproportionately high in neonates.[77,85] The reason for this is unknown, but it normalizes toward adult levels around 2 weeks of life.[77] Neonatal leptin levels have been shown to predict weight gains in infancy.[77,87]

GHRELIN

Ghrelin is an orexigenic peptide that was first identified in 1999 as the endogenous ligand for the growth hormone secretagogue receptor (GHSR).[88] Its central role in the stimulation of feeding was not appreciated until 2001.[89] Ghrelin is produced primarily in the stomach (X/A-like cells of the oxyntic glands) but also in the duodenum, jejunum, pituitary, kidney, placenta, and hypothalamus.[90] Although it is accepted that ghrelin-producing neurons exist in the hypothalamus, it is still controversial whether ghrelin is produced there in physiologically relevant amounts.[89,90] Regardless of the source, ghrelin can reach the mediobasal and mediolateral hypothalamus through the general circulation. It is unknown whether peripherally produced ghrelin can reach areas of the hypothalamus protected by the blood-brain barrier. Once ghrelin reaches the hypothalamus, the peptide targets ghrelin receptors present in various hypothalamic nuclei. Ghrelin then exerts its energy homeostatic effects through a central mechanism involving NPY[90,91] and AGRP.[90]

The effects of ghrelin on body metabolism are opposite those of leptin. However, ghrelin appears to be regulated more short term, unlike the more long-term regulation of leptin. During food deprivation, leptin levels fall, POMC production decreases, NPY and AGRP levels rise, and ghrelin levels increase.[92] In this situation, ghrelin serves as a hunger signal, trying to restore the body to a state of positive energy balance. On eating, increases in lower intestinal osmolarity (rather than direct effects of nutrients in the foregut) and insulin surges suppress postprandial ghrelin release.[93] Ghrelin levels drop after feeding, are decreased in obesity (though they are high in Prader-Willi syndrome), are increased in anorexia nervosa, and are low after gastric bypass surgery.[90,93,94] Ghrelin suppresses reproductive function, both centrally and through direct gonadal effects, in times of nutritional stress,[95] whereas leptin plays a permissive role during times of nutritional plenty.[96]

Apparently independently of its orexigenic effects, ghrelin stimulates growth hormone release. Because ghrelin and growth hormone–releasing hormone (GHRH) work through different receptors (GHSR and GHRH receptor, respectively), their stimulation of growth hormone secretion is synergistic.[97] GHSR type 1a is a G protein–coupled receptor that is mainly expressed in the pituitary and hypothalamus and mediates ghrelin's endocrine functions. Various related receptor subtypes are widely distributed in the central and peripheral tissues and mediate ghrelin's nonendocrine actions.[98] Short stature has been described in two unrelated families segregated with a missense mutation that decreased cell-surface expression of GHSR and selectively impaired constitutive activity of GHSR without it losing its ability to respond to ghrelin.[99] GHSR-null mice accumulated less body weight and adiposity than control mice when fed a high-fat diet,[100] similar to ghrelin-knockout mice.[101]

OTHER ADIPOKINES

Leptin has become the prototypic member of the adipokine family, a group of hormones produced primarily by adipose tissue that regulate energy homeostasis and affect other functions such as the reproductive, neuroendocrine, cardiovascular, and immune systems. Adipokines are reviewed extensively elsewhere.[102-105] Central actions, especially involving the hypothalamus, have been described as contributing mechanistically to adipokine effects on energy balance.[105] The most abundantly produced adipokine is adiponectin, a collagen-like molecule that decreases weight, fat, and eating; increases insulin sensitivity; and exerts antiatherogenic, antiangiogenic, and antitumor actions.[104-107] It was also found to regulate pituitary function—namely, inhibiting growth hormone and luteinizing hormone secretion in vitro.[108] The role of adiponectin in modulating pregnancy-related insulin resistance, fetal growth, and the metabolism of newborns and children is now being studied.[109,110]

DETERMINANT OF FUTURE—AS WELL AS CURRENT—HEALTH

The current obesity epidemic has spurred keen interest in the identification of precedent risk factors and the interplay between genetic and environmental traits in influencing human physical and metabolic development throughout the lifespan. In particular, nutritional status during the in utero and neonatal periods has been found to affect the risk for adiposity and metabolic syndrome later in life, even in adulthood.[111-113] A body of literature has emerged under the rubric of *fetal origins of adult disease*, extending beyond obesity and its comorbidities,[114-117] and the hypothalamus plays a prominent role. Because the hypothalamus integrates the various neuroendometabolic functions described in this chapter to maintain homeostasis, hypothalamic adaptations to in utero conditions mold the programming (i.e., setpoints and responsiveness) that will govern the homeostatic mechanisms throughout life.

ACKNOWLEDGMENT

The editors wish to thank authors Adda Grimberg and Jessica Katz Kutikov for their excellent contribution to this text in the fifth edition. This chapter has been reproduced here in the sixth edition essentially unchanged.

 A complete reference list is available at www.ExpertConsult.com.

SELECT REFERENCES

6. Swaab DF, Chung WC, Kruijver FP, et al. Structural and functional sex differences in the human hypothalamus. *Horm Behav*. 2001;40:93.
16. Negri-Cesi P, Colciago A, Celotti F, Motta M. Sexual differentiation of the brain: role of testosterone and its active metabolites. *J Endocrinol Invest*. 2004;27(suppl 6):120.
20. Michaud JL. The developmental program of the hypothalamus and its disorders. *Clin Genet*. 2001;60:255.
21. McClellan KM, Parker KL, Tobet S. Development of the ventromedial nucleus of the hypothalamus. *Front Neuroendocrinol*. 2006;27:193.
22. Koutcherov Y, Mai JK, Ashwell KW, Paxinos G. Organization of human hypothalamus in fetal development. *J Comp Neurol*. 2002;446:301.
24. Scully KM, Rosenfeld MG. Pituitary development: regulatory codes in mammalian organogenesis. *Science*. 2002;295:2231.
31. Kinney HC, Broadbelt KG, Haynes RL, et al. The serotonergic anatomy of the developing human medulla oblongata: implications for pediatric disorders of homeostasis. *J Chem Neuroanat*. 2011;41:182-199.
32. Serón-Ferré M, Torres-Farfán C, Forcelledo ML, Valenzuela GJ. The development of circadian rhythms in the fetus and neonate. *Semin Perinatol*. 2001;25:363.
36. Rivkees SA. Developing circadian rhythmicity in infants. *Pediatr Endocrinol Rev*. 2003;1:38.
37. Brooks E, Canal MM. Development of circadian rhythms: role of postnatal light environment. *Neurosci Biobehav Rev*. 2013;37:551-560.
38. Vanitallie TB. Sleep and energy balance: interactive homeostatic systems. *Metabolism*. 2006;55:S30.
42. DiPietro JA, Costigan KA, Pressman EK, Doussard-Roosevelt JA. Antenatal origins of individual differences in heart rate. *Dev Psychobiol*. 2000;37:221.
44. Suzuki T, Kimura Y, Murotsuki J, et al. Detection of a biorhythm of human fetal autonomic nervous activity by a power spectral analysis. *Am J Obstet Gynecol*. 2001;185:1247.
45. Boulant JA. Role of the preoptic-anterior hypothalamus in thermoregulation and fever. *Clin Infect Dis*. 2000;31(suppl 5):S157.
50. Lunze K, Hamer DH. Thermal protection of the newborn in resource-limited environments. *J Perinatol*. 2012;32:317-324.
51. Canteras NS. The medial hypothalamic defensive system: hodological organization and functional implications. *Pharmacol Biochem Behav*. 2002;71:481.
53. Bauer AM, Quas JA, Boyce WT. Associations between physiological reactivity and children's behavior: advantages of a multisystem approach. *J Dev Behav Pediatr*. 2002;23:102.
54. Ng PC. Effect of stress on the hypothalamic-pituitary-adrenal axis in the fetus and newborn. *J Pediatr*. 2011;158(suppl 2):e41-e43.
63. Ugrumov MV. Magnocellular vasopressin system in ontogenesis: development and regulation. *Microsc Res Tech*. 2002;56:164.
64. Brownstein MJ, Russell JT, Gainer H. Synthesis, transport, and release of posterior pituitary hormones. *Science*. 1980;207:373.
66. Morris JF, Pow DV. New anatomical insights into the inputs and outputs from hypothalamic magnocellular neurons. *Ann N Y Acad Sci*. 1993;689:16.
67. Dewey KG. Maternal and fetal stress are associated with impaired lactogenesis in humans. *J Nutr*. 2001;131:S3012.
69. Theodosis DT. Oxytocin-secreting neurons: a physiological model of morphological neuronal and glial plasticity in the adult hypothalamus. *Front Neuroendocrinol*. 2002;23:101.
72. Thompson C, Hoorn EJ. Hyponatraemia: an overview of frequency, clinical presentation and complications. *Best Pract Res Clin Endocrinol Metab*. 2012;26(suppl 1):S1-S6.
73. Kortenoeven ML, Fenton RA. Renal aquaporins and water balance disorders. *Biochim Biophys Acta*. 2014;1840:1533-1549.
74. Ervin MG. Perinatal fluid and electrolyte regulation: role of arginine vasopressin. *Semin Perinatol*. 1988;12:134.
76. Zhang Y, Proenca R, Maffei M, et al. Positional cloning of the mouse obese gene and its human homologue. *Nature*. 1994;372:425.
77. Park HK, Ahima RS. Physiology of leptin: energy homeostasis, neuroendocrine function and metabolism. *Metabolism*. 2015;64:24-34.
82. Ollmann MM, Wilson BD, Yang YK, et al. Antagonism of central melanocortin receptors in vitro and in vivo by agouti-related protein. *Science*. 1997;278:135.
84. Farooqi IS, O'Rahilly S. 20 years of leptin: human disorders of leptin action. *J Endocrinol*. 2014;223:T63-T70.
85. Tome MA, Lage M, Camiña JP, et al. Sex-based differences in serum leptin concentrations from umbilical cord blood at delivery. *Eur J Endocrinol*. 1997;137:655.
86. Hauguel-de Mouzon S, Lepercq J, Catalano P. The known and unknown of leptin in pregnancy. *Am J Obstet Gynecol*. 2006;194:1537.
88. Kojima M, Hosoda H, Date Y, et al. Ghrelin is a growth-hormone-releasing acylated peptide from stomach. *Nature*. 1999;402:656.
89. Nakazato M, Murakami N, Date Y, et al. A role for ghrelin in the central regulation of feeding. *Nature*. 2001;409:194.
90. Horvath TL, Diano S, Sotonyi P, et al. Minireview: ghrelin and the regulation of energy balance—a hypothalamic perspective. *Endocrinology*. 2001;142:4163.
91. Shintani M, Ogawa Y, Ebihara K, et al. Ghrelin, an endogenous growth hormone secretagogue, is a novel orexigenic peptide that antagonizes leptin action through the activation of hypothalamic neuropeptide Y/Y1 receptor pathway. *Diabetes*. 2001;50:227.
93. Cummings DE. Ghrelin and the short- and long-term regulation of appetite and body weight. *Physiol Behav*. 2006;89:71.
95. Fernandez-Fernandez R, Martini AC, Navarro VM, et al. Novel signals for the integration of energy balance and reproduction. *Mol Cell Endocrinol*. 2006;127:154-255.
97. Hataya Y, Akamizu T, Takaya K, et al. A low dose of ghrelin stimulates growth hormone (GH) release synergistically with GH-releasing hormone in humans. *J Clin Endocrinol Metab*. 2001;86:4552.
101. Wortley KE, del Rincon JP, Murray JD, et al. Absence of ghrelin protects against early-onset obesity. *J Clin Invest*. 2005;115:3573.
103. Rondinone CM. Adipocyte-derived hormones, cytokines, and mediators. *Endocrine*. 2006;29:81.
107. Qi Y, Takahashi N, Hileman SM, et al. Adiponectin acts in the brain to decrease body weight. *Nat Med*. 2004;10:524.
109. Mazaki-Tovi S, Kanety H, Sivan E. Adiponectin and human pregnancy. *Curr Diab Rep*. 2005;5:278.
111. Contreras C, Novelle MG, Leis R, et al. Effects of neonatal programming on hypothalamic mechanisms controlling energy balance. *Horm Metab Res*. 2013;45:935-944.
112. Roth CL, Sathyanarayana S. Mechanisms affecting neuroendocrine and epigenetic regulation of body weight and onset of puberty: potential implications in the child born small for gestational age (SGA). *Rev Endocr Metab Disord*. 2012;13:129-140.
113. McMillen IC, Edwards LJ, Duffield J, Muhlhausler BS. Regulation of leptin synthesis and secretion before birth: implications for the early programming of adult obesity. *Reproduction*. 2006;131:415.
114. Phillips DI, Jones A. Fetal programming of autonomic and HPA function: do people who were small babies have enhanced stress responses? *J Physiol*. 2006;572:45.
115. Braun T, Challis JR, Newnham JP, Sloboda DM. Early-life glucocorticoid exposure: the hypothalamic-pituitary-adrenal axis, placental function, and long-term disease risk. *Endocr Rev*. 2013;34:885-916.
116. Duthie L, Reynolds RM. Changes in the maternal hypothalamic-pituitary-adrenal axis in pregnancy and postpartum: influences on maternal and fetal outcomes. *Neuroendocrinology*. 2013;98:106-115.
117. Reynolds RM. Glucocorticoid excess and the developmental origins of disease: two decades of testing the hypothesis—2012 Curt Richter Award winner. *Psychoneuroendocrinology*. 2013;38:1-11.

Growth Factor Regulation of Fetal Growth

140

Colin P. Hawkes | Lorraine E. Levitt Katz

INTRODUCTION

Growth during fetal life is characterized by an early period of cell division and organogenesis, followed by a more prolonged period of growth and refinement of organ development. *Growth factors* are peptides or proteins that serve as key regulators of cell proliferation and differentiation that exert their effects by binding to specific receptors, which mediate signal transduction across cell membranes. This binding triggers a cascade of responses, including those involving second messengers, which ultimately result in cell mitogenesis or differentiation. Various growth factors are expressed in diverse tissues during embryonic life, which may have endocrine as well as autocrine-paracrine effects. Our understanding of growth factor regulation of fetal growth has developed through in vitro, animal, and clinical studies, which will be reviewed in this chapter.

INSULIN-LIKE GROWTH FACTOR AXIS

The primary regulator of postnatal somatic growth is growth hormone (GH). In the liver and other target cells, GH induces the production of insulin-like growth factors (IGFs), IGF-1 and IGF-2.[1] The IGFs, particularly IGF-1, have direct endocrine effects on somatic growth and on the proliferation of many tissues and cell types. Both IGF-1 and IGF-2 are expressed during fetal development in a GH-independent fashion. In addition to their anabolic effects, IGFs also are thought to be significant autocrine-paracrine factors involved in cellular and tissue function.[2,3] Locally produced IGFs have been demonstrated in nearly all tissue types, where they are considered to be responsible for cell growth and differentiation. GH is thought to play only a minor role in fetal growth, limited to the third trimester, and infants born with congenital GH deficiency are normally grown at birth.[4] This chapter presents evidence that the IGFs and their regulatory proteins play a central role in the regulation of fetal growth.

INSULIN-LIKE GROWTH FACTORS

IGF-1 and IGF-2 are two closely related peptide hormones approximately 7 kDa in size that share a high degree of structural similarity with proinsulin.[3] Like proinsulin, they are composed of A, B, and C domains; however, they also include a D domain. Together, these components form the mature IGF peptide. The IGFs are synthesized with an additional extension peptide known as the *E peptide,* which is removed during post-translational processing.[5] Both IGF-1 and IGF-2 are encoded by a single gene each, which by alternative splicing results in several messenger RNA (mRNA) species. The *IGF1* gene spans 95 kilobases (kb) on the long arm of chromosome 12 and contains 6 exons; the *IGF2* gene has a total genomic size of 35 kb and is made up of 9 exons. *IGF2* is located on the short arm of chromosome 11 (near the insulin gene), in an area that is paternally imprinted in all mammalian species. This paternal imprinting phenomenon is related to the fact that IGF-2 is a major fetal growth factor.

IGF RECEPTORS

The IGFs interact with specific receptors, designated type 1 and type 2 IGF receptors, as well as with the insulin receptor, which can bind IGF-1 and IGF-2, but with much lower affinity than for insulin.[3] The type 1 IGF receptor binds IGF-1 with high affinity, IGF-2 with slightly lower affinity, and insulin with low affinity. This receptor mediates the known mitogenic effects of the IGFs. The type 1 IGF receptor and the closely related insulin receptor are heterotetramers composed of two pairs of α and β subunits, the result of post-translational processing of a single gene product of a single gene that encodes for the entire receptor. The two α subunits, which are involved in ligand binding, are linked by disulfide bonds and are primarily extracellular (Fig. 140.1). The β subunits are connected to the α subunits by disulfide bonds and function as intracellular tyrosine kinases. On ligand binding, the subunits undergo a conformational change that enables them to bind ATP and become autophosphorylated. Subsequently, these kinases phosphorylate cytoplasmic molecules known as the *insulin receptor substrates* (IR[6,7] S-1 and -2), which are involved in mediating many of the effects of insulin and IGFs. IRS proteins couple insulin and IGF receptors to the phosphoinositide 3-kinase (PI3-kinase) and extracellular signal-regulated kinase (ERK) cascades. Products of PI3-kinase, including phosphatidylinositol-3,4-biphosphate and phosphatidylinositol 3,4,5-triphosphate, attract serine kinases to the plasma membrane, including the phosphoinositide-dependent kinase (PDK1 and PDK2) and at least three protein kinases B (PKB)/AKT isoforms. During co-localization at the plasma membrane, PDK1 or PDK2 phosphorylates and activates PKB-1, -2, or -3. The activated PKB/AKT phosphorylates many substrates to control various biologic signaling cascades, including glucose transport, protein synthesis, glycogen synthesis, and cellular proliferation and survival in various cells and tissues.[8]

The insulin receptor itself exists in two isoforms in humans, produced by tissue-specific alternative splicing of exon 11 of the insulin receptor gene, *IR*.[9] Relative expression of the different insulin receptor isoforms, the type A insulin receptor (IR-A) and type B insulin receptor (IR-B), is not only tissue-specific but also developmentally regulated, with IR-A preferentially expressed in fetal tissues.[10] In addition, IR-A binds IGF-2 with an affinity equal to that for insulin, whereas IR-B has less affinity for IGF-2. Insulin binding to IR-A stimulates the metabolic effects of insulin receptor activation, while IGF-2 binding to IR-A more effectively stimulates mitogenic processes.[10] This differential effect may result from less insulin receptor endocytosis following IGF-2 binding relative to insulin binding.[11,12]

The type 2 IGF receptor is structurally distinct from the type 1 receptor and the insulin receptor and primarily binds IGF-2.[2] Unlike the insulin receptor and the type 1 IGF receptor, the type 2 IGF receptor is not a tyrosine kinase. Instead, it is a monomeric receptor with a large extracellular domain made up of 15 repeat sequences and a small region homologous to the collagen-binding domain of fibronectin. The type 2 IGF receptor is 270 kDa in size and functions also as the cation-independent mannose-6-phosphate receptor.[13] The receptor does not have a signaling domain and is thought to be recycled between the

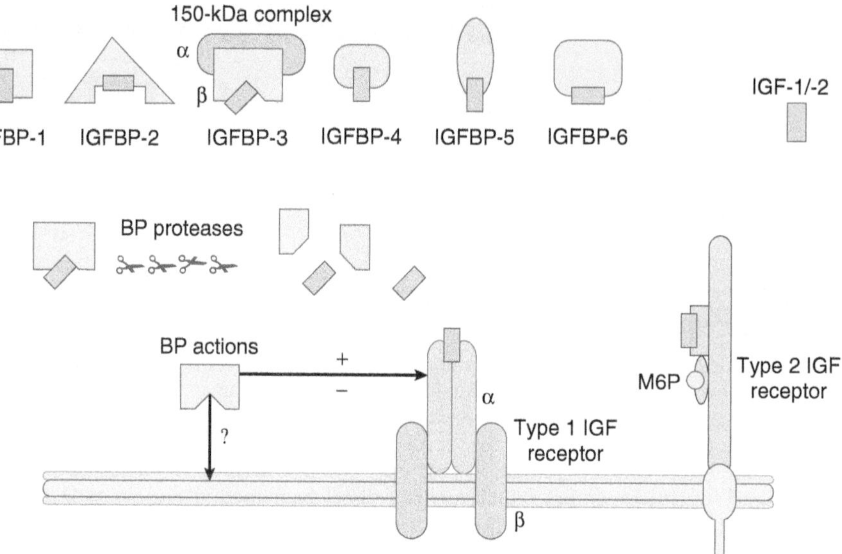

Fig. 140.1 The insulin-like growth factor *(IGF)* axis, including the IGFs, IGF-binding proteins *(IGFBP)*, and IGFBP proteases. The relationship of the components of the IGF axis is depicted. *BP,* Binding protein; *M6P,* mannose-6-phosphate.

plasma membrane and intracellular compartments. It also has been suggested that the type 2 IGF receptor targets excess IGF-2 for lysosomal destruction during fetal life. The type 2 receptor is maternally imprinted in mice but not in humans.[14]

Additional members of the class of receptors for the IGF-insulin family are less well characterized. One such receptor is composed of an insulin receptor α-β heterodimer binding to a type 1 IGF receptor α-β heterodimer and thus has been labeled the hybrid receptor.[15] Analysis of tissues in which this receptor appears to be common (such as placenta) and transfection experiments in cell lines have demonstrated two isoforms of this hybrid receptor—a hybrid receptor containing insulin receptor isoform A (Hybrid-Rs^A) and one containing insulin receptor isoform B (Hybrid-Rs^B). Hybrid-Rs^A has biologic properties intermediate between those of the insulin and the type 1 IGF receptor: It binds both insulin and IGFs with high affinity and stimulates cell proliferation and migration.[16] (By contrast, Hybrid-Rs^B binds IGF-1 with high affinity but IGF-2 with only low affinity, whereas insulin has little to no affinity at all.) The complementary DNA (cDNA) for an additional receptor has been cloned, and because of its high homology with the insulin receptor, it has been designated the ***insulin receptor-related receptor*** (IRR).[17] IRR has been regarded as an orphan receptor of the insulin receptor family that does not bind insulin or insulin-like peptide and can be expressed as variably spliced isoforms. IRR is expressed specifically in developing renal and neural tissues. IRR also is expressed in pancreatic islets, but the lack of this receptor in mice does not affect β cell development and function.[18] It is activated in mildly alkaline media and may play a role in acid-base balance.[19] An additional atypical IGF receptor with altered ligand binding also has been described.[20] This may represent a post-translationally modified type 1 IGF receptor of unclear function.

IGF BINDING PROTEINS

The IGF-binding proteins (IGFBPs), a family of proteins with high affinity for the IGFs, have been shown to be involved in the modulation of the mitogenic effects of IGFs on cells. In vivo, the IGFs are bound to this family of six structurally and evolutionarily related IGFBPs (IGFBP-1 to IGFBP-6). In serum, a majority (70% to 80%) of IGFs exist in a 150-kDa complex composed of one IGF molecule, IGFBP-3, and the acid-labile subunit (ALS). A smaller proportion (approximately 20%) of the IGFs are associated with other serum IGFBPs within a 50-kDa complex, and less than 5% of the IGFs are found in the free form of 7.5 kDa. ALS is a protein that binds to the IGF/IGFBP-3 binary complex, primarily in serum, prolonging the $t_{1/2}$ of serum IGFs and facilitating their endocrine actions. These IGFBPs appear to regulate the availability of free IGFs for interaction with the IGF receptors, as well as to interact directly with cell function.[21] They are part of a superfamily that comprises six high-affinity IGFBPs and at least four other low-affinity IGF binders, termed ***insulin-like growth factor–binding protein-related proteins (IGFBP-rPs)***.[22] In addition, the cell surface proteoglycan glypican-3 (GPC3) binds both IGF-2 and the type 1 IGF receptor, facilitating IGF-2 mediated signaling. Mutations of this causes the overgrowth syndrome known as *Simpson-Golabi-Behmel syndrome type 1*[23] and GPC3 may also have a role in oncogenesis.[24]

IGFBP-1 is a 25-kDa protein that is found in high concentrations in amniotic fluid; it also is secreted by hepatocytes under negative regulation by insulin. IGFBP-2 is a 31-kDa protein found in serum, cerebrospinal fluid, and seminal plasma. It is expressed in many fetal and adult tissues. IGFBP-3 is the major binding protein in postnatal serum and is synthesized by hepatocytes and other cells. In plasma, IGFBP-3 is found as part of a 150-kDa complex, which also includes an ALS and an IGF molecule, all of which are GH-dependent. IGFBP-4 is a 24-kDa protein that has been identified in serum, seminal plasma, and numerous cell types. IGFBP-5 appears to be an IGF-enhancing protein that is found in cerebrospinal fluid and serum. It also is observed in rapidly growing fetal tissues. IGFBP-6 has relative specificity for IGF-2 over IGF-1. It is found in cerebrospinal fluid and serum and is produced by many cells. The six cloned cDNAs for the IGFBPs show a high degree of structural similarity and sequence conservation across species. IGFBPs are tightly regulated by various endocrine factors and are uniquely expressed during ontogeny. Three possible models for the interaction of the IGFBPs with the IGFs and their receptors have been proposed.[25] The first is that these molecules limit the availability of free IGFs for interaction with the IGF receptors. For example, the addition of IGFBPs to many cell cultures in vitro results in the inhibition of IGF actions within these experimental systems.[26] However, in other systems, IGFBPs have been demonstrated to enhance IGF action under circumstances that may involve cellular processing of the IGFBPs.[21] Finally, as has been shown in several in vitro systems, IGFBPs may inhibit cell growth in an IGF-independent fashion, acting through their own receptors.[25,26]

IGFBP-3 is a mediator of apoptosis under the control of a number of cell cycle regulators.[27] In studies using specific antisense oligonucleotides and neutralizing anti-IGFBP-3 antibodies to block IGFBP-3 expression and action, IGFBP-3 was identified as the mediator of apoptosis induced by retinoic acid and transforming growth factor-β (TGF-β).

INSULIN-LIKE GROWTH FACTOR–BINDING PROTEIN PROTEASES

A group of enzymes that are capable of cleaving IGFBPs have been recognized as potential modulators of IGF action.[28] First identified in pregnancy serum, IGFBP-3 proteolytic activity is responsible for the disappearance of intact IGFBP-3 from the serum of pregnant women, with no change in IGFBP-3 immunoreactivity and an increase in lower-molecular-weight fragments.[29,30] IGFBP proteases also have been reported in the serum of severely ill patients in a state of cachexia, in critically ill neonates, in patients with GH receptor deficiency, and in patients with in prostate cancer and other malignancies.[31-33] Prostate-specific antigen was the first kallikrein protein demonstrated to be an IGFBP protease.[34] Subsequently, it has been determined that other members of the kallikrein family, such as nerve growth factor (NGF), also serve as specific IGFBP proteases.[35] Cathepsins are another class of IGFBP proteases that have been shown to be active in acid pH.[36] Finally, matrix metalloproteinases, which are known to cleave collagen and other extracellular matrix components, are a group of IGFBP proteases.[37] It has been speculated that the IGFBP proteases are important modulators of IGF bioavailability and bioactivity through their modification of the IGF carrier proteins. The proteolytic activity may play a role in regulating IGF availability at the tissue level by decreasing the affinity of the binding proteins for the growth factors, thereby releasing free IGFs and allowing increased receptor binding.[34,37,38] Mutations in pregnancy-associated plasma protein A2 (PAPP-A2), a protease that cleaves IGFBP-3 and -5, have recently been shown to cause short stature with elevated circulating IGF-1 concentrations and reduced free IGF-1 levels.[39,40] Although this confirms the role of proteases in modulating height in childhood and circulating bioavailable IGF-1, the role of these proteases in fetal growth is not known. Birth length was variable in the five reported children who had pathogenic PAPPA-A2 mutations, with Z-scores ranging from −0.07 to −2.75.[39] Low concentrations of IGFBP proteases have been described during the first trimester in pregnancies at higher risk of subsequent preeclampsia and growth restriction, suggesting that reduction in proteases in pregnancies may reduce IGF bioavailability for placental development.[41,42]

ADDITIONAL GROWTH-REGULATING PEPTIDES

FIBROBLAST GROWTH FACTOR FAMILY OF PEPTIDES AND RECEPTORS

Fibroblast growth factors (FGFs) are a family of peptide cytokines that are important in the regulation of many tissues. To date, 23 different FGFs have been identified, including the best-characterized acidic FGF (aFGF), or FGF1; basic FGF (bFGF), or FGF2; and keratinocyte growth factor (KGF), or FGF7. The FGFs exert their actions by binding to one of a family of four membrane-bound FGF receptors, FGFR1 to FGFR4, and a heparin sulfate proteoglycan co-receptor to form a three-part signaling complex.[43] FGFs appear to have primarily autocrine-paracrine functions in organ growth and differentiation, bone formation, and cell differentiation and migration, as well as in carcinogenesis.[44] The role of FGF in osteogenesis and growth initially was demonstrated by the discovery of a gain-of-function mutation in *FGFR3* as the cause of achondroplasia in humans.[45,46] Other forms of chondrodysplasia, as well as other skeletal dysplasias, were subsequently found to be caused by mutations in the FGFRs, further emphasizing the importance of FGF signaling in bone formation.[47]

NERVE GROWTH FACTORS

The complex array of cells that make up the nervous system is under the regulatory influence of specific growth factors, such as NGF, neurotensin, and the neural-derived growth factors (NDGFs). NGF is synthesized in peripheral cells and transported in retrograde fashion up the neuronal axis to the cell body—a process that suggests that NGF is a neurotropic agent directing neurons to sites of innervation.[48] NGF exerts its effects on cells derived from the neural crest, including central nervous system and peripheral nervous system neurons, and some non-neurons, such as immune cells and endocrine cells. NGF stimulates mitosis in some cell types and is capable of inducing differentiation events in neural tissue. NGF synthesis is controlled in part by hormones, such as testosterone and thyroxine. It also has been demonstrated that the γ subunit of NGF serves as an IGFBP protease.[35]

EPIDERMAL GROWTH FACTOR SYSTEM

Epidermal growth factors (EGFs) and their receptors are widespread in many tissues and participate in specific developmental processes such as neonatal eyelid opening and tooth eruption. EGFs have potent mitogenic actions that have been extensively explored in cell culture systems. The receptor for EGFs was characterized as a prototype model for signal transduction involving tyrosine kinases. EGFs have been identified in most body fluids of mammals, and extensive in vitro data indicate multiple cellular functions of EGFs. Members of the EGF family may have a role in embryogenesis and fetal growth, because receptors have been identified in fetal tissues. The mouse fetus expresses EGF receptors from 12 days onward,[49] and targeted mutation of the EGF receptor demonstrated its significance in fetal development and growth.[50] EGFs can induce tracheal branching morphogenesis in chick lung rudiments and stimulate epithelial maturation in the lung and other tissues in rabbits.[51] Although EGF transcripts have not been detected in the fetus, it is maternal EGF that appears to play a role in fetal growth, because maternal EGF deficiency leads to hypoglycemia and intrauterine growth restriction (IUGR) in offspring—an effect that is corrected by EGF administration.[52] Transforming growth factor-α (TGF-α) is a peptide that displays 30% homology with EGF and exerts effects through the EGF receptor.[50,53] It has been shown to be expressed in pre-implantation mouse embryos and decidua of rat and may therefore be important in fetal development.[54-56]

OTHER GROWTH-PROMOTING PEPTIDES

An increasing number of growth factors are being recognized as having growth-promoting activities in certain cell types. In general, these molecules appear to play important autocrine-paracrine as well as endocrine roles. Notable among these are groups of growth factors that have tissue-specific effects. Endothelin, platelet-derived growth factor (PDGF), and vascular epithelial growth factor (VEGF) regulate angiogenesis and other vascular processes, in addition to modulating the function of numerous cultured cells. PDGF acts in sequence with other growth factors to regulate entry into the cell cycle.[57] A variety of hematopoietic growth factors such as granulocyte colony-stimulating factor (G-CSF), macrophage colony-stimulating factor (M-CSF), erythropoietin, and thrombopoietin promote the growth of the different lineages of the precursor cells in the bone marrow. Growth of immune system cells is stimulated by an array of cytokines, including interleukins and interferons. Other growth factors, such as hepatocyte growth factor (HGF), that have been attributed to specific tissues are being recognized as having general growth-promoting effect in numerous tissues.

GROWTH INHIBITORY PEPTIDES

A particularly interesting class of cytokines that can negatively modulate cellular growth is the TGF-β family, members of which are structurally distinct from TGF-α. TGF-β can either act to mediate cellular growth and malignant transformation or act as a growth inhibitory substance with the potential for arresting the growth of normal and neoplastic cells. TGF-β transcripts have been detected in pre-implantation embryos.[55] This peptide is involved in mesodermal differentiation and organogenesis. It may stimulate some mesenchymal mitosis while inhibiting the proliferation of epithelial cells.

TGF-βs have both autocrine and paracrine effects. The response depends on the origin of the cell: In some cell types (e.g., hepatocytes, hematopoietic cells), cell growth is stimulated, whereas in other cell types (e.g., osteoblasts, granulocytes), growth is inhibited. During pregnancy, TGFs are important in the regulation of trophoblast invasion, decidualization, and placentation.[58] Mutations in the TGF-β family ligands are responsible for a number of human diseases, including hereditary chondrodysplasia.[59] Retinoic acid and other steroid hormones also have been shown to have inhibitory effects on cell growth. Tumor necrosis factors (TNFs) and other compounds have been described to have similar effects. These molecules may regulate the entry of cells into programmed cell death (apoptosis).

GROWTH FACTORS IN FETAL GROWTH: ANIMAL MODELS

In this section, comparisons are made with corresponding human mutations when appropriate.

IGF AXIS EXPRESSION

The embryo establishes its own IGF axis very early in gestation, providing evidence that this axis plays a functional role in fetal growth. The mRNAs for IGF-2, the type 2 IGF receptor, and IGFBP-2, -3, and -4 are among the earliest of fetal mouse transcripts and are detectable in two-cell murine embryos by reverse transcriptase-polymerase chain reaction analysis.[60,61] These transcripts become more abundant as gestation progresses. The distribution of the type 2 IGF receptor in tissues corresponds to that of IGF-2 mRNA. IGF-1 expression occurs somewhat later, by 7 to 8 days gestation in mouse embryos.[56] The type 1 IGF receptor is expressed in the eight-cell rat embryo, and its mRNA is widely distributed in various tissues by midgestation.[62]

Regulation of IGF expression in fetal life is not fully defined. Postnatal IGF synthesis is controlled by GH and by nutritional status, but IGF regulation in intrauterine life is less well understood and does not appear to be GH-dependent. Furthermore, evidence suggests that IGFs not only stimulate proliferation but also can induce differentiation events in some cells during organogenesis in an autocrine or paracrine manner. With regard to organ differentiation, these actions are probably tightly regulated within specific tissues and developmental stages during intrauterine life.

OVEREXPRESSION OF THE GH–IGF AXIS IN TRANSGENIC ANIMALS

OVEREXPRESSION OF GH AND IGF-1 AND -2

The creation of transgenic mice overexpressing GH-IGF axis molecules has furthered the understanding of the control of IGF-1 secretion and actions in fetal and postnatal growth (Table 140.1). Mice with GH overexpression display increased postnatal linear growth and dramatic weight gain to as much as twice the normal body weight with selective organ hypertrophy.[63,64] Acceleration of growth correlates with the onset of GH-dependent IGF-1 expression during the second to third postnatal week, suggesting that the growth-promoting properties of the transgene are mediated through the induction of IGF-1 expression postnatally. IGF-1 transgenic mice also are larger than normal, but their weight increase (to 30% over that of control mice), which occurs after 4 to 6 weeks of postnatal life, is more modest than that in the GH transgenic mice. This is probably related to the lower IGF levels seen with the former.[65] The brains and other organs of these animals demonstrate a large increase in weight relative to overall growth. IGF-1 levels in these mice are elevated but are lower than those seen in the GH-transgenic mice; endogenous GH and hepatic IGF-1 expression are suppressed by 60% to 75% (see Table 140.1).[66] IGF-2 transgenic mice are not bigger than normal, but in the existing models, the major portion of IGF-2 expression occurs postnatally.[67]

To separate out more completely the effects of endogenous GH and IGF-1 expression, IGF-1 transgenic mice were mated with a GH-deficient mouse strain.[68,69] The offspring displayed normal body weight and linear growth. Some non–GH-dependent effects of IGF-1 were present, including a disproportionate increase in brain weight, implying that these are local effects of IGF-1. The livers of these mice were hypoplastic (an effect seen in GH-deficient mice), an abnormality that was only partially corrected with IGF-1. Overall, the transgenic animal data confirm the role of GH and IGF-1 in postnatal growth and suggest that IGF-1 mediates a majority of GH effects, but that variations in local expression IGF-1 can result in altered growth of specific tissues.

OVEREXPRESSION OF IGFBPS

Mice overexpressing IGFBP-1 are similar in size to (or slightly smaller than) the wild type at birth.[70,71] Brain weights are decreased in these transgenic mice compared with wild-type mice.[72] It is generally thought that IGFBP-1 functions to inhibit IGF-1 action and thus may contribute to the impaired fetal brain development seen in these transgenic animals. Overexpression of IGFBP-2 in mice did not result in a different birth weight and was associated with a reduction of body weight gain only after the age of 3 weeks.[73] In two different IGFBP-3 transgenic mouse models, transgene expression resulted in a 10% reduction in birth weight, as well as organomegaly in body regions different from the major expression sites.[74-76] Total body weight in transgenic mice overexpressing IGFBP-4 is indistinguishable from that in control animals.[77]

INSULIN AND IGF AXIS–NULL MUTATIONS

Studies of null mutations (knockouts) created by homologous recombination in the genes encoding insulin, IGF-1, IGF-2, and the IGF receptors have enabled investigators to explore the role of the IGF axis in fetal growth. In all of the null mutations, body proportions are qualitatively normal.

IGF AND IGF RECEPTOR MUTATIONS

Mice in which the IGF-2 gene has been eliminated by targeted disruption exhibit severe growth restriction, to 60% of normal size at birth, with small placentas.[78-80] However, after birth, survival is normal, and the mice grow at a near-normal rate, although they remain small relative to normal littermates. In the heterozygous state, the IGF-2 knockout can manifest itself only if the paternal allele is targeted, elegantly demonstrating the paternal imprinting of the IGF-2 gene.[81] IGF-1 gene-targeted mice also are small (60% of normal) at birth, whereas the placentas are of normal size.[78,82,83] Furthermore, they display dramatic growth arrest postnatally (30% of normal). These mice also are more likely to die during the neonatal period; the increased death rate may be related to the poor development of diaphragm and lung.[80]

Postnatal development of surviving IGF-1–knockout mice has been analyzed in detail. At 2 months of age, IGF-1–deficient mice show extensive reductions in brain size, consistent with a role for IGF-1 in axon growth.[84] Morphologic and morphometric analyses of long bones in mice lacking IGF-1 indicate that IGF-1 promotes bone development by increasing cellular proliferation, without affecting differentiation. The growth plates are uniformly affected, with reductions in the resting, proliferative, and hypertrophic chondrocytes. As a result, the formation of secondary ossification centers is delayed.[85] Other reports have described homozygous IGF-1 mutations in humans, manifesting as severe prenatal and

Table 140.1 Physical and Biochemical Features of Various GH/IGF-1 Transgenic Mouse Models.

Transgene Model	Postnatal Growth (% normal)	GH	IGF-1	IGFBP-3	Brain Size	Liver Size
GH	200	↑↑	↑↑	—	Normal	↑↑
IGF-1	130	↓	↑	↑	↑↑	↑
GH^-	60	↓↓	↓↓	↓↓	↓	↓↓
$GH^-/IGF\text{-}1^+$	Normal	↓	Normal	Normal or ↓	↑	↓
IGFBP-3	80	—	↑↑	↑↑	↓	↑

GH, Growth hormone; *IGF-1*, insulin-like growth factor-1; *IGFBP-3*, insulin-like growth factor-binding protein-3.

postnatal growth failure, sensorineural deafness, and mental retardation.[86,87] Mice with null mutations of both IGF-1 and IGF-2 also displayed more severe IUGR (to 30% of normal size), and all of these mice died after birth from respiratory failure. Thus IGF-1 and IGF-2 appear to have independent growth-promoting activities that are compounded when both are absent. The results of the studies confirm that both IGF-1 and IGF-2 appear to be critical for fetal growth, whereas IGF-1 promotes postnatal growth as well. IGF-2 signaling may dictate the size of the placenta, thereby affecting fetal size.

Liver IGF-1-deficient (LID) mice grow normally despite a 75% reduction in serum IGF-1 levels.[88] In these mice, expression of IGF-1 in nonhepatic tissues is normal, suggesting that the normal growth exhibited by these animals may be mediated by autocrine-paracrine actions of IGF-1, as well as by some nonhepatic sources of circulating IGF-1. Similarly, ALS-knockout (ALSKO) mice demonstrate only a 10% reduction in body weight despite a 65% reduction in circulating IGF-1 levels.[89] More recent reports of human ALS mutations show similar findings: markedly reduced circulating total IGF-1 levels, undetectable ALS, but only mildly affected prenatal and postnatal growth.[90,91] These findings are consistent with the idea that locally synthesized IGF-1 plays a prominent role in somatic growth. LID + ALS double-knockout mice showed serum levels of IGF-1 reduced to approximately 10% to 15% of normal levels.[92] In these animals, GH levels were markedly increased and linear growth was severely attenuated (for a 30% reduction in body length and weight starting at the age of 2 to 3 weeks). Thus, the double-gene-disruption LID + ALSKO mouse model demonstrates that a threshold concentration of circulating IGF-1 is necessary for normal growth.

Gene targeting of the type 1 IGF receptor results in severe IUGR, with a phenotype similar to that seen in double–IGF-1/IGF-2 gene targeting.[82] These mice also die after birth, apparently from inadequate respiration. The results indicate that the mitogenic effects of IGF-1 and IGF-2 are mediated primarily through the type 1 IGF receptor. Although no humans have been identified with homozygous mutations, patients have been described with heterozygous mutations of the IGF-IR or the IGF-IR proreceptor, all with IUGR progressive postnatal growth failure.[93-95]

Although mice with disruption of the type 1 IGF receptor displayed growth failure, only the mice missing IGF-2 displayed decreased placental growth. Indeed, placenta-specific IGF-2 represents a major regulator of placental growth.[96] By controlling placental growth and ability to transport vital amino acids and glucose to the fetus, placental IGF-2 in turn affects fetal growth, especially in late gestation.[97,98] Furthermore, the fact that genetic IGF-2 deficiency has a phenotype independent of that associated with the type 1 and type 2 receptors suggests that an additional receptor mediates IGF-2 actions in fetal life. Gene targeting of the type 2 receptor results in mice that are 30% larger than littermates—a finding compatible with its negative growth-modulating effect.[99] This gene is maternally imprinted in mice but not in humans. Thus, those mice inheriting the maternal 2R allele lack functional 2R receptors and die shortly after birth. The levels of lysosomal enzymes in amniotic fluid are increased, and selective organ enlargement is apparent. It has been hypothesized that mice lacking the type 2R accumulate toxic levels of IGF-2.[99]

These studies provide supportive evidence that the IGF-2/mannose-6-phosphate (M6P) receptor may function primarily to degrade and remove IGF-2 from the extracellular environment. The opposite imprinting of IGF-2 and the type 2 IGF receptor may modulate fetal demand and maternal supply of nutrients.[100] The phenotype of mice lacking both type 1 IGF receptor and type 2 IGF receptor provides evidence for the ability of IGF-1 to signal through the insulin receptor, because these mice exhibit normal embryonic and postnatal growth. It has been shown that mice lacking the type 2 IGF receptor are rescued from perinatal lethality and undergo near-normal postnatal development when they carry null mutations of the type 1 IGF receptor. Triple mutants lacking IGF-2 and both IGF receptors exhibit only approximately 30% of normal weight, phenotypically indistinguishable from double mutants lacking IGF type 1 receptor and IGF-2 (Table 140.2).[101] Genetic evidence indicates that the receptor supporting somatic growth of the type 1–type 2 IGF receptor double mutants is the insulin receptor, because mice lacking all three genes (insulin receptor, type 1 IGF receptor, type 2 IGF receptor) are nonviable dwarfs that attain only 30% of normal size.[102]

To address the issue of the role of GH and IGF-1 in growth, Lupu and colleagues[85] have generated mice lacking both IGF-1 and GH receptor. Double-knockout mice exhibit a greater degree of growth restriction (to 17% of normal size) than that seen in mice lacking either gene alone, indicating that the two genes act both independently and synergistically to promote growth. Whereas IGF-1 promotes both prenatal and postnatal growth, GH appears to be required exclusively for postnatal growth, because the growth defect in GH receptor–deficient mice becomes apparent only after postnatal day 20.

INSULIN AND INSULIN RECEPTOR MUTATIONS

The generation of mice bearing insulin receptor mutations has been instrumental in delineating the pathogenesis of insulin resistance, diabetes, and obesity. In terms of somatic growth, mice lacking the insulin receptor are born at term with slight growth retardation (approximately 10%)[102]; inactivation of the two insulin genes also results in a slight impairment of embryonic growth, with a 15% to 20% decrease in birth weight.[103] The growth impairment observed in mice lacking the insulin genes indicates that the effect of insulin to promote mouse embryo growth is paltry compared with that of IGF-1 and IGF-2. Mutations of the insulin receptor in humans are phenotypically heterogeneous in terms of the metabolic consequences. As in mice, lack of the insulin receptor in humans is compatible with embryonic development and term birth. However, most strikingly, human infants lacking the insulin receptor demonstrate severe growth restriction at birth and gain little if any weight thereafter.[104] The most likely explanation of the difference between insulin receptor–deficient mice and children is that embryonic growth

Table 140.2 Physical and Biochemical Features of the Various GH/IGF1–Knockout Mouse Models.

Knockout Model	Birth Weight (% of Normal)	Other Features	Postnatal Course
IGF-1	60	Normal placenta; decreased brain size	Slow growth; death before adulthood
IGF-2	60	Small placenta	Normal growth rate
IGF-1 + IGF-2	30	Small placenta; no respirations	Immediate postnatal death
LID	Normal	75% reduction in serum IGF-1	Normal growth
ALSKO	Normal	65% reduction in serum IGF-1	10% reduction in body weight
LID + ALSKO[a]	Normal	85%–90% reduction in serum IGF-1; increased GH levels	30% reduction in body weight and length
IGF-1 receptor	45	No respirations	Immediate postnatal death
IGF-2 receptor	130	Edema, large placenta	Death in utero
IGF-1 receptor + IGF-2 receptor	100	Large placenta	Normal growth rate
IGF-1 receptor + IGF-2	30	Small placenta	
IGF-2 receptor + IGF-2	80	Small placenta	
IGF-1 receptor + IGF-2 receptor + IGF-2	30	Small placenta	
IGF-1 + GH receptor	17		Postnatal growth retardation
IRS-1	50–70	Insulin resistance	Survival with normal growth rate, but persistent small size (no catch-up growth)
IRS-2	90	Insulin resistance, pancreatic β cell failure	Development of diabetes
AKT-1	80	Normal glucose tolerance	Neonatal death in some animals Persistent small size in surviving pups
Insulin genes (Ins1 + Ins2)	80–85	Diabetes	Normal growth rate; early death from diabetes
Insulin receptor	90	Diabetes; hypotrophy of subcutaneous fat	Normal growth rate; early death from diabetes

[a]Double-knockout model.
ALSKO, acid-labile subunit knockout; *GH*, growth hormone; *IGF-1*, insulin-like growth factor-1; *IGFBP-3*, insulin-like growth factor-binding protein-3; *LID*, liver IGF-1–deficient.

in humans and that in rodents follow different patterns. During the last trimester of human gestation, corresponding to the first weeks of postnatal life in mice, a significant increase in adipose mass is seen. The adipose organ is exquisitely sensitive to insulin, as demonstrated by the excessive adiposity of fetuses exposed to high insulin concentrations in utero who are born large for gestational age (LGA) as a result of maternal diabetes[105,106] or hyperinsulinism.[107,108] Thus, in contrast with its role in mice, insulin is a fetal growth factor in humans. Null mutations of the human insulin gene have not been reported.

INSULIN-LIKE GROWTH FACTOR–BINDING PROTEIN MUTATIONS

When the knockout approach was applied to the IGFBPs, the results were surprisingly subtle: In IGFBP-2–knockout mice, a reduction in spleen weight of adult males was the only morphologic alteration.[107] IGFBP-4 mutants appear to be slightly smaller than their normal counterparts, and the genetic ablation of IGFBP-6 has not resulted in any apparent phenotypic manifestation.[109] A recently described IGFBP-3/IGFBP-4/IGFBP-5 triple-knockout mouse was shown to have a modest reduction in birth weight, similar to that for the IGFBP-4 single-gene mutant, and a moderate reduction in postnatal growth (78% of wild type).[110] It has been speculated that functional compensation by other members of the IGFBP family (including IGFBP-rPs) may prevent the appearance of dramatic phenotypes.[111]

INSULIN RECEPTOR SUBSTRATE AND AKT MUTATIONS

The two IRS proteins, IRS-1 and IRS-2, mediate many insulin and IGF responses, especially those associated with somatic growth and carbohydrate metabolism. The IRS-1 branch of the pathway plays a significant role in mediating the effects of IGF-1 on growth. Deletion of the *IRS1* gene in mice reduces embryonic and neonatal growth,[112] whereas deletion of *IRS2* barely reduces prenatal and early postnatal growth by 10%.[113]The *IRS1*-knockout mouse has been described as having a phenotype of fetal growth restriction to 50% to 70% normal size in the homozygous state.[112] Postnatally, these mice remain small (at 50% to 70% of normal weight), and catch-up growth does not occur. The offspring display no obvious developmental abnormalities and have normal bone development. Gene targeting of *IRS1* results in impairment of both growth and carbohydrate metabolism, compatible with its role in mediating both insulin and IGF-1 effects.[112,114] Growth is reduced 40% in *IRS2*-null mice that are also haploinsufficient for IRS-1, whereas growth is reduced 70% in *IRS1*-null mice also haploinsufficient for *IRS2*.[115] Thus IRS-2 cannot fully replace IRS-1 in this process. *IRS2*-null mice also exhibit a diabetic phenotype with peripheral insulin resistance and pancreatic beta cell failure.[113]

Downstream from IRS, *AKT1* and *AKT2* gene deletions also result in different phenotypes. Although *AKT2*-null mice exhibit insulin resistance,[116] at birth *AKT1*-null mice have a 20% reduction in body weight compared with wild-type mice.[117] The decrease in body weight in AKT-1–deficient mice persists throughout postnatal development regardless of sex, and glucose tolerance is normal.[117] These data demonstrate that AKT-1 is more important to the growth of the organism, both in utero and after birth, whereas AKT-2 is critical to insulin-dependent control of carbohydrate metabolism.

IGF axis gene knockouts are summarized in Table 140.2.

GROWTH FACTORS IN HUMAN FETAL GROWTH

PREGNANCY

During pregnancy, circulating levels of IGF-1 and IGF-2 rise in maternal serum and significantly in fetal serum,[118,119] and this may be regulated by placental GH, human placental lactogen (HPL), and nutritional factors.[120,121] Placental GH is not detected in the fetus, but HPL stimulates IGF-1 and IGF-2 production in fetal tissue.[122] As previously discussed, bioavailable IGF can be modulated by binding proteins, and significant changes in binding protein concentrations are seen in pregnancy. Maternal IGFBP-1 levels rise 5- to 10-fold during gestation,[118] probably as a manifestation of the insulin resistance of pregnancy. IGFBP-1 levels are substantial in amniotic fluid, where they may have a fetal renal or hepatic source. A negative correlation exists between term IGFBP-1 levels in maternal serum or IGFBP-1 levels in amniotic fluid at 16 weeks gestation and fetal weight.[30,123] IGFBP-1 phosphorylation increases its binding with IGF-1, reducing its bioavailability. Increased concentrations of phosphorylated IGFBP-1 in amniotic fluid is also associated with lower birthweight.[124] Thus IGFBP-1 in amniotic fluid may modulate fetal IGF action through altering its bioavailability.

Pregnancy-associated IGFBP-3 protease activity, which has been shown to appear after 6 weeks gestation, is responsible for the decrease in and progressive disappearance of intact IGFBP-3 on Western ligand blot analysis (without a change in IGFBP-3 immunoreactivity) and the appearance of lower-molecular-weight fragments of IGFBP-3 with a lower affinity for IGFs.[125,126] It has been demonstrated that IGFBP-2, IGFBP-4, and IGFBP-5 also undergo proteolysis during pregnancy.[29,30,127] Pregnancy serum protease may play a role in regulating IGF bioactivity by making IGFs more available to the cells.[128] Therefore it is possible that this proteolytic activity could affect placental and, consequently, fetal growth by releasing free IGFs and allowing increased receptor binding. This is supported by recent data showing reduced birth weight (*Z*-score ranging from −1.3 to −2.2) in infants with pathogenic mutations in *PAPPA2*.[39]

IGFBP-4 elevation in maternal serum in the first trimester is associated with fetal growth restriction, and it is postulated that IGFBP-4/IGF-2 complexes in the placental bed play a role in regulating placental development.[129] Protease processing of this complex may regulate IGF-2 bioavailability, explaining the fetal growth restriction associated with excess IGFBP-4 excess in humans or IGFBP-4 deficiency in the knockout mouse model.[130]

Other circulating maternal growth factors, including EGF, PDGF, FGF-2, FGF-4, and TGF-β, are also increased in pregnancy[131] and the potential mechanisms for each of these in promoting fetal and placental growth are discussed elsewhere in this chapter. FGF21 plays a role in regulating insulin, glucose, and lipid metabolism,[132] and its production in the placenta is associated with increased expression of glucose transporters in gestational diabetes.[133] Maternal serum FGF21 levels have been demonstrated to be increased in preeclampsia, suggesting a role in regulating placental metabolism.[134] However, further studies have not shown increased maternal levels or placental expression in preeclampsia.[135] Thus, although FGF21 appears to be negatively correlated with early infant growth,[136] its role in regulating fetal growth remains unclear.

IGF AXIS EXPRESSION BY THE FETUS

Available data regarding the earliest expression of the IGF axis in the human embryo are limited. The addition of growth factors to culture media for pre-implantation human embryos improve efficacy of in vitro fertilization, suggesting that the human embryo is responsive to these even at this early stage.[137] In the trophoblast, *IGF2* mRNA is detected by days 12 to 18,[138,139] and soon after, mRNA encoding the type 1 and 2 receptors also can be found.[140] The animal data demonstrating IGF-2 expression before that of IGF-1 indicate the importance of IGF-2 in early embryogenesis. Expression of IGFs is widespread in all human tissues during the second trimester.[141] Western immunoblotting techniques have demonstrated that type 2 IGF receptors are present in most human fetal tissues at 23 weeks.[142] The widespread expression and action of IGFs in embryogenesis are mostly autocrine-paracrine in nature and GH-independent. Although the control of IGF levels in the fetus is not well understood, IGF actions are thought to occur in concert with other hormones and growth factors and to be greatly influenced by the presence and distribution of IGFBPs. Techniques of immunocytochemistry, in situ hybridization, and Northern blot analysis have identified IGFBP-1 through IGFBP-6 in most fetal tissues.[143,144] Synthesis and secretion of IGFBPs are tissue-specific.[142]

In the third trimester, fetal serum IGF-1 concentrations steadily increase, correlating with the time of peak fetal weight gain. Although fetal serum IGF-1 levels are lower than those in adults, several investigators have reported that maternal and fetal cord serum IGF-1 levels correlated with birth weight,[145–149] suggesting co-regulation by nutritional factors. However, this correlation has not been a consistent finding in every study.[118] Insulin levels appear to affect IGF levels as well, although this effect may be secondary. Fetal IGF-2 levels have shown a correlation with birth weight in some studies but not in others.[145–148,150] The animal studies presented in the previous section indicate that IGFs are not under endocrine control prenatally and that GH deficiency, although affecting postnatal growth, does not result in significant prenatal growth retardation. Nevertheless, data from humans with hypopituitarism do support a role of GH in third-trimester fetal growth, because these infants, although demonstrating overall growth still within the normal range, often have mean birth lengths 0.8 to 1.7 standard deviation scores below the mean.[151,152] Furthermore, neonates with GH insensitivity (resulting in Laron syndrome) also are small at birth (−1.59 mean standard deviation score [SDS] for height), and their serum levels of IGF-1 and IGF-2 are low at birth as well.[153] The phenotype of severe IUGR in patients with mutations of the *IGF1* gene proves that IGF-1 plays a critical part in human fetal growth, independently of GH.[86,87,154]

The IGFBP profile for cord serum differs from that for adult serum. IGFBP-3 is low, with relative predominance of IGFBP-2.[146] Furthermore, IGFBP-1 levels in cord serum are up to 10 times higher than levels seen in adults and decline markedly during the first week of life. IGFBP-1 levels show a negative correlation with birth weight. In addition, correlation between IGFBP-1 and insulin level has been demonstrated both in infants who are born LGA and those with IUGR. In LGA infants born to nondiabetic mothers, significantly elevated insulin levels are associated with decreased IGFBP-1 levels; an opposite trend is seen in IUGR infants.[155] An alternative link has been proposed where maternal undernutrition is associated with reduced fetal hepatic mammalian target of rapamycin (mTOR)C1 activity, leading to IGFBP-1 hyperphosphorylation and fetal growth restriction.[156]

INTRAUTERINE GROWTH RESTRICTION

IUGR is defined by a birth weight or length 2 or more standard deviations below the mean (i.e., −2 SD) for gestational age and gender, a cutoff that corresponds approximately to the 3rd percentile for gestational age. A total of 3,957,577 infants were born in the United States in 2013; of these, approximately 91,000 were affected with IUGR, as determined using an overall prevalence rate of 2.3%.[157]

IUGR may result from diverse genetic and environmental influences on the developing fetus: chromosomal defects, maternal nutrition, genetics, or decreased uteroplacental blood flow. Disproportional IUGR can result from circulatory changes in the fetus that favor redistribution of blood flow to the heart and brain. In severe IUGR, head size is compromised as well. Endocrine factors appear to play a role in the pathogenesis of IUGR. Decreased levels of placental GH and maternal IGF-1 have been demonstrated in IUGR.[158] In both preterm and full-term infants, low birth weight is associated with low cord serum IGF-1, IGF-2, and IGFBP-3, and high IGFBP-1.[a] However, some investigators have demonstrated more variable IGF levels in infants with IUGR,[118] indicating that this single marker may underestimate the complexity of this condition and the heterogeneity of its causes. IGFBP-2 levels may be higher, similar to those seen in patients with hypopituitarism postnatally.[155] The increase in IGFBP-1 (mostly of hepatic origin) appears to be the result of inadequate nutrient supply, with resultant hypoinsulinemia.

It has been speculated that the elevated IGFBP-1 levels in these infants may induce sequestration of IGFs, thereby restricting fetal growth. Not only are alterations in IGF levels seen in children with IUGR, but also the IGF type 1 receptor affinity was reduced in a subgroup of patients with IUGR.[161] The finding of a homozygous deletions of *IGF1* in a handful of patients with severe IUGR[86,87,154] implicates IGF-1 in the etiology of this disorder, but larger studies looking for *IGF1* mutations in larger groups of children born with IUGR have failed to identify them, suggesting that these mutations are not a common cause of IUGR.[162–164] Conversely, an association between a polymorphism of the *IGF1* gene and low serum IGF-1 levels was found in a study involving children with short stature born small for gestational age (SGA), suggesting that genetically determined low serum IGF-1 levels may lead not only to reduction in birth length, weight, and head circumference but also to persistent short stature.[165] TGF-β also has been implicated in the pathogenesis of IUGR. TGF-β cord blood levels were found to be significantly lower in pregnancies complicated by IUGR than those in "control pregnancies," in which children were born at a weight appropriate for gestational age (AGA).[58]

A majority of children born with IUGR will experience adequate catch-up growth in length during the first 2 years of life. Postnatal catch-up growth usually begins immediately after birth, and in fact, most of the increases in SDS for height occur by 6 months of age.[166,167] McCowan and co-workers[168] showed that 40 of 203 infants (20%) born SGA remained short and 31 (16%) remained light at 6 months. Around 2 years of age, most children born SGA tend not to exhibit further catch-up growth, and approximately 10% will remain at −2 SD or below for height throughout childhood and adolescence and into adulthood, indicating a persistent failure to achieve normal linear growth. In one study of a large population of neonates with follow-up to adulthood, height was measured at the age of 20 to 21 years. Compared with an AGA control population, the SGA subjects were 4 to 6 cm shorter as adults.[169]

In 2001, the use of recombinant human GH was approved by the US Food and Drug Administration (FDA) for the long-term treatment of growth failure in children born SGA who fail to manifest catch-up growth by the age of 2 years. Multiple studies have demonstrated the efficacy of GH therapy in promoting catch-up growth in children born with IUGR.[170–177] Some of these studies also have demonstrated positive effects of GH therapy on body composition, blood pressure, and lipid metabolism.[b] Although decreased insulin sensitivity has been reported in SGA children on GH treatment, glucose tolerance remained normal,[183] and fasting insulin and glucose levels returned to the levels in control subjects after the discontinuation of treatment.[181] Thus far, the evidence suggests that GH therapy in short children born SGA is safe and efficacious.[181,183]

Growth restriction during the fetal period has been associated with a higher prevalence of such conditions as hypertension, cardiovascular disease, and type 2 diabetes in adult life.[184,185] These findings constitute the basis for the fetal origins of the adult disease hypothesis, which proposes that insults in utero lead to "reprogramming" of the endocrine system, which in turn predisposes infants born with IUGR to adverse health outcomes in adulthood. Lifelong programming of the IGF system by the intrauterine hormonal and nutritional environment has been suggested to be a key mediator of the link between small size at birth and cardiovascular disease in adulthood.[159] An increased prevalence of metabolic syndrome (consisting of obesity, cardiovascular disease, hypertension, and type 2 diabetes) has been reported among adults who were born SGA.[186] In addition to risk factors associated with IUGR, increasing evidence suggests that rapid postnatal catch-up growth further enhances risk for development of obesity and the metabolic syndrome.[187,188] Insulin resistance has been linked to thinness at birth followed by obesity in adulthood.[189,190]

MACROSOMIA

Alterations in the IGF axis also have been demonstrated in infants who are LGA, including those born to diabetic mothers (Fig. 140.2 and Table 140.3). In these infants, IGF-1, insulin, and IGFBP-3 levels are increased, whereas IGFBP-1 levels are significantly decreased.[155] Fetal hyperinsulinemia secondary to maternal diabetes mellitus results in increased body fat, with a more modest increase in body length. Insulin promotes fetal growth by permitting nutrient uptake, and increased

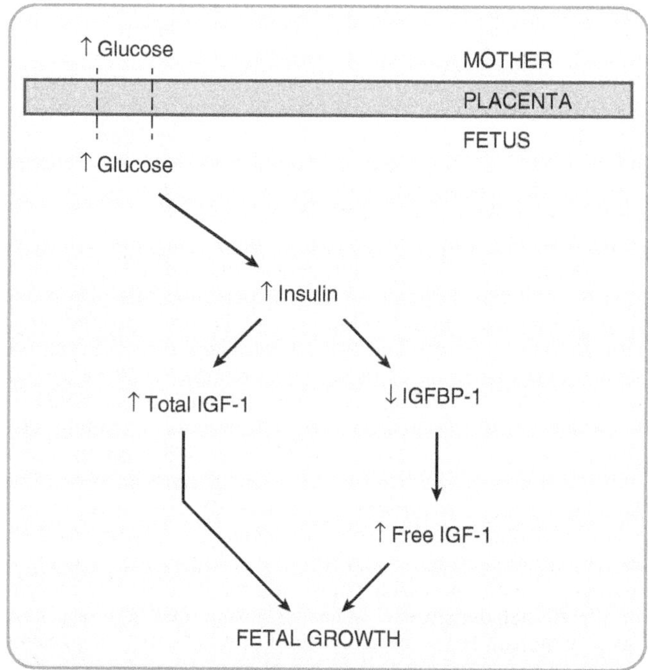

Fig. 140.2 The interrelationships among maternal and fetal glucose, insulin, insulin-like growth factor 1 *(IGF-1)*, and insulin-like growth factor binding protein 1 *(IGFBP-1)* levels in the regulation of fetal growth and the evolution of macrosomia.

Table 140.3 IGF Axis Findings Seen in Extremes of Human Fetal Growth.

Growth Pattern	IGF-1	IGF-2	IGFBP-1	IGFBP-2	IGFBP-3
Intrauterine growth restriction	↓	↓	↑	↑	↓
Large for gestational age	↑	Normal or ↑	↓	Normal	↑

IGF, Insulin-like growth factor; *IGFBP*, IGF-binding protein.

[a]References 123, 146, 147, 155, 159, 160.
[b]References 152, 153, 155, 176, 178–182.

IGF-1 production may be a result of the nutritional state of these infants.[191] The alterations in IGFBP-1 also appear to be secondary to the higher insulin levels, but IGF-1 levels and nutritional status also may play a role.

Infants with the Beckwith-Wiedemann syndrome have a doubling in *IGF2* gene dosage as a result of alterations at chromosomal locus 11p15.5. These infants are macrosomic and often demonstrate evidence of congenital hyperinsulinism. Placental hypertrophy is seen as well.[192] In the limited studies that have been performed, levels of IGF-2 are not increased in cord serum in these infants, but it is possible that *IGF2* gene dosage may increase fetal growth through the stimulation of placental growth.[193] These infants also are predisposed to the development of IGF-2-dependent neoplasms, such as Wilms tumor. In fact, in an analysis of birth weights for more than 1800 patients with Wilms tumor, the mean was significantly greater than the national average, especially for those with Beckwith-Wiedemann syndrome or hemihypertrophy, suggesting the presence of systemic growth effects of IGF-2 on both fetal size and the development of Wilms tumor.[194] Of interest, single-nucleotide polymorphisms in *H19*, a maternally imprinted gene implicated in translational regulation of *IGF2*, when identified in either offspring or maternal DNA, have been associated with elevated cord blood IGF-2 levels and higher birth weight.[195] This evidence suggests a role for *H19* in controlling fetal growth restraint through the regulation of IGF-2.

CONCLUSION

Local IGFs and IGFBPs are of prime importance in fetal and placental growth. Genetic manipulations of IGF axis components in fetal mice have further clarified the roles of these agents. Undoubtedly, the coming years will bring even more new information on the physiology and pathology of these key cellular regulators. These discoveries are likely to lead to the increasing use of diagnostic tests and to the recognition of genetic mutations of the GH-IGF axis in cases of IUGR, as well as to therapeutic applications of these agents.

 A complete reference list is available at www.ExpertConsult.com.

SELECT REFERENCES

1. Vottero A, Guzzetti C, Loche S. New aspects of the physiology of the GH-IGF-1 axis. *Endocr Dev*. 2013;24:96-105.
2. Cohen P. Overview of the IGF-I system. *Horm Res*. 2006;65(suppl 1):3-8.
3. Denley A, Cosgrove LJ, Booker GW, et al. Molecular interactions of the IGF system. *Cytokine Growth Factor Rev*. 2005;16:421-439.
4. Pena-Almazan S, Buchlis J, Miller S, et al. Linear growth characteristics of congenitally GH-deficient infants from birth to one year of age. *J Clin Endocrinol Metab*. 2001;86:5691-5694.
5. Philippou A, Maridaki M, Pneumaticos S, et al. The complexity of the IGF1 gene splicing, posttranslational modification and bioactivity. *Mol Med*. 2014;20:202-214.
6. Erondu NE, Dake BL, Moser DR, et al. Regulation of endothelial IGFBP-3 synthesis and secretion by IGF-I and TGF-beta. *Growth Regul*. 1996;6:1-9.
10. Frasca F, Pandini G, Scalia P, et al. Insulin receptor isoform A, a newly recognized, high-affinity insulin-like growth factor II receptor in fetal and cancer cells. *Mol Cell Biol*. 1999;19:3278-3288.
11. Giudice J, Barcos LS, Guaimas FF, et al. Insulin and insulin like growth factor II endocytosis and signaling via insulin receptor B. *Cell Commun Signal*. 2013;11:18.
12. Morcavallo A, Genua M, Palummo A, et al. Insulin and insulin-like growth factor II differentially regulate endocytic sorting and stability of insulin receptor isoform A. *J Biol Chem*. 2012;287:11422-11436.
14. Kalscheuer VM, Mariman EC, Schepens MT, et al. The insulin-like growth factor type-2 receptor gene is imprinted in the mouse but not in humans. *Nat Genet*. 1993;5:74-78.
15. Moxham CP, Duronio V, Jacobs S. Insulin-like growth factor I receptor beta-subunit heterogeneity. Evidence for hybrid tetramers composed of insulin-like growth factor I and insulin receptor heterodimers. *J Biol Chem*. 1989;264:13238-13244.
16. Pandini G, Frasca F, Mineo R, et al. Insulin/insulin-like growth factor I hybrid receptors have different biological characteristics depending on the insulin receptor isoform involved. *J Biol Chem*. 2002;277:39684-39695.
18. Kitamura T, Kido Y, Nef S, et al. Preserved pancreatic beta-cell development and function in mice lacking the insulin receptor-related receptor. *Mol Cell Biol*. 2001;21:5624-5630.
21. Firth SM, Baxter RC. Cellular actions of the insulin-like growth factor binding proteins. *Endocr Rev*. 2002;23:824-854.
22. Baxter RC, Binoux M, Clemmons DR, et al. Recommendations for nomenclature of the insulin-like growth factor binding protein (IGFBP) superfamily. *Growth Horm IGF Res*. 1998;8:273-274.
25. Cohen P, Lamson G, Okajima T, et al. Transfection of the human insulin-like growth factor binding protein-3 gene into Balb/c fibroblasts inhibits cellular growth. *Mol Endocrinol*. 1993;7:380-386.
27. Grimberg A, Liu B, Bannerman P, El-Deiry WS, Cohen P. IGFBP-3 mediates p53-induced apoptosis during serum starvation. *Int J Oncol*. 2002;21(2):327-335.
30. Giudice LC, Farrell EM, Pham H, et al. Insulin-like growth factor binding proteins in maternal serum throughout gestation and in the puerperium: effects of a pregnancy-associated serum protease activity. *J Clin Endocrinol Metab*. 1990;71:806-816.
32. Katz LEL, Cohen P, Rosenfeld RG. Clinical significance of IGF binding proteins. *Endocrinologist*. 1995;5(1):36-43.
38. Cohen P, Peehl DM, Graves HC, et al. Biological effects of prostate specific antigen as an insulin-like growth factor binding protein-3 protease. *J Endocrinol*. 1994;142:407-415.
39. Dauber A, Munoz-Calvo MT, Barrios V, et al. Mutations in pregnancy-associated plasma protein A2 cause short stature due to low IGF-I availability. *EMBO Mol Med*. 2016;8:363-374.
40. Fujimoto M, Hwa V, Dauber A. Novel modulators of the growth hormone - insulin-like growth factor axis: pregnancy-associated plasma protein-a2 and stanniocalcin-2. *J Clin Res Pediatr Endocrinol*. 2017;9:1-8.
42. Boldt HB, Conover CA. Pregnancy-associated plasma protein-A (PAPP-A): a local regulator of IGF bioavailability through cleavage of IGFBPs. *Growth Horm IGF Res*. 2007;17:10-18.
47. Ornitz DM. FGF signaling in the developing endochondral skeleton. *Cytokine Growth Factor Rev*. 2005;16:205-213.
50. Miettinen PJ, Berger JE, Meneses J, et al. Epithelial immaturity and multiorgan failure in mice lacking epidermal growth factor receptor. *Nature*. 1995;376:337-341.
52. Kamei Y, Tsutsumi O, Yamakawa A, et al. Maternal epidermal growth factor deficiency causes fetal hypoglycemia and intrauterine growth retardation in mice: possible involvement of placental glucose transporter GLUT3 expression. *Endocrinology*. 1999;140:4236-4243.
53. Lee DC, Rose TM, Webb NR, et al. Cloning and sequence analysis of a cDNA for rat transforming growth factor-alpha. *Nature*. 1985;313:489-491.
58. Ostlund E, Tally M, Fried G. Transforming growth factor-beta1 in fetal serum correlates with insulin-like growth factor-I and fetal growth. *Obstet Gynecol*. 2002;100:567-573.
59. Attisano L, Wrana JL. Signal transduction by the TGF-beta superfamily. *Science*. 2002;296:1646-1647.
61. Hahnel A, Schultz GA. Insulin-like growth factor binding proteins are transcribed by preimplantation mouse embryos. *Endocrinology*. 1994;134:1956-1959.
66. Camacho-Hubner C, Clemmons DR, D'Ercole AJ. Regulation of insulin-like growth factor (IGF) binding proteins in transgenic mice with altered expression of growth hormone and IGF-I. *Endocrinology*. 1991;129:1201-1206.
70. Dai Z, Xing Y, Boney CM, et al. Human insulin-like growth factor-binding protein-1 (hIGFBP-1) in transgenic mice: characterization and insights into the regulation of IGFBP-1 expression. *Endocrinology*. 1994;135:1316-1327.
74. Modric T, Silha JV, Shi Z, et al. Phenotypic manifestations of insulin-like growth factor-binding protein-3 overexpression in transgenic mice. *Endocrinology*. 2001;142:1958-1967.
78. Baker J, Liu JP, Robertson EJ, et al. Role of insulin-like growth factors in embryonic and postnatal growth. *Cell*. 1993;75:73-82.
79. DeChiara TM, Efstratiadis A, Robertson EJ. A growth-deficiency phenotype in heterozygous mice carrying an insulin-like growth factor II gene disrupted by targeting. *Nature*. 1990;345:78-80.
80. Yakar S, Adamo ML. Insulin-like growth factor 1 physiology: lessons from mouse models. *Endocrinol Metab Clin North Am*. 2012;41:231-247, v.
81. DeChiara TM, Robertson EJ, Efstratiadis A. Parental imprinting of the mouse insulin-like growth factor II gene. *Cell*. 1991;64:849-859.
82. Liu JP, Baker J, Perkins AS, et al. Mice carrying null mutations of the genes encoding insulin-like growth factor I (Igf-1) and type 1 IGF receptor (Igf1r). *Cell*. 1993;75:59-72.
89. Ueki I, Ooi GT, Tremblay ML, et al. Inactivation of the acid labile subunit gene in mice results in mild retardation of postnatal growth despite profound disruptions in the circulating insulin-like growth factor system. *Proc Natl Acad Sci U S A*. 2000;97:6868-6873.
90. Domene HM, Bengolea SV, Martinez AS, et al. Deficiency of the circulating insulin-like growth factor system associated with inactivation of the acid-labile subunit gene. *N Engl J Med*. 2004;350:570-577.
91. Hwa V, Haeusler G, Pratt KL, et al. Total absence of functional acid labile subunit, resulting in severe insulin-like growth factor deficiency and moderate growth failure. *J Clin Endocrinol Metab*. 2006;91:1826-1831.

93. Abuzzahab MJ, Schneider A, Goddard A, et al. IGF-I receptor mutations resulting in intrauterine and postnatal growth retardation. *N Engl J Med*. 2003;349:2211-2222.
95. Walenkamp MJ, van der Kamp HJ, Pereira AM, et al. A variable degree of intrauterine and postnatal growth retardation in a family with a missense mutation in the insulin-like growth factor I receptor. *J Clin Endocrinol Metab*. 2006;91:3062-3070.
96. Constancia M, Hemberger M, Hughes J, et al. Placental-specific IGF-II is a major modulator of placental and fetal growth. *Nature*. 2002;417:945-948.
99. Wang ZQ, Fung MR, Barlow DP, et al. Regulation of embryonic growth and lysosomal targeting by the imprinted Igf2/Mpr gene. *Nature*. 1994;372:464-467.
149. Hawkes CP, Grimberg A, Kenny LC, et al. The relationship between IGF-I and -II concentrations and body composition at birth and over the first 2 months. *Pediatr Res*. 2019;85:687-692.
150. Hawkes CP, Murray DM, Kenny LC, et al. Correlation of insulin-like growth factor-i and -ii concentrations at birth measured by mass spectrometry and growth from birth to two months. *Horm Res Paediatr*. 2018;89:122-131.
172. Ranke MB, Lindberg A. Growth hormone treatment of short children born small for gestational age or with Silver-Russell syndrome: results from KIGS (Kabi International Growth Study), including the first report on final height. *Acta Paediatr Suppl*. 1996;417:18-26.
193. Deal CL, Guyda HJ, Lai WH, et al. Ontogeny of growth factor receptors in the human placenta. *Pediatr Res*. 1982;16:820-826.

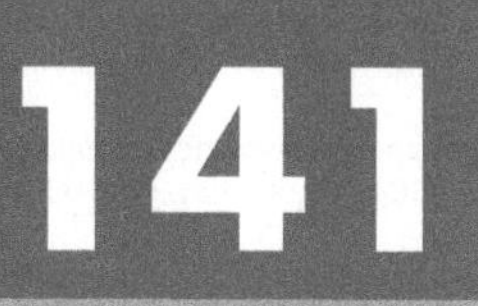

Growth Hormone, Prolactin, and Placental Lactogen in the Fetus and Newborn

Nursen Gurtunca | Mark A. Sperling

INTRODUCTION AND BACKGROUND

In the fully developed organism, growth hormone (GH), a 22-kDa molecule of 191 amino acids,[1] is synthesized by acidophil cells in the anterior pituitary gland under the direction of hypothalamic GH-releasing hormone,[2] which binds to its G protein–coupled receptor to stimulate GH secretion, and via somatotropin release–inhibiting factor, also known as *somatostatin,* an inhibitor of GH release in a "dominant negative" manner. The interplay of positive and negative signals results in a pulsatile release of GH.[2] In addition, the anterior pituitary contains a distinct and separate GH secretagogue receptor.[3] The endogenous ligand for GH secretagogue receptor is the gastric hormone ghrelin, which is released by the sensing of hunger, and acts to stimulate GH release[4] to mobilize fuels via metabolic effects on fat, muscle, and liver, and induce insulin resistance to diminish the risk for hypoglycemia. Sleep augments GH release by increasing the amplitude of pulses; increased secretion occurs during the first phase of slow-wave sleep (stages III to IV).[5] A variety of signals can augment GH secretion, including α-adrenergic stimuli,[6] dopa, opioids, sex hormones (primarily estrogen),[6] glucagon, and certain amino acids, especially arginine.[6] Glucocorticoids and hypothyroidism blunt GH secretion.[7]

Therefore, GH secretion is influenced by a variety of physiologic and nonphysiologic states that also form the basis for GH stimulation tests in the evaluation of GH reserves. The maturation of GH-releasing hormone secretion in the fetus precedes that of somatotropin release–inhibiting factor. Hence, GH secretion is stimulated in the absence of restraint by somatotropin release–inhibiting factor, and consequently, GH levels are high in the fetus and newborn infant and range from 20 to 50 ng/mL in the first few weeks of life. These levels gradually decline to below 10 ng/mL.[8] Normal functional maturation of pulsatile GH secretion is not attained until several months of postnatal life in the term infant.[9] High GH levels in the newborn may be partly related to diminished GH sensitivity and growth hormone receptor (GHR) immaturity.[10]

From a diagnostic point of view, this has the advantage that screening for GH deficiency in the newborn does not require stimulation tests. A random GH level of 10 ng/mL or lower in the newborn is virtually diagnostic of GH deficiency. GH deficiency may be associated with hypoglycemia, requires evaluation of other pituitary hormone deficiencies that provide clues to the genetic defect responsible, and requires magnetic resonance imaging for determination of anatomic maldevelopment. Genetic studies using sequencing techniques such as targeted exome sequencing can be utilized to make a specific molecular diagnosis.[11]

The gastric hormone ghrelin is also capable of directly stimulating GH release and increasing the GH response to GH-releasing hormone.[4] The role of ghrelin in fetal GH secretion is not known. GH secretion is also regulated in a negative feedback fashion by insulin-like growth factor 1 (IGF-1), a member of the insulin-like growth factor family of peptides.[12] In the fully mature organism, GH stimulates the production and release of IGF-1 from the liver after interacting with its cognate receptors, and this is the major source of circulating IGF-1; smaller amounts of IGF-1 may be produced after GH interacts with its receptors at local tissue sites, such as bone.[13]

The effects of GH on growth are mediated in part by direct effects on bone and via the generation of IGF-1 (Fig. 141.1). To do so, GH must interact with its cognate receptor, GHR, via a process mediated by the Janus kinase 2-signal transducer and activator of transcription 5 signaling cascade.[14] GHR belongs to the cytokine family of receptors. In humans, after binding GH, the extracellular binding domain of GHR is released into the circulation as GH-binding protein, which can be measured as an indirect reflection of GHR.[15] IGF-1 from the liver is coupled with a binding protein (insulin-like growth factor–binding protein 3) and the acid-labile subunit as a ternary complex transporting IGF-1 in the circulation.[12] IGF-1 also can be generated in bone, muscle, and fat, but the predominant source in the circulation is the liver.[16]

GH is so named because of its dramatic effects in those with excessive GH-secreting conditions, gigantism if onset is before closure of the epiphyses, and acromegaly if onset begins after puberty. This growth is caused in part by direct effects of GH itself and in part by a "second messenger," IGF-1. However,

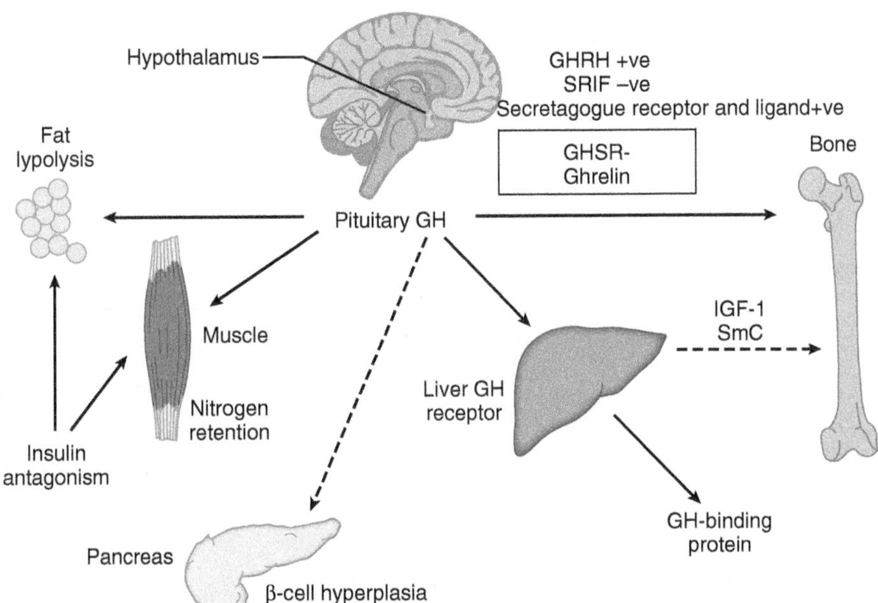

Fig. 141.1 Growth hormone secretion and action. *GH*, Growth hormone; *GHRH*, growth hormone–releasing hormone; *GHSR*, growth hormone secretagogue receptor; *IGF*, insulin-like receptor; *SmC*, somatomedin C; *SRIF*, somatotropin release–inhibiting factor.

GH has profound direct effects on metabolic functions. These include lipolysis with release of fatty acids and their subsequent mitochondrial conversion to ketone bodies that can be used as a source of energy,[17] as well as the augmentation of amino acid uptake and nitrogen retention by muscle.[18] In addition, GH induces resistance to insulin's effects on carbohydrate metabolism, which is compensated by an increase in pancreatic insulin secretion and hyperplasia of pancreatic β cells in young organisms.[19] However, pancreatic "exhaustion" can lead to various degrees of carbohydrate intolerance, including diabetes, in the older organism.[20] Notably, the resistance to insulin's effects on carbohydrate is not shared by muscle or fat[21]; GH has synergistic effects on muscle anabolism via insulin, as well as via sex steroids.[22] Thus GH, in addition to its growth-promoting effects, is a major regulator of metabolism, acting to counter insulin effects to avoid hypoglycemia (i.e., it is one of the counterregulatory hormones together with glucagon, catecholamines, and cortisol), promoting lipolysis in response to fasting, and regulating muscle anabolism.

The consequences of deficiency or excess of GH secretion and action become apparent from consideration of the growth-promoting and metabolic effects of this hormone system. Deficiency of GH promotes fasting hypoglycemia, poor muscle development, excessive body fat, poor growth, and diminished bone mass. Conversely, excessive secretion and action of GH result in rapid growth, well-developed muscles with large bones, increased lean body mass, and possibly impaired carbohydrate tolerance. The degree and severity of these features depend on the degree of deficiency/excess of the hormone and timing. The developmental aspects of these coordinated actions form the basis of this chapter.

DEVELOPMENTAL ASPECTS OF GROWTH HORMONE SECRETION AND ACTION

Growth of the human is fastest in fetal life and continues at a fast but rapidly decelerating rate in the neonatal period. Fetal growth is determined by genetic, nutritional, and environmental factors.[23] Maternal environmental influences are the most important determinant of fetal growth. However, several genetic conditions causing growth factor deficiencies may play a role in intrauterine growth retardation. *IGF1* mutations and deletions have been associated with intrauterine growth failure.[24] Genetic defects in *IGF2* have also been identified to cause both prenatal and postnatal growth failure due to insulin-like growth factor 2 (IGF-2) deficiency.[25] External environmental factors such as nutrition and good general health are the key factors in normal growth in early infancy. Although the GH-IGF-1 axis has significant roles in childhood growth, growth in the fetus and the newborn is not determined by GH because GHR is poorly expressed in fetal life and appears to become functional at approximately 3 to 6 months of life.[26] However, GH levels are high in the newborn, and although they assist in limiting hypoglycemia in the newborn, the full functional significance of these high concentrations is not clear.[27] Understanding the natural patterns of developmental and functional changes in pituitary hormone-producing cells during the fetal and perinatal period will help to differentiate normal and adverse development.

THE DEVELOPMENT OF THE HYPOTHALAMOPITUITARY AXIS

The pituitary gland is formed from two distinct embryologic sources.[28] Known as the *adenohypophysis*, the anterior pituitary gland is formed by an invagination of the oral cavity (stomodeal ectoderm) called *Rathke pouch*. The posterior pituitary originates from the floor of the forebrain (neural ectoderm) and is known as the *neurohypophysis*. The adenohypophysis constitutes 80% of the weight of the pituitary gland and comprises three parts: pars distalis, pars intermedia, and pars infundibularis. In humans, most of the hormone-producing cells are found in the pars distalis. The pars intermedia is rudimentary and largely disappears during embryogenesis. The pars infundibularis extends upwards to the pituitary stalk and may contain limited numbers of gonadotropin-producing cells. The pars distalis and pars intermedia are separated by a cleft, a rudimentary structure of Rathke pouch from which the anterior pituitary develops. This vestigial structure may often persist as a Rathke's cleft cyst. The neurohypophysis consists of the posterior lobe, infundibular stalk, and median eminence of the tuber cinereum. The posterior pituitary gland contains the terminal axons of the neurons from the paraventricular and supraoptic nuclei of the hypothalamus. These nuclei and neurons produce oxytocin, which has smooth muscle and vasoconstrictor properties required during childbirth and lactation, as well as vasopressin, which is required for osmotic regulation.

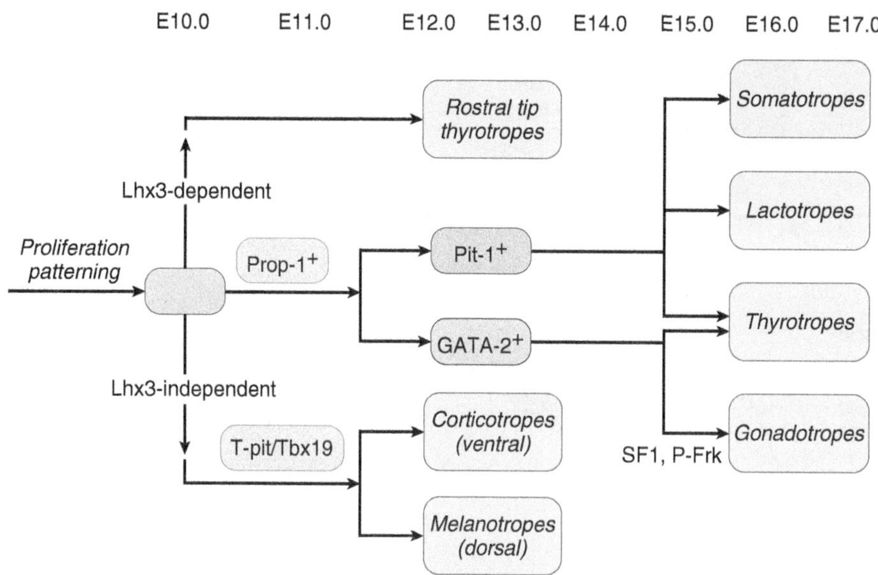

Fig. 141.2 Transcription factors and differentiation of cell lineage of the anterior pituitary in the mouse. Transcription factors are highlighted in *yellow.* Pluripotent cells are *gray*. Pituitary-specific positive transcription factor 1 *(Pit-1)*-positive cells in *pink* proliferate into three Pit-1-dependent cell types. GATA-2-positive cells in *blue* differentiate into gonadotrophs through activation of steroidogenic factor 1 *(SF1)* and the transcription factor pituitary forkhead factor *(P-Frk)*, and into thyrotrophs in the absence of SF1 and P-Frk. Terminal hormone-producing cells are *green,* with the hormones they produce superimposed on the cell types. *Lhx3,* LIM homeobox 3; *Prop-1,* prophet of pituitary-specific positive transcription factor 1; *Tbx19;* T-box 19. (From Scully KM, Rosenfeld MG. Pituitary development: regulatory codes in mammalian organogenesis. *Science* 2002;295:2231–2235.)

Rathke pouch is present as an indentation at the roof of the oral cavity by the third gestational week.[29] This indentation turns into Rathke pouch and completely disconnects from the oral ectoderm by the end of the sixth week of gestation. GH-producing cells can be identified by the ninth gestational week. The vascular connections between the anterior pituitary lobe and the hypothalamus that control anterior pituitary function develop at the same time. Apposition and interaction between oral ectoderm and neuroectoderm are critical for the initiation of anterior pituitary development, normal progression of development, and anterior pituitary cell differentiation. Although GH-producing cells, somatotrophs, are demonstrable from the anterior pituitary in the anencephalic newborn, initiation of development and normal differentiation and function of the hormone-producing cells are dependent on the interaction between the diencephalon and the oral ectoderm.

GH-, prolactin-, and thyroid-stimulating hormone–producing cells develop from common progenitor cells under the influence of the developmental cascade of genes and epigenetic mechanisms (Fig. 141.2).[30] Although Fig. 141.2 describes the genes and timing of events relevant to mouse development, similar processes apply to human development.

The expression of specific genes and the signaling through the transcription factors at each stage of development determine the fate of the progenitor cells.[31] Identification of the developmental cascade of genes implicated in human pituitary development clarifies the many congenital defects associated with pituitary development and function.[32] Advances in diagnostic genetic tools, such as next-generation sequencing including whole genome and exome sequencing, will uncover other genetic disorders that cause intrauterine growth retardation.[33] Knowledge of specific gene defects can direct the clinical options for management,[34] although phenotype and severity may be variable even with the same gene variants.[34a] Abnormalities in the *HESX1* gene (homeobox gene expressed in embryonic stem cells 1) give rise to hypoplasia/aplasia of the optic chiasm, as well as other anatomic midline defects that constitute the syndrome of septo-optic dysplasia, and may occur together with hypothalamic/pituitary dysfunction.[32] However, pituitary hormone deficiencies such as GH deficiency may not be apparent at birth. Nevertheless, a newborn with abnormalities of the eye or the optic nerve should be evaluated for pituitary hormone deficiencies. Adrenocorticotropic hormone deficiency and thyroid-stimulating hormone deficiency also need to be considered and determined early on, to prevent adrenal crisis and an unfavorable neurologic outcome, respectively.[32] Ectopic posterior pituitary and associated infundibular anomalies (interrupted, absent, or hypoplastic stalk) are classically associated with anterior pituitary hormone deficiencies and can be caused by defects in *HESX1* or *LHX4.* Typically, posterior pituitary function is preserved.[35]

Although GH does not play an important role in fetal growth,[36] the metabolic effects of GH deficiency can also have consequences in the newborn period, resulting in severe hypoglycemia, and prolonged jaundice with elevation of both indirect and direct bilirubin levels reflecting hepatocellular and obstructive liver injury. Gonadotropin (follicle-stimulating hormone and luteinizing hormone) deficiencies may present with micropenis in the newborn male because the pituitary-gonadal axis is functional in the third trimester.[37] Measurement of prolactin (PRL), another anterior pituitary hormone produced by acidophil cells that also produce GH, provides clues to the integrity of communication between the hypothalamus and the anterior pituitary gland, as PRL secretion is normally suppressed by hypothalamic L-dopa.[38] Hence, an elevated PRL level while GH levels are inappropriately low suggests a defect at the level of the hypothalamus, reducing the stimulation of pituitary GH by GH-releasing hormone, and reducing the inhibition of PRL provided by L-dopa. These hormonal abnormalities may or may not be clinically manifest at birth but can become progressively apparent subsequently.[38a]

The transcription factor prophet of pituitary-specific positive transcription factor 1 (PROP1) of the developmental cascade (see Fig. 141.2) further differentiates pituitary progenitor cells. Abnormalities of the *PROP1* gene result in combined pituitary hormone deficiencies with variable degrees of deficiencies of follicle-stimulating hormone, luteinizing hormone, GH, prolactin, thyroid-stimulating hormone, and at times adrenocorticotropic hormone.[39] *PROP1* mutations represent a relatively common cause

Table 141.1 Transcription Factors in Human Pituitary Development, Associated Deficiencies, and Their Inheritance Patterns.

Transcription Factor	Deficiencies/Syndrome	Inheritance
HESX1	Variable pituitary deficiency/septooptic dysplasia	Autosomal dominant or autosomal recessive
PROP1	Somatolactotroph, thyrotroph, gonadotroph, corticotroph/pituitary hyperplasia, or hypoplasia	Autosomal recessive
PIT-1	Somatolactotroph, thyrotroph/pituitary hypoplasia	Autosomal dominant or autosomal recessive
LHX3	Somatolactotroph, thyrotroph, gonadotroph/limited head and neck rotation	Autosomal recessive
LHX4	Variable pituitary deficiency/ectopic neurohypophysis; cerebellar abnormalities	Autosomal dominant

HESX1, Homeobox gene expressed in embryonic stem cells 1; *LHX3*, LIM homeobox 3; *LHX4*, LIM homeobox 4; *PIT-1*, pituitary-specific positive transcription factor 1; *PROP1*, prophet of pituitary-specific positive transcription factor 1.

of hypopituitarism.[40] PROP1 (also known as POU domain, class 1, transcription factor 1) is required for the differentiation of GH-, prolactin-, and thyroid-stimulating hormone–producing cells from a common progenitor (see Fig. 141.2). Therefore congenital and developmental abnormalities in one of these cell lines are likely associated with the defects in the other cell lines in distinct patterns that provide clues to the genetic defects.[41] Cells that are positive for the transcription factor GATA-2 (zinc finger transcription factor that binds nucleotide sequence GATA) are differentiated further to gonadotrophs.[42] GATA-2 also has a synergistic effect with PROP1 in the differentiation of thyrotrophs.[43] Table 141.1 presents transcription factor mutations associated with pituitary deficiencies and their inheritance pattern.

HYPOTHALAMIC-PITUITARY PORTAL SYSTEM

The portal circulatory system, which exists within the pituitary, is critical to normal pituitary function. The communication between the hypothalamus and anterior pituitary gland is through the pituitary portal circulatory system.[44] The main blood supply for the hypothalamic-pituitary portal system is derived from the superior and inferior hypophysial arteries, branches of the internal carotid artery. The anterior and posterior branches of the superior hypophysial artery terminate within the infundibulum and the proximal portion of the pituitary stalk and form the primary plexus of the hypophysial portal system. Peptides produced in hypothalamic neurons that terminate in the infundibulum enter the primary plexus of the hypophysial portal circulation and are transported by the hypophysial portal veins to the capillaries of the anterior pituitary gland. This portal system thus provides the important communication between hypothalamic neurons and the hormone-producing anterior pituitary cells. There is also communication between the different hormone-producing cells of the anterior pituitary, and this organized distribution of the hormone-producing cells facilitates the coordinated secretary pulses of hormones to their target tissues. The blood supply of the neurohypophysis comes from the inferior hypophysial artery, but posterior pituitary function is not regulated by the hypophysial portal circulation; there are direct neural connections from the diencephalon to the neurohypophysis that affect function.

GROWTH HORMONE

GH is secreted by the somatotrophs of the anterior pituitary gland.[45] Human GH is homologous with several other proteins produced by the pituitary or the placenta, including PRL, placental lactogen (chorionic somatomammotropin), and human GH variant (22 kDa) secreted only by the placenta.[46] The genes for these proteins share a common structural organization comprising four introns separating five exons and are probably descended from a common ancestral gene, though the genes are now located on different chromosomes; the *PRL* gene is located on chromosome 6 and the pituitary human GH (normal human GH) gene is located on chromosome band 17q24.2.[47] This locus contains four other related genes interspersed in the same transcriptional orientation thought to have evolved from a series of gene duplications.[47] Alternative splicing of these five GH variants provides a diversity of circulating isoforms.[47] These forms are expressed in the pituitary but not in the placenta.[47] The 217–amino acid GH precursor is produced in the somatotroph and is cleaved in the endoplasmic reticulum to its mature 191–amino acid 22-kDa single-chain, nonglycosylated protein.[48] The mature protein is transported to the Golgi apparatus and secretory granules. Zinc ions facilitate the formation of soluble GH dimer complexes for storage and secretion within the secretory granules.[49]

The importance of the pulsatile secretion of GH for its biologic action remains uncertain. GH can be detected in fetal serum by the end of the first trimester.[50] The levels of GH are higher in the preterm than the term infant, perhaps reflecting the maturation of the negative feedback from the higher IGF-1 concentrations in the term infant.[50] GH acts through its receptor (GHR), a class 1 hematopoietic cytokine receptor that is homologous to prolactin receptor (PRLR) and other cytokine receptors such as interleukins, interferon, granulocyte-macrophage colony-stimulating factor, erythropoietin, and leptin.[51] GHR is located on chromosome band 5p13-p12,[14] so deletions in this region will result in deficient GH action and variable degrees of GH insensitivity syndrome, including short stature postnatally, although similarly to GH deficiency, birth size is not greatly affected.[52] Binding of GH to its receptor induces intracellular Janus kinase 2–signal transducer and activator of transcription 5 and other signaling intermediates that result in its biologic action, including growth and other metabolic effects.[14] Anabolic effects of GH are partly mediated through IGF-1, located on chromosome band 12q23.2.[53] However, GH has a variety of effects that are independent of IGF-1, such as lipolysis, increased nitrogen retention, increased energy expenditure, and increased insulin resistance.[54] In fact, GH and IGF-1 have opposing effects on glucose metabolism; GH has "diabetogenic" action, whereas IGF-1 has "glucose-lowering" activity as a result of its insulin-like effects.[55] Although GH deficiency is associated with postnatal growth restriction, IGF-1 deficiency is associated with both prenatal and postnatal growth deficiency, in addition to neurodevelopmental delay. This implies an important role for IGF-1 in regulating fetal growth, as well as central nervous system development.[56,24] IGF-1 levels in the human fetal serum increase with advancing gestational age.[57] Because GH receptors are not fully developed and not functioning before birth, IGF-1 secretion in utero is likely regulated by nutrition and insulin.[57] IGF-1 acts through its receptor (IGF-1 receptor, located on 15q26.3), which is similar to the insulin receptor as both are composed of two α-subunits and two β-subunits.[58] The two α-subunits contain a ligand-binding domain and are extracellular. The β-subunits are intracellular and contain a tyrosine kinase domain. This homology in structure explains the ability of IGF-1 to bind to the insulin receptor and for insulin to bind to the IGF-1 receptor. The macrosomic effects of high intrauterine insulin exposure are evident in the infant of a diabetic mother[59] and in the genetic causes of hyperinsulinism most commonly involving inactivating mutations in the ATP-sensitive K^+ channel genes *KCNJ11* and *ABCC8*.[60] The recognition of the macrosomic infant and the metabolic consequences of severe hypoglycemia are crucial in the care of the newborn.

PROLACTIN

PRL is secreted mainly by lactotrophs of the anterior pituitary gland, but it is also found in various tissues, such as the mammary gland, ovary, kidney, and osteoblasts, where it may be synthesized locally and exert diverse functions. These functions include the enablement of milk production, metabolic effects, regulation of the immune system, pancreatic development, and regulation of blood vessel growth.[61,62] PRL is structurally and functionally similar to GH and placental lactogen but is encoded on chromosome 6 rather than 17q22-24 for the GH cluster.[63] It has several structural isoforms as a result of transcriptional and posttranslational modifications, such as glycosylation, which can explain the diversity of its functions.[61] PRL release by the lactotrophs is under the control of hypothalamic inhibition by dopamine, the putative prolactin release–inhibiting factor.[61] Thyroxine inhibits PRL release, whereas thyrotropin-releasing hormone stimulates PRL release.[64] Lactotroph growth and PRL secretion are stimulated by estrogen.[65] Suckling also has a stimulatory effect. PRL exerts its biologic actions through its receptor, PRLR, which, like GHR, is a cytokine receptor. The *PRLR* gene is on chromosome 5, close to the *GHR* gene.[61] Binding of PRL to PRLR causes activation of the Janus kinase/signal transducer and activator of transcription cell signaling pathways similarly to the activation induced by GH after binding to its receptor, GHR. Binding of PRL to its receptor also activates mitogen-activated protein kinases and Src kinase.[61] GH and placental lactogen bind to PRLR with high affinity in humans, but PRL does not bind to GHR.[61] PRL does not cross the placenta.[61] The fetus produces its own PRL early in gestation. The levels of PRL rise with gestational age; low levels are first detected at 12 weeks after conception and rise sharply at 26 weeks of gestation.[66] Umbilical cord blood levels are high in the term neonate (approximately 170 ng/mL) compared with normal adult levels of less than 20 ng/mL.[66] Umbilical cord blood levels of PRL correlate with gestational age. PRL levels decrease to the 90 to 100 ng/dL range in the first week of life in the term infant. This decline is delayed in premature babies.[67] The best understood function of PRL in humans is its role in milk secretion in the mother. In the fetus, PRL has been associated with lung maturation,[67] and it may also have a role in osmoregulation of amniotic fluid,[68] in bone formation and angiogenesis.[69,62]

PRL promotes angiogenesis, but PRL fragments generated by proteolytic processing, exert antiangiogenic, proapoptotic, vasoconstrictive, and anti-vasopermeability effects. Higher PRL and PRL fragments, the vasoinhibins, are associated with retinopathy of prematurity.[70]

HUMAN PLACENTAL LACTOGEN

Human placental lactogen, also known as *human chorionic somatomammotropin,* is produced and secreted by the syncytiotrophoblast of the placenta. It is structurally and functionally related to GH, exists in several forms, and its genes are encoded, together with the pituitary GH gene (normal GH) and the placental GH gene (GH variant), on chromosome band 17q22-24.[63] Human placental lactogen has more sequence homology with normal GH than with human prolactin and is first detected in the maternal circulation at 6 weeks of gestation; the levels rise progressively to concentrations in the 5 to 7 μg/mL range at term.[71] Only small amounts are believed to cross the placenta into the fetal circulation. Its prolactin-like properties are responsible for its lactogenic and mammogenic effects, although a role in human lactation is unclear. However, a major role is the GH-like effect in inducing resistance to insulin action in the mother. This limits maternal glucose utilization, while ensuring an appropriate supply of free fatty acids derived from lipolysis for the mother during fasting, sparing glucose for fetal energy needs to protect against fetal hypoglycemia. A possible role for human placental lactogen to promote fetal growth by stimulating amino acid uptake, DNA synthesis, and IGF-1 production has also been suggested.[72] Human placental lactogen does not possess a specific receptor but is capable of binding to both GHR and PRLR.[72]

The placental GH (GH variant) is produced only by the placental syncytiotrophoblast, beginning at approximately 24 weeks of gestation. Production continues until term, and gradually replaces pituitary GH expression in the mother. Secretion is continuous rather than pulsatile as occurs for pituitary GH secretion, and placental GH does not cross the placenta to the fetus. It is not regulated by hypothalamic control but is suppressed by high glucose concentrations. Its precise function is unknown, but it is believed to have metabolic effects like those of human placental lactogen, hence protecting the fetus from hypoglycemia.[72]

CONCLUSION

Human GH, human PRL, and human placental lactogen share an intricate evolutionary relationship that created a network of multiple related forms of these proteins likely arising from a common ancestral gene. All three hormones share structural homology in their protein sequence, and in their binding to their canonical receptors with significant cross reaction between each subtype. Both human GH and human PRL are produced and secreted by pituitary acidophil cells under a complex regulatory system that involves hypothalamic and other neural peptides, as well as metabolic regulators of secretion, and neither has all of the functions in the fetus and newborn that are typically seen in the adult. The formation of the pituitary is under a complex system of transcription and other factors, and mutations in the gene encoding these factors result in distinct patterns of hormone deficiencies that, in the case of human GH and human PRL, become apparent only after birth. Their role in fetal growth and mammary gland function is marginal. Both appear quite early in gestation, with high concentrations at birth that decline postnatally, as the inhibitory effects of somatotropin release–inhibiting factor and L-dopa and maturation of their receptors and signal transduction cascades become established over a period of 3 to 6 months. For "normal" pituitary GH, the primary role in the fetus and newborn appears to be the metabolic actions of lipolysis, amino acid incorporation into muscle, and "anti-insulin" effects that protect the fetus/newborn from hypoglycemia and ensure an adequate nutrient supply; this role is further magnified by human placental lactogen, and by human GH variant, both secreted by the syncytiotrophoblast. Human placental lactogen circulates in the mother at concentrations 10^3-fold higher than those of human GH and ensures fuel supplies to the fetus even under conditions of maternal nutritional deficiencies such as fasting; human GH variant plays a similar role. The functions of fetal human prolactin are poorly defined, although roles in regulating amniotic fluid osmolality, lung maturation, and angiogenesis have been proposed.

This chapter has summarized the embryonic development of the pituitary and the patterns of hormone deficiencies, which may arise as a result of mutations in the developmental cascade of genes and transcription factors that act to create the normal structure and function of this organ in the fetus and newborn. Whole exome sequencing has been instrumental as a research tool in identifying genetic associations in hormone deficiencies and structural abnormalities. This knowledge has proven invaluable in recognizing patterns of hormone deficiencies in the newborn; future studies may unravel the physiologic significance of their roles in the fetus and the newborn.

A complete reference list is available at www.ExpertConsult.com.

SELECT REFERENCES

1. Lewis UJ, et al. Human growth hormone: a complex of proteins. *Recent Prog Horm Res*. 1980;36:477–508.
2. Hartman ML, et al. Temporal structure of *in vivo* growth hormone secretory events in humans. *Am J Physiol*. 1991;260:E101–E110.
3. Bowers CY, et al. On the *in vitro* and *in vivo* activity of a new synthetic hexapeptide that acts on the pituitary to specifically release growth hormone. *Endocrinology*. 1984;114:1537–1545.
4. Kojima M, Hosoda H, Kangawa K. Purification and distribution of ghrelin: the natural endogenous ligand for the growth hormone secretagogue receptor. *Horm Res*. 2001;56(suppl 1):93–97.
5. Sassin JF, et al. Human growth hormone release: relation to slow-wave sleep and sleep-walking cycles. *Science*. 1969;165:513–515.
6. Mauras N, et al. Selective beta 1-adrenergic receptor-blockade with atenolol enhances growth hormone releasing hormone and mediated growth hormone release in man. *Metabolism*. 1987;36:369–372.
7. Korytko AI, Cuttler L. Thyroid hormone and glucocorticoid regulation of pituitary growth hormone-releasing hormone receptor gene expression. *J Endocrinol*. 1997;152:R13–R17.
8. Cornblath M, et al. Secretion and metabolism of growth hormone in premature and full-term infants. *J Clin Endocrinol Metab*. 1965;25:209–218.
16. Fan Y, et al. Liver-specific deletion of the growth hormone receptor reveals essential role of growth hormone signaling in hepatic lipid metabolism. *J Biol Chem*. 2009;284:19937–19944.
18. Mavalli MD, et al. Distinct growth hormone receptor signaling modes regulate skeletal muscle development and insulin sensitivity in mice. *J Clin Invest*. 2010;120:4007–4020.
19. Green H, Morikawa M, Nixon T. A dual effector theory of growth-hormone action. *Differentiation*. 1985;29:195–198.
20. Sherwin RS, et al. Effect of growth hormone on oral glucose tolerance and circulating metabolic fuels in man. *Diabetologia*. 1983;24:155–161.
21. Rosenfeld RG, et al. Both human pituitary growth hormone and recombinant DNA-derived human growth hormone cause insulin resistance at a postreceptor site. *J Clin Endocrinol Metab*. 1982;54:1033–1038.
22. Mauras N, et al. Sex steroids, growth hormone, insulin-like growth factor-1: neuroendocrine and metabolic regulation in puberty. *Horm Res*. 1996;45:74–80.
23. Gluckman PD, Pinal CS. Regulation of fetal growth by the somatotrophic axis. *J Nutr*. 2003;133(5 suppl 2):1741S–1746S.
26. Bernardini S, et al. Plasma levels of insulin-like growth factor binding protein-1, and growth hormone binding protein activity from birth to the third month of life. *Acta Endocrinol*. 1992;127:313–318.
27. Johnson JD, et al. Hypoplasia of the anterior pituitary and neonatal hypoglycemia. *J Pediatr*. 1973;82:634–641.
28. Asa SL, Kovacs K. Functional morphology of the human fetal pituitary. *Pathol Annu*. 1984;19:275–315.
29. Kaplan SL, Grumbach MM, Aubert ML. The ontogenesis of pituitary hormones and hypothalamic factors in the human fetus: maturation of central nervous system regulation of anterior pituitary function. *Recent Prog Horm Res*. 1976;32:161–243.
32. Kelberman D, Dattani MT. Role of transcription factors in midline central nervous system and pituitary defects. *Endocr Dev*. 2009;14:67–82.
36. Mehta A, et al. The role of growth hormone in determining birth size and early postnatal growth, using congenital growth hormone deficiency (GHD) as a model. *Clin Endocrinol*. 2005;63:223–231.
37. Salisbury DM, et al. Micropenis: an important early sign of congenital hypopituitarism. *Br Med J*. 1984;288:621–622.
38. Ben-Jonathan N, Hnasko R. Dopamine as a prolactin (PRL) inhibitor. *Endocr Rev*. 2001;22:724–763.
39. Wu W, et al. Mutations in PROP1 cause familial combined pituitary hormone deficiency. *Nat Genet*. 1998;18:147–149.
41. Pfäffle R, Klammt J. Pituitary transcription factors in the aetiology of combined pituitary hormone deficiency. *Best Pract Res Clin Endocrinol Metab*. 2011;25:43–60.
42. Rosenfeld MG, et al. Multistep signaling and transcriptional requirements for pituitary organogenesis *in vivo*. *Recent Prog Horm Res*. 2000;55:1–13.
46. Frankenne F, et al. The physiology of growth hormones (GHs) in pregnant women and partial characterization of the placental GH variant. *J Clin Endocrinol Metab*. 1988;66:1171–1180.
47. Cooke NE, et al. Human growth hormone gene and the highly homologous growth hormone variant gene display different splicing patterns. *J Clin Invest*. 1988;82:270–275.
48. de Vos AM, Ultsch M, Kossiakoff AA. Human growth hormone and extracellular domain of its receptor: crystal structure of the complex. *Science*. 1992;255:306–312.
49. Mullis PE, Deladoey J, Dannies PS. Molecular and cellular basis of isolated dominant-negative growth hormone deficiency, IGHD type II: insights on the secretory pathway of peptide hormones. *Horm Res*. 2002;58:53–66.
51. Kelly PA, et al. The prolactin/growth hormone receptor family. *Endocr Rev*. 1991;12:235–251.
52. Daughaday WH, Trivedi B. Absence of serum growth hormone binding protein in patients with growth hormone receptor deficiency (Laron dwarfism). *Proc Natl Acad Sci U S A*. 1987;84:4636–4640.
53. Brissenden JE, Ullrich A, Francke U. Human chromosomal mapping of genes for insulin-like growth factors I and II and epidermal growth factor. *Nature*. 1984;310:781–784.
54. Carrel AL, Allen DB. Effects of growth hormone on body composition and bone metabolism. *Endocrine*. 2000;12:163–172.
55. Haymond MW, Horber FF, Mauras N. Human growth hormone but not insulin-like growth factor I positively affects whole-body estimates of protein metabolism. *Horm Res*. 1992;38(suppl 1):73–75.
56. Woods KA, et al. Intrauterine growth retardation and postnatal growth failure associated with deletion of the insulin-like growth factor I gene. *N Engl J Med*. 1996;335:1363–1367.
57. Bennett A, et al. Levels of insulin-like growth factors I and II in human cord blood. *J Clin Endocrinol Metab*. 1983;57:609–612.
58. Werner H, Le Roith D. The insulin-like growth factor-I receptor signaling pathways are important for tumorigenesis and inhibition of apoptosis. *Crit Rev Oncog*. 1997;8:71–92.
59. Candido CS, Sperling M. Infants of mothers with diabetes. In: Lebovitz HE, ed. *Therapy for Diabetes Mellitus and Related Disorders*. 5th ed. Alexandria, VA: American Diabetes Association; 2009:64–74.
60. De Leon DD, Stanley CA. Mechanisms of disease: advances in diagnosis and treatment of hyperinsulinism in neonates. *Nat Clin Pract Endocrinol Metab*. 2007;3:57–68.
61. Harris J, et al. Prolactin and the prolactin receptor: new targets of an old hormone. *Ann Med*. 2004;36:414–425.
63. Owerbach D, et al. The prolactin gene is located on chromosome 6 in humans. *Science*. 1981;212:815–816.
64. Mitsuma T, Nogimori T. Changes in plasma thyrotrophin-releasing hormone, thyrotrophin, prolactin and thyroid hormone levels after intravenous, intranasal or rectal administration of synthetic thyrotrophin-releasing hormone in man. *Acta Endocrinol*. 1984;107:207–212.
65. Mulchahey JJ, et al. Hormone production and peptide regulation of the human fetal pituitary gland. *Endocr Rev*. 1987;8:406–425.
66. Suganuma N, et al. Ontogenesis of pituitary prolactin in the human fetus. *J Clin Endocrinol Metab*. 1986;63:156–161.
67. Gluckman PD, et al. Prolactin in umbilical cord blood and the respiratory distress syndrome. *J Pediatr*. 1978;93:1011–1014.
68. Pullano JG, et al. Water and salt conservation in the human fetus and newborn. I. Evidence for a role of fetal prolactin. *J Clin Endocrinol Metab*. 1989;69:1180–1186.
69. Seriwatanachai D, Krishnamra N, van Leeuwen JP. Evidence for direct effects of prolactin on human osteoblasts: inhibition of cell growth and mineralization. *J Cell Biochem*. 2009;107:677–685.
71. Kzhyshkowska J, et al. Alternatively activated macrophages regulate extracellular levels of the hormone placental lactogen via receptor-mediated uptake and transcytosis. *J Immunol*. 2008;180:3028–3037.
72. Handwerger S, Freemark M. The roles of placental growth hormone and placental lactogen in the regulation of human fetal growth and development. *J Pediatr Endocrinol Metab*. 2000;13:343–356.

142 Luteinizing Hormone and Follicle-Stimulating Hormone Secretion in the Fetus and Newborn Infant

Sumana Narasimhan | Ethel G. Clemente | Neha V. Vyas | T. Rajendra Kumar

INTRODUCTION

The pituitary gonadotropins, luteinizing hormone (LH) and follicle-stimulating hormone (FSH), influence the function of the differentiated gonad in utero and regulate gonadal function in later life. LH and FSH are glycoprotein hormones secreted by the same pituitary cell, the gonadotroph, under the influence of hypothalamic and other hormones. Glycoprotein hormones such as LH, FSH, thyroid-stimulating hormone (TSH), and human chorionic gonadotropin (hCG) are heterodimers composed of two non-covalently associated protein subunits α and β. The α subunits are identical but the β-subunits are unique and confer biologic specificity. The biologic specificity and mechanism of action of hCG, a placental glycoprotein, is mostly similar to that of LH.

Gonadotropin-releasing hormone (GnRH; also known as *LH-releasing hormone* or *LH-releasing factor*) is the main hypothalamic peptide controlling the secretion of LH and FSH. The major role of LH and FSH is to control steroidogenesis in the gonad and gametogenesis. Congenital abnormalities or mutations in the regulation of LH and FSH can therefore lead to abnormalities of phallic development, puberty, and fertility.

In this chapter, we review the anatomic development of key components of the gonadotropin regulatory axis (including the hypothalamus, pituitary, and portal circulation), the role of gonadotropins in the fetus and neonate, the factors that control gonadotropin secretion, and disorders in the development of the gonadotropin regulatory system.

DEVELOPMENT OF THE HYPOTHALAMUS AND PITUITARY

HYPOTHALAMUS

The hypothalamus (Table 142.1)[1-4] develops from the primitive forebrain (prosencephalon). By approximately the fifth week after conception, the forebrain differentiates into the cerebral hemispheres and the diencephalon; the ventral aspect of the diencephalon then develops into the hypothalamus. By 14 to 16 weeks gestation, hypothalamic nuclei and fiber tracts become differentiated.[5-9]

GnRH, the major secretagogue of pituitary LH and FSH, is a decapeptide released by specific neurosecretory cells in the hypothalamus and is carried by portal circulation to the pituitary. The hypothalamic content of GnRH has been reported to rise during the first half of gestation and GnRH has generally been reported to be similar in male and female fetuses,[10-13] with some exceptions.[14] Little is known about the early postnatal development of hypothalamic GnRH in humans, although an increase in immunoreactive GnRH neurons in the hypothalamuses of human neonates compared with those of late-gestation fetuses has been seen.[15] The *GNRH* gene is expressed in the hypothalamus during early stages of development. GnRH has been detected by radioimmunoassay as early as 4.5 weeks gestation.[16] GnRH has been identified within the hypothalamus by 8 to 13 weeks gestation[11,13,15-17] and by 16 weeks gestation, GnRH-containing neurons are known to terminate on portal vessels.[18]

As indicated above, GnRH neurons originate in the embryonic olfactory placode as early as 4.5 weeks gestation[19] and undergo a unique pattern of axophilic migration across the terminal nerve to their ultimate location in the hypothalamus by mid-gestation.[20-22] Then they extend axonal processes into the median eminence to establish neurovascular connections.

GnRH neuronal migration is complex and is influenced by many genes, proteins, and nuclear transcription factors (summarized in Table 142.2), and is essential for cell survival, growth, and differentiation. The chemical guidance for axonal routing and GnRH neuron migration is provided by axonal guidance molecules, extracellular matrix proteins, growth factors, and neurotransmitters. The molecular pathways involved in GnRH cell migration include the Rho GTPase family, phosphatidylinositol 3-kinase, mitogen-activated protein kinase, and the Ras family. For a detailed review of this process, the reader is referred to the articles by Tobet and colleagues,[3] Gonzalez-Martinez and colleagues,[23] and Wierman and colleagues.[24] Studies on human GnRH cells in long-term cell cultures have shown that GnRH can also modulate the differentiation and migration of GnRH-secreting neurons in an autocrine fashion.[25] Various genes that have been implicated in GnRH neuronal migration include the Kallmann syndrome gene (ANOS1) located on Xp22.3, *KAL2* (which encodes fibroblast growth factor receptor 1 [FGFR-1]),[26] and the G protein–coupled receptor 54 gene *(GPR54)*, also *(KISS1R)*.[27]

The *KAL1* gene and its product, anosmin,[28] are implicated in the X-linked form of Kallmann syndrome, whereas FGFR-1 is implicated in autosomal dominant hypothalamic hypogonadism seen in males and females.[26,29] FGFR-1 is a member of the receptor tyrosine kinase superfamily, and it regulates cell proliferation, migration, differentiation, and survival. Hence, mutations in *FGFR1* are associated with other congenital malformations in addition to hypogonadotropic hypogonadism and may explain some forms of Kallmann syndrome that are not associated with anosmia. *KISS1R* and its ligand kisspeptin have been described as major neuromodulators of the gonadotropic axis.[29-31]

Recently, a variety of strategies including high throughput genome and exome sequencing, functional phenotyping and genetic association studies using large cohorts of patients have resulted in identification of a number of genes regulating GnRH neuronal migration, synthesis, and release. Moreover, these studies have also identified that defects in GnRH regulation can result from multiple mutations in the same patient and manifest as diverse phenotypes.[32,33]

Complex molecular mechanisms are responsible for tissue-specific transcriptional activity of the *GNRH* gene. The human GnRH-encoding gene *(GnRH-I)*, located on 8p21-p11.2 and comprising three exons encoding a protein of 92 amino acids,[34,35] is the form found in hypothalamic neurons and regulates pituitary gonadotropins. A second gene, *GnRH-II*, encodes a decapeptide neurotransmitter in the midbrain. Other GnRH-encoding genes have been described in mammals and nonmammalian vertebrates.[36] The *GnRH-I* gene is thought to be targeted to hypothalamic neurons by enhancer and promoter elements acting in concert with the transcription factors Otx2, Brn-2, and Oct-1[37,38] and the pituitary octamer unc (POU) domain of the transcription factors SCIP, Pct-6, and Tst-1. A variety of hormones and second messengers also

Table 142.1 Luteinizing Hormone and Follicle-Stimulating Hormone in the Human Fetus and Neonate: Early Events in the Anatomic Development of the Hypothalamus and Pituitary Unit.

	Weeks Gestation	Comment	Reference
Hypothalamus			
Forebrain differentiates into cerebral hemispheres and diencephalon; the latter then develops into hypothalamus	3–5		Terasawa[1]
GnRH identified in whole-brain extract	4.5		Thliveris and Currie[2]
GnRH neurons found in olfactory placode	5.5		Tobet and Schwarting[3]
GnRH identified in hypothalamus	8–13		Grumbach[4]
Pituitary			
LH and FSH identified within the pituitary	9.5–11	Pituitary secretes LH and FSH in vitro at 5–7 wk	
Pituitary releases gonadotropins into the circulation	11–12		
Portal Circulation			
Intact	11.5–12		

FSH, Follicle-stimulating hormone; *GnRH,* gonadotropin-releasing hormone; *LH,* luteinizing hormone.

Table 142.2 Factors Implicated in Gonadotropin-Releasing Hormone Neuron Migration.

Cell Matrix/Adhesion	Neurotransmitters	Growth Factors	G Protein–Coupled Receptors	Transcription Factors	Other
Neural cell adhesion molecule	GABA/GABA-A and GABA-B	FGF8/FGFR1	PROK2/PROKR2	Ebf2	NELF
Cell surface proteoglycans (e.g., B3GNT1)	CCK8/CCK1R	Gas6/Axl and Tyro3	SDF1/CXCR4	Nhlh2	
Anosmin (KAL1)		HGF/Met	Kiss/KissR		
Heparan sulfate proteoglycans					
Ephrins/ephrin receptors					
Semaphorin 4D/plexin B1					
Semaphorin 3A/neuropilin 2/plexin A1					
Netrin/DCC					
Reelin/ApoER2/Lrp8					

ApoER2, Apolipoprotein E receptor 2; *B3GNT1*, βGal β-1,3-*N*-acetylglucosaminyltransferase 1; *CCK1R*, cholecystokinin 1 receptor; *CCK8*, cholecystokinin 8; *CXCR4*, chemokine (C-X-C motif) receptor 4; *DCC*, deleted in colorectal cancer gene; *Ebf2*, early B-cell factor 2; *FGF8*, fibroblast growth factor 8; *FGFR1*, fibroblast growth factor receptor 1; *GABA*, γ-aminobutyric acid; *Gas6*, growth arrest–specific gene 6; *HGF*, hepatocyte growth factor; *KAL1*, Kallmann 1; *Kiss*, kisspeptin; *KissR*, kisspeptin receptor; *Lrp8*, low-density lipoprotein receptor related protein 8; *NELF*, nasal embryonic luteinizing hormone–releasing hormone factor; *Nhlh2*, nescient helix-loop-helix 2; *PROK2*, prokineticin 2; *PROKR2*, prokineticin 2 receptor; *SDF1*, stromal cell–derived factor 1.
From Wierman ME, Kiseljak-Vassiliades K, Tobet S. Gonadotropin releasing hormone (GnRH) neuron migration, initiation, maintenance and cessation as critical steps to ensure normal reproductive function. *Front Neuroendocrinol*. 2011;31(1):43–52.

influence *GNRH* gene expression.[39] Nuclear receptors DAX-1 (dosage sensitive sex reversal, adrenal hypoplasia critical region, on chromosome X, gene 1) and splicing factor 1 (SF-1) have been shown to be important for the proper development and function of the entire hypothalamic-pituitary-gonadal (HPG) axis.[40,41]

PITUITARY

The pituitary gland arises from ectoderm, with the adenohypophysis (anterior pituitary) originating from oral ectoderm and the neurohypophysis (posterior pituitary) deriving from the neuroectoderm.[42] Pituitary development starts on embryonic day 8.5 in the mouse. In humans, terminal differentiation of cells is completed in the first trimester. Pituitary development has been identified in the human fetus by the third week of pregnancy, with Rathke pouch, the precursor of the anterior pituitary, developing as an evagination of the primitive stomodeum in the fourth week of gestation, with subsequent separation from the stomodeum by the fifth week of gestation.[43-45] The floor of the sella turcica forms by the seventh week of gestation, and, by the eighth week, the connection of the pouch with the oral cavity fully disappears.[46]

The anterior pituitary is populated in a temporally and spatially specific fashion by the corticotrophs (which secrete adrenocorticotropic hormone), the somatotrophs (which secrete growth hormone), the lactotrophs (which secrete prolactin), the thyrotrophs (which secrete TSH), and the gonadotrophs (which secrete LH and FSH).[42,47,48] Two important principles that have emerged from ongoing studies are (1) the differentiation of specific cell types in the pituitary follows a highly ordered sequence, and (2) the coordinated expression and down-regulation of homeodomain transcription factors plays a critical role in controlling the differentiation.[42,47,49] For example, rodent studies indicate that differentiation of all cell types requires transient expression of HESX homeobox 1 *(HESX1)* and paired-like homeodomain 1 *(PITX1)*, but then, on approximately embryonic day 10, the cells divide into LIM homeobox 3 (Lhx3)-dependent and Lhx3-independent lineages (Fig. 142.1).[48]

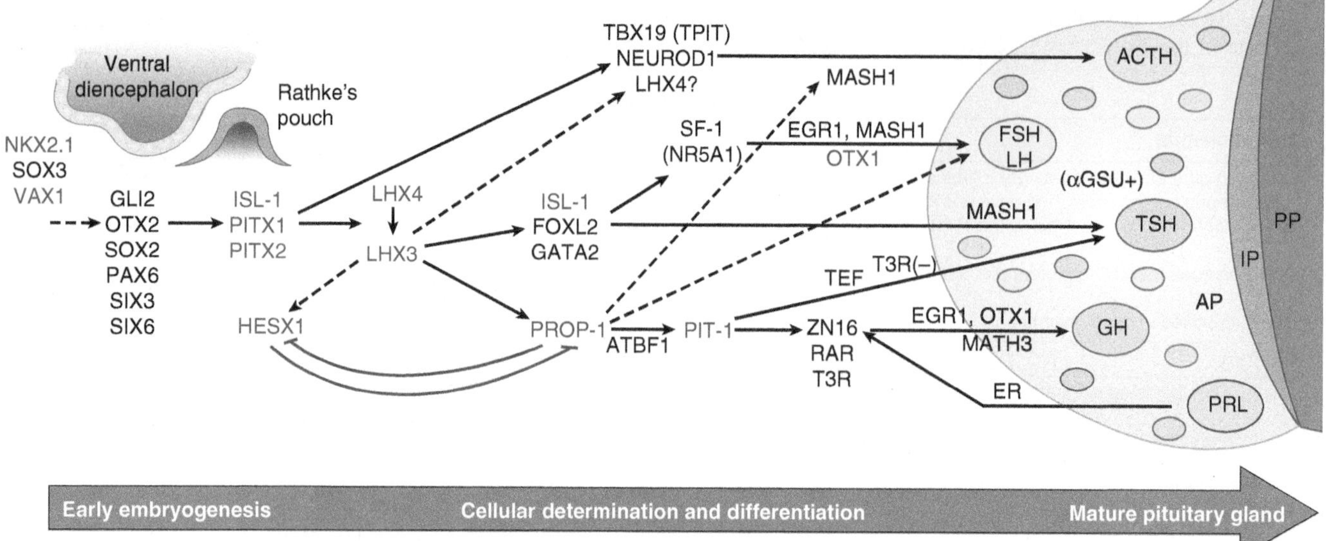

Fig. 142.1 Molecular regulation of anterior pituitary gland development. Multiple transcription factors contribute to the development of the pituitary gland and the subsequent differentiation of the five specialized hormone-secreting cell types of the mature anterior pituitary gland: corticotrophs (adrenocorticotropic hormone *[ACTH]*), gonadotrophs (follicle-stimulating hormone *[FSH]* and luteinizing hormone *[LH]*), thyrotrophs (thyroid-stimulating hormone *[TSH]*), somatotrophs (growth hormone *[GH]*), and lactotrophs (prolactin *[PRL]*). Homeodomain-containing transcription factors critical to this process are highlighted in *red. Arrows* indicate upstream relationships in molecular signaling pathways but do not necessarily imply direct activation. *Flat ars* denote repressive relationships. The placement of specific cell types in the diagram does not reflect their actual location within the anterior pituitary gland. *AP,* Anterior pituitary gland; *IP,* intermediate pituitary gland; *PP,* posterior pituitary gland. (From Prince KL, Walvoord EC, Rhodes SJ. The role of homeodomain transcription factors in heritable pituitary disease. *Nat Rev Endocrinol.* 2011;7:727–737.)

The main population of corticotrophs is Lhx3 independent and appears by embryonic day 12 or 13; the other cell lineages appear to be Lhx3 dependent. Under the influence of PROP paired-like homeobox 1 *(PROP1)*, the LHX3-dependent lineage further bifurcates into POU class 1 homeobox 1 (POUF1)-dependent and POUF1-independent pathways. The POUF1-dependent pathway leads to the differentiation of somatotrophs, lactotrophs, and thyrotrophs by embryonic day 16. The POUF1-independent pathway, under the influence of other factors, including SF-1, leads to differentiation of the gonadotrophs by embryonic day 17. In addition to intrinsic pituitary factors, there is evidence that, at distinct developmental stages, inductive processes from adjacent tissue are also important for proper cell differentiation and expansion of pituitary cell lineages.[46] In animal models, other signaling molecules, such as GNRH2, activin A receptor type 2A *(ACVR2)*, bone morphogenetic protein 4 *(BMP4)*, fibroblast growth factor (FGF), Wnt gene family (Wnt), and Sonic hedgehog *(SHH)*, have been found to be critical for pituitary development. Of note, *Insm1* has been shown to be required for differentiation of all endocrine cells in the pituitary gland, and mutation of this gene leads to a normal-sized anterior pituitary without the ability for hormone production.[50] Detailed discussion of this topic is available in the articles by Cohen and Radovick,[42] Zhu and colleagues,[47] and Quentien and colleagues.[51] Recent studies with human patients and genetically modified mouse models have identified putative pituitary stem cells/progenitors that give rise to multiple hormone-producing cell types. Two master regulators known as *Sox2* and *Prop1* orchestrate these developmentally regulated cell fate decisions.[52] The importance of these basic components of pituitary development to human physiology is emphasized by identification of corresponding human mutations that cause predictable pituitary cell phenotypes.[47,53]

The fetal pituitary secretes LH and FSH in culture at 5 to 7 weeks of gestation.[54,55] LH and FSH have been detected in the pituitary as early as 9.5 to 11 weeks of gestation.[56-60] The pituitary content of LH and FSH then rises sharply, with pituitary LH and FSH content peaking at 25 to 29 weeks of gestation in female fetuses and at 35 to 40 weeks of gestation in male fetuses.[59] The pituitary content of LH and FSH is higher in female fetuses than in male fetuses between approximately 10 and 25 weeks of gestation.[57,59-62] This sexual dimorphism may reflect testosterone production by the male fetus, with resulting inhibition of pituitary gonadotropin production during early pituitary development.[63]

Early in gestation, the predominant pituitary glycoprotein fraction is the common α-glycoprotein hormone subunit.[15,58,64] As gestation progresses, the relative amount of the β-subunit and intact gonadotropin appears to rise.[15,62,65] Kaplan and colleagues[12] found that the content and concentration of pituitary LH and FSH in 2- to 6-month-old infants were higher than in late-gestation female fetuses.

It is not clear to what extent GnRH normally contributes to the functional development of the gonadotroph. In vitro, GnRH can stimulate differentiation of fetal rat gonadotrophs[66,67] and LH synthesis in cultured fetal human pituitary cells.[68] Human anencephalic fetuses have reduced pituitary gonadotropin content,[12] as well as persistent predominant secretion of the α-glycoprotein hormone subunit,[64,65] suggesting that GnRH normally contributes to gonadotroph development and function. At 17 to 18 weeks of gestation, the number, size, and distribution of gonadotropin-containing cells was similar in anencephalic fetuses and normal fetuses. However, after 26 weeks of gestation, anencephalic fetuses appeared to have fewer cells containing SF-1 and the β-subunits of both LH and FSH than did normal fetuses.[69] The fetal pituitary also has potential for some differentiation in the absence of direct hypothalamic influences,[70] as suggested by studies on anencephalic fetuses[71-73] and transplanted rat pituitary.[74,75]

PORTAL CIRCULATION

Work using vascular casts suggests that the hypothalamic pituitary portal system is intact by 11.5 to 12 weeks of gestation,[2] earlier than originally estimated.[76-78] It has been suggested that local diffusion may allow communication between the hypothalamus and pituitary before that time.[12]

ROLE OF PITUITARY GONADOTROPINS IN THE FETUS AND NEONATE

Fetal pituitary LH and FSH are not required for sexual and gonadal differentiation. However, pituitary gonadotropins are required for normal function of the differentiated gonad. Because hCG can activate LH receptors, placental hCG leads to production of testosterone early in gestation,[63,79] and this testosterone production leads to normal formation of male external genitalia by 12 to 14 weeks of gestation. However, later in gestation, testosterone production by the fetal testes depends on fetal LH, which is responsible for growth of the formed phallus during the later stages of pregnancy. The increased incidence of a normally formed but small phallus (microphallus) and cryptorchidism in male infants with anencephaly or gonadotropin deficiency[4,80,81] supports the concept that pituitary gonadotropins influence testicular growth and function later in gestation, as does the finding that the testes of anencephalic fetuses are hypoplastic, with decreased numbers of testicular Leydig cells.[81-83] Female anencephalic fetuses have been reported to show small ovaries with hypoplasia of the primary follicles.[83] Some reports suggest that the ovaries are relatively normal until 34 to 36 weeks of gestation and only later show evidence of abnormal development.[84]

REGULATION OF PITUITARY LUTEINIZING HORMONE AND FOLLICLE-STIMULATING HORMONE SECRETION IN THE FETUS AND NEONATE

FACTORS THAT REGULATE PITUITARY LUTEINIZING HORMONE AND FOLLICLE-STIMULATING HORMONE SECRETION IN ADULTS

In adults, the secretion of pituitary LH and FSH involves the finely balanced interplay of several regulatory factors (Fig. 142.2). The major "centers" involved in this interplay are the hypothalamus, pituitary, and gonad (a unit referred to as the *hypothalamic-pituitary-gonadal or HPG axis*). The main stimulus for pituitary gonadotropin secretion is the hypothalamic decapeptide, GnRH. More than 16 GnRH peptides and several GnRH receptors have been identified in mammals and nonmammalian vertebrates.[85,86] The function and tissue specificity of these various peptides are still being elucidated, but the regulation of LH and FSH secretion seems to reside primarily with the originally identified molecular species.[85] At least two forms of GnRH and two GnRH receptors are expressed in humans.

Many afferent neurotransmitter systems from the brain stem, limbic system, and other areas of the hypothalamus convey information to the GnRH neurons. They may contain norepinephrine, dopamine, serotonin, γ-aminobutyric acid, glutamate, endogenous opioid peptides, neuropeptide Y, galanin, and other neuropeptides.[1,87,88] Glutamate and norepinephrine are stimulatory, whereas γ-aminobutyric acid and endogenous opioid peptides are inhibitory factors for GnRH secretion (see Fig. 142.2). Secretions from surrounding glial cells, such as transforming growth factor-α, can also stimulate GnRH release.[87,89] Steroid hormones such as estradiol and testosterone can alter the pattern of GnRH secretion by binding to steroid hormone receptors in the hypothalamus and pituitary, providing negative feedback. It is important to note that GnRH neurons themselves lack steroid hormone receptors; hence, the negative feedback of steroids at the level of the hypothalamus is mediated via actions on other neural systems that, in turn, input to the GnRH neurons.[87] In addition, glucose, thyroxine, glucocorticoids, leptin, and exogenous factors (e.g., stress, health, exercise, and nutrition) can also influence GnRH secretion.[90]

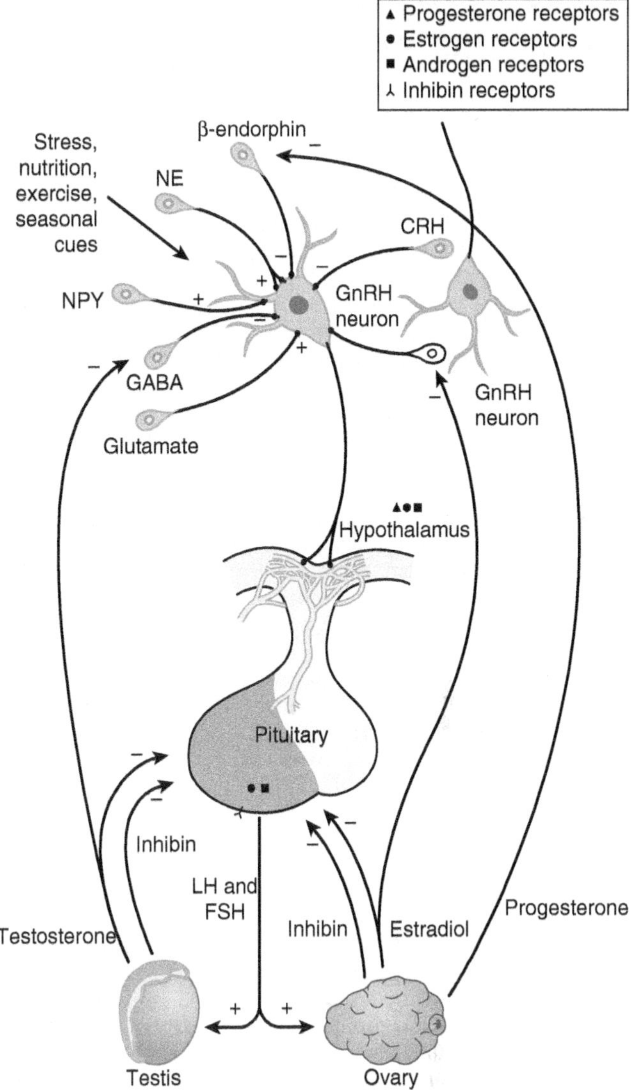

Fig. 142.2 The gonadotropin control system in adults. Feedback loops are indicated by *arrows*, *plus signs* indicate positive feedback loops, and *minus signs* indicate negative feedback loops. The principal sex steroids in females are estradiol and progesterone; in males, the principal sex steroid is testosterone. *CRH*, Corticotropin-releasing hormone; *FSH*, follicle-stimulating hormone; *GABA*, γ-aminobutyric acid; *GnRH*, gonadotropin-releasing hormone; *LH*, luteinizing hormone; *NE*, norepinephrine; *NPY*, neuropeptide Y. (From Cone RD, Low MJ, Elmguist JK, et al. Neuroendocrinology. In Larsen PR, Kronenberg HM, Melmed S, et al., eds. *Williams Textbook of Endocrinology.* 10th ed. Philadelphia: WB Saunders; 2003:132.)

The normal pulsatile secretion of LH is believed to be mediated directly by episodic release of GnRH, which is critical for the maintenance of gonadotropin secretion in adults. Animal studies have shown that different pulse frequencies of GnRH can lead to differential ratios of FSH and LH synthesis and or secretion.[87,91] Continuous administration of exogenous GnRH to adults leads to an initial increase in gonadotropin secretion, followed by prolonged suppression of gonadotropin secretion owing to down-regulation of the GnRH receptors in pituitary gonadotroph.[66,91,92] The rate of pulsatile GnRH secretion, along with ovarian hormone feedback, also influences the degree of glycosylation of LH and FSH, which can profoundly influence the physiologic function and stability, and consequently, the plasma half-life of these hormones in the circulation.[93,94]

GnRH is released into the hypophysial portal blood system and reaches the anterior pituitary, where it binds to GnRH receptors on the cell surface of gonadotrophs to stimulate gonadotropin release.[87,95] The human GnRH receptor gene *(GNRHR)* is localized on chromosome band 4q21.2. The GnRH receptor belongs to a family of G protein–coupled receptors, and ligand binding initiates several intracellular signaling pathways, including phospholipase C, inositol 1,4,5-triphosphate, protein kinase C, mitogen-activated protein kinase 1, calcium influx, and calcium release from intracellular stores.[96] The mobilization of intracellular calcium affects the initial burst of LH secretion, and the influx of extracellular calcium maintains sustained gonadotropin secretion.[97]

Another G protein–coupled receptor, *KISS1R*, and the corresponding ligand, kisspeptin have been extensively studied.[30,98-103] Kisspeptin, a product of the *KISS1* gene, is the key neuropeptide that gates puberty and maintains fertility by regulating the GnRH neuronal system in mammals.[100,101] Current understanding based on mouse studies indicates that kisspeptin stimulates GnRH secretion by a direct effect on GnRH neurons, most of which express *KISS1R*. Estradiol and testosterone inhibit *KISS1* messenger RNA (mRNA) expression in the arcuate nucleus, whereas these steroids induce *KISS1* mRNA expression in the anteroventral periventricular nucleus. Inactivating mutations in *KISS1*, as well as loss-of-function mutations of *KISS1R*, are associated with pubertal failure and infertility.[100,101]

Although implicated as a critical permissive signal triggering puberty, kisspeptin is paradoxically produced by neurons in the developing brain much before puberty onset.[102] Micropenis and bilateral cryptorchidism may be noted at birth in males with *KISS1R* mutations, indicating a role for kisspeptins in gonadotropic axis activation during fetal development. However, the timing of gonadotropic axis activation by kisspeptins in fetuses remains unknown.[100] In zebrafish, kisspeptin is the primary stimulator of GnRH3 neuronal development in the embryo and an activator of stimulating hypophysiotropic neuron activities in the adult.[101] In the female mouse embryo, kisspeptin-producing neurons in the arcuate nucleus communicate with a specific subset of GnRH neurons in utero. It was also demonstrated that neural circuits between arcuate nucleus kisspeptin and GnRH neurons are fully established and operative before birth, and that most GnRH neurons express the kisspeptin receptor GPR54 on circuit formation, suggesting that the signaling system implicated in gatekeeping puberty becomes operative in the embryo.[102] The ability of kisspeptin to stimulate GnRH neurons is proven, but the possibility of direct pituitary effects of kisspeptins in the control of gonadotropin secretion remains controversial.[103]

Gonadal secretions are also major physiologic regulators of LH and FSH secretion in adults and exert negative feedback (inhibitory) effects on gonadotropin release. In mature premenopausal women, estrogens can exert positive feedback, mediating the ovulatory surge of gonadotropins. The gonads also produce peptides, such as inhibins A and B, which selectively modulate FSH-secretion from gonadotroph cells. Although other regulators, such as activins and follistatin, are present in the peripheral circulation, these factors probably act locally within the gonadotroph in an autocrine/paracrine fashion, with activin stimulating FSH release and follistatin inhibiting FSH release by binding to activin. (See the articles by Cone and colleagues[87] and Kuohung and Kaiser[104] for further review.)

FACTORS THAT REGULATE PITUITARY LUTEINIZING HORMONE AND FOLLICLE-STIMULATING HORMONE RELEASE IN THE FETUS AND NEWBORN INFANT

GONADOTROPIN-RELEASING HORMONE

GnRH is present in the human fetal hypothalamus by 8 to 11 weeks of gestation.[11,13,15-17,105] The secretory pattern of GnRH during human fetal and early neonatal development is not known. However, GnRH neurons isolated from nonhuman primates secrete GnRH peptide in a pulsatile manner in vitro, suggesting that early intrinsic pulsatile secretion of GnRH may be independent of non-GnRH neuronal synaptic input.[1,106]

GnRH appears to influence gonadotropin release early in gestation. The human fetal pituitary in vitro releases LH or FSH, or both, in response to GnRH by approximately 13 to 19 weeks of gestation (Figs. 142.3-142.6).[107-109] By the second trimester, pretreatment with estradiol enhances the sensitivity of human fetal pituitaries to GnRH.[110] GnRH appears capable of influencing LH synthesis and secretion in this period of development.[68]

The human fetal pituitary releases gonadotropins in response to exogenous GnRH in vivo by the second trimester, and the increment in LH and FSH levels after GnRH administration is greater in the second trimester than in the third trimester.[111] These findings are supported by studies in monkeys[61,112,113] and sheep[114] that show the fetal gonadotroph is responsive to GnRH, with a declining response as gestational age advances.[114,115]

In human neonates[110,111,116] and infants,[116-119] exogenous GnRH also stimulates gonadotropin release. Tapanainen and colleagues[119] administered GnRH (50 μg/m² intravenously) to male infants who had undescended but palpable testes and whose age ranged from 3 to 390 days. GnRH stimulated LH and FSH release in all age groups, but peak gonadotropin release occurred at 1 to 3 months of age, with a subsequent decline from 3 to 12 months of age. A similar age-dependent change in LH response to GnRH was found in infant monkeys.[112]

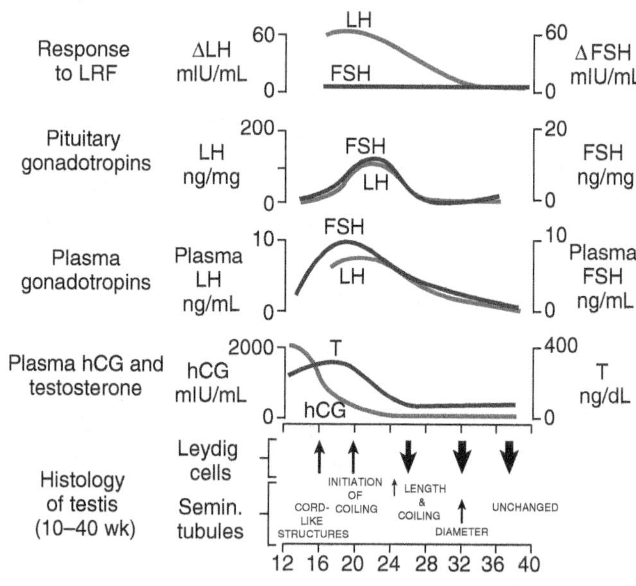

Fig. 142.3 Graphic comparison of gonadotropin response to gonadotropin-releasing hormone (also known as *luteinizing hormone–releasing factor [LRF]*), pituitary and plasma gonadotropins, and plasma human chorionic gonadotropin *(hCG)* and testosterone *(T)*, with histologic changes in the testis of the human male fetus during gestation. *FSH*, Follicle-stimulating hormone; *LH*, luteinizing hormone. (From Gluckman PD, et al. The human fetal hypothalamus and pituitary gland. In: Tulchinsky LD, Ryan KJ, eds. *Maternal-Fetal Endocrinology*. Philadelphia: WB Saunders; 1980:2423.)

Gonadotropin secretion is episodic in rhesus monkey[120] and ovine[121] fetuses, as well as in human, ovine,[122] and rhesus monkey[123] infants. In the ovine fetus, administration of a GnRH antagonist decreases LH pulse frequency.[121] Because pulsatile secretion of LH is believed to depend on pulsatile release of GnRH, these findings also suggest a role for endogenous GnRH in the regulation of LH release in the perinatal period.

The observation that the fetal pituitary releases gonadotropins in response to GnRH by the second trimester[107,109,111,124] suggests the presence of hypophysial GnRH receptors by that time. Studies on zebrafish indicate that *GNRHR* mRNA may be present as early as 36 to 56 hours after fertilization.[125] In rats, pituitary binding sites for GnRH have been detected by 13 days of gestation (term is 22 days),[126] with the pituitary GnRH receptor number increasing in the late prenatal and early postnatal period.[127] Postnatally, the concentration of GnRH receptors in rodents is highest between 15 and 20 to 30 days of age and decreases thereafter to reach adult levels by approximately 60 days of age.[95] Although GnRH has been detected in the placenta,[85,128] the role of the placental material in the physiologic regulation of pituitary gonadotropin release is uncertain. Anencephalic and gonadotropin-deficient fetuses are deficient in hypothalamic GnRH but are presumably not deficient in placental GnRH. The subnormal quantities of pituitary gonadotropins in most of these infants[12,129] suggests that placental GnRH may not be an important factor for the normal regulation of gonadotropin release in utero. The overall influence of neurotransmitters on gonadotropin release in the human fetus and neonate is not known, although some animal studies suggest that specific neurotransmitters such as endogenous opioids may be involved.[130]

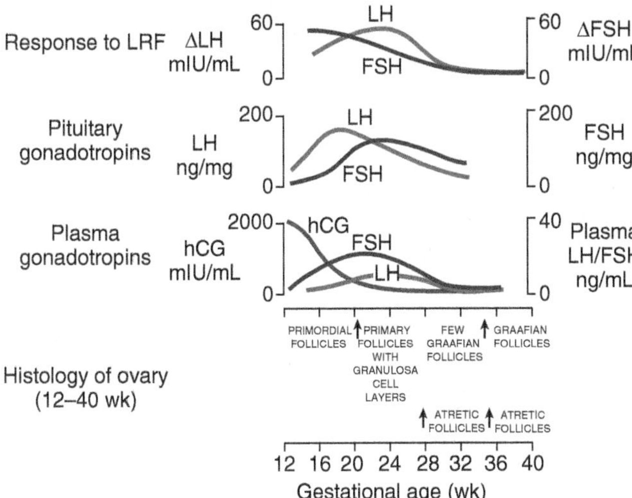

Fig. 142.4 Graphic comparison of gonadotropin response to gonadotropin-releasing hormone (also known as *luteinizing hormone–releasing factor [LRF]*), pituitary and plasma gonadotropins, and plasma human chorionic gonadotropin *(hCG)*, with histologic changes in the ovary of the human female fetus during gestation. *FSH,* Follicle-stimulating hormone; *LH,* luteinizing hormone. (From Gluckman PD, et al. The human fetal hypothalamus and pituitary gland. In: Tulchinsky LD, Ryan KJ, eds. *Maternal-Fetal Endocrinology*. Philadelphia: WB Saunders; 1980:2423.)

GONADAL STEROIDS

There is indirect evidence from animal studies that the capacity of gonadal steroids, especially testosterone, to inhibit gonadotropin release is present during fetal development. For example, castration of male rhesus monkey fetuses at approximately mid-gestation results in elevation of gonadotropin levels,[1,131,132] and early testosterone or dihydrotestosterone replacement prevents the rise of gonadotropin levels after castration.[132] These results suggest that functional negative feedback between the testes and the hypothalamic-pituitary axis is present by mid-gestation in rhesus monkey male fetuses. The role of fetal ovarian estrogen in regulating gonadotropin secretion is less clear, in part because both male and female fetuses develop in an environment that is rich in estrogens of fetoplacental origin. In rhesus monkey female fetuses, gonadectomy has had variable results on gonadotropin secretion.[131-133] Estradiol infusions blunt LH release in the late-gestation ovine fetus.[134] Gonadotropin levels, which rise in the early postnatal period, may reflect, in part, a

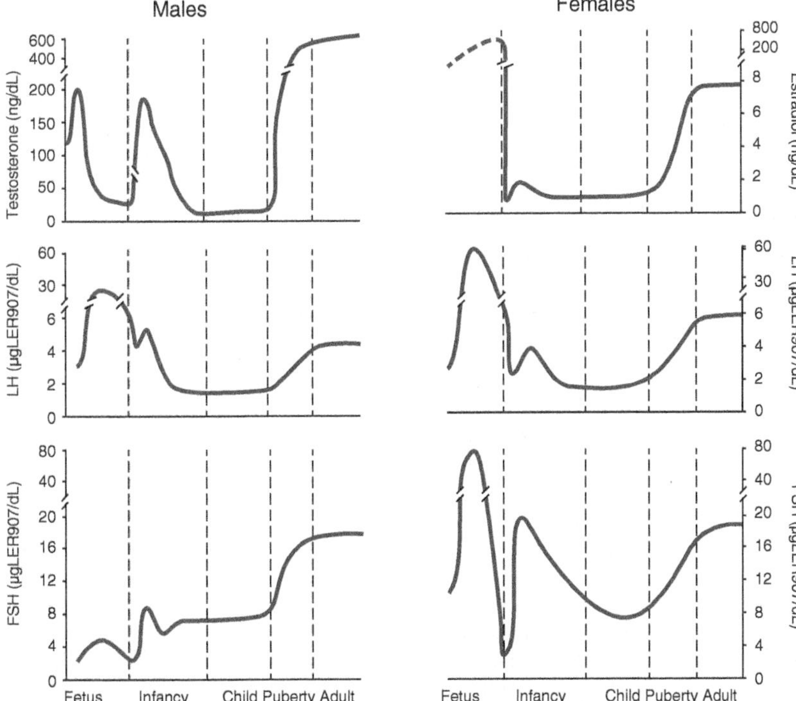

Fig. 142.5 Mean concentrations of serum luteinizing hormone *(LH)*, follicle-stimulating hormone *(FSH)*, and estradiol during human pregnancy and postnatal development. (From Winter JS, Hughes IA, Reyes FI, et al. Pituitary-gonadal relations in infancy: 2. Patterns of serum gonadal steroid concentrations in man from birth to two years of age. *J Clin Endocrinol Metab.* 1976;42:679.)

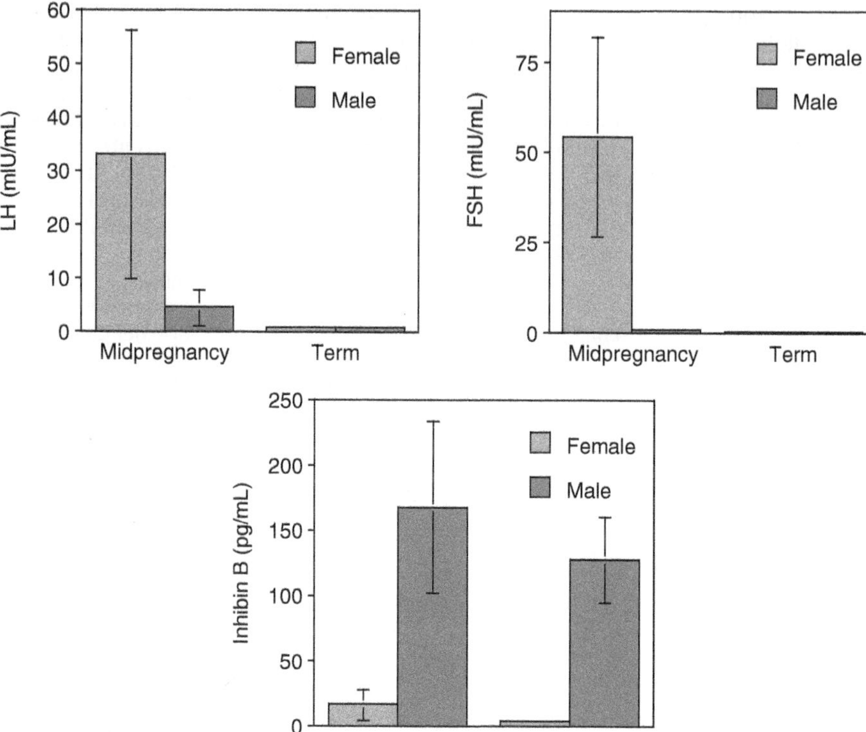

Fig. 142.6 Luteinizing hormone *(LH)*, follicle-stimulating hormone *(FSH)*, and inhibin B levels in human fetal female and male serum at midpregnancy and term (mean ± standard deviation). (From Debieve F, Beerlandt S, Hubinont C, et al. Gonadotropins, prolactin, inhibin A, inhibin B, and activin A in human fetal serum from midpregnancy and term pregnancy. *J Clin Endocrinol Metab.* 2000;85:270.)

release from negative feedback as sex steroids are removed from the fetal circulation.

Neonatally, gonadal steroids appear to suppress gonadotropin secretion in both sexes. Castration of newborn female rhesus monkeys results in elevation of FSH levels and, to a lesser extent, LH levels.[135] Orchiectomy of male monkey neonates also results in elevation of LH and FSH levels, suggesting that testosterone may influence early postnatal gonadotropin secretion in males.[133,135-137] The specific gonadotropin secretion pattern differs between neonatal castrated male and female monkeys, and it has been suggested that this reflects intrinsic sexual dimorphism of hypothalamic GnRH secretion.[135] Similarly, gonadal failure in human neonates leads to elevated gonadotropin levels,[138] indicating that gonadal factors normally suppress gonadotropin secretion even in the neonatal period. Further evidence for negative feedback by gonadal steroids derives from the observation that administration of estrogen and progesterone to extremely premature female infants suppresses LH and FSH secretion.[139]

However, castration-induced elevation of circulating gonadotropin levels is not fully sustained into late childhood, and gonadotropin levels in both experimental orchiectomy and in naturally occurring gonadal failure decline during infancy or early childhood (only to rise again in the peripubertal per iod).[133,136,138] However, the gonadotropin levels do not reach levels as low as those in children with normal gonads.[140] Taken together, these findings suggest that although gonadal steroids influence gonadotropin secretion in neonates, they are not the sole mediators of changing gonadotropin levels in infancy. The eventual decline in gonadotropin levels in late infancy and early childhood is due primarily to extragonadal and presumably central hypothalamic-pituitary factors in combination with some gonadal-derived inhibitory factors.[133,136,137]

INHIBIN

Inhibins are members of the transforming growth factor-β superfamily of polypeptides secreted by the Sertoli cells in the testis and by the granulosa cells in the ovary, which inhibit the release of FSH but not LH from the pituitary. Inhibin is a heterodimer of an α-subunit and either an activin βA or βB subunit, and accordingly termed as ***inhibin A*** or ***inhibin B***.[141,142] Inhibin is also synthesized by the placenta.[143] Biologically active inhibin is present in the fetus, and administration of inhibin suppresses serum FSH.[144] Apart from their essential role in the selective control of FSH secretion, inhibins are currently recognized as paracrine ovarian and testicular regulators and have multiple paracrine effects in the uteroplacental unit, representing a promising marker for male and female infertility and gynecologic and gestational diseases.[145,141,142]

Studies have shown the presence of inhibin B in male and female fetuses at mid-gestation, with higher levels in males than in females (Figs. 142.7 and 142.8, see also Fig. 142.6). Circulating inhibin levels are higher in premature infants than in term infants.[146] Inhibin B levels are higher in boys than in girls after birth.[147-149] In boys, the levels peak at approximately 3 to 12 months of age and remain elevated until approximately 15 months of age.[148] The production of inhibin during the first month of life may be enhanced by the postnatal surge in the levels of gonadotropins.[59,63] Although the precise role of inhibins in the fetus and neonate is not clear, these findings suggest that endogenous inhibin may play a physiologic role in suppressing FSH in fetal and neonatal animals.[144]

PLASMA GONADOTROPINS IN THE FETUS AND NEONATE

GENERAL PATTERN

Circulating immunoreactive FSH is detectable by the tenth to thirteenth week of gestation in human fetuses and rises to peak levels at approximately midgestation (see Figs. 142.3–142.6).[59,63] At that time, FSH concentrations are comparable to those of castrated animals. FSH levels then decline; by birth, they are low, similar to those of prepubertal children.[12,59,150,151] Circulating LH concentrations in the fetus follow a similar pattern.[59,60,63,151]

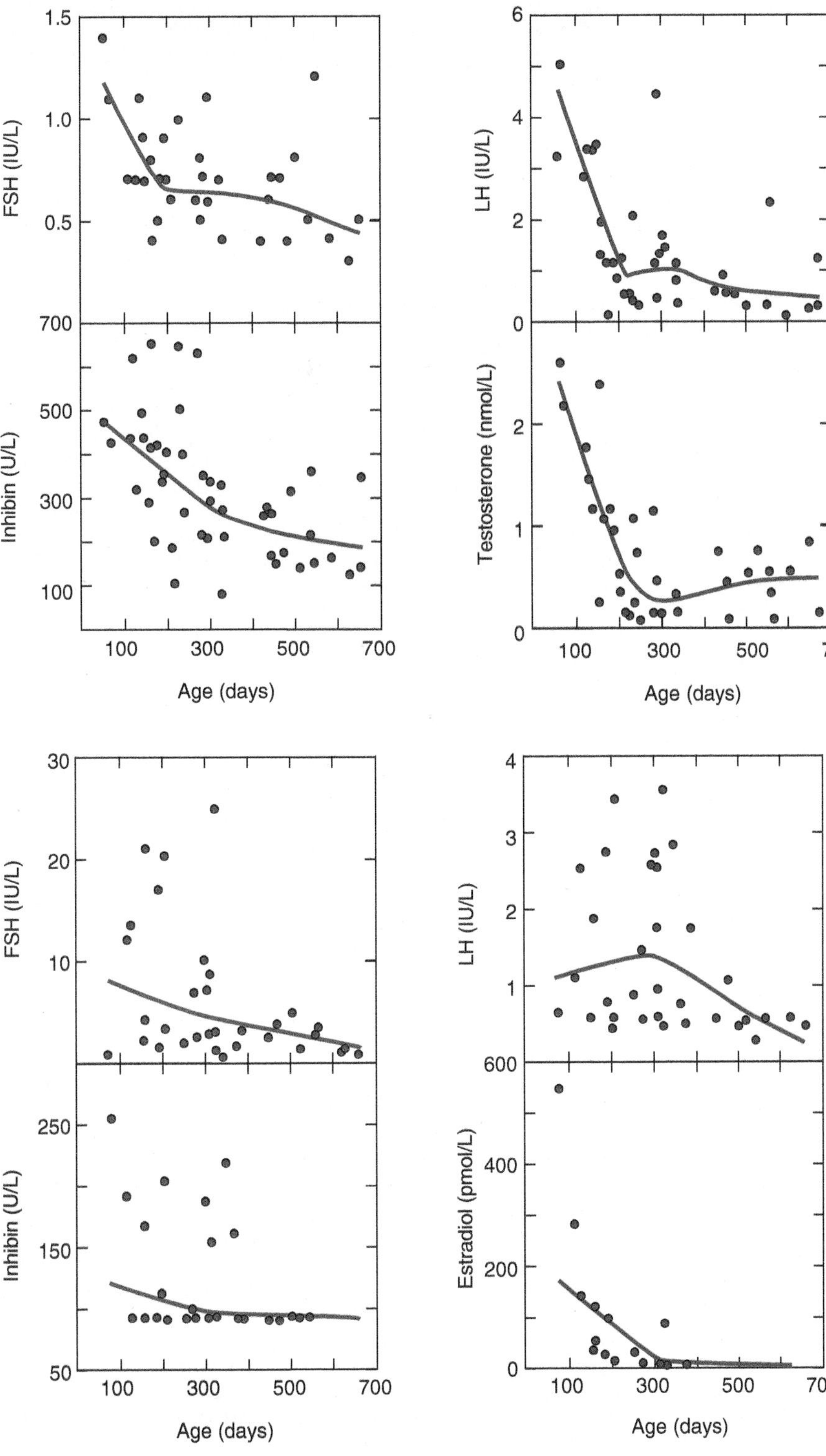

Fig. 142.7 Scatterplot matrix of hormone changes with age in boys. The *continuous line* represents the robust, locally weighted regression. *FSH,* Follicle-stimulating hormone; *LH*, luteinizing hormone. (From Burger HG, Yamada Y, Bangah ML, et al. Serum gonadotropin, sex steroid, and immunoreactive inhibin levels in the first two years of life. *J Clin Endocrinol Metab.* 1991;72:682.)

Fig. 142.8 Scatterplot matrix of hormone changes with age in girls. The *continuous line* represents the robust, locally weighted regression. *FSH,* Follicle-stimulating hormone; *LH*, luteinizing hormone. (From Burger HG, Yamada Y, Bangah ML, et al. Serum gonadotropin, sex steroid, and immunoreactive inhibin levels in the first two years of life. *J Clin Endocrinol Metab.* 1991;72:682.)

Studies in premature infants are consistent with studies in fetuses and show a decline in serum LH and FSH levels with advancing gestational age.[146]

Soon after birth, LH and FSH levels rise (see Fig. 142.5). Though reported patterns vary somewhat, this increase is sustained for weeks to months and is followed by a decline to prepubertal levels (see Figs. 142.5, 142.7, and 142.8).[131,152,153] The specific patterns also differ between boys and girls, as discussed in detail later.[149,153–155]

Pulsatile secretion of gonadotropins is a hallmark feature of the mature hypothalamic-pituitary axis. Studies in primate[120] and ovine[121,156] fetuses suggest that pulsatile secretion of gonadotropins may develop in utero. There is evidence that gonadotropin secretion in the 1- to 3-month-old human infant is also episodic.[157,158]

Circulating hCG, the placental glycoprotein, declines from high levels at 13 to 17 weeks of gestation to low levels at term (see Figs. 142.3 and 142.4)[59,60,111] and falls to undetectable levels by the fifth postnatal day.[111,155] Plasma levels of free α-subunit are high at mid-gestation and decline near term.[64,65,159] The α—glycoprotein hormone subunit may originate from cells that secrete LH, FSH, hCG, or TSH. The finding that the level of the α-subunit declines postnatally,[58,160] whereas plasma LH and FSH levels rise, suggests that most of the α-subunit that circulates in the fetus is derived from hCG.

SEXUAL DIMORPHISM

Sexual dimorphism characterizes both the prenatal and postnatal patterns of gonadotropin secretion.[161] In the fetus, FSH levels peak at mid-gestation in both sexes, but FSH levels at this time are higher in female fetuses than in male fetuses (see Figs. 142.3–142.6).[12,60,63,79,111,151,159] LH levels have also been reported to be higher at mid-gestation in females than in males[56,146,154] but not in all studies.[59,111] The subsequent decline in LH and FSH levels with advancing gestational age occurs in both sexes, and by term, the low FSH levels are similar in males and females (see Figs. 142.3–142.6). Umbilical cord blood concentrations of both LH and FSH are low.[63,161,162]

After birth, FSH levels rise markedly in girls and peak at approximately 3 months of age and usually decline to prepubertal levels by 6 to 9 months,[1] although elevated levels can persist up to 2 years.[147] In contrast, FSH levels of male infants have been reported to rise less briskly, peak at 1 week to 3 months of age at levels lower than those of females,[1,106,149,155,163] and more uniformly decline to prepubertal levels by approximately 4 to 9 months after birth.[147,155] LH levels peak in boys at approximately 1 to 3 months of age and decline to prepubertal levels by approximately 4 to 9 months.[147,155,164] Girls exhibit a similar pattern, but, in contrast to FSH, peak LH levels are generally lower than those of boys.[155] Similar patterns of gonadotropin secretion have been found in the ovine fetus[165] and in neonatal subhuman primates.[155,166,167]

MECHANISMS POSTULATED TO BE RESPONSIBLE FOR CHARACTERISTIC PATTERNS OF GONADOTROPIN LEVELS IN THE FETUS AND NEONATE

In the fetus, rising levels of LH and FSH at mid-gestation may reflect autonomous or unrestrained release of gonadotropins.[59,63] The later decline in gonadotropin levels with advancing gestational age may reflect increased sensitivity to the inhibitory effects of gonadal steroids (especially in males)[59,63]; rising levels of circulating fetal estrogen in both sexes[63]; and reduced GnRH secretion owing to central neuroinhibitory influences or maturation of sensitivity to sex steroids, or both.[63] Data from the study of 46,XY infants with androgen insensitivity syndrome suggest that the withdrawal from the negative feedback of androgens during the neonatal transition may play a critical role in the postnatal LH and testosterone surge.[66] In a longitudinal study, infants with partial androgen insensitivity syndrome mounted the expected postnatal surges, but LH and testosterone levels failed to increase in infants with complete androgen insensitivity syndrome.[168] The early postnatal rise in gonadotropin levels had been postulated to reflect the loss of the negative feedback effect previously exerted by maternal estrogens. This mechanism now seems less likely in 46,XY infants, but the roles that estradiol and androgens play in regulation of the postnatal surge in 46,XX infants remain unclear.[169]

After the postnatal surge, the reproductive endocrine axis enters a long period of relative, but not absolute, quiescence (often referred to as the *juvenile pause*) until GnRH secretion reemerges, leading to pubertal maturation. The factors causing the postnatal decline in gonadotropin levels are not clear. Several regulatory processes are likely involved, including central neuroinhibitory processes[136,137] and the potentially increased sensitivity of the hypothalamus and pituitary to the negative feedback effect of gonadal steroids.[63] Factors that may mediate the central inhibition include the relative predominance of γ-aminobutyric acid versus glutamate neurotransmitter activity and the inhibitory action of neuropeptide Y.[1,170]

CONDITIONS ASSOCIATED WITH ABNORMALITIES OF GONADOTROPIN SECRETION IN THE FETUS AND NEONATE

ANENCEPHALY

Anencephaly is a severe defect of neural tube development that is incompatible with long-term survival. Major portions of the nervous system including the hypothalamus are absent, usually. The pituitary gland is present but severely hypoplastic. Though the number and size of pituitary cells appear normal at week 17 or week 18 of gestation, by term, gonadotrophs are almost absent.[171] The pituitary content of LH and FSH appears reduced[12,129] and is comparable to that of 10- to 20-week fetuses.[12] The α-subunit appears to be the dominant glycoprotein present.[61,129]

Anencephalic male infants often have normally formed but small external genitalia and undescended testes. This likely reflects reduced testosterone synthesis in the latter part of gestation owing to gonadotropin deficiency. The testes have reduced numbers of Leydig cells, and the epididymis is underdeveloped.[81,82] Anencephalic female fetuses have normal external genitalia, consistent with the concept that gonadotropins and ovarian secretion products are not essential for female sexual differentiation. The ovaries are small, with reduced numbers of primary follicles.[83] In anencephalic newborn infants, basal plasma LH and FSH levels are generally low compared with levels in normal neonates,[12,162] and in a limited number of studies, LH and FSH levels failed to rise after administration of exogenous GnRH.[12,172,173]

Together, these characteristics of infants with anencephaly suggest that pituitary differentiation may occur even in the absence of normal GnRH production, but that full activity and maintenance of the immature gonadotroph normally requires endogenous GnRH.

CONGENITAL HYPOTHALAMIC AND PITUITARY ABNORMALITIES

Hypogonadotropic hypogonadism can be caused by genetic defects at the level of the hypothalamus or pituitary (Fig. 142.9). Kallmann syndrome is a genetically heterogeneous disorder of hypogonadotropic hypogonadism with hyposmia or anosmia. Various reports have indicated autosomal dominant, autosomal recessive, and X-linked transmission. Mutations in the *KAL1* gene have been found in 14% of familial and 11% of sporadic cases of hypogonadotropic hypogonadism in males. Other phenotypic features in males with *KAL1* mutations include delayed puberty, variable degrees of anosmia or hyposmia, and mirror movements and unilateral renal agenesis.[35,174] Female carriers have no specific phenotypic abnormalities. Several other mechanisms of inheritance and molecular mutations that result in congenital hypogonadotropic hypogonadism with anosmia/hyposmia are summarized in Table 142.3.[175]

In contrast to Kallman syndrome, patients with normosmic hypogonadotropic hypogonadism have normal sense of smell and tend not to have other clinical signs. Rare genetic abnormalities causing this condition are listed in Table 142.4.[175]

The *GPR54* gene and its ligand, kisspeptin, are important in the regulation of gonadotroph function.[31] The phenotypic features include normal sense of smell, as well as other manifestations of hypogonadism.[35] At the pituitary level, GnRH receptor mutations have been described in familial autosomal recessive, normosmic hypogonadotropic hypogonadism. They are predominantly missense mutations and result in loss of receptor function.[35] Mutations in various pituitary transcription factors can cause gonadotropin deficiency, which is usually associated with other pituitary hormone deficiencies. The reader is referred to the articles by Grumbach,[4] Baker and Jaffe,[56] and Valdes-Socin and

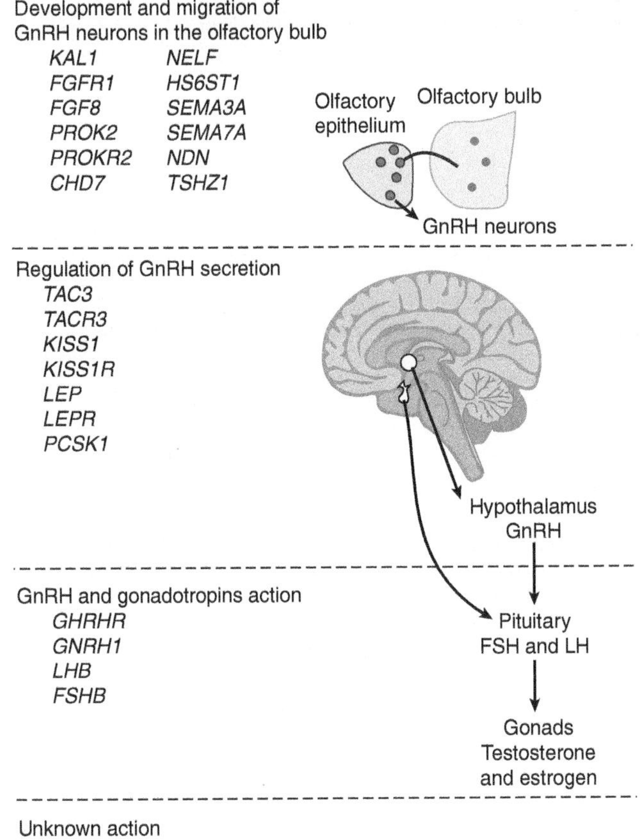

Fig. 142.9 Scheme of all human hypogonadotropic hypogonadism related genes involved at different steps in the hypothalamic-pituitary-gonadal axis development and functioning. *FSH*, Follicle-stimulating hormone; *GnRH*, gonadotropin-releasing hormone; *LH*, luteinizing hormone. (From Marino M, Moriondo V, Vighi E, et al. Central hypogonadotropic hypogonadism: genetic complexity of a complex disease. *Int J Endocrinol.* 2014;2014:649154.)

colleagues[175] for detailed descriptions. In syndromes such as CHARGE syndrome[176] or Noonan syndrome that are associated with hypogonadotropic hypogonadism, the exact molecular mechanism is not yet clear.

Many features of gonadotropin deficiency will not be apparent in the neonatal period. At birth, girls with congenital GnRH or gonadotropin deficiency have normal external genitalia because, as noted, female sexual differentiation does not appear to require GnRH, LH-FSH, or ovarian hormones. Males with congenital GnRH or gonadotropin deficiency (whether isolated or associated with other pituitary hormone deficiencies) tend to have microphallus and undescended testes.[4] Infants with Allman syndrome and other forms of gonadotropin deficiency have been reported to show low basal gonadotropin levels and subnormal gonadotropin responses to GnRH.[12,80,177] Male infants with LH receptor abnormalities are unable to fully stimulate testosterone production in response to LH or hCG signaling, and can present with phenotypes ranging from complete failure of virilization to hypospadias and/or microphallus.[40] Of note, because neonates with congenital growth hormone and adrenocorticotropic hormone deficiency are prone to develop hypoglycemia, the association of hypoglycemia and microphallus—particularly in a term infant—should alert the physician to the possibility of congenital panhypopituitarism.[4] The recent advances in gene editing/manipulation technologies provide rapid methods to design mutant mouse or zebra fish models and study the molecular basis of many of these human mutations and the resulting phenotypes.

GONADAL FAILURE

Gonadal differentiation and its abnormalities are described in Chapters 146 to 148. In this section, we refer to gonadal failure as absence of normal gonadal development or inability of the gonad to produce sex steroids, and we discuss the effects of such failure on gonadotropin secretion.

Elevated circulating levels of gonadotropins have been found in neonates and infants with gonadal failure.[138,140] For example, in cases of gonadal dysgenesis (Turner syndrome), levels of FSH and, to a lesser extent, LH are elevated above the normal range during infancy.[138] In Turner syndrome, gonadotropin levels decline after 4 years of age, even despite continuing gonadal failure,[138] suggesting that both central processes and gonadal factors contribute to the inhibition of gonadotropin secretion in the prepubertal child.

Similarly, elevation of basal and stimulated gonadotropin levels has been described in male infants with anorchia, rudimentary testes,[178] and other forms of primary testicular failure.[179] Boys with anorchia have elevated concentrations of basal gonadotropins, particularly FSH, from infancy to 4 years. The levels of gonadotropins then slightly decrease until 9 years of age, at which time they rise and remain elevated during adulthood. The levels of FSH are lower than those seen in girls with gonadal dysgenesis. This may be attributable to the effect of fetal testosterone on the fetal hypothalamus.[180] Male infants with certain forms of androgen resistance may have elevated LH levels.[181]

PREMATURITY AND SMALL-FOR-GESTATIONAL AGE STATUS

The effects of prematurity on gonadotropin secretion are not fully understood. In preterm females, umbilical cord blood levels of LH and FSH were found to be elevated and declined with advancing gestational age to term.[182,183] For the first 10 postnatal weeks, serum levels of LH and FSH are higher in premature infant girls than in term girls; no difference in gonadotropin levels between premature and term male infants has been noted.[182,184] Hypersecretion of FSH has been reported in infants born small for their gestational age.[184,185]

CONCLUSION

The coordinated regulation of the HPG axis during fetal and neonatal development is highly complex.[186] Defects in these critical early developmental events leads to various reproductive anomalies including anosmia, delayed/precocious puberty, pituitary agenesis/hyperplasia, gonadal dysgenesis, and other syndromes. While some of these anomalies can be explained by single gene mutations, some of these genetically inherited traits cold also result from oligo-or polygenic mutations in multiple loci.[187] Fetal and neonatal development of the pituitary and in particular, gonadotrope development is also dependent upon multiple signaling pathways that regulate cascades of transcription factors. Human mutations that result in aberrant regulation of some of these pathways have been identified and modeled in genetically engineered mouse models. Mechanisms of synthesis and secretion of gonadotropins during fetal and neonatal development are not yet fully identified. The molecular basis for sexual dimorphism in gonadotropin secretion is not yet known, and it may be

Table 142.3 Genes, Gene Products, Functions, and Phenotypes Associated With Congenital Hypogonadotropic Hypogonadism With Anosmia/Hyposmia.

Gene	Locus	Gene Product	Function	Inheritance	Type of Hypogonadism	Clinical Phenotype
KAL1 (Kallmann syndrome 1)	Xp22.3	Anosmin 1	Migration of GnRH and olfactory neurons	X-linked	Kallmann syndrome or normosmic IHH	Unilateral renal agenesis, synkinesia
FGF8 (Kallmann syndrome 6)	10q24	Fibroblast growth factor 8	Migration of GnRH neurons	Autosomal dominant	Kallmann syndrome or normosmic IHH	Cleft lip/relatively common (mid-line defects)
FGFR1 (Kallmann syndrome 2)	8p11.22		Fibroblast growth factor receptor	Migration of GnRH neurons	Autosomal dominant	Kallmann syndrome or normosmic IHH
FGF17	8p2.3	Fibroblast growth factor 17	Migration of GnRH neurons	Autosomal recessive	Kallmann syndrome or normosmic IHH	
FLRT3	20p12.1	Fibronectin-like domain–containing leucine-rich transmembrane protein 3	Interaction with FGFR	Complex trait	Kallmann syndrome	FGF network–knockout mouse is embryonic lethal
DUSP6	12q21.33	Dual specific inhibitor phosphatases	Inhibitor of MAPK pathway	Autosomal recessive	Kallmann syndrome	FGF network
IL17RD	3p14.3	Interleukin-17 receptor	Early stage of GnRH specification	Autosomal recessive	Kallmann syndrome	FGF network
SPRY4	5q31.3	Sprouty homologue interactor with FGFR1	Inhibitor of MAPK pathway	Autosomal recessive	Kallmann syndrome	FGF network
CHD7 (Kallmann syndrome 5)	8q12.1-12.2	Chromatin remodeling factor		Autosomal dominant	Kallmann syndrome or normosmic IHH	CHARGE syndrome
SEMA3A	7q21.11	Semaphorin 3A	Axonal path finding of GnRH neurons	Autosomal dominant	Kallmann syndrome	–
PROK2 (Kallmann syndrome 3)	3p21.1	Prokineticin 2	Migration of GnRH neurons	Autosomal dominant and recessive	Kallmann syndrome or normosmic IHH	Obesity, epilepsy, sleep disorders, fibrous dysplasia, and synkinesia
PROKR2 (Kallmann syndrome 4)	20p13	Prokineticin receptor		Kallmann syndrome or normosmic IHH		
NELF	9q34.3	Nasal embryonic LHRH factor	Migration of GnRH neurons	Digenic model (in association with *FGFR1* and *HS6ST1*)	Kallmann syndrome or normosmic IHH	–
WDR11	10q	WD repeat–containing protein family	Development of neuron	Autosomal dominant	Kallmann syndrome or normosmic IHH	–
HS6ST1	2q21	Heparan sulfate 6-*O*-sulfotransferase	Heparan sulfate modifier; regulates neural branching	Complex trait	Kallmann syndrome or normosmic IHH	–

FGF, Fibroblast growth factor; *FGFR,* fibroblast growth factor receptor; *GnRH,* gonadotropin-releasing hormone; *IHH,* idiopathic hypogonadotropic hypogonadism; *LHRH,* luteinizing hormone–releasing hormone; *MAPK,* mitogen-activated protein kinase.
From Valdes-Socin H, Rubio Almanza M, Tomé Fernández-Ladreda M, et al. Reproduction, smell and neurodevelopmental disorders: genetic defects in different hypogonadotropic hypogonadal syndromes. *Front Endocrinol.* 2014;5:109.

hypothesized that epigenetic factors may regulate this process. Finally, it is anticipated in the future that a combination of ex vivo models, stem cell-based in vitro organoid cultures, rapid genome editing techniques, sensitive hormone measurement assays, and high throughput genome sequencing technologies will all contribute to a better understanding of the physiologic regulation of gonadotropin secretion and in general the HPG axis during the fetal and neonatal period.

ACKNOWLEDGMENTS

Research work in the senior author's (TRK) laboratory is supported in part by the National Institutes of Health (AG056046, HD081162, AG029531, AG062319, HD097202) and The Makowski Family Endowment.

A complete reference list is available at www.ExpertConsult.com. 

Table 142.4 Genes and Phenotypes Related Only With Normosmic Idiopathic Hypogonadotropic Hypogonadism.

Gene	Locus	Inheritance	Comment
GNRH1	8p21-11.2	Autosomal recessive	Cryptorchidism
GNRHR	4q13.2-3		—
KISS1	1q32	Autosomal recessive	—
KISS1R	19p13.3		—
LEP	7q31.3	Autosomal recessive	Severe obesity
LEPR	1p31		
TAC3	12q13.3	Autosomal recessive	—
TACR3	4q25		—
DUSP6	12q21.33	Complex trait	—
LHB	19q13.32	Polymorphism and mutations (homozygous and heterozygous)	—
FSHB	11p13	Polymorphism and mutations	—

IHH, Idiopathic hypogonadotropic hypogonadism.
From Valdes-Socin H, Rubio Almanza M, Tomé Fernández-Ladreda M, et al. Reproduction, smell and neurodevelopmental disorders: genetic defects in different hypogonadotropic hypogonadal syndromes. *Front Endocrinol*. 2014;5:109.

SELECT REFERENCES

1. Terasawa E. Neurobiological mechanisms of the onset of puberty in primates. *Endocr Rev*. 2001;22:111.
2. Thliveris J, Currie R. Observations on the hypothalamo-hypophyseal portal vasculature in the developing human fetus. *Am J Anat*. 1980;157:441.
3. Tobet SA, Schwarting GA. Minireview: recent progress in gonadotropin-releasing hormone neuronal migration. *Endocrinology*. 2006;147:1159–1165.
4. Grumbach M. Commentary: a window of opportunity- the diagnosis of gonadotropin deficiency in the male infant. *JCEM*. 2005;90:3122–3127.
5. Hyyppa M. Hypothalamic monoamines in human fetuses. *Neuroendocrinology*. 1972;9:257.
6. Kuhlenbeck H. *The Human Diencephalon:A Summary of Development, Structure, Function and Pathology*. New York: Karger; 1954.
7. Lemire R. Embryology of the central nervous system. In: Davis J, Dobbins J, eds. *Scientific Foundations of Pediatrics*. Philadelphia: WB Saunders Co; 1974.
8. O'Rahilly R, Gardener E. The timing and sequence of events in the development of the human nervous system during the embryonic period proper. *Z Anat Entwicklungsgesch*. 1971;134:1.
9. Papez J. The embryonic development of the hypothalamic area in mammals. *Res Publ Assoc Nerv Ment Dis*. 1940;20:31.
10. Aksel S, Tyrey L. Luteinizing hormone-releasing hormone in the human fetal brain. *Fertil Steril*. 1977;28:1067.
11. Clements JA, et al. Ontogenesis of gonadotropin-releasing hormone in the human fetal hypothalamus. *Proc Soc Exp Biol Med*. 1980;163:437.
12. Kaplan SL, et al. The ontogenesis of pituitary hormones and hypothalamic factors in the human fetus: maturation of central system regulation of anterior pituitary function. *Recent Prog Horm Res*. 1976;32:161.
13. Aubert ML, et al. The ontogenesis of human fetal hormones: IV. Somatostatin, luteinizing hormone releasing factor, and thyrotropin releasing factor in hypothalamus and cerebral cortex of human fetuses 10–22 weeks of age. *JCEM*. 1977;44:1130.
14. Siler-Khodr TM. Studies in human fetal endocrinology: luteinizing hormone-releasing factor content of the hypothalamus. *Am J Obstet Gynecol*. 1978;130:795.
15. Bugnon C, et al. Cyto-immunological study of the ontogenesis of the gonadotropic releasing hormone in the human fetal hypothalamus. *J Steroid Biochem*. 1977;8:565.
16. Winters AJ, et al. Concentration and distribution of TRH and LRH in the human fetal brain. *JCEM*. 1974;39:960.
17. Gilmore DP, et al. Presence and activity of LH-RH in the mid term human fetus. *J Reprod Fertil*. 1978;52:355.
18. Asa SL, et al. Human fetal adenohypophysis: morphologic and functional analysis *in vitro*. *Neuroendocrinology*. 1991;53:562.
19. Verney C, et al. Comigration of tyrosine hydroxylase and gonadotropin releasing hormone immunoreactive neurons in the nasal area of human embryos. *Brain Res Dev Brain Res*. 1996;97:251–259.
20. Ronnekleiv OK, Resko JA. Ontogeny of gonadotropin-releasing-hormone-containing neurons in early development of rhesus macaques. *Endocrinology*. 1990;126:598.
21. Schwanzel-Fakuda M, Pfaff DW. Origin of luteinizing hormone-releasing hormone neurons. *Nature*. 1989;338:161.
22. Kim KH, et al. Gonadotropin-releasing hormone immunoreactivity in the adult and fetal human olfactory system. *Brain Res*. 1999;826:220.
23. Gonzalez-Martinez D, Hu Y, Bouloux PM. Ontogeny of GnRH and olfactory neuronal systems in man: novel insights from the investigation of inherited forms of Kallmann's syndrome. *Front Neuroendocrinol*. 2004;25:108–130.
24. Wierman ME, Kiseljak-Vassiliades K, Tobet S. Gonadotropin releasing hormone (GnRH) neuron migration: initiation, maintenance and cessation as critical steps to ensure normal reproductive function. *Front Neuroendocrinol*. 2011;32:43–52.
25. Romanelli R, Barni T, Maggi M, et al. Expression and function of GnRH receptor in human olfactory GnRH secreting neurons: an autocrine GnRH loop underlies neuronal migration. *J Biol Chem*. 2004;279:117–126.
26. Pitteloud N, Meysing A, Quinton R, et al. Mutations in fibroblast growth factor receptor-1 cause Kallmann syndrome with wide spectrum of reproductive phenotype. *Mol Cell Endocrinol*. 2006;254-255:60–69.
27. Gottsch ML, Clifton DK, Steiner RA. From KISS1 to kisspeptins: an historical perspective and suggested nomenclature. *Peptides*. 2009;1:4–9.
28. Soussi-Yanicostas N, de-Castro F, Julliard A, et al. Anosmin-1, defective in the X linked form of Kallmann's syndrome, promotes axonal branch formation from olfactory bulb output neurons. *Cell*. 2002;109.
29. Iovane A, Aumas C, De Roux N. New insights in the genetics of isolated hypogonadotropic hypogonadism. *Eur J Endocrinol*. 2004;151:U83–U88.
30. De Roux N, Genin E, Carel J, et al. Hypogonadotropic hypogonadism due to loss of function of the KiSS1-derived peptide receptor GPR54. *Proc Natl Acad Sci U S A*. 2003;100:10972–10976.
31. Seminara SB, et al. The GPR54 gene as a regulator of puberty. *N Engl J Med*. 2003;349:1614–1627.
32. Balasubramanian R, Crowley Jr WF. Isolated GnRH deficiency: a disease model serving as a unique prism into the systems biology of the GnRH neuronal network. *Mol Cell Endocrinol*. 2011;346:4–12.
33. Stamou MI, Cox KH, Crowley Jr WF. Discovering genes essential to the hypothalamic regulation of human reproduction using a human disease model: adjusting to life in the "omics" -era. *Endocrine Rev*. 2016:4–22.
34. Seeburg P, Adelman J. Characterization of cDNA for precursor of human luteinizing hormone-releasing hormone. *Nature*. 1984;311:666–668.
35. Karges B, De Roux N. Molecular genetics of isolated hypogonadotropic hypogonadism and Kallmann syndrome. *Endocr Dev*. 2005;8:67–80.
36. Fernald R, White R. Gonadotropin releasing hormone genes: phylogeny, structure and functions. *Front Neuroendocrinol*. 1999;20:224–240.
37. Kelley C. The Otx2 homeoprotein regulates expression from the gonadotropin-releasing hormone proximal promoter. *Mol Endocrinol*. 2000;14:1246.
38. Wolfe A. Identification of a discrete promoter region of the human GnRH gene that is sufficient for directing neuron specific expression: a role for POU homeodomain transcription factors. *Mol Endocrinol*. 2002;16:2002.
39. Nelson S, Eraly S, Mellon P. GnRH promoter: target of transcription factors, hormones and signaling pathways. *Mol Cell Endocrinol*. 1998;140:151–155.
40. Acherman JC. Genetic causes of human reproductive disease. *JCEM*. 2002;87:2447.
41. Iyer AK, McCabe ERB. Molecular mechanisms of DAX-1 action. *Mol Genet Metab*. 2004;83:60–73.
42. Cohen LE, Radovick S. Molecular basis of combined pituitary hormone deficiencies. *Endocr Rev*. 2002;23:431–442.
43. Atwell WJ. The development of the hypophysis cerebri in man, with special reference to the pars tuberalis. *Am J Anat*. 1926;37:159.
44. Conklin J. The development of the human fetal adenohypophysis. *Anat Rec*. 1968;160:79.
45. Daikoku S. Studies on the human foetal pituitary: 2. On the form and histological development, especially that of the anterior pituitary. *Tokushima J Exp Med*. 1958;5:214.
46. Mullis P. Transcription factors in pituitary development. *Mol Cell Endocrinol*. 2001;185:1.
47. Zhu X, Lin CR, Prefontaine GG, et al. Genetic control of pituitary development and hypopituitarism. *Curr Opin Genet Dev*. 2005;15:332–340.
48. Prince KL, Walvoord EC, Rhodes SJ. The role of homeodomain transcription factors in heritable pituitary disease. *Nat Rev Endocrinol*. 2011;7:727–737.
49. Scully K. Pituitary development: regulatory codes in mammalian organogenesis. *Science*. 2002;295:2231.
50. Welcker J, Hernandez-Miranda L, Paul F, et al. Insm1 controls development of pituitary endocrine cells and requires a SNAG domain for function and for recruitment of histone-modifying factors. *Development*. 2013;140:4947–4958.

143 Development of the Hypothalamus-Pituitary-Adrenal Axis in the Fetus

Brian J. Feldman | Abby Walch | Jennifer Zabinsky

INTRODUCTION

The development of the hypothalamus-pituitary-adrenal (HPA) axis begins early in gestation. Corticotropin-releasing hormone (CRH) is synthesized and secreted into the hypophyseal portal circulation by the paraventricular nucleus of the hypothalamus. CRH acts on corticotroph cells in the anterior pituitary gland to regulate the secretion of adrenocorticotropic hormone (ACTH). ACTH, in turn, stimulates cortisol secretion from the zona fasciculata of the adrenal cortex. ACTH is also an important stimulus for adrenal gland development and proliferation. The regulation of the secretion of these hormones is not fully established until late gestation, as demonstrated by the hormone levels seen in preterm neonates. This chapter reviews the basic development and regulation of the HPA axis, its interplay with the maternal HPA axis during fetal development, and the impact of fetal programming on the risk of chronic illnesses later in life.

DEVELOPMENT

Throughout pregnancy, significant changes in both the maternal and fetal HPA axis play crucial roles in the development and maturation of the fetus.

CORTICOTROPIN-RELEASING HORMONE

The hypothalamus develops from the ventral diencephalon and is differentiated by 9 to 10 weeks of gestation in the human fetus.[1] The anterior pituitary derives from the Rathke pouch, an invagination of oral ectoderm, and is present at approximately 5 weeks gestation. The neurovascular link between the hypothalamus and the pituitary is evident as early as 11 weeks of gestation. By 12 to 13 weeks of gestation, the fetal hypothalamus shows immunoactivity and bioactivity of CRH.[1] Therefore the fetal hypothalamus can provide the stimulus for ACTH secretion from the anterior pituitary starting from early in the second trimester. However, based on the hormone levels seen in preterm infants, the regulated axis of hypothalamic CRH, ACTH, and cortisol secretion (HPA) may not be fully developed until late gestation.[1]

CRH is a 41-amino acid neuropeptide synthesized in the paraventricular nucleus of the hypothalamus.[2,3] CRH is secreted, along with arginine vasopressin (AVP), into the hypophyseal portal blood and regulates the release of ACTH from the anterior pituitary gland. CRH acts by binding G protein–coupled receptors located on corticotroph cells of the anterior pituitary gland, leading to the activation of adenylate cyclase resulting in increased levels of intracellular cyclic adenine monophosphate (cAMP). The induction of cAMP activates protein kinase A, which ultimately stimulates the secretion of ACTH from the corticotroph cells.

Studies in fetal sheep reveal that there is a progressive elevation in CRH that is particularly notable during the second half of gestation.[4-6] The expression of hypothalamic CRH messenger RNA (mRNA) during this time appears to be regulated by a glucocorticoid-mediated negative feedback signal, as is the case postnatally.[7] However, the sensitivity of this feedback may decrease with increasing gestational age. This could explain how, despite the presence of high levels of cortisol that stimulate parturition, CRH-stimulated ACTH secretion persists in late-gestation fetuses.[8]

In addition to the central nervous system, CRH is produced in peripheral sites, including the adrenal medulla, ovaries, uterus, and placenta.[3] Placental expression of CRH is unique to primates and, as a source of both maternal and fetal serum CRH, has an important role in the development of the placenta and fetus and the progression to parturition.[9,10] Placental CRH increases exponentially during pregnancy, with expression increasing 100-fold during the last 6 to 8 weeks of pregnancy.[10] CRH from the placenta stimulates the production of fetal ACTH, leading to the production of dehydroepiandrosterone (DHEA) and cortisol by the fetal adrenal gland.[9,10] Fetal DHEA serves as the predominant precursor for the synthesis of estradiol by the placenta, which increases throughout the course of pregnancy up to the time of birth, when the rise in estrogen, particularly in amniotic fluid, promotes myometrial contractility.[3] This is essential because the primate placenta does not express significant levels of 17α-hydroxylase-17,20-lyase, which is required for conversion of progesterone to estrogen, as is seen in the placenta of other mammals.[9] In human pregnancies, the rise in estrogen comes from the conversion of DHEA secreted from the fetal adrenal.

The rise in placental CRH during pregnancy increases cortisol from both the fetal and maternal adrenal glands. In turn, placental CRH is paradoxically stimulated by cortisol such that a positive feedback system is created (Fig. 143.1). The surge in fetal cortisol secretion that precipitates parturition is crucial in fetal organ maturation, preparing the fetus for extrauterine life. Cortisol is of particular importance to maturation of the fetal lungs, as indicated by the frequent occurrence of respiratory distress syndrome in preterm infants and the risk of which is reduced by antenatal corticosteroids. Placental CRH stimulation of both cortisol and DHEA tethers the effects of cortisol on fetal organ maturation to the timing of parturition.[9,10]

Increasing placental CRH contributes to the rise in maternal serum CRH.[3,9] Maternal plasma levels of CRH increase steadily in the second trimester, reaching up to 1000-fold above the levels of nonpregnant women.[2,3] However, abnormally elevated maternal CRH levels are associated with complications during pregnancy, including preterm labor, preeclampsia, intrauterine growth restriction (IUGR), and postpartum depressive symptoms.[2,9,11,12] High levels of cortisol from prenatal maternal stress can stimulate placental CRH secretion, leading to premature birth.[3] Together, these clinical findings suggest that the timing of birth can be altered by modulation of the HPA axis.

ADRENOCORTICOTROPIC HORMONE

Maternal plasma ACTH levels increase moderately during pregnancy, with corresponding increases in cortisol concentrations.[3,13] By 16 weeks gestation, ACTH is detectable

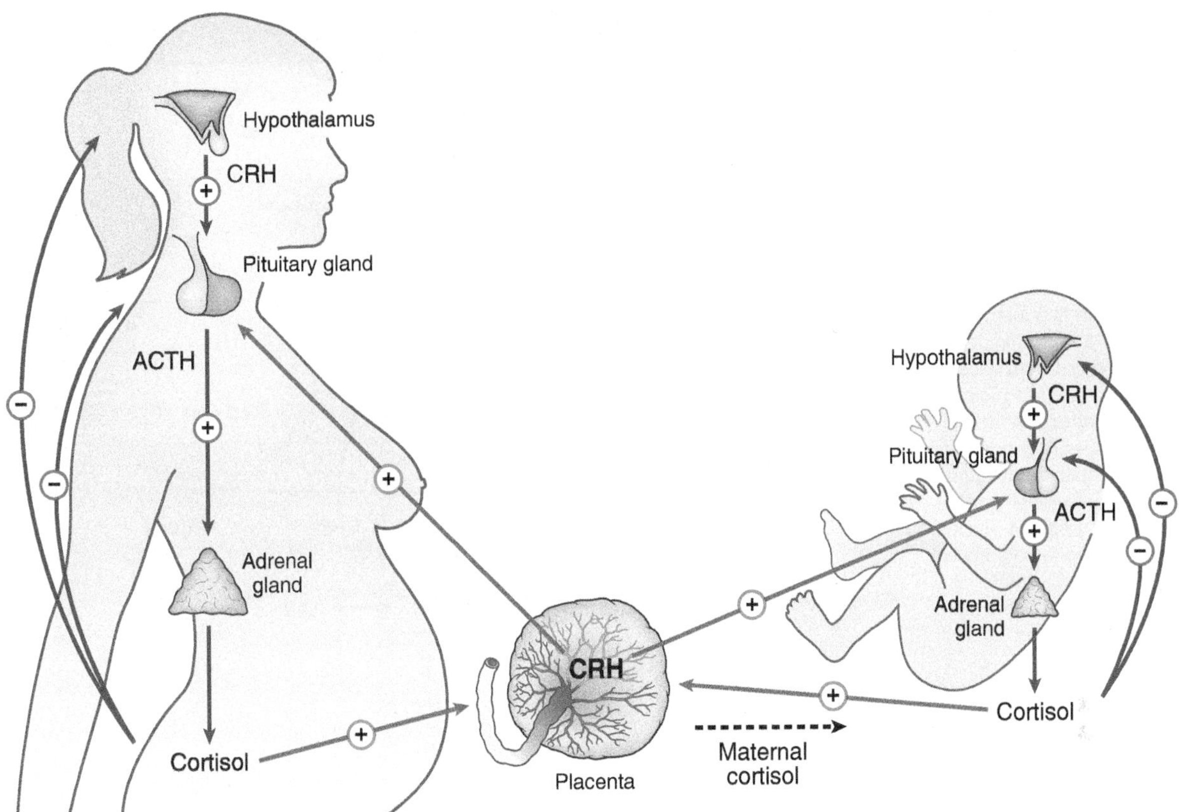

Fig. 143.1 Influence of placental corticotropin-releasing hormone *(CRH)* on both the maternal and fetal hypothalamus-pituitary-adrenal axes. *ACTH*, Adrenocorticotropic hormone. (Modified from Howland MA, Sandman CA, Glynn LM. Developmental origins of the human hypothalamic-pituitary-adrenal axis. *Expert Rev Endocrinol Metab.* 2017;12:321–339.)

in fetal blood, and studies report that levels of ACTH increase slightly as gestation progresses.[14,15] However, the extent of the increase in ACTH during pregnancy is disproportionate to the massive increase in circulating placental-derived CRH. ACTH is synthesized and secreted by corticotroph cells in the anterior pituitary gland, and it is a hormone end product of its precursor, proopiomelanocortin (POMC) (Fig. 143.2). Depending on the site of origin, POMC is converted, through a series of enzyme-induced cleavages, to various peptides. In the anterior pituitary, the enzyme prohormone convertase 1/3 acts on POMC to form pro-ACTH and β-lipotropin. Pro-ACTH is processed further to yield other peptides, including ACTH and α-melanocyte-stimulating hormone (αMSH).[15] The action of αMSH, through the melanocortin-1 receptor (MC1R), stimulates production of melanin, resulting in darkening of skin cells. This explains why individuals with primary adrenal insufficiency, such as Addison disease, develop hyperpigmentation. The loss of negative feedback from cortisol results in excessive production of ACTH along with other POMC peptides, including αMSH. It is also likely that the precursors of αMSH, including POMC, at high enough concentrations can act at the MC1R to cause hyperpigmentation.[16]

The action of ACTH occurs when the hormone binds to its receptor, the melanocortin-2 receptor (MC2R), located in all zones of the adrenal cortex. The primary site of ACTH action is in the zona fasciculata, where binding results in activation of the adenylate cyclase system, which induces the synthesis of cortisol.[17,18] Cortisol has negative feedback on its own secretion by fast inhibition of ACTH secretion and delayed inhibition of CRH and ACTH production. The stimulatory actions of ACTH at the fetal adrenal are also inhibited by other POMC peptides that contain the ACTH sequence, namely, POMC itself and pro-ACTH.[19] Consequently, the precursor peptide levels in the adrenal may be as important as levels of ACTH. Immunoreactive ACTH, as measured by some assays, may reflect levels of both ACTH and the precursors.

ACTH is required for normal structure and function of the adrenal cortex. In mice with complete absence of POMC, the adrenal glands fail to proliferate, resulting in atrophic adrenals. High-dose replacement of ACTH in these mice rescues the adrenal glands in terms of weight, morphology, and cortisol secretion, but this may be due to hypertrophy of the zona fasciculata, not full regeneration of the glands.[18] Similarly, human babies born with agenesis of the pituitary gland or hypopituitarism often have atrophic or malformed and unresponsive adrenal glands. In addition, the presence of excess exogenous or endogenous glucocorticoids suppresses ACTH secretion and can also cause atrophic and hyporesponsive adrenal glands.

REGULATION

Pituitary responsiveness to CRH increases during development, resulting in stimulation of ACTH secretion. Interesting, CRH appears to be the major driver of ACTH secretion in early fetal development, whereas responsiveness to AVP increases later in gestation, corresponding to increasing fetal cortisol levels. This association suggests that cortisol levels feedback to influence the CRH-ACTH axis in the pituitary and brain during fetal development. Consistent with this, the receptor for cortisol (glucocorticoid receptor [GR]) is expressed in the fetal pituitary, hypothalamus, and hippocampus as early as midgestation.

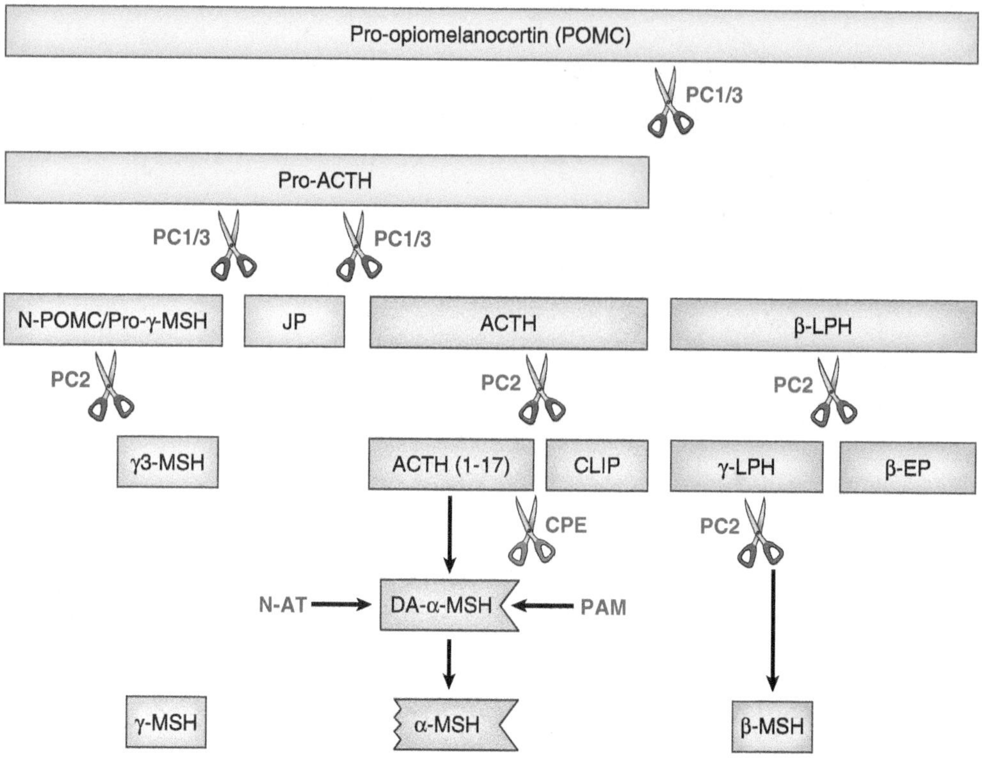

Fig. 143.2 Processing of proopiomelanocortin *(POMC)*. *ACTH*, Adrenocorticotropic hormone; *CLIP*, corticotropin-like intermediate peptide; *CPE*, carboxypeptidase E; *DA-αMSH*, des-acetyl αMSH; *EP*, endorphin; *JP*, joining peptide; *LPH*, lipotropic hormone; *MSH*, melanocyte-stimulating hormone; *N-AT*, N-acetyltransferase; *N-POMC*, amino-terminal end of POMC; *PAM*, peptidyl-glycine α-amidating monooxygenase; *PC1/3*, prohormone convertase 1/3; *PC2*, prohormone convertase 2. (Modified from Harno E, Gali Ramamoorthy T, Coll AP, et al. POMC: the physiological power of hormone processing. *Physiol Rev.* 2018;98:2381–2430.)

Immediately preceding parturition, there is an increase in ACTH levels. This surge is paradoxical to usual feedback mechanisms because cortisol levels are simultaneously elevated. Although unexplained, it is important to keep this process in mind when interpreting laboratory values in samples taken during this time.

ACTH stimulates synthesis of glucocorticoids in the adrenal cortex that are then released into the circulation to reach most cells in the body. Cortisol is the primary glucocorticoid generated in humans. After the neonatal period, basal secretion of ACTH and cortisol occur with a circadian rhythm, rising prior to waking and peaking approximately half an hour after waking in most diurnal individuals living with wake/sleep patterns that are concordant with the approximately 24-hour light/dark cycles of the planet. The precise timing of when this circadian rhythm develops remains undefined, and there is variability between individuals that are likely driven by diversity in when consistent sleep patterns develop. However, it appears to take months to develop and sustain a consistent circadian HPA axis pattern, and therefore measuring morning ACTH and cortisol levels in newborns is unlikely to be informative of the status of the HPA axis, as it is when this is done later in life. Furthermore, secretion of cortisol into the circulation is pulsatile and rapidly responsive to changes in the systemic environment such as stress and hypoglycemia. The physician must synthesize all of these factors when interpreting test results of glucocorticoid levels.

Glucocorticoids are so termed because of their major actions to increase plasma concentrations of glucose. This occurs by their induction of the transcription of the genes encoding the enzymes of the Embden-Meyerhof glycolytic pathway and other hepatic enzymes that divert amino acids, such as alanine, to the production of glucose. Virtually all of these actions are mediated through GRs, which are found in most cells. However, despite the initial simple appearance of the hormone-receptor relationship, receptor bound glucocorticoids exert surprisingly diverse context and cell-specific activities. Recent advances in the field have identified a variety of mechanisms by which this is accomplished, including context-specific allosteric changes in the receptor conformation that drive the formation of distinct transcriptional regulatory complexes.[20] This can be observed at the molecular level by comparing RNA expression profiles across different tissues and cell types in response to the same glucocorticoid signal. This plasticity has important physiologic implications, serving as the underpinning mechanism for the different tissue responses to glucocorticoids, including the promotion of visceral adipose tissue expansion while simultaneously inhibiting growth of muscle and bone.

The GR was the first nuclear hormone receptor to be cloned, which revealed a series of functional domains in the protein that turned out to be prototypical for the nuclear receptor family.[21] In particular, the ligand-binding domain (LBD) is located at the C-terminus of the protein, which is also a region for interaction with co-activator proteins. The LBD of the GR is particularly highly homologous to the mineralocorticoid receptor (MR). Subtle structural differences between MR and GR confer specificity for aldosterone binding to MR, but cortisol is able to bind to both receptors. Sensitive tissues, such as the kidney, express the enzyme 11-beta-hydroxysteroid dehydrogenase type 2 (11βHSD2), which converts cortisol into inactive cortisone, protecting MRs from being activated by cortisol. Other domains identified in the GR that are conserved across nuclear receptors include the DNA-binding domain (DBD), which is centrally located in the GR protein. The DBD facilitates receptor dimerization and also contains two zinc-finger motifs that can bind to the major groove of DNA. The N-terminal domain of GR is the least conserved and enables interactions with coregulators.

Unbound GRs exist predominantly in the cytoplasm of cells. When glucocorticoid levels increase, more GRs in cells become bound by hormone and translocate into the nucleus. Rather than being a passive process, the binding of glucocorticoids induces conformational changes in GR that expose nuclear localization motifs, promoting facilitated trafficking of the hormone-receptor complex into the nucleus. Once in the nucleus, the action of glucocorticoids/GR occurs by (1) occupancy of defined sequences of DNA designated as glucocorticoid response elements (GREs), (2) context-specific interactions with cofactors and coregulators, and (3) engagement with transcriptional machinery. The combinatorial sum of these actions modulates the expression of target genes. Glucocorticoid/GR access to GREs in the DNA can be gated by a variety of factors, including chromatin structure, contributing to cell-specific activity of glucocorticoids. Similarly, posttranslational modifications of the GR further refine glucocorticoid action on target genes. Together, these variables enable context and cell-specific glucocorticoid activity as well as a capacity for fine-tuned modulation of the transcription levels of target genes in response to dynamic physiologic needs.

FETAL PROGRAMMING AND THE HYPOTHALAMUS-PITUITARY-ADRENAL AXIS

Fetal programming refers to environmentally induced changes that occur in the fetus that fundamentally alter physiology and are sustained into adulthood.[22,23] The ability of fetal programming to modify HPA function in later adult life was first described more than 50 years ago.[24,25] Studies indicate that programming of the HPA axis occurring during the fetal and early postnatal environment can influence susceptibility to a range of psychologic, cardiovascular, infectious, metabolic, and inflammatory diseases.[24,26-29] It is important to note when assessing potential consequences of exposures that they can be highly variable, depending on the time of exposure, the sex of the individual, and the age at which they are being assessed.[30] Furthermore, once fetal programming has occurred, the changes can be passed down across multiple generations.[30] Largely unstudied is whether any changes might ultimately prove to be beneficial in later life.[31-37]

PROGRAMMING VARIABLES

Multiple variables in early development, including maternal psychologic and physiologic states during pregnancy, have effects on the development and function of the HPA axis.[24,38-40]

STEROIDS

Glucocorticoids are one of the proposed mechanisms that mediate fetal programming. The effect of glucocorticoids on fetal programming appears to be dependent upon the timing of exposure, endogenous versus exogenous steroid use, single versus multiple doses, and sex of the offspring.[1,30,41-50] In humans, placental 11βHSD2 only partially limits fetal exposure to maternal cortisol, with approximately 15% able to cross through the placenta unmetabolized.[51-54] The fetus is less protected from maternal cortisol during early and late gestation, when placental 11βHSD2 activity is lower.[51,55-59] Elevated maternal cortisol levels in late gestation can be beneficial as they promote fetal organ maturation and enhance neurodevelopment with lasting benefits including accelerated development over the first year of life and enhanced cognitive functioning when assessed at 6 to 9 years of age.[32,34-37] However, maternal cortisol levels during early to mid-gestation and prolonged exposure to high levels of cortisol may exert negative effects by suppressing fetal and placental growth and have been associated with neurologic and learning defects, cardiovascular disease, and metabolic disease later in life.[30,32,34-37,60-64]

Most synthetic glucocorticoids (including betamethasone), in contrast to maternal cortisol, are not metabolized by placental 11βHSD2 and readily cross into circulation of the developing fetus where they may program developing organ systems and dysregulate postnatal HPA axis function.[1,45-50,65] Synthetic glucocorticoids are the standard of care in the treatment of women at risk of preterm delivery to improve survival of preterm infants.[60,66] A single dose of a synthetic glucocorticoid prior to delivery accelerates fetal lung development and subsequently reduces the incidence and severity of respiratory distress syndrome, the most common cause of death in preterm infants.[60,66-69] This treatment has profoundly increased the survival rate of premature infants.[60,70] Increased glucocorticoid exposure may induce additional long-lasting beneficial effects in offspring by stimulating the differentiation of several tissues (Fig. 143.3).[70] In addition to these potential benefits, treatment with glucocorticoids likely have detrimental fetal programming effects on the HPA axis.[61,62,70-73] For example, neonates born prematurely following exposure to synthetic glucocorticoids in utero exhibited reduced basal cortisol levels at birth, and term-born infants exhibited heightened HPA reactivity.[30,74,75] Studies have also found that antenatal exposure to synthetic glucocorticoids have long-term effects on brain structure and behavior, as well as neurosensory, neuroendocrine, and cardiometabolic function.[30] Antenatal treatment with synthetic glucocorticoids has been associated with thinning of the anterior cingulate cortex, an increased risk for mental and somatic health disorders, an increased risk for the development of severe neurocognitive and neurosensory disability, and disruption in the circadian regulation of the HPA axis.[30,42,43,65]

As mentioned previously, clinicians should consider that fetal programming can have sexual dimorphic effects. Antenatal betamethasone was found to alter placental glucocorticoid metabolism in neonates in a sex-specific manner.[41] Males born following this treatment had increased 11βHSD2 levels, whereas females had decreased 11βHSD2 levels and activity, as well as reduced head circumferences. Female fetuses subsequently exposed to higher cortisol levels may benefit from accelerated organ maturation with a higher likelihood of survival in an adverse in utero environment.[41] However, this adaptive process does not come without the risk for impaired HPA axis development and vulnerability to anxiety and affective disorders later in life.[41] In contrast, males, possibly due to increased 11βHSD2 levels, are shielded from cortisol exposure but are then at higher risk of being less adapted to postnatal survival.[41]

MATERNAL PSYCHOLOGICAL DISTRESS

Substantial amounts of cortisol and CRH are produced by the maternal-placental-fetal steroidogenic unit in the antenatal period. Although these increases are normal and expected during the gestational period, the developing fetus remains vulnerable to stress-induced maternal increases in these hormones, which exert programming effects on the fetal HPA axis.[1] Reduced placental 11βHSD2 gene expression and activity are associated with prenatal maternal stress. Depressed enzymatic activity facilitates increased transfer of maternal cortisol across the placenta into fetal circulation.[1,15,51-53,76] Affected offspring have reduced birth weight, higher levels of anxiety and depression, and an increased risk of developing various diseases, including coronary artery disease and type 2 diabetes.[70,77,78] Overall, studies suggest that prenatal maternal stress resulted in heightened HPA axis activity during the neonatal period.[1] Reactivity of the HPA axis in toddlers exposed to antenatal maternal stress may depend on the type of maternal stress experienced (i.e., objective exposure vs. subjective stress) and the sex of the child.[31] An array of developmental outcomes in children may be affected by maternal stress during pregnancy, including temperament, cognition, language skills, and motor functioning.[31,79] In addition, HPA axis function in offspring affected by maternal stress throughout pregnancy may be a cause of increased vulnerability to behavioral and mental health problems; however, more studies are needed to further examine this relationship.[31,80] Furthermore, the long-term effects of maternal stress on the offspring's HPA axis reactivity has not yet been thoroughly studied.

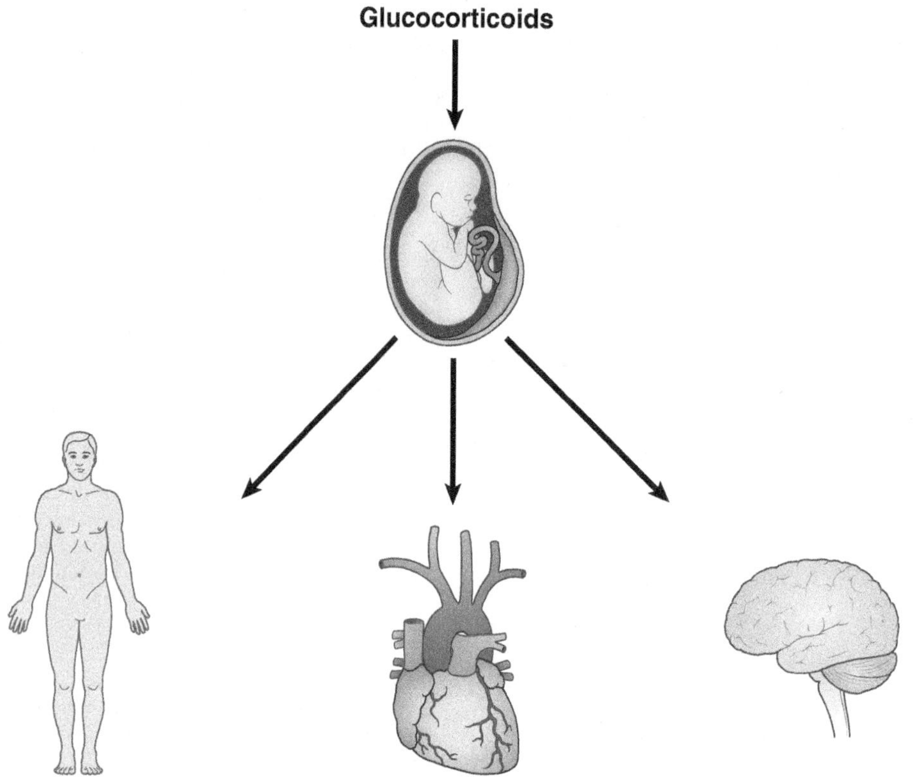
Glucocorticoids
Systemic effects:
• Promotion of organ maturation
• Suppression of fetal and placental growth
• Reduced birth weight and size
• Higher risk for metabolic disease
Cardiovascular effects:
• Increased risk for cardiovascular disease
• Enhanced blood pressure reponse to stress
Brain effects:
• Enhanced neurodevelopment and cognitive functioning
• Dysregulation of the HPA axis
• Changes in brain structure
• Neurologic and learning defects
• Increased risk for mental health disorders

Fig. 143.3 Beneficial and detrimental fetal programming effects of exposure to maternal glucocorticoids. *HPA*, Hypothalamus-pituitary-adrenal. (Modified from Joseph DN, Whirledge S. Stress and the HPA axis: balancing homeostasis and fertility. *Int J Mol Sci*. 2017;18:2224.)

MATERNAL DEPRESSION

Maternal depression appears to have programming effects on the developing fetal HPA axis. Some studies found that neonates exposed to greater maternal depressive symptoms in the second half of gestation had higher levels of ACTH versus infants exposed to fewer maternal depressive symptoms.[1,81] Two other investigations found that neonates born to mothers with elevated prenatal depressive symptoms had higher urinary cortisol levels.[82,83] Another study observed that 1-month-old infants born to mothers with depressive disorders had higher baseline salivary cortisol levels and greater salivary cortisol levels in response to a stressor compared with a control group.[84]

MATERNAL ANXIETY

Prenatal anxiety in mothers was found to be associated with higher infant baseline and stimulated cortisol levels compared with controls.[1,85,86] Maternal pregnancy-specific anxiety was associated with lower scores on the Bayley Scales of Infant Development at 12 months and increased negative temperament in children.[34,87]

MATERNAL LIPIDS

High maternal antenatal levels of triglycerides and total cholesterol have been associated with increased cortisol reactivity in the child, independent of maternal obesity and other confounders.[88]

ALCOHOL/NICOTINE/DRUGS

A meta-analysis of maternal alcohol, tobacco, and drug use found that all three variables have an effect on baseline and reactive cortisol secretion in early childhood.[85] Studies using rodent models revealed that prenatal nicotine exposure can increase the potential excitatory set point of the hypothalamus in offspring and result in increased HPA axis hypersensitivity in adulthood.[44] Prenatal ethanol exposure in rodent models was found to result in low basal activity but hyperresponsiveness of the HPA axis in offspring.[89]

POSTNATAL STEROID TREATMENT

Glucocorticoids are a commonly used treatment in the postnatal period for patients at risk for bronchopulmonary dysplasia (BPD) and in critically ill preterm infants.[90] Three Cochrane reviews have examined the relative benefits and adverse effects of systemic postnatal glucocorticoids administered to preterm infants.[90-92]

EARLY (≤7 DAYS)

Studies indicate that early (initiated in the first week of life) glucocorticoid treatment in preterm infants facilitated extubation and reduced the risk of BPD, patent ductus arteriosus (PDA), and retinopathy of prematurity (ROP). However, adverse effects of this treatment included gastrointestinal (GI) bleeding, intestinal perforation, hyperglycemia, hypertension, hypertrophic cardiomyopathy, and growth failure. In addition, long-term follow-up studies reported an increased risk of abnormal findings, including an increased risk of cerebral palsy, on neurologic examinations. There were no significant differences in mortality rates. Subgroup analyses by the type of glucocorticoid used revealed that dexamethasone was the most efficacious but also had the most significant adverse side effects. Hydrocortisone had little effect in most analyses, but it demonstrated some advantages in improving rates of mortality, extubation failure, and PDA with reduced long-term adverse effects compared with dexamethasone. However, hydrocortisone was associated with an increased occurrence of intestinal perforation. A review of the literature ultimately concluded that the benefits of early postnatal corticosteroids, particularly dexamethasone, may not outweigh real or potential adverse effects and suggested curtailing early corticosteroid treatment for prevention of BPD.[90]

LATE (>7 DAYS)

Late (initiated after the first week of life) use of glucocorticoids for preterm infants to treat evolving or established BPD resulted in reduced extubation failures, need for late rescue treatments with dexamethasone, discharges on home oxygen, and neonatal mortality at 28 days (but no reduction in mortality thereafter). Adverse effects included hyperglycemia, glycosuria, hypertension, and severe ROP. There were trends towards increased risk of infection, GI bleeding, and cerebral palsy or abnormal neurologic examination. There was no significant difference between steroid and control groups in major neurosensory disability, the combined rate of death or major neurosensory disability, or other outcomes in later childhood, including respiratory health or function, blood pressure, and growth. Ultimately, a review of the literature concluded that benefits of late glucocorticoid therapy may not outweigh actual or potential adverse effects, and it may be prudent to reserve this treatment for infants who cannot be weaned from mechanical ventilation via an endotracheal tube after the first week of life and to minimize both dose and duration for any course of treatment given.[91]

VERY LOW-BIRTH-WEIGHT INFANTS

A review of the literature found that the optimal type of glucocorticoid, dosage, and timing of initiation for the prevention of BPD in very low-birth-weight (VLBW) preterm infants could not be made based on the current level of evidence, and no change in the recommendations published in international guidelines of glucocorticoid use were made.[92] A systematic review and meta-analysis evaluated the efficacy of intratracheal administration of budesonide-surfactant in the prevention of BPD in VLBW infants.[93] The study found that infants who received intratracheal budesonide-surfactant mixture had a 43% reduction in the risk of BPD, although mortality was not affected. Larger trials are needed before this treatment can be recommended as a standard of care.[93]

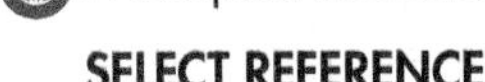

A complete reference list is available at www.ExpertConsult.com.

SELECT REFERENCES

1. Howland MA, Sandman CA, Glynn LM. Developmental origins of the human hypothalamic-pituitary-adrenal axis. *Expert Rev Endocrinol Metab*. 2017;12:321-339.
2. Reis FM, Fadalti M, Florio P, et al. Putative role of placental corticotropin-releasing factor in the mechanisms of human parturition. *J Soc Gynecol Investig*. 1999;6:109-119.
3. Mastorakos G, Ilias I. Maternal and fetal hypothalamic-pituitary-adrenal axes during pregnancy and postpartum. *Ann N Y Acad Sci*. 2003;997:136-149.
4. Currie IS, Brooks AN. Corticotrophin-releasing factors in the hypothalamus of the developing fetal sheep. *J Dev Physiol*. 1992;17:241-246.
5. Brieu V, Tonon MC, Lutz-Bucher B, et al. Corticotropin-releasing factor-like immunoreactivity, arginine vasopressin-like immunoreactivity and ACTH-releasing bioactivity in hypothalamic tissue from fetal and neonatal sheep. *Neuroendocrinology*. 1989;49:164-168.
6. Matthews SG, Challis JR. Regulation of CRH and AVP mRNA in the developing ovine hypothalamus: effects of stress and glucocorticoids. *Am J Physiol*. 1995;268:E1096-1107.
7. Reichardt HM, Schütz G. Feedback control of glucocorticoid production is established during fetal development. *Mol Med*. 1996;2:735-744.
8. Wood CE. Insensitivity of near-term fetal sheep to cortisol: possible relation to the control of parturition. *Endocrinology*. 1988;122:1565-1572.
9. Power ML, Schulkin J. Functions of corticotropin-releasing hormone in anthropoid primates: from brain to placenta. *Am J Hum Biol*. 2006;18:431-447.
10. Majzoub JA, Karalis KP. Placental corticotropin-releasing hormone: function and regulation. *Am J Obstet Gynecol*. 1999;180:S242-246.
11. Glynn LM, Sandman CA. Evaluation of the association between placental corticotrophin-releasing hormone and postpartum depressive symptoms. *Psychosom Med*. 2014;76:355-362.
12. Yim IS, Glynn LM, Dunkel-Schetter C, et al. Risk of postpartum depressive symptoms with elevated corticotropin-releasing hormone in human pregnancy. *Arch Gen Psychiatry*. 2009;66:162-169.
13. Sandman CA, Wadhwa PD, Chicz-DeMet A, et al. Maternal corticotropin-releasing hormone and habituation in the human fetus. *Dev Psychobiol*. 1999;34:163-173.
14. Rose J, Schwartz J, Young S. Development of corticotropin-releasing hormone-corticotropin/beta endorphin system in the mammalian fetus. In: Polin R, Fox W, Abman S, eds. *Fetal and Neonatal Physiology*. Philadelphia: WB Saunders; 2004:1097-1914.
15. Lockwood CJ, Radunovic N, Nastic D, et al. Corticotropin-releasing hormone and related pituitary-adrenal axis hormones in fetal and maternal blood during the second half of pregnancy. *J Perinat Med*. 1996;24:243-251.
16. Harno E, Gali Ramamoorthy T, Coll AP, et al. POMC: the physiological power of hormone processing. *Physiol Rev*. 2018;98:2381-2430.
17. Stevens A, White A. ACTH: cellular peptide hormone synthesis and secretory pathways. *Results Probl Cell Differ*. 2010;50:63-84.
18. Novoselova TV, King PJ, Guasti L, et al. ACTH signalling and adrenal development: lessons from mouse models. *Endocr Connect*. 2019;8:R122-R130.
19. Schwartz J, Kleftogiannis F, Jacobs R, et al. Biological activity of adrenocorticotropic hormone precursors on ovine adrenal cells. *Am J Physiol*. 1995;268:E623-629.
24. Kapoor A, Dunn E, Kostaki A, et al. Fetal programming of hypothalamo-pituitary-adrenal function: prenatal stress and glucocorticoids. *J Physiol*. 2006;572:31-44.
25. Levine S. Maternal and environmental influences on the adrenocortical response to stress in weanling rats. *Science*. 1967;156:258-260.
30. Constantinof A, Moisiadis VG, Matthews SG. Programming of stress pathways: a transgenerational perspective. *J Steroid Biochem Mol Biol*. 2016;160:175-180.
31. Van den Bergh BRH, van den Heuvel MI, Lahti M, et al. Prenatal developmental origins of behavior and mental health: the influence of maternal stress in pregnancy. *Neurosci Biobehav Rev*. 2020;117:26-64.
32. Davis EP, Head K, Buss C, et al. Prenatal maternal cortisol concentrations predict neurodevelopment in middle childhood. *Psychoneuroendocrinology*. 2017;75:56-63.
34. Davis EP, Sandman CA. The timing of prenatal exposure to maternal cortisol and psychosocial stress is associated with human infant cognitive development. *Child Dev*. 2010;81:131-148.
35. Buss C, Davis EP, Shahbaba B, et al. Maternal cortisol over the course of pregnancy and subsequent child amygdala and hippocampus volumes and affective problems. *Proc Natl Acad Sci U S A*. 2012;109:E1312-1319.
37. Davis EP, Glynn LM, Waffarn F, et al. Prenatal maternal stress programs infant stress regulation. *J Child Psychol Psychiatry*. 2011;52:119-129.
41. Braun F, Hardt AK, Ehrlich L, et al. Sex-specific and lasting effects of a single course of antenatal betamethasone treatment on human placental 11β-HSD2. *Placenta*. 2018;69:9-19.
45. Kajantie E, Raivio T, Jänne OA, et al. Circulating glucocorticoid bioactivity in the preterm newborn after antenatal betamethasone treatment. *J Clin Endocrinol Metab*. 2004;89:3999-4003.
50. Ashwood PJ, Crowther CA, Willson KJ, et al. Neonatal adrenal function after repeat dose prenatal corticosteroids: a randomized controlled trial. *Am J Obstet Gynecol*. 2006;194:861-867.
51. Benediktsson R, Calder AA, Edwards CR, et al. Placental 11 beta-hydroxysteroid dehydrogenase: a key regulator of fetal glucocorticoid exposure. *Clin Endocrinol (Oxf)*. 1997;46:161-166.
52. Gitau R, Cameron A, Fisk NM, et al. Fetal exposure to maternal cortisol. *Lancet*. 1998;352:707-708.
53. Gitau R, Fisk NM, Teixeira JM, et al. Fetal hypothalamic-pituitary-adrenal stress responses to invasive procedures are independent of maternal responses. *J Clin Endocrinol Metab*. 2001;86:104-109.
55. Beitins IZ, Bayard F, Ances IG, et al. The metabolic clearance rate, blood production, interconversion and transplacental passage of cortisol and cortisone in pregnancy near term. *Pediatr Res*. 1973;7:509-519.
58. McTernan CL, Draper N, Nicholson H, et al. Reduced placental 11beta-hydroxysteroid dehydrogenase type 2 mRNA levels in human pregnancies complicated by intrauterine growth restriction: an analysis of possible mechanisms. *J Clin Endocrinol Metab*. 2001;86:4979-4983.
60. Busada JT, Cidlowski JA. Mechanisms of glucocorticoid action during development. *Curr Top Dev Biol*. 2017;125:147-170.
63. Murphy KE, Hannah ME, Willan AR, et al. Multiple courses of antenatal corticosteroids for preterm birth (MACS): a randomised controlled trial. *Lancet*. 2008;372:2143-2151.

65. Edelmann MN, Sandman CA, Glynn LM, et al. Antenatal glucocorticoid treatment is associated with diurnal cortisol regulation in term-born children. *Psychoneuroendocrinology*. 2016;72:106-112.
66. Liggins GC, Howie RN. A controlled trial of antepartum glucocorticoid treatment for prevention of the respiratory distress syndrome in premature infants. *Pediatrics*. 1972;50:515-525.
68. Matsuzaki Y, Xu Y, Ikegami M, et al. Stat3 is required for cytoprotection of the respiratory epithelium during adenoviral infection. *J Immunol*. 2006;177:527-537.
69. Effect of corticosteroids for fetal maturation on perinatal outcomes. NIH Consensus Development Panel on the effect of corticosteroids for fetal maturation on perinatal outcomes. *JAMA*. 1995;273:413-418.
70. Joseph DN, Whirledge S. Stress and the HPA axis: balancing homeostasis and fertility. *Int J Mol Sci*. 2017;18:2224.
71. Nyirenda MJ, Lindsay RS, Kenyon CJ, et al. Glucocorticoid exposure in late gestation permanently programs rat hepatic phosphoenolpyruvate carboxykinase and glucocorticoid receptor expression and causes glucose intolerance in adult offspring. *J Clin Invest*. 1998;101:2174-2181.
81. Field T, Diego M, Dieter J, et al. Prenatal depression effects on the fetus and the newborn. *Infant Behav Dev*. 2004;27:216-229.
85. Pearson J, Tarabulsy GM, Bussières EL. Foetal programming and cortisol secretion in early childhood: a meta-analysis of different programming variables. *Infant Behav Dev*. 2015;40:204-215.
90. Doyle LW, Cheong JL, Ehrenkranz RA, et al. Early (< 8 days) systemic postnatal corticosteroids for prevention of bronchopulmonary dysplasia in preterm infants. *Cochrane Database Syst Rev*. 2017;10:Cd001146.
91. Doyle LW, Cheong JL, Ehrenkranz RA, et al. Late (> 7 days) systemic postnatal corticosteroids for prevention of bronchopulmonary dysplasia in preterm infants. *Cochrane Database Syst Rev*. 2017;10:CD001145.
92. Onland W, De Jaegere AP, Offringa M, et al. Systemic corticosteroid regimens for prevention of bronchopulmonary dysplasia in preterm infants. *Cochrane Database Syst Rev*. 2017;1:CD010941.

144 Fetal and Neonatal Adrenocortical Physiology

Kristi L. Watterberg | Louis J. Muglia

INTRODUCTION

The adrenal cortex undergoes remarkable growth and unique metamorphosis during the fetal and neonatal period. Its morphology, functions, and secretory product profiles are distinctly different during fetal and postnatal life. The major products of the fetal adrenal cortex, the weak androgens dehydroepiandrosterone (DHEA) and its sulfate (DHEAS), disappear almost completely after birth, reappearing years later at the onset of adrenarche. The functions of the adrenal cortex during fetal life—participation in the maintenance of pregnancy and initiation of parturition, as well as secretion of cortisol to promote organ maturation before birth—also change postnatally for the maintenance of homeostasis, particularly in the presence of stress, and modulation of inflammatory challenges.[1]

The cumulative work of many investigators has demonstrated that the structural and functional organization of the fetal adrenal cortex of humans and higher primates is unique.[2] In addition, a major regulator of fetal adrenal development, placental corticotropin-releasing hormone (CRH), is present only in humans and anthropoid primates.[3] Thus, although insights can be obtained from other animal models, caution must be exercised in applying such findings to human physiology. Wherever possible, this chapter will focus on studies of humans and other primates.

DEVELOPMENTAL HISTOLOGY

The primordial adrenal gland is first evident in humans as a distinct cluster of cells at 33 days postconception.[4] By 50 to 52 days postconception, steroidogenic activity can be detected within the nascent fetal zone.[5] The gland then grows exponentially, increasing 10-fold between 8 and 10 weeks postconception,[5] equaling the kidney in weight by 20 weeks of gestation, then doubling in size between 20 and 30 weeks, and doubling again by term, reaching a combined weight of approximately 8 g (Fig. 144.1).[6] After birth, the gland quickly involutes, shrinking to a combined weight of approximately 2 g by 1 year of age before beginning to grow again.

This remarkable growth during fetal life occurs through a combination of hyperplasia, hypertrophy, and reduced apoptosis. During the embryonic period, mitotic activity has been observed throughout the fetal adrenal cortex.[6] The cortex then quickly differentiates into two distinct zones: an outer definitive zone, composed of a thin layer of tightly packed small, basophilic cells with ultrastructural characteristics consistent with cellular proliferation, and a much larger inner fetal zone, containing large, eosinophilic cells with a steroid secreting phenotype.[4,7]

The ultrastructural appearance of these two zones led investigators to conclude that cells in the fetal zone did not divide. Using newer techniques, however, investigators have identified mitotic figures throughout the fetal zone, suggesting that it grows by hyperplasia as well as hypertrophy.[7] Because the mitotic index in the definitive zone exceeds that in the fetal zone, however, proliferation appears to occur predominantly in the definitive zone, with new cells migrating toward the center, where they undergo hypertrophy and terminally differentiate into steroid producing cells.[7] At the intersection of these two zones, a transitional zone appears and begins to secrete cortisol at week 22 to 24 of pregnancy.[4,8] This transitional zone expands through the latter part of gestation and becomes the cortisol-secreting zona fasciculata by term gestation; the outer, definitive zone becomes the zona glomerulosa, which secretes the mineralocorticoid aldosterone.[4,8]

Apoptotic nuclei have been identified primarily at the center of the cortex.[7] These nuclei are present in low but increasing numbers during gestation. After birth, maximal apoptosis is observed in the fetal zone, which subsequently disappears.[7] Several years later, the zona reticularis will appear at the site of the earlier fetal zone and begin to secrete DHEA and DHEAS, thus regulating the onset of adrenarche.[1]

ENZYMES AND SECRETORY PRODUCTS

The major secretory products of the adrenal cortex include weak androgens (DHEA and DHEAS), cortisol, and aldosterone. As shown in Fig. 144.2, steroidogenesis requires a series of enzymatic

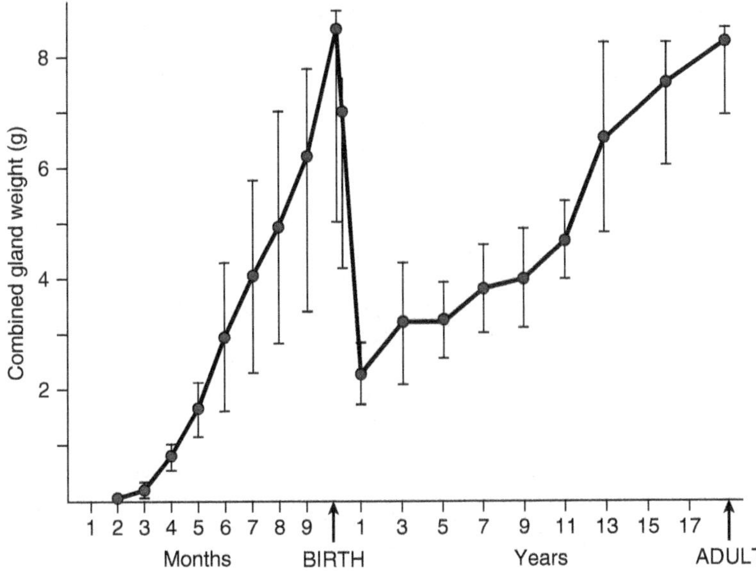

Fig. 144.1 Adrenal gland weights during human development. (From Neville AM, O'Hare MJ. *The human adrenal cortex*. Berlin: Springer-Verlag; 1982:12.)

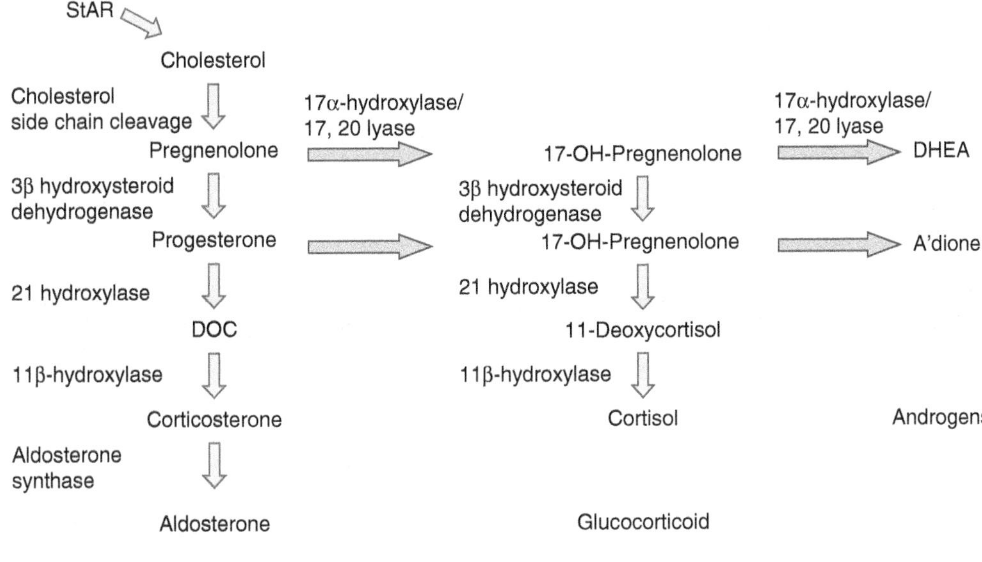

Fig. 144.2 Adrenal steroidogenesis. After the steroidogenic acute regulatory *(StAR)* protein-mediated uptake of cholesterol into mitochondria within adrenocortical cells, aldosterone, cortisol, and adrenal androgens are synthesized through the coordinated action of a series of steroidogenic enzymes in a zone-specific fashion. *A'dione,* Androstenedione; *DHEA,* dehydroepiandrosterone; *DOC,* deoxycorticosterone. (From Stewart PM. The adrenal cortex. In: Larsen PR, Kronenberg HM, Melmed S, Polonsky KS, eds. *Williams Textbook of Endocrinology.* Philadelphia: Saunders; 2003:495.)

steps, including four cytochrome P450 oxidase enzymes.[1] Two of these are located in the mitochondria (cholesterol side-chain cleavage enzyme [P450scc] and 11β-hydroxylase [P450C11]) and two are found in the endoplasmic reticulum (17α-hydroxylase/17,20-lyase [P450C17] and 21-hydroxylase [P450C21]).[9] The first, rate-limiting step in the synthesis of steroid hormones is the conversion of cholesterol to pregnenolone by P450scc, which is dependent on the delivery of cholesterol to the mitochondrion by the steroidogenic acute regulatory protein.[9] Absence of this regulatory protein impairs adrenal and gonadal steroidogenesis and is clinically manifested as congenital lipoid adrenal hyperplasia.[9] The critical branch point enzymes regulating steroidogenesis are 3β-hydroxysteroid dehydrogenase (type 2 isozyme, 3βHSD2) and P450C17. These two enzymes compete for substrate.[10] In tissues in which 3βHSD2 is highly expressed, cortisol is produced preferentially; low 3βHSD activity in conjunction with high P450C17 activity promotes DHEA production.[10,11]

After the embryonic period, the enzymes and secretory patterns of each zone within the adrenal cortex are distinct, and the specific steroidogenic enzymes within each zone determine the type of steroid produced in that zone.[4,8] The fetal zone contains P450C17 but lacks 3βHSD2, and thus secretes DHEA and DHEAS in massive amounts—up to 200 mg/day during the third trimester.[12] These adrenal androgens serve as substrates for placental aromatases, which convert them to the estrogens estriol, estradiol, and estrone (Fig. 144.3).[13,14] This process appears to be fundamental to the normal maintenance of pregnancy, as reviewed later in this chapter.

The transitional zone, which appears at 22 to 24 weeks gestation, contains 3βHSD2 and can therefore synthesize cortisol de novo from cholesterol (see Fig. 144.2).[1,8] Before the appearance of the transitional zone, however, cortisol may be produced by the fetus using placental progesterone as a substrate (see Fig. 144.3).[4] The outer, definitive zone of the cortex also begins to express 3βHSD2 toward the end of gestation, but this zone lacks P450C17 and therefore secretes the mineralocorticoid aldosterone (see Fig. 144.2).[4,8] The zona reticularis, which will not become morphologically apparent until adrenarche, appears to be analogous to the fetal adrenal cortex in that it lacks 3βHSD2 and secretes DHEA and DHEAS.[1]

Expression of these critical branch point enzymes very early in gestation, and their effects on early development have been unclear. 3βHSD2 was generally believed to be absent from the human fetal adrenal cortex in the undisturbed pregnancy until 22 to 24 weeks' gestation. However, an immunohistochemical study found transient staining for 3βHSD in numerous definitive zone cells and occasional fetal zone cells very early in development, which disappeared by 14 weeks postconception.[15] A subsequent study confirmed this transient expression of 3βHSD2, as well as its regulatory orphan nuclear receptor (nerve growth factor-induced clone B, or NGFIB), in human adrenal cortex during the embryonic period, and additionally documented a brief spike in adrenal cortisol content and secretion during this time (Fig. 144.4).[5,16] Biosynthesis was maximal at 8 to 9 weeks postconception, after which 3βHSD immunoreactivity and cortisol content decreased quickly, declining by half at 10 weeks and to undetectable levels by 14 weeks postconception. This early, transitory cortisol production was coincidental with the detection of adrenocorticotropic hormone (ACTH) in the same fetuses. In addition, these adrenocortical cells were responsive to ACTH, strongly suggesting that even at this early stage, adrenal cortical cells are regulated by ACTH secretion.[5]

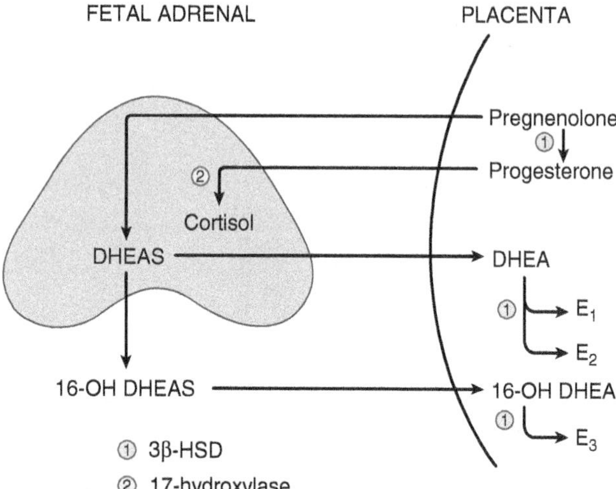

Fig. 144.3 Diagrammatic representation of the fetoplacental unit composed of the fetal adrenal cortex and the placenta. The placenta is deficient in 17-hydroxylase activity and cannot synthesize estrogens from progesterone. The fetal adrenal cortex has low 3β-hydroxysteroid dehydrogenase *(3βHSD)* and Δ4,5 isomerase activity and cannot synthesize progesterone. Sulfokinase activity is high in fetal adrenal tissue, and steroid sulfatase activity is high in placental tissue. Thus the placenta produces progesterone, which is predominantly converted to dehydroepiandrosterone *(DHEA)* by the fetal adrenal cortex; the DHEA can be sulfated to form dehydroepiandrosterone sulfate *(DHEAS)*. Part of this is 16-hydroxylated by the fetal liver, and both DHEA and DHEAS are used by the placenta as substrates for estrone *(E_1)* and estradiol *(E_2)* synthesis, respectively. Placental sulfatase converts DHEAS and 16-hydroxy-DHEAS to DHEA and 17-hydroxy-DHEA. The 16-hydroxy-DHEA is used for estriol *(E_3)* synthesis. (From Fisher DA. Endocrinology of fetal development. In: Larsen PR, Kronenberg HM, Melmed S, Polonsky KS, eds. *Williams Textbook of Endocrinology.* Philadelphia: Saunders; 2003:813.)

The thought-provoking work just described helps solve the puzzle of how female fetuses affected by P450C21-deficient congenital adrenal hyperplasia become virilized very early in gestation, at a time before the fetus had been thought to produce cortisol. Virilization occurs in congenital adrenal hyperplasia when the cortisol biosynthesis pathway is stimulated by ACTH, and cortisol production is blocked by the absence of P450C21 (see Fig. 144.2). This block in cortisol synthesis removes the normal negative feedback of cortisol to the pituitary and results in increased ACTH secretion. In this situation, continuing stimulation of the cortisol synthesis pathway leads to an accumulation of cortisol precursors, which are shunted into increased production of DHEA and DHEAS (see Fig. 144.2). Later in gestation, these increased fetal androgens will be converted to estrogens by placental aromatases (see Fig. 144.3), thus preventing accumulation in the fetus.[5,13,16] At this early stage of gestation, however, placental aromatase activity is low, resulting in an accumulation of androgens and virilization of the external female genitalia during differentiation—a process that occurs at 8 to 10 weeks postconception.[5]

REGULATION OF FETAL ADRENAL DEVELOPMENT

As befits an organ involved in the vital functions of maintaining the pregnancy, initiating parturition, and maturing fetal organs for extrauterine existence, the fetal adrenal cortex is regulated by an intricate web of factors from fetus, placenta, and mother. These factors combine to shield the fetus from premature exposure to excess cortisol early in gestation and then to stimulate the increased cortisol production essential for preparation for extrauterine survival. Normal fetal cortisol concentrations are low until well into the third

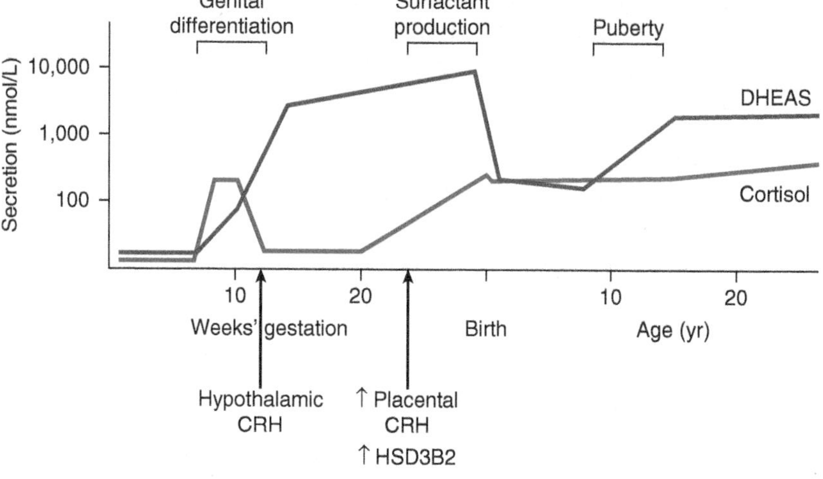

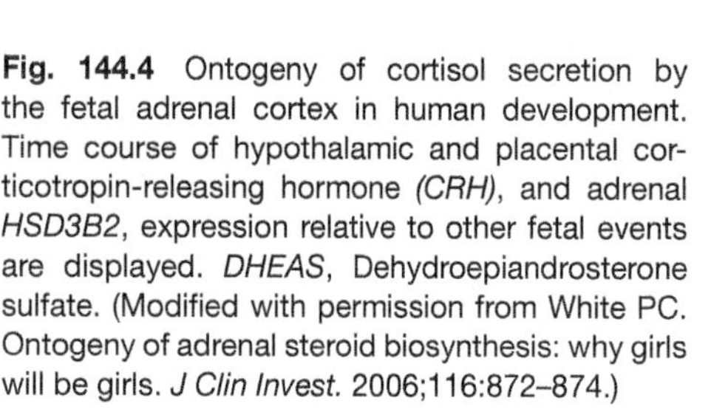

Fig. 144.4 Ontogeny of cortisol secretion by the fetal adrenal cortex in human development. Time course of hypothalamic and placental corticotropin-releasing hormone *(CRH)*, and adrenal *HSD3B2*, expression relative to other fetal events are displayed. *DHEAS*, Dehydroepiandrosterone sulfate. (Modified with permission from White PC. Ontogeny of adrenal steroid biosynthesis: why girls will be girls. *J Clin Invest.* 2006;116:872–874.)

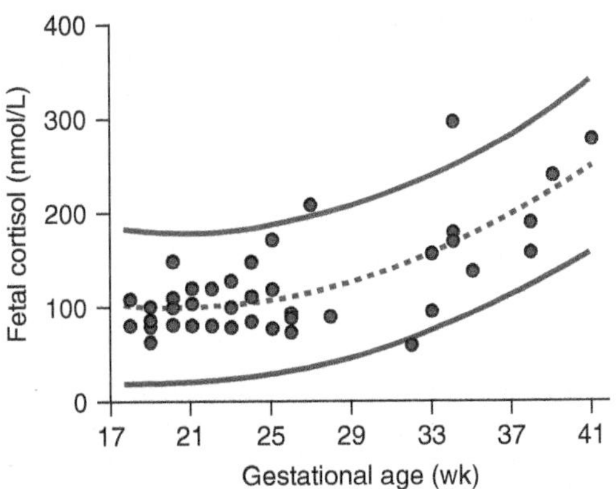

Fig. 144.5 Individual values and reference range (mean and 95% confidence intervals) of fetal serum cortisol throughout pregnancy. Regression line: $y = 0.339x^{-2} - 13.5 + 231$; $r = 0.72$; $P = .0001$. (From Donaldson A, Nicolini U, Symes EK, et al. Changes in concentrations of cortisol, dehydroepiandrosterone sulphate and progesterone in fetal and maternal serum during pregnancy. *Clin Endocrinol.* 1991;35:447.)

trimester of pregnancy (Fig. 144.5).[17] The profound effects of premature exposure of the fetus to increased glucocorticoid concentrations have been well documented in animal models, including decreased body, brain, and organ weights.[18,19]

FETAL FACTORS

ADRENOCORTICOTROPIC HORMONE

Stimulation of the adrenal cortex by ACTH from the fetal pituitary is necessary for its normal morphologic development and steroidogenic function. The effects of a lack of ACTH in the human are demonstrated in the anencephalic fetus. Stereologic studies of adrenal cortex structure in anencephalic fetuses have shown a striking decrease in both cell number and total volume of the fetal zone and transitional zone (zona fasciculata), with less effect on the zona glomerulosa.[20,21] Although ACTH has been detected in placental tissue,[22] outcomes such as these suggest that placental ACTH is insufficient for normal human adrenocortical growth and development.

The specific effects of ACTH on adrenocortical cells have been documented in primate models. Administration of exogenous ACTH or suppression of fetal cortisol synthesis with metyrapone results in hypertrophy of the transitional zone and early appearance of 3βHSD message in both the transitional and definitive zones.[2,23] Conversely, administration of betamethasone to suppress fetal ACTH secretion eliminates the transitional zone and decreases mRNA expression of both 3βHSD and the ACTH receptor.[23,24] Suppression of ACTH with betamethasone at mid-gestation also resulted in decreased adrenal weight and cell size, cellular disorganization, increased apoptosis, and reduction in expression of mRNA for the P450scc and P450C17 enzymes—effects that were reversed by concomitant treatment with ACTH.[25]

The expression of the ACTH receptor in the adrenal cortex increases through mid-gestation and then decreases substantially by term.[26] In addition, the responsiveness of the fetal and the developing transitional zones to ACTH appear to diverge during the second half of gestation. In the fetal zone, a selective decrease in ACTH receptor expression and a consequently decreased responsiveness to ACTH occurs; in the emerging transitional zone, an increase in ACTH receptor density and 3βHSD expression is seen.[26,27] The decline in ACTH responsiveness in the fetal zone may be due to suppression by increasing estrogen concentrations (see later discussion).[28] In contrast to the effects of ACTH on the fetal and transitional zones, the outer definitive zone, the future zona glomerulosa, may be less affected by exogenous ACTH or betamethasone.[23] This is consistent with findings in human anencephalic infants, in whom the growth of the zona glomerulosa is relatively unaffected by the absence of fetal ACTH.[20,21]

ACTH exerts its effects on adrenal cells at least in part through local growth factors, particularly insulin-like growth factor (IGF)-2. A polypeptide growth factor important in the regulation of fetal growth, IGF-2 is highly expressed in the fetal adrenal cortex, and its expression is stimulated by ACTH.[29] In turn, IGF-2 stimulates the proliferation of fetal adrenal cortical cells, increases steroid production, and augments the expression of steroidogenic enzymes.[29] IGF-2 appears to act through the IGF-1 binding protein, possibly in concert with other polypeptide growth factors that have been shown to be mitogenic for human fetal adrenal cells, particularly basic fibroblast growth factor and epidermal growth factor.[29-32]

Transcription of ACTH's effect on the fetal adrenal cortex appears to be modulated by members of the nuclear receptor superfamily. Several nuclear receptors essential for human adrenal cortex development have been implicated in the transcription of ACTH's effect, and it is likely that more will be identified. The orphan nuclear receptor steroidogenic factor (SF)-1 is expressed throughout the adrenal gland and participates in the activation of numerous enzymes in the steroid biosynthetic pathway.[33] Activation of ACTH-dependent signaling cascades has been shown to lead to the cyclic recruitment of SF-1 and multiple rounds of transcription.[33] Human mutations of SF-1 produce adrenal failure, indicating its importance in adrenal development.[33] Another orphan nuclear receptor responsive to ACTH stimulation is NGFIB. NGFIB shows differential expression in the different fetal adrenal zones and may play a crucial role in functional adrenal zonation by upregulating 3βHSD2 gene transcription in the transitional and definitive zones.[11] A third nuclear receptor, DAX-1 (dosage-sensitive sex reversal, adrenal hypoplasia congenita, critical region on X-chromosome, gene 1) appears to be an important negative modulator of ACTH-stimulated glucocorticoid synthesis, repressing SF-1–dependent activation.[34] ACTH has been shown to downregulate DAX-1 as well as stimulate SF-1, a potential mechanism for modulating cortisol production by the adrenal cortex.[35] Deletion or mutation of DAX-1 results in X-linked adrenal hypoplasia congenita, a disorder with profound hormonal deficiencies.[36]

ANGIOTENSIN II

Angiotensin II has been implicated in apoptosis of fetal adrenal cells, acting through its type 2 receptor (AT_2).[37] This receptor is most strongly expressed at the center of the fetal zone, which is also the location with the highest density of apoptotic figures. In cells cultured from second-trimester human adrenal glands, stimulation with angiotensin II produced changes consistent with apoptosis, including DNA fragmentation, interruption of the DNA repair mechanism, and reorganization of the actin cytoskeleton. This suggests that angiotensin II–related apoptosis contributes to the involution of the fetal zone seen after birth.[37]

LOCAL MICROENVIRONMENT/EXTRACELLULAR MATRIX

The regulation of zonal expression of enzymes within the adrenal cortex has been a major area of curiosity. That is, if the cells primarily originate from the definitive zone and then migrate inward, why do they express different enzyme profiles in different zones, resulting in the functional zonation observed in the gland?[8,38] Comparing in vivo with in vitro cellular function has strongly implicated a local regulation of the phenotype. For example, human fetal zone cells do not express 3βHSD in vivo; however, these cells quickly begin to produce 3βHSD in response to ACTH in vitro.[39] This functional zonation of the cortex may be regulated in part by the extracellular matrix of the local microenvironment, in particular type IV collagen, laminin, and fibronectin. Type IV collagen is present throughout the adrenal cortex and has been shown to promote cellular proliferation as well as increase cortisol secretion in response to ACTH.[40,41] Laminin is found primarily at the periphery of the gland and causes increased proliferation and decreased apoptosis in cultured human fetal adrenal cells.[41] In contrast, the fetal zone is rich in fibronectin, which does not promote proliferation, but facilitates migration and apoptosis, enhances DHEAS secretion, and decreases cortisol secretion in cell culture.[40,42] In addition, type IV collagen and fibronectin both have been shown to modulate the intracellular localization of DAX-1, which is likely to affect the function of this negative regulator of steroidogenesis.[43]

PLACENTAL FACTORS

A unique interactive relationship between the placenta and adrenal cortex in primate pregnancy appears to be vital to the maintenance of pregnancy, the development and maturation of the adrenal gland—and consequently other organs, such as the lung—and possibly the initiation of parturition. In addition, the interrelationship of the placenta and adrenal cortex serves to shield the fetus from premature exposure to excess cortisol.

ESTROGEN

Albrecht and Pepe have proposed a central integrative role for estrogen in regulating the maturation of both the placenta and the fetal hypothalamic-pituitary-adrenal (HPA) axis.[44] Their extensive studies of the baboon pregnancy demonstrated both the model's relevance to human pregnancy and the effects that estrogen exerts by (1) acting directly on the adrenal cortex, (2) regulating the expression of 11βHSD in the placenta, and (3) affecting placental progesterone production. Because fetal androgens are the primary substrate for placental estrogen production, the fetal adrenal cortex is central to these functions.

Estrogen appears to have a direct effect on the fetal adrenal cortex. In the baboon model, estrogen receptors α and β are expressed throughout the fetal adrenal cortex.[45] In this model, estrogen administration suppresses DHEA but not cortisol production in response to ACTH at mid-gestation.[44,45] Conversely, suppression of placental estrogen production during the second half of pregnancy significantly increases DHEA secretion and the size of the fetal zone; these effects are reversed by concomitant treatment with estradiol.[28] These findings are consistent with an inhibitory effect of estrogen on the fetal zone during the latter half of gestation. No such effect was observed in the transitional or definitive zone.[28] These data suggest that placental estrogen provides a feedback mechanism to restrain the growth of the fetal zone during the second half of pregnancy, thus providing a consistent but not deleteriously high estrogen exposure.[28]

Numerous studies have shown that estrogen also modulates the maturation of the primate fetal adrenal cortex through its regulation of the expression of placental 11β-hydroxysteroid dehydrogenase (11βHSD; Fig. 144.6).[44] This enzyme is widely distributed in the body and modulates local exposure to cortisol in many tissues, including lung and kidney.[46] 11βHSD exists in two forms: 11βHSD1, which converts biologically inactive cortisone to active cortisol, and 11βHSD2, which transforms cortisol into cortisone.[46] At mid-gestation, 11βHSD1 predominates in the placenta, allowing the transfer of some maternal cortisol to the fetus, suppressing the fetal HPA axis.[47] Later in gestation, however, 11βHSD2 predominates, transforming most maternal cortisol into the biologically inactive cortisone, thus releasing the fetal HPA axis from negative feedback and stimulating its maturation.[47] Estrogen appears to regulate this shift in the relative concentrations of 11βHSD2 and 11βHSD1 by late in gestation; suppression of placental estrogen synthesis with an aromatase inhibitor significantly decreases 11βHSD2 expression.[48]

The two different forms of 11βHSD also appear to localize to different membrane fractions of the syncytiotrophoblast: 11βHSD1 is abundant in the membranes closest to the maternal circulation, and 11βHSD2 is concentrated in the membranes facing fetal vasculature.[47] This organization creates a gradient favoring metabolism of maternal cortisol to cortisone as gestation progresses. Investigators have reported that during the final few days of gestation in both the baboon and human, the expression of placental 11βHSD2 again decreases, possibly providing brief exposure to additional maternal cortisol to further prepare the fetus for delivery.[49,50]

This changing pattern of placental 11βHSD expression would serve to first limit the exposure of the fetus to cortisol during most of the gestational period, permitting the necessary intense fetal growth and cellular proliferation, then subsequently stimulate the increased fetal adrenal cortisol production needed for maturation of vital organ systems before birth.[51] The importance of placental 11βHSD2 in limiting fetal exposure to cortisol is supported by several findings in the human. First, placentas from pregnancies complicated by intrauterine growth restriction and preeclampsia show decreased expression and activity of 11βHSD2, consistent with a role for placental 11βHSD2 in limiting exposure of the fetus to cortisol.[52,53] In addition, investigators found that placentas from preeclamptic pregnancies contained measurable amounts of cortisol, while those from normotensive pregnancies did not.[53] And finally, a genetic deficiency of 11βHSD2 significantly reduces birth weight.[54,55] Fetal growth restriction also has been correlated with higher cortisol but lower ACTH concentrations in the fetus, and with decreased response to ACTH stimulation in the preterm

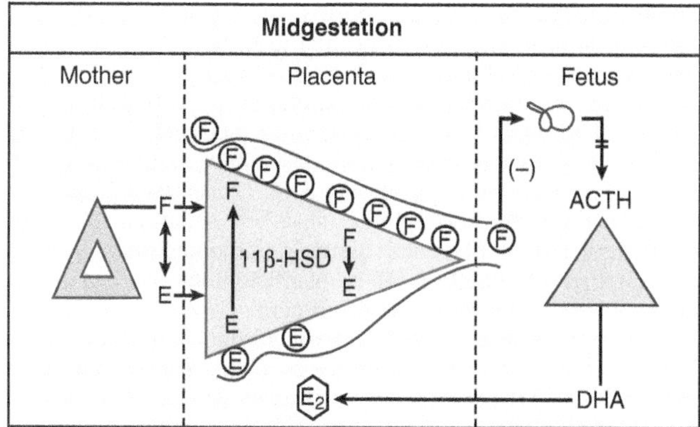

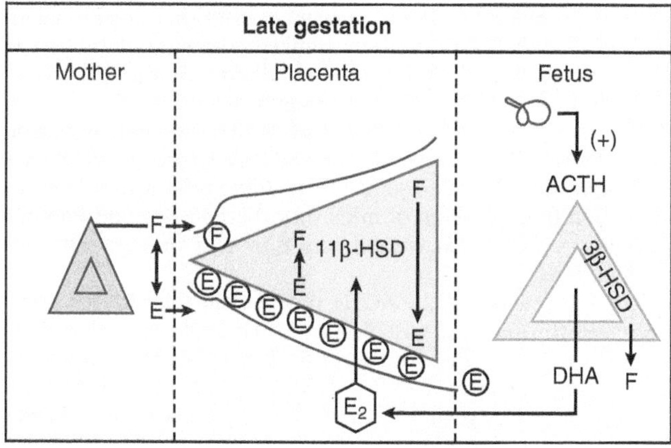

Fig. 144.6 The role of estrogen *(E_2)* on placental 11βHSD-catalyzed metabolism of cortisol *(F)* and cortisone *(E)* and regulation of the fetal pituitary-adrenocortical axis at mid-and late gestation in the baboon. *ACTH,* Adrenocorticotropic hormone. (From Albrecht ED, Pepe GJ. Central integrative role of oestrogen in modulating the communication between the placenta and fetus that results in primate fetal-placental development. *Placenta.* 1999;20:133.)

infant.[56,57] These findings are consistent with an increased exposure of the fetus to maternal cortisol in the face of decreased 11βHSD2 activity, with resulting passive suppression of the fetal HPA axis.

Estrogen also may play a part in maintaining pregnancy by increasing progesterone synthesis in the placenta. Estrogen promotes low-density lipoprotein uptake and P450scc activity by the placenta, rate-limiting steps for progesterone production.[58,59] Suppression of estrogen production has been shown to decrease placental uptake of low-density lipoprotein, placental P450scc activity, and peripheral progesterone concentrations in a dose-dependent manner.[58,59] However, when pregnant baboons were treated with a specific nonsteroidal aromatase inhibitor that substantially decreased maternal estrogen concentrations, maternal concentrations of progesterone were no different from untreated animals, leaving the effect of estrogen on progesterone concentrations in vivo open for further investigation.[60]

PLACENTAL CORTICOTROPIN-RELEASING HORMONE

CRH is produced by the placenta and fetal membranes in increasing amounts as gestation progresses, with exponentially increased production during the last 6 to 8 weeks of pregnancy.[61-63] Placental CRH stimulates the fetal HPA axis to increase fetal cortisol production.[62,64] However, in contrast to the hypothalamus, where cortisol suppresses CRH production, placental CRH production is stimulated by glucocorticoids.[62] A rise in placental CRH further stimulates fetal adrenal cortisol production, creating a so-called *feed-forward* loop that contributes to the maturation of the fetal adrenal cortex (Fig. 144.7).[4,62,64] CRH also stimulates DHEA/DHEAS production in the fetal adrenal, resulting in increased estrogen concentrations (see Fig. 144.3). The combination of increased estrogen, cortisol, and CRH, together with functional progesterone withdrawal, may contribute to the initiation of parturition.[4] CRH also directly stimulates parturition in part by stimulating the production of prostaglandins.[4] A premature rise in CRH in maternal serum has been associated with preterm delivery, leading to its putative role as a *placental time clock* for human gestation.[63] The magnitude of the increase in CRH during human pregnancy is much greater than in other primates,[65] which may limit the value of such models in describing this facet of human physiology.

MATERNAL FACTORS

Maternal circulating total and free cortisol increase throughout pregnancy.[66] As discussed previously, placental enzyme activity shields the fetus from exposure to excess cortisol concentrations. However, several maternal conditions can perturb that system. Notably, maternal malnutrition and stress during pregnancy have both been convincingly linked to decreased fetal growth and adverse outcomes later in life (i.e., fetal programming of adult disease).[54,67] Recent work in both mouse and baboon models show that maternal malnutrition results in activation of the fetal HPA axis and increased fetal exposure to glucocorticoid, perhaps reconciling the nutritional and the glucocorticoid hypotheses of fetal programming.[54,68] Stress can increase maternal cortisol directly, potentially increasing delivery of cortisol to the fetus; in addition, markers of social stress have been linked to decreased methylation of 11βHSD2, which may allow increased cortisol to reach the fetus.[69]

FUNCTIONS OF THE FETAL ADRENAL CORTEX

The fetal adrenal cortex appears to partner with the placenta to maintain pregnancy and initiate parturition and to provide the late-term cortisol surge necessary for maturation of organ systems in preparation for extrauterine life.

MAINTENANCE OF PREGNANCY AND INITIATION OF PARTURITION

As reviewed earlier, the fetal zone of the adrenal cortex secretes increasing amounts of DHEA and DHEAS through gestation, which serve as substrates for the synthesis of placental estrogens. Estrogen appears critical to the maintenance of primate pregnancy. In humans, a 50% spontaneous abortion rate has been reported in women who have a mutation of the estrogen receptor gene, and in baboons, administration of an aromatase inhibitor to suppress placental estrogen production resulted in miscarriage in 50% of pregnancies.[60] Although human pregnancies complicated by very low estrogen levels (e.g., placental sulfatase or aromatase deficiency) can result in term pregnancies, the investigators postulate that estradiol may be maintained in a low but bioactive range in these conditions.[60]

In contrast to its actions in sheep, the increase in cortisol concentration at term does not initiate labor in the primate.[51] However, through its unique relationship with the placenta, the fetal adrenal cortex appears directly involved in the cascade of events leading to parturition. In the rhesus monkey, infusion of androstenedione increases placental estradiol synthesis and induces premature labor.[65] Conversely, when the synthesis of estrogen from androstenedione is blocked by an aromatase inhibitor, the androgen-induced preterm labor is prevented.[70] Interestingly in this model, peripheral infusion of estrogen to the dam increased myometrial activity but did not result in fetal membrane changes or preterm birth, implicating a paracrine function of placental estrogen in the initiation of parturition.[70] Cortisol may also participate in the initiation of labor indirectly by competing with progesterone for binding to placental glucocorticoid receptors. Progesterone binding of the glucocorticoid receptor inhibits placental CRH production;

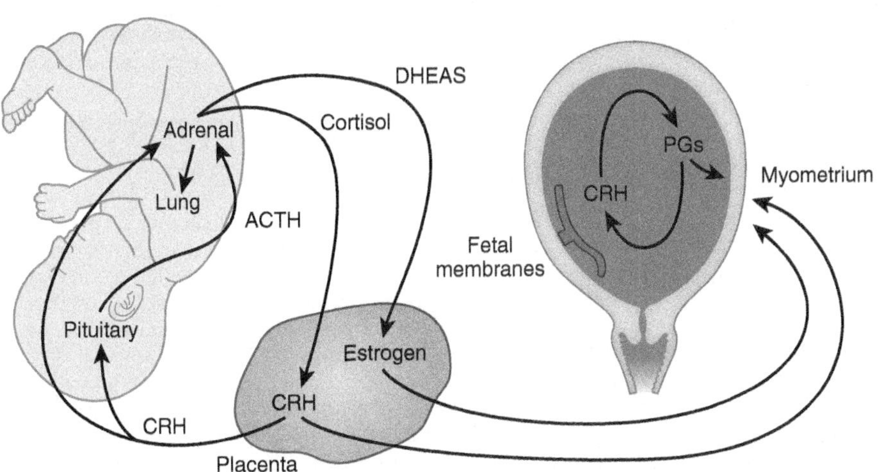

Fig. 144.7 Interacting positive-feedback hormonal loops in the fetal, amniotic, and maternal compartments that may promote the progression of fetal maturation and initiation of parturition in humans. Each of the *arrows* represents a stimulatory action of the indicated hormone. *ACTH,* Adrenocorticotropic hormone; *CRH,* corticotropin-releasing hormone; *DHEAS,* dehydroepiandrosterone sulfate; *PGs,* prostaglandins. (From McLean M, Smith R. Corticotrophin-releasing hormone and human parturition. *Reproduction.* 2001;121:496.)

as fetal cortisol concentrations rise late in gestation, cortisol can displace progesterone from the glucocorticoid receptor, further stimulating CRH production.[71,72]

MATURATION OF ORGANS AND ENZYME SYSTEMS

During most of gestation, low fetal cortisol concentrations permit necessary cellular growth and proliferation. Late in gestation, however, cortisol concentrations rise, promoting the cellular differentiation and organ maturation necessary to sustain independent existence (see Figs. 144.4 and 144.5).[17,51] A large body of literature supports the role of cortisol in regulating numerous maturational processes, particularly lung structure and function, kidney function, glycogen accumulation and gluconeogenesis in the liver, triiodothyronine and catecholamine production, regression of lymphoid tissue in spleen and thymus, and increased β-adrenergic receptor density in numerous tissues.[51]

NEONATAL ADRENAL CORTICAL FUNCTION

The sudden loss of placental and maternal protection at birth requires the newborn to provide its own homeostasis, for which the hormones of the adrenal cortex are essential. Cortisol regulates protein, carbohydrate, lipid, and nucleic acid metabolism; maintains cardiac and vascular response to vasoconstrictors; regulates extracellular water and promotes free water excretion; suppresses the inflammatory response and decreases capillary permeability during inflammation; and modulates central nervous system (CNS) processing and behavior.[73,74] Aldosterone regulates fluid and electrolyte homeostasis; deficiency produces hypovolemia, hyponatremia, and hyperkalemia.[75] In the absence of an enzyme deficiency that blocks glucocorticoid synthesis, the adrenal cortex of the newborn infant should be able to respond to ACTH stimulation with an appropriate rise in cortisol concentration. However, two circumstances may be exceptions to that statement: the first several days of transition to extrauterine life and preterm birth.

TRANSITION TO EXTRAUTERINE LIFE

After the surge of cortisol normally engendered by parturition,[14] cortisol concentrations in healthy infants may fall to very low levels without apparent clinical compromise.[76] However, several small studies have suggested that in the first days of life, apparently normal term infants may be unable to respond to critical illness with production of sufficient cortisol to maintain cardiovascular stability, resulting in a relative adrenal insufficiency similar to that seen in other critically ill patients.[77-84] One report found that critically ill term and near-term infants had low ACTH levels and low cortisol concentrations, but their cortisol response to exogenous ACTH stimulation was indistinguishable from that of healthy term infants.[85] These data suggest that the observed low cortisol concentrations result from an abnormality further upstream in the HPA axis.

A possible explanation for the finding of low cortisol values but adequate response to ACTH is the sudden withdrawal of the very high concentrations of CRH produced by the placenta at term. As reviewed earlier, CRH concentrations are low in nonpregnant individuals but reach very high concentrations in both maternal and fetal plasma before term or preterm delivery.[61-63] At birth, the major source of this CRH—the placenta—is removed, and maternal plasma concentrations again fall to undetectable levels within 24 hours.[61] A blunted ACTH response to CRH stimulation has been documented in women during the postpartum period.[86] It is not known whether the same phenomenon may exist in newborns, leading to a transient decrease in their ability to respond to stress.

PRETERM INFANTS

From the review of fetal adrenal cortical development, it would seem reasonable to postulate that highly preterm infants may not have sufficient functional adrenal capacity to respond to postnatal stress. In the undisturbed pregnancy, the transitional zone only begins to appear at 22 to 24 weeks' gestation, and 3βHSD expression then increases gradually until term.[4] However, most preterm deliveries result from a disordered pregnancy, which may alter adrenal development. For example, a large autopsy series found that premature infants exposed to prenatal inflammation from chorioamnionitis had larger adrenal glands than those not exposed, suggesting an effect of inflammation on adrenal development.[87] Consistent with these findings, infants exposed to chorioamnionitis have elevated cortisol values early in life.[88]

In the baboon model, a significant percentage of extremely preterm neonates have decreased cortisol production early in life, with associated cardiovascular dysfunction that can be reversed by hydrocortisone supplementation.[89] In human infants, a developing body of literature has shown that healthy preterm infants, similar to term infants, may have low serum cortisol values without apparent clinical compromise.[76] However, these infants may not respond to critical illness with increased cortisol production. Sick preterm infants and those receiving vasopressor support for hypotension have been shown to have lower cortisol concentrations than healthy infants, a reversal of the expected pattern of higher cortisol values with increasing illness.[90-93] Hydrocortisone treatment of infants with vasopressor-resistant hypotension results in amelioration of hypotension and weaning of vasopressor support.[94,95] In addition, extremely preterm infants have elevated cortisol precursors, consistent with a limited enzymatic capacity to synthesize cortisol.[96-98] Several studies have linked lower cortisol values or decreased cortisol response to ACTH and the development of bronchopulmonary dysplasia.[92,99-103]

These data support the possibility of a developmental adrenal insufficiency in the extremely preterm infant, with clinical consequences. The preponderance of these data might suggest a benefit to cortisol replacement in the extremely preterm infant; however, even low-dose hydrocortisone therapy in such infants was associated with a serious adverse effect: spontaneous gastrointestinal perforation.[104,105] Although this effect may have been due to an interaction with concurrent indomethacin or ibuprofen therapy, it emphasizes the need for caution in approaching the treatment of infants who, in utero, would be exposed to a much lower level of cortisol.[17] It is clear that extrauterine existence requires the extremely preterm infant to respond to significant stress and that both adrenal insufficiency and glucocorticoid excess are detrimental to homeostasis and neurologic development[73,74]; however, neither the most appropriate measures of adrenal function nor the most beneficial supportive therapies for preterm infants have yet been elucidated.

EFFECTS OF PREMATURELY INCREASED EXPOSURE TO GLUCOCORTICOIDS

Administration of synthetic glucocorticoids, primarily betamethasone or dexamethasone, to pregnant women at risk for preterm delivery clearly has been shown to provide a broad range of benefits to infants born prematurely.[106] However, antenatal exposure to synthetic glucocorticoids can increase placental 11βHSD2 expression and alter postnatal HPA function.[49,106-110] In addition, a large RCT comparing one course of prenatal steroids to repeated exposures at 2-week intervals found that repeated steroids did not result in any further reduction in a composite measure of morbidity, but did result in significantly lower birth weight and shorter gestation.[111]

Premature exposure to increased concentrations of endogenous cortisol may also have adverse short-term and long-term effects. Cortisol concentrations in extremely preterm infants in the first postnatal weeks are far higher than normal fetal concentrations,[104,112] and extremely preterm infants have been shown to also have higher cortisol concentrations at 8 and 18 months.[113] In turn, elevated cortisol concentrations in children and adults have been correlated with elevated blood pressure and increased insulin resistance, suggesting a long-term effect of HPA axis programming.[114]

CONCLUSION

The adrenal cortex undergoes remarkable growth and unique metamorphosis during the fetal and neonatal period. The structural and functional organization of the fetal adrenal cortex of higher primates is unique, with distinctly different morphology, functions, and secretory product profiles during fetal versus postnatal life. After the embryonic period, the enzymes and secretory patterns of each zone within the adrenal cortex are distinct, and the specific steroidogenic enzymes within each zone determine the type of steroid produced: DHEA from the fetal zone (which will reappear as the zona reticularis at adrenarche), cortisol from the transitional zone (the future zona fasciculata), and aldosterone from the definitive zone (the future zona glomerulosa). Prenatally, the adrenal gland participates in the vital functions of maintaining the pregnancy, initiating parturition, and maturing fetal organs for extrauterine existence, and is regulated by an intricate web of factors from fetus, placenta, and mother. Postnatally, cortisol is a critical regulator of protein, carbohydrate, lipid, and nucleic acid metabolism; cardiovascular response to vasoconstrictors; extracellular water and free water excretion; inflammatory response; and CNS processing and behavior, while aldosterone regulates fluid and electrolyte homeostasis. Preterm delivery may result in a developmental adrenal insufficiency, limiting the ability of the immature adrenal glands to perform these functions and resulting in clinical compromise. Conversely, exposure to increased concentrations of glucocorticoid, whether exogenous or endogenous, has long-term consequences, the scope and nature of which continue to be elucidated.

ACKNOWLEDGMENT

The editors wish to thank the authors for their valuable contributions to this chapter in the 5th edition. The chapter has been republished here virtually unchanged.

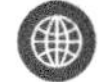

A complete reference list is available at www.ExpertConsult.com.

SELECT REFERENCES

4. Ishimoto H, Jaffe RB. Development and function of the human fetal adrenal cortex: a key component in the feto-placental unit. *Endocr Rev*. 2011;32:317.
5. Goto M, Hanley KP, Marcos J, et al. In humans, early cortisol biosynthesis provides a mechanism to safeguard female sexual development. *J Clin Invest*. 2006;116:953.
11. Bassett MH, Suzuki T, Sasano H, et al. The orphan nuclear receptor NGFIB regulates transcription of 3β-hydroxysteroid dehydrogenase: implications for the control of adrenal functional zonation. *J Biol Chem*. 2004;279:37622.
13. Pepe GJ, Albrecht ED. Actions of placental and fetal adrenal steroid hormones in primate pregnancy. *Endocr Rev*. 1995;16:608.
16. White PC. Ontogeny of adrenal steroid biosynthesis: why girls will be girls. *J Clin Invest*. 2006;116:872.
17. Donaldson A, Nicolini U, Symes EK, et al. Changes in concentrations of cortisol, dehydroepiandrosterone sulphate and progesterone in fetal and maternal serum during pregnancy. *Clin Endocrinol (Oxf)*. 1991;35:447.
18. Howard E. Reductions in size and total DNA of cerebrum and cerebellum in adult mice after corticosterone treatment in infancy. *Exp Neurol*. 1968;22:191.
19. Reinisch JM, Simon NG, Karow WG, Gandelman R. Prenatal exposure to prednisone in humans and animals retards intrauterine growth. *Science*. 1978;202:436.
23. Leavitt MG, Albrecht ED, Pepe GJ. Development of the baboon fetal adrenal gland: regulation of the ontogenesis of the definitive and transitional zones by adrenocorticotropin. *J Clin Endocrinol Metab*. 1999;84:3831.
25. Aberdeen GW, Leavitt MG, Pepe GJ, Albrecht ED. Effect of maternal betamethasone administration at midgestation on baboon fetal adrenal gland development and adrenocorticotropin receptor messenger ribonucleic acid expression. *J Clin Endocrinol Metab*. 1998;83:976.
28. Albrecht ED, Aberdeen GW, Pepe GJ. Estrogen elicits cortical zone-specific effects on development of the primate fetal adrenal gland. *Endocrinology*. 2005;146:1737.
29. Mesiano S, Katz SL, Lee JY, Jaffe RB. Insulin-like growth factors augment steroid production and expression of steroidogenic enzymes in human fetal adrenal cortical cells: implications for adrenal androgen regulation. *J Clin Endocrinol Metab*. 1997;82:1390.
32. Mesiano S, Jaffe RB. Role of growth factors in the developmental regulation of the human fetal adrenal cortex. *Steroids*. 1997;62:62.
38. Coulter CL, Jaffe RB. Functional maturation of the primate fetal adrenal in vivo: 3. Specific zonal localization and developmental regulation of CYP21A2 (P450c21) and CYP11B1/CYP11B2 (P450c11/aldosterone synthase) lead to integrated concept of zonal and temporal steroid biosynthesis. *Endocrinology*. 1998;139:5144.
42. Chamoux E, Otis M, Gallo-Payet N. A connection between extracellular matrix and hormonal signals during the development of the human adrenal gland. *Braz J Med Biol Res*. 2005;38:1495.
44. Albrecht ED, Pepe GJ. Central integrative role of oestrogen in modulating the communication between the placenta and fetus that results in primate fetal-placental development. *Placenta*. 1999;20:129.
46. Chapman K, Holmes M, Seckl J. 11β-hydroxysteroid dehydrogenases: intracellular gate-keepers of tissue glucocorticoid action. *Physiol Rev*. 2013;93:1139.
48. Pepe GJ, Burch MG, Albrecht ED. Estrogen regulates 11beta-hydroxysteroid dehydrogenase-1 and -2 localization in placental syncytiotrophoblast in the second half of primate pregnancy. *Endocrinology*. 2001;142:4496.
51. Liggins GC. The role of the hypothalamic-pituitary-adrenal axis in preparing the fetus for birth. *Am J Obstet Gynecol*. 2000;182:475.
52. McTernan CL, Draper N, Nicholson H, et al. Reduced placental 11beta-hydroxysteroid dehydrogenase type 2 mRNA levels in human pregnancies complicated by intrauterine growth restriction: an analysis of possible mechanisms. *J Clin Endocrinol Metab*. 2001;86:4979.
53. Aufdenblatten M, Baumann M, Raio L, et al. Prematurity is related to high placental cortisol in preeclampsia. *Pediatr Res*. 2009;65:198.
54. Cottrell EC, Holmes MC, Livingstone DE, et al. Reconciling the nutritional and glucocorticoid hypotheses of fetal programming. *FASEB J*. 2012;26:1866.
56. Economides DL, Nicolaides KH, Linton EA, et al. Plasma cortisol and adrenocorticotropin in appropriate and small for gestational age fetuses. *Fetal Ther*. 1998;3:158.
57. Bolt RJ, van Weissenbruch MM, Popp-Snijders C, et al. Fetal growth and function of the adrenal cortex in preterm infants. *J Clin Endocrinol Metab*. 2002;87:1194.
60. Albrecht ED, Aberdeen GW, Pepe GJ. The role of estrogen in the maintenance of primate pregnancy. *Am J Obstet Gynecol*. 2000;182:432.
61. Goland RS, Wardlaw SL, Blum M, et al. Biologically active corticotropin-releasing hormone in maternal and fetal plasma during pregnancy. *Am J Obstet Gynecol*. 1988;159:884.
62. Majzoub JA, Karalis KP. Placental corticotropin-releasing hormone: function and regulation. *Am J Obstet Gynecol*. 1999;180:242.
63. McLean M, Smith R. Corticotrophin-releasing hormone and human parturition. *Reproduction*. 2001;121:493.
66. Reynolds RM. Glucocorticoid excess and the developmental origins of disease: two decades of testing the hypothesis-2012 Curt Richter Award Winner. *Psychoneuroendocrinology*. 2013;38:1.
67. Cottrell EC, Seckl JR. Prenatal stress, glucocorticoids and the programming of adult disease. *Front Behav Neurosci*. 2009;3:19.
68. Li C, Ramahi E, Nijland MJ, et al. Up-regulation of the fetal baboon hypothalamo-pituitary-adrenal axis in intrauterine growth restriction: coincidence with hypothalamic glucocorticoid receptor insensitivity and leptin receptor down-regulation. *Endocrinology*. 2013;154:2365.
69. Appleton AA, Armstrong DA, Lesseur C, et al. Patterning in placental 11-B hydroxysteroid dehydrogenase methylation according to prenatal socioeconomic adversity. *PLoS ONE*. 2013;8:74691.
72. Challis JRG, Bloomfield FH, Bocking AD, et al. Fetal signals and parturition. *J Obstet Gynaecol Res*. 2005;31:492.
74. de Kloet ER. From receptor balance to rational glucocorticoid therapy. *Endocrinology*. 2014;155:2754.
81. Soliman AT, Taman KH, Rizk MM, et al. Circulating adrenocorticotropic hormone (ACTH) and cortisol concentrations in normal, appropriate-for-gestational-age newborns versus those with sepsis and respiratory distress: cortisol response to low-dose and standard-dose ACTH tests. *Metabolism*. 2004;53:209.
83. Cooper MS, Stewart PM. Adrenal insufficiency in critical illness. *J Intensive Care Med*. 2007;22:348.
84. Joosten KFM, de Kleijn ED, Westerterp M, et al. Endocrine and metabolic responses in children with meningococcal sepsis: striking differences between survivors and nonsurvivors. *J Clin Endocrinol Metab*. 2000;85:3746.
85. Fernandez EF, Watterberg KL. ACTH and cortisol response to stress in critically ill newborns. *J Perinatol*. 2008;28:797.
86. Thomson M. The physiological roles of placental corticotropin releasing hormone in pregnancy and childbirth. *J Physiol Biochem*. 2013;69:559.
90. Scott SM, Watterberg KL. Effect of gestational age, postnatal age, and illness on plasma cortisol concentrations in premature infants. *Pediatr Res*. 1995;37:112.

92. Huysman MW, Hokken-Koelega AC, De Ridder MA, Sauer PJ. Adrenal function in sick very preterm infants. *Pediatr Res*. 2000;48:629.
94. Higgins S, Friedlich P, Seri I. Hydrocortisone for hypotension and vasopressor dependence in preterm neonates: a meta-analysis. *J Perinatol*. 2010;30:373.
95. Ng PC, Lee CH, Bnur FL. A double-blind, randomized, controlled study of a "stress dose" of hydrocortisone for rescue treatment of refractory hypotension in preterm infants. *Pediatrics*. 2006;117:367.
98. Watterberg KL, Gerdes JS, Cook KL. Impaired glucocorticoid synthesis in premature infants developing chronic lung disease. *Pediatr Res*. 2001;50:190.
104. Watterberg KL, Gerdes JS, Cole CH, et al. Prophylaxis of early adrenal insufficiency to prevent bronchopulmonary dysplasia: a multicenter trial. *Pediatrics*. 2004;114:1649.
106. Braun T, Challis JR, Newnham JP, Sloboda DM. Early-life glucocorticoid exposure: the hypothalamic-pituitary-adrenal axis, placental function, and long-term disease risk. *Endocr Rev*. 2013;34:885.
108. Tegethoff M, Pryce C, Meinlschmidt G. Effects of intrauterine exposure to synthetic glucocorticoids on fetal, newborn, and infants hypothalamic-pituitary-adrenal axis function in humans: a systematic review. *Endocr Rev*. 2009;30:753.
109. Nykänen P, Raivio T, Heinonen K, et al. Circulating glucocorticoid bioactivity and serum cortisol concentrations in premature infants: the influence of exogenous glucocorticoids and clinical factors. *Eur J Endocrinol*. 2007;156:577.
111. Murphy KE, Willan AR, Hannah ME, et al. Effect of antenatal corticosteroids on fetal growth and gestational age at birth. *Obstet Gynecol*. 2012;119:917.
114. Clark PM. Programming of the hypothalamo-pituitary-adrenal axis and the fetal origins of adult disease hypothesis. *Eur J Pediatr*. 1998;157:7.

145 Fetal and Neonatal Thyroid Physiology

Andrew J. Bauer

INTRODUCTION

Normal embryonic development in vertebrates requires the highly coordinated action of thyroid hormones. In mammals, these iodothyronine hormones (T3 and T4) are derived from both maternal and fetal sources and regulate the proliferation, differentiation, and apoptosis of developing tissues in a temporally and anatomically precise manner. During most of gestation, extracellular concentrations of active thyroid hormones in the fetus are low (as compared with maternal serum) and the local action of thyroid hormones is regulated by the dynamic expression of cellular thyroid hormone transporters, metabolizing enzymes, and nuclear receptors. During the second trimester, concentrations of thyroid hormone in fetal serum rise, and after delivery the infant begins transitioning to an adult pattern of thyroid hormone metabolism over the ensuing 2 to 4 weeks. This transition may be altered by the gestational age at the time of delivery, illness, exogenous medications administered to the mother or infant, abnormal development of the hypothalamic-pituitary-thyroid (HPT) axis, or disorders of thyroid hormone production and/or metabolism.

Progress in human genetics has helped define many of the key mechanisms required for normal thyroid development, migration, and function and several of the transcription factors critical for thyroid gland development also play an important role in non-thyroid organogenesis (Table 145.1).[1,2] These patients have expanded our understanding of thyroid hormone physiology and underscore the role that local thyroid hormone signaling plays in fetal and neonatal development.

EMBRYOLOGY OF THE THYROID GLAND

The primordial thyroid begins as an involution of the foregut on the midline of the embryonic mouth referred to as the *median anlage*. In humans, this anlage appears at embryonic day 20 to 22 with caudal migration through the thyroglossal duct to its mature location at the base of the neck starting at embryonic day 30 to 40 (Fig. 145.1).[1] By embryonic day 50, migration is complete and the thyroglossal duct has involuted. Notably, thyroid follicular cells (the cell type that biosynthesizes thyroid hormones) arise from this median anlage.[1] The second secretory cell type found within the mature thyroid gland, the calcitonin-secreting para follicular or C cells, are believed to arise from the lateral anlages of the ultimobranchial bodies, a pair of embryonic structures that migrate from the fourth pharyngeal pouches and fuse into the definitive thyroid gland around embryonic day 60. Of note, more recent studies have raised the possibility that the C cells may arise in the endoderm germ layer.[3] Over this time, the embryonic thyroid gland begins to express thyroid-specific genes required for T4 and T3 biosynthesis. The mature anatomy of the thyroid gland is a bilobed structure with two lateral lobes connected by the isthmus. The pyramidal lobe of the thyroid gland is a normal anatomic variant found in up to 65% of patients that extends superiorly from the isthmus or lateral lobe.[4,5]

Thyroid dysgenesis (TD; abnormal development of the embryonic thyroid), including the most severe form, agenesis (the complete absence of the thyroid), is the most common cause of permanent hypothyroidism in humans, representing approximately 65% of the 1 in 3000 children who are born with congenital hypothyroidism (CH).[6] The remaining 35% of infants with CH have a eutopic thyroid (located in the correct anatomic position), with approximately 50% of these infants having an identifiable defect in thyroid hormone biosynthesis (thyroid dyshormonogenesis).[7] TD is typically considered a sporadic disease with ongoing investigation if familial cases follow an autosomal dominant, Mendelian mode of inheritance.[7,8] In contrast, the majority of germline mutations causing thyroid dyshormonogenesis are inherited in an autosomal recessive manner.[1,8]

The most common form of TD is thyroid ectopy (75% of cases) where the glandular tissue is located in the tongue (lingual thyroid)[9] or anywhere else along the normal migratory path (see Fig. 145.1).[6,10] The expression of the transcription factors *HHEX*, *NKX2-1*, *FOXE1*, and *PAX8* is critical for specification of the ventral endoderm cells that ultimately comprise the median and lateral anlagen, with *NKX2-1*, *FOXE1*, and *PAX8* critical for thyroid folliculogenesis (*NKX2-1* and *PAX8*) and migration (*FOXE1* and *CDCA8*/Borealin).[11,12] Several of these transcription factors are also involved in non-thyroid related organogenesis with mutations resulting in syndromic-forms of CH. As an example, expression of *NKX2-1* is critical in the development and function of interneurons in the central nervous system (CNS), surfactant producing cells in the lungs, and expression of thyroid

Table 145.1 Genes and Phenotype Associated With Thyroid Dysgenesis.

Gene (OMIM)	Name	Thyroid Phenotype	Additional Features
NKX2-1 (600635)	NK2 homeobox 1 or thyroid transcription factor 1	Thyroid hypoplasia, hemiagenesis, or athyreosis	Brain-lung-thyroid syndrome; benign hereditary chorea, infant respiratory distress syndrome (surfactant deficiency)
PAX8 (167415)	Paired box 8	Thyroid hypoplasia, ectopy, or athyreosis	Urogenital tract abnormalities
FOXE1 (602617)	Forkhead box protein E1 or thyroid transcription factor 2	Thyroid hypoplasia or athyreosis	Bamforth-Lazarus syndrome; cleft palate, choanal atresia, bifid epiglottis, and spiky hair
TSHR (603372)	Thyroid-stimulating hormone receptor	Thyroid hypoplasia	None
HHEX (604420)	Hematopoietically expressed homeobox	Thyroid hypoplasia and ectopy	None

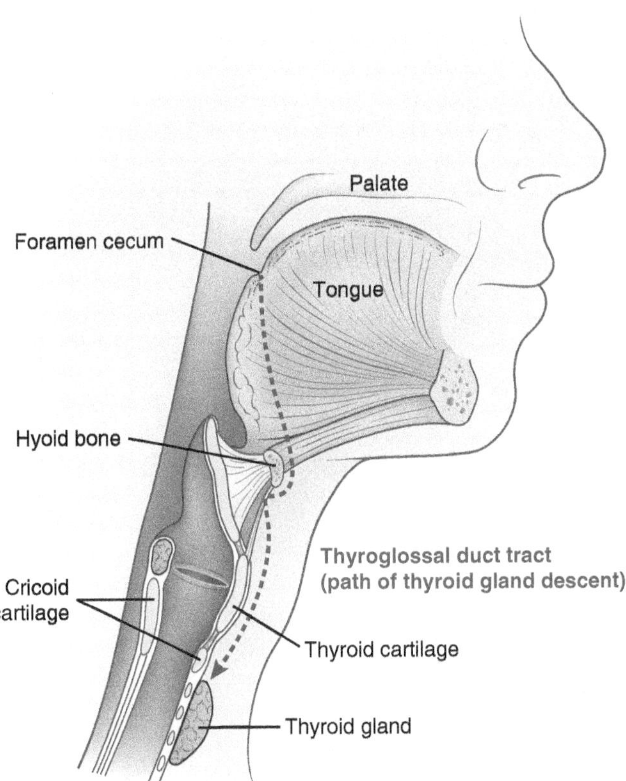

Fig. 145.1 The thyroid gland develops in the pharyngeal floor, migrating caudally through the foramen cecum along the thyroglossal duct tract to a location inferior to the cricoid cartilage by the seventh week of gestation. Failure to form (agenesis) or complete migration (dysgenesis with ectopic location) is the most common etiology of congenital hypothyroidism and may be secondary to mutations in several genes (see Table 145.1). (From Hanley P, Lord K, Bauer AJ. Thyroid disorders in children and adolescents: a review. *JAMA Pediatr.* 2016;170[1]:1008–1019. Reproduced with permission from *JAMA Pediatr.* 2016;170[1]:1008–1019. Copyright © 2021. American Medical Association. All rights reserved.)

peroxidase (TPO) and thyroglobulin. Mutations in *NKX2-1* are associated with brain-lung-thyroid syndrome characterized by benign hereditary chorea, infant respiratory distress syndrome, and CH secondary to varying severity of TD. Similarly, mutations in *FOXE1* are associated with craniofacial alterations, including bilateral choanal atresia, cleft palate, bifid epiglottis, spiky hair, and athyreosis (Bamforth-Lazarus syndrome; see Table 145.1).[1,10]

THYROID HORMONE BIOSYNTHESIS

The only biologically essential function of the thyroid gland is to produce adequate amounts of the iodothyronine hormones, 3′,3,5-triiodothyronine (T3) and tetra-iodothyronine (T4). Thyroid hormone producing cells are arranged as spheres or "follicles" in which the thyroid follicular cells surround a lumen of colloid. This structure facilitates a unique feature of the thyroid among endocrine glands, which is its ability to store large amounts of preformed hormone. This adaptation allows the thyroid to secrete adequate amounts of thyroid hormone during limited interruptions in dietary iodine intake. The thyroidal C-cells secrete calcitonin, a hormone involved in calcium balance through inhibition of osteoclast activity and decreased resorption of calcium in the kidneys. These activities oppose the action of parathyroid hormone; however, there is no significant bone morbidity or negative alternation in calcium homeostasis associated with the loss of endogenous calcitonin production in patients with thyroid agenesis or in patients who have undergone thyroidectomy.

Each thyroid follicular cell contains the machinery required for thyroid hormone synthesis (Fig. 145.2). Only T3 and T4 are capable of binding to the nuclear thyroid hormone receptors (TRs). T3 binds to the TRs with approximately 12-fold higher affinity compared to T4 and because of this T3 is accepted to be the active form of thyroid hormone and T4 its prohormone. Thyroid hormone synthesis requires the nutritional precursor of iodine, which is absorbed from the gut and circulates in plasma as iodide. Plasma iodide is actively transported or "trapped" into thyroid follicular cells through the sodium-iodine symporter (NIS). Using H_2O_2 generated by calcium-dependent dual oxidase (DUOX) enzymes, intracellular iodide in thyroid follicular cells is oxidized and then incorporated onto tyrosine residues within the thyroglobulin glycoprotein. The latter process is termed *iodine organification* and is catalyzed by the heme-containing TPO protein. The addition of a single iodine atom to tyrosine results in monoiodotyrosine (MIT), and the addition of two iodine atoms produces diiodotyrosine (DIT). Within the thyroglobulin protein, these iodotyrosine molecules fuse or "couple" to form either T3 (from DIT + MIT coupling) or T4 (from DIT + DIT coupling). This coupling reaction is also catalyzed by TPO.[6] The dietary requirements of iodine are based on age, with increased daily requirements from 150 μg/day for women during pre-pregnancy planning to 250 μg/day during pregnancy and lactation, secondary to increased maternal thyroid hormone production and fetal iodine requirements.[13,14]

The binding of thyroid stimulating hormone (TSH) to the TSH-receptor (TSHR) increases synthesis of iodothyronines as well as secretion of T3 and T4. At the apical membrane of the thyrocyte, colloid is endocytosed into the follicular cell and

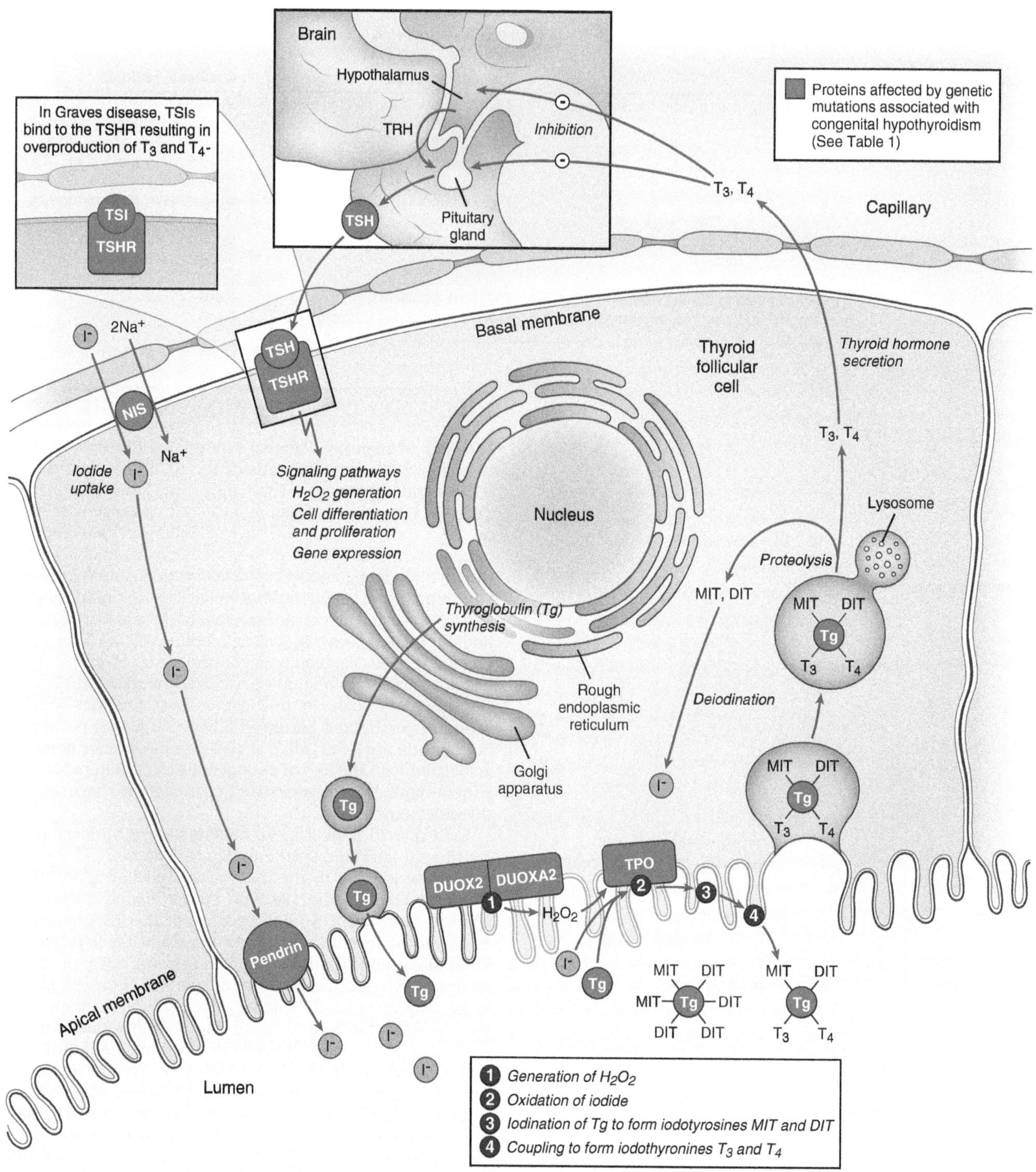

Fig. 145.2 Thyroid hormone synthesis begins with iodide uptake by the thyroid follicular cells via the sodium-iodide symporter *(NIS)*. Iodide is transported across the apical membrane via pendrin and subsequently oxidized by thyroid peroxidase *(TPO)* using endogenously generated H_2O_2. The TPO-mediated iodination of tyrosine residues on thyroglobulin *(Tg)* forms mono- and diiodotyrosinases (*MIT* and *DIT*), which then couple to form T3 or T4. Release of T3 and T4 occurs by endocytosis of stored thyroid hormone in the lumen (colloid) with subsequent proteolysis of bound Tg. Congenital hypothyroidism mutations in multiple genes associated with thyroid hormone biosynthesis, described as dyshormonogenesis, may result in a fetal goiter and congenital hypothyroidism (see Table 145.2). The top insert of the figure summarizes the hypothalamic-pituitary-thyroid axis regulatory feedback loop. *TRH*, Thyrotropin-releasing hormone; *TSHR*, TSH-receptor; *TSH*, thyroid-stimulating hormone; *TSI*, thyroid-stimulating immunoglobulin. (From Hanley P, Lord K, Bauer AJ. Thyroid disorders in children and adolescents: a review. *JAMA Pediatr.* 2016;170[1]:1008–1019. Reproduced with permission from *JAMA Pediatr.* 2016;170[1]:1008–1019. Copyright © 2021. American Medical Association. All rights reserved.)

Table 145.2 Genes and Phenotype Associated With Thyroid Dyshormonogenesis.

Gene (OMIM)	Name	Mode of Inheritance	Phenotype
TSHR (603372)	Thyroid-stimulating hormone receptor	AD	TSH resistance with elevated TSH and T4 in the normal range
SLC5A5 (601843)	NIS: sodium-iodide symporter	AR	Absent or low iodide uptake on scintigraphy with elevated serum thyroglobulin (Tg). Variable hypothyroidism and goiter
SLC26A4 (605646)	Pendrin: Anion transporter	AR	High level of uptake on scintigraphy with positive perchlorate discharge test and elevated serum Tg. Sensorineural hearing loss with enlarged vestibular aqueduct hypothyroidism and goiter
DUOX1/DUOX2 (606758/606759)	Dual oxydase 1 and 2	AR or AD	High level of uptake on scintigraphy with positive perchlorate discharge test and elevated serum Tg. Transient or permanent hypothyroidism and goiter
DUOXA2 (612772)	Dual oxidase associated protein	AR	High level of uptake on scintigraphy with positive perchlorate discharge test and elevated serum Tg. Transient or permanent hypothyroidism and goiter
TPO (606765)	Thyroid peroxidase	AR	High level of uptake on scintigraphy with positive perchlorate discharge test and elevated serum Tg. Severe hypothyroidism and goiter
Tg (188450)	Thyroglobulin	AR	Positive uptake on thyroid scintigraphy and low to undetectable serum Tg. Variable hypothyroidism and goiter
IYD/DEHAL1 (612025)	Iodotyrosine dehalogenase	AR	Positive uptake on thyroid scintigraphy and elevated serum Tg. Variable hypothyroidism and goiter
GNAS (139320)	Alpha subunit of the stimulatory guanine nucleotide-binding G-protein	Imprinted gene	Hypothyroidism with partial TSH resistance

AD, Autosomal dominant; *AR*, autosomal recessive; *TSH*, thyroid-stimulating hormone.

thyroglobulin undergoes lysosomal proteolysis to release T4 and T3 into the circulation. Uncoupled iodotyrosines are also released by proteolysis and then deiodinated by intracellular iodotyrosine dehalogenases, allowing their iodine to be recycled for new organification reactions. In a healthy, iodine-replete individual, the ratio of T4/T3 (T4:T3) secretion is approximately 14:1 with only 20% of circulating T3 originating from the thyroid; the remainder (80%) is converted from the prohormone T4 in peripheral tissues.[15]

Genetic alterations in the genes involved in thyroid hormone biosynthesis are collectively called *thyroid dyshormonogenesis* (Table 145.2). Loss of function mutations in the genes that encode NIS *(SLC5A5)*, pendrin *(SLC26A4)*, DUOX1/DUOX2 and DUOXA2, TPO *(TPO)*, thyroglobulin *(Tg)*, and iodotyrosine deiodinase or dehalogenase *(IYD)* are well recognized causes of dyshormonogenesis associated CH. The majority of these syndromes are inherited in an autosomal recessive pattern. Interestingly, mutations in TSHR may follow an autosomal dominant pattern, associated with TSH resistance (varying degrees of elevated TSH with normal to low T4), or an autosomal recessive pattern, associated with thyroid hypoplasia.[10]

The pattern and timing of hypothyroidism and goiter onset may vary based on the genetic etiology. Mutations in *Tg*[16], *TPO*[17], and *DUOXA2*[18] have been reported as etiologies of fetal goiter. Prenatal US in the second trimester is an accurate means of assessing for fetal thyroid volume, and treatment should be considered based on the severity and progression of polyhydramnios as well as concerns of premature labor and airway compromise after delivery. Mutations in *DUOX2* can cause either transient (monoallelic mutation) or permanent (biallelic mutation) CH,[19] and mutations in *SLC26A4* (pendrin)[20] and *IYD*[21] may present in early infancy or have delay in presentation into late childhood.

Under normal physiologic circumstances, thyroid hormone secretion is tightly regulated by the HPT axis (see Fig. 145.2). The hypothalamus secretes thyrotropin-releasing hormone (TRH), which stimulates the pituitary to secrete thyrotropin (also called *TSH*). Thyrotropin in turn stimulates the thyroid gland to secrete T4 and T3, both by stimulating hormone biosynthesis and by promoting the growth of thyroid tissue. Acting through the plasma membrane TSHR, TSH signals through phospholipase C, cyclic adenosine monophosphate, and inositol-phosphate diacylglycerol pathways to increase H_2O_2 production, iodine organification, iodide uptake, and the expression of *NIS, TPO,* and *Tg* (see Fig. 145.2). Postnatally, TRH and TSH secretion are negatively regulated by feedback from circulating T4 and T3.

Studies of fetal serum show that the secretion of fetal TSH is minimal until mid-gestation (18 to 20 weeks), when the fetal thyroid gland begins to concentrate iodine, with subsequent increases in T3 and T4 secretion between 20 weeks and term gestation (Fig. 145.3).[22] During the first trimester, maternal T4 production increases by approximately 20% under stimulation of placental human chorionic gonadotropin (hCG). Maternal T4 then crosses the placenta to drive fetal organogenesis and development after conversion to T3 by type 2 deiodination within fetal tissues.[23] In the early third trimester (25 weeks) the fetal pituitary response to TRH develops as well as maturation of the negative feedback control of pituitary TSH from T3 and T4. The ability of the fetal pituitary to both stimulate thyroid secretion and to sense negative feedback is intact prior to delivery, as has been demonstrated by (1) development of fetal goiter in the offspring of mothers with Graves disease overtreated with antithyroid medication (due to transplacental transfer of the antithyroid medication, blockade of fetal thyroid hormone production, and subsequent increase in fetal TSH), and (2) neonatal thyrotoxicosis with elevated T3 and T4 and suppressed TSH in infants born to mothers with Graves disease (due to transplacental transfer of maternal TSHR-stimulating antibodies).[7]

THYROID HORMONE METABOLISM

As mentioned above, most thyroid hormone secreted from the gland is in the form of T4 prohormone that is subsequently metabolized in peripheral tissues. In humans, the major pathway of thyroid hormone metabolism is sequential monodeiodination,

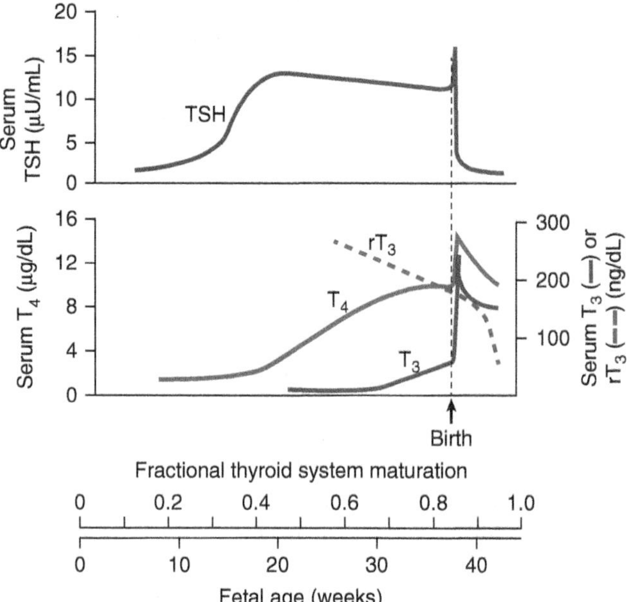

Fig. 145.3 Patterns of thyroid-stimulating hormone *(TSH)* and thyroid hormones in fetal and neonatal serum.

catalyzed by a family of enzymes called the *iodothyronine deiodinases*. There are three deiodinases: type 1 (D1), type 2 (D2), and type 3 (D3) deiodinase. All deiodinases are integral membrane proteins with a single transmembrane domain. They share approximately 50% sequence identity and are selenoproteins that require the amino acid selenocysteine for catalytic activity. Despite these similarities, each deiodinase possesses unique substrate affinities and tissue expression patterns that facilitate the tissue-specific metabolism of thyroid hormones.[24]

T4 is converted into the more biologically active T3 by the removal of an iodine atom from its "outer" phenolic ring. Conversely, both T4 and T3 are converted into inactive metabolites (reverse T3 (rT3) and T2, respectively) by "inner" tyrosyl ring deiodination (Fig. 145.4). D2 catalyzes outer-ring deiodination, and D3 is the primary inactivator of thyroid hormones. D1 is unique in its capacity to catalyze both outer- and inner-ring deiodination. However, its inactivating inner-ring deiodinase activity has minimal affinity for T4 or T3 unless these substrates are first sulfated. In addition to deiodination, the conjugation of the thyroid hormone phenolic hydroxyl group by sulfotransferases or glucuronidases are alternative pathways of thyroid hormone inactivation. Sulfation of T4 and T3 promotes their inactivation by D1-catalyzed inner-ring deiodination. Glucuronidation promotes the inactivation of thyroid hormones by biliary excretion.[24]

An important physiologic concept is that deiodination primarily occurs in peripheral tissues. This explains how standard monotherapy with levothyroxine (T4) restores normal serum and tissue levels of both T4 and T3 in infants with primary hypothyroidism. Furthermore, because the deiodinases are integral membrane proteins, their tissue-specific expression can induce and maintain local thyroid homeostasis in the tissue microenvironment. This local regulation of thyroid hormone signaling by deiodination is critical for embryonic development, as discussed above. While no disease-causing mutations in the deiodinases have been identified, missense mutations in the selenocysteine insertion sequence (SECIS)-binding protein 2 (*SECISBP*$_2$ or *SBP*$_2$), required for selenoprotein synthesis, have been shown to impair deiodinase expression and produce a phenotype that includes abnormal serum thyroid tests and psychomotor retardation.[25]

While individual deiodinases are dynamically expressed within fetal tissues during development, the uteroplacental unit as a whole functions as a potent inactivator of maternal thyroid hormone. Robust D3 expression in the placenta and fetal epithelium acts as a biochemical shield to protect the developing fetus from excessive transfer of maternal thyroid hormones in early gestation.[26] In addition, the combined high expression of thyroid hormone sulfotransferases and D1 within the fetal liver also promotes the inner-ring deiodination of extracellular T4 and T3. These deiodinase reactions also release free iodine to support endogenous T4 and T3 biosynthesis in the fetal thyroid.

THYROID HORMONE TRANSPORT

While it was once assumed that the hydrophobic properties of T4 and T3 allowed them to passively diffuse into cells through the lipid bilayer, it is now well established that the cellular uptake and efflux of thyroid hormone is mediated by specific transporter proteins.[27] Members of several transmembrane protein families have been shown to transport iodothyronines in vitro, including the monocarboxylate transporters (MCTs), the organic anion transporter polypeptides (OATPs), and the L-type amino acid transporters (LATs). Within this large group, three proteins, MCT8, MCT10, and OATP1C1, have been shown to be specific transporters for T4 and T3 and to be functionally significant in vivo, with MCT8 showing the highest specificity for TH transport.[27]

The specific expression of thyroid hormone transporters allows individual tissues to regulate intracellular thyroid hormone signaling by controlling the entry and efflux of thyroid hormones. This concept has been proven by showing tissue-specific derangements of thyroid hormone homeostasis in transgenic mice with MCT8, MCT10, or OATP1C1 deficiency.[28,29]

In humans, the *SLC16A2* gene that encodes MCT8 resides on the X chromosome and germline loss of function mutations result in the X-linked mental retardation syndrome of Allan Herndon-Dudley syndrome (AHDS; MCT8 deficiency).[27] Affected males have severe motor and neurocognitive delays that are attributed to cell-specific hypothyroidism in CNS neurons that normally rely upon MCT8 for T3 entry. Histologic analysis of a 30-week gestational male fetus with AHDS has documented prenatal brain damage (delayed cortical and cerebellar development and myelination with impaired axonal maturation),[30] illustrating that neuronal differentiation and myelination are T3-dependent processes that rely upon ligand transport during fetal development. However, while the majority of children will have evidence of delayed myelination on magnetic resonance imaging, the majority of patients have an uneventful fetal and early postnatal life, presenting with developmental delay and feeding problems in the first year of life. With advancing age, the central hypotonia persists with the onset of dyskinesia, dysmorphic features (elongated face, abnormal ear anatomy, and chest malformations), and evidence of peripheral hyperthyroidism (tachycardia, diaphoresis, and malnutrition).[27] Affected patients have normal to low serum T4 concentrations with elevated T3 concentrations. TSH is most commonly in the normal range.[27] The combination of hypotonia, developmental delay, and peripheral signs of hyperthyroidism (baseline tachycardia) in a male infant should raise suspicion for MCT8 deficiency; addition of T3 to the thyroid function assessment is critical for diagnosis. The presence of a non-elevated TSH in the presence of a low T4 should help to avoid a misdiagnosis of CH.

CELLULAR ACTIONS OF THYROID HORMONE

Intracellular T3 regulates the expression of thyroid hormone responsive genes through binding to the T3-responsive elements (TREs) of specific nuclear receptors, *THRA*[31] and *THRB*.[32] While

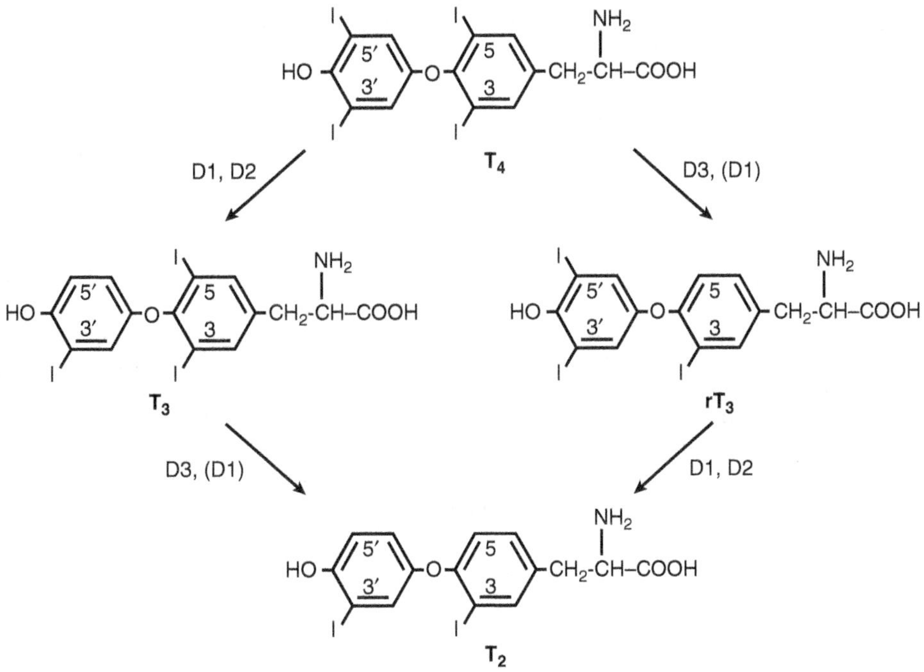

Fig. 145.4 Thyroid hormone deiodination.

these genes have high homology in the sequences encoding their DNA- and ligand-binding domains, each *THR* gene has a unique pattern of tissue expression and produces multiple protein products via alternative splicing. *THRA* produces one T3-binding product, Trα1, which is primarily expressed in the brain and heart.[33] *THRB* produces two major T3 binding products: TRβ1 (wide tissue expression) and TRβ2 (primarily expressed in the brain, retina, and cochlea).[33]

Upon ligand binding, TRs combine with co-activating factors and regulate the transcription of thyroid hormone responsive genes by binding to TRE sequences (Fig. 145.5).[33] Unique among other hormone nuclear receptors, TRs inhibit the expression of positively regulated target genes in the absence of ligand by constitutively binding repressive regulatory elements. Thus, in the absence of ligand, the expression of positively regulated thyroid hormone responsive genes is lower in the presence of TRs than in their absence. This explains why the phenotype of patients with germline thyroid hormone receptor mutations is similar to, but less severe than, the phenotype of untreated hypothyroidism.[33]

As with thyroid hormone metabolism and transport, TR expression represents another mechanism to control local thyroid hormone signaling. This selectively is achieved by the unique distribution of TR isoforms and co-activating transcription factors across different tissues and perhaps by the relative isoform specificity of certain TREs.[33] This concept of TR-mediated tissue specificity is illustrated by the differing clinical phenotypes of *THRA* versus *THRB* with dominant negative TR mutations. In such patients, the loss of TR function results in T3 insensitivity that is specific to the affected gene's normal distribution. The classic form of RTH (resistance to thyroid hormone) is due to dominant negative mutations in *THRB*, termed *RTHβ*.[32] The classic clinical phenotype reflects differences in the tissue-specific predominance of the TR isoforms and includes hypothyroidism features, such as decreased linear growth and hearing abnormalities, as well as goiter, resting tachycardia, and attention-deficit disorder. Because *THRB* is the predominant TR isoform expressed in the pituitary, affected individuals have nonsuppressed TSH secretion (inappropriately normal or high serum TSH concentrations) in the setting of increased T3 and T4.[32,33] The hyperthyroidism symptoms (tachycardia and ADD)

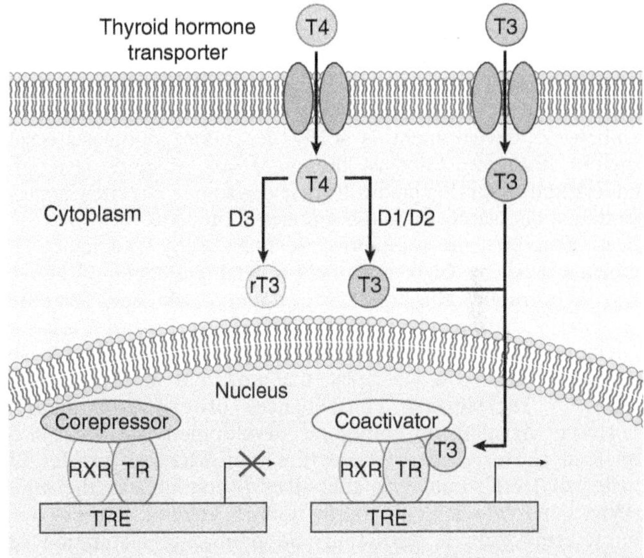

Fig. 145.5 Cellular thyroid hormone action. Extracellular thyroid hormones enter through cell membrane transporters and are metabolized by deiodinases (D1, D2, D3). Intracellular T3 is available to bind thyroid hormone receptors *(TR)*, which usually bind thyroid hormone response elements *(TRE)* of DNA as a heterodimer with retinoid X receptor *(RXR)*. (From Brent GA. Mechanisms of thyroid hormone action. *J Clin Invest.* 2012;122:3035–3043.)

occur secondary to the increased responsiveness of tissues that predominantly express *THRA* such as the brain and heart.[34]

In contrast to RTHβ, persons with RTH due to dominant negative *THRA* mutations (termed RTHα) display growth restriction, delayed bone development, mild developmental delay, and constipation, features that support important tissue-specific predominance of *THRA* in the bone, brain, and intestine.[31,34,35] Because *THRA* normally plays a minor role in pituitary feedback, individuals with RTHα have minimal impairment in thyroid hormone feedback and, in contrast to RTHβ patients, typically present with normal to low serum T4 concentrations accompanied by normal or low level of serum TSH. However, similar to patients with AHDS, patients with RTHα often have isolated elevations in T3 that may be secondary to increased hepatic D1 activity that augments conversion of T4 to T3 or reduced levels of D3 that decrease conversion of T3 to T2.[34] While RTHα and AHDS have similar biochemical findings (elevated T3, low T4, and normal TSH), one of the clinical features that distinguishes AHDS from RTHa is the presence of tachycardia in AHDS compared with bradycardia in patients with RTHα, because the thyroid-dependent impact on heart rate is mediated by THRA.

While it is generally accepted that most classic thyroid hormone actions are mediated through nuclear TRs, several studies have supported the existence of nongenomic actions of thyroid hormone at the plasma membrane. Early investigations of nongenomic thyroid hormone effects show their impact on Ca^{2+}-ATPase and Na,K-ATPase activities.[36] More recently, thyroid hormone binding to a cell surface receptor on integrin $\alpha_v\beta_3$ has been shown to have proangiogenic effects.[37]

MATERNAL-FETAL INTERACTIONS AND THE TRANSITION TO EXTRAUTERINE THYROID PHYSIOLOGY

Thyroid signaling in fetal tissues changes dynamically during normal pregnancy through precise interactions between the maternal and fetal endocrine axes. Fetal thyroid hormone is derived from both the transplacental transfer of maternal hormone and from the embryo's endogenous thyroid secretion. The relative contributions of these sources change during gestation. In the first trimester, when the fetal thyroid has minimal secretory capacity, embryonic development is solely dependent upon maternal thyroid hormone. Later, as the embryonic thyroid develops, endogenous secretion gradually increases to become the primary source of circulating thyroid hormones in the fetus.[23,38]

As described in the above sections, early pregnancy is characterized by high maternal to fetal gradients of active thyroid hormones. This protects developing fetal tissues from the temporally inappropriate action of excessive maternal thyroid hormone and is maintained by strong inner-ring deiodinase activities within the uteroplacental unit and in the embryo itself.[39,40] The adverse consequences of excessive thyroid hormone signaling on embryonic development are illustrated by fetal Graves disease, where the transplacental transfer of maternal TSHR-stimulating antibodies overstimulates the fetal thyroid and causes fetal hyperthyroidism. Affected fetuses have intrauterine growth restriction and premature maturation of skeletal structures (craniosynostosis) and CNS myelination that can result in neurodevelopmental delay.[41] Fetal thyrotoxicosis also increases the likelihood of miscarriage.

Thyroid hormone deficiency also has a negative impact on fetal development. In humans, this is most significantly illustrated by the permanent neurocognitive injury associated with combined maternal and fetal thyroid deficiency due to either profound, untreated maternal autoimmune hypothyroidism (Hashimoto's thyroiditis) or severe maternal iodine deficiency.[13,42] In other settings, where at least one thyroid axis is intact, the supply of thyroid hormones from either maternal or fetal secretion can function as a protective homeostatic mechanism for the fetus. Even with complete fetal athyreosis, maternal thyroid hormone alone is sufficient to support normal fetal development, as is illustrated by the normal growth and intellectual outcome of athyreotic children who receive adequate levothyroxine treatment from birth. The effective transplacental transfer of maternal thyroid hormone in this setting has been directly documented in humans by the demonstration of T4 and T3 in the serum of infants with complete organification defects or athyreosis prior to treatment.[43]

In contrast to the protection afforded by maternal thyroid hormones, fetal compensation for the converse pathophysiology of maternal hypothyroidism appears to be incomplete. Two large studies of pregnant women have associated maternal hypothyroxinemia with decreased intellectual outcome of the offspring, despite normal fetal thyroid function.[44,45] This indicates a risk of developmental injury from isolated maternal hypothyroidism. The risk is theoretically greatest in the first trimester, when the fetal thyroid has minimal secretory capacity and when maternal thyroid hormone requirements are typically increasing.[23] This is the rationale for current recommendations to monitor thyroid status frequently upon the diagnosis of pregnancy in women with preexisting hypothyroidism.[13] However, even in the unfortunate occurrence of untreated, overt maternal hypothyroidism discovered late in pregnancy (second or third trimester), aggressive thyroid hormone replacement therapy to achieve a maternal TSH less than 3 μU/mL can result in infants without significant cognitive delay.[46]

At birth, the neonate rapidly shifts to postnatal thyroid physiology. Thyroid secretion is acutely stimulated, with a rapid peak in TSH (as high as 60 to 80 μU/mL) approximately 30 to 60 minutes after delivery, followed by elevations in T4 and a decrease in reverse T3 levels.[47] The molecular regulators of this transition, termed the *neonatal thyroid surge*, are incompletely understood, but it is speculated that both TSH secretion and D2 expression within brown fat are stimulated by transition from the intrauterine environment to the colder extrauterine temperature and that the rapid suppression of fetal D3 expression is triggered by the acute rise in arterial partial pressure of oxygen (PO_2).[39] The TSH surge is transient, decreasing to around 20 μU/mL at 24 hours, with a continued, gradual decline over the first week.[48] Subsequent to the TSH surge, there is an increase in T4 levels, which peak about 3 days after delivery.[49,50] For the majority of healthy term infants, the serum concentration of TSH approximates adult levels within 2 weeks.[49] Serum T3 levels increase more slowly than T4 up to approximately 3 months of age, when both T3 and T4 begin to decrease toward adult levels.[51]

The above transition from fetal to neonatal thyroid physiology is altered in prematurely born infants. Neonates born before 28 weeks gestation often exhibit a blunted TSH and T4 surge, followed by a period of prolonged hypothyroxinemia (total T4) with inappropriately normal or low serum TSH concentrations.[52] A major contributor of the fall in T4 is loss of transplacental maternal T4 and iodine secondary to early parturition. Due to immaturity of the HPT axis, serum TSH does not increase (and may actually decrease) in response to the low T3 and T4 and may remain "inappropriately" low for 2 to 3 months until the HPT axis begins to mature.[53] A rise in serum T3 levels often lags compared to T4 secondary to low tissue type 1 and 2 deiodinase activity. This contributes to altered thermogenesis because expression of thermogenin (uncoupling protein 1 or UCP1) in brown adipose tissue (reduced in premature infants) is T3-dependent.

This pattern of *transient hypothyroxinemia of prematurity* has become the subject of intense research as the survival of premature neonates has increased. As briefly described above, the etiology of hypothyroxinemia in this population is multifactorial, reflecting persistence of the fetal thyroid hormone metabolic state (low T3 and T4 with elevated rT3), reduced maternal transfer of iodine and T4, and a lack of response of the neonatal HPT axis feedback loop to low T3 and T4 levels, which begins to mature at approximately 30 weeks adjusted gestational age. Nonthyroidal illness syndrome (the suppression of thyroid function that occurs in patients of all ages during critical illness), associated with administration of drugs known to suppress TSH release (dopamine, glucocorticoids) and/or production and secretion of T3 and T4 (iodine-containing antiseptics, amiodarone;

Wolff-Chaikoff effect), often complicates the interpretation of the thyroid axis and may prolong the period of HPT axis maturation. In this setting, hepatic thyroid binding globulin production is reduced, so free-T3 and free-T4 concentrations reflect thyroid gland production more accurately than total T3 or T4 levels. The severity of the transient hypothyroxinemia correlates with increased morbidity and decreased survival.[54-56] Although some studies have shown an association between the severity of this hypothyroxinemia and later intellectual outcome, none have demonstrated a consistent benefit of levothyroxine treatment.[57-60] Consequently, controversy exists regarding the appropriateness of treatment, and more research is needed to address this.

As the HPT axis matures, preterm infants may display a delayed elevation in TSH (dTSH).[61] The increase in TSH may be modest (between 5 and 15 μU/mL) or more significant (>25 μU/mL, rarely >100 μU/mL) and typically occurs between 2 weeks and 6 months of age, with a mean of 30 days.[48] While the majority of infants that develop dTSH have a normal thyroid on imaging and ultimately recover normal thyroid function, up to 25% may have permanent hypothyroidism.[62,63] In an effort to avoid missing appropriate treatment, serial thyroid hormone monitoring should be standardized for preterm infants, most notably in infants less than 1500 g at birth. Several protocols exist, with two examples including testing at (1) 48 hours, 2 weeks, 6 weeks, 10 weeks, or until the infant is greater than 1500 g,[64] or (2) 72 to 120 hours, 1 week, 2 weeks, 4 weeks, and at term-corrected gestational age.[62] There is no consensus on criteria for initiation of thyroid hormone replacement therapy, but treatment should be considered if the TSH is greater than 10 μU/mL.[48]

BIOLOGIC EFFECTS OF THYROID HORMONE SIGNALING ON FETAL AND NEONATAL HEALTH

T3 is a master regulator of cellular metabolism, proliferation, and differentiation. The absolute dependence of human neurodevelopment on these thyroid hormones is illustrated by the severe growth restriction and neurologic injury that results from untreated CH that is completely prevented by oral levothyroxine therapy (Fig. 145.6). More recently, the identification of patients with genetic defects in thyroid hormone metabolism, transport, and receptor action have shown that the derangement of local thyroid hormone signaling is sufficient to impair neurodevelopment and growth, even in the absence of primary thyroid disease.

In humans, thyroid hormone is present in fetal tissues throughout all three trimesters and the embryo expresses TRs, deiodinases, sulfotransferases, and transporters in temporally dynamic and tissue-specific patterns throughout gestation.[7,23,50] This suggests that the highly coordinated regulation of thyroid hormone signaling is critical for even the earliest phases of embryonic development. Supporting this, knockout mouse experiments have shown important effects of local T3 action on the early embryonic development of the photoreceptors, cochlea, and skeleton.[39,65]

Thyroid hormone also regulates multiple aspects of brain differentiation, including dendritic and axonal growth, neuronal migration, and myelination.[66,67] Most human research of thyroid hormone dependent development has focused on the endpoint of cognition, because it is the primary clinical morbidity associated with inadequately treated CH and because it exhibits a critical time dependence, where the loss of intellect incurred from infantile thyroid dysfunction cannot be recovered by later treatment.[68] Illustrating this, large studies of children with CH indicate that 3 to 5 IQ points are permanently lost for each month of untreated hypothyroidism during the first year of life. These

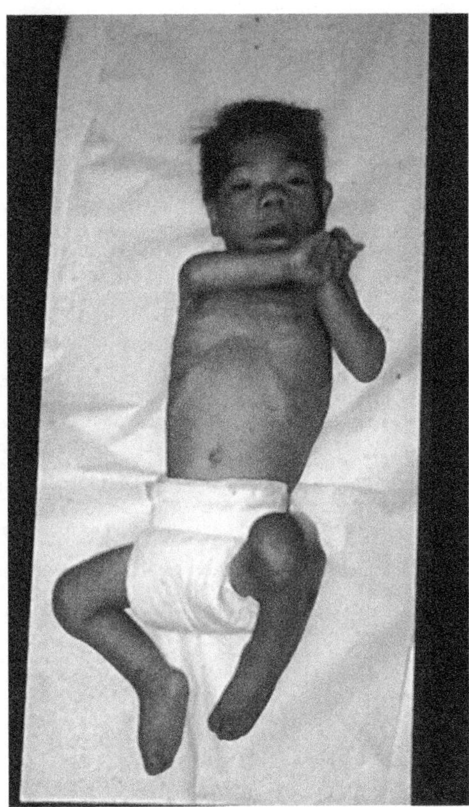

Fig. 145.6 Untreated congenital hypothyroidism. Owing to the unfortunate absence of treatment, this 17-year-old girl has the height and bone age of a 2-year-old. She has severe and irreversible mental retardation, shortened extremities, and dysmorphic facial features (wide-set eyes, poorly developed nasal bridge). Patients with congenital hypothyroidism who are optimally treated with oral levothyroxine have normal growth and neurodevelopment. (From Brent GA, Davies TF. Hypothyroidism and thyroiditis. In: Melmed S, Polonsky KS, Larsen PR, Kronenberg HM, eds. *Williams Textbook of Endocrinology*. 12th ed. Philadelphia: Elsevier Saunders; 2012:406–439.)

data drive the management of CH (which is based upon the goals of early treatment and rapid restoration of euthyroidism) and ongoing research to determine the potential neurologic impact of other hypothyroxinemic states, such as maternal hypothyroidism, transient hypothyroxinemia of prematurity, and nonthyroidal illness syndrome in critically ill newborns.

CONCLUSION

Abundant basic and clinical research demonstrates that thyroid hormone signaling is required for both fetal and pediatric development. In addition to novel animal studies, much of what we now know about fetal and neonatal thyroid physiology has been learned through the discovery and clinical characterization of patients with genetic defects in thyroid hormone physiology. The identification of genes critical for thyroid hormone metabolism, transport, and receptor function has revealed that derangement of local thyroid hormone signaling can impact development, even in the absence of primary thyroid disease. Further clinical research is needed to understand the consequences of fetal and neonatal hypothyroxinemia, especially for preterm and/or critically ill infants, to better understand the potential benefits and risks of treatment.

A complete reference list is available at www.ExpertConsult.com. 

SELECT REFERENCES

1. Fernandez LP, Lopez-Marquez A, Santisteban P. Thyroid transcription factors in development, differentiation and disease. *Nat Rev Endocrinol.* 2015;11:29-42.
2. Stoupa A, Kariyawasam D, Carre A, et al. Update of thyroid developmental genes. *Endocrinol Metab Clin North Am.* 2016;45:243-254.
3. Nilsson M, Williams D. On the origin of cells and derivation of thyroid cancer: C cell story revisited. *Eur Thyroid J.* 2016;5:79-93.
4. Gurleyik E, Gurleyik G, Dogan S, et al. Pyramidal lobe of the thyroid gland: surgical anatomy in patients undergoing total thyroidectomy. *Anat Res Int.* 2015;2015:384148.
5. Kovacic M, Kovadcic I. [Incidence and surgical importance of pyramidal lobe and tubercle of the thyroid gland: a prospective study]. *Lijec Vjesn.* 2015;137:357-360.
6. Hanley P, Lord K, Bauer AJ. Thyroid disorders in children and adolescents: a review. *JAMA Pediatr.* 2016;170:1008-1019.
7. Polak M, Luton D. Fetal thyroidology. *Best Pract Res Clin Endocrinol Metab.* 2014;28:161-173.
8. Sun F, Zhang JX, Yang CY, et al. The genetic characteristics of congenital hypothyroidism in China by comprehensive screening of 21 candidate genes. *Eur J Endocrinol.* 2018;178:623-633.
9. Carranza Leon BG, Turcu A, Bahn R, et al. Lingual thyroid: 35-year experience at a tertiary care referral center. *Endocr Pract.* 2016;22:343-349.
10. Mio C, Grani G, Durante C, et al. Molecular defects in thyroid dysgenesis. *Clin Genet.* 2020;97:222-231.
11. Nilsson M, Fagman H. Development of the thyroid gland. *Development.* 2017;144:2123-2140.
12. Carre A, Stoupa A, Kariyawasam D, et al. Mutations in BOREALIN cause thyroid dysgenesis. *Hum Mol Genet.* 2017;26:599-610.
13. Alexander EK, Pearce EN, Brent GA, et al. 2017 Guidelines of the American Thyroid Association for the diagnosis and management of thyroid disease during pregnancy and the postpartum. *Thyroid.* 2017;27:315-389.
14. Leung AM, Pearce EN, Braverman LE. Sufficient iodine intake during pregnancy: just do it. *Thyroid.* 2013;23:7-8.
15. Jonklaas J, Bianco AC, Bauer AJ, et al. Guidelines for the treatment of hypothyroidism: prepared by the American Thyroid Association task force on thyroid hormone replacement. *Thyroid.* 2014;24:1670-1751.
16. Vasudevan P, Powell C, Nicholas AK, et al. Intrauterine death following intraamniotic triiodothyronine and thyroxine therapy for fetal goitrous hypothyroidism associated with polyhydramnios and caused by a thyroglobulin mutation. *Endocrinol Diabetes Metab Case Rep.* 2017.
17. Borgel K, Pohlenz J, Holzgreve W, et al. Intrauterine therapy of goitrous hypothyroidism in a boy with a new compound heterozygous mutation (Y453D and C800R) in the thyroid peroxidase gene. A long-term follow-up. *Am J Obstet Gynecol.* 2005;193:857-858.
18. Tanase-Nakao K, Miyata I, Terauchi A, et al. Fetal goitrous hypothyroidism and polyhydramnios in a patient with compound heterozygous DUOXA2 mutations. *Horm Res Paediatr.* 2018;90:132-137.
19. Moreno JC, Bikker H, Kempers MJ, et al. Inactivating mutations in the gene for thyroid oxidase 2 (THOX2) and congenital hypothyroidism. *N Engl J Med.* 2002;347:95-102.
20. Wemeau JL, Kopp P. Pendred syndrome. *Best Pract Res Clin Endocrinol Metab.* 2017;31:213-224.
21. Moreno JC, Klootwijk W, van Toor H, et al. Mutations in the iodotyrosine deiodinase gene and hypothyroidism. *N Engl J Med.* 2008;358:1811-1818.
22. Thorpe-Beeston JG, Nicolaides KH, Felton CV, et al. Maturation of the secretion of thyroid hormone and thyroid-stimulating hormone in the fetus. *N Engl J Med.* 1991;324:532-536.
23. Patel J, Landers K, Li H, et al. Delivery of maternal thyroid hormones to the fetus. *Trends Endocrinol Metab.* 2011;22:164-170.
24. Bianco AC, Dumitrescu A, Gereben B, et al. Paradigms of dynamic control of thyroid hormone signaling. *Endocr Rev.* 2019;40:1000-1047.
25. Dumitrescu AM, Refetoff S. Impaired sensitivity to thyroid hormone: defects of transport, metabolism and action. In: Feingold KR, Anawalt B, Boyce A, et al., eds. *Endotext.* South Dartmouth, MA: MDText.com, Inc.; 2000.
26. Chapman AK, Farmer ZJ, Mastrandrea LD, et al. Neonatal thyroid function and disorders. *Clin Obstet Gynecol.* 2019;62:373-387.
27. Groeneweg S, van Geest FS, Peeters RP, et al. Thyroid hormone transporters. *Endocr Rev.* 2020;41.
28. Bernal J, Guadano-Ferraz A, Morte B. Thyroid hormone transporters–functions and clinical implications. *Nat Rev Endocrinol.* 2015;11:406-417.
29. Mayerl S, Muller J, Bauer R, et al. Transporters MCT8 and OATP1C1 maintain murine brain thyroid hormone homeostasis. *J Clin Invest.* 2014;124:1987-1999.
30. Lopez-Espindola D, Morales-Bastos C, Grijota-Martinez C, et al. Mutations of the thyroid hormone transporter MCT8 cause prenatal brain damage and persistent hypomyelination. *J Clin Endocrinol Metab.* 2014;99:E2799-E2804.
31. van Gucht ALM, Moran C, Meima ME, et al. Resistance to thyroid hormone due to heterozygous mutations in thyroid hormone receptor alpha. *Curr Top Dev Biol.* 2017;125:337-355.
32. Pappa T, Refetoff S. Human genetics of thyroid hormone receptor beta: resistance to thyroid hormone beta (rthbeta). *Methods Mol Biol.* 2018;1801:225-240.
33. Singh BK, Yen PM. A clinician's guide to understanding resistance to thyroid hormone due to receptor mutations in the TRalpha and TRbeta isoforms. *Clin Diabetes Endocrinol.* 2017;3:8.
34. Moran C, Chatterjee K. Resistance to thyroid hormone due to defective thyroid receptor alpha. *Best Pract Res Clin Endocrinol Metab.* 2015;29:647-657.
35. Ortiga-Carvalho TM, Sidhaye AR, Wondisford FE. Thyroid hormone receptors and resistance to thyroid hormone disorders. *Nat Rev Endocrinol.* 2014;10:582-591.
36. Davis PJ, Goglia F, Leonard JL. Nongenomic actions of thyroid hormone. *Nat Rev Endocrinol.* 2016;12:111-121.
37. Davis PJ, Sudha T, Lin HY, et al. Thyroid hormone, hormone analogs, and angiogenesis. *Compr Physiol.* 2015;6:353-362.
38. Polak M. Human fetal thyroid function. *Endocr Dev.* 2014;26:17-25.
39. Gereben B, Zavacki AM, Ribich S, et al. Cellular and molecular basis of deiodinase-regulated thyroid hormone signaling. *Endocr Rev.* 2008;29:898-938.
40. Huang SA, Dorfman DM, Genest DR, et al. Type 3 iodothyronine deiodinase is highly expressed in the human uteroplacental unit and in fetal epithelium. *J Clin Endocrinol Metab.* 2003;88:1384-1388.
41. Samuels SL, Namoc SM, Bauer AJ. Neonatal thyrotoxicosis. *Clin Perinatol.* 2018;45:31-40.
42. Stenzel D, Huttner WB. Role of maternal thyroid hormones in the developing neocortex and during human evolution. *Front Neuroanat.* 2013;7:19.
43. Vulsma T, Gons MH, de Vijlder JJ. Maternal-fetal transfer of thyroxine in congenital hypothyroidism due to a total organification defect or thyroid agenesis. *N Engl J Med.* 1989;321:13-16.
44. Haddow JE, Palomaki GE, Allan WC, et al. Maternal thyroid deficiency during pregnancy and subsequent neuropsychological development of the child. *N Engl J Med.* 1999;341:549-555.
45. Pop VJ, Kuijpens JL, van Baar AL, et al. Low maternal free thyroxine concentrations during early pregnancy are associated with impaired psychomotor development in infancy. *Clin Endocrinol.* 1999;50:149-155.
46. Downing S, Halpern L, Carswell J, et al. Severe maternal hypothyroidism corrected prior to the third trimester is associated with normal cognitive outcome in the offspring. *Thyroid.* 2012;22:625-630.
47. Segni M. Disorders of the thyroid gland in infancy, childhood and adolescence. In: Feingold KR, Anawalt B, Boyce A, et al., eds. *Endotext.* South Dartmouth, MA: MDText.com, Inc.; 2000.
48. LaFranchi SH. Screening preterm infants for congenital hypothyroidism: better the second time around. *J Pediatr.* 2014;164:1259-1261.
49. Fisher DA, Nelson JC, Carlton EI, et al. Maturation of human hypothalamic-pituitary-thyroid function and control. *Thyroid.* 2000;10:229-234.
50. Kratzsch J, Pulzer F. Thyroid gland development and defects. *Best Pract Res Clin Endocrinol Metab.* 2008;22:57-75.

Genetics of Sex Determination and Differentiation

146

Peter James Ivor Ellis

INTRODUCTION

The classical paradigm of mammalian, including human, sexual development postulates an initially "indifferent" (sexually undifferentiated) state that is transformed, in two major stages, into the sexually dimorphic male and female forms. The two stages are called *primary,* relating to the gonad, and *secondary,* referring to all other genital organs.[1] In the first stage, *primary sex determination,* specific sex-determining genetic factors that are present from conception drive the development of the gonad. In the second stage, *secondary sexual differentiation,* all other features of sexual dimorphism are established. In this concept, all features of both internal and external sexually dimorphic structures other than the gonads develop from the action of hormones produced in males by the testis, lack of these hormones (or production of other hormones) in females, and independently of the sex-determining gene(s). This paradigm is known as the *Jost principle*.[1] A large number of genetic pathways interact in a complex and, in part, overlapping and redundant manner to execute the genetic control of sexual development. In this chapter, we will describe this dynamic, sequential program as occurring in six stages as follows:

1. Chromosomal assignment of sex
2. Pregonadal sexual development and nongonadal sexual dimorphism
3. Formation and development of the indifferent gonad
4. Transformation of the indifferent gonad into a testis or an ovary
5. Lifelong maintenance of gonadal identity
6. Secondary sexual differentiation

THE JOST PRINCIPLE AND BEYOND

The primordial, indifferent gonad is situated in the gonadal (genital) ridge region of the intermediate mesoderm of the fetus. In genetic males, the indifferent gonad is induced to become a testis under the influence of male-determining genes. In the female, with no such genes present, the gonad remains uninduced and an ovary develops. The mesenchymal cells of the gonadal ridge and the neighboring metanephros give rise, in males, to androgen-producing Leydig cells of the testis or, in females, to the theca cells of the ovary and to connective tissue. The adjacent coelomic epithelium grows into the mesodermal mass to produce the Sertoli cells of the testicular seminiferous tubules, or the follicle cells of the ovary. In addition, primordial germ cells migrate to the developing gonad to give rise to sperm or egg cells.

Although current understanding builds on this framework, our knowledge has advanced considerably in recent years, leading to some modifications of the original paradigm. It is now known that "genetic maleness" in mammals is normally dependent on the presence of a sex-determining region of the Y chromosome and "genetic femaleness" is normally dependent on its absence. The identity of the testis-determining gene on the Y chromosome is known, as is the fact that the effect of this gene in formation of the testis is not direct, but rather is mediated by other, so-called downstream genes. Some of the latter have been identified. Also, the action of the Y-chromosomal region is preceded by "upstream" gene action that is evidently a prerequisite for Y-chromosomal function in gonadal determination. Furthermore, some sex-specific gene action, including but not limited to Y-chromosomal (male-specific) gene action, appears to influence the sexual phenotype either before gonadal development (i.e., at a "pregonadal" juncture) or later, but independently of hormonal action. Finally, we now better understand the development of the ovary as being not merely a passive, uninduced state, but also dependent on specific gene action. These findings necessitate modification of the Jost paradigm. Fig. 146.1 summarizes the original Jost paradigm (see Fig. 146.1A) and the updated version based on current understanding (see Fig. 146.1B).

CHROMOSOMAL ASSIGNMENT OF SEX

In 1923 it was demonstrated cytologically that humans have X and Y chromosomes.[2] By analogy with *Drosophila,* it was assumed that sex determination in mammals would be mediated by the ratio of the number of X chromosomes to the number of sets of autosomes. However, in 1959, it was discovered that an XO sex chromosome karyotype produced a predominantly female phenotype both in humans (Turner syndrome)[3] and in mice,[4] and XXY produced predominant maleness in humans (Klinefelter syndrome).[5,6] These observations demonstrated firstly that the presence of a Y chromosome resulted in the development of a predominantly male phenotype independently of the number of X chromosomes, and secondly that the absence of the Y chromosome resulted in the development of a predominantly female phenotype. Thus the Y chromosome appeared to possess a gene or genes, the presence or absence of which determined the destiny of the bipotential gonad as a testis or ovary, respectively, and, through this, the development of the dimorphic secondary sex characteristics.[1] In the human the hypothetical Y-chromosomal gene was named *testis-determining factor (TDF),* and in mice it was named *testis-determining gene on the Y (Tdy)*. Minor deviations of Klinefelter and Turner syndromes from the normal male and female phenotype, respectively, are probably due to the influence of other (non-*TDF*) sex-chromosomal factors (see later) on the sex differentiation pathway.

MAPPING OF TESTIS-DETERMINING FACTOR

The discovery that 46,XX males usually have translocations (transfers of chromosomal material) of Yp (where *p* indicates the short arm of a chromosome; *q* indicates the long arm) to one of their Xps was a major breakthrough in mapping *TDF* on the Y chromosome.[7,8] The X and Y chromosomes

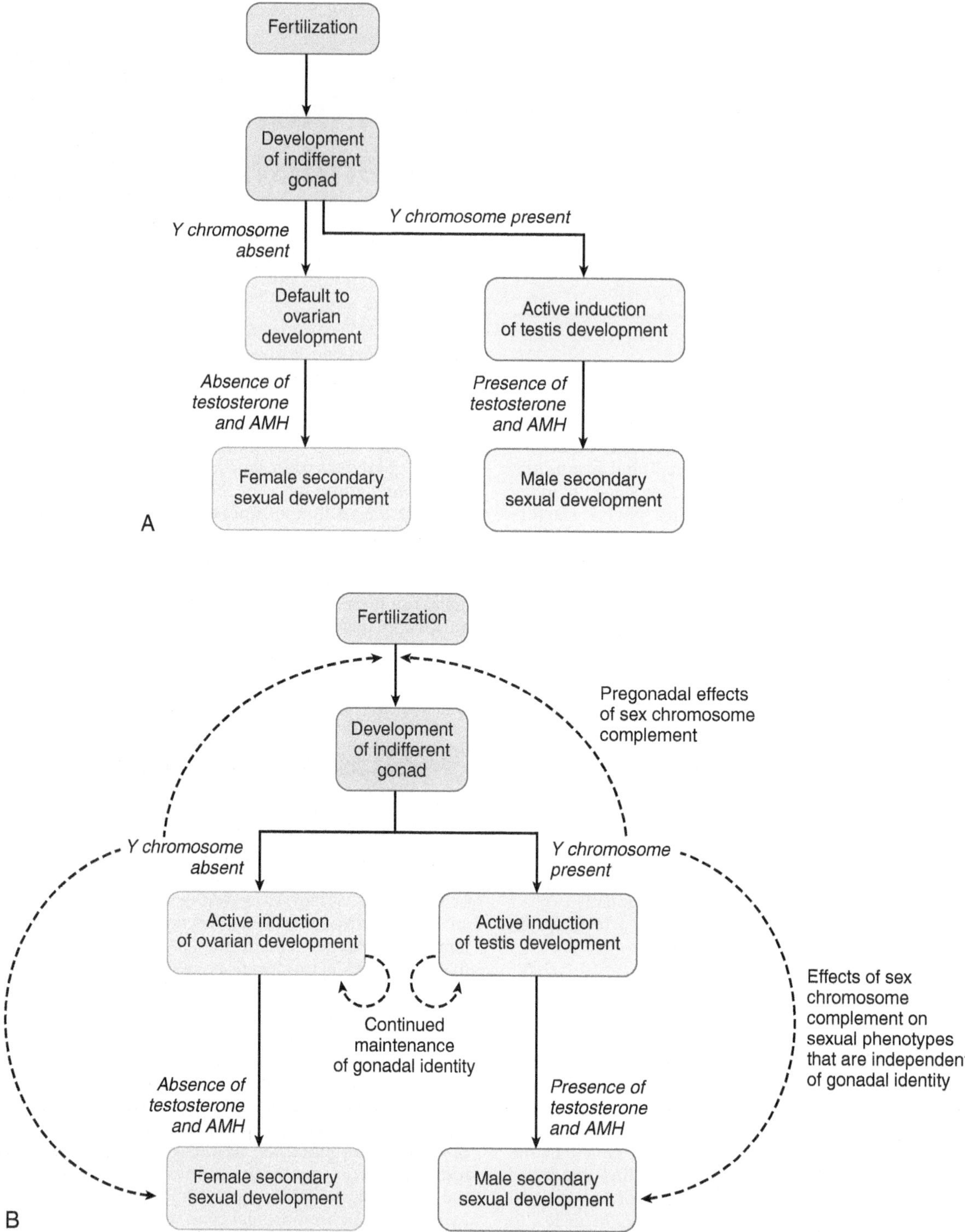

Fig. 146.1 Jost paradigm for sexual differentiation (A) as originally formulated and (B) as revised in the light of recent advances. *AMH,* Anti-müllerian hormone.

have homologous segments at the ends of their respective p arms, that pair during male meiosis. Because of genetic exchange between these segments, allelic variants located in this region appear to be inherited as if on autosomes. Accordingly, these regions are called *pseudoautosomal.* The occurrence of abnormal crossovers adjacent to the pseudoautosomal region can result in the illegitimate transfer of *TDF* to the X chromosome.[9,10] Molecular analyses in such patients permitted the construction of a deletion map of the Y chromosome[11,12] and showed that a small region of Yp adjacent to the pseudoautosomal region is essential for testicular differentiation. Finer mapping continued, and one candidate gene was mistakenly identified: Page and colleagues[13] found a highly conserved sequence that seemed to map with a male-determining Y fragment and named it *ZFY*. However, one of their XX males did not have *ZFY*, and the finding of more such patients[14,15] suggested that *ZFY* could not be *TDF*.

IDENTIFICATION OF *TDF/Tdy* AS THE GENE *SRY/Sry*

The resumed search for *TDF* was targeted on 35 kilobases (kb) of DNA between the proximal (i.e., towards the centromere of the chromosome) limit of the pseudoautosomal region of the Y chromosome and the breakpoint in XX males lacking *ZFY*. A subclone selected for its male specificity in mammals was found to encode a protein containing an 80-amino acid segment that was homologous to the mating-type protein in *Schizosaccharomyces pombe* and to a conserved 80-amino acid, DNA-binding motif present in the high mobility group (HMG) 1 transcription-regulating proteins.[16] Further analyses of a variety of tissues disclosed a transcript of this gene only in the testes. It was proposed that this gene, designated *sex-determining region, Y chromosome* (*SRY*), was *TDF*.[16] Soon thereafter, mutations in the *SRY* gene were found in some cases of XY, pure gonadal dysgenesis.[17-20] The mouse *Sry* gene was cloned at the same time as human *SRY*.[21] Some mice transgenic (i.e., in which a gene has been artificially transferred) for a fragment containing *Sry* showed 40,XX sex reversal—that is, mice otherwise destined to be female had a male appearance (although they were sterile).[21] Testes of these mice were histologically similar to those of human XX males. However, sex reversal did not always occur, and this incomplete penetrance may be related to the influence of genetic background on *Sry* transgene expression.[22] Genetic modifiers may also be the explanation for the multiple phenotypes seen with particular mutations in *SRY*. Interestingly, human *SRY* does not cause sex reversal in transgenic mice; it is not nearly as conserved in function as some human genes, a few of which can work even in *Drosophila*. The HMG boxes of *SRY* and its mouse homologue, *Sry*, are examples of so-called generalized HMG boxes.[23] It has been demonstrated that the SRY HMG box not only binds to synthetic DNA fragments of the sequence AACAAAG[24] but also to cruciform DNA structures irrespective of their sequence. Both targets adopt similar conformations in solution, in which state the binding of SRY induces a large conformational change in the DNA.[25] Some mutations in the SRY HMG box alter the DNA contact sites in such a way as to preclude the usual deformation of the DNA.[26]

The principal evidence in favor of *SRY/Sry* being *TDF/Tdy* is the following:

1. It is localized in the smallest region of chromosome Y capable of inducing testicular differentiation in humans[16] and mice.[21]
2. Some cases of XY, pure gonadal dysgenesis, have de novo mutations in the *SRY* gene.[17-20]
3. In the mouse, *Sry* expression correlates with the initiation of testicular determination in the gonadal ridge,[27] and in both the mouse and the human, its expression in the blastocyst corresponds to the more rapid growth of the Y-bearing blastocyst (see later).[28-31]
4. A fragment of DNA that includes the mouse gene is able to induce male-type development in some transgenic XX mice.[32]
5. It is an evolutionarily conserved gene on the Y chromosome of metatherian and eutherian mammals.[17,33]

PREGONADAL AND NONGONADAL SEXUAL DIMORPHISM

Pregonadal and nongonadal sexual dimorphism comprises those differences between individuals that are related to sex chromosome complement, but that either arise before (pregonadal) or are otherwise independent of (nongonadal) the presence of testes/ovaries and associated sex hormones.[34] Nongonadal sexually dimorphic phenotypes are outside the scope of this chapter, but interested readers are referred to a recent review.[34]

Marsupial mammals clearly have pregonadal sexual differentiation. In the tammar wallaby, some features of sexual dimorphism, including the scrotum in the male and the mammary glands in the female, appear before development of the gonads and independently of hormones.[35] Although these organs develop mainly under hormonal influence in placental (eutherian) mammals, evolutionary conservation of some pregonadal sex-determining gene expression has also occurred in mice. The anogenital distance, which is a measure of masculinization (and which is also the region in which the scrotum develops), is smaller in prepubertal and XX, *Sxr* pseudomales than in their normal, XY brothers.[36] These data suggest an effect of an effect of sex chromosome dosage on this secondary sex characteristic in mice, independent of any hormonal action.[37,38] These and other pregonadal sex differences might be controlled by sex chromosome to autosome or X to Y ratios: "Re-examination of the few known marsupial intersexes suggested that a gene on the X chromosome is responsible, with one X chromosome coding for a scrotum, and two X chromosomes for a pouch, regardless of the presence or absence of testes or ovaries."[39]

Since the technology was developed to identify the sex of preimplantation embryos by polymerase chain reaction, many studies on the differential rates of early embryo development have been performed. Conflicting results on which sex develops faster, and whether in vitro or in vivo, have been obtained. However, there is abundant evidence of sexual dimorphism. Yadav and colleagues,[40] studying in vitro fertilized and cultured bovine embryos, found that the first embryos performing the one cell division were significantly likelier to be male than female. This faster division rate has been confirmed in humans.[31] Preimplantation XY mouse embryos have been reported to be more advanced than XX embryos,[41] as have XY cattle embryos.[42,43] In contrast, Peippo and Bredbacka[44] found that among day 3 mouse embryos in vivo, females were more advanced, but during a subsequent 24-hour in vitro culture period the increase in cell numbers was greater in male embryos. They proposed that previous results suggesting increased rates of cell division in male embryos might be an artifact of in vitro culture. Larson and colleagues[45] showed no difference in the rates of development of male and female bovine embryos in vitro, but observed a sexual dimorphism in interferon-tau expression and a delay in expanded blastocyst formation of female embryos when using a rich culture medium. However, gene expression is altered when embryos are cultured in vitro. This has been particularly shown for *Igf1*, the expression of which is very significantly delayed with in vitro culture.[46]

On balance, therefore, most studies indicate that male embryos grow faster than female embryos throughout development, including before gonad formation. This faster growth is reflected at the transcriptional level: there are sexually dimorphic gene expression patterns in the pre-sex-specific gonadal embryo,[47] as early as day 7.5.[48]

ARE PREGONADAL AND NONGONADAL DIFFERENCES DUE TO *SRY/Sry* OR ARE THEY DUE TO OTHER GENES?

These differences between male and female embryos naturally raise the question as to whether they are mediated by an extragonadal role of *Sry*. Some studies on the expression of *Sry* did not show expression until day 10.5 (reviewed by Kanai and colleagues[49]); however, other studies have shown much earlier expression in preimplantation embryos. Polymerase chain reaction studies of mouse embryos from embryonic day 1.5 to embryonic day 4.5 found abundant evidence for the transcription of *Sry* from the two-cell stage to the blastocyst stage,[28] and this result was confirmed in human embryos.[29] Quantitation disclosed that there are approximately 40 to 100 copies of the messenger RNA (mRNA) per cell in a male blastocyst.[50] This is a much larger amount than could have been carried in with sperm.[51] An effect of SRY on preimplantation growth rate could potentially explain its rapid evolution.[52,53]

However, *SRY/Sry* is not the only potential candidate gene. One especially fruitful line of inquiry has been the comparison of chromosomally variant and/or consomic mice, in order to tease out the interacting effects of Y chromosome presence/absence, X chromosome dosage, and X chromosome parent of origin. Thornhill and Burgoyne[54] showed via comparison of X_mO and X_pO embryos that the presence of a paternal X (and absence of a maternal X) has a retarding effect on early embryonic growth, particularly of the ectoplacental cone, in XO mouse embryos, a finding that was subsequently confirmed by Jamieson and colleagues.[55] Although this was initially proposed as an explanation for growth rate differences between XY males and XX females (because only the latter have a paternal X), it is now believed that the effect is specific to XO conceptuses and reflects the paternal imprinting of Xp in rodent preimplantation embryos and extraembryonic tissue.[56]

In a comparison of consomic strains with different Y chromosomes, Burgoyne[57] found an accelerating effect of the Y chromosome on preimplantation growth in mouse embryos, which was polymorphic among different Y chromosomes. Further analyses by Burgoyne and colleagues[58] showed that for mid-gestation embryos (10.5 days after coitus), there are two competing effects on embryo size: an *Sry*-independent Y chromosome effect promotes faster growth of male embryos relative to female embryos, whereas a dosage-dependent effect of the X chromosome promotes faster female growth relative to male growth. This suggests that the gene modulating early embryonic growth may be an X-Y homologous gene escaping X inactivation, and that the variability in experimental data for male and female comparisons may relate to allelic differences segregating in different populations. An attractive candidate gene in this case is *Zfy*, because this has also been shown to be expressed in preimplantation embryos,[28] and the X-linked homologue *Zfx* is known to play a role in stem cell maintenance.[59] Set against this, in the mouse (although not in the human), *Zfx* is subject to X inactivation, and thus it is challenging to explain the effects of X dosage in this species.

Turning to later stages of gestation, Ishikawa and colleagues[56] showed that in late-gestation embryos there is a specific effect of X dosage on placental size, with a single X chromosome promoting late-onset placental hyperplasia independently of the parental origin of the X chromosome, fetal androgens, and the presence or absence of a Y chromosome. This effect is likely to be mediated by X-specific genes that escape X inactivation. These genes will be selected for female benefit and therefore may act to restrict fetal growth and reduce the demand on the mother, in accordance with the fetal-maternal conflict hypothesis.

DOWNSTREAM MECHANISMS GOVERNING PREGONADAL SEXUAL DIMORPHISM

A possible role of insulin-related growth factors for sex differences in preimplantation growth has been elucidated. Functional insulin receptor family members (insulin receptor [*Insr*], insulin receptor–related [*Insrr*], and insulin-like growth factor-1 [*Igf1r*]) are needed for male sexual differentiation since double knockouts (KOs) show partial, and triple KOs show complete XY sex-reversal.[60] *Insr*, *Insrr*, and *Igf1r* are expressed in preimplantation embryos,[61] and ablation of insulin/IGF signaling leads to a reduced proliferation rate of somatic progenitor cells in both XX and XY gonads prior to sex determination.[62] This proliferation defect slows but does not prevent female sexual development; however, it leads to complete failure of testis development (and a delayed switch to ovarian development) in XX embryos. Mittwoch[63] has long maintained that a fast growth rate actually leads to testis formation, and a slow growth rate leads to ovary formation. Scott and Holson[64] reported that male rat fetuses are larger than female rat fetuses and have a higher protein content at 12.5 days after coitus. We hypothesize that the mitogenic role of the insulin/IGF signaling pathway in embryos is involved in the more rapid growth of XY embryos and prepares them for further sexual differentiation at the gonadal stage of development.

EXPERIMENTAL MODELS TO INVESTIGATE PREGONADAL AND NONGONADAL SEXUAL DIMORPHISM

In recent years a number of studies have begun to take advantage of the so-called four core genotypes model, particularly for the study of behavioral and neuroendocrine phenotypes.[65,66] This experimental system uses a $Y^{\Delta Sry}$ chromosome with a small deletion that removes the *Sry* gene (meaning the $Y^{\Delta Sry}$ chromosome no longer confers maleness), combined with an autosomally borne *Sry* transgene (*Sry-tg*) complementing the deficiency. In a cross between $XY^{\Delta Sry}$, *Sry-tg* males and wild-type XX females, the transgene segregates independently of the Y chromosome, meaning the offspring comprise all four combinations of XX and $XY^{\Delta Sry}$ females and XX, *Sry-tg* and $XY^{\Delta Sry}$, *Sry-tg* males. This allows a balanced factorial experimental design, which separates the effects of maleness and X/Y chromosomal complement. In addition to the behavioral and metabolic study reviewed by Arnold,[34] this will be a very useful system to investigate questions of pregonadal and nongonadal effects of X- and Y-borne genes on sexual differentiation.

FORMATION AND DEVELOPMENT OF THE INDIFFERENT GONAD

A number of genes are expressed equally in both sexes in the gonadal ridge before *SRY* is expressed. Many are required for the development of the mesonephros, others are transcriptional activators of *SRY*, and some play both roles. Formation of the indifferent gonad both provides the necessary substrate for the testis-determining gene *SRY* to act on and initiates the upstream regulatory cascades that will activate *SRY* (if present) and permit testis differentiation. Failure of indifferent gonad formation leads to individuals that are neither gonadally male nor gonadally female but who (owing to the absence of male hormones) appear externally to be female; that is, sex reversal of a chromosomally male individual and sterility of a chromosomally female individual.

GENES CRITICAL FOR BOTH INDIFFERENT GONAD FORMATION AND *SRY* EXPRESSION: *WT1* AND *NR5A1*

The association between the *WT1* gene and testis development was recognized from investigations into Denys-Drash syndrome and WAGR syndrome. WAGR syndrome consists of Wilms tumor, aniridia, genitourinary anomalies, and mental retardation and is caused by deletions of 11p13 and hemizygosity in this region. Further, the phenotype caused by the deletions suggested that there was a tumor suppressor in this region related to Wilms tumor (for a review, see Hastie[67]). In Denys-Drash syndrome, there is a complex nephropathy and sexual ambiguity. Patients with WAGR syndrome may have undescended testes and hypospadias, whereas males with Denys-Drash syndrome may have female or ambiguous external genitalia with dysgenic gonads.

WT1 was found to code for a DNA-binding, zinc-finger transcription factor with several isoforms resulting from alternative splicing. High levels of *WT1* are expressed in the developing kidney, especially in glomeruli and mesangial cells that are involved in the above-mentioned nephropathy, and in the indifferent gonads, Sertoli cells, and granulosa cells. Mice transgenic for the Denys-Drash mutation in *Wt1* did not express androgen receptor or anti-müllerian hormone (*AMH*) in Sertoli cells.[68]

Differential splicing of WT1 generates at least 24 different isoforms, at least two of which show a functional difference. Alternative splice donor sites at the end of exon 9 lead to the inclusion or omission of three amino acids (Lys-Thr-Ser, KTS) between the third and fourth zinc finger, and both isoforms (WT1+KTS and WT1−KTS) are strongly evolutionarily conserved.[69] Children with Frasier syndrome, a variant of Denys-Drash syndrome, with late-onset glomerular nephropathy are mostly mutant for the splice site, which creates the longer transcript, and thus have a deficiency of the WT1+KTS isoform.[70] Hammes and colleagues[71] suggest that the WT1+KTS isoform may be an important activator of SRY in the developing gonad, and this seems to have been confirmed,[72] although Hossain and Saunders[73] have shown that only the WT1−KTS isoform could activate SRY. There may be an autoregulatory loop because *WT1* has been shown to be a target gene of *SRY* in vitro but not in vivo.[74] Thus Hastie[67] has argued that the frequent, but also frequently not complete, 46X,Y sex reversal seen in Frasier syndrome patients (where the levels of hWT1−KTS isoforms are increased 50%) makes an increase in the mWT1−KTS isoform unlikely to be the cause of the phenotype of the mWT1+KTS isoform knockout. In fact, because the WT1+KTS isoform has been shown to have a potential role in the regulation of *AMH*, one might anticipate less sexual ambiguity with increased expression of the WT1+KTS isoform.[75] However, SOX9 seems to be the most crucial transcriptional activator of *AMH* gene expression.[76]

Another gene whose absence prevents gonad formation is the steroidogenic factor 1 gene *Nr5a1*. *NR5A1* is homologous to the *Drosophila* gene *fushi tarazu transcription factor 1*, and sometimes is called *ftz-f1*; it is an orphan nuclear receptor that has been shown to be a key regulator of steroidogenic enzymes in adrenocortical cells[77]; it is also known as *SF1*. Developmental studies demonstrated that *Nr5a1* is expressed in the urogenital ridge of both sexes at embryonic day 9 to 9.5 in the mouse. This is at an early stage of organogenesis of the developing gonads and before *Sry* is expressed.[78] This result has been confirmed in humans.[79] The knockout of *Nr5a1* resulted in mice that died 8 days after birth.[80,81] The knockout mice lacked adrenal glands and gonads, and had a resulting deficiency in corticosterone that was the likely cause of death. Expression studies[82,83] have demonstrated a late sexually dimorphic expression pattern of *Nr5a1* with persistence in males and a discontinuation of expression in females, which was hypothesized to link the expression of *Sry* to that of AMH. NR5A1 was shown to regulate AMH expression in vitro[83] and in vivo.[84] However, another in vitro study could not demonstrate that NR5A1 could mediate between SRY and AMH,[85] whereas evidence for the interaction of homologues of NR5A1 and AMH has been found in zebrafish.[86] A direct role of Nr5a1 in *SRY* expression has been demonstrated in porcine cell culture.[87] Dramatic co-stimulation of the AMH promoter by WT1−KTS with NR5A1 has been demonstrated[88] and can be antagonized by Nr0b1; transcription of the Leydig insulin-like gene is also mediated.[89] Mutations in *NR5A1* can cause infertility in men.[90] A 46,XY female with adrenal failure at 2 weeks of life was found to have a 2-bp mutation at exon 3, resulting in a mutated glycine, which is an essential part of the zinc finger and is important for DNA binding.[91] Three other patients have now been described.[92-94]

GENES CRITICAL FOR INDIFFERENT GONAD FORMATION, BUT WITH NO KNOWN DIRECT EFFECT ON *SRY*: *Emx2*, *Pax2*, *Pax8*, *Lhx1*, AND *Tcf21* (*Pod1*)

The absence of these genes causes a lack of any visible gonadal development, with both male and female sterility, indicating that the disruption is at the level of the indifferent gonad rather than within the testicular or ovarian differentiation pathway. As for *WT1* and *NR5A1*, most of these genes are also implicated in development of other renal and adrenal structures. For example, *Emx2*-knockout mice do not have kidneys, ureters, gonads, or genital tracts.[95] Although *Wt1* and other genes that are normally expressed in the metanephric mesenchyme were initially expressed normally in these knockout mice, subsequent expression was greatly reduced, and degeneration and apoptosis occurred in the mesonephros.[95]

Pax2 and *Pax8* double-knockout mice fail to develop a pronephros[96] and fail to initiate *Lhx1* expression.[97] *Lhx* refers to the LIM homeobox family, a family of nongrouped homeobox-containing transcription factors.[98] *Lhx1* absence prevents kidney and gonad development.[99] *Lhx1* and *Lhx9* transcripts are present in the urogenital ridges of mice at embryonic day 9.5.[100] The *Lhx9*-knockout mouse fails to form a gonad because somatic cells of the genital ridge fail to proliferate despite normal germ cell migration.[100] Further, 40,XY mice with the knockout were phenotypically female and had no gonads. Presumably, cell migration from the mesonephros, an important source of cells in the developing gonad,[101] also did not occur. Importantly, evidence was also provided that *Nr5a1* expression (see later) was markedly decreased,[100] and a direct demonstration of *Lhx9* and *Wt1* in activating *Nr5a1* has been provided.[102] *Fgf8* and *Wnt4* are also upstream of *Lhx1*,[103,104] and HNF1β opposes *Pax8* and *Lhx1* function.[105] *Wnt4* appears to be involved in controlling the number of steroidogenic cells in the early gonadal ridge.[106]

Differential complementary DNA screening of embryonic day 13.5 male versus female gonads resulted in the discovery of *Tcf21*,[107] which might be involved in the regulation of *Nr5a1*. Its time course of expression is similar to that of *Nr5a1*, but the two do not colocalize. Co-transfection of *Tcf21* with *Nr5a1* resulted in the repression of *Nr5a1* expression.[107] However, the knockout of *Tcf21* resulted in ectopic expression of *Nr5a1*, misdirection of urogenital cells to a steroidogenic fate, and failure of development of both testes and ovaries.[108]

ADDITIONAL TRANSCRIPTIONAL REGULATORS OF *Sry*/*SRY*: *Gata4*, *Zfpm2*, AND *Cbx2* (*M33*)

These are transcriptional regulators expressed within the indifferent gonad and that act upstream of *Sry*/*SRY*, but that are not necessary for initial formation of the indifferent gonad itself. There is good evidence for transcriptional activation of *Sry* by GATA4 and its partner, ZFPM2 (also known as *FOG2*).[72,109] Additionally, mutations in genes involved in chromatin structure can also cause failure of *Sry* expression, together with partial or complete XY sex reversal. The knockout of *Cbx2* (also known as *M33*), the mouse homolog of *Drosophila* polycomb that regulates chromatin structure, results in hermaphroditism with intersex genitalia or complete male-to-female sex reversal.[110] The primordial gonad failed to grow at the normal time of *Sry* expression in mutants with a disrupted carboxyl-terminal domain, suggesting that *Cbx2* may be upstream of *Sry*. The primary role of *Cbx2* is probably in cell cycle control,[111] and the deficiency cannot be replicated simply with the use of histone deacetylase inhibitor.[112] Polycomb homologue complexes help to maintain the undifferentiated state of embryonic stem cells by inhibiting the expression of many genes,[113] and may similarly be involved in inhibiting premature expression of the sex determination cascade. Mutations in human *CBX2* were observed in a girl with XY sex reversal.[114] It is unclear whether the effects of *Cbx2* represent direct regulation of *Sry* or a more general effect on chromatin. Thus, NR5A1, GATA4 in a complex with FOG2, and WT1 appear to be the major transcriptional activators of *SRY.*

TRANSFORMATION OF THE INDIFFERENT GONAD INTO A TESTIS OR AN OVARY

In this section we discuss the differentiation of the indifferent gonad into a testis in response to the presence of *Sry/SRY* and review recent data on genes involved in the ovarian differentiation that occurs in the absence of *Sry/SRY*. The components of the human bipotential gonadal primordium were described in the introduction to this chapter. Migration of the primordial germ cells is completed in the sixth week of gestation, when the embryonic female or male gonads are indistinguishable. The absence of primordial germ cells is not compatible with ovarian differentiation but does not prevent testicular seminiferous tubule morphogenesis.[115] Evidence suggests that the initial stages of gonadal differentiation are realized in the supporting cells (pre-Sertoli or prefollicular cells),[116] but cell-to-cell interactions are critical for the function of *SRY* and, in general, for gonadal differentiation (Fig. 146.2).[117]

The data on transcription of *SRY* in human and mouse blastocysts, discussed earlier, suggest the possibility that there are pregonadal events that have set in motion biochemical pathways related to gonadal ridge differentiation. Nevertheless, the key event in testis differentiation is the expression of *Sry/SRY* in the developing Sertoli cells within the indifferent gonad, and the subsequent downstream pathways that complete the process of testicular differentiation. Conversely, for normal female sex determination to occur and the primitive gonad to differentiate to an ovary, a double dose of at least one X-chromosomal locus appears to be essential. Relatively little is known about genetic control of ovarian development. A possible candidate locus for a role is *DSS* (discussed later).[118]

INITIATION OF TESTIS DIFFERENTIATION BY *Sry/SRY*

The *SRY* gene has a simple structure, with only one exon and no introns. The 5′ flanking sequence does not contain TATA or CAAT boxes; it is GC rich and contains two tandem Sp1 recognition sites, a sequence known to potentiate transcription.[119] The region transcribed consists of 841 bp, resulting in a transcript of 1.1 kb, whereas the translated region consists of 612 bp, producing a protein of 204 amino acids with a molecular mass of 23.9 kDa. The *SRY* gene is flanked by two regions rich in adenine- and thymidine-containing inverted repeat sequences, suggesting that this gene has its origin in the retroposition of the transcript of some other gene during human evolution. The region that codes for the HMG box is located practically in the center of the *SRY* gene, at amino acids 57 to 137 of the protein.[120] The copy number of *Sry/SRY*, the copy number of the surrounding flanking DNA, and the characteristics of the flanking DNA vary greatly between species.[121] Thus conclusions about its control and function in mice cannot always be extended to humans.[72]

The HMG boxes of hSRY and mSRY correspond to generalized HMG boxes[24] and contain two nuclear localization signals.[122] Calmodulin has been implicated in *SRY* nuclear localization.[123] In addition to the HMG box, SRY contains a large glutamine

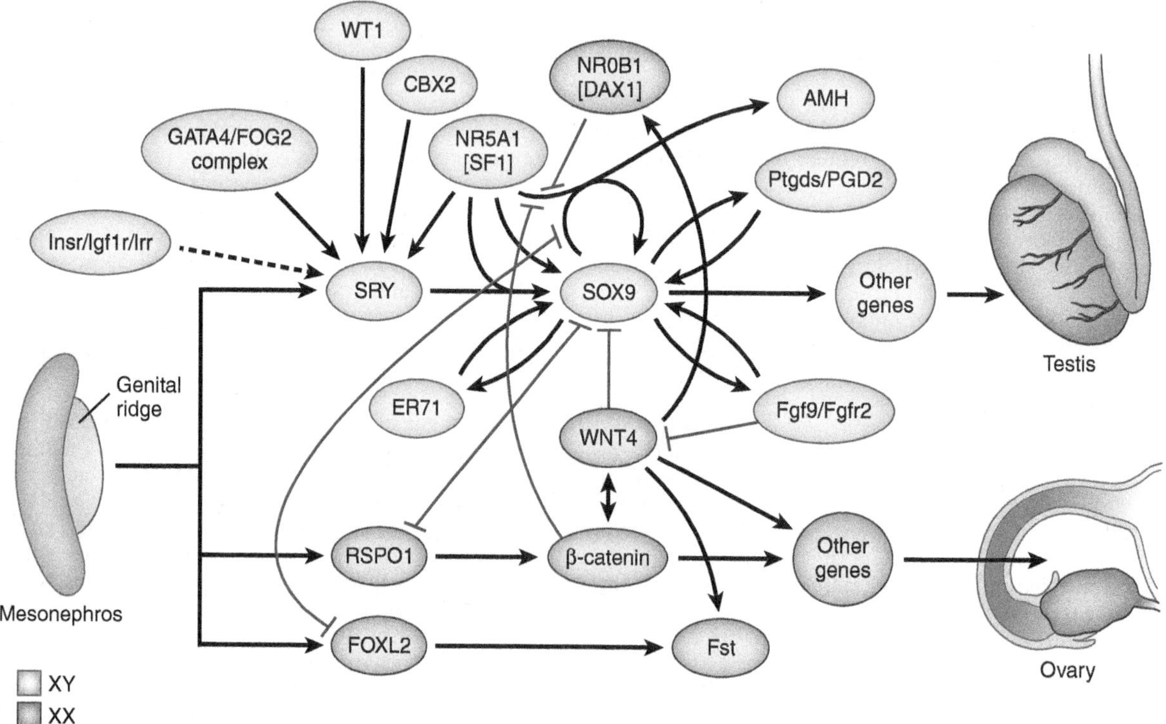

Fig. 146.2 In pre-Sertoli of cells *XY* individuals, direct *(solid arrows)* and indirect *(dashed arrow)* activation of *SRY*—the key Y-linked testis determining factor—triggers activation of *SOX9*, the master transcription factor of the testis developmental pathway. SOX9 activation is "locked in" via a series of autocrine and paracrine feedback loops, and also represses the ovarian determinants *RSPO1* and *FOXL2*. In XX individuals, the absence of SRY allows RSPO1 and FOXL2 to activate *WNT4*/β-catenin signaling. These are upstream activators of ovarian development and also repress SOX9 thus preventing testis development. *NR0B1 (DAX1)* is an X-linked dosage-sensitive regulator that fine-tunes the balance of this "see-saw" to ensure robust acquisition of a testis or ovary fate during development. (Modified from Narang K, Cope ZS, Teixeira JM. Developmental genetics of the female reproductive tract. In: *Human Reproductive and Prenatal Genetics*. Academic Press; 2019:129–153, Fig. 6.2.)

repeat region that is important for function in *Mus musculus* but not in other species of rodents.[124,125] SRY can be phosphorylated in vitro, and the phosphorylated form binds DNA more tightly.[72]

SRY and other SOX proteins have also been shown to be involved in pre-mRNA splicing, but the importance of this role is not yet clear.[126] HMG domain proteins in general appear to gain their DNA-binding specificity from protein cofactors (reviewed by Kamachi and colleagues).[127] A candidate for a coregulator protein for SRY, SLC9A3R2 (SIP-1), has been identified by a yeast two-hybrid screen,[128] but its role in sex determination is not yet known. More recent searches for SRY-interacting proteins have identified a splice variant of Zfp748 (known as *KRAB-only protein*, *KRAB-O*), that recruits the KAP1 corepressor machinery. The silencing of genes involved in the ovarian development pathway (e.g., *RSPO1*) is believed to be achieved by an SRY-KRAB-O-KAP1 complex.[129]

DIRECT TARGETS OF *Sry*

There are three well-known targets of *Sry*, these being (in order of identification) *Sox9*, *Cbln4*,[130] and *Etv2*.[131] Their temporal control is critical because expression of *Sry* is needed for only 6 hours in mouse development![132] It is unknown whether mutations in the latter two genes affect sex determination, but haploinsufficiency of *SOX9* (which leads to campomelic dysplasia) has long been known to have a major effect on human sexual determination, and sex reversal or sexual ambiguity is frequently seen in this condition. Strong evidence for the pivotal role of *Sox9* in sex determination is adduced by the controlled knockout of *Sox9*. This model, using the loxP system with Cre under the control of the cytokeratin 19 promoter to ablate *Sox9* expression in the gonadal anlagen, results in complete sex reversal.[133] Conversely, a new dominant insertional mutation, *Odsex* (Bishop and colleagues),[134] leads to the up-regulation of Sox9 expression in fetal gonads. *Odsex* represents a 150-kb deletion that maps approximately 10^6 bp upstream of *Sox9*, and 40,XX mice carrying *Odsex* develop as phenotypic males[134] on some genetic backgrounds. A second locus, *Odsml*, strongly influences the effect of *Odsex*[135] and is imprinted.[136] Long-range control of *SOX9* has also been shown in humans.[137]

Collectively these observations demonstrate that *Sox9* expression in developing gonads is both necessary and sufficient for testis development, independently of *Sry*, and it is therefore currently believed to be the most important (perhaps the *only* important) target of *Sry*. *Sry* regulates *Sox9* expression by binding to a 3.2-kb testis-specific enhancer sequence 13 kb upstream of the *Sox9* transcriptional start site.[138] This binding is dependent on *Nr5a1*, thus providing an explanation for the sex reversal effects of *Nr5a1* mutation (see earlier). A core region of the testis-specific enhancer (TESCO) is conserved in humans, mice, rats, and dogs, and a 180-bp element within TESCO is conserved in birds, reptiles, and amphibians.[138,139] This suggests that strong selective pressures maintain this region.

THE WIDER TRANSCRIPTIONAL NETWORK DOWNSTREAM OF *Sry* AND *Sox9*

SOX9 activity in the testis is associated with a shift from cytoplasmic to nuclear localization, this shift being seen only in the male gonad. SOX9 nuclear relocalization involves microtubule reorganization,[140] a possible target of prostaglandin D_2 (see later). In addition, in the human testes the time of activation of the targets of SOX9 corresponds to a time when SOX9 is found in the nucleus instead of the cytoplasm,[141] but inhibition of SOX9 nuclear export by leptomycin B in cultured mouse XX gonads resulted in a sex reversal phenotype.[142]

SOX8 is also expressed in the developing testis and may function redundantly with SOX9.[143] However, although *Sox9* can be partially substituted by *Sox8*,[144] the *Sox8*-knockout mouse does not show sex reversal[145] and *sox8* is not co-expressed with *sox9* in zebrafish, where *sox9* may also regulate AMH.[146] One interesting case of agonadism with other abnormalities has been described with a duplication 18 kb upstream of *SOX8* that also included *GNG13*, which is a candidate gene for ovarian development.[147] Thus SOX8 or GNG13 or both could be causal for the phenotype.

Pdgfra is also required for the migration of mesonephric cells into the early gonad, but the defect is in the cells of the gonad, not those of the mesonephros.[148] Desert hedgehog (DHH) is expressed in pre-Sertoli cells and is required for spermatogenesis[149]; a mutation in *DHH* was associated with partial gonadal dysgenesis.[150] It has long been known that deletions on distal 9p are frequently associated with 46,XY sex reversal. These were reviewed, and the essential chromosomal region was better defined by Flejter and colleagues.[151] A mammalian homologue of a DM domain-containing gene *(DMRT1)* shared by *Caenorhabditis elegans* and *Drosophila*, which is involved in their sex differentiation cascade, was found to map to this region.[152] This is particularly intriguing because conservation of sex determination pathways across such distantly related taxa has been an exception not a rule. Mutations in this highly conserved *DMRT1* gene are infrequent in 46,XY males. However, deletional mapping of the critical region on 9p includes both *DMRT1* and a paralogous gene, *DMRT2*,[153,154] and further homologues may be involved in sex differentiation.[155] Thus haploinsufficiency of one or both genes may contribute to 46,XY sex reversal.[156,157]

Microarray experiments have revealed other candidates for a role in the regulation or function of *Sry*. A search for the genes expressed differentially between the two sexes after overt gonad differentiation led to the identification of nexin 1 and vanin 1, which also show male-specific expression before this differentiation.[158,159] Of the two, vanin 1 is believed to be a downstream target of Sox9,[160] whereas only nexin 1, a serine protease inhibitor with a binding site for WT1 (see earlier) in its promoter,[161] is possibly expressed in time (at embryonic day 11.25) to influence *Sry* (onset at day 10.5 by the most sensitive techniques).[162] However, it seems more likely that nexin 1 is downstream of *Sry* and involved in the rapid proliferation of the male coelomic epithelium seen at this time.[163] This rapid enlargement of the gonad in males involves increased gonadal cell division and migration of cells from the adjacent mesonephros.[163,164]

Downstream targets of SOX9 are now being elucidated. SOX9 has been found to have a major effect on AMH transcription, whereas NR5A1 has only a minor effect in vivo.[76] GATA4 also plays a major role in stimulating transcription of AMH[165] and could be downstream, as well as upstream (see earlier), of SOX9. Although NR5A1 has earlier roles in gonadal development (see earlier), it is believed that NR5A1 is a key coactivator of AMH expression by SOX9. Both SOX9 and NR5A1 co-associate and, although their binding sites are 40 bp apart on the DNA, it has been proposed that the local bending of the DNA by SOX9 could contribute to stabilization of a transcriptional regulator form of NR5A1.[166] Thus NR5A1 may be a specific gonadal coactivator for SOX9, whereas some other coactivator—possibly including phosphorylation by protein kinase A[167]—is involved in promoting expression of the target of SOX9 in bone, COL2A1. AMH and the testosterone production by Leydig cells become the major downstream inducers of the male phenotype.

The role of AMH in development seems quite dependent on the signaling molecule Wnt7a. The *Wnt7a*-knockout mouse has postaxial hemimelia but otherwise is fully viable although sterile.[168] Studies on this mutant,[169,170] as well as on the spontaneous mutant in *Wnt7a* that is identified by a similar phenotype,[170] led to the recognition that males failed to undergo regression of the müllerian duct, whereas females show abnormal oviduct and uterine development. It was found that the AMH receptor was not being expressed in the males[170]; thus Wnt7a is essential for AMH function. In addition, *Hoxa10* and *Hoxa11* expression was abnormal postnatally in the female oviduct and uterus of these mutants,[169] indicating that Wnt7a is important for maintaining their expression.

As more powerful modern techniques are brought to bear on the question, it is likely that a flood of further downstream targets of *Sry* and *Sox9* will be identified. Efforts in this direction are already under way, with a ChIP/chip (chromatin immunoprecipitation on a chip) study[171] claiming 71 downstream binding targets for *Sry* and 109 targets for *Sox9*, with minimal overlap (5 genes only). However, a problem for such assays is the choice of targets represented on the array; for example, this study looked only at binding sites within 4 kb of transcription start sites, and thus the known shared target TESCO was not identified in this study because it lies 7 kb upstream of the *Sox9* transcriptional start site. This limitation will doubtless be lifted as array density increases. A more fundamental problem is that transcription regulation depends on combinatorial assembly of multiple transcription factors rather than simple binding by individual factors: in particular it appears that Nr5a1 is an important partner of Sry and Sox9. It is unknown how many of the sites identified in the study by Bhandari and colleagues[171] also bind *Nr5a1*.

X DOSAGE SENSITIVITY OF THE TESTIS-DETERMINING TRANSCRIPTIONAL CASCADE

A number of 46,XY individuals with sex reversal have partial duplications of Xp and an intact *SRY* gene. They usually have female external and internal genitalia with partial gonadal dysgenesis. Bernstein and colleagues[172] presented two cases and concluded that "testis-determining genes of the Y chromosome may be suppressed by regulatory elements of the X." XXY (Klinefelter syndrome) individuals do develop testes, but they are not normal, and these individuals have partially feminized phenotypes. Furthermore, some XXY triploids have shown sexual ambiguity[173]; lack of X inactivation in the triploids may be the cause.[174] Collectively, therefore, these observations indicate that there is at least one gene on the X chromosome that opposes testis determination and that it acts dose sensitively (i.e., the gene must escape X inactivation). Bardoni and colleagues[118] hypothesized a single gene in the Xp region of interest, and named it *dosage-sensitive sex reversal (DSS)*. This region includes *NR0B1*, formerly known as *DAX1* (*d*osage-sensitive sex reversal, *a*drenal hypoplasia congenita gene on the *X* chromosome gene *1*), gene defects of which cause adrenal hypoplasia.[175,176] *NR0B1* is a candidate for *DSS*. Swain and colleagues[177] have argued that an increased dosage of *NR0B1* would override the *SRY* signal for testis development.

NR0B1 is an orphan member of the nuclear hormone receptor family, meaning that its ligand is unknown. NR0B1 is related to NR5A1, which, as discussed earlier, is critical to both the initial activation of *Sox9* by *Sry* and the subsequent feedback autoactivation of *Sox9* itself. Competition between NR0B1 and NR5A1 for binding to testis-specific enhancer, shown by Ludbrook and colleagues,[178] provides a plausible mechanism whereby NR0B1 can interfere with the initiation and maintenance of the male transcriptional network centered on *Sox9*, and provides sound biochemical grounds for the dosage-sensitive nature of the phenotype. This hypothesis is supported by the fact that NR0B1 is normally down-regulated in the developing testis, whereas its expression persists in the developing ovary,[179] and overexpression in *Nrob1* transgenics delays testicular development and can result in sex reversal in the presence of weak-functioning (hypomorphic) *Sry*.[177]

POSITIVE FEEDBACKS AND THE "LOCKING IN" OF FATE CHOICE IN TESTIS DEVELOPMENT

As discussed already, the critical factor in *Sry*-mediated testis determination appears to be robust up-regulation of *Sox9* in the pre-Sertoli cells. Consistent with this, whereas *Sry* expression in the developing gonad is transient, *Sox9* expression is sustained after its initial induction by *Sry*. Moreover, whereas *Sry* expression is seen only in a subset of the supporting cells, all Sertoli cells subsequently become *Sox9* positive. Quinn and Koopman[180] liken *Sry* to a starter motor in a car: necessary to get things moving, but dispensable thereafter.

Maintenance of *Sox9* expression involves at least four positive feedback loops. Firstly, within the cell *SOX9* acts at the testis-specific enhancer in exactly the same manner as *SRY* and consequently stimulates its own transcription—this is doubtless why only transient *Sry* expression is required to trigger testis development. Secondly, there is a self-reinforcing feedback loop between *Er71* and *Sox9* whereby each reinforces expression of the other.[131] Thirdly, there is an autocrine feedback loop via fibroblast growth factor 9 and fibroblast growth factor receptor 2. Null mutations of both *Fgf9* and *Fgfr2* lead to loss of *Sox9* expression and sex reversal in the mouse,[139,181,182] and deletion of a region on chromosome band 10q26 encompassing *FGFR2* results in XY sex reversal.[183] Fourthly, at the paracrine level, SRY and SOX9 both induce prostaglandin D synthase,[184,185] and prostaglandin D_2 signaling induces neighboring cells to become SOX9 positive.

Collectively, these feedback loops constitute a highly redundant, robust developmental pathway and ensure that the fate choice for the indifferent gonad—the "switch" between the testicular and the ovarian developmental pathway—is a true binary choice and the potential for the development of infertile intersex phenotypes is minimized as far as possible.

DEVELOPMENT OF THE OVARY

As indicated in the introduction to this chapter, the idea that the ovary arises solely as an outcome of an "uninduced state" is being replaced as new data emerge that elucidate the existence of genes specifically involved in ovarian differentiation. Overexpression of *WNT4* (in transfection experiments with cultured Sertoli and Leydig cells) causes up-regulation of *NR0B1*, thus suggesting a correlation between these two genes such that each, in various circumstances, appears to promote ovarian development. Lack of *Wnt4* gives rise to masculinization of the XX gonad, although a study has shown that *Wnt4* also has a specific but different role in male gonadal development.[186] Nef and colleagues[47] used microarrays to compare gene expression patterns of XX and XY *Nr5a1*-positive gonadal cells and found that cyclin-dependent kinase inhibitors were overexpressed in XX gonads, a finding that could relate to the known difference in proliferation rates of XX and XY gonads discussed earlier. Jorgensen and Gao[187] demonstrated a sixfold ovary-specific enhancement of *Irx3* (Iroquois homeobox gene family member 3) at days 12 to 13.5 of murine development. This finding was independent of the presence of germ cells.

Early entry into meiosis is a key feature of female germ cells, and retinoic acid (RA) was initially identified as a trigger.[188] RA was thought to act through stimulation by retinoic acid gene 8 (*Stra8*), whereas it is degraded by a cytochrome P-450, CYP26B1, in fetal testis.[189] Kumar and colleagues challenged this model by generating mice deficient for RA production (*Aldh1a2*-knockout mice) in the mesonephros. In this knockout model, female embryos maintain *Stra8* expression[190] and initiate meiosis in the absence of detectable RA in the *Aldh1a2*$^{-/-}$ fetal ovary. Additionally, in males, ketoconazole inhibition of CYP26B1 in the *Aldh1a2*$^{-/-}$ testis promotes premature meiotic entry in the absence of RA. It is important to note that changes in *Stra8* expression in males are associated both with germline stem cell commitment to mitotic division and with the subsequent commitment to meiosis several days later, with DMRT1 being a further key player in the regulatory cascade.[191] These observations were resolved by the discovery that RA stimulation during early gonadal development is redundantly provided by *Aldh1a2* activity in the mesonephros and *Aldh1a1* activity in the fetal ovary.[192]

The female-to-male sex reversal seen in polled (hornless) goats (polled intersex syndrome [PIS]) has long been the subject of much interest, partly because the reversal trait occurs only in animals homozygous for the mutation (i.e., it is inherited as an autosomal recessive), whereas the trait of absence of horns behaves as an autosomal dominant. Research reviewed by Baron and colleagues[193] has revealed some fascinating insights and brought to light the existence of another gene involved in ovarian development in mammals, including humans.

The polled mutation in goats is an approximately 12-kb deletion from a *cis*-regulating region, on band q43 on goat chromosome 1, that controls the expression of three contiguous genes.[194] One of these three, *FOXL2*, which is highly conserved in vertebrates, appears to be an ovary-determining gene. Another of the three—*PISRT1* (*PIS*-related *t*ranscript, gene *1*)—is a regulatory element necessary for *FOXL2* expression in the ovary. In XY males, *SRY* evidently blocks *PISRT1* and thus prevents gonadal expression of *FOXL2* (and hence ovarian induction). However, *PISRT1* evidently also inhibits *SOX9*, thus suppressing testis formation. Fetal gonads of the polled goat (i.e., animals carrying the *PIS* deletion) show complete repression of both *FOXL2*, the ovarian inducer, and *PISTR1*, the suppressor of testis inducing *SOX9*,[194] thus accounting for the observed sex-reversal phenotype.

The genetics of the polled trait itself illuminates another intriguing feature of sexual development: the independence from hormonal influence of a feature of secondary sexual maturity. In wild-type fetuses, the PIS *cis*-regulating element suppresses the expression of the three adjacent genes in skin surrounding the future horn buds. The function of at least one of these is evidently to limit horn growth.[194] Other examples, in the XX *Sxr* pseudomale mouse and in the tammar wallaby, of such exceptions to the Jost principle were given earlier. The polled situation in which the PIS *cis*-regulating element controls the expression of an adjacent gene[194] might be a model to account for those other Jost principle exceptions.[35-37]

In humans, band q23 on chromosome 3 is homologous to the *FOXL2/PISRT1* region (q43) of goat chromosome 1. FOXL2 has been detected in the nuclei of human fetal granulosa cells but not in fetal or adult testes. Loss-of-function mutations in *FOXL2* in humans can be responsible for a syndrome of eyelid dysmorphism and ovarian dysgenesis that causes primary amenorrhea in 46,XX women.[195]

The mutual interrelationships of the different genes shown to be involved in ovarian development remain to be elucidated, but it is clear that clarification of this central piece of the sex determination paradigm is imminent.

LIFELONG MAINTENANCE OF GONADAL IDENTITY

It has become increasingly clear that there is not just a genetic pathway to develop a testis from a bipotential gonad but that additional genetic influences are required to maintain its identity as a testis. Despite the substantial array of positive feedbacks reinforcing *Sox9* expression (see earlier), maintenance of male gonadal identity is still not fixed and can be altered by perturbations acting in adult life, long after sex determination, particularly those involving DMRT1. As stated earlier, *DMRT1* codes for a DM domain-containing protein that is required for sexual differentiation in *Drosophila* and *C. elegans.* The mammalian homologue of *Dmrt1* may have some role in sexual differentiation in humans (see earlier), but the knockout of *Dmrt1* in mice does not prevent normal testis differentiation. However, research has shown that conditional knockout of *Dmrt1* in adult Sertoli cells induces them to transdifferentiate into granulosa cells.[196] *Dmrt1* knockout in the male germline induces precocious entry into meiosis (i.e., more similar to the female situation, where meiosis begins during fetal life); however, it cannot be concluded at this point whether this represents transdifferentiation of male germ cells into oocytes or simply a function of *Dmrt1* as a regulator of meiosis.[192]

Conversely, female gonadal identity is also not fixed, being dependent on continued expression of *Foxl2.* Conditional ablation of this gene leads to ectopic activation of *Sox9* and transdifferentiation of granulosa and theca cell lineages into Sertoli-like and Leydig-like cell lineages.[197] Thus, in contrast to Jost's original view of testis development being an active choice and ovarian development as "basal," it appears rather that this model really only applies to the initial SRY-dependent choice of the developmental trajectory, and that subsequently there is a lifelong balancing act played out between testis-fate-promoting and ovarian-fate-promoting gene networks, with both being mutable. Collectively, therefore, these findings indicate that much remains to be uncovered, and that the gene networks involved in the initial fate choice between testis and ovary may be to some degree distinct from those required to maintain gonadal identity in adult life (Fig. 146.3).

SECONDARY SEXUAL DIFFERENTIATION

The classical paradigm of sexual development introduced at the beginning of this chapter was formulated in principle by Alfred Jost[1] at the end of the 1940s to explain the results of his observation that extirpation of the gonads (ovaries or testes) of rabbits before sexual differentiation had occurred invariably resulted in the development of a basic, female-type pattern in the fetuses.[198] This and subsequent research established that although sex-determining genes are evidently responsible for directing the development of the gonad, secondary sexual differentiation of internal duct systems and external genitalia is under hormonal control in eutherian mammals, including humans.

Indifferent (bipotential) external structures are initially present in males and females. The testis produces androgens, which masculinize the labioscrotal folds to form a scrotum and the genital tubercle to form the penis. In the absence of the testis, and therewith of high levels of androgen molecules, the labioscrotal folds do not fuse and form labia, and the genital tubercle becomes the clitoris. Internally, the mesonephric (wolffian) and paramesonephric (müllerian) ducts will develop into male or female structures, respectively. Testicular androgen promotes development of the wolffian ducts into epididymides, vasa deferentia, and seminal vesicles, and absence of androgens leads to degeneration of the wolffian ducts. Also produced in the testis is AMH, which causes disintegration of the müllerian duct. In the female, in absence of AMH, the müllerian ducts become the uterine tubes, uterus, and upper part of the vagina. The possible place of the gene for AMH in the sequence of events downstream of *SRY*[85] was discussed earlier.

Information on genes controlling female secondary sexual development can be obtained from studies on patients with pseudohermaphroditism. In this group of conditions, the patient's primary and secondary sexual features are discordant. Thus in male pseudohermaphroditism, a genetic male, having a testis, has female or ambiguous external and/or internal genitalia.

For example, androgen insensitivity syndrome, an X-linked condition also known as *testicular feminization,* occurs in XY individuals and illustrates the above description of the main features of secondary sexual differentiation.[199] In androgen insensitivity syndrome, the Y-chromosomal testis-determining

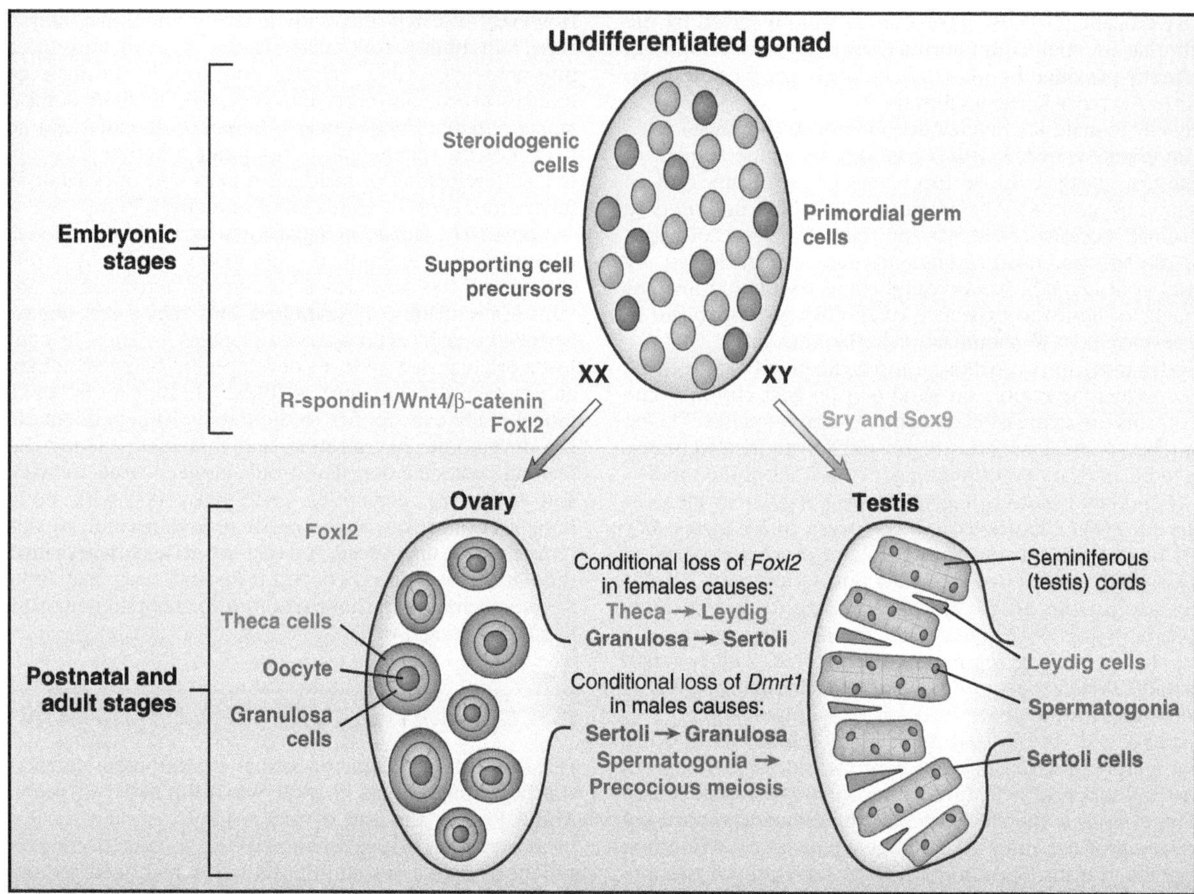

Fig. 146.3 Following gonad differentiation, testis/ovary identity is maintained by a competition between the male-promoting factor *DMRT1* and the female-promoting factor *FOXL2*. Although the details are currently poorly understood, it appears that conditional depletion of either gene in adult animals can lead to transdifferentiation of gonadal cell types, with consequent partial sex reversal of gonadal tissue. (Modified from Sinclair A, Smith C. Females battle to suppress their inner male. *Cell*. 2009;139(6), Fig. 1.)

mechanism is intact, and testes are present, but because the X-linked mutation renders tissues insensitive to androgens, the external genitalia fail to develop in a masculine direction. Instead, they retain the basic female configuration, and the sex of the individual is diagnosed as female at birth. The wolffian ducts also do not develop and, because the testis produces AMH, the müllerian ducts regress, so the individual does not have a uterus, uterine tubes, and the upper part of the vagina. At pubertal age, menarche fails to occur.

In female pseudohermaphroditism, individuals have ambiguous or male-type external genitalia with female gonads and karyotype. Perloff and colleagues[200] and others[201-204] have described a distinct form of female pseudohermaphroditism associated with malformations of the internal genital, urinary, and gastrointestinal tracts. They may occur in the apparent absence of testosterone or *SRY*.[205] Possible causes include a disturbance of a specific caudal developmental field,[202] a primary defect in the cloacal membrane,[204] and failed fusion of the urorectal septum with the cloacal membrane.[206] Some cases of penoscrotal transposition[207,208] and some cases of prune belly sequence and of bilateral renal agenesis[201,209] have similar patterns of caudal malformations. Furthermore, this pattern of dysmorphism, but without female pseudohermaphroditism, is found in the MURCS (*müllerian* duct aplasia-*r*enal aplasia-*c*ervicothoracic *s*omite dysplasia) association. This condition usually occurs sporadically in families. In most cases, the cause is unknown.

The role of growth factors in the differentiation of the genital tubercle has been explored in mice. The possible role of *Fgf9* in gonadal differentiation was mentioned earlier. *Fgf8* and *Fgf10* are implicated in external sexual differentiation; knockout of *Fgf10* results in marked sexual ambiguity.[210] A pathway initiated by sonic hedgehog *(Shh)*, and interactions of its product with a number of these factors, has been studied in organ cultures of murine genital tubercles.[211] *Shh*-knockout embryos showed no external genitalia at 12.5 days gestation and showed down-regulation of *Fgf8*. Cultured genital tubercle explants treated with antibody to Shh also showed no external genitalia at 12.5 days gestation and marked down-regulation of *Fgf10*. It has been shown that *Fgf8* also has a role upstream of *Shh*[212] and downstream of androgens.[213]

These findings are also relevant to the hypospadias seen in Smith-Lemli-Opitz syndrome; the developmental defects seen in this cholesterol synthesis deficiency may in part be due to altered Shh signaling. Holoprosencephaly, sometimes seen in Smith-Lemli-Opitz syndrome, occurs with *Shh* haploinsufficiency, whereas hypospadias does not. Shh is also required for prostate development.[214] In contrast, DHH is required to maintain germ cells in the testis.[215]

Although, as mentioned previously, *Wnt4* is implicated in gonadal differentiation, *Wnt5a* has also been implicated in genital tubercle development.[216] Furthermore, the role of AMH in development seems dependent on the signaling molecule *Wnt7a*. In *Wnt7a*-knockout mice, males fail to undergo regression of the müllerian duct, and females show abnormal oviduct/uterine development.[217,218] AMH receptor is not expressed in the males[217]; thus *Wnt7a* is essential for AMH function.

Multiple Hox genes, including the Hoxa and Hoxd groups, are involved in sexual differentiation. For example, compound double homozygous deficiency of *Hoxa13* and *Hoxd13* resulted in a complete absence of external genitalia.[219] Haploinsufficiency of the HOXD complex caused genital anomalies of a small phallus and no palpable testes in one case, and penoscrotal transposition with micropenis with multiple limb and other abnormalities in another.[220] Hand-foot-genital syndrome with male cryptorchidism and hypospadias is due to mutations in *HOXA13*.[221]

CONCLUSION

The classical paradigm of Jost, formulated in the 1940s, provides a starting point for present-day consideration of sexual development in humans. However, recent research requires modification of that framework. Although Jost regarded the establishment of genetic sex that occurs at conception, and the determination of the fate of the gonad, to constitute a single step, it is now known that much transpires between these two events. Furthermore, the Jost principle envisioned active induction of the testis only; the ovary developed by default in the absence of testis-determining factors. However, the existence of ovary-determining genes has now been established. The new paradigm, formulated here, proposes that primary sex determination comprises sex-chromosomal (X or Y) assignment of sex, pregonadal sexual development and sexual dimorphism, and gonadal (testicular or ovarian) development—the latter being necessarily dependent on correct formation of the indifferent gonad. Furthermore, the Jost principle envisioned that all development of sexual dimorphism other than that of the gonads was due to hormones and independent of genetic sex. It is now clear that the situation is more complex. The new paradigm recognizes that some features of secondary sexual differentiation are directly influenced by gene action that is independent of testicular (or ovarian) hormones. The sex determination pathway, like most developmental pathways, has a strong tendency to maintain its function (i.e., is homeostatic). Redundancy in pathways may be part of the mechanism by which the homeostatic continuation of sexual development occurs. One can surmise that a number of genes in the pathway might be up-regulated or down-regulated to compensate for deficiencies in other members of the pathway. Further understanding of the sex determination pathway will come from studies of altered gene expression in deficient states and the location and identification of modifier genes that alter the pathway.

A complete reference list is available at www.ExpertConsult.com.

SELECT REFERENCES

1. Jost A, Vigier B, Prépin J, Perchellet JP. Studies on sex differentiation in mammals. *Recent Prog Horm Res*. 1973;29:1-41.
3. Ford CE, Jones KW, Polani PE, et al. A sex chromosome anomaly in a case of gonadal dysgenesis (Turner's syndrome). *Lancet*. 1959;1:711.
4. Welshons WJ, Russell LB. The Y-chromosome as the bearer of male determining factors in the mouse. *Proc Natl Acad Sci U S A*. 1959;45:560.
10. Stalvey JR, Durbin EJ, Erickson RP. Sex vesicle "entrapment": translocation or nonhomologous recombination of misaligned Yp and Xp as alternative mechanisms for abnormal inheritance of the sex-determining region. *Am J Med Genet*. 1989;32:564.
11. Vergnaud G, Page DC, Simmler MC, et al. A deletion map of the human Y chromosome based on DNA hybridization. *Am J Hum Genet*. 1986;38:109.
15. Verga V, Erickson RP. An extended long-range restriction map of the human sex-determining region on Yp, including ZFY, finds marked homology on Xp and no detectable Y sequences in an XX male. *Am J Hum Genet*. 1989;44:756.
16. Sinclair AH, Berta P, Palmer MS, et al. A gene from the human sex-determining region encodes a protein with homology to a conserved DNA-binding motif. *Nature*. 1990;346:240.
17. Berta P, Hawkins JR, Sinclair AH, et al. Genetic evidence equating SRY and the testis-determining factor. *Nature*. 1990;348:448.
20. Affara NA, Chalmers IJ, Ferguson-Smith MA. Analysis of SRY in 22 sex-reversed XY females identifies four new point mutations in the conserved DNA binding domain. *Hum Mol Genet*. 1993;2:785.
28. Zwingman T, Erickson RP, Boyer T, Ao A. Transcription of the sex-determining region genes Sry and Zfy in the mouse preimplantation embryo. *Proc Natl Acad Sci U S A*. 1993;90:814.
32. Koopman P, Gubbay J, Vivian N, et al. Male development of chromosomally female mice transgenic for Sry. *Nature*. 1991;351:117.
39. Renfree M, Pask A, Shaw G. Reproduction down under: the marsupial mode. *Australian Biochemist*. 2011;42:16-19.
47. Nef S, Schaad O, Stallings NR, et al. Gene expression during sex determination reveals a robust female genetic program at the onset of ovarian development. *Dev Biol*. 2005;287:361-377.
52. Hurst LD. Embryonic growth and the evolution of the mammalian Y chromosome. I. The Y as an attractor for selfish growth factors. *Heredity*. 1994;73:223-232.
54. Thornhill AR, Burgoyne PS. A paternally imprinted X chromosome retards the development of the early mouse embryo. *Dev*. 1993;118:171-174.
56. Ishikawa H, Rattigan A, Fundele R, Burgoyne PS. Effects of sex chromosome dosage on placental size in mice. *Biol Reprod*. 2003;69(2):483-488.
57. Burgoyne PS. A Y-chromosomal effect on blastocyst cell number in mice. *Dev*. 1992;117:341-345.
58. Burgoyne PS, Thornhill AR, Kalmus Boudrean S, et al. The genetic basis of XX-XY differences present before gonadal sex differentiation in the mouse. *Philos Trans R Soc Lond B Biol Sci*. 1995;350:253-261.
60. Nef S, Verma-Kurvari S, Merenmies J, et al. Testis determination requires insulin receptor family function in mice. *Nature*. 2003;426:291-295.
65. De Vries GJ, Rissman EF, Simerly RB, et al. A model system for study of sex chromosome effects on sexually dimorphic neural and behavioural traits. *J Neurosci*. 2002;22:9005-9014.
66. Arnold AP, Chen X. What does the "four core genotypes" mouse model tell us about sex differences in the brain and other tissues? *Front Neuroend*. 2009;30(1):1-9.
67. Hastie ND. Life, sex, and WT1 isoforms: three amino acids can make all the difference. *Cell*. 2001;106:391-394.
72. Larney C, Bailey TL, Koopman P. Switching on sex: transcriptional regulation of the testis-determining gene *Sry*. *Dev*. 2014;141:2195-2205.
73. Hossain A, Saunders GF. The human sex-determining gene SRY is a direct target of WT1. *J Biol Chem*. 2001;276:16817-16823.
79. de Santa Barbara P, Bonneaud N, Boizet B, et al. Direct interaction of SRY-related protein SOX9 and steroidogenic factor 1 regulates transcription of the human anti-Müllerian hormone gene. *Mol Cell Biol*. 1998;18:6653.
87. Pilon N, Daneau I, Paradis V, et al. Porcine SRY promoter is a target for steroidogenic factor 1. *Biol Reprod*. 2003;68:1098-1106.
106. Jeays-Ward K, Dandonneau M, Swain A. Wnt4 is required for proper male as well as female sexual development. *Dev Biol*. 2004;276:431-440.
107. Tamura M, Kanno Y, Chuma S, et al. Pod-1/Capsulin shows a sex- and stage-dependent expression pattern in the mouse gonad development and represses expression of Ad4BP/SF-1. *Mech Dev*. 2001;102:135-144.
109. Tevosian SG, Albrecht KH, Crispino JD, et al. Gonadal differentiation, sex determination and normal Sry expression in mice require direct interaction between transcription factors GATA4 and FOG2. *Dev*. 2002;129:4627-4634.
118. Bardoni B, Zabaria E, Guioli S, et al. A dosage sensitive locus at chromosome Xp21 is involved in male to female sex reversal. *Nat Genet*. 1994;7:497-501.
119. Vilain E, Fellous M, McElreavey K. Characterization and sequence of the 5' flanking region of the human testis-determining factor SRY. *Methods Mol Cell Biol*. 1992;3:128-134.
121. Cortez D, Marin R, Toledo-Flores D, et al. Origin and functional evolution of Y chromosomes across animals. *Nature*. 2014;508:488-491.
132. Hiramatsu R, Matoba S, Danai-Azuma M, et al. A critical time window of *Sry* action in gonadal sex determination in mice. *Dev*. 2009;136:129-138.
133. Barrionuevo F, Bagheri-Fam S, Klattig J, et al. Homozygous inactivation of Sox9 causes complete XY sex reversal in mice. *Biol Reprod*. 2006;74:195-201.
135. Qin Y, Poirier C, Truong C, et al. A major locus on mouse chromosome 18 controls XX sex reversal in odd sex (Ods) mice. *Hum Mol Genet*. 2003;12:509-515.
138. Sekido R, Lovell-Badge R. Sex determination involves synergistic action of SRY and SF1 on a specific *Sox9* enhancer. *Nature*. 2008;453:930-934.
139. Bagheri-Fam S, Sinclair AH, Koopman P, Harley VR. Conserved regulatory modules in the Sox9 testis-specific enhancer predict roles for SOX, TCF/LEF, Forkhead, DMRT, and GATA proteins in vertebrate sex determination. *Int J Biochem Cell Biol*. 2010;42(3):472-477.
142. Gasca S, Canizares J, De Santa Barbara P, et al. Boizet-Bonhoure B: a nuclear export signal within the high mobility group domain regulates the nucleocytoplasmic translocation of SOX9 during sexual determination. *Proc Natl Acad Sci U S A*. 2002;99:11199-111204.
152. Raymond CS, Shamu CE, Shen MM, et al. Evidence for evolutionary conservation of sex-determining genes. *Nature*. 1998;391:691.
171. Bhandari RK, Haque MM, Skinner MK. Global genome analysis of the downstream binding targets of testis determining factor SRY and SOX9. *PloS One*. 2012;7(9):e43380.
177. Swain A, Narvaez V, Burgoyne P, et al. *Dax1* antagonizes *Sry* action in mammalian sex determination. *Nature*. 1998;391:761.
178. Ludbrook LM, Bernard P, Bagheri-Fam S, et al. Excess DAX1 leads to XY ovotesticular disorder of sex development (DSD) in mice by inhibiting steroidogenic factor-1 (SF1) activation of the testis enhancer of SRY-box-9 (Sox9). *Endocrinology*. 2012;153(4):1948-1958.
180. Quinn A, Koopman P. The molecular genetics of sex determination and sex reversal in mammals. *Semin Reprod Med*. 2012;30(5):351-363.
185. Wilhelm D, Martinson F, Bradford S, et al. Sertoli cell differentiation is induced both cell-autonomously and through prostaglandin signaling during mammalian sex determination. *Dev Biol*. 2005;287(1):111-124.

188. Bowles J, Knight D, Smith C, et al. Retinoid signaling determines germ cell fate in mice. *Science*. 2006;312:596-600.
189. Bowles J, Koopman P. Retinoic acid, meiosis and germ cell fate in mammals. *Dev*. 2007;134:3401-3411.
190. Kumar S, Chatzi C, Brade T, et al. Sex-specific timing of meiotic initiation is regulated by Cyp26b1 independent of retinoic acid signalling. *Nat Commun*. 2011;2:151.
191. Endo T, Mikedis MM, Nicholls PK, et al. Retinoic acid and germ cell development in the ovary and testis. *Biomolecules*. 2019;9(12):775.
192. Matson CK, Murphy MW, Griswold MD, et al. The mammalian doublesex homolog DMRT1 is a transcriptional gatekeeper that controls the mitosis versus meiosis decision in male germ cells. *Dev Cell*. 2010;19(4):612-624.
196. Matson CK, Murphy MW, Sarver AL, et al. DMRT1 prevents female reprogramming in the postnatal mammalian testis. *Nature*. 2011;476:101-105.
197. Uhlenhaut NH, Jakob S, Anlag K, et al. Somatic sex reprogramming of adult ovaries to testes by FOXL2 ablation. *Cell*. 2009;139:1130-1142.
198. Jost A. Problems of fetal endocrinology: the gonadal and hypophyseal hormones. *Recent Prog Horm Res*. 1953;8:379.
199. Hughes IA, Davies JD, Bunch TI, et al. Androgen insensitivity syndrome. *Lancet*. 2012;380:1419-1428.

147 Differentiation of the Ovary

Linn Salto Mamsen | Claus Yding Andersen | Andrew J. Childs | Richard A. Anderson

DEVELOPMENT OF A FUNCTIONAL OVARY

The follicle—the functional unit of the ovary—consists of an oocyte in the late prophase of the first meiotic division surrounded by granulosa cells enclosed by a basement membrane. Later, during follicle growth, it will become surrounded by theca cells.

Human gonads of both sexes are established at week 4 post conception (pc) and are intimately connected to the mesonephros throughout early differentiation. The gonads are populated by somatic cells deriving from the mesonephros, as well as cells from the coelomicepithelium.[1,2] The primordial germ cells (PGCs) are specified far from the gonad in embryonic epiblast.[3,4] The PGCs migrate initially to the yolk sac wall, then through the hindgut towards the gonads in week 4 to 5 pc mediated by chemotactic signals, active movement, and nerve fiber guidance, and populate the gonads at the ventrocranial aspect of the mesonephros in week 6.[5,6]

Three major events are prerequisites for the development of a functional ovary: (1) initiation of germ cell meiosis, (2) formation of follicles, and (3) differentiation of steroid-producing cells. In humans, as in many other mammalian species, these events begin during embryonic life, at a time when germ cells and somatic cells have populated the ovarian anlage.

Meiosis and follicle formation are interrelated processes, the first being the prerequisite for the second, which secures survival of the oocyte. The primordial follicles constitute the ovarian reserve, providing a steady number of growing follicles some of which will develop to antral and potentially ovulatory stages in adult life. The female reproductive life span is determined by the number of resting primordial follicles. The steroidogenic theca cells enclose the growing follicle and provide the androgen substrate, which is converted to estrogen by the granulosa cells.[7]

GONADAL SEX DETERMINATION

In most vertebrate classes, gonadal differentiation is the result of the genetic sex. In mammals, the gonads arise from thickenings of the coelomic epithelium and are initially bipotential, having the capacity to develop as testes or ovary. The fate of the indifferent gonad is dependent on the presence or absence of a Y chromosome: the gonad becomes a testis when a Y chromosome is present, and an ovary develops if this chromosome is absent, irrespective of additional sex chromosomes.[8-11] In 1990, the testes determining factor was identified as a single gene, named *Sex-Determining Region Y (SRY)*,[12,13] the expression of which is sufficient to direct the formation of testes in chromosomally female (XX) mice. SRY initiates a cascade of gene networks through the direct regulation of *Sox9* expression initiating differentiation of the supporting cells (i.e., Sertoli and Leydig cells), vasculature formation, and testis cord development. In the human embryonic testis *SRY* is activated in embryonic week 6 initiating the sex differentiation.[14] In the female embryo, the absence of *SRY* initiates alternative genetic cascades, including female sex-determining genes *RSPO1, Wnt4/β-catenin, Foxl2, Follistatin (Fst),* and *Gata4* leading to formation of the ovaries and including fallopian tubes, uterus, and upper part of the vagina.[9,15-17]

EARLY OVARIAN DIFFERENTIATION

In humans, PGCs arise from the cells of the embryonic epiblast, under the inductive action of Wnt3 and bone morphogenetic proteins (BMPs) 2, 4, and 8b. These signals induce expression of SOX17 and PRDM1 (BLIMP1) in a localized subset of epiblast cells, directing them to adopt a PGC fate and upregulate PGC-specific markers such as DPPA3 (STELLA).[18] Significant species-specific differences exist between PGC specification in humans (and most mammals) and rodent models: PGC specification in mice does not require SOX17, while PRDM14 is an essential regulator of the process in mice but appears to be dispensable in humans.

Proliferating PGCs migrate first to the extraembryonic mesoderm or dorsal yolk sac wall,[4] then along the hindgut, through the dorsal mesentery towards their final destination at the gonadal ridge.[19,20] The PGCs migrate along autonomic nerves to the gonad,[19] guided by chemotactic mediators such as the c-kit receptor and its ligand.[21-23] PGC migration is completed around the ninth week of fetal life.[20,24] Simultaneously, invading mesonephric cells accumulate in the central medullary region of the ovary, and form the intraovarian rete (Fig. 147.1). The proliferating germ cells (now termed oogonia) with intermingled somatic cells (precursors of the granulosa- and theca-cell populations) become separated from areas of somatic cells by a basement membrane. This prevents cell intermingling although the basement membrane-enclosed regions are open at the periphery of the ovary. Within these germ cell cords the germ cells divide with incomplete cytokinesis mediated by germ cell-specific factors including Tex14 and DAZL, giving rise to clusters of germ cells linked with intercellular bridges termed germ cell nests.[25-27] It appears that mouse germ cells receive organelles and cytoplasm from the surrounding nest cells to become oocytes,

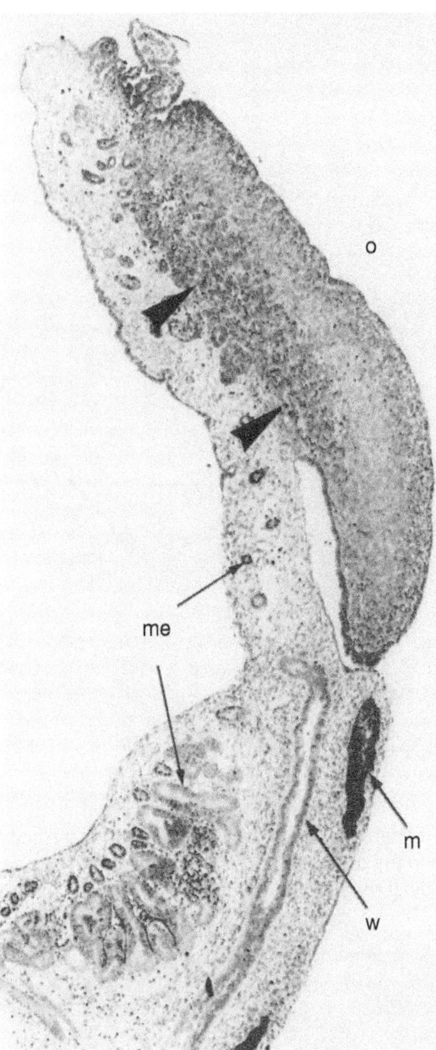

Fig. 147.1 Ovarian-mesonephric complex of an 11-week-old human fetal ovary. The mesonephric cells that invade the ovary are recognized as the dark cell mass *(arrowheads)* in the basal part of the ovary *(o)*. The Wolffian duct *(w)*, the müllerian duct *(m)*, and mesonephric tubules *(me)* are seen. (Original magnification ×200.) (From Byskov AG, Høyer PE. In: Knobil E, Neil J, eds. *The Physiology of Reproduction*. New York: Raven Press; 1988.)

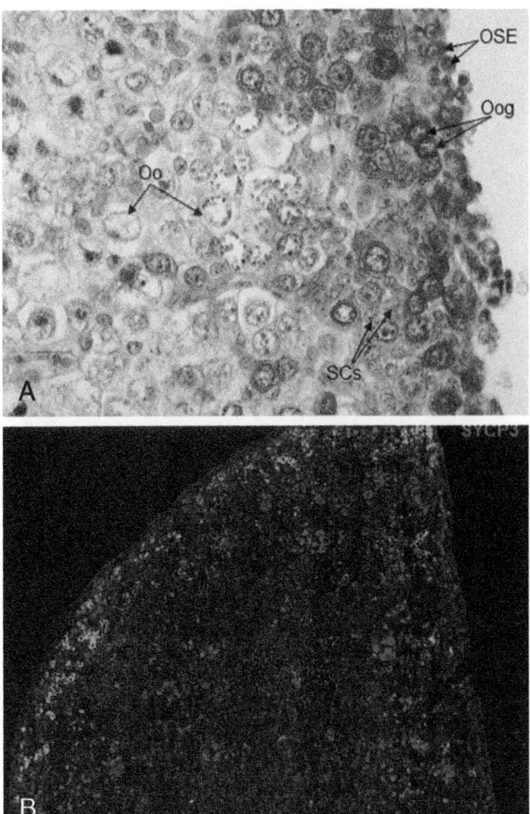

Fig. 147.2 Arrangement of germ cell populations in the human fetal ovary. (A) Photomicrograph of a section of 18 weeks gestation human fetal ovary, immunostained for the germline stem cell marker LIN28A *(brown)*. Small, mitotic, LIN28-expressing oogonia *(oog)* are located at the periphery of the ovary, under the ovarian surface epithelium *(OSE)*. As oogonia enter meiosis and become oocytes *(Oo)*, they move deeper into the ovary and extinguish LIN28A expression (note the characteristic meiotic chromatin arrangement in the nuclei of these cells *(asterisks)*). Somatic cells *(SCs)* are interspersed between germ cells (see References 12 and 21 for further details). (B) Fluorescent micrograph of a section of 15 weeks gestation human fetal ovary, showing the radial arrangement of germ cell populations at different states of maturation. Pre- and early-meiotic oocytes expressing DAZL *(green)* are located towards the periphery of the ovary. Oocytes in mid- and late-meiotic prophase express BOLL and SYCP3, and are located more centrally, towards the ovarian medulla, where germ cell nest breakdown and primordial follicle formation occurs (see References 73 and 79 for further details).

whereas the donor germ cells die.[28] The formation of intercellular bridges between germ cells is, however, not essential for the oocyte competence, since *Tex14*- or *DAZL*-deficient mice develop functional oocytes in the absence of bridge formation (albeit in reduced numbers).[26,27] Oogonia continue to express pluripotency markers such as OCT4 and LIN28 during proliferation in the primitive ovary, but these factors are lost shortly before or at the initiation of meiosis (Fig. 147.2).[29]

By morphologic criteria, the ovary is usually recognizable at a later stage of gonadal differentiation than the testis. The first indications that the indifferent gonad is becoming a testis are the formation of the testicular cords enclosing the germ cells[30] and the rounding up of the organ.[31] In the human testis, these events take place at the sixth week of fetal life.

Cords enclosing the germ cells are, however, also seen at early stages of ovarian differentiation in some mammalian species (e.g., the pig and the sheep). In other species (e.g., the mouse and the hamster), the germ cells are not confined to cords and the germ cells are more evenly distributed throughout the ovary.[5,32] These different patterns of germ cell location within the ovary are closely related to the onset of meiosis—in all females the cords disappear when meiosis starts. In species in which germ cell cords are formed, meiosis is delayed until the cords dissolve, whereas in species without cord formation, meiosis proceeds immediately.[32] During the delay period, transitory ovarian steroidogenesis takes place (see later). This is analogous to early testicular differentiation, in which steroidogenesis begins immediately after testicular cords are formed.[32,33] It has been proposed that enclosure of germ cells into specific germ cell compartments, either as temporarily formed cords or as follicles, is a prerequisite for the start of steroid production in the developing gonads.[32]

Morphologically and functionally, the human fetal ovary represents an intermediate type between immediate and delayed meiosis. Although germ cells appear in clusters during fetal life, well-defined cords are not formed (Figs. 147.3 and 147.4).[34] Nonetheless, the delay period lasts for a relatively long

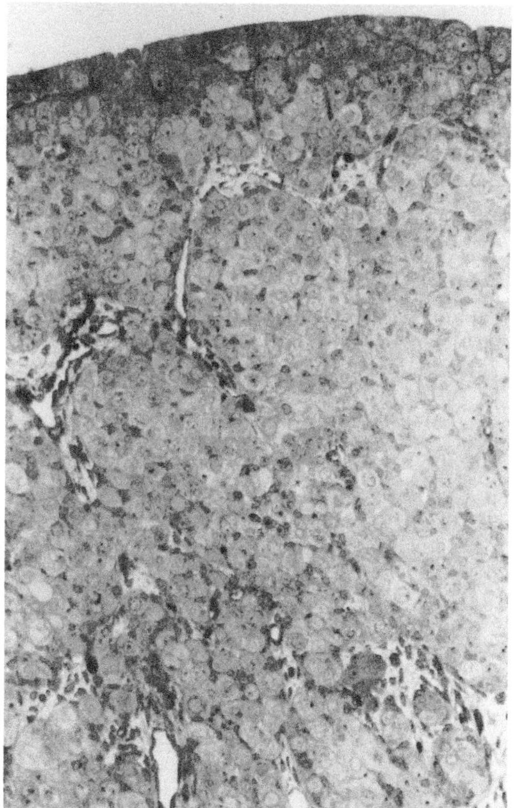

Fig. 147.3 Human fetal ovary, 21st week, with clusters of oocytes in different stages of meiosis in the inner part of the cortex, in connection with an intraovarian rete cord *(arrow)*. (Original magnification ×600.)

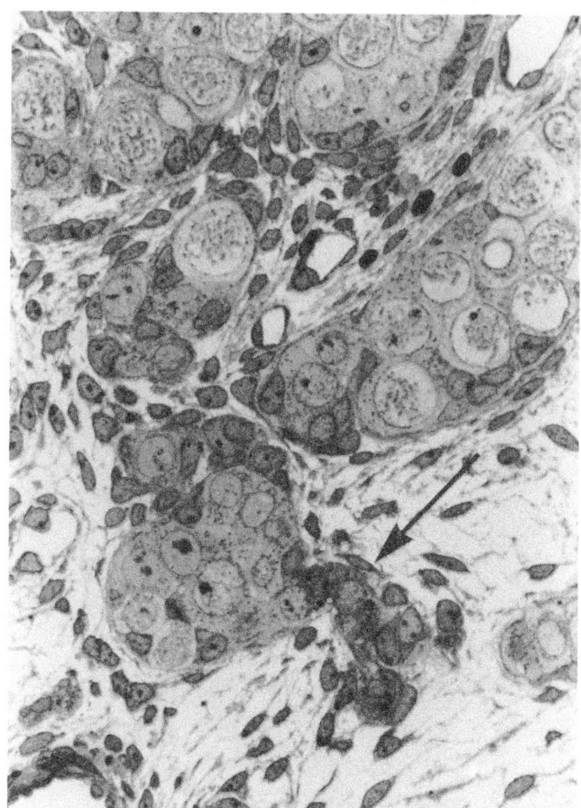

Fig. 147.4 Human fetal ovary, 21st week, showing the cortex packed with oogonia in the outermost part of the cortex and oocytes towards medulla. (Original magnification ×300.)

time, from the onset of sex differentiation at approximately the sixth week of fetal life until the ninth week, when meiosis starts.[35,36] Although the aromatizing enzyme system is present by the sixth week of fetal life, few or no steroids are produced by human ovaries during the delay period.[37] Interstitial cells with ultrastructural resemblance to steroid-producing cells have been recognized from the 13th week of fetal life (Fig. 147.5).[38]

The origin of the somatic cell population of the cortex is uncertain, and different theories have been proposed. Generally, the following sources for their origin have been suggested: the surface epithelium,[1,39] the mesonephros, or a combination of the two.[34,40] A 2018 review suggests that the granulosa cells derive from the somatic progenitor cells located in the gonadal ridge, whereas theca cells derive from at least two progenitor populations: the majority deriving from the gonadal ridge and a smaller population deriving from the mesonephros.[2] Analysis of bovine ovarian development has identified a putative cell termed the *gonadal ridge epithelial-like (GREL)* cell, which derived from the surface epithelium of the mesonephros and penetrate, intermingled with oogonia, into the ovary giving rise to the granulosa cells population.[41]

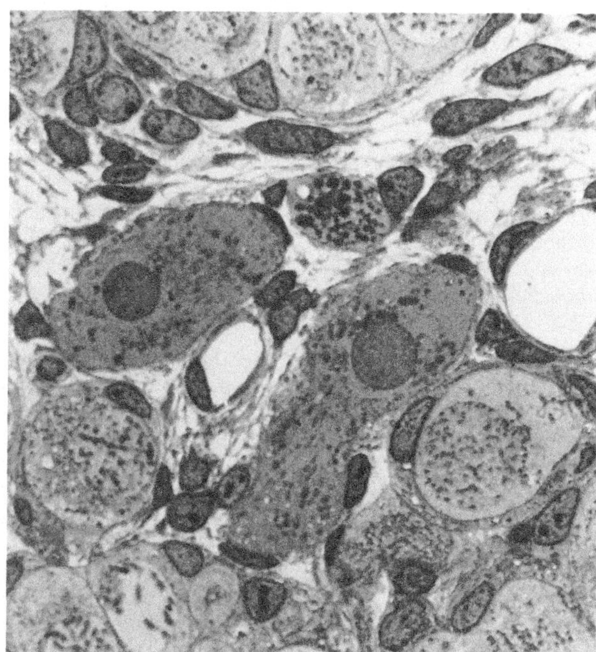

Fig. 147.5 Two interstitial cells in the inner part of the ovarian cortex from a fetal human ovary, 21 weeks old. (Original magnification ×900.)

MEIOTIC PROPHASE OF OOCYTES

The number of mitotically dividing *oogonia* increases exponentially from approximately 25,000 in the 6-week-old human embryo to approximately 250,000 in the 9th week,[36,42,43] reaching a maximum of around 7 million in the 20th week (Fig. 147.6).[43,44] When the oogonia stop mitotic divisions and enter meiosis, they are termed *oocytes*. The first meiotic stages can be identified in week 9 pc.[36] The term *oogenesis* denotes the transformation of an oogonium into an oocyte, and maturation into a fertilizable oocyte. Extensive degeneration, however,

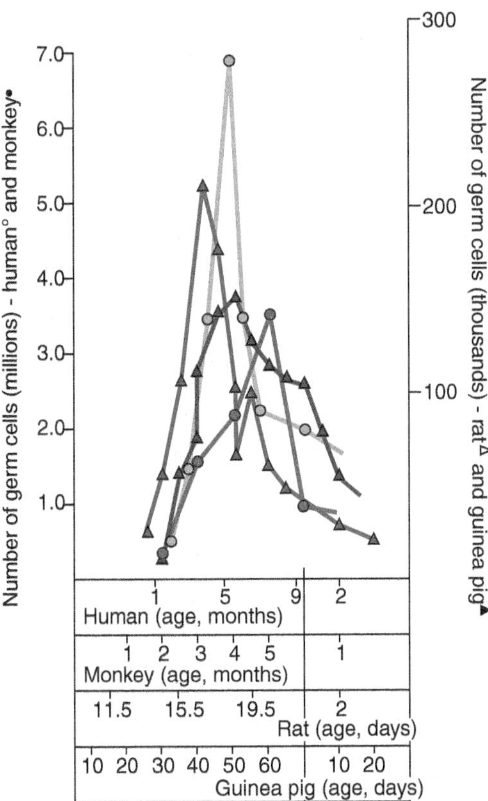

Fig. 147.6 Number of germ cells in fetal and neonatal ovaries of human, monkey, rat, and guinea pig. (From Baker TG: In Balin H, Glasser SR, eds. *Reproductive Biology.* Amsterdam: Excerpta Medica; 1973.)

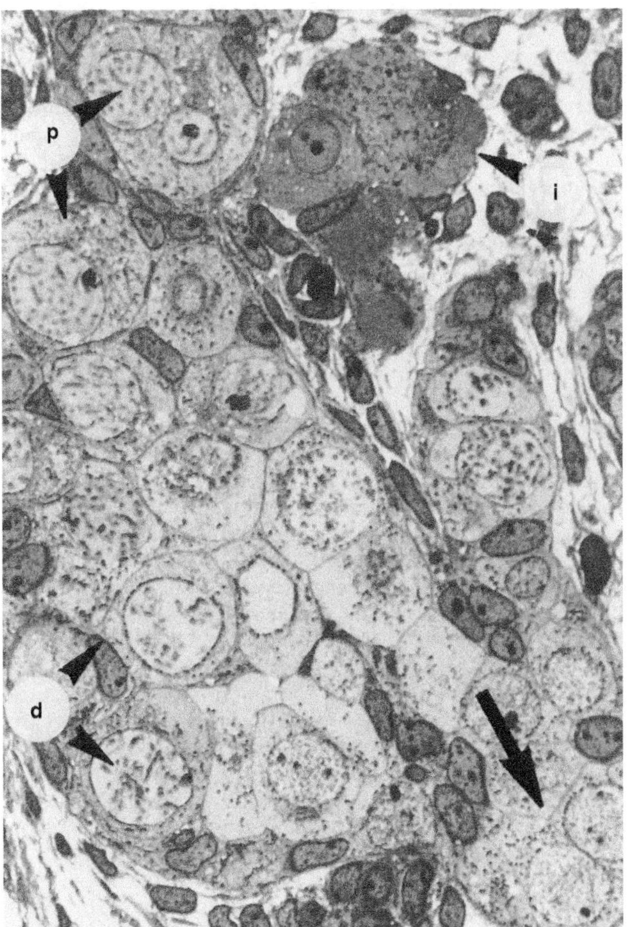

Fig. 147.7 Inner part of the ovarian cortex of a human ovary, 21-week-old fetus, showing different stages of meiosis and interstitial cells *(arrow) d,* Early diplotene; *i,* interstitial cells; *p,* pachytene. (Original magnification ×900.)

reduces the number of germ cells drastically during the rest of fetal life, leaving only 300,000 to 2.5 million oocytes in the ovaries of the newborn girl.[44-46]

In the mammalian ovary, meiosis commences with a round of pre-meiotic DNA replication, doubling the DNA content of the germ cell from 2c (i.e., copies of) DNA to 4c. This DNA must last until the oocyte has been successfully ovulated and fertilized, which in humans may occur up to 40 years later. The absence of detectable DNA synthesis in germ cells in the postnatal ovary has been taken as evidence that neoformation of oocytes does not occur later in life; that is, the entire pool of oogonia initiate meiosis and differentiate into oocytes before or around birth.[47-50] However, the ovaries of adult prosimians (lower primates) are an exception to this rule, wherein DNA synthesis can be detected in oogonia-like germ cells.[51,52] In the postnatal and adult mouse oogonial stem cells have been identified[53,54] and subsequently in human ovaries as well.[55,56] Isolation of these stem cells in mice can generate new oocytes and even support the development of live offspring when reintroduced into a donor ovary,[55,57] challenging the concept that postnatal neoformation of oocytes does not occur in most mammals. There is an increasing body of evidence that demonstrates the existence of stem cells with germ cell-like characteristics in the adult ovary in some species,[58] but whether such ovarian stem cells contribute new oocytes to the follicle pool under normal conditions in vivo remains a matter of intense debate.[57-66]

Pre-meiotic DNA replication is followed by the transitory stages of the first meiotic prophase: preleptotene-leptotene-zygotene, pachytene, and diplotene (Fig. 147.7). During the first meiotic prophase, maternal and paternal genetic material is exchanged through the process of recombination between homologous chromosomes, a unique characteristic of meiotic cell division (for review see Cohen and colleagues).[67] Once the diplotene stage of the first meiotic prophase is complete, oocyte progression through meiosis becomes arrested at the dictyate stage. Oocytes are maintained in this state until the oocyte resumes meiosis (just before ovulation) or degenerates. At resumption of meiosis, the first meiotic prophase is completed and the oocyte proceeds through the first meiotic division, during which the homologous chromosomes are separated into two daughter cells, each containing one set of chromosomes with duplicated DNA. At the second meiotic division, which in the human takes place at fertilization, the replicated chromosomes termed *chromatids* split up hereby halving the DNA content of the germ cell again and (in humans) yielding one haploid oocyte and excess DNA material is extruded in polar bodies.

The different transitory stages of the first meiotic prophase are identifiable by the extent to which the synaptonemal complex (SC)—a proteinaceous structure that mediates the pairing of, and recombination between, homologous chromosomes—has been assembled.[68] SC assembly begins at leptotene and is completed in the pachytene stage.[67] Recombination is the exchange of genetic material between homologous chromosomes. Recombination is completed by the diplotene stage, at which the SC is disassembled, although homologous chromosomes remain linked at the sites of recombination, known as chiasmata.[67] During the diplotene stage, the oocyte and its nucleus enlarge, and the chromosomes decondense, thus making the nucleus faintly stainable. Handel and Schimenti provide an excellent review of the genetic control of meiotic prophase, recombination, and the consequences of mutations in genes that regulate these processes.[69]

INITIATION AND REGULATION OF MEIOSIS

The time of onset of meiosis in the females varies among different mammalian species but occurs always at an early stage of development, often in fetal life. In the testis, by contrast, initiation of meiosis is postponed until puberty in all species. These discrepancies led to the hypothesis that an internal clock within germ cells determined the onset of meiosis, independent of external factors.[70] However, premature entry into meiosis can in human fetal male germ cells be induced when exposed to a meiosis-inducing substance (MIS) before the testis is sex differentiated,[32] suggesting that the transition from mitotic proliferation to meiotic differentiation may not be governed entirely by the germ cells themselves, but may be subject to the influence of external stimuli. In mammals, germ cells enter meiosis in waves starting from the rete ovarii located in the innermost part of the cortex. The rete ovarii is considered to be of mesonephric origin, and therefore it has been proposed that mesonephric-derived substances in the ovary trigger the onset of meiosis.[71] In vitro experiments using fetal mouse gonads suggest that the mesonephros produces a diffusible substance that promotes and induces meiosis in both sexes.[72,73] This substance was termed the *meiosis-inducing substance* and proposed to be a lipid.[73,74]

Observations of the behavior of germ cells in the fetal mouse ovary are consistent with this hypothesis. The fetal mouse gonad is connected to the mesonephros by the mesonephric tubules, which link the two organs at the anterior end of the gonad. Germ cells in the fetal mouse ovary enter meiosis in a wave that spreads along the long axis of the gonad over a period of 3 to 4 days, which is initiated at the anterior end of the organ.[75,76] This is consistent with a model of a diffusible mesonephros-derived MIS that enters the gonad at the anterior end, and diffuses along it, inducing germ cells to enter meiosis as it progresses.[77,78] Mice studies have shown that ectopic germ cells can enter meiosis.[70,79,80] However, more recent studies have in mouse models demonstrated that aberrant development of gonadal somatic cells leads to abnormal meiotic initiation and meiotic arrest before prophase I in both sexes, suggesting the gonadal somatic cells are essential for normal meiotic initiation.[81]

Extensive work has in mice identified retinoic acid, an active derivative of vitamin A, as the MIS,[73,77,82] consistent with the proposal made 40 years ago that the MIS is likely to be a lipid. Consistent with the observation that germ cells enter meiosis in an anterior-to-posterior wave in the fetal mouse ovary, retinoic acid is synthesized and secreted by the mesonephros in fetal mice of both sexes.[77] However, in the developing testis retinoic acid is converted into inactive products by the enzyme Cyp26b1, which is expressed by the testicular somatic cells.[77,82] Disruption of Cyp26b1 function in the fetal testis (either genetically or pharmacologically) results in germ cells being exposed to the meiosis-inducing action of retinoic acid, causing them to initiate meiosis.[77,82,83] The gonads of both sexes initially express Cyp26b1, but its expression is down-regulated in the ovary just prior to the onset of meiosis, leaving germ cells unshielded from the meiosis-inducing action of retinoic acid.[77,78,82] Retinoic acid activates two independent gene expression programs within the germ cells. Firstly, RA triggers expression of *Stimulated by Retinoic Acid Gene 8* (*Stra8*),[77,82] which is required for pre-meiotic DNA replication and the initiation of meiosis in both sexes.[84,85] Secondly, RA promotes expression of Rec8, a component of the cohesion complex that holds the chromatids together through meiosis and beyond, and other structural proteins important for the progression through meiosis.[86]

In the human fetal gonad, the regulation of meiotic initiation appears more complex. In contrast to the fetal testis-specific expression of *Cyp26b1* at the time of meiotic entry in mice, the human fetal ovary and testis express similar levels of *CYP26B1* mRNA at the time of meiosis initiation,[87,88] in contrast to the male-specific expression of *Cyp26b1* in the fetal mouse testis.[77,82,89] Furthermore, the genes encoding retinoic acid synthesis enzymes are expressed at similar levels in human fetal gonads and mesonephros, suggesting that the human fetal ovary may itself be a site of retinoic acid synthesis.[87,88] Together, these data indicate that retinoic acid produced and metabolized locally within the gonad itself may be important in regulating the progressive entry of germ cells into meiosis in the human fetal ovary, rather than the process being driven by retinoic acid from the mesonephros.[87,88] Such a model may explain how mitotic oogonia persist in the human fetal ovary for several weeks after the first oocytes have initiated meiosis.[29,90–92]

In addition to the extrinsic retinoic acid signal, germ cells must express intrinsic factors that enable them to respond appropriately to meiosis-inducing cues. The fetal germ cells of mice that lack the germ cell-specific RNA-binding protein DAZL (Deleted in Azoospermia-Like) fail to upregulate Stra8 expression and initiate meiosis in response to retinoic acid,[93] and instead remain in a sexually-undifferentiated state similar to early PGCs.[94] This has led to the hypothesis that the expression of DAZL by germ cells confers upon them "meiotic competence": the ability of a germ cell to respond appropriately to meiosis-inducing signals.[93] In the human fetal ovary germ cells fail to initiate meiosis in response to retinoic acid treatment prior to 12 weeks gestation,[87] around the time at which the expression of DAZL increases markedly, and when DAZL protein translocates from the nucleus of germ cells to the cytoplasm.[90,95] In the human fetal ovary DAZL is suggested to regulate several functions in oocytes at the time when meiosis starts and may have a key role in determining oocyte quality.[96] How the expression of DAZL itself is activated within PGCs at the gonadal ridge is unclear but is likely stimulated by extrinsic signals from the gonadal microenvironment. In genetically-modified mouse models in which the gonads fail to form, the PGCs migrate to the appropriate site within the embryo, but in the absence of gonadal somatic cells they fail to initiate the expression of DAZL and remain unresponsive to meiotic cues.[97]

FOLLICULOGENESIS

Folliculogenesis is the process during which the diplotene oocyte becomes surrounded by a single layer of granulosa cells and enclosed by an intact basal lamina, thus forming a specific germ cell compartment (Fig. 147.8).

The separation of the diplotene oocyte from the surrounding tissue secures its survival and creates a unique environment, which is necessary to sustain further growth and differentiation. If the oocyte in the diplotene stage fails to be enclosed in a follicle, it invariably degenerates. Some follicles die as a result of specific programmed cell death, or *apoptosis*.[98–100] In the human fetal ovary, *naked oocytes* (diplotene oocytes without a granulosa layer) are often seen, but they always appear to be degenerating. Such oocytes are never seen later in life.[101]

The first follicles are encountered in the human ovary at approximately the 14th week of fetal life, and follicle formation is completed immediately after birth.[102] The formation of the primordial follicle pool is largely driven by the interaction between the germ cell and its surrounding somatic environment.[103] The transforming growth factor beta (TGF-β) family members, activins, and BMPs signal primarily from germ cell to somatic cell and vice versa and are important mediators of follicle formation. Also kit ligand/C-kit and neurotrophin signaling is essential for normal follicle formation.[104] Within the germ cell, oocyte-specific transcription factors including Figla, Nobox, and Sohlh2 are necessary for follicle formation.[1,105]

Forkhead box protein L2 (FOXL2) is expressed by pre-granulosa cells prior to and on initiation of follicle formation. Mutations in the *FOXL2* gene in humans are associated with a congenital abnormality characterized with underdeveloped eyelids and premature ovarian insufficiency (POI).[106] Studies in goat have

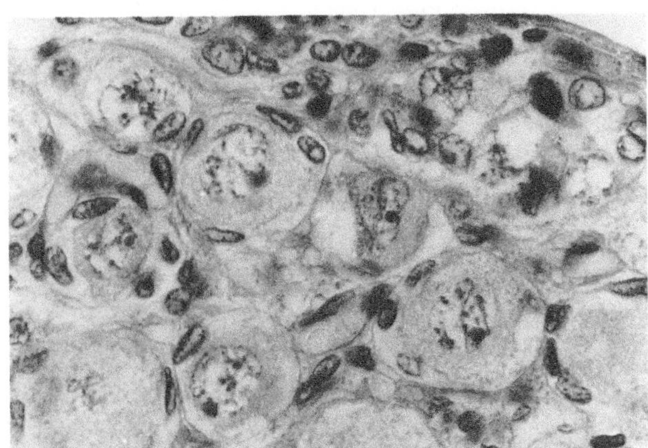

Fig. 147.8 Primordial follicles in the ovarian cortex of a 30-week-old human fetus. (Original magnification ×560.)

shown that FOXL2 may be a female sex-determining gene, as without it XX females develop testis.[107] In mice, FOXL2 may not be involved in phenotypic sex-reversal, but it is necessary for correct follicle development and thus for the maintenance of the adult female fertility.[108] There appear to be two waves of follicle formation, at least in the mouse, the first generating primordial follicles located in the medulla that subsequently activate growth prepubertally before degeneration, and the second, cortical population, underpinning adult fertility. The relevance of this to human ovarian development is unclear: the ovaries of children contain a large proportion of abnormal follicles that are lost by puberty,[109] which may potentially represent the second of these two populations.

The appearance and growth of the first follicles coincides with the increase of fetal gonadotropins. Whether these two events are causally related is uncertain, but it is perhaps of relevance that sex steroids, particularly estrogen, have been implicated in the timing of follicle formation in several species, including the bovine and baboon.[110,111] Human fetal oogonia also express estrogen receptor beta at this stage of development.[112] Androgen action in the ovary may also be important at this stage of development and has been proposed to be involved in the etiology of polycystic ovary syndrome.[113] It is believed that antral follicular somatic cells (i.e., mural granulosa-, cumulus-, and theca cells) produce cAMP that is transferred to the oocyte keeping it inactive. This inactivation results in the fully-grown oocyte arrest in the diplotene state until the pituitary-derived LH surge that leads to meiosis resumption and triggers ovulation.[103]

OVARIAN STEROIDOGENESIS

EARLY STEROID PRODUCTION BY THE OVARY

The progenitor cells and the mechanisms that regulate differentiation of the hormone-producing somatic cells of the differentiated gonad of both sexes and of the adrenal gland is far from being fully elucidated. In vivo studies in mice using conditional knockout of *Nr5a1* (which encodes the transcription factor Steroidogenic Factor 1 [SF-1]) in differentiated steroid-producing cells have shown that SF-1 is a regulator of the expression of steroidogenic genes in ovaries, testis, and adrenal organs[114] and that the testis as such become permanently disrupted in the presence of reduced levels of SF-1.[115] Human testicular steroidogenesis initiates in embryonic week 7.5[14] that contrast the ovarian steroidogenesis, which is first seen when the follicles begin to grow in late fetal life. Stanniocalcin 1 and 2 exert a number of functions including Ca^{2+} homeostasis, but have been shown to be specific inhibitors of the metalloproteinase pregnancy associated pregnancy protein A (PAPP-A), which specifically cleave the IGF binding proteins IGFBP4 and IGFBP5 and is therefore intimately involved in regulation of the activity of IGF1 and IGF2.[116,117] Stanniocalcin 1 and 2 are expressed in the mesonephros and genital ridge prior to differentiation in mice[116] and have shown to affect steroidogenesis. It has been suggested that stanniocalcins may be implicated in the differentiation of steroid-producing cells.[118]

In vitro studies of human fetal ovaries have shown that the capacity to aromatase testosterone starts as early as week 6 to 8.[37] However, it does not appear that the enzyme, P450c17, converting pregnenolone to androgens is expressed until around week 12 to 18, and therefore the ovary does not possess a capacity to produce estrogens de novo until around mid-gestation. While P450c17 in the adult ovary is specifically expressed in interstitial and theca cells, it appears to be expressed also in oocytes and somatic cells in second trimester human ovaries, albeit at low levels localized to isolated cell clusters.[112] In first trimester human ovaries P450c17 is not expressed.[14]

Although cells with ultrastructural characteristics of steroid-producing cells are noted from the 12th week of gestation in the human ovary,[5] hardly any estradiol synthesis is observed in fetal ovaries from mid- to late gestation[119,120] illustrating that the whole chain of enzymes necessary for converting cholesterol to estradiol is not properly expressed in sufficient quantities until just before birth. Fetal blood does, however, contain large amounts of estrogens, thus providing an exogenous source.[121,122]

Small antral follicles from adult women have the capacity to metabolize androgens to oestrogens.[123] Primordial/primary follicles and follicles up to a diameter of 200 μm all showed gene expression of the enzyme 17β-hydroxysteroid dehydrogenase 1 (17β-HSD1) converting androstenedione to testosterone and aromatase converting both androstenedione and testosterone to estrogens, while expression of 3β-hydroxysteroid dehydrogenase 1 and 2 (3β-HSD1 and 2) initiating the first enzymatic conversion of steroidogenesis were absent. This demonstrates that conversion of androgens to estrogens is feasible in small antral human follicles, while de novo synthesis of estrogens from cholesterol will not take place.[123] By mid-gestation, theca interna cells start to differentiate and express 3β-HSD1.[124] This agrees with a immunohistochemical study showing a robust staining of 3β-HSD2 just prior to mid-gestation, while only a diffuse staining was observed from week 12 to 16.[112]

Interestingly, the development of aromatizing capacity of the fetal ovary develops simultaneously with testosterone secretion from the newly differentiated testis, suggesting that the two sexes at least in this respect have a conserved temporal development. In mammals the steroidogenic activity of the ovary is related to the initiation of meiosis. In species with delayed meiosis, such as the sheep,[125] rabbit,[126] and cow,[127] considerable amounts of estradiol are secreted during a limited premeiotic period (the delay period) of fetal life. In the rabbit, it has been shown by quantitative cytochemistry that the intraovarian rete cells of the medulla exhibit activity of 3β-HSD during the delay period.[128] It is likely that these cells are responsible for the synthesis of the steroids.[124] However, in species with immediate meiosis (i.e., mouse and humans), steroid production is low or undetectable during early stages of development. In human, the early interstitial cells are located in the inner part of the ovarian cortex close to the developing follicles, but they never make contact with the oocytes (see Fig. 147.5).

The mechanisms that trigger differentiation of the steroid-producing cells and initiation of steroid production are unknown. In the human fetal pituitary gland, the production of luteinizing hormone (LH) and follicle-stimulating hormone (FSH) reaches a peak between the 16th and 20th weeks of gestation and then levels off and remains low until puberty.[129,130] Thus the peak production of gonadotropins occurs several weeks before the start of ovarian steroidogenesis. Moreover, once started, a slight increase of ovarian steroidogenesis (i.e., estrogen production) is seen throughout late fetal life when fetal gonadotropin secretion decreases. It therefore seems unlikely that pituitary gonadotropins control the onset of fetal ovarian steroidogenesis.

FORMATION OF THE THECA LAYER AND EARLY FOLLICULAR STEROIDOGENESIS

In the human ovary from late fetal life and until the follicle pool is exhausted, theca cells differentiate around the late preantral or early antral follicles (Fig. 147.9).[101] Spindle-shaped hypotrophic cells encircle the basement membrane delineating the follicle, together with blood vessels and nerves, and subsequently the theca cells acquire the ultrastructural and biochemical characteristics of steroid-producing cells. The origin of the theca cells has not been definitively identified.[131,132] It has in mice been suggested that theca cells derive from two sources: (1) *Wt1* positive cells indigenous to the ovary and (2) *Gli1* positive mesenchymal calls migrated from the mesonephros.[131] The specification into theca cells requires multicellular interactions via both oocyte and granulosa cells. The progenitor cells acquire the theca cells marker *Gli1* in response to paracrine Desert hedgehog signaling (Dhh) from granulosa cells and the Dhh signaling requires growth differentiation factor 9 (GDF9) from the oocyte.[131]

The late fetal ovary and the ovary during childhood contain numerous small antral follicles with well-differentiated theca cells. However, throughout childhood, serum levels of estrogens and other steroids remain low, probably because of lack of sufficient gonadotropic stimulation during this period.

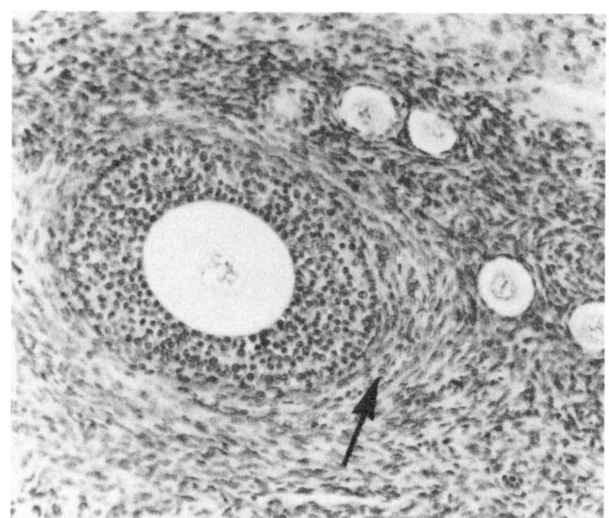

Fig. 147.9 Inner part of the ovarian cortex of a 32-week-old human fetus showing a growing preantral follicle with a differentiating theca layer *(arrow)* and some primordial follicles. (Original magnification ×450.)

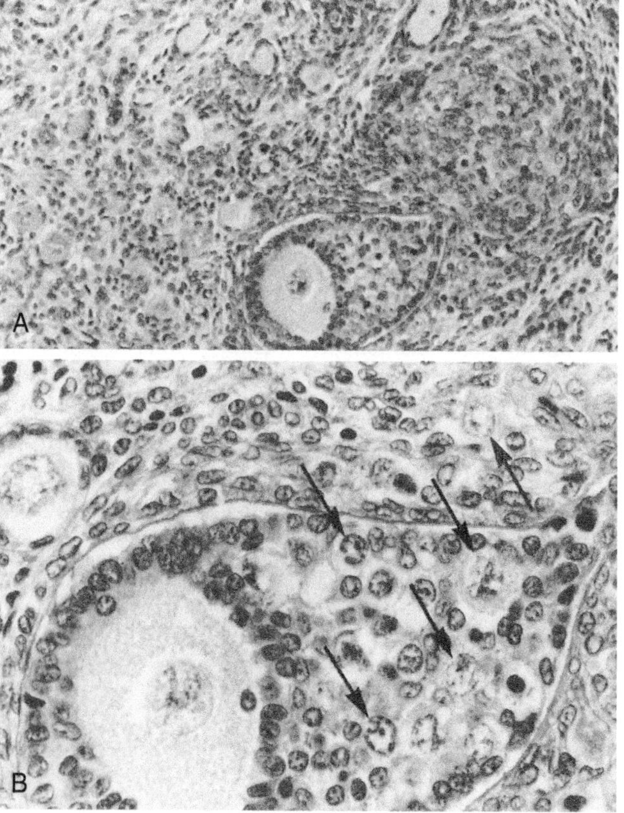

Fig. 147.10 Abnormal follicle of a human fetal ovary, 33 weeks old. (A) Besides a large oocyte, the granulosa layer contains numerous small oocytes and oogonia, some of which are degenerating. The granulosa layer opens up into a "nest" of small oocytes tightly packed with somatic cells. (Original magnification ×400.) (B) Higher magnification of A. The *arrows* point at some of the small oocytes.

FOLLICULAR GROWTH DURING CHILDHOOD

Birth itself is not a landmark in ovarian development and differentiation. Follicular growth starts in the early mid-trimester, and antral follicles are often seen 1 month before birth. Therefore the ovaries of newborn girls contain preantral and antral follicles, at different stages of growth and atresia, and a large pool of primordial follicles.[45] Growing follicles are normal in the ovary of the newborn girl (Fig. 147.10).[101,133] The peri- and postnatal increase in human gonadotropins, decline only after the third month of age, and sometimes cause development of ovarian cysts a few months later. This phenomenon is normal and is most often unrecognized. However, if the cysts are larger than 5 cm in diameter, intervention may be needed to prevent adnexal torsion.[134] In addition to gonadotropins and steroids, small antral follicles accumulate anti-müllerian hormone (AMH) in very high concentrations (two- to three-fold higher than in circulation). This suggests that these hormones also play important intrafollicular functions in follicles from the ovaries of young girls.[135,136] It has it has been suggested that the high intrafollicular concentrations of AMH act as an aromatase inhibitor limiting granulosa cell synthesis of estradiol.[137]

All follicles that start to grow during childhood are destined to undergo atresia at some stage of development, because no ovulations occur before menarche (Fig. 147.11). Although follicles may reach 6 mm in diameter during childhood, the size of the largest healthy, growing follicle does not generally exceed 10 mm.[138] The number of antral follicles also increases with age. In newborn girls, three to five follicles larger than 1 mm in diameter may be present, whereas, in 8-year-old girls, the number is often 10 or more (Fig. 147.12). This increase in the number of antral follicles is probably caused by the simultaneous increase in the basal levels of FSH and LH.[139] Little is known about the developmental potential of follicles that initiate growth during childhood. A higher fraction of abnormal non-growing follicles are found in prepubertal ovaries with a

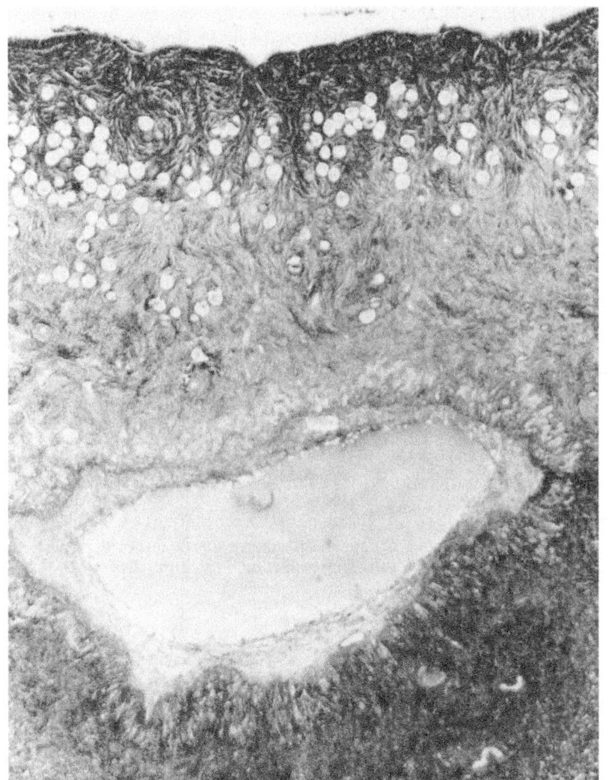

Fig. 147.11 Cortex of an ovary from a 4-year-old child. Many small oocytes populate the area below the dense tunica albuginea. Remnants of a collapsing antral follicle occupy the lower part of the figure. (Original magnification ×280.)

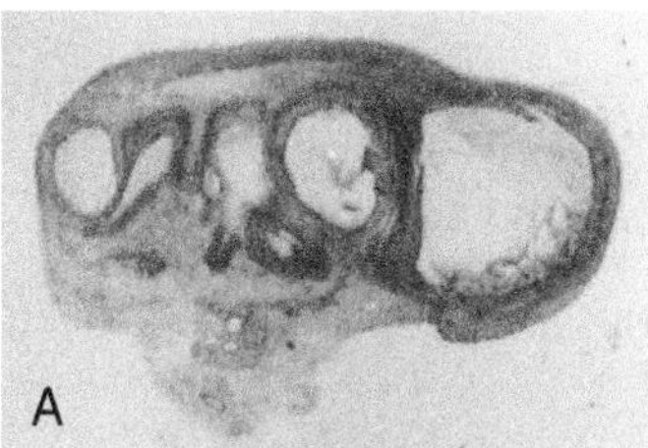

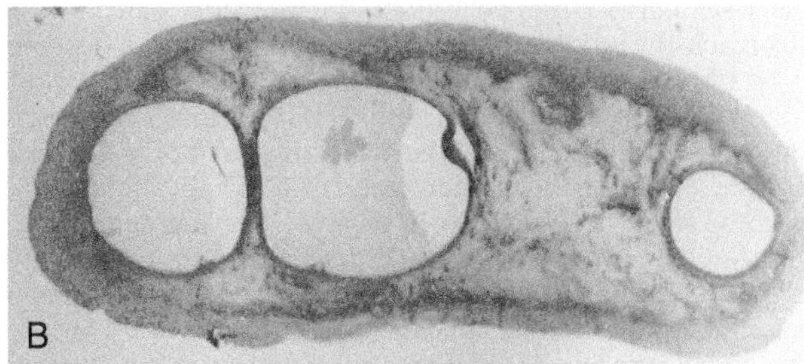

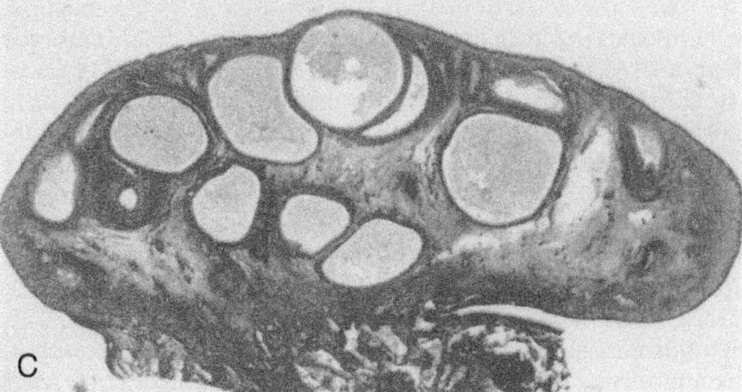

Fig. 147.12 Human ovaries of young children, all with several antral follicles, none of which exceed 6 mm in diameter. (Original magnification ×5.) (A) 2 months old. (B) 4 years old. (C) 7 years old.

reduced capacity for in vitro growth compared to follicles from adult ovaries, indicating that there are maturational processes occurring in the ovary through childhood and adolescence, which involve the loss of abnormal follicles, and increasing follicle developmental competence.[109] This is supported by a 2019 study that found chromosome errors and aneuploidy in human oocytes to be highest during childhood and at the end of reproductive life and lowest in women in their twenties, determining the curve of natural fertility.[140] Knowledge of the follicle development during childhood becomes clinically relevant as fertility preservation is increasingly offered to children undergoing gonadotoxic treatment or who have a diagnosis that in itself may thread the fertility potential (i.e., Turner syndrome, thalassemia, and galactosemia). The aim here is to replace the tissue in adult life and evidence thus far indicates that transplanted prepubertal ovarian tissue has the capacity for steroid production and when transplanted in adult life can regain fertility and give rise to healthy livebirths.[141,142]

A complete reference list is available at www.ExpertConsult.com. 

SELECT REFERENCES

1. Mork L, Maatouk DM, McMahon JA, et al. Temporal differences in granulosa cell specification in the ovary reflect distinct follicle fates in Mice1. *Biol Reprod*. 2012;86(2):37.
4. Popovic M, Bialecka M, Gomes Fernandes M, et al. Human blastocyst outgrowths recapitulate primordial germ cell specification events. *Mol Hum Reprod*. 2019;25(9):519-526.
5. Byskov AG, Høyer PE. Embryology of mammalian gonads and ducts. *Physiol Reprod*. 1994:487-540.
9. Kobayashi A, Behringer RR. Developmental genetics of the female reproductive tract in mammals. *Nat Rev Genet*. 2003;4(December):969-980.
12. Sinclair AH, Berta P, Palmer MS, et al. A gene from the human sex-determining region encodes a protein with homology to a conserved DNA-binding motif. *Nature*. 1990;346(6281):240-244.
14. Mamsen LS, Ernst EH, Borup R, et al. Temporal expression pattern of genes during the period of sex differentiation in human embryonic gonads. *Nat Sci Reports*. 2017;7(15961):1-16.
19. Mamsen LS, Brøchner CB, Byskov AG, Møllgard K. The migration and loss of human primordial germ stem cells from the hind gut epithelium towards the gonadal ridge. *Int J Dev Biol*. 2012;56:771-778.
25. Lei L, Spradling AC. Mouse primordial germ cells produce cysts that partially fragment prior to meiosis. *Development*. 2013;140(10):2075-2081.
28. Lei L, Spradling AC. Mouse oocytes differentiate through organelle enrichment from sister cyst germ cells. *Science*. 2016;352(6281):95-99.
29. Childs AJ, Kinnell HL, He J, Anderson RA. LIN28 is selectively expressed by primordial and pre-meiotic germ cells in the human fetal ovary. *Stem Cells Dev*. 2012;21(0):2343-2349.
32. Byskov AG. Primordial germ cells and regulation of meiosis. *Germ Cell Fertil*. 1982;1-17.
34. Wartenberg H. Development of the early human ovary and role of the mesonephros in the differentiation of the cortex. *Anat Embryol*. 1982;165(2):253-280.
35. Gondos B, Westergaard L, Byskov AG. Initiation of oogenesis in the human fetal ovary: ultrastructural and squash preparation study. *Am J Obstet Gynecol*. 1986;155(1):189-195.
38. Gondos B, Hobel CJ. Interstitial cells in the human fetal ovary. *Endocrinology*. 1973;93(3):736-739.
43. Mamsen LS, Lutterodt MC, Andersen EW, Byskov AG, Andersen CY. Germ cell numbers in human embryonic and fetal gonads during the first two trimesters of pregnancy: analysis of six published studies. *Hum Reprod*. 2011;26(8).
44. Baker T, Sum W. Development of the ovary and oogenesis. *Clin Obstet Gynaecol*. 1976;3(1):3-26.
46. Wallace WHB, Kelsey TW. Human ovarian reserve from conception to the Menopause. *PloS One*. 2010;5(1):e8772.
53. Johnson J, Canning J, Kaneko T, Pru J, Tilly J. Germline stem cells and follicular renewal in the postnatal mammalian ovary. *Nature*. 2004; 428(6979):145-150.
55. White Y, Woods D, Takai Y, et al. Oocyte formation by mitotically active germ cells purified from ovaries of reproductive-age women. *Nat Med*. 2012;18(3):413-421.
67. Cohen PE, Pollack SE, Pollard JW. Genetic analysis of chromosome pairing, recombination, and cell cycle control during first meiotic prophase in mammals. *Endocr Rev*. 2006;27(4):398-426.
69. Handel MA, Schimenti JC. Genetics of mammalian meiosis: regulation, dynamics and impact on fertility. *Nat Rev Genet*. 2010;11(2):124-136.
73. Byskov AG, Saxén L. Induction of meiosis in fetal mouse testis in vitro. *Dev Biol*. 1976;52(2):193-200.
74. Andersen C, Byskov A, Grinsted J. Partial purification of the meiosis inducing substance (MIS). *Dev Funct Reprod Organs*. 1981:73-80.
77. Bowles J, Knight D, Smith C, et al. Retinoid signaling determines germ cell fate in mice. *Science*. 2006;312(2006):596-600.

79. McLaren A, Southee D. Entry of mouse embryonic germ cells into meiosis. *Dev Biol*. 1997;187(1):107-113.
82. Koubova J, Menke D, Zhou Q, et al. Retinoic acid regulates sex-specific timing of meiotic initiation in mice. *Proc Natl Acad Sci U S A*. 2006;103(8):2474-2479.
88. Childs AJ, Cowan G, Kinnell HL, Anderson RA, Saunders PTK. Retinoic acid signalling and the control of meiotic entry in the human fetal gonad. *PloS One*. 2011;6(6):e20249.
90. Anderson RA, Fulton N, Cowan G, Coutts S, Saunders PT. Conserved and divergent patterns of expression of DAZL, VASA and OCT4 in the germ cells of the human fetal ovary and testis. *BMC Dev Biol*. 2007;7:136.
93. Lin Y, Gill M, Koubova J, Page D. Germ cell-intrinsic and -extrinsic factors govern meiotic initiation in mouse embryos. *Science*. 2008;322(5908):1685-1687.
95. He J, Stewart K, Kinnell HL, Anderson RA, Childs AJ. A developmental stage-specific switch from DAZL to BOLL occurs during fetal oogenesis in humans, but not mice. *PloS One*. 2013;8(9):e73996.
99. Tilly JL, Kowalski KI, Johnson AL, Hsueh AJW. Involvement of apoptosis in ovarian follicular atresia and postovulatory regression. *Endocrinology*. 1991;129(5):2799-2801.
101. Peters H, Byskov AG, Grinsted J. Follicular growth in fetal and prepubertal ovaries of humans and other primates. *Clin Endocrinol Metab*. 1978;7(3):469-485.
103. Pan B, Li J. The art of oocyte meiotic arrest regulation. *Reprod Biol Endocrinol*. 2019;17(1):8.
109. Anderson RA, McLaughlin M, Wallace WHB, Albertini DF, Telfer EE. The immature human ovary shows loss of abnormal follicles and increasing follicle developmental competence through childhood and adolescence. *Hum Reprod*. 2014;29(1):97-106.
110. Pepe GJ, Billiar RB, Albrecht ED. Regulation of baboon fetal ovarian folliculogenesis by estrogen. *Mol Cell Endocrinol*. 2006;247(1-2):41-46.
112. Fowler PA, Anderson RA, Saunders PT, et al. Development of steroid signaling pathways during primordial follicle formation in the human fetal ovary. *J Clin Endocrinol Metab*. 2011;96(6):1754-1762.
113. Abbott DH, Barnett DK, Bruns CM, Dumesic DA. Androgen excess fetal programming of female reproduction: a developmental aetiology for polycystic ovary syndrome? *Hum Reprod Update*. 2005; 11(4):357-374.
114. Buaas FW, Gardiner JR, Clayton S, Val P, Swain A. In vivo evidence for the crucial role of SF1 in steroid-producing cells of the testis, ovary and adrenal gland. *Development*. 2012;139(24):4561-4570.
116. Jepsen MR, Kløverpris S, Mikkelsen JH, et al. Stanniocalcin-2 inhibits mammalian growth by proteolytic inhibition of the insulin-like growth factor axis. *J Biol Chem*. 2015;290(6):3430-3439.
122. Fowler PA, Childs AJ, Dé Rique Courant F, et al. In utero exposure to cigarette smoke dysregulates human fetal ovarian developmental signalling. *Hum Reprod*. 2014;29(7):1471-1489.
128. Byskov AG, Hoyer PE, Westergaard L. Origin and differentiation of the endocrine cells of the ovary. *J Reprod Fertil*. 1985;75(1):299-306.
131. Liu C, Peng J, Matzuk MM, H-C Yao H. Lineage specification of ovarian theca cells requires multi- cellular interactions via oocyte and granulosa cells. *Nat Commun*. 2015;6(6934):1-19.
133. Gougeon A. Regulation of ovarian follicular development in primates: facts and hypotheses. *Endocr Rev*. 1996;17(2):121-155.
137. Jeppesen J, Anderson RA, Kelsey TW, et al. Which follicles make the most anti-Müllerian hormone in humans? Evidence for an abrupt decline in AMH production at the time of follicle selection. *Mol Hum Reprod*. 2013;19(8): 519-527.

148 Testicular Development and Descent

Mary M. Lee

INTRODUCTION

Male specification of the primordial germ cells and gonadal somatic cells, and ensuing differentiation and descent of the testis, are critical determinants of adult reproductive function and fertility. During embryogenesis, the expression of sex-determining region Y gene *(SRY)* in males along with a transcriptional regulatory network are required for testis determination.[1-3] Although chromosomal/genetic sex (46,XX or 46,XY) is established at the time of fertilization, the gonads and embryonic precursors of the genitalia are initially identical in male and female embryos. *SRY* activation serves as a master switch to initiate testis determination and male-specific development of the embryo, with differentiation of the somatic cells of the gonad as Leydig and Sertoli cells and virilization of the internal and external genitalia (reviewed by Makela et al.[4]). In a series of testicular grafting experiments, Jost[5] first demonstrated in the 1940s that two distinct testicular hormones direct differentiation along the male pathway. During embryogenesis, the secretion of testosterone by Leydig cells and anti-müllerian hormone (AMH) by Sertoli cells are critical for male sex differentiation.[2,3,6,7]

TESTIS DETERMINATION

Three to four weeks after conception, primitive germ cells are first detected in the dorsal endoderm of the yolk sac. These germ cells migrate to the hindgut epithelium, then spread dorsally along the mesentery and the body wall mesenchyme in response to chemotactic signals to populate the primitive gonad in the urogenital ridge.[3,7] The germ cells proliferate during their migration from the yolk sac endoderm to the urogenital ridge. Epithelial cells delaminate from the coelomic epithelium, enter the urogenital ridge, and enclose the germ cells to form the primary sex cords. Germ cells along the migratory pathway that fail to reach the ridge undergo degeneration; those that persist may be the embryonic precursors of teratomas.[8] Transcription factors such as steroidogenic factor 1 (SF1), homeobox genes (*Lhx9*, *Lhx1*, and *Emx2*), and the Wilms tumor suppressor gene *(Wt1)* are essential for gonadogenesis.[9-12] Some of the genes critical for testis development have other developmental roles. For example, children with *WT1* mutations may have both gonadal dysgenesis and renal impairment, whereas *SF1* mutations manifest as adrenal and gonadal dysgenesis.[9,13-15]

The gonad remains undifferentiated until 6 weeks gestational age, when the activation of *SRY*, a single-exon Y chromosome gene, initiates the male developmental pathway in 46,XY embryos (Fig. 148.1A).[1-3,6,7,16] *SRY* is a member of the SOX family of transcription factors that share a high mobility group DNA-binding motif.[16] The sexually dimorphic expression of SRY is transcriptionally regulated by WT1, GATA4 and its partner FOG2, and NR5A1 via distinct pathways that converge on the SRY promoter. Activation of a transient but precise spatiotemporal pattern of SRY expression in pre-Sertoli cells leads to hypomethylation of CpG sites in the SRY promoter and demethylation of histone H3K9.[17] SRY induces the expression of *SOX9* (17q24.3-25.1), an autosomal sex-determining gene that is initially expressed in the supporting cell lineage in both males and females.[18,19] After

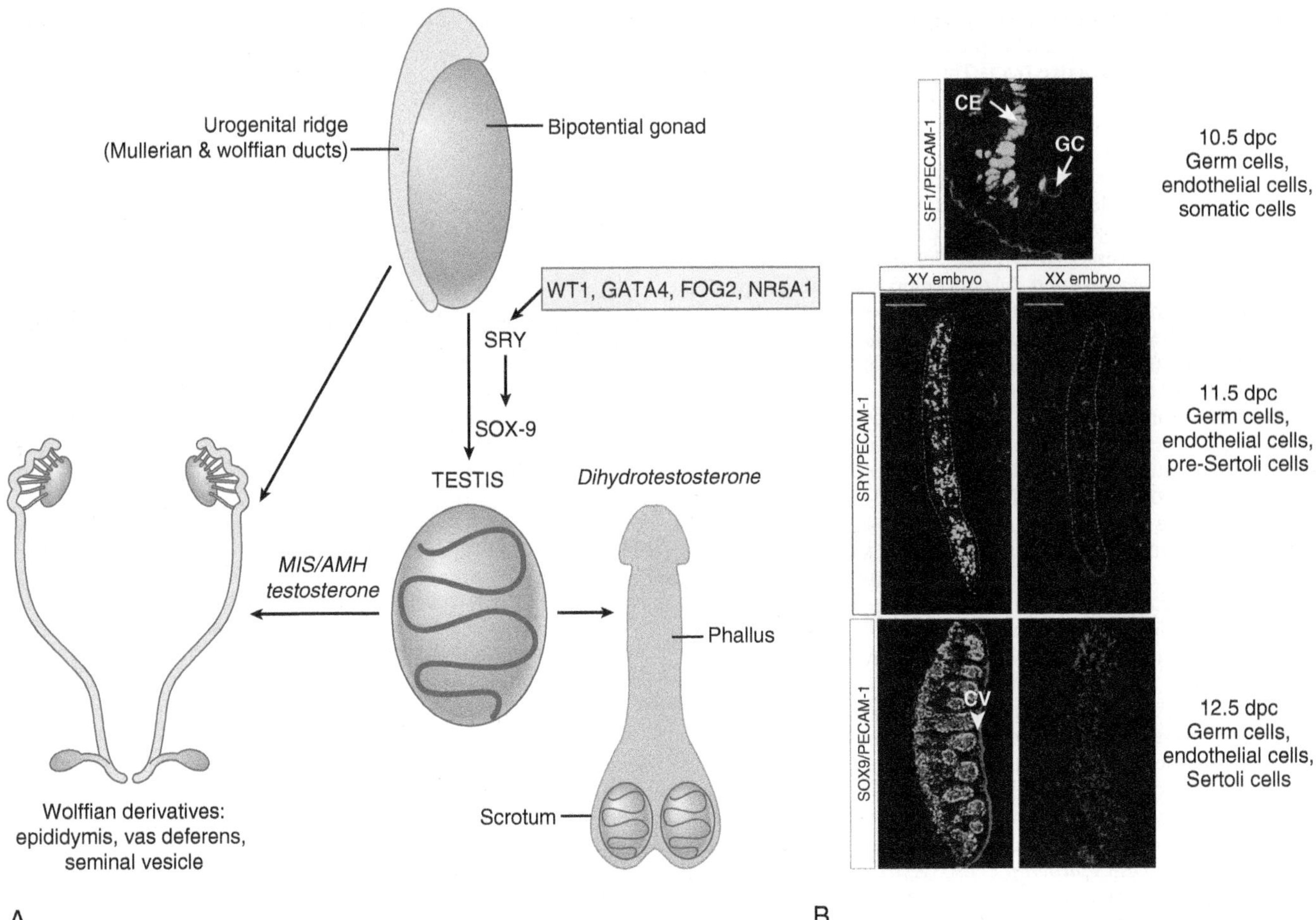

Fig. 148.1 Testis determination and male sex differentiation. (A) The bipotential gonad develops as a testis when sex-determining region Y gene *(SRY)* is activated. The testis secretes anti-müllerian hormone *(AMH),* or müllerian inhibiting substance (MIS) which induces regression of the female müllerian ducts and testosterone, which stimulates male differentiation of the internal (wolffian ducts) and external genitalia. (B) Confocal images showing the sex-specific changes in gonadal morphology and gene expression during this early stage of gonadal development. *CE,* Coelomic epithelium; *CV,* coelomic vessel; *dpc,* days post coitum; *GC,* germ cells. (From Polanco JC, Koopman P. Sry and the hesitant beginnings of male development. *Dev Biol.* 2007;302:13.)

induction of *SRY* expression in males, *SOX9* expression increases and shifts from a cytoplasmic to a nuclear distribution.[20,21] In females, the absence of SRY down-regulates the expression of *SOX9*. Patients with loss-of-function mutations in either *SRY* or *SOX9* have variable degrees of testicular dysgenesis.[19–22] In the mouse, *SRY* activation induces the desert hedgehog gene *(Dhh)* in pre-Sertoli cells and its receptor *Patched 1 (Ptch1)* in peritubular cells and Leydig cell precursors.[23,24] The expression of *Dhh* is not essential for initial testicular determination but is critical for subsequent somatic cell differentiation, steroidogenesis, and cord formation. Targeted deletion of *Dhh* disrupts early cord formation and severely impairs spermatogenesis and fetal Leydig cell differentiation. Additional autosomal genes located within chromosomal deletions, such as 9p24 and 10q, are also associated with sex reversal or partial gonadal dysgenesis.

SRY expression in pre-Sertoli cells stimulates their proliferation and differentiation to the Sertoli cell lineage signified by their synthesis of AMH and other Sertoli cell–specific genes.[2,3,7,25] *Sry* also stimulates migration of peritubular myoid and endothelial cells from the mesonephros into the urogenital ridge—an essential step in the formation of testicular cords.[26] Shortly after Sertoli cell differentiation, male-specific vascularization of the gonad occurs with organization of the gonad into discrete cords (see Fig. 148.1B). The coelomic vessel is formed with a network of branching capillaries restricted to the interstitial space. These capillaries eventually drain into venules in the mesonephros and are thought to be important for rapid distribution of testicular hormones into the systemic circulation. Concurrently, fetal steroidogenic Leydig cells differentiate from the interstitial mesenchymal cells between the testicular cords. The interstitium also contains endothelial cells, macrophages, and fibroblasts. The testicular cords separate from the overlying epithelium when a dense layer of fibroblastic cells forms the tunica albuginea. During this period the primordial germ cells within the testicular cords differentiate and proliferate to increase in number from 3000 to 30,000 by 9 weeks' gestation.[27] In contrast to ovarian development, the presence of germ cells is not necessary for testicular morphogenesis to proceed. By the ninth week, the rete testis, the anastomosing ends of the cords near the testicular hilum, extends into the mesonephric ridge and connects to the remaining mesonephric tubules to form the ductus deferens.

INTERNAL REPRODUCTIVE TRACTS AND EXTERNAL GENITALIA

The urogenital ridge arises from the intermediate mesoderm as bilateral thickenings at the ventrolateral surface of the mesonephros. Many genes that are critical for formation of the bipotential gonad are also essential for formation of the urogenital ridge. Mice with null deletions of *Lhx1, Lhx9,* and *Emx2* have defects in urogenital ridge development and gonadal agenesis.[10,12,23-25] All embryos initially have embryonic ductal precursors for both male and female internal reproductive tracts. The wolffian, or mesonephric, duct arises as the caudal extension of the pronephric excretory duct. The müllerian (paramesonephric) duct develops in close proximity to the wolffian duct by invagination of the coelomic epithelium to form a tube surrounded by mesenchymal cells. Sexually dimorphic development of the primitive ducts in the undifferentiated urogenital ridge is dependent on the local hormonal milieu. In mice with *Pax2* deletions, the gonads form normally, but the genital ducts fail to develop, suggesting a specific role for *Pax2* in controlling differentiation of the intermediate mesoderm.[28] *Pax2* may also have a secondary role in wolffian duct differentiation as it localizes to the wolffian duct at later stages of genital tract development.

Paracrine hormones from the testis play critical roles in mediating the sexually dimorphic differentiation of the wolffian (male) and müllerian (female) internal genital ducts. Male differentiation of the internal and external genital structures requires that the testis secretes AMH and testosterone in a specific temporal pattern and that their downstream signaling pathways are functional. A number of genes, such as *SRY, SOX9, SF1, GATA4,* and *WT1,* have been shown in vitro to act cooperatively or synergistically to activate AMH expression in Sertoli cells.[29,30] AMH, a 140-kDa glycoprotein in the transforming growth factor (TGF) β family of cellular growth and transcription factors, is produced as a prohormone requiring proteolytic cleavage to generate a bioactive hormone.[29-31] AMH binds to cell-surface serine-threonine kinase receptors and signals through the Sma- and Mad-related pathways. Although AMH receptors localize to the *mesenchymal* cells surrounding the müllerian duct, epithelial-mesenchymal interactions culminate in apoptotic cell death of the adjacent *epithelial* cells.[32] AMH-induced regression of the müllerian ducts occurs at gestational weeks 8 to 12, leaving a vestigial remnant that persists as the prostatic utricle. Androgens have no independent effect on the müllerian duct, but act synergistically with AMH to promote full regression, whereas estrogens inhibit AMH-mediated ductal involution.

Testosterone-stimulated differentiation and growth of the wolffian structures (epididymis, vas deferens, seminal vesicles) occurs between 9 and 14 weeks of embryonic life.[2,3,6,7] *SF1* induces the expression of steroidogenic pathway genes: acute steroidogenic regulatory protein, the cytochrome P-450 steroid hydroxylases, and 3β-hydroxysteroid dehydrogenase to initiate testosterone biosynthesis in Leydig cells.[15] Virilization of the external genitalia is also androgen dependent but requires enzymatic reduction of testosterone to its more active metabolite, dihydrotestosterone, by 5α-reductase, an enzyme present on genital skin.

LEYDIG CELLS

The Leydig stem cells are believed to migrate from either the mesonephrogenic mesenchyme or coelomic epithelium to the gonadal ridge, where they localize to the interstitial space of the developing testis.[15,25,33] The initial differentiation of fetal Leydig cells and onset of androgen production occurs at 7 to 8 weeks' gestation—before the onset of pituitary secretion of luteinizing hormone (LH) and prior to expression of the LH receptor in the testis, and thus is considered LH independent.[33,34] Factors secreted by Sertoli cells, such as desert hedgehog, and genes expressed in Leydig cell precursors, such as the platelet-derived growth factor receptor α gene and the GATA4 gene, play key roles in modulating differentiation of fetal Leydig cells. *SF1,* a gene expressed downstream of *SRY,* has a pivotal role in gonadal and adrenal organogenesis, as well as transcriptionally activating steroid hydroxylases and other genes that are

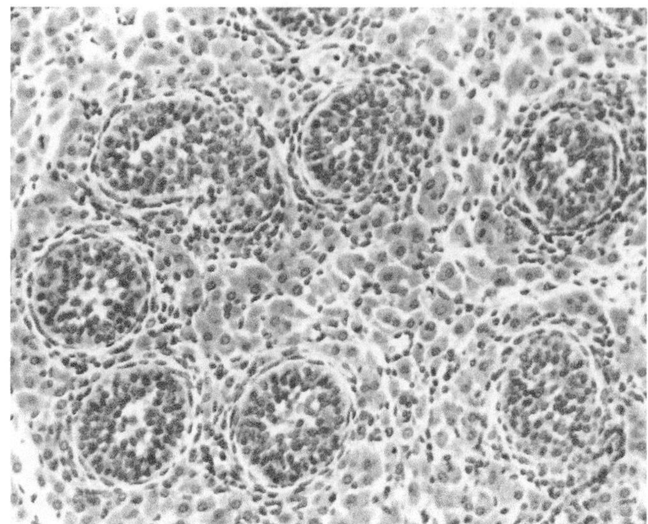

Fig. 148.2 Human fetal testis histology. Section of testis at 12 weeks' gestation showing the seminiferous cords and abundant Leydig cells in the interstitial spaces (×250). (From Aslan AR, Kogan BA, Gondos B. Testicular development. In: Polin RA, Fox WW, Abman SH, eds. *Fetal and Neonatal Physiology*. 3rd ed. Philadelphia: WB Saunders; 2004:1956–1960.)

essential for androgen biosynthesis.[15] Disruption of the GATA-FOG2 interaction results in reduced expression of male-specific genes in the somatic cell lineages and in aberrant Leydig cell differentiation.[35]

Fetal Leydig cells progressively increase in number to reach a maximum of 48×10^6 cells per pair of testes at week 14. The increase in Leydig cell numbers is attributed to proliferation of the precursor cells because differentiated steroidogenic Leydig cells no longer divide. From week 12 to 18, the Leydig cells appear hyperplastic and constitute the largest relative percentage of the testicular volume during fetal development. During this period, the fetal Leydig cells are in their most active phase of testosterone production and serum testosterone concentrations reach peak levels (Fig. 148.2). In the third trimester, fetal Leydig cells decline in number and mass through degeneration to reach their lowest number of 18×10^6 cells per pair of testes just before birth.[33,36,37] The decrease in Leydig cell numbers is accompanied by a parallel decline in their production of androgen.[33,35,37]

Androgen biosynthesis and secretion by fetal Leydig cells is essential for virilization of the internal and external genitalia. The hallmark of a terminally differentiated Leydig cell is the acquisition of steroidogenic capacity.[33,37] As the testis organizes into cords, 3β-hydroxysteroid dehydrogenase starts to be expressed in somatic interstitial cells that are distinguishable as steroidogenic Leydig cells by their ultrastructural features. The biosynthesis of testosterone commences at week 7 or 8 and thereafter increases markedly to reach peak rates at 14 to 16 weeks. During the critical window of sex differentiation from week 8 to 12, the production of testosterone and its conversion to its more active metabolite dihydrotestosterone are gonadotropin independent.[34,35] By the second trimester, androgen biosynthesis becomes gonadotropin dependent as Leydig cells start to express the LH receptor and respond to the high concentrations of placental human chorionic gonadotropin in the intrauterine environment. Along with the induction of LH receptor expression, pituitary secretion of LH increases during the latter half of gestation. Fetal Leydig cells are not subject to negative feedback by LH and have a greater response to its stimulatory effects, in contrast to the robust negative feedback by LH on postnatal adult Leydig cells. Thus, the steroidogenic capacity per fetal Leydig cell is higher than that of adult Leydig cells.[37] Nevertheless, before birth, both the total number of Leydig cells and the steroid content per fetal Leydig cell decreases (perhaps as a result of inhibitory paracrine hormones) and circulating testosterone concentrations are much lower.

Studies on the regulation of fetal Leydig cell steroidogenesis have yielded discrepant findings. Fetal Leydig cells are insensitive to the inhibitory effects of estrogens, a property that would enable the fetus to circumvent the high concentrations of maternal estrogens that are present in the intrauterine milieu.[38] Conversely, studies have also shown that estrogens inhibit testosterone production in cultured Leydig cells and inhibit Leydig cell proliferation. Other regulators of fetal steroidogenesis include two paracrine factors, AMH and TGF-β, that both inhibit androgen biosynthesis.[39]

After birth, a transient neonatal activation of the hypothalamic-pituitary-gonadal axis at 2 to 4 months of age stimulates an increase in Leydig cell numbers and a robust rise in androgen production.[40] This is followed by dedifferentiation and/or degeneration of the fetal Leydig cells and a marked decline in androgen production to the low levels that persist until the onset of puberty. Very few differentiated Leydig cells are present in the prepubertal testis. The interstitial space contains predominantly mesenchymal cells that are precursors of the postnatal adult Leydig cells. These "infantile" Leydig cells have a multilobed nucleus and little smooth endoplasmic reticulum. The mesenchymal cells proliferate and increase in number during childhood, then differentiate at puberty to adult steroid-secreting cells with a large polygonal configuration, eccentric nuclear position, abundant smooth endoplasmic reticulum, pleomorphic mitochondria, and well-developed Golgi apparatus. LH, in concert with other hormones that stimulate androgen production, promotes maturation of the steroidogenic enzymes to progressively increase androgen production. The secretion of testosterone by mature adult Leydig cells is required for spermatogenesis and secondary sexual maturation. Morphologically, adult Leydig cells can be distinguished from fetal Leydig cells by the presence of Reinke crystals, which are of unknown function but specific to mature Leydig cells. The number of mature Leydig cells in the adult testis is relatively static as the terminally differentiated cells do not divide, although a limited number of Leydig cells may arise de novo from mesenchymal precursors in the interstitial space.

SERTOLI AND GERM CELLS

As the primordial germ cells migrate to the urogenital ridge, they are enclosed by fetal Sertoli cells and organized into seminiferous cords (see Figs. 148.1 and 148.3). The Sertoli cells are considered the "nurse" or supporting cells for the germ cells and regulate many germ cell functions. A deficiency in Sertoli cell number will impact the number and quality of sperm in the mature testis. The relative numbers of Sertoli and germ cells within the seminiferous tubules vary throughout the stages of reproductive development, with the predominance being Sertoli cells initially.[41,42] The high fetal testosterone concentration from week 8 to 22 of gestation stimulates germ cell proliferation and reverses the ratio of germ cells to immature Sertoli cells. As testosterone production declines during the third trimester, however, germ cell mitotic activity also declines, resulting in fewer germ cells than Sertoli cells at birth. During the neonatal "minipuberty," germ cells proliferate transiently, then stop dividing. The Sertoli cells divide rapidly during childhood until pubertal onset, when they differentiate, form tight junctions, and no longer undergo cell division.[42] At that time, the germ cells proliferate to equalize the number of germ cells and Sertoli cells in the pubertal testis.

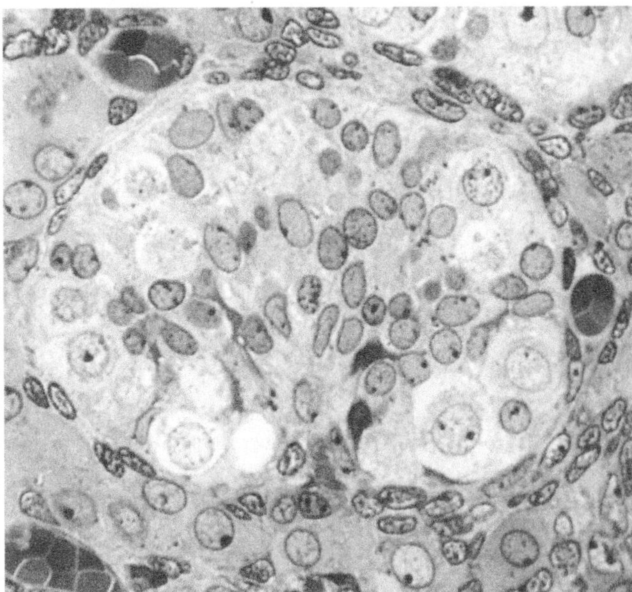

Fig. 148.3 Seminiferous cords in human fetal testis with Sertoli cells and round immature germ cells at the periphery. (Toluidine blue, ×500.) (From Aslan AR, Kogan BA, Gondos B. Testicular development. In: Polin RA, Fox WW, Abman SH, eds. *Fetal and Neonatal Physiology*. 3rd ed. Philadelphia: WB Saunders; 2004:1956–1960.)

In the immature testis, round to oval gonocytes are located centrally within the tubules. As they mature to prespermatogonia, they shift to the periphery of the tubules near the basal lamina. The prespermatogonia are connected by residual cytoplasmic bridges that remain after incomplete cytokinesis during mitosis. These interconnections between differentiating spermatogonia enable synchronized maturation of adjacent germ cells. Each germ cell division replenishes the spermatogonial pool and generates a germ cell that undergoes spermatogenetic maturation. Spermatogonia are classified by their morphology, maturational stage, position within the germinal epithelium, and variations in nuclear chromatin precipitation.[43] More immature spermatogonia are found along the basement membrane, whereas mature forms reside closer to the tubular lumen. Type A spermatogonia, divided into dark type A (Ad) and pale type A (Ap) groups, are considered part of the spermatogonial stem pool. Progressive differentiation to type B spermatogonia represents the first step of spermatid formation. Sequential stages of spermatogenesis can be identified within a testis, including from the least mature to the most mature forms: Ad spermatogonia; Ap spermatogonia; type B spermatogonia; primary spermatocytes (leptotene, zygotene, and pachytene); secondary spermatocytes, Sa, Sb1, Sb2, Sc, Sd1, and Sd2 spermatids; and mature spermatozoa. In men who had orchidopexy before the age of 2 years, the risk for infertility correlated with the presence of Ad spermatogonia at the time of orchidopexy; it has been proposed that increased testosterone levels during the minipuberty of infancy may be essential for transformation of germ cells to Ad spermatogonia.[44]

The development of germ cells occurs in parallel with the maturation of Sertoli cells. Fetal Sertoli cells have round to elliptical nuclei and small nucleoli. They have minimal smooth endoplasmic reticulum but contain abundant ribosomes and rough endoplasmic reticulum.[45] At puberty the immature Sertoli cells differentiate and develop tight junctions that form the blood-testis barrier. This unique characteristic enables the Sertoli cells to establish a microenvironment to control the biochemical milieu within the cords as well as to facilitate the migration of germ cells within the seminiferous tubules.

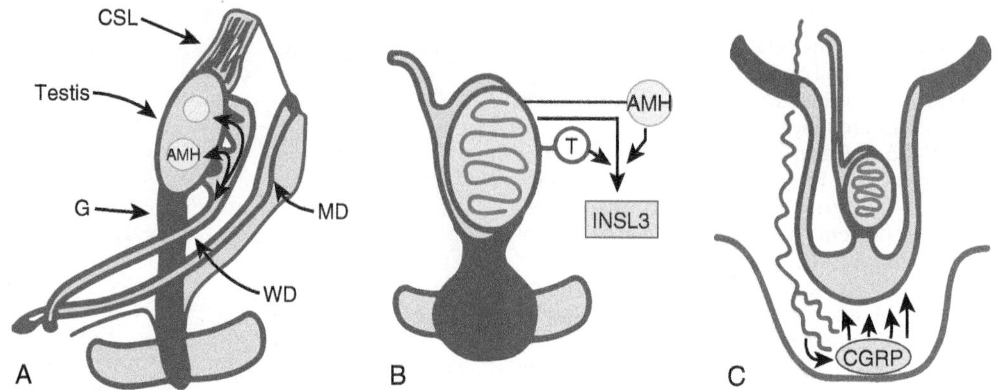

Fig. 148.4 The two phases of testicular descent. (A) Initial intraabdominal position of the gonads, wolffian duct *(WD)*, müllerian duct *(MD)*, cranial suspensory ligament *(CSL)*, and gubernaculum *(G)*. (B) The transabdominal phase of testicular descent is mediated primarily by insulin-like factor 3 (INSL3). (C) The inguinal scrotal phase of testicular descent is an androgen-dependent process. *AMH*, Anti-müllerian hormone; *CGRP*, calcitonin gene–related peptide; *T*, testosterone. (From Hutson JM, Hasthorpe S. Testicular descent and cryptorchidism: the state of the art in 2004. *J Pediatr Surg.* 2005;40:297.)

Although the number of Sertoli cells is static during pubertal maturation, they occupy a relatively smaller area of the tubules as the tubules elongate and enlarge due to active germ cell proliferation.[45] During testis determination, the first hormone secreted by the Sertoli cell is AMH, the hormone responsible for inducing regression of müllerian duct structures in males during normal embryogenesis. Mutations of AMH or its type II receptor result in retained müllerian structures in males, a condition termed *persistent müllerian duct syndrome.* Although müllerian duct regression is complete by the second trimester, AMH has paracrine modulatory actions on germ cell maturation and Leydig cell development and continues to be abundantly produced throughout gestation and after birth.[37,39,45,46]

The Sertoli cells also secrete inhibin, a related hormone in the TGF-β family that down-regulates pituitary secretion of follicle-stimulating hormone (FSH).[47,48] Similarly to the other members of this gene family, inhibin consists of two subunits—inhibin A and inhibin B—and undergoes proteolytic processing. Inhibin indirectly regulates spermatogenesis through its modulation of FSH and is also believed to have direct paracrine effects on spermatogenesis.

BLOOD-TESTIS BARRIER

The Sertoli cells develop tight junctions that create a physical barrier between the bloodstream and the testicular tubules.[49,50] In rats the blood-testis barrier is not fully developed until puberty; in humans the age at which the barrier becomes fully functional is not known. The blood-testis barrier helps maintain the microenvironment of the apical adluminal compartment of the seminiferous tubules. The tight junctions prevent passage of large tracers from the interstitium to the apically located tubular lumen, whereas smaller tracers are incompletely excluded. This physical barrier enables the Sertoli cell to maintain the microenvironment of the tubular lumen to support spermatogenesis. The blood-testis barrier also has an immunoprotective role to prevent autoimmune destruction of differentiating germ cells. A number of extracellular matrix proteins and ectoplasmic specialization proteins are critical for the structural and functional integrity of the blood-testis barrier. In the rat testis, inhibitors of protein phosphatase disrupt the barrier, whereas pretreatment with protein tyrosine kinase inhibitors can prevent this effect. Similarly, both protein kinase A activator and protein kinase C inhibitors perturb the Sertoli cell tight junctions, indicating a regulatory role for protein kinases. Formation of the barrier can be disrupted by certain toxins, hormonally active compounds such as diethylstilbestrol, and heavy metals such as cadmium.

Immature spermatogonia (spermatogonia and preleptotene spermatocytes) are located close to the basement membrane, whereas more mature, differentiating spermatocytes and spermatids are found in the adluminal compartment. During the meiotic phase of spermatogenesis, the remodeling of the intercellular junctions enables migration of the preleptotene and leptotene spermatocytes across the barrier into the adluminal compartment. The spermatogonia complete maturation on the apical side of the tubules and are released from the seminiferous epithelium. The regulation of this process is not fully understood, but cytokines are known to have a role in the restructuring of the tight junctions that is essential during spermatogenesis.[49,50]

PERITUBULAR STRUCTURES

The peritubular structures impart structural integrity to the seminiferous tubules. In humans the lamina propria contains five to seven layers separating the seminiferous tubules from the interstitium.[51] The external one or two layers consist of fibroblastic cells that form the adventitia and provide structural support for the tubules. The middle layers contain myoid cells with fibroblastic characteristics that help create the blood-testis barrier. These myofibroblasts are contractile and may therefore facilitate movement of spermatozoa from the tubules to the rete testis. In experimentally created cryptorchidism, there is thickening of the peritubular structures that may interrupt the movement of the differentiating germ cells and contribute to the associated infertility. The collagen-rich innermost layer is immediately adjacent to the basal membrane of the tubules. This cellular layer secretes paracrine growth factors and extracellular matrix proteins for structural support of the basement membrane.

Complex cell-to-cell interactions and signaling pathways are used to establish the organizational structure of the testes and to complete the maturational processes that are needed for virilization of the genitalia and reproductive competence. The descent of the testes from an intraabdominal to a scrotal position is an important early developmental step to attain reproductive competence.

REGULATION OF TESTICULAR DESCENT

In parallel with in utero testicular development and somatic and germ cell differentiation, the fetal testis undergoes anatomic changes in its position. The regulation of testicular descent from an abdominal to a scrotal position has been well studied in rodents, with complementary insights gained from detailed assessments to help clarify this process during human development. Differences among species in timing, anatomy and final testicular position, and hormonal milieu limit the ability to fully extrapolate observations in animal models to human testicular descent. For example, in humans, testes move into the scrotum during late gestation, whereas testicular descent occurs at puberty in rodents, when the pouchlike processus vaginalis is formed.

In humans, testicular descent is considered to be a biphasic process comprising two distinct phases—a transabdominal step and an inguinoscrotal step (Fig. 148.4).[52,53] The developing testes remain attached to the posterior abdominal wall by the cranial suspensory ligament and caudally by the genitoinguinal ligament (or the gubernaculum). During the transabdominal phase of descent from week 10 to 15 of gestation, the cranial suspensory ligament regresses under the influence of androgens, whereas the caudal end of the gubernaculum enlarges in a "swelling reaction" to form an outgrowth. The testes are anchored by the gubernaculum to the abdominal wall near the site of the future inner ring of the inguinal canal. As the abdominal cavity enlarges during the second trimester, the testes remain in the lower abdomen and eventually assume a position lateral to the inferior pole of the kidneys. Insulin-like factor 3 (INSL3), also known as *relaxin-like factor,* a member of the insulin-like superfamily produced in Leydig cells, has been identified as a key hormone responsible for the gubernacular swelling.[52] INSL3 signals through its receptor, relaxin-family peptide receptor 2 (RXFP2), on gubernacular cells to stimulate gubernacular differentiation and growth. The gubernacular outgrowth ("swelling") is characterized by hyperplasia and hypertrophy of the mesenchymal cells due to an increase in the levels of glycosaminoglycans and hyaluronic acid that promotes water retention and makes the gubernaculum gelatinous. Male mice with a null mutation of *Insl3* have a poorly developed gubernacular bulb, intact cranial suspensory ligament, and undescended testes,[54,55] whereas overexpression of *Insl3* in females results in descent of the ovaries to the inguinal region.[56] Mutations in *INSL3* and *RXFP2* have been reported in only a small subset of patients with cryptorchidism; therefore the cause of undescended testes in humans appears to be multifactorial.[52-55,57]

The regression of the cranial suspensory ligaments during the transabdominal phase of testicular descent is thought to be under androgen control and necessary for full abdominal descent. In rodents, prenatal antiandrogen treatment prevents complete regression of the cranial suspensory ligaments whereas prenatal androgen treatment induces regression of the ligaments and partial ovarian descent.[52,57,58] In the absence of androgen action, such as in androgen-insensitive testicular feminizing mice and in humans with androgen insensitivity syndrome (AIS), the cranial suspensory ligaments do not regress and the gubernacular bulb is smaller.[52,57] In humans with AIS, the testes are located either in the inguinal region (suggesting that androgens are not essential for the transabdominal phase of descent) or midway down the abdomen (suggesting a supportive role for androgens).[59]

Androgens mediate testicular movement from the inguinal region through the inguinal canal into the scrotum during the inguinoscrotal phase of testicular descent. From week 25 to 35 of gestation, the testes shift from their intraabdominal position at the level of the anterior iliac spine through the internal and external rings of the inguinal canal into the scrotal sacs.[52,53,57,60] The gubernacular bulb lengthens and the peritoneum protrudes through the developing scrotal sac to form the processus vaginalis, which facilitates movement of the testes through the inguinal canal. Subsequent shortening of the proximal part of the gubernaculum and involution of the caudal bulb facilitates movement of the testes from the external inguinal ring to the bottom of the scrotal sacs. In addition to hormonal regulators, intraabdominal pressure is also believed to play a role in this final stage of testicular descent.

Androgen action is essential for the inguinoscrotal phase of testicular descent. Cryptorchidism is a cardinal feature of a number of animal models and human disorders associated with either inadequate androgen action or perturbation of the hypothalamic-pituitary-gonadal axis.[52,53,57,59,60] Several animal models of experimentally induced cryptorchidism can be reversed by administration of exogenous testosterone, confirming its critical role. Moreover, patients with hypothalamic hypogonadism or other forms of secondary testosterone deficiency have an increased rate of inguinal testes. Undescended testes are also a common finding in undervirilized infants with AIS or defects in testosterone biosynthesis.[60] Although 5α-reductase activity is present in the rat gubernaculum, finasteride, a 5α-reductase inhibitor, has little effect on testicular descent; therefore the reduction of testosterone to dihydrotestosterone does not appear to be essential.

Animal studies have also explored the adjunct role of other hormones on this complex process. In rodents, testicular descent into the scrotum occurs at puberty rather than in utero; thus rodent models are not directly applicable to human testicular descent. For example, in postnatal rats, removal of the salivary glands, the major source of epidermal growth factor (EGF), compromises testicular descent and administration of EGF prevents cryptorchidism induced by flutamide (an antiandrogen). The role of EGF in human testicular descent, however, is unknown. Administration of estrogenic agents, endocrine-disrupting compounds, and antagonists or antibodies that block LH, INSL3, and/or testosterone can all inhibit testicular descent.

Boys with cryptorchidism have been reported to have lower serum AMH and inhibin values and higher FSH values,[61,62,64,66] whereas no consistent pattern has been reported for LH or testosterone values in cryptorchid boys compared with controls.[62-65]

Animal models suggest that the effects of androgens on testicular descent are mediated both directly through androgen receptors expressed on mesenchymal cells found in the muscle and also indirectly via androgen stimulation of a neuropeptide, calcitonin gene-related peptide (CGRP), from sensory neurons in the genitofemoral nerve.[52,57] The key role of the genitofemoral nerve was recognized via rodent experiments demonstrating that transection of the genitofemoral nerve early in gestation inhibited gubernacular development and the testes remained in an inguinal position.[52] Receptors for CGRP are expressed on embryonic myotubules found within the gubernacular cells in the developing cremasteric muscle. CGRP stimulates rapid rhythmic contractions of the gubernaculum that may be important for its migration to the scrotum. In vitro, CGRP has been shown to act as a chemotactic and proliferative signal to stimulate caudal migration of the gubernacular cells. Exogenous treatment with a synthetic CGRP antagonist (CGRP 8 to 37) has been shown to delay testicular descent in rats, whereas administration of CGRP stimulated testicular descent in cryptorchid pigs. The data supporting a role of CGRP in human testicular descent are limited to evidence that CGRP is able to stimulate fusion of inguinal hernia sacs in organ culture.[67] Although indirect, this serves as a model for one of the events that occur during testicular descent, the obliteration of the processus vaginalis.

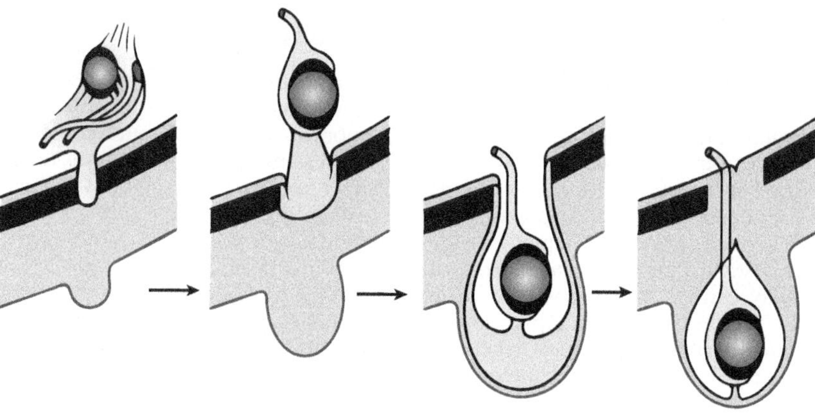

Fig. 148.5 Fetal stages of testicular descent. In humans, the process of testicular descent occurs in two phases: the transabdominal and inguinoscrotal stages. The gubernaculum undergoes a "swelling reaction" bringing the testes into a lower abdominal position. As the gubernacular bulb protrudes into the scrotum, the testes are drawn through the inguinal canal to the bottom of the scrotal sac. The extracellular matrix and cranial suspensory ligaments regress after the testes have descended into the scrotum, and the processus vaginalis closes to prevent an inguinal hernia. (From Hutson JM, Baskin LS, Risbridger G, et al. The power and perils of animal models with urogenital anomalies: handle with care. *J Pediatr Urol.* 2014;10:699–705.)

THE DIAGNOSIS AND INCIDENCE OF CRYPTORCHIDISM

Clinical disorders of testicular descent are the most common minor congenital abnormality in male newborns.[68] The term for this condition, *cryptorchidism,* is derived from the Greek words *kryptos* and *orchis* for *hidden gonad.* Most commonly, the undescended testes are found in the inguinal region, stemming from a disruption of the more complex inguinoscrotal phase of descent involving the slower process of migration from the external ring to the scrotum. The testes, however, can be asymmetrically positioned and found anywhere along the path of embryologic testicular descent, even in ectopic locations (Fig. 148.5).

The cause of cryptorchidism is unknown in most cases and appears to be multifactorial.[52,53,57,69] Only a minority of cases are known to be caused by a specific genetic or endocrine disorder, although the likelihood of finding a specific cause increases if associated anomalies are present. Epidemiologic studies have demonstrated geographic differences in the prevalence of cryptorchidism and other male reproductive disorders, such as hypospadias and decreased fertility, suggesting that underlying genetic or environmental factors may play a causative role.[57,68,70] Some studies have also reported a secular rise in the incidence of these conditions over the past century.[70,71] A unified hypothesis of a testicular dysgenesis syndrome due to embryonic disturbance in testicular formation or function has been proposed to explain these findings.[71]

One of the major obstacles to determining the exact prevalence of cryptorchidism is the lack of specificity in the diagnosis. Although the distinction between a completely nonpalpable, intraabdominal testis and a scrotal testis is readily appreciated, the difficulty lies in distinguishing inguinal undescended testes from those that are retractile. This becomes even more difficult later in infancy and childhood, when the cremasteric reflex is more active; therefore, there is high interobserver variability with the diagnosis of cryptorchidism.[72] The cremasteric reflex is easily triggered during an examination when the scrotum is exposed to cold and the child is apprehensive, leading to misdiagnosis of a retracted normally descended testis as being undescended. The erroneous classification of a retractile testis as cryptorchid and the different criteria used by investigators to define a cryptorchid testis may account for inconsistencies in the prevalence data among centers. This lack of standardization in the diagnosis of cryptorchidism and the potential for misdiagnosis also contribute to the discrepant data on the efficacy of different modes of management.

A systematic review of the literature found a rate of undescended testes that ranged from 1.0% to 4.6% in newborn infants with birth weight greater than 2.5 kg, and a rate of 1.1% to 45.3% in preterm infants weighing less than 2.5 kg.[68] At 1 year of age, the rate of undescended testes in the term infants had decreased to 1.0% to 1.5%, consistent with previous reports of spontaneous descent in the first year in 50% to 75% of cases, with most occurring in the first 3 months. Prevalence rates in school-aged children were more variable—6-year-olds had a rate of 0% to 2.6%, and 11-year-olds had a rate of 0% to 6.6%. One longitudinal study reported that most cryptorchid testes underwent spontaneous descent by 9 months of age, with an incidence at birth of 2.7% decreasing to 0.8% by 1 year of age.[73] An increase in prevalence noted in some school studies has been attributed to acquired ascent of the testes during childhood as a result of inadequate elongation of the spermatic cord.[74,75] Prematurity and low birth weight are both significant risk factors for cryptorchidism, and a family history of cryptorchidism also increases the relative risk for cryptorchidism—in one study, the relative risk was 10.1% for twins and 3.52% for siblings.[76] Despite familial risk for cryptorchidism and the identification of genes critical for this process, studies have shown that a specific genetic cause is found in a minority of patients. Epidemiologic and animal studies have increasingly shown an association of cryptorchidism with intrauterine factors, including environmental exposure such as to endocrine-disrupting compounds.

CONCLUSION

The testis initially forms as an undifferentiated gonad that arises from the urogenital ridge. It is the activation of *SRY,* the sex-determining gene, that signals testis determination and development of the testis, internal reproductive tracts, and external genitalia along a male developmental pathway. The genetic and signaling pathways for testicular somatic and germ cell differentiation and genital development have been mapped, and many of the genes have been identified. Testicular and genital morphogenesis is complete by the end of the first trimester. Thereafter, the testis descends into the lower abdominal cavity by thickening of the caudally positioned gubernaculum and regression of the cranial suspensory ligament for the first phase of testicular descent. The second, inguinoscrotal phase occurs during the last trimester as the gubernaculum lengthens and the processus vaginalis forms into the scrotum to mediate movement of the testes into the scrotal sacs. Elucidation of the developmental process of testicular morphogenesis and descent provides insights into understanding the causes of cryptorchidism and may have relevance for pubertal and adult reproductive health.

A complete reference list is available at www.ExpertConsult.com. 

SELECT REFERENCES

1. Larney C, Bailey T, Koopman P. Switching on sex: transcriptional regulation of the testis-determining gene Sry. *Development*. 2014;141:2195.
2. Ono M, Harley V. Disorders of sex development: new genes, new concepts. *Nat Rev Endocrinol*. 2013;9:79–91.
3. Wilhelm D, Palmer S, Koopman P. Sex determination and gonadal development in mammals. *Physiol Rev*. 2007;87:1.
4. Makela JA, Koskenniemi JJ, Virtanen HE, et al. Testis development. *Endocrine Rev*. 2019;40:857.
5. Jost A. A new look at the mechanisms controlling sex differentiation in mammals. *Johns Hopkins Med J*. 1972;130:38.
6. Warr N, Greenfield A. The molecular and cellular basis of gonadal sex reversal in mice and humans. *Wiley Interdiscip Rev Dev Biol*. 2012;1:559.
7. Cederroth CR, Pitetti JL, Papaioannou MD, et al. Genetic programs that regulate testicular and ovarian development. *Mol Cell Endocrinol*. 2007;265:3.
8. Oosterhuis JW, Stoop H, Honecker F, et al. Why human extragonadal germ cell tumours occur in the midline of the body: old concepts, new perspectives. *Int J Androl*. 2007;30:256.
9. Achermann JC, Meeks JJ, Jameson JL. Phenotypic spectrum of mutations in DAX-1 and SF-1. *Mol Cell Endocrinol*. 2001;151:17.
10. Birk OS, Casiano DE, Wassif CA, et al. The LIM homeobox gene Lhx9 is essential for mouse gonad formation. *Nature*. 2000;403:909.
11. Bruening W, Bardeesy N, Silverman BL, et al. Germline intronic and exonic mutations in the Wilms' tumour gene (WT1) affecting urogenital development. *Nat Genet*. 1992;1:144.
12. Miyamoto N, Yoshida M, Kuratani S, et al. Defects of urogenital development in mice lacking Emx2. *Development*. 1997;124:1653.
13. Coppes MJ, Huff V, Pelletier J. Denys-Drash syndrome: relating a clinical disorder to genetic alterations in the tumor suppressor gene WT1. *J Pediatr*. 1993;123:673.
14. Little M, Wells C. A clinical overview of WT1 gene mutations. *Hum Mutat*. 1997;9:209.
15. Parker KL, Rice DA, Lala DS, et al. Steroidogenic factor 1: an essential mediator of endocrine development. *Recent Prog Horm Res*. 2002;57:19.
16. Sinclair AH, Berta P, Palmer MS, et al. A gene from the human sex-determining region encodes a protein with homology to a conserved DNA-binding motif. *Nature*. 1990;346:240.
17. Tachibana M. Epigenetic regulation of mammalian sex determination. *J Med Invest*. 2015;62:19.
18. Morais da Silva S, Hacker A, Harley V, et al. Sox9 expression during gonadal development implies a conserved role for the gene in testis differentiation in mammals and birds. *Nat Genet*. 1996;14:62.
19. Clarkson MJ, Harley VR. Sex with two SOX on: SRY and SOX9 in testis development. *Trends Endocrinol Metab*. 2002;13:106.
20. Foster JW, Dominguez-Steglich MA, Guioli S, et al. Campomelic dysplasia and autosomal sex reversal caused by mutations in an SRY-related gene. *Nature*. 1994;372:525.
21. Hawkins JR, Taylor A, Berta P, et al. Mutational analysis of SRY: nonsense and missense mutations in XY sex reversal. *Hum Genet*. 1992;88:471.
22. Wagner T, Wirth J, Meyer J, et al. Autosomal sex reversal and campomelic dysplasia are caused by mutations in and around the SRY-related gene SOX9. *Cell*. 1994;79:1111.
23. Clark AM, Garland KK, Russell LD. Desert hedgehog (Dhh) gene is required in the mouse testis for formation of adult-type Leydig cells and normal development of peritubular cells and seminiferous tubules. *Biol Reprod*. 2000;63:1825.
24. Yao HH, Whoriskey W, Capel B. Desert hedgehog/Patched 1 signaling specifies fetal Leydig cell fate in testis organogenesis. *Genes Dev*. 2002;16:1433.
25. Lin YT, Capel B. Cell fate commitment during mammalian sex determination. *Curr Opin Genet Dev*. 2015;1:144.
26. Tilmann C, Capel B. Mesonephric cell migration induces testis cord formation and Sertoli cell differentiation in the mammalian gonad. *Development*. 1999;126:2883.
27. Bendsen E, Byskov AG, Laursen SB, et al. Number of germ cells and somatic cells in human fetal testes during the first weeks after sex differentiation. *Hum Reprod*. 2003;18:13.
28. Torres M, Gomez-Pardo E, et al. Pax-2 controls multiple steps of urogenital development. *Development*. 1995;121:4057.
29. Lasala C, Carre-Eusebe D, Picard JY, et al. Subcellular and molecular mechanisms regulating anti-Mullerian hormone gene expression in mammalian and nonmammalian species. *DNA Cell Biol*. 2004;23:572.
30. Visser JA. AMH signaling: from receptor to target gene. *Mol Cell Endocrinol*. 2003;211:65.
31. Teixeira J, Maheswaran S, Donahoe PK. Mullerian inhibiting substance: an instructive developmental hormone with diagnostic and possible therapeutic applications. *Endocr Rev*. 2001;22:657.
32. Xavier F, Allard S. Anti-Mullerian hormone, beta-catenin and Mullerian duct regression. *Mol Cell Endocrinol*. 2003;211:115.
33. Teerds K, Huhtaniemi I. Morphological and functional maturation of Leydig cells: from rodent models to primates. *Hum Reprod Update*. 2015;0:1-19.
34. Majdic G, Saunders PT, Teerds KJ. Immunoexpression of the steroidogenic enzymes 3-beta hydroxysteroid dehydrogenase and 17 alpha-hydroxylase, C17,20 lyase and the receptor for luteinizing hormone (LH) in the fetal rat testis suggests that the onset of Leydig cell steroid production is independent of LH action. *Biol Reprod*. 1998;58:520.
35. Migrenne S, Pairault C, Racine C, et al. Luteinizing hormone-dependent activity and luteinizing hormone-independent differentiation of rat fetal Leydig cells. *Mol Cell Endocrinol*. 2001;172:193.
36. Bielinska M, Seehra A, Toppari J, et al. GATA-4 is required for sex steroidogenic cell development in the fetal mouse. *Dev Dyn*. 2007;236:203.
37. Wu X, Wan S, Lee MM. Key factors in the regulation of fetal and postnatal Leydig cell development. *J Cell Physiol*. 2007;213:429.
38. Abney TO. The potential roles of estrogens in regulating Leydig cell development and function: a review. *Steroids*. 1999;64:610.
39. Rey R, Lukas-Croisier C, Lasala C, et al. AMH/MIS: what we know already about the gene, the protein and its regulation. *Mol Cell Endocrinol*. 2003;211:21.
40. Forest MG, Sizonenko PC, Cathiard AM, et al. Hypophyso-gonadal function in humans during the first year of life. 1. Evidence for testicular activity in early infancy. *Clin Res*. 1974;53:819.
41. Muller J, Skakkebaek NE. Quantification of germ cells and seminiferous tubules by stereological examination of testicles from 50 boys who suffered from sudden death. *Int J Androl*. 1983;6:143.
42. Hilscher B, Engemann A. Histological and morphometric studies on the kinetics of germ cells and immature Sertoli cells during human prespermatogenesis. *Andrologia*. 1992;24:7.
43. Clermont Y. Kinetics of spermatogenesis in mammals: seminiferous epithelium cycle and spermatogonial renewal. *Physiol Rev*. 1972;52:198.
44. Hadziselimovic F, Herzog B. The importance of both an early orchidopexy and germ cell maturation for fertility. *Lancet*. 2001;358:1156.
45. Petersen C, Soder O. The sertoli cell—a hormonal target and 'super' nurse for germ cells that determines testicular size. *Horm Res*. 2006;66:153.
46. Lee MM, Donahoe PK, Hasegawa T, et al. Mullerian inhibiting substance in humans: normal levels from infancy to adulthood. *J Clin Endocrinol Metab*. 1996;81:571.
47. Wu X, Arumugam R, Baker SP, et al. Pubertal and adult Leydig cell function in Mullerian inhibiting substance-deficient mice. *Endocrinology*. 2005;146:589.
48. de Kretser DM, Buzzard JJ, Okuma Y, et al. The role of activin, follistatin and inhibin in testicular physiology. *Mol Cell Endocrinol*. 2004;225:57.
49. Wong CH, Cheng CY. The blood-testis barrier: its biology, regulation, and physiological role in spermatogenesis. *Curr Top Dev Biol*. 2005;71:263.
50. Lui WY, Cheng CY. Regulation of cell junction dynamics by cytokines in the testis: a molecular and biochemical perspective. *Cytokine Growth Factor Rev*. 2007;18:299.

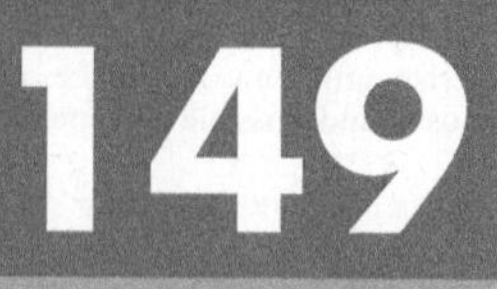

149 The Pathophysiology of Twin-Twin Transfusion Syndrome, Twin-Anemia Polycythemia Sequence, and Twin-Reversed Arterial Perfusion

Christoph Wohlmuth

INTRODUCTION

Twin pregnancies account for 3.7% of all births in the United States, and the incidence has increased over the past decades.[1] From a developmental and genetic perspective, twins are characterized either as *dizygotic*, arising from two eggs fertilized by two different sperm, or *monozygotic*, resulting from the division of one zygote, whereby both halves generally carry the same genetic information and are of the same sex.[2,3]

From a (patho)physiologic and management perspective, however, it is more important to determine chorionicity and amniocity (Fig. 149.1).[4-6] Dizygotic twins are generally dichorionic-diamniotic (DCDA). In monozygotic twins, it depends on the timing of separation: (1) if separation occurs early, the embryos are DCDA; (2) with later separation, the inner cell mass has already formed, resulting in monochorionic-diamniotic (MCDA) embryos that share a common placenta; (3) if the separation occurs after the amnion has been formed, the embryos are monochorionic-monoamniotic (MCMA); and (4) in the rare case where splitting occurs even later—after the embryonic disc has formed—conjoined twins result.[2,3]

THE PHYSIOLOGY AND PATHOPHYSIOLOGY OF THE PLACENTAL CIRCULATION

In monochorionic twin pregnancies, only one placenta comprising two vascular beds is formed. It has been shown that more than 95% of all monochorionic pregnancies have placental vascular anastomoses that connect the fetal circulations.[7-10] It has been shown that more than 95% of all monochorionic pregnancies have placental vascular anastomoses that connect the circulations of the two fetuses; these can be arteriovenous (AV), arterioarterial (AA) or veno-venous (VV)[6-10] (Fig. 149.2).

AA and VV anastomoses are typically superficial on the chorionic plate, although partially hidden anastomoses have been reported in 3% to 5%.[11] These end-to-end anastomoses allow blood flow in both directions.[6,11] Placental injection studies have shown that an AA anastomosis is present in more than 90% of uncomplicated pregnancies, and these are thought to compensate for hemodynamic imbalances from AV anastomoses.[12]

VV anastomoses are present in only around 20% of MCDA placentas.[7,13] Their role is not fully clarified. Although an increase in perinatal mortality and MCDA complications has been reported by some, others have found that VV anastomoses may equilibrate pressure differences, and their presence may protect from volume overload.[7,14-16]

In contrast to these superficial connections, AV anastomoses are formed when a cotyledon is supplied by an artery of one twin and blood is drained through a vein of the other twin, permitting only unidirectional blood flow.[6,7] The majority of monochorionic placentas have a combination of (several) AV anastomoses and superficial (AA, VV) anastomoses.[17]

The occurrence of placental anastomoses and their specific constellation is associated with complications unique to monochorionic pregnancies. When AV anastomoses permit unidirectional flow that is not compensated by other anastomoses, fluid is shifted chronically from one fetal circulation to its twin's circulation. On the other hand, bidirectional (AA and VV) anastomoses may permit drastic fluid shifts during brief episodes of bradycardia or hypotension of one fetus, where a large volume may be shifted from the fetus with the normal circulation to the bradycardic/hypotensive fetus within a short period of time, potentially leading to brain injury or single/dual fetal demise.[6,18]

THE PATHOPHYSIOLOGY OF TWIN-TWIN TRANSFUSION SYNDROME

Chronic net transfusion of fluid from one fetus to its twin through AV anastomoses that is not compensated by AA anastomoses or oppositely directed AV anastomoses causes hypervolemia in one (the "recipient" fetus) and hypovolemia in the other (the "donor" fetus). This triggers a cascade of events in both twins that ultimately result in twin-twin transfusion syndrome (TTTS), a complication that occurs in approximately 10% of all MCDA twin pregnancies.[19] TTTS typically occurs in midtrimester, between 16 and 26 weeks of gestation.[20]

The fluid overload in the recipient causes cardiac stretch, resulting in the secretion of atrial and b-type natriuretic peptides. These increase the glomerular filtration rate, decrease tubular reabsorption, and thereby foster polyuria and polyhydramnios.[6,21-23]

In the donor fetus, hypovolemia results in centralization of the circulation and hypoperfusion of the kidneys. This activates the renin-angiotensin-aldosterone system (RAAS), as shown by increased renin mRNA expression in donor kidneys.[24,25] In turn, angiotensin II is secreted to maintain the blood pressure in the volume-depleted donor circulation. In addition, aldosterone is secreted in response to renin and increases the tubular

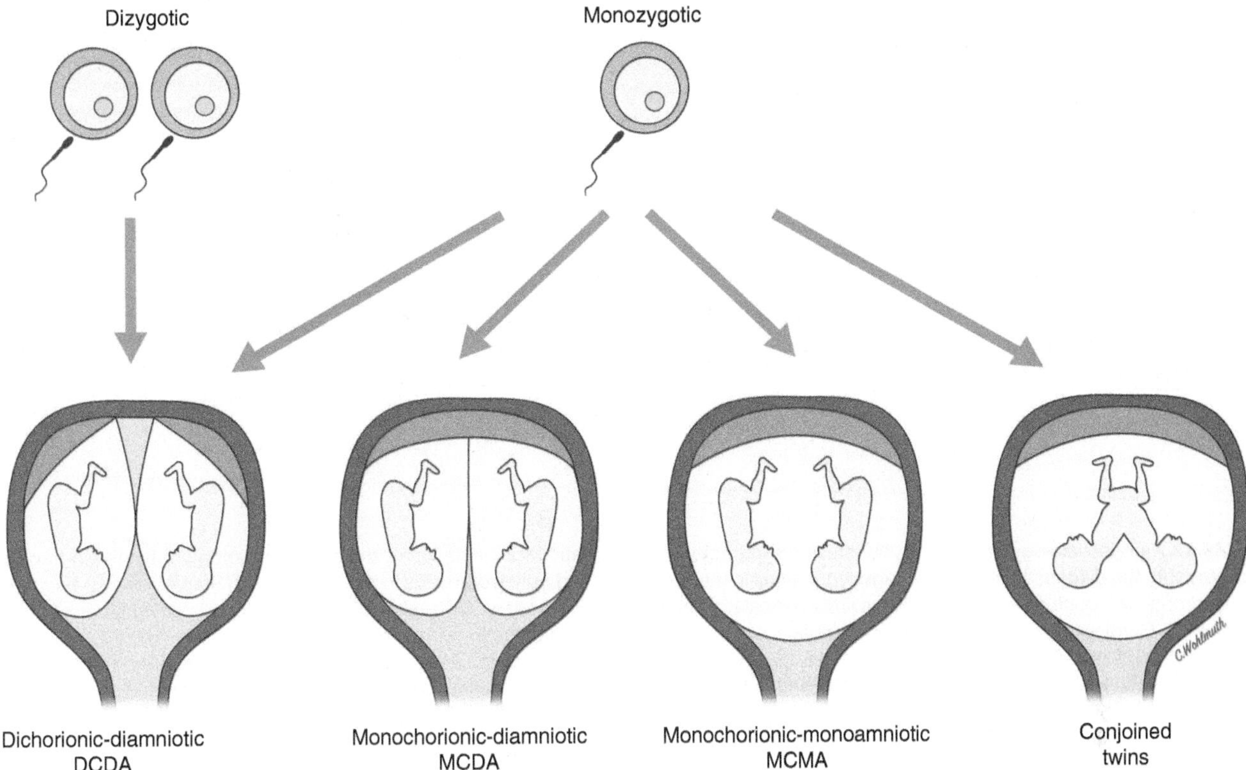

Fig. 149.1 Monozygotic and dizygotic twinning. The relations between zygosity and chorionicity/amniocity are shown. Dizygotic twins are generally dichorionic-diamniotic *(DCDA)*. Monozygotic twins can be DCDA, monochorionic-diamniotic *(MCDA)*, monochorionic-monoamniotic *(MCMA)*, or rarely conjoined.

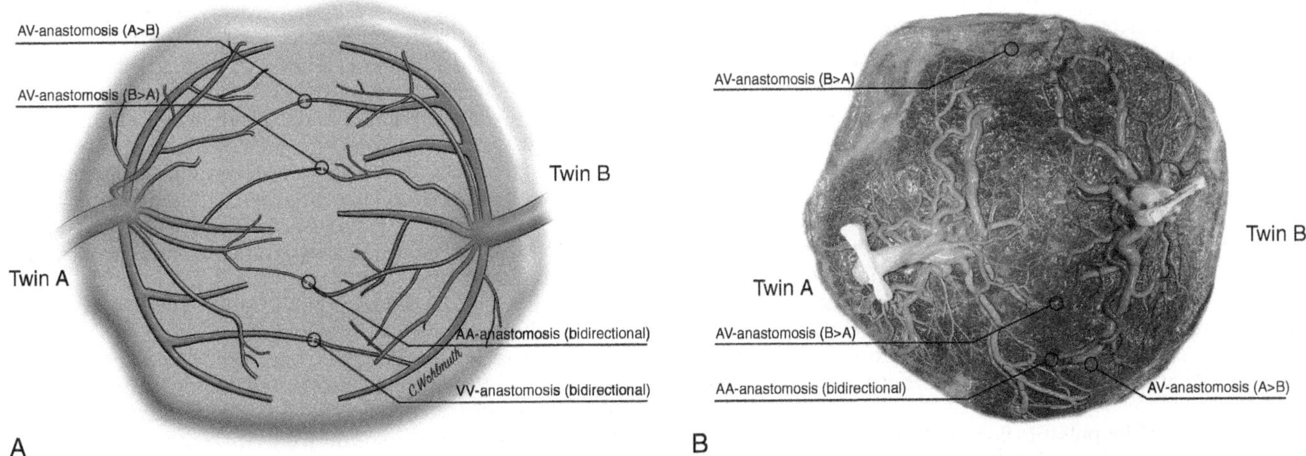

Fig. 149.2 Placental vascular anastomoses. (A) Schematic representation of a monochorionic placenta. More than 95% of all monochorionic placentas show anastomoses along the vascular equator, which can be bidirectional (arterio-arterial *[AA]* and venovenous *[VV]*) or unidirectional (arteriovenous *[AV]*). (B) Postnatal placental injection study of a monochorionic pregnancy delivered at 37 weeks of gestation in a pregnancy without complications. *A>B*, Flow from twin A to B; *B>A*, flow from twin B to A.

reabsorption of sodium and fluid, which—in combination with the renal hypoperfusion—results in oliguria and oligohydramnios.[25,26] Polyhydramnios in the recipient and oligohydramnios in the donor is sometimes referred to as twin-oligo-polyhydramnios sequence (TOPS) and constitute the diagnostic criterion for TTTS. This is usually quantified by measuring the deepest vertical pocket of amniotic fluid for both fetuses. Most centers use a cutoff of 2 cm or less for oligohydramnios and 8 cm or more for polyhydramnios independent of gestational age.[4]

In the recipient kidney, the RAAS system is downregulated as a result of the hypervolemia, with virtually no mRNA expression found in immunohistochemical studies.[24] However, when renin levels are measured in the umbilical cord, they are elevated in both the recipient and the donor. This provides evidence that renin is transferred from the donor to the recipient via placental vascular anastomoses.[25,27,28] The continuing shift of volume and vasoactive mediators aggravates the circulation of both the recipient and donor, resulting in a vicious cycle that can cause renal failure in the donor, heart failure, hydrops, and ultimately fetal demise for one or both twins. Quintero developed a staging system based on a hypothetical sequence of observed events that continues to be used, although it has been shown

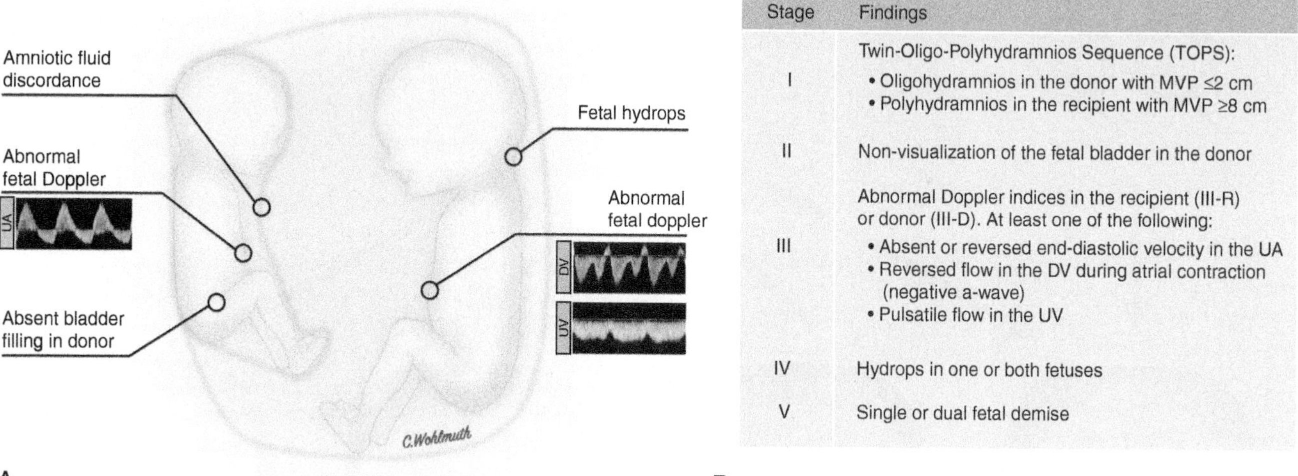

Stage	Findings
I	Twin-Oligo-Polyhydramnios Sequence (TOPS): • Oligohydramnios in the donor with MVP ≤2 cm • Polyhydramnios in the recipient with MVP ≥8 cm
II	Non-visualization of the fetal bladder in the donor
III	Abnormal Doppler indices in the recipient (III-R) or donor (III-D). At least one of the following: • Absent or reversed end-diastolic velocity in the UA • Reversed flow in the DV during atrial contraction (negative a-wave) • Pulsatile flow in the UV
IV	Hydrops in one or both fetuses
V	Single or dual fetal demise

Fig. 149.3 Pathophysiology of twin-twin transfusion syndrome. (A) Schematic representation of the pathophysiology of twin-twin transfusion syndrome with the diagnostic criterion of oligohydramnios in the donor twin and polyhydramnios in the recipient. (B) Staging of twin-twin transfusion syndrome *DV*, Ductus venosus; *MVP*, maximal vertical pocket; *UA*, umbilical artery; *UV*, umbilical vein. (A, Reproduced with permission from Wohlmuth C, Gardiner HM, Diehl W, Hecher KF, et al. Cardiovascular hemodynamics in twin-twin transfusion syndrome. *Acta Obstet Gynecol Scand.* 2016;95[6]:664–671. https://doi.org/10.1111/aogs.12871. B, Based on the suggested sequence of events by Quintero RA, Morales WJ, Allen MH, Bornick PW, Johnson PK, Kruger M. Staging of twin-twin transfusion syndrome. *J Perinatol.* 1999;19[8 Pt 1]:550–555.)

that TTTS does not necessarily follow this sequence. Although regression of stage I occurs in more than 40% of cases, stages can be skipped and hydrops and fetal demise can develop rapidly (Fig. 149.3).[29-31]

CARDIOVASCULAR HEMODYNAMICS IN TWIN-TWIN TRANSFUSION SYNDROME

Abnormal echocardiographic findings can be observed in up to 70% of all recipients with TTTS.[32] These pathologic changes include altered preload and afterload as well as compromised cardiac function.[33-35]

With the chronic volume shift across placental anastomoses, the venous flow in the recipient's umbilical vein increases and the venous compartment accommodates large amounts of the increased intravascular volume.[36] The ductus venosus (DV) connects the intra-abdominal umbilical vein to the inferior vena cava at its inlet to the heart.[37,38] Its trumpet-shaped geometry and narrow configuration result in the acceleration of blood and phasic flow patterns that provide information on cardiac preload and atrial pressure-volume changes during the cardiac cycle.[37-40]

Assessment of the pulsatile flow in the DV using the pulsatility index for veins (PIV) or qualitatively grading flow during atrial contraction (forward/absent/reversed a-wave) is an established standard of clinical practice to predict adverse perinatal outcome. More recently, however, parameters for DV time intervals have been developed to refine the assessment of pressure-volume changes (Fig. 149.4).[33,41]

A study has shown that findings of abnormal cardiac filling and volume overload were present in future recipients even before the diagnostic criteria of TTTS were met. The use of DV time intervals could identify pregnancies that developed TTTS with a sensitivity of 73% and a specificity of 67% when used as an isolated parameter.[33] The traditional sign of absent or reversed flow in the a-wave of the DV was present only in advanced disease stages.[33] Diastolic dysfunction usually occurs earlier and is more pronounced than systolic dysfunction.[6] Monophasic ventricular filling with fusion of E and A waves is observed in 20% to 30%, often with a significant shortening of the ventricular filling time resulting from increased ventricular pressure. This can cause atrioventricular valve regurgitation, which is observed in 23% of recipients in early-stage and 50% of advanced-stage TTTS.[6,34,42-44] In addition, the isovolumic relaxation time is prolonged, thereby increasing the myocardial performance (Tei) index, a sign of abnormal global cardiac function.[34,45,46]

Studies using tissue Doppler imaging of the recipient heart have confirmed that signs of elevated ventricular filling pressures are evident at early stages of TTTS.[34] During fetal life, the ventricles operate physiologically near the Frank-Starling limit[38]; with increasing severity of TTTS, systolic function is reduced.[34] This was confirmed by studies assessing long-axis function and ventricular speckle tracking techniques revealing reduced cardiac contractility in recipients with TTTS.[19,47] In severe cases cardiac function can deteriorate and lead to functional pulmonary atresia and heart failure.[6]

As outlined in the last section, TTTS is not merely a condition of fluid shift from one fetus to the other. The pathophysiology is much more complex, where the donor releases vasoactive mediators in response to protracted hypovolemia, mediators that are transferred to the recipient through vascular anastomoses. It was hypothesized that the combination of hypervolemia and vasoactive mediators results in significant hypertension in the recipient.[6,35] However, owing to the lack of accessibility to fetal blood pressure, this could not be directly proven. Two studies have suggested increased intraventricular pressures measured from peak velocities of atrioventricular valve regurgitation jets using the modified Bernoulli equation.[34,48] More recently, aortic fractional area change (AFAC), a measure of the aortic distension waveform, has been used as a surrogate for pulse pressure. Invasive fetal lamb models have shown that increased distensibility reflects a higher pulse pressure amplitude and blood pressure.[49,50] A study of monochorionic twin pregnancies has shown that AFAC was significantly increased in recipients and reduced in donor twins, whereas no intertwin pair differences were seen in a control group of uncomplicated monochorionic pregnancies. AFAC correlated with left and right ventricular filling pressures, and cardiac output correlated positively with AFAC when

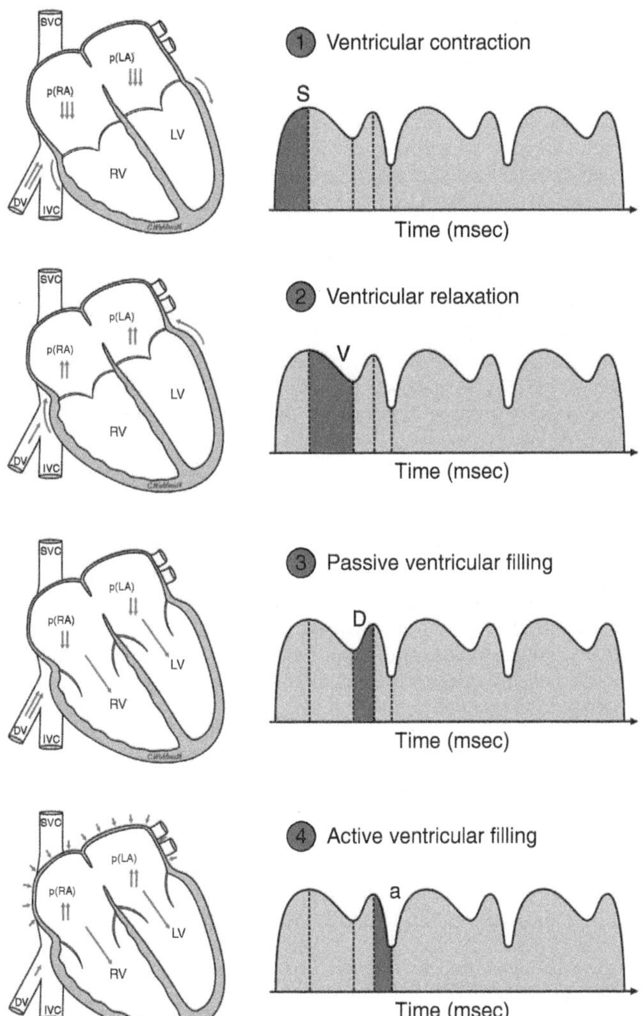

Fig. 149.4 Ductus venosus reflecting the pressure-volume changes of the fetal heart. The phasic flow profile of the ductus venosus reflects the ventricular contraction *(S)*, ventricular relaxation *(V)*, and passive *(D)* and active ventricular filling *(a)*. The base of the heart descends with ventricular contraction. This causes a pressure drop in the atria, resulting in the acceleration of flow in the ductus venosus *(DV)* (S). During ventricular relaxation, the base ascends, resulting in a relative atrial pressure increase and a decrease in forward flow in the DV (V). The opening of the atrioventricular valves results in a rapid decrease in atrial pressure, causing a second acceleration of the DV flow (D). Finally, atrial contraction augments and completes ventricular filling and causes increased atrial pressure, resulting in the second and more pronounced decrease in DV flow (a). *IVC*, Inferior vena cava; *LV*, left ventricle; *p(LA)*, pressure in the left atrium; *p(RA)*, pressure in the right atrium; *RV*, right ventricle.

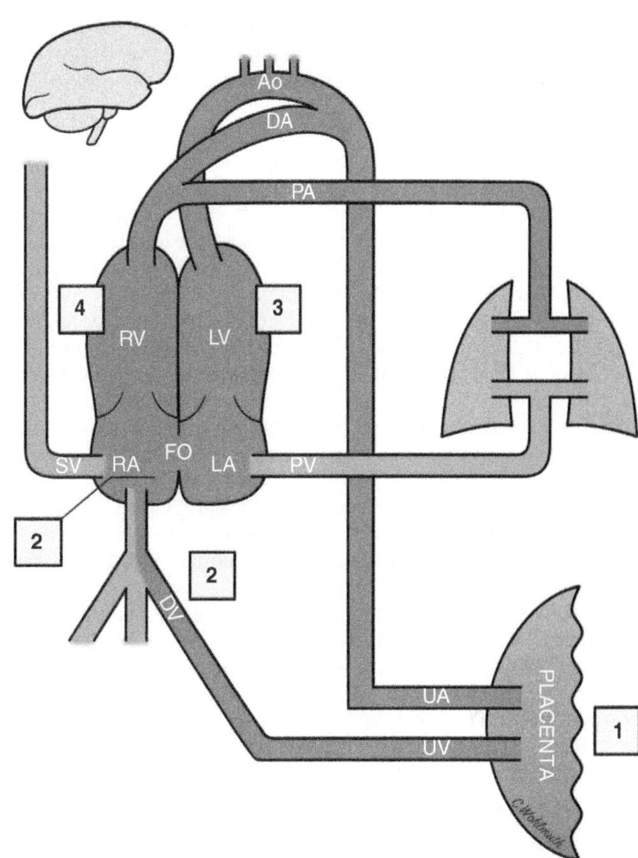

Fig. 149.5 Recipient pathophysiology in twin-twin transfusion syndrome. Proposed pathophysiology of twin-twin transfusion syndrome in the recipient twin. *(1)* Vasoactive factors and fluid are transferred from the donor through vascular anastomoses and cause increased recipient blood pressure. *(2)* Altered ductus venosus *(DV)* filling times and decreased right-to-left shunting are observed. *(3)* Altered ventricular function and, ultimately, *(4)* bilateral atrioventricular valve regurgitation and ventricular hypertrophy are seen, which can lead to functional pulmonary atresia in extreme cases of cardiac dysfunction. *Ao*, Aorta; *DA*, ductus arteriosus; *FO*, foramen ovale; *LA*, left atrium; *PA*, pulmonary arteries; *PV*, pulmonary veins; *RA*, right atrium; *RV*, right ventricle; *SVC*, superior vena cava; *UA*, umbilical artery; *UV*, umbilical vein. (Reproduced and modified with permission from Wohlmuth C, Boudreaux D, Moise KJ, et al. Cardiac pathophysiology in twin-twin transfusion syndrome: new insights into its evolution. *Ultrasound Obstet. Gynecol.* 2018;51[3]:341–348. doi:10.1002/uog.17480.)

AFAC was in physiologic ranges; however, it became negative when it exceeded 70%, similar to a Frank-Starling response.[35] Interestingly, the intertwin differences in AFAC, and therefore blood pressure, were present at the early stages of TTTS. These findings are supported by observations of increased umbilical cord coiling seen during fetoscopy and quantified by ultrasound. Increased intravascular pressure in the umbilical arteries may lead to arterial lengthening and hypercoiling.[51] A summary of the proposed pathophysiology of the recipient twin in twin-twin transfusion syndrome is shown in Fig. 149.5.

Although the recipient twin shows evident signs of cardiovascular distress even at early stages of TTTS, donors usually have normal echocardiographic parameters at the time of diagnosis. Approximately 10% to 15% show abnormal peripheral Doppler waveforms, depending on the disease stage.[34,44] As a result of hypovolemia, the inlet of the DV dilates and allows more shunting of blood through it. This promotes increased transmission of the pulse wave into the umbilical vein, which may become apparent as umbilical venous pulsations.[37] Unequal placental sharing in combination with hemodynamic imbalance may cause absence or reversal of end-diastolic velocities in the umbilical artery.[44]

IMPACT OF LASER SURGERY ON CARDIOVASCULAR PATHOPHYSIOLOGY

If left untreated, TTTS is associated with a mortality of 80% to 100%.[52] Before the invention of fetoscopy, serial amnioreductions were performed to remove excess amniotic fluid from the recipient's amniotic cavity. This alleviated maternal symptoms of excess polyhydramnios, decreased the risk of premature contractions, and hypothetically improved placental blood flow by decreasing the pressure on the chorionic plate.[6]

Fetoscopic laser photocoagulation (FLP) disrupts the underlying pathophysiology and treats the cause rather than the symptoms of TTTS. A randomized controlled trial directly comparing serial amnioreduction to FLP showed significantly improved survival and better neurologic outcome for pregnancies treated by FLP.[53] FLP has now become the standard of care for the treatment of TTTS stages II through IV, whereas its role in stage I remains unclear and the results of a separate randomized controlled trial are awaited.[54,55] Timely FLP can result in the survival of at least one twin in 87% and dual survival in 69% of pregnancies with TTTS.[56]

Studies comparing echocardiographic parameters before and after FLP have shown that cardiovascular readaptation occurs within days after the procedure.[34,46,57,58] Recipient cardiac contractility and global cardiac function significantly improve after FLP[34,46]; with improved systolic function and reduced afterload, normalization of functional pulmonary atresia can be observed.[6,34,58]

In the donor, the weight-corrected umbilical venous flow is increased by more than 50% within 48 hours of FLP and increased ventricular filling pressures can be measured by tissue Doppler.[34,59] The rapid increase in preload may result in increased DV pulsatility and transient hydrops that are sometimes observed after FLP.[59,60] With increased preload, improved combined cardiac output can be seen in ex-donor fetuses.[34]

LONG-TERM IMPLICATIONS FOR THE CARDIOVASCULAR SYSTEM

With the implementation of FLP, the duration of disease in utero was significantly shortened compared with serial amnioreduction, where TTTS was sometimes managed for weeks. Therefore the impact on the cardiovascular system seems to have decreased compared with the early reports of myocardial hypertrophy, severe tricuspid regurgitation, and pulmonary valve stenosis requiring postnatal balloon valvuloplasty.[48,61,62] Long-term follow-up studies 10 years after delivery have been reassuring, with only mild alterations in diastolic function.[63,64] However, obstruction of the right ventricular outflow tract is overrepresented, affecting up to 10% of children after TTTS.[63] Therefore long-term follow-up and targeted echocardiography are warranted.

THE PATHOPHYSIOLOGY OF TWIN-ANEMIA-POLYCYTHEMIA SEQUENCE

Twin-anemia-polycythemia sequence (TAPS) is a complication in monochorionic pregnancies that is characterized by a marked intertwin hemoglobin difference. It develops from unbalanced transfusion through minuscule AV anastomoses, leading to anemia in the donor and polycythemia in the recipient.[65,66] Unlike the case in TTTS, the transfusion occurs slowly, with modeled blood flow between 5 and 15 mL per 24 hours through the anastomoses.[66,67] The slower rate of transfusion may allow for hemodynamic equilibration, likely explaining the lack of oligohydramnios and polyhydramnios that is characteristic for TTTS.[68]

TAPS can develop spontaneously in 3% to 5% of monochorionic pregnancies or may arise iatrogenically following incomplete ablation of placental vascular anastomoses in 2% to 16% of laser photocoagulations performed for TTTS.[66] The prenatal diagnosis is based on the blood velocimetry of the middle cerebral artery (MCA), which is also used to diagnose hemolytic anemia.[69] An increased peak systolic velocity of the MCA has been shown to be predictive of anemia in TAPS.[70,71] A diagnostic cutoff of the MCA peak systolic velocity of 1.5 multiples of the median (MoM) or greater in the anemic and 0.8 MoM or less in the polycythemic twin was originally suggested as a diagnostic criterion and recently agreed to by leading experts using a Delphi procedure.[72,73] However, studies have shown that sensitivity and specificity are improved when an intertwin difference of 0.5 MoM or greater, rather than the previously mentioned criteria, is used.[74,75]

With increasing severity of TAPS, the donor becomes progressively more anemic. This can result in an increasing cardiac output and ultimately high-output cardiac failure. A recent study has found cardiomegaly in 40% of early-stage TAPS. In addition, placental dichotomy, which is thought to represent placental edema, was observed with increasing severity.[76] More severe disease stages can result in abnormal fetal Doppler flow profiles, hydrops, and single or dual fetal demise.[66] In the recipient, polycythemia may lead to hyperviscosity syndrome, and rare cases of skin necrosis and cerebral injury from severe polycythemia have been reported.[72,77]

Randomized trials are lacking, and there is no universal agreement on the optimal management of TAPS.[73] Although expectant management for mild cases and preterm delivery for TAPS in advanced gestational age seem to be reasonable options, intrauterine transfusions (IUTs), FLP, and selective feticide can be considered in more severe cases encountered at earlier gestational ages.[78,79] Although it is technically the same, laser surgery is more challenging in TAPS owing to the absence of polyhydramnios and the presence of minuscule anastomoses that are harder to visualize. IUTs are not a causal treatment and may have to be repeated during pregnancy. In addition, IUTs can worsen recipient polycythemia, which may be reduced by performing a partial exchange in the recipient.[79] The required transfusion volume (VT) and exchange volume can be calculated using the following formulas[79]:

Anemic Twin

$$VT = CBV \times \frac{F_{Htc} - I_{Htc}}{PRBC_{Htc}}$$

$$CBV = EFW_{Ultrasound} \times 150$$

CBV, Circulating blood volume; $PRBC_{Htc}$, hematocrit of packed red blood cell unit; $EFW_{Ultrasound}$, estimated fetal weight in kilograms measured by ultrasound; F_{Htc}, desired final hematocrit (ideally 40%); I_{Htc}, anemic twin's initial hematocrit.

Polycythemic Twin

$$EV = CBV \times \frac{C_{Htc} - D_{Htc}}{C_{Htc}}$$

$$CBV = EFW_{Ultrasound} \times 150$$

CBV, Circulating blood volume; C_{Htc}, current hematocrit of the polycythemic twin; D_{Htc}, desired hematocrit (ideally 50%); $EFW_{Ultrasound}$, estimated fetal weight in kilograms as measured by ultrasound.

Postnatally, TAPS is diagnosed by an intertwin hemoglobin difference of 8 g/dL or greater and intertwin reticulocyte ratio of 1.7 or greater.[66,73] Although data are still limited, TAPS seems to be associated with significant risks of neurodevelopmental impairment, especially in the ex-donors.[80]

THE PATHOPHYSIOLOGY OF TWIN REVERSED ARTERIAL PERFUSION

Twin reversed arterial perfusion (TRAP) is a distinctive complication unique to monochorionic pregnancies. Reports suggest that TRAP complicates 1% to 3% of all monochorionic twin pregnancies.[81,82] Although the exact initiating mechanisms remain unknown, the presence of an AA and a VV anastomosis is a prerequisite. A hemodynamic advantage arises for one twin (pump twin), causing a reversal of the circulation in the second twin. Thereby the pump twin perfuses the other twin with deoxygenated blood through an AA anastomosis and its umbilical artery in a reverse manner (Fig. 149.6). This allows the perfused twin's body to grow despite the lack of important cardiac activity.[83] It is hypothesized that the lower oxygen saturation contributes to the serious derangement of normal organogenesis and growth and may lead to the characteristic amorphous and bizarre appearance of the acardiac twin.[83]

The pump twin is often morphologically and genetically normal (although a 9% risk for chromosomal abnormalities has been described in a small series[84]) and shows normal growth and development during the first trimester. However, while the fetus maintains its own circulation, increasing cardiac output is required to supply the growing acardiac mass. Thus the pump twin is exposed to a significant risk of high-output cardiovascular failure. If left untreated, the mortality for TRAP can be as high as 50%.[82] Echocardiographic studies in pump twins have shown that the global heart size is increased and atrioventricular valve regurgitation is commonly observed. Indexed cardiac output was used in an attempt to identify fetuses at high risk for cardiovascular compromise and unfavorable outcome.[85,86] However, measured cardiac output is a rather crude estimate of the true cardiac output, as it is based on the diameter of the semilunar valves and the velocity-time integral of the outflow Doppler and heart rate; moreover, the first two parameters are prone to measurement errors during fetal echocardiography.[87] Van Gemert and colleagues have developed a mathematical model using diameter measurements of the umbilical vein that reflect the excess cardiac output required to perfuse the acardiac twin.[88] Although this model was tested in a small series of fetuses with TRAP and sacrococcygeal teratoma, its prospective validation is pending.[89,90] TRAP can be successfully treated by interrupting the blood flow to the perfused twin with minimally invasive techniques using radiofrequency ablation (RFA), bipolar cord occlusion (BCO), or interstitial laser, leading to a significant reduction in mortality.[82,91–97] A systematic review and meta-analysis on RFA versus BCO has shown that overall survival is very similar for the two procedures.[98] Studies have shown that the interruption of blood flow to the acardiac twin leads to normalization of the high-output state, and cases with resolution of hydrops fetalis have been reported.[93,95,96] The current surgical approaches, despite their minimally invasive nature, are performed at the expense of iatrogenic complications in the pump twin, including preterm premature rupture of membranes and preterm delivery.[98] Therefore patient selection and timing of the intervention remain critical but as yet unanswered questions. The TRAPIST trial, a multicenter randomized controlled trial comparing early versus late intervention in TRAP, is recruiting patients as of 2020.[99]

CONCLUSION

Monochorionic pregnancies are unique in that the fetal circulations are connected through placental vascular anastomoses that permit the transfer of fluid and substances from one fetus to its twin. In the majority of pregnancies, this exchange remains balanced. Unbalanced transfer can lead to TTTS, TAPS, and TRAP, all of which are associated with significant morbidity and mortality. A profound understanding of the underlying pathophysiology can facilitate early detection and guide timely treatment.

A complete reference list is available at www.ExpertConsult.com. 

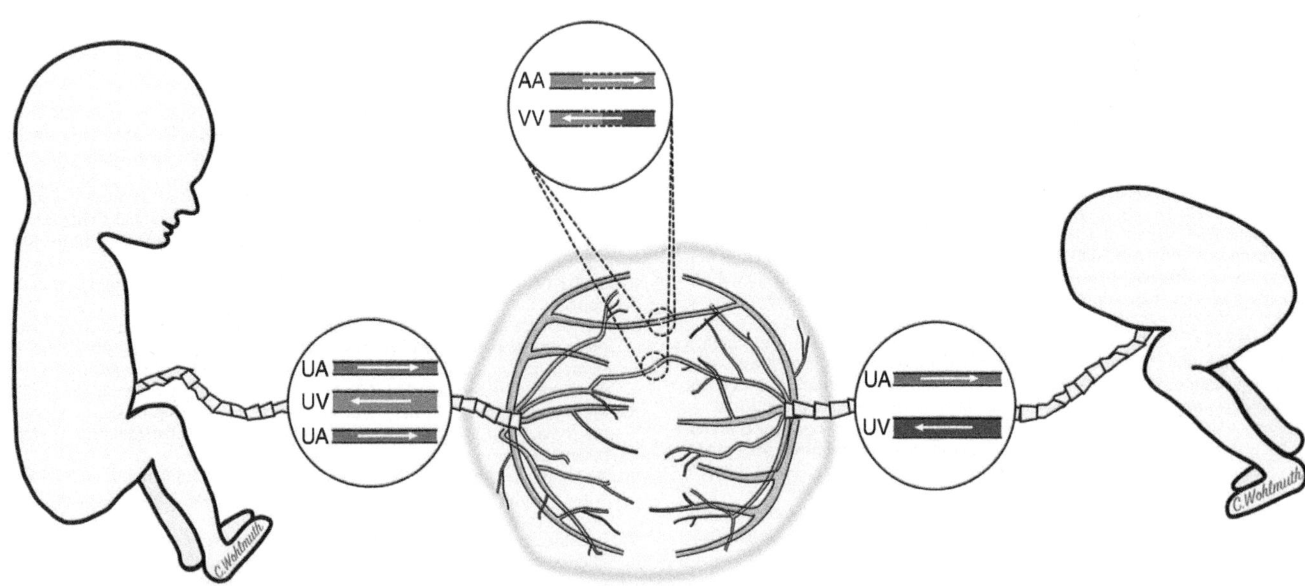

Fig. 149.6 Pathophysiology of twin reversed arterial perfusion. Schematic representation of the pathophysiology of twin reversed arterial perfusion with regular antegrade perfusion of the pump twin's circulation and no (relevant) cardiac activity in the acardiac twin. The pump twin perfuses the acardiac twin with deoxygenated blood through an arterio-arterial anastomosis. In the acardiac twin, the circulation is reversed, with blood flow through the umbilical arteries allowing the perfused twin's body to grow. The further deoxygenated blood is transferred retrograde through the venous system and the umbilical vein through a venovenous (*VV*) anastomosis back to the pump twin. *AA*, Arterio-arterial anastomosis; *UA*, umbilical artery; *UV*, umbilical vein.

SELECT REFERENCES

2. Hall JG. Developmental biology IV twinning. *Lancet*. 2003;362:735–743. https://doi.org/10.1016/S0140-6736(03)14237-7.
4. Khalil A, Rodgers M, Baschat A, et al. ISUOG Practice Guidelines: role of ultrasound in twin pregnancy. *Ultrasound Obstet Gynecol*. 2016;47(2):247–263. https://doi.org/10.1002/uog.15821.
5. Committee on Practice Bulletins—Obstetrics, Society for Maternal–Fetal Medicine. Practice bulletin No. 169: multifetal gestations: twin, triplet, and higher-order multifetal pregnancies. *Obstet Gynecol*. 2016;128(4):e131–e146. https://doi.org/10.1097/AOG.0000000000001709.
6. Wohlmuth C, Gardiner HM, Diehl W, Hecher K. Fetal cardiovascular hemodynamics in twin-twin transfusion syndrome. *Acta Obstet Gynecol Scand*. 2016;95(6):664–671. https://doi.org/10.1111/aogs.12871.
7. Denbow ML, Cox P, Taylor M, Hammal DM, Fisk NM. Placental angioarchitecture in monochorionic twin pregnancies: relationship to fetal growth, fetofetal transfusion syndrome, and pregnancy outcome. *Am J Obstet Gynecol*. 2000;182(2):417–426. https://doi.org/10.1016/S0002-9378(00)70233-X.
10. Wohlmuth C. Placental anastomoses in a spontaneous monochorionic-triamniotic triplet pregnancy. *Am J Obstet Gynecol*. 2019;221(3):280. https://doi.org/10.1016/j.ajog.2019.01.207.
17. Lewi L, Cannie M, Blickstein I, et al. Placental sharing, birthweight discordance, and vascular anastomoses in monochorionic diamniotic twin placentas. *Am J Obstet Gynecol*. 2007;197(6):587.e1–e8. https://doi.org/10.1016/j.ajog.2007.05.009.
18. Lewi L, Deprest J, Hecher K. The vascular anastomoses in monochorionic twin pregnancies and their clinical consequences. *Am J Obstet Gynecol*. 2013;208(1):19–30. https://doi.org/10.1016/j.ajog.2012.09.025.
19. Wohlmuth C, Agarwal A, Stevens B, et al. Fetal ventricular strain in uncomplicated and selective growth-restricted monochorionic diamniotic twin pregnancies and cardiovascular response in pre-twin-twin transfusion syndrome. *Ultrasound Obstet Gynecol*. 2020;56(5):694–704. https://doi.org/10.1002/uog.21911.
25. Mahieu-Caputo D, Muller F, Joly D, et al. Pathogenesis of twin-twin transfusion syndrome: the renin-angiotensin system hypothesis. *Fetal Diagn Ther*. 2001;16(4):241–244. https://doi.org/10.1159/000053919.
28. Galea P, Barigye O, Wee L, Jain V, Sullivan M, Fisk NM. The placenta contributes to activation of the renin angiotensin system in twin-twin transfusion syndrome. *Placenta*. 2008;29(8):734–742. https://doi.org/10.1016/j.placenta.2008.04.010.
29. Quintero RA, Morales WJ, Allen MH, Bornick PW, Johnson PK, Kruger M. Staging of twin-twin transfusion syndrome. *J Perinatol*. 1999;19(8 Pt 1):550–555.
30. O'Donoghue K, Cartwright E, Galea P, Fisk NM. Stage I twin-twin transfusion syndrome: rates of progression and regression in relation to outcome. *Ultrasound Obstet Gynecol*. 2007;30(7):958–964. https://doi.org/10.1002/uog.5189.
33. Wohlmuth C, Osei FA, Moise KJ, et al. Changes in ductus venosus flow profile in twin-twin transfusion syndrome: role in risk stratification. *Ultrasound Obstet Gynecol*. 2016;48(6):744–751. https://doi.org/10.1002/uog.15916.
34. Wohlmuth C, Boudreaux D, Moise KJ, et al. Cardiac pathophysiology in twin-twin transfusion syndrome: new insights into its evolution. *Ultrasound Obstet Gynecol*. 2018;51(3):341–348. https://doi.org/10.1002/uog.17480.
35. Wohlmuth C, Osei FA, Moise KJ, et al. Aortic distensibility as a surrogate for intertwin pulse pressure differences in monochorionic pregnancies with and without twin-twin transfusion syndrome. *Ultrasound Obstet Gynecol*. 2016;48(2):193–199. https://doi.org/10.1002/uog.15836.
37. Kiserud T. The ductus venosus. *Semin Perinatol*. 2001;25(1):11–20.
38. Kiserud T. Physiology of the fetal circulation. *Semin Fetal Neonatal Med*. 2005;10(6):493–503. https://doi.org/10.1016/j.siny.2005.08.007.
39. Kiserud T, Eik-Nes SH, Blaas HG, Hellevik LR. Ultrasonographic velocimetry of the fetal ductus venosus. *Lancet*. 1991;338(8780):1412–1414.
41. Bensouda B, Fouron JC, Raboisson MJ, Lamoureux J, Lachance C, Leduc L. Relevance of measuring diastolic time intervals in the ductus venosus during the early stages of twin-twin transfusion syndrome. *Ultrasound Obstet Gynecol*. 2007;30(7):983–987. https://doi.org/10.1002/uog.5161.
45. Wohlmuth C, Gardiner HM. Evaluation of fetal cardiac function – techniques and implications. In: Yagel S, Silverman NH, Gembruch U, eds. *Fetal Cardiology: Embryology, Genetics, Physiology, Echocardiographic Evaluation, Diagnosis, and Perinatal Management of Cardiac Diseases*. 3rd ed. CRC Press; 2018.
47. Taylor-Clarke MC, Matsui H, Roughton M, Wimalasundera RC, Gardiner HM. Ventricular strain changes in monochorionic twins with and without twin-to-twin transfusion syndrome. *Am J Obstet Gynecol*. 2013;208(6):462.e1–e6. https://doi.org/10.1016/j.ajog.2013.02.051.
50. Wohlmuth C, Moise Jr KJ, Papanna R, et al. The influence of blood pressure on fetal aortic distensibility: an animal validation study. *Fetal Diagn Ther*. 2018;43(3):226–230. https://doi.org/10.1159/000477396.
51. Donepudi R, Mann LK, Wohlmuth C, et al. Recipient umbilical artery elongation (redundancy) in twin-twin transfusion syndrome. *Am J Obstet Gynecol*. 2017;217(2):206.e1–206.e11. https://doi.org/10.1016/j.ajog.2017.04.024.
53. Senat MV, Deprest J, Boulvain M, Paupe A, Winer N, Ville Y. Endoscopic laser surgery versus serial amnioreduction for severe twin-to-twin transfusion syndrome. *N Engl J Med*. 2004;351(2):136–144. https://doi.org/10.1056/NEJMoa032597.
54. Khalil A, Cooper E, Townsend R, Thilaganathan B. Evolution of Stage 1 Twin-to-Twin Transfusion Syndrome (TTTS): systematic review and meta-analysis. *Twin Res Hum Genet*. 2016;19(3):207–216. https://doi.org/10.1017/thg.2016.33.
57. Fratelli N, Pedretti C, Gerosa V, et al. Changes in ductus venosus velocity ratios after fetoscopic laser surgery for twin-twin transfusion syndrome. *Ultrasound Obstet Gynecol*. 2018;52(6):802–803. https://doi.org/10.1002/uog.19020.
60. Gratacós E, Van Schoubroeck D, Carreras E, et al. Transient hydropic signs in the donor fetus after fetoscopic laser coagulation in severe twin-twin transfusion syndrome: incidence and clinical relevance. *Ultrasound Obstet Gynecol*. 2002;19(5):449–453. https://doi.org/10.1046/j.1469-0705.2002.00642.x.
63. Herberg U, Bolay J, Graeve P, Hecher K, Bartmann P, Breuer J. Intertwin cardiac status at 10-year follow-up after intrauterine laser coagulation therapy of severe twin-twin transfusion syndrome: comparison of donor, recipient and normal values. *Arch Dis Child Fetal Neonatal Ed*. 2014;99(5):F380–F385. https://doi.org/10.1136/archdischild-2013-305034.
64. Gardiner HM, Matsui H, Roughton M, et al. Cardiac function in 10-year-old twins following different fetal therapies for twin-twin transfusion syndrome. *Ultrasound Obstet Gynecol*. 2014;43(6):652–657. https://doi.org/10.1002/uog.13279.
65. Lopriore E, Middeldorp JM, Oepkes D, Kanhai HH, Walther FJ, Vandenbussche FPHA. Twin anemia-polycythemia sequence in two monochorionic twin pairs without oligo-polyhydramnios sequence. *Placenta*. 2007;28(1):47–51. https://doi.org/10.1016/j.placenta.2006.01.010.
66. Tollenaar LSA, Slaghekke F, Middeldorp JM, et al. Twin anemia polycythemia sequence: current views on pathogenesis, diagnostic criteria, perinatal management, and outcome. *Twin Res Hum Genet*. 2016;19(3):222–233. https://doi.org/10.1017/thg.2016.18.
67. van den Wijngaard JPHM, Lewi L, Lopriore E, et al. Modeling severely discordant hematocrits and normal amniotic fluids after incomplete laser therapy in twin-to-twin transfusion syndrome. *Placenta*. 2007;28(7):611–615. https://doi.org/10.1016/j.placenta.2006.10.002.
69. Mari G, Deter RL, Carpenter RL, et al. Noninvasive diagnosis by Doppler ultrasonography of fetal anemia due to maternal red-cell alloimmunization. Collaborative Group for Doppler Assessment of the Blood Velocity in Anemic Fetuses. *N Engl J Med*. 2000;342(1):9–14. https://doi.org/10.1056/NEJM200001063420102.
70. Slaghekke F, Pasman S, Veujoz M, et al. Middle cerebral artery peak systolic velocity to predict fetal hemoglobin levels in twin anemia-polycythemia sequence. *Ultrasound Obstet Gynecol*. 2015;46(4):432–436. https://doi.org/10.1002/uog.14925.
72. Robyr R, Lewi L, Salomon LJ, et al. Prevalence and management of late fetal complications following successful selective laser coagulation of chorionic plate anastomoses in twin-to-twin transfusion syndrome. *Am J Obstet Gynecol*. 2006;194(3):796–803. https://doi.org/10.1016/j.ajog.2005.08.069.
75. Tollenaar LSA, Lopriore E, Middeldorp JM, et al. Improved prediction of twin anemia-polycythemia sequence by delta middle cerebral artery peak systolic velocity: new antenatal classification system. *Ultrasound Obstet Gynecol*. 2019;53(6):788–793. https://doi.org/10.1002/uog.20096.
76. Tollenaar LSA, Lopriore E, Middeldorp JM, et al. Prevalence of placental dichotomy, fetal cardiomegaly and starry-sky liver in twin anemia polycythemia sequence. *Ultrasound Obstet Gynecol*. 2019;56(3):395–399. https://doi.org/10.1002/uog.21948.
78. Slaghekke F, Zhao DP, Middeldorp JM, et al. Antenatal management of twin-twin transfusion syndrome and twin anemia-polycythemia sequence. *Expert Rev Hematol*. 2016;9(8):815–820. https://doi.org/10.1080/17474086.2016.1200968.
80. Tollenaar LSA, Lopriore E, Slaghekke F, et al. High risk of long-term impairment in donor twins with spontaneous twin anemia polycythemia sequence. *Ultrasound Obstet Gynecol*. 2019;55(1):39–46. https://doi.org/10.1002/uog.20846.
82. Moore TR, Gale S, Benirschke K. Perinatal outcome of forty-nine pregnancies complicated by acardiac twinning. *Am J Obstet Gynecol*. 1990;163(3):907–912. https://doi.org/10.1016/0002-9378(90)91094-S.
85. Byrne FA, Lee H, Kipps AK, Brook MM, Moon-Grady AJ. Echocardiographic risk stratification of fetuses with sacrococcygeal teratoma and twin-reversed arterial perfusion. *Fetal Diagn Ther*. 2011;30(4):280–288. https://doi.org/10.1159/000330762.
87. Mielke G, Benda N. Cardiac output and central distribution of blood flow in the human fetus. *Circulation*. 2001;103(12):1662–1668.
88. van Gemert MJC, Pistorius LR, Benirschke K, et al. Hypothesis acardiac twin pregnancies: pathophysiology-based hypotheses suggest risk prediction by pump/acardiac umbilical venous diameter ratios. *Birth Defects Res Part A Clin Mol Teratol*. 2016;106(2):114–121. https://doi.org/10.1002/bdra.23467.
89. Wohlmuth C, Bergh E, Bell C, et al. Clinical monitoring of sacrococcygeal teratoma. *Fetal Diagn Ther*. 2019;46(5):333–340. https://doi.org/10.1159/000496841.
90. Wohlmuth C, Boudreaux D, Van Gemert MJC, et al. High-output states: know when to fold' em. *International Fetal Medicine and Surgery Society - 35th Annual Meeting*. 2016.
91. Bebbington MW, Danzer E, Moldenhauer J, Khalek N, Johnson MP. Radiofrequency ablation vs bipolar umbilical cord coagulation in the management of complicated monochorionic pregnancies. *Ultrasound Obstet Gynecol*. 2012;40(3):319–324. https://doi.org/10.1002/uog.11122.
96. Quintero R, Chmait RH, Murakoshi T, et al. Surgical management of twin reversed arterial perfusion sequence. *Am J Obstet Gynecol*. 2006;194(4):982–991. https://doi.org/10.1016/j.ajog.2005.10.195.
97. Roman A, Papanna R, Johnson A, et al. Selective reduction in complicated monochorionic pregnancies: radiofrequency ablation vs. bipolar cord coagulation. *Ultrasound Obstet Gynecol*. 2010;36(1):37–41. https://doi.org/10.1002/uog.7567.
98. Gaerty K, Greer RM, Kumar S. Systematic review and metaanalysis of perinatal outcomes after radiofrequency ablation and bipolar cord occlusion in monochorionic pregnancies. *Am J Obstet Gynecol*. 2015;213(5):637–643. https://doi.org/10.1016/j.ajog.2015.04.035.

Physiology of Neonatal Resuscitation

150

Stuart B. Hooper | Arjan B. te Pas

INTRODUCTION

The transition to newborn life represents one of the greatest physiologic challenges that humans face during their lives. Before birth, the future airways of the lungs are liquid-filled and the lungs play no role in gas exchange.[1] Instead, gas exchange occurs across the placenta and the majority of right ventricular output bypasses the lungs and passes through the ductus arteriosus (DA) to enter the descending aorta (Fig. 150.1). As much of this blood is directed through the placenta, the right ventricle provides the majority of blood flow through the organ of gas exchange in the fetus, just as it does in the adult (lung).[2] Similarly, much of the umbilical venous blood returning from the placenta passes through the ductus venosus (DV) and foramen ovale (FO) to directly enter the left atrium.[2] Thus, the left ventricle in the fetus receives highly oxygenated blood from the organ of gas exchange, just as occurs in adults (see Fig. 150.1). As such, the transition to newborn life at birth primarily involves transferring the role of gas exchange from the placenta to the lungs, which requires a major reorganization of the circulatory system. Both of these physiologic changes are interlinked, commencing with lung aeration, which then triggers the circulatory transition by increasing pulmonary blood flow (PBF).[2]

Considering the complexities involved, it is remarkable that most infants easily make the transition to life after birth. Nevertheless, approximately 20% of infants need some form of respiratory support at birth, and a small percentage require significant intervention. While assisting infants at birth is commonly referred to as *neonatal resuscitation*, the need for "resuscitation" is rare. Instead, most infants usually just require assistance to transition from a physiologic state consistent with in utero life into one consistent with ex utero life. As such, the phrase *neonatal stabilization* rather than *neonatal resuscitation* is probably more appropriate, to avoid the impression that intervention is required when it is only assistance and support that are needed.

The type and degree of assistance infants require at birth can vary considerably depending on the degree of development the infant has achieved at delivery and whether the infant has been exposed to adverse conditions, such as severe asphyxia, prior to birth. As our understanding of the physiologic challenges infants face at birth has improved, it has become clear that extrapolating treatments from one group of infants to another is inappropriate. For instance, the approaches required to assist asphyxiated term infants are very different to those required for very preterm infants, particularly as the physiologic challenges facing term and preterm infants are fundamentally different.

In this chapter, we discuss the general physiologic principles of the fetal-to-neonatal transition, before discussing how these principles are differentially affected by lung immaturity, abnormal lung development, and severe birth asphyxia.

NORMAL PHYSIOLOGIC TRANSITION

LUNG AERATION AT BIRTH

AIRWAY LIQUID BEFORE BIRTH

Before birth, the future airways of the lung are liquid-filled.[3] This liquid is secreted by the lung, enters the airways across the distal airway surface and leaves the lungs by flowing out of the trachea, whereby it is either swallowed or enters the amniotic sac.[1,4] Liquid efflux from the lungs is mostly unidirectional, flowing out of the lungs primarily during fetal breathing movements (FBMs) when the glottis is open and upper airway resistance is low.[1,4] While liquid can enter the upper airways, this is uncommon, with significant volumes only entering the airways during periods of prolonged hypoxia, thereby facilitating meconium entry into the lower airways before birth.[5] During fetal apnea (approximately 50% of the time) the fetal glottis adducts, which restricts the efflux of liquid from the airways. This plays a vital role in fetal lung growth and development as the retention of liquid within the airways maintains the lung in a distended state (see Chapter 57).[4] Increasing the degree of lung distension is a potent stimulus for fetal lung growth, whereas a reduction in lung expansion causes fetal lung growth to cease (see Chapter 57).[4] However, at birth this liquid must be cleared from the airways to allow the entry of air and the onset of pulmonary gas exchange.

Airway liquid has a profound effect on respiratory function at birth, with the lung passing through two distinct phases before it starts to function like a newborn lung.[6] During the first phase, which is usually quite short (30 to 60 seconds), the airways are liquid-filled, which prevents pulmonary gas exchange and greatly increases airway resistance. During the second phase, the liquid has been cleared from the airways into the surrounding lung tissue, but still remains within the thoracic cavity.[7] As the liquid can take 4 to 6 hours to clear from lung tissue, it can adversely influence respiratory function well into the newborn period, which is a largely unrecognized problem.[6]

PHASE 1: AIRWAY LIQUID CLEARANCE AND LUNG AERATION AT BIRTH

Phase contrast (PC) x-ray imaging (Figs. 150.2 and 150.3) has led to a new understanding of the timing and mechanisms of airway liquid clearance by visualizing the air entering the lungs at birth.[8,9] Indeed, it is now clear that airway liquid clearance does not simply result from Na^+ reabsorption induced by the stress of labor. Instead, up to three mechanisms are involved, with the primary mechanism depending upon the timing and mode of delivery.[6] Two of the mechanisms are active during labor, and the third is active after birth (see below). More importantly, only one of these mechanisms results in the loss of liquid from the respiratory system, as the other two involve the reabsorption of liquid into lung tissue, which may interfere with lung function after birth.

Some have argued that liquid clearance begins days to weeks before labor onset,[3] but the evidence supporting this concept was questioned when the relationship between reduced amniotic fluid volumes and reduced lung liquid volumes was fully explored.[10,11] Nevertheless, it is clear that the volume of liquid present in the airways before birth varies considerably between individuals and largely depends on the available intrauterine space. Reducing this space, as occurs with reduced amniotic fluid volumes and uterine contractions, reduces fetal lung liquid volumes due to increased spinal flexion (Fig. 150.4).[10] Other factors, such as a twin, may have a similar effect.

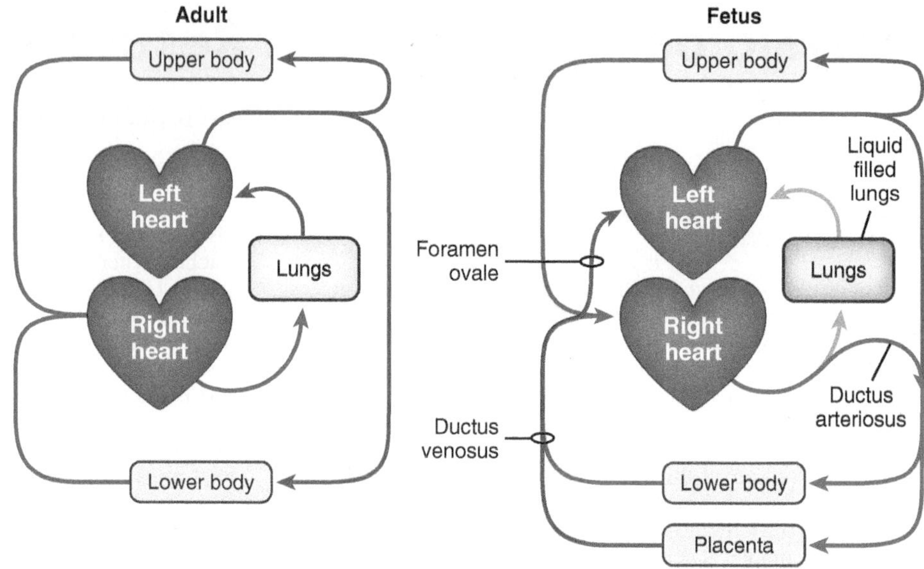

Fig. 150.1 Schematic diagram of the circulation in the adult and fetus. While the fetal circulation is structurally more complex than the adult, the two circulations are functionally similar, differing only due to the different sites of gas exchange in the fetus and adult. In the fetus, the right ventricle provides the majority of blood flow to the organ of gas exchange (placenta), as occurs in adults (lung), due to the ductus arteriosus that shunts blood from the pulmonary artery into the descending aorta. Similarly, the left ventricle receives most of its venous return from the organ of gas exchange, as occurs in adults, which passes from the umbilical vein through the ductus venosus and foramen ovale directly into the left atrium.

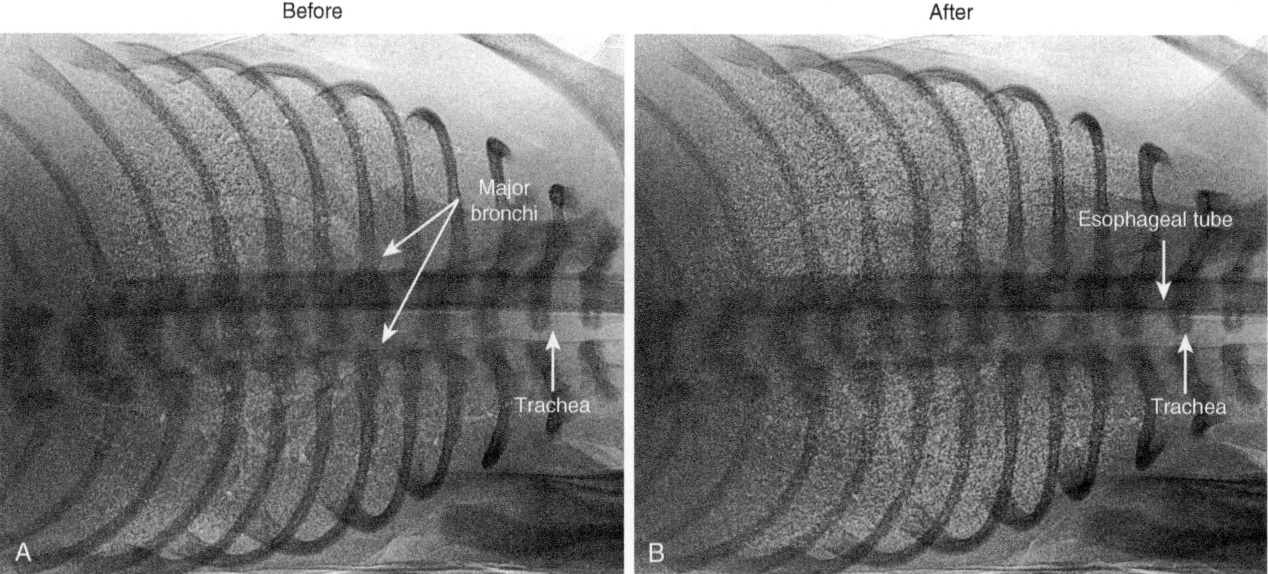

Fig. 150.2 Phase contrast x-ray images of a near-term (30 days) newborn rabbit acquired at rest immediately before (A) and after (B; approximately 600 ms later) a single breath during lung aeration. The trachea and major bronchi are clearly visible in both images, and the degree of lung aeration in the distal airways is evident by the degree of "speckle" in the image (refer also to Fig. 150.3). Note that aeration in the nondependent lung is greater than in the dependent lung in the image acquired before the breath (A) and that the chest wall has expanded after the breath compared with before the breath. The *dark* tubular structure in both images is an esophageal tube used to measure reductions in intrathoracic pressure and assess breathing activity.

AIRWAY LIQUID CLEARANCE BEFORE BIRTH; SODIUM REABSORPTION

The stress of labor (particularly during vaginal delivery of the head) is thought to stimulate fetal adrenaline release, which acts on β-adrenoceptors located on the basolateral surface of alveolar epithelial cells to increase intracellular cyclic adenosine monophosphate (cAMP) concentrations.[3,12] This stimulates opening of luminal surface Na^+ channels (ENaCs), leading to increased Na^+ and Na-linked Cl^- transport from the lung lumen into lung tissue.[3,12] This reverses the osmotic gradient across the lung epithelium, leading to liquid reabsorption from the airways. However, Na^+-induced liquid reabsorption is slow (maximum rates of 10 mL/kg/h), only develops late in gestation, and requires high levels of adrenaline, which must remain elevated well (hours) into the newborn period to clear all of the liquid.[12-14] Thus, this mechanism is not active in preterm infants and if adrenaline levels were to remain elevated for hours after birth, this should be reflected by elevated heart rates. However, heart rate nomograms over the newborn period are not consistent with this concept[15] and if airway liquid clearance occurred by Na^+ reabsorption alone, it would take hours before gas exchange could occur in term infants and preterm infants would not be able to aerate their lungs.

PC x-ray imaging has demonstrated that Na^+ channel blockade (with amiloride) does not affect the extent or the

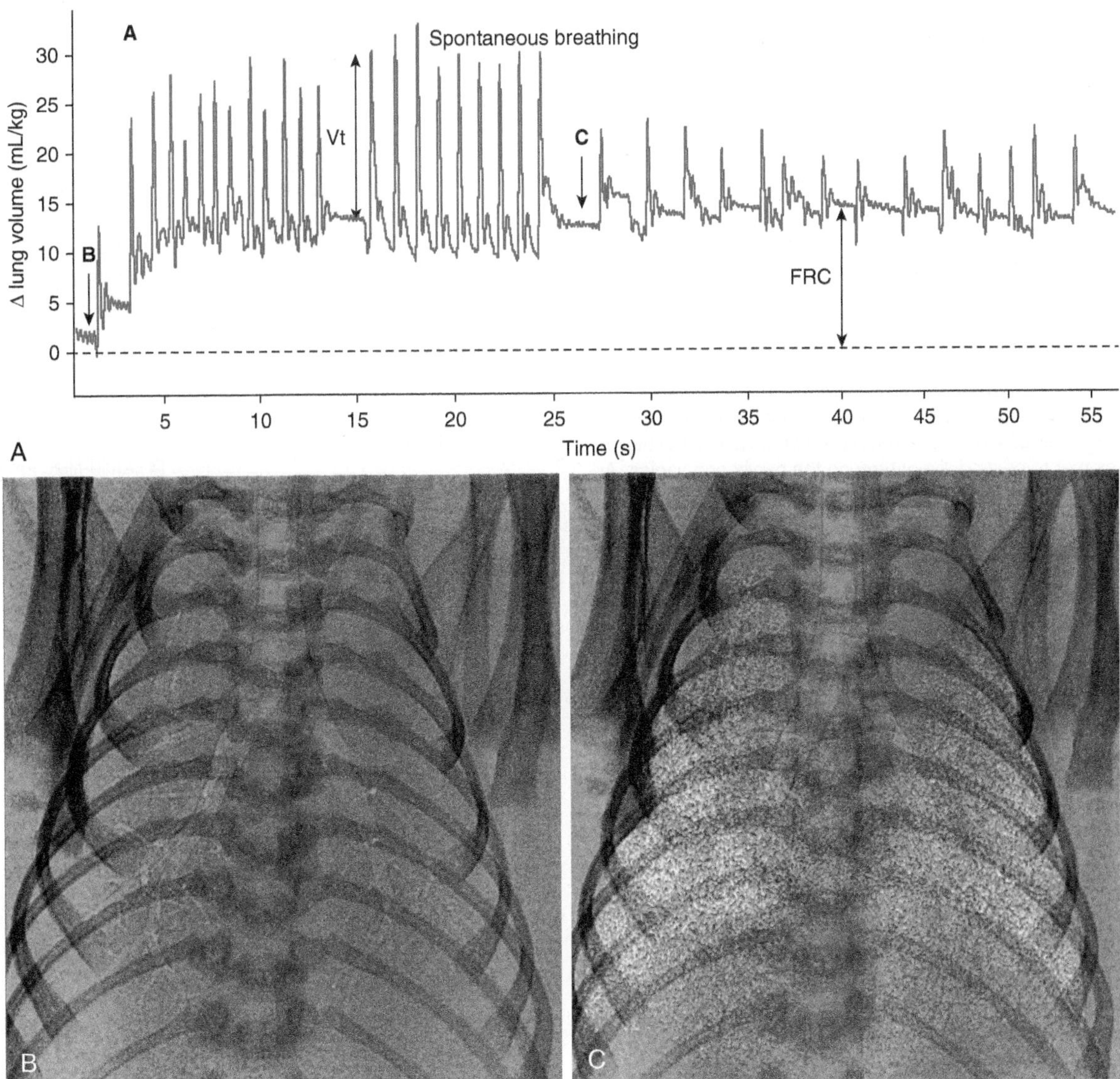

Fig. 150.3 (A) Lung gas volumes measured using a plethysmograph in a spontaneously breathing near term (31 days) newborn rabbit. Simultaneous phase contrast x-ray images were acquired near the beginning of lung aeration (B) and approximately 40 seconds later after the recruitment of a functional residual capacity *(FRC)* of approximately 15 mL/kg (C). The times at which each image was acquired are indicated by *arrows* on the plethysmograph recording. Initially, the tidal volume *(Vt)* of the initial spontaneous breaths was large (approximately 15 mL/kg), but this gradually reduced as the lung aerated.[23] (Data and images from Hooper SB, Kitchen MJ, Wallace MJ, et al. Imaging lung aeration and lung liquid clearance at birth. *FASEB J.* 2007;21:3329-3337; and redrawn.)

spatial and temporal pattern of airway liquid clearance after birth.[16] However, it did increase the rate of airway liquid re-entry between inflations, indicating that Na^+ reabsorption may help to keep liquid out of the airways following its clearance,[16] but the ongoing need for increased adrenaline levels to sustain this role is unclear. There is also much confusion over whether adrenaline levels are consistently increased during delivery and whether the mode of delivery (vaginal vs. cesarean section [CS]) influences adrenaline levels. The commonly cited reference[17] found no increase in cord blood adrenaline levels and no difference between vaginally or CS-delivered infants. In contrast, asphyxiated and breech-delivered infants had markedly elevated adrenaline levels.[17] Similarly, while knockout of the *αENaC* gene, but not the *βENaC* or *δENaC* genes, causes apparent respiratory failure and death within 40 hours of birth,[18] these newborn mice also had poor respiratory efforts.[19] Furthermore, increased wet lung tissue weights after death were cited as evidence for airway liquid retention,[18] but this is a poor indicator of airway liquid retention, as it does not distinguish between liquid in the tissue or the airways or postmortem movement between the two.

AIRWAY LIQUID CLEARANCE BEFORE BIRTH; FETAL POSTURE

Forces imposed on the infant during uterine contractions (see Fig. 150.4) can also cause liquid to exit the lungs via the nose and mouth.[10] Gushes of liquid from the nose and mouth have been observed upon delivery of the head, which likely results from increased dorsoventral flexion (knees to chest) causing compression of the fetal abdomen and chest during vaginal delivery (see Fig. 150.4).[20,21] Increased spinal flexion increases abdominal pressure and elevates the diaphragm, which increases transpulmonary pressure and forces liquid to leave the lung via the trachea.[10] As the fetal respiratory system is highly compliant, only small increases in transpulmonary pressure are required to displace large volumes of liquid.[22] However, the contribution of this mechanism to airway liquid clearance at birth is difficult to quantify and likely varies between individuals. For instance, infants

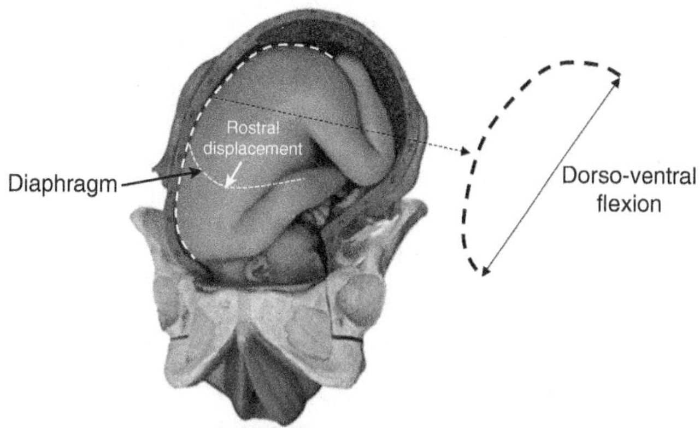

Fig. 150.4 Diagrammatic representation of a human fetus in a dorsoventrally flexed (knees to chest flexion) position as a result of uterine contractions that force its delivery through the cervix and vagina. An increase in spinal curvature increases abdominal pressure, which increases rostral displacement of the diaphragm and forces liquid to leave the lungs via the nose and mouth.

delivered vaginally and exposed to strong uterine contractions during a protracted labor could lose large volumes of lung liquid via this mechanism.[6] However, infants delivered by elective CS without labor may lose little or no liquid via this mechanism. Nevertheless, it is important to note that this mechanism of airway liquid clearance is the only known mechanism whereby liquid is completely lost from the respiratory system as a result of its clearance from the airways. Both other mechanisms (Na^+ reabsorption and inspiratory efforts, see below) involve the clearance of liquid into lung tissue, before it is eventually cleared from the tissue hours after birth.[6]

AIRWAY LIQUID CLEARANCE AFTER BIRTH

Imaging studies have demonstrated that, after birth, the pressure gradients generated by inspiration rapidly and efficiently clear the airways of liquid (see Figs. 150.2 and 150.3), resulting in full aeration within 3 to 5 breaths (<30 seconds) in term newborns.[9,23] The calculated rates of liquid clearance during inspiration are very large (approximately 32 L/h/kg) and explain why infants can rapidly initiate pulmonary gas exchange after birth, even in infants born by CS without labor.[9,23] The air/liquid interface moves distally through the airways in a stepwise manner with each inspiration, with little or no distal movement between breaths (see Fig. 150.3). Some proximal movement can occur between breaths (see Fig. 150.3), which is considered to result from liquid re-entry into the airways.[9,23] Inspiration generates the pressure gradients that drive liquid movement distally through the airways and across the distal airway wall by reducing interstitial tissue pressures, a mechanism first described in humans.[24] The resulting hydrostatic pressure gradient between the tissue and airways causes liquid to move out of the airways into the surrounding lung tissue. As similar pressure gradients can be generated by applying positive pressures to the airways, positive pressure ventilation can also rapidly clear airway liquid.[16,25,26] While this confirms the rationale for providing positive pressure ventilation to infants at birth, deciding the best way to provide this support is unclear, but understanding the physiology provides important clues.

The initial resistance to air entry into the lung at birth is primarily governed by the resistance to moving liquid through the airways and across the distal airway wall.[6] As lung liquid has a viscosity that is approximately 70× greater than air, the initial resistance is considerably (approximately 100-fold) greater than it is following lung aeration, and it rapidly decreases (approximately 100-fold) as the lung aerates (Fig. 150.5).[27] Preterm infants have smaller

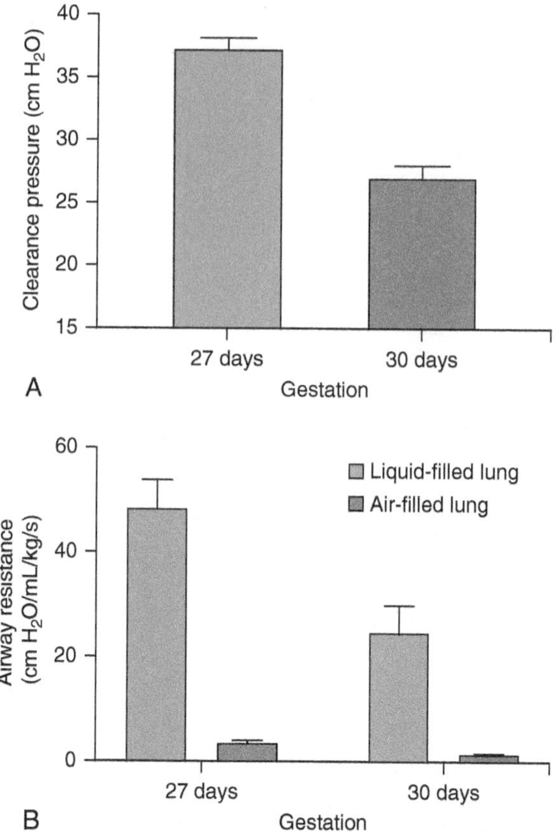

Fig. 150.5 (A) The inflation pressure required to initiate airway liquid clearance (clearance pressure) is considerably greater in extremely preterm (27 days; *blue bar*) compared with near term (30 days; *black bar*) newborn rabbits. (B) Airway resistance of the liquid-filled lung (*blue bars*) is considerably greater than the air-filled (*black bars*) lung, although the resistance of both the liquid and air-filled lung decreases with gestational age. (Data from te Pas AB, Kitchen MJ, Lee K, et al. Optimizing lung aeration at birth using a sustained inflation and positive pressure ventilation in preterm rabbits. *Pediatr Res.* 2016;80[1]:85–91; and redrawn.)

airways and, as the resistance increases exponentially (fourth power) with decreasing airway radius, the initial resistance to moving liquid through the airways is significantly greater in preterm compared to term newborns (see Fig. 150.5).[27] Similarly, as the surface area of the distal airways increases exponentially with increasing gestational age (Fig. 150.6), preterm infants have a markedly reduced distal airway surface area, which must increase the resistance for liquid movement across the distal airway wall into lung tissue.[27] Despite the smaller airways and a reduced gas exchange surface area, it is recommended that very preterm infants are ventilated with starting pressures that are much lower than term infants at birth.[28] While this may be protective for an immature lung that is well aerated, it is questionable whether this approach is relevant for an immature liquid-filled lung.

As the cross-sectional surface area of the airways increases exponentially with increasing airway generation number, airway resistance decreases exponentially as the air/liquid interface moves distally. Indeed, the huge reduction in airway resistance during lung aeration (see Fig. 150.5) can be very rapid (seconds) and follows an exponential function that is difficult to predict. As a result, large changes in respiratory mechanics (e.g., 10-fold increase in lung compliance) can occur on a breath-by-breath basis.[27] Thus, use of a single set inflation pressure during intermittent positive pressure ventilation (iPPV) at birth may initially produce small tidal volume changes, but result in

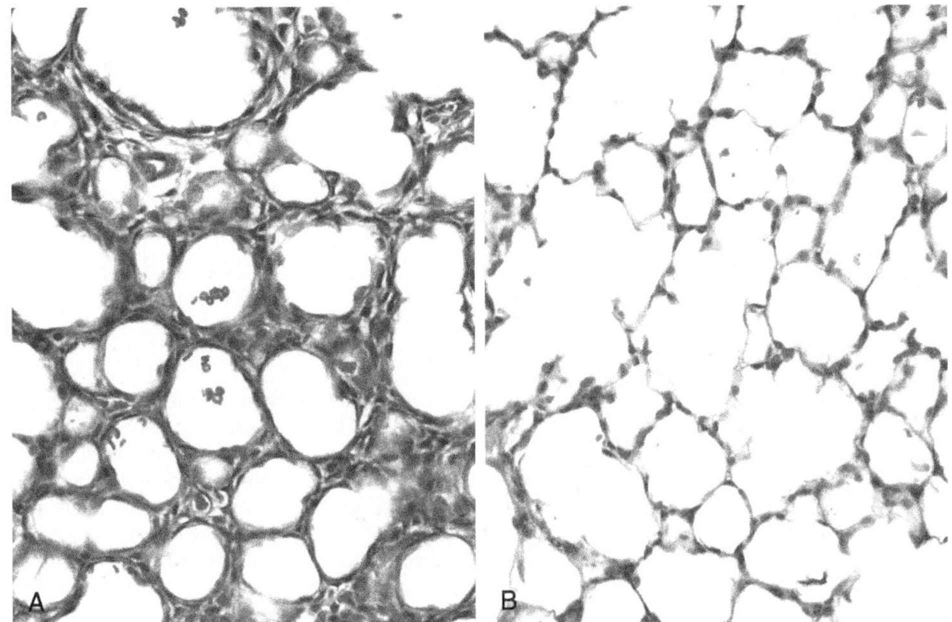

Fig. 150.6 Histologic sections of the lung collected from fetal sheep at approximately 60% (90 days; A) and near term (140 days; B) of gestation (term = approximately 147 days). Note that the immature lung (A) has simplified airway structures, with considerable amounts of lung tissue *(magenta)* separating the airways. Cell nuclei are stained a *darker purple* and red blood cells, most located in the blood vessels are stained a *lighter red*. Note that few blood vessels lie adjacent to the airway wall in the immature lung, whereas they lie in close apposition to the airspaces in the mature lung (B), thereby greatly reducing the air/blood gas barrier.

progressively larger tidal volumes as the lung aerates, which risk overexpanding and injuring the lung.[25] As such, it is difficult to understand why highly sophisticated ventilators that can monitor and respond to breath-by-breath changes in respiratory mechanics are commonly used in the neonatal intensive care unit (NICU), but not in the delivery room. Indeed, respiratory mechanics have usually stabilized by the time the infant reaches the NICU, whereas in the delivery room, the changes are rapid and complex.[24,29] Despite this, ventilation in the delivery room most commonly involves the use of rudimentary devices (T-piece devices or resuscitation bags) that are incapable of automatically adjusting ventilation parameters to take into account rapidly changing respiratory mechanics. This may partly explain the large variation in tidal volumes measured in preterm infants at birth.[30,31]

PHASE 2: EFFECT OF AIRWAY LIQUID WITHIN LUNG TISSUE

As indicated above, only one mechanism of airway liquid clearance (fetal postural changes) results in liquid loss from the chest as it leaves the airways via the nose and mouth. The other two mechanisms (Na^+ reabsorption and pressures generated by inspiration) involve liquid clearance into the lung's interstitial tissue.As this tissue compartment has a fixed volume (see Fig. 150.6), the entry of liquid into the interstitial tissue increases pressures from approximately 0 to 6 cm H_2O.[32] This causes a form of pulmonary edema that persists for 4 to 6 hours after birth while the liquid is gradually cleared from the tissue.[32,33]

The presence of airway liquid in lung tissue potentially has major implications for the infant's respiratory function after birth. For instance, while the liquid moves from the airways into lung tissue to allow the entry of air, it still remains within the chest. As a result, the chest wall must expand to temporarily accommodate both the liquid and the incoming volume of air, which also causes the diaphragm to flatten (Fig. 150.7).[7,9] This explains why the chest wall must be highly compliant at birth, allowing it to easily expand and accommodate both the liquid and incoming air after birth. If the chest wall is stiff, its ability to expand is reduced, leading to much greater interstitial tissue pressures. Increased interstitial tissue pressure

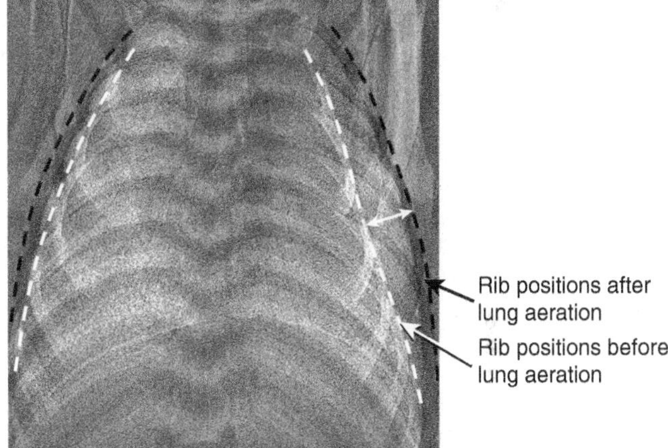

Fig. 150.7 Lung aeration increases chest wall expansion. Superimposition of two phase contrast x-ray images (contrast is inverted in one image) collected before *(white ribs)* and after *(black ribs)* lung aeration in a spontaneously breathing near-term newborn rabbit acquired between breaths (i.e., at functional residual capacity [FRC]). Following lung aeration, the chest wall significantly expands to accommodate both the air that forms the FRC after birth and the liquid that has moved from the airways into lung tissue but still remains in the chest. Chest wall expansion is also clearly evident in Fig. 150.2. (From Hooper SB, Kitchen MJ, Wallace MJ, et al. Imaging lung aeration and lung liquid clearance at birth. *FASEB J.* 2007;21:3329-3337; and modified.)

increases the pressure gradient for liquid to re-enter the airways at end-expiration. While this liquid may be re-cleared during the next breath/inflation,[16] the functional residual capacity (FRC) is reduced. Furthermore, the presence of this liquid in lung tissue reduces lung compliance,[7] making the lungs more difficult to inflate. Currently, there is very little understanding of how this consequence of airway liquid clearance contributes to respiratory morbidity in newborn infants.[6] However, an expanded chest wall and flattened diaphragm, along with a stiffer lung, will increase the work of breathing and limit tidal volumes, leading to tachypnea and labored breathing. In addition, a reduction in FRC usually induces expiratory braking (glottis closure during expiration) in the newborn, or grunting. All of these signs are evident in infants with transient tachypnea of the newborn (TTN).

CARDIOVASCULAR CHANGES AT BIRTH

FETAL CARDIOVASCULAR PHYSIOLOGY

The fetal circulation is considerably more complex than that of the adult (see Fig. 150.1). Like adults, fetuses have both a pulmonary and a systemic circulation, but also have a placental circulation connected in parallel across the lower body. Furthermore, unlike the adult, all of these circulations are interconnected due to the presence of multiple shunts,[34] which include the DV, FO, and the DA (see Fig. 150.1). The DV allows approximately 50% of umbilical venous blood to flow directly into the inferior vena cava (IVC, in sheep) or right atrium (in humans). The other 50% passes into the hepatic portal system and eventually back into the IVC. Much of the blood passing through the DV also passes through the FO to directly enter the left atrium, thereby bypassing the right atrium, right ventricle, and pulmonary circulation.[34] Of the blood that does enter the right atrium and right ventricle, the majority (80% to 90%) bypasses the lungs and flows from the pulmonary artery into the descending aorta via the DA.

While anatomically distinct (see Fig. 150.1), the fetal and adult circulations are functionally similar, differing only because the placenta, rather than the lung, is the fetal organ of gas exchange. As the DA shunts blood from the pulmonary artery into the aorta, the right ventricle provides the majority of blood flow to the organ of gas exchange (placenta) in the fetus,[34] just like it does in the adult. Similarly, due to the presence of the DV and FO, highly oxygenated umbilical venous blood passes directly into the left atrium and left ventricle.[34] Thus, blood returning from the gas exchange organ provides the majority of preload for the left ventricle in the fetus, just like it does in the adult.[2,35,36] As the lungs must take over the role of the gas exchange at birth, the circulation has to undergo a massive re-organization so that the lungs can (1) become the sole recipient of blood exiting the right ventricle and (2) become the sole provider of preload (venous return) for left ventricular output. It is very important not to overlook this second role, as it is critical for cardiac function after birth.

PERINATAL CARDIOVASCULAR PHYSIOLOGY

At birth, lung aeration decreases pulmonary vascular resistance (PVR), which increases PBF and redirects right ventricular output through the lungs.[34] As a result, right-to-left shunting of blood through the DA decreases and flow in the umbilical artery also decreases,[37] if the cord remains unclamped (Fig. 150.8; see below). In effect, the lung and placenta compete with one another for both right and left ventricular output due to the ongoing presence of the DA (see Fig. 150.8).[37] If the decrease in PVR precedes umbilical cord clamping (UCC), UCC greatly increases PBF due to a large increase in left-to-right shunting through the DA.[2,35,36] This results from the loss of the low-resistance placental circulation, which increases systemic vascular resistance and promotes blood flow from the systemic into the pulmonary circulation. This reversal in DA blood flow (Fig. 150.9) is a normal feature of the cardiovascular transition at birth, irrespective of the timing of cord clamping (see below) but is transient (1 to 2 hours) in normal healthy infants.[38] Nevertheless, the DA blood flow profile after birth is very dynamic and bidirectional, depending upon the phase of the cardiac cycle.[38-40] While it is mostly left-to-right (see Fig. 150.9), during early systole the flow is right-to-left but becomes left-to-right during late systole and throughout diastole.[38-40] During early systole, the pressure wave emanating from the right ventricle reaches the pulmonary artery end of the DA

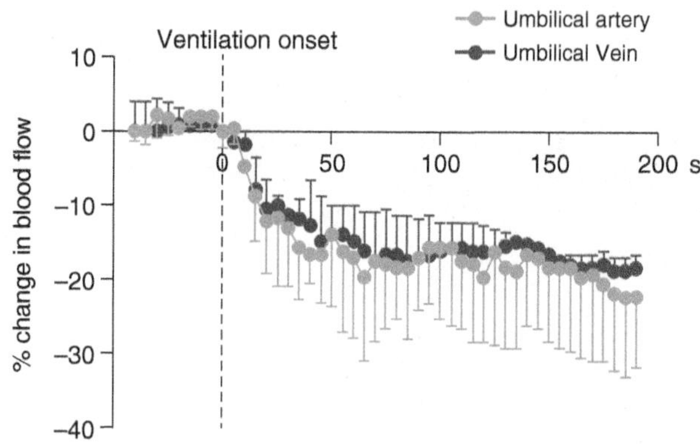

Fig. 150.8 Changes in umbilical artery and venous blood flow in response to ventilation onset and the decrease in pulmonary vascular resistance (PVR) following delivery, but before umbilical cord clamping. The decrease in PVR redirects right ventricular output through the lungs and initiates left-to-right shunting across the ductus arteriosus. As a result, the increase in PBF "steals" blood flow from the placenta and the lung acts as a competitive (to the placenta) low-resistance pathway for blood flow derived from both right and left ventricles. *PBF*, Pulmonary blood flow. (Data from Blank DA, Polglase GR, Kluckow M, et al. Haemodynamic effects of umbilical cord milking in premature sheep during the neonatal transition. *Arch Dis Child Fetal Neonatal Ed.* 2018;103:F539-F546; and redrawn.)

before the pressure wave emanating from the left ventricle reaches the aortic end (see Fig. 150.1). As a result, the pressure gradient across the DA is initially higher at the pulmonary end, resulting in right-to-left flow, but rapidly reverses as the pressure wave from the left ventricle reaches the aortic end of the DA (see Fig. 150.9). The continued left-to-right flow during diastole reflects the lower resistance to blood flow through the pulmonary circulation, compared with the systemic circulation, and significantly contributes to PBF (up to 50% of flow) in the immediate newborn period.[38]

Umbilical venous return is lost following UCC and so the left ventricle becomes solely dependent upon pulmonary venous return for preload.[35] While this has implications for the timing of UCC in relation to lung aeration (see below), the large contribution of left-to-right shunting through the DA to PBF immediately after birth (see Fig. 150.9) indicates that the left ventricle contributes to its own preload.[38] That is, shortly after birth, a left ventricle, DA, lung, left ventricle short circuit develops (see Fig. 150.1). While this is commonly referred to as "ductal steal" when the DA persists into the newborn period, it is a normal feature of the fetal to neonatal cardiovascular transition immediately after birth.[38-40] The significance of this is unclear, but as the "short circuit" includes all preductal arteries (see Fig. 150.1), it would appear that these vessels retain a privileged position within the newborn circulation. It may also offer an opportunity for the output of both ventricles to gradually come into balance before the DA closes and the circulations separate.

In view of the large amount of left-to-right shunting in the DA (see Fig. 150.9), venous return to the right ventricle must decrease, which may induce left-to-right shunting through the FO. While it is widely assumed that flow through the FO is unidirectional,[41] bidirectional flow has been observed in fetal sheep following cord clamping, and left-to-right shunting has been observed in premature infants (Fig. 150.10).[42] This may also help balance preload and output from both ventricles before the two circulations eventually separate. On the other hand, left-to-right shunting through the FO can only occur if left atrial pressure exceeds right atrial pressure, which is thought to be the primary mechanism driving closure of the FO.[41] As such, the contribution

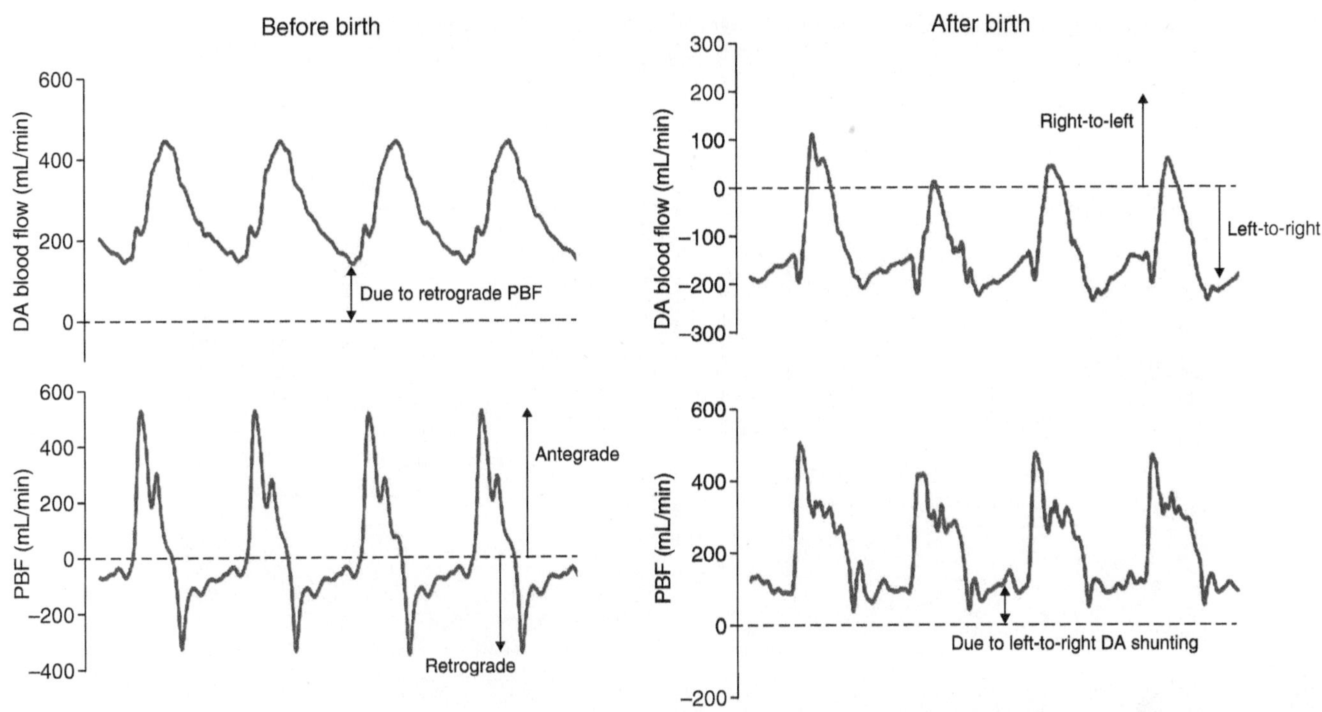

Fig. 150.9 Blood flow profiles in the left pulmonary artery *(bottom panels)* and in the ductus arteriosus (*DA*; *top panels*) throughout four consecutive cardiac cycles before birth *(left panels)* and after birth, following lung aeration, in a newborn lamb. Before birth, retrograde (away from the lungs) pulmonary blood flow *(PBF)* is represented by negative PBF values and contributes to significant levels of right-to-left flow in the DA during diastole. As a result, continuous flow through the DA (right-to-left) occurs throughout the cardiac cycle. After birth and lung aeration, a decrease in pulmonary vascular resistance (PVR) causes a large increase in PBF, resulting in a loss of retrograde flow during diastole and the onset of left-to-right shunting through the DA. While DA flow is predominantly left-to-right, it is bidirectional. It is briefly right-to-left during early systole before reversing and becoming left-to-right in late systole and throughout diastole, when it significantly contributes to PBF.[38] This bidirectional pattern of DA flow is thought to result from the pressure wave emanating from the ventricle reaching the pulmonary artery end of the DA before the pressure wave arising from the left ventricle reaches the aortic end of the DA. As a result, the pressure gradient across the DA is initially right-to-left but then rapidly reverses to become left-to-right throughout most of the cardiac cycle.

of the left ventricle and left-to-right shunting through the DA to PBF (see Fig. 150.9) and pulmonary venous return would help to increase left atrial pressure above right atrial pressure and facilitate closure of the FO.

INCREASE IN PULMONARY BLOOD FLOW AT BIRTH

The large and rapid decrease in PVR at birth is triggered by the one event that cannot occur before birth: lung aeration (Figs. 150.11 and 150.12).[2] The precise mechanisms involved have been a matter of debate for decades. Increased vasodilator release, particularly nitric oxide (NO), in response to an increase in oxygenation is thought to be the primary mechanism that triggers the decrease in PVR in response to lung aeration.[43] Indeed, oxygenation is an important regulator of PBF in adults, being largely responsible for ventilation/perfusion matching in the lung. However, while increasing oxygen levels can increase fetal PBF, the effect of oxygen is not sustained[43] and ventilation of the lung with a gas devoid of oxygen (i.e., 100% nitrogen) or with low oxygen levels, can trigger a large increase in PBF.[44,45] Thus, other mechanisms are also involved. These may include an increase in lung recoil caused by the formation of an air/liquid interface and the creation of surface tension within the lung following aeration.[46] However, while deflating the fetal lung increases PBF, the increase is considerably smaller than the increase in PBF at birth.[46]

While investigating the spatial relationship between lung aeration and the increase in PBF at birth, imaging experiments (see Fig. 150.12) have demonstrated a previously unknown mechanism for the aeration-induced increase in PBF.[47-49] In view of the effects of oxygenation and lung recoil on PBF, it was hypothesized that the increase in PBF at birth would be restricted to aerated lung regions.[49] However, partial lung aeration caused a global increase in PBF (see Fig. 150.12), which occurred equally and simultaneously in all parts of the lung, irrespective of their aerated state. Further, partial aeration of the lung with a gas devoid of oxygen (100% nitrogen) also caused a global increase in PBF,[47] demonstrating that the global response was unrelated to oxygenation. However, as partial lung aeration with 100% oxygen caused a larger PBF increase in aerated lung regions,[47] the effect of increased oxygenation is localized to aerated lung regions.

Recent experimental evidence indicates that a neural reflex may mediate the lung aeration-induced increase in PBF, explaining simultaneous PBF increases in aerated and nonaerated lung regions.[48] In the adult lung, juxtacapillary receptors (J-receptors) are responsive to lung edema, are thought to be located within juxtacapillary tissue between alveoli, signal via afferent C-fibers within the vagal trunk, and, when activated, trigger tachypnea.[50] As lung aeration at birth involves liquid leaving the distal airways and entering perialveolar tissue, liquid accumulation within lung tissue (see Fig. 150.6) simulates lung edema and may activate these receptors, which then signal via the vagus to initiate global pulmonary vasodilation. This hypothesis is consistent with the finding that bilateral transection of the vagus nerves (vagotomy) blocked the global increase in PBF caused by partial lung aeration.[48] Interestingly, following vagotomy, partial lung aeration with

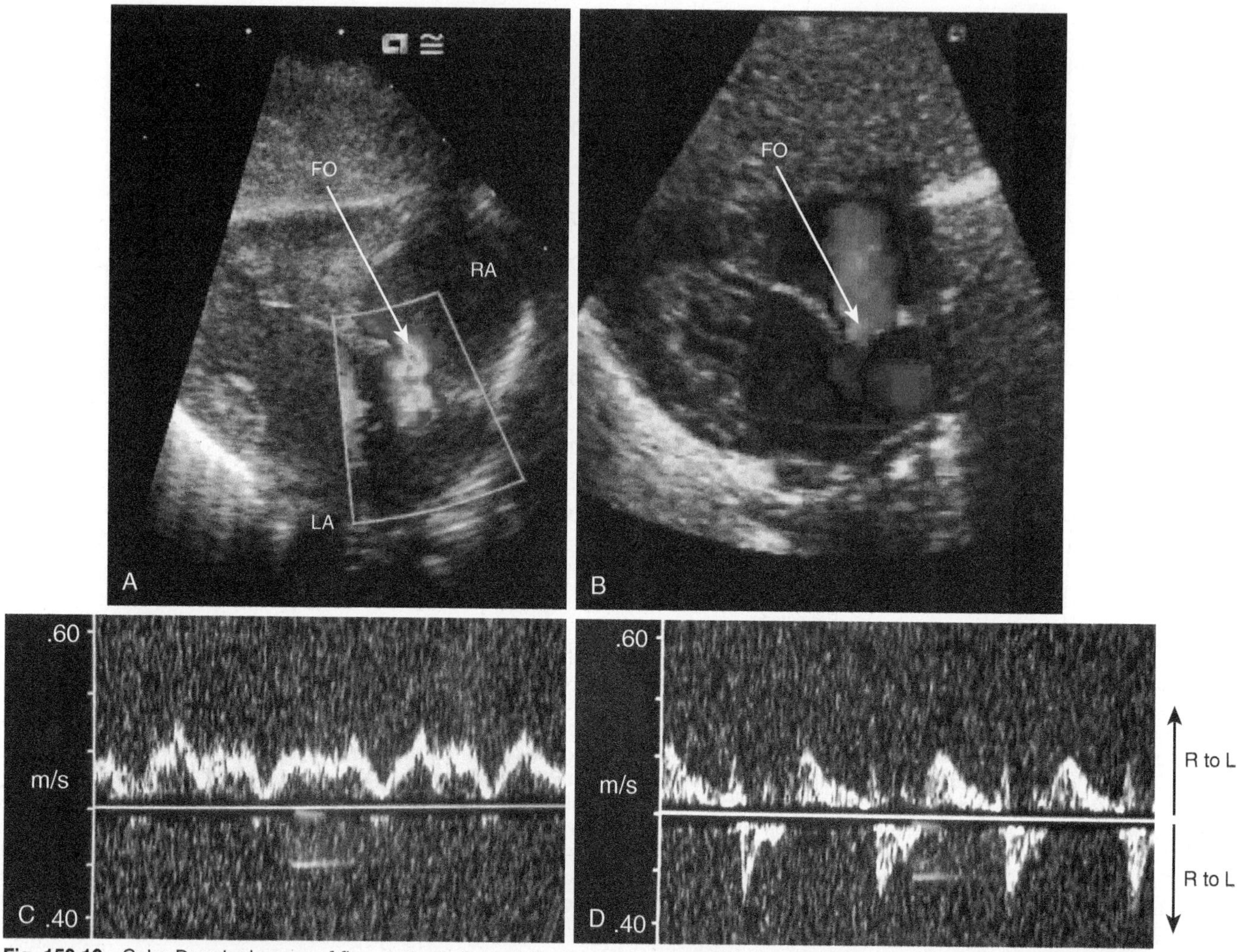

Fig. 150.10 Color Doppler images of flow patterns through the foramen ovale *(FO)* in human infants after birth (A and B) showing both right-to-left (A; R-to-L) and left-to-right (B; L-to-R) shunting. *LA,* Left atrium, *RA,* right atrium. Panels C and D show Doppler flow velocity waveforms through the FO in a newborn lamb immediately before (C) and after (D) umbilical cord clamping. Before cord clamping (C) the flow is almost entirely right-to-left, decreasing to zero during atrial contractions, whereas after clamping (D), the flow initially decreases to zero before becoming bidirectional. (Doppler images courtesy Prof. Martin Kluckow, University of Sydney, Sydney, Australia; and Dr. Andrew Gill, The University of Western Australia, Perth, Australia.)

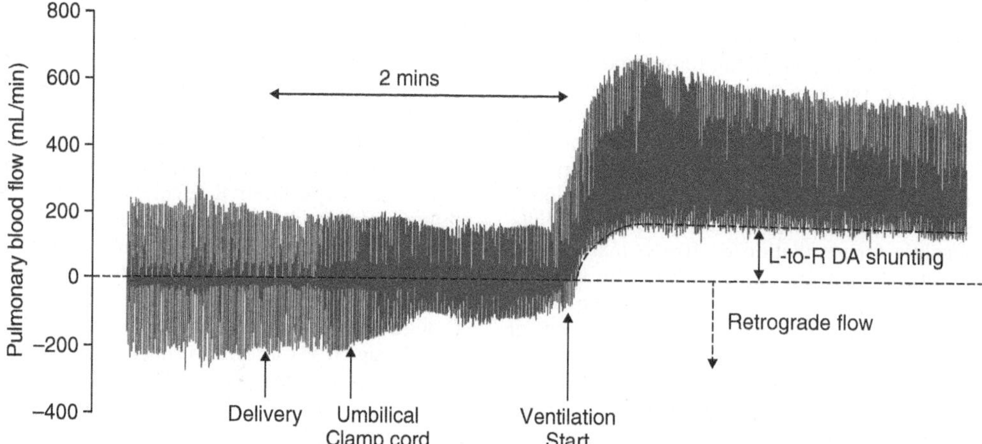

Fig. 150.11 Pulmonary blood flow (PBF) measured in the left pulmonary artery before delivery, after delivery and before cord clamping, after cord clamping and before ventilation onset, and then after ventilation onset in a newborn preterm lamb. Before delivery, PBF oscillates around zero throughout the cardiac cycle (see also Fig. 150.9), with negative PBF indicating retrograde flow of blood away from the lungs during diastole. While delivery has no effect on this blood flow profile, clamping the umbilical cord reduces the amplitude of the waveform due to a reduction in right ventricular stroke volume.[38] Ventilation onset reduces pulmonary vascular resistance and causes a large positive shift in the wave form, with elevated diastolic flows resulting from the onset of left-to-right shunting through the ductus arteriosus. *DA,* Ductus arteriosus.

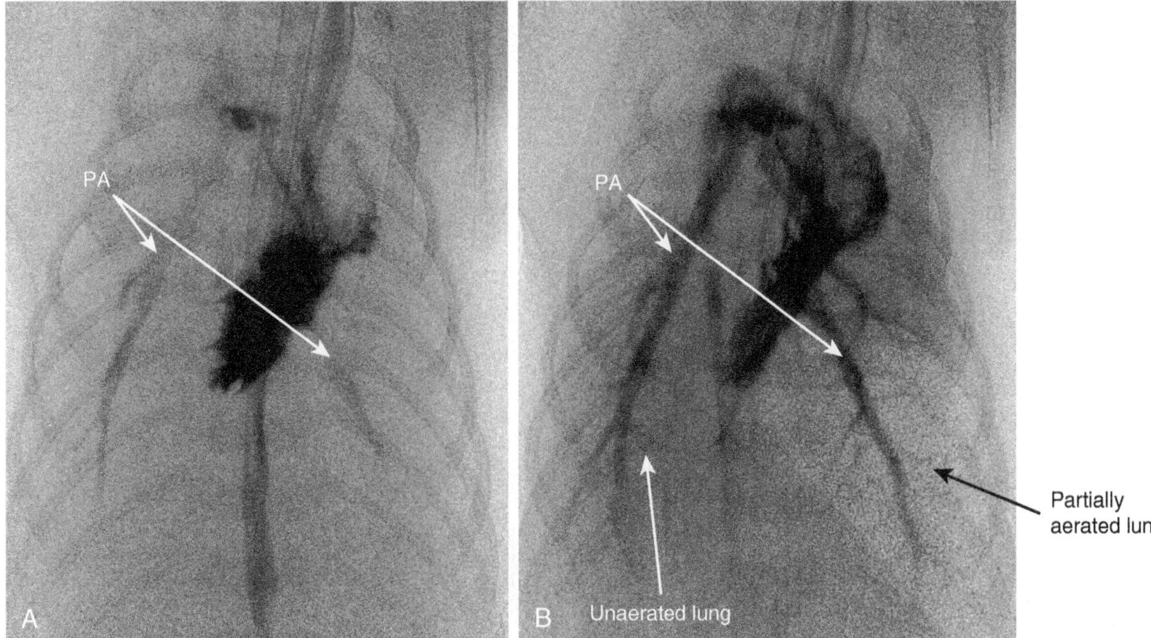

Fig. 150.12 Simultaneous phase contrast and angiographic images acquired before lung aeration (A) and after partial lung aeration (B). A radio-opaque iodine-based contrast agent was administered intravenously to highlight the pulmonary blood vessels. When the entire lung is liquid-filled, very little contrast agent enters the left and right pulmonary arteries (*PA*; *white arrows*), with most of the contrast agent flowing across the ductus arteriosus and down the dorsal aorta. This is due to a high pulmonary vascular resistance (PVR) and continuation of the low PBF characteristic of the "fetal state." Following partial lung aeration *(black arrow)*, PBF markedly increased and the increase was similar in both PAs, irrespective of which lung was partially aerated, demonstrating a marked ventilation/perfusion mismatch in the unaerated lung. This demonstrates that partial lung aeration causes a global decrease in PVR and that the increase in PBF at birth is not spatially related to aerated lung regions. *PBF*, Pulmonary blood flow. (Data from the study of Lang JA, Pearson JT, te Pas AB, et al. Ventilation/perfusion mismatch during lung aeration at birth. *J Appl Physiol*. 2014;117[5]:535–543; and modified.)

100% oxygen increased PBF in aerated lung regions, indicating that the oxygen-mediated increase in PBF was not affected.[48] Thus, the increase in PBF at birth in response to lung aeration likely results from a hierarchy of mechanisms that have either global or localized effects. For instance, the initial movement of liquid out of the airways into lung tissue may activate a global increase in PBF that is modulated at a local level by increased oxygenation, mediated by NO release.[2]

VENTILATION/PERFUSION MATCHING IN THE LUNG AT BIRTH

Ventilation/perfusion matching is a well-described characteristic of the healthy adult lung.[51] This plays an important role in optimizing the lung's gas exchange potential by ensuring that ventilation within lung regions is "matched" with blood flow to those regions. In the diseased lung, ventilation/perfusion "mismatches" can occur whereby lung regions with little or no ventilation receive high blood flow, which is commonly referred to as a "pulmonary shunt" that reduces the lung's gas exchange efficiency.

While a ventilation/perfusion "mismatch" is thought to be problematic in adults, the presence of a large pulmonary shunt in newborns at birth can be viewed differently.[49] Indeed, while survival at birth is not dependent upon the entire lung being ventilated, good cardiac output is essential for preventing hypoxic-ischemic brain injury during periods of reduced oxygenation, which is relatively common at birth.[52] Thus, as a high PBF is essential to maintain left ventricular output, it is important that the increase in PBF is not limited by whether or not the lung is fully aerated. As lung aeration can be delayed in some infants, particularly very preterm infants, it is logical that cardiac output is not limited by the degree of lung aeration.[2]

CARDIOVASCULAR EFFECTS OF UMBILICAL CORD CLAMPING AT BIRTH

During fetal life, PBF is low and contributes little to the supply of preload for the left ventricle, which instead primarily comes from umbilical venous return.[34,53] Thus, after birth the supply of preload for the left ventricle must switch from umbilical venous to pulmonary venous return.[2] However, before this can happen, the lungs must aerate so that PBF can increase.[35,38] As such, when UCC occurs before the lungs have aerated, the loss of umbilical venous return causes a loss of preload and a sudden reduction in cardiac output.[35] Cardiac output remains low until the lungs aerate and PBF increases to restore venous return to the left ventricle.[35] In addition, due to the loss of the low-resistance placental circulation, UCC rapidly increases systemic vascular resistance (Fig. 150.13), causing a rapid increase in arterial pressure (30% increase in four heartbeats).[35] As a result, UCC before lung aeration not only causes a loss in ventricular preload, but also causes a large increase in afterload, which likely contributes to the reduction in cardiac output.[35]

The question of whether immediate UCC before lung aeration could impact cardiac output at birth was first raised by a study detailing the heartrate changes from birth in normal healthy well-oxygenated infants.[15] Up to 50% of normal healthy infants were found to be bradycardic (heart rate <100) within the first minute of birth, which was difficult to explain by a hypoxia-mediated bradycardia.[15] Instead, they suggested that loss of umbilical venous return due to UCC reduced cardiac output, which was reflected by a decrease in heart rate.[15] This suggestion was subsequently confirmed in animal studies, which also demonstrated that if lung aeration and the increase in PBF occurs before UCC, the reduction in cardiac output is avoided.[35] This is now referred to as physiologic-based cord clamping (PBCC) and provides an additional or alternative explanation for the benefits of delayed UCC.[2,36,54]

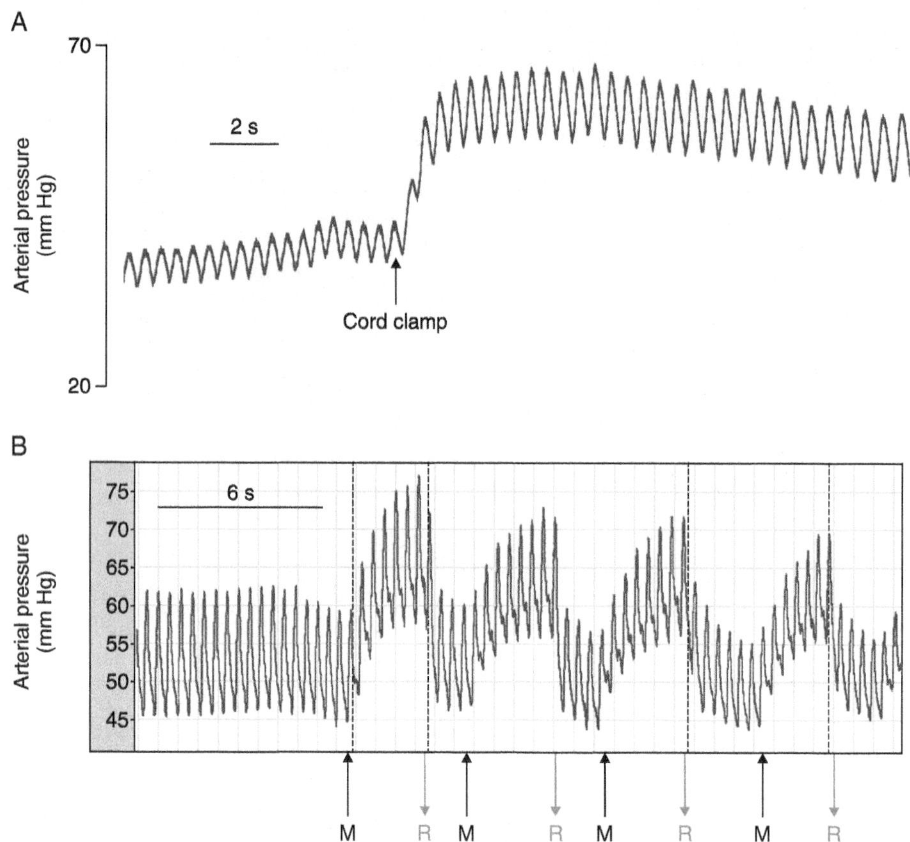

Fig. 150.13 Rapid increases (within four heart beats) in carotid arterial pressure caused by umbilical cord clamping (A) or umbilical cord milking (B) when clamping/milking occurs before ventilation onset. In B, each "milk" *(M)* of the cord simulates the effect of cord clamping on arterial blood pressure, with pressures rapidly returning to base line during the "release" phase *(R)*, before increasing again during the subsequent "milk." The resulting "sawtooth" blood pressure pattern is at high risk of causing cerebral vascular damage and may explain the increased rates of intraventricular hemorrhage observed in extremely preterm infants receiving cord milking.[74] (Data from Bhatt S, Alison B, Wallace EM, et al. Delaying cord clamping until ventilation onset improves cardiovascular function at birth in preterm lambs. *J Physiol.* 2013;591:2113-2126; and Blank DA, Polglase GR, Kluckow M, et al. Haemodynamic effects of umbilical cord milking in premature sheep during the neonatal transition. *Arch Dis Child Fetal Neonatal Ed.* 2018;103:F539-F546; and redrawn.)

DELAYED UMBILICAL CORD CLAMPING AND PLACENTAL TRANSFUSION

Until recently, the benefits of delaying or deferring UCC (DCC) after birth entirely centered around the concept of placental transfusion.[55,56] This refers to the net shift of blood out of the placenta into the infant in a time-dependent manner after birth if the cord remains unclamped.[57] Compared with immediate UCC, the infant body weight gains associated with placental transfusion during DCC[55] are consistent with the reduction in birth weights found in meta-analyses comparing active versus expectant management of the third stage of labor[58]; immediate UCC is one of three components of the active management strategy. As such, the evidence for "placental transfusion" is compelling,[59] but as yet there is still no scientific data explaining how this occurs, and it is possible that the word "transfusion" is misleading.

Placental transfusion can only result if umbilical venous flow into the fetus exceeds umbilical artery flow leaving the fetus. While this could result from large compliance changes in either the placental or the fetal circulations, in almost every instance examined, reducing umbilical artery flow also reduces umbilical venous flows to a similar degree (see Fig. 150.8). Indeed, placental transfusion is unlikely to be gravity related,[60,61] as flows in both umbilical vessels are affected to a similar degree when the newborn is held above or below the introitus.[61] Similarly, uterine contractions do not "squeeze" blood out of the placenta, but instead reduce flows in both vessels and can cause a complete cessation of umbilical flows. While this explanation is regularly used to explain placental transfusion, it is at odds with the known effects of uterine contractions on umbilical blood flows, which underpins our understanding of fetal heart rate monitoring during labor.[62]

Increased compliance of the fetal circulation caused by a large decrease in PVR and the stealing of blood away from the umbilical artery also cannot explain placental transfusion. Although the decrease in PVR causes flow from both the right and left ventricles to be redirected though the lungs, umbilical artery and venous flow decrease to a similar degree (see Fig. 150.8).[37] Similarly, while the decrease in PVR causes a 30 to 40-fold increase in PBF, the associated increase in total pulmonary blood volume is small (approximately 40%) and cannot explain placental transfusion.[63] This is because the volume of a vessel only increases with increasing radius squared (r^2) whereas the resistance decreases with increasing radius to the fourth power (r^4). Furthermore, as the pulmonary circulation is a low-volume, high-flow circuit, this increase (40%) only amounts to a very small proportion of total body blood volume (approximately 2 mL/kg or approximately 2%).[63]

An alternative explanation for placental transfusion is that it reflects rebalancing of blood volume between the fetal and placental circulations following vaginal delivery. That is, blood may shift out of the infant and into the placenta during vaginal birth, which then shifts back into the infant as the circulations "rebalance" after delivery. Indeed, increased dorso-ventral flexion of the fetus may not only result in the loss of lung liquid from the airways (see above), but may also shift blood volume into the placenta. However, this explanation needs verification.

Nevertheless, unfortunately the focus on "placental transfusion" has meant that the vast majority of clinical trials on DCC have used a time-based approach and have ignored the physiologic state of the infant.[55,56] However, we now know that a time-based approach makes little biologic sense and is less than ideal, particularly for infants requiring respiratory support after birth.[36,54] Indeed, under current recommendations, those infants will either receive immediate UCC or have their respiratory support delayed so that they can receive a "placental transfusion." As indicated above and below, the science is very clear and predicts that both strategies are not ideal, particularly the latter.

PHYSIOLOGIC BASED CORD CLAMPING

At birth, if the lung aerates and PBF increases before the cord is clamped, then PBF is able to immediately take over the role of providing preload for the left ventricle following cord clamping.[2,35] This avoids the reduction in cardiac output caused by the loss of umbilical venous return with UCC.[35] In addition, cord clamping after lung aeration mitigates the increase in arterial pressure caused by UCC, because the lung becomes an alternate low-resistance pathway for blood flow.[35,38] As a result, left-to-right shunting through the DA increases, leading to a further increase in PBF and venous return to the left ventricle.[38] On the other hand, immediate UCC after birth causes a reduction in cardiac output that is sustained until the lungs aerate and PBF increases.[35] Thus, if lung aeration is delayed, cardiac output will remain reduced, which increases the risk of hypoxic-ischemic brain injury if the infant is hypoxic. Then, after lung aeration, cardiac output is rapidly restored, causing a rebound in arterial pressure and a large increase in cerebral blood flow.[35] It is not surprising, therefore, that one of the noted benefits of DCC is a reduction in intraventricular hemorrhage (IVH).[59]

The logistics of helping infants, particularly very preterm infants, aerate their lungs with an intact umbilical cord was, until recently, thought to be unfeasible. However, recent feasibility studies have demonstrated that the logistical issues are not insurmountable.[64,65] One study (Baby-directed umbilical cord clamping study; Baby-DUCC) assessed the feasibility of stabilizing preterm infants (>32 weeks) with the cord intact by placing the baby on the mother's legs.[66] They found that stabilizing infants, as indicated by regular stable breathing, with the cord intact, prevented the bradycardia evident in normal healthy infants immediately after birth. Another study (ABC) has used a purpose-built resuscitation table (Concord table, Concord Neonatal, the Netherlands) that allows for more extensive resuscitation and monitoring of the infant while the umbilical cord remains intact.[64,65] Recent safety and feasibility studies in very preterm infants (<30 weeks) have shown that all necessary interventions for cardiopulmonary stabilization can be performed while the infant remains attached to the umbilical cord.[64,65] They also observed less bradycardia and hypoxia at birth, supporting the concept of a more stable hemodynamic transition. As the average cord clamping time was over 4 minutes,[64,65] this approach also allows preterm infants to maximally benefit from placental transfusion, while not delaying the onset of resuscitation. Trials are now focusing on PBCC, rather than a time-based approach, in subgroups of infants that will likely experience a long delay between birth and lung aeration. These include very preterm infants (<28 weeks) and newborns with a congenital diaphragmatic hernia.[67-69]

UMBILICAL CORD MILKING

It has been suggested that the "placental transfusion" associated with DCC can be replicated, over a much shorter time period, by milking the umbilical cord.[70-72] Umbilical cord milking (UCM) involves squeezing the cord between thumb and finger and then "milking" the cord towards the infant, forcing blood in the cord to move into the infant. This procedure can occur once or several times along a segment of cord (up to 20 cm long).[70] It has been suggested that UCM may be an alternative to DCC and may benefit infants needing resuscitation at birth, allowing them to get a "transfusion" without the delay.[70] However, this assumes that placental transfusion is the only benefit of DCC, which is incorrect.[2,36] Furthermore, recent scientific evidence indicates that UCM is potentially worse than immediate UCC, particularly if it is done several times.[37] That is, consecutive milks result in large fluctuations in blood pressure and cerebral blood flow that are potentially injurious (see Fig. 150.13),[37] particularly if the infant is hypoxic at birth and has a vasodilated cerebral vascular bed. Furthermore, whether UCM results in a net "transfusion" of blood into the infant depends on the milking procedure, because retrograde flow from the infant can occur between milks.[37]

Numerous trials have not detected any harmful effects of UCM in infants,[70] and the European resuscitation guidelines suggest that it may be an alternative to DCC in emergency situations.[73] However, this is in stark contradiction to what is predicted by the science.[37] More recently, a trial (PREMOD2) in very preterm infants was stopped early due to an increase in IVH rates in UCM infants (22% vs. 6%).[74] This indicates that, while it is safe in some infants, it increases the risk of cerebral vascular damage in others. This can be explained by the fact that lung aeration prior to cord clamping (i.e., PBCC) greatly reduces the increase in arterial blood pressure caused by cord clamping.[35] As UCM simulates cord clamping (see Fig. 150.13), if it occurs after breathing onset, its effect on arterial blood pressure will be minimal, whereas if it occurs before breathing onset, it will cause large fluctuations in pressure.[37] Until recently, most trials examining the effects of UCM occurred in healthy near-term infants.[72,75] As these infants usually commence breathing immediately after birth, the pressure fluctuations caused by UCM are likely to be minimal. In contrast, those infants requiring resuscitation at birth were mostly excluded from the trials. However, as very preterm infants have difficulty in aerating their lungs at birth, most will not have aerated their lungs before UCM. As such, these infants are at high risk of being exposed to the large arterial pressure surges associated with UCM (see Fig. 150.13).[37] Nevertheless, until the science has been thoroughly investigated, it seems prudent to avoid UCM, particularly in infants requiring resuscitation at birth.

ASSISTING INFANTS' TRANSITION AT BIRTH

The challenges faced by infants as they transition to newborn life can vary depending upon the infant's level of maturity and lung development and whether or not they were exposed to significant periods hypoxia/asphyxia before or during birth. As such, the type of assistance applied should be tailored towards the needs of the individual. In particular, it should not be assumed that a uniform approach that covers all infants is best, due to its ease and simplicity of implementation. We will discuss the physiologic challenges faced by different subgroups of infants in order to understand the approaches that may best assist these infants.

STABILIZING VERY PRETERM INFANTS AT BIRTH

The primary challenge facing very or extremely preterm infants at birth is immaturity of their respiratory system (see Fig. 150.5), but considerable variability exists among preterm infants due to a variety of factors.[76] These include the presence/absence of antenatal corticosteroids and the presence/absence of comorbidities such as chorioamnionitis and fetal growth restriction. As such, treating this subgroup of infants as a uniform group is also likely to be problematic.

LUNG IMMATURITY

Chapter 57 provides a detailed description of the factors regulating normal and abnormal development of the lung and, in particular, the stage of lung development attained at the time of premature birth. In short, very or extremely preterm infants have immature and underdeveloped lungs that are in the canalicular or early saccular stages of development. While most conducting airways will have formed, the distal gas exchange regions exist as rudimentary sac-like structures with limited surface area for gas exchange (see Fig. 150.6). The mesenchymal tissue surrounding the distal airways is relatively thick and the penetration of capillaries around these structures is limited, resulting in large gas diffusion distances between airspaces and capillaries (i.e., large air/blood gas diffusion barrier). Extremely preterm infants will have few, if any, differentiated type-I and type-II alveolar epithelial cells, making the lungs surfactant deficient. While the consequences of this for postnatal respiratory function can be partially mitigated with exogenous surfactant, surfactant deficiency may also adversely affect lung aeration (see below).

PHYSIOLOGIC CONSEQUENCES OF LUNG IMMATURITY

PRESSURE- VERSUS VOLUME-CONTROLLED VENTILATION IN THE DELIVERY ROOM

After birth, the dynamics of lung aeration are determined by the distal movement of liquid through the airways and then across the distal airway walls into the surrounding lung tissue. The resistance to this liquid movement is determined by the total cross-sectional area of the conducting airways at each generation and the surface area of the distal airways, which are both reduced in preterm infants. As such, the resistance to moving liquid through the airways during lung aeration is considerably greater in preterm newborns, thereby requiring higher pressure gradients (see Fig. 150.5).[27] Despite this, current resuscitation guidelines recommend the initial use of lower inflation pressures in preterm (20 to 25 cm H_2O) compared to term (25 to 30 cm H_2O) infants.[28] This reflects a high degree of caution, as high tidal volumes are known to cause lung injury.[77,78] However, these pressure ranges are an estimate of what is needed to achieve tidal volumes within the desired range of 4 to 8 mL/kg,[79,80] but assume that lung compliances are static and similar in the liquid and air-filled lungs. However, lung compliances are not static and increase exponentially as the lung aerates, a fact that appears to have been overlooked. While this holds true for both term and preterm infants, it is particularly relevant in very preterm infants as it is important to keep tidal volumes within a narrow margin of safety. This raises the vexed question as to why airway pressures are universally measured in the delivery room, whereas the routine measurement of tidal volumes is largely restricted to research active institutions. As the tidal volume range is the targeted outcome and as the airway pressures required to achieve these volumes will markedly change as the lung aerates and compliances increase, directly measuring tidal volumes is the most logical approach.

SURFACTANT ADMINISTRATION IN THE DELIVERY ROOM

As surfactant is normally released into lung liquid before birth and enters amniotic fluid, measurement of the lecithin-sphingomyelin (LS) ratio has been used as an indicator of lung development near term.[81] Nevertheless, evidence suggests that prenatal surfactant release may benefit lung aeration by enhancing the uniformity of lung aeration. PC x-ray imaging studies in preterm rabbits found that when surfactant is administered prior to lung aeration, the entry of air was evenly distributed across all lung quadrants, which was maintained throughout lung aeration.[82] In the absence of surfactant, different lung regions aerated at different rates, leading to nonuniform ventilation, which is potentially injurious. This effect of surfactant was thought to result from its ability to reduce surface tension at the air/liquid interface. Thus, as the air/liquid interface moves distally through the airways, when it reaches a branching point, a reduced surface tension increases the likelihood that air will pass down both daughter airways. However, if surface tensions are high, small differences in airway dimensions may encourage air to only enter and move down the larger of the two airways. The ability of surfactant to improve the uniformity of lung aeration likely explains its ability to protect the lung from injury to high tidal volumes[78] by facilitating a more even distribution of ventilation across the lung, but also increases the surface area for gas exchange by increasing the proportion of lung aerated. This likely contributes to the well-known effect of surfactant on oxygenation in the first few hours after birth in very preterm infants.[83]

CLINICAL APPLICATIONS OF THE KNOWN PHYSIOLOGY

SUSTAINED INFLATIONS

As the lung must pass through two distinct phases before it stabilizes into a functional gas exchange organ after birth (see above), it is logical to tailor the respiratory support provided to the lung's physiology at any moment in time.[6] For instance, during phase 1, when the distal airways are liquid-filled, the lung is incapable of gas exchange. As such, the concept of applying tidal ventilation, to get oxygen in and carbon dioxide out of the lung, is illogical.[6] Indeed, while the inflation component of the positive pressure cycle will aid airway liquid clearance, the expiration component provides little or no benefit when there is no CO_2 exchange. This logic underpins the rationale for applying an initial sustained inflation (SI) at birth, whereby the expiration component is abandoned, because it is thought to serve no function.[6] Studies in animal models have detailed how a SI can improve the rate and spatial pattern of lung aeration at birth, without having any adverse effect on pulmonary physiology,[26,45,84] although there is some evidence that it increases the risk of lung injury.[85] Furthermore, as the inflation pressures and inflation durations required to aerate the lung of very preterm infants are interrelated and vary considerably between individuals, it is evident that inflating the lung to a fixed volume is the best approach.[27,86] However, any benefit of an SI is rapidly lost, if the SI is followed by iPPV without a positive end-expiratory pressure (PEEP), due to airway reflooding.[26] This indicates that, by itself, SI is not a solution to the pulmonary ventilation problems faced by preterm infants after birth, but may be effective for initiating homogenous ventilation and pulmonary gas exchange.

Clinical trials, including the SAIL trial, have failed to confirm the benefits of SI at birth in very preterm infants.[87-89] Indeed, the SAIL trial was stopped early due to an increase in adverse outcomes in the treatment group.[89] While it is not clear why an SI was found to be beneficial in experimental studies but not in human trials, the approach used in the human trials did not replicate the approach used in the animal studies.[87-89] In all animal studies, the newborns were intubated and so the inflation pressures were directly applied to the lungs. However, in all human trials,[87-89] the SI was applied noninvasively (mostly via a face mask) and so whether or not the inflation pressure was applied to the airways depended upon face mask leak and whether the upper airway, including the larynx, was patent.[87] As the larynx is closed at birth if the infant is apneic or has an irregular or unstable breathing pattern (see below), this precludes gas from entering the lungs during the SI. Thus, to duplicate the successful findings in animal studies, it is likely that any future SI trial should be restricted to intubated infants. Nevertheless, realization that the glottis is likely to be closed at birth in apneic infants has far-reaching implications for noninvasive ventilation (NIV) in the delivery room.

NONINVASIVE VENTILATION

NIV, usually applied via a face mask or nasal prongs, is currently the recommended "first choice" approach for providing respiratory assistance to very preterm infants at birth.[28,73] This is because intubation in the delivery room is thought to be difficult, stressful for inexperienced caregivers, invasive for the infant, and mechanical ventilation increases the risk of lung injury. However, NIV has been largely adopted under the assumption that it interacts with the infant in exactly the same way as intubation and mechanical ventilation, except in a less invasive way. As such, many assume that iPPV using a face mask can take over the role of breathing in apneic nonintubated infants, just like mechanical ventilation does in intubated infants. However, this assumption has major caveats. Indeed, supporting infants in the delivery room with NIV requires a different approach to intubation and mechanical ventilation, unless the infant is severely asphyxiated. In particular, during NIV, the focus should be on supporting and encouraging spontaneous breathing[73] rather than trying to take over the role of breathing.

As indicated above, the fetal larynx plays an important role in fetal lung development. Closure of the larynx during apnea greatly reduces the loss of fetal lung liquid via the trachea, causing it to accumulate within the future airways, thereby maintaining the lungs in a distended state.[1,4] As lung distension is the primary stimulus for fetal lung growth (see Chapter 57), bypassing the larynx or a loss of laryngeal function causes lung growth to essentially cease.[1,4] During FBMs, the larynx opens in phase with the diaphragm and remains mostly open during continuous, vigorous FBMs.[90] This causes a reduction in the resistance to liquid efflux from the trachea and explains the accelerated rate of liquid loss from the lungs during FBMs compared to apnea.[91] Thus, the fetal larynx is closed during apnea, opens briefly during a breath when breathing is irregular, and is mostly open when FBMs are continuous and regular.

As preterm infants are essentially exteriorized fetuses, it should not be surprising that, at birth, the larynx will close and only open during a breath in preterm infants who are apneic or have an irregular breathing pattern. This has been observed in preterm newborn rabbits[92] and explains why iPPV given noninvasively is often ineffective (Fig. 150.14). As closure of the larynx prevents gas from entering the sublaryngeal airways,[92] inflation pressures applied noninvasively via a face mask cannot ventilate the lung. However, the factors regulating opening or closure of the larynx are numerous and complex, and so, even if the infant is in a stable breathing pattern, the larynx can close during expiratory braking maneuvers, postural changes (e.g., lifting its legs), swallowing, and crying. On the other hand, during irregular breathing the larynx will open briefly during a breath.[92] While the glottis likely opens if the infant becomes so hypoxic and bradycardic that it loses tone and laryngeal reflexes, ideally it is best to avoid this level of hypoxia and bradycardia. As such, the success of NIV at birth is largely dependent on the presence of spontaneous breathing, when the larynx is predominantly open (see Fig. 150.14).

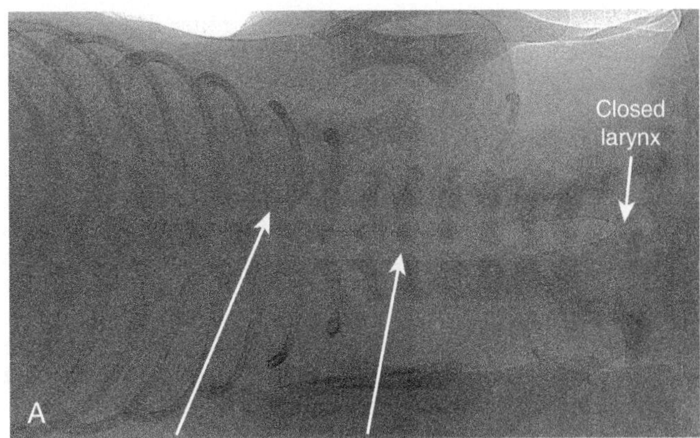

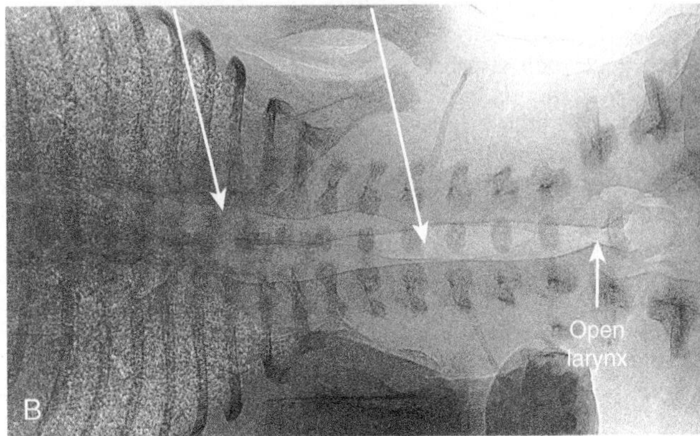

Fig. 150.14 Phase contrast x-ray images of (A) an apneic preterm rabbit with a closed larynx and (B) a spontaneously breathing preterm rabbit with an open larynx. Very little of the lung is aerated in the apneic newborn rabbit, and as a result the apnea and closed larynx was likely in response to hypoxia. In contrast, the spontaneously breathing newborn rabbit had a stable regular breathing pattern, and as a result the lung was well aerated and the larynx remained open throughout the respiratory cycle. Each of the preterm newborn rabbits received 5 cm H_2O via a face mask. (From Crawshaw JR, Kitchen MJ, Binder-Heschl C, et al. Laryngeal closure impedes non-invasive ventilation at birth. *Arch Dis Child Fetal Neonatal Ed*. 2017;103[2]:F112–F119.)

STIMULATING BREATHING AT BIRTH

Studies in preterm rabbits have confirmed that, at birth, the larynx will close during apnea, but will be mostly open if the newborn has a stable and continuous breathing pattern (see Fig. 150.14).[92] Furthermore, if the newborn is in a regular stable breathing pattern and then becomes progressively hypoxic, the period of time the larynx is open decreases, and eventually it closes when the newborn becomes apneic (unpublished observations). Clearly, therefore, as the efficacy of NIV is reliant on the infant breathing so that the larynx is open, it is important to focus on stimulating breathing in the newborn and avoiding factors, like hypoxia, that inhibit breathing.[93] This may explain why the use of low inspired oxygen levels (FiO_2) have failed to meet expectations in reducing morbidity and mortality in very preterm infants and have even been associated with worse outcomes (see below). On the other hand, physical stimulation is a well-established method for stimulating infants at birth.[94,95] Recent studies in both animals and infants have shown that physical stimulation at birth increases minute volume and oxygenation and reduces the risk of apnea.[95,96] However, it is unclear how much stimulation is required and how it should be applied.

While hypoxia is potent inhibitor of FBM, it is not the only factor that influences FBM. For instance, both prostaglandin E_2 (PGE_2) and adenosine inhibit FBM and are released from the placenta into the fetal circulation during development.[97,98] The release of both are increased in response to hypoxia and while the hypoxia-induced inhibition of FBM is very potent, the inhibitory effects of PGE_2 and adenosine may also have a major impact.[99,100] Similarly, chorioamnionitis is a common antecedent of preterm birth and a major cause of antenatal inflammation, leading to the release of pro-inflammatory cytokines, such as PGE_2.[101] Thus, it is possible that spontaneous breathing may be reduced or inhibited in very preterm infants at birth exposed to antenatal inflammation associated with chorioamnionitis. As the lung becomes a major site of prostaglandin metabolism after birth,[102] the rapid and large increase in PBF would be expected to rapidly decrease circulating PGs, thereby mitigating some of the inhibitory effect on breathing. However, PGE_2 is also produced locally within the respiratory center and so may act locally to inhibit breathing.

Caffeine is widely used to stimulate breathing in very preterm infants and acts as a competitive adenosine antagonist within the respiratory center, a known inhibitor of breathing.[103]

While caffeine is commonly used to treat apnea of prematurity, treatment usually commences 1 to 2 hours after birth.[93] A small clinical trial has shown that caffeine, given via a butterfly needle directly into the umbilical vein within 1 to 2 minutes of birth, increased breathing efforts in preterm infants.[104] The finding that the stimulatory effect of caffeine on breathing was gestational age-dependent (greater in older infants), raises several interesting considerations that require investigation. For instance, (1) do younger infants require a higher dose of caffeine, (2) how does placentally derived adenosine, particularly following antenatal hypoxia, influence the dose of caffeine required to stimulate breathing at birth, and (3) as caffeine crosses the placenta, can maternal caffeine administration prior to birth enhance breathing in very preterm infants at birth?

ROLE OF OXYGEN AT BIRTH

In 2010, the revised resuscitation guidelines recommended that respiratory support for very preterm infants should commence with air or a gas mixture with a low FiO_2 (0.3).[105] This recommendation was based on decades of research, showing that high inspired FiO_2 levels are injurious to the lung, may impede transition in term infants, and are not necessarily required to resuscitate preterm infants.[106] However, much of this research was based on animal studies exposed to prolonged periods (days to weeks) of high oxygen levels[107] and on infants that were intubated and mechanically ventilated. Nevertheless, it was concerning when, following the guideline change in 2010, studies emerged showing an increase in morbidity and mortality in very preterm infants and higher mortality rates in infants randomized to receiving respiratory support with a low FiO_2.[108,109] While a subsequent meta-analysis has failed to confirm the higher mortality in preterm infants commencing with a low FiO_2,[110] from a physiologic point of view, the finding is explainable.

The recommendation for using a low FiO_2 to resuscitate very preterm infants at birth coincided with a wider acceptance for using NIV instead of intubation and mechanical ventilation.[105] As NIV is largely dependent on the infant breathing (see above), the initial use of low FiO_2 levels may have increased the risk of hypoxia-induced inhibition of breathing, causing closure of the glottis. This suggestion has been confirmed by studies in both animals and infants, which compared the initiation of respiratory support at birth with high (100%) and low (30%) FiO_2 levels.[111,112] Resuscitation with a high FiO_2 significantly increased breathing rates, minute volumes, and oxygenation levels in both very preterm infants and rabbits and reduced the incidence of apnea.[111,112] Interestingly, as the FiO_2 was rapidly titrated in infants based on oxygenation levels, infants starting with a high FiO_2 had an overall oxygen exposure that was not different from the low FiO_2 group.[112] This confirms the influence of oxygen, or lack thereof, on breathing in premature newborns at birth, with low FiO_2 levels increasing the risk of apnea and/or irregular breathing. This finding can be explained by the fact that the lung of very preterm infants is likely to be poorly aerated immediately after birth. As such, the surface area available for gas exchange will be reduced and so a high oxygen concentration gradient is required initially to oxygenate the infant. However, as the lung aerates the gas exchange surface area increases exponentially,[113] even in the very immature lung, and so the oxygen concentration requirement rapidly diminishes. As a result, while the oxygen requirement is initially high, following lung aeration, oxygenation can be sustained with a lower FiO_2 due to the larger gas exchange surface area.

SUMMARY

An infant's physiology at birth is distinctly different from its physiology hours to days later, mostly because the lung is liquid-filled at birth. As lung aeration is the trigger for the transition to newborn life, failure to aerate the lung not only prevents pulmonary gas exchange but also prevents the increase in PBF, causing a loss of venous return and cardiac output if the umbilical cord is clamped. This explains the neonatologist's mantra that "pulmonary ventilation is the cornerstone of neonatal resuscitation." However, as the immature lung of very preterm infants is highly prone to injury, assisting infants to aerate their lungs without causing injury is a difficult and challenging "balancing act." Indeed, to aerate the lung and oxygenate the infant may initially require high pressures and a high FiO_2 because the airways are either fully or partially liquid-filled. But, as lung compliance and gas exchange surface area markedly increase as the lung aerates, the required airway pressures and FiO_2 rapidly decrease. As such, unless the infant's tidal volume and oxygenation level are carefully monitored, there is a significant risk of either injuring the lung, due to over-expansion, or causing hyperoxia as the infant's physiology transitions into a state compatible with life after birth.

NIV is now the preferred approach for assisting very preterm infants at birth as it is less injurious to the immature lung, but spontaneous breathing is required for this approach to be effective so that the larynx does not close. Thus, when using this approach, the focus should be on stimulating and supporting spontaneous breathing rather than attempting to replace breathing with iPPV. Although it is still unclear how this is best achieved in different subgroups of infants, it is well established that physical stimulation and respiratory stimulants, while avoiding inhibitory factors like hypoxia, are quite effective.

RESPIRATORY DISTRESS IN TERM INFANTS

Respiratory distress in term or near-term infants is a growing clinical problem, accounting for 33% of all infants admitted into intensive care for respiratory problems.[114] This is partly due to increasing CS rates, as 7% to 10% of infants delivered by elective CS develop respiratory distress.[115,116] Many of these infants are diagnosed with TTN. However, this diagnosis is imprecise, is often made retrospectively, and because it is usually self-resolving, TTN is commonly regarded as a minor issue. Nevertheless, it results in the unexpected admission of large numbers of otherwise healthy infants into intensive care within hours of birth, and a small number of infants go onto to develop severe and protracted respiratory distress as well as pulmonary hypertension.[116]

As airway liquid loss from the nose and mouth during vaginal delivery is the only mechanism that results in liquid loss from the respiratory system at birth,[6] if this mechanism is not activated, all liquid in the airways must be cleared into lung tissue. Thus, in infants born by elective CS without labor, the majority of airway liquid must be cleared by the pressures generated during inspiration, and all of this liquid must enter lung tissue (Fig. 150.15).[6] In contrast, infants delivered vaginally can lose significant volumes of liquid via the nose and mouth during delivery.[117] As a result, the volume of liquid that must be cleared into lung tissue after birth is considerably less (see Fig. 150.15). Thus, near-term respiratory distress in otherwise healthy infants may be caused by larger volumes of airway liquid at the onset of breathing.[6,7] As this liquid must be cleared into lung tissue, larger volumes must increase the degree of lung tissue "edema" following lung aeration (see Fig. 150.15).[32,33] This is a very different explanation to the widespread prevailing view that TTN is caused by a failure to clear airway liquid due to the absence of the stress of labor.[3,118]

Experimental studies have simulated the influence of labor (reduced lung liquid) and absence of labor (increased lung liquid) on respiratory function and mechanics immediately after birth.[7,27] Increasing lung liquid volumes at birth reduces lung compliance and FRC and causes the chest wall to expand further and the diaphragm to flatten.[7] These changes readily explain the respiratory symptoms characterized by infants diagnosed with

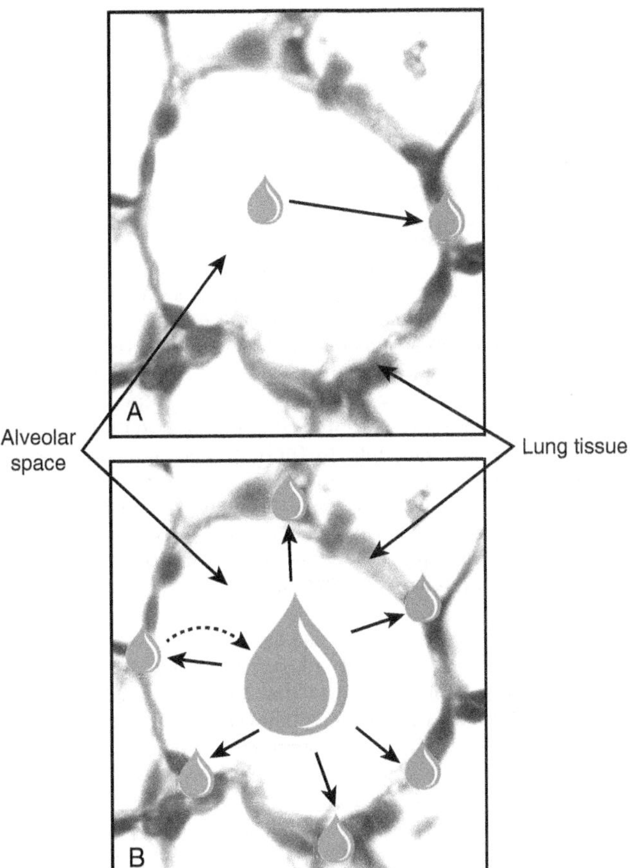

Fig. 150.15 Diagrammatic representation indicating how the movement of elevated airway liquid volumes into lung tissue may cause lung tissue edema. (A) Smaller volumes of airway liquid at breathing onset requires the accommodation of less liquid within the thin ribbons of tissue surrounding the airways of the mature lung near term. (B) Larger airway liquid volumes at breathing onset increases the amount of liquid that must be accommodated within lung tissue, leading to edema and an increase in lung interstitial tissue pressure.

TTN. The reduction in FRC explains the expiratory grunting, which is caused by closure of the glottis during expiration and is commonly used by newborns to preserve FRC after birth.[23] On the other hand, chest wall expansion and flattening of the diaphragm (see Fig. 150.7) reduces inspiratory reserve volumes and, when combined with a lower lung compliance, restricts tidal volumes. Thus, to sustain alveolar ventilation, respiratory rates increase, which explains the tachypnea and labored breathing.

While there are likely to be many causes of respiratory distress in near-term infants at birth, whether or not excess lung liquid and the resulting pulmonary edema is a central underlying cause warrants closer examination. Infants diagnosed with TTN are commonly regarded as a separate subgroup of infants, simply because their form of respiratory morbidity is usually milder and self-limiting, with the latter being a major contributing factor to the diagnosis. However, how should infants who initially show TTN-like symptoms, but then develop more severe and protracted respiratory distress, be diagnosed? It is possible that the underlying morbidity has similar origins and that the morbidity varies from mild to severe respiratory distress depending on the volume of airway liquid present at breathing onset and the availability and timely use of treatments like continuous positive airway pressure (CPAP).[119] Indeed, accommodating large volumes of liquid in lung tissue may cause lung injury and further respiratory distress due to a continuous cycle of airway liquid clearance and then re-entry with each breath.[23] As end-expiratory pressures provide a positive pressure gradient that opposes airway liquid re-entry during expiration,[25,26] this may explain why CPAP is an effective treatment for TTN. However, prevention is better than treatment and so fully understanding the mechanism of near-term respiratory distress may help to develop delivery techniques at elective CS that simulate the liquid loss during vaginal delivery.

RESUSCITATION OF SEVERELY ASPHYXIATED INFANTS AT BIRTH

The term ***birth asphyxia*** is commonly used to describe severely asphyxiated infants that are bradycardic (detected by ECG), apneic, have little or no tone, and may lack a detectable pulse. However, asphyxia is a continuum that ranges from mild to the very severe, and the type of assistance an infant requires likely depends on where it is along that continuum. For instance, mildly asphyxiated infants may only need physical stimulation to commence breathing and aerate their lungs to increase oxygenation and heart rate.[95] However, as the asphyxia deepens, physical stimulation may be insufficient to stimulate breathing and so iPPV is required.[120] When the asphyxia is severe and protracted, myocardial contractility diminishes and arterial blood pressures decrease with decreasing cardiac output.[121,122] In newborn lambs, positive pressure ventilation alone is sufficient to aerate the lungs, oxygenate the newborn, and restore cardiac output if mean arterial pressures remain above approximately 20 mm Hg.[121] However, when blood pressures decrease below approximately 15 mm Hg, chest compressions and epinephrine are required to restore oxygenation and cardiac output.[123]

Research using experimental animal models has investigated approaches that can be used to resuscitate asphyxiated infants at birth. However, many of these studies have used newborns hours to days after birth,[124,125] largely because the logistics of performing these studies in large animal species at birth is difficult and expensive.[121] Nevertheless, the underlying physiologic state of animals is very different at birth from what it is hours to days after birth. Indeed, newborns at birth have liquid-filled lungs, a functional DA allowing bidirectional shunting between the pulmonary and systemic circulations, and may or may not have the placental circulation attached (see above). As such, the relevance of the conclusions drawn from these studies should be viewed with this difference in mind, particularly the ventilation strategies examined and the approaches used to restore spontaneous circulation.

While heart rate is universally used as a clinical indicator of birth asphyxia, by itself it is a very poor discriminator for determining mild or severe asphyxia at birth.[121] An infant may have a vagal-mediated bradycardia (<100 bpm), due to a rapid and transient decrease in oxygenation, but otherwise have good blood pressure and cardiac output.[126,127] Indeed, this rapid, vagal-mediated bradycardia, originally described by Dawes,[120] is much less pronounced if the newborns face is not covered by liquid, indicating that the "diving reflex" may contribute to the response in utero.[128] Nevertheless, it indicates that the heart rate response to the same level of asphyxia differs before (in utero) and after birth (ex utero). On the other hand, a similar level of bradycardia can be accompanied with myocardial anoxia and severe hypotension as a result of little or no cardiac output[121]; this is commonly referred to as a pulseless ECG. Furthermore, a bradycardia at birth can also be caused by a loss of left ventricular preload due to cord clamping before lung aeration,[35] as shown in the heart rate nomograms in healthy term infants.[15] This was confirmed in newborn rabbits ventilated with a gas devoid of oxygen (100% nitrogen), showing that lung aeration, even in the absence of oxygen, can increase both PBF and heart rate after birth.[47] Nevertheless, apnea accompanies both mild and severe asphyxia, and so asphyxiated infants will almost certainly require iPPV to aerate their lungs and increase oxygenation. However, it is unclear how asphyxiated infants should be ventilated at birth and whether an elevated FiO_2 is required.

VENTILATION OF THE ASPHYXIATED INFANT

In newborn lambs with severe asphyxia at birth, a SI is superior to both conventional iPPV and multiple, short SIs (5 × 3 seconds) at restoring heart rate and blood pressure and recruitment of tidal volume, leading to a more rapid increase in blood pressures, cerebral perfusion, and cerebral oxygenation.[129] To clarify whether the more rapid cardiovascular response with a SI resulted from a more rapid increase in PBF or oxygenation in response to better lung aeration, severely asphyxiated lambs were given a SI using gases containing, 0% (100% nitrogen), 5%, 21% (air), or 100% oxygen.[130] While a SI with 0% oxygen had little effect on heart rate and blood pressure, a gas containing 5% oxygen was able to increase heart rate, blood pressure, and PBF almost as effectively as air, which was not different from 100% oxygen.[130] At the very least, this indicates that resuscitation of severely asphyxiated term infants may not require 100% oxygen, and that only a small amount of oxygen is required to improve myocardial function. These studies also showed that while the very rapid cardiovascular response induced by an SI was associated with a greater rebound hypertension, higher cerebral blood flows, and oxygen delivery, it also appeared to be associated with increased cerebral vascular damage.[121] Thus, it is possible that a more rapid restoration and a greater post-asphyxial rebound response is injurious to the brain.[131] Indeed, as the cerebral vascular bed maximally vasodilates in response to the asphyxia, a rapid and large increase in blood pressure gives little opportunity for the cerebral vasculature to invoke autoregulatory mechanisms and vasoconstrict in order to protect the cerebral microvasculature from high pressures. Thus, while heart rates and blood pressure recovered more rapidly with a 30-second SI, it was also associated with a greater post-asphyxia rebound response and an increase in cerebral vascular damage.[121] This raises the very important question as to whether the post-asphyxial response may contribute to the overall cerebral injury suffered by infants exposed to birth asphyxia.[131] These studies also indicate that resuscitation with 100% oxygen confers no clear benefits over air and may cause excess cerebral oxygen delivery in the immediate post-asphyxia period.

CHEST COMPRESSIONS AND RESTORATION OF SPONTANEOUS CIRCULATION

While bradycardia is an early sign of asphyxia, if the asphyxia is protracted, myocardial anoxia causes a loss in cardiac contractility, resulting in a gradual reduction in blood pressure. As newborn lambs can take 15 to 20 minutes from asphyxia onset to a complete loss of cardiac function (indicated by very low blood pressures and little to no ventricular outputs), the fetal heart must have significant oxygen reserves.[123,131] When measured by ECG, heart rates can stay relatively constant at 60 to 70 beats/minute throughout this time and continue at this rate even in the absence of a detectable pulse.[121] When newborn lambs reach this level of asphyxia (mean arterial pressures <15 mm Hg), lung aeration and pulmonary ventilation along with chest compressions and epinephrine are required to restore spontaneous circulation.[123] However, many questions still remain as to how this is most effectively applied. For instance, it is unclear what ventilation mode (SI vs. conventional iPPV), chest compression rate, synchronization between chest compressions and iPPV, and administration route for epinephrine (e.g., intravenous, intratracheal, intraosseous, and intranasal) are best. Nevertheless, to achieve ROSC, it is clear that during chest compressions, diastolic pressures need to increase above 15 to 20 mm Hg. While epinephrine is one way of achieving this, it is unclear whether other mechanisms may be equally effective.[123] It is also unclear why this level of diastolic pressure is required, but in the absence of this pressure, chest compressions cause large oscillations in flow.[123] As a result, the net flow into vital organs (e.g., brain) is effectively zero as the forward flow into the organ is counterbalanced by retrograde flow out during the relaxation phase. In contrast, higher diastolic pressures prevent or greatly reduce the retrograde flow, thereby increasing net flow through vital organs such as the heart.

POST-ASPHYXIAL REBOUND HYPERTENSION

It is largely assumed that the brain injury commonly associated with birth asphyxia entirely results from hypoxic/ischemic brain injury. However, asphyxial episodes are commonly followed by a large "rebound" hypertension that is mediated by increased sympathetic drive. Indeed, the systolic pressures measured during the first 10 minutes of the post-asphyxial period can be very high (approximately 120 mm Hg), but the potential of these high pressures to contribute to the cerebral injury associated with severe asphyxia is unclear. As this response is so rapid in onset, the cerebral resistance vessels, which normally protect the microvasculature from high blood pressures, should still be dilated. If so, these high pressures could be directly transmitted onto the cerebral microvasculature and tissue, potentially causing injury.

A recent study in severely asphyxiated lambs has shown that it is possible to mitigate the post-asphyxial hypertension by resuscitating lambs with the umbilical cord intact.[131] The original hypothesis was that severely asphyxiated lambs could not be resuscitated while their umbilical cords remained intact because the low resistance placental circulation would prevent chest compressions and epinephrine from increasing diastolic pressures needed for ROSC. While the presence of an intact cord had no effect on ROSC, the presence of the low-resistance placental circulation was found to greatly reduce the rebound hypertension (by 20 to 30 mm Hg). The caveat to this finding was that if UCC was only delayed for a minute or two, and therefore occurred during the peak of the rebound sympathetic response, the hypertension tended to be worse.[131] Nevertheless, these studies have highlighted the concept that the post-asphyxial rebound response may contribute to the brain injury (and seizures) associated with severe birth asphyxia. Furthermore, it raises the possibility that if the post-asphyxial rebound response can be avoided, its contribution (if any) to brain injury may also be avoided.

CONCLUSION

In order to improve the assistance provided to infants as they transition to newborn life, we need to better understand the physiologic changes that must occur as they pass through this very challenging phase of life. In particular, we need to understand that the physiology of infants at birth is very different from the physiology of children and adults and even from the same infant hours to days after birth. As such, extrapolating physiologic concepts and knowledge from children or adults into the newborn (particularly respiratory physiology) is inappropriate and potentially dangerous. Indeed, the physiology of infants at birth is much more akin to that of fetuses that are at different intermediary stages along the continuum between a fetus and newborn. Similarly, assuming that the difficulties faced by different subgroups of infants are similar at birth is also misguided. As such, the type of assistance provided needs to be targeted to the specific needs of the individual. Over the last 2 decades, an increasing interest in perinatal physiology has re-emerged and provided an understanding for why modern medicine has been unable to make a major impact on reducing neonatal morbidity and mortality despite an enormous investment in time, money and energy. As a result, we have a much better understanding of (1) how the lung aerates at birth and what strategies can be used to assisted this, (2) how the timing of cord clamping in regard to lung aeration can improve cardiac function throughout transition, (3) why noninvasive positive pressure ventilation is fundamentally different from intubation and mechanical ventilation and why spontaneous breathing is essential for the success of noninvasive respiratory support, and (4) the physiology underpinning the return of spontaneous circulation in severely asphyxiated newborns and how the rebound hypertension and tachycardia can be managed.

 A complete reference list is available at www.ExpertConsult.com.

SELECT REFERENCES

1. Harding R, Hooper SB. Regulation of lung expansion and lung growth before birth. *J Appl Physiol*. 1996;81:209-224.
2. Hooper SB, te Pas AB, Lang J, et al. Cardiovascular transition at birth: a physiological sequence. *Pediatr Res*. 2015;77:608-614.
3. Olver RE, Walters DV, Wilson SM. Developmental regulation of lung liquid transport. *Annu Rev Physiol*. 2004;66:77-101.
6. Hooper SB, te Pas AB, Kitchen MJ. Respiratory transition in the newborn: a three-phase process. *Arch Dis Child Fetal Neonatal Ed*. 2016;101:F266-F271.
9. Hooper SB, Kitchen MJ, Wallace MJ, et al. Imaging lung aeration and lung liquid clearance at birth. *FASEB J*. 2007;21:3329-3337.
10. Harding R, Hooper SB, Dickson KA. A mechanism leading to reduced lung expansion and lung hypoplasia in fetal sheep during oligohydramnios. *Am J Obstet Gynecol*. 1990;163:1904-1913.
15. Dawson JA, Kamlin CO, Wong C, et al. Changes in heart rate in the first minutes after birth. *Arch Dis Child Fetal Neonatal Ed*. 2010;95:F177-F181.
23. Siew ML, Wallace MJ, Kitchen MJ, et al. Inspiration regulates the rate and temporal pattern of lung liquid clearance and lung aeration at birth. *J Appl Physiol*. 2009;106:1888-1895.
24. Vyas H, Field D, Milner AD, et al. Determinants of the first inspiratory volume and functional residual capacity at birth. *Pediatr Pulmonol*. 1986;2:189-193.
26. te Pas AB, Siew M, Wallace MJ, et al. Establishing functional residual capacity at birth: the effect of sustained inflation and positive end expiratory pressure in a preterm rabbit model. *Pediatr Res*. 2009;65:537-541.
28. Perlman JM, Wyllie J, Kattwinkel J, et al. Part 7: neonatal resuscitation: 2015 international consensus on cardiopulmonary resuscitation and emergency cardiovascular care science with treatment recommendations. *Circulation*. 2015;132:S204-S241.
29. Vyas H, Milner AD, Hopkin IE. Intra-thoracic pressure and volume changes during the spontaneous onset of respiration in babies born by cesarean-section and by vaginal delivery. *J Pediatr*. 1981;99:787-791.
30. Schmolzer GM, Kamlin OC, O'Donnell CP, et al. Assessment of tidal volume and gas leak during mask ventilation of preterm infants in the delivery room. *Arch Dis Child Fetal Neonatal Ed*. 2010;95:F393-F397.
32. Miserocchi G, Poskurica BH, Del Fabbro M. Pulmonary interstitial pressure in anesthetized paralyzed newborn rabbits. *J Appl Physiol*. 1994;77:2260-2268.
33. Bland RD, McMillan DD, Bressack MA, et al. Clearance of liquid from lungs of newborn rabbits. *J Appl Physiol Respir Environ Exerc Physiol*. 1980;49:171-177.
35. Bhatt S, Alison B, Wallace EM, et al. Delaying cord clamping until ventilation onset improves cardiovascular function at birth in preterm lambs. *J Physiol*. 2013;591:2113-2126.
37. Blank DA, Polglase GR, Kluckow M, et al. Haemodynamic effects of umbilical cord milking in premature sheep during the neonatal transition. *Arch Dis Child Fetal Neonatal Ed*. 2018;103:F539-F546.
38. Crossley KJ, Allison BJ, Polglase GR, et al. Dynamic changes in the direction of blood flow through the ductus arteriosus at birth. *J Physiol*. 2009;587:4695-4704.
43. Gao Y, Raj JU. Regulation of the pulmonary circulation in the fetus and newborn. *Physiol Rev*. 2010;90:1291-1335.
44. Teitel DF, Iwamoto HS, Rudolph AM. Changes in the pulmonary circulation during birth-related events. *Pediatr Res*. 1990;27:372-378.
47. Lang JA, Pearson JT, Binder-Heschl C, et al. Increase in pulmonary blood flow at birth: role of oxygen and lung aeration. *J Physiol*. 2016;594:1389-1398.
55. McDonald SJ, Middleton P, Dowswell T, et al. Effect of timing of umbilical cord clamping of term infants on maternal and neonatal outcomes. *Cochrane Database Syst Rev*. 2013;7:CD004074.
56. Fogarty M, Osborn DA, Askie L, et al. Delayed vs early umbilical cord clamping for preterm infants: a systematic review and meta-analysis. *Am J Obstet Gynecol*. 2018;218:1-18.
59. Niermeyer S, Velaphi S. Promoting physiologic transition at birth: re-examining resuscitation and the timing of cord clamping. *Semin Fetal Neonatal Med*. 2013;18:385-392.
62. Westgate JA, Wibbens B, Bennet L, et al. The intrapartum deceleration in center stage: a physiologic approach to the interpretation of fetal heart rate changes in labor. *Am J Obstet Gynecol*. 2007;197:236.e231-211.
63. Walker AM, Alcorn DG, Cannata JC, et al. Effect of ventilation on pulmonary blood volume of the fetal lamb. *J Appl Physiol*. 1975;39:969-975.
64. Brouwer E, Knol R, Vernooij ASN, et al. Physiological-based cord clamping in preterm infants using a new purpose-built resuscitation table: a feasibility study. *Arch Dis Child Fetal Neonatal Ed*. 2019;104:F396-F402.
66. Blank DA, Badurdeen S, Omar FKC, et al. Baby-directed umbilical cord clamping: a feasibility study. *Resuscitation*. 2018;131:1-7.
67. Kashyap AJ, Hodges RJ, Thio M, et al. Physiologically based cord clamping improves cardiopulmonary haemodynamics in lambs with a diaphragmatic hernia. *Arch Dis Child Fetal Neonatal Ed*. 2019.
69. Lefebvre C, Rakza T, Weslinck N, et al. Feasibility and safety of intact cord resuscitation in newborn infants with congenital diaphragmatic hernia (CDH). *Resuscitation*. 2017;120:20-25.
70. Katheria AC. Umbilical cord milking: a review. *Front Pediatr*. 2018;6:335.
74. Katheria A, Reister F, Essers J, et al. Association of umbilical cord milking vs delayed umbilical cord clamping with death or severe intraventricular hemorrhage among preterm infants. *J Am Med Assoc*. 2019;322:1877-1886.
77. Bjorklund LJ, Ingimarsson J, Curstedt T, et al. Manual ventilation with a few large breaths at birth compromises the therapeutic effect of subsequent surfactant replacement in immature lambs. *Pediatr Res*. 1997;42:348-355.
82. Siew ML, Te Pas AB, Wallace MJ, et al. Surfactant increases the uniformity of lung aeration at birth in ventilated preterm rabbits. *Pediatr Res*. 2011;70:50-55.
83. Polin RA, Carlo WA, Committee on F, et al. Surfactant replacement therapy for preterm and term neonates with respiratory distress. *Pediatrics*. 2014;133:156-163.
87. van Vonderen JJ, Hooper SB, Hummler HD, et al. Effects of a sustained inflation in preterm infants at birth. *J Pediatr*. 2014;165. 903-908 e901.
89. Kirpalani H, Ratcliffe SJ, Keszler M, et al. Effect of sustained inflations vs intermittent positive pressure ventilation on bronchopulmonary dysplasia or death among extremely preterm infants: the SAIL Randomized Clinical Trial. *J Am Med Assoc*. 2019;321:1165-1175.
92. Crawshaw JR, Kitchen MJ, Binder-Heschl C, et al. Laryngeal closure impedes non-invasive ventilation at birth. *Arch Dis Child Fetal Neonatal Ed*. 2018;103:F112-F119.
95. Dekker J, Hooper SB, Martherus T, et al. Repetitive versus standard tactile stimulation of preterm infants at birth - a randomized controlled trial. *Resuscitation*. 2018;127:37-43.
104. Dekker J, Hooper SB, van Vonderen JJ, et al. Caffeine to improve breathing effort of preterm infants at birth: a randomized controlled trial. *Pediatr Res*. 2017;82:290-296.
106. Vento M, Moro M, Escrig R, et al. Preterm resuscitation with low oxygen causes less oxidative stress, inflammation, and chronic lung disease. *Pediatrics*. 2009;124:e439-e449.
110. Oei JL, Vento M, Rabi Y, et al. Higher or lower oxygen for delivery room resuscitation of preterm infants below 28 completed weeks gestation: a meta-analysis. *Arch Dis Child Fetal Neonatal Ed*. 2017;102:F24-F30.
112. Dekker J, Martherus T, Lopriore E, et al. The effect of initial high vs. low F_iO_2 on breathing effort in preterm infants at birth: a randomized controlled trial. *Front Pediatr*. 2019;7:504.
113. Hooper SB, Fouras A, Siew ML, et al. Expired CO_2 levels indicate degree of lung aeration at birth. *PloS One*. 2013;8:e70895.
115. Morrison JJ, Rennie JM, Milton PJ. Neonatal respiratory morbidity and mode of delivery at term: influence of timing of elective caesarean section. *Br J Obstet Gynaecol*. 1995;102:101-106.
118. Jain L, Eaton DC. Physiology of fetal lung fluid clearance and the effect of labor. *Semin Perinatol*. 2006;30:34-43.
121. Klingenberg C, Sobotka KS, Ong T, et al. Effect of sustained inflation duration; resuscitation of near-term asphyxiated lambs. *Arch Dis Child Fetal Neonatal Ed*. 2012.
124. Dannevig I, Solevag AL, Wyckoff M, et al. Delayed onset of cardiac compressions in cardiopulmonary resuscitation of newborn pigs with asphyctic cardiac arrest. *Neonatology*. 2011;99:153-162.
128. Ong T, Sobotka KS, Siew ML, et al. The cardiovascular response to birth asphyxia is altered by the surrounding environment. *Arch Dis Child Fetal Neonatal Ed*. 2016.
131. Polglase GR, Blank DA, Barton SK, et al. Physiologically based cord clamping stabilises cardiac output and reduces cerebrovascular injury in asphyxiated near-term lambs. *Arch Dis Child Fetal Neonatal Ed*. 2018;103:F530-F538.

151 Pathophysiology of Neonatal Sepsis

James L. Wynn

INTRODUCTION

A successful immune response is critically necessary to eradicate infectious challenges and prevent dissemination of the infection throughout the host. However, if inflammation is not limited and becomes generalized, it can result in the constellation of signs and symptoms of a systemic inflammatory response syndrome (SIRS). If the infection is not contained, the spread of the pathogen from its local origin through the blood may result in systemic endothelial activation and precipitate sepsis or septic shock. Progression of sepsis to shock may lead to multi-organ dysfunction syndrome (MODS) and ultimately to death.

Host immunity is divided into innate and adaptive immune systems for purposes of discussion and teaching, but there is a great deal of interaction between the two systems. Innate immunity is rapid, largely nonspecific, and is composed of barriers, phagocytic cells, the complement system, and other soluble components of inflammation. Following breech of physical barriers, cellular elements of the innate immune response are the first line of defense against the development and progression of infection. Adaptive immunity, which is antigen-specific, long-lived, and often takes several days to develop, provides immunologic specificity and memory. These systems work together to protect the host from pathogenic challenge but may also precipitate host injury through aberrant responses. The outcome of infection is dependent on at least five major factors: (1) the pathogen, (2) the pathogen load, (3) the site of infection, (4) the host response, and (5) the underlying health status of the host. For a number of reasons, less is known about the host response in neonates compared to adults—the principal reason being the highly variable definition of sepsis.

Our understanding of the pathophysiology of sepsis largely owes to investigations in adult populations among both humans and animals. There is clear evidence from both preclinical models of sepsis that neonates manifest different host immune responses compared to adults.[1-5] Even among children, neonates manifest a unique host immune response to sepsis and septic shock.[5,6] Thus, neonatal-specific clinical investigations, particularly in the very preterm infant, are required to improve both survival and long-term outcomes for these populations. By parallel processing of observational human studies with mechanistic investigations that leverage preclinical sepsis modeling, we can tap the power of transgenic approaches to tease out which elements are critical for survival and more clearly describe the pathophysiology.[2,7-10] A better understanding of the pathophysiology will uncover new opportunities for interventional studies ultimately aimed at improving outcomes. To this end, in this chapter, we explore the pathophysiology of sepsis in the neonate with special attention to the immunobiology of sepsis.

THE DEFINITION OF SEPSIS

A discussion of the pathophysiology of sepsis must begin with a definition of sepsis. Adult and pediatric intensivists currently use consensus definitions for sepsis for goal-based therapeutic interventions.[11-14] In 2016, a third iteration for the consensus definition of sepsis in adults was established and supported by 31 professional societies.[15] The definition of sepsis is "life-threatening organ dysfunction caused by a dysregulated host response to infection." Organ dysfunction indicates a pathobiology more complex than simple infection plus an accompanying inflammatory response. Neonatal sepsis has been variably defined based on a number of clinical and laboratory criteria that make the study of this condition and the description of the pathophysiology very difficult.[16] Diagnostic challenges and uncertain disease epidemiology necessarily result from a variable definition of disease. The distinction of infection from sepsis is not widely recognized in the neonatal intensive care unit (NICU). By contrast to the definitions of sepsis in adults and children, the definitions of sepsis commonly used in neonatology are not only variable but also heavily predicated on the isolation of pathogens from blood and/or the associated length of prescribed antimicrobial treatment.[16] Meningitis, soft-tissue (omphalitis), osteomyelitis, pneumonia, and perforated bowel (spontaneous intestinal perforation [SIP] or necrotizing enterocolitis [NEC]) are frequently associated with negative blood cultures in all populations.[6,16-18]

The presence of life-threatening organ dysfunction is demonstrated using a sequential organ failure assessment (SOFA) to determine risk of intensive care unit (ICU) admission or mortality. Because admission to a NICU for preterm infants is not optional, ICU admission is not applicable in this population. To define sepsis in neonates therefore requires an operational definition of organ dysfunction applicable specifically to this population (neonatal SOFA [nSOFA]) that predicts mortality in the setting of presumed infection. The progression of organ failure in neonates with lethal late-onset sepsis (LOS) was shown in a large retrospective cohort.[19] The need for mechanical ventilation, oxygen requirement, requirement for cardiovascular support in the form of vasoactive drugs, and the prevalence of thrombocytopenia all significantly increased during the progression to mortality with LOS. Guided by those data, an objective, electronic health record (EHR)-automated, nSOFA scoring system was developed and tested that predicted LOS mortality in premature very low-birth-weight infants.[20,20a]

EPIDEMIOLOGY AND RISK FACTORS FOR DEVELOPMENT OF NEONATAL SEPSIS

Sepsis or serious infection within the first 4 weeks of life kills in excess of 1 million newborns worldwide annually.[21,22] The incidence of neonatal sepsis is variable (from <1% to >35% of live births) based on gestational age and time of onset (early onset sepsis [EOS], <72 hours after birth or late onset sepsis [LOS], ≥72 hours after birth).[23-29] Preterm neonates suffer the greatest sepsis incidence and mortality among all age groups (Fig. 151.1).[30-35]

Risk factors for developing sepsis in neonates, particularly the very premature, have been well described.[23,24,36-42] Maternal factors that contribute to the risk of neonatal sepsis have been identified. Prematurity, low birth weight (<2500 g, LBW), a positive maternal vaginal culture for group B streptococcus (GBS), prolonged rupture of membranes, maternal intrapartum

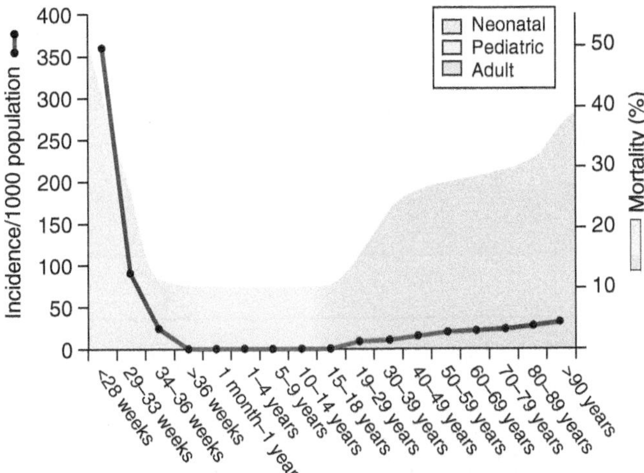

Fig. 151.1 Incidence and mortality of sepsis in humans across developmental age groups. Incidence (*line*, left y-axis), mortality (*shade*, right y-axis).

fever, and chorioamnionitis (intraamniotic infection) are strongly associated with GBS EOS.[39] Chorioamnionitis is associated with the greatest risk of subsequent clinically or culture-proven sepsis.[38] Studies demonstrate the risk of sepsis in clinical chorioamnionitis-exposed newborns is strongly dependent on gestational age, with minimal risk in neonates 35 weeks and older and greater risk with increasing degrees of prematurity.[43-50] The risk of neonatal sepsis conferred by maternal GBS colonization[38] is significantly reduced with adequate intrapartum antibiotic prophylaxis.[51] Despite the efficacy of this intervention, the incidence of invasive GBS disease in African American neonates is rising[51] as is the incidence of *Escherichia coli* sepsis in preterm and term neonates.[52] Vaginal delivery in the presence of maternal active primary herpes simplex virus (HSV) significantly increases the risk for neonatal HSV, which often has a fulminant course and high mortality.[53-55] Preexisting maternal immunodeficiency or sepsis also increases the risk for sepsis in the neonate.[56] Factors immediately after delivery and in the postnatal period influence the risk for the development of sepsis. Nonmodifiable risk factors such as gender (male), extremely low birth weight (ELBW) less than 1000 g and gestational age less than 30 weeks increase risk for the development of sepsis.[57] In contrast, risk is increased by clinical interventions such as parenteral alimentation, intubation and mechanical ventilation, and central venous access.[23,24]

Metabolic demands may represent a substantial risk factor for the development of infection and sepsis in neonates.[58,59] The neonatal immune response is consistent with disease tolerance (minimizing harm from immunopathology), whereas a disease resistance strategy (minimizing harm from pathogens) predominates in adults.[60] Increased resistance to disease requires substantial energy, and thus host metabolism is inexorably connected to host inflammatory responses.[59] Accordingly, immunometabolism is an area of intense research across multiple disciplines and disease states including cancer, sepsis, and autoimmunity.[61] Neonates, particularly those born extremely preterm, have daily caloric needs that are at least fivefold greater than adults (150 kcal/kg vs. 25 kcal/kg). In conjunction with a lack of functional fat stores, the critical differences in metabolic demand and substrate utilization between neonates and adults severely restrict the capacity for a preterm neonate to mount a disease resistance response. Importantly, although a state of "metabolic bankruptcy" may be reached early after infectious challenge in the neonate, adults with chronic infection/critical illness may also demonstrate similar metabolic deficits that contribute to a persistent immune-catabolism syndrome (PICS).[62]

PRIMARY SOURCE OF INFECTION

Because sepsis definitions in neonates are largely predicated on the isolation of a pathogen from blood rather than the presence of life-threatening organ dysfunction, studies that describe the primary source of infection in the absence of bacteremia are frequently considered as separate clinical entities, e.g., meningitis, pneumonia, peritonitis (SIP/NEC), urinary tract infection (UTI), soft-tissue/skin. For example, among 1961 adults with severe sepsis, the most common primary sites in order were lung, abdominal, genitourinary, and skin/soft tissue.[63] Among patients aged greater than 55 years admitted to an surgical ICU with a diagnosis of severe sepsis or septic shock, the most common primary sites in order were abdominal, lung, necrotizing soft tissue, and UTI.[64] A prevalence study of 569 children with severe sepsis in pediatric ICUs worldwide revealed the order of primary site infections was lung (40%), blood (19%), abdominal (8%), central nervous system (CNS) (4%), genitourinary (4%), skin (4%), and unknown (16%) (18). Among 429 neonates with late-onset infection, the causes were blood (primary [38%] and central line-associated bloodstream infection [29%]), urine (8%), lung (6%), CNS (6%), peritonitis (6%), and other (ear, nose, and throat infection, bone and joint infection, or skin and soft tissue infection [7%]).[65] An understanding of the primary sources for sepsis across populations is necessary to inform relevant and effective strategies for intervention.

THE IMPACT OF SEPSIS

Common potential consequences of infection in very low-birth-weight (VLBW) infants (<1500 g) include prolonged hospital stay, need for intubation and surfactant therapy, prolonged mechanical ventilation, chronic lung disease, severe intraventricular hemorrhage, delayed initiation of enteral feedings and prolonged parenteral nutrition, extended need for central venous lines, need for umbilical, or peripheral arterial access, and patent ductus arteriosus (PDA).[24,25,40,66,67]

Four out of 10 neonates that develop sepsis die or experience major morbidity[68] including neurodevelopmental impairment (NDI) as well as impairment of hearing and vision.[69-73] Studies of children at 9 and 10 years of age after preterm birth and LOS reveal persistently increased risks for motor impairment, attention-deficit hyperactivity disorder, and intellectual impairments compared to their preterm peers without sepsis.[74,75] Sepsis-associated NDI was associated with a higher prevalence of white matter abnormality compared to nonseptic controls.[76] Seventy-three percent of ELBW infants that develop Candidiasis suffer death or NDI[77] including retinopathy.[78] Outcomes are worse following neonatal septic shock. The composite of death or severe sequelae (cerebral palsy, severe developmental delay, hearing impairment, blindness, or short bowel syndrome) occurred in 52% of all neonates with septic shock, and only 28% of all neonates were alive and considered normal at 18 months of age.[57] Septic shock mortality was greatest in ELBW infants (71%).

MOLECULAR EVENTS DURING EARLY INFECTION

PATHOGEN RECOGNITION

Once the local barrier function (skin and mucosal surfaces) has been compromised (Fig. 151.2), pathogen recognition by local immune sentinel cells is the first step toward development of

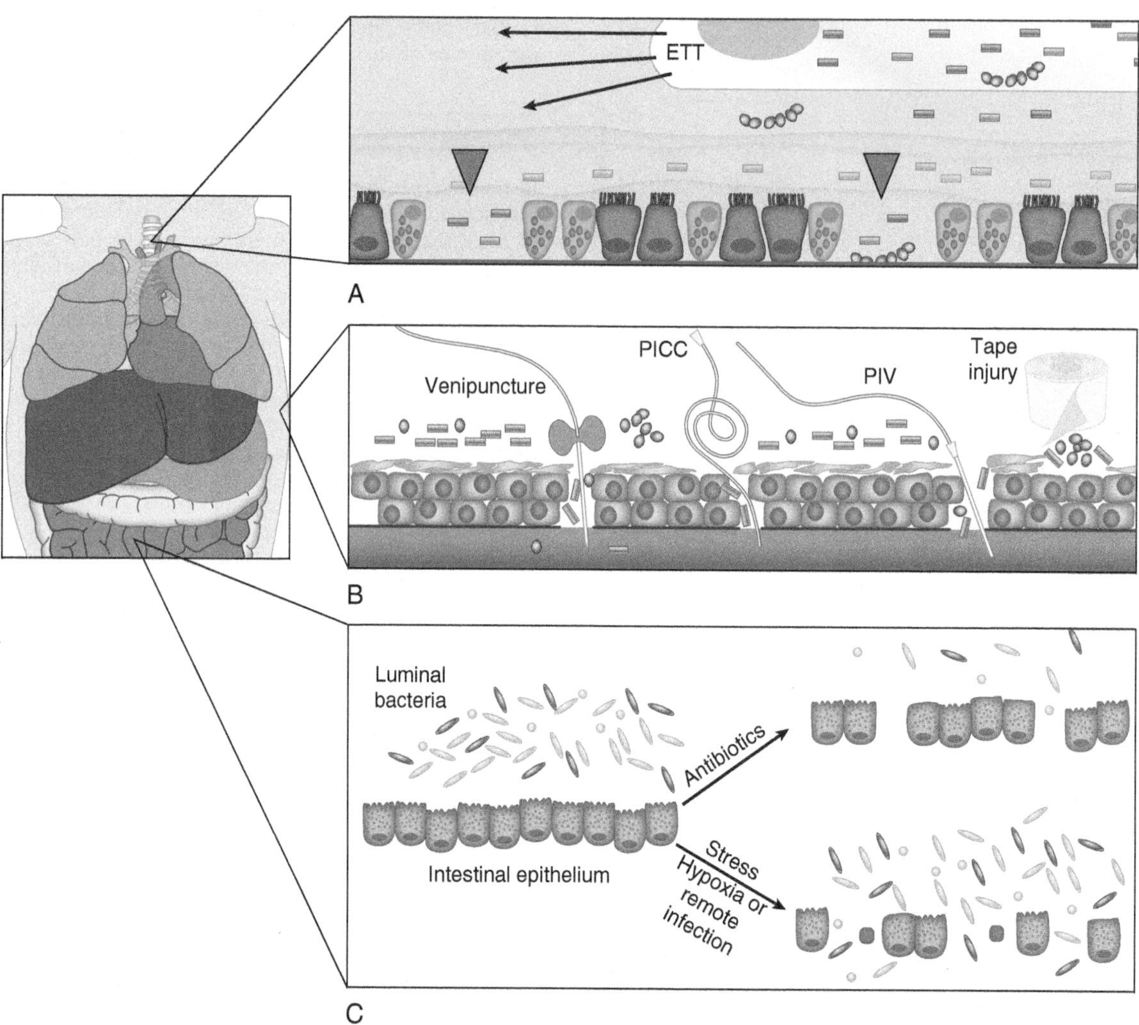

Fig. 151.2 Physical barriers. (A) *Respiratory mucosa*: A foreign body (ETT) and/or positive pressure can irritate and injure the respiratory epithelium (ciliated cells, gray arrowheads denote denuded areas). Increased goblet cells (blue cells with inclusions) with decreased mucociliary clearance of airway further increases the likelihood of infection (bacteria represented by purple spherical chains and blue/pink rods). (B) *Skin*: Disruptions associated with trauma (venipuncture or heelstick), PICC, PIV, or tape-related abrasions compromise the skin barrier (bacteria represented by clusters of purple spheres and green rods). (C) *Gastrointestinal mucosa*: Luminal bacteria (microbiota) are a valuable component of the mucosal barrier. The interaction between intestinal bacteria and intestinal epithelium is necessary for homeostasis and normal function of repair mechanisms. Disruption of this interaction, through the use of antibiotics or via stress to the organism (e.g., hypoxia or remote infection such as sepsis or pneumonia) results in loss of homeostasis and degradation of the intestinal boundaries with subsequent microbial translocation. *ETT*, Endotracheal tube; *PICC*, peripherally inserted central catheter; *PIV*, peripheral intravenous (line).

an immune response (Fig. 151.3). Elegant sensing mechanisms have evolved to facilitate detection of potentially pathogenic microorganisms. Since Dr. Charles Janeway predicted their existence,[79] multiple classes of pathogen recognition receptors (PRRs) have been discovered that serve as detectors of pathogen-associated molecular patterns (PAMPs) including cell wall and membrane components, flagellum, nucleic acids, and carbohydrates. A litany of PRR classes have been discovered including the Toll-like receptors (TLRs), nucleotide-binding oligomerization domain (NOD)-like receptors (NLRs), retinoic-acid-inducible protein I (RIG-I)-like receptors (RLRs), peptidoglycan recognition proteins (PGRPs), β_2-integrins, and C-type lectin receptors (CLRs). The TLRs, β_2-integrins, and CLRs detect pathogens on the cell surface and in the endosome, whereas RLRs and NLRs detect pathogens intracellularly. The discovery that TLR4 was integral for a robust lipopolysaccharide (LPS)-mediated inflammatory response that occurs with gram-negative sepsis may be why TLRs have been more thoroughly investigated in the setting of sepsis than have other PRRs.[80] Each of the 10 known TLRs in humans, present on and within multiple cell types, recognizes extracellular and intracellular pathogens via specific PAMPs.[81,82] Multiple TLRs may be activated in concert by intact or partial microorganisms and activate multiple second messenger pathways simultaneously.[82,83]

LPS is the prototypic mediator of systemic inflammation and generates many of the clinical findings of sepsis and septic shock including MODS and death.[84] LPS signals through TLR4 in conjunction with the adaptor proteins CD14 and myeloid differentiation factor-2 (MD-2).[85] A study in adults demonstrated a reduction in mortality and improvement in hemodynamics when serum LPS was reduced.[86] LPS is elevated in blood from septic neonates and those with NEC even in the absence of gram-negative bacteremia.[87] High levels of circulating endotoxin found during sepsis and NEC are associated with multiple organ failure, thrombocytopenia, neutropenia, and death.[87] Administration of anti-LPS antibodies to small numbers of neonates with sepsis (n = 16) and endotoxemia reduced the time to recovery, but not mortality compared to placebo-treated

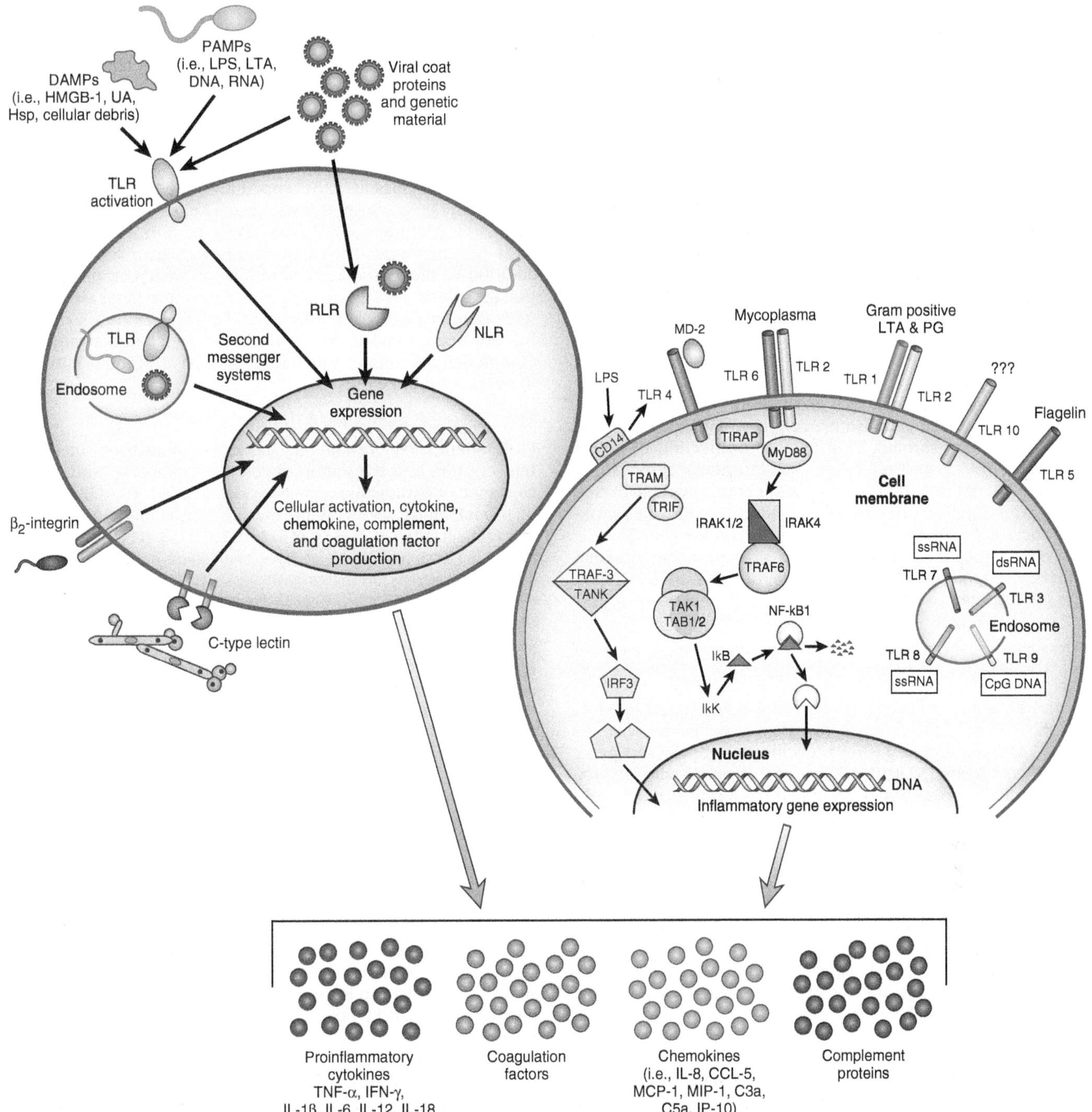

Fig. 151.3 Activation of sentinel immune cells. Sentinel cells (e.g., monocyte, macrophage) sense pathogens via pathogen associated molecular patterns *(PAMPs)* or damage-associated molecular patterns *(DAMPs)* binding to PRRs. Pathogen recognition receptors (PRRs) include *TLRs* (toll-like receptor), *RLRs* (RIG-1-like receptors), *NLRs* (NOD-like receptors), CLRs (C-type lectin receptors), and β_2-integrins. PAMPs include *LPS* (lipopolysaccharide), *LTA* (lipoteichoic acid), *DNA*, and *RNA*. DAMPs can also be sensed through TLRs and include uric acid *(UA)*, heat shock proteins *(Hsp)*, and HMGB1. Signaling occurs through a series of second messengers and results in transcription and translation of cytokines and chemokines that amplify the immune response. Additional detail is shown for TLR signaling. TLR3 is TRIF-dependent, TLR4 signals through TRIF and MyD88, and the remaining TLRs signal through MyD88. The details for TLR4 signaling are shown. LPS is shuttled to the TLR4/MD-2 complex via CD14. MyD88 signaling utilizes toll-interleukin 1 receptor domain containing adaptor protein *(TIRAP)*, Interleukin-1 receptor-associated kinases (IRAK1, IRAK2, IRAK4), tumor necrosis factor receptor-associated family *(TRAF)* 6, transforming growth factor *(TGF)* β-activated kinase *(TAK)* 1, and TGF-β activated kinase 1 binding protein *(TAB)* 1 and 2, ultimately leading to destruction of IκBα and translocation of NF-κB to the nucleus. TRIF-dependent signaling from TLR4 proceeds via TRAF 3 and TRAF-associated NF-κB activator *(TANK)*, interferon regulatory factor *(IRF)* 3, which dimerizes and subsequently translocates to the nucleus.

neonates.[88] Reduction of serum LPS by exchange transfusion in infected neonates (n = 10) may be associated with improved survival.[89]

Bacterial cell wall components (e.g., lipoteichoic acid) signal primarily through TLR1/2/6, flagellin through TLR5, and CpG double-stranded DNA through TLR9. Common viral PAMPs such as double-stranded RNA or single-stranded RNA signal through TLR3 and TLR7/8, respectively (see Fig. 151.3). Agonist-TLR binding results in a signaling cascade of intracellular second messenger proteins ultimately leading to production of cytokines and chemokines as well as activation of other antimicrobial effector mechanisms.[81] Key intracellular messengers critical for effective TLR signaling include myeloid differentiation factor 88 (MyD88), Toll/IL-1 receptor domain (TIR) containing adaptor protein (TIRAP), TIR domain containing adapter-inducing interferonβ (TRIF), TRIF-related adaptor molecule (TRAM), IL-1 receptor-associated kinase (IRAK)-1 and IRAK-4, and nuclear factor of κ light polypeptide gene enhancer in B cells 1 (NF-κB). Signaling through MyD88 typically leads to the production of NF-κB-dependent inflammatory cytokines/chemokines, whereas signaling through TRIF induces production of type I interferons (IFN) as well as NF-κB-related inflammatory cytokines. Upregulation of TLR2 and TLR4 mRNA in neonates occurs during gram-positive and gram-negative infection, respectively, across gestational ages.[90] Dysregulation or overexpression of TLR4 is involved in the development of NEC in experimental animal models,[91] implicating the importance of TLRs in the initial immune response to pathogens and their role in neonatal sepsis.

NLRS, RLRS, CLRS, β_2-INTEGRINS

Beyond TLRs, other important intracellular PRRs include NLRs and RLRs. For NLRs, multiple cytosolic proteins are able to act as PAMP sensors (e.g., NOD leucine rich repeat and pyrin domain containing [NLRP]1, NLRP3) and coalesce with adaptor proteins and pro-caspase-1 (CASP1) to form a multimeric protein complex termed the *inflammasome*.[92] The formation of the inflammasome activates CASP1 that cleaves the inactive precursor proteins of IL-1β and IL-18 to their active forms.[92] Small molecular NLR inhibitors are available and could be beneficial if aberrant NLR signaling was shown to contribute to neonatal sepsis outcomes.[93] RLRs are cytoplasmic RNA helicases that, like TLR3, sense double-stranded RNA of viral origin and induce type I IFN production and NF-κB activation.[82] To date, the impact of RLR and NLR signaling has not been specifically examined in neonates with sepsis.

In addition to its roles in leukocyte adhesion, phagocytosis, migration and activation, and complement binding, the β_2-integrin complement receptor 3 (CR3), also known as *MAC-1* and *CD11b/CD18*, functions as a pathogen sensor on the surface of phagocytes. CR3 binds LPS as well as a broad range of other microbial products, in cooperation with or independent of CD14, leading to upregulation of inducible nitric oxide (NO) synthase (iNOS) and NO production.[94] Diminished expression of L-selectin and CR3 on stimulated neonatal neutrophils (PMN) impairs neonatal PMN and monocyte activation and accumulation at sites of inflammation.[95-97] Decreased expression of L-selectin and CR3 persists for at least the first month of life in term infants, possibly contributing to an increased risk for infection.[98] The expression of CR3 (CD11b) may be reduced further in preterm neonates compared to term neonates.[99] In umbilical cord blood from neonates less than 30 weeks' gestation, PMN CR3 content was similar to levels found in patients with type 1 leukocyte adhesion deficiency (failure to express CD18).[95,96] Thus, decreased leukocyte CR3 surface expression increases the likelihood of suboptimal pathogen detection and cellular activation, particularly in the preterm neonate.

CLRs are PRRs that recognize bacterial, viral, fungal, and parasitic carbohydrate moieties. CLRs may be expressed on the cell surface (e.g., macrophage mannose receptor, Mincle [CLR], dectin-1/2 [transmembrane PRRs]) or secreted as soluble proteins (e.g., mannose-binding lectin [MBL]) as one of the acute phase reactants (APRs). Once bound to its carbohydrate ligand, MBL initiates activation of complement via the lectin pathway to promote opsonization and phagocytic clearance of pathogens. Plasma MBL concentrations are low at birth (especially in preterm infants), but rise steadily throughout infancy and childhood.[100] Low levels of MBL are associated with the increased incidence of sepsis in neonates.[101-103] In addition to decreased concentrations at birth, certain genetic polymorphisms of MBL, namely MBL2, have also been associated with an increased risk of infection.[102] However, this association has not been found in all studies.[104-106] M-ficolin activates the complement system in a manner similar to MBL and is elevated in neonates with sepsis.[107]

THE ROLE OF INFLAMMATION

PRR stimulation results in rapid inflammatory mediator transcription and translation directed at cellular activation and clearance of pathogenic organisms (see Fig. 151.3).[108] Elevations of pro-inflammatory cytokines during sepsis and septic shock, including IL-1β, IL-6, IL-8 (CXCL8), IL-12, IL-18, IFN-γ, and tumor necrosis factor-α (TNF-α),[109] have been identified. Compared to adults with sepsis, neonates with sepsis produce less IL-1β, TNF-α, IFN-γ, and IL-12.[110-115] The decreased cytokine production is due in part to decreased production of important intracellular mediators of TLR signaling including MyD88, interferon regulatory factor 5 (IRF5), and p38, which exhibit gestational age-specific diminution.[116] Studies have demonstrated impaired inflammasome activation and mature IL-1β production by neonatal mononuclear cells.[117,118] In a comprehensive study (>140 analytes) of serum from neonates evaluated for LOS, IL-18 emerged as a predictive biomarker to differentiate infected from noninfected neonates,[119] similar to data from adults with sepsis.[120] IL-18 reduces PMN apoptosis,[121] drives IFN-γ production,[122] and induces production of TNF-α, IL-1β, and CXCL8.[123] IL-18 primes PMNs for degranulation with production of reactive oxygen intermediates (ROI) on subsequent stimulation.[124] Dysregulation of many of these functions linked to IL-18 are seen in sepsis and septic shock. Increased IL-18 has been demonstrated in premature neonates with brain injury[125] and also an experimental model of NEC,[126-128] highlighting a common pathway activated with states of ischemia and inflammation. IL-18-null neonatal mice are highly protected from polymicrobial sepsis, whereas replenishing IL-18 increased lethality of sepsis or endotoxemia.[129] IL-18-augmented sepsis mortality depended on IL-1R1 signaling but not adaptive immunity. IL-18 administration in sepsis increased IL-17A production by murine intestinal γδT cells as well as Ly6G$^+$ myeloid cells, and blocking IL-17A reduced IL-18-potentiated mortality to both neonatal sepsis and endotoxemia. Excessive levels of IL-1β, TNF-α, IL-6, CXCL8, IL-10, and IL-18, such as those seen with advanced stage NEC, severe sepsis or septic shock, correlate with poor survival.[87,130-133] Altered cytokine levels (increased IL-10 and IL-6, and decreased CCL5) may identify those neonates at highest risk for the development of sepsis-associated disseminated intravascular coagulation (DIC).[134]

Pro-inflammatory cytokine production leads to activation of endothelial cells including increased expression of cellular adhesion molecules (CAMs) that facilitate leukocyte recruitment and diapedesis (Fig. 151.4). Upregulation of CAMs (soluble intercellular CAM [sICAM], vascular CAM [VCAM], L-, P-, and E-selectins, and CD11b/CD18) during sepsis facilitates rolling and extravascular migration of leukocytes.[135-138] Decreased neonatal PMN and monocyte L-selectin and MAC-1 expression impairs PMN accumulation at sites of inflammation.[95,96]

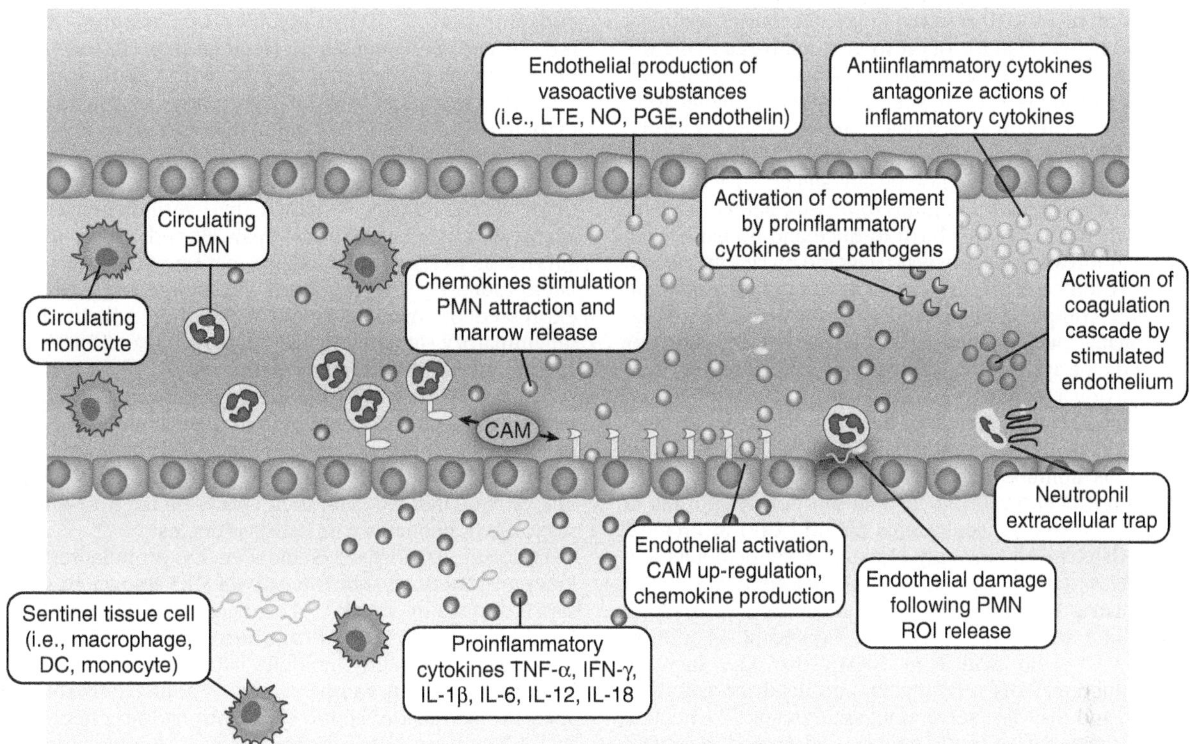

Fig. 151.4 Cellular recruitment and endothelial activation following pathogen detection. Pathogen-stimulated tissue/blood monocytes, dendritic cells *(DC)*, and macrophages release proinflammatory cytokines that activate the surrounding endothelium. Endothelial activation results in upregulation of cell adhesion molecules *(CAM)*, production of chemokines and vasoactive substances, activation of complement, and development of a procoagulant state. Recruitment of PMNs occurs along the chemokine gradient surrounding the area of inflammation. Antiinflammatory cytokines counter the actions of proinflammatory cytokines to prevent excessive cellular activation and recruitment that can result in tissue damage and systemic inflammation. Endothelium can be damaged when PMNs release reactive oxygen intermediates *(ROI)* or from neutrophil extracellular traps (NETs). *LTE,* Leukotriene; *NO,* nitric oxide; *PGE,* prostaglandin E; *PMN,* neutrophil.

Chemokine gradients produced by endothelial cells and local macrophages are necessary in addition to CAM interactions for effective and specific leukocyte attraction and accumulation (see Fig. 151.4). Without adequate leukocyte recruitment, there is increased risk for propagation from a local to a systemic infection. Although poor cellular chemotaxis in the neonate has been observed, it is not likely a result of reduced serum concentrations of chemokines, as baseline levels are similar in preterm and term neonates compared to adults.[139] Suboptimal cellular chemotaxis may be related to other mechanisms such as poor CR upregulation following stimulation,[97] deficiencies in another downstream signaling process,[140] or inhibition by bacterial products.[141] A wide variety of chemokines are increased during sepsis, including CCL2, CCL3, CCL5, CXCL8, and CXCL10.[142] Other chemo-attractive molecules also increase with sepsis, including complement proteins C3a and C5a, antimicrobial proteins and peptides (APPs), including cathelicidins and defensins, as well as components of invading bacteria themselves.[109,119] The importance of chemo-attractive substances in the pathogenesis of severe sepsis is highlighted by studies showing that CXCL8 can be used as a stratifying factor for survival in children,[143] and C5a is implicated in sepsis-associated organ dysfunction in adults.[84] Chemokine investigations in septic neonates revealed that CXCL10 is a sensitive early marker of infection,[142] and low CCL5 levels may predict development of DIC.[134]

Damage-associated molecular patterns (DAMPs or alarmins), such as intracellular proteins or mediators released by dying or damaged cells including IL-1α, high mobility group box (HMGB)-1, IL-33, and S100 proteins, may also activate PRRs and thus play a critical role in the amplification of the host immune response. Neonatal mice that lack IL-1 receptor 1 (IL-1R1; cognate receptor for IL-1α and IL-1β) had improved sepsis survival and attenuated plasma inflammatory mediator production compared with wild-type (WT) septic mice.[144] The survival benefit in IL-1R1 knockout mice was not replicable with pharmacologic use of an IL-1R antagonist in WT mice and furthermore was restricted to mice that lacked IL-1α specifically. Taken together, these data highlight the importance of rapid, tissue-level DAMP-signaling in the pathophysiology of sepsis.

HMGB1 is involved in the progression of sepsis to septic shock in adults.[84,145] Macrophages or endothelial cells stimulated with LPS or TNF-α produce HMGB1, which signals through TLR2, TLR4, and receptor for advanced glycation end products (RAGE).[146] HMGB1 results in cytokine production, activation of coagulation, and PMN recruitment.[145,147] HMGB1 mediates disruption of epithelial junctions within the gut via the induction of reactive nitrogen intermediates (RNIs), leading to increased bacterial translocation.[148] The role of HMGB1 and RAGE signaling in human neonates with sepsis has not been well characterized, but has been shown to be involved in the pathophysiology of NEC in a preclinical model.[149] Significantly lower soluble RAGE (sRAGE) was found in human fetuses that mounted robust inflammatory responses and HMGB1 levels correlated significantly with levels of IL-6 and S100β in fetal circulation.[150]

S100 proteins A8/A9 are highly elevated in the plasma of human newborns for several days after birth. The heterodimer S100A8/A9 specifically programs human neonatal monocytes at birth by inducing MyD88-dependent gene programs via NF-κB and IRF5 activation, without influencing TRIF-dependent genes.[151]

Genetic deletion of S100A9 resulted in greater murine neonatal mortality and a hyperinflammatory response compared to the WT neonatal mouse. The net effect of birth-associated programming by these S100 proteins was prevention of hyperinflammation via a selective, transient microbial unresponsiveness while allowing for sufficient immunologic protection. Myeloid-derived suppressor cells (MDSCs), phenotypically similar to PMNs and monocytes, have significant immunosuppressive activity and are present in high numbers after birth in mice and humans.[152] In mice, MDSC suppressive activity was triggered by lactoferrin and mediated by S100A8 and S100A9 as well as NO and prostaglandin (PG) E_2. A more complete understanding of the mechanisms that underlie neonatal-specific inflammatory responses may allow for precision-medicine approaches in the future that address specific deficits in individual patients.

Other specific DAMPs, including heat shock proteins (Hsps) and uric acid, may also stimulate TLRs, regulate PMN function, and function as immune adjuvants. Hsp production in septic neonates has not been evaluated to date but polymorphisms in Hsps increase the risk for acute renal failure (ARF) in preterm neonates.[153] Hsps are significantly elevated in septic adults and children.[154] Elevated Hsp60 and Hsp70 measured within 24 hours of pediatric ICU admission were associated with septic shock, and there was a trend toward a significant association with death.[155,156] Uric acid is a DAMP that can increase cytokine production, PMN recruitment, and dendritic cell (DC) stimulation[157] and may also serve as an antioxidant.[158] Uric acid is reduced in the serum of septic neonates compared to control neonates.[159]

In addition to facilitating leukocyte attraction, pro-inflammatory stimuli result in production of vasoactive substances that decrease or increase vascular tone and alter vascular permeability (see Fig. 151.4). These include platelet-activating factor (PAF), thromboxane (TBX), leukotrienes (LTE), NO, PG histamine, and bradykinin.[160,161] These substances are produced predominantly by host endothelium and mast cells. Activated PMNs produce phospholipase A2 (PLA_2), which is increased in the serum of neonates with sepsis[162] and leads to generation of vasoactive substances including PGE and LTE. TBX produced by activated platelets and endothelin (ET-1) produced by activated endothelium[163] are potent vasoconstrictors that participate in the development of pulmonary hypertension.[164-167] Systemic overproduction of cytokines and vasoactive substances is associated with circulatory alterations and organ failure seen in severe sepsis and septic shock (Fig. 151.5).[11,168-171]

THE ANTIINFLAMMATORY RESPONSE

If the pathogen is not contained locally and inflammatory homeostasis is not restored, SIRS may develop, persist, and lead to MODS and death (see Fig. 151.5).[172] The traditional paradigm for understanding the host-response to sepsis consists of an intense pro-inflammatory response, or SIRS temporally followed by a compensatory antiinflammatory response syndrome. This paradigm has been challenged by the failure of multiple antiinflammatory strategies to improve sepsis outcomes in in adults.[173] New data in adults and children demonstrate a simultaneous pro/antiinflammatory response where the magnitude of either response may determine outcome.[174,175] Near simultaneous increases in antiinflammatory cytokine production (transforming growth factor [TGF]-β, IL-4, IL-10, IL-11, and IL-13) countering the actions of pro-inflammatory cytokines[109,176,177] occur in neonates during infection. These mediators blunt activation and recruitment of phagocytic cells, block fever, modify coagulation factor expression, and decrease production of ROI/RNI, NO, and other vasoactive mediators.[178-183]

Soluble cytokine and receptor antagonists produced during sepsis also modulate pro-inflammatory mediator action. Elevations of TNF receptor 2 (TNFR2), which regulates the concentration of TNF-α, soluble IL-6 receptor, soluble IL-2 (sIL-2), and endogenous IL-1Rantagonist (IL-1ra) have been documented in neonatal sepsis, with resolution following effective treatment.[177,184,185] The role of these regulatory cytokine inhibitors in the immune response to neonatal sepsis and septic shock has been incompletely characterized. sRAGE competes with cell-bound RAGE for the binding of HMGB1 and other RAGE ligands.[186] sRAGE has antiinflammatory effects, is elevated in adults during sepsis,[187] and results in improved survival as well as reduced inflammation when given to infected adult rodents.[188] Serum levels of soluble triggering receptor expressed on myeloid cells-1 (sTREM-1), which may reduce inflammatory signaling by the unknown ligand for TREM-1, may predict mortality in preterm neonates.[189]

MicroRNAs (miRNAs) may regulate inflammation at the level of gene expression via several putative mechanisms.[190] Several pilot studies in rodents and humans have demonstrated regulatory functions for miRNA in neonates.[191-196] The impact of regulatory microRNAs (miRNAs) and their effects on the host inflammatory response in neonates with sepsis is unclear.

Endogenous cortisol is induced by proinflammatory cytokines and attenuates the intensity of SIRS associated with severe sepsis and septic shock.[197] Low-dose cortisol treatment in conjunction with standard of care measures was associated with a reduction in mortality in adults with septic shock and adrenal insufficiency.[198] In another study of adults, cortisol treatment sped the reversal of septic shock but had no effect on mortality.[199] Newborn cortisol production is significantly increased early in shock.[200] However, very preterm neonates may have relative adrenal insufficiency that may contribute to hemodynamic instability and hypotension. Cortisol replacement may be critical in these infants and deserves further study.[201] It should be kept in mind, however, that in children with septic shock adjunctive corticosteroids are associated with repression of gene programs corresponding to the adaptive immune system.[202]

THE IMPACT OF GENETICS IN SEPSIS-ASSOCIATED INFLAMMATORY SIGNALING

A twin study that assessed frequency of infections among monozygotic and dizygotic prematurely born twins identified 49.0% (P = .002) of the variance in susceptibility to LOS was due to genetic factors alone, and 51.0% (P = .001) the result of residual environmental factors.[203] The impact of genetics in the host response is also underscored by the increased risk of death from infection seen with African American race or male gender among low-birth-weight infants.[204] An ethnically unique single nucleotide polymorphism (SNP) in the TLR4 promoter region was significantly associated with preterm neonatal gram-negative bacterial infections.[205] Several neonatal studies have demonstrated an association between SNPs and infection development and outcomes.[104,206-210]

Because TLRs play an essential role in recognition and response to pathogens, alterations in their expression, structure, signaling pathways, and function can have consequences for host defense. Polymorphisms or mutations in TLRs are associated with increased risk for infection in adults[211-214] and in children[215-217] but are less well characterized in neonates. After controlling for confounders, the presence of a TLR4 SNP was associated with a threefold increase in the risk of gram-negative infections in VLBW infants.[210] Polymorphisms in *TLR2, TLR5, IL10,* and PLA_2 *(PLA2G2A)* genes were associated with the development of neonatal sepsis.[206]

Modifications in expression or function of co-stimulatory molecules necessary for TLR activation are also associated with an increased risk for infection. For example, LPS (endotoxin)

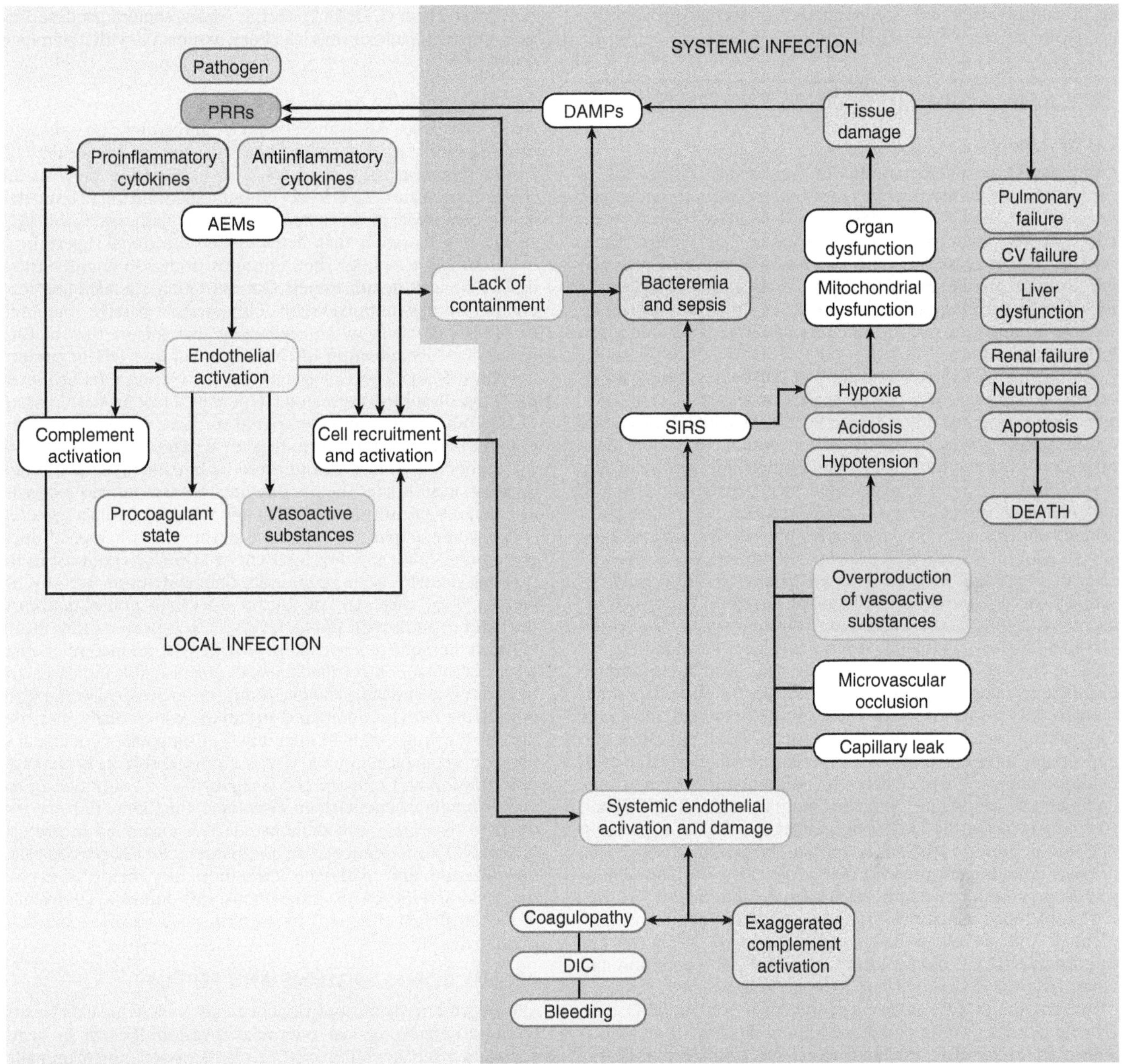

Fig. 151.5 Pathophysiology of neonatal sepsis and septic shock. *AEMs,* Antimicrobial effector mechanisms; *CV,* cardiovascular; *DAMPs,* damage-associated molecular patterns; *DIC,* disseminated intravascular coagulation; *PRRs,* pattern recognition receptors; *SIRS,* systemic inflammatory response syndrome.

binding protein (LBP) (which binds intravascular LPS) and the LPS co-receptor CD14 are both increased during neonatal sepsis,[218-220] and genetic variations in these proteins have been associated with increased risk for sepsis in adults.[221-223] Gene polymorphisms in MD-2, a small protein involved in LPS signaling through TLR4, increase the risk for organ dysfunction and sepsis in adults,[224] but the significance in neonates is unknown. Polymorphisms in post-TLR activation intracellular signaling molecules, including MyD88,[225] IRAK-4,[226] and NF-κB essential modulator (NEMO),[227] are associated with invasive bacterial infection in older populations. Identification of additional genetic polymorphisms in intracellular second messenger inflammatory signaling systems with impact on neonatal sepsis risk and progression are likely to be uncovered with the implementation of biobanking and mining of stored samples.

Mutations have been identified in NLRs that are involved in the pathogenesis of Crohn's disease (NOD2),[228] and neonatal-onset multisystem inflammatory disease (NLRP3).[229] Investigation for mutations in specific domains of NLRs has been performed to identify potential causes of abnormal inflammatory signaling and involvement with the development of NEC, but no associations have been found.[230] Further investigation of these signaling pathways in neonates is warranted. RLR mutations have been identified but have an unknown clinical significance.[231] The role played by intracellular PRRs, including NLRs, is of particular interest given that *Listeria monocytogenes*, a pathogen with a history of virulence in neonates, can be recognized by NLRs.[232] Polymorphisms in cytokines and their receptors as well as pathogen recognition system proteins have been evaluated for association with neonatal sepsis but have not yielded consistent results due to relatively small sample sizes and a general lack of formal prospective validation studies.[208,221-223,233-244]

INFLAMMATORY RESPONSE PROTEINS

COMPLEMENT

Complement is an extraordinarily important component of early innate immunity that facilitates killing of bacteria through opsonization and direct microbicidal activity. Complement components also possess chemotactic or anaphylactic activity that increase leukocyte aggregation and local vascular permeability at the site of invasion. Furthermore, complement reciprocally activates a number of other important processes such as coagulation, proinflammatory cytokine production, and leukocyte activation.[84]

Complement-mediated activation of leukocytes during sepsis occurs via upregulation of cell surface receptors CR1 (CD35) and CR3 (Mac-1, CD11b/CD18).[245,246] C3b and C5a facilitate opsonization (primarily C3b), redistribution of blood flow, increased inflammation, platelet aggregation, and release of ROI (primarily C5a).[247,248] C5a-mediated local leukocyte activation also results in increased cytokine production with subsequent upregulation of adhesion molecules on vascular endothelium allowing for increased cell recruitment to the site of infection.[249] Data in adults link elevated C5a levels with multiple facets of sepsis-associated pathology such as the development of DIC via increased tissue factor expression, cardiomyopathy, increased pro-inflammatory cytokine levels, and the development of SIRS, apoptosis of adrenal medullary cells leading to adrenal insufficiency, and PMN dysfunction.[84] Septic shock in adult humans was associated with extensive complement activation, C-reactive protein (CRP)-dependent loss of C5aR on PMNs, and appearance of circulating C5aR in serum, which correlated with a poor outcome.[250] Deficiencies in C5aR found in term neonates compared to adults may limit the ability to respond to C5a and therefore increase the likelihood of infection.[251] The expression of C5aR on preterm PMNs is unknown. The extent to which C5a or other complement proteins play a role in the development of pathology in septic neonates remains to be determined.

Complement regulatory proteins modify the effects of complement and prevent potential damage due to over-activation. In particular, CD59 blocks formation of C9 polymerization and target lysis, CD55 destabilizes CR1 (CD35) as well as C3 and C5 convertases, and CR1 accelerates the deactivation of C3b.[252] Dysregulation of complement activation can lead to a vicious activation cycle that results in excessive cellular stimulation, cytokine production, endothelial cell activation, and local tissue damage promulgating SIRS and septic shock (see Fig. 151.5).[253]

ACUTE PHASE REACTANTS

In addition to the initial inflammatory response, molecular detection of PAMPs drives elevation of IL-1β and IL-6 that in turn promulgate increases in multiple other innate proteins that serve to reduce pathogen load.[254] APR proteins, produced predominantly in the liver, include the pentraxins CRP (opsonin) and serum amyloid A (SAA, cellular recruitment), lactoferrin (reduce available iron/antimicrobial peptide-lactoferricin), procalcitonin (unknown function), haptoglobin, fibronectin (opsonic function), pentraxin 3 (binds C1q and activates classical complement pathway), MBL, and LBP, among many others.[109,218,219,254-259] Of note, APRs have been studied in neonates with sepsis primarily to assess for diagnostic utility, rather than immunologic function. In particular, elevated plasma concentrations of CRP and LBP are often associated with EOS.[219,260] Levels of IL-10 and CRP found on the initial evaluation as well as 24 hours later were significantly higher in non-survivors with sepsis, pneumonia, or NEC.[261] A lack of sustained increase in APR production (CRP, SAA) during sepsis, sometimes described as immune exhaustion, has also been associated with a fulminant course.[262]

PASSIVE IMMUNOGLOBULIN

Neonates have passively acquired antibodies via placental transfer with a significant increase beginning around 20 weeks gestation. As a result of a shorter period of gestation, preterm neonates have lower immunoglobulin (Ig) G subclass levels compared to term neonates, particularly IgG1 and IgG2 subclasses.[263] A study that characterized the global repertoire of maternal IgG to 93,904 viral epitopes from 206 unique viruses in 78 neonates demonstrated that extremely preterm and term children are equipped with comparable passive immunity to viruses at birth, with repertoires that mirror that of their mothers.[264] Examination of the impact of low IgG in preterm neonates 24 to 32 weeks gestational age (serum total IgG levels <400 mg/dL at birth) revealed an increased risk for development of LOS but not mortality compared to those with levels greater than 400 mg/dL after controlling for gestational age. There was a 15% increase in LOS risk in these infants for every 100 mg/dL decrease in serum IgG below baseline that was not reduced with intravenous IgG infusion.[265,266] In line with this finding, IgG titers and opsonic activity to coagulase negative Staphylococci were not predictive for the development of LOS.[267] In contrast to the preterm neonate with profoundly deficient serum IgG1 (<100 mg/dL),[268,269] there are significant infectious consequences in the child or adult with similar levels.[270] Reliance on other means of innate immune defense likely provides the premature neonate with microbial control mechanisms. Despite APR increases and the presence of maternally derived Ig, neonates exhibit impaired opsonizing activity compared to adults, which likely increases the risk for progression of infection.[271] Complement, deficient in preterm neonatal plasma,[272] plays a critical role in Ig-mediated opsonization and effector cell phagocytosis.[273] Although Ig has many putative beneficial immunologic functions, the majority of these have not been demonstrated or examined in preterm infants.[274] The dependence on complement for effective Ig-based opsonization and pathogen clearance may help to explain the lack of efficacy of intravenous IgG infusion (polyclonal, monoclonal, IgM-enriched) to prevent sepsis or sepsis mortality in neonates.[68,275-280]

ANTIMICROBIAL PROTEINS AND PEPTIDES

APPs represent the most phylogenetically ancient means of innate immune defense against microbial invasion. Present in nearly every organism including bacteria, plants, insects, non-mammalian vertebrates, and mammals, these small, often cationic peptides are capable of killing microbes of multiple types including viruses, bacteria, parasites, and fungi largely by disruption of the pathogen membrane.[281] Constitutive expression of APPs occurs in humans on barrier areas with consistent microbial exposure such as skin and mucosa. Following microbial stimulation, both release of pre-formed APPs as well as inducible expression are thought to contribute to early host defense.[282] Importantly, there is no evidence to date for the development of microbial resistance to APPs that target fundamental components of the microbial cell wall. Some APPs can bind and neutralize microbial components such as endotoxin, precluding engagement with TLRs and other PRRs and thereby reducing inflammation. Many APPs can potentially reduce the intensity of the inflammatory response associated with the presence of bacterial toxins.[283-285] Because endotoxemia is an important contributor to neonatal MODS and mortality with sepsis and NEC,[87] LPS-binding/blocking strategies including synthetic APPs may have a significant positive impact on outcomes.[283,286]

Bactericidal/permeability-increasing protein (BPI) is a 55 kDa protein present in the respiratory tract, PMN primary granules, and blood plasma. BPI exerts selective cytotoxic, anti-endotoxic, and opsonic activity against gram-negative bacteria.[283] Plasma BPI concentrations in critically ill children with sepsis syndrome or organ system failure both had higher median plasma BPI concentrations than critically ill controls without sepsis or organ failure. Plasma BPI concentrations were also positively associated with the Pediatric Risk of Mortality Score.[254] PMNs from term neonates are deficient in BPI, potentially contributing to the increased risk for infection.[287] While term neonates demonstrate upregulation of plasma BPI during infection, premature neonates showed a decreased ability to mobilize BPI upon stimulation,[288] which may contribute to their risk for infection with gram-negative bacteria. Polymorphisms in BPI increase the risk for gram-negative sepsis in children, but the impact of these polymorphisms in neonates is unknown.[289] PMNs from term neonates produce similar concentrations of defensins but reduced BPI and elastase compared to adults.[287,290,291] Recombinant BPI ($rBPI_{21}$) treatment was associated with improved functional outcome, reduced amputation, but no difference in mortality in a multicenter study of children with severe systemic meningococcal disease.[292]

Lactoferrin is the major whey protein in mammalian milk (in particularly high concentrations in colostrum) and is important in innate immune host defense. Lactoferrin is present in tears and saliva and has antimicrobial activity both via binding iron and by direct membrane disruption activity via a portion of its N-terminus lactoferricin.[293] Lactoferrin is also an alarmin (e.g., HMGB1 or IL-33), capable of activating leukocytes, binding endotoxin, and modifying the host response by acting as a transcription factor that regulates mRNA decay.[294,295] These many beneficial biologic activities may contribute to the reductions in bacterial and fungal sepsis[296,297] as well as NEC[298] seen with oral bovine lactoferrin supplementation. However, a large (n = 2203) multicenter placebo-controlled randomized trial of enteral bovine lactoferrin in preterm infants aged less than 32 weeks did not reduce the risk of late-onset infection compared to placebo.[299]

Lysozyme is present in tears, tracheal aspirates, skin, and in PMN primary and secondary granules and contributes to degradation of peptidoglycan of bacterial cell walls. Secretory PLA_2 ($sPLA_2$) can destroy gram-positive bacteria through hydrolysis of their membrane lipids.[162] PMN elastase is a serine protease released by activated PMNs with microbicidal function and is believed to play a role in the inflammatory damage seen with PMN recruitment, particularly in the lung.[99,119] Cathelicidin (LL-37) and the defensins are other APPs that possess antimicrobial properties.[300] LL-37 is present in the amniotic fluid, vernix, skin, saliva, respiratory tract, and leukocytes (PMNs, B cells, T cells, monocytes, and macrophages). α-Defensins are cysteine-rich 4 kDa peptides expressed in the amniotic fluid, vernix, spleen, cornea, thymus, Paneth cells, and leukocytes (PMNs, monocytes, macrophages, and lymphocytes). β-defensins are found in skin, gastrointestinal tract (salivary gland, tonsil, gastric antrum, stomach, liver, pancreas, small intestine, colon), reproductive organs and urinary tract (placenta, uterus, testes, kidney), respiratory tract, breast milk and mammary gland, and thymus. In addition to microbicidal action, APPs possess a wide range of immunomodulatory functions on multiple cell types from both the innate and adaptive immune system.[282,301,302] Immunomodulatory effects on macrophages, DC, monocytes, mast cells, PMNs, and epithelia attributed to APPs include altered cytokine and chemokine production, improved cellular chemotaxis and recruitment, improved cell function (maturation, activation, phagocytosis, ROI production), enhancement of wound healing (neovascularization, mitogenesis), and decreased apoptosis. It is unclear what effect APPs have on sepsis risk or progression of infection in neonates.

The cytosolic granules of PMN are rich in APPs that can be released upon stimulation into the extracellular space including α-defensins, lactoferrin, lysozyme, LL-37, $sPLA_2$, and BPI. Gestational age-related decreases in the cord blood concentration of several APPs (LL-37, BPI, Calprotectin, $sPLA_2$, α-defensins) were described in comparison to maternal serum levels.[303] Plasma APP deficiencies may contribute to the increased risk of infection associated with prematurity, and their absence may increase the risk of excessive levels of bacterial toxins. Preterm neonates show lower human β-defensin-2 levels in cord blood compared with term neonates.[304] Upregulation of APPs (defensins) occurs in blood of infected adults[305] and children (defensins, lactoferrin).[306] The effect of sepsis on the production of plasma APPs in neonates has not been investigated in detail.

COAGULATION

Development of a pro-coagulant state in the surrounding microvasculature allows for trapping of invading pathogens and prevents further dissemination (see Fig. 151.5). In general, the intrinsic pathway amplifies coagulation following initiation by the extrinsic pathway.[307] Important differences exist in children compared to adults in the coagulation system. Reduced vitamin K-dependent factors (Factor II, VII, IX, X), thrombin generation, consumption of platelets with formation of microthrombi, and counterregulatory elements (inhibitors) increase the risk for bleeding in pediatric patients.[308] A microvascular pro-coagulant state develops via stimulation of monocytes, PMNs, platelets, and endothelium resulting in expression of tissue factor.[309,310] Tissue factor-mediated activation of the coagulation cascade results in activation of thrombin-antithrombin complex, plasminogen activator inhibitor type-1 (PAI-1), and plasmin-a2-antiplasmin complex,[311] as well as inactivation of protein S and depletion of anticoagulant proteins including antithrombin III and protein C.[312-314] Decreased activated protein C (aPC) levels were associated with increased risk of death from sepsis in preterm neonates.[315] A multinational, placebo-controlled, randomized trial of aPC revealed no change in mortality among pediatric patients with sepsis but term infants less than 60 days old experienced increased bleeding.[316]

The coagulation cascade is intimately tied to inflammation, including complement activation.[84] Cytokine production increases expression of endothelial PAI-1. PAI-1 inhibits fibrinolysis by inhibiting the conversion of plasminogen to plasmin that in turn is important for the breakdown of fibrin. Deposition of fibrin in small vessels leads to inadequate tissue perfusion and organ failure.[317] Increased PAI-1 activity levels are associated with increasing IL-6, nitrite and nitrate levels (metabolites of NO production), the development of organ failure (cardiovascular, renal, hepatic, coagulopathy), and mortality.[317] Sepsis is associated with thrombocytopenia in neonates[318] and is attributed to reduced megakaryopoiesis in the setting of consumption with clot formation.[319] Simultaneous measurements of serum thrombopoietin levels and reticulated platelet percentage may be helpful in discriminating hyperdestructive from hypoplastic thrombocytopenia among septic neonates.[320] Decreased platelet function in preterm neonates with sepsis further increases the risk for bleeding.[321] In ELBW infants, platelets are hyporeactive for the first few days after birth, complicating the ability of the immune system to contain a microbiologic threat and increasing the risk for hemorrhage.[322] Clotting can lead to propagation of inflammation via thrombin-induced production of PAF. PAF-activated or platelet TLR4-activated PMNs may then contribute to further endothelial injury and dysfunction leading to the development of a vicious clotting-inflammation-clotting cycle. Activated platelets may be consumed in clot formation and/or may also be removed from the circulation by the liver,[323] potentially resulting in thrombocytopenia, particularly during gram-negative and fungal infections.[184,318,324]

Systemic activation of coagulation is associated with consumption of clotting factors and increased risk of bleeding, prolonged proinflammatory responses, and DIC.[110,134,325] This finding is consistent with the elevated serum levels of IL-6[326] and high frequency of DIC seen with disseminated HSV infection[327] which may explain why pentoxifylline, which reduces IL-6, reduced DIC in neonates.[328] Evolution of DIC to purpura fulminans is uncommon in septic neonates but has been reported with methicillin-resistant *Staphylococcus aureus* sepsis.[329] The protease-activated receptor (PAR)-1 also played a major role in orchestrating the interplay between coagulation and inflammation in adult mice.[330] PAR-1 may modify the endothelial response during neonatal sepsis and thus represent a target for therapeutic intervention.

ROLE OF VASCULAR ENDOTHELIUM

Recent studies have shown the critical importance of vascular endothelial activation in the early recognition and containment of microbial invasion. Through the use of transgenic mice, it has been shown that pulmonary endothelial cells sense bloodborne bacteria and their products,[141] while alveolar macrophages patrol the air spaces.[331] These data illustrate the role of endothelium and help in part to explain the occurrence of acute respiratory distress syndrome (ARDS) and pulmonary hypertension associated with severe sepsis in the absence of a primary pulmonary infectious focus. Expression of TLRs allows endothelium to become activated in the presence of microbial components, leading to production of cytokines and chemokine gradients, as well as adhesion molecules (e.g., VCAM, ICAM, L-, P-, and E-selectins). These substances are all necessary to attract immune cells (primarily PMNs) to the site of infection and to facilitate pathogen containment.[135-138,141] Vasoactive substances released from activated leukocytes, platelets, and endothelial cells include PAF, TBX, LTE, NO, histamine, bradykinin, and PGE.[160,161] The balance of NO and ET-1, a vasoconstrictor, may be disrupted with endothelial damage, favoring the constrictive effects of ET-1 leading to ischemia and injury.[163] This phenomenon may explain in part why NO inhibitors increased mortality in adults with septic shock.[332] Stimulated endothelium can be a double-edged sword, however, because excessive activation can lead to systemic overproduction of cytokines and vasoactive substances (including NO). Endothelial cell apoptosis, detachment from the lamina, and alterations in vascular tone combine to promote capillary leak of proteins and fluid leading to hypovolemia, shock, and organ failure (see Fig. 151.5).[141,333,334] Release of microparticles from PMNs may also injure surrounding endothelium via myeloperoxidase.[335] Activated or damaged endothelium establishes a prothrombotic environment that can result in local microvascular occlusion[310] or progression to DIC.[336]

The glucocorticoid receptor is the target for the endogenous, adrenally produced steroid cortisol. Endothelial glucocorticoid receptor is a critical negative regulator of iNOS expression and NF-κB activation,[337] demonstrating its effects on endothelium toward protection of the host during sepsis. Recent studies revealed a potential role of plasma angiopoietin protein during pediatric septic shock.[338] Angiopoietin-1 (protects against vascular leak) was reduced while angiopoietin-2 (promotes vascular permeability) was elevated, highlighting a novel potential therapeutic opportunity to reduce end organ injury with pediatric septic shock. The roles for endothelial glucocorticoid receptor and angiopoietin-1 in neonatal sepsis are unknown.

The role of endothelium activation during sepsis and septic shock in neonates, particularly in the premature, has been less well investigated. Toxins from GBS have been shown to damage pulmonary endothelium[339] and likely participate in pulmonary complications associated with GBS pneumonia such as ARDS and the development of pulmonary hypertension.[340] The adhesion molecules E- and P-selectin, expressed and secreted by activated endothelium, are increased in the serum of septic neonates[119] and likely reflect significant endothelial activation. Activation of endothelial TLR4 impaired intestinal perfusion with experimental NEC via endothelial NOS-nitrite-NO signaling.[341]

INNATE IMMUNE CELLULAR CONTRIBUTIONS

The PMN is the primary effector of innate immune cellular defense. Endothelial cells produce activating cytokines and chemokine gradients that recruit circulating PMNs to the site of infection. Expression of cell adhesion molecules by PMNs and endothelium allows cells to roll and extravasate into surrounding tissues. Activated PMNs phagocytose and kill pathogens via oxygen-dependent and oxygen-independent mechanisms. IL-1β is produced by activated PMNs largely via an NLRP3/apoptosis-associated speck-like protein containing a C-terminal caspase-recruitment domain (ASC)/CASP1-dependent mechanism that amplifies the recruitment of additional PMNs from the bone marrow to the site of infection.[342]

Activated PMNs may release RNI, ROI, and proteolytic enzymes extracellularly via activation of membrane-associated nicotinamide adenine dinucleotide phosphate (NADPH) oxidase. These reactive intermediates and enzymes can lead to destruction of non-phagocytized bacteria but can also cause local tissue destruction, including neonatal endothelial and lung injury as well as surfactant inactivation,[99,343] and thus play a role in progression from sepsis to MODS.

Neonatal PMNs exhibit quantitative and qualitative deficits compared to adult cells.[290,344] PMN respiratory burst activity is suppressed during sepsis and may contribute to poor microbicidal activity.[345-347] Compared to adult PMNs, neonatal PMNs exhibit delayed apoptosis[348,349] as well as sustained capacity for activation (CD11b upregulation) and cytotoxic function (ROI production) that contributes to tissue damage.[350] Reduced apoptosis with prolonged survival of PMNs may result in improved bacterial clearance but may also paradoxically increase the risk for sustained PMN-mediated tissue damage. Consistent with these findings, increased serum PMN elastase, urokinase plasminogen activator, and urokinase plasminogen activator receptor are found at presentation in infected neonates.[119]

With PMN death, the DNA (chromatin), histone, and APPs may be expelled into the environment and serve to trap bacteria (neutrophil extracellular traps [NETs]).[351] The formation of NETs can occur following activation of platelet TLR4[352] and may lead to excessive local inflammation and tissue damage.[353] High early levels of circulating free PMN-derived DNA produced by NETs are associated with MODS and death[354] potentially through the clogging of capillary networks.[355] NETs contain destructive proteases capable of bacterial killing even after the PMN dies.[356] Formation of NETs is reduced in PMNs from preterm neonates and nearly absent in term neonates.[357] Decreased NET formation is secondary to high, but transient, concentrations of NET inhibitors,[358] but NETs may be produced even under these conditions with sustained cellular stimulation.[359] PMNs may form NETs more readily, with collateral damage to surrounding tissues, when the target microbe is too large to effectively phagocytose (e.g., fungal hyphae).[360] The contribution of NET production toward detrimental outcomes in septic neonates is unknown, but excessive NET formation with collateral tissue injury may contribute to the poor outcomes seen in preterm neonates with fungal infections.[361]

Rapid depletion of bone marrow PMN reserves during infection, particularly in neonates,[362] can lead to neutropenia with consequent impaired antimicrobial defenses and significantly increased risk for death.[363] Neutropenia and metabolic acidosis were associated with fatal neonatal sepsis by multivariate analysis.[364] Neutropenia is particularly common in gram-negative sepsis in neonates.[365] Release of immature PMN forms (bands), which have greater dysfunction than mature PMNs,[366] may further predispose to adverse outcomes. Murine neonates with experimental sepsis exhibit delayed emergency myelopoiesis (the process by which the host repopulates peripheral myeloid cells lost early during sepsis) independent of TRIF and MyD88.[367] Interventions aimed at addressing reduced PMN numbers in neonates have included provision of mature PMNs[368] and prophylaxis or treatment with colony-stimulating factors (CSFs). Despite strong biologic plausibility, these interventions have been unsuccessful in reducing neonatal infectious burden.[369-371] In a meta-analysis, treatment with granulocyte CSF (G-CSF) or granulocyte-monocyte CSF (GM-CSF) therapy in a subgroup (n = 97) of neutropenic (absolute neutrophil count <1700/μL) neonates with culture-positive sepsis (largely gram-negative and GBS) significantly reduced the risk of death (relative risk [RR] = 0.34; 95% confidence interval [CI] 0.12–0.92).[370] Therefore, stimulation of granulopoiesis could be beneficial under these specific circumstances, although further studies are needed focused on whether to use G-CSF or GM-CSF and what subpopulations to use.

Irreversible aggregation and accumulation of newborn PMNs in the vascular space following stimulation leads to decreased diapedesis, rapid depletion of bone marrow reserves, vascular crowding,[372] and increased likelihood of microvascular occlusion.[373] Neonatal PMN deformation is reduced at baseline compared to adults, which also increases the risk of occlusion.[372] Furthermore, low blood pressure/flow states seen during septic shock further exacerbate existing microvascular ischemia.[290] In combination with NET formation and chromatin clogging of capillary networks, these features increase the propensity for systemic spread of infection and set the stage for microvascular occlusion and tissue ischemia.

OTHER INNATE CELLULAR CONTRIBUTIONS

Many other cells besides PMNs are involved in the development of an immune response to infection. Monocytes, macrophages, and DCs amplify cellular recruitment through production of inflammatory mediators and activation of endothelium, phagocytosis and killing of pathogens, and antigen presentation to T and B cells of the adaptive immune system. The primary functions of monocytes are the synthesis of crucial proteins in the inflammatory response and antigen presentation to naïve CD4⁺ T cells. Examples of important products from monocytes following stimulation include complement components, extracellular matrix proteins, coagulation factors, and cytokines (both pro- and antiinflammatory).[374]

Patterns of cytokine production can promote the differentiation of naïve $CD4^+$ T cells into distinct subtypes of T cells that serve important roles in the clearance of pathogens. For example, T-helper 1 (T_H1) cells are produced from naïve $CD4^+$ T cells following exposure to IFN-γ and IL-12, and support cell-mediated immunity against intracellular pathogens through production of IFN-γ, TNF-α, and lymphotoxin. T_H2 cells arise in the presence of IL-2 and IL-4, produce IL-4, IL-5, IL-13, downregulate T_H1 responses, and support humoral immunity as well as defense against extracellular parasites. A third subset of T_H cells, T_H17 cells, are produced in the presence of TGF-β, IL-6, IL-21, IL-23, produce IL-17, IL-22, and are important for defense against extracellular bacteria and fungi. Neonatal mononuclear cells exhibit a bias away from T_H1 cell-polarizing activity via increased IL-6 and low TNF-α production.[375] Proposed benefits of this phenomena are a mobilization of antiinfective proteins/peptides that serve to protect the newborn during microbial colonization[255] and perhaps a role in immune tolerance.[344] The consequence is a reduced ability to respond to infection with microorganisms; particularly intracellular pathogens such as *Listeria*[376] and mycobacteria.[377] Preterm infants (<30 weeks) may have greater attenuation of TNF-α and IL-6 secretion compared to term infants and adults.[273]

Monocyte recruitment to sites of inflammation or infection may be decreased in neonates compared to adults due to decreased chemotactic ability.[378] Although peripheral monocytes decrease early during sepsis (between 60 and 120 hours), likely secondary to extravasation and differentiation into macrophages, sepsis-related elevation of monocyte-CSF (M-CSF)[379] results in a late increase in the number of peripheral monocytes (>120 hours).[380] In addition to altered cytokine production and suboptimal recruitment, monocyte phagocytic function during sepsis is also reduced from baseline.[381] Antigen presentation to naïve $CD4^+$ T cells is an important immune function performed by monocytes. The decrease in relative monocytic antigen presenting function compared to adult cells is in part due to decreased major histocompatibility complex (MHC) class 2 molecule expression[382] and decreased costimulatory molecules including CD86 and CD40.[383]

Monocytes leave the blood stream, enter the tissues, and can differentiate into macrophages and DCs following exposure to maturing cytokines. Monocytes and macrophages are closely related to PMNs (i.e., they share a common myeloid progenitor) and can kill pathogens by similar means. Important substances produced by stimulated monocytes/macrophages that may contribute to sepsis and septic shock include complement components, cytokines (both pro- and anti-inflammatory), coagulation factors, and extracellular matrix proteins.[374] Present just below epithelial borders, macrophages encounter pathogens immediately after entry. Macrophages are avidly phagocytic and generate APPs to reduce bacterial burden such as lactoferrin, defensins, transferrin, and lysozyme. In addition, macrophages play an important role in the amplification of the immune response through the production of cytokines and chemokines as well as in antigen presentation to naïve $CD4^+$ T-cells. Macrophages are poorly responsive to several TLR agonists.[384]

Eosinophils phagocytose antigen-antibody complexes, release cytokines (TNF-α, IFN-γ, IL-1, IL-2, IL-4, IL-6, CXCL8, IL-10), chemokines (CCL3, CCL5), cytotoxic molecules (eosinophil peroxidase), APPs (major basic protein, eosinophil cationic protein, eosinophil-derived neurotoxin), and other substances (PGE, TBX, LTE) when stimulated.[385] Eosinophilia is associated with neonatal sepsis due to *Candida* spp.[386] and bacteria,[387] and is seen in infants with NEC.[385] In infants less than 26 weeks gestation, eosinophilia (absolute eosinophil count >1000/μL) may predict bacterial sepsis.[387] Eosinophilia in premature infants is not associated with production of IgE.[388] Examination of eosinophils demonstrated an integral role in adult intestinal integrity and revealed a novel innate bactericidal non-phagocytic function via extracellular catapulting of mitochondrial DNA nets with associated bound toxic proteins.[389] The precise role of eosinophils in the neonatal immune response to sepsis as well as in maintenance of intestinal integrity has yet to be determined.

Mast cells play a role in the response to pathogen invasion as part of the innate cellular immune system via production of histamines (which promote vasodilation and upregulation of P-selectin), cytokines (TNF-α, IL-1α/β, IL-17), PMN recruitment, direct bacterial phagocytosis, and antigen presentation.[390,391] Mast cell involvement was demonstrated in erythema toxicum, where mast cell recruitment, degranulation, and expression of APPs occurs.[392] Interestingly, adult rodents deficient in mast cells exhibit impaired PMN influx,[393] clearance of enteric organisms, and decreased sepsis survival,[394] demonstrating the critical role of mast cells in PMN recruitment. Mast cell production of histamine likely contributes to the vasodilation associated with sepsis and septic shock. Like eosinophils and PMNs, mast cells are also capable of bacterial killing via generation of extracellular traps in adults.[395] This means of immune protection has not been investigated in neonates. Mast cells may also alter adaptive immune function by patterning the T_H2 immunophenotype seen in the neonate and therefore contribute to the increased risk of infection. Immature DCs exposed to histamine during maturation (with LPS) exhibit altered T-cell polarizing activity with predominance toward T_H2 phenotype via increased production of IL-10 and decreased IL-2 production.[396] Furthermore, mast cells from neonates were shown to secrete significantly more histamine following stimulation compared to adults[397] and may contribute to vasodilation and the development of shock.[398]

The role of natural killer (NK) cells in neonatal bacterial sepsis is incompletely defined. NK cell numbers increase with gestational age[399] and a reduced percentage of NK cells present at birth can be associated with LOS in preterm infants.[400] Numbers of circulating NK cells may not be different in either preterm or term neonates with or without antenatal or postnatal infection.[401,402] Circulating NK cells are decreased with neonatal shock.[403] Mechanisms used by NK cells to destroy bacteria include APPs (defensins), direct contact and lysis, antibody-dependent cellular cytotoxicity (ADCC), as well as cytokine (IFN-γ) production.[404]

Neonatal NK cell activation in bacterial sepsis is evidenced by upregulation of CD69.[2,405] Despite activation, NK cytotoxicity is deficient in both sepsis and recurrent infections.[402,404] Although neonatal macrophages exhibit impaired baseline activation in response to IFN-γ,[344] NK-mediated production of IFN-γ potentially activates macrophages and can enhance their phagocytic capability. Further studies are necessary to more clearly define the role of NK cells in neonatal bacterial sepsis.

$CD71^+Ter119^+$ (erythroid) cells may contribute to the increased susceptibility of the neonate to infection as a consequence of reducing the inflammatory response associated with bacterial colonization of the gut. TNF-α production by stimulated adult effector cells was reduced in the presence of murine neonatal splenic $CD71^+$ erythroid cells via an arginase-2-dependent mechanism.[406] The $CD71^+$ erythroid population represents a large portion of murine fetal liver, neonatal spleen/bone marrow, and adult bone marrow.[407-409] The murine neonatal spleen contains large numbers of colony-forming progenitor cells for 2 to 3 weeks after birth.[410] Of note and in stark contrast to the lymphoid and reticuloendothelial system roles of the spleen in the healthy adult, the spleen is normally a major site of erythropoiesis during fetal and neonatal life to support the rapid fetal and postnatal growth rate in the setting of significantly reduced erythroid reservoirs compared to the adult.[409,411,412] Accordingly, a subsequent study demonstrated that survival rates after endotoxin challenge and polymicrobial sepsis in murine neonates were not affected by adoptive transfer, depletion, or depletion-repletion of neonatal $CD71^+$ erythroid cells. The ex vivo immunomodulatory effects attributed to $CD71^+$ cells also occurred with hematopoietic tissue from neonatal and adult bone marrow. Enhanced bacterial clearance following anti-CD71 treatment was the result of immune priming rather than a reduction in immunosuppressive cells.[413]

ADAPTIVE IMMUNE SYSTEM CONTRIBUTIONS

The contribution of the adaptive immune system in the neonatal host response to sepsis is uncertain. The 5 to 7 days required for development of an adaptive immune response, namely the selection and amplification of specific clones of lymphocytes (B cells and T cells) that results in immunologic memory, argues against a central role for adaptive immunity in the protective response to early neonatal bacterial sepsis. As a result, the neonate is thought to largely depend on innate immunity for protection from infection during the first days of life. In adults, absence or dysfunction of the adaptive immune system has a profound impact on survival in preclinical models.[414] B cells (and in particular B-cell cytokine production) and not T cells were shown to be important in the early host response to experimental sepsis.[415] Interestingly, experimental data using neonatal mice that lack an adaptive immune system (recombination-activating gene-1 null [$RAG\text{-}1^{-/-}$]) showed no difference in polymicrobial sepsis survival compared to WT animals with a normal adaptive immune system.[3] Furthermore, many quantitative and qualitative differences in lymphocytes are present compared to adults,[416] each with respective proposed clinical impact.[417] As these findings illustrate, the contribution of adaptive immunity for protection and response against sepsis, and in particular which components are protective, is unclear in the most immature and requires further investigation.

Peripheral blood examination has yielded inconsistent changes in the percentage, number, and type of circulating lymphocytes during neonatal sepsis.[401,418-423] Furthermore, the duration of alterations in peripheral circulating cells, if present, is not known. Moreover, changes in lymphocyte representation related to the timing of sepsis onset (EOS or LOS) and prematurity have been incompletely characterized. Regulatory T cells (T_{REG}) are abundant and potent at birth, facilitating inhibition of T_H1 cell immunity,[424] and perhaps mediating a state of immunologic tolerance.[425] Although splenic T_{REG} are increased in septic murine neonates and adults, T_{REG} depletion had no effect on adult murine sepsis survival.[2,426] Alterations in T_{REG} number or function in human neonatal sepsis have not been reported.

Examination of peripheral blood to identify markers of sepsis has yielded a number of lymphocyte cell-surface molecules that increase during sepsis. Activation of neonatal T cells is evidenced by increased CD45RO expression (present on T cells following antigenic stimulation), at the time of sepsis diagnosis,[419,427,428] and with congenital infection[429] although changes may take several days to occur after stimulation.[430] Other markers of lymphocyte activation may be found at different time points during the course of infection. For example, expression of the activation marker CD69 is high on T cells ($CD4^+$) early during infection, whereas CD25 and CD45RO expression persist for several days.[405] Increased $CD4^+$T-cell CD66a expression with LOS in preterm infants may contribute to sepsis-associated immune suppression.[431] HLA-DR expression is increased on multiple cell types including T cells during neonatal sepsis.[405] In contrast to adults, a large portion of neonatal T cells produce CXCL8 that activates PMN and γδT cells.[432] These data show neonatal T cells are activated and are capable of playing a role in the host response to bacterial sepsis in vivo.

Neonatal lymphocyte function is skewed toward T_H2 responses setting the stage for immune tolerance (T_H2) rather than immune priming for infection (T_H1).[416] Multiple maternal immunologic factors contribute to the neonate's immunopolarization that is directed largely at prevention of fetal rejection.[433] The residual effects of that necessary immune modulation in utero are what the newborn must overcome in order to mount effective responses to specific infectious challenges as well as appropriate responses to vaccination. An example of the impact of this immunopolarization include decreased IFN-γ production by $CD4^+$ and $CD8^+$ T cells compared to children and adults.[434,435] Furthermore, during the initial response to microorganisms, antigen presenting cells can facilitate polarization and function of T-cell responses via secretion of cytokines such as IFN-γ (T_H1) or IL-10 (T_H2).[436] The likely significance of decreased IFN-γ production is a reduction in activation of other immune cells such as macrophages.

Reports of lymphocyte function in septic newborns are very limited. Expansion of lymphocytes following antigenic stimulation is important for development of sustained immunity. Decreased lymphocyte proliferative responses have been shown during the first 8 weeks of life in VLBW neonates[421] and may predispose the premature neonate to development of LOS. T-Lymphocyte function was depressed in septic newborns, and especially in those with multiorgan failure, versus healthy term or growing preterm infants.[437] The production of lymphocyte-associated cytokines following GBS stimulation of cord blood mononuclear cells was significantly deficient for both preterm and term infants compared to levels for adults.[273] Cytomegalovirus (CMV) infection in utero leads to the expansion and the differentiation of mature CMV-specific $CD8^+$ T cells, which have similar characteristics to those detected in adults.[438] These cells showed potent perforin-dependent cytolytic activity and produced antiviral cytokines which highlights the potential for adult-like immunocompetence of neonatal T cells under specific circumstances.

An important location for effective lymphocytic function during systemic bacterial infection is the spleen. The marginal zone of the spleen facilitates the clearance of bacteria, particularly encapsulated organisms, from the bloodstream. These functions are accomplished via the interaction of multiple leukocytes including macrophages, DCs, B cells, and T cells within follicles of the spleen. The neonatal splenic marginal zone is immature due to a lack of antecedent antigen exposure and is virtually devoid of $CD21^+$ B cells.[411] As a result of this functional asplenia, there is decreased clearance of pathogens from the blood and potential for a more fulminant course with bacteremia.[439,440]

Among classic lymphocyte populations, B cells are critically important in the adult host response to sepsis. Both treatment of B cell-deficient mice with serum from WT mice and repletion of RAG-$1^{-/-}$ mice with B cells improve sepsis survival, which suggests antibody-independent and antibody-dependent roles for B cells in the outcome to sepsis.[415] Studies that have deciphered the role of B cells in neonatal sepsis are very limited, and thus the role that B cells play in the neonatal host response is unclear. In contrast to T cells, alterations in the number of circulating peripheral blood B cells have not been described during neonatal sepsis.[418,419] IgM production was found after GBS meningitis, which suggests that neonatal B cells can and do respond to pathogenic challenge.[441] Premature neonates with perinatal infection or nosocomial infection may show signs of humoral immunoparalysis manifested by decreased IgM/IgG production ex vivo compared to their healthy age-matched counterparts.[442] Sepsis in early life did not reduce serum antibody titers after completing the series for pneumococcal conjugate vaccine (PCV7) (by World Health Organization standard) in preterm infants but was associated with a reduced opsonization titer to a single serotype, which suggests that the capacity to respond to vaccination or other immune challenge may be altered.[443]

In the setting of reduced classic adaptive immune function seen in early life compared to adults, innate lymphoid populations (which lack B-cell receptor and T-cell receptor) may play a significant role in protecting the neonate from infectious challenge.[444-452] Examples of innate lymphoid cells (ILCs) include γδT cells, ILCs, invariant NK T cells (iNKT), mucosa-associated invariant T cells, and B1 cells. Mechanistic investigations that fully explore the role of these newly discovered populations in the neonatal host response to sepsis are likely to uncover novel therapeutic opportunities.[453]

IMPACT OF SYSTEMS BIOLOGY APPROACHES

Systems biology and the use of "omic" approaches have the potential to produce significant yields in understanding sepsis pathogenesis. Genomic and proteomic approaches have yielded important data associated with septic shock in older populations.[454-462] The utilization of these modern techniques in the study of neonatal immunity, inflammation, and response to pathogen challenge has only just begun.[119,186,264,463-466] The ability to profile genome-wide expression has significantly enhanced our understanding of the complexity of the host immune response to sepsis in children.[6,454,455,458,467] For example, genome-wide expression profiling (GWEP) revealed zinc homeostasis as an important feature of pediatric sepsis.[455,458,468] Prophylactic zinc supplementation reduced bacterial load and mortality in a murine model of peritoneal sepsis.[469] However, oral zinc supplementation did not alter mortality in neonates with probable sepsis.[470]

In addition to the wealth of data derived using a genome-wide transcriptomic approach, this and other high-throughput molecular techniques have the potential to greatly amplify noise and heterogeneity among the groups being compared. Thus, for optimal analysis and interpretation of the findings, groups under investigation must be very clearly delineated, with unequivocal disease and minimal confounding clinical factors, such as timing of sepsis (EOS vs. LOS), congenital and chromosomal anomalies, or postoperative assessments.

In a study of pediatric ICU patients that met criteria for septic shock,[11] a unique whole blood transcriptomic response was found for neonates compared to infants, toddlers, and school-age children. Direct comparisons demonstrated minimal differences between infant, toddler, and school-age groups. In contrast, neonates manifested the largest number of uniquely regulated genes, representing both innate and adaptive immune system pathways, and showed a predominance of downregulated transcripts representing adaptive immune system.[6] The number of upregulated genes increased in proportion to developmental age. This study highlighted that, for the host response to septic shock, neonates are not small children and age-specific study of neonates is required. Investigation of the murine circulating leukocyte transcriptome revealed significant differences in the host immune response to sepsis across the age spectrum (neonate, young adult, elderly), *despite similar increases in mortality* among the neonates and elderly mice compared to young adult mice.[1] These data underscore the impact of developmental age on the host immune response and suggest that interventional therapeutics, which may have efficacy in older populations, may be ineffective or possibly detrimental to neonates. A study of VLBWs with blood culture-proven LOS (59% coagulase negative staphylococcus) identified a 554-gene signature associated with sepsis with increased expression of TNF-α network including MMP-8 and CD177 among the top upregulated genes.[471] Elevated MMP-8 mRNA expression and activity in septic shock correlated with decreased survival and increased organ failure in pediatric patients. MMP-8 is a direct activator of NF-κB.[472] Inhibition (genetic or pharmacologic) of MMP-8 leads to improved survival and a blunted inflammatory profile in a murine model of sepsis. Subsequently, a 52-gene network was uncovered and validated that accurately identified infected infants represented by increased expression of genes for innate immune and metabolic pathways with decreased adaptive immune transcripts.[473] In a whole-blood genome-wide transcriptomic study of preterm infants evaluated and empirically treated for sepsis, principal component analyses revealed significant differences between patients with early (<3 days after birth) or late (>3 days after birth) sepsis compared to their age-matched uninfected infants despite the presence of similar key immunologic pathway aberrations in both groups.[474] The uninfected state and host response to sepsis were significantly affected by timing relative to birth. This study showed future therapeutic approaches may need to be tailored, not only to the developmental age (preterm neonate, term neonate, infant, toddler, child, adolescent, adult, elderly), but also to the timing of the infectious event based on postnatal age. In a comparison of nine human whole-blood gene expression to sepsis datasets (636 patients), adults and neonates manifested a reduced response magnitude (fold-change) overall compared to children and infants.[5] Neonates showed reduced inflammatory recognition and signaling pathways compared to all other age groups. The number of dysregulated genes was proportional to age, and 167 genes were dysregulated across all age groups. The latter finding highlights the possibility to improve diagnostic testing across all populations by targeting a shared and specific gene set. New RNA analysis platforms can deliver transcript results in a few hours, and an 11-gene panel has shown promise.[475,476] A proteomics approach revealed proapolipoprotein CII and a des-arginine variant of SAA as promising biomarkers for LOS and NEC.[477] It is very likely that implementation of unbiased "omic" approaches will reveal critical age-appropriate pathways and opportunities for therapeutic interventions aimed at improving neonatal sepsis outcomes.

SEPSIS-ASSOCIATED ORGAN FAILURE

Sepsis that leads to shock and organ failure carries the worst prognosis. SIRS contributes to the development of organ failure in neonates (see Fig. 151.5).[133,169,326,478] Persistent decreases in capillary perfusion are associated with MODS and death in adults.[479] Lethargy, shock, and VLBW were independent predictors of sepsis mortality.[480] In neonates, impairment of the cardiovascular system, manifested by poor perfusion o2r hypotension, is invariably associated with septic shock. Sustained poor organ perfusion in neonatal sepsis and septic shock due to cardiovascular dysfunction is associated with MODS affecting the kidney,[481,482] liver,[483] gut,[484] and CNS (see Fig. 151.5).[485] The mechanism of organ failure may be decreased oxygen utilization associated with mitochondrial dysfunction rather than poor oxygen delivery to tissue. Based on available evidence, it has been speculated that the prolonged SIRS associated with severe sepsis and shock leads to organ failure via a cessation of energy consuming processes.[486,487] The development of severe NEC is also associated with severe sepsis, shock, MODS, and death.[87,488] Risk factors for sepsis-related death include the need for intubation, initiation of vasoactive medications, hypoglycemia and thrombocytopenia, increased prothrombin time, and excessive bleeding as presenting laboratory signs of sepsis.[364,484,489] Independent predictors of in-hospital LOS mortality during the birth hospitalization were presence of congenital anomalies (odds ratio [OR] = 4.12; 95% confidence interval [CI] 1.60–10.60), neuromuscular comorbidities (OR = 3.34; 95% CI 1.66–6.73), and secondary pulmonary hypertension with or without cor pulmonale (OR = 23.48; 95% CI 5.96–92.49),[490] underscoring the impact of organ level comorbidities that increase neonatal sepsis mortality.

CARDIOVASCULAR DYSFUNCTION

Cardiovascular dysfunction associated with sepsis may lead to shock that is a composite of hypovolemic, cardiogenic, and distributive shock. Distributive shock is related to endothelial NO production that leads to excessive vasodilation. Cardiogenic shock may be related to mitochondrial death (induced by RNI and ROI) with subsequent myocardial dysfunction. Peripheral vasoregulation abnormalities and myocardial dysfunction may play a larger role in hemodynamic derangements in pediatric patients, especially infants and neonates. Factors that contribute to developmental differences in hemodynamic responses include altered structure and function of cardiomyocytes, limited ability to increase stroke volume and contractility, and contributions of the transition from fetal to neonatal circulation.[4,491] Abnormal peripheral vasoregulation with or without myocardial dysfunction is the primary mechanism for the hypotension accompanying septic shock in the neonate.[492] Therefore, septic neonates can present with hypotension and adequate perfusion (warm shock) or inadequate perfusion (cold shock). Myocardial dysfunction can lead to ventricular wall stretch that in turn elevates B-type natriuretic peptide (BNP). BNP is elevated in children with septic shock[493] and concentrations have utility as prognostic indicators of mortality[494] in older patients with sepsis as well as in postoperative children.[495] The utility of BNP or NT-proBNP in neonatal sepsis is unknown. Plasma NO is elevated in neonates with sepsis and shock compared to those with shock alone.[170]

Preterm neonates with sepsis have relatively high left and right cardiac outputs and low SVRs. A decrease in right ventricular output (RVO) or left ventricular output (LVO) greater than 50% compared with the initial measurement is associated with increased mortality from neonatal sepsis.[496] Elevated LVO but normal ejection fraction in preterm neonates with septic shock suggests that septic shock increases RVO predominantly by an increase in heart rate.[497] Neonatal sepsis may or may not be associated with left ventricular diastolic dysfunction, but evidence of cardiac injury was present in septic neonates as manifested by elevated cardiac troponin T.[498,499]

PULMONARY DYSFUNCTION

Acute hypoxic respiratory failure, ARDS, and acute lung injury are the most common organ dysfunctions associated with neonatal sepsis. Destruction of the alveolar capillary membrane leads to refractory hypoxemia. Following direct or indirect insults to the lung, alveolar macrophages produce chemokines that mediate PMN influx to lung parenchyma. Activated PMNs release ROI/RNI that damage endothelial and epithelial barriers leading to leakage of protein-rich edema fluid into the air spaces. Other pulmonary complications with severe sepsis may include secondary surfactant deficiency,[500] primary or secondary pneumonia,[501] and reactive pulmonary hypertension.[491,502] Murine neonatal sepsis-induced lung injury was attenuated via peptide-mediated blockade of cold-inducible RNA binding protein receptor.[503] This receptor is important for TNFα production, and inhibition of receptor-interacting protein kinase isoforms, important in necroptosis.[504,505]

CENTRAL NERVOUS SYSTEM

The detrimental neurodevelopmental long-term impact of sepsis has been demonstrated in multiple studies and has been reviewed in detail.[72,506-509] CNS injury is predominantly white-matter injury (loss of preoligodendrocytes), manifested by focal cystic periventricular leukomalacia, diffuse necrosis, or a combination of these entities.[76,510] CNS injury is, in part, mediated by inflammation with or without direct pathogen invasion.[125,511-513] The impact of sepsis on CNS injury is intensified in infants with lower gestational ages, highlighting the detrimental effects of sepsis on the developing brain.[76] The importance of evaluating the preterm infant for disseminated infection that may include meningitis cannot be overemphasized. Almost one-third of the cases of culture-positive meningitis in VLBWs are associated with negative concurrent blood cultures.[514] Clinically apparent seizures may occur in 25% of VLBW preterm infants with meningitis.[514] Low voltage background pattern, sleep-wake cycling, and seizure activity on a EEG may be helpful to predict neurologic outcome in infants with sepsis or meningitis.[515] Significantly lower resistance, vasodilatation, and higher blood flow were noted in the cerebral arteries of septic infants. Furthermore, the increase in cerebral blood flow velocity was correlated with elevated IL-6 concentrations.[516] Alterations in blood flow in preterm infants, in addition to factors associated with sepsis such as respiratory distress, hypercarbia, hypotension, and PDA, contribute to the risk of intracerebral hemorrhage.

OTHER ORGAN SYSTEM CONTRIBUTIONS

Endocrine abnormalities associated with sepsis may include altered thyroid function[517] and adrenal insufficiency associated with refractory hypotension.[518] Induced by proinflammatory cytokines, cortisol production in the neonate may be significantly increased early in septic shock.[200] However, very preterm neonates can have relative adrenal insufficiency that may contribute to hemodynamic instability and hypotension. An inadequate adrenocortical response is associated with increased mortality.[519,520] In many clinical practices, hydrocortisone is the third-line agent in treatment of neonatal shock after volume resuscitation and dopamine.[492,521,522] Hydrocortisone has not been evaluated in prospective randomized clinical trials for the treatment of septic shock in the neonate, but it has been shown to increase blood pressure, decrease heart rate, and decrease vasoactive medication requirements in preterm and term neonates in addition to cytokine-suppressing effects.[521,523,524]

Sepsis was the most common etiology (78%) of acute kidney injury (AKI) in term neonates and was associated with high mortality (37%; $n = 49$).[525] Neutrophil gelatinase-associated lipocalin (NGAL) has been evaluated as a marker of AKI but may be a less specific marker of the severity of inflammation.[526] Among infants with MODS, renal failure is among the first presenting signs after edema.[527] The frequency of ARF, defined as blood urea nitrogen greater than 20 mg/dL in septic neonates, was 26% and oliguria occurred in 15% of ARF cases.[528] AKI, defined as an increase of serum creatinine levels ≥0.3 mg/dL compared to basal values in preterm neonates, was associated with high mortality.[529]

Hepatic injury and dysfunction are frequent associations with severe sepsis. Mechanisms include reduced hepatic perfusion associated with septic shock and mitochondrial energy failure. Reductions in coagulation and complement factors, APRs, as well as increases in transaminases and bilirubin are commonly seen especially with decreased perfusion states. Increased energy expenditure and oxygen consumption during sepsis[530] and decreased mitochondrial oxidative function precipitated by hypoxia and the presence of ROI may lead to impaired growth, caloric deficiency, and energy failure.[531,532]

IMMUNE SYSTEM

Following severe sepsis or septic shock, there is an increased risk of subsequent infection and mortality in children and adults. This phenomenon is termed *immunoparalysis* and is associated with reduced MHC class 2 expression and TNF-α production by mononuclear cells following endotoxin stimulation. In addition to altered monocytic responses, there is significant loss of lymphoid $CD4^+$ T and B cells via caspase-dependent apoptotic pathways.[414,533] Whether by clonal selection, apoptosis, or elevated endogenous glucocorticoid levels,[534-536] lymphocyte loss may lead to a state of immune compromise following the acute phase of sepsis.[411,534,536-540] New data suggest that IL-7 may play an important role in promoting T-cell activation and the prevention of apoptosis.[541] The importance of immunoparalysis has been convincingly demonstrated in infected adults[542-545] and children.[546] However, while immunoparalysis may occur following sepsis in neonates,[547] it does not have the same degree of clinical impact in the preterm neonate in whom adaptive immune function is less well developed.[548,549]

In examinations of peripheral blood and postmortem spleens from septic adults, there is significant loss of B and $CD4^+$ T lymphocytes as well as DCs,[533,550] resulting in decreased antigen presentation, antibody production, and macrophage activation.[551] Circulating peripheral absolute lymphocyte counts (ALC) can drop significantly in the septic adult, but this phenomenon is also seen in the nonseptic critically ill adult.[552] Sustained lymphopenia significantly increases the risk for secondary infection, MODS, and death in children.[540] In line with findings in septic adults, extensive loss of lymphocytes (both B and T) has been described post mortem in thymic and splenic tissues from preterm and term infants with sepsis.[411,534,536-539] The number and the size of follicles in the spleen decreased significantly, and the total number of cells decreased more than three times; similar changes were found in lymph nodes.[553] However, these histopathologic splenic findings are in contradiction to earlier reports where no differences were described between septic and nonseptic infants.[411] Although splenic histologic changes may occur with sepsis, sepsis-associated splenomegaly was not apparent in bacterial EOS but was significant in LOS and was due to splenic congestion in the absence of hyperplasia of white pulp.[537]

Mechanisms behind sepsis and post-sepsis immune alterations are beginning to emerge. The intensity of the inflammatory response may be modified by neural-based mechanisms.[554] T-cell-secreted acetylcholine acts on macrophages to reduce production of TNF, IL-1, IL-18, HMGB1, and other cytokines.[555] The role of vagal tone in the neonatal host response to sepsis is unclear.

Discovery and characterization of the impact of epigenetic-mediated immune system functional alterations following sepsis is an area of intense research. DNA methylation as well as posttranslational modification of histone proteins (methylation, acetylation, phosphorylation, ubiquitination, sumoylation) may occur after sepsis.[108,556] These DNA alterations may modify transcription factor access of gene-specific promoter regions ultimately leading to short- and long-term changes in gene expression and immune function. DNA methylation pattern in the promoter region of the calcitonin-related polypeptide α-gene varies in different types of bacterial sepsis in preterm infants, suggesting a potential use as an epigenetic biomarker.[557]

Trained immunity, the term coined to describe an adaptive innate immune response, may also be a positive or negative consequence of sepsis in early life.[558] Mechanisms that underlie trained immunity are beginning to emerge and include DNA methylation and modification of energy utilization pathways.[559,560] Nonspecific vaccine benefits and resistance to subsequent pathogen challenge following innate immune priming or previous infection are likely manifestations of trained immunity in neonates.[3,549,561] The cell types, extent, and duration of trained immunity-based modifications in neonates with sepsis have not been studied. MDSCs manifest immunosuppressive activity with sepsis[562] and were described in neonates. MDSCs are present at high frequency at birth and decline with postnatal age. They inhibit T-cell proliferative responses and IFN-γ production.[563] In addition to host-mediated immunosuppression, reactivation of viral infection that may contribute to morbidity and mortality has been demonstrated in adults with sepsis.[564] The impact, if any, of viral reactivation in neonates is unknown.

MULTI-ORGAN FAILURE/DYSFUNCTION

Sepsis that leads to MODS carries a dismal prognosis. Inadequate cardiac output and microcirculatory failure, which may be combined with formation of microthrombi and DIC, can lead to poor perfusion to the kidney,[481,482] liver,[483] gut,[484] and CNS.[133,169,326,478,485] Studies suggest that the mechanism of organ failure in sepsis may relate to decreased oxygen utilization associated with mitochondrial dysfunction rather than or in addition to poor oxygen delivery to tissues.[486,487] Mitochondrial dysfunction can initiate activation of cell death pathways including apoptosis, pyroptosis, necrosis, and NETosis (i.e., cell death mediated by NETs). DAMPs, including nucleosomes and microparticles, created by activation of these cell death programs further amplify the host inflammatory response.

Free radicals play an important role in the inflammatory process of sepsis.[565] In a piglet neonatal sepsis model, edaravone, a novel free radical scavenger, increased mean arterial pressure and cardiac output, lowered hydroperoxide, nitrite, and nitrate levels, delayed the TNF-α surge, prevented HMGB1 elevation, and was associated with longer survival times.[566] Elevated plasma nitrite/nitrates and increased organ failure scores are present in children with sepsis with an exaggerated proinflammatory state and a robust antiinflammatory response.[567] Increased plasma nitrite and nitrate concentrations are associated with the development of multiple organ failure in pediatric sepsis[568] but have not been investigated in neonates.

FUTURE CONSIDERATIONS

The incidence of neonatal sepsis remains high and outcomes remain poor despite considerable technologic advances in the field of neonatology. Much remains to be learned about the impact of developmental age on host response in the host response to sepsis and what facets are critically important. Key considerations for future investigations include the implementation of a consensus definition for neonatal sepsis, the use of homogeneous systems (only neonatal components) for human ex vivo studies, the use of transgenic approaches in preclinical models alongside observational studies in humans to ensure meaningful findings, and clinical trials using precision medicine to reduce the deficits that occur secondary to sepsis in neonates.

ABBREVIATIONS

ADCC: antibody–dependent cell–mediated cytotoxicity
AKI: acute kidney injury
APR: acute phase reactant
ARDS: acute respiratory distress syndrome
ARF: acute renal failure
ASC: apoptosis-associated speck-like protein containing a c-terminal caspase-recruitment domain
BNP: b-type natriuretic peptide
BPI: bactericidal/permeability-increasing protein
CAM: cell adhesion molecule
CASP-1: caspase 1
CD: cluster of differentiation
CI: confidence interval
CNS: central nervous system
CoNS: coagulase negative staphylococcus
CR3: complement receptor 3
CRP: C-reactive protein
DAMPs: Damage-associated molecular patterns
DC: dendritic cell
DIC: disseminated intravascular coagulation
ELBW: extremely low birth weight
eNOS: endothelial nitric oxide synthase
EOS: early-onset sepsis
ET-1: endothelin-1
GBS: Group B streptococcus
G-CSF: granulocyte colony stimulating factor
GM-CSF: granulocyte monocyte colony stimulating factor
GWEP: genome-wide expression profiling
HLA: human leukocyte antigen
HMGB-1: high mobility group binding protein 1
HSP: heat shock protein
HSV: herpes simplex virus
ICAM: intercellular adhesion molecule
ICU: intensive care unit
IFN: interferon
Ig: immunoglobulin
IL: interleukin
IL-1ra: IL-1 receptor antagonist
iNKT: invariant natural killer T cell
IRAK: IL-1 receptor-associated kinase
IRF5: interferon regulatory factor 5
LBP: lipopolysaccharide binding protein
LBW: low birth weight
LOS: late-onset sepsis
LPS: lipopolysaccharide
LTE: leukotriene
LVO: left ventricular outflow
MBL: mannose-binding lectin
MDSCs: myeloid-derived suppressor cell
MHC: major histocompatibility complex
miRNA: microRNA
MMP: matrix metalloproteinase
MODS: multi-organ dysfunction syndrome
MyD88: myeloid differentiation factor 88
NADPH: nicotinamide adenine dinucleotide phosphate
NDI: neurodevelopmental impairment
NEC: necrotizing enterocolitis
NEMO: NF-κ-B essential modulator
NET: neutrophil extracellular trap
NF-κB: nuclear factor kappa B
NGAL: neutrophil gelatinase associated-lipocalin
NICU: neonatal intensive care unit
NK: natural killer cell
NLR: nucleotide-binding oligomerization domain-like receptors
NLRP: NOD leucine rich repeat and pyrin domain containing
NO: nitric oxide
NOD: nucleotide-binding oligomerization domain
nSOFA: neonatal sequential organ failure assessment
OR: odds ratio
PAF: platelet activating factor
PAI-1: plasminogen activator inhibitor-1
PAMPs: pathogen-associated molecular patterns
PCV: pneumococcal conjugate vaccine
PDA: patent ductus arteriosus
PGE: prostaglandin E
PICS: persistent inflammation, immunosuppression, and catabolism syndrome
PICU: pediatric ICU
PLA2: phospholipase A2
PMN: polymorphonuclear cell; neutrophil
PPHN: persistent pulmonary hypertension
PRRs: pathogen recognition receptors
RAG-1: recombinase activating gene-1
RAGE: receptor for advanced glycation end products
RCT: randomized clinical trial
RIG: retinoic acid-inducible gene-I
RLR: RIG-like receptors
RNI: reactive nitrogen intermediates
ROI: reactive oxygen intermediates
RVO: right ventricular output
SAA: serum amyloid A
SICU: surgical ICU
sIL-2: soluble IL-2
SIP: spontaneous intestinal perforation
SIRS: systemic inflammatory response syndrome
SNPs: single nucleotide polymorphism
SOFA: sequential organ failure assessment
sRAGE: soluble RAGE
sTREM-1: soluble triggering receptor expressed on myeloid cells-1
TBX: thromboxane
TGF: transforming growth factor
TIR: Toll/IL-1 receptor
TLR: Toll-like receptor
TNF: tumor necrosis factor
TNFR2: TNF receptor 2

TRAM: TRIF related adaptor molecule
TREM-1: triggering receptor expressed on myeloid cells-1
TRIF: TIR-domain-containing adapter-inducing interferon-β
UTI: urinary tract infection
VCAM: vascular cell adhesion molecule
VLBW: very low birth weight
WHO: World Health Organization
WT: wild-type

ACKNOWLEDGMENT

I am indebted to Professor Hector Wong for his assistance with the prior iteration of this chapter.

 A complete reference list is available at www.ExpertConsult.com.

SELECT REFERENCES

1. Gentile LF, Nacionales DC, Lopez MC, et al. Protective immunity and defects in the neonatal and elderly immune response to sepsis. *J Immunol.* 2014;192(7):3156-3165.
2. Wynn JL, Scumpia PO, Delano MJ, et al. Increased mortality and altered immunity in neonatal sepsis produced by generalized peritonitis. *Shock.* 2007;28(6):675-683.
3. Wynn JL, Scumpia PO, Winfield RD, et al. Defective innate immunity predisposes murine neonates to poor sepsis outcome but is reversed by TLR agonists. *Blood.* 2008;112(5):1750-1758.
4. Wynn J, Cornell TT, Wong HR, Shanley TP, Wheeler DS. The host response to sepsis and developmental impact. *Pediatrics.* 2010;125(5):1031-1041.
5. Raymond SL, Lopez MC, Baker HV, et al. Unique transcriptomic response to sepsis is observed among patients of different age groups. *PLoS One.* 2017;12(9):e0184159.
6. Wynn JL, Cvijanovich NZ, Allen GL, et al. The influence of developmental age on the early transcriptomic response of children with septic shock. *Mol Med.* 2011;17(11-12):1146-1156.
7. Byun HJ, Jung WW, Lee JB, et al. An evaluation of the neonatal immune system using a listeria infection model. *Neonatology.* 2007;92(2):83-90.
8. Venkatesh MP, Pham D, Fein M, Kong L, Weisman LE. Neonatal coinfection model of coagulase-negative Staphylococcus (Staphylococcus epidermidis) and Candida albicans: fluconazole prophylaxis enhances survival and growth. *Antimicrob Agents Chemother.* 2007;51(4):1240-1245.
9. Echeverry A, Schesser K, Adkins B. Murine neonates are highly resistant to Yersinia enterocolitica following orogastric exposure. *Infect Immun.* 2007;75(5):2234-2243.
10. Pedras-Vasconcelos JA, Goucher D, Puig M, et al. CpG oligodeoxynucleotides protect newborn mice from a lethal challenge with the neurotropic Tacaribe arenavirus. *J Immunol.* 2006;176(8):4940-4949.
11. Goldstein B, Giroir B, Randolph A. International pediatric sepsis consensus conference: definitions for sepsis and organ dysfunction in pediatrics. *Pediatr Crit Care Med.* 2005;6(1):2-8.
12. Bone RC, Balk RA, Cerra FB, et al. Definitions for sepsis and organ failure and guidelines for the use of innovative therapies in sepsis. The ACCP/SCCM Consensus Conference Committee. American College of Chest Physicians/Society of Critical Care Medicine. *Chest.* 1992;101(6):1644-1655.
13. Brierley J, Carcillo JA, Choong K, et al. Clinical practice parameters for hemodynamic support of pediatric and neonatal septic shock: 2007 update from the American College of Critical Care Medicine. *Crit Care Med.* 2009;37(2):666-688.
14. Dellinger RP, Levy MM, Carlet JM, et al. Surviving Sepsis Campaign: international guidelines for management of severe sepsis and septic shock: 2008. *Intensive Care Med.* 2008;34(1):17-60.
15. Singer M, Deutschman CS, Seymour CW, et al. The Third International Consensus Definitions for Sepsis and Septic Shock (Sepsis-3). *JAMA.* 2016;315(8):801-810.
16. Wynn JL, Wong HR, Shanley TP, Bizzarro MJ, Saiman L, Polin RA. Time for a neonatal-specific consensus definition for sepsis. *Pediatr Crit Care Med.* 2014;15(6):523-528.
17. Gupta S, Sakhuja A, Kumar G, McGrath E, Nanchal RS, Kashani KB. Culture-negative severe sepsis: nationwide trends and outcomes. *Chest.* 2016;150(6):1251-1259.
18. Weiss SL, Fitzgerald JC, Pappachan J, et al. Global epidemiology of pediatric severe sepsis: the sepsis prevalence, outcomes, and therapies study. *Am J Respir Crit Care Med.* 2015.
19. Wynn JL, Kelly MS, Benjamin DK, et al. Timing of multiorgan dysfunction among hospitalized infants with fatal fulminant sepsis. *Am J Perinatol.* 2017;34(7):633-639.
20. Wynn JL, Polin RA. A neonatal sequential organ failure assessment score predicts mortality to late-onset sepsis in preterm very low birth weight infants. *Pediatr Res.* 2019.
21. Liu L, Johnson HL, Cousens S, et al. Global, regional, and national causes of child mortality: an updated systematic analysis for 2010 with time trends since 2000. *Lancet.* 2012;379(9832):2151-2161.
22. Lawn JE, Cousens S, Zupan J. 4 million neonatal deaths: when? Where? Why? *Lancet.* 2005;365(9462):891-900.
23. Stoll BJ, Hansen N, Fanaroff AA, et al. Changes in pathogens causing early-onset sepsis in very-low-birth-weight infants. *N Engl J Med.* 2002;347(4):240-247.
24. Stoll BJ, Hansen N, Fanaroff AA, et al. Late-onset sepsis in very low birth weight neonates: the experience of the NICHD Neonatal Research Network. *Pediatrics.* 2002;110(2 Pt 1):285-291.
25. Stoll BJ, Hansen NI, Higgins RD, et al. Very low birth weight preterm infants with early onset neonatal sepsis: the predominance of gram-negative infections continues in the National Institute of Child Health and Human Development Neonatal Research Network, 2002-2003. *Pediatr Infect Dis J.* 2005;24(7):635-639.
26. Haque KN, Khan MA, Kerry S, Stephenson J, Woods G. Pattern of culture-proven neonatal sepsis in a district general hospital in the United Kingdom. *Infect Control Hosp Epidemiol.* 2004;25(9):759-764.
27. Klinger G, Levy I, Sirota L, Boyko V, Lerner-Geva L, Reichman B. Outcome of early-onset sepsis in a national cohort of very low birth weight infants. *Pediatrics.* 2010;125(4):e736-e740.
28. Boghossian NS, Page GP, Bell EF, et al. Late-onset sepsis in very low birth weight infants from singleton and multiple-gestation births. *J Pediatr.* 2013;162(6):1120-1124.4 e1.
29. Stoll BJ, Hansen NI, Sanchez PJ, et al. Early onset neonatal sepsis: the burden of group b streptococcal and E. coli disease continues. *Pediatrics.* 2011;127(5):817-826.
30. Barton L, Hodgman JE, Pavlova Z. Causes of death in the extremely low birth weight infant. *Pediatrics.* 1999;103(2):446-451.
31. Cohen-Wolkowiez M, Moran C, Benjamin DK, et al. Early and late onset sepsis in late preterm infants. *Pediatr Infect Dis J.* 2009;28(12):1052-1056.
32. Girard TD, Opal SM, Ely EW. Insights into severe sepsis in older patients: from epidemiology to evidence-based management. *Clin Infect Dis.* 2005;40(5):719-727.
33. Martin GS, Mannino DM, Moss M. The effect of age on the development and outcome of adult sepsis. *Crit Care Med.* 2006;34(1):15-21.
34. Stoll BJ, Hansen NI, Bell EF, et al. Neonatal outcomes of extremely preterm infants from the NICHD Neonatal Research Network. *Pediatrics.* 2010;126(3):443-456.
35. Watson RS, Carcillo JA, Linde-Zwirble WT, Clermont G, Lidicker J, Angus DC. The epidemiology of severe sepsis in children in the United States. *Am J Respir Crit Care Med.* 2003;167(5):695-701.
36. Shah GS, Budhathoki S, Das BK, Mandal RN. Risk factors in early neonatal sepsis. *Kathmandu Univ Med J (KUMJ).* 2006;4(2):187-191.
37. Salem SY, Sheiner E, Zmora E, Vardi H, Shoham-Vardi I, Mazor M. Risk factors for early neonatal sepsis. *Arch Gynecol Obstet.* 2006;274(4):198-202.
38. Yancey MK, Duff P, Kubilis P, Clark P, Frentzen BH. Risk factors for neonatal sepsis. *Obstet Gynecol.* 1996;87(2):188-194.
39. Benitz WE, Gould JB, Druzin ML. Risk factors for early-onset group B streptococcal sepsis: estimation of odds ratios by critical literature review. *Pediatrics.* 1999;103(6):e77.
40. Fanaroff AA, Korones SB, Wright LL, et al. Incidence, presenting features, risk factors and significance of late onset septicemia in very low birth weight infants. The National Institute of Child Health and Human Development Neonatal Research Network. *Pediatr Infect Dis J.* 1998;17(7):593-598.
41. Schuchat A, Zywicki SS, Dinsmoor MJ, et al. Risk factors and opportunities for prevention of early-onset neonatal sepsis: a multicenter case-control study. *Pediatrics.* 2000;105(1 Pt 1):21-26.
42. Escobar GJ, Li DK, Armstrong MA, et al. Neonatal sepsis workups in infants >/=2000 grams at birth: a population-based study. *Pediatrics.* 2000;106(2 Pt 1):256-263.
43. Gagliardi L, Rusconi F, Bellu R, Zanini R, Italian Neonatal N. Association of maternal hypertension and chorioamnionitis with preterm outcomes. *Pediatrics.* 2014;134(1):e154-e161.
44. Garcia-Munoz Rodrigo F, Galan Henriquez G, Figueras Aloy J, Garcia-Alix Perez A. Outcomes of very-low-birth-weight infants exposed to maternal clinical chorioamnionitis: a multicentre study. *Neonatology.* 2014;106(3):229-234.
45. Jackson GL, Engle WD, Sendelbach DM, et al. Are complete blood cell counts useful in the evaluation of asymptomatic neonates exposed to suspected chorioamnionitis? *Pediatrics.* 2004;113(5):1173-1180.
46. Jackson GL, Rawiki P, Sendelbach D, Manning MD, Engle WD. Hospital course and short-term outcomes of term and late preterm neonates following exposure to prolonged rupture of membranes and/or chorioamnionitis. *Pediatr Infect Dis J.* 2012;31(1):89-90.
47. Kiser C, Nawab U, McKenna K, Aghai ZH. Role of guidelines on length of therapy in chorioamnionitis and neonatal sepsis. *Pediatrics.* 2014;133(6):992-998.
48. Pappas A, Kendrick DE, Shankaran S, et al. Chorioamnionitis and early childhood outcomes among extremely low-gestational-age neonates. *JAMA pediatrics.* 2014;168(2):137-147.
49. Soraisham AS, Singhal N, McMillan DD, Sauve RS, Lee SK, Canadian Neonatal N. A multicenter study on the clinical outcome of chorioamnionitis in preterm infants. *Am J Obstet Gynecol.* 2009;200(4):372.e1-e6.
50. Garcia-Munoz Rodrigo F, Galan Henriquez GM, Ospina CG. Morbidity and mortality among very-low-birth-weight infants born to mothers with clinical chorioamnionitis. *Pediatr Neonatol.* 2014;55(5):381-386.

152 Pathophysiology of Neonatal Hypoglycemia

Colin P. Hawkes | Diana E. Stanescu | Charles A. Stanley

INTRODUCTION

Hypoglycemia in neonates has been a topic of major concern and of controversy for many decades. These arise from two competing clinical issues. On the one hand, for a small number of infants born with persistent forms of hypoglycemia, there is the serious risk of seizures and permanent brain injury if not detected early and treated adequately. For example, over half of the children with genetic forms of congenital hyperinsulinism suffer from seizures and permanent brain injury[1-3] that could have been prevented if their hypoglycemia had been diagnosed and treated before discharge from the newborn nursery. On the other hand, there is a competing need to avoid overdiagnosis and unnecessary interventions, because hypoglycemia to varying degrees is common in normal infants during the first days of life and usually has no apparent consequence. For example, in normal newborns, mean plasma glucose concentrations transiently drop by 25 to 40 mg/dL from the fetal range of 70 to 100 mg/dL to a nadir of approximately 55 to 65 mg/dL immediately after birth; glucose levels then quickly rise within 1 to 2 days back again into the normal range for infants, children, and adults of 70 to 100 mg/dL.[4-8] This *transitional neonatal hypoglycemia in normal newborns* can create confusion in recognizing cases with permanent or persistent hypoglycemia disorders. Contributing to the difficulty in balancing concerns about persistent, potentially damaging forms of hypoglycemia and the commonness of transitional hypoglycemia in normal newborns is the imbalance in our understanding of these conditions. The persistent forms of hypoglycemia that can present in the newborn have been well described and their diagnosis and treatment well defined. However, the mechanism(s) and management of transitional neonatal hypoglycemia remain poorly understood, further complicating efforts to distinguish the etiology of hypoglycemia in individual cases. The purposes of this chapter are (1) to review the pathophysiology of neonatal hypoglycemia with an emphasis on the mechanism underlying transitional neonatal hypoglycemia in normal newborns; (2) to describe the severe prolonged hyperinsulinism disorder that frequently occurs in neonates with perinatal stress such as birth asphyxia or intrauterine growth retardation; and (3) to outline the diagnosis and management of the major genetic or other persistent hypoglycemia disorders, which are most likely to be encountered in the neonatal period.

BACKGROUND

MECHANISMS OF GLUCOSE HOMEOSTASIS

Since glucose is an obligate fuel for brain metabolism and serves as the predominant fuel for the rest of the body, plasma glucose concentrations must be controlled within narrow limits at all times. The major elements of glucose homeostasis include (1) the **glucose set-point** (the target glucose concentration that maintains normal physiology); (2) various **glucose thresholds** (levels at which individual hormonal and neural glucoregulatory signaling factors are activated or inhibited to raise or lower plasma glucose levels); and (3) **glucose sensor(s)** that responds to glucose level to transmit a signal to control glucoregulatory factors.

As shown in Fig. 152.1, in children and adults, the **glucose set-point** is approximately 5 mmol/L, which represents the normal range of plasma glucose in both intrauterine and extrauterine life of 70 to 100 mg/dL. Plasma glucose levels are tightly maintained at this set-point by the counter-balancing glucose-lowering actions of insulin, which is suppressed below a **glucose threshold** of approximately 4 mM (70 mg/dL), and the glucose-raising actions of various counterregulatory factors with individual glucose thresholds ranging from 65 to 55 mg/dL, including especially glucagon and the sympathetic nervous system, as well as the more long-term effects of cortisol and growth hormone. The major **glucose sensor** for maintaining glucose homeostasis is glucokinase, a form of hexokinase expressed specifically in pancreatic islets and liver. Glucokinase is a low-affinity glucose-phosphorylating enzyme, which unlike the forms of hexokinase in all other tissues, becomes highly active only at glucose levels above 4 mM and thus sets the glucose threshold for insulin release by pancreatic islets. As evidence of the important role of this enzyme as the key glucose sensor for insulin secretion, glucokinase loss of function mutations result in diabetes and mutations (or drugs) that increase glucokinase activity cause hyperinsulinemic hypoglycemia.

The set-point for glucose reflects the glucose concentration required for optimal rates of energy production in the brain and other tissues. Newborns in the first few days of life have a transitional period of hypoglycemia, where the blood glucose is not maintained at the normal set-point level, for reasons that have not been clearly defined, but, as discussed in the section "Transitional Neonatal Hypoglycemia in Normal Newborns," are most likely due to persistence of the fetal lower β cell threshold for insulin release.

SOURCES OF GLUCOSE AND OTHER FUELS DURING THE TRANSITION FROM FED TO FASTED STATE

The changes in source of substrates for brain metabolism during increasing periods of fasting are shown in Fig. 152.2A and B. Following a meal, brain metabolism initially depends on glucose released from hepatic glycogen stores (**glycogenolysis**) and then on hepatic glucose synthesis (**gluconeogenesis**) using substrates such as amino acids generated by protein turnover in peripheral tissues, especially muscle. As fasting is extended and hepatic glycogen reserves become depleted, glucose production declines and free fatty acids, derived from the release of triglycerides stored in adipose tissue (**lipolysis**), become the major fuel for peripheral tissues, such as muscle. Although the brain cannot oxidize fatty acids directly, it can use fat stores indirectly after conversion of free fatty acids to ketones (β-hydroxybutyrate and acetoacetate) by hepatic **ketogenesis**; these ketones serve as a major fuel for the brain when their plasma concentrations become elevated, and can partially replace the need for glucose.

DEFINITION OF HYPOGLYCEMIA

Clinical hypoglycemia is a plasma glucose concentration low enough to cause signs or symptoms of impaired brain function. Recognition of clinical hypoglycemia is most reliably made by Whipple's Triad (symptoms compatible with hypoglycemia, associated with a low plasma glucose concentration, and relief of symptoms when glucose concentration is restored to normal). Recognition of hypoglycemia may be difficult when the patient cannot communicate symptoms (e.g., young infants and neonates).

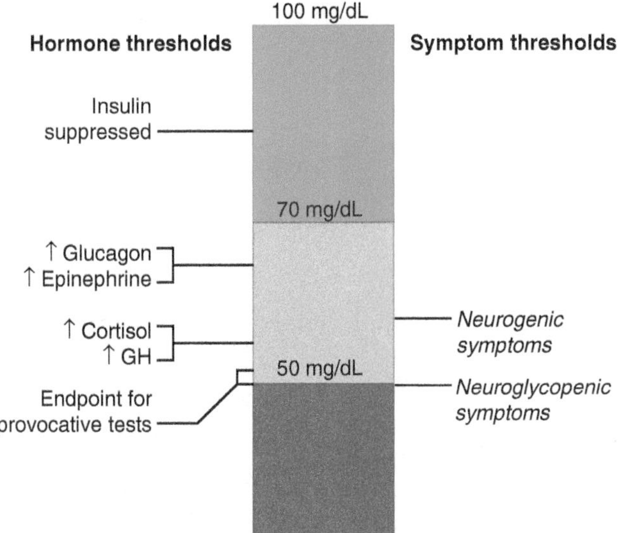

Fig. 152.1 Glucose thresholds for neuroendocrine and neuroglycopenic responses to hypoglycemia. As plasma glucose decreases towards 70 mg/dL, insulin secretion is suppressed. With further reductions in plasma glucose, glucagon and epinephrine secretion is increased, before growth hormone and cortisol secretion increases. Note that the thresholds for symptomatic hypoglycemia are lower than many of the thresholds for hormonal responses to reducing plasma glucose. *GH,* Growth hormone. (Modified from Shwartz NS, Cutter WE, Shah SD, et al. Glycemic thresholds for activation of glucose counterregulatory systems are higher than the threshold for symptoms. *J Clin Invest.* 1987;79:777–781; Heller SR, Cryer PE. Reduced neuroendocrine and symptomatic responses to subsequent hypoglycemia after 1 episode of hypoglycemia in nondiabetic humans. *Diabetes.* 1991;40:223–226; and Cryer PE, Gerich JE. Glucose counterregulation, hypoglycemia, and intensive insulin therapy in diabetes mellitus. *N Engl J Med.* 1985;313:232–241.)

The **glucose set-point** (the physiologically normal range of plasma glucose) appears to be the same across all ages from the fetus to adulthood (70 to 100 mg/dL, 3.9 to 5.6 mmol/L, Fig. 152.1).

It must be emphasized that clinical hypoglycemia cannot be defined as a specific plasma glucose value. This is because (1) as shown in Fig. 152.1, the various neural and endocrine responses to hypoglycemia occur across a range of plasma glucose concentrations,[9] (2) brain responses may be altered by availability of alternative fuels (ketones), and (3) brain injury from low glucose concentrations depends on both the degree and duration of hypoglycemia. In addition, there are many potential artifacts in measuring plasma glucose concentrations: (1) venous and capillary blood have lower glucose concentrations than the concentration of arterial plasma glucose to which the brain is exposed,[10] (2) the glucose concentration in plasma is approximately 15% higher than in whole blood due to the volume occupied by red blood cells, (3) glucose concentrations in whole blood specimens decline rapidly with delays in processing due to consumption by red and white blood cells,[11] and (4) glucose measurements by bedside glucometer testing inherently have a 15% imprecision and are also highly susceptible to multiple artifacts of sampling and operator errors.

SYMPTOMS OF HYPOGLYCEMIA

The symptoms of hypoglycemia reflect brain responses to glucose deprivation. These are not specific to hypoglycemia and fall into two categories. **Neurogenic symptoms** are caused by the activation of sympathetic nervous system discharge triggered by hypoglycemia. These include both adrenergic symptoms (tachycardia, palpitations, tremor, anxiety) and cholinergic symptoms (sweating, hunger, paresthesias). Awareness of hypoglycemia depends on perception of these neurogenic responses. **Neuroglycopenic symptoms** reflect brain dysfunction due to deficient glucose supply. The glucose threshold for neurogenic responses to hypoglycemia can be impaired by previous episodes of hypoglycemia for 24 hours or more (hypoglycemia unawareness or hypoglycemia-associated autonomic failure [HAAF]).[12] However, the glucose threshold for neuroglycopenia is not affected by prior exposure to hypoglycemia. In patients with diabetes, HAAF is associated with increased risk of brain damage due to impairment of counter-regulatory responses to hypoglycemia and may also be a risk factor for hypoglycemic injury in neonates with persistent hypoglycemia disorders.

As mentioned, normal newborns in the first 2 days of life routinely have plasma glucose concentrations below the glucose set-point of the body, which is determined by the glucose utilization rates of peripheral tissues. The impact of this transient difference between glucose levels and glucose set-point in normal newborns is not known but is generally assumed to not have permanent adverse consequences if only mild and of brief duration.

DIAGNOSIS OF HYPOGLYCEMIA BASED ON FASTING METABOLIC FUEL RESPONSES

The integrity of the various metabolic and endocrine systems required for glucose homeostasis can be most readily tested by examining changes in the plasma levels of the major fuels at the end of a fasting test when plasma glucose concentrations have fallen toward 50 mg/dL (Fig. 152.2A).[13-16] As shown in Fig. 152.3, measurement of lactate (a major gluconeogenic substrate), β-hydroxybutyrate (the major ketone), and free fatty acids (released by lipolysis from adipose tissue) provides a robust foundation for the differential diagnosis of hypoglycemia disorders. Normally, at the time plasma glucose has fallen toward 50 mg/dL, plasma lactate remains low (<2.0 mM), but plasma levels of free fatty acids have increased several-fold to greater than 1 to 1.5 mM and levels of β-hydroxybutyrate have risen 10- to 20-fold to greater than 2.0 mM. Because plasma insulin concentrations are frequently not elevated enough to diagnose hyperinsulinism, the diagnosis of hyperinsulinism is most reliably based on evidence of excessive insulin effects, including inappropriate suppression of the levels of free fatty acids and, especially, of β-hydroxybutyrate. Confirmation of hyperinsulinism can be readily done by demonstrating inappropriate conservation of liver glycogen reserves during hypoglycemia as reflected by an inappropriately large (>30 mg/dL) glycemic response to injection of glucagon.[17] It is important to note that plasma cortisol and growth hormone levels are often not high enough to rule out pituitary deficiency and, therefore, specific diagnostic testing for these hormones is frequently necessary.[18,19]

FETAL GLUCOSE REGULATION

Prior to birth, fetal metabolism is supported almost entirely by oxidation of glucose. Fetal glucose is derived via passive transport across the placenta from the maternal plasma, where its concentration is under the control of maternal insulin secretion. This constant supply of maternal glucose means that fetal glucose homeostasis does not depend on the fetal metabolic and endocrine systems. Fetal insulin secretion is responsive to changes in fetal glucose concentrations, but since the concentrations of fetal plasma glucose are determined by maternal levels, the function of fetal insulin secretion is primarily to regulate growth, rather than glucose levels in the fetus. For example, mothers with inactivating mutations of glucokinase (maturity onset diabetes of the young [MODY] type 2) have mild persistent hyperglycemia that leads to increased insulin secretion by the unaffected fetus and approximately 0.25 kg increased birth weight.[20] Conversely, fetuses with a glucokinase

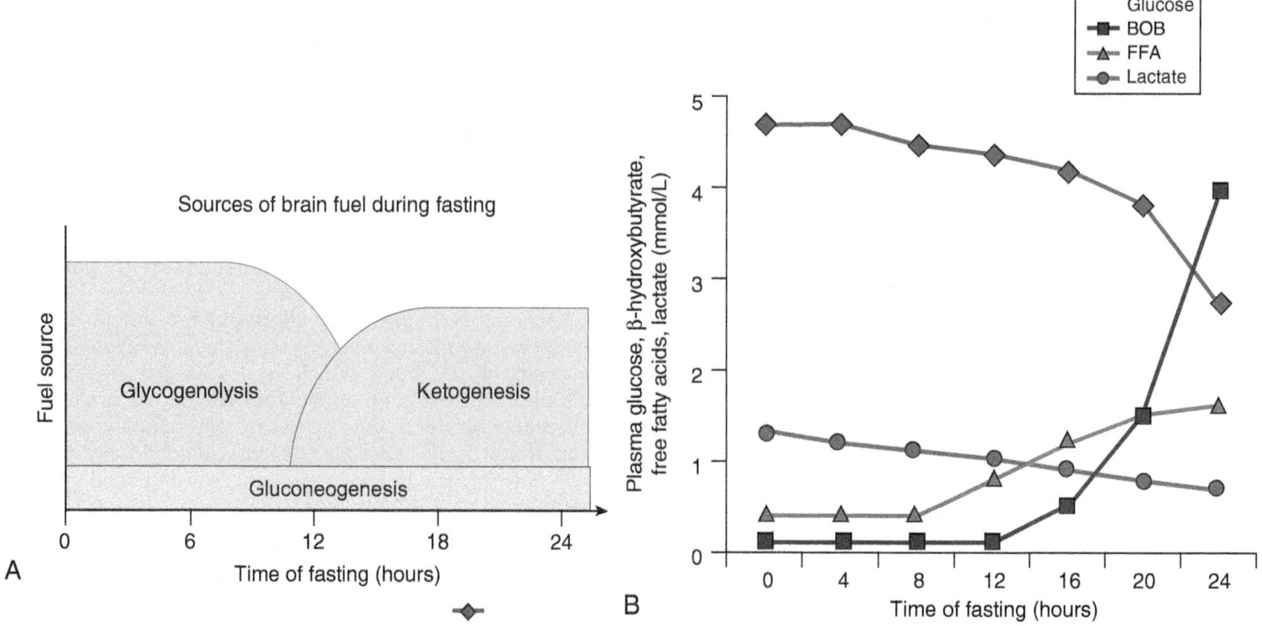

Fig. 152.2 The metabolic fuel response to fasting. (A) shows the shows the predominant fuel sources as the duration of fasting increases. Plasma glucose, β-hydroxybutyrate, free fatty acid, and lactate levels during fasting are shown in (B). Plasma glucose falls as liver glycogen stores become depleted. Lactate, as a representative gluconeogenic substrate declines slightly as glycogen stores become depleted and generation of gluconeogenic precursors diminishes. Free fatty acid concentrations rise as insulin secretion declines with the fall in plasma glucose, followed by a sharp increase in plasma ketones as hepatic fatty acid oxidation rises and serve to provide an alternative fuel for the brain in compensation for the reduced supply of plasma glucose. *BOB,* Beta-hydroxybutyrate; *FFA,* free fatty acids.

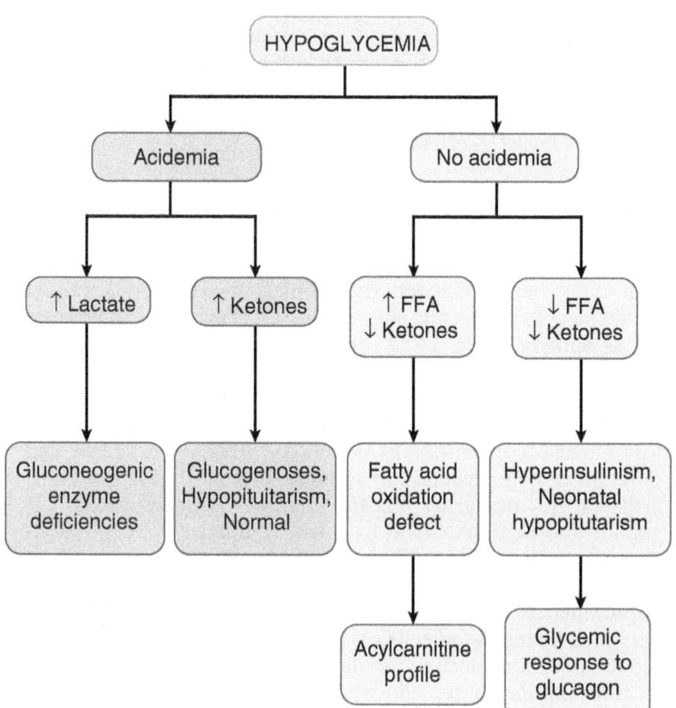

Fig. 152.3 Use of the "Critical Sample" to diagnose the etiology of hypoglycemia. Note that hypoketotic hypoglycemia in hypopituitarism is only seen in neonatal hypopituitarism, and the older child with hypopituitarism generally has ketotic hypoglycemia. Confirmatory testing for hyperinsulinism includes a glycemic response to glucagon, although neonatal hypopituitarism can sometimes also have a positive response (possibly related to perinatal stress hyperinsulinism, see text). Acylcarnitine profile is a confirmatory test for suspected fatty acid oxidation defects. Examples of gluconeogenic enzyme deficiencies include glucose-6-phosphatase, fructoes-1,6-bisphosphatase, pyruvate carboxylase. *FFA,* Free fatty acids.

inactivating mutation, but an unaffected mother, have reduced insulin secretion resulting in approximately 0.4 kg lower birthweight. Early in gestation, the fetal brain is perfused with plasma glucose concentrations that are essentially identical to maternal levels. Fetal plasma glucose levels near term fall slightly below maternal values, reflecting the limitation of placental glucose transport.[4] However, the difference between maternal and fetal plasma glucose concentrations at birth remains very small (approximately 9 mg/dL [0.5 mmol/L]).[21]

TRANSITIONAL NEONATAL HYPOGLYCEMIA IN NORMAL NEWBORNS

PLASMA GLUCOSE CONCENTRATIONS IN NORMAL NEWBORNS AFTER BIRTH

Fig. 152.4 illustrates the changes in mean glucose concentrations in newborn infants during the transition from intrauterine to extrauterine life (similar data has been reported in many other

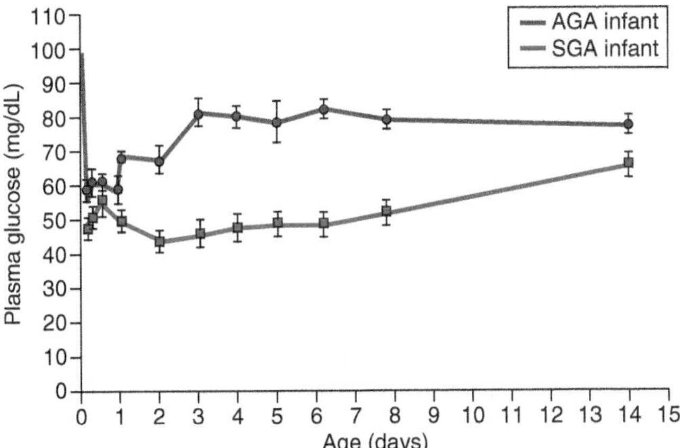

Fig. 152.4 In the first 3 days of life, plasma glucose after 3 to 4 hours of fasting can be lower than in older infants. In AGA infants, glucose concentrations after the third day are relatively consistent with levels seen in older infants. In infants born SGA, these glucose concentrations can take longer to reach the levels seen in older infants. *AGA,* Appropriate for gestational age; *SGA,* small for gestational age. (Some data from Cornblath M, Reisner SH. Blood glucose in the neonate and its clinical significance. *N Engl J Med.* 1965;273:378–381.)

cross-sectional studies).[22-24] In normal newborns, mean plasma glucose quickly falls from levels prior to delivery that are close to maternal glucose levels and similar to the normal levels of infants, children, and adults (approximately 80 mg/dL); mean glucose quickly drops to reach a mean (SD) of approximately 57 (13) mg/dL by 0 to 4 hours after delivery before rising by the third or fourth day after birth back into the normal range of 70 to 100 mg/dL for children and adults.[8] This short period of hypoglycemia immediately after birth in normal newborns has been termed *transitional neonatal hypoglycemia*. Certain high-risk groups of newborn infants (illustrated as "low birth weight" in Fig. 152.4) may have a more pronounced and more prolonged "dip" in plasma glucose concentrations after birth and can remain hypoglycemic for several weeks. This group of "low birthweight" infants would now be categorized as being small for gestational age (SGA) due to intrauterine growth restriction. They illustrate a common type of neonatal hypoglycemia associated with high-risk factors and will be discussed separately as "perinatal-stress hyperinsulinism" or "prolonged neonatal hyperinsulinism."

Fig. 152.5 illustrates the distribution of plasma glucose concentrations in various groups of newborn infants at the nadir of hypoglycemia prior to a first feeding at 8 hours of age.[23] In the term-AGA group, 80% dropped their plasma glucose concentrations below the range of 70 to 100 mg/dL, which is normal for the fetus prior to birth and for older infants, children, and adults. The mean glucose concentration in the term-AGA group was 54 mg/dL, similar to values in the transition period after birth in normal neonates found in many other studies.[24] Note that the distribution of glucose values in the term-AGA groups is skewed to the left; this reflects an excess of low or very low glucose values in neonates who had evidence of perinatal stress[23] such as birth asphyxia, maternal hypertension, or low weight for length consistent with late fetal growth deceleration (see later section on **perinatal stress hyperinsulinism**). The frequency of severe hypoglycemia was more marked in the other groups of neonates shown in Fig. 152.5, being especially high in SGA infants (perinatal stress) and in the LGA group (partly due to inclusion of infants with maternal diabetes). The SGA groups, in particular, show a bimodal distribution, with those having more evidence of perinatal stress also having more severe hypoglycemia. Of importance, the high frequency of hypoglycemia after birth quickly resolved: in this study, while 36% of the term-AGA neonates had glucose concentrations less than 50 mg/dL at 8 hours of age, none had glucose less than 50 mg/dL on day 2 to 3 and only 1% of the infants in the other groups had glucose levels less than 50 mg/dL after the first day.

That the glucose values shown in Fig. 152.5 are not normally distributed is noteworthy, because, in the past, it had been a long-standing practice in neonatology to try to create a "statistical" definition of neonatal hypoglycemia. This statistical definition of hypoglycemia was based on a value two SD below the mean (originally a whole blood glucose <30 mg/dL in "normal weight" and <20 mg/dL in "low birth weight" neonates, i.e., plasma glucose values <35 mg/dL and <25 mg/dL, respectively). In addition to this approach not being valid for data that are not normally distributed, the fallacy of such "statistical" definitions is now well appreciated; what is statistically "normal" only refers to what is "most common" and does not represent what is physiologically normal. As pointed out earlier in the chapter, hypoglycemia cannot be defined by any specific single value for plasma glucose concentration. As shown below, there is no evidence that the newborn brain has any special protection against the consequences of glucose deprivation.

While transitional neonatal hypoglycemia is common, other more persistent disorders of glucose metabolism may present similarly. A key differentiating factor is that the expected duration of transitional hypoglycemia should not exceed 48 hours.[25] It is critical to differentiate transitional hypoglycemia from persistent forms of neonatal hypoglycemia prior to hospital discharge,[26] since the latter conditions are associated with increased risks of adverse neurodevelopmental outcomes. Characteristics of infants who require monitoring for neonatal hypoglycemia and for whom a persistent disorder of hypoglycemia should be excluded prior to discharge are summarized in Box 152.1. Subsequent sections of this chapter describe these persistent disorders of hypoglycemia in detail.

MECHANISM OF TRANSITIONAL NEONATAL HYPOGLYCEMIA

PLASMA GLUCOSE CONCENTRATIONS ARE LOW, BUT STABLE DURING THE PERIOD OF TRANSITIONAL NEONATAL HYPOGLYCEMIA

There are few longitudinal studies of plasma glucose concentrations in individual newborn infants; however, there is strong evidence that the low levels of plasma glucose in normal newborns are remarkably stable and not much affected by the duration of postnatal fasting.[24] This had been demonstrated in older studies when normal nursery practice was to withhold feedings for 24 hours or more after delivery. For example, Desmond and colleagues in 1950 reported mean glucose levels in normal term neonates who were fasted for 24 hours after birth of 57 to 69 mg/dL (2.8 to 3.3 mM), which is almost identical to that seen in Fig. 152.5 after fasting for only 8 hours after birth.[27] Similarly, breast-fed neonates consume very few calories during the first few days of life and have mean plasma glucose concentrations that are similar to those of formula-fed infants.[6,28,29]

The remarkably stable low glucose concentrations on the first day after birth suggests that transitional hypoglycemia in normal newborns does not reflect a block in any of the specific metabolic systems (e.g., hepatic glycogenolysis, gluconeogenesis, or ketogenesis). Rather, it behaves like a controlled process where the mean concentration of plasma glucose is initially regulated at 55 to 60 mg/dL immediately after birth, but then increases to greater than 70 mg/dL (>3.9 mmol/L) by 2 to 3 days of age. This conclusion deserves emphasis, because previous efforts to understand neonatal hypoglycemia have focused on developmental studies of hepatic enzymatic pathways in various animal models. For example, studies in rodent models have shown developmental changes in the expression or activities of the enzymes of hepatic gluconeogenesis (especially PEP-CK) and hepatic ketogenesis (especially CPT-1 and HMG-CoA synthase).[30,31] However, deficiencies of these pathways cannot adequately explain the glucose patterns seen in the newborn

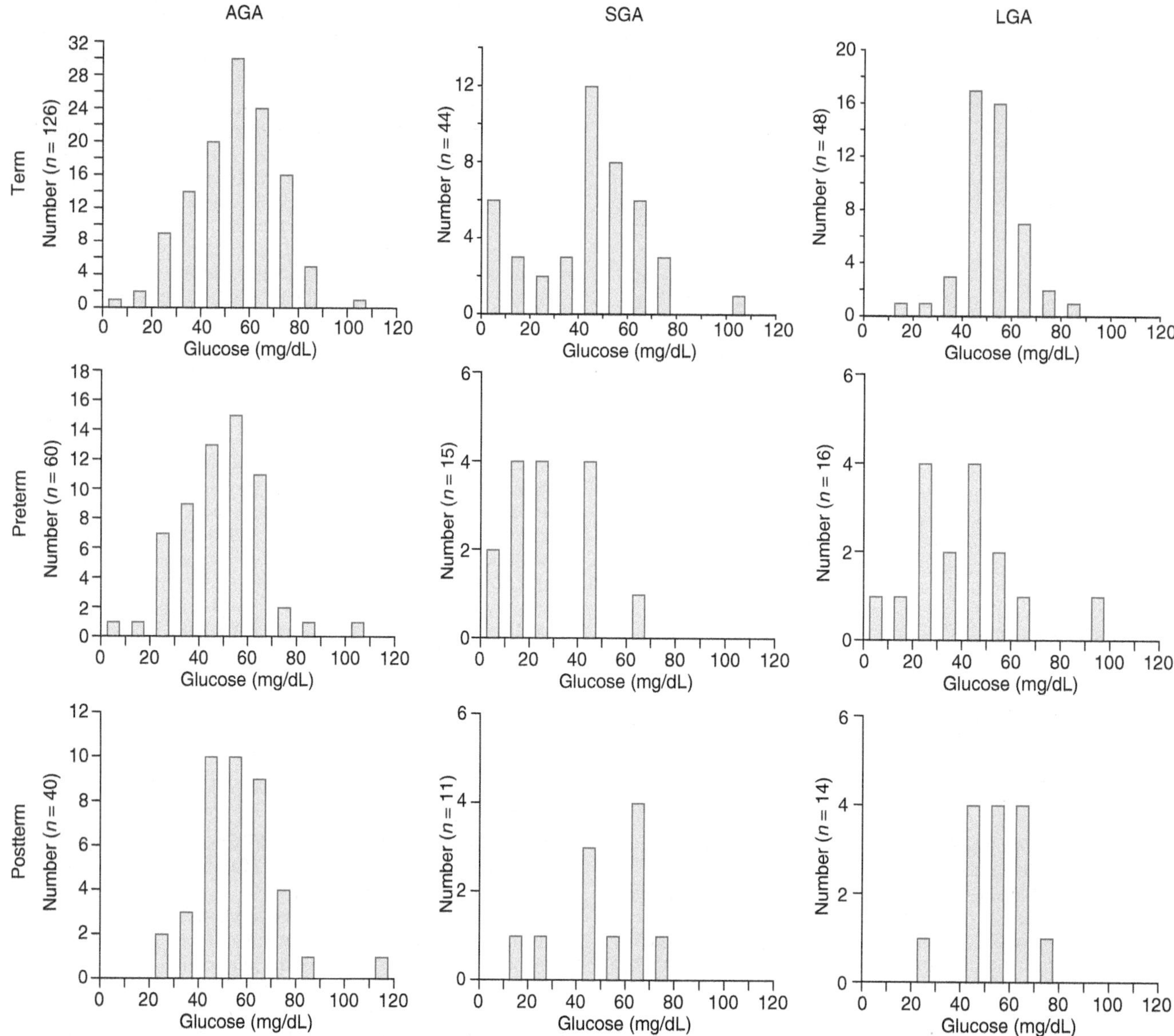

Fig. 152.5 Fasting glucose at 3 to 6 hours of age. Distribution of blood glucose categorized according to gestational age (Preterm, Term, and Post term) and birth weight (small for gestational age *[SGA]*, appropriate for gestational age *[AGA]*, and large for gestational age *[LGA]*). Note that there is a bimodal pattern in the SGA infants, with those with lowest blood glucose in this group likely having perinatal stress. (Some data from Lubchenco LO, Bard H. Incidence of hypoglycemia in newborn infants classified by birth weight and gestational age. *Pediatrics.* 1971;47:831–838.)

(especially since clinical experience with genetic defects in these pathways indicates that, unlike normal newborns with transitional neonatal hypoglycemia, affected patients maintain normoglycemia during fasting initially and then, only after glucose reserves become exhausted, show a rapid fall in glucose to profoundly hypoglycemic levels).

TRANSITIONAL NEONATAL HYPOGLYCEMIA IN NORMAL NEWBORNS IS A HYPOKETOTIC HYPOGLYCEMIA

The fasting systems approach outlined in Fig. 152.3 has been applied in studies of hypoglycemia in normal newborns in three separate studies that provide insight into the underlying mechanism of transitional neonatal hypoglycemia. These studies show that transitional neonatal hypoglycemia is associated with suppressed plasma concentrations of ketones (β-hydroxybutyrate and acetoacetate) during the first 1 to 2 days of life.[24,32] This is illustrated in Table 152.1 by data from Stanley and colleagues on fuel responses to hypoglycemia in groups of normal neonates compared to the normal responses to fasting hypoglycemia seen in older children and to the responses seen in children with hypoglycemia due to hyperinsulinism. Note that both neonates with severe hypoglycemia (<40 mg/dL) and those with milder hypoglycemia (mean 61 ± 2 mg/dL, mean ± SEM) had mean levels of total ketones that were 10-fold lower than those of hypoglycemic normal children (0.37 and 0.18 compared to 2.7 mmol/L). Suppression of ketones during hypoglycemia on the first day after birth in normal newborns has been reported by Hawdon and colleagues[32] and by Haymond and colleagues[33] and in SGA and other neonates by several other groups.[24,34,35] Suppressed ketone production is a more sensitive marker of hyperinsulinism than insulin measurement, likely due to hemolysis during phlebotomy or hepatic clearance leading to the failure to detect elevated plasma insulin levels.[36] Since ketone production by the liver and utilization by the brain are both linearly related to plasma concentrations, these very low levels of ketones indicate a marked suppression of ketogenesis. The low levels also highlight the fact that ketones cannot compensate as a fuel for the brain when newborns are hypoglycemic. As shown in Fig. 152.6, the inability to increase ketone production during hypoglycemia is a feature of SGA and premature neonates, as well as normal term-AGA infants.

Parenthetically, it should be noted that surveys of ketone levels in neonates over the first weeks of life have demonstrated mild increases in plasma levels on day 3 to 5 after birth in breast-fed, but not in formula-fed neonates. This was originally interpreted as a "suckling ketosis," similar to what occurs in rodents and some other species due to the high fat content of their milk. However, the transient elevation of ketones in breast-fed human infants is most likely due to a combination of not yet having achieved full calorie intake, together with the resolution of transitional neonatal hyperinsulinism releasing the inhibition of ketone production by insulin.

Box 152.1 Pediatric Endocrine Society Guidelines for Evaluation and Management of Persistent Hypoglycemia

Neonates Requiring Glucose Screening

1. Clinical signs of hypoglycemia
2. Large for gestational age (with or without maternal diabetes)
3. Perinatal stress:
   a. Birth asphyxia; cesarean delivery for fetal distress
   b. Maternal preeclampsia/eclampsia or hypertension
   c. Intrauterine growth restriction (small for gestational age)
   d. Meconium aspiration syndrome, erythroblastosis fetalis, polycythemia, hypothermia
4. Premature or postmature delivery
5. Infant of diabetic mother
6. Family history of a genetic form of hypoglycemia
7. Congenital syndromes (e.g., Beckwith-Wiedemann), abnormal physical features (e.g., midline facial malformations, microphallus)

Neonates for Whom Persistent Hypoglycemia Should Be Excluded Before Discharge

1. Severe hypoglycemia (e.g., episode of symptomatic hypoglycemia or need for IV dextrose to treat hypoglycemia)
2. Inability to consistently maintain preprandial plasma glucose concentrations >50 mg/dL up to 48 hours of age and >60 mg/dL after 48 hours of age
3. Family history of a genetic form of hypoglycemia
4. Congenital syndromes (e.g., Beckwith-Wiedemann), abnormal physical features (e.g., midline facial malformations, microphallus)

Adapted from Thornton PS, Stanley CA, De Leon DD, et al. Recommendations from the Pediatric Endocrine Society for evaluation and management of persistent hypoglycemia in neonates, infants, and children. *J Pediatr.* 2015;167(2):238–245.

TRANSITIONAL NEONATAL HYPOGLYCEMIA IS ASSOCIATED WITH CONSERVATION OF LIVER GLYCOGEN STORES

During fasting, liver glycogen stores normally become depleted before plasma glucose falls to the level of hypoglycemia. The glycemic response to administration of glucagon or epinephrine can be used to estimate liver glycogen reserves. Thus, a glycemic response to glucagon injection of greater than 30 mg/dL at a time of hypoglycemia provides evidence of an inappropriate liver glycogen reserve in the setting of hypoglycemia and, as shown in Fig. 152.3, provides a simple test for confirmation of hyperinsulinism.[17]

In 1950, Desmond and colleagues studied the glycemic response to epinephrine in normal infants during the first several days after birth. During the first 24 hours after delivery, no feedings were given according to the usual practice at that time. At 24 hours of age, epinephrine produced a brisk rise in glucose levels from a mean of approximately 50 mg/dL to a mean of approximately 85 mg/dL.[27] Similar brisk glycemic responses have been reported in normal newborns using glucagon as a stimulus for glycogenolysis[37,38] and also in hypoglycemic premature and SGA infants.[39,40] These studies of the glycemic response to glucagon and epinephrine in newborn infants during the first two days after birth provide evidence that insulin is the mechanism of transitional neonatal hypoglycemia in normal newborns.

INSULIN SECRETION IS NOT COMPLETELY SUPPRESSED DURING TRANSITIONAL NEONATAL HYPOGLYCEMIA

As shown in Table 152.1, plasma insulin concentrations are slightly higher in term-AGA neonates compared to normal older children with hypoglycemia, suggesting that neonatal hypoglycemia is accompanied by incomplete suppression of insulin secretion. Fig. 152.6 provides further evidence that insulin secretion is suppressed at lower glucose levels in neonates compared to older children. In Fig. 152.6B, betahydroxybutyrate levels rise as plasma glucose falls in normal infants but not in hyperinsulinism. Normal and SGA infants do not have a rise in betahydroxybutyrate concentrations as plasma glucose falls. This hypoketonemia is a marker of excess insulin in these neonates.[41,42] Whereas insulin levels in normal children were suppressed completely at plasma glucose concentrations below 4.0 to 4.5 mmol/L (70 to 75 mg/dL),[42] complete suppression of insulin did not occur in term and preterm neonates until plasma glucose levels were below 2 to 3 mmol/L (35 to 55

Table 152.1 Response of Normal Neonates to 8 Hour Fast After Delivery.

	Term, AGA (n = 20) (glucose >40 mg/dL)	Term, AGA (n = 4) (glucose <40 mg/dL)	Normal Children (n = 7) (after 24 h of fasting)	Hyperinsulinism (n = 7) (when hypoglycemic)
Length of Fast (h)	7.6 ± 0.1	3.8 ± 1.4	24	6.4 ± 1.9
Plasma Glucose (mg/dL)	61 ± 2	38 ± 1.4	52 ± 4.5	29 ± 5
β-Hydroxybutyrate (mmol/L)	0.31 ± 0.04	0.16 ± 0.03	2.5 ± 0.5	0.6 ± 0.2
Acetoacetate (mmol/L)	0.06 ± 0.01	0.02 ± 0.01	0.2 ± 0.1	0.1 ± 0.08
Free Fatty Acids (mmol/L)	1.4 ± 0.07	1.3 ± 0.23	1.6 ± 0.2	0.5 ± 0.2
Plasma Insulin (μU/mL)	10 ± 1	10.3 ± 3	6.8 ± 1.3	15 ± 3.5

All values mean ± SEM. Adapted from Stanley et al.[24,42] with permission.

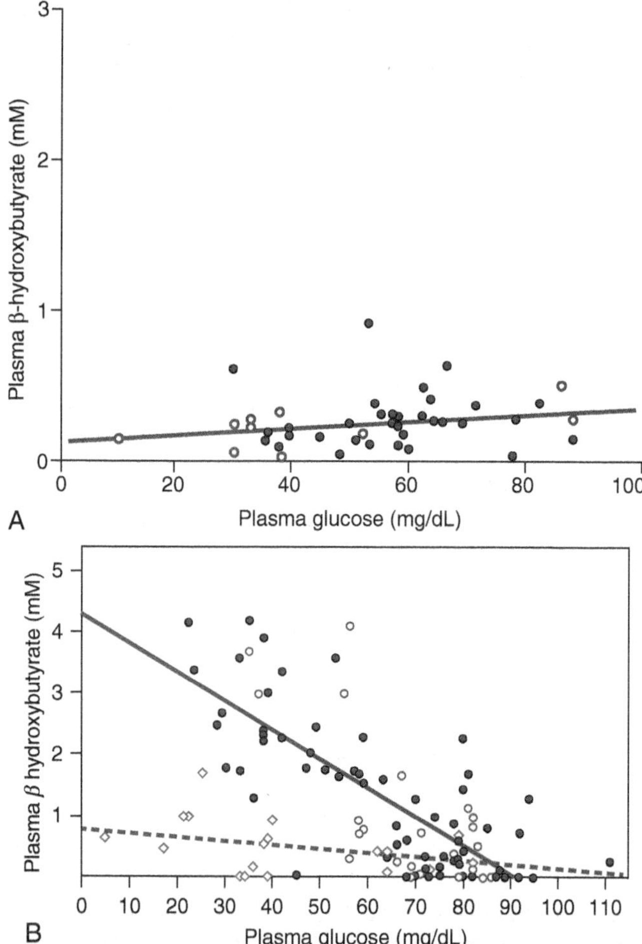

Fig. 152.6 Plasma glucose and β-hydroxybutyrate levels at the end of fasting studies. (A) Postnatal fasts in appropriate-for-gestational-age infants *(solid circles)* and small-for-gestational-age infants *(open circles)*. In the first 8 hours after birth, appropriate-for-gestational-age *(solid circles)* and small-for-gestational-age *(open circles)* newborn infants (age <8 hours) had suppressed ketones during hypoglycemia. (From Stanley CA, Anday EK, Baker L, et al. Metabolic fuel and hormone responses to fasting in newborn infants. *Pediatrics.* 1979;64:613–619). B, Fasting infants with hyperinsulinism (diamonds), control infants *(open circles)*, and children with ketotic hypoglycemia *(closed circles)*. The hypoketotic hypoglycemia seen in the first few hours after birth (A) is similar to that seen in older infants (age 4 ± 1 months) with congenital hyperinsulinism, and is not hyperketotic as in older control infants (age 10 ± 3 months). (From Stanley CA, Baker L. Hyperinsulinism in infancy: diagnosis by demonstration of abnormal response to fasting hypoglycemia. *Pediatrics.* 1976;57:702–711.)

mg/dL). These data are also consistent with a study of basal and glucose-stimulated insulin secretion in normal newborns immediately after delivery, which indicated that portal vein insulin concentrations were not suppressed (49 ± 29 μU/mL) at mean plasma glucose of 44 ± 20 mg/dL;[43] this contrasts with older infants in whom portal vein insulin levels were normally suppressed at glucose levels of 35 to 50 mg/dL.[43] Note that although plasma insulin levels at times of hypoglycemia are not dramatically elevated in neonates, the same is also true of infants with genetic forms of congenital hyperinsulinism (see Table 152.1).[42,44] Therefore, the problem with insulin secretion in congenital hyperinsulinism is not primarily due to hypersecretion, but rather a failure to turn off insulin secretion adequately at low glucose; this is also true during transitional neonatal hypoglycemia in normal newborns.

POTENTIAL MECHANISMS FOR TRANSITIONAL NEONATAL HYPOGLYCEMIA IN NORMAL NEWBORNS

The above cardinal features of transitional neonatal hypoglycemia in normal term, AGA newborns show that it is caused by hyperinsulinism. This transient postnatal hyperinsulinism is most likely an extension of the fetal pattern of insulin secretion into the early neonatal period. As discussed above, persistent fetal insulin secretion, in spite of fetal normoglycemia, is required to preserve fetal growth. Hence it is necessary for fetal and early neonatal islets to have a lower glucose threshold for insulin secretion than islets from mature individuals. In support of this concept, studies in rodents have shown that the glucose threshold for insulin release is lower in islets isolated from newborn rats on postnatal day 1 (2.8 mmol/L) compared to islets from mature animals (5 mmol/L).[45] Similarly, limited studies in human fetal islets show increased insulin secretion at 2.8 mM glucose.[46] There have been several suggested mechanisms to explain the low glucose threshold for insulin secretion in the fetus: (1) developmental differences in forbidding β-cell expression of lactate dehydrogenase *(LDH)* or monocarboxylic transporter *(SLC16A1)* could allow other fuels to stimulate insulin secretion in addition to glucose;[47] (2) expression of hexokinase isoforms with high affinity for glucose *(HK1, HK3)*, which permit stimulation of insulin secretion at low glucose concentrations; (3) differences in Ca^{2+} sensitivity of insulin granule release, leading to increased insulin secretion by fetal and neonatal mouse islets.[48] Further studies are needed on the mechanisms that control insulin secretion during the fetal to newborn transition period, and of the signals that allow rapid adaptation of β function during the first 1 to 3 days of life.

PERINATAL STRESS HYPOGLYCEMIA (PROLONGED NEONATAL HYPERINSULINISM)

In contrast to transitional neonatal hypoglycemia, which is mild and usually of very short duration, certain groups of newborns are at high risk for developing a more severe and more prolonged form of hypoglycemia, which can persist for several weeks after birth before resolving. This is illustrated in Fig. 152.5 from Lubchenco and Bard, where extremely low plasma glucose levels were associated with perinatal stresses, including late intrauterine growth retardation and birth asphyxia.[23] Similarly, in Fig. 152.4, the group labeled low birth weight infants (i.e., SGA) had lower mean glucose levels, which persisted until 2 weeks after birth.[5]

Severe and prolonged hypoglycemia in high-risk neonates caused by hyperinsulinism was first described in the 1980s and is commonly referred to as either *perinatal stress hypoglycemia* or *prolonged neonatal hyperinsulinism*. Collins and Leonard initially described perinatal stress hyperinsulinism in 1984 in six neonates,[49] three of whom had perinatal hypoxia and three who were SGA. These infants had severe hypoglycemia and symptoms, including seizures, and diagnostic features of hyperinsulinism; their hypoglycemia was controllable with diazoxide, a drug that acts by suppressing insulin release, and eventually resolved after several weeks. These authors subsequently described additional cases of SGA neonates with severe hyperinsulinism who required diazoxide treatment for several weeks to control their hypoglycemia before it resolved.[49] In 2006, Hoe et al.[50] described a larger group of 26 infants with prolonged neonatal hyperinsulinism. As shown in Table 152.1, associated risk factors included male gender (81%), cesarean delivery (62%), perinatal stress (35%), poor intrauterine growth (27%), prematurity (23%), and maternal hypertension (12%). In one fifth of the infants, no specific perinatal stresses or risk factors were identified. Infants with erythroblastosis fetalis are also known to be at high risk of transient hyperinsulinemic hypoglycemia at birth, which may be secondary to perinatal hypoxia due to their extreme anemia.[51-53]

Perinatal stress hypoglycemia/prolonged neonatal hyperinsulinism, is a relatively common occurrence in the newborn period and much more common than the genetic or syndromic forms of hypoglycemia that are described in a following section. Mizumoto and colleagues, in Japan, described cases of perinatal stress hypoglycemia/prolonged neonatal hyperinsulinism occurring among approximately 10% of infants admitted to a neonatal intensive care unit.[54] Palloto and Simmons have estimated that perinatal stress hypoglycemia persists beyond one week after birth in 8% of SGA infants.[55]

The clinical severity and duration of hyperinsulinism in infants with prolonged neonatal hyperinsulinism is variable and not predictable by the degree of perinatal stress. While a mechanistic link between hyperinsulinism in perinatal stress and transitional neonatal hypoglycemia in normal neonates has not been established, it is tempting to speculate that the two share a common mechanism and that perinatal stresses simply cause a prolongation of the normal period of transitional hyperinsulinism after birth. Although most cases of perinatal stress hypoglycemia respond well to diazoxide treatment, some of the more severe cases may have extremely high glucose requirements and may not respond to diazoxide. In these exceptional cases, support with supplemental glucose may be required for a prolonged period after birth until the hyperinsulinism resolves.

PERMANENT HYPOGLYCEMIC DISORDERS THAT PRESENT IN THE NEONATE

This section will briefly review the most common types of persistent hypoglycemia disorders that can present in the newborn period: genetic and syndromic forms of congenital hyperinsulinism and congenital pituitary deficiency. It is extremely important to identify patients with these hypoglycemia disorders prior to discharge home from the nursery, since they are at very high risk of seizures and brain injury, especially if diagnosis and treatment are delayed.[2] Transitional neonatal hypoglycemia can interfere with recognition of these disorders during the first 1 to 2 days after birth. However, after the third day after birth, plasma glucose concentrations and insulin secretion in normal newborns should be similar to the normal range for older children and evaluation and treatment should be considered for any neonate with recurrent hypoglycemia that persists beyond 3 days of age.[56]

GENETIC FORMS OF CONGENITAL HYPERINSULINISM

The incidence of the severe form of congenital hyperinsulinism ranges from an estimated 1 in 40,000 births in Europe to 1 in 2500 in Saudi Arabia;[57,58] if the milder forms of hyperinsulinism are included, the total incidence may be as high in 1 in 10,000 to 1 in 20,000 births. Congenital persistent hyperinsulinism is both clinically and genetically heterogeneous. The clinical manifestations range from extremely severe, life-threatening disease immediately after birth to very mild clinical symptoms, which may sometimes be difficult to identify until several weeks or months of age. Furthermore, responsiveness to medical and surgical management is variable and may be genotype-specific.[59]

As shown in Fig. 152.7, 16 different genetic loci have been associated with congenital hyperinsulinism and more are likely to be discovered. These occur in the major pathways for triggering insulin secretion by the major nutrients, glucose and amino acids. Some of these defects are recessive, but some are dominant and frequently appear to be sporadic rather than familial. The most frequent causes of congenital hyperinsulinism are loss of function mutations in either of the two subunits of the β cell adenosine triphosphate (ATP)-sensitive potassium channel (K_{ATP}), consisting of sulfonylurea receptor (SUR1) encoded by ABCC8 and inward-rectifying potassium channel (Kir 6.2) encoded by KCNJ11.[60] The second most common defect associated with hyperinsulinism is a dominant gain of function mutations of glutamate dehydrogenase (GDH, encoded by GLUD1), which cause a diazoxide responsive protein-sensitive form of hyperinsulinism associated with persistent mild hyperammonemia (HI-HA syndrome). The third most common

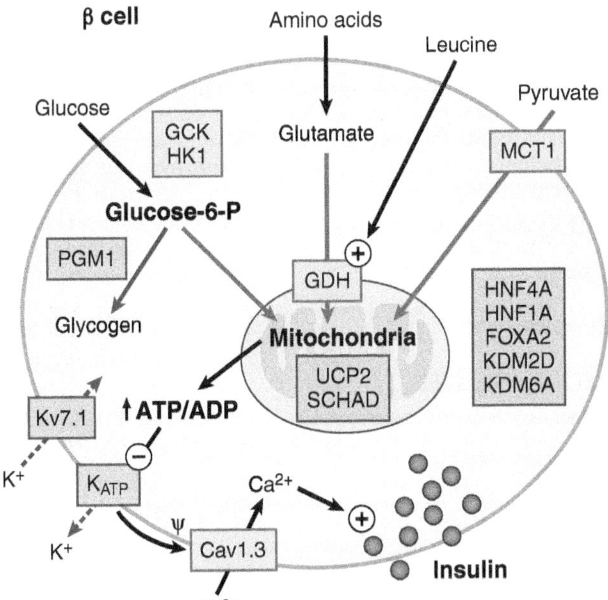

Gene	Protein	
ABCC8 *KCNJ11*	K_{ATP}	ATP-sensitive potassium channel
GLUD1	GDH	Glutamate dehydrogenase
GCK	GCK	Glucokinase
HNF4A *HNF1A*	HNF4A HNF1A	Hepatocyte nuclear factor 4a Hepatocyte nuclear factor 1a
KDM2D *KDM6A*	KDM2D KDM6A	Histone-lysine N-methyltransferase 2d Histone-lysine N-methyltransferase 6a
HADH	SCHAD	Short-chain3-hydroxyacyl-CoA dehydrogenase
PGM1	PGM1	Phosphoglucomutase 1
HK1	HK1	Hexokinase 1
SLC16A1	MCT1	Monocarboxylic transporter 1
UCP2	UCP2	Uncoupling protein 2
CACNA1D	Cav1.3	Voltage-dependent calcium channel
KCNQ1	Kv7.1	Voltage-gated potassium channel
FOXA2	FOXA2	Forkhead box A2

Fig. 152.7 Fuel-mediated insulin secretion by the pancreatic β cell. Glucose stimulates insulin secretion through its oxidation, which increases levels of intracellular adenosine triphosphate *(ATP)*, which in turn inhibits potassium efflux through the K_{ATP} potassium channel. Closure of the K_{ATP} channel depolarizes the plasma membrane, which activates voltage-gated calcium channels to increase cytosolic calcium and trigger exocytosis of insulin granules. Mutations in proteins associated with congenital hyperinsulinism are shown in boxes. Mutations that lead to functional activation are depicted in *green* and mutations that lead to functional inactivation are depicted in *red*.

genetic form of congenital hyperinsulinism is caused by dominant gain of function mutations of glucokinase (encoded by GCK) and is often not responsive to diazoxide. The remaining genetic loci shown in Fig. 152.7 are much rarer, and each account for only 1% to 2% of the total number of hyperinsulinism cases.[61-64] In as many as 50% of the cases of congenital hyperinsulinism, no genetic defect has (yet) been demonstrated.[65]

In addition to the congenital forms of hyperinsulinism associated with genetic defects in the pathways of insulin secretion shown in Fig. 152.7, which have manifestations largely limited to pancreatic islets, several syndromes associated with hyperinsulinism and other systemic features may present in newborn infants. These include infants with Beckwith-Wiedemann syndrome, which is associated with large for gestational age birth weight, hemihypertrophy, organomegaly, large tongue, umbilical hernia, and ear lobe creases. Approximately half of infants with Beckwith-Wiedemann syndrome have hyperinsulinemic hypoglycemia of varying severity and duration after birth. While some may be responsive to diazoxide, some (particularly those with mosaic isodisomy for the paternally derived 11p region[66]) may have very severe hyperinsulinism that does not respond to diazoxide and may persist for several years. Other syndromes associated with hyperinsulinism include the Kabuki-makeup syndrome, Turner syndrome, and certain of the congenital disorders of glycosylation.

The mainstay of medical therapy for congenital hyperinsulinism is diazoxide, which activates the K_{ATP} channel to suppress insulin release by binding to the SUR1 subunit (see Fig. 152.7). In most patients with hyperinsulinism due to mutations in either of the two subunits of the K_{ATP} channel, diazoxide has no effect, and many may require near-total pancreatectomy to control hypoglycemia. Of special importance, however, about half of the K_{ATP} channel cases of diazoxide-unresponsive hyperinsulinism can have a surgically curable focal form of hyperinsulinism. These focal lesions of islet adenomatosis are caused by a loss of the maternal chromosome 11p region in combination with isodisomy for a paternally transmitted recessive K_{ATP} mutation. Fluid retention is commonly seen with diazoxide use, and diuretics are often prescribed prophylactically in infants at the time of starting treatment, especially in patients requiring high rates of intravenous dextrose fluids. Other reported complications of diazoxide use include pulmonary hypertension in 2.4%, neutropenia in 15.6%, thrombocytopenia in 4.7%, and hyperuricemia in 5%.[67] Hypertrichosis is common in infants treated with diazoxide,[68] and parents should be counseled regarding this likely side effect. All of these side effects of diazoxide are part of the Cantu syndrome, which is caused by activating mutations of SUR2.[69] This suggests that the side effects of diazoxide represent off-target actions on the alternative SUR2 subunit in various peripheral tissues.

CONGENITAL HYPOPITUITARISM

The clinical presentation of neonates with panhypopituitarism can include features of severe hypoglycemia, which are identical to those seen in congenital hyperinsulinism. These include a high glucose requirement to maintain euglycemia, inappropriate hypoketonemia, and a positive glycemic response to glucagon at the time of hypoglycemia. Plasma insulin concentrations may be elevated or normal. The hyperinsulinism may represent a form of perinatal stress-induced hyperinsulinism peculiar to the newborn period, since hypoglycemia seen with pituitary deficiency in older infants and children is associated with hyperketonemia (see Fig. 152.3). Usually the pituitary deficiency associated with neonatal hypoglycemia involves multiple deficiencies of cortisol and growth hormone, with or without concomitant secondary hypothyroidism. The hyperinsulinemic hypoglycemia of neonatal panhypopituitarism responds poorly to treatment with diazoxide but is readily controlled with treatment that replaces all of the deficient hormones (including thyroxine, in addition to cortisol and growth hormone). Physical features, such as micropenis or midline facial malformations (such as cleft palate or microphthalmia), should suggest the possibility of pituitary deficiency as the cause of neonatal hypoglycemia, but some patients may lack abnormal physical features.[70] Neonatal hypopituitarism sometimes is associated with cholestatic jaundice, which often does not improve until hormone deficiencies are corrected.[71]

As emphasized above, low cortisol or growth hormone levels during hypoglycemia are not sufficient for diagnosis of deficiency of these hormones.[18,19] Specific stimulation testing of these hormones is recommended if there is clinical suspicion. In regions where only thyroid stimulating hormone and not thyroxine concentrations are measured, central hypothyroidism may not be detected on the newborn screen.

CONCLUSION

Prompt recognition and treatment of hypoglycemia disorders in neonates is essential to prevent the possibility of seizures and permanent brain injury. This is complicated by the need to consider three broad categories of hypoglycemia immediately after birth. First is transitional neonatal hypoglycemia, which is common to all normal newborns and reflects persistence of the fetal pattern of insulin regulation; the hypoglycemia is usually mild and fully resolves within 2 to 3 days after birth. Second is perinatal stress-induced hypoglycemia, which is a more severe and more prolonged period of hyperinsulinemic hypoglycemia commonly associated with perinatal stresses such as intrauterine growth restriction, birth asphyxia, maternal preeclampsia, etc.; this disorder may reflect an exaggeration of normal transitional neonatal hyperinsulinism, but some cases can cause seizures and brain damage, and many require treatment for weeks to months after birth. The third category includes the congenital or genetic disorders of hypoglycemia that will require life-long treatment, and in which maintaining normoglycemia may be very difficult. Although these disorders are uncommon, genetic and syndromic forms of congenital hyperinsulinism and congenital hypopituitarism are the most urgent to recognize before discharge from the nursery, since the risk of permanent hypoglycemic brain damage is high. During the first 2 days after birth, it is often difficult to determine in which category an infant belongs: transitional; perinatal stress hyperinsulinism; or persistent hypoglycemia. However, a definitive determination of transient or persistent hypoglycemia usually becomes feasible by 3 to 4 days of age and should be made prior to discharge from the nursery.

A complete reference list is available at www.ExpertConsult.com. 

SELECT REFERENCES

1. Meissner T, Wendel U, Burgard P, Schaetzle S, Mayatepek E. Long-term follow-up of 114 patients with congenital hyperinsulinism. *Eur J Endocrinol.* 2003;149(1):43–51.
2. Menni F, de Lonlay P, Sevin C, et al. Neurologic outcomes of 90 neonates and infants with persistent hyperinsulinemic hypoglycemia. *Pediatrics.* 2001;107(3):476–479.
3. Steinkrauss L, Lipman TH, Hendell CD, Gerdes M, Thornton PS, Stanley CA. Effects of hypoglycemia on developmental outcome in children with congenital hyperinsulinism. *J Pediatr Nurs.* 2005;20(2):109–118.
4. Bozzetti P, Ferrari MM, Marconi AM, et al. The relationship of maternal and fetal glucose concentrations in the human from midgestation until term. *Metabolism.* 1988;37(4):358–363.
5. Cornblath M, Reisner SH. Blood glucose in the neonate and its clinical significance. *N Engl J Med.* 1965;273(7):378–381.
6. Hoseth E, Joergensen A, Ebbesen F, Moeller M. Blood glucose levels in a population of healthy, breast fed, term infants of appropriate size for gestational age. *Arch Dis Child Fetal Neonatal Ed.* 2000;83(2):F117–F119.

7. Srinivasan G, Pildes RS, Cattamanchi G, Voora S, Lilien LD. Plasma glucose values in normal neonates: a new look. *J Pediatr*. 1986;109(1):114-117.
8. Harris D, Weston P, Harding J. Glucose profiles in healthy term babies in the first five days: the glucose in well babies (GLOW) study. *J Paediatr Child Health*. 2019;55(S1):23-23.
9. Schwartz NS, Clutter WE, Shah SD, Cryer PE. Glycemic thresholds for activation of glucose counterregulatory systems are higher than the threshold for symptoms. *J Clin Invest*. 1987;79(3):777-781.
12. Heller SR, Cryer PE. Reduced neuroendocrine and symptomatic responses to subsequent hypoglycemia after 1 episode of hypoglycemia in nondiabetic humans. *Diabetes*. 1991;40(2):223-226.
13. Chaussain JL. Glycemic response to 24 hour fast in normal children and children with ketotic hypoglycemia. *J Pediatr*. 1973;82(3):438-443.
14. Chaussain JL, Georges P, Calzada L, Job JC. Glycemic response to 24-hour fast in normal children: III. Influence of age. *J Pediatr*. 1977;91(5):711-714.
15. Chaussain JL, Georges P, Olive G, Job JC. Glycemic response to 24-hour fast in normal children and children with ketotic hypoglycemia: II. Hormonal and metabolic changes. *J Pediatr*. 1974;85(6):776-781.
16. van Veen MR, van Hasselt PM, de Sain, van der Velden MG, et al. Metabolic profiles in children during fasting. *Pediatrics*. 2011;127(4):e1021-e1027.
17. Finegold DN, Stanley CA, Baker L. Glycemic response to glucagon during fasting hypoglycemia: an aid in the diagnosis of hyperinsulinism. *J Pediatr*. 1980;96(2):257-259.
18. Kelly A, Tang R, Becker S, Stanley CA. Poor specificity of low growth hormone and cortisol levels during fasting hypoglycemia for the diagnoses of growth hormone deficiency and adrenal insufficiency. *Pediatrics*. 2008;122(3):e522-e528.
19. Hawkes CP, Grimberg A, Dzata VE, De Leon DD. Adding glucagon-stimulated GH testing to the diagnostic fast increases the detection of GH-sufficient children. *Horm Res Paediatr*. 2016;85(4):265-272.
22. Desmond MM. Observations related to neonatal hypoglycemia. *J Pediatr*. 1953;43(3):253-262.
23. Lubchenco LO, Bard H. Incidence of hypoglycemia in newborn infants classified by birth weight and gestational age. *Pediatrics*. 1971;47(5):831-838.
24. Stanley CA, Anday EK, Baker L, Delivoria-Papadopolous M. Metabolic fuel and hormone responses to fasting in newborn infants. *Pediatrics*. 1979;64(5):613-619.
25. Stanley CA, Rozance PJ, Thornton PS, et al. Re-evaluating "transitional neonatal hypoglycemia": mechanism and implications for management. *J Pediatr*. 2015;166(6):1520-1525.e1521.
26. Thornton PS, Stanley CA, De Leon DD, et al. Recommendations from the Pediatric Endocrine Society for evaluation and management of persistent hypoglycemia in neonates, infants, and children. *J Pediatr*. 2015;167(2):238-245.
27. Desmond MM, Hild JR, Gast JH. The glycemic response of the newborn infant to epinephrine administration: a preliminary report. *J Pediatr*. 1950;37(3):341-350.
28. Diwakar KK, Sasidhar MV. Plasma glucose levels in term infants who are appropriate size for gestation and exclusively breast fed. *Arch Dis Child Fetal Neonatal Ed*. 2002;87(1):F46-F48.
30. Thumelin S, Forestier M, Girard J, Pegorier JP. Developmental changes in mitochondrial 3-hydroxy-3-methylglutaryl-CoA synthase gene expression in rat liver, intestine and kidney. *Biochem J*. 1993;292(Pt 2):493-496.
32. Hawdon JM, Ward Platt MP, Aynsley-Green A. Patterns of metabolic adaptation for preterm and term infants in the first neonatal week. *Arch Dis Child*. 1992;67(4 Spec No):357-365.
33. Haymond MW, Karl IE, Pagliara AS. Increased gluconeogenic substrates in the small-for-gestational-age infant. *N Engl J Med*. 1974;291(7):322-328.
35. Anday EK, Stanley CA, Baker L, Delivoria, Papadopoulos M. Plasma ketones in newborn infants: absence of suckling ketosis. *J Pediatr*. 1981;98(4):628-630.
36. Ferrara C, Patel P, Becker S, Stanley CA, Kelly A. Biomarkers of insulin for the diagnosis of hyperinsulinemic hypoglycemia in infants and children. *J Pediatr*. 2016;168:212-219.
37. Hawdon JM, Aynsley-Green A, Ward Platt MP. Neonatal blood glucose concentrations: metabolic effects of intravenous glucagon and intragastric medium chain triglyceride. *Arch Dis Child*. 1993;68(3 Spec No):255-261.
40. Jackson L, Burchell A, McGeechan A, Hume R. An inadequate glycaemic response to glucagon is linked to insulin resistance in preterm infants? *Arch Dis Child Fetal Neonatal Ed*. 2003;88(1):F62-F66.
41. Hawdon JM, Aynsley-Green A, Alberti KG, Ward Platt MP. The role of pancreatic insulin secretion in neonatal glucoregulation. I. Healthy term and preterm infants. *Arch Dis Child*. 1993;68(3 Spec No):274-279.
42. Stanley CA, Baker L. Hyperinsulinism in infancy: diagnosis by demonstration of abnormal response to fasting hypoglycemia. *Pediatrics*. 1976;57(5):702-711.
44. Stanley CA, Baker L. Hyperinsulinism in infants and children: diagnosis and therapy. *Adv Pediatr*. 1976;23:315-355.
50. Hoe FM, Thornton PS, Wanner LA, Steinkrauss L, Simmons RA, Stanley CA. Clinical features and insulin regulation in infants with a syndrome of prolonged neonatal hyperinsulinism. *J Pediatr*. 2006;148(2):207-212.
56. Harris D, Weston P, Harding J. Glucose profiles in healthy term babies in the first five days: the glucose in well babies (GLOW) study. *J Paediatr Child Health*. 2019;55(S1):23-23.
59. Stanley CA. Hyperinsulinism in infants and children. *Pediatr Clin North Am*. 1997;44(2):363-374.
63. Hussain K, Clayton PT, Krywawych S, et al. Hyperinsulinism of infancy associated with a novel splice site mutation in the SCHAD gene. *J Pediatr*. 2005;146(5):706-708.
66. Kalish JM, Boodhansingh KE, Bhatti TR, et al. Congenital hyperinsulinism in children with paternal 11p uniparental isodisomy and Beckwith-Wiedemann syndrome. *J Med Genet*. 2016;53(1):53-61.
67. Herrera A, Vajravelu ME, Givler S, et al. Prevalence of adverse events in children with congenital hyperinsulinism treated with diazoxide. *J Clin Endocrinol Metab*. 2018;103(12):4365-4372.
68. Baker L, Kaye R, Root AW, Prasad ALN. Diazoxide treatment of idiopathic hypoglycemia of infancy. *J Pediatr*. 1967;71(4):494-505.

Pathophysiology of Cardiomyopathies 153

Hugo R. Martinez | Thomas D. Ryan | Jeffrey A. Towbin

INTRODUCTION

Cardiomyopathies constitute a group of heterogenous disorders in which the muscle of the heart (myocardium) remodels and becomes structurally and functionally abnormal. This pathophysiology can potentially lead to progressive systolic and/or diastolic heart failure, thus representing a cause of morbidity and mortality during the neonatal period.[1,2] Cardiomyopathies are frequently caused by pathogenic gene variants, in addition to other triggers such as the presence of anatomic anomalies, dysrhythmias, infectious and environmental exposures, and underlying systemic disorders (metabolic, neuromuscular, mitochondrial).[1-3] Unfortunately, not all neonates present with obvious signs and symptoms of heart failure, making the diagnosis more challenging when compared with patients at other pediatric ages.[4] In 2006, a classification scheme included five types of cardiomyopathy: dilated cardiomyopathy (DCM), hypertrophic cardiomyopathy (HCM), restrictive cardiomyopathy (RCM), arrhythmogenic cardiomyopathy (ACM), and noncompaction cardiomyopathy (NCM); which can be further classified into genetic/inherited and acquired/noninherited diseases.[2,3,5] An estimated incidence of cardiomyopathy in children has been reported by the Pediatric Cardiomyopathy Registry as 1.13 per 100,000.[6] However, the overall incidence of cardiomyopathy in the neonatal period has not been completely elucidated, mainly because of the high incidence of unknown diagnoses in sudden unexpected infant deaths and the lack of recognition of this disease before death.[7] This chapter provides information regarding the molecular structure of the cardiomyocytes and describes the pathophysiology of the most common types of neonatal cardiomyopathies (DCM, HCM, RCM, NCM). ACM is a group

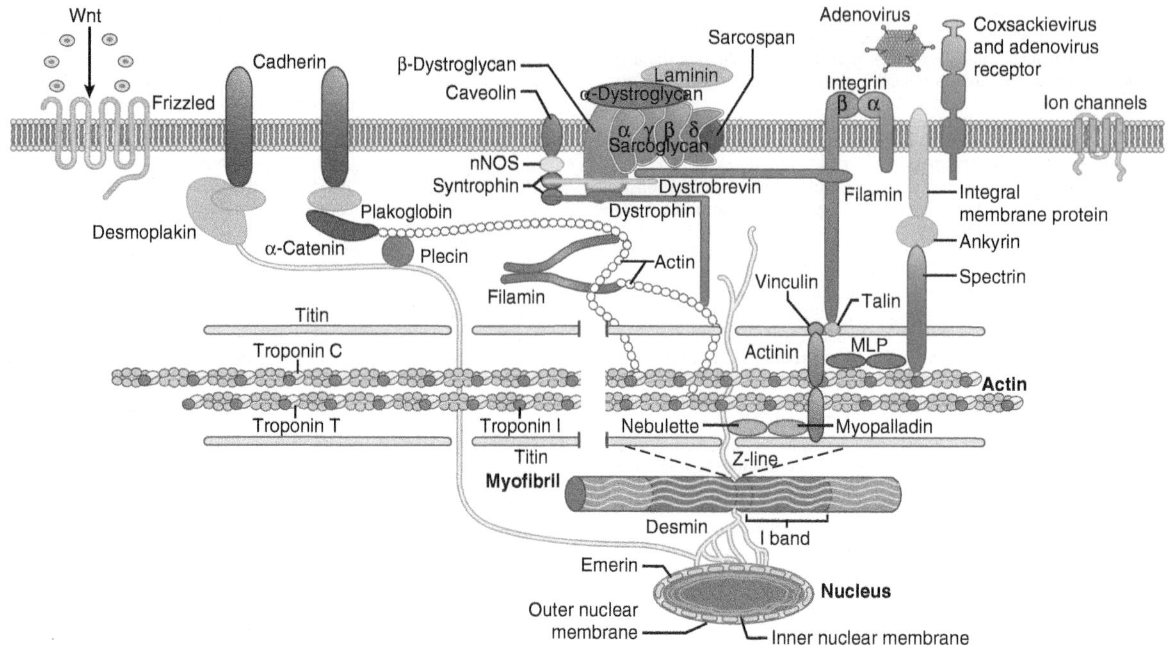

Fig. 153.1 Cardiac myocyte cytoarchitecture. The interactions between dystrophin and the dystrophin-associated proteins in the sarcolemma and intracellular cytoplasm (dystroglycans, sarcoglycans, syntrophins, dystrobrevin, sarcospan) at the carboxy-terminal end of dystrophin. The integral membrane proteins interact with the extracellular matrix via α-dystroglycan–α_2-laminin connections. The amino terminus of dystrophin binds actin and connects dystrophin with the sarcomere intracellularly, the sarcolemma, and the extracellular matrix. Additional sarcolemmal proteins include ion channels, adrenergic receptors, integrins, and the Coxsackie virus and adenovirus receptor. Cell-cell junctions, including cadherins, the plakin, and other desmosomal family proteins, are also notable. Also shown is the interaction between intermediate filament proteins (i.e., desmin) with the nucleus. *MLP*, Muscle LIM protein; *nNOS*, neuronal nitric oxide synthase; *Wnt*, wingless-related integration 1 site.

of cardiomyopathies associated with early-onset arrhythmias (ventricular tachycardia or fibrillation, atrioventricular block, etc.) and can affect the right ventricle, the left ventricle, or have biventricular disease. Right ventricular ACM is almost always identified in late adolescence or in young adults and is rarely described before 10 years of age; thus, it will not be addressed in detail in this chapter.[5] Additionally, transient conditions that mimic cardiomyopathy, such as diabetic cardiomyopathy, will not be covered.

NORMAL CARDIAC STRUCTURE

Cardiac muscle fibers are composed of separate cellular units or myocytes connected in series.[8] In contrast to skeletal muscle fibers, cardiac fibers do not assemble in parallel arrays but bifurcate and recombine to form a complex three-dimensional network. Cardiac myocytes are joined at each end to adjacent myocytes at the intercalated disk, the specialized area of interdigitating cell membrane (Fig. 153.1). The intercalated disk contains gap junctions (containing connexins) and mechanical junctions, composed of adherens junctions (consisting of N-cadherin, catenins, and vinculin) and desmosomes (containing desmin, desmoplakin, desmocollin, desmoglein, and junctional plakoglobin). Cardiac myocytes are surrounded by a thin membrane (sarcolemma), and the interior of each myocyte contains bundles of longitudinally arranged myofibrils. The myofibrils are formed by repeating sarcomeres, the basic contractile units of cardiac muscle composed of interdigitating thin (actin) and thick (myosin) filaments (see Fig. 153.1), which give the muscle its characteristic striated appearance.[9,10] The thick filaments are composed primarily of myosin but additionally contain myosin-binding proteins C, H, and X. The thin filaments are composed of cardiac actin, α-tropomyosin, and troponins T, I, and C. In addition, myofibrils contain a third filament formed by the giant filamentous protein titin, which extends from the Z disk to the M line and acts as a molecular template for the layout of the sarcomere. The Z disk at the borders of the sarcomere is formed by a lattice of interdigitating proteins that maintain myofilament organization by crosslinking antiparallel titin and thin filaments from adjacent sarcomeres (Fig. 153.2). Other proteins in the Z disk include α-actinin, nebulette, telethonin, muscle LIM protein (MLP; encoded by *CSRP3*, and also known as *cysteine- and glycine-rich protein 3*), myopalladin, myotilin, cardiac ankyrin repeat protein (CARP; encoded by *ANKRD1*, and also known as *ankyrin repeat domain 1*), cypher (encoded by *LDB3* and also known as *LIM domain-binding 3* and *ZASP*), filamin, nexilin, and filamin, actinin, and *FATZ*.[8,10,11]

Finally, the extra-sarcomeric cytoskeleton, a complex network of proteins linking the sarcomere with the sarcolemma and the extracellular matrix, provides structural support for subcellular structures and transmits mechanical and chemical signals within and between cells. The extra-sarcomeric cytoskeleton has intermyofibrillar and subsarcolemmal components, with the intermyofibrillar cytoskeleton composed of intermediate filaments, microfilaments, and microtubules.[12-14] Desmin intermediate filaments form a three-dimensional scaffold throughout the extra-sarcomeric cytoskeleton with desmin filaments surrounding the Z disk, allowing longitudinal connections to adjacent Z disks and lateral connections to subsarcolemmal costameres.[11,13] Microfilaments composed of nonsarcomeric actin (mainly γ-actin) also form complex networks linking the sarcomere (via α-actinin) to various components of the costameres. Costameres are subsarcolemmal domains located in a periodic, grid-like pattern, flanking the Z disks and overlying the I band, along the cytoplasmic side of the sarcolemma. These costameres are sites of interconnection between various cytoskeletal networks linking the sarcomere and the sarcolemma and are thought to function as anchor sites for stabilization of the sarcolemma and for integration

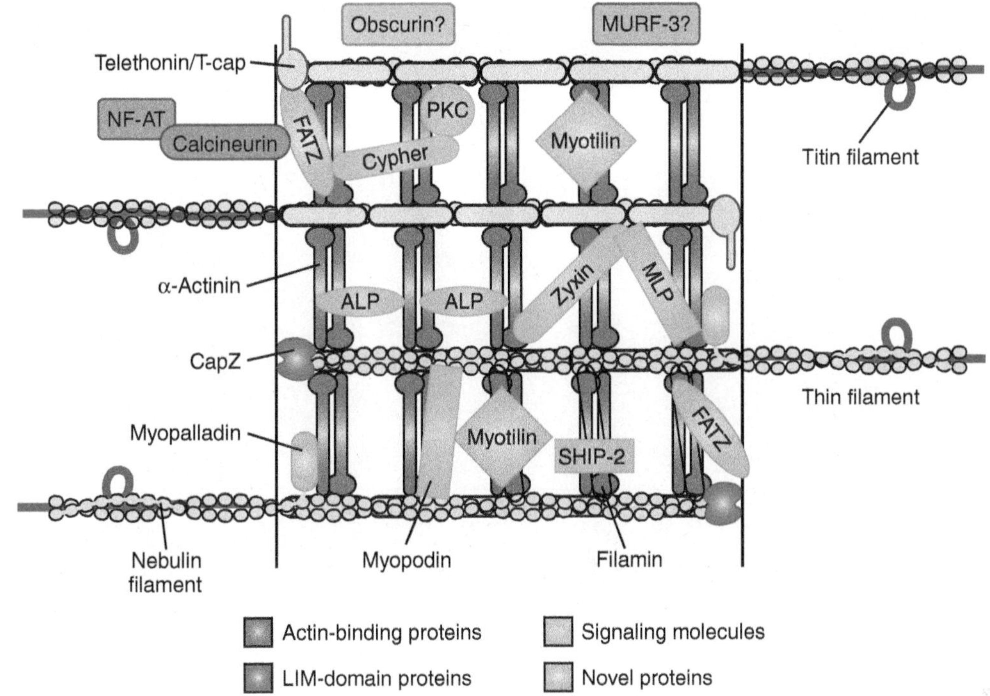

Fig. 153.2 Z-disk architecture. The Z disk of the sarcomere is composed of multiple interacting proteins that anchor the sarcomere. *MLP*, Muscle LIM protein. (From Clark KA, McElhinny AS, Beckerle MC, et al. Striated muscle cytoarchitecture: an intricate web of form and function. *Annu Rev Dev Biol.* 2002;18:637–706.)

of pathways involved in mechanical force transduction. Costameres contain three principal components: the focal adhesion-type complex, the spectrin-based complex, and the dystrophin-associated protein complex.[15,16] The focal adhesion-type complex, composed of cytoplasmic proteins (i.e., vinculin, talin, tensin, paxillin, and zyxin), connects with cytoskeletal actin filaments and with the transmembrane proteins α-dystroglycan, β-dystroglycan, α-sarcoglycan, β-sarcoglycan, γ-sarcoglycan, δ-sarcoglycan, dystrobrevin, and syntrophin. Several actin-associated proteins are located at sites of attachment of cytoskeletal actin filaments. The carboxyl terminus of dystrophin binds β-dystroglycan (see Fig. 153.1), which in turn interacts with α-dystroglycan to link to the extracellular matrix (via α_2-laminin).[8,14,16,17] The amino terminus of dystrophin interacts with actin. Also notable, voltage-gated sodium channels colocalize with dystrophin, β-spectrin, ankyrin, and syntrophins, and potassium channels interact with the sarcomeric Z disk and intercalated disks.[8,14,18] Because arrhythmias and conduction system diseases are common in children and adults with DCM, it is likely that functional disturbance of these ion channels could play an important role in the development of the arrhythmia phenotype commonly associated with DCM. Hence, disruption of the links from the sarcolemma to the extracellular matrix at the dystrophin carboxyl terminus and those to the sarcomere and nucleus via amino-terminal dystrophin interactions could lead to a domino effect disruption of systolic function and the development of arrhythmias.[19]

DILATED CARDIOMYOPATHY

CLINICAL FEATURES OF DILATED CARDIOMYOPATHY

DCM is characterized by LV dilation, relatively decreased LV wall thickness, and systolic dysfunction in the absence of either pressure or volume overload or coronary artery disease sufficient to explain the dysfunction (Fig. 153.3). Arrhythmias, biventricular dilation, and/or diastolic dysfunction may also be appreciated.[20] DCM is the most common form of CM, and it may be secondary to genetic, infectious, metabolic, systemic, and/or toxic etiologies.[21-23] In children, the annual incidence of DCM is 0.57 cases per 100,000 but is higher in boys than in girls, higher in blacks than in whites, and higher in infants (younger than 1 year) than in older children.[23] Most children (66%) are thought to have idiopathic disease.[23] Although such rigorous data are not available in adult populations, it is believed that the incidence is much higher than that seen in children, possibly being as high as 1 in 250 individuals.[21,23] There is also an important distinction in adults not generally applicable in children: ischemic versus nonischemic DCM.

Presentation of symptomatic DCM in the neonatal and pediatric patient usually involves irritability, difficulty feeding, and poor weight gain. Physical examination findings may include tachycardia, gallop rhythm, jugular venous distension, hepatomegaly, and a murmur consistent with mitral valve regurgitation. Testing can reveal cardiomegaly and pulmonary edema on chest x-ray; sinus tachycardia, conduction system disease, ST-segment changes, and atrial or ventricular arrhythmias on electrocardiography; and a dilated, poorly functioning left ventricle on echocardiography, with or without mitral regurgitation or pericardial effusion.[21,23] Elevation of serum biomarkers of heart failure (troponins, soluble-ST2, BNP, and NT-ProBNP) also can be considered in the diagnosis, prognosis, and management.[24] Patients with DCM, or any cardiomyopathy, can be further stratified by their degree of heart failure. Adult classification schemes, such as the scheme from the NYHA, are often inappropriate or useless in pediatric patients, particularly neonates. Because of this, the modified Ross classification of heart failure was developed for pediatric patients (Table 153.1).[25] Further, use of the ACC/AHA staging of heart failure is also generally applicable in pediatric cardiology (Table 153.2).[26]

The overall mortality rate in the United States resulting from cardiomyopathy is greater than 10,000 deaths per annum, with DCM being the major contributor.[26] DCM has among the highest death rates for any pediatric heart disease. Fortunately, survival appears to be improving, and since the 1990s the 1- and 5-year survival rates for all individuals with DCM have been 90% and

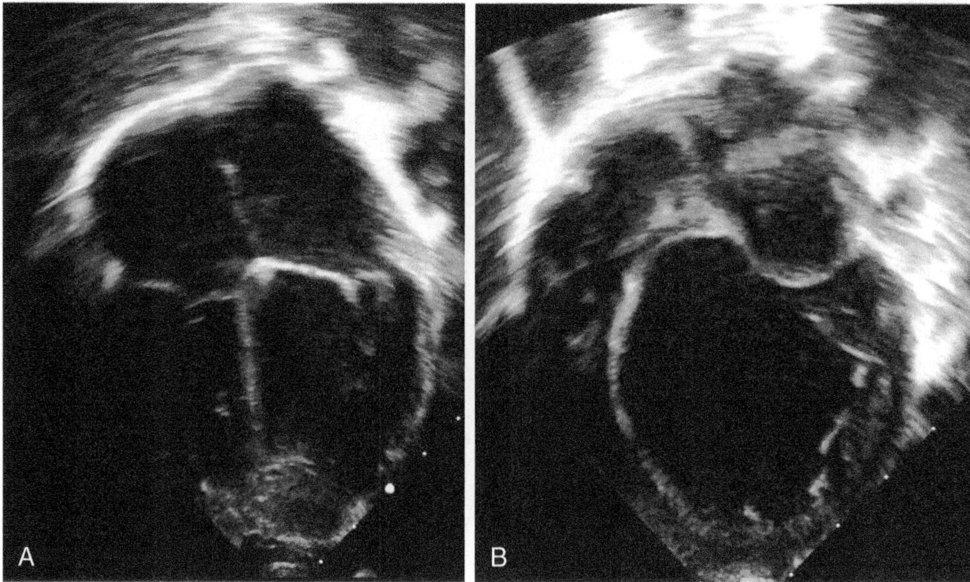

Fig. 153.3 Echocardiographic features of dilated cardiomyopathy. From a classic apical four-chamber view, 2-D echocardiography shows on the left (A), a normal triangular-shaped left ventricular chamber. On the right (B), echocardiography displays an enlarged and globular-shaped left ventricle with relative wall thinning to the chamber diameter, making the diagnosis of dilated cardiomyopathy.

Table 153.1 Modified Ross Scoring System for Heart Failure in Infants.

Scoring	0	1	2
Feeding History			
Volume consumed (oz)	>3.5	2.5–3.5	<2.5
Time taken per feeding (min)	<40	>40	–
Physical Examination			
Respiratory rate per minute	<50	50–60	>60
Heart rate per minute	<160	160–170	>170
Respiratory pattern	Normal	Abnormal	–
Peripheral perfusion	Normal	Decreased	–
S3 or diastolic rumble	Absent	Present	–
Liver edge from costal margin (cm)	<2	2–3	>3

Adapted from Ross RD. The Ross classification for heart failure in children after 25 years: a review and an age-stratified revision. *Pediatr Cardiol*. 2012;33:1295–1300.[25]

83%, respectively.[21,23,24] In a study of 1803 children with DCM by the Pediatric Cardiomyopathy Registry Investigators, the 5-year incidence rates were 29% for heart transplantation, 2.4% for SCD, and 12.1% for non-SCD.[27]

CAUSES OF DILATED CARDIOMYOPATHY

The clinical appearance of DCM, a dilated left ventricle with poor contractile performance, has various causes. Acquired forms of disease include myocarditis; intrauterine disorders such as placental insufficiency and nonimmune hydrops, postpartum cardiomyopathy, dysfunction in the setting of systemic disease such as renal or hepatic failure, toxic exposures, neonatal myocarditis, and acute stress such as hypoxia. These disorders are not the focus of this chapter. Alternatively, DCM can develop because of genetic-based disease, either familial or nonfamilial. These genetic disorders include inherited forms of disease, cardioskeletal disease such as muscular dystrophies, and metabolic forms of disease.[21,24,27]

CLINICAL GENETICS OF DILATED CARDIOMYOPATHY

DCM was initially believed to be an inherited disorder in a small percentage of cases, but it has been estimated that between 20% and 40% patients with idiopathic DCM have a positive family history, suggesting primary genetic etiologies, with autosomal dominant inheritance being the predominant pattern of transmission; X-linked, autosomal recessive, and mitochondrial (maternal) patterns of inheritance are less commonly encountered.[28,29]

MOLECULAR GENETICS OF DILATED CARDIOMYOPATHY

DCM has become a popular target of research during the past few decades, with numerous genes being identified (Table 153.3). Studies have demonstrated that there is a significant amount of overlap in the genes identified as important for all types of cardiomyopathy.[24] The advent of next-generation sequencing technologies expedited gene screening studies and brought fresh perspectives on DCM genetics. Commercially available gene testing for cardiomyopathy includes tests for more than 75 genes, with the option to analyze a nearly unlimited number of genes by means of current next-generation sequencing approaches. The genes important in DCM appear to encode two major subgroups: cytoskeletal and sarcomeric proteins. Additionally, ion channels, mitochondrial proteins, desmosomal proteins, nuclear envelope proteins, and an assortment of other protein-encoding genes also have been found associated with DCM.[2,30] Despite this wide genetic variation, the individuals with DCM and HCM in whom a genetic cause is identified have mutations in the genes encoding myosin-binding protein C, β-myosin heavy chain, cardiac troponin I, cardiac troponin T, and α-tropomyosin in more than 95% of cases.[2,30] Gene discovery efforts will continue to elucidate additional pathogenic gene variants and comprehensive assessment of transcription factors, noncoding sequencing tracks, gene copy number variants, and other key factors involved in heritable myocardial disease and epigenetics. Currently, in most cases of DCM the cause cannot be determined by genetic testing, with a diagnostic rate of approximately 40%.[31,32]

Table 153.2 American College of Cardiology/American Heart Association Staging System of Heart Failure.

At Risk for Heart Failure		Heart Failure	
Stage A	**Stage B**	**Stage C**	**Stage D**
At high risk for HF but without structural heart disease or symptoms of HF	Structural heart disease but without signs or symptoms of HF	Structural heart disease with prior or current symptoms of HF	Refractory HF

HF, Heart failure.

Adapted from Jessup M, Abraham WT, Casey DE, et al. 2009 focused update: ACCF/AHA Guidelines for the Diagnosis and Management of Heart Failure in Adults: a report of the American College of Cardiology Foundation/American Heart Association Task Force on Practice Guidelines: developed in collaboration with the International Society for Heart and Lung Transplantation. *Circulation*. 2009;119:1977–2016.[26]

Acquired forms of DCM can encompass the same clinical features as genetically determined disease, including symptomatic heart failure, arrhythmias, and conduction block.[32,33] The most common causes of myocarditis are viral, including the enteroviruses (Coxsackie virus and echovirus), adenoviruses, parvovirus B19, and Epstein-Barr virus, among other cardiotropic viruses.[23,27]

Initial progress in the understanding of familial forms of DCM came from study of families with X-linked forms of the disease, XLCM, which presents in adolescence and young adults. Barth syndrome is most frequently identified in infancy, while Danon disease typically presents with HCM with later onset of DCM, although this presentation can be variable.[22,23]

BARTH SYNDROME

Barth syndrome is a rare, X-linked mitochondrial disease. Mutations in the tafazzin gene on chromosome Xq28 lead to a loss of function in the tafazzin protein responsible for cardiolipin maturation. The defect in cardiolipin maturation/metabolism has been shown to impact the integrity and functions of the mitochondria.[34] Barth syndrome typically presents in male infants as heart failure associated with cyclic neutropenia and 3-methylglutaconic aciduria.[35] The most widely recognized features of this mitochondrial disease are cardiomyopathy, skeletal myopathy, neutropenia, fatigue (especially exertional fatigue), and growth delay.[34,35] In fact, analysis of the Barth Syndrome Registry reveals a history of cardiomyopathy in 69 of 73 individuals.[35] Echocardiographically, infants with Barth syndrome typically have LV dysfunction with LV dilation and hypertrabeculation, with or without endocardial fibroelastosis.[34] A HCM may also be seen. In some cases, the cardiomyopathy affecting these patients exhibits an "undulating cardiac phenotype" with a mixed dilated and hypertrophic left ventricle.[34,36] Some neonates succumb because of heart failure/sudden death, ventricular tachycardia/ventricular fibrillation, or sepsis caused by leukocyte dysfunction.[37] In some cases, cardiac transplantation has been performed.[36] Although rare, Barth syndrome should be considered in young males presenting with cardiomyopathy.

DANON DISEASE

Another form of X-linked disease associated with DCM is Danon disease, which is discussed in the section entitled "Hypertrophic Cardiomyopathy Associated With Infiltrative and Systemic Diseases."

AUTOSOMAL DOMINANT DILATED CARDIOMYOPATHY

The most common form of inherited DCM is the autosomal dominant form.[23,29] Patients typically present with classic "pure" DCM or DCM associated with ECSD, such as tachyarrhythmias and atrioventricular blocks.[22,23,27] DCM usually presents late in the course, but is out of proportion to the degree of conduction delay and is considered a form of ACM. The echocardiographic and histologic findings in both subgroups are classic for DCM, although the conduction system may be fibrotic in patients with ECSD. In both groups of patients with DCM, ventricular tachycardia, ventricular fibrillation, or torsades de pointes can occur and may result in sudden death.[21,23,27]

Genetic heterogeneity exists for autosomal dominant DCM, with at least 30 genes identified for pure DCM and five genes for ECSD.[30] Some of the most common pathogenic variants have been associated with genes encoding δ-sarcoglycan; α-sarcoglycan; β-sarcoglycan, γ-sarcoglycan; α-actinin 2; ZASP/LBD3; actin; desmin; troponins C, I, and T; β-myosin heavy chain; myosin-binding protein C; myosin light chains 2 and 3; α-tropomyosin; titin; lamin A/C; CARP; metavinculin; MLP/CSRP3; telethonin; myopalladin; nebulette; voltage-gated sodium channel, phospholamban, and RB20 (see Table 153.3).[29,30,38–42]

CYTOSKELETAL PROTEINS

Most DCM-associated genes identified to date encode either cytoskeletal or sarcomeric proteins (see Table 153.3). In the case of cytoskeletal proteins, defects of force transmission are considered to result in the DCM phenotype, whereas defects of force generation have been speculated to cause sarcomeric protein–induced DCM.[41] Desmin is a cytoskeletal protein that forms intermediate filaments specific for muscle.[40] This muscle-specific 53-kDa subunit of class III intermediate filaments forms connections between the nuclear and plasma membranes of cardiac, skeletal, and smooth muscle. Desmin is found at the Z lines and intercalated disk of muscle, and its role in muscle function appears to involve attachment or stabilization of the sarcomere. Mutations in the desmin gene appear to cause abnormalities of force and signal transmission similar to those believed to occur with actin gene mutations (see later).[43,44]

Another DCM-causing gene encodes δ-sarcoglycan, a member of the sarcoglycan subcomplex of the dystrophin-associated protein complex. The gene encodes a protein involved in stabilization of the myocyte sarcolemma as well as signal transduction. Mutations identified in familial and sporadic cases resulted in reduction of the expression of protein within the myocardium. In the absence of δ-sarcoglycan, the remaining sarcoglycans (δ, β, γ, Σ) cannot assemble properly in the endoplasmic reticulum.[39] Mouse models of δ-sarcoglycan deficiency demonstrate dilated HCM, sarcolemmal fragility, and disrupted vascular smooth muscle, which leads to vascular spasm, including coronary spasm.[45,46]

Laminins are extracellular proteins that interact with cellular integrins, allowing communication between the cell and its extracellular matrix environment. Mutations in the genes *LAMA* and *ILK*, which connect integrins and the actin cytoskeleton, lead to severe cardiac dysfunction in mice. This was the impetus to look for, and find, mutations in the human genes in patients with DCM.[47–49]

Table 153.3 Genes Associated With Cardiomyopathy.

Gene	Protein	Pattern of Inheritance	Disease Association	OMIM#	Locus
ABCC9	ATP-binding cassette, subfamily c, member 9	AD	DCM	601439	12p12.1
ACTC1	Actin, α, cardiac muscle	AD	HCM, DCM, NCM, ACM	102540	15q14
ACTN2	Actinin, α-2	AD	HCM, DCM	102573	1q42-q43
AKAP9	A-kinase anchor protein 9	AD	DCM	604001	7q21.2
ALMS1	Centrosome and basal body associated protein	AR	DCM	606844	2p13.1
ALPK3	α kinase 3	AR	HCM, DCM	617608	
ANKRD1	Ankyrin repeat domain-containing protein 1	AD	HCM, DCM	609599	10q23.3
ARVD3	Arrhythmogenic right ventricular dysplasia, familial, 3	AD	ACM	602086	14q12-q22
ARVD4	Arrhythmogenic right ventricular dysplasia, familial, 4	AD	ACM	602087	2q32.1-q32.3
ARVD6	Arrhythmogenic cardiomyopathy, familial, 6	AD	ACM	604401	10p14-p12
BAG3	Bcl2-associated athanogene 3	AD	HCM, DCM, RCM	603883	10q25.2-q26.2
BRAF	V-Raf murine sarcoma viral oncogene homolog B1	AD	HCM	164757	
CASQ2	Calsequestrin 2	AR, AD	NCM	114251	1p13.1
CAV3	Caveolin 3	AD	HCM, DCM	601253	3p25.3
CHRM2	Cholinergic receptor, muscarinic, 2	AD	DCM	118493	7q33
CRYAB	Crystallin, α-B	AD	DCM	123590	11q23.1
CSRP3	Cysteine- and glycine-rich protein 3	AD	DCM, HCM	600824	11p15.1
CTF1	Cardiotrophin 1		DCM	600435	16p11.2
CTNNA3	Catenin α 3	AD	ACM	607667	10q21.3
DES	Desmin	AD,AR	DCM, ACM, RCM	125660	2q35
DMD	Dystrophin	XL	DCM	300377	Xq21.2-p21.1
DOLK	Dolichol kinase	AR	DCM	610746	9q34.11
DSC2	Desmocollin 2	AD, AR	DCM, ACM	600271	18q12.1
DSG2	Desmoglein 2	AD	DCM, ACM	125671	18q12.1
DSP	Desmoplakin	AD, AR	DCM, ACM	125485	4q21.3
DTNA	Dystrobrevin, α	AD	NCM	601239	18q12.1
EMD	Emerin	XL	DCM	300384	Xq28
EYA4	Eyes absent, drosophila, homolog of, 4	AD	DCM	603550	6q23.2
FHL1	Four-and-a-half LIM domains 1	XL	HCM	300163	Xq26.3
FHL2	Four-and-a-half LIM domains 2	Unknown	DCM	602633	2q12.2
FKRP	Fukutin related protein	AR	DCM	606596	19q13.32
FKTN	Fukutin	AR	DCM	607440	9q31.2
FLNC	Filamin C	AD	RCM, HCM, ACM, DMC	102565	7q32.1
GAA	Glucosidase, α, acid	AR	HCM	606800	17q25.3
GATA4	Gata-binding protein 4	AD	DCM	600576	8p23.1
GATAD1	Gata zinc finger domain-containing protein 1	AR	DCM	614518	7q21-q22
GLA	Galactosidase, α	XL	HCM	300644	Xq22
HCN4	Hyperpolarization-activated cyclic nucleotide-gated potassium channel 4	AD	NCM	605206	15q24.1
HRAS	V-Ha-Ras Harvey rat sarcoma viral oncogene homolog	AD	HCM	190020	11p15.5
ILK	Integrin-linked kinase	AD	DCM	602366	11p15.4
JPH2	Junctophilin 2	AD	HCM	605267	20q13.12
JUP	Junction plakoglobin	AD, AR	ACM	173325	17q21
KRAS	V-Ki-Ras2	AD	HCM	190070	12p12.1
LAMA4	Laminin, α-4	AD	DCM	600133	6q21
LAMP2	Lysosome-associated membrane protein 2	XL	HCM, DCM	309060	Xq24
LDB3	Lim domain-binding 3	AD	HCM, DCM, NCM, ACM	605906	10q22.3-q23.2
LMNA	Lamin A/C	AD, AR	DCM, NCM, ACM, HCM	150330	1q22
LRRC10	Leucine-rich repeat-containing protein 10	AD, AR	DCM	610846	12q15
MAP2K1	Mitogen-activated protein kinase kinase 1	AD	HCM	176872	15q22.31
MAP2K2	Mitogen-activated protein kinase kinase 2	AD	HCM	601263	19p13.3
MIB1	E3 ubiquitin protein ligase 1	AD	NCM	608677	18q11.2
MURC/CAVIN4	Muscle-related coiled-coil protein/caveolae-associated protein 4	AD	DCM	617714	9q31.1
MYBPC3	Myosin-binding protein C, cardiac	AD	HCM, DCM, NCM, RCM	600958	11p11.2
MYH6	Myosin, heavy chain 6, cardiac muscle, α	AD	HCM, DCM	160710	14q12
MYH7	Myosin, heavy chain 7, cardiac muscle, β	AD	HCM, DCM, NCM, RCM	160760	14q12
MYL2	Myosin, light chain 2, regulatory, cardiac, slow	AD	HCM	160781	12q24.11
MYL3	Myosin, light chain 3, alkali, ventricular, skeletal, slow	AD, AR	HCM, RCM	160790	3p21.3-p21.2

Table 153.3 Genes Associated With Cardiomyopathy.—cont'd

Gene	Protein	Pattern of Inheritance	Disease Association	OMIM#	Locus
MYLK2	Myosin light chain kinase 2	AD	HCM	606566	20q13.31
MYOM1	Myomesin 1	AD	HCM	603508	18p11.31
MYOT	Myotilin	AD	DCM	604103	5q31.2
MYOZ2	Myozenin 2	AD	HCM, DCM, RCM	605602	4q26-q27
MYPN	Myopalladin	AD	HCM, DCM, RCM	608517	10q21.3
NEBL	Nebulette	AD	DCM	605491	10p12
NEXN	Nexilin (F actin binding protein)	AD	HCM, DCM	613121	1p31.1
NKX2-5	Nk2 homeobox 5	AD	DCM	600584	5q35.1
NRAS	Neuroblastoma Ras viral oncogene homolog	AD	HCM	164790	1p13.2
PDLIM3	Pdz and Lim domain protein 3	AD	HCM, DCM	605899	4q35.1
PKP2	Plakophilin 2	AD	DCM, ACM	602861	12p11
PLN	Phospholamban	AD	HCM, DCM, ACM	172405	6q22.1
PRDM16	Pr domain-containing protein 16	AD	DCM, NCM	605557	1p36.32
PRKAG2	Protein kinase, amp-activated, noncatalytic, gamma-2	AD	HCM	602743	7q36.1
PTPN11	Protein-tyrosine phosphatase, nonreceptor-type, 11	AD	HCM	176876	12q24.13
RAF1	V-Raf-1 murine leukemia viral oncogene homolog 1	AD	HCM	164760	3p25.2
RBM20	Rna-binding motif protein 20	AD	DCM	613171	10q25.2
RIT1	Ras-like without Caax 1	AD	HCM	609591	1q22
RYR2	Ryanodine receptor 2 (cardiac)	AD	HCM, ACM	180902	1q43
SCN5A	Sodium channel, voltage-gated, type V, α subunit	AD	DCM, ACM	600163	3p21
SGCA	Sarcoglycan α	AR	LGMD	600119	17q21.33
SGCB	Sarcoglycan β	AR	LGMD	600900	4q12
SGCD	Sarcoglycan, δ (35 kDa dystrophin-associated glycoprotein)	AD, AR	DCM	601411	5q33-q34
SHOC2	Soc-2 homolog	AD	HCM	602775	10q25.2
SLC25A4	Solute carrier family 25, member 4 (mitochondrial carrier adenine nucleotide translocator)	AD, AR	DCM	103220	5q31.1
SOS1	Son of sevenless, drosophila, homolog 1	AD	HCM	182530	2p22.1
TAZ	Tafazzin	AR, XL	DCM, NCM	300394	Xq28
TBX20	T-Box 20	AD	DCM, NCM	606061	7p14.2
TCAP	Titin-Cap (Telethonin)	AR	HCM, DCM	604488	17q12
TGFB3	Transforming growth factor β 3	AD	ACM	190230	14q24.3
TMEM43	Transmembrane protein 43	AD	ACM	612048	3p25.1
TMPO	Thymopoietin	AD	DCM	188380	12q23.1
TNNC1	Troponin C type 1 (slow)	AD	HCM, DCM	191040	3p21.1
TNNI3	Troponin I type 3 (cardiac)	AD	HCM, DCM, RCM	191044	19q13.4
TNNT2	Troponin T type 2 (cardiac)	AD	HCM, DCM, NCM, RCM	191045	1q32
TOR1AIP1	Torsin-1a-interacting protein 1	AR	DCM	614512	1q25.2
TPM1	Tropomyosin 1 (α)	AD	HCM, DCM, RCM	191010	15q22.1
TRDN	Triadin	AR	DCM	603283	6q22.31
TTN	Titin	AD, AR	HCM, DCM, ACM	188840	2q31
TTR	Transthyretin	AD	HCM	176300	18q12.1
TXNRD2	Thioredoxin reductase 2	AD, AR	DCM	606448	22q11.21
VCL	Vinculin	AD	HCM, DCM, NCM	193065	10q22.2

ACM, Arrhythmogenic cardiomyopathy; *AD*, autosomal dominant; *AR*, autosomal recessive; *ATP*, adenosine triphosphate; *DCM*, dilated cardiomyopathy; *HCM*, hypertrophic cardiomyopathy; *LGMD*, limb girdle muscular dystrophy; *NCM*, noncompaction cardiomyopathy; *OMIN*, Online Mendelian Inheritance in Man; *RCM*, restrictive cardiomyopathy; *XL*, X-linked.

Dystrophin is a vital protein complex that connects the cytoskeleton of a muscle fiber to the surrounding extracellular matrix through the cell membrane. This complex is variously known as the *costamere* or the *dystrophin-associated protein complex*. Many muscle proteins, such as α-dystrobrevin, syncoilin, synemin, sarcoglycan, dystroglycan, and sarcospan, colocalize with dystrophin at the costamere. Pathogenic gene variants in the dystrophin gene causes various degrees of deficiency. When this protein is abnormally expressed or deficient, it results in a constellation of symptoms characterized by muscular dystrophy, DCM, heart failure, and arrhythmias typically seen in the first or second decades of life.[50]

The final cytoskeletal protein-encoding gene, *VCL*, encodes vinculin and its splice variant metavinculin. Vinculin is ubiquitously expressed, and metavinculin is coexpressed with vinculin in heart, skeletal, and smooth muscle. The protein complex is localized to subsarcolemmal costameres in the heart, where it interacts with α-actinin, talin, and γ-actin to form a microfilamentous network linking cytoskeleton and sarcolemma.[51,52] In addition, these proteins are present in adherens junctions in intercalated disks and participate in cell-cell adhesion. Mutations in metavinculin have been shown to disrupt the intercalated disks and alter actin filament crosslinking.[51-53]

SARCOMERIC PROTEINS

Mutations in the sarcomere may produce HCM, DCM, or NCM. In the latter case, abnormalities in force generation or transmission are thought to contribute to the development of this phenotype.[30,41] Cardiac actin is a sarcomeric protein that is a member of the sarcomeric thin filament interacting with tropomyosin and the troponin complex. As previously noted, actin plays a significant role in linking the sarcomere to the sarcolemma. The mutations in actin that resulted in DCM, as described by Olson and colleagues,[54] appear to be directly involved in the binding of dystrophin. Further, actin interacts in the sarcomere with cardiac troponin T and β-myosin heavy chain, the products of two other genes resulting in either DCM or HCM depending on the position of the mutation.[55-57]

In addition to mutations in the thin filament protein actin, mutations in the thick filament protein-encoding gene β-myosin heavy chain and myosin binding protein C3 have been shown to cause DCM with associated sudden death in at least one infant, as well as DCM in older children and adults.[55-57] Mutations in this gene are thought to perturb the actin-myosin interaction and force generation or alter cross-bridge movement during contraction.

Mutations in all three cardiac troponin types (C, I, and T) have been speculated to disrupt calcium-sensitive troponin C binding.[55,58-60] Recessive mutation in troponin I is thought to impair the interaction with troponin T, and α-tropomyosin mutations also have been identified and were predicted to alter the surface charge of the protein, leading to impaired interaction with actin.[61,62] Mutations in phospholamban have also been identified that further support calcium handling as a potentially important mechanism in the development of DCM.[63]

An area of interest for evaluation at the molecular level has been the Z disk. Knoll and colleagues identified mutations in the *CSRP3* gene and demonstrated that this results in defects in the interaction of MLP with telethonin.[64] Mutations in *CSRP3* also have been shown to result in abnormalities in the T-tubule system and Z-disk architecture by electron microscopy, which correlates with the histopathologic findings in *CSRP3*-knockout mice.[65] In addition, mutations in α-actinin 2, which is involved in crosslinking actin filaments and shares a common actin-binding domain with dystrophin, were also identified in familial DCM; these mutations in α-actinin 2 disrupt its binding to MLP.[55,66,67]

A number of other sarcomeric proteins also have been shown involved in DCM. Titin is a giant sarcomeric cytoskeletal protein that contributes to the maintenance of the sarcomere organization and myofibrillar elasticity, and interacts with these proteins at the Z disk–I band transition zone.[64,65,68] Mutations in the titin gene have been identified in familial DCM, and it is thought to be the most common gene mutated, as it is estimated to be seen in 20% of affected individuals.[69,70] The titin splicing factor RNA-binding motif protein 20 has a role in posttranslational modifications which appear to alter the mechanics of titin,[69] and mutations are likewise associated with DCM. Purevjav and colleagues[71] showed that mutations in myopalladin, an immunoglobulin-domain family member protein that works as an intermediate in sarcomere/Z-disk assembly, were present in several patients with DCM and HCM, and animal models revealed various pathways of cellular disturbance based on specific mutations. Finally, CARP, encoded by *ANKRD1*, also interacts with myopalladin and titin and may be mutated in both DCM and HCM.[72,73]

LAMIN A/C

The lamins are located in the nuclear lamina at the nucleoplasmic side of the inner nuclear membrane, and lamins A and C are expressed in heart and skeletal muscle.[74] Mutations in the *LMNA* gene were initially reported to cause electrical conduction system disease.[75] Also, they have been found to cause a form of autosomal dominant limb girdle muscular dystrophy (type 1B), which is also associated with electrical conduction system disease.[76] The mechanism responsible for the development of DCM and conduction system abnormalities and for the development of skeletal myopathy is being determined, with recent evidence suggesting a role for the interactions between lamin A/C and emerin, the protein responsible for X-linked Emery-Dreifuss muscular dystrophy.[75,77,78] Emerin alone has also been found to cause isolated cardiomyopathy.[79]

MUSCLE IS MUSCLE: CARDIOMYOPATHY AND SKELETAL MYOPATHY GENES OVERLAP

Nearly all of the genes identified for inherited DCM are also known to cause skeletal myopathy in humans and/or mouse models. Well-described examples include the genes encoding dystrophin, δ-sarcoglycan, and lamin A/C. Mutations in the genes encoding desmin, tafazzin, α-dystrobrevin, ZASP/LBD3, MLP/CSRP3, α-actinin 2, and titin also result in an associated skeletal myopathy. This suggests that cardiac and skeletal muscle function is interrelated and that the skeletal muscle fatigue seen in patients with DCM may be due to primary skeletal muscle disease and not simply the cardiac dysfunction.

HYPERTROPHIC CARDIOMYOPATHY

CLINICAL FEATURES OF HYPERTROPHIC CARDIOMYOPATHY

HCM is the second most prevalent type of cardiomyopathy in children representing around 40% of cases with an estimated incidence of about 0.47 in 100,000 children.[1,3,24,80] HCM is more prevalent in boys than in girls, is more common in black children than in white or Hispanic children, and the incidence of diagnosis is 10 times greater in patients under the age of 1 year compared with older children.[80] In adults, similarly to DCM, HCM is much more prevalent and occurs at a rate of 1 in 500 people or greater.[26] HCM is a primary myocardial disorder with an autosomal dominant pattern of inheritance that is characterized by hypertrophy of the left ventricle (with or without hypertrophy of the right ventricle) with histologic features of myocyte hypertrophy, myofibrillar disarray, and interstitial fibrosis. LV hypertrophy occurs in either a symmetric or, more commonly, an asymmetric pattern (Fig. 153.4).[80,81] As with DCM, HCM can occur in isolation or in association with systemic disorders. However, the major impact of this disorder on human health is its reputation as the most common cause of sudden death in young, healthy, athletic individuals and its potential to cause heart failure.[80,81] Heart failure can occur because of diastolic factors or because of the development of systolic dysfunction, so-called *burned-out HCM*.[82,83]

In the pediatric age range, the causes of HCM and the variable age range of onset differentiate further the neonatal and childhood form of disease from the adolescent and adult counterpart.[84] Overwhelmingly, the cause has been reported to be idiopathic (75%), with the remainder of cases evenly distributed between inborn errors of metabolism, malformation syndromes, and neuromuscular disorders.[84-86] Recent evidence suggests that familial HCM, separate from malformation syndromes and metabolic disorders, is common among infants and children primarily through mutations in the sarcomeric genes, which is similar to what is found in adult and adolescent populations. In our experience in the past 10 years, approximately 70% of noninfantile individuals have an identifiable mutation in a sarcomere-encoding gene, whereas mutation is identified in fewer infants (more typically in the 20% range).

HCM can be detected in asymptomatic individuals with a family history, at the time of an SCD event, or in patients with signs of heart failure (with or without preserved systolic function). Presentation at

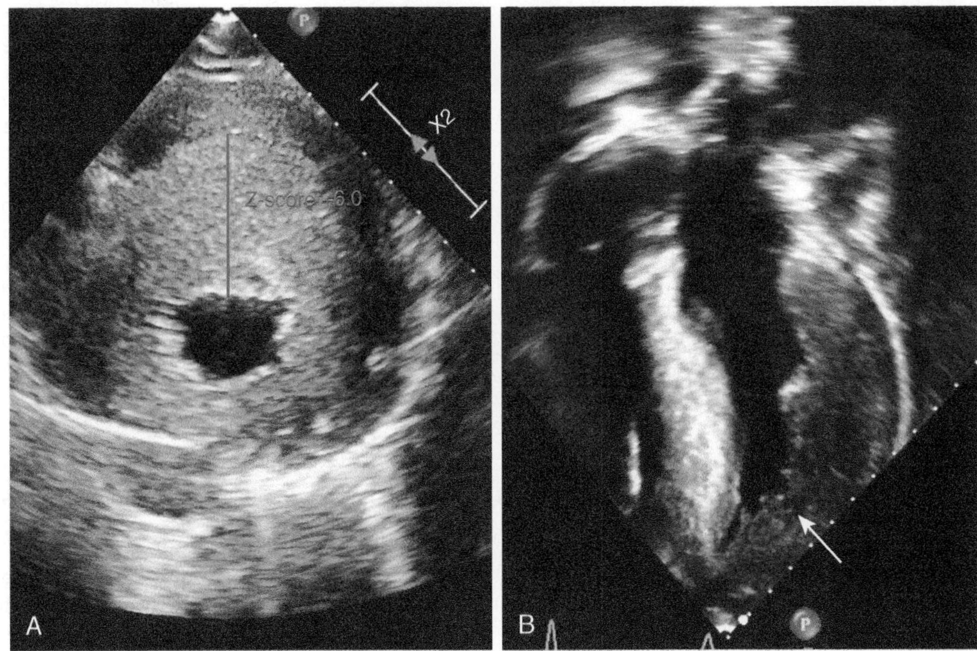

Fig. 153.4 Echocardiographic features of hypertrophic cardiomyopathy; (A) from a parasternal short axis view (a transecting view through the middle of the left ventricle) displays an out of proportion hypertrophy of the interventricular septum at the end of diastole representing a Z-score of +6.0 *(arrow)*; (B) from a classic apical four-chamber view, echocardiography shows asymmetric hypertrophy of the interventricular septum, pathognomonic findings in the diagnosis of HCM. *HCM,* Hypertrophic cardiomyopathy.

less than 1 year of age due to symptoms portends a poor outcome but is uncommon.[84,85,87-89] Presenting signs and symptoms may be secondary to many different physiologic disturbances, including LV outflow tract obstruction, LV dysfunction (systolic or diastolic), and/or arrhythmias. The physical examination findings are often normal unless there is outflow tract obstruction leading to a murmur, mitral regurgitation causing a murmur, or diastolic dysfunction leading to a pathologic gallop. Radiography may show cardiomegaly.[87,88] Electrocardiography can demonstrate left axis deviation, repolarization changes manifested by abnormal Q wave patterns, atrial enlargement, inversion of the T waves, and LV hypertrophy that can then be confirmed by noninvasive imaging. Echocardiography is essential for the assessment of LV thickness and the septal shape, diastolic and systolic dysfunction, outflow track obstruction, mitral valve abnormalities, and the overall progression of disease.[87] Utilization of CMR is useful for further characterization of the disease, for patients with inadequate echocardiographic images,[90] and for the assessment of myocardial fibrosis.

Survival for patients with HCM is dependent on the cause and age at diagnosis, although there are notably worse outcomes with presentation at <1 year of age and in certain associated disorders, in particular Noonan syndrome.[84,87,89,91,92]

CAUSES OF HYPERTROPHIC CARDIOMYOPATHY

The causes of HCM can be subdivided into sarcomeric and syndromic. Most of the disease-causing gene variants implicated in the sarcomeric HCM include mutations in the *MYH7* and the *MYBPC3* genes. These two mutated genes account individually for approximately 40% of the total diagnosed cases. The remaining sarcomeric genes such as *TNNT2, TPM1, ACTC1, TNNI3, TTN,* and *MYL2* account collectively for a small percentage of the cases.[62,80,93] Those cases attributed to syndromic HCM usually have systemic manifestations in addition to cardiovascular involvement, such as mitochondrial disease, Fabry disease, Noonan syndrome, Pompe disease, and Friedreich ataxia.[94]

The first clinical description of HCM was reported in 1868 in France,[95] and was recognized to be a genetic disorder in the late 1950s. Since then, numerous clinical and pathology studies of HCM have been performed. During the last 25 years, molecular-genetic studies have provided important insights into the pathogenesis of HCM and have provided a new perspective for the diagnosis of HCM and the treatment of patients with this disorder.[96] Evidence suggests that a genetic cause may account for half of presumed sporadic cases and two thirds of familial cases of pediatric HCM.[97,98]

GENETICS OF FAMILIAL HYPERTROPHIC CARDIOMYOPATHY

From the genetic point of view, more than 90% of HCM is inherited as an autosomal dominant disease with variable expressivity and age-related penetrance. Hence, the offspring of an affected individual have a 50% probability of inheriting a mutation and risk for HCM. Furthermore, a recent study identified a mutation in the gene encoding the four-and-a-half LIM domain 1 (FHL1) protein responsible for HCM, suggesting an X-linked inheritance.[93,99,100] Alternatively, sporadic HCM cases may be due to de novo mutations in the proband (absent in the parents).

Most of the disease-causing genes identified to date code for proteins that are part of the sarcomere, which is a complex structure with an exact stoichiometry and multiple sites of protein-protein interactions.[101-103] To date, around 1400 mutations have been identified as being responsible for HCM and about 70% of these mutations are in the sarcomere genes encoding MYH7 and cardiac myosin binding MYBPC3.[104,105] Other causative genes include myosin light chains (thick filament); actin (thin filament); α-tropomyosin (thin filament); troponins T, C, and I (thin filament); myopalladin (Z disk); CARP (Z disk); titin (Z-disk); myozenin 2 (Z-disk); α-actinin (Z disk); ankyrin repeat domain 2 (Z disk); telethonin (Z disk); MLP (Z disk); and nexilin (Z disk).[88,99,104,105] Moreover, 5% of patients with familial HCM are heterozygous carriers, carrying up to three distinct mutations that are associated with a poorer prognosis.[104] In addition, the phenotypic heterogeneity of HCM within families suggests an environmental role and epigenetics in onset of the disease.[105]

SARCOMERE GENE MUTATIONS

The β isoform of myosin heavy chain, the major isoform in the human ventricle and in slow-twitch skeletal fibers, is encoded by MYH7. This gene appears to be the most commonly mutated

HCM gene, and hot spots for mutations have been identified.[103,106] Most of the mutations are missense mutations located either in the head or in the head-rod junction of the molecule. On the basis of their structural location in the myosin head, most of the mutations are likely to disrupt both mechanical and catalytic components of actin-myosin interaction, resulting in reduced force generation. Sarcomere assembly is also likely to be disrupted. Mutations in the light meromyosin domain have also been identified, and Blair and colleagues[107] speculated that HCM develops in this case because of abnormalities of myosin filament assembly or interactions with thick filament binding proteins.

Involvement of the myosin heavy chain α isoform is much less common than that of the β isoform. Mutations in the *MYH6* and *MYH7* genes have been identified in patients with both DCM and HCM.[108] Merlo and colleagues[109] reported poorer outcomes in patients with rare variants in *MYH6* when compared with more common mutations, a finding also described for *MYH7*, *MYBPC3*, *TNNT2*, and *TTN*. In addition to the role of *MYH6* in cardiomyopathy, functional alterations in *MYH6* and *MYH7* have been found associated with a wide spectrum of congenital cardiac malformations, particularly as an underappreciated cause of secundum atrial septal defects. This is in direct contrast to the other sarcomeric proteins investigated, none of which were found to be abnormal in a cohort of patients with atrial septal defect.[110,111] The myosin light chain isoforms are expressed in the ventricular myocardium and in the slow-twitch muscles and are the so-called ventricular myosin regulatory light chains encoded by *MYL2* and the ventricular myosin essential light chain encoded by *MYL3*.[110,111] The myosin light chains are thought to influence the mechanical efficiency of cross-bridge cycling and the speed of contraction. It is believed that these proteins regulate power output via a calcium-dependent mechanism, and disruption has been shown in patients with HCM.[110,111] Mutations in *MYL2* and *MYL3* have been identified in cases of infantile HCM.[112,113] Myosin-binding protein C is a myosin-associated protein that binds at 43-nm intervals along the myosin thick filament backbone within the C region of the sarcomere A band. For more than a decade, evidence has existed indicating both structural and regulatory roles. Partial extraction of cardiac myosin-binding protein C from rat skinned cardiac myocytes and rabbit skeletal muscle fibers alters Ca^{2+}-sensitive tension,[114,115] and it has shown that phosphorylation of cardiac myosin-binding protein C alters myosin cross-bridges in native thick filaments, suggesting that myosin-binding protein C can modify force production in activated cardiac muscles. The cardiac isoform is encoded by the *MYBPC3* gene, mutations in which have been characterized by specific clinical features with a mild phenotype in young individuals, a delayed age at the onset of symptoms, and a favorable prognosis before the age of 40 years.[115,116]

The thin filament contains actin, the troponin complex, and tropomyosin. The troponin complex and tropomyosin constitute the Ca^{2+}-sensitive switch that regulates the contraction of cardiac muscle fibers. Mutations have been found in α-tropomyosin and in all three of the subunits of the troponin complex: cardiac troponin C, responsible for calcium binding; cardiac troponin I, the inhibitory subunit; and cardiac troponin T, the tropomyosin-binding subunit.

α-Tropomyosin is encoded by *TPM1*, and mutations in *TPM1* have long been known to be a cause of familial HCM; it is believed that some mutations in this gene could alter tropomyosin binding to actin.[117-119]

Cardiac troponin T is encoded by the *TNNT2* gene. In human cardiac muscle, multiple isoforms of cardiac troponin T have been described that are expressed in the fetal, adult, and diseased heart and that result from alternative splicing of the single gene *TNNT2*.[117,120] The precise physiologic relevance of these isoforms is poorly understood. Mutations in the *TNNT2* gene are predicted to influence the inhibitory regulatory effect of the tropomyosin-troponin complex. *TNNI3* encodes cardiac troponin I. The cardiac troponin I isoform is expressed only in cardiac muscles.[120-124] Cooperative binding of cardiac troponin I to actin-tropomyosin is a unique property of the cardiac variant; it is thought that mutations disrupt the calcium-sensitive switch mediated by this protein, resulting in increased calcium sensitivity and reduced maximum tension.[120-124] Cardiac troponin T is encoded by *TNNC1*. The primary role for this protein is calcium sensing. Mutations in a number of the proteins already described appear to affect the function of cardiac troponin C in HCM through alterations in calcium sensitivity. Mutations in the *TNNC1* gene have been described with prevalence similar to those of mutations in other well-documented sarcomeric genes known to cause HCM.[125-127] Functional studies of these variants showed increased calcium sensitivity consistent with the phenotype of mutations in other sarcomeric proteins.

CYTOSKELETAL GENE MUTATIONS

Despite the predominance of sarcomeric protein mutations in HCM, there is evidence for a role of cytoskeletal proteins as well. A mutation in desmin, which links the plasma and nuclear membranes, has been demonstrated to cause an HCM phenotype.[128,129] Additional cytoskeletal proteins with potential roles in HCM, described earlier for their roles in DCM, include integrin-linked protein kinase,[130] junctophillin 2,[131] PDZ and LIM domain protein 3,[132] and vinculin/metavinculin.[133,134]

OTHER PROTEINS

Mutations in the Z-disk protein-encoding genes *TTN* and *CSRP3* have been identified as causes of HCM, suggesting that the Z disk is also important in the development of HCM.[135,136] More recently, mutations in the genes encoding ZASP/LBD3, telethonin, α-actinin 2,[115,137] myozenin,[138] myopalladin,[139] and nexilin[140] have also been demonstrated to cause HCM.

HYPERTROPHIC CARDIOMYOPATHY ASSOCIATED WITH INFILTRATIVE AND SYSTEMIC DISEASES

A variety of disorders that have apparent LV hypertrophy and features of HCM occur in the setting of systemic disease. This includes infiltrative disease, mitochondrial disorders, and malformations syndromes.

POMPE DISEASE (TYPE II GLYCOGEN STORAGE DISEASE)

Pompe disease is a genetic deficiency of acid α-1,4-glucosidase, an enzyme involved in the breakdown of glycogen to glucose, resulting in a wide clinical spectrum ranging from the rapidly fatal infantile onset of type II glycogen storage disease to a slowly progressive adult-onset myopathy. This rare inborn error of glycogen metabolism occurs in less than 1 per 100,000 births. Massive glycogen accumulation occurs, leading to the clinical findings of enlarged tongue, striking hepatomegaly, hypotonia with decreased deep tendon reflexes, and cardiomyopathy (usually HCM) with congestive heart failure. The glycogen accumulation can be noted histologically in skeletal muscle, liver, and heart.[141,142] The gene coding for the lysosomal enzyme was originally mapped to chromosome 17 at 17q23-q25, and the disease has autosomal recessive inheritence.[141] The infantile-onset form (Pompe disease) typically manifests itself during the first 5 months of life, and patients usually die before their second year.[143] Children usually die in the first 2 years of life unless enzyme replacement therapy, which appears to be an increasingly rare commodity, is commenced. The diagnosis may be predicted from the nearly pathognomonic electrocardiogram, with a short PR interval and prominent QRS voltages (Fig. 153.5).[142]

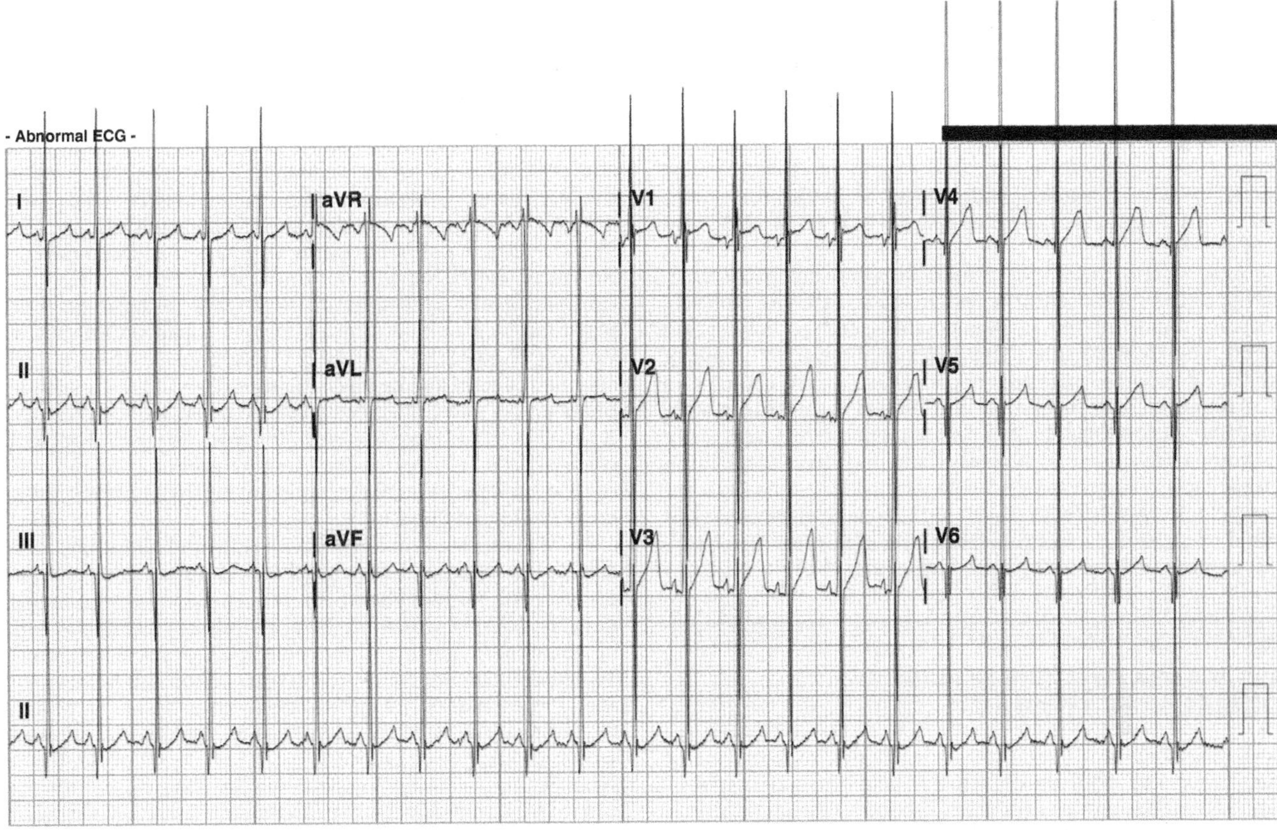

Fig. 153.5 Electrocardiographic features of Pompe disease. As a severe form of hypertrophic cardiomyopathy, an electrocardiogram displays short PR intervals, prominent right and left ventricular voltages, in addition to ST-segment and T-wave abnormalities. *aVF,* Augmented vector foot lead; *aVL,* augmented vector left lead; *aVR,* augmented vector right lead.

FABRY DISEASE

Fabry disease is an X-linked recessive disorder caused by deficiency of the enzyme α-galactosidase. Mild expression of the disorder is occasionally seen in carrier females. Young adults may be prone to renal failure and myocardial infarctions. Fabry disease usually has its onset in adolescence and manifests itself with sensations of burning pain in the hands and feet. With increasing age, multiple angiokeratomas become noticeable, especially around the umbilicus and genitalia. Corneal opacities are often noted. Progressive renal failure develops with age. Central nervous system manifestations include seizures and headaches. There is an increased risk for stroke, which may result in hemiplegia. The primary cardiac manifestations in affected males are HCM and mitral insufficiency, which is diagnosed by echocardiography. The LV myocardium and mitral valve tend to be areas of greatest storage of lipid material. On the electrocardiogram, the PR interval is usually short.[144]

DANON DISEASE

Danon disease is an X-linked dominant disorder characterized by intracytoplasmic vacuoles containing autophagic material and glycogen in cardiac and skeletal muscle cells, cardiomyopathy, and skeletal myopathy (with or without a conduction defect, Wolff-Parkinson-White syndrome, or mental retardation).[145] The underlying abnormality affects lysosomal function and is due to mutations in the gene encoding *LAMP2*.[145] The clinical phenotypic expression of Danon disease is variable. Charron and colleagues screened 50 individuals with HCM for *LAMP2* mutations and identified mutations in two patients with HCM and skeletal myopathy.[146] Both of these individuals presented with Danon disease during their teenage years; however, other individuals in the family were identified as young as 7 years of age. Wolff-Parkinson-White syndrome, high-voltage QRS complexes on the electrocardiogram, and high plasma creatine kinase levels were notable in affected individuals. LV dilation and dysfunction occurred later with symptoms of heart failure. Atrial and ventricular arrhythmias and conduction disease were notable, along with death during their 20s. A visual acuity abnormality was also common, because of choriocapillary ocular atrophy. In at least one family, XLCM was the presenting form of Danon disease despite a family history of the more commonly associated HCM. A *LAMP2* mutation, as opposed to a dystrophin gene mutation, was identified as the cause of DCM in these patients.[147] Danon disease appears to be underrecognized and may play a significant role in pediatric heart failure.

ADENOSINE MONOPHOSPHATE–ACTIVATED PROTEIN KINASE

Adenosine monophosphate–activated protein kinase, encoded by the γ_2 regulatory subunit of the *PRKAG2* gene on chromosome band 7q31, is an enzyme that modulates glucose uptake and glycolysis.[148] Dominant mutations in this gene were first identified in individuals with HCM, Wolff-Parkinson-White syndrome preexcitation, and atrioventricular block.[148,149] Cardiac disease differed from that in other forms of HCM, with pronounced formation of vacuoles that were filled with glycogen-associated granules, but no myocyte and myofibrillar disarray.[150]

MITOCHONDRIAL CARDIOMYOPATHIES

The normal function of the heart relies on a series of complex metabolic processes orchestrating the proper generation and use of energy. Mitochondria serve a crucial role as a platform for energy (ATP) to the varying demand of cardiomyocytes. The failure of these processes results in structural and functional deficiencies of the cardiac muscle, including inherited cardiomyopathies.[151,152] Cardiac disease is most commonly seen with respiratory chain defects.[153] Ragged red fibers are present in muscle biopsy specimens almost invariably when the molecular defect involves mitochondrial DNA, except in infants.[154] The cardiac diseases associated with mutations in the respiratory chain and mitochondrial transfer RNA include HCM, DCM, and NCM.[153,155,156]

Kearns-Sayre syndrome is a mitochondrial myopathy characterized by ptosis, chronic progressive external ophthalmoplegia, abnormal retinal pigmentation, cardiac conduction defects, and DCM. Channer and colleagues reported a case of rapidly developing progressive congestive heart failure and DCM requiring transplantation in a patient with Kearns-Sayre syndrome. Approximately 20% of patients with Kearns-Sayre syndrome have cardiac involvement, and most have conduction defects causing progressive heart block.[157,158]

Myoclonic epilepsy with ragged red muscle fibers syndrome is caused by a single nucleotide substitution in transfer RNA lysine that interferes with mitochondrial translation.[159,160]

DISORDERS OF THE RAS-MITOGEN-ACTIVATED PROTEIN KINASE SIGNALING PATHWAY

The RASopathies are a group of disorders due to variations of genes associated with the Ras/MAPK pathway and represent one of the largest groups of genetic disorders, with an estimated prevalence of approximately 1 in 1000. Some of the most frequent RASopathies include neurofibromatosis type 1 (the first syndrome identified) caused by mutation of a gene in the Ras/MAPK pathway,[161,162] and Noonan syndrome, caused by pathogenic gene variants in PTPN11, SOS1, RAF1, KRAS, NRAS, SHOC2, or CBL. Noonan syndrome, the second most common syndromic cause of congenital heart disease, includes pulmonary valvular stenosis (50% to 60%), atrial septal defects (10% to 25%), ventricular septal defects (5% to 20%), and HCM (12% to 35%).[163-166]

Noonan syndrome with multiple lentigines is caused by mutations in *PTPN11* and *RAF1*. Approximately 85% of affected individuals present with HCM (typically appearing during infancy) and pulmonary valve stenosis.[167-169] Capillary malformation-arteriovenous malformation syndrome is caused by haploinsufficiency of *RASA1*.[170]

Cardiac abnormalities in Costello syndrome, caused by pathogenic gene variations in *HRAS*, include supraventricular tachycardia, structural heart defects, and HCM.[171] Cardio-facio-cutaneous syndrome is caused by alteration of MAPK pathway activation by activating mutations in *BRAF, MAP2K1*, and *MAP2K2*. Cardiac abnormalities include structural heart defects and HCM.[172,173] Legius syndrome is caused by pathogenic gene variants in *SPRED1*.[162,164,165,174] Because of the widespread involvement of the RAS-MAPK pathway in a number of functions, the RASopathies have overlapping clinical phenotypes.[161,166]

NONCOMPACTION CARDIOMYOPATHY

NCM was previously considered a rare disease identified by a variety of names, including *spongy myocardium, fetal myocardium*, and *noncompaction of the LV myocardium*.[175] Despite its name, NCM may affect the right ventricle as well.[176] The abnormality is believed to represent an arrest in the normal process of myocardial compaction, the final stage of myocardial morphogenesis, resulting in persistence of multiple prominent ventricular trabeculations and deep intertrabecular recesses.[177] This cardiomyopathy is somewhat difficult to diagnose unless the physician has a high level of suspicion during echocardiographic and cardiac magnetic resonance evaluation.[90] In fact, on careful review of echocardiograms and other clinical data, it appears that NCM is relatively common in children and is also seen in adults.[178] Adult echocardiographic laboratories have reported the prevalence of isolated NCM to be between 0.014% and 1.3%,[177,179] and it is identified in approximately 5% of patients in the Pediatric Cardiomyopathy Registry.[180] In the most recent American Heart Association/American College of Cardiology cardiomyopathy classification, NCM was recognized for the first time as a unique form of cardiomyopathy. Clinically, nine variants of NCM are described: (1) isolated NCM with normal systolic function and cardiac structure; (2) NCM arrhythmogenic phenotype; (3) NCM dilated phenotype; (4) NCM hypertrophic type; (5) NCM mixed/undulating type; (6) NCM restrictive phenotype; (7) biventricular noncompaction phenotype; (8) right ventricular noncompaction; and (9) NCM associated with congenital heart disease (Fig. 153.6).[176]

NCM may present in infancy with signs and symptoms of heart failure, but some patients are identified during later childhood, adolescence, or adulthood. In the Pediatric Cardiomyopathy Registry, NCM represented 5% of all primary cardiomyopathies in children.[181] Pignatelli and colleagues reported findings in 36 children identified over a 5-year period, with the median age at presentation being 90 days (range 1 day to 17 years). In that study, 40% of the children presented with low cardiac output or congestive heart failure and one child presented with syncope. The most common presenting sign, other than heart failure, was asymptomatic electrocardiographic or radiographic abnormalities in 42% of patients. In addition, 14% of children had associated dysmorphic features, and 19% of affected children had first-degree relatives with cardiomyopathy.[178]

In another single-center study report of 242 children with NCM, which excluded patients with concomitant congenital heart disease, 31 patients (12.8%) had died, 13 (5.4%) underwent transplantation, and more than half of the patients developed evidence of LV systolic dysfunction.[182] In the National Australian Childhood Cardiomyopathy Study, symptomatic children with NCM presented early in infancy and there was lower freedom from death and/or transplantation at 15 years after diagnosis in the subjects with the DCM form of NCM versus DCM.[183] Predictors of mortality were myocardial dysfunction, arrhythmias, and repolarization abnormalities on the electrocardiogram. Those children with normal systolic function and no evidence of arrhythmias were at very low risk for sudden death.[178,180,183]

CAUSES OF NONCOMPACTION CARDIOMYOPATHY

During human embryogenesis, from week 5 through week 8, the loss of LV trabeculations, known as *compaction*, starts at the base of the heart and moves towards the apex.[184] NCM is a proposed disruption of this process resulting in two distinct layers of myocardium: a thin layer of compact epicardium and an overlying layer of noncompacted myocardium.[185] The typical modes of inheritance in pediatric patients include autosomal dominant (most common type), mitochondrial, X-linked, and recessive.[176,180,185]

Bleyl and colleagues[186] identified mutations in the *TAZ* gene, the gene also causative for Barth syndrome, as the first specific cause of isolated NCM. Since then, a number of genes have been identified as important in autosomal dominant forms of NCM, including that in patients with congenital heart disease and NCM. Overall, current genetic testing identifies mutations in 35% to 40% of patients tested.[187] However, the yield can vary

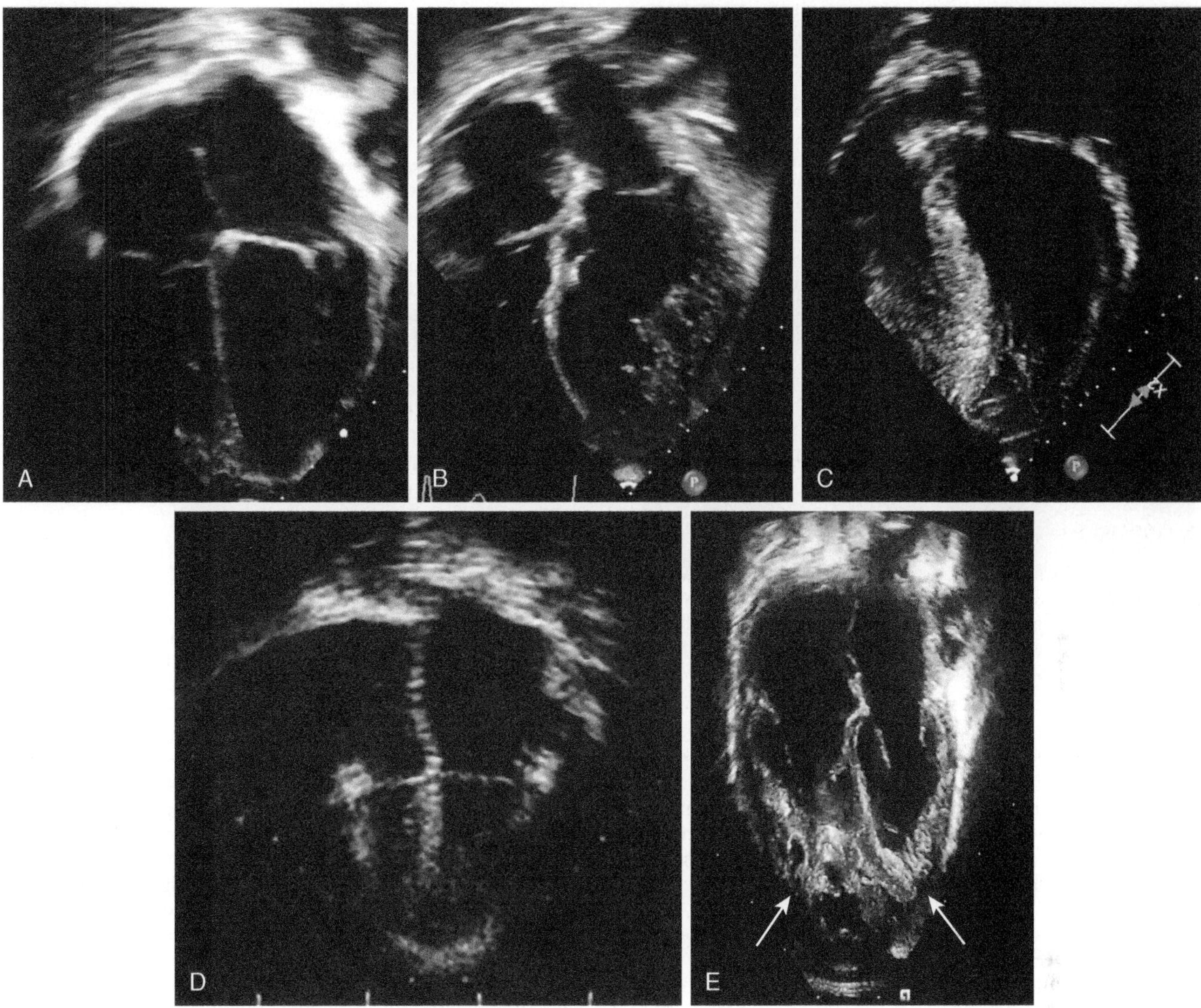

Fig. 153.6 Sub phenotypes of noncompaction cardiomyopathy (NCM). From a typical four-chamber view, echocardiography displays: (A) a normal baseline cardiac structure; (B) NCM with dilated phenotype; (C) NCM with hypertrophic subtype; (D) NCM with restrictive subtype; (E) NCM with biventricular involvement. *Arrows* indicate the presence of hypertrabeculations at the apical portion of the ventricular chambers.

significantly whether the NCM is isolated (i.e., normal ventricular function) or associated with another cardiomyopathy.[188] The cytoskeletal protein α-dystrobrevin is mutated in patients with NCM and hypoplastic left heart syndrome; mutations in *NKX2-5* gene are found in children with NCM and atrial septal defect; and *MYH7* is disrupted in patients with NCM and Ebstein's anomaly.[176,177,185,187] In NCM without congenital heart disease, mutations in the Z-disk gene *LDB3*, the nuclear envelope protein lamin A/C, and several sarcomeric genes (*MYH7*, *ACTC1*, *TNNT2*, *MYBPC3*, *TMP1*, and *TNNI3*) account for 20% or more of NCM.[185,187,189] Additional mutations identified in other cardiomyopathies may account for a smaller portion of cases and include mutations in the sodium channel gene *SCN5A* (associated with NCM and rhythm disturbance)[190]; dystrophin gene mutations in boys with NCM and Duchenne muscular dystrophy/Becker muscular dystrophy[191]; mutations in the desmosomal protein-encoding gene *DSP* (desmoplakin), also known to cause AVC and DCM,[192] and mitochondrial genome mutations.[192] Chromosomal abnormalities and syndromic patients have also been identified with NCM, including 1p36 deletion, 7p14.3p14.1 deletion, 18p subtelomeric deletion, 22q11.2 deletion, distal 22q11.2, trisomies 13 and 18, 8p23.1 deletion, tetrasomy 5q35.2-5q35, Coffin-Lowry syndrome (*RPS6KA3* mutation), Sotos syndrome (*NSD1* mutation), and Charcot-Marie-Tooth disease type 1A (*PMP22* duplication).[181,184,193-197]

RESTRICTIVE CARDIOMYOPATHY

CLINICAL FEATURES OF RESTRICTIVE CARDIOMYOPATHY

RCM is a physiologic, rather than anatomic, diagnosis. Although it is the rarest form of cardiomyopathy, at approximately 2% to 5% of cases, it accounts for 10% to 15% of heart transplants in pediatric patients.[198,199] RCM represents diastolic dysfunction of the myocardium, usually with preserved systolic function. Because of the subsequent elevated filling pressures, hearts often develop atrial enlargement, which is considered a hallmark of the disease (Fig. 153.7). SCD or a life-threatening cardiac event due to ventricular arrhythmias or heart block is common, as is heart failure; death occurs within a few years of diagnosis and there is no medical treatment.[200-202] The clinical manifestations in advanced disease are secondary to diastolic dysfunction and include pulmonary edema, pulmonary hypertension, and decreased myocardial reserve. Some reports suggest clinical overlap between RCM and HCM; however, patients younger

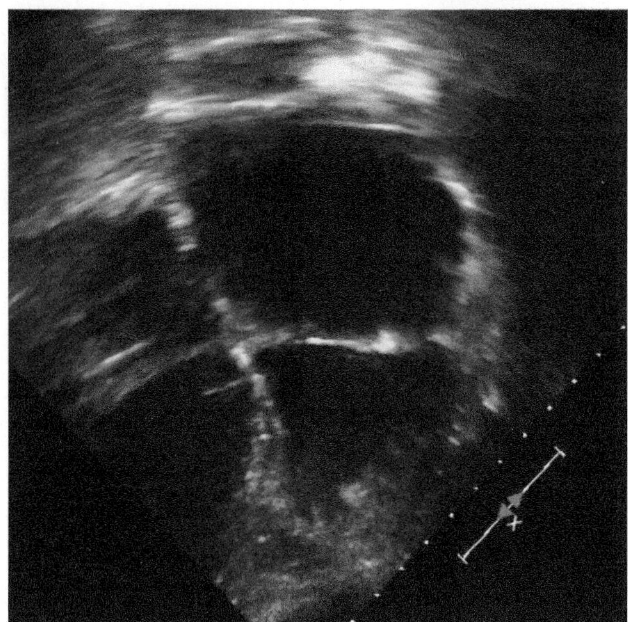

Fig. 153.7 Echocardiographic features of restrictive cardiomyopathy. From a typical four-chamber view, two-dimensional echocardiography displays disproportionately enlarged atria relative to the ventricular chamber size.

than 1 year of age are more likely to present with an HCM/RCM phenotype compared to pure RCM, and for all age groups pure RCM has poorer outcomes compared to the combined type. A substantial proportion of arrhythmic events in RCM may be bradycardic or asystolic in nature, as opposed to ventricular tachycardia. This has allowed the use of defibrillators/pacemakers as prophylactic management in appropriate cases.[200,203]

CAUSES OF RESTRICTIVE CARDIOMYOPATHY

RCM in children is much different from that of adults. Many adults with RCM have amyloidosis or a type of endocardial fibroelastosis, but most still have an idiopathic and/or presumptively familial disease.[198,200] The most common acquired cause in children is exposure to radiation or an underlying storage disease such as Gaucher or Hurler syndrome, but as with adults most cases are idiopathic and/or familial.[200]

RCM usually has autosomal dominant inheritance but autosomal recessive, X-linked, and mitochondrial-transmitted forms have been described. As would be suspected by the overlap with HCM, most identified genes encode sarcomeric proteins, such as *TNNI3*, *TNNT2*, *MYH7*, *ACTC1*, *TPM1*, *MYL3*, and *MYL2* (see Table 153.3).[198,200,202] Z-disk protein-encoding genes, including *MYPN*, *TTN*, and *BAG3*, also have been identified.[187,202] Variants in *DES* have been identified in several families with desmin-related myopathy, which can present with RCM, with or without skeletal myopathy and/or atrioventricular block.[200]

FINAL COMMON PATHWAYS

During the past decades, genes responsible for the development of many different cardiomyopathies have been identified. In an attempt to target genes for study, we developed the *final common pathway hypothesis*, which states that genes encoding proteins with similar functions or involved in the same pathway are responsible for a particular disease or syndrome phenotype.[19] In other situations, multiple mutations in the same gene (compound heterozygosity) or in different genes (digenic heterozygosity) may lead to a phenotype that may be classic, more severe, or even overlapping with other disease forms.

As a result, we, along with others, have identified structure-function similarities of proteins encoded by genes that, when disrupted, lead to a somewhat predictable gross clinical phenotype. For instance, the genes identified as causative for inherited arrhythmia disorders tend to encode ion channels, those identified as causative for HCM encode tend to encode sarcomeric proteins, and those identified to be causative for ACM tend to encode cell-cell junction proteins. The information gained from the studies on XLCM, Duchenne muscular dystrophy, and Becker muscular dystrophy led us to hypothesize that DCM is a disease of the cytoskeleton/sarcolemma that affects the sarcomere, a final common pathway of DCM.[19] It appears that the proteins disturbed by a mutated gene directly disrupt the normal function of the structures in which they are integrated most commonly but, in some instances, disrupt a binding partner protein that causes downstream disturbance of the final common pathway.

CONCLUSION

Pediatric cardiomyopathies, while not common, are a significant cause of morbidity and mortality in afflicted neonates. Dilated forms are the most common, followed by hypertrophic, ventricular noncompaction, arrhythmogenic, and RCM. Cardiomyopathies appear to occur because of disruption of final common pathways. These disruptions may be due to purely genetic causes, such as mutations in a single gene that result in a dysfunctional protein, which leads to a domino effect of downstream protein interaction abnormalities and ultimately a phenotype. In some cases, different intersecting pathways may become disturbed, resulting in complex phenotypes. Further, acquired causes may play a role by causing disruption of these functional pathways. Fortunately, novel therapies have resulted from the improved understanding of this clinical phenotype, as noted earlier. The development of novel targeted therapies has been somewhat slow in coming but is expected to increase soon. The future of cardiomyopathy care is poised to shift in the next decade because of these new developments, as well as the growing science of stem cell therapy. Because children have pure disease states, unfettered by comorbidities, the dream of cures of muscle will likely be realized more fully in this population.

ABBREVIATIONS

2D: Two-dimensional
ABCC9: ATP-binding cassette, subfamily C, member 9
ACC: American College of Cardiology
ACM: Arrhythmogenic cardiomyopathy
ACTC1: Actin, alpha, cardiac muscle
ACTN2: Actinin-alpha-2 protein
AD: Autosomal dominant
AHA: American Heart Association
AKAP9: A-kinase anchor protein 9
ALMS1: Centrosome and basal body associated
ALPK3: Alpha kinase 3
ANKRD1: Ankyrin repeat domain-containing protein 1
AR: Autosomal recessive
ARVD3: Arrhythmogenic right ventricular dysplasia, familial, 3
ARVD4: Arrhythmogenic right ventricular dysplasia, familial, 4
ARVD6: Arrhythmogenic cardiomyopathy, familial, 6
BAG3: Bcl2-associated athanogene 3
BNP: Brain natriuretic peptide
BRAF: V-Raf murine sarcoma viral oncogene homolog B1

CARP: Cardiac adriamycin-responsive protein
CASQ2: Calsequestrin 2
CAV3: Caveolin 3
CHRM2: Cholinergic receptor, muscarinic, 2
CM: Cardiomyopathy
CMR: Cardiac magnetic resonance
CNG: Cyclic nucleotide-gated
CRYAB: Crystallin, alpha-B
CSRP3: Cysteine- and glycine-rich protein 3
CTF1: Cardiotrophin 1
CTNNA3: Catenin alpha 3
DAPC: Dystrophin-associated protein complex
DCM: Dilated cardiomyopathy
DES: Desmin
DMD: Dystrophin
DOLK: Dolichol kinase
DSC2: Desmocollin 2
DSG2: Desmoglein 2
DSP: Desmoplakin
DTNA: Dystrobrevin, alpha
ECSD: Electrical conduction system disease
EMD: Emerin
EYA4: Eyes absent, drosophila, homolog of, 4
FHL1: Four-and-a-half LIM domains 1
FHL2: Four-and-a half LIM domains 2
FKRP: Fukutin related protein
FKTN: Fukutin
FLNC: Filamin C
GAA: Glucosidase, alpha, acid
GATA4: Gata-binding protein 4
GATAD1: Gata zinc finger domain-containing protein 1
GLA: Galactosidase, alpha
HCM: Hypertrophic cardiomyopathy
HCN4: Hyperpolarization-activated
HRAS: V-Ha-Ras Harvey rat sarcoma viral oncogene homolog
ILK: Integrin-linked protein kinase
ILK: Integrin-linked kinase
JPH2: Junctophilin 2
JUP: Junction plakoglobin
KRAS: V-Ki-Ras2
LAMA4: Laminin α4 subunit
LAMA4: Laminin, alpha-4
LAMP2: Lysosome-associated membrane protein 2
LDB3: Lim domain-binding 3
LMNA: Lamin A/C
LRRC10: Leucine-rich repeat-containing protein 10
LV: Left ventricular
MAP2K1: Mitogen-activated protein kinase kinase 1
MAP2K2: Mitogen-activated protein kinase kinase 2
MIB1: E3 ubiquitin protein ligase 1
MURC/CAVIN4: Muscle-related coiled-coil protein/caveolae-associated protein 4
MYBPC3: Cardiac myosin-binding protein C3
MYBPC3: Myosin-binding protein C, cardiac
MYH6: Myosin, heavy chain 6, cardiac muscle, alpha
MYH7: Myosin heavy chain 7
MYH7: Myosin, heavy chain 7, cardiac muscle, beta
MYL2: Myosin, light chain 2, regulatory, cardiac, slow
MYL3: Myosin, light chain 3, alkali, ventricular, skeletal, slow
MYLK2: Myosin light chain kinase 2
MYOM1: Myomesin 1
MYOT: Myotilin
MYOZ2: Myozenin 2
MYPN: Myopalladin
NCM: Noncompaction cardiomyopathy
NEBL: Nebulette
NEXN: Nexilin (F actin binding protein)
NKX2-5: Nk2 homeobox 5
NRAS: Neuroblastoma Ras viral oncogene homolog
NT-ProBNP: N-Terminal Pro Brain Natriuretic Peptide
NYHA: New York Heart Association
PC4: Potassium channel 4
PDLIM3: Pdz and Lim domain protein 3
PKP2: Plakophilin 2
PLN: Phospholamban
PRDM16: Pr domain-containing protein 16
PRKAG2: Protein kinase, Amp-Activated, noncatalytic, gamma-2
PTPN11: Protein-tyrosine phosphatase, nonreceptor-type, 11
RAF1: V-Raf-1 murine leukemia viral oncogene homolog 1
RBM20: Rna-binding motif protein 20
RCM: Restrictive cardiomyopathy
RIT1: Ras-like without Caax 1
RVNC: Right ventricular noncompaction
RYR2: Ryanodine receptor 2 (cardiac)
SCD: Sudden cardiac death
SCN5A: Sodium channel, voltage-gated, type v, alpha subunit
SGCA: Sarcoglycan alpha
SGCB: Sarcoglycan beta
SGCD: Sarcoglycan dDelta
SHOC2: Soc-2 homolog
SLC25A4: Carrier, adenine nucleotide translocator
SOS1: Son of sevenless, drosophila, homolog 1
TAZ: Tafazzin
TAZZ: Tafazzin gene
TBX20: T-Box 20 gene
Tcap: Telethonin
TCAP: Titin-Cap (telethonin)
TGFB3: Transforming growth factor beta 3
TMEM43: Transmembrane protein 43
TMPO: Thymopoietin
TNNC1: Troponin C type 1 (slow)
TNNI3: Troponin I type 3 (cardiac)
TNNT2: Troponin T type 2 (cardiac)
TOR1AIP1: Torsin-1a-interacting protein 1
TPM1: Tropomyosin 1 (Alpha)
TRDN: Triadin
TTN: Titin
TTR: Transthyretin
TXNRD2: Thioredoxin reductase 2
VCL: Vinculin protein
XLCM: X-linked cardiomyopathy

A complete reference list is available at www.ExpertConsult.com.

SELECT REFERENCES

1. Lee TM, Hsu DT, Kantor P, et al. Pediatric cardiomyopathies. *Circ Res.* 2017;121:855–873.
2. Hershberger RE, Givertz MM, Ho CY, et al. Genetic evaluation of cardiomyopathy: a clinical practice resource of the American College of Medical Genetics and Genomics (ACMG). *Genet Med.* 2018;20:899–909.
3. Maron BJ, Towbin JA, Thiene G, et al. Contemporary definitions and classification of the cardiomyopathies: an American Heart Association Scientific Statement from the Council on Clinical Cardiology, Heart Failure and Transplantation Committee; Quality of Care and Outcomes Research and Functional Genomics and Translational Biology Interdisciplinary Working Groups; and Council on Epidemiology and Prevention. *Circulation.* 2006;113:1807–1816.
4. Ware SM. Evaluation of genetic causes of cardiomyopathy in childhood. *Cardiol Young.* 2015;25(suppl 2):43–50.
5. Towbin JA, McKenna WJ, Abrams DJ, et al. 2019 HRS expert consensus statement on evaluation, risk stratification, and management of arrhythmogenic cardiomyopathy. *Heart Rhythm.* 2019;16(11):e301–e372.
6. Lipshultz SE, Sleeper LA, Towbin JA, et al. The incidence of pediatric cardiomyopathy in two regions of the United States. *N Engl J Med.* 2003;348:1647–1655.
7. Centers for Disease Control and Prevention. In: *Sudden Unexpected Infant Death and Sudden Infant Death Syndrome*. CDC Website; 2017.
8. Schwartz SM, Duffy JY, Pearl JM, et al. Cellular and molecular aspects of myocardial dysfunction. *Crit Care Med.* 2001;29:S214–S219.
9. Fritz-Six KL, Cox PR, Fischer RS, et al. Aberrant myofibril assembly in tropomodulin1 null mice leads to aborted heart development and embryonic lethality. *J Cell Biol.* 2003;163:1033–1044.

10. Clark KA, McElhinny AS, Beckerle MC, et al. Striated muscle cytoarchitecture: an intricate web of form and function. *Annu Rev Cell Dev Biol*. 2002;18:637-706.
11. Wang J, Shaner N, Mittal B, et al. Dynamics of Z-band based proteins in developing skeletal muscle cells. *Cell Motil Cytoskeleton*. 2005;61:34-48.
12. Gul IS, Hulpiau P, Saeys Y, et al. Evolution and diversity of cadherins and catenins. *Exp Cell Res*. 2017;358:3-9.
13. Capetanaki Y. Desmin cytoskeleton: a potential regulator of muscle mitochondrial behavior and function. *Trends Cardiovasc Med*. 2002;12:339-348.
14. Capetanaki Y. Desmin cytoskeleton in healthy and failing heart. *Heart Fail Rev*. 2000;5:203-220.
15. Sharp WW, Simpson DG, Borg TK, et al. Mechanical forces regulate focal adhesion and costamere assembly in cardiac myocytes. *Am J Physiol*. 1997;273:H546-H556.
16. Rando TA. The dystrophin-glycoprotein complex, cellular signaling, and the regulation of cell survival in the muscular dystrophies. *Muscle Nerve*. 2001;24:1575-1594.
17. Sciandra F, Bozzi M, Bianchi M, et al. Dystroglycan and muscular dystrophies related to the dystrophin-glycoprotein complex. *Ann Ist Super Sanita*. 2003;39:173-181.
18. Kucera JP, Rohr S, Rudy Y. Localization of sodium channels in intercalated disks modulates cardiac conduction. *Circ Res*. 2002;91:1176-1182.
19. Bowles NE, Bowles KR, Towbin JA. The "final common pathway" hypothesis and inherited cardiovascular disease. The role of cytoskeletal proteins in dilated cardiomyopathy. *Herz*. 2000;25:168-175.
20. Merlo M, Cannata A, Gobbo M, et al. Evolving concepts in dilated cardiomyopathy. *Eur J Heart Fail*. 2018;20:228-239.
21. Silva JN, Canter CE. Current management of pediatric dilated cardiomyopathy. *Curr Opin Cardiol*. 2010;25:80-87.
22. Jefferies JL, Towbin JA. Dilated cardiomyopathy. *Lancet*. 2010;375:752-762.
23. Towbin JA, Lowe AM, Colan SD, et al. Incidence, causes, and outcomes of dilated cardiomyopathy in children. *J Am Med Assoc*. 2006;296:1867-1876.
24. Everitt MD, Wilkinson JD, Shi L, et al. Cardiac biomarkers in pediatric cardiomyopathy: study design and recruitment results from the Pediatric Cardiomyopathy Registry. *Prog Pediatr Cardiol*. 2019;53:1-10.
25. Ross RD. The Ross classification for heart failure in children after 25 years: a review and an age-stratified revision. *Pediatr Cardiol*. 2012;33:1295-1300.
26. Jessup M, Abraham WT, Casey DE, et al. Focused update: ACCF/AHA Guidelines for the diagnosis and management of heart failure in adults: a report of the American College of Cardiology Foundation/American Heart Association Task Force on practice guidelines: developed in collaboration with the International Society for Heart and Lung Transplantation. *Circulation*. 2009;119:1977-2016.
27. Pahl E, Sleeper LA, Canter CE, et al. Incidence of and risk factors for sudden cardiac death in children with dilated cardiomyopathy: a report from the Pediatric Cardiomyopathy Registry. *J Am Coll Cardiol*. 2012;59:607-615.
28. Towbin JA, Bowles NE. The failing heart. *Nature*. 2002;415:227-233.
29. Petretta M, Pirozzi F, Sasso L, et al. Review and metaanalysis of the frequency of familial dilated cardiomyopathy. *Am J Cardiol*. 2011;108:1171-1176.
30. Fatkin D, Huttner IG, Kovacic JC, et al. Precision medicine in the management of dilated cardiomyopathy: JACC State-of-the-Art Review. *J Am Coll Cardiol*. 2019;74:2921-2938.
31. Weischenfeldt J, Symmons O, Spitz F, et al. Phenotypic impact of genomic structural variation: insights from and for human disease. *Nat Rev Genet*. 2013;14:125-138.
32. Minoche AE, Horvat C, Johnson R, et al. Genome sequencing as a first-line genetic test in familial dilated cardiomyopathy. *Genet Med*. 2019;21:650-662.
33. Morita H, Seidman J, Seidman CE. Genetic causes of human heart failure. *J Clin Invest*. 2005;115:518-526.
34. Jefferies JL. Barth syndrome. *Am J Med Genet C Semin Med Genet*. 2013;163C:198-205.
35. Roberts AE, Nixon C, Steward CG, et al. The Barth Syndrome Registry: distinguishing disease characteristics and growth data from a longitudinal study. *Am J Med Genet*. 2012;158A:2726-2732.
36. Hanke SP, Gardner AB, Lombardi JP, et al. Left ventricular noncompaction cardiomyopathy in Barth syndrome: an example of an undulating cardiac phenotype necessitating mechanical circulatory support as a bridge to transplantation. *Pediatr Cardiol*. 2012;33:1430-1434.
37. Barth PG, Scholte HR, Berden JA, et al. An X-linked mitochondrial disease affecting cardiac muscle, skeletal muscle and neutrophil leucocytes. *J Neurol Sci*. 1983;62:327-355.
38. Gigli M, Merlo M, Graw SL, et al. Genetic risk of arrhythmic phenotypes in patients with dilated cardiomyopathy. *J Am Coll Cardiol*. 2019;74:1480-1490.
39. Tsubata S, Bowles KR, Vatta M, et al. Mutations in the human delta-sarcoglycan gene in familial and sporadic dilated cardiomyopathy. *J Clin Invest*. 2000;106:655-662.
40. Li D, Tapscoft T, Gonzalez O, et al. Desmin mutation responsible for idiopathic dilated cardiomyopathy. *Circulation*. 1999;100:461-464.
41. Kamisago M, Sharma SD, DePalma SR, et al. Mutations in sarcomere protein genes as a cause of dilated cardiomyopathy. *N Engl J Med*. 2000;343:1688-1696.
42. Misaka T, Yoshihisa A, Takeishi Y. Titin in muscular dystrophy and cardiomyopathy: urinary titin as a novel marker. *Clin Chim Acta*. 2019;495:123-128.
43. Brodehl A, Gaertner-Rommel A, Milting H. Molecular insights into cardiomyopathies associated with desmin (DES) mutations. *Biophys Rev*. 2018;10:983-1006.
44. Ripoll-Vera T, Zorio E, Gamez JM, et al. Phenotypic patterns of cardiomyopathy caused by mutations in the desmin gene. A clinical and genetic study in two inherited heart disease units. *Rev Esp Cardiol*. 2015;68:1027-1029.
45. Campbell MD, Witcher M, Gopal A, et al. Dilated cardiomyopathy mutations in delta-sarcoglycan exert a dominant-negative effect on cardiac myocyte mechanical stability. *Am J Physiol Heart Circ Physiol*. 2016;310:H1140-H1150.
46. Mitsuhashi S, Saito N, Watano K, et al. Defect of delta-sarcoglycan gene is responsible for development of dilated cardiomyopathy of a novel hamster strain, J2N-k: calcineurin/PP2B activity in the heart of J2N-k hamster. *J Biochem*. 2003;134:269-276.
47. Lee YK, Lau YM, Cai ZJ, et al. Modeling treatment response for lamin a/c related dilated cardiomyopathy in human induced pluripotent stem cells. *J Am Heart Assoc*. 2017;6.
48. Perez-Serra A, Toro R, Campuzano O, et al. A novel mutation in lamin a/c causing familial dilated cardiomyopathy associated with sudden cardiac death. *J Card Fail*. 2015;21:217-225.
49. Tesson F, Saj M, Uvaize MM, et al. Lamin A/C mutations in dilated cardiomyopathy. *Cardiol J*. 2014;21:331-342.
50. Hoffman EP, Brown Jr RH, Kunkel LM. Dystrophin: the protein product of the Duchenne muscular dystrophy locus. *Cell*. 1987;51:919-928.

154 Pathophysiology of Persistent Pulmonary Hypertension of the Newborn

Satyan Lakshminrusimha | Robin H. Steinhorn

INTRODUCTION

Persistent pulmonary hypertension of the newborn (PPHN) is a syndrome of failed circulatory adaptation at birth, which is seen in about 2 in 1000 live-born infants; the incidence has not changed significantly over the last 20 years.[1,2] The syndrome is characterized by a sustained elevation of pulmonary vascular resistance (PVR) and is often associated with normal or low systemic vascular resistance (SVR). Consequently these infants exhibit extrapulmonary right-to-left shunting across persistent fetal channels (patent ductus arteriosus and patent foramen ovale), leading to labile hypoxemia. PPHN was previously referred to as *persistent fetal circulation*.[3] Although it is seen mostly in term and late-preterm infants, it is recognized in up to 2% of premature infants with respiratory distress syndrome (RDS).[4,5] Most commonly, PPHN is secondary to delayed or impaired relaxation of the pulmonary vasculature and associated with a diverse group of pulmonary pathologies (e.g., meconium aspiration syndrome [MAS], congenital diaphragmatic hernia [CDH], pneumonia, and RDS). This chapter reviews the applied pathophysiology of fetal pulmonary circulation, pulmonary vascular transition at birth, hemodynamic and biochemical changes associated with PPHN, and the physiologic basis of various therapeutic interventions.

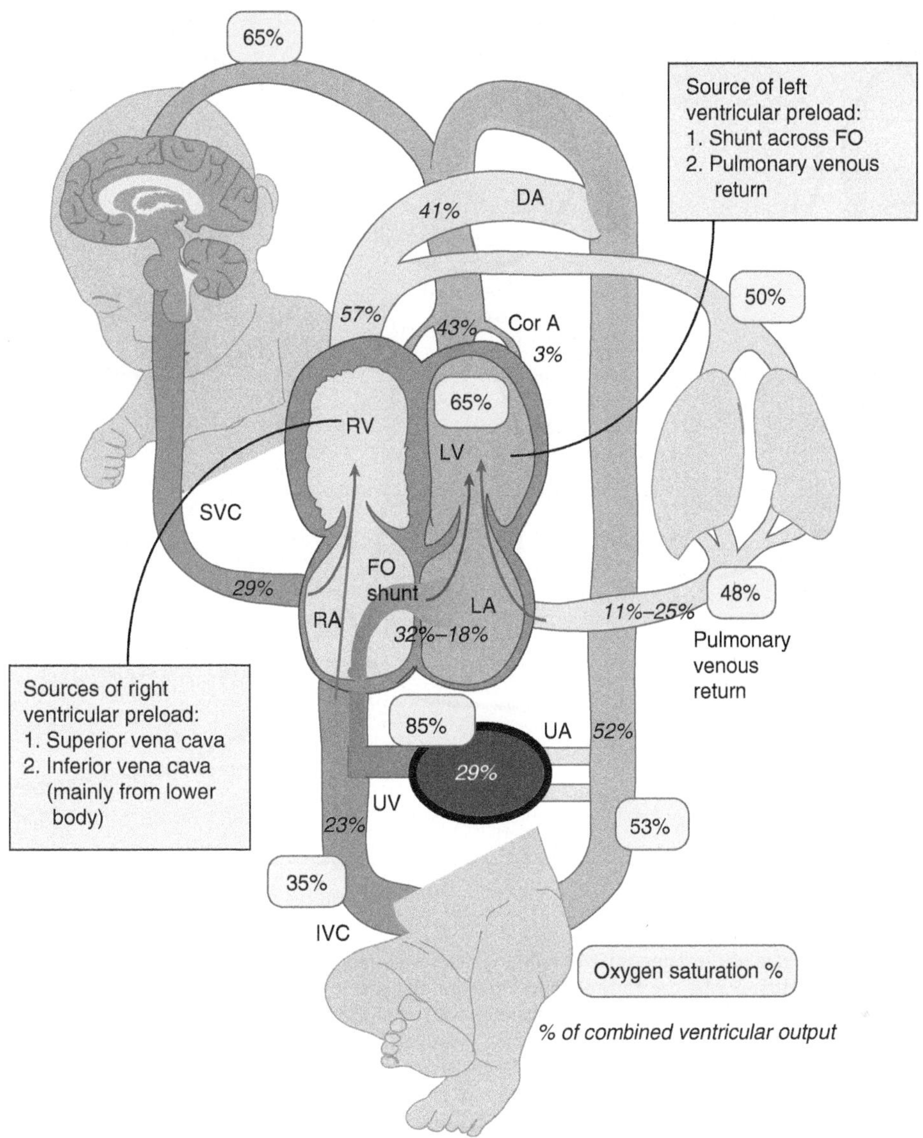

Fig. 154.1 Fetal circulation. Circulatory pattern in a normal human fetus at late gestation. The numbers shown as percentages in italics represent percentage of combined ventricular output based on data from human fetuses. The numbers in *light green boxes* represent oxygen saturation based on data from fetal lambs. The *blue shade* indicates lower oxygen saturation.[12,13,228,229] *Cor A,* Coronary arteries; *DA,* ductus arteriosus; *FO,* foramen ovale; *IVC,* inferior vena cava; *LA,* left atrium; *LV,* left ventricle; *RA,* right atrium; *RV,* right ventricle; *SVC,* superior vena cava; *UA,* umbilical arteries; *UV,* umbilical vein. (Copyright 2020, Lakshminrusimha and Steinhorn.)

FETAL PULMONARY CIRCULATORY PHYSIOLOGY

The fetus is in a state of physiologic pulmonary hypertension. In the fetal lamb, the pulmonary arterial blood has a partial pressure of oxygen (Po_2) of approximately 18 mm Hg and oxygen saturation (So_2) of 50%.[6] The PVR is high partly secondary to hypoxic pulmonary vasoconstriction. The pattern of blood flow in a normal fetus is shown in Fig. 154.1. Our understanding of human fetal hemodynamics has improved secondary to cine cardiovascular magnetic resonance imaging (MRI) techniques. The opposing magnetic properties of oxy- and deoxyhemoglobin can quantify blood oxygenation.[7] Human fetal studies demonstrate higher cerebral and pulmonary blood flow (PBF) and lower umbilical flow compared with sheep studies.[7] The blood is oxygenated in the placenta and returns to the body through the umbilical vein (So_2 ~ 82% to 88% and Po_2 32 to 35 mm Hg in lambs).[6] The umbilical venous return is preferentially directed through the ductus venosus and left lobe of the liver to form a high-velocity stream (with a velocity three to four times higher velocity than that of the flow in the inferior vena cava [IVC]; 59 to 71 cm/s vs. 16 cm/s)[8] in the leftward posterior aspect of the IVC,[9] which is directed toward the foramen ovale and the left ventricle (see Fig. 154.1).[6,10] This mechanism maintains a higher oxygen content of the blood in the left heart (~65% with higher glucose content—which supplies cerebral and coronary circulation, and approximately 15% higher saturation than pulmonary arterial and umbilical arterial saturation ~50% to 52%). The same streaming mechanism results in deoxygenated blood shunted to the placenta via the ductus arteriosus. ***This umbilical venous oxygenated blood shunting through the foramen ovale is an important component of left ventricular preload in the fetus.*** Because of high PVR, only about 16% of the combined ventricular output (11% to 25% in various studies)[11-13] is directed to the lungs; the remainder passes through the ductus arteriosus to the descending aorta. The difference in So_2 (a measure of oxygen uptake from the organ of gas exchange) between the

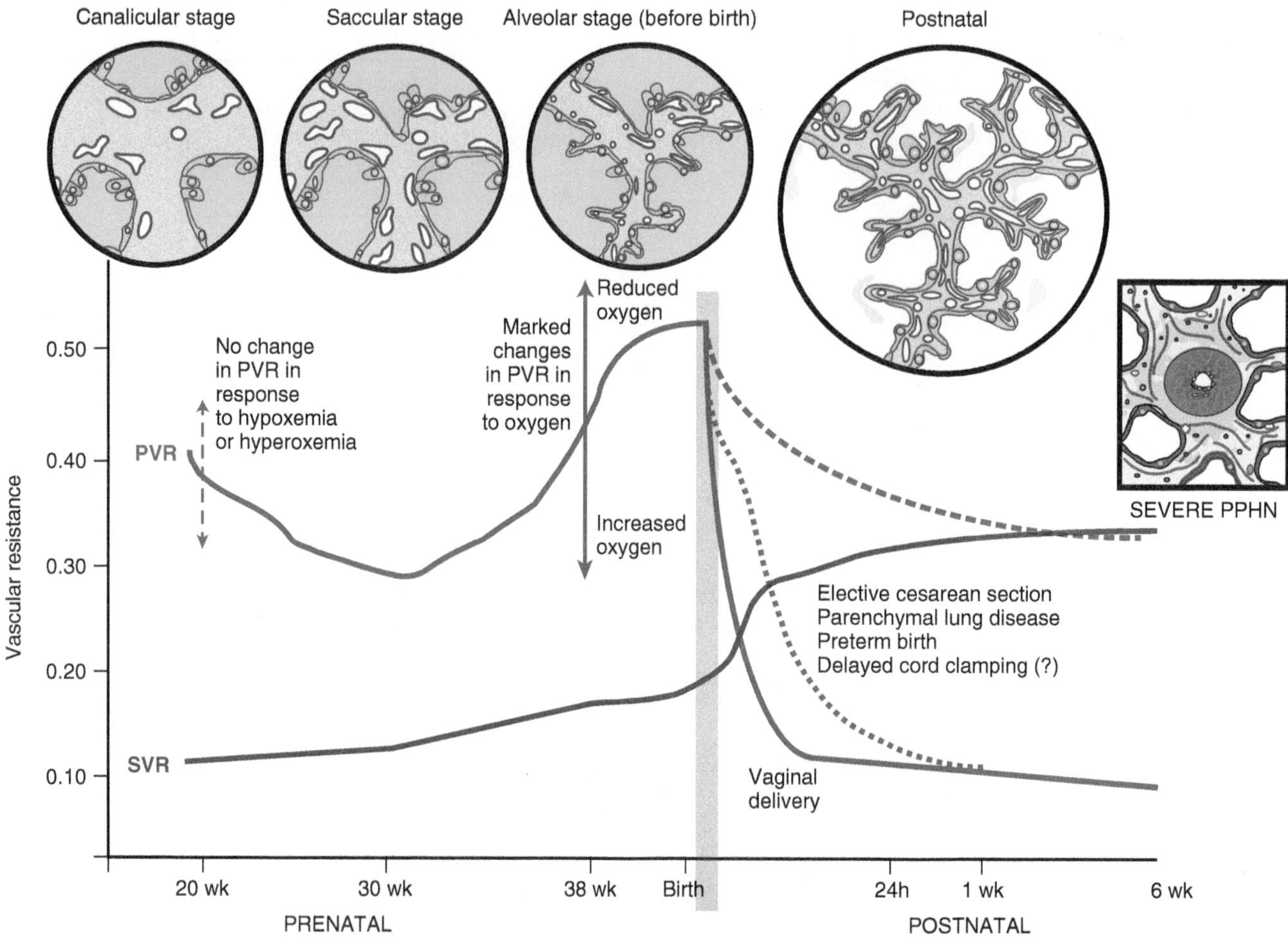

Fig. 154.2 Changes in pulmonary vascular resistance (*PVR, blue line*) and systemic vascular resistance *(red line)* during the last half of gestation and postnatal period in a human fetus. During the early second trimester, the pulmonary vasculature does not respond to changes in oxygen tension *(dashed black arrows).* During the third trimester, PVR changes with changes in oxygen tension (*solid black arrows*). The *dotted PVR line* represents the delayed decrease of PVR observed following elective cesarean section, preterm birth, parenchymal lung disease, and possibly delayed cord clamping. The *dashed PVR line* represents severe PPHN where PVR is closed to systemic vascular resistance. *PPHN*, Persistent pulmonary hypertension of the newborn. (Copyright 2020, Lakshminrusimha and Steinhorn.)

umbilical vein (85%) and umbilical artery (52%) during fetal life (see Fig. 154.1) is similar to the difference between the pulmonary vein/aorta (95% to 100%) and pulmonary artery (60% to 70%) in an adult. The fetus achieves normal oxygen delivery at low Po_2 levels (<35 mm Hg) compared with the postnatal period, thus limiting the risk of oxygen toxicity.

CHANGES IN PULMONARY VASCULAR RESISTANCE AND PULMONARY BLOOD FLOW WITH GESTATION

Rasanen and colleagues[12] used direct measurements of PBF in the right and left pulmonary arteries and found that it is approximately 21% of combined ventricular output by 38 weeks in human fetuses. Phase-contrast cine-MRI[13] in late-gestation human fetuses demonstrated that PBF is 74 ± 43 mL/kg/min or approximately 16% ± 9% of combined ventricular output. There was a 10-fold difference in PBF between subjects (2% to 30% of combined ventricular output). It is possible that PBF is dynamic[14] and varies between different fetal subjects, at different times within the same subject, and with advancing gestation.[12]

Doppler flow studies in human fetuses have demonstrated that flow into the left and right pulmonary arteries is 13% of combined ventricular output at 20 weeks of gestation (canalicular stage); it increases to 25% at 30 weeks (saccular stage) and decreases to 21% at 38 weeks (alveolar stage) (Fig. 154.2).[12] The fetal PVR is high during the canalicular stage secondary to the paucity of a pulmonary vascular network, leading to a reduced cross-sectional area of the immature pulmonary vascular bed. Experiments in fetal lambs have shown that the PBF does not increase in response to hyperoxia at 94 to 101 days' gestation (term ~147 days).[15] At this gestation, fetal hypoxia results in very minimal change in PVR.[16] Similarly, Rasanen and colleagues demonstrated that, between 20 and 26 weeks of gestation, maternal hyperoxygenation using 60% oxygen by face mask does not result in pulmonary vasodilation in the human fetus.[17] These findings suggest a lack of sensitivity to oxygen and high PVR in early gestation. Interestingly, birth at this gestational age (23 to 26 weeks in humans) is associated with a much higher risk (2%) of pulmonary hypertension compared with term gestation (0.2%)[4,5] and high rates of clinical use of inhaled nitric oxide (iNO).[18-20] In an Australia-New Zealand database of neonatal intensive care unit admissions requiring invasive ventilation, the U-shaped curve of PVR during fetal life (see Fig. 154.2) resembled the U-shaped curve of iNO (Fig. 154.3) use: 15.4% at 24 to 25 weeks, 3.8% at 30 to 31 weeks, and 19% at 37 to 44 weeks of gestational age at birth.[19,21] Similar trends in iNO use were observed among preterm infants in the Ohio Perinatal Network (17.5% at 22 to 24 weeks and 3.7% at 31 to 33 weeks' gestational age at birth)[18] and California Perinatal Quality Care (4.9% at 22 to 24 weeks, 1.1% at 31 to 33 weeks, and 6.2% at 38 to 43 weeks).[20] During the early saccular stage, the rapid proliferation of pulmonary vessels decreases fetal PVR; during late

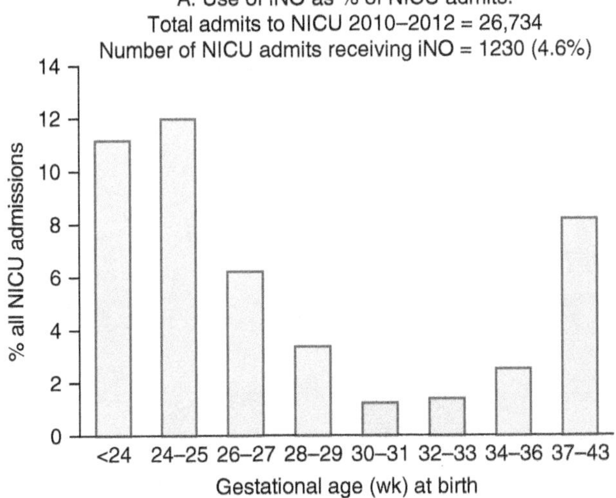

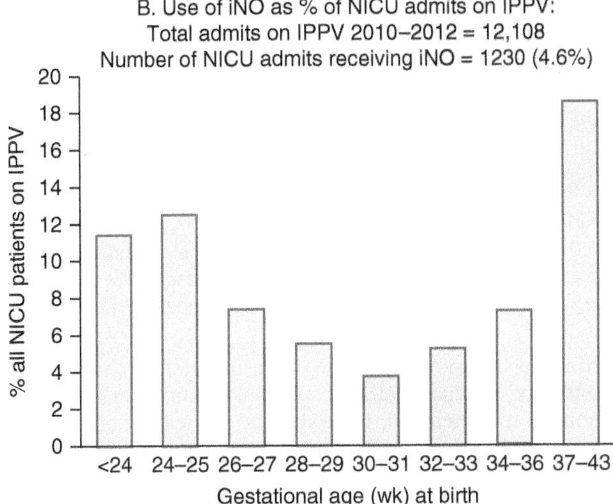

Fig. 154.3 The use of inhaled nitric oxide based on gestational age at birth from 2010 to 2012 derived from the reports of the Australian and New Zealand Neonatal Network (ANZNN). The top graph is the percentage of all eligible admissions to the neonatal intensive care units *(NICUs)* at that specific gestational age group. The bottom graph is the percentage of all admits who received at least 4 hours of intermittent positive pressure ventilation. Note that the last two columns (34 to 36 weeks and 37 to 43 weeks of gestation) may not represent all births in that gestational age group, indicating only admissions to the NICU that met ANZNN registration criteria. Both of these curves demonstrate a U-shaped pattern with few infants receiving inhaled nitric oxide at 30 to 31 weeks' gestation. (With permission from the ANZNN.)

gestation, there is a marked increase in cross-sectional area of the pulmonary vascular bed. However, pulmonary vessels become more sensitive to vasoconstrictive mediators such as endothelin and hypoxia during this period, resulting in active pulmonary vasoconstriction (see Fig. 154.2)[16,22] and dilation in response to increased oxygen.[23,24] In late-gestation lambs (136 to 146 days of gestation), maternal hyperbaric hyperoxia increased pulmonary arterial Po_2 from 19 ± 1.5 to 48 ± 9 mm Hg, leading to an increase in PBF from 34 ± 3.3 to 298 ± 35mL/kg per minute.[15] Similarly, maternal hyperoxygenation increased PBF in late-gestation (31 to 36 weeks) human fetuses.[17] The maternal hyperoxygenation test (administered with 60% oxygen by face mask) has been proposed to measure the ability of fetal pulmonary arteries to vasodilate in response to oxygen in late gestation and predict pulmonary vascular reactivity and survival in cases of CDH.[25]

In fetal lambs, pulmonary vasodilation in response to endothelium-independent mediators such as NO precedes response to endothelium-dependent mediators such as acetylcholine and oxygen. Response to NO is dependent on activity of its target enzyme, soluble guanylate cyclase (sGC), in the smooth muscle cell (Fig. 154.4). In the ovine fetus, sGC mRNA levels are low during early preterm (126 days) gestation and increase markedly during late preterm and early term gestation (137 days).[26] Low levels of pulmonary arterial sGC activity during the late canalicular and early saccular stages of lung development may partly explain the poor response to iNO observed in some extremely preterm infants.[4]

FETAL GROWTH RESTRICTION AND PULMONARY BLOOD FLOW

Fetal growth restriction is associated with chronic hypoxia and reductions in umbilical venous So_2 and flow.[27] Lower So_2 in the ascending aorta is associated with higher superior vena caval flow ("brain-sparing physiology"). In contrast, lower So_2 in pulmonary arteries is associated with decreased PBF.[7] Pulmonary hypertension with bronchopulmonary dysplasia (BPD) is associated with fetal growth restriction in preterm infants and with a trend toward higher morbidity and mortality during longitudinal follow-up.[28] In the SUPPORT trial, randomization to a lower So_2 target was associated with increased mortality in growth-restricted infants with RDS and BPD as leading causes.[29] However, individual patient data meta-analysis of all the oxygen saturation trials in preterm infants did not show a similar association.[30] Other mechanisms in addition to hypoxemia may also contribute to a higher incidence of PPHN in growth-restricted infants.[31]

FETAL PULMONARY VASCULAR RESISTANCE AND LEFT VENTRICULAR FILLING

The shunt across the foramen ovale and PBF are the two sources of left ventricular filling during fetal life (see Fig. 154.1). Left ventricular preload is an important determinant of blood flow to the heart and brain and of left ventricular development. Prsa et al. found a strong inverse correlation between foramen ovale shunt and PBF in human fetuses.[12,13] The physiologic mechanism behind this finding is not clear. One potential explanation is that fetal PVR is very sensitive to small changes in Po_2. Arraut et al., working with nonhuman primate fetuses, evaluated the effect of maternal hypoxemia (by the administration of 12% oxygen) and hyperoxemia (by the administration of 100% oxygen) on the fetal right pulmonary arterial pulsatility index (PI) (PI = [peak systolic velocity − end-diastolic velocity] ÷ time-averaged maximum velocity over the cardiac cycle).[14] An increase in right pulmonary arterial PI suggests an increase in peripheral pulmonary vasoconstriction with decreased flow. Maternal hypoxemia increased the fetal right pulmonary arterial PI fivefold, suggesting fetal pulmonary vasoconstriction. Maternal hyperoxemia decreased the right pulmonary arterial PI fourfold and also decreased blood flow through the ductus arteriosus. Maternal oxygenation status did not affect the umbilical arterial or ductus venosus PI, suggesting that umbilical flow is neither influenced by nor regulates fetal oxygenation.[14] Similarly, Konduri et al. showed that an increase in pulmonary arterial Po_2 of 7 mm Hg resulted in a threefold increase in PBF in fetal lambs.[32] However, the variability of PI changes in response to maternal hyperoxygenation have limited the utility of PI as a diagnostic tool.[33]

These studies indicate that fetal PVR is dynamic and an important regulator of the distribution of cardiac output and the relative contributions of the pulmonary circulation and foramen ovale shunt to left ventricular filling. The So_2 of blood

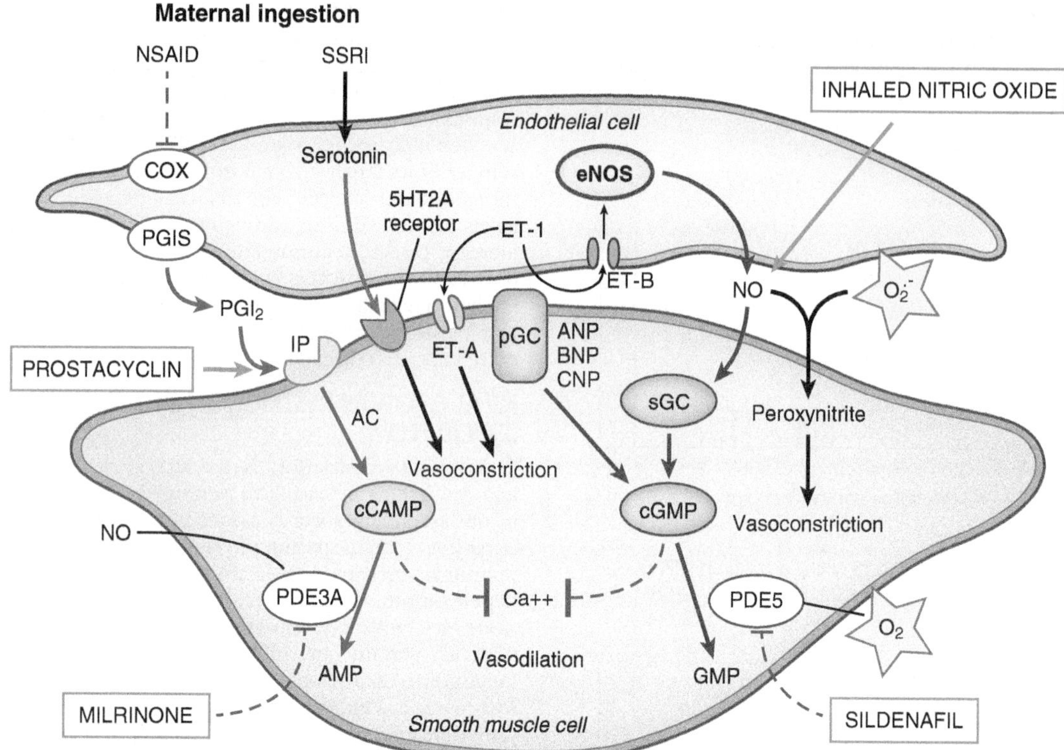

Fig. 154.4 Endothelium-derived vasodilators. Prostacyclin *(PGI₂)*, nitric oxide *(NO)*, and vasoconstrictor (endothelin *[ET-1]*) pathways. Therapeutic interventions are shown in black boxes. *AC,* Adenylate cyclase; *ANP,* atrial natriuretic peptide; *BNP,* brain type natriuretic peptide; *CNP,* C-type natriuretic peptide; *COX,* cyclooxygenase; *eNOS,* endothelial nitric oxide synthase; *PDE,* phosphodiesterase; *pGC,* particulate guanylate cyclase; *PGIS,* prostacyclin synthase; *sGC,* soluble guanylate cyclase.[119,166,167] (Copyright 2020, Lakshminrusimha and Steinhorn.)

in the left atrium (and left ventricle) is dependent on the relative contributions of oxygenated blood from the foramen ovale and deoxygenated blood from the pulmonary veins. The mean value is usually around 65%. During periods of hypoxemia, fetal PVR increases markedly[34,35] and the left ventricle is filled with better oxygenated umbilical venous blood shunted across the foramen ovale (see Fig. 154.1). Conversely, during maternal hyperoxemia, PBF increases and flow through the ductus arteriosus and foramen ovale decreases.[17,36] These changes in PVR will determine the distribution of fetal cardiac output[12] and oxygen delivery to the brain and heart.[37] Furthermore, reduced pulmonary venous return and left ventricular filling in fetuses with CDH may contribute to left ventricular hypoplasia, emphasizing the role of PBF during fetal life.[38,39]

FACTORS CONTRIBUTING TO FETAL PULMONARY VASCULAR RESISTANCE

Numerous factors—such as mechanical factors (compression of the small pulmonary arterioles by the fluid-filled alveoli and a lack of rhythmic distension) and a relative lack of vasodilators—contribute to the high PVR in utero.[40] Low oxygen tension and elevated levels of vasoconstictor mediators, such as endothelin-1 (ET-1) and thromboxane, play a crucial role in maintaining the elevated fetal PVR.[40]

MODULATION OF FETAL PULMONARY VASCULAR RESISTANCE

Conditions such as CDH, antenatal closure of the ductus arteriosus, and idiopathic PPHN are often associated with vascular remodeling and elevated PVR during fetal life. Studies in animal models and human populations have suggested that maternal therapy can alter fetal PVR. Two classes of medications, selective serotonin receptor inhibitors (SSRIs) and nonsteroidal antiinflammatory agents (NSAIDs), have been relatively well studied.

Serotonin infusions increase PVR in fetal lambs,[41,42] and exposure of pregnant rats to the SSRI fluoxetine produced pulmonary hypertension, hypoxia, and increased mortality in rat pups.[43,44] The use of SSRIs during the last half of pregnancy has been associated with an increased incidence of PPHN in at least three human studies.[45-48] Although the mechanism by which SSRIs induce pulmonary hypertension in the newborn is not known, it is speculated that drug-induced elevation in serotonin levels results in pulmonary vasoconstriction. Some studies have questioned the association between maternal SSRI intake and PPHN.[49,50] Furthermore, the severity of PPHN has not been well described; a report observed no differences in right pulmonary artery Doppler PI in fetuses of mothers exposed to SSRI antidepressants.[51] In addition, the risk appears to be more with exposure beyond 20 weeks of gestation. Alternate antidepressants, such as selective serotonin norepinephrine reuptake inhibitors (SNRIs), are not well studied, and their association with PPHN in offspring is not known at this time.[52] At present, maternal physical and psychological well-being should be the primary factor guiding antidepressant therapy during pregnancy and the postpartum period.

Ingestion of NSAIDs such as aspirin during late gestation may be associated with closure of the fetal ductus arteriosus.[53] Experimental ligation or constriction of the ductus arteriosus in lambs during fetal life is associated with the rapid development of pulmonary vascular remodeling and PPHN.[54] Prostaglandins maintain ductal patency in utero and are important mediators of pulmonary vasodilation in response to ventilation at birth. Pharmacologic blockade of prostaglandin production by NSAIDs can result in PPHN. Analysis of meconium from newborn infants with PPHN revealed the presence of a NSAID in approximately half of the samples,[55] linking antenatal NSAID exposure to PPHN. This association has been questioned,[56] although aspirin use during late pregnancy remains a risk factor for PPHN.

Maternal medications also have the potential to correct pathologic fetal vascular development. Maternal betamethasone reduced oxidative stress and improved the relaxation response to adenosine triphosphate and NO donors in fetal lambs with PPHN induced by ductal ligation.[57] In fetal rats with nitrofen-induced CDH, antenatal administration of sildenafil to the dam improved lung structure (decreased mean linear intercept) and reduced pulmonary hypertension (decreased right ventricle/left ventricle + septum ratio).[58] However, the use of sildenafil during pregnancy may be associated with adverse effects on the fetus. The Sildenafil TheRapy in dismal prognosis early onset fetal growth restriction (STRIDER), an international consortium of randomized placebo-controlled trials, explored the effects of sildenafil for treatment of fetal growth restriction in four trials. The Dutch STRIDER trial was suspended evoking significant global interest in media reports due to a signal of potential harm relating to increased PPHN and a nonsignificant trend towards an increase in neonatal death. In contrast, the UK and New Zealand/Australia STRIDER trials found no evidence of PPHN or neonatal death but did not find any beneficial effect of sildenafil therapy on fetal growth restriction. This consortium strongly recommends not to prescribe sildenafil for fetal growth restriction outside clinical trials until more data are available.[59]

TRANSITION AT BIRTH

After birth and following initiation of air breathing, PBF markedly increases,[40,60] resolving fetal physiologic pulmonary hypertension.[61] In some infants with adverse in utero events or with abnormalities of pulmonary transition at birth, pulmonary hypertension persists into the newborn period, resulting in PPHN and hypoxemic respiratory failure (HRF).[62,63]

A series of circulatory events take place at birth to ensure a smooth transition from fetal to extrauterine life. Clamping of the umbilical cord removes the low resistance placental circulation, increasing SVR (see Fig. 154.2). Simultaneously, various mechanisms operate to rapidly reduce pulmonary arterial pressure and increase PBF. Of these, the most important stimuli appear to be ventilation of the lungs and an increase in oxygen tension.[60] The vascular endothelium releases several vasoactive products that play a critical role in achieving rapid pulmonary vasodilation. Pulmonary endothelial NO production increases markedly at the time of birth. Oxygen is believed to be an important catalyst for this increased NO production, although the precise mechanism is not clear. NO exerts its action through sGC and cyclic guanosine monophosphate (cGMP) (see Fig. 154.4). Bloch et al. reported that expression of sGC peaks in late gestation in rats,[64] which may explain the better response to NO at birth in neonates than in any other reported age group. Phosphodiesterase 5 (PDE5) catalyzes the breakdown of cGMP (see Fig. 154.4). Similar to sGC, expression of PDE5 in the lungs peaks in the immediate newborn period in sheep and rats.[65,66] The recognition of the role of NO in mediating pulmonary vascular transition at birth[67] has led to the development of iNO as a therapeutic strategy in PPHN.

The arachidonic acid–prostacyclin pathway also plays an important role in the transition at birth. The cyclooxygenase enzyme acts on arachidonic acid to produce prostaglandin endoperoxides. Prostaglandins activate adenylate cyclase to increase cAMP concentrations in vascular smooth muscle cells. Phosphodiesterase 3A (PDE3A) catalyzes the breakdown of cAMP (see Fig. 154.4).

CIRCUMSTANCES THAT RESULT IN ABNORMAL VASCULAR TRANSITION AT BIRTH

CESAREAN SECTION

Vaginal delivery is associated with a reduction in fetal PVR at birth. In comparison, delivery by elective cesarean section[68–70] delays the decrease in pulmonary arterial pressure (see Fig. 154.2), as evidenced by prolonged right-sided systolic time intervals and increases the risk of PPHN.[71] Compared with matched control subjects, infants with PPHN are more likely to have been delivered by cesarean section.[49,72]

EARLY VERSUS DELAYED CORD CLAMPING

Early clamping of the umbilical cord before the first breath results in a decrease in heart size during the first 3 or 4 cardiac cycles, presumably due to decreased left ventricular filling.[73] In preterm lambs, delaying cord clamping for 3 to 4 minutes until after ventilation is established improves cardiovascular function by increasing PVR and left ventricular filling before the cessation of umbilical venous return.[74] The precise effect of delayed cord clamping on pulmonary vascular transition is not clear. Interestingly, Arcilla et al. demonstrated increased pulmonary arterial pressure following late cord clamping in newborn infants nearly 50 years ago by catheterizing the pulmonary artery.[75] There are no reports of increased incidence of PPHN associated with delayed cord clamping. In lambs with CDH, a condition commonly associated with PPHN, delayed cord clamping after onset of effective ventilation results in a threefold decrease in PVR.[76] Two delivery room trials have demonstrated the feasibility of this technique without any negative consequences.[77,78] Larger trials are needed to confirm the benefits of delayed cord clamping in CDH. Similarly, it is possible that a slower decrease in PVR may offer circulatory stability in extremely preterm infants.

EXTREME PRETERM BIRTH

The decrease in pulmonary arterial pressure after birth is significantly slower in preterm infants (especially if associated with RDS) than in term infants.[79] The pulmonary arterial pressure is increased relative to the systemic arterial pressure, and such elevation may persist for a few days in extremely preterm infants with respiratory disease.[80,81] Skimming et al. have questioned whether the naturally increased PVR affords benefit to the preterm infant by reducing the ductal steal and stabilizing systemic circulation.[82] Such delay in decrease in PVR may contribute to the high incidence of PPHN in extremely preterm infants.[83]

ASPHYXIA

Perinatal asphyxia interferes with the mechanisms of pulmonary transition at birth and modifies this complex adaptation by impeding the fall in PVR and increasing the risk for PPHN.[84] A wide variety of pathophysiologic processes cause respiratory failure and increase PVR, including fetal hypoxemia, ischemia, meconium aspiration, ventricular dysfunction, and fetal acidosis.[84] Acute asphyxia is associated with reversible pulmonary vasoconstriction,[85] but chronic in utero asphyxia with or without meconium aspiration may be associated with vasoconstriction and vascular remodeling.[86]

There was considerable concern that therapeutic hypothermia in asphyxiated infants with moderate to severe hypoxic-ischemic encephalopathy (HIE) would increase the risk of PPHN. Induction of severe hypothermia in 1- to 3-day-old lambs (decreasing temperature from 40°C to 30°C) increased mean pulmonary arterial pressure from 29 to 40 mm Hg.[87] However, the effect of moderate hypothermia (33.5°C) on PVR is not known. Pooled analysis of randomized trials has not shown an increased incidence of PPHN (25% in moderate hypothermia vs. 20% in normothermia) with hypothermia in this population.[88] The type of cooling (selective head cooling vs. whole-body cooling) does not alter the incidence of PPHN.[89] In infants with moderate to severe HIE, the presence of PPHN significantly increases mortality (~27% vs. 16% in a study from the Neonatal Research Network).[90]

OXYGEN DURING NEONATAL RESUSCITATION

The use of 100% oxygen during initial ventilation of normal lambs at birth results in a small but significantly greater decrease in PVR during the first few minutes of life compared with 21% or 50% oxygen.[91] However, ventilation with 100% oxygen at birth impairs subsequent relaxation to iNO and acetylcholine, probably due to the formation of reactive oxygen species (ROS). Similar results were observed in lambs with PPHN and remodeled pulmonary vasculature.[92] In lambs with asphyxia induced by umbilical cord occlusion, PVR was lower at 1 minute of age when 100% oxygen was used for resuscitation compared with 21% oxygen; by 2 minutes, however, PVR was similar in both groups. These findings suggest that optimal ventilation (and not hyperoxygenation) is the key to reducing PVR.[93] Thirty minutes of resuscitation with 100% oxygen increased pulmonary arterial contractility and superoxide anion formation in pulmonary arteries. Therefore the use of 100% oxygen has transient advantages in rapidly reducing PVR; however, it increases the formation of ROS, increases pulmonary arterial contractility, and impairs vasodilation to endothelium-dependent (acetylcholine) and endothelium-independent (iNO) agents. These findings support the neonatal resuscitation guidelines that recommend the use of room air for the initial resuscitation of asphyxiated newborn term infants.[94]

In one study involving extremely preterm infants, the use of room air for initial resuscitation was associated with increased mortality from respiratory causes.[95] It is possible that higher levels of inspired oxygen may be necessary to mediate pulmonary vasodilation due to factors such as mask leaks, immature alveolar architecture, and a high alveolar-arterial gradient in extremely preterm infants.[96,97]

CLASSIFICATION OF PULMONARY HYPERTENSION

During the sixth World Symposium of Pulmonary Arterial Hypertension held in 2018 in Nice, France, the classification of pulmonary arterial hypertension (PAH) was updated.[98] The basic outline of the Nice classification is shown in Table 154.1.[99] Owing to its particular anatomic and physiologic nature, PPHN has been moved to a separate subcategory, 1.7. In group 3.5, developmental lung diseases are listed because of growing recognition of the important role of abnormal pulmonary vascular growth in the pathogenesis of pulmonary hypertension and impaired lung structure in these disorders. CDH, BPD, and several other developmental disorders—such as surfactant protein deficiencies and alveolar capillary dysplasia (ACD)—are now included as relatively rare but important causes of pulmonary hypertension. Rare variants in the T-box transcription factor 4 gene *(TBX4)* have recently been recognized as an emerging cause of pediatric pulmonary hypertension, although its contribution to PPHN is not known.[100]

A more commonly used classification of PPHN is based on etiology. *Primary or idiopathic PPHN* refers to the absence of parenchymal lung disease to explain elevated pulmonary arterial pressure and implies intrauterine pulmonary vascular remodeling. About 10% of cases of PPHN are idiopathic, with no associated pulmonary airspace pathology. However, PPHN is usually associated with other acute respiratory conditions—such as MAS, RDS, pneumonia, or CDH—and is referred to as secondary PPHN. In these cases, it can be more difficult to separate chronic intrauterine remodeling from acute pulmonary vasoconstriction due to parenchymal lung disease.

PATHOPHYSIOLOGY OF PERSISTENT PULMONARY HYPERTENSION OF THE NEWBORN AND PHYSIOLOGIC BASIS OF CURRENT AND FUTURE THERAPIES

The pathophysiology of PPHN is based on changes in pulmonary vascular structure and function. Four patterns of pulmonary

Table 154.1 Updated Classification of Pulmonary Hypertension.[98,99]

1. Pulmonary arterial hypertension (PAH)
   - 1.1 Idiopathic PAH
   - 1.2 Heritable PAH *(BMP2; TBX4 and ACVRL1 mutations common in children)*
   - 1.3 Drug and toxin induced (e.g., diazoxide use in neonates with hypoglycemia)
   - 1.4 Associated with connective tissue disease (1.4.1), HIV infection (1.4.2), portal hypertension (1.4.3), congenital heart diseases (1.4.4—includes transient pulmonary hypertension associated with repair of congenital heart disease and infants with Eisenmenger physiology), and schistosomiasis (1.4.5)
   - 1.5 PAH long-term responders to calcium channel blockers
   - 1.6 PAH with overt features of venous/capillary involvement (pulmonary veno-occlusive disease and/or pulmonary capillary hemangiomatosis)
   - 1.7 Persistent pulmonary hypertension of the newborn (PPHN)

Associated disorders:

Idiopathic PPHN, myocardial dysfunction (asphyxia, infection), Down syndrome, structural heart disease, meconium aspiration syndrome, respiratory distress syndrome, transient tachypnea of the newborn, pneumonia/sepsis, developmental lung disease, perinatal stress, hepatic and cerebral arteriovenous malformations, associations with placental dysfunction, metabolic disease or maternal drug use or smoking

2. Pulmonary hypertension due to left-sided heart disease
   - 2.1 Pulmonary hypertension due to heart failure with preserved left ventricular ejection fraction
   - 2.2 Pulmonary hypertension due to heart failure with reduced left ventricular ejection fraction
   - 2.3 Valvular heart disease
   - 2.4 Congenital/acquired cardiovascular conditions leading to postcapillary pulmonary hypertension (includes pulmonary venous stenosis) isolated or associated with BPD and prematurity, cor triatrium, obstructed pulmonary venous return, mitral/aortic stenosis (including supra/subvalvular), and coarctation of the aorta
3. Pulmonary hypertension due to lung diseases and/or hypoxia
   - 3.1 Obstructive pulmonary disease
   - 3.2 Restrictive lung disease
   - 3.3 Other pulmonary diseases with mixed restrictive and obstructive pattern
   - 3.4 Hypoxia without lung disease
   - 3.5 Developmental lung diseases (CDH, BPD, ACD, ACD with misalignment of pulmonary veins), lung hypoplasia, surfactant protein (SP) abnormalities–SPB deficiency, SPC deficiency, ATP-binding cassette A3 mutation, thyroid transcription factor 1/Nkx2.1 *homeobox* mutation, TBX4, pulmonary interstitial glycogenosis, pulmonary alveolar proteinosis, pulmonary lymphangiectasia
4. Pulmonary hypertension due to pulmonary artery obstructions
   - 4.1 Chronic thromboembolic pulmonary hypertension
   - 4.2 Other pulmonary artery obstructions
5. Pulmonary hypertension with unclear and/or multifactorial mechanisms
   - 5.1 Hematologic disorders: chronic hemolytic anemia, myeloproliferative disorders, splenectomy
   - 5.2 Systemic and metabolic disorders: sarcoidosis, pulmonary histiocytosis, glycogen storage disease, Gaucher disease, thyroid disorders
   - 5.3 Others: tumoral obstruction, fibrosing mediastinitis, chronic renal failure, segmental PH
   - 5.4 Complex congenital heart disease: includes segmental pulmonary hypertension (isolated pulmonary artery of ductal origin, absent pulmonary artery, pulmonary atresia with ventricular septal defect and major aorto-pulmonary collateral arteries, hemitruncus, etc.), single ventricle (unoperated or operated) and Scimitar syndrome

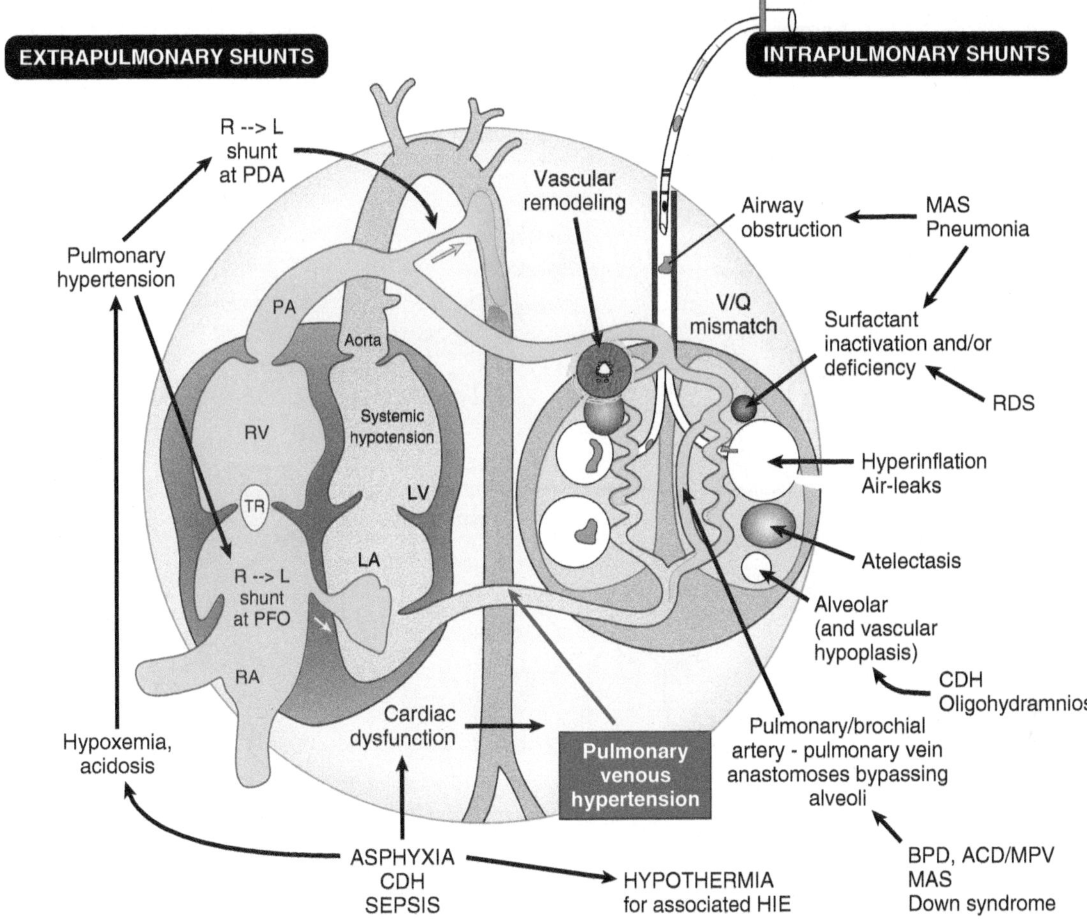

Fig. 154.5 Various etiologic factors causing persistent pulmonary hypertension of the newborn *(PPHN)* and hemodynamic changes in PPHN/hypoxemic respiratory failure. *CDH,* Congenital diaphragmatic hernia; *LA,* left atrium; *LV,* left ventricle; *MAS,* meconium aspiration syndrome; *PA,* pulmonary artery; *PDA,* patent ductus arteriosus; *PFO,* patent foramen ovale; *RA,* right atrium; *RDS,* respiratory distress syndrome; *RV,* right ventricle; *TR,* tricuspid regurgitation; *TTN,* transient tachypnea of the newborn; *V/Q,* ventilation/perfusion. (Copyright 2020, Lakshminrusimha and Steinhorn.)

vascular changes are predominantly associated with neonatal HRF. Elevated PVR may result from (1) pulmonary vasoconstriction, (2) structural remodeling of the pulmonary vasculature, (3) intravascular obstruction from increased viscosity of blood as in polycythemia, and (4) lung (alveolar and vascular) hypoplasia. An elevated pulmonary-to-SVR ratio (PVR/SVR) resulting from one or more of these patterns (Fig. 154.5) can lead to right-to-left shunting of blood across the foramen ovale and ductus arteriosus, resulting in severe hypoxemia. Recent recommendations from the European Pediatric Pulmonary Vascular Disease Network (EPPVDN)[101] and the American Thoracic Society (ATS)/American Heart Association (AHA) guide the diagnosis and treatment of PPHN.[102]

Hypoxemia results from PPHN due to intrapulmonary shunting secondary to ventilation/perfusion (V/Q) mismatch and/or extrapulmonary right-to-left shunting of blood. In some newborns, a single mechanism predominates (e.g., extrapulmonary right-to-left shunting in idiopathic PPHN). However, more commonly, several of these mechanisms contribute to hypoxemia. For instance, in MAS, obstruction of the airways by meconium decreases V/Q matching and increases intrapulmonary right-to-left shunt. Other segments of the lungs may be overventilated relative to perfusion, increasing the physiologic dead space. The same patient may also exhibit severe hypoxemia due to extrapulmonary right-to-left shunting at the ductus arteriosus and foramen ovale. As such, the PPHN in MAS may result from the alveolar hypoxia, from inflammatory mediators, or from abnormal pulmonary vascular muscularization. The presence of anastomoses from the pulmonary/bronchial artery to the pulmonary vein (intrapulmonary bronchopulmonary anastomoses, or IBA) that bypass alveolar gas exchange contributes to hypoxemia (intrapulmonary shunts) that does not respond to pulmonary vasodilators (Fig. 154.5). Such anastomoses have been described in Down syndrome,[103] CDH,[104] ACD,[105] and BPD.[106]

CHANGES IN THE NITRIC OXIDE CGMP PATHWAY IN PERSISTENT PULMONARY HYPERTENSION OF THE NEWBORN

ENDOTHELIAL NITRIC OXIDE SYNTHASE AND SOLUBLE GUANYLATE CYCLASE

Decreased expression of endothelial nitric oxide synthase (eNOS)[107] and reduced levels of NO metabolites in urine[108] have been noted in infants with PPHN. Most of the information on changes in vasoactive mediators in PPHN is derived from animal models.[109] In fetal lambs, disruption of the NO pathway by chronic in utero inhibition of NOS results in the physiologic characteristics of PPHN.[110] Either partial[111] or complete ductal ligation[54] during fetal life increases pulmonary arterial pressure without sustained elevation in PBF or in utero hypoxemia.[112] Endothelial dysfunction (Fig. 154.6) rapidly emerges and results in poor response to endothelium-dependent vasodilators such as oxygen and acetylcholine, along with decreased expression and activity of pulmonary eNOS.[113] This model[54] was utilized for preclinical studies to evaluate iNO in PPHN.[114]

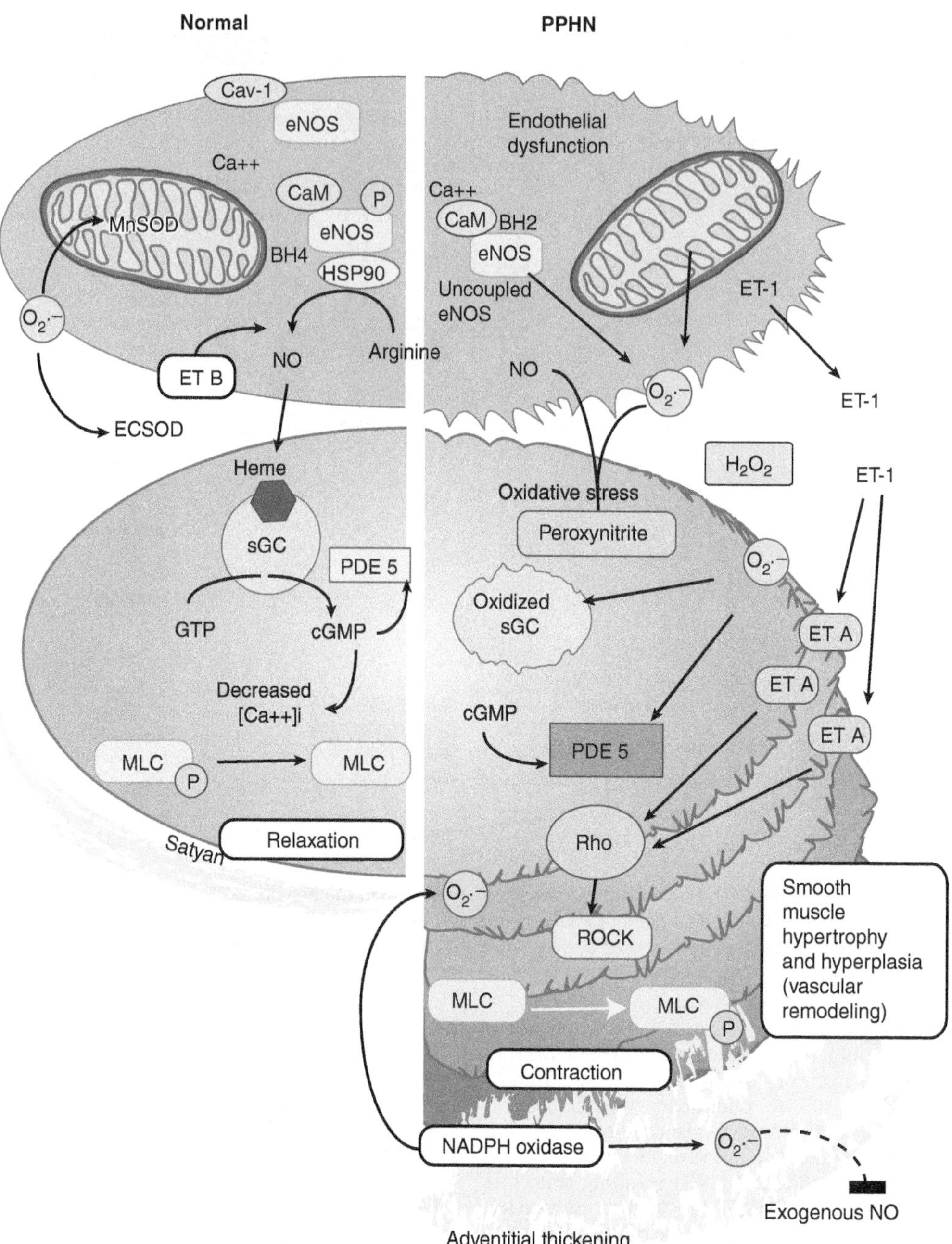

Fig. 154.6 Biochemical and enzymatic pathways in normal pulmonary arteries and those affected by persistent pulmonary hypertension of the newborn *(PPHN)*. Pulmonary arteries from human neonates and animal models of PPHN demonstrate thickening of the muscular layer and adventitia. The normal pulmonary arterial endothelium produces nitric oxide *(NO)* from phosphorylated endothelial nitric oxide synthase *(eNOS)* coupled to heat-shock protein 90 (HSP90) with tetrahydrobiopterin *(BH_4)* as a cofactor with adequate supply of arginine as substrate. The eNOS protein is bound to caveolin-1 *(Cav-1)* before its release by a calcium-calmodulin *(CaM)*-dependent process. Endothelin acting through endothelin-B receptor *(ET_B)* on the endothelium stimulates NO production. Manganese superoxide dismutase (MnSOD or SOD-2) is present in the mitochondria and scavenges superoxide anions. Extracellular superoxide dismutase *(ecSOD)* limits the interaction (and inactivation) of NO with superoxide anions in the endothelial-smooth muscle interface. NO reaches the smooth muscle cell and binds to reduced soluble guanylate cyclase (sGC), which in turn catalyzes the conversion of GTP to cGMP. Cyclic GMP is an important second messenger that reduces the cytosolic concentration of ionic calcium $[Ca^{2+}]_i$. Reduced concentration of ionic calcium leads to dephosphorylation of myosin light chains *(MLCs)*, resulting in smooth muscle relaxation. In PPHN, endothelial dysfunction leads to uncoupling of eNOS. Low levels of MnSOD and possibly ecSOD increase oxidative stress and formation of superoxide anions ($O_2^{\cdot-}$). Superoxide anions inactivate NO resulting in the formation of toxic peroxynitrite. Oxidized sGC cannot be activated by NO to produce cGMP. Superoxide anions stimulate phosphodiesterase 5 *(PDE5)* activity and enhance breakdown of cGMP. Pulmonary arterial endothelial cells from PPHN pulmonary arteries produce increased levels of endothelin-1 (ET-1), a powerful pulmonary vasoconstrictor. ET-1 acts through the ET_A receptor and stimulates Rho-A; the Rho-kinase *(ROCK)* pathway leads to phosphorylation of MLC and smooth muscle contraction. The pulmonary arterial endothelial cells have low levels of ET_B receptors. The net effect is reduced cGMP (vasodilator second messenger) and sensitization of the smooth muscle to ionic calcium. (Copyright 2020, Lakshminrusimha and Steinhorn.)

NO produced by the endothelium stimulates sGC in the pulmonary arterial smooth muscle cell (PASMC) to produce cGMP. Soluble GC is a heme-containing enzyme that can be inactivated by a variety of conditions. Abnormal vasodilator responses to NO secondary to impaired sGC activity are well described in animal models of neonatal pulmonary hypertension[115] and CDH.[116] PASMCs from fetal lambs with PPHN have normal or increased sGC expression but lower levels of basal cGMP,[117,118] possibly secondary to oxidization of sGC that renders it insensitive to NO (see Fig. 154.6). Cinaciguat, an sGC activator, stimulates oxidized sGC, increases cGMP in PASMC, and induces pulmonary vasodilation.[117] Because NO and cGMP both vasodilate and inhibit vascular smooth muscle growth, it is possible that the combination of diminished eNOS expression, inactivation of sGC, and reduced cGMP levels contribute to both abnormal vasoreactivity and excessive muscularization of pulmonary vessels in PPHN.

PHOSPHODIESTERASE 5

Increased PDE5 activity results in catabolism of cGMP and limitation of NO-induced vasodilation. Ventilation with high concentrations of inspired oxygen and exposure to ROS stimulates PDE5 activity[119] and decreases cGMP levels (see Figs. 154.4 and 154.6). Inhibition of PDE5 with the use of sildenafil is a promising strategy in the treatment of PPHN.[120,121] Sildenafil has been studied in the acute phase of PPHN (especially in situations without access to iNO or extracorporeal membrane oxygenation [ECMO]) and in patients with chronic pulmonary hypertension.[122] In a dose-finding study, intravenous sildenafil improved oxygenation as a primary agent (without the use of iNO).[121] Sildenafil may also augment the effect of iNO in patients with partial or poorly sustained responses to iNO; it may be particularly effective in patients following prolonged hyperoxic ventilation, which increases production of superoxide anions and stimulates PDE5 activity.[119] Oral sildenafil has been used in infants with prolonged pulmonary hypertension associated with BPD.[123,124]

OXIDATIVE STRESS

ROS such as hydrogen peroxide, superoxide, and peroxynitrite cause pulmonary vasoconstriction and play a role in the pathogenesis of PPHN. Increased superoxide levels have been demonstrated in the pulmonary arteries from the fetal lamb model of PPHN.[125,126] Superoxide may scavenge NO and disrupt its signaling pathway.[127] In addition to direct inactivation of NO, ROS can decrease eNOS and sGC activity and increase PDE5 activity,[128] resulting in decreased cGMP levels (see Fig. 154.6). Increased ROS can be secondary to exposure to high concentrations of oxygen[93]; reduced levels of antioxidant enzymes such as superoxide dismutase, catalase, and glutathione peroxidase[129]; and increased activity of prooxidant enzymes such as NADPH oxidase (Nox).[125] Oxidative stress can be minimized by judicious use of inspired oxygen or possibly by the use of targeted antioxidants.

Oxygen is a specific and potent pulmonary vasodilator and increased oxygen tension is a central mediator of the reduction in PVR at birth. Alveolar hypoxia and hypoxemia increase PVR and contribute to the pathophysiology of PPHN. Furthermore, animal studies demonstrate exaggerated hypoxic pulmonary vasoconstriction with pH below 7.25, suggesting that acidosis should be avoided.[130] Avoiding hypoxemia by mechanical ventilation with high concentrations of oxygen is a mainstay of PPHN management. However, exposure to extreme hyperoxia promotes the formation of ROS and may lead to lung injury. Brief exposure to 100% oxygen in newborn lambs increases the contractility responses of pulmonary arteries[131] and the formation of superoxide anions[93] while reducing the response to inhaled NO.[91,92]

The optimal Pa_{O_2} in the management of PPHN is not clear. Wung and colleagues have suggested that gentle ventilation with avoidance of hyperoxia and hyperventilation results in good outcomes for neonates with respiratory failure.[132] Decreasing Pa_{O_2} below 45 to 50 mm Hg results in increased PVR in newborn calves[130] and lambs.[92] In contrast, maintaining Pa_{O_2} above 80 mm Hg does not result in any additional decrease in PVR in either control lambs or lambs with PPHN. Maintaining preductal oxygen saturations in the range between 90% to 97% appears to maximize the drop in PVR in the ductal ligation model of PPHN. Current guidelines recommend maintaining preductal SpO_2 between 91% and 95%.[101] In aggregate, these studies show that hypoxemia results in pulmonary vasoconstriction; normoxemia reduces PVR; but hyperoxemia does not enhance pulmonary vasodilation. Furthermore, ventilation with 100% oxygen in PPHN lambs prevents the normal postnatal increase in eNOS expression in pulmonary arteries[133] and increases PDE5 activity. However, to date, randomized studies comparing different Pa_{O_2} targets have not been conducted in infants with PPHN. Randomized trials in preterm infants have demonstrated that a similar target (91% to 95%) is associated with a lower mortality but also increased the need for therapy of retinopathy of prematurity when compared with a target of 85% to 89%.[134] However, there are no trials targeting Sp_{O_2} among preterm infants with PPHN. Based on the current evidence from translational studies, it appears that avoiding hyperoxia is as important as avoiding hypoxia in the management of PPHN.

ANTIOXIDANTS

Elevations of ROS in the pulmonary artery have been observed in the lamb model of PPHN induced by antenatal ductal ligation.[125,135,136] Although animal trials provide encouraging evidence that antioxidants such as recombinant superoxide dismutase (rhSOD) or catalase improve oxygenation and reduce vascular reactivity, success in finding clinical applications has been quite limited. Antioxidants may be ineffective once the disease has progressed beyond a critical stage, suggesting that prevention of oxidant stress could be key to improving outcomes. ROS scavenging may also interfere with normal redox signaling pathways in the developing lung. Furthermore, oxidant stress is often localized to specific subcellular compartments in disease states, which may limit the clinical efficacy of nonspecific antioxidants such as rhSOD. Thus highly targeted therapies may be required to maximize the potential of antioxidants in the treatment of hypertensive diseases.

ABNORMALITIES OF THE ENDOTHELIN PATHWAY

ET-1 synthesized by vascular endothelial cells is a potent vasoconstrictor[137] and acts through two receptors: ET_A and ET_B (see Figs. 154.4 and 154.6). The ET_A receptor plays a critical role in vasoconstriction, whereas the endothelin-B receptor (ET_B) receptor promotes vasodilation[138,139] mediated by endothelium-derived NO.[140,141] Selective blockade of the ET_A receptor causes fetal pulmonary vasodilation.[142] ET-1 gene expression and levels are increased[143] in the lungs and pulmonary arterial endothelial cells in the fetal lamb model of PPHN,[143,144] whereas ET_B protein is decreased in pulmonary artery endothelial cells isolated from lambs with PPHN.[144] Chronic intrauterine ET_A receptor blockade following ductal ligation decreases pulmonary arterial pressure and distal muscularization of small pulmonary arteries in utero, decreases right ventricular hypertrophy, and increases the fall in PVR at delivery in newborn lambs with PPHN.[145] Thus ET-1 acting through the ET_A receptor might contribute to the pathogenesis and pathophysiology of PPHN. Bosentan, a nonspecific ET-1 receptor blocker, has been used mainly to treat PH in adults. Two trials showed that bosentan is well tolerated in neonates with PPHN, although its efficacy is variable, possibly owing to inconsistent intestinal absorption.[146,147]

ABNORMALITIES IN THE Rho-KINASE PATHWAY

Vascular smooth muscle contraction is regulated by cytosolic Ca^{2+} levels $[Ca^{2+}]_I$. With an elevation of $[Ca^{2+}]_I$, formation of the calcium-calmodulin complex increases, and myosin light-chain kinase (MLCK) is activated (see Fig. 154.6). MLCK phosphorylates the myosin light chain (MLC), enhancing cross-bridge cycling and inducing vascular smooth muscle contraction.[148] On the other hand, decreases in $[Ca^{2+}]_I$ reduce MLCK activity leading to dephosphorylation of MLC and vasorelaxation (see Fig. 154.6). RhoA, a small guanosine triphosphase (GTP)-binding protein, increases Rho-kinase (ROCK) activity, leading to the phosphorylation of MLC and vascular contraction. The RhoA-ROCK pathway "sensitizes" the contractile proteins to $[Ca^{2+}]_I$ and plays an important role in hypoxic pulmonary vasoconstriction.[148,149] RhoA-ROCK is an important mediator of elevated myogenic tone, which contributes to high PVR in fetal lambs.[150] PPHN induced by partial constriction of the ductus arteriosus in fetal lambs is associated with increased ROCK activity in pulmonary arterial endothelial cells and contributes to impaired angiogenesis.[151] Furthermore, endothelin activates the RhoA-ROCK pathway in pulmonary arterial endothelial cells isolated from lambs with PPHN.[144]

CHANGES IN THE PROSTAGLANDIN-cAMP PATHWAY

Prostacyclin (PGI_2) mediates vasodilation by activating adenylate cyclase and increasing cAMP in the PASMC (see Fig. 154.4). PGI_2 partly mediates pulmonary vasodilation at birth in response to ventilation of the lungs; it does not play a significant role in vasodilation in response to oxygenation.[152-154] In lambs with PPHN induced by ductal ligation, pulmonary PGI_2 synthase and PGI_2 receptor protein levels in the lung were decreased, but the adenylate cyclase and PDE3A levels were not altered.[155]

PGI_2 analogs administered by the intravenous route are the mainstay of pulmonary vasodilator therapy in adults with PAH. Inhaled PGI_2 (epoprostenol) is commonly used in the adult intensive care unit setting and improves oxygenation in PPHN.[156,157] In anecdotal studies, intravenous epoprostenol has been shown to improve oxygenation in some infants with iNO-resistant PPHN.[158] PGI_2 may act synergistically with iNO and prevent rebound hypertension seen while weaning iNO. Use of inhaled iloprost has also been reported in combination with iNO for intractable PPHN.[159] A major side effect of iloprost is bronchoconstriction, which limits its utility for infants with pulmonary hypertension secondary to BPD. As there are no randomized controlled trials evaluating the effect of prostaglandin vasodilators, their use remains limited.

MILRINONE

An alternate method of enhancing cAMP levels is through inhibition of its metabolism by PDE3A. Milrinone inhibits PDE3A activity in pulmonary arterial smooth muscle and increases cAMP, resulting in pulmonary vasodilation (see Fig. 154.4). In addition, milrinone enhances the heart's inotropic effect through inhibition of cardiac PDE3A and is considered an inodilator.[160,161] In some infants with PPHN, left ventricular dysfunction or hypoplasia (due to CDH, asphyxia, or sepsis) results in elevation of left atrial pressures and pulmonary venous hypertension. Administration of iNO to a patient with pulmonary venous hypertension may flood the pulmonary capillary bed and worsen pulmonary edema, resulting in clinical deterioration.[162]

Three case series have demonstrated the effectiveness of milrinone in improving oxygenation in iNO-resistant PPHN.[163-165] The pulmonary vasodilatory response to milrinone is proportional to PDE3A activity in PASMCs. Interestingly, exposure to NO donors increases PDE3A expression in rat PASMCs,[166] and ventilation of newborn lambs with iNO increases PDE3A activity in resistance-level pulmonary arteries compared with ventilation using oxygen alone.[167] These studies suggest that exposure to iNO increases PDE3A activity and that milrinone may be especially effective in promoting pulmonary vasodilation and improving oxygenation in iNO-resistant PPHN.[163,164]

HISTOLOGIC CHANGES IN PERSISTENT PULMONARY HYPERTENSION OF THE NEWBORN

Information on histologic changes in the pulmonary vasculature is obtained from fatal cases (usually due to meconium aspiration or idiopathic PPHN) of PPHN in term infants.[168,169] In two autopsy series of patients with PPHN, remodeling resulted in the extension of muscle into small arteries. Alveolar duct and wall arteries (<30 μM external diameter), normally nonmuscular, were fully muscularized.[86,169] In addition, the medial wall thickness of the normally muscular intra-acinar arteries was doubled. These findings suggest that in fatal cases of PPHN, structural maldevelopment of the peripheral pulmonary arterial bed was initiated in utero and does not merely represent a failure of the fetal pattern to regress. Similar changes are observed in animal models of PPHN, including the lamb model of antenatal ductal ligation.[54]

In addition to changes in the muscular medial layer, adventitial thickening is observed in PPHN (Fig. 154.7)[54] and contributes

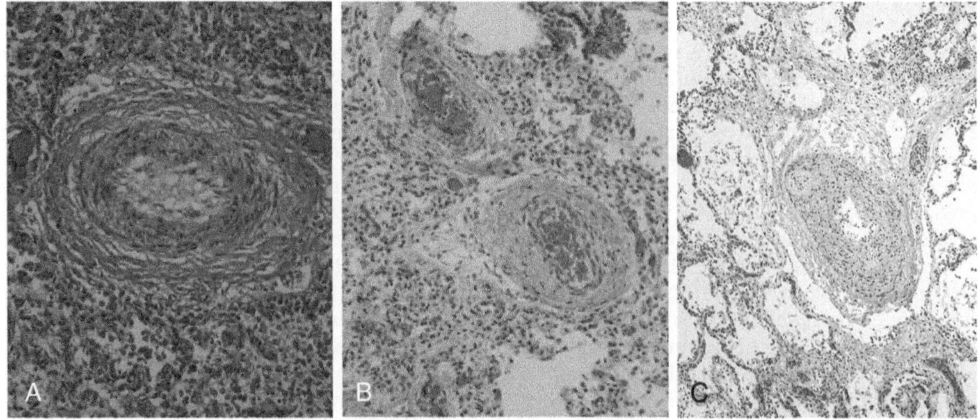

Fig. 154.7 Vascular remodeling in neonatal pulmonary hypertension. Histology of pulmonary arteries in lung sections from three patients with pulmonary hypertension. (A) A 14-day-old infant with trisomy 21 who was born at 37 weeks of gestation. (Note the significant thickening of the medial and adventitial layers.) (B) A 5-day-old preterm infant with pulmonary hypertension and severe hypoxemic respiratory failure who was born at 25 weeks of gestation. (C) A 4-month-old infant with bronchopulmonary dysplasia and pulmonary hypertension who was born at 23 weeks of gestation. (Copyright 2020, Lakshminrusimha and Steinhorn.)

to pulmonary artery stiffness.[170] The adventitial cells (fibroblasts, pericytes, progenitor cells, etc.) appear to be a critical regulator of vascular wall function from the outside in.[171,172] NO relaxes vessels only when administered to the endothelial side but not the adventitial side in rabbits,[173] rats,[174] and lambs.[175] Recent evidence suggests that constitutively active NADPH oxidase is located in adventitia and is an important source of superoxide anions, creating a barrier to NO-induced vasodilation (see Fig. 154.6).

Intrapulmonary shunts connecting pulmonary and bronchial arteries to pulmonary veins have been observed in autopsy samples from patients with ACD, CDH, BPD, and Down syndrome.[103-106] These shunts contribute to hypoxemia that is refractory to pulmonary vasodilators.

GENETICS AND PERSISTENT PULMONARY HYPERTENSION OF THE NEWBORN

Many gene mutations including those in the gene-coding bone morphogenic protein receptor type 2 *(BMPR2)* and related genes have been identified in adults with PAH. Additional genes and mutations *(CAV1, KCNK3, EIF2AK4)* associated with familial and nonfamilial forms of PAH have been discovered.[176] In contrast, limited data are available on genetic mutations associated with PPHN. Unlike the case in adults, no association between PPHN and the *BMPR2* gene has been detected.[177] Abnormalities in the *TBX4* gene have been associated with neonatal and pediatric pulmonary hypertension.[100]

GLUCOCORTICOIDS AND PERSISTENT PULMONARY HYPERTENSION OF THE NEWBORN

Interestingly, PPHN is significantly associated with genetic variants in corticotropin-releasing hormone (CRH) receptor 1 and CRH-binding protein.[177] The CRH-binding protein decreases the bioavailability of CRH, diminishes the activity of the hypothalamic-pituitary-adrenal axis, and may affect either fetal lung functional development or the capacity to adequately transition to ex utero life. Additionally, CRH receptor 1 single nucleotide polymorphisms are located close to the transcription factor binding site for peroxisome proliferator-activated receptor-γ (PPAR-γ). PPAR-γ is an essential regulator of PASMC proliferation and vascular tone.

Together, these findings suggest that glucocorticoids may have a role in prevention and management of PPHN and HRF.[177-182] In neonatal lambs with PPHN, postnatal administration of hydrocortisone improved oxygenation, sGC activity, and cGMP concentrations. A recent single-center study reported improvement in oxygenation and weaning of inotropes with hydrocortisone therapy in PPHN.[183]

NITRIC OXIDE PATHWAY GENES IN PERSISTENT PULMONARY HYPERTENSION OF THE NEWBORN

Although eNOS mRNA expression was found to be reduced or absent in umbilical venous endothelial cells of infants with PPHN,[107] a candidate gene analysis did not identify any polymorphisms of the eNOS gene in infants with PPHN.[177] However, other genetic abnormalities of the NO pathway have been associated with PPHN. Endothelial cells generate NO from the precursor L-arginine, an amino acid supplied by the urea cycle. Carbamoyl-phosphatase synthetase (CPS) catalyzes the first, rate-determining step of the urea cycle.[108] Infants with PPHN were observed to have lower plasma concentration of arginine and NO metabolites compared to control infants with respiratory distress without PPHN. Compared with the general population, infant groups with respiratory distress (with or without PPHN) exhibited a skewed distribution of the genotypes for the CPS variants.[108] Others have reported that a single nucleotide polymorphism of the arginase I gene was associated with lower risk of pulmonary hypertension with BPD.[184]

TRISOMY 21 AND PULMONARY HYPERTENSION

Trisomy 21 with or without congenital heart disease is strongly associated with pulmonary hypertension.[185-187] In newborns with trisomy 21, the elevated PVR persists longer. The incidence of PPHN is estimated to be 1% to 5% in trisomy 21 versus 0.1% to 0.2% in the general population.[188,185] In the presence of atrioventricular septal defects in trisomy 21, the left-to-right shunting is delayed (secondary to a slow drop in PVR) in the neonatal period; however, pulmonary hypertension develops earlier and Eisenmenger syndrome is observed more frequently[189] than in genetically normal children. Respiratory abnormalities such as pulmonary hypoplasia, upper airway obstruction and intrapulmonary shunts may promote development of hypoxemia and pulmonary hypertension in trisomy 21.

CAUSES OF PULMONARY HYPERTENSION IN NEONATES WITH POOR RESPONSE TO CONVENTIONAL MANAGEMENT

The conventional and advanced management of PPHN is outlined in Fig. 154.8. The class of recommendation (COR) and level of evidence (LOE) are color coded in this figure.

PRETERM INFANTS WITH EARLY PULMONARY HYPERTENSION (PRETERM PERSISTENT PULMONARY HYPERTENSION OF THE NEWBORN)

Following early preterm birth, PVR decreases at a slower rate than it does in term neonates.[79] Extremely preterm infants (born at <26 weeks' gestation) with prolonged rupture of membranes and chorioamnionitis are at high risk of early pulmonary hypertension.[4,5] Furthermore, these infants are at high risk of mortality (~48%) and brain injury.[190] The use of iNO in extremely low-birth-weight infants with HRF has resulted in contradictory responses,[191,192] but overall it has not improved mortality or neurologic outcomes.[190] Based on these results and systematic reviews[193] and metaanalyses,[194,195] the American Academy of Pediatrics has stated that the current evidence does not support treating preterm infants with respiratory failure with iNO for rescue or routine use to improve survival.[196,197] Despite these recommendations, the use of iNO among extremely low-birth-weight infants remains high[20] (approximately 8% of infants less than 29 weeks' gestation in the Eunice Kennedy Shriver National Institute of Child Health and Human Development network[198] and 7.2% of infants less than 34 weeks' gestation in the Ohio Perinatal network[18]).

There appears to be a subset of preterm infants with pulmonary hypertension who respond well to iNO.[199] These infants have preterm prolonged rupture of membranes with oligohydramnios and some degree of pulmonary hypoplasia.[200] Preterm infants with prolonged rupture of membranes presenting with HRF were noted to have low levels of nitrate/nitrite in the tracheal aspirate, suggesting a specific deficiency of NO; these infants responded well to iNO.[5] The ATS/AHA,[102] EPPVDN,[101] and Pediatric Pulmonary Hypertension Network[201] recommend iNO in selected preterm infants with hypoxemia secondary to PPHN physiology or with clinical/echocardiographic confirmation of PPHN.

BRONCHOPULMONARY DYSPLASIA WITH PULMONARY HYPERTENSION

Pulmonary hypertension is observed in approximately 25% to 37% of infants with moderate to severe BPD.[202,203] Severity of BPD, antenatal growth failure,[204] and oligohydramnios are associated with development of pulmonary hypertension. The

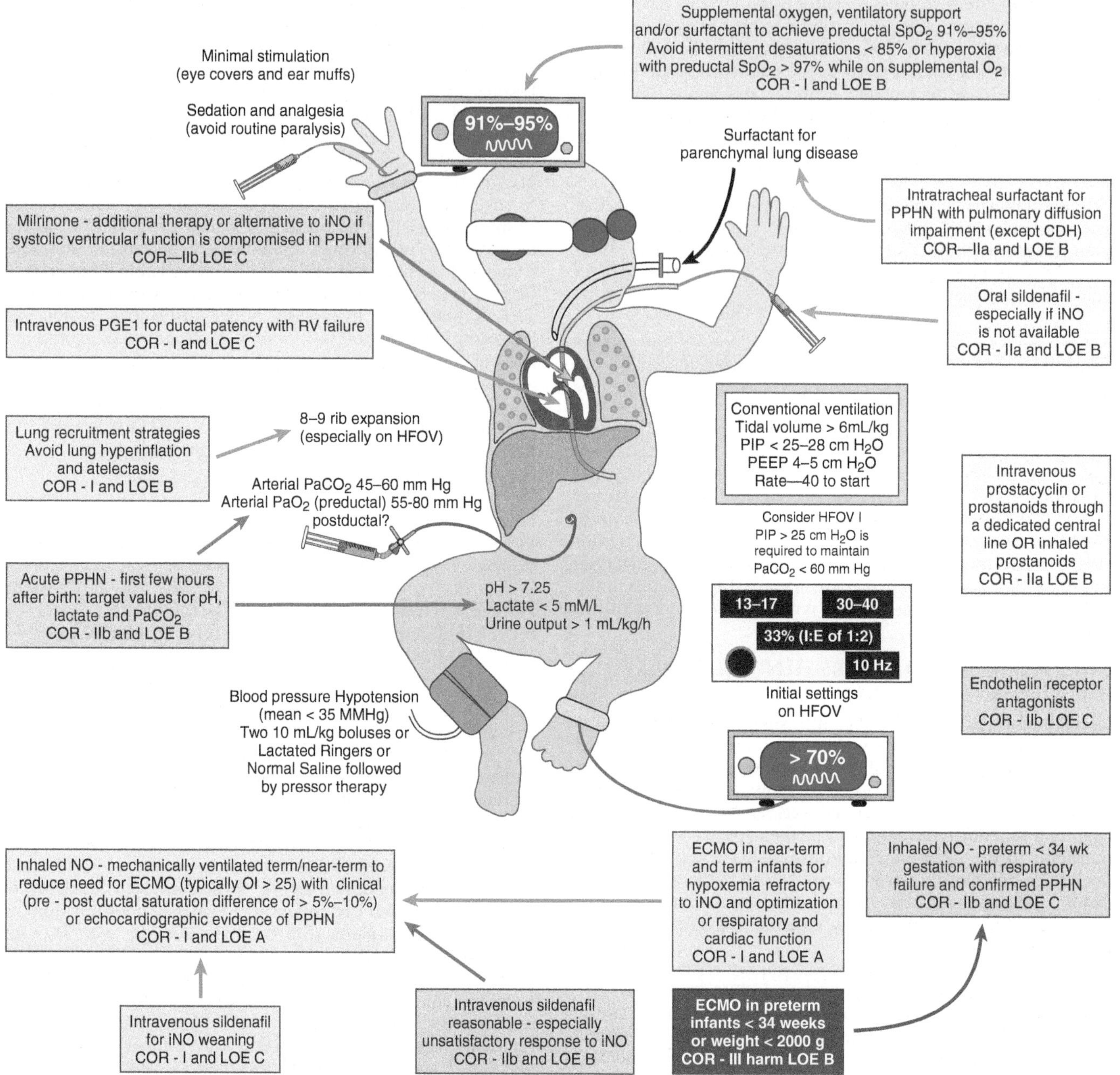

Fig. 154.8 Recommendations for supportive measures and pharmacotherapy in persistent pulmonary hypertension of the newborn. The class of recommendation *(COR)* and level of evidence *(LOE)* are based on AHA definitions. Recommendations with class I (benefits > risk are shown in a *green box*), Class IIa (benefit > risk) is shown in the *yellow box*, class IIb (benefit ≥ risk) is shown in the *orange box*, and class III (no benefit or harm) is shown in the red box. (Based on Abman et al.[102] and Hansmann et al.[101] Copyright 2020, Lakshminrusimha.)

pathophysiology of pulmonary hypertension in these infants is a combination of simplified lung parenchyma and impaired vascular development. BPD is associated with reduced cross-sectional perfusion area with decreased arterial density and abnormal muscularization of peripheral pulmonary arteries.

The onset of pulmonary hypertension in BPD is variable and can be as late as 3 to 4 months of age.[205] Delayed diagnosis is often associated with progressive pulmonary vascular disease, cor pulmonale, and high mortality. Echocardiographic screening starting as early as 7 days of postnatal age[206] is the best way to estimate pulmonary artery pressures and possibly identify infants with evolving pulmonary hypertension, but results may be misleading.[207]

The optimal interventions for reversing early pulmonary hypertension or treating established pulmonary hypertension in BPD are not clear. Preventing periods of hypoxemia is important to prevent further progression of pulmonary hypertension. This may require setting higher oxygen saturation targets, providing long-term mechanical ventilator support, and minimizing gastroesophageal reflux in the most severely affected infants. Multiple vascular therapies such as inhaled NO, sildenafil, PGI_2, and endothelin receptor antagonists have been tried anecdotally with mixed results. A stepwise algorithm using inhaled NO and sildenafil has been proposed.[208] Mourani and colleagues demonstrated improvement in echocardiographic parameters in 88% of patients given sildenafil therapy.[124,208] However, a

US Food and Drug Administration notice warned of increased mortality among children (1 to 17 years of age) treated with chronic sildenafil for pulmonary hypertension due to congenital heart disease or idiopathic causes. This warning has likely limited the use of PDE inhibitors in the management of infants with BPD and pulmonary hypertension.[209-211] The importance of multidisciplinary care and nutritional interventions to foster lung development and healing in these patients cannot be overemphasized. At this time, prevention remains the best strategy, and lung protective strategies employed very early in the neonatal course may decrease the incidence of BPD-associated pulmonary hypertension. A review of current recommendations for BPD-associated pulmonary hypertension from Pediatric Pulmonary Hypertension Network have been published.[212]

CONGENITAL DIAPHRAGMATIC HERNIA

Of the various causes of PPHN in term and late-preterm infants, CDH is associated with the most intractable pulmonary hypertension and is now the leading respiratory indication for ECMO. Recent data from the Extracorporeal Life Support Organization registry shows that CDH survival following ECMO is only 48% compared with 95% with MAS.

Inhaled NO has not been effective in decreasing the incidence of death or ECMO in infants with CDH.[213] There are two animal models of CDH—the rat model created by maternal ingestion of the herbicide nitrofen and surgical creation of a diaphragmatic defect in fetal lambs. Abnormalities in NOS expression,[214] along with abnormal sGC and PDE5 function,[116] have been observed in these models. These latter abnormalities, in addition to left ventricular hypoplasia,[38,39] may contribute to poor response to iNO in CDH.

A systematic review of best practice has identified key elements of respiratory care in infants with CDH that are associated with improved outcomes.[215,216] Gentle ventilation with permissive hypercapnia is advocated to avoid high peak inspiratory pressures and reduce volutrauma to the hypoplastic lungs. The goal is to achieve preductal saturations equal to or greater than 85%, $Paco_2$ equal to or greater than 65 mm Hg, pH equal to or greater than 7.25, and adequate tissue perfusion by monitoring pH and lactate levels.[217,218] Studies of infants with PPHN maintained at $Paco_2$ levels slightly above normal (40 to 60 mm Hg) indicate similar or better outcomes with less chronic lung disease in infants with CDH.[132,219] Maintaining patency of the ductus arteriosus can also provide a "pop-off" that may protect the right ventricle from acute strain. Trials evaluating milrinone[220] and sildenafil versus iNO[221] in CDH are currently recruiting patients.

ALVEOLAR CAPILLARY DYSPLASIA

ACD (with or without misalignment of the pulmonary veins) is a rare form of interstitial and vascular lung disease that presents as severe pulmonary hypertension and refractory hypoxemia early in life.[222] The etiology of ACD is not well understood, but it is believed that a genetic defect or an early antenatal insult prevents normal development of the pulmonary capillary bed. These early events produce remodeling of the pulmonary arterioles, simplification of the alveolar architecture, and development of congested misaligned pulmonary veins residing in the same adventitial sheath. No long-term survivors of ACD have yet been reported despite treatment with all known modalities, including extracorporeal support. Other anomalies of the genitourinary, cardiovascular, and gastrointestinal systems are seen in up to half of infants with ACD. The diagnosis can be confirmed only based on microscopic examination of the lung. Therefore a complete postmortem evaluation should be recommended for all newborns who die as a result of unexplained pulmonary hypertension, and a lung biopsy should be considered in all infants with prolonged, refractory PPHN.

Although ACD classically presents in the neonatal period, a late presentation at several months of life has been reported. Approximately 10% of reported ACD cases are familial, indicating a probable genetic component. In 40% of infants with ACD, mutations or deletions in the *FOXF1* transcription factor gene or deletions upstream to *FOXF1* are identified.[223] A recent report of a French cohort of 21 patients provided a description of diagnosis and course of ACD in the era of genetic diagnosis. These patients were born at a mean gestation of 37.6 weeks and were symptomatic by a median postnatal age of 2.5 hours. Most of the patients (20 of 21) had PPHN and two patients survived to 3.3 and 14 months. The diagnosis was established by evaluation of lung tissue at autopsy (12 patients) or by percutaneous biopsy (6 patients). Unlike previous reports, a higher number of patients (17, or 71%) had abnormal FOXF1 (eight deletions and seven point mutations). This study emphasizes the importance of using a combined genetic and histologic approach for early diagnosis of ACD.[224] A murine model of *FOXF1* deficiency has been described, and it has further demonstrated the importance of the Foxf1 protein in embryonic development of the pulmonary vasculature.[225]

CONCLUSION

Increased understanding of the pathophysiologic changes in pulmonary circulation in neonatal HRF and PPHN over the last two decades has led to improved management of PPHN and a substantial decrease in the number of neonatal respiratory patients requiring ECMO. However, the mortality among infants with PPHN that require positive pressure ventilator support (invasive or noninvasive) continues to be high at approximately 10%.[226] Animal models have contributed significantly to our understanding of fetal circulation, pulmonary vascular transition at birth, and hemodynamic and biochemical abnormalities associated with PPHN. Further basic, translational, and clinical research into pulmonary vasodilator therapy and reversal of remodeling in the pulmonary vasculature is crucial. Two unmet challenges are particularly apparent in the field of PPHN: CDH and the premature infant with pulmonary hypertension.[227] Further research to evaluate and develop appropriate strategies to ameliorate pulmonary vascular disease in these conditions is warranted.

A complete reference list is available at www.ExpertConsult.com. 

SELECT REFERENCES

1. Walsh-Sukys MC, Tyson JE, Wright LL, et al. Persistent pulmonary hypertension of the newborn in the era before nitric oxide: practice variation and outcomes. *Pediatrics*. 2000;105(1 Pt 1):14-20.
3. Gersony WM. Persistence of the fetal circulation: a commentary. *J Pediatr*. 1973;82(6):1103-1106.
4. Kumar VH, Hutchison AA, Lakshminrusimha S, et al. Characteristics of pulmonary hypertension in preterm neonates. *J Perinatol*. 2007;27(4):214-219.
5. Aikio O, Metsola J, Vuolteenaho R, et al. Transient defect in nitric oxide generation after rupture of fetal membranes and responsiveness to inhaled nitric oxide in very preterm infants with hypoxic respiratory failure. *J Pediatr*. 2012;161(3):397-403.e391.
6. Rudolph AM. Aortopulmonary transposition in the fetus: speculation on pathophysiology and therapy. *Pediatr Res*. 2007;61(3):375-380.
8. Kessler J, Rasmussen S, Hanson M, et al. Longitudinal reference ranges for ductus venosus flow velocities and waveform indices. *Ultrasound Obst Gynecol*. 2006;28(7):890-898.
9. Edelstone DI, Rudolph AM. Preferential streaming of ductus venosus blood to the brain and heart in fetal lambs. *Am J Physiol*. 1979;237(6):H724-H729.
10. Rudolph AM. In: *Congenital Diseases of the Heart: Clinical-Physiological Considerations*. 3rd ed. West Sussex: John Wiley and Sons; 2009.
11. Mielke G, Benda N. Cardiac output and central distribution of blood flow in the human fetus. *Circulation*. 2001;103(12):1662-1668.
12. Rasanen J, Wood DC, Weiner S, et al. Role of the pulmonary circulation in the distribution of human fetal cardiac output during the second half of pregnancy. *Circulation*. 1996;94(5):1068-1073.
13. Prsa M, Sun L, van Amerom J, et al. Reference ranges of blood flow in the major vessels of the normal human fetal circulation at term by phase-contrast magnetic resonance imaging. *Circ Cardiovasc Imaging*. 2014;7(4):663-670.

40. Lakshminrusimha S, Steinhorn RH. Pulmonary vascular biology during neonatal transition. *Clin Perinatol*. 1999;26(3):601-619.
41. Delaney C, Gien J, Grover TR, et al. Pulmonary vascular effects of serotonin and selective serotonin reuptake inhibitors in the late-gestation ovine fetus. *Am J Physiol Lung Cell Mol Physiol*. 2011;301(6):L937-L944.
42. Delaney C, Gien J, Roe G, et al. Serotonin contributes to high pulmonary vascular tone in a sheep model of persistent pulmonary hypertension of the newborn. *Am J Physiol Lung Cell Mol Physiol*. 2013;304(12):L894-L901.
60. Teitel DF, Iwamoto HS, Rudolph AM. Changes in the pulmonary circulation during birth-related events. *Pediatr Res*. 1990;27(4 Pt 1):372-378.
67. Abman SH, Chatfield BA, Hall SL, et al. Role of endothelium-derived relaxing factor during transition of pulmonary circulation at birth. *Am J Physiol*. 1990;259(6 Pt 2):H1921-H1927.
74. Bhatt S, Alison BJ, Wallace EM, et al. Delaying cord clamping until ventilation onset improves cardiovascular function at birth in preterm lambs. *J Physiol*. 2013;591(Pt 8):2113-2126.
84. Lapointe A, Barrington KJ. Pulmonary hypertension and the asphyxiated newborn. *J Pediatr*. 2011;158(suppl 2):e19-e24.
89. Sarkar S, Barks JD, Bhagat I, et al. Pulmonary dysfunction and therapeutic hypothermia in asphyxiated newborns: whole body versus selective head cooling. *Am J Perinatol*. 2009;26(4):265-270.
91. Lakshminrusimha S, Russell JA, Steinhorn RH, et al. Pulmonary hemodynamics in neonatal lambs resuscitated with 21%, 50%, and 100% oxygen. *Pediatr Res*. 2007;62(3):313-318.
92. Lakshminrusimha S, Swartz DD, Gugino SF, et al. Oxygen concentration and pulmonary hemodynamics in newborn lambs with pulmonary hypertension. *Pediatr Res*. 2009;66(5):539-544.
99. Rosenzweig EB, Abman SH, Adatia I, et al. Paediatric pulmonary arterial hypertension: updates on definition, classification, diagnostics and management. *Eur Respir J*. 2019;53(1).
108. Pearson DL, Dawling S, Walsh WF, et al. Neonatal pulmonary hypertension—urea-cycle intermediates, nitric oxide production, and carbamoyl-phosphate synthetase function. *N Engl J Med*. 2001;344(24):1832-1838.
109. Steinhorn RH, Morin III FC, Fineman JR. Models of persistent pulmonary hypertension of the newborn (PPHN) and the role of cyclic guanosine monophosphate (GMP) in pulmonary vasorelaxation. *Semin Perinatol*. 1997;21(5):393-408.
110. Fineman JR, Wong J, Morin III FC, et al. Chronic nitric oxide inhibition in utero produces persistent pulmonary hypertension in newborn lambs. *J Clin Invest*. 1994;93(6):2675-2683.
111. Abman SH, Accurso FJ. Acute effects of partial compression of ductus arteriosus on fetal pulmonary circulation. *Am J Physiol*. 1989;257(2 Pt 2):H626-H634.
116. de Buys Roessingh A, Fouquet V, Aigrain Y, et al. Nitric oxide activity through guanylate cyclase and phosphodiesterase modulation is impaired in fetal lambs with congenital diaphragmatic hernia. *J Pediatr Surg*. 2011;46(8):1516-1522.
117. Chester M, Seedorf G, Tourneux P, et al. Cinaciguat, a soluble guanylate cyclase activator, augments cGMP after oxidative stress and causes pulmonary vasodilation in neonatal pulmonary hypertension. *Am J Physiol Lung Cell Mol Physiol*. 2011;301(5):L755-L764.
118. Farrow KN, Lakshminrusimha S, Czech L, et al. SOD and inhaled nitric oxide normalize phosphodiesterase 5 expression and activity in neonatal lambs with persistent pulmonary hypertension. *Am J Physiol Lung Cell Mol Physiol*. 2010;299(1):L109-L116.
121. Steinhorn RH, Kinsella JP, Pierce C, et al. Intravenous sildenafil in the treatment of neonates with persistent pulmonary hypertension. *J Pediatr*. 2009;155(6):841-847.
130. Rudolph AM, Yuan S. Response of the pulmonary vasculature to hypoxia and H+ ion concentration changes. *J Clin Invest*. 1966;45(3):399-411.
144. Gien J, Tseng N, Seedorf G, et al. Endothelin-1 impairs angiogenesis in vitro through Rho-kinase activation after chronic intrauterine pulmonary hypertension in fetal sheep. *Pediatr Res*. 2013;73(3):252-262.
165. McNamara PJ, Shivananda SP, Sahni M, et al. Pharmacology of milrinone in neonates with persistent pulmonary hypertension of the newborn and suboptimal response to inhaled nitric oxide. *Pediatr Crit Care Med*. 2013;14(1):74-84.
172. Stenmark KR, Yeager ME, El Kasmi KC, et al. The adventitia: essential regulator of vascular wall structure and function. *Annu Rev Physiol*. 2013;75:23-47.
177. Byers HM, Dagle JM, Klein JM, et al. Variations in CRHR1 are associated with persistent pulmonary hypertension of the newborn. *Pediatr Res*. 2012;71(2):162-167.
182. Perez M, Lakshminrusimha S, Wedgwood S, et al. Hydrocortisone normalizes oxygenation and cGMP regulation in lambs with persistent pulmonary hypertension of the newborn. *Am J Physiol Lung Cell Mol Physiol*. 2012;302(6):L595-L603.
185. Weijerman ME, van Furth AM, van der Mooren MD, et al. Prevalence of congenital heart defects and persistent pulmonary hypertension of the neonate with Down syndrome. *Eur J Pediatr*. 2010;169(10):1195-1199.
194. Askie LM, Ballard RA, Cutter GR, et al. Inhaled nitric oxide in preterm infants: an individual-patient data meta-analysis of randomized trials. *Pediatrics*. 2011;128(4):729-739.
206. Mourani PM, Sontag MK, Younoszai A, et al. Early pulmonary vascular disease in preterm infants at risk for bronchopulmonary dysplasia. *Am J Respir Crit Care Med*. 2015;191(1):87-95.
213. The Neonatal Inhaled Nitric Oxide Study Group N. Inhaled nitric oxide and hypoxic respiratory failure in infants with congenital diaphragmatic hernia. The Neonatal Inhaled Nitric Oxide Study Group (NINOS). *Pediatrics*. 1997;99(6):838-845.
217. Reiss I, Schaible T, van den Hout L, et al. Standardized postnatal management of infants with congenital diaphragmatic hernia in Europe: the CDH EURO Consortium consensus. *Neonatology*. 2010;98(4):354-364.
218. van den Hout L, Tibboel D, Vijfhuize S, et al. The VICI-trial: high frequency oscillation versus conventional mechanical ventilation in newborns with congenital diaphragmatic hernia: an international multicentre randomized controlled trial. *BMC Pediatr*. 2011;11:98.
219. Dworetz AR, Moya FR, Sabo B, et al. Survival of infants with persistent pulmonary hypertension without extracorporeal membrane oxygenation [comment]. *Pediatrics*. 1989;84(1):1-6.
222. Bishop NB, Stankiewicz P, Steinhorn RH. Alveolar capillary dysplasia. *Am J Resp Crit Care Med*. 2011;184(2):172-179.
223. Stankiewicz P, Sen P, Bhatt SS, et al. Genomic and genic deletions of the FOX gene cluster on 16q24.1 and inactivating mutations of FOXF1 cause alveolar capillary dysplasia and other malformations. *Am J Hum Genet*. 2009;84(6):780-791.
225. Kalinichenko VV, Lim L, Stolz DB, et al. Defects in pulmonary vasculature and perinatal lung hemorrhage in mice heterozygous null for the Forkhead Box f1 transcription factor. *Dev Biol*. 2001;235(2):489-506.
227. Aschner JL, Fike CD. New developments in the pathogenesis and management of neonatal pulmonary hypertension. In: Bancalari E, ed. *The Newborn Lung*. Philadelphia: Saunders Elsevier; 2008:241-299.
228. Kiserud T. Physiology of the fetal circulation. *Semin Fetal Neonatal Med*. 2005;10(6):493-503.
229. Rudolph AM, Heymann MA. The fetal circulation. *Annu Rev Med*. 1968;19:195-206.

155 Pathophysiology of Shock in the Fetus and Neonate

Shahab Noori | Philippe S. Friedlich | Istvan Seri

INTRODUCTION

Cardiovascular compromise in the fetus and neonate often leads to severe organ injury or death, and the success of therapeutic interventions is limited by difficulties with accurate and timely detection of the condition, especially in the fetus, and the sensitivity of the developing organism to alterations in blood and oxygen (O_2) supply. Studies using animal models of fetal or neonatal shock have investigated the cause-specific pathophysiologic changes in the cardiovascular system and, although in much less detail, the cardiovascular response to therapeutic interventions. However, little is known about the cellular effects of shock in the developing animal, and virtually no data exist for the human fetus and neonate. Extrapolation of adult data to the fetus or neonate must be done with caution, and because of the unpredictable impact of interspecies differences on organ development and maturational processes, extrapolation of data obtained in animal models of fetal and neonatal shock to the human fetus and neonate may be even more prone to error.

CARDIOVASCULAR COMPROMISE IN THE FETUS

In the fetus, inadequate tissue O_2 delivery is most often caused by decreased blood flow to the uterus, the placenta, or fetus. In addition, circulatory failure resulting from developmental abnormalities, infections, cardiac arrhythmias, and decreased O_2 carrying capacity of the blood may lead to development of hydrops, and ultimately, the fetus may die. Studies on fetal shock have primarily used experimental models of decreased blood flow or O_2 delivery, or both, and most of these studies have used the pregnant sheep model.

DEVELOPMENTAL CHANGES IN FETAL GAS PARAMETERS

The average measured partial pressures of oxygen in umbilical artery and vein are approximately 20 and 30 mm Hg, respectively.[1,2] As a result of the higher affinity of fetal hemoglobin for oxygen, the hemoglobin O_2 saturations in the fetal umbilical artery and vein are approximately 50% and 75%, respectively.[2] Thus the fetus is exposed to lower levels of oxidant stress compared with the newborn. Fetal O_2 tension (PO_2) and pH decrease and carbon dioxide tension (PCO_2) increases with advancing gestational age.[3-5] These changes are primarily driven by increased O_2 consumption and associated CO_2 production by the growing fetus. The fall in the pH is secondary to the higher CO_2 production as gestational age progresses. Because O_2 carrying capacity also increases, total O_2 content in the fetal blood remains stable throughout gestation. Although controversial,[5] fetal O_2 saturation has been reported to decrease with advancing gestational age.[6] The decrease in fetal O_2 saturation is thought to result both from the effect of decreasing pH and increasing PCO_2 on the hemoglobin-O_2 dissociation curve and the drop in PO_2.[6]

OXYGEN DELIVERY, OXYGEN CONSUMPTION, AND OXYGEN EXTRACTION IN THE FETUS

Delivery of O_2 depends on blood O_2 content and cardiac output. In the fetus, regional O_2 delivery is unique because the O_2 content of blood flowing to different organs varies significantly. Under physiologic conditions, despite the low fetal $PO_{2\,value}$, O_2 delivery exceeds the metabolic demand of the tissues. The high cardiac index and hematocrit, the increased O_2 affinity of fetal hemoglobin, and the balanced distribution of cardiac output between the placenta and fetus ensure adequate O_2 delivery to the fetal organs.[2] In addition, tight regulation of uterine and umbilical blood flow plays a major role in ensuring appropriate fetal O_2 uptake. Reductions in uterine blood flow are relatively well tolerated by the fetus, and, in the sheep, decreasing uterine blood flow by as much as 50% does not adversely affect fetal blood gas parameters.[7] An increase in O_2 extraction is an immediate and effective mechanism compensating for the decrease in O_2 delivery in cases of reduced uterine blood flow.[8] *O_2 extraction,* defined as the ratio between O_2 consumption and O_2 delivery, is approximately 0.3 in the animal fetus.[9,10] Data obtained from umbilical vessels at the time of delivery suggest a higher extraction in the human fetus (0.52 to 0.62).[6,11] Because of lower O_2 consumption in the immature compared with the more mature fetus, O_2 extraction is significantly lower during early gestation.[6,12] When O_2 consumption is increased up to 28% higher than baseline levels in the fetus by the infusion of norepinephrine or thyroid hormone, arterial or venous blood gas values remain unaffected.[13] This finding underscores that, despite the low PaO_2, the fetus is able to adapt to conditions associated with significant increases in O_2 consumption without evidence of disturbances in oxidative metabolism in the tissues.

FETAL RESPONSE TO HYPOXEMIA

LACTIC ACIDOSIS IN FETAL HYPOXEMIA

Under physiologic conditions, lactate levels are higher in the fetal than the maternal circulation. The increase in fetal lactate levels is the result of enhanced placental lactate production and decreased fetal gluconeogenic utilization of lactate.[2] Lactic acidosis develops under pathologic conditions when compensatory increases in O_2 extraction and cardiac output have reached the limit of their capacity to satisfy tissue O_2 demand. Critical O_2 delivery in fetal sheep appears to be at 12 mL/kg/min, and decrements in O_2 delivery to less than this value are associated with impaired oxidative metabolism and accumulation of lactic acid in the fetal tissues and blood.[14] Indeed, elevated plasma lactate has been shown to be a good indicator of fetal hypoxemia. In addition to the significant correlation between umbilical lactate levels and other measures of acidosis, a recent meta-analysis also found that plasma lactate levels predict neurologic outcome including hypoxic-ischemic encephalopathy.[15] After 4 to 5 hours of fetal hypoxemia, blood lactate reaches a plateau despite continued anaerobic metabolism. Placental clearance of lactate is responsible for this phenomenon.[8] Thus, despite ongoing fetal anaerobic metabolism in cases of chronic and severe fetal hypoxemia, the fetal serum lactate level does not increase beyond the point of equilibrium.[8]

The fetus responds differently to various levels of severity of hypoxia. Maternal hypoxia-induced mild fetal hypoxia does not alter fetal acid-base balance when fetal arterial O_2 saturations remain in the 40% range even when the hypoxemia persists for 24 hours.[16] However, when fetal hypoxia results in fetal arterial O_2 saturations of less than 30%, metabolic acidosis develops.[17] Human data are consistent with the results of animal studies indicating that arterial oxygen saturation of 30% is the threshold for developing metabolic acidosis.[18,19] Thus the *critical threshold of arterial O_2 saturation,* defined as the arterial O_2 saturation below which metabolic acidosis develops, is approximately 30% in the maternal hypoxia-induced fetal hypoxia model in sheep. It appears that susceptibility of the fetus to hypoxia is developmentally regulated; the preterm fetus is less sensitive to the effects of maternal hypoxia than the term counterpart.[17,20] For instance, when maternal hypoxia results in fetal arterial O_2 saturations of less than 30%, the preterm ovine fetus develops metabolic acidosis at a much slower pace than that described for the fetus near or at term.[20]

The fetus also appears to respond differently to various causes of hypoxia.[21] Due to compensatory mechanisms within the placenta, placental oxygenation is protected from maternal hypoxia to a certain degree.[22] When fetal hypoxemia is induced by umbilical cord occlusion, the fetal response differs from that seen with maternal hypoxia.[23] When fetal hypoxemia is caused by umbilical cord occlusion, metabolic acidosis develops more rapidly compared with maternal hypoxia-induced fetal hypoxemia.[20] The lack of placental compensatory mechanisms in the cord occlusion model may be responsible for this difference. Finally, the fetal response to hypoxemia is also altered when hypoxia is caused by decreased uterine blood flow. In this model, the critical threshold of arterial O_2 saturation is lower than observed in the maternal hypoxia or cord occlusion models; rapid lactate accumulation and fall in pH only occur when fetal O_2 saturation is in the 15% to 20% range.[24] This finding suggests that placental compensatory mechanisms remain effective when blood flow to the uterus is decreased. Because of interspecies differences, these findings obtained in the sheep should be translated to the human fetus with caution.

ENDOCRINE RESPONSES TO FETAL HYPOXEMIA

In the fetus, acute hypoxemia is associated with an increase in plasma concentration of several hormones, including adrenocorticotropic hormone,[25-27] β-endorphin,[28,29] vasopressin,[30-32] glucocorticoids,[25-27] norepinephrine, and epinephrine.[24,32,33] This stress hormone response facilitates fetal adaptation to hypoxemia in part by ensuring the redistribution of blood flow to vital organs.[34]

However, the effectiveness of the fetal stress hormone response is limited by the developmentally regulated immaturity of certain endocrine organs and the cellular mechanisms of end-organ responses. For instance, although the fetal adrenal gland increases cortisol secretion in response to hypoxemic stress, the increase in the cortisol level is significantly less than occurs in mature animals, whereas the increase in the catecholamine levels is similar to that seen in the mature animal.[24] In addition, expression of the cardiovascular adrenergic receptors and second-messenger systems is developmentally regulated, contributing to the observed differences in the stress response between the fetus and the mature animal.

The exact mechanisms of the 50- to 1000-fold increase in fetal catecholamine release to fetal stress remain to be clarified. Cohn and colleagues[35] investigated the effect of metabolic acidosis on adrenal catecholamine secretion. In an effort to avoid the adrenal stimulatory effect of hypoxemia associated with acidosis-induced rightward shift in oxyhemoglobin dissociation curve, 100% O_2 was administered to the pregnant ewe during the infusion of 30% lactic acid to the fetus. Under these experimental circumstances, metabolic acidosis in the absence of hypoxia did not stimulate adrenal catecholamine secretion. Conversely, studies investigating fetal catecholamine release in the presence of hypoxemia have reported increased catecholamine and vasopressin secretion in the presence or absence of associated metabolic acidosis.[30,36]

CARDIOVASCULAR EFFECTS OF FETAL HYPOXEMIA

In the fetus, the right and left ventricles work in parallel, and therefore the combined left and right cardiac output is considered the total cardiac output. In the fetal lamb, the combined cardiac output is 450 mL/kg/min, to which the right and left ventricles contribute 300 and 150 mL/kg/min, respectively.[37] Similarly, in the human fetus, the contribution of the right ventricle to the combined cardiac output is significantly higher than that of the left ventricle. Data obtained by echocardiography show the combined cardiac output in human fetus to be similar to that of fetal sheep; however, the right ventricle contributes only approximately 60% of the combined output.[38,39]

In the fetal lamb, the cardiovascular response to acute hypoxemia is characterized by the rapid development of hypertension, bradycardia, increased peripheral vascular resistance, and a 15% to 20% decrease in the cardiac output. The decrease in cardiac output is primarily the result of the increased peripheral vascular resistance (afterload), bradycardia, vagal stimulation, and myocardial depression. However, significant myocardial depression occurs only if the hypoxemia is severe or prolonged or is associated with metabolic acidosis.[36] In the fetus, adenosine may play an important modulatory role in the previously described cardiovascular "maladaptation" by influencing fetal autonomic and glycolytic responses to hypoxia. In the sheep, blockade of adenosine receptors during fetal hypoxia significantly attenuates the development of hypertension (systemic vascular resistance [SVR] increase), bradycardia, and metabolic acidosis.[40,41] The fetal cardiovascular response to prolonged hypoxemia is different from that seen in acute hypoxemia models. In fetal sheep with sustained hypoxemia, cardiac output drops progressively to 38%, and, not unexpectedly, right ventricular output is compromised earlier than the left ventricular output.[42] Similarly, in a fetal lamb model using intermittent umbilical cord occlusions, metabolic acidosis is more severe with moderate variable heart rate decelerations in the chronically hypoxic fetus compared with the normoxic fetal sheep model.[43] In addition, the recovery time from acidosis is longer in chronically hypoxic fetus.

In response to fetal hypoxemia, distribution of cardiac output and venous return is altered in an effort to maintain perfusion and O_2 delivery to the vital organs such as the heart, brain, and adrenal glands.[9,44,45] During induced maternofetal hypoxia, the percentage of systemic venous blood recirculated to the fetal body and not sent to the placenta is decreased, whereas the proportion of umbilical venous blood contributing to fetal cardiac output is increased from 27% to 39%.[44] As mentioned earlier, there are differences in the fetal response, including the distribution of cardiac output, venous return, and O_2 delivery among the different models of fetal hypoxia. However, regardless of the cause of hypoxia, the blood flow and O_2 delivery to the heart, brain, and adrenal glands are maintained, and the proportion of umbilical venous blood bypassing the liver through the ductus venosus is increased in all cases.[9,44,45]

Finally, the fetal cardiovascular and endocrine response to acute hypoxemia is altered when repeated hypoxic events occur. This is important because recurrence of hypoxic insults to the fetus may not be infrequent in human pregnancies in which blood flow to the uterus, placenta, or the fetus is repeatedly compromised. It appears that hypoxemia sensitizes the cardiac and vasoconstrictor chemoreflex responses to repeated episodes of hypoxemia. For example, enhanced femoral vasoconstriction and marked elevation in plasma norepinephrine and vasopressin have been demonstrated in response to acute hypoxemia in fetal sheep that had been previously exposed to sustained hypoxemia.[46]

RENAL RESPONSES TO HYPOXEMIA

Although the placental-maternal unit performs most of the effective compensatory functions,[47] the fetal kidney has the ability to contribute to the maintenance of fetal acid-base balance. For instance, ammonium excretion and hence generation of bicarbonate, as well as sodium excretion, increase during the recovery period from hypocapnic-hypoxia in the fetal sheep.[48] The presence of hypocapnia appears to be a key determinant in the timing of fetal renal responses. Because fetal P_{CO_2} is low as a result of maternal compensatory hyperventilation in response to hypoxia in this model and because CO_2 is required for bicarbonate absorption in the proximal tubule, bicarbonate reabsorption and acid excretion in the fetus are delayed until hypoxemia subsides and maternal, and thus fetal, P_{CO_2} returns to normal.

In addition to the effects of hypoxemia on the renal compensatory mechanisms to maintain fetal acid-base balance, other changes in renal function are induced by hypoxemia. Fractional excretion of sodium is increased by a decrease in proximal tubule sodium reabsorption.[48,49] Urine osmolality also increases, and free water clearance drops secondary to increases in vasopressin release.[48,50] Finally, like the other organs, the immature kidney is also less susceptible to hypoxemia than the mature kidney.[51] The renal response to lactic acidosis induced by acid infusion in the fetal sheep is confined to tubular adaptive responses with decreases in urine pH and increases in ammonium and titratable acid excretion without changes in glomerular filtration rate.[52]

CARDIOVASCULAR COMPROMISE IN THE NEONATE

DEFINITION AND PHASES OF NEONATAL SHOCK

Shock develops when O_2 delivery to the tissues is inadequate to satisfy cellular metabolic demand. Independent of the origin, there are three phases of shock, and each phase is characterized by unique pathophysiologic changes.

In the *compensated phase*, vital organ function is maintained by intrinsic neurohormonal compensatory mechanisms resulting in distribution of organ blood flow primarily to the heart, brain, and adrenal glands and away from other, "nonvital," organs. Several hormones and local factors affecting myocardial function, organ blood flow distribution, capillary integrity, systemic and pulmonary vascular resistance, and cellular metabolism are released during this phase. Stroke volume, central venous pressure, and urine output all decrease. However, blood pressure remains within normal limits because the increases in myocardial contractility and heart rate maintain cardiac output close to the normal range. Because blood pressure is the function of blood flow and SVR, blood pressure may not always appropriately reflect the status of organ blood flow in this phase. This observation may be especially relevant for the nonacidotic extremely low-birth-weight preterm neonate with immature myocardium and compensated shock during the first postnatal day.[53,54] Importantly, the developing cerebral cortex of the extremely low-birth-weight preterm neonate may function as a "nonvital" organ (similar to the skin, muscle, kidney, liver, and mesentery) with a low-priority circulation resulting in vasoconstriction and decreased cortical perfusion in cases with low cardiac output.[55] Thus, in these patients, blood flow to only the brain stem and not to the entire brain may be maintained during the compensated phase of shock.

If the circulatory compromise is not recognized and treated, neonatal shock will enter the *uncompensated phase,* in which failure of the intrinsic neurohormonal compensatory mechanisms results in decreased microvascular perfusion, myocardial contractility, stroke volume, and blood pressure, with ensuing significant decreases in organ blood flow and tissue perfusion; ultimately lactic acidosis develops. If treatment is delayed or the condition is prone to rapid deterioration, such as in fulminant sepsis, myocarditis, or asphyxia with multiorgan failure, neonatal shock will enter the final and *irreversible phase,* in which cellular damage leading to complete organ failure dominates the clinical picture, and death invariably occurs.

FACTORS IN THE PATHOPHYSIOLOGY OF SHOCK AT THE CELLULAR AND MOLECULAR LEVEL

REACTIVE OXYGEN SPECIES

These molecules are involved in initiation and amplification of cellular injury in shock. Under normal conditions, the redox coupling reactions generate water as a result of complete O_2 reduction with only minimal (1%) univalent O_2 reduction to superoxide anion ($O \bullet_2^-$).[56] However, in shock, $O \bullet_2^-$ is significantly increased.[57] Ischemia and hypoxia result in accumulation of electron donor compounds such as reduced nicotinamide adenine dinucleotide (NADH) secondary to impairment of oxidative phosphorylation in the mitochondria.[57] Subsequent reperfusion then leads to enhanced production of reactive O_2 species because of increased availability of the electron acceptor O_2. The excess and dysregulated nitric oxide (NO) production in shock (see later) promotes reaction with superoxide anion producing the potent oxidant species peroxynitrite, which contributes to development of cardiovascular dysfunction.[58]

Anaerobic metabolism leads to inadequate production of adenosine triphosphate (ATP); as a result, hypoxanthine and xanthine accumulate. Under normal physiologic conditions, hypoxanthine is oxidized to urate by xanthine oxidoreductase. This enzyme exists in two forms, xanthine dehydrogenase and xanthine oxidase, with the latter generating $O \bullet_2^-$ and H_2O_2 as byproducts. During ischemia-reperfusion, cellular changes favor hypoxanthine oxidation by xanthine oxidase, with a resultant increase in the production of reactive O_2 species. Reactive O_2 species cause cellular injury through their adverse effects on cellular structures that lead to polysaccharide depolymerization, lipid peroxidation,[59] alterations in the primary structure of amino acids,[60] and nucleic acid oxidation.[61] These effects impair the cellular adhesion and receptor physiology, disrupt cell membrane integrity[59] and the function of many enzymes,[60] and damage DNA.[61] The fetus and neonate are prone to develop severe cellular injury during the ischemia-reperfusion cycle because they have immature antioxidant defenses.

NITRIC OXIDE

Under physiologic conditions, NO plays an important role in the regulation of vascular tone. However, under pathologic conditions, inducible NO synthase (iNOS) is up-regulated by endotoxin and proinflammatory cytokines, and large amounts of NO are produced.[62,63] Overproduction of NO by iNOS has been implicated in the pathogenesis of shock in pediatric patients, including newborn infants.[64,65] Excessive production of NO then leads to hypotension, decreased vascular response to vasoconstrictor hormones, and myocardial dysfunction.[62] In addition to the adverse cardiovascular effects, NO can cause direct cellular injury through formation of reactive free radicals such as peroxynitrite[66] and by inhibiting mitochondrial respiratory function.[67]

Because excess NO is involved in the pathogenesis of shock, studies have focused on testing therapeutic modalities that inhibit NOS as a possible treatment strategy, especially in septic shock. However, the use of nonselective NOS inhibitors that inhibit both endothelial NO synthase (eNOS) and iNOS has resulted in deleterious effects in immature[68] and mature animal models of shock and increased mortality in human adults with septic shock.[69,70] While excessive NO production in septic shock adversely affects hemodynamics and cellular functions, at the level of the microcirculation, reduced eNOS activity and NO availability may impair the microcirculation.[71] Therefore, further reduction of eNOS by nonselective NOS inhibition likely contributed to the observed poor outcome. In contrast, selective inhibition of iNOS improves lactic acidosis and circulatory function in the mature canine and sheep models of septic shock.[72,73] Despite observation that the use of selective iNOS inhibitors might be promising, to date none of these agents has been approved in humans.[74] As such, whether selective iNOS inhibition would be helpful in the treatment of neonatal shock remains to be elucidated.[65,75]

PLATELET-ACTIVATING FACTOR

This phospholipid mediator has been implicated in the pathogenesis of shock in both animal models[76,77] and adult subjects.[78,79] In animal models of septic shock, animals treated with a platelet-activating factor antagonist showed improvement in their cardiovascular status.[80,81] However, a randomized controlled trial (RCT) of a platelet-activating factor antagonist in adults with severe sepsis did not show any improvement in 28-day mortality.[82]

Although there is no study on the role of platelet-activating factor in neonatal shock, it may be important in the pathogenesis of necrotizing enterocolitis.[83,84]

EICOSANOIDS

In inflammation, arachidonic acid derived from cell membrane phospholipids is metabolized by cyclooxygenase or lipoxygenase to produce inflammatory mediators such as prostaglandins, thromboxanes, and leukotrienes. More recently, eicosanoids derived from the cytochrome P450 pathway of arachidonic acid such as hydroxyeicosatetraenoic acid and epoxyeicosatrienoic acid have also been shown to play a role in the inflammation associated with septic shock.[85] Although eicosanoids have been implicated in the pathogenesis of organ failure and shock, their exact role remains to be elucidated. Rats deficient in essential fatty acids, and thus unable to produce significant amounts of eicosanoids, are much less susceptible to endotoxic shock and have significantly improved survival rates compared with wild-type rats.[86]

Vasodilating eicosanoids, such as prostacyclin and prostaglandin E_2, and the vasoconstrictor thromboxane A_2, play an important role in the regulation of vascular tone. Some eicosanoids (thromboxane A_2) induce platelet and neutrophil aggregation and thus have significant proinflammatory effects, whereas others, such as prostaglandin E_2, also exert an antiinflammatory action by down-regulating cytokine release by macrophages and lymphocytes. Indeed, there are both animal and human data supporting the role of prostaglandins as both proinflammatory and antiinflammatory agents. In animals with hypovolemic shock, administration of prostacyclin or prostaglandins E_1 and E_2 improves cardiovascular status.[87-89] Furthermore, in the infected human and animal, studies have shown that inhibition of cyclooxygenase may improve both the cardiovascular status and survival especially in animal models of septic shock.[90-93]

Studies in animal models and humans have also shown that the levels of thromboxane B_2, a metabolite of thromboxane A_2, are increased in septic shock.[94,95] In addition to its proinflammatory and vasoconstrictor effects, thromboxane A_2 may have a direct myocardial depressant effect, and therefore it may significantly compromise cardiac output.[94]

K_{ATP} CHANNELS

Among the various potassium channels, ATP-dependent potassium (K_{ATP}) channel has emerged as the key channel through which many modulators exert their action on vascular smooth muscle tone. These channels are located in cell membrane of vascular smooth muscle cells. Under hypoxic conditions, reduction in ATP and increase in lactate level activate K_{ATP} channels, leading to efflux of K^+. The resultant hyperpolarization of the cell membrane decreases vascular tone by decreasing intracellular calcium concentrations through inhibition of voltage-gated calcium channels.[96]

K_{ATP} channels have been implicated in the pathogenesis of vasodilatory shock.[71,97] Some of the mediators of septic shock, such as NO, are known to activate K_{ATP}.[98] Animal studies have shown an improvement in blood pressure in response to K_{ATP} blockers,[99,100] but small human trials failed to show any benefit of the administration of the K_{ATP} channel inhibitor glibenclamide in adults with septic shock.[101,102]

OTHER FACTORS

Among other factors with potential clinical importance in shock, nuclear factor-κB (NF-κB, a nuclear transcription factor) has been suggested to have prognostic value. In patients with septic shock, higher peripheral mononuclear cell NF-κB activity is associated with increased mortality.[103] It is not known whether this is an association or a causative relationship.

DOWN-REGULATION OF ADRENERGIC RECEPTORS

Down-regulation of the adrenergic receptors and second-messenger systems in neonates[104] and adults[105] with critical illness, those receiving exogenous catecholamine administration,[106] as well as neonates with a relative or absolute adrenal insufficiency,[107] have emerged as probable causative factors for development of pressor-resistant shock. Because expression of the cardiovascular adrenergic receptors and some components of their second-messenger systems is inducible by glucocorticoids,[108] steroid administration offers a powerful clinical tool to reverse the effects of adrenergic receptor down-regulation.[104,105] These genomic effects of steroids resulting in the synthesis and membrane assembly of new receptor proteins require at least several hours to take place. However, improvement in cardiovascular function occurs within 1 to 2 hours following hydrocortisone administration to neonates.[104] This rapid therapeutic response may occur because steroids also have certain nongenomic actions, which affect the cardiovascular system without delay. Glucocorticoids inhibit catechol-*O*-methyltransferase, the rate-limiting enzyme in catecholamine metabolism, and decrease the reuptake of norepinephrine by the sympathetic nerve endings, leading to increases in the plasma concentration of catecholamines.[109] Physiologic doses of mineralocorticoids and, to a lesser degree, pharmacologic doses of glucocorticoids also instantly increase cytosolic calcium availability in myocardial and vascular smooth muscle cells by acting through putative cell membrane-bound specific steroid receptors.[109] In addition, steroids inhibit prostacyclin production and the induction of iNOS,[110] and limit the pathologic vasodilation associated with the nonspecific or specific inflammatory responses. Finally, by improving capillary integrity, steroid administration may also increase the effective circulating blood volume in neonates with capillary leak.[111,112]

PHYSIOLOGY OF NEONATAL CIRCULATION

CARDIAC OUTPUT

Under physiologic conditions, tissue perfusion is maintained by the provision of uninterrupted blood flow through the microcirculation. An intact microcirculation, in turn, depends on organ perfusion pressure maintained by the interaction among cardiac output, preload, and afterload. *Cardiac output* is the product of stroke volume and heart rate and is determined by the amount of blood returning to the heart (preload), the strength of myocardial contractility, and the resistance against which the heart must pump (afterload). When myocardial function is intact, cardiac output depends solely on preload and afterload, according to the relationships described by the Starling curve.

Normal ranges for left and right ventricular output for preterm and term neonates have been reported between 150 and 300 mL/kg/min.[113,114] In the transitional circulation of the newborn infant, in whom ventricular output does not consistently reflect systemic blood flow because of the shunts across the fetal channels,[114] superior vena cava (SVC) blood flow can be measured and used as a surrogate for systemic blood flow.[54] Normal values for SVC blood flow in well preterm neonates range between 40 and 120 mL/kg/min, with the median value rising from 70 mL/kg/min at 5 hours of age to 90 mL/kg/min at 48 hours.[54] However, further validation of the use of SVC blood flow as a measure of systemic blood flow is needed because a study using magnetic resonance imaging as the "gold standard" of cardiac output and blood flow measurement has cast some doubt on the accuracy of SVC blood flow measurement by echocardiography.[115]

The strength of myocardial contractility depends on the filling volume and pressure and on the maturity and integrity of the myocardium. Thus decreases in preload (e.g., hypovolemia or cardiac arrhythmia), as well as prematurity and hypoxic or infectious insults, all decrease contractility and lead to decreases in cardiac output.

If the systemic or pulmonary vascular resistance (afterload) is too high, the ability of the myocardium to pump against the increased resistance may become compromised and cardiac output will fall.[116] In the neonate, significant increases in afterload may occur with enhanced endogenous catecholamine release during the period of immediate postnatal adaptation, with volume overload, during hypothermia, and following administration of high doses of vasopressors to a patient with intact cardiovascular adrenoreceptor responsiveness. Depending on which circulation (systemic or pulmonary) is more severely affected, high afterload can impair the function of either ventricle. However, through the ensuing decrease in blood return to the initially unaffected ventricle, reduction in the output of one of the ventricles will influence the function of the other ventricle.

In the immediate postnatal period, shunts through the patent ductus arteriosus or foramen ovale may compromise the circulation.[117] During the first 20 minutes of normal transition following delivery, net blood flow through the ductus arteriosus becomes increasingly left to right.[118] In term neonates, the ductus arteriosus constricts in the first few hours and the shunt is closed by the second or third day. On the other hand, normal postnatal closure of these fetal channels frequently fails in the extremely low-birth-weight neonate. Therefore, as the right-sided pressures fall, pulmonary edema may rapidly develop, further compromising the hemodynamic status.[117]

SYSTEMIC BLOOD PRESSURE

Systemic blood pressure is the product of cardiac output and SVR. The gestational and postnatal age-dependent normal ranges for systemic blood pressure in neonates have been described in the literature.[119-121] Although blood pressure only weakly correlates with blood flow in the critically ill extremely low-birth-weight neonate during the period of immediate postnatal adaptation,[54,116] there is an association between low blood pressure and early central nervous system injury in this patient population.[122,123] However, a more recent study failed to show any association between hypotension in first 3 postnatal days (as defined by three commonly used thresholds) and brain injury diagnosed by ultrasound obtained before 10 postnatal days in preterm infants.[124] Data indicate that only when mean blood pressures in extremely low-birth-weight neonates are less than or equal to 20 mm Hg or greater than or equal to 40 mm Hg, blood pressure becomes a more accurate indicator of abnormal and normal systemic blood flow.[125,126] Thus, in extremely preterm neonates with mean blood pressures between 20 and 40 mm Hg in the immediate postnatal period, the state of systemic blood flow is unclear, and the situation may be clarified by obtaining additional information on cardiac function and organ blood flow using echocardiography, electrical impedance velocimetry, and near infrared spectroscopy. However, evidence for potential utility of such monitoring techniques has only recently started to emerge.

In contrast to extremely preterm infants, in more mature preterm and term neonates, blood pressure and organ blood flow appear to have a better correlation. Studies have provided some insights into the possible lower blood pressure limit of the cerebral blood flow autoregulatory curve. In extremely low-birth-weight infants during the transitional period (first 2 postnatal days), cerebral blood flow was maintained if mean blood pressure was greater than 29 mm Hg.[127] Interestingly, cerebral blood flow autoregulation in the frontal cortex assessed by near infrared spectroscopy became pressure-passive once mean blood pressure decreased to less than 29 mm Hg. Similarly, Børch and colleagues demonstrated that blood flow autoregulation in the white matter is also lost with mean blood pressure less than 29 mm Hg.[128] However, even if this cutoff value holds true in larger studies, lower blood pressures do not necessarily result in ischemic cerebral injury because compensatory mechanisms provide some degree of protection. Indeed, in one study, cerebral function as assessed by electroencephalogram was affected only when mean blood pressure decreased to less than 23 mm Hg.[129]

It has been postulated that by impairing cerebral blood flow, hypotension contributes to poor long-term neurodevelopmental outcome in the preterm infants. Indeed, numerous studies have shown a better outcome for normotensive compared with hypotensive preterm infants.[130,131] However, as hypotension is commonly treated, it is unclear whether the observed association between hypotension and poor outcome is primarily due to the underlying pathology, hypotension itself or the treatment used to "normalize blood pressure." This uncertainty has led to a call for less aggressive treatment of hypotension during the last decade. Indeed, some have even advocated to disregard the numeric value of blood pressure and to use clinical and laboratory makers of poor tissue perfusion to assess the adequacy of cardiovascular function.[132] As the approach has been adopted by some clinicians, this has provided an opportunity to evaluate the effect of "isolated" hypotension (i.e., no clinical or laboratory evidence of impaired tissue hypoperfusion but low blood pressure value). In a recent analysis of the French national prospective population-based cohort study, 119 extremely preterm infants with untreated "isolated" hypotension (defined as mean blood pressure <gestational age [GA]) were matched with 119 preterm neonates who received treatment for "isolated" hypotension during the first 3 postnatal days.[133] In this study, the treated group had a higher rate of survival without severe morbidity and lower rate of severe intraventricular hemorrhage (IVH) and cerebral injury. Interestingly, the association between treatment and better outcome was even stronger when hypotension was defined as mean arterial pressure (MAP)<GA−5 mm Hg. This dose-effect relationship strengthens the likelihood for causality.

ORGAN BLOOD FLOW AND ITS AUTOREGULATION

Most extremely immature preterm neonates are able to autoregulate their cerebral blood flow (Fig. 155.1).[123,134-136] However, autoregulation of organ blood flow is impaired in some preterm neonates, especially in those with birth asphyxia, acidosis, infection, tissue ischemia, and sudden alterations in arterial P_{CO_2}, rendering these patients at higher risk for cerebral injury. As mentioned earlier, the cortical vessels of extremely low-birth-weight neonates may be regulated as low-priority vessels, and thus blood is shifted away from the immature cerebral cortex during periods of circulatory compromise, as it is in other low-priority organ systems.[9,34,44,45] It is likely that the development of compensated shock and relative cortical ischemia is part of the transition to extrauterine life in most extremely low-birth-weight neonates.[137-141] The cortical ischemia then sets the stage for reperfusion injury (intracranial hemorrhage or periventricular white matter injury) once myocardial function and organ perfusion improve.[142,143] Several studies using different methodologies have shown that cerebral blood flow is low during first postnatal day in a subset of extremely preterm infants who later develop peri(P)/IVH.[137,138,142-145] This period is also associated with low cardiac output.[143] Subsequently, on day 2 or 3, after recovery of cardiac function and increase in cardiac output, cerebral blood flow increases significantly. The cycle of ischemia-reperfusion during postnatal transition has been postulated to be one of the pathophysiologic factors contributing to the development of P/IVH.[143,146] The cause of the initial low cardiac output is not clear. It has been suggested that the immature myocardium may not able to handle the suddenly increased afterload following removal of the low-resistance placental circulation at the time of cord clamping. Although there is some evidence to support this hypothesis,[147] poor contractility as measured by conventional echocardiographic techniques has not been consistently reported in this patient population.[143]

PATHOGENESIS OF NEONATAL SHOCK

The clinical presentation, pathophysiology, and treatment of neonatal shock are significantly affected by the primary cause of the condition.[148] Hypovolemia, myocardial dysfunction, and abnormal regulation of peripheral vascular tone are the primary etiologic factors leading to shock in the neonate. In the critically ill neonate, more than one of these factors may be involved. For instance, in a newborn with septic shock, capillary leak–induced hypovolemia, direct myocardial injury, and abnormal regulation of vascular tone may all contribute to development of the circulatory compromise.

HYPOVOLEMIA

Hypovolemia is an uncommon primary cause of neonatal shock, especially during the first postnatal days. In preterm newborns, there is little evidence that hypotensive babies as a group are hypovolemic,[149] which may, at least in part,

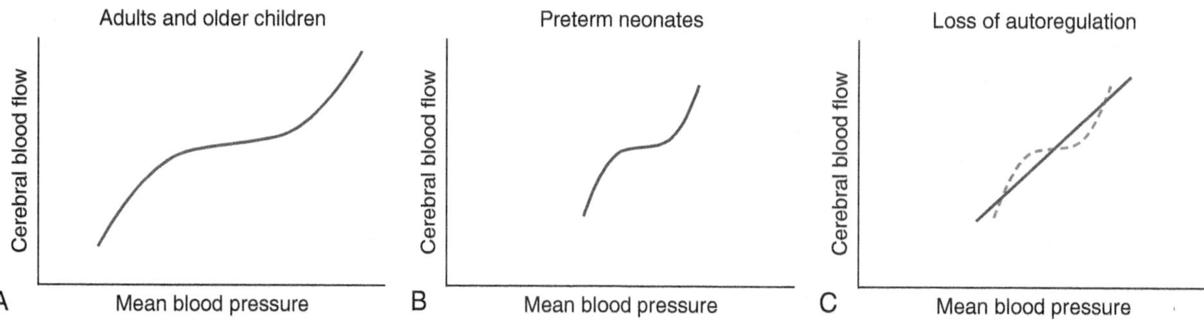

Fig. 155.1 The schematic drawings illustrate the concept of cerebral blood flow (CBF) autoregulation. If autoregulation is intact, within the autoregulatory range of blood pressure, CBF is maintained relatively constant. Note, that the blood flow regulatory function is far from being perfect as the autoregulatory CBF slope is approximately 10 degrees rather than 0 degree. Compared with adults and older children (A), preterm infants have a narrow autoregulatory blood pressure range (B). Therefore preterm infants are more likely to experience CBF fluctuations when their blood pressure changes (i.e., to have a pressure passive CBF). In sick preterm infants the autoregulation can be completely lost (C), in which case the risk of ischemia-reperfusion injury increases even further.

explain the absent, weak, or inconsistent responses to volume expanders.[150] However, the findings of improved hemodynamics following delayed compared with immediate cord clamping in preterm infants suggest a possible role for hypovolemia in the development of cardiovascular compromise during postnatal transition.[151,152] Although the hemodynamic impact of delayed cord clamping likely extends beyond the increase in intravascular volume (e.g., a more gradual increase in left ventricular afterload), the finding of improved blood pressure and decreased need for vasopressors/inotropes with cord milking[153,154] suggests that volume expansion is the primary mechanism responsible for hemodynamic improvement.

Hypovolemia causes low cardiac output and hypotension by decreasing preload. Hypovolemia can result from loss of circulating blood volume after hemorrhage (absolute hypovolemia) or from inappropriate increases in the capacitance of the blood vessels as in vasodilatory shock (relative hypovolemia). In addition, the positive intrathoracic pressure associated with positive pressure mechanical ventilation reduces venous return and hence preload and cardiac output in ventilated preterm and term neonates.[155]

Absolute hypovolemia in the neonate can be caused by intrapartum fetal blood loss resulting from a hemorrhage from the fetal side of the placenta, from acute fetomaternal hemorrhage, or from acute fetoplacental hemorrhage. The latter may occur in neonates with breech presentation or a tight nuchal cord, in whom the umbilical cord comes under significant pressure.[156] Postnatal hemorrhage may occur from or at any site and is frequently associated with endothelial damage and disseminated intravascular coagulation induced by sepsis or asphyxia. Acute abdominal surgical problems accompanied by peritonitis and conditions associated with increased capillary leak with loss of fluid into the interstitium can also lead to significant decreases in the circulating blood volume.

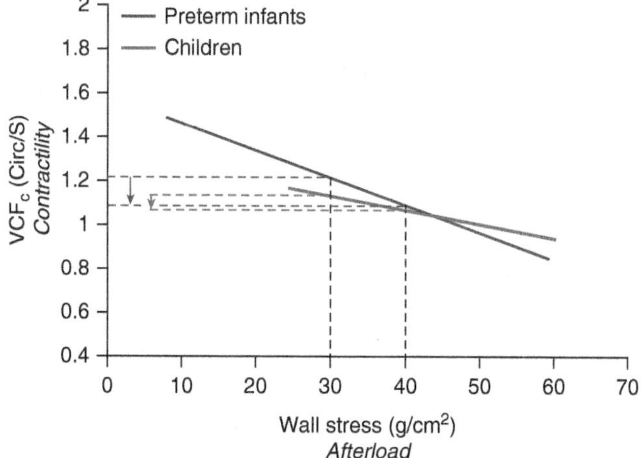

Fig. 155.2 The immature myocardium is more sensitive to afterload. The *green line* represents the normal inverse relationship that exists between myocardial contractility (heart rate–corrected velocity of circumferential fiber shortening *[VCFc]*) and afterload (wall stress) in children. In both term and preterm infants, the slope of this line is steeper (*red line* represents data from preterm infants during the transitional period). Accordingly, if, for example, afterload increases from 30 to 40 g/cm^2, myocardial contractility decreases far more in preterm infants (*red arrow*) than in older children (*green arrow*). (Data from Rowland DG, Gutgesell HP. Noninvasive assessment of myocardial contractility, preload, and afterload in healthy newborn infants. *Am J Cardiol.* 1995;75[12]:818–821; and Noori S, Wu T-W, Seri I. pH effects on cardiac function and systemic vascular resistance in preterm infants. *J Pediatr.* 2013;162[5]:958–963.e1. doi:10.1016/j.jpeds.2012.10.021)

MYOCARDIAL DYSFUNCTION AND STRUCTURAL HEART DISEASE

There are significant differences in myocardial structure and function between the immature myocardium of neonates and the mature myocardium of older children and adults.[148,157] Of particular interest among the differences are the greater dependence of the immature myocardium on extracellular calcium concentration and its greater sensitivity to an increase in afterload (Fig. 155.2). Therefore the neonate is more prone to develop myocardial dysfunction and decreased cardiac output in response to increased afterload compared with a child or an adult. Unfortunately, conditions that can lead to increase in afterload are not uncommon in the immediate postnatal period. With the cessation of low resistance placental flow after delivery, the SVR increases. The rise in SVR can lead to an increase in left ventricular afterload, with resultant decrease in cardiac output, and development of shock, primarily in the more immature preterm neonate during the transitional period. In one study, approximately half of the preterm infants with hypotension or metabolic acidosis exhibited myocardial dysfunction.[158] In addition, the myocardium in preterm infants with a low SVC flow (used as a surrogate of upper body blood flow) appears to be more sensitive to afterload than those with a normal SVC flow.[147] This finding suggests that developmentally regulated dysfunction of the immature myocardium plays a potential role in the development of poor organ perfusion. However, this phenomenon needs to be more extensively investigated because a study did not find that poor contractility was the underlying cause of low cardiac output associated with a low cerebral blood flow.[143] Interestingly, even though the myocardium takes months to mature, myocardial dysfunction of immaturity does not play a significant role in pathogenesis of neonatal shock beyond the transitional period.

Other than myocardial immaturity, perinatal asphyxia and prolonged septic shock (see under "Sepsis") are the major causes of myocardial dysfunction. Asphyxia significantly affects the cardiovascular system. Although the mechanisms of myocardial injury are not fully understood, degradation of contractile proteins such as myosin light chains and troponin I is known to be a major contributing factor. Hypoxia-ischemia followed by reperfusion increases reactive oxygen species, such as peroxynitrite, which can modify myosin light chains and lead to poor myocardial contractility.[159-161] However, studies evaluating cardiac function in asphyxiated neonates have shown variable results, in part due to the variability of the population studied in terms of severity of the perinatal hypoxic-ischemic event and the temporal relation between the event and patient assessment. Systolic function, as assessed by shortening and ejection fractions, has been shown to be decreased or unchanged. Newer echocardiographic modalities such as tissue Doppler and speckle tracking are more sensitive than the conventional method in detecting abnormal myocardial function in asphyxiated neonates. Although there is some variability on myocardial function in asphyxia among studies, markers of myocardial injury such as troponin T and I have been consistently found to be elevated.[162-164]

Even in neonates with mild perinatal depression, troponin T and I can be helpful in identifying the patient population with the highest likelihood of myocardial injury.[165] However, although cardiac troponin T and I may be more sensitive than echocardiography in detecting myocardial injury, the clinical significance of the elevation of troponins in the absence of echocardiographically diagnosed myocardial dysfunction remains unclear.

In addition to the impact of perinatal asphyxia on cardiac function, the standard treatment (therapeutic hypothermia) also affects cardiovascular function. During therapeutic hypothermia, cardiac output is reduced primarily due to a reduction in heart rate.[166,167] The reduction in cardiac output may also lead to reduction in perfusion of nonvital organs.[167]

Preterm infants who undergo ductal ligation may also develop myocardial dysfunction in the immediate postoperative period.[168-170] The cause of this phenomenon is unclear. It is possible that the acute decrease in myocyte fiber length due to the decrease in left ventricular preload following the removal of the left-to-right shunt by ligation of the ductus arteriosus plays a role. Myocardial function generally improves as the myocardium resets to the new loading condition.[168] Clinically, approximately one third of the patients undergoing patent ductus arteriosus (PDA) ligation exhibit some degree of cardiovascular compromise including hypotension.[171] Findings of studies suggest that myocardial dysfunction is the underlying etiologic factor in cases presenting with mild to moderate hypotension, whereas poor vascular tone, frequently associated with adrenal insufficiency, is the predominant underlying pathophysiologic factor in patients with severe hypotension refractory to vasopressor administration.[172,173] Interestingly, the significantly lower rate of hypotension and the need for vasopressors/inotropes with transcatheter device closure of PDA[174,175] suggest that surgical ligation itself and/or the stress associated with the procedure are among the important underlying causes of the postligation hemodynamic instability.

Finally, structural heart defects that result in ductal-dependent systemic circulation (hypoplastic left heart syndrome, critical coarctation of aorta, and critical aortic stenosis), and infants with an anomalous left coronary artery, myocarditis, or tachyarrhythmias can also present in early neonatal life with cardiogenic shock.

ABNORMAL PERIPHERAL VASOREGULATION AND NEONATAL SHOCK WITH COMPLEX PATHOGENESIS

Extreme Prematurity

The transitional circulatory changes in the first 12 to 24 hours after birth represent a period of unique circulatory vulnerability for the extremely preterm infant. During the period of immediate postnatal adaptation, the left ventricle has to double its output. As described in the section on organ blood flow autoregulation, the extremely premature infant has significant difficulties in transition to extrauterine life and is prone to develop reperfusion injury in the brain.[116,142,143] Under these conditions, blood pressure in the low-normal to normal range does not necessarily translate into normal organ blood flow and tissue perfusion.[54,116]

In the transitional circulation of the preterm infant, neither right nor left ventricular output will consistently reflect systemic blood flow because of the shunts across the ductus arteriosus and foramen ovale.[114] Consequently, measurement of either ventricular output can overestimate systemic blood flow by more than 100% in some cases.[114] As mentioned earlier, SVC flow has been used as a marker of total systemic blood flow,[55] and serial measurements of SVC flow have been used to describe the natural history of systemic blood flow changes in preterm neonates in the early postnatal period.[142,176] At least one third of preterm neonates born before 30 weeks gestation have a period of low systemic blood flow, mostly during the first 12 hours after birth.[54,142] Gestational age is the dominant predictor of the development of the low-flow state; 70% of babies born before 26 weeks gestation have a period of low systemic flow compared with approximately 10% at 29-weeks' gestation. However, a study by the authors of the original publication on the presence and incidence of low systemic blood flow found the incidence of low SVC flow to be only 19%, an incidence much lower than that in the original study.[177] Thus the development of a low-flow state with compensated neonatal shock appears to be part of the adaptation process in the extremely low-birth-weight patient population immediately after birth. Although myocardial dysfunction and disturbed cerebral autoregulation may be predisposing factors for central nervous system injury, iatrogenic factors such as inappropriately high mean airway pressure and/or hypocarbia may also decrease cardiac output and lower cerebral blood flow. The low-flow state can persist for up to 24 hours but usually improves thereafter. As noted earlier, there is a strong relationship between recovery from the low-flow state and subsequent IVH.[142,143] Furthermore, the low-flow state itself has also been identified as a significant risk factor for poor neurodevelopmental outcome.[131]

Sepsis

Endotoxin or lipopolysaccharide plays a major role in the pathophysiology of septic shock caused by gram-negative organisms. Lipopolysaccharide induces the production of proinflammatory cytokines such as tumor necrosis factor-α (TNF-α) and interleukin-1. In addition to activating the inflammatory response, TNF-α also induces apoptosis.[178] NF-κB, a nuclear transcriptional factor, mediates the inflammatory response induced by TNF-α.[179] TNF-α is a potent stimulator of iNOS, and overproduction of NO causes vasodilatation and systemic hypotension, and generates reactive free radicals such as peroxynitrite. In gram-negative septic shock, myocardial dysfunction develops, at least in part because of the effect of up-regulated TNF-α production.[180] In critically ill adults with sepsis, improvements in cardiac function have been noted following the administration of anti-TNF-α antibody.[181] Finally, TNF-α, by up-regulating tissue factor production in endothelial cells, also activates the extrinsic coagulation pathway and contributes to the generation of thrombi in the microcirculation.[182]

The triggers of inflammation and the host response in septic shock caused by gram-positive organisms are less well defined.

However, cell wall components such as peptidoglycans and lipoteichoic acid, as well as exotoxins, have been implicated in the induction of the cytokine cascade.[183] Regardless of the trigger, endothelial damage appears to be a key factor in the pathogenesis of sepsis and the development of shock.[184]

Although clinical evidence of circulatory compromise is a feature of many infectious processes in the newborn, the hemodynamics in neonatal septic shock have not been well studied. In older subjects, two distinct hemodynamic patterns occur. *Warm shock* is characterized by loss of vascular tone, increased systemic blood flow, and low blood pressure; it is difficult to recognize initially unless the blood pressure is closely monitored. Conversely, *cold shock* is characterized by increased vascular tone, low systemic blood flow, and eventually falling blood pressure and has been well described in the newborn.[185] In pediatric patients, both systolic and diastolic myocardial dysfunction are common in septic shock.[186] Myocardial dysfunction is more likely to occur in the more severe cases and in the more advanced stages of shock.[187,188] A recent study of 78 children with fluid- and catecholamine-refractory septic shock found the rate of left and right ventricular dysfunction to be 72% and 63%, respectively.[188] Left ventricular dysfunction was associated with a higher severity of illness and use of vasoactive medications, whereas right ventricular systolic dysfunction was associated with cold shock. The prevalence of myocardial dysfunction in neonatal septic shock is unclear. One study showed a high cardiac output in preterm infants with sepsis.[189] Another study demonstrated a higher left ventricular output (LVO) and incidence of PDA in preterm infants with septic shock compared with control infants, but right ventricular output (RVO) and ejection fraction were similar.[190] Interestingly, there was evidence of peripheral vasoconstriction (cool peripheries, poor peripheral pulses) in the majority of patients with septic shock.[190] A more recent study found high LVO and low SVR in neonates (mean gestational age of 30 weeks) with fluid-refractory septic shock.[191] However, the high rate of PDA (50%) in this study may in part explain high LVO and calculated low SVR. In summary, although overall evidence points to warm shock as the more common initial presentation of septic shock in neonates, data indicate that cold shock is commonly observed.

VASOPRESSOR-RESISTANT SYSTEMIC HYPOTENSION IN NEONATES

As discussed in the section on down-regulation of adrenergic receptors, vasopressor-resistant hypotension in preterm and term infants is now a well-recognized condition.[104,192] The underlying systemic hemodynamic changes appear to be similar to those seen in adult vasodilatory shock, with normal to high systemic blood flow and often supernormal cardiac outputs.[193] Neonates with this condition are more likely to be critically ill or extremely premature (≤27 weeks) or have suffered from perinatal asphyxia. Potential mechanisms for the uncontrolled vasodilation include dysregulated cytokine release, excess NO synthesis, vasopressin deficiency, overactivation of the potassium-ATP channels in the vascular smooth muscle cell membrane in response to tissue hypoxia, and down-regulation of the cardiovascular adrenergic receptors and the renin-angiotensin system.[104] In the neonate, the foregoing mechanisms may be exacerbated by immaturity, relative adrenal insufficiency,[107,194] and preceding asphyxia, or they may be secondary to the transitional circulatory failure of the extremely low-birth-weight neonate. Recently, a polymorphism in the glucocorticoid receptor gene was shown to be associated with refractory hypotension in premature infants.[195] Accordingly, the differences in glucocorticoid receptors sensitivity to glucocorticoids among different patients has been attributed to receptor gene polymorphisms. The genotype C/G of the *BclI* polymorphism was associated with higher rate of refractory hypotension and a need for higher doses of vasopressors/inotropes and hydrocortisone in preterm infants during first 48 hours after birth.[195]

CONCLUSION

In utero environment is characterized by significant hypoxemia compared with the normal level of oxygenation during extrauterine life. However, the fetus is well equipped to ensure adequate oxygen delivery for growth and development via, among others, higher cardiac output, differential oxygen saturation to selected organs, higher oxygen carrying capacity, and higher oxygen affinity of fetal hemoglobin. Depending on the cause of the decrease in oxygenation below the physiologic fetal levels, animal models indicate that the fetus has the capacity to compensate up to a certain degree. For instance, the fetus can divert a greater proportion of the better oxygenated blood of the umbilical vein away from the liver into ductus venosus and also can preferentially perfuse the vital organs. The process of transition from the parallel circulation of fetal life to that of a circulation in series after birth may be impaired in a subset of neonates, especially in the extremely preterm infant. Developmental characteristics of the circulatory system and vulnerability of the immature organs put the neonate at increased risk for morbidity and mortality when faced with pathologic processes such as neonatal sepsis.

A complete reference list is available at www.ExpertConsult.com. 

SELECT REFERENCES

1. Nye GA, et al. Human placental oxygenation in late gestation: experimental and theoretical approaches. *J Physiol (Lond.)*. 2018;596:5523–5534.
2. Rothstein R, Longo L. Respiration in the fetal-placental unit. In: Cowett R, ed. *Principles of Perinatal-Neonatal Metabolism*. Vol 451. New York:Springer-Verlag; 1998.
3. Nicolaides KH, Economides DL, Soothill PW. Blood gases, pH, and lactate in appropriate- and small-for-gestational-age fetuses. *Am J Obstet Gynecol*. 1989;161:996–1001.
4. Weiner CP, Sipes SL, Wenstrom K. The effect of fetal age upon normal fetal laboratory values and venous pressure. *Obstet Gynecol*. 1992;79:713–718.
5. Arikan GM, et al. Low fetal oxygen saturation at birth and acidosis. *Obstet Gynecol*. 2000;95:565–571.
6. Richardson B, et al. Fetal oxygen saturation and fractional extraction at birth and the relationship to measures of acidosis. *Am J Obstet Gynecol*. 1998;178:572–579.
7. Ehrenkranz RA, Walker AM, Oakes GK, McLaughlin MK, Chez RA. Effect of ritodrine infusion on uterine and umbilical blood flow in pregnant sheep. *Am J Obstet Gynecol*. 1976;126:343–349.
8. Hooper SB. Fetal metabolic responses to hypoxia. *Reprod Fertil Dev*. 1995;7:527–538.
9. Itskovitz J, LaGamma EF, Rudolph AM. Effects of cord compression on fetal blood flow distribution and O2 delivery. *Am J Physiol*. 1987;252:H100–H109.
10. Smolich JJ. NO modulates fetoplacental blood flow distribution and whole body oxygen extraction in fetal sheep. *Am J Physiol*. 1998;274:R1331–R1337.
11. Rurak D, Selke P, Fisher M, Taylor S, Wittmann B. Fetal oxygen extraction: comparison of the human and sheep. *Am J Obstet Gynecol*. 1987;156:360–366.
12. Bell AW, Kennaugh JM, Battaglia FC, Makowski EL, Meschia G. Metabolic and circulatory studies of fetal lamb at midgestation. *Am J Physiol*. 1986;250:E538–E544.
13. Lorijn RH, Longo LD. Clinical and physiologic implications of increased fetal oxygen consumption. *Am J Obstet Gynecol*. 1980;136:451–457.
14. Edelstone DI, Darby MJ, Bass K, Miller K. Effects of reductions in hemoglobin-oxygen affinity and hematocrit level on oxygen consumption and acid-base state in fetal lambs. *Am J Obstet Gynecol*. 160:820-826; discussion 826-828 (1989).
15. Allanson ER, Waqar T, White C, Tunçalp Ö, Dickinson JE. Umbilical lactate as a measure of acidosis and predictor of neonatal risk: a systematic review. *BJOG*. 2017;124:584–594.
16. Towell ME, Figueroa J, Markowitz S, Elias B, Nathanielsz P. The effect of mild hypoxemia maintained for twenty-four hours on maternal and fetal glucose, lactate, cortisol, and arginine vasopressin in pregnant sheep at 122 to 139 days' gestation. *Am J Obstet Gynecol*. 1987;157:1550–1557.

17. Nijland R, Jongsma HW, Nijhuis JG, van den Berg PP, Oeseburg B. Arterial oxygen saturation in relation to metabolic acidosis in fetal lambs. *Am J Obstet Gynecol.* 1995;172:810-819.
18. Dildy GA, Thorp JA, Yeast JD, Clark SL. The relationship between oxygen saturation and pH in umbilical blood: implications for intrapartum fetal oxygen saturation monitoring. *Am J Obstet Gynecol.* 1996;175:682-687.
19. Kühnert M, Seelbach-Göebel B, Butterwegge M. Predictive agreement between the fetal arterial oxygen saturation and fetal scalp pH: results of the German multicenter study. *Am J Obstet Gynecol.* 1998;178:330-335.
20. Matsuda Y, Patrick J, Carmichael L, Challis J, Richardson B. Effects of sustained hypoxemia on the sheep fetus at midgestation: endocrine, cardiovascular, and biophysical responses. *Am J Obstet Gynecol.* 1992;167:531-540.
21. Ross MG, Gala R. Use of umbilical artery base excess: algorithm for the timing of hypoxic injury. *Am J Obstet Gynecol.* 2002;187:1-9.
22. Arthuis CJ, et al. Real-time monitoring of placental oxygenation during maternal hypoxia and Hyperoxygenation using photoacoustic imaging. *PloS One.* 2017;12:e0169850.
23. Ball RH, Parer JT, Caldwell LE, Johnson J. Regional blood flow and metabolism in ovine fetuses during severe cord occlusion. *Am J Obstet Gynecol.* 1994;171:1549-1555.
24. Paulick R, Kastendieck E, Weth B, Wernze H. [Metabolic, cardiovascular and sympathoadrenal reactions of the fetus to progressive hypoxia–animal experiment studies]. *Z Geburtshilfe Perinatol.* 1987;191:130-139.
25. Jones CT, Boddy K, Robinson JS, Ratcliffe JG. Developmental changes in the responses of the adrenal glands of foetal sheep to endogenous adrenocorticotrophin, as indicated by hormone responses to hypoxaemia. *J Endocrinol.* 1977;72:279-292.
26. Challis JR, Richardson BS, Rurak D, Wlodek ME, Patrick JE. Plasma adrenocorticotropic hormone and cortisol and adrenal blood flow during sustained hypoxemia in fetal sheep. *Am J Obstet Gynecol.* 1986;155:1332-1336.
27. Challis JR, Fraher L, Oosterhuis J, White SE, Bocking AD. Fetal and maternal endocrine responses to prolonged reductions in uterine blood flow in pregnant sheep. *Am J Obstet Gynecol.* 1989;160:926-932.
28. Wardlaw SL, Stark RI, Daniel S, Frantz AG. Effects of hypoxia on beta-endorphin and beta-lipotropin release in fetal, newborn, and maternal sheep. *Endocrinology.* 1981;108:1710-1715.
29. Skillman CA, Clark KE. Fetal beta-endorphin levels in response to reductions in uterine blood flow. *Biol Neonate.* 1987;51:217-223.
30. Raff H, Kane CW, Wood CE. Arginine vasopressin responses to hypoxia and hypercapnia in late-gestation fetal sheep. *Am J Physiol.* 1991;260:R1077-R1081.
31. Stark RI, Daniel SS, Husain MK, Tropper PJ, James LS. Cerebrospinal fluid and plasma vasopressin in the fetal lamb: basal concentration and the effect of hypoxia. *Endocrinology.* 1985;116:65-72.
32. Sameshima H, Ikenoue T, Kamitomo M, Sakamoto H. Vasopressin and catecholamine responses to 24-hour, steady-state hypoxemia in fetal goats. *J Matern Fetal Med.* 1996;5:262-267.
33. Cohen WR, Piasecki GJ, Jackson BT. Plasma catecholamines during hypoxemia in fetal lamb. *Am J Physiol.* 1982;243:R520-R525.
34. Cohn HE, Sacks EJ, Heymann MA, Rudolph AM. Cardiovascular responses to hypoxemia and acidemia in fetal lambs. *Am J Obstet Gynecol.* 1974;120:817-824.
35. Cohn HE, Piasecki GJ, Cohen WR, Jackson BT. The adrenal secretion of catecholamines during systemic metabolic acidosis in fetal sheep. *Biol Neonate.* 1997;72:125-132.
36. Faucher DJ, et al. Vasopressin and catecholamine secretion during metabolic acidemia in the ovine fetus. *Pediatr Res.* 1987;21:38-43.
37. Fineman J, Clyman R, Heymann M. Fetal cardiovascular physiology. In: Creasy R, Resnik R, Iams J, eds. *Maternal-Fetal Medicine: Principles and Practice.* Vol 169. Philadelphia: WB Saunders Co; 2004.
38. Rasanen J, Wood DC, Weiner S, Ludomirski A, Huhta JC. Role of the pulmonary circulation in the distribution of human fetal cardiac output during the second half of pregnancy. *Circulation.* 1996;94:1068-1073.
39. Mielke G, Benda N. Cardiac output and central distribution of blood flow in the human fetus. *Circulation.* 2001;103:1662-1668.
40. Koos BJ, Chau A, Ogunyemi D. Adenosine mediates metabolic and cardiovascular responses to hypoxia in fetal sheep. *J Physiol (Lond.).* 1995;488(Pt 3):761-766.
41. Koos BJ, Maeda T. Adenosine A(2A) receptors mediate cardiovascular responses to hypoxia in fetal sheep. *Am J Physiol Heart Circ Physiol.* 2001;280:H83-H89.
42. Kamitomo M, Longo LD, Gilbert RD. Cardiac function in fetal sheep during two weeks of hypoxemia. *Am J Physiol.* 1994;266:R1778-R1785.
43. Amaya KE, et al. Accelerated acidosis in response to variable fetal heart rate decelerations in chronically hypoxic ovine fetuses. *Am J Obstet Gynecol.* 2016;214:270.e1-270.e8.
44. Reuss ML, Rudolph AM. Distribution and recirculation of umbilical and systemic venous blood flow in fetal lambs during hypoxia. *J Dev Physiol.* 1980;2:71-84.
45. Jensen A, Roman C, Rudolph AM. Effects of reducing uterine blood flow on fetal blood flow distribution and oxygen delivery. *J Dev Physiol.* 1991;15:309-323.
46. Gardner DS, Fletcher AJW, Bloomfield MR, Fowden AL, Giussani DA. Effects of prevailing hypoxaemia, acidaemia or hypoglycaemia upon the cardiovascular, endocrine and metabolic responses to acute hypoxaemia in the ovine fetus. *J Physiol (Lond.).* 2002;540:351-366.
47. Blechner JN. Maternal-fetal acid-base physiology. *Clin Obstet Gynecol.* 1993;36:3-12.
48. Gibson KJ, McMullen JR, Lumbers ER. Renal acid-base and sodium handling in hypoxia and subsequent mild metabolic acidosis in foetal sheep. *Clin Exp Pharmacol Physiol.* 2000;27:67-73.
49. Cock ML, Wlodek ME, McCrabb GJ, Harding R. Alterations in fetal urine production during prolonged hypoxaemia induced by reduced uterine blood flow in sheep: mechanisms. *Clin Exp Pharmacol Physiol.* 1996;23:57-63.
50. Wintour EM, Congiu M, Hardy KJ, Hennessy DP. Regulation of urine osmolality in fetal sheep. *Q J Exp Physiol.* 1982;67:427-435.

Pathophysiology of Apnea of Prematurity 156

Lisa J. Mitchell | Peter M. MacFarlane | Ryan W. Bavis | Richard J. Martin

EPIDEMIOLOGY AND DEFINITION OF APNEA

DEFINITION

Apnea is an almost universal manifestation of immature respiratory control in premature infants. Such infants may experience respiratory pauses of varying duration, with decreasing gestational age increasing vulnerability to such events. Short respiratory pauses may be self-limiting, while longer episodes may necessitate intervention, especially in the most immature infants. Apnea has traditionally been defined as a respiratory pause lasting at least 20 seconds, or a pause accompanied by bradycardia, cyanosis, or pallor. However, shorter apnea events (e.g., 15 seconds in duration), if recurrent, may also require clinical intervention, particularly if they result in hypoxemia.

Apnea should be distinguished from periodic breathing, in which the infant exhibits regular cycles of rapid respiration for approximately 10 seconds interspersed with pauses of similar duration, in a recurring pattern (≥3 cycles). Periodic breathing has been considered to represent a benign respiratory pattern in the premature or young term infant, although there may be

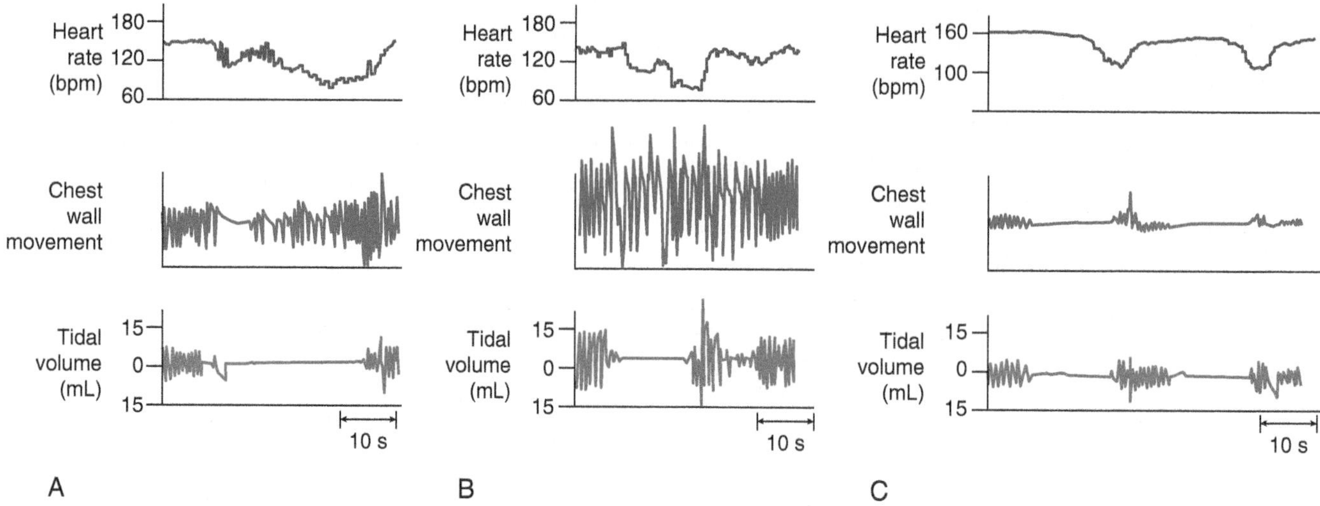

Fig. 156.1 (A) Mixed apnea. Obstructed breaths precede and follow a central respiratory pause. (B) Obstructive apnea. Breathing efforts continue, although no nasal airflow occurs. (C) Central apnea. Both nasal airflow and breathing efforts cease simultaneously. (From Miller MJ. In Edelman N, Santiago T, eds. *Breathing Disorders of Sleep*. New York: Churchill Livingstone; 1986.)

accompanying hypoxemia and bradycardia. The respiratory pause of apnea, unlike that of periodic breathing, may not be self-limiting and may produce significant physiologic changes. Such changes are considered in detail in the following discussion.

CLASSIFICATION

Apneic events are distinguished not only by their duration but also by the presence or absence of airway obstruction during the episode of apnea. Thach and Stark[1] initially described an increase in the frequency of apnea when the premature infant's neck was flexed. Subsequently, upper airway obstruction was found to accompany apnea in preterm babies, even though neck flexion was not present.[2] The location within the upper airway at which obstruction occurs is usually within the pharynx but may vary between pharyngeal and laryngeal structures.

The presence or absence of upper airway obstruction forms the basis of the classification of apnea into three types (Fig. 156.1). Mixed apnea is the most commonly observed clinically significant event in small premature infants and consists of obstructed inspiratory efforts as well as a central pause (see Fig. 156.1A). In obstructive apnea, obstructed breaths characterized by chest wall motion without nasal airflow continue throughout the entire apnea (see Fig. 156.1B). In central apnea, inspiratory efforts cease entirely, and obstructed breaths are not observed (see Fig. 156.1C). Mixed apnea accounts for approximately 50% to 75% of all instances of apnea in premature infants; obstructive apnea, 10% to 20%; and central apnea, 10% to 25%.[3] The longer an apneic event lasts, the more likely that it is a mixed-type apnea rather than a purely centrally mediated event.

Apnea duration and classification also may correlate with the infant's neurologic status. Apnea in a subset of infants may possibly be a sign of a diffuse neurologic insult in prenatal or postnatal life that leads to disordered control of breathing. In most infants, however, an underlying neuropathologic process is unlikely, because apnea frequency decreases as the infant matures. Whether apnea with accompanying hypoxemia and bradycardia contributes to later adverse outcome remains speculative. Hypothetically, apnea may resolve when central and peripheral chemoreceptors develop to the point at which appropriate responses to change in blood gas status can occur, possibly with accompanying arousal. A further important developmental contribution to resolution of apnea may be the increasing ability of medullary respiratory control centers to activate upper airway–dilating musculature in synchrony with increasing ventilatory drive.

Hypoxemic events resembling apneic spells also occur in intubated, mechanically ventilated preterm infants. Bolivar and co-workers[4] described episodes of hypoxemia preceded by an increase in total pulmonary resistance, a decrease in compliance, and apnea in intubated infants. Furthermore, Dimaguila and colleagues[5] reported that such episodes may be preceded by subtle spontaneous movement and are characterized by both central respiratory depression and obstruction to airflow (the latter features being analogous to mixed apnea). These hypoxemic episodes in intubated infants are a consequence of hypoventilation and are frequently associated with arousal.[6] They further illustrate the vulnerability of premature infants to imbalance of central respiratory control and altered pulmonary function.

PHYSIOLOGIC EFFECTS

Cessation of respiration during apnea has significant ventilatory and reflex cardiovascular consequences for the preterm infant. Both hypoxemia and hypercarbia accompany prolonged apnea. The decrease in oxygenation with apnea may be directly related to the duration of the apnea and baseline respiratory status (Fig. 156.2). The reflex effects of apnea include characteristic changes in heart rate. Bradycardia may begin within seconds of the onset of the apneic episode (Fig. 156.3). The bradyarrhythmia most often is sinus in character, with an occasional infant showing a nodal escape. Dorostkar and associates[7] have observed that 1.8% of preterm infants may even have asystolic events during apnea, defined as absence of QRS complex for more than 3 seconds during apnea. This subgroup of infants appears to have a benign clinical outcome. Henderson-Smart and co-workers[8] noted a significant correlation between the decrease in oxygen saturation and heart rate and postulated that bradycardia during apnea could result from hypoxic stimulation of the carotid body chemoreceptors.

The relationship between reflex control of heart rate and breathing is complex. When ventilation is allowed to increase in response to hypoxia, tachycardia occurs. When this reflex increase in ventilation is prevented, bradycardia results. At the onset of apnea, at which time cessation of ventilation and onset of hypoxemia occur almost simultaneously, hypoxemia would be expected to produce bradycardia.

Other reflex input may accentuate the bradycardia during hypoxemia. For example, the reflex effects of apnea in infants also have been likened to the physiologic responses in diving mammals. During reflex apnea in these animals, upper airway afferent input from superior laryngeal and trigeminal nerve

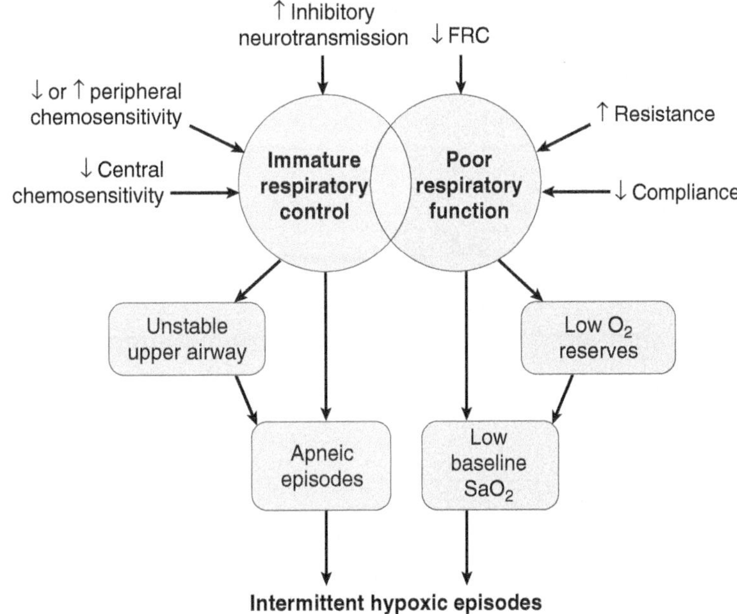

Fig. 156.2 Overview of the various contributors to vulnerability of neonatal respiratory control superimposed on impaired respiratory function in preterm infants. *FRC,* Functional residual capacity; *Sao_2,* arterial oxygen saturation.

stimulation may produce greatly enhanced bradycardia. The contribution of upper airway reflexes to the bradycardia that occurs during apnea is difficult to study in human infants. In summary, the rapid onset of bradycardia during apnea may be a complex reflex deriving from multiple sources, including trigeminal receptors and carotid chemoreceptors.

A change in blood pressure also accompanies apnea in newborn infants. The decrease in heart rate during apnea may be accompanied by a concomitant rise in pulse pressure, usually owing to an increase in systolic pressure, occasionally accompanied by a fall in diastolic pressure. During bradycardia, filling volume of the heart may increase, leading to a rise in stroke volume and pulse pressure in accordance with the Starling law. With prolonged apnea and more severe bradycardia (less than 80 beats/min), a decrease in systemic blood pressure may occur, accompanied by a fall in cerebral diastolic and systolic blood flow velocity. In premature infants with poor cerebrovascular autoregulation, cerebral blood flow may mirror systemic blood flow, and cerebral perfusion may decrease during prolonged apnea, although potential consequences remain speculative. Resolution of apnea may then be accompanied by cerebral hyperperfusion.

INTERMITTENT HYPOXEMIA

Continuous recording of oxygen saturations via pulse oximetry has revealed a much higher incidence of intermittent hypoxemic (IH) events associated with apnea than was previously thought, and permitted analysis of high-risk IH patterns that correlate with undesirable clinical outcomes. Previous studies examining the long-term effects of apnea may in fact be proxy for the effects of IH. IH events are associated with multiple negative outcomes including retinopathy of prematurity (ROP), bronchopulmonary dysplasia (BPD), sleep-disordered breathing, wheezing, unfavorable neurodevelopmental outcomes, and death, but it can be difficult to separate the effects of IH itself from the therapies, such as oxygen, used to treat it. Furthermore, the association between IH events and adverse outcomes may not be causal. Although the mechanisms underlying the pathologic correlates of IH are still under investigation, there is evidence from rodent models that IH causes changes in inflammatory signaling[9] and generation of reactive oxygen species.[10] Normally only a small amount of oxygen is incompletely reduced to form reactive oxygen species, which in most cases are neutralized by endogenous antioxidants and free radical scavengers. However, preterm infants do not have well-developed antioxidant defenses, and under metabolically stressful situations the free radicals generated could cause direct tissue damage and trigger proinflammatory and proapoptotic pathways. ATP is exhausted during hypoxia, leading to the generation of purine derivatives (e.g., hypoxanthine); upon reoxygenation, oxidases that metabolize these derivatives are reactivated and generate a burst of superoxide anion.[11]

IH exposure appears to have different effects depending on the specific developmental window in which it occurs. For example, a higher incidence of IH within the first 3 days of life is associated with increased risk of airway hyperreactivity, whereas increased frequency of IH events after 21 days of life (especially in infants with intrauterine growth restriction [IUGR]) is associated with development of BPD.[11] Increased frequency of IH episodes in the first 8 weeks of life (especially after 5 weeks of age) in preterm infants is associated with severe ROP requiring laser surgery.[12] The pattern of IH events appears significant, as well; the relationship between IH and severe ROP was even stronger when there was a time interval of at least one minute between events, possibly reflecting the time interval required for development of oxidative stress affecting neovascularization.[13] In addition, BPD is associated with more frequent, longer, but less severe IH events, combined with exposure to increased oxygen within the first 26 days after birth.[14] Prolonged IH episodes lasting at least one minute in the first 2 to 3 months of life were associated with worse outcomes (late death or disability) at 18 months of age. Isolated bradycardic events were not prognostically significant.[15] Interestingly, not all IH patterns are detrimental. Some rodent studies have shown improved long-term spatial learning and memory with brief, mild hypoxic exposures.[16,17] The most damaging IH events appear to be those that last longer than 1 minute and are 1 to 20 minutes apart.

EPIDEMIOLOGY

In defining the epidemiology and developmental correlates of apnea, part of the difficulty lies in the numerous definitions of apnea that have been used by various investigators. However, some trends do emerge. Apnea is more frequent in more immature infants, and almost all who weigh less than 1000 g will experience apnea during the neonatal period. Onset of apnea

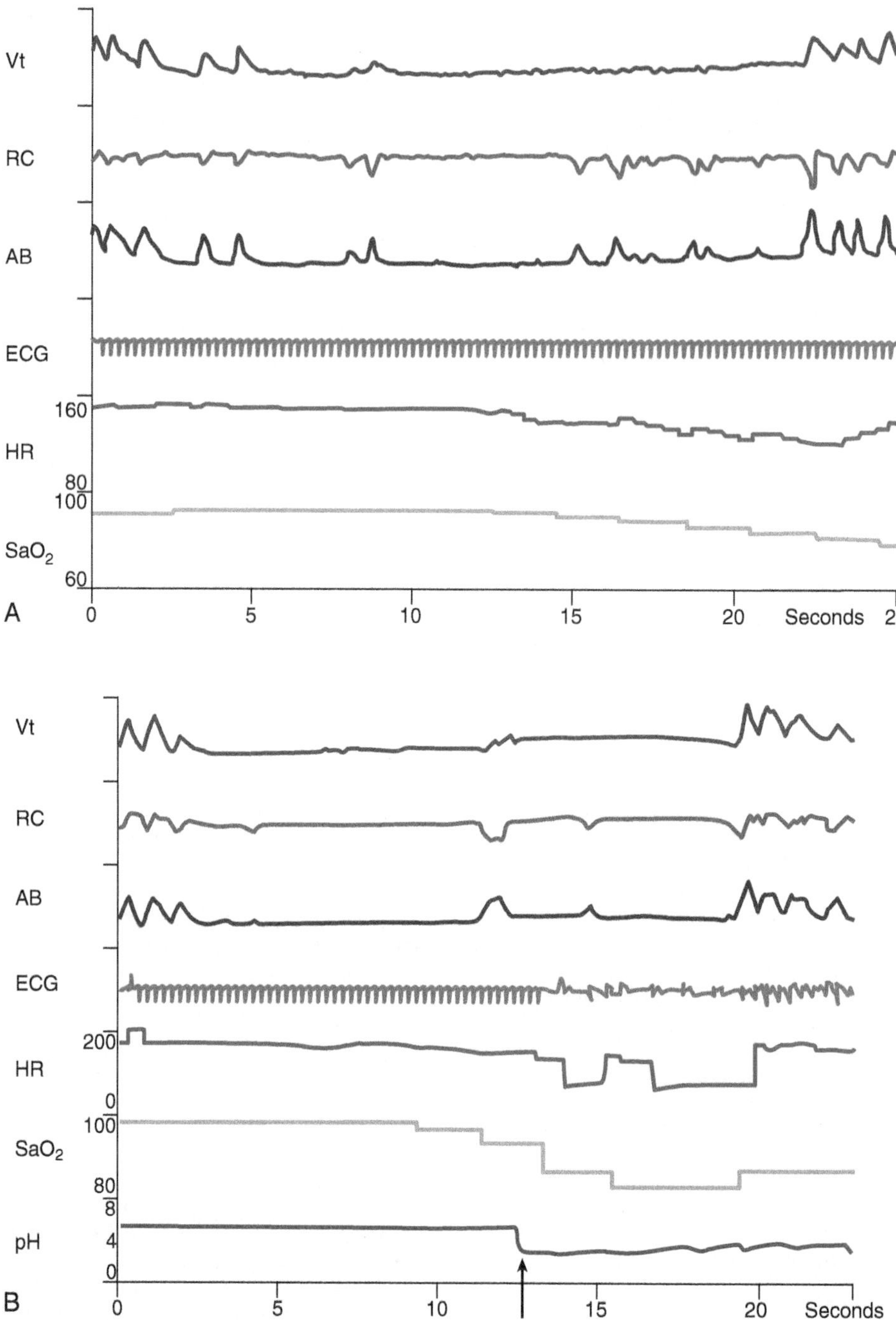

Fig. 156.3 (A) Relationship between apnea and bradycardia. During this mixed apnea, the heart rate *(HR)* begins to decrease approximately 5 seconds after the apnea begins. Timing of the relationship between bradycardia and hypoxemia onset is difficult to assess because of pulse oximeter averaging. (B) Relationship between apnea and gastroesophageal reflux. Reflux occurs after the onset of apnea, as indicated by the decrease in lower esophageal pH *(arrow)*. Most apnea events are not preceded by reflux; when there is an association as seen in this infant, the apnea may precede reflux. *AB,* Abdomen motion; *ECG,* electrocardiogram; *RC,* rib cage motion; *Sao_2,* arterial oxygen saturation; *Vt,* tidal volume (estimated).

may be as early as day 1 of life in infants without respiratory distress syndrome. By contrast, spontaneously breathing infants with respiratory distress syndrome may show a delay in the peak frequency of apnea. Consistent with this observation, Di Fiore and associates have shown that IH episodes in very preterm infants are infrequent in the first week, followed by a progressive increase over weeks 2 to 4 before decreasing in weeks 6 to 8.[12] Thereafter, both the frequency and duration of apnea and IH events decrease with advancing postnatal age (Fig. 156.4). These observations serve to emphasize the developmental immaturity of respiratory control that underlies infantile apnea, as well as the resolution of this disorder over time. Idiopathic apnea and IH events are thought to be related to prematurity. In rare infants, however, an underlying specific familial neuropathology may be identified. Disorders affecting the brain stem that may manifest with apnea include olivopontocerebellar atrophy, myotonic dystrophy, and syringobulbia, as well as brain stem infarction resulting from asphyxia.

Apnea can recur in premature infants after the neonatal period in response to specific clinical situations in which respiratory drive

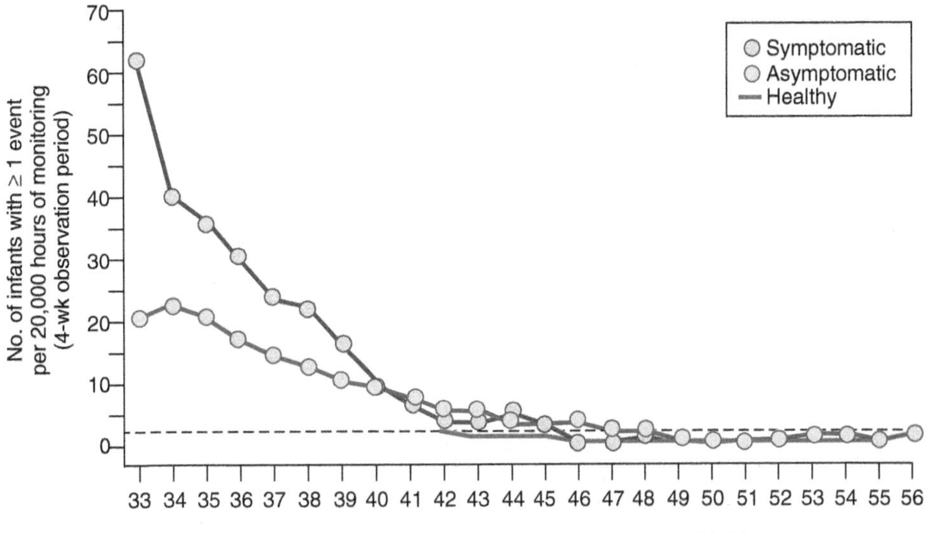

Fig. 156.4 The number of infants who experienced at least one apneic episode lasting 30 seconds accompanied by bradycardia decreased with advancing postmenstrual age *(PMA)*. Data are presented for symptomatic and asymptomatic preterm infants, depending on the persistence of cardiorespiratory events before discharge, and for healthy term infants. (From Ramanathan R, Corwin MJ, Hunt CE, et al. Cardiorespiratory events recorded on home monitors: comparison of healthy infants with those at increased risk for SIDS. *JAMA*. 2001;285:2199.)

is altered. Respiratory syncytial viral infection is well known to elicit apnea. These spells may be severe, necessitating endotracheal intubation. The cause of respiratory depression in respiratory syncytial viral infection is unknown; however, inhibitory reflexes from upper airway afferents have been implicated.

Former premature infants also may experience apnea during recovery from anesthesia. This form of apnea most commonly occurs in the first few months of life, particularly when general anesthesia is used during surgery. For this reason, in former preterm infants, cardiorespiratory monitoring during the acute postoperative period is an important part of their care. Routine care of the premature infant before discharge includes several practices that may cause temporary recurrence of apnea. For example, eye examination for retinopathy of prematurity may be associated with cyanosis, apnea, and gastrointestinal side effects. Immunization also has been found to be associated with apnea, bradycardia, and desaturation. With such practices, therefore, infants require continued monitoring until they are stable, but evidence of a subsequent detrimental effect is lacking.

PHYSIOLOGIC FACTORS

ALTERATION IN CENTRAL DRIVE

Immaturity or depression of central inspiratory drive to the muscles of respiration is accepted as a key factor in the pathogenesis of apnea of prematurity. Vulnerability of the bulbopontine respiratory centers in the brain stem to inhibitory mechanisms could explain why apneic episodes are precipitated in preterm infants by such a wide diversity of specific clinicopathologic events. In other words, apnea may represent the final common response of incompletely organized and interconnected respiratory neurons to a multitude of afferent stimuli. It has been proposed that immature circuits within neuronal networks may be highly susceptible to inhibitory neurotransmitters and neuroregulators such as adenosine, γ-aminobutyric acid (GABA), and endogenous opiates. Unfortunately, the maturation of central respiratory integrative mechanisms and of their biochemical neurotransmitters is inaccessible to study in human infants, and no ideal animal model of spontaneous apnea has been identified for study in the nonanesthetized state.

Brain stem conduction times of auditory evoked responses are longer in infants with apnea than in matched premature infants without apnea. This observation provides indirect evidence that infants with apnea exhibit greater-than-expected immaturity of brain stem function on the basis of postmenstrual age and supports the concept that stability of central respiratory drive improves as dendritic and other synaptic interconnections multiply in the maturing brain.

The absence of respiratory muscle activity during central apnea unequivocally points to the depression of respiratory center output. In support of this concept, Gauda and co-workers[18] documented a decrease in diaphragmatic activity using electromyography (EMG) during spontaneously obstructed inspiratory efforts that characterize mixed apnea. Thus both central and mixed apneic episodes share an element of decreased respiratory center output to the respiratory muscles. The role played by the balance of neurotransmitter substances in modulating this inhibition is not yet known. GABA is considered a ubiquitous major inhibitory neurotransmitter within the brain. Physiologic studies in neonatal animal models have implicated GABA in inhibition of respiratory frequency and decreased ventilatory responses during hypercapnia, hypoxia, and superior laryngeal nerve stimulation.[19] GABA thus has the potential to play a key role in the vulnerability of preterm infants to apnea.

Infants with sepsis are prone to respiratory compromise, including apnea. The proinflammatory cytokine IL-1β may be released in response to infection, and animal studies have shown that IL-1β can depress respiration by way of a prostaglandin E_2-related mechanism. Thus activation of this pathway may trigger apnea in the infant with infection.[20] Chorioamnionitis is a major precipitant of preterm birth and is associated with neonatal brain injury in the form of periventricular leukomalacia and chronic neonatal lung disease in the form of BPD. It is possible that antenatal or postnatal exposure of the lung to a proinflammatory stimulus may activate brain circuits via vagally mediated processes. Lipopolysaccharides (LPSs) instilled into the trachea of 10- to 12-day-old rat pups increased inflammatory cytokine gene expression in the medulla oblongata and attenuated both the immediate and late hypoxic ventilatory response when animals were tested within 3 hours of treatment.[21] This brain stem response to intrapulmonary LPS was diminished after

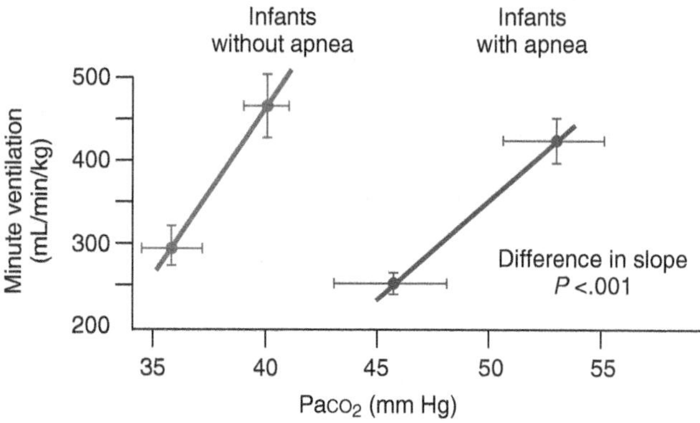

Fig. 156.5 Comparison of carbon dioxide sensitivity obtained from ventilatory responses to changing alveolar partial pressure of carbon dioxide ($Paco_2$) in preterm infants with and without apnea. Note the less steep ventilatory response in the apneic group. (From Gerhardt T, Bancalari E. Apnea of prematurity. I. Lung function and regulation of breathing. *Pediatrics.* 1984;74:58. Reproduced by permission of *Pediatrics*.)

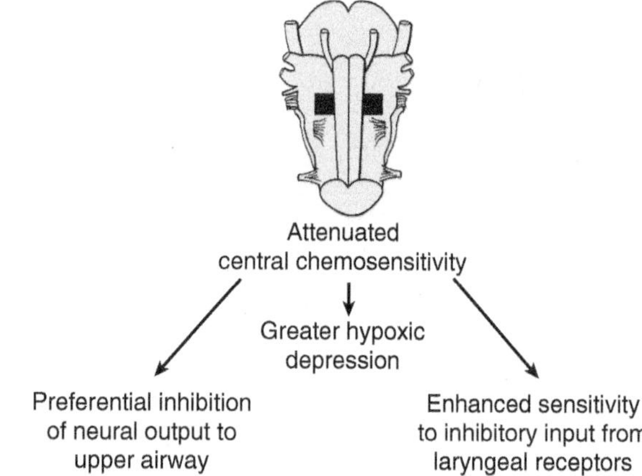

Fig. 156.6 Hypothetical framework for mechanisms whereby attenuated central (carbon dioxide) chemosensitivity enhances vulnerability to neonatal apnea. The *black squares* indicate the intermediate area of the ventral medullary surface of the brain stem.

vagotomy, suggesting a lung-to-brain stem communication via vagal afferents.

It became apparent in the mid-1970s that central respiratory control is influenced by sleep state in infants. Apnea was observed to occur more commonly during active (or rapid eye movement) and indeterminate (or transitional) sleep, when respiratory patterns are irregular in both timing and amplitude. Apnea is less commonly observed during quiet sleep, when respiration is characteristically regular with little breath-by-breath change in tidal volume or respiratory frequency, although periodic breathing may actually occur predominantly in quiet sleep. In term neonates, respiratory variability alone can be used to stage sleep with a high degree of accuracy. However, sleep state is not easily definable by any criteria before 32 weeks of gestation, when apnea occurs most frequently.

INFLUENCE OF CHEMORECEPTORS AND MECHANORECEPTORS

The ventilatory and respiratory muscle responses to increases in inspired carbon dioxide (CO_2) reflect predominantly central chemoreceptor activity and are less well developed in the immature infant before 33 weeks of postmenstrual age.[22]

The reduced ventilatory response to CO_2 in small preterm infants is primarily the result of decreased central chemosensitivity; however, mechanical factors preventing an appropriate increase in ventilation may contribute. Unlike adults, preterm infants do not tend to increase frequency of ventilation during hypercapnia. In these infants, hypercapnia may be accompanied by prolongation of expiratory duration.[23] The CO_2 response curve has a decreased slope (indicating a less steep ventilatory response to increasing CO_2 concentrations) in preterm infants who exhibit apnea (Fig. 156.5).[24] However, a cause-and-effect relationship between decreased CO_2 responsiveness and apnea of prematurity has not been clearly established. Both entities may simply reflect decreased respiratory drive. Administration of CO_2 at low inspiratory concentrations would be expected to relieve apnea, as it does periodic breathing; this approach has been investigated but may not be therapeutically feasible in human infants. Interestingly, the hypercapnic response of infants born to smoking and substance-abusing mothers is reduced, which may contribute to vulnerable respiratory control in this population.[25]

A newborn piglet model has been used to identify the physiologic consequences of decreased central (CO_2) chemosensitivity by cooling a discrete area (the intermediate area) of the ventral medullary surface.[26] Cooling at this site (or microinjection of inhibitory neurotransmitters) inhibits central chemosensitivity, possibly by directly affecting chemosensitive cells, but also by inhibiting neural transmission between central chemosensitive cells and respiratory rhythm generators situated in the brain stem. Obvious limitations arise in extrapolating data from anesthetized newborn piglets to apneic human infants. Nonetheless, as seen in Fig. 156.6, attenuated central chemosensitivity may underlie some of the physiologic characteristics of neonatal respiratory control, including preferential inhibition of neural output to the upper airway muscles compared with the diaphragm, enhanced sensitivity to inhibitory afferents from upper airway (e.g., laryngeal) receptors, and greater hypoxic depression of breathing.

It has been known for many years that infants respond to a fall in inspired oxygen concentration with a transient increase in ventilation over approximately 1 minute, followed by a return to baseline or even depression of ventilation. The characteristic response to low oxygen in infants appears to result from initial peripheral chemoreceptor stimulation, followed by overriding depression of the respiratory center as a result of hypoxemia. This biphasic response has been described in term infants up to 6 months of age, but is more pronounced in the preterm infant, leading to worse arterial desaturations.[27] One study of the hypoxic ventilatory response in convalescing premature infants found that those with the most markedly increased ventilatory response to hypoxia also had more apneic events recorded at baseline, suggesting that enhanced peripheral chemoreceptor activity in these infants causes respiratory control instability and contributes to apnea of prematurity.[28] In very low-birth-weight infants (<1500 g), the biphasic response may be absent, and such infants show only a sustained decrease in ventilation in response to hypoxia.[29] Such hypoxic respiratory depression may be useful in the hypoxic intrauterine environment where respiratory activity is only intermittent and not contributing to gas exchange. Consistent with these findings is the observation that a progressive decrease in inspired oxygen concentration causes a significant flattening of CO_2 responsiveness in preterm infants. This unstable response to low inspired oxygen concentration may play an important role in the origin of neonatal apnea. It offers a physiologic rationale for the decreased incidence of apnea observed when a slightly increased concentration of inspired oxygen is administered to apneic infants. However, this approach to treat apnea should not be recommended because of potential adverse effects of hyperoxemia. Prolonged vulnerability of respiratory control to hypoxic stress in preterm infants is consistent with persistence of the characteristic biphasic ventilatory response to hypoxia into the second month of postnatal life.

The effects of hypoxia on respiratory control are critically dependent on the timing and duration of hypoxia. Exposure of

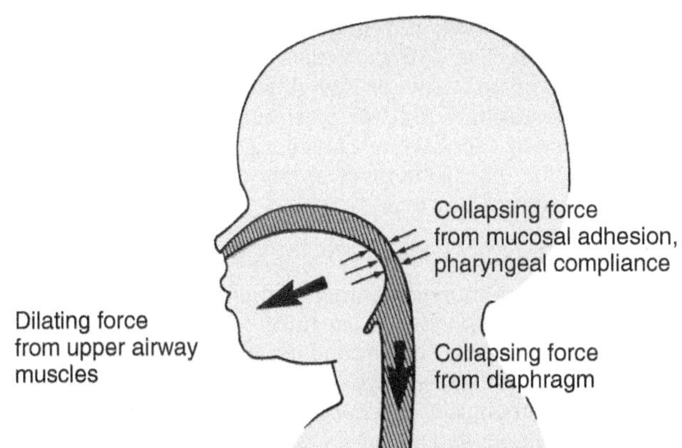

Fig. 156.7 Sagittal section of the upper airway, demonstrating various forces operating either to collapse the pharynx or to maintain its patency during normal respiration. (Modified from Thach BT. The role of pharyngeal airway obstruction in prolonging infantile apneic spells. In: Tildon JT, Roeder L, Steinschneider A, et al, eds. *Sudden Infant Death Syndrome.* New York: Academic Press; 1983.)

rat pups to sustained hypoxia during a window (11 to 15 days of age) was lethal (84% mortality, versus very little with earlier or later exposures), suggesting a heightened vulnerability of the respiratory control system to prolonged hypoxia during a critical developmental window characterized by complex changes in brainstem neurotransmitter expression.[30] The combination of sustained hypoxia and IH to which preterm infants may be exposed has barely been addressed. Mayer and associates have documented in rat pups that when an initial postnatal exposure to sustained hypoxia is followed by a period of IH, the hypoxic ventilatory response to subsequent hypoxic exposures is profoundly suppressed.[31]

Afferent neural input from pulmonary stretch receptors is capable of substantially modulating respiratory timing in human neonates. This vagally mediated response, called the *Hering-Breuer reflex,* acts to inhibit inspiration, prolong expiration, or both, in response to increasing lung volume, thereby limiting lung overinflation. Active shortening of expiratory duration with decrease in lung volume may similarly provide a neonatal breathing strategy to preserve functional residual capacity in the presence of a highly compliant chest wall. Another manifestation of this reflex response to lung inflation is that inspiratory duration is typically prolonged after end-expiratory airway obstruction when lung inflation is prevented. This ability of neonates to increase the duration of an obstructed inspiratory effort appears to be an appropriate compensatory mechanism during airway occlusion, and may be limited in preterm infants. More important, upper airway obstruction contributes substantially to the initiation of apneic episodes in preterm infants, and upper airway muscles show preferential reflex activation in response to airway obstruction in infants.

DIFFERENTIAL RESPONSES OF UPPER AIRWAY AND CHEST WALL MUSCLES

Because premature infants exhibit pharyngeal or laryngeal obstruction during spontaneous apnea, much interest has focused on the interactions among the various respiratory muscle groups in maintaining airway patency. A model was proposed for the pathogenesis of neonatal apnea by Thach,[32] a modification of which is shown in Fig. 156.7. According to this model, negative luminal pressures generated in the upper airway during inspiration predispose a compliant pharynx to collapse. Patency can be maintained by activation of upper airway muscles, which may increase tone within the extrathoracic airway through tonic or phasic contraction in synchrony with the chest wall muscles. The relative roles played by active upper airway muscle contraction and passive rigidity of the anatomic framework of the upper airway in maintaining pharyngeal patency in preterm infants are unclear.

Whereas many upper airway muscles, including the alae nasi, laryngeal abductor, and adductor muscles, modulate patency of the extrathoracic airway, failure of genioglossus activation has been most widely implicated in mixed and obstructive apnea in both adults and infants. Carlo and co-workers[33] compared activity of the genioglossus muscle with that of the diaphragm in response to hypercapnic stimulation. Consistent with data obtained in animal models, genioglossus activation in preterm infants was delayed for approximately 1 minute after initiation of CO_2 rebreathing and occurred only after an end-tidal P_{CO_2} threshold of approximately 45 mm Hg had been reached.[33] By contrast, diaphragmatic EMG activity increased linearly with progressive hypercapnia. Thus it is possible that an absent, small, or delayed upper airway muscle response to hypercapnia may result in upper airway instability when accompanied by a linear increase in chest wall activity. This instability may predispose affected infants to obstruction of inspiratory efforts after a period of central apnea. Consistent with this hypothesis is the observation that short apneic episodes are more likely to be central, and longer episodes (lasting longer than 15 seconds) are more likely to be accompanied by obstructed breaths. Furthermore, airway obstruction often occurs toward the end of the longer episodes of mixed apnea, when diaphragmatic activity may be enhanced before that of the upper airway muscles.

Gauda and co-workers[34] used sublingual surface electrodes (placed over the insertion of the genioglossus within the mandible) to compare the genioglossus responses with end-expiratory airway occlusion in preterm infants with mixed and obstructive apnea and in nonapneic control infants. In both groups, genioglossus EMG activity was typically absent during unobstructed breathing. Occlusion resulted in immediate release of this inhibition, with resultant augmentation of the genioglossus activity in the nonapneic infants. In infants with apnea, however, activation of the genioglossus in response to occlusion was significantly delayed.

Subsequently, Gauda and co-workers[18] evaluated the activity of the genioglossus and diaphragm during spontaneously occurring mixed and obstructive apneic episodes. During mixed apnea, the amplitude of the diaphragmatic EMG activity decreased on the initial obstructed inspiratory effort and did not exceed that for the breath preceding apnea until flow was reestablished (Fig. 156.8). Genioglossus activity accompanied approximately 20% of breaths immediately preceding spontaneous apnea; this frequency did not increase significantly until resolution of the apnea, with genioglossus activity present during 40% of breaths associated with reestablishing airflow. Thus, decreased diaphragmatic activity is a major component of spontaneous apnea associated with airway obstruction, and neither diaphragm nor genioglossus activity is increased until resolution of apnea. These findings suggest that central, mixed, and obstructive apneas are caused by a common mechanism—a reduction in central drive affecting the diaphragm and dilating muscles of the upper airway. However, the finding that only 40% of spontaneous apneic episodes were terminated with genioglossus activation indicates that this is not the sole mechanism by which upper airway obstruction is relieved in premature infants.

GASTROESOPHAGEAL REFLUX

Although pharyngeal and laryngeal stimulation may trigger apnea, caution should be exercised before apnea is attributed to gastroesophageal reflux. Despite the frequent coexistence of apnea and gastroesophageal reflux in preterm infants, investigations into the timing of reflux in relation to apneic events indicate that they are not commonly temporally related.[35] Monitoring studies demonstrate that when a relationship between reflux and apnea is observed, apnea may precede

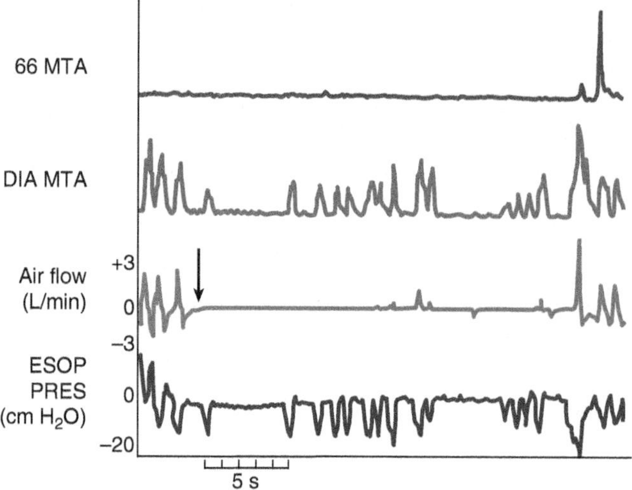

Fig. 156.8 A representative tracing of the genioglossus muscle (GG) and diaphragm *(DIA)* electromyographic activity during spontaneous apnea. The *arrow* denotes the onset of mixed apnea. The diaphragmatic amplitude of the initial obstructed inspiratory effort is less than the diaphragmatic amplitude of the breath preceding apnea, whereas the diaphragmatic amplitude of the breath at resolution of the apnea exceeds that of the preapneic breath. Electromyographic activity of the genioglossus muscle appears only at resolution of the apnea. The moving time averaged *(MTA)* signals are depicted for both the genioglossus and diaphragm. *ESOP PRES,* Esophageal pressure. (From Gauda EB, Miller MJ, Carlo WA, et al. Genioglossus and diaphragm activity during obstructive apnea and airway occlusion in infants. *Pediatr Res.* 1989;26:583.)

rather than follow reflux, as seen in Fig. 156.2.[36] This finding suggests that loss of respiratory neural output during apnea may be accompanied by a decrease in lower esophageal tone and gastroesophageal reflux. Such a phenomenon is supported by data from a newborn piglet model, in which apnea was accompanied by a fall in lower esophageal sphincter pressure.[37] Although physiologic experiments in animals reveal that reflux of gastric contents to the larynx induces reflex apnea, no clear evidence is available showing that treatment of reflux will affect frequency of apnea in most preterm infants.[38] Therefore pharmacologic management of reflux with agents that decrease gastric acidity or enhance gastrointestinal motility should only be used in rare preterm infants with severe gastroesophageal reflux disease, regardless of whether apnea is present. As acid suppression therapy increases the risk of neonatal sepsis, such treatment should be discontinued in the absence of clear clinical benefit.

PHYSIOLOGIC BASIS FOR THERAPIES

NONPHARMACOLOGIC APPROACHES

CONTINUOUS POSITIVE AIRWAY PRESSURE

Continuous positive airway pressure (CPAP) has been a relatively safe and effective therapy for 40 years. It has a dual function to stabilize lung volume and improve airway patency by limiting upper airway closure. Because longer episodes of apnea frequently involve an obstructive component, CPAP appears to be effective by "splinting" the upper airway with positive pressure and decreasing the risk of pharyngeal or laryngeal obstruction.[3] At the lower functional residual capacity, which accompanies many preterm infants with residual lung disease, pulmonary oxygen stores are probably reduced and there is a very short time from cessation of breathing to onset of desaturation and bradycardia. Therefore CPAP is likely to reduce this vulnerability to episodic desaturation (see Fig. 156.2). Nasal CPAP is well tolerated by most preterm infants. Low- or high-flow nasal cannula therapies are being increasingly used as treatment modalities that may allow delivery of CPAP while enhancing mobility of the infant; equivalence for management of apnea of prematurity has not been demonstrated, however.[39]

OPTIMIZATION OF MECHANOSENSORY INPUTS

The respiratory rhythm-generating circuitry within the central nervous system depends on intrinsic rhythmic activity and sensory afferent inputs to generate breathing movement. Bloch-Salisbury and colleagues have demonstrated that their novel technique of stochastic mechanosensory stimulation, using a mattress with imbedded actuators, is able to stabilize respiratory patterns in preterm infants as manifested by a decrease in apnea and an almost three-fold decrease in percentage of time with oxygen saturations below 85%.[40] Interestingly, the level of stimulation employed was below the minimum threshold for behavioral arousal to wakefulness, thus inducing no apparent state change in the infants, and the effect could probably not be attributed to the minimal increase in sound level associated with stimulation. Such an approach is clearly worthy of future study.

OPTIMIZATION OF BLOOD GAS STATUS

IH episodes are almost always the result of respiratory pauses, apnea, or ineffective ventilation. Targeting lower baseline oxygen saturation has been associated with persistence of intermittent hypoxic episodes.[41] It is unclear whether this lower baseline oxygen saturation increases the incidence of apnea with resultant hypoxemia (via hypoxic depression of breathing), or whether the incidence of apnea is comparable between oxygen targets, but the lower oxygen saturation baseline predisposes to more frequent or profound intermittent hypoxemia. Similarly, it is unclear whether the beneficial effect of packed red cell transfusion is secondary to improved respiratory control or better delivery of oxygen to the central nervous system.[42] However, given the potential oxidative stress associated with clinically significant intermittent hypoxic episodes, the latter are probably best avoided.[43]

Automated control of inspired oxygen is generating increasing interest and is being used clinically in some European centers. This automated technique has been compared to manual adjustments of inspired oxygen in preterm infants. Initial studies were more successful in preventing hyperoxia than in reducing hypoxic episodes with automated FiO_2 control, but more recent studies have shown increased time within the targeted SpO_2 range.[44-47] However it should be noted that although time spent within the target range was statistically greater in the automated group relative to the manual group, the difference was minimal,[44-47] underscoring the inherent difficulty in maintaining stable oxygen saturations in preterm infants even with automated control.

PHARMACOLOGIC APPROACHES

METHYLXANTHINE THERAPY

Methylxanthine therapy has been used to prevent and treat apnea of prematurity since the 1970s. Xanthines are nonspecific adenosine receptor inhibitors. Their primary mechanism of action in the perinatal period is thought to be blockade of inhibitory adenosine A_1 receptors with resultant excitation of respiratory neural output (Fig. 156.9).[48] An alternative mechanism of caffeine action is blockade of excitatory adenosine A_{2A} receptors at GABAergic neurons and resultant decrease in GABA output, resulting in excitation of respiratory neural output.[49] The xanthines also inhibit phosphodiesterase, which normally breaks down cyclic adenosine monophosphate (cAMP), although the relationship of cAMP accumulation to relief of apnea in infants is questionable.

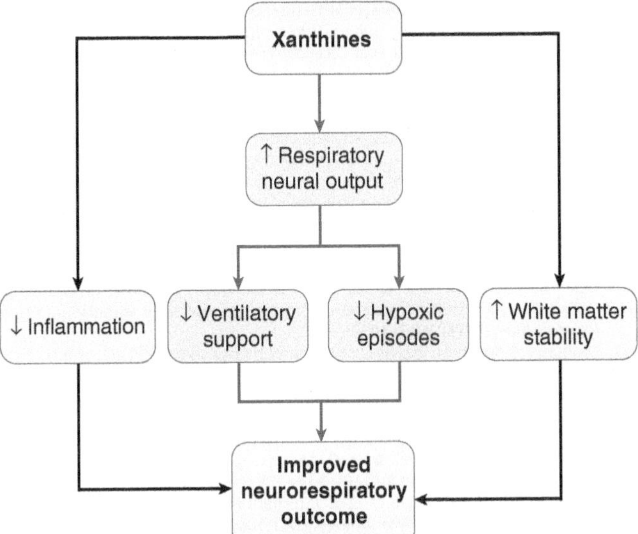

Fig. 156.9 Proposed mechanisms whereby xanthine therapy benefits neurorespiratory outcome in preterm infants.

The complex neurotransmitter interactions elicited by caffeine led to concerns regarding its safety. A large multicenter trial, however, demonstrated that caffeine treatment (used to treat apnea or enhance extubation) is effective in decreasing the rate of BPD and improving neurodevelopmental outcome at 18 to 21 months, especially in those receiving respiratory support.[50,51] There is also evidence for reduction in developmental coordination disorder in the caffeine-treated cohort at 5 years of age,[52] and reduced risk of motor impairment at 11 years of age, without clear academic benefit.[53] This benefit may be secondary to decrease in apnea and resultant IH episodes; however, that is speculative (see Fig. 156.9).

Xanthines appear to have the ability to increase central respiratory drive[54] in the neonatal period without an overall increase in arousal or change in sleep patterns, which is surprising, given the relatively high caffeine levels to which these infants are exposed. Earlier physiologic studies in the neonatal period have documented an increase in minute ventilation with xanthines, associated with shift of the CO_2 response curve to the left and a decrease in hypoxic respiratory depression. Rodent studies suggest relative importance of adenosinergic modulation of breathing changes over the course of prenatal and postnatal development.[55,56] No studies have shown attenuation of caffeine's effectiveness in treating apnea of prematurity in neonates of different gestational ages, but its metabolism is known to increase with maturation, and older infants may require larger doses to achieve the same trough serum concentration.[57,58]

Recent data in neonatal rodents demonstrate an antiinflammatory effect of caffeine in proinflammatory states elicited by postnatal hyperoxia or antenatal endotoxin exposure.[59-62] In these studies, improved lung pathology and respiratory system mechanics were observed after caffeine treatment. In contrast, other data raise concerns about potential adverse effects of neonatal caffeine exposure in various animal models.[63,64] Data on the effects of caffeine on the developing brain are controversial and include no effect in an ovine model,[65] a protective effect on hypoxia-induced perinatal white matter injury,[66] and improved white matter structural development in preterm infants.[67]

These conflicting data in the face of clinical benefit suggest that changes in dosing and indications for caffeine that deviate from proven beneficial protocols should proceed with caution. Prophylactic use of methylxanthines use is widespread, especially in Europe.[67] Initial studies suggested that very early initiation of caffeine therapy results in improved outcome; however, these findings are based on retrospective review with potential confounders.[68,69] A recent randomized controlled trial on early caffeine initiation in mechanically ventilated infants was stopped early due to concern for a nonsignificant trend toward increased mortality in the early group.[70] More importantly, this study showed no ability of early caffeine to enhance successful extubation or prevent BPD. Patel and colleagues,[71] working with a large data set from the Pediatrix Medical Group Clinical Data Warehouse, showed that caffeine started on the day of birth also did not decrease the incidence of CPAP failure. Finally, the extended use of caffeine to 40 weeks' postmenstrual age was associated with a decrease in IH among a cohort of preterm infants;[72] however, the relationship between long-term morbidity, and this type of IH remains unclear. The longer-term effects of this changing therapeutic landscape are unknown.

CONCLUSION

Delayed or impaired maturation of neonatal respiratory control continues to play a central role in clinical practice. Both the consequences of and therapeutic modalities employed to avoid these cardiorespiratory events secondary to decreased respiratory neural output are not yet fully understood. Ongoing investigation of the neurorespiratory axis during early development should generate important insight into the ongoing morbidity to which former preterm infants may be predisposed.

A complete reference list is available at www.ExpertConsult.com. 

SELECT REFERENCES

1. Thach BT, Stark AR. Spontaneous neck flexion and airway obstruction during apneic spells in preterm infants. *J Pediatr*. 1979;94(2):275-281.
2. Milner AD, Boon AW, Saunders RA, et al. Upper airways obstruction and apnoea in preterm babies. *Arch Dis Child*. 1980;55(1):22-25.
3. Miller MJ, Carlo WA, Martin RJ. Continuous positive airway pressure selectively reduces obstructive apnea in preterm infants. *J Pediatr*. 1985;106(1):91-94.
4. Bolivar J, Gerhardt T, Gonzalez A, et al. Mechanisms for episodes of hypoxemia in preterm infants undergoing mechanical ventilation. *J Pediatr*. 1995;127(5):767-773.
5. Dimaguila MA, Di Fiore JM, Martin RJ, et al. Characteristics of hypoxemic episodes in intubated very low birthweight infants. *J Pediatr*. 1997;130(4):577-583.
6. Lehtonen L, Johnson MW, Bakdash T, et al. Relation of sleep state to hypoxemic episodes in ventilated extremely-low-birth-weight infants. *J Pediatr*. 2002;141(3):363-368.
7. Dorostkar PC, Arko MK, Baird TM, et al. Asystole and severe bradycardia in preterm infants. *Biol Neonate*. 2005;88(4):299-305.
8. Henderson-Smart DJ, Butcher-Puech MC, Edwards DA. Incidence and mechanism of bradycardia during apnoea in preterm infants. *Arch Dis Child*. 1986;61(3):227-232.
9. Del Rio R, Moya EA, Iturriaga R. Differential expression of pro-inflammatory cytokines, endothelin-1 and nitric oxide synthases in the rat carotid body exposed to intermittent hypoxia. *Brain Res*. 2011;1395:74-85.
10. Yang CH, Shen YJ, Lai CH, et al. Inflammatory role of ROS-sensitive AMP-activated protein kinase in the hypersensitivity of lung vagal C fibers induced by intermittent hypoxia in rats. *Front Physiol*. 2016;7:263.
11. Di Fiore JM, Vento M. Intermittent hypoxemia and oxidative stress in preterm infants. *Respiratory Physiol&Neurobiol*. 2019;266:121-129.
12. Di Fiore JM, Bloom JN, Orge F, et al. A higher incidence of intermittent hypoxemic episodes is associated with severe retinopathy of prematurity. *J Pediatr*. 2010;157(1):69-73.
13. Di Fiore JM, Kaffashi F, Loparo K, et al. The relationship between patterns of intermittent hypoxia and retinopathy of prematurity in preterm infants. *Pediatr Res*. 2012;72:606-612.
14. Raffay TM, Dylag AM, Sattar A, et al. Neonatal intermittent hypoxemia events are associated with diagnosis of bronchopulmonary dysplasia at 36 weeks postmenstrual age. *Pediatr Res*. 2019;85:318-323.
15. Poets CF, Roberts RS, Schmidt B, et al. Association between intermittent hypoxemia or bradycardia and late death or disability in extremely preterm infants. *J Am Med Assoc*. 2015;314:595-603.
16. Martin N, Pourie G, Bossenmeyer-Pourie C, et al. Conditioning-like brief neonatal hypoxia improves cognitive function and brain tissue properties with marked gender dimorphism n adult rats. *Semin Perinatol*. 2010;34:193-200.

17. Zhang JX, Chen XQ, DU JZ, et al. Neonatal exposure to intermittent hypoxia enhances mice performance in water maze and 8-arm radial maze tasks. *J Neurobiol.* 2005;65:72-84.
18. Gauda EB, Miller MJ, Carlo WA, et al. Genioglossus and diaphragm activity during obstructive apnea and airway occlusion in infants. *Pediatr Res.* 1989;26(6):583-587.
19. Abu-Shaweesh JM, Dreshaj IA, Haxhiu MA, et al. Central GABAergic mechanisms are involved in apnea induced by SLN stimulation in piglets. *J Appl Physiol.* 2001;90(4):1570-1576.
20. Olsson A, Kayhan G, Lagercrantz H, et al. IL-1β depresses respiration and anoxic survival via a prostaglandin-dependent pathway in neonatal rats. *Pediatr Res.* 2003;54(3):326-331.
21. Balan KV, Kc P, Hoxha Z, et al. Vagal afferents modulate cytokine-mediated respiratory control at the neonatal medulla oblongata. *Respir Physiol Neurobiol.* 2011;178(3):458-464.
22. Rigatto H, Brady JP, de la Torre Verduzco R. Chemoreceptor reflexes in preterm infants: II. The effect of gestational and postnatal age on the ventilatory response to inhaled carbon dioxide. *Pediatrics.* 1975;55(5):614-620.
23. Noble LM, Carlo WA, Miller MJ, et al. Transient changes in expiratory time during hypercapnia in premature infants. *J Appl Physiol.* 1987;62(3):1010-1013.
24. Gerhardt T, Bancalari E. Apnea of prematurity. I. Lung function and regulation of breathing. *Pediatrics.* 1984;74(1):58-62.
25. Ali K, Wolff K, Peacock JL, et al. Ventilatory response to hypercarbia in newborns of smoking and substance-misusing mothers. *Ann Am Thorac Soc.* 2014;11(6):933-938.
26. Martin RJ, Dreshaj IA, Miller MJ, et al. Hypoglossal and phrenic responses to central respiratory inhibition in piglets. *Respir Physiol.* 1994;97(1):93-103.
27. Verbeek MM, Richardson HL, Parslow PM, et al. Arousal and ventilatory responses to mild hypoxia in sleeping preterm infants. *J Sleep Res.* 2008;17(3):344-353.
28. Nock ML, Difiore JM, Arko MK, et al. Relationship of the ventilator response to hypoxia with neonatal apnea in preterm infants. *J Pediatr.* 2004;144(3):291-295.
29. Alvaro R, Alvarez J, Kwiatkowski K, et al. Small preterm infants (≤1500g) have only a sustained decrease in ventilation in response to hypoxia. *Pediatr Res.* 1992;32:403-406.
30. Mayer CA, Di Fiore JH, Martin RJ, MacFarlane PM. Vulnerability of neonatal respiratory neural control to sustained hypoxia during a uniquely sensitive window of development. *J Appl Physiol.* 2014;116(5):514-521.
31. Mayer CA, Ao J, Di Fiore JM, et al. Impaired hypoxic ventilatory response following neonatal sustained and subsequent chronic intermittent hypoxia in rats. *Respir Physiol Neurobiol.* 2013;187(2):167-175.
32. Thach BT. The role of pharyngeal airway obstruction in prolonging infantile apneic spells. In: Tilden JT, Roeder L, Steinschneider A, eds. *Sudden Infant Death Syndrome.* New York: Academic Press; 1983:279.
33. Carlo WA, Martin RJ, Difiore JM. Differences in CO2 threshold of respiratory muscles in preterm infants. *J Appl Physiol.* 1988;65(6):2434-2439.
34. Gauda EB, Miller MJ, Carlo WA, et al. Genioglossus response to airway occlusion in apneic versus nonapneic infants. *Pediatr Res.* 1987;22(6):683-687.
35. Di Fiore J, Arko M, Herynk B, et al. Characterization of cardiorespiratory events following gastroesophageal reflux in preterm infants. *J Perinatol.* 2010;10:683-687.
36. Omari TI. Apnea-associated reduction in lower esophageal sphincter tone in premature infants. *J Pediatr.* 2009;154(3):374-378.
37. Kiatchoosakun P, Dreshaj IA, Abu-Shaweesh JM, et al. Effects of hypoxia on respiratory neural output and lower esophageal sphincter pressure in piglets. *Pediatr Res.* 2002;52(1):50-55.
38. Wheatley E, Kennedy KA. Cross-over trial of treatment for bradycardia attributed to gastroesophageal reflux in preterm infants. *J Pediatr.* 2009;155(4):516-521.
39. Manley BJ, Arnolda GRB, Wright IMR, et al. Nasal high-flow therapy for newborn infants in special care nurseries. *N Engl J Med.* 2019;380(21):2031-2040.
40. Bloch-Salisbury E, Indic P, Bednarek F, et al. Stabilizing immature breathing patterns of preterm infants using stochastic mechanosensory stimulation. *J Appl Physiol.* 2009;107(4):1017-1027.
41. Di Fiore JM, Walsh M, Wrage L, et al. On behalf of the SUPPORT group of the Eunice Kennedy Shriver National Institute of Child Health and Human Development Neonatal Research Network: low oxygen saturation target range is associated with increased incidence of intermittent hypoxemia. *J Pediatr.* 2012;161(6):1047-1052.
42. Zagol K, Lake DE, Vergales B, et al. Anemia, apnea of prematurity, and blood transfusions. *J Pediatr.* 2012;161(3):417-421.
43. Martin RJ, Wang K, Köroğlu Ö, et al. Intermittent hypoxic episodes in preterm infants: do they matter? *Neonatology.* 2011;100(3):303-310.
44. Gajdos M, Waitz M, Mendler MR, et al. Effects of a new device for automated closed loop control of inspired oxygen concentration on fluctuations of arterial and different regional organ tissue oxygen saturations in preterm infants. *Arch Dis Child Fetal Neonatal Ed.* 2019;104:F360-F365.
45. Waitz M, Schmid MB, Fuchs H, et al. Effects of automated adjustment of inspired oxygen on fluctuations of arterial and regional cerebral tissue oxygenation in preterm infants with frequent desaturations. *J Pediatr.* 2015;166:240-244.
46. Van Kaam AH, Hummler HD, Wilinska M, et al. Automated versus manual oxygen control with different saturation targets and modes of respiratory support in preterm infants. *J Pediatr.* 2015;167:545-550.
47. Claure N, Bancalari E. Targeting arterial oxygen saturation by closed-loop control of inspired oxygen in preterm infants. *Clin Perinatol.* 2019;46(3):567-577.
48. Herlenius E, Aden U, Tang LQ, et al. Perinatal respiratory control and its modulation by adenosine and caffeine in the rat. *Pediatr Res.* 2002;51(1):4-12.
49. Mayer CA, Haxhiu MA, Martin RJ, et al. Adenosine A_{2A} receptors mediate GABAergic inhibition of respiration in immature rats. *J Appl Physiol.* 2006;100(1):91-97.
50. Davis PG, Schmidt B, Roberts RS, et al. Caffeine for apnea of prematurity trial: benefits may vary in subgroups. *J Pediatr.* 2010;156(3):382-387.

157 Pathophysiology of Respiratory Distress Syndrome

Alan H. Jobe

INTRODUCTION

Respiratory distress syndrome (RDS) in preterm infants is the disease most identified with the development of neonatal intensive care. Before the late 1960s, the only therapy for preterm infants who developed progressive respiratory failure shortly after birth was supplemental oxygen; most of these infants died. At autopsy the lungs were atelectatic and had epithelial injury with hyaline membranes, resulting in the name *hyaline membrane disease* (HMD). Avery and Mead[1] reported in 1959 that saline extracts of lungs of infants with HMD had high minimum surface tensions in contrast to lungs of infants without HMD. The HMD lungs also inflated poorly and collapsed to low volumes at low transpulmonary pressures.[2] Saline lavages of the air spaces recovered small amounts of surfactant lipids that had poor function in vitro.[3] Although mechanical ventilation was used in the 1960s, the mortality rate was high. The first successful therapy was continuous positive airway pressure (CPAP) first described by Gregory and colleagues in 1971.[4] Concurrently, antenatal tests to predict the risk of what is now called *RDS* were developed using amniotic fluid.[5] Liggins and Howie[6] reported that the risk of having RDS could be decreased with antenatal corticosteroid treatments. These innovations, together with the development of infant ventilators, a better understanding of their use and the physiology of the preterm lung, and improved intensive care for preterm infants (temperature control, nutrition, infection control), resulted in a striking decline in deaths from RDS in the United States from 1970 to 1990 (Fig. 157.1).[7] The care of infants with RDS was simplified and mortality further decreased after 1990 with surfactant therapy[8] (reviewed in Chapter 79) and with the widespread use of antenatal corticosteroids (ANS).[9] The strikingly improved outcomes for infants with RDS is the great success story in neonatology. By 2015 and after, an infant in the United States should not die of RDS unless the disease is complicated by severe prematurity or other lung pathologies.

EPIDEMIOLOGY OF RESPIRATORY DISTRESS SYNDROME

RDS is closely associated with preterm birth, with the incidence increasing as gestational age decreases. The standard diagnosis for RDS requires progressive respiratory failure beginning at or shortly after birth. The respiratory failure is characterized by respiratory distress, clinically identified by tachypnea, grunting, nasal flaring, and chest wall retractions and an increasing oxygen requirement. The chest film shows poor inflation with a uniform hazy and granular appearance on air bronchograms. The odds ratio for RDS at 34 weeks' gestational age is 40 relative to term infants (Fig. 157.2A).[10] The risk is much higher and approaches 100% at gestations below 34 weeks (see Fig. 157.2B). Furthermore, the risk of RDS is inversely proportional to the lecithin/sphingomyelin ratio.[11,12] The human lung is not sufficiently consistently mature to avoid RDS until a gestational age of about 35 weeks, but in clinical practice the incidence of RDS at 35 weeks is only about 20%. This discrepancy is explained by the human lung's remarkable capacity to induce lung maturation, driven either by abnormalities associated with preterm birth or in response to antenatal corticosteroid treatments.[13]

New approaches to the diagnosis of RDS are point-of-care ultrasound of the newborn lungs,[14] analysis of gastric aspirates for indications of surfactant,[15] or (in the future) maternal plasma blood to identify mRNA indications of lung maturation.[16] Amniotic fluid can be used to determine mRNA markers of lung maturation.[17]

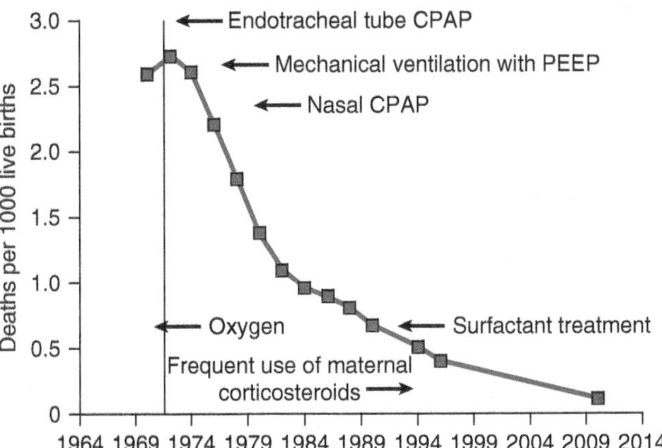

Fig. 157.1 Deaths from respiratory distress syndrome (RDS) in the United States from 1968 to 2010. The curve shows deaths from RDS in preterm infants per 1000 live births. The curve for the striking decrease in death is annotated for innovations that improved outcomes for infants with RDS. The infants who died in the 1960s and 1970s were larger and more mature than the few infants who now die of RDS. *CPAP,* Continuous positive airway pressure; *PEEP,* positive end-expiratory pressure. (Redrawn and annotated from Lee K, , Khoshnood B, Wall SN, et al. Trend in mortality from respiratory distress syndrome in the United States, 1970–1995. *J Pediatr.* 1999;134[4]:434–440.)

DOSING OF ANTENATAL CORTICOSTEROIDS

ANS are standard of care at 24 to 37 weeks for women at risk of preterm delivery.[18] However, the standard-of-care treatment is the dosing initially used in 1972 by Liggins and Howie.[6] There has not been an interest in evaluating the treatment, as it is off label and not FDA approved.[18] We have been concerned that the dose is too high and have formally tested lower doses in fetal sheep and rhesus macaque models, together with pharmacokinetic (PK) and pharmacodynamic (PD) studies in reproductive-age, nonpregnant women in India.[19] The concern is to model development of the human fetus for developmental disorders of health and disease (DoHAD)—for very delayed effects on cardiovascular function and metabolic syndrome, as occur in animal models.[20] Fig. 157.3 is a sketch of maternal blood levels for the frequently used treatments.[21] The standard of care in the United States is a 2 to 12 mg dose of a 1:1 mixture of β phosphate + betamethasone acetate (BetaAc). The BetaAc functions as a slow-release reservoir of betamethasone. We tested only the BetaAc form of betamethasone, which is effective for lung maturation in fetal sheep and monkeys, as is the betamethasone phosphate, which yields much higher fetal plasma levels.[22] Therefore, phosphorylated betamethasone or dexamethasone simply exposes the fetus to excess drug. Using infusions of betamethasone phosphate, we determined that fetal exposure of 1 ng/mL was sufficient for lung maturation[23] in sheep or monkeys. A durable response requires greater than 48 hours exposure for lung maturation to have a permanent effect.[23] The exposure needs to be continuous for 48 hours or longer without interruption.[24,25] Of interest for low- and middle-income countries (LMIC), oral doses of very inexpensive and stable oral drugs are as effective as intramuscular injections.[24-26] A concern for the drug used routinely in the United States is that betamethasone is measurable in the maternal blood for greater than 14 days, causing prolonged adrenal suppression and fetal exposures.[19,27] To change standard of care, new lower dosing strategies will need to be tested. Our conclusion is that we have used the wrong dose of the wrong drug for 40 years.

This epidemiology and the diagnosis of RDS can be confounded by a number of factors frequently encountered in neonatal practice. Low-birth-weight infants at high risk of RDS often are intubated in the delivery room and treated with surfactant, which prevents a diagnosis of surfactant-deficiency RDS. The management strategy of initiating CPAP therapy in the delivery room to

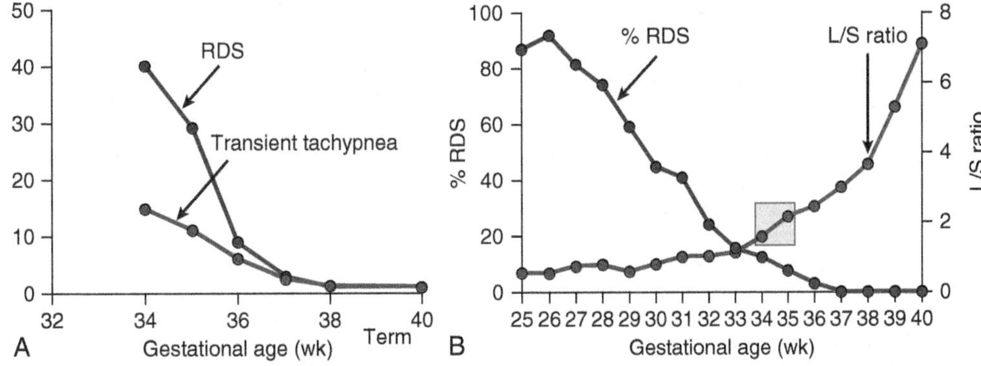

Fig. 157.2 (A) Odds ratios for respiratory morbidities diagnosed as respiratory distress syndrome *(RDS)* or transient tachypnea for 180,000 births from 2002 to 2008 relative to birth at 40 weeks' gestational age.[10] (B) Curve for percent infants with RDS versus gestational age in comparison to curve for lecithin/sphingomyelin *(L/S ratio)* values for normal pregnancies. The *box* highlights the L/S ratio measured on amniotic fluid that reliably predicts RDS if delivery were to occur. (A, Data from Consortium on safe labor, respiratory morbidity in late preterm births. *JAMA.* 2010;304:419. B, Data from Chang E, Menard K, Vermillion S, et al. The association between hyaline membrane disease and pre-eclampsia. *Am J Obstet Gynecol.* 2004;191:1414; and Gluck L, Kulovich M, Borer R, et al. The interpretation and significance of the lecithin-sphingomyelin ratio in amniotic fluid. *Am J Obstet Gynecol.* 1974;120:142.)

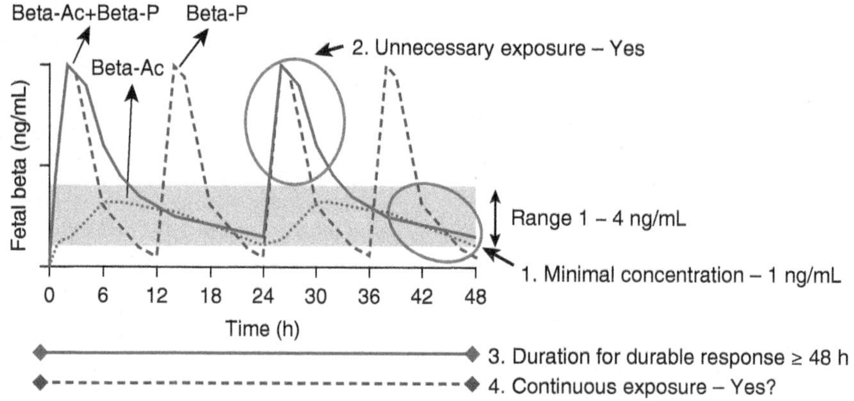

Fig. 157.3 Sketch of fetal blood levels after several of the standard treatments for antenatal steroids, Beta-P is shown here as betamethasone phosphate *(BetaP)* given as 12 mg every 24 hours × 2 doses. Beta-acetate + beta-phosphate *(BetaAc + BetaP)* is 12 mg of a 1:1 mixture of betamethasone acetate and betamethasone phosphate given twice at a 24 hour interval and BetaAc is a dose of 6 mg betamethasone acetate given twice at a 24 hour interval. Beta Ac is not available as a single component drug. The given green band is the concentration of betamethasone in the fetus that causes lung maturation, based on cord blood values with questions about dose in the figure. (Adapted from a sketch by Ballard PL, Ballard RA. Scientific basis and therapeutic regimens for use of antenatal glucocorticoids. *Am J Obstet Gynecol.* 1995;173[1]:254–262.)

Box 157.1 Fetal and Newborn Conditions That May Confound to a Diagnosis of Respiratory Distress Syndrome

1. Fetal growth restriction/preeclampsia
2. Chorioamnionitis/fetal lung inflammation
3. Neonatal pneumonia
4. Pulmonary hypoplasia
5. Transient tachypnea of the newborn

assist newborn transition can mitigate the early respiratory distress and the need for oxygen.[28,29] Further, for epidemiologic purposes, the NICHD Neonatal Research Network (NRN) has simplified the clinical diagnosis of RDS. For the interval 1997 to 2002, the NRN diagnosis of RDS required oxygen use for the interval of 6 to 24 hours after birth with some respiratory support to 24 hours and a chest film consistent with RDS.[30] In that era, the incidence of RDS was 63% for infants weighing 500 to 1000 g. In contrast, for the years 2003 to 2007, the diagnosis of RDS was given to 95% of 22 to 28 weeks' gestational age infants based only on the need for oxygen for more than the first 6 hours of life.[31] In contrast, 69% of 309 patients with birth weights of 0.5 to 1 kg were successfully managed with CPAP and without surfactant in South Africa.[32] The delivery room management of the very preterm infant with CPAP likely can decrease the frequency of the diagnosis of RDS. In contrast, intubation and ventilation in the delivery room are likely to result in a diagnosis of RDS even if the infant has relatively clear lungs and no oxygen requirement. Further, the smallest and most immature infants may need CPAP to maintain functional residual capacity (FRC) and to decrease apnea.[33] These infants may be given a diagnosis of RDS even if surfactant is adequate.

RDS is a diagnosis of exclusion, particularly in the very preterm infant (Box 157.1). Very preterm infants are born because the pregnancy is not normal. A frequent cause of very preterm birth is preeclampsia, which can result in fetal growth restriction and abnormal lung parenchymal and microvascular development in animal models and in infants.[34] The associated respiratory abnormalities may coexist or may mimic RDS. Severe pulmonary hypoplasia is a distinct diagnosis resulting from space-occupying masses in the chest, which inhibit fetal breathing, or a lack of amniotic fluid (Potter syndrome, prolonged rupture of membranes). However, milder variants of pulmonary hypoplasia are probably frequent and difficult to distinguish from RDS. The majority of preterm infants born at less than 30 weeks' gestational age will have been exposed to histologic chorioamnionitis,[35] and the inflammation in amniotic fluid results in inflammation in the fetal lungs even if frank pneumonia or positive cultures are not identified.[36] Tracheal aspirates of these infants contain inflammatory cells and increased levels of cytokines. The organisms are often low-grade pathogens such as *Ureaplasma* that do not grow using standard microbiologic techniques (see Chapter 79).

Proinflammatory mediators such as lipopolysaccharide, interleukin-1, or live organisms can inhibit alveolar development and cause microvascular injury in the preterm fetal lung.[37] Similarly, ANS inhibit saccular and alveolar development in multiple animal models.[38] In fetal sheep some inflammatory stimuli and ANS increase surfactant and thus mature the fetal lungs.[39] However, the adverse effects of inflammation and interference with lung structural development may contribute to the variable presentations and progression of RDS. Some infants will have frank pneumonia at birth from pathogens such as Group B streptococcus and *Escherichia coli* with clinical presentations that mimic severe RDS.

The incidence of the diagnosis of transient tachypnea of the newborn increases as gestational age decreases (see Fig. 157.2A). Transient tachypnea is respiratory distress resulting from delayed clearance of fetal lung fluid from the airways and lung parenchyma. This abnormality is diagnosed primarily in moderately preterm infants or term infants delivered by cesarean section before labor.[40] However, the sodium transporters that help keep the air space free of excess fluid following delivery are developmentally regulated, and low function in the preterm lung likely contributes to RDS.[41] Gastric aspirates from infants with a diagnosis of transient tachypnea also have decreased lamellar body counts and surfactant function.[42] Therefore, RDS likely includes the pathophysiology of delayed fluid clearance and may be indistinguishable from severe transient tachypnea.

RDS is in part a diagnosis of exclusion because the clinician relies only on clinical and radiologic findings. Any cause of respiratory compromise will result in tachypnea, retractions, and flaring in the term and preterm infant. The hazy lungs by radiologic assessment can reflect surfactant deficiency, pneumonia, hypoplasia, or excess fluid, or simply the lungs imaged on expiration in the early hours of life. Although not widely used, a more specific diagnosis can result from analyses of gastric fluid aspirated soon after birth by counting lamellar bodies or measuring the stability of bubbles.[43,44] For infants thought to have RDS, perhaps the best diagnostic test is the clinical response to surfactant treatment characterized primarily by an acute increase in oxygenation. Infants can have

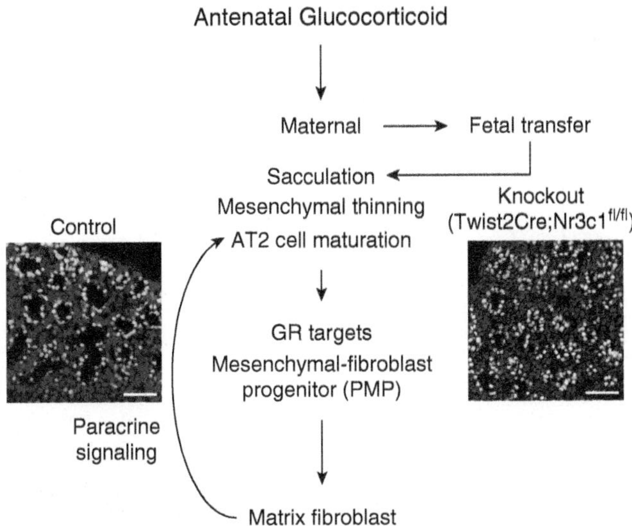

Fig. 157.4 Antenatal glucocorticoid signaling of fetal lung maturation. Based on new information from transgenic mouse models.[47] The figure illustrates that the induction of lung maturation primarily is through a newly identified mesenchymal precursor cell through a mesenchymal fibroblast to the surfactant producing Type 2 cells. Sketch based on.[47] Tissue was stained for Thyroid transcription factor-1 (TTF-1) in epithelial cells *(green)*, Glucocorticoid receptor *(GR)* in red and DAPI dye for nuclei. (Modified from Bridges JP, Sudha P, Lipps D, et al. Glucocorticoid regulates mesenchymal cell differentiation required for perinatal lung morphogenesis and function. *Am J Physiol Lung Cell Mol Physiol*. 2020;319(2):L239–L255.

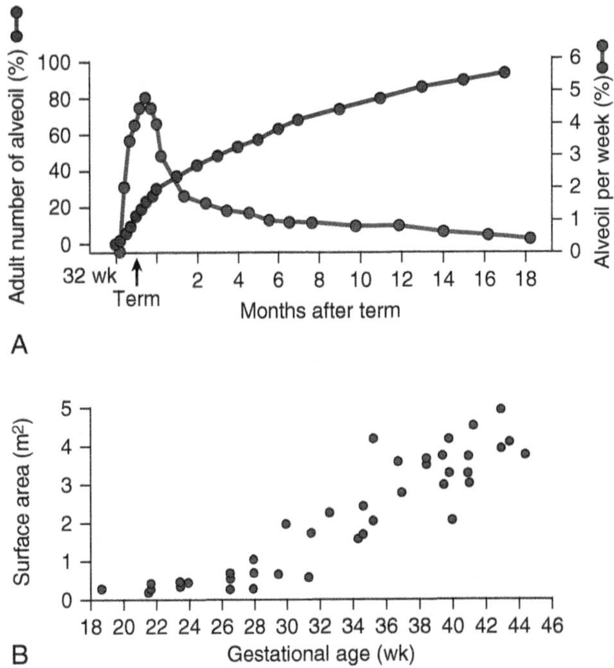

Fig. 157.5 Lung structural maturation. (A) Alveolar number and weekly rate of accumulation of alveoli are expressed as percentage of the adult number of alveoli. The curves assume that the term infant has 30% of the adult number of alveoli. (B) The large increase in lung surface area does not occur until after the saccular lung begins to alveolarize. (A, Modified from Hislop AA, Wigglesworth JS, Desai R. Alveolar development in the human fetus and infant. *Early Hum Dev.* 1986;13:1. B, Modified from Langston C, Kida D, Reed M, et al. Human lung growth in late gestation and in the neonate. *Am Rev Respir Dis.* 1984;129:607.)

RDS and other lung abnormalities at the same time. For example, fetuses exposed to chorioamnionitis and funisitis—an indicator of a fetal inflammatory response—will have decreased clinical response to surfactant treatment.[45]

LUNG STRUCTURE OF THE PRETERM LUNG WITH RESPIRATORY DISTRESS SYNDROME/EFFECT OF ANTENATAL CORTICOSTEROID THERAPY

Great progress has been made in elucidating the molecular mechanisms mediating the effects of antenatal glucocorticoids on lung maturation. Transgenic manipulation of gene expression in mouse models has been used to identify cell-specific pathways activated by glucocorticoid signals, which activate fetal lung fibroblasts, in a paracrine fashion, to induce perinatal lung maturation. Likewise, cellular and molecular insights into the pathogenesis of congenital lung malformations[46] and large airway developmental abnormalities are enabled by recent technical advances in cell and molecular biology. Relevant to the effects of ANS are recent data demonstrating that glucocorticoids signal differentiation through a newly identified pulmonary mesenchymal progenitor cell (PMP), which differentiates into matrix fibroblasts by modulation of *VEGF, JAK-STAT,* and *WNT* pathways to signal, in a paracrine fashion, to *SOX9*+-alveolar epithelial progenitor cells to enhance maturation of alveolar type 2 (AT2) cells and alveolar type 1 (AT1) cells in the fetal lung (Fig. 157.4).[47] This sequence of paracrine signaling differs from previous concepts that considered AT2 epithelial cells as the primary target of ANS to increase surfactant synthesis—an effect on surfactant pool sizes that requires several days.[48] The initial increases in lung gas volume caused by ANS result primarily from the direct effects of glucocorticoids on lung mesenchymal cells.[48]

The lung undergoes dramatic changes in cell number, differentiation, and structure in late gestation, a process that continues after birth. The lung of the term infant contains approximately 30% of the 500 million alveoli that are present in the adult lung (Fig. 157.5).[49-51] At the margin of viability at 24 weeks' gestation, the lung has just matured beyond the canalicular stage to the early saccular stage of development.[52] The saccular lung has undifferentiated distal air saccules with a poorly developed capillary microvasculature. The potential surface area for gas exchange of the developing human lung does not increase much before 30 weeks' gestation. Septation of the distal saccules to form alveoli does not begin until after 34 weeks. The rate of septation to form alveoli is high until term. After birth, the rate of alveolar septation decreases through early infancy, but alveolar development and remodeling probably continue at a slow rate throughout life.[53] Precocious maturation that commonly occurs in preterm infants with maternal glucocorticoid treatment or after exposure to chorioamnionitis accelerates mesenchymal involution and increases surfactant synthesis, but may disrupt alveolar septation, a process with potential long-term consequences on lung growth and structure.[54,55]

LUNG INJURY WITH MECHANICAL VENTILATION

A major factor determining how the preterm lung responds to treatment and injury is the structural maturation of the lung at delivery.[56] The preterm lung with RDS has lung gas pressure-volume characteristics quite distinct from the term or adult lung. As illustrated in Fig. 157.6, all lung volume variables are less for the preterm infant with RDS than in the adult lung. FRC and total lung capacity (TLC) are lower. Pressures needed to achieve lung opening and TLC are higher for the premature lung. Pressure-volume characteristics resulting from the immature air space structure explain why the preterm lung is more easily injured by mechanical ventilation.

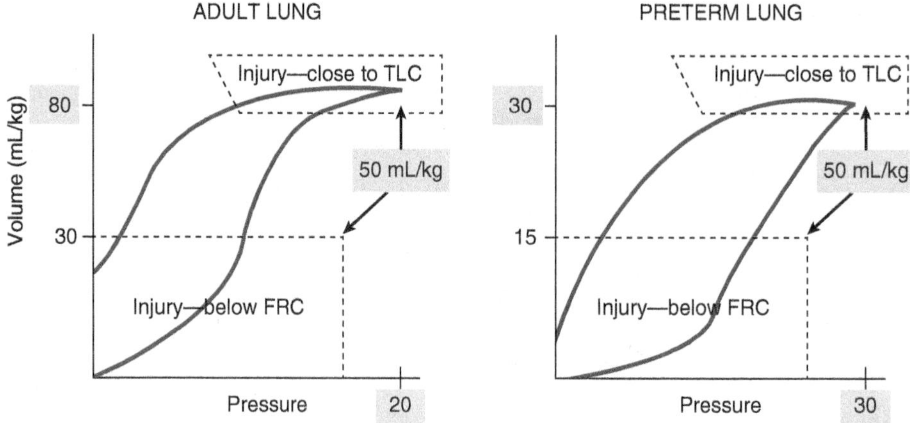

Fig. 157.6 Pressure-volume relationships for the lung with premature respiratory distress syndrome (RDS) and the adult lung. The preterm lung requires higher pressures to inflate to achieve a lower total lung capacity (TLC) than the adult lung. The premature lung also has a lower functional residual capacity (FRC) than the adult lung. The lung is likely to be injured if ventilation volumes are below FRC or encroach on TLC as indicated by the *injury boxes.*

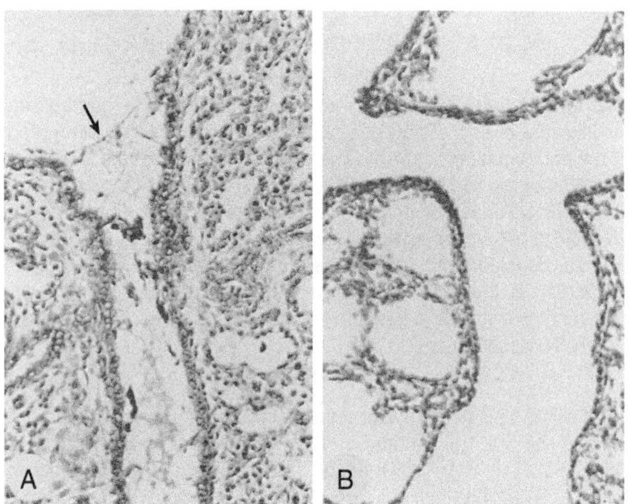

Fig. 157.7 Bronchiolar-epithelial injury in respiratory distress syndrome. (A) Lungs from preterm ventilated rabbits had fluid-filled airways with epithelial tears in the absence of surfactant treatment. *Arrow indicates air fluid interface in small airway.* (B) With surfactant treatments, the bronchiolar epithelium remained intact, and fluid was cleared from the airways and alveoli. (From Lachmann B, Berggren P, Curstedt T, et al. Combined effects of surfactant substitution and prolongation of inspiration phase in artificially ventilated premature newborn rabbits. *Pediatr Res.* 1982;16:921.)

The lungs of infants who have died from RDS are atelectatic with evidence of alveolar and interstitial edema, hyaline membranes, hemorrhage in distal saccules, and distorted small airways. Hyaline membranes are coagula of cell debris, surfactant, and serum proteins caused by epithelial injury, and result in large amounts of soluble and insoluble proteins in the air spaces. The earliest anatomic lesion identified in the lungs of infants who died of RDS shortly after birth is epithelial disruption in the small airways.[57] In preterm surfactant-deficient rabbits, bronchiolar epithelial injury develops within minutes of delivery and ventilation. This injury can be prevented with surfactant treatment (Fig. 157.7).[58] The epithelial damage occurs because the small airways of the immature lung are compliant and distort during ventilation. Lung fluid clearance is not complete, and small airways are fluid-filled at end-expiration.[41] Ventilation requires high peak pressures in the noncompliant lung to achieve relatively normal tidal volumes and carbon dioxide removal.

The preterm lung has both endothelial and epithelial abnormalities that cause proteinaceous pulmonary edema after delivery and ventilation.[59] In preterm lambs ventilated for the first 3 hours of life, 11.5% per hour of the labeled albumin mixed with the fetal lung fluid at birth left the lung, and 1.7% per hour of the labeled albumin given intravascularly at birth was recovered from the air spaces, demonstrating the bidirectional movement of albumin across an injured alveolar epithelium.[60] The protein in the alveolar washes increased more than fourfold, indicating that the net protein movement was from the intravascular compartment to the air spaces. The rate of protein accumulation in the air spaces was striking in preterm ventilated rabbits. Approximately 2% to 3% of the intravascularly injected and labeled albumin was recovered from the air spaces within 20 minutes of birth. The leakage was not homogeneous.[61] Leakage involved an increasing number of saccules with time and appeared to occur directly into the alveoli rather than at the bronchiolar level.

Lung gas volumes of infants with RDS can be low because the lung has not yet developed sufficiently to hold much gas, or because distal air spaces are uninflated (see Fig. 157.6). Another cause of the volume loss in the lungs of infants with RDS is alveolar edema. After 3 hours of ventilation, the TLC was 48 mL/kg in preterm monkeys without RDS and 19 mL/kg for monkeys with RDS.[62] The flash-frozen lungs, evaluated by light and scanning electron microscopy, of animals with RDS had overexpanded distal airways and underexpanded and fluid-filled alveolar spaces (Fig. 157.8).[63] By scanning electron microscopy, the alveoli of animals with RDS were filled with proteinaceous liquid, and the interstitium was swollen by edema fluid (Fig. 157.9).[63] The lungs of monkeys with RDS exhibit alveolar and interstitial edema because of the slow clearance of fetal lung fluid after birth and the entrance of proteinaceous edema into the air spaces.

Five clinical variables are important determinants of the amount of edema formation: gestational age, tidal volume, positive end-expiratory pressure (PEEP), antenatal corticosteroid treatment, and surfactant treatment. In preterm animal models, protein leaks from the vascular space to the alveolar space and from the alveolar space to the vascular space increase as gestation decreases (Fig. 157.10).[64] The pressure needed to achieve an adequate tidal volume and gas exchange decreases as gestational age increases. Therefore, a possible explanation of the increased leak is the barotrauma caused by the ventilatory requirements needed to support the more immature lung. In the mature lung, pulmonary edema occurs after lung overdistension[65] using high tidal volumes (volutrauma). High pressures or volumes are not required to injure the immature surfactant-deficient lung because nonuniform inflation causes focal overdistension. Without surfactant treatment, pulmonary edema occurs with relatively low tidal volume ventilation.[66] The end-expiratory volume of the preterm lung also is an important injury variable.[67] Ventilation of preterm lambs with the same

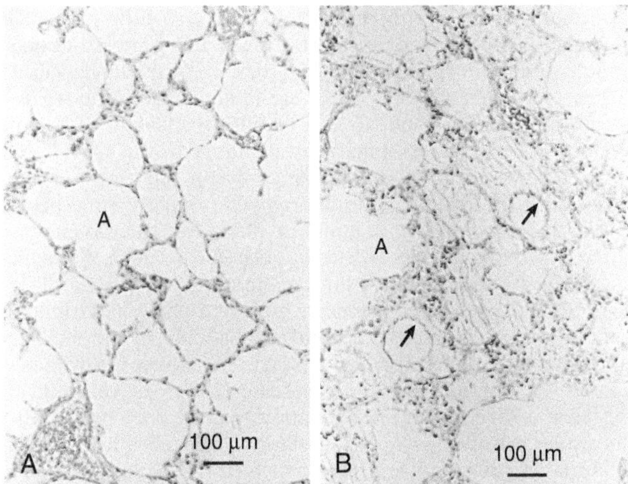

Fig. 157.8 Fluid-filled alveoli with respiratory distress syndrome (RDS). (A) Light micrograph of flash-frozen lung tissue from a preterm monkey without RDS. The alveoli and alveolar ducts (indicated by *A*) are air-filled. (B) In contrast, lung tissue from a monkey with RDS has some air-filled alveoli, and other alveoli are completely or partially filled with proteinaceous material. The *arrows* indicate partially filled alveoli. (From Jackson JC, Truog WE, Standaert TA, et al. Effect of high-frequency ventilation on the development of alveolar edema in premature monkeys at risk for hyaline membrane disease. *Am Rev Respir Dis.* 1991;143:865.)

tidal volume results in different amounts of protein recovery from the airways, depending on the PEEP used to support end-expiratory lung volume.[68] Antenatal treatment with ANS also can greatly decrease injury and edema.[69,70]

These observations describe outcomes of preterm animals ventilated from birth for several hours. The preterm lung may be most easily injured with the initiation of ventilation at birth because the air spaces are fluid-filled and the clinician wants to establish gas exchange quickly. Tidal volumes increased to 15 mL/kg severely injure the airways of preterm lambs, and subsequent ventilation amplifies and propagates that injury to the lung parenchyma (Fig. 157.11).[71,72] The injury can be decreased with lower tidal volumes, the use of PEEP to maintain FRC, and surfactant treatment.[73] These experiments in animal models provide the context for understanding why the gentle recruitment of tidal volume in the delivery room when supported by CPAP can decrease the number of infants diagnosed with RDS.[29]

An integrated perspective on the major variables that determine the pathophysiology of RDS is shown in Fig. 157.12. Lung development as modified by gestational age and exposures such as ANS, inflammation, and growth restriction determine the lung structure and the amount of surfactant that the preterm infant has at birth. The preterm lung structure can be injured to alter tissue function, primarily by epithelial disruption causing pulmonary edema. An inadequate surfactant pool can be corrected with surfactant treatment. The integration of these variables primarily determines the severity of RDS.

OVERVIEW OF SURFACTANT METABOLISM IN RESPIRATORY DISTRESS SYNDROME

Surfactant metabolism in the adult lung is the basis for the discussion of surfactant metabolism in the preterm lung with RDS (Fig. 157.13).[74] Extensive descriptions of the surfactant lipids and proteins, the biophysics of surfactant function, and regulation of synthesis and secretion are found in Chapters 73 through 80. Surfactant lipids are synthesized from glucose and

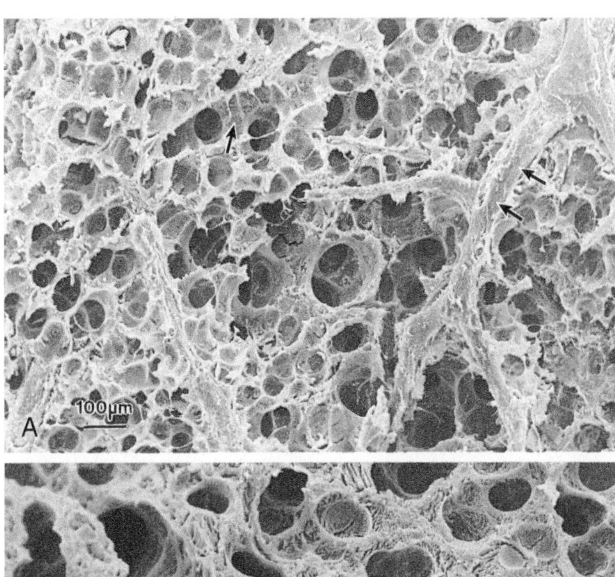

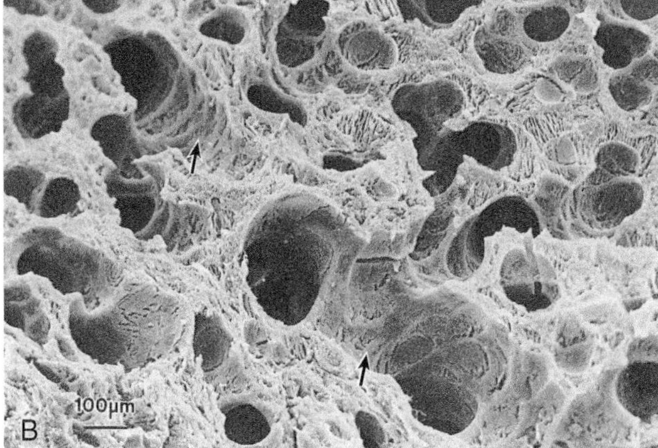

Fig. 157.9 Scanning electron micrographs from a preterm monkey without respiratory distress syndrome (RDS; A) and a preterm monkey at the same gestational age with RDS (B). The lung from the RDS animal has dilated alveolar ducts and interstitial and alveolar edema as indicated by *arrow*. (From Jackson JC, Truog WE, Standaert TA, et al. Effect of high-frequency ventilation on the development of alveolar edema in premature monkeys at risk for hyaline membrane disease. *Am Rev Respir Dis.* 1991;143:865.)

lipid precursors by type II cells in the alveoli. The lipids are processed via the Golgi to multivesicular bodies that aggregate the lipids with the surfactant protein SP-B and SP-C. The surfactant is stored in membrane-enclosed lipid and protein structures called *lamellar bodies* in the type II cells. Lamellar bodies are secreted by exocytosis either constitutively or when type II cells are stimulated by secretagogues such as β-agonists and purines or by mechanical stretch. The other SPs, SP-A and SP-D, are primarily secreted by type II cells independently of the lamellar bodies.

Surfactant has an extracellular life cycle once secreted to the thin fluid hypophase lining the alveoli and small airways of the healthy lung. The SP-A associates in the hypophase with the lipids plus SP-B and SP-C to form tubular myelin and other loose lipid arrays that are macroaggregated lipoprotein forms.[75] These large lipoprotein aggregates are the forms of surfactant that adsorb to the air-water interface. The surfactant film is multilayered and continuously replenished from surfactant in the hypophase.[76] Lipids are cleared from the air spaces as small liposomal vesicles that contain the phospholipids but essentially no SPs. The SPs are cleared separately by macrophages and type II cells. Approximately half of the surfactant components are catabolized by alveolar macrophages, and the other half are catabolized by type II cells in the adult mouse lung.[77] However, the type II cells also take up phospholipids, SP-B, SP-C, and SP-A and recycle them via multivesicular bodies back to lamellar bodies for resecretion. At steady state, the alveolar surfactant pool

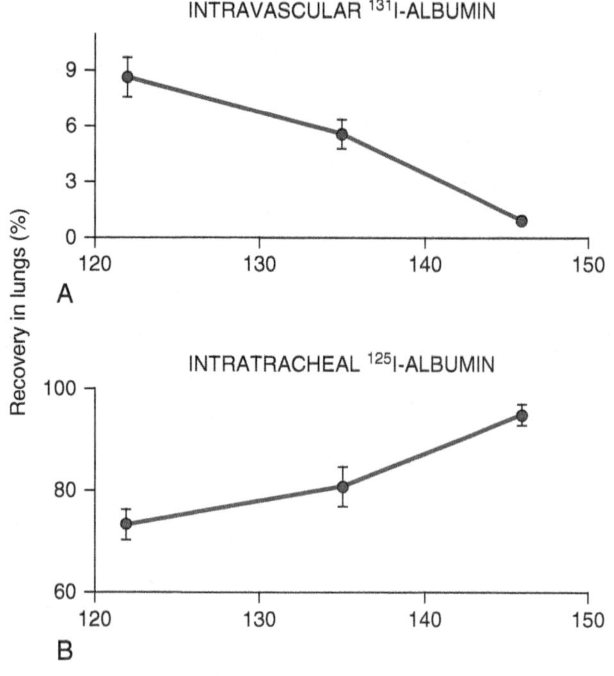

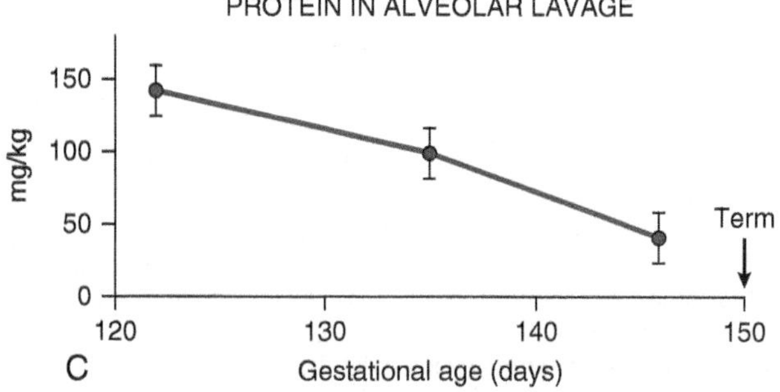

Fig. 157.10 Effect of gestational age on the movement of labeled albumin and protein in and out of the air spaces of preterm lambs. Peak ventilatory pressures were held constant at the three gestational ages for 3 hours of ventilation. The more-preterm lambs were treated with surfactant to achieve similar ventilatory pressures. (A) ^{131}I-albumin was given into the vascular space, and the net recovery in alveolar washes and in the total lung (sum of parenchyma plus alveolar wash) decreased as gestational age increased toward term. (B) ^{125}I-albumin was given into the airways at birth and the amount that was lost from the lungs decreased as gestation increased. (C) The total amount of protein in alveolar washes decreased as gestation increased. (Data from Jobe A, Jacobs H, Ikegami M, et al. Lung protein leaks in ventilated lambs: effects of gestational age. *J Appl Physiol.* 1985;58:1246.)

is very metabolically active and is replaced every 5 hours.[78] The airway clearance rates and efficiencies of recycling for SP-A, -B, and -C are similar to the lipids.[79]

CHARACTERISTICS OF SURFACTANT IN THE PRETERM LUNG

COMPOSITION

The surfactant that is recovered from the air spaces of preterm animals with RDS has less saturated phosphatidylcholine relative to total phospholipids.[80] The reduced amount of saturated phosphatidylcholines results in a surfactant with decreased surface activity. The surfactant of a mature animal or human contains approximately 8% phosphatidylglycerol and little phosphatidylinositol. In contrast, surfactant from the preterm contains much more phosphatidylinositol than phosphatidylglycerol.[81] These two acidic phospholipids are interchangeable in terms of surfactant function, but the lack of phosphatidylglycerol in surfactant indicates lung immaturity or injury to the type II cells. The changes in the lecithin/sphingomyelin (L/S) ratio in amniotic fluid with advancing gestation result primarily from the mixing of fetal lung fluid with amniotic fluid. The L/S ratio increases after approximately 34 weeks of gestation in normal pregnancies, indicating progressive lung maturation (see Fig. 157.2).[12,28] The L/S ratio measures primarily saturated phosphatidylcholine relative to sphingomyelin, a lipid not specific to the fetal lung surfactant. In the normal pregnancy, the phosphatidylinositol content of amniotic fluid increases after 28 weeks' gestation and peaks at 35 weeks, and phosphatidylglycerol does not begin to increase until after 34 weeks' gestation.[81] Infants with early lung maturation caused by fetal stress or fetal exposure to inflammation can increase the amounts of saturated phosphatidylcholine, decrease phosphatidylinositol, and increase phosphatidylglycerol in amniotic fluid, resulting in a surfactant composition comparable to a mature lung. Infants recovering from RDS have increasing amounts of phosphatidylglycerol in the surfactant. In contrast, RDS that progresses to bronchopulmonary dysplasia (BPD) results in surfactant with a delayed appearance of phosphatidylglycerol, presumably because of injury to type II cells.[82]

The surfactant-specific protein content of surfactant from the preterm lung is low relative to the amount of lipid. Type II cells with lamellar bodies appear in the human lung after approximately 22 weeks, but very little SP-A or -B mRNA is expressed until later in gestation. The timing of gene expression and protein secretion in the normal human preterm fetus can be inferred from the increases in the proteins in amniotic fluid.[83] SP-A increases after 32 weeks' gestation, and SP-B increases after 34 weeks. SP-B protein must be extensively processed before it enters lamellar bodies. With induced lung maturation in fetal sheep, both the mRNA and the protein processing of SP-B increase in parallel.[84] SP-D mRNA in the lung is also low until late gestation, and amniotic fluid levels of SP-D do not change much with advancing gestation.[85] SP-A and SP-D in amniotic fluid may also come from nonpulmonary sources, because these innate host defense proteins are made in locations other than the lung.

In contrast to other SPs, SP-C mRNA is highly expressed at the tips of branching airways during early lung development.[86] SP-C mRNA also is expressed in the developing type II cells before SP-C is found in the fetal airways. Expression of all the SPs is increased by fetal exposure to ANS and to intraamniotic inflammation.[39]

SURFACTANT POOL SIZE

During normal gestation, the lungs store progressively larger amounts of surfactant in the maturing type II cells. The appearance of surfactant in fetal air spaces lags behind the accumulation of surfactant in fetal lung tissue. After approximately 34 weeks' gestation, surfactant is secreted by the normal fetus, and large amounts of surfactant can be isolated from amniotic fluid at term. The term infant has a large excess of surfactant that facilitates rapid pulmonary adaptation to air breathing. The amount of surfactant in the lung saccules in infants younger than 32 weeks and in the developing alveoli and small airways after 32 weeks depends on the physiologic events experienced by the fetus or newborn. With labor and the stress of delivery, some of the lamellar bodies are secreted into the fetal lung fluid, and surfactant concentration increases as fetal lung fluid volume decreases.[87] More surfactant is secreted after the initiation of ventilation in response to stretch, increased catecholamines, and purinoceptor agonists. In the preterm sheep, the fetal surfactant stores in the type II cells are secreted within approximately 30 minutes of ventilation after birth.[88]

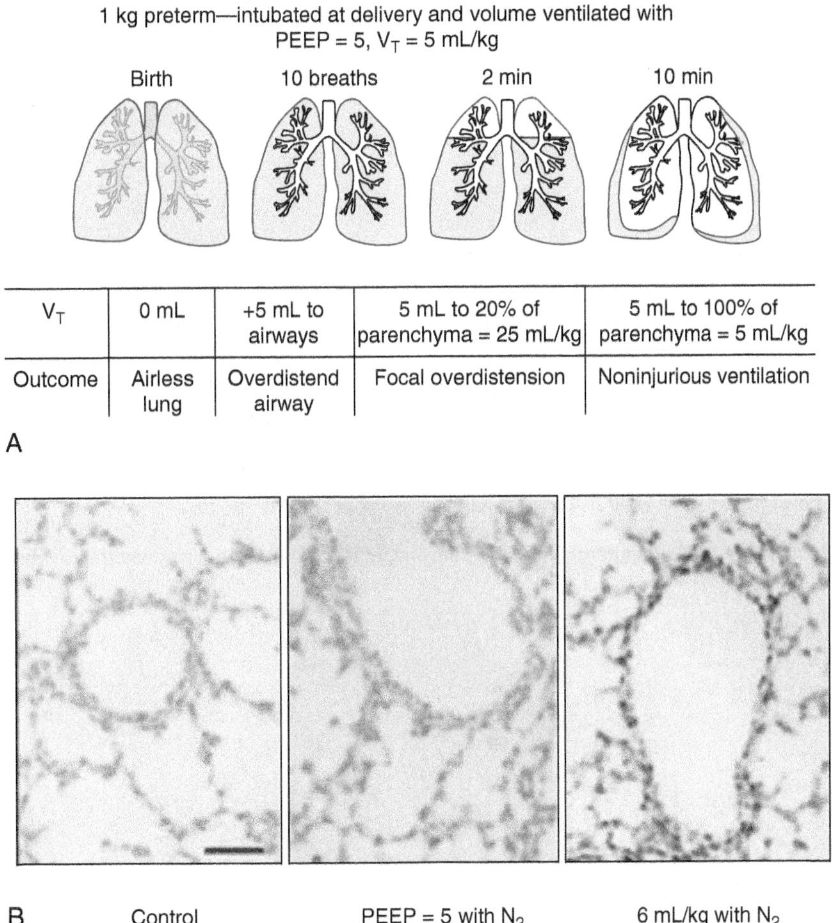

Fig. 157.11 (A) Hypothetical effects of initiating mechanical ventilation at birth for a 1-kg preterm using volume-targeted ventilation of 5 mL/kg and a positive end-expiratory pressure (PEEP) of 5 cm H_2O. The volume will overdistend the airways with the initial breaths. The volume then may cause focal overdistension if the lung is only partially recruited at 2 min. By 10 min the lung is uniformly distended, but airway and focal overdistension may have injured the lung during recruitment. (B) Expression of mRNA for Egr-1 occurs primarily in the wall of the bronchioles. Fetal sheep were exteriorized from the uterus and ventilated with nitrogen at a tidal volume of 6 mL/kg for 15 min. Egr-1 mRNA expression was increased in the bronchiole by the tidal volume, but not by a positive end expiratory pressure of 5 cm H_2O. (A, Modified from Kramer BW, Jobe AH. The clever fetus: responding to inflammation to minimize lung injury. *Biol Neonate.* 2005;88[3]:202–207. B, Modified from Hillman N, Moss T, Nitsos I, et al. Moderate tidal volumes and oxygen exposure during initiation of ventilation in preterm fetal sheep. *Pediatr Res.* 2012;72:593.)

The only direct measurements of surfactant pool sizes of infants were made by alveolar lavage of lungs of infants who died of RDS soon after birth in the era before mechanical ventilation.[89] The lavages contained approximately 5 mg/kg surfactant. Measurements by bronchoalveolar lavage in preterm rabbits and lambs with severe RDS yield values less than 3 mg/kg. Preterm lambs can be supported with CPAP if their surfactant pool size is greater than about 4 mg/kg (Fig. 157.14).[90] Smaller pool sizes result in severe respiratory failure. The differences in phospholipid composition between exogenous surfactant used for treatment of RDS and the endogenous surfactant were used to estimate the pool size in infants with RDS. By measuring the change in phosphatidylglycerol composition, Hallman and colleagues[91] estimated a surfactant pool size of approximately 9 mg/kg for infants with RDS. Similar measurements by Griese and colleagues[92] yielded a surfactant pool size estimate of 20 mg/kg. Measurements using stable isotope-labeled dipalmitoylphosphatidylcholine yielded a value of 5.6 mg/kg.[93] These techniques assume that there is good mixing of the treatment surfactant with the endogenous pool, that there is no loss of the treatment surfactant from the alveolar pool, and that airway aspirates represent what is in the distal lung. These assumptions are not strictly valid, and the techniques used clinically will overestimate the endogenous pool size by at least twofold.[94]

The endogenous pool size of surfactant is the major determinant of lung compliance in preterm animals (see Fig. 157.14).[95,96] Very preterm infants with severe RDS probably have surfactant pools of less than 5 mg/kg. Although not measured in humans, term newborn animals have surfactant pools of approximately 100 mg/kg. In contrast, the surfactant pool size in the adult human is only approximately 4 mg/kg.[97] Therefore, preterm infants have perhaps 5% of the amount of surfactant in the term newborn lung, but they have amounts comparable to the healthy adult human. This inconsistency will be addressed relative to surfactant function later in this chapter.

CHANGES IN SURFACTANT POOL SIZE AFTER BIRTH

The pool sizes of surfactant that can be recovered by alveolar lavage increase slowly after birth in preterm ventilated monkeys and sheep. In monkeys recovering from RDS, surfactant increases from approximately 5 mg/kg toward term values by 3 to 4 days of age (Fig. 157.15).[98,99] No direct measurements of surfactant pool sizes as infants recover from RDS are available. The changes in surfactant concentration in airway samples will, in part, reflect pool sizes. The concentration of surfactant was similar for infants without RDS and for infants with RDS who were treated with surfactant.[100] Infants with RDS had a progressive increase in surfactant concentration during approximately 4 days.

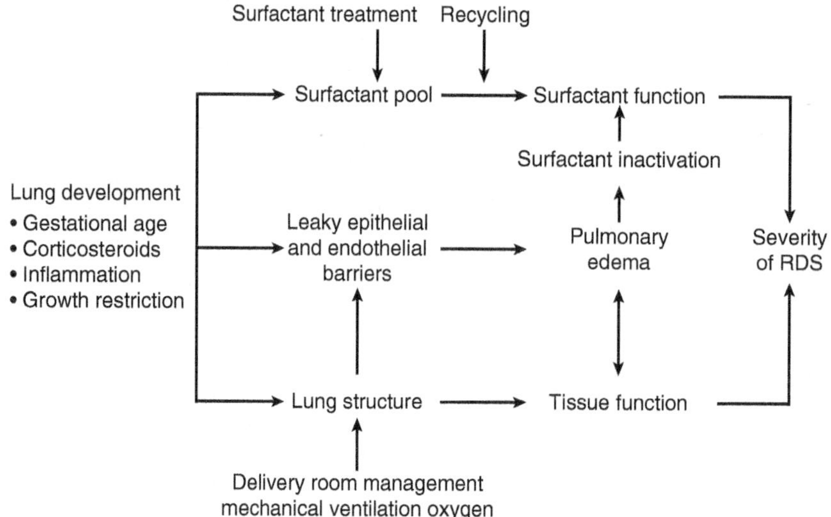

Fig. 157.12 Flow diagram of major variables that contribute to the severity of respiratory distress syndrome *(RDS)*.

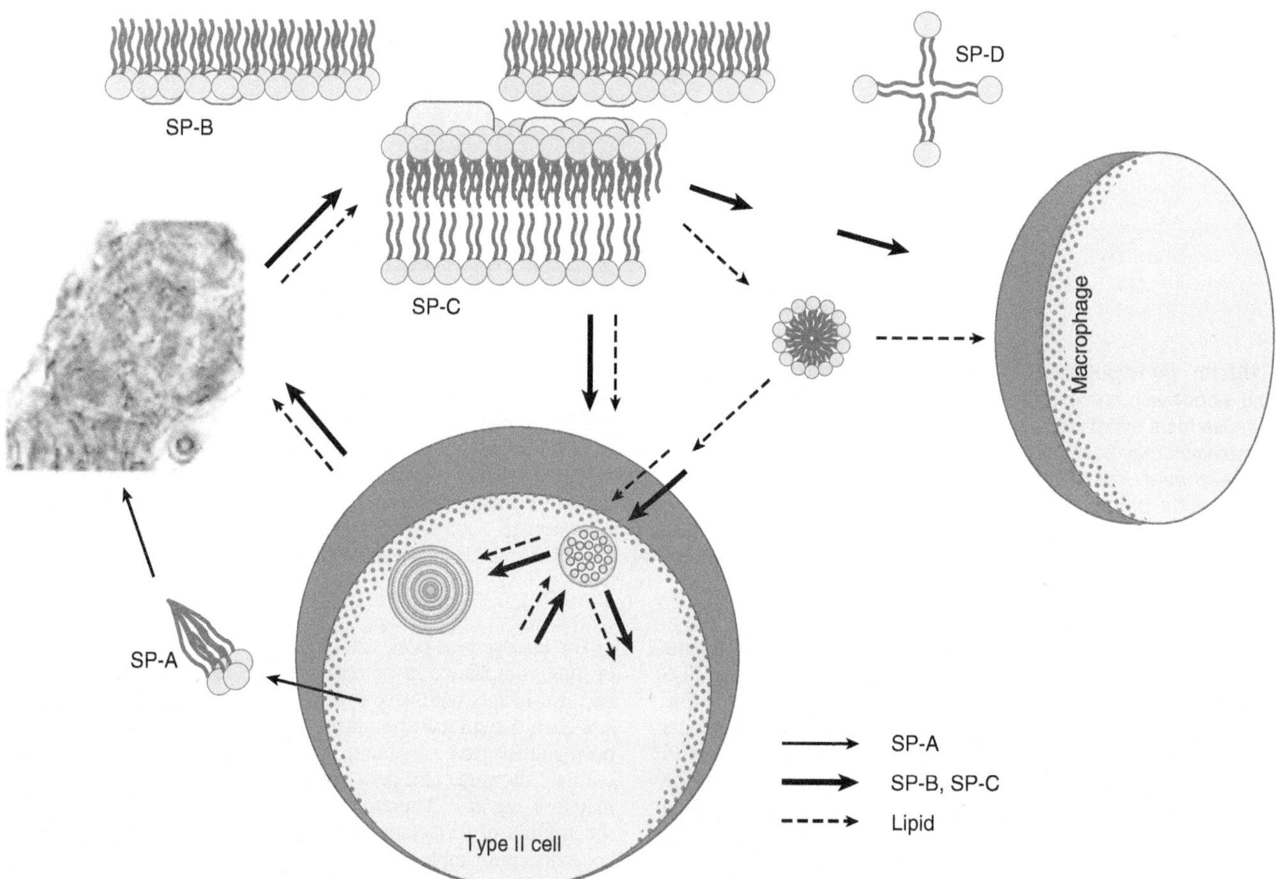

Fig. 157.13 Major metabolic pathways of surfactant. Surfactant components are synthesized and packaged into lamellar bodies in type II cells. The lamellar bodies are secreted to the hypophase and surfactant is adsorbed to the air fluid interface. Surfactant components are cleared from the air spaces primarily by type II cells and macrophages. *SP,* Surfactant-associated protein.

Surfactant treatments with the commonly used dose of 100 mg/kg do not result in large or sustained increases in alveolar surfactant pool size. For example, in sheep only approximately 25% of the treatment dose is recovered 5 hours after treatment.[101] In preterm ventilated baboons, approximately 20% of the treatment amount of surfactant was recovered 24 hours later.[102] Infants with RDS had a mean surfactant pool size estimated with stable isotopes of 17 mg/kg, 33 hours after an initial 100 mg/kg surfactant treatment.[93] The increase in alveolar surfactant that accompanies the resolution of RDS does not occur in preterm ventilated baboons that are developing BPD.[103] The alveolar pool size after surfactant treatment at birth and 6 days of ventilation was approximately 30 mg/kg, which was not increased after a second surfactant treatment and a further 8 days of ventilation. The alveolar content of the SP-A and SP-D also were low in preterm baboons developing BPD.[104] Nevertheless, the lung tissue content of saturated phosphatidylcholine increased approximately fourfold, and the tissue content of SP-A and SP-D increased, indicating a defect in surfactant processing and secretion in the early phases of BPD.

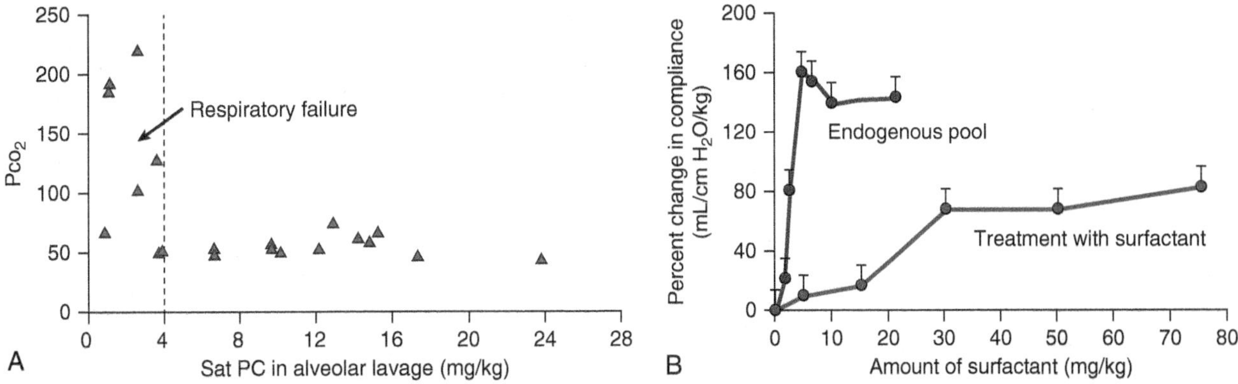

Fig. 157.14 Relationship between surfactant pool sizes and lung function. (A) Preterm lambs were delivered and supported with continuous positive airway pressure (CPAP) for 2 hours. Lambs with surfactant pool sizes estimated by alveolar wash to be greater than about 4 mg/kg could maintain Pco_2 values on CPAP.[90] (B) The curve for the endogenous pool was estimated by alveolar wash of ventilated preterm rabbits that were 27 to 29 days' gestational age. The increase in compliance includes increased surfactant and spontaneous lung structural maturation that occurred over the 2-day interval. The curve for treatment with surfactant gives the dose-response curve for ventilated 27-day gestation rabbits. (Data from Ikegami M, Jobe AH, Yamada T, et al. Relationship between alveolar saturated phosphatidylcholine pool sizes and compliance of preterm rabbit lungs, the effect of maternal corticosteroid treatment. *Am Rev Respir Dis.* 1989;139:367; and Seidner S, Pettenazzo A, Ikegami M, et al. Corticosteroid potentiation of surfactant dose response in preterm rabbits. *J Appl Physiol.* 1988;64:2366.)

SURFACTANT METABOLISM IN THE PRETERM

To understand how the alveolar surfactant pool is maintained in the lung, it is helpful to divide metabolism into the anabolic components of synthesis and secretion and the catabolic activities of uptake, degradation, and recycling. In clinical studies, surfactant components labeled with stable isotopes were used to evaluate surfactant metabolism in infants. Most metabolic studies have focused on saturated phosphatidylcholine because it is the major component of surfactant and is primarily responsible for the biophysical properties of surfactant. Measurements of synthesis of surfactant phospholipids generally involve the intravascular injection of labeled precursors. The labeled precursors are taken up by type II cells and incorporated into phosphatidylcholine, which is transacylated to increase the amount of saturated phosphatidylcholine. The surfactant lipids together with SP-B and SP-C are processed and packaged via multivesicular bodies to become the storage-secretion granule, the lamellar body (see Fig. 157.13). Secretion can be measured by recovering the labeled surfactant components from the air spaces, which aids in evaluating the overall kinetics of synthesis and secretion. The absolute amount of a surfactant component that is synthesized cannot be easily determined, because the radiolabeled precursor is diluted into the plasma pool and is further diluted by the precursor pool in the type II cell. However, the net kinetics of synthesis and secretion provide critical information for understanding why surfactant deficiency requires days to resolve in infants with RDS.

After term delivery and ventilation of lambs, an intravascular injection of radiolabeled palmitic acid is incorporated into lung phosphatidylcholine within minutes.[105] However, radiolabeled surfactant is not detected in the air spaces for approximately 5 hours, and the amount of radiolabeled surfactant continues to accumulate in the air spaces for 30 to 40 hours (Fig. 157.16).[106] A similar curve for accumulation of de novo synthesized surfactant was measured for ventilated preterm lambs with mild RDS. Subsequent surfactant treatment of these preterm lambs caused a large dilution of the endogenous surfactant. After a ^{13}C-glucose infusion, surfactant lipids labeled with ^{13}C-glucose could not be detected in airway samples of surfactant-treated very preterm baboons until 24 hours of age.[107] The peak accumulation of ^{13}C-glucose in phosphatidylcholine was at approximately 100 hours. The curve for preterm baboons has a longer delay in detection than the curve for preterm sheep because the radiolabel was not given as a pulse label and time was required to get enough label into the air space to be detected. Preterm surfactant-treated infants with RDS given infusions of ^{13}C-palmitic acid and ^{13}C-glucose have curves similar to baboons for surfactant lipids in airway samples (see Fig. 157.16).[108] The conclusion is that secretion is delayed for hours after synthesis, and surfactant made shortly after birth is secreted gradually over a prolonged period of time. The curves are not altered much by surfactant treatment or by age after birth when the labeled precursor is given.[107] Antenatal glucocorticoids may increase lipid synthesis after several days.[108] Surfactant treatment does not inhibit de novo synthesis of lipids or the SPs in the preterm lungs. Surfactant treatment also does not alter the ultrastructure of type II cells or the volume fraction of lamellar bodies in type II cells.[109] The timing of phosphatidylcholine secretion measured with stable isotopes was similar for infants with RDS ventilated with conventional or high-frequency oscillatory ventilation.[110]

The other half of the metabolic equation is the loss of surfactant from the lung. This measurement has two components that include uptake and catabolism of surfactant components from the air space by type II cells and macrophages and recycling by type II cells. Little surfactant is lost from adult lungs to the lymph or vascular space unless the lung is injured, and minimal amounts of surfactant are lost by suctioning the airways, unless edema fluid is present. In the term lamb, a trace dose of surfactant given at birth had a half-life of approximately 6 days, which is longer than values of approximately 10 hours for adult animals.[111] Almost all of a trace dose of surfactant given to preterm lambs with mild RDS was recovered in the lungs after 24 hours of ventilation, demonstrating minimal catabolism (Fig. 157.17).[112] However, only 20% of the labeled surfactant was still in the air spaces, and 80% was associated with lung tissue. Similar measurements in preterm lambs with more severe RDS that were treated with surfactant demonstrated a 30% loss of surfactant used for treatment by 24 hours and only 14% of the surfactant recovered by alveolar lavage.[113] This rate of loss of surfactant from the lungs yielded a biologic half-life of approximately 48 hours. The percentage of a treatment dose of surfactant that was lost from the air spaces was similar with high tidal volume ventilation or with high-frequency oscillatory ventilation in preterm lambs[66,114] Surfactant-treated and ventilated preterm baboons that were developing BPD retained only 4% of the treatment in the airspaces, and approximately 80% of the surfactant was lost from the lungs by 6 days, yielding a half-life of approximately 60 hours.[102] These results indicate that the term and preterm lung degrades surfactant lipids slowly and that injury can increase the loss of surfactant from the lungs.

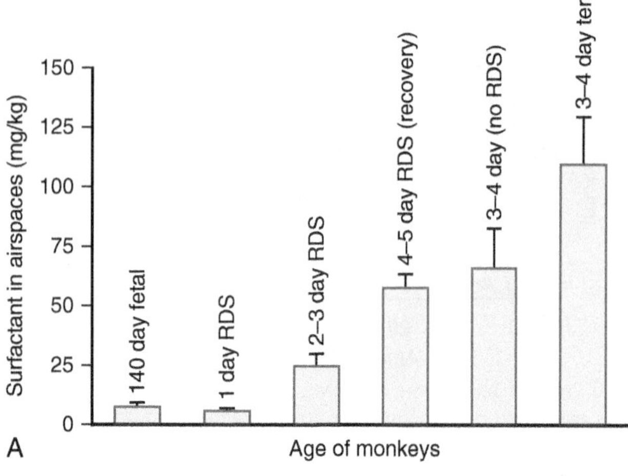

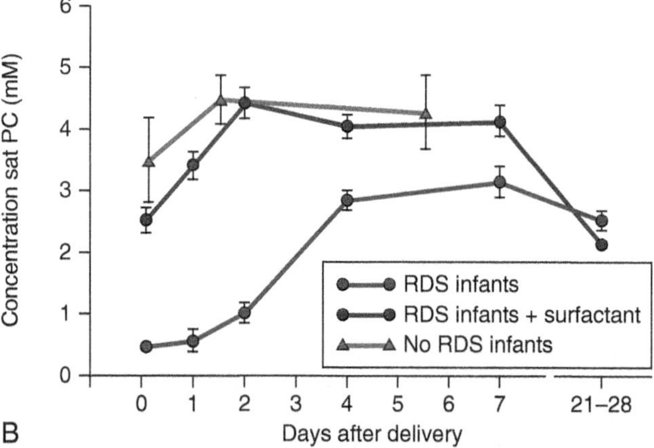

Fig. 157.15 Surfactant pool sizes with resolution of respiratory distress syndrome *(RDS)*. (A) The amount of surfactant recovered by alveolar lavage from mechanically ventilated preterm monkeys with RDS is shown relative to age and stage of the disease. (B) The concentrations of saturated phosphatidylcholine *(sat PC)* in airway samples from infants with RDS, infants with RDS treated with surfactant, and infants without RDS are graphed relative to age from birth. The concentrations of sat PC approached values for healthy preterm infants by 4 to 7 days. (A, Data from Jackson JC, Palmer S, Truog WE, et al. Surfactant quantity and composition during recovery from hyaline membrane disease. *Pediatr Res.* 1986;20:1243; and Jackson JC, Palmer S, Flandaert T. Developmental changes of surface active material in newborn non-human primates. *Am Rev Respir Dis.* 1984;129:A204. (B) Data from Hallman M, Merritt TA, Akino T, et al. Surfactant protein-A, phosphatidylcholine, and surfactant inhibitors in epithelial lining fluid: correlation with surface activity, severity of respiratory distress syndrome, and outcome in small premature infants. *Am Rev Respir Dis.* 1991;144:1376.)

No information is available about where degradation of surfactant occurs in the preterm. The normal preterm lung at birth contains few macrophages and essentially no granulocytes. However, inflammation and injury will rapidly recruit inflammatory cells to the lung, which may then increase the loss of surfactant. A significant amount of a treatment dose of surfactant that becomes associated with the lung tissue probably is in type II cells. In the term newborn rabbit, more than 90% of the surfactant phospholipids are recycled back into the type II cells for resecretion.[115] In the only estimate available, ventilated preterm lambs with mild RDS had a turnover time for surfactant phosphatidylcholine of approximately 13 hours.[112] These animals had no measurable surfactant catabolism, indicating efficient recycling.

The only practical measurement of surfactant pool size and biologic half-life in the human is to give a trace or treatment dose of surfactant containing a stable isotope and to follow the change in concentration of the label in the surfactant sampled by aspiration of the air spaces. This measurement gives an integrated assessment of the mixing of the exogenous label with the endogenous air space surfactant and tissue pools of surfactant. A decrease in the concentration of the label in the airway sample represents dilution of the label with surfactant from the lung, but it does not necessarily measure catabolism. Such measurements have been made in surfactant-treated preterm ventilated baboons and infants with RDS (see Fig. 157.17).[93,102] In baboons the concentration of labeled lipid (specific activity) did not change for approximately 24 hours, indicating that little endogenous surfactant was present. However, independent data from preterm lambs and baboons indicate that only approximately 20% of the surfactant would have been in the air spaces at 24 hours, and 25% of the surfactant would have been lost from the lung compartment.[112,113] Subsequently the specific activity decreased exponentially, yielding a biologic half-life of approximately 30 hours. The biologic half-life values for infants with RDS measured with ^{13}C-dipalmitoylphosphatidylcholine were 34 ± 9 hours after surfactant treatment at a mean of 4.6 hours of age, and they were similar after a second dose of surfactant given at a mean age of 37 hours. The consistency of the indirect measurements in humans and animals indicates that surfactant catabolism is slow in the preterm with RDS. The treatment dose of surfactant does not remain in the air space but becomes part of the overall metabolic pool of surfactant. Measurements with stable isotopes in preterm infants also indicate that surfactant catabolism is increased, and recycling efficiency is decreased with lung injury and development of BPD.

The SPs (SP-A, SP-B, and SP-C) are cleared from the air spaces and the lung compartment of adult animals in parallel with the surfactant lipids.[79] The proteins are recycled with an efficiency somewhat lower than the lipids, and degradation of SP-A occurs approximately equally in macrophages and type II cells.[77] The preterm ventilated lamb lung clears SP-A from the air spaces more rapidly than the lipids.[116] The lipophilic proteins SP-B and SP-C are cleared from the air spaces and from the lung compartment similarly to saturated phosphatidylcholine in ventilated preterm lamb lungs.[101,114] SP-B clearance is similar in lambs ventilated with a conventional style of ventilation or with high-frequency oscillatory ventilation. In the only measurement in humans, SP-B secretion paralleled saturated phosphatidylcholine and clearance was somewhat faster..[117]

SURFACTANT FUNCTION IN THE ALVEOLUS

SURFACTANT FORMS

Surfactant is in the alveolus in different structural forms that have different characteristics and functions.[118] After secretion, the lamellar bodies unravel to form the elegant structure called *tubular myelin*. This lipoprotein array has SP-A at the corners of the lattice and requires at least SP-A, SP-B, and the phospholipids for its unique structure. Tubular myelin and other loose surfactant lipoprotein arrays in the hypophase generate the surface film within the alveolus and small airways. New surfactant enters the surface film and "used" surfactant leaves as small vesicles, which then are cleared from the air spaces. The major differences in composition between the surface-active tubular myelin and the biophysically inactive small vesicles are that the small forms contain little SP-A, SP-B, or SP-C.

Surfactant is secreted to yield an alveolar pool that is primarily lamellar bodies and tubular myelin. During neonatal transition to air breathing, the percent of surface-active forms falls as the small vesicular forms increase (Fig. 157.18).[119] At steady state, approximately 50% of the surfactant in the air spaces is in a

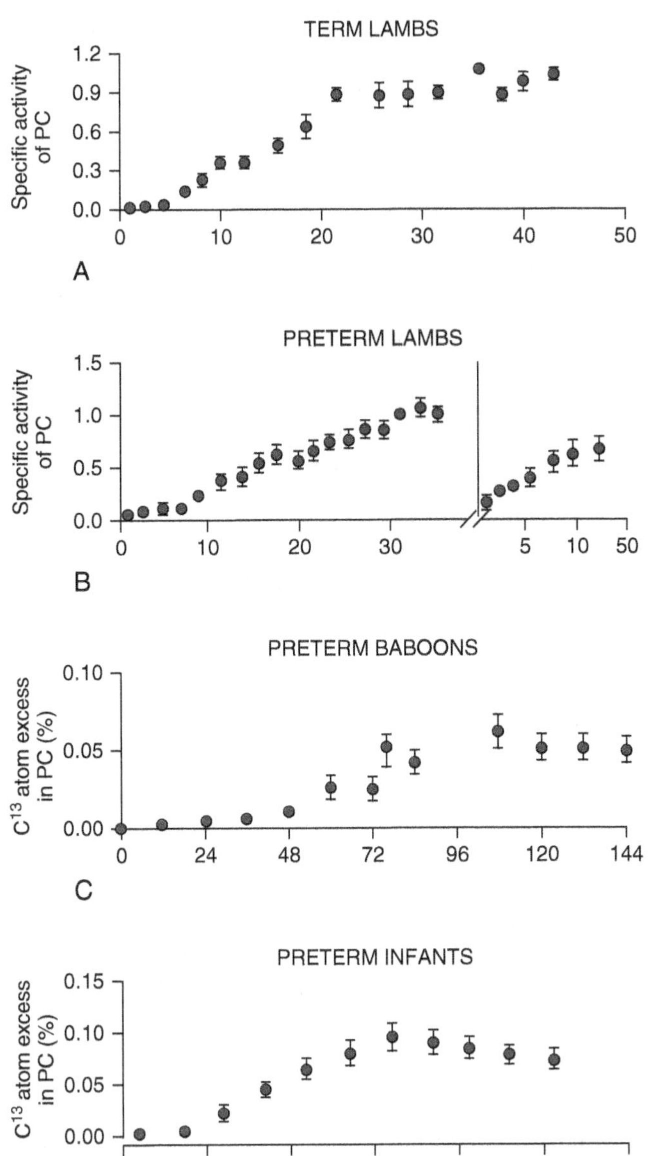

Fig. 157.16 Time course of appearance of de novo synthesized surfactant phosphatidylcholine (PC) in airway samples of term lambs, preterm lambs, preterm baboons, and preterm infants. (A) Radiolabeled saturated PC in airway samples of ventilated term lambs given ^{3}H-palmitic acid as a bolus intravascular injection at birth. Data are mean ± standard error of specific activities (counts/min/μmol PC) normalized to the maximal values for each animal. (B) Labeled saturated PC in airway samples of ventilated preterm lambs given a single intravascular injection of ^{3}H-palmitic acid at birth and not treated with surfactant until approximately 38 hours of age. The discontinuity in the curve demonstrates the fall in the specific activity after treatment with surfactant (dilution of surfactant pool with treatment dose of surfactant). (C) Labeling of PC in airway samples of preterm surfactant-treated baboons that were ventilated for 6 days. The animals received ^{13}C-glucose by intravascular infusion for the first 24 hours of age and the ^{13}C in the palmitate of PC is expressed as ^{13}C-atom percent excess. (D) Labeling of PC in airway samples of surfactant treated and mechanically ventilated infants with RDS following an intravascular infusion of ^{13}C-glucose for the first 24 hours of life. The label in the PC is expressed as atom percent excess. (A and B, Data from Jobe AH, Ikegami M, Glatz T, et al. Saturated phosphatidylcholine secretion and the effect of natural surfactant on premature and term lambs ventilated for 2 days. *Exp Lung Res.* 1983;4:259. C, Data from Bunt JE, Carnielli VP, Seidner SR. Metabolism of endogenous surfactant in premature baboons and effect of prenatal corticosteroids. *Am J Respir Crit Care Med.* 1999;160:1481. D, Data from Bunt JE, Carnielli VP, Darcos Wattimena JL, et al. The effect in premature infants of prenatal corticosteroids on endogenous surfactant synthesis as measured with stable isotopes. *Am J Respir Crit Care Med.* 2000;162:844.)

surface-active form, and 50% is in the inactive vesicular form. The total surfactant pool size is not equivalent to the amount of active surfactant. The maintenance of surfactant function depends on the preservation of the active forms of surfactant in the air space.

SURFACTANT INACTIVATION

Surfactant inactivation or inhibition is a complex concept because it is the integrated result of multiple factors that can alter the alveolar forms and biophysical properties of the surfactant in the air spaces (Box 157.2).[120] The net effects can be a decrease in the effective pool size, a degradation of the surface tension–lowering properties of the surfactant, or both. Injury to the alveolar epithelium and edema change the environment where surfactant acts. The mechanisms that contribute to surfactant inactivation will vary with the type of lung injury. The biophysically active surfactant pool can be depleted by an increased rate of conversion to the inactive vesicular forms. This conversion is accelerated by proteinaceous edema and inflammatory products, probably because proteases degrade SPs.[121] Ventilation styles that use large tidal volumes and no PEEP can deplete the active surfactant pool and high-frequency oscillatory ventilation can preserve surfactant in adult animal models.[122] However, in surfactant-treated preterm lambs, ventilation with high-frequency oscillation did not have an advantage over conventional ventilation.[114] Meconium and bilirubin can accelerate the conversion to inactive surfactant forms, and surfactant with less SP will be inactivated more quickly.

Another mechanism of inactivation is the removal of the surfactant by sequestration into clots or hyaline membranes. Surfactant is a thromboplastin and will activate clotting, and in vitro the clot will capture much of the alveolar pulmonary surfactant.[120] Although most soluble proteins can interfere with surface adsorption and film formation, the products of clot lysis are particularly inhibitory.[123] Albumin is not as inhibitory as fibrinogen, although it is the protein that is in the highest concentration in edema and inflammatory fluid. Hemoglobin and other protein products of lung injury also are inhibitors. The phenomenon of interference with film formation by soluble proteins is dependent on both the relative and absolute concentrations of the surfactant and the inhibiting proteins.[124] If surfactant concentrations are high, potent inhibitors at high concentration have little adverse effect when tested in vitro. However, when surfactant concentrations are low, low concentrations of inhibitors can severely degrade surfactant function. Surfactants that contain low amounts of SPs also are more sensitive to inactivation by soluble proteins.

Lung function will deteriorate when inactivation interferes with enough surfactant to alter the function of the surfactant at the air-fluid interface. Therefore, inactivation can be a severe problem when the surfactant pool size is small, as in RDS. Airway samples taken at the time of intubation from infants with RDS had high minimal surface tensions (Fig. 157.19).[125] Inhibition of surfactant function contributed to the problem because the airway samples contained surfactant with good function that could be isolated by centrifugation. The soluble proteins from these airway samples inhibited natural surfactant more than did proteins from airway samples from infants without RDS. The importance of surfactant inactivation can be demonstrated using a preterm ventilated lamb model of RDS (Fig. 157.20).[126]

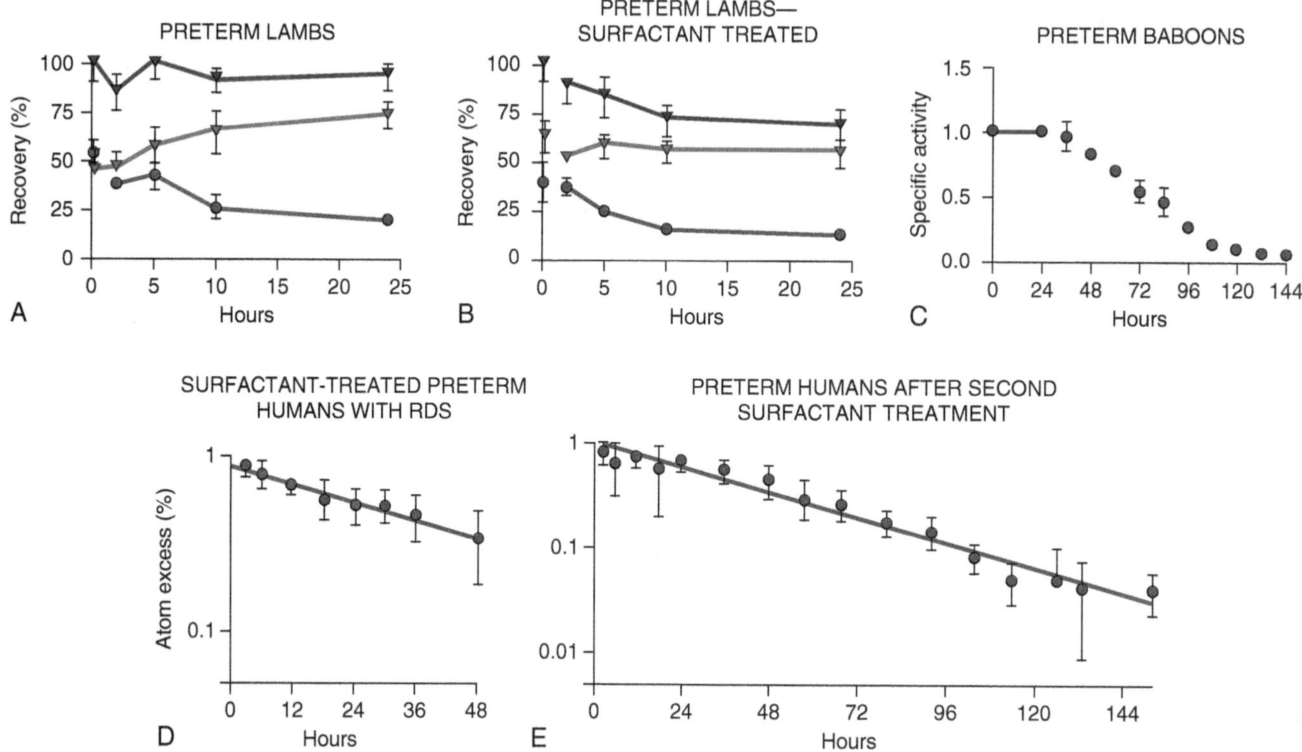

Fig. 157.17 Loss of labeled phosphatidylcholine (PC) given into the airways of preterm lambs not treated with surfactant (A); preterm lambs treated with surfactant (B); preterm surfactant-treated baboons (C); and surfactant-treated preterm infants (D and E). All animals and infants were mechanically ventilated and had respiratory distress syndrome. (A) The preterm lambs received a trace dose of natural sheep surfactant labeled with ^{3}H-dipalmitoylphosphatidylcholine. Recoveries in alveolar washes, lung tissue, and total lungs (alveolar + tissue) were measured 2, 5, 10, and 24 hours after birth. (B) Preterm lambs were treated at birth with 100 mg/kg of natural sheep surfactant, containing radiolabeled phosphatidylcholine and the lambs were ventilated for periods up to 24 hours for measurements of the percent recovery of the phosphatidylcholine from the surfactant used for treatment. (A and B) *Green line,* Lung tissue; *red line,* alveolar wash; *purple line,* total lung. (C) Curve for specific activity of phosphatidylcholine in airway samples of preterm baboons treated at birth with ^{14}C-dipalmitoylphosphatidylcholine–labeled surfactant. The specific activities were normalized to the values for the surfactant used to treat the baboons. (D) Curve for atom percent excess in airway samples for ^{13}C-dipalmitoylphosphatidylcholine–labeled surfactant used to treat preterm ventilated infants with RDS. The atom percent excess in the initial surfactant dose given after delivery fell exponentially for 48 hours. (E) A second dose given at approximately 2 days of age resulted in a similar curve. (A, Data from Jobe AH, Ikegami M, Seidner SR, et al. Surfactant phosphatidylcholine metabolism and surfactant function in preterm, ventilated lambs. *Am Rev Respir Dis.* 1989;139:352. B, Data from Ikegami M, Jobe A, Yamada T, et al. Surfactant metabolism in surfactant-treated preterm ventilated lambs. *J Appl Physiol.* 1989;67:429. C, Data from Seidner SR, Jobe AH, Coalson JJ, et al. Abnormal surfactant metabolism and function in preterm ventilated baboons. *Am J Respir Crit Care Med.* 1998;158:1982. D and E, Data from Torresin M, Zimmermann LJ, Cogo PE, et al. Exogenous surfactant kinetics in infant respiratory distress syndrome: a novel method with stable isotopes. *Am J Respir Crit Care Med.* 2000;161:1584.)

Ventilation for 30 minutes caused severe lung injury in preterm lambs with surfactant pools of less than 1 mg/kg. Surfactant treatment resulted in improved oxygenation and a fall in minimal surface tensions of the surfactant in airway samples. However, decreased oxygenation recurred because these animals had progressive lung injury and surfactant inhibition.

These inhibitory effects explain the progressive deterioration in lung function after birth in infants with RDS. Surfactant function may initially be adequate but with low surfactant pool sizes (creating a honeymoon period). Spontaneous or mechanical ventilation can cause edema, inflammation, and progressive lung injury. The combination of clot formation (hyaline membranes) and increased soluble inhibitory proteins depletes the small functional surfactant pool, which results in progressive respiratory failure.

Inactivation phenomena depend on the type of surfactant being tested. The animal-source surfactants in clinical use have in common organic solvent extraction steps that remove nonspecific contaminating proteins, SP-A and SP-D. SP-B and SP-C are retained in the surfactant extract in variable amounts with the phospholipids and neutral lipids. The only functional abnormality in surfactant from mice that lack SP-A is increased sensitivity to inhibition.[127] The addition of SP-A to an organic solvent-extracted surfactant made that surfactant less sensitive to inactivation by albumin and fibrinogen.[128] The potent inactivation of surfactant by fibrinogen was reversed by 0.5% SP-A. Addition of SP-A to SP-B and SP-C–containing surfactant preserved the in vivo function of the surfactant in the presence of plasma when the mixture was used to treat preterm rabbits.[129,130] These observations may have direct clinical relevance because Hallman and colleagues[91] reported that soluble proteins in airway samples from infants with RDS were much more inhibitory to surfactant samples with low SP-A-to-saturated-phosphatidylcholine ratios than were surfactant samples with higher ratios.

SP-B and SP-C also influence the sensitivity of lipid mixtures to inactivation.[131] Synthetic surfactants that lack these SPs are sensitive to inactivation by albumin or fibrinogen. Addition of native SP-B and SP-C improved resistance to inactivation.[132] Recombinant SP-C and lipids and mixtures of SP-B and SP-C and lipids are less sensitive to protein inactivation than are lipid mixtures alone.

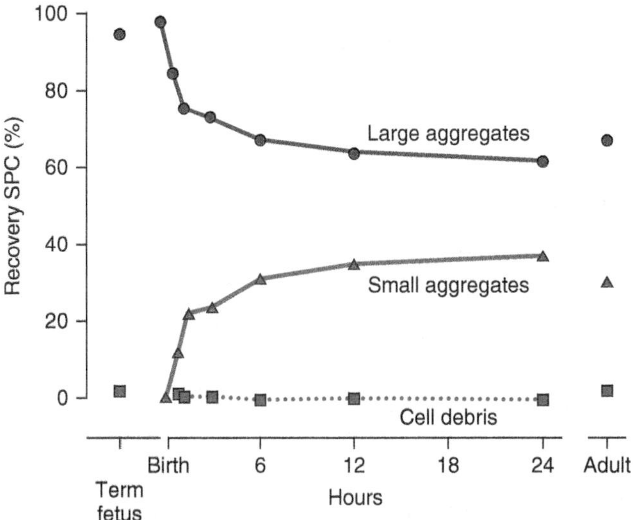

Fig. 157.18 Changes in surfactant aggregate size distribution with time after birth. Surfactant suspensions recovered by alveolar wash from term rabbit fetuses and at various ages after birth were fractionated by centrifugation. The distribution of saturated phosphatidylcholine (SPC) in fractions is also indicated for alveolar washes from adult rabbits. (Modified from Bruni R, Baritussio A, Quaglino D, et al. Postnatal transformations of alveolar surfactant in the rabbit: changes in pool size, pool morphology and isoforms of the 32 to 38 kDa apolipoprotein. *Biochim Biophys Acta.* 1988;958:255.)

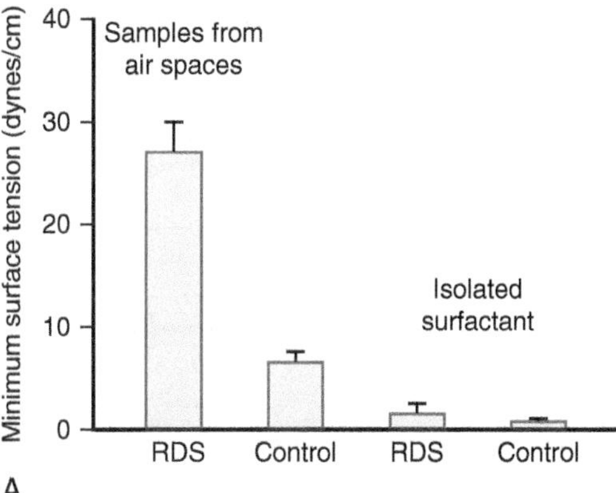

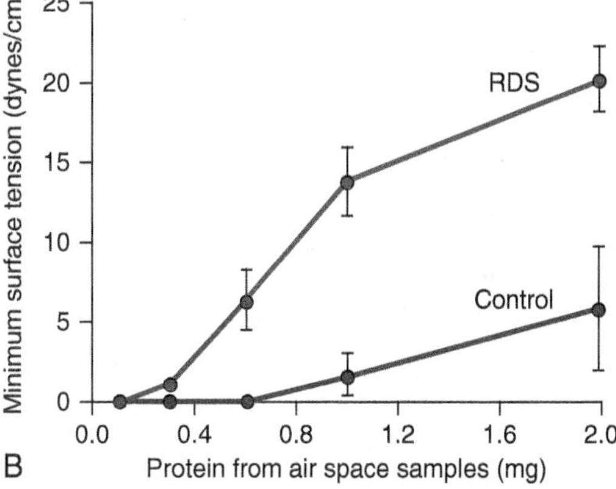

Fig. 157.19 Minimum surface tensions of airway samples from infants with respiratory distress syndrome (*RDS*; A) and control infants and inhibition of surfactant by proteins (B). (A) Samples from infants with RDS had high minimum surface tensions, whereas control samples had low minimum surface tensions. After isolation of surfactant by centrifugation, the surfactants from RDS and control infants had low minimum surface tensions. (B) Supernatant protein fractions from airway samples were added to a constant amount of natural sheep surfactant. Protein fractions from infants with RDS had higher inhibitory activity than proteins from the control infants. (From Ikegami M, Jacobs H, Jobe AH. Surfactant function in the respiratory distress syndrome. *J Pediatr.* 1983;102:443.)

Box 157.2 Mechanisms of Surfactant Inactivation and Substances That Contribute to Inactivation

Form Conversions in Air Spaces

- Normal process of alveolar metabolism
- Increased conversion with proteinaceous edema (proteases?)
- Ventilation, meconium, decreased surfactant protein content

Removal of Surfactant From Alveolar Pool

- Clots and hyaline membranes

Inhibitors of Adsorption and Film Stabilization

- Proteins
- Edema fluid
- Plasma
- Fibrinogen, monomers
- Albumin
- Laminin
- Hemoglobin
- Lipids
- Lysophosphatidylcholine
- Cholesterol
- Red cell membranes

Other Inactivators

- Meconium
- Bilirubin
- Oxidizing agents
- Amino acids

QUALITY OF SURFACTANT IN THE PRETERM INFANT

The preterm infant with RDS has surfactant with properties that are inferior to surfactant from the mature lung, which compounds the problem of a small pool size of surfactant.[80] Surfactant from the preterm lung with RDS has a different composition from surfactant from the mature or adult lung. The phosphatidylglycerol content is lower, the phosphatidylinositol content is higher, and the percent-saturated phosphatidylcholine is lower. The alveolar pool from preterm lambs with RDS has a higher percentage of the surfactant in inactive forms than more mature lambs, and in vitro conversion rates from active to inactive forms are more rapid. Preterm surfactant is also more sensitive to inactivation in vitro by soluble proteins, most likely because of a lower SP content. Furthermore, when surfactants from preterm lambs or baboons were tested in preterm surfactant-deficient rabbit lungs, they were less effective at improving compliance than surfactant from term animals.[80,102] Therefore, surfactant from the preterm lung is intrinsically less effective and more susceptible to inactivation than surfactant from the mature lung.

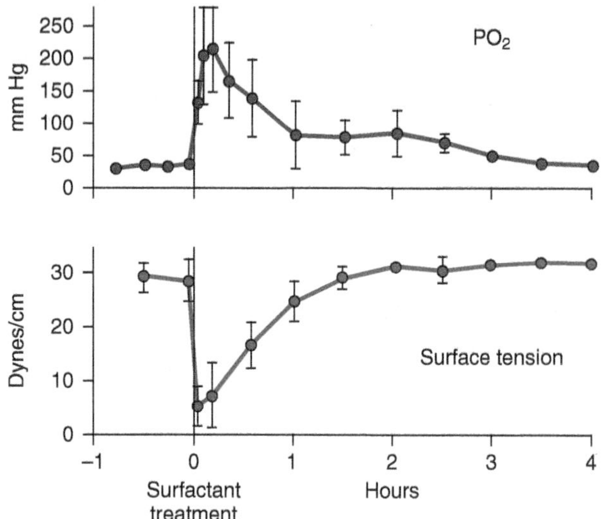

Fig. 157.20 Surface tension and clinical response to surfactant treatment. Immature lambs had severe respiratory failure despite ventilatory support and 100% O_2. With surfactant treatment at approximately 45 minutes of age, Po_2 values increased and surface tensions of airway samples decreased. Subsequently the respiratory function of the lambs deteriorated as minimum surface tension values increased in the airway samples. (From Ikegami M, Jobe A, Jacobs H, et al. A protein from airways of premature lambs that inhibits surfactant function. *J Appl Physiol.* 1984;57:1134.)

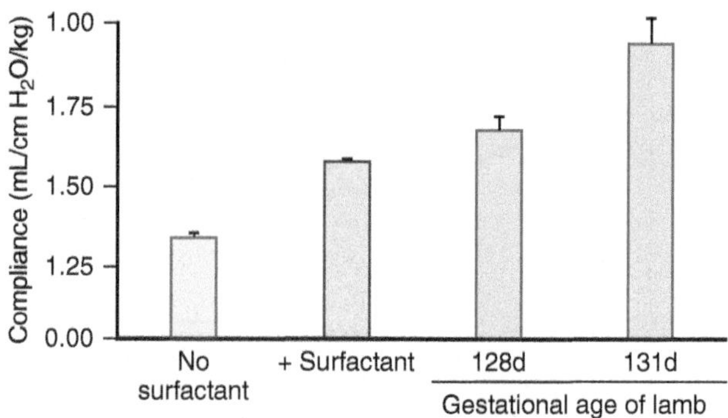

Fig. 157.21 Surfactant function after surfactant treatment. Preterm lambs were treated with 100 mg/kg surfactant and ventilated for several hours. Surfactant was recovered by alveolar wash and used to treat preterm surfactant-deficient rabbits. The surfactant from the more mature lambs at 131 days of gestation had enhanced function relative to the surfactant used to treat the lambs. (Modified from Ikegami M, Ueda T, Absolom D, et al. Changes in exogenous surfactant in ventilated preterm lamb lungs. *Am Rev Respir Dis.* 1993;148:837.)

SURFACTANT FUNCTION WITH SURFACTANT TREATMENT (REVIEWED IN CHAPTER 79)

The surfactants used clinically are organic solvent extracts of alveolar washes or lung tissue from pig or calf lungs. These surfactants contain no SP-A, the amount of SP-B and SP-C is variable, and processing and sterilization disrupt the lipoprotein structure. The clinical surfactants are more sensitive to inactivation by plasma proteins than natural surfactant. However, surfactant can have improved function after exposure to the preterm lung. When surfactant is recovered by alveolar wash after surfactant treatment of preterm lambs with RDS, the surfactant has enhanced function.[133] This improved function can be demonstrated by comparing the surfactant used to treat the lambs with the surfactant recovered from the lambs for treatment responses in surfactant-deficient rabbit lungs (Fig. 157.21). The very preterm lung cannot improve the function of surfactant used for treatment; the more mature lung can. The mechanism for the enhanced function probably is the mixing of the surfactant used for treatment with small amounts of endogenous surfactant lipids and proteins. Many hours after treatment, the enhanced function of surfactant can occur by recycling of components from the surfactant used for treatment through the type II cells. The sensitivity to inactivation of the surfactants used clinically also can be modulated after exposure to the preterm lung.[134] The surfactants become less susceptible to inactivation if mixed with 5% or 10% by weight natural surfactant. Therefore, small endogenous surfactant pools can interact with the large doses of surfactant used clinically to result in improved function of surfactant. This activation phenomenon will not occur if the lung is injured.

SURFACTANT AND INNATE HOST DEFENSES

The lung of the infant with RDS is not inflamed at birth unless chorioamnionitis and infection were present before birth. However, the initiation of ventilation and oxygen initiates inflammation in the preterm lung.[67] The ventilation results in nonuniform inflation of the surfactant-deficient lung and stretch-mediated injury. If the tidal volume is high or the FRC is too high or too low, further lung injury will occur. Supplemental oxygen also may initiate an inflammatory response. Surfactant treatment decreases the severity of this initial inflammation, in part by its mechanical effects on the lungs to make lung inflation more uniform at lower pressures. However, surfactant also can have effects on the inflammatory response because of its multiple innate host defense functions.[135] The preterm lung is severely deficient in SP-A and SP-D. These proteins opsonize a variety of organisms and promote phagocytosis and suppress inflammation in the adult lung. Addition of recombinant SP-D to surfactant prevented the systemic shock caused by intratracheal endotoxin in preterm ventilated sheep.[136] The commercial surfactants do not contain SP-A or SP-D. The hydrophobic proteins SP-B and SP-C also have antiinflammatory properties and can mitigate oxidant-induced injury. The potential for surfactant components to modulate the inflammation that accompanies RDS has not been tested clinically.

CONCLUSION

Modern neonatology has conquered the initial management of RDS in infants of reasonable size and gestational age who do not have other abnormalities that degrade lung function (see Fig. 157.1). That success has resulted from the general improvements in obstetrics and neonatal care for the preterm infant and the specific therapies of CPAP, improved ventilation strategies, ANS, and surfactant treatment. Therapies to improve outcomes depend on meticulous efforts to prevent lung injury. Progress is being made with noninvasive methods of respiratory support from the delivery room and new strategies for the timing and methods of surfactant treatment. The imprecision of the diagnosis of RDS, particularly in extremely low-birth-weight infants, confounds epidemiologic documentation of the incidence of RDS and its severity. A remaining concern is that improvements in the initial management of RDS and decreases in mechanical ventilation have not translated into decreases in BPD. New synthetic surfactants will become available, but they likely will not have substantial outcome benefits over those currently available. The core problem for the very preterm infant with RDS is not the treatment of RDS, but rather subsequent lung development. Fortunately, the human preterm lung seems to have the capacity to grow and remodel to compensate for early lung immaturity and injury.[53]

A complete reference list is available at www.ExpertConsult.com. 

SELECT REFERENCES

1. Avery ME, Mead J. Surface properties in relation to atelectasis and hyaline membrane disease. *AMA J Dis Child*. 1959;97:517-523 (5, Part 1).
3. Adams FH, Fujiwara T, Emmanouilides G, Scudder A. Surface properties and lipids from lungs of infants with hyaline membrane disease. *J Pediatr*. 1965;66:357-364.
4. Gregory GA, Kitterman JA, Phibbs RH, Tooley WH, Hamilton WK. Treatment of the idiopathic respiratory-distress syndrome with continuous positive airway pressure. *N Engl J Med*. 1971;284(24):1333-1340.
5. Gluck L, Kulovich MV, Borer Jr RC, Brenner PH, Anderson GG, Spellacy WN. Diagnosis of the respiratory distress syndrome by amniocentesis. *Am J Obstet Gynecol*. 1971;109(3):440-445.
6. Liggins GC, Howie RN. A controlled trial of antepartum glucocorticoid treatment for prevention of the respiratory distress syndrome in premature infants. *Pediatrics*. 1972;50(4):515-525.
7. Lee K, Khoshnood B, Wall SN, Chang Y, Hsieh HL, Singh JK. Trend in mortality from respiratory distress syndrome in the United States, 1970-1995. *J Pediatr*. 1999;134(4):434-440.
8. Jobe AH. Pulmonary surfactant therapy. *N Engl J Med*. 1993;328(12):861-868.
9. Roberts D, Dalziel S. Antenatal corticosteroids for accelerating fetal lung maturation for women at risk of preterm birth. *Cochrane Database Syst Rev*. 2006;(3):CD004454.
10. Consortium on Safe L, JU H, Wilkins I, et al. Respiratory morbidity in late preterm births. *J Am Med Assoc*. 2010;304(4):419-425.
11. Chang EY, Menard MK, Vermillion ST, Hulsey T, Ebeling M. The association between hyaline membrane disease and preeclampsia. *Am J Obstet Gynecol*. 2004;191(4):1414-1417.
17. Kamath-Rayne BD, Du Y, Hughes M, et al. Systems biology evaluation of cell-free amniotic fluid transcriptome of term and preterm infants to detect fetal maturity. *BMC Med Genomics*. 2015;8:67.
18. Brownfoot FC, Gagliardi DI, Bain E, Middleton P, Crowther CA. Different corticosteroids and regimens for accelerating fetal lung maturation for women at risk of preterm birth. *Cochrane Database Syst Rev*. 2013;(8):CD006764.
19. Jobe AH, Milad MA, Peppard T, Jusko WJ. Pharmacokinetics and pharmacodynamics of Intramuscular and oral betamethasone and dexamethasone in reproductive age women in India. *Clin Transl Sci*. 2019;13(2):391-399.
20. Jobe AH. Antenatal corticosteroids-a concern for Lifelong outcomes. *J Pediatr*. 2020;217:184-188.
26. Kemp MW, Schmidt AF, Jobe AH. Optimizing antenatal corticosteroid therapy. *Semin Fetal Neonatal Med*. 2019;24(3):176-181.
27. Gyamfi C, Mele L, Wapner RJ, et al. The effect of plurality and obesity on betamethasone concentrations in women at risk for preterm delivery. *Am J Obstet Gynecol*. 2010;203(3):e1-5. 219.
29. Schmolzer GM, Kumar M, Pichler G, Aziz K, O'Reilly M, Cheung PY. Non-invasive versus invasive respiratory support in preterm infants at birth: systematic review and meta-analysis. *BMJ*. 2013;347:f5980.
30. Fanaroff AA, Stoll BJ, Wright LL, et al. Trends in neonatal morbidity and mortality for very low birthweight infants. *Am J Obstet Gynecol*. 2007;196(2):147. e1-8.
33. Bancalari EH, Jobe AH. The respiratory course of extremely preterm infants: a dilemma for diagnosis and terminology. *J Pediatr*. 2012;161(4):585-588.
35. Goldenberg RL, Culhane JF, Iams JD, Romero R. Epidemiology and causes of preterm birth. *Lancet*. 2008;371(9606):75-84.
36. Watterberg KL, Demers LM, Scott SM, Murphy S. Chorioamnionitis and early lung inflammation in infants in whom bronchopulmonary dysplasia develops. *Pediatrics*. 1996;97(2):210-215.
46. Sinner DI, Carey B, Zgherea D, et al. Complete tracheal ring deformity. A translational genomics approach to pathogenesis. *Am J Respir Crit Care Med*. 2019;200(10):1267-1281.
47. Bridges J, Sudha P, Lipps D, et al. Glucocorticoid regulates mesenchymal cell differentiation required for perinatal lung morphogenesis and function. *Am J Physiol Lung Cell Mol Physiol*. 2020;319(2):L239-L255.
52. Burri P. Stuctural aspects of prenatal and postnatal development and growth of the lung. In: McDonald J, ed. *Lung Growth and Development*. New York: Marcel Dekker; 1997:1-35.
54. Massaro D, Massaro G. The regulation of the formation of pulmonary alveoli. In: Bland R, Coalson J, eds. *Chronic Lung Disease in Early Infancy*. New York: Marcel Dekker; 2000:479-492.
56. Hillman NH, Kallapur SG, Jobe AH. Physiology of transition from intrauterine to extrauterine life. *Clin Perinatol*. 2012;39(4):769-783.
62. Jackson JC, MacKenzie AP, Chi EY, Standaert TA, Truog WE, Hodson WA. Mechanisms for reduced total lung capacity at birth and during hyaline membrane disease in premature newborn monkeys. *Am Rev Respir Dis*. 1990;142(2):413-419.
71. Kramer BW, Jobe AH. The clever fetus: responding to inflammation to minimize lung injury. *Biol Neonate*. 2005;88(3):202-207.
74. Whitsett JA, Wert SE, Weaver TE. Alveolar surfactant homeostasis and the pathogenesis of pulmonary disease. *Annu Rev Med*. 2010;61:105-119.
80. Ueda T, Ikegami M, Jobe AH. Developmental changes of sheep surfactant: in vivo function and in vitro subtype conversion. *J Appl Physiol*. 1994;76(6):2701-2706.
81. Hallman M, Kulovich M, Kirkpatrick E, Sugarman RG, Gluck L. Phosphatidylinositol and phosphatidylglycerol in amniotic fluid: indices of lung maturity. *Am J Obstet Gynecol*. 1976;125(5):613-617.
100. Hallman M, Merritt TA, Akino T, Bry K. Surfactant protein A, phosphatidylcholine, and surfactant inhibitors in epithelial lining fluid. Correlation with surface activity, severity of respiratory distress syndrome, and outcome in small premature infants. *Am Rev Respir Dis*. 1991;144(6):1376-1384.
102. Seidner SR, Jobe AH, Coalson JJ, Ikegami M. Abnormal surfactant metabolism and function in preterm ventilated baboons. *Am J Respir Crit Care Med*. 1998;158(6):1982-1989.
108. Bunt JE, Carnielli VP, Darcos Wattimena JL, Hop WC, Sauer PJ, Zimmermann LJ. The effect in premature infants of prenatal corticosteroids on endogenous surfactant synthesis as measured with stable isotopes. *Am J Respir Crit Care Med*. 2000;162(3 Pt 1):844-849.
109. Pinkerton KE, Ikegami M, Dillard LM, Jobe AH. Surfactant treatment effects on lung structure and type II cells of preterm ventilated lambs. *Biol Neonate*. 2000;77(4):243-252.
115. Jacobs H, Jobe A, Ikegami M, Conaway D. The significance of reutilization of surfactant phosphatidylcholine. *J Biol Chem*. 1983;258(7):4159-4165.
118. Wright JR, Dobbs LG. Regulation of pulmonary surfactant secretion and clearance. *Annu Rev Physiol*. 1991;53:395-414.
120. Jobe A. Surfactant-edema interactions. In: Weir E, JT R, eds. *The Pathogenesis and Treatment of Pulmonary Edema. Armonk*. New York: Futura Publishing; 1998:113-131.
121. Ueda T, Ikegami M, Jobe A. Surfactant subtypes. In vitro conversion, in vivo function, and effects of serum proteins. *Am J Respir Crit Care Med*. 1994;149(5):1254-1259.
123. Gunther A, Seeger W. Resistance to surfactant inactivation. In: Robertson B, Taeusch H, eds. *Surfactant Therapy for Lung Disease*. New York: Marcel Dekker; 1995:269.
125. Ikegami M, Jacobs H, Jobe A. Surfactant function in respiratory distress syndrome. *J Pediatr*. 1983;102(3):443-447.
127. Korfhagen TR, Bruno MD, Ross GF, et al. Altered surfactant function and structure in SP-A gene targeted mice. *Proc Natl Acad Sci U S A*. 1996;93(18):9594-9599.
129. Rider ED, Ikegami M, Whitsett JA, Hull W, Absolom D, Jobe AH. Treatment responses to surfactants containing natural surfactant proteins in preterm rabbits. *Am Rev Respir Dis*. 1993;147(3):669-676.
130. Yukitake K, Brown CL, Schlueter MA, Clements JA, Hawgood S. Surfactant apoprotein A modifies the inhibitory effect of plasma proteins on surfactant activity in vivo. *Pediatr Res*. 1995;37(1):21-25.
131. Seeger W, Gunther A, Thede C. Differential sensitivity to fibrinogen inhibition of SP-C- vs. SP-B-based surfactants. *Am J Physiol*. 1992;262(3 Pt 1):L286-L291.
133. Ikegami M, Ueda T, Absolom D, Baxter C, Rider E, Jobe AH. Changes in exogenous surfactant in ventilated preterm lamb lungs. *Am Rev Respir Dis*. 1993;148(4 Pt 1):837-844.
134. Chen CM, Ikegami M, Ueda T, Polk DH, Jobe AH. Exogenous surfactant function in very preterm lambs with and without fetal corticosteroid treatment. *J Appl Physiol*. 1995;78(3):955-960.
135. Crouch EC. Collectins and pulmonary host defense. *Am J Respir Cell Mol Biol*. 1998;19(2):177-201.
136. Ikegami M, Carter K, Bishop K, et al. Intratracheal recombinant surfactant protein d prevents endotoxin shock in the newborn preterm lamb. *Am J Respir Crit Care Med*. 2006;173(12):1342-1347.

158 Pathophysiology of Meconium Aspiration Syndrome

Jason Gien | John P. Kinsella

INTRODUCTION

Meconium aspiration syndrome (MAS) follows fetal hypoxic/ischemic stress that leads to intestinal peristalsis, meconium release, contamination of the amniotic fluid, and gasping respirations, which causes aspiration of noxious meconium-stained fluid deep into the fetal lung. Aspiration of meconium manifests as airway obstruction with trapping of gas in the lung during exhalation, chemical pneumonitis, and surfactant inactivation with decreased lung compliance. The newborn typically presents with respiratory distress shortly after birth with or without evidence of pulmonary hypertension.

Observation of meconium-stained amniotic fluid (MSAF) is essential for the diagnosis of MAS. With changes in obstetric practice, specifically reducing delivery after 41 weeks gestation, the incidence of MSAF in the United States has decreased from 10% to 15% of all live births to less than 1%, with MAS occurring in approximately 2.5 infants per 1000 live births. In addition, as a result of advances in neonatal care, MAS mortality has improved from approximately 4% to 7% to less than 1%.[1-4] Several risk factors for MAS have been identified. MSAF and MAS occur with a higher frequency in post-term infants; approximately 30% of infants greater than 41 weeks are born through MSAF. Some 20% to 33% of MAS cases are associated with nonreassuring fetal heart tones and perinatal depression.[5-7] Fetal distress is associated with acidosis and decreased muscle tone. Vagal stimulation and parasympathetic tone increase with repeated cord compression, leading to evacuation of meconium. In addition, hypoxia causes fetal gasping, which results in aspiration of MSAF into the lungs.[2,8-10]

A recent report assessed the relationship between umbilical cord lactate levels and outcomes in infants with MAS.[11] The presence of lactate in both serum and urine can be a sign of asphyxia in neonates; however, the prognostic significance has not been evaluated. In this report the authors found that a serum lactate of 4.1 mmol/L could discriminate between the presence of thin and thick MSAF, with thick MSAF more frequently associated with pulmonary hemorrhage, persistent pulmonary hypertension of the neonate (PPHN), intraventricular hemorrhage, and respiratory failure requiring ventilation support. In addition, infants with thick MSAF had higher gestational age, lower Apgar scores, greater base deficit, higher P_{CO_2}, lower P_{O_2}, and a lower pH. These findings suggest an association between MSAF and asphyxia, with umbilical cord lactate predictive of severity and adverse neonatal outcomes. Finally, published studies have also confirmed an association between MSAF and oligohydramnios.[4]

Meconium is a thick, black-green, odorless material first demonstrable in the fetal intestine during the third month of gestation. The characteristics of meconium are key to understanding the pathophysiology of MAS. Meconium results from the accumulation of debris, including desquamated cells from the intestine and skin, gastrointestinal mucin, lanugo hair, fatty material from the vernix caseosa, amniotic fluid, and intestinal secretions, leading to the formation of a viscous, adhesive substance. Meconium also contains blood group-specific glycoproteins and a small amount of lipid and protein that decreases during gestation.[12,13] The black-green color results from bile pigments. Meconium may or may not be sterile, but free fatty acids, bile salts, and pancreatic phospholipases in meconium are responsible for the adverse effect on surfactant function. When aspirated into the lung, meconium results in decreased pulmonary function and compliance with secondary surfactant inactivation and small airway obstruction with ball-valve or check-valve phenomena leading to atelectasis or air trapping within the alveoli and bronchioles.[6,14,15] Progressive hyperinflation ensues, which increases the risk for pneumothoraces. Patients with severe disease are at risk for respiratory failure necessitating intubation and mechanical ventilation (Fig. 158.1).

Inflammation is central to the pathogenesis of MAS, as meconium stimulates production of cytokines and other vasoactive substances that lead to cardiovascular and inflammatory responses in the fetus and newborn.[16,17] These secondary effects develop almost immediately after birth and worsen over the first 24 hours of life. Severe pulmonary hypertension develops in 20% to 40% of patients with MAS. Mechanisms responsible for the development of pulmonary hypertension are the release of inflammatory cytokines, hypoxia, hypercarbia, acidosis, and poor lung recruitment. Remodeling of the pulmonary vasculature in utero in severe cases of MAS also contributes to the development of pulmonary hypertension and suggests that chronic intrauterine stress may further account for the severity of cardiopulmonary disease at birth in the setting of MAS.

PATHOPHYSIOLOGY OF MECONIUM ASPIRATION SYNDROME

In addition to the mechanical ball-valve/check-valve effects on the airway and lung parenchyma and inflammation, there are several other mechanisms by which meconium results in respiratory failure after birth. Meconium directly alters pulmonary function, produces a chemical pneumonitis, inactivates surfactant, predisposes to infection, and contributes to the development of PPHN.

LUNG FUNCTION

Lung function in MAS is characterized by both hyperinflation and volume loss, with both adversely effecting pulmonary function and gas exchange. Airway obstruction is a major contributor to both hyper- and hypoinflation and is central to the pathogenesis of MAS. Airway obstruction can be complete or partial and occurs by several mechanisms. Meconium induces apoptosis of the airway epithelium, resulting in sloughing of cellular debris from apoptotic cells into the airway and causing airway obstruction and inflammation. In addition, meconium is proinflammatory, further exacerbating airway inflammation. Airway inflammation results in increased mucus production as well as narrowing of the caliber of the airways. Inflammation of the airways also increases resistance and contributes to the development of atelectasis. Another mechanism by which airway obstruction occurs is through particulate meconium, which can completely or partially occlude the airway. Complete obstruction produces a ball-valve effect preventing the passage of air into the lung, leading to distal atelectasis. Partial airway obstruction occurs when the airway diameter is larger in inspiration and gas can enter around the partial obstruction. However, as the airway narrows during

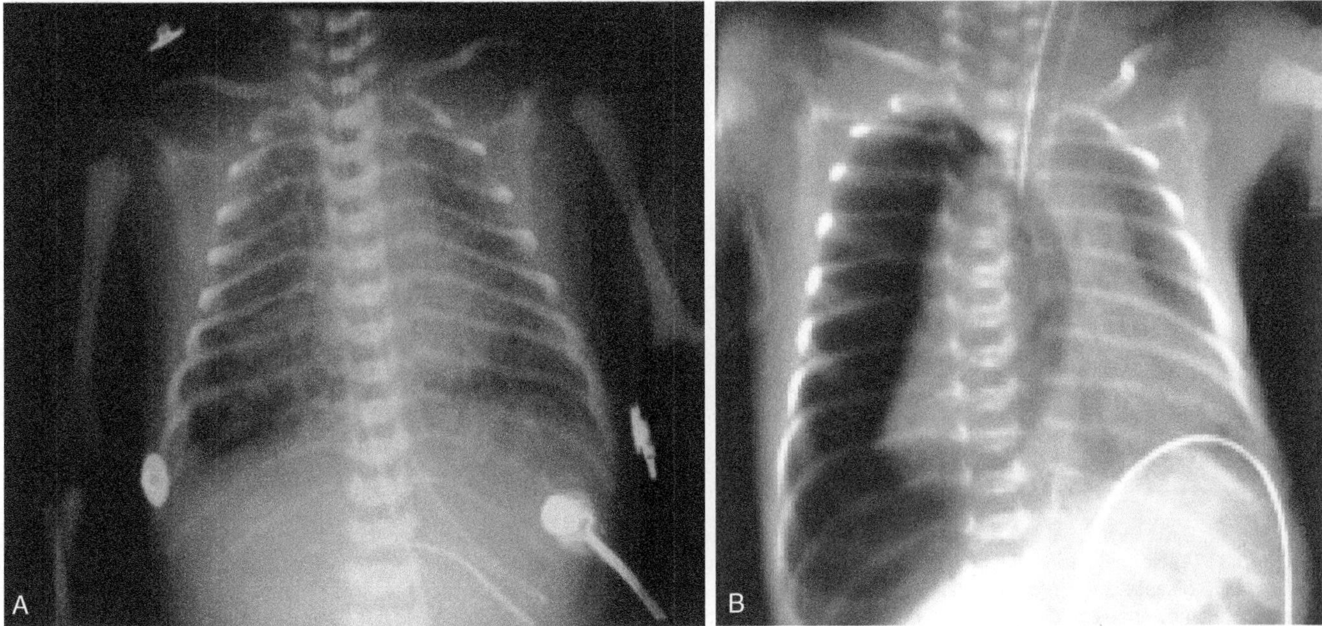

Fig. 158.1 (A) Chest radiograph demonstrating meconium aspiration syndrome with bilateral patchy infiltrates and hyperinflation at the right base. (B) Interval development of a tension pneumothorax.

exhalation, the meconium plug occludes the airway completely, trapping the gas distally. This process is consistent with a check-valve effect and can lead to overdistension of the lung and alveolar rupture, with a resulting pneumothorax or other air leak complications. This check-valve effect is responsible for air leak in 10% to 30% of infants with MAS.[6,14,15] Overdistension of the lung with progressive hyperinflation also results in difficulty with carbon dioxide (CO_2) elimination.

In addition to the lung function abnormalities that result secondary to airway inflammation, decreased pulmonary compliance secondary to surfactant inactivation also contributes to hypoinflation and atelectasis in MAS. Fig. 158.2 demonstrates the relationship between lung compliance and functional residual capacity (FRC) in infants with MAS and control patients.[18] FRC was determined by a closed loop helium method, and compliance was determined using a pneumotachograph, an esophageal pressure probe, and a pressure manometer. When the FRC was low and compliance remained low, the patients were found to be atelectatic on chest x-ray. However, when the FRC was high, they were hyperinflated. These changes in lung function ultimately lead to ventilation/perfusion (V/Q) mismatch and worsening hypoxia and hypercarbia.

More recent reports have evaluated the sensitivity of lung ultrasound for the detection of MAS.[19] The following ultrasound findings were observed: (1) B-pattern (alveolar-interstitial syndrome [AIS]) either coalescent or sparse; (2) lung consolidation with irregular edges; (3) atelectasis and air bronchograms. The latter ultrasound findings reliably predicted the presence of MAS when compared to a routine chest x-ray. A follow-up study on a larger cohort of 117 patients demonstrated that consolidation with irregular edges, disappearance of the pleural or A line, and/or the presence of AIS or B-line in the nonconsolidation area predicted the presence of MAS with 100% sensitivity and specificity (Fig. 158.3).[20]

The airway inflammation in MAS may persist for weeks, after the parenchymal disease has recovered, with resultant airways reactivity and wheezing. Steroids and bronchodilator therapy are often effective in this setting of prolonged airway hyperresponsiveness.[21,22]

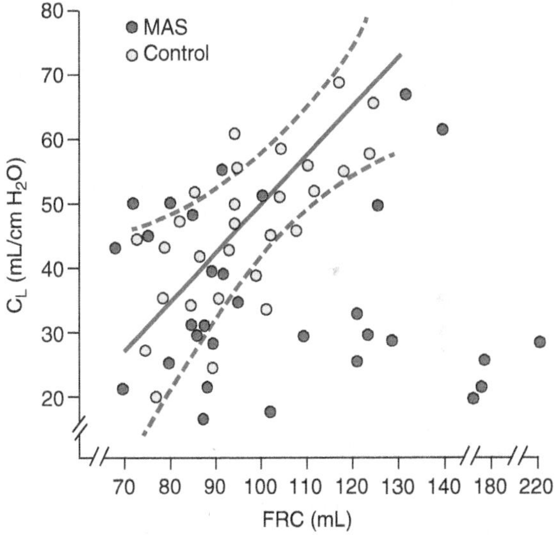

Fig. 158.2 Lung compliance in relation to functional residual capacity *(FRC)*. The *dashed lines* indicate the 95% confidence interval for normal patients. Each *blue circle* represents one test period for the 12 patients, and the *gray circles* are the control patients. As demonstrated, when the FRC was low and compliance remained low, the patients were found to be atelectatic on chest x-ray. However, when the FRC was high, patients were hyperinflated on chest x-ray. *MAS*, Meconium aspiration syndrome.

CHEMICAL PNEUMONITIS

Aspiration of meconium into the lung also results in a chemical pneumonitis, which occurs secondary to macrophage and neutrophil activation.[23,24] Influx of macrophages and neutrophils influx results in increased free radical formation and the production of cytokines, interleukin (IL-1), IL-6, IL-8, and tumor necrosis factor-α.[20,25,26] Increased production of proinflammatory cytokines causes an exudative and inflammatory pneumonitis with epithelial disruption, proteinaceous exudation with alveolar collapse, and cellular necrosis. Cytokine production is central to the pathogenesis of MAS, such that improvement in pulmonary function directly correlates with a fall in proinflammatory cytokines over the first 96 hours of life.[25] MAS also results in activation of the arachidonic acid pathway and through

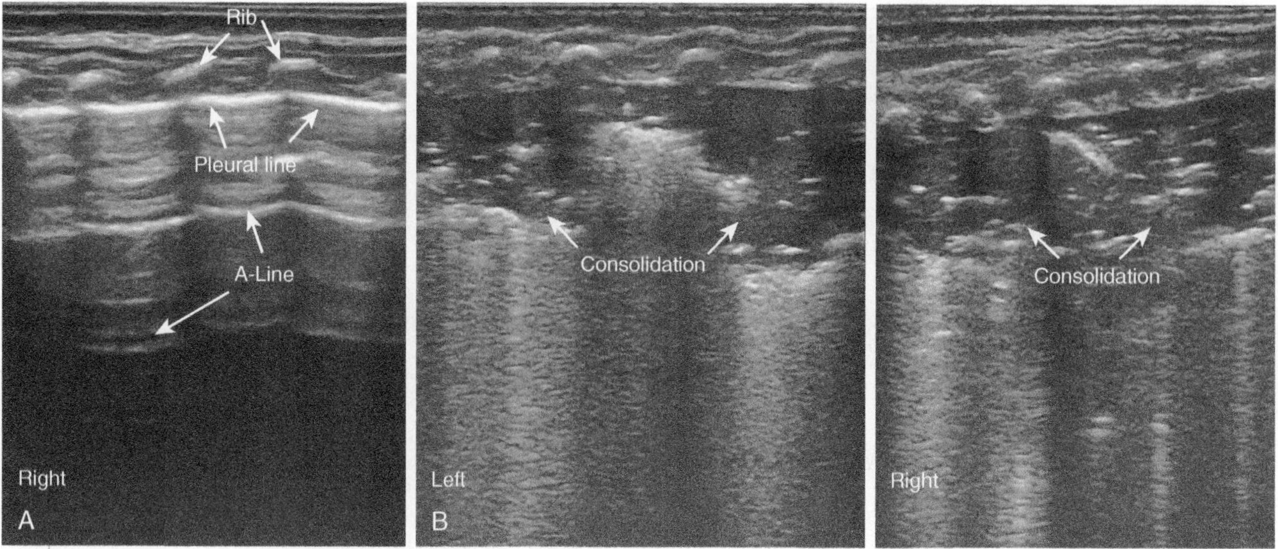

Fig. 158.3 (A) Normal neonatal lung ultrasonographic appearance of the right lung of a newborn in the control group. In normal newborns without lung disease, the lungs were hypoechoic; the pleural line and *A-line* were hyperechoic, clear, smooth, regular, and parallel and equally spaced, and the echoes gradually became weaker and eventually disappeared as the pleural line and the *A-line* extended deep into the lungs. (B) Lung ultrasonographic findings in a newborn with neonatal meconium aspiration syndrome. This patient had large areas of pulmonary consolidation with air bronchogram shown on lung ultrasonography; two consolidation areas of different sizes are shown in the right lung, the pleural line blurred or disappeared, and the A-line disappeared.

cycloxygenase-2 results in the release of thromboxanes and leukotrienes. Meconium can also activate the complement system, which exacerbates inflammation and results in further tissue damage. In addition to its proinflammatory effect, meconium induces apoptosis on airway epithelium as well as type 2 pneumocytes in the lung.[27,28] In the first 24 hours after aspiration of meconium, caspase 3 activity—a direct marker for apoptotic activity—increases with peak expression seen at 8 hours.[17,25,26] Cellular debris from apoptotic cells sloughs off and is released into the airway, exacerbating airway obstruction and inflammation.

INFECTION

While meconium is usually sterile, the presence of meconium in the lung predisposes to the development of infection. The mucopolysaccharide component provides an excellent growth medium for microorganisms, especially *Escherichia coli.*[29] However, two recent review articles evaluated the efficacy and safety of antibiotics for the prevention of infection, morbidity, and mortality among infants born through MSAF who were both asymptomatic at birth or had signs and symptoms compatible with MAS.[30,31] Prior to these reviews antimicrobial administration was recommended for all symptomatic patients with MAS. While the evidence was weak, in both reviews the antibiotics did not decrease the risk of thromboxane's early- and late-onset neonatal sepsis in neonates who were either asymptomatic or symptomatic with a diagnosis of MAS. In addition, there were no significant differences in mortality or duration of hospital stay between groups given antibiotics and control groups.

SURFACTANT INACTIVATION

Surfactant is a macroaggregate molecule secreted by type 2 pneumocytes as the infant approaches term gestation. Surfactant is made up of 90% phospholipid and 10% proteins (surfactant protein [SP] A, B, C, and D). The primary function of surfactant is to reduce surface tension in the lung. Dipalmitoyl phosphatidylcholine (DPPC) is the key phospholipid in surfactant for lowering surface tension. SP-B and SP-C are also hydrophobic and necessary for lowering surface tension in the lung. By lowering surface tension in the lung, surfactant prevents alveolar collapse during expiration, thus maintaining FRC and improving compliance of the lung. The estimated surfactant stores of term infants is approximately 100 mg/kg compared with preterm infants who have approximately 4 to 5 mg/kg. Surfactant deficiency results in respiratory distress syndrome (RDS), which can occur due to primary deficiency such as occurs with prematurity or to inactivation, as seen with MAS, pneumonia, asphyxia, etc. In addition to reducing surface tension in the lung, surfactant plays a key role in regulating the immune response in the lungs, with SP-A and SP-D primarily responsible. A deficiency in SP-A or SP-D predisposes to the development of pulmonary infection. There are several mechanisms by which meconium interferes with surfactant function. Meconium directly decreases the synthesis and secretion of surfactant by alveolar type 2 cells, disrupts formation of the lamellar layer,[32] and increases metabolism and degradation of phospholipases. Rodent studies have confirmed decreased SP-A and SP-B in the setting of MAS,[33] and a more recent human study confirmed decreases in DPPC in infants with MAS needing extracorporeal membrane oxygenation therapy (ECMO).[34]

Free fatty acids and bile salts are theorized to be key ingredients of meconium, which contribute to surfactant dysfunction. Palmitic, stearic, and oleic acids are commonly found in meconium. In experimental studies, when these substances were administered by bronchoalveolar lavage, they were found to significantly increase surface tension by stripping surfactant from the alveolar wall.[35] In addition, free fatty acids produce a fluidizing effect that interferes with the ability of spread surfactant films to reach low surface tensions.[36]

Bilirubin present in meconium also inhibits surfactant in a dose-dependent manner, by altering the effects of SP-B and SP-C.[37] Pancreatic phospholipases, especially phospholipase A2, are present in meconium and have been investigated for their role in surfactant degradation. Their unique properties allow them to hydrolyze phospholipids, including DPPC in surfactant, and induce type II pneumocyte apoptosis.[27,28] In addition, meconium stimulates inflammatory cells such as macrophages and neutrophils to produce oxidative damage through the formation of peroxynitrite and hypochlorous acid, with resultant type 2 pneumocyte apoptosis and surfactant breakdown.[26,34,38] In these studies, protein carbonyl concentration, previously shown to correlate with the severity of bronchopulmonary dysplasia in preterm infants[39] was used as a marker of oxidative damage.

Minimal amounts of cholesterol are normally present in surfactant, and it is required for natural pulmonary surfactant membranes to adopt their structure and dynamics.[40] Meconium contains a substantial amount of cholesterol, and exposure to meconium results in incorporation of cholesterol into surfactant membranes and films.[41] Elevated cholesterol may form complexes with surfactant phospholipids, thus increasing the surfactant film fluidity. Higher fluidity results in collapse rather than multilayer formation during lateral compression in breathing cycle.[40] Besides enabling the insertion of cholesterol into surfactant membranes, bile acids in lungs lead to a decrease in DPPC portion and shift in the ratio between phosphatidylglycerol and sphingomyelin.[41] Taurocholic acid, one of the most abundant bile acids in humans, was found to affect the structure of both surfactant monolayers at the interface and surfactant aggregates in solution[42,43] thus contributing to loss of surfactant function.

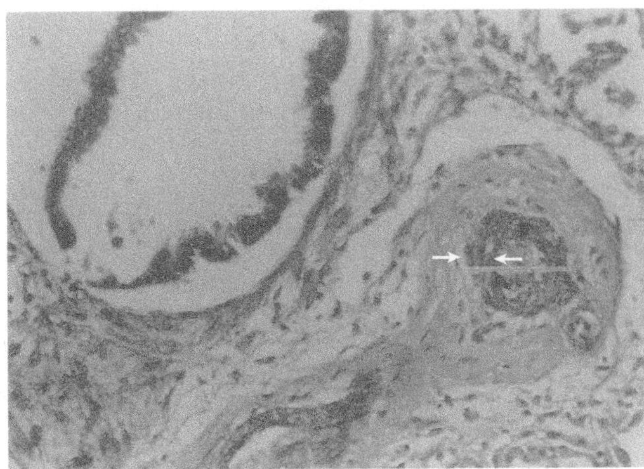

Fig. 158.4 Pulmonary artery bronchiole. *Arrows,* pulmonary artery wall thickness. Hematoxylin and eosin stain. Original magnification ×200. (Reprinted with permission from Thureen PT, Hall DM, Hoffenberg A, et al. Fatal meconium aspiration in spite of appropriate perinatal airway management: pulmonary and placental evidence of prenatal disease. *Am J Obstet Gynecol.* 1997;176:967–975.)

PERSISTENT PULMONARY HYPERTENSION OF THE NEWBORN

PPHN is a failure to transition from intrauterine to extrauterine life, with persistent right-to-left shunting through fetal conduits (patent ductus arteriosus [PDA] and patent foramen ovale [PFO]) and resultant hypoxemia. PPHN occurs in 20% to 40% of infants with MAS. Several mechanisms contribute to the development of PPHN in MAS. Parenchymal lung disease with poor alveolar recruitment and decreased FRC or hyperinflation with increased FRC contribute to elevations in pulmonary vascular resistance (PVR). In addition, hypercarbia, hypoxemia, and acidosis lead to vasoconstriction and increased PVR. The release of chemically vasoactive mediators, such as endothelin-1 (ET-1), thromboxane-A2 (TX-A2), and prostaglandins, has also been shown to contribute to the development of PPHN in MAS.[44] ET-1 is a potent vasoconstrictor that is released by endothelial cells, macrophages, and neutrophils. Experimental studies of meconium aspiration in newborn piglets have demonstrated a direct correlation between ET-1 concentrations and PVR.[44] Human infants with MAS also demonstrate increased serum ET-1 levels.[45] TX-A2, another potent vasoconstrictor, is released from the epithelium after exposure to meconium.[46] Meconium aspiration also has been associated with the development of vascular remodeling with hyperplasia of the vascular media and interstitium, narrowing of the vessel lumen, tortuosity of the arteries, and muscularization of the alveolar septal arterioles. These changes likely develop in utero, impair the response to pulmonary vasodilator therapy, and contribute to significant morbidity after birth (Fig. 158.4).[47,48]

PROMINENT INTRAPULMONARY ANASTOMOTIC VESSELS

Infants with MAS often present with severe hypoxemia that cannot be explained by the presence of extrapulmonary shunting through fetal conduits (PDA, PFO) as seen with PPHN. Historically the presence of an intrapulmonary shunt secondary to V/Q mismatch has been thought to account for the hypoxemia. Recently the presence of intrapulmonary anastomotic vessels (IPAVs) was described in the lungs of infants dying with congenital diaphragmatic hernia, alveolar-capillary dysplasia,[49,50] and MAS.[51] In animal and human fetal lungs, preacinar IPAVs exist under normal conditions connecting the pulmonary and systemic (bronchial) circulations.[47,52,53] These anastomoses form vascular pathways through which blood potentially can be directed away from smaller arteries and capillaries associated with distal airspaces through communications between the bronchial circulation and pulmonary veins. The potential exists that under pathologic conditions IPAVs may persist after birth and potentially contribute to hypoxemia in MAS (Fig. 158.5).

EXTRAPULMONARY CLINICAL MANIFESTATIONS

CARDIAC

Left ventricular (LV) or right ventricular (RV) dysfunction commonly occurs in the setting of MAS. Predisposing factors are birth depression, peri- or postnatal hypoxemia, acidosis, and electrolyte disturbance (hypocalcemia). In infants with PPHN, RV dysfunction predominates. Infants with LV dysfunction present with signs of poor end-organ perfusion, shock, and cardiovascular collapse. Echocardiography is necessary to make the diagnosis and inotropic agents are often needed for cardiac support.

SHOCK

Hemodynamic instability with hypotension and shock is frequently seen in the setting of MAS. The etiology of shock in MAS is multifactorial, with LV dysfunction, vasoplegia secondary to sepsis or hypoxemia, adrenal insufficiency, and vascular leak, all contributing to the hypotension.

NEUROLOGIC

Approximately 20% to 30% of infants with MAS have associated birth depression, and these infants may present with variable degrees of encephalopathy. Encephalopathy may be mild with the infant presenting in a hyperalert state, with increased muscle tone and irritability (Sarnat stage 1), or more severe with the infant presenting with marked hypotonia, apnea, and seizures (Sarnat stage 2 or 3). In all infants with MAS, a thorough history and assessment should be performed to determine if the infant would benefit for induced hypothermia as treatment for birth depression. Independent of a history of birth depression, all infants with MAS should be monitored closely for seizures, as

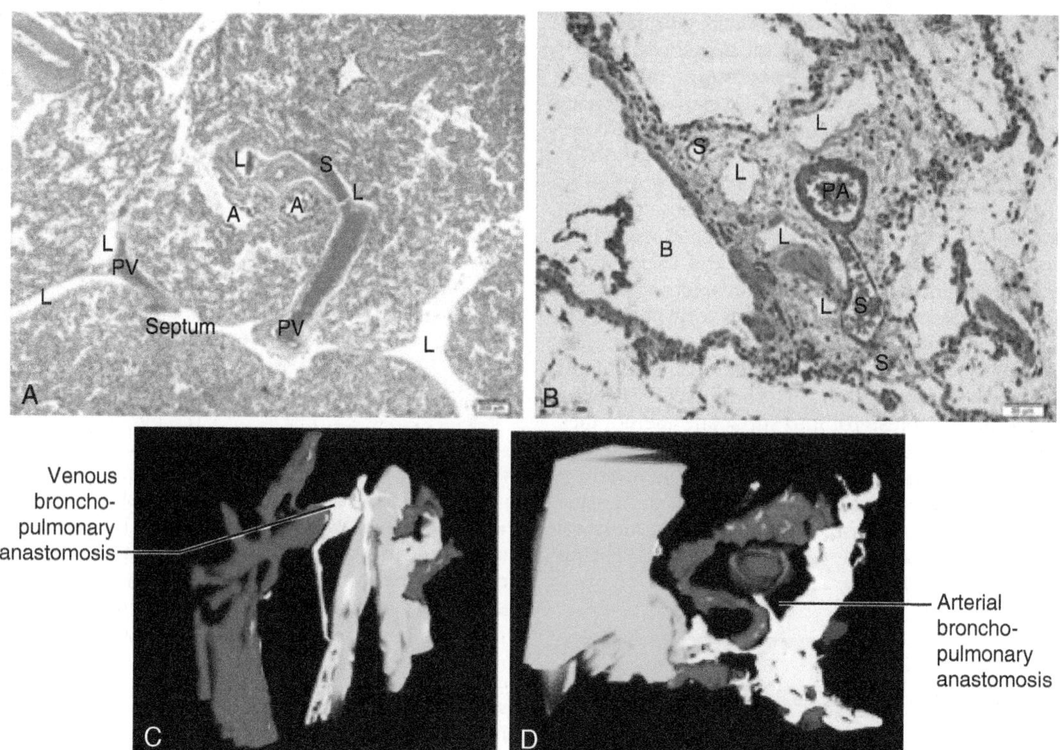

Fig. 158.5 (A) Venous intrapulmonary anastomotic vessels (IPAVs), or shunt vessels, appear as thin-walled vessels that bridge pulmonary veins and microvessels. (B) Arterial IPAVs are connections between pulmonary arteries *(PAs)* and bronchial arteries *(BAs)*. *A,* Airspace; *B,* bronchus; *L,* lymphatic; *S,* shunt vessel. (C and D) Three-dimensional reconstruction images of venous (C) and arterial bronchopulmonary anastomotic or "shunt" (D) vessels. Color key: *aqua,* PA wall: *green,* airway; *purple,* lymphatic; *red,* PA endothelium; *yellow,* shunt vessel. (Reprinted with permission from Acker SN, Mandell EW, Sims-Lucas S, et al. Histologic identification of prominent intrapulmonary anastomotic vessels in severe congenital diaphragmatic hernia. *J Pediatr.* 2015;166:178–183.)

they will occur in 20% of affected infants.[54] This association suggests that in the setting of MAS, seizures may be related to a more remote preexisting injury or a nonhypoxic mechanism.

MULTIORGAN FAILURE

As 20% to 30% of cases of MAS occur in the setting of birth depression, multiorgan failure with shock, disseminated intravascular coagulation, and renal dysfunction complicating the course. In addition, infants with MAS are often hypoxemic and acidotic after birth, which may contribute to end-organ dysfunction.

DELIVERY ROOM MANAGEMENT IN THE PRESENCE OF MECONIUM-STAINED AMNIOTIC FLUID

Prior to 2016, the Neonatal Resuscitation Program recommendation for the nonvigorous infant born through MSAF was to perform endotracheal intubation and, with the use of a meconium aspirator, suction for meconium below the cords. With the latest edition of neonatal resuscitation protocol (NRP) the approach to the nonvigorous infant born through MSAF was revised to state that resuscitation of infants with MSAF should follow the same principles as for those with clear fluid, but an individual skilled in tracheal intubation should be present at the time of birth. If a baby is born through MSAF and has depressed respirations or poor muscle tone, the baby is to be placed on the radiant warmer and initial steps of newborn care implemented. This recommendation was changed to minimize the risks of intubation and to decrease the time to positive pressure ventilation for the compromised infant, given the lack of evidence to support benefit from routine tracheal suctioning. Since the implementation of the guideline, several studies have addressed the implications, with two recent publications showing an increase in length of hospital stay and a trend towards an increased incidence of MAS and increased respiratory admissions to the neonatal intensive care unit (NICU) in nonvigorous infants without routine tracheal suctioning.[55-57] However, a more recent study queried a large multicenter database of nearly 2 million births and 50,000 NICU admissions and could not confirm the above observation, supporting the current NRP recommendations.[58] In addition, since implementation of the new guideline, fewer infants were noted to require ECMO; both in this dataset as well as the most recent report from the extracorporeal life support organization registry.[58,59] Whether this decline is secondary to the initiation of prompt resuscitation and ventilation in 2017 compared with previous years cannot be determined.

SURFACTANT ADMINISTRATION IN MECONIUM ASPIRATION SYNDROME

As noted, there are several mechanisms by which meconium interferes with surfactant function. Meconium directly decreases the synthesis and secretion by alveolar type 2 cells, disrupts formation of the lamellar layer,[32] and increases metabolism and degradation of phospholipases. In addition, the release of proinflammatory cytokines results in an exudative and inflammatory pneumonitis with epithelial disruption, proteinaceous exudation, and alveolar collapse secondary to surfactant inactivation. After aspiration of meconium, inflammatory cells (e.g., macrophages and neutrophils) are recruited and produce oxidative damage through the formation of peroxynitrite and hypochlorous acid with resultant type 2 pneumocyte apoptosis and surfactant breakdown.[26,34,37] Decreased surfactant production, increased breakdown, and inactivation of secreted surfactant all provide the rationale for surfactant replacement in MAS.

Administration of surfactant as a bolus or by lavage has been studied in infants with MAS. Surfactant lavage utilizes its detergent properties to remove meconium from the airways and lung parenchyma. In addition to removing noxious stimuli, surfactant administration by lavage has the potential to replace marginalized surfactant stores and to improve the natural history of the disease.

In 1996, the first randomized trial of surfactant administration in MAS was published.[51] Forty infants with moderate MAS were randomized to receive beractant (Survanta) 150 mg/kg (6 mL/kg) or air placebo. Infants were less than 6 hours old at the time of enrollment. Surfactant was administered as a bolus and then received up to four doses every 6 hours if the patient still met inclusion criteria. Surfactant administration resulted in significant improvement in the oxygenation index with decreased risk for air leaks, duration of mechanical ventilation and oxygen therapy, and length of hospitalization. There were no significant complications with surfactant administration. Three subsequent studies confirmed a decreased need for ECMO, but they did not find a difference in air leaks, duration of mechanical ventilation, oxygen therapy, and length of hospitalization.[60-62] In these studies surfactant was administered later (15.6 ± 13 hours[60] and 29 ± 21 hours[61]) after birth, possibly explaining the differences in outcome.

An alternative approach to bolus surfactant treatment of MAS is dilute surfactant lavage. The rationale for lavage is to wash out the particulate meconium from the airways and deliver the surfactant more effectively. Paranka and colleagues showed that surfactant lavage caused short-term improvement in oxygenation in a piglet model of MAS.[63]

Cochrane and colleagues instilled meconium into the airway of newborn rabbits to study the effects of surfactant bolus versus lavage treatment.[64] The animals were then randomly assigned to four groups: surfactant lavage (20 mL/kg) of diluted surfactant divided into two equal portions; saline lavage of a similar volume; surfactant bolus; and control. The first lavage removed 29% of the instilled meconium; the second lavage removed 7.5% more; and the third lavage less than 5%. In both the surfactant and saline lavage groups, there was less meconium present in the lungs. The surfactant lavage reduced inflammation, as demonstrated by decreased numbers of polymorphonuclear neutrophils, red blood cells, and metaloperoxidases. In addition, oxygenation improved in both the lavage and bolus surfactant groups; however, surfactant lavage had a lasting response with sustained improvement in Pao_2. With bolus therapy, the modest improvement in Pao_2 was not sustained.

The randomized clinical trial of Dargaville and colleagues compared surfactant lavage with standard care in 65 ventilated newborns with moderate to severe MAS.[65] There were no statistically significant benefits in mortality and common comorbidities. Several complications occurred during the treatment: bradycardia (2 patients), coughing (2 patients), hypoxia less than 80% Spo_2 at 10 minutes (5 patients), and hypotension (6 patients, requiring increased inotrope or fluid bolus). One patient died 3 hours after lavage of intractable PPHN. Therefore, surfactant lavage for MAS remains experimental with the risks potentially outweighing the benefits. The large volume of diluted surfactant to be administered increases the risks of hypoxia and may exacerbate PPHN.

More recent studies have evaluated the effect of hypothermia on surfactant function, as a follow-up to animal studies, which demonstrated reduced inflammation and improved surfactant function with hypothermia.[66] Whole body hypothermia is the mainstay of therapy for neonatal birth depression; however, the majority of studies have focused on long-term neurologic function as an outcome measure.[67] The initial observation in 2014 in a subset of 31 patients undergoing whole body cooling for birth depression, the fraction of inspired oxygen, the mean airway pressure (MAP), the oxygenation index, and the alveolar-arterial gradient decreased during the induction of hypothermia and tended to increase during rewarming.[68] This was followed-up in two subsequent studies that evaluated surfactant function and lung cytokines with whole body hypothermia.[69,70] In these reports the authors demonstrated improved surfactant function at 48 hours and reduced levels of proinflammatory cytokines (IL-6, IL-8). Following this in the largest cohort studied to date, the TOBY (total body hypothermia) investigators compared a cohort of patients with MAS treated with hypothermia according to TOBY trial criteria[71] to a subset of patients with MAS in whom whole body hypothermia criteria were not met.[72] A total of 108 neonates were enrolled (43 cooled; 65 uncooled); the cohorts were similar for basic data other than SNAPPEII score (Score for Neonatal Acute Physiology—Perinatal Extension II), which was adjusted for in the analysis. Infants undergoing therapeutic hypothermia demonstrated improved oxygenation and required fewer days of mechanical ventilation, and shorter NICU and hospital stays. The authors concluded that while limited evidence exists, based on their report and the underlying biologic plausibility, whole body hypothermia should be considered as an adjunctive therapy for MAS, after careful risk/benefit ratio evaluation, and when other respiratory therapies have been already optimized. As therapeutic hypothermia becomes standard of care for neonatal birth depression, tracking pulmonary outcomes, especially in the setting of MAS, will be relevant and important.

MECHANICAL VENTILATION IN MECONIUM ASPIRATION SYNDROME

Approximately 30% of patients with MAS require mechanical ventilation due to respiratory failure.[5,73] Indications for intubation and positive pressure ventilation are hypercarbic respiratory failure, pulmonary hypertension, and birth depression necessitating head or selective body cooling.[74] For patients requiring assisted ventilation, synchronized intermittent mandatory ventilation is usually chosen as the initial mode. Infants with MAS are often tachypneic and prone to ventilator asynchrony.

Optimizing the approach to mechanical ventilation in MAS involves an assessment of the underlying pathophysiology. For example, the level of positive end-expiratory pressure (PEEP) used must balance the interaction between preventing end-expiratory collapse and avoiding overdistension secondary to the airways disease and meconium plugs. Early observations suggested that the greatest benefit of PEEP was achieved with pressures ranging between 4 and 7 cm H_2O; higher PEEP settings (8 to 14 cm H_2O) increased oxygenation minimally.[75] In the setting of regional or global hyperinflation, a lower PEEP (3 to 4 cm H_2O) may be more effective.[74]

As with PEEP, setting inspiratory time in MAS must take into account the balance between atelectasis and overdistension. Term infants generally have longer time constants than preterm infants with RDS[76] and thus require a longer inspiratory time (around 0.5 seconds). Even longer inspiratory times may be useful for lung recruitment during inspiration if atelectasis is prominent. In the setting of airways disease and high airways resistance, longer inspiratory times allow for better gas distribution. However, it is important to remember that a sufficient expiratory time is needed to allow for adequate emptying of the lung in the setting of meconium plugging.

Central to the pathophysiology of MAS are air trapping and expiratory airflow limitation, which are caused by large and small airways inflammation and meconium plugs. An optimal conventional ventilation rate in MAS requires the use of a relatively low ventilator rate (<40) to allow for a longer expiratory time. This will help to avoid inadvertent PEEP, secondary to stacking of breaths. As the resultant minute ventilation must be sufficient to produce adequate CO_2 clearance, a higher tidal volume may be needed. Hyperventilation-induced alkalosis, which anecdotally appeared to reduce the need for ECMO in infants with PPHN,[77] is no longer practiced due to the risk of sensorineural hearing loss[78] and the widespread availability of inhaled nitric oxide (iNO) as a potent and selective pulmonary vasodilator. In infants failing conventional mechanical ventilation, high-frequency oscillation ventilation (HFOV) may be needed.

Early reports of iNO use in the setting of MAS demonstrated that HFOV could augment the response to iNO in patients who did not initially respond to iNO therapy.[79] This was evident especially in patients with parenchymal lung disease (MAS or RDS). This report and others highlighted the importance of effective lung recruitment to ensure adequate iNO delivery. When to transition from conventional mechanical ventilation to HFOV in the setting of MAS is unclear. As noted above, air trapping and expiratory airflow limitation are central to the pathophysiology of MAS. Airway obstruction secondary to large and small airways inflammation and meconium plugs limits exhalation, necessitating the use of a relatively low ventilator rate (<40) to allow for a longer expiratory time. This will help to avoid inadvertent PEEP, secondary to stacking of breaths. With the use of HFOV the same principles apply. As a surrogate to the use of a lower rate on conventional ventilation, a lower frequency of 6 Hz or less is recommended when utilizing HFOV ventilation. Another challenge with HFOV is the heterogeneity of the lung disease with MAS. MAS is characterized by both hyperinflation and volume loss, with differential compliance in these heterogenous areas of the lung. High rate ventilation with HFOV predisposes to over inflation of the more compliant lung segments without recruitment of the atelectatic lung segments. The MAP applied to the lung should account for this heterogeneity, and utilizing the lowest MAP that allows for adequate oxygenation is recommended. Aggressive lung recruitment strategies will predispose to the development of air leak, with overdistension of the more compliant lung segments or gas trapping in segments with expiratory airflow limitation.

EXPERIMENTAL THERAPIES IN MECONIUM ASPIRATION SYNDROME

Research studies are evaluating several therapeutic options as adjuvant therapy for MAS. More specifically antioxidant and antiinflammatory therapy.[80,81] In two separate studies utilizing the rabbit model of meconium aspiration, N acetylcysteine and NFκβ inhibitors were administered intravenously in combination with intratracheal administration of surfactant. When compared to either therapy alone, combination therapy improved oxygenation, prevented the development of pulmonary edema with improved lung wet:dry ratios, and reduced the neutrophil influx into the lung and proinflammatory cytokine levels. In addition to these therapies, the efficacy of inhalational gasses has been explored for the treatment of MAS. While extensive experience exists with the use of inhaled nitric oxide in MAS, attention has turned to the use of novel inhalational gasses such as helium, xenon, and hydrogen. In 2011, Heliox ventilation was utilized to treat a small number of infants with MAS and demonstrated improved lung compliance, pulmonary mechanics, and oxygenation.[82] Xenon and hydrogen are being extensively explored in animal models of asphyxia; however, their utility in the primary management of MAS has yet to be explored.

CONCLUSION

MAS follows fetal hypoxic/ischemic stress that leads to intestinal peristalsis, meconium release with contamination of the amniotic fluid, and gasping respirations, which cause aspiration of noxious meconium-stained fluid deep into the fetal lung. MAS occurs most frequently in the setting of fetal distress, and postdates delivery. Aspiration of meconium manifests as airway obstruction with the trapping of gas in the lung during exhalation, chemical pneumonitis, and surfactant inactivation with decreased lung compliance. Decreased lung compliance leads to atelectasis, and gas trapping produces hyperinflation, such that lung disease in MAS is characterized by marked heterogeneity. Patients typically present with respiratory distress shortly after birth with or without evidence of pulmonary hypertension. Extrapulmonary manifestations are cardiac dysfunction, shock, neonatal ischemic encephalopathy, and—in rare cases—multiorgan failure. Management is supportive and includes mechanical ventilation for respiratory failure, surfactant replacement, hemodynamic support with inotropes, and screening for neonatal ischemic encephalopathy and multiorgan failure. In rare cases, ECMO may be needed for pulmonary or hemodynamic support.

A complete reference list is available at www.ExpertConsult.com. 

SELECT REFERENCES

1. Yeh T. Core concepts: meconium aspiration syndrome: pathogenesis and current management. *NeoReviews*. 2010;11:e503.
2. Yoder BA, Kirsch EA, Barth WH, Gordon MC. Changing obstetric practices associated with decreasing incidence of meconium aspiration syndrome. *Obstet Gynecol*. 2002;99(5 Pt 1):731.
5. Cleary GM, Wiswell TE. Meconium-stained amniotic fluid and the meconium aspiration syndrome. An update. *Pediatr Clin North Am*. 1998;45(3):511.
6. Wiswell TE, Tuggle JM, Turner BS. Meconium aspiration syndrome: have we made a difference? *Pediatrics*. 1990;85(5):715.
7. Wiswell TE, Bent RC. Meconium staining and the meconium aspiration syndrome. Unresolved issues. *Pediatr Clin North Am*. 1993;40(5):955.
8. Miller FC. Meconium staining of the aminiotic fluid. *Clin Obstet Gynaecol*. 1979;6(2):359.
9. Yeomans ER, Gilstrap III LC, Leveno KJ, Burris JS. Meconium in the amniotic fluid and fetal acid-base status. *Obstet Gynecol*. 1989;73(2):175.
10. Lucas A, Christofides ND, Adrian TE, et al. Fetal distress, meconium, and motilin. *Lancet*. 1979;1(8118):718.
12. Rapoport S, Buchanan DJ. The composition of meconium; isolation of blood-group-specific polysaccharides; abnormal compositions of meconium in meconium ileus. *Science*. 1950;112(2901):150.
13. Côté RH, Valet JP. Isolation, composition and reactivity of the neutral glycoproteins from human meconiums with specificities of the ABO and Lewis systems. *Biochem J*. 1976;153(1):63.
14. Tran N, Lowe C, Sivieri EM, Shaffer TH. Sequential effects of acute meconium obstruction on pulmonary function. *Pediatr Res*. 1980;14(1):34–38.
15. Kinsella JP. Meconium aspiration syndrome. *Am J Respir Crit Care Med*. 2003;168:413–414.
16. Sienko A, Altshuler G. Meconium-induced umbilical vascular necrosis in abortuses and fetuses: a histopathologic study for cytokines. *Obstet Gynecol*. 1999;94(3):415.
17. Hsieh TT, Hsieh CC, Hung TH, et al. Differential expression of interleukin-1 beta and interleukin-6 in human fetal serum and meconium-stained amniotic fluid. *J Reprod Immunol*. 1998;37(2):155.
18. Yeh TF, Harris V, Srinivasan G, et al. Roentgenographic findings in infants with meconium aspiration syndrome. *J Am Med Assoc*. 1979;242:60.
23. Yamada T, Minakami H, Matsubara S, et al. Meconium-stained amniotic fluid exhibits chemotactic activity for polymorphonuclear leukocytes in vitro. *J Reprod Immunol*. 2000;46(1):21.
24. de Beaufort AJ, Pelikan DM, Elferink JG, Berger HM. Effect of interleukin 8 in meconium on in-vitro neutrophil chemotaxis. *Lancet*. 1998;352(9122):102.
25. Cayabyab RG, Kwong K, Jones C, et al. Lung inflammation and pulmonary function in infants with meconium aspiration syndrome. *Pediatr Pulmonol*. 2007;42(10):898.
26. Vidyasagar D, Zagariya A. Studies of meconium-induced lung injury: inflammatory cytokine expression and apoptosis. *J Perinatol*. 2008;28(suppl 3):S102–S107.
27. Schrama AJ, de Beaufort AJ, Sukul YR, et al. Phospholipase A2 is present in meconium and inhibits the activity of pulmonary surfactant: an in vitro study. *Acta Paediatr*. 2001;90:412–416.
28. Soukka H, Kääpä P. Phospholipase A2 in meconium-induced lung injury. *J Perinatol*. 2008;28:S120–S122.
29. Bryan CS. Enhancement of bacterial infection by meconium. *John Hopkins Med J*. 1967;121:9.
32. Bae C, Takahashi A, Chida S, Sasaki M. Morphology and function of pulmonary surfactant inhibited by meconium. *Pediatr Res*. 1998;44:187–191.
33. Cleary GM, Antunes MJ, Ciesielka DA, et al. Exudative lung injury is associated with decreased levels of surfactant proteins in a rat model of meconium aspiration. *Pediatrics*. 1997;100:998–1003.

34. Janssen DJ, Carnielli VP, Cogo P, et al. Surfactant phosphatidylcholine metabolism in neonates with meconium aspiration syndrome. *J Pediatr*. 2006;149:634-639.
35. Clark DA, Nieman GF, Thompson JE, et al. Surfactant displacement by meconium free fatty acids: an alternative explanation for atelectasis in meconium aspiration syndrome. *J Pediatr*. 1987;110:765-770.
37. Amato M. Mechanisms of bilirubin toxicity. *Eur J Pediatr*. 1995;154(9 suppl 4):S54.
38. Taeusch HW. Treatment of acute (adult) respiratory distress syndrome. The holy grail of surfactant therapy. *Biol Neonate*. 2000;77:2-8.
39. Ballard PL, Truog WE, Merrill JD, et al. Plasma biomarkers of oxidative stress: relationship to lung disease and inhaled nitric oxide therapy in premature infants. *Pediatrics*. 2008;121(3):555-561.
44. Zagariya A, Doherty J, Bhat R, et al. Elevated immunoreactive endothelin-1 levels in newborn rabbit lungs after meconium aspiration. *Pediatr Crit Care Med*. 2002;3(3):297-302.
45. Yigit S, Tekinalp G, Oran O, et al. Endothelin 1 concentrations in infants with meconium stained amniotic fluid. *Arch Dis Child Fetal Neonatal Ed*. 2002;87(3):F212-F213.
46. Khan AM, Lally KP, Larsen GL, Colasurdo GN. Enhanced release of thromboxane A(2) after exposure of human airway epithelial cells to meconium. *Pediatr Pulmonol*. 2002;33(2):111-116.
47. Thureen PJ, Hall DM, Hoffenberg A, Tyson RW. Fatal meconium aspiration in spite of appropriate perinatal airway management: pulmonary and placental evidence of prenatal disease. *Am J Obstet Gynecol*. 1997;176(5):967-975.
48. Murphy JD, Vawter GF, Reid LM. Pulmonary vascular disease in fatal meconium aspiration. *J Pediatr*. 1984;104(5):758-762.
49. Acker SN, Mandell EW, Sims-Lucas S, et al. Histologic identification of prominent intrapulmonary anastomotic vessels in severe congenital diaphragmatic hernia. *J Pediatr*. 2015;166(1):178-183.
50. Galambos C, Sims-Lucas S, Ali N, et al. Intrapulmonary vascular shunt pathways in alveolar capillary dysplasia with misalignment of pulmonary veins. *Thorax*. 2015;70(1):84-85.
51. Ali N, Abman SH, Galambos C. Histologic evidence of intrapulmonary bronchopulmonary anastomotic pathways in neonates with meconium aspiration syndrome. *J Pediatr*. 2015;167(6):1445-1447.
52. Robertson B. Anastomoses in the human lung: postnatal formation and obliteration of arterial anastomoses in the human lung: a microangiographic and histologic study. *Pediatrics*. 1969;43:971.
53. Wilkinson MJ, Fagan DG. Postmortem demonstration of intrapulmonary arteriovenous shunting. *Arch Dis Child*. 1990;65:435-437.
54. Blackwell SC, Moldenhauer J, Hassan SS, et al. Meconium aspiration syndrome in term neonates with normal acid-base status at delivery: is it different? *Am J Obstet Gynecol*. 2001;184(7):1422-1425, discussion 1425-1426.
60. Findlay RD, Taeusch HW, Walther FJ. Surfactant replacement therapy for meconium aspiration syndrome. *Pediatrics*. 1996;97:48-52.
61. Chinese Collab: Chinese Collaborative Study Group for Neonatal Respiratory Diseases. Treatment of severe meconium aspiration with porcine surfactant: a multicentre, randomized, controlled trial. *Acta Paediatr*. 2005;94:896-902.
62. Lotze A, Mitchell BR, Bulas DI, et al. Multicenter study of surfactant (beractant) use in the treatment of term infants with severe respiratory failure. *J Pediatr*. 1998;132:40-47.
63. Maturana A, Torres-Pereyra J, Salinas R, et al. *The Chile Surf Group: A Randomized Trial of Natural Surfactant for Moderate to Severe Meconium Aspiration Syndrome*. Washington, DC: Abstract presented at the Pediatric Academic Societies Annual Meeting; 2005.
64. Paranka MS, Walsh WF, Stancombe BB. Surfactant lavage in a piglet model of meconium aspiration syndrome. *Pediatr Res*. 1992;31(6):625-628.
65. Cochrane CG, Revak SD, Merritt TA, et al. Bronchoalveolar lavage with KL4-surfactant in models of meconium aspiration syndrome. *Pediatr Res*. 1998;44(5):705-715.
73. Dargaville PA, Copnell B, Mills JF, et al. Randomized controlled trial of lung lavage with dilute surfactant for meconium aspiration syndrome. *J Pediatr*. 2011;158(3):383-389.
74. van Ierland Y, de Boer M, de Beaufort AJ. Meconium-stained amniotic fluid: discharge vigorous newborns. *Arch Dis Child Fetal Neonatal Ed*. 2010;95:F69.
75. Goldsmith JP. Continuous positive airway pressure and conventional mechanical ventilation in the treatment of meconium aspiration syndrome. *J Perinatol*. 2008;28(suppl 3):S49-S55.

Pathophysiology of Bronchopulmonary Dysplasia 159

Eduardo H. Bancalari | Deepak Jain

INTRODUCTION

More than half a century after its first description by Northway and colleagues, bronchopulmonary dysplasia (BPD) continues to be the most common respiratory morbidity in extremely preterm infants surviving after different modes of respiratory support.[1] Over the years, the epidemiologic, clinical, and pathologic picture of this condition has changed remarkably. In its current form, BPD is the end result of various antenatal and postnatal factors that interfere with the normal progression of development of lung parenchyma, vasculature, and airways, leading to varying degrees of respiratory failure. This complex, multifactorial pathogenesis has provided unique challenges to not only fully understand the pathophysiology but also to devise effective prevention and treatment strategies for BPD.

BPD, as originally described by Northway and colleagues, resulted from severe injury to the developing lung in the presaccular phase of development, secondary to prolonged mechanical ventilation with high pressures and inspired oxygen concentrations. This resulted in a grossly distorted pathologic picture characterized by emphysema, fibrosis, and marked vascular and airway epithelial changes.[1] Since then, changes in clinical practices such as widespread use of antenatal steroids, exogenous surfactant, and less invasive respiratory support have led to a reduction in injury to the developing lung. In addition, advances in neonatal care have improved the survival of extremely premature infants whose lungs are at the late canalicular or early saccular phase of development exposing them to various antenatal and postnatal factors that can disrupt normal alveolar and vascular development. Hence the pathologic picture of this new form of chronic lung disease, "new BPD," is markedly different and is characterized by alveolar simplification with fewer and dysmorphic capillaries, but less evidence of emphysema, airway damage, vascular remodeling, and pulmonary hypertension.[2]

PATHOPHYSIOLOGIC FACTORS ASSOCIATED WITH LUNG INJURY AND IMPAIRED DEVELOPMENT

Human lung development is a complex process comprising of anatomic structure development, histologic differentiation, and biochemical maturation in conjunction with vascular development. These mechanisms are discussed in detail in other chapters. There are multiple factors that can contribute to an aberration in the normal lung development, including prenatal factors such as genetic predisposition and exposure to maternal smoking, antenatal conditions associated with or resulting in

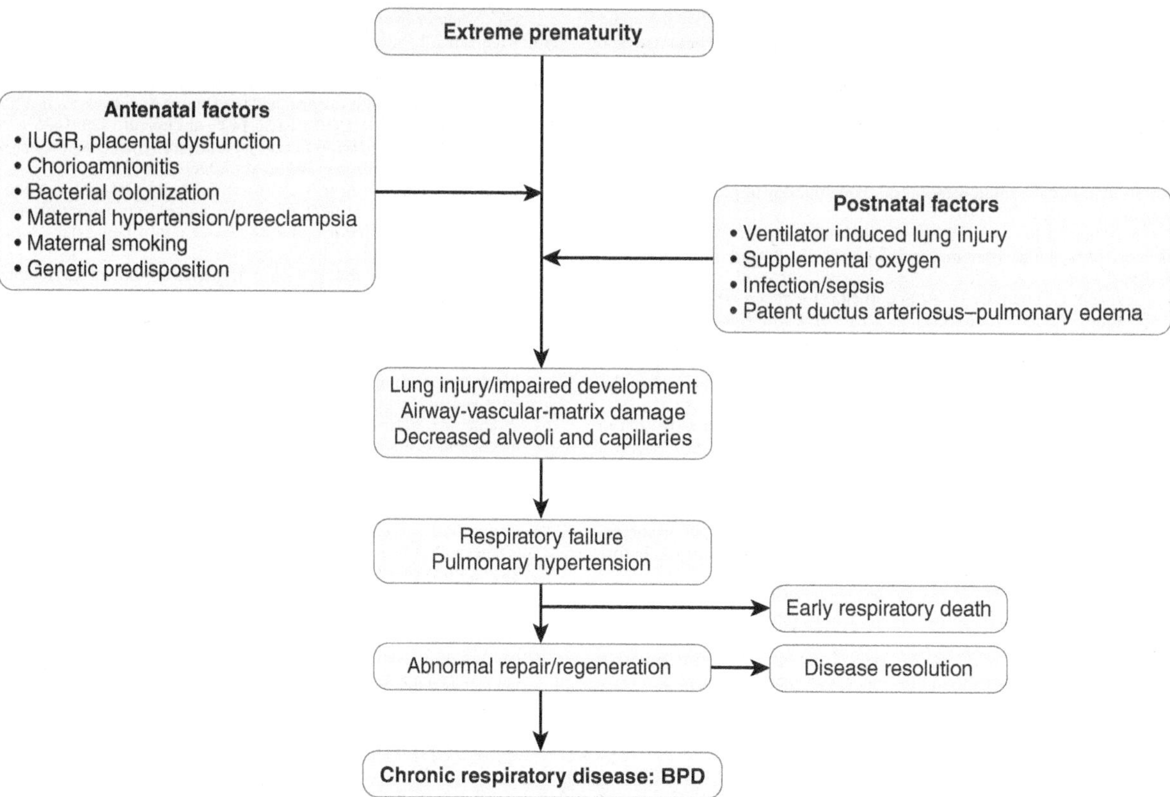

Fig. 159.1 Pathogenesis of bronchopulmonary dysplasia *(BPD)*. *IUGR,* Intrauterine growth retardation.

preterm birth, untoward effects of life-sustaining procedures like mechanical ventilation or oxygen supplementation, as well as associated complication such as infections or nutritional deficiencies (Fig. 159.1).

While gestational age at birth continues to be the most significant determinant for the risk of most of the sequelae of prematurity, including BPD,[3] other conditions can have a significant effect on lung development and risk for BPD. One of the more studied in-utero exposures is cigarette smoking. In addition to epidemiologic studies suggesting an association between maternal smoking and increased risk of BPD,[4] several animal models have shown exposure to nicotine in-utero results in abnormal airway branching with increased smooth muscle thickness and collagen deposition.[5-7]

Lung angiogenesis is one of the critical components of alveolar development, with increasing evidence that conditions affecting primarily angiogenesis may also contribute to abnormal alveolar development.[8] Disorders affecting placental function, such as gestational hypertension, preeclampsia, and intrauterine growth restriction, have also been associated with impaired vascular growth, with evidence that suggests these effects are mediated by an imbalance in pro- and anti-angiogenic factors.[9-11] Impaired vascular growth and function may disrupt distal airspace development (the "vascular hypothesis" of BPD).[12-14]

Exposure of the fetal lung to infection has been shown to result in inflammation and lung injury,[15,16] as well as enhanced lung maturation.[17] It is likely that chorioamnionitis has variable effects, depending on the fetal inflammatory response, the organism causing the infection, exposure to antenatal steroids, and the severity and duration of infection.[18,19]This is supported by clinical evidence from several studies suggesting an increased risk for BPD in infants born to mothers with evidence of chorioamnionitis[20,21]; others, however, have failed to show this association.[22]

Preterm birth interrupts normal fetal lung development, leading to a premature infant who is exposed to multiple life-saving therapies that are likely to cause lung injury.The relative contribution of different factors has evolved over time, with newer strategies such as less invasive respiratory support and judicious use of supplemental oxygen most likely being responsible for the reduced severity of the chronic lung injury. The two main mechanisms of lung injury from mechanical ventilation are volutrauma,[23,24] due to excessive stretching of tissues from over inflation, and atelectotrauma, caused by repetitive opening of closed lung units resulting in shear injury. These can result in damage to the alveolar-capillary barrier, exudation of intravascular fluid resulting in pulmonary edema, release of cytokines, chemokines, and proteases, as well as recruitment and activation of inflammatory molecules.[25,26] Oxidative stress continues to be a significant risk factor for lung injury in preterm infants due to a combination of factors, including the transition from a fetal low oxygen environment to a postnatal high oxygen environment, need for supplemental oxygen, as well as inadequate antioxidant mechanisms.[27] The resultant generation of reactive oxygen species may cause lipid peroxidation with cell membrane damage, apoptosis and cell death, surfactant inactivation, protein and DNA damage, as well as activation of inflammatory cascade.[28] The effect of patent ductus arteriosus (PDA) on lung injury has been debated for a long time. As a consequence of the left-to-right shunting through the PDA, pulmonary blood flow and lung fluid increase, negatively affecting lung mechanics and gas exchange and thereby increasing the need for more aggressive mechanical ventilation and the risk for BPD.[29-31] Furthermore, simultaneous occurrence of both infection and PDA leads to a synergistic interaction that may further increase the risk for developing BPD.[32]

PATHOPHYSIOLOGIC PROCESSES IN THE DEVELOPMENT OF LUNG INJURY

Inflammation continues to be considered as a major mediator in the pathogenesis of lung injury.[15,33] The pulmonary inflammatory response can be triggered prior to birth, as in the setting of antenatal infection,[34] or postnatally by a number of factors, including ventilation with excessive tidal volumes,[25,35] oxygen free radicals,[36,37] and postnatal infections.[38]

A significant increase in inflammatory cells (macrophages, neutrophils), eicosanoids, and various cytokines (IL-1β, IL-6, IL-8, tumor necrosis factor-α) has been demonstrated in the airways of infants in whom BPD develops subsequently.[39–41] The increase in cytokine concentrations has been documented early after birth, supporting the contention that in many infants the insult may start during fetal life or in the early postnatal period.[42] There is evidence of pulmonary alveolar macrophage (PAM) activation in infants who later develop BPD, and these activated PAMs have been suggested as a source of neutrophil chemo attractants, especially when exposed to high oxygen concentrations.

Alterations in alveolar and vascular development is one of the hallmarks of bronchopulmonary dysplasia. The interaction between epithelium and mesenchyme is critical for lung development, with multiple signaling pathways playing important roles during different stages of lung development.[43] These include members of transforming growth factor (TGF)-β,[44,45] bone morphogenic protein (BMP),[46] vascular endothelial growth factor (VEGF),[10,47] fibroblast growth factor (FGF),[48] sonic hedgehog (SHH),[49] platelet-derived growth factor,[50,51] Wnt,[52] and insulin growth factor (IGF).[53]

Lung injury and repair mechanisms play a key role in the development of BPD. While effective repair helps preserve structure and cellular function, defective tissue repair can contribute to the impaired lung function seen in BPD. Connective tissue growth factor (CTGF) is one of the downstream mediators of lung injury, with increased expression seen in infants with BPD as well as different animal models of lung injury.[54] Overexpression of CTGF in neonatal mice results in thickened alveolar septae, decreased alveolarization, reduced capillary density, and pulmonary hypertension.[55] An increase in elastase and an imbalance between elastase and α_1 proteinase inhibitor in the lung has also been postulated as a possible mechanism for neonatal lung injury.[56,57]

The major obstacle in preventing BPD is that as lung damage progresses, the deterioration in lung mechanics and gas exchange requires an increase in respiratory support and use of higher inspired oxygen concentrations. A vicious cycle is thereby created in which the required interventions to improve respiratory failure, mechanical ventilation, and increased inspired oxygen induce more lung damage and exacerbate the respiratory impairment.

PATHOPHYSIOLOGIC BASIS FOR THERAPIES FOR BRONCHOPULMONARY DYSPLASIA

Since BPD is a multifactorial disease process, there are several potential prevention strategies. So far, the majority of the prevention and treatment strategies, like less invasive respiratory support, prevention of infection, or judicious use of oxygen supplementation, aim to reduce iatrogenic injury to the developing lung. Additional therapies like corticosteroids have multiple potential effects, including antiinflammatory activity, reduction of lung mesenchyme resulting in improved lung function, and maturation of surfactant system.[58,59]

Caffeine, a nonselective inhibitor of adenosine receptor commonly used for treatment or prevention of apnea of prematurity, has also been shown to have an antiinflammatory effect in newborn animals and possibly reduce BPD in infants.[60] Nitric oxide (NO) is another drug that has been tried for the prevention of BPD, with inconclusive results. NO has multiple potential mechanisms of actions, including having antiinflammatory effects; serving as a mediator for several angiogenic factors, including VEGF; and reducing pulmonary vascular tone.[61]

Specific interventions to modulate growth factors or target inflammatory pathways have been used in animal models of BPD with variable success. These include administration of molecules to antagonize the effect of IL-1, such as receptor antagonist (IL-1Ra), competitive inhibitor anakinra, or upstream pathways inhibiting the production of IL-1β.[62,63] Other pathways that have been targeted include CTGF pathway with inhibition of β catenin signaling,[64] Fgf10 pathway with micro RNA-421 inhibition,[65] recombinant Club cell-10Kilodalton protein (CC-10) as an immunomodulatory agent,[66] and recombinant IGF-1[53], with some success. There continues to be concern regarding the effects of these drugs on other organ systems, as well as the differentiation between physiologic need and the pathologic role in the disease process.

There is increasing evidence of the repairability of the lung following injurious stimuli, and endogenous stem cells play an important role in this process.[67,68] In contrast to full-term infants, stem cells in preterm infants at risk for BPD have impaired replication and differentiation potential, possibly contributing to the pathogenesis of BPD.[69] This has resulted in concerted efforts to explore stem cell treatment for the prevention and treatment of BPD in animal models of hyperoxia-induced lung injury, showing reduced lung inflammation, attenuation of fibrosis, improved lung alveolar and vascular structure, and improved lung function with the use of mesenchymal stem cells (MSCs).[70,71] It is increasingly clear that the mechanism of action of stem cells is not mainly by engrafting and replacement of damaged cells but by paracrine effect with secretion of antiinflammatory and trophic factors. Extracellular vesicles (EVs), small nano-sized particles secreted by the MSC, are responsible for these paracrine effects.[72] MSC-derived EVs have been shown to have similar beneficial effects on the prevention as well as treatment of hyperoxia-induced lung injury in neonatal animal models.[73]

PULMONARY FUNCTION IN INFANTS WITH BRONCHOPULMONARY DYSPLASIA

The alterations in pulmonary function in infants with BPD are nonspecific and result from the severe disruption of lung development and architecture that occurs in these infants. The degree of abnormality in lung function may range from mild to severe, paralleling the clinical and radiographic presentation. Few studies have described the early changes in lung function in infants who subsequently develop BPD or have longitudinally followed the course of lung function in these infants.

LUNG FUNCTION IN EARLY BRONCHOPULMONARY DYSPLASIA

Infants who develop BPD have more severe respiratory failure and worse lung function early in their evolution than infants who recover without lung sequelae. Studies from the presurfactant era have shown higher airway resistance during the first weeks of life in infants in whom BPD developed subsequently compared to infants who recovered without lung damage,[74,75] suggesting that early airway obstruction may be a marker or a predisposing factor for the development of more severe pulmonary damage. Studies evaluating longitudinal lung function in preterm infants in the post-surfactant era have shown decreased lung compliance and functional residual capacity (FRC), but no difference in resistance between infants who go on to develop BPD versus those who did not.[76] These results are consistent with the pathologic picture of new BPD, which is characterized by alveolar simplification but less airway injury. Lung mechanics measurements during the first week of life have been used to improve the accuracy of BPD prediction models with inconsistent results,[77-79] likely reflecting differing severities of disease and different methods used to assess lung function. The worse initial respiratory function observed in infants who subsequently develop BPD most likely reflects the more severe initial respiratory illness in these infants.

LUNG FUNCTION IN ESTABLISHED BRONCHOPULMONARY DYSPLASIA

VENTILATION

Tidal volume is normal or reduced and respiratory rate is increased in most of the infants with severe BPD, resulting in a normal or increased minute ventilation.[80] The increased dead space ventilation that results from this contributes to the hypercapnia observed in infants with severe BPD.

DISTRIBUTION OF VENTILATION

The morphologic alterations in the lungs of infants with severe BPD result in a significant disruption of the relationship between ventilation and perfusion. The damage to the small airways produces different time constants in different areas of the lungs, thereby altering the distribution of the inspired gas. The disturbed ventilation-perfusion relationships lead to an increased arterial-alveolar gradient for carbon dioxide (CO_2) in areas that are ventilated but poorly perfused (high V_A/Q ratio) and an increased alveolar-arterial oxygen gradient caused by poorly or nonventilated areas that receive blood flow (low V_A/Q ratio).[81,82]

LUNG VOLUME

Lung volume measurements in infants with BPD have yielded variable results, depending on age. FRC values below normal have been reported during the first month of life, but values increased to above normal by the age of 6 to 16 months.[83-86] The increase in lung volume in infants with BPD may reflect gas trapping, secondary to progressive small airway obstruction.

LUNG COMPLIANCE

Dynamic lung compliance is consistently decreased in infants with BPD (Fig. 159.2).[86] This decrease may reflect changes in the elastic properties of the lung secondary to fibrosis and interstitial fluid accumulation. Compliance also may be reduced by alterations in surfactant metabolism, which have been described in infants with BPD.[87] The decrease in dynamic compliance also reflects the increase in small airway resistance that produces frequency dependence of compliance. Overdistension of portions of the lung from gas trapping can further contribute to the decrease in compliance.

AIRWAY RESISTANCE

A consistent alteration in lung function in infants with severe BPD is increased airway resistance (see Fig. 159.2). This can lead to severe maldistribution of the inspired gas, lung overdistension from gas trapping, and hypoventilation with hypercapnia secondary to the increased work required for breathing.

The mechanisms for increased airway resistance include several factors that contribute to airway damage and obstruction. During the initial stages of severe BPD, histopathologic changes include epithelial cell damage with hyperplasia and squamous metaplasia of the airway epithelial lining. Infection and inflammatory reaction in the airways increase mucus secretion. In addition, clearance of mucus may be decreased as a result of depression of ciliary activity during prolonged intubation. Infants with severe BPD can exhibit hypertrophy of airway smooth muscle.[1] This plays an important role in the increased airway resistance and airway hyperreactivity observed in these infants. Increased production of inflammatory mediators, such as leukotrienes and PAF, also may contribute to airway smooth muscle constriction and increased pulmonary resistance.[88,89] A more frequent family history of asthma in infants with BPD raises the possibility that a genetically determined airway hyperreactivity may also contribute to the development of BPD in some cases.[90,91] The increase in airway resistance is not specific to infants with BPD but is observed in most premature infants who receive prolonged mechanical ventilation, regardless of whether or not they develop BPD. The increase in airway resistance combined with lower compliance is responsible for a marked increase in the work of breathing and for the alveolar hypoventilation and CO_2 retention that are characteristic of these infants. The degree of airway damage is not uniform throughout the lung, and this contributes to the abnormal distribution of ventilation and the development of areas of overdistension, alternating with areas of collapse observed in cases of severe BPD.

The exact location of the obstruction has not been defined, but forced expiratory flows at FRC are decreased, suggesting that the main obstruction is at the level of the small airways.[85,92,93] In infants with severe BPD, large airways also are compromised and may demonstrate increased collapsibility that manifests during active expiration as a result of tracheomalacia or bronchomalacia.[94,95] This alteration is responsible for the severe deterioration in gas exchange observed in some of these infants during periods of agitation, which results in the generation of positive intrathoracic pressure. These episodes can be ameliorated by sedation and by maintaining a relatively high positive end-expiratory airway pressure, 6 to 10 cm H_2O, until the episode is over.[96,97]

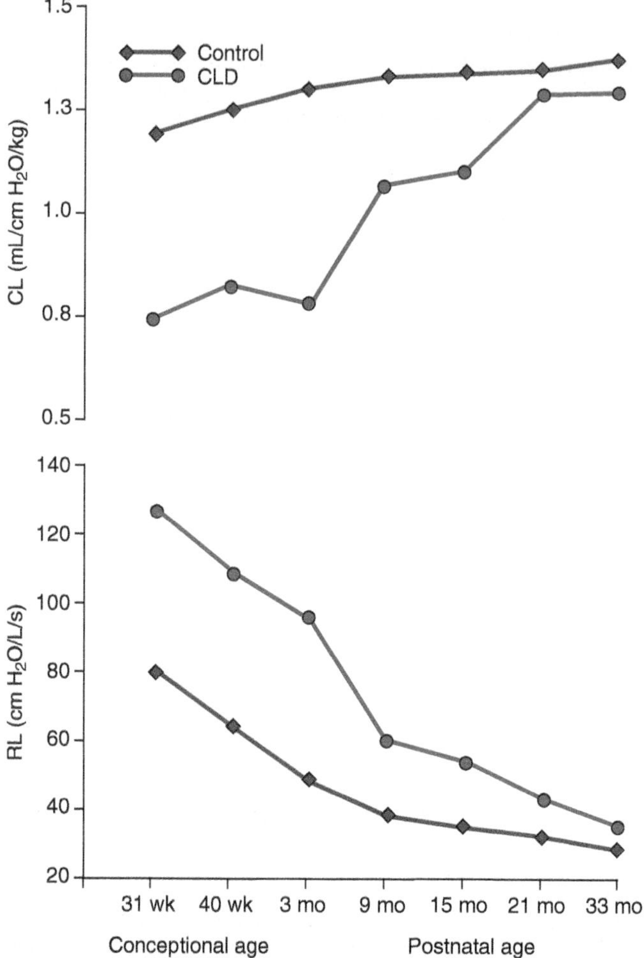

Fig. 159.2 Sequential measurements of lung compliance *(CL)* and lung resistance *(RL)* in infants with chronic lung disease *(CLD)* and in normal control subjects. (Modified from Gerhardt T, Hehre D, Feller R, et al. Serial determination of pulmonary function in infants with chronic lung disease. *J Pediatr.* 1987;110:448.)

Of interest are observations that demonstrate increased airway resistance in infants with BPD in response to a reduction in the inspired oxygen concentration.[98,99] This physiologic response also might explain the episodic airway obstruction often observed in infants with BPD. Cold air or methacholine challenge also produces a marked increase in pulmonary resistance in these patients.[100-102]

The increased airway resistance in infants with BPD is in some cases partially reversible with bronchodilators[103-105] and diuretic therapy.[106,107] This suggests that the increased airway resistance is due to a combination of airway hyperreactivity and interstitial pulmonary edema, both of which may play a role in the obstruction of the small airways. The administration of systemic or inhaled steroids has also been demonstrated to reduce airway obstruction in some infants with BPD.[108,109]

Because most of the definitions of BPD are based on oxygen requirement at an arbitrary time point, it is possible that the addition of lung function evaluation may predict long-term respiratory outcomes more accurately.[110] Several studies have tried to evaluate this possibility, but results have been inconsistent.[111-114] In addition, because most of the lung function studies require special equipment, expertise, and sedation, they are not used in clinical practice.[115]

GAS EXCHANGE

Most infants with severe BPD exhibit marked hypoxemia and hypercapnia and require supplemental oxygen to maintain normal oxygenation. This hypoxemia is mainly due to a reduced ventilation-perfusion ratio and alveolar hypoventilation.[81] The oxygen requirement decreases gradually as the disease process subsides but may increase during sleep, feedings, agitation, or during episodes of pulmonary infection or edema. Infants with BPD, and preterm infants in general, have lower diffusion capacity as measured by diffusion of CO when compared to healthy controls.[116]

The increased $Paco_2$ frequently observed in infants with BPD is secondary to alveolar hypoventilation and to an increased arterial-alveolar CO_2 gradient produced by a mismatch of ventilation and perfusion and increased alveolar dead space. The chronic hypercapnia is often accompanied by an increase in serum bicarbonate concentration that compensates for the respiratory acidosis. This increase in plasma base is frequently exaggerated by the administration of diuretics, which are commonly used in infants with BPD.

METABOLIC RATE

Infants with BPD have an increased metabolic rate.[117] This increase in oxygen consumption is due, at least in part, to the increased work of breathing and is one of the factors that may interfere with normal growth in these infants.[118] The increased metabolic rate also can impose an extra load on the respiratory system, contributing to respiratory failure in infants with severe BPD. This impairment may become evident when CO_2 production is suddenly increased, such as during glucose loading, which in theory can worsen hypercapnia in these infants.[119]

BPD PHENOTYPES

Based on pulmonary function abnormalities, patients with BPD can present with different phenotypes.[120] These can be primarily obstructive, restrictive, or mixed. The obstructive phenotype is most prevalent and is observed in infants with greater birth weight. The purely alveolar or restrictive phenotype is less common, and these patients may be weaned relatively quickly from mechanical ventilation. The level and type of respiratory support for infants with BPD may be optimized, based on the type of alteration in lung mechanics. Initially, the main abnormality is low lung compliance, with a relatively homogeneous lung and low airway resistance. At this stage, the ventilator support strategy should include fast-rate, low-tidal volumes and relatively short inspiratory times. Later, the changes are dominated by high airway resistance, gas trapping, and heterogeneous aeration, which leads to diverse time constants. At this stage, a slow-rate, high tidal volume and prolonged inspiratory time strategy may be the most appropriate to achieve better ventilation and oxygenation. At this stage, hypercarbia is common, with radiographic findings of hyperinflation alternating with areas of atelectasis.[97] During these later phases, infants with more severe BPD frequently develop a phenotype that is predominantly vascular and characterized by severe pulmonary hypertension, and the management needs to be focused on the control of their pulmonary hypertension.

Other alterations that may be combined with the previous phenotypes include tracheomalacia or bronchomalacia, obstructive sleep apnea, and control of breathing issues. Addressing each of these phenotypes with individualized care is critical to improving long-term respiratory outcomes in later life.[121]

LONG-TERM LUNG FUNCTION IN INFANTS WITH BRONCHOPULMONARY DYSPLASIA

As more preterm infants with BPD survive, there is increasing information on the long-term consequences of early lung damage in these infants. However, there is still a paucity of evidence on the respiratory outcomes of adult survivors of the new milder forms of BPD. Because the initial damage occurs at a critical time when the lung is in one of the most rapid phases of growth and development, many of the alterations in lung structure and function may persist through adulthood.

Infants with BPD are more susceptible to lower respiratory tract diseases in childhood, resulting in increased rates of rehospitalization.[122,123] Although rates of hospitalizations decrease with age, these children continue to have more respiratory symptoms. In a group of infants with BPD born in the surfactant era, at about 9 years of age, these children had increased respiratory symptoms, use of asthma medications, and lung function abnormalities indicating airway obstruction.[124] Cough, wheeze, and dyspnea are also more common in adult survivors of BPD.[125]

There is increasing evidence that preterm infants, even in the absence of significant neonatal respiratory disease, have impaired lung development resulting in altered pulmonary functions when compared with term control subjects.[126-128] These studies have shown decreased expiratory flow rates suggesting small airway dysfunction, which is generally more severe in infants with a history of BPD. There is some evidence of improvement in pulmonary function with time in these infants. Serial pulmonary function evaluations for up to 3 years in a group of infants who had relatively mild BPD showed gradual improvement over time; at the end of the follow-up period, the values for compliance and resistance were close to the normal range (see Fig. 159.2). In more severe lung damage, the increased airway resistance and flow limitation seem to persist longer and through adulthood (Fig. 159.3).[129-134] The degree of flow limitation at the age of 11 years has been correlated with the duration and amount of supplemental oxygen received during the neonatal period (Fig. 159.4).[129] Surprisingly, despite these persistent abnormalities in lung function, most survivors with BPD do not exhibit a significant reduction in exercise capacity when compared with healthy term infants or preterm babies without lung disease.[135,136]

Infants with a history of BPD have decreased pulmonary diffusing capacity but similar alveolar volume in infancy and early childhood when compared with term infants, suggesting impaired alveolar development (Fig. 159.5).[137] A reduced soluble gas transfer at rest and during exercise has been reported in school-age children with a history of BPD.[138]

Study or subgroup	BPD group Mean	BPD group SD	BPD group Total	Term group Mean	Term group SD	Term group Total	Weight	Mean difference IV, random, 95% CI
1997 Giacoia	72.7	21.131	12	97.2	15.9349	12	2.0%	−24.50 [−39.47, −9.53]
1998 Gross	83	17	43	97	12	108	10.4%	−14.00 [−19.56, −8.44]
1998 Jacob	63.6	20.6	15	94.3	8.3	13	3.4%	−30.70 [−42.06, −19.34]
2002 Mieskonen	73.5	12	9	101.7	8.4	14	5.1%	−28.20 [−37.19, −19.21]
2003 Kilbride	72	15	16	91	9	25	5.9%	−19.00 [−27.15, −10.85]
2004 Korhonen	82	13	10	99	11	33	5.2%	−17.00 [−25.89, −8.11]
2005 Halvorsen	81.4	10.7	24	98.6	9.9	81	12.6%	−17.20 [−21.99, −12.41]
2006 Doyle	81.1	13.7	89	97.9	11.8	208	18.3%	−16.80 [−20.07, −13.53]
2007 Palta	78	13	59	97	12	360	17.1%	−19.00 [−22.54, −15.46]
2010 Fawke	80	13	129	100	12	161	20.0%	−20.00 [−22.91, −17.09]
Total (95% CI)			**406**			**1015**	**100.0%**	**−18.92 [−21.14, −16.70]**

Heterogeneity: $Tau^2 = 4.20$; $Chi^2 = 14.51$, df = 9 ($P = .110$); $I^2 = 38\%$

Test for overall effect: $Z = 16.74$ ($P < .00001$)

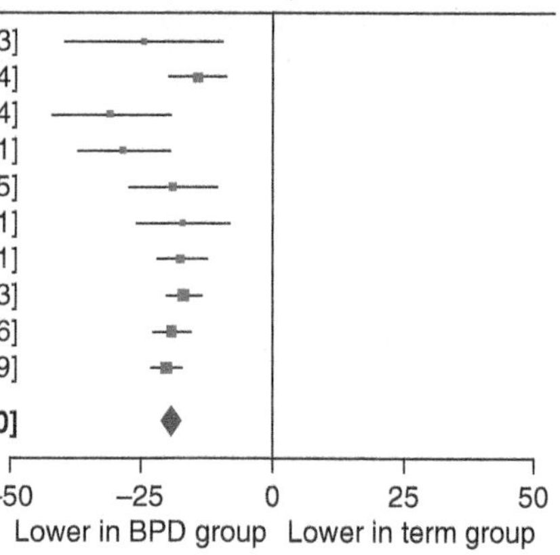

Mean difference IV, random, 95% CI

−50 −25 0 25 50

Lower in BPD group Lower in term group

Fig. 159.3 Percentage of predicted forced expiratory volume in 1s (%FEV_1) in the bronchopulmonary dysplasia *(BPD)* group (oxygen dependency at 36 weeks of postmenstrual age) compared with the term control group. *CI,* Confidence interval; *IV,* intravenous; *SD,* standard deviation. (From Kotecha SJ, Edwards MO, Watkins WJ, et al. Effect of preterm birth on later FEV_1: a systematic review and meta-analysis. *Thorax.* 2013;68[8]:760–766.)

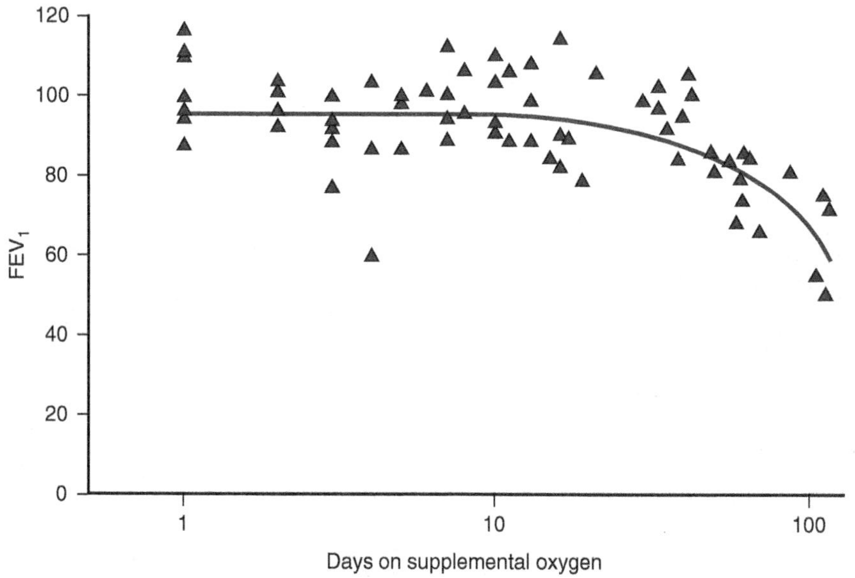

Fig. 159.4 Relation between forced expiratory volume in 1 second *(FEV_1)* and duration of supplemental oxygen (in log days) during the neonatal period. *Solid line* shows fitted values derived by use of the power function $FEV_1 = \beta 0 + \beta 1r$ (days on oxygen). (Modified from Kennedy JD, Edward LJ, Bates DJ, et al. Effects of birthweight and oxygen supplementation on lung function in late childhood in children of very low birth weight. *Pediatr Pulmonol.* 2000;30:32.)

Morphometric studies in lungs from children who died with severe BPD between the ages of 2 and 28 months revealed a striking reduction in the number of alveoli when compared with the lungs of control subjects.[139] However, there is increasing evidence that alveolar growth occurs beyond infancy through adolescence.[140,141] A study of alveolar structure using helium-3 magnetic resonance in school-age children with a history of BPD showed alveolar size similar to infants without BPD, suggesting catch-up alveolarization resulting in the normalization of deranged alveolar structure in infants with a history of BPD.[142]

CARDIOVASCULAR FUNCTION IN INFANTS WITH BRONCHOPULMONARY DYSPLASIA

PULMONARY VASCULAR DISEASE AND PULMONARY HYPERTENSION

Altered alveolar development in BPD is also associated with abnormalities in growth, structure, and function of pulmonary vasculature resulting in pulmonary vascular disease.[14] The pathogenesis is complex and multifactorial, with genetic and epigenetic factors acting in conjunction with prenatal and postnatal factors, including alveolar hypoxia and hypercapnia, increased alveolar pressure and overdistension, infection, and release of mediators of inflammation, such as PAF and leukotriene B_4, which are also pulmonary vasoconstrictors.[143] There is increasing evidence that pulmonary vascular disease can be diagnosed soon after birth and may correlate not only with risk for BPD but as well late respiratory outcomes.[144,145]

Pulmonary hypertension is commonly observed in infants with severe BPD and has been associated with increased mortality and long-term morbidities.[146,147] A postmortem study of infants with BPD showed abnormal distribution of pulmonary vasculature with dysmorphic capillaries in thickened alveolar septa and decreased expression of messenger RNA (mRNA) for VEGF and angiogenic receptors.[148] In addition, the media of small pulmonary arteries may undergo smooth muscle cell

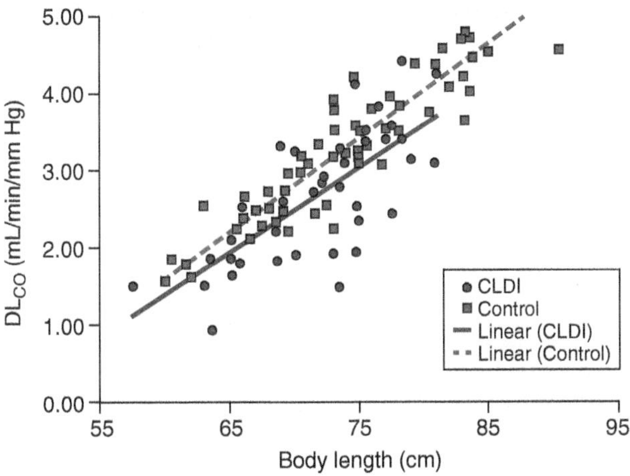

Fig. 159.5 Pulmonary diffusing capacity, DL_{CO} (mL/min/mm Hg) versus body length (cm). Individual data for subjects with chronic lung disease of infancy *(CLDI) (red circles)* and control subjects *(blue squares)* are presented, as well as the linear regressions for each group. DL_{CO} was significantly lower for subjects with CLDI compared with control subjects when adjusted for body length by analysis of covariance (P = .0004). (Reprinted with permission of the American Thoracic Society. Copyright © 2015 American Thoracic Society. From Balinotti JE, Chakr VC, Tepper RS, et al. Growth of lung parenchyma in infants and toddlers with chronic lung disease of infancy. *Am J Respir Crit Care Med.* 2010;181:1093–1097. The *American Journal of Respiratory and Critical Care Medicine* is an official journal of the American Thoracic Society.)

proliferation and incorporation of fibroblasts into the vessel wall. Some cases of pulmonary hypertension also show evidence of thromboembolism in the lumina of pulmonary vessels.[149] The bronchial arteries in infants with BPD are abnormally prominent, and communications may exist between those arteries and the pulmonary circulation through precapillary collaterals. These systemic-to-pulmonary communications may aggravate the existing pulmonary hypertension. The pulmonary vasculature in infants with BPD is also characterized by enhanced vasoreactivity, as shown by an increased vasoconstrictor response to acute hypoxia.[150,151]

Pulmonary hypertension is commonly diagnosed indirectly by echocardiography and in selected cases directly by cardiac catheterization, which remains the gold standard. Cardiac catheterization also enables the detection of lesions such as pulmonary vein stenosis and systemic-pulmonary collateral vessels. Many therapeutic agents, including inhaled NO and phosphodiesterase inhibitors, have been used in infants with BPD to decrease pulmonary vascular resistance and improve ventilation-perfusion matching, but clear evidence of improved outcome has not been shown. Although results have not been consistent, some studies have shown an improvement in oxygenation during NO administration.[152-154] In animal models, impaired endogenous NO production contributes to the pathogenesis of BPD, and administration of low-dose NO attenuates the effects of interventions causing BPD in these models.[155,156] Early administration of NO in preterm infants with respiratory failure has resulted in reduced incidence of BPD in some studies,[157,158] but these results have not been consistent enough to recommend routine administration of NO in high-risk preterm infants.[159,160] Phosphodiesterase inhibitors are commonly used as a second-line treatment of pulmonary hypertension, with some evidence of hemodynamic improvement with prolonged use.[161]

SYSTEMIC VASCULAR EFFECTS

Systemic hypertension has been described in infants with BPD.[162,163] The mechanism for the systemic hypertension is not entirely clear, but altered systemic vascular structure and function in response to inflammation and oxidative stress are some of the potential pathophysiologic mechanisms. There is also evidence of increased aortic stiffness and abnormal vasomotor tone in infants with severe BPD.[164] A decreased pulmonary vascular clearance of catecholamines was reported in infants with severe BPD and may also contribute to the systemic hypertension observed in some of these patients.[165] The resultant increase in left ventricular afterload may contribute to the left ventricular dysfunction and hypertrophy observed in many of these patients.[166] Right ventricular hypertrophy can also interfere with left ventricular function, contributing to the hypertrophy of the left ventricle.

Left-sided dysfunction seen in infants with BPD can contribute to pulmonary venous congestion, resulting in an increase in pulmonary hypertension and impaired right-sided cardiac function.[167] These abnormalities are not amenable to treatment with conventional pulmonary vasodilators like NO, which may in fact worsen the condition.[168] In long-term studies, prematurity has been associated with higher systolic and diastolic blood pressures in adults.[169] The impact of BPD on longer-term systemic cardiovascular health needs to be further elucidated.[170]

CONCLUSION

With the increasing survival of extremely low gestational age infants, there has been a continued evolution of BPD as a disease process. This has led to key changes in almost all aspects of this disease, including the pathogenesis and pathology of the lung injury, thereby altering its clinical presentation and effect on short-term and long-term pulmonary function. These changes have led to the reexamination of the basic question "How should we define BPD?" so that it better reflects the disease process.

There are increasing efforts to elucidate the normal mechanisms of alveolar and vascular development, which may provide answers to the pathways through which various antenatal and postnatal factors interfere with normal lung development.[171] This knowledge can potentially help us better delineate the type of lung injury and develop specific prevention and treatment strategies for individual patients.

A complete reference list is available at www.ExpertConsult.com. 

SELECT REFERENCES

1. Northway Jr WH, Rosan RC, Porter DY. Pulmonary disease following respirator therapy of hyaline-membrane disease. Bronchopulmonary dysplasia. *N Engl J Med*. 1967;76(7):357-368.
2. Coalson JJ. Pathology of bronchopulmonary dysplasia. *Semin Perinatol*. 2006;30(4):179-184.
3. Travers CP, et al. Mortality and pulmonary outcomes of extremely preterm infants exposed to antenatal corticosteroids. *Am J Obstet Gynecol*. 2018;218(1):130.e1-130.e13.
4. Morrow LA, et al. Antenatal determinants of bronchopulmonary dysplasia and late respiratory disease in preterm infants. *Am J Respir Crit Care Med*. 2017;196(3):364-374.
5. Wongtrakool C, et al. Nicotine alters lung branching morphogenesis through the alpha7 nicotinic acetylcholine receptor. *Am J Physiol Lung Cell Mol Physiol*. 2007;293(3):L611-L618.
6. McEvoy CT, Spindel ER. Pulmonary effects of maternal smoking on the fetus and child: effects on lung development, respiratory morbidities, and life long lung health. *Paediatr Respir Rev*. 2017;21:27-33.
7. Kuniyoshi KM, Rehan VK. The impact of perinatal nicotine exposure on fetal lung development and subsequent respiratory morbidity. *Birth Defects Res*. 2019;111(17):1270-1283.
8. Stenmark KR, Abman SH. Lung vascular development: implications for the pathogenesis of bronchopulmonary dysplasia. *Annu Rev Physiol*. 2005;67:623-661.

9. Mestan KK, et al. Cord blood biomarkers of placental maternal vascular underperfusion predict bronchopulmonary dysplasia-associated pulmonary hypertension. *J Pediatr*. 2017;185:33-41.
10. Tang JR, et al. Excess soluble vascular endothelial growth factor receptor-1 in amniotic fluid impairs lung growth in rats: linking preeclampsia with bronchopulmonary dysplasia. *Am J Physiol Lung Cell Mol Physiol*. 2012;302(1):L36-L46.
11. Torchin H, et al. Placental complications and bronchopulmonary dysplasia: EPIPAGE-2 cohort study. *Pediatrics*. 2016;137(3):e20152163.
12. Sehgal A, et al. Preterm growth restriction and bronchopulmonary dysplasia: the vascular hypothesis and related physiology. *J Physiol*. 2019;597(4):1209-1220.
13. Abman SH. Bronchopulmonary dysplasia: "a vascular hypothesis." *Am J Respir Crit Care Med*. 2001;164(10 Pt 1):1755-1756.
14. Thebaud B. Abman SH, Bronchopulmonary dysplasia: where have all the vessels gone? Roles of angiogenic growth factors in chronic lung disease. *Am J Respir Crit Care Med*. 2007;175(10):978-985.
15. Kramer BW, et al. Prenatal inflammation and lung development. *Semin Fetal Neonatal Med*. 2009;14(1):2-7.
16. Novy MJ, et al. Ureaplasma parvum or Mycoplasma hominis as sole pathogens cause chorioamnionitis, preterm delivery, and fetal pneumonia in rhesus macaques. *Reprod Sci*. 2009;16(1):56-70.
17. Willet KE, et al. Intra-amniotic injection of IL-1 induces inflammation and maturation in fetal sheep lung. *Am J Physiol Lung Cell Mol Physiol*. 2002;282(3): L411-L420.
18. Kuypers E, et al. Intra-amniotic LPS and antenatal betamethasone: inflammation and maturation in preterm lamb lungs. *Am J Physiol Lung Cell Mol Physiol*. 2012;302(4):L380-L389.
19. Kallapur SG, et al. Fetal immune response to chorioamnionitis. *Semin Reprod Med*. 2014;32(1):56-67.
20. Villamor-Martinez E, et al. Association of chorioamnionitis with bronchopulmonary dysplasia among preterm infants: a systematic review, meta-analysis, and metaregression. *JAMA Netw Open*. 2019;2(11):e1914611.
21. Hartling L, Liang Y, Lacaze-Masmonteil T. Chorioamnionitis as a risk factor for bronchopulmonary dysplasia: a systematic review and meta-analysis. *Arch Dis Child Fetal Neonatal Ed*. 2012;97(1):F8-f17.
22. Nasef N, et al. Effect of clinical and histological chorioamnionitis on the outcome of preterm infants. *Am J Perinatol*. 2013;30(1):59-68.
23. Bjorklund LJ, et al. Manual ventilation with a few large breaths at birth compromises the therapeutic effect of subsequent surfactant replacement in immature lambs. *Pediatr Res*. 1997;42(3):348-355.
24. Hillman NH, et al. Brief, large tidal volume ventilation initiates lung injury and a systemic response in fetal sheep. *Am J Respir Crit Care Med*. 2007;176(6):575-581.
25. Hillman NH, et al. Inflammation and lung maturation from stretch injury in preterm fetal sheep. *Am J Physiol Lung Cell Mol Physiol*. 2011;300(2):L232-L241.
26. Kneyber MC, Zhang H, Slutsky AS. Ventilator-induced lung injury. Similarity and differences between children and adults. *Am J Respir Crit Care Med*. 2014;190(3):258-265.
27. Perez M, et al. Oxygen radical disease in the newborn, revisited: oxidative stress and disease in the newborn period. *Free Radic Biol Med*. 2019;142:61-72.
28. Saugstad OD, et al. Oxygen therapy of the newborn from molecular understanding to clinical practice. *Pediatr Res*. 2019;85(1):20-29.
29. Clyman RI. Patent ductus arteriosus, its treatments, and the risks of pulmonary morbidity. *Semin Perinatol*. 2018;42(4):235-242.
30. Gerhardt T. Bancalari E Lung compliance in newborns with patent ductus arteriosus before and after surgical ligation. *Biol Neonate*. 1980;38(1-2):96-105.
31. McCurnin D, et al. Ibuprofen-induced patent ductus arteriosus closure: physiologic, histologic, and biochemical effects on the premature lung. *Pediatrics*. 2008;121(5):945-956.
32. Gonzalez A, et al. Influence of infection on patent ductus arteriosus and chronic lung disease in premature infants weighing 1000 grams or less. *J Pediatr*. 1996;128(4):470-478.
33. Shahzad T, et al. Pathogenesis of bronchopulmonary dysplasia: when inflammation meets organ development. *Mol Cell Pediatr*. 2016;3(1):23.
34. Viscardi RM, et al. Antenatal Ureaplasma urealyticum respiratory tract infection stimulates proinflammatory, profibrotic responses in the preterm baboon lung. *Pediatr Res*. 2006;60(2):141-146.
35. Bose CL, et al. Systemic inflammation associated with mechanical ventilation among extremely preterm infants. *Cytokine*. 2013;61(1):315-322.
36. Buczynski BW, Maduekwe ET, O'Reilly MA. The role of hyperoxia in the pathogenesis of experimental BPD. *Semin Perinatol*. 2013;37(2):69-78.
37. Saugstad OD. Oxygen and oxidative stress in bronchopulmonary dysplasia. *J Perinat Med*. 2010;38(6):571-577.
38. Kelly MS, et al. Postnatal Cytomegalovirus infection and the risk for bronchopulmonary dysplasia. *JAMA Pediatr*. 2015;169(12):e153785.
39. Jonsson B, et al. Early increase of TNF alpha and IL-6 in tracheobronchial aspirate fluid indicator of subsequent chronic lung disease in preterm infants. *Arch Dis Child Fetal Neonatal Ed*. 1997;77(3):F198-F201.
40. Groneck P, et al. Association of pulmonary inflammation and increased microvascular permeability during the development of bronchopulmonary dysplasia: a sequential analysis of inflammatory mediators in respiratory fluids of high-risk preterm neonates. *Pediatrics*. 1994;93(5):712-718.
41. Speer CP. Pulmonary inflammation and bronchopulmonary dysplasia. *J Perinatol*. 2006;26(suppl 1):S57-S62; discussion S63-S64.
42. Leroy S, et al. A time-based analysis of inflammation in infants at risk of bronchopulmonary dysplasia. *J Pediatr*. 2018;192:60-65.e1.
43. Desai TJ, Cardoso WV. Growth factors in lung development and disease: friends or foe? *Respir Res*. 2002;3:2.
44. Alejandre-Alcazar MA, et al. TGF-beta signaling is dynamically regulated during the alveolarization of rodent and human lungs. *Dev Dyn*. 2008;237(1):259-269.
45. Kotecha S, et al. Increase in the concentration of transforming growth factor beta-1 in bronchoalveolar lavage fluid before development of chronic lung disease of prematurity. *J Pediatr*. 1996;128(4):464-469.
46. Alejandre-Alcazar MA, et al. Hyperoxia modulates TGF-beta/BMP signaling in a mouse model of bronchopulmonary dysplasia. *Am J Physiol Lung Cell Mol Physiol*. 2007;292(2):L537-L549.
47. Levesque BM, et al. Low urine vascular endothelial growth factor levels are associated with mechanical ventilation, bronchopulmonary dysplasia and retinopathy of prematurity. *Neonatology*. 2013;104(1):56-64.
48. Danopoulos S, Shiosaki J, Al Alam D. FGF signaling in lung development and disease: human versus mouse. *Front Genet*. 2019;10:170.
49. Fernandes-Silva H, Correia-Pinto J, Moura RS. Canonical sonic hedgehog signaling in early lung development. *J Dev Biol*. 2017;5(1).
50. Popova AP, et al. Reduced platelet-derived growth factor receptor expression is a primary feature of human bronchopulmonary dysplasia. *Am J Physiol Lung Cell Mol Physiol*. 2014;307(3):L231-L239.

160 Pathophysiology of Ventilator-Dependent Infants

Howard B. Panitch

GENERAL CONSIDERATIONS

The respiratory system comprises an organ for gas exchange (the lung) and structures that move air into the lung (the respiratory pump). The lung includes the airways, alveoli, and blood vessels. The respiratory pump contains the respiratory muscles, the central nervous system and peripheral chemoreceptors that modulate pump output, and the structural tissues of the chest wall, including the ribs, cartilage, spine, and abdominal wall. Successful gas exchange requires the output of the respiratory pump to equal or exceed the load placed upon it by the lung and chest wall. Thus, respiratory failure occurs when the pump,

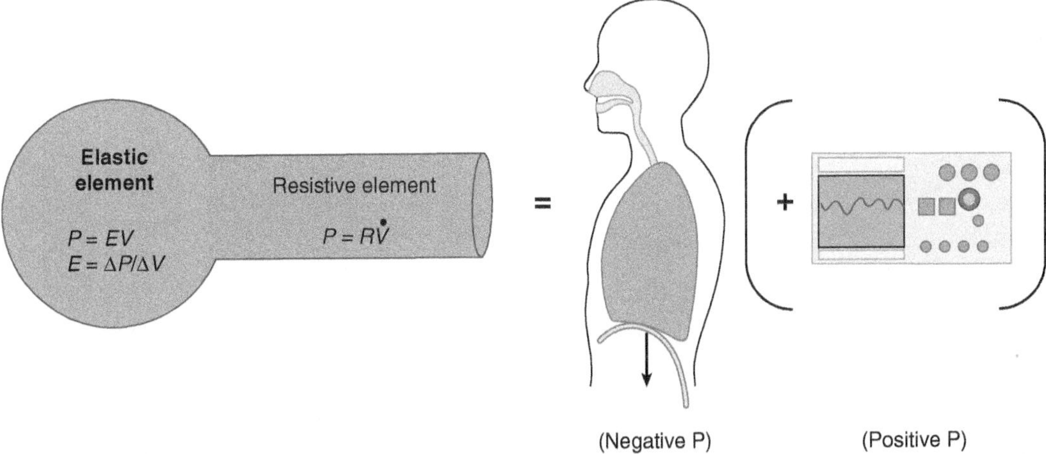

Fig. 160.1 Graphic depiction of the series elastic-resistive model of the respiratory system upon which the equation of motion of the respiratory system is based. The respiratory muscles (together with a mechanical ventilator in the case of a ventilator-assisted individual) must generate enough pressure to overcome resistive forces of moving air through the airways and forces related to stretching the elastic elements of the lung for ventilation to occur. The pressure cost of overcoming the resistive component is proportional to the flow through the airways, and the pressure needed to stretch the elastic elements is determined by the elastance of the tissues and the magnitude of the desired volume change. Respiratory muscles exert a negative pressure while positive pressure ventilators apply positive pressure; therefore accurate measurement of the necessary pressure to move air requires that the ventilator or the respiratory muscles be at rest for the measurement.

the lung itself, or both become dysfunctional. When respiratory pump output is insufficient for the imposed load, the primary gas exchange abnormality will be hypercapnia. However, if the partial pressure of arterial carbon dioxide ($Paco_2$) becomes high enough, hypoxemia will also occur. Alternatively, when the major problem involves the lung parenchyma, the resulting blood gas abnormality typically is hypoxemia.[1]

For purposes of understanding the forces involved in breathing, the respiratory system can be modeled as an elastic element (lung parenchyma) and a resistive element (airways) in series with each other. This model can be likened to a balloon attached to a straw (Fig. 160.1). A tissue's compliance (ΔV/ΔP) describes how easily it can be stretched for a given pressure change. The reciprocal of compliance, or elastance (E), describes how much a tissue withstands being stretched. Greater pressure must be applied to a balloon with high elastance compared with one with lower elastance to expand it, and the applied pressure will also be proportional to the desired volume change above the resting volume. Pressure must also be applied to the system to move air through the straw. The amount of pressure necessary to generate flow will be directly related both to how quickly air flows through the straw and to the resistance of the straw itself.

In the lung, therefore, the pressures required to move air into the alveoli include the pressure necessary to stretch the lung and chest wall above their resting volumes, described by the respiratory system's elastance, and the pressure necessary to overcome the resistance forces associated with flow through the airways. A third pressure that must be overcome relates to the cost of accelerating the gas through the airways *(inertance)*, but at normal respiratory rates this value is quite small and can be ignored. However, under conditions of high-frequency ventilation, the inertance pressure will predominate. When breathing at respiratory rates of less than 100 breaths/min, the forces involved with breathing can be described by a simplified *equation of motion of the respiratory system:*

$$\text{Pmus} = \text{EV} + \text{R}\dot{\text{V}} \qquad [160.1]$$

Or

$$\text{Pmus} = (1/\text{C})\text{V} + \text{R}\dot{\text{V}}$$

where Pmus is the total pressure that must be developed by the respiratory muscles, E is the respiratory system elastance (or 1/compliance), V is the volume to be moved, R is the airway resistance, and $\dot{V}$ is flow.

When the equation of motion is applied to patients supported by mechanical ventilation, special considerations must be recognized. The pressure generated to create adequate movement of gas for ventilation now represents a combination of pressures from the muscles (Pmus) that lower intrapleural pressure and positive pressure from the ventilator (Pvent) applied directly to the airway:

$$\text{Pmus} + \text{Pvent} = \text{EV} + \text{R}\dot{\text{V}} \qquad [160.2]$$

Although both pressures work on the respiratory system to expand the lungs, they do so in opposite directions. Thus to measure pressure exerted during mechanical ventilation based on the readings from a ventilator accurately, Pmus must equal zero; that is, the patient should be relaxed or paralyzed and not contribute to the breathing effort. In addition, the changes in pressure, flow, and volume considered are referenced to end-expiratory conditions (e.g., not to atmospheric pressure but to positive end-expiratory pressure [PEEP]). When the only pressure applied to the respiratory system comes from the ventilator, then inferences about respiratory system mechanics can be made using data from the ventilator's pressure and flow sensors. It is also important to recognize that resistance of the endotracheal tube contributes to the resistance of the airways. If the endotracheal tube is small relative to the infant's natural airway, it can become the predominant resistance in the system.

The two points used to calculate the pressure cost of breathing reflect only those structures between them. For instance, when an esophageal balloon is inserted to estimate pleural pressure and the pressure difference is measured between airway opening pressure and pleural pressure, the derived pressure is the *transpulmonary pressure*.[2] This includes pressure applied to the airways and lung parenchyma, and any mechanics measurements derived from these pressures will reflect the properties of the lung (i.e., lung compliance [C_L] or resistance [R_L]). If, however, the pressures are measured at the airway opening and at the body surface (as is usually done for patients supported by positive pressure ventilation), the intervening structures will include the chest wall in addition to the airways (including the artificial airway) and lung parenchyma, so that the resulting applied pressures will relate to respiratory system mechanics (i.e.,

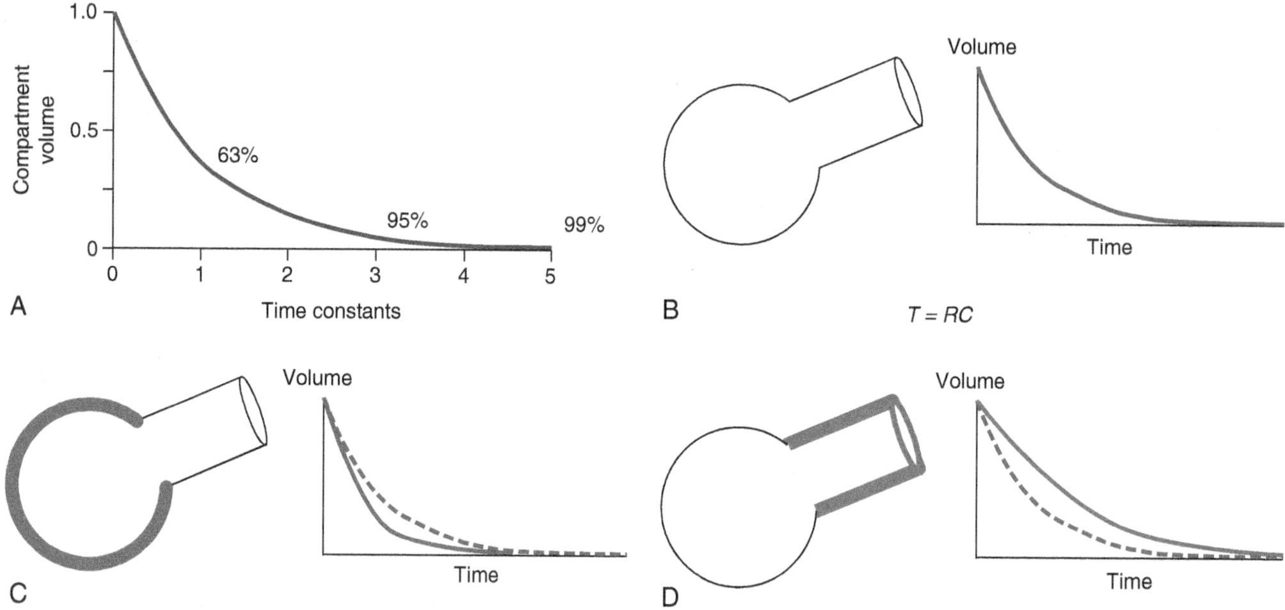

Fig. 160.2 (A) A time constant reflects the amount of time required for a compartment to empty or fill. The illustration reflects emptying of a compartment. One time constant results in a 63% decrease from the original volume, three time constants result in a 95% decrease, and five time constants result in a 99% decrease. (B) In the lung, a time constant is the product of a unit's resistance and compliance ($T = RC$). (C) A decrease in compliance results in a shorter time constant and faster emptying. (D) An increase in resistance results in a longer time constant and slower emptying.

respiratory system compliance [C_{RS}] or resistance [R_{RS}]). Because the chest wall is normally much more compliant than the lung in neonates, its addition to these calculations does not greatly alter the necessary applied pressure. However, that assumption is obviated if the chest wall becomes abnormally stiff, as it does in infants with anasarca or marked abdominal distension. If the pressure transducer of the ventilator, which is used to measure airway opening pressure, is housed within the body of the ventilator instead of at the patient's Y-piece, then the compliance and resistance of the ventilator circuit will also become a part of the measurements.

The same balloon-and-straw model used for the entire respiratory system can be used to describe a single alveolus and the airway that supplies it. The compliance of the balloon and resistance of the associated airway influence how quickly the unit fills and empties with pressure changes. The time required for such a unit to fill or empty following a step-change in pressure is described by its time constant (Fig. 160.2). During exhalation, for example, one time constant represents the time it takes for a unit to empty by 63%; a compartment will empty 95% in three time constants and 99% in five time constants. The time constant of a lung unit can be represented by the equation:

$$\tau = RC$$

where τ is the time constant, R is the resistance of the airway, and C is the compliance of the alveolus. When the characteristics of the lung are regionally uniform, the entire lung can be described by a single τ.[3] When used to describe a phenomenon associated with mechanical ventilation, τ refers to the time course response of the passive respiratory system for either emptying or filling after a step change in pressure. Because $\tau = RC$, the effects of altering resistance or compliance can be anticipated (see Fig. 160.2). If the balloon is made stiffer (compliance decreased, as in fibrosis), the elastic recoil will be greater, and τ will be shorter. However, if the straw is narrowed, the resistance will be greater and τ will be longer.

In conditions in which there are compartments with widely differing time constants, lung compliance will decrease as the respiratory rate increases. This *frequency dependence of compliance* occurs because those units with longer time constants fill and empty at slower rates, and as the frequency increases, they become progressively more distended. In turn, they will compress areas with shorter time constants, making it harder for them to fill. The sum result is a decrease in overall compliance.

Respiratory failure is a common problem for neonates admitted to the neonatal intensive care unit (NICU). Preterm infants often demonstrate abnormalities of parenchymal function because of surfactant deficiency or structural problems such as lung hypoplasia. Term infants can also experience lung parenchymal respiratory failure in the setting of pneumonia, aspiration syndromes, or pulmonary hemorrhage. The neonatal respiratory pump has a limited ability to compensate for an increased load because of its structural and compositional immaturity. When respiratory failure ensues, mechanical ventilation can be life-saving, but often the very modalities used to support adequate gas exchange impose additional damage to airways and lung parenchyma. A brief review of the maturational aspects of the respiratory system is helpful in understanding the neonate's predisposition to respiratory failure and the expected mechanical alterations of the injured lung. This in turn provides a basis for determining the most appropriate type of mechanical ventilatory support to be used.

THE NEONATAL RESPIRATORY PUMP

There are important maturational differences in the structure and function of the neonatal respiratory pump compared with that of the older child or adult. The passive properties of the chest wall, expressed as its compliance, are determined by the stiffness of the rib cage and the tissue-elastic properties of the intercostal and ventral abdominal muscles. An inverse relationship exists between age and chest wall compliance, with a gradual reduction of compliance of the chest wall between birth and 3.5 years of age.[4] Furthermore, a similar relationship exists between gestational age and chest wall compliance, so that the younger the gestational age, the greater the chest wall compliance.[5] Chest wall compliance has been calculated to be three times greater than lung compliance at term, and it remains greater than lung compliance in healthy children beyond the first year of age.[4] This relationship results in a reduction in lung volume at the passive end-expiration lung volume and favors alveolar collapse. When positive pressure is applied to the lung during assisted ventilation, the more compliant chest wall is also less able to protect alveoli from overdistension and injury than a stiff chest wall can.[2,6]

Parenchymal diseases that result in an additional reduction in lung compliance or increase in airway resistance exacerbate the disparity between chest wall and lung compliance. The clinical manifestation of this imbalance is chest wall distortion with sternal retractions and paradoxical movement of the thoracic cage and abdomen. The movement of the thoracic and abdominal compartments relative to each other can be described in terms of their phase angle. When an infant's chest wall and abdomen move in the same direction simultaneously, breathing is synchronous; a phase angle of 0 degrees reflects this synchrony, whereas a phase angle of 180 degrees reflects complete paradoxical motion or "see-saw" breathing.[7] Term infants demonstrate fairly synchronous breathing, whereas preterm infants demonstrate moderate thoracoabdominal asynchrony. To illustrate, a recent study of tidal breathing patterns in preterm and term infants showed that the 18 term infants had a phase angle of 14.0 ± 6.8 degrees compared with a phase angle of 79.1 ± 45.6 degrees among 537 preterm infants born at 26.9 ± 1.4 weeks gestation and studied at 37.5 ± 2 weeks postmenstrual age (PMA).[8] Among the group of preterm infants, there was no difference in phase angles between those who went on to develop bronchopulmonary dysplasia (BPD) and those who did not. In contrast, thoracoabdominal asynchrony was worse in a group of 10 infants with established BPD studied at 49 ± 3.2 weeks PMA, in whom the phase angle was 102 ± 16 degrees, with some infants demonstrating frank paradox.[9] Furthermore, the degree of thoracoabdominal asynchrony correlated directly with pulmonary resistance and inversely with pulmonary compliance.[9] The inward movement of the chest wall during inspiration in such infants results in loss of thoracic volume during each breath, thereby making breathing less efficient. This imposes additional work on the diaphragm: diaphragm displacement is doubled in preterm neonates recovering from respiratory distress syndrome (RDS) in order for them to maintain an adequate tidal volume in the face of a reduction in thoracic volume.[10] Similarly, electrical activity of the diaphragm, which correlates with work of breathing, increases in preterm infants being weaned from nasal continuous positive airway pressure (CPAP) to low flow nasal cannula therapy, and the amplitude of diaphragmatic electromyogram activity is higher in those infants failing such a wean in therapy compared with those who succeed.[11] If chest wall distortion is excessive, hypoventilation and eventual respiratory failure can ensue. Preterm infants subjected to inspiratory resistive loading demonstrate greater thoracoabdominal asynchrony than term infants, and they are unable to maintain tidal volume and minute ventilation under the imposed load.[12]

Anatomic differences related to maturation also place the respiratory pump at a mechanical disadvantage. The shape of the mature thoracic cavity in axial section is elliptical, with a smaller anterior-posterior diameter than lateral diameter. Additionally, the ribs are caudally declined. In the infant, the thorax is more circular, and the ribs are positioned more horizontally.[13] The main function of the intercostal muscles in older children and adults is to elevate the rib cage and increase thoracic volume, whereas in the neonate, intercostal muscle contraction conserves tidal volume by stiffening the chest wall and diminishing chest wall distortion. The anatomic arrangements in the infant limit the potential for thoracic expansion by rib elevation with intercostal contractions, making the infant more reliant on diaphragm function to generate an adequate tidal volume.

There are also critical differences between infants and adults in the relationship of the diaphragm with the chest wall. In the adult, during quiet breathing the diaphragm fibers run parallel with the inner thoracic wall over approximately one-quarter to one-third of the rib cage.[14] Contraction of the diaphragm results not only in a reduction of intrapleural pressure, but also in an increase in intraabdominal pressure through this area of apposition. The increase in abdominal pressure is applied to incompressible abdominal viscera residing within the lower rib cage, and these in turn act as a fulcrum to elevate the lower rib cage within the zone of apposition. In contrast, the infant appears to have less of an area of apposition, with insertion of the diaphragm onto the chest wall at a more acute angle.[15] This arrangement makes the neonatal diaphragm less efficient in expanding the lower rib cage. Additionally, if air trapping occurs because of lung disease, the diaphragm is caudally displaced, and the area of apposition is further reduced: contraction of the diaphragm will reduce rather than expand the lower rib cage (Hoover sign) and compromise tidal volume.

The types of muscle fibers composing the diaphragm and intercostal muscles change throughout gestation and into infancy.[16,17] The proportion of high oxidative or fatigue-resistant muscle fibers is low in preterm infant ventilatory muscles but increases throughout late gestation and through 8 months of age. This suggests that the preterm infant is more prone to develop respiratory muscle fatigue when a load is imposed. However, other studies in nonhuman primates demonstrate that although the fibers of ventilatory muscles undergo maturational changes in a similar time course to those of humans, other fiber types are present that confer high oxidative capacity to the preterm diaphragm and intercostal muscles, making them relatively fatigue resistant.[18,19] These differences may be the result of species differences, alterations in tissue sampling among biopsy or necropsy specimens, or differences in the histochemical techniques used to identify the oxidative capacity of the muscle fibers. However, premature birth alone can interfere with the normal postnatal growth of diaphragm muscle fibers, as evidenced by a decrease in the cross-sectional area of diaphragm muscle fibers 10 days after birth in a preterm baboon model.[18] That lack of continued growth of diaphragm fibers makes the ventilatory muscles less able to meet the demand of spontaneous breathing. In human neonates, as little as 12 days of continuous mechanical ventilation produced marked diaphragmatic atrophy.[20] Older children undergoing mechanical ventilation for acute respiratory failure also demonstrated diaphragmatic atrophy with a 3.4% daily reduction in diaphragm thickness, and the degree of diaphragmatic atrophy was accentuated in those subjects treated with neuromuscular blockade.[21] Thus mechanical ventilation schemes that inhibit spontaneous breathing efforts likely enhance the disruption of normal diaphragm development and promote atrophy.

RESPIRATORY CONTROL

Peripheral chemoreceptor responses to hypoxia, central nervous system chemoreceptor responses to carbon dioxide, and brainstem respiratory rhythmogenesis are all immature in preterm infants. Furthermore, they demonstrate developmental plasticity so that perinatal exposure to hyperoxia or hypoxia can lead to lasting changes in response well beyond the newborn period.[22] Carotid body sensitivity to hyperoxia and hypoxia increases over the first 10 weeks of life in healthy term infants.[23] However, preterm infants of 27 weeks gestational age (range 25 to 32 weeks) who required at least 1 week of mechanical ventilation and supplemental oxygen beyond 28 days of age demonstrated a blunted ventilatory response to hypoxia or hyperoxia at 93 ± 14 days compared with preterm infants of

30 weeks gestational age (range 28 to 36 weeks) who required no supplemental oxygen or mechanical ventilation studied at 38 ± 6 days.[24] Animal models suggest that moderate exposure of the preterm infant to hyperoxia for days to weeks during the period of maturation of the respiratory control system can lead to long-lasting hypoventilation and diminished responses to acute hypoxia.[25] There is also a suggestion that intermittent periods of hypoxia predispose the preterm neonate to episodes of apnea by sensitizing the carotid body chemoreceptor to hypoxia, leading to hyperventilation followed by periods of apnea and respiratory instability on subsequent exposure to hypoxic stimuli.[26,27] Among 37 of 49 preterm infants who failed a physiologic challenge involving a reduction in supplemental oxygen or augmented airflow at 36 weeks PMA, 16 (43.2%) demonstrated an increase in periodic breathing leading to sustained or severe drops in SpO_2, reflecting unstable ventilatory control.[28] Maturational effects on the ventilatory response to hypercapnia are not well understood. However, chronic carbon dioxide retention eventually blunts central drive to hypercapnia; this can, in turn, make the preterm infant with chronic hypercapnia more reliant on already-impaired peripheral chemoreceptors for ventilatory control.[26] This subsequently could lead to episodes of apnea when the infant is exposed to hyperoxia.

PULMONARY PARENCHYMA AND AIRWAYS

The gas exchange region of the lung undergoes significant changes during the latter part of gestation. Respiratory mechanics of an infant born prematurely precariously balance the system between respiratory success and failure as the lungs continue to undergo changes that would otherwise occur in late gestation. Airway resistance is higher,[29] while total lung volume is much lower[30] in the preterm than in the term infant. Over the last trimester, saccules subdivide, causing lung volume to almost triple between 30 and 40 weeks gestation[29]; the growth of the airways proceeds more slowly, in a linear fashion.[31] In a rabbit model, premature birth without any postnatal exposure to positive pressure ventilation or supplemental oxygen results in smaller pups with smaller lungs and lower alveolar surface area, as well as alterations in lung function including decreased dynamic compliance and increased tissue resistance.[32] It is likely that the normal progression of air space development is also altered in infants who survive extremely premature birth even without the development of BPD because the factors that result in premature birth also tend to cause the lung to mature more rapidly.[33,34] The result is a preterm lung with fewer, larger alveoli, thinned air space walls, and increases in the quantity of pulmonary surfactant.

Elastin deposition provides a scaffolding for saccular development[35] so that as the number of saccules increases, the amount of elastin in the lung also increases. The volume of elastin in the lung doubles between 22 and 30 weeks gestation and doubles again over the next 20 weeks.[36] The lower amount of elastin in the saccules and alveolar ducts of the preterm lung predisposes them to overdistension with the application of some positive pressure ventilation strategies.[36] The reduced elastin content also causes the preterm lung to have a lower elastic recoil pressure than the lung of a term infant or child.[37] Elastic recoil pressure (Pel) is the transmural pressure across the alveolus, or alveolar pressure (Palv) minus pleural pressure (Ppl) as in the equation:

$$\text{Pel} = \text{Palv} - \text{Ppl}$$

Lung elastic recoil, along with the outward recoil of the chest wall, provides a tethering effect on small airways that causes them to dilate at a higher lung volume.[38-40] The elastin fibers within the saccule walls create a meshwork that surrounds intraparenchymal airways and creates the structure through which elastic recoil exerts its outward pull on small airways. Because alveolar multiplication is largely a postnatal event, there are fewer alveolar wall attachments on small airways in the preterm lung. Furthermore, perinatal insults can contribute to these developmental alterations; hyperoxia-exposed neonatal mice show a significant reduction in bronchiolar-alveolar attachments in adulthood compared with mice that breathed room air over the first week of life.[41] In addition, the highly compliant neonatal chest wall adds little to the outward traction on airways. Along with the lower elastic recoil of the preterm lung, these issues cause the tethering effect to be less pronounced on preterm small airways, making them less stable and more prone towards closure at lower lung volumes.[42] The tendency for airways to close, combined with the absence of structures like pores of Kohn or canals of Lambert to provide collateral ventilation,[42] increases the risk for atelectasis in the infant lung.

The lung has a tendency to recoil inward, resulting from both its elastic properties and surface tension forces. The presence of surfactant in the newborn minimizes surface tension forces, but the inward tissue forces of the lung remain greater than the outward recoil forces of the highly compliant neonatal chest wall.[4] If left to the passive balance of forces, this combination would result in an equilibrium end-expiratory lung volume that is proportionally lower in infants compared with that of older children and adults. Furthermore, if the neonate were to rely on the balance of these forces to establish the end-expiratory lung volume or functional residual capacity (FRC), airway closure would occur during normal exhalation, and gas exchange would be compromised.[43] Instead, the infant uses several strategies to maintain FRC above the equilibrium resting lung volume. These include adduction of the laryngeal muscles (laryngeal braking), postinspiratory contraction of the inspiratory muscles to slow expiratory flow, and employment of an expiratory time that is shorter than the time it would take the respiratory system to empty.[11,44-48] Endotracheal intubation or tracheostomy placement negates the ability of laryngeal muscles to retard expiratory flow and promotes a decrease in resting lung volume and the development of atelectasis if PEEP is not applied to the airway opening.

AIRWAYS

All preacinar airways are formed by 16 weeks gestation, but the airways continue to undergo structural maturation throughout gestation.[49] Although differentiation of airway structures into muscle and cartilage occurs at an early gestational age, the tissues that comprise the airways continue to undergo changes that result in a marked reduction in airway compliance throughout the latter part of gestation. Cartilage is first identified in the trachea and main bronchi by 10 weeks gestation, and new cartilage continues to appear in more peripheral segmental airways until approximately 25 weeks gestation.[49] The cartilage first appears as precartilage, after which it undergoes transformation to cartilage by deposition of ground substance.[49,50] Thus some of the cartilage present in the more peripheral airways at 25 weeks gestation is still in precartilage form. The consequence of this maturational process is that there is a five-fold reduction in tracheal compliance throughout the last trimester, and the airways continue to stiffen postnatally.[51-54] The mechanical properties of the individual components of the airway wall (i.e., cartilage and smooth muscle) parallel the changes in tracheal compliance, becoming stiffer throughout gestation.[55,56]

As a result of its increased compliance, the preterm trachea is easier to deform when exposed to positive pressure than is a term or adult trachea.[57] Even brief periods of exposure to positive pressure results in a marked increase in resting volume of the extremely immature airway. Furthermore, the degree of deformation is related to the degree and duration of pressure applied.[58] Acquired tracheomegaly has been described in infants 27 ± 0.6 weeks gestation exposed to positive pressure ventilation of 15 to 25 cm H_2O for 25.4 ± 4.9 days.[59] The preterm airway is also more collapsible than more mature airways, and resistance through preterm tracheal segments exposed to modest positive pressure ventilation for as little as 2 hours resulted in a significantly higher resistance through the ventilated segments than through unventilated segments.[60] The highly compliant nature of preterm central airways translates clinically into tracheomalacia or bronchomalacia, especially in premature neonates who go on to develop BPD.[61-65] Although the prevalence of tracheobronchomalacia (TBM) among infants with BPD is not well described, it was found in 36.2% of 974 neonates with BPD who were entered into a multicenter database over a 5-year period and who underwent bronchoscopy.[66]

Therefore the physiologic properties of the extremely preterm airway that has been exposed to mechanical ventilation can affect gas exchange significantly. The increase in size of the airway after it has been deformed increases dead space, and the increased tendency for the airway to collapse on exhalation can lead to prolonged expiratory times and air trapping. Such expiratory events occasionally lead to acute episodes of hypoxemia, cyanosis, and respiratory distress ("BPD spells") and require application or increased amounts of expiratory distending pressure and occasionally sedation or pharmacologic paralysis. The presence of significant TBM also can alter the amount of PEEP used to prevent airway collapse.[67,68] In a retrospective analysis, those BPD infants diagnosed with TBM were found to have a longer and more complicated neonatal course, were more likely to undergo tracheostomy placement, and required a longer course of mechanical ventilation than those with noncollapsible airways.[66] Among 17 infants with BPD who underwent ultrashort echo-time magnetic resonance imaging (MRI) sequence to evaluate their central airways, those with severe BPD (n = 11) had a significantly greater range of airway narrowing compared with those with mild/moderate BPD or controls.[69]

However, the finding of significant central airway collapse in neonates with severe lung disease may not always be a primary abnormality of the central airways. The presence of large airway collapse represents a balance between the intrinsic stiffness of the airway wall and the magnitude of the transmural pressure exerted across the airway wall (Fig. 160.3). Healthy infants, for instance, can narrow the airway by as much as 50% with crying or straining, reflecting an increase in transmural pressure.[70] In contrast, some infants with lung disease will have abnormally compliant airway segments that collapse when transmural pressure is normal or low. However, others can have large airway collapse as a secondary manifestation of small airway obstruction. Elevated peripheral airway resistance not only will accentuate the intraluminal pressure drop from alveolus to mouth, but also will often cause the neonate to use abdominal accessory muscles to exhale forcefully to overcome the obstruction.[70] The resulting lower intraluminal pressure within larger airways and higher pleural pressure occurring from accessory muscle use greatly increases collapsing transmural pressure. Because the neonatal airway is already a highly compliant structure, the resulting applied pressure can cause localized or diffuse central airway collapse. In adults, this phenomenon is referred to as "excessive dynamic airway collapse" (EDAC) and is distinguished from TBM because the cartilaginous rings retain their shape while there is significant invagination of the pars membranacea (posterior membrane); in contrast, TBM refers to collapse of the cartilaginous portion of the airway.[71] However, given the highly compliant nature of neonatal airways, such a distinction can be difficult to make.

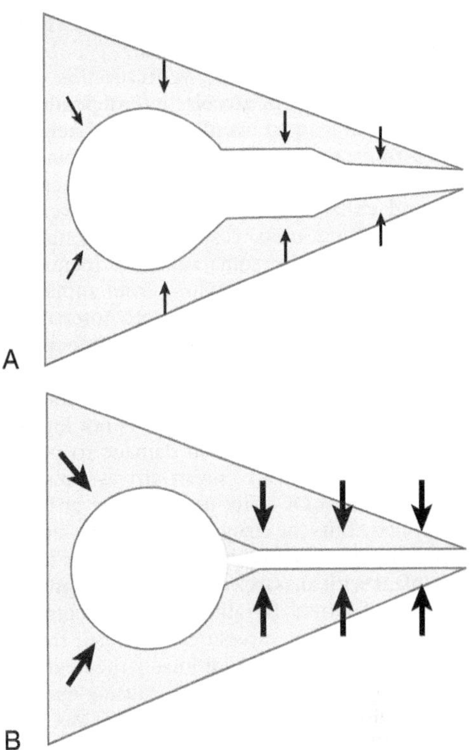

Fig. 160.3 (A) In an infant with tracheomalacia or bronchomalacia, central airway collapse occurs even when collapsing (transmural) pressure is low because of the abnormal compliance of the airway wall. (B) The central airways can appear abnormally collapsible in the presence of peripheral airway obstruction because the infant must exert higher pleural pressures *(heavy arrows)* to overcome the obstruction. Intraluminal pressure also falls more quickly than normal because of resistive losses, accentuating the collapsing transmural pressure across airway walls.

Treatment with distending pressure can reduce airway collapse by at least two mechanisms.[64,72] The pressure applied at the airway opening can redistribute the intraluminal pressure gradient from alveolus to mouth, thereby decreasing transmural pressure across the collapsible segment. Alternately, the distending pressure can raise lung volume, which in turn dilates smaller airways and reduces resistance. This would also serve to decrease transmural pressure and might decrease the need for forceful exhalation.

ACUTE RESPIRATORY FAILURE

Preterm infants with RDS who require mechanical ventilation have surfactant deficiency.[73] Additionally, processes like sepsis or pneumonia can render any surfactant that is present nonfunctional. Thus, in addition to the developmental structural disadvantages noted previously, surface tension forces that are created once an air-liquid interface is established greatly increase elastic recoil pressure and favor alveolar and small airway collapse, especially at end-expiration. The increased recoil pressure presents an increased load to a respiratory pump that cannot compensate for it. Furthermore, surface tension is greater in poorly expanded alveoli and favors collapse of those lung units; in addition, according to the law of Laplace, the poorly expanding lung units will require much higher pressures for expansion. The lungs may also be filled with fluid because of infection or inadequate clearance of fetal lung fluid, further compromising lung inflation.[74-76] The normal FRC cannot be established, and gas exchange is compromised.[77] In this setting, it has long been recognized that continuous distending pressure (CPAP or PEEP) can be used to establish an effective FRC.[78]

In the absence of surfactant, ventilation is regionally inhomogeneous.[79] Because of alveolar interdependence, collapse of some alveoli will lead to overdistension of neighboring lung units. When positive pressure is applied to the airways to facilitate ventilation, the cyclic opening and closing of lung units during inspiration and exhalation and the regional overdistension of more compliant lung units result in iatrogenic lung injury, including barotrauma, volutrauma, and atelectrauma.[80-84]

Barotrauma, or lung injury resulting from application of high airway pressures, results in air leak into interstitial tissues.[85] The clinical result is pneumomediastinum, pneumothorax, and pulmonary interstitial emphysema. In neonates, application of positive pressure also can cause airway deformation and lead to excessive central airway collapse.[57,59] It is not known whether the critical pressure to cause such damage to parenchyma or airways is the peak pressure, mean airway pressure, or end-expiratory pressure.[85] Of note, it is not the absolute positive pressure applied, but the magnitude of the transpulmonary pressure that determines the degree of alveolar distension.[83,85] As such, an infant with anasarca or massive abdominal distension, whose chest wall would be abnormally noncompliant, would tolerate higher inflating pressures because transpulmonary pressure would still be low.[83] Additionally, the degree of regional overdistension is the critical factor in causing air leaks, not the magnitude of airway pressure applied.[83] Thus experimental mechanical ventilation of animals with 45 cm H_2O whose chests and abdomens were strapped to limit the degree of alveolar expansion resulted in protection against epithelial disruption, air leak, or the development of pulmonary edema.[86] In contrast, ventilating animals either with the same high positive pressure and high tidal volume (40 ± 3 mL/kg) or with negative pressure to achieve the same high tidal volume resulted in lung injury with epithelial disruption and pulmonary edema.[86] This type of lung injury resulting from overdistension of lung units has been coined *volutrauma.*

The effect of cyclical overdistension of lungs of adults with acute respiratory distress syndrome (ARDS) on subsequent lung injury and ultimately on mortality was demonstrated first in single-center studies and then in a large multicenter study.[87-89] Outcomes of adults with ARDS who received mechanical ventilation with the traditional approach of supplying tidal volumes of 12 mL/kg of predicted body weight and 50 cm H_2O or less airway pressure after a 0.5-second pause (plateau pressure) were compared with those of patients who received a low tidal volume strategy of 6 mL/kg of predicted body weight and 30 cm H_2O or less plateau pressure; the mortality rate was 22% lower, and there were more ventilator-free days during hospitalization in the low tidal volume group.[87]

The rationale underlying low tidal volume ventilation is that the lung disease in ARDS is heterogeneous and that a substantial proportion of the total lung volume reflects diseased lung. As a consequence, only a small percentage of the lung has relatively normal characteristics. Application of higher pressures or higher set tidal volumes would perhaps not only ventilate diseased areas of the lung, but also overdistend those areas of the lung with more normal compliance and resistance characteristics. Although no similar studies have been conducted in neonates or children, the concept of low tidal volume ventilation using 3 to 6 mL/kg tidal volumes has been widely adopted in the care of neonates with RDS as part of a lung-protective strategy.[90] This adjustment of tidal volume for weight has been further refined, recognizing that all of the lung is not available for ventilation because of regional collapse and overdistension. More recent studies in adults with ARDS have normalized delivered tidal volume to C_{RS}, using the ratio as an index of functional lung size.[91] This ratio yields the "driving pressure" (DP = V_T/C_{RS}), which is also equal to the inspiratory plateau pressure—PEEP. In a multilevel mediation analysis of nine trials of lung protective strategies in adults with ARDS, DP was the variable most strongly associated with survival at 60 days.[91] However, significant differences in biologic and physiologic pulmonary responses to lung stretch exist between infants and adults, making direct extrapolation of adult mechanical ventilation practices to neonates difficult.[90]

In a surfactant-deficient lung, a low volume and pressure ventilation strategy can lead to another type of lung injury when unstable lung units repeatedly collapse and are reopened by positive pressure breaths. Upon reopening, a bubble of air is pushed through the collapsed airway, leading to epithelial sloughing, pulmonary edema formation, and hyaline membranes.[83,92] This form of lung injury has been called *atelectrauma.*[85] In lungs in which marked heterogeneity in time constants exists, the effects of atelectrauma can be magnified. Because of the interdependence of lung units, regions of atelectasis surrounded by a fully expanded lung would be exposed to considerably higher distending pressures. Mead and co-workers estimated that at a transpulmonary pressure of 30 cm H_2O, an atelectatic region surrounded by fully expanded lung would be exposed to a distending pressure of 140 cm H_2O.[93] The deleterious effects of atelectrauma are amplified when volutrauma is also applied to the lung.

A fourth type of lung injury arises from the inflammatory response to mechanical damage of airway and alveolar epithelium, known as *biotrauma.*[80,81,83,94,95] When injurious mechanical ventilation causes necrosis of cells or disruption of epithelial and endothelial barriers without cellular destruction, it can also induce or perpetuate the recruitment of neutrophils and activation of alveolar macrophages.[96] Cellular necrosis causes the direct release of preformed proinflammatory mediators and destructive cellular enzymes. Macrophage activation results in the release of cytokines that in turn stimulate vascular endothelial cells to express vascular adhesion molecules. In response, circulating neutrophils adhere to vascular endothelial cells and transmigrate into alveolar and interstitial spaces. Activated macrophages and neutrophils directly damage epithelial and endothelial cells, as well as matrix glycoproteins like elastin and collagen. Mechanical ventilation that causes disruption of epithelial or endothelial barriers also results in the release of intracellular proinflammatory mediators. However, excessive stretch of lung tissue that does not disrupt plasma membranes also can be injurious by causing activation of signaling cascades for inflammatory mediator release through a process called *mechanotransduction.*[84,96] Mechanical ventilation can also promote the release of inflammatory mediators or transcription factors that result in induction of genes that advance an inflammatory cascade associated with changes in perfusion pressure and vascular shear stress.[84,96] In addition to the physical stimuli related to mechanical ventilation that create inflammatory injury, the use of supplemental oxygen also contributes to lung injury by overproduction of superoxide, hydrogen peroxide, and perhydroxyl radicals. This is especially problematic in preterm infants because antioxidant enzyme levels do not increase until the last 10% to 15% of gestation.[97,98]

MECHANICAL VENTILATION IN ACUTE RESPIRATORY FAILURE

In the surfactant-deficient neonatal lung, surface tension forces are elevated, leading to areas of alveolar collapse. Atelectasis occurs in some areas with overdistension of air spaces in others, and there is increased lung water resulting from retained fetal lung fluid and inflammation.[74-76] Consequently, ventilation becomes regionally heterogeneous.[99] The FRC and lung compliance are reduced.[100-105] Respiratory system resistance is elevated in neonates who require mechanical ventilation,[3,106] but the reduction in lung compliance must be the predominant alteration in mechanics because the time constant of the respiratory system is shorter in infants who require positive pressure ventilation compared with neonates who do not require respiratory support or those supported with CPAP.[3]

CONTINUOUS POSITIVE AIRWAY PRESSURE AND POSITIVE END-EXPIRATORY PRESSURE

Ever since the initial description that application of distending pressure improved oxygenation in neonates with severe RDS,[78] use of CPAP has been a mainstay of therapy for neonates with acute respiratory failure. Application of CPAP or PEEP for infants receiving positive pressure ventilation not only can restore FRC and improve oxygenation, but also can reduce damage resulting from the cyclic opening and closing of lung units when applied at the appropriate pressure.[107,108] It can also lower driving pressure by placing the lung on a more favorable position on its pressure-volume (P-V) curve.[109] The level of PEEP is often arbitrarily set in neonates with RDS and may be more reflective of center practice than of the neonate's physiologic requirement.[110-112] The aim of therapy is to recruit collapsed alveoli without overdistending already-open lung units.[81] Attempts to individualize or determine optimal PEEP or CPAP have used as endpoints measures of homogeneity of ventilation as determined by electrical impedance tomography,[113] an increase in blood oxygenation with or without an accompanying increase in esophageal pressure[114-116] or measures of lung mechanics derived by creating quasistatic P-V relationships of the lung.[117] In children and adults, measures of transpulmonary pressure by esophageal manometry have also been used to calculate driving pressure at different levels of PEEP to establish the best level of distending pressure to minimize lung injury.[2,118]

When a P-V curve is generated with brief pauses in inspiratory and expiratory flow or with extremely low flow rates, then the pressure cost is assumed to relate only to lung stretch and not to frictional resistive forces. Most studies using this technique outside of adults with ARDS have used animals, as the subject is usually pharmacologically paralyzed, must be able to tolerate a prolonged apnea, and is theoretically at greater risk to develop air leak as the lung is inflated to total lung capacity.[119] The point on the inspiratory limb of the P-V curve where the slope abruptly increases has been called the lower inflection point (LIP) and was frequently considered to be the critical pressure at which previously closed alveoli are recruited, making compliance greater above this point (Fig. 160.4).[120] Conversely, the LIP was also initially considered to be the volume below which cyclic closing and reopening of lung units, and therefore atelectrauma, occurs. Thus, investigators have recommended setting PEEP 1 or 2 cm H_2O above the LIP.[121] More recently, investigators have argued that because derecruitment occurs during exhalation, the important pressure about which to set PEEP occurs as a downward inflection on the expiratory quasistatic P-V curve.[122] Lung volume is greater at the expiratory inflection point than at the inspiratory LIP, and the lung requires more inspiratory pressure to achieve the same expiratory volume throughout the inspiratory P-V maneuver; the pressure difference causing this hysteresis is the pressure required to overcome surface tension forces, tissue resistance, and re-expansion of collapsed alveoli.[123] Furthermore, recent investigations have demonstrated that alveolar recruitment in adults with ARDS occurs not only around the LIP, but also throughout the inspiratory P-V curve.[123] Regardless, at volumes greater than the LIP, respiratory system compliance is greatest, so a desired tidal volume can be delivered at lower pressure, thereby minimizing barotrauma. Others have used different measures of lung mechanics that are more readily accomplished at the bedside, like static compliance after an inspiratory hold, to determine the best PEEP.[124,125]

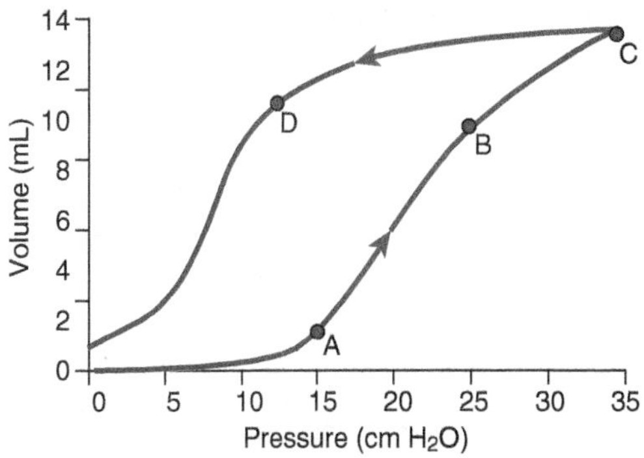

Fig. 160.4 Idealized quasistatic pressure-volume (P-V) curve of the respiratory system. *Arrows* represent direction of pressure change. Point *A* represents the lower inflection point, often considered to be the volume at which the majority of alveolar recruitment occurs; the segment *A-B* represents the portion of the inspiratory P-V curve at which compliance is greatest; point *B* marks the upper inflection point, where compliance decreases, reflecting lung overdistension (segment *B-C*). Point *D* is the expiratory upper inflection point and is considered to be the point below which derecruitment occurs. (From Monkman S, Kirpalani H. PEEP—a "cheap" and effective lung protection. *Paediatr Respir Rev.* 2003;4:15–20.)

Effects of PEEP must be balanced against possible side effects of the therapy, including lung overdistension with increases in air leak,[126,127] decreased cardiac venous return, reduction of lymphatic drainage with development of pulmonary edema,[128,129] and increased right ventricular afterload.[126,130,131] The lung disease in RDS is not homogeneous, and not all lung units may be recruitable.[132] Application of excessive PEEP in such circumstances will overdistend more normal lung units without necessarily recruiting more diseased areas of the lung.

INSPIRATORY TIME

Although ventilation has been shown to be regionally heterogeneous in the RDS lung,[79,99,133] regional time constants (ventral vs. dorsal regions) were not markedly different from each other in preterm infants with RDS studied within 72 hours of birth and before exogenous surfactant administration.[134] Similarly, a single time constant can be used to describe the respiratory system of most neonates with RDS,[3,134] which both fills and empties quickly in the presence of surfactant deficiency. The inspiratory time constant of a neonate with RDS is approximately 0.05 seconds, whereas that of a normal neonate is 0.25 seconds.[135] As a result, the recommendation for ventilation of neonates with acute respiratory failure is to use a short (0.25 to 0.4 seconds) inspiratory time[112,136]; even at a high mandatory rate set on the ventilator (e.g., 60 breaths/min), an inspiratory time of 0.3 seconds allows for enough expiratory time (0.7 seconds in this example) for the lung to empty by at least three time constants, or by 95%. Excessively long inspiratory times can cause active exhalation during inspiration and other types of patient-ventilator asynchrony.[137] A meta-analysis of five studies involving 694 neonates with acute respiratory failure compared long (0.66 to 2.0 seconds) versus short (0.33 to 1.0 seconds) inspiratory times and demonstrated a significantly increased risk for pulmonary air leak (relative risk [RR], 1.56 [95% confidence interval (CI), 1.25 to 1.94]; number needed to treat [NNT], 8 [95% CI, 5 to 14]) and a borderline statistically significant increase in mortality before discharge (RR, 1.26 [95% CI, 1.00 to 1.59]) among infants receiving long inspiratory times.[135] The long inspiratory time in a lung with short time constants will cause overdistension of more compliant lung units. If the set ventilator rate is high relative to the long inspiratory time so that there is inadequate time for the lung to empty fully during the expiratory phase, dynamic hyperinflation can occur and will be another cause of overdistension.[138]

TIDAL VOLUME

Neonates with respiratory failure have some lung units that do not participate in gas exchange. Until those units are recruited, the volume of lung available for ventilation will be less than normal, and any additional volume applied to the lung will overdistend more normal lung units. If the lung becomes overstretched as it is distended during application of a tidal volume, there will be an abrupt reduction in compliance that appears as a sudden decrease in the slope of the P-V curve (Fig. 160.5). This upper inflection point or "beaking" of the tidal volume P-V loop marks the development of lung overdistension, or *volutrauma*. Its presence can be quantified by comparing the compliance over the last 20% of the tidal volume (C_{20}) with the total compliance over the entire breath (C): a C_{20}/C ratio of less than 0.8 denotes overdistension, whereas a ratio of more than 1.0 reflects a normal P-V loop.[139]

The concept that the pathophysiologic processes present in ARDS lead to a marked reduction in normally aerated lung, coined *baby lung*,[140] was the impetus for adopting the low tidal volume strategy of 6 mL/kg in ARDS.[87,88] A similar strategy has been adopted for neonates with RDS, for whom tidal volumes of 3 to 6 mL/kg are recommended.[136] However, too small a tidal volume is deleterious. In a study of 30 preterm infants with RDS ventilated with tidal volumes of either 5 mL/kg (n = 15) or 3 mL/kg (n = 15), evidence of pulmonary inflammation, reflected in levels of interleukin-8 and tumor necrosis factor-α in tracheal aspirates at 7 days of age, was greater in the infants receiving the smaller tidal volumes.[141] The infants receiving 3 mL/kg tidal volumes also required significantly longer (16.8 ± 4 vs. 9.2 ± 4 days, P = .05) duration of mechanical ventilation. The authors speculated that the 3-mL/kg strategy did not allow for adequate lung recruitment in the acute phase of RDS, leading to more atelectrauma.

Instrumentation can also affect the size of the tidal volume chosen, especially in extremely low-birth-weight infants, as the fixed dead space of the flow sensor used in flow-triggered ventilation adds substantially to the overall dead space. A retrospective analysis of tidal volumes, calculated dead space, and $Paco_2$ values in 47 preterm infants weighing less than 800 g within the first 2 days of life who were mechanically ventilated for RDS showed an inverse relationship between birth weight and the tidal volume per kg of body weight (V_T/kg) required for normocapnia.[142] Those infants with a birth weight of 500 g or less required a V_T/kg of 5.92 ± 0.30 mL compared with those infants with a birth weight of 700 g or more, who required a V_T/kg of 4.69 ± 0.45 mL (P < .001). The authors reasoned that this relationship reflected the effect of the fixed instrumental dead space.

The earliest positive pressure ventilators used to support neonates provided a large preset tidal volume at low rates. Subsequently, neonatal ventilators were made that delivered machine-triggered, time-cycled, and pressure-controlled breaths with no servo-mechanisms to monitor the delivered tidal volume.[137] The advent of microprocessor technology allowed for better monitoring of patient-ventilator interactions and the use of volume-targeted ventilation in neonates. As a result, investigators have questioned whether volume-targeted ventilation is superior to pressure-limited ventilation in neonates with RDS.[143,144] The rationale is that pressure-limited ventilation could result in lung overdistension as compliance or resistance improves, as endotracheal tube leak changes, or as the neonate's contribution to a delivered breath changes.[145] Several studies have been conducted addressing this question, and a recent meta-analysis of 16 randomized parallel trials and 4 crossover trials involving 977 and 88 infants, respectively, concluded that volume-targeted ventilation was associated with a reduction in the combined

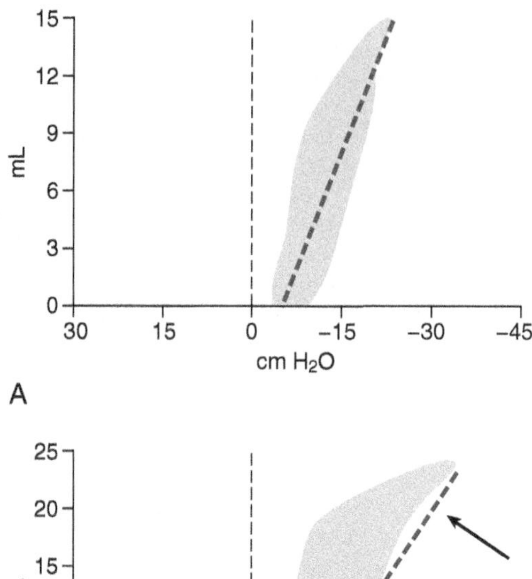

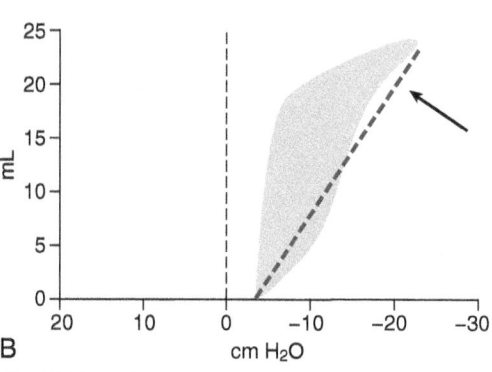

Fig. 160.5 (A) Normal pressure-volume (P-V) curve in a neonate requiring positive pressure ventilation. (B) "Beaking" of the P–V curve, reflecting overdistension during a tidal breath of another infant receiving positive pressure ventilation. The *dotted lines* represent lung compliance over the entire breath. (From Fisher JB, Mammel MC, Coleman JM, et al. Identifying lung overdistention during mechanical ventilation by using volume-pressure loops. *Pediatr Pulmonol.* 1988;5:10–14.)

outcome of death or BPD at 36 weeks PMA (typical RR, 0.73 [95% CI, 0.59 to 0.89]; NNT, 8 [95% CI, 5 to 20]), incidence of pneumothorax (typical RR, 0.52 [95% CI, 0.31 to 0.87]; NNT, 20 [95% CI, 12 to 100]), and hypocarbia ($Paco_2$ < 35 torr) (typical RR, 0.49 [95% CI, 0.33 to 0.72]; NNT, 3 [95% CI, 2 to 5]), among other important outcomes.[146] There was no difference between the two modalities in the primary outcome, which was death before hospital discharge. However, there are different ways in which ventilators target and adjust for alterations in the delivered tidal volume, by monitoring either the inflation tidal volume or the exhaled tidal volume.[145] Each has its strengths and weaknesses, and to date there are no studies that demonstrate the superiority of one method of volume targeting over others.

CHRONIC RESPIRATORY FAILURE

Most neonates with acute respiratory failure from RDS or pneumonia recover after several days and can be weaned from mechanical ventilation. However, depending on gestational age, as many as 40% to 55% develop BPD[147] and those with the most severe disease will continue to require mechanical ventilatory support for weeks to months. A review of registry data from 18 centers in the Neonatal Research Network showed that among 2677 neonates born at less than 32 weeks' gestation who survived to 36 weeks PMA, 9% continued to require mechanical ventilation at 36 weeks PMA.[148]

Several investigators have measured lung mechanics in ventilator-dependent infants who then go on to develop severe BPD, both before and after the era of surfactant and prenatal steroid administration. Although there is not complete concordance among studies, several have demonstrated that lung or respiratory system resistance is elevated within the first 2 weeks of life among ventilator-dependent infants who go on to develop BPD compared with those who do not.[149-153] Others have demonstrated a reduction in lung or respiratory system compliance.[149,150,153,154] Whether or not such abnormal mechanics predict the development of BPD, the described alterations in elastic and resistive properties of the lung affect the way in which the lung fills and empties. The respiratory system time constant (τ_{RS}) of 24 infants who were mechanically ventilated for 38 ± 4 days and then developed BPD increased from 0.14 ± 0.01 seconds at 10 to 20 days of life to 0.33 ± 0.02 seconds at 6 months, 0.48 ± 0.03 seconds at 1 year, and 0.50 ± 0.03 seconds at 2 years ($P < .0001$).[149] In another study, the passive flow-volume curve of six ventilator-dependent infants at 26 ± 16 days was curvilinear towards the volume axis rather than straight, suggesting that there was regional heterogeneity of time constants and that the lung no longer emptied as a single compartment.[155] These authors modeled the lungs into a two-compartment model, with a faster, more normal emptying compartment and a second slower one. These findings likely reflect the obstructive lung disease and air trapping that occurs in infants with BPD. In fact, when lung volumes are determined by dilutional methods in infants with BPD, values often are lower than normal in the first 6 months of life but become greater than normal by 1 year of age.[149,150] This is because dilutional methods detect only lung units that are in communication with the airway opening. When both dilutional and plethysmographic methods are used to measure lung volume, the plethysmographic method is significantly greater[156]; this is because the plethysmographic method measures both lung units in communication with the airway opening and those that are obstructed; the difference between the two techniques reflects the amount of gas trapping. Ultrashort echo time pulmonary MRI of neonates with BPD at 35 to 42 weeks PMA demonstrated hyperinflation that increased with the increasing severity of BPD.[157]

The hallmark of the BPD lung in the postsurfactant era is alveolar simplification, with fewer and larger air spaces and less septal fibrosis than was noted in classic BPD.[158] However, the few studies that examined the effect of mechanical ventilation on the conducting airways demonstrate that they are also affected in these infants. Within the first month of life, airway smooth muscle of the central airways in BPD infants was increased,[159] and in BPD infants 33 weeks to 22 months of age, both central and peripheral airway smooth muscle was increased compared with age-matched infants who died of sudden infant death syndrome.[160] In that study, peripheral airway epithelium of BPD infants was intact, but its height was considerably greater than that of controls, further reducing airway lumen size. Experimentally, even brief periods of mechanical ventilation during the canalicular period can induce persistent increases in epithelial height, airway smooth muscle hypertrophy, and collagen deposition in peripheral airway walls.[161] The combination of thickened airway walls and smooth muscle hypertrophy, together with fewer alveolar wall attachments because of alveolar simplification, contributes to airway narrowing, increased airway resistance, regionally heterogeneous ventilation with prolonged time constants of lung units, and air trapping.

MECHANICAL VENTILATION IN CHRONIC RESPIRATORY FAILURE

There are no studies that examine the best way to mechanically ventilate newborn infants who develop chronic respiratory failure. However, the alterations in mechanics and histopathology of the lung noted previously offer an insight into why authors suggest that these infants should be supported with lower mandatory rates, longer inspiratory times, and larger tidal volumes.[136,162]

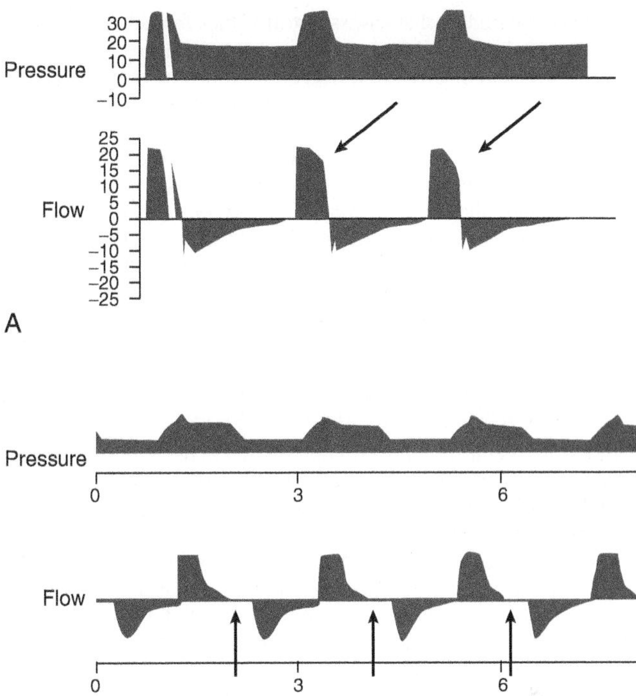

Fig. 160.6 (A) Truncated inspiratory flow *(arrow)* in a patient receiving an inspiratory time of 0.55 second to facilitate adequate expiratory time. (B) Prolonged inspiratory time (0.9 second) in an infant with bronchopulmonary dysplasia undergoing mechanics measurements, resulting in a period of lung inflation without flow *(arrow)*.

INSPIRATORY TIME

Because of regional heterogeneity and the longer time constant of the respiratory system in infants with BPD, it will take longer to fill the lung. Short inspiratory times will preferentially ventilate lung units with short time constants, whereas those units with longer time constants will not have the opportunity to fill and will contribute to the physiologic dead space. This will result in worsening hypercapnia and will also promote a rapid shallow breathing pattern that can lead to dynamic hyperinflation as the expiratory time becomes too short for adequate emptying. BPD infants with chronic respiratory failure typically require an inspiratory time of 0.6 to 0.9 seconds to maximize ventilation. The flow-time tracing presented as part of the ventilator graphics package can guide the practitioner in determining whether the inspiratory time is too short (truncated flow) or too long (a period of 0 flow appears before the ventilator cycles to exhalation) (Fig. 160.6).

TIDAL VOLUME

At some time in the first month of life, as the inflammatory processes that were present at birth subside and the reparative phase of BPD begins, the infant requires a larger tidal volume, in the order of 8 to 12 mL/kg. This not only allows for more efficient ventilation as the dead space–tidal volume ratio decreases, but also it allows the infant to breathe at a slower rate and to allow more time for emptying to avoid dynamic hyperinflation. The size of the tidal volume breath is occasionally limited by the pressure required to achieve it, as some practitioners set arbitrary limits as to the peak pressure they will tolerate. Because of air trapping or hyperinflation, the infant with chronic respiratory failure may be breathing at the flat upper end of the lung P-V curve, so that small volume changes require considerably more pressure. However, there are no studies that assess cutoff values for peak or plateau pressures in infants with chronic respiratory failure.

With the advent of patient-triggered modes of ventilation like pressure support, the rate of mandatory breaths can be set fairly low so that the infant can have more control over the respiratory pattern. Whether the mandatory rate is used to provide occasional "sigh" breaths or is set at a rate that dictates the breathing pattern, there must be adequate expiratory time to allow for complete emptying. This requires three to five time constants, or an expiratory time of approximately 2 to 3 seconds. This means that the tidal volume must be set high enough to accomplish an adequate minute ventilation, usually at a respiratory rate of less than 30 breaths/min.

POSITIVE END-EXPIRATORY PRESSURE OR CONTINUOUS POSITIVE AIRWAY PRESSURE

There are several pathophysiologic issues that might dictate the baseline level of distending pressure required. A slightly higher end-distending pressure than used in the newborn with acute respiratory failure will increase elastic recoil and can help reduce some of the small airway obstruction present in BPD infants. However, there are few trials that assess different levels of PEEP in BPD infants.[110] Some infants with BPD develop tracheomalacia or bronchomalacia and require higher levels of distending pressure to maintain airway patency and to promote adequate emptying.[61,64,67,72] Whether the application of distending pressure works by stenting the airway open[64,67] or by raising lung volume[72] is not entirely clear, but often the magnitude of pressure required to maintain airway patency is much greater than that required to maintain an appropriate FRC, with the result of causing significant overdistension in an effort to eliminate or ameliorate acute obstructive events (BPD spells).

Occasionally, the combination of a BPD infant's respiratory mechanics and his respiratory drive result in inadequate emptying time, and the infant develops dynamic hyperinflation and intrinsic PEEP (PEEPi or autoPEEP).[163] Dynamic hyperinflation can be readily identified using the flow-time tracing on the ventilator graphic menu and is present when expiratory flow does not reach zero before the next breath is delivered.[164] PEEPi can be detected by imposing an expiratory hold; that is, manually keeping the expiratory valve open for 3 or 4 seconds in an infant who is paralyzed or heavily sedated and not making inspiratory efforts (Fig. 160.7). If PEEPi is present, the baseline pressure will increase by the amount of PEEPi.[165] In nonparalyzed infants, esophageal manometry can be used to identify PEEPi while the infant breathes spontaneously (Fig. 160.8).[163] PEEPi not only can cause profound hemodynamic consequences including reduced venous return and increased right ventricular afterload, but it also can impose tremendous work on the infant, make it difficult or impossible for the infant to generate spontaneous breaths, and exacerbate patient-ventilator dyssynchrony.[163,166-168] This is because for the infants to trigger the ventilator, they must first generate enough pleural pressure to lower alveolar pressure by the amount of PEEPi; only then will additional negative pressure be rewarded with inspiratory flow. In such circumstances, setting the applied PEEP close to the measured PEEPi level can improve the infant's ability to trigger the ventilator, reduce work, and restore patient-ventilator synchrony.[163] Thus even in an infant who appears markedly hyperinflated radiographically, the amount of PEEP might have to be increased to improve mechanics and overall function if PEEPi is present (Fig. 160.9).

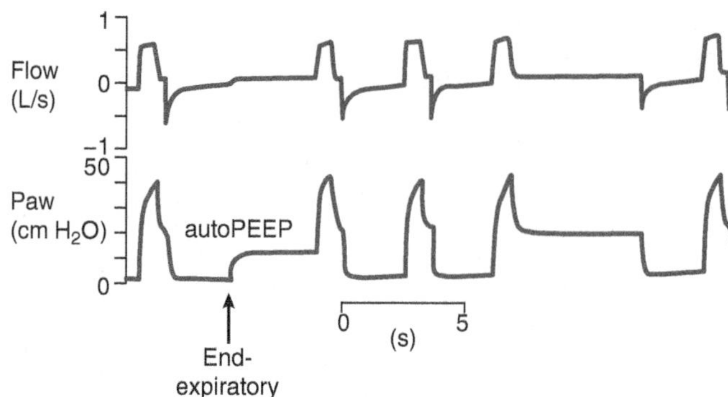

Fig. 160.7 Determination of intrinsic positive end-expiratory pressure *(PEEPi)*. The clinician performs an expiratory hold maneuver, and in the presence of PEEPi, airway opening pressure will equilibrate with alveolar pressure. The increase in pressure following the end-expiratory hold reflects the magnitude of PEEPi. (From Blanch L, Bernabe F, Lucangelo U. Measurement of air trapping, intrinsic positive end-expiratory pressure, and dynamic hyperinflation in mechanically ventilated patients. *Respir Care.* 2005;50:110–123; discussion 23–24.)

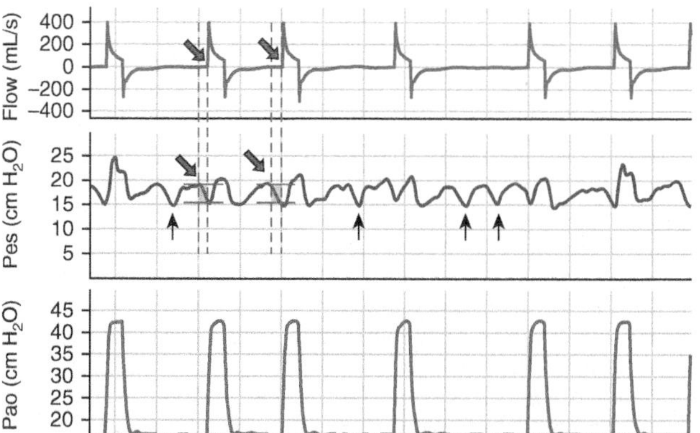

Fig. 160.8 Graphic tracings from a mechanically ventilated infant with severe bronchopulmonary dysplasia and intrinsic positive end-expiratory pressure (PEEPi) who is breathing spontaneously, receiving pressure-supported breaths. The top tracing represents flow at the airway opening; the middle tracing reflects esophageal pressure *(Pes)*, and the bottom tracing represents airway opening pressure *(Pao)*. Downward deflections of esophageal pressures signify inspiratory efforts. There are several wasted efforts *(black arrows)* where lowering pleural pressure does not trigger the ventilator and no inspiratory flow occurs. Two inspiratory efforts demonstrate a trigger delay between the patient's inspiratory effort *(blue arrows)* and onset of inspiratory flow from the ventilator *(green arrows)*. The drop in esophageal pressure between the patient's effort and onset of flow *(parallel horizontal blue lines, shaded area)* represents the magnitude of PEEPi the infant has to overcome to generate flow adequate enough (0.2 L/min) to trigger the ventilator. (From Napolitano N, Jalal K, McDonough JM, et al. Identifying and treating intrinsic PEEP in infants with severe bronchopulmonary dysplasia. *Pediatr Pulmonol.* 2019;54:1045–1051.)

CONCLUSION

The pathophysiologic processes that result in neonatal acute respiratory failure also help to determine appropriate strategies for newborns who require mechanical ventilation. The overarching goal of ventilatory support for neonates with acute respiratory failure is to support vital functions while protecting the lung from further injury as much as possible. As the processes that result in respiratory failure move from the acute inflammatory stage to the reparative stage, lung mechanics change. As a result, alterations in the style of ventilation are required to prevent complications and delayed

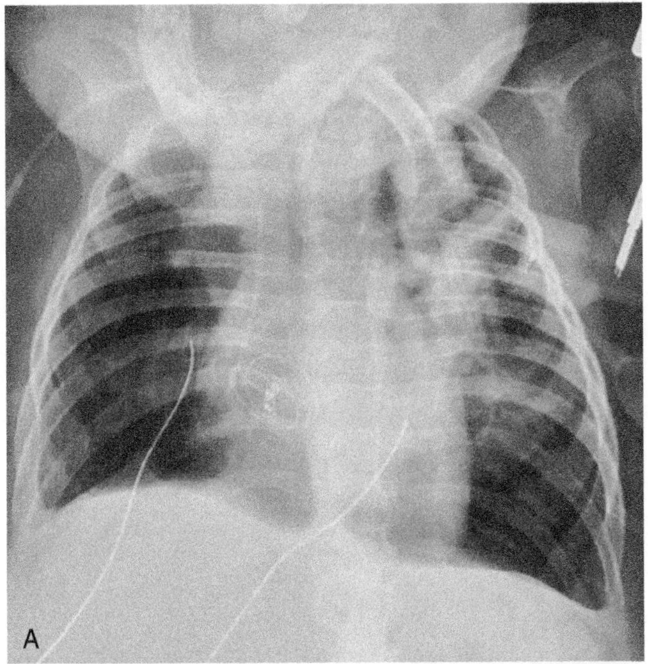

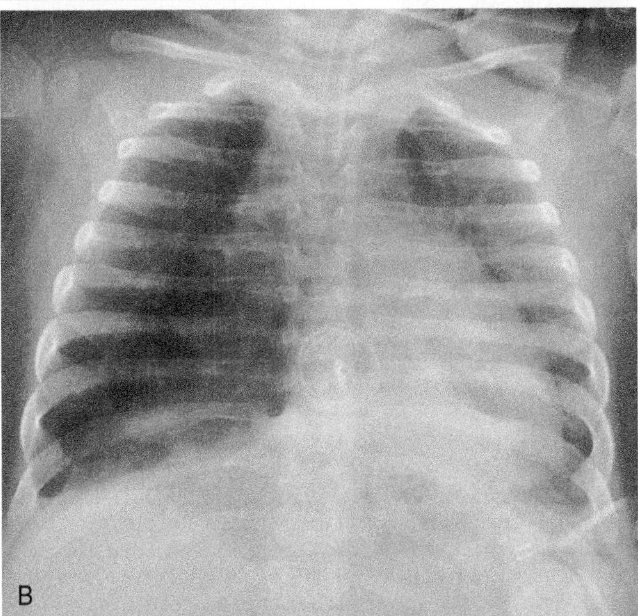

Fig. 160.9 (A) Chest radiograph of an 8.6-kg infant with bronchopulmonary dysplasia who was supported by positive pressure ventilation with the following settings: rate 30 breaths/min, tidal volume 50 mL, inspiratory time 0.5 second, positive end-expiratory pressure (PEEP) 7 cm H_2O, and pressure support 20 cm H_2O over PEEP. The radiograph demonstrates marked hyperinflation and hyperlucent right middle and left lower lobes. Evaluation of respiratory system mechanics disclosed an intrinsic PEEP of 11 cm H_2O. (B) The same patient 24 hours after ventilator settings were adjusted by increasing PEEP to 11 cm H_2O, decreasing the rate to 20 breaths/min, increasing the inspiratory time to 0.7 second, and increasing the tidal volume to 100 mL. Hyperinflation has decreased, despite the increase in PEEP.

weaning from support. Controlled trials addressing the best methods for supporting neonates with chronic respiratory failure are desperately needed to enhance the outcomes for those infants.

 A complete reference list is available at www.ExpertConsult.com.

SELECT REFERENCES

1. Roussos C, Macklem PT. The respiratory muscles. *N Engl J Med.* 1982;307(13):786-797.
4. Papastamelos C, Panitch HB, England SE, Allen JL. Developmental changes in chest wall compliance in infancy and early childhood. *J Appl Physiol (1985).* 1995;78(1):179-184.
6. Hernandez LA, Peevy KJ, Moise AA, Parker JC. Chest wall restriction limits high airway pressure-induced lung injury in young rabbits. *J Appl Physiol (1985).* 1989;66(5):2364-2368.
8. Ren CL, Feng R, Davis SD, et al. Tidal breathing measurements at discharge and clinical outcomes in extremely low gestational age neonates. *Ann Am Thorac Soc.* 2018;15(11):1311-1319.
9. Allen JL, Greenspan JS, Deoras KS, Keklikian E, Wolfson MR, Shaffer TH. Interaction between chest wall motion and lung mechanics in normal infants and infants with bronchopulmonary dysplasia. *Pediatr Pulmonol.* 1991;11(1):37-43.
11. Kraaijenga JV, de Waal CG, Hutten GJ, de Jongh FH, van Kaam AH. Diaphragmatic activity during weaning from respiratory support in preterm infants. *Arch Dis Child Fetal Neonatal Ed.* 2017;102(4):F307-F311.
17. Polla B, D'Antona G, Bottinelli R, Reggiani C. Respiratory muscle fibres: specialisation and plasticity. *Thorax.* 2004;59(9):808-817.
21. Glau CL, Conlon TW, Himebauch AS, et al. Progressive diaphragm atrophy in pediatric acute respiratory failure. *Pediatr Crit Care Med.* 2018;19(5):406-411.
26. Bates ML, Pillers DA, Palta M, Farrell ET, Eldridge MW. Ventilatory control in infants, children, and adults with bronchopulmonary dysplasia. *Respir Physiol Neurobiol.* 2013;189(2):329-337.
28. Coste F, Ferkol T, Hamvas A, et al. Ventilatory control and supplemental oxygen in premature infants with apparent chronic lung disease. *Arch Dis Child Fetal Neonatal Ed.* 2015;100(3):F233-F237.
31. Hislop AA, Haworth SG. Airway size and structure in the normal fetal and infant lung and the effect of premature delivery and artificial ventilation. *Am Rev Respir Dis.* 1989;140(6):1717-1726.
38. Moreno RH, Hogg JC, Pare PD. Mechanics of airway narrowing. *Am Rev Respir Dis.* 1986;133(6):1171-1180.
39. Plopper CG, Nishio SJ, Schelegle ES. Tethering tracheobronchial airways within the lungs. *Am J Respir Crit Care Med.* 2003;167(1):2-3.
51. Bhutani VK, Rubenstein SD, Shaffer TH. Pressure-volume relationships of tracheae in fetal newborn and adult rabbits. *Respir Physiol.* 1981;43(3):221-231.
57. Bhutani VK, Rubenstein D, Shaffer TH. Pressure-induced deformation in immature airways. *Pediatr Res.* 1981;15(5):829-832.
64. Panitch HB, Allen JL, Alpert BE, Schidlow DV. Effects of CPAP on lung mechanics in infants with acquired tracheobronchomalacia. *Am J Respir Crit Care Med.* 1994;150(5 Pt 1):1341-1346.
66. Hysinger EB, Friedman NL, Padula MA, et al. Tracheobronchomalacia is associated with increased morbidity in bronchopulmonary dysplasia. *Ann Am Thorac Soc.* 2017;14(9):1428-1435.
68. Wiseman NE, Duncan PG, Cameron CB. Management of tracheobronchomalacia with continuous positive airway pressure. *J Pediatr Surg.* 1985;20(5):489-493.
78. Gregory GA, Kitterman JA, Phibbs RH, Tooley WH, Hamilton WK. Treatment of the idiopathic respiratory-distress syndrome with continuous positive airway pressure. *N Engl J Med.* 1971;284(24):1333-1340.
81. Clark RH, Gerstmann DR, Jobe AH, Moffitt ST, Slutsky AS, Yoder BA. Lung injury in neonates: causes, strategies for prevention, and long-term consequences. *J Pediatr.* 2001;139(4):478-486.
82. Dreyfuss D, Saumon G. Ventilator-induced lung injury: lessons from experimental studies. *Am J Respir Crit Care Med.* 1998;157(1):294-323.
83. Slutsky AS, Ranieri VM. Ventilator-induced lung injury. *N Engl J Med.* 2013;369(22):2126-2136.
87. Acute Respiratory Distress Syndrome N, Brower RG, Matthay MA, et al. Ventilation with lower tidal volumes as compared with traditional tidal volumes for acute lung injury and the acute respiratory distress syndrome. *N Engl J Med.* 2000;342(18):1301-1308.
88. Amato MB, Barbas CS, Medeiros DM, et al. Effect of a protective-ventilation strategy on mortality in the acute respiratory distress syndrome. *N Engl J Med.* 1998;338(6):347-354.
90. Kneyber MC, Zhang H, Slutsky AS. Ventilator-induced lung injury. Similarity and differences between children and adults. *Am J Respir Crit Care Med.* 2014;190(3):258-265.
91. Amato MB, Meade MO, Slutsky AS, et al. Driving pressure and survival in the acute respiratory distress syndrome. *N Engl J Med.* 2015;372(8):747-755.
95. Curley GF, Laffey JG, Zhang H, Slutsky AS. Biotrauma and ventilator-induced lung injury: clinical implications. *Chest.* 2016;150(5):1109-1117.
99. Adams EW, Counsell SJ, Hajnal JV, et al. Magnetic resonance imaging of lung water content and distribution in term and preterm infants. *Am J Respir Crit Care Med.* 2002;166(3):397-402.
102. Dreizzen E, Migdal M, Praud JP, et al. Passive total respiratory system compliance and gas exchange in newborns with hyaline membrane disease. *Pediatr Pulmonol.* 1989;6(1):2-7.
108. Thome U, Topfer A, Schaller P, Pohlandt F. The effect of positive endexpiratory pressure, peak inspiratory pressure, and inspiratory time on functional residual capacity in mechanically ventilated preterm infants. *Eur J Pediatr.* 1998;157(10):831-837.

110. Bamat N, Fierro J, Wang Y, Millar D, Kirpalani H. Positive end-expiratory pressure for preterm infants requiring conventional mechanical ventilation for respiratory distress syndrome or bronchopulmonary dysplasia. *Cochrane Database Syst Rev*. 2019;2:CD004500.
112. Carlo WA, Ambalavanan N. Conventional mechanical ventilation: traditional and new strategies. *Pediatr Rev*. 1999;20(12):e117-e126.
120. Harris RS. Pressure-volume curves of the respiratory system. *Respir Care*. 2005;50(1):78-98; discussion 98-9.
123. Gattinoni L, Carlesso E, Cressoni M. Selecting the 'right' positive end-expiratory pressure level. *Curr Opin Crit Care*. 2015;21(1):50-57.
127. Simbruner G. Inadvertent positive end-expiratory pressure in mechanically ventilated newborn infants: detection and effect on lung mechanics and gas exchange. *J Pediatr*. 1986;108(4):589-595.
129. Maybauer DM, Talke PO, Westphal M, et al. Positive end-expiratory pressure ventilation increases extravascular lung water due to a decrease in lung lymph flow. *Anaesth Intensive Care*. 2006;34(3):329-333.
132. Gattinoni L, Caironi P, Cressoni M, et al. Lung recruitment in patients with the acute respiratory distress syndrome. *N Engl J Med*. 2006;354(17):1775-1786.
133. Armstrong RK, Carlisle HR, Davis PG, Schibler A, Tingay DG. Distribution of tidal ventilation during volume-targeted ventilation is variable and influenced by age in the preterm lung. *Intensive Care Med*. 2011;37(5):839-846.
136. Ambalavanan N, Carlo WA. Ventilatory strategies in the prevention and management of bronchopulmonary dysplasia. *Semin Perinatol*. 2006;30(4):192-199.
137. Brown MK, DiBlasi RM. Mechanical ventilation of the premature neonate. *Respir Care*. 2011;56(9):1298-1311; discussion 1311-1293.
139. Fisher JB, Mammel MC, Coleman JM, Bing DR, Boros SJ. Identifying lung overdistention during mechanical ventilation by using volume-pressure loops. *Pediatr Pulmonol*. 1988;5(1):10-14.
140. Gattinoni L, Pesenti A. The concept of "baby lung. *Intensive Care Med*. 2005;31(6):776-784.
146. Klingenberg C, Wheeler KI, McCallion N, Morley CJ, Davis PG. Volume-targeted versus pressure-limited ventilation in neonates. *Cochrane Database Syst Rev*. 2017;10:CD003666.
148. Jensen EA, Dysart K, Gantz MG, et al. The diagnosis of bronchopulmonary dysplasia in very preterm infants. An evidence-based approach. *Am J Respir Crit Care Med*. 2019;200(6):751-759.
152. Lui K, Lloyd J, Ang E, Rynn M, Gupta JM. Early changes in respiratory compliance and resistance during the development of bronchopulmonary dysplasia in the era of surfactant therapy. *Pediatr Pulmonol*. 2000;30(4):282-290.
158. Husain AN, Siddiqui NH, Stocker JT. Pathology of arrested acinar development in postsurfactant bronchopulmonary dysplasia. *Hum Pathol*. 1998;29(7):710-717.
163. Napolitano N, Jalal K, McDonough JM, et al. Identifying and treating intrinsic PEEP in infants with severe bronchopulmonary dysplasia. *Pediatr Pulmonol*. 2019;54(7):1045-1051.

161 Pathophysiology of Gastroesophageal Reflux

Sudarshan Rao Jadcherla

INTRODUCTION

Gastroesophageal reflux (GER) is defined as a retrograde movement of gastric contents into the esophagus; it is a normal physiologic phenomenon across the age spectrum. Importantly, the physical and chemical properties of the gastric contents vary with an infant's feeding cycle and activity state.[1] Therefore the symptoms resulting from provocation during esophageal distension also vary. When the symptoms become troublesome, it is called *gastroesophageal reflux disease (GERD)*. No single aerodigestive symptom or sign is specific to GER or other related aerodigestive pathology, and there is no simple method that can provide clues to aerodigestive pathophysiology.

In this chapter, pertinent to GER, we clarify (1) developmental biology of gastroesophageal junction, (2) physiologic mechanisms of GER, and (3) pathophysiologic considerations of GER.

DEVELOPMENTAL BIOLOGY OF GASTROESOPHAGEAL JUNCTION

EMBRYOLOGY OF THE AERODIGESTIVE APPARATUS

Embryologic origins and the neuroanatomic relationships between the airway and foregut are intricate and develop from adjacent segments of the primitive foregut (Fig. 161.1).[2-5] The tracheobronchial diverticulum, the pharynx, the esophagus, the stomach, and the diaphragm are all derived from the primitive foregut and/or its mesenchyme and share similar control systems. By 4 weeks of embryonic life, tracheobronchial diverticulum appears at the ventral wall of the foregut, with left vagus nerve being anterior and right vagus being posteriorly located. The stomach is a fusiform tube with the dorsal side growth rate greater than the ventral side, thus creating greater and lesser curvatures. At 7 weeks of embryonic life, the stomach also rotates 90 degrees clockwise, with the greater curvature displaced to the left. The left vagus innervates the stomach anteriorly, and the right vagus innervates the posterior aspect. At 10 weeks, the esophagus and the stomach are properly positioned; the circular and longitudinal muscle layers and the ganglion cells are in place. The true vocal cords begin as glottal folds. By the sixth or seventh week of gestation, a structure superior to the true vocal cords evolves to protect the vocal cords and lower airway. This superior structure consists of the epiglottis, aryepiglottic folds, false vocal cords, and the laryngeal ventricles. The epiglottis starts as a hypobranchial eminence behind the future tongue and by week 7, the epiglottis is separated from the tongue. At the same time, two lateral folds connect to the base of the epiglottis, which develop into the arytenoids cartilages at the distal end. The larynx begins as a groove in the primitive foregut, which folds upon itself to become the laryngotracheal bud, the subsequent divisions of which form the bronchopulmonary segments. From this phase, 20 generations of conducting airways form. The first 8 generations constitute bronchi and acquire cartilaginous walls; the next 9 to 20 generations comprise the nonrespiratory bronchioles, which are not cartilaginous and contain smooth muscle. Subsequent divisions form the bronchopulmonary segments.

Thus, congenital anomalies of the aerodigestive tract and gastroesophageal junction can result in situations predisposing to GER. Such conditions may include but are not limited to craniofacial anomalies, airway anomalies, esophageal atresia and tracheoesophageal fistula, congenital diaphragmatic hernia, hiatal hernia, abdominal wall defects, malrotation, atresias, and duplication of the small intestine.

NEUROMUSCULAR COMPONENTS OF GASTROESOPHAGEAL JUNCTION

The pharynx, upper esophageal sphincter (UES), and proximal esophagus are composed of striated muscle. The distal esophagus and the lower esophageal sphincter (LES) are composed of smooth muscle with an inner layer consisting of circular

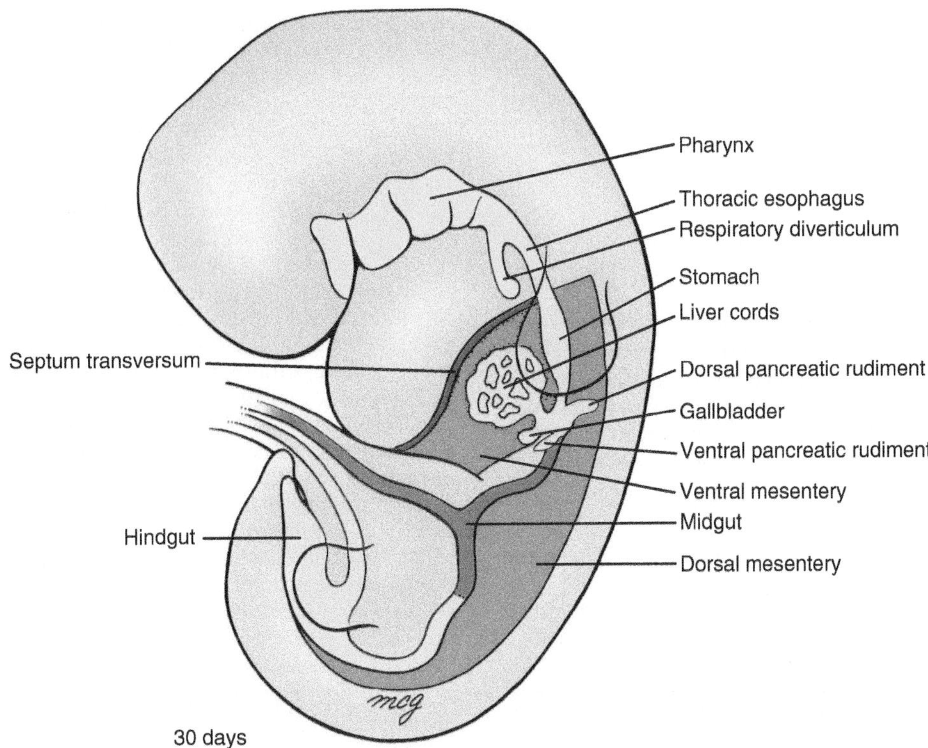

Fig. 161.1 Three subdivisions of the gut tube. The foregut consists of the pharynx, located cranial to the respiratory diverticulum, the thoracic esophagus, and the abdominal foregut. The abdominal foregut forms the abdominal esophagus, stomach, and half of the duodenum; it gives rise to the liver, gallbladder, pancreas, and their associated ducts. The midgut forms half of the duodenum, the jejunum and ileum, the ascending colon, and about two thirds of the transverse colon. The hindgut forms one third of the transverse colon, the descending colon, and the sigmoid colon and the upper two thirds of the anorectal canal. The abdominal esophagus, stomach, and superior part of the duodenum are suspended by dorsal and ventral mesenteries; the abdominal gut tube excluding the rectum is suspended in the abdominal cavity by a dorsal mesentery only. (From Schoenwolf GC, Bleyl SB. *Larsen's Human Embryology*. 5th ed. Philadelphia, PA: Churchill Livingstone, an imprint of Elsevier, Inc; 2015:341–374. Fig. 14-4.)

muscle cells and an outer layer consisting of longitudinal muscle cells with a myenteric plexus in between. The UES high-pressure zone is a constriction between the pharynx and the proximal esophagus generated by the cricopharyngeus (the principal muscle), proximal cervical esophagus, and inferior pharyngeal constrictor.[6] The LES is an autonomous sphincter composed chiefly of circular smooth muscle; the integrity of the gastroesophageal junction is further augmented by (1) diaphragmatic crural fibers and (2) the intraabdominal part of esophagus and sling fibers of the stomach.[7] The UES is innervated by (1) the vagus via the pharyngoesophageal, superior laryngeal, and recurrent laryngeal branches; (2) the glossopharyngeal nerve; and (3) sympathetic nerve fibers via the cranial cervical ganglion. The LES is an autonomous contractile apparatus that is tonically active and relaxes periodically to facilitate bolus transit. Although the LES is considered to be an important functional segment in preventing GER, other neighboring structures including oblique sling fibers of the stomach, the musculofascial diaphragmatic sling, and intraabdominal esophagus also contribute to this function.[8]

The musculature of the larynx is derived from the mesenchyme of the fourth and sixth pharyngeal arches. Laryngeal muscles are innervated by branches of the tenth cranial nerve. The superior laryngeal nerve innervates the derivatives of the fourth pharyngeal arch (cricothyroid, levator palatini, and constrictors of pharynx), and the recurrent laryngeal nerve innervates derivatives of the sixth pharyngeal arch (intrinsic muscles of the larynx).

The airways and esophagus share common innervations.[6,8,9] Foregut afferents are derived from both vagal and dorsal root ganglions with cell bodies in the nodose ganglion. This afferent apparatus conveys signals to the neurons in the nucleus tractus solitarius, located in the dorsomedial medulla oblongata. These signals are integrated in a specific terminal site of the nucleus tractus solitarius, the subnucleus centralis, which is the sole point of termination of esophageal afferents. After sensory integration in the nucleus tractus solitarius, the signals in turn activate airway motor neurons in the nucleus ambiguus and the dorsal motor nucleus of the vagus, producing an efferent parasympathetic response and or nonadrenergic, noncholinergic response mediated via vasoactive intestinal polypeptide or nitric oxide.[10-12]

Thus anomalies of the aerodigestive tract and anomalies of the neuromuscular apparatus predispose one to GER and/or its consequences.

PHYSIOLOGY OF GASTROESOPHAGEAL JUNCTION, ESOPHAGUS, AND STOMACH

Normally, intragastric pressure is higher and is highly variable; the gastric contractility is dependent on the phases of interdigestive motility cycle, feeding intervals, and antral contractions. This occurs regardless of the activity or sleep states. On the other hand, basal intraesophageal pressures during normal breathing reflect intrathoracic pressures; pressures are negative or more negative during inspiration and less negative or positive during expiration. Thus at rest, a pressure gradient exists between the stomach and the esophagus. In the absence of other factors, this pressure difference should propel gastric contents into the esophagus. However, the gastroesophageal junction, a tonically active high-pressure zone, acts as a protective barrier and regulates to-and-fro bolus movement between the esophagus and stomach.[7] This

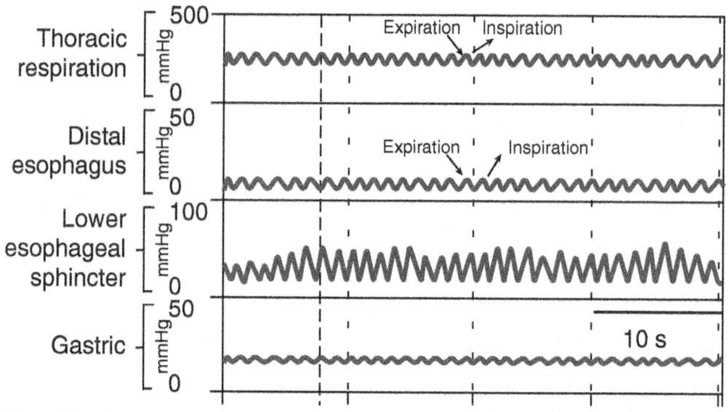

Fig. 161.2 Lower esophageal sphincter (LES) respiratory fluctuations. Shown is an example of how the LES is heavily influenced by diaphragm movements during inspiration and expiration utilizing pharyngoesophageal motility methods. (Courtesy S.R. Jadcherla.)

high-pressure zone at the gastroesophageal junction reflects the combined activities of two sphincter subsystems: the LES and the crural diaphragm. The activities of these two subsystems are constantly changing to prevent reflux despite changes in gastric, abdominal, and thoracic pressures. The LES muscle is thicker than muscle in the more proximal esophagus or adjoining stomach and has specialized neural innervation.[13] The myocytes of LES have unique mechanical, electrical, and neurotransmitter-related response characteristics.[10,14-16] In contrast to the adjacent esophagus, in which the plexus lies only between the circular and longitudinal muscle layers,[15] the innervation of the LES is unique in that the myenteric plexus occupies multiple muscle planes. As shown in Fig. 161.2, at normal tidal breathing, the high-pressure zone is characterized by a tonically elevated basal pressure contributed by intrinsic LES and respiratory-induced pressure oscillations contributed by active contractions in the diaphragmatic crura, both of which are of greater magnitude than the pressure simultaneously found in the adjacent stomach and esophagus.[17,18]

The crural diaphragm is distinguished from the costal diaphragm by its attachment to the vertebral column rather than the rib cage. Because the esophagus passes through the crural diaphragm, diaphragmatic contractions create an external sphincter mechanism at the gastroesophageal junction. The activity of the crural diaphragm varies with the respiratory cycle, thereby compensating for variations in thoracic and abdominal pressure that would otherwise favor GER during inspiration (see Fig. 161.2). Another important contributory factor to the integrity of the gastroesophageal junction comes from the smooth muscle fibers of the stomach, constituting a sling around the greater curvature of the stomach.[19] Although they are not strictly part of the LES, the sling fibers help to prevent reflux by acting as a flap valve during fundal distension, pressing the closed end of the sling against the distal esophagus.[20]

MATURATIONAL PHYSIOLOGY OF THE GASTROESOPHAGEAL JUNCTION

The high-pressure zone of the gastroesophageal junction must also relax to allow passage of material across the gastroesophageal junction during swallowing, vomiting, eructation, reflux, and esophageal distension. As shown in Figs. 161.3 and 161.4, this high-pressure zone changes with pressure gradient to allow for basal deglutition, pharyngeal stimulation, esophageal distension, abdominal strain, and GER. The neural pathways controlling such rapid changes in LES tone have been characterized.[6,15,20-22] For example, during swallowing, afferent signals from the pharynx ascend to nucleus solitarius in the medulla. Efferent outputs from the adjacent dorsal vagal nucleus and the nucleus ambiguus descend through the vagus nerve to the esophagus, thereby mediating both esophageal peristalsis and LES relaxation to propel swallowed material into the stomach. During this phase (see Fig. 161.3), the onset of the pharyngeal contractile waveform is immediately followed by UES and LES relaxation. This results from cessation of excitatory output to the UES and an increase in inhibitory output to the LES, both favoring sphincteric relaxation at the skeletal and smooth muscles, respectively.

In mammals, swallowing, distension of the esophagus, eructation, vomiting, regurgitation, and rumination are all associated with an inhibition of diaphragmatic electrical activity, thereby facilitating passage of material through the gastroesophageal junction.[6,21-25] During bolus transit through the gastroesophageal junction, inhibition of the crural diaphragm occurs to a much greater degree than that of the costal diaphragm. Swallowing and esophageal distension result in concurrent relaxation of the LES and inhibition of crural inspiratory activity.[22,23,26,27] The respiratory-induced oscillations in the high-pressure zone are abolished as a result of inhibition of crural inspiratory activity, whereas relaxation of the LES results in a decrease in baseline end-expiratory pressure. Costal diaphragmatic activity remains unchanged and allows continued ventilation with little change in the respiratory rate or intrapleural pressure (Fig. 161.5). During periods of increased intraabdominal pressure, such as the Valsalva maneuver, coughing, straight-leg raising, or abdominal compression, an increase occurs in crural diaphragmatic tone, thereby compensating for the increased pressure gradient favoring GER.[21]

In summary, the high-pressure zone at the gastroesophageal junction depends on the tone generated by the intrinsic LES and also on the magnitude of crural diaphragmatic contraction. Transit of material through the gastroesophageal junction is most likely to occur during simultaneous relaxation of the LES and inhibition of the crural diaphragm, but is also dependent on the pressure gradients across the stomach and esophageal lumina.

PHYSIOLOGIC MECHANISMS OF GASTROESOPHAGEAL REFLUX

During GER, movement of refluxate from the stomach into the esophagus occurs when the pressure gradient between the stomach and the esophagus is wider and the LES tone is less. Changes in the tone at the gastroesophageal junction (relaxation of the high-pressure zone, either transiently or prolonged) weaken the barrier function; when coupled with retrograde movement of bolus from stomach into the esophagus, this results in elevation of the gastroesophageal pressure gradient and culminates in reflux. Therefore possible mechanisms of GER (see Fig. 161.4) include (1) transient LES relaxation (TLESR)—this is the presumed mechanism in 80% to 90% of episodes, (2) an increase in intraabdominal pressure greater than that of the LES, (3) a hypotonic LES, (4) multiple swallows associated with prolonged LES relaxation as may happen during feeding, and (5) structural deficits in the apparatus at the gastroesophageal junction (e.g., hiatal hernia or congenital anomalies of the esophagus and diaphragm). Regardless of all these subtypes, a decrease in LES tone and relaxation of the sphincter is of paramount importance.

TRANSIENT RELAXATION OF THE LOWER ESOPHAGEAL SPHINCTER IS THE MOST FREQUENT MECHANISM FOR GASTROESOPHAGEAL REFLUX

Most episodes of GER occur during transient relaxation of the high-pressure zone (see Fig. 161.4A) when an abrupt collapse of pressure in the high-pressure zone exists in the absence of a pharyngeal swallow, primary esophageal peristalsis, or secondary esophageal peristalsis (Fig. 161.6).[28-32] Pressure in the LES

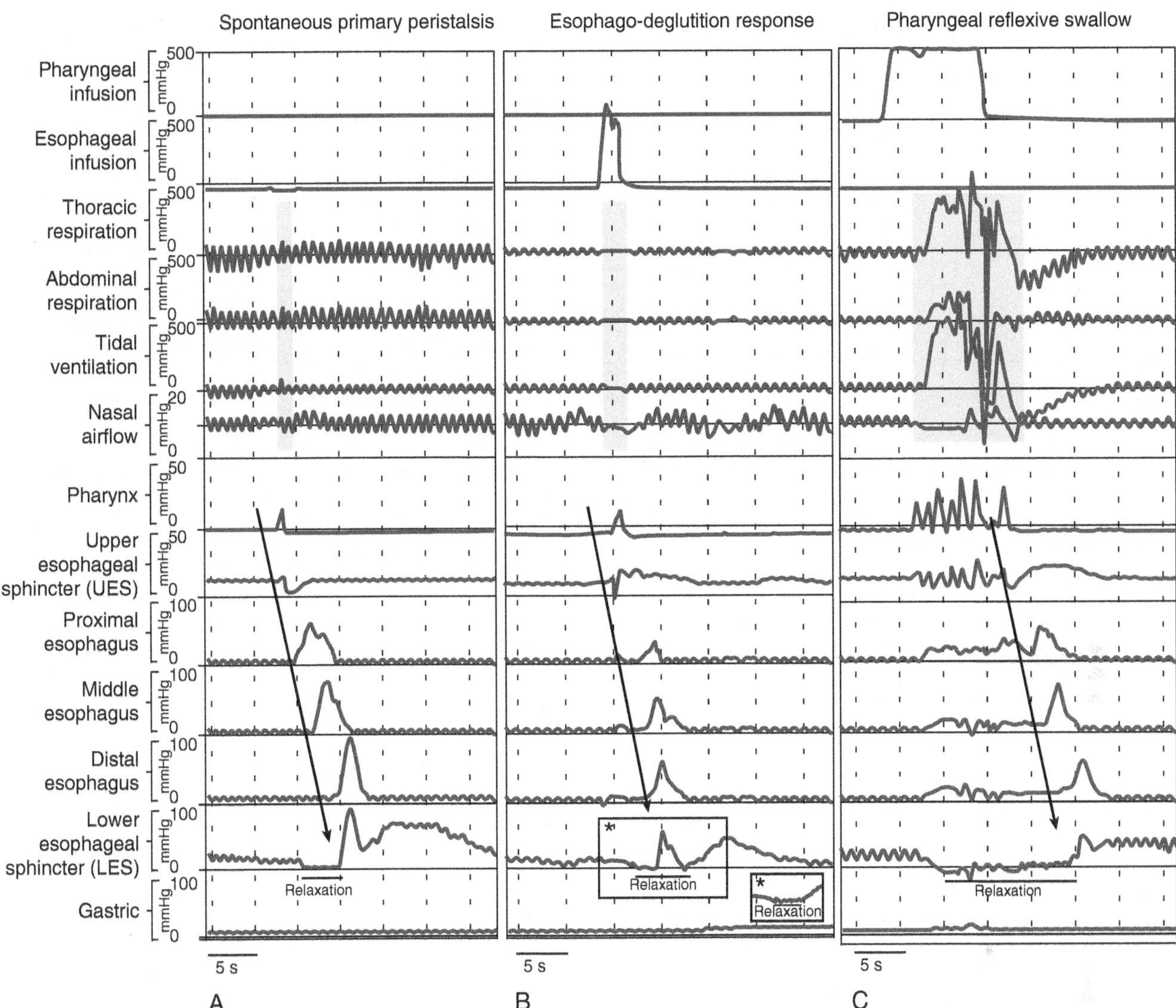

Fig. 161.3 Occurrences of pharyngeal swallowing. Swallow-associated apnea (deglutition apnea) protects against anterograde aspiration during pharyngeal swallowing. (A) Spontaneous primary peristalsis functions to clear the oropharyngeal region of secretions. (B) Esophago-deglutition response (EDR) arises in response to midesophageal stimulation as would occur during gastroesophageal reflux. EDR functions to clear refluxed material back into the stomach. *Due to the sleeve technology in the LES, reflection of the distal esophageal contraction is frequently noted during LES relaxation. The inset visualizes LES relaxation without this esophageal artifact. (C) Pharyngeal reflexive swallows (PRS) arise in response to pharyngeal stimulation as would occur during feeding. PRS functions to clear material from the esophagus and airway into the stomach. (Courtesy S.R. Jadcherla.)

high-pressure zone before and immediately after these episodes is always greater than gastric pressure (see Fig. 161.6).The pressure profile of the high-pressure zone during transient relaxation is similar to that observed during a swallow and is characterized by decreases in both LES activity and crural diaphragm activity.[23] The physiologic role of transient relaxations is to allow eructation (belching) to occur; this is consistent with the finding that gastric distension can trigger transient relaxations.[33-38]

Other mechanisms for LES relaxation may include those events induced by a swallow or esophageal bolus or fundal distension. Relaxations of the high-pressure zone are identical manometrically, and in humans, relaxations frequently occur within a few seconds of a previous swallow-induced relaxation or in association with an incomplete peristaltic sequence.[7,36-38] In the opossum, transient LES relaxations have been produced by subthreshold stimuli, a stimulus that did not induce a fully propagated deglutition sequence or secondary esophageal peristalsis.[39,40] Dose-dependent pharyngeal stimulation with sterile water or liquids causes pharyngeal reflexive swallowing; the swallows are often multiple and vary with dose (see Fig. 161.3C).[6,40-42] During this process, LES relaxation is prolonged.

Electrical stimulation of the central end of the superior laryngeal nerve (vagal afferent stimulation) or the peripheral end of the cervical vagus (vagal efferent stimulation) at high frequencies results in a normal deglutition sequence, whereas stimulation at low frequencies results in isolated LES relaxation.[7] Studies in humans have shown that transient relaxation is frequently associated with mylohyoid and pharyngeal activity of a much lower magnitude than that observed during a swallow or with a nonperistaltic esophageal contraction.[38] As a result of these studies, it has been suggested that transient relaxations occur by the same neural pathways as swallowing-associated relaxation (see earlier) and may be induced by a long train of subthreshold stimuli originating in the pharynx.[39]

Using manometric methods, it has become clear that most GER is associated with a transient relaxation of the high-pressure zone involving decreased activity in both the LES and the crural diaphragm. However, the converse is not true—that is,

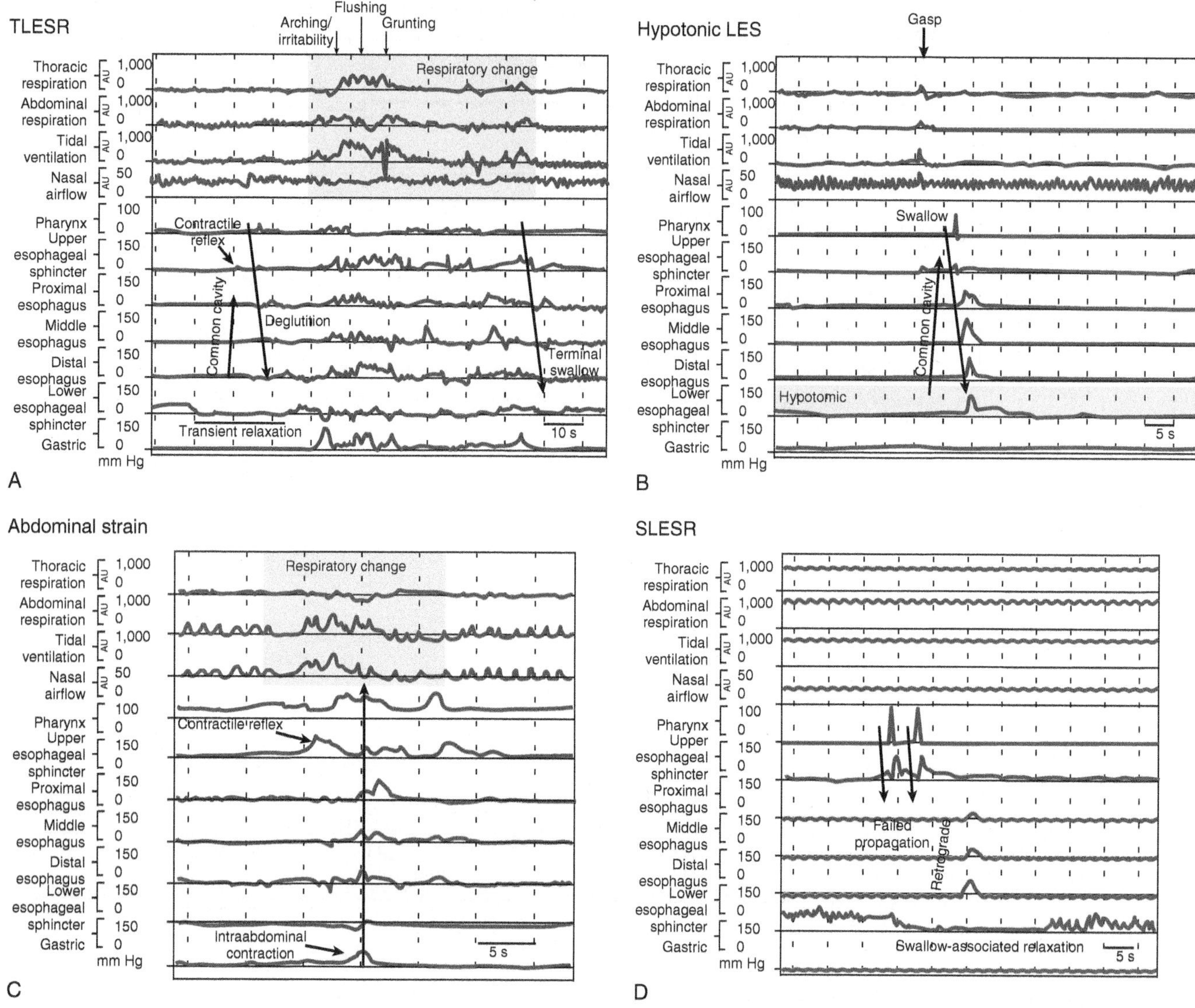

Fig. 161.4 Markers of reflux mechanisms utilizing pharyngoesophageal motility. (A) The lower esophageal sphincter *(LES)* transiently relaxes for more than 10 seconds *(TLESR)*, followed by esophageal common cavity and the upper esophageal sphincter *(UES)* contractile reflex. Following the reflux event are symptoms and multiple swallowing attempts to clear the refluxate until a terminal swallow that restores respiratory and digestive normalcy. (B) A chronically hypotonic LES makes the infant more susceptible to pathologic reflux due to an inadequate pressure barrier between the stomach and esophagus. Similar to TLESR, reflux is observed by common cavity in the esophageal body and followed by a swallow. Also note the presence of a gasp preceding the common cavity. (C) During an episode of TLESR, an abdominal contraction causes gastric contents to be expelled into the esophagus. Note the UES contraction to protect the infant from aspiration, in addition to the respiratory change during the event. (D) Swallow-associated LES relaxation *(SLESR)* occurs with multiple swallow attempts. Reflux caused by SLESR can occur when multiple swallows are present without esophageal body propulsion, thus allowing retrograde movement of material from the stomach into the esophagus. (Courtesy S.R. Jadcherla.)

most transient relaxations are not associated with reflux events. Transient relaxations of the high-pressure zone can occur in normal subjects and is a common finding in healthy individuals. However, it appears that those with GERD have both a higher frequency of relaxations and an increased rate of reflux per episode of relaxation. Other factors, therefore, must also play a role in the pathogenesis of GERD, such as transient increases in intraabdominal pressure, impaired clearance of refluxed material, presence of hiatal hernia or structural deficits, abrupt distension of the gastric fundus, TLESR during postural changes, and prolonged acid clearance with inadequate buffering mechanisms.[1,43,44]

Studies in both normal subjects and in patients with GERD have shown that most reflux episodes occur during transient relaxations.[34-37] Although transient relaxations of the high-pressure zone may last from 10 to 45 seconds, the actual episodes of reflux occur only during the period when the baseline high-pressure zone pressure is zero and respiratory-related pressure oscillations are absent. Studies of transient relaxations in patients with and without reflux symptoms have found only a slight increase in the frequency of relaxations in those with symptoms of reflux.[36] Some of these patients, children in particular, may have delayed gastric emptying resulting in gastric distension, which in turn may produce transient relaxations of the LES.[28,29,31,45,46] A more important difference appears to be an increase in the percentage of transient relaxations that result in reflux from 40% to 50% in physiologically normal persons to 60% to 70% in patients with GERD.[36]

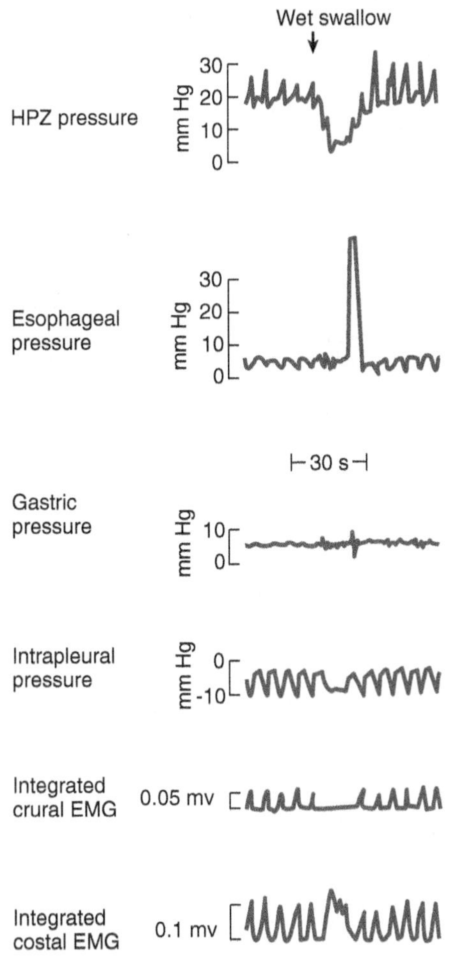

Fig. 161.5 Effect of a wet swallow on high-pressure zone *(HPZ)* pressure and diaphragmatic activity. The wet swallow was induced by a bolus injection of water into the posterior pharynx. The swallow results in an esophageal contraction, with a simultaneous relaxation of the intrinsic LES and inhibition of integrated crural electromyographic *(EMG)* activity. The combination of these events results in end-expiratory HPZ pressure decreasing to gastric baseline and an absence of respiratory-induced oscillations in HPZ pressure. The costal diaphragm remains active during the swallow, thus allowing ventilation to continue. (From Altschuler SM, Boyle JT, Nixon TE, et al. Simultaneous reflex inhibition of lower esophageal sphincter and crural diaphragm in cats. *Am J Physiol.* 1985;249:G586–G591.)

OTHER MECHANISMS AND RISK ASSOCIATIONS FOR THE OCCURRENCE OF GASTROESOPHAGEAL REFLUX

Increased intraabdominal pressure transients occur during coughing, straining, and changes in position, and an increase in crural diaphragm activity during these events is thought to prevent episodes of GER.[21] In contrast, during passive abdominal compression, crural diaphragmatic activity is inhibited, and the tonic activity of the LES is increased, thus leaving the LES as the sole barrier to GER (Fig. 161.7).[47] This adaptive response involves a vagally mediated increase in LES pressure in excess of the transmitted pressure increase in the stomach.[47]

A decrease in LES pressure resulting from immaturity of the gastroesophageal junction has been attributed to a hypotonic intrinsic LES, which permits retrograde movement of gastric contents into the esophagus.[48,49] Although LES resting pressure is lower in infants than in adults, the LES resting pressure increases with maturation.[29,50,51] Similarly, the length of the esophagus and the length of the physiologically active high-pressure zone increase with growth.[50] However, LES hypotonia has been observed in neurologically impaired individuals.[30,32] An alteration in central neural input to the LES or an impairment of the contractile function of the LES muscle is likely present in these patients.[7,33]

Esophageal dysmotility and impaired clearance permit prolonged contact within the esophagus.[43,44] Such events happen during prolonged repetitive swallowing bursts or result from a primary gastroesophageal refluxate that has not been cleared. Such situations can result in prolonged LES relaxation and can lead to recurrence of GER or prolonged duration of GER. Both acid clearance time and bolus clearance time are prolonged under such circumstances (Fig. 161.8). The cause of esophageal dysmotility and the presence of symptoms can be difficult to clarify because the aerodigestive symptoms can be nonspecific. In general, inflammation by itself can cause esophageal dysmotility. Esophageal dysmotility and inflammation can coexist or occur independently in infants with hiatal hernia, congenital foregut anomalies (e.g., esophageal atresia and trachea-esophageal fistula), diaphragmatic defects and hernias, and abdominal wall defects and may be secondary to esophageal shortening.[7,52]

Delayed gastric emptying or *gastroparesis* are also potential mechanisms for GER because they favor a prolonged dwell of the feeds and fundal distension, which in turn can trigger an LES relaxation response. Such phenomena can coexist with structural anomalies of the stomach and proximal small bowel, malrotation, hypertrophic pyloric stenosis, prolonged gastrointestinal stasis, and delayed transit. In such situations, a hypotonic LES can be a contributing factor.

RISK FACTORS, POSITIONS, AND GASTROESOPHAGEAL REFLUX MECHANISMS UNIQUE TO NEONATES AND INFANTS

TLESR remains the most common mechanism in neonates and infants.[53,54] Regurgitation is very common in this age group; 40% to 60% of normal 0- to 4-month-old infants regurgitate some amount of their feedings. Basic mechanical considerations provide some explanation for the high frequency of regurgitation in infants.[55-61] Newborns sleep or spend most of their time in the supine position, a position that is protective against sudden infant death syndrome (SIDS). Supine and right lateral positions increase the risk of GER, whereas prone and left lateral positions are associated with less GER but an increased rate of SIDS.[55,62-64] The length of the infant's esophagus and LES are short and increase with maturation.[50] A term infant's esophagus may be only 8 to 10 cm; the intraabdominal esophagus grows during the first 6 months of life. Thus refluxed material has a greater chance of extending to a more proximal extent than that seen in older infants (Fig. 161.9).

Manometric studies in both premature and term neonates have confirmed normal primary esophageal peristalsis. However, premature infants at 30 to 34 weeks' gestational age have lower esophageal peristaltic velocity and amplitude than term infants,[27,65] and preterm infants as young as 33 weeks' postmenstrual age have a lower esophageal high-pressure zone, which increases with age.[29,30,51] In response to midesophageal liquid infusion, premature infants have a longer delay to LES relaxation, but once the relaxation occurs, it is of a longer duration than that seen in term infants.[26] Premature infants have an elevated frequency of synchronous (i.e., nonperistaltic) esophageal contractions in the absence of a swallow, and this lack of coordination may lead to inadequate clearance of refluxed material.[29,51] As in adults, it appears that transient relaxations of the high-pressure zone are the primary mechanism of GER in neonates.[29,31,51]

In summary, the most frequent mechanism for GER is TLESR, a common mechanism in neonates and adults. Factors unique to neonates include anatomic factors, position, feeding methods,

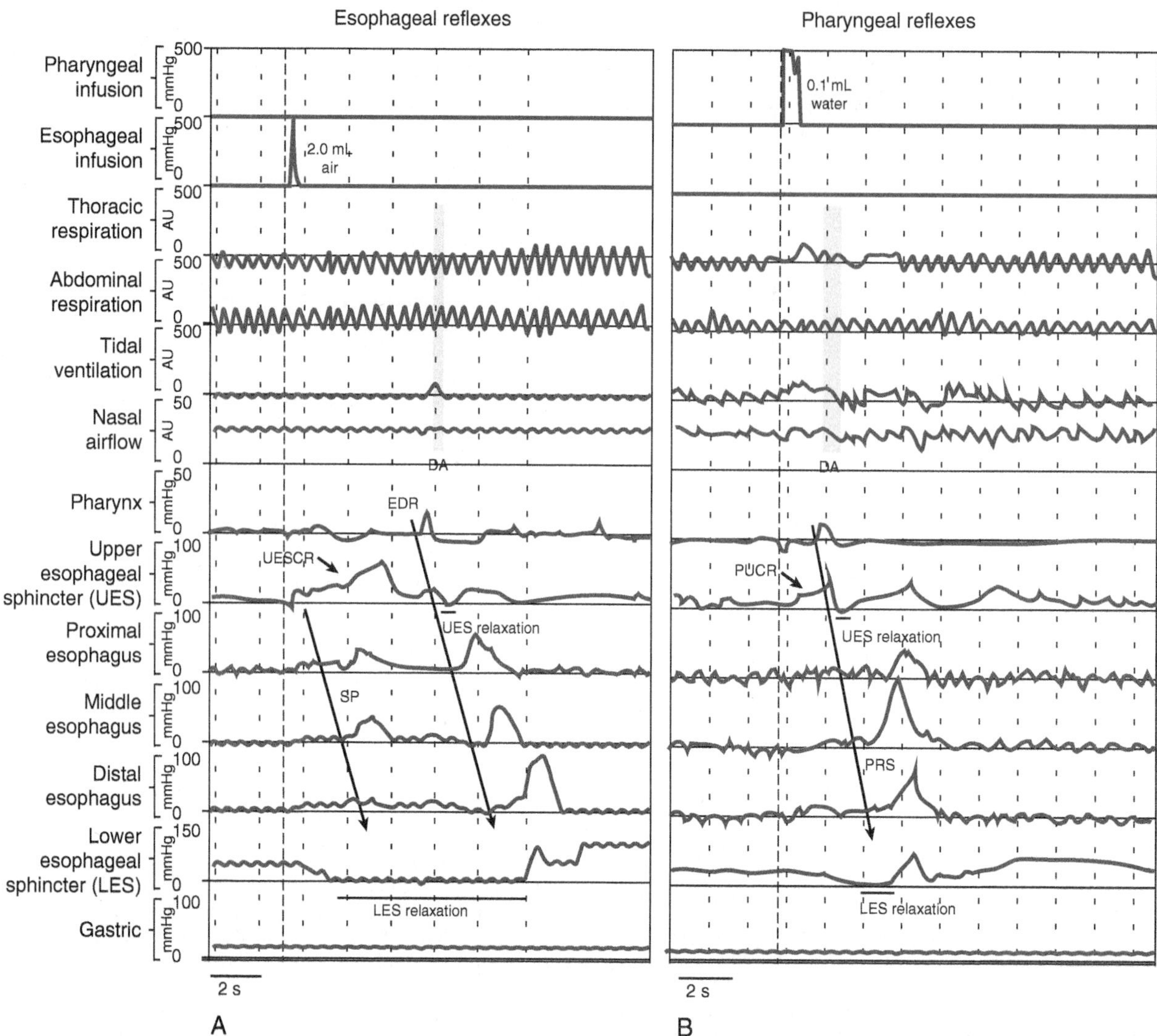

Fig. 161.6 Classification of esophageal and pharyngeal reflexes. (A) Upon midesophageal provocation (to simulate reflux), there are two possible distinct reflexes: secondary peristalsis *(SP)* or esophago-deglutition response *(EDR)*. SP is associated with upper esophageal sphincter *(UES)* contractile reflex *(UESCR)* to protect the airway, esophageal body *(EB)* peristalsis, and lower esophageal sphincter *(LES)* relaxation. EDR is associated with pharyngeal contraction, UES relaxation, EB peristalsis, and LES relaxation. (B) Similarly, upon pharyngeal provocation (to simulate oral bolus), there are two possible distinct reflexes. Pharyngo-UES contractile reflex *(PUCR)* occurs without EB peristalsis or LES relaxation as is more commonly seen in adults. Pharyngeal reflexive swallow *(PRS)* is similar to EDR in the fact that pharyngeal contraction occurs along with UES and LES relaxation and EB peristalsis. A swallow-associated apnea (deglutition apnea; *DA*) occurs during pharyngeal swallowing, signaling a break in respiratory rhythm and thus protecting against anterograde aspiration during deglutition. (Courtesy S. R. Jadcherla.)

inflammation, anomalies, immaturity, and esophageal clearance mechanisms.

PATHOPHYSIOLOGIC CONSIDERATIONS OF GASTROESOPHAGEAL REFLUX

MANIFESTATIONS OF GASTROESOPHAGEAL REFLUX IN THE NEONATE

Neonatal GER is considered pathologic if it is associated with growth failure due to poor feeding, excessive regurgitation, pulmonary complications, or neurobehavioral manifestations, such as severe irritability or Sandifer syndrome. In these cases, the diagnosis is made on the basis of a clear temporal association of the symptoms with feeding times or episodes of regurgitation. The relationship between GER and apnea of prematurity is now clearer. Although it had been assumed that apnea of prematurity is caused at least in part by GER, several studies using combined pH monitoring, multichannel intraluminal impedance, and polysomnography have demonstrated that apnea is no more likely to occur after a reflux event (either acid or non-acid) than during a reflux-free period.[66-75] Therefore measures directed towards modifying GER events or refluxate characteristics will be less effective in reducing the frequency or severity of apnea of prematurity.

SYMPTOMATOLOGY

Aerodigestive symptoms provide clues to GER, and persistence of troublesome symptoms in the presence of chronic GER constitutes GERD. *Dysphagia*, or abnormalities of swallowing in its various phases (oral, pharyngeal, esophageal, or gastric phase), can be related to esophageal pathology. GER or GERD are commonly suspected to be causes of swallowing problems. These entities range from simple regurgitation or physiologic reflux in healthy-appearing, thriving infants (see Fig. 161.8) to troublesome symptoms (Fig. 161.10; see Fig. 161.9) seen in the pathologic form of GERD. The signs and symptoms of GERD and its complications commonly include arching, irritability, throat clearing, autonomic signs (e.g., facial flushing, tearing, and cardiorespiratory changes), hoarse cry, choking, coughing and stridor, airway and respiratory compromise, retrograde aspiration, and bronchospasm. The symptoms in GERD can be due to abnormalities of refluxate clearance or abnormalities of aerodigestive protective functions.

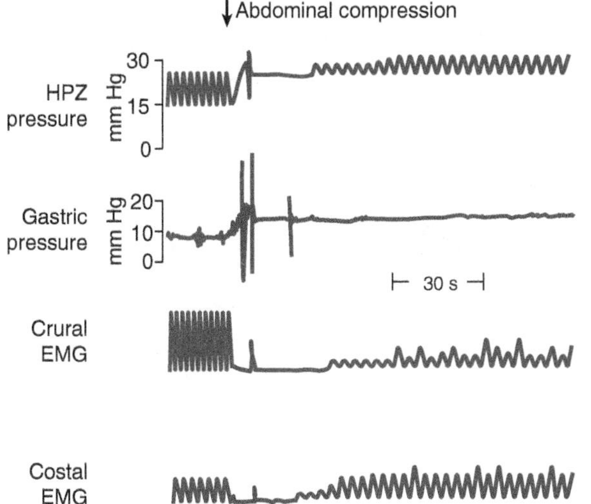

Fig. 161.7 Effect of abdominal compression on the high-pressure zone *(HPZ)* pressure profile. With the onset of abdominal compression, end-expiratory HPZ pressure increases, and crural and costal diaphragmatic electromyographic *(EMG)* activity decreases. The crural diaphragmatic EMG activity remains inhibited for the duration of the stimulus, whereas costal activity returns to baseline levels. As a result of the inhibition of crural EMG activity, a decrease occurs in the magnitude of the respiratory-induced oscillations in HPZ pressure. The increase in end-expiratory HPZ pressure is greater than the increase in gastric pressure induced by the abdominal compression, a finding indicating that the lower esophageal sphincter has undergone an adaptive response during the period of abdominal compression. (From Boyle JT, Altschuler SM, Nixon TE, et al. Responses of feline gastroesophageal junction to changes in abdominal pressure. *Am J Physiol.* 1987;253:G315–G322.)

PATHOPHYSIOLOGIC BASIS FOR SYMPTOMS IN GASTROESOPHAGEAL REFLUX DISEASE

The aerodigestive symptoms result either from neural reflexes evoked in response to spread of the refluxate along the esophagus or from respiratory compromise when the refluxate reaches the pharynx. Owing to the variable composition of refluxed material, symptoms can vary and depend on the spatial and temporal characteristics of its spread, chemical, and volume clearance.[1,43,44] For example, the refluxate has (1) variable physical characteristics (the contents may be gas, liquid, mixed, or semisolid); (2) variable chemical characteristics (the contents may be acid, weakly acid, nonacid, or alkaline); (3) variability of constituents (milk, partially digested milk, enzymes, bacteria, and saliva); and (4) variability of its most proximal extent (the distal esophagus, midesophagus, proximal esophagus, pharynx, nasopharynx, or oropharynx could be the targets for provoking symptoms).

Thus GER symptoms result from activation of afferent and efferent nerves subserving that route of spread of refluxate. For example, when the most proximal extent is the pharynx, there is predominance of respiratory symptoms; however, when the most proximal extent is the distal esophagus, there is predominance of sensory symptoms.[43,44]

Posture has an important bearing on GER and therefore the symptoms associated with the events. This is because (1) the angle at gastroesophageal junction (angle of His) is obtuse (contrasting with acute angle in adults) and is altered in different postures, (2) the relationship of the fundus to the esophageal body is modified, and (3) protective mechanisms can be recruited differently.[1,60,61,76–78] The effects of posture are summarized and referenced as follows:

1. Supine posture is the recommended posture to prevent SIDS (as per the American Academy of Pediatrics' Back to Sleep campaign). GER occurs more frequently in this position because the angle of His at the gastroesophageal junction becomes more obtuse. Notably, airway protection mechanisms are also more favorable in the supine position.[79-82]
2. Prone posture is associated with more acute angulation at the gastroesophageal junction, thus preventing GER. However, aerodigestive clearance and protection mechanisms are impaired under these conditions. In extreme cases of GERD, this position is permissible under inpatient monitored conditions.[58,60,83,84]
3. Left lateral posture is associated with less GER.[60,85]

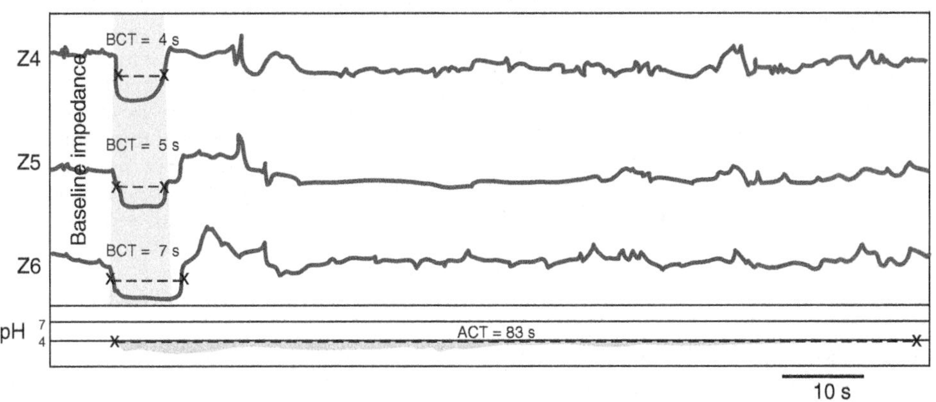

Fig. 161.8 Physical and chemical characteristics of refluxate. Depicted is an example of acid (pH<4) gastroesophageal reflux utilizing pH/impedance methods. Note the presence of liquid bolus in the impedance sensors (Z4, Z5, Z6) with the corresponding bolus clearance time *(BCT)* defined as the duration (seconds) from when the baseline impedance drops by 50% and returns to 50% of the baseline impedance. Similarly, note the acid clearance time *(ACT)* in the pH sensor defined as the duration from pH of less than 4 to pH of 4 or greater, with magnitude measured as the lowest pH reached. Also, notice that BCTs are often shorter in duration than ACT. (Courtesy S.R. Jadcherla.)

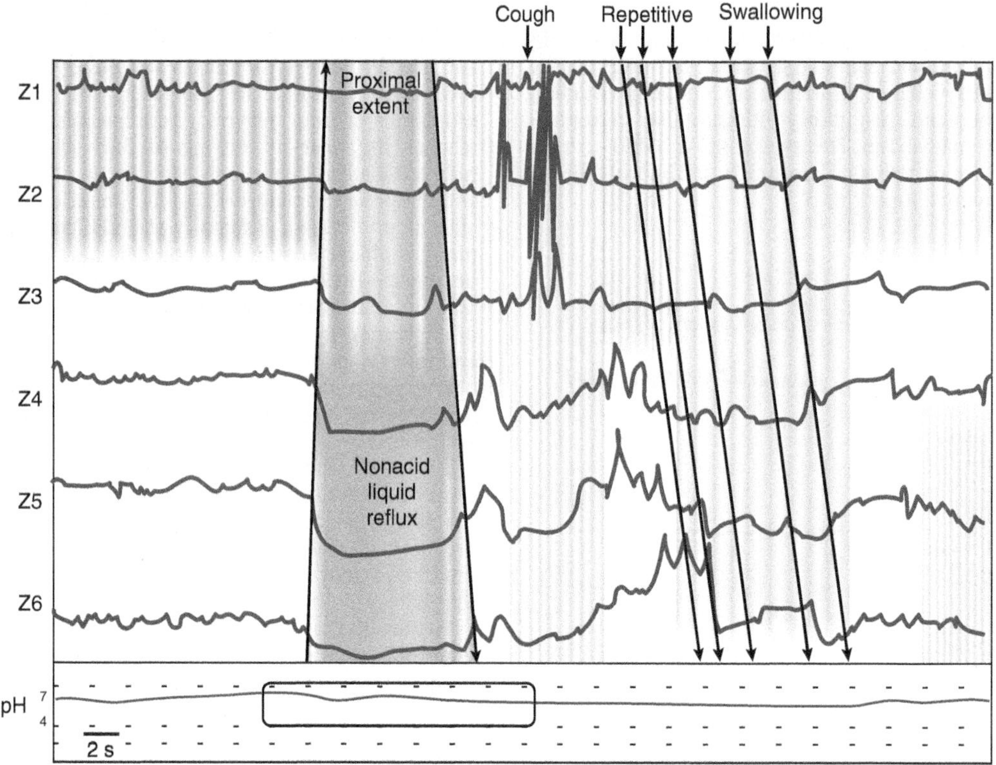

Fig. 161.9 Symptomatic nonacid reflux. Depicted is an example of nonacid (pH>4) reflux utilizing pH/impedance methods. Impedance *(Z)* sensors range from the proximal *(Z1)* to distal *(Z6)* esophagus, with *gray shade* representing liquid. Note that nonacid reflux ascends through the proximal esophagus and pharynx (Z1) and is followed by cough and multiple swallow attempts to clear the reflux. (Courtesy S.R. Jadcherla.)

4. Right lateral posture is associated with better gastric emptying, but more GER, thus implying that GER and gastric emptying can be unrelated.[61]

CAUSAL MECHANISMS OF GASTROESOPHAGEAL REFLUX IN THE NEONATE CAN BE DISTINCT

GER occurs more frequently in neonates and young infants than in individuals of any other age owing to the following mechanisms:

1. GER occurs most commonly due to transient LES relaxation in response to esophageal or gastric distension.[86] As noted previously, transient LES relaxations are mediated by the vagus nerve. A variety of neurotransmitters have been implicated including vasoactive intestinal peptide, nitric oxide, cholecystokinin, and acetylcholine. In contrast, gamma-aminobutyric acid (targeting GABA-B receptors) and opioids inhibit TLESR.[87-89]
2. Inflammation in infants with GERD increases TLESR and decreases resting LES tone.
3. Premature infants have a reduced stomach capacity, shorter esophageal length, and shorter intraabdominal part of the LES.
4. With TLESR, the crural diaphragm is inhibited concurrent with LES relaxation. Thus, the antireflux barrier is weakened.[7,90]

PROTECTIVE MECHANISMS AGAINST GASTROESOPHAGEAL REFLUX AND ASPIRATION

There are several hierarchical tiers of protective mechanisms against GER and its consequences.

1. When the esophagus is provoked due to refluxate, regional reflexes are activated, facilitating upstream protection (UES contractile reflex and secondary peristalsis), hypervigilant airway reflexes (esophagoglottal closure reflex and bronchospasm), and downstream clearance (secondary peristalsis and LES relaxation reflex).[26,91-95] In situations when refluxate ascends to the pharynx, repetitive deglutition sequences occur (see Fig. 161.3C).
2. When the pharynx is provoked by refluxate, it initiates reflexive swallowing, the pharyngoglottal closure reflex, and modulation of respiratory rhythms to clear the pharynx and protect the airway.[40,96,97] Persistent and repetitive events such as these may lead to swallowing dysfunction.
3. When the laryngeal airway is provoked, it initiates the glottic-closure reflex, cough reflex, prolonged exhalation, bronchospasm, and repetitive swallowing to clear the airway of the stimulus. During this sequential phenomenon, airway adaptation and modulation of breathing ensues. Persistent and recurrent events may lead to airway inflammation, laryngeal penetration, laryngeal aspiration, atelectasis, bronchospasm, and changes in pulmonary function.
4. GER events during sleep are associated with arousals and changes in sleep stages, thus supporting a hypervigilant state.[95,98] During these occurrences, modulation of breathing also ensues, and restoration of respiratory and sleep rhythms occur upon peristalsis and esophageal clearance. Persistent and recurrent situations lead to disruption of sleep cycles and life-threatening events. Examples of causal and protective mechanisms are shown in Figs. 161.4 and 161.6.

RECENT ADVANCES IN GER OR GERD RESEARCH

Coexisting morbidities, along with factors that influence extrauterine maturation of sensory-motor behaviors, may increase the risk of GERD, and these may include but are not limited to congenital anomalies, chronic lung disease in infants, or neuropathology.[99,100] The use of acid-suppressive therapies, caffeine, and bronchodilators may not help

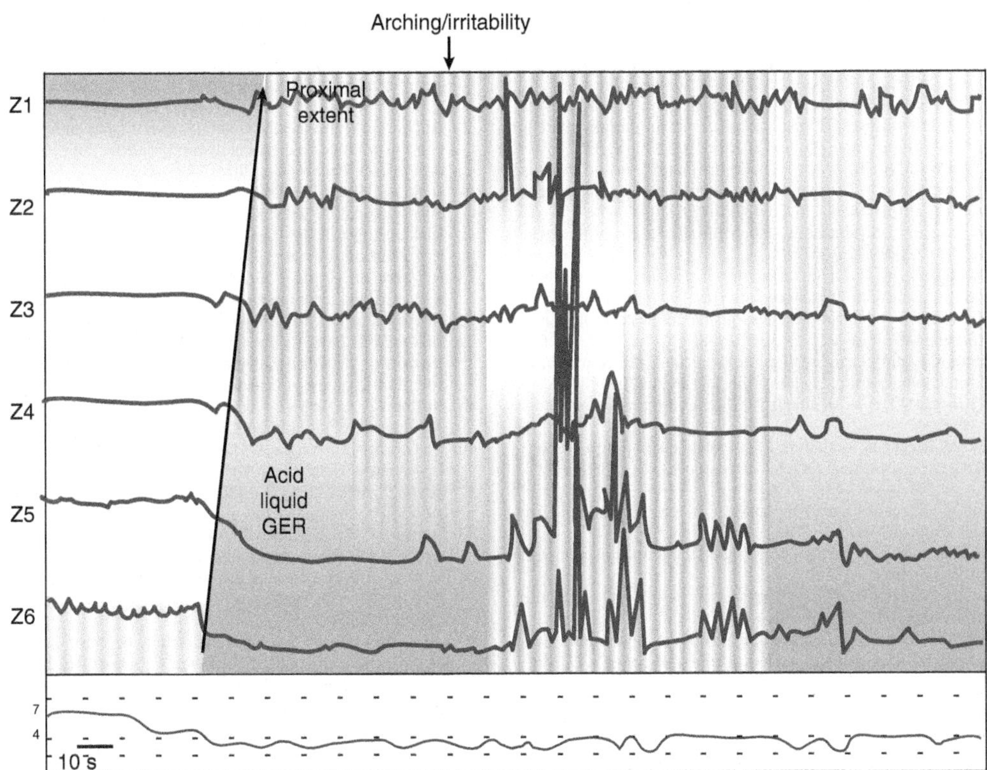

Fig. 161.10 Symptomatic acid reflux. Depicted is an example of acid (pH<4) gastroesophageal reflux *(GER)* utilizing pH/impedance methods. Impedance *(Z)* sensors range from the proximal *(Z1)* to distal *(Z6)* esophagus, with *gray shading* representing liquid. Note the acid GER migrates to the proximal extent (Z1) and is followed by arching/irritability; clearance is delayed. (Courtesy S. R. Jadcherla.)

with GERD management, or may even worsen GERD due to altering gastric pH and therefore its sensitivity in the esophagus; furthermore, changes in LES tone or responses to esophageal provocation can be altered.[101,102] Symptom-based clinical management alone is not ideal unless the basis for symptoms is determined. The latter may include examining for heightened visceral or somatic sensitivity, acid neutralization delays, pharyngoesophageal clearance, foregut dysmotility, inflammation, or impaired pharyngoesophageal-cardiorespiratory reflexes.[103,104] True causality needs to be determined prior to subjecting infant for medical or surgical therapies for ameliorating GERD.

ACKNOWLEDGMENTS

Dr. Jadcherla's efforts are supported in part by NIH grants RO1 DK 068158 and PO1 DK 068051. We are grateful to Kathryn Hasenstab, BS, BME, for assistance with manuscript submission, and creating figures and artwork.

 A complete reference list is available at www.ExpertConsult.com.

SELECT REFERENCES

1. Jadcherla SR, Chan CY, Moore R, et al. Impact of feeding strategies on the frequency and clearance of acid and nonacid gastroesophageal reflux events in dysphagic neonates. *JPEN J Parenter Enteral Nutr*. 2012;36:449–455.
2. Mansfield LE. Embryonic origins of the relation of gastroesophageal reflux disease and airway disease. *Am J Med*. 2001;111:3S–7S.
3. Miller JL, Sonies BC, Macedonia C. Emergence of oropharyngeal, laryngeal and swallowing activity in the developing fetal upper aerodigestive tract: an ultrasound evaluation. *Early Hum Dev*. 2003;71:61–87.
4. Sadler TW. Respiratory system. *Langman's Medical Embryology*. 7th ed. Baltimore: Williams & Wilkins; 1995:232–241.
5. Sadler TW. Digestive system. *Langman's Medical Embryology*. 7th ed. Baltimore: Williams & Wilkins; 1995:208–229.
6. Lang IM, Shaker R. Anatomy and physiology of the upper esophageal sphincter. *Am J Med*. 1997;103:50S–55S.
7. Mittal RK, Balaban DH. The esophagogastric junction. *N Engl J Med*. 1997;336:924–932.
8. Goyal R, Sivarao D. *Functional Anatomy and Physiology of Swallowing and Esophageal Motility*. Philadelphia: Lippincott Williams & Wilkins; 1999.
9. Goyal RK, Padmanabhan R, Sang Q. Neural circuits in swallowing and abdominal vagal afferent-mediated lower esophageal sphincter relaxation. *Am J Med*. 2001;111:95S–105S.
10. Rattan S, Goyal RK. Neural control of the lower esophageal sphincter: influence of the vagus nerves. *J Clin Invest*. 1974;54:899–906.
11. Biancani P, Zabinski M, Kerstein M, Behar J. Lower esophageal sphincter mechanics: anatomic and physiologic relationships of the esophagogastric junction of cat. *Gastroenterology*. 1982;82:468–475.
12. Behar J, Kerstein M, Biancani P. Neural control of the lower esophageal sphincter in the cat: studies on the excitatory pathways to the lower esophageal sphincter. *Gastroenterology*. 1982;82:680–688.
13. Liu JB, Miller LS, Goldberg BB, et al. Transnasal US of the esophagus: preliminary morphologic and function studies. *Radiology*. 1992;184:721–727.
14. Goyal RK, Rattan S. Genesis of basal sphincter pressure: effect of tetrodotoxin on lower esophageal sphincter pressure in opossum in vivo. *Gastroenterology*. 1976;71:62–67.
15. Sengupta A, Paterson WG, Goyal RK. Atypical localization of myenteric neurons in the opossum lower esophageal sphincter. *Am J Anat*. 1987;180:342–348.
16. Hillemeier C, Gryboski J, McCallum R, Biancani P. Developmental characteristics of the lower esophageal sphincter in the kitten. *Gastroenterology*. 1985;89:760–766.
17. Pope 2nd CE. A dynamic test of sphincter strength: its application to the lower esophageal sphincter. *Gastroenterology*. 1967;52:779–786.
18. Welch RW, Gray JE. Influence of respiration on recordings of lower esophageal sphincter pressure in humans. *Gastroenterology*. 1982;83:590–594.
19. Liebermann-Meffert D, Allgower M, Schmid P, Blum AL. Muscular equivalent of the lower esophageal sphincter. *Gastroenterology*. 1979;76:31–38.
20. Goyal RK, Rattan S. Nature of the vagal inhibitory innervation to the lower esophageal sphincter. *J Clin Invest*. 1975;55:1119–1126.
21. Mittal RK, Fisher M, McCallum RW, et al. Human lower esophageal sphincter pressure response to increased intra-abdominal pressure. *Am J Physiol*. 1990;258:G624–G630.
22. Mittal RK, Fisher MJ. Electrical and mechanical inhibition of the crural diaphragm during transient relaxation of the lower esophageal sphincter. *Gastroenterology*. 1990;99:1265–1268.
23. Altschuler SM, Boyle JT, Nixon TE, et al. Simultaneous reflex inhibition of lower esophageal sphincter and crural diaphragm in cats. *Am J Physiol*. 1985;249:G586–G591.

24. Harding R, Titchen DA. Oesophageal and diaphragmatic activity during sucking in lambs. *J Physiol*. 1981;321:317-329.
25. Duron B. Proceedings: inhibitory reflex from the oesophagus to the crura of the diaphragm. *Bull Physio-Pathol Respir (Nancy)*. 1975;11:105P-106P.
26. Pena EM, Parks VN, Peng J, et al. Lower esophageal sphincter relaxation reflex kinetics: effects of peristaltic reflexes and maturation in human premature neonates. *Am J Physiol Gastrointest Liver Physiol*. 2010;299:G1386-G1395.
27. Gupta A, Gulati P, Kim W, et al. Effect of postnatal maturation on the mechanisms of esophageal propulsion in preterm human neonates: primary and secondary peristalsis. *Am J Gastroenterol*. 2009;104:411-419.
28. Werlin SL, Dodds WJ, Hogan WJ, Arndorfer RC. Mechanisms of gastroesophageal reflux in children. *J Pediatr*. 1980;97:244-249.
29. Omari TI, Miki K, Davidson G, et al. Characterisation of relaxation of the lower oesophageal sphincter in healthy premature infants. *Gut*. 1997;40:370-375.
30. Kawahara H, Dent J, Davidson G. Mechanisms responsible for gastroesophageal reflux in children. *Gastroenterology*. 1997;113:399-408.
31. Omari T, Barnett C, Snel A, et al. Mechanism of gastroesophageal reflux in premature infants with chronic lung disease. *J Pediatr Surg*. 1999;34:1795-1798.
32. Werlin SL, Dodds WJ, Hogan WJ, et al. Mechanisms of gastroesophageal reflux in children. *J Pediatr*. 1980;9(2):244-249.
33. Holloway RH, Hongo M, Berger K, McCallum RW. Gastric distention: a mechanism for postprandial gastroesophageal reflux. *Gastroenterology*. 1985;89:779-784.
34. Kahrilas PJ, Dodds WJ, Dent J, et al. Upper esophageal sphincter function during belching. *Gastroenterology*. 1986;91:133-140.
35. Wyman JB, Dent J, Heddle R, et al. Control of belching by the lower oesophageal sphincter. *Gut*. 1990;31:639-646.
36. Mittal RK, Holloway RH, Penagini R, et al. Transient lower esophageal sphincter relaxation. *Gastroenterology*. 1995;109:601-610.
37. Mittal RK, McCallum RW. Characteristics and frequency of transient relaxations of the lower esophageal sphincter in patients with reflux esophagitis. *Gastroenterology*. 1988;95:593-599.
38. Mittal RK, McCallum RW. Characteristics of transient lower esophageal sphincter relaxation in humans. *Am J Physiol*. 1987;252:G636-G641.
39. Paterson WG, Rattan S, Goyal RK. Experimental induction of isolated lower esophageal sphincter relaxation in anesthetized opossums. *J Clin Invest*. 1986;77:1187-1193.
40. Jadcherla SR, Shubert TR, Gulati IK, et al. Upper and lower esophageal sphincter kinetics are modified during maturation: effect of pharyngeal stimulus in premature infants. *Pediatr Res*. 2015;77:99-106.
41. Shaker R, Hogan WJ. Reflex-mediated enhancement of airway protective mechanisms. *Am J Med*. 2000;108:8S-14S.
42. Shaker R, Ren J, Xie P, et al. Characterization of the pharyngo-UES contractile reflex in humans. *Am J Physiol*. 1997;273:G854-G858.
43. Jadcherla SR, Gupta A, Fernandez S, et al. Spatiotemporal characteristics of acid refluxate and relationship to symptoms in premature and term infants with chronic lung disease. *Am J Gastroenterol*. 2008;103:720-728.
44. Jadcherla SR, Peng J, Chan CY, et al. Significance of gastroesophageal refluxate in relation to physical, chemical, and spatiotemporal characteristics in symptomatic intensive care unit neonates. *Pediatr Res*. 2011;70:192-198.
45. Sutphen JL, Dillard VL. Dietary caloric density and osmolality influence gastroesophageal reflux in infants. *Gastroenterology*. 1989;97:601-604.
46. Di Lorenzo C, Piepsz A, Ham H, Cadranel S. Gastric emptying with gastro-oesophageal reflux. *Arch Dis Child*. 1987;62:449-453.
47. Boyle JT, Altschuler SM, Nixon TE, et al. Responses of feline gastroesophageal junction to changes in abdominal pressure. *Am J Physiol*. 1987;253:G315-G322.
48. Biancani P, Walsh JH, Behar J. Vasoactive intestinal polypeptide. A neurotransmitter for lower esophageal sphincter relaxation. *J Clin Invest*. 1984;73:963-967.
49. Strawczynski H, McKenna RD, Nickerson GH. The behavior of the lower esophageal sphincter in infants and its relationship to gastroesophageal regurgitation. *J Pediatr*. 1964;64:17-23.
50. Gupta A, Jadcherla SR. The relationship between somatic growth and in vivo esophageal segmental and sphincteric growth in human neonates. *J Pediatr Gastroenterol Nutr*. 2006;43:35-41.

162 Pathophysiology and Prevention of Neonatal Necrotizing Enterocolitis

Misty Good | Michael Caplan

INTRODUCTION

Neonatal necrotizing enterocolitis (NEC) is a common and devastating gastrointestinal disease that primarily afflicts premature neonates after the initiation of enteral feeding.[1,2] Despite the significant morbidity and mortality associated with NEC, the pathophysiology has remained poorly understood. The disease is seen clinically in premature neonates with variable signs, including intestinal bleeding, emesis, abdominal distension and tenderness, lethargy, apnea and bradycardia, thrombocytopenia, metabolic acidosis, respiratory failure, and, if severe, shock.[3] Clues to the origin are suggested by the pathologic changes observed in surgical specimens and autopsy material, including coagulation necrosis, inflammation (acute or chronic), and less commonly ulceration, hemorrhage, reparative change, bacterial overgrowth, edema, and pneumatosis intestinalis.[1,4]

Although most cases of NEC are diagnosed in premature neonates, term infants with specific underlying risk factors are at risk for this disease.[5] Previous studies have identified birth asphyxia, polycythemia, exchange transfusion, intrauterine growth restriction, cyanotic congenital heart disease, myelomeningocele, gastroschisis, and intrauterine cocaine exposure as potential events leading to the development of intestinal injury.[6] Nonetheless, the presentation of NEC in these cases is typically different from that in premature infants, with the onset in the first days after delivery and the course often less dramatic. For these reasons, the pathophysiology in term infants may be quite different from that in the premature neonate and is therefore not considered further in this chapter.

PREMATURITY: THE MAJOR RISK FACTOR FOR NECROTIZING ENTEROCOLITIS

The multifactorial theory of NEC pathogenesis was previously suggested to explain the pathophysiology of neonatal NEC and purports that several risk factors (prematurity, formula feeding, ischemia or asphyxia, and bacterial colonization) result in the final common pathway of bowel necrosis.[7] More than 90% of cases of NEC occur in premature infants, whereas stratification studies have shown that gestational age and birth weight inversely correlate with a higher incidence of disease, with the highest incidence of NEC at 28 to 32 weeks corrected age.[8] Epidemiologic observations suggest a relationship between intestinal ischemia, infection, and formula feeding on the development of NEC; however, the presence of these factors is less consistent than the presence of prematurity. Although there are many differences between preterm and term neonates, the specific underlying mechanisms responsible for the predilection of NEC for the premature condition remain incompletely elucidated and are an area of intense investigation. Studies in humans and animals have identified alterations in multiple components of intestinal host

Box 162.1 Premature Infants

Factors That May Increase Their Susceptibility to Necrotizing Enterocolitis

1.1 Compromised Intestinal Host Defense
1.2 Physical Barriers
- Skin
- Mucous membranes
- Epithelia and microvilli
- Tight junctions
- Mucin

1.3 Immune Factors
- Neutrophils
- Macrophages
- Eosinophils
- Lymphocytes (including intraepithelial lymphocytes)
- Secretory IgA

1.4 Biochemical Factors
- Antimicrobial proteins (trefoil factor, defensins, and cryptdins)
- Oligosaccharides
- Glutamine
- Lactoferrin
- Polyunsaturated fatty acids
- Nucleotides
- Growth factors (EGF, TGF, IGF, erythropoietin)
- Gastric acid
- Cytokines

1.5 Intestinal Dysmotility
- Migratory motor complexes

1.6 Bacteria
- Patterns of colonization or overgrowth
- Pathogenicity of organisms

1.7 Altered Autoregulation of Intestinal Circulation
- Basal vascular resistance
- Response to stress

1.8 Disordered Inflammatory Response
- Increased proinflammatory response to stimuli
- Suppressed antiinflammatory components

EGF, Epidermal growth factor; *Ig,* immunoglobulin; *IGF,* insulin-like growth factor; *TGF,* transforming growth factor.

defense,[9] motility,[10-12] bacterial colonization,[13-15] blood flow regulation,[16-18] and inflammatory response,[19,20] which may all contribute to the development of intestinal injury in this unique population (Box 162.1).

HOST DEFENSE

Intestinal host defense involves a complex combination of factors that function to prevent intraluminal pathogens and toxins from resulting in disease while allowing for normal absorption of nutrients. This intricate system includes the following: (1) physical barriers such as skin, mucous membranes, intestinal epithelia and microvilli, epithelial cell tight junctions, and mucin; (2) immune cells such as polymorphonuclear leukocytes, macrophages, eosinophils, lymphocytes, as well as secretory immunoglobulin A (IgA); and (3) several biochemical factors shown to impact the development of NEC.[21-26] Many of these important functions appear to be abnormal in the premature infant and may, therefore, put this population at risk for NEC. Intestinal permeability to macromolecules including immunoglobulins, proteins, and carbohydrates is known to be greater in neonates compared with older children and adults, and in premature infants, this permeability is more pronounced.[27] Although mucosal permeability is beneficial for developing animals to augment passive immunity and nutrient absorption, the precise mechanisms accounting for these differences are poorly understood. The intestinal tight junctions that maintain the gut barrier may also be deficient in the premature infant.[28,29] It is known that intestinal mucus (a complex gel consisting of water, electrolytes, mucins, glycoprotein, immunoglobulins, and glycolipids) protects against bacterial and toxin invasion and the thickness of the mucus layer and expression of mucus glycoproteins are reduced in developing animals.[30-32] In addition, key bacteriostatic proteins are secreted from epithelium, which bind to or inactivate the function of invading organisms. Intestinal trefoil factor is one such molecule that appears to be developmentally regulated and therefore deficient in the premature neonate.[33] Human defensins (or cryptdins) are bacteriostatic proteins synthesized and secreted from Paneth cells that protect against bacterial translocation, and their expression is significantly decreased (200-fold lower) in the intestine of a premature infant compared to adults.[34,35] In contrast, during surgical NEC, the small intestinal mRNA expression of defensins 5 and 6 were upregulated compared to controls, which may perhaps be due to the timing of the resection relative to epithelial healing.[35-38]

Immunologic host defense is abnormal in developing animals. For example, intestinal lymphocytes are decreased in neonates (B and T cells) and do not approach adult levels until 3 to 4 weeks of life.[39,40] Newborns also have markedly reduced secretory IgA in salivary samples, reflecting the decreased activity presumed in the intestine.[41] Breast-milk feeding provides multiple immune factors; formula-fed neonates have impaired intestinal humoral immunity, and this deficiency may predispose to the increased incidence of NEC.[24,42] A complete review of the importance of breast milk in immunologic host defense can be found in Chapters 23 and 122 of this textbook.

Several biochemical factors that are present in the intestinal milieu play an important role in the maintenance of gut health and integrity. Examples are substances such as lactoferrin[43] and glutamine,[44] growth factors such as epidermal growth factor (EGF),[45] transforming growth factor-β,[46] and erythropoietin.[47,48] Lactoferrin is present in high concentrations in human milk and has been shown to reduce NEC severity in animal models of NEC,[49] but did not prevent NEC in a large randomized controlled trial (RCT) of over 2000 infants.[50] Interestingly, a meta-analysis that included six RCTs found that administration of lactoferrin decreased late-onset sepsis and Bell's Stage II or III NEC, but the evidence was deemed low in quality.[51] Another important component of human milk is the amino acid glutamine; higher concentrations of this can lead to increased weight gain and length in infants.[52,53] As with lactoferrin, glutamine also demonstrated efficacy in a neonatal rat model of NEC[54] and can play a role in maintaining the integrity of the gut barrier,[55] but in large RCTs failed to show a benefit against NEC in humans.[56] An area of intense interest in preclinical studies has been the use of growth factors to attenuate intestinal inflammation in animal models of NEC. Treatment with EGF and heparin-bound EGF have been shown to protect against gut barrier failure in experimental NEC,[57-59] decreased intestinal epithelial cell apoptosis,[45,60,61] and enhanced epithelial cell proliferation.[45,62] These studies suggest that growth factor administration may be beneficial in protecting against intestinal inflammation during NEC. In addition, other substances such as gastric acid,[63] oligosaccharides,[64] polyunsaturated fatty acids,[65] and many others affect mucosal barrier function, intestinal inflammation, and the viability of intraluminal bacteria. Many of these factors are deficient or absent in the preterm neonate, especially in those patients not receiving breast-milk feedings. Intensive research is ongoing to define the specific role of each in gut barrier integrity and the development of intestinal inflammation and necrosis.

MOTILITY

The premature infant has altered gastrointestinal motility; term newborn motility patterns or "migratory motor complexes" do not appear until 34 to 35 weeks' gestation.[10,66] Abnormal peristaltic activity may allow for bacterial overgrowth that could increase endotoxin exposure and predispose the infant to NEC.[67] Furthermore, dysmotility can cause intestinal dilatation and compromised intestinal blood flow, as demonstrated in a premature rabbit model of NEC.[68]

BACTERIAL COLONIZATION/INTESTINAL DYSBIOSIS

Premature infants hospitalized in the neonatal intensive care unit have different patterns of gut bacterial colonization than healthy breast-fed term infants.[15,69,70] Although epidemics of NEC have been described associated with specific bacteria (e.g., *Clostridia* spp., *Escherichia coli*, *Klebsiella* spp., *Staphylococcus epidermidis*), most cases occur endemically and are not associated with one specific bacteria in the stool.[71] Blood cultures are positive in only 20% to 30% of affected cases, and this likely represents the degree of mucosal damage at presentation. At birth, the intestine is a relatively sterile environment, and although there are several reports of low concentrations of bacteria in meconium present prior to delivery, no cases of NEC have been described in utero, a finding supporting the importance of bacterial colonization in the pathophysiology. Colonization develops with several species in breast-fed infants by 1 week of age that include probiotic (bacteria defined to confer a benefit to the host) organisms such as *Bifidobacteria* spp. and *Lactobacillus* spp., whereas the intestine in the hospitalized, extremely premature infant has less species diversity and fewer facultative anaerobes. This imbalance is referred to as *intestinal dysbiosis* and may allow for pathologic proliferation, binding, and invasiveness of otherwise nonpathogenic intestinal bacteria. In early DNA-focused microbiologic assessments, it was shown that extremely low-birth-weight infants have very different patterns of intestinal colonization compared to full-term infants.[69] Further, preterm infants afflicted with NEC appear to have different microbial ecology compared to preterm infant controls without NEC, at the time of disease onset and within 72 hours of developing disease.[15,72-74] Intestinal diversity was reduced in those patients who developed NEC, and those with disease had an increase and/or a preponderance of colonization by *Proteobacteria* phyla, gram-negative enteric pathogens that have been associated with the development of NEC. It has been shown that probiotic organisms can modulate the inflammatory response and improve mucosal barrier function by multiple mechanisms that can contribute to overall intestinal health.[75,76] It remains unclear whether bacterial translocation into submucosa is a prerequisite for NEC or, rather, the activation of the Toll-like receptors (TLRs) from endotoxin and other pathogen-associated molecular patterns is adequate to initiate the final common pathway of intestinal injury.[19,20,77] Nonetheless, certain bacteria contribute to the pathology seen in many animal models of NEC.[78] Furthermore, multiple reports have suggested that early enteral supplementation of probiotics (e.g., *Bifidobacterium* and *Lactobacillus*) reduces the risk of NEC in infants.[79,80] Probiotic trials have enrolled over 10,000 infants and even with clinical heterogeneity in each study, meta-analysis demonstrates a significant reduction in the incidence of NEC with a relative risk of 0.53; 95% confidence interval 0.42 to 0.66.[79] It is important that, in the context of neurodevelopmental outcomes and very low-birth-weight infants, an RCT of 400 infants demonstrated that administration of the probiotic *Lactobacillus reuteri* did not demonstrate differences in adverse neurocognitive outcomes compared to infants that received placebo.[79] Due to the clinical heterogeneity of each trial, it is imperative to consider each study and each strain independently. A strain-specific review was performed by van den Akker and colleagues and showed that relative risks for NEC are significantly decreased with seven probiotic treatments, specifically, *B. lactis*, *L. reuteri*, *L. rhamnosus GG*; the combination of *B. bifidum*, *B. infantis*, *B. longum*, and *L. acidophilus*; the combination of *B. infantis* and *L. acidophilus*; the combination of *B. infantis*, *B. lactis*, and *S. thermophilus*; and the combination of *B. longum* and *L. rhamnosus GG*.[81] In contrast, the Probiotics in Very Preterm Infants (PiPS) trial is the largest single trial to date, which demonstrated no difference in the risk of NEC between premature infants treated with the strain *Bifidobacterium breve* compared to placebo.[82] In addition, quality control and safety of these bacteria in immune-compromised high-risk infants must be confirmed.[83] While it is known that very low-birth-weight infants are at high risk for bacterial infection, it must also be noted that in premature infants a dose-response relationship to exposure to antibiotics results in an increased risk of NEC.[84] In summary, altered bacterial colonization patterns are an important factor in the initiation of intestinal injury, and additional studies demonstrate that microbial replacement is an effective preventive strategy for NEC.

INTESTINAL BLOOD FLOW REGULATION

Early observations of bowel wall perfusion using color Doppler ultrasonography suggested that profound intestinal ischemia was present in infants with NEC compared to similarly aged control infants.[85] Murdoch and colleagues demonstrated that high resistance patterns of Doppler flow velocity in the superior mesenteric artery just after birth increased an infant's risk for developing NEC.[86] Several groups have hypothesized that, in periods of stress, blood flow gets diverted away from the splanchnic circulation, with resultant intestinal mucosal injury and necrosis. In animal models, studies have shown that the reperfusion after intestinal ischemia is required for the cell death seen in experimental NEC, and therefore investigations of the role of intestinal ischemia in the pathophysiology of NEC are focused on this construct.[87]

Intestinal and somatic growth is dramatic in developing animals, and therefore providing sufficient blood flow is mandatory. Neonatal animals have been shown to have differences in the intestinal circulation that may predispose them to NEC. The basal intestinal vascular resistance is elevated in the fetus and decreases significantly after birth, thus allowing for a rapid increase in intestinal blood flow.[88] It has been shown that this change in the resting vascular resistance is dependent on the balance between the dilator (nitric oxide) and constrictor (endothelin) molecules and the myogenic response.[89,90] In findings perhaps more relevant than basal vascular tone, studies have shown that the newborn has alterations in response to circulatory stress, resulting in compromised intestinal flow and altered vascular resistance. In response to hypotension, studies demonstrate that newborn animals (3-day-old but not 30-day-old swine) appear to have defective pressure-flow autoregulation, resulting in compromised intestinal oxygen delivery and tissue oxygenation.[88,91,92] In addition, in the presence of arterial hypoxemia, the newborn intestinal circulatory response differs from that in older animals. Although intestinal vasodilation and increased intestinal perfusion occur after modest hypoxemia, severe hypoxemia causes vasoconstriction, intestinal ischemia, and hypoxia, mediated in part by the loss of nitric oxide production.[18] Multiple chemical mediators (nitric oxide, endothelin, substance P, norepinephrine, and angiotensin) affect intestinal vasomotor tone, and, in the stressed newborn, abnormal production of these mediators can result in compromised circulatory autoregulation, leading to the perpetuation of intestinal ischemia and tissue necrosis.[93,94]

ENTERAL ALIMENTATION

Enteral alimentation has long been considered a significant risk factor in the initiation of NEC; more than 90% of cases occurred in premature infants after feedings were introduced. The timing of disease onset occurs after the first feeding and typically ten days after birth in premature infants.[95] The relationship between enteral feedings and NEC has been well studied, and several investigators have identified the importance of breast milk (vs. formula), osmolality, and substrate fermentation as important factors.[42,96]

Donor breast-milk feeding has been shown in early human studies to reduce the incidence of NEC by six to ten times compared to infants fed formula.[96] Breast milk contains multiple bioactive factors that influence host immunity, inflammation, and mucosal protection including secretory IgA, leukocytes, lactoferrin, lysozyme, mucin, cytokines, growth factors, enzymes, oligosaccharides, and polyunsaturated fatty acids, which are absent in or recently added to (e.g., polyunsaturated fatty acids) neonatal formula preparations.[42] Specific intestinal host defense factors acquired from breast milk such as growth factors (EGF,[45] heparin-binding EGF,[97] transforming growth factor β,[46] and erythropoietin[47]), polyunsaturated fatty acids,[98] oligosaccharides,[17,99] platelet-activating factor (PAF) acetylhydrolase,[100] IgA,[24] and macrophages are effective in reducing the incidence of disease in animals.[22] Previous studies and a recent Cochrane review suggest that an exclusively milk-based diet reduces the risk of disease (human milk with human milk–based fortification versus human milk with bovine-based fortifiers).[101-103] Because most premature infants receive breast milk by the nasogastric route after artificial collection by mothers and subsequent freezing, it has been suggested that the methods of collection and feeding interfere with the immune properties of breast milk. Additionally, the presence of a nasogastric tube can lead to colonization of opportunistic pathogens and can constitute an infectious risk factor to consider when evaluating feeding strategies in premature infants.[104-106]

Specific components of milk feedings have been implicated in causing mucosal injury in the high-risk neonate. Studies have shown that hyperosmolar formulas resulted in NEC, and the addition of medication to feedings can markedly increase osmolality.[107] Animal studies have shown that the fat composition in infant formula, specifically the long-chain triglyceride-containing unsaturated fatty acids, can damage the developing intestine and lead to oxidative stress.[65] Additional research is needed to determine the mechanisms by which different components of formula lead to intestinal injury in premature infants.

Different approaches to feeding have been associated with the initiation of NEC. Early studies suggested that rapid volume increases with full-strength formula increased the incidence of disease, and protocols were designed to limit feeding advancement. However, several studies have now shown that early trophic feedings are safe and improve gastrointestinal function in very low-birth-weight infants.[108] The rate of feeding advancement is not a significant contributing factor to the risk of NEC.[108]

In summary, the premature neonate has several unique features that may increase susceptibility to NEC. Still, the precise interrelationship of these factors in the final common pathway of intestinal necrosis remains unclear.

FINAL COMMON PATHWAY: THE INFLAMMATORY CASCADE

Based on a growing body of evidence obtained from humans, and from animal and tissue experimentation, the final common pathway of intestinal injury appears to result from a disordered intestinal microbiome initiating the activation of the inflammatory cascade.[3] This cascade involves a complex balance of pro-inflammatory and antiinflammatory endogenous mediators, receptors, signaling pathways, second messengers, and a variety of downstream effects that ultimately results in end-organ damage in certain circumstances (Fig. 162.1). Inflammation can be initiated by a variety of factors, most notably the exposure to the bacterial cell wall product endotoxin,[109] and as previously mentioned, there is significant evidence that increased intestinal colonization of gram-negative pathogenic organisms precedes the diagnosis of NEC.[13,15] After endotoxin stimulation of the TLR family in animals, tissue, or cells, several mediators are rapidly produced, including PAF, tumor necrosis factor, and interleukin (IL)-1.[110] With the use of a neonatal mouse model of NEC that resembles the human condition after exposure to formula feeding and asphyxial stress, it was shown that the interaction of endotoxin with TLR4 is a critical determinant of disease pathogenesis.[19,20,31] In the intestine, subsequent events lead to chemotaxis, transmigration, and activation of leukocytes and the synthesis and release of many products from epithelial and inflammatory cells such as IL-6, IL-8, IL-10, IL-18, thromboxanes, leukotrienes, prostaglandins, nitric oxide, endothelin-1, and oxygen-free radicals.[9] In addition, evidence demonstrates that TLR responses are dependent on β-catenin signaling and HSP70 expression.[111,112] If counterregulatory responses are insufficient, pathologic changes to gut mucosa occur and may include accentuated apoptosis and autophagy of epithelial cells, perturbation of tight junctional proteins and complexes, increased mucosal permeability, bacterial translocation, alterations of vascular tone and microcirculation, and additional immune cell infiltration and accumulation.[17,18,113-115] The process may then be perpetuated by the activation of the secondary inflammatory response (Fig. 162.2), and the final common pathway will result in intestinal necrosis. Although these events remain localized in some cases, in others, this activation results in the systemic inflammatory response syndrome, in which patients have capillary leak, hypotension, metabolic acidosis, thrombocytopenia, renal failure, respiratory failure, and, often, death.

Evidence suggests that the premature neonate may have an abnormal balance between pro-inflammatory and antiinflammatory mediator production, thereby increasing the neonate's predisposition for diseases such as NEC.[116] PAF is a potent phospholipid inflammatory mediator that is associated with NEC in several experimental models and human analyses.[117,118] PAF infusion causes intestinal necrosis in animals, and PAF receptor antagonists prevent injury after hypoxia, endotoxin challenge, tumor necrosis factor infusion, and ischemia-reperfusion.[119] It has been shown that neonates are markedly deficient in their ability to degrade PAF because of decreased activity of the PAF-specific enzyme PAF acetylhydrolase.[120] PAF acetylhydrolase is present in breast milk but absent in commercial formula, and this may in part explain the beneficial effects of breast-milk feeding. IL-10 is an antiinflammatory cytokine thought to be important in reducing intestinal inflammation and possibly NEC in animals and humans.[121] In neonatal rats, maternal milk feedings increased ileal IL-10 expression and reduced the incidence of NEC,[122] whereas deficiency in this important cytokine increased experimental NEC severity.[123] Moreover, studies in infants with NEC demonstrated that serum IL-10 concentrations of over 250 pg/mL had a sensitivity of 100% and a specificity of 90% to identify Bell's stage III NEC.[121] Studies have compared pro-inflammatory responses to endotoxin in different cell lines and have found that the IL-8 response is significantly higher in fetal intestinal epithelium compared with mature adult intestine.[124] Additional studies have shown persistent activation of a key pro-inflammatory transcriptional regulator, nuclear factor κ beta (NF-κB), in premature or neonatal intestine compared with more mature samples.[125] These findings suggest that the balance of

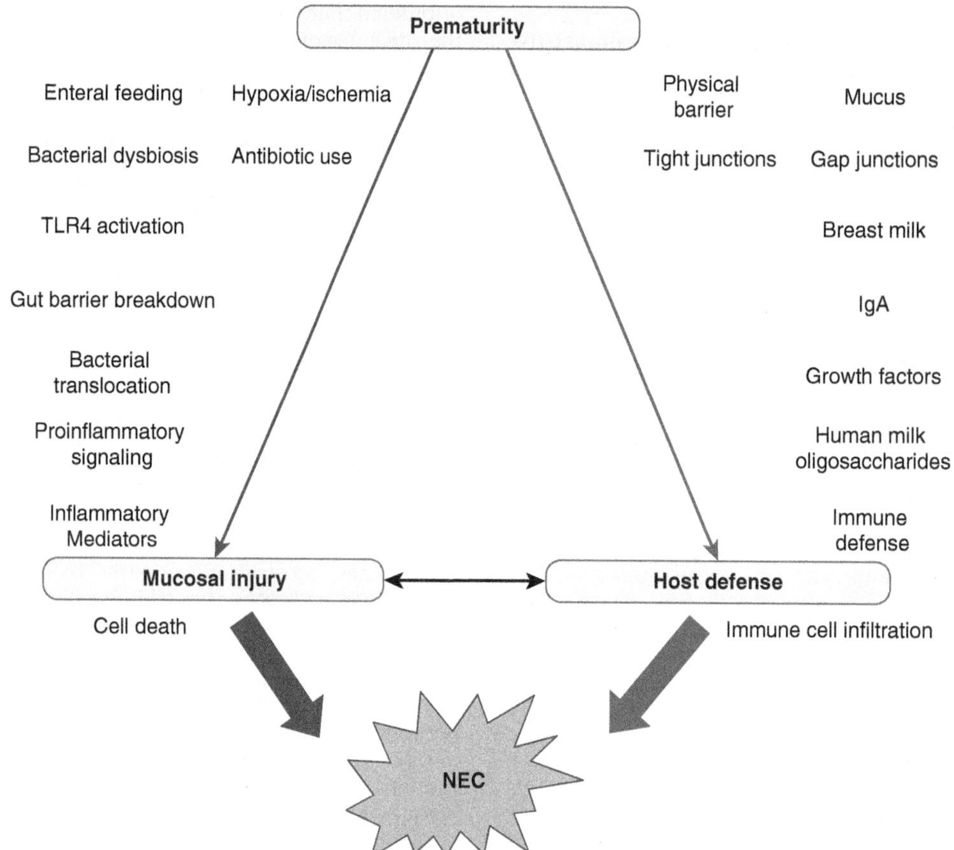

Fig. 162.1 Conditions related to prematurity can lead to the activation of signaling pathways and the release of proinflammatory mediators resulting in cell death, gut barrier breakdown, and the mucosal injury seen in necrotizing enterocolitis *(NEC)*. Host defense mechanisms, including mucus production, secretory immunoglobulin A *(IgA)*, and tight junctions, can protect premature infants from NEC. *TLR*, Toll-like receptor.

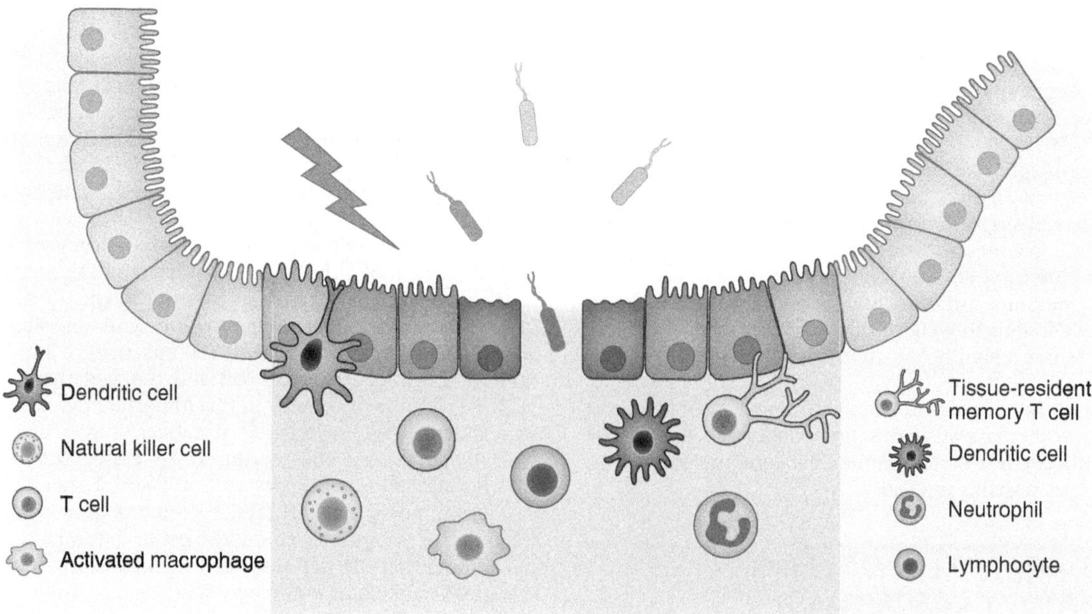

Fig. 162.2 When host defense responses are insufficient, pathologic changes to gut mucosa occur and may include apoptosis of epithelial cells, disruption of tight junction proteins, increased mucosal permeability, bacterial translocation, and subsequent immune cell infiltration, which can result in intestinal necrosis and injury. (Created in coordination with Biorender.com.)

the inflammatory response in the neonate may be weighted toward the pro-inflammatory side and more likely to result in the pathologic outcome of NEC.

CONCLUSION

NEC results from an exaggerated immune response to a bacterial dysbiosis in the premature intestine.The well-described epidemiologic risk factors, including bacterial dysbiosis, intestinal ischemia or hypoxia, and formula feeding, stimulate a final common pathway that results in intestinal injury in a susceptible premature host. Premature infants differ from term infants and older patients in multiple ways, including the complex system of intestinal host defense, intestinal motility, bacterial colonization patterns, autoregulation of splanchnic blood flow, and the regulation of the inflammatory cascade. Recent evidence suggests that an altered intestinal microbiome initiates a pro-inflammatory response that ultimately results in intestinal injury. Because each case of NEC is different, and the importance of each of the complex factors may vary between cases, no single approach has been entirely successful in eradicating this disease, although several prospects in animal models are compelling. Carefully controlled trials in high-risk premature infants will be needed to significantly reduce this morbidity and mortality that currently plagues neonatal intensive care units worldwide.

A complete reference list is available at www.ExpertConsult.com.

SELECT REFERENCES

1. Neu J, Walker WA. Necrotizing enterocolitis. *N Engl J Med*. 2011;364:255-264.
2. Patel RM, Kandefer S, Walsh MC, et al. Causes and timing of death in extremely premature infants from 2000 through 2011. *N Engl J Med*. 2015;372:331-340.
3. Frost BL, Caplan MS. Necrotizing enterocolitis: pathophysiology, platelet-activating factor, and probiotics. *Semin Pediatr Surg*. 2013;22:88-93.
4. Ballance WA, Dahms BB, Shenker N, Kliegman RM. Pathology of neonatal necrotizing enterocolitis: a ten-year experience. *J Pediatr*. 1990;117:S6-S13.
5. Overman Jr RE, Criss CN, Gadepalli SK. Necrotizing enterocolitis in term neonates: a different disease process? *J Pediatr Surg*. 2019;54:1143-1146.
6. Lopez SL, Taeusch HW, Findlay RD, Walther FJ. Time of onset of necrotizing enterocolitis in newborn infants with known prenatal cocaine exposure. *Clin Pediatr (Phila)*. 1995;34:424-429.
7. Kliegman RM, Fanaroff AA. Necrotizing enterocolitis. *N Engl J Med*. 1984;310:1093-1103.
8. Yee WH, Soraisham AS, Shah VS, et al. Incidence and timing of presentation of necrotizing enterocolitis in preterm infants. *Pediatrics*. 2012;129:e298-e304.
9. Hodzic Z, Bolock AM, Good M. The role of mucosal immunity in the pathogenesis of necrotizing enterocolitis. *Front Pediatr*. 2017;5:40.
10. Berseth CL. Gut motility and the pathogenesis of necrotizing enterocolitis. *Clin Perinatol*. 1994;21:263-270.
11. Berseth CL. Neonatal small intestinal motility: motor responses to feeding in term and preterm infants. *J Pediatr*. 1990;117:777-782.
12. Koike Y, Li B, Lee C, et al. Gastric emptying is reduced in experimental NEC and correlates with the severity of intestinal damage. *J Pediatr Surg*. 2017;52:744-748.
13. Mai V, Young CM, Ukhanova M, et al. Fecal microbiota in premature infants prior to necrotizing enterocolitis. *PloS One*. 2011;6:e20647.
14. Wang Y, Hoenig JD, Malin KJ, et al. 16S rRNA gene-based analysis of fecal microbiota from preterm infants with and without necrotizing enterocolitis. *ISME J*. 2009;3:944-954.
15. Warner BB, Deych E, Zhou Y, et al. Gut bacteria dysbiosis and necrotising enterocolitis in very low birthweight infants: a prospective case-control study. *Lancet*. 2016;387:1928-1936.
16. Nowicki PT, Minnich LA. Effects of systemic hypotension on postnatal intestinal circulation: role of angiotensin. *Am J Physiol*. 1999;276:G341-G352.
17. Good M, Sodhi CP, Yamaguchi Y, et al. The human milk oligosaccharide 2'-fucosyllactose attenuates the severity of experimental necrotising enterocolitis by enhancing mesenteric perfusion in the neonatal intestine. *Br J Nutr*. 2016;116:1175-1187.
18. Yazji I, Sodhi CP, Lee EK, et al. Endothelial TLR4 activation impairs intestinal microcirculatory perfusion in necrotizing enterocolitis via eNOS-NO-nitrite signaling. *Proc Natl Acad Sci U S A*. 2013.
19. Jilling T, Simon D, Lu J, et al. The roles of bacteria and TLR4 in rat and murine models of necrotizing enterocolitis. *J Immunol*. 2006;177:3273-3282.
20. Leaphart CL, Cavallo J, Gribar SC, et al. A critical role for TLR4 in the pathogenesis of necrotizing enterocolitis by modulating intestinal injury and repair. *J Immunol*. 2007;179:4808-4820.
21. Dvorak B. Milk epidermal growth factor and gut protection. *J Pediatr*. 2010;156:S31-S35.
22. MohanKumar K, Namachivayam K, Chapalamadugu KC, et al. Smad7 interrupts TGF-beta signaling in intestinal macrophages and promotes inflammatory activation of these cells during necrotizing enterocolitis. *Pediatr Res*. 2016;79:951-961.
23. Ravisankar S, Tatum R, Garg PM, Herco M, Shekhawat PS, Chen YH. Necrotizing enterocolitis leads to disruption of tight junctions and increase in gut permeability in a mouse model. *BMC Pediatr*. 2018;18:372.
24. Gopalakrishna KP, Macadangdang BR, Rogers MB, et al. Maternal IgA protects against the development of necrotizing enterocolitis in preterm infants. *Nat Med*. 2019;25:1110-1115.
25. Egan CE, Sodhi CP, Good M, et al. Toll-like receptor 4-mediated lymphocyte influx induces neonatal necrotizing enterocolitis. *J Clin Invest*. 2016;126:495-508.
26. Grothaus JS, Ares G, Yuan C, Wood DR, Hunter CJ. Rho kinase inhibition maintains intestinal and vascular barrier function by upregulation of occludin in experimental necrotizing enterocolitis. *Am J Physiol Gastrointest Liver Physiol*. 2018;315:G514-G528.
27. van Elburg RM, Fetter WP, Bunkers CM, Heymans HS. Intestinal permeability in relation to birth weight and gestational and postnatal age. *Arch Dis Child Fetal Neonatal Ed*. 2003;88:F52-F55.
28. Bein A, Eventov-Friedman S, Arbell D, Schwartz B. Intestinal tight junctions are severely altered in NEC preterm neonates. *Pediatr Neonatol*. 2018;59:464-473.
29. Hogberg N, Stenback A, Carlsson PO, Wanders A, Lilja HE. Genes regulating tight junctions and cell adhesion are altered in early experimental necrotizing enterocolitis. *J Pediatr Surg*. 2013;48:2308-2312.
30. Johansson ME, Ambort D, Pelaseyed T, et al. Composition and functional role of the mucus layers in the intestine. *Cell Mol Life Sci*. 2011;68:3635-3641.
31. Sodhi CP, Neal MD, Siggers R, et al. Intestinal epithelial Toll-like receptor 4 regulates goblet cell development and is required for necrotizing enterocolitis in mice. *Gastroenterology*. 2012;143:708-718.e1-e5.
32. Zhang K, Dupont A, Torow N, et al. Age-dependent enterocyte invasion and microcolony formation by Salmonella. *PLoS Pathog*. 2014;10:e1004385.
33. Stanford AH, Gong H, Noonan M, et al. A direct comparison of mouse and human intestinal development using epithelial gene expression patterns. *Pediatr Res*. 2019.
34. Mallow EB, Harris A, Salzman N, et al. Human enteric defensins. Gene structure and developmental expression. *J Biol Chem*. 1996;271:4038-4045.
35. Salzman NH, Polin RA, Harris MC, et al. Enteric defensin expression in necrotizing enterocolitis. *Pediatr Res*. 1998;44:20-26.
36. Jenke AC, Zilbauer M, Postberg J, Wirth S. Human beta-defensin 2 expression in ELBW infants with severe necrotizing enterocolitis. *Pediatr Res*. 2012;72:513-520.
37. Lueschow SR, Stumphy J, Gong H, et al. Loss of murine Paneth cell function alters the immature intestinal microbiome and mimics changes seen in neonatal necrotizing enterocolitis. *PloS One*. 2018;13:e0204967.
38. Chen L, Lv Z, Gao Z, et al. Human beta-defensin-3 reduces excessive autophagy in intestinal epithelial cells and in experimental necrotizing enterocolitis. *Sci Rep*. 2019;9:19890.
39. Kuo S, El Guindy A, Panwala CM, Hagan PM, Camerini V. Differential appearance of T cell subsets in the large and small intestine of neonatal mice. *Pediatr Res*. 2001;49:543-551.
40. Dimmitt RA, Staley EM, Chuang G, Tanner SM, Soltau TD, Lorenz RG. Role of postnatal acquisition of the intestinal microbiome in the early development of immune function. *J Pediatr Gastroenterol Nutr*. 2010;51:262-273.
41. Rogier EW, Frantz AL, Bruno ME, et al. Secretory antibodies in breast milk promote long-term intestinal homeostasis by regulating the gut microbiota and host gene expression. *Proc Natl Acad Sci U S A*. 2014;111:3074-3079.
42. Nolan LS, Parks OB, Good M. A review of the immunomodulating components of maternal breast milk and protection against necrotizing enterocolitis. *Nutrients*. 2019;12.
43. He Y, Cao L, Yu J. Prophylactic lactoferrin for preventing late-onset sepsis and necrotizing enterocolitis in preterm infants: a PRISMA-compliant systematic review and meta-analysis. *Medicine (Baltim)*. 2018;97:e11976.
44. El-Shimi MS, Awad HA, Abdelwahed MA, Mohamed MH, Khafagy SM, Saleh G. Enteral L-arginine and glutamine supplementation for prevention of NEC in preterm neonates. *Int J Pediatr*. 2015;2015:856091.
45. Good M, Sodhi CP, Egan CE, et al. Breast milk protects against the development of necrotizing enterocolitis through inhibition of Toll-like receptor 4 in the intestinal epithelium via activation of the epidermal growth factor receptor. *Mucosal Immunol*. 2015;8:1166-1179.
46. Maheshwari A, Kelly DR, Nicola T, et al. TGF-beta2 suppresses macrophage cytokine production and mucosal inflammatory responses in the developing intestine. *Gastroenterology*. 2011;140:242-253.
47. Shiou SR, Yu Y, Chen S, et al. Erythropoietin protects intestinal epithelial barrier function and lowers the incidence of experimental neonatal necrotizing enterocolitis. *J Biol Chem*. 2011;286:12123-12132.
48. Yu Y, Shiou SR, Guo Y, et al. Erythropoietin protects epithelial cells from excessive autophagy and apoptosis in experimental neonatal necrotizing enterocolitis. *PloS One*. 2013;8:e69620.
49. Liu J, Zhu HT, Li B, et al. Lactoferrin reduces necrotizing enterocolitis severity by upregulating intestinal epithelial proliferation. *Eur J Pediatr Surg*. 2020;30:90-95.
50. Griffiths J, Jenkins P, Vargova M, et al. Enteral lactoferrin to prevent infection for very preterm infants: the ELFIN RCT. *Health Technol Assess*. 2018;22:1-60.

163 Pathophysiology of Kernicterus

Thor Willy Ruud Hansen

INTRODUCTION

Jaundice is a common transitional phenomenon in newborn infants and may have been first described in the Chinese textbook *On the Origins and Symptoms of Diseases* written in CE 610.[1] It is not clear when the association between neonatal jaundice and yellow staining of the brain was first noticed, but the staining phenomenon later known as *kernicterus* was first described in 1875 by Johannes Orth,[2] who had performed an autopsy on an infant that died at 2 days of age with very intense jaundice. The term *kernicterus*, the German word for jaundice of the nuclei (or basal ganglia), was coined by Christian Georg Schmorl,[3] in a landmark article in 1904. Of the 120 jaundiced infants he had autopsied, 114 had jaundiced brains, but only 6 of the 120 exhibited a pattern of more intense yellow color of the basal ganglia and medulla oblongata, which gave rise to the term. More than 100 years have passed since then, but the explanation for this localization phenomenon still eludes medical researchers.

In addition to severe jaundice and lethargy progressing to stupor and coma, the clinical picture in the infants who died included hypotonia, increasing tone in extensor groups, retrocollis/opisthotonos, seizures, ophthalmoplegia (paresis of upward gaze), fever, high-pitched cry, and poor sucking. During the first half of the 20th century it became clear that the pathoanatomic finding of jaundiced brain nuclei had a clinical correlation in infants who survived extreme jaundice. Clinical manifestations that appeared to evolve during the first days/weeks to 2 to 3 months of life included hypertonicity, opisthotonos, absent Moro reflex, high-pitched cry, and poor feeding.[4] From then on until approximately 2 years of age, marked delay of motor development became obvious, with decreased muscle tone, hyperreflexia, and persistence of immature postural patterns. Athetosis could begin towards the end of the second year of life but might not become apparent until 8 to 9 years of age. The degree of athetosis was quite variable, from hardly detectable (except to the trained observer) to completely disabling. Some degree of hearing loss was present in most patients. Paresis of upward gaze appears to be fairly obligate in kernicterus but is rare in other types of cerebral palsy. Intellectual deficits were not necessarily present, and only a minority of the patients had developmental delay. The sequelae of bilirubin encephalopathy may present a many-faceted picture,[5] and a proposal for updated nomenclature that incorporates these aspects is discussed below.

There appears to be general agreement among present-day bilirubin researchers that the toxic influence of bilirubin on brain cells is the primary and causative factor in kernicterus. However, as yet no agreement exists on which mechanism(s) might mediate brain bilirubin toxicity. This chapter provides an overview of research on the effects and interactions of bilirubin with the brain, and discusses the relative merits and weaknesses of several theories on the "basic mechanism of bilirubin neurotoxicity."

BILIRUBIN BRAIN TOXICITY—NOMENCLATURE AND CLASSIFICATION

Kernicterus, strictly speaking, refers to the pathoanatomic finding of intense yellow coloring of the basal ganglia and associated structures superimposed on a paler yellow background as first described by Orth[2] and Schmorl.[3] When Georg Schmorl coined the term *kernicterus*, the term *kern* (i.e., basal ganglia) probably included most of the subcortical structures of forebrain grey matter. Present-day neuroanatomists use the term *basal ganglia* more to describe a set of functionally related cell groups rather than in a strictly topographic sense, a concept illustrated in Figs. 163.1 and 163.2.[6] This evolving terminology should be kept in mind when considering the study of Zuelzer and Mudgett, who compared the frequency of staining of brain areas/structures in kernicterus cases.[7] In descending order of frequency, they found that stained areas included the hippocampus, thalamus, hypothalamus, corpus striatum, medulla, olives, pons, and dentate nucleus.[7] In these areas ultrastructural findings have included membrane alterations, dense cytoplasmic bodies thought to represent degenerated mitochondria, and calcium granules.[8] Changes of this nature are likely to be irreversible and to represent the pathoanatomic correlate of the chronic, clinical after effects of bilirubin brain toxicity, until recently called *kernicterus.* Thus, a discussion of the mechanisms of bilirubin-induced brain injury must necessarily include events that cause or are associated with cell death.

With modern imaging techniques, such as magnetic resonance imaging, lesions may be seen in both the globus pallidus and the subthalamic nucleus. Lesions in the globus pallidus tend to be more intense than those in the subthalamic nucleus, whereas lesions in the auditory brain stem nuclei and cerebellum are often not noted on routine magnetic resonance imaging scans.[9] Magnetic resonance imaging scans done within a few weeks of the neurotoxic jaundice episode in babies who develop chronic sequelae tend to show bilateral hyperintensities in the globus pallidus on T1 weighting, without change on T2 weighting. Subsequently, the magnetic resonance imaging scan may become apparently normal, but later T2 and fluid-attenuated inversion recovery images become hyperintense.[9]

However, bilirubin effects on the brain often appear to be transitory. Thus, neonates with significant jaundice frequently exhibit lethargy or drowsiness, hypotonia, and feeding problems.[10] Evoked response studies, both in human infants and experimental animals, have given more objective evidence of such reversible toxicity,[11-15] although permanent changes have been found in some subjects.[16,17] The increased incidence of apnea in jaundiced premature infants, as compared with less jaundiced controls, appears to abate after the first week of life and is associated with progression of changes in the auditory brain stem response.[18] This type of reversible toxicity is not *kernicterus,* yet there is little doubt that it reflects bilirubin effects on the brain.

Recently a group of bilirubin experts proposed a revision of the terminology used to describe and classify bilirubin effects on the brain.[19] They introduced *kernicterus spectrum disorder* (KSD) as an overarching term to reflect the range of bilirubin effects, which includes both acute and chronic signs as well as type and severity of damage. Proposed modifier terms include mild, moderate, and severe. Subtypes may then be described in terms of auditory (auditory-predominant), motor (motor-predominant), and classical (involving both auditory and motor dysfunction). Further, the authors suggest retaining the term *acute bilirubin*

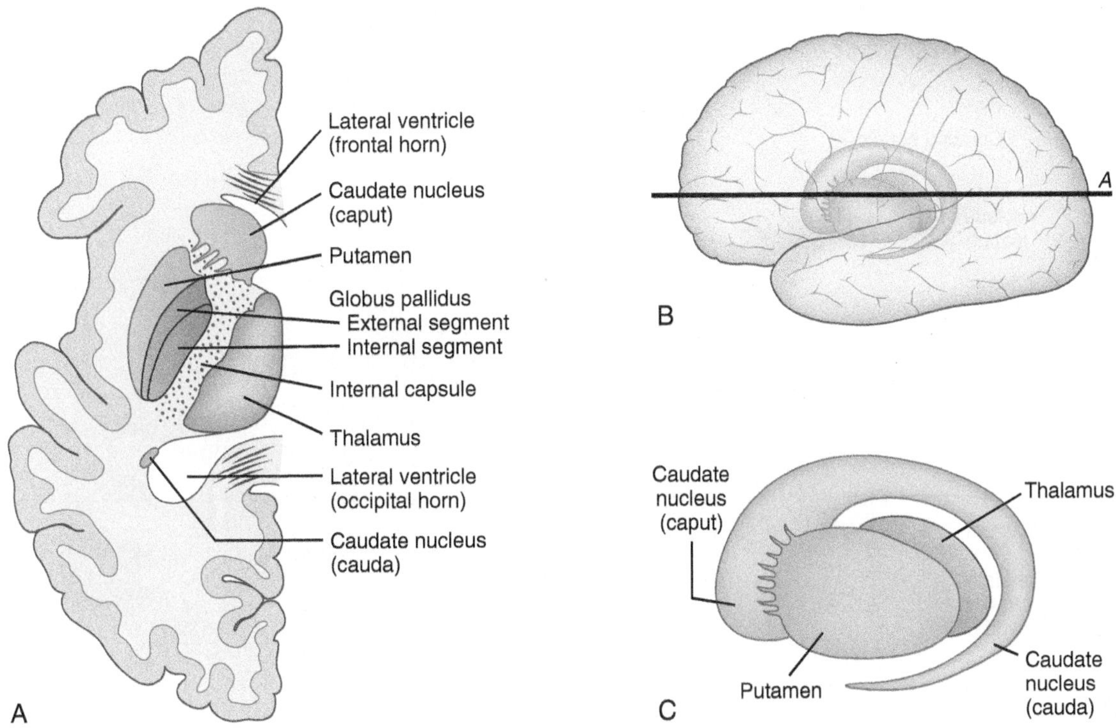

Fig. 163.1 Shape and position of the basal ganglia. (A) Part of a horizontal section through the hemisphere, as shown (B) with a line in the drawing of the hemisphere. (C) Left putamen and caudate nucleus; lateral aspect. (From Brodal P. *The Central Nervous System*. 5th ed. Oxford, UK: Oxford University Press; 2016:fig. 23.3.)

encephalopathy (ABE), as it correctly describes the neurologic effects of ongoing bilirubin exposure. However, the term *chronic bilirubin encephalopathy* (CBE) should be discarded in favor of KSD, because CBE may be misinterpreted to suggest that bilirubin exposure is still happening, although the signs and symptoms we observe are in fact the long-term sequelae of an acute, time-limited bilirubin exposure that happened in the past.[19] Similarly the term *bilirubin-induced neurologic dysfunction* (BIND) has been used both as a scoring system and as a descriptive term for a range of bilirubin effects on brain function and should be abandoned in favor of KSD.[20] The authors also proposed a set of guidelines to define levels of severity for motor and auditory sequelae.

It is not clear whether ABE and KSD represent the extreme ends of a continuum of toxicity, or whether separate and distinct mechanisms are involved in cell death versus a transitory disturbance in neuronal signaling.[21] Even moderate degrees of hyperbilirubinemia may have discernible long-term effects on behavior,[22] and questions relating to the sensitivity and specificity of the tools used to study the long-term effects of neonatal jaundice will have to be resolved before we can determine what effects are reversible. This chapter therefore discusses bilirubin-induced brain injury in a wide sense, including bilirubin effects on processes that may not result in cell death and residual damage. Whether such effects may permanently alter cell functions without causing cell death is at present not known.

BILIRUBIN CHEMISTRY AND SOLUBILITY

Certain aspects of bilirubin chemistry and solubility are inextricably linked to bilirubin neurotoxicity and therefore are briefly discussed here. The main bilirubin isomer in humans is bilirubin IXα (*Z,Z* isomer), which exists either as a charged dianion or as bilirubin acid. The eight hydrophilic groups of the dianion impart some water solubility at neutral pH, whereas the presence of intramolecular hydrogen bonds in the bilirubin acid results in near-insolubility in water.[23,24] The hydrophobic bilirubin IXα isomer appears to be responsible for the toxic effects, whereas the water-soluble isomers are believed to be nontoxic.[25-27] Bilirubin becomes water soluble when it is conjugated to glucuronic acid in the hepatocytes, and when bound to albumin for transport in serum.[28] Isomerization of the bilirubin molecule during phototherapy also results in molecules that are more polar (photoisomers).[29]

Bilirubin experts disagree on the issue of bilirubin solubility and its impact on studies of bilirubin brain toxicity, hence the claims that many experiments on bilirubin toxicity have been done at nonphysiologic concentrations, and thus the results may not be relevant.[30] Others argue that concentrations of bilirubin for in vitro studies must mimic those found in the brains of infants with kernicterus,[31] as well as those found in experimental animals with clinically relevant levels of serum bilirubin.[32-34]

Bilirubin IXα (*Z,Z*) is an amphipathic molecule but, with respect to membranes, behaves as lipophilic; thus it binds to and crosses phospholipid membranes.[35-37] It is presumably this characteristic that enables bilirubin IXα (*Z,Z*) to cross the intact blood-brain barrier and enter the brain.[38] A minute amount of bilirubin (in the nanomolar range) is always present in plasma as "free" or unbound bilirubin. According to the "free bilirubin theory," it is this unbound bilirubin moiety that enters the brain to produce neuronal injury.[39-41] Increased concentrations of unbound bilirubin in the blood will, by the laws of equilibrium, shift more bilirubin into tissues, including the brain. Bilirubin is bound to albumin at primary and secondary binding sites, with higher affinity at the primary site, such that the concentrations of unbound bilirubin in serum are normally very low.[23,28,36] Factors that increase the concentrations of unbound bilirubin, and thus augment bilirubin entry into brain, include altered albumin characteristics,[42] changes in pH, and the presence of exogenous or endogenous binding competitors.[42-44] An epidemic of kernicterus occurred in the 1950s and was shown to be related

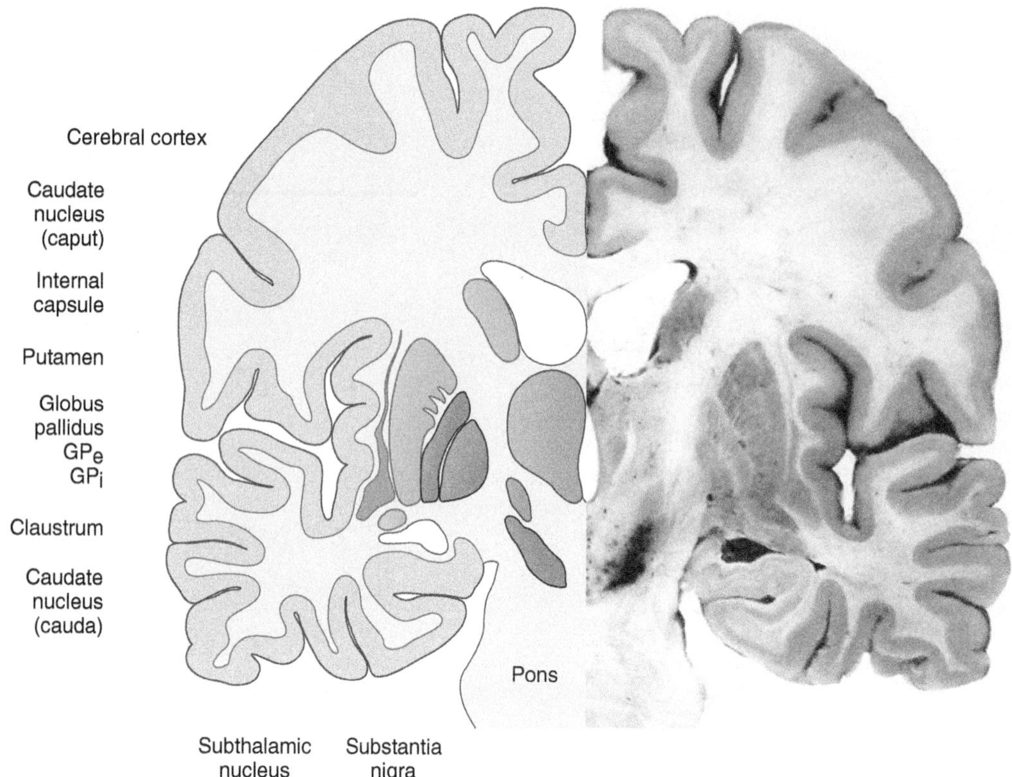

Fig. 163.2 The basal ganglia seen in the frontal plane. (Reproduced with permission from Brodal P. *The Central Nervous System*. 5th ed. Oxford, UK: Oxford University Press; 2016:Fig. 23.4.)

to the use of sulfisoxazole.[45] In subsequent years it was shown that many drugs compete with bilirubin for binding to serum albumin.[46] Bilirubin "displacers" are now well recognized to increase the risk of bilirubin neurotoxicity in jaundiced infants, and this has significantly influenced the use and choice of drugs in neonatal medicine. Numerous animal studies show that the blood-brain equilibrium for bilirubin is shifted towards the brain when bilirubin-displacing substances are administered.[44,47–50]

The water solubility of bilirubin photoisomers raises questions regarding their neurotoxicity. McDonagh and Lightner[51] proposed decades ago that bilirubin photoisomers ought to be less toxic than the predominant IXα *(Z,Z)* isomer. Also, by virtue of their polarity the photoisomers should not easily cross the blood-brain barrier, lacking a specific transporter. Thus, the theoretical arguments are chemically and physiologically coherent.[52] The reports of apparent reversibility of acute intermediate-to-advanced stage bilirubin encephalopathy with timely aggressive therapy may also be interpreted to support this hypothesis.[53,54] Unfortunately, experimental models to test this hypothesis have been hard to devise. Thus many of the in vitro studies of bilirubin photoisomers in cultured cells have methodologic issues that limit the conclusions that can be drawn.[55] However, a recent well-controlled study exposed a human neuroblastoma cell line (SH-SY5Y) to bilirubin-IXα (Z,Z), or lumirubin, or a mixture of bilirubin-IXα (Z,E/E,Z) isomers.[56] These had been carefully prepared and purified. While the cells exposed to the IXα (Z,Z) isomer exhibited significant loss of viability that increased with time, viability was not affected in cells exposed to photoisomers.

THE BLOOD-BRAIN AND BLOOD-CEREBROSPINAL FLUID BARRIERS AND BILIRUBIN-BRAIN KINETICS

Entry of bilirubin into brain is a sine qua non for neurotoxicity. An unstable state of equilibrium appears to exist between bilirubin in the blood and bilirubin in the brain, an equilibrium influenced by a number of factors (Fig. 163.3). The blood-brain gradient of bilirubin is high; in experimental animals with an intact blood-brain barrier the brain bilirubin concentrations are only 1% to 2% of the serum bilirubin concentrations.[47–50] Molecules that can cross the blood-brain barrier appear to share certain characteristics, including (1) low molecular weight (<400 daltons), (2) increased lipid solubility, and (3) not being a substrate for an efflux transporter.[57] Bilirubin has a molecular weight of 585; its lipid solubility depends on the isomeric form,[23,24] and it is a substrate for an efflux transporter (P-gp).[58] Thus, native bilirubin really does not satisfy any of these criteria. This may explain why bilirubin entry into brain is limited. The blood-brain barrier may be more permeable to bilirubin in neonates than in mature subjects, and in studies with experimental animals the brain-to-blood ratios appear to be higher in subcortical regions in immature organisms, suggesting the possibility that the subcortical areas may be more accessible to bilirubin entry. On the other hand, albumin permeability is equally restricted in both young and old subjects.[59–61] Studies involving P-gp (a bilirubin transporter) indicate that expression of this efflux pump for bilirubin in endothelial cells increases with maturation and may contribute to the perceived immaturity of the blood-brain barrier in the newborn.[62]

Bilirubin may interact with biologic membranes in a way that affects their function,[63–65] thus it seems reasonable to ask whether bilirubin could also affect the blood-brain barrier. In that regard, perturbation of blood-brain barrier function by bilirubin might be secondary to the toxic effects of bilirubin on glial cells.[66,67] Studies addressing the question of direct bilirubin effects on the blood-brain barrier found that pre-exposure to bilirubin increased the permeability of the blood-brain barrier both to a dye and to bilirubin itself.[68,69]

P-gp is a member of the adenosine triphosphate (ATP)-binding cassette superfamily of membrane transporters, which are expressed both in normal and in diseased tissues and appear

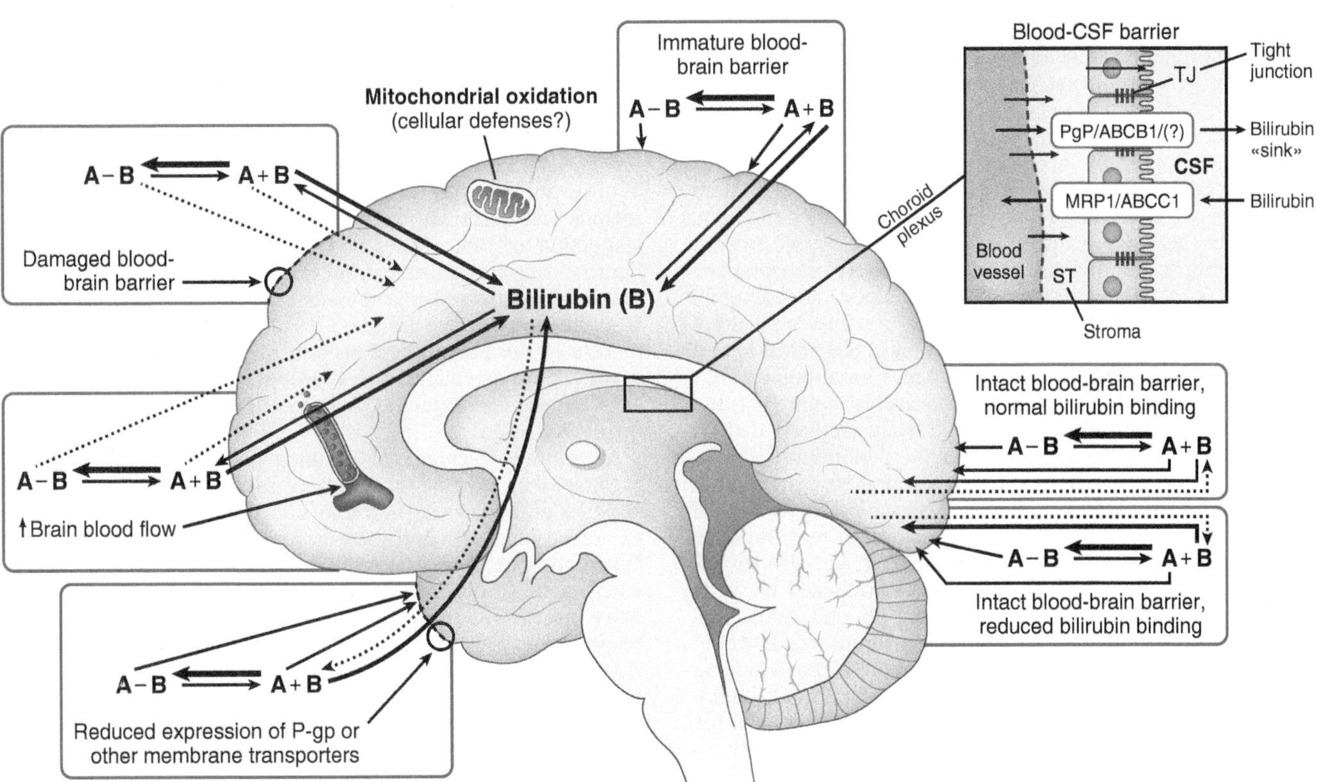

Fig. 163.3 Factors that modulate the bilirubin-brain equilibrium. A number of factors can modulate bilirubin uptake into and clearance from brain. These include the avidity of bilirubin binding to serum albumin, the presence of competitors for the albumin binding site, immaturity or other factors that may affect blood-brain permeability, the presence and activity or expression of membrane pumps in the blood-brain barrier, and brain blood flow. *A,* Albumin; *A-B,* albumin-bound bilirubin; *B,* (unbound) bilirubin; *BV,* blood vessel; *CSF,* cerebrospinal fluid; *MRP1,* multidrug resistance–associated protein 1 (also referred to as ATP binding cassette subfamily C member 1 [ABCC1); *P-gp,* phosphoglycoprotein (also referred to as multidrug resistance protein 1 *[MDR1]* or ATP-binding cassette subfamily B member 1 [ABCB1]); *ST,* stroma; *TJ,* tight junction.

to limit the entry of xenobiotics into cells.[70] P-gp (encoded by *ABCB1*) is localized on the luminal (blood) side of the blood-brain barrier.[71] Bilirubin is a substrate for P-gp and may also inhibit P-gp function.[72,73] This has several interesting implications for the interaction between bilirubin and brain. Brain bilirubin content in P-gp-deficient mice after an intravenous bilirubin bolus was almost twofold higher than in wild-type mice.[58] Drugs known to inhibit P-gp significantly enhanced bilirubin entry into rat brain after an intravenous bilirubin bolus.[74] P-gp function appears to be regulated by phosphorylation, and phosphorylation has been linked to enhanced activity of P-gp.[75,76] This provides a possible link to understanding how bilirubin might increase blood-brain barrier permeability,[68,69] as bilirubin has been shown to inhibit phosphorylation of a wide range of protein-peptide substrates.[77,78]

In astrocytes, which are important for blood-brain barrier function, bilirubin appears to mediate up-regulation of multidrug resistance-associated protein 1 (MRP1) (a member of the ATP-binding cassette transporter superfamily), resulting in decreased sensitivity to bilirubin toxicity.[79] However, other findings suggest that astrocytes are sensitive to toxicity, and particularly that immature cells are more vulnerable than mature cells.[80,81] In mouse embryo fibroblasts, intracellular accumulation of [^{3}H] bilirubin, as well as cytotoxicity, were significantly greater in cells from MRP1-deficient mice than in cells from wild-type controls.[82] The implications of these findings remain to be elucidated and clearly need further study.

Opening of the blood-brain barrier by radiation, inflammation, asphyxia/hypoxia, hyperosmolality, and hypercarbia has been shown to increase bilirubin entry into the brain in a number of studies.[47,49,50,83,84] The latter three conditions may occur quite frequently in sick neonates and appear to be relevant for clinical management of jaundice in neonatal intensive care unit (NICU) infants. In hypercarbia, most, but not all, of the bilirubin enters brain as the unbound molecule; however, with hyperosmolality considerable entry of albumin into the brain also occurs, and in the jaundiced individual a large proportion of this albumin will carry bilirubin.[47] In hypercarbia the rapid entry of bilirubin into the brain is increased compared to control conditions, but clearance is also rapid.[50] In contrast, with hyperosmolality it appears that bilirubin remains in the brain significantly longer than under control conditions.[50] Whether such prolonged exposure is associated with an increased risk of toxicity is speculation, but some clinical data suggest that not only the level of serum bilirubin but also the duration of exposure is associated with risk of neurologic sequelae.[85]

Opening of the blood-brain barrier may contribute to or exacerbate bilirubin neurotoxicity.[83,84,86] In vitro studies suggest that albumin blocks the toxic effects of bilirubin when present in equimolar concentrations.[64,87,88] Opening of the blood-brain barrier (e.g., with hyperosmolality) permits the entry of albumin-bound, as well as unbound, bilirubin, and, because the equilibrium balance in serum is heavily tilted towards albumin-bound bilirubin, the observation of increased toxicity in vivo is somewhat surprising. Earlier studies had suggested that signs of toxicity might best be predicted by total brain bilirubin content, and enhanced binding to albumin appeared to be protective.[84] More recently, Daood and Watchko[34] demonstrated an association between calculated free bilirubin levels in brain and signs of toxicity in a Gunn rat pup model.

The role of brain blood flow may be best illustrated by studies of hypercarbia, which results in increased brain blood flow.[47,50,61,89] These studies show that increased brain blood flow in experimental animals is associated with increased entry of bilirubin into brain. One may speculate that with increased brain blood flow each circulating bilirubin molecule passes the blood-brain barrier more often and thus has more opportunity to equilibrate with bilirubin in the brain.

If we accept the likelihood that bilirubin IXα (*Z,Z* isomer), in the presence of an intact blood-brain barrier, enters the brain primarily in the unbound form, it is reasonable to ask in what form bilirubin is found in the brain. The majority of cerebrospinal fluid (CSF) proteins originate from blood, and albumin constitutes 35% to 80% of CSF proteins[90,91]; thus we cannot rule out the possibility that a small fraction of the bilirubin that enters the brain in a jaundiced newborn may be albumin-bound. The experimental studies that have measured brain bilirubin concentrations have mostly been done using methods that do not distinguish between bound and unbound bilirubin.[47,48]

Several groups have studied the relationship between bilirubin in serum and bilirubin in CSF, as well as bilirubin and protein (or albumin) in CSF.[92-95] CSF-unconjugated-bilirubin was found to correlate with total serum bilirubin (TSB),[92,96] and also to CSF total protein or albumin,[97] although one study failed to verify the CSF bilirubin-to-protein relationship.[98] In one study, CSF-bilirubin was also found to correlate with serum free bilirubin measurements.[99] Meisel and colleagues measured CSF bilirubin in jaundiced newborns and found a mean value of 4.5 ± 3.1 μmol/L in the presence of a mean total serum bilirubin value of 221 ± 130 μmol/L. Thus, the CSF bilirubin value was approximately 2% of the serum bilirubin value.[95] Several other groups also found CSF bilirubin concentrations in the low micromolar range.[92,93] The bilirubin:albumin (B:A) ratio in CSF was 0.32 ± 0.22, and Meisel and colleagues suggested that the concentration of free bilirubin in CSF must be low.[95] However, given the brain-CSF barrier and the hypothesized role of CSF as a "sink" for brain bilirubin, it is not clear that these findings can be directly related to the question of bilirubin in brain tissue. Interpretation of these data is further complicated by the fact that within the CSF space there is a gradient of blood-derived proteins from the ventricles to the lumbar space, which for albumin is 2.5-fold.[91] Applied to the data from Meisel and colleagues,[95] the albumin concentration in the ventricles would be only 40% of that in the lumbar CSF, bringing the B:A ratio in the ventricular space to approximately 0.8, assuming that CSF bilirubin content is uniformly distributed within the CSF space. Whether this latter assumption holds is unknown. However, this question seems worthy of further investigation, as a higher B:A ratio in the ventricular CSF would theoretically be accompanied by a higher concentration of free bilirubin.

Daood and Watchko have calculated unbound bilirubin levels in the central nervous system (CNS) of homozygous Gunn rat pups after administration of sulfadimethoxine, using published in vivo albumin-bilirubin binding constants, and found a value that appears to be approximately two-thirds of the measured bilirubin content in whole brain.[34] Their calculations assumed that in situ flushing of the brain vasculature completely clears these blood vessels of blood, thus also removing intravascular bilirubin as well as albumin. However, an earlier study had examined this assumption, using approximately the same volume-for-weight to flush the rat brain vasculature in situ, and using both ^{51}Cr-labeled erythrocytes and ^{125}I-IgM to estimate brain blood volume.[100] Approximately 30% to 40% of pre-flushing brain blood volume was still present after flushing. Applying this correction to Daood's and Watchko's data would probably change their estimate. Thus, the question of binding of bilirubin in brain warrants further study.

Organic anion transporters, such as MRPs, may play a role in limiting bilirubin accumulation in the CSF and in keeping bilirubin out of brain.[101] Preliminary data appear compatible with a role for MRP1 (encoded by *ABCC1*), which appears to be localized on the basolateral face of the choroid plexus epithelium of the blood-CSF barrier.[71,102]

The question of how bilirubin localizes to the basal ganglia will be addressed here, although whether the localization phenomenon is related to bilirubin entry into or clearance from brain is not clear. The predilection of bilirubin for certain brain regions was described early and was primarily based on visual inspection of brain slices.[2,3] However, more objective, albeit limited, data are available from human subjects. Claireaux and colleagues extracted bilirubin from the brains of four infants who died with severe jaundice.[31] They found approximately 35 nmol/g in the nuclear regions and 8 nmol/g in the remainder of the brains, speculating that bilirubin concentrations may have been several-fold higher in the most intensely stained areas of the nuclei.

Attempts to recreate this staining pattern in animal models have met with variable success. Burgess and colleagues[33,89] found regional differences in bilirubin concentrations in piglets that had received a [^{3}H]bilirubin infusion and were exposed either to hypercarbia or hyperosmolality. However, the question remains whether these differences were due to variations in bilirubin entry into or disappearance from brain, or whether they might be related to redistribution or binding to specific tissue or cell elements. Cannon and colleagues examined regional bilirubin concentrations in 15- to 19-day-old Gunn rat pups pretreated with sulfadimethoxine and found significant differences in bilirubin localization.[103] The cerebellar bilirubin concentration was 18.9 μg/g, whereas the brain stem and cortex contained 10.7 and 4.7 μg/g, respectively. These numbers are overall surprisingly similar to those previously found in human brains.[31] The brain bilirubin concentrations were higher in the male pups, suggesting that sex may modulate brain bilirubin uptake or clearance. However, no clear explanation was offered for how these regional differences arose, nor could they be said to mimic a typical kernicteric pattern. Attempts to recreate a kernicteric staining pattern in Sprague Dawley rats through infusion of bilirubin and manipulations of bilirubin binding, blood-brain barrier opening, and brain blood flow have not been succesful.[47-50] These studies also failed to show interregional differences between bilirubin uptake into or clearance from brain. Other studies have examined bilirubin metabolism in brain, and, although differences were found, the findings did not conform to or explain the staining pattern of kernicterus.[104] Although, as previously discussed, membrane transporters may play a role in extruding bilirubin from brain and in modulating toxicity, there is no evidence for region-specific differences in the expression of either *ABCB1* or *ABCC1*.[105]

Hemolysis is believed to be implicated in the mechanisms underlying bilirubin neurotoxicity, and this is reflected in most therapeutic guidelines, which call for more aggressive management in the presence of hemolysis.[106,107] However, the mechanisms underlying this increased toxicity are not known.[108] In rats with a chemically induced hemolytic anemia neither entry into nor clearance of bilirubin from the brain were different from that in control rats after an intravenous bolus of bilirubin.[109] This obviously does not model the immunologic aspects of anemia in infants with blood group incompatibility and thus cannot discount the possibility that blood-brain barrier permeability may be affected by such mechanisms. However, immunology is not involved in the hemolysis of glucose 6-phosphate dehydrogenase deficiency, where increased risk of kernicterus is well described.[110] Rhesus incompatibility with a hematocrit less than 35% had an odds ratio of 48.6 (95% confidence interval, 14 to 168) for ABE and/or death, or a pathologic neurologic examination at discharge in infants admitted to Cairo University Children's Hospital.[111] However, ABO incompatibility with a similarly low hematocrit was not associated with ABE or neurologic abnormalities at discharge in this population.[111] In other studies both ABO and Rh incompatibility were risk factors for KSD.[112,113] Whether other products of hemolysis than bilirubin could increase bilirubin neurotoxicity has apparently not been studied.

INHIBITION-UNCOUPLING OF OXIDATIVE PHOSPHORYLATION: "THE CLASSIC STORY"

The first in vitro experimental studies of bilirubin toxicity were performed in 1954 and showed that bilirubin inhibited respiration in a rat brain homogenate.[114] In rat liver mitochondria in vitro, bilirubin 300 μmol/L partially inhibited respiration, and phosphorylation was nearly completely inhibited.[115] The interpretation was that bilirubin uncoupled oxidative phosphorylation. This, for many years, was the prevailing theory for the basic mechanism of bilirubin toxicity. A number of in vitro studies also lend some credence to the role of mitochondria in bilirubin toxicity. Thus, bilirubin can affect the mitochondrial membrane, resulting in increased membrane permeability, decreased membrane potential, release of cytochrome *c*, and triggering of apoptosis.[116–118] An illustration depicting some of the many different effects and interactions of bilirubin with cells and cellular processes is shown in Fig. 163.4.

Some in vivo data also support the role of mitochondria. Thus, ultrastructural changes were found in the mitochondria of Gunn rats with bilirubin encephalopathy.[119,120] Rats with infusion-induced extreme hyperbilirubinemia exhibited significantly decreased phosphocreatine and ATP levels in the brain, but only after opening the blood-brain barrier with hyperosmolality.[121] In a study of magnetic resonance spectroscopy in infants with severe neonatal jaundice, one of five infants had an abnormally high ratio of lactate to *N*-acetylaspartate.[122] This was the only infant who also exhibited abnormalities in the basal ganglia on magnetic resonance imaging and one of two who had evidence of KSD during follow-up. The elevated ratio of lactate to *N*-acetylaspartate may have been the result of changes in mitochondrial function.

However, these data do not unequivocally confirm a role for mitochondria as the primary targets of bilirubin toxicity in vivo. Early electron-microscopic observations in Gunn rats suggested that the mitochondrial changes might result from earlier effects in the cytoplasm.[119] When the effects of bilirubin on L-929 cells in culture were compared with those of known uncouplers of oxidative phosphorylation and inhibitors of reduced nicotinamide adenine dinucleotide oxidase, the results were more indicative of membrane perturbation than of toxic effects on the respiratory chain.[64] Studies in newborn pigs, who received intravenous infusions of bilirubin, failed to show changes in cerebral oxygen, glucose, and lactate metabolism compatible with perturbation of mitochondrial function.[123] Furthermore, bilirubin has been found to affect neurotransmitter metabolism in permeabilized synaptosomes in vitro (synaptic nerve endings that retain their function in vitro) in the presence of high ATP concentrations, so depletion of endogenous ATP could not have contributed to the observed effects.[124] In a

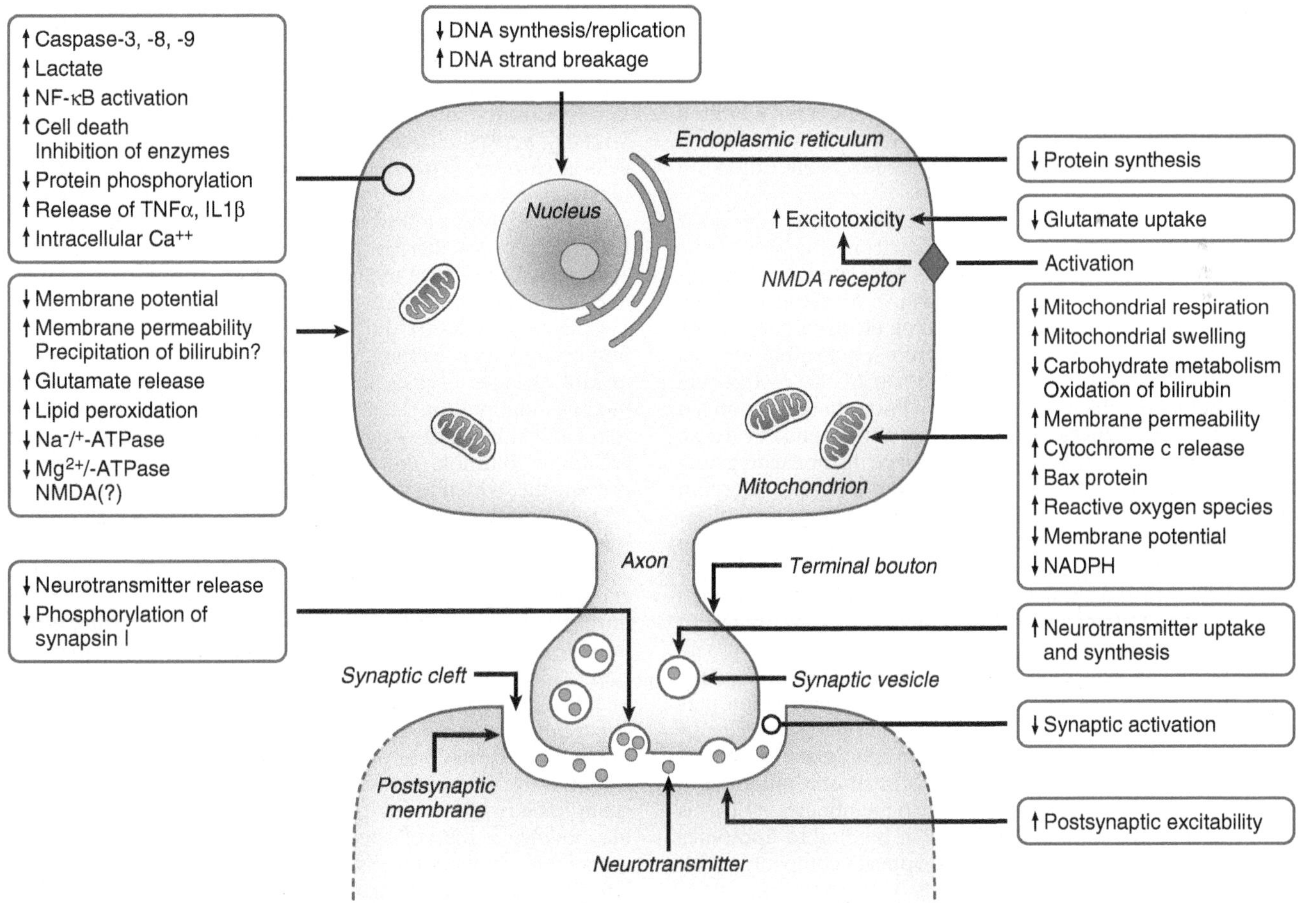

Fig. 163.4 Interactions of bilirubin with cells and cellular processes. Bilirubin has been shown to interact with many different cellular processes and reactions. Although several of the studies have been performed in nonneuronal cells, in this figure these processes and reactions are depicted in a schematic and simplified neuron. *IL,* Interleukin; *NADPH,* dihydronicotinamide-adenine dinucleotide phosphate; *NF-κB,* nuclear factor kappa-light-chain-enhancer of activated B cells; *NMDA, N*-methyl-D-aspartate; *TNF,* tumor necrosis factor.

study of six infants with extreme jaundice, of whom four were neurologically abnormal at 1 year of age, none demonstrated elevated brain lactate levels.[125] In fact, the findings in that study were more compatible with changes in *N*-methyl-D-aspartate (NMDA) receptor sensitivity.

For bilirubin to perturb mitochondrial function, it needs to be present in concentrations sufficient to cause toxicity. Whether this is the case has been addressed by only one study, in which [^{3}H]bilirubin was given as an intravenous bolus to rats. The rats were killed after 10 or 30 minutes, and their brains were subjected to subcellular fractionation.[126] Although absolute values for bilirubin could not be computed, the bilirubin content relative to protein in mitochondria was much less than that in the cytoplasm and membrane fractions. In conclusion, whether the mitochondria are the primary targets for bilirubin neurotoxicity remains a theory for which some experimental support exists, but a number of studies point to other possibilities.

INTERACTION WITH MEMBRANES

There is ample evidence that bilirubin may interact with biologic membranes.[63-65] Some of these findings were discussed in the section entitled "The Blood-Brain and Blood-CSF Barriers and Bilirubin-Brain Kinetics." Bilirubin content in rat brains subjected to subcellular fractionation was higher in the myelin (membrane) compartment than in any of the other compartments.[126] In brain slices exposed to [^{3}H]bilirubin, bilirubin appeared to bind more avidly to neurons, suggesting a particular affinity for neuronal cell membranes.[127] An important question regarding the interaction of bilirubin with membranes is whether such interaction is primarily a phenomenon of physicochemical binding with perturbation of membrane integrity and potentials or whether it is associated with more specific effects on membrane-located enzymes, pumps, channels, or transporters. While some of the membrane effects of bilirubin appear to be reversible, others are not so.

It has been suggested that interaction of bilirubin with polar lipids may play an important role in the toxicity mechanism.[128]The addition of bilirubin to cell cultures was associated with leakage of cytosolic enzymes into the medium.[64] Erythrocytes from jaundiced neonates examined by scanning electron microscopy demonstrated a crenated surface structure, compatible with an interaction of bilirubin with the outer half of the erythrocyte plasma membrane bilayer complex.[25] Phototherapy reversed the membrane changes. Others have also found evidence for crenation of the red cell outer surface in nonaggregating conditions in the presence of clinically relevant bilirubin concentrations.[129] Bilirubin appears to have a high affinity for the phospholipids in cell membranes, and there is some evidence that it may form complexes with these phospholipids.[23,130,131] Partitioning into membranes was increased if they contained proteins but the effect of proteins could not be attributed to specific binding sites.[131]

Bilirubin in its acid conformation may possibly precipitate, particularly in the presence of acidosis, when aggregation may be irreversible.[36,132] Precipitation of bilirubin aggregates remains a theory that is supported by some investigators.[101] Others have proposed that bilirubin in the form of the monovalent anion of the acid might bind reversibly to membranes.[133] This is consistent with the finding that bilirubin binding to liposomes and red blood cells is reversible[133] and appears compatible with the known reversibility of milder signs of bilirubin toxicity.[134] However, reversibility of membrane changes caused by bilirubin appears to be dependent on model and experimental conditions. In an erythrocyte model, washing with albumin could not fully reverse such membrane changes.[135] Inherent in the proposed model of reversible bilirubin binding to membranes is also the possibility that decreasing pH could result in irreversible aggregation of bilirubin in tissues.[133]

Some effects of bilirubin on cell membranes may also reflect interaction with membrane-localized enzymes, pumps, channels, or transporters. Bilirubin decreased the "break temperature" (point at which the enzyme denatures) for sodium-potassium adenosine triphosphatase (Na^+, K^+-ATPase) from young rat brains, whereas the break temperature for the enzyme from adult rats was unaffected.[136] Bilirubin also inhibited Na^+, K^+-ATPase activity in human erythrocyte membranes with stronger inhibition at lower temperature.[137] This suggests an interaction between the enzyme, bilirubin, and the surrounding membrane lipid environment. Changes in the transition temperature under the influence of bilirubin have also been found for brain nitric oxide synthase (NOS).[138] Bilirubin-induced changes in NOS activity may be attenuated by 7-nitroindazole, a specific inhibitor of neuronal NOS.[139] After intraperitoneal or intravenous administration of bilirubin boluses, Na^+, K^+-ATPase, and acetylcholinesterase activities were more strongly inhibited in young versus adult rat brains.[140] However, the activity Mg^{2+}-ATPase was not affected.

Bilirubin has been shown to inhibit the enzymes involved in the transfer of reducing equivalents across the inner mitochondrial membrane[141] and to inhibit vasopressin-stimulated water and Na^+ transport across the toad bladder membrane,[142] showing that bilirubin may exert a tissue-specific effect on membrane transport mechanisms. Inhibition of membrane ion transport, accompanied by increased water retention, is another bilirubin-associated perturbation of membrane function.[143]

The NMDA receptor is a glutamate receptor and ion channel protein localized to nerve cell membranes and is important during development.[144,145] Activation permits positively charged ions to flow through the cell membrane, thus it plays an important role in membrane function. Bilirubin-induced apoptosis in developing rat brain neurons was reduced by the NMDA blocker MK-801.[146-148] Similar results were found in human neuron-like cells in vitro.[149,150] In young pigs NMDA affinity for MK-801 was increased by a bilirubin infusion,[151] and in homozygous Gunn rats who received a bilirubin binding competitor to induce acute brain toxicity, MK-801 treatment reduced clinical symptoms,[152] suggesting that NMDA-mediated excitotoxicity may be involved in bilirubin encephalopathy (see Fig. 163.4).

Conversely, MK-801 did not prevent bilirubin toxicity in rat hippocampal cell cultures, nor did it prevent the development of ABR changes in jaundiced Gunn rat pups given a bilirubin binding competitor.[153] Further, in transverse hippocampal slices and Müller cells studied acutely in vitro using a cell clamp technique, bilirubin did not affect the NMDA receptor.[154] At present the evidence for involvement of the NMDA receptor in acute bilirubin neurotoxicity appears contradictory, and further studies are needed to elucidate its role.

Voltage-gated calcium channels are found in cell membranes of excitable cells such as neurons, glia, and muscle cells.They open during depolarizing membrane potentials, allowing entry of Ca^{2+} into the cell, resulting in excitation of neurons, for example. In rat pup ventral cochlear nucleus bushy cells, acute administration of bilirubin increased voltage-gated calcium channel currents, apparently involving Ca^{2+}- and calmodulin-dependent mechanisms.[155] Neonatal neurons possess more P/Q-subtype calcium channels than more mature cells. Hence, the vulnerability to bilirubin toxicity of neurons, both in auditory and other brain cells, may involve a subtype-specific increase of P/Q-type Ca^{2+} currents.[155] Further evidence supporting a role for Ca^{2+} channels in bilirubin neurotoxicity was obtained from studies of recombinant Cav2.3 + β3 channel complexes as well as ex vivo electroretinograms from wild-type and Cav2.3-deficient mice.[156] In this model, 10 μM bilirubin caused changes in the voltage-dependence of activation as well as pre-pulse inactivation. In mouse retina exposed to bilirubin, the responses from the inner retina of wild-type mice were suppressed compared to retina from Cav2.3-deficient mice. In addition, recovery after washout was more rapid and complete in retinae that did not have Cav2.3 channels.[156]

Depression of the membrane potential of synaptosomes by bilirubin pointed to a mechanism involving alterations in ion permeability.[65] Perturbation of membrane function has been proposed as the triggering event in a cascade leading to excitotoxicity and mitochondrial energy failure.[157] However, it is not clear that such perturbation is an essential element in bilirubin toxicity. In a model involving synaptosomes permeabilized with streptolysin O, thus excluding the importance of plasma membrane polarity, bilirubin was shown to inhibit Ca^{2+}-dependent neurotransmitter exocytosis and, at higher concentrations, to disrupt vesicular norepinephrine storage.[124]

NEUROTRANSMITTER METABOLISM AND SYNAPTIC FUNCTION

Both the inhibitory effects of bilirubin on evoked potentials and the reversible inhibition of synaptic activation in rat transverse hippocampal slices[158] suggested that neurotransmitter metabolism might be affected by bilirubin. Phosphorylation of synapsin I is an important step in neurotransmitter release at the synapse, and the ability of bilirubin to inhibit synapsin I phosphorylation[77] might therefore also predict bilirubin effects on neurotransmitter cycling.

Studies in synaptosomes showed that bilirubin was both able to inhibit the uptake of tyrosine, a precursor of dopamine, and to inhibit the formation of dopamine in these nerve endings.[159] Other studies showed that bilirubin inhibited direct uptake of dopamine into synaptosomes but not its release.[160] However, using a different stimulus for release, other investigators observed the inhibition of dopamine release by bilirubin.[161] The release of endogenous acetylcholine was also inhibited by bilirubin, and depolarization of the synaptosomal membrane was observed.[161]

Another contribution to decreased synaptic function in the jaundiced brain might be the inhibitory interaction between bilirubin and transport proteins in synaptic vesicle membranes, leading to inhibition of neurotransmitter uptake into these vesicles.[162] It was noteworthy in the studies cited above that uptake of dopamine and uptake of glutamate into synaptic vesicles were equally inhibited, although these are presumed to be driven by two different mechanisms (proton gradient and membrane potential, respectively). In a further attempt to delineate the relative importance of membrane potential versus energy metabolism, permeabilized synaptosomes were used to study the release of norepinephrine, showing that bilirubin inhibited both exocytotic release and synaptic vesicular storage of brain catecholamines independently of ATP and in the absence of a membrane potential.[124]

Exposure of rat hippocampal slice cultures to bilirubin for 24 or 48 hours resulted in impairment of CA1 long-term potentiation and long-term depression induction in a time- and concentration-dependent manner.[146] Hippocampal slice cultures stimulated with bilirubin showed no changes in the secretion profiles of proinflammatory cytokines, interleukin (IL)-1β and tumor necrosis factor-α (TNF-α), or propidium iodide uptake (to quantitatively assess DNA content). However, bilirubin treatment produced a significant decrease in the levels of NR1, NR2A, and NR2B (subunits of NMDA) receptors through a calpain-mediated proteolytic cleavage mechanism. Pretreatment of hippocampal slice cultures with NMDA receptor antagonist or calpain inhibitors effectively prevented the bilirubin-induced impairment of long-term potentiation and long-term depression.

In an in vitro study of neurons that were mechanically dissociated from lateral superior olive nuclei of 2-week old rats, a brainstem auditory nucleus that is vulnerable to bilirubin, 10 μM bilirubin increased the frequency, but not the amplitudes, of spontaneous inhibitory postsynaptic currents, suggesting a presynaptic point of action.[163] This effect was independent of voltage-activated Na^+ and Ca^{2+} channels, but not of presynaptic $Ca^{2+}{}_i$, and increased with bilirubin concentration and exposure time. This may have implications for understanding the impairment of transduction of signals in acute bilirubin auditory neurotoxicity.[163] The mechanisms of γ-aminobutyric acid (GABA)/glycinergic synaptic transmission were explored further in the same lab, using rat ventral cochlear nucleus neurons from 10- to 12-day old rats.[164] These neurons were studied with voltage-clamp technique in whole-cell mode. Similar to the findings in their previous study, bilirubin increased miniature inhibitory postsynaptic current frequencies, but not amplitudes. Pretreatment with forskolin, an activator of phosphokinase A (PKA), blocked the bilirubin effect. Chelerythrine, an inhibitor of phosphokinase C (PKC), increased the current frequency, and adding bilirubin increased the frequency further. As in the previous study,[163] the sum of findings here also pointed to a presynaptic locus. Taken together, their data showed that both PKA and PKC can modulate GABA and glycine release in rat ventral cochlear nucleus neurons, and that bilirubin facilitated transmitter release through presynaptic activation of PKA. In a follow-up study using the same model, the above effects of bilirubin were confirmed.[165] However, pretreatment with minocycline, shown in other studies to protect against or ameliorate bilirubin neurotoxicity,[105,166-168] did not abolish bilirubin effects in this model. Thus, minocycline protection against bilirubin neurotoxicity is likely to involve other mechanisms than those of neuronal hyperexcitation.

Exposure of astrocytes, microglia, and neurons in culture to bilirubin was followed by release of glutamate and cell death.[169-171] Immature cells were more vulnerable to loss of glutamate. Glutamate uptake in rat cortical astrocytes was also inhibited by bilirubin.[172] L-carnitine, which protects neurons in culture from glutamate toxicity, has been shown to significantly reduce bilirubin toxicity in cerebellar granule cells in culture, further pointing to the role of glutamate and excitotoxicity in bilirubin neurotoxicity.[173]

The relevance of these in vitro studies for the situation in human brain was supported by findings in specimens from kernicteric brains, reflecting both acute and chronic cases.[174] Thus, in specimens from cases who had died with ABE as newborns, tyrosine hydroxylase expression was reduced both in the globus pallidus and in the putamen. In specimens from patients who had died later with signs of KSD, tyrosine hydroxylase expression was also found to be lower in the globus pallidus, but not in the putamen. Another brain area where findings were similar in both acute and KSD specimens concerned the external segment of the globus pallidus, where the expression of methionine-enkephalin was reduced. Immunoreactivity for substance P was significantly reduced both in the internal and external segments of the globus pallidus in specimens from KSD, but expression was only marginally lowered in specimens from cases who had died during ongoing ABE as newborns.[174]

BILIRUBIN METABOLISM IN BRAIN

Bilirubin that enters the brain is also cleared from the brain. The half-life of bilirubin in brain was first estimated at 1.7 hours; the clearance rate from blood was 1.6 hours.[61] Later work yielded the much lower estimated half-life of 16 to 18 minutes during baseline conditions[48] and 38 minutes during hyperosmolality.[50] A meta-analysis of these data indicated that clearance from brain may be more rapid than from blood, suggesting that additional mechanisms might be operating to remove bilirubin from brain.[104] Brodersen and Bartels described an enzyme localized on the inner mitochondrial membrane of brain cells, as well as in other tissues, capable of oxidizing bilirubin.[175] Others have also found bilirubin-oxidizing activity in brain mitochondria.[104,176-180] This enzyme appears to have some of the characteristics of the cytochrome P-450 oxidases, although it has not been unequivocally identified.[180] Cytochrome P-450 2A5 may play an important role in hepatic oxidation of bilirubin,[181] but hepatic and brain metabolic pathways may not be the same. The activity of this enzyme in the brain is lower in the immature organism and in neurons versus glia.[177] These data are compatible with the clinical impressions of greater vulnerability to bilirubin toxicity in infants than in older children and adults, and in brain neurons versus glia. The activity is also subject to genetic variability,[178] and one may speculate as to whether apparent inter-individual differences in vulnerability to bilirubin neurotoxicity may, perhaps in part, have a genetic basis.[182]

Gazzin and colleagues showed that there was a close inverse relationship between brain bilirubin content and expression of cytochrome P-450 mRNA.[183] Some brain regions affected in kernicterus demonstrated delayed induction of cytochromes P-450. Whether these findings can be reconciled with the above-mentioned studies of a mitochondrial enzyme that oxidizes bilirubin,[176-180] deserves further study. Thus, although cytochromes P-450 in liver are typically associated with microsomes and the endoplasmic reticulum, cytochrome P-450 activity in brain is mainly found in the mitochondrial subcellular fraction.[184] Additionally, messenger RNA levels do not necessarily predict protein levels, and in the central nervous system a protein and its messenger RNA are not necessarily expressed in the same part of the cell.[184]

Currently there appears to be three groups working on bilirubin oxidation in brain.[176-180,183,185-187] Their observations are in some ways discrepant, and it appears possible that there may be more than one enzyme involved in bilirubin brain oxidation. One difference between the apparent enzyme activities that have been studied is that while one needed NADPH as a cofactor in oxidation reactions,[185] the other activity needed neither NAD, NADP, NADH, NADPH, GSH, nor GSSH for bilirubin oxidation to take place.[179] The latter enzyme was cytochrome c dependent, and could be inhibited by clotrimazole and ketoconazole, which are both cytochrome P450 oxidase (CYP) inhibitors.[179] Data obtained with enzyme from a pure glial source also appeared compatible with CYP activity, specifically CYPs 1A1 and 1A2.[185,186] However, inhibitors of CYPs 1A1 and 1A2 (omeprazole and fluvoxamine) did not inhibit the activity in brain mitochondrial membranes from a mixed glial and neuronal source.[180] CYP1A2 mRNA levels appear to increase with maturation in rat brain and liver microsomes.[187] However, microsomes had no effect on bilirubin or bilirubin metabolites. Thus, this CYP may not have a physiologic role in bilirubin oxidation.[187] We have recently attempted to purify the mixed mitochondrial enzyme activity by salt fractionation.[180] Fractions that came out at around 205 mM NaCl showed the highest activity. Proteomics data from salt-separated fractions, among many other proteins/peptides, also pointed to cytochrome oxidases. So far attempts to block activity with currently available antibodies has not allowed for a conclusion.[180]

The fact that bilirubin oxidation appears to take place in brain, does not necessarily imply that this activity is physiologically important, nor that it plays a protective role against bilirubin neurotoxicity. Thus, the clinical implications of bilirubin metabolism in brain are at present unknown, and more studies are needed to understand this phenomenon. However, the term *bilirubin oxidase* probably does not denote the activity described above.[105] The enzyme commercially available as *bilirubin oxidase* (EC 1.3.3.5) clearly has characteristics different from those of the mitochondrial enzyme discovered by Brodersen and Bartels[175] and studied by Hansen and colleagues,[104,176-180] and there is no evidence that this enzyme is responsible for bilirubin metabolism in brain.

APOPTOSIS AND NECROSIS

Cell death is clearly involved in the devastating effects of bilirubin neurotoxicity seen in victims of kernicterus[188] and is observed in the brains of Gunn rats, where both Purkinje and granular cells appear vulnerable.[189-194] Since the development of methods to study cell death processes in detail, many studies have addressed the question of how cells die when exposed to bilirubin toxicity.

In vitro cell cultures have been especially useful, and several different cell lines have been used. In rat cerebellar granule cells, bilirubin causes apoptosis, which can be blocked by RNA and protein synthesis inhibitors. This suggests that execution of the death process requires de novo synthesis of RNA and protein.[194] In embryonic rat forebrain neurons in culture, apoptosis caused by toxicity was dependent on bilirubin dose and was blocked by an NMDA receptor antagonist, suggesting a role for NMDA receptors.[147]

In a comparison of bilirubin effects on rat brain astrocytes and neurons, toxicity was evident in both cell types but required higher bilirubin concentrations to injure the astrocytes.[195] In addition, glutamate uptake and 3-(4,5-dimethylthiazol-2-yl)-2,5-diphenyltetrazolium bromide (MTT) reduction (a measure of cell function), exhibited greater inhibition in astrocytes, whereas neurons exhibited a greater tendency for necrosis and apoptosis. Apoptosis was preceded by signs of impaired mitochondrial metabolism and membrane perturbation in the form of altered lipid polarity and fluidity, protein order, and redox status.[116] However, when neurons and astrocytes from young and old rats were compared, immature cells were more susceptible to the toxic effects of bilirubin, although mitochondria from the younger rats were more resistant.[196] This suggests that although mitochondrial injury may play a role in mediating bilirubin toxicity, it is not likely to be the sole, nor probably the primary, mechanism.

In murine hepatoma cells, bilirubin also appeared to have an effect on cell membranes, possibly involving the aryl hydrocarbon receptor.[197] In rat oligodendrocytes, bilirubin-induced apoptotic cell death was associated with induction of NOS.[198] Additional studies in rat neurons suggested that apoptosis triggered by mitochondrial depolarization and Bax (a pro-apoptotic member of the B-cell lymphoma 2 family) translocation could be prevented by ursodeoxycholate.[116] It is noteworthy that hyperphosphorylation of enzyme activity (p38 mitogen-activated protein kinase) as a trigger for bilirubin-induced neuronal death was observed in rat cerebellar granule cells.[199] This finding is intriguing in light of other evidence that bilirubin appears to have inhibitory effects on protein-peptide phosphorylation.[77,78,200,201] Minocycline, which acts partly by inhibiting glial caspase 1 and inducible NOS activity, appears to block bilirubin toxicity in rat cerebellar granule cells in vitro and largely prevents loss of Purkinje cells and cerebellar hypoplasia in homozygous Gunn rat pups.[202] Somewhat surprisingly, phototherapy, which might also have been posited to be neuroprotective because of the formation of presumably nontoxic water-soluble photoisomers, appears to accentuate bilirubin toxicity in cultured cells.[203] However, in vitro studies of bilirubin photoisomer toxicity in cell cultures are fraught with methodologic challenges, as previously discussed.[55]

Although the studies just mentioned were performed in cells of animal origin, a human neuron-like cell line (NT2-N neurons) has been used to assess bilirubin's ability to cause apoptosis or necrosis. It has been shown that the induction of apoptosis as opposed to necrosis may depend on bilirubin concentration, such that high bilirubin concentrations induce early necrosis, whereas low-to-moderate concentrations predominantly induce delayed apoptosis.[204] Further studies with a specific caspase 3 inhibitor, a general caspase inhibitor, and an NMDA receptor antagonist indicated that both NMDA receptor-mediated and caspase-mediated pathways may be involved in bilirubin-induced cell death.[149] Concomitant inhibition of both pathways resulted in synergistic protection. However, in follow-up studies examining recovery after short-term bilirubin exposure in NT2-N cells, caspase inhibition did not have a positive impact on cell survival, whereas NMDA blockade significantly increased the number of undamaged nuclei, without impacting cell viability.[150] However, as discussed above, the evidence that NMDA receptors have a role in bilirubin toxicity is equivocal.

INFLAMMATION AND INFECTION

Neonatal jaundice in the presence of infection has been believed to increase the risk of ABE and KSD, this is supported by several clinical studies.[111,205] Others, however, have failed to confirm this association.[206] In a rat model, endotoxemia was found to increase the net accumulation of bilirubin in brain, apparently by increasing both total and unbound bilirubin.[207] This is compatible with data from infected human infants, who had a lower reserve albumin binding capacity for bilirubin.[208] It is also possible that inflammatory cytokines may increase blood-brain barrier permeability, and this might facilitate bilirubin passage into the brain.[209] Such barrier permeability changes may be disruptive or nondisruptive and, in the latter case, may also involve cytokines.[210] Microglia exposed to bilirubin in vitro were activated and released high levels of TNF-α, IL-1β, and IL-6, also supporting the idea that bilirubin-induced cytokine production can exacerbate neurotoxicity.[169] However, endotoxemia or sepsis did not affect bilirubin metabolism in rat brain.[176]

In astrocytes exposed to bilirubin in conditions that induced less than 10% cell death, the release of TNF-α and IL-1β was significantly enhanced, whereas the production of IL-6 was inhibited.[171] Young astrocytes in culture were more prone to bilirubin-induced cell death and exhibited a greater inflammatory response than older cells, and bilirubin cytotoxicity was increased by endotoxin, a finding confirmed by other studies.[170] Astrocytes exposed to bilirubin 50 μM in a 1:2 molar ratio with human serum albumin demonstrated a rapid rise in the levels of TNFα receptor 1, followed by activation of p38 mitogen-activated protein kinase and nuclear factor κB (NF-κB).[171] However, inhibition of the NFκB signal transduction pathway reduced the loss of cell viability as well as cytokine secretion. This suggests that NF-κB may play a role in the astroglial response to bilirubin involving inflammatory pathways.

The interaction of bilirubin with the immunologic cascade may be very complex, and not all of the data appear to agree. Thus, in apparent contradiction to the findings discussed above, others working with in vivo animal models found no effect of bilirubin on NF-κB or p38 mitogen-activated protein kinase. To the contrary, in a rat model of endotoxemia involving infusion of lipopolysaccharide, bilirubin treatment was followed by improved survival and attenuation of liver injury.[211] The authors suggested that bilirubin may exert a cytoprotective effect through inhibition of expression of inducible NOS and, possibly, through stimulation of local prostaglandin E_2 production.[211] In another study, jaundiced rats were shown to be more resistant to endotoxin-induced hypotension or death compared with nonjaundiced controls and exhibited reduced expression of inducible NOS.[212]

In a mouse model acute/transient hyperbilirubinemia and neurotoxicity were induced by intraperitoneal administration of bilirubin and sulfadimethoxine.[213] Cerebellar and auditory brainstem tissue were investigated with whole genome gene expression followed by immunoblotting, and showed that endoplasmic reticulum stress and inflammation were important contributors to bilirubin auditory neurotoxicity. Antiinflammatory drugs that inhibit NF-κB and TNFα signaling protected the auditory pathway against bilirubin toxicity.[214]

Innate immunity signaling may ameliorate bilirubin neurotoxicity. In a genetic mouse model (UGT1A1*28), the Toll-like receptor 2 signaling pathway appeared to protect against the effects of severe hyperbilirubinemia.[214] Thus, jaundiced hUGT1A1*28/Tlr22/2 mice pups who failed to activate glial cells, proinflammatory cytokines, and stress response genes had significantly increased mortality rates.[214] It also appears that bilirubin may have antiinflammatory effects in the brain. In mouse experimental autoimmune encephalomyelitis, bilirubin injections that caused TSB levels of ~60 μmol/L half an hour after injection delayed the onset and reduced the severity of chronic encephalomyelitis, while depletion of endogenous bilirubin exacerbated the disease.[215]

Thus, while the evidence suggests a role for inflammation and/or infection in the pathophysiology of bilirubin encephalopathy, and the possibility that bilirubin may modulate immune mechanisms in the brain, many questions remain unresolved.

EFFECTS OF BILIRUBIN IN OTHER SYSTEMS

Some investigators have studied the effect of bilirubin on enzyme activity. A 1979 review listed 25 separate enzymes and four pathways that bilirubin appeared to inhibit.[216] A number of other enzymes and pathways have subsequently been studied, and with few exceptions the effects of bilirubin are inhibitory.[136,141,200,217-219] The inhibitory effects of bilirubin on protein kinases are discussed elsewhere in this chapter.[77,78,220]

Several studies have found that bilirubin inhibits protein synthesis,[63,221-223] although at least one study reached the opposite conclusion.[148] Inhibition of DNA synthesis,[63,224,225] and increased strand breakage in DNA in combination with phototherapy,[226,227] have also been described. Finally, several older studies documented bilirubin inhibitory effects on carbohydrate metabolism.[228,229]

PROTEIN PHOSPHORYLATION

Protein/peptide phosphorylation may regulate the function of some enzymes,[77,78] but very limited research efforts have been directed towards understanding how bilirubin exerts its effects on enzymes. Lysine appears to be present on the active sites of several of the enzymes whose activity seems to be modulated by bilirubin. Although a parallel to the binding of bilirubin to lysine on albumin may be suggested,[230] there is no direct evidence to support a role in enzyme inhibition. Thus, more research is needed.

Bilirubin toxicity has been described across a wide range of biologic reactions and systems. It is not clear that these reactions or systems are actually implicated in the bilirubin effects we observe in jaundiced infants. Also, no agreement exists as to which of these reactions/systems might be the principal or basic mechanism for bilirubin neurotoxicity, although several of the bilirubin effects described in the preceding sections have been proposed for this role.

Therefore energy failure through inhibition of oxidative phosphorylation was first proposed as the basic mechanism of bilirubin toxicity,[114,115] and this theory continues to have support.[101] However, it seems reasonable to ask whether the many apparently divergent toxic and inhibitory effects of bilirubin may have something in common and whether bilirubin inhibition of such a putative basic reaction might explain the wide range of bilirubin toxicity. Protein-peptide phosphorylation has been shown to be an important regulatory mechanism for many cell processes.[72,75,76,231-233] Current knowledge regarding the many bilirubin-affected processes suggests that regulation by protein-peptide phosphorylation might constitute a common theme.

Early studies showed that bilirubin inhibited the binding of cyclic adenosine monophosphate (cAMP) to protein kinase, as well as the phosphorylation of histone.[200] Protein phosphorylation in cell-free preparations from newborn rabbit brains was inhibited by bilirubin given intravenously before the rabbits were killed.[201] In vitro, bilirubin inhibits phosphorylation of endogenous proteins in fibroblasts.[234] Bilirubin inhibits phosphorylation of synapsin I, a protein that is preferentially localized to presynaptic vesicles.[77] Dephosphorylated synapsin I inhibits neurotransmitter release. This observation might explain why bilirubin inhibits synaptic activation in transverse rat hippocampal slices, and why jaundiced infants are drowsy and evince changes in brain stem auditory evoked responses.[11,12,14,158] Several protein-kinase interactions are similarly inhibited by bilirubin, suggesting that inhibition of protein-peptide phosphorylation might explain the effects of bilirubin in many biologic systems.[78]

An intriguing new perspective may link the role of P-gp as a membrane-localized pump that may limit the intracellular and intracerebral accumulation of bilirubin (see earlier),[72,74,75] with its regulation by phosphorylation.[76,231-233] Although no studies that directly address the impact of bilirubin on P-gp phosphorylation have been published, the fact that both protein kinase A and protein kinase C are involved in P-gp phosphorylation and that bilirubin has been shown to inhibit the interaction between these two kinases and other peptide-protein substrates suggests that P-gp phosphorylation may have a role in bilirubin toxicity.[78]

BILIRUBIN BINDING

Bilirubin binds to albumin in serum, as well as to glutathione *S*-transferase (previously known as *ligandin*) in hepatocytes. Lysine seems to be common to both binding sites,[230,235] and to the active sites in many of the reactions perturbed by bilirubin, including ATP-binding subdomain II of the protein kinase family.[236] Lysine-containing peptides were shown to modulate the toxic effects of bilirubin in a model peptide-kinase system.[237] Thus binding of bilirubin to lysine may play a role in the mediation and/or modulation of bilirubin neurotoxicity.

A "PROMISCUOUS INHIBITOR"?

McDonagh expressed a note of caution regarding the many in vitro studies of bilirubin toxicity. He suggested that bilirubin might be a "promiscuous inhibitor."[238] The concept of promiscuous inhibition evolved from automated in vitro screening of potential new drugs, where some compounds that showed strong activity against many protein receptor targets did not show "drug-like" activity on further testing.[239,240] Along with bilirubin these promiscuous inhibitors share the following characteristics: high hydrophobicity, high molecular flexibility, and the ability to form microaggregates. A hypothesis casting bilirubin as a promiscuous inhibitor is consistent with observations that bilirubin inhibits a wide variety of enzymes in vitro, with no notable effect on them in vivo.[241] Therefore, as pointed out by McDonagh, "deducing the biochemical pathways of kernicterus from the numerous in vitro studies is fraught with risk."[238]

BILIRUBIN CELL TOXICITY: SELECTIVITY VERSUS GLOBAL EFFECTS

Although bilirubin appears to be toxic in all cell systems that have been studied in vitro, some cell types seem to be more vulnerable than others, and the age of the cells also modulates toxicity. This is in accordance with clinical data. Thus, although cerebellar affection is rare when KSD results from severe neonatal jaundice,[242,243] cerebellar symptoms have been reported in persons with Crigler-Najjar syndrome type 1 who were neurologically normal in early life but developed signs of KSD later on.[244]

Bilirubin toxicity was seen in neuroblastoma cells, but not in glial cells from rodents.[222] Mitochondria from rodent glial cells oxidize bilirubin at a greater rate than mitochondria from a pure neuronal source, and thus may have greater ability to protect themselves against bilirubin toxicity.[177] A greater affinity for neurons was suggested by binding of [^{3}H]bilirubin to hippocampal pyramidal and granule cells as well as to Purkinje cells in rat brain slices.[127]

Differences between neurons and glia in reactions to bilirubin exposure may not be simply one of tolerance versus sensitivity. Apoptosis, cytoskeleton disassembly, and membrane leakage were greater in rat neurons than in astrocytes exposed to bilirubin 85.5 μmol/L, while inhibition of MTT metabolism and glutamate uptake were more pronounced in astrocytes.[195] Classes of glia may also react differently. Thus, microglia may be more sensitive to bilirubin toxicity than astrocytes.[169] However, cells exposed to a lower bilirubin concentration became increasingly apoptotic if treated with a MRP1-blocking agent (MK571), suggesting that variable expression of membrane "flippases" such as MRP1 might modulate sensitivity to bilirubin toxicity.

Neuroblastoma cells exposed to prostaglandin E_1 and cAMP during differentiation lost their sensitivity to bilirubin toxicity,[222] and rat astrocytes exposed to dibutyryl cAMP evinced a similar reaction.[245] Both prostaglandin E_1 and cAMP stimulate phosphorylation of a membrane glycoprotein in human platelets.[246,247] MRP1 and P-gp are expressed in cultured rat astrocytes,[248,249] and human studies showed that drug treatment may lead to overexpression of P-gp[250] and may even cause therapy resistance in epilepsy.[251] MRP1 and P-gp are expressed in different brain cells with a different pattern of distribution.[252] Thus, further studies of regulation of membrane transporter expression may shed light on differences in vulnerability to bilirubin toxicity.

Resistance to bilirubin toxicity increased from day 2 to day 12 in rat glial cells in culture, suggesting that immature cells are more vulnerable.[67] This finding was also confirmed with different cells and techniques.[170] The expression of P-gp in rodent brain increases with maturation.[249,253] As increased expression of MRPs may protect cells against bilirubin cytotoxicity,[82] decreasing sensitivity to bilirubin toxicity with increasing age may, at least in part, be tied to increasing membrane transporter expression. Increased bilirubin oxidation by more mature brain cells might also confer protection, although no direct proof of this is available.[177]

Ngai and colleagues compared neuroblastoma and glioblastoma cells with fibroblasts and liver cells.[254] With increasing bilirubin-albumin ratio, CNS cells were clearly more vulnerable. However, when comparing the two neuronal cell lines NBR10A and N115, the latter were more resistant to bilirubin toxicity.[225] Pathoanatomic data from kernicterus patients and from Gunn rats clearly show that not all neurons are damaged by bilirubin. The reasons for such differences in sensitivity are not clear. Although both P-gp and MRP1 may be expressed in neurons in experimental or refractory epilepsy,[255,256] they do not appear to be generally expressed in neurons.[257] Other MRPs may be found in neurons,[258,259] but the implications for bilirubin neurotoxicity are unknown.

INTERINDIVIDUAL DIFFERENCES IN SENSITIVITY TO BILIRUBIN TOXICITY

Clinical data suggest a wide interindividual disparity in sensitivity to bilirubin neurotoxicity.[110,260-264] Whereas some infants may tolerate serum bilirubin levels in excess of 500 to 600 μmol/L, the literature has reported cases of kernicterus in term infants with serum bilirubin levels barely in excess of 350 μmol/L,[265,266] and at even lower levels in preterm infants.[267]

There has been considerable discussion among bilirubin experts regarding this phenomenon. Although immaturity and diseases may explain vulnerability in some cases, kernicterus has occurred in apparently healthy, term infants at serum bilirubin levels that many others tolerate without evidence of ABE or KSD. The explanation for this remains speculative. Future research should probably investigate genetic differences in the expression of membrane transporters, as well as how their expression may be modulated by factors such as disease, drugs, and even bilirubin itself.[182] Bilirubin oxidation in brain may be hypothesized to be protective, but this remains to be proven. Whether genetic differences in such oxidation, as suggested by animal studies,[178] might play a role in humans, is also awaiting further studies.

CONCLUSION

Our understanding of the mechanism(s) of kernicterus and bilirubin encephalopathy is far from complete, and the challenge of translating these data into clinical guidelines has been daunting. Thus, there is great variability in practice; guidelines vary between countries and even individual NICUs.[106,268] Although our current state of knowledge regarding the mechanism(s) of bilirubin neurotoxicity does provide some input into the practical management of a newborn with jaundice, further work is needed to precisely understand bilirubin's neurotoxic mechanisms in the developing human infant brain. Such information is likely to be helpful in elaborating more consistent and robust clinical protocols to prevent the devastating effects of bilirubin toxicity on long-term neurodevelopmental outcomes in human neonates.

 A complete reference list is available at www.ExpertConsult.com.

SELECT REFERENCES

3. Schmorl C. Zur Kenntnis des Ikterus neonatorum, insbesondere der dabei auftretenden Gehirnveränderungen. *Verh Dtsch Pathol Ges*. 1904;6:109-115.
18. Amin SB, Charafeddine L, Guillet R. Transient bilirubin encephalopathy and apnea of prematurity in 28 to 32 weeks gestational age infants. *J Perinatol*. 2005;25:386-390.
19. Le Pichon JB, Riordan SM, Watchko J, Shapiro SM. The neurological sequelae of neonatal hyperbilirubinemia: definitions, diagnosis and treatment of the kernicterus spectrum disorders (KSDs). *Curr Pediatr Rev*. 2017;13:199-209.
22. Soorani-Lunsing I, Woltil HA, Hadders-Algra M. Are moderate degrees of hyperbilirubinemia in healthy term neonates really safe for the brain? *Pediatr Res*. 2001;50:701-705.
23. Brodersen R. Bilirubin: solubility and interaction with albumin and phospholipids. *J Biol Chem*. 1979;254:2364-2369.
28. Brodersen R. Binding of bilirubin to albumin. *Crit Rev Clin Lab Sci*. 1980;11:305-399.
29. Maisels MJ, McDonagh AF. Phototherapy for neonatal jaundice. *N Engl J Med*. 2008;358:920-928.
31. Claireaux AE, Cole PG, Lathe GH. Icterus of the brain in the newborn. *Lancet*. 1953;2:1226-1230.
34. Daood MJ, Watchko JF. Calculated *in vivo* free bilirubin levels in the central nervous system of Gunn rat pups. *Pediatr Res*. 2006;60:44-49.
42. Cashore WJ, Horwich A, Karotkin EH, Oh W. Influence of gestational age and clinical status on bilirubin-binding capacity in newborn infants. *Am J Dis Child*. 1977;131:898-901.
46. Maruyama K, Harada S, Nishigori H, Iwatsuru M. Classification of drugs on the basis of bilirubin-displacing effect on human serum albumin. *Chem Pharm Bull*. 1984;32:2414-2420.
50. Hansen TWR. Bilirubin entry into and clearance from rat brain during hypercarbia and hyperosmolality. *Pediatr Res*. 1996;39:72-76.
51. McDonagh AF, Lightner DA. 'Like a shrivelled blood orange'—bilirubin, jaundice, and phototherapy. *Pediatrics*. 1985;75:443-445.
53. Hansen TWR, Nietsch L, Norman E, et al. Apparent reversibility of acute intermediate phase bilirubin encephalopathy. *Acta Paediatr*. 2009;98:1689-1694.
54. Harris MC, Bernbaum JC, Polin JR, et al. Developmental follow-up of breastfed term and near-term infants with marked hyperbilirubinemia. *Pediatrics*. 2001;107:1075-1080.
55. Hansen TWR. Biology of bilirubin photoisomers. *Clin Perinatol*. 2016;43:277-290.
56. Jasprova J, Dal Ben M, Vianello E, et al. The biological effects of bilirubin photoisomers. *PloS One*. 2016;11:e0148126.
58. Watchko JF, Daood MJ, Hansen TW. Brain bilirubin content is increased in P-glycoprotein-deficient transgenic null mutant mice. *Pediatr Res*. 1998;44:763-766.
62. Tsai CE, Daood MJ, Lane RH, et al. P-glycoprotein expression in mouse brain increases with maturation. *Biol Neonate*. 2002;81:58-64.
71. Gazzin S, Strazielle N, Schmitt C, et al. Differential expression of the multidrug resistance-related proteins ABCb1 and ABCc1 between blood-brain interfaces. *J Comp Neurol*. 2008;510:497-507.
78. Hansen TWR, Mathiesen SB, Walaas SI. Bilirubin has widespread inhibitory effects on protein phosphorylation. *Pediatr Res*. 1996;39:1072-1077.
80. Fernandes A, Falcão AS, Silva RF, et al. Inflammatory signalling pathways involved in astroglial activation by unconjugated bilirubin. *J Neurochem*. 2006;96:1667-1679.
82. Calligaris S, Cekic D, Roca-Burgos L, et al. Multidrug resistance associated protein 1 protects against bilirubin-induced cytotoxicity. *FEBS Lett*. 2006;580:1355-1359.
101. Ostrow JD, Pascolo L, Shapiro SM, Tiribelli C. New concepts in bilirubin encephalopathy. *Eur J Clin Invest*. 2003;33:988-997.
102. Pascolo L. Protective role of MRP1/mrp1 (ABCC1/abcc1) in bilirubin neurotoxicity. In Tiribelli C, Ostrow JD (eds): The Molecular Basis of Bilirubin Encephalopathy and Toxicity: Report of an EASL Single Topic Conference, Trieste, Italy 1-2 October, 2004. *J Hepatol*. 2005;43:156-166.
103. Cannon C, Daood MJ, O'Day TL, Watchko JF. Sex-specific regional brain bilirubin content in hyperbilirubinemic Gunn rat pups. *Biol Neonate*. 2006;90:40-45.
105. Watchko J, Tiribelli C. Bilirubin-induced neurologic damage—mechanisms and management approaches. *N Engl J Med*. 2013;369:2021-2030.
107. American Academy of Pediatrics Subcommittee on Hyperbilirubinemia. Management of hyperbilirubinemia in the newborn infant 35 or more weeks of gestation. *Pediatrics*. 2004;114:297-316.
112. Ip S, Chung M, Kulig J, et al. An evidence-based review of important issues concerning neonatal hyperbilirubinemia. *Pediatrics*. 2004;114:e130-e153.
114. Day RL. Inhibition of brain respiration *in vitro* by bilirubin: reversal of inhibition by various means. *Am J Dis Child*. 1954;88:504-506.
115. Zetterström R, Ernster L. Bilirubin, and uncoupler of oxidative phosphorylation in isolated mitochondria. *Nature*. 1956;178:1335-1337.
118. Rodrigues CM, Solá S, Brito MA, et al. Bilirubin directly disrupts membrane lipid polarity and fluidity, protein order, and redox status in rat mitochondria. *J Hepatol*. 2002;36:335-341.
124. Hansen TWR, Mathiesen SB, Sefland I, Walaas SI. Bilirubin inhibits Ca^{2+}-dependent release of norepinephrine from permeabilized nerve terminals. *Neurochem Res*. 1999;24:733-738.
126. Hansen TW, Tommarello S, Allen J. Subcellular localization of bilirubin in rat brain after in vivo i.v. administration of [^{3}H]bilirubin. *Pediatr Res*. 2001;49:203-207.
147. Grojean S, Koziel V, Vert P, Daval JL. Bilirubin induces apoptosis via activation of NMDA receptors in developing rat brain neurons. *Exp Neurol*. 2000;166:334-341.
149. Hankø E, Hansen TW, Almaas R, et al. Synergistic protection of a general caspase inhibitor and MK-801 in bilirubin-induced cell death in human NT2-N neurons. *Pediatr Res*. 2006;59:72-77.
152. McDonald JW, Shapiro SM, Silverstein FS, Johnston MV. Role of glutamate receptor-mediated excitotoxicity in bilirubin-induced brain injury in the Gunn rat model. *Exp Neurol*. 1998;150:21-29.
157. Watchko JF. Kernicterus and the molecular mechanisms of bilirubin-induced CNS injury in newborns. *NeuroMolecular Med*. 2006;8:513-529.
170. Falcão AS, Fernandes A, Brito MA, et al. Bilirubin-induced immunostimulant effects and toxicity vary with neural cell type and maturation state. *Acta Neuropathol*. 2006;112:95-105.
171. Fernandes A, Silva RF, Falcão AS, et al. Cytokine production, glutamate release and cell death in rat cultured astrocytes treated with unconjugated bilirubin and LPS. *J Neuroimmunol*. 2004;153:64-75.
175. Brodersen R, Bartels P. Enzymatic oxidation of bilirubin. *Eur J Biochem*. 1969;10:468-473.
177. Hansen TWR, Allen JW. Oxidation of bilirubin by brain mitochondrial membranes—dependence on cell type and postnatal age. *Biochem Mol Med*. 1997;60:155-160.
179. Hansen TW, Allen JW, Tommarello S. Oxidation of bilirubin in the brain—further characterization of a potentially protective mechanism. *Mol Genet Metab*. 1999;68:404-409.
180. Hansen TWR, Whitin JC, Pierce NW, et al. Studies on bilirubin metabolism in the brain. *Acta Paediatr*. 2017;106:14-15.
182. Riordan SM, Bittel DC, Le Pichon J-B, et al. A hypothesis for using pathway genetic load analysis for understanding complex outcomes in bilirubin encephalopathy. *Front Neurosci*. 2016;10:376.

183. Gazzin S, Zelenka J, Zdrahalova L, et al. Bilirubin accumulation and Cyp mRNA expression in selected brain regions of jaundiced Gunn rat pups. *Pediatr Res.* 2012;71:653-660. [Erratum, Pediatr Res 71:731, 2012.]

195. Silva RF, Rodrigues CM, Brites D. Rat cultured neuronal and glial cells respond differently to toxicity of unconjugated bilirubin. *Pediatr Res.* 2002;51: 535-541.

230. Jacobsen C. Lysine residue 240 of human serum albumin is involved in high-affinity binding of bilirubin. *Biochem J.* 1978;171:453-459.

238. McDonach AF. Controversies in bilirubin biochemistry and their clinical relevance. *Semin Fetal Neonatal Med.* 2010;15:141-147.

262. Ebbesen F. Recurrence of kernicterus in term and near-term infants in Denmark. *Acta Paediatr.* 2000;89:1213-1217.

164 Pathophysiology of Neonatal Acute Kidney Injury

David T. Selewski | David J. Askenazi | Jennifer R. Charlton | Jennifer G. Jetton

INTRODUCTION

In recent years, there has been an exponential expansion of our understanding of the epidemiology and adverse outcomes associated with neonatal acute kidney injury (AKI). From a multitude of single-center studies and in the recent multicenter Assessment of Worldwide Acute Kidney Injury Epidemiology in Neonates (AWAKEN) study, AKI is now known to be associated with several adverse outcomes (increased length of stay, length of mechanical ventilation, mortality) in a variety of neonatal populations.[1-6] Furthermore, neonatal AKI may increase the risk of chronic kidney disease (CKD) later in life. AKI can no longer be viewed as an incidental finding, but rather an independent risk factor for poor outcomes.

Neonates are vulnerable to AKI secondary to maternal, neonatal, and perinatal risk factors associated with the transition from intrauterine to extrauterine life (e.g., perinatal asphyxia, sepsis, nephrotoxic medications).[7] Subsequently, factors associated with critical illness will predominate the risk for AKI.[8] Finally, neonatal AKI may differ and have differing long-term implications, depending on the neonate's gestational age, as nephrogenesis continues until 32 to 36 weeks of gestation.[9-11] AKI in premature infants, in particular, may therefore have significant implications for long-term renal health and the development of CKD.

Future strategies to prevent and treat AKI will require a better understanding of the pathophysiology of neonatal AKI, risk factors associated with AKI, and more sensitive and specific methods for the detection of AKI. The purpose of this chapter is to describe the pathophysiology of neonatal AKI, identify associated risk factors, highlight recent epidemiology studies, and discuss the gaps in knowledge that need to be filled to improve outcomes.

NEONATAL PHYSIOLOGY, PATHOPHYSIOLOGY, AND ACUTE KIDNEY INJURY

The unique and rapidly changing physiology surrounding birth and the first few months of life creates challenges in the diagnosis of neonatal AKI. Many aspects of physiology unique to term or premature neonates pertinent to the study of AKI predispose them to AKI or create challenges for the rapid identification of an episode of neonatal AKI by clinicians.

NEPHROGENESIS, PREMATURITY, AND THE IMPACT ON RISK OF ACUTE KIDNEY INJURY

Nephrogenesis begins at the fifth week of gestation and continues until 34 to 36 weeks gestation,[9] yielding the adult complement of 200,000 to 2.7 million nephrons at the time of term delivery.[12,13] Autopsy data of full-term, generally healthy neonates provide evidence that the wide variation in nephron endowment is established early in life.[10,14] With nearly two-thirds of nephron formation occurring during the third trimester, nephrogenesis may be limited and disrupted by preterm birth. Rodriguez and colleagues found that premature infants who survived to 40 days of age had fewer layers of glomeruli than their term counterparts.[15] When stratified for AKI status, those infants exposed to AKI had fewer glomerular layers than those without AKI. Sutherland and colleagues noted that premature infants seemed to have accelerated maturation of the glomeruli, with a smaller nephrogenic zone, suggesting early cessation of nephrogenesis, as well as signs of glomerular hypertrophy, dilation of Bowman space, and shrunken glomerular tufts.[16] The concept of nephron loss during nephron development was evaluated in a recent rat study where unilateral nephrectomy during nephrogenesis led to a greater degree of glomerular and tubular damage in adulthood, as compared to the group that underwent nephrectomy after the epoch of nephrogenesis.[17] Given their decreased number of filtration units, premature and very low-birth-weight (VLBW) infants have less renal reserve and are particularly susceptible to various renal insults encountered in the neonatal intensive care unit (NICU).[3,18]

RENAL BLOOD FLOW, PERFUSION, AND ISCHEMIA

The newborn kidney undergoes important hemodynamic changes in the perinatal period. In contrast to adult kidneys, which receive 20% to 30% of cardiac output, the developing fetal kidney receives only 2.5% to 4% of cardiac output. Over time, the proportion of renal cardiac output seen by the kidney increases from 6% at 24 hours to 10% at 1 week and 15% to 18% at 6 weeks of age.[19-21] Changes in renal perfusion pressure after birth occur because of *increasing peripheral* vascular resistance, coupled with *decreasing renal* vascular resistance. The decreased renal vascular resistance is driven by two main factors: a redistribution of renal blood flow within the kidney from the medulla and inner cortex during the fetal period to the outer cortex after birth, and a change in the balance of vasoconstrictive and vasodilatory factors affecting glomerular arteriolar resistance (Fig. 164.1).[22]

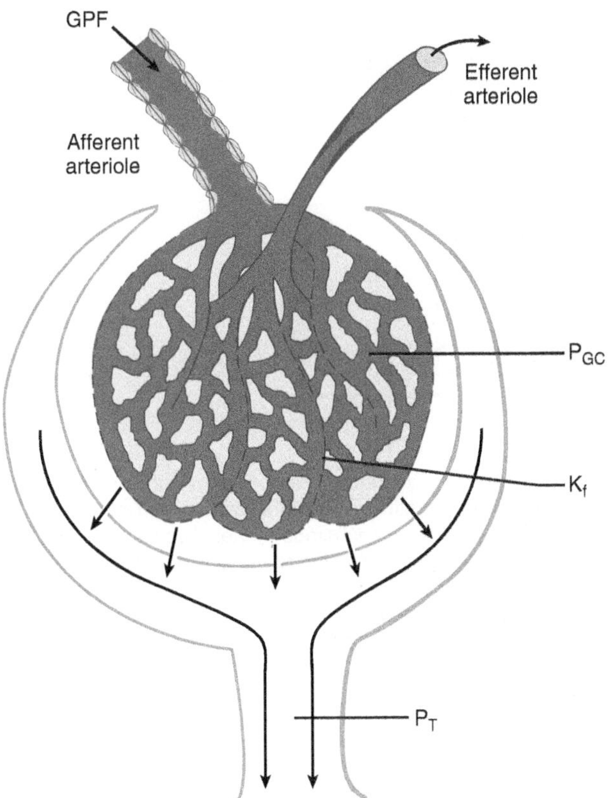

Fig. 164.1 The glomerular filtration process. Glomerular filtration is determined by the rate of glomerular plasma flow *(GPF)* entering the afferent arteriole, hydraulic pressure within the glomerular capillary *(P_{GC})* minus hydraulic pressure in proximal tubule *(P_T)*, and the glomerular capillary ultrafiltration coefficient *(K_f)*, which describes the permeability properties of the glomerular capillary membrane. (Modified from Winkler D, Elger M, Sakai T, et al. Branching and confluence pattern of glomerular arterioles in the rat. *Kidney Int.* 1991;39[suppl 32]:S2.)

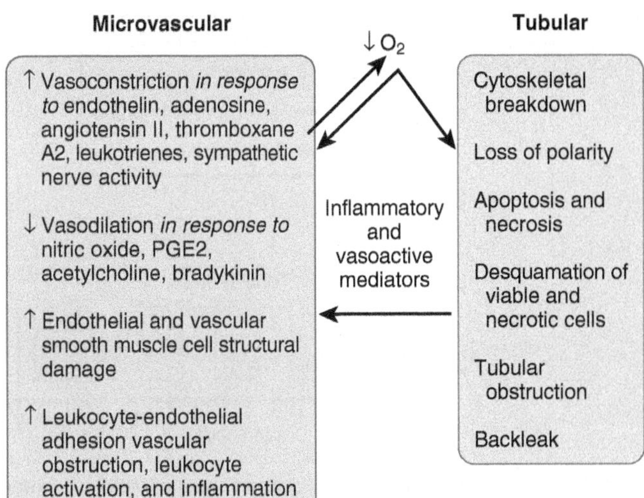

Fig. 164.2 Interacting microvascular and tubular events contributing to the pathophysiology of ischemic acute kidney injury. *PGE2*, Prostaglandin E_2. (Modified from Bonventre JV, Weinberg JM. Recent advances in the pathophysiology of ischemic acute renal failure. *J Am Soc Nephrol.* 2003;14:2200.)

The renin-angiotensin-aldosterone system is a primary determinant of renal vasoconstriction and a key mechanism for maintaining the glomerular filtration rate (GFR) in the newborn. This pathway is active throughout fetal development and in the newborn period. Angiotensin II acts via the AT_1 receptor, causing vasoconstriction at the afferent and efferent arterioles.[23] Angiotensin II increases GFR by a causing greater degree of constriction of and increase in resistance at the efferent arteriole relative to the afferent arteriole, increasing GFR. Other important renal vasoconstrictors active in the newborn period include endothelin,[24] adenosine, and sympathetic innervation.[25,26]

Vasodilators, including prostaglandins and atrial natriuretic peptide, increase renal blood flow by causing vasodilatation of the afferent arteriole. They counterbalance the effects of angiotensin II, catecholamines, and other vasoconstrictive substances in the neonatal kidney.[27,28] It follows then that nonsteroidal antiinflammatory drugs such as indomethacin, a potent prostaglandin inhibitor used to treat patent ductus arteriosus in premature infants, can cause severe, though usually reversible, acute kidney injury (AKI). Maternal exposure to nonsteroidal antiinflammatory drugs also predisposes neonates to decreased renal perfusion and AKI.[29]

A delicate balance of homeostatic mechanisms in the neonate is required to maintain renal perfusion and GFR in the postnatal period. Although it rises quickly after birth, the GFR of the newborn infant is still low compared with that of older children and will not reach the level associated with normal renal function in adults until 18 to 24 months of age.[30-32]A number of maternal exposures and perinatal events can disrupt the homeostatic balance and lead to decreased renal blood flow, impaired renal perfusion, and AKI. Common causes of renal hypoperfusion in the NICU include low intravascular volume from fluid losses such as insensible losses, chest tubes, blood loss, nasogastric suction, abdominal drains, and chronic diuretic use. Poor cardiac preload can occur from high mean airway pressures or congenital heart disease; congestive heart failure can also lead to poor perfusion. Low oncotic pressure can lead to low intravascular volume. Correction of the underlying problem with restoration of adequate renal blood flow is critical for the normalization of renal function.

Prolonged renal hypoperfusion or severe acute hypoperfusion events from perinatal asphyxia, poor cardiac function, hypoalbuminemia, or hypotension can cause inadequate oxygen delivery resulting in cellular injury and more pronounced organ dysfunction, such as acute tubular necrosis. A series of important events have been well described in the course of ischemic AKI.[33] These include epithelial cell injury with subsequent structural changes and in some cases cell death, endothelial injury and dysfunction, inflammation, and repair (Fig. 164.2). These events correspond with the phases of ischemic AKI classically described as the initiation, extension, maintenance, and recovery.[34] Decreased renal blood flow leads to inadequate intracellular ATP levels and subsequent cellular injury or death depending on the severity of the insult (initiation phase). The areas that have the highest metabolic demand and decreased ability to convert to anaerobic metabolism (including the proximal tubule and the medullary thick ascending limb) are particularly susceptible to hypoxic-ischemic injury.[35] In the proximal tubule, the apical brush border is lost through the detachment of the microvilli that subsequently form membrane-bound "blebs," which are released into the tubular lumen.[36]

The actin cytoskeleton, a key element for maintaining cell structure and function, also undergoes important structural changes after the loss of intercellular adhesion junctions that anchor the epithelial cells to the basement membranes. These structural elements normally serve important roles in paracellular transport, cell polarity, and cell morphology.[37] Loss of their integrity allows back-leak of the glomerular filtrate into the interstitium, as well as sloughing of the epithelial cells into

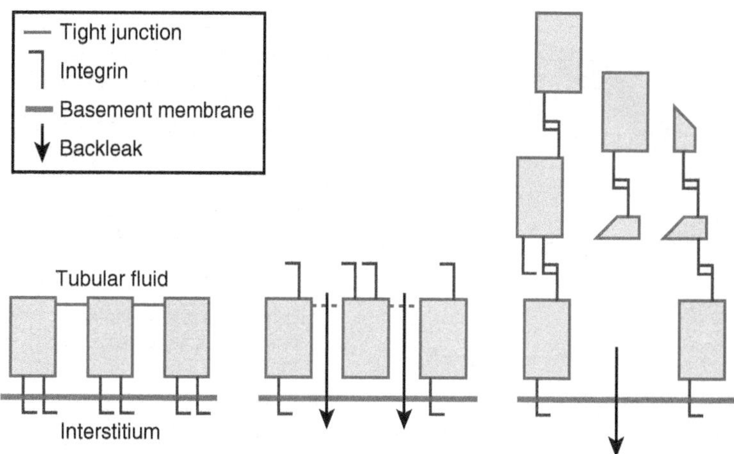

Fig. 164.3 The role of intratubular obstruction and back-leak in acute kidney injury. *Left,* Normal tubular cells linked by tight junctions into an epithelial sheet that forms a selective barrier between the tubular fluid compartment and the interstitium. The tight junction regulates cell polarity, segregating molecules such as the integrins to the basal plasma membrane, forming the adhesive anchorage of the cell basement membrane junction. *Middle,* Ischemia-induced tight junction dysfunction leads to a loss of barrier function contributing to the loss of polarity and integrin migration to the apical surface, as well as leakage of glomerular filtrate back into the interstitium. *Right,* Loss of basal anchorage molecules allows cells or cell fragments to exfoliate into the tubular lumen and adhere and aggregate with other exfoliated cells or fragments, contributing to an increase in tubular pressure proximal to the obstruction. Tubular obstruction will oppose glomerular filtration, as well as accelerate back-leak of tubular fluid across the denuded basement membrane. (Modified from Lee DBN, Huang E, Ward HJ. Tight junction biology and kidney dysfunction. *Am J Physiol Renal Physiol.* 2006;290:F26.)

the tubular lumen.[38] Detached cells, cellular debris, and microvilli blebs may form granular casts that obstruct the tubular lumen and lead to loss of function.[39]

The disruption of the actin cytoskeleton results in changes in cell polarity and function. Na^+-K^+-ATPase pumps normally found on the basolateral membrane redistribute to the apical membrane and allow bidirectional transport of sodium and water.[40] As a result, cellular sodium may be transported back into the tubular lumen, resulting in a high fractional excretion of sodium characteristic of acute tubular necrosis. Further decline in GFR may then result from the activation of tubuloglomerular feedback by the delivery of high sodium concentrations to the distal tubule (Fig. 164.3).[41]

The impact of the ischemic injury on tubular epithelial cells depends on the severity and duration of the event. If the underlying condition is corrected in a timely fashion and adequate perfusion is restored, cells may demonstrate structural and functional recovery. With more severe injury, cells may undergo either apoptosis or necrosis.[42]

In addition to tubular injury, ischemia results in endothelial cell dysfunction that in turn perpetuates ongoing ischemia and further renal injury (extension phase).[34] As noted previously, certain segments of the nephron are more profoundly affected by poor perfusion than others. Ischemia may persist in those areas even after renal blood flow has been restored, highlighting the important concept that ischemic AKI is driven by changes in the microcirculation and not solely by systemic pressure or global renal blood flow.[43] The endothelium undergoes loss of structural integrity that results in increased microvascular permeability.[34] Vascular permeability allows the passage of chemokines and cytokines between the blood compartment and adjacent renal tubules, promoting inflammation in both regions. In addition, ischemia induces a prothrombotic environment, leading to microvascular congestion and dysfunction.[33]

Endothelial dysfunction and damage have implications for long-term kidney outcomes, as data suggest that the vasculature does not regenerate or recover in the way that the tubular epithelial cells can.[44] This lack of recovery, or "vascular dropout," and subsequent scar formation may be key risk factors for the development of CKD after AKI[44,45] (see the section entitled "Long-Term Outcomes and Progression to Chronic Kidney Disease" later in this chapter).

Inflammation plays an important role in the perpetuation of tubular and endothelial injury, resulting in apoptosis and necrosis (maintenance phase). A number of inflammatory cells and chemical mediators influence this process.[46] Toll-like receptors 2 and 4, components of the innate immune system, have been identified as important components in the development of AKI. These proteins are expressed on the renal epithelium and are upregulated during ischemic AKI, further amplifying the inflammatory process. Moreover, the deletion of *TLR2* or *TLR4* protects against renal injury in animal models.[47,48]

The kidney has many mechanisms responsible for protection, repair, and recovery (recovery phase). Restoration of blood flow is followed by repair of cells with mild injury; cells with more severe injury go through a process of dedifferentiation during which they appear flattened with an ill-defined brush border.[36] Cells that have not undergone necrosis or apoptosis are able to proliferate across the basement membrane and undergo restoration of the cytoskeleton and proper cell polarity.[49] Cell recovery is also aided by the heat shock proteins, a system that assists recovery in the proper folding of both denatured and newly synthesized proteins.[50,51] An association between genetic polymorphisms that result in low HSP72 protein expression and increased risk of AKI in VLBW neonates was demonstrated in a Hungarian neonatal cohort.[51] Heme oxygenase 1, an enzyme with antiinflammatory effects, conferred resistance to apoptosis in an in vitro study.[52] Kidney injury molecule 1 and transmembrane glycoprotein nonmetastatic melanoma B (NMB) have been identified in animal models as phagocytic proteins that promote cell repair and remodeling through the removal of apoptotic cellular debris.[53,54]

The tubular and endothelial cell damage that occurs during ischemic AKI leads not only to dysfunction within the kidney but also to a systemic inflammatory response that may impact distant organs. This inflammatory dysregulation is partly due to dysfunctional immune, inflammatory, and soluble mediator metabolism.[55,56] Thus AKI can lead to pulmonary inflammation, brain injury, and cardiac dysfunction.

SYSTEMIC EFFECTS OF ACUTE KIDNEY INJURY

AKI in the context of multiorgan dysfunction is of growing interest because AKI portends poor clinical outcomes independently of the severity of illness and comorbid conditions. AKI may play an important role in modulating the inflammatory response in critically ill patients. Proinflammatory mechanisms, including neutrophil migration, cytokine expression, and oxidative stress, increase the risk of injury to other organs in the setting of AKI.[55] Brain and lung development are of particular interest in the neonatal population; thus the impact of AKI on these organ systems is described as follows.

LUNG

The negative impact of AKI is particularly profound when coupled with comorbid lung injury. Indeed, the kidney plays an important role in the physiologic processes that directly and indirectly influence the ability of the lungs to deliver oxygen. The kidney has an important impact on fluid balance, vascular tone (renin-angiotensin system), acid/base status, and hormone production (erythropoietin).[57] Large observational studies in critically ill adults have shown mortality rates of more than 80% when AKI is complicated by respiratory failure or vice versa.[58,59] AKI occurs in up to 82% of critically ill children who require ventilator support,[60] and those with AKI have worse lung function, a higher number of ventilator days, and a poorer oxygenation index than similar children without AKI.[61,62] Recent data from the AWAKEN study demonstrate similar findings in neonates.[63,64]

The interaction between lung and kidney injury may be particularly important for premature infants who are at risk of the development of bronchopulmonary dysplasia. Data in preterm neonates, along with near term/term neonates, are becoming available, suggesting a link between fluid balance/AKI and respiratory outcomes. Data from the AWAKEN study show that the peak fluid balance during the first postnatal week and the fluid balance on postnatal day 7 were independently associated with the need for mechanical ventilation on postnatal day 7 in both preterm[64] and near-term neonates.[63] This association persisted even after adjusting for AKI, suggesting an independent impact of fluid on outcomes. In addition, data from the AWAKEN cohort also show that AKI is independently associated with chronic lung disease in premature[65] and near-term/term neonates.[66]

Several animal models have shown that the association between AKI and lung disease is not just about fluid overload. AKI has been shown to impact the lungs by influencing vascular permeability, cytokine profiles, and cellular immunity.[57,67-69] The integrity of the lung epithelium is dependent on tight junctions and channels involved in water and sodium transport, including epithelial sodium channels and aquaporins. Animal models of bilateral nephrectomized mice show a downregulation of these channels in the alveolar epithelium.[70] Animal models of nonoliguric AKI show pulmonary inflammation characterized by an abundance of inflammatory cells and abnormal lung permeability.[59,71] Proinflammatory cytokines such as IL-6 and IL-1β triggered by an AKI episode contribute to lung injury.[68,72,73] AKI has been shown to influence cellular immunity in the lungs, including T-cell handling of antigens and neutrophil migration.[74,75] Notably, fluid overload was not a factor in these animal models, suggesting that AKI may lead to abnormal lung function and architecture independently of the effects of volume status. Although the association of AKI with lung injury has been reported in preterm neonates, it is uncertain if the increased risk of bronchopulmonary dysplasia is due to fluid overload or intrinsic lung damage.[76,77]

BRAIN

Both animal and human data, including data from several studies in neonates, have demonstrated an association between AKI and brain injury in the setting of hypoxic-ischemic AKI. In a mouse model of ischemia-reperfusion injury, Liu and colleagues demonstrated a broad range of inflammatory changes and abnormalities in the brain after a severe ischemic AKI event.[78] Specifically, the brains of mice in the study group had higher levels of inflammatory markers, more extensive cellular inflammation, greater injury to susceptible areas of the brain as shown by increased numbers of pyknotic neuronal cells in the hippocampus, and microvascular dysfunction with disruption of the blood-brain barrier. In addition, the mice in the ischemic AKI group demonstrated decreased locomotor activity (behavioral dysfunction) after the AKI event. Several single-center studies have shown an association between AKI during perinatal asphyxia and subsequent neurologic outcomes.[79,80] Furthermore, recent data in a single-center study[81] and in the AWAKEN cohort[82] suggest that AKI is independently associated with intraventricular hemorrhage. The authors postulate that this could be due to vasoactive hormone release during AKI, hypertension from fluid overload, or inflammatory mediators that impact the blood-brain barrier.

RISK FACTORS FOR ACUTE KIDNEY INJURY

Critically ill neonates experience multiple events that put them at risk for the development of AKI, including hypotension, exposure to nephrotoxic drugs (e.g., indomethacin, gentamicin), and severe infections (e.g., sepsis).[7,8] Specific neonatal cohorts at high risk of AKI include those undergoing cardiac surgery or needing extracorporeal membrane oxygenation (ECMO), sick term/premature infants, low-birth-weight babies, neonates with hypoxic-ischemic encephalopathy, and neonates with necrotizing enterocolitis (Tables 164.1 and 164.2).

SEPSIS

Sepsis is a cause of significant morbidity and mortality in critically ill neonates and is a known risk factor for AKI.[83-85] Mathur and colleagues found that 26% of infants with sepsis developed AKI.[86] Neonates that develop sepsis are classically thought to be predisposed to AKI secondary to the hypotension associated with systemic inflammation as well as nephrotoxic medications administered as treatment. Studies have challenged this mantra, as there appears to be a direct impact of the systemic inflammatory process on the kidneys that occurs in the absence of hypotension.[87] To this point, biopsy data have shown that sepsis-associated AKI is histologically distinct from acute tubular necrosis.[88] Large animal models of septic shock from gram-negative bacterial organisms have clearly shown that AKI occurs in the setting of *increased* cardiac output and *increased* renal blood flow.[89,90] Animal studies have also suggested that direct damage to the kidney microvasculature may be an important pathophysiologic mechanism of sepsis-associated AKI.[87,91-93]

NEPHROTOXIC MEDICATIONS

Nephrotoxic medication exposures represent a common cause of AKI across medicine and a potentially modifiable risk factor for AKI. Nephrotoxic medications are widely used in the NICU (Table 164.3) and are associated with AKI in neonates.[29,94,95] In a study of 107 VLBW infants, Rhone and colleagues demonstrated that exposure to one or more of these medications was nearly universal, with 87% of neonates receiving at least one nephrotoxic medication (most commonly gentamicin).[95] On average these neonates were exposed to nephrotoxic medications for 14 days during their NICU stay. Nephrotoxic medications can cause AKI in a variety of ways, including decreased renal perfusion (nonsteroidal antiinflammatory drugs, diuretics, angiotensin-converting enzyme inhibitors), direct tubular injury (aminoglycosides, amphotericin B, vancomycin, nonsteroidal

Table 164.1 Studies Evaluating Risks for Neonatal Acute Kidney Injury.

Study	Population	Incidence of AKI	Risk Factors for AKI
Askenazi et al.[146]	Very low-birth-weight infants (*N* = 195)	Matched case-control study	Receive chest compressions, receive cardiac drugs, intraventricular hemorrhage
Gadepalli et al.[2]	CDH on ECMO (*N* = 68)	71%	Lower 5-min Apgar score, AKI correlated with left-sided CDH
Kaur et al.[4]	Perinatal asphyxia (*N* = 36)	41.7%	Severe asphyxia (Apgar score <3 at 1 min)
Koralkar et al.[5]	Very low-birth-weight infants (*N* = 229)	18%	Lower birth weight, lower gestational age, lower Apgar scores, umbilical artery catheter, mechanical ventilation, inotrope support
Askenazi et al.[147]	Sick near-term neonates (*N* = 58)	15.6%	Lower birth weight, male, lower 5-min Apgar score, lower umbilical cord pH, mechanical ventilation
Alabbas et al.[148]	Cardiac surgery <28 days (*N* = 122)	62%	Open heart surgery, cardiopulmonary bypass time ≥120 min, ECMO, vasopressor use
Selewski et al.[6]	Perinatal asphyxia (*N* = 96)	38%	Asystole at the time of birth, clinical seizures before cooling, persistent pulmonary HTN, elevated gentamicin or vancomycin levels, pressor support, transfusions
Zwiers et al.[109]	ECMO <28 days (*N* =242)	64%	Younger age at initiation, lack of pre-ECMO inhaled nitric oxide
Rhone et al.[95]	Very low-birth-weight infants (*N* = 107)	26.2%	Nephrotoxic exposure
Morgan et al.[149]	Cardiac surgery ≤6 wk (*N* = 264)	64%	Lower age, longer cardiopulmonary bypass time, hypothermic circulatory arrest, type of repair, lower gestational age, and preoperative ventilation
Carmody et al.[18]	Very low-birth-weight infants (*N* = 455)	39.8%	Lower gestational age, lower birth weight, lower Apgar scores (1 and 5 min), higher CRIB II score
Constance et al.[150]	Infants with PDA and received gentamicin (*n* = 594)	12%	NSAID therapy increases risk of AKI
Weintraub et al.[151]	Infants admitted to NICU (*N* = 357)	30.3%	GA, initial Cr, maternal magnesium, and volume resuscitation were associated with early AKI. Volume resuscitation, umbilical arterial line, and receipt of NSAIDs for PDA were associated with intermediate AKI. GA, steroid use for hypotension, NEC, and sepsis were associated with late AKI.
Velazquez et al.[152]	Preterm infants admitted to NICU who received PDA screening (*N* = 151)	27%	Preterm infants with hemodynamically significant PDA had similar rates of AKI as those with non-hemodynamically significant PDAs.
Lee et al.[100]	ELBW (*N* = 276)	56%	AKI associated with lower GA, high-frequency ventilation support, the presence of PDA, and inotropic agent use
Carmody et al.[101]	VLBW infants (*N* = 140)	25%	VLBW infants who are exposed to caffeine are less likely to experience AKI than unexposed infants
Harer et al.[102]	Secondary analysis of the AWAKEN Study. Infants <33 wk gestational age (*N* = 675)	18.1%	Caffeine administration in preterm neonates is associated with reduced incidence and severity of AKI

AKI, Acute kidney injury; AWAKEN, Assessment of Worldwide Acute Kidney Injury Epidemiology in Neonates; *CDH*, congenital diaphragmatic hernia; *CRIB*, clinical risk index for babies; *ECMO*, extracorporeal membrane oxygenation; *ELBW*, extremely low birth weight; *HTN*, hypertension; *NEC*, necrotizing enterocolitis; *NICU*, neonatal intensive care unit; *PDA*, patent ductus arteriosus.

antiinflammatory drugs), or tubular obstruction (acyclovir; see Table 164.3).

Gentamicin, an aminoglycoside, is one of the most widely used antibiotics in the NICU because of its excellent antimicrobial activity in patients who are at high risk of sepsis and sepsis-related death.[96] Gentamicin is filtered at the glomerulus and then taken up in the proximal tubule epithelial cells via endocytosis by the megalin receptor. Accumulation of the drug in the proximal tubules can lead to mitochondrial dysfunction resulting in apoptosis and/or necrosis.[97] Nephrotoxicity is increased in patients with preexisting renal dysfunction, concomitant nephrotoxic medication use, or poor renal perfusion.

Prevention of AKI due to nephrotoxic medications may have an important role in reducing both short- and long-term adverse outcomes. In a single-center NICU quality improvement study, Stoops and colleagues described the implementation of a standardized, pharmacist-led initiative to reduce harm from nephrotoxic medications. They showed the combination of a computer-assisted screening protocol for nephrotoxic medications and daily discussion on rounds reduced the number of exposures to nephrotoxic medication, occurrence of AKI, and the number of days with AKI. This suggests that a systematic surveillance program can prevent AKI due to nephrotoxic medications.[98]

EPIDEMIOLOGY AND OUTCOMES ASSOCIATED WITH NEONATAL ACUTE KIDNEY INJURY

In recent years, there has been a rapid expansion of our knowledge of the epidemiology and outcomes associated with neonatal AKI (see Table 164.2). This has culminated with the publication of the international multicenter AWAKEN study, which evaluated the impact of AKI across neonatal populations. This work supports detailed work in specific neonatal populations including preterm neonates (VLBW and extremely low birth weight (ELBW), neonates with perinatal asphyxia, and neonates with concurrent disease processes or treatments (e.g., necrotizing enterocolitis, ECMO). In different neonatal populations, AKI is common and associated with adverse outcomes.

GENERAL NEONATAL INTENSIVE CARE UNIT POPULATION

In 2017 the AWAKEN study was published and provided a comprehensive evaluation of the epidemiology and outcomes

Table 164.2 Epidemiology and Outcomes of Acute Kidney Injury in Specific Neonatal Populations.

Study	Population *(n)*	% Patients With AKI	Findings
General NICU			
Jetton et al.[3]	AWAKEN Study. All neonates admitted to one of 24 participating centers over a 3-mo (*N* = 2022)	29.9%	AKI is associated with increased mortality and longer hospital stay.
Starr et al.[66]	Secondary analysis of the AWAKEN Study. Infants ≥32 wk gestational age (*N* = 1348)	24%	Infants with AKI had an almost fivefold increased odds of chronic lung disease/death
Premature, VLBW, ELBW			
Chowdhary et al.[153]	ELBW (*N* = 483)	60%	AKI is associated with increased mortality, prolonged NICU stay, and poor growth
Srinivasan et al.[154]	VLBW (*N* = 457)	19.5%	AKI is associated with BPD, longer NICU stay, and increased mortality
Maqsood et al.[155]	ELBW (*N* = 222)	50%	Infants with severe AKI (Stage 2 or 3) have higher diastolic BP at discharge. ELBW infants are at risk for CKD at ≥2 yr of life.
Stoops et al.[81]	Premature infants (*N* = 125)	30.5%	Infants with AKI were more likely to develop ≥grade 2 IVH
Askenazi et al.[156]	Premature infants (*N* = 122)	30%	AKI is associated with BPD and mortality
Carmody et al.[18]	VLBW infants (*N* = 455)	39.8%	AKI is associated with increased mortality and length of stay adjusted for severity of illness.
Rhone et al.[95]	VLBW infants (*N* = 107)	26.2%	AKI is associated with nephrotoxic medication exposure.
Starr et al.[157]	Secondary analysis of the AWAKEN Study. Infants <32 wk gestation (*N* = 546)	33.1%	Those born between 29 and 32 wk who develop AKI had a higher likelihood of moderate or severe BPD/death than those without AKI
Lee et al.[100]	ELBW (*N* = 276)	56%	AKI associated with higher mortality before the postmenstrual age of 36 wk
Stoops et al.[82]	Secondary analysis of the AWAKEN Study. Infants <33 wk gestational age (*N* = 825)	22.2%	Independent association between AKI and IVH.
Perinatal Asphyxia			
Chock et al.[158]	Infants with moderate to severe HIE (*N* = 38)	39%	During therapeutic hypothermia, infants with AKI had higher renal saturations measured by NIRS than those without AKI.
Sarkar et al.[79]	Infants with HIE (*N* = 88)	39%	AKI is independently associated with hypoxic-ischemic lesions on brain MRI at 7–10 days of life
Selewski et al.[6]	Infants with HIE (*N* = 96)	38%	AKI predicted prolonged mechanical ventilation and length of stay
Necrotizing Enterocolitis			
Criss et al.[106]	Infants with NEC (*N* = 181)	54%	AKI is common in infants with NEC and is associated with increased mortality.
Bakhoum et al.[107]	Premature infants with NEC (*N* = 77)	42.9%	AKI increases mortality significantly. Severe NEC puts patients at higher risk for AKI.
ECMO			
Zwiers et al.[109]	ECMO-treated infants (*N* = 242)	64%	Those with severe AKI have increased risk of mortality.

AKI, Acute kidney injury; *AWAKEN*, Assessment of Worldwide Acute Kidney Injury Epidemiology in Neonates; *BP*, blood pressure; *BPD*, bronchopulmonary dysplasia; *CKD*, chronic kidney disease; *ECMO*, extracorporeal membrane oxygenation; *ELBW*, extremely low birthweight; *HIE*, hypoxic ischemic encephalopathy; *NEC*, necrotizing enterocolitis; *NICU*, neonatal intensive care unit; *NIRS*, near-infrared spectroscopy; *VLBW*, very-low-birth-weight.

associated with neonatal AKI.[3,99] This study included all neonates admitted to one of 24 participating centers over a 3-month period who met criteria. Approximately half of the screened subjects did not meet criteria; the majority did not receive intravenous fluids for greater than 48 hours. The incidence of AKI was 30% in the 2022 neonates in the study. The incidence of AKI differed by gestational age (48% <29 weeks, 18% in ≥29 to <36 weeks, and 37% in ≥36 weeks). In a multivariable analysis, AKI was associated with mortality after adjusting for potential confounding variables (adjusted odds ratio [aOR] = 4.6 [95% confidence interval (CI) 2.5 to 8.3; $P < .0001$]) and increased length of stay by 8.8 days (95% CI 6.1 to 11.5; $P < .0001$). These associations held true for subgroups of neonates stratified by gestational age. This multicenter study confirms the findings of smaller single-center studies in high-risk populations outlined as follows.[3]

VERY LOW-BIRTH-WEIGHT AND EXTREMELY LOW-BIRTH-WEIGHT INFANTS

In two large single-center studies evaluating AKI in neonates (500 to 1500 g), the incidence of AKI was reported to be 18% to 40%, with a concomitant increase in morbidity and mortality.[5,18] In a prospective study of 229 VLBW infants followed up from birth until 36 weeks postmenstrual age, the mortality in infants with AKI was significantly higher than in those without AKI (42% vs. 5%, $P < .001$), with the highest mortality risk in those with stage 3 AKI (adjusted hazard ratio 3.1, 95% CI 1.1 to 8.9). In a retrospective study of 455 VLBW infants, Carmody and colleagues showed that AKI was independently associated with increased mortality (OR 4.00, 95% CI 1.4 to 11.5) and increased hospital length of stay (11.7 hospital days, 95% CI 5.1 to 18.4).[18] In a recent study of

Table 164.3 Commonly Used Drugs Known to Cause Nephrotoxicity in Neonates.

	Proposed Mechanisms			Clinical Aspects	
Medication	**Vasculature**	**Proximal Tubule**	**Tubule**	**Features**	**Electrolyte Abnormalities**
Acyclovir		Directly toxic to the proximal tubules	Urinary precipitation can result in crystal-induced AKI resulting from obstruction	Can be prevented by good hydration and slowed infusions; oliguric AKI	
Aminoglycosides	Intrarenal vasoconstriction	Freely filtered and transported into the proximal tubule by megalin-mediated endocytosis, leading to lysosomal accumulation, disruption of protein sorting and mitochondrial function, cell death	May cause direct tubular toxicity (metabolites)	Gradual rise in serum creatinine level, classically nonoliguric AKI	Hypokalemia, hypomagnesemia, hypocalcemia, and hypophosphatemia
Amphotericin B	Renal vasoconstriction leading to decreased GFR		Direct tubular toxicity: insertion into cell membranes to create pores, resulting in increased membrane permeability (driving electrolyte disturbances)	Polyuria and impaired urinary concentrating ability, volume expansion can mitigate decline in GFR, newer lipid-based preparations decrease nephrotoxicity but do not eliminate it	Hypokalemia, hypomagnesemia, metabolic acidosis: distal renal tubular acidosis
Angiotensin-converting enzyme inhibitors	Decreased angiotensin II production leading to reduction in GFR via decreased efferent arteriolar vasoconstriction			Increased risk of nephrotoxicity with volume depletion, renal ischemia, reduced renal blood flow (e.g., renal artery stenosis)	Associated with hyperkalemia independently of AKI
Nonsteroidal antiinflammatory drugs	Decreased prostaglandin production resulting in afferent arteriole vasoconstriction and reduced GFR, reduced renal blood flow			Oliguria, increased risk of nephrotoxicity with volume depletion, renal ischemia, reduced renal blood flow (e.g., renal artery stenosis)	
Radiocontrast agents	Intrarenal vasoconstriction		Tubular injury: free radical production, direct cytotoxic effects	SCr rise 24–48 h after exposure, classically non-oliguric AKI but may develop oliguria, may be prevented with adequate volume before exposure	
Vancomycin			Unclear cause, possibly related to the generation of reactive oxygen species, tubular injury	Additive nephrotoxicity with aminoglycosides, unclear clinical nephrotoxicity profile: studies have not convincingly demonstrated nephrotoxicity due to vancomycin alone	

AKI, Acute kidney injury; *GFR*, glomerular filtration rate; *SCr*, serum creatinine.

276 ELBW infants, the incidence of AKI was reported to be 56% with higher mortality before the postmenstrual age (PMA) of 36 weeks (adjusted HR 5.34, 95% CI 1.21 to 23.53; $P = .027$).[100]

In premature neonates, the role of caffeine in preventing AKI has recently been studied. In a study of 140 VLBW neonates at a single center, exposure to caffeine was associated with lower rates of AKI (aOR 0.21).[101] In a secondary analysis of 675 premature neonates in the AWAKEN study, caffeine administration reduced the odds of developing AKI (aOR, 0.20) in a very similar manner.[102] These studies suggest that caffeine may play a role in preventing AKI in preterm neonates, but further study is warranted.

PERINATAL ASPHYXIA

AKI commonly in neonates suffering from perinatal asphyxia with a reported incidence of up to 60%.[6,80] In each of these studies, those with AKI have been shown to have adverse outcomes. A single-center randomized controlled trial has suggested that therapeutic hypothermia may ameliorate the development of AKI in asphyxiated newborns with the rates of AKI significantly lower in those treated with therapeutic hypothermia (32% vs. 60%, $P < .05$).[103] Seven small randomized trials have shown that a single dose of theophylline given within 6 hours of birth decreases the rates of AKI and oliguria in asphyxiated newborns.[104] This has yet to be studied in a cohort undergoing therapeutic hypothermia.

As discussed earlier, AKI often is associated with detrimental impacts on distant organs. Recent epidemiologic work has shown an association of AKI during perinatal asphyxia with adverse neurologic outcomes. In a retrospective study of 88 asphyxiated newborns, brain magnetic resonance imaging (MRI) findings consistent with hypoxic-ischemic injury were more frequent in neonates with AKI than in neonates with no AKI (73% vs. 46%). Furthermore, those with AKI had 3.2 higher odds of abnormal MRI findings (95% CI 1.3 to 8.2; $P = .012$).[79] Gupta and colleagues performed a prospective study of 70 asphyxiated infants and 28 healthy controls and found that patients with higher grades of hypoxic-ischemic injury had higher serum creatinine (SCr) levels than the controls and those with grade 1 hypoxic-ischemic encephalopathy.[80] In a prospective observational study of 101 neonates receiving therapeutic hypothermia for perinatal asphyxia, AKI was associated with a poor composite outcome (death or disability) at 24 months.[105]

NEONATES WITH SPECIFIC DISEASE PROCESSES

In critically ill neonates, there is a multitude of comorbid conditions that can increase the risk of developing AKI. Here we will focus on necrotizing enterocolitis and neonates treated with ECMO. The incidence and impact of AKI in other high-risk populations (e.g., intraventricular hemorrhage, patent ductus arteriosus) are outlined in Table 164.2.

Necrotizing enterocolitis has been recognized as a risk factor for the development of AKI in critically ill neonates. AKI in this population is multifactorial, stemming from a number of factors, including hypotension, sepsis, systemic inflammation, and nephrotoxic medications.[106-108] Recent reports have evaluated the incidence and impact of AKI in populations with necrotizing enterocolitis and have shown the incidence to be as high as 40% to 60%. In a single-center study of 77 preterm neonates with necrotizing enterocolitis, AKI was strongly associated with mortality (adjusted HR = 20.3 [95% CI 2.5 to 162.8]; $P = .005$).[107] Recent work has suggested that caffeine exposure in preterm neonates with necrotizing enterocolitis may help protect against the development of AKI.[108]

Neonates treated with ECMO are particularly prone to the development of AKI. The pathophysiology of AKI in this population is multifactorial, with contributions from underlying illness, nephrotoxic exposures, systemic inflammation, and elements intrinsic to the ECMO circuit. The incidence of AKI in this population is as high as 72%.[2] Zwiers and colleagues published a comprehensive evaluation of the incidence of and impact of AKI in a single-center experience with 242 neonates. In this study, 64% of neonates developed AKI and those with the highest stage of AKI had significantly decreased survival.[109] Other single-center studies have yielded similar results.

ACUTE KIDNEY INJURY BIOMARKERS, DIAGNOSTIC FRAMEWORKS, AND DEFINITION

As described already, there have been major advances in our understanding of AKI through basic science and clinical research. However, there is still much work to be done to optimize our ability to detect AKI in neonates and intervene early enough to improve outcomes. Importantly, there have been fundamental changes in the terminology and diagnostic frameworks used to describe AKI. The dated description *acute renal failure* has now been supplanted by the new term AKI to highlight the dynamic nature of this complex syndrome and the importance of early recognition at the time of *injury* rather than at the time of complete *organ* failure.[110] There is also recognition that the traditional framework for classifying AKI events anatomically as *prerenal azotemia*, *intrinsic renal failure*, and *postrenal obstruction*, though simple to use at the bedside, is imprecise in its ability to describe adequately the mechanism of injury and the appropriate therapeutic intervention.[111]

A major advance in the field of AKI research has been the development of multidimensional, categoric AKI definitions for use in adult, pediatric, and now neonatal populations, based on incremental increases in SCr concentration or decreases in urine output.[60,110,112] These definitions have driven clinical research by allowing comparison of patients and outcomes across studies. In multiple critically ill pediatric and adult cohorts, even mild forms of AKI (SCr concentration increases as low as 0.3 mg/dL) are associated with increased morbidity and mortality.[113] Those with increasing degrees of AKI have increasingly worse outcomes. Investigators have proposed a neonatal AKI definition (Table 164.4).[114] Small single-center studies and the recent multicenter AWAKEN study have shown trends in neonatal morbidity and mortality similar to those seen in pediatric and adult patients.[3]

Despite the use of the neonatal Kidney Disease: Improving Global Outcomes (KDIGO) AKI definition by us and others, it is important to recognize that this empiric definition represents

Table 164.4 Proposed Definition for Acute Kidney Injury in Neonates.

Stage of Severity	Criteria
No AKI	No SCr concentration change or rise in SCr concentration of <0.3 mg/dL from a previous trough
Stage 1	Increase in SCr concentration of 0.3 mg/dL or by 150%–200% (1.5–2 times) from a previous trough
Stage 2	Increase in SCr concentration by 200%–300% (2–3 times) from a previous trough
Stage 3	Increase in SCr concentration by 300% (3 times) from a previous trough or SCr concentration ≥2.5 mg/dL or receipt of dialysis for AKI

AKI, Acute kidney injury; *SCr*, serum creatinine.
Modified from Jetton JG, Askenazi DJ. Update on acute kidney injury in the neonate. *Curr Opin Pediatr.* 2012;24:191–196.

the first step in an iterative process in defining neonatal AKI.[115] The use of SCr to define AKI is particularly challenging in the first postnatal week as neonatal SCr reflects maternal SCr. During the days that follow, neonates establish their own SCr steady-state, which is primarily determined by innate kidney function. As kidney function varies greatly by gestational age, so will the SCr trajectories and steady-state levels.[116,117] As a result, a refined definition of neonatal AKI may need to take into account factors such as gestational age.

In an extremely premature infant, it may be appropriate to have a slight rise in SCr after birth as the infant finds its own steady-state creatinine. In one study of ELBW infants, 89% had a rise in SCr of 0.3 mg/dL or more.[18] On the other hand, a healthy term neonate with normal kidney function should have a steady decline in SCr after birth. The absence of this normal trajectory or "failure of SCr to decline" could signify a substantial injury, but this is not accounted for in the current KDIGO definition. Gupta and colleagues reported on term asphyxiated neonates and showed that infants with abnormal SCr trajectories (failure to drop) were more similar to those with AKI than to those who had normal SCr trajectory in clinical parameters (e.g., receipt of hemodynamic support, time on ventilators, length of hospital stay, and urine kidney injury biomarkers).[118] This suggests that term infants with an abnormal SCr decline, or any SCr increase, during the first postnatal week may have experienced a significant kidney injury that is not detected by the neonatal KDIGO definition.

Using the AWAKEN database, we have challenged the neonatal modified KDIGO AKI definition and have shown that the absolute SCr changes are superior to the percentage change in SCr in predicting important outcomes associated with AKI such as mortality.[119] In addition, this study showed that a rise in SCr of 0.3 mg/dL is highly specific (but not sensitive) to predict mortality in those greater than 29 weeks GA. In those less than 29 weeks GA, a rise in SCr of 0.3 mg/dL is highly sensitive (but not specific) to predict mortality. The SCr rise cutoff that maximizes the high specificity of morality for those greater than 29 weeks was 0.6 mg/dL or greater.[119] Further work with large prospective data is needed to validate these findings, and we anticipate these studies will allow for fine-tuning of the neonatal AKI definition. Until such work is completed, the neonatal modified KDIGO definition of AKI remains the standard to be utilized.

Another priority in AKI research is the development of more timely and accurate AKI biomarkers. Changes in SCr and/or urine output are late indicators that an AKI event has occurred. Changes in either SCr concentration or urine output alert the clinician only to changes in kidney function, not to damage. In addition, the handling of SCr and free water by the neonatal kidney makes the application of modern AKI definitions difficult.

Interpretation of changes in urine output as an indicator of AKI is problematic in neonates as well. The newborn infant has an excess of total body water at birth. After delivery, the term infant typically loses 5% to 10% of body weight over the first few days of life; premature and low-birth-weight infants may lose as much as 15%.[120] Concentrating ability due to an immature response to antidiuretic hormone in the cortical collecting duct and low tonicity in the interstitium are impaired in term and especially premature infants.[121,122] Levels of atrial natriuretic peptide are also elevated in the newborn and likely contribute to the postnatal diuresis.[123,124] However, this impaired concentrating ability may increase the risk of hypovolemia in critically ill neonates, as well as limit the ability of clinicians to recognize a change in urine output as an indication that AKI has occurred. In a retrospective cohort study of 312 premature and term infants, Bezerra and colleagues found an association between reduction in urine output (i.e., AKI) and mortality, but only a few patients had urine output less than 0.5 mL/kg/h, the traditional threshold for oliguria in older children and adults.[125] Stepwise increase in mortality was associated with incremental decreases in urine output, though with a higher threshold of 1.5 mL/kg/h. Patients with the severest oligo/anuria had the highest risk of mortality (aOR 23.3), though again, these patients accounted for a very small percentage of the sample.

Immaturity in tubular function also helps explain some of the subtleties of urinary findings in neonatal AKI that differ from those in older children. For example, fractional excretion of sodium is often used in older patients to help distinguish hypoperfusion events from acute tubular necrosis. Premature infants have higher rates of urinary sodium excretion at the baseline and thus exhibit a higher fractional excretion of sodium independently of the level of renal perfusion.

There has been much interest in novel urine and serum biomarkers that would have the ability to detect AKI earlier in the process, identify the site of injury (e.g., the proximal tubule, distal tubule, vasculature), help elucidate the underlying cause, and help predict outcomes.[126] The prognostic and diagnostic utility of a number of these, including neutrophil gelatinase-associated lipocalin, uromodulin, kidney injury molecule 1, cystatin C, osteopontin, β_2-microglobulin, epidermal growth factor, and albumin, have been studied in low-birth-weight, critically ill neonates.[127] Infants in this cohort with AKI had lower uromodulin and epidermal growth factor levels and higher cystatin C levels during the first few days of life compared with infants without AKI. Other studies in VLBW infants,[128] infants undergoing cardiopulmonary bypass,[129-131] and other sick newborns[127] cared for in the NICU suggest that a variety of biomarkers can detect infants who will later have a rise in SCr levels. Although these novel biomarkers continue to show promise, they have not yet been validated in large studies. Consequently, measurement of SCr levels remains the gold standard for the diagnosis of AKI in all populations.

LONG-TERM OUTCOMES AND PROGRESSION TO CHRONIC KIDNEY DISEASE

CHRONIC KIDNEY DISEASE AFTER PRETERM BIRTH

The dramatic improvement in the survival of even the smallest infants is among the greatest successes in modern medicine. As survival rates have improved, former premature infants entering into childhood and adulthood may have an increased risk of developing CKD.

Premature infants have substantially higher rates of albuminuria, hypertension, and CKD later in life.[132] In 2009, a meta-analysis by White and colleagues showed that low birth weight (<2500 g) is associated with increased odds of albuminuria, a low GFR, and end-stage kidney disease in later life.[133] Of the 489 subjects enrolled in the NIH-sponsored Chronic Kidney Disease in Children (CKiD) study,[134] 17% were low birth weight (<2500 g), 13% were of low gestational age, 15% were small for their gestational age, and 41% had been admitted to an NICU; each of these rates is increased compared with those in the general population. In 2019 Crump and colleagues published data from Sweden's nationwide birth registry demonstrating the risk for CKD was two- to threefold higher in the preterm and extremely preterm population at the age of 30 years.[135] The risk for CKD is not only detectable in adulthood, but a population-based case-control study demonstrated nearly three times increased odds of CKD in children who were born with low birth weight, potentially representing a surrogate for preterm birth.[136] In follow-up studies of a shorter duration, hypertension, decreased glomerular filtration, small kidneys, and albuminuria can be detected in children as young as 2 years of age, as well as in adolescents born preterm.[137-139]

RISK OF CHRONIC KIDNEY DISEASE AFTER AN ACUTE KIDNEY INJURY EPISODE

Previously, it was assumed that those who survive an episode of AKI would recover kidney function without long-term sequelae; however, in the last decade, epidemiologic data from critically ill children[140] and adults[141] with AKI suggest that survivors are indeed at risk of the development of CKD.

A meta-analysis by Coca and colleagues showed that adults with AKI have a higher risk of developing incident CKD (pooled adjusted HR 8.8, 95% CI 3.1 to 25.5), end-stage kidney disease (pooled adjusted HR 3.1, 95% CI 1.9 to 5.0), and death (pooled adjusted HR 2.0, 95% CI 1.3 to 3.1) compared with adults without AKI.[142] Mammen and colleagues reported the largest long-term follow-up study of AKI in children, which included 126 critically ill children with AKI but lacking detectable preexisting CKD.[143] At 1 to 3 years of follow-up, 13 of 126 children (10%) developed CKD, as defined by an estimated GFR of less than 60 mL/min/1.73 m^2 or persistent albuminuria. In addition, 59 of 126 patients (47%) were considered at risk of CKD, as defined by an estimated GFR of 60 to 90 mL/min/1.73 m^2, hyperfiltration (estimated GFR of more than 150 mL/min/1.73 m^2), or hypertension.

These clinical data are supported by animal models showing that AKI causes long-term kidney-related sequelae. After ischemia-reperfusion injury, there is substantial damage to tubular and endothelial cells,[34] leading to vascular injury and dropout, as well as tubulointerstitial fibrosis.[144] The vascular dropout after AKI results from an endothelial phenotypic transition combined with an impaired regenerative capacity, which might contribute to progressive CKD.[145]

Although animal models of AKI may not fully reflect neonatal AKI, the combination of these animal data and the data from epidemiology studies provide evidence that children with AKI are at risk of CKD and should be monitored and treated for CKD-related problems. Despite the growing evidence showing a strong association between AKI and CKD, further work is necessary to fully understand this relationship and the mechanisms involved in the progression from one to the other. For the clinicians, the challenge going forward is determining which babies need to be followed, how frequently, and for how long.

CONCLUSION

AKI has important implications for clinical outcomes, both short-term and long-term, in critically ill neonates. Further research is needed to develop better AKI definitions and more accurate and timely AKI biomarkers to allow earlier diagnosis. Advances in these areas will ultimately allow the development of therapeutics and other interventions to mitigate the impact of AKI on these patients as well as their long-term risk of CKD.

CONFLICTS OF INTEREST

Drs. Jetton and Selewski have no conflicts of interest relevant to this article. Dr. Askenazi is a consultant for Baxter, Medtronic, and CHF solutions. He has grant support from Baxter and CHF solutions. He has submitted patent applications to improve kidney support therapy and urine collection systems in neonates. Dr. Charlton is co-owner of Sindri Technologies, LLC.

A complete reference list is available at www.ExpertConsult.com.

SELECT REFERENCES

3. Jetton JG, Boohaker LJ, Sethi SK, et al. Incidence and outcomes of neonatal acute kidney injury (AWAKEN): a multicentre, multinational, observational cohort study. *Lancet Child Adolesc Health*. 2017;1:184-194.
5. Koralkar R, Ambalavanan N, Levitan EB, et al. Acute kidney injury reduces survival in very low birth weight infants. *Pediatr Res*. 2011;69:354-358.
6. Selewski DT, Jordan BK, Askenazi DJ, et al. Acute kidney injury in asphyxiated newborns treated with therapeutic hypothermia. *J Pediatr*. 2013;162: 725-729.e721.
7. Charlton JR, Boohaker L, Askenazi D, et al. Incidence and risk factors of early onset neonatal AKI. *Clin J Am Soc Nephrol*. 2019;14:184-195.
8. Charlton JR, Boohaker L, Askenazi D, et al. Late onset neonatal acute kidney injury: results from the AWAKEN Study. *Pediatr Res*. 2019;85:339-348.
18. Carmody JB, Swanson JR, Rhone ET, et al. Recognition and reporting of AKI in very low birth weight infants. *Clin J Am Soc Nephrol*. 2014;9:2036-2043.
31. Vieux R, Hascoet JM, Merdariu D, et al. Glomerular filtration rate reference values in very preterm infants. *Pediatrics*. 2010;125:e1186-e1192.
32. Abitbol CL, Seeherunvong W, Galarza MG, et al. Neonatal kidney size and function in preterm infants: what is a true estimate of glomerular filtration rate? *J Pediatr*. 2014;164:1026-1031.e1022.
57. Basu RK, Wheeler DS. Kidney-lung cross-talk and acute kidney injury. *Pediatr Nephrol*. 2013;28:2239-2248.
63. Selewski DT, Akcan-Arikan A, Bonachea EM, et al. The impact of fluid balance on outcomes in critically ill near-term/term neonates: a report from the AWAKEN study group. *Pediatr Res*. 2019;85:79-85.
64. Selewski DT, Gist KM, Nathan AT, et al. The impact of fluid balance on outcomes in premature neonates: a report from the AWAKEN study group. *Pediatr Res*. 2020;87:550-557.
65. Starr MC, Boohaker L, Eldredge LC, et al. Acute kidney injury and bronchopulmonary dysplasia in premature neonates born less than 32 weeks' gestation. *Am J Perinatol*. 2020;37:341-348.
66. Starr MC, Boohaker L, Eldredge LC, et al. Acute kidney injury is associated with poor lung outcomes in infants born >/=32 weeks of gestational age. *Am J Perinatol*. 2020;37:231-240.
79. Sarkar S, Askenazi DJ, Jordan BK, et al. Relationship between acute kidney injury and brain MRI findings in asphyxiated newborns after therapeutic hypothermia. *Pediatr Res*. 2014;75:431-435.
81. Stoops C, Sims B, Griffin R, et al. Neonatal acute kidney injury and the risk of intraventricular hemorrhage in the very low birth weight infant. *Neonatology*. 2016;110:307-312.
82. Stoops C, Boohaker L, Sims B, et al. The association of intraventricular hemorrhage and acute kidney injury in premature infants from the assessment of the worldwide Acute Kidney Injury Epidemiology in Neonates (AWAKEN) Study. *Neonatology*. 2019;116:321-330.
83. Stojanovic V, Barisic N, Milanovic B, et al. Acute kidney injury in preterm infants admitted to a neonatal intensive care unit. *Pediatr Nephrol*. 2014;29:2213-2220.
95. Rhone ET, Carmody JB, Swanson JR, et al. Nephrotoxic medication exposure in very low birth weight infants. *J Matern Fetal Neonatal Med*. 2014;27:1485-1490.
96. Murphy HJ, Thomas B, Van Wyk B, et al. Nephrotoxic medications and acute kidney injury risk factors in the neonatal intensive care unit: clinical challenges for neonatologists and nephrologists. *Pediatr Nephrol*. 2019.
98. Stoops C, Stone S, Evans E, et al. Baby NINJA (Nephrotoxic Injury Negated by Just-in-Time Action): reduction of nephrotoxic medication-associated acute kidney injury in the Neonatal Intensive Care Unit. *J Pediatr*. 2019;215. 223-228 e226.
100. Lee CC, Chan OW, Lai MY, et al. Incidence and outcomes of acute kidney injury in extremely-low-birth-weight infants. *PLoS One*. 2017;12:e0187764.
101. Carmody JB, Harer MW, Denotti AR, et al. Caffeine exposure and risk of acute kidney injury in a retrospective cohort of very low birth weight neonates. *J Pediatr*. 2016;172:63-68.e61.
102. Harer MW, Askenazi DJ, Boohaker LJ, et al. Association between early caffeine citrate administration and risk of acute kidney injury in preterm neonates: results from the AWAKEN Study. *JAMA Pediatr*. 2018;172:e180322.
104. Bellos I, Pandita A, Yachha M. Effectiveness of theophylline administration in neonates with perinatal asphyxia: a meta-analysis. *J Matern Fetal Neonatal Med*. 2019:1-9.
105. Cavallin F, Rubin G, Vidal E, et al. Prognostic role of acute kidney injury on long-term outcome in infants with hypoxic-ischemic encephalopathy. *Pediatr Nephrol*. 2020;35:477-483.
106. Criss CN, Selewski DT, Sunkara B, et al. Acute kidney injury in necrotizing enterocolitis predicts mortality. *Pediatr Nephrol*. 2018;33:503-510.
107. Bakhoum CY, Basalely A, Koppel RI, et al. Acute kidney injury in preterm infants with necrotizing enterocolitis. *J Matern Fetal Neonatal Med*. 2018:1-6.
108. Aviles-Otero N, Kumar R, Khalsa DD, et al. Caffeine exposure and acute kidney injury in premature infants with necrotizing enterocolitis and spontaneous intestinal perforation. *Pediatr Nephrol*. 2019;34:729-736.
109. Zwiers AJ, de Wildt SN, Hop WC, et al. Acute kidney injury is a frequent complication in critically ill neonates receiving extracorporeal membrane oxygenation: a 14-year cohort study. *Crit Care*. 2013;17:R151.
114. Jetton JG, Askenazi DJ. Update on acute kidney injury in the neonate. *Curr Opin Pediatr*. 2012;24:191-196.
115. Zappitelli M, Ambalavanan N, Askenazi DJ, et al. Developing a neonatal acute kidney injury research definition: a report from the NIDDK neonatal AKI workshop. *Pediatr Res*. 2017;82:569-573.
117. Thayyil S, Sheik S, Kempley ST, et al. A gestation- and postnatal age-based reference chart for assessing renal function in extremely premature infants. *J Perinatol*. 2008;28:226-229.

119. Askenazi D, Abitbol C, Boohaker L, et al. Optimizing the AKI definition during first postnatal week using Assessment of Worldwide Acute Kidney Injury Epidemiology in Neonates (AWAKEN) cohort. *Pediatr Res*. 2019;85:329–338.
132. Carmody JB, Charlton JR. Short-term gestation, long-term risk: prematurity and chronic kidney disease. *Pediatrics*. 2013;131:1168–1179.
135. Crump C, Sundquist J, Winkleby MA, et al. Preterm birth and risk of chronic kidney disease from childhood into mid-adulthood: national cohort study. *BMJ*. 2019;365:l1346.
136. Hsu CW, Yamamoto KT, Henry RK, et al. Prenatal risk factors for childhood CKD. *J Am Soc Nephrol*. 2014;25:2105–2111.
146. Askenazi DJ, Griffin R, McGwin G, et al. Acute kidney injury is independently associated with mortality in very low birthweight infants: a matched case-control analysis. *Pediatr Nephrol*. 2009;24:991–997.
147. Askenazi DJ, Koralkar R, Hundley HE, et al. Fluid overload and mortality are associated with acute kidney injury in sick near-term/term neonate. *Pediatr Nephrol*. 2013;28:661–666.
148. Alabbas A, Campbell A, Skippen P, et al. Epidemiology of cardiac surgery-associated acute kidney injury in neonates: a retrospective study. *Pediatr Nephrol*. 2013;28:1127–1134.
149. Morgan CJ, Zappitelli M, Robertson CM, et al. Risk factors for and outcomes of acute kidney injury in neonates undergoing complex cardiac surgery. *J Pediatr*. 2013;162:120–127.e121.
150. Constance JE, Reith D, Ward RM, et al. Risk of nonsteroidal anti-inflammatory drug-associated renal dysfunction among neonates diagnosed with patent ductus arteriosus and treated with gentamicin. *J Perinatol*. 2017;37:1093–1102.
151. Weintraub AS, Connors J, Carey A, et al. The spectrum of onset of acute kidney injury in premature infants less than 30 weeks gestation. *J Perinatol*. 2016;36:474–480.
152. Velazquez DM, Reidy KJ, Sharma M, et al. The effect of hemodynamically significant patent ductus arteriosus on acute kidney injury and systemic hypertension in extremely low gestational age newborns. *J Matern Fetal Neonatal Med*. 2018:1–6.
153. Chowdhary V, Vajpeyajula R, Jain M, et al. Comparison of different definitions of acute kidney injury in extremely low birth weight infants. *Clin Exp Nephrol*. 2018;22:117–125.
154. Srinivasan N, Schwartz A, John E, et al. Acute kidney injury impairs postnatal renal adaptation and increases morbidity and mortality in very low-birth-weight infants. *Am J Perinatol*. 2018;35:39–47.
155. Maqsood S, Fung N, Chowdhary V, et al. Outcome of extremely low birth weight infants with a history of neonatal acute kidney injury. *Pediatr Nephrol*. 2017;32:1035–1043.
156. Askenazi D, Patil NR, Ambalavanan N, et al. Acute kidney injury is associated with bronchopulmonary dysplasia/mortality in premature infants. *Pediatr Nephrol*. 2015;30:1511–1518.
157. Starr MC, Boohaker L, Eldredge LC, et al. Acute kidney injury and bronchopulmonary dysplasia in premature neonates born less than 32 weeks' gestation. *Am J Perinatol*. 2020;37:341–348.
158. Chock VY, Frymoyer A, Yeh CG, et al. Renal saturation and acute kidney injury in neonates with hypoxic ischemic encephalopathy undergoing therapeutic hypothermia. *J Pediatr*. 2018;200. 232–239.e231.

165 Pathophysiology of Edema

David P. Carlton

GENERAL CONSIDERATIONS

Edema is the clinical term used to describe excessive fluid accumulation in the adventitial tissue spaces of the body. Excess fluid accumulates when the net rate of transvascular fluid filtration from the microcirculation is exceeded by the rate of fluid removal from the interstitial space, usually as a result of lymphatic clearance. Postnatally, edema occurs in the neonate in association with a variety of conditions, including respiratory failure, sepsis, and renal failure. Underlying all circumstances in which edema is present, a disturbance in the normal balance of total body salt and water occurs either as a primary (e.g., anuria) or secondary (e.g., retention of fluid to preserve circulating volume) event.[1] Although renal or hormonal abnormalities may not be directly responsible for edema formation, nearly all conditions associated with edema have disturbances in these systems, and the resolution of edema ultimately occurs when normal renal and hormonal control of fluid and salt balance is established.

Total body water balance is a dynamic process during fetal development.[2] Early in gestation, the total body water content is approximately 95% of total body weight, decreasing to approximately 75% of body weight at term, and then to approximately 60% of body weight by the end of the first year after birth. Similarly, the fraction of total body water that comprises interstitial fluid declines during fetal development.

TRANSVASCULAR FLUID FILTRATION

Fluid movement across the endothelium is driven by forces that regulate fluid flux across a semipermeable membrane.[3] These forces are the hydrostatic and protein osmotic, or oncotic, pressures of the intravascular and interstitial spaces. The ostensibly quantitative expression of how these forces influence fluid filtration is shown in the equation.

$$J_v = K\ [(P_{mv} - Pi)\ - \sigma\ (\pi_{mv} - \pi_i)] \qquad [165.1]$$

where J_v represents net transvascular fluid flow, K is a coefficient that accounts for the permeability of the barrier and surface area for filtration, σ is the reflection coefficient of the barrier to protein, P_{mv} and P_i are the hydrostatic pressures of the microvascular compartment and interstitium, respectively, and π_{mv} and π_i are the osmotic pressures generated by the protein in the microvascular and interstitial spaces, respectively. For a barrier that is completely impermeable to protein, σ would assume the value of 1, and for a barrier across which protein moves without restriction, σ would assume the value of 0. The most complete analysis of fluid filtration across the endothelium would include values for σ that are specific for each plasma protein.

Countless attempts have been made to quantify each of the variables in Eq. 165.1 for different organs in animals and in man. All experimental approaches involve assumptions about the validity of the values measured, and thus all values so measured lack a sense of finality, particularly in the fetus and newborn.[4,5]

Under usual circumstances J_v is greater than 0 in most tissue spaces. That is, the sum of forces regulating fluid filtration result in a net movement of fluid out of the microcirculation.[6] However, it is important to recognize that fluid filtration processes are dynamic and at any one time, in any specific section of the microcirculation, filtration forces may not result in fluid moving into the interstitium, even though the net J_v of the tissue or organ is greater than 0. For instance, the return of lung liquid into the circulation that occurs after birth takes place predominantly across the microcirculation and not by lymphatic channels.[7]

Intravascular pressure in the microcirculation, P_{mv}, can be measured directly using micropuncture or indirectly techniques using isogravimetric methods.[8] It is unlikely that intravascular pressure remains constant across the entire fluid-exchanging surface because resistance to flow along the vessel results in a drop in pressure over the length of the vessel. Thus P_{mv} is understood to be the net hydrostatic force for the surface area involved in fluid exchange, even if the hydrostatic pressure at the arterial end of the vessel results in fluid filtration, and hydrostatic pressure at the venous end results in fluid reabsorption.

P_{mv} is influenced by the relative vascular resistances in the circulation before and after the fluid-exchanging regions.[9] An increase in upstream resistance or a decrease in downstream resistance reduces P_{mv} and fluid filtration, and a decrease in upstream resistance or an increase in downstream resistance has the opposite effect. The importance of considering the profile of vascular resistance distribution is that the effect of a change in arterial pressure on fluid filtration cannot be predicted with certainty. The redistribution of vascular resistance in response to an intervention or a change in condition ultimately determines whether transvascular fluid filtration is affected, and because resistance cannot be assessed clinically, the ability to predict whether a change in transvascular filtration will occur is difficult. For instance, alveolar hypoxia increases pulmonary arterial pressure in both adults and neonates, but alveolar hypoxia affects transvascular fluid filtration only in the newborn.[10-12]

Interstitial pressure, P_i, has been assessed by several different techniques, including porous capsule embedment, direct micropuncture, and cotton wick insertion into the adventitial space.[8] It is not possible to assign a general value to P_i because it assumes different values depending on the tissue bed under study. Values that exceed atmospheric pressure, and those that are subatmospheric have been measured.[13] Although P_i often assumes a value near 0 mm Hg, changes in interstitial pressure in response to physiologic disturbances can be dramatic. For example, in tissue that has suffered thermal trauma, P_i may decrease many folds over baseline, thus contributing, in part, to the rapid accumulation of interstitial fluid seen with burn injuries.[14] The molecular mechanisms underlying control of interstitial pressure are not clear, but the binding of collagen molecules on the surface of adventitial cells may play a role, because antibodies to the β_1-integrin lower interstitial pressure and prompt edema formation.[15]

Microvascular protein osmotic pressure, π_{mv}, has been the focus of investigation and clinical study to understand better whether changing this value can improve total body fluid balance.[16,17] In the strictest analysis, π_{mv} should be measured for each plasma protein constituent, along with the corresponding σ, but like the aforementioned P_{mv}, a net value of osmotic pressure generated by the sum of plasma proteins suffices to account qualitatively for the relative importance of plasma oncotic pressure to transvascular fluid filtration. The osmotic force of all components of the extracellular fluid is on the order of 5000 to 6000 mm Hg. However, because these components pass unimpeded across the endothelial barrier of the microcirculation (i.e., they have a reflection coefficient of 0), they do not affect fluid flux.[18] In contrast, plasma proteins do not move with complete freedom across the circulation and have a significant effect on fluid filtration despite an osmotic pressure in plasma being in the range of 10 to 20 mm Hg.

Interstitial protein osmotic pressure, π_i, has been measured by direct micropuncture, implanted tissue capsules, and absorbent materials placed within the tissue space.[8,18] In vivo measurements of π_i have relied on collection of lymph from organs of interest, with the assumption that the protein concentration of lymph is equivalent to that of interstitial fluid (this is likely to be a safe assumption under steady-state conditions when lymph is collected from afferent lymphatics).

The membrane parameter, σ, represents the sieving ability of a semipermeable membrane for protein. High values of σ imply that osmotic pressure differences across the vascular barrier will exert a greater effect on fluid flux than will lower values of σ. One can measure σ in vitro as the ratio between the measured and expected osmotic pressure generated by the protein of interest. Furthermore, the value of this coefficient can be estimated in vivo from experiments in which transvascular fluid filtration is maximized (i.e., under conditions in which protein flow is nearly all convective).

Eq. 165.1 describes the driving forces for transvascular fluid movement, but a different mathematical relationship exists for describing transvascular protein movement. This relationship contains two components, one describing flow of protein as a result of convective movement:

$$J_s = (1-\sigma)\ PJ_v \quad [165.2]$$

where J_s is transvascular protein flow, σ is the protein reflection coefficient, P is the concentration of protein in the vasculature, and J_v represents net transvascular fluid movement. The second relationship describes the flow of protein as a result of diffusion:

$$J_s = K\ (P-L) \quad [165.3]$$

where K is the product of the permeability and surface area of the microcirculation, and P and L represent the concentration of protein in the vasculature and lymph (interstitium), respectively. Combining these two equations yields the equation that describes net total transvascular protein movement:

$$J_s = (1-\sigma)\ PJ_v + K\ (P-L) \quad [165.4]$$

Under steady-state conditions, lymph contains all the transvascular protein filtered if no metabolism occurs in the interstitium, and thus J_s is reduced to LJ_v. In this analysis, J_v is equal to lymph flow and L is equal to lymph protein concentration. Rearranging the above equation, simplifying it, and arranging experimental conditions in which lymph flow is maximized yields the equation $\sigma = 1 - L/P$.[19] When measured experimentally, σ is well over 0.5 in most tissue beds and usually in the range of 0.75 to 0.90, even in the neonate.[20] Capillary beds that contain fenestrations, as in the liver, represent little restriction to transvascular protein movement, and under such conditions σ would be low. Capillaries in other vascular beds contain few if any discontinuous regions, and σ under these circumstances would be closer to 1. The closer σ is to unity, the greater the influence of plasma proteins on fluid filtration.[19]

The lower the value of σ, the less able proteins are to generate a force counteracting fluid filtration. This arises for two reasons. First, with a less restrictive barrier, π_i increases numerically toward π_{mv} because the sieving quality of the membrane is diminished. Second, any difference between π_{mv} and π_i is minimized as σ decreases. Thus, under conditions in which the vascular barrier is injured, allowing a greater degree of protein leak, administration of protein intravenously to augment vascular protein osmotic pressure and to reduce edema formation theoretically should have little, if any, effect. The administration of protein to affect fluid balance in some other fashion (e.g., on barrier function per se or to provide other favorable effects unrelated to fluid balance [e.g., to maintain plasma drug binding]) may subserve a clinical benefit, but such a rationale would be independent of the presumed advantage of an increase in microvascular protein osmotic pressure on transvascular fluid filtration.

Finally, the coefficient K represents the product of barrier hydraulic conductivity and the surface area available for fluid filtration.[16] These two components of K are difficult to separate experimentally. Hydraulic conductivity itself is predominantly a function of the density of the pathways for liquid and solute movement, and is not necessarily a measure of protein permeability. That is, more pathways, or pores, for solute and liquid exchange might exist under different conditions without the individual pathways being more permeable. Thus changes in K may occur with true alterations in liquid and solute permeability (i.e., pathways that allow passage of larger proteins), but changes in K may occur simply with an alteration in the density of pathways for liquid and solute movement or with changes in surface area for filtration, as would occur when unperfused capillaries are filled.

Consideration of Eq. 165.1 allows several general statements about fluid filtration under normal conditions during steady-state.[19] First, because some degree of sieving always occurs across the microvascular barrier, the protein concentration in the interstitium is less than that in the vascular space. This difference in protein concentration yields a difference in protein osmotic pressures that is subtracted from the hydrostatic pressure difference term. In this sense, protein osmotic pressure attempts to balance the "edema-promoting" effect of microvascular hydrostatic pressure. Second, because a net exit of fluid from the circulation occurs, the hydrostatic pressure difference term in Eq. 165.1 must exceed the difference in osmotic pressure term when total body fluid balance is under consideration. No experimental evidence exists that indicates the presence of net "active" transport of water and solute across the endothelium that would influence transvascular fluid flux.

Although the concepts expressed in Eq. 165.1 serve physiologists and clinicians well when considering fluid balance in a general sense, the equation does not always allow a precise calculation of the change in fluid filtration (J_v), even when only one variable in the equation changes. This arises because a change in one of the variables in Eq. 165.1 usually results in a change in one of the other variables, even if such a change is unexpected. For instance, under conditions in which microvascular hydrostatic pressure is increased, one might assume that transvascular flow will increase by an amount that can be arrived at arithmetically from Eq. 165.1. When P_{mv} increases in the presence of a stable vascular barrier, J_v increases, but as it does, the interstitial protein concentration decreases. This occurs because the driving force for liquid exceeds the bulk flow of protein across the barrier (because σ is greater than 0 for protein); there is no sieving of water. When interstitial protein concentration is reduced, the protein osmotic pressure difference between the vascular and interstitial spaces increases. Thus, from Eq. 165.1, J_v will increase in response to an increase in P_{mv}, but as $(\pi_{mv} - \pi_i)$ becomes larger, J_v assumes a new steady-state value that is less than that predicted by the increase in P_{mv} alone. Additionally, if excess fluid expands the interstitium, interstitial pressure increases to some extent, although the magnitude of this change is not predictable because tissue space compliance is not linear in the presence of increasing interstitial edema. This increase in tissue hydrostatic pressure also acts to slow transvascular fluid movement. Changes that occur in driving forces for filtration that counteract the change in the "edema-promoting" variable are referred to as the *edema safety factors*. The implication of the edema safety factors is that increases in transvascular filtration are blunted because of the countervailing changes seen in other variables in Eq. 165.1.[8,16,18,19]

LYMPH FLOW MODULATION OF EDEMA

An increase in interstitial fluid volume can be conceptually understood as an inability of the lymphatic system to remove fluid at the same rate as that being filtered across the microcirculation. Lymphatics are present in most but not all tissue beds; brain, specific areas of the eye, and bone marrow are examples of organs that do not contain lymphatics.[19] With regard to fluid balance, lymphatics serve to return not only water but also protein into the circulation. Without the return of protein to the circulation, protein concentration differences between the interstitium and circulation narrow.

Lymphatics are located primarily in loose connective tissue spaces and appear to end bluntly. Like blood vessel capillaries, the smallest terminal lymphatics do not contain smooth muscle, but the presence of actin filaments in lymphatic endothelium suggests that the initial lymphatics may possess some limited contractile properties. As the lymphatic vasculature is traced centrally, valves appear, and smooth muscle cells surrounding the lymphatics are more consistently observed. Lymphatics ultimately drain into the central circulation through the thoracic and right lymphatic ducts.

The movement of interstitial fluid from the tissue space into the terminal lymphatics requires a driving force. Experimental evidence points to the importance of both interstitial pressure and interstitial volume in modulating lymph flow. However, an increase in interstitial pressure alone, in the absence of a change in interstitial volume, would be unlikely to result in a hydrostatic pressure gradient sufficient to account for lymphatic filling. It is the combination of anchoring filaments attached to the external wall of the lymphatics and an increase in interstitial volume that results in a pressure gradient sufficient to account for initial lymphatic filling.[18,19]

Lymph drainage is not constant but varies with changes in filtration driving force[16]; therefore lymph drainage can also be considered an edema safety factor. Interstitial pressure is closely associated with lymph flow, but the relationship between interstitial pressure and lymph flow is not linear over all tissue pressures. Although an association exists between interstitial pressure and lymph flow, other factors also influence lymphatic clearance. One of the most important is the presence of valves within the lymphatics that provide directionality to flow.[19] Valves also reduce the direct influence of downstream outflow pressure on transendothelial fluid movement into the terminal lymphatics. Lymph is propelled centrally by extrinsic and intrinsic factors. Extrinsic forces include both passive and active muscular movement. Intrinsic forces are those associated with spontaneous lymph vessel contraction and relaxation. Motion associated with respiration and blood vessel pulsation also contributes to lymphatic movement.

EFFECT OF OUTFLOW PRESSURE ON LYMPHATIC DRAINAGE

Lymph from the large lymphatic collecting vessels ultimately drains into the central circulation. If lymph drainage is obstructed, interstitial tissue volume increases and edema becomes obvious, implying that outflow pressure is an important variable influencing the effectiveness of lymph drainage.[21] Because the thoracic duct empties into the central venous circulation, an increase in central venous pressure should be an important factor influencing lymph drainage. Experimental evidence from fetal and adult animals confirms this notion.[22-24]

MOVEMENT OF PROTEIN ACROSS THE MICROVASCULAR BARRIER

The specific site of fluid and protein transfer along the circulation is likely to be variable within an organ and among tissues. Venules, arterioles, and capillaries may each contribute to transvascular fluid filtration. Molecular size plays a role in transvascular filtration, with ease of transport into the interstitium being inversely proportional to size.[17] Proteins cross the endothelium through channels or pores and by transcytosis, but the magnitude of each to total transvascular protein movement is debated.[25] The importance of protein movement through pores of various sizes in the vascular barrier is highlighted by studies that show that movement of protein into the interstitium is closely linked to the flow of liquid; that is, movement occurs by convection or bulk flow. In the lung, inhibitors of transcytosis do not significantly decrease transvascular protein transport, casting doubt on the importance of transcytosis as an important pathway for transvascular protein movement involved in fluid balance.[26]

The morphologic basis for an increase in microvascular permeability is not completely resolved. Under some conditions, gaps between endothelial cells can be seen microscopically, but this is not a consistent observation.[25] Intercellular proteins between endothelial cells are linked to actin and other intracellular structures that are thought to regulate microvascular protein permeability by rearrangement of the cytoskeleton. Cellular contraction is thought to be the means by which intercellular gaps are formed and thus permeability is regulated.[27]

The molecular basis for changes in permeability is also not completely understood.[28-31] Clinically, inflammatory processes are frequently associated with changes in permeability. The molecular initiation of permeability occurs, at least in a number of circumstances, as a result of calcium-dependent events. Calcium entry appears to be regulated, in part, by potassium modulation of transmembrane potential and not through voltage-regulated calcium channels. An increase in intracellular calcium is thought to promote myosin light-chain phosphorylation by kinases and thus initiate contraction. The evidence that intracellular calcium may be influenced by novel means is shown by experiments in which surface molecules, not thought to be receptors for the typical inflammatory ligands, influence vascular permeability. A well-studied example is the ligation of the luminal surface integrin, $\alpha_v\beta_3$, on the microvasculature, which increases transcapillary liquid flux.[32] An increase in intracellular calcium also modulates nitric oxide synthesis and the generation of cyclic guanosine monophosphate (cGMP). These mediators are known to affect vascular permeability, but the mechanism by which this occurs is unclear. Their effect may be indirect, perhaps by modulating the concentration of intracellular cyclic adenosine monophosphate (cAMP); cAMP blunts cell contraction and myosin light-chain phosphorylation, but it also may influence the expression of molecules important in intercellular binding and thus limit the ability of the cytoskeleton to influence permeability.[25]

SPECIFIC CLINICAL CONSIDERATIONS: CHANGES IN TRANSVASCULAR FLUID FILTRATION WITH INTRAVENOUS PROTEIN INFUSIONS

Intravenous infusions of solutions containing protein or dextran are frequently administered to patients with edema to increase plasma protein osmotic pressure. The expectation is that transvascular fluid filtration will decrease as plasma protein concentration increases. However, experiments have not supported that practice. For example, infusing albumin in sufficient quantities to increase plasma albumin concentration by as much as 20% or infusing dextran in sufficient quantity to increase plasma osmotic pressure by more than twofold, has little effect on steady-state lymph flow.[33,34] However, if microvascular hydrostatic pressure is then increased, the additional plasma osmotic pressure blunts the expected increase in transvascular fluid filtration. The explanation for this response is not completely clear, but probably results from changes in hydraulic conductivity and from changes in the distribution of vascular resistance, both of which could result in changes in effective P_{mv}.

Experiments evaluating hypoproteinemia in the neonate predictably show that lymph flow increases when protein is removed from the circulation.[20,35] The explanations for this response are conflicting, but at least in the newborn lamb increases appear to result from a decrease in transvascular protein osmotic pressure difference and an increase in vessel hydraulic conductivity, but not from an increase in protein permeability. Whether albumin plays some role in maintaining the health of the barrier wall is uncertain. In vitro data suggest that albumin per se favorably influences the endothelial barrier.[36]

The preceding discussion examines the issue of plasma proteins and fluid balance in the context of a normally permeable microvascular barrier. When barrier integrity is compromised, the movement of protein is less restricted, the reflection coefficient is reduced, and any effect of protein osmotic pressure on fluid movement is minimized. Consistent with this theoretical assumption, experiments in which the lung microvasculature has been injured show no change in fluid egress from the pulmonary circulation with the infusion of albumin.[37] Thus, any favorable effect of plasma protein osmotic pressure on transvascular fluid balance depends on the extent to which the endothelial barrier remains intact.

SPECIAL CONSIDERATIONS OF EDEMA IN THE FETUS

An edematous fetus, regardless of the etiology of the edema, is labeled with the diagnosis of hydrops fetalis. Numerous medical conditions are associated with hydrops, but the pathophysiologic link between the condition and edema formation is not clear in many of these patients.[38] Approximately 75% of the cases of nonimmune hydrops in the United States occur in association with an identifiable disorder, and in the remainder the condition is labeled idiopathic.[39]

PROPOSED MECHANISMS OF EDEMA FORMATION IN PATIENTS WITH HYDROPS

As outlined above, edema may form if the driving forces for fluid filtration or vascular permeability increase without a concomitant increase in lymphatic drainage. Although disturbances in microvascular permeability could be relevant in explaining some cases of fetal hydrops, vascular protein permeability seems to be independent of overall body water content or maturation.[7,40,41]

A variety of hypotheses might explain the pathophysiology of hydrops, but one that is most compatible with the current experimental evidence is that the elevation of central venous pressure is a critical element in the pathogenesis of fetal edema. Conditions that elevate central venous pressure are common in hydropic infants and thus provide a compelling clinical link for this hypothesis. An elevation in central venous pressure increases microvascular pressure upstream and thus enhances transvascular fluid movement. An increase in central venous pressure also impairs lymphatic drainage into the central circulation and thus increases interstitial fluid volume. If lymphatic drainage is completely interrupted (a limiting-case example of increased central venous pressure), the fetus becomes hydropic.[21] In experiments designed to evaluate more modest effects of disturbances in central venous pressure on lymph drainage, thoracic duct lymph flow was found to be inversely proportional and linearly related to outflow pressure. In these studies, increasing central venous pressure by only 5 mm Hg reduced the rate of lymph drainage by nearly 50%.[24]

A helpful model that clarifies total body fluid dynamics in the presence of elevated central venous pressure is the fetal lamb that undergoes rapid atrial pacing. When fetal sheep are paced at rates of 300 to 320 per minute, central venous pressure nearly doubles, without changes in systemic arterial pressure, plasma albumin concentration, or vascular protein permeability.[42,43] Fetal edema occurs quickly, sometimes within 12 to 24 hours, indicating excessive transvascular fluid filtration, impaired lymphatic clearance, or both. Thoracic duct lymph flow increases by nearly

50% when measured at an outflow pressure equivalent to central venous pressure under baseline conditions, but when measured at the central venous pressure induced by pacing, lymph flow is significantly reduced. Thus in conditions that increase central venous pressure, hydrops may be caused, or at least aggravated, by two distinct mechanisms: increased transvascular fluid entry and impaired interstitial fluid clearance.

Anemia is another human fetal condition often associated with hydrops. An exchange transfusion in fetal lambs sufficient to reduce hematocrit from 32% to 12% produces hydrops, but only if the anemia is associated with an increase in central venous pressure.[44] Whether edema develops may depend to a large extent on whether lymph drainage can accommodate the increase in fluid filtration.

In newborn sheep made hypoproteinemic, plasma protein osmotic pressure reduces and transvascular fluid filtration increases, but no increase in interstitial fluid volume occurs, at least in the lung, because lymph flow increases to match transvascular filtration.[20,35] Likewise, in fetal sheep, simply lowering plasma protein oncotic pressure by removing protein from the circulation has no effect on total body water.[45] The lack of effect of hypoproteinemia on edema formation is likely to be a result of increased lymphatic drainage back into the central circulation. In isolated fetal hypoproteinemia, central venous pressure does not increase, and thus there is no impediment to lymph drainage back into the central circulation. The increase in fetal lymph flow is approximately 40%, similar to that seen in newborn lambs made hypoproteinemic.[20,34] Because fetal lymph flow can increase two- to fourfold over baseline values, increases in transvascular filtration prompted by hypoproteinemia can be easily accommodated by increases in fetal lymph flow.

ACKNOWLEDGMENT

The editors thank David P. Carlton for his excellent work on this chapter in the fifth edition. It has been republished here essentially unchanged.

REFERENCES

1. Witte CL, Witte MH. On the causation of edema: a lymphologic perspective. *Perspect Biol Med*. 1997;41:86.
2. Simpson J, Stephenson T. Regulation of extracellular fluid volume in neonates. *Early Hum Dev*. 1993;34:179.
3. Joles JA, et al. Plasma volume regulation: defenses against edema formation (with special emphasis on hypoproteinemia). *Am J Nephrol*. 1993;13:399.
4. Gold PS, Brace RA. Fetal whole-body permeability—surface area product and reflection coefficient for plasma proteins. *Microvasc Res*. 1988;36:262.
5. Brace RA, Gold PS. Fetal whole-body interstitial compliance, vascular compliance, and capillary filtration coefficient. *Am J Physiol*. 1984;247:800.
6. Nicoll PA, Taylor AE. Lymph formation and flow. *Annu Rev Physiol*. 1977;39:73.
7. Bland RD, et al. Lung fluid balance in lambs before and after birth. *J Appl Physiol*. 1982;53:992.
8. Taylor AE. Capillary fluid filtration. Starling forces and lymph flow. *Circ Res*. 1981;49:557.
9. Cope DK, et al. Pulmonary capillary pressure: a review. *Crit Care Med*. 1992;20:1043.
10. Bland RD, et al. Lung fluid balance in hypoxic, awake newborn lambs and mature sheep. *Biol Neonate*. 1980;38:221.
11. Bressack MA, Bland RD. Alveolar hypoxia increases lung fluid filtration in unanesthetized newborn lambs. *Circ Res*. 1980;46:111.
12. Bland RD, et al. Effects of alveolar hypoxia on lung fluid and protein transport in unanesthetized sheep. *Circ Res*. 1977;40:269.
13. Reed RK, et al. Control of interstitial fluid pressure: role of beta1-integrins. *Semin Nephrol*. 2001;21:222.
14. Lund T, et al. Acute postburn edema: role of strongly negative interstitial fluid pressure. *Am J Physiol*. 1988;255:1069.
15. Reed RK, et al. Blockade of beta1-integrins in skin causes edema through lowering of interstitial fluid pressure. *Circ Res*. 1992;71:978.
16. Taylor AE. The lymphatic edema safety factor: the role of edema-dependent lymphatic factors (EDLF). *Lymphology*. 1990;23:111.
17. Renkin EM. Some consequences of capillary permeability to macromolecules: Starling's hypothesis reconsidered. *Am J Physiol*. 1986;250:706.
18. Aukland K, Nicolaysen G. Interstitial fluid volume: local regulatory mechanisms. *Physiol Rev*. 1981;61:556.
19. Aukland K, Reed RK. Interstitial-lymphatic mechanisms in the control of extracellular fluid volume. *Physiol Rev*. 1993;73:1.
20. Hazinski TA, et al. Effect of hypoproteinemia on lung fluid balance in awake newborn lambs. *J Appl Physiol*. 1986;61:1139.
21. Andres RL, Brace RA. The development of hydrops fetalis in the ovine fetus after lymphatic ligation or lymphatic excision. *Am J Obstet Gynecol*. 1990;162:1331.
22. Laine GA, et al. Effect of systemic venous pressure elevation on lymph flow and lung edema formation. *J Appl Physiol*. 1986;61:1634.
23. Brace RA. Effects of outflow pressure on fetal lymph flow. *Am J Obstet Gynecol*. 1989;160:494.
24. Gest AL, et al. The effect of outflow pressure upon thoracic duct lymph flow rate in fetal sheep. *Pediatr Res*. 1992;32:585.
25. Michel CC, Curry FE. Microvascular permeability. *Physiol Rev*. 1999;79:703.
26. Rippe B, Taylor A. NEM and filipin increase albumin transport in lung microvessels. *Am J Physiol Heart Circ Physiol*. 2001;280:34.
27. Dudek SM, Garcia JG. Cytoskeletal regulation of pulmonary vascular permeability. *J Appl Physiol*. 2001;91:1487.
28. Lum H, Malik AB. Mechanisms of increased endothelial permeability. *Can J Physiol Pharmacol*. 1996;74:787.
29. Lum H, Malik AB. Regulation of vascular endothelial barrier function. *Am J Physiol*. 1994;267:223.
30. Stevens T, et al. Mechanisms regulating endothelial cell barrier function. *Am J Physiol Lung Cell Mol Physiol*. 2000;279:419.
31. Mehta D, et al. Novel regulators of endothelial barrier function. *Am J Physiol Lung Cell Mol Physiol*. 2014;307:924–935.
32. Tsukada H, et al. Ligation of endothelial alphav beta3 integrin increases capillary hydraulic conductivity of rat lung. *Circ Res*. 1995;77:651.
33. Wareing TH, et al. Increased plasma oncotic pressure inhibits pulmonary fluid transport when pulmonary pressures are elevated. *J Surg Res*. 1989;46:29.
34. Demling RH, et al. Effect of albumin infusion on pulmonary microvascular fluid and protein transport. *J Surg Res*. 1979;27:321.
35. Cummings JJ, et al. Hypoproteinemia slows lung liquid clearance in young lambs. *J Appl Physiol*. 1993;74:153.
36. Schneeberger EE, Hamelin M. Interaction of serum proteins with lung endothelial glycocalyx: its effect on endothelial permeability. *Am J Physiol*. 1984;247:206.
37. Nanjo S, et al. Concentrated albumin does not affect lung edema formation after acid instillation in the dog. *Am Rev Respir Dis*. 1983;128:884.
38. Jones DC. Nonimmune fetal hydrops: diagnosis and obstetrical management. *Semin Perinatol*. 1995;19:447.
39. Carlton DP, et al. Nonimmune hydrops fetalis: a multidisciplinary approach. *Clin Perinatol*. 1989;16:839.
40. Carlton DP, et al. Lung vascular protein permeability in preterm fetal and mature newborn sheep. *J Appl Physiol*. 1994;77:782.
41. Phibbs RH, et al. Cardiorespiratory status of erythroblastotic newborn infants. II. blood volume, hematocrit, and serum albumin concentration in relation to hydrops fetalis. *Pediatrics*. 1974;53:13.
42. Gest AL, et al. Thoracic duct lymph flow in fetal sheep with increased venous pressure from electrically induced tachycardia. *Biol Neonate*. 1993;64:325.
43. Gest AL, et al. Atrial tachycardia causes hydrops in fetal lambs. *Am J Physiol*. 1990;258:1159.
44. Blair DK, et al. Hydrops in fetal sheep from rapid induction of anemia. *Pediatr Res*. 1994;35:560.
45. Moise AA, et al. Reduction in plasma protein does not affect body water content in fetal sheep. *Pediatr Res*. 1991;29:623.

Pathophysiology of Retinopathy of Prematurity

166

M. Elizabeth Hartnett

INTRODUCTION

Retinopathy of prematurity (ROP) is a leading cause of blindness in children worldwide and is increasing in emerging countries able to save premature infants but without resources to provide optimal care.[1,2] ROP, first identified as *retrolental fibroplasia* (RLF) in the United States, was reported by Terry[3] as a white mass behind the lens, which likely represented fibrovascular tissue and an underlying total retinal detachment. The cause was unknown, and studies in animals were done to understand causes.[4] It was not until the 1950s that Arnall Patz[5] observed that use of high oxygen concentrations in preterm infants without respiratory distress was associated with RLF. He performed a small clinical trial followed by a multicenter trial with Kinsey that showed high unregulated oxygen in preterm infants at birth was one cause of RLF.[5a] When oxygen was regulated, RLF virtually disappeared. However, additional advances in neonatology permitted ever smaller and younger preterm infants to survive, and the newly termed *ROP* reemerged[6] with earlier stages identified and classified.[7] We have since come to realize that high oxygen at birth is not the only factor in the pathophysiology of ROP in extremely premature infants nowadays.

ANATOMY AND GENERAL PHYSIOLOGY OF THE RETINA

The eye has unique optical properties allowing light to be focused onto the photoreceptors, which are deep within the layers of the neural retina (Fig. 166.1A). Two-thirds of the focusing power of the eye is attributed to the cornea and one-third to the lens. The cornea, lens, vitreous, and neural retina are transparent aside from retinal vessels that cast shadows on the retina and can be appreciated by optical coherence tomography (OCT), which provides structure of the retinal layers in vivo (see Fig. 166.1B). Once light is processed by photoreceptors through phototransduction, the signal is synaptically transmitted from the photoreceptors to bipolar cells and then from the bipolar cells to the ganglion cells. The axons of the ganglion cells create the optic "nerve," which comprises approximately 1 million nerve fibers that transmit the visual message through bundles and pathways in the brain to the occipital cortex, where the message is interpreted as vision. Signal processing through synaptic communication occurs within the retina through multiple distinct classes of cells that include different types of bipolar cells, amacrine cells, horizontal cells, and glia to result in increased synaptic gain (see Fig. 166.1A).[8]

The inner retina includes nine layers extending from the inner limiting membrane to the photoreceptors. The photoreceptor outer segments interact with the apical processes of a monolayer of epithelial cells, called the *retinal pigment epithelium (RPE)*, which has tight junctions and makes up the outer blood-retinal barrier. The basal side of the RPE rests on a collagen and elastin sandwich called *Bruch membrane* that includes the cell membranes of the fenestrated choriocapillaris (see Fig. 166.1C). The RPE performs multiple processes, including transport of substances from the inner retina to the outer choroidal circulation and from the choroid to the retina, important steps in the visual cycle; phagocytosis of the outer segments of the photoreceptors; and secretion of factors.[9]

On the scleral-most side of the Bruch membrane is the choriocapillaris. The choriocapillaris is one of three layers of the choroid, which has one of the highest blood flows of any tissue in the body, estimated to be 500 to 2000 mL/min/100 g tissue. The high flow of the choroid is believed to provide a heat sink for metabolic activities performed by the RPE. Besides heat, photooxidation in the outer retina also may increase oxidative stress. Mechanisms to reduce reactive oxygen are believed to include antioxidative properties of melanin within the RPE, inner retinal macular pigment (lutein and zeaxanthin), and absorbed ascorbate, tocopherol, and glutathione.

The photoreceptors are normally avascular and obtain nutrients and oxygen from the choroid. Based on studies in cats[10] and macaques,[11] the PO_2 of the retinal layers was determined. During dark adaption, approximately 90% of the oxygen to the photoreceptors is from choroid and 10% from the retina, whereas in light-adapted states, the choroid provides 100% of the oxygenation.[11] The retinal vasculature provides oxygenation of the inner retina from the ganglion cell layer to the inner nuclear layer and makes up the inner blood retinal barrier (see Fig. 166.1A). In adults, the retinal vasculature accounts for approximately 4% of the ocular blood flow (estimates of 40.8 to 52.9 μL/min).[12] The inner retinal oxygenation ranges from approximately 10 mm Hg in the light-adapted retina to approximately 20 mm Hg in the dark-adapted retina.[10] In the fovea, where the retina is thinner and devoid of vessels and inner retinal neurons, the oxygen consumption is lower than in the parafoveal region, where interneural connections exist, and suggests that interneural synaptic connections consume additional oxygen (see Fig. 166.1A).

DEVELOPMENT OF THE RETINA AND OCULAR VASCULATURES

Much of the understanding of the development of the retina and ocular circulations is assimilated from studies in human tissue, other species, and embryology.[13] Studies using animal models or genetically modified mice provide a deeper understanding of molecular mechanisms involved, although differences between human and other species need to be considered. An important difference is that the retinal vasculature is complete by term birth in the human but is incomplete in rodents, and for this reason full-term rodents are often exploited in studies related to vascular development and ROP. In human, immunohistochemical studies are helpful, but it is difficult to obtain autopsy tissue from preterm infant eyes that may characterize changes after birth and before the development of ROP, which occurs often 1 to 2 months after birth.

EMBRYOLOGY

The retina is first recognized as the optic pit in the anterior neuroectoderm at day 23 of gestation and develops into a two-layered structure of neural retina and the RPE known as the optic cup, which remains attached to the brain by an optic stalk. Continued growth of the optic cup causes the formation of a

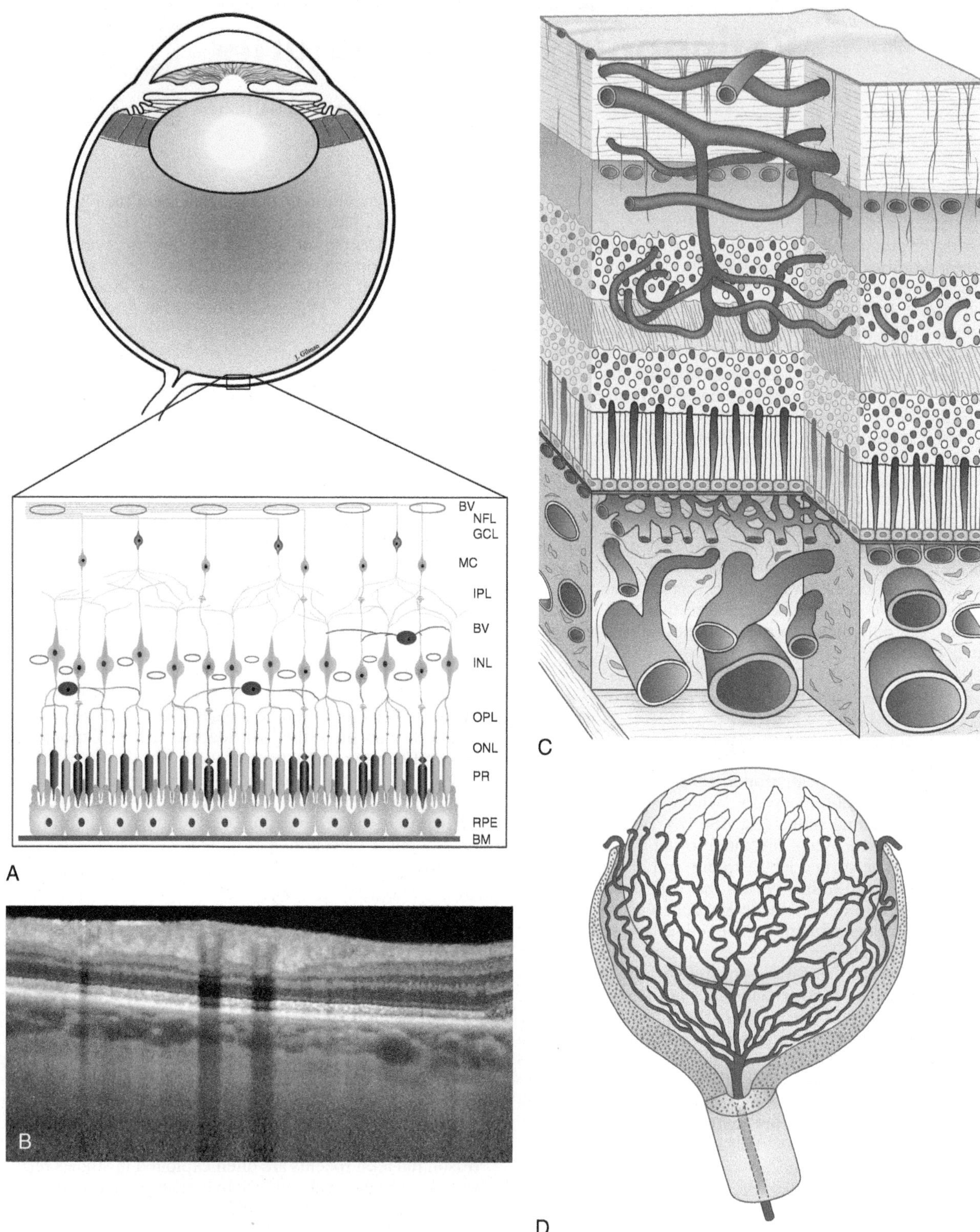

Fig. 166.1 (A) Cross sectional diagram *(bottom)* of the retina showing different layers of neurons and main two plexi of the retinal circulation. (B) Optical coherence tomography of retina showing shadowing of the deeper layers of retina by the retinal vessels. (C) Artist rendition of retinal and choroidal circulations. (D) Artist rendition of hyaloidal circulation. *BM*, Bruch membrane; *BV*, blood vessels; *GCL*, ganglion cell layer; *INL*, inner nuclear layer; *IPL*, inner plexiform layer; *MC,* Müller cells; *NFL*, nerve fiber layer; *ONL*, outer nuclear layer; *OPL*, outer plexiform layer; *PR*, photoreceptors; *RPE*, retinal pigment epithelium. Produced by James Gilman, CRA, FOPS. (A and B, Courtesy M. Elizabeth Hartnett, MD. Produced by James Gilman, CRA, FOPS. C and D, Illustrations adapted from Mann I. *Development of the Human Eye*. 3rd ed. Australia: Grune & Stratton; 1964.)

fissure that ultimately closes around day 33 and through which the hyaloidal artery enters the eye. The process is complicated and involves many coordinated cellular and molecular events. As neural layers form, synapses between retinal cells develop, and these processes drive metabolism and the need for oxygen.

OCULAR CIRCULATIONS

Oxygen is provided through the help of several circulations, the hyaloidal circulation, the choroidal circulation, and the retinal circulation. Each develops through one or more processes, namely hemovasculogenesis, vasculogenesis, or angiogenesis. Hemovasculogenesis is the development of vessels and all components of the blood system, including the hematopoietic and erythropoietic ones, from a common precursor called a *hemangioblast*. Vasculogenesis is the de novo development of vessels from mesenchymal precursor cells called *angioblasts*. Angiogenesis is the formation of vasculature by budding from existing vessels.

As the optic fissure closes, the hyaloidal circulation and primary vitreous form at approximately 4 to 5 weeks of age through hemovasculogenesis,[14,15] which becomes maximal at 2 to 3 months of age and then regresses by approximately 36 weeks gestation (see Fig. 166.1D). Several mechanisms involved in hyaloid regression were determined in murine eyes and included angiopoieitin-2–induced Wnt7b production by macrophages leading to endothelial cell arrest along with angiopoietin-2 suppression of Akt survival signaling[16] and neuronal activation of vascular endothelial growth factor receptor 2 (VEGFR2), thereby reducing the supply of vascular endothelial growth factor (VEGF) to maintain the hyaloid.[17] As the hyaloidal circulation regresses, the retinal vasculature begins to develop at about 12 to 14 weeks gestation.

The choroid also begins by hemovasculogenesis at close to the time of the hyaloidal circulation, approximately 5 weeks of age.[18,19] The choroid has three layers, the choriocapillaris, Sattler layer, and Haller layer. The choriocapillaris becomes fenestrated at 24 to 26 weeks gestation. The choroid matures from posterior (near the optic nerve) to the peripheral eye.

Finally, the retinal vasculature develops as the hyaloidal vessels regress. The retina initially develops by vasculogenesis, which is believed to support the posterior retina around the optic nerve (called the *posterior pole*) up to approximately 22 weeks gestational age (GA). Initially, angioblasts migrate toward the inner retina from the outer neuroblastic layer and express CD39 and CXCR4, which is the receptor for a stromal cell–derived factor (SDF-1).[14] Following vasculogenesis, the ensuing retina is vascularized by angiogenesis. Astrocytes and their precursors are also believed to be important, having been identified in advance of human retinal vessels.[20,21] These $PAX2^+$ nonendothelial cells migrate out and sense physiologic hypoxia. In response to hypoxia, the astrocytes upregulate VEGF, which is important in angiogenesis and in the development of the inner retinal vascular plexus that extends out to the ora serrata by 36 weeks gestation nasally and 40 weeks temporally (Fig. 166.2A).[22,23] The retinal circulation includes three main plexi, but other plexi have been identified in adults using OCT angiography. The inner plexus is completed prior to the deeper plexi. Müller cell glia are believed important in the development of the deeper retinal plexi.[24] These three vasculatures are tightly regulated to ensure oxygenation of the developing eye.

PATHOPHYSIOLOGY OF RETINOPATHY OF PREMATURITY

ASHTON'S ORIGINAL TWO-PHASED HYPOTHESIS

When RLF was identified in the United States, scientists exposed full-term healthy newborn animals to various stresses that premature infants then experienced to find out the cause. Several individuals are credited for identifying high oxygen at birth as damaging to newly developed retinal capillaries and include Michaelson, Campbell, and Ashton.[4] Ashton found that full-term newborn animals in 70% to 80% inspired oxygen (FiO_2) delivered continuously for 4 days developed "vasoobliteration" of newly formed capillaries. Weaning to ambient air led to "vasoproliferation" of endothelial cells onto the vitreous collagen (intravitreal neovascularization). Later fibrovascular contraction between the retina and vitreous led to complex retinal detachments.[25] Ashton's observations created the initial two-phase hypothesis of the pathogenesis of ROP: high oxygen caused phase I "vasoobliteration" and subsequent weaning to room air led to relative hypoxia and stimulation of phase II "vasoproliferation" from an angiogenic factor or factors. (We now know that hypoxia-inducible factors [HIFs] are stabilized in hypoxia and translocate to cell nuclei to transcribe a number of angiogenic factors,[26] most notably VEGF, erythropoietin, and angiopoietins.) Following seminal clinical trials by Patz and Kinsey,[5a] high oxygen at birth was found to cause RLF. With advancements in neonatal care, including the ability to regulate and monitor oxygen, RLF virtually disappeared, but with later survival of extremely premature infants, ROP reemerged.[6]

REFINED TWO-PHASED HYPOTHESIS OF CURRENT DAY RETINOPATHY OF PREMATURITY

A number of factors led to the need for a refined hypothesis of ROP. The adoption of indirect ophthalmoscopy by Schepens led to greater ability to examine the peripheral infant retina.[28] It became appreciated that extremely preterm infants born at or less than 28 weeks GA and who survived to develop ROP had incompletely vascularized retinas, which was expected because retinal vascular development is not complete until 36 to 40 weeks of gestation. In addition, other stresses besides high oxygen at birth were associated with ROP, including oxygen fluctuations, poor growth, and oxidative stress, and these factors were associated with delayed retinal vascular development.[29] Therefore the refined hypothesis includes phase I as not only high oxygen–induced damage to newly developed capillaries (compromised physiologic vascularity), but also delayed physiologic retinal vascular development, and phase II as vasoproliferation.[30]

DIFFERENCES IN RETINOPATHY OF PREMATURITY IN EMERGING COUNTRIES

The refined hypothesis relates to most developed countries that have resources for optimal prenatal and perinatal care, including the monitoring and regulation of oxygen. However, in emerging countries, ROP is on the rise because there are resources to save preterm infants but not to provide optimal prenatal nutrition, perinatal care, and regulate oxygen.[1,2] ROP then can have a component of oxygen-induced vasoobliteration,[31] also known as aggressive retinopathy of prematurity (A-ROP) for its rapidity of progression, as well as delayed physiologic retinal vascular development in phase I followed by vasoproliferation in phase II.

TWO-PHASE HYPOTHESIS AND CLINICAL CLASSIFICATION OF RETINOPATHY OF PREMATURITY

The two-phased hypothesis of ROP was formed 30 years before the International Classification of Retinopathy of Prematurity (ICROP) developed a clinical classification of stages of severity of disease, zone of ROP location on the retina, and vascular activity or Plus disease (Fig. 166.3).[7] This classification is used to describe levels of severity of disease, test treatments, and assess outcomes in clinical trials.

The ICROP terms can be related to the phases of ROP, including the refined hypothesis. Phase I corresponds to incomplete vascular development of the retina (no ROP) or stages 1 to 2 ROP without vascular activity. Phase II is vascular

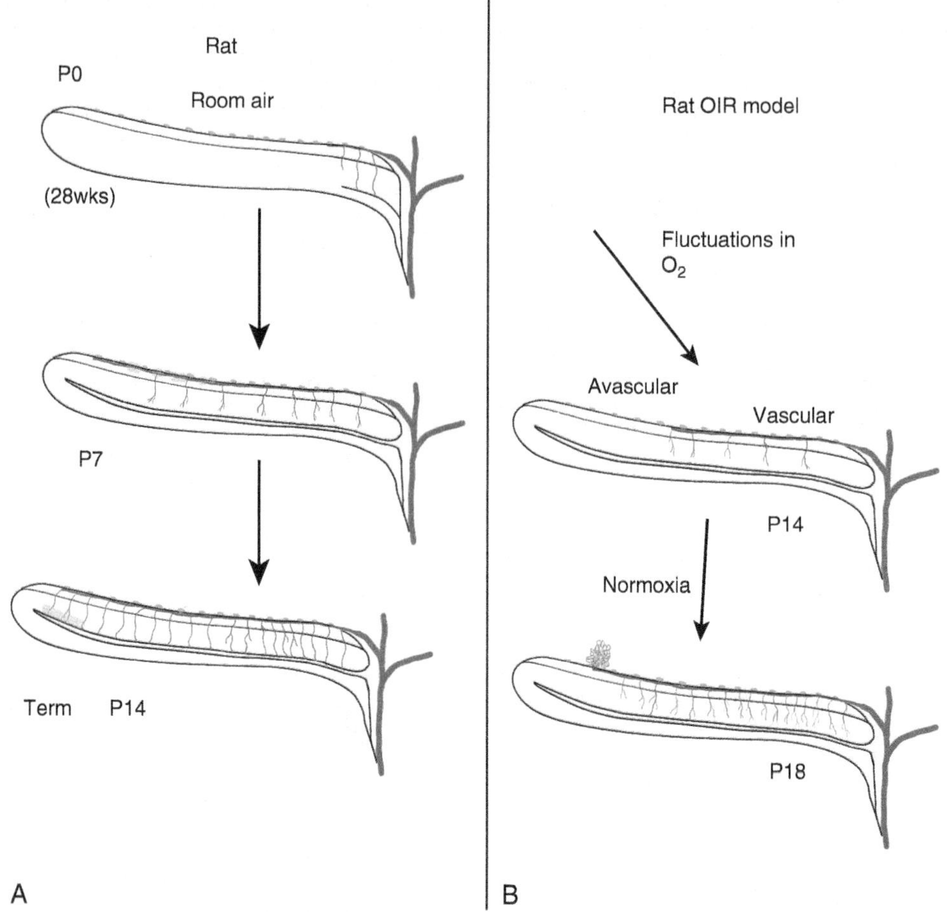

Fig. 166.2 (A) Retinal angiogenesis in a room air–raised rat extending to the ora serrata at several postnatal days designated by "P." (B) The rat oxygen-induced retinopathy *(OIR)* model shows compromised physiologic vascularity and peripheral avascular retina after repeated fluctuations in oxygen at P14, followed by intravitreal neovascularization at the junction of the vascularized and avascular retina at P18. (A, Courtesy M. Elizabeth Hartnett, MD. Produced by James Gilman, CRA, FOPS.)

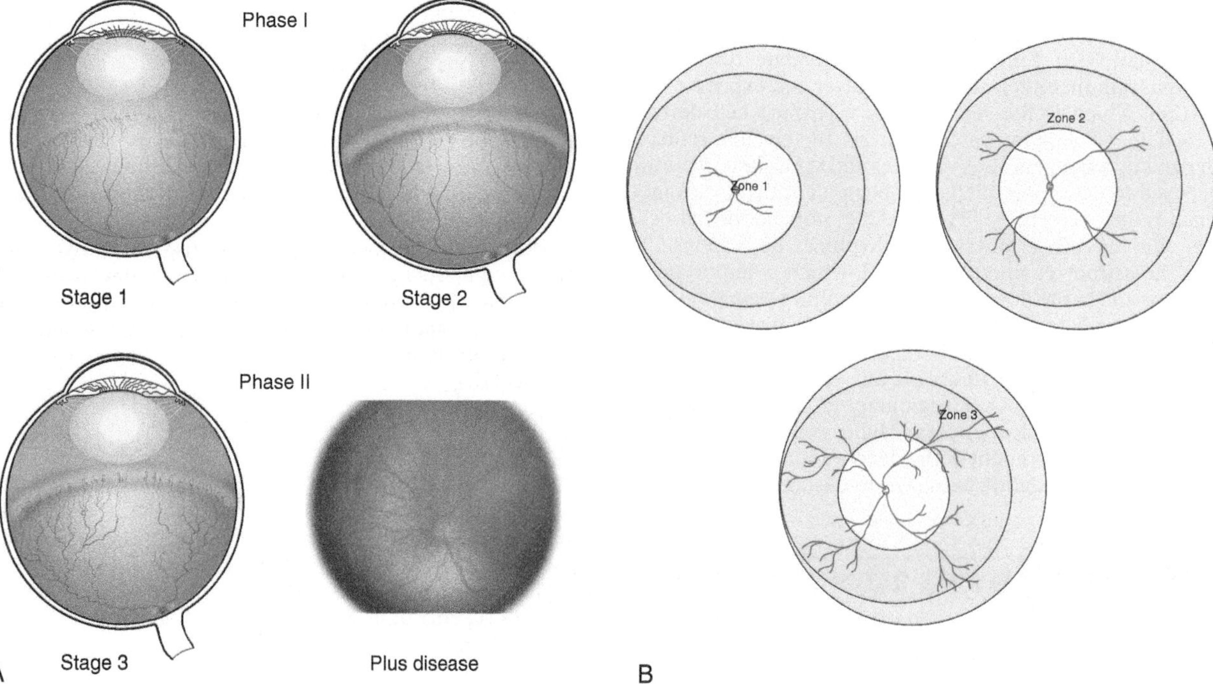

Fig. 166.3 (A) Clinical stages and phases of retinopathy of prematurity (ROP) of refined hypothesis. (B) Zones represent the extent of physiologic retinal vascular development and are used to describe the location of the stage of ROP. (Courtesy M. Elizabeth Hartnett, MD. Produced by James Gilman, CRA, FOPS.)

activity and/or stage 3 ROP (intravitreal neovascularization) (see Fig. 166.3). Animal models generally do not model stages 4 and 5 ROP, which describe different degrees of retinal detachment. The International Classification of ROP Study Group is revising the classification of ROP (ICROP3) to include new features, knowledge from imaging modalities and concepts of regression, and reactivation after treatment.

MODELS TO STUDY PATHOPHYSIOLOGY OF RETINOPATHY OF PREMATURITY

It is not possible to study molecular mechanisms of ROP in the human premature infant retina, so besides some studies in human tissue, others are performed in animals exposed to stresses similar to those experienced by premature infants.[32] Although there are similarities between models and human ROP, there are limitations. First, all animals used are full term. Second, there are not currently large animal models. Preterm lambs, which are intubated and maintained under conditions similar to a neonatal intensive care unit and used to study complications of prematurity,[33] do not develop ROP (personal observation).

Early studies in cats and current models in mice and beagles use constant high inspiratory oxygen concentrations, similar to ROP/RLF of the 1950s and are generally avoided nowadays. The mouse model of oxygen-induced retinopathy (OIR) exposes 7-day-old mice to constant 75% inspired oxygen (75% FiO_2) for 5 days, leading to central vasoobliteration of newly formed capillaries[34] followed by vasoproliferation upon return to room air. Because 7-day-old mice have most of their retinas already vascularized, this model does not test the effect of factors on peripheral retinal vascular development[34] but has the advantage of genetic manipulation to study mechanisms of high oxygen-induced vascular loss and angiogenesis. The rat model of OIR exposes newborn rats within approximately 6 hours of birth to FiO_2 fluctuating between 50% and 10% every 24 hours for 14 days, followed by room air exposure.[32] The animals develop compromise of the newly developed retinal vasculature (compromised physiologic vascularity) and delayed vascularization of the peripheral retina (see Fig. 166.2B). The rat OIR model has features representative of human ROP[35]: PaO_2 levels in the pups mimic extremes of transcutaneous oxygen measurements in human infants at risk of ROP[36]; pups experience poor postnatal growth similar to poor growth in human preterm infants at risk of ROP[37,38]; and the phases are similar to current day human ROP. The beagle OIR model also recapitulates the phases of ROP, including vasoobliteration and delay in physiologic retinal vascular development, and also includes a fibrovascular component of stage 4 ROP that cannot be created in other OIR models.[39–41] However, it exposes beagles to high constant oxygen, which is generally avoided in developed countries currently.

FACTORS AND MOLECULAR SIGNALING IN RETINOPATHY OF PREMATURITY PATHOPHYSIOLOGY

OXYGEN

Oxygen Levels in the Fetus and Preterm Infant

Estimates of normal oxygenation of the blood in the fetus are complex and have been based on animal studies. The umbilical artery blood has a PaO_2 of 15 to 25 mm Hg, and the umbilical vein is as high as 55 mm Hg.[42] Mixing of blood returning from the placenta with the inferior and superior vena cava through the foramen ovale and the less oxygenated blood from the pulmonary veins reduce oxygenation further. If an infant is resuscitated in 100% oxygen, there is a tremendous difference in oxygen levels compared with in utero. Even resuscitation in room air causes a change in oxygenation from the in utero environment. An FiO_2 of 80% is believed to be high enough to damage the newly developed capillaries of the retina.[43]

After birth, it is difficult to know the oxygenation of the retina in a preterm infant at any time, because there is currently not a method to measure this. For the past 7 months of gestation and up to 6 months postnatal life, fetal hemoglobin (HbF) is the primary oxygen transport protein in red blood cells. HbF has higher affinity for oxygen so that release of oxygen requires a lower tissue oxygenation than adult hemoglobin. Red blood cell HbF content in the infant differs by gestational and chronologic age and the number of blood transfusions received (which contain adult hemoglobin). There are also changes in cardiovascular parameters, heart rate, and blood flow, as well as pH, temperature, and anemia, which alter tissue extraction and delivery of oxygen. Finally, the retinal vasculature is developing and with fluctuations of oxygenation, there is a delay in physiologic retinal vascular development.[44]

Delivery of High Oxygen Concentrations at Birth

Although high concentrations of oxygen at birth are generally avoided, it continues to be a factor in emerging countries with the resources to save preterm infants but not the technology to monitor and regulate oxygen to the infants.[1,45] Preterm infants in these emerging countries at risk of ROP are often larger and of older GAs than those in the United States and developed countries, suggesting a repeat of what occurred in the United States in the 1940s.[45,46]

Evidence suggests high oxygen levels cause death of newly developed endothelial cells by apoptosis. In the mouse OIR model, the angiogenic factor VEGF appears to be a survival factor for newly developed capillaries when delivered during hyperoxia in phase I.[47] However, during relative retinal hypoxia, stimulation of VEGF expression causes vasoproliferation in phase II.[48] Thus VEGF is important for ongoing retinal vascular development in the human infant but also leads to vasoproliferation in phase II.

Clinical trials to target lower oxygen saturation have not yielded universal support. Three international randomized, controlled trials evaluated the effects of targeting an oxygen saturation of 85% to 89% SaO_2 compared with a range of 91% to 95% SaO_2 on disability-free survival at 2 years in infants born before 28 weeks gestation. In the Surfactant, Positive Pressure, and Pulse Oximetry Randomized Trial (SUPPORT) study, there was variability in overall survival of infants among various neonatal intensive care units (NICUs), suggesting differences in treatment interventions, the genetics, or other characteristics of the populations of premature infants.[49,50] In two of the trials (BOOST II and the Canadian Oxygen Trial),[51–53] the oximeter-calibration algorithm was revised halfway through the studies. Both the BOOST II and SUPPORT studies found reduced ROP but increased infant mortality in the infants in the 85% to 89% SaO_2 groups, and recruitment was stopped early in the BOOST II trial when an interim analysis showed an increased rate of death at 36 weeks in the group with a lower oxygen saturation target range.

A retrospective review of biphasic oxygen targets based on use of low oxygen saturation targets at postmenstrual ages less than 34 weeks and higher oxygen saturation targets after 34 weeks found reduced ROP compared to infants in static 91% to 95% SaO_2.[54] The study compared infants pre-SUPPORT and those post-SUPPORT, so there were also potential temporal differences in the infants in the two groups. However, further study of the effect of biphasic oxygen targets in a prospective trial is potentially warranted.

Fluctuations in Oxygenation

Treatment-warrantied ROP is associated with other risks besides high oxygen at birth and include fluctuations in transcutaneous and arterial oxygen.[36,55] The rat OIR model uses oxygen fluctuations in the newborn rat.[32] In the model, it was found that not only changes in retinal oxygenation affected the expression of angiogenic factors and inhibitors[56] but also that the repeated changes in oxygen levels activated oxidative signaling pathways. The activated pathways included nicotinamide adenine dinucleotide phosphate (NADPH) oxidase, in which generated reactive oxygen species led to angiogenesis.[57,58] The changes in oxygen levels in the retina changed the expression of VEGF with increased expression in hypoxia and reduced expression in hyperoxia. The expression of the angiostatic factor pigment epithelial-derived factor (PEDF) was not significantly changed by different oxygen levels in the rat ROP model.[59] At the time of phase I, delayed physiologic retinal vascular development and compromised physiologic vascularity, the VEGF/PEDF ratio unexpectedly favored angiogenesis. The VEGF/PEDF ratio also favored angiogenesis during phase II, vasoproliferation.[59] From these studies, VEGF appeared involved in both phases of OIR.

A study testing the expression of messenger RNA (mRNA) splice variants of VEGF found that repeated fluctuations in oxygen as opposed to a single episode of hypoxia increased the expression of the more prevalent $VEGF_{164}$ variant, whereas hypoxia increased $VEGF_{120}$.[60] Subsequent OIR studies that knocked down the full-length VEGF with lentiviral-delivered short hairpin RNAs (shRNAs) using cell specific promoters to Müller cells found evidence suggesting greater retinal neural damage than with partial knockdown of VEGF forms by targeting $VEGF_{164}$.[61] These studies supported others[62] in which VEGF was found to be neuroprotective to retina, but in this case in the setting of exposure to fluctuations in oxygenation. This line of evidence supports the line of thinking that a low dose of anti-VEGF to reduce intravitreal neovascularization but not damage the neural retina may be efficacious and safe in the treatment of ROP.

Hypoxia

Hypoxia stabilizes HIFs, which translocate to the nucleus to transcribe a number of angiogenic factors.[63] HIFs are degraded by prolyl hydroxylases; inhibiting prolyl hydroxylase during phase I in the murine OIR model reduced avascular retina from oxygen stresses and did not increase vasoproliferation.[64] HIFs may mediate protection against high oxygen-induced vascular loss, in part, by a change from oxidative to glycolytic metabolism that occurs in the liver.[65]

Oxidative Stress

The transition from a relatively hypoxic to a hyperoxic environment at birth increases the susceptibility to oxidative stress. Full-term birth increases oxidative stress, and the preterm infant is more susceptible because of insufficient development of antioxidant defenses and responses.[66,67] Antioxidant responses are reduced due to insufficient fetal availability, as well as lack of maternal sources often provided during the third trimester. Preterm infants also have lower mitochondrial function and are believed to require more glutathione. Therefore the premature infant has much oxidative susceptibility related to changes in oxygen content from in utero to post birth and also has fewer antioxidant reserves.[68]

Although both high oxygen and hypoxia can affect oxidation, the superoxide radical that forms in high oxygen is highly damaging. Hyperoxia-induced apoptosis has been identified in experimental models of OIR[69,70] and through inflammation mediated by leukocytes.[71] High oxygen can also interact with nitric oxide to produce damaging peroxynitrite.[72] However, nitric oxide can be beneficial as a vasodilator.

Besides the finding that oxidative compounds can damage tissue and cells, reactive oxygen species also act as signaling factors and trigger pathways to affect biologic outcomes.[73] A consequence of this is that systemic antioxidants that do not access intracellular compartments may not affect signaling mechanisms related to increased intracellular oxidative stress. This observation has been recognized with several studies testing antioxidants on ROP (e.g., n-acetylcysteine,[74] vitamin E[75]), in which there was limited effect. Some of the antioxidants, including vitamin E (tocopherol), had toxicity.[76]

One method being studied to stimulate oxidant defenses is the use of nuclear factor (erythroid-derived 2)-like 2 (Nrf2) agonists, which translocate to the DNA and are important in transcription of a number of antioxidant enzymes. Inhibition of NADPH oxidase has been associated with reduction in the area of avascular retina and in apoptosis in animal models.[77] NADPH oxidase has also been implicated in later aberrant angiogenesis through a pathway that involved endothelial cell STAT3, potentially independent from VEGF signaling.[57,78] Lutein and zeaxanthin reduce oxidative stress and provide macular pigment to the macula.[79]

Vascular Endothelial Growth Factor

Besides its role in pathologic retinovascular diseases in adults, VEGF is also important in both phases I and II in the murine, rat, and beagle OIR models.[40,41,48] In addition, VEGF expression has also been identified in a human preterm infant retina with ROP.[80] However, VEGF also is important in normal retinal vascular development. Therefore, VEGF inhibition may reduce both pathologic and developing physiologic angiogenesis and have more of an adverse effect than in adult retinovascular diseases. Because there are no large animal models of ROP that would better reflect human infant ROP, the rat model of OIR provides a model that represents several characteristics in human preterm infants at risk of severe ROP and that allows an understanding of the pathophysiology of ROP.

In the rat model of OIR, the expression of VEGF was increased by stresses that also affect premature infants at risk of ROP, including hypoxia, repeated oxygen fluctuations, and oxidative stress.[60,77,78,81,82] Furthermore, the retinal mRNAs of VEGF splice variants and VEGFR2, but not VEGFR1, were increased at time points in the rat model corresponding to phases I and II. By in situ hybridization, VEGF splice variants were localized to layers of the retina of the rat OIR model where Müller cell nuclei existed. Cell-specific promoters that drove shRNAs to knock down VEGF in Müller cells reduced retinal VEGF protein to levels similar to rats in room air of the same developmental ages and reduced phase II vasoproliferation without increasing phase I peripheral avascular retina. Endothelial cell-specific knockdown of VEGFR2 reduced phase II vasoproliferation and, surprisingly, reduced phase I peripheral avascular retina, thus increasing physiologic retinal vascularization.[82a] These findings provided evidence that inhibition of the angiogenic factor VEGF was associated with reduced vasoproliferation but also increased physiologic angiogenesis. The results also aligned with observations in some infants treated with intravitreal anti-VEGF agents.[83]

A single allele knockout of VEGF or a receptor is lethal. Thus an embryonic stem cell model with a knockout of VEGFR1 was used to cause VEGF to overactivate VEGFR2. Compared with control, dividing endothelial cells were disordered, causing a pattern similar to phase II vasoproliferation. The pattern was rescued with a transgene that expressed VEGFR1 in endothelial cells and normalized activation of VEGFR2. These data supported the concept that regulation of overactive VEGFR2 ordered developmental angiogenesis and provided an understanding of how VEGFR2 regulation would reduce pathologic angiogenesis and promote physiologic angiogenesis in ROP. Clinically, intravitreal neutralizing antibodies to VEGF are being studied in human ROP. However, the effect of an intravitreal antibody to neutralize VEGF is not specific to endothelial cell VEGFR2 but affects VEGF binding VEGFR2 on neurons and glia, where it may have a protective role. Studies of safety in premature infants are ongoing in clinical trials in the RAINBOW study[84] and the PEDIG studies of deescalating dose studies for bevacizumab.[85,86]

INFLAMMATION

Inflammation has been reported in association with ROP, and there are links between inflammatory cytokines and pathways related to oxidative stress. Staniocalcin-1 is a neuroprotective protein with both antiinflammatory and antioxidative properties that affect OIR-induced vasoproliferation by regulating VEGF.[87] Inflammatory or oxidative pathways can lead to pathology that predispose to angiogenesis or directly trigger signaling of angiogenic pathways.[88] The interleukin-1 receptor has been involved in vascular pathology in experimental models of OIR.[89,90]

POSTNATAL GROWTH AND NUTRITION/METABOLISM

Insulin-like Growth Factor-1

Insulin-like growth factor-1 (IGF-1), which is suppressed during starvation, is essential for muscle, bone, neural, and vascular growth during fetal life and for growth and remodeling postnatally, mediated mainly through the IGF-1 receptor (IGF-1R) and regulated by at least six IGF-binding proteins (BPs).[91]

IGF-1 is part of a family of polypeptides that are implicated in human fetal retinal neurovascular growth. IGF-1 serum levels fall rapidly after preterm birth due to loss of the maternal-fetal interaction.[91] The role of IGF-1 in retinal angiogenesis is supported by the observation that IGF-1 is required for maximum VEGF activation of vascular endothelial cell proliferation and survival pathways.[92,93] Replacement of IGF-1 to in utero levels in preterm infants may restore normal retinal neurovascular growth and prevent phase I (and thereby prevent phase II) of ROP. A phase II study of IGF-1 replacement (www.clinicaltrials.gov;#NCT01096784) was reported. The findings were encouraging for reducing lung disease and intraventricular hemorrhage but did not show reduced ROP. However, the supplementation of IGF-1 did not meet the target levels for individual infants and may have affected the outcomes on ROP. Additional study is planned.[94]

Role of Maternal Preeclampsia

Maternal preeclampsia increases the morbidity and mortality rates of infants and mothers.[95] It has been associated with increased risk of preterm birth, but there is conflicting evidence as to its role in ROP. Studies reported that preeclampsia was associated with either increased or decreased risk of ROP. Studies differ by the degree of prematurity of infants and how the analyses were performed. Because preeclampsia is closely aligned with preterm birth and preterm birth is necessary for the diagnosis of ROP, there also can be collider bias.[96,97] In a retrospective analysis of 290,992 live births over 10 years, preeclampsia was found to increase risk of ROP when births included all live births (preterm or full term) of mothers with or without preeclampsia. However, when a restricted subset of only preterm infants was included from the full cohort, preeclampsia appeared protective.[97] In an experimental model of uteroplacental insufficiency in rat dams followed by OIR in rat pups, retinopathy was less severe compared with dams undergoing anesthesia only. Further analysis found that erythropoietin was increased in the serum and kidneys of pups to a greater degree than was VEGF suggesting a potential protective effect from endogenous erythropoietin or other effects associated with ischemic preconditioning.[98] These findings suggest that some infants who are able to invoke protective mechanisms may not develop severe signs of ROP. These findings also highlight differences in preeclampsia associated with full-term compared with preterm birth.

Erythropoietin

Erythropoietin has been proposed to have neuroprotective effects and is being tested in human trials of premature infants. However, erythropoietin can increase angiogenesis and may worsen outcomes by increasing vasoproliferation in phase II. Some studies have found independent data of the use of erythropoietin in causing ROP.[99] However, a meta-analysis of studies has not found evidence for reduced or increased risk of ROP,[100] except for a trend toward stage 3 ROP if erythropoietin is given late in the neonatal course, but the quality of the data analyzed in the meta-analysis was deemed poor.[101] The Preterm Erythropoietin Neuroprotection Trial (PENUT) reported no difference in ROP outcomes in 24 to 27 6/7 week GA preterm infants who received erythropoietin (Epo, 6 doses of 1000U/kg at 48 hour intervals within the first 24 hours of birth), followed by subcutaneous Epo (400U/kg/dose three times a week until 32 6/7 weeks) compared with vehicle control.[101a]

Metabolism in Retinopathy of Prematurity

Enhancing retinal endothelial glycolysis by inhibiting the uncoupling protein 2 with a systemically delivered UCP2 inhibitor, genipin, was found to promote physiologic retinal vascular development experimentally.[102] This finding supports a role of energy regulation on retinal vascularization, an energy requiring process.

ω-3 Polyunsaturated Fatty Acids

Polyunsaturated fatty acids (PUFAs), both ω-3 and ω-6, have been studied with respect to the development of the brain and vision as well as of ROP.[103] Like IGF-I, ω-3 PUFA is depleted in preterm infants, who miss the normal massive transfer of PUFAs in the third trimester from mother to infant.[104] ω-3 PUFA is not found in most parenteral nutrition formulas given to preterm infants. Premature baboons showed declines in docosahexaenoic acid (DHA), which is one form of ω-3 PUFAs, and arachidonic acid (AA), a form of ω-6 PUFAs, in the retina, brain, liver, and plasma. Formula supplemented with DHA and AA significantly reduced declines in these tissues associated with premature birth compared with formula without supplementation.[105] These studies provide evidence that nutritional supplementation affects target tissues. ω-3 Fatty acids can reduce phase I and phase II in the mouse OIR model and may play a role in human infants,[104] and supplementation with both ω-3 and ω-6 PUFAs may offer a promising new therapy for the prevention of ROP.[106,106a]

GENETICS

There have been many studies assessing genetic variants associated with ROP. Studies are difficult to compare because they differ in the level of prematurity determined by GA and/or birth weight of infants. An infant with a genetic variant may not survive if born at a young GA and might at an older GA and then develop ROP. A number of candidate gene studies were done in small samples of infants in various locations throughout the world. Variants in *EPAS* (transcribes erythropoietin), several members of the Wnt signaling pathway, VEGF, superoxide dismutase, and others were identified in association with ROP. Variants of *FZD4* were also associated with larger infants having extremely severe ROP.[107] Variants in the Wnt signaling pathway can be associated with retinopathies that occur in full-term infants and include Norrie disease (variants in *NDP*, a ligand for the Wnt pathway) or familial exudative vitreoretinopathy (variants in *NDP*, or the co-receptors, *FZD4*, *LRP5* or a tetraspanin, *TSPAN12*). Therefore some infants with variants in genes of the Wnt signaling pathway may be predisposed to more severe ROP if they are born premature. In a study that analyzed blood spots from 1000 extremely premature infants in the Neonatal Research Network in the United States, variants in the intronic region of brain-derived neurotrophic factor *(BDNF)* were noted in association with ROP and severe ROP requiring treatment.[108,109]

LIGHT

Light and phototransduction are important in vision. Light also may increase oxidative stress. However, the retina is more metabolically active in the dark. A clinical trial tested the effect of light within the first 4 weeks of life or until 31 weeks postmenstrual age (the sum of gestational and chronologic ages in weeks) and did not find an effect on ROP by wearing of goggles that reduced visible light 97% and ultraviolet light by 100%.[110] A Cochrane review found no effect on ROP by light within the first week of life.[111]

Experimental studies have found that light through the maternal wall of a mouse dam can stimulate melanopsin-expressing ganglion cells and increase retinal hypoxia-induced

VEGF expression, which then leads to persistence of the hyaloid that affects physiologic retinal vascular development in the pups.[112] Neuropsin-dependent retinal light responses reduce vitreous dopamine and the regulation of VEGFR2 to interfere with hyaloid regression.[113] These studies show a potential role for light affecting retinal vascular development in the fetal eye. A retrospective study was performed in Cincinnati, which is located in a region of the world where the average light varies depending on the season.The investigators tested the hypothesis that infants in gestation with longer daylight would have more normal retinal vascular development (greater physiologic retinal vascular development in phase I) and therefore less hypoxia-induced vasoproliferation in phase II. A retrospective multiple logistic regression analysis of 343 premature infants found higher average day length reduced the likelihood of having severe ROP significantly.[114] Further study is warranted.

Some clinical studies have tried to incorporate a number of changes to reduce phase II ROP by optimizing hematocrit, affecting light and increasing oxygen to saturations just below 100% to reduce VEGF expression,[115] but controlled clinical trials are lacking to date.

CONCLUSION

The understanding of the pathophysiology of ROP requires review of the development of the retina, the intersection of development or regression of the ocular circulations and stresses associated with premature infant birth and perinatal course. The two-phased hypothesis of phase I, vasoobliteration, and phase II, vasoproliferation, has been refined with the survival of extremely low-birth-weight infants to include phase I, compromised physiologic vascularity and delayed physiologic retinal vascular development, and phase II, vasoproliferation. Although many external factors and molecular mechanisms are involved, VEGF remains an important angiogenic factor in both vasoproliferation and normal vascular development. Based on representative experimental models of human ROP, regulation of signaling in endothelial cell VEGFR2 both inhibits pathologic vasoproliferation and supports physiologic retinal vascular development, whereas broad inhibition of the ligand, VEGF, with intravitreal neutralizing antibodies may have adverse effects on the neural or glial retina. Other factors such as IGF-1 or nutritional supplements including ω-3 and ω-6 polyunsaturated fatty acids may be neuroprotective or provide support to the development of the retina. The complexity and changing environment of the premature infant make the area of study challenging and constantly evolving.

ACKNOWLEDGMENTS

The authors thank Maria Isabel Gomez for her expert help in organization and formatting the manuscript.

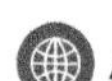
A complete reference list is available at www.ExpertConsult.com.

SELECT REFERENCES

2. Gilbert C, Malik ANJ, Nahar N, et al. Epidemiology of ROP update - Africa is the new frontier. *Semin Perinatol*. 2019;43:317-322.
4. Hartnett ME. Advances in understanding and management of retinopathy of prematurity. *Surv Ophthalmol*. 2017;62:257-276.
5. Kinsey VE. Retrolental fibroplasia: cooperative study of retrolental fibroplasia and the use of oxygen. *AMA Arch Ophthalmol*. 1956;56(4):481-543.
7. International Committee for the Classification of Retinopathy of Prematurity. The international classification of retinopathy of prematurity revisited. *Arch Ophthalmol*. 2005;123:991-999.
10. Linsenmeier RA, Braun RD. Oxygen distribution and consumption in the cat retina during normoxia and hypoxemia. *J Gen Physiol*. 1992;99:177-197.
12. Riva CE, Alm A, Pournaras CJ. Ocular circulation. In: Levin LA, Ver Hoeve J, Wu SM, eds. *Adler's Physiology of the Eye*. Philadelphia: Elsevier; 2011: 243-273.
13. Mann I. *Development of the Human Eye*. 3rd ed. Australia: Grune & Stratton; 1964.
19. Lutty GA, McLeod DS. Development of the hyaloid, choroidal and retinal vasculatures in the fetal human eye. *Prog Retin Eye Res*. 2018;62:58-76.
20. Chan-Ling T, McLeod DS, Hughes S, et al. Astrocyte-endothelial cell relationships during human retinal vascular development. *Invest Ophthalmol Vis Sci*. 2004;45:2020-2032.
22. Chan-Ling T, Stone J. Retinopathy of prematurity: origins in the architecture of the retina. *Prog Retin Eye Res*. 1993;12:155-178.
25. Ashton N, Ward B, Serpell G. Effect of oxygen on developing retinal vessels with particular reference to the problem of retrolental fibroplasia. *Br J Ophthalmol*. 1954;38:397-432.
26. Semenza GL. Hypoxia-inducible factor 1 and the molecular physiology of oxygen homeostasis. *J Lab Clin Med*. 1998;131:207-214.
27. Kinsey VE, Arnold HJ, Kalina RE, et al. PaO2 levels and retrolental fibroplasia: a report of the cooperative study. *Pediatrics*. 1977;60:655-668.
29. Hartnett ME. Discovering mechanisms in the changing and diverse pathology of retinopathy of prematurity: the Weisenfeld Award Lecture. *Invest Ophthalmol Vis Sci*. 2019;60:1286-1297.
30. Hartnett ME, Penn JS. Mechanisms and management of retinopathy of prematurity. *N Engl J Med*. 2012;367:2515-2526.
32. Penn JS, Tolman BL, Lowery LA. Variable oxygen exposure causes preretinal neovascularisation in the newborn rat. *Invest Ophthalmol Vis Sci*. 1993;34:576-585.
35. Hartnett ME. Pathophysiology and mechanisms of severe retinopathy of prematurity. *Ophthalmology*. 2015;122:200-210.
36. Cunningham S, Fleck BW, Elton RA, et al. Transcutaneous oxygen levels in retinopathy of prematurity. *Lancet*. 1995;346:1464-1465.
37. Lofqvist C, Andersson E, Sigurdsson J, et al. Longitudinal postnatal weight and insulin-like growth factor I measurements in the prediction of retinopathy of prematurity. *Arch Ophthalmol*. 2006;124:1711-1718.
39. Lutty GA, McLeod DS, Bhutto I, et al. Effect of VEGF trap on normal retinal vascular development and oxygen-induced retinopathy in the dog. *Invest Ophthalmol Vis Sci*. 2011;52:4039-4047.
42. Murphy PJ. The fetal circulation. *CEACCP*. 2005;5:107-112.
43. Flynn JT, Bancalari E, Snyder ES, et al. A cohort study of transcutaneous oxygen tension and the incidence and severity of retinopathy of prematurity. *N Engl J Med*. 1992;326:1050-1054.
47. Alon T, Hemo I, Itin A, et al. Vascular endothelial growth-factor acts as a survival factor for newly formed retinal-vessels and has implications for retinopathy of prematurity. *Nat Med*. 1995;1:1024-1028.
49. SUPPORT Study Group of the Eunice Kennedy Shriver NICHD Neonatal Research Network, Carlo WA, Finer NN, et al. Target ranges of oxygen saturation in extremely preterm infants. *N Engl J Med*. 2010;362:1959-1969.
50. Alleman BW, Bell EF, Li L, et al. Individual and center-level factors affecting mortality among extremely low birth weight infants. *Pediatrics*. 2013;132:e175-e184.
51. Schmidt B, Whyte RK, Asztalos EV, et al. Effects of targeting higher vs lower arterial oxygen saturations on death or disability in extremely preterm infants: a randomized clinical trial. *J Am Med Assoc*. 2013;309:2111-2120.
53. BOOST II United Kingdom Collaborative Group, BOOST II Australia Collaborative Group, BOOST II New Zealand Collaborative Group, et al. Oxygen saturation and outcomes in preterm infants. *N Engl J Med*. 2013;368:2094-2104.
55. York JR, Landers S, Kirby RS, et al. Arterial oxygen fluctuation and retinopathy of prematurity in very-low-birth-weight infants. *J Perinatol*. 2004;24:82-87.
56. Werdich XQ, McCollum GW, Rajaratnam VS, et al. Variable oxygen and retinal VEGF levels: correlation with incidence and severity of pathology in a rat model of oxygen-induced retinopathy. *Exp Eye Res*. 2004;79:623-630.
57. Saito Y, Uppal A, Byfield G, et al. Activated NAD(P)H oxidase from supplemental oxygen induces neovascularization independent of VEGF in retinopathy of prematurity model. *Invest Ophthalmol Vis Sci*. 2008;49:1591-1598.
58. Hartnett ME. The effects of oxygen stresses on the development of features of severe retinopathy of prematurity: knowledge from the 50/10 OIR model. *Doc Ophthalmol*. 2010;120:25-39.
60. McColm J, Geisen P, Hartnett M. VEGF isoforms and their expression after a single episode of hypoxia or repeated fluctuations between hyperoxia and hypoxia: relevance to clinical ROP. *Mol Vis*. 2004;10:512-520.
61. Becker S, Wang H, Simmons AB, et al. Targeted knockdown of overexpressed VEGFA or VEGF164 in Muller cells maintains retinal function by triggering different signaling mechanisms. *Sci Rep*. 2018;8:2003.
62. Nishijima K, Ng YS, Zhong LC, et al. Vascular endothelial growth factor-A is a survival factor for retinal neurons and a critical neuroprotectant during the adaptive response to ischemic injury. *Am J Pathol*. 2007;171:53-67.
63. Semenza GL. Hydroxylation of HIF-1: oxygen sensing at the molecular level. *Physiology*. 2004;19:176-182.
70. Uno K, Merges CA, Grebe R, et al. Hyperoxia inhibits several critical aspects of vascular development. *Dev Dyn*. 2007;236:981-990.
73. Wang H, Zhang SX, Hartnett ME. Signaling pathways triggered by oxidative stress that mediate features of severe retinopathy of prematurity. *JAMA Ophthalmol*. 2013;131:80-85.
77. Saito Y, Geisen P, Uppal A, et al. Inhibition of NAD(P)H oxidase reduces apoptosis and avascular retina in an animal model of retinopathy of prematurity. *Mol Vis*. 2007;13:840-853.
78. Byfield G, Budd S, Hartnett ME. The role of supplemental oxygen and JAK/STAT signaling in intravitreous neovascularization in a ROP rat model. *Invest Ophthalmol Vis Sci*. 2009;50:3360-3365.
83. Mintz-Hittner HA, Kennedy KA, Chuang AZ, et al. Efficacy of intravitreal bevacizumab for stage 3+ retinopathy of prematurity. *N Engl J Med*. 2011;364:603-615.

84. Stahl A, Lepore D, Fielder A, et al. Ranibizumab versus laser therapy for the treatment of very low birthweight infants with retinopathy of prematurity (RAINBOW): an open-label randomised controlled trial. *Lancet*. 2019;394:1551-1559.
86. Wallace DK, Dean TW, Hartnett ME, et al. A dosing study of bevacizumab for retinopathy of prematurity: late recurrences and additional treatments. *Ophthalmology*. 2018;125:1961-1966.
91. Hard AL, Smith LE, Hellstrom A. Nutrition, insulin-like growth factor-1 and retinopathy of prematurity. *Semin Fetal Neonatal Med*. 2013;18:136-142.
96. Shulman JP, Weng C, Wilkes J, et al. Association of maternal preeclampsia with infant risk of premature birth and retinopathy of prematurity. *JAMA Ophthalmol*. 2017;135:947-953.
97. Greene T, Hartnett ME. Programming error led to underestimate of effect sizes in study of association of maternal preeclampsia and risk of infant retinopathy of prematurity. *JAMA Ophthalmol*. 2019;137:119.
98. Becker S, Wang H, Yu B, et al. Protective effect of maternal uteroplacental insufficiency on oxygen-induced retinopathy in offspring: removing bias of premature birth. *Sci Rep*. 2017;7:42301.
103. Connor KM, SanGiovanni JP, Lofqvist C, et al. Increased dietary intake of omega-3-polyunsaturated fatty acids reduces pathological retinal angiogenesis. *Nat Med*. 2007;13:868-873.
109. Hartnett ME, Morrison MA, Smith S, et al. Genetic variants associated with severe retinopathy of prematurity in extremely low birth weight infants. *Invest Ophthalmol Vis Sci*. 2014;55:6194-6203.
112. Rao S, Chun C, Fan J, et al. A direct and melanopsin-dependent fetal light response regulates mouse eye development. *Nature*. 2013;494:243-246.
115. Gaynon MW, Wong RJ, Stevenson DK, et al. Prethreshold retinopathy of prematurity: VEGF inhibition without VEGF inhibitors. *J Perinatol*. 2018;38:1295-1300.

Pathophysiology of Neonatal Hypoxic-Ischemic Brain Injury

167

Vadim S. Ten

INTRODUCTION

The pathophysiology of neonatal hypoxic-ischemic (HI) brain injury or hypoxic-ischemic encephalopathy (HIE) defines the response of central nervous system (CNS) to ischemia and reperfusion. Neonatal HI brain injury usually occurs due to a collapse of systemic circulation at or near birth or during the neonatal period. If not interrupted, HI insult can be lethal. If the systemic circulation is restored in timely fashion, then full or partial recovery of the brain and other organs is expected. The extent of this recovery will determine the absence or presence, as well as the severity of HIE. Thus the return of the systemic and cerebral circulation (reperfusion) defines the disease state following HI insult. Because the brain is extremely sensitive to ischemic injury, neurologic outcome following neonatal HI remains a major clinical concern. What determines the risk for HIE?

Analysis of neonatal outcomes of cesarean deliveries associated with maternal cardiovascular crisis revealed that, when delivered within 5 minutes of maternal circulatory arrest, 70% of infants were free of neurologic sequelae. However, if the delivery was delayed by 6 to 10 minutes, only 13% of infants developed normally.[1] Models of neonatal asphyxia and cerebral ischemia-reperfusion demonstrated that the length of ischemia is the most critical determinant of severity of injury.[2-4] The quality of reperfusion also has significant impact on the extent of cerebral damage. Even brief ischemic insults followed by suboptimal oxygen redelivery upon reperfusion may cause surprisingly extensive cerebral tissue loss.[5] On the other hand, when the length of neonatal ischemic event extends over 5 to 7 minutes at physiologic temperature,[6,7] reperfusion contributes to both cellular recovery and injury via mechanisms driven by reintroduction of oxygen and energy substrates (e.g., oxidative stress and apoptosis). Thus, two interconnected biologic processes, ischemia and reperfusion, serve as pathologic ground for evolution of HIE. A pathophysiologic essence of ischemia is primary energy failure driven by acute oxygen and substrate deprivation. The pathophysiology of reperfusion is more complex, as reperfusion initiates both cellular recovery and may be detrimental to cellular recovery mechanisms (Fig. 167.1).

ISCHEMIA: PRIMARY ENERGY FAILURE AND METABOLIC CHANGES

Primary energy failure is characterized by acute depletion of high-energy phosphates, adenosine triphosphate (ATP) and phosphocreatine (PCr) in the brain. Absence of the oxygen results in cessation of electron transport in the mitochondrial respiratory chain (Fig. 167.2). Therefore, mitochondrial complexes cannot pump out protons from the matrix space into intermembrane space and maintain a proton gradient (proton motive force) across the inner mitochondrial membrane. Without this proton motive force, phosphorylation of adenosine-diphosphate (ADP) to ATP by ATP-synthase is impossible. This defines an energy failure state. Once circulation is failed, a bioenergetic crisis develops very quickly; significant depletion of PCr, ATP, and elevation of ADP and adenosine monophosphate (AMP) occurs in 10 seconds and profound depletion of energy charges ensures within 5 to 7 minutes of an acute ischemic insult.[5] For a short time, hydrolysis of residual ATP stores and the use of PCr for phosphorylation of ADP partially supports cellular energy demand. Meanwhile, anaerobic glycolysis becomes the main mechanism of energy production. In neonates, cerebral immaturity is associated with poorer efficiency of glycolysis compared to the mature brain. Neonatal rats subjected to HI demonstrated limited activation of anaerobic glycolysis in their brains due to developmental deficiency of the glucose transporter proteins.[8] This suggests that in the developing brain, the acuity of primary energy failure may be greater compared to the mature CNS. The immediate sequelae of primary bioenergetic crisis is a failure of cellular structure and function-maintaining ion pumps, such as $Na\text{-}K^+$ ATPase, leading to a loss of ion gradient across cellular membrane, depolarization, and cytotoxic swelling. Experimental and clinical research offers clear evidence for a strong association between the severity of primary bioenergetic crisis and poor neurologic prognosis following neonatal asphyxia.[9-11] In addition to primary energy failure, other fundamental biochemical responses to ischemia extend their contribution to injury into the reperfusion stage of the disease.

Acute oxygen deprivation results in a complete reduction of the electron-transferring components; flavins; iron-sulfur clusters; coenzyme Q; and cytochromes *a*, *b*, and *c*, in the mitochondrial

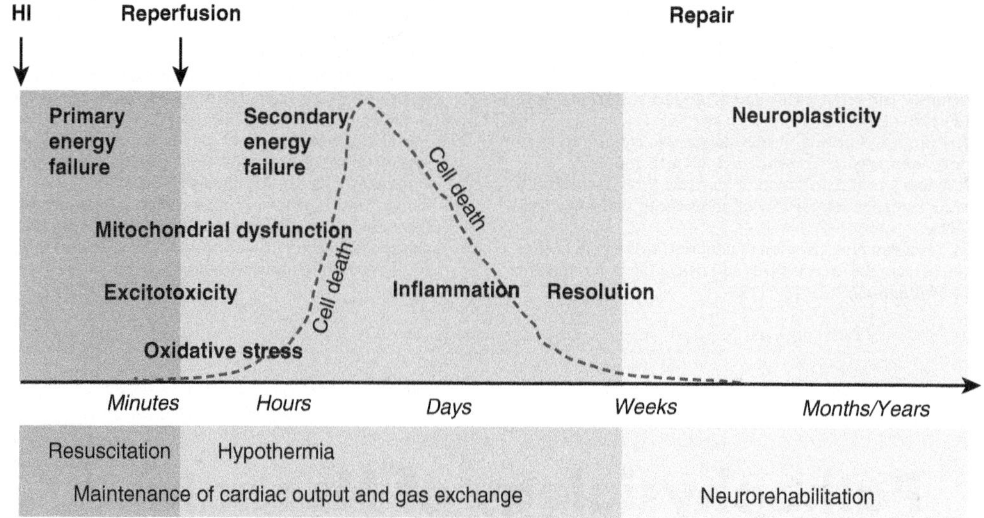

Fig. 167.1 Schematic evolution of neonatal hypoxic-ischemic *(HI)* injury with depicting stages and major events participating in cellular death and cerebral recovery.

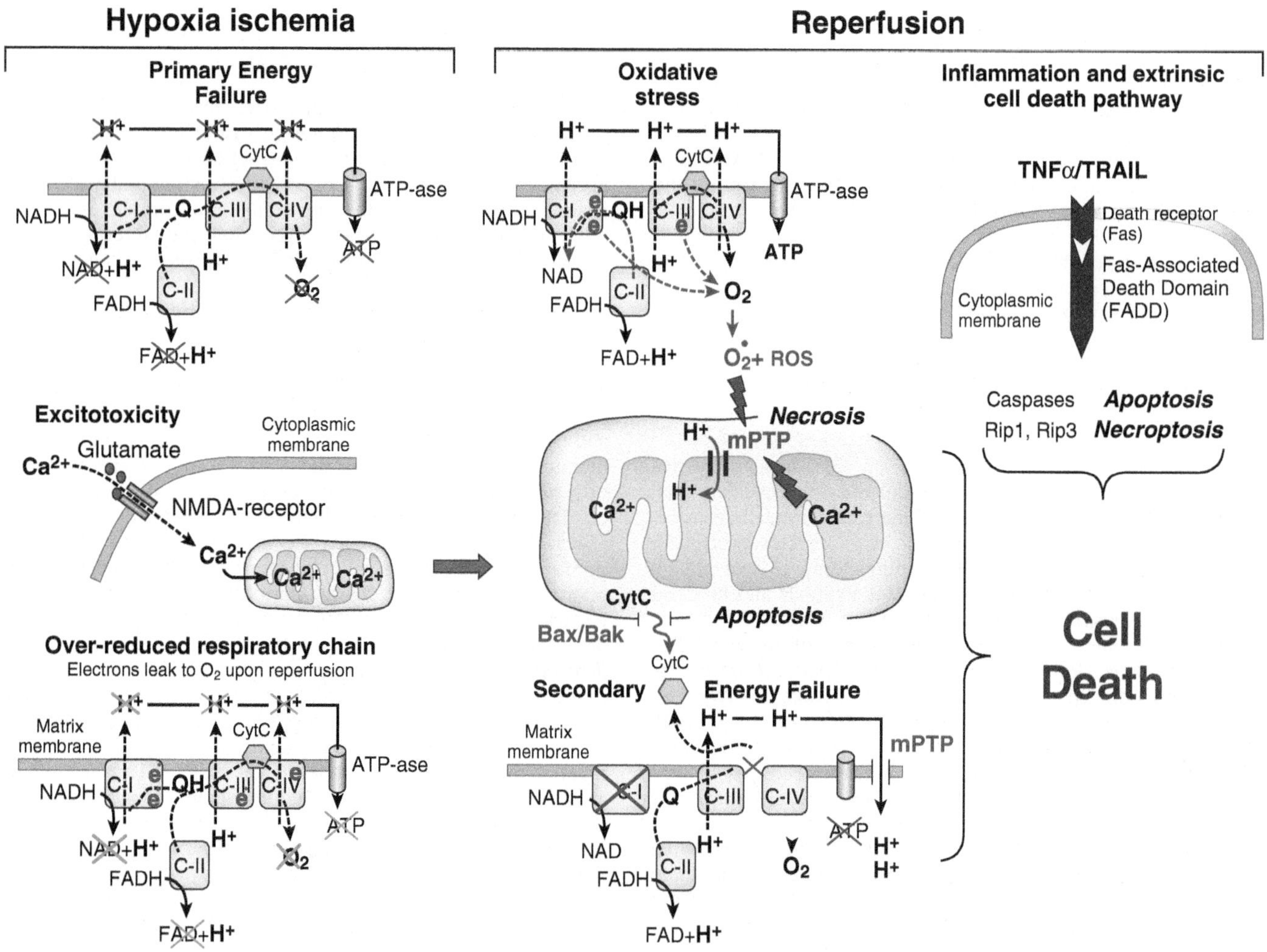

Fig. 167.2 The diagram of major events connecting proposed mechanisms of cellular death during neonatal hypoxia ischemia and reperfusion. *ATP*, Adenosine triphosphate; *FADH*, flavin adenine dinucleotide + $2H^+$; *mPTP*, mitochondrial permeability transition pore; *NADH*, nicotinamide adenine dinucleotide + H^+; *NMDA*, *N*-methyl-D-aspartate; *ROS*, reactive oxygen species.

respiratory chain (see Fig. 167.2). Primary Krebs cycle electron donors (NADH and $FADH_2$) are also fully reduced. Ischemic over-reduction of NAD^+ to NADH contributes to inhibition of glycolytic ATP generation, as oxidation of glyceraldehyde 3-phosphate requires NAD^+. Next, upon reperfusion-driven reintroduction of oxygen, in special circumstances, fully reduced redox centers (electron carriers), like flavins and quinones, may leak electrons onto oxygen, producing superoxide.[12] Thus over-reduction of electron carriers during ischemia predisposes the respiratory chain to excessive electron leak and formation of oxidative radicals during reperfusion (see Fig. 167.2).

Anaerobic glycolysis produces not only ATP but also lactate, as the ischemia inhibits pyruvate dehydrogenase complex[13] and inhibits the respiratory chain. As a result, pyruvate cannot be utilized in the Krebs cycle and is shunted into lactic acid. Even in the absence of any substrate delivery, the preischemic glucose and glycogen levels are sufficient to increase tissue lactate from 1.5 to 12 to 14 μmole/g within 2 to 3 minutes.[14] In isolated brain mitochondria, lactic acidosis inhibits the respiratory chain,[15] contributing to ischemic bioenergetic collapse. In developing and mature brains, ischemia also results in a dramatic (approximately 30-fold) accumulation of succinate, while the levels of other Krebs cycle intermediates are depleted.[16-18] These metabolic changes has been proposed as mechanistic factors predisposing to oxidative stress upon reperfusion.[18,19]

On a cellular level, ischemia causes over-excitation of neurons and oligodendrocytes, the event driven by excessive release of neurotransmitters (glutamate) and bioenergetic failure of glutamate reuptake.[20] Glutamate release and activation of the glutamate receptors, *N*-methyl-D-aspartate (NMDA) and AMPA, α-amino-3-hydroxy-5-methyl-4-isoxazolepropionic acid, initiates an excitotoxic cascade where downstream cellular Ca^{2+} influx plays a central role in cellular damage during reperfusion.[21-23] Thus in addition to primary energy failure, ischemia sets in motion biochemical changes that limit cellular bioenergetic restoration and cellular recovery upon reperfusion.

REPERFUSION: SECONDARY ENERGY FAILURE

The concept of secondary energy failure rests on experimental and clinical data demonstrating brisk, near-full or partial restoration of high-energy phosphates in the ischemic brain upon reperfusion.[10,24-26] These data imply that upon oxygen and substrates redelivery, postischemic mitochondria are capable of ATP generation. However, following few hours of reperfusion, 6 to 8 hours in human neonates,[27] cerebral bioenergetics progressively decline, evidenced by secondary depletion of high-energy charges in the postischemic brain. The mechanism of secondary energy failure closely relates to changes in mitochondrial capacity to generate ATP during reperfusion. In the Rice-Vannucci model of neonatal HI-brain injury (ligation of the common carotid artery and exposure to hypoxia), cerebral mitochondria, isolated immediately after the insult, exhibited significantly decreased respiratory control ratio (a measure of mitochondrial coupling) mostly due to inhibited phosphorylating respiration.[28,29] At 3 hours postreperfusion, the mitochondrial phosphorylating respiration and respiratory control ratio had partially recovered.[28] In the same mouse model, when tested at 30 minutes of reperfusion, post-HI mitochondria exhibited near-full restoration of their ADP-phosphorylating capacity.[29] In mature gerbils, after 30 minutes of global brain ischemia, at 5 to 30 minutes of reperfusion, mitochondrial respiration fully regained their capacity to phosphorylate ADP, which was significantly depressed immediately after ischemic insult. However, at 120 minutes of reperfusion there was a secondary decline in mitochondrial phosphorylating activity.[30] These reperfusion-associated changes in mitochondrial respiration were paralleled by similar changes in enzymatic activities of respiratory chain complexes I to III, but not complex IV.[19,30] Regardless of the extent of mitochondrial functional recovery, these and other studies[31] have shown reproducible restoration of oxidative phosphorylation after HI followed by a progressive decline of mitochondrial function after few hours of reperfusion (i.e., secondary energy failure).

To understand a pathogenic significance of secondary energy failure, we need to determine whether secondary bioenergetics crisis contributes to the evolution of cellular injury or simply reflects metabolic shutdown in the dying tissue. Vannucci and colleagues examined temporal changes in the brain high-energy phosphates reserves and markers of neuronal damage during post-HI reperfusion. Based on the close association of PCr levels with the loss of neuronal protein markers and cerebral injury scores at 6 to 18 and at 24 to 48 hours of reperfusion, the authors proposed that secondary energy failure represents the consequence, rather than the cause of ultimate cellular death.[26] Others also reported a temporal association between neuronal protein (microtubule-associated protein 2 [MAP2]) loss, caspase 3 activation, and secondary mitochondrial dysfunction. Importantly, caspase 3 activation was detected at the time-point of reperfusion, when mitochondria exhibited near-normal respiratory activity, suggesting that activation of this cell death pathway precedes secondary mitochondrial dysfunction.[28] To link the evolution of HI brain injury to cellular bioenergetics, the mitochondrial morphologic and functional changes in the brains that ultimately developed infarcts were analyzed. Immediately after the HI-insult, mice exhibited no injury and electron microscopy of mitochondria isolated from the same postischemic hemisphere demonstrated no readily detectable morphologic changes compared to controls (Fig. 167.3B). However, mitochondrial phosphorylating respiration was significantly depressed compared to control organelles (see Fig. 167.3C). At 30 minutes of reperfusion, in the absence of detectable damage, mitochondria isolated from ischemic hemisphere exhibited near-full recovery of ADP-phosphorylating respiration (see Fig. 167.3C). Electron microscopy, however, revealed pathologic swelling of some organelles. At 4 hours of reperfusion, tri-phenyl-tetrazolium chloride staining detected an evolving brain infarct (see Fig. 167.3B). This was coupled with secondary depression of mitochondrial respiration (see Fig. 167.3C) and a loss of mitochondrial matrix integrity and swelling. At 12 hours, there was a clearly identified infarct, severely depressed mitochondrial respiration, and extensive organelle disintegration (see Fig. 167.3B and C). Close temporal relationships between mitochondrial swelling, the secondary decline in mitochondrial phosphorylating respiration, and evolution of the infarct suggests that secondary mitochondrial dysfunction may contribute to the reperfusion brain injury following HI insult. Of note, neuroprotective action post-HI hypothermia has been linked to a decreased cellular energy demand in asphyxiated neonates.[32] To clarify the role of secondary energy failure in HI brain injury we need better understanding the mechanisms of secondary mitochondrial dysfunction.

MITOCHONDRIAL PERMEABILITY TRANSITION PORE AND SECONDARY ENERGY FAILURE

Mitochondrial matrix content is isolated from cytosol by two membranes, the ion-impermeable inner membrane and outer mitochondrial membrane, which is ion-permeable via voltage-dependent anion-selective channel (VDAC) (see Fig. 167.3A).[33] The import of nuclear-coded proteins for mitochondria is assisted by the translocase of the outer membrane (TOM) and by the translocase of the inner membrane (TIM). These translocases control movement of proteins through the mitochondrial membranes. Impermeability of the inner mitochondrial membrane for ions/protons supports the proton motive force for ATP-synthase

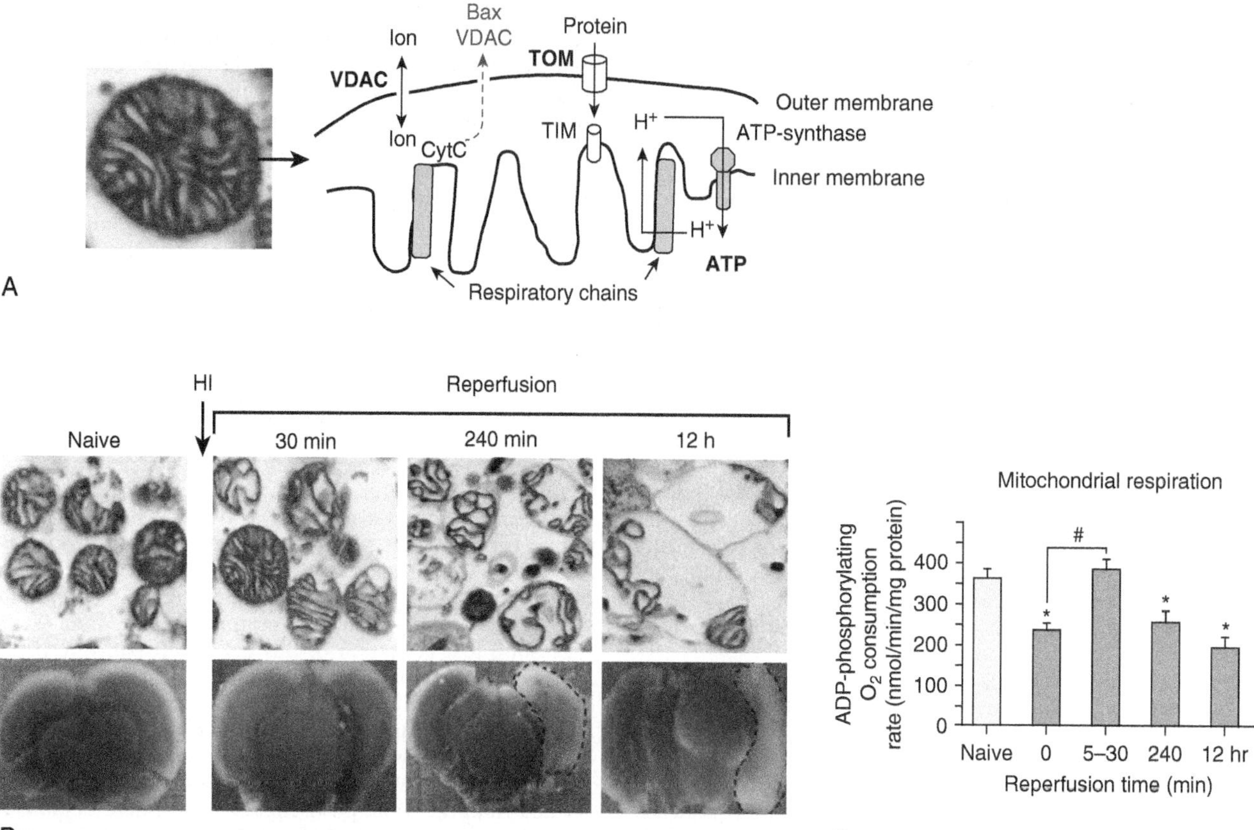

Fig. 167.3 Schema of mitochondrial intermembrane space with systems providing ion exchange (*VDAC*, voltage dependent anion channel), protein import (translocator of the outer and inner membrane, *TOM/TIM*), matrix located structures for oxidative phosphorylation. Pathologic Bax/VDAC interaction driven permeabilization of the outer membrane is colored in *red* (A). Electron microscopy of mitochondria isolated from the injured hemisphere with outlined infarcts during reperfusion (B) and adenosine-diphosphate *(ADP)*-phosphorylating respiration rates in mitochondria isolated from the injured hemisphere (C).

activity and mitochondrial membrane potential (ψm). The ion/proton leakage of the inner mitochondrial membrane may occur due to action of ionophores (e.g., free fatty acids) or due to an opening of ion/proton permeable channel/pore, which allows H^+ protons backflow into matrix, bypassing ATP-synthase. Therefore, activation of mitochondrial permeability transition pore (mPTP) renders mitochondria incapable of ATP production due to proton leak known as the *state of uncoupled mitochondrial respiration*. Thus if during reperfusion, brain mitochondria activate mPTP, then uncoupling of mitochondrial respiration explains secondary mitochondrial dysfunction (see Fig. 167.2). Why does the matrix membrane leak?

In the brain, HI-insults results in excessive release of glutamate, activation of NMDA, and AMPA glutamate receptors (see Fig. 167.2). The primary detrimental mechanism, downstream to glutamate-NMDA and AMPA interaction, is excessive intracellular Ca^{2+} flux.[20,34] Mitochondria are the organelles that actively regulate Ca^{2+} level in the cytosol by quickly taking Ca^{2+} up into their matrix via a mitochondrial Ca^{2+} uniporter and slowly exporting Ca^{2+} by Ca^{2+}/Na^+ and H^+/Ca^{2+} exchangers.[35,36] Mitochondrial Ca^{2+} buffering prevents cell damage caused by toxic effects of excessive Ca^{2+}. However, when mitochondria become Ca^{2+} overloaded, inner mitochondrial membrane may activate an opening of the pore, which freely releases Ca^{2+} out, but the same process dissipates a proton motive force. This mechanism of Ca^{2+} release via transient activation of mPTP has been reported in physiologic conditions in cardiomyocytes and other cells.[37,38] Following acute ischemia in the heart, brain, liver, or kidney, a massive Ca^{2+} overload results in Ca^{2+}-induced permanent opening of mPTP. Compared to physiologic transient activation of the low-conductance mPTP, postischemic mPTP has been characterized as a permanent formation of high-conductance channel causing mitochondrial swelling and tissue necrosis.[39] A useful framework concept for the mPTP-driven evolution of reperfusion brain injury can be stated as: *Ischemic glutamate-receptor activation → excessive Ca^{2+} cellular/mitochondrial influx → Ca^{2+} dependent opening of permanent mPTP → mitochondrial uncoupling and swelling that eventuates in mitochondrial matrix disintegration* (see Fig. 167.2). This concept explains reasonably well the mechanisms for secondary inhibition of mitochondrial ATP production, mPTP-dependent necrosis, and activation of the apoptotic cell-death pathway. Opening of mPTP and mitochondrial swelling promotes a release of cytochrome *c* and other mitochondrial apoptosis-inducing components into the cytosol. A loss of cytochrome *c* also interrupts electron transfer in the respiratory chain contributing to malfunction.[40,41] Thus the concept of permanent mPTP activation considers mitochondrial dysfunction as the event initiating necrotic and apoptotic cellular death pathways in ischemia-reperfusion injury.[42] Several reports demonstrating cerebral and cardiac protection afforded by inhibition of mPTP opening following ischemia and reperfusion in mature and immature animals support a central role of mPTP in mediating cellular injury.[39,43,44] There are, however, very important unresolved questions. Firstly, the molecular identity of mPTP remains cryptic. Secondly, studies addressing the role of mPTP are conflicting. Some authors have reported beneficial or partially beneficial effect of blockage of Ca^{2+}-dependent mPTP opening with cyclosporin A.[45,46] In contrast, mPTP inhibition with

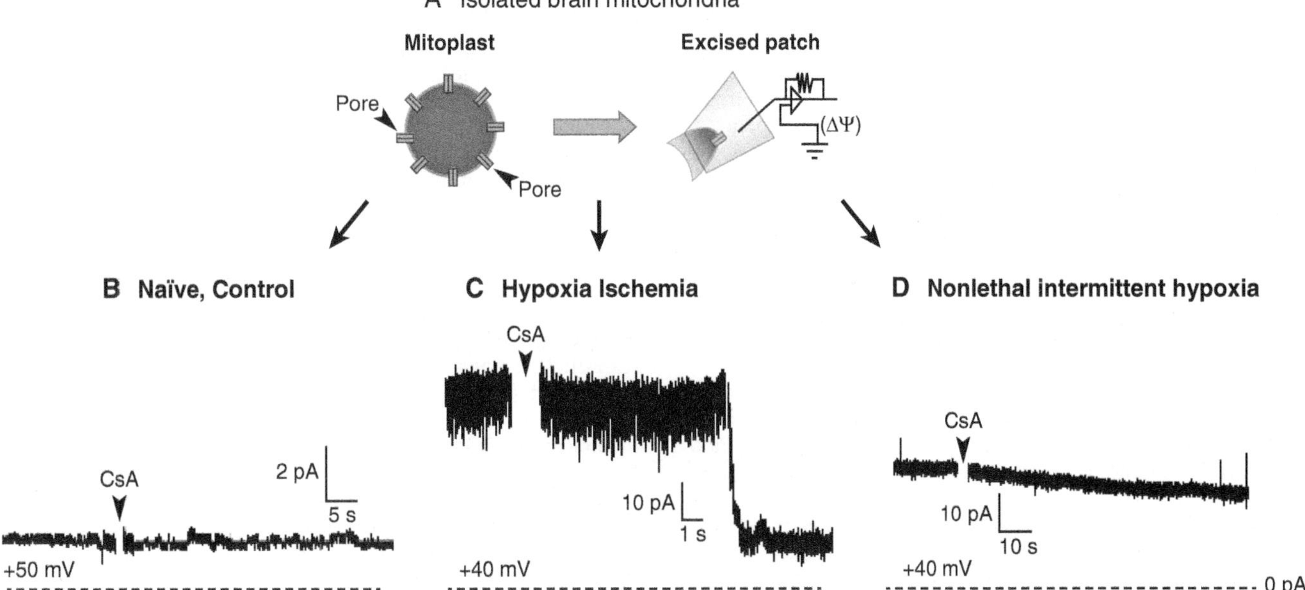

Fig. 167.4 The diagram of excised mitochondrial patch-clamp technique (A) and representative electrical conductance tracings obtained in mitoplasts from different mouse brains (B–D). *CsA*, Cyclosporin A (2 μM).

different inhibitor (GNX-4728) in the same model failed to afford neuroprotection.[47] Cyclosporin A is a nonspecific inhibitor of the cyclophilin D, the protein that is well-characterized as a critical component of mPTP activation. A pathogenic contribution of the cyclophilin D-dependent mPTP opening in focal ischemic brain injury has been strongly supported by significant attenuation of brain injury in cyclophilin D knock-out mature mice.[43] In contrast, cyclophilin D-deficient immature mice exhibited exacerbation of the brain injury following HI-insult, yet mature cyclophilin D-deficient mice, subjected to the same model were protected.[48] These data suggest that the effects of cyclophilin D relevant to the cellular fate following ischemic insult may be completely different depending upon the developmental stage of the brain. Conflicting data with the use of mPTP inhibitors in the same species and in the same model challenge a fundamental role mPTP in pathophysiology of ischemia-reperfusion injury. Given that the initial effect of mPTP is proton leak, it is important to note that studies on mitochondrial respiration, conducted during different time-points of reperfusion, did not reveal excessive proton leak, consistent with elevated resting respiration rate.[28,29] Using isolated brain mitochondria from neonatal animals exposed to hypoxia-ischemia and reperfusion, we found a presence of high-conductance, cyclosporin A-sensitive ion leak, consistent with mPTP opening in the inner membrane (Fig. 167.4B). Organelles from control animals were free of membrane leakage (see Fig. 167.4A). Furthermore, cerebral mitochondria isolated from the mice exposed to cell nonlethal intermittent hypoxic stress[49] also demonstrated cyclosporin A-sensitive ion leak but of low electrical conductance (see Fig. 167.4D). Chronic sublethal and nonlethal intermittent hypoxemia stress driven by apnea of prematurity, bronchopulmonary dysplasia is associated with diffuse white matter injury (WMI) and neurodevelopmental impairment.[49a] The mechanisms of diffuse WMI, however, relate to maturation failure of oligodendrocyte lineage cells, rather than a massive cellular loss characteristic for an ischemic insult.[49b] Therefore it is intriguing that following either hypoxia-ischemia or nonlethal hypoxia, isolated mitochondria exhibit active ion leak of various intensity (conductance) depending on a severity of the insult. Lethal insult is coupled with high-conductance mPTP activation; nonlethal hypoxia is accompanied by a low-conductance ion leak. Thus the role of mPTP in the pathogenesis of ischemia-reperfusion injury in immature brain, especially with regard to secondary energy failure, requires further study.

DYSFUNCTION OF RESPIRATORY CHAIN AND SECONDARY ENERGY FAILURE

Ischemic inhibition of mitochondrial respiration, detected at the onset of cerebral reperfusion in neonatal rodents, has been reported and interpreted as depressed activity of the respiratory chain.[29,31,50,51] Indeed, in immature and mature animals, cerebral ischemic insult significantly decreased activity of complex I, mildly inhibited complexes II to III, and did not affect complex IV.[19,30] Thus, ischemia mostly affects enzymatic activity of complex I and to a lesser extent, complexes II to IV. Thus, when supported by substrates (e.g., succinate) generating electron flux via complex II to IV, postischemic mitochondria exhibited near-normal ADP-phosphorylating oxygen consumption rates. In contrast, the same organelles fueled with complex I-dependent substrates displayed significantly poorer respiration rates.[19,52] One of the potential explanations for ischemic inhibition of complex I has been based on the existence of complex I active/deactive (A/D) transition in hypoxia.[53-55] Functional A/D transition of complex I in response to a lack of oxygen has been linked to structural rearrangements of ND3 and NDUFA9 subunits of the complex I characterized by exposure of ND3 Cys39 thiol groups detectable only in the D-form.[56-58] Upon reoxygenation, the D-form converts back into the A-form, which restores complex I enzymatic activity. Indeed, in few minutes of established reperfusion, mitochondrial respiration fueled with complex I-linked substrates always quickly recovers. The pathogenic relevance of this in vitro phenomenon to neonatal HI brain injury has been recently reported.[19,59] Theoretically, the D-form of complex I is susceptible to oxidative modification of the critical Cys39. If this thiol is oxidized, reactivation of complex I via retransition of the D-form to the A-form during reperfusion would be arrested. Because reperfusion state is known to be associated with an oxidative stress, it is possible that reactivation of complex I is limited by an oxidative modification of Cys39.[54,60-62]

Another potential mechanism for complex I inactivation during ischemia relates to over-reduction of complex I electron carriers, specifically, flavin mononucleotide (FMN). In vitro, fully reduced FMN ($FMNH_2$) is released from complex I, and this negatively affects the electron transferring capacity of the complex I. This mechanism of complex I inhibition has been described in isolated brain mitochondria, when over-reduction of FMN was achieved by stimulation of reverse electron transfer (RET).[63,64] RET occurs only during complex II-dependent mitochondrial respiration, when electrons flow from complex II toward complex I and eventually reduce NAD^+ (see Fig. 167.2, oxidative stress). During RET, electron transferring components of complex I are fully reduced and $FMNH_2$ may escape complex I, thereby limiting its capacity to transfer electrons from NADH to ubiquinone (coenzyme Q). An existence of reperfusion-activated RET and its pathogenic role has been reported in the models of ischemia-reperfusion injuries of the heart and mature and immature brains.[18,19,29]

Another mechanistic concept for secondary inhibition of mitochondrial respiratory chain relates to activation of mPTP, which contributes to cytochrome *c* release together with Bax/Bak-induced mitochondrial outer membrane permeabilization (see Fig. 167.2). Cytochrome *c* release, in addition to driving necrosis and apoptosis, disrupts electron transfer in the respiratory chain due to the depletion of this electron carrier between complexes III and IV.[65] Experimental evidence for existence of this mechanism was collected in a model of cardiac ischemia-reperfusion injury. For neonatal HI brain damage, this concept requires further experimental support.

While the exact mechanisms of secondary energy failure are still not well understood, existing data clearly demonstrate a reperfusion-driven nature of secondary mitochondrial dysfunction. This dysfunction is characterized by progressive inhibition of respiratory chain and mitochondrial uncoupling after transient near-full recovery of oxidative phosphorylation. If reintroduction of oxygen and nutrients following an ischemic event revives cerebral bioenergetics, then why this recovery is not sustainable, and what is the mitochondria-deleterious mechanism of reoxygenation?

REPERFUSION: OXIDATIVE STRESS

One of the central roles in reperfusion injury is played by an oxidative stress, the event driven by excessive production of reactive oxygen species (ROS). ROS or free radicals are molecules that carry unpaired electron/s in their outer orbit. ROS are highly aggressive molecules and can oxidize structural and functional cellular components. Among ROS, superoxide, hydrogen peroxide, hydroxyl radicals, peroxynitrite, and others are proposed as the major contributors to the oxidative injury in neonatal HI brain injury.[66] Primary deleterious actions of ROS are peroxidation of lipids, oxidation/nitration of proteins, inactivation of enzyme's iron-sulfur clusters, and DNA damage. Severe oxidative stress is capable of massive tissue damage even without ischemia and reperfusion. In neonatal HI brain injury, the severity of oxidative stress, the sources of ROS, and most importantly, the mechanisms of reperfusion injury that are initiated and driven by the ROS are yet to be determined.

ROS are constantly produced not only in a disease but in a healthy state and play a major role in intracellular redox signaling. Normally, antioxidant systems, enzymatic (e.g., Cu/Zn or Mn superoxide dismutase, catalase) and nonenzymatic (e.g., glutathione), support a balance of pro/antioxidant states. In neonates, antioxidant systems are still developing and display a limited ROS scavenging capacity.[67] For example, while upregulation of Cu/Zn superoxide dismutase (cytosolic enzyme converting superoxide into H_2O_2) exacerbated HI brain injury in neonatal rats,[68] transgenic mice overexpressing glutathione peroxidase, which converts H_2O_2 into H_2O, were protected against HI insult.[69] These data not only highlight the detrimental role of hydrogen peroxide in pathophysiology of post-HI cerebral damage, but also demonstrate an importance of glutathione system. The relevance of this experimental information is supported by the observation of a significant depletion of reduced glutathione in the brains of human neonates following HI insult.[70] Pathogenic contribution of peroxynitrite and reactive nitric oxide (NO) species were highlighted by neuroprotection in animals with inhibition of neuronal NO synthase (nNOS) or nNOS-deficient mice.[71,72]

The existing clinical strategies addressing an oxidative stress are based on our general understanding that oxygen is an indispensable component of ROS. This tempered the enthusiasm for the use of pure oxygen in neonatal resuscitation. Clinical trials demonstrated that in the majority of depressed infants, resuscitation could be successful with the use of room air,[73,74] and reported lower level of circulating markers of oxidative stress in neonates resuscitated with room air, compared to infants resuscitated with the 100% oxygen.[75] It is important to note that in preclinical studies reporting detrimental outcomes of reoxygenation with 100% O_2, asphyxiated animals received pure oxygen for 30 to 60 minutes of the initial reperfusion, causing extreme hyperoxemia.[76-78] Given that the ultimate goal of resuscitation is the return of spontaneous circulation (ROSC), experiments with hyperoxic support beyond the time-point of ROSC have limited translational value. Importantly, the equal efficacy of resuscitation with room air or with 100% O_2 following severe (Apgar score = 0 to 1) asphyxia is not yet proven. In newborn piglets, resuscitation with room air or 100% O_2 resulted in similar rates of ROSC following 1-minute cardiac arrest.[79] The same authors also reported a dramatic shortening of the time to ROSC when suboptimal (2% of the baseline minute ventilation) positive pressure ventilation was supplemented with 100% oxygen but not with room air.[80] Following a lethal HI insult with arrested circulation, the use of hyperoxic-reoxygenation restricted to the time required to achieve ROSC significantly improved survival of neonatal mice.[81] Thus the extent of oxygen redelivery is very important for successful resuscitation and cannot be sacrificed in an attempt to alleviate an oxidative stress. However, hyperoxemia during reperfusion once ROSC is achieved should be prevented. The simplicity of this clinical concept underscores the state of mechanistic understanding of oxidative stress in HI brain injury.

During a simulated HI insult (oxygen-glucose deprivation) and reperfusion, in cultured neurons, three distinct ROS generating systems have been identified: (1) mitochondrial respiratory chain, (2) xanthine oxidase, and (3) nicotinamide adenine dinucleotide phosphate (NADPH) oxidase.[82] In immature animals and humans with HI brain injury, elevated levels of hypoxanthine have been detected and proposed as the evidence for the pathogenic role of xanthine oxidase.[83,84] However, an inhibition of xanthine oxidase with oxypurinol or allopurinol failed to reduce lipid peroxidation and did not protect the brain in the rat model of HI injury[85] or in human neonates with an HI insult.[86] Earlier, pretreatment with allopurinol significantly decreased the extent of HI brain injury in neonatal rats and preserved energy metabolism during the HI insult.[87,88] Interestingly, newborn piglets subjected to HI and posttreated with allopurinol, at 24 hours of reperfusion, exhibited attenuation of secondary energy failure, yet the extent of cellular degeneration in their brains did not differ from the vehicle-treated animals.[89] Furthermore, while inhibition of NADPH oxidase also did not exert neuroprotection in different models of perinatal HI brain injury,[90] the role of NADPH-derived ROS in autophagosome formation in neonatal HI brain injury has been reported.[91] Thus data on pathogenic contribution of NADPH oxidase or xanthine oxidase to an oxidative brain damage following neonatal HI are not yet definitive.

Several reports proposed a mechanistic role for ROS originating in the mitochondrial respiratory chain following neonatal HI brain injury.[19,66,92] In the models of ischemia-reperfusion injury of mature and immature brains, regardless of the affected organ and the developmental stage, one of the mechanisms for excessive ROS production during reperfusion has been linked to a dramatic accumulation of succinate (flavin adenine dinucleotide [FAD]-linked substrate), which fuels RET in mitochondria upon reperfusion (see Fig. 167.2).[18,19,29,59] RET generates the highest rate of ROS release in coupled mitochondria.[12,93,94] A beneficial effect of inhibition of RET-dependent ROS release from complex I during reperfusion in ischemic brain and heart in adult and neonatal rodents has been reported.[18,29,95] A detailed mechanism for elevated ROS production during RET is not yet clear, but complex I is an established source of free radicals generated in this process. Compared to RET, forward electron transfer (FET) produces negligible amount of ROS. Experimental conditions for demonstration of elevated FET-driven ROS generation in complex I and complex III requires the use of complex inhibitors in order to initiate electron escape and form superoxide.[96] Therefore, translational significance of FET-supported mitochondrial ROS production is limited to conditions in which complex I or complex III is affected by genetic or acquired defects.[97-99] Given that complex III activity is spared after neonatal HI[19] and complex I activity recovers very quickly upon reperfusion, one may propose the RET as the main pathway for excessive ROS production in reperfusion. This mechanism is transient and limited by availability of succinate which normalizes within 30 minutes of reperfusion.[17] Theoretical challenge to the concept of the RET-driven oxidative stress in ischemia-reperfusion relates to mitochondrial depolarization caused by the activation of mPTP,[100] because accelerated ROS production during RET requires well-polarized mitochondria.[101] Nevertheless, there is a body of data proposing the mitochondrial respiratory chain as a primary source of excessive ROS production in the ischemic brain upon reperfusion.

In addition to oxidation of cellular structures, reperfusion-associated oxidative stress can potentiate specific mechanisms of postischemic injury. For example, activation of the Ca^{2+}-induced mPTP is known to be triggered by free radicals.[102] A pathogenic role of ROS originating in mitochondrial respiratory chain in seizure-induced excitotoxic limbic neuronal death has been reported. Developmental or fat-diet induced overexpression of uncoupling protein 2 (UCP2) was associated with limited ROS generation in mitochondria and greater resistance to seizure-induced excitotoxic neuronal death compared to cells normally expressing UCP2.[103]

REPERFUSION: EXCITOTOXICITY

Excitotoxicity is an accepted cell death mechanism in neonatal HI brain injury. This mechanism relates to excessive neuronal neurotransmitter-receptor interactions in excitatory synapses.[104] The dominant neurotransmitter exerting excitotoxicity is glutamate. Glutamate interacts with multiple subtypes of glutamate receptors, NMDA, AMPA, and kainic acid, which represent three major types of ionotropic glutamate receptors in postsynaptic membrane. Metabotropic glutamate receptors (mGluR) are members of the G-protein (guanine nucleotide-binding protein) coupled receptor superfamily and mediate slow synaptic glutamate effects. Normally, glutamate is released from the presynaptic terminal in response to neuronal activation/depolarization and interacts with receptors, inducing transient intracellular Ca^{2+} flux via NMDA and Ca^{2+}-permeable AMPA receptors channels.[20] Glutamate is then rapidly removed by astroglia to set the stage for next transmission. Astroglia, using glutamate transporters, take up neurotransmitter and convert it into glutamine. Finally, neuronal transporters transfer the glutamine back into neurons for recycling.[105] Glutamate upload by astrocytes uses a Na^+-K^+ ATPase dependent electrochemical Na^+ gradient,[106] and glutamate-glutamine conversion is an energy-dependent process. Because up to 90% of total cortical glucose metabolism is coupled with the energy demand of glutamatergic neurons,[107] it is expected that during HI insult, primary energy failure triggers a massive glutamate release by depolarized neurons along with astroglial failure to upload and convert glutamate into glutamine. Interestingly, in hippocampal slices exposed to severe anoxia, the primary role in both neuronal depolarization and extracellular glutamate release was assigned to the reverse action of neuronal glutamate uptake transporters.[108] Regardless of the mechanisms of glutamate release, extracellular accumulation of glutamate is one of the metabolic hallmarks of post-HI brain in immature animals[20,109] and human infants.[110] Primary detrimental effect of excessive glutamate-receptor interaction is continuous intracellular Ca^{2+} flux via NMDA and Ca^{2+}-permeable AMPA channels (see Fig. 167.2). Excessive intracellular Ca^{2+} flux leading to mitochondrial Ca^{2+} load triggers activation of mPTP. This sequence of events, termed *Ca^{2+} deregulation*, eventuates in mitochondrial depolarization, dysfunction, swelling, and disintegration. In addition, cytosolic Ca^{2+} flux activates calpain (a calcium-dependent protease) and nNOS, both of which have been implicated in HI neuronal damage.[71,111,112] Thus, intracellular Ca^{2+} flux could be considered as a central point converging several mechanisms of neuronal death in neonatal HI (see Fig. 167.2).

Excitotoxicity affects cell types other than neurons. In the developing brain, immature oligodendrocytes (pre-OL) are rich in expression of Ca^{2+}-permeable AMPA and NMDA receptors. This makes pre-OL highly sensitive to excitotoxic mechanisms of ischemic injury.[113,114] In a model of oxygen-glucose deprivation, a glutamate scavenging maneuver (glutamate-pyruvate transaminase plus pyruvate) attenuated pre-OL injury. In contrast, normoxic pre-OL were resistant to glutamate excitotoxicity at lower concentrations, but not at high glutamate concentrations. However, using a mitochondrial respiratory chain inhibitor or uncoupler, glutamate excitotoxicity was unmasked in the glutamate exposed normoxic cells.[115] Thus there is a mechanistic link between glutamate excitotoxicity and mitochondrial dysfunction in pre-OL injury following simulated ischemia-reperfusion. Indeed, when pre-OL were pretreated with nontoxic doses of a mitochondrial uncoupler or respiratory chain inhibitor, their death rate increased in response to simulated ischemia-reperfusion (oxygen glucose deprivation); the AMPA receptor antagonist, NBQX, abrogated this effect.[115] Thus the mechanistic sequence of glutamate excitotoxicity following HI insult involves other mechanisms of cellular injury (e.g., mitochondrial dysfunction). It has to be noted that delayed mechanisms of cellular death are also initiated in reperfusion and drive the cellular death continuum.

CELL DEATH PATHWAYS

APOPTOSIS

Compared to the mature brain, neonatal HI brain damage activates apoptotic death pathway to greater extent due to developmental overexpression of caspase 3-dependent apoptosis.[116] In neonatal rodents, caspase 3 activation peaks at 24 hours of reperfusion[117] and apoptosis-induced degeneration is detected for weeks following an acute HI insult.[118] Apoptosis following HI is mostly triggered intracellularly (intrinsic pathway) by a release of apoptosis-activating proteins from the mitochondrial intermembrane space including, cytochrome *c*, apoptosis-inducing factor (AIF), second mitochondria-derived activator of caspases (SMAC), and endonuclease G. The primary initiator of cell death in the intrinsic pathway is believed to be cytochrome *c* release, which in the cytosol activates caspases 9-3 (aspartate-specific proteases). The intrinsic pathway relies on permeabilization of mitochondrial outer membrane, which is regulated by the Bcl-2 protein family. Members of Bcl-2 family fall into three subclasses: the pro-apoptotic BH3-only proteins; the pro-survival Bcl-2-like proteins; and pro-apoptotic pore-forming Bax and Bak proteins.[119] By binding to BH3-only proteins or to activated Bax/Bak homologies, pro-survival proteins can block propagation of apoptosis. Normally, inactive Bax and Bak are located in the cytosol with a small portion being in the endoplasmic reticulum; part of the Bak family is inserted into outer mitochondrial membrane.[120-122] If not sequestered by binding to pro-survival proteins, activated Bax/Bak proteins translocate to mitochondria and form a pore (nonphysiologic, opened conformation of VDAC) in the outer membrane, causing a release of pro-apoptotic proteins (see Figs. 167.2 and 167.3A).[123] While VDAC normally functions as a gatekeeper for the exit and entry of ions, upon interaction with Bax, it forms the channel that is not voltage dependent and allows passage of positively charged cytochrome *c*. Indeed, supplementation of cytochrome *c* decreased electrical conductance of this channel.[124] Bax-inhibiting strategies afforded significant neuroprotection in rodent models of HI.[125] Bad and Bim are also Bcl-2 family members that activate apoptosis. Selective contribution of Bad and Bim to neonatal HI brain injury has also been reported.[117] Interestingly, an inhibition of Bax significantly reduced the extent of HI-brain injury in neonatal mice but not in adult mice, while genetic deletion of cyclophilin D (mPTP promoter) was protective in adult HI-mice, but exacerbated injury in neonates.[48] This suggests that, compared to the adult brain, the Bax-dependent apoptotic pathway of cellular death in the immature brain dominates over mPTP-driven necrosis or apoptosis. Another argument for Bax-mediated apoptosis as the principal mode of cell death in neonatal HI-brain is a robust neuroprotection afforded by either overexpression of Bcl-xL or by TAT-protein transduction induced systemic delivery of Bcl-xL.[126,127] Bcl-xL is an antiapoptotic member of the Bcl-2 family. It is noteworthy that overexpression of Bcl-2 members also inhibits necrotic cell death in hepatocytes and neurons, possibly by inhibiting activation of mPTP,[128,129] suggesting that apoptosis and necrosis share some cell death pathways. For example, mitochondrial translocation of Bax and release of cytochrome *c* without caspase 3 activation has been shown to cause liver necrosis in animals.[130,131] Bax interacts with mPTP to facilitate cytochrome *c* release from isolated mitochondria.[132] In addition to pro-apoptotic mitochondrial release of cytochrome *c*, cyclophilin A-facilitated translocation of AIF from mitochondria to nucleus also contributes to neuronal degeneration in HIE.[133] However, based on morphologic characteristics of dying cells, this pathway has been considered as a regulated necrotic mechanism of cell death, termed *parthanatos*.[134] In the rodent models of ischemia-reperfusion injury in immature brains, a predominant role for the apoptotic cell-death pathway has been generally accepted.[135] However, in piglets subjected to transient hypoxia-ischemia, the preferential mode of cellular damage depended upon the cell types and the extent of cellular maturation.[136]

NECROSIS

Necrosis is the term often used in reference to a nonapoptotic, accidental cell death.[137] In various organs, ischemia-reperfusion has been accepted as a cause for necrotic cell death. Generally, ischemic ATP depletion causes ion pumps failure that leads to cellular and mitochondrial swelling, dilatation of the endoplasmic reticulum, and formation of plasma membrane protrusions (*blebs*) due to dysfunctional cellular volume control.[137,138] Because ischemic cell death is accompanied by swelling, the term *oncotic necrosis* (from *onkos*, meaning swelling) has been proposed for this condition.[139] Another characteristic of oncotic necrosis is the associated inflammatory response secondary to release of cellular contents into interstitial space. While in the ischemia-reperfusion models of the mature brains, the mechanisms of injury generally assume oncotic necrosis, abundance of apoptotic markers in the same models, together with reports on predominance of apoptosis in the developing brain injury seems to be confusing. Part of the confusion concerning the roles of apoptosis and necrosis in ischemia-reperfusion injury arises from the assumption that apoptotic and necrotic mechanisms are distinct when, in fact, these mechanisms can be shared.[140] It is generally accepted that necrotic cell death represents an acute bioenergetics crisis when cells disintegrate due to nearly a complete loss of ATP. In turn, ATP is required for execution of apoptosis,[141] which implies that apoptosis cannot be active in energy depleted tissue. Indeed, when piglets were subjected to mild or severe transient HI insult, cells were dying by both modes, apoptosis and necrosis. Very little necrosis was seen after mild HI, but approximately 50% of cells were necrotic after severe HI.[142] Thus postischemic bioenergetic state may define cellular death mode. Furthermore, there are molecular signals, which shift the mode of neuronal death following ischemia from necrosis toward apoptosis.[143,144] The Northington group reported the relevance of another cell death pathway, necroptosis or programmed necrosis to neonatal HI injury.[145] The evidence for participation of this pathway in mechanisms of cellular degeneration include neuroprotection afforded by inhibition of receptor-interacting protein 1 (Rip1) kinase by necrostatin in a mouse model of HI brain damage.[146] This group has proposed the term *cell-death continuum*, pointing out the crosstalk between cell death pathways. This implies that inhibition of necroptotic cellular death pathway can decrease the extent of the ultimate tissue loss possibly by shifting cellular death pathway from programmed necrosis toward apoptosis.[147] Indeed, genetic loss or pharmacologic inhibition of caspase 3 activity led to either partial neuroprotection or exacerbation of injury in neonatal mice and rats,[148,149] displaying mostly necrotic cell death markers in caspase inhibited animals.[150] The cell death continuum concept opens a new therapeutic prospective: development of approaches aimed at switching cells death modes in addition to inhibiting certain pathways. In this respect, the report that in vitro hyperglycemia shifts apoptotic degeneration toward necroptosis and in vivo aggravates HI brain injury in neonatal mice deserves attention.[151] Other cell-death pathways (ferroptosis, autophagy, pyroptosis, parthanatos, lysosome-dependent autolysis) may be active following ischemia-reperfusion injury in the developing brain.[91,152-154]

NEUROINFLAMMATION

In the developing brain, HI activates the immune system, which results in a neuroinflammatory response. On the cellular level, this response activates local micro and astroglia,[155,156] mast cells,[157] and promotes cerebral infiltration with circulating neutrophils and myeloid cells[158-160] and T-lymphocytes.[161] Infiltration of the postischemic brain with circulating cells implies impaired permeability of the blood-brain barrier (BBB). In rodents, after neonatal HI, a disrupted BBB integrity was evidenced by extravasation of large molecules such as IgG or albumin.[162,163] Clinical studies also showed elevated CSF/blood ratios of albumin content, which positively correlated with clinical severity of asphyxia.[164,165] In contrast, in the neonatal rat model of focal brain ischemia, BBB permeability was minimally affected.[166] The exact mechanisms behind this important observation are not clear. It is possible that compromised BBB function following HI brain injury, which is the part of systemic ischemia, is caused by circulating inflammatory mediators interacting with postischemic cerebral vasculature. Generalized inflammation can produce cerebral endothelial activation, disrupting BBB integrity.[167,168]

The inflammation following HI insult is initiated once the pattern recognition receptors of innate immune system sense damaged molecules expressed by destructed cells. These receptors are not specific and recognize "non-self" structures, including bacterial and viral antigens. In the mouse models of neonatal HI, upregulation of Toll-like receptors (TLRs, the member of pattern recognition receptors family) 1, 2, and 7 has been demonstrated, and genetic deletion of TLR2 decreased the extent of injury.[169] The same model demonstrated extensive deposition of activated complement components in the injured areas of the brain suggesting a role of the innate immune system in recognition of stressed cells.[31,170] Either pharmacologic complement depletion prior to HI or genetic ablation of the initial component of the classical complement activation pathway (C1q) resulted in neuroprotection.[31,170] However, genetic ablation of the essential component of the complement membrane attack complex, C6, failed to confer neuroprotection.[31] This argues against the terminal complement contribution to reperfusion injury. While these reports highlight a pathogenic role of activated innate immune system in the evolution of neonatal HI damage, the mechanisms of detrimental action are not clear. For example, hippocampal neuroprotection associated with canonical overexpression of C3a (an activated C3 component of the complement) in astrocytes following HI[171] suggests that different activated complement components act on mechanisms of cellular injury or adaptation in this disease.

In addition to activation of innate immune systems, activated local and infiltrating immune cells produce pro- and antiinflammatory mediators. At a cellular level, blockage of mast cell degranulation after HI, or neutrophil depletion before HI, confers significant neuroprotection.[157,172] Antibody-driven depletion of circulating myeloid cells, monocytes, and granulocytes, also conferred protection, but only in male neonatal mice.[159] In contrast, depletion of peripheral T-cells significantly exacerbated neonatal HI injury in mice.[173] Similarly, microglial depletion aggravated injury in neonatal and adult focal ischemia-reperfusion injury models.[174,175] There is also a line of experimental evidence supporting a detrimental role of activated microglia in the evolution of HIE. Minocycline-afforded neuroprotection was strongly associated with blunted microglial activation in HI.[176] In human infants with HIE, postmortem exam of the dentate gyrus revealed significantly greater microglial infiltration compared to children suffering from sepsis or trauma.[177]

Detrimental action of activated microglia and infiltrating myeloid cells has been assigned to a release of proinflammatory mediators. Human infants who suffered from HIE exhibited greater circulating and CSF levels of tumor necrosis factor (TNF-α), interleukin (IL)-1β, which positively correlated with a severity of brain injury.[178-180] Genetic or pharmacologic blockade of these mediators and their receptors improved neurologic outcome in rodent models of neonatal HI[181-183] and adult stroke.[184] Furthermore, TNF-α, and IL-1β are capable of producing brain injury without HI insult[185] via activation of extrinsic apoptotic pathways (see Fig. 167.2). Compelling evidence for the detrimental effect of systemic and focal CNS inflammation has been shown in experiments where pretreatment and posttreatment with lipopolysaccharide (endotoxin) significantly exacerbated HI brain injury in newborn rodents and pigs.[186-188] In neonates with birth asphyxia, CSF IL-6 concentrations are elevated and have been associated with worse neurologic outcomes[189]; circulating levels of IL-6 exhibit a biphasic pattern, showing early and delayed peaks.[190] Compared to newborns with adverse outcome of HIE, the serum levels of IL-6, IL-1β, and IL-2 measured at 24 hours of therapeutic hypothermia were significantly reduced in infants with favorable outcome.[191] While these clinical data suggest that IL-6 contributes to HI brain injury, in experimental HI, IL-6 enhanced the antiapoptotic activity of astrocytes. Similarly, IL-6–deficient mice or mice treated with anti–IL-6R antibody exhibited exacerbated brain injury following focal stroke.[192-194] Thus neuroinflammation following neonatal HI brain injury governs both pro-survival and pro-death mechanisms. The mechanisms driving aggravation of injury are linked to excessive generation of ROS/NOS (activated microglia and neutrophils),[195-197] activation of the extrinsic apoptotic pathway (TNF1α-TNF1α receptor 1, TNF-related apoptosis inducing ligand [TRAIL] receptors, Fas/FasL, IL-1b, see Fig. 167.2),[198,199] potentiation of glutamate excitotoxicity, inhibition of mitochondrial ADP-phosphorylating respiration (TNF-1α),[200,201] and phagocytosis of injured yet still viable cells.[153] The protective action of inflammation includes microglial production of neurotrophic and growth factors, phagocytosis of toxic cellular debris,[202-204] and benefits related to control (IL-10) propagation or resolution of inflammation.[205,206] The benefit of the inflammation-resolving strategy in neonatal HI brain injury is supported by the neuroprotective action of the docosahexaenoic acid (DHA)[207] and DHA metabolites,[208] which can act as inflammation resolving mediators.[209] Analysis of current data suggests that the early stage of reperfusion accentuates mostly the detrimental side of inflammation, while at the later stage (weeks) after HI insult, the inflammation becomes beneficial and plays an important role in resolution of injury and healing.

RESOLUTION OF INJURY AND FUNCTIONAL RECOVERY

Resolution of HI brain could be viewed as a completion of cellular degeneration with formation of glial scar or cystic substitution of the lost brain tissue. The process of recovery falls into two categories: restitution and substitution.[210] Restitution occurs when the damaged brain heals, and neural pathways are reactivated leading to at least partially restored functions. Axonal sprouting could be viewed as an example of restitution. Although the ischemic insult can result in widespread neuronal death, many neurons will only be partially damaged or undamaged, with axons having the potential for sprouting and re-innervating new target cells.[211] However, only a subset of axons will reach their appropriate destinations, leading to incomplete or even maladaptive recovery. Sprouting occurs early and is complete in a matter of weeks, with some evidence of behavioral improvement.[212] Substitution refers to recovery via transfer of functions from damaged areas to intact sites. Interhemispheric transfer is probably the best example of substitution, when the contralateral hemisphere has some capacity to restore skills lost due to unilateral brain damage, like hemispherectomy for intractable epilepsy[213] or cerebral palsy, following unilateral lesions.[214,215] Functional imaging studies in humans have shown that, following early brain insult, there is potential for relocation of language skills or at least recruitment of the nondominant hemisphere.[216] The process of functional recovery following acute brain injury has been attributed to plasticity of the CNS.

Plasticity of the brain may refer either to normal state[217] or to a disease state, when plasticity represents reparative processes of the injured brain, remyelination, reorganization of circuits, and/or neural and behavioral compensation.[218] In respect to neonatal injury, brain plasticity is often referred to a greater ability of immature brain in functional recovery, compared to mature brain.[219] The concept of developmental advantage of the immature brain in functional recovery has been proposed by Margaret Kennard. In 1930s and 1940s she compared a recovery of function in monkeys with premotor lesions produced in infancy, adolescence, and adulthood and reported that unilateral motor cortex injury in infancy resulted in better outcomes than those seen in adults (reviewed in Anderson and colleagues[220]). Subsequent animal studies also demonstrated a better functional recovery from frontal cortex lesions acquired during infancy compared to the outcome of the same lesion acquired in the adulthood.[221,222] Over time, however, animal research has painted a less clear picture than early studies predicted. It has been found that the extent of functional recovery closely relates to the developmental stage of the injured area. The injury sustained during migration or early synaptogenesis led to permanent behavioral impairment, but those produced later in synaptogenesis were associated with better recovery.[223] After decades of research, Dr. Kolb, the expert in the developing brain plasticity, concluded that functional recovery following a focal brain lesion is closely related to age at lesion, with poorest recovery from lesions sustained around birth (in human terms).[224] Indeed, children with prenatal lesions and perinatal bilateral or diffuse pathology commonly experience severe and permanent neurologic impairment.[225-227] Studies of long-term outcomes of diffuse early brain insult suggest that the extent of the deficits decreases as the age at the insult and the maturity of the brain increases.[228-230] Thus, while results of early animal research have been interpreted as evidence for the benefits of immaturity in terms of enhanced adaptive plasticity after brain insult, findings provide support for the unique vulnerability of the developing brain, which ultimately defines the extent of the handicap. Furthermore, the degree of structural plasticity may not always correlate with a better neurofunctional recovery. For example, more extensive structural plasticity after lesions in the immature midbrain compared to that in the mature midbrain was associated with poorer neurologic outcome.[231] Brain plasticity itself is neutral and "intends" no particular outcome, which may be either adaptive or maladaptive.[232] Many plasticity mechanisms are not intrinsically tied to age, and even adaptive outcomes often come with developmental impairment not observed with advanced age at injury.[232]

NEUROPROTECTIVE STRATEGIES: HYPOTHERMIA AND ERYTHROPOIETIN

HYPOTHERMIA

Since ancient times, people have noticed the beneficial effects of hypothermia. Hippocrates advised snow and ice packing to alleviate hemorrhage and noticed a better survival of infants exposed to open in the winter than in the summer.[233,234] Preclinical and clinical trials have reproducibly demonstrated a neuroprotective effect of mild hypothermia applied after an ischemic insult,[235-238] and therapeutic hypothermia has become the standard of clinical care for near-term and term infants with HI brain injury. Nevertheless, the exact mechanism of hypothermia in cerebral protection against reperfusion injury remains unclear.

Cerebral metabolic rate decreases by about 6% to 7% for every 1°C drop in the body temperature,[239] which proportionally decreases cerebral oxygen demand. In canine brains, systemic hypothermia significantly decreases cerebral blood flow and the oxygen consumption rate, while the difference between arterial-venous oxygen contents remains unchanged.[240] Supported by clinical data,[241] this suggests that well-coupled oxygen demand and oxygen delivery could be achieved during hypothermia. Poorly coupled oxygen redelivery to oxygen demand during reperfusion contributes to reperfusion brain injury.[5] In rats following cardiac arrest, a secondary decline in the cerebral blood flow, termed *no-reflow*, was associated with exacerbated brain injury.[242] Mechanisms implicated in this secondary ischemia include perivascular edema,[242] vasoconstriction and compromised microcirculation driven by endothelial activation,[243,244] decreased cerebral perfusion pressure due to cytotoxic brain edema and hypercapnia-induced elevation of intracranial pressure,[245,246] and poor cerebral blood flow autoregulation.[247,248] By decreasing cerebral metabolic rate, post-HI hypothermia can alleviate the severity of secondary ischemia in reperfusion. In addition, in asphyxiated fetal sheep, hypothermia decreased the extent of cytotoxic edema assessed by cortical impedance.[249] The initial reperfusion stage is characterized by a brief period (minutes) of reactive hyperemia or hyperperfusion, which is not defined by the increased oxygen or substrate demand,[250] but is driven by abnormal vascular reactivity in the postischemic brain.[251] This hyperemia is detrimental for cellular survival, and the length of reactive hyperemia is proportional to the length of the ischemia.[250] In mature rats subjected to focal stroke, pre- and intra-ischemic cerebral hypothermia did not attenuate the extent, but significantly shortened the hyperemic stage of reperfusion.[252] Postischemic local hypothermia significantly decreased the reactive hyperemic response to reperfusion.[253] Both regimens of therapeutic hypothermia attenuated brain injury, suggesting improved oxygen delivery and reduced metabolic demand in the postischemic neurovascular unit. However, when cooling is initiated before 6 hours of reperfusion (current practice), it can only partially count on addressing secondary ischemia and miss reactive hyperemia. When hypothermia was initiated later (6 to 24 hours after birth), the beneficial effects were inconclusive.[254] In contrast, even brief (1 hour) hypothermia initiated immediately after resuscitation of asphyxiated piglets attenuated neuronal loss but lost its protective effect with a 30-minute delay.[255,256] Interestingly, hypothermia was not associated with differences between groups in the duration, severity of brain acidosis, and concentrations of phosphorylated metabolites.[255] Pericranial hypothermia applied during global brain ischemia afforded robust neuroprotection, yet the duration of hippocampal neuronal depolarization (evidence of bioenergetic collapse) was equivalent (9 minutes) in normothermic and hypothermic rats.[257] These data suggest that therapeutic mechanisms of hypothermia may not be limited only to a hypothermic reduction in cerebral metabolic demand in reperfusion.[249] Neuroprotective effect of postischemic hypothermia has been linked to inhibition of extrinsic and intrinsic apoptosis,[258-260] attenuation of NMDA receptor hyperactivity,[249] salvage of neurons from delayed calcium influx via metabotropic glutamate receptor 2,[261] increased level of the brain-derived neurotrophic factor,[262] attenuation of a reperfusion-driven ROS production,[263] and decreased microglial activation and neuroinflammation.[264,265] Such a long list of potential mechanistic actions of hypothermia underscores (1) an associative relationship between hypothermia-induced neuroprotection and molecular changes and (2) suggests a nonspecific nature of proposed molecular mechanisms that could be the downstream effects of improved coupling between oxygen redelivery and metabolic demand achieved by hypothermia in the brain.

Clinical strategy for the use of postischemic cooling is still developing. Studies addressing therapeutic mechanisms will optimize our current use of hypothermia and improve the current long-term neurologic outcome of postischemic hypothermia. At 6 to 7 years of age, compared to the normothermic group, the children with perinatal depression treated with whole-body cooling exhibited no neurologic benefit (IQ score <70, P = .51). Only combined (Death + IQ <70) outcome demonstrated a strong tendency (P = .06) toward improvement.[266] The follow-up of infants enrolled in the Cool-Cap trial demonstrated a strong association of favorable neurodevelopmental outcome assessed at 18 months with favorable outcome at school age (6 to 8 years), underscoring a predictive power of neurologic assessment at 18 months in this cohort. However, although underpowered, comparative analysis revealed an absence of a beneficial neurologic effect of hypothermia assessed at school-age.[267] In contrast, Total Body Hypothermia for Neonatal Encephalopathy (TOBY) trial demonstrated significantly greater survival with an IQ score 85 or greater and significant reductions in the risk of cerebral palsy at 6 to 7 years.[268] Overall, to date, therapeutic hypothermia has proven to be moderately effective, which requires further research efforts to optimize this clinically effective strategy.

ERYTHROPOIETIN

Erythropoietin (Epo) is a 30.4 kDa glycoprotein that regulates mammalian erythropoiesis.[269] It has become increasingly evident that Epo has significant biologic effects apart from modulation of red cell production. These are inhibition of apoptosis, neurotrophic, angiogenic, and antiinflammatory actions and attenuation of an oxidative stress.[270] In the brain, Epo and erythropoietin receptor (EpoR) mRNAs are widely expressed throughout development.[271] Primary cultured neurons in the presence of Epo exhibited resistance to NMDA receptor-mediated glutamate excitotoxicity and Epo-treated gerbils were protected against global brain ischemia-reperfusion.[272,273] Epo treatment has received significant attention due to neuroprotection afforded in neonatal rodent models of HI and focal brain injury,[274,275] and this has translated into clinical trials.[276] While recent phase I/II trials demonstrated good tolerance of high doses of recombinant human Epo in conjunction with hypothermia,[277,278] and improved neurologic outcome in a small cohort of patients,[242,279] the question whether the combination of the Epo treatment with hypothermia demonstrates an additive protective effect in the infants with HIE is being addressed in several on-going trails. Preclinical studies are somewhat conflicting and report either an absence of additive neuroprotective action of Epo in the hypothermia-treated rodents with cerebral HI injury,[280,281] exacerbation of the HI brain damage in mice overproducing H_2O_2,[282] or dramatic improvement of neurologic outcome in nonhuman primates treated with hypothermia + Epo compared to the hypothermia-only-treated animals.[283]

CONCLUSION

The pathophysiology of neonatal HI brain injury reflects the evolution of two fundamental biologic processes: (1) the mechanisms of cellular damage driven by ischemia-reperfusion and (2) the brain developmental stage-specific alterations in mechanisms of postischemic brain injury and recovery. Current progress in the field remains relatively stagnant.This is evidenced by the absence of clinically proven therapeutic strategies directly addressing known mechanisms of HI brain injury proposed in the preclinical studies. It is still unclear what is the exact mechanism of the only clinically proven strategy, post-HI hypothermia, and the emerging neuroprotective strategy, Epo administration.[284,285] All neuroprotective strategies proposed for neonatal HIE can be divided into three main categories: (1) those addressing the physiology of oxygen delivery during ischemia and reperfusion, (2) those addressing proposed mechanisms of postischemic cellular death and survival, and (3) exploratory neuroprotective strategies with no specifically targeted mechanism. In preclinical research, the balance has been markedly tipped toward addressing specific molecular mechanisms of injury and toward testing exploratory neuroprotective strategies in which mechanistic explanations are limited to nonspecific antiapoptotic, antioxidative, or antiinflammatory properties of the tested compound. However, current clinical practice still operates on our knowledge of physiology of oxygen delivery, metabolism, and growth. Perhaps more preclinical and clinical research addressing the mechanistic link between oxygen delivery, demand, energy metabolism at the initial stage of reperfusion, and neurodevelopmental outcomes[286,287] will demonstrate a better clinical utility. For example, epidemiologic data suggest that there is considerable room for improvement in the resuscitation of severely asphyxiated infants (5 minute Apgar score ≤3).[288] Clinical consensus is yet to be reached on how to address a cold stress during post-HI hypothermia, the optimal cerebral oxygenation and cerebral perfusion pressure, the best combination of energy substrates, and the utility of sedation and analgesia at the initial hours of reperfusion. If we believe that the mechanisms of cellular injury are not completely overlapping and evolve to a certain extent sequentially, then each mechanism, therapeutically, should be prioritized at each stage of postresuscitation care. Overall, it is clear that the field requires more research efforts addressing pathophysiology of the developing brain HI injury, perhaps matching the efforts devoted to the mechanisms of neurodegeneration in the ageing brain.A simple literature search (on February 10, 2020) revealed 12,762 publications under key words "neonatal HI brain injury," while the search under "Alzheimer disease" displayed 87,000 scientific reports.

ACKNOWLEDGMENT

This work was partially supported by NIH grants NS 100850, NS 099109, NS 088197.

GLOSSARY

Bax, Bak, Bim, Bad: Pro-apoptotic proteins and Bcl-XL is an antiapoptotic protein of the nuclear coded Bcl-2 gene protein family that controls cell death by regulating cytochrome *c* release from mitochondria.

Flavin adenine dinucleotide + 2H⁺($FADH_2$): Reducing agent. In quinone form, donates electrons to complex II in mitochondria.

Mitochondrial respiration: O_2 consumption rate by mitochondrial respiratory chain during pumping of H+ out from the matrix into intermembrane space. During the resting state (ADP-nonphosphorylating state), mitochondria consume minimal amounts of O_2. During the ADP-phosphorylating state or uncoupled respiration, oxygen consumption rates are the greatest, as mitochondria compensate for a loss of proton motive force used either by ATP-synthase or due to leakage of the inner mitochondrial membrane.

Mitochondrial respiratory chain: The main structure generating proton motive force for oxidative phosphorylation.

Mitochondrial uncoupling: An imbalance between rates of O_2 consumption and ADP-phosphorylation results in decreased ATP production per atom of consumed oxygen.

Nicotinamide adenine dinucleotide + H^+ (NADH): Reducing agent. Donates electrons to complex I in mitochondria.

***N*-methyl-D-aspartate (NMDA) receptor and α-amino-3-hydroxy-5-methyl-4-isoxazolepropionic acid (AMPA) receptor:** Glutamate receptors-channels regulating Ca^{2+} influx for neurotransmission.

Proton motive force: H^+ gradient across the inner mitochondrial membrane. This gradient is known as proton motive force that drives ATP-synthase activity.

Reduction/oxidation: Reduction is the reaction of gaining electrons (reduced). Fully reduced substances can generate superoxide by donating electrons to O_2. Oxidation is the reaction of electron release.

A complete reference list is available at www.ExpertConsult.com. 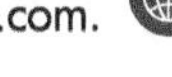

SELECT REFERENCES

5. Siesjö BK, Wieloch T. Cerebral metabolism in ischaemia: neurochemical basis for therapy. *Br J Anaesth*. 1985;57:47–62.
9. Yager JY, Brucklacher RM, Vannucci RC. Cerebral energy metabolism during hypoxia-ischemia and early recovery in immature rats. *Am J Physiol*. 1992;262:H672–H677.
18. Chouchani ET, et al. Ischaemic accumulation of succinate controls reperfusion injury through mitochondrial ROS. *Nature*. 2014;515:431–435.
19. Kim M, et al. Attenuation of oxidative damage by targeting mitochondrial complex I in neonatal hypoxic-ischemic brain injury. *Free Radic Biol Med*. 2018;124:517–524.
20. Johnston MV. Excitotoxicity in perinatal brain injury. *Brain Pathol*. 2005;15:234–240.

22. Schinder AF, Olson EC, Spitzer NC, Montal M. Mitochondrial dysfunction is a primary event in glutamate neurotoxicity. *J Neurosci*. 1996;16:6125-6133.
24. Palmer C, Brucklacher RM, Christernsen MA, Vannucci RC. Carbohydrate and energy metabolism during the evolution of hypoxic-ischemic brain damage in the immature rat. *J Cereb Blood Flow Metab*. 1990;10:227-235.
26. Vannucci RC, Towfighi J, Vannucci SJ. Secondary energy failure after cerebral hypoxia-ischemia in the immature rat. *J Cereb Blood Flow Metab*. 2004;24:1090-1097.
28. Puka-Sundvall M, et al. Impairment of mitochondrial respiration after cerebral hypoxia-ischemia in immature rats: relationship to activation of caspase-3 and neuronal injury. *Brain Res Dev Brain Res*. 2000;125:43-50.
29. Niatsetskaya ZV, et al. The oxygen free radicals originating from mitochondrial complex I contribute to oxidative brain injury following hypoxia-ischemia in neonatal mice. *J Neurosci*. 2012;32:3235-3244.
31. Ten VS, et al. Complement component C1q mediates mitochondria-driven oxidative stress in neonatal hypoxic-ischemic brain injury. *J Neurosci*. 2010;30:2077-2087.
39. Nakagawa T, et al. Cyclophilin D-dependent mitochondrial permeability transition regulates some necrotic but not apoptotic cell death. *Nature*. 2005;434:652-658.
43. Schinzel AC, et al. Cyclophilin D is a component of mitochondrial permeability transition and mediates neuronal cell death after focal cerebral ischemia. *Proc Natl Acad Sci U S A*. 2005;102:12005-12010.
48. Wang X, et al. Developmental shift of cyclophilin D contribution to hypoxic-ischemic brain injury. *J Neurosci*. 2009;29:2588-2596.
52. Sims NR. Selective impairment of respiration in mitochondria isolated from brain subregions following transient forebrain ischemia in the rat. *J Neurochem*. 1991;56:1836.
61. Chouchani ET, et al. Cardioprotection by S-nitrosation of a cysteine switch on mitochondrial complex I. *Nat Med*. 2013;19:753-759.
65. Halestrap AP, Richardson AP. The mitochondrial permeability transition: a current perspective on its identity and role in ischaemia/reperfusion injury. *J Mol Cell Cardiol*. 2015;78:129-141.
68. Ditelberg JS, Sheldon RA, Epstein CJ, Ferriero DM. Brain injury after perinatal hypoxia-ischemia is exacerbated in copper/zinc superoxide dismutase transgenic mice. *Pediatr Res*. 1996;39:204-208.
73. Saugstad OD, Rootwelt T, Aalen O. Resuscitation of asphyxiated newborn infants with room air or oxygen: an international controlled trial: the Resair 2 study. *Pediatrics*. 1998;102:e1.
80. Linner R, Cunha-Goncalves D, Perez-de-Sa V. One oxygen breath shortened the time to return of spontaneous circulation in severely asphyxiated piglets. *Acta Paediatr Int J Paediatr*. 2017;106:1556-1563.
82. Abramov AY, Scorziello A, Duchen MR. Three distinct mechanisms generate oxygen free radicals in neurons and contribute to cell death during anoxia and reoxygenation. *J Neurosci*. 2007;27:1129-1138.
86. Chaudhari T, McGuire W. Allopurinol for preventing mortality and morbidity in newborn infants with suspected hypoxic-ischaemic encephalopathy. *Cochrane Database Syst Rev*. 2008;CD006817.
90. Doverhag C, et al. Pharmacological and genetic inhibition of NADPH oxidase does not reduce brain damage in different models of perinatal brain injury in newborn mice. *Neurobiol Dis*. 2008;31:133-144.
96. Brand MD. The sites and topology of mitochondrial superoxide production. *Exp Gerontol*. 2010;45:466-472.
104. Johnston MV, Trescher WH, Ishida A, Nakajima W, Zipursky A. Neurobiology of hypoxic-ischemic injury in the developing brain. *Pediatric Research*. 2001;49:735-741.
113. Jensen FE. The role of glutamate receptor maturation in perinatal seizures and brain injury. *Int J Dev Neurosci*. 2002;20:339-347.
115. Deng W, Yue Q, Rosenberg PA, Volpe JJ, Jensen FE. Oligodendrocyte excitotoxicity determined by local glutamate accumulation and mitochondrial function. *J Neurochem*. 2006;98:213-222.
116. Johnston MV, Nakajima W, Hagberg H. Mechanisms of hypoxic neurodegeneration in the developing brain. *Neuroscientist*. 2002;8:212-220.
118. Nakajima W, et al. Apoptosis has a prolonged role in the neurodegeneration after hypoxic ischemia in the newborn rat. *J Neurosci*. 2000;20:7994-8004.
123. Shimizu S, Narita M, Tsujimoto Y. Bcl-2 family proteins regulate the release of apoptogenic cytochrome c by the mitochondrial channel VDAC. *Nature*. 1999;399:483-487.
125. Wang X, et al. Neuroprotective effect of Bax-inhibiting peptide on neonatal brain injury. *Stroke*. 2010;41:2050-2055.
132. Narita M, et al. Bax interacts with the permeability transition pore to induce permeability transition and cytochrome c release in isolated mitochondria. *Proc Natl Acad Sci U S A*. 1998;95:14681-14686.
133. Zhu C, et al. Apoptosis-inducing factor is a major contributor to neuronal loss induced by neonatal cerebral hypoxia-ischemia. *Cell Death Differ*. 2007;14:775-784.
135. Thornton C, et al. Cell death in the developing brain after hypoxia-ischemia. *Front Cell Neurosci*. 2017;11:248.
136. Yue X, et al. Apoptosis and necrosis in the newborn piglet brain following transient cerebral hypoxia-ischaemia. *Neuropathol Appl Neurobiol*. 1997;23:16-25.
140. Jaeschke H, Lemasters JJ. Apoptosis versus oncotic necrosis in hepatic ischemia/reperfusion injury. *Gastroenterology*. 2003;125:1246-1257.
146. Northington FJ, et al. Necrostatin decreases oxidative damage, inflammation, and injury after neonatal HI. *J Cereb Blood Flow Metab*. 2011;31:178-189.
147. Northington FJ, Chavez-Valdez R, Martin LJ. Neuronal cell death in neonatal hypoxia-ischemia. *Ann Neurol*. 2011;69:743-758.
149. West T, Atzeva M, Holtzman DM. Caspase-3 deficiency during development increases vulnerability to hypoxic-ischemic injury through caspase-3-independent pathways. *Neurobiol Dis*. 2006;22:523-537.
162. Ek CJ, et al. Brain barrier properties and cerebral blood flow in neonatal mice exposed to cerebral hypoxia-ischemia. *J Cereb Blood Flow Metab*. 2015;35:818-827.
166. Fernández-López D, et al. Blood-brain barrier permeability is increased after acute adult stroke but not neonatal stroke in the rat. *J Neurosci*. 2012;32:9588-9600.
170. Cowell RM, Plane JM, Silverstein FS. Complement Activation Contributes to Hypoxic-Ischemic Brain Injury in Neonatal Rats. *J Neurosci*. 2003;23:9459-9468.
171. Jarlestedt K, et al. Receptor for complement peptide C3a: a therapeutic target for neonatal hypoxic-ischemic brain injury. *FASEB J*. 2013;27:3797-3804.
172. Palmer C, Roberts RL, Young PI. Timing of neutrophil depletion influences long-term neuroprotection in neonatal rat hypoxic-ischemic brain injury. *Pediatr Res*. 2004;55:549-556.
175. Jin WN, et al. Depletion of microglia exacerbates postischemic inflammation and brain injury. *J Cereb Blood Flow Metab*. 2017;37:2224-2236.
177. Bigio MRD, Beckery LE. Microglial aggregation in the dentate gyrus: a marker of mild hypoxic–ischaemic brain insult in human infants. *Neuropathol Appl Neurobiol*. 1994;20:144-151.
184. Hallenbeck JM. The many faces of tumor necrosis factor in stroke. *Nature Medicine*. 2002;8:1363-1368.
220. Anderson V, Spencer-Smith M, Wood A. Do children really recover better? Neurobehavioural plasticity after early brain insult. *Brain*. 2011;134:2197-2221.
221. Kolb B, Gibb R. Possible anatomical basis of recovery of function after neonatal frontal lesions in rats. *Behav Neurosci*. 1993;107:799-811.
230. Anderson V, Catroppa C, Morse S, Haritou F, Rosenfeld J. Functional plasticity or vulnerability after early brain injury? *Pediatrics*. 2005;116:1374-1382.
232. Dennis M, et al. Age, plasticity, and homeostasis in childhood brain disorders. *Neurosci Biobehav Rev*. 2013;37:2760-2773.
284. Matsushita H, Johnston MV, Lange MS, Wilson MA. Protective effect of erythropoietin in neonatal hypoxic ischemia in mice. *Neuroreport*. 2003;14:1757-1761.
286. Bainbridge A, et al. Brain mitochondrial oxidative metabolism during and after cerebral hypoxia-ischemia studied by simultaneous phosphorus magnetic-resonance and broadband near-infrared spectroscopy. *NeuroImage*. 2014;102:173-183.

168 Pathophysiology of Neonatal Acute Bacterial Meningitis

Rodrigo Hasbun | Allan Collodel | Tatiana Barichello

BACTERIAL MENINGITIS

Meningitis is a life-threatening infection of the central nervous system (CNS) that affects the pia mater, the arachnoid, and the subarachnoid space. The microorganisms can activate the host immune response, and both inflammatory mediators and microorganisms can break down the blood-brain barrier, allowing the influx of fluid and solutes into the brain, triggering the brain edema. This infection is a significant cause of morbidity and mortality worldwide, primarily in neonates, in whom it is associated with long-term neurologic sequelae in up to 50% of the survivors.[1-3] In Europe and North America, *Streptococcus agalactiae* (group B *Streptococcus*) is the most common etiologic agent of neonatal meningitis, followed by *Escherichia coli*.[4-6] The remaining agents include *Listeria monocytogenes*, *Streptococcus pneumoniae*, and *Neisseria meningitidis*.[5]

The multiplication of bacteria within the subarachnoid space occurs concomitantly with the release of bacterial products, such as peptidoglycan, lipoteichoic acid (a constituent of the cell wall of gram-positive bacteria; e.g., *S. agalactiae*, *S. pneumoniae*, and *Listeria* spp.), lipopolysaccharide (LPS, a constituent of the cell wall of gram-negative bacteria; e.g., *E. coli*), lipooligosaccharide (a constituent of the cell wall of *N. meningitidis*), flagellum (motility, e.g., *E. coli* and *Listeria* spp.), pilus (mediating the attachment of the bacteria on cells, e.g., *S. agalactiae*, *E. coli*, and *N. meningitidis*), DNA, and cell wall fragments.[7-9] These bacterial compounds are all denoted as pathogen-associated molecular patterns (PAMPs).[10,11] These PAMPs are recognized by pattern-recognition receptors (PRRs) and non-PRRs, which are essential constituents of the immune system.[12,13] PRRs include several families, including Toll-like receptors (TLRs), nucleotide-binding oligomerization domain (NOD)-like receptors (NLRs), retinoic acid-inducible gene I (RIG-I)-like receptors (RLRs), C-type lectin receptors (CLRs), and intracellular DNA-sensing molecules. The non-PRRs receptors include receptors for advanced glycation end products (RAGEs), triggering receptors expressed on myeloid cells (TREMs), and G-protein-coupled receptors (GPCRs).[14] The sensing of PAMPs by immune receptors triggers a cascade of signaling pathways that activate several transcription factors and promote the production of proinflammatory mediators. The inflammatory mediators include cytokines, chemokines, and antimicrobial peptides, which are necessary to eliminate the invading pathogens.[15]

Endogenous molecules that are released from stressed or injured cells during meningitis infection also trigger the innate immune system. These molecules are recognized by PRRs and non-PRRs and are known as *damage-associated molecular patterns (DAMPs)*.[16,17] Among the DAMPs identified, there are cellular proteins and nucleic acid–related molecules, such as the heat shock protein (HSP), the high mobility group box-1 (HMGB-1) protein, members of the S-100 family, cytochrome-c, nucleic acids, and adenosine triphosphate.[16,18,19] Thus the development of brain damage during bacterial meningitis results from the combined effects of both the pathogen and the innate immune response. The recognition of PAMPs and DAMPs by immune receptors result in amplification of the proinflammatory response and can lead to long-term cognitive impairment in survivors of neonatal meningitis.[9,20]

COLONIZATION

S. agalactiae is a gram-positive diplococcus, and it is categorized according to capsular antigens such as Ia, Ib, II, III, IV, V, VI, VII, VIII, and IX.[21,22] Although all of the serotypes can cause infections, in North America, serotypes Ia, Ib, II, III, and V are most frequently associated with invasive disease.[23] However, in other studies, the most frequent serotype associated with invasive disease was type III, demonstrating that the dominant serotypes vary regionally and differ by invasive and colonizing isolates.[24] This microorganism is considered part of the healthy microflora in the vagina in up to 10% to 30% of healthy women, and it is a risk factor for early-onset meningitis due to *S. agalactiae*.[25,26] The adherence of the microorganism to epithelial cells has shown to be an essential factor in the colonization of the mucous membranes of both the human rectum and vagina.[27] The pathogens can also attach to the placental membranes, respiratory tract epithelium, and blood-brain barrier endothelium.[28]

The human placenta does not present a microbiome and also does not have evidence for the presence of bacteria in complicated and uncomplicated pregnancies.[29] The neonatal infection occurs when the infant is exposed during the birth process to a large number of pathogens that can be transmitted through the vagina to ruptured amniotic membranes, or due to contact of the infant during passage through the birth canal. In addition, *S. agalactiae* can be aspirated into the fetal lungs and transferred haematogenously into the CNS.[30,31] The colonization of *S. agalactiae* is associated with their ability to bind to extracellular matrix proteins, predominantly to human fibrinogen. Fibrinogen is a glycoprotein present in the bloodstream and on the surface of the cells and tissues.[32] *S. agalactiae* interactions with fibrinogen are linked with the expression of the cell wall-anchored LPXTG protein fibrinogen-binding protein-A (FbsA) and the secreted protein FbsB, which promote invasion of epithelial cells. The LPXTG glycoproteins including Srr1 and Srr2also contribute to fibrinogen binding. In addition, Srr1 and FbsC can mediate the microorganism invasion of brain vascular endothelial cells and the translocation through the blood-brain barrier.[33,34] Another critical pathogenic mechanism for *S. agalactiae* is the production of the β-hemolysin. This toxin is cytolytic for brain endothelial cells and causes a disruption of the blood-brain barrier. This inflammatory mechanism also induces the production of interleukin (IL)-8 and the neutrophil receptor intercellular adhesion molecule-1 (ICAM-1), thereby promoting neutrophil migration across microvascular endothelial cells, suggesting that this toxin is crucial to the invasion of *S. agalactiae* into the CNS.[31]

E. coli colonizes the digestive tract of humans and animals, and it is the most common gram-negative microorganism that causes neonatal meningitis. In 80% of gram-negative neonatal meningitis cases, *E. coli* with K1 capsular polysaccharides are isolated in the cerebrospinal fluid (CSF).[24] E. coli K1 colonizes the gastrointestinal mucosa and translocates from the lumen of the small intestine or colon into the systemic circulation before entering into the CNS across the blood-brain barrier.[35] In an experimental meningitis model, the oral administration of E. coli K1 resulted in stable and persistent gastrointestinal colonization in newborn rats.[36] Using the same experimental model in a different study, *E. coli* K1 colonized the gut and then crossed the gastrointestinal barrier. With *the microorganism* present in the blood circulation and brain tissue, the neonatal rats developed a lethal systemic infection.[37]

L. monocytogenes is a facultative anaerobic, intracellular gram-positive bacillus that is motile by the use of its peritrichous flagella. This microorganism is a foodborne pathogen that can grow at low temperatures and cause meningitis, sepsis, and meningoencephalitis in neonates, pregnant women, and immunocompromised patients.[38] Maternal bacteremia can lead to fetal intrauterine infection; however, *L. monocytogenes* can also gain access to the neonate via oral exposure during the passage through the birth canal. An elevated concentration of this pathogen was found in the lung and gastrointestinal tract, suggesting that this infection can also be acquired in utero via the inhalation and ingestion of infected amniotic fluid and via the hematogenous route cross the blood-brain barrier.[39] In a preclinical model, 2 days after the oral inoculation with *L. monocytogenes* into pregnant guinea pigs, the pathogen was isolated from the placenta, fetal liver, and fetal brain.[40]

S. pneumoniae is a gram-positive lancet-shaped diplococcus arranged in pairs. The human nasopharynx is the main reservoir of *S. pneumoniae*, which usually leads to asymptomatic colonization. This microorganism is transferred between people by coughing and sneezing.[13,24] Pneumococcus colonizes the human nasopharynx through the degradation of mucus by several enzymes, such as neuraminidase A, β-galactosidase A, β-acetylglucosaminidase, and neuraminidase B.[41] Moreover, this microorganism is capable of expressing more than 90 serotypes based on differences in their capsular polysaccharides.[42] The expression of a polysaccharide capsule is required for the full pathogenicity of *S. pneumoniae* because the capsule can repulse the sialic acid residues of mucus, thereby decreasing the probability of pneumococcal immobilization.[43] Another virulence factor is a pore-forming toxin known shown as *pneumolysin*. This enzyme can induce pores in cholesterol-rich membranes and decrease cell ciliary beating to further activate the host immune response.[44,45] The pneumolysin can activate TLR 4 and NLRP3 (a PRR) and increase the proinflammatory response.

N. meningitidis is a gram-negative diplococcus that colonizes the nasopharynx of up to 35% of healthy individuals.[46,47] This pathogen presents 13 different capsular polysaccharide structures; however, only A, B, C, W-135, Y, and X cause the most life-threatening disease.[48] This microorganism may be acquired through the inhalation of respiratory droplets. *N. meningitidis* colonizes the nonciliated mucosal epithelial cells of the upper respiratory tract, where it can enter cells briefly before migrating back to the apical surfaces of the cells for the propagation to a new host.[49] The pathogen uses the polysaccharide capsules, pili, and outer membrane adhesion to develop an interface between the host and meningococcus. Thus, after the microorganism gains access to the bloodstream, it can multiply and disseminate into various tissues, thereby causing sepsis, purpura fulminans, and meningitis.[50]

CENTRAL NERVOUS SYSTEM BACTERIAL INVASIONS

MECHANISMS IMPLICATED IN MICROBIAL TRAVERSAL OF BLOOD-BRAIN BARRIER

The passage of microorganisms across the blood-brain barrier is a vital step in the development of meningitis.[51] The pathogens can cross the blood-brain barrier via the following different mechanisms: transcellular traversal, paracellular traversal, or Trojan-horse (microorganism inside of phagocytes).[52,53] Transcellular traversal occurs when the microorganism penetrates the cells without any traces or intracellular tight-junction disruption. In paracellular traversal, the microorganism penetrates between cells with or without evidence of tight-junction disruption, and by Trojan-horse, the microorganism crosses endothelial cells transmigrating into phagocytes.[52]

The microbial traversal of the blood-brain barrier occurs via an interaction between the microorganisms and host receptors.[54] *S. agalactiae* binds to the microvascular endothelial cells via the laminin-binding protein (LmB), FbsA, pilus tip adhesion (Pil-A), and invasion protein regulator (IagA) through lipoteichoic acid anchoring.[54] Pil-A binds to collagen, which promotes the *S. agalactiae* interaction with the $\alpha_2\beta_1$ integrin. Experimental meningitis in Pil-A–deficient mutant mice exhibited delayed mortality, a decrease in leukocyte infiltration, and bacterial dissemination into the CNS.[55] The FbsA binds with the Fn-integrin; the antifibronectin antibody that blocks fibronectin binding to integrins reduced the invasion of the wild-type *S. agalactiae*.[56]

E. coli K1 interacts with CD48 on brain microvascular endothelial cells through a type 1 fimbrial adhesion (FimHa bacterial adhesin), an outer-membrane protein A (OmpA) through *N*-acetylglucosamine (GlcNAc) or glucose-regulated protein-96 (Gp96), and cytotoxic-necrotizing factor 1 (CNF1) through the laminin receptor (LR).[52] CNF1 is a bacterial virulence factor that is primarily related to *E. coli* strains that cause meningitis.[57] This toxin contributes to the *E. coli* K1 invasion of brain endothelial cells in vitro and the traversal of the blood-brain barrier in a neonatal experimental meningitis model. Furthermore, an isogenic mutant lacking CNF1 was less invasive in brain endothelial cells and less able to penetrate the brain in vivo.[58] In vitro, a double-knockout mutant with deleted OmpA and CNF1 genes was less invasive in human brain microvascular endothelial cells.[59]

L. monocytogenes can cause life-threatening meningitis, and during this process, the pathogen crosses the blood-brain barrier by paracellular, transcellular, and intracellular mechanisms or within infected phagocytes.[52,60] The intracellular *L. monocytogenes* escapes from the phagosome by disrupting the phagosome membrane secreting the phosphatidylinositol-specific phospholipase C (Pic)-A and PlcB phospholipases, and the toxin listeriolysin O. Ultimately, the bacteria are released and multiply in the cytoplasm and disseminate into adjacent cells.[61] Another mechanism of invasion for this microorganism involves the functions of its surface proteins, internalin (Inl)-A and Inl-B. These proteins bind with the receptor for the globular head of the complement component C1q (gC1qR) or vascular endothelial (VE)-cadherin on endothelial cells.[60,62] The deletion of either or both of the proteins leads to decreased invasion, suggesting an interdependency of Inl-A and Inl-B during the invasion of choroid plexus epithelial cells.[62]

S. pneumoniae adheres to the blood-brain barrier endothelium before causing meningitis. This adhesion occurs when the pneumococcal surface protein C (PspC) interacts with the laminin receptor or the polymeric immunoglobulin receptor (pIgR) on brain endothelial cells.[13,63] *S. pneumoniae* adhesion is associated with pIgR on brain endothelial cells, and blocking the pIgR reduces the pneumococcal adhesion on endothelial cells.[63] Another interaction is between the cell-wall phosphorylcholine and the platelet-activating-factor receptor (PAFr) on endothelial cells.[52] The PAFr knockout mice showed an impaired ability to support bacterial translocation from the blood to the brain.[64] *S. pneumoniae* may penetrate the CSF intracellularly by disrupting tight intraepithelial junctions or by the transcellular mechanism.[13,52]

The *N. meningitidis* interaction involves numerous microbial structures and proteins, such as type IV pili, the CD147 receptor, and the β2-adrenoceptor (β2AR) on endothelial cells. CD147 is a receptor for the type IV pilus that facilitates the adhesion of meningococci on endothelial cells and in the brain. The pilin subunits PilE and PilV activate β2AR, thereby promoting endothelial cell signaling and facilitating the passage of the microorganisms through the blood-brain barrier.[50,65] This interaction between meningococcal ligands and the cellular host receptor is essential for *N. meningitidis* adhesion to human endothelial cells. Interfering with this interaction could prevent meningococcus-induced vascular dysfunctions (Fig. 168.1).[50]

RECOGNITION OF BACTERIAL INFECTION BY INNATE IMMUNE SENSORS

TOLL-LIKE RECEPTOR-SENSING BACTERIA

The innate immune system detects pathogens via several receptor families. TLRs recognize molecular motifs that are expressed by pathogens or endogenous ligands released by tissue insult.[66] TLRs trigger the immune response during meningitis, with TLR signaling representing a pivotal role in innate immune function.[67] The TLR receptors are organized into two broad categories: one group of receptors is expressed at the cell surface for extracellular ligand recognition (TLR1, TLR2, TLR4, TLR5, TLR6, and TLR10), and the other group is localized in intracellular endosomal compartments to recognize pathogen nucleic acids (TLR3, TLR7, TLR8, and TLR9) (see Fig. 168.1).[18]

TLR2 recognizes bacterial compounds, such as lipoproteins, peptidoglycan, and lipoteichoic acid.[68,69] In vitro, *L. monocytogenes* cell wall components were recognized by TLR2 with the help of CD14 and TLR6[70–72]; the lack of TLR2 was associated with a diminished bacterial clearing and impaired host resistance to *S. agalactiae* infection.[73] LPS is the significant component of the outer membrane of gram-negative bacteria, such as *E. coli*, which is recognized by TLR4; however, HMGB1, HSP, hyaluronic

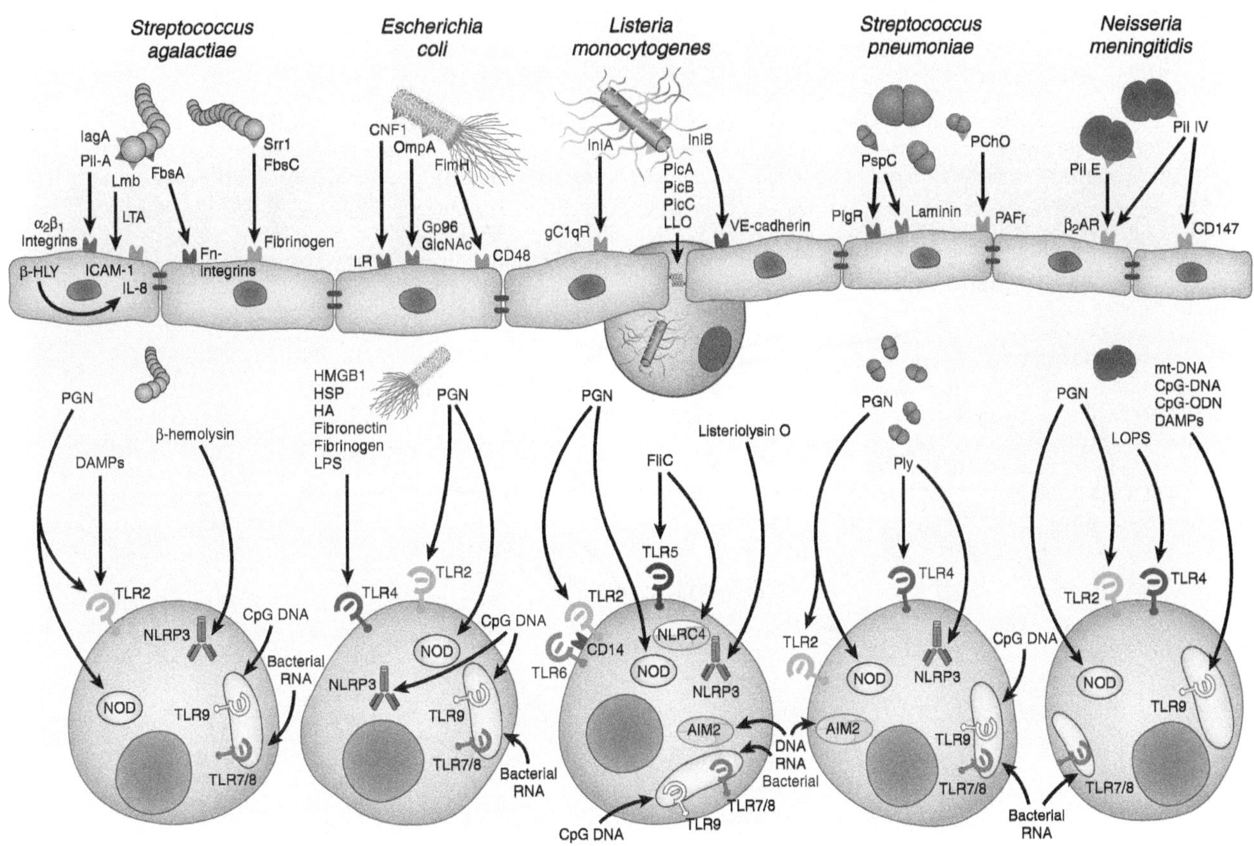

Fig. 168.1 Mechanisms involved in the microbial traversal of the blood-brain barrier.

acid, fibronectin, and fibrinogen are also recognized by TLR4.[14,74] In a preclinical study, the prestimulation of TLR4 increased the phagocytosis of *E. coli* strains by murine microglial cells.[75] Similarly, brain abscess caused by *E. coli* in a twin pair of neonatal patients was associated with a TLR4 gene mutation.[76] The important exotoxin pneumolysin produced by *S. pneumoniae* is recognized by TLR4 and confers resistance to pneumococcal infection.[77] Gram-positive and gram-negative bacteria can also have a flagellin protein, which is a component of the flagella, and TLR5 recognizes this protein.[78] TLR9 is a receptor for oligodeoxy nucleotides that contain unmethylated CpG motifs (CpG-ODN)[79,80] and recognizes bacterial cytosine-guanine (CpG)-containing DNA, mitochondrial DNA (mtDNA), and DAMPs.[81]

TLR signaling is initiated by the dimerization and recruitment of adaptor proteins. TLR1, TLR2, and TLR6 signal via myeloid differentiation factor 88 (MyD88) and the Toll/IL-1 receptor (TIR)-containing adaptor protein (TIRAP). TLR3 recruits the TIR domain–containing adaptor protein inducing interferon-β (TRIF). TLR5, TLR7, and TLR9 recruit only the MyD88 adaptor. TLR4 can signal through four of the adaptor molecules. TLR4 uses the TIRAP to bind MyD88 and the TRIF-related adaptor molecule (TRAM) to bind TRIF to stimulate the production of proinflammatory mediators.[10,82] *E. coli, S. pneumoniae,* and *N. meningitidis* are sensed by TLR4, thereby initiating a potent immune response through the four adaptors. Based on this feature, *N. meningitides, S. pneumoniae,* and *E. coli* can rapidly lead to a fatal septic shock.[4,50] After the recruitment by TLRs, the MyD88 adaptor molecule associates with IL-1 receptor-associated kinase-4 (IRAK-4), which is a serine/threonine kinase that phosphorylates IRAK-1 and IRAK-2.[83] Subsequently, IRAK interacts with the receptor-associated factor (TRAF) family and provides a link to the TAK1/TAB1/TAB2/TAB3 complex.[66] TAK1 phosphorylates the IKK complex, which in turn phosphorylates IKQ, resulting in the release and nuclear translocation of the transcription factor, nuclear factor-κB (NF-κB). NF-κB is a transcriptional activator of various genes involved in the pathogenesis of meningitis, such as tumor necrosis factor-alpha (TNF-α), IL-1β–inducible nitric oxide synthase (iNOS), and ICAMs.[84,85] TAK1 activation is also associated with the mitogen-activated protein kinase (MAPK) pathway. In addition, MAPKK-3/6, MAPKK-4/7, and MEK-1/2 induce the activation of p38, c-jun N-terminal kinase (JNK), and extracellular signal-regulated (ERK-1/2), respectively. These cascades lead to the translocation of protein-1 (AP-1) to the nucleus, thus promoting the transcription of inflammatory cytokines (Fig. 168.2).[66]

Among patients with a MyD88 deficiency or an IRAK-4 deficiency, 68% presented with invasive pneumococcal disease, and 45% presented with meningitis.[86,87] IRAK-4 and MyD88 deficiencies predispose patients to recurrent life-threatening bacterial infections in infancy and early childhood, resulting in minimal clinical features despite invasive bacterial infection.[88,89] According to the aforementioned studies in humans, in experimental pneumococcal meningitis, MyD88-deficient mice presented with a decrease of pleocytosis, proinflammatory mediators, cytokines, and chemokines in the CNS. Nevertheless, MyD88 deficiency was associated with severe bacteremia.[90] Similarly, in *E. coli* K1 neonatal meningitis, MyD88-deficient mice were unable to control meningitis, demonstrating that MyD88 has a critical role in early host defense.[91] In mice, vulnerability to neurologic morbidity changes intensely during the first few weeks of life. This may elucidate why the neonatal brain is particularly sensitive to infection and why infection during this time can lead to long-term neurologic sequelae.[92]

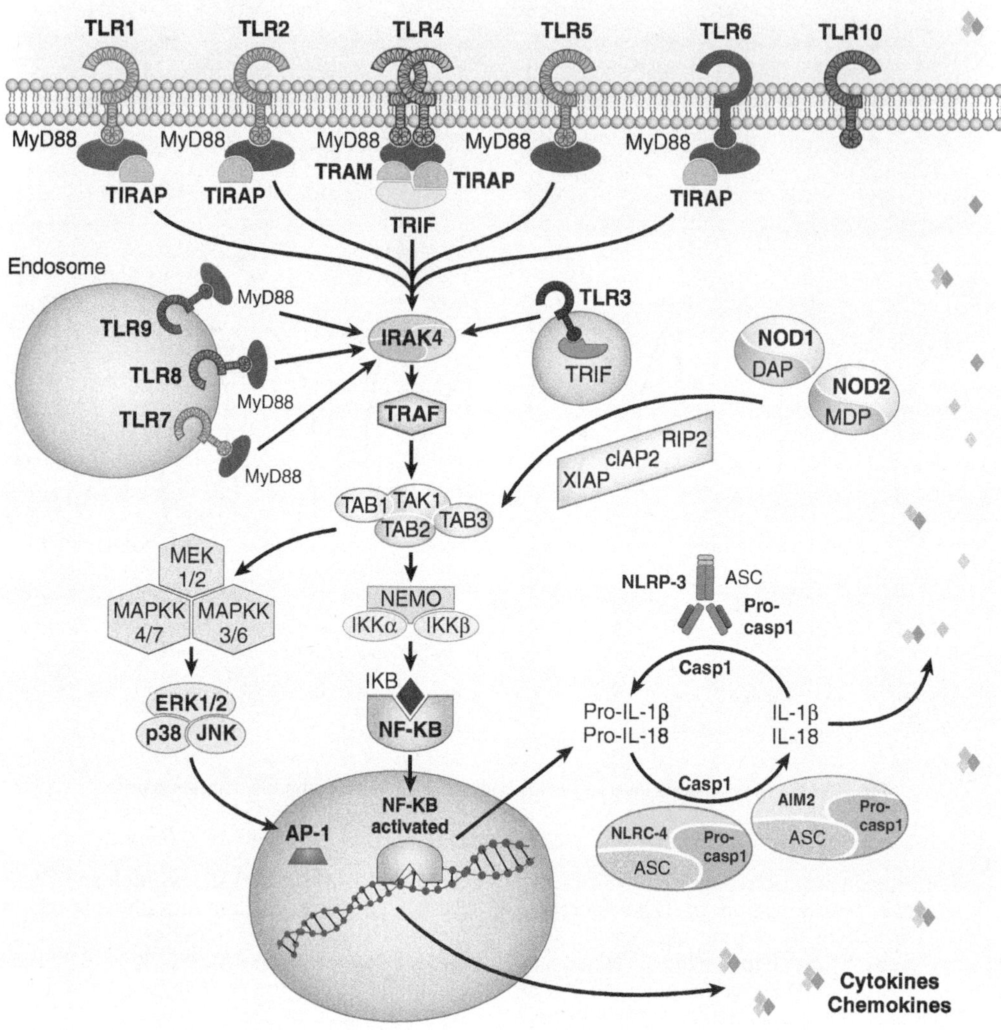

Fig. 168.2 Recognition of bacterial compounds by innate immune sensors.

NOD1 AND NOD2 SIGNALING

NLRs belong to a family of cytosolic sensors that are involved in the detection of different pathogens and the detection of DAMPs.[18] NLR intracellular proteins are characterized by their C-terminal leucine-rich repeat (LRR) domains and central NACHT nucleotide-binding domains (NBDs).[93] One group includes NOD1 (CARD4) and NOD2 (CARD15), which activates several transcription factors to trigger the production of proinflammatory mediators.[94] The second group operates through the formation of a multiprotein complex called the *inflammasome*, in which the components signal for the activation of procaspase-1 and the maturation of the IL-1 family of cytokines.[10] NOD1 and NOD2 identify peptidoglycan remains from gram-positive and gram-negative bacteria. The peptidoglycans are abundant constituents of bacterial cell walls and exhibit numerous immunobiologic activities.[95] NOD1 binds to γ-D-glutamyl-Meso-diaminopimelic acid (DAP), and NOD2 is activated by the muramyl dipeptide (MDP).[94] After the recognition of the bacterial peptidoglycan, cytosolic NOD1/2 receptors recruit the receptor-interacting protein-2 (RIP2), cellular inhibitor of apoptosis-2 (cIAP2), and X-linked inhibitor of apoptosis protein (XIAP). This cascade provides a link to the TAK1/TAB1/TAB2/TAB3 complex and IKK complex, which phosphorylate IKB, resulting in the release and nuclear translocation of the transcription factor, NF-κB and MAPK, to induce the transcription of IL-1 cytokines.[10,96] Rodents lacking NOD1 were susceptible to both gram-positive microorganisms and early pneumococcal sepsis.[97] In vitro, NOD2 mediated the high inflammatory responses of primary murine glia to *S. pneumoniae*.[98] Otherwise, NOD2 knockout mice showed similar levels of bacteremia and survival rates compared with a control group using a model of infection by *S. agalactiae*.[99]

NLRP3 INFLAMMASOME-SENSING BACTERIA

The NLRP3 inflammasome is composed of NOD-like receptor 3 (NLRP3), pro-caspase-1, and the adaptor protein apoptosis-associated speck-like protein comprising a caspase recruitment domain (ASC).[10] The NLRP3 inflammasome oligomerization is activated by a large number of stimuli, such as bacterial toxins, β-hemolysin, pneumolysin, listeriolysin O, bacterial compounds, and DAMPs. Pneumolysin, the exotoxin from pneumococcus can activate NLRP3 and AIM2 (absent in melanoma-2)[100] and β-hemolysin, a vital virulence factor *S. agalactiae* can activate

NLRP3. NLRP3 has also been associated with the responses to several microorganisms, such as *Staphylococcus aureus* (hemolysin O), *L. monocytogenes* (listeriolysin O), *Klebsiella pneumoniae,* and *E. coli*.[101] *Listeria* sp. infection is also sensed by AIM2 and NLRC-4,which, with NLRP-3, orchestrate a strong caspase-1 activation and proinflammatory response.[102] Upon activation, NLRP3 oligomerizes with ASC and pro-caspase 1. Procaspase-1 is converted to activated caspase-1, which subsequently matures and secretes the proinflammatory cytokines IL-1β and IL-18 in their mature form.[103]

The NLPR3 inflammasome is responsible for the production of critical proinflammatory cytokines that are well known in the CSF of patients with bacterial meningitis. IL-1β and IL-18 levels in the CSF are associated with unfavorable disease outcomes in patients with bacterial meningitis.[104] In a murine model of pneumococcal meningitis, NLRP3 induced caspase-1 activation. In addition, NLRP3 and ASC inhibition were associated with reduced clinical and histologic disease severity and decreased brain inflammation.[105] In another experimental study, NLRP3- and ASC-deficient mice displayed a decrease in systemic inflammatory responses. However, the same animals exhibited an increase in cerebral neutrophil infiltration and cerebral hemorrhages compared with wild-type mice.[104] Mice lacking NLRP3, ASC, or caspase-1 were more susceptible to *S. agalactiae* infection compared with wild-type mice.[106] The challenge lies in identifying when the immune response is essential to eliminate the microorganism versus when it is activated to cause impairment to the host.

CENTRAL NERVOUS SYSTEM IMMUNE RESPONSE

PROINFLAMMATORY CYTOKINES

The CSF of neonates with bacterial meningitis contains high levels of TNF-α, IL-1β, and IL-6.[107,108] Likewise, children with bacterial meningitis exhibited an increase in TNF-α, IL-6, and IL-8 concentrations in the CSF.[109] Tang and coworkers identified IL-1β and TNF-α in the CSF of children with bacterial meningitis, with 78% and 74% sensitivity and 96% and 81% specificity, respectively.[110] In a meta-analysis, the TNF-α and IL-1β levels were identified as useful markers for the prediction of bacterial meningitis.[111] It was suggested that the levels of these cytokines, particularly TNF-α and IL-1β, are useful markers for distinguishing bacterial meningitis from aseptic meningitis.

In experimental neonatal meningitis caused by *S. agalactiae*, the levels of TNF-α, IL-1β, IL-6, and cytokine-induced neutrophil chemoattractant-1 (CINC-1), an analogue of human IL-8, were detectable in the first 24 hours post infection. These cytokines were increased simultaneously with the blood-brain barrier disruption.[112] The same result was found in rodents subjected to *E. coli* K1 meningitis[113] and in experimental pneumococcal meningitis infection during the neonatal period of life.[114] The time-dependent association between the complex interactions among cytokines and chemokines could be responsible for the blood-brain barrier breakdown and the severity of neonatal meningitis. Differences in brain inflammation responses were found between neonatal and weanling rodents. Neonatal and weanling mice were inoculated intracerebrally with LPS, the ligand for TLR4, or the ligand for TLR9. IL-1α, IL-1β, IL-2, IL-5, IL-6, TNF-α, CC chemokine ligand-2 (CCL-2), CCL3, and CXCL9 were significantly higher in the neonatal brain than in the weanling brain tissue in response to LPS. The TLR4 ligand also induced higher levels of IL-2, IL-5, TNF, CCL2, and CXCL9 in the neonatal brain tissue compared with the levels in the weanling mice brain.[92]

TNF-α and IL-1β are important early proinflammatory response cytokines for adequate host response to an infection. The administration of TNF-α or recombinant human IL-1 intracerebrally in rodents resulted in inflammation and blood-brain barrier breakdown, and these pathophysiologic changes were similar to that of bacterial meningitis infection.[115,116] On the contrary, mice deficient in TNF-α that were subjected to pneumococcal meningitis showed an increase in mortality and memory impairment.[117] Likewise, mice deficient in interleukin-1 receptor (IL-1R) type I gene showed higher mortality and an earlier course of pneumococcal meningitis.[118] The TNF-α antibody was not as effective as adjunctive therapy in attenuating acute inflammatory responses and improving brain injury in neonatal *E. coli* meningitis.[119] Thus these cytokines were responsible for the complications of the inflammatory response in several rodent models of meningitis but are simultaneously essential for an adequate host immune response.

IL-6 is produced in response to infections and tissue injuries and contributes to the host immune defense through the stimulation of acute phase proteins, fever, leukocytosis, and the activation of the complement cascade.[120] In patients with acute bacterial meningitis, the IL-6 concentrations in the CSF[121,122] and the serum were significantly elevated.[123] Moreover, although IL-6 was elevated in the CSF of pediatric patients with bacterial meningitis, this cytokine was not associated with bacteremia, neurologic complications, or sequelae in these patients.[124] In experimental meningitis, mice that lacked IL-6 presented with an increase in the inflammatory response in the CSF; however, there was also a reduction of vascular permeability, intracranial pressure, and blood-brain barrier disruption during the bacterial meningitis infection.[125] In experimental models, IL-6 has shown a dual role as both a proinflammatory and antiinflammatory cytokine.[125,126]

IL-8 is a potent chemoattractant for polymorphonuclear leukocytes and helps to direct these cells to the site of inflammation.[127] The IL-8 concentration in the CSF of infants with purulent meningitis was significantly higher compared with infants without meningitis. Furthermore, after the initiation of antibiotic therapy in bacterial meningitis, the levels of this cytokine decreased rapidly.[128] In a study that included children up to 14 years of age with meningitis, the CSF level of IL-8 showed a sensitivity and specificity of 80.7% and 86.7%, respectively.[109] Another study evaluated the role of the CSF IL-8 in differentiating acute bacterial meningitis from aseptic meningitis. The IL-8 levels in the CSF were higher in bacterial meningitis compared with aseptic meningitis, suggesting that IL-8 could be an essential biomarker to differentiate bacterial meningitis from aseptic meningitis.[129] The cytokine CINC-1 is the rat homologue to human IL-8, and in experimental neonatal meningitis induced by *S. agalactiae*, *E. coli* K1, or *S. pneumoniae*, CINC-1 was produced primarily during the first 6 hours in the hippocampus and cortex.[113,114,130] The CINC-1 levels showed an increase in the jugular veins rather than the arterial plasma, suggesting their production in the brain.[131] In a rabbit model of pneumococcal meningitis, a monoclonal antibody to IL-8 administered intravenously attenuated the pleocytosis in the CSF.[132] Thus CINC-1 seems to be relevant in the early stage of bacterial meningitis because of its ability to promote leukocyte migration.[131]

Due to the production of cytokines, leukocytes are attracted from the bloodstream to the site of infection.[133] Initially, the interaction between leukocytes and endothelial cells is mediated by the endothelial adhesion molecules E-selectin and P-selectin with their leukocyte counterparts, L-selectin and P-selectin glycoprotein ligand (PSGL)-1.[134] Selectins also recognize the fucose-containing tetrasaccharide sialyl-Lewis X attached to glycoproteins and glycolipids on endothelial cells.[135] This connection becomes stronger when IL-8 binds to its specific receptor on leukocytes, triggering the production of the integrin lymphocyte function-associated antigen-1 (LFA-1). Inflammatory cytokines such as TNF-α are necessary to induce the expression of the adhesion molecules ICAM-1 and ICAM-2. The link between the endothelial cells and ICAM-1 allows the passage of leukocytes in the direction of the gradient of chemoattractant substances.[136,137]

OXIDATIVE DAMAGE

During bacterial meningitis, oxidative and nitrogen species are produced by immune cells as part of the host response in an attempt to inhibit the invading microorganism.[13,138] The simultaneous production of superoxide anion radicals ($O_2^{-\bullet}$) and nitric oxide (NO) leads to the formation of peroxynitrite ($ONOO^-$), which is a strong oxidant.[139] The $ONOO^-$ can cause injury in neurons and glial cells through lipid peroxidation, cell membrane destabilization, and DNA disintegration, which leads to a cell energy reduction and death.[140] Furthermore, other chemical reactions can produce several toxic agents; $O_2^{-\bullet}$ is transformed by the enzyme superoxide dismutase into hydrogen peroxide (H_2O_2).[141,142] The peroxidase enzyme can transform H_2O_2 in the presence of Fe^{2+} into hypochlorite (OCl^-) and hydroxyl radicals ($^\bullet OH$).[139,142,143] As a consequence, oxidative stress leads to the activation of cytokines, lipid peroxidation, mitochondrial injury, activation of matrix metalloproteinases (MMPs), increased blood-brain barrier permeability, and the development of long-term neurologic damage.[9,139]

The evidence for the relevance of oxidative stress in meningitis came from CSF and blood sample studies. The biomarkers of oxidative damage (i.e., malondialdehyde [lipid peroxidation], protein carbonyl, and nitrite) showed elevated levels in the plasma and the CSF of children with bacterial meningitis, whereas the antioxidant defense concentrations of ascorbic acid, glutathione, and superoxide dismutase levels were significantly decreased.[144] In another study, a positive correlation was found between the NO index and white blood cells and malondialdehyde in the CSF of children with bacterial meningitis compared to a control group.[145] In preclinical experiments, a similar result was found in neonatal meningitis induced by different microorganisms. The protein carbonyl and malondialdehyde levels increased in the hippocampus; however, the superoxide dismutase activity decreased in the same brain structure in meningitis induced by *S. agalactiae* and *S. pneumoniae*.[112,114] The infant animals also had a loss of the cortical concentrations of the endogenous antioxidant ascorbate and reduced glutathione (GSH) and presented a moderate increase in their malondialdehyde levels in the cortex after pneumococcal meningitis.[146] Reactive oxygen species contribute to necrotic and apoptotic neuronal injury in an infant rodent model of meningitis due to group B streptococci. Treatment with the radical scavenger α-phenyl-tert-butyl nitrone (PBN) eliminated ROS detection and prevented neuronal injury in the cortex and hippocampus.[147] Another consequence of oxidative stress production is an increase in the blood-brain barrier permeability. The breakdown of the blood-brain barrier occurs with a decrease in enzymatic defense, oxidative damage, and cytokine production after neonatal meningitis induced by *S. agalactiae* and *S. pneumoniae*.[112,114] Oxidative and nitrosative stress have been implicated as mediators of blood-brain barrier breakdown,[139] suggesting that an increase of the blood-brain barrier permeability appears to be related to the presence of $NO^\bullet$ and $O_2^{-\bullet}$.[148] This unbalances between an increase in the production of reactive oxygen species, and a decrease of antioxidant defenses is defined as oxidative stress[149] and can be associated with the long-term consequences of bacterial meningitis.

KYNURENINE PATHWAY

Tryptophan is an essential amino acid that serves as a substrate for the production of numerous bioactive compounds involved in the host immune response, inflammatory mediators, and neurotransmission.[150] The kynurenine pathway of tryptophan degradation metabolizes most of the concentration of tryptophan ingested, and approximately 60% of kynurenine and its metabolites are transported across the blood-brain barrier and are degraded via the kynurenine pathway.[150,151] Upon entering the kynurenine pathway, tryptophan is converted to N-formyl-L-kynurenine by tryptophan 2,3-dioxygenase and indoleamine 2,3-dioxygenase (IDO).[152] Enzymes then metabolize kynureninein, a sequence of new compounds that have neurotoxic (quinolinic acid and 3-hydroxykynurenine) or neuroprotective properties (kynurenic acid, picolinic acid, and nicotinamide-adenine-dinucleotide [NAD]$^+$).[153] The neurotoxic effect of the intermediates 3-hydroxykynurenine and 3-hydroxyanthranilic acid involves the generation of $O_2^{-\bullet}$ and H_2O_2, which contribute to the oxidative processes implicated in the pathophysiology of the meningitis.[154] The proinflammatory environment during bacterial meningitis is a potent inducer of IDO.[153] Patients with bacterial meningitis exhibited an increase in kynurenic acid, anthranilic acid, and IDO activity in the CSF,[151] corroborating the findings from animal models.[153,155] The levels of IL-1β, IL-6, TNF-α, IFN-γ, IL-10, and IL-1Ra were significantly up-regulated in CSF during bacterial meningitis when compared with the nonmeningitis control group. The INF-γ and IL-1Ra cytokines presented a positive correlation with IDO activity. In addition, TNF-α and IL-10 showed a positive association with kynurenine and kynurenic acid. The L-tryptophan-kynurenine pathway produces neuroprotective as well as neurotoxic metabolites. In this study, the CSF of the patients with bacterial meningitis presented increased levels of kynurenic acid. This acid acts as an antiexcitotoxic and anticonvulsant by blocking excitatory amino acid receptors. The levels of kynurenine and anthranilic acid and the activity of IDO were also increased compared with the nonmeningitis group, demonstrating that bacterial meningitis activates the L-tryptophan-kynurenine pathway.[156]

In a neonatal rat model of pneumococcal meningitis, there was an activation of the kynurenine pathway through the production of the neurotoxic metabolites 3-hydroxykynurenine and 3-hydroxyanthranilic acid in the cortex and hippocampus. There was also a positive correlation between the concentration of 3-hydroxykynurenine and hippocampal apoptosis.[153] In an adult rodent model of pneumococcal meningitis, the inhibition of IDO decreased TNF-α, CINC-1, and leukocytes in the CSF and prevented long-term cognitive impairment.[157] IDO has been identified as having critical immunomodulatory properties, primarily immunosuppressive effects, in the kynurenine pathway.[158,159] In another study, the inhibition of kynurenine 3-hydroxylase and kynureninase led to decreased cellular NAD levels and increased apoptosis in the hippocampus, suggesting that the activation of the kynurenine pathway could be neuroprotective by compensating for an increased NAD demand caused by infection and inflammation.[155]

MICROGLIA AND MENINGITIS

Microglia cells are the resident macrophages of the CNS; they originate from the yolk sac or bloodstream and help to regulate inflammation in the brain.[160] When in a resting/inactive state, microglia present a ramified morphology and exhibit an extensive surface area to assess and control the changes in their environment; activated microglia modify their phenotype depending on the type of stimulus and the environment. Typically, the amoeboid microglia shape appears in response to infection, trauma, and infarction of the CNS.[161] Thus the microglial response has been proposed to mediate a myriad of aspects of neuroinflammation, and these various functions are associated with numerous phenotypes that can induce different signaling cascades involved in chemotaxis, phagocytosis, and the production of neurotoxic and antiinflammatory mediators.[162,163] Activated microglia release IL-1α, TNF-α, and C1q, and these proinflammatory mediators can induce reactive astrocytes, called A1. The A1 astrocytes lose their ability to promote neuronal survival, outgrowth, synaptogenesis, and phagocytosis, and produce a neurotoxin that can induce the death of neurons and oligodendrocytes.[164] Microglial cells can also identify neuronal damage and neurodegeneration-associated molecular patterns (NAMPs), via specific receptors (TREM2 and purinergic receptors) demonstrating a possible protective role in neurodegenerative diseases.[165] A heightened neonatal microglia activation was found in the CNS in response to TLR4 and TLR9 stimulation. The expression of the gene markers CD11, CD172, and F4/80 was increased in the microglia cells of rodent neonates.[92] In another study, neonatal rats that received stimulation from LPS injected into the brain presented in their adulthood with an increase in the number of activated microglial cells in the hippocampus and other brain regions, such as the cerebral cortex and thalamus. The microglial activation was identified through the ionized calcium-binding adaptor molecule 1 (Iba1), a microglial marker.[166] The activation of microglia coincided with the intense production of TNF-α, IL-1β, and IL-6 and oxidative damage in the same brain structure in experimental *K. pneumoniae* meningitis.[167]

DAMPS AND BACTERIAL MENINGITIS

Bacterial meningitis and the host immune response generated by meningitis disease can damage or distress cells, which led to these cells or damaged tissues to release several endogenous molecules that can activate the classical PRRs and non-PRRs receptors, and DAMPs.[168] The DAMPs can activate the immune response by binding to TLRs, NOD-like receptors, RIG-I, CLRs, RAGE, TREMs, and CPCRs (Table 168.1).

The HMGB1 protein is a nonhistone chromosomal protein that forms an integral part of the architectural protein repertoire to support chromatin structure in the cell nucleus.[169] During meningitis, HMGB1 is likely released from dying cells, and it also presents a role as a cytokine and elicits variable immunologic responses. HMGB1 is recognized by TLR2, TLR4, TLR9, and RAGE, activating the immune response as a central propagator of inflammation in bacterialmeningitis.[170,171] The CSF levels of HMGB1 and HSP-72 were higher in children with a variety of kinds of bacterial and viral meningitis compared with controls, and CSF levels of HMGB1 levels were four times higher in children with bacterial meningitis compared with aseptic meningitis.[172] The HMGB1 is a central propagator of inflammation in bacterial meningitis.[170] Another DAMP, HSP, is produced by cells following intense heat or other severe stresses; during normal physiologic conditions, they are not synthesized. The TLR2 and TLR4 recognize the HSPs by activating the immune system. The HSP72 levels were higher in the CSF of children with bacterial meningitis compared with controls.[173] In another study, the CSF level of HSP70 was higher in the CSF of purulent meningitis, viral meningitis, and tuberculous meningitis compared with the control group.[174] The S-100 protein is localized in the cytoplasm and nucleus of a wide variety of cells, and members of this protein family are implicated in intracellular and extracellular regulatory effects.[175] Low levels of S-100B (which is trophic to neural cells) under normal physiologic conditions have been shown to decrease microglial activation via the STAT3 pathway. Moreover, during inflammation, there are increases of the S-100B and the S-100B receptor, RAGE, in neural and inflammatory cells that can activate microglia via NF-κB- and AP-1-dependent pathways.[175] The concentration of the S-100B protein in the CSF of patients appeared to be related to the clinical severity of the bacterial meningitis infection.[176] CSF S-100B levels were evaluated in children with CNS infections and children as a control group. CSF S-100B levels in the encephalitis group were higher than the meningitis group and the control group at each age range.[177] S-100B also presented higher levels in the CSF of children with bacterial meningitis compared with healthy children.[145] Other studies have corroborated this findings.[178]

NEURONAL BRAIN DAMAGE

Apoptosis of the neurons in the dentate gyrus was observed in 70% of autopsy cases of bacterial meningitis.[179] The axonal injury was also found in the white matter in all autopsy cases.[180] The same findings were identified in animal models of bacterial meningitis. In the experimental rodent model, the histomorphologic brain damage was characterized by necrotic tissue damage in the cortex and apoptosis of neurons in the hippocampal dentate gyrus.[181,182] Apoptosis in the dentate gyrus of infant mice infected with *S. pneumoniae* showed a peak at 30 hours after infection.[182] The bacteremia occurring during meningitis also plays an essential role in the development of the hippocampal apoptosis injury in experimental pneumococcal meningitis,[183] and there is an association between the extent of apoptotic neuronal injury in the dentate gyrus and reduced learning capacities of the animals.[184] Bacterial meningitis injures hippocampal stem and progenitor cells, a finding that may explain the persistence of the neurofunctional deficits after bacterial meningitis.[185]

Reactive oxygen intermediates contributed to necrotic and apoptotic neuronal damage in an infant rodent model of bacterial meningitis caused by *S. agalactiae*.[147] Similarly, NO played a vital role in the hippocampal caspase-3 activation during pneumococcal meningitis. The inactivation of iNOS resulted in a reduction of caspase-3 activation in experimental murine pneumococcal meningitis.[186] The brain is vulnerable to oxidative damage primarily because of its high oxygen consumption, presence of iron, relatively low expression of antioxidant defenses,[187] and significant presence of polyunsaturated fatty acids.[139] Furthermore, the production of toxic species such as H_2O_2 and pneumolysin can cause neuronal cell death through mitochondrial damage,[188,189] leading to the release of the apoptosis-inducing factor (AIF) into the cytosol and subsequently inducing apoptosis by a caspase-independent pathway.[189] The impairment of mitochondrial function was induced by the pore-forming toxin produced by *L. monocytogenes* (listeriolysin O).[190] *S. agalactiae* also produces a critical pore-forming cytolytic toxin, β-hemolysin. This toxin is responsible for causing damage in brain endothelial cells and macrophages[191] and also induces neuronal apoptosis independently of caspase activation that was not preventable by the broad-spectrum caspase inhibitor in experimental neonatal meningitis.[192]

Bacterial meningitis causes the secretion of proinflammatory cytokines, chemokines, and other chemotactic stimuli, followed by the recruitment of leukocytes into the CNS.[193] Infants with bacterial meningitis had an increase in white blood cells in the CSF compared with infants without meningitis.[194,195] Invading peripheral immune cells into the brain and microglial activation may induce caspase-independent apoptosis during pneumococcal meningitis.[13] Thus leukocytes activate the tumor suppressor protein (p53) and the ataxia telangiectasia-mutated (ATM) kinase, which induce mitochondria to release cytochrome-c. The cytochrome-c, apoptotic protease-activating factor-1 (Apaf-1), and deoxyadenosine triphosphate (dATP) are required to form the apoptosome. The apoptosome is a protein complex that activates caspase-9, which results in the activation of caspase-3 and apoptosis.[189,196]

LONG-TERM BEHAVIORAL SEQUELAE

In neonatal meningitis, half of the children who survived presented with long-term impairment in learning, hearing, and memory.[1-3] The disabilities found included developmental delay, cerebral palsy, decreased visual acuity, and sensorineural deafness.[3,20] The pathophysiologic mechanisms of neonatal meningitis leading to long-term behavioral compromise occur

Table 168.1 Pathogen-Associated Molecular Patterns and Damage-Associated Molecular Patterns Associated With Bacterial Meningitis and Their Receptors in Central Nervous System.

Microorganism	PAMPs	DAMPs	Receptors	PRRs in CNS human cells	Refs
Streptococcus agalactiae	Triacylated lipoproteins		TLR1/2	Microglia and neuron	67
	Lipoteichoic acid	HMGB-1, HSPs, histone	TLR2	Microglia, oligodendrocyte, neuron	14,18,67,203,204
	Diacylated lipoproteins		TLR2/6		
		HMGB1, HSP60, HSP70, hyaluronic acid, fibronectin, fibrinogen	TLR4	Microglia, astrocyte, neuron	168
	Bacterial RNA	MicroRNAs	TLR7/8	Microglia and neuron	67,205
	CpG DNA	HMGB1, mtDNA	TLR9	Microglia, astrocyte, and neuron	67,79,168
	DAP		NOD1	Microglia	10,18,206
	MDP		NOD2		
	β-hemolysin	ATP, Amyloid-β, ROS	NLRP3	Microglia, astrocyte, and neuron	10,106
		HMGB-1, Amyloid-β, S-100β	RAGE	Microglia, astrocyte, and neuron	14,207
Escherichia coli	Triacylated lipoproteins		TLR1/2	Microglia and neuron	67
	Diacylated lipoproteins	HMGB-1, HSPs, histone	TLR2	Microglia, oligodendrocyte, neuron	67
	Diacylated lipoproteins		TLR2/6		
	Lipopolysaccharide	MRP8, MRP14, HMGB1, HSP60, HSP70, hyaluronic acid, fibronectin, fibrinogen	TLR4	Microglia, astrocyte, and neuron	67,208
	Bacterial flagellin		TLR5	Microglia, astrocyte, and neuron	209
	Bacterial RNA		TLR7/8		
	Bacterial CpG DNA	HMGB1, mtDNA	TLR9	Microglia, astrocyte and neuron	14,67,79
	DAP		NOD1	Microglia	10,18,206
	MDP		NOD2		
	Bacterial DNA	ATP, Amyloid-β, ROS	NLRP3	Microglia, astrocyte, and neuron	10,210
		HMGB-1, Amyloid-β, S-100β	RAGE	Microglia, astrocyte, and neuron	14,207
			TREM1		211,212
Listeria monocytogenes	Triacylated lipoproteins		TLR1/2	Microglia and neuron	67
	Listeria lipoprotein, lipoteichoic acid	HMGB-1, HSPs, histone	TLR2	Microglia, oligodendrocyte, neuron	67,203,213
		HMGB1, HSP60, HSP70, hyaluronic acid, fibronectin, fibrinogen	TLR4	Microglia, astrocyte, neuron	
	Protein flagellin		TLR5	Microglia, neuron	67,78
	Diacylated lipoprotein		TLR2/6	Microglia, neuron	67
	Bacterial RNA		TLR7/8		
	Bacterial CpG DNA	HMGB1, mtDNA	TLR9	Microglia, astrocyte and neuron	168
	Listeria DNA		AIM2	Microglia, astrocyte, and neuron	214
	DAP		NOD1	Microglia	10,18,206,215
	MDP		NOD2		
	Listeria pedtidoglycan				
	Listeria DNA/toxin listeriolysin O	Cathepsin B, ATP, Amyloid-β, ROS	NLRP3	Microglia, astrocyte, and neuron	10,202
	Listeria monomeric flagellin		NLRC4		214
		HMGB1, Amyloid-β	RAGE	Microglia	216
Streptococcus pneumoniae	Triacylated lipoproteins		TLR1/2	Microglia and neuron	67
	Peptidoglycan, lipoteichoic acid	HMGB-1, HSPs, histone	TLR2	Microglia, oligodendrocyte, neuron	217
	Diacylated lipoproteins		TLR2/6		
	Pneumolysin	MRP14, HMGB1, HSP60, HSP70, hyaluronic acid, fibronectin, fibrinogen	TLR4	Microglia, astrocyte, neuron	67,77,218
	Bacterial RNA		TLR7/8		
	Pneumococcal CpG DNA	HMGB-1, mtDNA	TLR9	Microglia, astrocyte and neuron	67,69,79,168
	Pneumococcal DNA		AIM2	Microglia, astrocyte and neuron	100
	DAP		NOD1	Microglia	10,18,206,215
	MDP		NOD2		
	Pneumolysin, bacterial DNA, muramyl dipeptide	ATP, Amyloid-β, ROS	NLRP3	Microglia, astrocyte, and neuron	10,210
	PCho-bearing teichoic acids		PAFr	Microglia, neurons	217
		HMGB-1, Amyloid-β, S-100β	RAGE	Microglia, astrocyte, and neuron	14,170,219
			TREM1	Microglia	211

Table 168.1 Pathogen-Associated Molecular Patterns and Damage-Associated Molecular Patterns Associated With Bacterial Meningitis and Their Receptors in Central Nervous System—cont'd

Microorganism	PAMPs	DAMPs	Receptors	PRRs in CNS human cells	Refs
Neisseria meningitidis	Triacylated lipoproteins		TLR1/2	Microglia and neuron	
	Peptidoglycan	HMGB-1, HSPs, histone	TLR2	Microglia, oligodendrocyte, neuron	67,203
	Lipooligosaccharide	HMGB1, HSP60, HSP70, hyaluronic acid, fibronectin, fibrinogen	TLR4	Microglia, astrocyte, and neuron	67,220,221
	Bacterial RNA		TLR7/8		
	Bacterial CpG DNA	HMGB1, mtDNA	TLR9	Microglia, astrocyte, and neuron	67,69,79,168
	DAP		NOD1	Microglia	10,18,206,215
	MDP		NOD2		
		ATP, Amyloid-β, ROS	NLRP3	Microglia, astrocyte, and neuron	10,210
		HMGB-1, Amyloid-β, S-100β	RAGE	Microglia, astrocyte, and neuron	14,207
			TREM1		211

AIM, Apoptosis inhibitor of macrophages receptor; *ATP,* adenosine triphosphate; *CNS,* central nervous system; *CpG,* Unmethylated cytosine-phosphate-guanine; *DAMP,* damage-associated molecular pattern; *DAP,* d-glutamyl-Meso-diaminopimelic acid; *HSPs,* Heat-shock proteins; *HMGB1,* High mobility group box 1 protein; *mtDNA,* mitochondrial DNA; *MDP,* Muramyl dipeptide; *MRP,* myeloid-related protein; *NLR,* NOD-like receptor; *NLRP3,* NOD-like receptor 3; *NOD,* nucleotide-binding oligomerization domain; *PAFr,* platelet-activating factor receptor; *PAMP,* pathogen-associated molecular pattern; *PCho,* phosphocholine; *ROS,* reactive oxygen species; *RAGE,* receptor for advanced glycation end products; *TLR,* Toll-like receptor; *TREM,* triggering receptor expressed on myeloid cells.

through a combination of several factors.[181] During replication, the microorganisms release their bacterial components, which are highly immunogenic and may lead to an increase in the inflammatory response in the host.

As a consequence, immune cells are recruited from the bloodstream to the site of infection producing proinflammatory mediators and phagocytosing the invasive pathogen. During phagocytosis, high amounts of reactive oxygen and nitrogen species are produced in an attempt to eliminate the microorganism invasion, which subsequently leads to lipid peroxidation, protein oxidation, mitochondrial damage, blood-brain barrier breakdown, and release of DAMPs. This inflammatory and activated state contributes to brain cell injury during bacterial meningitis.[11,51,197,198] Thus the development of brain damage results from the combined effects of pathogen-derived factors and the host immune response.[9,24]

Experimental rodent models of neonatal meningitis induced by different microorganisms have demonstrated the consequences of neurologic sequelae in adulthood. Neonatal rats that received an intrahippocampal injection of LPS demonstrated behavioral alterations (e.g., deficits in social interaction, did not recognize a novel object, anxiety- and depression-like behavior) and microglial cell activation in adulthood.[166] Similarly, adult rats survivors of neonatal meningitis by *S. agalactiae* showed a decrease in the brain-derived neurotrophic factor (BDNF) levels in the hippocampus and impairment of learning and memory.[199] The same impairment of learning and memory has also been shown in rodents subjected to neonatal meningitis by *S. pneumoniae*. The decrease of hippocampal BDNF levels was correlated with memory impairment in adult animals subjected to experimental meningitis during the neonatal period.[200] *E. coli* K1 neonatal meningitis triggered an impairment of habituation and aversive memory in the adult life of rodents. The animals needed a significant increase in training tasks to learn when compared with the control group.[113] In an attempt to minimize the long-term cognitive impairment, infant animals that were subjected to bacterial meningitis were exposed to environmental enrichment until adulthood. The environmental enrichment included an altered housing condition in which the animals were kept, which contained spacious cages with toys, running wheels, climbing ropes, and several objects with different shapes and textures.[201] In adult life, these animals demonstrated preservation of aversive and habituation memory when compared with survivors of neonatal meningitis placed in a usual cage.[202]

CONCLUSION

Neonatal bacterial meningitis is a life-threatening infection that is associated with long-term cognitive impairment in many survivors. Neonatal infection occurs primarily when the microorganism ascends from the vagina and traverses the placental membrane. The fetus is infected within the amniotic cavity, inducing a placental membrane rupture or triggering premature delivery. Moreover, the bacteria can be aspirated into the lungs and transferred hematogenously into the CNS. The bacteria enter the CNS following a direct interaction with the luminal side of the cerebral endothelium.

As a consequence, the replication of bacteria within the subarachnoid space occurs concomitantly with the release of their compounds, which are shown as PAMPs. These PAMPs are recognized by PRRs, which are essential constituents of the innate immune system. The sensing of PAMPs by PRRs triggers a cascade of signaling pathways that activate several transcription factors and promote the production of proinflammatory mediators, such as cytokines, chemokines, and antimicrobial peptides. These proinflammatory mediators are necessary to eliminate the invading pathogens.

Consequently, leukocyte cells are recruited from the bloodstream to the site of infection. High amounts of reactive oxygen and nitrogen species are produced, which lead to lipid peroxidation, mitochondrial damage, and blood-brain barrier breakdown. These cascades contribute to brain cell injury during bacterial meningitis and neuronal sequelae. Thus the development of long-term impairment results from the combined effects of pathogen-derived factors and the host immune response.

GLOSSARY

AIF: Apoptosis-inducing factor. AIF is involved in starting a caspase-independent pathway of apoptosis by producing DNA fragmentation and chromatin condensation. This protein triggers programmed cell death.

AIM2: Absent in melanoma-2. AIM2 is a class of pattern-recognition receptors (PRRs) associated with cytosolic and nuclear pathogen DNA recognition.

AP-1: Activator protein-1. AP-1 is a transcription factor that plays a crucial role in the maintenance of cellular homeostasis.

Apaf-1: Apoptotic protease-activating factor-1. Apaf-1 is a protein that binds to pro-caspases, developing an ATP-dependent oligomeric complex that triggers protease activation.

ASC: Apoptosis-associated speck-like protein containing a C-terminal caspase recruitment domain. The adaptor protein ASC contributes to innate immunity through the assembly of caspase-1-activating inflammasome complexes.

ATM: Ataxia telangiectasia-mutated kinase. It is a DNA damage-inducible protein kinase.

ATP: Adenosine triphosphate. ATP is a complex organic chemical that delivers energy to living cells.

BDNF: Brain-derived neurotrophic factor. It is a neurotrophin involved in neuronal development, synaptic plasticity, and cognitive function.

CCL: CC: chemokine ligand. CCL-2 and CCL-3 belong to the CC-chemokine family, and these chemokines recruit immune cells to the site of inflammation or infection. CCL9 attracts dendritic cells that possess the cell surface molecule CD11b and the chemokine receptor CCR1.

CD: Cluster of differentiation. CD is used for the identification of cell surface molecules providing targets for immunophenotyping of cells.

cIAP2: Cellular inhibitor of apoptosis protein-2. cIAP2 is an inhibitor of apoptosis.

CINC-1: Cytokine-induced neutrophil chemoattractant-1. CINC-1 is an acute phase protein induced by endogenous and exogenous pyrogens, and this chemokine also promotes the migration of neutrophils to the site of inflammation.

CLRs: C-type lectin receptors. CLRs are involved in fungal recognition and the modulation of the innate immune response.

CNF1: Cytotoxic-necrotizing factor 1. CNF1 is a toxin produced by uropathogenic *Escherichia coli*.

CNS: Central nervous system.

CpG: Unmethylated cytosine-phosphate-guanine. CpG oligodeoxynucleotides are motifs in bacterial DNA. The motifs interact with a protein and can be organized into several categories according to their function: chromosome replication, repair, and organization.

CpG-ODN: CpG-oligodeoxynucleotide. They contain unmethylated CpG motifs. The CpG-ODN sculpts the bacterial chromosome.

CSF: Cerebrospinal fluid. It is a clear, colorless body fluid found surrounding the brain and spinal cord.

CXCL: CX chemokine ligand. Chemokine (C-X-C motif) ligand (CXCL) is a group of secreted growth factor that signals through a G protein, and CXCL protein family members play essential roles in inflammation.

DAMPs: Damage-associated molecular patterns. DAMPs are molecules released by stressed cells that act as endogenous signals to trigger and intensify the host inflammatory response.

DAP: Diaminopimelic acid. It is a characteristic of cell walls of certain bacteria

DNA: Deoxyribonucleic acid. DNA contains the genetic instructions that coordinate the development and functioning of all living things.

ERK: Extracellular signal-regulated kinase. They are the intracellular protein kinases that are involved in cellular functions such as regulation of meiosis, mitosis, and postmitotic phases.

Fbs: Fibrinogen-binding protein. It is a protein presented on the outer surface of *Staphylococcus aureus* that binds to fibrinogen and fibronectin.

FimH: Type 1 fimbrial adhesin. Type 1 fimbriae are filamentous appendages that confer bacterial binding to glycoproteins with terminally exposed mannose. FimH is localized in the fimbrial tip attached to the fimbrial rod.

gC1qR: Globular head of the complement component C1q. It is similar to the domains found within the tumor necrosis factor.

GlcNAc: *N*-acetylglucosamine. GlcNAc is a component of bacterial cell wall peptidoglycan and fungal cell wall that stimulates the cell surface signaling proteins.

Gp96: Glucose-regulated protein-96. Gp96 is a stress-inducible molecular chaperone that belongs to the heat shock protein (HSP) family.

GPCRs: G-protein-coupled receptors. GPCRs are cell surface receptors of the membrane in eukaryotes that act as a door for messages in the form of peptides, lipids, carbohydrates, and proteins.

GSA-IB4: Griffonia-simplicifolia isolectin-B4. It is a useful cell marker that binds to cell membrane glycoconjugates bearing terminal alpha-D-galactose in macrophages.

GSH: Glutathione. It is a water-soluble antioxidant, recognized as the most essential nonprotein thiol in living systems.

H_2O_2: Hydrogen peroxide. It is a chemical compound with the formula H_2O_2.

HMGB-1: High mobility group box-1 protein. It is a nuclear protein that can bind to DNA and act as a cofactor for gene transcription.

HSP: Heat shock protein. They are a family of proteins that are produced by cells in response to exposure to stressful conditions.

IagA: Invasion protein regulator. It is an invasion protein regulator.

Iba1: Ionized calcium-binding adaptor molecule 1. It is a 147-amino-acid calcium-binding protein widely in use as a marker for microglia.

ICAM: Intercellular adhesion molecule. This gene encodes a cell surface glycoprotein that is typically expressed in endothelial cells and immune cells.

IDO: Indoleamine 2,3-dioxygenase. It is one of the three enzymes that catalyze the first and rate-limiting step in the kynurenine pathway.

IKK: Inhibitor of NF-κB kinase. It is a small molecule that can specifically inhibit the IκB phosphorylation and degradation and the subsequent nuclear translocation of NF-κB.

IL: Interleukin. They are a group of cytokines that were first seen to be expressed by white blood cells.

Inl: Internalin. They are surface proteins found on *Listeria monocytogenes*.

iNOS: Inducible nitric oxide synthase. They are a family of enzymes that catalyze nitric oxide production.

IRAK-4: Interleukin-1 receptor-associated kinase 4. It is a protein kinase involved in signaling innate immune responses from Toll-like receptors.

IκB: Inhibitor of NF-κB. They are the transcription factors that regulate several critical physiologic processes, including inflammation and immune responses

JNKs: c-Jun N-terminal kinases. JNKs are a family of mitogen-activated protein kinase (MAPK) family that controls a range of biologic processes implicated in gene expression, neuronal plasticity, regeneration, and cell death.

LFA-1: Lymphocyte function-associated antigen-1. It plays a crucial role in emigration, which is the process by which the leukocytes leave the bloodstream to enter the tissues.

LmB: Laminin-binding adhesin. LmB is an adhesin from *Streptococcus* sp., specifically to adhere to the human extracellular matrix protein laminin.

LPS: Lipopolysaccharide. It is the major component of the outer membrane of gram-negative bacteria, contributing significantly to the structural integrity of the bacteria and protecting the membrane from certain kinds of chemical attacks.

LR: Laminin receptor. It is a nonintegrin protein, which binds to both laminin-1 of the extracellular matrix and prion protein that holds a central role in prion diseases.

LRR: Leucine-rich repeat. It is a protein structural motif that forms an α/β horseshoe fold.

LTA: Lipoteichoic acid. It is a significant constituent of the cell wall of gram-positive bacteria.

MAPK: Mitogen-activated protein kinase. It is a type of protein kinase that is specific to the amino acids serine and threonine.

MDP: Muramyl dipeptide. MDP is a peptidoglycan component of both gram-positive and gram-negative bacteria.

MMPs: Matrix metalloproteinases. They are a group of enzymes that in concert are responsible for the degradation of most extracellular matrix proteins during organogenesis, growth, and normal tissue turnover.

MRP: Myeloid-related protein. It is secreted by activated monocytes via a novel, tubulin-dependent pathway during inflammation.

mtDNA: Mitochondrial DNA. It is the DNA located in mitochondria.

MyD88: Myeloid differentiation primary response 88. It is a pivotal signaling component of the innate immune response, serving as an adaptor for the interleukin-1 receptor and the majority of Toll-like receptors (TLRs).

NAD: Nicotinamide-adenine-dinucleotide. It is an organic compound (the active form of vitamin B3) found in the cells of all living things and used as an "electron transporter" in metabolic oxy-reduction reactions.

NAMPs: Neurodegeneration-associated molecular patterns. They are danger signals that are present in neurodegenerative diseases and are recognized by microglial cell receptors.

NBDs: Nucleotide-binding domains. NBDs provide the energy necessary for transport by binding and hydrolyzing molecules of ATP.

NEMO: NF-κB essential modulator. NEMO is known as an inhibitor of NF-κB kinase subunit gamma (IKK-γ).

NF-κB: Nuclear factor-κB. NF-κB is a protein complex that controls the transcription of DNA, cytokine production, and cell survival.

NLRC4: NLR family CARD domain containing protein 4. The NLRC4 inflammasome is activated as part of the innate immune response to a variety of invasive intracellular pathogens.

NLRP3: nucleotide-binding domain, leucine-rich-containing family, N-terminal pyrin domain-containing (PYD)-3 or Nod-like receptor protein 3. The NLRP3 inflammasome oligomerization is activated by bacterial toxins, bacterial compounds, and DAMPs. NLRP3 matures and secretes the IL-1β and IL-18 cytokines.

NLRs: The Nod-like receptor family of proteins. NLRs are located in the cytosol of the cells and regulate inflammation and apoptosis pathways.

NO: Nitric oxide. NO is also produced in phagocytic cells by NO synthase to eliminate the pathogen. NO is also a neurotransmitter.

NOD: Nucleotide-binding oligomerization domain receptors. NOD-like receptors (NLRs) are intracellular sensors of PAMPs, DAMPs, and NAMPs.

$O_2^{-\bullet}$: Superoxide anion radicals. It is an inorganic radical anion, oxygen radical, and a member of reactive oxygen species.

OCl^-: Hypochlorite ion. The OCl^- is produced in phagocytic leukocytes by myeloperoxidase to eliminate the pathogen.

$OH^\bullet$: Hydroxyl radicals. The $OH^\bullet$ radical is the neutral form of a hydroxide ion and is an extremely reactive free radical.

OmpA: Outer-membrane protein A. The OmpA is a protein found in the C-terminal region of gram-negative bacteria outer membrane proteins.

$ONOO^-$: Peroxynitrite. The $ONOO^-$ is a nitric oxide-derived molecule that causes nitration of proteins.

PAFr: Platelet-activating-factor receptor. The PAFr is a GPCR present in the plasma and nuclear membranes of the innate immune system that activates inflammation.

PAMPs: Pathogen-associated molecular patterns. The PAMPs bind to the pattern-recognition receptors (PRRs) to induce host immune response.

PBN: α-Phenyl-*N*-tert-butyl nitrone. The PBN is a free radical spin trap.

pIgR: Polymeric immunoglobulin receptor. The pIgR mediates the transport of secretory immunoglobulins and binds polymeric IgA and IgM.

Pil-A: Pilus tip adhesin. It contributes to Group B streptococcus adherence to the blood-brain barrier endothelium.

PI-PLC: Phosphatidylinositol-specific phospholipase C. It is an intracellular enzyme that plays an essential role in signal transduction processes.

PRRs: Pattern-recognition receptors. They are the proteins capable of recognizing molecules frequently found in pathogens (PAMPs), or molecules released by damaged cells (DAMPs).

PSGL: P-selectin glycoprotein ligand. It is a dimeric mucin-like 120-kDa glycoprotein on leukocyte surfaces that binds to P- and L-selectin and promotes cell adhesion in the inflammatory response.

PspC: Pneumococcal surface protein C. It is the protein primarily responsible for binding human lactoferrin to the pneumococcal cell surface.

RAGE: Receptor for advanced glycation end products. It is a multiligand receptor that propagates cellular dysfunction in several inflammatory disorders.

RIG-I: Retinoic acid-inducible gene I. RIG-I is an intracellular molecule that responds to viral nucleic acids, triggering the induction of the type I interferon (IFN) family.

RIP2: Receptor-interacting protein-2. It is serine/threonine kinase with the C-terminal caspase activation and recruitment domain.

RLRs: Retinoic acid-inducible gene I-like receptors. They are another family of cytosolic pattern-recognition receptors (PRRs) that activate the inflammasome and can detect the presence of RNA from a broad range of viruses.

RNA: Ribonucleic acid. It is a polymeric molecule essential in various biologic roles in coding, decoding, regulation, and expression of genes.

ROS: Reactive oxygen species. They are generated during mitochondrial oxidative metabolism as well as in cellular response to xenobiotics, cytokines, and bacterial invasion.

SRRPs: Serine-rich repeat proteins. They are a family of surface-expressed proteins found in numerous gram-positive pathogens.

STAT: Signal transducers and activators of transcription. They are transcription factors that work via the JAK/STAT pathway regulating the expression of genes involved in cell survival, proliferation, differentiation, development, and immune response, among other essential biologic functions.

TAB: Transforming growth factor-β-activated protein kinase 1 (TAK1)-binding protein. It is a protein -coding gene, and it is related pathways are activated TLR4 signaling and IL-1 family signaling pathways.

TAK: Transforming growth factor-β-activated kinase. It is an indispensable signaling intermediate in tumor necrosis factor (TNF), interleukin 1, and Toll-like receptor signaling pathways.

TIR: Toll/interleukin-1 receptor. It is an intracellular signaling domain found in MyD88, interleukin-1 receptors, and Toll receptors.

TIRAP: Toll-interleukin 1 receptor (*TIR*) domain-containing adaptor protein. It is an adapter molecule associated with Toll-like receptors.

TLRs: Toll-like receptors. They are a class of proteins that play a vital role in the innate immune system.

TNF-α: Tumor necrosis factor-α. It is a cell-signaling protein (cytokine) involved in systemic inflammation and is one of the cytokines that make up the acute phase reaction.

TRAF: TNF receptor-associated factor. They are a family of proteins primarily involved in the regulation of inflammation, antiviral responses, and apoptosis.

TRAM: TRIF-related adaptor molecule. TRAM is the fourth Toll/IL-1 resistance domain-containing adaptor to be described that participates in TLR signaling.

TREM: Triggering receptors expressed on myeloid cells. They are a family of activating receptors with some homology with activating natural killer cell receptors.

TRIF: TIR-domain-containing adapter inducing interferon-β. It is an adapter in responding to the activation of TLRs.

XIAP: X-linked inhibitor of apoptosis protein. It is a gene that encodes a protein that belongs to a family of apoptotic suppressor proteins.

A complete reference list is available at www.ExpertConsult.com. 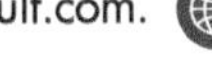

SELECT REFERENCES

1. Klinger G, Chin CN, Beyene J, Perlman M. Predicting the outcome of neonatal bacterial meningitis. *Pediatrics*. 2000;106:477–482.
2. de Louvois J, Halket S, Harvey D. Neonatal meningitis in England and Wales: sequelae at 5 years of age. *Eur J Pediatr*. 2005;164:730–734. https://doi.org/10.1007/s00431-005-1747-3.
3. Heath PT, Okike IO, Oeser C. Neonatal meningitis: can we do better? *Adv Exp Med Biol*. 2011;719:11–24. https://doi.org/10.1007/978-1-4614-0204-6_2.

4. Gaschignard J, et al. Neonatal bacterial meningitis: 444 cases in 7 years. *Pediatr Infect Dis J*. 2011;30:212-217.
5. Okike IO. *et al.* Incidence, etiology, and outcome of bacterial meningitis in infants aged <90 Days in the United Kingdom and republic of Ireland: prospective, enhanced, national population-based surveillance. *Clin Infect Dis*. https://doi.org/10.1093/cid/ciu514.
6. Thigpen MC, et al. Bacterial meningitis in the United States, 1998-2007. *N Engl J Med*. 2011;364:2016-2025. https://doi.org/10.1056/NEJMoa1005384.
7. Mitchell AM, Mitchell TJ. Streptococcus pneumoniae: virulence factors and variation. *Clin Microbiol Infect*. 2010;16:411-418. https://doi.org/10.1111/j.1469-0691.2010.03183.x.
8. Kim KS. Current concepts on the pathogenesis of Escherichia coli meningitis: implications for therapy and prevention. *Curr Opin Infect Dis*. 2012;25:273-278. https://doi.org/10.1097/QCO.0b013e3283521eb0.
9. Barichello T, et al. Pathophysiology of neonatal acute bacterial meningitis. *J Med Microbiol*. 2013;62:1781-1789. https://doi.org/10.1099/jmm.0.059840-0.
10. Kumar S, Ingle H, Prasad DV, Kumar H. Recognition of bacterial infection by innate immune sensors. *Crit Rev Microbiol*. 2013;39:229-246. https://doi.org/10.3109/1040841x.2012.706249.
11. Heckenberg SG, Brouwer MC, van de Beek D. Bacterial meningitis. *Handb Clin Neurol*. 2014;121:1361-1375. https://doi.org/10.1016/b978-0-7020-4088-7.00093-6.
12. Sellner J, Täuber MG, Leib SL. In: Roos Karen L, Tunkel Allan R, eds. *Handbook of Clinical Neurology*. Vol 96. Elsevier; 2010:1-16.
13. Mook-Kanamori BB, Geldhoff M, van der Poll T, van de Beek D. Pathogenesis and pathophysiology of pneumococcal meningitis. *Clin Microbiol Rev*. 2011;24:557-591. https://doi.org/10.1128/cmr.00008-11.
14. Gong T, Liu L, Jiang W, Zhou R. DAMP-sensing receptors in sterile inflammation and inflammatory diseases. *Nat Rev Immunol*. 2019. https://doi.org/10.1038/s41577-019-0215-7.
15. Iwasaki A, Medzhitov R. Regulation of adaptive immunity by the innate immune system. *Science*. 2010;327:291-295. https://doi.org/10.1126/science.1183021.
16. Wiersinga WJ, Leopold SJ, Cranendonk DR, van der Poll T. Host innate immune responses to sepsis. *Virulence*. 2014;5:36-44. https://doi.org/10.4161/viru.25436.
17. Lu B, et al. Molecular mechanism and therapeutic modulation of high mobility group box 1 release and action: an updated review. *Expet Rev Clin Immunol*. 2014;10:713-727. https://doi.org/10.1586/1744666x.2014.909730.
18. Kigerl KA, de Rivero Vaccari JP, Dietrich WD, Popovich PG, Keane RW. Pattern recognition receptors and central nervous system repair. *Exp Neurol*. 2014;258:5-16. https://doi.org/10.1016/j.expneurol.2014.01.001.
19. Kataoka H, Kono H, Patel Z, Rock KL. Evaluation of the contribution of multiple DAMPs and DAMP receptors in cell death-induced sterile inflammatory responses. *PloS one*. 2014;9:e104741. https://doi.org/10.1371/journal.pone.0104741.
20. Baud O, Aujard Y. Neonatal bacterial meningitis. *Handb Clin Neurol*. 2013;112:1109-1113. https://doi.org/10.1016/b978-0-444-52910-7.00030-1.
21. Slotved HC, Kong F, Lambertsen L, Sauer S, Gilbert GL. Serotype IX, a Proposed New Streptococcus agalactiae Serotype. *J Clin Microbiol*. 2007;45:2929-2936. https://doi.org/10.1128/jcm.00117-07.
22. Dutra VG, et al. Streptococcus agalactiae in Brazil: serotype distribution, virulence determinants and antimicrobial susceptibility. *BMC Infect Dis*. 2014;14:323. https://doi.org/10.1186/1471-2334-14-323.
23. Raabe VN, Shane AL. Group B Streptococcus (Streptococcus agalactiae). *Microbiol Spectr*. 2019;7. https://doi.org/10.1128/microbiolspec.GPP3-0007-2018.
24. Sellner J, Tauber MG, Leib SL. Pathogenesis and pathophysiology of bacterial CNS infections. *Handb Clin Neurol*. 2010;96:1-16. https://doi.org/10.1016/s0072-9752(09)96001-8.
25. Colbourn T, Gilbert R. An overview of the natural history of early onset group B streptococcal disease in the UK. *Early Hum Dev*. 2007;83:149-156. https://doi.org/10.1016/j.earlhumdev.2007.01.004.
26. Tazi A, et al. Group B Streptococcus surface proteins as major determinants for meningeal tropism. *Curr Opin Microbiol*. 2012;15:44-49. https://doi.org/10.1016/j.mib.2011.12.002.
27. Bodaszewska-Lubas M, et al. Adherence of group B streptococci to human rectal and vaginal epithelial cell lines in relation to capsular polysaccharides as well as alpha-like protein genes - pilot study. *Pol J Microbiol*. 2013;62:85-90.
28. Doran KS, Nizet V. Molecular pathogenesis of neonatal group B streptococcal infection: no longer in its infancy. *Mol Microbiol*. 2004;54:23-31. https://doi.org/10.1111/j.1365-2958.2004.04266.x.
29. de Goffau MC, et al. Human placenta has no microbiome but can contain potential pathogens. *Nature*. 2019;572:329-334. https://doi.org/10.1038/s41586-019-1451-5.
30. Pong A, Bradley JS. Bacterial meningitis and the newborn infant. *Infect Dis Clin*. 1999;13:711-733. https://doi.org/10.1016/S0891-5520(05)70102-1.
31. Maisey HC, Doran KS, Nizet V. Recent advances in understanding the molecular basis of group B Streptococcus virulence. *Expert Rev Mol Med*. 2008;10:e27. https://doi.org/10.1017/s1462399408000811.
32. Adams RA, Schachtrup C, Davalos D, Tsigelny I, Akassoglou K. Fibrinogen signal transduction as a mediator and therapeutic target in inflammation: lessons from multiple sclerosis. *Curr Med Chem*. 2007;14:2925-2936.
33. Seo HS, Mu R, Kim BJ, Doran KS, Sullam PM. Binding of glycoprotein Srr1 of Streptococcus agalactiae to fibrinogen promotes attachment to brain endothelium and the development of meningitis. *PLoS Patho*. 2012;8:e1002947. https://doi.org/10.1371/journal.ppat.1002947.
34. Buscetta M, et al. FbsC, a Novel Fibrinogen-binding Protein, Promotes Streptococcus agalactiae-Host Cell Interactions. *J Biol Chem*. 2014;289:21003-21015. https://doi.org/10.1074/jbc.M114.553073.
35. Birchenough GM, et al. Altered innate defenses in the neonatal gastrointestinal tract in response to colonization by neuropathogenic Escherichia coli. *Infect Immun*. 2013;81:3264-3275. https://doi.org/10.1128/iai.00268-13.
36. Pluschke G, Mercer A, Kusecek B, Pohl A, Achtman M. Induction of bacteremia in newborn rats by Escherichia coli K1 is correlated with only certain O (lipopolysaccharide) antigen types. *Infect Immun*. 1983;39:599-608.
37. Zelmer A, et al. Differential expression of the polysialyl capsule during blood-to-brain transit of neuropathogenic Escherichia coli K1. *Microbiology (Reading)*. 2008;154:2522-2532. https://doi.org/10.1099/mic.0.2008/017988-0.
38. Mateus T, Silva J, Maia RL, Teixeira P. Listeriosis during pregnancy: a public health concern. *ISRN Obstet Gynecology*. 2013;2013:851712. https://doi.org/10.1155/2013/851712.
39. Posfay-Barbe KM, Wald ER. Listeriosis. *Semin Fetal Neonatal Med*. 2009;14:228-233. https://doi.org/10.1016/j.siny.2009.01.006.
40. Williams D, Dunn S, Richardson A, Frank JF, Smith MA. Time course of fetal tissue invasion by Listeria monocytogenes following an oral inoculation in pregnant guinea pigs. *J Food Protect*. 2011;74:248-253. https://doi.org/10.4315/0362-028x.jfp-10-163.
41. King SJ, Hippe KR, Weiser JN. Deglycosylation of human glycoconjugates by the sequential activities of exoglycosidases expressed by Streptococcus pneumoniae. *Mol Microbiol*. 2006;59:961-974. https://doi.org/10.1111/j.1365-2958.2005.04984.x.
42. Porter BD, Ortika BD, Satzke C. Capsular Serotyping of Streptococcus pneumoniae by Latex Agglutination. *J Vis Exp*. 2014. https://doi.org/10.3791/51747.
43. Nelson AL, et al. Capsule enhances pneumococcal colonization by limiting mucus-mediated clearance. *Infect Immun*. 2007;75:83-90. https://doi.org/10.1128/iai.01475-06.
44. Feldman C, et al. The effect of Streptococcus pneumoniae pneumolysin on human respiratory epithelium in vitro. *Microb Pathog*. 1990;9:275-284.
45. Marriott HM, Mitchell TJ, Dockrell DH. Pneumolysin: a double-edged sword during the host-pathogen interaction. *Curr Opin Infect Dis*. 2008;8:497-509.
46. Caugant DA, Maiden MC. Meningococcal carriage and disease--population biology and evolution. *Vaccine*. 2008;27(suppl 2):B64-B70. https://doi.org/10.1016/j.vaccine.2009.04.061.
47. Claus H, et al. Genetic analysis of meningococci carried by children and young adults. *J Infect Dis*. 2005;191:1263-1271. https://doi.org/10.1086/428590.
48. Strelow VL, Vidal JE. Invasive meningococcal disease. *Arq Neuropsiquiatr*. 2013;71:653-658. https://doi.org/10.1590/0004-282x20130144.
49. Virji M. Pathogenic neisseriae: surface modulation, pathogenesis and infection control. *Nat Rev Microbiol*. 2009;7:274-286. https://doi.org/10.1038/nrmicro2097.
50. Bernard SC, et al. Pathogenic Neisseria meningitidis utilizes CD147 for vascular colonization. *Nat Med*. 2014;20:725-731. https://doi.org/10.1038/nm.3563.

Pathophysiology of Neural Tube Defects

169

Andrew J. Copp | Nicholas D.E. Greene

INTRODUCTION

Neural tube defects (NTDs) are among the commonest and most severe birth anomalies, second only in frequency to congenital heart defects. Worldwide, around 300,000 to 500,000 new cases of NTD are thought to arise each year, representing not only a significant challenge for the affected individuals and their families, but also a major financial burden for health services. For example, 166,000 people are estimated to live with spina bifida in the United States alone, with average lifetime medical and nonmedical costs for each affected person of around $560,000, not counting their "lost" earnings.[1]

NTDs affect the central nervous system and axial skeleton and can vary from fatal to asymptomatic. The severe end of the spectrum is represented by defects of the cranial region: anencephaly and craniorachischisis (CRN), which are both incompatible with survival beyond birth, and encephalocele, which can be lethal depending on the extent of brain damage. Somewhat less severe NTDs affect the spine, of which open spina bifida (often called myelomeningocele) is usually not lethal but can be a cause of multiple disabilities throughout life. At the mild end of the NTD spectrum is closed spinal dysraphism (or lipomyelomeningocele), which can cause lower limb weakness and urologic disorders but is often clinically undetectable.

EPIDEMIOLOGY

NTDs exhibit an average worldwide prevalence of 0.5 to 2 per 1000 births, but this varies markedly with geographic location and ethnic origin.[2] For example, more abundant NTDs were observed in previous decades in Ireland, South Wales, and Northern China, and an especially high prevalence (6 to 13 per 1000 births) was reported recently in Ethiopia.[3,4] Differences in NTD prevalence between different ethnic groupings have been described: for example, people of Hispanic origin in the United States exhibit higher rates than those of white ancestry, with African Americans showing the lowest frequencies.[5] Rates of NTDs are higher among miscarried fetuses,[6] suggesting that the true incidence may be greater than is typically recorded from studies of late-stage pregnancies, planned abortions, and still/live births. Confirmed epidemiologic conditions associated with NTDs include low socioeconomic status, maternal obesity and/or diabetes, suboptimal folate status, and anticonvulsant medication usage.[7-9] Female fetal sex is strongly associated with anencephaly.[10]

NORMAL DEVELOPMENT OF THE NEURAL TUBE

Neurulation is the process by which the neural tube, the precursor of the brain and spinal cord, is formed during embryogenesis. Key events in this process include induction of neural identity in the embryonic epiblast, convergent extension (CE) cell rearrangements that produce an elongated, mediolaterally narrowed neural primordium, and conversion of this primordium into a neural tube. Two successive phases of neural tube formation occur, involving neural plate bending and fusion in the dorsal midline (primary neurulation) followed by canalization of a neural primordium in the caudal region (secondary neurulation).

CLOSURE INITIATION SITES

Primary neurulation begins at several discrete points along the rostro-caudal axis,[11] in a pattern that varies somewhat between mammals. In rodents (Fig. 169.1A), where neurulation has been most intensively studied, closure begins at the boundary between the future hindbrain and cervical spine (termed Closure 1). Twelve hours later, closure initiates independently at the forebrain/midbrain boundary (Closure 2) and, soon after, at a third initiation site at the rostral extremity of the forebrain (Closure 3). Recently, a further caudal initiation site (Closure 5) was described during the final stages of spinal closure.[12] In human embryos (see Fig. 169.1B), only two closure initiation sites have been described, termed α and β,[13] which are equivalent to Closures 1 and 3 respectively in rodents. Closure 2 does not appear to occur in humans, and it is not yet clear whether an equivalent of Closure 5 may exist.

ZIPPERING AND NEUROPORES

The open regions of neural folds between the different closure initiation sites are termed neuropores; they close progressively by "zippering" along the body axis (see Fig. 169.1). Mouse embryos have three neuropores: the anterior and hindbrain neuropores complete closure within a few hours of Closures 2 and 3, whereas spinal neurulation continues zippering over a much longer period, along the growing spinal region, until the posterior or caudal neuropore (PNP) completes its closure in the upper sacral region. This marks the end of mouse primary neurulation, a process that takes ~40 hours, between embryonic days (E) 8.5 and 10. Because human embryos lack Closure 2, they exhibit only single anterior (rostral) and posterior (caudal) neuropores. Human neural tube closure begins around 22 days post-fertilization and is completed by 26 days (i.e., between Carnegie Stages 10 and 12).

SECONDARY NEURULATION

This is the process of neural tube formation in the lower sacral and coccygeal regions,[14] and is part of "secondary body" development that also forms caudal notochord, somites and postcloacal gut. It begins at Carnegie stage 12 and follows on seamlessly from primary neurulation, so that ultimately the primary and secondary neural tubes have no obvious boundary between them. The caudal end of the embryo comprises the tail bud (also called the caudal eminence), which contains self-renewing, multipotent progenitor cells whose derivatives condense into longitudinal cell masses. The dorsal mass then undergoes canalization to form the hollow secondary neural tube, while the ventral mass canalizes to form the tail gut. The longitudinal structure lying between neural tube and gut forms the solid notochord. A multipotent stem cell population, the "neuro-mesodermal progenitors" (NMPs), is present in the tail

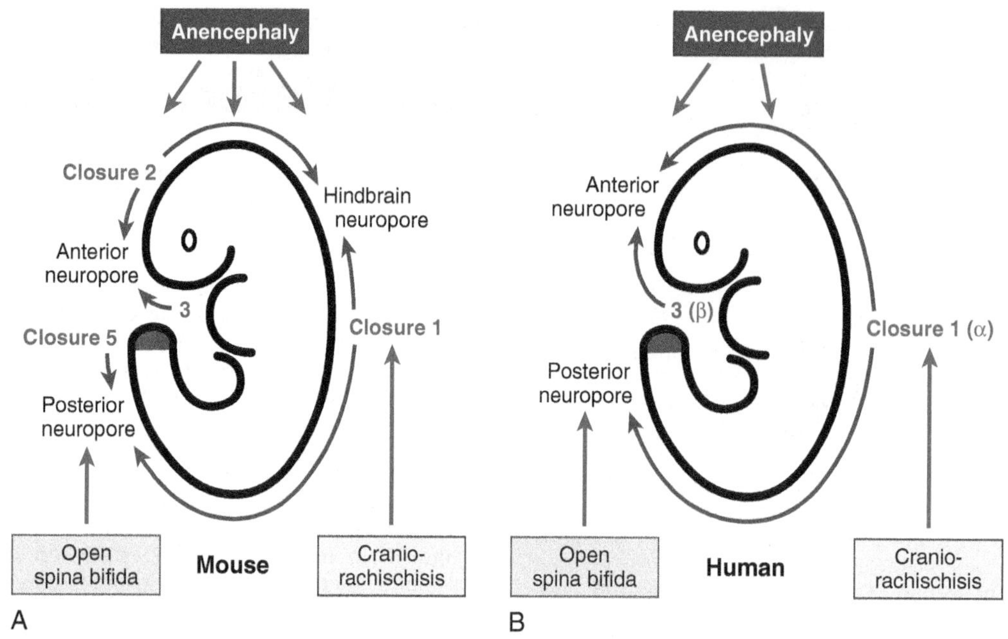

Fig. 169.1 Schematic of neural tube closure and the origin of neural tube defects (NTDs) in mouse and human embryos. (A) In mice, closure initiates sequentially at four separate sites: *Closures 1, 2, 3, and 5*. Note that *Closure 4* was postulated in the hindbrain,[11] but this not been confirmed. Zippering occurs from the initiation sites, to complete closure at the three neuropores: anterior, hindbrain, and posterior. From *Closure 1*, zippering progresses in a rostral direction into the hindbrain and simultaneously in a caudal direction along the spinal region. From *Closure 2*, bi-directional zippering occurs rostrally into the forebrain and caudally into the midbrain and then hindbrain. From *Closure 3*, unidirectional (caudal) zippering occurs through the forebrain. (B) In humans, two initiation sites occur: site α (*Closure 1* equivalent) and site β (*Closure 3* equivalent). Zippering from site α progresses in a rostral direction, into the hindbrain and then midbrain, and in a caudal direction along the spine. From site β, closure occurs in a caudal direction through the forebrain. Closure is completed at two neuropores: anterior (rostral) and posterior (caudal). In both mice and humans, secondary neurulation occurs in the tail-bud (caudal eminence) to elongate the neural tube caudal to the upper sacral level, where primary neurulation finishes. The neurulation events whose failure gives rise to the main NTD types are indicated. (Adapted with permission from Copp AJ, Greene ND. Neural tube defects—disorders of neurulation and related embryonic processes. *WIREs Dev Biol*. 2013;2:213–217.)

bud at this stage, and NMPs give rise to all nonepidermal tissues of the lower body, including neural tube and vertebrae.[15] Possibly for this reason, malformations and tumors (e.g., sacrococcygeal teratoma) of the lower body often embrace several tissue types.

REGRESSION OF THE NEURAL TUBE

In the mouse and rat, the entire tail region (~50% of the total body axis) is originally occupied by secondary neural tube. Following completion of tail formation at E13.5 (i.e., three days after the end of primary neurulation), the neural tube and tail gut regress with cells dying by apoptosis.[16] In contrast, the notochord (around which the vertebral centra develop) and somitic derivatives (the future vertebrae and tendons) persist in the tail. Human secondary body formation ceases much earlier than in embryos of long-tailed rodents; the tail structure subsequently regresses completely, so that all tissues, not just the neural tube and tail gut, are "reabsorbed" into the upper body.[17] The human secondary neural tube contributes to the lowest part of the spinal cord: the conus medullaris, cauda equina, and filum terminale.

ASCENT OF THE CORD

While the neural tube and somitic (prevertebral) segments are in register at the time of their formation during neurulation, the growth of the somitic system outstrips the neural tube postneurulation, so that the caudal end of the neural tube appears to "ascend"; by birth, the conus lies at the level of the L3 vertebra and in the adult at the L1 level.[18] This is important in NTDs, as "tethering" of the cord, which happens in both open and closed low-spinal defects, prevents ascent of the cord and causes symptomatic stretching of the spinal nerves.

CLASSIFICATION OF NEURAL TUBE DEFECTS

The clinical classification of NTDs is inconsistent and confusing, with variation in terminology even between medical specialties. For example, public health studies typically refer to "NTDs" or "ASB" (anencephaly and spina bifida), whereas pediatric neurosurgeons use "dysraphism" to denote both open and closed spinal lesions. In this chapter, NTDs are classified based on their developmental (embryonic and fetal) origins. While this system can be applied with some degree of confidence to NTDs where human defects are modeled faithfully in an animal model (thereby allowing longitudinal and experimental studies), it is more hazardous for NTDs that have no animal models. Speculation on the "embryological" origin of NTDs without experimental evidence is rife in the neurosurgical literature but can be highly misleading and is best avoided.

OPEN NEURAL TUBE DEFECTS: DISORDERS OF PRIMARY NEURULATION

Failure of any aspect of the complex primary neurulation process can yield an open NTD.

CRANIORACHISCHISIS

This prenatally lethal NTD, whose name means "brain and spine open," arises when Closure 1 fails, so that the neural tube remains open from mid/hindbrain level to the end of the spine. The open neural tube degenerates due to prolonged exposure to amniotic fluid, with loss of neural tissue, absence of dorsal skull and vertebral structures, and angioma-like formations.[19] The independent closure initiation site at the rostral end of the neural tube (site β or Closure 3), generally does not fail in CRN, so forebrain closure occurs relatively normally and there are distinct optic vesicles. This contrasts with another dramatic brain defect, holoprosencephaly,[20] where the most severe manifestation is univentricular forebrain and fused optic vesicles (cyclopia). A high prevalence of CRN has been seen in some geographical locations: for example on the Texas-Mexico border, where CRN comprised 3.8% of NTDs, in contrast to the usual 1% of NTDs.[21] In a north Chinese region 18.8% of NTDs were CRN,[22] with an overall NTD frequency that was six times the world average (5.7/1000 births in N. China, vs. 1/1000 worldwide). The origin of CRN is closely linked to faulty function of the planar cell polarity (PCP) signaling pathway, and harmful PCP genetic variants are associated with CRN in humans and mice.[23]

ANENCEPHALY

This is the most common cranial NTD, characterized by congenital absence of a major portion of the brain, skull, and scalp. It accounts for around 40% of all NTDs and shows a strong female preponderance,[10] with an average sex ratio of 2 to 3:1. It is uniformly fatal, and is invariably detected by prenatal ultrasound examination, in countries where this test is available. Most affected fetuses are spontaneously aborted, are stillborn, or die within the first week after birth. Anencephaly arises when some aspect of cranial closure fails, most commonly faulty completion of anterior (rostral) neuropore closure in humans. Holoanencephaly is a severe form that extends through the level of the foramen magnum whereas meroanencephaly is a less extensive form. In anencephaly, the calvarium is hypoplastic or absent, the base of the skull is thick and flattened, and there is a constant anomaly of the sphenoid bone resembling "a bat with folded wings."[19] The orbits are well formed, as in CRN, but are shallow, causing protrusion of the eyes. Attached to the skull base is a dark reddish irregular mass of vascular tissue with multiple cavities containing cerebrospinal fluid (CSF), the area cerebrovasculosa. The mass is cystic with a midline dorsal aperture opening to the exterior. No recognizable neural tissue can be found in the anterior and middle fossae except for the trigeminal ganglia and limited lengths of the 2nd to 5th cranial nerves. A hypoplastic anterior pituitary is present in a shallow sella, but the intermediate and posterior pituitary lobes are missing. Other terms, including acrania and cranioschisis, are sometimes used to describe anencephaly.

EXENCEPHALY

Confusion exists over this condition, in which the brain fails to close and neural tissue (often voluminous) projects from the top of the embryonic head. Some authors have suggested it to be a rare condition, distinct from anencephaly, whereas longitudinal studies of rodent NTD models[24,25] show clearly that exencephaly is the embryonic forerunner of anencephaly. Hence, the embryonic and fetal pathogenesis of anencephaly begins with failure of cranial closure (Fig. 169.2A), which is followed by eversion of the neural folds, giving the "overgrown" exencephalic appearance (see Fig. 169.2B). Subsequently, the toxic effects of amniotic fluid exposure cause the protruding neural tissue to degenerate, leading ultimately to the absent brain phenotype, anencephaly (see Fig. 169.2C). Exencephaly can be missed in humans as it occurs early and is usually converted to anencephaly (see Fig. 169.2D) by the late fetal stages when detailed observations are made of the fetal head.

OPEN SPINA BIFIDA

This is often used synonymously with myelomeningocele (also called myelodysplasia and "open spinal dysraphism"). It is a nonlethal NTD that has a similar prevalence to anencephaly and comprises around 40% of NTDs. It arises due to a primary neurulation defect in the spinal region, with failure of the posterior neuropore to complete its zippering closure. Open spina bifida has two typical clinical manifestations: (1) the common cystic myelomeningocele lesion (spina bifida cystica) in which the open portion of neural tube (often called the placode) is located on the surface of a meningeal sac that comprises CSF within the subarachnoid space (Fig. 169.3A and B), and (2) the less common myelocele or myeloschisis defect in which a CSF-containing sac is absent, and the open spinal cord is exposed on the back of the fetus or child (see Fig. 169.3C and D).

The spinal neuroepithelium in open spina bifida is initially healthy and undergoes normal differentiation and spinal nerve development, with onset of lower sensory and motor function in both humans and mice.[26] However, neurodegeneration then intervenes, due to prolonged exposure of the neuroepithelium to amniotic fluid, in the same way as for open cranial defects; by birth, neurologic function has been lost from the rostral level of the lesion downward. One rationale for the fetal surgical approach to spina bifida management, therefore, is to cover the lesion as early in pregnancy as possible, in order to minimize exposure to CSF and the spinal neurodegeneration that leads to disability. Patients with "high" lesions (e.g., open from thoracic to low spine) typically exhibit lower limb paralysis and incontinence, whereas those with "low" lesions (e.g., confined to low lumbar or sacral regions) often have preserved limb function, although continence can still be affected. Following postnatal surgical closure, the 40-year survival is significantly lower for individuals with high spina bifida than for those with low lesions.[27]

CHIARI II MALFORMATION

While not an NTD itself, the Chiari II malformation is present in around 90% of open spina bifida cases and can be a life-threatening complication: brainstem compression may lead to respiratory distress and death. An abnormally small posterior skull fossa is associated with herniation of the cerebellar vermis and brain stem (including the fourth ventricle) into the spinal canal, through an enlarged foramen magnum. Associated brain anomalies include agenesis of the corpus callosum, enlargement of the massa intermedia, cortical heterotopia, and polymicrogyria.[28] While the developmental origin of Chiari II has not been experimentally determined, the predominant hypothesis considers chronic leakage of CSF from the open spina bifida lesion as the primary causal factor.[29] Hydrostatic pressure is reduced in the developing ventricular system, producing a relatively "deflated" hindbrain that induces formation of a small posterior skull fossa. This cannot accommodate the enlarging hindbrain, leading to herniation. Fetal surgery to close the open spina bifida lesion in utero is associated with a high frequency of resolution of Chiari II hindbrain herniation.[30] Since the surgery includes sealing the site of CSF leakage, this provides support for the "hydrostatic pressure" hypothesis.

HEALTH CHALLENGES IN OPEN SPINA BIFIDA

For infants born with open spina bifida, whether the lesion is closed surgically before or after birth, a number of lifelong disabilities are typically encountered. Paraplegia and sensory loss in the lower body, together with neurogenic bladder and sexual dysfunction, are direct sequelae of the neurologic defect in the lower spinal cord. Urinary incontinence is common, with the need for children to learn "clean intermittent self-catheterization" early in life. Nevertheless, many individuals progress to chronic kidney disease with renal failure as a common cause of death. The development of latex sensitization, which affects around half of individuals with open spina bifida, may be related to this frequent instrumentation, although more fundamental immunologic causation has not been ruled out. Other morbidities include hydrocephalus, for which CSF shunt

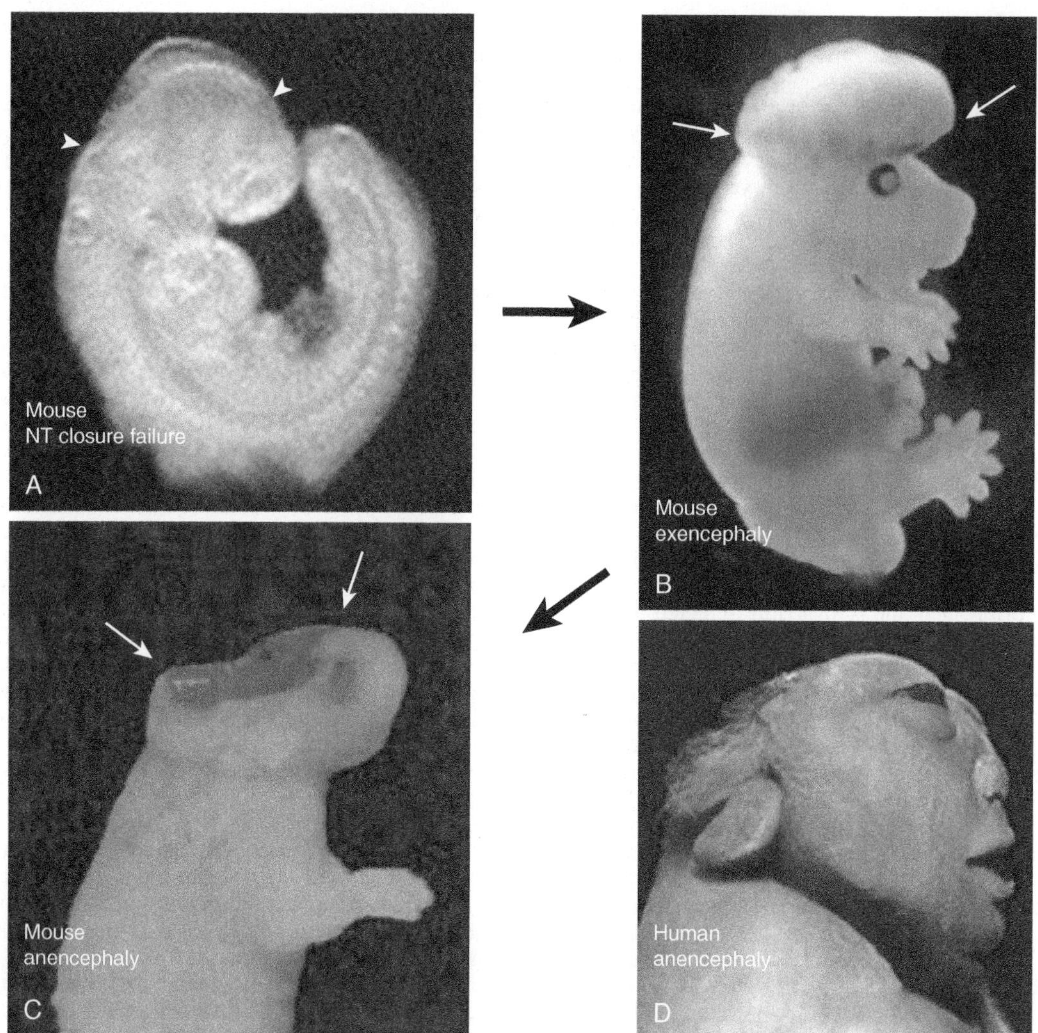

Fig. 169.2 Embryonic and fetal development of anencephaly. (A–C) Events in the mouse beginning with failed closure of the cranial neural tube (NT) at E9.5 (between *arrowheads* in A), then eversion of the initially healthy neural tissue as exencephaly at E13.5 (between *arrows* in B) and finally degeneration of the exposed neural tissue resulting in anencephaly in the newborn (between *arrows* in C). (D) Human anencephaly viewed from the right side in a stillborn fetus. (A, Reproduced with permission from Dunlevy LPE, Burren KA, Chitty LS, et al. Excess methionine suppresses the methylation cycle and inhibits neural tube closure in mouse embryos. *FEBS Lett*. 2006;580:2803–2807. B, Reproduced with permission from Copp AJ, Greene NDE, Murdoch JN. The genetic basis of mammalian neurulation. *Nat Rev Genet*. 2003;4:784–793. C, Reproduced with permission from Copp AJ. Neurulation in the cranial region—normal and abnormal. *J Anat*. 2005;207:623–635. D, Copp AJ, Stanier P, Greene ND. Neural tube defects: recent advances, unsolved questions, and controversies. *Lancet Neurol*. 2013;12:799–810.)

insertion is often required, pulmonary and bowel dysfunction, and skeletal deformations. A significant proportion of individuals with open spina bifida exhibit cognitive impairment. Hence, establishment of an independent lifestyle for these individuals can be extremely challenging. With optimum health and social care support systems in place, life expectancy for a person with open spina bifida can be 30 to 40 years or more, although this varies widely depending on the degree of disability.

CLOSED NEURAL TUBE DEFECTS: HERNIATION DISORDERS

Encephalocele and meningocele are usually included within the spectrum of NTDs, and yet they have a different embryonic pathogenesis from the open NTDs.

ENCEPHALOCELE

This defect comprises around 10% of all NTDs, and is characterized by herniation of the meninges, with or without brain tissue, outside the skull. This exposes the brain to potential damage both pre- and postnatally and, despite surgical repair, later health problems are common, including hydrocephalus, epilepsy, and learning difficulties. Encephaloceles emerge along the skull midline, with fronto-ethmoidal, parietal, occipital, and cervical forms regularly encountered. They have been variously reported as primary neurulation defects,[31] or defects of skull development with secondary brain herniation.[32] However, recent studies in a mouse genetic model of parieto-occipital encephalocele show that cranial neurulation is completed before the onset of brain herniation, which occurs due to rupture of the future epidermal layer that normally covers the closed brain.[33] A skull defect develops later, overlying the herniated region, to generate the appearance as seen in the "mature" encephalocele lesion.

MENINGOCELE

This defect involves herniation of meninges through a dorsal bony defect, usually involving 2 to 3 vertebrae. It is typically located in the lumbosacral region but can occur elsewhere along the body axis. The meningocele sac comprises both arachnoid and dural meninges and contains CSF and often neural elements. Meningocele is often mistaken for cystic myelomeningocele, but

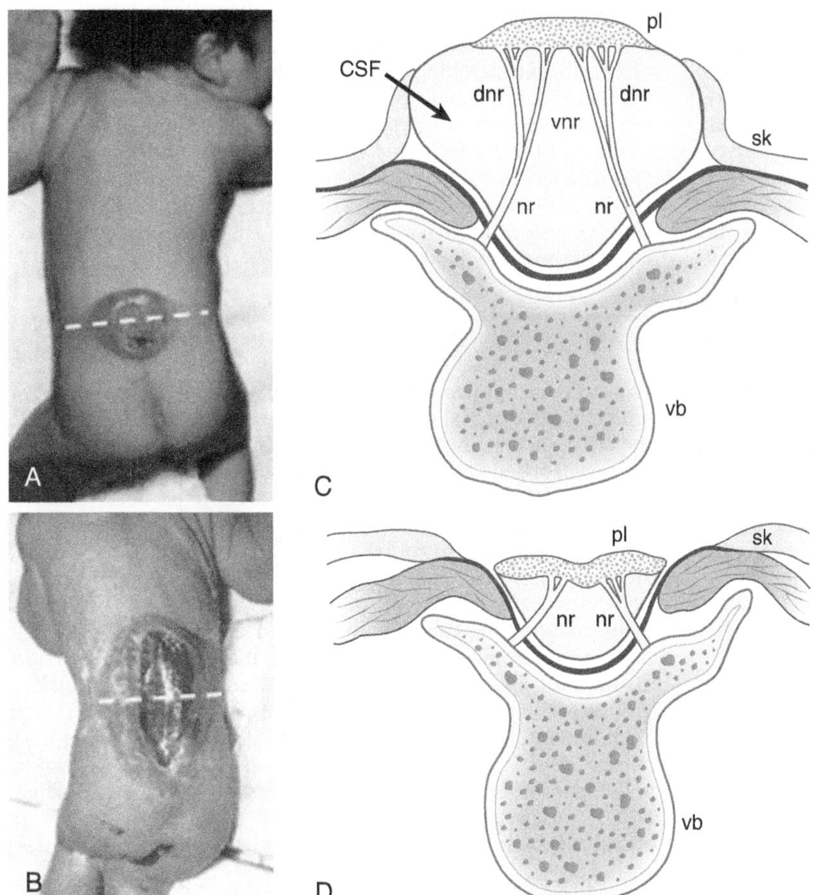

Fig. 169.3 The two main forms of open spina bifida. (A) Myelomeningocele (spina bifida cystica), showing the cystic lesion on the back of the newborn baby. (B) Myelocele, showing an open neural tube on the surface of the newborn baby's back with no cystic lesion. (C and D) Schematic cross-sections through myelomeningocele (A) and myelocele (B) lesions, at levels indicated by *dashed lines* in A and B. Note the differing relationships of the open spinal cord (*pl*, placode) to the associated tissues, owing to the presence or absence of the cerebrospinal fluid *(CSF)*-containing sac. *dnr*, Dorsal nerve roots; *nr*, nerve roots; *sk*, skin; *vb*, vertebral body; *vnr*, ventral nerve roots. (B, Reproduced with permission from Copp AJ, Harding BN. Neural tube defects. In: Adle-Biassette H, Harding BN, Golden J, eds. *Developmental Neuropathology*. 2nd ed. Hoboken, NJ: Wiley; 2018:13–28. https://doi.org/10.1002/9781119013112. C and D, Adapted from Caldarelli M, Rocco CD. Myelomeningocele primary repair surgical technique. In: Memet Özek M, Cinalli G, Maixner WJ, eds. *The Spina Bifida: Management and Outcome*. Milano: Springer Milan; 2008:143–155.)

close examination reveals a closed neural tube, demonstrating this is not a defect of primary neurulation, but rather a result of herniation following normal neural tube closure. In keeping with this, affected infants are neurologically intact, and have an excellent outlook, requiring surgery only to remove the herniated meninges. There is no well characterized mouse model of meningocele, and hence the embryonic pathogenesis of the defect is poorly understood.

CLOSED (SKIN-COVERED) SPINAL NEURAL TUBE DEFECTS: DISORDERS OF SECONDARY BODY AXIS FORMATION

This is the least severe and most poorly defined group of NTDs, often referred to as spinal dysraphism. A prenatal origin is suggested by the frequent occurrence in fetuses and young children, and mostly the defects appear to be "malformations" resulting from disturbed low spinal and vertebral development. However, an acquired pathogenesis, for example involving vascular insults later in gestation, could apply in some cases. Closed spinal NTDs are by definition skin-covered, in contrast to the open defects of primary neurulation. Skeletal development is often disturbed, with vertebral fusions or other malformations such as a midline bony spur. In its least severe form, the only defect may be absence of 1 to 2 neural arches from the lumbar vertebrae, an asymptomatic variant called spina bifida occulta which is present in around 10% of people.

Abnormalities of the spinal cord include overdistension of the central canal (hydromyelia), longitudinal duplication or splitting (diplomyelia, diastematomyelia), and tethering of the cord's lower end. Low spinal/vertebral defects are also regularly associated with anorectal abnormalities including anal stenosis or atresia. The clinical effects of closed spinal NTDs vary widely, depending on the precise nature of the defects, and can include lower limb weakness, sensory disturbance, and bladder dysfunction. There may be gradual progression of symptoms and presentation only in late childhood or adulthood. However, many cases remain asymptomatic throughout the person's life.

Terminal myelocystocele is a rare condition in which a CSF-containing cyst is associated with the end of the spinal cord, and adherent to the subcutaneous fat. The cyst is lined by glial tissue, not neuroepithelium or ependyma, and may also contain fat or neural tissue.[34] It has been likened to the expanded end of the chick secondary neural tube, which itself is transiently attached to surface ectoderm (future epidermis). Whereas the cyst detaches and disappears during chick development,[35] the pathologic cyst in humans is suggested to persist, leading to myelocystocele. To date, however, there have been no findings of a transient cyst at the end of the secondary neural tube in humans, unlike in the chick embryo.

LIPOMA-ASSOCIATED NEURAL TUBE DEFECTS

A striking and unexplained association of these low skin-covered spinal disorders is with adipose tissue (spinal lipoma, lipomyelomeningocele) which can be present within or attached to the spinal cord or filum terminale, and are frequent causes of symptomatic spinal cord tethering.[36] Adipocytes make up the majority of the lipoma tissue but, in contrast to lipomas elsewhere in the body, there is also frequent connective tissue, nerve fibers, abnormal blood vessels and glial tissue,[37] consistent with a different pathogenesis.

PATHOGENESIS OF CLOSED NEURAL TUBE DEFECTS

The lack of animal models exhibiting closed spinal NTDs has meant that little experimental evidence exists on the developmental origin of closed spinal lesions. It seems most likely that abnormalities of secondary body formation (including secondary neurulation) are responsible for closed spinal NTDs, in view of their low spinal location and skin-covered nature. In recent years, a population of self-renewing progenitor cells has been identified in the caudal region of vertebrate embryos, now termed NMPs. These cells give rise during development to both neural and mesodermal tissue types, and very likely also endoderm of the tail-gut.[15] It has proven possible to generate and further differentiate cells resembling NMPs starting with mouse or human embryonic stem cells (ESCs), and applying treatments with specific growth factors in vitro.[38,39] It seems likely, therefore, that the aberrant cell differentiation observed in closed spinal NTDs, with formation of lipoma and other tissues, may arise from faulty NMP development. However, other possibilities also exist: for example, neural crest (NC) cells arising from the neural tube have the ability to form multiple tissue types, representing a different potential pathogenic route towards spinal dysraphism. It is currently unclear, however, whether the mammalian secondary neural tube actually generates multipotential NC cells. In the chick embryo, such cells arise but have a limited differentiative capacity, with no neuronal derivatives.[40]

OTHER DEFECTS OFTEN CLASSIFIED WITH NEURAL TUBE DEFECTS

Several other rare defects are often classified with the NTDs. Iniencephaly is a usually lethal abnormality characterized by extreme cervicothoracic spinal retroflexion as a result of anomalous cervical vertebrae. In affected infants, an encephalocele or spina bifida is often associated with malformations in other body systems: for example, hydronephrosis, cardiovascular malformations, single umbilical artery, diaphragmatic hernia, facial clefts, omphalocele, and clubfoot.[41] A causal link with open NTDs is suggested by the higher prevalence of iniencephaly in locations where NTDs are more abundant[22] and the recent finding that two of eight infants with iniencephaly had a sibling or a cousin with anencephaly.[42] Sacrococcygeal teratoma is an often massive, benign tumor of the low spinal region that typically contains many cell types. It may be isolated or associated with other defects of the lower body.[43] While sometimes described as a "germ cell tumor," by analogy with testicular and ovarian teratomas, its caudal location is strongly suggestive of an embryonic origin from cells of the embryonic tail-bud: the NMPs. In sacro-caudal agenesis (also called caudal regression syndrome), the sacral and coccygeal elements are missing. This can be isolated, associated with maternal diabetes mellitus, or part of a syndrome including OEIS complex, VACTERL association, and Curriano triad.[44] In mice, continued proliferation of the NMP cell population is vital for axial elongation, and failure of canonical Wnt or fibroblast growth factor (FGF) signaling leads to body axis truncation, as does excessive retinoid (vitamin A derivative) exposure or loss of the retinoid metabolizing enzyme Cyp26a1.[45] Pathogenesis of human sacral agenesis could also involve one or more of these mechanisms.

CAUSATION OF NEURAL TUBE DEFECTS

Two NTD categories can be distinguished: (1) "isolated" NTDs which are associated only with disorders resulting directly from the NTD, such as hydrocephalus and Chiari II malformation, and (2) "nonisolated" NTDs, which are associated with birth defects that do not result directly from the NTD (e.g., heart defects, omphalocele, kidney defects). Nonisolated NTD-malformation associations may correspond to a known syndrome: for example, Meckel syndrome, characterized by occipital encephalocele, polycystic kidneys, and polydactyly. Or the pattern of malformations may appear unique and not correspond to any known syndrome. Epidemiologically, the two categories are distinct, for example, with marked differences between ethnic groups in the prevalence of isolated but not nonisolated NTDs.[46] Such findings led to the idea that isolated NTDs, which comprise at least 75% of all NTDs, result largely from multifactorial (genetic and environmental) causation, whereas the rarer, nonisolated NTDs are highly heterogeneous with a variety of different causations, including single gene and chromosomal abnormalities.

ENVIRONMENTAL (NONGENETIC) FACTORS IN NEURAL TUBE DEFECTS

Nongenetic factors play a significant role in the origin of many NTDs, especially isolated cases with multifactorial causation. A variety of specific malformation-causing (teratogenic) agents can cause NTDs in mice and rats,[47] with a smaller number also implicated in humans (Table 169.1). The anticonvulsant valproic acid (VPA) increases risk of spinal NTDs 10-fold when taken early in pregnancy,[48] with a primary effect on epigenetic gene regulation (see below). Similar teratogenicity is seen with the anticonvulsant carbamazepine, although the mechanism in this

Table 169.1 Environmental Factors Linked to the Causation of Human Neural Tube Defects.

Category	Teratogenic Agent	Proposed Teratogenic Mechanism	References
Anticonvulsants	Valproic acid	Histone deacetylase inhibition leading to disruption of key signaling pathways in neurulation	48
	Carbamazepine	Inhibition of cellular folate uptake	180
Maternal glycemic dysregulation	Hyperglycemia (poorly controlled type I maternal diabetes)	Altered gene expression and/or oxidative damage leading to increased cell death in embryonic tissues	51
	Maternal obesity (type II diabetes)	Unknown	53
Micronutrient deficiencies	Folate	Disturbance of FOCM	181
	Inositol	Disturbance of phosphorylation events downstream of protein kinase C	182
	Vitamin B12	Disturbance of FOCM	181
	Zinc	Unknown	183
Thermal dysregulation	Hyperthermia (e.g., maternal fever in weeks 3–4 of pregnancy)	Altered gene expression and/or oxidative damage leading to increased cell death in embryonic tissues	184
Toxic exposures	Fumonisin	Disturbance of sphingolipid biosynthesis and metabolism with effects on signaling pathways in neurulation	50

FOCM, Folate one-carbon metabolism.

case is unclear. The fungal toxin fumonisin, which contaminates tortilla flour on a seasonal basis, was responsible for a 2-fold increase in NTD prevalence along the Texas-Mexico border in the early 1990s.[49] Fumonisin causes NTDs in mice, with marked effects on sphingolipid metabolism that likely disturb downstream embryonic gene expression.[50] In addition to those drugs and toxins, a number of maternal factors lead to a uterine environment that predisposes to NTDs. These include maternal diabetes mellitus,[51] maternal obesity,[52] and exposure to high temperatures during early pregnancy.[53] While hyperglycemia and hyperthermia are both proven NTD-causing teratogens in animal models, the precise mechanisms by which types I and II diabetes in particular predispose to human NTDs remains unclear.

Environmental causes are perhaps the most preventable of predisposing factors, but very few congenital defects overall have a known environmental cause: among European pregnancies, environmental causes could be identified in only 0.12 cases per 1000 births (0.5% of all birth defects).[54] Moreover, genetic variation plays an important role in determining the susceptibility of a particular pregnancy to a particular environmental factor. For example, marked differences in NTD frequency are routinely observed when different inbred mouse strains (with different genotype) are exposed to teratogenic factors including VPA and fumonisin.[55,56]

CHROMOSOMAL DISORDERS INVOLVING NEURAL TUBE DEFECTS

Abnormalities of chromosome number or structure (aneuploidy) are especially prevalent among nonisolated NTDs, which occur in up to 10% of first trimester miscarriages: a 10-fold higher frequency than in later pregnancies and live births. Among miscarried NTD-affected embryos, 70% to 100% are aneuploidy,[57] whereas aneuploidy is less common in later-stage NTDs. Triploidy occurs in 30% to 40% of miscarried NTDs and in up to 50% of miscarried open spina bifida cases,[58] but in less than 20% of later-stage NTDs. Aneuploidy is more common in open spina bifida than in anencephaly, with the most prevalent defects being trisomy 18 (Edwards syndrome; open spina bifida) and trisomy 13 (Patau syndrome; open spina bifida, and encephalocele).

Structural chromosome anomalies in NTDs are mostly copy number variants (CNVs): duplications or deletions of specific chromosomal regions.[59] For example, analysis by array-CGH (comparative genomic hybridization) of a fetus prenatally diagnosed with open spina bifida, facial dysmorphism, and cleft palate (i.e., nonisolated NTD), revealed a 5.6 Mb interstitial deletion of the long arm of chromosome 2 (2q36).[60] Of 17 genes in the deleted region, one was *PAX3* which causes Waardenburg syndrome types I and III in humans and results in NTDs in mice.[61] Haplo-insufficiency for *PAX3* may have caused this fetal NTD, but the deletion also removed the *EPHA4* gene which may play a role in mouse spinal closure.[62] Hence, this case could represent a "contiguous gene deletion syndrome," where two or more genes, physically linked to the same CNV, contribute to the phenotype.

NEURAL TUBE DEFECTS AS SINGLE GENE DISORDERS

ENCEPHALOCELE

This is the most strongly syndromic NTD type, with a number of genes implicated in its causation.[63] These include *COL18A1* in Knobloch syndrome (Table 169.2), *FGFR2* in Apert syndrome and *FGFR3* in thanatophoric dysplasia. Occipital encephalocele is best known as part of Meckel syndrome (overlapping with Joubert syndrome), in which individuals also exhibit polydactyly, polycystic kidneys, and biliary defects. A number of genes with autosomal recessive inheritance have been identified (see Table 169.2),[64] and the encoded proteins play a key role in the structure and function of primary cilia, protrusions of the cell surface that are rooted in the centrosome and undergo a disassembly and reassembly cycle as the cell proliferates.[65] Hence, Meckel syndrome is now classified as a *ciliopathy*. How encephalocele results from disordered ciliary function is unknown.

OTHER NEURAL TUBE DEFECTS

Single gene defects that are associated with spina bifida include *PAX3*, mutated in Waardenburg syndrome types I and III, in which NTDs occur in a few patients who are likely *PAX3* homozygotes. Mutations of the sonic hedgehog (SHH) pathway repressors *PTCH1*, *PTCH2*, or *SUFU* cause Gorlin syndrome, in which occasional NTDs are observed,[66] which might relate to proliferative effects of SHH in neural tube formation. Increased dosage of *SOX3* has been described in a case of human spina bifida.[67]

EVIDENCE FOR GENETIC CAUSATION IN NONSYNDROMIC, ISOLATED NEURAL TUBE DEFECTS

The commonest NTDs, anencephaly and open spina bifida, occur sporadically and are rarely found as multiple cases in families, making single gene causation unlikely. Most (~70%) of the variance in prevalence of such sporadic NTDs appears genetic,[7] as judged by the increased recurrence risk for siblings of index cases (2% to 5%) compared with the 0.1% risk in the general population; risk decreases progressively in more distant relatives. Women with two or more affected pregnancies have a higher risk (~10%) of further recurrence. NTD prevalence is greater in like-sex twins (assumed to include all monozygotic cases) compared with unlike-sex pairs, consistent with a significant genetic component. Together, this evidence suggests a multifactorial oligogenic or polygenic inheritance pattern, with an important role for nongenetic factors interacting with the genetic predisposition.[68]

CLUES FROM MOUSE GENETIC MODELS OF NEURAL TUBE DEFECT

More than 300 different genes yield open NTDs when individually inactivated in mice,[69,70] attesting to the genetic complexity of neural tube closure. Exencephaly is the most common NTD observed, while a smaller number of mutants yield open spina bifida, often with tail flexion defects. Genes that function in the PCP pathway are required for initiation of neural tube closure, and mutants develop CRN.[23] In contrast, only a few mouse mutants display encephalocele,[33] and there are essentially no models of skin-covered low spinal NTDs. Mouse NTDs were originally identified in single gene homozygotes, but gene-gene and gene-environment interactions are also being increasingly described. These most accurately model the multifactorial risk (genes plus environment) that applies to human NTDs.

GENE-GENE INTERACTIONS

Some pairs of genes with close functional relationships need to be inactivated simultaneously to elicit NTDs, as with *Cdx1/Cdx2* double knockouts.[71] Pairwise heterozygous combinations of genes in the PCP signaling pathway (see below) produce CRN,[72] while genes from overtly different genetic pathways can interact to generate NTDs, as with *Pax3/Shmt1* compound heterozygotes.[73] NTD penetrance and expressivity also varies between inbred strains of mice, which differ at many ("modifier") genetic loci.[74] For example, the high rate of exencephaly resulting from *Cecr2* mutation on the BALB/c inbred background is almost abolished on the FVB/N background.[75]

GENE-ENVIRONMENT INTERACTIONS

Teratogens often produce NTDs of differing frequency and severity, depending on the mouse genetic strain background, as observed for VPA[55] and fumonisin.[76] Moreover, specific genes can interact with teratogenic or other environmental factors to modify the frequency of NTDs: for example, arsenic

Table 169.2 Categories of Genes Associated With Human Neural Tube Defects.[a]

Function	Genes (Variants)	Inheritance/Occurrence	Human NTDs[b]	Mouse NTD Models	Refs.[c]
Cilia function	*MKS1, TMEM216, TMEM67, CEP290, RPGRIP1L, CC2D2A NPHP3, TCTN2, B9D1, B9D2, TMEM231*	Autosomal recessive	ENC (occipital) as part of Meckel syndrome	No encephalocele in gene knockouts studied to date	64
Diabetes and obesity related	*FTO, LEP, GLUT2*	Maternal risk reduced by rare FTO variants and increased by rare LEP variants	OSB	No NTDs reported for these genes. NTDs increased in maternal type 1 diabetes	98,97
Extracellular matrix	*COL18A1*	Autosomal recessive	ENC (occipital) as part of Knobloch syndrome	No encephalocele in Col18a1 knockout	185
Folate metabolic enzymes, cytoplasmic	*MTHFR (C677T), MTHFD1 (G1958A), MTRR (A66G)*	Increased frequency in NTD cases (MTHFR-TT) and in NTD mothers (MTHFR-TT; MTHFD1-AA; MTRR-GG)	ANEN, OSB; sporadic cases	No NTDs in Mthfr or Mthfd1 knockouts. NTDs in mice with severely reduced Mtrr expression	85
Folate metabolic enzymes, mitochondrial	*MTHFD1L, GLDC, AMT*	Variants mostly unique to NTD patients; cases homozygous	ANEN, OSB; sporadic cases	Cranial NTDs in homozygotes	93,186
Planar Cell Polarity (PCP) pathway core components	*VANGL1, VANGL2, DVL1, DVL2, CELSR1, SCRIB*	Variants mostly unique to NTD patients; cases heterozygous; often transmitted from unaffected parent	CRN, ANEN, OSB; sporadic cases	Craniorachischisis in homozygotes and compound heterozygotes. Spinal NTDs at low frequency in some heterozygotes	23
Platelet derived growth factor receptor	*PDGFRA*	Haplotypes promoting high PDGFRA expression enriched in NTDs among European Caucasians	OSB	Spina bifida occulta in Pdgfra mutants (Patch); open spina bifida in Pdgfra/Pax1 double mutants	187,188
Sonic hedgehog pathway inhibitors	*PTCH1, PTCH2, SUFU*	Autosomal dominant	Occasional SBO as part of Gorlin (Basal Cell Nevus) syndrome	Craniorachischisis in Ptch1 and SUFU homozygotes	115
Transcription factors	*GRHL3, PAX3*	GRHL3 variants mostly unique to NTD patients; cases heterozygous; Many PAX3 variants: autosomal recessive for NTDs	ANEN, OSB; with GRHL3 variants; Occasional ANEN and OSB as part of Waardenburg syndromes I and III with PAX3 mutations	Open cranial & spinal NTDs in Grhl3 and Pax3 homozygotes and occasionally in heterozygotes	189

[a]Only genetic variants that show reproducible association with human NTDs are shown.
[b]NTD abbreviations: *ANEN*, Anencephaly; *CRN*, craniorachischisis; *ENC*, encephalocele; *OSB*, open spina bifida; SBO, spina bifida occulta.
[c]Key references only are shown. These should be consulted for additional references to the gene(s) and NTDs.
NTD, Neural tube defect.

interacts with the *Pax3 (splotch)* mutation[77] while hydroxyurea, mitomycin C, and retinoic acid all interact with the *Grhl3 (curly tail)* mutation.[78]

GENES ASSOCIATED WITH THE RISK OF HUMAN NEURAL TUBE DEFECTS

Although much evidence supports a multifactorial predisposition to NTDs, involving genetic and nongenetic influences, relatively few individual NTD risk genes have so far been definitively identified, despite increasing application of next-generation DNA sequencing methods (Box 169.1). Two criteria are useful in indicating whether a gene has a true causal relationship with NTDs. Reproducibility of findings between individual, often small-scale, human genetic studies can be tested by *systematic review and statistical meta-analysis*, in which multiple existing data sets are combined to give an overall significance value. Moreover, human genetic data can be compared with the *phenotypes of mice* deficient or otherwise abnormal for the corresponding gene, to determine whether NTDs or related defects occur in the model system. Genes that best satisfy these criteria are included in the list of likely NTD risk genes and variants (see Table 169.2).

Folate one-carbon metabolism (FOCM) generates purines and pyrimidines for DNA synthesis during cell replication, and methyl groups for regulation of gene, protein and lipid function (Fig. 169.4). Genetic variants that reduce FOCM efficiency might increase NTD risk by compromising cell proliferation, gene expression, or both. Cell lines from NTD fetuses showed disordered folate metabolism, as indicated by diminished thymidylate biosynthesis,[79] suggesting that FOCM-related genetic factors do indeed play a role in NTDs.

Folate uptake and transport would appear likely candidates for genetic variants affecting human NTD risk, but few positive findings have emerged.[80] Some women with NTD-affected pregnancies exhibit circulating autoantibodies that block binding

Box 169.1 Sex Differences in the Prevalence of Neural Tube Defects

Anencephaly is 2–3 times more common in females than males[170] whereas spina bifida affects males and females more equally. Mice of several different mutant mouse strains also show a female excess in anencephaly.[171] This sex difference is unlikely to result from hormonal influences, as sex hormones do not begin secretion from the embryonic gonad until after neural tube closure is complete.[172] While prenatal loss of anencephalic males is theoretically possible, it is not observed in mice. Hence, there appears to be a greater susceptibility to failure of cranial neural tube closure in females than males. It was suggested that female embryos develop more slowly than males, and so experience a longer time window for neurulation disturbance.[173] However, female and male mouse embryos actually develop at the same rate during neurulation,[174] although males are developmentally ahead of females due to a growth advantage that arises in the preimplantation period.[175] Genetic analysis in mice shows the predisposition to exencephaly of female embryos results from possession of two X chromosomes, whereas a Y chromosome is not protective.[176] Female cells inactivate one of their X chromosomes from early in the postimplantation period, a process that consumes methyl groups which "coat" the inactive X chromosome.[177] Hence, it has been suggested that female neurulation-stage embryos may experience a shortage of methyl groups compared with males, and this may disrupt the epigenetic regulation of genes required for cranial neural tube closure.[10] This hypothesis is compelling, but has not yet been tested experimentally. Strikingly, analysis of sex ratios in human neural tube defects (NTDs) in both Latin America[178] and China[179] have found a larger decrease in anencephaly rate in females than males, following fortification or supplementation with folic acid. As folates provide methyl groups to the cell, this supports the idea that cranial NTD preponderance in females may be related to a shortage of intracellular methylation potential.

of folates to their cellular receptors, and diminish uptake, which could produce embryonic folate deficiency in the absence of transporter gene mutations. However, original positive findings in an American NTD population[81] were not reproduced in Irish mothers with NTDs.[82]

Enzymes of cytoplasmic FOCM have been analyzed extensively for genetic association with NTDs, and best known is the C677T polymorphism of methylene tetrahydrofolate reductase (*MTHFR*), which is reproducibly associated with a 1.5- to 2-fold increased risk of NTDs in cases and mothers in non-Hispanic populations (see Table 169.2). However, *MTHFR* inactivation in mice does not lead to NTDs,[83,84] questioning the specificity of the *MTHFR* association with NTDs. Other genes with consistent human NTD associations include *MTHFD1*, *MTRR*, *SHMT1* and *TS* (see Table 169.2). Variant alleles are most commonly increased among mothers of NTD pregnancies, although some associations with NTD cases have also been found, especially for pregnancies where folate intake was judged to be suboptimal, based on dietary questionnaires.[85] In mice, *SHMT1* null mouse embryos develop NTDs under folate-deficient conditions[86] and mice with reduced *MTRR* function have severe defects including NTDs, an effect that has intriguing transgenerational features.[87]

Mitochondrial enzymes of FOCM generate formate that exits the mitochondrion and supplies the majority of 1-C units for cytoplasmic FOCM (see Fig. 169.4).[88] An intronic polymorphism in *MTHFD1L* that influences splicing efficiency in generating alternate mRNA transcripts is associated with increased risk of NTDs in an Irish population.[89] Moreover, in mice, MTHFD1L loss of function causes severe, fully penetrant NTDs even under folate-replete nutritional conditions.[90] Two enzymes of the glycine cleavage system (GCS; see Fig. 169.4), aminomethyltransferase (AMT) and glycine decarboxylase (GLDC), have been found to harbor a number of missense (i.e., amino acid–changing) genomic alterations in NTD cases, but not in unaffected controls.[91,92] These *GLDC* variants diminish enzyme activity, indicating a functional effect on mitochondrial FOCM. In mice, *Amt* and *Gldc* mutants both display NTDs and, strikingly, supply of exogenous formate to pregnant females prevented NTDs in *Gldc* mutant embryos,[93] positively implicating disturbed FOCM in NTD causation.

PLANAR CELL POLARITY PATHWAY GENES

These genes participate in an evolutionarily conserved, Wnt-frizzled-disheveled intracellular signaling cascade that does not involve stabilization of β-catenin (i.e., a noncanonical pathway). Mice lacking function of any of the transmembrane PCP proteins *VANGL2*, *CELSR1*, *PTK7* and *FZD3/6* (double mutant), or the cytoplasmic proteins *DVL1/2/3* and *SCRIB*, develop CRN, with failure of Closure 1 during primary neurulation.[72] In humans, missense variants in the orthologues of most core PCP genes or PCP-related genes (see Table 169.2) have been found in small numbers of patients with NTDs, but not in unaffected control individuals. The patients are usually heterozygous for a variant, which is often transmitted from an unaffected parent.[23] Hence, the combined mouse and human data make it very likely that PCP gene variants contribute to the risk of NTD in some individuals, probably through interaction with other as yet unidentified predisposing gene mutations.

DIABETES-RELATED GENETIC EFFECTS

Type I diabetes has long been known to associate with an elevated NTD risk[94] and, more recently, maternal obesity with its type II diabetes connection has also been linked to NTDs by meta-analysis.[95,96] There is a reduced risk of NTD-affected pregnancy in mothers carrying less common variants of the *FTO* (fat mass and obesity-associated) gene,[97] *LEP* (leptin) variants are associated with increased maternal NTD risk even in nonobese women,[98] and *GLUT2* variants are associated with individual NTD risk.[99] Hence, genetic variants affecting glucose homeostasis may modify a woman's risk of having an NTD-affected pregnancy.

EPIGENETIC CONTRIBUTIONS TO NEURAL TUBE DEFECTS

In addition to genomic sequence risk factors, it is possible that the causation of NTDs may also involve epigenetic changes. For example, methylation and acetylation of DNA or its associated histone proteins, and larger-scale remodeling of chromatin, can all regulate gene expression.[100] Moreover, environmental influences can alter gene expression via epigenetic mechanisms. Indeed, methylation of a class of genomic sequences (LINE-1 elements) is reduced in the DNA of fetuses with anencephaly[101] although methylation of such elements did not respond to folate supplementation in the peri-conceptional period.[102] Moreover, CpG methylation in newborn cord blood shows a primarily inverse correlation with maternal plasma folate levels,[103] suggesting a possibly complex relationship between folate availability and DNA methylation. In mice, several NTD-associated genes play key roles in epigenetic regulation, including *DNMT3b* (DNA methyl-transferase 3b), the histone acetyltransferase genes *p300*, *GCN5*, and *CITED2*, and the chromatin remodeling genes *CECR2*, *SMARCA4*, and *SMARCA1*.[104] The anticonvulsant VPA, a well-known risk factor for human spina bifida, is a potent histone deacetylase (HDAC) inhibitor.[105] Hence, epigenetic regulation of gene expression may play an important role in NTD causation.

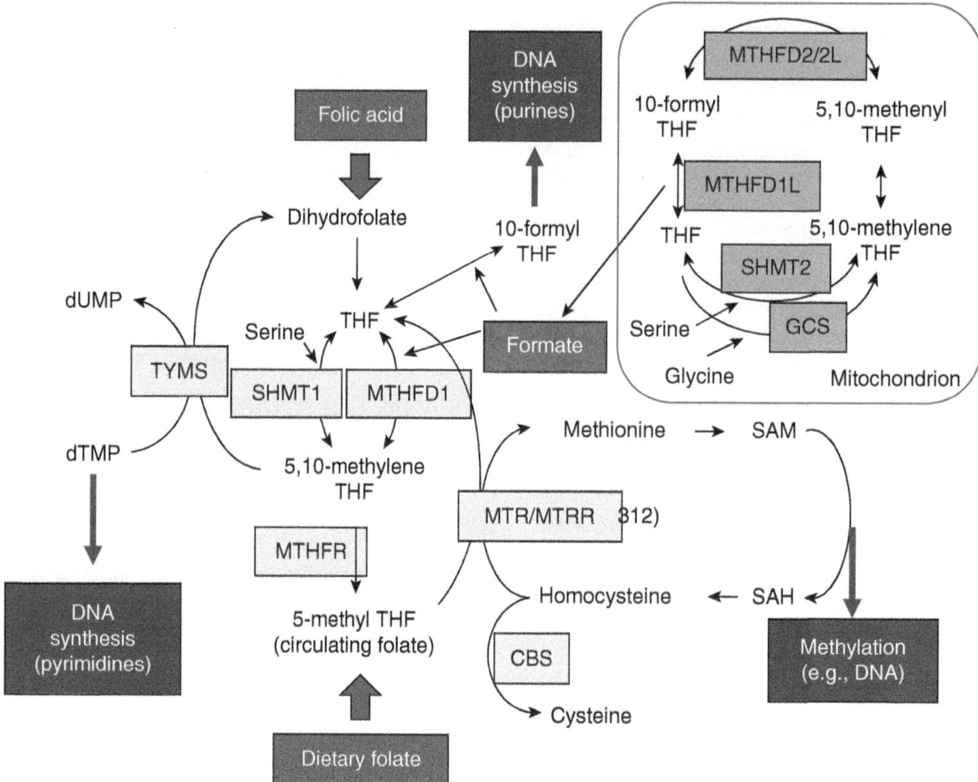

Fig. 169.4 Pathways of folate one-carbon metabolism showing the key cytoplasmic *(yellow)* and mitochondrial *(orange)* enzymes/genes that have been implicated in neural tube defect (NTD) causation. Inputs to the pathways are either as folic acid or dietary folate *(green)*. Outputs are DNA synthesis or methylation of DNA and other macromolecules *(red)*. Formate export from the mitochondrion *(purple)* supplies a significant proportion of one-carbon units to the cytoplasm. (Adapted with permission from Copp AJ, Stanier P, Ne NDE. Genetic basis of neural tube defects. In: Di Rocco C, Pang D, Rutka JT, editors. *Textbook of Pediatric Neurosurgery*. Online: Springer International Publishing AG; 2020:1–28.)

EMBRYONIC PATHOGENESIS OF NEURAL TUBE DEFECTS

Neurulation can become disrupted at various positions along the body axis, yielding NTDs of the cranial region, upper/lower spinal region, or both. This generates the spectrum of NTD anomalies that is seen clinically. An understanding of the cellular and molecular mechanisms that intervene between the etiologic factors (genes and environment) and the NTDs themselves may suggest targets for new therapeutic interventions to prevent NTDs. Mechanistic evidence, mostly from animal models, so far exists mainly for primary neurulation, where several key sequential embryonic processes are recognized, supported by experimental studies that have yielded information on their molecular pathogenesis.

CONVERGENT EXTENSION: SHAPING THE NEURAL PLATE

In all vertebrate species that undergo neural tube closure (amphibians, birds, mammals), the onset of neurulation is marked by medio-lateral convergence and rostro-caudal extension of the body axis. This CE is a process by which the neural plate becomes shaped,[106] converting it from an ovoid structure prior to gastrulation to the keyhole-shaped neurula, with an enlarged rostral region (future brain) and narrow trunk region (future spine). During CE, cells move medio-laterally relative to each other, with intercalation in the midline to extend the body axis. CE depends on function of the noncanonical Wnt/PCP pathway: defective CE in the embryonic midline of PCP mutants causes the neural plate to remain too wide for the neural folds to meet and fuse, resulting in an embryo with short, broad body axis and the severe NTD CRN.[107,108] Although embryos completely lacking PCP function cannot progress in neurulation beyond Closure 1, it is possible that partial loss of PCP function can result in later-stage neurulation defects, including open spina bifida.[109] This is in agreement with the finding of PCP genetic variants in humans with either spina bifida or CRN.[23]

NEURAL FOLD ELEVATION: BENDING OF THE NEURAL PLATE

During primary neurulation, the neural folds elevate bilaterally and approach each other in the dorsal midline, a process that differs in morphology between cranial and spinal regions. The mouse midbrain neural folds are initially biconvex with their tips orientated away from the midline (Fig. 169.5A). Subsequently, dorsolateral bending occurs, converting the folds to a biconcave morphology and orienting the tips towards the midline for fusion (see Fig. 169.5B and C).[110] This biphasic sequence results from an initial expansion of the underlying cranial mesoderm, which produces the biconvex neural fold morphology.[111] Apical constriction of neuroepithelial cells, involving actomyosin contraction, causes bending near the fold tips that generates the biconcave morphology.[112]

In the spinal region, by contrast, the neural folds bend only at focal sites, which are located at the midline (the MHP, or median hinge point) and dorsolaterally (DLHPs, or paired dorsolateral hinge points) (see Fig. 169.5D–F). As the wave of closure progresses along the spinal region, bending shifts from MHP-mediated to DLHP-mediated.[113] DLHP bending is regulated by mutually inhibitory interactions between BMP2 and its antagonist Noggin, both secreted from dorsal cells, and by SHH secreted from the ventrally located notochord.[114] SHH inhibits DLHPs at high spinal levels, but declines in activity further down the spine, allowing DLHP-mediated bending to complete spinal closure. Over-activation of the SHH signaling pathway, as seen in

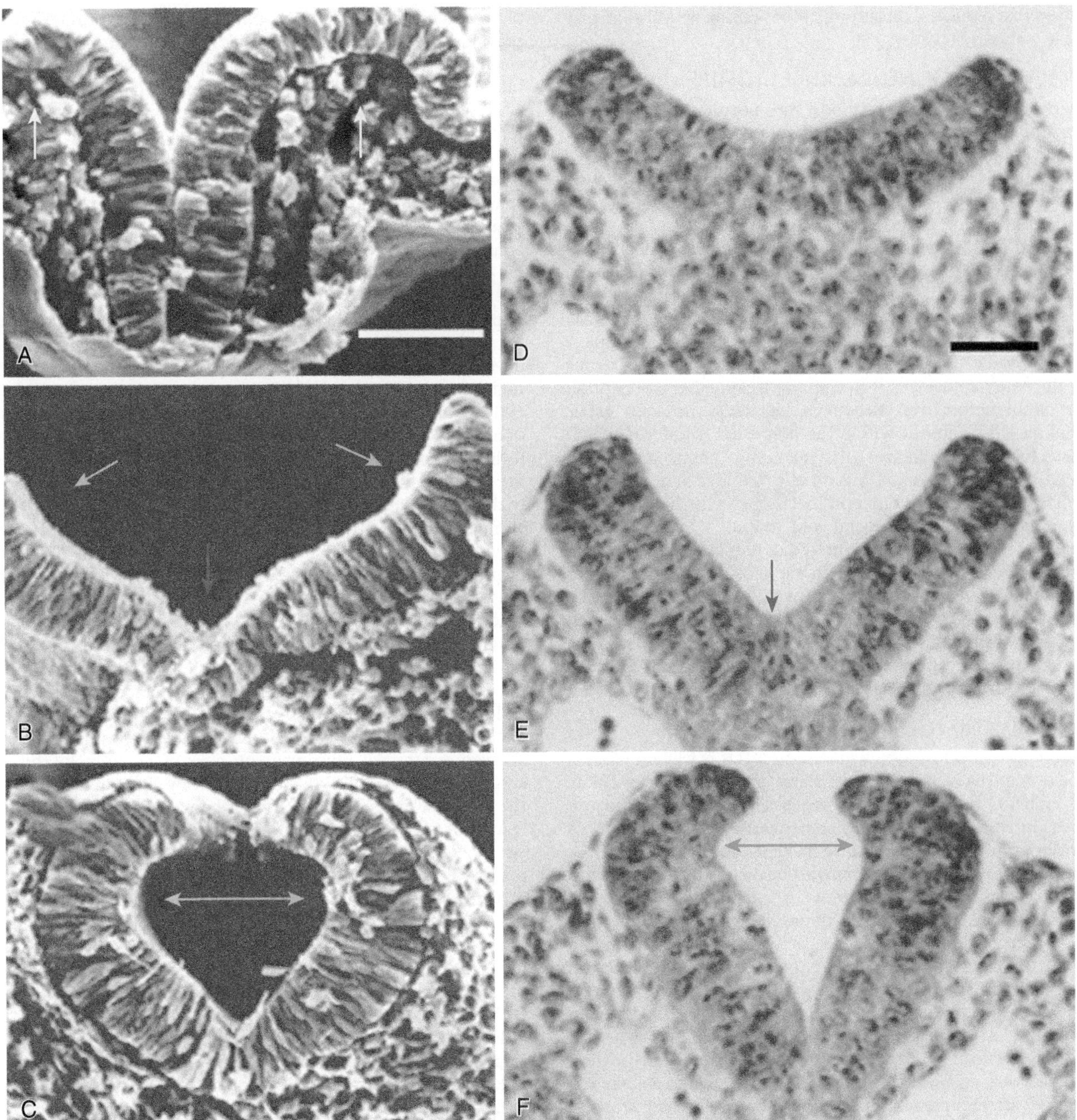

Fig. 169.5 Morphology of cranial and spinal neural tube closure in rodent embryos. (A–C) Cranial closure in transverse scanning electron micrographs of the midbrain region of E9 rat embryos. The neural folds show initial convex bending (*yellow arrows* in A) before onset of dorsolateral bending (*green arrows* in B and C) that brings the neural fold tips together. (D–F) Spinal closure in H&E stained transverse sections along the closing region of a mouse embryo (E9.5). There is no convex stage (D and E), although midline bending is prominent as in the cranial region *(red arrows)*. Dorsolateral hinge points (*blue arrows* in F) develop and bring the neural fold tips together in the low spinal region. Scale bars represent 50 μm, *white* (A–C), *black* (D–F). (A–C, Reproduced with permission from 110. Morriss-Kay GM. Growth and development of pattern in the cranial neural epithelium of rat embryos during neurulation. *J Embryol Exp Morphol*. 1981;65(suppl):225–241. D–F, Reproduced with permission from Shum ASW, Copp AJ. Regional differences in morphogenesis of the neuroepithelium suggest multiple mechanisms of spinal neurulation in the mouse. *Anat Embryol*. 1996;194:65–73.)

PTCH and SUFU mutants, represses DLHP formation and leads to NTDs in both cranial and spinal regions.[115]

FUSION AND REMODELING OF THE NEURAL FOLDS

Completion of neural tube closure involves "fusion" of the elevated neural fold tips to create the closed neural tube covered by nonneural ectoderm (future epidermis). Considerable remodeling of tissue layers is involved, and this coincides with plentiful programmed cell death (apoptosis) at the fusion site.[116] However, pharmacologic inhibition of apoptosis does not prevent fusion or remodeling,[117] and it remains unclear why cell death occurs at this site. Neural fold fusion is mediated by cellular protrusions that arise from the neural fold tips, and form the first points of attachment across the midline gap.[118] The protrusions are actomyosin-containing, highly motile structures that in other cell types are regulated by small GTPases: Rho, Rac, and Cdc42. Indeed, ablation of Rac1 from the neural fold tips results in spina bifida, with absent protrusions.[119] It remains to be determined whether variants of *RAC1*, or other genes within the pathways that regulate cellular protrusions during neurulation, may underlie NTDs in humans.

BIOMECHANICS OF NEURAL TUBE CLOSURE

Biomechanical factors are critical in morphogenetic events. For example, shaping, bending, and fusion of the neural folds, and the propagation of closure along the body axis, all involve biomechanical forces. These may arise from the underlying cellular processes or, conversely, biomechanical influences may feedback onto cells, changing gene expression and modulating cell shape, proliferation, and survival. In mouse embryos, simple biomechanical impediments such as increased ventral curvature of the caudal body axis can lead to failed neural tube closure and spina bifida.[120] During normal spinal closure, use of laser ablation methods has shown that the entire closing region is biomechanically coupled, in part by force transmission through an actin cable that runs along the neural fold edges.[12] In embryos lacking the transcription factor Grhl2, actomyosin structures, including the actin cable, are diminished or absent within the nonneural ectoderm, which biomechanically destabilizes the elevating neural folds and prevents closure.[121] Overexpression of *Grhl2* is also incompatible with closure, but due to a different mechanism, which may involve faulty remodeling during neural fold fusion.[121] Propagation of closure by "zippering" along the body axis requires dynamic shape changes as cells transition through the closure site. Interaction of extracellular matrix fibronectin with cell surface receptor integrins is necessary for these cell shape changes, as evidenced by integrin β1 mutants which fail in zippering, leading to spina bifida.[122] Hence, a variety of biomechanical mechanisms underlie NTDs arising from particular genetic and nongenetic influences.

FOLIC ACID AND NEURAL TUBE CLOSURE

The preventive effect of folic acid (FA) on NTDs is well established (see below) and FA is known to have a direct effect on the neurulation-stage embryo, as treatment of genetically predisposed mouse embryos in vitro can normalize neural tube closure.[123] FOCM, has two main outputs: production of pyrimidines and purines for DNA replication during cell proliferation, and donation of methyl groups to macromolecules including DNA, proteins, and lipids (see Fig. 169.4). Cell proliferation is highly active during neural tube closure and, indeed, a recent study found specific effects on the cell cycle of mouse embryos during FA-mediated prevention of NTDs.[124] Methylation of genomic DNA and histones is also central to the (epigenetic) regulation of gene expression,[104] and impaired methylation related to dysregulation of folate metabolism could contribute to some NTDs. Direct effects of impaired folate metabolism on methylation of proteins that play a key role in neurulation, such as F-actin and tubulins,[125] are also possible. It remains to be determined precisely how FA can prevent a proportion of human NTDs.

TREATMENT AND PREVENTION OF NEURAL TUBE DEFECTS

Surgery in the early postnatal period, and increasingly during the fetal period, is the mainstay of treatment for children with spinal NTDs. In addition, two modes of NTD "prevention" are now widely used. Secondary prevention, through abortion following prenatal diagnosis, is the routine practice in many countries and has led to major reductions in the birth prevalence of the most severe NTDs. In parallel, primary prevention by nutritional supplementation, in particular using peri-conceptual FA, has been implemented worldwide, and is estimated to have prevented around 50,000 NTDs in 2017.[126]

POSTNATAL SURGICAL REPAIR

This is usually performed within 1 to 3 days of birth and involves untethering the placode and covering the lesion. The aim is to preserve residual neurologic function and to minimize the risk of ascending infection, which can lead to infant death.[127] It was previously suggested that neurologic outcome can be improved if elective cesarean delivery is undertaken for fetuses with open spina bifida, perhaps by avoiding injury to the exposed neural tissue during labor and vaginal delivery.[128] However, this finding has not been replicated in more recent studies,[129] and vaginal delivery is currently not contraindicated in spina bifida pregnancies. Subsequent to surgical repair, children with open spina bifida often receive implantation of ventriculo-peritoneal shunts, to treat hydrocephalus, and undergo other surgical and nonsurgical treatments in response to the wide array of medical problems that they typically face throughout life.[130]

FETAL SURGICAL REPAIR

Repair of the open spina bifida lesion in utero has been practiced for more than 20 years in the United States, following method development in a large animal model[131] and through pioneering human surgical studies.[132,133] While the earliest reports employed endoscopic surgery, the most widely adopted method involves an open surgical approach. Recently, endoscopic surgery has begun to be re-explored as a less invasive alternative.[134] A landmark in the field was the publication of a randomized, double-blind clinical trial, the Management of Myelomeningocele Study (MOMS), which compared child and maternal outcomes in matched groups of fetal and postnatal surgical repair operations.[30] Selective eligibility criteria were applied so that, of 1083 women screened for possible fetal surgery, only 183 (17%) actually underwent randomization while 345 (32%) failed to meet the inclusion criteria, the commonest reason being a maternal body mass index of 35 or more. The results showed a significant reduction in the need for ventriculo-peritoneal shunt placement at 1 year of age in children who received fetal surgery (40% vs. 82% after postnatal surgery). Overall neuromotor function at 30 months of age also showed substantial improvement; 42% of children in the fetal surgery group were walking independently compared with 21% in the postnatal surgery group. Importantly, hindbrain herniation (a feature of Chiari II malformation) was reduced in the fetal surgery group; herniation was absent in 36% of infants after fetal surgery compared with only 4% of postnatally operated infants.

Against these positive child outcomes, there were increased risks for mothers who received fetal surgery: spontaneous rupture of membranes, oligohydramnios and preterm delivery were all more frequent. A quarter of the mothers showed thinning of the uterine wound, with 10% having variable degrees of dehiscence at the hysterotomy site.[30]

Follow-up of the children and mothers in the MOMS trial is now underway, with the aim of comparing the long-term effects of prenatal versus postnatal surgery on the adaptive behavior, physical and cognitive function, health, and well-being of children with spina bifida, and on the future reproductive health of their mothers. Urologic outcomes have been compared in young school-age children, with the finding of a significantly lower rate of clean intermittent catheterization and a higher rate of volitional voiding in children who received fetal surgery compared with the postnatal surgery group.[135] Hence, there is convincing evidence from the MOMS trial that prenatal surgery, in cases that satisfy the rather stringent entry criteria, can be beneficial for a range of childhood outcomes, compared with standard postnatal surgery. However, the increased risks for the mother must be balanced against these fetal benefits.

PRENATAL DIAGNOSIS OF NEURAL TUBE DEFECTS

Ultrasound examination in the second trimester is the gold-standard method for NTD prenatal diagnosis.[136] Anencephaly is diagnosed with almost 100% efficiency, whereas detection of open spina bifida is more challenging. The majority of cases are identified when the fetal spine is scanned in all three planes: sagittal, axial, and coronal, from the late first trimester onwards. In addition, the "lemon" and "banana" cranial signs can aid diagnosis. The lemon sign refers to loss of the convex outward shape of the frontal bones and is present in almost all affected fetuses at 16 to 24 weeks gestation. The banana sign refers to the shape of the cerebellum and is likely due to presence of the Chiari II malformation; it is generally used at 14 to 24 weeks' gestation. Using this combination of features, more than 90% of open spina bifida cases are detectable by ultrasound.

Methods for prenatal diagnosis of open NTDs, developed in the 1970s, were initially based on measurement of alpha fetoprotein (AFP), and later acetylcholinesterase, in the amniotic fluid.[137-139] These amniocentesis-dependent methods enabled diagnosis in pregnancies at high risk of NTD, whereas detection of elevated AFP concentration in maternal blood produced a more generally applicable screening tool.[140] While prenatal ultrasound examination has to a large extent supplanted serum AFP measurement as the primary method of prenatal diagnosis for NTDs, there are still indications for biochemical screening: for example, in maternal obesity where detailed ultrasound examination of the fetal anatomy can be problematic.[141] Moreover, a prenatal diagnosis system that combines ultrasound and serum AFP was found to be more efficient than one based on ultrasound alone.[142] Hence, both biochemical and sonographic diagnosis are used together in many health systems.

A systematic review of abortion following prenatal diagnosis,[143] using data collected during the 1990s and 2000s, found that 83% (range 59% to 100%) of anencephalic pregnancies were terminated in the group of countries for which studies had been performed: Brazil, Canada, China, Germany, Italy, Netherlands, Sweden, Switzerland, UK, United States. For spina bifida, 63% (range 31% to 97%) of pregnancies were terminated. In other countries, the percentage is much lower, or even zero, for example where abortion is illegal or prenatal diagnostic services are unavailable. Hence, "secondary" prevention of NTD births by termination of pregnancy is variably practiced across the world.

PRIMARY PREVENTION BY FOLIC ACID

In the 1970s, reductions in the serum concentrations of several vitamins (e.g., folate, riboflavin, vitamin C) were noted in mothers pregnant with NTD fetuses.[144] This stimulated a UK-based intervention trial of a multivitamin supplement containing 0.36 mg FA (Pregnavite Forte F) during the periconceptional period: that is, several weeks prior to conception and continuing until the 12th week of pregnancy. NTD recurrence in women with a history of NTD-affected pregnancy was significantly lower in those who took supplements.[145] However, the Pregnavite Forte F study was not randomized, and its findings were not universally accepted as definitive evidence of prevention.[146] Subsequently, a randomized, double-blind study (the Medical Research Council [MRC] Vitamin Study) assessed 4 mg FA separately from multivitamins, and FA was shown to be the essential factor for significant prevention of NTD recurrence.[147] A randomized clinical trial in Hungary then found that a multivitamin containing 0.8 mg FA could significantly reduce first occurrence of NTDs,[148] an important finding considering that 95% of all NTDs occur in women with no previous history of the condition. In China, a dramatic fall in NTD prevalence was noted, subsequent to introduction of FA supplements in both high- and low-prevalence regions.[149]

FOOD FORTIFICATION WITH FOLIC ACID

The MRC trial led to the recommendation that all women planning a pregnancy should consume 0.4 mg FA per day, and that women at high risk of NTD should receive 4 to 5 mg per day. Moreover, to enhance the folate status of women prior to pregnancy, a number of countries introduced mandatory fortification of bread or tortilla flour with FA.[150,151] Comparisons between countries that have fortified the staple food supply with FA (e.g., United States, Canada, South American countries), and those that rely on voluntary FA supplementation (e.g., UK) shows that the fortification route is effective, with a sizeable reduction in NTD prevalence compared with prefortification values,[152] whereas voluntary supplementation has been associated with relatively small changes in NTD prevalence over the same period (Fig. 169.6).[153] In the light of recent findings of extremely high NTD frequencies in some locations (e.g., India, Ethiopia), there is an impetus to extend FA fortification to such areas, perhaps with new fortification vehicles, including iodized salt.[154]

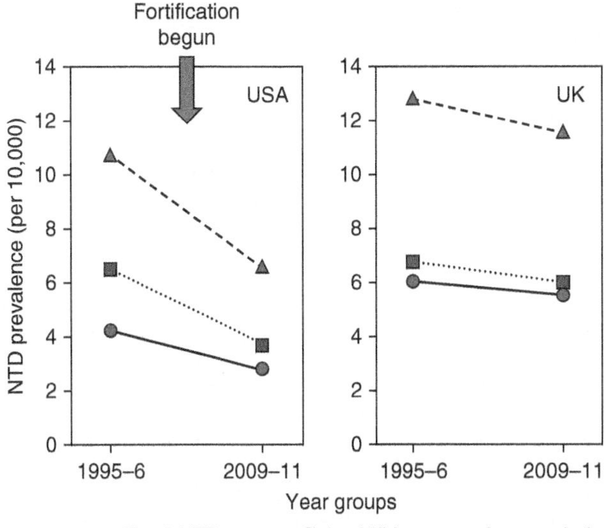

Fig. 169.6 Neural tube defect *(NTD)* prevalence trends since the 1990s: (A) in United States of America *(USA)* before and after introduction of folic acid fortification of bread flour; (B) in United Kingdom *(UK)* over the same time period, in the absence of food fortification. NTD prevalence values include numbers at birth and in terminations of pregnancy. (Data from Williams J, Mai CT, Mulinare J, et al. Updated estimates of neural tube defects prevented by mandatory folic acid fortification—United States, 1995–2011. *MMWR Morb Mortal Wkly Rep*. 2015;64:1–5 and EUROCAT [https://eu-rd-platform.jrc.ec.europa.eu/eurocat/eurocat-data].)

FOLIC ACID (NONRESPONSIVE NEURAL TUBE DEFECTS)

While NTD rates have declined following food fortification, the drop in prevalence in most countries has been smaller than expected from the MRC recurrence trial.[147] Hence, a proportion of NTD cases, perhaps on average ~0.5 per 1000 pregnancies, persist regardless of FA usage. Little additional benefit seems likely to accrue from a further increase in FA dose level.[155,156] A "FA-non-responsive" sub-group of NTDs is well established in mouse models of NTDs where some genetic types are FA-preventable while others are not.[157] Use of molecules that are related to folate metabolism, such as formate or nucleotides, to prevent NTDs in FA-resistant mouse models suggest that additional approaches may be beneficial.[84,158] Another potential adjunct therapy that has arisen from the mouse studies is use of inositol supplementation, which is effective in preventing a large proportion of spinal NTDs in the *curly tail* (*GRHL3* hypomorphic) mouse mutant, where FA is ineffective.[159] Uniquely among vitamins, inositol deficiency leads to NTDs in rodent embryos.[160] A pilot clinical trial to evaluate inositol in human pregnancies at high risk of NTD recurrence yielded results consistent with a greater preventive effect of inositol + FA, compared with FA alone.[161] A large-scale clinical trial is now needed to determine whether inositol could be added to FA supplements in future, for improved prevention of NTDs.

CONCLUSION

NTDs represent arguably the best understood category of human birth defects. Several decades of multidisciplinary research—spanning areas including epidemiology, developmental biology, neuropathology, metabolism, clinical trials, and clinical medicine/surgery—have led to significant advances in our knowledge of different aspects of this multifaceted group of disorders. Genetic causation is among the most studied but least well advanced areas of NTD research and, while there is no doubt that genetic factors play a key (perhaps predominant) role in etiology, we are yet to define exactly how genetic variation influences human NTD risk. An improved understanding of NTD genetics should enable etiologic (as opposed to purely morphological) subtypes to be distinguished, which could allow predictive genetic testing to be implemented. In terms of primary prevention, much work remains to be done both in terms of maximizing the impact of folate primary prevention and bringing into clinical practice other preventive strategies to target NTDs that escape folate prevention. A multidisciplinary approach remains a key factor in unraveling the remaining complexities of NTDs.

GENE/PROTEIN ABBREVIATIONS

AFP: Alpha fetoprotein (gene, protein)
AMT: Aminomethyltransferase (gene, protein)
B9D1/2: B9 domain containing 1 or 2 (gene, protein)
BALB/c: Bagg Albino, mouse inbred genetic background
CC2D2A: Coiled coil and C2 domain protein 2A (gene, protein)
CDC42: Cell division cycle 42 (gene, protein)
CDX1/2: Caudal type homeobox 1 or 2 (gene, protein)
CE: Convergent extension
CECR2: Cat eye syndrome chromosome region, candidate 2 (gene, protein)
CELSR1: Cadherin, epidermal growth factor, laminin G seven-pass G-type receptor 1 (gene, protein)
CEP290: Centrosomal protein 290 (gene, protein)
CGH: Comparative genomic hybridization
CITED2: Cyclic adenosine monophosphate binding protein (CREB)/p300-interacting transactivator, with Glu/Asp-rich carboxy-terminal domain 2 (gene, protein)
CNV: Copy number variant
COL18A1: Collagen type XVIII alpha 1 chain (gene, protein)
CpG: Cytosine phosphate guanine binucleotide
CRN: Craniorachischisis
CSF: Cerebrospinal fluid
CYP26a1: Cytochrome P450 type 26a1 (gene, protein)
DLHP: Dorsolateral hinge point
DNA: Deoxyribose nucleic acid
DVL1/2: Disheveled 1 or 2 (gene, protein)
EPHA4: Ephrin type A receptor 4 (gene, protein)
ESC: Embryonic stem cell
EUROCAT: European Concerted Action on Congenital Anomalies and Twins
FA: Folic acid
FGF: Fibroblast growth factor (gene, protein)
FGFR2: Fibroblast growth factor receptor 2 (gene, protein)
FOCM: Folate one-carbon metabolism
FTO: Fat mass and obesity-associated protein (gene, protein)
FVB/N: Friend leukemia virus susceptible, mouse inbred genetic background
GCN5: Histone acetyltransferase GCN5 (gene, protein)
GLDC: Glycine decarboxylase (gene, protein)
GLUT2: Glucose transporter 2 (gene, protein)
GRHL2/3: Grainyhead-like 2 or 3 (gene, protein)
GTPase: Guanosine triphosphatase
HDAC: Histone deacetylase
LEP: Leptin (gene, protein)
LINE-1: Long interspersed element 1
MHP: Median hinge point
MKS1: Meckel syndrome 1 (gene, protein)
MOMS: Management of Myelomeningocele Study
MRC: Medical Research Council UK
MTHFD1: Methylenetetrahydrofolate dehydrogenase, cyclohydrolase and formyltetrahydrofolate synthetase 1 (gene, protein)
MTHFD1L: Methylenetetrahydrofolate dehydrogenase, cyclohydrolase and formyltetrahydrofolate synthetase 1-like (gene, protein)
MTHFR: Methylenetetrahydrofolate reductase (gene, protein)
MTRR: 5-Methyltetrahydrofolate-homocysteine methyltransferase reductase (gene, protein)
NC: Neural crest
NMP: Neuro-mesodermal progenitor
NPHP3: Nephronophthisis 3 (gene, protein)
NTD: Neural tube defect
OEIS: Syndrome of omphalocele, exstrophy of the cloaca, imperforate anus, and spine abnormalities
p300: Histone acetyltransferase protein 300 (gene, protein)
PAX3: Paired box 3 (gene, protein)
PCP: Planar cell polarity
PDGFRA: Platelet-derived growth factor receptor A (gene, protein)
PTCH1/2: Patched 1 or 2 (gene, protein)
RAC1: Ras-related C3 botulinum toxin substrate 1 (gene, protein)
RHO: Rho GTPase (gene, protein)
RPGRIP1L: Retinitis pigmentosa GTPase regulator-interacting protein 1-like (gene, protein)
SCRIB: Scribble (gene, protein)
SHH: Sonic hedgehog (gene, protein)
SHMT1: Serine hydroxymethyltransferase 1 (gene, protein)
SMARCA1/4: Switch/sucrose non-fermentable related (SWI/SNF), matrix associated, actin dependent regulator of chromatin, subfamily A, member 1 or 4 (gene, protein)
SOX3: SRY-related HMG-box 3 (gene, protein)
SUFU: Suppressor of fused (gene, protein)
TCTN2: Tectonic family member 2 (gene, protein)
TMEM67/216/231: Transmembrane protein 67, 216 or 231
VACTERL: Syndrome of vertebral defects, anal atresia, cardiac defects, tracheo-esophageal fistula, renal anomalies, and limb abnormalities
VANGL1/2: Van Gogh-like planar cell polarity 1 or 2 (gene, protein)
WNT3a: Wingless and Int-1 type 3a (gene, protein)

ACKNOWLEDGMENTS

The authors' research on neurulation and NTDs is supported by grants from the Medical Research Council, Wellcome, NC3Rs, Sparks, Newlife, Action Medical Research, the Bo Hjelt Spina Bifida Foundation, Great Ormond Street Hospital Children's Charity, and the National Institute for Health Research, Biomedical Research Centre, at Great Ormond Street Hospital for Children, NHS Foundation Trust, and University College London.

A complete reference list is available at www.ExpertConsult.com. 

SELECT REFERENCES

2. Zaganjor I, Sekkarie A, Tsang BL, et al. Describing the prevalence of neural tube defects worldwide: a systematic literature review. *PloS One*. 2016;11:e0151586.
8. Mitchell LE. Epidemiology of neural tube defects. *Am J Med Genet*. 2005;135C:88–94.
10. Juriloff DM, Harris MJ. Hypothesis: the female excess in cranial neural tube defects reflects an epigenetic drag of the inactivating X chromosome on the molecular mechanisms of neural fold elevation. *Birth Defects Res A Clin Mol Teratol*. 2012;94:849–855.
15. Henrique D, Abranches E, Verrier L, Storey KG. Neuromesodermal progenitors and the making of the spinal cord. *Development*. 2015;142:2864–2875.
23. Juriloff DM, Harris MJ. A consideration of the evidence that genetic defects in planar cell polarity contribute to the etiology of human neural tube defects. *Birth Defects Res A Clin Mol Teratol*. 2012;94:824–840.
27. Oakeshott P, Hunt GM, Poulton A, Reid F. Open spina bifida: birth findings predict long-term outcome. *Arch Dis Child*. 2012;97:474–476.

29. McLone DG, Knepper PA. The cause of Chiari II malformation: a unified theory. *Pediatr Neurosci*. 1989;15:1-12.
30. Adzick NS, Thom EA, Spong CY, et al. A randomized trial of prenatal versus postnatal repair of myelomeningocele. *N Engl J Med*. 2011;364:993-1004.
33. Rolo A, Galea GL, Savery D, Greene NDE, Copp AJ. Novel mouse model of encephalocele: post-neurulation origin and relationship to open neural tube defects. *Dis Model Mech*. 2019;12:dmm040683.
45. Wilson V, Olivera-Martinez I, Storey KG. Stem cells, signals and vertebrate body axis extension. *Development*. 2009;136:1591-1604.
46. Khoury MJ, Erickson JD, James LM. Etiologic heterogeneity of neural tube defects: clues from epidemiology. *Am J Epidemiol*. 1982;115:538-548.
70. Harris MJ, Juriloff DM. An update to the list of mouse mutants with neural tube closure defects and advances toward a complete genetic perspective of neural tube closure. *Birth Defects Res A Clin Mol Teratol*. 2010;88:653-669.
84. Leung KY, Pai YJ, Chen QY, et al. Partitioning of one-carbon units in folate and methionine metabolism is essential for neural tube closure. *Cell Rep*. 2017;21:1795-1808.
91. Narisawa A, Komatsuzaki S, Kikuchi A, et al. Mutations in genes encoding the glycine cleavage system predispose to neural tube defects in mice and humans. *Hum Mol Genet*. 2012;21:1496-1503.
104. Greene ND, Stanier P, Moore GE. The emerging role of epigenetic mechanisms in the aetiology of neural tube defects. *Epigenetics*. 2011;6:875-883.
108. Ybot-Gonzalez P, Savery D, Gerrelli D, et al. Convergent extension, planar-cell-polarity signalling and initiation of mouse neural tube closure. *Development*. 2007;134:789-799.
114. Ybot-Gonzalez P, Gaston-Massuet C, Girdler G, et al. Neural plate morphogenesis during mouse neurulation is regulated by antagonism of BMP signalling. *Development*. 2007;134:3203-3211.
115. Murdoch JN, Copp AJ. The relationship between Hedgehog signalling, cilia and neural tube defects. *Birth Defects Res A Clin Mol Teratol*. 2010;88:633-652.
119. Rolo A, Savery D, Escuin S, et al. Regulation of cell protrusions by small GTPases during fusion of the neural folds. *Elife*. 2016;5:e13273.
126. Kancherla V, Wagh K, Johnson Q, Oakley Jr GP. A 2017 global update on folic acid-preventable spina bifida and anencephaly. *Birth Defects Res*. 2018;110:1139-1147.
130. Sandler AD. Children with spina bifida: key clinical issues. *Pediatr Clin North Am*. 2010;57:879-892.
142. Chan A, Robertson EF, Haan EA, Ranieri E, Keane RJ. The sensitivity of ultrasound and serum alpha-fetoprotein in population-based antenatal screening for neural tube defects. South Australia 1986-1991. *Br J Obstet Gynaecol*. 1995;102:370-376.
143. Johnson CY, Honein MA, Dana Flanders W, Howards PP, Oakley Jr GP, Rasmussen SA. Pregnancy termination following prenatal diagnosis of anencephaly or spina bifida: a systematic review of the literature. *Birth Defects Res A Clin Mol Teratol*. 2012;94:857-863.
145. Smithells RW, Sheppard S, Schorah CJ, et al. Apparent prevention of neural tube defects by periconceptional vitamin supplementation. *Arch Dis Child*. 1981;56:911-918.
147. MRC-Vitamin-Study-Research-Group. Prevention of neural tube defects: results of the medical research council vitamin study. *Lancet*. 1991;338:131-137.
149. Berry RJ, Li Z, Erickson JD, et al. Prevention of neural-tube defects with folic acid in China. *N Engl J Med*. 1999;341:1485-1490.
157. Copp AJ, Greene NDE, Murdoch JN. The genetic basis of mammalian neurulation. *Nat Rev Genet*. 2003;4:784-793.
162. Copp AJ, Greene ND. Neural tube defects - disorders of neurulation and related embryonic processes. *WIREs Dev Biol*. 2013;2:213-217.
165. Copp AJ, Stanier P, Greene ND. Neural tube defects: recent advances, unsolved questions, and controversies. *Lancet Neurol*. 2013;12:799-810.
170. Carter CO. Clues to the aetiology of neural tube malformations. *Dev Med Child Neurol*. 1974;16(suppl.32):3-15.
181. Kirke PN, Molloy AM, Daly LE, Burke H, Weir DG, Scott JM. Maternal plasma folate and vitamin B_{12} are independent risk factors for neural tube defects. *Q J Med*. 1993;86:703-708.
189. Greene ND, Copp AJ. Neural tube defects. *Annu Rev Neurosci*. 2014;37:221-242.

Pathophysiology of Preeclampsia 170

Sarosh Rana | S. Ananth Karumanchi

INTRODUCTION

Preeclampsia is a multiorgan disease specific to pregnancy most often characterized by hypertension and proteinuria occurring after 20 weeks gestation.[1] It is among the most common medical complication of pregnancy and is a leading cause of maternal/fetal morbidity and mortality highest in the developing nations.[2] Although the eclamptic convulsion may have been recognized 4000 years ago and the term *"eclampo"* signifying "lightning" used to describe both the puerperal convulsion and epilepsy can be found in Greek writings, eclampsia as a convulsion specific to pregnancy appears only in the 18th century. Preeclampsia, the preconvulsive stage of the disorder, was not recognized until after an apparatus for blood pressure measurements was perfected at the dawn of the 20th century. In this respect, recognizing, classifying, and understanding the hypertensive disease that precedes the eclamptic convulsion are relatively recent historically. It is currently believed that preeclampsia has its origin in a disorder in development of the placenta, which in turn leads to widespread maternal endothelial effects. In this chapter, we will focus on recent evidence that aberrant placental production of antiangiogenic factors is a major pathophysiologic mechanism that underlies preeclampsia.[3]

EPIDEMIOLOGY AND CLINICAL SPECTRUM OF PREECLAMPSIA

INCIDENCE AND RISK FACTORS

Preeclampsia complicates 3% to 6% of all pregnancies throughout the world.[4] Rates of severe preeclampsia are steadily increasing in the United States, likely related to increasing obesity and invitro fertilization.[5] In developed countries, maternal lives are saved at the cost of premature delivery of the neonate. There are disproportionately higher rates of preeclampsia with morbidity and mortality among African American women, even after controlling for confounders; however, the reasons for this racial disparity remain unclear.[6,7] In countries where access to health care is limited, preeclampsia is a leading cause of maternal mortality, with estimates of greater than 60,000 maternal deaths/year.[2]

The epidemiology of preeclampsia provides hints about its pathophysiology that are still being deciphered. Although there are several risk factors for preeclampsia, most cases of preeclampsia occur in healthy nulliparous women.[8] Associations between preeclampsia and nulliparity, change in paternity from a previous pregnancy,[9] short or long interpregnancy interval (less than 2 years or more than 10 years),[10,11] use of barrier contraception,[12] and assisted reproductive technologies[13] implicate a possible immunogenic exposure to paternal antigen as a predisposing factor. Genetic factors may also contribute, because both a maternal and paternal family history of the disease predisposes to preeclampsia.[14] A woman's risk for severe preeclampsia is increased two- to four-fold if she has a first-degree relative with a history of preeclampsia. There is a seven-fold risk of recurrence of preeclampsia for women who have had the condition in a previous pregnancy.[8] Genome-wide association study of neonates from 4380 cases of preeclampsia and 310,238 controls found a genome-wide susceptibility locus near the FMS-like tyrosine kinase 1 *(FLT1)* gene, the protein product of which is a well-established pathogenetic factor in preeclampsia.[15] Multiple gestation is an additional risk factor, with triplet gestation carrying a greater risk than twin gestation; this suggests that increased placental mass may play a role.[16] Other risk factors include advanced maternal age, insulin resistance, obesity, systemic inflammation, and chronic hypertension.[17-19] The only known factor that is associated with reduced risk for preeclampsia is, paradoxically, cigarette smoking, which is directly associated with fetal growth restriction.[20]

CLINICAL FEATURES

Preeclampsia is not only a hypertensive disorder but a multisystem disease. In addition to the vascular system and kidney involvement, preeclampsia includes dysfunction of the liver, hemolysis and thrombocytopenia, an increased risk of abruption, and eclamptic seizures.[21] One feature of the disorder is how rapidly it can evolve when a seemingly stable patient with mild hypertension and minimal proteinuria suddenly develops marked liver involvement and extreme hemolysis with thrombocytopenia (HELLP syndrome [*H*emolysis *E*levated *L*iver enzymes and *L*ow *P*latelets]). Other aspects of the preeclampsia's spectrum includes cardiac dysfunction described as subtle diastolic dysfunction[22,23] or frank heart failure and cardiomyopathy,[24,25] thrombotic microangiopathy leading to disseminated intravascular coagulopathy, and a variety of forms of liver dysfunction including subcapsular hematomas.[21] The cerebral effects in addition to severe headache include cerebral edema, intracranial hemorrhage, and even blindness. Magnetic resonance imaging (MRI) studies have revealed that the cerebral edema is often localized to the posterior cerebrum and has been labeled as posterior reversible encephalopathy syndrome (PRES).[26] This is believed to be a result of endothelial damage and loss of myogenic tone in the cerebral vasculature.[27] Severe preeclampsia is associated with intrauterine growth restriction (IUGR) of the fetus and oligohydramnios.[28,29] Neonatal morbidity is most often due to the sequelae of prematurity and low birth weight, including prolonged neonatal intensive care unit stays, respiratory distress, necrotizing enterocolitis, intraventricular hemorrhage, sepsis, and death.[30]

The exact diagnostic criteria for preeclampsia are not agreed upon worldwide in part due to a plethora of national guidelines.[31] In United States, we adhere mainly to the American College of Obstetrics task force criteria that included appearance of hypertension (systolic or diastolic at or above 140 and 90 mm Hg, respectively) and new-onset proteinuria (at or greater than 300 mg/24 hours of protein, or a protein to creatinine ratio in a spot urine of 0.3 [mg/dL] after 20 weeks of gestation).[32,33] In the absence of proteinuria the diagnosis should be made when any other of the multisystem aspects are present, such as new-onset thrombocytopenia, liver function abnormalities, pulmonary edema, and cerebral and visual system abnormalities (Table 170.1).[32,33] The task force also maintained as a classification gestational hypertension, a designation when hypertension alone appeared de novo after mid-pregnancy without proteinuria or any severe features.[32] However, such patients contain a mixture of different pathologies. In some it is chronic previously undiagnosed hypertension masked by the normal decrease in blood pressure that occurs in early gestation. In others it may be subclinical preeclampsia that may progress to full-blown disease with advancing gestational age.

Table 170.1 Diagnostic Criteria for Preeclampsia.

Diagnostic Criteria for Preeclampsia	
Hypertension	• ≥140 mm Hg systolic or ≥ 90 mm Hg diastolic after 20 weeks gestation on two occasions at least 4 h apart in a woman with a previously normal blood pressure
	OR
	• With blood pressures ≥160 mm Hg systolic or ≥105 mm Hg diastolic, hypertension can be confirmed within a short interval (minutes) to facilitate timely antihypertensive therapy
and	
Proteinuria	• ≥300 mg/24 h (or this amount extrapolated from a timed collection)
	OR
	• Protein/Creatinine ratio ≥0.3 mg protein/mg creatinine
	OR
	• Dipstick 1+ (used only if other quantitative methods not available)
Or in the absence of proteinuria, new-onset hypertension with the new onset of any of the following:	
Thrombocytopenia	• ≤100,000 platelets/mL
Renal insufficiency	• Serum creatinine concentrations greater than 1.1 mg/dL or a doubling of the serum creatinine concentrations in the absence of other renal disease
Impaired liver function	• Elevated blood concentrations of liver transaminases to twice normal concentrations
Pulmonary edema	
Cerebral or visual symptoms	
Diagnostic Criteria for Superimposed Preeclampsia	
Hypertension	• A sudden increase in blood pressure in a woman with chronic hypertension that was previously well controlled or escalation of antihypertensive medications to control blood pressure
OR	
Proteinuria	• New onset of proteinuria in a woman with chronic hypertension or a sudden increase in proteinuria in a woman with known proteinuria before or in early pregnancy

Adapted from Report of the American College of Obstetricians and Gynecologists' Task Force on Hypertension in Pregnancy. *Obstet Gynecol.* 2013;122:1122–1131.

MANAGEMENT OF PREECLAMPSIA

The most reliable treatment of preeclampsia is delivery. Removal of the placenta usually results in prompt improvement, although in a few cases, in which the disease has been explosive, symptoms may progress for several days even after delivery. By 6 weeks after delivery, hypertension and proteinuria have usually disappeared, but in unusual cases, this may take 3 or 4 months. The hypertension of preeclampsia usually responds to pharmacologic treatment. Prompt lowering of the blood pressure is important to reduce the risk of cerebral edema, cerebral hemorrhage, and eclampsia.[34] Although proteinuria may lessen as the blood pressure decreases, renal function may not improve and the levels of creatinine, urea, and uric acid in the serum continue to increase slowly even

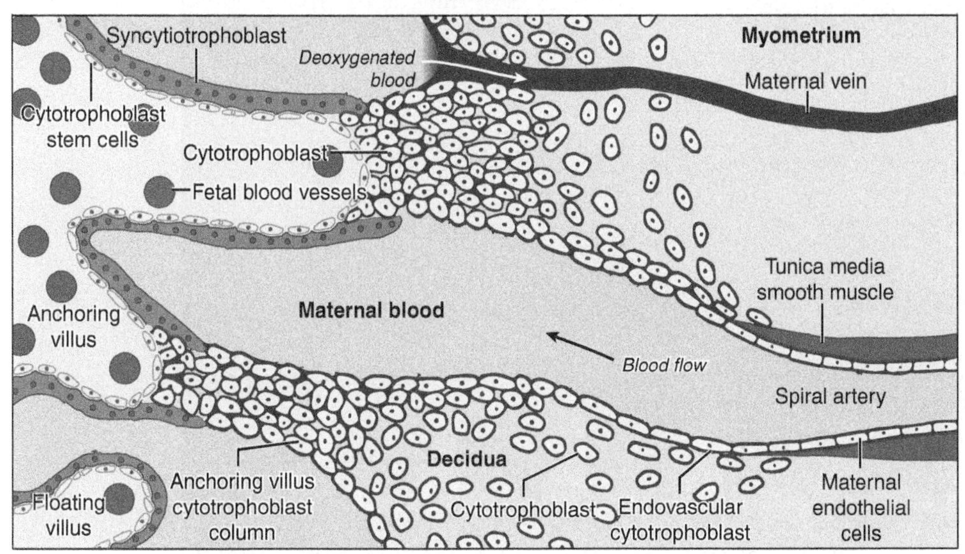

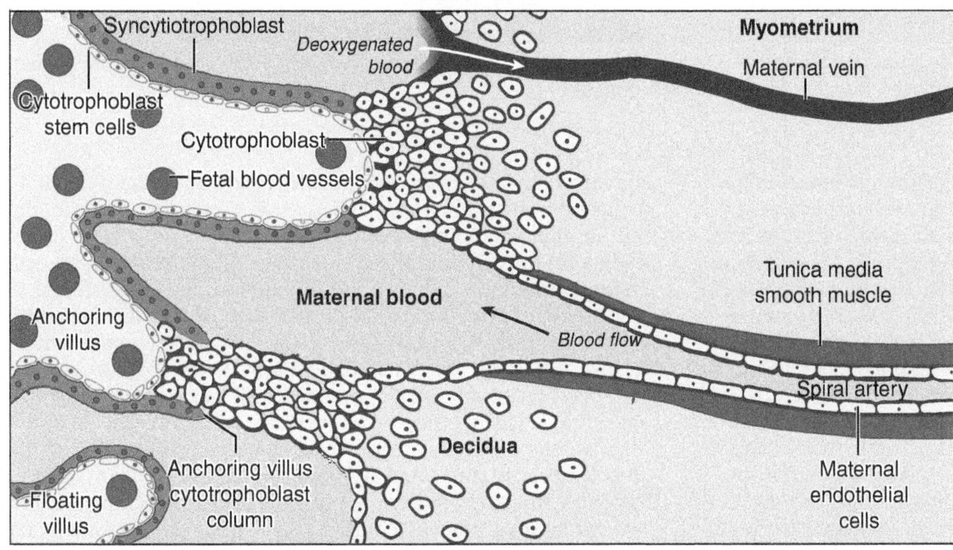

Fig. 170.1 Spiral artery defects in preeclampsia. Exchange of oxygen, nutrients, and waste products between the fetus and the mother depends on adequate placental perfusion by maternal vessels. In normal placental development, invasive cytotrophoblasts of fetal origin invade the maternal spiral arteries, transforming them from small-caliber resistance vessels to high-caliber capacitance vessels capable of providing placental perfusion adequate to sustain the growing fetus. During the process of vascular invasion, the cytotrophoblasts differentiate from an epithelial phenotype to an endothelial phenotype, a process referred to as *pseudovasculogenesis (upper panel)*. In preeclampsia, cytotrophoblasts fail to adopt an invasive endothelial phenotype. Instead, invasion of the spiral arteries is shallow, and they remain small caliber, resistance vessels leading to placental ischemia *(lower panel)*. (Reproduced with permission from Lam C, Lim KH, Karumanchi SA. Circulating angiogenic factors in the pathogenesis and prediction of preeclampsia. *Hypertension.* 2005;46[5]:1077–1085.)

after delivery. The mother remains at risk for development of the HELLP syndrome and the fetus for intrauterine death or placental abruption. Infusions of magnesium sulfate are effective in preventing epileptic seizures.[21] At high concentrations, magnesium ions depress all neural activity, including that of the respiratory center, and infusions of magnesium should not be given if the deep tendon reflexes (e.g., patellar reflex) cannot be elicited or if magnesium levels in the serum are greater than 9 mg/dL. Women with decreased renal function are at increased risk of magnesium toxicity, and it should be used with caution in those patients. Preterm delivery and IUGR are the two most common problems for infants who deliver to women with preeclampsia. Appropriate timing of delivery is a difficult decision, with the goal of balancing the infant's risk for complications related to prematurity versus maternal morbidity and mortality with continued pregnancy. Although several strategies to prevent preeclampsia have been proposed, none have been proven to be unequivocally effective.

PREECLAMPSIA PREVENTION

A meta-analysis of more than 30,000 patients from several trials found a 17% reduction in risk of preeclampsia associated with use of low-dose aspirin.[35] In a large multicenter randomized control trial including approximately 1800 European women, use of aspirin (150 mg) for preeclampsia prevention among women at high risk based on biomarker and imaging data resulted in 62% reduction in preterm preeclampsia.[36] However, because biomarker testing and uterine artery doppler studies are not routinely performed in the United States, the American College of Obstetricians and Gynecologists and the Society for Maternal-Fetal Medicine support use of low-dose aspirin (81 mg/day) prophylaxis in women at high risk of preeclampsia based on historic and demographic risk factors. This should be initiated between 12 and 28 weeks of gestation (optimally before 16 weeks) and continued daily until delivery.[37]

MOLECULAR MECHANISMS OF PREECLAMPSIA

ABNORMAL PLACENTATION IN PREECLAMPSIA

Preeclampsia is primarily a placental disease, with the disease characterized by shallow invasion of the cytotrophoblast into the

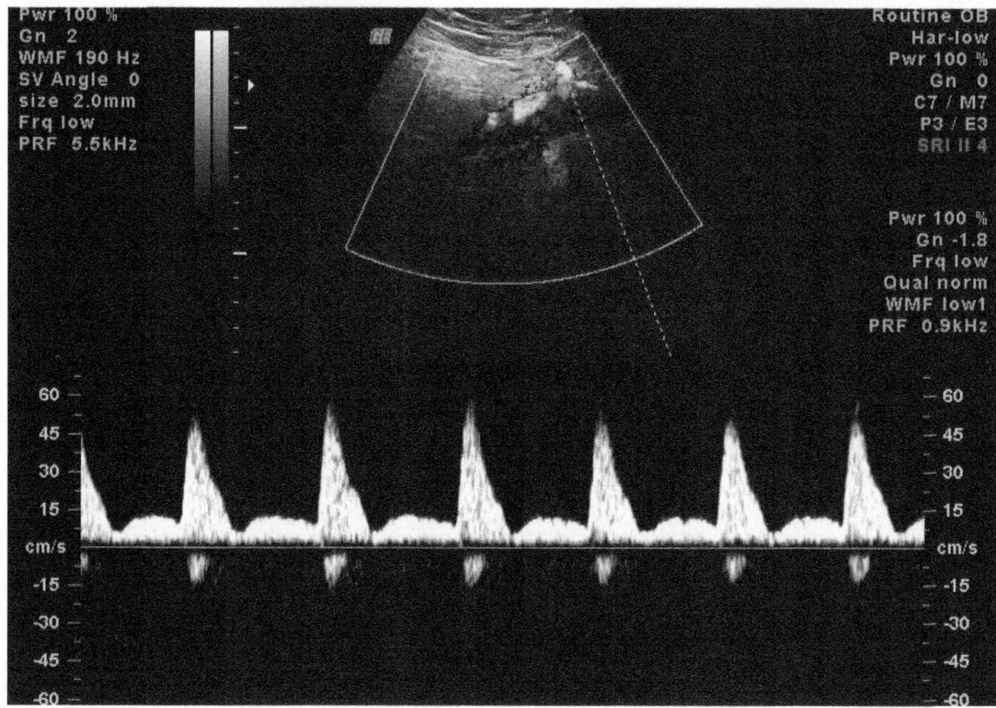

Fig. 170.2 Uterine artery notching of preeclampsia. Panel shows impaired uterine arterial flow on Doppler studies in a high-risk woman during third trimester as evidenced by notching between the systolic and diastolic phases.

maternal vasculature (Fig. 170.1). This shallow implantation leads to release of circulating factors but also causes derangement of the placenta.[3,38] Patients with preeclampsia are shown to have small placental weights at birth, but more importantly these patients have been shown to have abnormal uterine artery dopplers in early pregnancy.[39] Failed vascular remodeling leads to increased flow resistance within uterine arteries, which is represented by either an increased resistance index, or pulsatility index, or by the persistence of a unilateral or bilateral diastolic notch (Fig. 170.2).[40]

The characteristic placental lesion in severe preeclampsia is a diminution in endovascular invasion by cytotrophoblasts and a decrease in remodeling of the uterine spiral arterioles.[41] Cytotrophoblast invasion is limited to the proximal decidua, and the myometrial segments of the spiral arteries remain narrow and undilated, resulting in uterine hypoperfusion (see Fig. 170.1).[42] Fisher and colleagues have shown that invasive cytotrophoblasts down-regulate the expression of adhesion molecules characteristic of their epithelial cell origin and adopt a cell-surface adhesion phenotype typical of endothelial cells, a process referred to as *pseudovasculogenesis*.[43,44] They hypothesized and confirmed that, in preeclampsia, cytotrophoblast cells fail to undergo the switching of cell-surface integrins and adhesion molecules.[44] This work suggests that cytotrophoblast differentiation is abnormal in severe preeclampsia and may be an early defect that eventually leads to placental ischemia.

Impaired corin expression in the pregnant uterus has been suggested as another mechanism for failed spiral artery remodeling.[45] Local atrial natriuretic peptide (ANP) production by corin, a cardiac protease that activates ANP, promoted trophoblast invasion and spiral artery remodeling in a mouse model. However, ANP levels are higher in patients with preeclampsia,[46] and therefore it is unclear if corin deficiency is critical in most cases of preeclampsia. There is also emerging evidence that decidual natural killer (NK) cells play a critical role in the physiologic vascular remodeling during normal pregnancy.[47] Human studies have suggested that the susceptibility to preeclampsia may be influenced by polymorphic human leucocyte antigen-C (HLA-C) ligands on trophoblasts and their NK cell receptors killer-cell immunoglobulin-like receptors (KIR).[48] However, more studies are needed to evaluate the nature of the decidual NK cell dysfunction in preeclampsia and other placentation disorders.

Inadequate placentation due to deficient trophoblast invasion of uterine spiral arteries can lead to placental hypoxia, which in turn leads to abnormal expression of angiogenic factors that play a central role in the pathogenesis of the maternal syndrome.[49] The hypothesis that defective trophoblastic invasion with accompanying uteroplacental hypoperfusion may lead to preeclampsia is supported by both animal and human studies. Placentas from pregnancies with advanced preeclampsia often have numerous placental infarcts and sclerotic narrowing of arterioles. Uteroplacental blood flow is usually diminished, and uterine vascular resistance increased in preeclamptic women (see Fig. 170.2). Placental ischemia induced by mechanical constriction of the uterine arteries or aorta produces hypertension, proteinuria, and glomerular endotheliosis in pregnant rats and baboons.[50,51] However, placental ischemia alone, as seen in many cases of IUGR, does not appear to be sufficient to produce preeclampsia. A secondary insult in the syncytiotrophoblast layer of the placenta that occurs following placental ischemia may be critical for the development of the maternal syndrome.[52,53] Abnormalities in syncytialization and placental microparticle release have been reported in preeclampsia but not in IUGR.[54] Studies have shown that during preeclampsia, there is increased release of placental syncytiotrophoblast extracellular vesicles (STBEVs), which can transfer placenta-specific functional miRNAs mediating effects on gene regulation in the endothelial cells. Thus STBEVs may cause endothelial damage and contribute to the endothelial dysfunction typical for preeclampsia.[55] More studies are needed to understand the molecular apparatus that drives the formation of the syncytium and how placental ischemia may lead to shedding of placental microparticles into the systemic circulation.

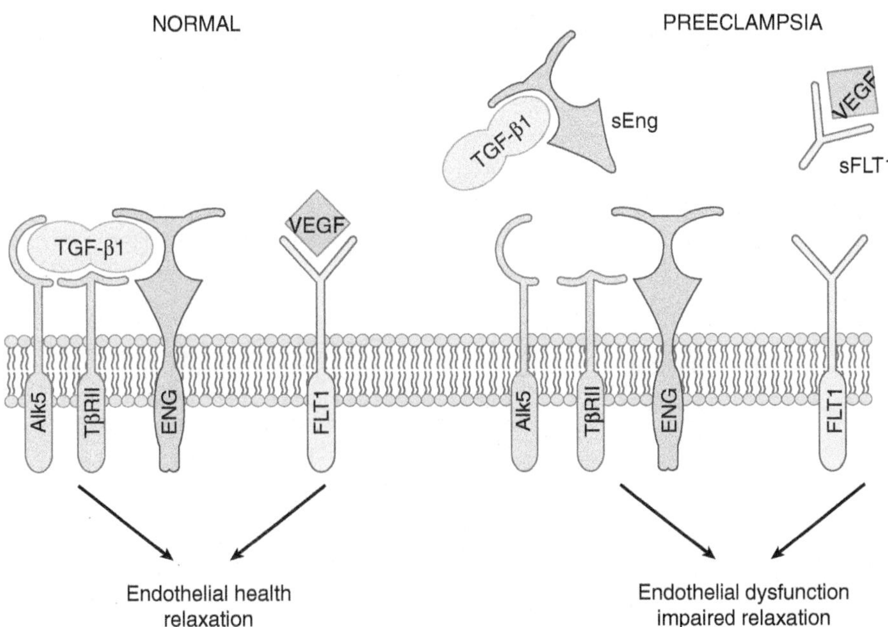

Fig. 170.3 *sFlt1* and *sEng* causes endothelial dysfunction by antagonizing *VEGF* and *TGF-β1* signaling. There is mounting evidence that VEGF and TGF-β are required to maintain endothelial health in several tissues, including the kidney and perhaps the placenta. During normal pregnancy, vascular homeostasis is maintained by physiologic levels of VEGF and TGF-β signaling in the vasculature. In preeclampsia, excess placental secretion of sFlt1 and sEng (two endogenous circulating antiangiogenic proteins) inhibits VEGF and TGF-β signaling, respectively, in the vasculature. This results in endothelial cell dysfunction, including decreased prostacyclin, nitric oxide production, and release of procoagulant proteins. *sEng,* Soluble endoglin; *sFlt1,* soluble fms-like tyrosine kinase 1; *TGF,* transforming growth factor; *VEGF,* vascular endothelial growth factor. (Reproduced with permission from Powe CE, Levine RJ, Karumanchi SA. Preeclampsia, a disease of the maternal endothelium: the role of antiangiogenic factors and implications for later cardiovascular disease. *Circulation.* 2011;123[24]:2856-2869.)

THE ROLE OF ANGIOGENIC FACTORS IN THE MATERNAL SYNDROME

All of the clinical manifestations of preeclampsia can be attributed to endothelial dysfunction leading to end-organ damage and hypoperfusion. Because the placenta plays an important role in the pathogenesis of preeclampsia, researchers have focused their search for identification of such factors primarily on the placenta. With the advent of more sensitive molecular technology, it has been possible to use small amounts of placental material to learn which genes or proteins are expressed by the placenta during healthy or complicated pregnancy. Using microarray technology, new genes were discovered that play an important role in placental biology. These include two antiangiogenic proteins, soluble fms-like tyrosine kinase 1 (sFlt1) and soluble endoglin (sEng) that have been causally linked with the pathogenesis of the maternal syndrome of preeclampsia (Fig. 170.3).[3]

Placental production of all the isoforms of sFlt1 are increased during preeclampsia.[56-59] sFlt1 acts by adhering to the receptor-binding domains of placental growth factor (PlGF) and vascular endothelial growth factor (VEGF), preventing their interaction with the cell surface endothelial receptors, and thus inducing endothelial dysfunction.[60,61] Circulating concentrations of sFlt1 are increased and free PlGF and free VEGF are decreased during active disease and several weeks before onset of symptoms.[62-66] When administered to pregnant animals, sFlt1 produces a syndrome of hypertension, proteinuria, and glomerular endotheliosis that mimics the human syndrome of preeclampsia.[58,67] VEGF or PlGF therapy or lowering of sFlt1 ameliorates preeclampsia phenotype in rodent models.[68-70] sEng, another candidate pathogenic antiangiogenic protein, is up-regulated in preeclampsia and acts by disrupting transforming growth factor-β signaling in the vasculature (see Fig. 170.3).[71,72] In rodent studies it was reported that sEng may act in concert with sFlt1 to induce a severe preeclampsia-like illness.[72,73] The main source of sFlt1 and sEng in pregnancy is the placenta.[52,74] sFlt1 and sEng are highly overexpressed in preeclamptic placentas, in particular in syncytial knots. Additional sources such as peripheral blood mononuclear cells have been described,[75] but the clinical significance is unknown.

The studies on sFlt1 and other angiogenic factors in preeclampsia biology have also led to new insights into basic biology of vascular and placental homeostasis in health and disease. The microvasculature of organs affected in preeclampsia, such as the glomeruli and hepatic sinusoidal vasculature, are more permeable due to the presence of intracellular perforations referred to as *fenestrations*. Although it was previously known that VEGF induces endothelial fenestrae in culture,[76] experimental data in VEGF knockout mice demonstrated that fenestral density is regulated by constitutive expression of VEGF.[77] Therefore it is not surprising that the microvascular damage in preeclampsia is largely concentrated in vasculature that constitutively express VEGF and that loss of endothelial fenestrae in preeclampsia is due to excess circulating sFlt1. Interestingly, preeclampsia-like signs and symptoms have been reported in cancer patients receiving anti-VEGF drugs, including the renal histopathologic lesion characteristic of preeclampsia, glomeruloendotheliosis.[78-80] Functional characterization of sFlt1 actions during pregnancy has also helped to elucidate the role of preeclampsia as an important risk factor for neonatal respiratory distress syndrome and bronchopulmonary dysplasia (BPD).[81,82] Prior studies had suggested that BPD is characterized by impaired angiogenesis in the lung.[83] In humans with preeclampsia, amniotic fluid sFlt1 is markedly elevated, in parallel with maternal serum concentrations, and this amniotic fluid sFlt1 bathes the developing fetal lungs leading to impaired angiogenesis. Intraamniotic sFlt1 infusion in pregnant rats during late gestation led to BPD and pulmonary hypertension.[84] These studies suggest a novel molecular target and strategy for the prevention of BPD.

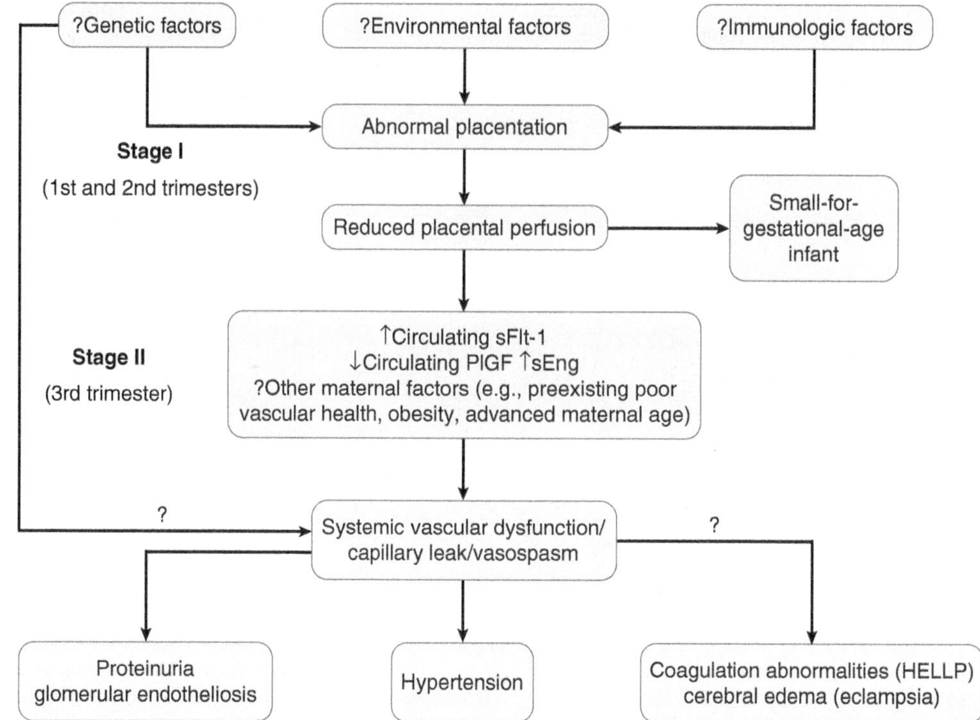

Fig. 170.4 Summary of the pathogenesis of preeclampsia. Placental dysfunction from immunologic and genetic factors leads to the release of antiangiogenic factors (e.g., *sFlt1* and *sEng*), which synergize with maternal risk factors such as obesity to induce preeclampsia. *sEng,* Soluble endoglin; *sFlt1,* soluble fms-like tyrosine kinase 1.

OTHER PATHWAYS

Increased sensitivity to the vasopressor effects of angiotensin is a well-established feature of preeclampsia.[85] Wallukat and colleagues noted increased concentrations of agonistic antibodies to the angiotensin AT-1 receptor (AT1-AA) in women with preeclampsia.[86] These autoantibodies may induce the production of reactive oxygen species and induce hypertension and a preeclampsia-like state in pregnant mice.[87] Alterations in the regulator of G protein signaling 5 were found to be critical determinant of angiotensin II sensitivity and preeclampsia phenotype in pregnant mice.[88] Recent preclinical studies on the hypersensitivity of the AT1 receptor when complexed with the bradykinin B2 receptor provide compelling evidence for another model for the activation of angiotensin II sensitivity in the setting of down-regulated renin.[89] Using a new transgenic mouse model with maternal, systemically up-regulated smooth muscle AT1B2 complexes, the group was able to replicate the preeclampsia syndrome, with pregnant animals developing hypertension, proteinuria, low platelets, increased sFlt1-1, AT1-AA, and endothelin 1, smaller litter sizes, IUGR, lower renin levels, and a decreased placental labyrinth layer. Furthermore, when heteromerized with B2, ATI appears independently sensitive to angiotensin II and mechanostimulation, which, the authors suggest, may evolve with an increase in fetal-placental mass regardless of renin activity.[89] Additional human studies are required to assess applicability of this model to the biology of preeclampsia. It would also be critical to evaluate whether these factors synergize with known mediators of preeclampsia such as sFlt1 and sEng to induce severe disease.

In summary, abnormal placentation during early pregnancy leads to secretion of antiangiogenic factors such as sFlt1 and sEng into maternal circulation. These antiangiogenic factors synergize with other maternal risk factors such as obesity and insulin resistance and induce maternal endothelial dysfunction and the clinical signs and symptoms of preeclampsia (Fig. 170.4). It would also be critical to evaluate other synergistic factors such as AT1-AA that may act in concert with sFlt1 and sEng to induce severe disease.

ANGIOGENIC FACTORS AS BIOMARKERS AND THERAPEUTIC TARGETS

ANGIOGENIC MARKERS AS AN AID IN THE PREDICTION OF PREECLAMPSIA

There is a large body of literature demonstrating that maternal serum levels of sFlt1, PlGF, and sEng correlate with preeclampsia disease activity and are altered well before onset of clinical signs and symptoms.[62,64,65,71,90] Elevated sFlt1 and depressed PlGF are more dramatically altered in preterm preeclampsia and/or in preeclampsia complicated by fetal growth restriction.[71,91] The ratio of sFlt1/PlGF has been proposed as an index of antiangiogenic activity, which reflects alterations in both biomarkers and is a better predictor of preeclampsia than either measure alone (Fig. 170.5). Adding sEng to the equation, (sFlt1+sEng): PlGF ratio was more strongly predictive of preeclampsia than were individual biomarkers.[71] Kusanovic and colleagues measured sFlt1, PlGF, and sEng in 1622 consecutive singleton pregnant women during early pregnancy and in mid-trimester and found superior performances for the PlGF/sEng ratio during mid-trimester, with sensitivity of 100% and a specificity of 98% for early-onset preeclampsia.[92] Serum levels of PlGF tend to be lower in women who go on to develop preeclampsia from the first or early second trimester.[93,94] Because PlGF alterations occur early in first trimester, PlGF has been tested alone and in combination with other biomarkers as a potential predictive test. In a large prospective clinical study involving nearly 8000 subjects, Poon and colleagues demonstrated that a combination of angiogenic factors (PlGF), pregnancy associated plasma protein A (PAPP-A), and uterine artery Doppler velocimetry in the first trimester can predict the subsequent development of early-onset preeclampsia in a low-risk population, with a sensitivity of 93% at a 5% false-positive rate.[95] This suggests that screening for early-onset preeclampsia in the general population is possible and that one in five pregnancies that had a positive screen would develop preeclampsia. More prospective studies are needed to confirm this observation and to evaluate whether accurate prediction

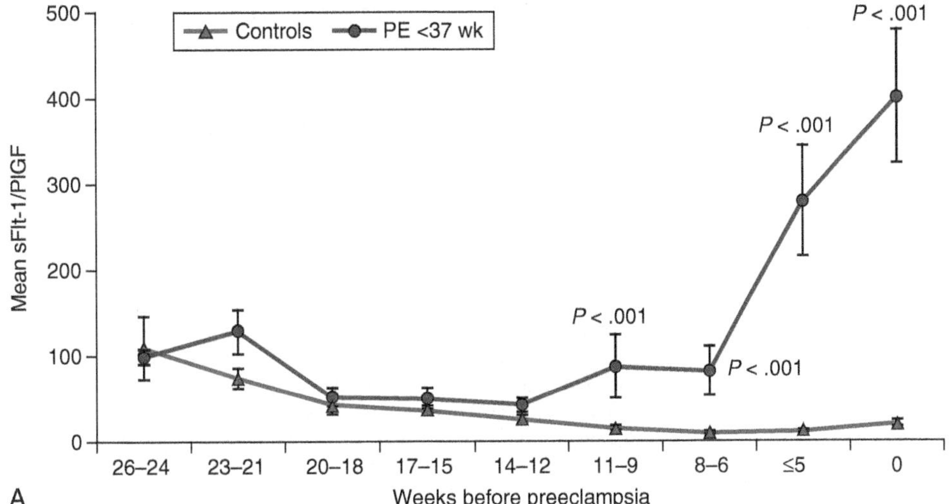

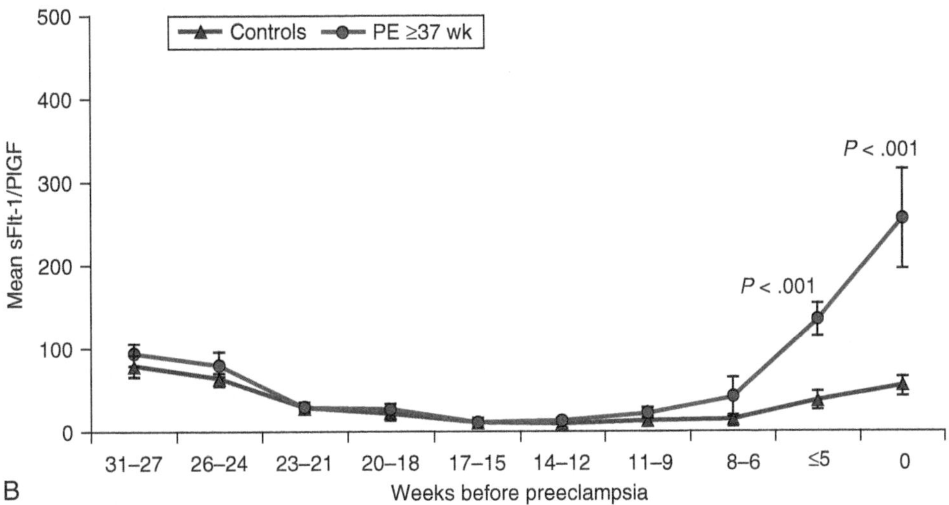

Fig. 170.5 Mean serum *sFlt-1/PlGF* in the weeks prior to the onset of clinical signs and symptoms of preeclampsia. Figure shows the mean sFlt-1/PlGF ratios before and after the onset of preterm *(panel A)* and term *(panel B)* preeclampsia according to the weeks before preeclampsia. *PlGF,* Placental growth factor; *sFlt1,* soluble fms-like tyrosine kinase 1. (Reproduced with permission from Hagmann H, Thadhani R, Benzing T, Karumanchi SA, Stepan H. The promise of angiogenic markers for the early diagnosis and prediction of preeclampsia. *Clin Chem.* 2012;58[5]:837-845.)

of early-onset preeclampsia can be followed by interventions or close follow-up that improve maternal and/or fetal outcome.

ANGIOGENIC FACTORS AS AN AID IN DIAGNOSIS AND PROGNOSIS OF PREECLAMPSIA

Given the nonspecific nature of clinical signs and symptoms necessary for diagnosis of preeclampsia, it is important to develop tests that are specific to preeclampsia such that pregnancy can perhaps be continued in patients with unclear diagnosis and with normal angiogenic profiles. With the availability of automated assays to measure sFlt1 and PlGF, several studies have confirmed that plasma or serum measurements of sFlt1 and PlGF have sensitivities and specificities of approximately 95% as an aid in diagnosis of preterm preeclampsia.[96-99] Several groups have demonstrated that sFlt1 and PlGF levels can be used to differentiate preeclampsia from diseases that mimic preeclampsia such as chronic hypertension, gestational hypertension, kidney disease, and gestational thrombocytopenia.[100-104] Moreover, angiogenic factors can also be used as an aid in predicting short-term adverse outcomes, including preterm delivery. In a large prospective study, it was demonstrated that the plasma sFlt1/PlGF ratio among women with suspected preeclampsia predicts adverse maternal and perinatal outcomes (occurring within 2 weeks) in the preterm setting.[105] This ratio alone outperformed standard clinical diagnostic measures including blood pressure, proteinuria, uric acid, and others. Importantly, sFlt1/PlGF levels in the triage setting correlated with preterm delivery (Fig. 170.6), an observation that has now been confirmed by several groups.[106-108] In a similar but more recent large prospective multisite observational study enrolling approximately 1000 women with suspected preeclampsia, an sFlt1/PlGF ratio of less than 38 showed a negative predictive value of 99.3% for development of preeclampsia within 1 week.[109] Another study evaluating the time to delivery ($n = 753$) in women with signs or symptoms of preeclampsia compared with women with normal PlGF levels found that those women with PlGF of 100 pg/mL or less had an HR of 7.17 in Cox regression for time to delivery after adjustment for both gestational age at enrollment and the final diagnosis of preeclampsia.[110] In addition, studies have shown that women diagnosed with preeclampsia, but with a normal plasma angiogenic profile, are not at risk for adverse maternal or fetal outcomes.[111] These observations have led to incorporation of angiogenic factors for prediction of preeclampsia in countries where these assays are available, such as the National Institute for Health and Care Excellence in the United Kingdom and many parts of Europe.[112]

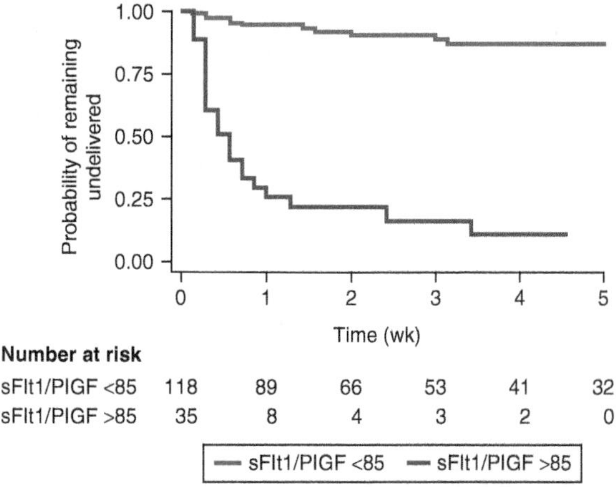

Fig. 170.6 Angiogenic factors as prognostic markers in preeclampsia. Kaplan-Meier survival function for time to delivery in patients with suspected preeclampsia presenting less than 34 weeks gestation. *PlGF,* Placental growth factor; *sFlt1,* soluble fms-like tyrosine kinase 1. (Reproduced with permission from Rana S, Powe CE, Salahuddin S, et al. Angiogenic factors and the risk of adverse outcomes in women with suspected preeclampsia. *Circulation.* 2012;125[7]:911-919.)

Because most studies showing association between angiogenic factors and preeclampsia are observational, randomized trials are now being done to determine if information about plasma angiogenic factors in real time will improve patient outcomes. A recent multicenter, pragmatic, stepped-wedge cluster-randomized controlled trial enrolling approximately 1000 women with suspected preeclampsia evaluated the effect of knowledge of PlGF on clinicians' decision making. The median time to preeclampsia diagnosis was 4.1 days with concealed testing versus 1.9 days with revealed testing. There was a small but significant difference in maternal severe adverse outcomes; however, there was no difference in perinatal outcomes or gestational age of delivery.[113] Another prospective, interventional, parallel-group, randomized clinical trial evaluated the knowledge of sFlt-1/PlGF ratio on hospitalization within 24 hours of the test. The study found that use of the sFlt-1/PlGF ratio significantly improved clinical precision but did not change the admission rate.[114] Further trials are ongoing to determine the clinical utility of angiogenic biomarkers for prediction and diagnosis of preeclampsia.

THERAPEUTIC STUDIES

Human and animal studies as outlined earlier have strongly suggested that targeting angiogenic factors and in particular sFlt1 may be a viable strategy to prevent or treat preeclampsia.[115] Thadhani and colleagues translated some fundamental discoveries to the bedside.[116] Taking advantage of the positive charge of sFlt1, they used a negatively charged dextran sulfate cellulose column for extracorporeal removal of sFlt1. In two studies including women with preterm preeclampsia, dextran sulfate apheresis lead to a reduction in sFlt-1 levels and improvement in proteinuria and blood pressure, without evident adverse effects to the mother and fetus. In all of these cases, there was evidence of continued fetal growth and prolongation of pregnancy.[116,117] Other modalities for targeting the angiogenic imbalance are administration of agents that scavenge sFlt1, such as sFlt1 antibodies, PlGF, or VEGF. Strategies aimed at decreasing sFlt1 production by siRNA strategies or small molecules are currently being evaluated in the preclinical settings.[115,118] Compounds that up-regulate proangiogenic factors such as statins also have been demonstrated to reverse preeclampsia in animal models[69] and has prolonged pregnancy in few cases of severe preterm preeclampsia.[119,120] A clinical trial to test the safety of statins in women with established preeclampsia has been initiated in the United States.[121]

LONG-TERM COMPLICATIONS OF PREECLAMPSIA

Although delivery of the placenta resolves the immediate preeclamptic episode, women with preeclampsia are at significantly higher risk of developing postpartum hypertension (within 6 weeks of delivery). The continued crisis after birth has led to labeling the time after delivery as *fourth trimester of pregnancy*. The rates of postpartum hypertension can vary based on definitions, and limited data exist about etiology of hypertension persisting after delivery.[122-124]

Women affected by hypertensive disorders of pregnancy are at risk for developing long-term complications such as chronic hypertension, ischemic heart disease, and stroke many years postpartum.[125] A large meta-analysis by Bellamy and colleagues in 2007 of prospective and retrospective cohort studies dating as far back as the 1960s found an increased relative risk of developing hypertension after a hypertensive pregnancy of 3.39 (95% confidence interval [CI], 2.7 to 5.05).[126] It has been known for some time that women with preeclampsia have poor long-term cardiovascular outcome, but there is emerging evidence suggesting that the impact of preeclampsia on maternal health is more immediate and profound than previously suspected. A prospective observational cohort (The Nulliparous Pregnancy Outcomes Study Monitoring Mothers-to-be Heart Health Study) that followed 4484 women for 2 to 7 years after the first pregnancy affected by adverse pregnancy outcomes (defined as hypertensive disorders of pregnancy, small-for-gestational-age birth, preterm birth, and stillbirth) found that the rates of hypertension were higher among with these women; the risk of developing hypertension was approximately four times higher if the pregnancy was complicated by indicated preterm birth and hypertensive disorder of pregnancy.[127] In addition, studies have also shown that women diagnosed with hypertensive complication during pregnancy have a two-fold risk of future ischemic heart disease and stroke.[128-130] Whether these long-term effects reflect preexisting risk factors (given multiple shared risk factors), or whether they are a result of preeclampsia itself, is unknown.

The pervading theory to explain enhanced cardiovascular disease (CVD) risk in women with a history of preeclampsia is that pregnancy is a "stress test" and the development of hypertensive disorders during pregnancy identifies women destined to develop CVD.[131] Both cardiovascular and preeclampsia share risk factors, including shared genetic factors, diabetes, hypertension, increased insulin resistance, and increased homocysteine concentration. Whether these common associations are causative or correlative is difficult to discern. Using longitudinal data from two consecutive studies, Romunstad and colleagues noted that women with a history of preeclampsia or gestational hypertension also had substantially higher body mass index and systolic and diastolic blood pressures and unfavorable lipids compared with those with normotensive pregnancies.[132] After adjustment for prepregnancy risk factors, the correlation with body mass index was attenuated by more than 65%, and the increase in blood pressure following preeclampsia was attenuated by approximately by 50%.[132] These data provide support for the theory that the association of preeclampsia may be due to shared risk factors.

An emerging alternate hypothesis is that preeclampsia enhanced cardiovascular risk may be secondary to permanent vascular damage sustained during the preeclamptic episode from inflammatory stress, coagulation dysregulation, and endothelial damage.[125] Experimental studies in animals suggest that vessels exposed to preeclampsia retain a persistently enhanced vascular responsiveness to injury despite complete recovery of cardiovascular function after delivery.[133] Women with preeclampsia show evidence of cardiac dysfunction when evaluated by an echocardiogram during pregnancy, and these changes persist postpartum.[23,134-136] Animal studies have also shown evidence of cardiac dysfunction and impaired global longitudinal strain in models of preeclampsia.[137] Animals exposed to preeclampsia-like illness also develop long-term changes in the global plasma protein profile (proteome) that correlate with changes associated with CVD.[138] Absence of hypertension in the siblings of women with preeclampsia who might be expected to have more similar risk of CVD based on genetic and other environmental factors supports this theory.[139] Recurrent preeclampsia is associated with an even greater CVD risk,[140,141] and women who have had preeclampsia before 34 weeks or preeclampsia associated with fetal growth restriction[142,143] have a risk of death from CVD that is four to eight times the risk of women who had a normal pregnancy. These studies support the idea that preeclampsia per se may contribute directly to the progression of CVD.

Although cardiac changes in pregnancy have been associated with levels of antiangiogenic proteins (including sFlt1 and sEng),[144] the levels of these proteins decline to normal levels after delivery. Perhaps, a persistent and subtle antiangiogenic milieu may contribute to lasting endothelial dysfunction and an elevated risk of CVD in women with a history of preeclampsia. Human studies suggested that women with a history of a hypertensive pregnancy disorder demonstrate increased Ang II sensitivity as evidenced by increased pressor, adrenal, and sFlt1 responses to infused Ang II in low-sodium balance.[145] If these observations are confirmed, therapies to block Ang II signaling may provide a novel mechanistic target to prevent future hypertension and CVD in these high-risk women.[145] Studies have suggested that Activin A (a marker for cardiac fibrosis) is also associated with postpartum cardiac dysfunction in women with hypertensive disorders of pregnancy.[146] Further studies are needed to find novel biomarkers for prediction of CVD among women with preeclampsia, leading to early diagnosis and intervention. Pulmonary and systemic vascular dysfunction in young offspring of mothers with preeclampsia has also been described[147]; however, the mechanisms mediating these phenotypes are largely unknown. Children born to women with preeclampsia have an increased risk of CVD[148]; this may be related to "Barker hypothesis" that suggests that growth restriction and the abnormal uterine environment increase susceptibility to CVD.[149]

CONCLUSION

In summary, preeclampsia and eclampsia have a large burden of disease throughout the world and are leading causes of maternal and infant morbidity. In areas where access to prenatal care is limited, patients present late with advanced disease and suffer from severe complications. The search for the ability to better diagnose, predict, and prevent preeclampsia and the mechanisms of its pathogenesis, to develop a therapy that safely prolongs gestation has been extensive. Exciting data on angiogenic factors as central contributors to the pathogenesis of preeclampsia, candidate biomarkers, and therapeutic targets have opened clinically meaningful options for patients in the near future. Women with history of preeclampsia are at increased risk for developing future CVD. Identification of novel biomarkers and systematic management of women in postpartum period hold the key for improved long-term outcomes in these women.

 A complete reference list is available at www.ExpertConsult.com.

SELECT REFERENCES

3. Powe CE, Levine RJ, Karumanchi SA. Preeclampsia, a disease of the maternal endothelium: the role of antiangiogenic factors and implications for later cardiovascular disease. *Circulation*. 2011;123(24):2856-2869.
5. Ananth CV, Keyes KM, Wapner RJ. Pre-eclampsia rates in the United States, 1980-2010: age-period-cohort analysis. *BMJ*. 2013;347:f6564.
6. Breathett K, Muhlestein D, Foraker R, Gulati M. Differences in preeclampsia rates between African American and Caucasian women: trends from the National Hospital Discharge Survey. *J Womens Health*. 2014;23(11):886-893.
11. Skjaerven R, Wilcox AJ, Lie RT. The interval between pregnancies and the risk of preeclampsia. *N Engl J Med*. 2002;346(1):33-38.
15. McGinnis R, Steinthorsdottir V, Williams NO, et al. Variants in the fetal genome near FLT1 are associated with risk of preeclampsia. *Nat Genet*. 2017;49(8):1255-1260.
22. Buddeberg BS, Sharma R, O'Driscoll JM, Kaelin Agten A, Khalil A, Thilaganathan B. Cardiac maladaptation in term pregnancies with preeclampsia. *Pregnancy Hypertens*. 2018;13:198-203.
24. Bello N, Rendon IS, Arany Z. The relationship between pre-eclampsia and peripartum cardiomyopathy: a systematic review and meta-analysis. *J Am Coll Cardiol*. 2013;62(18):1715-1723.
26. Schwartz RB, Feske SK, Polak JF, et al. Preeclampsia-eclampsia: clinical and neuroradiographic correlates and insights into the pathogenesis of hypertensive encephalopathy. *Radiology*. 2000;217(2):371-376.
27. Cipolla MJ, Vitullo L, Delance N, Hammer E. The cerebral endothelium during pregnancy: a potential role in the development of eclampsia. *Endothelium*. 2005;12(1-2):5-9.
28. Odegard RA, Vatten LJ, Nilsen ST, Salvesen KA, Austgulen R. Preeclampsia and fetal growth. *Obstet Gynecol*. 2000;96(6):950-955.
32. American College of O, Gynecologists, Task Force on Hypertension in P. Hypertension in pregnancy. Report of the American College of Obstetricians and Gynecologists' Task Force on Hypertension in Pregnancy. *Obstet Gynecol*. 2013;122(5):1122-1131.
33. ACOG Practice Bulletin No. 202. Gestational hypertension and preeclampsia. *Obstet Gynecol*. 2019;133(1):e1-e25.
34. Easterling TR. Pharmacological management of hypertension in pregnancy. *Semin Perinatol*. 2014;38(8):487-495.
36. Rolnik DL, Wright D, Poon LC, et al. Aspirin versus placebo in pregnancies at high risk for preterm preeclampsia. *N Engl J Med*. 2017;377(7):613-622.
37. ACOG Committee Opinion No. 743. Low-dose aspirin use during pregnancy. *Obstet Gynecol*. 2018;132(1):e44-e52.
44. Zhou Y, Damsky CH, Fisher SJ. Preeclampsia is associated with failure of human cytotrophoblasts to mimic a vascular adhesion phenotype. One cause of defective endovascular invasion in this syndrome? *J Clin Invest*. 1997;99(9):2152-2164.
47. Moffett A, Colucci F. Uterine NK cells: active regulators at the maternal-fetal interface. *J Clin Invest*. 2014;124(5):1872-1879.
53. Redman CW, Sargent IL. Latest advances in understanding preeclampsia. *Science*. 2005;308(5728):1592-1594.
58. Maynard SE, Min JY, Merchan J, Lim KH, Li J, Mondal S, et al. Excess placental soluble fms-like tyrosine kinase 1 (sFlt1) may contribute to endothelial dysfunction, hypertension, and proteinuria in preeclampsia. *J Clin Invest*. 2003;111(5):649-658.
62. Chaiworapongsa T, Romero R, Kim YM, et al. Plasma soluble vascular endothelial growth factor receptor-1 concentration is elevated prior to the clinical diagnosis of pre-eclampsia. *J Matern Fetal Neonatal Med*. 2005;17(1):3-18.
64. Levine RJ, Maynard SE, Qian C, et al. Circulating angiogenic factors and the risk of preeclampsia. *N Engl J Med*. 2004;350(7):672-683.
65. Noori M, Donald AE, Angelakopoulou A, Hingorani AD, Williams DJ. Prospective study of placental angiogenic factors and maternal vascular function before and after preeclampsia and gestational hypertension. *Circulation*. 2010;122(5):478-487.
69. Kumasawa K, Ikawa M, Kidoya H, et al. Pravastatin induces placental growth factor (PGF) and ameliorates preeclampsia in a mouse model. *Proc Natl Acad Sci U S A*. 2011;108(4):1451-1455.
71. Levine RJ, Lam C, Qian C, et al. Soluble endoglin and other circulating antiangiogenic factors in preeclampsia. *N Engl J Med*. 2006;355(10):992-1005.
72. Venkatesha S, Toporsian M, Lam C, et al. Soluble endoglin contributes to the pathogenesis of preeclampsia. *Nat Med*. 2006;12(6):642-649.
73. Maharaj AS, Walshe TE, Saint-Geniez M, et al. VEGF and TGF-beta are required for the maintenance of the choroid plexus and ependyma. *J Exp Med*. 2008;205(2):491-501.
80. Vigneau C, Lorcy N, Dolley-Hitze T, et al. All anti-vascular endothelial growth factor drugs can induce 'pre-eclampsia-like syndrome': a RARe study. *Nephrol Dial Transplant*. 2014;29(2):325-332.
81. Hansen AR, Barnes CM, Folkman J, McElrath TF. Maternal preeclampsia predicts the development of bronchopulmonary dysplasia. *J Pediatr*. 2010;156(4):532-536.
82. Wang A, Holston AM, Yu KF, et al. Circulating anti-angiogenic factors during hypertensive pregnancy and increased risk of respiratory distress syndrome in preterm neonates. *J Matern Fetal Neonatal Med*. 2012;25(8):1447-1452.
83. Baker CD, Abman SH. Impaired pulmonary vascular development in bronchopulmonary dysplasia. *Neonatology*. 2015;107(4):344-351.

84. Tang JR, Karumanchi SA, Seedorf G, Markham N, Abman SH. Excess soluble vascular endothelial growth factor receptor-1 in amniotic fluid impairs lung growth in rats: linking preeclampsia with bronchopulmonary dysplasia. *Am J Physiol Lung Cell Mol Physiol*. 2012;302(1):L36-46.
91. Romero R, Nien JK, Espinoza J, et al. A longitudinal study of angiogenic (placental growth factor) and anti-angiogenic (soluble endoglin and soluble vascular endothelial growth factor receptor-1) factors in normal pregnancy and patients destined to develop preeclampsia and deliver a small for gestational age neonate. *J Matern Fetal Neonatal Med*. 2008;21(1):9-23.
92. Kusanovic JP, Romero R, Chaiworapongsa T, et al. A prospective cohort study of the value of maternal plasma concentrations of angiogenic and anti-angiogenic factors in early pregnancy and midtrimester in the identification of patients destined to develop preeclampsia. *J Matern Fetal Neonatal Med*. 2009;22(11):1021-1038.
95. Poon LC, Kametas NA, Maiz N, Akolekar R, Nicolaides KH. First-trimester prediction of hypertensive disorders in pregnancy. *Hypertension*. 2009;53(5): 812-818.
98. Verdonk K, Visser W, Russcher H, Danser AH, Steegers EA, van den Meiracker AH. Differential diagnosis of preeclampsia: remember the soluble fms-like tyrosine kinase 1/placental growth factor ratio. *Hypertension*. 2012;60(4):884-890.
99. Verlohren S, Galindo A, Schlembach D, et al. An automated method for the determination of the sFlt-1/PIGF ratio in the assessment of preeclampsia. *Am J Obstet Gynecol*. 2010;202(2):161.e1-e11.
105. Rana S, Powe CE, Salahuddin S, et al. Angiogenic factors and the risk of adverse outcomes in women with suspected preeclampsia. *Circulation*. 2012;125(7):911-919.
107. Chappell LC, Duckworth S, Seed PT, et al. Diagnostic accuracy of placental growth factor in women with suspected preeclampsia: a prospective multicenter study. *Circulation*. 2013;128(19):2121-2131.
109. Zeisler H, Llurba E, Chantraine F, et al. Predictive value of the sFlt-1:PlGF ratio in women with suspected preeclampsia. *N Engl J Med*. 2016;374(1):13-22.
112. Stepan H, Herraiz I, Schlembach D, et al. Implementation of the sFlt-1/PlGF ratio for prediction and diagnosis of pre-eclampsia in singleton pregnancy: implications for clinical practice. *Ultrasound Obstet Gynecol*. 2015;45(3): 241-246.
116. Thadhani R, Kisner T, Hagmann H, et al. Pilot study of extracorporeal removal of soluble fms-like tyrosine kinase 1 in preeclampsia. *Circulation*. 2011;124(8):940-950.
117. Thadhani R, Hagmann H, Schaarschmidt W, et al. Removal of soluble fms-like tyrosine kinase-1 by dextran sulfate apheresis in preeclampsia. *J Am Soc Nephrol*. 2016;27(3):903-913.
118. Turanov AA, Lo A, Hassler MR, et al. RNAi modulation of placental sFLT1 for the treatment of preeclampsia. *Nat Biotechnol*. 2018;10.
122. Goel A, Maski MR, Bajracharya S, et al. Epidemiology and mechanisms of de novo and persistent hypertension in the postpartum period. *Circulation*. 2015;132(18):1726-1733.
125. Chen CW, Jaffe IZ, Karumanchi SA. Pre-eclampsia and cardiovascular disease. *Cardiovasc.Res*. 2014;101(4):579-586.
133. Pruthi D, Khankin EV, Blanton RM, et al. Exposure to experimental preeclampsia in mice enhances the vascular response to future injury. *Hypertension*. 2015;65(4):863-870.
141. Wikstrom AK, Haglund B, Olovsson M, Lindeberg SN. The risk of maternal ischaemic heart disease after gestational hypertensive disease. *BJOG*. 2005;112(11):1486-1491.
147. Jayet PY, Rimoldi SF, Stuber T, et al. Pulmonary and systemic vascular dysfunction in young offspring of mothers with preeclampsia. *Circulation*. 2010;122(5):488-494.
148. Davis EF, Lazdam M, Lewandowski AJ, et al. Cardiovascular risk factors in children and young adults born to preeclamptic pregnancies: a systematic review. *Pediatrics*. 2012;129(6):e1552-e1561.
149. Barker DJ, Osmond C. Infant mortality, childhood nutrition, and ischaemic heart disease in England and Wales. *Lancet*. 1986;1(8489):1077-1081.

171 Pathophysiology of Preterm Birth

David A. MacIntyre | Shirin Khanjani | Phillip R. Bennett

INTRODUCTION

Although clinically managed as if it were a single disease, preterm birth is increasingly recognized as a syndrome secondary to multiple causative mechanisms and etiologies. In this chapter, we discuss the epidemiology of preterm birth, the endocrinology and physiology of parturition, and current practice in prediction and prevention of preterm labor (PTL).

EPIDEMIOLOGY OF PRETERM BIRTH

PTL is defined as the onset of labor before 37 completed weeks of gestation. Preterm birth may follow spontaneous or induced labor, or a planned cesarean section due to maternal or fetal complications.[1] It is estimated that between 30% and 40% of all cases are induced or elective with remaining 60% to 70% occurring spontaneously.[2] In most developed nations the rate of preterm birth is below 10%; the UK rate is around 7% and in the USA the rate fluctuates between 9% and 12% and varies by geographic location and ethnicity. Many low-income nations have preterm birth rates exceeding 15%. Preterm birth accounts for more than 75% of all perinatal deaths. Epidemiologic studies of PTL vary in terms of categorization. Generally, delivery prior to 23 to 24 weeks is considered pre-viable, although in the developed world survival after birth at 23 weeks is improving. "Viability" is often a legally defined limit, being, for example, 24 weeks in the United Kingdom but 20 weeks in the United States. The World Health Organization defines subcategories of preterm birth, based on gestational age as "extremely preterm" (<28 weeks), "very preterm" (28 to 32 weeks), and "moderate to late preterm" (32 to 37 weeks).[3] The proportion of preterm births in each gestational age week epoque increases almost exponentially from approximately 32 weeks. The majority of preterm births are therefore at later gestational ages.

Preterm delivery is a major cause of neonatal morbidity and mortality, accounting for 65% of neonatal deaths and 50% of childhood neurologic disabilities. Prematurity is the biggest single cause of death within the first year of life. Survival rates are determined by gestation and birth weight.[4] Intraventricular hemorrhages occur in 25% to 30% of very low-birth-weight neonates, compared to 3% to 4% of term babies.[5] Those infants with higher grade hemorrhages are at risk to develop cerebral palsy, hydrocephalus, and seizures.[6] The risks of major long-term morbidities following preterm birth after 34 weeks are considered to be comparable to those after 37 weeks' gestation, although a significant risk of minor morbidities remains, and late preterm birth represents a much larger proportion of overall preterm births.[5,7] While a reduction in the rate of "extremely preterm" and "very preterm" births would significantly reduce the societal burden in the developed world, the greatest benefit in the developing world would be obtained by reducing the burden of "moderate-to-late preterm" births.

Although not identifiable in a significant proportion of women with preterm labor, risk factors include primigravida pregnancy, cervical incompetence or insufficiency, uterine distension (multiple pregnancy or polyhydramnios), infection, uterine and placental abnormalities, a previous history of preterm birth or second trimester pregnancy loss, advanced age, race, socioeconomic status, and body mass index (BMI).[1] In the United Kingdom, the risk of preterm birth is 6% in white Europeans but 10% in Africans or Afro-Caribbeans.[8] Similarly, African American women are overrepresented in rates of preterm birth in the United States. A poorer socioeconomic status in such groups and other minority groups adds environmental causes to probable genetic causes of preterm birth (i.e., polymorphisms in tumor necrosis factor α, TNF-α, a proinflammatory cytokine).[9] Other environmental factors include poor nutrition, smoking, substance abuse, and psychosocial factors.[1]

There are strong associations with preterm birth in women with diabetes, a low BMI, poor weight gain, or excess weight gain and obesity.[10,11] Alcohol consumption, smoking, and cocaine exposure all increase the risk of preterm birth. Dose-response effects have been described in alcohol consumption in various European studies, as well as increased risks from low-to-moderate and heavy smoking.[12-14] Maternal stress is considered to increase the risk of preterm birth via a neuroendocrine pathway that activates the maternal-placental-fetal endocrine systems that promote parturition via immune and/or inflammatory pathway activation.[15]

There is a clear role for genetics in the regulation of length of pregnancy and in the risk of preterm birth.[16] The risk of a woman having a preterm delivery is increased if her mother, sisters, or maternal half-sisters have had preterm deliveries, but not if her paternal half-sisters or members of her partner's family have preterm deliveries. Being a preterm baby increases a woman's own risk of preterm delivery and having a previous preterm delivery confers an increased risk of recurrent preterm delivery. Therefore, the genetic traits linked to preterm birth are principally transmitted in a matrilineal manner. The candidate gene approach has suggested a potential association between preterm birth and polymorphisms in the β2-adrenergic receptor gene, which promotes smooth muscle relaxation in the uterus. Other commonly studied candidate genes are those involved in immunity and inflammation, such as tumor necrosis factor, interleukins, other cytokines, and their receptors. Although some studies have detected polymorphisms in these genes that alter the risk for preterm birth in either the mother or fetus in specific cohorts, the results have generally failed to be replicated or generalized across populations. The use of genome-wide association studies (GWAS) in preterm birth is affected by the heterogeneity of preterm birth etiology, by the arbitrary definition of the outcome and by limited availability of suitable cohorts. However, sample-size limitations have been to some extent overcome by using genomic data from a large cohort of women of European ancestry who had undergone commercial "recreational genetics." This has identified maternal genomic loci associated with length of pregnancy linked to genes whose functions are consistent with a role in the timing of birth.[17]

MAINTENANCE OF HUMAN PREGNANCY AND THE ONSET OF PARTURITION

Human pregnancy lasts for approximately 280 days (from last menstrual period, or 266 days from conception) with minor variations between ethnic groups.[18] For the majority of pregnancy, the uterus remains quiescent yet expands to accommodate the growing fetus. At the same time, the cervix remains rigid and closed to retain the developing fetus within the uterus and to prevent ascending infection. Throughout pregnancy "pro-pregnancy" factors, such as progesterone and prostacyclin, inhibit myometrial contractility. At the end of pregnancy, "pro-labor" factors begin to mediate remodeling of the cervix and the uterus is stimulated to begin coordinated contractions. It has been suggested that labor results from the activation of a "cassette of contraction-associated proteins" (CAPs), which convert the myometrium from a quiescent to a contractile state.[19] CAPs include gap junction proteins, oxytocin (OT) and prostanoid receptors, enzymes for prostaglandin synthesis, and cell signaling proteins. The latter mediate the uterine response to receptor activation. Activation of myometrial contractility, cervical remodeling, and fetal membrane rupture mark the initiation of parturition that culminates in the expulsion of the fetus and the placenta. It is thought that a combination of maternal and fetal signals contributes toward the timing of labor.[20,21]

ENDOCRINOLOGY OF PARTURITION

An intricate interplay of endocrine, paracrine, and autocrine factors from both fetal and maternal origin has been proposed to play important modulatory roles in regulating the onset of human parturition. The most well characterized factors are considered here.

PROGESTERONE

In many species, progesterone acting through progesterone receptor (PR) inhibits labor-associated biochemical changes, and labor is heralded by withdrawal of the suppressive effects of progesterone. Unlike most mammals, circulating progesterone levels and PRs in the uterus do not fall with the onset of human labor. However, administration of PR antagonists (e.g., RU486) as well as inhibitors of progesterone synthesis can be used to ripen the cervix and induce labor in humans and primates. These findings indicate that removal of the progesterone "block" is still an important facet of human parturition. In the absence of a demonstrable fall in progesterone concentrations, a number of possible mechanisms of "functional progesterone withdrawal" have been postulated. First, progesterone action may be functionally mediated by alterations in the levels of different PR isoforms.[22] PR-A and PR-B are the two major PR isoforms in human and are both capable of binding to progesterone response elements (PREs) in DNA. However, PR-A lacks one of the three activation domains, present in PR-B, and has been reported to suppress PR-B activity in certain gene contexts and cells.[23-26] Second, increased metabolism of progesterone in the placenta and other gestational tissues at the time of parturition onset could lead to reduced functionality of progesterone.[27] In mice, the onset of labor is associated with an increase in expression of 5α-reductase type I and 20α-hydroxysteroid dehydrogenase (20α-HSD) in the cervix[28,29] and uterus, respectively.[21] Both enzymes are involved in the metabolism of progesterone. Third, it has been proposed that progesterone action may be regulated by interaction between PR and nuclear factor kappa B (NF-κB). A mutual inhibitory interaction between the RelA (p65) subunit of NF-κB and PR has been reported in Hela cells; PR transcriptional activity is inhibited by the activation of NF-κB while PR also represses TNF-α induced NF-κB activity.[30] Finally, altered expression of PR co-activators and co-repressors may lead to a functional withdrawal of progesterone.[31]

ESTROGEN

Similar to progesterone, circulating concentrations of estrogens steadily rise during pregnancy and promote a labor phenotype by stimulating the expression of pro-contractile factors such as prostaglandins, gap junction proteins (e.g., connection 43), and the oxytocin receptor (OTR). The action of estrogen is largely regulated by nuclear estrogen receptors (ERs) and a seven-transmembrane G protein-coupled receptor (GPCR) known as GPR30. In humans, the uterus is exposed to high levels of estrogens (mainly estradiol, estrone, and estriol) for most of pregnancy. Although poorly understood, it is thought that the modulation of ERs permits the uterus to be largely refractory to the pro-labor actions of estrogens during pregnancy but then increase the responsiveness to estrogens at the time of parturition. Therefore, functional withdrawal of progesterone's action, combined with increased estrogen responsiveness, would promote the transformation of the uterus to a contractile phenotype.

CORTICOTROPHIN-RELEASING HORMONE; A PLACENTAL CLOCK

In the sheep, corticotrophin-releasing hormone (CRH) is released by the fetal hypothalamus and helps regulate the timing of labor.[32] In the human however, it is proposed that placental CRH is part of a mechanism that acts as a clock, controlling the length of pregnancy.[33] Indeed, women destined to have preterm delivery show elevated plasma CRH levels and a more rapid rise in CRH during pregnancy.[34] Humans produce a circulating binding protein for CRH (CRHBP) and toward the end of the pregnancy the levels of CRHBP fall, thus increasing the available or free, bioactive CRH at term.[35] In contrast to hypothalamic CRH, placental CRH is stimulated by glucocorticoids, providing a positive feed-forward system.[36] Moreover, the modulation of parturition onset by CRH may occur indirectly by establishing a variety of positive feedback mechanisms involving other regulatory factors including adrenal steroids, prostaglandins, and OT.[37] Direct modulation of labor onset by CRH may also be achieved through its interaction with its receptors that are expressed in the uterus (CRHR1 and CRHR2). When the receptor is bound, it stimulates production of the myometrial relaxant cyclic adenosine monophosphate (cAMP).[38,39]

OXYTOCIN

OT is a nonapeptide produced by the posterior pituitary, known to have a potent contractile activity on the pregnant uterus. However, it does not seem to be essential for normal parturition, as there is no increase in circulating OT in the mother or fetus with the onset of labor. Moreover, normal parturition has been observed in cases of pituitary gland dysfunction.[30] However, the expression of the OTR does increase in the pregnant uterus. An up-regulation by two orders of magnitude has been demonstrated leading to a strong increase in sensitivity to OT.[40] Comparable increases in OTR mRNA concentrations in the myometrium are associated with this up-regulation of OT binding sites.[32] Postdelivery, myometrial OT binding sites rapidly decrease, whereas the expression of OTR remains high in the mammary gland throughout lactation.[40]

The human OTR couples to Gαq/11 and Gαi/o G-proteins.[7] Gαq/11 signaling in myometrium leads to phospholipase C (PLC)-mediated increases in intracellular Ca^{2+} via inositol triphosphate (IP3) and contractions; signaling through Gαi/o inhibits adenylate cyclase activity and reduces cAMP.[41]

CERVICAL RIPENING

Appropriate and timely cervical ripening is required for vaginal delivery. The transformation of the cervix from a closed firm structure to one that opens adequately for birth is a dynamic process that precedes the onset of labor. Cervical remodeling can be split into four overlapping phases termed *softening*, *ripening*, *dilation*, and *postpartum repair*. Softening can be defined as the first measurable decline in the tensile strength. This phase is distinct from the subsequent two phases in that softening is a relatively slow and incremental process that takes place in a progesterone- and prostaglandin-rich environment. Following softening, cervical ripening occurs in the weeks or days preceding birth and is a more accelerated phase characterized by maximal loss of tissue compliance and integrity. Upon initiation of uterine contractions, the ripened cervix can dilate sufficiently to allow passage of a fetus. The final phase of remodeling, termed *postpartum repair*, ensures recovery of tissue integrity and competency. Cervical ripening is thought to be an inflammatory process in both term and preterm deliveries.[42,43]

MYOMETRIAL CONTRACTILITY

The final pathway of labor culminates in the myometrium with the initiation of sustained, rhythmic, coordinated contractions. This involves precise regulation of myometrial intracellular calcium concentrations, increased electrical excitability and connectivity between myocytes, and modulation of the cellular cytoskeletal architecture.[44] The basic functional unit of the myometrium is the smooth muscle cells, which are in turn arranged into bundles of approximately 300 ± 100 μm in diameter. Each bundle is surrounded by connective tissue interspersed with microvasculature. The bundles are further organized into fasciculi, which are covered by a dense collagen matrix and the major vasculature of the myometrium.[45] Therefore, this structure enables the uterus to generate an expulsive force dependent on the orientation of these fibers relative to the cervix. Uterine contractions are then initiated by the propagation of action potentials within these defined vectors of muscle bundles.[46] The intracellular basis for contraction is via the cyclical attachment and detachment of cross-bridges between myosin and actin filaments, triggered via activation of the regulatory 20 kDa chain of myosin molecules. Myosin light chain is activated by phosphorylation by myosin light chain kinase, which, in turn, is activated by calmodulin.[47] It is through the actions of calmodulin, that during an action potential, the calcium influx can be connected with a contraction; a process known as excitation-contraction coupling.[48] Once the uterus has been activated, the myometrium is susceptible to stimulation by a number of different agonists, primarily prostaglandins and OT.

INFLAMMATION

One of the consistent features of labor is an intense inflammatory infiltration into the myometrium. Infection and associated inflammation is the only pathologic process that has a firm causal link with PTL.[49] A substantial body of evidence supports the link between increased cytokine synthesis and both term and PTL.[50,51] Prior to the onset of uterine contractions, activated inflammatory cells infiltrate the cervix and fetal membranes, which extends during labor to involve the myometrium.[52,53] The influx of activated inflammatory cells results in an increase in the synthesis and release of cytokines and chemokines[54–56]; the former promote the synthesis of prostaglandins and the latter increase the infiltration of inflammatory cells.[54–56]

It is currently unclear to what extent activation of inflammation is a cause or a consequence of labor. In the mouse it seems that a final precision timing of parturition is signaled by the mature fetus, through surfactant protein release into amniotic fluid, which also activates inflammation associated transcription factors NF-κB and activation protein 1 (AP-1) through Toll-like receptors.[57] This drives the production of prostaglandins and other proinflammatory effectors, which down-regulate choriodecidual prostaglandin dehydrogenase, and contributes to NF-κB and AP-1 activation in the fetal membranes, decidua and myometrium further stimulating production of pro-labor and prostaglandin synthetic proteins, and influx of inflammatory cells. However, labor can be induced in the mouse by inhibition of PR function using drugs such as mifepristone. In this situation there is little activation of downstream inflammatory mediators, suggesting that it is the effect of inflammation associated transcription factors in mediating completion of progesterone withdrawal rather than the downstream mediators that is required.[57,58] PTL may also be induced in the mouse using bacterial lipopolysaccharides, but neutrophil depletion in this context does not delay induced preterm birth.[59]

CYTOKINES AND CHEMOKINES

A comparison of the changes in myometrial gene expression between mouse and human suggests that human labor more closely resembles lipopolysaccharide-induced PTL in the mouse, supporting an essential role for inflammatory mediators in human.[58] Accumulating evidence suggests that, in the human, proinflammatory cytokines are causal, rather than a consequence, of labor onset. The production of secondary mediators of inflammation such as interleukin (IL)-8 and prostaglandins in human fetal membranes and myometrial cells is induced by IL-1β and TNF-α in vitro.[55,60–62] In an infection-induced model of parturition in the rhesus monkey, an increase in amniotic fluid levels of IL-1β, TNF-α, and IL-6 was found to precede increases in amniotic fluid levels of prostaglandins and IL-8.[63] Prostaglandins and IL-8, in turn, act synergistically to promote cervical ripening and dilation.[64,65]

Chemokines dominate all inflammatory responses, controlling leukocyte recruitment, activation, degranulation, proliferation, and survival. Prior to and during labor it is likely that specific subsets of proinflammatory chemokines direct uterine and cervical leukocyte homing and site-specific action. Increased expression of chemokines is a prominent feature of the myometrium and cervix before and after the onset of labor.[66] IL-8, a chemokine, is believed to have an important role in preterm and term birth.[52,61,67,68] Similarly, monocyte chemoattractant protein (MCP)-1 expression is also increased in amniotic fluid and cervical excretion in both term and preterm deliveries.[69,70] Levels of the antiinflammatory cytokine IL-10 are elevated in amniotic fluid, in both term and PTL with and without infection.[71] However, CXCL-6—another potent chemokine—does not appear to have a role in spontaneous term parturition but plays a role in the deployment of an antiinflammatory response as its concentration increases in amniotic fluid with an intraamniotic infection.[72]

PROSTAGLANDINS

Prostaglandins are synthesized from a common precursor, arachidonic acid, by the action of a central enzyme known as cyclooxygenase (COX). COX exists in two major isoforms, COX-1, which is constitutively expressed in all cell types, and COX-2, which is inducible and is mostly found at sites of inflammation.[73] There is substantial evidence for the importance of the COX-2 isoform in human labor. The amnion is a major source of prostaglandins, and there is a marked increase in prostaglandin E_2 (PGE_2) synthesis at the time of labor onset.[74] This is associated with the selective induction of COX-2 expression.[75,76] Similarly upregulation of COX-2, but not COX-1, expression is observed in the chorion in association with labor.[76,77]

Although both $PGF_2\alpha$ and PGE_2 induce contractions, PGE_2 binds its myometrial receptors more avidly, and is 10-fold more potent in stimulating contractions. PGE_2 activates four members of the GPCR superfamily (EP1–EP4). EP2 and EP4 are classically thought to maintain uterine relaxation during pregnancy via Gαs-cAMP signaling, while myometrial contractions in labor are thought to arise via activation of Gαq/11-PLC-Ca^{2+} pathways by EP1 and EP3. Studies have revealed that EP3, not EP1, mediates PGE_2-induced contractility in human term pregnant myometrium. Furthermore, EP2 (but not EP4) activation not only stimulates cAMP signaling and reduces contractility, but contrastingly, induces a pro-labor response by increasing COX-2 and PGE_2 production via activation of Gαq/11-mediated Ca^{2+}. EP2-mediated cAMP signaling is severely attenuated in laboring myometrium, thereby favoring COX-2 synthesis.[78] Overall, studies suggest that PGE_2 receptors induce complex signaling responses mediating inflammation and contractility.

INFLAMMATORY TRANSCRIPTION FACTOR ACTIVATION

NF-κB is a cytokine-inducible transcription factor activated in response to infection and proinflammatory cytokines, which regulates many proinflammatory and labor-associated genes.[25] In most cells, NF-κB exists in an inactive form in the cytoplasm, bound to an inhibitory protein, such as IκBα. Three distinct NF-κB signaling pathways have been identified to date.[79] Labor is associated with an increase in the baseline level of NF-κB DNA binding and transcriptional activity in the human amnion. Because NF-κB downregulates PR function, it seems to be related to a "functional progesterone withdrawal" in the human myometrium.[80] CCAAT/enhancer-binding proteins (C/EBP) is a family of transcription factors that regulate a variety of genes including genes for acute phase response proteins; however, the number of studies investigating the role of C/EBP in parturition is limited. Lee and colleagues demonstrated that in primary human amnion cells, C/EBP DNA-binding sites are crucial for the function of the COX-2 gene promoter.[81] OTR promoter also contains putative binding sites for C/EBP, and the OTR promoter activity is synergistically upregulated by NF-κB and C/EBP.[82] AP-1 transcription factors are early response genes involved in a diverse set of transcriptional regulatory processes. AP-1 is a dimeric complex composed of members of the Fos and Jun protein families.[83] NFκB and AP-1 drive human myometrial IL-8 gene expression.[84] A study showed that while NFκB activation is not a functional requirement for infection/inflammation-induced PTL in mice, AP-1 activation is sufficient to drive inflammatory pathways that cause PTL.[85]

MECHANISMS OF PRETERM LABOR

Approximately one-third of preterm births are medically indicated, usually because of maternal complications including preeclampsia, diabetes, and renal disease, or fetal complications, principally intrauterine growth restriction. A discussion of the etiology and management of these conditions is beyond the scope of this chapter; however, while spontaneous and iatrogenic preterm birth are clearly distinguishable, there is growing evidence that common pathways may underlie both. Fetal growth restriction is associated with some of the same biomarkers as spontaneous preterm birth.[86] There is a well-known association between spontaneous preterm birth and growth restriction in utero. In general, preterm babies tend to be small for gestational age.[87] It seems probable that implantation and early pregnancy events causing inadequate placental function may lead to either spontaneous or medically indicated preterm birth.

UTERINE STRETCH

A further factor influencing the length of human pregnancy is mechanical signal transduction. The myometrium undergoes changes in phenotype throughout pregnancy, characterized by an early proliferation, then cellular hypertrophy and matrix elaboration, a third phase in which the cells assume a contractile phenotype, and then final phase of labor. In animal and human cell in vitro studies stretch leads to activation of inflammatory mediators and up-regulation of contraction associated proteins. This is opposed by progesterone, which acts to stimulate growth and remodeling of the myometrium during pregnancy, associated with increased synthesis of extra cellular matrix (ECM) proteins and integrin receptors. Near to term there is decrease in expression of fibrillar collagens and increased expression of basement membrane components associated with increased mechanical tension, which then commits these cells to the labor phenotype, with increased responsiveness to agonists and effective coupling of the myocytes. Unsurprisingly, pathologic stretch of the uterus, through twin or higher order multiple pregnancy, or through polyhydramnios, associated with certain fetal abnormalities, leads to PTL. It is also probable that syndromes, which prevent the uterus from expanding appropriately such as congenital uterine anomalies, and fibroids may also associate with PTL through mechanical signal transduction.

VAGINAL MICROBIOTA

The vagina plays host to populations of microbiota that have a critical role in maintaining reproductive health. The cervix, the cervical mucous plug, and the presence of a population of generally harmless and potentially beneficial microorganisms, collectively referred to as the microbiome, protect the growing fetus from infection throughout the pregnancy. During healthy pregnancy, vaginal microbiota communities shift to become more dominated by *Lactobacillus* species, which are thought to inhibit the growth of potential pathogens through the production of lactic acid and the release of antibacterial bacteriocins.[88] Vaginal microbiome dysbiosis is associated with a risk of preterm birth.[89] For example, bacterial vaginosis (BV) is a risk factor for PTL and histologic chorioamnionitis and is characterized by reduced numbers of *Lactobacillus*, higher pH, and increased abundance of potential pathogens including *Gardnerella vaginalis*, Group B *Streptococcus*, *Escherichia coli*, and *Peptostreptococcus* and *Bacteroides* species. The combination of BV and maternal carriage of a single nucleotide polymorphism (SNP) in the TNF-α promoter increases the risk of PTL fourfold, suggesting that maternal genetic/inflammatory interaction with the vaginal microbiome can influence risk of PTL.[9] Studies of the human microbiome have been accelerated by the development of DNA sequencing-based approaches that enable identification of almost all bacteria in any biologic sample and comparison of relative abundance between taxa, including those species not normally amenable to culture. These approaches have now been widely applied to women in pregnancy and shown that specific bacterial community structures and species are associated with relative risk of preterm birth. A consistent finding across most studies is the protective effect of *Lactobacillus crispatus*. A longitudinal study of UK women throughout pregnancy showed that pregnancy induces a shift in vaginal microbiota profiles from temporally dynamic communities toward more stable, *Lactobacillus* spp. dominance and that the postpartum period is associated with a reduced *Lactobacillus* spp. and increased diversity of BV-associated bacteria.[90] This provides further evidence for the role of estrogen in modulating the vaginal microbiome during pregnancy and provides new understanding of the role bacteria play in post-delivery complications such as endometritis.[91] A study from the United States also found that the vaginal microbiome shifts during pregnancy toward *Lactobacillus*-dominated profiles at the expense of taxa often associated with vaginal dysbiosis. The shifts occurred early in pregnancy and followed predictable patterns. Furthermore, they were associated with simplification of the metabolic capacity of the microbiome but were significant only in women of African or Hispanic ancestry.[92] In a UK-based general population, *Lactobacillus* depletion and a high diversity microbiome is a rare finding; however, women with *Lactobacillus-iners*-dominant vaginal bacterial communities at 16 weeks of gestational age are more likely to have a short cervix and are at increased risk of early but not late preterm birth.[93] In contrast, *L. crispatus* dominance early in pregnancy is highly predictive of term birth. *L. iners* dominance is associated with higher rates of shifting toward a high-diversity microbiota typically enriched with potentially pathogenic bacteria including *Gardnerella*, *Atopobium*, *Streptococcus*, and *Staphylococcus* species. In populations from the United States, *Lactobacillus* depletion and a high-diversity microbiome associated with *Gardnerella* spp. is seen more commonly and is a risk factor for preterm birth in especially populations of white women, but not in all populations of black women.[92] In another cohort of women predominantly of African ancestry, those who delivered preterm exhibited significantly lower vaginal levels of *L. crispatus* and higher levels of BVAB1, *Sneathia amnii*, TM7-H1, a group of *Prevotella* species, and nine other taxa, and this was associated with evidence of activation of inflammation.[94] There are clearly geographic, ethnic, and probably genetic and immunologic factors that influence both the vaginal microbiome itself and the host response to a change in flora. Preterm premature rupture of membranes (PPROM) is associated with second trimester instability of bacterial community structure during pregnancy and a shift toward reduced *Lactobacillus* spp. abundance and higher diversity characterized by increased relative abundance of potentially pathogenic species including *Prevotella*, *Peptoniphilus*, *Streptococcus*, and *Dialister*.[95,96] Approximately 50% of women who experience PPROM have a dysbiotic vaginal microbiome just prior to and after the rupture event. This suggests at least two etiologic groups, related and unrelated to the genital tract microbiota. The composition of the vaginal microbiome is therefore likely to be a critical determinant of PTB in a significant number of women and may be a critical determinant of PPROM, the risk of subsequent ascending infection, and the ultimate outcome of the neonate.[97]

CURRENT PREDICTION OF PRETERM LABOR

As precise disease mechanisms behind preterm birth are not so well understood, clinical predictive tests and preventative treatments remain limited. However, if women who are at high risk of spontaneous preterm birth in early pregnancy can be identified, they may be targeted for more intensive antenatal care and prophylactic interventions. A history of previous preterm birth, second trimester loss, or induced abortion is a noninvasive, simple, cost-effective way to identify women who may benefit from more intensive screening (Fig. 171.1). There is a weak association between cervical intraepithelial neoplasia (CIN, the precursor to cervical cancer) and a stronger association between treatment of CIN by cone biopsy or by large loop excision of the transformation zone of the cervix (LLETZ) and risk of preterm birth.[98] Once individuals have been identified as at-risk, further

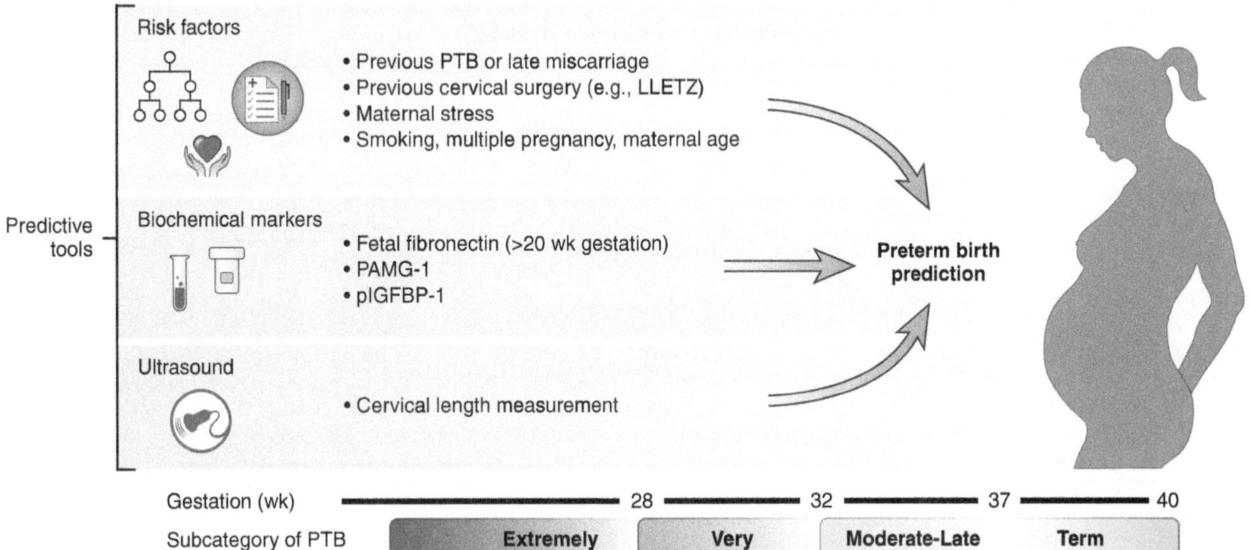

Fig. 171.1 Current tools for the prediction of preterm birth. *LLETZ*, Large loop excision of the transformation zone of the cervix; *PAMG-1*, placental alpha microglobulin-1; *pIGFBP-1*, phosphorylated insulin-like growth factor binding protein-1.

assessment can be made by the use of ultrasonographic cervical length measurement, and/or cervical-vaginal fetal fibronectin (fFN) screening.

Women admitted to hospital with a history of preterm uterine contractions mostly do not deliver preterm. However, there is clear benefit from antenatal administration of high-dose corticosteroids to the mother at least 24 hours prior to preterm birth, for in utero transfer to a hospital with neonatal intensive care faculties for the baby, and for administration of magnesium sulfate to the mother at the time of delivery. Differentiation between those women with contractions who are or who are not likely to deliver preterm can also be achieved by the use of ultrasonographic cervical length measurement, and/or cervical-vaginal fFN screening.

FETAL FIBRONECTIN AND OTHER CERVICAL-VAGINAL FLUID BIOMARKERS

fFN is an extracellular matrix found in the deciduas basalis next to the placental intervillous space. It forms attachments between the fetal membranes and the decidua, and when mechanical or inflammatory changes occur, it leaks into the cervical-vaginal fluid. It can be measured quantitatively in cervico-vaginal secretions, obtained from the posterior fornix when performing an internal examination with a speculum. Commercial kits are now available that give a positive/negative result, reporting positive when concentrations are greater than 50 ng/mL. Commercial bedside kits are also available that report quantitative data. fFN is normally present in cervical secretions up to 20 weeks of pregnancy. Therefore, fFN testing is of poor predictive value before 20 weeks. At present, it is widely accepted as a good test for excluding preterm birth in those presenting with threatened PTL due to its strong negative predictive value: only 0.5% of women deliver within 7 to 10 days after a negative test.[99] A positive result is associated with the greatest odds ratio for preterm delivery before 35 weeks gestation.[100] Although not yet widely adopted, the use of quantification of fibronectin leads to improvements in the positive predictive value for fibronectin testing while maintaining a good negative predictive value.[101] Recently, two other bedside tests have become available to predict preterm delivery. These measure placental α microglobulin-1 (PAMG-1) and phosphorylated insulin-like growth factor binding protein-1 (pIGFBP-1 protein) but are currently much less studied than fFN.[102]

CERVICAL LENGTH MEASUREMENT

Iams and colleagues[103] were the first to demonstrate that the risk of PTL is inversely proportional to the length of the cervix between 24 and 28 weeks gestation. Ultrasonographic cervical length measurement is a reproducible method of assessing the cervix, with little inter- and intraobserver error. A transvaginal probe is used to obtain the length between the internal and external os. The risk of preterm delivery increases exponentially with decreasing length, from less than 1% at 30 mm to 80% at 5 mm.[104] In women with symptoms of PTL, it is estimated that 50% of women with a cervical length of less than 15 mm deliver within 7 days.[105,106]

CURRENT MANAGEMENT OF PRETERM LABOR

The management of preterm birth can be divided into two strategies: (1) Primary prevention, which is aimed at averting the onset of PTL, and (2) secondary prevention, which refers to therapeutic interventions to stop PTL once it has started (Fig. 171.2).

PRIMARY PREVENTION

Primary prevention of preterm delivery is more desirable but is hindered by a lack of reliable predictors of PTL. Progesterone, as discussed, is important in maintaining uterine quiescence, and therefore there is an interest in the use of progesterone or progesterone analogs as prophylaxis for preterm delivery. Both natural progesterone given by vaginal pessary and intramuscular 17-hydroxyprogesterone caproate have been extensively trialed in women at high risk for preterm delivery. The current evidence more strongly supports the use of natural progesterone given by vaginal pessary over intramuscular 17-hydroxyprogesterone caproate, and this is specifically in the context of a short cervix, measured by transvaginal ultrasound. It has been suggested that healthcare agencies should introduce routine screening for PTL by transvaginal ultrasound measurement of cervical length followed by vaginal progestogen treatment in those women in whom it is found to be short. However, both the effectiveness of cervical length measurements in predicting preterm birth and the effectiveness of transvaginal progesterone in preventing it vary dramatically from population to population, and so this

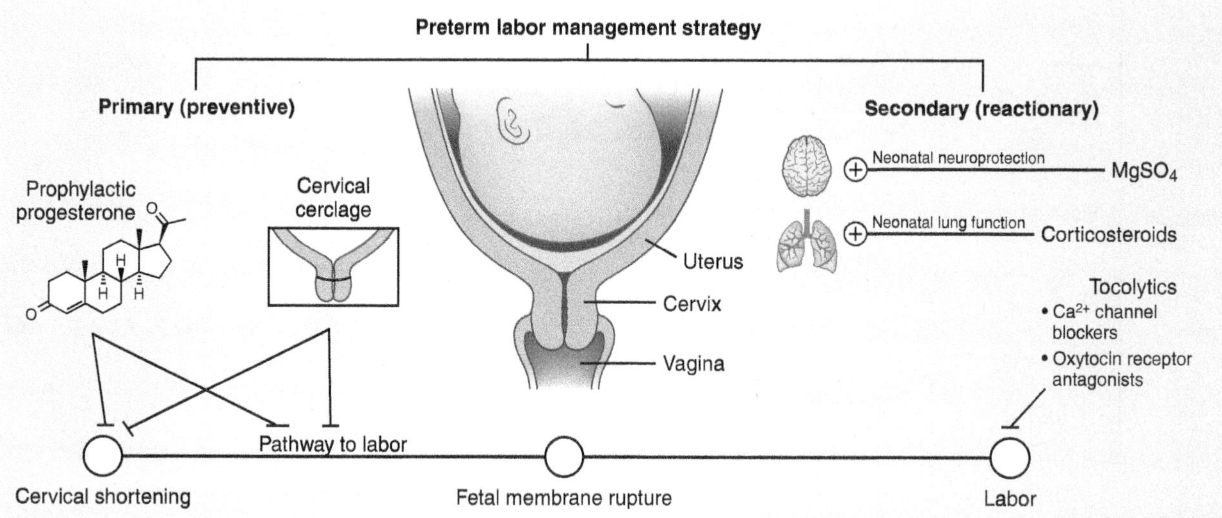

Fig. 171.2 Current clinical management strategies for preterm labor.

approach would need to be assessed based upon individual local regional or national data.

Surgical intervention is widely used to tackle PTL related to cervical insufficiency, which is identified by early cervical changes, such as funneling or dilation. The placement of a cerclage in patients with cervical shortening results in an increase in cervical length. However, the evidence to support either prophylactic or therapeutic use of cervical cerclage is limited.[107] The current evidence suggests that cervical cerclage may improve outcome in women who have both a short cervix and another risk factor, such as pervious preterm birth or previous LLETZ.

SECONDARY PREVENTION AND MANAGEMENT

The main rationale for the use of tocolytics (drugs intended to inhibit uterine contractions) is to delay delivery long enough for corticosteroid administration to improve neonatal lung function[108,109] and for in utero transfer to an appropriate neonatal special care unit. Antenatal administration of corticosteroids to the mothers of fetuses at risk of preterm delivery is associated with a reduction in the risk of neonatal respiratory distress syndrome and a substantial reduction in mortality and intraventricular hemorrhage. The benefits of a single course of steroid given at between 24 and 34 weeks of pregnancy to women who are in suspected, diagnosed, or established PTL outweigh the potential risks. These benefits include giving maternal corticosteroids to women are having a planned preterm birth or have PPROM. A single course of steroids becomes effective within 24 to 48 hours and is generally accepted to continue to confer benefit for up to 7 days. However, administration of multiple courses may be associated with adverse effects upon fetal growth. It is also established that neonatal outcome is better if the potentially preterm baby is transferred in utero to a hospital with an appropriate neonatal special care unit rather than being transferred after birth. To correctly target these interventions requires better diagnostic accuracy for PTL than is achieved simply from observing contractions. This can be undertaken either by fibronectin (or other biomarkers) testing, which is popular in the United Kingdom, or by measurement of cervical length by transvaginal ultrasound, which is popular in the United States. In some regions both techniques are used together.

Tocolytic drugs have distinct modes of action, but all target uterine contractility. They include β-sympathomimetics, calcium channel blockers, OT antagonists, magnesium sulfate, and nitric oxide donors.[110] With the exception of nifedipine, no tocolytic has been shown to significantly improve neonatal outcome and there is currently no evidence that any tocolytic drug improves long-term outcomes. Current UK guidelines suggest that if tocolytics are administered for the medical treatment of PTL, the first choice should be a calcium channel blocker (nifedipine) or if that is contraindicated, an OT receptor antagonist is indicated (atosiban; currently not available in the United States). Use of β-sympathomimetics has been largely discontinued because of the poor maternal side effect profile.

There is great deal of evidence suggesting that the OT receptor has an important role in the onset of labor. The myometrium becomes increasingly sensitive to OT in late pregnancy, and this is directly related to an increase in OT receptor density.[111] Atosiban is a synthetic OT analogue and represents a competitive antagonist of OT and vasopressin. Administration of atosiban results in a dose-dependent inhibition of uterine contractility and OT mediated prostaglandin release. Based on data from randomized clinical trials, the efficacy of atosiban is similar to betamimetics. However, the OT antagonist is much better tolerated and side effects are significantly more common with β-agonists. A study by Romero and colleagues[112] comparing atosiban with placebo showed that more patients allocated to atosiban remained undelivered at 24 hours, 48 hours, and 7 days.

The effects of calcium channel blockers in decreasing contractions of the human myometrium have been known for several years. Nifedipine is a calcium channel blocker originally developed in the 1960s as a treatment for angina pectoris. Calcium channel blockers exert their effect by binding to L-type channels and reducing intracellular levels of calcium. Nifedipine is able to block the flow of extracellular calcium into myometrial cells and in this way decreases contractions. Although there are no trials in which calcium channel blockers were compared with placebo, nifedipine has been compared with the β-sympathomimetic ritodrine in a number of randomized trials. A Cochrane meta-analysis[113] compared the effects of calcium channel blockers with β-sympathomimetics on maternal, fetal, and neonatal outcome. Calcium channel blockers were shown to reduce the number of preterm births within 7 days of starting treatment. Adverse drug reactions, discontinuation due to side effects, respiratory distress syndrome, necrotizing enterocolitis, intraventricular hemorrhage, and hyperbilirubinemia were all less with the use of calcium channel blockers than with β-sympathomimetics. There is some evidence that antenatal nifedipine exposure may provide some protection against neonatal morbidity and mortality.[114]

Pharmacologic compounds that inhibit prostaglandin synthesis have also been used as tocolytics in the treatment of PTL. A meta-analysis of 13 trials concluded that inhibition of prostaglandin synthesis decreased the incidence of preterm birth and had fewer maternal side effects than other tocolytic drugs, but did not improve neonatal outcome.[115] However, prostaglandin synthesis inhibitors are not widely used, because they are associated with premature constriction of the ductus arteriosus and reduced fetal renal function, which become more significant with advancing gestational age.

Intrauterine infection has long been recognized as a major cause of PTL[116-119]; therefore antibiotics have been used in the treatment of PTL. A meta-analysis of 14 trials showed that administration of antibiotics, specifically erythromycin, following PPROM delayed delivery and improved maternal and neonatal outcomes.[120] In contrast, a meta-analysis of 11 trials showed that the use of antibiotics in PTL with intact membranes did not have any benefits.[121] Furthermore, administration of antibiotics in that population was associated with a higher risk of cerebral palsy.[108] Inconsistent results in such trials likely reflect differences in underlying causes of pathology and highlight problems with a "one size fits all" approach to treatment strategy. For example, it has recently been shown that vaginal dysbiosis increases the risk of PPROM, and that approximately half of all women with PPROM have vaginal dysbiosis.[96] In the women with PPROM who do not have vaginal dysbiosis, treatment with erythromycin leads to development of vaginal dysbiosis. Overall, in all cases of PPROM, vaginal dysbiosis associated with increased risk of early onset neonatal sepsis. Improved outcome in PPROM may therefore come from the development of bedside tests capable of discriminating a healthy vaginal microbiota (in which antibiotics might be contraindicated) from vaginal dysbiosis in which antibiotics might be beneficial.

Neuroprotection using intravenous magnesium sulfate is a relatively recent addition to the obstetrician's armamentarium. The value of an antenatal infusion of magnesium sulfate in reducing the risk of subsequent cerebral palsy in babies born preterm has been sufficiently proven. An important difference between antenatal corticosteroid therapy and magnesium sulfate therapy is that magnesium sulfate has been shown to be beneficial even if it is administered for the first time very close to the time of delivery. While the effect of corticosteroids on surfactant production generally requires 24 to 48 hours to enhance the metabolic pathways in the lung, the mechanism of action of magnesium sulfate is thought to occur immediately via a number of potential pathways such as stabilization of cerebral circulation, prevention of hypoxic damage and free radical activity, and inhibition of excitatory injury through blocking of neurotransmitters such as glutamate release and *N*-methyl-D-aspartic acid (NMDA) receptors on oligodendrocytes, which are implicated in periventricular white matter injury in preterm infants.[122-124] While antenatal corticosteroids may have adverse maternal effects particularly in a diabetic woman, generally the intramuscular administration of steroids does not cause maternal complications and does not require any particular monitoring thereafter. However, magnesium sulfate needs to be given as a single bolus followed by a continuous infusion, and because magnesium may be toxic to the mother, it requires close monitoring. Magnesium sulfate would therefore be given if it is expected that delivery would be genuinely "imminent," that is to say within a few hours. The various studies of magnesium sulfate for neuroprotection have suggested that infusions should be planned for 12 to 24 hours, and then discontinued if preterm birth has not occurred. The available evidence is that magnesium sulfate is effective even if it is only administered for an hour or so prior to preterm birth, or during established PTL.[125]

CONCLUSION

Pregnancy involves a remarkable transformation of the uterus, which at the time of parturition sees it undergo a process of activation that facilitates a switch from a nonresponsive organ to one that is very sensitive to uterotonins and capable of intense, rhythmic contractions characteristic of labor. Substantial research effort is providing insight into the underlying mechanisms of these processes, which involve complex integration of endocrine and mechanical stimuli. Although strategies have been developed for primary and secondary prevention of preterm birth, the complex nature and uniqueness of human parturition and the multiple etiologies that might lead to PTL mean that preventing preterm birth remains a major unmet healthcare need.

A complete reference list is available at www.ExpertConsult.com. 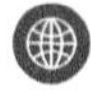

SELECT REFERENCES

1. Murphy DJ. Epidemiology and environmental factors in preterm labour. *Best Pract Res Clin Obstet Gynaecol*. 2007;21(5):773-789.
2. Khan KS, Honest H. Risk screening for spontaneous preterm labour. *Best Pract Res Clin Obstet Gynaecol*. 2007;21(5):821-830.
9. Macones GA, Parry S, Elkousy M, Clothier B, Ural SH, Strauss 3rd JF. A polymorphism in the promoter region of TNF and bacterial vaginosis: preliminary evidence of gene-environment interaction in the etiology of spontaneous preterm birth. *Am J Obstet Gynecol*. 2004;190(6):1504-1508; discussion 3A.
10. Norman JE, Morris C, Chalmers J. The effect of changing patterns of obstetric care in Scotland (1980-2004) on rates of preterm birth and its neonatal consequences: perinatal database study. *PLoS Medicine*. 2009;6(9):e1000153.
16. Muglia LJ, Katz M. The enigma of spontaneous preterm birth. *N Engl J Med*. 2010;362(6):529-535.
18. Steer P. The epidemiology of preterm labour. *BJOG An Int J Obstet Gynaecol*. 2005;112(suppl 1):1-3.
22. Mesiano S, Chan EC, Fitter JT, Kwek K, Yeo G, Smith R. Progesterone withdrawal and estrogen activation in human parturition are coordinated by progesterone receptor A expression in the myometrium. *J Clin Endocrinol Metabol*. 2002;87(6):2924-2930.
25. Pieber D, Allport VC, Bennett PR. Progesterone receptor isoform A inhibits isoform B-mediated transactivation in human amnion. *Euro J Pharmacol*. 2001;427(1):7-11.
26. Pieber D, Allport VC, Hills F, Johnson M, Bennett PR. Interactions between progesterone receptor isoforms in myometrial cells in human labour. *Mol Human reprod*. 2001;7(9):875-879.
31. Condon JC, Jeyasuria P, Faust JM, Wilson JW, Mendelson CR. A decline in the levels of progesterone receptor coactivators in the pregnant uterus at term may antagonize progesterone receptor function and contribute to the initiation of parturition. *Proc Natl Acad Sci U S A*. 2003;100(16):9518-9523.
33. Smith R. *Parturition. N Engl J Med*. 2007;356(3):271-283.
34. McLean M, Bisits A, Davies J, Woods R, Lowry P, Smith R. A placental clock controlling the length of human pregnancy. *Nat Med*. 1995;1(5):460-463.
36. Robinson BG, Emanuel RL, Frim DM, Majzoub JA. Glucocorticoid stimulates expression of corticotropin-releasing hormone gene in human placenta. *Proc Natl Acad Sci U S A*. 1988;85(14):5244-5248.
40. Soloff MS, Alexandrova M, Fernstrom MJ. Oxytocin receptors: triggers for parturition and lactation? *Science*. 1979;204(4399):1313-1315.
47. Word RA, Stull JT, Casey ML, Kamm KE. Contractile elements and myosin light chain phosphorylation in myometrial tissue from nonpregnant and pregnant women. *J Clin Invest*. 1993;92(1):29-37.
48. Blanks AM, Zhao ZH, Shmygol A, Bru-Mercier G, Astle S, Thornton S. Characterization of the molecular and electrophysiological properties of the T-type calcium channel in human myometrium. *J Physiol*. 2007;581(Pt 3):915-926.
52. Osman I, Young A, Ledingham MA, et al. Leukocyte density and pro-inflammatory cytokine expression in human fetal membranes, decidua, cervix and myometrium before and during labour at term. *Mol Human Reprod*. 2003;9(1):41-45.
54. Elliott CL, Slater DM, Dennes W, Poston L, Bennett PR. Interleukin 8 expression in human myometrium: changes in relation to labor onset and with gestational age. *Am J Reprod Immunol*. 2000;43(5):272-277.
56. Shynlova O, Tsui P, Dorogin A, Lye SJ. Monocyte chemoattractant protein-1 (CCL-2) integrates mechanical and endocrine signals that mediate term and preterm labor. *J Immunol*. 2008;181(2):1470-1479.

58. Migale R, MacIntyre DA, Cacciatore S, et al. Modeling hormonal and inflammatory contributions to preterm and term labor using uterine temporal transcriptomics. *BMC Med.* 2016;14(1):86.
60. Sooranna SR, Engineer N, Loudon JA, Terzidou V, Bennett PR, Johnson MR. The mitogen-activated protein kinase dependent expression of prostaglandin H synthase-2 and interleukin-8 messenger ribonucleic acid by myometrial cells: the differential effect of stretch and interleukin-1{beta}. *J Clin Endocrinol Metabol.* 2005;90(6):3517-3527.
66. Bollopragada S, Youssef R, Jordan F, Greer I, Norman J, Nelson S. Term labor is associated with a core inflammatory response in human fetal membranes, myometrium, and cervix. *Am J Obstet Gynecol.* 2009;200(1):104.e1-e11.
68. Elliott CL, Loudon JA, Brown N, Slater DM, Bennett PR, Sullivan MH. IL-1beta and IL-8 in human fetal membranes: changes with gestational age, labor, and culture conditions. *Am J Reprod Immunol.* 2001;46(4):260-267.
74. Bennett PR, Slater D, Sullivan M, Elder MG, Moore GE. Changes in amniotic arachidonic acid metabolism associated with increased cyclo-oxygenase gene expression. *Br J Obstet Gynaecol.* 1993;100(11):1037-1042.
75. Hirst JJ, Teixeira FJ, Zakar T, Olson DM. Prostaglandin endoperoxide-H synthase-1 and -2 messenger ribonucleic acid levels in human amnion with spontaneous labor onset. *J Clin Endocrinol Metabol.* 1995;80(2):517-523.
76. Slater D, Allport V, Bennett P. Changes in the expression of the type-2 but not the type-1 cyclo-oxygenase enzyme in chorion-decidua with the onset of labour. *Br J Obstet Gynaecol.* 1998;105(7):745-748.
78. Kandola MK, Sykes L, Lee YS, Johnson MR, Hanyaloglu AC, Bennett PR. EP2 receptor activates dual G protein signaling pathways that mediate contrasting proinflammatory and relaxatory responses in term pregnant human myometrium. *Endocrinology.* 2014;155(2):605-617.
81. Lee YS, Terzidou V, Lindstrom T, Johnson M, Bennett PR. The role of CCAAT/enhancer-binding protein beta in the transcriptional regulation of COX-2 in human amnion. *Mol Human Reprod.* 2005;11(12):853-858.
82. Terzidou V, Lee Y, Lindstrom T, Johnson M, Thornton S, Bennett PR. Regulation of the human oxytocin receptor by nuclear factor-kappaB and CCAAT/enhancer-binding protein-beta. *J Clin Endocrinol Metabol.* 2006;91(6):2317-2326.
84. Khanjani S, Terzidou V, Johnson MR, Bennett PR. NFkappaB and AP-1 drive human myometrial IL8 expression. *Mediat Inflam.* 2012;2012:504952.
85. MacIntyre DA, Lee YS, Migale R, et al. Activator protein 1 is a key terminal mediator of inflammation-induced preterm labor in mice. *FASEB J.* 2014;28(5):2358-2368.
88. Verstraelen H, Verhelst R, Claeys G, De Backer E, Temmerman M, Vaneechoutte M. Longitudinal analysis of the vaginal microflora in pregnancy suggests that L. crispatus promotes the stability of the normal vaginal microflora and that L. gasseri and/or L. iners are more conducive to the occurrence of abnormal vaginal microflora. *BMC Microbiology.* 2009;9:116.
90. MacIntyre DA, Chandiramani M, Lee YS, et al. The vaginal microbiome during pregnancy and the postpartum period in a European population. *Sci Rep.* 2015;5:8988.
93. Kindinger LM, Bennett PR, Lee YS, et al. The interaction between vaginal microbiota, cervical length, and vaginal progesterone treatment for preterm birth risk. *Microbiome.* 2017;5(1):6.
94. Fettweis JM, Serrano MG, Brooks JP, et al. The vaginal microbiome and preterm birth. *Nat Med.* 2019;25(6):1012-1021.
96. Brown RG, Marchesi JR, Lee YS, et al. Vaginal dysbiosis increases risk of preterm fetal membrane rupture, neonatal sepsis and is exacerbated by erythromycin. *BMC Med.* 2018;16(1):9.
98. Kyrgiou M, Athanasiou A, Paraskevaidi M, et al. Adverse obstetric outcomes after local treatment for cervical preinvasive and early invasive disease according to cone depth: systematic review and meta-analysis. *BMJ.* 2016;354:i3633.
99. Honest H, Bachmann LM, Gupta JK, Kleijnen J, Khan KS. Accuracy of cervicovaginal fetal fibronectin test in predicting risk of spontaneous preterm birth: systematic review. *BMJ.* 2002;325(7359):301.
101. Abbott DS, Hezelgrave NL, Seed PT, et al. Quantitative fetal fibronectin to predict preterm birth in asymptomatic women at high risk. *Obstet Gynecol.* 2015;125(5):1168-1176.
102. Melchor JC, Khalil A, Wing D, Schleussner E, Surbek D. Prediction of preterm delivery in symptomatic women using PAMG-1, fetal fibronectin and phIGFBP-1 tests: systematic review and meta-analysis. *Ultrasound Obstetr Gynecology.* 2018;52(4):442-451.
103. Iams JD, Goldenberg RL, Meis PJ, et al. The length of the cervix and the risk of spontaneous premature delivery. National Institute of Child Health and Human Development maternal fetal medicine unit network. *N Engl J Med.* 1996;334(9):567-572.
108. Roberts D, Dalziel S. Antenatal corticosteroids for accelerating fetal lung maturation for women at risk of preterm birth. *Cochrane Database Syst Rev.* 2006;3:CD004454.
111. Fuchs AR, Fuchs F, Husslein P, Soloff MS. Oxytocin receptors in the human uterus during pregnancy and parturition. *Am J Obstet Gynecol.* 1984;150(6):734-741.
113. King JF, Flenady VJ, Papatsonis DN, Dekker GA, Carbonne B. Calcium channel blockers for inhibiting preterm labour. *Cochrane Database Syst Rev.* 2003;1:CD002255.
115. King J, Flenady V, Cole S, Thornton S. Cyclo-oxygenase (COX) inhibitors for treating preterm labour. *Cochrane Database Syst Rev.* 2005;(2):CD001992.
120. Kenyon S, Boulvain M, Neilson J. Antibiotics for preterm rupture of the membranes: a systematic review. *Obstet Gynecol.* 2004;104(5 Pt 1):1051-1057.
121. King J, Flenady V. Prophylactic antibiotics for inhibiting preterm labour with intact membranes. *Cochrane Database Syst Rev.* 2002;4:CD000246.
122. Doyle LW, Crowther CA, Middleton P, Marret S, Rouse D. Magnesium sulphate for women at risk of preterm birth for neuroprotection of the fetus. *Cochrane Database Syst Rev.* 2009;(1):CD004661.
123. Rouse DJ, Hirtz DG, Thom E, et al. A randomized, controlled trial of magnesium sulfate for the prevention of cerebral palsy. *N Engl J Med.* 2008;359(9):895-905.

Pathophysiology of Chorioamnionitis: Host Immunity and Microbial Virulence

Thomas A. Hooven | Tara M. Randis

INTRODUCTION

Approximately 1% to 10% of all births in the United States are complicated by chorioamnionitis,[1-3] but the incidence varies significantly by study population, gestational age at presentation, and diagnostic criteria.[4] *Histologic chorioamnionitis* is a pathologic term that refers to an influx of maternal inflammatory cells (neutrophils, macrophages, and T cells) into the placental membranes.[3] The term *clinical chorioamnionitis* is used when overt signs of intraamniotic infection—such as maternal fever, leukocytosis, and uterine tenderness—are present.[4] Although histologic and clinical chorioamnionitis frequently occur together in response to invading microorganisms, histologic chorioamnionitis is three times more common.[5] It is therefore possible to have pathologically significant inflammatory lesions in the placenta with no intrapartum clinical signs and a negative amniotic fluid culture. Furthermore, only about two-thirds of women with suspected clinical chorioamnionitis have histologic evidence of placental inflammation.[6] A recent update to clinical guidelines issued by the American College of Obstetrics and Gynecology acknowledges the potential gaps between isolated maternal fever, suspected intraamniotic infection (maternal fever with one or more additional signs of chorioamnionitis), and confirmed intraamniotic infection (confirmation is achieved by laboratory testing of the amniotic fluid).[7] Invading pathogens differ in their ability to induce a host inflammatory response; some organisms cause a more chronic subclinical infection, whereas others induce a robust, clinically apparent inflammatory syndrome.[8] *Intrauterine infection and/or inflammation (III)* is sometimes used as an alternative diagnostic term to more precisely describe the clinical spectrum of chorioamnionitis.[9]

Intrauterine infections are almost always polymicrobial and often involve fastidious organisms, making culture-based identification unreliable. The use of molecular-based techniques for microbial detection, most notably broad-range16s rDNA polymerase chain reaction (PCR), has provided a more accurate estimate of the frequency of microbial invasion of the amniotic cavity[10] and may explain some of the disparity in the reported frequencies of clinical infection versus histologic inflammation. Although the presence of microbial DNA in amniotic fluid has been associated with increased proinflammatory signaling and adverse pregnancy outcomes,[10] data obtained using these highly sensitive detection methods raise the question of whether the presence of microbes in the intrauterine space is always pathogenic.[11-14]

Invading pathogens most frequently access the intrauterine cavity by ascending through the cervix from the lower genital tract. Organisms may also gain entry via hematogenous transmission through the placenta, retrograde migration from the abdominal cavity through the fallopian tubes, and iatrogenic introduction during amniocentesis or chorionic villus sampling.[15] This chapter reviews what is known about the anatomic and immunologic barriers that function to protect the developing fetus from intrauterine pathogens along each of these routes of infection and the microbial virulence mechanisms that have evolved to escape these host defenses. The specific fetal and maternal inflammatory responses to intrauterine infection are discussed in detail in Chapter 12.

HOST BARRIERS (FIG. 172.1)

THE LOWER GENITAL TRACT

The vast majority of intrauterine infections are caused by bacteria that first colonize or invade the vaginal epithelium and then ascend through the cervix into the upper genital tract. Therefore the epithelial cells of vaginal mucosa serve as the first line of

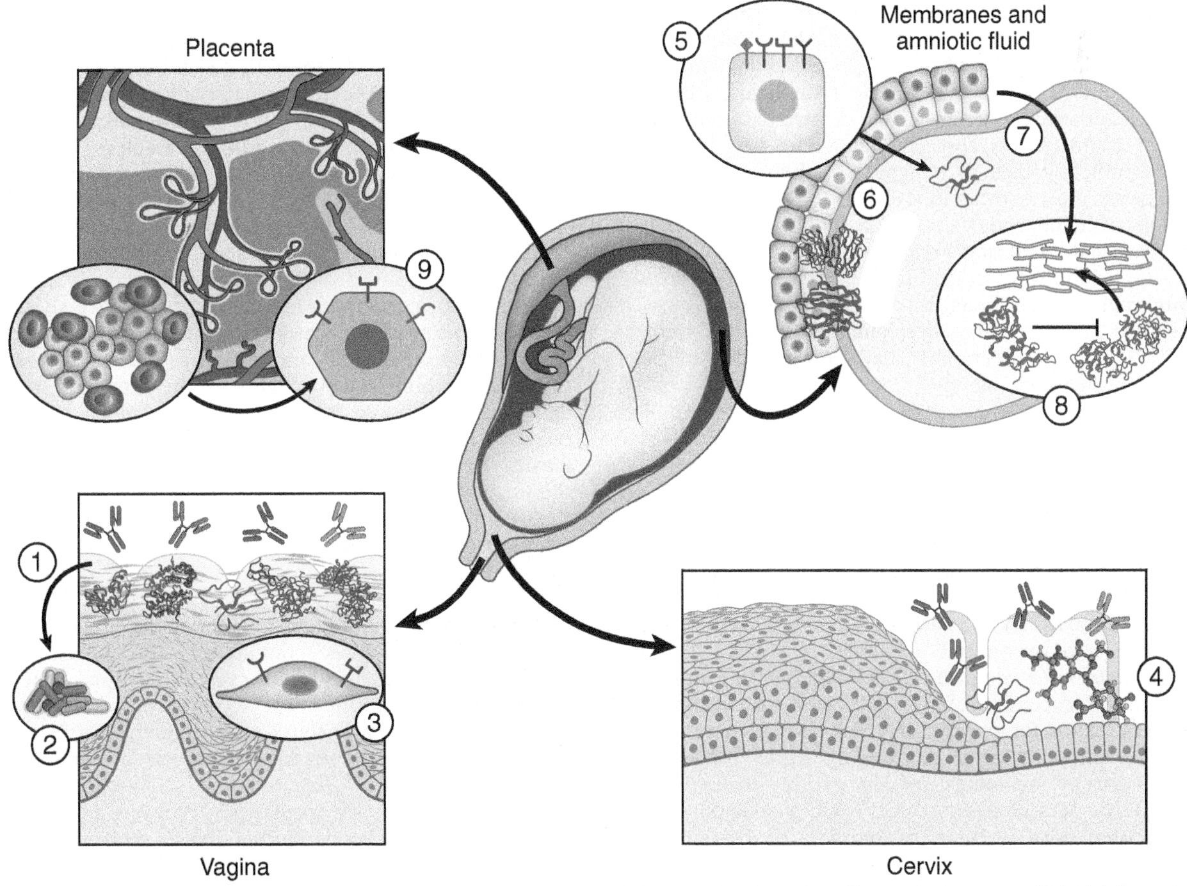

Fig. 172.1 The fetus has multiple anatomic and immune-mediated protections against infection. The vaginal mucosa (1) is rich in secreted IgA and multiple antimicrobial proteins and peptides including (from left to right) lysozyme, calprotectin, defensins, secretory leukocyte protease inhibitor, and lactoferrin. The vaginal microbiome (2) normally exerts a physiologic homeostatic role that helps to protect against dysbiosis and infection. The vaginal epithelial cells (3) express Toll-like receptors (TLRs) that, when stimulated, can activate innate immune factors to clear pathogenic organisms. The cervical mucous plug (4) is also enriched with protective immunoglobulins and defensins. Hyaluronan in the cervix contributes to a flexible barrier against ascending infection. The chorioamniotic membranes are composed of juxtaposed epithelia of maternal and fetal origins that express TLR-2, -4, -5, and -6 (5) and galectin-1 and -3 (6), both of which modulate fetal innate immunity. Secreted defensins (7) contribute to the antimicrobial properties of amniotic fluid. The physical barrier of the extracellular matrix of the membranes is continuously remodeled throughout pregnancy by matrix-metalloproteinases, whose activity is regulated by tissue inhibitors of metalloproteinase (8). In the placenta, where trophoblastic proximity to maternal cells and blood create potential for hematogenous or intercellular vertical transmission, trophoblastic TLR expression serves a protective function (9).

defense, functioning as a physical barrier that inhibits the passage of pathogens to underlying tissues. In addition, the vaginal epithelium is coated with a thin layer of mucus that not only traps infectious agents but also contains immunoglobulin (Ig)[16] and several antimicrobial peptides (AMPs), including defensins, secretory leukocyte protease inhibitor, calprotectin, lysozyme, and lacteroferrin.[17] Finally, vaginal epithelial cells express several Toll-like receptors (TLRs) and therefore are capable of sensing and rapidly responding to a wide spectrum of pathogens.[18]

THE VAGINAL MICROBIOTA

The microbial inhabitants of the female genital tract play a critical role in maintaining reproductive health. It has long been recognized that *Lactobacillus* spp. are the dominant members of the vaginal microbiota[19]; when these organisms are diminished in number or absent, the risk of acquiring urogenital infections increases. Lactobacilli protect against colonization and overgrowth of potentially pathogenic organisms through numerous mechanisms. They compete for nutrients and receptors at the epithelial surface and produce a variety of antimicrobial substances, including lactic acid (which maintains the vaginal tract at an acidic pH), bacteriocins, and hydrogen peroxide.[20] In addition, vaginal lactobacilli are capable of modulating innate immune responses in the female genital tract via the production of TLR ligands and short-chain fatty acids.[21,22] For example, exposure of a multilayer vaginal epithelial cell culture to lactobacilli significantly reduced proinflammatory cytokine secretion in an isolate-specific fashion following TLR stimulation.[22] Although there are ample in vitro data supporting the role of *Lactobacillus* spp. in maintaining vaginal health, there are conflicting data as to which of these antimicrobial mechanisms are most relevant in vivo.[23,24]

Although both the composition and stability of the vaginal microbiota is altered during pregnancy, *Lactobacillus* species remain the dominant constituents.[25-27] A *Lactobacillus*-dominant vaginal microbiota is associated with a reduced incidence of miscarriage, chorioamnionitis, and preterm delivery.[28-33] These observations have prompted numerous clinical trials investigating the potential preventative and/or therapeutic effects of administering lactobacilli-containing probiotics during pregnancy.[34-37] However, the data thus far are insufficient to incorporate this into clinical practice.[38] Of note, not all *Lactobacillus* spp. may be regarded as beneficial; *L. iners*, in particular, may destabilize the microbiota, predisposing to colonization with potentially pathogenic organisms during pregnancy and may be an independent risk factor for preterm birth.[39-41]

Bacterial vaginosis (BV) is a dysbiosis characterized by a loss of lactobacilli and overgrowth of other anaerobic microbes including *Gardnerella vaginalis*, *Bacteroides* spp., *Mobiluncus* spp., *Peptostreptococcus* spp., and *Mycoplasma hominis*. BV is a known risk factor for preterm delivery and miscarriage.[42,43] However, the physiologic mechanisms by which BV leads to adverse pregnancy outcomes remain poorly understood. It is possible that replacement of the *Lactobacillus*-dominated microbial community with an overgrowth of BV-associated organisms stimulates a local or systemic inflammatory response that ultimately reaches the intrauterine environment. Although increases in local cytokine concentrations have been documented during BV, several studies have shown that circulating levels of serum cytokines remain unchanged.[44-46] BV has been associated with endometritis,[47,48] which may in itself predispose to early pregnancy loss or subsequent intrauterine infection.[49] It is plausible that the direct ascension of BV-associated bacteria into the intrauterine space may be responsible for observed pregnancy complications.[50,51] A 2015 study of otherwise healthy nonpregnant women (without BV) undergoing hysterectomy demonstrated that the upper genital tract is routinely colonized with vaginal species that generally do not elicit a strong proinflammatory response.[52,53] Hillier and colleagues reported that BV was significantly associated with the isolation of microorganisms from the chorioamnion.[53] DiGiulio and colleagues, using both standard culture and broad-range PCR to analyze the amniotic fluid of women in spontaneous preterm labor with intact membranes, documented the presence of *G. vaginalis* and other BV-associated organisms.[10]

Aerobic vaginitis (AV) is another type of vaginal dysbiosis in which there is a decreased abundance of lactobacilli and a predominance of aerobic microflora composed largely of enteric commensals or pathogens (e.g., *Escherichia coli*, *Staphylococcus aureus*, and group B *Streptococcus* [GBS]).[54] In contrast to BV, AV is characterized by the presence of toxic-appearing leukocytes and parabasal cells, which are considered to be indicative of severe epithelial inflammation. This robust local inflammatory response is associated with significantly increased interleukin (IL)-6 and IL-1β concentrations in vaginal fluid.[54] Given that many of these enteric organisms are often associated with chorioamnionitis, it is not surprising that some investigators have demonstrated an association between a diagnosis of AV during the first trimester of pregnancy and an increased risk of preterm birth, chorioamnionitis, and fetal funisitis.[32,55]

Because of the consistent association of these vaginal dysbioses (BV and AV) with adverse pregnancy outcomes, some hypothesize that the risk of ascending infection and preterm birth is secondary to the absence of lactobacilli rather than to the presence of other potentially pathogenic microorganisms.[29,56] However, investigations using non-culture based methodologies are not supportive of this hypothesis. Romero and colleagues demonstrated that there were no differences in the relative abundance of microbial phylotypes between women who had a spontaneous preterm delivery and those who delivered at term.[57] Furthermore, in both of these patient groups, the composition of the vaginal microbiota during pregnancy changes as a function of gestational age, with an increase in the relative abundance of *Lactobacillus* species as gestation advances.[57] Data from another study suggest that the composition of intestinal, rather than vaginal, microbiota is associated with the likelihood for preterm delivery.[58] This is an interesting finding, given the extensive remodeling of the intestinal microbiota that is reported to occur during the course of pregnancy.[59] Our overall understanding of the impact of the human microbiota on pregnancy outcome is clearly in its infancy, and this topic represents fertile ground for future research.

THE CERVIX

Cervical mucus, an important component of defense against mucosal pathogens, is continuously produced at a rate determined by the menstrual cycle in nonpregnant women. During pregnancy, the rate of cervical mucus production decreases secondary to the waning influence of estrogen, and the mucus becomes increasingly more viscous due to increasing progesterone.[60] The resultant cervical mucous plug (CMP) may be considered "the gatekeeper," because both its physical and immunologic properties function to prevent the ascent of microbes into the intrauterine space.[61]

The CMP is primarily composed of mucin produced by secretory cells that reside within the glandlike crypts of the cervical canal.[62,63] Mucins provide the basic structural framework and confer important rheologic properties to the cervical plug, thereby contributing to the structural barrier function.[61,64] In addition, mucins exhibit a number of critical immune functions, including serving as ligands for cytokines, lectins, and adhesion molecules.[65] Although the distal segment of the CMP contains relatively few cells, the proximal portion is rich in neutrophils, macrophages, and epithelial cells that secrete immunologically important proteins and peptides. IgG and IgA concentrations in the CMP are significantly higher than those found in the cervical mucus of nonpregnant women,[66] and numerous AMPs are present within the CMP at concentrations believed to be bactericidal to common intrauterine pathogens.[67] One recent study examining the antimicrobial properties of proteins extracted from human CMP specimens failed to demonstrate direct bactericidal activity against GBS.[68] However, CMP-derived proteins augmented the opsonophagocytic killing of GBS. In addition, the CMP appeared to function as a biologic reservoir for parenterally administered antibiotics.

Elevated concentrations of proinflammatory cytokines in the cervicovaginal secretions are associated with intraamniotic infection and subsequent preterm birth.[69-71] It is unclear whether these cytokines are merely a marker for an existing intrauterine infection or somehow predispose the host to subsequent microbial invasion. It has been hypothesized that an exaggerated local inflammatory response may lead to microscopic disruption in the amniotic membranes, thus permitting the entry of microorganisms.[72] Conversely, other investigators have observed that low concentrations of cervical cytokines are associated with an increased risk of subsequent chorioamnionitis[73] and preterm birth.[74] Generalized immune hyporesponsiveness of the host may create a permissive environment for ascending infection during pregnancy.[73] Taken together, these disparate findings suggest that women who are at either extreme of immune responsiveness may be at risk for infection- and inflammation-mediated adverse obstetric events.[73]

The extracellular matrix of the cervical tissues also contributes to its barrier function. Hyaluronan (hyaluronic acid) is a large linear polysaccharide found ubiquitously in the extracellular matrix of all mammalian tissues. Throughout pregnancy, hyaluronan levels increase within the cervix[75] and are critical to the process of cervical remodeling/ripening just before parturition.[76,77] Evidence shows that hyaluronan also contributes to cervical epithelial barrier function and functions to protect against infection-mediated preterm birth. Specifically, depletion of hyaluronan in the vagina and cervix resulted in substantially increased preterm birth in a mouse model of ascending *E. coli* infection.[78] GBS and other gram-positive pathogens secrete hyaluronidases that aid in tissue invasion.[79]

FETAL MEMBRANES

The chorioamniotic membranes, derived from extraembryonic tissues of the zygote, surround and protect the developing fetus, and represent the final physical barrier against intraamniotic bacteria. The amnion has an inner layer of epithelial cells characterized by tight intercellular junctions that are in direct contact with amniotic fluid (Fig. 172.2).[80] These epithelial cells are planted on a basement membrane that is connected to a thin but strong connective tissue layer rich in collagen. With advancing gestation, the expanding amnion becomes functionally fused to the chorion, although it remains anatomically separated by a spongy layer of extracellular matrix. Adjacent to this is the tough fibrous tissue layer of the chorionic membrane. The outermost surface of the chorion contains a highly variable layer of trophoblast cells that persist until term.[81]

The connective tissue layers of the chorioamnion provides the tensile strength and elastic recoil needed as fetal growth and movement increase with gestation. The matrix-metalloproteinases (MMPs) are a family of zinc-dependent endopeptidases that are responsible for remodeling of the physiologic membrane as needed throughout pregnancy as well as for the activation of labor at term.[82] Control of MMP activity is complex and tightly regulated at the transcriptional, translational, and posttranslational levels.[83-85] Furthermore, specific inhibitors known as *tissue inhibitors of metalloproteinases (TIMPs)* are present in the tissues and provide local regulation of MMPs activity. Disruption of the MMP/TIMP balance may result in weakening of the chorioamnion's extracellular matrix via increased collagen degradation. This weakening may predispose to preterm premature rupture of membranes (pPROM), thereby exposing the fetus to intrauterine or cervical microbes. Early investigation of using MMP levels in maternal plasma as a potential biomarker for pPROM has shown signs of promise.[86]

Although bacterial invasion of the amniotic cavity is an expected consequence of membrane rupture, there are

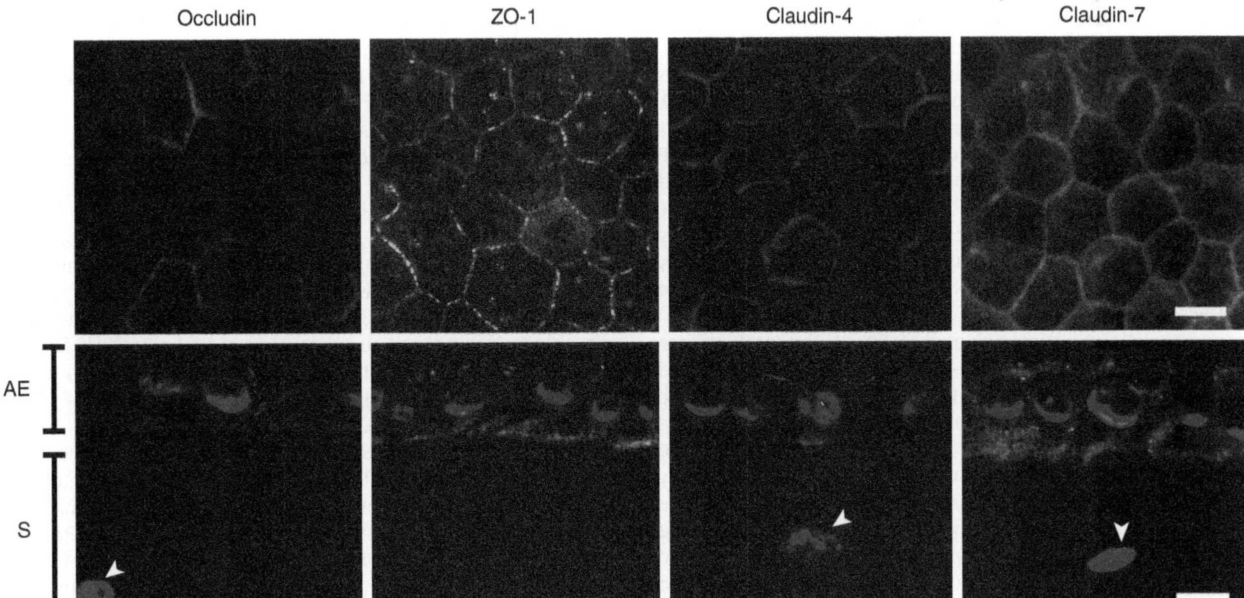

Fig. 172.2 Tight junctions along the inner surface of the amnion epithelium. Fluorescent immunostaining of human fetal membranes shows expression of four tight junction proteins in cells of the amnion epithelium *(AE)* in parallel *(top row)* and cross-sectional *(bottom row)* orientations but not in stromal *(S)* tissue. Blue coloration is DAPI staining of nucleic acid. *White arrowheads* show fibroblasts existing in the stromal tissue. Scale bars = 10 μm. (From Kobayashi K, Kadohira I, Tanaka M, et al. Expression and distribution of tight junction proteins in human amnion during late pregnancy. *Placenta*. 2010;31:158–162.)

sufficient data to conclude that pathogens and the subsequent host response together play a causative role. Numerous bacterial products (enzymes and toxins) may directly disrupt or weaken the chorioamnion.[87] Proinflammatory signaling cascades triggered by invading pathogens are characterized by the production of cytokines that are known to induce the production of MMPs and apoptotic signaling within the membranes (reviewed in detail in Chapter 12).[88,89]

The chorioamniotic membranes not only provide a physical barrier to organisms ascending from the lower genital tract but also directly contribute to innate immunity. Studies using human amniotic epithelial cell culture reveal that amniotic epithelial cells express several TLRs, including TLR-2, TLR-4, TLR-5, and TLR-6.[90,91] Stimulation of these receptors by their respective agonists leads to a diverse array of downstream effects that include activation of NF-κB signaling pathways, stimulation of cytokine secretion, recruitment and activation of neutrophils, upregulation of MMP activity, and induction of apoptosis.[92,93] Interestingly, membrane expression of TLRs and subsequent signaling cascades vary by race[94] and by specific pathogen exposure,[95-97] suggesting that there may be heterogeneity in the mechanisms by which infection-associated pregnancy complications such as pPROM and preterm birth arise. Immunohistochemical staining of membranes of women in preterm labor without chorioamnionitis has revealed that TLR-2 expression specifically was polarized to the basal rather than apical surface of the amniotic epithelial cells.[96] Because the most common pathway of intrauterine infection is via the ascension of organisms from the lower genital tract, invading pathogens will first interact with the decidua, chorion, and basal surface of the amniotic epithelium. Thus this geographic distribution of TLR-2 may potentially maximize the engagement of the innate immune system in cases of ascending infection.[96]

In addition to their ability to induce proinflammatory signaling via TLR stimulation, fetal membranes also exhibit intrinsic antimicrobial properties.[98] Chorioamniotic membranes obtained from healthy women at term exhibited an inhibitory effect on the growth of a variety of bacterial species in vitro, including GBS, group A *Streptococcus*, *S. aureus*, and *Staphylococcus saprophyticus*.[99] The mechanisms underlying the inhibition of bacterial growth are relatively unknown. However, evidence suggests that membrane production of soluble factors such as AMPs may be responsible. Cultured extraplacental membranes have been shown to express human β-defensin (HBD)-1, HBD-2, HBD-3, and lactoferrin.[100] Furthermore, exposure of these tissues to pathogenic bacteria such as GBS and *E. coli* induces AMP expression. Exposure to GBS specifically results in increased expression of HBD-2 and HBD-3.[100-102] Because of these intrinsic antimicrobial properties, amniotic membranes have been widely used as biologic dressings in a multitude of surgical applications; they have been shown to reduce bacterial counts and promote wound healing.[103]

The epithelial and mesenchymal cells of the amnion are of particular interest because they have several observed antiinflammatory properties. Studies of human amniotic membrane tissues have demonstrated the expression of proinflammatory cytokine receptor antagonists,[104] active secretion of TIMPs,[105] and mechanical trapping of inflammatory cells within the matrix.[106] The vast majority of these data come from the field of ophthalmology, where amniotic membrane transplantation is used for a wide spectrum of ophthalmic indications including corneal and conjunctival injuries.[107] The potential contribution of these antiinflammatory amniotic cells to the development of maternal-fetal immune tolerance is an intriguing but relatively unexplored concept.

A demonstration that immunomodulatory galectin (Gal) proteins 1 and 3 are expressed on the amniotic epithelium and chorioamniotic mesoderm has led some to hypothesize such a role for these molecules.[108] Gal-1 is a carbohydrate-binding lectin known to inhibit neutrophil extravasation, reduce the release of proinflammatory cytokines from T cells, and aid in establishment and maintenance of T-cell tolerance. Interestingly, in patients with pPROM, galectin-1 mRNA expression in the fetal membranes was found to be higher in those women with histologic chorioamnionitis than in those without.[109] These data suggest that Gal-1 may also contribute to the fetal antiinflammatory response in the setting of intrauterine infection.

Gal-3 has a more proinflammatory valence and has been implicated in rheumatologic disease, cardiovascular disease, and cancer.[110-112] Gal-3 expression has been demonstrated on amniotic epithelial cells in the setting of pPROM with histologic chorioamnionitis[113] and has been shown to be upregulated in a mouse model of gingival infection associated with preterm birth.[114] Together, these studies suggest a possible role for the balance between Gal-1 and Gal-3 (perhaps with other immunomodulators expressed in the chorioamniotic membranes) on the stability of the membrane barrier.

PLACENTAL BARRIERS

Pathogens may reach the placenta through maternal blood or via ascension from the lower genital tract. Hematogenous transmission may occur during episodes of transient bacteremia, and recent work has shown differences between the blood microbiome of pregnant women who deliver prematurely and those who carry their pregnancies to term.[115] The transit of pathogens from mother to fetus can occur at two distinct sites in the placenta where there is direct contact between maternal cells and fetal trophoblast cells: (1) the uterine implantation site, where maternal immune and endothelial cells are juxtaposed to extravillous trophoblasts (EVTs), and (2) the maternal blood surrounding the syncytiotrophoblasts (Fig. 172.3).[116]

The syncytiotrophoblast, or syncytium, is the largest maternal-fetal interface and is composed of a continuous layer of fused multinucleated trophoblasts that are bathed in maternal blood. The syncytium mediates the exchange of nutrients and gases between the mother and fetus. The human syncytium demonstrates a unique resistance to both viral and bacterial pathogens through a variety of mechanisms. The formation of a fused multinucleate syncytium foregoes the need for intercellular junctions, which may be used by pathogens to breach cellular barriers.[117] The multinucleate syncytium may therefore have evolved as a defense mechanism.[118] This lack of intercellular junctions has been postulated to play a role in placental resistance to herpes simplex virus[119] and cytomegalovirus[120] infections. The basal surface of the syncytium has a dense cytoskeletal network that functions as a biophysical barrier against pathogen invasion.[121]

The second point of direct contact between maternal and fetal cells is formed by EVTs invading deep into the uterine implantation site, which contains an abundance of maternal leukocytes. Most pathogens that invade the placenta and/or fetus are able to infect them and to survive in leukocytes.[118] Data from animal models and primary human placental organ cultures suggest that the implantation site is the preferred site of entry for *Listeria monocytogenes*.[122-124]

Trophoblasts express a variety of pattern recognition receptors (PRRs) that allow them to respond to the presence of viral and bacterial pathogens. The expression of TLRs in the placental tissues varies throughout gestation, as does their differential responses to stimulation.[125] TLR-2 and TLR-4 proteins are highly expressed by EVTs in the first trimester but not by the syncytiotrophoblast cells. By the third trimester, TLR-2 and TLR-4 are expressed in the outer syncytiotrophoblast layer as well. It has been hypothesized that this altered pattern of TLR expression may reflect changes in placental function as gestation progresses.[92] Upon stimulation, trophoblast TLRs may produce a number of antimicrobial products that may inhibit invading

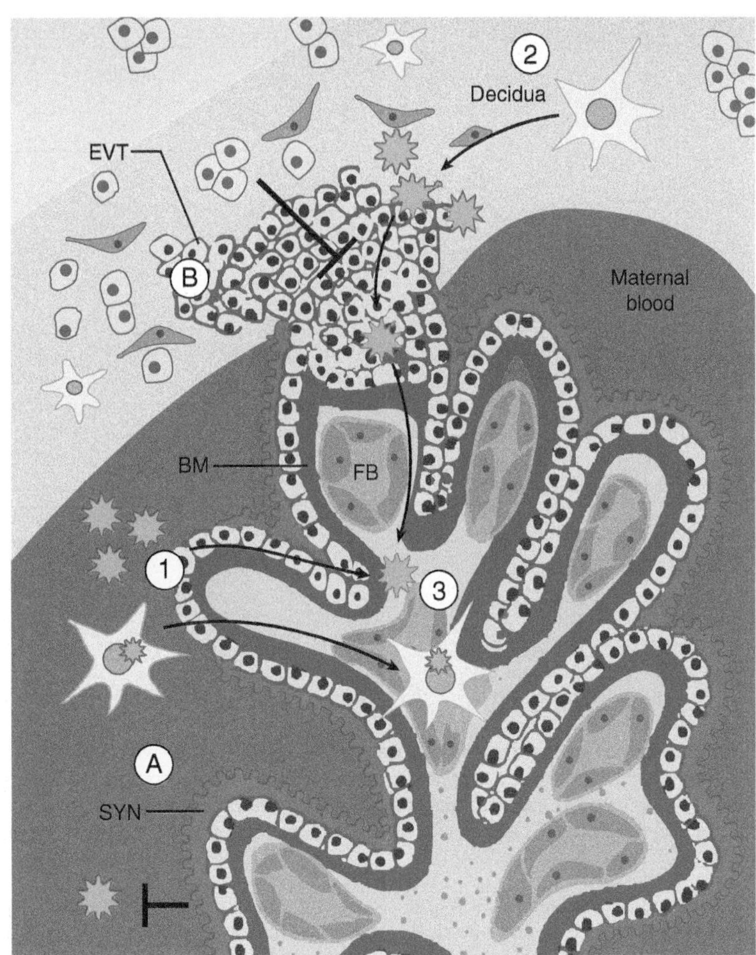

Fig. 172.3 The human maternal–fetal interface. The two sites of direct contact between maternal and fetal cells are the syncytiotrophoblasts *(SYN)* (A) and the extravillous trophoblast *(EVT)* (B). The basement membrane *(BM)*, located below the trophoblast, presents an additional physical barrier. Damage of the syncytiotrophoblast enables pathogens *(green stars)* that are free in maternal blood or inside maternal leukocytes *(yellow cells)* to cross into fetal tissues *(1)*. Most placental infections originate in the uterine decidua *(2)*, which is minimally accessible from the maternal blood. Pathogens can reach the decidua only by dissemination in maternal cells, most likely leukocytes. If the defense mechanisms of the EVT are overcome, the infection may spread to the fetal blood *(FB) (3)*. (From Robbins JR, Bakardjiev AI. Pathogens and the placental fortress. *Curr Opin Microbiol.* 2012;15:36–43.)

pathogens.[126,127] Trophoblasts also express cytoplasmic-based PRRs known as *Nod-like receptors (NLRs)*.[128] Stimulation of NLRs by intracellular bacterial cell products activates inflammasomes, triggering subsequent proinflammatory response. Therefore NLRs may provide a second line of defense, facilitating trophoblast responses to microorganisms that have gained access to the cell's intracellular space.[129]

AMNIOTIC FLUID

The antibacterial properties of amniotic fluid are well characterized.[130] Numerous AMPs and proteins are present in amniotic fluid throughout gestation, including human neutrophil peptides 1, 2, and 3, lysozyme, bactericidal/permeability-increasing protein, LL-37, calprotectin, macrophage inhibitory factor, ubiquitin, hyaluronan, β_2 microglobulin, and lactoferrin.[131-133] These potent antimicrobials exhibit broad-spectrum activity against bacteria, fungi, and viruses. Soluble receptors, including a truncated form of TLR-2 (sTLR-2) and TNF receptors (sTNFR1, sTNFR2), are also present and may function as decoy ligands, dampening the inflammatory response to microbial pathogens.[134,135] The primary sources of these molecules are believed to be amniotic epithelial cells, fetal skin, and lung. In the setting of inflammation, fetal neutrophils also contribute (Fig. 172.4).[136] Elevated concentrations of these peptides have been documented in the setting of infection, preterm parturition, and pPROM, highlighting the capacity of the fetal innate immune system to react and respond (Fig. 172.5).[132,137,138] Recent investigations characterizing the amniotic fluid proteome and metabolome have identified novel candidate biomarkers for adverse pregnancy outcomes.[139,140] The fetal inflammatory response is characterized by the presence of several proinflammatory cytokines and chemokines in the amniotic fluid (discussed in detail in Chapter 121). This amniotic fluid cytokine profile has both diagnostic and prognostic utility in the setting of chorioamnionitis and fetal infection.

MECHANISMS OF MICROBIAL VIRULENCE

Stimulation of maternal and fetal innate immune systems by pathogen-association molecular patterns is fundamental to the pathogenesis of intrauterine infection and subsequent preterm birth. Components of the bacterial cell wall or outer cell membrane—including lipoteichoic acid, peptidoglycan, and lipopolysaccharide—are potent inducers of innate immune signaling, as they are recognized by PRRs located throughout the

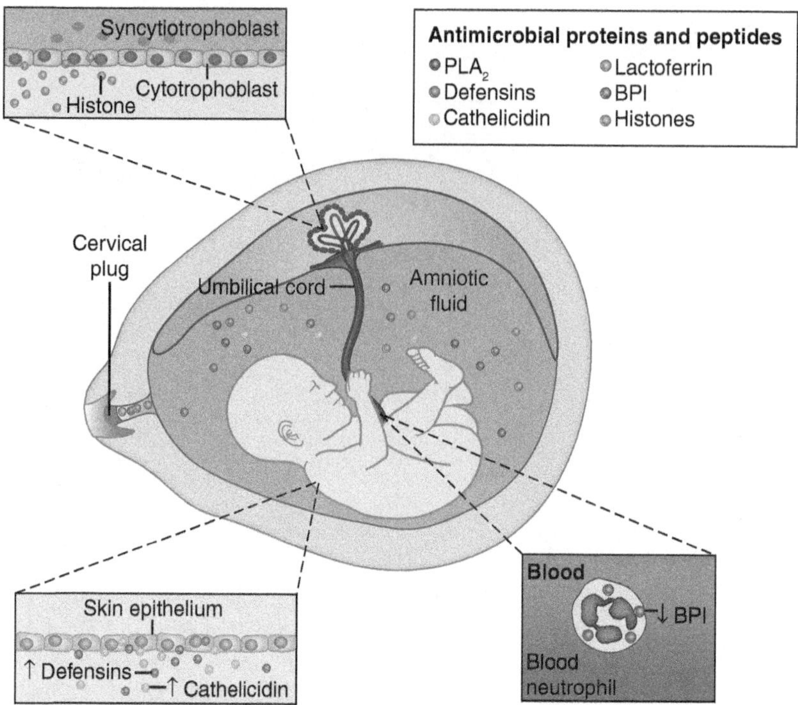

Fig. 172.4 Antimicrobial proteins and peptides within the amniotic cavity. The cervical plug, which contains many antimicrobial molecules, serves to separate potential pathogens colonizing the vaginal epithelium from the intrauterine compartment. The maternal-fetal membranes of the placenta and fetus secrete various antimicrobial peptides into the amniotic fluid. *BPI*, Bactericidal/permeability-increasing protein; *PLA₂*, phospholipase A2. (From Levy O. Innate immunity of the newborn: basic mechanisms and clinical correlates. *Nat Rev Immunol.* 2007;7:379–390.)

female genital tract, placental tissues, and fetal membranes. Many of these bacterial products have been utilized in animal models of intrauterine infection and have shed considerable light on the mechanistic link between maternal-fetal inflammation and preterm delivery. The use of live organisms in both animal models and tissue culture models has yielded considerable data regarding specific bacterial virulence factors that promote invasion of the amniotic cavity and evasion of host immune responses. Those virulence factors are discussed in detail further on.

PORE-FORMING TOXINS

Several intrauterine pathogens are known to produce pore-forming toxins (*E. coli*, *L. monocytogenes*, *G. vaginalis*, and GBS). Although the mechanistic contribution of most of these toxins to the pathogenesis of intrauterine infection is largely unknown, investigations highlight their importance in breaching maternal-fetal barriers and resisting immune clearance.

GBS produces β-hemolysin/cytolysin (βH/C), a surface-associated pore-forming toxin that is cytolytic for eukaryotic cells. Biochemically, βH/C is an ornithine rhamnolipid that is responsible for both the characteristic pigment of GBS colonies as well as the surrounding zone of β hemolysis observed when they are grown on blood-containing agar.[141] In addition to its cytolytic activity, βH/C induces apoptosis, recruits neutrophils, stimulates cytokine release, and enhances bacterial intracellular invasion.[142] βH/C plays a critical role in invasive GBS neonatal diseases including sepsis, pneumonia, and meningitis.[143-145] Several lines of evidence suggest that this toxin is essential in the pathogenesis of intrauterine infection as well.

In vitro data demonstrate that βH/C production is necessary for GBS penetration of chorioamniotic membranes and that it promotes invasion of human amniotic epithelial cells.[141] Furthermore, GBS is capable of inducing trophoblast cell death in a βH/C-dependent manner.[146] βH/C contributes to GBS evasion of the host immune responses by enhancing survival within macrophages and neutrophils, thereby avoiding phagocytic clearance[147] and stimulating the release of the antiinflammatory cytokine IL-10. In a murine model of ascending GBS infection during pregnancy, GBS strains expressing the βH/C toxin exhibit a significant competitive colonization advantage over a toxin-deficient mutant strain.[148] Once in the intrauterine space, βH/C induces robust placental inflammation and subsequent fetal infection, culminating in preterm delivery or intrauterine fetal demise.[148]

Lysteriolysin O (LLO) is a cholesterol-dependent pore-forming toxin produced by *L. monocytogenes*, a facultative intracellular pathogen. It enters host cells via phagocytosis or is internalized via interaction of bacterial surface proteins with host-cell receptors. Successful intracellular replication of this organism then relies upon the escape of the bacteria from the acidified vacuole or phagosome into the cytoplasm.[149] Because LLO exhibits maximal activity at an acidic pH, it ruptures the vacuole, thus enabling the release of bacteria into the neutral cytosolic environment without subsequent damage to the plasma membrane.[150,151] Recent work has shown that LLO also prevents host-cell mitophagy (cellular consumption of its own mitochondria) in order to promote bacterial intracellular survival.[152] The specific role of LLO in intrauterine infection is not well understood. Transmission of *L. monocytogenes* from mother to fetus occurs via hematogenous spread to the placenta with subsequent invasion of EVTs. In primary human EVT cultures, *L. monocytogenes* becomes trapped inside the vacuoles despite the production of LLO.[153] This apparent bottleneck in *L. monocytogenes* transmission at the level of the EVT is a distinctly unique aspect of the maternal-fetal interface. In vivo investigations by Le Monnier and colleagues yield contradictory data. Using a murine model of placental infection, they demonstrated that LLO is absolutely required for bacterial growth in murine trophoblastic cells and subsequent fetal invasion.[154]

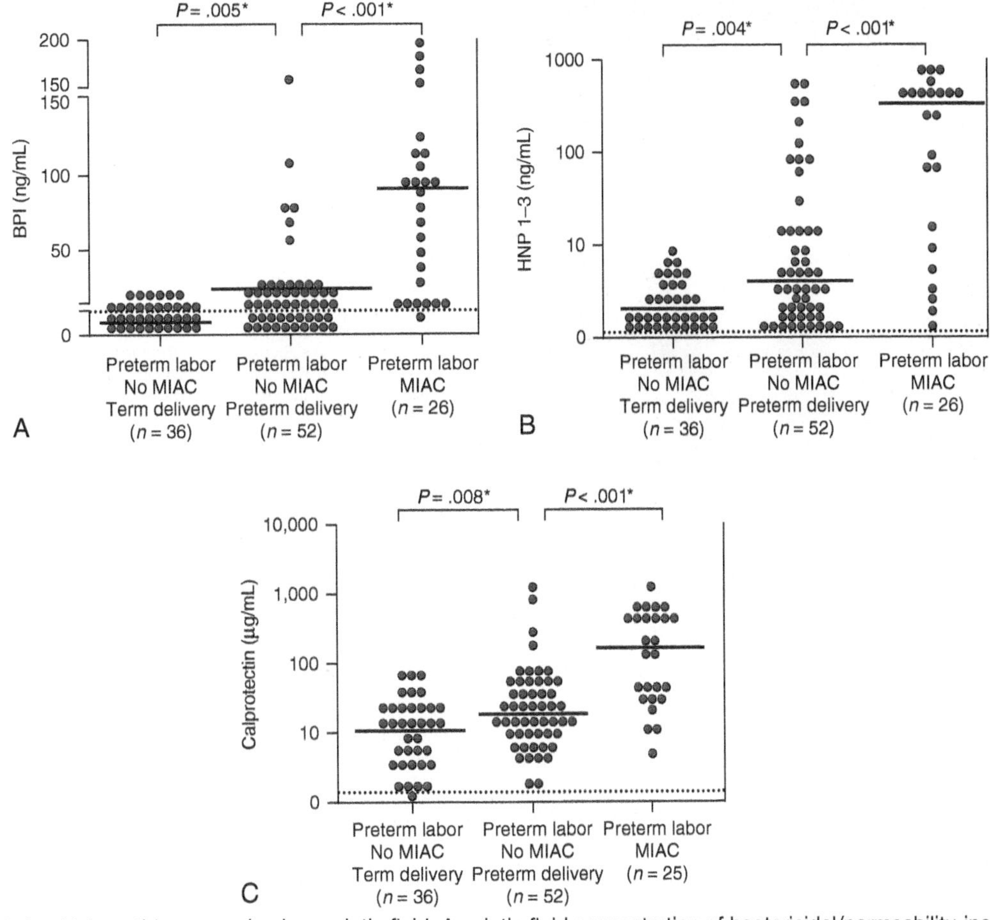

Fig. 172.5 Antimicrobial peptide expression in amniotic fluid. Amniotic fluid concentration of bactericidal/permeability-increasing protein *(BPI)* (A), human neutrophil defensins *(HNP)* 1–3 (B), and calprotectin (C) in women with preterm labor and intact membranes. *Dotted lines* indicate detection limits. *MIAC*, Microbial invasion of the amniotic cavity. (From Espinoza J, Chaiworapongsa T, Romero R, et al. Antimicrobial peptides in amniotic fluid: defensins, calprotectin and bacterial/permeability-increasing protein in patients with microbial invasion of the amniotic cavity, intra-amniotic inflammation, preterm labor and premature rupture of membranes. *J Matern Fetal Neonatal Med*. 2003;13:2–21.)

CELLULAR TARGETING AND TRANSMISSION

The tropism of *L. monocytogenes* for fetoplacental tissues raises the possibility that a specific mechanism may be responsible for targeting bacteria to the maternal-fetal barrier.[155] Previous data demonstrate that internalization of *L. monocytogenes* into nonphagocytic cells is mediated by the interaction of a bacterial surface protein known as *internalin*, with its human receptor, E-cadherin.[156] The internalin-E-cadherin interaction is necessary for *L. monocytogenes* to cross the intestinal epithelium and blood-brain barriers to cause gastroenteritis and meningitis, respectively.[155] This same mechanism is exploited by *L. monocytogenes* to target and cross the human placental tissues. Investigation of the cellular patterns of expression of E-cadherin at the maternal-fetal interface demonstrated that it is located on the basal and apical plasma membranes of syncytiotrophoblasts and on villous cytotrophoblasts.[155] Primary trophoblast cultures and placental villous explants have demonstrated that bacterial entry into syncytiotrophoblasts occurs via the apical membrane in a manner dependent on internalin-E-cadherin.[155]

Another unique feature of *L. monocytogenes* is that it can spread directly from cell to cell without leaving the cytoplasm. Mechanistically, this occurs because of the actions of the actin assembly-inducing protein (ActA).[157] This protein induces actin polymerization on the bacterial surface, thereby generating an actin "comet tail" that serves to propel the organism through the cytoplasm and into neighboring cells.[158] ActA-mediated cell-to-cell spreading promotes vertical transmission of *L. monocytogenes* to the fetus by allowing bacteria to pass through trophoblast and endothelial cell layers in a murine model.[154]

BIOFILM FORMATION

The formation of biofilms is a major microbial survival strategy, promoting bacterial recalcitrance to both antibiotic therapy and host immune responses. Biofilm formation by bacteria colonizing the lower genital tract may displace healthy flora, alter the local vaginal epithelial cell microenvironment, and lead to chronic dysbioses. Many organisms associated with ascending intrauterine infection during pregnancy are capable of biofilm formation, including *G. vaginalis*, *Ureaplasma* spp., *Mycoplasma* spp., and GBS.[159-162] *G. vaginalis*, in particular, forms adherent biofilms to the vaginal epithelium and is a major contributor to treatment failure and recurrent disease in women with BV.[162] Investigations using fluorescence in situ hybridization (FISH) demonstrate the presence of structured polymicrobial *G. vaginalis*-dominated biofilms that extend into the endometrium and fallopian tubes of pregnant women (Fig. 172.6).[48] The extension of biofilms into the upper genital tract has significant implications for our understanding of pathogenesis infection-related adverse pregnancy outcomes.

Sonographic imaging during pregnancy occasionally reveals the presence of particulate matter in amniotic fluid near the cervix, a finding that is commonly referred to as amniotic fluid "sludge." This sludge is hypothesized to represent clusters of bacteria and inflammatory cells and may be indicative of chronic

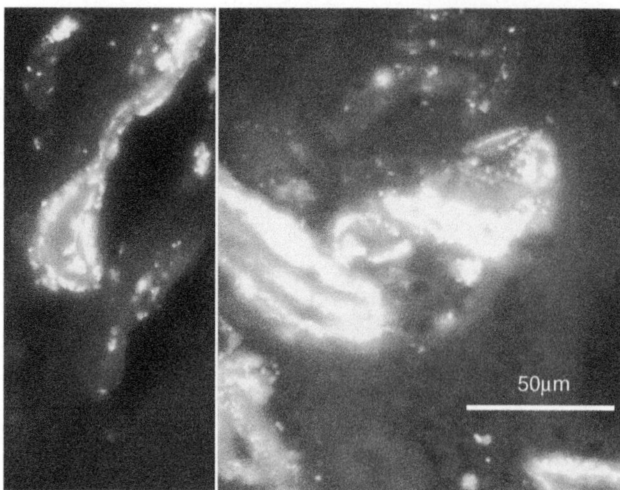

Fig. 172.6 *Gardnerella*-dominated polymicrobial biofilm extends into the uterine cavity. Fluorescent in situ hybridization (FISH) reveals a *Gardnerella*-dominated biofilm within follicular *(left panel)* and luteal *(right panel)* endometrium. Hybridization is performed with a *Gard C3* orange fluorescence FISH probe at magnification ×1000. (From Swidsinski A, Verstraelen H, Loening-Baucke V, et al. Presence of a polymicrobial endometrial biofilm in patients with bacterial vaginosis. *PLoS One*. 2013;8:e53997.)

intraamniotic infection.[163,164] Investigations using scanning electron microscopy and FISH to examine this particulate matter have confirmed the presence of bacterial cells as well as an exopolymeric matrix material that is typical of microbial biofilms.[165] Several epidemiologic studies and case reports demonstrate an association between the presence of sludge and adverse pregnancy outcomes.[163,164,166]

CONCLUSION

The innate immune system of the female reproductive tract consists of highly specialized mechanical, chemical, and cellular components capable of rapidly detecting and responding to invading pathogens throughout pregnancy. Commensal bacteria that colonize the female genital tract are capable of modulating these responses, although the mechanisms by which this occurs are poorly understood. Stimulation of proinflammatory signaling cascades by pathogenic bacteria or their products is fundamental to the pathogenesis of intrauterine infection and subsequent preterm birth. In vivo animal modeling has enabled the exploration of specific microbial virulence factors that promote invasion of maternal-fetal barriers and enhance escape from host immune cell clearance. These factors may serve as candidate targets in the development of novel strategies to reduce the incidence of intrauterine infection and prevent associated maternal and neonatal morbidities.

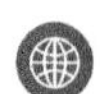 A complete reference list is available at www.ExpertConsult.com.

SELECT REFERENCES

3. Redline RW. Placental inflammation. *Semin Neonatol*. 2004;9:265–274.
8. Goldenberg RL, Hauth JC, Andrews WW. Intrauterine infection and preterm delivery. *N Engl J Med*. 2000;342:1500–1507.
10. DiGiulio DB, Romero R, Amogan HP, et al. Microbial prevalence, diversity and abundance in amniotic fluid during preterm labor: a molecular and culture-based investigation. *PLoS One*. 2008;3:e3056.
12. Aagaard K, Ma J, Antony KM, et al. The placenta harbors a unique microbiome. *Sci Transl Med*. 2014;6:237ra265.
14. de Goffau MC, Lager S, Sovio U, et al. Human placenta has no microbiome but can contain potential pathogens. *Nature*. 2019;572:329–334.
15. Goldenberg RL, Culhane JF, Iams JD, et al. Epidemiology and causes of preterm birth. *Lancet*. 2008;371:75–84.
22. Rose 2nd WA, McGowin CL, Spagnuolo RA, et al. Commensal bacteria modulate innate immune responses of vaginal epithelial cell multilayer cultures. *PLoS One*. 2012;7:e32728.
25. Serrano MG, Parikh HI, Brooks JP, et al. Racioethnic diversity in the dynamics of the vaginal microbiome during pregnancy. *Nat Med*. 2019;25:1001–1011.
26. Romero R, Hassan SS, Gajer P, et al. The composition and stability of the vaginal microbiota of normal pregnant women is different from that of non-pregnant women. *Microbiome*. 2014;2:4.
33. Elovitz MA, Gajer P, Riis V, et al. Cervicovaginal microbiota and local immune response modulate the risk of spontaneous preterm delivery. *Nat Commun*. 2019;10:1305.
37. Othman M, Neilson JP, Alfirevic Z. Probiotics for preventing preterm labour. *Cochrane Database Syst Rev*. 2007:CD005941.
39. Callahan BJ, DiGiulio DB, Goltsman DSA, et al. Replication and refinement of a vaginal microbial signature of preterm birth in two racially distinct cohorts of US women. *Proc Natl Acad Sci U S A*. 2017;114:9966–9971.
42. Hillier SL, Nugent RP, Eschenbach DA, et al. Association between bacterial vaginosis and preterm delivery of a low-birth-weight infant. The Vaginal Infections and Prematurity Study Group. *N Engl J Med*. 1995;333:1737–1742.
48. Swidsinski A, Verstraelen H, Loening-Baucke V, et al. Presence of a polymicrobial endometrial biofilm in patients with bacterial vaginosis. *PLoS One*. 2013;8:e53997.
50. Krohn MA, Hillier SL, Nugent RP, et al. The genital flora of women with intraamniotic infection. Vaginal Infection and Prematurity Study Group. *J Infect Dis*. 1995;171:1475–1480.
57. Romero R, Hassan SS, Gajer P, et al. The vaginal microbiota of pregnant women who subsequently have spontaneous preterm labor and delivery and those with a normal delivery at term. *Microbiome*. 2014;2:18.
61. Becher N, Adams Waldorf K, Hein M, et al. The cervical mucus plug: structured review of the literature. *Acta Obstet Gynecol Scand*. 2009;88:502–513.
67. Hein M, Valore EV, Helmig RB, et al. Antimicrobial factors in the cervical mucus plug. *Am J Obstet Gynecol*. 2002;187:137–144.
69. Goepfert AR, Goldenberg RL, Andrews WW, et al. The Preterm Prediction Study: association between cervical interleukin 6 concentration and spontaneous preterm birth. *Am J Obstet Gynecol*. 2001;184:483–488.
73. Simhan HN, Caritis SN, Krohn MA, et al. Decreased cervical proinflammatory cytokines permit subsequent upper genital tract infection during pregnancy. *Am J Obstet Gynecol*. 2003;189:560–567.
78. Akgul Y, Word RA, Ensign LM, et al. Hyaluronan in cervical epithelia protects against infection-mediated preterm birth. *J Clin Invest*. 2014;124:5481–5489.
90. Gillaux C, Mehats C, Vaiman D, et al. Functional screening of TLRs in human amniotic epithelial cells. *J Immunol*. 2011;187:2766–2774.
92. Abrahams VM. Pattern recognition at the maternal-fetal interface. *Immunol Invest*. 2008;37:427–447.
95. Waring GJ, Robson SC, Bulmer JN, et al. Inflammatory signalling in fetal membranes: increased expression levels of TLR 1 in the presence of preterm histological chorioamnionitis. *PLoS One*. 2015;10:e0124298.
108. Than NG, Romero R, Erez O, et al. Emergence of hormonal and redox regulation of galectin-1 in placental mammals: implication in maternal-fetal immune tolerance. *Proc Natl Acad Sci U S A*. 2008;105:15819–15824.
113. Stefanoska I, Tadic J, Vilotic A, et al. Histological chorioamnionitis in preterm prelabor rupture of the membranes is associated with increased expression of galectin-3 by amniotic epithelium. *J Matern Fetal Neonatal Med*. 2017;30:2232–2236.
114. Miyauchi M, Ao M, Furusho H, et al. Galectin-3 plays an important role in preterm birth caused by dental infection of *Porphyromonas gingivalis*. *Sci Rep*. 2018;8:2867.
116. Robbins JR, Bakardjiev AI. Pathogens and the placental fortress. *Curr Opin Microbiol*. 2012;15:36–43.
117. Greber UF, Gastaldelli M. Junctional gating: the Achilles' heel of epithelial cells in pathogen infection. *Cell Host Microbe*. 2007;2:143–146.
118. Zeldovich VB, Bakardjiev AI. Host defense and tolerance: unique challenges in the placenta. *PLoS Pathog*. 2012;8:e1002804.
121. Zeldovich VB, Clausen CH, Bradford E, et al. Placental syncytium forms a biophysical barrier against pathogen invasion. *PLoS Pathog*. 2013;9:e1003821.
122. Robbins JR, Skrzypczynska KM, Zeldovich VB, et al. Placental syncytiotrophoblast constitutes a major barrier to vertical transmission of *Listeria monocytogenes*. *PLoS Pathog*. 2010;6:e1000732.
125. Koga K, Mor G. Expression and function of toll-like receptors at the maternal-fetal interface. *Reprod Sci*. 2008;15:231–242.
129. Abrahams VM. The role of the Nod-like receptor family in trophoblast innate immune responses. *J Reprod Immunol*. 2011;88:112–117.
134. Dulay AT, Buhimschi CS, Zhao G, et al. Soluble TLR2 is present in human amniotic fluid and modulates the intraamniotic inflammatory response to infection. *J Immunol*. 2009;182:7244–7253.
136. Levy O. Innate immunity of the newborn: basic mechanisms and clinical correlates. *Nat Rev Immunol*. 2007;7:379–390.
138. Espinoza J, Chaiworapongsa T, Romero R, et al. Antimicrobial peptides in amniotic fluid: defensins, calprotectin and bacterial/permeability-increasing protein in patients with microbial invasion of the amniotic cavity, intra-amniotic inflammation, preterm labor and premature rupture of membranes. *J Matern Fetal Neonatal Med*. 2003;13:2–21.
141. Whidbey C, Harrell MI, Burnside K, et al. A hemolytic pigment of Group B *Streptococcus* allows bacterial penetration of human placenta. *J Exp Med*. 2013;210:1265–1281.

147. Liu GY, Doran KS, Lawrence T, et al. Sword and shield: linked group B streptococcal beta-hemolysin/cytolysin and carotenoid pigment function to subvert host phagocyte defense. *Proc Natl Acad Sci U S A*. 2004;101:14491-14496.
148. Randis TM, Gelber SE, Hooven TA, et al. Group B Streptococcus beta-hemolysin/cytolysin breaches maternal-fetal barriers to cause preterm birth and intrauterine fetal demise in vivo. *J Infect Dis*. 2014;210:265-273.
152. Zhang Y, Yao Y, Qiu X, et al. *Listeria* hijacks host mitophagy through a novel mitophagy receptor to evade killing. *Nat Immunol*. 2019;20:433-446.
155. Lecuit M, Nelson DM, Smith SD, et al. Targeting and crossing of the human maternofetal barrier by Listeria monocytogenes: role of internalin interaction with trophoblast E-cadherin. *Proc Natl Acad Sci U S A*. 2004;101:6152-6157.
162. Swidsinski A, Mendling W, Loening-Baucke V, et al. An adherent *Gardnerella vaginalis* biofilm persists on the vaginal epithelium after standard therapy with oral metronidazole. *Am J Obstet Gynecol*. 2008;198:97.
165. Romero R, Schaudinn C, Kusanovic JP, et al. Detection of a microbial biofilm in intraamniotic infection. *Am J Obstet Gynecol*. 2008;198:135.

Pathophysiology of Genetic Neonatal Disease

173

Katrina A. Andrews | Sarah A. Bowdin

INTRODUCTION

Genetic diseases are a leading cause of neonatal morbidity and mortality. Estimates of the incidence of genetic disease in neonates admitted to intensive care units have historically been based on targeted genetic testing of cohorts selected to have a high pretest probability, such as those with multiple congenital anomalies. However, the neonatal presentation of many thousands of genetic diseases overlaps with common, typically nongenetic conditions such as sepsis, hypoxic ischemic encephalopathy, and in utero infections. It is now possible to explore the potential for many nonspecific, life-threatening neonatal presentations (e.g., seizures, hypotonia, respiratory and cardiac failure) to have a monogenic or genomic etiology. This has become possible with the availability of clinical grade genome-wide sequencing technologies (whole exome sequencing [WES] or whole genome sequencing [WGS]). A recent study from regional neonatal intensive care units (NICUs) in the United States estimated that the minimum incidence of genetic disease is 14%, and highlighted the benefits of ultra-rapid diagnostic testing in a subset of neonates who were gravely ill and in whom individualized management may change the outcome.[1] This study added to the increasing body of evidence to support the use of WES or WGS as a first-line test for critically ill neonates, in whom a genetic condition is suspected.[2,3] However, optimizing the clinical utility of such tests is dependent on healthcare providers understanding their strengths and limitations, as well as defining which patients will benefit, and at what point the test should be integrated into their care.

Healthcare policy makers worldwide are beginning to make decisions about the availability of, and eligibility for, neonatal genomic tests. It has never been more important for healthcare professionals who care for critically ill neonates to become familiar with the scientific rationale for the use of these evolving genomic technologies, as well as the ethical issues surrounding their implementation.

GENETIC LANDSCAPE OF NEONATAL GENETIC DISEASE

Genetic disease presenting in the neonatal intensive care unit represents the severe end of a spectrum of human genetic disease. Gains or losses of chromosome material, ranging in size from microdeletions to aneuploidies, affect the function of multiple genes required for health and development and have a tendency to present as severe prenatal or neonatal phenotypes. Because of this, the International Standard Cytogenomic Array (ISCA) Consortium recommends that a chromosomal microarray be used as a first-tier clinical diagnostic test in individuals with congenital anomalies or developmental disabilities.[4] One study of chromosome microarrays in 638 neonates with birth defects found that 2.5% had aneuploidies and 12.7% had other copy number variants (CNVs).[5] In recent years it has become possible, but is not yet routine, to detect CNVs by WES or WGS. A small but highly impactful number of diagnoses of CNVs are found in neonates in most large WES/WGS studies,[2,3,6] even though, in many centers, sick neonates would have had a chromosome microarray prior to consideration for recruitment to these studies.

With regard to genomic sequence variants, there is a preponderance towards de novo autosomal dominant and autosomal recessive disorders in neonates. As many neonatal genetic disorders affect life span and reproductive fitness, a relatively low proportion of diagnoses are likely to be explained by inherited autosomal dominant disorders with similar phenotypes across multiple generations. In large studies of whole genome or exome sequencing in neonates,[1,6,7] 46% to 84% of genetic diagnoses were autosomal dominant, 11% to 42% autosomal recessive, and 5% to 15% X-linked. In these studies, the majority (66% to 100%) of the autosomal dominant disorders were de novo rather than inherited. When a dominant genetic condition is proven to have occurred de novo in an affected neonate, there will be no family history consistent with similarly affected family members. However, there may be a history of older paternal age at conception, due to the mechanism discussed in the later section "Origin of Single Nucleotide Variants."

A similar pattern of enrichment for de novo dominant disorders is seen in larger cohorts of infants with developmental disorders, perhaps with a lower rate of diagnosis of autosomal recessive disease than in neonates. In a trio WES study of 6040 families of children with developmental disorders (Deciphering Developmental Disorders), an estimated 42% of cases can be explained by de novo coding mutations, and just 3.6% by autosomal recessive disease (in patients with European ancestry).[8,9]

Some autosomal dominant disorders exhibit remarkable differences in degrees of penetrance or expression, where the same pathogenic variant can leave the parents relatively healthy

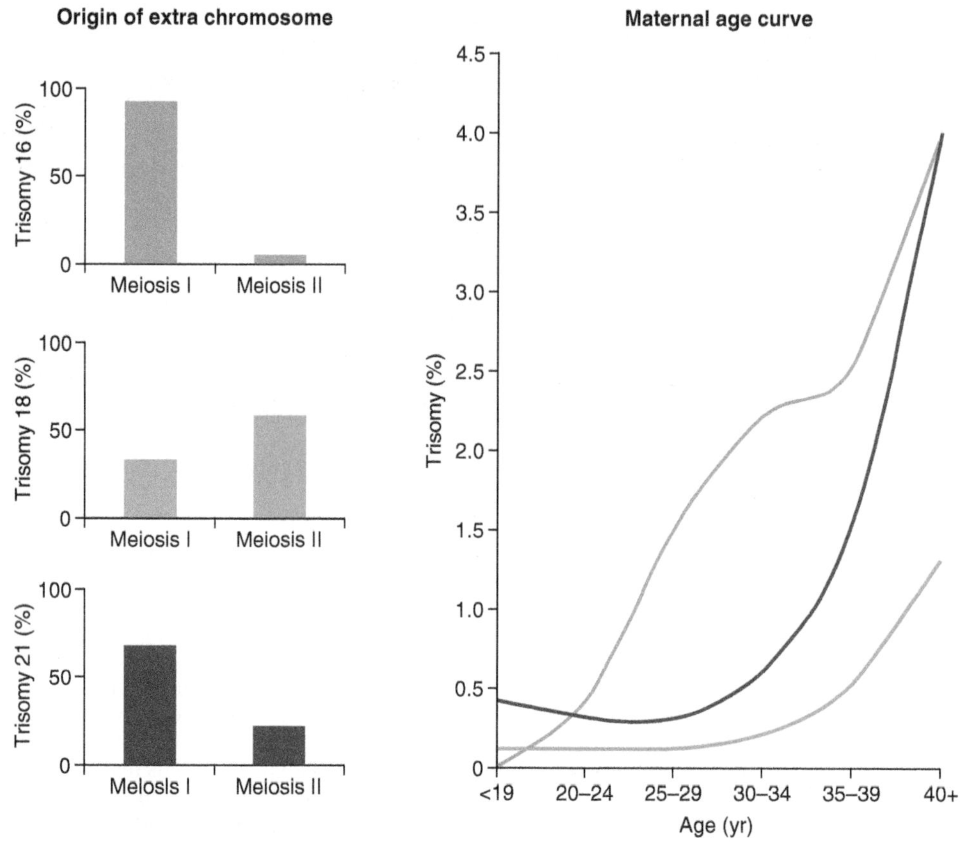

Fig. 173.1 The relative contribution of meiosis I and meiosis II errors to trisomy formation, and the relationship with maternal age, varies by chromosome. (Modified from Nagaoka SI, Hassold TJ, Hunt PA. Human aneuploidy: mechanisms and new insights into an age-old problem. *Nat Rev Genet*. 2012;13[7]:493–504. Published 2012 Jun 18. https://doi.org/10.1038/nrg3245.)

but the neonate very sick. In such instances, a detailed personal medical history and examination of the parents with additional enquiry regarding the family history can be critical.

For example, pathogenic variants in the *SCN5A* gene cause Brugada syndrome. This can predispose an individual to early-onset dangerous arrhythmias, whilst others with the same variant can remain free of arrhythmias until adulthood or for their entire lifetime.[10] The family history in this instance may be as subtle as relative or relatives who drowned or had an unexplained road traffic accident. Another example is *NOTCH1* pathogenic variants, which predispose to congenital heart disease (CHD). Penetrance is variable and can range from severe neonatal disease through to completely healthy adults.[11] In this case the phenotype is predominantly congenital and, if survived, will usually result in a healthy adult life with reproductive fitness.

It is unclear why there can be such a wide spectrum of severity for many genetic disorders, even from the same pathogenic variant within the same family. The likelihood is that other genetic and environmental factors are acting to modify the phenotype.

ORIGIN OF PATHOGENIC GENETIC VARIANTS

Many pathogenic genetic variants in neonates arise de novo rather than being inherited from a parent. The mechanism by which these copying errors arise when a sperm or oocyte is being formed are linked to parental age.

ORIGIN OF ANEUPLOIDY

Aneuploidy is present in greater than 35% of spontaneous abortions, 4% of stillbirths, and around 0.3% of live-born neonates, reflecting the severe phenotypes and embryonic lethality of many of the aneuploidies.[12]

Aneuploidy originates during cell division when the chromosomes do not separate equally (nondisjunction). If this occurs in the germ cell lineage during meiosis, it can result in oocytes or sperm with an aberrant number of chromosomes and so result in an aneuploid embryo. The origin of aneuploidy is predominantly from oocytes. Around 10% to 35% of human oocytes and 1% to 4% of sperm are aneuploid.[13] The incidence of aneuploidy increases with maternal age.[14] The precise mechanism by which aging oocytes are prone to aneuploidy is unclear and likely multifactorial. Indeed, the relationship between maternal age and aneuploidy is different for different chromosomes, suggesting multiple pathways at play (Fig. 173.1).

Nondisjunction can occur at the first or the second cell division of meiosis (meiosis I or meiosis II—Fig. 173.2). Oocytes have a fundamentally different mechanism of meiosis from sperm, which have symmetric cell divisions and proceed swiftly through meiosis. Oocytes are arrested in prophase I from embryonic development until puberty. At this point, luteinizing hormone stimulates the resumption of meiosis. At anaphase I, homologous chromosomes separate; one remains in the oocyte and the other forms the first polar body. The ovulated oocyte is arrested in metaphase II. Fertilization triggers the second meiotic division with separation of the sister chromatids: one in the oocyte and the other into a second polar body. As this process of a single meiotic division lasts decades in oocytes, this provides opportunities for segregation errors to occur.

The relative contribution of meiosis I errors and meiosis II errors in oocytes varies according to the chromosome in question, but in general meiosis I errors are more common in natural pregnancies[13]—see Fig. 173.1. Failure of meiotic recombination

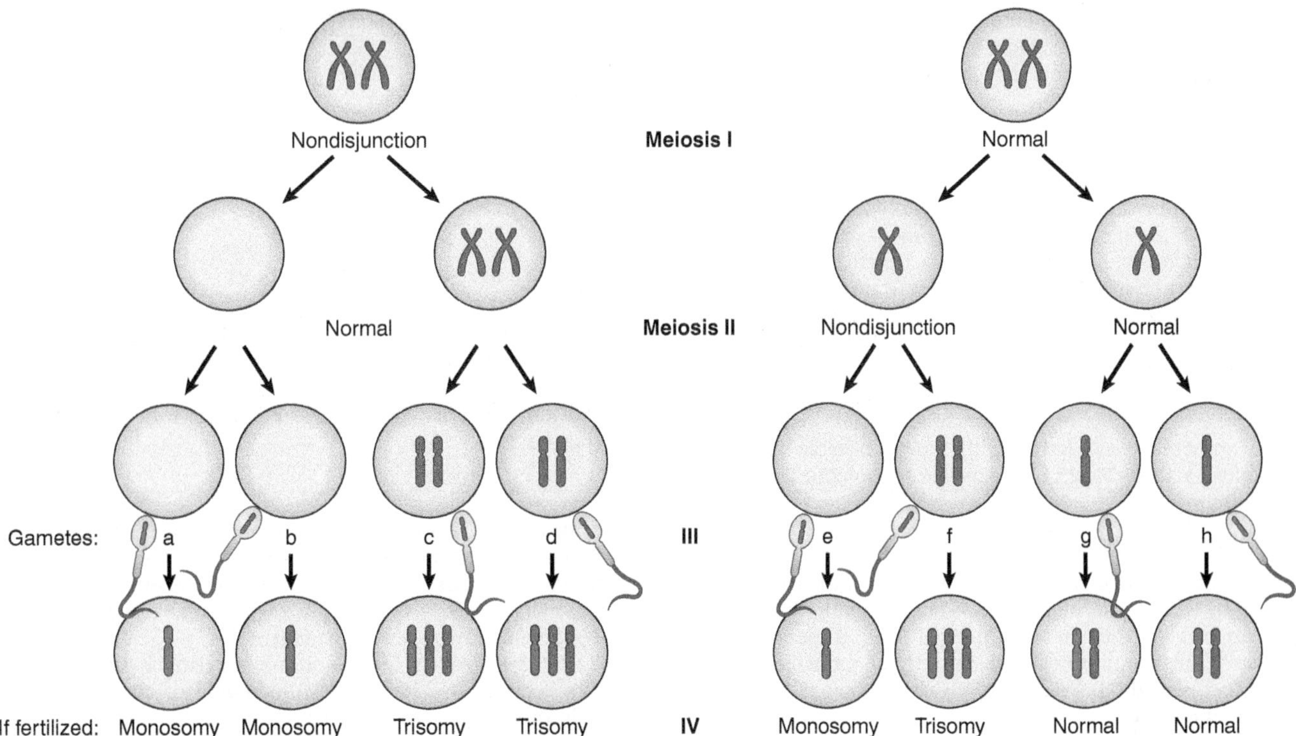

Fig. 173.2 Meiosis involves two cell divisions to create haploid gametes with one copy of each chromosome. Nondisjunction at the first (meiosis I) or second (meiosis II) cell division result in aneuploidy.

or suboptimal location of crossover points predisposes to aneuploidy, and aging oocytes suspended in meiosis suffer a loss of sister chromatic cohesion.[14]

Embryos mosaic for aneuploidy can also form (with a mixture of aneuploidy and euploid cells). There is evidence that aneuploidy cells can suffer apoptosis and proliferative defects, meaning that the proportion of aneuploid cells becomes progressively depleted as the embryo develops. This happens—to a lesser extent—in placental tissue compared to fetal tissue,[15] meaning that prenatal tests that sample placental DNA (including chorionic villus sampling and free fetal DNA sequencing) may overestimate the degree of mosaic aneuploidy in the fetus.

ORIGIN OF SINGLE NUCLEOTIDE SEQUENCE VARIANTS

In contrast to aneuploidies, germline sequence variants predominantly originate from the sperm rather than oocytes, with a ratio of around 3.5:1.[16] The rate of de novo genetic variants in sperm increases as a male ages. This is because, in contrast with oocytes, which are produced early in life and have a fixed number of replication cycles, sperm continue to undergo cell divisions throughout a male's reproductive lifetime. Each cell division requires copying of the DNA and a chance for replication errors. Sperm have undergone approximately 160 replications in a 20-year-old man, and this increases to 610 in a 40-year-old man.[17] Each sperm carries two to three additional de novo sequence variants per additional year of paternal age (Fig. 173.3).[16,18]

Some genetic variants give sperm cells a survival or proliferation advantage. Sperm with these variants will drift upwards in frequency as they form a rapidly dividing clone within the testis. An example is the *FGFR2* p.Ser252Trp mutation, which is seen in 62% to 71% of cases of Apert syndrome.[19] The frequency with which sperm are seen with this point mutation is far higher than would be expected due to chance as *FGFR2* is a growth factor receptor and activating mutations will cause greater growth and proliferation of the sperm.

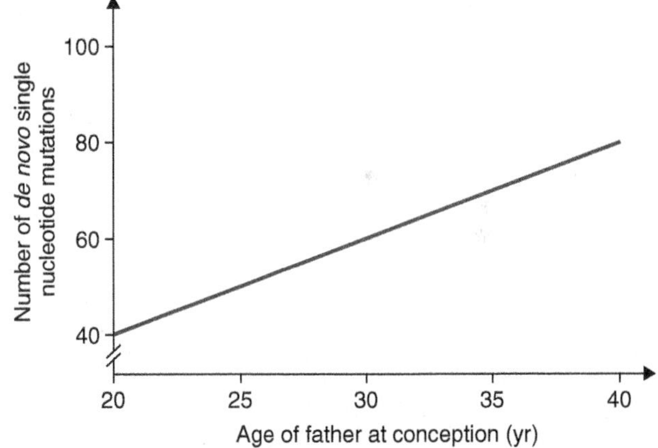

Fig. 173.3 De novo mutation rate in offspring increases as a father ages. (Data from Rahbari R, Wuster A, Lindsay S, et al. Timing, rates and spectra of human germline mutation. *Nat Genet*. 2016;48:126–133. https://doi.org/10.1038/ng.3469; and Kong A, Frigge M, Masson G, et al. Rate of de novo mutations and the importance of father's age to disease risk. *Nature*. 2012:488:471–475. https://doi.org/10.1038/nature11396.)

The origin of de novo large CNVs is currently less clear. Some studies have suggested a bias towards paternal origin of deletions, and a maternal origin of duplications.[20,21]

MECHANISM OF DISEASE IN ANEUPLOIDY AND COPY NUMBER VARIATION

CNVs are deletions or duplications of a large number (usually at least 1000) of DNA base pairs. CNVs have traditionally been detected using a chromosome microarray: a first-line genetic test in the context of multiple congenital anomalies. The ability of

WGS/WES technologies to detect CNVs is improving, and more CNVs are likely to be diagnosed this way in the future, using WGS/WES as a combined test for both CNVs and sequence variants.

As CNVs usually disrupt the expression of a number of genes, they frequently have multiple phenotypes of early or congenital onset.The severity of the phenotype will depend on a number of factors, not only the size of the CNV but also its location. Some genomic loci are more gene-rich or contain genes more critical to health and development than others. Deletions tend to have a more severe phenotypic effect than duplications as many genes are "haploinsufficient"—a single copy of the gene is insufficient to produce enough protein product to allow the cell to function normally.

The most extreme example of CNVs are the aneuploidies—where there is a gain or loss of whole chromosomes. Most of these are embryonic lethal with a few notable exceptions: trisomies 13, 18, or 21, sex chromosome aneuploidies, and mosaic aneuploidies.

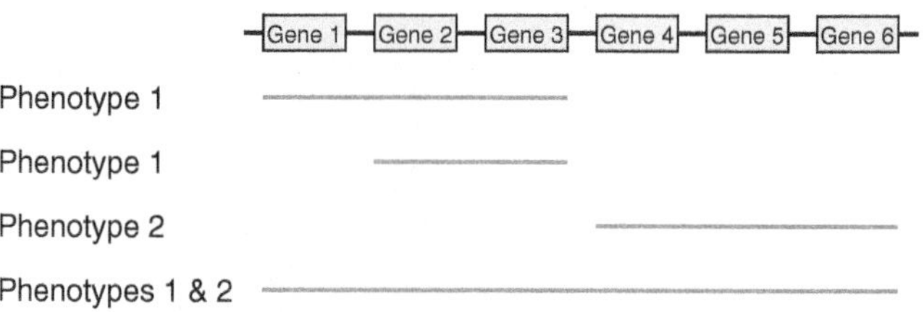

Fig. 173.4 The concept of a minimally deleted/duplicated region. This figure shows the deletion sizes for four patients with deletions in the same region. It is likely that genes 2 and/or 3 are responsible for phenotype 1, and that genes 4 and/or 5 and/or 6 are responsible for phenotype 2.

TRISOMY OF CHROMOSOME 21

Down syndrome affects 1 in 1000 live births in Europe[22] and is caused by a duplication of chromosome 21. Phenotypic features can present in the prenatal period (e.g., increased nuchal thickness), neonatal period (e.g., congenital anomalies), infancy (e.g., learning difficulties), and adulthood (e.g., early-onset Alzheimer disease).

The relationship between genotype and phenotype is complex.[23] Chromosome 21 is the smallest human chromosome: approximately 46 million base pairs long and with approximately 200 to 300 genes.This is likely to explain why trisomy 21 is one of only a few chromosome aneuploidies that are compatible with survival into adulthood in the nonmosaic form. However, the impact of duplication of such a large number of genes is extensive and results in a genome-wide shift in gene expression patterns.

The majority of chromosome 21 genes are overexpressed in cells with trisomy 21.[24] Chromosome 21 contains a number of transcription factors each of which can control the expression of hundreds or even thousands of other genes across the genome. Studies in mouse embryonic stem cells have revealed 1229 high-confidence binding sites across the genome for the chromosome 21 encoded transcription factor SIM2 alone.These binding sites overlap with master transcription factors such as SOX2 and OCT4, key regulators of embryonic development.[25]

There are also noncoding RNA (nc-RNA) transcripts on chromosome 21 that can control gene expression. For example, miR-155 can downregulate expression of the AGTR1 gene (located on chromosome 3).This is the gene for the angiotensin receptor 1, and its dysregulation may be responsible for the relatively low blood pressure found in trisomy 21.[26]

Efforts to narrow down the critical genes responsible for the majority of phenotypes in Down syndrome initially focused on studies of individuals with Down syndrome phenotypes but only partial trisomy 21 (smaller chromosome 21 duplications).There are approximately 200 such case reports.[27] One systematic comparison of cases of partial trisomy 21 with useable mapping data has indicated a very small Down syndrome critical region (DSCR) at 21q22.13. At just 34 kb in size, this represents only 0.07% of chromosome 21.The authors conclude that this small section of chromosome 21 is likely to be responsible for the key features of intellectual disability and characteristic dysmorphic facial features.[27]

22Q11.2 DELETION SYNDROME

The 22q11.2 deletion syndrome (22q11.2DS) is the most common microdeletion syndrome, with an estimated prevalence of 1 in 5950 births.[28] The neonatal phenotypic presentation of this syndrome is variable, with major clinical manifestations including CHD, immune deficiency, and palatal abnormalities. However, any organ system can be involved with structural or functional anomalies, resulting in a wide range of recommended evaluations following initial diagnosis.[29]

22q11.2 microdeletion syndrome is relatively common due to the genomic architecture of this region of chromosome 22, which predisposes to unequal crossing over during meiotic recombination. The typically deleted region is 3Mb in size and contains a number of genes that are known or hypothesized to contribute to the phenotypic expression of this deletion. For example, haploinsufficiency for the transcription factor *TBX1* is associated with congenital heart defects. More than 85% of individuals with 22q11DS have the same 3Mb deletion; however, the remainder have either a smaller deletion "nested" within the typically deleted region, or they have variant deletion end points. There is clinical relevance of knowing which size deletion is present in any individual patient, since the genetic content of the deletion will inform the patient's initial management and allow more accurate discussion of the likely evolution of the phenotype.

MINIMALLY DELETED/DUPLICATED REGIONS

This refers to the concept of defining and comparing the exact gene content of a deleted or duplicated region in patients who have pathogenic, overlapping genomic copy number variation, with the aim of explaining phenotypic variability (Fig. 173.4). Some microdeletions and microduplications are relatively common and recurrent in terms of genomic region involved, such as the 22q11.2DS, while others are rare or even unique to the individual. In all neonatal cases involving copy number variation, peer-reviewed literature and/or the known gene content of the variant region should inform the initial investigations. It is now possible to accurately compare the genomic region involved in rare but overlapping CNVs using chromosome microarray analysis, with the aim of defining genotype-phenotype correlations. In some recurrent CNV "syndromes," it has been proved that there is only one gene that causes the most clinically impactful part of the phenotype, whereas in other CNVs there is multigenic contribution. An example of the latter is 22q11.2DS, in which at least three genes other than *TBX1* contribute to the phenotype. In contrast, Smith-Magenis syndrome (SMS) is usually caused by a recurrent 3.5Mb deletion of chromosome 17p11.2 including the gene *RAI1*. However, some individuals who have features consistent with SMS do not have the typical 3.5Mb microdeletion but have a pathogenic variant in the gene *RAI1,* which is now understood to cause most features of SMS except for short stature and visceral anomalies.[30]

MECHANISM OF DISEASE IN MONOGENIC DISORDERS

Monogenic diseases exhibit extreme variability in the mechanisms by which they disrupt cellular or molecular pathways, ultimately leading to the disease state. The mechanisms can be described at the level of the gene and the pathway in which the gene product normally functions. For example, a single nucleotide variant may code for an early stop codon in a gene whose normal product functions as a tumor suppressor, leading to the development of a cancer.

The most common mechanisms by which genetic variants lead to disease include haploinsufficiency (loss of function of one allele and therefore a reduction in the amount of gene product), hypomorphic alleles with decreased function, gain of function alleles (constitutive protein activity), neomorphic alleles (new function such as altered substrate specificity), and dominant-negative mechanisms (toxic effects of an altered protein interferes with the wild-type protein). The reader is referred to Emery and Rimoin's Principles and Practice of Medical Genetics[31] for an in-depth review of these and other less common disease-causing mechanisms.

The mechanism of disease in monogenic disorders can also be sub-classified according to the cellular structure or function that is affected, termed a *pathway-based* classification. Pathway-based analysis has become possible due to the concurrent increase in our contemporary understanding of molecular genetics and molecular biology. Many monogenic diseases disrupt unique pathways, leading to a common phenotypic spectrum shared amongst genetically related disorders. An example is a group of conditions termed the *disorders of transcriptional regulation*. These are genetic disorders caused by mutations in genes encoding components of the cellular transcriptional machinery, which are characterized at the cellular level by global transcriptional dysregulation. Transcription of genes must be co-ordinated precisely in space and time, for normal embryonic development to occur. The overlapping phenotype of patients affected by dysregulation of this most basic cellular function includes growth restriction, multiple physical differences, and intellectual disability.[32] However, disorders of transcriptional regulation exhibit allelic heterogeneity due to the hundreds of genes involved in this pathway. Understanding the common pathophysiology of this group of conditions allows supportive and preemptive patient management to occur once such a molecular diagnosis is made, which is a key component of precision medicine.

Elucidating the pathway(s) within which a gene functions may allow gene-disease associations to be predicted even where a gene has no currently known human phenotype. However, one gene may be associated with multiple, nonoverlapping human disorders depending on the impact or location of the variant in the gene (termed *allelic heterogeneity*). An example is the gene *FBN1*, which is not only the cause of classical Marfan syndrome, but also has seven additional disease phenotypes listed in Online Mendelian Inheritance in Man (OMIM), some of which have no overlapping phenotypic features. Such allelic heterogeneity can be caused by variants affecting different functional regions of the protein, or by the contrast between a dominant negative effect of an abnormal protein versus haploinsufficiency of the same protein.

Allelic heterogeneity contributes to a proportion of genome-wide clinical tests in which no genomic diagnosis is made. If the patient's phenotype does not overlap with the stated gene-disease association, a variant in the gene may be disregarded as a possible cause of disease. To increase the diagnostic rate for rare and ultra-rare diseases, a crucial component remains international data sharing to enable exact genotype-phenotype matches, which then provide strong evidence for the gene-disease association.

MECHANISM OF DISEASE IN POLYGENIC DISORDERS

Polygenic disorders are those influenced by variation in multiple genes and usually also the environment. These are not inherited in a classic mendelian way. Often each individual genetic variant has a modest impact on risk of developing the disorder and has a low penetrance. This is in contrast to monogenic disorders that are caused by a single gene defect with high penetrance.

In reality, there is a continuous spectrum from monogenic to polygenic disorders.[33] A genetic variant may give a 1% increased risk of a given phenotype and represent part of an individual's polygenic and environmental risk. Another genetic variant may give a 100% risk of a given phenotype and represent an archetypal monogenic disorder; for example, trisomy 21 has complete penetrance for the phenotype of developmental delay intellectual disability (albeit of variable severity) and dysmorphic features.

However, there are also genetic variants that may give say a 50% chance of developing a given phenotype. These may be regarded as monogenic with reduced penetrance, but in reality there is no clear-cut line where a disease is no longer "monogenic" and often penetrance is overestimated in classical genetic studies because of ascertainment bias—the individuals with the genetic variant who do not develop the phenotype are never discovered and sequenced.[34]

Many phenotypes that present in neonatal life can have a spectrum of causes, ranging from environmental to polygenic to monogenic. CHD, for example, can be the result of an environmental insult in utero such as a teratogen or maternal diabetes. Some genetic variants can give a modest increased risk of CHD, and others can give a dramatically elevated risk such as trisomy 18 (Edwards syndrome), which is estimated to have an 80% penetrance for CHD.[35]

A large WES study[36] of 1891 individuals with CHD found a significant enrichment of de novo protein truncating variants in syndromic CHD, suggesting highly penetrant disorders abound in this group. In nonsyndromic CHD, in contrast, the authors found a significant enrichment of *inherited* protein truncating variants. As variants were inherited from unaffected parents, this suggests a prominent role of incompletely penetrant genetic variants in the causation of nonsyndromic CHD.

Hirschsprung disease is an example of a congenital anomaly which is strongly inherited, but usually not in a monogenic manner. A recent study of 190 patients with Hirschsprung disease[37] found a mixture of common noncoding variants, rare coding variants, and CNVs, with a huge variation in estimated penetrance. For example, those with risk alleles in an important region of noncoding variation influencing the expression of their RET gene had an odds ratio for developing Hirschsprung of between 2 (for 3 risk alleles) and 24 (for 7 to 8 risk alleles). The authors identified more than one genetic risk factor in 21% of patients.

Epilepsies are another phenotype with a range of genetic and environmental causes. Some highly penetrant monogenetic disorders, particularly pathogenic genetic variants in ion channels essential to neuronal activity, cause early-onset seizures and encephalopathy.[38] In other instances, seizures can cluster in families but without a clear mendelian inheritance pattern and often as a result of oligogenic or polygenic inheritance.

One study of WES in 743 individuals with epileptic or developmental and epileptic encephalopathy[39] found an enrichment of damaging ultra-rare genetic variants even in a subset of individuals who already had a diagnostic mutation, strongly suggesting that their "diagnostic" genetic variant was not the only contributing genetic factor to their seizures. Another large study[40] found a convergence in the genetics of severe and less severe epilepsies, with an enrichment of ultra-rare deleterious variants, traditionally associated with early-onset epilepsy/encephalopathy, in individuals with more mild or later-onset epilepsy phenotypes. In this era of widespread genetic testing for neonates, caution is indicated in assuming a single genetic variant is the sole cause of the neonate's phenotype, or assuming that it is fully penetrant.

Genetic testing is often useful when it reveals a highly penetrant monogenic cause for a neonate's condition. This information is useful in predicting prognosis and recurrence risk in future pregnancies, for example. However, the identification of lower penetrance genetic variants is sometimes of questionable utility for the neonate and for the family. It can also be challenging to predict the prognosis for the neonate, or the phenotype of future family members, if the genetic condition identified is rare. In such instances there may be limited information available regarding the penetrance and phenotypic spectrum of the disorder.

NONCODING GENETIC VARIATION

Interpretation of a genetic sequence in the clinical genomics laboratory setting is mainly focused upon the coding regions of DNA (the parts of the genome that code for protein). This makes up just 1.3% of the human genome. It is relatively easy to predict the consequence of such genetic variants on protein production and protein structure. However, there has been much interest in recent years regarding pathogenic genetic variation in noncoding regions of the genome, many of which play a role in the control of gene activity. This type of genetic variation is best interrogated with WGS.

TYPES OF NONCODING VARIATION

Some noncoding DNA immediately surrounding each gene has a relatively conserved sequence, the function of which has been known about for decades. For example, immediately prior to and following each exon is a "splice site"—a region of DNA where the spliceosome will bind so that introns can be removed from mRNA before translation (see Genetic Principles chapter). Genetic variants in these regions can cause incorrect splicing and a nonfunctional protein. Analysis of the splice sites of each exon of the gene(s) beings sequenced forms part of routine diagnostic sequencing in most genetic laboratories.

Another example of a relatively well-characterized noncoding genetic element is the promoter region immediately upstream of the coding region, responsible for RNA polymerase and associated protein binding to initiate transcription (see Genetic Principles chapter). CNVs have frequently been identified in this region and can influence gene expression (reviewed here[41]).

The 5′ and 3′ untranslated regions of genes, transcribed into mRNA but not part of the final protein coding sequence, have an important role in transcript stability. They are also involved in the control of mRNA localization, stability, and the rate of translation.[42]

These localized and highly conserved noncoding parts of each gene are the tip of the iceberg in terms of range of noncoding elements that can influence gene expression. Many genes have enhancer or repressor sequences—some located mega-bases away from the gene itself—which can increase or decrease gene expression. There are also regions of the genome that code for RNA transcripts that do not make proteins but are functional in their own right: nc-RNAs. It can be difficult to predict if and how genetic variation in these distant noncoding regions are linked to disease.

ENHANCER ELEMENT GENETIC VARIATION

Noncoding elements that influence gene expression can do so in a tissue specific or developmental stage specific manner, creating even greater complexity for scientists involved in variant interpretation.

Take the *SOX9* gene, for example. Pathogenic genetic variants in the coding region of this gene cause campomelic dysplasia, a severe skeletal dysplasia with phenotypic features including Pierre Robin sequence and sex reversal. There is evidence that noncoding variation in a mandibular enhancer for this gene can cause isolated Pierre Robin sequence without other features of campomelic dysplasia, presumably because this enhancer influences *SOX9* gene expression only in (or predominantly in) the developing mandible.[43] Duplications upstream of *SOX9* have been associated with a female-to-male sex reversal phenotype,[44] while a de novo deletion upstream of *SOX9* has been associated with XY male to female sex reversal syndrome.[45]

There are multiple other examples where pathogenic genetic variants in enhancers can cause some but not all of the phenotypes that manifest of the protein coding region of the gene itself.[46]

GENETIC VARIATION IN NONCODING RNA

Please see "Structure of Genes" subsection of Chapter 1 for a summary of the types of ncRNA. An astonishingly high proportion of the nonprotein-coding genome is transcribed and is highly conserved across mammalian species and therefore likely to be functional.[47] Pathogenic genetic variants affecting ncRNAs that are critical to health and development can cause genetic disease in neonates.

One example is deletions in the 16p24.1 region. Deletions here are associated with alveolar capillary dysplasia with misalignment of pulmonary veins, a severe congenital lung disorder. Interrogation of the minimally deleted region revealed that the deletion included lung-specific ncRNA genes that play a role in regulating the gene *FOXF1*. Pathogenic single nucleotide variants in *FOXF1* cause the same disease.[48] It is important to bear in mind complex mechanisms like this when a patient is "mutation negative" in the protein coding gene expected to cause their disorder.

THE BURDEN OF NONCODING VARIATION IN NEONATAL GENETIC DISEASE

Historically, the low rates of diagnosis of pathogenic noncoding genetic variation in cohorts of patients with severe genetic disorders was assumed to be because of a lack of interrogation of noncoding regions: most diagnoses were achieved through techniques of single gene sequencing, panel sequencing, and WES, all of which interrogate the coding sequence and canonical splice sites only. With the advent of more affordable WGS, there is a new opportunity to search the noncoding DNA for pathogenic variants.

Large studies have attempted to estimate the contribution of noncoding genetic variation to human disease. In the Deciphering Developmental Disorders study of 7930 individuals with a severe undiagnosed developmental disorder, the authors found an enrichment of de novo genetic variants in evolutionarily conserved noncoding elements that they were able to interrogate with WES data. From this, they estimate that 1% to 3% of patients without a diagnostic coding variant have a pathogenic de novo mutations in fetal brain-active regulatory element.

Most large sequencing studies of neonates have not reported diagnoses of noncoding pathogenic genetic variants, even when WGS has been used.[1,6] This gap in rates of diagnosis of coding versus noncoding pathogenic genetic variants could be because of a relative lack of knowledge regarding how to interpret noncoding genetic variation, or could be because noncoding variation plays a less prominent role in the severe and early-onset phenotypes of neonatal genetic disease.

THE DIAGNOSTIC ROLE OF WHOLE GENOME VERSUS WHOLE EXOME SEQUENCING

There is currently much debate as to whether WGS should be used instead of WES to diagnose a sick neonate. WGS has the advantage of including noncoding regions of DNA (98% of the genome), some of which can contain diagnostic pathogenic genetic variation. In addition, the advent of polymerase chain reaction (PRC)-free library preparation in WGS can overcome some of the technical artefacts that are problematic in exome sequencing.

One randomized, controlled trial of WGS versus WES in 213 infants showed a similar diagnostic performance: 18 diagnoses in 94 infants (19%) versus 19 diagnoses in 95 infants (20%).[1] This was despite the WGS picking up more genetic variants, including 12% more coding variants and twice as many variants annotated as pathogenic or likely pathogenic in the database ClinVar.[49] While this study highlighted the superiority of WGS for variant detection even in coding regions, this did not translate into more diagnoses in a cohort of this size.

Other nonrandomized cohort studies have compared WES and WGS and reported a 4% to 7% increased diagnostic yield with

WGS.[50-53] Variants detected by WGS but missed by WES include noncoding variants, CNVs, mitochondrial DNA variants, and exonic single nucleotide variants in areas with poor coverage by WES.

The choice between WES and WGS will in the future be driven by the relative cost and yield, with current data indicating a small but modestly improved diagnostic yield from the more expensive WGS.

VARIANT INTERPRETATION

The typical unique human genome differs from the reference genome at 4 to 5 million sites.[54] When a neonate has a genome-wide genetic test to look for the cause of their illness, millions of genetic variants will be found. One of these many variants may be the disease-causing variant. Most will be harmless. Some may be "incidental findings"; for example, the neonate may be a carrier for a recessive disorder or have a genetic variant that will put them at a higher risk of certain cancer types in adult life. There is currently much debate about if and how incidental findings, particularly of adult-onset disorders, should be fed back to the carers of neonates.[55]

However, categorizing these millions of variants into disease causing, harmless, or incidental findings can be challenging. The process of variant interpretation begins with bioinformatic pipelines that aim to automatically exclude as many harmless variants as possible. It ends with manual curation by a clinical scientist, often in consultation with a clinical geneticist. At the end of this process some genetic findings may be described as "variants of uncertain significance"—not clearly pathogenic or benign. It is important to note that for a given variant these labels can change with time as more evidence becomes available to support the assertion that the variant is benign or pathogenic.

Genetic variants are currently classified into one of five categories indicating the probability that the variant is disease causing (Table 173.1).

Table 173.1 Classification of Genetic Variants in a Five-Tier Terminology System as Recommended by the American College of Medical Genetics.[56]

Class 1—Benign
Class 2—Likely benign
Class 3—Variants of uncertain significance
Class 4—Likely pathogenic
Class 5—Pathogenic

To classify a variant in to one of these categories, bioinformaticians have developed algorithms to assist scientists to integrate different types of evidence to create a combined score.[56,57] For example, if the variant is common in the general population, then it is more likely to be benign. If the variant has been seen previously in individuals with the same disease as the patient in question, then it is more likely to be pathogenic. Evidence from other patients with the same variant is gathered from publications, and from large, collaborative databases such as ClinVar[49] and Decipher.[58]

The process of variant interpretation is different for CNVs versus sequence variants but follows similar principles. Tables 173.2 and 173.3 show some categories of evidence that are taken into account when classifying a variant according to the American College of Medical Genetics criteria for classification of sequence variants and CNVs.

Robust variant classification is critical. Incorrectly assuming a variant is pathogenic can lead to incorrect management decisions for the neonate, misleading future prenatal tests for their parents, and potentially misleading genetic test information and management decisions for the wider family.

To help aid variant interpretation, many centers have variant interpretation meetings where candidate diagnostic variants can be discussed with a multidisciplinary team including clinical geneticists and clinical genetic scientists. Patients should always be advised that variant interpretation and genetic diagnoses can change as more evidence comes to light, particularly for class 2/3/4 variants.

SINGLETON VERSUS TRIO WHOLE EXOME SEQUENCING/WHOLE GENOME SEQUENCING

In dominant genetic disorders, variant interpretation in neonatal genetic disease often hinges on determining if a genetic variant has occurred de novo or if it has been inherited from a parent. A candidate dominant genetic variant in a sick neonate with multisystem involvement is far less likely to be causative if it has been inherited from a healthy parent, although the possibility of extreme phenotypic variability or reduced penetrance must always be considered before discarding the variant as being causative of the neonate's phenotype.

In addition, information about inheritance is useful when investigating the pathogenicity of recessive genetic variants as it enables the determination of phase: whether the two candidate genetic variants are both on the same allele (both inherited from

Table 173.2 Categories of Evidence Used When Classifying the Pathogenicity of a Sequence Variant.

Type of Evidence	Example
Population data	Absence of the genetic variant in large databases of healthy individuals would make it more likely to be pathogenic
Computational and predictive data	Computational tools can predict what impact the genetic variant will have on the protein structure and function
Functional data	Laboratory data may show the impact of the genetic variant on the function of the protein, for example, in an animal or cellular model
Segregation data	If the genetic variant is present in multiple affected members of the same family, and absent in healthy members of the family, this would make it more likely to be pathogenic
De novo data	If a genetic variant is de novo, then this would make it more likely to be pathogenic than if it was inherited from a healthy parent
Allelic data	For recessive disorders, a genetic variant detected on the different allele (in trans) from a pathogenic variant would make it more likely to itself be pathogenic
Other database	If another source (e.g., a curated database) asserts that the variant is pathogenic, then this can be taken into account
Other data	If a patient's phenotype or family history are highly specific for a particular gene and this gene has been sequenced then any variants found in this gene are more likely to be pathogenic

De novo = A genetic variant that occurs for the first time in that individual (is not present in either parent).

Table 173.3 Categories of Evidence Used When Classifying the Pathogenicity of a Copy Number Variant.

Type of Evidence	Example
Genomic content initial assessment	If the region of DNA that is deleted or duplicated does not contain any genes or known functionally important elements then it is less likely to be pathogenic
Overlap with established or predicted dosage sensitive genes or genomic regions	A deletion of a gene that is known to be "haploinsufficient" (the body is predicted to need both copies to be transcribed) is more likely to be pathogenic, as is a deletion in a region of the genome known to be associated with a particular syndrome
Evaluation of gene number	The higher the number of genes in the region that is deleted/duplicated, the more likely it is to be pathogenic
Evidence from published literature, public databases, and/or internal lab data	Reported probands from the literature may have a copy number variant that is similar to or overlaps with that of the probands in question. If they have similar phenotypes, this supports the assertion that the variant is pathogenic
Evaluation of inheritance pattern/family history	If the copy number variant is de novo or is present in other family members with a similar phenotype and is absent from healthy family members, then this supports the assertion that the variant is pathogenic

De novo = A genetic variant that occurs for the first time in that individual (is not present in either parent).

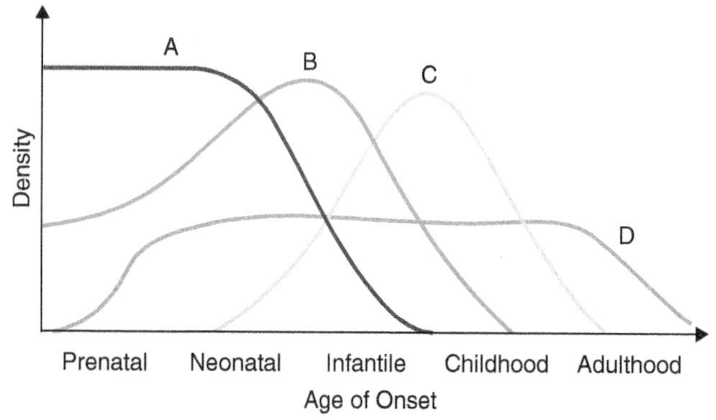

Examples of distributions of age of onset:

A–Mostly prenatal with some neonatal onset e.g., Campomelic dysplasia (SOX9 mutations)

B–Mostly later prenatal and neonatal onset e.g., Osteogenesis imperfecta (COL1A1/2 glycine substitution mutations)

C–Mostly infantile/childhood onset e.g., Osteogenesis imperfecta (COL1A1/2 truncating mutations)

D–Broad range of onset from neonate to adulthood (and rarely prenatal) e.g., Marfan syndrome (FBN1 mutations)

Fig. 173.5 Age of onset varies widely in different genetic conditions. Different classes of mutation in the same gene (in this case COLA1/2) can cause widely different age of onset distributions.

the same parent) or whether they are on different alleles (one variant inherited from each parent). Pathogenic recessive genetic variants would have to be on different alleles to disrupt the function of both copies of the same gene.

Having parental samples is therefore very useful and often critical for rapid and accurate variant interpretation. It is possible to perform WES/WGS on probands only, and then use cheaper Sanger sequencing to investigate if a candidate genetic variant is present in parental samples. An alternative approach is to perform WES/WGS on the child and both parents in parallel (trio WES/WGS). The latter means that inheritance information can be taken into account in the interpretation of every genetic variant identified, which will aid variant prioritization.

In a meta-analysis of the diagnostic utility of genome sequencing in children with suspected genetic diseases, trio genome sequencing gave twice the odds of achieving a diagnosis compared to singleton genome sequencing (odds ratio 2.04, 95% confidence interval, 1.62 to 2.56, $P < .0001$).[59]

However, in a recent large study of WES/WGS in neonates, the incremental diagnostic yield of pursuing trio sequencing after negative proband analysis was just 0.7% (1 additional diagnosis out of 147).[1] In this study the inheritance of the variants found in the singleton proband WES/WGS analysis were individually confirmed by Sanger sequencing. Therefore, the addition of trio WES/WGS gave less additional information that in other studies. However, the authors did note that pursuing trio WES/WGS from the outset saves around 5 days in comparison to singleton WES/WGS with confirmatory Sanger sequencing of parent samples. Such delays could be critical if the diagnosis is important for management of the patient or making the decision to pursue palliative care.

CONCLUSION

Genetic disease is an important cause of neonatal morbidity and mortality, and experienced neonatologists have fundamental knowledge and first-hand experience of the breadth of genetic conditions that present in the prenatal and neonatal period. Monogenic causes of conditions that were previously thought to be multifactorial, such as cerebral palsy, are now being discovered. These apparently rare and esoteric discoveries are contributing towards a greater understanding of the pathophysiology of neonatal disease and lead us towards cellular pathways that may become drug targets of the future. Any neonatologist who has a concern that their patient has a genetic disorder is encouraged to pursue their instincts further; an accurate molecular diagnosis may change the patient's disease trajectory as well as contributing towards a greater global understanding of the disease in question.

The landscape of genetic mutations in neonates differs from children and adults with enrichment for aneuploidy, very large/destructive CNVs, and mutations in genes critical for development without which multiple congenital anomalies will occur (Fig. 173.5). For a minority of genetic diseases, there is an exact genotype–phenotype correlation that allows individualized prediction of the severity of the condition, whereas for many other genetic and genomic disorders it is currently unclear how the same CNV or single nucleotide variant can cause a severe neonatal onset disorder in one patient and a more mild or later-onset disorder in another family member. However, an exact molecular or genomic diagnosis has a value beyond prognostication or management decisions, and in many cases relieves the burden of guilt felt by many parents if they are able to accept that they are not to blame for their child's condition. Clinical Geneticists often spend time in consultations discussing such issues, and Genetic Counsellors are invaluable if a genetic diagnosis has been made and the family wishes to discuss their reproductive choices.

WGS/WES is likely to become a first-line diagnostic investigation in neonatal units in the near future with increasing evidence for high diagnostic yields, cost effectiveness, and genetic diagnoses resulting in change in management. Neonatologists have a major role to play in deciding the "right time" to employ such a broad test and will be best-placed to take into account the welfare of the neonate as well as the wishes of the parents in choosing if or when to use such a test. The future of effective, individualized healthcare relies on early, accurate diagnosis and the availability of disease-modifying treatments. Fundamental to the progress of developing new treatments is the understanding of the pathophysiology of disease, and genetic pathology has a huge role to play in furthering this aspect of scientific knowledge. The future of neonatal healthcare is likely to include emerging technologies within the next 5 years, such as gene editing and mutation-specific drug treatments.

 A complete reference list is available at www.ExpertConsult.com.

SELECT REFERENCES

1. Kingsmore SF, Cakici JA, Clark MM, et al. A randomized, controlled trial of the analytic and diagnostic performance of singleton and trio, rapid genome and exome sequencing in ill infants. *Am J Hum Genet*. 2019;105(4):719-733.
2. Van Diemen CC, Kerstjens-Frederikse WS, Bergman KA, et al. *Rapid Targeted Genomics in Critically Ill Newborns*. [Internet]. Available from: www.aappublications.org/news.
3. Farnaes L, Hildreth A, Sweeney NM, et al. Rapid whole-genome sequencing decreases infant morbidity and cost of hospitalization. *NPJ Genomic Med [Internet]*. 2018;3:10.
4. Miller DT, Adam MP, Aradhya S, et al. Consensus statement: chromosomal microarray is a first-tier clinical diagnostic test for individuals with developmental disabilities or congenital anomalies. *Am J Hum Genet*. 2010;86(5):749-764.
5. Lu X-Y, Phung MT, Shaw CA, et al. Genomic imbalances in neonates with birth defects: high detection rates by using chromosomal microarray analysis. *Pediatrics*. 2008;122(6):1310-1318.
6. French CE, Delon I, Dolling H, et al. Whole genome sequencing reveals that genetic conditions are frequent in intensively ill children. *Intensive Care Med*. 2019;45(5):627-636.
7. Meng L, Pammi M, Saronwala A, et al. Use of exome sequencing for infants in intensive care units ascertainment of severe single-gene disorders and effect on medical management. *JAMA Pediatr*. 2017;171(12):1-10.
8. McRae JF, Clayton S, Fitzgerald TW, et al. Prevalence and architecture of de novo mutations in developmental disorders. *Nature*. 2017;542(7642):433-438.
9. Martin HC, Jones WD, McIntyre R, et al. Quantifying the contribution of recessive coding variation to developmental disorders. *Science (80-)*. 2018;362(6419):1161-1164.
10. Giuseppe C, Egle C, Antonio C, et al. Update on Brugada syndrome 2019. *Curr Probl Cardiol*. 2021;46(3):100454.
11. Kerstjens-Frederikse WS, Van De Laar IMBH, Vos YJ, et al. Cardiovascular malformations caused by NOTCH1 mutations do not keep left: data on 428 probands with left-sided CHD and their families. *Genet Med*. 2016;18(9):914-923.
12. Hassold T, Abruzzo M, Adkins K, et al. Human aneuploidy: incidence, origin, and etiology. *Environ Mol Mutagen*. 1996;28(3):167-175.
13. Nagaoka SI, Hassold TJ, Hunt PA. Human aneuploidy: mechanisms and new insights into an age-old problem. *Nat Rev Genet*. 2012;13(7):493-504.
14. Hassold T, Hunt P. To err (meiotically) is human: the genesis of human aneuploidy. *Nat Rev Genet*. 2001;2:280-291.
15. Bolton H, Graham SJL, Van Der Aa N, et al. Mouse model of chromosome mosaicism reveals lineage-specific depletion of aneuploid cells and normal developmental potential. *Nat Commun*. 2016;7:1-12.
16. Rahbari R, Wuster A, Lindsay SJ, et al. Timing, rates and spectra of human germline mutation. *Nat Genet*. 2016;48(2):126-133.
17. Wilson Sayres MA, Makova KD. Genome analyses substantiate male mutation bias in many species. *Bioessays*. 2011;33(12):938-945.
18. Kong A, Frigge ML, Masson G, et al. Rate of de novo mutations and the importance of father's age to disease risk. *Nature*. 2012;488.
19. Aslam AZ, Waseem R, Yaqoob M, Abbas A, Noor T, Rauf MA. Apert syndrome. *Pakistan Paediatr J*. 2015;39(1):53-56.
20. Hehir-Kwa JY, Rodríguez-Santiago B, Vissers LE, et al. De novo copy number variants associated with intellectual disability have a paternal origin and age bias. *J Med Genet*. 2011;48(11):776-778.
21. Ma R, Deng L, Xia Y, et al. A clear bias in parental origin of de novo pathogenic CNVs related to intellectual disability, developmental delay and multiple congenital anomalies. *Sci Rep*. 2017;7(1):1-9.
22. Khoshnood B, Greenlees R, Loane M, Dolk H. Paper 2: EUROCAT public health indicators for congenital anomalies in Europe. *Birth Defects Res A Clin Mol Teratol*. 2011;91(Suppl 1):S16-S22.
23. Antonarakis SE. Down syndrome and the complexity of genome dosage imbalance. *Nat Publ Gr*. 2016;18.
24. Olmos-Serrano JL, Kang HJ, Tyler WA, et al. Down syndrome developmental brain transcriptome reveals defective oligodendrocyte differentiation and myelination. *Neuron*. 2016;89(6):1208-1222.
25. Letourneau A, Cobellis G, Fort A, et al. HSA21 Single-minded 2 (SIM2) binding sites co-localize with super-enhancers and pioneer transcription factors in pluripotent mouse ES cells. *PloS One*. 2015;10(5):1-21.
26. Sethupathy P, Borel C, Gagnebin M, et al. Human microRNA-155 on chromosome 21 differentially interacts with its polymorphic target in the AGTR1 3 untranslated region: a mechanism for functional single-nucleotide Polymorphisms related to phenotypes. *Am J Hum Genet*. 2007;81:405-13.
27. Pelleri MC, Cicchini E, Locatelli C, et al. Systematic reanalysis of partial trisomy 21 cases with or without Down syndrome suggests a small region on 21q22.13 as critical to the phenotype. *Hum Mol Genet*. 2016;25(12):ddw116.
28. Botto LD, May K, Fernhoff PM, et al. A population-based study of the 22q11.2 Deletion: phenotype, incidence, and contribution to major birth defects in the population. *Pediatrics*. 2003;112(1 I):101-107.
29. Fung WLA, Butcher NJ, Costain G, et al. Practical guidelines for managing adults with 22q11.2 deletion syndrome. *Genet Med*. 2015;17(8):599-609.
30. Girirajan S, Elsas LJ, Devriendt K, Elsea SH. RAI1 variations in Smith-Magenis syndrome patients without 17p11.2 deletions. *J Med Genet [Internet]*. 2005;42(11):820-828.
31. Rimoin D, Pyeritz R, Korf B, eds. *Emery and Rimoin's principles and practice of medical genetics and genomics*. Cambridge, MA: Academic Press; 2013.
32. Izumi K. *Disorders of Transcriptional Regulation: An Emerging Category of Multiple Malformation Syndromes. Mol Syndromol*. 2016;7(5):262-73.
33. Boyle EA, Li YI, Pritchard JK. An expanded view of complex traits: from polygenic to omnigenic. *Cell*. 2017;169(7):1177-1186.
34. Wright CF, West B, Tuke M, et al. Assessing the pathogenicity, penetrance, and expressivity of putative disease-causing variants in a population setting. *Am J Hum Genet [Internet]*. 2019;104(2):275-286.
35. Springett A, Wellesley D, Greenlees R, et al. Congenital anomalies associated with trisomy 18 or trisomy 13: a registry-based study in 16 European countries, 2000-2011. *Am J Med Genet Part A*. 2015;167(12):3062-3069.
36. Sifrim A, Hitz M-P, Wilsdon A, et al. Distinct genetic architectures for syndromic and nonsyndromic congenital heart defects identified by exome sequencing. *Nat Genet*. 2016;48(9):1-9.
37. Tilghman JM, Ling AY, Turner TN, et al. Molecular genetic anatomy and risk profile of Hirschsprung's disease. *N Engl J Med*. 2019;380(15):1421-1432.
38. Allen AS, Berkovic SF, Cossette P, et al. De novo mutations in epileptic encephalopathies. *Nature*. 2013;501(7466):217-221.
39. Takata A, Nakashima M, Saitsu H, et al. Comprehensive analysis of coding variants highlights genetic complexity in developmental and epileptic encephalopathy. *Nat Commun*. 2019;10(1).
40. Feng Y-CA, Howrigan DP, Abbott LE, et al. Ultra-rare genetic variation in the epilepsies: a whole-exome sequencing study of 17,606 individuals. *Am J Hum Genet*. 2019:1-16.
41. Zhang F, Lupski JR. Non-coding genetic variants in human disease. *Hum Mol Genet*. 2015;24(R1):R102-R110.
42. Pesole G, Mignone F, Gissi C, Grillo G, Licciulli F, Liuni S. *Structural and Functional Features of Eukaryotic Mrna Untranslated Regions. Gene*. Philadelphia: Elsevier; 2001:73-81.
43. Benko S, Fantes JA, Amiel J, et al. Highly conserved non-coding elements on either side of SOX9 associated with Pierre Robin sequence. *Nat Genet*. 2009;41(3):359-64.
44. Cox JJ, Willatt L, Homfray T, Woods CG. A SOX9 duplication and familial 46, XX developmental testicular disorder. *N Engl J Med*. 2011;364(1):91-93.
45. Pop R, Conz C, Lindenberg KS, et al. Screening of the 1 Mb SOX9 5' control region by array CGH identifies a large deletion in a case of campomelic dysplasia with XY sex reversal. *J Med Genet*. 2004;41(4):e47.
46. Gordon CT, Lyonnet S. Enhancer mutations and phenotype modularity. *Nat Genet*. 2014;46(1):3-4.
47. Khalil AM, Guttman M, Huarte M, et al. Many human large intergenic noncoding RNAs associate with chromatin-modifying complexes and affect gene expression. *Proc Natl Acad Sci U S A*. 2009;106(28):11667-11672.
48. Szafranski P, Dharmadhikari A V, Brosens E, et al. Small noncoding differentially methylated copy-number variants, including lncRNA genes, cause a lethal lung developmental disorder. *Genome Res*. 2013;23(1):23-33.
49. Landrum MJ, Lee JM, Benson M, et al. ClinVar: improving access to variant interpretations and supporting evidence. *Nucleic Acids Res*. 2018;46(D1):D1062-D1067.
50. Lionel AC, Costain G, Monfared N, et al. Improved diagnostic yield compared with targeted gene sequencing panels suggests a role for whole-genome sequencing as a first-tier genetic test. *Genet Med*. 2018;20(4):435-443.

174 Genetic Variants and Neonatal Disease

Jennifer L. Cohen | C. Michael Cotten

INTRODUCTION

Infants with complex phenotypes and infants born at early gestational age are two of the most challenging groups of patients cared for in neonatal intensive care units (NICUs). Since the initial reports of the sequence of the human genome,[1,2] clinicians have hoped that the "genomic revolution" would lead to increasing likelihood of diagnoses for infants with complex phenotypes and identification of common variants associated with prematurity-associated morbidities. In both situations, identification of variants linked with disease would hopefully lead to novel, genetically informed prevention and treatment strategies. Progress in molecular methodologies coupled with collaborative efforts to compile, link, and analyze phenotype and genomic data from large cohorts is enabling identification of rare genetic variants that are likely causative of disease, and is informing care in many patient populations.[3] These efforts, with validated clinical data, collaborative data accumulation, and advanced analysis approaches, have improved the identification of variations in the genome that are likely to contribute to or cause disease and malformations in neonates.[4,5] For preterm infants, there has been limited success in identifying common genetic variants with associations to common complex morbidities such as retinopathy of prematurity (ROP), intraventricular hemorrhage (IVH), necrotizing enterocolitis (NEC), and bronchopulmonary dysplasia (BPD) that would provide insights into pathophysiology for most infants with these problems. In this chapter, we will discuss (1) the expanding application of genetic testing in infants in the NICU with complex phenotypes and (2) the ongoing investigations to identify genetic risk factors for common morbidities seen in extremely preterm infants.

GENETIC DISEASE IN NEONATES WITH COMPLEX PHENOTYPES

Congenital malformations and genetic disorders have long been recognized as major contributing factors to pediatric hospitalization, morbidity, and mortality,[6-8] and this finding extends to the patient population treated in the NICU.[9-12] Gene discovery for ultra-rare Mendelian disorders is ongoing, and large-scale genomic technologies and international collaborative efforts have allowed for advancement in this field.[13] Along with simply identifying phenotype—genotype associations, rapid detection of genetic disorders through more expansive genomic sequencing has changed medical management of neonates with suspected genetic disease and presents new possibilities and challenges. As genomic medicine and technology improve, the efficiency with which we are able to conduct precision pediatric medicine—accurate diagnosis followed by tailored management based on this growing amount of genomic information linked with clinical phenotypes—has improved and has reminded us of the importance of multidisciplinary teams at the diagnostic and subsequent care stages for these infants.[5,14] As an indicator of the rapid increase in knowledge since publication of the first draft of the human genome, as of October 2001, the Online Mendelian Inheritance in Man (OMIM) database included approximately 2610 disorders with associated genetic loci.[15] OMIM now encompasses approximately 6500 Mendelian phenotypes for which over 4300 genes have been identified.[16]

CURRENT GENETIC TESTING APPROACHES IN THE NEONATAL INTENSIVE CARE UNIT AND THEIR EVOLUTION

Initially, cytogenetic and molecular (DNA-based) genetic testing were considered separate specialties, but with the advent of new sequencing technologies, the boundaries between fields have blurred. Traditionally, cytogenetic tests focused on aneuploidies and large structural chromosomal rearrangements—both balanced and unbalanced—and used techniques such as G-banding karyotype (often referred to clinically as a "karyotype") and fluorescence in situ hybridization (FISH). The development of chromosomal microarrays (CMA) in the early 2000s maintained the ability to detect aneuploidies and unbalanced chromosomal rearrangements but provided the added ability to detect large regions of homozygosity and smaller copy number abnormalities such as microdeletions and microduplications, and refined the positions of breakpoints for all chromosomal alterations. CMA is still largely applied as a first-tier test in clinical cases of multiple congenital anomalies, developmental delay, intellectual disability, and behavioral differences like autism spectrum disorder.[17,18] In order to find even smaller insertions and deletions (indels) at the exon level and simultaneously uncover single-nucleotide variants (SNVs), DNA-based sequencing technology is required. Initially, this was accomplished through Sanger sequencing, and later, next-generation sequencing (NGS). In high-resource settings, providers can order these DNA-based tests in the clinical setting as phenotype-specific gene sequencing panels with copy number variant (CNV) analysis, thus merging the realms of cytogenetics and molecular genetics. When the phenotype is both complex and broad, the same technology can be used in a test known as whole exome sequencing (WES) to investigate almost all known genomic exons and a limited number of introns (altogether accounting for approximately 1.5% to 2% of the genome). WES will detect the majority of known disease-causing variant types (SNVs, indels, and CNVs).[14,19]

WES can be coupled with CMA to ensure fuller coverage of exon-level copy number changes. In the clinical setting, WES can also be ordered simultaneously with sequencing of the patient's mitochondrial DNA, if indicated. The main purpose of these tests is to investigate for monogenic disorders in which a pathogenic variant or biallelic pathogenic variants confirm a clinical diagnosis. CMA and gene sequence panels currently maintain an active role in the field of neonatology for well-characterized genetic diseases (e.g., autosomal trisomies and microdeletion syndromes), or a phenotypic presentation with a targeted differential diagnosis (e.g., skeletal dysplasias or seizures); in these cases, a precise test may still be an efficient path toward diagnosis, if the expense for WES is prohibitively high and time to result for a center's currently available WES test platforms remains weeks to months. Another consideration that has become available in addition to the gene sequencing panels based on specific phenotypes and WES is whole genome sequencing (WGS) as a clinical test.[4]

Recognizing the possible prolonged time-to-result and resource-related hurdles of WES and WGS, a study to test the potential for applying a broad sequencing panel to patients with suspected genetic disease was conducted among 20 NICU patients who had been referred to the medical genetics or metabolic inpatient consult services and had features suggesting an underlying genetic or metabolic condition. Twelve infants had been discharged from the NICU, and eight were enrolled prospectively. Subjects underwent a broad genomic sequencing panel identifying sequences of 4813 "disease-relevant" genes that had known associated clinical phenotypes either in OMIM or the United Kingdom's Human Gene Mutation Database (www.hgmd.cf.ac.uk/ac/index.php).[20] The investigators found a diagnostic rate of 40%, suggesting analysis of a broad list of Mendelian genes can produce high diagnostic yields at reduced costs. Of note, only 2 of the 8 infants had genetic diagnoses made by standard clinical approaches inclusive of sequencing of one suspected gene in one patient, and studying a limited panel of 18 sequenced genes in the other.[21] These authors cite another report of 35 infants less than 4 months old in a single tertiary center with suspected genetic conditions in whom 57% had genetic diagnoses from rapid WGS and data analysis.[22] With costs associated with sequencing and data storage decreasing and the speed of performing testing and analyzing results increasing, the field of genomic medicine has been moving toward WES and WGS analyses.[4] The widespread adoption of these technologies has led to gene discovery and novel syndrome characterization and has broadened the phenotypic spectrum of known disorders. The increasing efficiency with which these tests are able to produce a diagnosis has also allowed for individual changes in medical management including earlier administration of targeted therapeutics or enrollment in clinical trials/experimental therapeutics in some instances.[22-25] While there are many diagnostic and clinical advantages to broader tests such as WES and WGS, aspects to consider and plan for include pretest counseling for secondary and incidental findings, how patient data can be used for data reanalysis and research, or the impact testing could have on future insurance discrimination.[26-28]

UTILIZATION AND SUCCESS RATES OF VARIOUS GENETIC TESTING METHODOLOGIES IN THE NEONATAL INTENSIVE CARE UNIT

In a study aimed solely at detecting chromosomal abnormalities through array-based comparative genomic hybridization (a type of CMA analysis), investigators reported a detection rate of 17% for clinically significant chromosomal alterations among neonates with birth defects.[29] Studies aimed at identifying pathogenic variants in the protein coding regions of Mendelian genes with broad NGS technology—WES or WGS—cite diagnostic rates ranging from approximately 35% to 60%. A study of ultra-rapid exome sequencing, with a goal of return of results within 5 days, in critically ill patients where the median age was 28 days cited a diagnostic rate of 51%.[30] WES in critically ill children mostly less than 1 month old found a diagnosis in 43%.[5] Infants less than 100 days old in intensive care units demonstrated a 36.7% diagnostic yield with WES.[31] Acutely ill children with median age 28 days showed a diagnostic rate of 52.5% with WES.[32] Infants less than 2 years old, not necessarily in an acute care setting, demonstrated a diagnostic rate of 57.5%.[33] In a report on 307 infants from 3 tertiary centers in Shanghai, China, WES or sequence panels identified pathogenic genetic etiologies in over 40% of the patients, including genetic etiologies identified in over 60% of the infants who died during the 180-day follow-up period. Of note, and indicative of the importance of selection criteria for application of WES or WGS, four clinical traits had higher likelihood of identifying genetic diagnoses: integument abnormalities, complex immune-related phenotypes, mixed nervous system phenotypes and congenital anomalies, and mixed metabolism and nervous system phenotypes.[34]

WGS studies in the critically ill infant cite diagnostic yields ranging from 20% to more than 50%.[22,24,35,36] A study of critically ill infants and children cited a 42% diagnostic rate.[37] Pediatric patients less than 18 years old in the Hospital for Sick Children in Toronto, Ontario, Canada, not necessarily in the critical care setting, were found to have WGS diagnostic rates of 41%.[38] In the report by Lionel and colleagues, testing 103 children in non-genetic service clinics, all with conditions suspected to be genetically related, all the subjects with molecular diagnoses eventually made by conventional methods were captured by WGS. The 18 new diagnoses made with WGS and not by conventional methods included structural and non-exonic sequence variants not detectable with WES, which were confirmed in gene-disease associations that had been recently identified, highlighting the importance of periodically reviewing a patient's WGS and WES results. This review of results, along with new laboratory-based genomic technologies, can help account for recent gene discovery and new evidence linking variants and disease.[38] In another study of 100 pediatric patients referred for genetic testing, WGS identified genetic variants meeting clinical diagnostic criteria in 34% of cases, compared to 8% identified by CMA alone and 13% identified by CMA plus targeted sequencing of a small number of suspect genes. WGS identified all rare clinically significant CNVs that were detected by CMA.[39] A recent meta-analysis of 37 studies compared the diagnostic rate of the broadest NGS technologies—WES and WGS—with chromosomal microarray and concluded that WGS/WES should be considered as a first-line genetic test in children, based on the greater diagnostic and clinical utility of both, when compared to chromosomal microarray (<20% diagnostic yield).[14] Interestingly, this analysis also found that the diagnostic utility of WGS (41%) was not significantly different than WES (36%). Not surprisingly, the meta-analysis found that availability of parental samples for "trio" analysis and hospital-based interpretation (deep phenotypic information and communication between clinician and lab) enhanced diagnostic utility.[14] Other studies have shown higher diagnostic rates for WGS among pediatric patients when parental samples are available and when the test is performed on samples obtained from a hospitalized patient.[40] Further work is required to fully elucidate optimal testing inclusion criteria and algorithms, to determine high-yield disease presentations most likely to benefit from WES and WGS, given the variations in cost, reimbursement, and turn-around time.

While WGS and WES categorically appear to be advantageous, the ability to complete accurate sequencing as well as gene-variant characterization and clinical interpretation utilizing publicly available databases in less than 3 days, as first reported in 2012, provides compelling evidence for considering this approach as a first-line test, in sites where this approach is available.[41] A well-cited advantage for rapid WES or WGS is a curtailment of the diagnostic odyssey and the ability to forgo the previously utilized stepwise approach of increasingly broader testing if initial laboratory investigations are non-diagnostic or inconclusive.[41,42] The theoretical diagnostic advantages of WGS compared to WES are that through examination of greater than 90% of the genome, it has the capability to: discover a greater percentage of single-exon CNVs, uncover balanced chromosomal structural variations, diagnose repeat expansions important to specific disorders such as congenital myotonic dystrophy, and discover non-exonic regulatory and splicing variations, all of which can theoretically increase the diagnostic yield.[14,43,44] At present, however, not all clinical WGS is validated to diagnose certain genetic disorders—namely repeat expansion disorders, genes with a known pseudogene, or imprinting disorders that rely on methylation analysis, for instance.[18,26] The technology is moving toward capturing some of these capabilities (specifically the repeat expansion disorders and pseudogenes) as additional positive cases become available for test validation and new software tools are developed.[43,44] Therefore, WGS will likely be able to deliver the advantages of WES while still providing crucially important genomic information typically uncovered by cytogenetic techniques like CMA, which can be absent/incomplete from WES.[14,18,45] In one study comparing WGS and WES, 25.7% of patients who had a negative exome analysis were found to have a diagnostic variant on subsequent WGS.[38] Additionally, the raw data generated for a single patient through WGS is more comprehensive than the data generated by WES. This allows for future reanalysis that may be beneficial, as our knowledge of the genome increases to include a fuller understanding of the non-exonic regions.[19] Thinking toward the future, a patient's RNA may be used to conduct clinical RNA sequencing, which may one day complement DNA analysis and help elucidate certain diagnoses.[46-49]

One of the highest hurdles that remains with such broad testing is the large number of genomic variants uncovered by sequencing and the associated time- and labor-intensive variant analysis and interpretation. Researchers are actively pursuing ways to partially automate this process and decrease the turnaround time by utilizing clinical natural language processing to parse the clinical phenotype from the patient's electronic medical record.[4] Studies conducted within the NICU patient population have thus far reported successful outcomes, quoting diagnostic percentages of 42% to 57%, clinical management alterations (as a result of the diagnosis) in 30% to 72%, and change in outcomes experienced by 24% to 34% of patients in the studies who receive rapid WGS.[4,22,24,35,37]

IMPLEMENTATION AND IMPLICATIONS OF BROADER GENOMIC TESTING

A concern that arises is that the cost and informatics demands of broader genomic technologies like WES and WGS remain greater than more targeted NGS or cytogenetic testing.[50] Research has shown, however, that rapid use of these broader technologies when implemented with some degree of automation to their variant interpretation may reduce overall costs for healthcare systems.[24] Recent studies have replicated a net healthcare cost savings with the use of rapid WES.[51] Savings have been directly related to speed with which a diagnosis is made, providing additional evidence that utilization of rapid WGS in the critically ill infant as a first-tier test may have economic as well as clinical benefits. Many of the diagnoses discovered by rapid WES or WGS are rare genetic diseases, in which there are few reported cases and published literature, and for which a targeted differential diagnosis or curated NGS gene panel may simply not exist. For patients without a diagnosis following the broader tests of WGS or WES, having the ability to periodically repeat analysis of the patient's WGS or WES data in the setting of expanding genotype-phenotype databases is another benefit of these broader genomic tests being performed early in life. Online networks such as GeneMatcher (see Table 174.1 for this and other useful genomic websites) allow providers to submit through an online portal a candidate gene (a gene of uncertain clinical significance) in an attempt to connect with other providers and researchers who may have a patient that matches their own patient's phenotype and has the same gene affected. In this way, patient cohorts can be collected and functional studies regarding the gene can be undertaken to determine whether the candidate gene is responsible for human disease, and ultimately may lead to characterization of new ultra-rare Mendelian conditions. Separately, progress regarding the genomic variants associated with more common medical concerns such as preterm birth may also result from assembling accurately phenotyped cohorts inclusive of thousands of unaffected infants and affected newborns, and applying some of these more advanced genomic technologies such as WGS, RNA sequencing, and DNA methylation analyses to these patients on a broad scale.[52]

As has been noted, WGS is only as useful as the clinical phenotypic description provided, the molecular methodologies used, and the variant analysis and interpretation conducted. Genetics and genomics resources are growing, but the growth and availability of tests and support staff inevitably falls short of demand, creating limited access to testing which leads to healthcare inequities.[21,27] Researchers are working on methods to overcome some of these limitations, in part by creating partially automated methods for phenotyping.[53] Another aspect of inequity currently inherent in all NGS-based testing is the reliance, in part, on large population databases and variant frequency in determining pathogenicity of a particular variant. Large population databases have an underrepresentation of ethnic minority groups, often leaving patients from underrepresented minorities with a higher percentage of variants of uncertain significance (VUS) on their clinical test report, and oftentimes leading to a non-diagnostic test result.[54-57] As broad NGS technology becomes more widely available, laboratories will have a greater number of control data that may help begin to resolve some of these VUS. Additionally, new methodologies are being actively pursued that may further enhance our ability to resolve variants.[58]

The effort to build consistency into up-to-date classification of the gene-disease and variant-disease relationship is through the National Human Genome Research Institute (NHGRI)-funded Clinical Genome Resource (ClinGen).[59] ClinGen's mission is to define the clinical relevance of genes and variants to be used in research and precision medicine (Fig. 174.1). ClinGen has developed tools to evaluate clinical validity of gene-disease associations and pathogenicity of genetic variants for use in clinical care as well as educational material for clinicians and patients to better understand the process of curation of gene- and variant-disease associations. Curation is a term used to describe the analysis of the existing data and evidence about a specific gene or gene variant and its relation to a specific phenotype. The tools used allow for a quantitative approach to weighing the evidence supporting gene-disease and variant-disease associations to reach summary categories: pathogenic, likely pathogenic, uncertain significance, likely benign, and benign. ClinGen's work and impact is made directly available on their website (https://clinicalgenome.org/) and additionally, via another resource, ClinVar. ClinVar is the NCBI archival database that aggregates information about genomic variation and relationships to human health that are provided by researchers, clinical laboratories conducting sequencing, expert groups, clinics, and patient registries (listed in Table 174.1). In addition, with genomeconnect.org (an online registry designed by ClinGen), patients may also submit their clinical genetic test reports and health information to increase researchers' and healthcare providers' overall understanding of the relationship between genetics and health. While single investigators may submit a variant suspected of association with specific disease, ClinVar submissions are scored based on the number and types of sources submitting the same data, and validation by working groups and expert panels that examine the genetic epidemiologic evidence as well as supportive evidence from experimental model systems. These curations, as well as user interfaces, are constantly evolving, as data from multiple sources become available for consideration by expert panels.[60,61] Currently there are over 20 working groups, 30 gene curation panels, and over 30 variant curation panels working within the broader ClinGen effort (https://clinicalgenome.org/). The ClinGen website includes links to multiple educational modules and publicly available browser tools (Fig. 174.2). Clinicians should be aware that different automated curation tools in use in academic and commercial laboratories may make different "calls" of significance of associations between specific variants and disease. Clinicians should also be aware that data continue to accumulate, and the number of expert panels that have been trained using ClinGen programs is also growing, with the aim to decrease the heterogeneity of interpretation about significance of gene/variant/disease associations. As the legitimacy of the

Table 174.1 Web Resources Providing Genetic and Genomic Information and Training.

ClinGen: a National Institutes of Health (NIH)-funded resource dedicated to building a central resource that defines the clinical relevance of genes and variants for use in precision medicine and research: https://clinicalgenome.org/

ClinVar: freely accessible, public archive of reports of the relationships among human variations and phenotypes, with supporting evidence: https://www.ncbi.nlm.nih.gov/clinvar/

Database of Genotype and Phenotype (dbGaP): an archive of data from genome-wide association studies on a variety of diseases and conditions accessible through this NCBI: https://www.ncbi.nlm.nih.gov/gap/

DECIPHER: a database of reported copy number variants and linked phenotypes: https://decipher.sanger.ac.uk/

Ensembl: a genome browser for vertebrate genomes that supports research in comparative genomics, evolution, sequence variation, and transcriptional regulation. Ensembl annotates genes, computes multiple alignments, predicts regulatory function, and collects disease data: https://www.ensembl.org/index.html

GeneMatcher: website that enables connections between clinicians who have a patient with a candidate or ultra-rare gene and researchers who have an interest in that gene: https://genematcher.org/

GeneReviews: a clinical resource for many genetic conditions that provides clinically actionable information including diagnosis, inheritance, and management as well as a differential diagnosis of related conditions: https://www.ncbi.nlm.nih.gov/books/NBK1116/

GenomeConnect: GenomeConnect is an online registry designed by the Clinical Genome Resource (ClinGen) for people who are interested in sharing de-identified genetic and health information to improve understanding of genetics and health: https://www.genomeconnect.org/

Online Mendelian Inheritance in Man (OMIM): a searchable database of clinical features, phenotypes, and genes: https://omim.org/

Unique: a website with patient-/family-facing resources regarding chromosome and gene disorders: https://www.rarechromo.org/

University of California Santa Cruz Genome Browser: a website created initially to ensure public access to the initial human genome assembly; has now evolved to include a broad collection of vertebrate and model organism assemblies and annotations, along with a large suite of tools for viewing, analyzing, and downloading data: https://genome.ucsc.edu/

databases increases with replication, clinicians must continue to be vigilant and cautious, as increasing knowledge may sometimes lead to a change in the classification of a variant. As a cautionary example, a recent report analyzing variants that had been classified as pathogenic or likely pathogenic, and also occurred in more than 0.5% of the population, found that of 217 variants in 173 genes that were selected for curation, 87 (40%) of the variants were downgraded to benign, likely benign, or variant of uncertain significance.[62]

Obtaining informed consent prior to testing is critical for the purpose of educating patients and families about possible testing outcomes.[27,63,64] Some outcomes can cause unexpected difficulties including incidental but clinically relevant findings not related to the phenotype that prompted the test but linked with adult onset diseases; VUSs, which can lead to unanswerable questions and possible frustration; and candidate gene discovery that may require many years of research-based functional analysis before the gene's relevance to human disease is conclusively determined.

The case for the adoption of widespread WGS will arise from its successful utilization across a variety of clinical indications and patient cohorts. As researchers who have successfully built the infrastructure to support effective application of this technology continue to expand their networks, patients, families, and caregivers may begin to see the benefit of this testing through earlier diagnosis and potentially a change in clinical management. These tests will also necessitate continued monitoring of variants either for evolving evidence of clinical significance, in the case of variants of unknown significance, or the confirmation of persistent classification among variants determined to cause disease.[65]

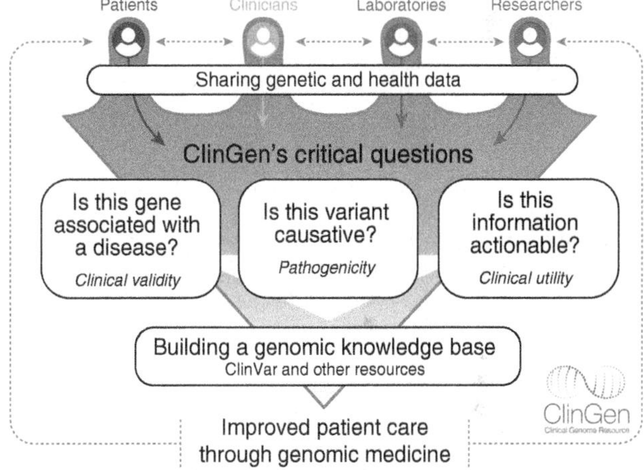

Fig. 174.1 Clinical genomic *(ClinGen)* resource framework. ClinGen's overall mission is to build a genomic knowledge base to improve patient care. The ClinGen framework provides a semiquantitative measurement for the strength of evidence of a gene-disease relationship that correlates to a qualitative classification: "Definitive," "Strong," "Moderate," "Limited," "No Reported Evidence," or "Conflicting Evidence." Within the ClinGen structure, classifications derived with this framework are reviewed and confirmed or adjusted based on clinical expertise of appropriate disease experts. Detailed guidance for utilizing this framework and access to the curation interface is available on the ClinGen website.[122] (From https://clinicalgenome.org/start/#loc_1550536143-7476-1. Accessed December 2020.)

GENOMICS OF COMMON COMPLEX DISEASES ASSOCIATED WITH PREMATURITY

While NGS-based testing continues to inform clinicians and families about the genes and variants that contribute to complex, severe phenotypes in NICU patients, identifying genes and variants associated with the more common complex disorders of prematurity such as ROP, IVH, NEC, and BPD remains a challenge.

Why look for genetic variants? Morbidities of prematurity are strongly associated with mortality and longer-term neurodevelopmental disabilities.[66–68] Identifying whether genetic variations play a role in the pathophysiology of these diseases could allow for development of mechanistic, individualized prevention and treatment approaches based on the individual patient's genotype. Dosing and treatment strategies based on genotype exist in several diseases usually associated with adult diseases, including cancer, with various tumor genotypes guiding therapeutic decisions.[69] In addition, when management trials targeting these morbidities are undertaken, taking into account genetic variation as a potential confounder on the effect of specific management strategies may be important, as in the interactions of certain *CYP2C19* genotypes in combination with clopidogrel and aspirin in adults with minor stroke and transient ischemic

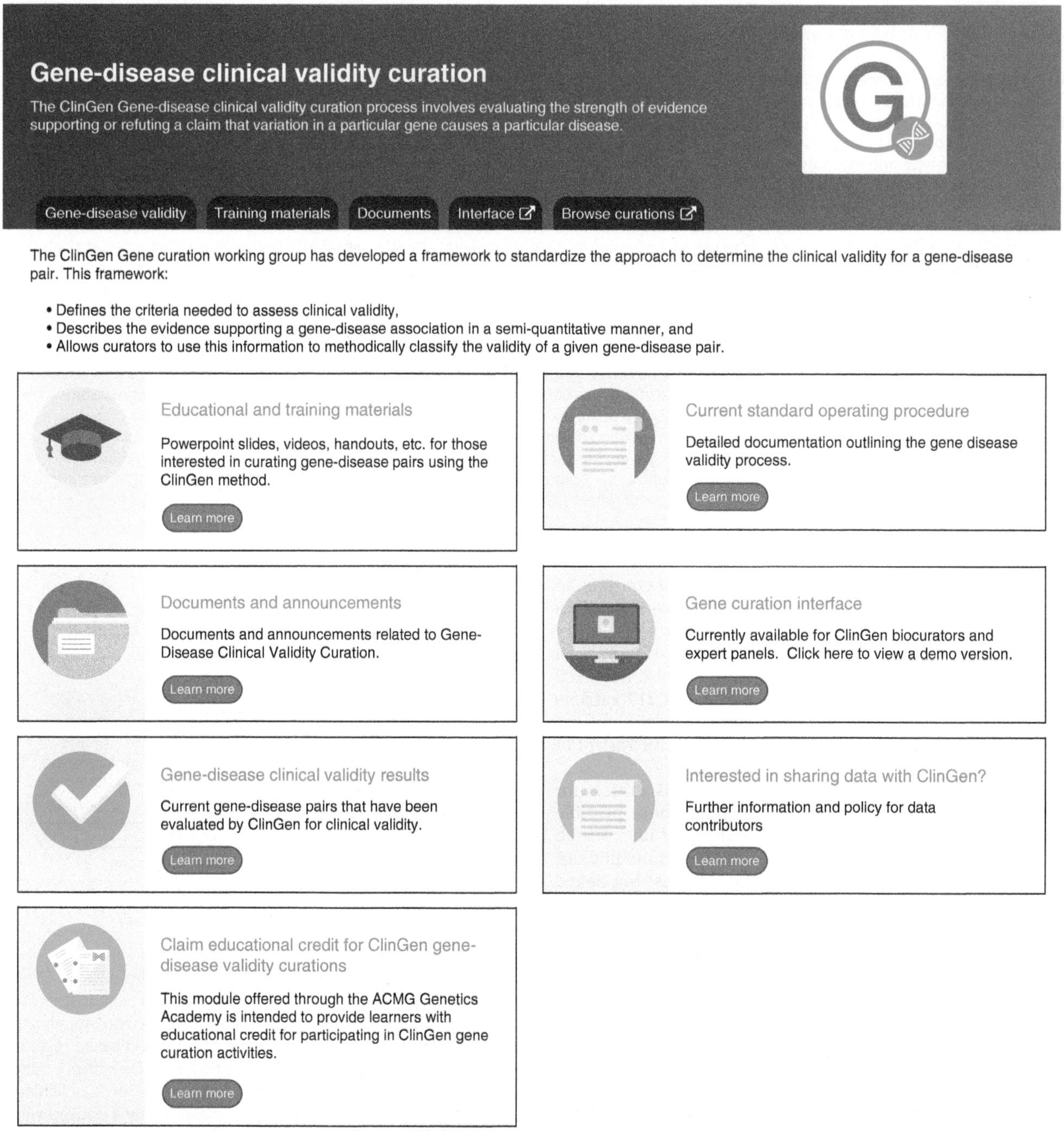

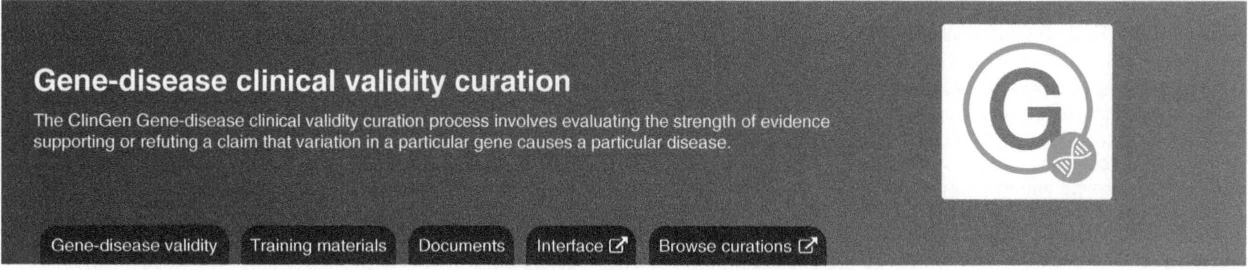

Gene-disease clinical validity curation
The ClinGen Gene-disease clinical validity curation process involves evaluating the strength of evidence supporting or refuting a claim that variation in a particular gene causes a particular disease.
Gene-disease validity
Training materials
Documents
Interface
Browse curations

The ClinGen Gene curation working group has developed a framework to standardize the approach to determine the clinical validity for a gene-disease pair. This framework:

- Defines the criteria needed to assess clinical validity,
- Describes the evidence supporting a gene-disease association in a semi-quantitative manner, and
- Allows curators to use this information to methodically classify the validity of a given gene-disease pair.

Educational and training materials

Powerpoint slides, videos, handouts, etc. for those interested in curating gene-disease pairs using the ClinGen method.

Learn more

Current standard operating procedure

Detailed documentation outlining the gene disease validity process.

Learn more

Documents and announcements

Documents and announcements related to Gene-Disease Clinical Validity Curation.

Learn more

Gene curation interface

Currently available for ClinGen biocurators and expert panels. Click here to view a demo version.

Learn more

Gene-disease clinical validity results

Current gene-disease pairs that have been evaluated by ClinGen for clinical validity.

Learn more

Interested in sharing data with ClinGen?

Further information and policy for data contributors

Learn more

Claim educational credit for ClinGen gene-disease validity curations

This module offered through the ACMG Genetics Academy is intended to provide learners with educational credit for participating in ClinGen gene curation activities.

Learn more

Fig. 174.2 ClinGen resource link page. Publicly accessible web resource with links to explanation of the process for gene and variant disease curation. The links bring users to manuals and training resources related to ClinGen's gene curation process, which is designed to aid in evaluating the strength of a gene-disease relationship based on publicly available evidence. Genetic, experimental, and contradictory evidence curated from the literature is compiled and used to assign a clinical validity classification per criteria established by the ClinGen Gene Curation Working Group.[122,123] (From www.clinicalgenome.org. Accessed December 2020.)

attack.[70,71] Of note, for preterm infants, there is suggestion, but not definitive evidence of genotypic influence on response to medical therapy for the patent ductus arteriosus.[72,73]

The first mandatory steps to investigate before going to the trouble of testing genetic variants for associations with disease include testing whether or not inherited factors are likely contributing to risk of specific disease, either directly or via genetics-environment interactions. Quantitatively, this association is measured as heritability, which is a quantitative measure of the extent to which genetic factors account for the phenotypic variance. The process, which includes testing disease prevalence among monozygotic versus dizygotic twins, has been carefully outlined by Bhandari and Gruen.[74] In studies with mono- and dizygotic twins, significant heritability has been identified for ROP, NEC, sepsis, IVH, and BPD.[75-80]

With establishment of an inherited basis for these common complex diseases, researchers started to test associations between relatively common variants, known as "single nucleotide polymorphisms" or "SNPs" that have been identified in 1% or more of tested populations. Having the minor (less common) allele can sometimes increase or decrease the functionality of the gene product. Because they are relatively common, methodologies to genotype SNPs were characterized fairly early in the "genomics era" after the successful sequencing of the entire human genome. Much of the early work on diseases in neonatology focused on assessing associations between SNPs in genes for TNFα or IL-6, which are associated with immune response or regulation of inflammation, and diseases such as BPD or late onset sepsis, often with disparate results for the same SNP.[81,82] Tests for associations with a handful of SNPs in relatively small cohorts dominated early reports, and some identified associations with statistical significance with $P < 0.05$; however, with 3 billion nucleotides comprising the genome, over 30 million known SNPs, thousands of variants in the genome of any one individual, and relatively small sample sizes, replication has proven difficult, and the concept of the candidate gene analysis, or, more specifically, candidate SNP analysis, approach was called into question unless study cohorts included thousands of cases and controls.[83,84]

With early evidence encouraging a more agnostic approach, broader arrays of genes and variants were developed and multiple candidate genes across the genome could be tested. With knowledge of the genome expanding, SNPs that are in linkage disequilibrium (the occurrence of a set of of SNPs forming a haplotype) could be predicted accurately without actually genotyping every SNP. This allows for "imputation" of multiple "tagSNPs," in which actual genotyping of one SNP allows prediction of the genotypes of 5 to 10 neighboring SNPs (i.e., haplotype).[85] In the genome-wide association studies (GWAS) approach, hundreds of thousands, even millions, of SNPs are genotyped and tagSNPs imputed, and then individually tested for association in well-phenotyped cohorts (Fig. 174.3). Statistical approaches have had to be adapted to the millions of tested associations using GWAS. The standard has been to determine "genome-wide significance" when the P values identified with the comparison reached lower than 5×10^{-8}, much lower than the conventional $P < 0.05$ used with debatable authority in many epidemiology studies and clinical trials.[86-88] To realistically test hypotheses using GWAS, large cohorts with thousands of subjects with the disease phenotype are ideal, as have been used for multiple complex common diseases of adulthood, such as prostate cancer and Alzheimer disease.[89,90] GWAS studies in the NICU population have numbered in the hundreds and rarely thousands, much smaller than the adult cohorts.[91-96] As a comparison, in a GWAS of 2727 cases and 3336 controls for Alzheimer disease, *APOE* gene variants, were found to be associated with Alzheimer disease with a P value of 2.52×10^{-53}.[97]

An additional challenge for genomic analysis among extremely preterm cohorts are the differences in minor allele frequency among study cohorts of differing ancestry. While studies on samples from relatively homogenous nations, such as Iceland, may produce fairly homogenous, replicable results, results from cohorts of mixed ancestry, which is more common in the United States, present challenges to analyzing associations between variants that differ in prevalence in cohorts of different ancestry. Acknowledging those strategies and challenges, studies in cohorts of premature infants for genetic associations using candidate gene and SNP analyses and more agnostic GWAS approaches have produced some findings of interest that reach genomic significance within the study cohort. These results, while encouraging, continue to be only tempting because of the severe limitation of examining relatively small cohorts compared to the more typical larger population analyses that can be done for common, complex diseases that emerge later in life.[98,99]

RETINOPATHY OF PREMATURITY

Recent reviews of genetic risk factors for ROP document the lack of any emergent, identifiable strongly associated genetic variants with severe ROP risk among preterm infants. Certainly, ROP-like phenotypes are linked with rare inherited variants or spontaneous mutations causing diseases like familial exudative vitreoretinopathy (FEVR) and Kabuki syndrome, but for the vast majority of premature infants, candidate gene/SNP studies have not identified variants with genome-wide significance. Multiple attempts have been made to identify associations that are plausibly associated with the pathophysiologic mechanisms of ROP, including VEGF and VEGF receptors. One report, which tested a panel of over 1000 variants in over 100 genes related to inflammation and organ development, identified two intronic variants in the brain-derived neurotrophic factor *(BDNF)* gene with severe ROP versus non-severe or no ROP with a P value of less than 5×10^{-7}.[100] Lower serum levels of BDNF have been associated with higher likelihood of ROP in reports testing associations of serum levels of various cytokines and growth factors with outcomes in premature infants. This adds some plausibility to an association with *BDNF* variants that might influence expression, or an association with some other gene product/component of a pathway important for neurovascular development that includes BDNF.[101-103] While this is promising, the impact of specific variants on BDNF circulating levels, or in situ levels in the developing retina, have not been described. More recently, analysis beyond genotyping has identified placental CpG methylation, a measure of epigenetic modification, of 12 different genes is associated with development of pre-threshold ROP. Interestingly, the genes with methylation changes associated with ROP included BDNF.[104] No GWAS has been done to examine ROP to date.

NECROTIZING ENTEROCOLITIS

In a cohort study using a GWAS approach, minor allele(s) in a cluster of SNPs spanning a 43-kb region of chromosome 8 (8q23.3) conferred an odds ratio of 4.72 (95% confidence interval [CI]: 2.51 to 8.88) for elevated risk of NEC, with multiple SNPs associated with $P < 10^{-8}$ (Fig. 174.4). To date, in the GWAS analyses of morbidities associated with prematurity, this is the only gene region to reach genome-wide significance. Two smaller clusters on chromosome 14 and chromosome 11 exhibited P values of 10^{-7} to 10^{-8}. Like many gene association studies done in the extremely preterm population, this analysis was limited by a small sample size ($n = 751$, only 30 with surgical NEC), from multiple sites in the United States, with significant ancestry admixture. Interestingly, the increased risk was similar for all three genetic ancestries represented in this population.[105] The investigators attempted to validate the associations of the SNPs in the chromosome 8 region with NEC in a separate cohort ($N = 1018$, 26 with surgical NEC) of premature infants enrolled in a study using GWAS to identify variants associated with severe intraventricular hemorrohage.[94] In that cohort, one of the SNPs (rs13252246) was associated with NEC with a P value of < 0.02. In in silico analysis, a term that means use of computer modeling systems to predict gene products and their potential activities and pathologies, the NEC-associated region of chromosome 8 appears to be evolutionarily conserved, but without any previously identified genes. Pathway analysis, testing variants in multiple pathway-linked genes for associations with NEC, identified associations with over 50 pathways, including pathways involved with immune response, growth regulation, and G-protein signaling. Interestingly, the *LTB4R* gene close to the chromosome 14 region with strong association with surgical NEC encodes an eicosanoid receptor. Eicosanoid receptor signaling was found to be the second most prominent pathway affected by NEC-associated SNPs. In terms of physiological plausibility, *LBT4* plays a significant role in a toll-like receptor 4 and cyclooxygenase-2 mediated mechanism of intestinal ischemia/reperfusion injury.[105]

INTRAVENTRICULAR HEMORRHAGE

Several candidate gene studies have been conducted in relatively small cohorts testing associations between SNPs in inflammation, complement, and coagulation pathways.[106,107] One case report of two preterm siblings suggested a novel mutation in the collagen 4 A1 gene may be associated with severe IVH.[108] In the precursor to a GWAS study, the Gene Targets for Intraventricular Hemorrhage study group conducted a candidate gene study of SNPs in 7 genes, in 224 preterm infants with grade III-IV IVH, and 389 matched controls. Only SNPs in the methylenetetrahydrofolate reductase *(MTHFR)* gene gave even equivocal results of associations with severe IVH.[109] In the GWAS analysis, the group tested over 600,000 SNPs in 458 inborn appropriate for gestational age neonates with severe IVH and 866 infants without IVH, from US and Scandinavian cohorts.[94] No individual SNP reached genome-wide significance; however, a 10-SNP haplotype ranging from the intergenic region of *GM140* and *CACNA1E* to the intron region of *CACNA1E* had a *P* value of 7.16×10^{-10}. *CACNA1E* (calcium channel, voltage-dependent, R type, α 1E subunit) is mutated in a Mendelian form of hemiplegic migraine, a known vascular phenotype, as well as various epilepsies.[110] None of the prior candidate individual SNPs reached genome-wide association significance. Like many similar endeavors, the summary of the report of results of this GWAS for severe IVH concluded, "Because common variants have small-to-moderate effects, a large-scale neonatal genomic medicine network must be developed with the infrastructural capacity to host an accessible database of sequence variants, their phenotypic associations and environmental risk factors."[94]

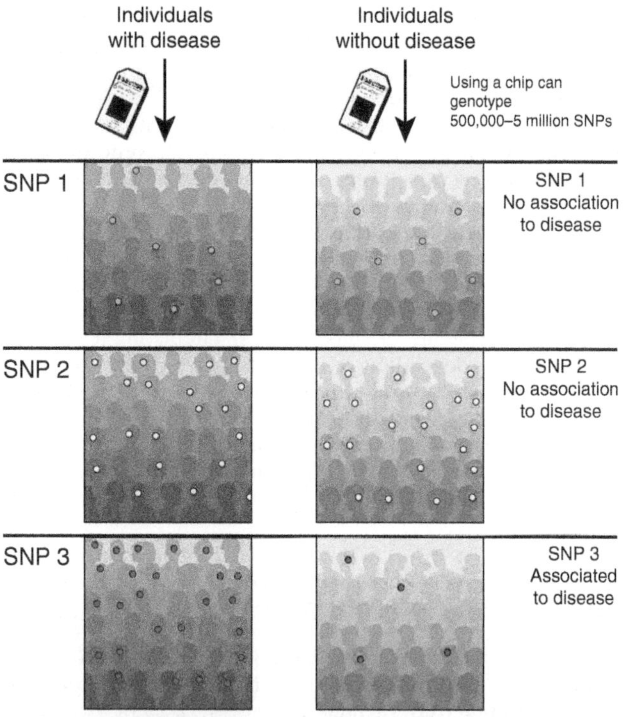

Fig. 174.3 Genome wide association studies. In genome-wide association studies (GWAS), genotypes of single nucleotide polymorphisms, that is, loci with variants identified in 1% or more of the population, are identified across the entire genome. Prevalence of the variants among individuals with a condition is compared with prevalence among individuals without the condition to identify candidate genes and variants associated with disease. *SNP*, Single nucleotide polymorphism. (From www.genome.gov/about-genomics/fact-sheets/Genome-Wide-Association-Studies-Fact-Sheet. Accessed December 2020.)

BRONCHOPULMONARY DYSPLASIA

Of the morbidities of extreme prematurity, BPD is the most common.[111,112] While severe ROP, NEC, and severe IVH have phenotypes that are usually defined by imaging or direct visualization, BPD is defined usually by some level of respiratory support, making the anatomic and physiologic details of the phenotype that might be influenced by genetic variations somewhat challenging.[113,114] In part because of relatively small sample sizes, and the limitations related to phenotype definitions that are not anatomically or physiologically defined, the five groups that have used an agnostic GWAS approach to try to identify variants or groups of variants in genes and pathways associated with epidemiologically defined BPD have met with limited success.[91-93,95,96] Hadchouel and colleagues studied 418 premature neonates (gestational age below 28 weeks, 22% with BPD, and a replication cohort of 213 Finnish neonates, 26% with BPD) and identified SNPs in the *SPOCK2* gene associated with BPD in the discovery cohorts (of African and Caucasian ancestry) and the replication cohort.[91] Wang and colleagues

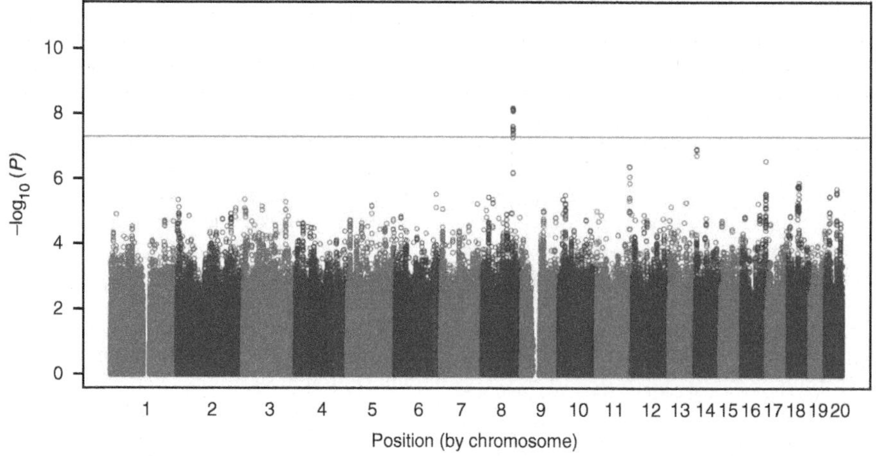

Fig. 174.4 Necrotizing enterocolitis (NEC) genome-wide association studies (GWAS) result. "Manhattan Plot" of over 7 million genotyped and imputed single nucleotide polymorphisms tested in the GWAS for surgical NEC versus controls. Data shown are –log *P* values on the Y axis versus chromosome locations along the X axis. The region on chromosome 8 at the location 8q23.3 shows the strongest association with the incidence of NEC (see Fig. 174.4).[105]

studied over 2000 very low-birth-weight infants born in California and did not identify genomic loci or pathways associated with moderate to severe BPD with genome-wide significance.[92] In the study of Ambalavanan and colleagues, which included 751 infants with birthweights ranging between 401 and 1000 g (428 diagnosed with BPD or who died), no SNPs achieved genome-wide significance. Pathways of lung development and repair and novel molecules and pathways (adenosine deaminase, targets of microRNA or miR-219) were associated with BPD. Pathways associated with mild BPD were different from the pathways associated with severe BPD. In addition, the variants/pathways associated with BPD varied by ancestry.[93,115] In the fourth study, GWAS was performed in a Finnish discovery cohort of 60 cases with moderate-to-severe BPD and 114 controls. The SNP flanking the C-reactive protein gene had strongest association with BPD ($P = 3.4 \times 10^{-6}$), and in multivariate logistic regression this SNP was associated with BPD in two replication cohorts (one Finnish and one comprised of European and African individuals).[95] In the most recent GWAS study, which tested 9 million genotypes and imputed variants from 387 preterm infants who participated in the Trial of Late Surfactant (TolSURF) study for associations with BPD, no individual SNPs were associated with BPD with genome-wide significance. Similar to the study by Ambalavanan, which demonstrated variation by ancestry in pathways associated with BPD, this group reported that genetic ancestry was associated with the degree of survival without BPD. The associations between genetic ancestry and BPD suggest patterns of genetic variation in infants with or without BPD are likely to differ by continental origin.[96] Ultimately, the five GWAS studies failed to identify a specific gene or variant in a gene to be specifically and convincingly associated with BPD; however, the studies, individually and collectively, are limited by small sample sizes and high levels of phenotype variation.

Investigators have also applied WES to BPD, with hopes that by much more extensive sequencing, which includes rare variants, that the collective influence of these rare variants may be detected.[116–118] Carrera and colleagues studied 26 unrelated infants with severe BPD from Italian NICUs. Identified variants were classified as likely to have high, moderate, or low impact based on predicted protein effects, and whether or not they were novel variants in genes with occurrence in more than one subject. As expected, each subject had approximately 200,000 identified variants, with about 10% of all variants identified from all subjects as possibly having moderate or high impact. In each sample, approximately 100 variants were identified that were hypothesized by structural predictive analysis to have an impact on protein structure. Two subjects had novel missense mutations in *ABCA3*, which is a gene responsible for transporting phospholipids to lamellar bodies in type II alveolar cells. Rare and novel variants in *NOS2* and toll-receptor genes and C-reactive protein were also identified in this cohort with BPD.[116] Li and colleagues used newborn screening samples from the state of California for exome sequencing of 50 twin pairs, including 51 infants with BPD. The accumulated variants in 258 genes in the subjects with BPD had a significantly higher haploinsufficiency score (haploinsufficiency can be defined as the situation when one copy of a gene is either deleted or has a loss-of-function variant, and dosage of the gene product is reduced enough to affect function[119]). Variants clustered in genes in pathways involved in embryonic epithelial development, organization of collagen, and Wnt-signaling were increased among the infants with BPD compared with non-BPD infants. This group also looked at tissue expression in human tissue from patients with BPD, and in lung tissue from the hyperoxic mouse model of BPD, and detected increased expression in the exome-identified BPD candidate genes in hyperoxia exposed animals.[117] Most recently Hamvas and colleagues studied 146 subjects (85 with BPD and 61 unaffected) enrolled in the Prematurity and Respiratory Outcomes Program (PROP) with WES. This group tested for associations between disease status and individual common (minor allele frequency >0.05) and rare variants, in affected or unaffected subjects. Three hundred forty-five genes with extremely rare, non-synonymous variants, that is, variants that would lead to a change in the amino acid sequence of the gene product, were identified only in the BPD-affected subjects. This study, the largest to date, replicated 28 genes with extremely rare variants in patients with BPD that were previously associated with BPD in the California cohort reported by Li and colleagues.[118]

In summary, no genes have been identified to be associated with BPD with genome-wide significance, so there is not likely to be a highly prevalent "BPD gene." The complexities of the phenotype combined with the relatively small size of the study populations to date are significantly limiting factors. The GWAS and WES studies to date are also limited in their ability to identify rare variants in noncoding regions that may be of importance to the pathogenesis of BPD; however, the WES approach has identified associations with genes containing rare variants and candidate pathways, and the WGS approach has yet to be tested.

CONCLUSION

Twenty years ago, the ability to clinically utilize the genetic sequence of a NICU patient with a complex disorder, to have the informatics and genomic analysis bandwidth to determine within 48 hours whether the patient likely possesses a pathogenic genetic variant that may direct care, and to have access to a growing database of genotypes and associated phenotypes to help guide our knowledge, were only possible in our imaginations. Since then, application of genomic technology and methodologies in the NICU has become more of a reality, particularly with the emerging reports of utilization of WES and WGS with rapid turnaround times relevant to care in the NICU. With the growing availability of these types of tests, NICU clinicians will grapple with challenges related to the follow-up of unexpected findings and VUS. Clinicians must remain aware of the very real possibility of modifications to the results of these tests, as more information may arise to either validate a variant's pathogenicity or shift a particular variant's classification toward benign. Because of the complexity and potential for new findings in the future, it is imperative that NICU providers caring for these infants and ordering these tests connect with providers who have the expertise and ability to stay up to date with accumulating gene-disease association data and the ability to clinically follow and manage the patients and families long term. The increasing knowledge of the genome, as well as multiple other "-omics" related sciences such as proteomics and metabolomics, as well as studies of the microbiome, are elucidating mechanisms of the more common complex diseases of prematurity like BPD,[120] as well as preterm birth itself.[121] While the impact of this latter work is felt less at the clinical level currently, it continues to inform or affirm studies regarding mechanisms of disease and disease prevention and therapy.

A complete reference list is available at www.ExpertConsult.com. 

SELECT REFERENCES

4. Clark MM, Hildreth A, Batalov S, et al. Diagnosis of genetic diseases in seriously ill children by rapid whole-genome sequencing and automated phenotyping and interpretation. *Sci Transl Med*. 2019;11(489):eaat6177.
5. Freed AS, Clowes Candadai SV, Sikes MC, et al. The impact of rapid exome sequencing on medical management of critically ill children [published online ahead of print, 2020 Jun 15]. *J Pediatr*. 2020;S0022-3476(20):30721-30726.
12. Michel MC, Colaizy TT, Klein JM, Segar JL, Bell EF. Causes and circumstances of death in a neonatal unit over 20 years. *Pediatr Res*. 2018;83(4):829-833.
14. Clark MM, Stark Z, Farnaes L, et al. Meta-analysis of the diagnostic and clinical utility of genome and exome sequencing and chromosomal microarray in children with suspected genetic diseases. *NPJ Genom Med*. 2018;3:16.
18. Lalonde E, Rentas S, Lin F, Dulik MC, Skraban CM, Spinner NB. Genomic diagnosis for pediatric disorders: revolution and evolution. *Front Pediatr*. 2020;8:373.

19. Bick D, Jones M, Taylor SL, Taft RJ, Belmont J. Case for genome sequencing in infants and children with rare, undiagnosed or genetic diseases. *J Med Genet.* 2019;56(12):783-791.
24. Farnaes L, Hildreth A, Sweeney NM, et al. Rapid whole-genome sequencing decreases infant morbidity and cost of hospitalization. *NPJ Genom Med.* 2018;3(10).
25. Ceyhan-Birsoy O, Murry JB, Machini K, et al. Interpretation of genomic sequencing results in healthy and Ill newborns: results from the babyseq PROJECT. *Am J Hum Genet.* 2019;104(1):76-93.
27. Gyngell C, Newson AJ, Wilkinson D, Stark Z, Savulescu J. Rapid Challenges: Ethics and Genomic Neonatal Intensive Care. *Pediatrics.* 2019;143(suppl 1):S14-S21.
28. Smith EE, du Souich C, Dragojlovic N, CAUSES Study, RAPIDOMICS Study, Elliott AM. Genetic counseling considerations with rapid genome-wide sequencing in a neonatal intensive care unit. *J Genet Couns.* 2019;28(2): 263-272.
35. Petrikin JE, Cakici JA, Clark MM, et al. The NSIGHT1-randomized controlled trial: rapid whole-genome sequencing for accelerated etiologic diagnosis in critically ill infants. *NPJ Genom Med.* 2018;3:6.
38. Lionel AC, Costain G, Monfared N, et al. Improved diagnostic yield compared with targeted gene sequencing panels suggests a role for whole-genome sequencing as a first-tier genetic test. *Genet Med.* 2018;20(4):435-443.
41. Saunders CJ, Miller NA, Soden SE, et al. Rapid whole-genome sequencing for genetic disease diagnosis in neonatal intensive care units. *Sci Transl Med.* 2012;4(154):154ra135.
60. Landrum MJ, Kattman BL. ClinVar at five years: delivering on the promise. *Hum Mutat.* 2018;39(11):1623-1630.
61. Landrum MJ, Chitipiralla S, Brown GR, et al. ClinVar: improvements to accessing data. *Nucleic Acids.*
64. Lantos JD. Ethical and psychosocial issues in Whole Genome Sequencing (WGS) for newborns. *Pediatrics.* 2019;143(suppl 1):S1-S5.
74. Bhandari V, Gruen JR. What is the basis for a genetic approach in neonatal disorders? *Semin Perinatol.* 2015;39(8):568-573.
85. Hirschhorn JN, Daly MJ. Genome-wide association studies for common diseases and complex traits. *Nat Rev Genet.* 2005;6(2):95-108.
87. Ioannidis JPA, Khoury MJ. Evidence-based medicine and big genomic data. *Hum Mol Genet.* 2018;27(R1):R2-R7.
91. Hadchouel A, Durrmeyer X, Bouzigon E, et al. Identification of SPOCK2 as a susceptibility gene for bronchopulmonary dysplasia. *Am J Respir Crit Care Med.* 2011;184(10):1164-1170.
92. Wang H, St Julien KR, Stevenson DK, et al. A genome-wide association study (GWAS) for bronchopulmonary dysplasia. *Pediatrics.* 2013;132(2): 290-297.
93. Ambalavanan N, Cotten CM, Page GP, et al. Integrated genomic analyses in bronchopulmonary dysplasia. *J Pediatr.* 2015;166(3):531-537.e13.
94. Ment LR, Ådén U, Bauer CR, et al. Genes and environment in neonatal intraventricular hemorrhage. *Semin Perinatol.* 2015;39(8):592-603.
95. Mahlman M, Karjalainen MK, Huusko JM, et al. Genome-wide association study of bronchopulmonary dysplasia: a potential role for variants near the CRP gene. *Sci Rep.* 2017;7(1):9271.
96. Torgerson DG, Ballard PL, Keller RL, et al. Ancestry and genetic associations with bronchopulmonary dysplasia in preterm infants. *Am J Physiol Lung Cell Mol Physiol.* 2018;315(5):L858-L869.
98. Ioannidis JP, Ntzani EE, Trikalinos TA. Racial' differences in genetic effects for complex diseases. *Nat Genet.* 2004;36(12):1312-1318.
99. Popejoy AB, Fullerton SM. Genomics is failing on diversity. *Nature.* 2016;538(7624):161-164.
105. Jilling T, Ambalavanan N, Cotten CM, et al. Surgical necrotizing enterocolitis in extremely premature neonates is associated with genetic variations in an intergenic region of chromosome 8. *Pediatr Res.* 2018;83(5):943-953.
116. Carrera P, Di Resta C, Volonteri C, et al. Exome sequencing and pathway analysis for identification of genetic variability relevant for bronchopulmonary dysplasia (BPD) in preterm newborns: a pilot study. *Clin Chim Acta.* 2015;451(Pt A):39-45.
117. Li J, Yu KH, Oehlert J, et al. Exome sequencing of neonatal blood spots and the identification of genes implicated in bronchopulmonary dysplasia. *Am J Respir Crit Care Med.* 2015;192(5):589-596.
118. Hamvas A, Feng R, Bi Y, et al. Exome sequencing identifies gene variants and networks associated with extreme respiratory outcomes following preterm birth. *BMC Genet.* 2018;19(1):94.
120. Lal CV, Bhandari V, Ambalavanan N. Genomics, microbiomics, proteomics, and metabolomics in bronchopulmonary dysplasia. *Semin Perinatol.* 2018;42(7):425-431.

Index

Page numbers followed by *f* indicate figure, by *t* table, and by *b* box.

C

J

M

O

P

Q

R

S

W